Nelson Textbook of Pediatrics

15TH EDITION

Nelson Textbook of Pediatrics

SENIOR EDITOR
Waldo E. Nelson, MD

EDITED BY
Richard E. Behrman, MD
Director, Center for the Future of Children
The David and Lucile Packard Foundation
Clinical Professor of Pediatrics
Stanford University and
University of California, San Francisco;
Attending Physician,
Lucile Salter Packard Children's Hospital at Stanford;
Stanford, California

Robert M. Kliegman, MD
Professor and Chairman
Department of Pediatrics
Medical College of Wisconsin
Pediatrician-in-Chief
Children's Hospital of Wisconsin
Milwaukee, Wisconsin

Ann M. Arvin, MD
Professor of Pediatrics and
Microbiology/Immunology
Associate Chair for Academic Affairs
Department of Pediatrics
Stanford University School of Medicine
Chief, Infectious Diseases
Lucile Salter Packard Children's Hospital at Stanford
Stanford, California

W.B. SAUNDERS COMPANY
A Division of Harcourt Brace & Company
Philadelphia London Toronto Montreal Sydney Tokyo

W.B. SAUNDERS COMPANY
A Division of Harcourt Brace & Company

The Curtis Center
Independence Square West
Philadelphia, Pennsylvania 19106

Library of Congress Cataloging-in-Publication Data

Nelson textbook of pediatrics.—15th ed. / edited by Richard E. Behrman, Robert M. Kliegman, Ann M. Arvin; senior editor, Waldo E. Nelson.

p. cm.

Includes bibliographical references and index.

ISBN 0–7216–5578–5

1. Pediatrics. I. Behrman, Richard E. II. Kliegman, Robert. III. Nelson, Waldo E. (Waldo Emerson). IV. Title: Textbook of pediatrics. [DNLM: 1. Pediatrics. WS 100 N432 1996]

RJ45.N4 1996 618.92—dc20

DNLM/DLC 95–1789

Nelson Textbook of Pediatrics ISBN 0–7216–5578–5
International Edition ISBN 0–7216–6766–X

Printed in The United States of America

Last digit is the print number: 9 8 7 6 5 4 3 2 1

DEDICATION

This edition is dedicated to the physicians and nurses who care for children in many different circumstances throughout the world and who, by their efforts and commitment, make the world a better place for children.

Contributors

RAYMOND D. ADELMAN, M.D.
Professor and Chairman, Department of Pediatrics, Eastern Virginia Medical School; Senior Vice President for Academic Affairs, Children's Hospital of The King's Daughters, Norfolk, Virginia
Part VII: Pathophysiology of Body Fluids

WILLIAM ALBRITTON, M.D., Ph.D.
Formerly, Professor of Pediatrics; Director, Provincial Laboratory of Public Health, University of Alberta, Edmonton, Alberta, Canada
Chapter 188: Yersinia; Chapter 189: Tularemia; Chapter 190: Brucellosis; Chapter 191: Listeriosis

ALIA Y. ANTOON, M.D.
Assistant Clinical Professor of Pediatrics, Harvard Medical School; Shriner Burn Institute, Boston, Massachusetts
Chapter 60: Pediatric Critical Care

JAMES E. ARNOLD, M.D.
Associate Professor of Otolaryngology–Head and Neck Surgery, Assistant Professor of Pediatrics, Case Western Reserve University School of Medicine; Director, Pediatric Otolaryngology, Rainbow Babies and Children's Hospital, Cleveland, Ohio
Part XIX: The Respiratory System; Section 2: Upper Respiratory Tract; Part XXX: The Ear

STEPHEN S. ARNON, M.D.
Senior Investigator and Chief, Infant Botulism Prevention Program, California Department of Health Services, Berkeley, California
Chapter 192: Botulism; Chapter 193: Tetanus; Chapter 194: Anaerobic Infections

STEPHEN C. ARONOFF, M.D.
Professor of Pediatrics, Microbiology, and Immunology, West Virginia University; Section Chief, Infectious Disease and Pediatrics, West Virginia University Hospitals, Morgantown, West Virginia
Chapter 229: Candida; Chapter 230: Aspergillosis; Chapter 231: Histoplasmosis; Chapter 232: Blastomycosis; Chapter 234: Cryptococcosis; Chapter 235: Mucormycosis; Chapter 236: Sporotrichosis; Chapter 244: Protozoan Diseases; Chapter 667: Nonbacterial Food Poisoning; Chapter 669: Mammalian Bites

ANN M. ARVIN, M.D.
Professor of Pediatrics and Microbiology/Immunology; Associate Chair for Academic Affairs, Department of Pediatrics, Stanford University School of Medicine; Chief, Infectious Diseases, Lucile Salter Packard Children's Hospital at Stanford, Stanford, California
Part XVII: Infectious Diseases; Section 1: General Considerations; Chapter 184: Escherichia Coli, Aeromonas, *and* Plesiomonas; *Chapter 213: Varicella-Zoster Virus; Chapter 249: Infection Control*

DAVID M. ASHER, M.D.
Medical Officer, National Institutes of Health, Bethesda, Maryland
Chapter 228: Slow Viral Infections of the Human Nervous System

SHAI ASHKENAZI, M.D., M.Sc.
Senior Lecturer, Sackler School of Medicine, Tel Aviv University; Attending Physician, Children Medical Center, Petah Tiqua, Israel
Chapter 182: Salmonella Infections; Chapter 186: Campylobacter

JANE T. ATKINS, M.D.
Assistant Professor of Pediatrics, The University of Texas Health Science Center at Houston, Texas
Chapter 187: Helicobacter

JOHN AUCOTT, M.D.
Assistant Professor of Medicine, Case Western Reserve University School of Medicine; Section Head, General Internal Medicine, Cleveland Veterans Administration Medical Center, Cleveland, Ohio
Chapter 244: Protozoan Diseases

PARVIN H. AZIMI, M.D.
Clinical Professor of Pediatrics, University of California, San Francisco; Director of Infectious Diseases, Children's Hospital, Oakland, California
Chapter 201: Spirochetal Infections

ROBERT L. BAEHNER, M.D.
Professor of Pediatrics, University of Southern California School of Medicine; USC/LAC Women's and Children's Hospital, Los Angeles, California
Chapter 122: The Phagocytic System; Chapter 123: Neutrophilia; Chapter 124: Neutropenia; Chapter 125: Adhesion Deficiency Disorders; Chapter 126: Neutrophil Granule Defects; Chapter 127: Chédiak-Higashi Syndrome; Chapter 128: Disorders of Cell Motility and Chemotaxis; Chapter 129: Chronic Granulomatous Disease; Chapter 130: Disorders of Neutrophil Oxidative Metabolism Other Than CGD; Chapter 131: Inherited Leukocyte Abnormalities

WILLIAM F. BALISTRERI, M.D.
Director, Division of Pediatric Gastroenterology and Nutrition; Dorothy M.M. Kersten Professor of Pediatrics,

University of Cincinnati School of Medicine; Director, Division of Pediatric Gastroenterology and Nutrition, Children's Hospital Medical Center, Cincinnati, Ohio
Chapter 300: Development and Function; Chapter 301: Manifestations of Liver Disease; Chapter 302: Cholestasis; Chapter 303: Metabolic Diseases of the Liver; Chapter 304: Liver Abscess; Chapter 305: Liver Disease Associated With Systemic Disorders; Chapter 306: Reye Syndrome and "Reye-like" Diseases

LEWIS A. BARNESS, M.D.
Professor of Pediatrics, University of South Florida College of Medicine; Staff Pediatrician, Tampa General Hospital, Tampa, Florida
Part VI: Nutrition

KENNETH J. BART, M.D.
National Vaccine Program, Rockville, Maryland
Chapter 247: Immunization Practices

DORSEY M. BASS, M.D.
Assistant Professor of Pediatrics (Gastroenterology and Nutrition), Stanford University School of Medicine, Stanford, California
Chapter 222: Rotavirus and Other Agents of Viral Gastroenteritis

HOWARD BAUCHNER, M.D.
Associate Professor of Pediatrics, Boston University School of Medicine; Director, Division of General Pediatrics, Boston City Hospital, Boston, Massachusetts
Chapter 39: Failure to Thrive

RICHARD E. BEHRMAN, M.D.
Director, Center for the Future of Children, David and Lucile Packard Foundation; Clinical Professor of Pediatrics, Stanford University and UCSF; Attending Physician, Lucile Salter Packard Children's Hospital at Stanford, Stanford, California
Chapter 1: Overview of Pediatrics; Chapter 42: Children at Special Risk

CHARLES B. BERDE, M.D., Ph.D.
Associate Professor of Anaesthesia (Pediatrics), Harvard Medical School; Director, Pain Treatment Service; Senior Associate in Anesthesia, Children's Hospital, Boston, Massachusetts
Chapter 61: Anesthesia and Perioperative Care

JERRY M. BERGSTEIN, M.D.
Professor, Department of Pediatrics, Indiana University School of Medicine; Director, Section of Nephrology, James Whitcomb Riley Hospital for Children, Indianapolis, Indiana
Part XXIII: Nephrology

DANIEL BERNSTEIN, M.D.
Associate Professor of Pediatrics, Stanford University; Chief, Division of Pediatric Cardiology, Lucile Salter Packard Children's Hospital at Stanford, Palo Alto, California
Part XX: The Cardiovascular System

RONALD BLANTON, M.D.
Assistant Professor, Case Western Reserve University School of Medicine; Physician, University Hospitals of Cleveland, Cleveland, Ohio
Chapter 245: Helminthic Diseases

THOMAS F. BOAT, M.S., M.D.
Professor and Chairman, Department of Pediatrics, University of Cincinnati College of Medicine; Physician-In-Chief, Children's Hospital Medical Center, Cincinnati, Ohio
Chapter 362: Chronic or Recurrent Respiratory Symptoms; Chapter 363: Cystic Fibrosis; Chapter 364: Primary Ciliary Dyskinesia

DOROTHY BOLDING, Dr.P.H., M.S.W.
Assistant Professor of Psychiatry, Tulane University School of Medicine; Clinical Social Worker, Children's Neuropsychiatric Inpatient Unit, Tulane University Hospital, New Orleans, Louisiana
Chapter 33: Foster Care; Chapter 37: Impact of Violence

ROBERT BONOMO, M.D.
Assistant Professor, Case Western Reserve University School of Medicine; Assistant Professor, Division of Geriatrics, Department of Medicine, University Hospitals of Cleveland, Cleveland, Ohio
Chapter 244: Protozoan Diseases; Chapter 246: Antiparasitic Drugs for Children; Chapter 248: Health Advice for Traveling Children

LAURA C. BOWMAN, M.D.
Associate Professor, Department of Pediatrics, University of Tennessee College of Medicine; Associate Member, Department of Hematology-Oncology, St. Jude Children's Research Hospital, Memphis, Tennessee
Chapter 457: Neoplasms of the Liver

J. TIMOTHY BOYLE, M.D.
Associate Professor of Pediatrics, Case Western Reserve University School of Medicine; Chief, Division of Pediatric Gastroenterology and Nutrition, Rainbow Babies and Children's Hospital, Cleveland, Ohio
Chapter 287: Chronic Diarrhea

W. TED BROWN, M.D., Ph.D.
Chair, Department of Human Genetics, Institute of Basic Research, Staten Island, New York
Chapter 659: Progeria

DENA BROWNSTEIN, M.D.
Assistant Professor of Pediatrics, University of Washington; Attending Physician, Emergency Services, Children's Hospital and Medical Center, Seattle, Washington

Chapter 58: Injury Control; Chapter 59: Emergency Medical Services for Children

REBECCA H. BUCKLEY, M.D.
J. Buren Sidbury Professor of Pediatrics, Professor of Immunology, Duke University Medical Center; Chief, Division of Allergy and Immunology, Department of Pediatrics, Duke University Medical Center, Durham, North Carolina
Chapter 116: T-, B-, and NK-Cell Systems; Chapter 117: Primary B-Cell Diseases; Chapter 118: Primary T-Cell Disease; Chapter 119: Combined B- and T-Cell Diseases

BRUCE M. CAMITTA, M.D.
Professor of Pediatrics, Director of Hematology-Oncology, Medical College of Wisconsin; Director, Midwest Children's Cancer Center; Chief, Pediatric Hematology-Oncology, Children's Hospital of Wisconsin, Milwaukee, Wisconsin
Chapter 405: The Anemias; Part XXI: Diseases of the Blood; Section 4: Polycythemia; Section 8: The Spleen; Section 9: The Lymphatic System

JENNIFER PRATT CHENEY, M.D.
Assistant Professor, George Washington University School of Medicine; Co-Director, Pediatric Emergency Medicine Fellowship Program; Children's National Medical Center, Washington, D.C.
Chapter 60: Pediatric Critical Care

RUSSELL W. CHESNEY, M.D.
Le Bonheur Professor and Chair, The University of Tennessee and Le Bonheur Children's Medical Center, Memphis, Tennessee
Chapter 483: Renal Tubular Acidosis; Part XXXII: Bone and Joint Disorders; Section 3: Metabolic Bone Disease

CHING-HON PUI, M.D.
Professor of Pediatrics, University of Tennessee, College of Medicine; Vice Chairman for Research, Department of Hematology-Oncology, St. Jude Children's Research Hospital, Memphis, Tennessee
Chapter 449: The Leukemias

ROBERT D. CHRISTENSEN, M.D.
Professor of Pediatrics, Chief, Division of Neonatology, University of Florida College of Medicine; Attending Physician, Shands Teaching Hospital, Gainesville, Florida
Part XXI: Diseases of the Blood; Section 1: Development of the Hematopoietic System

THOMAS G. CLEARY, M.D.
Professor of Pediatrics, The University of Texas Medical School, Houston, Texas
Chapter 182: Salmonella Infections; Chapter 183: Shigella; Chapter 184: Escherichia coli, Aeromonas, and Plesiomonas; Chapter 185: Cholera; Chapter 186: Campylobacter; Chapter 187: Helicobacter

DAVID F. CLYDE, M.D., Ph.D., D.T.M. & H.
Adjunct Professor, Johns Hopkins University School of Hygiene and Public Health; Research Professor of Medicine, University of Maryland School of Medicine, Baltimore, Maryland
Chapter 244: Protozoan Diseases

PAUL M. COATES, Ph.D.
Research Professor of Pediatrics, University of Pennsylvania School of Medicine, Philadelphia, Pennsylvania; NIDDM Research Program Director, National Institute of Diabetes & Digestive & Kidney Diseases, National Institutes of Health, Bethesda, Maryland
Chapter 72: Defects in Metabolism of Lipids

HARVEY R. COLTEN, M.D.
Professor and Chairman, Department of Pediatrics, Washington University School of Medicine; Pediatrician-in-Chief, St. Louis Children's Hospital, St. Louis, Missouri
Chapter 350: Pulmonary Alveolar Proteinosis

JAMES J. CORRIGAN, M.D.
Dean and Professor of Pediatrics, Section of Pediatric Hematology-Oncology, Tulane University School of Medicine; Attending Physician, Tulane University Hospital and Clinics, Charity Hospital of New Orleans, New Orleans, Louisiana
Part XXI: Diseases of the Blood; Section 7: Hemorrhagic and Thrombotic Diseases

JEAN A. CORTNER, M.D.
Emeritus Professor of Pediatrics, University of Pennsylvania School of Medicine; Professor of Pediatrics, Division of Gastroenterology and Nutrition, The Children's Hospital of Philadelphia, Philadelphia, Pennsylvania
Chapter 72: Defects in Metabolism of Lipids

WILLIAM M. CRIST, M.D.
Professor, Department of Pediatrics, University of Tennessee, College of Medicine; Deputy Director and Chairman, Department of Hematology/Oncology, St. Jude Children's Research Hospital, Memphis, Tennessee
Part XXII: Neoplastic Diseases and Tumors; Chapter 445: Epidemiology; Chapter 447: Principles of Diagnosis; Chapter 448: Principles of Treatment; Chapter 449: The Leukemias; Chapter 453: Soft Tissue Sarcomas

JOHN S. CURRAN, M.D.
Professor of Pediatrics, University of South Florida College of Medicine; Chief of Pediatrics, Tampa General Hospital, Tampa, Florida
Part VI: Nutrition

RICHARD DALTON, M.D.
Professor of Psychiatry and Pediatrics, Tulane University School of Medicine, New Orleans, Louisiana
Part III: Psychologic Disorders; Chapter 32: Adoption; Chap-

ter 34: Effects of Mobile Society; Chapter 36: Separation and Death

GARY L. DARMSTADT, M.D.
Fellow, Department of Dermatology, Stanford University School of Medicine, Stanford, California
Part XXI: The Skin

ROBERT DAUM, M.D., C.M.
Professor of Pediatrics, University of Chicago; Chief, Pediatric Infectious Diseases, University of Chicago, Wyler Children's Hospital, Chicago, Illinois
Chapter 177: Haemophilus influenzae

FRANKLIN L. DeBUSK, M.D.
Professor of Pediatrics, University of Florida College of Medicine; Staff Member, Shands Hospital, Gainesville, Florida
Chapter 659: Progeria

DAPHNE E. DeMELLO, M.D.
Professor of Pathology and Pediatrics, Department of Pathology, St. Louis University School of Medicine, St. Louis, Missouri
Chapter 350: Pulmonary Alveolar Proteinosis

ANGELO M. DiGEORGE, M.D.
Professor Emeritus of Pediatrics, Temple University School of Medicine; Section of Endocrinology, Diabetes, and Metabolism, St. Christopher's Hospital for Children, Philadelphia, Pennsylvania
Part XXVI: The Endocrine System; Section 1: Disorders of the Hypothalamus and Pituitary Gland; Section 2: Disorders of the Thyroid Gland; Section 3: Disorders of the Parathyroid Glands; Section 4: Disorders of the Adrenal Glands; Section 5: Disorders of the Gonads

J. STEPHEN DUMLER, M.D.
Assistant Professor of Pathology, University of Maryland School of Medicine; Lecturer in Pathology, The Johns Hopkins University School of Medicine; Associate Director of Clinical Microbiology and Staff Pathologist, University of Maryland Medical Systems Hospital, Baltimore, Maryland
Part XVII: Infectious Diseases; Section 6: Rickettsial Infections

PAUL H. DWORKIN, M.D.
Professor and Associate Chairperson of Pediatrics; Head, Division of General Pediatrics, University of Connecticut School of Medicine, Farmington; Director/Chairperson, Department of Pediatrics, St. Francis Hospital and Medical Center, Hartford, Connecticut
Chapter 35: Child Care

MICHELE ESTABROOK, M.D.
Assistant Professor of Pediatrics, Case Western Reserve University; Division of Infectious Diseases, Rainbow Babies and Children's Hospital, Cleveland, Ohio
Chapter 178: Meningococcal Infections; Chapter 179: Gonococcal Infections

KENNETH FIFE, M.D., Ph.D.
Professor of Medicine, Microbiology and Immunology, and Pathology, Indiana University School of Medicine, Indianapolis, Indiana
Chapter 224: Human Papillomavirus

TIMOTHY FLANIGAN, M.D.
Assistant Professor of Medicine, Brown University; Director, Division of Geographic Medicine and Clinical Immunology, Miriam Hospital, Providence, Rhode Island
Chapter 244: Protozoan Diseases

J. JULIO PÉREZ FONTÁN, M.D.
Associate Professor of Pediatrics and Anesthesiology, Washington University School of Medicine; Director, Division of Pediatric Critical Care Medicine and Pediatric Intensive Care Unit, St. Louis Children's Hospital, St. Louis, Missouri
Chapter 60: Pediatric Critical Care; Chapter 319: Development of the Respiratory System

MARC A. FORMAN, M.D.
Professor of Psychiatry and Pediatrics and Director, Division of Child and Adolescent Psychiatry; Vice Chairman, Department of Psychiatry and Neurology, Tulane University School of Medicine, New Orleans, Louisiana
Chapter 18: Assessment and Interviewing; Chapter 19: Psychiatric Considerations of Central Nervous System Injury; Chapter 20: Psychosomatic Illness; Chapter 24: Mood Disorders; Chapter 27: Attention Deficit Hyperactivity Disorder (ADHD); Chapter 29: Psychosis in Childhood; Chapter 32: Adoption; Chapter 33: Foster Care; Chapter 36: Separation and Death; Chapter 37: Impact of Violence

NORMAN FOST, M.D., M.P.H.
Professor, Pediatrics and History of Medicine; Director, Program in Medical Ethics, University of Wisconsin School of Medicine; Pediatrician, University of Wisconsin Hospital, Madison, Wisconsin
Chapter 3: Ethics in Pediatric Care

JAMES FRENCH, M.D.
Pediatric Hematology-Oncology Fellow and Instructor in Pediatrics, Medical College of Wisconsin, Children's Hospital of Wisconsin, Milwaukee, Wisconsin
Part XXI: Diseases of the Blood; Section 8: The Spleen

LUIGI GARIBALDI, M.D.
Associate Professor of Pediatrics, Division of Pediatric Endocrinology, St. Louis University Health Sciences Center; Associate Professor, Cardinal Glennon Children's Hospital, St. Louis, Missouri
Chapter 516: Physiology of Puberty; Chapter 517: Disorders of Pubertal Development

J. CARLTON GARTNER, JR., M.D.
Professor of Pediatrics; Vice Chairman, Department of Pediatrics, University of Pittsburgh School of Medicine; Director, Diagnostic Referral Service; Director, Pediatric Residency Program, Children's Hospital of Pittsburgh, Pittsburgh, Pennsylvania
Chapter 313: Liver Transplantation

JEFFREY L. GOLDHAGEN, M.D., M.P.H.
Associate Professor of Pediatrics, University of Florida; Director, Duval County Public Health Unit, Jacksonville, Florida
Chapter 6: Child Health in the Developing World

HENRY F. GOMEZ, M.D.
Assistant Professor of Pediatrics, University of Texas, Houston, Houston Medical School, Houston, Texas
Chapter 183: Shigella; Chapter 185: Cholera

RICARDO GONZALEZ, M.D.
Professor of Urology, Wayne State University; Chief, Pediatric Urology, Children's Hospital of Michigan, Detroit, Michigan
Chapter 101: Urinary Tract Infections; Part XXIV: Urologic Disorders in Infants and Children

SAMUEL P. GOTOFF, M.D.
The Woman's Board Professor; Professor and Chair of Pediatrics, Rush Medical College, Chicago, Illinois
Part XII: Infections of the Neonatal Infant; Section 1: Unique Aspects of Infection; Chapter 98: Neonatal Sepsis and Meningitis

GREGORY A. GRABOWSKI, M.D.
Professor, Department of Pediatrics, University of Cincinnati; Director, Division of Human Genetics, Children's Hospital Medical Center, Cincinnati, Ohio
Chapter 68: Gene Therapy

CHARLES GROSE, M.D.
Professor of Pediatrics and Director of Infectious Disease, University of Iowa College of Medicine, Iowa City, Iowa
Chapter 96: Intrauterine Infection and Prenatal Diagnosis; Chapter 97: Viral Infections of the Fetus and Newborn

GABRIEL G. HADDAD, M.D.
Professor of Pediatrics and Cellular and Molecular Physiology; Director, Section of Respiratory Medicine, Department of Pediatrics, Yale University School of Medicine; Chief of Service, Respiratory Medicine; Attending Physician, Yale–New Haven Hospital, New Haven, Connecticut
Chapter 319: Development of the Respiratory System; Chapter 320: Regulation of Respiration; Chapter 321: Respiratory Function and Approach to Respiratory Disease; Chapter 322: Respiratory Failure; Chapter 323: Defense Mechanisms and Metabolic Function of the Lung; Chapter 330: Obstructive Sleep Apnea and Hypoventilation in Children; Chapter 377: Central Hypoventilation Syndromes

BRYAN HALL, M.D., F.A.A.P.
Professor of Pediatrics; Chief, Division of Genetics and Dysmorphology, University of Kentucky, Lexington, Kentucky
Part XXXII: Bone and Joint Disorders; Section 2: Genetic Skeletal Dysplasias

JUDITH G. HALL, M.D., F.R.C.P.C., F.A.A.P., F.C.C.M.G., F.A.B.M.G.
Professor and Head, Department of Pediatrics, University of British Columbia; Head, Department of Pediatrics, British Columbia's Children's Hospital, Vancouver, British Columbia, Canada
Chapter 67: Chromosomal and Clinical Abnormalities; Chapter 69: Genetic Counseling

SCOTT HALSTEAD, M.D.
Deputy Director, Health Sciences Division, The Rockefeller Foundation, New York, New York
Chapter 225: Arboviruses; Chapter 226: Hantavirus Pulmonary Syndrome

DAVIDSON H. HAMER, M.D.
Assistant Professor of Medicine, Tufts University School of Medicine; Director, Traveler's Health Service, Division of Geographic Medicine and Infectious Diseases, New England Medical Center, Boston; Project Scientist, Applied Diarrheal Disease Research Project, Harvard Institute for International Development, Cambridge, Massachusetts
Chapter 244: Protozoan Diseases

MARGARET R. HAMMERSCHLAG, M.D.
Professor of Pediatrics and Medicine, SUNY Health Science Center at Brooklyn; Co-Director, Pediatric Infectious Diseases, University Hospital of Brooklyn, Kings County Hospital Center, Brooklyn, New York
Chapter 197: Chlamydia

GARY E. HARTMAN, M.D.
Associate Professor of Surgery and Pediatrics, The George Washington University School of Medicine; Attending Surgeon, Children's National Medical Center, Washington, D.C.
Chapter 289: Acute Appendicitis; Chapter 317: Diaphragmatic Hernia; Chapter 318: Epigastric Hernia

ROBERT H. A. HASLAM, M.D., F.A.A.P., F.R.C.P.C.C.
Professor and Chairman, Department of Pediatrics, Professor of Medicine (Neurology), University of Toronto; Pediatrician-in-Chief, Hospital for Sick Children, Toronto, Ontario, Canada
Part XXVII The Nervous System

PETER L. HAVENS, M.S., M.D.
Associate Professor of Pediatrics and Epidemiology, Medical College of Wisconsin; Director, Pediatric HIV Program, Children's Hospital of Wisconsin, Milwaukee, Wisconsin
Chapter 2: Evaluating Medical Literature: Clinical Epidemiology

JOHN J. HERBST, M.D.
Professor of Pediatrics; Chief, Section Gastroenterology/Nutrition, Louisiana State University School of Medicine, Shreveport, Louisiana
Part XVIII: The Digestive System; Section 3: The Esophagus

JOHN T. HERRIN, M.B.B.S., F.R.A.C.P.
Associate Clinical Professor of Pediatrics, Harvard Medical School; Director, Clinical Service, Division of Nephrology, Children's Hospital, Boston, Massachusetts
Chapter 60: Pediatric Critical Care

HELEN HESLOP, M.D., F.R.A.C.P., F.R.C.P.A.
Associate Professor of Pediatrics, University of Tennessee; Associate Member, Division of Bone Marrow Transplantation, St. Jude Children's Research Hospital, Memphis, Tennessee
Chapter 447: Principles of Diagnosis; Chapter 448: Principles of Treatment; Chapter 449: The Leukemias

WILLIAM H. HETZNECKER, M.D.
Clinical Professor of Psychiatry, Temple University School of Medicine, Philadelphia, Pennsylvania
Chapter 18: Assessment and Interviewing

GEORGE R. HONIG, M.D., Ph.D.
Professor and Head, Department of Pediatrics, University of Illinois at Chicago College of Medicine; Professor and Head, Department of Pediatrics, University of Illinois Hospital, Chicago, Illinois
Chapter 419: Hemoglobin Disorders

R. RODNEY HOWELL, M.D.
Professor and Chairman, University of Miami School of Medicine; Pediatrician-in-Chief, Children's Hospital at University of Miami/Jackson Memorial Hospital, Miami, Florida
Chapter 75: Defects in Metabolism of Purines and Pyrimidines

MELISSA M. HUDSON, M.D.
Assistant Professor of Pediatrics, University of Tennessee; Assistant Member, Department of Hematology/Oncology, St. Jude Children's Research Hospital, Memphis, Tennessee
Chapter 450: Lymphoma

WALTER HUGHES, M.D.
Professor of Pediatrics, University of Tennessee College of Medicine; Chairman, Department of Infectious Diseases, St. Jude Children's Research Hospital, Memphis, Tennessee
Chapter 173: Infections in the Compromised Host; Chapter 237: Pneumocystis carinii Pneumonitis (Interstitial Plasma Cell Pneumonitis)

CARL E. HUNT, M.D.
Professor and Chairman of Pediatrics, The Medical College of Ohio, Toledo, Ohio
Chapter 657: Sudden Infant Death Syndrome

JEFFREY S. HYAMS, M.D.
Professor of Pediatrics, University of Connecticut School of Medicine, Farmington; Director, Division of Pediatric Gastroenterology and Nutrition, Hartford Hospital, Hartford, Connecticut
Chapter 314: Malformations; Chapter 315: Ascites; Chapter 316: Peritonitis

LILLY CHENG IMMERGLUCK, M.D.
Fellow in Pediatric Infectious Diseases, University of Chicago, Chicago, Illinois
Chapter 177: Haemophilus influenzae

RICHARD F. JACOBS, M.D., F.A.A.P.
Horace C. Cabe Professor of Pediatrics, University of Arkansas for Medical Sciences; Chief, Pediatric Infectious Diseases, Arkansas Children's Hospital, Little Rock, Arkansas
Chapter 202: Actinomycosis; Chapter 203: Nocardiosis

HAL B. JENSON, M.D.
Associate Professor and Chief, Pediatric Infectious Diseases, Departments of Pediatrics and Microbiology, University of Texas Health Science Center at San Antonio; Attending Physician, University Hospital and Santa Rosa Children's Hospital, San Antonio, Texas
Chapter 215: Epstein-Barr Virus; Chapter 661: Chronic Fatigue Syndrome

DAVID C. JOHNSEN, D.D.S., M.S.
Professor of Pediatric Dentistry, Case Western Reserve University; Attending Pediatric Dentist, Rainbow Babies and Children's Hospital, Cleveland, Ohio
Part XVIII: The Digestive System; Section 2: The Oral Cavity

CHARLES F. JOHNSON, M.D.
Professor of Pediatrics, The Ohio State University College of Medicine; Director, Child Abuse Program, Children's Hospital, Columbus, Ohio
Chapter 38: Abuse and Neglect of Children

RICHARD B. JOHNSTON, JR., M.D.
Adjunct Professor, Chief, Section of Pediatric Immunology, Yale University School of Medicine, New Haven, Connecticut; Medical Director, March of Dimes Birth Defects Foundation, White Plains, New York

Chapter 120: The Complement System; Chapter 121: Diseases of the Complement System

KENNETH LYONS JONES, M.D.
Professor of Pediatrics, University of California School of Medicine, San Diego; UCSD Medical Center, La Jolla, California
Chapter 86: Dysmorphology

HARRY J. KALLAS, M.D.
Assistant Professor of Pediatrics, University of California, Davis; Associate Director, Pediatric Critical Care Medicine, U.C. Davis Medical Center, Sacramento, California
Chapter 60: Pediatric Critical Care

JAMES W. KAZURA, M.D.
Professor of Medicine and International Health, Case Western Reserve University School of Medicine; Physician, University Hospitals of Cleveland, Cleveland, Ohio
Chapter 245: Helminthic Diseases

CHARLES H. KING, M.D.
Associate Clinical Professor of Medicine, Division of Geographic Medicine, Case Western Reserve University, Cleveland, Ohio
Chapter 245: Helminthic Diseases

ROBERT M. KLIEGMAN, M.D.
Professor and Chairman, Department of Pediatrics, Medical College of Wisconsin; Pediatrician-in-Chief, Children's Hospital of Wisconsin, Milwaukee, Wisconsin
Chapter 73: Defects in Metabolism of Carbohydrates; Part XI: The Fetus and the Neonatal Infant

WILLIAM C. KOCH, M.D.
Assistant Professor of Pediatrics, Children's Medical Center, Department of Pediatrics, Division of Infectious Diseases, Medical College of Virginia/Virginia Commonwealth University; Medical College of Virginia Hospitals, Richmond, Virginia
Chapter 210: Parvovirus B19

STEVE KOHL, M.D.
Professor of Pediatrics, University of California, San Francisco; Chief, Pediatric Infectious Diseases, Moffitt Long Hospital, San Francisco General Hospital, San Francisco, California
Chapter 211: Herpes Simplex Virus; Chapter 212: Human Herpesvirus 6

ROBERT A. KRANCE, M.D.
Vice Chairman, Clinical Affairs, and Director, Department of Hematology/Oncology, St. Jude Children's Research Hospital, Memphis, Tennessee
Chapter 449: The Leukemias

STEPHAN LADISCH, M.D.
Professor of Pediatrics and Biochemistry/Molecular Biology, The George Washington University School of Medicine and Health Sciences; Director, Center for Cancer and Transplantation Biology, Children's Research Institute, Washington, D.C.
Chapter 660: Histiocytosis Syndromes of Childhood

STEPHEN LaFRANCHI, M.D.
Professor, Department of Pediatrics; Head, Pediatric Endocrinology, Oregon Health Sciences University; Staff Physician, Doernbecher Children's Hospital, Portland, Oregon
Part XXVI: The Endocrine System; Section 2: Disorders of the Thyroid Gland; Section 3: Disorders of the Parathyroid Gland

GEORGE H. LAMBERT, M.D.
Associate Professor of Pediatrics; Director, Division of Pediatric Pharmacology and Toxicology, Department of Pediatrics, Robert Wood Johnson Medical School, University of Medicine and Dentistry of New Jersey, New Brunswick, New Jersey
Chapter 664: Mercury Exposure and Intoxication

ALFRED T. LANE, M.D.
Associate Professor of Dermatology and Pediatrics; Acting Chairman, Department of Dermatology, Director of Pediatric Dermatology, Stanford University School of Medicine; Stanford University Hospital, Lucile Salter Packard Children's Hospital, California
Part XXXI: The Skin

MARGARET W. LEIGH, M.D.
Associate Professor, Pediatrics Chief, Division of Pulmonary Medicine and Allergy, University of North Carolina at Chapel Hill; Attending Staff, UNC Hospitals, Chapel Hill, North Carolina
Chapter 658: Sarcoidosis

LENORE S. LEVINE, M.D.
Professor of Pediatrics, College of Physicians and Surgeons, Columbia University; Deputy Director, Pediatrics, St. Luke's–Roosevelt Hospital Center, New York, New York
Part XXVI: The Endocrine System; Section 4: Disorders of the Adrenal Glands

MELVIN D. LEVINE, M.D.
Professor of Pediatrics, University of North Carolina; Director, The Clinical Center for the Study of Development and Learning, Chapel Hill, North Carolina
Chapter 31: Neurodevelopmental Dysfunction in the School-Aged Child

GEORGE LISTER, M.D.
Professor of Pediatrics and Anesthesiology, Director, Division of Pediatric Critical Care Medicine, Yale University School of Medicine; Director, Pediatric Intensive Care Unit, Children's Hospital at Yale–New Haven, New Haven, Connecticut
Chapter 60: Pediatric Critical Care

IRIS F. LITT, M.D.
Professor of Pediatrics, Stanford University School of Medicine; Director, Division of Adolescent Medicine, Lucile Salter Packard Children's Hospital, Stanford, California
Part XIII: Special Health Problems During Adolescence

SARAH S. LONG, M.D.
Professor of Pediatrics, Temple University School of Medicine; Chief, Section of Infectious Diseases, St. Christopher's Hospital for Children, Philadelphia, Pennsylvania
Chapter 180: Diphtheria; Chapter 181: Pertussis

ADEL A. F. MAHMOUD, M.D., Ph.D.
Chairman and Professor of Medicine, Case Western Reserve University; Chairman of Medicine and Physician in Chief, University Hospitals of Cleveland, Cleveland, Ohio
Part XVII: Infectious Diseases; Section 7: Parasitic Infections

YVONNE MALDONADO, M.D.
Assistant Professor of Pediatrics, Stanford University School of Medicine; Attending Physician, Lucile Salter Packard Children's Hospital at Stanford, Palo Alto, California
Chapter 206: Measles; Chapter 207: Rubella; Chapter 208: Mumps

ANDREW M. MARGILETH, M.D., F.A.A.P., F.A.C.P.
Clinical Professor of Pediatrics, University of Virginia Medical Center, Charlottesville, Virginia; Chairman, Department of Pediatrics, Volunteers in Medicine Clinic, Hilton Head Island, South Carolina
Chapter 205: Cat Scratch Disease

NEYSSA MARINA, M.D.
Department of Pediatrics, University of Tennessee; Assistant Member, Department of Hematology/Oncology, St. Jude Children's Research Hospital, Memphis, Tennessee
Chapter 454: Neoplasms of Bone; Chapter 456: Gonadal and Germ Cell Neoplasms

MELVIN MARKS, M.D.
Professor and Vice Chair, Department of Pediatrics, University of California, Irvine, School of Medicine; Medical Director/Administrator, Memorial Miller Children's Hospital, Long Beach, California
Chapter 172: Osteomyelitis and Septic Arthritis

REUBEN K. MATALON, M.D., Ph.D.
Professor of Pediatrics, State University of New York Health Science Center, Brooklyn, New York; Professor, Department of Biology, College of Health, Florida International University; Director of Research Institute and Division of Genetics and Metabolism, Miami Children's Hospital, Miami, Florida
Chapter 71: Defects in Metabolism of Amino Acids; Chapter 72: Defects in Metabolism of Lipids; Chapter 74: Disorders of Mucopolysaccharide Metabolism

PAUL L. McCARTHY, M.D.
Professor of Pediatrics, Yale University School of Medicine; Head, Division of General Pediatrics, The Children's Hospital at Yale–New Haven, New Haven, Connecticut
Chapter 7: The Well Child; Chapter 57: Evaluation of the Sick Child in the Office and Clinic

MARCIA J. McDUFFIE, M.D.
Associate Professor of Pediatrics, University of Virginia School of Medicine, Charlottesville, Virginia
Chapter 146: Autoimmunity

KENNETH McINTOSH, M.D.
Professor of Pediatrics, Harvard Medical School; Chief, Division of Infectious Diseases, Children's Hospital, Boston, Massachusetts
Chapter 218: Respiratory Syncytial Virus; Chapter 219: Adenoviruses; Chapter 220: Rhinovirus

RIMA McLEOD, M.D.
Professor of Medicine, Immunology, Microbiology and Genetics; Lecturer in Medicine and Immunology, The University of Illinois at Chicago; Attending Physician, Michael Reese Hospital and Medical Center, Chicago, Illinois
Chapter 244: Protozoan Diseases

DEBORAH P. MERKE, M.D.
Clinical Associate, National Institute of Child Health and Human Development, Developmental Endocrinology Branch, Bethesda, Maryland
Chapter 662: Radiation Injury

WILLIAM MEYER, M.D.
Professor, Department of Pediatrics, University of Tennessee; Member and Vice-Chairman, Department of Hematology/Oncology, St. Jude Children's Research Hospital, Memphis, Tennessee
Chapter 454: Neoplasms of Bone

ROBERT W. MILLER, M.D., Dr.P.H.
Scientist Emeritus, Clinical Genetics Branch, National Cancer Institute, National Institutes of Health, Bethesda, Maryland
Chapter 662: Radiation Injury; Chapter 663: Chemical Pollutants

ABRAHAM MORAG, M.D.
Associate Professor (Clinical Virology), The Hebrew University–Hadassah Medical School; Head, Clinical Virology Unit, Hadassah University Medical Center, Jerusalem, Israel
Chapter 209: Enteroviruses

ARDYTHE L. MORROW, Ph.D., M.Sc.
Associate Professor of Pediatrics, Center for Pediatric Research, Eastern Virginia Medical School; Epidemiologist, Children's Hospital of The King's Daughters, Norfolk, Virginia
Chapter 250: Child Day Care and Communicable Diseases

HUGO W. MOSER, M.D.
University Professor of Neurology and Pediatrics, The Johns Hopkins University; Department Director, Neurogenetics, Kennedy Krieger Institute, Baltimore, Maryland
Chapter 72: Defects in Metabolism of Lipids

NANDINI NARASIMHAN, M.D.
Fellow, Pediatric Infectious Diseases, University of California, Irvine; Memorial Miller Children's Hospital, Long Beach, California
Chapter 172: Osteomyelitis and Septic Arthritis

ROBERT D. NEEDLMAN, M.D.
Assistant Professor of Pediatrics, Case Western Reserve University School of Medicine; Director, Continuity Training, Rainbow Babies and Children's Hospital, Cleveland, Ohio
Part II: Growth and Development

LEONARD B. NELSON, M.D.
Co-Director, Pediatric Ophthalmology, Wills Eye Hospital; Associate Professor of Ophthalmology and Pediatrics; Jefferson Medical College of Thomas Jefferson University, Philadelphia, Pennsylvania
Part XXIX: Disorders of the Eye

JOHN F. NICHOLSON, M.D.
Associate Professor of Pediatrics and Pathology, Columbia University College of Physicians and Surgeons; Associate Attending Pediatrician, Presbyterian Hospital, New York, New York
Chapter 670: Laboratory Testing and Reference Values (Table 670–2) for Infants and Children

MICHAEL E. NORMAN, M.D.
Clinical Professor of Pediatrics, University of North Carolina School of Medicine, Chapel Hill; Chairman, Department of Pediatrics, Carolinas Medical Center, Charlotte, North Carolina
Chapter 483: Renal Tubular Acidosis

PEARAY L. OGRA, M.D.
John Sealy Distinguished Chair and Professor, Department of Pediatrics, University of Texas Medical Branch; Pediatrician-in-Chief, Children's Hospital, University of Texas Medical Branch, Galveston, Texas
Chapter 209: Enteroviruses

ROBIN K. OHLS, M.D.
Assistant Professor of Pediatrics, Division of Neonatalogy, University of New Mexico, Albuquerque, New Mexico
Part XXI: Diseases of the Blood; Section 1: Development of the Hematopoietic System

DAVID M. ORENSTEIN, M.D.
Professor of Pediatrics, School of Medicine; Professor of Health, Physical, and Recreation Education and Exercise Physiology, School of Education, University of Pittsburgh; Director, Cystic Fibrosis/Pulmonary Disease Center, Children's Hospital of Pittsburgh, Pittsburgh, Pennsylvania
Chapter 332: Acute Inflammatory Upper Airway Obstruction; Chapter 333: Foreign Bodies in the Larynx, Trachea, and Bronchi; Chapter 334: Subglottic Stenosis; Chapter 338: Bronchiolitis; Chapter 339: Bronchiolitis Obliterans; Chapter 340: Aspiration Pneumonias and Gastroesophageal Reflux–Related Respiratory Disease; Chapter 354: Emphysema and Overinflation; Chapter 355: Pulmonary Edema; Chapter 362: Chronic or Recurrent Respiratory Symptoms; Part XIX: The Respiratory System; Section 4: Diseases of the Pleura; Section 5: Neuromuscular and Skeletal Diseases Affecting Pulmonary Function

P. PEARL O'ROURKE, M.D.
Associate Professor, Anesthesia (Pediatrics), University of Washington; Director, Pediatric Intensive Care Unit, Children's Hospital and Medical Center, Seattle, Washington
Chapter 60: Pediatric Critical Care

LUCY M. OSBORN, M.D., M.S.P.H.
Associate Vice President of Health Sciences, Professor of Pediatrics, University of Utah Health Science Center, Salt Lake City, Utah
Chapter 5: Preventive Pediatrics

LEE M. PACHTER, D.O.
Assistant Professor of Pediatrics and Anthropology, University of Connecticut School of Medicine, Farmington; Associate Director, Pediatric Inpatient Services, The Center for Children's Health and Development, Saint Francis Hospital and Medical Center, Hartford, Connecticut
Chapter 4: Cultural Issues in Pediatric Care

DEMOSTHENES PAPPAGIANIS, M.D., Ph.D.
Professor, Department of Medical Microbiology and Immunology, University of California School of Medicine, Davis, California
Chapter 233: Coccidioidomycosis (San Joaquin Fever, Valley Fever, Desert Rheumatism, Coccidioidal Granuloma)

ALBERTO S. PAPPO, M.D.
Assistant Professor of Pediatrics, The University of Tennessee, College of Medicine; Assistant Member, St. Jude Children's Research Hospital, Memphis, Tennessee
Chapter 453: Soft Tissue Sarcomas; Chapter 461: Benign Tumors

JOHN S. PARKS, M.D., Ph.D.
Professor of Pediatrics, Associate Professor of Biochemistry, Emory University School of Medicine, Atlanta, Georgia
Part XXVI: The Endocrine System; Section 1: Disorders of the Hypothalamus and Pituitary Gland; Chapter 512: Hypopituitarism

WADE PARKS, M.D., Ph.D.
Professor and Chairman, Department of Pediatrics, New York University School of Medicine, New York, New York
Chapter 223: Human Immunodeficiency Virus

ALBERTO PEÑA, M.D.
Professor of Surgery, Albert Einstein College of Medicine, New York; Chief of Pediatric Surgery, Schneider Children's Hospital Long Island Jewish Medical Center, New Hyde Park, New York
Chapter 281: Anorectal Malformations; Chapter 290: Surgical Conditions of the Anus, Rectum, and Colon

JAMES M. PERRIN, M.D.
Associate Professor of Pediatrics, Harvard Medical School; Director, Ambulatory Care Programs and General Pediatrics, Children's Service, Massachusetts General Hospital, Boston, Massachusetts
Chapter 40: Developmental Disabilities and Chronic Illness: An Overview

MICHAEL A. PESCE, Ph.D.
Associate Professor of Clinical Pathology, Columbia University College of Physicians and Surgeons; Director, Clinical Chemistry Laboratory, Columbia-Presbyterian Medical Center, New York, New York
Chapter 670: Laboratory Testing and Reference Values (Table 670–2) for Infants and Children

LARRY K. PICKERING, M.D.
Professor of Pediatrics, Eastern Virginia Medical School; Director, Center for Pediatric Research, Children's Hospital of The King's Daughters, Norfolk, Virginia
Chapter 100: Hepatitis in Neonates; Chapter 171: Gastroenteritis; Chapter 221: Hepatitis A Through B; Chapter 250: Child Day Care and Communicable Diseases

SERGIO PIOMELLI, M.D.
James A. Wolff Professor of Pediatrics, Columbia University College of Physicians and Surgeons; Director, Pediatric Hematology-Oncology, Babies and Children's Hospital of New York, New York, New York
Chapter 665: Lead Poisoning

PHILIP A. PIZZO, M.D.
Chief of Pediatrics and Head, Infectious Disease Section, National Cancer Institute, National Institutes of Health, Bethesda, Maryland
Part XXI: Diseases of the Blood; Section 5: The Pancytopenias

STANLEY A. PLOTKIN, M.D.
Emeritus Professor of Pediatrics, University of Pennsylvania, Philadelphia, Pennsylvania; Medical and Scientific Director, Sérum et Vaccins, Pasteur-Mérieux, Marnes-la-Coquette, France
Chapter 227: Rabies

DWIGHT A. POWELL, M.D.
Professor of Pediatrics, The Ohio State University; Chief, Section of Infectious Diseases, Children's Hospital, Columbus, Ohio
Chapter 196: Mycoplasmal Infections; Chapter 200: Nontuberculous Mycobacteria

KEITH R. POWELL, M.D.
Professor and Associate Chair of Pediatrics, University of Rochester School of Medicine and Dentistry; Attending Pediatrician, Strong Memorial Hospital, Rochester, New York
Chapter 167: Fever Without a Focus; Chapter 168: Sepsis and Shock

CHARLES B. PRATT, M.D.
Professor of Pediatrics, University of Tennessee, Memphis, College of Medicine; Member, Department of Hematology/Oncology, St. Jude Children's Research Hospital, Memphis, Tennessee
Chapter 455: Retinoblastoma; Chapter 458: Gastrointestinal Neoplasms; Chapter 459: Carcinomas; Chapter 460: Cancer of the Skin

CHARLES G. PROBER, M.D.
Professor of Pediatrics, Medicine, Microbiology, and Immunology; Associate Chairman, Department of Pediatrics, Stanford University School of Medicine; Attending Physician, Lucile Salter Packard Children's Hospital at Stanford, Stanford, California
Chapter 99: Pneumonia in the Neonate; Chapter 169: Infections of the Central Nervous System; Chapter 170: Pneumonia

ALBERT W. PRUITT, M.D.
Dean and Professor of Pediatrics, College of Medicine, and Vice President for Medical Affairs, University of South Alabama, Mobile, Alabama
Chapter 404: Systemic Hypertension

MICHAEL D. REED, Pharm.D.
Associate Professor of Pediatrics, Case Western Reserve University School of Medicine; Director, Pediatric Clinical Pharmacology/Toxicology, Rainbow Babies and Children's Hospital, Cleveland, Ohio
Chapter 63: Principles of Drug Therapy

JACK S. REMINGTON, M.D.
Professor of Medicine, Division of Infectious Diseases and Geographic Medicine, Stanford University School of Medicine, Stanford; Marcus A. Krupp Research Chair and Chairman, Department of Immunology and Infectious Diseases, Research Institute, Palo Alto Medical Foundation, Palo Alto, California
Chapter 244: Protozoan Diseases

IRAJ REZVANI, M.D.
Acting Chairman and Professor of Pediatrics, Temple University School of Medicine; Chief, Section of Endocrinology, Diabetes and Metabolism, St. Christopher's Hospital for Children, Philadelphia, Pennsylvania
Chapter 70: An Approach to Inborn Errors of Metabolism; Chapter 71: Defects in Metabolism of Amino Acids

THOMAS B. RICE, M.D.
Associate Professor of Pediatrics; Chief, Pediatric Pulmonary/Critical Care Section, Medical College of Wisconsin; Director of Critical Care, Children's Hospital of Wisconsin, Milwaukee, Wisconsin
Chapter 60: Pediatric Critical Care

FREDERICK P. RIVARA, M.D., M.P.H.
George Adkins Professor of Pediatrics, Adjunct Professor of Epidemiology, University of Washington; Director, Harborview Injury Prevention and Research Center, Seattle, Washington
Chapter 58: Injury Control; Chapter 59: Emergency Medical Services for Children

KENT A. ROBERTSON, M.D., Ph.D.
Assistant Professor of Pediatrics; Investigator, Herman B. Wells Center for Pediatric Research, Department of Pediatrics, Division of Pediatric Hematology and Oncology, Stem Cell Transplantation Program, Indiana University School of Medicine, James Whitcomb Riley Hospital for Children, Indianapolis, Indiana
Chapter 132: Bone Marrow Transplantation

LUTHER K. ROBINSON, M.D.
Associate Professor of Pediatrics, State University of New York at Buffalo School of Medicine and Biomedical Sciences; Director, Dysmorphology and Clinical Genetics, Children's Hospital of Buffalo, Buffalo, New York
Chapter 646: Marfan Syndrome

ALICE ROCK, M.D.
Assistant Professor of Pediatrics, Medical College of Wisconsin, Milwaukee, Wisconsin
Part XXI: Diseases of the Blood; Section 9: The Lymphatic System

CAROL L. ROSEN, M.D.
Associate Professor, Department of Pediatrics, Section of Respiratory Medicine, Yale University School of Medicine; Medical Director, Children's Sleep Center, Attending Physician, Yale–New Haven Hospital, New Haven, Connecticut
Chapter 330: Obstructive Sleep Apnea and Hypoventilation in Children

DAVID S. ROSENBLATT, M.D.
Professor, Department of Human Genetics, Departments of Medicine and Medical Genetics, University of Montreal, Montreal, Quebec, Canada
Chapter 70: An Approach to Inborn Errors of Metabolism

BARRY H. RUMACK, M.D.
Clinical Professor of Pediatrics, Director Emeritus, Rocky Mountain Poison and Drug Center, University of Colorado School of Medicine, Denver, Colorado
Chapter 666: Chemical and Drug Poisoning

NURIA SABATÉ, M.D.
Assistant Professor of Psychiatry, and Training Director in Child Psychiatry, University of Puerto Rico School of Medicine, San Juan, Puerto Rico
Chapter 20: Psychosomatic Illness; Chapter 34: Effects of Mobile Society

ROBERT A. SALATA, M.D.
Associate Professor of Medicine, Case Western Reserve University School of Medicine; Associate Chief and Clinical Program Director—Division of Infectious Disease, Hospital Epidemiologist, University Hospitals of Cleveland, Cleveland, Ohio
Chapter 244: Protozoan Diseases; Chapter 246: Antiparasitic Drugs for Children; Chapter 248: Health Advice for Traveling Children

JOHN T. SANDLUND, M.D.
Associate Professor, University of Tennessee; Assistant Member, St. Jude Children's Research Hospital, Memphis, Tennessee
Chapter 450: Lymphoma

JOSEPH S. SANFILIPPO, M.D.
Professor of Obstetrics and Gynecology, University of Louisville School of Medicine; President, Adult Health Services; Alliant Health System, Louisville, Kentucky
Part XXV: Gynecologic Problems of Childhood

VICTOR M. SANTANA, M.D.
Associate Professor of Pediatrics, University of Tennessee; Associate Member, Department of Hematology/Oncology, St. Jude Children's Research Hospital, Memphis, Tennessee
Chapter 451: Neuroblastoma

HARVEY B. SARNAT, M.D.
Professor of Pediatrics (Neurology) and Pathology (Neuropathology), University of Washington School of Medicine; Head, Division of Pediatric Neurology, Children's Hospital and Medical Center, Seattle, Washington
Part XXVIII: Neuromuscular Disorders

SHIGERU SASSA, M.D., Ph.D.
Associate Professor and Physician; Head, Laboratory of Biochemical Hematology, The Rockefeller University, New York, New York
Chapter 76: The Porphyrias

JANE GREEN SCHALLER, M.D.
Professor and Chair, Department of Pediatrics, Tufts University and New England Medical Center, Boston, Massachusetts
Part XVI: Rheumatic Diseases of Childhood (Inflammatory Diseases of Connective Tissue, Collagen Diseases)

WILLIAM S. SCHECHTER, M.D.
Instructor in Anaesthesia, Harvard University; Associate-in-Anesthesia; Director, Post-anesthesia Care Unit, Children's Hospital, Boston, Massachusetts
Chapter 61: Anesthesia and Perioperative Care

ELIAS SCHWARTZ, M.D.
Professor and Chairman, Department of Pediatrics, University of Pennsylvania School of Medicine; Physician-in-Chief, Werner and Gertrude Henle Chair, The Children's Hospital of Philadelphia, Philadelphia, Pennsylvania
Part XXI: Diseases of the Blood; Section 2: Anemias of Inadequate Production

PETER V. SCOLES, M.D.
Professor of Orthopedics and Pediatrics, Case Western Reserve University School of Medicine, Cleveland, Ohio
Part XXXII: Bone and Joint Disorders; Section 1: Orthopedic Problems

GEORGE B. SEGEL, M.D.
Professor of Pediatrics, Medicine and Genetics; Director, Division of Pediatric Genetics; Associate Chair for Academic Affairs, Department of Pediatrics, University of Rochester; Pediatrician and Physician, Strong Memorial Hospital, Rochester, New York
Part XXI: Diseases of the Blood; Section 3: Hemolytic Anemias

GLORIA L. SELLMAN, M.D.
Staff Anesthesiologist, Children's Hospital of Birmingham, Birmingham, Alabama
Chapter 62: Pain Management

DAVID N. SHAPIRO, M.D.
Associate Professor, Department of Pediatrics, University of Tennessee College of Medicine; Associate Member, Departments of Experimental Oncology and Hematology/Oncology, St. Jude Children's Research Hospital, Memphis, Tennessee
Chapter 446: Molecular Pathogenesis

EUGENE D. SHAPIRO, M.D.
Professor of Pediatrics and Epidemiology, Children's Clinical Research Center and Yale University School of Medicine; Attending Pediatrician, Children's Hospital at Yale–New Haven, New Haven, Connecticut
Chapter 198: Lyme Disease (Lyme Borreliosis)

LARRY J. SHAPIRO, M.D.
Professor and Chairman, Department of Pediatrics, University of California, San Francisco, School of Medicine, San Francisco, California
Chapter 64: The Molecular Basis of Genetic Disorders; Chapter 65: Molecular Diagnosis; Chapter 66: Inheritance Patterns

PATRICIA D. SHEARER, M.D.
Assistant Professor, The University of Tennessee; Assistant Member, St. Jude Children's Research Hospital, Memphis, Tennessee
Chapter 452: Neoplasms of the Kidney

STEPHEN J. SHOCHAT, M.D.
Professor of Surgery, University of Pennsylvania; Senior Associate, Children's Hospital of Philadelphia, Philadelphia, Pennsylvania
Chapter 292: Inguinal Hernias

JACK P. SHONKOFF, M.D.
Samuel F. and Rose B. Gingold Professor of Human Development; Dean of the Florence Heller Graduate School, Brandeis University, Waltham; Consultant in Medicine, Children's Hospital, Boston, Massachusetts
Chapter 40: Developmental Disabilities and Chronic Illness: An Overview

R. MICHAEL SLY, M.D.
Professor of Pediatrics, The George Washington University School of Medicine and Health Sciences; Chairman, Allergy and Immunology, Children's National Medical Center, Washington, D.C.
Part XV: Allergic Disorders

JOHN D. SNYDER, M.D.
Associate Professor of Pediatrics, University of California School of Medicine, San Francisco, California
Chapter 100: Hepatitis in Neonates; Chapter 171: Gastroenteritis; Chapter 221: Hepatitis A Through B

MICHAEL J. SOLHUNG, M.D.
Associate Professor of Pediatrics; Assistant Professor of Physiology, Eastern Virginia Medical School; Director, Pediatric Nephrology, Children's Hospital of The King's Daughters, Norfolk, Virginia
Part VII: Pathophysiology of Body Fluids

MARK A. SPERLING, M.D.
Professor and Chair, Department of Pediatrics, University of Pittsburgh School of Medicine and Children's Hospital of Pittsburgh, Pittsburgh, Pennsylvania

Chapter 77: Hypoglycemia; Part XXVI: The Endocrine System; Section 6: Diabetes Mellitus

SERGIO STAGNO, M.D.
Professor and Chairman, Department of Pediatrics, University of Alabama at Birmingham; Physician-in-Chief, The Children's Hospital of Alabama, Birmingham, Alabama
Chapter 214: Cytomegalovirus

CHARLES A. STANLEY, M.D.
Professor of Pediatrics, University of Pennsylvania School of Medicine; Senior Endocrinologist, Children's Hospital of Philadelphia, Philadelphia, Pennsylvania
Chapter 72: Defects in Metabolism of Lipids

JEFFREY R. STARKE, M.D.
Associate Professor of Clinical Pediatrics, Baylor College of Medicine; Director, Children's Tuberculosis Clinic, Houston, Texas
Chapter 199: Tuberculosis

BARBARA W. STECHENBERG, M.D.
Associate Professor of Pediatrics, Tufts University School of Medicine, Boston; Vice Chairman and Director, Pediatric Infectious Diseases, Baystate Medical Center Children's Hospital, Springfield, Massachusetts
Chapter 204: Bartonellosis

ROBERT C. STERN, M.D.
Professor of Pediatrics, Case Western Reserve University School of Medicine; Associate Pediatrician, Rainbow Babies and Children's Hospital, Cleveland, Ohio
Chapter 331: Congenital Anomalies; Chapter 335: Trauma to the Larynx; Chapter 336: Neoplasms of the Larynx; Chapter 337: Bronchitis; Chapter 341: Silo Filler Disease; Chapter 342: Paraquat Lung; Chapter 343: Hypersensitivity to Inhaled Materials; Chapter 344: Pulmonary Aspergillosis; Chapter 345: Loeffler Syndrome (Eosinophilic Pneumonia); Chapter 346: Pulmonary Involvement in Collagen Diseases; Chapter 347: Desquamative Interstitial Pneumonitis; Chapter 348: Hypostatic Pneumonia; Chapter 349: Pulmonary Hemosiderosis; Chapter 351: Idiopathic Diffuse Interstitial Fibrosis of the Lung (Hamman-Rich Syndrome); Chapter 352: Pulmonary Alveolar Microlithiasis; Chapter 353: Atelectasis; Chapter 356: Pulmonary Embolism and Infarction; Chapter 357: Bronchiectasis; Chapter 358: Pulmonary Abscess; Chapter 359: Lung Hernia; Chapter 360: Pulmonary Tumors; Chapter 361: Hiccup (Singultus)

RONALD G. STRAUSS, M.D.
Professor of Pathology and Pediatrics, University of Iowa College of Medicine; Medical Director, DeGowin Blood Center, University of Iowa Hospitals and Clinics, Iowa City, Iowa
Part XXI: Diseases of the Blood; Section 6: Blood and Blood Fraction Transfusions

FREDERICK J. SUCHY, M.D.
Professor of Pediatrics; Chief, Pediatric Gastroenterology/Hepatology; Yale University School of Medicine, New Haven, Connecticut
Chapter 307: Chronic Hepatitis; Chapter 308: Drug- and Toxin-Induced Liver Injury; Chapter 309: Fulminant Hepatic Failure; Chapter 310: Cystic Diseases of the Biliary Tract and Liver; Chapter 311: Diseases of the Gallbladder; Chapter 312: Portal Hypertension and Varices

ANDREW M. TERSHAKOVEC, M.D.
Assistant Professor, Department of Pediatrics, University of Pennsylvania School of Medicine; Assistant Physician, Division of Gastroenterology and Nutrition, The Children's Hospital of Philadelphia, Philadelphia, Pennsylvania
Chapter 72: Defects in Metabolism of Lipids

GEORGE H. THOMPSON, M.D.
Professor of Orthopaedics and Pediatrics, Case Western Reserve University School of Medicine; Director, Pediatric Orthopaedics, Rainbow Babies and Children's Hospital, Cleveland, Ohio
Part XXXII: Bone and Joint Disorders; Section 1: Orthopedic Problems

JAMES TODD, M.D.
Professor of Pediatrics, Microbiology, and Preventive Medicine, University of Colorado School of Medicine; Director of Epidemiology and Clinical Microbiology, Children's Hospital, Denver, Colorado
Chapter 174: Staphylococcal Infections; Chapter 175: Streptococcal Infections; Chapter 176: Pneumococcal Infections

LUCY TOMPKINS, M.D., Ph.D.
Associate Professor, Departments of Medicine (Infectious Diseases and Geographic Medicine) and Microbiology and Immunology, Stanford University School of Medicine; Director, Clinical Microbiology Laboratory; Director, Infection Prevention Program, Stanford University Medical Center, Stanford, California
Chapter 195: Legionella

MARTIN ULSHEN, M.D.
Professor of Pediatrics, Professor of Nutrition, University of North Carolina School of Medicine; Chief, Division of Pediatric Gastroenterology; North Carolina Children's Hospital, Chapel Hill, North Carolina
Part XVIII: The Digestive System; Section 1: Clinical Manifestations of Gastrointestinal Disease; Chapter 274: Normal Development, Structure, and Function; Chapter 282: Ulcer Disease; Chapter 283: Inflammatory Bowel Disease; Chapter 284: Dietary Protein Intolerance (Food Allergy); Chapter 285: Eosinophilic Gastroenteritis; Chapter 286: Malabsorptive Disorders; Chapter 288: Recurrent Abdominal Pain of Childhood; Chapter 291: Tumors of the Digestive Tract

RODRIGO E. URIZAR, M.D.
Professor of Pediatrics and Associate Professor of Medicine, Albany Medical College; Attending Physician, Departments of Pediatrics and Medicine; Medical Director, Pediatric Dialysis Services, Albany Medical Center Hospital, Albany, New York
Chapter 490: Renal Transplantation

VICTOR C. VAUGHAN, III, M.D.
Clinical Professor of Pediatrics, Stanford University School of Medicine; Voluntary Clinical Faculty, Lucile Salter Packard Children's Hospital, Stanford, California
Chapter 41: Care of the Child with a Fatal Illness

KENNETH H. WEBB, M.D.
Assistant Clinical Professor of Pediatrics, Tufts University School of Medicine, Boston; Attending Physician, Baystate Medical Center, Springfield, Massachusetts
Chapter 668: Envenomations

MARTIN WEISSE, M.D.
Assistant Professor, Department of Pediatrics, Sections of Infectious Diseases and General Pediatrics, West Virginia University School of Medicine, Morgantown, West Virginia
Chapter 229: Candida; Chapter 244: Protozoan Diseases

STEVEN L. WERLIN, M.D.
Professor of Pediatrics, Medical College of Wisconsin; Director of Gastroenterology, Children's Hospital of Wisconsin, Milwaukee, Wisconsin
Part XVIII: The Digestive System; Section 5: Exocrine Pancreas

JEFFREY A. WHITSETT, M.D.
Professor, Department of Pediatrics, University of Cincinnati; Director, Division of Pulmonary Biology, Children's Hospital Medical Center, Cincinnati, Ohio
Chapter 68: Gene Therapy

JUDITH A. WILIMAS, M.D.
Professor, The University of Tennessee; Member, St. Jude Children's Research Hospital, Memphis, Tennessee
Chapter 452: Neoplasms of the Kidney

DONALD K. WINSOR, Ph.D.
Instructor, The University of Texas Medical School, Houston, Texas
Chapter 184: Escherichia coli, Aeromonas, *and* Plesiomonas

ROBERT E. WOOD, Ph.D., M.D.
Professor of Pediatrics, University of North Carolina School of Medicine, Chapel Hill, North Carolina
Chapter 324: Diagnostic Procedures

PETER WRIGHT, M.D.
Professor of Pediatrics and Professor of Microbiology and Immunology, Vanderbilt University School of Medicine; Head, Pediatric Infectious Diseases, Vanderbilt Medical Center, Nashville, Tennessee
Chapter 216: Influenza Viral Infections; Chapter 217: Parainfluenza Virus

DAVID WYLER, M.D.
Professor of Medicine and of Molecular Biology and Microbiology, Tufts University School of Medicine; Founder and Former Director, Travelers' Health Service; Physician, New England Medical Center, Boston, Massachusetts
Chapter 244: Protozoan Diseases

ROBERT WYLLIE, M.D.
Head, Section of Pediatric Gastroenterology and Nutrition, Cleveland Clinic Foundation, Cleveland, Ohio
Chapter 275: Pyloric Stenosis and Other Congenital Anomalies of the Stomach; Chapter 276: Intestinal Atresia, Stenosis, and Malrotation; Chapter 277: Intestinal Duplications, Meckel Diverticulum, and Other Remnants of the Omphalomesenteric Duct; Chapter 278: Motility Disorders and Hirschsprung Disease; Chapter 279: Ileus, Adhesions, Intussusception, and Closed-Loop Obstructions; Chapter 280: Foreign Bodies and Bezoars

BASIL J. ZITELLI, M.D.
Professor of Pediatrics, University of Pittsburgh School of Medicine; Staff Pediatrician, Diagnostic Referral Service, Children's Hospital of Pittsburgh, Pittsburgh, Pennsylvania
Chapter 313: Liver Transplantation

Preface

The publication of the Fifteenth Edition of *Nelson Textbook of Pediatrics* reflects an era of accelerating growth in our basic knowledge of human biology and further understanding about health and disease in children. These advances are being translated into a broad spectrum of new diagnostic, treatment, and prevention modalities. Nevertheless, many children are still deprived of the opportunity to fulfill their potential by death or disability that we have the means, but not the political will or wisdom, to prevent, ameliorate, or cure.

In this edition, we address the broad range of problems related to the health and welfare of infants, children, and adolescents that are faced by practitioners, house staff, and medical students. Our goal is to be comprehensive, concise, and reader friendly within one volume. We have tried to do this in a manner that acknowledges both the science and the art of pediatrics.

This Fifteenth Edition represents a major revision and reorganization of the textbook based on a complete review of the field of pediatrics. It includes many new chapters as well as a substantial modification and expansion of others. Practically no area of the book has been left untouched and, we hope, no chapter unimproved. Although to an affected child and family and their physician even the rarest disorder is of vital importance, it is not possible to cover all health problems in the same degree of detail in a general textbook of pediatrics. Therefore, leading articles and subspecialty texts are included in the references and should be consulted when more information is desired. We are indebted to our contributors whose hard work, knowledge, thought, and judgment have resulted in completeness, relevance, and conciseness. A very special thanks to Lisette Bralow at W. B. Saunders Company. We have all worked to produce an edition that will continue to be helpful to those who provide care for children or to those wishing to know more about them.

Since the last edition, we have lost one contributor through death. Brigid Leventhal is greatly missed.

In this edition, we have had informal assistance from faculty and house staff of the departments of pediatrics at Stanford University and the Medical College of Wisconsin. The help of these individuals and the numerous pediatricians elsewhere in the United States and around the world who have taken time to offer thoughtful suggestions is greatly appreciated.

We especially wish to express our appreciation to Ann Behrman, Sharon Kliegman, and Matthew and Timothy Arvin-Shechmeister for their patience and understanding, without which this textbook would not have been possible.

RICHARD E. BEHRMAN, M.D.
ROBERT M. KLIEGMAN, M.D.
ANN M. ARVIN, M.D.

Contents

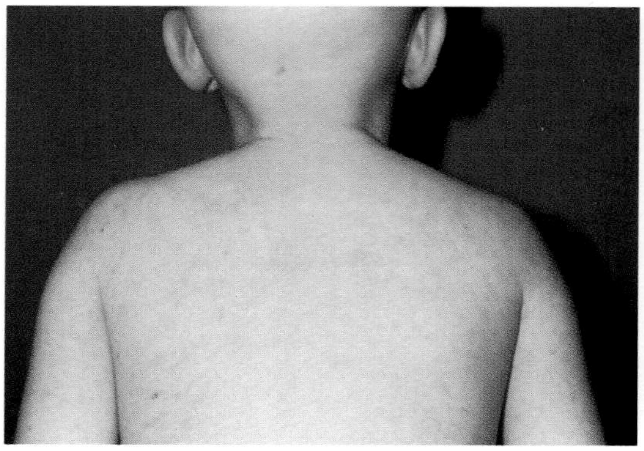

Figure 132–4

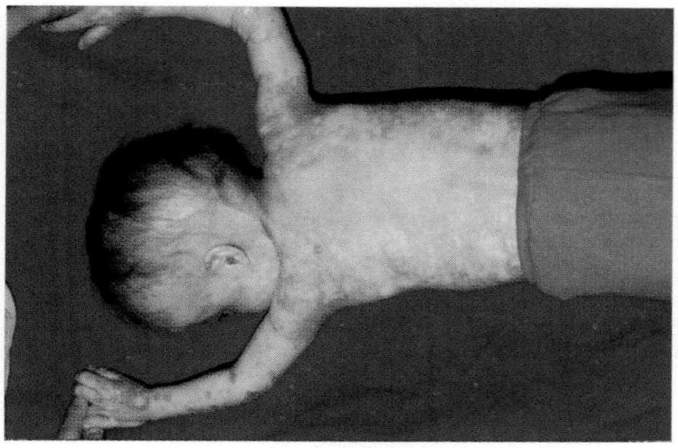

Figure 132–5

A

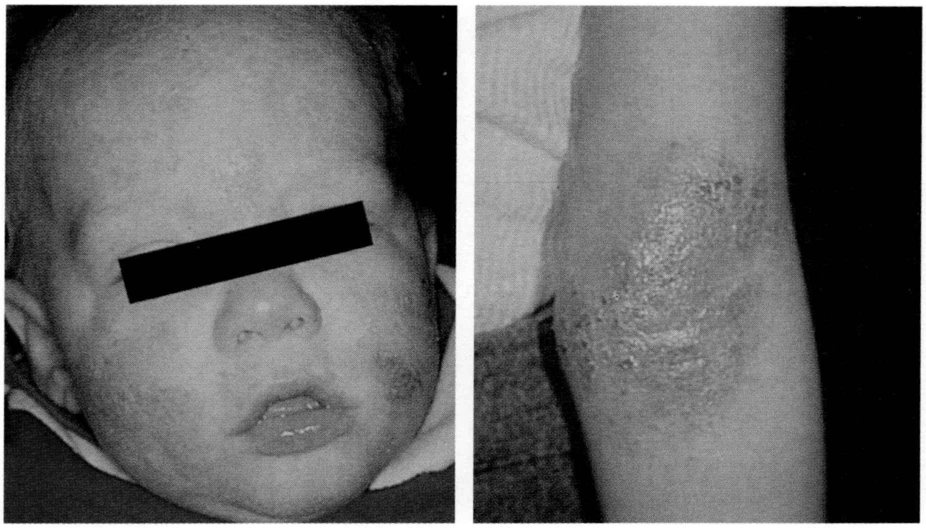

B

Figure 138–1

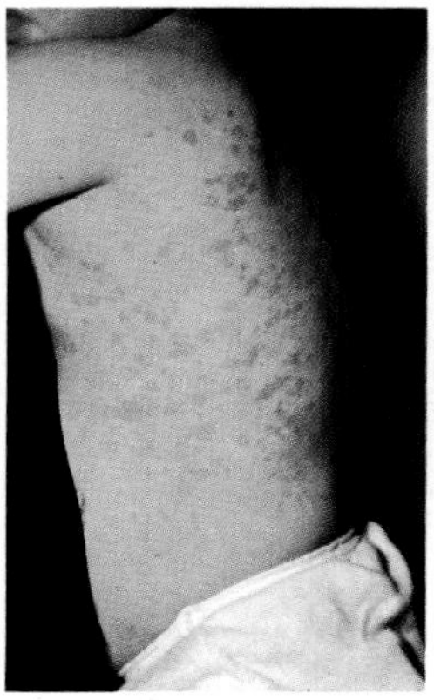

Figure 148–8

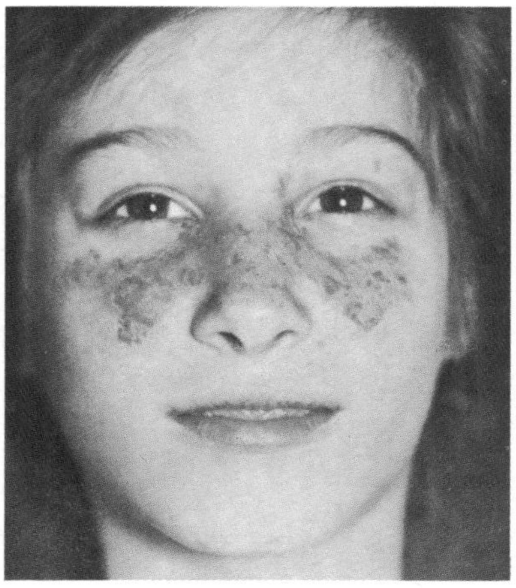

Figure 150–1

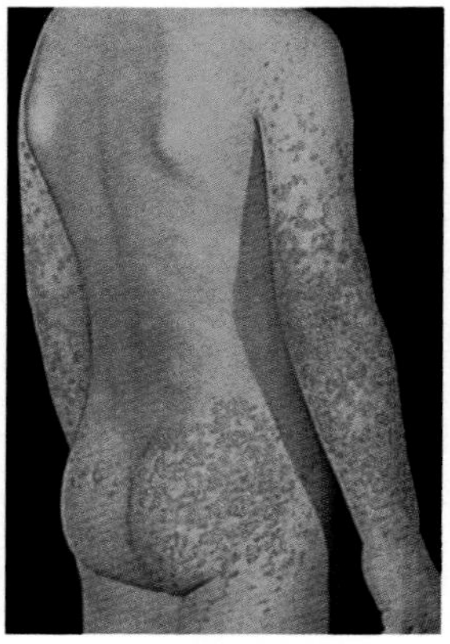

Figure 152–1

Figure 132–4. Acute graft-versus-host disease of the skin with ear, arm, shoulder, and trunk involvement. (Courtesy of Evan Farmer, MD.)

Figure 132–5. Chronic graft-versus-host disease of the skin with sclerodermoid changes. (Courtesy of Evan Farmer, MD.)

Figure 138–1. *A–B,* Infantile atopic dermatitis begins typically as a pruritic, erythematous, papulovesicular eruption over the cheeks but may also involve the wrists and extensor aspects of the extremities or may become generalized, usually sparing the diaper area. By 2 yr of age, involvement of antecubital and popliteal spaces, neck, wrists, and ankles is common with scaling, excoriations, lichenification, and hyperpigmentation. Crusting indicates superimposed infection. (From The Dermatologic Dozen, 1980. Used with permission of Westwood Pharmaceuticals, Inc.)

Figure 148–8. Rash of rheumatoid arthritis.

Figure 150–1. The butterfly rash of systemic lupus erythematosus.

Figure 152–1. Henoch-Schönlein purpura (anaphylactoid purpura). (From Korting GW: Hautkrankheiten bei Kindern und Jugendlichen, 3rd ed. Stuttgart, Germany, FK Schattauer Verlag, 1982.)

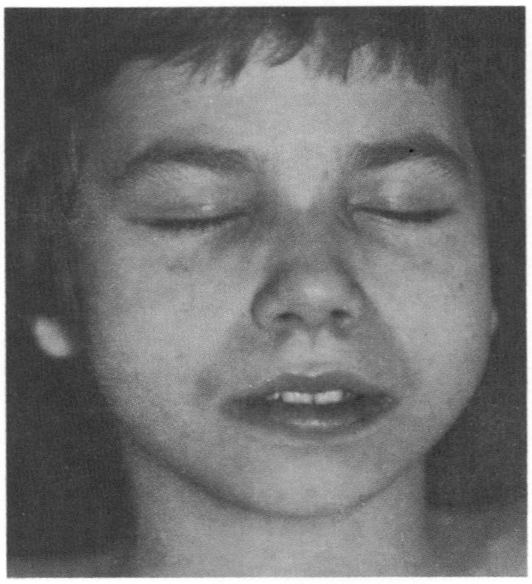

Figure 153–1

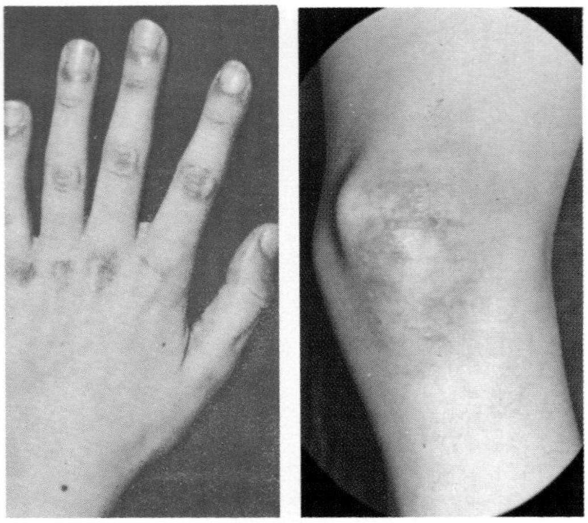

Figure 153–2

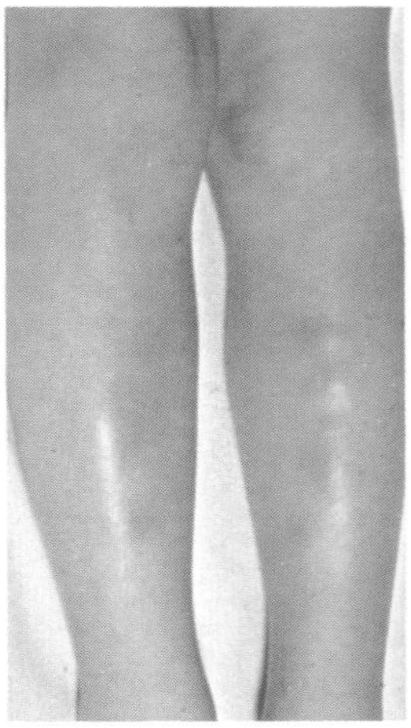

Figure 156–1

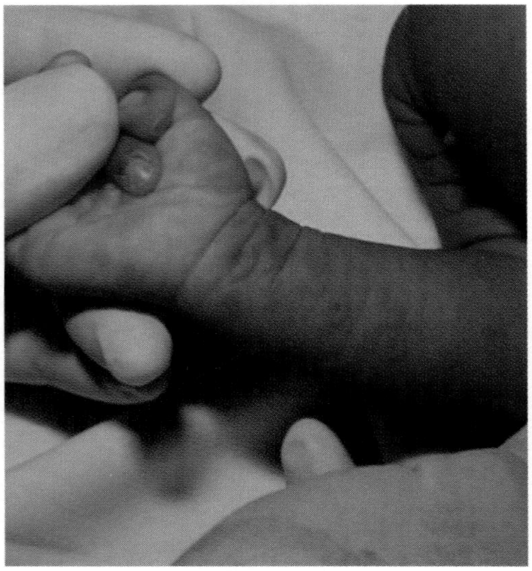

Figure 201–2

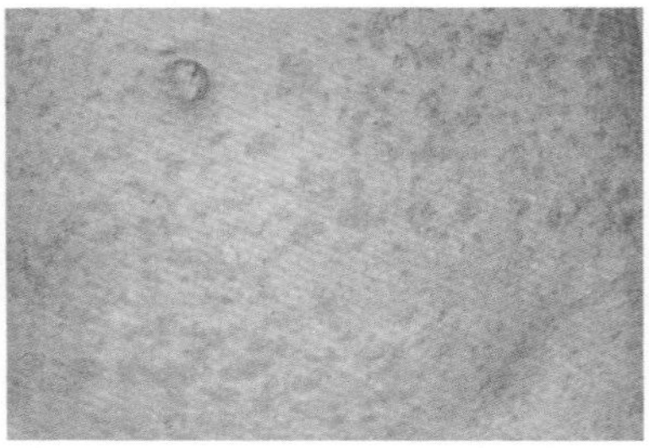

Figure 206–1

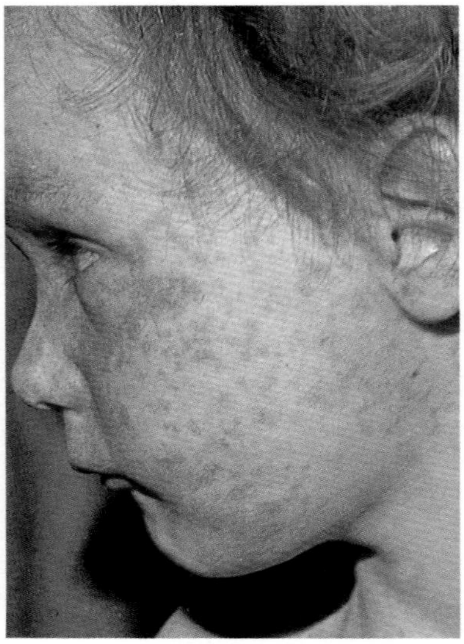

Figure 207–1

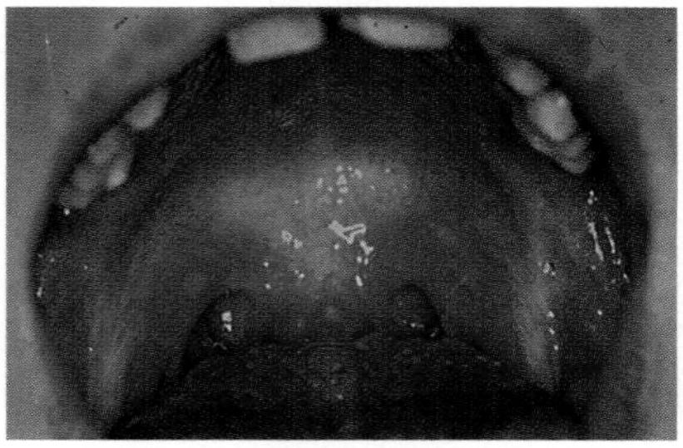

Figure 209–3

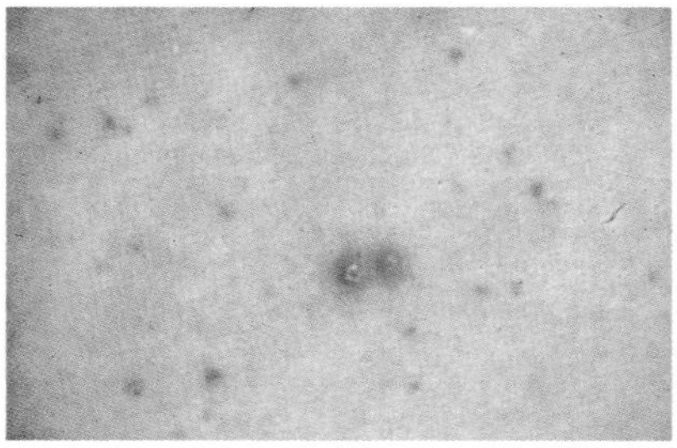

Figure 213–1

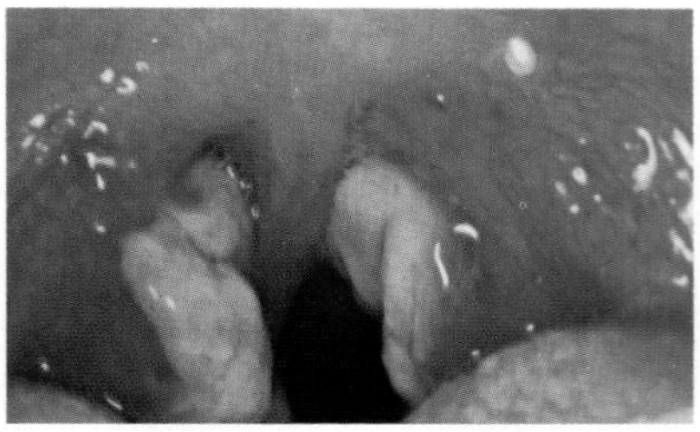

Figure 215–1

Figure 153–1. The facial rash of dermatomyositis. Notice the faint erythema over the bridge of the nose and malar areas and the heliotropic discoloration of the upper eyelids.

Figure 153–2. Rash of dermatomyositis. Notice the skin changes over the knuckles *(left)* and over the knee *(right)*.

Figure 156–1. Erythema nodosum.

Figure 201–2. The mucocutaneous rash of congenital syphilis.

Figure 206–1. Maculopapular rash of measles. (From Korting GW: Hautkrankheiten bei Kindern und Jugendlichen, 3rd ed. Stuttgart, Germany, FK Schattauer Verlag, 1982.)

Figure 207–1. Rash of rubella (German measles). (From Korting GW: Hautkrankheiten bei Kindern und Jugendlichen, 3rd ed. Stuttgart, Germany, FK Schattauer Verlag, 1982.)

Figure 209–3. Herpangina. This enanthem is predominantly a disease of children and is caused by group A coxsackieviruses. These lesions resemble the ones caused by herpes simplex virus. (From Edmond's Color Atlas of Infectious Diseases. Wolfe Medical Publishers, 1990, p 313.)

Figure 213–1. Skin lesions of chickenpox. Note the varying stages of development (macules, papules, and vesicles) present at the same time. (Courtesy of PF Lucchesi, M.D.)

Figure 215–1. Tonsillitis with membrane formation in infectious mononucleosis. (Courtesy of Alex J. Steigman, M.D.)

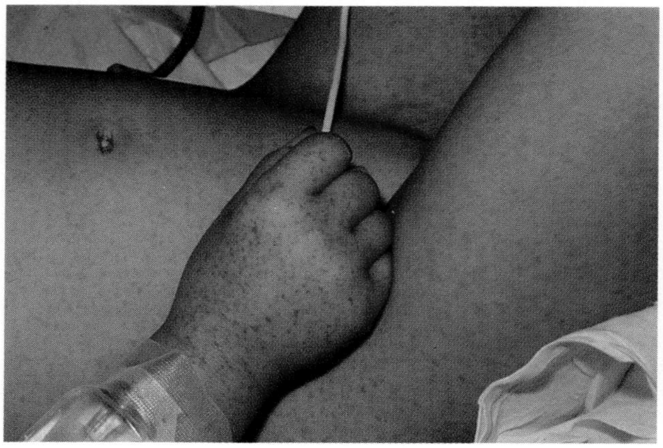

Figure 239–1

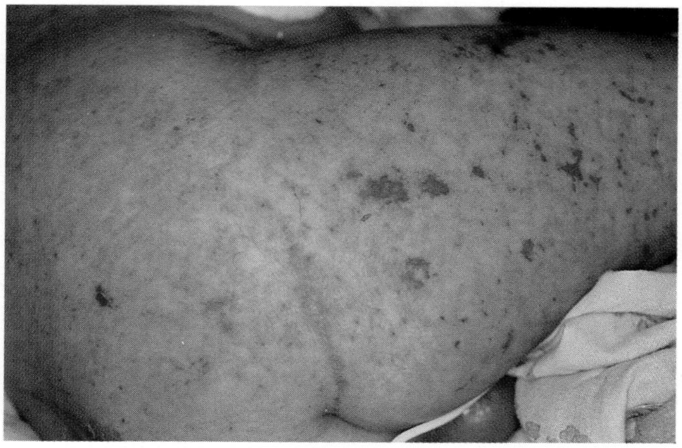

Figure 239–2

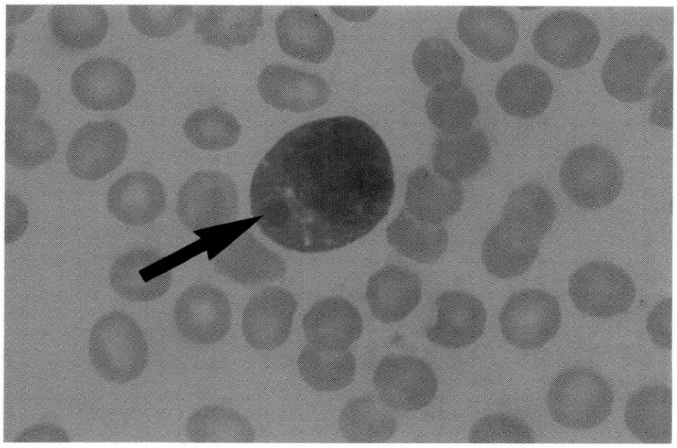

Figure 242–1

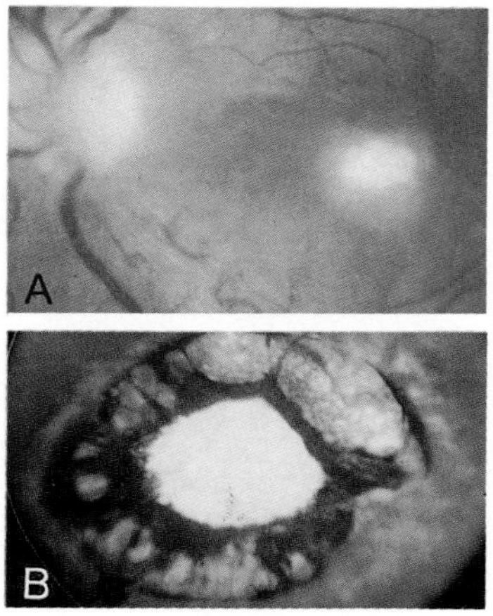

Figure 244–4

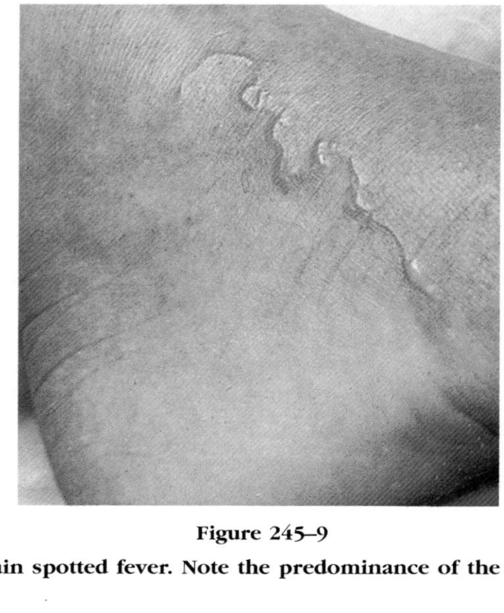

Figure 245–9

Figure 239–1. Patient with Rocky Mountain spotted fever. Note the predominance of the rash on the extremities. (Courtesy of Debra Karp Skopicki, M.D., Baltimore.)

Figure 239–2. Later in the course of Rocky Mountain spotted fever the rash may become hemorrhagic or purpuric. (Courtesy of Debra Karp Skopicki, M.D., Baltimore.)

Figure 242–1. *Ehrlichia* morula in a peripheral blood leukocyte: morula *(arrow)* containing *Ehrlichia chaffeensis* in a monocyte (Wright's stain, original magnification ×1,200). *Ehrlichia chaffeensis* and the human granulocytic ehrlichia have similar morphologies but are serologically and genetically distinct.

Figure 244–4. Toxoplasmic chorioretinitis. *A,* Active acute lesion by indirect ophthalmoscopy. *B,* Old, quiescent lesion. (*B,* adapted from Desmonts G, Remington J: Congenital Toxoplasmosis. *In:* Remington J, Klein J (eds): Infectious Diseases of the Fetus and Newborn Infant, 3rd ed. Philadelphia, WB Saunders, 1991.)

Figure 245–9. Creeping eruption of cutaneous larva migrans. (From Korting GW: Hautkrankheiten bei Kindern und Jugend-lichen. Stuttgart, Germany, FK Schattauer Verlag, 1969.)

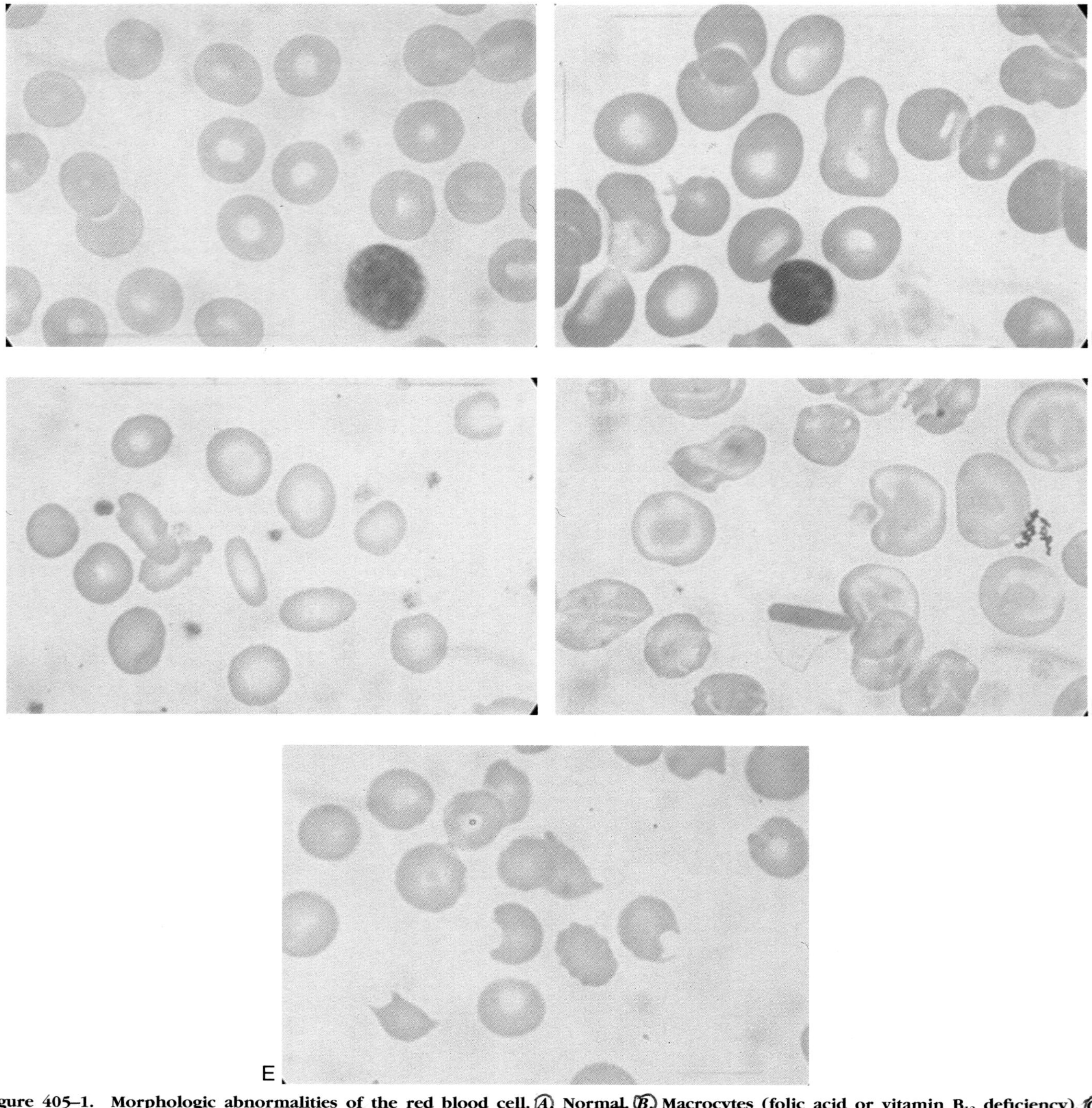

A B C D E

Figure 405–1. Morphologic abnormalities of the red blood cell. *A,* Normal. *B,* Macrocytes (folic acid or vitamin B_{12} deficiency). *C,* Hypochromic microcytes (iron deficiency). *D,* Target cells (Hb CC disease). *E,* Schizocytes (hemolytic-uremic syndrome). (Provided by Dr. E. Schwartz.)

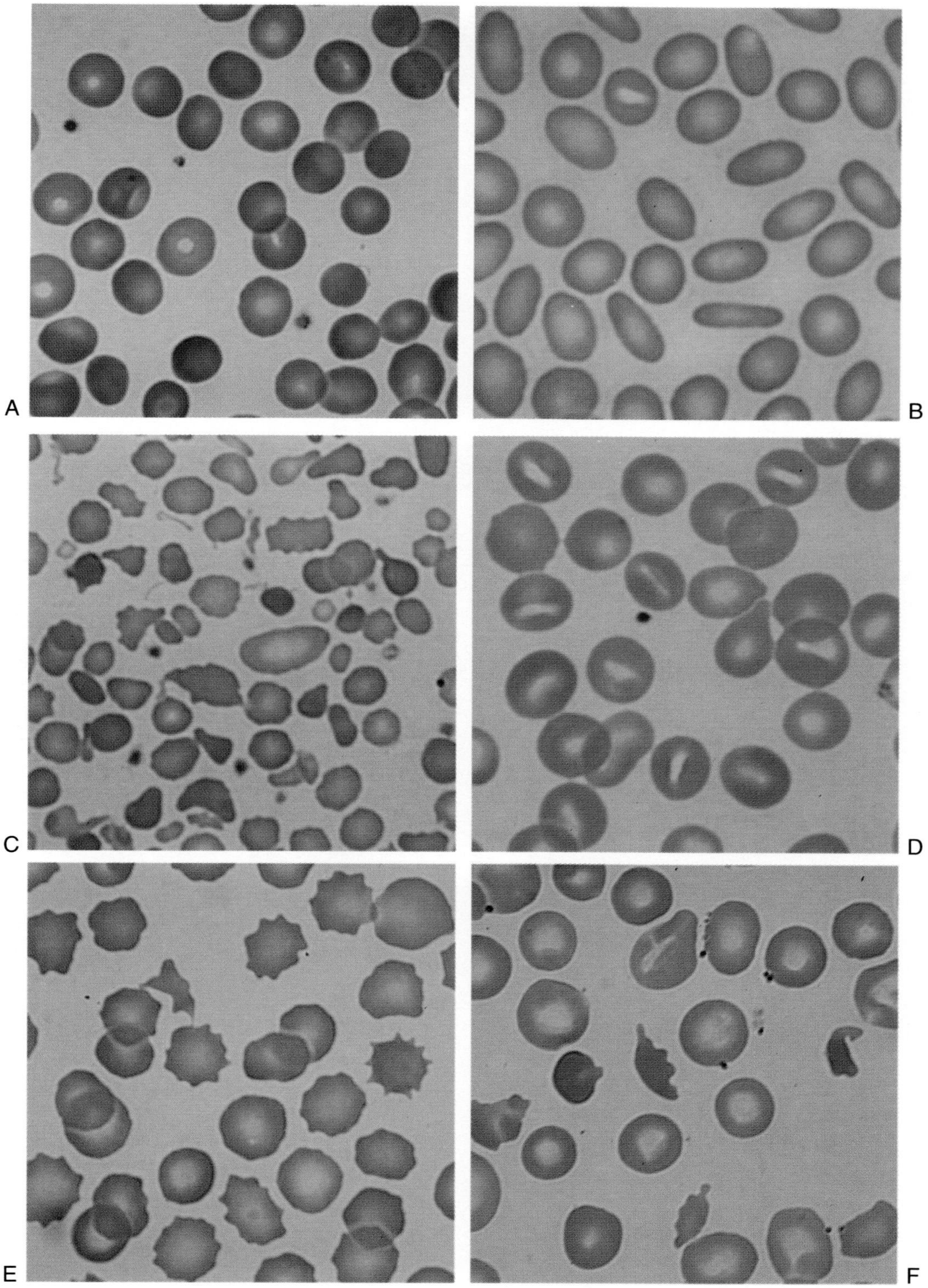

Figure 415–2. Morphology of abnormal red cells. ***A,*** **Hereditary spherocytosis;** ***B,*** **hereditary elliptocytosis;** ***C,*** **hereditary pyropoikilocytosis;** ***D,*** **hereditary stomatocytosis;** ***E,*** **acanthocytosis;** ***F,*** **fragmentation hemolysis.**

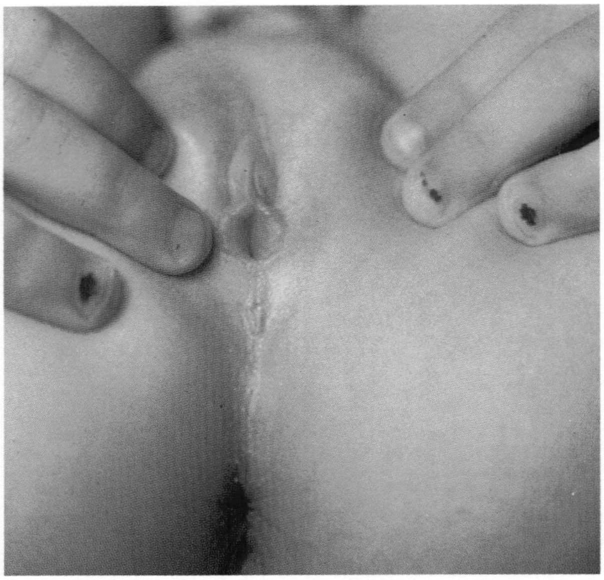

Figure 503–1

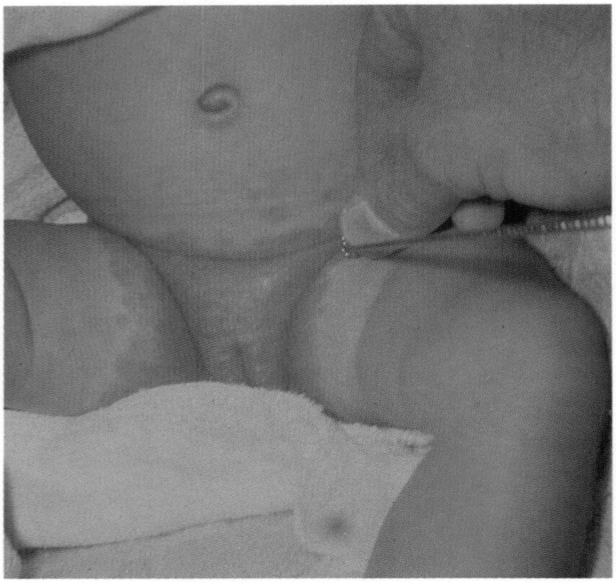

Figure 503–3

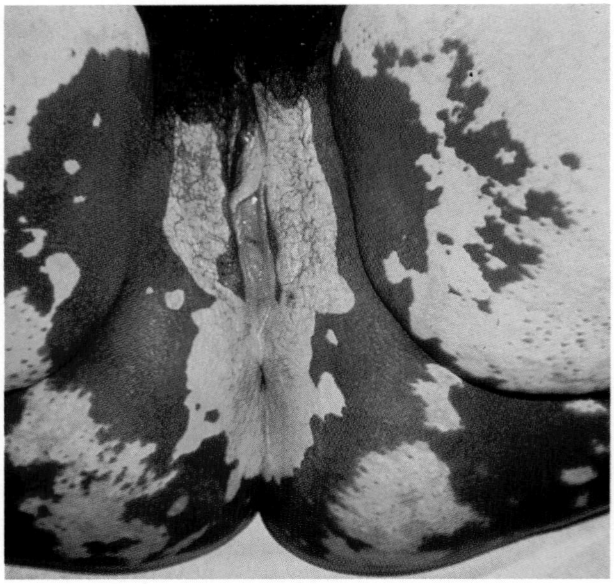

Figure 503–4

Figure 503–1. Labial adhesions.

Figure 503–3. Vulvar psoriasis.

Figure 503–4. Vitiligo.

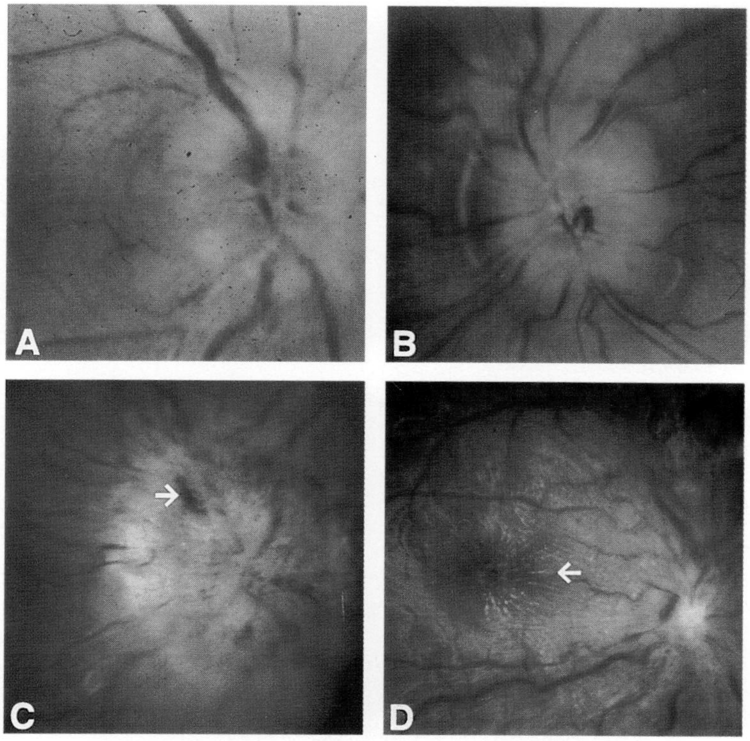

Figure 541–1

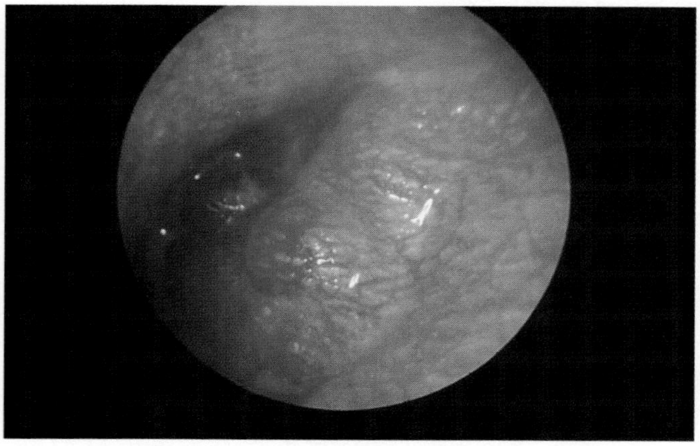

Figure 590–1

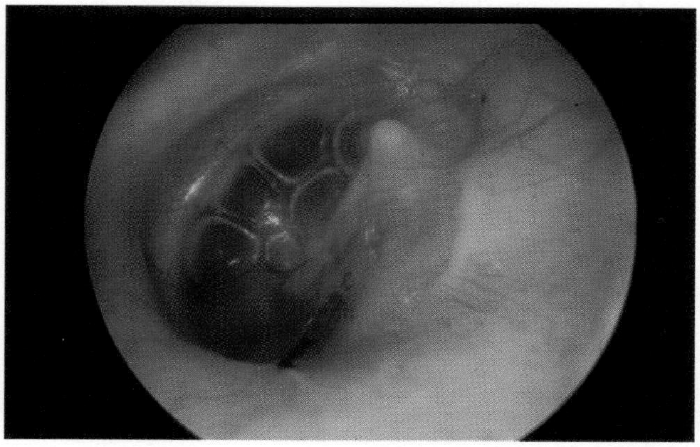

Figure 590–3

Figure 541–1. *A*, Mild papilledema. Blurred disc margins and venous congestion. *B*, Moderate papilledema. Disc edematous and raised. Vessels buried within substance of nerve tissue. *C*, Severe papilledema. Hemorrhages are evident within disc *(arrow)*, and there are microinfarcts (soft exudates) in the nerve fiber layer. *D*, Macular star *(arrow)* with edema residues distributed within the Henle layer of the macula.

Figure 590–1. Acute left otitis media.

Figure 590–3. Otitis media with effusion of left ear. Retracted ear drum, prominent short process of malleus, and air bubbles seen anteriorly through the tympanic membrane.

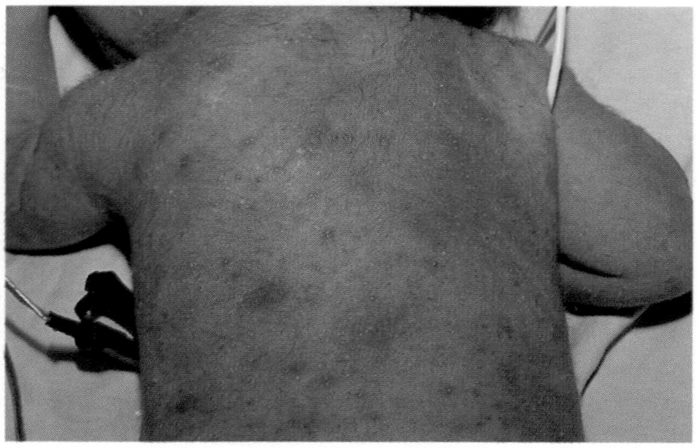

Figure 597–1

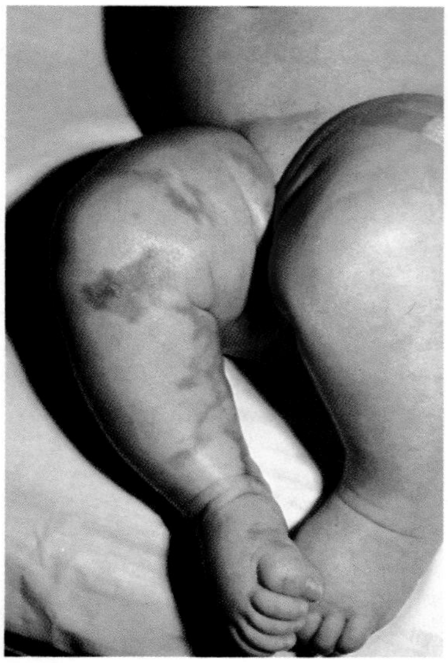

Figure 600–4

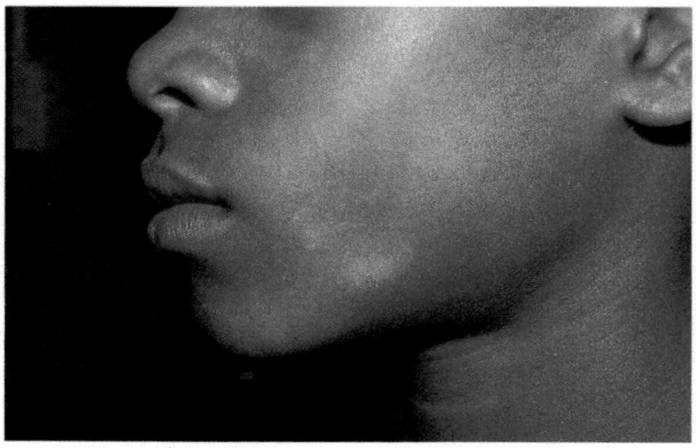

Figure 605–3

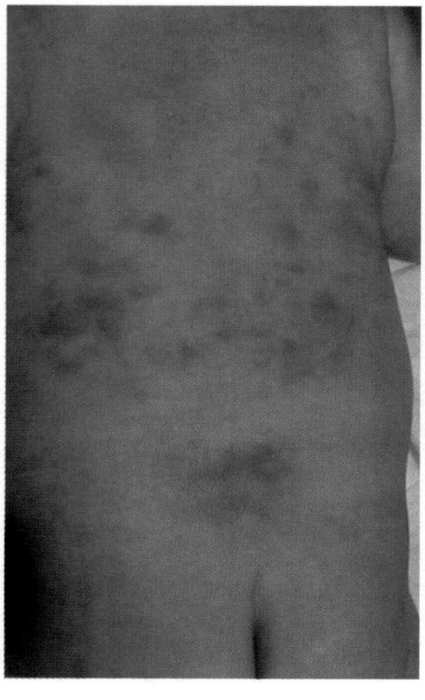

Figure 610–1

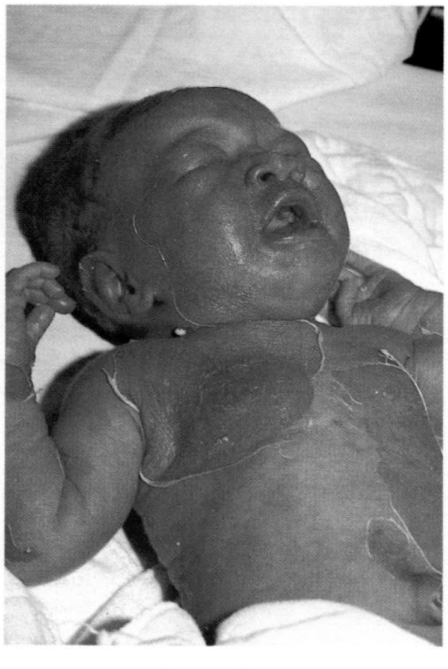

Figure 615–2

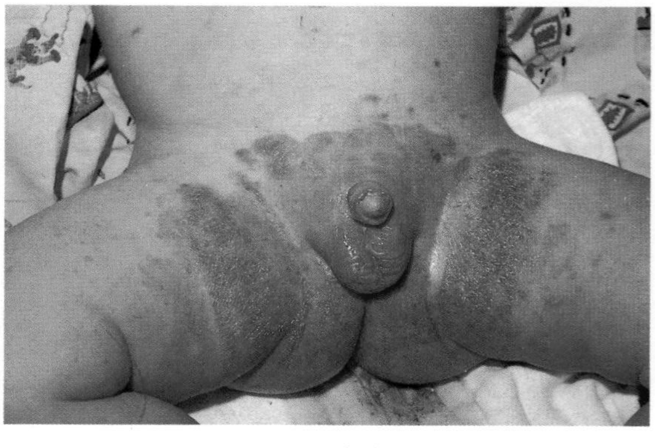

Figure 616–5

Figure 597–1. Erythema toxicum on the trunk of a newborn infant.

Figure 600–4. Marbled pattern of cutis marmorata telangiectatica congenita on the right leg.

Figure 605–3. Patchy hypopigmented lesions with diffuse borders characteristic of pityriasis alba.

Figure 610–1. Red-purple nodular infiltration of skin of back caused by subcutaneous fat necrosis.

Figure 615–2. Infant with staphylococcal scalded skin syndrome.

Figure 616–5. Erythematous confluent plaque with satellite pustules caused by candidal infection.

PART I

The Field of Pediatrics

CHAPTER 1

Overview of Pediatrics

*Richard E. Behrman**

Pediatrics is concerned with the health of infants, children, and adolescents, their growth and development, and their opportunity to achieve full potential as adults. As physicians who assume a responsibility for children's physical, mental, and emotional progress from conception to maturity, pediatricians must be concerned with social or environmental influences, which have a major impact on the health and well-being of children and their families, as well as with particular organ systems and biologic processes. The young are often among the most vulnerable or disadvantaged in society, and thus their needs require special attention.

SCOPE AND HISTORY OF PEDIATRICS

Over a century ago, pediatrics emerged as a medical specialty in response to an increasing awareness that the health problems of children differ from those of adults and that the child's response to illness and stress varies with age. The emphasis and scope of pediatrics continue to change, but these basic observations remain valid.

The health problems of children vary widely among the nations of the world depending on a number of factors, which are often interrelated. These factors include (1) the prevalence and ecology of infectious agents and their hosts; (2) climate and geography; (3) agricultural resources and practices; (4) educational, economic, social, and cultural considerations; (5) stage of industrialization and urbanization; and (6), in many instances, the gene frequencies for some disorders.

Not only do problems differ in various parts of the world, but priorities do also, because they must reflect local concerns, resources, and needs. The assessment of the state of health of any community must begin with a description of the incidence of illness and must continue with studies that show the changes that occur with time and in response to programs of prevention, case finding, therapy, and adequate surveillance. As contemporary problems in any community yield to study and to improved management, new problems become the foci of the attention and efforts of pediatric clinicians and research workers. Accordingly, with time, there may be major changes in the relative importance of the various causes of childhood morbidity and mortality.

In the late 19th century in the United States, of every 1,000 children born alive 200 might be expected to die before the age of 1 yr of conditions such as dysentery, pneumonia, measles, diphtheria, and whooping cough. The efforts of pediatricians, combined with those of scientists and pioneers in public health, have led to such better understanding of the origin and management of many problems of infants that in the past half century the infant mortality in the United States has fallen from around 75/1,000 live births in 1925 to approximately 8.3 in 1993. Both neonatal (<1 mo) and postneonatal (1–11 mo) mortality have had major reductions. The majority of deaths of infants under 1 yr of age occur within the first 28 days of life, most of these within the first 7 days; moreover, a large proportion of those within the first 7 days occur within the 1st day. However, an increasing number of severely ill infants born at low birthweight survive the neonatal period and die later in infancy from neonatal disease, its sequelae, or its complications. Table 1–1 shows the persistent disproportionately high death rate within the 1st yr, compared with the remainder of childhood.

Postneonatal infant mortality for the United States in 1993 was 3.1/1,000 live births (6.3/1,000 for black infants and 2.8/1,000 for white infants in 1991). The leading cause of death in this age group was the sudden infant death syndrome (SIDS), followed in order by congenital anomalies, perinatal conditions, respiratory system diseases, accidents, and infectious and parasitic diseases. Maternal risk characteristics, such as unmarried status, teenage, high parity, and less than 12 yr of education, are correlated significantly with increased risk of postneonatal mortality and morbidity and low birthweight.

In developed countries early in the 20th century, efforts at control of infectious disease began to be complemented by better understanding of nutrition. New and continuing discoveries in these areas led to establishment of public well child clinics for low-income families. Along with acute infections and the chronic disturbances associated with deficits of calories, vitamins, minerals, or proteins, the acute nutritional and metabolic disturbances that accompany acute diarrhea received attention.

In the middle years of the 20th century, a profound revolution in child health was brought about by the introduction of antibacterial chemicals and antibiotic agents. With improved control of infectious disease through both prevention and treatment and with other scientific and technical advances, pediatric medicine turned its attention increasingly to conditions affecting relatively small numbers of children. These included both potentially lethal conditions and temporarily or permanently handicapping conditions; among these disorders were leukemia, cystic fibrosis, diseases of the newborn infant, congenital heart disease, mental retardation, genetic defects, rheumatic diseases, renal diseases, and metabolic and endocrine disorders.

The last two decades of this century have been marked by accelerated understanding of and new approaches to the management of many disorders as a consequence of advances in molecular biology and genetics and in immunology. Increasing attention also has been given to behavioral and social aspects of child health, ranging from a re-examination of child-rearing practices to the creation of major programs aimed at

*Modified from the original version of this chapter in the 13th edition written by Victor C. Vaughan.

ing to adoption or to placement with foster families (Chapters 32 and 33). For handicapped children the massive centralized institutions of past years are being replaced by community-centered arrangements offering a better opportunity for these children to achieve their maximal potential. Pediatricians have been involved in shaping these and other institutions that provide services to children, and their insights and active contributions will continue to be needed.

COSTS OF HEALTH CARE

The growth of high technology, the redesign of health institutions (particularly with respect to the needs for and the uses of personnel), the public's demand for medical services, and the manner in which the costs of health care are paid (by public or private insurance programs based on fee for service) have driven the costs of health care in the United States up to a point at which they represent a significant proportion of the gross national product. Although children (0–18 yr) represent about 30% of the population, they account for only about 14% of the personal health care expenditures, or about 60% of adult per capita expenditures. Efforts to contain costs have led to revisions of the way in which physicians and hospitals are paid for services. Limits have been set on the fees for some services, capitated prepayment and a variety of managed care systems flourish, a program of reimbursement (diagnosis-related groups [DRGs]) based on the diagnosis rather than on the particular services rendered to the individual patient has been implemented, and a relative value scale for varying rates of payment among different physician services has been implemented. These changes in the system of financing health services raise important ethical issues for pediatricians to address (Chapter 3).

EVALUATION OF HEALTH CARE

The shaping of health care systems to meet the needs of children and their families requires accurate statistical data and difficult decisions in the setting of priorities. Along with growing concerns about the design and cost of health care systems and the ability to equitably distribute health services has come increasing concern about the quality of health care and about its efficiency and its effectiveness. There are large local and regional variations among similar populations of children in the rates of use of procedures and of hospital admissions. These variations require continuing evaluation and explanation in terms of the actual impact of medical and surgical services on health status and the outcome of illness. The need for technology assessment is increasing.

GROWTH OF SPECIALIZATION

The amount of information relevant to child health care is rapidly expanding, and no person can become master of it all. Physicians are increasingly dependent on one another for the highest quality of care for their patients; group practices in pediatrics are common in the United States and, although the vast majority of pediatricians are primary care generalists, as many as 25% claim an area of special knowledge and skill.

The growth of specialization within pediatrics has taken a number of different forms: Interests in problems of *age groups* of children have created neonatology and adolescent medicine; interests in *organ systems* have created pediatric cardiology, allergy, hematology, nephrology, gastroenterology, pulmonology, endocrinology, and specialization in metabolism and genetics; interests in the *health care system* have created pediatricians devoted to ambulatory care on the one hand or to intensive care on the other; and finally, multidisciplinary subspecialties have grown up around the problems of *handicapped children*, to which pediatrics, neurology, psychiatry, psychology, nursing, physical and occupational therapy, special education, speech therapy, audiology, and nutrition all make essential contributions. This growth of specialization has been most conspicuous in university-affiliated departments of pediatrics and medical centers for children.

NEED FOR CONTINUING SELF-EDUCATION

The explosion of information has also created a need for continuing education, which was felt much less keenly in earlier years, when the new information in any field of medicine was easily accessible through a relatively small number of journals, texts, or monographs. Now, relevant information is so widely scattered among the many published journals that elaborate electronic data systems are necessary to make it accessible. New auditory and visual aids to learning abound as well as postgraduate courses through which the participating physician can be brought up to date on various aspects of child health care. The American Board of Pediatrics and the American Academy of Pediatrics have arranged for the close linkage of continuing education of pediatricians to recertification in pediatrics.

There is no touchstone through which physicians can ensure that the process of their own continuing education will keep them abreast of advancing knowledge in the field, but they must find a way if they are to discharge their responsibility to their patients. An essential element of this process may be for the physician to take an *active* role, such as participating in medical student and resident education. Efforts in continuing self-education will also be fostered, for example, if clinical problems can be made a stimulus for a review of standard literature, alone or in consultation with an appropriate colleague or consultant. This continuing review will do much to identify those inconsistencies or contradictions that will indicate, in the ultimate best interest of the patient, that things are not what they seem or have been said to be. Physicians still learn most from their patients, but this will not be the case if they fall into the easy habit of accepting their patients' problems casually or at face value because they appear to be simple.

The tools that the physician must use in dealing with the problems of children and their families fall into three main categories: *cognitive* (up-to-date factual information regarding diagnostic and therapeutic issues, available on recall or easily found in readily accessible sources); *interpersonal or manual* (e.g., the ability to carry out a productive interview, execute a reliable physical examination, perform a deft venipuncture, or manage cardiac arrest or the resuscitation of a depressed newborn infant); and *attitudinal* (the physician's commitment to fullest possible implementation of knowledge and skills on behalf of children and their families in an atmosphere of empathetic sensitivity and concern). With regard to this last category, it is important that children participate with their families in informed decision-making about their own health care in a manner appropriate to their stage of development and the nature of the particular health problem.

The workaday needs of professional persons for knowledge and skills in care of children vary widely. The primary care physician needs depth in developmental concepts and in the ability to organize an effective system for achieving quality and continuity in assessing and planning for health care during the entire period of growth. There may often be little or no need for immediate recall of esoterica. On the other hand, the consultant or subspecialist not only needs a comfortable grasp of esoterica within his or her field and perhaps within related fields but also must be able to cope with controversial issues, with flexibility that will permit adaptation of a variety of points of view to the best interest of his or her unique patient.

At whatever level of care (primary, secondary, or tertiary),

PART I

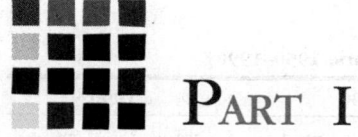

The Field of Pediatrics

CHAPTER 1

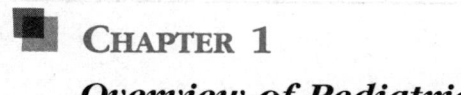

Overview of Pediatrics

Richard E. Behrman*

Pediatrics is concerned with the health of infants, children, and adolescents, their growth and development, and their opportunity to achieve full potential as adults. As physicians who assume a responsibility for children's physical, mental, and emotional progress from conception to maturity, pediatricians must be concerned with social or environmental influences, which have a major impact on the health and well-being of children and their families, as well as with particular organ systems and biologic processes. The young are often among the most vulnerable or disadvantaged in society, and thus their needs require special attention.

SCOPE AND HISTORY OF PEDIATRICS

Over a century ago, pediatrics emerged as a medical specialty in response to an increasing awareness that the health problems of children differ from those of adults and that the child's response to illness and stress varies with age. The emphasis and scope of pediatrics continue to change, but these basic observations remain valid.

The health problems of children vary widely among the nations of the world depending on a number of factors, which are often interrelated. These factors include (1) the prevalence and ecology of infectious agents and their hosts; (2) climate and geography; (3) agricultural resources and practices; (4) educational, economic, social, and cultural considerations; (5) stage of industrialization and urbanization; and (6), in many instances, the gene frequencies for some disorders.

Not only do problems differ in various parts of the world, but priorities do also, because they must reflect local concerns, resources, and needs. The assessment of the state of health of any community must begin with a description of the incidence of illness and must continue with studies that show the changes that occur with time and in response to programs of prevention, case finding, therapy, and adequate surveillance. As contemporary problems in any community yield to study and to improved management, new problems become the foci of the attention and efforts of pediatric clinicians and research workers. Accordingly, with time, there may be major changes in the relative importance of the various causes of childhood morbidity and mortality.

In the late 19th century in the United States, of every 1,000 children born alive 200 might be expected to die before the age of 1 yr of conditions such as dysentery, pneumonia, measles, diphtheria, and whooping cough. The efforts of pediatricians, combined with those of scientists and pioneers in public health, have led to such better understanding of the origin and management of many problems of infants that in the past half century the infant mortality in the United States has fallen from around 75/1,000 live births in 1925 to approximately 8.3 in 1993. Both neonatal (<1 mo) and postneonatal (1–11 mo) mortality have had major reductions. The majority of deaths of infants under 1 yr of age occur within the first 28 days of life, most of these within the first 7 days; moreover, a large proportion of those within the first 7 days occur within the 1st day. However, an increasing number of severely ill infants born at low birthweight survive the neonatal period and die later in infancy from neonatal disease, its sequelae, or its complications. Table 1–1 shows the persistent disproportionately high death rate within the 1st yr, compared with the remainder of childhood.

Postneonatal infant mortality for the United States in 1993 was 3.1/1,000 live births (6.3/1,000 for black infants and 2.8/1,000 for white infants in 1991). The leading cause of death in this age group was the sudden infant death syndrome (SIDS), followed in order by congenital anomalies, perinatal conditions, respiratory system diseases, accidents, and infectious and parasitic diseases. Maternal risk characteristics, such as unmarried status, teenage, high parity, and less than 12 yr of education, are correlated significantly with increased risk of postneonatal mortality and morbidity and low birthweight.

In developed countries early in the 20th century, efforts at control of infectious disease began to be complemented by better understanding of nutrition. New and continuing discoveries in these areas led to establishment of public well child clinics for low-income families. Along with acute infections and the chronic disturbances associated with deficits of calories, vitamins, minerals, or proteins, the acute nutritional and metabolic disturbances that accompany acute diarrhea received attention.

In the middle years of the 20th century, a profound revolution in child health was brought about by the introduction of antibacterial chemicals and antibiotic agents. With improved control of infectious disease through both prevention and treatment and with other scientific and technical advances, pediatric medicine turned its attention increasingly to conditions affecting relatively small numbers of children. These included both potentially lethal conditions and temporarily or permanently handicapping conditions; among these disorders were leukemia, cystic fibrosis, diseases of the newborn infant, congenital heart disease, mental retardation, genetic defects, rheumatic diseases, renal diseases, and metabolic and endocrine disorders.

The last two decades of this century have been marked by accelerated understanding of and new approaches to the management of many disorders as a consequence of advances in molecular biology and genetics and in immunology. Increasing attention also has been given to behavioral and social aspects of child health, ranging from a re-examination of child-rearing practices to the creation of major programs aimed at

*Modified from the original version of this chapter in the 13th edition written by Victor C. Vaughan.

■ **TABLE 1–1 Death Rates* for All Causes, According to Sex, Race, and Age: United States, Selected Years, 1950–1990†**

	1950		1960		1970		1980		1990	
	White	Black	White	Black	White	Black	White	Black	White	Black
Male										
<1 yr	3,401	1,413	2,694	5,307	2,113	4,299	1,230	2,587	896	2,112
1–4 yr	136		105	209	84	151	66	111	46	86
5–14 yr	67	95	53	75	48	67	35	47	26	41
15–24 yr	152	290	144	212	171	321	167	209	131	252
Female										
<1 yr	2,567	1,139	2,008	4,162	1,615	3,369	963	2,124	690	1,736
1–4 yr	112		85	173	66	129	49	84	36	68
5–14 yr	45	73	35	54	30	44	23	31	18	28
15–24 yr	72	213	55	108	62	112	56	71	46	69

*Death rates per 100,000 population.
†Adapted from Table 119. Statistical Abstract of the United States 1993, 113th ed. Lanham, MD, Berman Press, 1993.*

prevention and management of abuse and neglect of infants and children. Developmental psychologists, child psychiatrists, neuroscientists, sociologists, anthropologists, ethnologists, and others have brought us new insights into human potential, including new views of the importance of the environmental circumstances during pregnancy, surrounding birth, and in the early years of child rearing. However, during these latter years of the 20th century there has also been a resurgence of some of the infectious diseases previously controlled in developed countries, such as tuberculosis and syphilis; the emergence of new infectious pathogens, such as the human immunodeficiency virus (HIV); and the recognition of new disorders related to innovative therapies. In addition, in developing countries many of the disorders facing children earlier in this century persist, sometimes aggravated by war and famine.

Table 1–2 shows the five leading causes of death in various age groups in 1993. The problems of these children have changed significantly in the United States over a generation. Table 1–2 highlights the impact of violent deaths on mortality in older children, adolescents, and young adults.

Table 1–1 shows that the nonwhite children of the United States have not fully benefited from the changes in infant mortality in this century owing to a variety of socioeconomic and other disadvantages that have resisted the efforts of many who have struggled to reduce this disparity, including many pediatricians. Similar disparities between races occur in several indices of health, such as rates of diseases of the heart and homicides.

In the United States, existing programs for meeting child health problems are not available to all families in need, with gaps between eligibility for public support and parents' ability to pay for services. Needed services are often either nonexistent or fragmented among programs, agencies, or policies. Programs are often poorly coordinated and the data collection is inadequate. The resources available for maternal and child health care services are also generally inadequate. These findings reflect a need, not just in the United States but in many other parts of the world as well, for continuing re-examination and revision of the system of health care, especially with regard to its impact on the health status of children.

These problems are exacerbated by social and demographic changes in the United States. By 1991, 25.5% (16.6 million) of all children under 18 yr of age were living with one parent, about twice the number of such children in 1970. Of these one-parent families, 88% consisted of children living with their mother. There are substantial differences among children: 57.5% of black, 29.8% of Hispanic, and 19.5% of white children live with one parent. Furthermore, in 1993, 59% of black and white mothers with children under 6 yr of age and about 75% of mothers of children 6–17 yr of age worked full time or part time outside the home. In 1990, about 31% of children under 5 yr whose mothers worked outside the home were in day care. One in five children were living in poverty (13.6 million under 18 yr) in 1991 and a black or Hispanic child was more than two to three times as likely to be living in poverty as a white child. This increase in childhood poverty in the United States has been accompanied by a large increase in the number of children without adequate health insurance; by 1993 about 9 million children (0–17 yr) had no health insur-

■ **TABLE 1–2 Causes of Death and Age**

Rank	Causes	Subrank	Rate
	Under 1 Yr: All Causes*		845†
1	Perinatal conditions		
	Intrauterine growth, retardation/low birthweight	1	
	Respiratory distress syndrome	2	
	Newborn affected by maternal complications of pregnancy	3	
	Newborn affected by complications of placenta, cord, and membranes	4	
	Others	5	
2	Congenital anomalies		
3	Sudden infant death syndrome		
4	Infections		
5	Accidents and adverse events		
	1–4 Yr: All Causes§		44†
1	Injuries		
2	Congenital anomalies		
3	Malignant neoplasms		
4	Homicide and legal intervention		
5	Diseases of the heart‖		
	5–9 Yr: All Causes§		23†¶
1	Injuries		
2	Malignant neoplasms		
3	Congenital anomalies		
4	Homicide		
5	Diseases of the heart‖		
	10–14 Yr: All Causes§		23†¶
1	Injuries		
2	Malignant neoplasms		
3	Suicide		
4	Homicide		
5	Congenital anomalies		
	15–24 Yr:** All Causes§		98†
1	Injuries		
2	Homicide		
3	Suicide		
4	Malignant neoplasms		
5	Diseases of heart‖		

**Adapted from Monthly Vital Statistics Report 42(11)15. 1994. Rates are for 1993. Ranking is for 1990. Source U.S. National Center for Health Statistics.
†Rate per 100,000 population.
§Leading causes of death by age, 1990. National Center for Health Statistics.
‖Excludes congenital heart anomalies.
¶Mortality rate per 100,000 population ages 5–14 yr for 1993 (Prov.).
**Ranking is for ages 15–19 in 1990.*

ance for the year and an additional 7 million lacked insurance at some point during the year.

The aforementioned findings have generated three sets of goals. The first set included that all families have access to adequate perinatal, preschool, and family-planning services; that governmental activities be effectively coordinated at national and local levels; that services be so organized that they reach populations at special risk; that there be no insurmountable or inequitable financial barriers to adequate care; that the health care of children have continuity from prenatal through adolescent age periods; and that ultimately every family have access to *all* necessary services, including dental, genetic, and mental health services. A second set of goals addresses the needs for reducing accidents and environmental risks, for meeting nutritional needs, and for health education aimed at fostering health-promoting lifestyles. A third set of goals covers needs for research in biomedical and behavioral science, in fundamentals of bioscience and human biology, and in the particular problems of mothers and children.

The unfinished business in the quest for physical, mental, and social health in the community is illustrated by the disparities with which deaths due to disease, to accidents, and to violence are distributed between white and nonwhite children. Homicide has become a major cause of adolescent deaths and has increased in rate also among the very young, in whom the increase may in part represent the more accurate identification of child abuse (Chapter 38); among adolescents it may reflect unresolved social tensions, the epidemic of substance abuse (especially cocaine and crack), and an unhealthy preoccupation in our society with violence. Some of the issues underlying these problems are discussed in Chapters 25, 37, 42 and Part XII.

PATTERNS OF HEALTH CARE

In 1991, children (0–21 yr) made up 31.9% (80.3 million) of the population of the United States. The number of births has been increasing since 1976 and is expected to continue to increase at 1–2% annually. There were 4,111,000 live births in 1991. Table 1–3 indicates the distribution of children in the population by age. The population of children less than 5 yr of age has been increasing since 1980. The adolescent population (15–19 yr of age) will reach a crest in 2005, reflecting the peak of younger children. However, the proportion of children is decreasing relative to the adult population.

There were 141 million office visits to physicians by children aged 0–21 yr in 1990. About 62% of these children were examined by pediatricians, with the greatest number of visits being by children under 5 yr (69.4%) and the least by older children (4.7% of 15–21-yr-olds). The rate of office visits per 100 children per year decreases with age (272 for 5 yr and under, 80 for 6–10 yr, 49 for 11–14 yr, and 17 for 15–21 yr). Nonwhite children are more likely than are white children to use hospital facilities for their ambulatory care.

Hospitals, particularly in urban areas, are sources of both routine and intensive child care, with medical and surgical services that may range from immunization and developmental counseling to open heart surgery and renal transplantation. Clinical conditions and procedures requiring intensive care are likely to be clustered in university-affiliated centers serving as regional resources. The hospitalization rates for children (excluding newborn infants) are less than those of adults under 65 yr of age, except during the first year of life. In 1991, the rates per 1,000 population were: under 1 yr, 200.8; 1–4 yr, 48.3; 5–14 yr, 26.7; 15–19 yr, 17.4 (excluding obstetrics). The rates of hospitalization and lengths of hospital stay have declined significantly for children and adults over the past decade. Children represent less than 8% of the total acute hospital discharges, and in children's hospitals about 70% of admissions are for chronic conditions.

■ **TABLE 1–3 Distribution of Children by Age in the United States in 1991***

Age (yr)		Number (Resident Population)	
<1		4011	
1		3969	
2		3806	
3		3718	
4		3717	
	<5		19,222
5		3702	
6		3681	
7		3575	
8		3512	
9		3767	
	5–9		18,237
10		3703	
11		3662	
12		3484	
13		3414	
14		3409	
	10–14		17,671
15		3293	
16		3362	
17		3360	
18		3383	
19		3808	
	15–19		17,205
20		4080	
21		3969	
0–21		80,384	

**Source: U.S. Bureau of the Census.*

PLANNING AND IMPLEMENTING A SYSTEM OF CARE

Physicians caring for children have been increasingly called upon to advise in the management of disturbed behavior or in relationships between child and parent, child and school, or child and community and are increasingly concerned with problems of mental, social, and societal health. There is also an increasing concern with disparities in how the benefits of what we know about child health reach various groups of children. Just as in many developing countries, so in the United States the health of children lags far behind what it could be if the means and will to apply current knowledge could be brought to bear. The medical problems of the children are often intimately related to problems of mental and social health. The children most at risk are disproportionately represented among ethnic minority groups. Pediatricians have a responsibility to address themselves aggressively to problems such as these.

Linked with these views of the broad scope of pediatric concern is the concept that access to at least a basic level of services to promote health and treat illness is a right of every person. The failure of health services and health benefits to reach all who need them has led to re-examination of the design of health care systems in many countries; but unresolved problems remain in most health care systems, such as the maldistribution of physicians, institutional unresponsiveness to the perceived needs of the individual, failure of medical services to be adapted to the need and convenience of the patient, and deficiencies in health education. Efforts to make the delivery of health care more efficient and effective have led imaginative pediatricians to create new categories of health care providers, such as pediatric nurse practitioners, and to participate in new organizations for providing care to children, such as a variety of managed care arrangements.

New insights into the needs of children have reshaped the child health care system in other ways. Growing understanding of the need of the infant for certain qualities of stimulation and care has led to restudy and revision of the care of the newborn infant (Chapters 10 and 79) and of procedures leading to adoption or to placement with foster families (Chapters 32 and 33). For handicapped children the massive centralized institutions of past years are being replaced by community-centered arrangements offering a better opportunity for these children to achieve their maximal potential. Pediatricians have been involved in shaping these and other institutions that provide services to children, and their insights and active contributions will continue to be needed.

COSTS OF HEALTH CARE

The growth of high technology, the redesign of health institutions (particularly with respect to the needs for and the uses of personnel), the public's demand for medical services, and the manner in which the costs of health care are paid (by public or private insurance programs based on fee for service) have driven the costs of health care in the United States up to a point at which they represent a significant proportion of the gross national product. Although children (0–18 yr) represent about 30% of the population, they account for only about 14% of the personal health care expenditures, or about 60% of adult per capita expenditures. Efforts to contain costs have led to revisions of the way in which physicians and hospitals are paid for services. Limits have been set on the fees for some services, capitated prepayment and a variety of managed care systems flourish, a program of reimbursement (diagnosis-related groups [DRGs]) based on the diagnosis rather than on the particular services rendered to the individual patient has been implemented, and a relative value scale for varying rates of payment among different physician services has been implemented. These changes in the system of financing health services raise important ethical issues for pediatricians to address (Chapter 3).

EVALUATION OF HEALTH CARE

The shaping of health care systems to meet the needs of children and their families requires accurate statistical data and difficult decisions in the setting of priorities. Along with growing concerns about the design and cost of health care systems and the ability to equitably distribute health services has come increasing concern about the quality of health care and about its efficiency and its effectiveness. There are large local and regional variations among similar populations of children in the rates of use of procedures and of hospital admissions. These variations require continuing evaluation and explanation in terms of the actual impact of medical and surgical services on health status and the outcome of illness. The need for technology assessment is increasing.

GROWTH OF SPECIALIZATION

The amount of information relevant to child health care is rapidly expanding, and no person can become master of it all. Physicians are increasingly dependent on one another for the highest quality of care for their patients; group practices in pediatrics are common in the United States and, although the vast majority of pediatricians are primary care generalists, as many as 25% claim an area of special knowledge and skill.

The growth of specialization within pediatrics has taken a number of different forms: Interests in problems of *age groups* of children have created neonatology and adolescent medicine; interests in *organ systems* have created pediatric cardiology, allergy, hematology, nephrology, gastroenterology, pulmonology, endocrinology, and specialization in metabolism and genetics; interests in the *health care system* have created pediatricians devoted to ambulatory care on the one hand or to intensive care on the other; and finally, multidisciplinary subspecialties have grown up around the problems of *handicapped children,* to which pediatrics, neurology, psychiatry, psychology, nursing, physical and occupational therapy, special education, speech therapy, audiology, and nutrition all make essential contributions. This growth of specialization has been most conspicuous in university-affiliated departments of pediatrics and medical centers for children.

NEED FOR CONTINUING SELF-EDUCATION

The explosion of information has also created a need for continuing education, which was felt much less keenly in earlier years, when the new information in any field of medicine was easily accessible through a relatively small number of journals, texts, or monographs. Now, relevant information is so widely scattered among the many published journals that elaborate electronic data systems are necessary to make it accessible. New auditory and visual aids to learning abound as well as postgraduate courses through which the participating physician can be brought up to date on various aspects of child health care. The American Board of Pediatrics and the American Academy of Pediatrics have arranged for the close linkage of continuing education of pediatricians to recertification in pediatrics.

There is no touchstone through which physicians can ensure that the process of their own continuing education will keep them abreast of advancing knowledge in the field, but they must find a way if they are to discharge their responsibility to their patients. An essential element of this process may be for the physician to take an *active* role, such as participating in medical student and resident education. Efforts in continuing self-education will also be fostered, for example, if clinical problems can be made a stimulus for a review of standard literature, alone or in consultation with an appropriate colleague or consultant. This continuing review will do much to identify those inconsistencies or contradictions that will indicate, in the ultimate best interest of the patient, that things are not what they seem or have been said to be. Physicians still learn most from their patients, but this will not be the case if they fall into the easy habit of accepting their patients' problems casually or at face value because they appear to be simple.

The tools that the physician must use in dealing with the problems of children and their families fall into three main categories: *cognitive* (up-to-date factual information regarding diagnostic and therapeutic issues, available on recall or easily found in readily accessible sources); *interpersonal or manual* (e.g., the ability to carry out a productive interview, execute a reliable physical examination, perform a deft venipuncture, or manage cardiac arrest or the resuscitation of a depressed newborn infant); and *attitudinal* (the physician's commitment to fullest possible implementation of knowledge and skills on behalf of children and their families in an atmosphere of empathetic sensitivity and concern). With regard to this last category, it is important that children participate with their families in informed decision-making about their own health care in a manner appropriate to their stage of development and the nature of the particular health problem.

The workaday needs of professional persons for knowledge and skills in care of children vary widely. The primary care physician needs depth in developmental concepts and in the ability to organize an effective system for achieving quality and continuity in assessing and planning for health care during the entire period of growth. There may often be little or no need for immediate recall of esoterica. On the other hand, the consultant or subspecialist not only needs a comfortable grasp of esoterica within his or her field and perhaps within related fields but also must be able to cope with controversial issues, with flexibility that will permit adaptation of a variety of points of view to the best interest of his or her unique patient.

At whatever level of care (primary, secondary, or tertiary), only a very small volume of urine so that water can be retained in the body; the urine is also highly concentrated with ions. In addition, marine fishes drink seawater. The ingested salt is eliminated across the gills by active transport.

Exchanges Due to Feeding Because foods contain salts and water, eating also involves an obligatory exchange of these substances. Some plant products are over 95% water by weight, and other foods may contain high amounts of Na^+ or other ions. Therefore, the type of diet an animal consumes determines how much salt and water it ingests.

When food molecules are metabolized to provide energy that will be stored in the chemical bonds of ATP, oxygen captures electrons and combines with hydrogen ions, thereby making water (refer back to Figure 6.18). This water is sometimes called "metabolic water" to indicate its origin and, in some animals, is all the additional water they need to survive.

Exchanges Due to Evaporation of Water Endotherms use body water to cool off (refer back to Chapter 31). For example, sweating and panting are used to cool the body. These behaviors use the evaporation of water to draw heat out of the body. In the process, however, the animal loses water and, in sweat, some ions.

Other than perspiration and panting, very little water is gained or lost directly across the body surface of most terrestrial vertebrates (with the exception of amphibians), because their skin is impermeable to water. In invertebrates, the rate of water loss across the body surface depends on whether the animal is soft-bodied, like worms, or covered in a waxy, water-impermeable cuticle, like most insects.

The significance of obligatory exchanges and their effects on homeostasis was dramatically illustrated by a long-term investigation by a research team at the University of Florida, as described next. Their discovery would lead to a revolution in our understanding of exercise physiology in humans.

FEATURE INVESTIGATION

Cade and Colleagues Discovered Why Athletes' Performances Wane on Hot Days

On a typically hot summer day in the mid-1960s in Gainesville, Florida, the University of Florida football team was practicing in full equipment. The players were becoming dehydrated and, unbeknownst to them, the osmolarity of their body fluids was increasing as their bodies produced copious amounts of sweat in an effort to maintain body temperature. The athletes became aware of two things. First, they discovered that they did not need to urinate for long periods after a tough practice session, and second, their performance on the field suffered as they became increasingly fatigued and more susceptible to severe muscle cramps. Occasionally, players would require medical treatment for their symptoms. In extreme cases, athletes exercising in these conditions have been known to occasionally develop seizures—uncontrolled activity of neurons in the brain. This situation did not escape the notice of the team physicians and, notably, university faculty member and kidney specialist Robert Cade.

Many of the symptoms experienced by the players could be readily explained. The fatigue was directly related to loss of water from the body, which put a strain on the circulatory system and reduced blood flow to muscles and other organs. It was worsened by a decrease in blood glucose concentrations that were not being replenished during the long periods of strenuous activity. The muscle cramps and even occasional seizures arose from an imbalance in extracellular ions—notably Na^+ and K^+—which are secreted outside the body by sweat glands in the process of perspiration. Sweat is a hypo-osmotic solution relative to body fluids, and consequently sweating results in an imbalance in extracellular ion concentrations. In the athletes, this caused a change in the electrical potential across muscle and neuronal cell membranes, which triggered the symptoms. Lastly, the decreased urine production is one of the body's mechanisms for reducing fluid loss when body water is decreasing.

Cade and his colleagues rejected the prevailing view that drinking any fluids during heavy exercise somehow contributed to cramps and other problems. Instead, they hypothesized that the best way to maintain ion and water homeostasis in a profusely sweating person is to restore to the body exactly what was lost; that is, the person should drink a solution that resembles sweat!

The first thing Cade did was analyze how much Na^+, K^+, and other ions are present in sweat. Fortunately, he had an abundance of human sweat at his disposal to analyze. Once the players left the field, their jerseys were wrung out, and the composition of the collected sweat was determined with an ion analyzer such as the flame spectrophotometer shown in **Figure 38.3**. The concentrations could then be compared with known values of ion concentrations in human blood. Today, we know that the composition of human sweat can change under certain conditions and can vary among people, but Cade's results were typical. The athletes' sweat contained mostly Na^+, K^+, and Cl^- at concentrations that indicated the solution was dilute compared with blood. Once Cade completed this analysis, he simply made an artificial solution of a composition similar to human sweat. The next step was to have the players drink the solution before and during the practice sessions and games. Improving its taste—adding some lemon flavoring and sugar—removed any inhibitions the players may have had about drinking it, while also providing an energy boost.

For the first trial, Cade gave the solution to the freshman players during an intrasquad scrimmage against the more experienced varsity B-team, whose members received only pure water to drink as a control. At first, the freshman team appeared overmatched by the B-team, as might be expected. In the second half of the scrimmage, however, the freshman team vastly outperformed the more experienced players and did not suffer the characteristic late-game fatigue the B-team experienced. Based on this test, the varsity A-team was given a similar solution to drink the next day during a game against a heavily favored opponent, whom they beat handily on a hot 39°C (102°F) day. In subsequent years, Cade and other researchers would conduct carefully controlled experiments with humans and laboratory animals to confirm that a balanced solution of salts similar to that present in sweat effectively improves exercise performance and reduces the possibility of dehydration and its consequences. Because the solution was envisioned as "aid" for the team known as the University of Florida "Gators," the drink eventually came to be called Gatorade.

The story of Gatorade is one of a practical application based on solid scientific principles of osmolarity and ion and water homeostasis. You can now understand why drinking a dilute salt solution (in any of numerous sports drinks) during strenuous exercise is better than drinking water. Although drinking pure water prevents dehydration, if drunk in excess, it will actually reduce plasma ion concentrations to below normal. In other words, it will replace one type of ion imbalance with another.

Experimental Questions

1. What symptoms are sometimes seen in athletes after prolonged, strenuous exercise, particularly in hot weather? How are these symptoms related to water loss during exercise, and what did Cade and his colleagues hypothesize about this?
2. How did the researchers test their hypothesis?
3. What was the result of consuming the drink during exercise?

Figure 38.3 **Cade and colleagues discovered a way to improve athletic performance and prevent ion and water imbalance during strenuous exercise.**

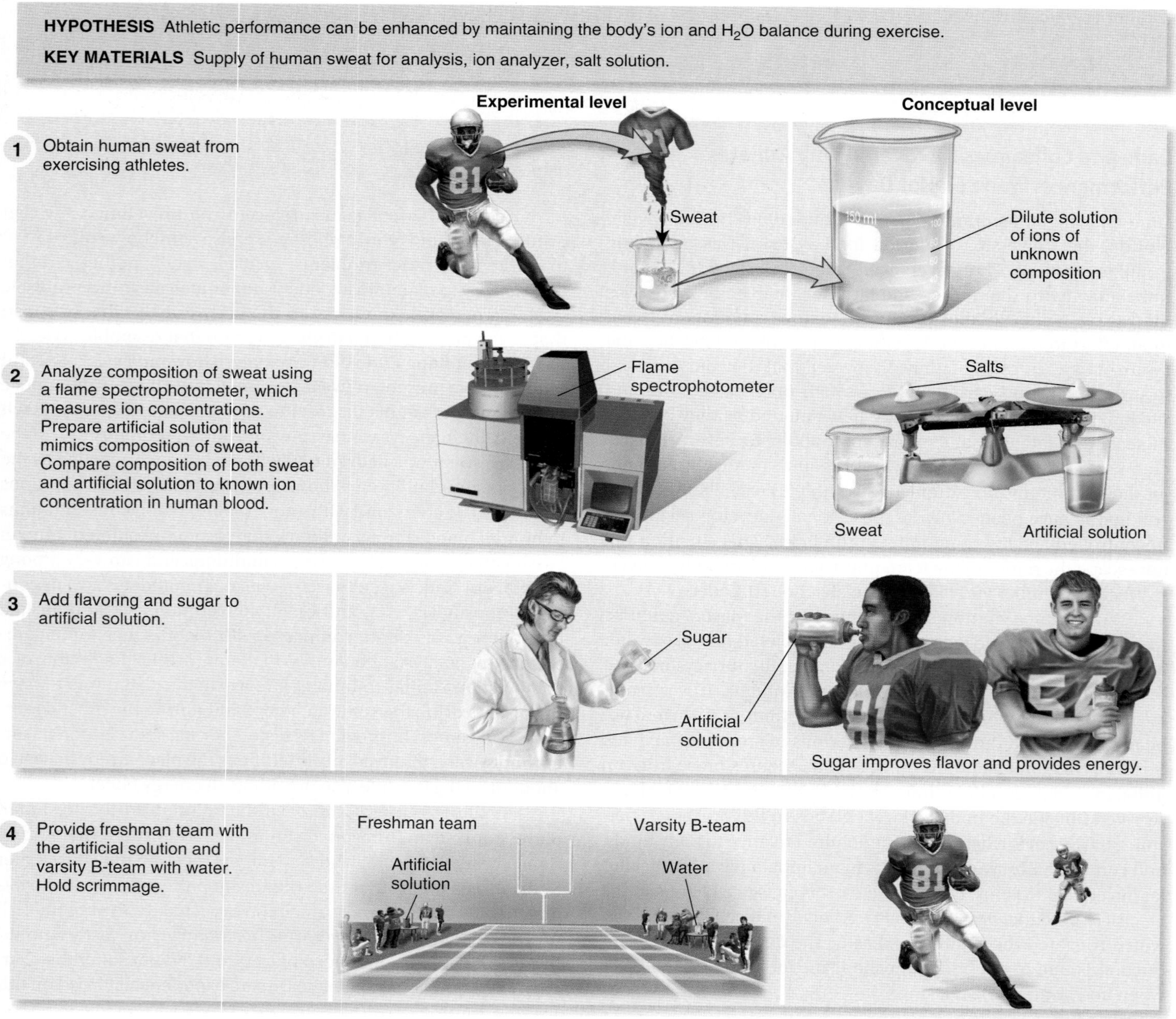

HYPOTHESIS Athletic performance can be enhanced by maintaining the body's ion and H_2O balance during exercise.
KEY MATERIALS Supply of human sweat for analysis, ion analyzer, salt solution.
Experimental level
Conceptual level
1 Obtain human sweat from exercising athletes.
Sweat
Dilute solution of ions of unknown composition
2 Analyze composition of sweat using a flame spectrophotometer, which measures ion concentrations. Prepare artificial solution that mimics composition of sweat. Compare composition of both sweat and artificial solution to known ion concentration in human blood.
Flame spectrophotometer
Salts
Sweat
Artificial solution
3 Add flavoring and sugar to artificial solution.
Sugar
Artificial solution
Sugar improves flavor and provides energy.
4 Provide freshman team with the artificial solution and varsity B-team with water. Hold scrimmage.
Freshman team
Varsity B-team
Artificial solution
Water

5 **THE DATA**

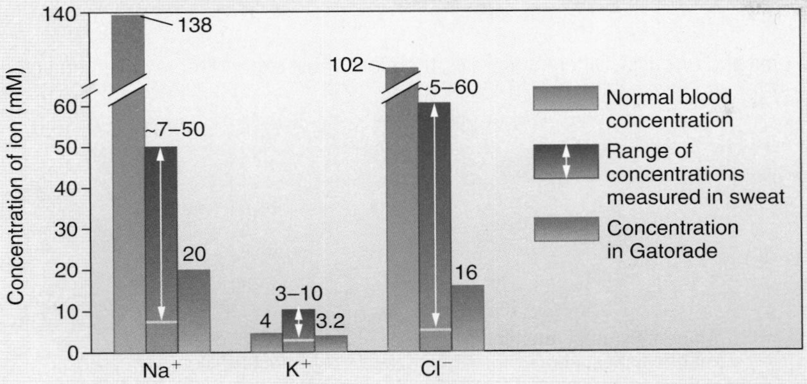

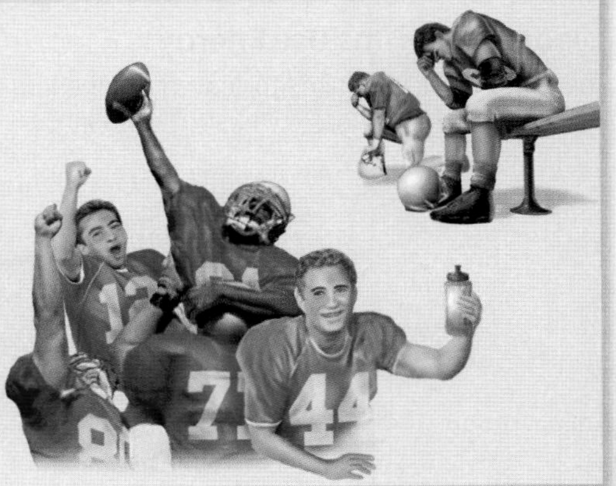

6 **CONCLUSION** Replacement of fluid with solute concentrations similar to those found in human sweat improves athletic performance compared with water replacement alone.

7 **SOURCE** Most of the original studies described here were published in expanded form in a later report. See Cade, R. et al. 1972. Effect of fluid, electrolyte, and glucose replacement during exercise on performance, body temperature, rate of sweat loss, and compositional changes of extracellular fluid. *Journal of Sports Medicine and Physical Fitness* 12:150–156.

38.1 Reviewing the Concepts

- Exchanges of ions and water with the environment resulting from vital processes, such as respiration or the elimination of wastes, are called obligatory exchanges (Figure 38.1).
- The solute concentration of a solution of water is known as the solution's osmolarity. Fishes and other water-breathing animals that live in fresh water and those that live in salt water face opposite osmoregulatory challenges (Figure 38.2).
- Robert Cade and coworkers discovered that fluid replacement during exercise is particularly beneficial if the fluid contains solutes at concentrations similar to those in sweat (Figure 38.3).

38.1 Testing Your Knowledge

1. A man eats several slices of a pizza topped with pepperoni and sausage. What might follow?
   a. The sodium concentration of his extracellular fluids will decrease.
   b. Water will move by osmosis out of his cells into his extracellular fluid.
   c. Cells will swell.
   d. Cells will shrink.
   e. b and d
2. Which is false?
   a. Sweat has a lower solute concentration than internal body fluids such as blood.
   b. Some animals can survive without drinking water.
   c. A solution of 1000 mOsm/L is hyperosmotic relative to the body fluids of a fish.
   d. Marine fishes, but not freshwater fishes, drink the water they swim in.
   e. A 300 mOsm/L solution of NaCl contains 300 mM Na^+ and 300 mM Cl^-.

38.2 Comparative Excretory Systems

Learning Outcomes:

1. Describe the forms of nitrogenous wastes generated by animals.
2. Describe the general processes of filtration, reabsorption, secretion, and excretion.
3. Identify several invertebrate osmoregulatory organs, and compare and contrast the process of elimination in each.
4. List the general features of kidneys that are common to all vertebrates.

Animals make use of one or more different organs to rid themselves of metabolic wastes, excess water and ions, and toxins from their environment. Most excretory organs contain tubular structures lined with epithelial cells that have the capacity to actively transport ions and other substances across their membranes. Wastes are excreted out of the body by means of these tubes.

Biology Principle

Living Organisms Use Energy

Energy from ATP is required to convert nitrogenous wastes into urea and uric acid. Different animals, therefore, must expend more or less energy each day to rid themselves of toxic nitrogenous wastes.

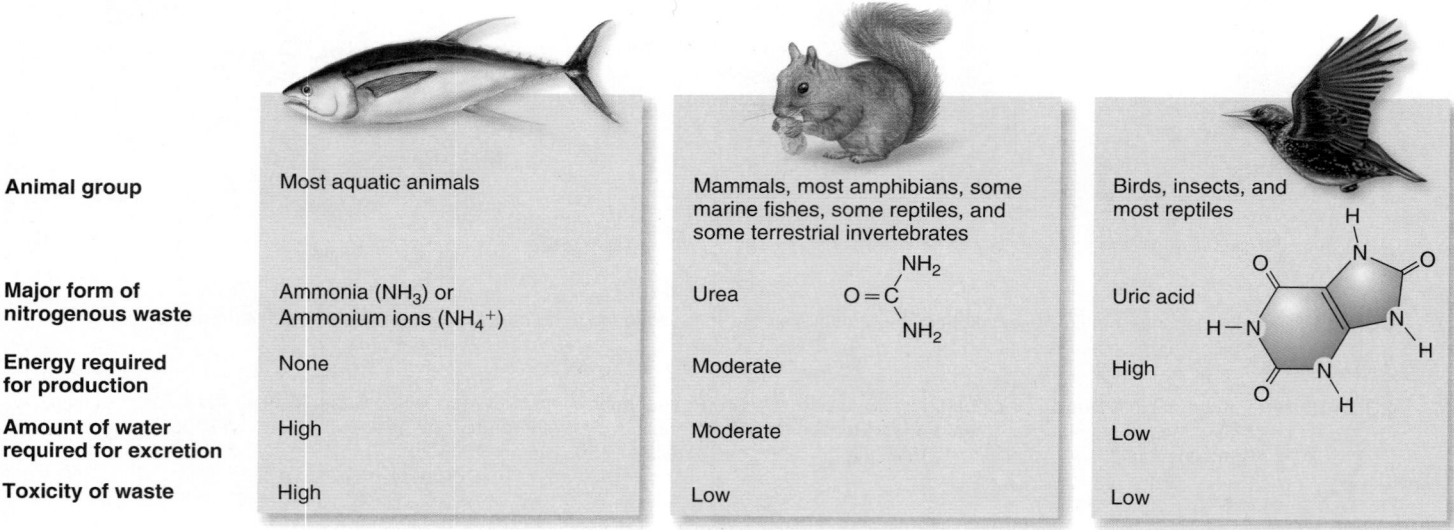

Animal group	Most aquatic animals	Mammals, most amphibians, some marine fishes, some reptiles, and some terrestrial invertebrates	Birds, insects, and most reptiles
Major form of nitrogenous waste	Ammonia (NH_3) or Ammonium ions (NH_4^+)	Urea $O=C(NH_2)_2$	Uric acid 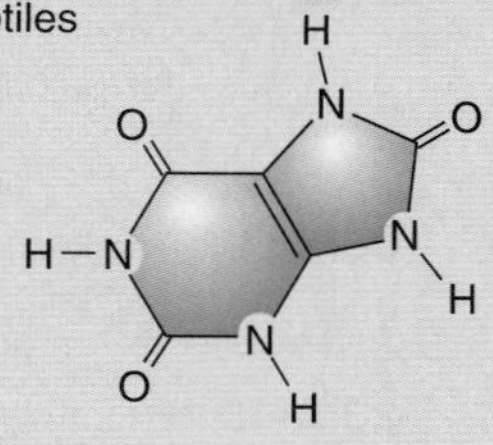
Energy required for production	None	Moderate	High
Amount of water required for excretion	High	Moderate	Low
Toxicity of waste	High	Low	Low

Figure 38.4 Nitrogenous wastes produced by different animal groups. The three forms of nitrogenous wastes, which are derived from the breakdown of proteins or nucleic acids, have different properties.

In some cases, animals may have considerable ability to regulate the rate at which waste is excreted and how much water is lost in the process. For example, even though a thirsty mammal on a hot, sunny day must continue to rid its body of soluble waste products, it must also conserve water. In this section, we consider the structure and function of invertebrate and vertebrate excretory organs. First, we examine the major forms of nitrogenous wastes generated in animals.

Nitrogenous Wastes Are Found in Three Major Forms

Nitrogenous wastes are usually found in three forms—ammonia (or ammonium ions), urea, or uric acid (Figure 38.4), depending on the species and the environment in which they live.

- **Ammonia (NH_3)** and **ammonium ions (NH_4^+)** are the most toxic of the nitrogenous wastes because they disrupt pH, ion electrochemical gradients, and many chemical reactions that involve oxidations and reductions. With some exceptions, animals that excrete wastes in this form typically live in water, where the ammonia is rapidly diluted. These animals generally excrete the ammonia as soon as it is formed, via the skin, gills, or kidneys. The chief advantage of excreting nitrogenous wastes as NH_3 or NH_4^+ is that energy is not required for their conversion to a less toxic product.
- **Urea** is produced and excreted in all mammals, most amphibians, some marine fishes, some reptiles, and some terrestrial invertebrates. It is less toxic than NH_3, and thus animals can tolerate some accumulation of urea in their blood, tissues, and storage organs such as the urinary bladder. As a result, unlike ammonia, urea does not need to be constantly excreted. One drawback of producing urea is that the enzymatic conversion of NH_3 into urea requires a moderate expenditure of ATP and thus consumes part of an animal's total daily energy budget.
- **Uric acid** is the major form of nitrogenous waste produced in birds, insects, and most reptiles. Like urea, it is less toxic than ammonia, but is even more energetically costly to synthesize. However, because it is poorly soluble in water, uric acid is not excreted in a watery urine but instead is packaged with other waste products and excess salts into a semisolid, partly dried precipitate that is excreted. The energy investment required to produce uric acid, therefore, is balanced against the water conserved by excreting nitrogenous wastes in this form.

Excretory Systems Use Four Processes to Cleanse Body Fluids of Nitrogenous and Other Wastes

Most excretory systems function by using one or more of four processes, as shown in Figure 38.5.

1. **Filtration:** In **filtration,** an organ acts like a filter or sieve, removing some of the water and its small solutes from the blood, interstitial fluid, or hemolymph, while excluding

or in whatever role (as student, as pediatric nurse practitioner, as resident pediatrician, as a practitioner of pediatrics or of family medicine, or as a pediatric or other subspecialist), professional persons dealing with children must be able to identify their roles of the moment and their levels of engagement with a child's problem; each must determine whether his or her experience and other resources at hand are adequate to deal with this problem and must be ready to seek other help when they are not. Among the necessary resources will be general textbooks, more detailed monographs in subspecialty areas, selected journals, audiovisual materials, and, above all, colleagues with exceptional or complementary experience and expertise. The intercommunication of all these levels of engagement with medical and health problems of children offers the best hope of bringing us closer to the goal of providing the opportunity for all children to achieve their maximum potential.

Advance Data, Nos. 208, 227, and 229. National Center for Health Statistics. 1992, 1993.
Advance Report of Final Natality Statistics, 1993. Monthly Vital Statistics Report 42(12), May 13, 1994. Washington, DC, US Department of Health and Human Services. Public Health Service, Centers for Disease Control.
Boyle CA, Decougle P, Yeargin-Allsopp M: Prevalence and health impact of developmental disabilities in U.S. children. Pediatrics 93:399, 1994.
Child Health USA, 1991. US Department of Health and Human Services.
Health Care Reform. The Future of Children 3(2):4–214, 1993.
Kins NMP, Cross AW: Children as decision makers: Guidelines for pediatricians. J Pediatr 115:10, 1989.
Morbidity and Mortality Weekly Report 43(16), April 29, 1994.
Statistical Abstract of the United States, 1993, 113th ed. Dept of Commerce.
The Child Welfare Stat Book, 1993. Child Welfare League of America.
U.S. Health Care System For Children. The Future of Children 2(2):1–191, 1992.

CHAPTER 2

Evaluating Medical Literature: Clinical Epidemiology

Peter L. Havens

Clinical epidemiology, a system of thought, can be used to solve problems that arise in clinical medicine. The major focus of epidemiologic thought in the analysis of medical literature is avoidance of systematic error (bias) and identification of confounding effects between variables. Statistics offers methods of computation and numbers manipulation that can assess the effects of random error and control for confounding variables in the analysis. Knowing where to look for errors as well as what kind of errors are possible makes it more likely that those errors will be found when reading pertinent literature. Finding errors in study design, implementation, or analysis is crucial to avoid mistakes in inferences made as the results of published clinical studies are applied to problems in patient management.

Table 2–1 outlines a series of questions that may be helpful in addressing five major issues important in evaluating the relevance of a clinical study to decisions about particular patients. These are (1) What population was studied? (2) What measurements were made? (3) What was the design of the study that related the measurements to the population? (4) What nonrandom errors were made in selection of study subjects (selection bias) or in measurements performed on those subjects (observation/measurement bias); and what hidden errors might there have been (confounding)? (5) What

■ TABLE 2–1 Questions to Ask of a Report of a Clinical Study: Outline for a Study Critique

Collection of Data
Why was the study done (and who paid for it)? What were the prior hypotheses?
What type of study was done?
How was the size of the study population determined?
How was the ratio of cases to controls determined?
Could there have been bias in the selection of study subjects? How might selection bias affect the data?
Could there have been bias in the collection of information and performance of measurements? How might observation or measurement bias affect the data?
What provisions were made to minimize confounding?

Analysis of Data
What methods were used to measure the association between exposure and disease?
What methods were used to measure the stability of the association between exposure and disease?
What methods were used to control for confounding?

Interpretation of Data
What were the major results of the study?
How might bias have affected these results?
How might random misclassification have affected these results?
To whom may the results of this study be generalized?
Is the interpretation of the data conservative?

Modified from Monson RR: Occupational Epidemiology, 2nd ed. Boca Raton, FL, CRC Press, 1990.

statistical techniques were used in the analysis of the study to report the main results, and what techniques were used to assess the effects of both random and systematic error on those results?

STUDY POPULATIONS. The actual patients in a study may differ dramatically from what was initially conceptualized as the intended population. These differences may be important as one tries to interpret the study's results. One approach to understanding problems associated with study populations is shown in Figure 2–1.

When starting to design a study, the investigator may plan to study everyone with a given disease, the "target population," e.g., "all children with otitis media." The investigator begins by exactly specifying the members of this group, both clinically and demographically. However, all children with otitis media are not available to any single investigator. Therefore, an investigator studies the subjects available, both in

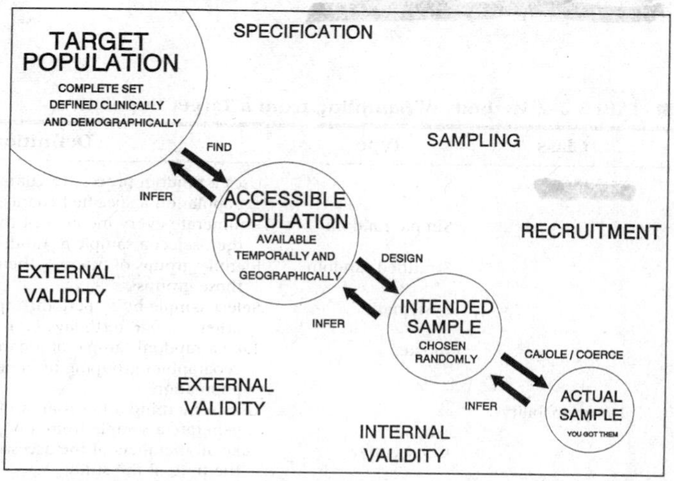

Figure 2–1. Subjects actually enrolled in a study may differ in important ways from the population that the investigators initially intended to study. Nonrandom errors in subject selection are called selection bias; they can produce studies that lead to improper inferences when study results are applied to populations other than the study population.

time and place. The population that is accessible may differ dramatically from the conceptualized target population, and understanding those differences is important in interpreting study results. A study performed with subjects with otitis media at a university hospital emergency room may be different from one performed at a suburban private practice.

Even the accessible population may be too large to study completely. Therefore, investigators often study a sample of the accessible population. The most ideal method of sampling the accessible population is random sampling, since all statistical tests of significance assume that the method of sampling was random. Methods of sampling from a population are outlined in Table 2–2. After the accessible population is sampled, one has the intended sample of study subjects. For example, they might all be patients with otitis media coming to the emergency room over a 1-year period. This study sample may not be particularly representative of the initially conceptualized target population. The generalizability, *external validity,* of a study is a measure of how representative the intended sample is of the target population. The results of a study of otitis media in patients who come to a subspecialty otorhinolaryngology clinic for evaluation may not be very generalizable to care of patients with otitis media seen in a primary care office practice. The subspecialty clinic patient sample could have many different problems from those of patients seen in a general office practice. Such a study would be said to have low generalizability or poor external validity.

Once an investigator has defined the population sample intended for study, the subjects must be recruited into a study. The differences between the intended sample and the actual sample can be significant. What leads people to refuse participation in a study may not be random; rather, there may be certain recurring problems that lead to the study of a biased sampling of intended study subjects. *Internal validity* is a measure of how representative the actual sample is compared with the intended sample. If sampling at this level is unbiased, the study is said to have good internal reliability. However, if all patients with severe otitis media refuse to enter a study, while patients with mild otitis media agree to be in a study, the subjects actually in the study would be different from those initially intended for inclusion. This would result in a systemic error in choosing study subjects, *selection bias,* even if the intended sample had been an unbiased representative sample of the population of interest. Such a study has poor internal validity, and the results would be only poorly generalizable to a different population of patients.

MEASUREMENTS

Variables. After a sample population is identified for study, the investigator decides on the variables to be measured. The conceptual definition of the variables of interest may differ from the operational definition of the actual measurements. The relationship between these two definitions also affects the internal validity of the study. In the theoretical study of otitis media, the child with ear pain and a bulging, opaque, immobile eardrum constitutes the conceptual definition of otitis media. The operational definition may include agreement on diagnostic criteria between two certified otoscopists, or it may involve tympanometry, as a way to objectively standardize the definition of otitis media. Understanding the differences between the conceptual definition and operational definition used in a study is important as one tries to generalize the results of a study to clinical practice. Operational definitions of disease used for clinical trials may be much narrower than definitions used for diagnosis in clinical practice, limiting the external validity of some trials.

There are several types of variables with different attributes. Truly continuous variables have an infinite number of potential values (age, weight, and blood pressure). Other types of continuous variables (ordered discrete variables) are different from truly continuous variables. Even though they represent ordered categories with quantifiable intervals between the categories, there is not an infinite number of potential values between each ordered discrete variable. An example of such a variable would be the number of feedings per day. Categorical variables sort study subjects into different unordered groups. Examples of categorical variables are gender, race, and vital status (dead or alive). Ordinal variables are a special type of categorical variable that sort study subjects into categories that have some relative ranking. An example of such a variable is an asthma score that might identify patients with mild, moderate, or severe asthma. Categorical variables are often used to measure and report the presence of disease in populations. Measures of disease frequency are reported as rates.

The information content of the statement "Ten people died of this illness" is greatly enhanced by adding the number of people at risk of the illness as well as the time period over which the risk was present. The *incidence rate* has as its numerator the number of newly affected individuals and as its denominator the person-time of observation (number of people at risk for the disease for a certain duration). The *cumulative incidence rate* has the number of newly affected in the numerator and the number at risk in the denominator. Time is not

■ **TABLE 2–2 Methods of Sampling from a Target Population***

Class	Type	Definition	Problems/Benefits
Probability		Uses a random process to guarantee each unit of population a specified chance of selection	The only valid method if you are expecting to do significance tests
	Simple random	Enumerate every member of the population, and then select a sample at random	Requires enumeration of the entire population, minimizes potential for sampling bias
	Stratified random	Identify groups of interest, then randomize within those groups	A good, nonbiased way to increase precision in subgroup analyses
	Systematic	Select sample by a "periodic" approach (e.g., every other . . . odd birthdays . . .)	No advantages over random number table, not really random, open to alteration and bias
	Cluster	Take a random sample of a natural (temporal or geographic) grouping of members of the population	Biased if the "natural grouping" is not representative of whole population
Nonprobability		Uses something other than a random process to generate a sample from a population	All are open to bias and diminish applicability of statistical tests of significance
	Consecutive	Take all members of the accessible population over the time of the study	Easy, but may not be a representative sample if the time of the study is short
	Convenience	Use members of the accessible population who are the easiest to get to	Strong potential for bias, volunteers are healthier than others
	Judgmental	Include those you want, and exclude the ones you don't want	Very little relation to a random probability sample, don't you think? The potential for systematic error is enormous

**All statistical significance tests depend on choosing a random probability sample from a population of interest.*

explicitly stated in the cumulative incidence rate, but it is often an annual rate. Incidence rates reflect new cases. *Prevalence rates* have the total number of cases in the numerator (independent of time of disease onset) and total number at risk in the denominator. In diseases for which the exact onset cannot be determined (cancers), it may be difficult to distinguish between incident and prevalent cases.

The *mortality rate* is a special kind of cumulative incidence rate, with deaths in the numerator and population in the denominator. The *case-fatality rate,* another special type of cumulative incidence rate, has deaths in the numerator and number of people with a specific disease in the denominator.

In the same way that selection bias can lead to errors in choosing study subjects, nonrandom or systematic errors can be a problem in measurements performed on study subjects. The degree to which a measurement actually represents what it was intended to represent is called *accuracy* or *validity.* Nonrandom systematic error in measurement that may lead to the wrong answer is called *measurement bias.* Special types of measurement bias are *observer bias,* which is a consistent distortion in the perception or reporting of the measurement by an observer, and *subject bias,* which is a consistent distortion of the measurement by the study subject. Comparing results of one study with a gold standard measurement is necessary to assess the accuracy of a study. Random errors that lead to finding an association when none actually exists are called *alpha errors.*

The *precision (reliability)* of a variable is an indicator of the extent to which a measurement gives the same results when performed several times. Problems with precision result in random errors. This type of error may lead to finding "no association" even when an association may exist. This is called *beta error.* A pictorial interpretation of the relationship between precision and accuracy as well as the importance of these concepts in design and interpretation of clinical studies is presented in Figure 2–2. It is possible to have a precise answer that is the wrong answer. It has been thought that it is better to find "no difference" (even if one exists) than to precisely describe an inaccurate answer. While precision is helpful, accuracy is the most important consideration.

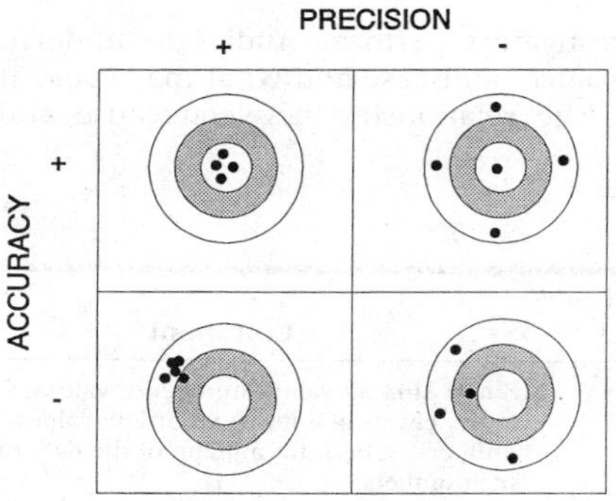

Precision and Accuracy of Measurement Variables

	Precision (Random Error)	Accuracy (Systematic Error; Bias)
Definition	The degree to which a variable has nearly the same value when measured several times	The degree to which a variable actually represents what it is supposed to represent
Assessment	Use statistical analysis to compare variation between repeated measurements. Look for standard deviation or 95% confidence interval.	Use epidemiologic thought. Compare measurements with a reference standard.
Importance	Allows detection of differences between groups at "statistically significant" levels	Allows detection of "clinically significant" differences between groups and identification of studies in which bias leads to the wrong answer.

Figure 2–2. The difference between precision and accuracy of measurements.

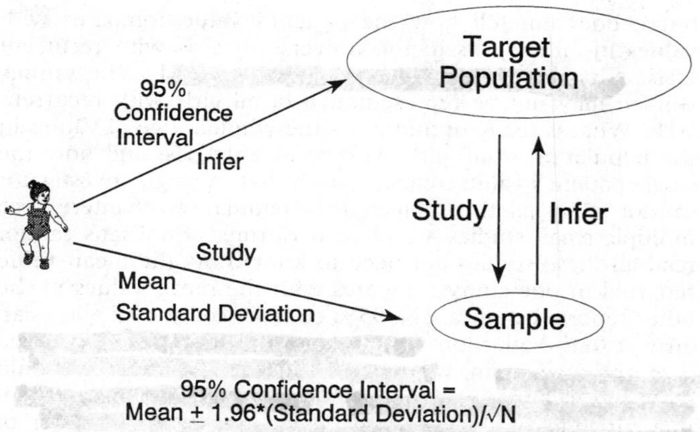

Figure 2–3. From the results of a study we know the mean and standard deviation of a measurement in the study sample. From this we make inferences about the mean in the target population. It is the 95% confidence interval that allows this inference to be made.

Statistical Inference for Nonstatisticians. Epidemiology is useful to control or identify nonrandom error, and statistics is important to control the effects of random error in a study. Each time a clinician evaluates a patient it is somewhat akin to performing a clinical trial, with a sample size of one. Clinicians are often in the position of comparing what happens with a patient to what has been reported in the literature. Inferences about a patient are based on comparing measured patient variables with reported reference values. The validity of the inference from reported value to single patient data depends in part on how well the reference study was designed and implemented and on how closely the patient in question matches the subjects in the comparison study. Deciding whether a single patient is significantly different from those reported in the literature also requires an understanding of statistical inference.

Suppose that there is an 8-yr-old female patient with recurrent urinary tract infections (UTIs). A clinician measures the blood pressure and wants to know if that measurement is higher than usual for other girls with her condition. There is no study that has evaluated all other such girls. There may be a study in which an investigator measures the blood pressure in a sample of 10 subjects from the universe of girls with recurrent UTIs (Fig. 2–3). The individual blood pressure values are summed and divided by the number of subjects in the study, and the mean blood pressure in those 10 girls is reported. The mean value from the subjects in the study sample estimates the mean blood pressure in the target population. It is called the point estimate of the main result of the study. The standard deviation of the sample mean is also calculated, as a way to describe the variability (*random error*) associated with the measurement. To measure the single patient value against those of the 10 patients in the study, the clinician compares the patient value with the mean blood pressure value in the study sample. If it is higher than the mean, the patient's value is then compared with the range of values encompassed by the standard deviation reported in the study. If the single patient's value falls within the range of values reported in the study, that is reassuring.

Finding a patient's blood pressure within the range of values encompassed by the standard deviation of the blood pressure of the 10 study subjects may be reassuring as far as it goes, but it does not tell how the patient's value compares with values in all subjects in the universe of girls with recurrent UTIs. A study with 10 subjects is a small study. The sample studied may not be representative of all girls with recurrent UTIs. What is really of interest is the whole range of values in the population of all girls with recurrent UTIs, and how the single patient's value compares with that. A single investigator cannot study all the subjects in a population of interest, so multiple small studies are often performed. Clinicians cannot read all these studies but need to know how the mean value reported in one study compares with the mean values in the other reported studies. The 95% confidence interval allows an answer to the question "If the same study were to be repeated over and over again, what is the range of answers that would be found 95 times out of 100?" The 95% confidence interval is a function of the standard deviation and the number of patients in a study and is calculated as

$$\text{mean} \pm 1.96^* \text{ (standard deviation) } / \sqrt{N}$$

where N is the number of subjects in the study.

Studies with many subjects (large N) will have narrower 95% confidence intervals than smaller studies. As the standard deviation increases (random variation in measurements increases) so does the length of the 95% confidence interval. If an investigator utilizes a precise measurement that reproducibly gives the same result with very little error, and there is little variability in the population sample being studied, a precise measure of the main effect, with a narrow 95% confidence interval, can be obtained using very few subjects. If the method of measurement is not very precise or if there is wide variability in the sample being studied, the 95% confidence limit will be very wide.

The example above uses a continuous variable. The summary statistic used to report the point estimate of the main effect in a study with a single continuous variable is the mean or median. The estimate of the uncertainty associated with that point estimate is the standard deviation or 95% confidence interval (Table 2–3). Studies with a categorical variable as their main measurement report a rate of illness as the point estimate of the main result. Estimates of rates have the potential for error and need to be reported with a 95% confidence interval. The 95% confidence interval has the same meaning with a categorical variable as it does with a continuous variable: If the study were repeated many times, the risk estimate generated by each of those studies would fall within the range of values encompassed by the 95% confidence interval 95 times out of 100.

Studies are often performed to measure differences between subjects in two groups. Such studies have main effects that report the size of the difference between the groups. This is called the effect size. Examples of various summary statistics are given in Table 2–3. The 95% confidence interval suggests the range that would include the point estimate of the main effect found in a study were the study to be performed over and over again. Many studies compare findings in two groups, when the question of interest is stated "Is the value in group 1 so much different than the value in group 2 that the populations from which they were sampled are really different?" The probability that the samples in the two groups came from the same target population is called the p value (for probability). When the p value is <0.05, it is inferred that the probability that the study group values were sampled from the same population is $<5\%$. There is a statistically significant difference between the values in the two groups, because they were distinct enough that they probably represent samples of different target populations.

Statistical significance depends on the same parameters as the 95% confidence interval: the standard deviation and the sample size. Studies with smaller standard deviations or more subjects in each group are more likely to be able to show differences than are studies with larger standard deviations or fewer subjects. A study with a precise measurement and many subjects may find a "statistically" significant difference between two groups, but the size of the difference itself may be very small. Such a small difference may not be "clinically" significant.

CAUSATION, CONFOUNDING, AND CLINICAL TRIAL DESIGN

Clinical investigators perform studies to understand what causes the presence of disease and what may cause the disease to get better. The relationship between cause and effect is

■ **TABLE 2–3 Reporting Results of Measurements**

Variable Type	Number of Groups	Estimate of Main Effect	Measurement of Variability of the Main Effect Estimate	Comment
Continuous	Single group	Mean	Standard deviation, 95% confidence interval	Mean = sum all values/number of values. Sensitive to the effects of a few high or low values (outliers). Check for a graph of the data to identify such outliers.
		Median	Range, interquartile range	Median = value in the middle of a range of values (half above, and half below the median). For data that are not uniformly distributed, the median is a more accurate representation of central tendency than the mean.
	Two groups	Mean difference	95% confidence interval	Mean difference = group 1 mean − group 2 mean.
Categorical	Single group	Rate (risk)	95% confidence interval	Rate = # affected / # at risk. If the 95% confidence interval includes 0, the risk is not significantly different from 0.
	Two groups	Risk difference	95% confidence interval	Risk difference = rate 1 − rate 2. If the 95% confidence interval includes 0, the risk is not statistically significantly different between the two groups being compared.
		Relative risk (rate ratio)	95% confidence interval	Relative risk = rate 1 / rate 2. If the 95% confidence interval includes 1, the risk is not statistically significantly different between the two groups being compared.
		Odds ratio	95% confidence interval	Odds ratio is calculated from data collected in a case control study. Closely approximates the relative risk for rare outcomes. If the 95% confidence interval includes 1, the risk is not statistically significantly different between the two groups being compared.

sometimes unclear. Finding an association between variable A and outcome B does not establish that variable A causes outcome B. The association may not be real. Such a spurious association may be caused by the presence of bias in sampling or measurement. Likewise, false associations can be caused by random error. Alternatively, some studies find associations that really do exist. The challenge is understanding the precise relationship between variable A and outcome B. Often the question is "Does A cause B?"

Criteria exist that can be applied to an association to assess the possibility that variable A causes outcome B (Table 2–4). If some or all of these criteria are met, it is likely that the identified association represents a causative link. Even if the criteria outlined in Table 2–4 are met, however, one major barrier to establishing a cause and effect relationship still exists. This is the possibility of a confounding variable that might explain the apparent relationship.

A *confounding variable* is one that is associated with the predictor variable and with the outcome variable (independent of its association with the predictor variable) and is not an intermediate in the causal pathway from exposure to disease (Miettinen). In the presence of confounding variable C, variable A appears to be associated with outcome B. In fact, the illusion of an association occurs only because the confounding variable C is associated independently with both A and B. It is often difficult to identify confounding variables in a study. One needs to critically examine every reported association and carefully consider the possibility that an association between two variables may be caused by their mutual relationship with a third, possibly unidentified, variable. Certain clinical studies are more likely than others to have problems with confounders.

There are multiple potential *clinical trial designs*. Three major design types are cohort studies, cross-sectional studies, and case control studies. Study design type affects the ability to infer causality from any association that might be found and can also affect the likelihood that apparent associations suffer from bias or confounding.

■ **TABLE 2–4 Criteria for Assessing Causation**

Criterion	Comment
Strength	Exposures that are very strongly associated with an outcome are more likely to be causal than are exposures that are weak.
Consistency	Associations that are consistently found in many different settings, and by many different investigators, are more likely to be causal.
Specificity	If a variable is associated with only one outcome, and the outcome is associated with only a single possible cause, then the relationship is more likely causal.
Temporality	Causes must precede effects. This is the only one of these criteria that is absolutely necessary to suggest causation.
Biologic gradient	If an increasing amount of exposure is associated with an increased rate or severity of disease, then a dose-response relationship exists and causality is more likely.
Plausibility	It is always encouraging if your hypotheses sound reasonable. However, some epidemiologic findings are truly new, in which case biologic knowledge may need to expand to be able to explain the relationship.
Coherence	A causal association is strengthened if data from epidemiology fit in with data from other areas (e.g., pathology).
Experiment	If a possible cause is removed from a population and disease frequency declines, the likelihood of a causal link is strengthened.
Analogy	If a similar association has been shown to be causal, then the association under investigation may be more likely to be causal.

From Hill AB: The environment and disease: Association or causation? Proc Soc Med 58:295, 1965.

An *experimental study* (Fig. 2–4, Table 2–5) is a special type of cohort study in which an investigator first chooses a sample population to study and then assigns subjects to exposed or unexposed categories. A randomized clinical trial identifies a group of willing participants and randomly assigns them to treatment A or treatment B. Such experiments give information about cause and effect that may be impossible to ascertain from other study designs. This design minimizes the potential for confounding because exposure category assignment is carried out by the investigator in a random fashion and not left to the will of study subjects. Selection bias is low, and measurement bias can be reduced by blinding investigators and study subjects to the group assignments. Such experiments are expensive to perform, and if there is a long delay between exposure and disease, subjects may be lost to follow-up. Experimental studies may be poorly generalizable, since subjects who are willing to participate in a randomized trial may differ from the general population. Therapies used in a clinical trial might be applied with more rigor than in usual clinical practice, further diminishing generalizability. The ethics of withholding therapy from one group in an experiment sometimes block investigators from performing randomized trials.

In a *prospective cohort study* (see Fig. 2–4; Table 2–5), subjects in the study sample are divided based on the presence or absence of an exposure or risk factor. Subjects in an observational cohort study have chosen their exposure category prior to the study. Subjects in the two groups are followed forward in time, and the presence or absence of the outcome of interest is assessed. At the end of a prospective cohort study, one can estimate the cumulative incidence rate of disease in the population of interest and measure the frequency of disease in exposed and unexposed subjects. Comparison of disease rates in exposed and unexposed subjects can be made using the relative risk or risk difference (see Table 2–3). Prospective cohort studies can show a clear temporal relationship between exposure and outcome. Selection bias and measurement bias in assessing exposure group are minimal. If the investigator who makes the outcome determination is blinded to the exposure group of the subjects, the possibility of measurement bias in assessing outcome is likewise minimal. Prospective cohort studies have high costs in both time and money. Since the investigator does not control membership in the exposed or unexposed category, confounding is possible. Loss to follow-up may be significant in a cohort study of a disease that progresses slowly from exposure to outcome determination. Loss to follow-up can lead to bias.

Cohort studies can be performed retrospectively as well. Subjects are identified by the presence or absence of exposure that occurred in the past, but in a retrospective cohort study, both exposure and disease occurred prior to the study's being performed. Retrospective cohort studies are less expensive and less time-consuming than prospective cohort studies but have problems of recall bias and confounding.

Subjects in a *case control study* are separated into two groups based on the presence or absence of disease (see Fig. 2–4; Table 2–5). Subjects in each group are evaluated for risk factors for diseases, and the association between risk factors and disease is measured using the odds ratio. Case control studies are useful for studying rare diseases and are inexpensive. The possibility of selection bias and bias in risk factor measurement (recall bias) is large in case control studies, at times limiting their usefulness. When carefully designed and performed, case control studies are useful for hypothesis generation and for examining the possibility of multiple risk factor associations with the disease. For rare diseases, the odds ratio that is generated by a case control study is a good estimate of the relative risk that might be generated by a cohort study.

Sampling bias is one of the major threats to validity of a case control study. Cases are easy to identify because the subjects

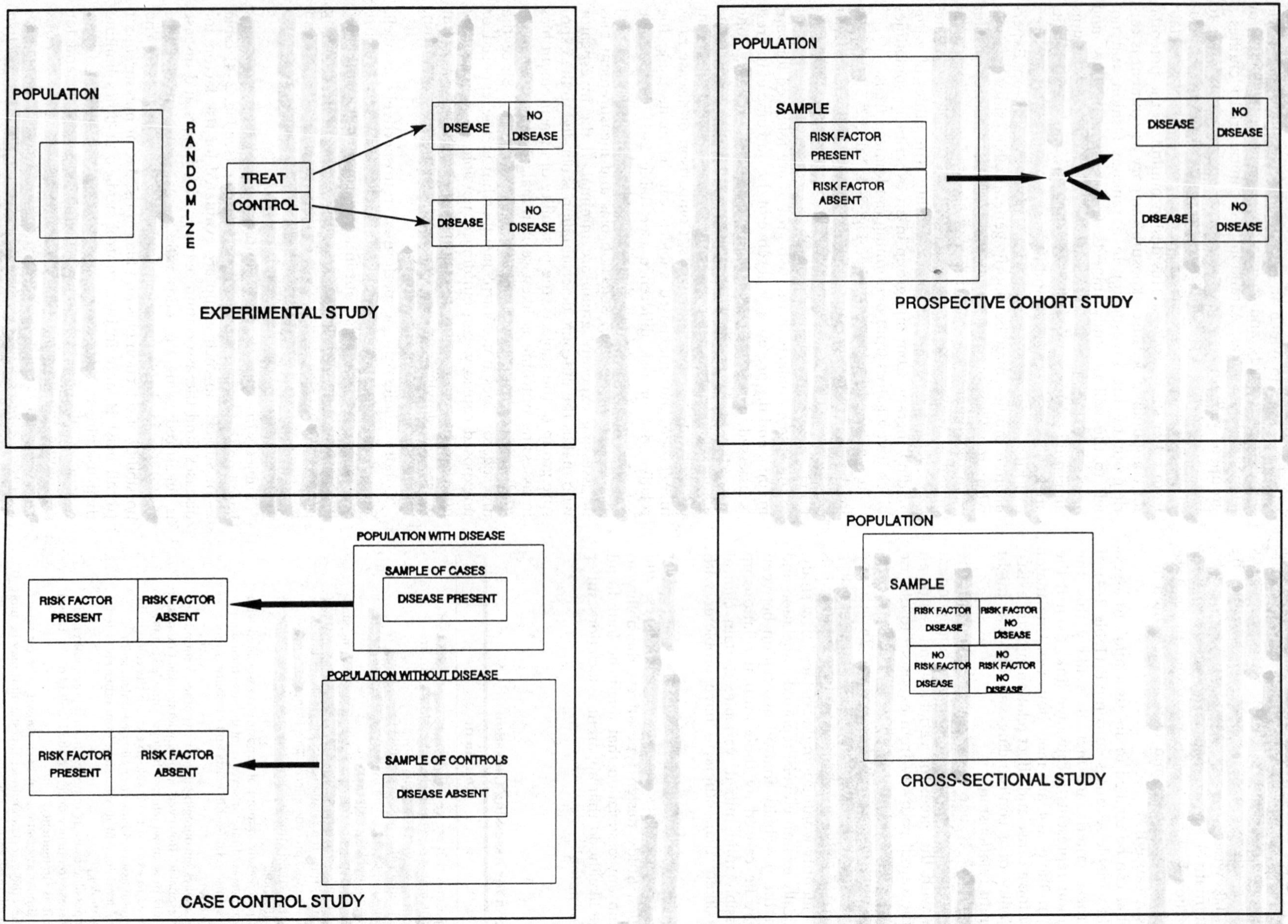

Figure 2–4. The major types of clinical study designs. (After Hulley SB, Cummings SR: Designing Clinical Research: An Epidemiologic Approach. Baltimore, Williams & Wilkins, 1988.)

■ **TABLE 2–5 Advantages and Disadvantages of the Major Types of Observational Studies**

	Prospective Cohort	Retrospective Cohort	Cross-sectional	Case Control	Nested Case Control
Sequence of events clear	yes	(yes)	no	no	yes?
Sampling (selection) bias	no	no	no	yes	no
Bias in risk factor measurement (recall bias)	no	maybe	yes	yes	no
Survivor bias	no	no	yes	yes	yes
Loss to follow-up	yes	yes	no	no	yes
Hypothesis generation	no	no	yes	yes	no
Examine multiple associations	yes	yes	yes	yes	no
Examine >1 outcome	yes	yes	yes	no	no
Study rare diseases	no	no	no	yes	yes
Cost in time	large	less	cheap	cheap	cheap
Cost in money	large	less	cheap	cheap	cheap
Statistic generated	incidence rate	incidence rate	prevalence rate	odds ratio	odds ratio

should have the specific disease. An appropriate control group is often difficult to identify. Subjects in the control group must have the same potential to develop the disease as the case subjects. Making this determination is sometimes very difficult. If an investigator has already done a cohort study, it is possible to do a case control study within the same sample. Since these subjects were all chosen as members of a single population group, the chance for sampling bias is diminished. Such a study is called a *nested case control study*; it combines the advantages of a cohort study and a case control study.

A *cross-sectional study* (see Fig. 2–4; Table 2–5), sometimes called a prevalence study, samples from a population of interest and simultaneously measures the presence of risk factors and outcomes. A cross-sectional study can calculate prevalence rates and compare the prevalence of disease in exposed and unexposed subjects. Since time does not pass between assessment of exposure and disease, the temporal relationship between exposure and disease is unclear. Assessing the causal nature of associations found in a prevalence study is often difficult. Cross-sectional studies are inexpensive and are useful to generate hypotheses and examine multiple associations between potential risk factors and the disease of interest. Cross-sectional studies are susceptible to a specific type of bias called incidence-prevalence bias. A cross-sectional survey is more likely to identify prevalent disease than incident disease, especially if people with the disease live a long time. This is important to remember in interpreting the results of cross-sectional studies.

DIAGNOSTIC TESTS. The study performed to identify the usefulness of a diagnostic test is a special form of cross-sectional study. Such studies measure the ability of a test to identify patients with a specific disease. The generalized form of the results of such a study are shown in Figure 2–5. The *sensitivity* of a test is the measurement that answers the question "Of all people with disease, how many will have a positive test?" The *specificity* answers the question "Of all people without disease, how many will have a negative test?" The *positive predictive value* answers the question "Of all people with a positive test, how many will have the disease?" The *negative predictive value* answers the question "Of all people with a negative test, how many will not have the disease?"

Developers of diagnostic tests often focus on maximizing either sensitivity or specificity. The decision to call a diagnostic test positive is somewhat arbitrary, especially for continuously varying laboratory values. Deciding on the cutoff value that defines a positive test is a tradeoff between increasing sensitivity at the expense of specificity, or vice versa. For example, if an elevated serum ALT concentration is used to define liver toxicity from a given therapeutic agent, the question becomes "How high an ALT really defines 'toxic'?" Choosing a very high cutoff value may increase the specificity of the test at the expense of sensitivity. This relationship is shown graphically in Figure 2–6, which plots sensitivity by specificity for a theoretical diagnostic test. Figure 2–6 demonstrates that as a cutoff value is chosen to increase sensitivity, the specificity will diminish. The curve in Figure 2–6 is called a *receiver operating characteristic* (ROC) curve. The area under the ROC curve is an excellent indicator of the total usefulness of the specific diagnostic test. Diagnostic tests with a sensitivity of 1 and a specificity of 1 have an area under the ROC curve of 1.

An important aspect of the choice of the cutoff value that defines a positive test is related to the situations in which the test results will be applied. Screening tests for identification of HIV infection are designed to be very sensitive, to screen out HIV-infected persons from the blood donor pool. A sensitive cutoff is thus chosen to ensure that all potentially positive samples are identified. Although choosing a low cutoff for the determination of a positive screening test increases the sensitivity, it results in decreased specificity and leads to identifying some persons as positive even though they are not truly HIV-infected. That is why all HIV screening tests need to be followed by a very specific test (the Western blot) to distinguish true from false-positive screening results.

Users of diagnostic tests often need to know the test's positive and negative predictive values as much as their sensitivity and specificity. Clinicians may find a positive test result and ask how likely it is that this patient with a positive test result actually has the disease. Unfortunately, the positive predictive value alone cannot answer that question. For a diagnostic test of given sensitivity and specificity, the positive predictive value of the test can be calculated only for the population in which the data were generated. The positive predictive value may be

	Disease Present	Disease Absent	
Test Positive	a	b	a + b
Test Negative	c	d	c + d
	a + c	b + d	

a = true positives

b = false positives

c = false negatives

d = true negatives

Sensitivity = a / a + c

Specificity = d / b + d

Positive Predictive Value = a / a + b

Negative predictive value = d / c + d

Figure 2–5. Results of a cross-sectional study to evaluate a diagnostic test.

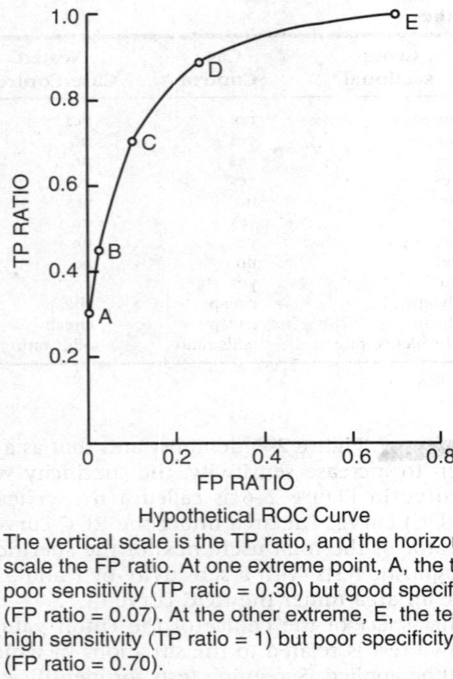

Figure 2–6. A hypothetical Receiver Operating Characteristic (ROC) Curve. The vertical scale is the sensitivity (true-positive ratio), and the horizontal scale is (1 − specificity), the false-positive ratio. At one extreme point, A, the test has poor sensitivity but good specificity. At the other extreme, E, the test has high sensitivity but poor specificity. (From McNeil BJ, Keeler E, Adelstein SJ: Primer on certain elements of medical decision making. N Engl J Med 293:211, 1975.)

different in another population, since the prevalence of disease in a population sample influences the positive predictive value of a diagnostic test. The relationship between prevalence and positive predictive value is described by Bayes' theorem and is shown in Figure 2–7. The test's positive predictive value is lower in a population with a low disease prevalence than it is in a population in which the disease is very common. The

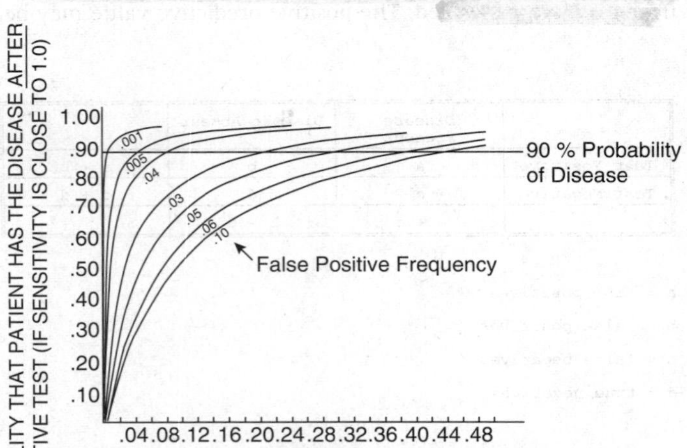

Figure 2–7. The relationship between positive predictive value and prevalence (prior probability) of disease. (From Katz MA: A probability graph describing the predictive value of a highly sensitive diagnostic test. N Engl J Med 291:1115, 1974.)

population prevalence of disease is called the prior probability of disease, a number used to estimate how likely it is that a patient has a disease before the test is performed.

Studies evaluating diagnostic tests are at risk of the same errors as other cross-sectional studies. Selection bias is a common problem: Initial studies of a test are performed in populations of patients with a high prevalence of disease, resulting in overestimation of the usefulness of the test when it is applied to patients in a population with a lower prevalence of disease. Error can also be made in the determination of diseased subjects. The best studies are those in which a true gold standard measurement exists for comparison with the new test.

Hill AB: The environment and disease: Association or causation? Proc Soc Med 58:295, 1965.
Hulley SB, Cummings SR: Designing Clinical Research: An Epidemiologic Approach. Baltimore, Williams & Wilkins, 1988.
Katz MA: A probability graph describing the predictive value of a highly sensitive diagnostic test. N Engl J Med 291:1115, 1974.
MacMahon B, Pugh TF: Epidemiology: Principles and Methods. Boston, Little, Brown, 1970.
McNeil BJ, Keeler E, Adelstein SJ: Primer on certain elements of medical decision making. N Engl J Med 293:211, 1975.
Miettinen O: Confounding and effect modification. Am J Epidemiol 100:350, 1974.
Sackett DL, Haynes RB, Buyatt GH, et al: Clinical Epidemiology: A Basic Science for Clinical Medicine, 2nd ed. Boston, Little Brown, 1991.
Streiner DL, GR Norman GR, Blum HM: PDQ Epidemiology. Toronto, BC Decker, 1989.
Users' Guides to the Medical Literature. Evidence-Based Medicine Working Group: JAMA 270:2093, 2098, 1993; 271:59, 389, 703, 1615, 1994; 272:234, 1994.

CHAPTER 3

Ethics in Pediatric Care

Norman Fost

Ethical issues permeate all interactions between physicians and patients: How much information should be disclosed? Is this patient consuming an unfair share of the physician's or society's resources? Should clinical decisions be made by the patient, the parent, or the physician? In pediatrics, these familiar dilemmas are compounded by the variable competence of the patient, the sometimes competing interests of parents and children, and the long-standing tradition of treating children more paternalistically than is acceptable for adult patients.

The following sections review the major conceptual principles in medical ethics; identify the central issues in the common clinical/ethical dilemmas involving children; identify areas of apparent consensus; and suggest a procedural approach to ethical decision-making.

3.1 Conceptual Issues

AUTONOMY. This is a central principle in contemporary medical ethics. Its purpose is to allow competent patients to make their own health care decisions, based on their own values. In the United States and many other nations, a competent patient has almost an absolute right to decide what shall be done to his or her own body. This right is not contingent on the patient making rational decisions. Thus, a patient may permissibly refuse lifesaving care for religious or other reasons, even though others may believe that he or she is making a foolish or unwise decision. This principle is particularly relevant in adolescence, when a patient's competence begins to resemble that of an adult, but younger children are also sometimes competent to make their own health care decisions.

COMPETENCE. The principle of autonomy is intertwined inextricably with the concept of competence, because only competent patients are granted the right to make their own health care decisions. The most common definition of competence is based on the patient's ability to understand the possible consequences of his or her decision and the available alternatives. Many adolescents meet this standard, creating potential conflicts when they are still under the supervision of their parents.

BENEFICENCE. This refers to the duties to avoid harm as well as to advance the welfare of others. It was at the root of the ancient nostrum "Do no harm"—an obvious oversimplification, since little medical benefit can be gained without the risk of harm. A more complete principle would include some sense of not causing harm without a likelihood of compensating good, but individuals vary as to what they consider a harm or a good and how much harm they are willing to risk in exchange for a potential benefit. The primacy of autonomy in the United States has led to a widespread, though not unanimous, view that competent patients should be allowed to decide for themselves how to balance harms and goods. Interference in these decisions is often based on claims of justified paternalism.

PATERNALISM. This is defined as interfering with the liberty of another person for his or her own benefit. It is generally considered to be a duty of parents, although this assumption has been questioned, and is morally unjustified with regard to competent patients, with limited exceptions. Physicians have historically believed that they had a right and duty to be paternalistic, based on the claim that their responsibility is *beneficence*—to promote the patient's health, not his or her autonomy. There is general support for the opinion that paternalism is justified at least when there is a high probability of serious harm; when interference with the patient's liberty is likely to prevent the harm; and when there is a reasonable likelihood that the patient would want to be treated in this manner or will appreciate it later on. This view of paternalism provides the justification for many intrusions done for the benefit of children over their apparent objection, such as surgery for suspected appendicitis or immunizations against serious diseases, but raises questions about the appropriateness of intrusions of uncertain effectiveness, particularly if the child objects or of intrusions for the purpose of preventing uncertain or minimal harms.

TRUTH TELLING. The duty to tell the truth is a requisite for any moral community. It has special importance in the physician-patient relationship, in which trust is essential because of unequal power and because of the serious consequences of medical decisions. Failure to respect this principle occurs by active lying, which is wrong under almost all circumstances in the health care setting, or by omission of information. Omissions should not be made for the purpose of deception or of manipulating the patient's response. Some consider that all intentional deceptions are examples of lying, which is justified only under exceptional circumstances.

CONFIDENTIALITY. Patients need to trust their physicians not to disclose private information to others because confidentiality facilitates full disclosure of information relevant for providing effective personal health care, may prevent disorders that threaten others in the community, and possibly reduces the total human and financial cost of illness and related disability through early treatment. There is an implied promise by the physician not to disclose information except with the consent of the patient, or his or her representative, or when required by law. Exceptions to this principle are generally limited to circumstances in which there is a high risk of serious physical harm to others that is most likely to be prevented only by unconsented disclosure (e.g., reporting suspected child abuse on the basis of information obtained from the potential abuser in what was presumed to be a confidential relationship).

CONFLICTS OF INTEREST. Because the child/patient is usually represented by someone else, there is an increased potential for the pediatrician to perceive the best interests of the child differently from the way in which they are perceived by the parent(s) or guardian(s). In addition, the physician's sense of responsibility for the rest of the family may result in conflicts between the interests of the family and the interests of the child patient (e.g., see the following section on "Baby Doe").

3.2 Withholding and Withdrawing Life Support

This is one of the most important ethical dilemmas that physicians have to deal with. In pediatrics, these issues arise most commonly in the newborn period, involving infants with limited prospects for survival without significant lifelong morbidity. These cases, however, are only one part of the general question of the justifications for withholding or withdrawing life support from children with a variety of illnesses from birth through adolescence (see also Chapter 41).

There is a strong ethical consensus in the United States that a competent person has an almost absolute right to determine what shall be done with his or her own body. This implies a right to refuse health care, even if the patient has excellent prospects for long-term survival and death is the certain result of refusing treatment. There is a similar tradition in the law. A familiar example is the common occurrence of a Jehovah's Witness refusing a lifesaving blood transfusion; religious justifications are not an essential aspect of this ethical or legal principle. Accordingly, an adolescent patient who is competent in the sense of understanding the consequences of his or her decision, including the prospects for survival and the likely quality of life if treatment is accepted and the certainty of death if treatment is withheld, should play a major role in such decisions. The more problematic cases involve younger adolescents at the boundary of competence and disorders with limited prospects for long-term survival.

Most pediatric patients are clearly not competent to make their own decisions with regard to the termination of care. Although parents have traditionally made such decisions on behalf of their children with little controversy, there has been increased questioning of the limits of such authority. This has occurred primarily in decisions involving handicapped or critically ill newborns—the so-called Baby Doe controversy.

"BABY DOE" DILEMMA. This term arose in a 1982 conflict over an infant with Down syndrome and esophageal atresia who was allowed to die at 6 days of age at the parents' request. The case was similar to many others that had occurred during the preceding decade, particularly involving undertreatment of newborns with Down syndrome and spina bifida. Many of these children appeared to have excellent prospects for long, happy lives, suggesting that the decisions were not being made in the interests of the children. Furthermore, in two large surveys, most pediatricians supported parental control of such decisions; some pediatricians stated that they considered their duty was not to serve the interests of their patient but rather to serve the interests of the parents. These problems were compounded by the fact that many decisions were being based on erroneous medical assumptions, including inappropriately pessimistic prognoses.

As a consequence of concern about this issue in the United

woman refuses standard, effective treatment essential for the benefit of a fetus/infant who is at high risk of death or serious disability, such as refusal of cesarean section for placenta previa in a voluntary pregnancy near term involving a presumably normal fetus/infant. Courts in the United States have sometimes decided that a woman can be required to undergo such a procedure when the benefit to the emergent child is clear. A federal court decided that such an order was inappropriate in a case involving a 26-wk-old fetus and, by implication, other cases in which the benefit of intervention was in doubt. Pediatricians may be required in such cases prenatally to initiate or support court proceedings in the interests of the future child or to consider postnatal sanctions, including reporting of child abuse or neglect.

Child abuse statutes have also been invoked in attempts to modify the behavior of women who ingest alcohol or illicit drugs during pregnancy and expose the fetus/infant to harm. The pediatrician considering reporting such cases must consider the likelihood of benefit from reporting, the harms to the child as well as to the mother if criminal charges or custody changes are sought, and the possible effects that reporting may have in driving pregnant women away from the health care system, particularly from prenatal care.

3.7 Access to Health Care; Rationing

(Distributive Justice)

The most serious ethical problem in health care in the United States may be the inequality in access to care. No other major industrial country rations basic health care on the basis of ability to pay. Approximately 10 million children are estimated to lack adequate health insurance, with serious consequences in terms of death, disability, and suffering. The central ethical principle at stake is fair opportunity to participate in the benefits of society; preventable death and disability undermine the claim that the society is one of equal opportunity. Another aspect of the claim of unfairness is that the present system is maintained by those who are already advantaged because of financial or social status, thereby aggravating existing inequalities.

Rationing of health care can be defined as limiting access to wanted and needed services of known benefit. It is increasingly recognized that no society can provide all beneficial services to all its citizens; rationing is therefore unavoidable. The question is not whether to ration health care services but how to do so fairly. Other ways of rationing are based on cost/benefit analysis, age, or likely effects on quality of life.

Beauchamp T, Walters L: Contemporary Issues in Bioethics, 3rd ed. Belmont, CA, Wadsworth Pub Co, 1989.

Culver CM, Gert B: The justification of paternalistic behavior. *In*: Philosophy in Medicine: Conceptual and Ethical Issues in Medicine and Psychiatry. New York, Oxford University Press, 1982.

Daniels N: Why saying no to patients in the United States is so hard: cost containment, justice and provider autonomy. New Engl J Med 312 (21):1380, 1986.

Fost N. Genetic diagnosis and treatment: ethical considerations. Am J Dis Child 147:1190, 1993.

Gaylin W, Macklin R (eds): Who Speaks for the Child?: The Problems of Proxy Consent. New York, Plenum Press, 1982.

Holder AR: Legal Issues in Pediatric and Adolescent Medicine, 2nd ed. New Haven, Yale Press, 1985.

Levine R: Ethics and Regulation of Clinical Research, 2nd ed. Baltimore, Urban and Schwarzenberg, 1986.

Menzel PT: Strong Medicine: The Ethical Rationing of Health Care. Oxford, New York, 1990.

O'Neill O, Ruddick W: Having Children: Philosophical and Legal Reflections of Parenthood. New York, Oxford University Press, 1979.

Weir R: Selective Nontreatment of Handicapped Newborns: Moral Dilemmas in Neonatal Medicine. New York, Oxford University Press, 1984.

CHAPTER 4
Cultural Issues in Pediatric Care

Lee M. Pachter

The physician who takes care of children and families from diverse ethnic backgrounds needs to be aware of cultural variations in the ways in which individuals deal with health, illness, and the health care system. Although biomedicine is often the dominant medical belief system, people may combine biomedicine with other beliefs and behaviors that may be individually, socially, or culturally based. This pluralistic approach to health and illness occurs to some extent with all individuals. See Chapters 7 and 18.

Special attention to these issues is needed when working with patients and families from ethnic minorities because as the "cultural distance" between patient and physician increases, the chance for miscommunication and harm increases as well. This miscommunication is more than linguistic; it may include the very essence of how one perceives and defines health and illness. Culturally sensitive health care acknowledges and respects that health and illness are, in large part, molded by variables such as ethnic values, cultural orientation and attitudes, religious beliefs, and linguistic considerations and that the culturally constructed meaning of illness is an important clinical concern. It also includes a sensitivity to variations in beliefs and practices within a group and avoids labeling and stereotyping.

Three steps are necessary to provide health care that is culturally sensitive. First, the pediatrician needs to become aware of the commonly held cultural beliefs and culturally normative interactive styles in the patient population. Next, he or she needs to assess the effects of these beliefs and behaviors on a particular patient or family. Finally, the physician should try to negotiate between the ethnocultural beliefs and practices of the patient and the culture of biomedicine for the benefit of the child. This chapter discusses specific issues and strategies for providing culturally sensitive pediatric care. Also see Chapter 42.

INTRACULTURAL DIVERSITY. Because individuals subscribe to group norms to varying degrees and are also influenced by personal experiences, not all people from a particular cultural heritage think and act in the same manner. The degree of adherence to cultural standards is related in part to the individual's *acculturation*—the changes in cultural beliefs due to contact with the "mainstream" culture—such as acceptance of the Western biomedical culture. Acculturation has been positively correlated with (1) length of residency in the host cultural area; (2) second generation or greater in the host cultural area; (3) level and location of formal education; (4) ease with which one speaks the host language; (5) residence outside an ethnic enclave; (6) reduced contact with the cultural area of origin; and (7) family composition (with older, more traditional relatives present, cultural transmission increases and acculturation decreases). When the social history is being taken, the patient's or parent's level of acculturation should be assessed by asking questions that pertain to these variables. When less acculturated families are identified, the clinician should ask about specific beliefs and practices concerning health care.

CULTURE AND CHILD BEHAVIOR AND DEVELOPMENT. Culture affects infant and childhood behavior and development by its influence on family structure, parental expectations, caretaking and child-rearing practices, the variety of individuals that infants and children are exposed to during the developmental process, and the stimuli that are presented to the infant and child at different ages. These issues, including the definition of roles and responsibilities of family members, have a profound influence on the social, cognitive, and emotional development of the infant and child. The physician needs to be sensitive to the important roles of individuals other than parents and siblings in many cultural groups.

The cultural environment also influences what is considered normal development. For example, in the United States and other industrialized countries the normal sleeping pattern of infants during the first year of life is that as the infant ages, the sleeping interval lengthens. Studies from rural East Africa show that the sleep/wake pattern for infants there is quite different—the average sleeping period up until 8 months of age remains at about 3 hours. These differences are not due to any underlying difference in neurologic maturation between American and East African infants but are probably secondary to the different spatial and social context of infant sleeping in these cultures.

Cultural values also affect parental expectations regarding a child's behavior and temperament. Studies have shown that Puerto Rican and Anglo-American mothers have different perspectives on what is considered positive and negative behavioral traits in children. Anglo mothers place greater positive value on an individualistic orientation and qualities that allow the child to become autonomous. Puerto Rican mothers place value on a more "sociocentric" orientation and qualities of respectfulness in social situations. The same behavior may be interpreted differently by mothers from different ethnocultural backgrounds. In part, this may explain studies showing different prevalences of childhood behavioral disorders (such as attention deficit disorder) in various cultural groups.

SICKNESS AND ITS CAUSES. Physicians and patients may conceptualize a sickness episode differently. Clinical miscommunication may occur if the physician addresses only disease-related issues (etiology, diagnosis, treatment) while the patient's concerns are more centered around illness issues (the perception of not being well and how this affects the individual as a social as well as biologic entity). This is an issue in all physican-patient relationships, but it may be exacerbated when the physician and patient are from different cultures, especially when the patient's cultural heritage includes nonbiomedical beliefs and practices.

Different cultural groups also may have theories and explanations for *illness causation* that do not fit into the biomedical paradigm. Some cultures believe that health is a product of a state of *natural balance* and that illness and disease result from a disruption of this balance. The Oriental belief in *yin* and *yang* and the *humoral* (or hot/cold) theory of illness found in many Latino cultures (which has its historical roots in the Hippocratic belief in the four cardinal humors) are examples of this concept. Individuals in some cultures may consider that illness is a *retribution for sins,* and some distinguish natural and supernatural causes of illness. These categorizations often have implications for the type of healer consulted for treatment. For example, sometimes patients go to a physician for relief of *symptoms* while at the same time consulting a folk healer to identify a spiritual or supernatural cause. Physicians should become familiar with the common beliefs that are held in the cultural groups that he or she serves and should inquire nonjudgmentally about the patient's or parent's thoughts concerning the cause of the illness. If the parent relates beliefs that are inconsistent with the biomedical explanatory model but that will have no adverse effect on the outcome of the illness, it is best not to contradict him or her but to offer the biomedical explanation *in addition.* Attempts to change long-held beliefs in a brief clinical visit will most likely fail.

Many cultures also have strict rules regarding conduct during times when the body is thought to be susceptible to illness. For example, many ethnic groups believe that the postpartum period is a critical time in which the newborn and mother are at risk for illness. The mother and infant are often kept at home in isolation for a period of time and may have special dietary restrictions, such as in traditional Haitian and Mexican cultures (e.g., *la cuarentena* and *la dieta* in Mexico). Another time of presumed increased susceptibility in many cultures is the menstrual period. Appointments for well child care during this time may be missed for fear of having the mother go outside the home.

FOLK ILLNESS AND FOLK HEALERS. Folk illnesses are culturally defined illness episodes that may be related or unrelated to a biomedical diagnostic category. Thus, the Mexican folk illness *caida de mollera* or "fallen fontanel" probably represents dehydration. *Mal de ojo* (in Latin America), *malocchio* (in Italy), and other "evil-eye" beliefs (in Europe and the Middle East) do not fit into a medical disease category. These are believed to be brought on by a spell placed on the child by someone who secretly covets him or her. Adults who display excessive attention to or direct strong glances at the child may be thought by the parents to be casting a spell. In the Puerto Rican culture, saying the words "Dios le (la) bendiga" ("God bless him [her]") will dispel concerns of malevolence. Although parents may present their child for medical care, they often do not express their thoughts about folk illness to the physician, and a cycle of miscommunication may result. Assessing the level of acculturation may provide insight into which parents believe in folk illnesses; another clue may be the display of protective objects, such as charms and amulets, attached to the baby's clothing or worn on chains. If the physician is concerned about injury caused by necklaces or bracelets on an infant, he or she should recommend that the object be safely attached to underclothing rather than being removed.

If the physician diagnoses "nothing wrong" or a self-limiting illness that requires no treatment, it is possible that the patient may seek further care with a *folk healer*—a culturally sanctioned healer who treats illness. Examples of folk healers include Mexican *curanderos,* African-American root doctors, Southeast Asian and Chinese herbalists, Puerto Rican *espiritistas* and *santiguadoras,* and Navajo singers. Some patients may present for medical care and at the same time use the services of a folk healer. As long as the healer is not providing therapies that are harmful or contradictory to medical management, they should not be disparaged.

Most folk remedies are not harmful. If biomedical therapy is necessary, the pediatrician should attempt to add it to the cultural practices. This will place the biomedical treatment within the cultural context and lifestyle of the patient and family and may help improve compliance with therapy. It also shows the family that the physician respects their beliefs. If there are folk remedies that are determined to be harmful, the physician should discourage their use. It is often possible and desirable to replace a harmful folk therapy with another practice that fits within the patient's cultural system. Other folk practices cause concern because they produce ecchymosis and scarring that can be mistaken for signs of child abuse, e.g., *coining* (rubbing oiled skin with the side of a coin or spoon), *cupping* (placing a heated cup on the skin), and *moxabustion* (touching the skin with burning herbs or incense).

PHYSICIAN-PATIENT INTERACTION. Different interactive styles may result in cross-cultural miscommunication. For example, many people display a deferential style when interacting with strangers, elders, and those of higher education and social class. This is often seen in traditional Puerto Ricans (who call it *respeto*), Asians, and Native Americans as well as others. Part of this behavioral style includes reticence in asking questions of authority figures. Other cultural groups display a more inquisitive and openly questioning style that may be mistaken for hostility. In some cultures the maintenance of eye contact with the patient is regarded as exhibiting caring and understanding, whereas in other cultures eye contact may be considered challenging or aggressive (especially from the opposite sex). Physical contact can also be interpreted as showing care by some groups and as culturally inappropriate behavior by others.

Some cultures also have strict definitions of appropriate topics of conversation with members of the opposite sex (e.g., traditional Chinese, Italian, Mexican-American, and Puerto Rican cultures). For example, a mother who is concerned about the foreskin care of her newborn son or masturbatory behavior in her preschool daughter, or an adolescent presenting with penile or vaginal discharge or for contraceptive planning, may, at the sight of a physician of the opposite sex, not reveal the true reason for the visit. If these concerns exist, the physician may need to elicit help from health care workers of the opposite sex and attempt to involve both parents in the history taking and treatment plan.

Clinicians working in the multicultural setting often find themselves in situations in which the patient or parents are not sufficiently fluent in the language of the physician to communicate adequately. Even if the patient is partially fluent in the physician's language, he or she may want to describe the important issues concerning health and illness in his or her native tongue. The physician who makes an effort to learn the language of his or her patients will meet with increased acceptance, but effective communication may require an interpreter. A professional interpreter should be fluent in both languages, have a basic knowledge of medical terminology, and have a good understanding of the interactive style and rules of communication in the cultural group. When a professional interpreter is not available, try to choose an interpreter who is similar to your patient population with regard to social class, area of origin, and cultural background and ask for a very literal translation.

COMPLIANCE. The acknowledgment of culturally mediated health beliefs and behaviors and their incorporation into the medical care plan, when appropriate, may improve compliance. Many cultural groups consider certain numbers and colors to have magical or religious connotations; administering medications on a schedule that incorporates these also may improve compliance. For example, in traditional gypsy culture the color red and the number 3 are considered beneficial. Prescribing a pink antibiotic three times a day for otitis media, (instead of a white antibiotic four times a day) utilizes traditional cultural beliefs to increase acceptance of medical therapy. Compliance may also be increased by administering medications with culturally appropriate foods or incorporating nonharmful folk remedies into the medical treatment plan. For example, telling a Puerto Rican mother to massage her baby's stomach during an episode of viral gastroenteritis will do no harm and will allow the mother to help actively manage her child's illness in a culturally acceptable way.

Buchwald D, Panwala S, Hooton TM: Use of traditional health practices by Southeast Asian refugees in a primary care clinic. West J Med 156:507, 1992.
Harkness S: The infant's niche in rural Kenya and metropolitan America. *In:* Adler LL (ed): Cross Cultural Research at Issue. New York, Academic Press, 1982, p 47.
Harwood A (ed): Ethnicity and Medical Care. Cambridge, Harvard University Press, 1981.
Harwood R: The influence of culturally derived values on Anglo and Puerto Rican mothers' perceptions of attachment behavior. Child Dev 63:822, 1992.
Kleinman A, Eisenberg L, Good B: Culture, illness, and care. Clinical lessons from anthropologic and cross-cultural research. Ann Intern Med 88:251, 1978.
Pachter LM: Culture and clinical care: Folk illness beliefs and behaviors and their implications for health care delivery. JAMA 271:690, 1994.
Pachter LM, Weller SC: Acculturation and compliance with medical therapy. J Dev Behav Pediatr 14:163, 1993.
Snow L: Walkin' Over Medicine: Traditional Health Practices in African-American Life. Boulder, CO: Westview Press, 1993.
Trotter RT II: The cultural parameters of lead poisoning: A medical anthropologist's view of intervention in environmental lead exposure. Environ Health Perspect 89:79, 1990.
Trotter RT II: Folk medicine in the Southwest: Myths and medical facts. Postgrad Med 78:167, 1985.

CHAPTER 5

Preventive Pediatrics

Lucy M. Osborn

Many of the conditions that affect health, such as peace, shelter, education, food, income, a stable ecosystem, sustainable resources, social justice, and equity, are not readily amenable to intervention through the health care system. In developing countries, contaminated water and lack of sewage systems, malnutrition, overpopulation, and poor housing are some of the major threats to health. In developed countries, such as the United States, major health problems are more likely to be related to lifestyle, i.e., accidents, alcohol and drug abuse, tobacco use, and violence, or to toxic effects of environmental pollution. Poverty is a threat to health in all societies.

In the United States the remarkable improvements in child health since the beginning of the 20th century, with dramatic decreases in mortality and morbidity, are the result of a combination of social and economic changes, advances in therapeutic medicine and surgery, and implementation of public health measures, including preventive pediatrics. The latter consists of efforts by physicians, especially pediatricians, to avoid, rather than cure, disease and disability in children through health promotion and prevention activities.

As mortality from infectious diseases was controlled through good sanitation, effective public health measures, and immunizations, the concept of health promotion has expanded to include the emotional and mental well-being of children and families. Emotional and behavioral problems among children are exceedingly common, with a prevalence of diagnosable disorders of about one in five. If the definition of "behavior problem" is expanded to mean undesirable behaviors that adversely influence the parent-child relationship or that can be disruptive of the child's relationships with peers, then virtually all families will be affected.

Preventive pediatric health care is a continuum that includes primary, secondary, and tertiary prevention. Primary preventive measures are directed at avoiding disorders before they begin, often with a special emphasis on those who are at increased risk to develop a condition or a disease. Examples are chlorination and fluoridation of water, tetanus immunization, and counseling the parents of toddlers about keeping poisons and drugs out of reach. Primary prevention is usually most successful when measures are based on an understanding of the etiology, pathogenesis, and natural course of the disease. Secondary preventive measures are those in which a condition or its precursor is identified early and effective treatment instituted for remediation of the condition before progression or for elimination of the precursor. Screening programs for blood lead levels and adolescent scoliosis are examples. Tertiary prevention is directed at ameliorating or halting disabilities from established diseases. An example is providing chest physiotherapy for a child with cystic fibrosis. These preventive interventions can occur at the level of the individual child, the family, or the community. The greatest benefits of prevention come from risk reduction that keeps those who are at low or medium risk to develop a condition from entering the high-risk or diseased categories. Pediatricians can play an integral part in protecting children's health at all three levels: (1) as direct providers of clinical prevention services; (2) as coordinators of services; (3) as leaders in developing community-based programs; and (4) as advocates for child health. In order to successfully fulfill these roles, physicians must have a basic knowledge of the principles of prevention, an understanding of epidemiology, and an appreciation of the program-planning process and the essentials of effective child advocacy.

PRINCIPLES OF PREVENTION

Effective prevention programs are usually dependent on understanding the epidemiology of disease and the medical and social factors that contribute to disease. Last has recently defined epidemiology as ". . . the study of the distribution and determinants of health-related states and events in specified populations and the application of this study to the control of health problems." Distribution of disease refers to the relationship of time, place, and person to the health problems in the population. Determinants of disease include both etiology and the factors that influence the risk of acquiring diseases. The epidemiologic sequence, scientific methods for ascertaining the distribution and determinants of disease, includes (1) observation of diseases and disease sequence; (2) counting cases or events; (3) relating observations to the population at risk; (4) making comparisons; (5) developing hypotheses regarding the relationship of disease to causal factors; (6) testing the hypothesis; (7) making scientific inferences; (8) conducting experimental studies; and (9) intervention and evaluation.

All practitioners eventually apply this epidemiologic sequence to their practices. Because astute clinicians are good observers, they will, without additional training, apply the first step of the epidemiologic sequence. They will rapidly discern that the patients they care for have certain health problems in common. This will be related to the ethnic and demographic distribution of their parents and their living conditions. The second step of the epidemiologic sequence means determining the incidence and prevalence of disease (see Chapter 2). *Incidence rates* refer to the number of persons developing a disease or having a condition or factor within a population at risk over a unit of time. An example of an incidence rate would be the number of children in a practice who received all needed vaccinations within a calendar year. *Prevalence rates* refer to the number of persons with a disease, condition, or factor compared with the total number of persons in a group. In the case of immunizations, an example of a prevalence rate would be the number of 2-yr-olds within a practice who are fully immunized. The next step (3) relates a patient to the population at risk, or case finding. With experience, clinicians are able to understand the characteristics of the populations they serve. To use the example of lead screening, if over time the number of truly positive lead screens in their practices is low, clinicians will interpret the results of a positive screen to a parent accordingly—by offering reassurance and saying that the test is likely to be a false-positive while still ordering the appropriate follow-up tests. On the other hand, if the prevalence of high lead levels is increased, clinicians may indicate to parents that getting the child retested is a reasonably urgent matter. The fourth step is that of making comparisons, such as determining whether the frequency of elevated lead levels in the clinician's community is higher than average. The next steps, development of hypotheses regarding causal factors and testing of the hypothesis, are illustrated by the example of querying patients who are late in getting immunizations. If most reply that they cannot afford the shots, then clinicians in their roles as developers of community programs might work with the county health department to designate all physicians' offices as county immunization clinics. A simple follow-up study of immunization rates in the community and in the clinician's practice would be good indicators of the effectiveness of such an intervention. The last phase of the epidemiologic sequence, intervention and its evaluation, should be increasingly emphasized, since all care should be efficiently and capably delivered. Prevention services will be judged in terms of efficacy, effectiveness, and efficiency. Although researchers are more likely to address these issues and use these concepts, individual clinicians must consider their activities in terms of effectiveness, framing every prevention visit as an "experiment of one." The latter must carefully consider what needs to be accomplished during a visit, how they can achieve their goals, and what outcomes they can examine to know whether they have attained those goals.

SCREENING

Screening is part of the counting process. In order for practitioners to know whether patients are at risk for a disease, they must screen the population they serve. The purpose of screening for preventable conditions is to detect individuals with early, mild, and asymptomatic disease. In order for screening to be most beneficial the disease should be common in the screened population, the morbidity and mortality from the untreated condition should be substantial, and the screening should ideally be done within a medical care program in which appropriate treatment is provided. In order for these conditions to be met, diseases must have a preclinical stage and must be detectable through the use of an accurate test; there must also be a cost-effective treatment available that is acceptable and results in better outcomes when used in a preclinical phase than therapy given after symptoms develop. Difficulties with implementing nationwide recommendations for screening are often due to the fact that these principles are ignored. The lack of universal screening for blood lead levels is an example. If the prevalence of elevated lead levels is low in a particular population, or if there are no acceptable treatments or interventions, physicians are unlikely to implement the recommended procedures. Also see Chapter 3.3.

Screening is usually population-based and attempts to diagnose conditions among basically healthy groups of people. Activities that are undertaken in an office setting are more appropriately termed case finding; the clinician is able to gather other information that can increase the efficiency of screening procedures. Unless the difference between screening and case finding is appreciated, understanding essential concepts of sensitivity and specificity is difficult. While an understanding of sensitivity and specificity is essential for choosing the appropriate test for a screening program, these characteristics are only marginally important for clinical interpretation of the results. Accurate interpretation of results is dependent upon derivatives of these test characteristics: their positive and negative predictive value (see Chapter 2).

Sensitivity refers to the proportion of individuals with the disease who are detected by the test; specificity refers to the proportion without the disease who will be correctly categorized by the test. The positive predictive value is the proportion of patients with a positive test who have the disease, whereas the negative predictive value is the proportion with negative tests who do not have the disease. Predictive values are dependent both on the characteristics of the test and on the prevalence of the disease in the population. If a test is highly sensitive, the negative predictive value will be good, i.e., the better the test, the more the practitioner can believe a negative result. Very specific tests mean that individuals with positive tests are likely to have the disease. However, with rare conditions, the major factor relating to the positive predictive value of a test is the prevalence of the disease in the population. In other words, if the disease is rare and a patient has a positive test, no matter how specific the test is, the result is more likely to

■ TABLE 5–1 Preventive Evaluation at Specific Ages*

Activity	1st week	1 mo	2 mo	4 mo	6 mo	9 mo	12 mo	15 mo	18 mo	2 yr	3 yr	4 yr	5 yr	6 yr	8 yr	10 yr	11–14 yr	15–17 yr	18–21 yr
Interview (for special attention)	√	√	√	√	√	√	√	√		√	√	√	√	√	√	√	√	√	√
Family history	√	√	√											√				√	
Pregnancy and delivery	√																		
Neonatal course	√	√																	
Developmental evaluation	√	√	√	√	√	√	√	√	√	√	√	√	√	√	√	√	√	√	√
Anticipatory guidance	√	√	√	√	√	√	√	√	√	√	√	√	√	√	√	√	√	√	√
Body systems																			
(for special attention)																			
Hearing/vision	√	√	√	√	√	√	√		√	√	√	√	√		√	√	√	√	
CNS (including sleep)	√	√	√	√	√	√	√		√	√	√	√							
Gastrointestinal/feeding	√	√	√	√	√	√	√		√	√	√	√	√		√	√	√	√	
Urinary	√									√									
Dental care							√	√	√	√	√	√	√	√	√	√	√	√	
Drugs, alcohol, tobacoo															√	√	√	√	√
Pica							√	√	√	√	√	√							
Sexual behavior															√	√	√	√	√
Physical Examination (complete) (for special attention)	√	√	√	√	√	√	√	√	√	√	√	√	√	√	√	√	√	√	√
Parent-child interaction	√	√	√	√	√	√	√	√	√	k	√	√	√	√	√	√			
Height and weight	√	√	√	√	√	√	√	√	√	√	√	√	√	√	√	√	√	√	√
Head circumference	√	√	√	√	√	√	√	√											
Blood pressure											√	√	√	√	√	√	√	√	√
Acne																	√	√	√
Vision																			
Tear ducts	√	√																	
Fixed eyes	√	√																	
Red reflex	√	√	√	√	√	√	√												
Fundus	√				√														
Strabismus	√	√	√	√	√	√				√									
Hearing	√	√	√			√	√	√	√	√	√	√	√	√					
Speech			√	√	√	√	√	√	√	√	√	√	√	√					
Neurologic problems			√	√	√	√	√												
Cardiac murmurs	√	√	√	√		√	√												
Abdominal masses	√	√	√																

Hip dysplasia	√	√	√	√	√	√	√		√	√									
Gait							√	√	√		√								
Metatarsus addictus			√																
Sexual development															√	√	√	√	
Scoliosis															√	√	√	√	√
Evidence of neglect/abuse		√	√	√	√	√	√	√	√	√	√	√	√	√	√	√	√	√	
Counseling (for special attention)																			
Diet	√	√	√	√	√	√	√	√	√	√	√					√	√	√	√
Sleep	√	√	√	√	√		√		√	√	√			√		√	√	√	√
Toilet training								√	√	√	√								
Accidents										√	√	√	√	√	√	√	√	√	√
Child care		√	√	√	√	√	√	√	√	√	√		√						
School problems													√	√	√	√	√	√	√
Puberty and sexuality															√	√	√	√	√
Substance abuse															√	√	√	√	√
Laboratory																			
Hgb/Hct					√ or	√ or	√			√					√		√	√	
Urinalysis					√					√					√				
Urine culture (girls)							√						√			√	√		
Tuberculin						√ or	√			√				√	√	√	√	√	√
Screening																			
Lipids										√	or	√		√		√	√	√	√
Metabolic	√																		
Lead			√		√ or	√ or	√ or	√		√	√		√						
Audiometer	√ (Prior to 3 mo)												√	√					
Snellen chart											√		√	√		√			
STD																	√	√	√
Immunizations (see Chapter 244 for details)	√	√	√	√	√	√	√	√	√			√ or	√				√		

**These suggestions or guidelines represent an analysis of recommendations by the American Academy of Pediatrics and Bright Futures. They are not intended to be all-inclusive but rather to serve as reminders for some of the important preventive and health promotion activities that should be considered at various ages when physician-patient encounters may occur. The content and timing of visits will need to be altered according to special needs and the presence or absence of risk factors for the child and his or her family.*

be a false-positive than an indication that the individual actually has the condition (see Fig. 2–5). The efficiency of this process is increased by a clinician's clinical acumen as he or she goes through the process of case finding. As physicians use other information to make decisions regarding whether or not a test is indicated, they are actually targeting a population with a higher prevalence of the disease, thus increasing the positive predictive value of the test ordered. The clinician can improve the quality and decrease the costs of clinical prevention services by using judgment in screening.

CLINICIANS AS PROVIDERS AND COORDINATORS OF PREVENTIVE SERVICES

Pediatricians spend 25–40% of their time in the delivery of clinical preventive services. Although many have contended that well child care has not been proved to be effective, there is increasing evidence that with well-designed programs, improved health outcomes are realized. The wise use of preventive interventions is a very complex matter that requires consideration not only of health care but also of the context in which the care is given. Personal care (such as well child care or child health supervision) provided in an office setting is one method of delivering preventive interventions. Because 80% of children in the United States receive their medical care through a private practice or a health maintenance organization, this is a reasonable approach to delivering prevention services to this population.

One of the problems facing the provider of preventive services is that the format needed to deliver "health services" does not conform to the traditional one used for other types of medical encounters. Prevention must be considered a constant, ongoing process rather than an episodic one. Therefore, preventive visits must be described both in terms of the individual visit and within the context of continuing care, through promotion of health within the family and community. The preventive health visit has three separate components, and each must be carefully considered and systematically delivered: (1) screening; (2) health promotion and disease prevention; and (3) patient management and follow-up (Table 5–1).

Screening has been described in detail earlier. In the well child visit, routine activities that can be considered screening procedures include gathering of historical data, physical examination including vision and hearing testing, observation of the patient and his or her parents, and laboratory testing (see Table 5–1). Screening questionnaires that parents can complete in the waiting room have also been shown to be useful. The purpose of screening is to define a population that needs further evaluation. If an interval history or a test reveals a problem that could require intervention, the clinician should then go through a logical process of decision making: Is the positive screen a true measure of risk? Is the perceived threat to health immediate and urgent? Is further evaluation necessary for confirmation of the problem? Should the positive screen simply be noted and followed up at the next visit? Can a simple intervention be made at this visit? An example of an urgent problem is a determination during the history that a child is at high risk of being abused. If the threat is urgent, the health promotion visit must be interrupted and "converted" to an acute care or intervention visit. An example of a positive screen that might be noted and simply followed in subsequent visits is a minor spinal curvature found on examination of a toddler. An adolescent's positive response to questions regarding drug use may require further evaluation and referral, whereas discovery of an asymptomatic ear infection can be treated during the visit. In each of these cases, health promotion must not be forgotten. If the visit is used to address the specific problem and the process of health promotion and disease prevention is interrupted, the patient should be rescheduled for the well child visit.

Health promotion and disease prevention are directed toward the determinants or causes of health and disease. Although in their roles as caregivers clinicians can do little to affect the overall environment in which children live or the organization of health care, in the office setting they can effectively address issues related to human biology and lifestyle. Disease prevention, introduced though a biologic approach, is accomplished through case finding and treatment as well as through delivery of immunization. Both the efficiency and the effectiveness of disease prevention are easier to measure because of its biologic basis.

Health promotion has been defined in *Healthy People* as "the development of community and individual measures which can help [people] to develop lifestyles that can maintain and enhance the state of well-being." Health promotion activities, because they involve lifestyle, are virtually always related to behavior. Because the results of lifestyle alteration are often not immediately seen, the effectiveness of health promotion programs is more difficult to measure. However, recent studies have indicated that health promotion strategies by medical personnel involving counseling patients regarding necessary behavioral changes can be successful.

Health promotion activities should be determined by the needs of the child and the family and considered in the context of the community as a whole. Counseling regarding good parenting practices or physical fitness constitutes health promotion. However, because the roots of disease are multifactorial, more sophisticated techniques may be needed for health promotion. Common, simple proscriptions and advice-giving are unlikely to significantly alter some factors that affect health. Clinicians must give careful consideration to those factors that can most be effectively addressed in the practice setting. These are (1) the formation of a therapeutic alliance and assurance of comprehensive care for children; (2) care for children's physical health through case finding, diagnosis and management of acute and chronic illnesses, provision of immunizations, and lifestyle counseling; (3) promotion of safety within the home and the community; and (4) support for families in their parenting roles. Each of these activities is complex. Table 5–1 lists recommended opportunities for preventive interventions and health promotion during office visits.

Patient management and follow-up constitute the portion of the visit in which care is coordinated. If no problems are detected during the screening procedures, the clinician can progress to health promotion counseling. Often, however, a complex or time-consuming intervention is needed. It is then that the provider assumes the role of coordinator of services, either rescheduling the patient for a return visit and providing the necessary care or referring the patient to the appropriate resource. An intimate knowledge of patients' health care needs, including their insurance and financial status; an understanding of the physical, emotional, and organizational barriers to patients' attaining care; and a thorough comprehension of available community resources (as well as the efficacy of programs) are necessary for clinicians to successfully fulfill this essential role.

CLINICIANS AS PROGRAM DEVELOPERS AND ADVOCATES FOR CHILDREN'S HEALTH NEEDS

Measures to prevent disease at the community level have had an enormous effect on childhood morbidity and mortality in the United States: sewage disposal and water sanitation; hygienic control of food, including pasteurization of milk and ionization of salt; control of arthropod vectors of disease such as the mosquito; fluoridation of public water supplies to decrease dental caries; establishment of poison control centers; infant car seat laws; childproof containers; flame-resistant fabrics for children's clothes; safe spacing of crib rails; and bicycle lanes. Despite these important successes in improving the welfare of children, there are still disturbing inadequacies (see Chapters 1 and 42). Health indicators, such as infant mortality and immunization rates, indicate that the United States is far behind other industrialized nations in the health status of children. Many of the environmental and social factors that affect child health are not amenable to intervention at the clinical level. Those prerequisites for health that can be achieved only through development of community-wide programs or advocacy include peace, shelter, education, income, a stable ecosystem, sustainable resources, social justice, and equity.

Community programs require a shift in perspective and use of a different set of analytic skills from those used directly with patients. Large-scale programs require more planning and coordination. Because more time, effort, and funds are concentrated in a single program, careful needs assessment and intervention planning are essential. Green and Kreuter have developed a methodology for community health promotion planning that involves an evaluation of the community health needs, description of the behavioral and environmental factors that affect the health variable determined in the needs assessment, consideration of the factors that either predispose individuals to the disease or enable or reinforce positive lifestyle change, and implementation of the intervention. In some cases, the intervention may be political, e.g., enactment of a bicycle helmet use law. These authors also point out the essential need for program evaluation. For clinicians to be effective advocates for child health, they must have access to data that both document the depth and pervasiveness of the health problems that face children and measure the effectiveness of intervention programs.

Although the design and implementation of a community program may seem overwhelming when first considered, most clinicians have the skills to do so and the American Academy of Pediatrics has assisted in such efforts. One example is the CATCH (Community Access to Child Health) program that supports local efforts to increase children's access to care. Funding for community programs can also often be found through local health departments and bureaus of maternal-child health. Local, state, and national governments can most rapidly institute programs that can affect the determinants of health. However, formulating and initiating public programs to benefit children require a process of sophisticated coalition building with coordination of health care providers and children's interest groups. The roots of pediatrics as a discipline were, in part, related to the creation of community programs to address pressing child health needs and the advocacy for implementation and maintenance of those programs. There is a continuing need for pediatric leaders who will devote time and attention to prevention as caregivers and coordinators and as community advocates for children.

Bright Futures: National Guidelines for Health Supervision of Infants, Children, and Adolescents. Arlington, VA, National Center for Education in Maternal and Child Health, 1994.

Committee on Psychosocial Aspects of Child and Family Health: Guidelines for Health Supervision II. Elk Grove, IL, American Academy of Pediatrics, 1988.

Green LW, Kreuter MW: Health Promotion Planning: An Educational and Environmental Approach, 2nd ed. Mountain View, CA, Mayfield Publishing Company, 1991.

Healthy People: The Surgeon General's Report on Health Promotion and Disease Prevention. Washington, DC, US Department of Health, Education, and Welfare. Publication No. 79–550701, 1979.

Last JM (ed): A Dictionary of Epidemiology. New York, Oxford University Press, 1983.

Public Health Service: Healthy People: National Health Promotion and Disease Prevention Objectives for the Year 2000. Washington DC, US Department of Health and Human Services, Public Health Service, 1990. DHHS Publication No. (PHS) 90–50212.

Tyler CW, Last JM: Epidemiology. *In*: Last JM, Wallace RB (eds): Maxcy-Rosenau-Last Public Health & Preventive Medicine, 13th ed. Norwalk, CT, Appleton & Lange, 1992, pp 11–39.

CHAPTER 6

Child Health in the Developing World

Jeffrey L. Goldhagen

More than 90% of the world's children are born each year in the developing world. Thirty-five thousand of them die each day, most from common and preventable problems. Health and illness for these children are the result of a complex dynamic of environmental, social, political, and economic factors. No single intervention will successfully interrupt the cycles of morbidity and mortality that plague them.

Much has been learned and many successes achieved over the past several decades with regard to the health needs of these children. Eighty per cent of children throughout the world are being immunized, and a decrease in measles has already been reported. Polio has been eradicated in the entire Western hemisphere. Use of oral rehydration therapy (ORT) saves more than 1 million child lives each year, and death due to diarrhea is no longer their primary cause of mortality.

The relevance of this experience to health service strategies in the United States and other developed countries has gained acceptance. This is due in part to increasing inequities in minority child health status. The United States has adopted Year 2000 goals patterned after those delineated by the United Nations International Children's Emergency Fund (UNICEF) and the World Health Organization (WHO) in 1978.

PRINCIPLES OF CHILD HEALTH IN DEVELOPING COUNTRIES. Approaches to child health evolved rapidly after the Second World War. This was due to the efforts of UNICEF and WHO, the emergence of Non-Government Relief and Development Organizations (NGOs), and changing strategies for international development assistance.

Trickle-down economics was the primary development strategy through the 1950s and early 1960s. However, increased per capita gross national products (GNPs) did not necessarily improve the social and health status of all population strata. Essential requirements for development, such as adequate shelter, safe water, and education, were identified, and a basic needs strategy was adopted to focus development efforts and resources. This strategy evolved through the 1970s, culminating in the 1977 Thirtieth World Health Assembly and the 1978 Alma Ata International Conference on Primary Health Care. The World Health Assembly established the main goal of WHO to be the attainment, by all people of the world, of a level of health that would permit them to lead a socially and economically productive life by the year 2000.

The Declaration of Alma Ata asserted primary care to be the key strategy for attaining Year 2000 goals and has had a profound impact on the structure and function of health systems in all regions of the world. It established 10 precepts for the definition of primary care: (1) Health is a state of complete well-being and not merely the absence of disease or infirmity; (2) inequities of health within and between countries is unacceptable and of global concern; (3) economic and social development are reciprocally tied to health development; (4) people have the right to participate in their own health care; (5) individuals' health should permit socially and economically productive lives; (6) primary health care is essential for overall social and economic development; (7) components of primary health care include personal health services, nutrition, safe water and sanitation, maternal and child health, immunization, essential drugs, and related sectors including agriculture, housing, public works, and so forth; (8) national policies should support comprehensive intersectoral health systems; (9) all countries should cooperate in a global health strategy; and (10) better use of resources, including diversion of those involved in military pursuits, would facilitate attaining Year 2000 goals.

International debate has focused on the balance between two approaches to achieving Year 2000 goals. An emphasis on developing comprehensive primary care systems is based on long-term strategies to build equitable systems that address all the health issues of a community. Alternatively, UNICEF, WHO, and developed countries, which contribute most of the world's assistance funds, have argued for more selective programs whose outcomes and cost can be readily measured. Selective strategies for the Child Survival Revolution were implemented after the Alma Ata conference using simple methods of *G*rowth monitoring, *O*ral rehydration, *B*reast-feeding, and *I*mmunization (GOBI). Later, categories of *F*ood, *F*emale education, and *F*amily planning were added (GOBI-FFF). GOBI-FFF has remained the developed world's primary strategy for health development.

Expanded funding for child survival programs has resulted in numerous innovative approaches. Networks of indigenous health workers have been established and health professionals trained to manage them. Social marketing strategies, operations and evaluation research, rapid assessment techniques, and so forth, have been developed. The role of women, the primacy of the household, and the importance of female education, family planning, and birth spacing have been better defined and related strategies integrated into health programs.

The knowledge and experience accrued over the past several decades provide reasons for optimism. The dramatic decrease in childhood mortality in the developed world prior to the delivery and use of antibiotics and vaccines is evidence of the importance of basic public health programs and their potential to improve the lives of all children everywhere.

BASIC HEALTH INDICATORS. Despite many successes, great disparity exists among nations in the health status of children. Annual health statistics and related indicators are reported in UNICEF's The State of the World's Children. Average infant and under-5-yr mortality rates (U5MR) range from 115 and 180 per 1,000 in least developed countries (34) to 9 and 11 per 1,000 in developed countries. The average annual rate of reduction in the U5MR is only 1.1% in countries with a very high U5MR (34) compared with 4.7% in low U5MR countries (33). Among the same countries: (1) 16% vs 7% of infants are born small for gestational age (SGA); (2) 34% vs 0% of children under 5 yr are moderately to severely malnourished; (3) the average annual population growth rate is 3% vs 0.7%; and (4) the crude birth and total fertility rates are 47, and 6.6 vs 14, and 1.8. With respect to women: (1) the contraceptive prevalence is 6% in developing countries vs 72% in wealthier nations; (2) maternal mortality rates are 640 vs 12 (per 100,000 live births); and (3) in the developing world only 28% of pregnant women are immunized against tetanus.

Key environmental and education indices related to health outcomes in very high U5MR countries demonstrate similar disparities. Only 43% of the population in these countries have access to safe water and adequate sanitation. Adult literacy rates are 59% and 37% for males and females. Less than one half of children are enrolled in primary school, and only 55% of these children complete it. Economic indices reveal increasing inequities between countries and predict potential deterioration in the health status of poorer nations. The per capita GNP (US$) in least developed (34) and developing (99) countries is $240 and $805 vs $14,710 in developed countries (30). The per capita average annual growth rate over the past decade is 0.1%, 2.2%, and 2.4%, respectively, while the rate of inflation is 23% and 62% in least developed and developing countries and only 5% in developed countries. Fifty-five per cent and 70% of the urban and rural population in least developed countries have lived in poverty over the past decade.

Trends in the health indices are a cause for both optimism and pessimism. Under 5-yr mortality rates have fallen by more than 50% over the past 30 years, with the most significant decrease registered over the past decade. Adult literacy and school enrollment rates have more than doubled. Crude birth and death rates have fallen by almost 50%, and life expectancy has increased from 39 to 50 years.

Despite these improvements, increasing disparity in economic indicators is a cause for alarm. In developing nations the average annual per cent growth rates in per capita GNP have remained stagnant or dropped over the past decade relative to the previous 15–20 years. Debt service has risen by 30% (as a percentage of exports of goods and services). Fertility rate reduction has remained virtually unchanged, and average annual population growth rates have actually increased over the past decade. Population growth in combination with deteriorating economic conditions portend increased difficulties for children in affected countries.

EPIDEMIOLOGY OF ILLNESS AND SPECIFIC INTERVENTION STRATEGIES. Each year 12.9 million children die: 28% of deaths are caused by pneumonia, 23% by diarrheal diseases, and 16% by vaccine-preventable diseases. Simple and affordable interventions, e.g., vaccines, antibiotics, ORT, contraceptives, could prevent 25% to 90% of deaths due to specific causes. Overall, 65% of child deaths are preventable at low cost.

Pneumonia. Pneumonia causes the majority of child deaths. Pathogens in developing countries are similar to those in economically advanced nations, but the frequency of primary and secondary bacterial infections is much greater. Respiratory viruses, in particular respiratory syncytial virus (RSV), cause the majority of acute lower respiratory tract infections (ALRTI). *Streptococcus pneumoniae, Haemophilus influenzae, Moraxella catarrhalis,* and *Staphylococcus aureus* account for the majority of bacterial infections. Cytomegalovirus, *Chlamydia, Mycoplasma pneumoniae,* and *Mycobacterium tuberculosis* are also common pathogens.

Vitamin A deficiency is clearly associated with increased incidence, morbidity, and mortality of respiratory tract disease (see Chapter 45.3). Vitamin A stabilizes the structure and function of mucosal surfaces and is involved with immune response (particularly T-cell function) and mucus production. There is at least a 2-fold increase in the incidence of respiratory disease and a 4- to 12-fold increase in mortality in children with even mild vitamin A deficiency. This explains the association of measles with vitamin A deficiency, xerophthalmia, respiratory and diarrheal diseases, and increased child mortality. Supplementation with as little as a single 200,000 IU vitamin A capsule per year has been shown to decrease childhood mortality by at least 49%. Treatment of measles with vitamin A supplementation is now recommended by the American Academy of Pediatrics.

Primary malnutrition can result in vitamin A deficiency, which increases the child's susceptibility to respiratory and diarrheal diseases. Viral and bacterial infections can also lead to vitamin A deficiency and further malnutrition. This vicious circle of malnutrition and infection is the principal cause of child deaths in the developing world.

Other simple interventions can decrease mortality due to pneumonia. Breast milk provides the required vitamin A through the first 6 months of life and most of the requirement until 2 yr of age. Prevention of hypothermia through continuous skin-to-skin contact of babies with their parents or surrogates (the kangaroo method) can prevent hypothermia in premature and SGA infants. Oiling the skin can also prevent body heat and moisture loss.

National acute respiratory infection (ARI) programs have been established in all regions of the world. Millions of mothers have learned to recognize respiratory distress by counting respirations and identifying chest indrawing and fever. Use of antibiotics at home for children identified by parents as having moderately severe ARIs and referral to health care facilities for those with severe disease have reduced mortality and the inappropriate use of antibiotics. National ARI programs train parents, supervise health workers, ensure adequate distribution of essential drugs and access of families to health facilities, monitor and evaluate programs, and provide ongoing surveillance for drug resistance.

Diarrheal Diseases (also see Chapter 171). The epidemiology of diarrheal disease in developing nations is similar to that in economically advanced countries. Rotavirus and other enteric viruses are the principal pathogens. Bacterial disease is most routinely caused by *Salmonella* and *Shigella.* Parasitic infections are endemic but generally result in nutritional deficiencies and not acute diarrheal disease. Cholera remains a problem throughout all regions of the developing world.

Oral rehydration solution (ORS) saves the lives of millions of children and adults each year. When given in the right proportion (3.5 g NaCl, 2.5 g $NaHCO_3$, 1.5 g KCl, and 20 g glucose in 1 L clean water), electrolytes and water will be absorbed across the intestine despite ongoing diarrhea. Hundreds of millions of ORS packets containing electrolytes and carbohydrates in powder form have been distributed worldwide. The content of oral rehydration solutions has evolved to include indigenous and culturally acceptable sources of carbohydrate as well as homemade recipes that use appropriate finger measurements for locally available containers. UNICEF and WHO's child survival strategy utilizes ORT (and breast-feeding) as two of its four pillars.

Diarrheal disease programs have significantly reduced mortality. International promotion of breast-feeding has included strict restrictions on advertising and sale of formula, development of baby-friendly hospitals, and extensive social marketing campaigns. Diarrheal disease programs also have had an important impact on the structure and function of national health service delivery systems. Effective, inexpensive, and simple therapies for diarrhea provide an example of how health can be promoted. Networks of indigenous health workers have been developed to teach people about the cause, prevention, and treatment of diarrhea.

These networks have served as the foundation for other health initiatives and have had a profound impact on the culture of many communities. Women, who have been traditionally denied access to important community roles, and traditional healers, who have been generally kept out of "mainstream" governmental initiatives, have been integrated into health systems. The fundamental role of women and the concept of health as a product generated in the context of a household have been recognized. The importance of female education has been appreciated and educational opportunities expanded.

Immunization-Preventable Diseases (also see Chapters 247 and 248). The six immunization-preventable diseases (measles, polio, diphtheria, pertussis, tetanus, and tuberculosis) kill, blind, cripple, and cause mental damage to some 10 million children each year. Complete immunization of all the world's children as well as eradication of diseases that have humans as their sole host is an international priority. The Expanded Program on Immunization (EPI) is the joint effort of WHO and UNICEF to attain these goals.

Dramatic successes have been achieved. The cold chain, necessary for the preservation of heat-intolerant vaccines, reaches virtually everywhere on the globe; effective evaluation and surveillance techniques to ensure vaccine viability have been implemented; new vaccines (HIB, HEP-B) have been introduced in some parts of the world, and others, including a vaccine for malaria and dengue fever, are under development; multiple antigen and new single-dose and heat-resistant vaccines have been introduced or are in final stages of development; new vaccine delivery systems and practices to minimize missed opportunities to vaccinate have been implemented; EPI funding resources and personnel have been expanded; management techniques for a global eradication strategy are being perfected; communication, computer, and surveillance systems have been introduced; and the commitment of virtually every nation in the world has been secured.

MALNUTRITION. Malnutrition is a primary cause of morbidity and mortality and a complicating factor for other illnesses. In utero caloric deprivation results in some SGA births. Subsequent protein, calorie, and micronutrient malnutrition results in moderate to severe stunting in 50% of children, with concomitant deficiencies in cognitive development. Susceptibility to infectious diseases is increased. Acute and chronic infections may further exacerbate a child's nutritional deficiencies and often result in the child's death. Anorexia and inaccessible tertiary care make nutritional resuscitation difficult or impossible.

In addition to unavailability of food and chronic parasitic infestation, malnutrition sometimes results from cultural food practices. Use of foods with low protein and calorie content as weaning foods, early displacement of infants from the breast (due often to the belief that infants should not be nursed if the mother is pregnant), and failure to initiate or early cessation of breast-feeding are common causes of primary malnutrition. Female education, family planning, and birth spacing are among the most effective strategies to prevent malnutrition.

OTHER CHILD HEALTH ISSUES. Malaria, schistosomiasis, and dengue fever are examples of other infectious diseases common to children in developing countries. However the medical, psychologic, and social impact of AIDS and violence may soon eclipse all other causes of morbidity and mortality in all regions of the world. In areas of Central Africa as many as 40% of women are infected with HIV. Approximately 25% of their offspring will contract HIV through vertical transmission. Uninfected children are often left orphaned and potentially without the support and nurturing required for normal early childhood development. The personal effect on families is complicated by the economic impact of the death of productive individuals on whole communities.

War has always had a disproportionate effect on children. Conflicts persist in all regions of the world, exposing children to acts of violence and traumatic stress disorders. The susceptibility of children through normal play to land mine injuries has spawned an international movement to limit their distribution and production. Violence directed at children, however, is not limited to war. Street children are routinely tortured and often killed; widespread childhood prostitution and forced labor persist, particularly in Southeast Asia and India; and patterns of abuse continue in all countries.

WORLD SUMMIT FOR CHILDREN AND CONVENTION ON THE RIGHTS OF THE CHILD. In response to the acute needs of children throughout the world, the 1990 United Nations World Summit for Children was convened to establish national programs of action for achieving basic health and social goals. These goals include control of major childhood diseases, a halving of child malnutrition, a one-third reduction in under 5-yr mortality rates, a halving of maternal mortality rates, the provision of safe water to all communities, universal availability of family planning, and basic education for all children. The Summit also urged the ratification of the Convention on the Rights of the Child. The Convention established standards for survival, protection, and development of all children. To date, 156 countries have signed the Convention. The United States remains the only major developed country that has not signed the Convention.

Bertrand W, Walmus B: Maternal knowledge, attitudes and practice as predictors of diarrhoeal disease in young children. Int J Epidemiol 12(2):205, 1983.
Bloom A, Reid J: Anthropology and primary health care in developing countries. Soc Sci Med 19(3):183, 1984.
Forgie I, O'Neill K, Lloyd-Evans N, et al: Etiology of acute lower respiratory tract infection in Gambian children: II. Acute lower respiratory tract infection in children ages one to nine years presenting at the hospital. Pediatr Infect Dis J 10(1):42, 1991.
Forgie I, O'Neill K, Lloyd-Evans N, et al: Etiology of acute lower respiratory tract infections in infants presenting at the hospital. Pediatr Infect Dis J 10(1):33, 1991.
Grant J: The State of the World's Children. Oxford, Oxford University Press, 1993.
Mandl P: A Child Survival and Development Revolution, 2nd ed. Geneva, United Nations Children's Fund, 1983.
Morley D, Lovel H: My Name is Today. London, Macmillan, 1986.
Mulholland K, Weber M: Recognising causes and signs of pneumonia. ARI News 24(11):2, 1992.
Oplatka E: Vitamin A treatment of measles. AAP News 9(4):7, 1993.
Pebley A, Millman S: Birth spacing and child survival. Healthy People 2000 12(3):71, 1986.
Sommer A, Katz J, Tarwotjo I: Increased risk of respiratory disease and diarrhea in children with preexisting mild vitamin A deficiency. Am J Clin Nutr 40(11):1090, 1984.
Werner D, Bower B: Helping Health Workers Learn. Palo Alto, CA, The Hesperian Foundation, 1984.

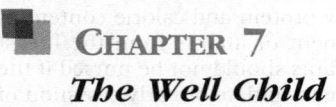

CHAPTER 7
The Well Child

Paul L. McCarthy

The most powerful diagnostic maneuver available to the pediatrician is the clinical evaluation: the process of observing the child, taking a history, and performing the physical examination. In order for the pediatrician to maximize the benefit of the clinical evaluation, some of the complexities of this process must be appreciated. Also see Chapter 4.

UNIQUE CHARACTER OF THE PEDIATRIC CLINICAL EVALUATION. This evaluation involves the physician, the parent(s), and the child. Historical information is often taken from the parents, and it is not until the child reaches later developmental stages that he or she can contribute information about symptoms more actively. These considerations change the manner in which the pediatrician gathers data about symptoms. Rather than asking, for example, if the child has abdominal pain, the physician asks questions that focus on the manner in which abdominal pain would present to an observer. Thus, questions about loss of appetite, sudden episodes of crying and drawing the legs up in a fetal position, or the child's crying when the parent has placed pressure on the abdomen are appropriate. The 24-mo-old child with a sore throat often does not complain of this but rather is observed by the parents to have more difficulty handling oral secretions, refuses solids, and has a foul breath odor. Questions are tailored to elicit this information.

As the child becomes older, he or she may begin to add historical information that expresses symptoms in unique ways. At times the information provided by the child suggests the diagnosis precisely, but at other times the child's information may reflect a less developed sense of cause-and-effect relationships and be at variance with the data provided by the parents. Thus, the 4-yr-old child with a urinary tract infection may be observed by the parent to be holding his or her abdomen and to have a subtle change in the frequency of urination. The child, on the other hand, may perceive that his or her abdominal complaints are related to a specific food that was ingested just prior to the onset of symptoms. In this instance, the pediatrician may conclude that the parent's history suggests the correct diagnosis (a urinary tract infection) by eliciting further information about, for example, discomfort when urinating.

PARENTS AND CHILD AS PARTICIPANTS IN THE CLINICAL EVALUATION. It is often left to the judgment of parents whether clinical symptoms should be brought to the attention of a physician. Moreover, children's interpretation of symptoms is intimately related to their developmental stage; this also influences the manner in which they transmit clinical information to the physician. Both parents and children must believe that the pediatrician is interested in their concerns, and that interactions with the pediatrician provide them support and enhance the acuity of their clinical perceptions. This process occurs at both well and sick child visits. At well child visits the parent or child might describe a specific behavior or symptom. The pediatrician demonstrates concern by listening attentively and by asking follow-up questions demonstrating that the behavior or symptom has been understood. These follow-up questions provide an opportunity for the parent or child to explore his or her own interpretation of these behaviors or symptoms, to explore what emotional response they have had, and to learn from the interpretation provided by the physician. For example, parents reporting that their 9-mo-old child cries when being put to bed and has difficulty falling asleep offers an opportunity for the pediatrician to explore their interpretations of this behavior, to discuss their response to it, and to discuss the developmental dimensions of individuation. Based on this discussion and a more precise appreciation of the meaning of that behavior, strategies can evolve as an appropriate response to that behavior.

The same interaction and education process occur during sick child visits (see Chapter 57). Upper respiratory symptoms may concern parents. The pediatrician's discussing the predominance of nasal breathing in younger children, the more prominent symptoms that arise from nasal stuffiness because of this, and the absence of other evidence of serious pulmonary involvement, such as tachypnea, enhance parents' abilities to interpret respiratory symptoms during subsequent upper respiratory infections. Similarly, the pediatrician can explain cause-and-effect relationships between infection and symptoms to the older child. Such encounters, during both well and ill child visits, serve to enhance the confidence of parents and children in their role as participants in the clinical evaluation. Studies have demonstrated the ability of parents to evaluate clinical data reliably and the ability of children, when given developmentally appropriate information, to improve their understanding of clinical causality.

DEVELOPMENTAL DIMENSIONS. The data generated from observation, history (see earlier), and physical examination are greatly influenced by the child's developmental stage. A portion of the observational assessment of a child focuses on signs related to specific organ systems that are intimately related to age. The child of 1 mo has a more rapid respiratory rate (30 breaths/min) than the 3-yr-old child. The infant's respiratory rate is more sensitive to other influences, such as gastric pressure on the diaphragm caused by the recent ingestion of a meal, than that of the older child. Other portions of observational assessment focus on data that are indicators of the child's overall state of well-being or functional status, such as how the child responds visually to the environment. The pediatrician should not only be aware that visual responses undergo developmental change but also be aware of the manner in which stimuli should be presented to elicit the child's optimal visual response at different developmental stages. The 1-mo-old infant, for example, is more nearsighted and tends to focus on objects held within 1 to 2 ft of the face; objects presented in the peripheral fields of vision may be ignored. The ability of the young infant to maintain attention on a visual stimulus is less developed than in the older child. Thus, the pediatrician must be aware of the developmental dimensions of observing children in order to gather and interpret clinical information accurately.

The data generated during the physical examination are also closely linked to the child's stage of development. Specific findings may be normal in one age group and abnormal in another. For example, the 1-mo-old child normally has a rooting reflex, which facilitates suckling. On the other hand, a rooting reflex found in a 2-yr-old child indicates central nervous system abnormalities. Not only do specific findings differ in different age groups, but the manner in which physical examination findings are elicited varies from one developmental stage to another. The 8-mo-old child, for example, is beginning to develop a sense of individuality and is aware of strangers and frightened by separation. To elicit accurate physical examination data, the child should remain cooperative and not resist the examination, especially during auscultation of the chest and heart. Based on an appreciation of the developmental stage of an 8-mo-old, the examiner should allow the child to remain close to the parent and make his or her approach as unobtrusively as possible. Factors that would lessen the strangeness of a situation, such as the warmth of the room, the stethoscope, and the examiner's voice, help facilitate data gathering. The older child is usually more comfortable with strangers and in separating from the parents, and hence, after initial assurances, the physical examination may be done on the examination table.

The pediatric clinical evaluation is a complex interaction because of the manner in which information flows among the participants, and because of the influence of developmental trends on gathering and interpreting the observation, history, and physical examination data.

GUIDELINES FOR EVALUATION. During the clinical encounter it is often difficult to separate each component of the evaluation. As the physician is taking a history from the parent, he or she is observing the child and observing the interaction with the parent; as the physician performs the physical examination, he or she is evaluating the child's global responses to the specific maneuver being performed. Nevertheless, certain guidelines can be followed during each part of the evaluation.

Observation is best done with the younger child in a comfortable position, usually on the parent's lap. Upset and anxiety on the parent's part are easily transmitted to the child; thus the parent and child must be placed at ease with a greeting and reassuring words. The tone of the examiner's voice is important and should convey a willingness to listen and a sensitivity to concerns being expressed. The manner in which the examiner is oriented to the parent and child is also important: If the examiner sits in one corner and regards only the notation page, a sense of unwillingness to communicate is conveyed. Sitting close to the parents and child and facing them directly is more effective. The examiner should observe the manner in which the parent and child are interacting—how are the parents responding to the child's needs and, in turn, how is the child responding to the parents? The pediatrician can modulate the stimuli in this situation to gather important information by observation. The child may initially be clinging to the parent, so the pediatrician should interact with the child, offer the child an object, or attempt some separation of the child and parent to observe the child's response.

The history is best taken with the child in a comfortable position. If the child is quiet and comfortable, the parent can focus better on specific questions. Physicians vary in their amount of note taking during the history. Some prefer to write the history directly to progress notes; others note only key words and, at the end of the examination, transfer the information to the medical record. Whichever technique is used, it is critical that the physician remain responsive to the information being presented. If highly sensitive information is being conveyed and the parent or child is responding emotionally, the physician must convey empathetic understanding. This is impossible, however, if note taking continues without interruption. Additional note taking during this critical moment can interfere with important observations about the parent and child and their interaction.

The precision and clarity with which parents and children describe symptoms vary. Ongoing interaction with the family over a period of time enables the pediatrician to learn how clinical information is perceived and transmitted within each family. If, for example, the parents perceive the child as vulnerable, minor symptoms may be overemphasized; the pediatrician can adjust the assessments accordingly.

The portions of the physical examination that require optimal cooperation are completed initially—the blood pressure measurement, pulmonary and cardiac examinations, and evaluations of the eyes and central nervous system. The younger child may be held by the parent or seated on the parent's lap for these parts of the examination. The older child can be seated on the examination table. The pattern and rate of respirations are evaluated initially. Is there tachypnea? Is there increased work of breathing, as manifested by subcostal, intercostal, and/or supraclavicular retractions? Is there an expiratory grunt indicating that the child is expiring against a closed glottis to keep the small airways open longer? What are the colors of the skin, nails, and mucous membranes? After these assessments have been made, the physician may proceed to palpation, percussion (if indicated), and auscultation. It is not uncommon for the younger child to cry as the stethoscope is placed on the chest, but this can usually be overcome by patience and by increasing the child's comfort, such as offering the infant a bottle. The same sequence may be followed for the cardiac examination. The ophthalmologic examination requires that the child be quietly wakeful; ophthalmoscopy can be done with the child in the parent's lap or as the child is being carried over the parent's shoulder. Sometimes the other parent can provide visual stimuli; the retina can be seen more easily as the child focuses on such stimuli. Many portions of the neurologic examination, such as eliciting reflexes, also require cooperation and a state of quiet wakefulness. In the older child this can be accomplished with the child on the examination table, but it is usually more helpful for the younger child to remain on the parent's lap.

After these portions of the examination the examiner proceeds to the parts of the examination that are usually more bothersome to the child. The abdominal examination requires that the child be on the examination table. It is helpful to have the parent hold a younger patient's hand and speak reassuringly. Thus, the child does not tense the abdominal musculature unnecessarily, as might occur during crying. After the abdominal examination, the pulses may be palpated, the genitalia examined, and the hips and extremities evaluated for clinical abnormalities. It is at this time that the examiner proceeds to the most intrusive portions of the examination, the evaluation of the ear canals and tympanic membranes and the examination of the oropharynx. During the ear examination, the parent may hold the child's head to minimize movement against the otoscope. The examiner should recognize that the ear canals are highly sensitive, and the speculum should be introduced gently. The free hand of the examiner can be used to put gentle traction on the pinna to straighten the canal. A portion of the hand holding the otoscope, usually the 5th finger, should rest against the head so that the otoscope moves with the head. At times, depending on the level of cooperation, the ears may be examined with the child in the parent's lap and the head resting against the parent's shoulder. The oropharyngeal examination is performed last, and the tongue blade is introduced gently.

The sequence of performing those portions of the physical

examination that require inspection, palpation, percussion, and auscultation (pulmonary, cardiac, and abdominal) varies according to organ system. The most bothersome maneuvers are performed last. For example, during the cardiac examination, inspection can be followed by palpation and percussion and then by auscultation. For the abdominal examination, inspection should be followed by auscultation before percussion and palpation are completed.

With appropriate sensitivity to the child and the parent, an appreciation of the child's developmental stage, and concern for minimizing the discomfort of an examination, the pediatrician can almost always obtain accurate clinical information and not cause undue upset to the child.

WELL CHILD EVALUATION. The broad principles of clinical data gathering outlined earlier apply to the clinical evaluation during the well child examination. Well child visits are recommended prenatally, in the newborn period, at 2 wk, 2, 4, 6, 9, 12, 15, 18, and 24 mo, annually between 3 and 6 yr, and every 2 yr thereafter (see Table 5–1). For children with chronic or intercurrent problems, this sequence can vary. Certain considerations should be addressed at each visit.

Open-Ended Questions. The physician should ask general questions that allow the parent or child to voice concerns that might not be raised if questions were too specific. Open-ended questions such as "How are you?" or "How is the baby?" transmit an interest in the general well-being of the child and family, as do the behavioral clues that were outlined previously. When such open-ended questions are asked, it is important that the physician explore the leads provided by the parents or child; ending the interaction prematurely, without appropriate follow-up questions, is frustrating to the parents and child and sends a mixed message about the physician's interest and concern.

Development. Each well child visit should determine the child's developmental achievements, such as by the widely used Denver Developmental Screening Test. Questions in the gross motor, person-social, language, and fine motor–adaptive realms can be presented and scored. Previous scores serve as a reference point for future visits; the rate of change in specific dimensions, such as language, can be more easily appreciated. As the child matures beyond 5 and 6 yr of age, questions that focus on school performance and talented accomplishments can be substituted for the Denver test. Reviewing developmental milestones provides the parents with a sense of satisfaction in their child's progress and reinforces the efforts they are making to nurture and teach their children. Reviewing the older child's accomplishments is an important demonstration of support for these activities.

Feeding and Diet. Many changes occur in the dietary intake of those in the pediatric age group, and these should be reviewed with the parents and children. During the first 12 mo of life, for example, breast milk or infant formula is the major source of calories and nutrients. The introduction of infant cereals, strained, then junior foods, and finally table foods, the change from formula to milk, and the use of vitamins and fluoride are issues of daily concern for parents. In the older child the intake of excessive salt, carbohydrates, or cholesterol can affect health adversely. If the rationale underlying the introduction of certain foods and dietary changes is discussed with parents and children, they can more easily play an active role in and feel comfortable with this process.

Accident Prevention. At each well child care visit accident prevention should be reviewed. Potential hazards around the home are emphasized as well as the importance of car safety measures. Syrup of ipecac is provided at the 6-mo visit, and the phone number of the local Poison Control Center should be given to the parents. In order for the parents and older children to participate more fully in this process, the developmental aspect of accident prevention should be stressed. For example, the child's ability to crawl and to grasp and place objects in the mouth make the issue of poison prevention especially critical when these developmental milestones have been reached. The necessity for having ipecac in the house and for "accident-proofing" the home then becomes clearer.

Growth. At each well child visit the height, weight, and head circumference are measured. These are plotted on standard graphs, such as those provided by the National Center for Health Statistics (see Chapter 13). It is important to review growth parameters with parents and children, because these are objective indicators of the child's progress. If abnormalities in the rate of growth are noted, the clinical evaluation can focus on possible causes. When interpreting these data the pediatrician must focus on what is normal for this child, given the family background. Growth charts rely on normative data from populations with selected growth characteristics; thus, if both parents are slightly below the 3rd percentile for height, these normative data require appropriate interpretation to allay undue concern in regard to this child's growth.

Family and Social Relations. To grow and develop normally, children rely on the support and nurturance provided by their family and the social environment (see Chapter 8). They are sensitive to disturbances in these supports, which can lead to nonoptimal growth, altered development, and adverse behavioral changes. The pediatrician should assess these supports by observation and questions. Observations can include the hygiene of the child and the child's general level of interest and response to people. How do the parents respond to the child's needs? What is the tone of parents' voices as they discuss the child? In what terms do the parents describe the child? If the child begins crying or is disruptive, how do the parents respond? Do the parents face the young child or do they show lack of interest or concern? Does the child appear depressed or inappropriately anxious? Specific questions from the pediatrician may elucidate other stresses or strengths in the environment. Is there an extended network of friends and family that provides support to the children and parents? Is the family under significant stress, such as through illness or loss of a job? The pediatrician's willingness to gather information about these issues and to address them demonstrates a realistic attitude toward what constitutes health or dysfunction for the child and family.

A particular challenge to all who care for children is represented by the special needs of children who live in impoverished environments (see Chapter 42). Empathizing with the difficulties of raising children in these circumstances and recognizing the obstacles that such children often face in realizing their potential are major concerns of pediatric care. Demonstrating a willingness to assist parents and children in resolving some of these adversities can provide them with a sense of hope and optimism about the future.

Anticipatory Guidance. Based on a developmental orientation, the physician should be aware of issues that might present problems or questions for the parents or child between the current and next visits. For example, the rate of growth of the 24-mo-old lessens compared with that of previous months, and this results in a diminished appetite. Rather than have the parents be unnecessarily concerned about this, it is prudent to preview the child's rate of growth in the next 6 mo and to discuss its impact on food intake. The developmental achievements that the parents might expect over the next several months and the type of activities that facilitate these developments can also be discussed. For example, the 12-mo-old's ability to grasp and bring objects to the mouth makes finger foods an option for the child at this age. In addition, this ability points out the necessity of removing small objects (e.g., peanuts) from the environment to minimize choking and aspiration hazards. The anticipatory guidance that is provided should also review issues in daily caretaking, such as hygiene and sleep patterns.

Again, every effort should be made to integrate these caretaking issues into a wider developmental perspective.

Other Concerns. At the initial well child visit, data should be entered into the medical record about the family medical history and the prenatal and perinatal history. At each well child visit, the physician should record and provide a record of immunizations to parents. Notes should be made about any intercurrent illness, such as otitis media or bronchitis. At each well child visit, a review of systems is carried out to ascertain whether there have been any symptoms related to specific organ systems, such as the gastrointestinal or neurologic. Finally, a flow sheet of laboratory screening tests, such as hemoglobin level, should be updated.

After the aforementioned considerations have been addressed and the physical examination completed, the pediatrician should summarize the child's health status. The parents should be complimented on their strengths as caregivers and the child complimented about his or her achievements and progress. It is also important to recognize problems and to express a willingness to work on these together with the family. The pediatrician's availability, if problems arise before the next visit, should be stressed. In this way the parents and child are reassured about the pediatrician's involvement in ongoing care. Parents and children should again be given an opportunity to ask questions or raise concerns about any aspect of the well child visit.

American Academy of Pediatrics: Guidelines for Health Supervision. Elk Grove Village, IL, American Academy of Pediatrics Press, 1985.

Green J: Pediatric interview and history. *In*: Haggerty R. Green M (eds): Ambulatory Pediatrics, 4th ed. Philadelphia, WB Saunders, 1990.

McCarthy PL: Demographic, clinical and psychosocial predictors of the reliability of mothers' clinical judgements. Pediatrics 88:1041, 1991.

PART II

Growth and Development

Robert D. Needlman

CHAPTER 8

Overview and Assessment of Variability

The pediatrician needs to understand both the general course of growth and development and the forces that shape each child's direction. Growth and development include a variety of processes: the formation of tissues; the enlargement of head, trunk, and limbs; the progressive increases in strength and ability to control large and small muscles; the development of social relatedness, thought, and language; and the emergence of personality. The unfolding of these processes and their interactions depends both on the child's biologic endowment and on the physical and social environment.

An understanding of development not only permits early detection of delays or deviance but also allows the pediatrician to help parents understand their observations. Parents and professionals create or adopt explanatory models or hypotheses about development. These models include implicit or explicit beliefs about the nature of children, the preferred characteristics of adults, and the processes that control the transformation from child to adult. For example, many parents see children as naturally dependent and see self-sufficiency as a preferred adult attribute. The belief that children learn self-sufficiency by coping with stress might lead such parents to wait before picking up a crying child. The opposing belief, that children learn self-sufficiency by internalizing the experience of being cared for, might lead other parents to pick up the child right away. To provide useful counseling, the pediatrician needs to understand the developmental models of parents as well as the models supported by scientific evidence.

BIOPSYCHOSOCIAL MODELS OF DEVELOPMENT

The debate between nature and nurture is age old. In the former model, the forces that determine development reside within the child; biology is destiny. In the latter, development is determined by forces outside of the individual; the child is infinitely mutable, a "blank slate." Biopsychosocial models, now widely accepted, recognize the importance of both intrinsic and extrinsic forces. Height, for example, is a function of the child's genetic endowment (biologic), personal habits of eating (psychological), and access to nutritious food (social). Biologic, psychological, and social influences on development are the focus, respectively, of the major theoretical perspectives described next.

BIOLOGIC INFLUENCES. Biologic influences on development include genetics, in utero exposure to teratogens, postpartum illnesses, exposure to hazardous substances, and maturation. Twin studies have established that a large part of the variance in IQ scores and various personality characteristics can be accounted for by genetic endowment. The developmental (biologic) correlates of prenatal exposure to teratogens such as mercury and alcohol and to postpartum medical problems such as meningitis have been extensively studied. Chronic illness affects growth and development; a particular illness may have specific developmental correlates.

Physical and neurologic maturation propels the child forward and sets lower limits for the emergence of most abilities. The age at which children walk independently is similar around the world, despite great variability in child-rearing practices. Other attainments (e.g., the acquisition of toilet training or of two-word sentences) are less tightly bound to a maturational schedule. Maturational changes also create the potential for behavioral problems at predictable times. For example, decrements in growth rate and sleep requirements around 2 yr of age often generate concerns about poor appetite and refusal to nap.

In addition to physical changes in size, body proportions, and strength, maturation is associated with hormonal influences. Sexual differentiation, both somatic and neurologic, begins in utero. Behavioral effects of testosterone may be evident even in young children and continue to be salient throughout life, particularly in the association between male gender and aggression.

A biologic influence of particular clinical importance is temperament. *Temperament* refers to the child's characteristic style of responding. There are nine proposed parameters of temperament (Table 8–1). Temperament, in this model, is intrinsic to the child and relatively resistant to modification by parenting practices. Most temperamental characteristics show only modest stability over time. Active, intense 2-yr-olds, for example, do not necessarily grow into active, intense 22-yr-olds.

Clinically, the concept of temperament is useful in two ways. First, it can help parents understand and accept the characteristics of their children without feeling responsible for having caused them. Second, behavioral and emotional problems tend to occur when the temperamental characteristics of children and parents conflict. Active children may be especially problematic for low-key parents; outgoing parents may pressure a child who is "slow to warm up" and create unnecessary upset; parents who lead highly structured lives may fare poorly with children whose biologic needs occur on a less regular schedule. "Goodness of fit" between the child and parents may be a powerful predictor of outcome.

PSYCHOLOGICAL INFLUENCES: ATTACHMENT AND CONTINGENCY. Despite the recognized importance of inborn traits, the influence of the child-rearing environment dominates most current models of development. Erik Erikson identified the 1st yr of life as a time when "basic trust" was established, based on the mother's consistent responsiveness to the child's needs. Studies of infants in hospitals and foundling homes documented the devas-

■ TABLE 8–1 Temperamental Characteristics: Descriptions and Examples

Characteristic	Description	Example*
Activity level	Amount of gross motor movement	"She ran before she walked." "He would rather sit still than run around."
Rhythmicity	Regularity of biologic cycles	"He is never hungry at the same time each day." "You could set a watch by her nap."
Approach and withdrawal	Typical response to a new stimulus	"She rejects every new food at first." "He loves new people."
Adaptability	How long it takes to adapt to novel stimulus	"Changes upset him." "She adjusts to new people quickly."
Threshold of responsiveness	How intense do stimuli need to be to evoke a response (e.g., feel, sound, light)	"Underwear and socks bother him; he does not like anything touching his skin." "She will eat anything, wear anything, do anything."
Intensity of reaction	How much energy the child puts out in emotions and actions	"She shouts when she is happy and wails when she is sad." "He never cries much."
Quality of mood	Usual disposition (e.g., pleasant, glum)	"He does not laugh much." "It seems like she is always happy."
Distractibility	How easily diverted from ongoing activity	"Her mind is always wandering." "He will listen through a whole story."
Attention span and persistence	How long the child pays attention and "sticks with" difficult tasks	"He goes from toy to toy every minute." "She will keep at a puzzle until she has mastered it."

Typical statements of parents, reflecting the range for each characteristic from very little to very much.

tating effects of maternal deprivation and pointed to the importance of attachment. Attachment refers to a biologically determined tendency of the young child to seek proximity with the parent during times of stress. Children who are securely attached are able to use their parents to re-establish a sense of well-being after a stressful experience, such as a physical examination or immunization. Insecure attachment may signal dysfunction in the parent-child relationship and may be predictive of later behavioral and learning problems.

At all stages of development, and across multiple developmental lines, progress is fostered by adult caregivers who observe the child's verbal and nonverbal cues and respond accordingly. In early infancy, such contingent responses of caregivers to signs of over- or underarousal help maintain infants in the state of quiet alertness and may foster autonomic self-regulation. Contingent responses to nonverbal gestures create the groundwork for the shared attention and reciprocity critical for later language and social development. At all stages, learning is fostered when new challenges are made contingent on the child's current level of competence, being just slightly harder than what has already been mastered. Such optimal tasks fall within the "zone of proximal development."

SOCIAL FACTORS: FAMILY SYSTEMS AND THE ECOLOGIC MODEL. Contemporary models of child development recognize the critical importance of influences *outside* of the mother-child dyad. These influences may be conceived of as contributing to a higher or lower level of stress that then impacts on the mother-child relationship. An abusive spousal relationship may exacerbate maternal depression, thus impairing the mother's ability to respond contingently to her child.

Families function as systems, with more or less rigidly defined boundaries, subsystems, roles, and rules for interaction. The impact of these forces on development is often subtle but powerful. In families with rigidly defined parental subsystems, children may be denied any decision making at all, exacerbating rebelliousness. If the parent-child boundary is overly porous, children may be "parentified," required to take on responsibilities beyond their years or recruited to play a spousal role.

Individuals within systems adopt implicit roles. One child is the "troublemaker," another is the "negotiator," another is "quiet." Changes in an individual's behavior affect every other member of the system; roles change until a new equilibrium is found. After a divorce, an older child may take on a more parentified role and become the "man of the family," whereas a younger child may take over the role of an irresponsible rebel. The birth of a new child, attainment of developmental milestones such as independent walking or the onset of nighttime fears, and the death of a grandparent are all changes that require renegotiation of roles within the family and have the potential for healthy adaptation or dysfunction.

The family system, in turn, functions within the larger systems of extended family, subculture, culture, and society. The ecologic model depicts these relationships as concentric circles, with the parent-child dyad at the center and the larger society at the periphery. Changes at any level are reflected in the levels above and below. The disappearance of well-paying blue-collar jobs from central cities is an obvious example of a societal change with profound effects on the family and children.

UNIFYING CONCEPTS: THE TRANSACTIONAL MODEL, RISK, AND RESILIENCE. Current thought has focused on understanding how biology and social interactions influence development. The transactional model proposes that the child's status at any point in time is a function of both biologic and social influences. The influences are bidirectional: biologic factors such as temperament and health status both affect the child-rearing environment and are affected by it (Fig. 8–1). For example, a premature infant may cry little and sleep for long periods; the infant's depressed parent may welcome this "good" behavior, setting up a cycle that leads to poor nutrition and slow growth. The child's "failure to thrive" may reinforce the parent's sense of failure as a parent. At a later stage, impulsivity and inattention associated with chronic undernutrition may interact with the parent's depression, leading to a referral for aggressive behavior. The "cause" of the aggression is not the prematurity, the undernutrition, or the maternal depression, but the interaction of all these factors.

Conversely, children with biologic risk factors may nevertheless do well developmentally if the child-rearing environment is supportive. For example, premature infants with electroencephalographic evidence of neurologic immaturity may be at increased risk of cognitive delay. However, this relationship

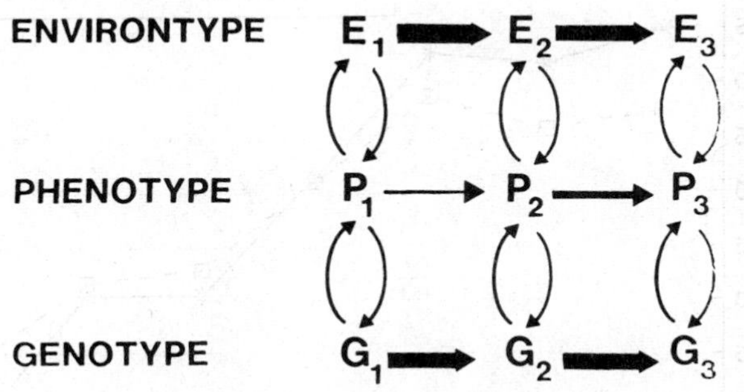

Figure 8–1. Transactional developmental model integrating environmental, genetic, and individual regulating systems. (From Sameroff AJ. *In:* Zeanah C [ed]: Handbook of Infant Mental Health. New York, Guilford Press, 1993, pp 29–41.)

will be true only when there is coexisting poor parent-child interaction. When parent-child interactions are optimal, the risk of developmental disability may be the same regardless of prematurity.

One implication of this model is that developmental assessment at any single point in time has limited ability to predict later outcome because at every stage the developmental trajectory is affected by both past and present conditions. To the extent that certain measures, such as IQ, tend to remain stable over time, this stability may well reflect the continuity of environmental conditions as much as it does the continuity of factors intrinsic to the child. The optimistic interpretation is that change is possible. Such an interpretation conflicts with popular tendencies to see certain early conditions, such as prenatal drug exposure, as "marking" children for life. Children growing up in poverty may be at "double jeopardy" because they face increased biologic risk factors such as lead poisoning, prematurity, and undernutrition as well as increased social risk factors such as overcrowding, lower maternal education, and exposure to violence (see Chapter 42).

The relative importance of environmental factors can be illustrated by a longitudinal study in which developmental outcome at age 13 yr was directly related to the number of social and family risk factors (Fig. 8–2). As the number of risk factors increases, the percentage of children who developmentally thrive decreases but never drops to zero. Protective factors may make some children resilient although not "invulnerable." These factors, like risk factors, may be either biologic (temperamental persistence, athletic talent) or social. The personal histories of children who "made it" despite great risks generally include at least one trusted adult—often a parent, grandparent, or teacher—with whom the child had a close relationship. The clinical assessment should include an enumeration not only of risk factors but of protective strengths as well.

DEVELOPMENTAL DOMAINS AND THEORIES OF EMOTION AND COGNITION. Another approach to child development tracks development within particular domains such as gross motor, fine motor, social, emotional, language, and cognition. Within each of these categories are developmental lines or sequences of changes leading up to particular attainments. One such line, leading from rolling to creeping to independent walking, is widely accepted. Others, such as the line leading to the development of conscience, are less recognized and more controversial.

The concept of a developmental line implies that the child passes though successive stages. The psychoanalytic theories of Sigmund Freud and Erik Erikson and the cognitive theory of Jean Piaget share the idea of stages as qualitatively different epochs in the development of emotion and cognition (Table 8–2). In contrast, the behavioral theory of Skinner relies less on qualitative change and more on the gradual modification of behavior or accumulation of knowledge.

Psychoanalytic Theories. At the core of Freudian theory is the idea of biologically determined drives. The core drive is sexual, broadly defined to include sensations that involve excitation or tension and satisfaction or release. The focus of the sexual drive shifts with maturation, defining discrete stages: oral (1st yr of life), anal (toddlerhood), oedipal (preschool), and genital (puberty and beyond) (see Table 8–2). At each stage, the drive comes into conflict with the social demands of civilization. The emotional health of the child and adult depends on the adequate resolution of these conflicts. The phase of *latency*, corresponding to middle childhood, is relatively free of psychosexual conflict, as the sexual drive is redirected (sublimated) to the achievement of social or external goals.

Controversy remains about many points. Latency may not be as conflict-free as once supposed. The nature of aggression is unclear: is it a primary drive or the result of frustration or feared loss? The consequences of unresolved early conflicts may or may not be lifelong, and progress may or may not require their "working through." Nonetheless, the Freudian legacy includes several concepts that are central to an understanding of emotional development: the importance of the child's inner life and sexuality; the normative existence of emotional conflict during childhood; and the possibility of emotional disturbance.

Erikson's chief contribution was to recast Freud's stages in terms of the emerging personality (see Table 8–2). The crisis that establishes the child's internal sense of either autonomy or shame and guilt corresponds with Freud's anal stage; the crisis that establishes a sense of either identity or role diffusion corresponds with Freud's genital stage (puberty). The stages mark the emergence of different issues as salient, although earlier issues remain important. Erikson recognized that these stages arise in the context of Western European societal expectations; in other cultures, the salient issues may be quite different.

One lasting contribution of Erikson's work is to call attention to the intrapersonal challenges facing children at different ages in a way that facilitates professional intervention. For example, knowing that the salient issue for school-age children is industry versus inferiority, the pediatrician can inquire about the child's experiences of mastery and failure and suggest ways to ensure adequate successes.

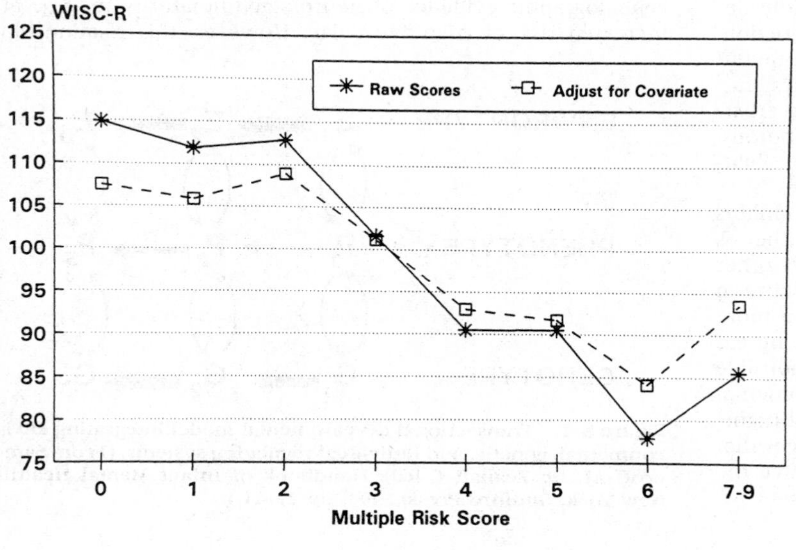

Figure 8–2. Relationship between mean IQ scores at 13 yr (both raw and adjusted for covariation of mother's IQ), as related to the number of risk factors. (From Sameroff AJ, Seifer R, Baldwin A, Baldwin C: Stability of intelligence from preschool to adolescence: the influence of social and family risk factors. Child Dev 64[1], 80–97, 1993, pp 29–41.)

■ **TABLE 8–2 Classic Stage Theories**

Theory	0–1 Infancy	2–3 Toddlerhood	3–6 Preschool	6–12 School Age	12–20 Adolescence
Freud: psychosexual	Oral	Anal	Oedipal	Latency	Adolescence
Erikson: psychosocial	Basic trust	Autonomy versus shame and doubt	Initiative versus guilt	Industry versus inferiority	Identity versus identity diffusion
Piaget: cognitive	Sensorimotor (stages I–IV)	Sensorimotor (stages V, VI)	Preoperational	Concrete operations	Formal operations

Piaget is synonymous with the study of cognitive development. A central tenet of Piagetian thought is that cognition is qualitatively different at different stages of development (see Table 8–2). During the *sensorimotor* stage, thoughts about the nature of objects and their relationships are acted out and tied to immediate sensations and manipulation. With the arrival of language, the nature of thinking changes dramatically; symbols increasingly take the place of things and actions. Preoperational, concrete operational, and formal operational stages correspond with the major periods of childhood: preschool, school age, and adolescence. At all stages, children are not passive recipients of knowledge but actively seek out experiences (assimilation) and use them to build implicit theories about how things work. Periodically, the child reorganizes these theories to fit the incoming data better (accommodation). The stages of cognitive reorganization can be mapped by observing children and by asking open-ended questions that make the implicit theories explicit.

Challenges to Piaget have included questions about the timing of various stages, the role of formal teaching, and the extent to which context may affect conclusions about cognitive stage. For example, children's thinking in the context of sibling relationships may be considerably more advanced than their thinking about inanimate objects; in many children formal operations appear well before puberty, the age postulated by Piaget. Of undeniable importance are Piaget's focus on cognition as a subject of empirical study, the universality of the progression of cognitive stages (even if details of timing are controversial), and the image of the child as actively and creatively interpreting the world.

Piaget's work is of special importance to pediatricians for three reasons: (1) it helps make sense of many common behaviors of infancy, such as the common exacerbations of sleep problems at 9 and 18 mo of age; (2) Piagetian observations often lend themselves to quick replication in the office, with little special equipment; and (3) open-ended questioning, based on Piaget's work, can provide insights into children's understanding of illness and hospitalization.

Behavioral Theory. The last major theory distinguishes itself by its complete lack of concern with the child's experience. Its sole focus is on observable behaviors and measurable factors that either increase or decrease the frequency with which these behaviors occur. No stages are implied: children, adults, and indeed animals all respond the same. In its simplest form, the behaviorist orientation asserts that behaviors that are positively reinforced occur more frequently; behaviors that are negatively reinforced or ignored occur less frequently.

The strengths of this position are its simplicity, wide applicability, and conduciveness to scientific verification. Environmental manipulation designed to reward wanted behaviors and punish or ignore unwanted ones may be the therapy of choice for behavior problems in cognitively limited children. A behavioral approach also lends itself to readily taught interventions for a variety of problems such as temper tantrums and nocturnal enuresis. In cases in which misbehavior is symptomatic of an underlying cognitive or emotional problem, however, an exclusive reliance on behavior therapy risks leaving the cause untreated.

Beckwith L, Parmelee A: EEG patterns of preterm infants, home environment, and later IQ. Child Dev 57:777, 1986.

Bronfenbrenner U: The Ecology of Human Development: Experiments by Nature and Design. Cambridge, MA, Harvard University Press, 1979.

Chess S, Thomas A: Temperament in Clinical Practice. New York, Guilford Press, 1986.

Erikson EH: Childhood and Society, 2nd ed. New York, WW Norton, 1963.

Hobson PR: Piaget: On the ways of knowing in childhood. *In:* Rutter M, Hersov L (eds): Child and Adolescent Psychiatry: Modern Approaches. Oxford, England, Blackwell Scientific, 1985, pp 191–203.

Parker S, Greer S, Zuckerman B: Double jeopardy: The impact of poverty on early child development. Pediatr Clin North Am 35:1227, 1988.

Vygotsky LS: Mind in Society: The Development of Higher Psychological Processes. Cambridge, MA, Harvard University Press, 1978.

CHAPTER 9

Fetal Growth and Development

The most dramatic events in growth and development occur before birth. These changes are overwhelmingly somatic: the transformation of a single cell into an infant. Behavioral and psychological developments in the fetus and the parents are also significant. The uterus, while offering a degree of protection, is permeable to social, psychological, and environmental influences such as maternal drug use. The complex interplay between these forces and the physical transformations occurring in utero shapes infants, as they appear at birth and throughout infancy, and parents.

SOMATIC DEVELOPMENT

Embryonic Period. Milestones of prenatal development are presented in Table 9–1. By 6 days postconceptual age, as implantation begins, the embryo consists of a spherical mass of cells with a central cavity (the blastocyst). By 2 wk, implantation is complete and the uteroplacental circulation has begun; the

■ **TABLE 9–1 Milestones of Prenatal Development**

Week	Developmental Events
1	Fertilization and implantation; beginning of embryonic period
2	Endoderm and ectoderm appear (bilaminar embryo)
3	First missed menstrual period; mesoderm appears (trilaminar embryo); somites begin to form
4	Neural folds fuse; folding of embryo into human-like shape; arm and leg buds appear; crown-rump length, 4–5 mm
5	Lens placodes, primitive mouth, digital rays on hands
6	Primitive nose, philtrum, primary palate; crown-rump length, 21–23 mm
7	Eyelids begin
8	Ovaries and testes distinguishable
9	*Fetal* period begins; crown-rump length, 5 cm; weight, 8 g
10	External genitalia distinguishable
20	Usual lower limit of viability; weight, 460 g; length, 19 cm
25	Third trimester begins; weight, 900 g; length, 25 cm
28	Eyes open; fetus turns head down; weight, 1,300 g
38	Term

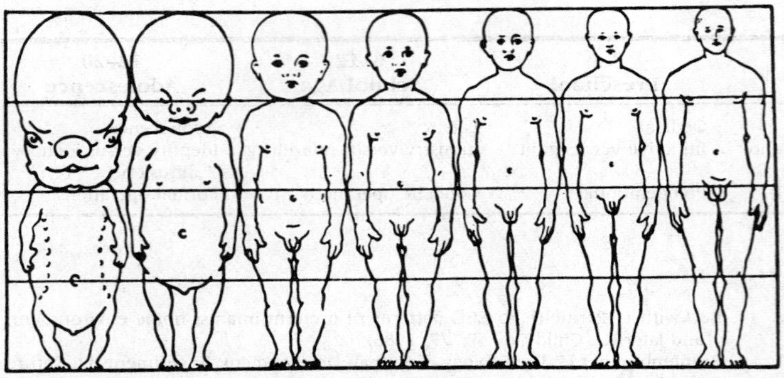

Figure 9–1. Changes in body proportions from the 2nd fetal mo to adulthood. (From Robbins WJ, Brody S, Hogan AG, et al: Growth. New Haven, Yale University Press, 1928. By permission of publisher.)

embryo has two distinct layers, endoderm and ectoderm, and the amnion has begun to form. By 3 wk, the third primary germ layer (mesoderm) has appeared, along with primitive neural tube and blood vessels. Paired heart tubes have begun to pump.

During the 4th through 8th wk, lateral folding of the embryologic plate, followed by growth at the cranial and caudal ends and the budding of arm and leg produces a human-like shape. Precursors of skeletal muscle and vertebrae (somites) appear, along with the branchial arches that will form the mandible, maxilla, palate, external ear, and other head and neck structures. Lens placodes appear, marking the site of future eyes; the brain grows rapidly. By the end of the 8th wk, as the embryonic period closes, the rudiments of all major organ systems have developed; the average embryo weighs 9 g and has a crown-rump length of 5 cm.

Fetal Period. From the 9th wk on (the fetal period), fetal somatic changes consist of increases in cell number and size and structural remodeling of several organ systems. Changes in body proportion are depicted in Figure 9–1. By 10 wk, the face is recognizably human. The midgut returns from the umbilical cord into the abdomen, rotating counterclockwise to bring the stomach, small intestine, and large intestine into their normal positions. By 12 wk, the gender of the external genitalia becomes clearly distinguishable. Lung development proceeds with the budding of bronchi, bronchioles, and successively smaller divisions. By 20–24 wk, primitive alveoli have formed and surfactant production has begun; before that time, the absence of alveoli renders the lung useless as an organ of gas exchange.

During the 3rd trimester, weight triples and length doubles as body stores of protein, fat, iron, and calcium increase (see Chapter 81). Low birthweight may be due to prematurity, intrauterine growth retardation (small for dates), or both (see Chapter 82.1).

NEUROLOGIC DEVELOPMENT. During the 3rd wk, a neural plate appears on the ectodermal surface of the trilaminar embryo. Infolding produces a neural tube that will become the central nervous system (CNS) and a neural crest that will become the peripheral nervous system. Neuroectodermal cells differentiate into neurons, astrocytes, oligodendrocytes, and ependymal cells, whereas microglial cells are derived from mesoderm. By the 5th wk, the three main subdivisions of forebrain, midbrain, and hindbrain are evident. The dorsal and ventral horns of the spinal cord have begun to form, along with the peripheral motor and sensory nerves. Myelinization begins at midgestation and continues throughout the 1st 2 yr of life.

By the end of the embryonic period (wk 1–8), the gross structure of the nervous system has been established. On a cellular level, the growth of axons and dendrites and the elaboration of synaptic connections continue at a rapid pace, making the CNS vulnerable to teratogenic or hypoxic influences throughout gestation. Rates of increase in DNA (a marker of cell number), overall brain weight, and cholesterol (a marker of myelinization) are shown in Figure 9–2. The prenatal and postnatal peaks of DNA probably represent rapid growth of neurons and glia, respectively.

BEHAVIORAL DEVELOPMENT. Muscle contractions first appear around 8 wk, soon followed by lateral flexion movements. By 13–14 wk, breathing and swallowing motions appear, and

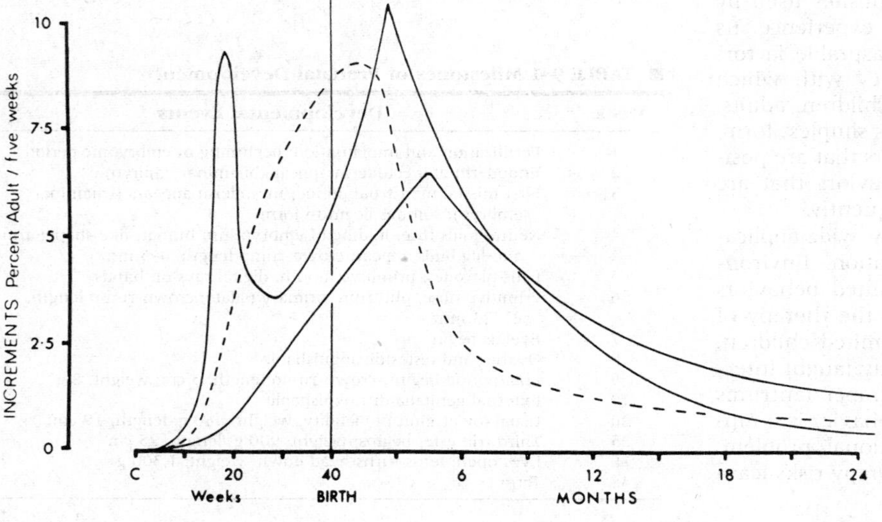

Figure 9–2. Velocity curves of the various components of human brain growth. Solid line with 2 peaks = DNA; dashed line = brain weight; single peak solid line = cholesterol. (From Brasel JA, Gruen RK. *In:* Falkner F, Tanner JM [eds]: Human Growth: A Comprehensive Treatise. New York, Plenum Press, 1986, pp 78–95.)

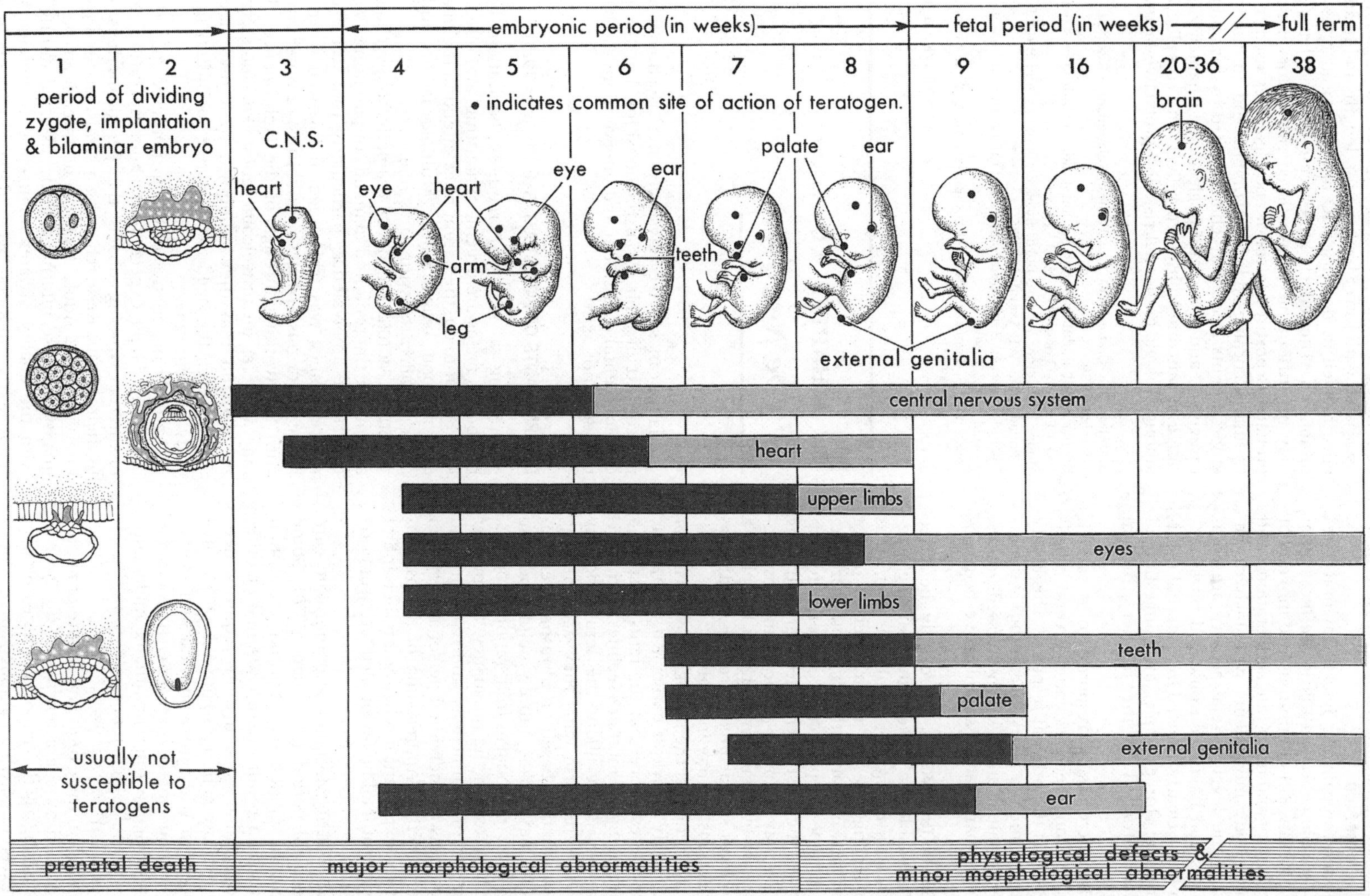

Figure 9–3. Schematic illustration of the sensitive or critical periods in prenatal development. Dark boxes denote highly sensitive periods; light boxes indicate states that are less sensitive to teratogens. (From Moore KL: Before We are Born: Basic Embryology and Birth Defects, 2nd ed. Philadelphia, WB Saunders, 1977.)

tactile stimulation elicits graceful movements. The grasp reflex appears at 17 wk and is well developed by 27 wk. Eye opening occurs around 26 wk. By midgestation, the full range of newborn movements can be observed.

During the 3rd trimester, three distinct fetal behavioral states have been described: (1) quiescence with little eye movement and little heart rate variability, (2) continuous eye movement with bursts of somatic activity and heart rate accelerations, and (3) continuous eye and body movements with tachycardia. Individual differences in the level of fetal activity are commonly noted by mothers and have been observed ultrasonographically. Fetal behavior is clearly affected by maternal medications and diet, increasing, for example, after ingestion of caffeine, and may be entrained to the mother's diurnal rhythms.

Fetal movement also increases in response to a sudden sound with a specific tone and decreases after several repetitions; a different tone elicits the original response. This ability to habituate to repeated stimuli, a form of learning, is diminished in neurologically impaired or physically stressed fetuses. Similar responses to visual and tactile stimuli have been observed.

PSYCHOLOGICAL CHANGES IN THE PARENTS. There may be three stages in the mother's psychological development during pregnancy. Stage 1 begins when the mother first learns that she is pregnant. Ambivalent feelings are the norm whether or not the pregnancy was planned. Elation at the thought of producing a baby and the wish to be the perfect parent compete with fears of inadequacy and of the lifestyle changes that mothering will impose. Old conflicts may resurface as the woman psychologically identifies with her own mother and with herself as a child. The father-to-be faces similar mixed feelings, and problems in the parental relationship may intensify.

Stage 2 begins with awareness of the infant's movements, or quickening, at approximately 20 wk or earlier with ultrasonic visualization. This palpable evidence that the fetus exists as a separate being often heightens the mother's feelings, both positive and negative. Parents worry about the fetus's healthy development and mentally rehearse what they will do if the child is malformed. Reassurances based on ultrasound examinations or amniocentesis may not be entirely helpful because the fears arise as much from irrational as from rational sources. During stage 3, toward the end of the pregnancy, the mother becomes aware of patterns of fetal activity and reactivity and begins to ascribe to her fetus an individual personality and an ability to survive independently. Appreciation of the psychological vulnerability of the expectant mother and father and of the powerful contribution of fetal behavior facilitates supportive clinical intervention.

THREATS TO FETAL DEVELOPMENT. Mortality and morbidity are highest during the prenatal period (see Chapter 78). Some 30% of pregnancies end in spontaneous abortion, most often during the 1st trimester as a result of chromosomal or other abnormalities. Major congenital malformations requiring neonatal surgical intervention occur in approximately 2% of live births. Teratogens associated with gross physical and mental abnormalities include various infectious agents (toxoplasma, rubella, syphilis), chemical agents (mercury, thalidomide, antiepileptic medications, ethanol), high temperature, and radiation (see Chapters 81 and 94).

For any potential teratogen, the extent and nature of teratogenic effects are determined by characteristics of the host as well as the dose and timing of the exposure. Rates of fetal alcohol syndrome are exceptionally high among Native Americans, for example, because of a possible inherited metabolic vulnerability. Organ systems are most vulnerable during periods of maximum growth and differentiation, generally during the first trimester (organogenesis). Figure 9–3 depicts sensitive periods during gestation for various organ systems.

Teratogenic effects may include not only gross physical malformation but also decreased growth and later cognitive or behavioral deficits. Prenatal exposure to cigarette smoke is associated with lower birthweight, length, and head circumference as well as decreased IQ and increased rates of learning disabilities. The effects of cocaine on the fetus and infant may be attributable to associated risk factors including other prenatal exposures (alcohol and cigarettes used in high doses by many cocaine-addicted women) and to "toxic" postnatal environments frequently characterized by instability, multiple caregivers, and abuse and neglect (see Chapter 92). The wide range of outcomes observed reflects the complex interactions among biologic and social risk and protective factors.

Brazelton TB, Cramer BG: The Earliest Relationship. Reading, MA, Addison-Wesley, 1990.

Hepper PG, Shahidullah S: Habituation in normal and Down's syndrome fetuses. Q J Exp Psychol *44*:305, 1992.

Moore KL: Before We Are Born: Basic Embryology and Birth Defects, 2nd ed. Philadelphia, WB Saunders, 1972.

Pillai M, James D: Behavioural states in normal mature human fetuses. Arch Dis Child *65*:39, 1990.

Zuckerman B, Frank D. Prenatal cocaine exposure: Nine years later. J Pediatr *124*:731, 1994.

CHAPTER 10
The Newborn

Infants can survive physically and psychologically only in the context of their social relationships. For the purposes of developmental assessment and intervention, the baby in isolation does not exist!

DETERMINANTS OF PARENTING (See Chapter 79.5)

Parenting a newborn requires dedication because the newborn's needs are urgent, exhausting, and often unclear. To know what to do, the parent must attend to the infant's signals and respond empathically. Multiple factors influence the parent's ability to assume this role.

PRENATAL FACTORS. Pregnancy is a period of psychological preparation for the profound demands of parenting. Most mothers experience ambivalence, particularly (but not exclusively) if the pregnancy was unplanned. If financial worries, physical illness, prior miscarriages or stillbirths, or other crises interfere with the working through of the ambivalence, the neonate may arrive as an unwelcome guest. For adolescent mothers, the demand that they relinquish their own developmental agenda (e.g., the need for an active social life) may be especially burdensome.

The early experience of being mothered may establish unconsciously held expectations about nurturing relationships, or internal working models, that permit mothers to "tune in" to their infants. Research using a semistructured psychological interview (the Adult Attachment Interview) has linked the quality of these internal models, assessed during pregnancy, with the quality of later infant-parent interactions. Mothers whose early childhoods were marked by traumatic separations, abuse, or neglect may find it especially difficult to provide consistent, responsive care. These mothers may re-enact their childhood experiences with their own infants as if they cannot conceive of the mother-child relationship any other way.

Social support during pregnancy is also important. A supportive relationship with the child's father predicts satisfaction in mothering. At the other extreme, conflict or abandonment by the father during pregnancy may undermine the mother's ability to become absorbed in her infant. After delivery, anticipation of an early return to work may make committing to the task at hand more difficult. A guarantee of 6 mo of unpaid maternity leave from work may help, although career and financial pressures often force an earlier return.

PERI- AND POSTPARTUM INFLUENCES. The continuous presence during labor of a woman trained to offer friendly support and encouragement (a doula) results in shorter labor, fewer obstetric complications, and reduced postpartum hospital stays. Skin-to-skin contact between mothers and infants immediately after birth may correlate with increases in the incidence of breastfeeding and duration of lactation. Increased contact over the succeeding several days may correlate with improved mother-infant interaction and decreased child abuse in the long term, although research findings have been inconclusive. The separation of mothers and infants does not inevitably lead to failed infant-parent relationships. Many fail-safe mechanisms may allow the mother-infant bond to survive separations in the early days and weeks. Early discharge from the maternity ward, often within the first 24 hr after delivery, may undermine bonding in cases in which the new mother is required to resume full responsibility for a busy household. Most new parents value even a brief period of uninterrupted time in which to get to know their new infants.

THE INFANT'S CONTRIBUTION

INTERACTIONAL ABILITIES. Almost immediately after birth, the neonate looks alert and readily suckles if given the opportunity. This first alert-awake period may be adversely modified by some maternal analgesics and anesthetics or fetal hypoxia. Nearsighted, the neonate has a fixed focal length of 8–12 in, approximately the distance from the breast to the mother's face, as well as an inborn visual preference for faces. Hearing is well developed, and infants preferentially turn toward a female voice. These innate abilities and predilections ensure that, when the mother gazes at her newborn, the gaze is likely to be returned. The initial period of social interaction, usually lasting about 40 min, is followed by a period of somnolence. After that, briefer periods of alertness or excitation alternate with sleep. If the mother misses the first alert-awake period (because she has been anesthetized), she may not experience as long a period of social interaction for several days.

MODULATION OF AROUSAL. Adaptation to extrauterine life requires rapid and profound physiologic changes, including aeration of the lungs, rerouting of the circulation, and activation of the intestinal tract. The necessary behavioral changes are no less profound. To obtain nourishment, to avoid hypo- or hyperthermia, and to ensure safety, the newborn must react appropriately to an expanded range of sensory stimuli. To do so, the infant must become aroused in response to stimulation but not so overaroused that behavior becomes random. Underaroused infants are not able to feed and interact; overaroused infants show signs of autonomic instability, including flushing or mottling, perioral pallor, hiccoughing, vomiting, uncontrolled limb movements, or inconsolable crying. The need to balance responsiveness to the external world against internal stability poses the central behavioral challenge for the newborn.

BEHAVIORAL STATES. The organization of infant behavior into discrete behavioral states may reflect the infant's inborn ability to regulate arousal. Six states have been described: quiet sleep, active sleep, drowsy, alert, fussy, and crying. In the alert state, infants visually fixate on objects or faces and follow them horizontally and (within a month) vertically; they also reliably turn toward a novel sound, as if searching for its source. When overstimulated, they may calm themselves by looking away, yawning, or sucking on their lips or hands, thereby increasing parasympathetic activity and reducing sympathetic nervous activity. The behavioral state determines the infant's muscle tone, spontaneous movement, electroencephalogram pattern, and response to stimuli. In active sleep, for example, the infant may show progressively less reaction to a repeated heel prick (habituation), whereas in the drowsy state the same stimulus may push the child into fussing or crying.

MUTUAL REGULATION. Parents actively participate in the infant's state regulation, alternately stimulating or soothing to prolong the social interaction. In turn, the parents are regulated by the infant's signals, responding, for example, with a letdown of milk (or with a bottle) in response to cries of hunger. Such interactions constitute a system directed toward furthering the infant's physiologic homeostasis and physical growth. At the same time, they form the basis for the emerging psychological relationship between parent and child. The infant comes to associate the presence of the parent with the pleasurable reduction of tension (as in feeding) and shows this preference by calming more quickly for the mother than for a stranger. This response, in turn, strengthens the mother's sense of efficacy and connection with her baby.

CLINICAL IMPLICATIONS: THE PHYSICIAN'S ROLE

Pediatric interventions to support healthy newborn development include (1) promoting optimal medical practices before, during, and after delivery; (2) assessing parent-infant interactions; and (3) teaching parents about their newborn's individual competencies and vulnerabilities.

OPTIMAL PRACTICES. A prenatal pediatric visit allows the pediatrician to assess potential problems of bonding (a tense spousal relationship) and sources of social support and to try to allay unrealistic fears. Supportive hospital policies include use of birthing rooms rather than sterile-looking delivery rooms; encouragement for the father or a trusted relative or friend to remain with the mother during labor or provision of a professional support person or doula; the practice of giving the newborn infant to the mother immediately after delivery or after brief stabilization and assessment; and placement of the newborn in the mother's room rather than in a central nursery. After discharge (often within 24 hr of delivery), home visits by nurses and lactation counselors may minimize early feeding problems and allow assessment of medical conditions that arise within the first week. Such family-focused policies may be particularly important for ill infants. For example, infants requiring transport to another hospital should be brought to see the mother first if at all possible. On discharge home, fathers can play an important role in protecting mothers from unnecessary visits and calls and in taking over household duties to allow the mothers to get to know their new infants without distractions.

ASSESSING PARENT-INFANT INTERACTIONS. Observation during a feeding or when infants are alert and "face to face" with parents can be revealing. It is normal for infants and parents to appear absorbed in one another. Infants who become overstimulated by the mother's voice or activity may turn away or appear to fall asleep, leading to a premature termination of the encounter. Alternatively, the infant may be alert and ready to interact, whereas the mother appears preoccupied.

TEACHING ABOUT INDIVIDUAL COMPETENCIES. The Newborn Behavior Assessment Scale (NBAS) provides a formal measure of the infant's neurodevelopmental competencies, including state control, autonomic reactivity, reflexes, habituation, and orientation (the ability to turn toward auditory and visual stimuli). This examination can also be used to demonstrate to the parents the infant's capabilities and vulnerabilities. Parents might learn that they need to undress the infant to increase the level of arousal or to swaddle the infant to contain random arm movements and reduce overstimulation. The NBAS can support the development of positive early parent-infant relationships and may prevent early problems that arise from misinterpretation of the infant's behavior. The effects of such early intervention, as with early physical contact, may be long term. Demonstration of the NBAS in the 1st wk of life has been shown to correlate with improvements in the care-taking environment months later.

Brazelton TB: The Neonatal Behavioral Assessment Scale. Philadelphia, JB Lippincott, 1973.
Klaus MH, Kennell JH: Bonding: The Beginnings of Parent-Infant Attachment. St. Louis, MO, CV Mosby, 1983.
Lyons-Ruth K, Zeanah CH: The family context of infant mental health: I. Affective development in the primary caregiving relationship. *In:* CH Zeanah (ed): Handbook of Infant Mental Health. New York, Guilford Press, 1993, pp 14–37.
MacFarlane JA, Smith DM, Garrow DH: The relationship between mother and neonate. *In:* Kitzinger S, Davis JA (eds): The Place of Birth. New York, Oxford University Press, 1978, pp 175–220.
Winnicott DW: The Maturational Processes and the Facilitating Environment. New York, International Universities Press, 1965.

CHAPTER 11

The First Year

Physical growth, maturation, acquisition of competence, and psychological reorganization occur rapidly during the 1st yr. These changes do not occur smoothly over time but rather in discontinuous bursts that qualitatively change the child's behavior. Physical growth during this period is rapid; growth parameters and normal ranges for attainable weight, length, and head circumference can be estimated as noted in Tables 11–1 and 11–2. Table 11–3 presents an overview of milestones in the domains of gross motor, fine motor, and cognitive development. Table 11–4 presents similar information arranged cross-sectionally. However, development in each domain affects the others.

AGE 0–2 MO

The biologic and psychological challenges facing neonates and their parents were described in Chapter 10. These consist of establishing effective feeding and a predictable sleep-wake cycle. In the course of accomplishing these tasks, infants and parents engage in significant social interaction, laying the foundation for cognitive and emotional development.

PHYSICAL DEVELOPMENT. The newborn's weight may drop 10% below birthweight in the 1st wk as a result of the excretion of excess extravascular fluid and possibly poor intake. Intake improves as colostrum is replaced by higher fat milk, as infants learn to latch on and suck more efficiently, and as mothers become more comfortable with feeding techniques. Infants should regain or exceed birthweight by 2 wk of age and should grow at approximately 30 g (1 oz)/day during the 1st mo (Table 11–5). Movements are largely uncontrolled, with the exception of eye gaze, head turning, and sucking. Smiling occurs involuntarily. Crying occurs in response to stimuli that may be obvious (a soiled diaper) but are often obscure. Crying normally peaks at about 6 wk of age, when healthy infants cry up to 3 hr a day, then decreases to 1 hr or less by 3 mo.

Behavioral states have been described (see Chapter 9). Initially, sleep and wakefulness are evenly distributed over the 24 hr (Fig. 11–1). Neurologic maturation accounts for the consolidation of sleep periods into longer and longer blocks. Learning plays a role as well. Infants whose parents are consistently more interactive and stimulating during the day learn to concentrate their sleeping during the night. By 2 mo of age, most infants are waking briefly two or three times to feed; some sleep 6 hr or more at a stretch.

COGNITIVE DEVELOPMENT. Caretaking activities provide visual, tactile, olfactory, and auditory stimuli; all of these stimuli play an important role in the development of cognition. Studies of habituation and gaze preference provide insights into how infants interpret these stimuli. Infants habituate to the familiar, attending less and less to a stimulus that is repeated multiple times and then increasing their attention when the stimulus changes. Experiments using habituation and renewed attention as outcomes show that infants can differentiate among similar patterns, colors, and consonants. They can recognize facial expressions (smiles) as similar, even when they appear on different faces. They also can match abstract properties of stimuli, such as contour, intensity, or temporal pattern across sensory modalities. For example, 3-wk-old infants can tell whether a spoken voice corresponds with the movements of the lips on a videotape. Blindfolded and given a bumpy pacifier to suck, they subsequently gaze longer at the bumpy pacifier than at a smooth one when both are presented visually.

Such studies suggest that infants are able to perceive objects and events as coherent, even while noting aspects that are discrepant. These abilities allow infants to sort stimuli into meaningful sets: a set of stimuli that correspond to sucking as well as others that correspond to sucking a bottle, sucking a pacifier, and sucking a finger. Infants appear to seek stimuli actively as though satisfying an innate need to make sense of the world.

EMOTIONAL DEVELOPMENT. Basic trust, the first of Erikson's psychosocial stages, develops as infants learn that their urgent needs are regularly met. The consistent availability of a trusted adult creates the conditions for a secure attachment. Infants who are consistently picked up and held in response to distress cry less at 1 yr and show less aggressive behavior at 2 yr.

The emotional significance of any experience depends on the individual child's temperament as well as the parent's responses. Consider the impact of different feeding schedules. Hunger generates increasing tension; as the urgency peaks, the infant cries, the parent arrives with a bottle or breast, and the tension dissipates. Infants fed "on demand" consistently experience this link between their distress, the arrival of the parent, and the relief from hunger. Most infants fed on a fixed schedule quickly adapt their hunger cycle to the schedule. Those who cannot because they are temperamentally prone to irregular biologic rhythms experience periods of unrelieved hunger as well as unwanted feedings when they already feel full. Similarly, infants fed at the parent's convenience, with neither attention to the infant's hunger cues nor a fixed sched-

■ **TABLE 11–1 Formulas for Approximate Average Height and Weight of Normal Infants and Children**

Weight	Kilograms	(Pounds)
(a) At birth	3.25	(7)
(b) 3–12 mo	$\frac{\text{age (mo)} + 9}{2}$	(age [mo] + 11)
(c) 1–6 yr	age (yr) × 2 + 8	(age [yr] × 5 + 17)
(d) 7–12 yr	$\frac{\text{age (yr)} \times 7 - 5}{2}$	(age [yr] × 7 + 5)
Height	**Centimeters**	**(Inches)**
(e) At birth	50	(20)
(f) At 1 yr	75	(30)
(g) 2–12 yr	age (yr) × 6 + 77	(age [yr] × 2½ + 30)

■ TABLE 11–2 Length, Weight, and Head Circumference by Age for Boys and Girls: Birth to 36 Mo

	Boys: Percentiles								Girls: Percentiles						
	5th	*10th*	*25th*	*50th*	*75th*	*90th*	*95th*	**Measurement**	*5th*	*10th*	*25th*	*50th*	*75th*	*90th*	*95th*
	46.4	47.5	49.0	50.5	51.8	53.5	54.4	Length, mm	45.4	46.5	48.2	49.9	51.0	52.0	52.9
	(18¼)	(18¾)	(19¼)	(20)	(20½)	(21)	(21½)	(in)	(17¾)	(18¼)	(19)	(19¾)	(20)	(20½)	(20¾)
Birth	2.54	2.78	3.00	3.27	3.64	3.82	4.15	Weight, kg	2.36	2.58	2.93	3.23	3.52	3.64	3.81
	(5½)	(6¼)	(6½)	(7¼)	(8)	(8½)	(9¼)	(lb)	(5¼)	(5¾)	(6½)	(7)	(7¾)	(8)	(8½)
	32.6	33.0	33.9	34.8	35.6	36.6	37.2	Head C, cm	32.1	32.9	33.5	34.3	34.8	35.5	35.9
	(12¾)	(13)	(13¼)	(13¾)	(14)	(14½)	(14¾)	(in)	(12¾)	(13)	(13¼)	(13½)	(13¾)	(14)	(14¼)
	50.4	51.3	53.0	54.6	56.2	57.7	58.6	Length, cm	49.2	50.2	51.9	53.5	54.9	56.1	56.9
	(19¾)	(20¼)	(20¾)	(21½)	(22¼)	(22¾)	(23)	(in)	(19¼)	(19¾)	(20½)	(21)	(21½)	(22)	(22½)
1 mo	3.16	3.43	3.82	4.29	4.75	5.14	5.38	Weight, kg	2.97	3.22	3.59	3.98	4.36	4.65	4.92
	(7)	(7½)	(8½)	(9½)	(10½)	(11¼)	(11¾)	(lb)	(6½)	(7)	(8)	(8¾)	(9½)	(10¼)	(10¾)
	34.9	35.4	36.2	37.2	38.1	39.0	39.6	Head C, cm	34.2	34.8	35.6	36.4	37.1	37.8	38.3
	(13¾)	(14)	(14¼)	(14¾)	(15)	(15¼)	(15½)	(in)	(13½)	(13¾)	(14)	(14¼)	(14½)	(15)	(15)
	56.7	57.7	59.4	61.1	63.0	64.5	65.4	Length, cm	55.4	56.2	57.8	59.5	61.2	62.7	63.4
	(22¼)	(22¾)	(23½)	(24)	(24¾)	(25½)	(25¾)	(in)	(21¾)	(22¼)	(22¾)	(23½)	(24)	(24¾)	(25)
3 mo	4.43	4.78	5.32	5.98	6.56	7.14	7.37	Weight, kg	4.18	4.47	4.88	5.40	5.90	6.39	6.74
	(9¾)	(10½)	(11¾)	(13¼)	(14½)	(15¾)	(16¼)	(lb)	(9¼)	(9¾)	(10¾)	(12)	(13)	(14)	(14¾)
	38.4	38.9	39.7	40.6	41.7	42.5	43.1	Head C, cm	37.3	37.8	38.7	39.5	40.4	41.2	41.7
	(15)	(15¼)	(15¾)	(16)	(16½)	(16¾)	(17)	(in)	(14¾)	(15)	(15¼)	(15½)	(16)	(16¼)	(16½)
	63.4	64.4	66.1	67.8	69.7	71.3	72.3	Length, cm	61.8	62.6	64.2	65.9	67.8	69.4	70.2
	(25)	(25¼)	(26)	(26¾)	(27½)	(28)	(28½)	(in)	(24¼)	(24¾)	(25¼)	(26)	(26¾)	(27¼)	(27¾)
6 mo	6.20	6.61	7.20	7.85	8.49	9.10	9.46	Weight, kg	5.79	6.12	6.60	7.21	7.83	8.38	8.73
	(13¾)	(14½)	(15¾)	(17¼)	(18¾)	(20)	(20¾)	(lb)	(12¾)	(13½)	(14½)	(16)	(17¼)	(18½)	(19¼)
	41.5	42.0	42.8	43.8	44.7	45.6	46.2	Head C, cm	40.3	40.9	41.6	42.4	43.3	44.1	44.6
	(16¼)	(16½)	(16¾)	(17¼)	(17½)	(18)	(18¼)	(in)	(15¾)	(16)	(16½)	(16¾)	(17)	(17¼)	(17½)
	68.0	69.1	70.6	72.3	74.0	75.9	77.1	Length, cm	66.1	67.0	68.7	70.4	72.4	74.0	75.0
	(26¾)	(27¼)	(27¾)	(28½)	(29¼)	(30)	(30¼)	(in)	(26)	(26½)	(27)	(27¾)	(28½)	(29¼)	(29½)
9 mo	7.52	7.95	8.56	9.18	9.88	10.49	10.93	Weight, kg	7.00	7.34	7.89	8.56	9.24	9.83	10.17
	(16½)	(17½)	(18¾)	(20¼)	(21¾)	(23¼)	(24)	(lb)	(15½)	(16¼)	(17½)	(18¾)	(20¼)	(21¾)	(22½)
	43.5	44.0	44.8	45.8	46.6	47.5	48.1	Head C, cm	42.3	42.8	43.5	44.3	45.1	46.0	46.4
	(17¼)	(17¼)	(17¾)	(18)	(18¼)	(18¾)	(19)	(in)	(16¾)	(16¾)	(17¼)	(17½)	(17¾)	(18)	(18¼)
	71.7	72.8	74.3	76.1	77.7	79.8	81.2	Length, cm	69.8	70.8	72.4	74.3	76.3	78.0	79.1
	(28¼)	(28¾)	(29¼)	(30)	(30½)	(31½)	(32)	(in)	(27½)	(27¾)	(28½)	(29¼)	(30)	(30¾)	(31¼)
12 mo	8.43	8.84	9.49	10.15	10.91	11.54	11.99	Weight, kg	7.84	8.19	8.81	9.53	10.23	10.87	11.24
	(18½)	(19½)	(21)	(22½)	(24)	(25½)	(26½)	(lb)	(17¼)	(18)	(19½)	(21)	(22½)	(24)	(24¾)
	44.8	45.3	46.1	47.0	47.9	48.8	49.3	Head C, cm	43.5	44.1	44.8	45.6	46.4	47.2	47.6
	(17¾)	(17¾)	(18¼)	(18½)	(18¾)	(19¼)	(19½)	(in)	(17¼)	(17¼)	(17¾)	(18)	(18¼)	(18½)	(18¾)
	77.5	78.7	80.5	82.4	84.3	86.6	88.1	Length, cm	76.0	77.2	78.8	80.9	83.0	85.0	86.1
	(30½)	(31)	(31¾)	(32½)	(33¼)	(34)	(34¾)	(in)	(30)	(30½)	(31)	(31¾)	(32¾)	(33½)	(34)
18 mo	9.59	9.92	10.67	11.47	12.31	13.05	13.44	Weight, kg	8.92	9.30	10.04	10.82	11.55	12.30	12.76
	(21¼)	(21¾)	(23½)	(25¼)	(27¼)	(28¾)	(29½)	(lb)	(19¾)	(20½)	(22¼)	(23¾)	(25½)	(27)	(28¼)
	46.3	46.7	47.4	48.4	49.3	50.1	50.6	Head C, cm	45.0	45.6	46.3	47.1	47.9	48.6	49.1
	(18¼)	(18½)	(18¾)	(19)	(19½)	(19¾)	(20)	(in)	(17¾)	(18)	(18¼)	(18½)	(18¾)	(19¼)	(19¼)
	82.3	83.5	85.6	87.6	89.9	92.2	93.8	Length, cm	81.3	82.5	84.2	86.5	88.7	90.8	92.0
	(32½)	(32¾)	(33¾)	(34½)	(35½)	(36¼)	(37)	(in)	(32)	(32½)	(33¼)	(34)	(35)	(35¾)	(36¼)
24 mo	10.54	10.85	11.65	12.59	13.44	14.29	14.70	Weight, kg	9.87	10.26	11.10	11.90	12.74	13.57	14.08
	(23¼)	(24)	(25¾)	(27¾)	(29¾)	(31½)	(32½)	(lb)	(21¾)	(22½)	(24½)	(26¼)	(28)	(30)	(31)
	47.3	47.7	48.3	49.2	50.2	51.0	51.4	Head C, cm	46.1	46.5	47.3	48.1	48.8	49.6	50.1
	(18½)	(18¾)	(19)	(19¼)	(19¾)	(20)	(20¼)	(in)	(18¼)	(18¼)	(18½)	(19)	(19¼)	(19½)	(19¾)
	87.0	88.2	90.1	92.3	94.6	97.0	98.7	Length, cm	86.0	87.0	88.9	91.3	93.7	95.6	96.9
	(34¼)	(34¾)	(35½)	(36¼)	(37¼)	(38¼)	(38¾)	(in)	(33¾)	(34¼)	(35)	(36)	(37)	(37¾)	(38¼)
30 mo	11.44	11.80	12.63	13.67	14.51	15.47	15.97	Weight, kg	10.78	11.21	12.11	12.93	13.93	14.81	15.35
	(25¼)	(26)	(27¾)	(30¼)	(32)	(34)	(35¼)	(lb)	(23¾)	(24¾)	(26¾)	(28½)	(30¾)	(32¾)	(33¾)
	48.0	48.4	49.1	49.9	51.0	51.7	52.2	Head C, cm	47.0	47.3	48.0	48.8	49.4	50.3	50.8
	(19)	(19)	(19¼)	(19¾)	(20)	(20¼)	(20½)	(in)	(18½)	(18½)	(19)	(19¼)	(19½)	(19¾)	(20)
	91.2	92.4	94.2	96.5	98.9	101.4	103.1	Length, cm	90.0	91.0	93.1	95.6	98.1	100.0	101.5
	(36)	(36½)	(37)	(38)	(39)	(40)	(40½)	(in)	(35½)	(35¾)	(36¾)	(37¾)	(38½)	(39¼)	(40)
36 mo	12.26	12.69	13.58	14.69	15.59	16.66	17.28	Weight, kg	11.60	12.07	12.99	13.93	15.03	15.97	16.54
	(27)	(28)	(30)	(32½)	(34½)	(36¾)	(38)	(lb)	(25½)	(26½)	(28¾)	(30¾)	(33¼)	(35¼)	(36½)
	48.6	49.0	49.7	50.5	51.5	52.3	52.8	Head C, cm	47.6	47.9	48.5	49.3	50.0	50.8	51.4
	(19¼)	(19¼)	(19½)	(20)	(20¼)	(20½)	(20¾)	(in)	(18¾)	(18¾)	(19)	(19½)	(19¾)	(20)	(20¼)

These data are those of the National Center for Health Statistics (NCHS), Health Resources Administration, Department of Health, Education, and Welfare. They were based on studies of The Fels Research Institute. Yellow Springs, Ohio. Metric data have been smoothed by a least-squares cubic spline technique. For details see Hamill PVV, Drizd TA, Johnson CL, et al: NCHS growth curves for children, birth–18 yr. United States Vital Health Statistics 1977 (Nov 165):1–1V, pp 1–74, 1979.

■ TABLE 11–3 Developmental Milestones in the First 2 Yr of Life

Milestone	Average Age of Attainment (mo)	Developmental Implications
Gross Motor		
Head steady in sitting	2.0	Allows more visual interaction
Pull to sit, no head lag	3.0	Muscle tone
Hands together in midline	3.0	Self-discovery
Asymmetric tonic neck reflex gone	4.0	Child can inspect hands in midline
Sits without support	6.0	Increasing exploration
Rolls back to stomach	6.5	Truncal flexion, risk of falls
Walks alone	12.0	Exploration, control of proximity to parents
Runs	16.0	Supervision more difficult
Fine Motor		
Grasps rattle	3.5	Object use
Reaches for objects	4.0	Visuomotor coordination
Palmar grasp gone	4.0	Voluntary release
Transfers object hand to hand	5.5	Comparison of objects
Thumb-finger grasp	8.0	Able to explore small objects
Turns pages of book	12.0	Increasing autonomy during book time
Scribbles	13.0	Visuomotor coordination
Builds tower of two cubes	15.0	Uses objects in combination
Builds tower of six cubes	22.0	Requires visual, gross, and fine motor coordination
Communication and Language		
Smiles in response to face, voice	1.5	Child more active social participant
Monosyllabic babble	6.0	Experimentation with sound, tactile sense
Inhibits to "no"	7.0	Response to tone (nonverbal)
Follows one-step command with gesture	7.0	Nonverbal communication
Follows one-step command without gesture (e.g., "Give it to me")	10.0	Verbal receptive language
Speaks first real word	12.0	Beginning of labeling
Speaks 4–6 words	15.0	Acquisition of object and personal names
Speaks 10–15 words	18.0	Acquisition of object and personal names
Speaks two-word sentences (e.g., "Mommy shoe")	19.0	Beginning grammaticization, corresponds with 50+ word vocabulary
Cognitive		
Stares momentarily at spot where object disappeared (e.g., yarn ball dropped)	2.0	Lack of object permanence (out of sight, out of mind)
Stares at own hand	4.0	Self-discovery, cause and effect
Bangs two cubes	8.0	Active comparison of objects
Uncovers toy (after seeing it hidden)	8.0	Object permanence
Egocentric pretend play (e.g., pretends to drink from cup)	12.0	Beginning symbolic thought
Uses stick to reach toy	17.0	Able to link actions to solve problems
Pretend play with doll (gives doll bottle)	17.0	Symbolic thought

ule, cannot consistently experience feeding as the pleasurable reduction of tension. These infants often show increased irritability and physiologic instability (spitting, diarrhea, poor weight gain) as well as later behavioral problems.

Implications for Parents and Pediatricians. Success or failure in establishing feeding and sleep cycles determines parents' feelings of efficacy despite the unquestionable importance of infant temperament. When things go well, anxiety, ambivalence, and the exhaustion of the early weeks relent. With physical recovery from delivery and endocrinologic normalization, the mild postpartum depression that affects some 50% of mothers ("baby blues") passes. If sad, overwhelmed, anxious feelings persist, the possibility of true postpartum depression needs to be considered.

AGE 2–6 MO

At about 2 mo, the emergence of voluntary (social) smiles and increasing eye contact mark a change in the parent-child relationship, heightening the parents' sense of being loved back. Over the next months, the infant's range of motoric and social control and cognitive engagement increases dramatically. Mutual regulation takes the form of complex social interchanges.

PHYSICAL DEVELOPMENT. Between 3 and 4 mo, the rate of growth slows to approximately 20 g/day (see Table 11–5 and Figs. 12–1 and 12–2). Early reflexes that limited voluntary movement recede. The disappearance of the asymmetric tonic neck reflex means that infants can roll over and also begin to examine objects in the midline and manipulate them with both hands. The waning of the early grasp reflex allows them both to hold objects and voluntarily to let them go. A novel object may elicit purposeful, although inefficient, reaching. Increasing control of truncal flexion makes intentional rolling possible. Head control improves, allowing the infant to gaze across at things rather than merely up and also to begin taking food from a spoon. At the same time, maturation of the visual system allows much greater depth of field.

Total sleep requirements are approximately 14–16 hr/day, with about 9–10 hr concentrated at night; about 70% of infants sleep for a 6- to 8-hr stretch by age 6 mo (see Fig. 11–1). By 4–6 mo, the sleep electroencephalogram shows a mature pattern, with demarcation of rapid eye movement (REM) and four stages of non-REM sleep. The sleep cycle remains short, only 50–60 min, compared with the adult cycle, approximately 90 min. As a result, infants rise to light sleep or wake frequently during the night, setting the stage for behavioral sleep problems.

COGNITIVE DEVELOPMENT. The overall effect of these developments is a qualitative change in the infant. Four-mo-old infants are described as "hatching" socially, becoming interested in a wider world. During feeding, the infant no longer focuses

■ **TABLE 11–4 Emerging Patterns of Behavior During the 1st Yr of Life***

	Neonatal Period (1st 4 Wk)
Prone:	Lies in flexed attitude; turns head from side to side; head sags on ventral suspension
Supine:	Generally flexed and a little stiff
Visual:	May fixate face or light in line of vision; "doll's-eye" movement of eyes on turning of the body
Reflex:	Moro response active; stepping and placing reflexes; grasp reflex active
Social:	Visual preference for human face
	At 4 Wk
Prone:	Legs more extended; holds chin up; turns head; head lifted momentarily to plane of body on ventral suspension
Supine:	Tonic neck posture predominates; supple and relaxed; head lags on pull to sitting position
Visual:	Watches person; follows moving object
Social:	Body movements in cadence with voice of other in social contact; beginning to smile
	At 8 Wk
Prone:	Raises head slightly farther; head sustained in plane of body on ventral suspension
Supine:	Tonic neck posture predominates; head lags on pull to sitting position
Visual:	Follows moving object 180 degrees
Social:	Smiles on social contact; listens to voice and coos
	At 12 Wk
Prone:	Lifts head and chest, arms extended; head above plane of body on ventral suspension
Supine:	Tonic neck posture predominates; reaches toward and misses objects; waves at toy
Sitting:	Head lag partially compensated on pull to sitting position; early head control with bobbing motion; back rounded
Reflex:	Typical Moro response has not persisted; makes defensive movements or selective withdrawal reactions
Social:	Sustained social contact; listens to music; says "aah, ngah"
	At 16 Wk
Prone:	Lifts head and chest, head in approximately vertical axis; legs extended
Supine:	Symmetric posture predominates, hands in midline; reaches and grasps objects and brings them to mouth
Sitting:	No head lag on pull to sitting position; head steady, tipped forward; enjoys sitting with full truncal support
Standing:	When held erect, pushes with feet
Adaptive:	Sees pellet, but makes no move to it
Social:	Laughs out loud; may show displeasure if social contact is broken; excited at sight of food
	At 28 Wk
Prone:	Rolls over; pivots; crawls or creep-crawls (Knobloch)
Supine:	Lifts head; rolls over; squirming movements
Sitting:	Sits briefly, with support of pelvis; leans forward on hands; back rounded
Standing:	May support most of weight; bounces actively
Adaptive:	Reaches out for and grasps large object; transfers objects from hand to hand; grasp uses radial palm; rakes at pellet
Language:	Polysyllabic vowel sounds formed
Social:	Prefers mother; babbles; enjoys mirror; responds to changes in emotional content of social contact
	At 40 Wk
Sitting:	Sits up alone and indefinitely without support, back straight
Standing:	Pulls to standing position; "cruises" or walks holding on to furniture
Motor:	Creeps or crawls
Adaptive:	Grasps objects with thumb and forefinger; pokes at things with forefinger; picks up pellet with assisted pincer movement; uncovers hidden toy; attempts to retrieve dropped object; releases object grasped by other person
Language:	Repetitive consonant sounds (mama, dada)
Social:	Responds to sound of name; plays peek-a-boo or pat-a-cake; waves bye-bye
	At 52 Wk (1 Yr)
Motor:	Walks with one hand held (48 wk); rises independently, takes several steps (Knobloch)
Adaptive:	Picks up pellet with unassisted pincer movement of forefinger and thumb; releases object to other person on request or gesture
Language:	A few words besides "mama," "dada"
Social:	Plays simple ball game; makes postural adjustment to dressing

**Data are derived from those of Gesell (as revised by Knobloch), Shirley, Provence, Wolf, Bailey, and others.*

■ **TABLE 11–5 Growth and Caloric Requirements**

Age	Approximate Daily Weight Gain (g)	Approximate Monthly Weight Gain	Growth in Length (cm/mo)	Growth in Head Circumference (cm/mo)	Recommended Daily Allowance (kcal/kg/day)
0–3 mo	30	2 lb	3.5	2.00	115
3–6 mo	20	1¼ lb	2.0	1.00	110
6–9 mo	15	1 lb	1.5	0.50	100
9–12 mo	12	13 oz	1.2	0.50	100
1–3 yr	8	8 oz	1.0	0.25	100
4–6 yr	6	6 oz	3 cm/yr	1 cm/yr	90–100

Adapted from National Research Council, Food and Nutrition Board: Recommended Daily Allowances. Washington, DC, National Academy of Sciences, 1989; Frank D, Silva M, Needlman R: Failure to thrive: Myth and method. Contemp Pediatr 10:114, 1993.

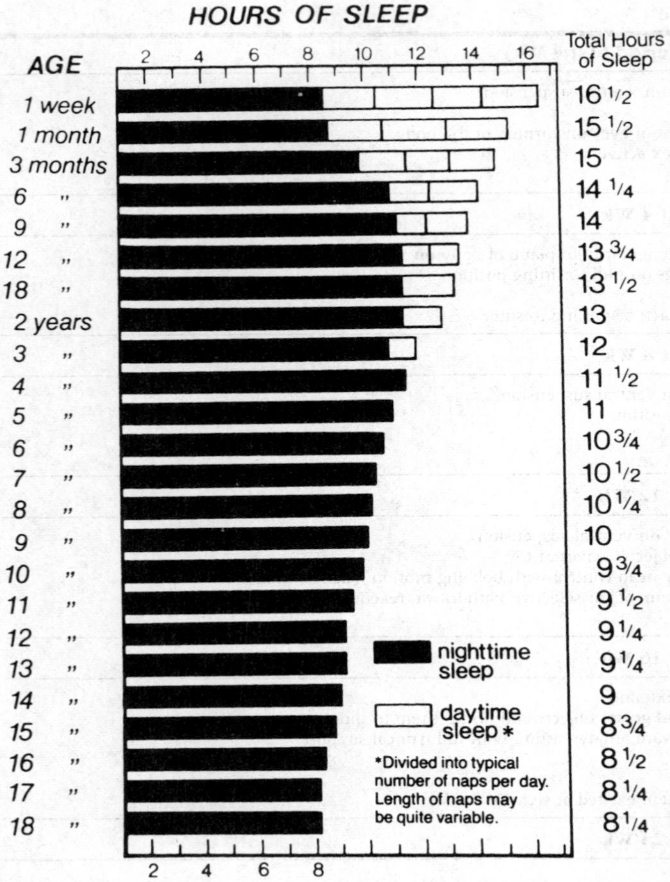

Figure 11–1. Typical sleep requirements in childhood. (From Ferber R: Solve Your Child's Sleep Problems. New York, Simon and Schuster, 1985.)

exclusively on the mother but becomes distracted; in the mother's arms, the infant may literally turn around, preferring to face outward.

Infants at this age also explore their own bodies, staring intently at their hands, vocalizing, blowing bubbles, and touching their ears, cheeks, or genitals. These explorations represent an early stage in the understanding of cause and effect as the infant learns that voluntary muscle movements generate predictable tactile and visual sensations. They also play a role in the emergence of a sense of self. Through frequent repetition, the infant comes to link certain sensations. The feeling of holding up the hand and wiggling the fingers always accompanies the sight of the fingers moving. Such "self" sensations are consistently linked and reproducible at will. In contrast, sensations that come to be classed as "nonself" occur intermittently and in varying combinations. The sound, smell, and feel of mother sometimes appears promptly in response to crying but sometimes does not.

EMOTIONAL DEVELOPMENT AND COMMUNICATION. The outward-looking baby interacts with increasing sophistication and range. The primary emotions of anger, joy, interest, fear, disgust, and surprise appear in appropriate contexts as distinct facial expressions. Face to face with a trusted adult, the infant and adult match affective expressions about 30% of the time; the intensity of their smiling, eye widening, and lip puckering rises and falls together. Every few seconds, as excitement builds, the infant turns away, settles, and then returns to the interaction. If the parent turns away, the infant leans forward, reaches, or in other ways tries to get the adult involved again; if that fails, the infant cries angrily.

Infants of depressed parents show a different pattern, spending less time in coordinated movement with their parents and making fewer efforts to re-engage. Rather than anger, they show sadness and a loss of energy when the parents continue to be unavailable. Such face-to-face behavior reveals the infant's ability to share emotional states, the first step in the development of communication; it also shows infants' (and parents') developing expectations about social relationships.

IMPLICATIONS FOR PARENTS AND PEDIATRICIANS. Motoric and sensory maturation makes the infant at 3–6 mo an exciting interactive partner, at once cuter and more appealing but also more separate. Some parents experience the 4-mo-old's outward turning as a rejection, secretly fearing that their infants no longer love them. For most parents, however, this is a happy period. The intensely cute infant of the baby food advertisements, pictured prone with the head and chest held up, is about 5 mo old. Most parents excitedly report that they can hold "conversations" with their infants, taking turns vocalizing and listening. Pediatricians share in the enjoyment, as the 4-mo-old flirts and coos. If this visit does not feel joyful and relaxed,

■ TABLE 11–6 Chronology of Human Dentition of Primary or Deciduous and Secondary or Permanent Teeth*

	Calcification		Age at Eruption		Age at Shedding	
Primary Teeth	*Begins at*	*Complete at*	*Maxillary*	*Mandibular*	*Maxillary*	*Mandibular*
Central incisors	5th fetal mo	18–24 mo	6–8 mo	5–7 mo	7–8 yr	6–7 yr
Lateral incisors	5th fetal mo	18–24 mo	8–11 mo	7–10 mo	8–9 yr	7–8 yr
Cuspids (canines)	6th fetal mo	30–36 mo	16–20 mo	16–20 mo	11–12 yr	9–11 yr
First molars	5th fetal mo	24–30 mo	10–16 mo	10–16 mo	10–11 yr	10–12 yr
Second molars	6th fetal mo	36 mo	20–30 mo	20–30 mo	10–12 yr	11–13 yr
Secondary Teeth						
Central incisors	3–4 mo	9–10 yr	7–8 yr	6–7 yr		
Lateral incisors	Max, 10–12 mo Mand, 3–4 mo	10–11 yr	8–9 yr	7–8 yr		
Cuspids (canines)	4–5 mo	12–15 yr	11–12 yr	9–11 yr		
First premolars (bicuspids)	18–21 mo	12–13 yr	10–11 yr	10–12 yr		
Second premolars (bicuspids)	24–30 mo	12–14 yr	10–12 yr	11–13 yr		
First molars	Birth	9–10 yr	6–7 yr	6–7 yr		
Second molars	30–36 mo	14–16 yr	12–13 yr	12–13 yr		
Third molars	Max, 7–9 yr Mand, 8–10 yr	18–25 yr	17–22 yr	17–22 yr		

Max = maxillary; Mand = mandibular.
**Adapted from chart prepared by PK Losch, Harvard School of Dental Medicine, who provided the data for this chart.*

causes such as social stress, family dysfunction, parental mental illness, or problems in the infant-parent relationship should be sought.

AGE 6–12 MO

Months 6–12 bring increased mobility and exploration of the inanimate world, advances in cognitive understanding and communicative competence, and new tensions around the themes of attachment and separation. The infant develops will and intentions, characteristics that most parents welcome but still find challenging to manage.

PHYSICAL DEVELOPMENT. Growth slows more (see Table 11–5 and Figs. 12–1 and 12–2). The ability to sit unsupported (about 7 mo) and to pivot while sitting (around 9–10 mo) provides increasing opportunities to manipulate several objects at a time and to experiment with novel combinations of objects. These explorations are aided by the emergence of a pincer grasp (around 9 mo). Many infants begin crawling and pulling to stand around 8 mo and walk before their first birthday either independently or in a walker. Motor achievements correlate with increasing myelinization and cerebellar growth. These ambulatory achievements expand the infant's exploratory range and create new physical dangers as well as opportunities for learning. Tooth eruption occurs, usually starting with the mandibular central incisors (Table 11–6). Tooth development also reflects, in part, skeletal maturation and bone age (Table 11–7).

COGNITIVE DEVELOPMENT. At first, everything goes into the mouth; in time, novel objects are picked up, inspected, passed from hand to hand, banged, dropped, and then mouthed. Each action represents a nonverbal idea about what things are for (in Piagetian terms, a *schema*). The complexity of the infant's play, how many different schemata are brought to bear, is a good index of cognitive development at this age. The pleasure, persistence, and energy with which infants tackle these challenges suggest the existence of an intrinsic drive, or mastery motivation. Mastery behavior occurs when infants feel secure; those with less secure attachments show limited experimentation and less competence.

A major milestone is the achievement (about 9 mo) of *object constancy,* the understanding that objects continue to exist even when not seen. At 4–7 mo, the infant looks down for a yarn ball that has been dropped but quickly gives up if it is not seen. With object constancy, the infant persists in searching, finding objects hidden under a cloth or behind the examiner's back.

EMOTIONAL DEVELOPMENT. The advent of object constancy corresponds with qualitative changes in social and communicative development. The infant looks back and forth between an approaching stranger and a parent, as if to contrast known from unknown, and may cling or cry anxiously. Separations often become more difficult. Infants who have been sleeping through the night for months begin to awaken regularly and cry, as though remembering that parents are in the next room.

At the same time, a new demand for autonomy emerges. The infant no longer consents to be fed but turns away as the spoon approaches or insists on holding it him- or herself. Self-feeding with finger foods allows the infant to exercise newly acquired fine motor skills (the pincer grasp); it may be the only way to get the child to eat. Tantrums make their first appearance as the drives for autonomy and mastery come in conflict with parental controls and with the infant's still-limited abilities.

COMMUNICATION. The infant at 7 mo is adept at nonverbal communication, expressing a range of emotions and responding to vocal tone and facial expressions. Around 9 mo, the infant becomes aware that emotions can be shared between people; he or she shows parents toys gleefully, as if to say, "When you see this thing, you'll be happy, too!" Between 8 and 10 mo, babbling takes on a new complexity, with multiple syllables ("ba-da-ma") and inflections that mimic the native language. At the same time, the infant loses the ability to distinguish between vocal sounds that are undifferentiated in the native language. The first true word, that is, a sound used consistently to refer to a specific object or person, appears in concert with the infant's discovery of object constancy.

At this age, picture books provide an ideal context for verbal language acquisition. With a familiar book as a shared focus of attention, the parent and child engage in repeated cycles of pointing and labeling, with elaboration and feedback by the parent.

Implications for Parents and Pediatricians. With the developmental reorganization around 9 mo, previously resolved issues of feeding and sleeping re-emerge. Pediatricians can prepare parents at the 6-mo visit so that these problems can be understood as the results of developmental progress and not regression. Parental ambivalence about separation can express itself in a delay in introducing finger foods or drinking from a cup (usually before the first birthday) or an intrusive, overly neat approach to meal times. Poor weight gain at this age often

■ **TABLE 11–7 Time of Appearance in Roentgenograms of Centers of Ossification in Infancy and Childhood**

Boys—Age at Appearance*	Bones and Epiphyseal Centers	Girls—Age at Appearance*
3 wk	*Humerus, head*	3 wk
	Carpal bones	
2 mo ± 2 mo	Capitate	2 mo ± 2 mo
3 mo ± 2 mo	Hamate	2 mo ± 2 mo
30 mo ± 16 mo	Triangular†	21 mo ± 14 mo
42 mo ± 19 mo	Lunate†	34 mo ± 13 mo
67 mo ± 19 mo	Trapezium†	47 mo ± 14 mo
69 mo ± 15 mo	Trapezoid†	49 mo ± 12 mo
66 mo ± 15 mo	Scaphoid†	51 mo ± 12 mo
No standards available	Pisiform†	No standards available
	Metacarpal bones	
18 mo ± 5 mo	II	12 mo ± 3 mo
20 mo ± 5 mo	III	13 mo ± 3 mo
23 mo ± 6 mo	IV	15 mo ± 4 mo
26 mo ± 7 mo	V	16 mo ± 5 mo
32 mo ± 9 mo	I	18 mo ± 5 mo
	Fingers (epiphyses)	
16 mo ± 4 mo	Proximal phalanx, 3rd finger	10 mo ± 3 mo
16 mo ± 4 mo	Proximal phalanx, 2nd finger	11 mo ± 3 mo
17 mo ± 5 mo	Proximal phalanx, 4th finger	11 mo ± 3 mo
19 mo ± 7 mo	Distal phalanx, 1st finger	12 mo ± 4 mo
21 mo ± 5 mo	Proximal phalanx, 5th finger	14 mo ± 4 mo
24 mo ± 6 mo	Middle phalanx, 3rd finger	15 mo ± 5 mo
24 mo ± 6 mo	Middle phalanx, 4th finger	15 mo ± 5 mo
26 mo ± 6 mo	Middle phalanx, 2nd finger	16 mo ± 5 mo
28 mo ± 6 mo	Distal phalanx, 3rd finger	18 mo ± 4 mo
28 mo ± 6 mo	Distal phalanx, 4th finger	18 mo ± 5 mo
32 mo ± 7 mo	Proximal phalanx, 1st finger	20 mo ± 5 mo
37 mo ± 9 mo	Distal phalanx, 5th finger	23 mo ± 6 mo
37 mo ± 8 mo	Distal phalanx, 2nd finger	23 mo ± 6 mo
39 mo ± 10 mo	Middle phalanx, 5th finger	22 mo ± 7 mo
152 mo ± 18 mo	Sesamoid (adductor pollicis)	121 mo ± 13 mo
	Hip and knee	
Usually present at birth	Femur, distal	Usually present at birth
Usually present at birth	Tibia, proximal	Usually present at birth
4 mo ± 2 mo	Femur, head	4 mo ± 2 mo
46 mo ± 11 mo	Patella	29 mo ± 7 mo
	Foot and ankle‡	

Values represent mean ± standard deviation, when applicable.

**To nearest month.*

†Except for the capitate and hamate bones, the variability of carpal centers is too great to make them very useful clinically.

‡Standards for the foot are available, but normal variation is wide, including some familial variants, so that this area is of little clinical use.

The norms present a composite of published data from the Fels Research Institute, Yellow Springs, Ohio (Pyle SI, Sontag L: Am J Roentgenol 49:102, 1943), and unpublished data from the Brush Foundation, Case Western Reserve University, Cleveland, OH, and the Harvard School of Public Health, Boston, MA. Compiled by Lieb, Buehl, and Pyle.

reflects a struggle between the infant and parent over control of the infant's eating. Discussions about the infant's drive for autonomy and need for limited choices may avert such problems.

The infant's wariness of strangers often makes the 9-mo examination difficult, particularly if the infant is temperamentally prone to react negatively to unfamiliar situations. Time spent talking with the mother and playing with the child will be rewarded by more cooperation.

Brazelton TB: Touchpoints: The Essential Reference. Reading, MA, Addison-Wesley, 1992.

Cohn JF, Tronick EZ: Three-month-old infants' reactions to simulated maternal deprivation. Child Dev *54*:185, 1983.

Lyons-Ruth K, Zeanah CH: The family context of infant mental health: I. Affective development in the primary caregiving relationship. *In:* Zeanah CH (ed): Handbook of Infant Mental Health. New York, Guilford Press, 1993, pp 14–37.

Mahler MS, Pine S, Bergman A: The Psychological Birth of the Infant. London, Hutchinson, 1975.

Needlman R, Zuckerman B: Fight illiteracy: Prescribe a book! Contemp Pediatr 9:41, 1992.

Stern D: The Interpersonal World of the Infant. New York, Basic Books, 1985.

Zuckerman BS, Frank DA: Infancy and toddler years. *In:* Levine MD, Carey WB, Crocker AC (eds): Developmental-Behavioral Pediatrics. Philadelphia, WB Saunders, 1992, pp 27–38.

CHAPTER 12
The Second Year

At approximately 18 mo, the emergence of symbolic thought causes a reorganization of behavior with implications in multiple developmental domains.

AGE 12–18 MO

PHYSICAL DEVELOPMENT. The growth rate slows further in the 2nd yr of life (see Table 11–5) and appetite declines. "Baby fat" is burned up by increased mobility; an exaggerated lumbar lordosis makes the abdomen protrude. Brain growth continues, with myelinization throughout the 2nd yr (see Fig. 9–2).

Most children begin to walk independently near their first birthday; some do not walk until 15 mo. Highly active, fearless infants tend to walk earlier; less active, more timid infants and those who are preoccupied with exploring objects in detail walk later. Early walking is not associated with advanced development in other domains.

At first, infants "toddle" with a wide-based gait, knees bent, and arms flexed at the elbow; the entire torso rotates with each stride; the toes may point in or out and the feet strike the floor flat. Subsequent refinements lead to greater steadiness and energy efficiency. After several months of practice, the center of gravity shifts back and the torso stays more stable, while knees extend and arms swing at the sides for balance. The toes are held in better alignment, and the child is able to stop, pivot, and stoop without toppling over.

COGNITIVE DEVELOPMENT. Object exploration accelerates because reaching, grasping, and releasing are nearly fully mature and walking increases access to interesting things. The toddler combines objects in novel ways to create interesting effects, such as stacking blocks or putting things into the videocassette recorder slot. Playthings are also more likely to be used for their intended purposes (combs for hair, cups for drinking). Imitation of parents and older children is an important mode of learning. Make-believe play centers on the child's own body (pretending to drink from an empty cup) (Table 12–1; see also Table 11–3).

EMOTIONAL DEVELOPMENT. Infants developmentally approaching the milestone of their first steps may be irritable. Once they start walking, their predominant mood changes markedly. Toddlers are described as "intoxicated" with their new ability and with the power to control the distance between themselves

■ TABLE 12–1 Emerging Patterns of Behavior from 1 to 5 Yr of Age*

15 Mo	
Motor:	Walks alone; crawls up stairs
Adaptive:	Makes tower of 3 cubes; makes a line with crayon; inserts pellet in bottle
Language:	Jargon; follows simple commands; may name a familiar object (ball)
Social:	Indicates some desires or needs by pointing; hugs parents
18 Mo	
Motor:	Runs stiffly; sits on small chair; walks up stairs with one hand held; explores drawers and waste baskets
Adaptive:	Makes a tower of 4 cubes; imitates scribbling; imitates vertical stroke; dumps pellet from bottle
Language:	10 words (average); names pictures; identifies one or more parts of body
Social:	Feeds self; seeks help when in trouble; may complain when wet or soiled; kisses parent with pucker
24 Mo	
Motor:	Runs well; walks up and down stairs, one step at a time; opens doors; climbs on furniture; jumps
Adaptive:	Tower of 7 cubes (6 at 21 mo); circular scribbling; imitates horizontal stroke; folds paper once imitatively
Language:	Puts 3 words together (subject, verb, object)
Social:	Handles spoon well; often tells immediate experiences; helps to undress; listens to stories with pictures
30 Mo	
Motor:	Goes up stairs alternating feet
Adaptive:	Tower of 9 cubes; makes vertical and horizontal strokes, but generally will not join them to make a cross; imitates circular stroke, forming closed figure
Language:	Refers to self by pronoun "I"; knows full name
Social:	Helps put things away; pretends in play
36 Mo	
Motor:	Rides tricycle; stands momentarily on one foot
Adaptive:	Tower of 10 cubes; imitates construction of "bridge" of 3 cubes; copies a circle; imitates a cross
Language:	Knows age and sex; counts 3 objects correctly; repeats 3 numbers or a sentence of 6 syllables
Social:	Plays simple games (in "parallel" with other children); helps in dressing (unbuttons clothing and puts on shoes); washes hands
48 Mo	
Motor:	Hops on one foot; throws ball overhand; uses scissors to cut out pictures; climbs well
Adaptive:	Copies bridge from model; imitates construction of "gate" of 5 cubes; copies cross and square; draws a man with 2 to 4 parts besides head; names longer of 2 lines
Language:	Counts 4 pennies accurately; tells a story
Social:	Plays with several children with beginning of social interaction and role-playing; goes to toilet alone
60 Mo	
Motor:	Skips
Adaptive:	Draws triangle from copy; names heavier of 2 weights
Language:	Names 4 colors; repeats sentence of 10 syllables; counts 10 pennies correctly
Social:	Dresses and undresses; asks questions about meaning of words; domestic role-playing

**Data are derived from those of Gesell (as revised by Knobloch), Shirley, Provence, Wolf, Bailey, and others. After 5 yr the Stanford-Binet, Wechsler-Bellevue, and other scales offer the most precise estimates of developmental level. In order to have their greatest value, they should be administered only by an experienced and qualified person.*

and their parents. Toddlers often "orbit" around their parents, like planets around the sun, moving away, looking back, moving farther, and then returning for a reassuring touch. In unfamiliar surroundings, with temperamentally timid children, such orbits might be small or nonexistent; in familiar ones, a bold child might "orbit" out of sight (see Table 12–1).

The ability of the child to use the parent as a "secure base" for exploration depends on the attachment relationship. Attachment can be assessed by having the parents leave the child in an unfamiliar playroom, the "strange situation." When their parents leave, most children stop playing, cry, and try to follow. The outcome of greatest interest, however, is the response of the child on the parents' return. *Securely attached* children instantly go to their parents to be picked up, are comforted, and then are able to return to play. Children with *ambivalent* attachments go to their parents but then resist being comforted and may hit at their parents in anger. Children categorized as *avoidant* may not protest when the parents leave and may turn away from the parent on the return. Insecure response patterns may represent strategies infants develop to cope with punitive or unresponsive parenting styles and may predict later cognitive and emotional problems. Controversy continues about how infant temperament and prior experience of separations might affect interpretation of strange situation results.

LINGUISTIC DEVELOPMENT. Receptive language precedes expressive. By the time infants speak their first words, around 12 mo, they already respond appropriately to several simple statements such as "no," "bye-bye," and "give me." By 15 mo, the average child points to major body parts and uses four to six words spontaneously and correctly, including proper nouns. The toddler also enjoys polysyllabic jargoning (see Tables 11–3 and 12–1) but does not seem upset that no one understands. Most communication of wants and ideas continues to be nonverbal.

Implications for Parents and Pediatricians. Parents who cannot recall any other milestone tend to remember when their child began to walk perhaps because of the symbolic significance of walking as an act of independence. The child's ability to wander out of sight also obviously increases the difficulty of providing supervision and the risks of injury. When walking is precluded by physical disability, parents and care providers should facilitate exploration and help the child attain greater control over separation and proximity.

Patterns of response similar to those rated in the strange situation procedure may be observable in the pediatric clinic. Many toddlers are comfortable exploring the examination room but cling to the parents under the stress of the examination. Infants who become more, not less, distressed in their parents' arms or who avoid their parents at times of stress may be insecurely attached. Young children who, when distressed, turn to strangers for comfort rather than to parents are particularly worrisome.

AGE 18–24 MO

PHYSICAL DEVELOPMENT. Motor development is incremental at this age, with improvements in balance and agility and the emergence of running and stair climbing. Height and weight increase at a steady rate, although head growth slows slightly (Figs. 12–1 and 12–2; see also Table 11–5).

COGNITIVE DEVELOPMENT. At approximately 18 mo, several cognitive changes come together to mark the conclusion of the sensorimotor period. Object permanence is firmly established; the toddler anticipates where an object may have been moved to even though the object was not visible while it was being moved. Cause and effect are better understood, and the toddler demonstrates flexibility in problem solving, using a stick to obtain a toy out of reach and figuring out how to wind a mechanical toy. Symbolic transformations in play are no longer tied to the toddler's own body, so that a doll can be "fed" from an empty plate. Like the reorganization at 9 mo, the cognitive changes at 18 mo correlate with important changes in the emotional and linguistic domains (see Table 12–1).

EMOTIONAL DEVELOPMENT. In many children, the relative independence of the preceding period gives way to increased clinginess around 18 mo. This stage, described as *rapprochement*, may be a reaction to growing awareness of the possibility of separation. Many parents report that they now cannot go anywhere without having a small child attached to them. Separations at bedtime are often difficult, with frequent false starts and tantrums. Many children use a special blanket or stuffed toy as a transitional object: something that functions as a symbol of the absent parent (in psychoanalytic terms, the object). The transitional object remains important until the transition to symbolic thought has been completed and the symbolic presence of the parent has been fully internalized.

Self-conscious awareness and internalized standards of evaluation first appear at this age. Toddlers looking in a mirror will, for the first time, reach for their own face rather than the mirror image if they notice a red dot on their nose or some other unusual appearance. They begin to recognize when toys are broken and may hand them to parents to fix. When tempted to touch a forbidden object, they may tell themselves "no, no," evidence of internalization of standards of behavior. That they often proceed to touch the object demonstrates the relative strength of internalized inhibitions (see Table 12–1).

LINGUISTIC DEVELOPMENT. Perhaps the most dramatic developments in this period are linguistic. Labeling of objects coincides with the advent of symbolic thought. Children may point at things with the index finger rather than the whole hand as though calling attention to objects not for the purpose of having them but of finding out their names. When this protolinguistic naming is accompanied by the phrase, "Whazzat?" the child's intentions are clear. After the realization that words can stand for things, the child's vocabulary balloons from 10–15 words at 18 mo to 100 or more at 2 yr. After acquiring a vocabulary of about 50 words, the toddler begins to combine them to make simple sentences, the beginning of grammar. At this stage, the toddler understands two-step commands, such as "Give me the ball, and then get your shoes." The emergence of verbal language marks the end of the sensorimotor period. As the toddler learns to use symbols to express ideas and solve problems, the need for cognition based on direct sensation and motoric manipulation wanes (see Table 12–1).

Implications for Parents and Pediatricians. With increasing mobility, physical limits on children's explorations become less effective; words become increasingly important for behavior control as well as cognition. Children with delayed language acquisition often have greater behavior problems. Language development is facilitated when parents and caregivers use clear, simple sentences, ask questions, and respond to children's incomplete sentences and gestural communication with the appropriate words. Regular periods of looking at picture books together continue to provide an ideal context for language development.

Pediatricians can help parents understand the resurgence of problems with separation and the appearance of a treasured blanket or teddy bear as a developmental phenomenon. Management of difficult behavior and assessment of children with delayed speech are discussed in Chapter 13.

Ainsworth MDS, Blehar MC, Waters E, et al: Patterns of Attachment: A Psychological Study of the Strange Situation. Hillsdale, NJ, Erlbaum, 1978.

Bates E, O'Connell B, Share C: Language and communication in infancy. *In:* Osofsky J (ed): Handbook of Infant Development. New York, Wiley, 1987.

Fraiberg S: The Magic Years. New York, Scribner's, 1959.

Kagan J: The Nature of the Child. New York, Basic Books, 1984.

Mahler MS, Pine S, Bergman A: The Psychological Birth of the Infant. London, Hutchinson, 1975.

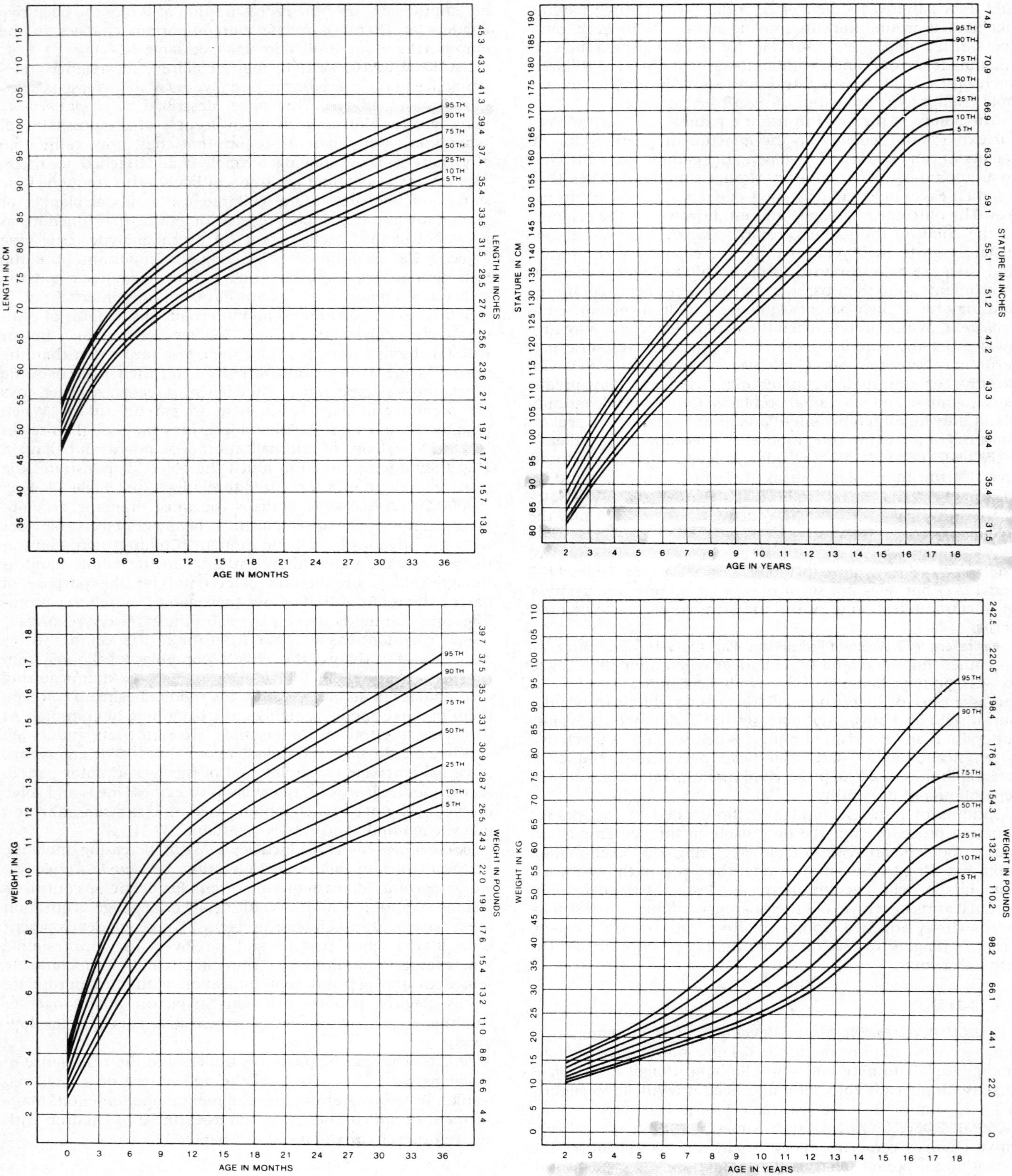

A

Figure 12–1. ***See legend on opposite page***

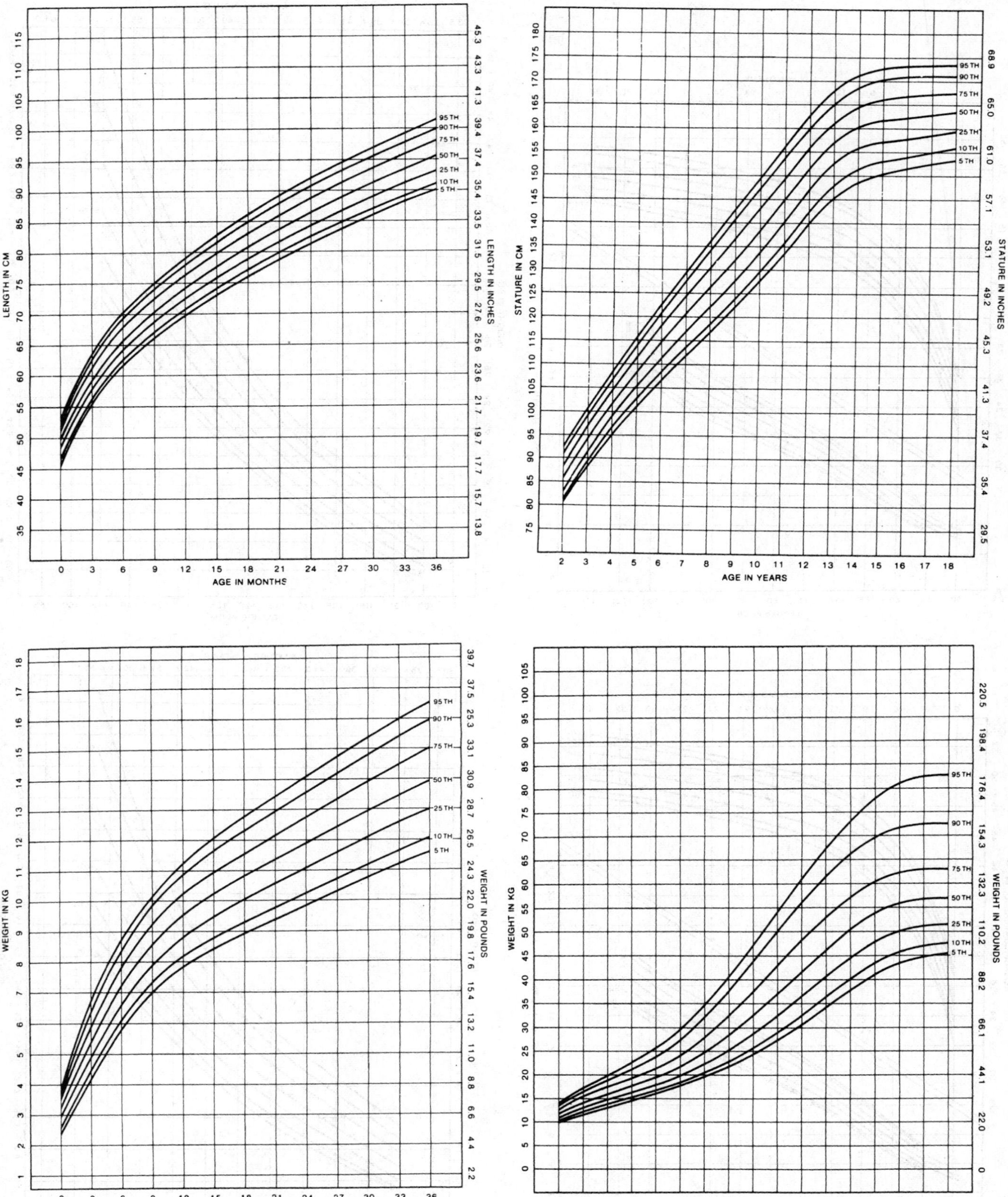

B

Figure 12–1. *A* and *B*. Charts for BOYS *(A)* and GIRLS *(B)* of length (or stature) by age *(upper curves)* and weight by age *(lower curves)*, each curve corresponding to the indicated percentile level. These charts are based on the data in Tables 11–2 and 13–1. (*A* and *B*, From Hamill PVV, Drizd TA, Johnson CL, et al: Physical growth: National Center for Health Statistics percentiles. Am J Clin Nutr 32:609–610, 1979.)

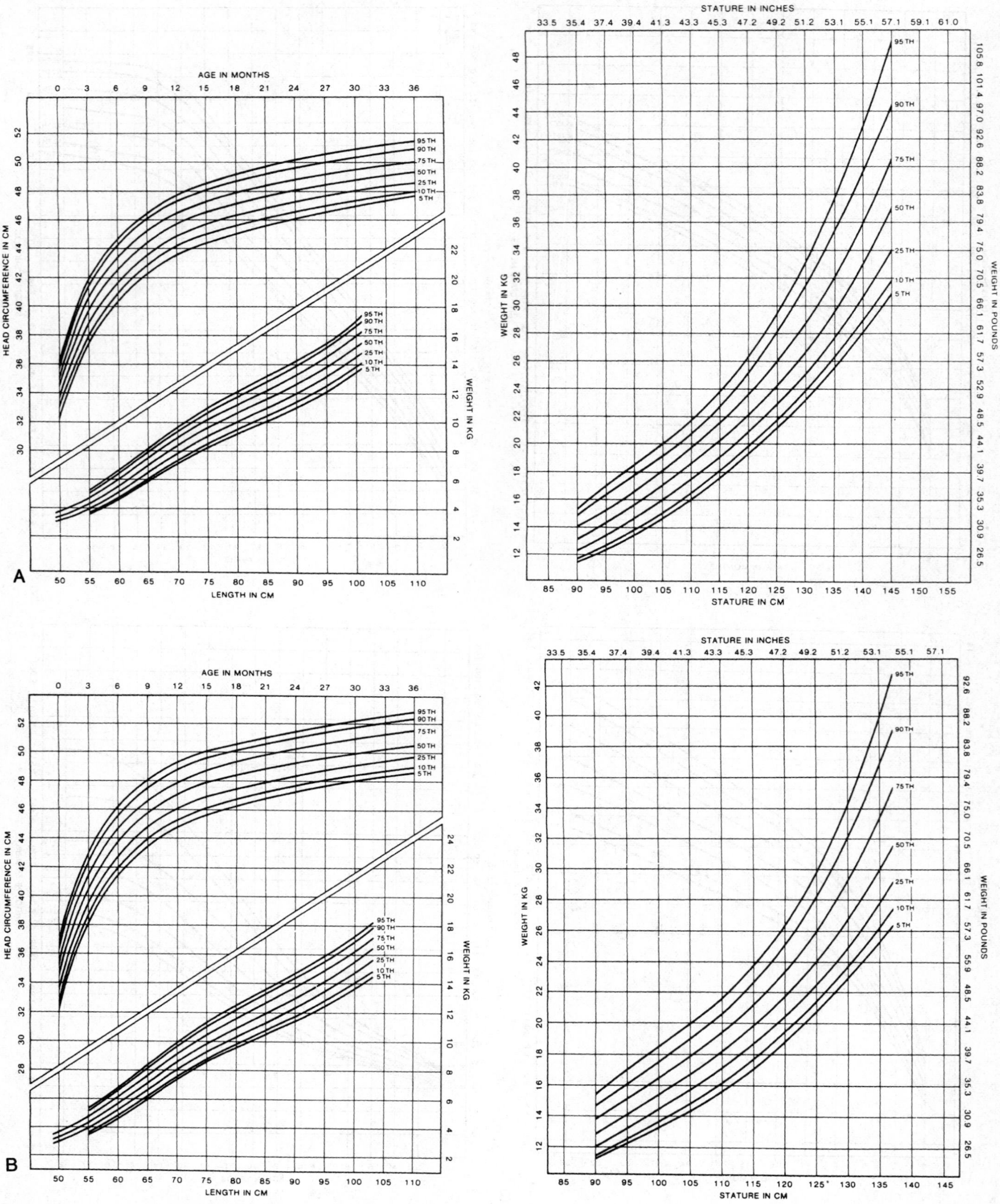

Figure 12–2. Charts for BOYS *(A)* and for GIRLS *(B)* of weight by length (or stature), for infants and young children (left), and for older (prepubertal) children (right). *Head circumference by age* is given for infants and young children (upper left). These charts are based on the data in Tables 11–2 and 13–1. (*A* and *B*, From Hamill PVV, Drizd TA, Johnson CL, et al: Physical growth: National Center for Health Statistics percentiles. Am J Clin Nutr 32:614, 1979.)

CHAPTER 13
Preschool Years

Between 2 and 5 yr of age, developmental challenges from earlier periods are played out in the context of a widening social sphere and reshaped by increasingly sophisticated language. An example is the challenge of self-regulation in the face of potentially overwhelming stimuli. This issue, dating from earliest infancy, re-emerges as the child confronts a busy playground or preschool classroom. Tension between the child's growing sense of autonomy and both internal and external limitations defines the central dynamic of this age. This tension is affected by and in turn affects development in multiple domains.

PHYSICAL DEVELOPMENT (Tables 13–1 and 13–2)

By the end of the 2nd yr, somatic and brain growth slows, with corresponding decreases in nutritional requirements and in appetite (see Table 11–5). Between the ages of 2 and 5 yr, the average child gains approximately 2 kg in weight and 7 cm in height per year. The toddler's prominent abdomen flattens and the body becomes leaner. Physical energy peaks, and the need for sleep declines to 11–13 hr/24 hr, usually including one nap (see Fig. 11–1). Visual acuity reaches 20/30 by age 3 yr and 20/20 by age 4. All 20 primary teeth have erupted by 3 yr of age (see Table 11–6).

Gross and fine motor milestones are presented in Table 11–4. Most children walk with a mature gait and run steadily before the end of their 3rd yr. Beyond this basic level, there is wide variation in ability as the range of motoric activities expands to include throwing, catching and kicking balls, riding on bicycles, climbing on playground structures, dancing, and other complex-pattern behaviors. Stylistic features of gross motor activity, such as tempo, intensity, and cautiousness, also vary largely because of inborn predilection.

The effects of such individual differences on cognitive and emotional development depend in part on the demands of the social environment. Energetic, coordinated children may thrive emotionally with parents who stress competitiveness and provide many opportunities for physical activity; lower energy, more cerebral children may thrive with parents who stress quiet play.

Handedness is usually established by the 3rd yr. Frustration may result from attempts to change children's hand preference. Variations in fine motor development reflect both individual proclivities and different opportunities for learning. Children who are seldom allowed to use crayons, for example, develop mature pencil grasp later.

Implications for Parents and Pediatricians. The normal decrease in appetite at this age often arouses worry about nutrition. For the most part, parents can be reassured that if growth is normal the child's intake is adequate. Usually, the parent is responsible for providing wholesome, age-appropriate food and deciding on the time and place; the child is responsible for determining the quantity of intake. Children normally modulate their food intake to match their somatic needs according to feelings of hunger or satiety. Daily intake fluctuates, at times widely, but intake over the period of a week is relatively stable. Parental attempts to control the child's intake interfere with this self-regulatory mechanism as the child must either accede to or rebel against the pressure. The result is either over- or undereating.

Motorically precocious, highly active children face increased risks of injury. Parents of such children benefit from early guidance about the need for childproofing the home, constant supervision, and bicycle helmet use (beginning with the tricycle). Parental concerns about possible "hyperactivity" may reflect inappropriate expectations, heightened fears, or true overactivity. Children who engage in reckless, uncontrollable activity with no apparent regard for personal safety need a safe environment with appropriate limits and very close supervision. Psychotherapy and medication may also be helpful. This pattern of indiscriminate activity is sometimes seen among children who have suffered abuse or neglect.

LANGUAGE, COGNITION, AND PLAY

These three domains all involve the symbolic function, a mode of dealing with the world that becomes increasingly important during the preschool period.

LANGUAGE. Language development occurs most rapidly between 2 and 5 yr of age. Vocabulary increases from 50–100 words to more than 2,000. Sentence structure advances from "telegraphic" two- and three-word phrases to sentences incorporating all of the major grammatical rules. An important distinction is between speech, the production of intelligible sounds, and language, the underlying mental act. Language includes both expressive and receptive functions. Generally, problems of speech are more amenable to therapy than are problems of language. Receptive language (understanding) varies less than expressive language and, therefore, is a more reliable target for assessment. Language assessment is described more fully in Chapters 17 and 31.

Language acquisition depends on both environmental and intrinsic factors. The manner in which adults address children, how they ask questions and give commands, the extent to which they engage in language teaching, and expectations for language competence vary from culture to culture. Children do not simply imitate adult speech. Rather, they abstract the complex rules of grammar from the ambient language by generating implicit hypotheses and modifying them progressively. Overgeneralization, such as the indiscriminate addition of the "s" sound at the end of a word to signify the plural or the "ed" sound to signify the past ("we seed lots of mouses"), gives evidence for the existence of such implicit rules.

Despite the importance of language exposure, there is increasing evidence that the basic mechanism for language acquisition is "hard-wired" into the brain. The inborn propensity to create language is illustrated by a study of deaf orphans raised by nonsigning adults; the orphans invented their own sign language, including all of the essential grammatical rules.

Language is a critical barometer of both cognitive and emotional development. Mental retardation may first become apparent with delayed speech at approximately 2 yr, although earlier signs may have been overlooked. Child abuse and neglect are correlated with delayed language, particularly the ability to convey emotional states. Conversely, such delays may contribute to problems of behavior, socialization, and learning. Language plays a critical role in the regulation of behavior first through the child's understanding of adult demands and limits and later through internalized "private speech" in which the child repeats adult prohibitions first audibly and then mentally. Language also allows the child to express feelings, such as anger or frustration, without acting them out; consequently, language-delayed children show higher rates of tantrums and other externalizing behaviors.

Preschool language development lays the foundation for later success in school. Approximately 35% of children in the United States may enter school lacking the language skills that are the prerequisites of literacy acquisition. Although most children learn to read and write in elementary school, critical foundations for literacy are established during the preschool years. Through repeated early exposure to written words, chil-

■ **TABLE 13–1 Percentiles of Stature and Weight by Age***

Age (Yr)	5th		10th		25th		50th		75th		90th		95th	
Boys: 2–18 Yr														
2.0†	82.50	(32½)	83.50	(32¾)	85.30	(33½)	86.80	(34¼)	89.20	(35)	92.00	(36¼)	94.40	(37¼)
	10.49	(23¼)	10.96	(24¼)	11.55	(25½)	12.34	(27¼)	13.36	(29½)	14.38	(31¾)	15.50	(34¼)
2.5†	85.40	(33½)	86.50	(34)	88.50	(34¾)	90.40	(35½)	92.90	(36½)	95.60	(37¾)	97.80	(38½)
	11.27	(24¾)	11.77	(26)	12.55	(27¾)	13.52	(29¾)	14.61	(32¼)	15.71	(34¾)	16.61	(36½)
3.0	89.00	(35)	90.30	(35½)	92.60	(36½)	94.90	(37¼)	97.50	(38½)	100.10	(39½)	102.00	(40¼)
	12.05	(26½)	12.58	(27¾)	13.12	(29¾)	14.62	(32¼)	15.78	(34¾)	16.95	(37¼)	17.77	(39¼)
3.5	92.50	(36½)	93.90	(37)	96.40	(38)	99.10	(39)	101.70	(40)	104.30	(41¼)	106.10	(41¾)
	12.84	(28¼)	13.41	(29½)	14.46	(32)	15.68	(34½)	16.90	(37¼)	18.15	(40)	18.98	(41¾)
4.0	95.80	(37¾)	97.30	(38¼)	100.00	(39¼)	102.90	(40½)	105.70	(41½)	108.20	(42½)	109.90	(43¼)
	13.64	(30)	14.24	(31½)	15.39	(34)	16.69	(36¾)	17.99	(39¾)	19.32	(42½)	20.27	(44¾)
4.5	98.90	(39)	100.60	(39½)	103.40	(40¾)	106.60	(42)	109.40	(43)	111.90	(44)	113.50	(44¾)
	14.45	(31¾)	15.10	(33¼)	16.30	(36)	17.69	(39)	19.06	(42)	20.50	(45¼)	21.63	(47¾)
5.0	102.00	(40¼)	103.70	(40¾)	106.50	(42)	109.90	(43¼)	112.80	(44½)	115.40	(45½)	117.00	(46)
	15.27	(33¾)	15.96	(35¼)	17.22	(38)	18.67	(41¼)	20.14	(44½)	21.70	(47¾)	23.09	(51)
5.5	104.90	(41¼)	106.70	(42)	109.60	(43¼)	113.10	(44½)	116.10	(45¾)	118.70	(46¾)	120.30	(47¼)
	16.09	(35½)	16.83	(37)	18.14	(40)	19.67	(43¼)	21.25	(46¾)	22.96	(50½)	24.66	(54¼)
6.0	107.70	(42½)	109.60	(43¼)	112.50	(44¼)	116.10	(45¾)	119.20	(47)	121.90	(48)	123.50	(48½)
	16.93	(37¼)	17.72	(39)	19.07	(42)	20.69	(45½)	22.40	(49½)	24.31	(53½)	26.34	(58)
6.5	110.40	(43½)	112.30	(44¼)	115.30	(45½)	119.00	(46¾)	122.20	(48)	124.90	(49¼)	126.60	(49¾)
	17.78	(39¼)	18.62	(41)	20.02	(44¼)	21.74	(48)	23.62	(52)	25.76	(56¾)	28.16	(62)
7.0	113.00	(44½)	115.00	(45¼)	118.00	(46½)	121.70	(48)	125.00	(49¼)	127.90	(50¼)	129.70	(51)
	18.64	(41)	19.53	(43)	21.00	(46¼)	22.85	(50¼)	24.94	(55)	27.36	(60¼)	30.12	(66½)
7.5	115.60	(45½)	117.60	(46¼)	120.60	(47½)	124.40	(49)	127.80	(50¼)	130.80	(51½)	132.70	(52¼)
	19.52	(43)	20.45	(45)	22.02	(48½)	24.03	(53)	26.36	(58)	29.11	(64¼)	32.73	(72¼)
8.0	118.10	(46½)	120.20	(47¼)	123.20	(48½)	127.00	(50)	130.50	(51½)	133.60	(52½)	135.70	(53½)
	20.40	(45)	21.39	(47¼)	22.09	(51)	25.30	(55¾)	27.91	(61½)	31.06	(68½)	34.51	(76)
8.5	120.50	(47½)	122.70	(48¼)	125.70	(49½)	129.60	(51)	133.20	(52½)	136.50	(53¾)	138.80	(54¾)
	21.31	(47)	22.34	(49¼)	24.21	(53¼)	26.66	(58¾)	29.61	(65¼)	33.22	(73¼)	36.96	(81½)
9.0	122.90	(48½)	125.20	(49¼)	128.20	(50½)	132.20	(52)	136.00	(53½)	139.40	(55)	141.80	(55¾)
	22.25	(49)	23.33	(51½)	25.40	(56)	28.13	(62)	31.46	(69¼)	35.57	(78½)	39.58	(87¾)
9.5	125.30	(49¼)	127.60	(50¼)	130.80	(51½)	134.80	(53)	138.80	(54¾)	142.40	(56)	144.90	(57)
	23.25	(51¼)	24.38	(53¾)	26.88	(58¾)	29.73	(65½)	33.46	(73¾)	38.11	(84)	42.35	(93¼)
10.0	127.70	(50¼)	130.10	(51¼)	133.40	(52½)	137.50	(54¼)	141.60	(55¾)	145.50	(57¼)	148.10	(58¼)
	24.33	(53¾)	25.52	(56¼)	28.07	(62)	31.44	(69¼)	35.61	(78½)	40.80	(90)	45.27	(99¾)
10.5	130.10	(51¼)	132.60	(52¼)	136.00	(53½)	140.30	(55¼)	144.60	(57)	148.70	(58½)	151.50	(59¾)
	25.51	(56¼)	26.78	(59)	29.59	(65¼)	33.30	(73½)	37.92	(83½)	43.63	(96¼)	48.31	(106½)
11.0	132.60	(52¼)	135.10	(53¼)	138.70	(54½)	143.33	(56½)	147.80	(58¼)	152.10	(60)	154.90	(61)
	26.80	(59)	28.17	(62)	31.25	(69)	35.30	(77¾)	40.38	(89)	46.57	(102¾)	51.47	(113½)
11.5	135.00	(53¼)	137.70	(54½)	141.50	(55¾)	146.40	(57¾)	151.10	(59½)	155.60	(61¼)	158.50	(62½)
	28.24	(62¼)	29.72	(65½)	33.08	(73)	37.46	(82½)	43.00	(94¾)	49.61	(109¼)	54.73	(120¾)
12.0	137.60	(54¼)	140.30	(55¼)	144.40	(56¾)	149.70	(59)	154.60	(60¾)	159.40	(62¾)	162.30	(64)
	29.85	(65¾)	31.46	(69¼)	35.09	(77¼)	39.78	(87¾)	45.77	(101)	52.73	(116¼)	58.09	(128)
12.5	140.20	(55¼)	143.00	(56¼)	147.40	(58)	153.00	(60¼)	158.20	(62¼)	163.20	(64¼)	166.10	(65½)
	31.64	(69¾)	33.41	(73¾)	37.31	(82¼)	42.27	(93¼)	48.70	(107¼)	55.91	(123¼)	61.52	(135¾)
13.0	142.90	(56¼)	145.80	(57½)	150.50	(59¼)	156.50	(61½)	161.80	(63¾)	167.00	(65¾)	169.80	(66¾)
	33.64	(74¼)	35.60	(78½)	39.74	(87½)	44.95	(99)	51.79	(114¼)	59.12	(130¼)	65.02	(143¼)
13.5	145.70	(57¼)	148.70	(58½)	153.60	(60½)	159.90	(63)	165.30	(65)	170.50	(67¼)	173.40	(68¼)
	35.85	(79)	38.03	(83¾)	42.40	(93½)	47.81	(105½)	55.02	(121¼)	62.35	(137½)	68.51	(151)
14.0	148.80	(58½)	151.80	(59¾)	156.90	(61¾)	63.10	(64¼)	168.50	(66¼)	173.80	(68½)	176.70	(69½)
	38.22	(84¼)	40.64	(89½)	45.21	(99¾)	50.77	(112)	58.31	(128½)	65.57	(144½)	72.13	(159)
14.5	152.00	(59¾)	155.00	(61)	160.10	(63)	166.20	(65½)	171.50	(67½)	176.60	(69½)	179.50	(70½)
	40.66	(89¾)	43.34	(95½)	48.08	(106)	53.76	(118½)	61.58	(135¾)	68.76	(151½)	75.66	(166¾)
15.0	155.20	(61)	158.20	(62¼)	163.30	(64¼)	169.00	(66½)	174.10	(68½)	178.90	(70½)	181.90	(71½)
	43.11	(95)	46.06	(101½)	50.92	(112¼)	56.71	(125)	64.72	(142¾)	71.91	(158½)	79.12	(174½)

■ **TABLE 13–1 Percentiles of Stature and Weight by Age*** *Continued*

Age (Yr)	5th	10th	25th	50th	75th	90th	95th
15.5	158.30 (62¼) 45.50 (100¼)	161.20 (63½) 48.69 (107¼)	166.20 (65½) 53.64 (118¼)	171.50 (67½) 59.51 (131¼)	176.30 (69½) 67.64 (149)	180.80 (71¼) 74.98 (165¼)	183.90 (72½) 82.45 (181¾)
16.0	161.10 (63½) 47.74 (105¼)	163.90 (64½) 51.16 (112¾)	168.70 (66½) 56.16 (123¾)	173.50 (68¼) 62.10 (137)	178.10 (70) 70.26 (155)	182.40 (71¾) 77.97 (172)	185.40 (73) 85.62 (188¾)
16.5	163.40 (64¼) 49.76 (109¾)	166.10 (65½) 53.39 (117¾)	170.60 (67¼) 58.38 (128¾)	175.20 (69) 64.39 (142)	179.50 (70¾) 72.46 (159¾)	183.60 (72¼) 80.84 (178¼)	186.60 (73½) 88.59 (195¼)
17.0	164.90 (65) 51.50 (113½)	167.70 (66) 55.28 (121¾)	171.90 (67¾) 60.22 (132¾)	176.20 (69¼) 66.31 (146¼)	180.50 (71) 74.17 (163½)	184.40 (72½) 83.58 (184¼)	187.30 (73¾) 91.31 (201¼)
17.5	165.60 (65¼) 52.89 (116½)	168.50 (66¼) 56.78 (125¼)	172.40 (67¾) 61.61 (135¾)	176.70 (69½) 67.78 (149½)	181.00 (71¼) 75.32 (166)	185.00 (72¾) 86.14 (190)	187.60 (73¾) 93.73 (206¾)
18.0	165.70 (65¼) 53.97 (119)	168.70 (66½) 57.89 (127½)	172.30 (67¾) 62.61 (138)	176.80 (69½) 68.88 (151¾)	181.20 (71¼) 76.00 (167¾)	185.30 (73) 88.41 (195)	187.60 (73¾) 95.76 (211)
Girls: 2 to 18 Yr							
2.0	81.60 (32¼) 9.95 (22)	82.10 (32¼) 10.32 (22¾)	84.00 (33) 10.96 (24¼)	86.80 (34¼) 11.80 (26)	89.30 (35¼) 12.73 (28)	92.00 (36¼) 13.58 (30)	93.60 (36¾) 14.15 (31¼)
2.5	84.60 (33¼) 10.80 (23¾)	85.30 (33½) 11.35 (25)	87.30 (34½) 12.11 (26¾)	90.00 (35½) 13.03 (28¾)	92.50 (36½) 14.23 (31¼)	95.00 (37½) 15.16 (33½)	96.60 (38) 15.76 (34¾)
3.0	88.30 (34¾) 11.61 (25½)	89.30 (35¼) 12.26 (27)	91.40 (36) 13.11 (29)	94.10 (37) 14.10 (31)	96.60 (38) 15.50 (34¼)	99.00 (39) 16.54 (36½)	100.60 (39½) 17.22 (38)
3.5	91.70 (36) 12.37 (27¼)	93.00 (36½) 13.08 (28¾)	95.20 (37½) 14.00 (30¾)	97.90 (38½) 15.07 (33¼)	100.50 (39½) 16.59 (36½)	102.80 (40½) 17.77 (39¼)	104.50 (41¼) 18.59 (41)
4.0	95.00 (37½) 13.11 (29)	96.40 (38) 13.84 (30½)	98.80 (39) 14.80 (32¾)	101.60 (40) 15.96 (35¼)	104.30 (41) 17.56 (38¾)	106.60 (42) 18.93 (41¾)	108.30 (42¾) 19.91 (44)
4.5	98.10 (38½) 13.83 (30½)	99.70 (39¼) 14.56 (32)	102.20 (40¼) 15.55 (34¾)	105.00 (41¼) 16.81 (37)	107.90 (42½) 18.48 (40¾)	110.20 (43½) 20.06 (44¼)	112.00 (44) 21.24 (46¾)
5.0	101.10 (39¾) 14.55 (32)	102.70 (40½) 15.26 (33¾)	105.40 (41½) 16.29 (36)	108.40 (42¾) 17.66 (39)	111.40 (43¾) 19.39 (42¾)	113.80 (44¾) 21.23 (46¾)	115.60 (45½) 22.62 (49¾)
5.5	103.90 (41) 15.29 (33¾)	105.60 (41½) 15.97 (35¼)	108.40 (42¾) 17.05 (37½)	111.60 (44) 18.56 (41)	114.80 (45¼) 20.36 (45)	117.40 (46¼) 24.48 (49½)	119.20 (47) 24.11 (53¼)
6.0	106.60 (42) 16.05 (35½)	108.40 (42¾) 16.72 (36¾)	111.30 (43¾) 17.86 (39¼)	114.60 (45) 19.52 (43)	118.10 (46½) 21.44 (47¼)	120.80 (47½) 23.89 (52¾)	122.70 (48¼) 25.75 (56¾)
6.5	109.20 (43) 16.85 (37¼)	111.00 (43¾) 17.51 (38½)	114.10 (45) 18.76 (41¼)	117.60 (46¼) 20.61 (45½)	121.30 (47¾) 22.68 (50)	124.20 (49) 25.50 (56¼)	126.10 (49¾) 27.59 (60¾)
7.0	111.80 (44) 17.71 (39)	113.60 (44¾) 18.39 (40½)	116.80 (46) 19.78 (43½)	120.60 (47½) 21.84 (48¼)	124.40 (49) 24.16 (53¼)	127.60 (50¼) 27.39 (60½)	129.50 (51) 29.68 (65½)
7.5	114.40 (45) 18.62 (41)	116.20 (45¾) 19.37 (42¾)	119.50 (47) 20.95 (46¼)	123.50 (48½) 23.26 (51¼)	127.50 (50¼) 25.90 (57)	130.90 (51½) 29.57 (65¼)	132.90 (52¼) 32.07 (70¾)
8.0	116.90 (46) 19.62 (43¼)	118.70 (46¾) 20.45 (45)	122.20 (48) 22.26 (49)	126.40 (49¾) 24.84 (54¾)	130.60 (51½) 27.88 (61½)	134.20 (52¾) 32.04 (70¾)	136.20 (53½) 34.71 (76½)
8.5	119.50 (47) 20.68 (45½)	121.30 (47¾) 21.64 (47¾)	124.90 (49¼) 23.70 (52¼)	129.30 (51) 26.58 (58½)	133.60 (52½) 30.08 (66¼)	137.40 (54) 34.73 (76½)	139.60 (55) 37.58 (82¾)
9.0	122.10 (48) 21.82 (48)	123.90 (48¾) 22.92 (50½)	127.70 (50¼) 25.27 (55¾)	132.20 (52) 28.46 (62¾)	136.70 (53¾) 32.44 (71½)	140.70 (55½) 37.60 (83)	142.90 (56¼) 40.64 (89½)
9.5	124.80 (49¼) 23.05 (50¾)	126.60 (49¾) 24.29 (53½)	130.60 (51½) 26.94 (59½)	135.20 (53¼) 30.45 (67¼)	139.80 (55) 34.94 (77)	143.90 (56¾) 40.61 (89½)	146.20 (57½) 43.85 (96¾)
10.0	127.50 (50¼) 24.36 (53¾)	129.50 (51) 25.76 (56¾)	133.60 (52½) 28.71 (63¼)	138.30 (54½) 32.55 (71¾)	142.90 (56¼) 37.53 (82¾)	147.20 (58) 43.70 (96¼)	149.50 (58¾) 47.17 (104)
10.5	130.40 (51¼) 25.75 (56¾)	132.50 (52¼) 27.32 (60¼)	136.70 (53¾) 30.57 (67½)	141.50 (55¾) 34.72 (76½)	146.10 (57½) 40.17 (88½)	150.40 (59¼) 46.84 (103¼)	152.80 (60¼) 50.57 (111½)
11.0	133.50 (52½) 27.24 (60)	135.60 (53½) 28.97 (63¾)	140.00 (55) 32.49 (71¾)	144.80 (57) 36.95 (81½)	149.30 (58¾) 42.84 (94½)	153.70 (60½) 49.96 (110¼)	56.20 (61½) 54.00 (119)
11.5	136.60 (53¾) 28.83 (63½)	139.00 (54¾) 30.71 (67¾)	143.50 (56½) 34.48 (76)	148.20 (58¼) 39.23 (86½)	152.60 (60) 45.48 (100¼)	156.90 (61¾) 53.03 (117)	159.50 (62¾) 57.42 (126½)
12.0	139.80 (55) 30.52 (67¼)	142.30 (56) 32.53 (71¼)	147.00 (57¾) 36.52 (80½)	151.50 (59¾) 41.53 (91½)	155.80 (61¼) 48.07 (106)	160.00 (63) 55.99 (123½)	162.70 (64) 60.81 (134)

Table continued on following page

■ **TABLE 13–1 Percentiles of Stature and Weight by Age*** *Continued*

Age (Yr)	5th		10th		25th		50th		75th		90th		95th	
12.5	142.70	(56½)	145.40	(57¼)	150.10	(59)	154.60	(60¾)	158.80	(62½)	162.90	(64½)	165.60	(65¼)
	32.30	(71¾)	34.42	(76)	38.59	(85)	43.84	(96¾)	50.56	(111½)	58.81	(129¾)	64.12	(141¼)
13.0	145.20	(57¼)	148.00	(58¼)	152.80	(60¼)	157.10	(61¾)	161.30	(63½)	165.30	(65)	168.10	(66¼)
	34.14	(75¼)	36.35	(80¼)	40.55	(89½)	46.10	(101¾)	52.91	(116¾)	61.45	(135½)	67.30	(148¼)
13.5	147.20	(58)	150.00	(59)	154.70	(61)	159.00	(62½)	163.20	(64¼)	167.30	(65¾)	170.00	(67)
	35.98	(79¼)	38.26	(84¼)	42.65	(94)	48.26	(106½)	55.11	(121½)	63.87	(140¾)	70.30	(155)
14.0	148.70	(58½)	151.50	(59¾)	155.90	(61½)	160.40	(63¼)	164.60	(64¾)	168.70	(66½)	171.30	(67½)
	37.76	(83¼)	40.11	(88½)	44.54	(98¼)	50.28	(110¾)	57.09	(125¾)	66.04	(145½)	73.08	(161)
14.5	149.70	(59)	152.50	(60)	158.80	(61¾)	161.20	(63½)	165.60	(65¼)	169.80	(66¾)	172.20	(67¾)
	39.45	(87)	41.83	(92¼)	46.28	(102)	52.10	(114¾)	58.84	(129¾)	67.95	(149¾)	75.59	(166¾)
15.0	150.50	(59¼)	153.20	(60¼)	157.20	(62)	161.80	(63¾)	166.30	(65¼)	170.50	(67¼)	172.80	(68)
	40.99	(90¼)	43.38	(95¾)	47.82	(105½)	53.68	(118¼)	60.32	(133)	69.54	(153¼)	77.78	(171½)
15.5	151.10	(59½)	153.60	(60½)	157.50	(62)	162.10	(63¾)	166.70	(65¾)	170.90	(67¼)	173.10	(68¼)
	42.32	(93¼)	44.72	(98½)	49.10	(108¼)	54.96	(121¼)	61.48	(135½)	70.79	(156)	79.59	(176½)
16.0	151.60	(59¾)	154.10	(60¾)	157.80	(62¼)	162.40	(64)	166.90	(65¾)	171.10	(67¼)	173.30	(68¼)
	43.41	(95¾)	45.78	(101)	50.09	(110½)	55.89	(123¼)	62.29	(137¼)	71.68	(158)	80.99	(178½)
16.5	152.20	(60)	154.60	(60¾)	158.20	(62¼)	162.70	(64)	167.10	(65¾)	171.20	(67½)	173.40	(68¼)
	44.20	(97½)	46.54	(102½)	50.75	(112)	56.44	(124½)	62.75	(138¼)	72.18	(159¼)	81.93	(180½)
17.0	152.70	(60)	155.10	(61)	158.70	(62½)	163.10	(64¼)	167.30	(65¾)	171.20	(67½)	173.50	(68¼)
	44.74	(98¾)	47.04	(103¾)	51.14	(112¾)	56.69	(125)	62.91	(138¾)	72.38	(159½)	82.46	(181¾)
17.5	153.20	(60¼)	155.60	(61¼)	159.10	(62¾)	163.40	(64¼)	167.50	(66)	171.10	(67¼)	173.50	(68¼)
	45.08	(99½)	47.33	(104¼)	51.33	(113¼)	56.71	(125)	62.89	(138¾)	72.37	(159½)	82.62	(182¼)
18.0	153.60	(60½)	156.00	(61½)	159.60	(62¾)	163.70	(64½)	167.60	(66)	171.00	(67¼)	173.60	(68¼)
	45.26	(99¾)	47.47	(104¾)	51.39	(113¼)	56.62	(124¾)	62.78	(138½)	72.25	(159¼)	82.47	(181¾)

Stature measured in centimeters (inches); weight measured in kilograms (pounds).

**Data are those of the National Center for Health Statistics, Health Resources Administration, Department of Health, Education, and Welfare, collected in its Health Examination Surveys. Metric data have been smoothed by the least-squares cubic spline technique. For details see footnote to Table 11–2.*

†Stature data for 2.0–3.0 yr include some recumbent length measurements, which make values slightly higher than if all measurements had been of stature.

dren learn about the uses of writing (telling stories or sending messages) and about its form (left to right, top to bottom). Early errors in writing, like errors in speaking, reveal that literacy acquisition is an active process involving hypothesis generation and revision. One hypothesis is that words that take longer to say ("big words") have more letters in them regardless of what the letters are. At a later stage, letters may be assigned one to a syllable, such as GNYS to spell "genius."

Picture books play a special role not only in familiarizing young children to the printed word but also in the development of verbal language. Reading aloud with a young child is an interactive process in which the parent focuses the child's attention on a particular picture, requests a response (by asking, "What's that?"), and then gives the child feedback ("Right, it's a dog."). This question-feedback routine is repeated multiple times in the course of reading the book. As the child's sophistication grows, the parent increases the complexity of the task, requesting descriptions ("What color is the dog?") and later projections ("What's that dog going to do?"). The elements of shared attention, active participation, immediate feedback, repetition, and graduated difficulty make such routines ideal for language learning.

COGNITION. The preschool period corresponds to Piaget's preoperational (prelogical) stage, characterized by magical thinking, egocentrism, and thinking that is dominated by perception (see Table 8–2). Magical thinking includes a confusion of coincidence for causality, animism (attributing motivations to inanimate objects and events), and unrealistic beliefs about the power of wishes. The child might believe that people cause it to rain by carrying umbrellas, that the sun goes down because "it's tired," or that feeling resentment toward a sibling can actually make that sibling sick. Egocentrism refers to the child's inability to take another's point of view and does not connote selfishness. The child might try to comfort an upset adult by bringing a favorite stuffed animal.

Piaget demonstrated the dominance of perception over logic by a famous series of "conservation" experiments. In one, water was poured back and forth from a tall, thin vase to a low, wide dish and children were asked which container had more water. Invariably, they chose the one that looked larger (usually the tall vase), even when the examiner pointed out that no water had been added or taken away. Such misunderstandings reflect young children's developing hypotheses about the nature of the world as well as their difficulty in attending simultaneously to multiple aspects of a situation.

PLAY. During the preschool period, play is marked by increasing complexity and imagination, from simple scripts replicating common experiences such as shopping and putting baby to bed (age 2 or 3 yr) to more extended scenarios involving singular events such as going to the zoo or going on a trip (age 3 or 4 yr) to creation of scenarios that have only been imagined, such as flying to the moon (age 4 or 5 yr). A similar progression in socialization moves from minimal social interaction with peers during play (solo or parallel play, age 1 or 2 yr) to cooperative play such as building a tower of blocks together (age 3 or 4 yr) to organized group play with distinct role assignments, as in playing "house." Play also becomes increasingly rule governed, from early rules about asking (rather than taking) and sharing (age 2 or 3 yr) to rules that change from moment to moment according to the desires of the players (ages 4 and 5 yr) to the beginning of the recognition of rules as relatively immutable (age 5 yr and beyond).

■ TABLE 13–2 Weight by Length*

Recumbent Length	Boys: Weight Percentiles, kg and (lb)							Girls: Weight Percentiles, kg and (lb)						
	5th	*10th*	*25th*	*50th*	*75th*	*90th*	*95th*	*5th*	*10th*	*25th*	*50th*	*75th*	*90th*	*95th*
Boys and Girls Younger Than 4 Years†														
48–50 cm (19–19¾ in)			2.86 (6¼)	3.15 (7)	3.50 (7¾)					3.02 (6¾)	3.29 (7¼)	3.59 (8)		
50–52 cm (19¾–20½ in)			3.16 (7)	3.48 (7¾)	3.86 (8½)					3.25 (7¼)	3.55 (7¾)	3.89 (8½)		
52–54 cm (20½–21¼ in)			3.25 (7¾)	3.88 (8½)	4.28 (9½)					3.56 (7¾)	3.89 (8½)	4.26 (9½)		
54–56 cm (21¼–22 in)	3.49 (7¼)	3.65 (8)	3.95 (8¾)	4.34 (9½)	4.76 (10½)	5.13 (11¼)	5.33 (11¾)	3.54 (7¾)	3.64 (8)	3.93 (8¾)	4.29 (9½)	4.70 (10¼)	5.02 (11)	5.21 (11½)
56–58 cm (22–22¾ in)	3.90 (8½)	4.09 (9)	4.43 (9¾)	4.84 (10¾)	5.29 (11¾)	5.69 (12½)	5.88 (13)	3.93 (8¾)	4.05 (9)	4.37 (9¾)	4.76 (10½)	5.20 (11½)	5.55 (12¼)	5.77 (12¾)
58–60 cm (22¾–23½ in)	4.37 (9¾)	4.58 (10)	4.94 (11)	5.38 (11¾)	5.84 (12¾)	6.28 (13¾)	6.47 (14¼)	4.38 (9¾)	4.50 (10)	4.85 (10¾)	5.27 (11½)	5.73 (12¾)	6.12 (13½)	6.36 (14)
60–62 cm (23½–24½ in)	4.88 (10¾)	5.10 (11¼)	5.49 (12)	5.94 (13)	6.42 (14¼)	6.88 (15¼)	7.08 (15½)	4.85 (10¾)	4.99 (11)	5.37 (11¾)	5.82 (12¾)	6.30 (14)	6.70 (14¾)	6.95 (15¼)
62–64 cm (24½–25¼ in)	5.43 (12)	5.65 (12½)	6.05 (13¼)	6.52 (14¼)	7.02 (15½)	7.50 (16½)	7.72 (17)	5.35 (11¾)	5.50 (12)	5.91 (13)	6.39 (14)	6.89 (15¼)	7.30 (16)	7.55 (16¾)
64–66 cm (25¼–26 in)	5.99 (13¼)	6.20 (13¾)	6.62 (14½)	7.11 (15¾)	7.63 (16¾)	8.13 (18)	8.36 (8½)	5.87 (13)	6.03 (13¼)	6.47 (14¼)	6.97 (15¼)	7.48 (16½)	7.90 (17½)	8.15 (18)
66–68 cm (26–26¾ in)	6.55 (14½)	6.76 (15)	7.19 (15¾)	7.70 (17)	8.23 (18¼)	8.75 (19¼)	8.99 (19¾)	6.38 (14)	6.56 (14½)	7.02 (15½)	7.55 (16¾)	8.07 (17¾)	8.50 (18¾)	8.75 (19¼)
68–70 cm (26¾–27½ in)	7.10 (15¾)	7.31 (16)	7.75 (17)	8.27 (18¼)	8.82 (19½)	9.35 (20½)	9.62 (21¼)	6.89 (15¼)	7.08 (15½)	7.56 (16¾)	8.11 (17¾)	8.64 (19)	9.08 (20)	9.33 (20½)
70–72 cm (27½–28¼ in)	7.63 (16¾)	7.84 (17¼)	8.28 (18¼)	8.82 (19½)	9.39 (20¾)	9.93 (22)	10.21 (22½)	7.37 (16¼)	7.58 (16¾)	8.08 (17¾)	8.64 (19)	9.18 (20¼)	9.63 (21¼)	9.88 (21¾)
72–74 cm (28¼–29¼ in)	8.13 (18)	8.33 (18¼)	8.78 (19¼)	9.33 (20½)	9.92 (21¾)	10.48 (23)	10.77 (23¾)	7.82 (17¼)	8.05 (17¾)	8.56 (18¾)	9.14 (20¼)	9.68 (21¼)	10.15 (22½)	10.41 (23)
74–76 cm (29¼–30 in)	8.58 (19)	8.78 (19¼)	9.24 (20¼)	9.81 (21¾)	10.43 (23)	10.99 (24¼)	11.29 (25)	8.24 (18¼)	8.49 (18¾)	9.00 (19¾)	9.59 (21¼)	10.14 (22¼)	10.63 (23½)	10.91 (24)
76–78 cm (30–30¾ in)	9.00 (19¾)	9.21 (20¼)	9.68 (21¼)	10.27 (22¾)	10.91 (24)	11.48 (25¼)	11.78 (26)	8.62 (19)	8.90 (19½)	9.42 (20¾)	10.02 (22)	10.57 (23¼)	11.08 (24½)	11.39 (25)
78–80 cm (30¾–31½ in)	9.40 (20¾)	9.62 (21¼)	10.09 (22¼)	10.70 (23½)	11.36 (25)	11.94 (26¼)	12.25 (27)	8.99 (19¾)	9.29 (20½)	9.81 (21¾)	10.41 (23)	10.97 (24¼)	11.51 (25¼)	11.85 (26)
80–82 cm (31½–32¼ in)	9.77 (21½)	10.01 (22)	10.49 (23¼)	11.12 (24½)	11.80 (26)	12.39 (27¼)	12.69 (28)	9.34 (20½)	9.67 (21¼)	10.19 (22½)	10.80 (23¾)	11.37 (25)	11.93 (26¼)	12.29 (27)
82–84 cm (32¼–33 in)	10.14 (22¼)	10.39 (23)	10.88 (24)	11.53 (25½)	12.23 (27)	12.83 (28¼)	13.13 (29)	9.68 (21¼)	10.04 (22¼)	10.57 (23¼)	11.18 (24¾)	11.75 (26)	12.35 (27¼)	12.72 (28)
84–86 cm (33–33¾ in)	10.49 (23¼)	10.76 (23¾)	11.27 (24¾)	11.93 (26¼)	12.65 (28)	13.26 (29¼)	13.56 (30)	10.03 (22)	10.41 (23)	10.94 (24)	11.56 (25½)	12.15 (26¾)	12.76 (28¼)	13.15 (29)
86–88 cm (33¾–34¾ in)	10.85 (24)	11.14 (24½)	11.67 (25¾)	12.34 (27¼)	13.07 (28¾)	13.69 (30¼)	14.00 (30¾)	10.39 (23)	10.78 (23¾)	11.33 (25)	11.95 (26¼)	12.55 (27¾)	13.19 (29)	13.57 (30)
88–90 cm (34¾–35½ in)	11.22 (24¾)	11.53 (25½)	12.08 (26¾)	12.76 (28¼)	13.50 (29¾)	14.13 (31¼)	14.44 (31¾)	10.76 (23¾)	11.17 (24½)	11.74 (26)	12.36 (27¼)	12.98 (28½)	13.63 (30)	14.01 (31)
90–92 cm (35½–36¼ in)	11.60 (25½)	11.94 (26¼)	12.52 (27½)	13.20 (29)	13.94 (30¾)	14.58 (32¼)	14.90 (32¾)	11.16 (24½)	11.58 (25½)	12.17 (26¾)	12.80 (28¼)	13.45 (29¾)	14.10 (31)	14.45 (31¾)
92–94 cm (36¼–37 in)	12.00 (26½)	12.37 (27¼)	12.97 (28½)	13.65 (30)	14.40 (31¾)	15.05 (33¼)	15.39 (34)	11.59 (25½)	12.02 (26½)	12.63 (27¾)	13.27 (29¼)	13.95 (30¾)	14.61 (32¼)	14.92 (33)
94–96 cm (37–37¾ in)	12.42 (27½)	12.81 (28¼)	13.45 (29¾)	14.14 (31¼)	14.88 (32¾)	15.54 (34¼)	15.90 (35)	12.05 (26½)	12.48 (27½)	13.12 (29)	13.77 (30¼)	14.48 (32)	15.14 (33½)	15.42 (34)
96–98 cm (37¾–38½ in)	12.88 (28½)	13.28 (29¼)	13.96 (30¾)	14.66 (32¼)	15.39 (34)	16.06 (35½)	16.43 (36¼)	12.55 (27¾)	12.98 (28½)	13.64 (30)	14.31 (31½)	15.04 (33¼)	15.71 (34¾)	15.99 (35¼)
98–100 cm (38½–39¼ in)	13.37 (29½)	13.78 (30½)	14.50 (32)	15.21 (33½)	15.94 (35¼)	16.62 (36¾)	17.00 (37½)	13.10 (29)	13.51 (29¾)	14.19 (31¼)	14.87 (32¾)	15.63 (34½)	16.32 (36)	16.64 (36¾)
100–102 cm (39¼–40¼ in)	13.90 (30¾)	14.30 (31½)	15.06 (33¼)	15.81 (34¾)	16.54 (36½)	17.22 (38)	17.60 (38¾)	13.68 (30¼)	14.08 (31)	14.77 (32½)	15.46 (34)	16.25 (35¾)	16.96 (37½)	17.39 (38¼)
102–104 cm (40¼–41 in)	14.48 (32)	14.85 (32¾)	15.65 (34½)	16.45 (36¼)	17.18 (37¾)	17.87 (39½)	18.24 (40¼)							

Table continued on following page

■ **TABLE 13–2 Weight by Length*** *Continued*

Recumbent Length	Boys: Weight Percentiles, kg and (lb)							Girls: Weight Percentiles, kg and (lb)						
	5th	*10th*	*25th*	*50th*	*75th*	*90th*	*95th*	*5th*	*10th*	*25th*	*50th*	*75th*	*90th*	*95th*
Boys and Girls: Prepubescent‡														
90–92 cm (35½–36¼ in)	11.70 (25¾)	11.97 (26½)	12.59 (27¾)	13.41 (29½)	14.35 (31¾)	15.25 (33½)	15.72 (34¾)	11.45 (25¼)	11.67 (25¾)	12.28 (27)	13.14 (29)	14.11 (31)	14.98 (33)	15.74 (34¾)
92–94 cm (36¼–37 in)	12.07 (26½)	12.36 (27¼)	13.03 (28¾)	13.89 (30½)	14.84 (32¾)	15.87 (35)	16.41 (36¼)	11.86 (26¼)	12.10 (26¾)	12.74 (28)	13.63 (30)	14.63 (32¼)	15.57 (34¼)	16.42 (36¼)
94–96 cm (37–37¾ in)	12.46 (27½)	12.77 (28¼)	13.49 (29¾)	14.38 (31¾)	15.34 (33¾)	16.45 (36¼)	17.06 (37½)	12.26 (27)	12.53 (27½)	13.21 (29)	14.12 (31¼)	15.14 (33½)	16.13 (35½)	17.05 (37½)
96–98 cm (37¾–38½ in)	12.87 (28¼)	13.21 (29)	13.98 (30¾)	14.89 (32¾)	15.87 (35)	17.01 (37½)	17.69 (39)	12.66 (28)	12.97 (28½)	13.70 (30¼)	14.62 (32¼)	15.66 (34½)	16.69 (36¾)	17.65 (39)
98–100 cm (38½–39¼ in)	13.31 (29¼)	13.67 (30¼)	14.48 (32)	15.43 (34)	16.41 (36¼)	17.56 (38¾)	18.29 (40¼)	13.06 (28¾)	13.42 (29½)	14.19 (31¼)	15.13 (33¼)	16.19 (35¾)	17.24 (38)	18.23 (40¼)
100–102 cm (39¼–40¼ in)	13.77 (30¼)	14.15 (31¼)	15.00 (33)	15.98 (35¼)	16.98 (37½)	18.11 (40)	18.89 (41¾)	13.48 (29¾)	13.88 (30½)	14.69 (32½)	15.65 (34½)	16.73 (37)	17.80 (39¼)	18.80 (41½)
102–104 cm (40¼–41 in)	14.25 (31½)	14.65 (32¼)	15.54 (34¼)	16.65 (36½)	17.57 (38¾)	18.67 (41¼)	19.50 (43)	13.91 (30¾)	14.36 (31¾)	15.21 (33½)	16.20 (35¾)	17.28 (38)	18.38 (40½)	19.38 (42¾)
104–106 cm (41–41¾ in)	14.76 (32½)	15.18 (33½)	16.10 (35½)	17.13 (37¾)	18.18 (40)	19.25 (42½)	20.12 (44¼)	14.36 (31¾)	14.85 (32¾)	15.75 (34¾)	16.75 (37)	17.86 (39¼)	18.98 (41¾)	19.98 (44)
106–108 cm (41¾–42½ in)	15.30 (33¾)	15.73 (34¾)	16.68 (36¾)	17.74 (39)	18.82 (41½)	19.86 (43¾)	20.76 (45¾)	14.84 (32¾)	15.37 (34)	16.30 (36)	17.33 (38¼)	18.46 (40¾)	19.62 (43¼)	20.61 (45½)
108–110 cm (42½–43¼ in)	15.85 (35)	16.31 (36)	17.28 (38)	18.37 (40½)	19.49 (43)	20.51 (45¼)	21.45 (47¼)	15.35 (33¾)	15.91 (35)	16.87 (37¼)	17.94 (39½)	19.09 (42)	20.30 (44¾)	21.29 (47)
110–112 cm (43¼–44 in)	16.43 (36¼)	16.91 (37¼)	17.90 (39½)	19.02 (42)	20.18 (44½)	21.22 (46¾)	22.18 (49)	15.90 (35)	16.48 (36¼)	17.47 (38½)	18.56 (41)	19.76 (43½)	21.03 (46¼)	22.03 (48½)
112–114 cm (44–45 in)	17.04 (37½)	17.53 (38¾)	18.54 (40¾)	19.70 (43½)	20.91 (46)	21.98 (48½)	22.98 (50¾)	16.48 (36¼)	17.09 (37¾)	18.08 (39¾)	19.22 (42¼)	20.47 (45¼)	21.81 (48)	22.84 (50¼)
114–116 cm (45–45¾ in)	17.66 (39)	18.18 (40)	19.20 (42¼)	20.39 (45)	21.66 (47¾)	22.82 (50¼)	23.85 (52½)	17.11 (37¾)	17.72 (39)	18.72 (41¼)	19.91 (44)	21.23 (46¾)	22.67 (50)	23.73 (52¼)
116–118 cm (45¾–46½ in)	18.32 (40½)	18.85 (41½)	19.89 (43¾)	21.11 (46½)	22.45 (49½)	23.73 (52¼)	24.80 (54¾)	17.77 (39¼)	18.40 (40½)	19.40 (42¾)	20.64 (45½)	22.04 (48½)	23.60 (52)	24.71 (54½)
118–120 cm (46½–47¼ in)	18.99 (41¾)	19.55 (43)	20.60 (45½)	21.85 (48¼)	23.28 (51¼)	24.73 (54½)	25.83 (57)	18.48 (40¾)	19.11 (42¼)	20.11 (44¼)	21.42 (47¼)	22.92 (50½)	24.62 (54¼)	25.81 (57)
120–122 cm (47¼–48 in)	19.70 (43½)	20.28 (44¾)	21.34 (47)	22.63 (50)	24.15 (53¼)	25.80 (57)	26.96 (59½)	19.22 (42¼)	19.85 (43¾)	20.87 (46)	22.25 (49)	23.88 (52¾)	25.73 (56¾)	27.03 (59½)
122–124 cm (48–48¾ in)	20.43 (45)	21.03 (46¼)	22.11 (48¾)	23.45 (51¾)	25.07 (55¼)	26.96 (59½)	28.18 (62¼)	19.99 (44)	20.64 (45½)	21.68 (47¾)	23.13 (51)	24.91 (55)	26.95 (59½)	28.37 (62½)
124–126 cm (48¾–49½ in)	21.20 (46¾)	21.82 (48)	22.92 (50½)	24.32 (53½)	26.05 (57½)	28.18 (62¼)	29.50 (65)	20.80 (45¾)	21.47 (47¼)	22.54 (49¾)	24.09 (53)	26.05 (57½)	28.27 (62¼)	29.87 (65¾)
126–128 cm (49½–50½ in)	21.99 (48½)	22.64 (50)	23.77 (52½)	25.24 (55¾)	27.10 (59¾)	29.48 (65)	30.92 (68¼)	21.65 (47¾)	22.34 (49¼)	23.47 (51¾)	25.11 (55¼)	27.28 (60¼)	29.71 (65½)	31.51 (69½)
128–130 cm (50½–51¾ in)	22.82 (50¼)	23.50 (51¾)	24.67 (54½)	26.22 (57¾)	28.21 (62¼)	30.86 (68)	32.44 (71½)	22.53 (49¾)	23.25 (51¼)	24.46 (54)	26.22 (57¾)	28.63 (63)	31.28 (69)	33.33 (73½)
130–132 cm (51¼–52 in)	23.69 (52¼)	24.59 (53¾)	25.62 (56½)	27.26 (60)	29.41 (64¾)	32.31 (71¼)	34.07 (75)	23.44 (51¾)	24.22 (53½)	25.52 (56¼)	27.40 (60½)	30.09 (66¼)	32.99 (72¾)	35.33 (78)
132–134 cm (52–52¾ in)	24.59 (54¼)	25.32 (55¾)	26.62 (58¾)	28.38 (62½)	30.68 (67¾)	33.82 (74½)	35.81 (79)	24.38 (53¾)	25.22 (55½)	26.66 (58¾)	28.68 (63¼)	31.68 (69¾)	34.84 (76¾)	37.53 (82¾)
134–136 cm (52¾–53½ in)	25.53 (56¼)	26.30 (58)	27.68 (61)	29.58 (65¼)	32.05 (70¾)	35.40 (78)	37.67 (83)	25.35 (56)	26.28 (58)	27.88 (61½)	30.06 (66¼)	33.41 (73¾)	36.84 (81¼)	39.93 (88)
136–138 cm (53½–54¼ in)	26.51 (58½)	27.32 (60¼)	28.80 (63½)	30.86 (68)	33.51 (74)	37.05 (81¾)	39.65 (87½)	26.34 (58)	27.39 (60½)	29.19 (64¼)	31.54 (69½)	35.29 (77¾)	39.01 (86)	42.54 (93¾)
138–140 cm (54¼–55 in)	27.53 (60¾)	28.38 (62½)	29.99 (66)	32.23 (71)	35.08 (77¼)	38.77 (85½)	41.74 (92)							
140–142 cm (55–56 in)	28.59 (63)	29.48 (65)	31.25 (69)	33.70 (74¼)	36.75 (81)	40.55 (89½)	43.97 (97)							
142–144 cm (56–56¾ in)	29.70 (65½)	30.64 (67½)	32.58 (71¾)	35.27 (77¾)	38.54 (85)	42.39 (93½)	46.32 (102)							
144–146 cm (56¾–57½ in)	30.86 (68)	31.85 (70¼)	34.00 (75)	36.95 (81½)	40.45 (89¼)	44.29 (97¾)	48.80 (107½)							

**Data are those of the National Center for Health Statistics (NCHS), Health Resources Administration, Department of Health, Education, and Welfare.*
†Data are based on studies of the Fels Research Institute, Yellow Springs, OH.
‡Data are based on the Health Examination Surveys of the NCHS. For details see footnote to Table 11–2.

Play allows children to experience mastery by solving puzzles, practicing adult roles, assuming the aggressor role rather than the victim (spanking a doll), taking on super powers (dinosaur and super hero play), and obtaining things that are denied in real life (a make-believe friend or stuffed pet). Drawing, painting, and other artistic activities are forms of play in which the creative motivation is most evident. The seeming immaturity of young children's art reflects, in part, the child's willingness to assign symbolic significance rather than perceptual or technical deficits. The child who chooses to let a big circle with sticks represent a body and limbs knows that real bodies do not actually look like that and may create a much more lifelike body in clay. Like other play, visual art often becomes increasingly rule governed with age.

Moral thinking mirrors and is constrained by the child's cognitive level. In its early stages rules tend to be absolute, with guilt assigned for bad outcomes regardless of intentions. In keeping with the child's inability to focus on more than one aspect of a situation at a time, fairness is taken to mean equal treatment regardless of circumstantial differences. Empathic responses to others' distress arise during the 2nd yr of life, but the ability to cognitively consider another child's point of view remains limited throughout the preschool period.

Implications for Parents and Pediatricians. The significance of language as a target for assessment and intervention cannot be overestimated because of its central role as an indicator of cognitive and emotional development and as a key factor in behavioral regulation and later school success. Detection and assessment of language delays, a critical part of preventive care, is discussed in Chapters 17 and 31. Parents can support emotional development by using words that describe the child's feeling states ("You sound angry right now.") and by urging the child to use words to express feelings rather than acting the feelings out.

Parents should have a regular time each day for reading or looking at books with their children. Programs in which pediatricians give out picture books along with appropriate guidance during primary care visits have been effective in increasing reading aloud, particularly in lower income families.

Preoperational thinking dictates the child's understanding of experiences of illness and treatment. Many children perceive needles as huge objects that threaten to puncture them like a balloon. Verbal explanation is often not as reassuring as giving the child an opportunity to administer "shots" to a doll and see, repeatedly, that nothing horrible happens. Explanations that involve multiple contradictory aspects ("This will hurt a little, but it will keep you from getting sick.") will be lost on most preoperational children; the immediate presence of a calm parent is more comforting. Children with precocious language development may elicit overly complex explanations from adults who assume incorrectly that their cognitive sophistication matches their verbal skill.

The imaginative intensity that fuels play and the magical, animist thinking characteristic of preoperational cognition also generate intense fears. More than 80% of parents report at least one fear in their preschool children and nearly 50% report seven or more fears. Refusal to take baths or to sit on the toilet may arise from the fear of being washed or flushed down, reflecting the child's immature appreciation of relative size. Attempts to demonstrate rationally that there are no monsters in the closet often fail, as the fear arises from prerational thinking. Reassurances that parents will use their "great power" (e.g., monster spray, tape) to guarantee the child's safety may be more effective because they appeal to the child's magical thinking.

EMOTIONAL DEVELOPMENT

Emotional challenges facing the preschool child include accepting limits while maintaining a sense of self-direction, reigning in aggressive and sexual impulses, and interacting with a widening circle of adults and peers. At age 2 yr, behavioral limits are predominantly external; by age 5 yr, these controls need to be internalized if the child is to function in a typical classroom. Success in achieving this goal relies on prior emotional development, particularly the ability to use internalized images of trusted adults to provide security in times of stress. Children need to believe themselves worthy of adult approval to be willing to work for it.

Children learn what behaviors are acceptable and how much power they wield vis-à-vis important adults by testing limits. Testing increases when it elicits an exceptional amount of attention, even though that attention is often negative, and when limits are inconsistent. Testing often arouses parental anger or inappropriate solicitude as the child's struggle to separate gives rise to a corresponding challenge for the parents: letting go. Excessively tight limits can undermine the child's sense of initiative, whereas overly loose limits can provoke anxiety in a child who feels that there is no one in control.

Control is a central issue. Inability to control some aspect of the external world, such as what to buy or when to leave, often results in a loss of internal control, that is, a *temper tantrum*. Fear, overtiredness, or physical discomfort can also evoke tantrums. When they are reinforced by intermittent rewards, as when the parent occasionally gives in to the child's demands, tantrums can also become an entrenched strategy for exerting control. Tantrums lasting more than 15 min or regularly occurring more than three times a day may reflect underlying medical, emotional, or social problems. Tantrums normally appear toward the end of the 1st yr of life and peak in prevalence between ages 2 and 4 yr. Frequent tantrums after age 5 yr tend to persist throughout childhood.

Preschool children normally experience complicated feelings toward their parents: intense love and jealousy and resentment and fear that angry feelings might lead to abandonment. The swirl of these emotions, most beyond the child's ability to analyze or express, often finds expression in highly labile moods. The resolution of this "crisis" (a process extending over years) involves the child's unspoken decision to emulate the parents rather than compete with them. Play and language foster the development of emotional controls by allowing children to express emotions and to enjoy gratifications (power or intimacy with parents) that are taboo in real life.

Curiosity about genitalia and adult sexual organs is normal as is masturbation. Modesty appears gradually between age 4 and 6 yr, with wide variations among cultures and families. Masturbation that has a compulsive quality or that interferes with the child's normal activities, acting out of sexual intercourse in doll play or with other children, extreme modesty, or mimicry of adult seductive behavior all suggest the possibility of sexual abuse.

Implications for Parents and Pediatricians. Most parents find it difficult to understand their preschool children at least some of the time. Rapid shifts between clinging dependence and defiant independence, between sophisticated sounding language and infantile helplessness, and between angelic joy and uncontrollable rage can erode parents' self-confidence and patience. Guidance emphasizing appropriate expectations for behavioral and emotional development and acknowledging normal parental feelings of anger, guilt, and confusion can help lessen parents' worries both about their children and about themselves. Many parents fail to raise such concerns during pediatric visits because they feel embarrassed or because they do not think the pediatrician can help. Pediatricians need to let parents know that the child's behavior and the parents' reactions are appropriate topics for discussion.

It may be difficult to decide whether a particular child's behavior is normally challenging or indicative of a true problem. "Red flags" include parents who do not volunteer any positive statements about their children, the existence of problems (especially tantrums) in day care or preschool, and evidence of threatening or overtly punitive discipline. The presence of chronic medical problems, developmental delays, or unusual family stresses signals the need for more detailed assessment. Even apparently normal behavior constitutes a problem if it arouses sufficient parental concern. An extended visit devoted to the issue or referral to a mental health professional is appropriate.

Corporal punishment is accepted in many traditional cultures but may be inappropriate in the modern context in which most families now live. There is no evidence that spanking per se is harmful. Regular use of corporal punishment often reflects a desperate attempt by parents to assert control. Parents usually claim that they do not like spanking but feel that "nothing else works." The pediatrician can point out that the spanking is not working either, or it would not have to be used so often. As children habituate to repeated spanking, parents are forced to spank ever harder to get the desired response, increasing the risk of serious injury. Sufficiently harsh punishment can probably inhibit any behavior but at great psychological cost. Children mimic the corporal punishment they receive and it is not uncommon for preschool-age children to strike their parents back. Parents may be helped to renounce spanking or at least reserve it for extreme circumstances if they learn more effective discipline techniques including consistent limit setting, clear communication, and frequent approval. "Time-out" periods of short duration, on a chair or in a room (specific place), are useful first attempts at noncorporal discipline.

Anderson RC, Hiebert EH, Scott JA, et al: Becoming a Nation of Readers: The Report of the Commission on Reading. Washington, DC, The National Institute of Education, 1985.

Faber A, Mazlish E: How to Talk So Kids Will Listen & Listen So Kids Will Talk. New York, Avon, 1980.

Ginsburg H, Opper S: Piaget's Theory of Intellectual Development. Englewood Cliffs, NJ, Prentice-Hall, 1969.

Richman N, Stevenson J, Graham PJ: Pre-School to School: A Behavioral Study. London, Academic Press, 1982.

Satter E: Child of Mine: Feeding with Love and Good Sense. Palo Alto, CA, Bull Publishing, 1986.

Schickedanz JA: More Than the ABCs: The Early Stages of Reading and Writing. Washington, DC, National Association for the Education of Young Children, 1986.

CHAPTER 14

Early School Years

The child between the ages of 6 and 12 yr, a period sometimes referred to as middle childhood or latency, has new challenges. The cognitive power to consider multiple factors simultaneously gives school-age children the ability to evaluate themselves and perceive others' evaluations of them. As a result, self-esteem becomes a central issue. Unlike infants and preschoolers, school-age children are judged according to their ability to produce socially valued outputs, such as good grades or home runs. Accordingly, Erikson identified the central psychosocial issue of this period as the crisis between industry and inferiority. Healthy development requires increasing separation from parents and the ability to find acceptance in the peer group and to negotiate challenges in the outside world.

PHYSICAL DEVELOPMENT

Growth during the period averages 3–3.5 kg (7 lb) and 6 cm (2.5 in) per year (see Figs. 12–1 and 12–2 and Table 13–1). The head grows only 2–3 cm in circumference throughout the entire period, reflecting slowed brain growth, because myelinization is complete by 7 yrs of age. Body habitus (endomorphic, mesomorphic, or ectomorphic) tends to remain relatively stable throughout middle childhood.

Growth of the midface and lower face occurs gradually. Loss of deciduous (baby) teeth is a more dramatic sign of maturation, beginning about age 6 yr after eruption of the 1st molars. Replacement with adult teeth occurs at a rate of about 4/yr. Lymphoid tissues hypertrophy, often giving rise to impressive tonsils and adenoids, which occasionally require surgical treatment.

Muscular strength, coordination, and stamina increase progressively, as does the ability to perform complex-pattern movements such as dancing, shooting basketballs, or playing the piano. Such higher order motor skills are the result of both maturation and training; the degree of accomplishment reflects wide variability in innate skill, interest, and opportunity. Epidemiologic studies report a general decline in physical fitness among school-age children. Sedentary habits at this age are associated with increased lifetime risk of obesity and cardiovascular disease.

The sexual organs remain physically immature, but interest in gender differences and sexual behavior remain active in many children and increase progressively until puberty. Masturbation is common, if not universal. In more permissive cultures, sexual experimentation often occurs among prepubertal children.

Implications for Parents and Pediatricians. "Normality" encompasses a wide range of physical sizes, shapes, and abilities in school-age children. Just as importantly, children's feelings about their physical attributes range from pride to shame to apparent nonchalance. Fears of being "defective" can lead to avoidance of situations in which physical differences might be revealed, such as gym class or medical examinations. Children with actual physical disabilities may face special stresses because of their difference. The routine physical examination provides an opportunity to elicit concerns and allay fears.

Girls, in particular, often worry that they are overweight and many engage in unhealthy dieting to achieve an abnormally thin cultural ideal. Shortness, particularly in boys, is associated with decreased educational attainment and increased risks for behavior problems. The child's physical appearance may also evoke strong feelings in parents. These feelings often complicate parents' efforts to foster their children's physical development without undercutting their self-esteem on the one hand and encouraging vanity on the other. Pediatricians can help parents distinguish between true health risks and individual variations that should be accepted. The availability of recombinant human growth hormone raises the possibility of medical treatment for short children who may not have documentable hormone deficiency. The decision to treat, with its attendant cost and discomfort, needs to be made in view of the meaning of shortness for the individual child (see Chapter 512).

A description of regular physical activities should be part of the medical history for health supervision visits. Participation in organized sports can foster skill, teamwork, and fitness, but excessive pressure to compete often has negative effects. Prepubertal children should not engage in high-stress, high-impact sports such as power lifting or football because skeletal immaturity increases the risk of injury.

COGNITIVE AND LANGUAGE DEVELOPMENT

The thinking of young school-age children differs qualitatively from that of children just 1 or 2 yr younger. In place of magical, egocentric, and perception-bound cognition, school-age children increasingly apply rules based on observable phenomena, factor in multiple dimensions and points of view, and interpret their perceptions in view of realistic theories about physical laws. This shift from "preoperational" to "concrete logical operations" was documented by Piaget in a series of "conservation" experiments (see Chapter 13). For example, 5-yr-olds who watch a ball of clay being rolled into a snake might insist that the snake has "more" because it is longer. Seven-year-olds typically reply that the ball and snake must weigh the same because nothing has been added or taken away or because the snake is both longer and thinner. This cognitive reorganization occurs at different rates in different contexts. In the context of social interactions with siblings, young children often demonstrate an ability to understand multiple points of view long before they demonstrate that ability in their thinking about the physical world.

School makes increasing cognitive demands. Mastery of the elementary curriculum requires that a large number of perceptual, cognitive, and language processes work efficiently (Table 14–1). Attention and receptive language affect each other as well as every other aspect of learning. One cannot attend to what one cannot understand or understand without first paying attention. By third grade, children need to be able to sustain attention through a 45-min period.

The first 2 yr of elementary school are devoted to acquiring the fundamentals: reading, writing, and basic mathematics skills. By third or fourth grade, the curriculum requires that children use those fundamentals to learn increasingly complex materials. The goal of reading a paragraph is no longer to decode the words but to understand the content; the goal of writing is no longer spelling or penmanship but composition. The volume of work rises along with the complexity. Children can meet these demands only if they have mastered the basic skills to the point at which they become automatic. Children who have to think about how to shape each letter or who have to recalculate basic mathematics facts each time they attempt to solve a word problem fall behind.

Cognitive abilities interact with a wide array of attitudinal and emotional factors in determining classroom performance. A partial list of such factors includes eagerness to please adults, cooperativeness, competitiveness, willingness to work for a delayed reward, belief in one's abilities, and ability to risk trying when success is not ensured. Success predisposes to success, whereas failure undercuts the child's ability to take cognitive-emotional risks in the future.

Children's intellectual activity extends beyond the classroom. Beginning in third or fourth grade, children increasingly enjoy strategy games and word play (puns and insults) that exercise growing cognitive and linguistic mastery. Many become experts on subjects of their own choosing, such as sports trivia or stamps. Others become avid readers.

Implications for Parents and Pediatricians. Children in the cognitive stage of concrete logical operations can understand simple explanations for illnesses and necessary treatments, although they may revert to prelogical thinking under stress (as may adults). A child with pneumonia may be able to explain about white cells fighting the "germs" in the lungs but still secretly harbor the belief that the sickness is a punishment for not having obeyed the parents.

Academic and classroom behavior problems, like fever, are symptoms that require diagnosis. Among the broad range of possible causes are deficits in specific cognitive, perceptual, or linguistic functions (specific learning disabilities); global cognitive delay (mental retardation); primary attention deficit; and attention deficits secondary to emotional preoccupation, depression, anxiety, or any chronic illness. Commonly, the cause is a combination of several such factors. Assessment of school problems is discussed in Chapters 27 and 31.

Remedial approaches depend on the underlying problem or problems. Children who are inattentive because of receptive language disability will benefit more from language therapy than from stimulant medication. Similarly, psychotherapy is generally less helpful for primary attention deficits than are medication and environmental modifications aimed at increasing structure and decreasing distractions. Simply having a child repeat a failed grade rarely has any beneficial effect and often seriously undercuts the child's self-esteem. See Chapter 31

■ **TABLE 14–1 Selected Perceptual, Cognitive, and Language Processes Required for Elementary School Success**

Process	Description	Associated Problems
Perceptual		
Visual analysis	Ability to break a complex figure into components and understand their spatial relationships	Persistent letter confusion (e.g., between *b, d,* and *g*); difficulty with basic reading and writing and limited "sight" vocabulary
Proprioception and motor control	Ability to obtain information about body position by feel and unconsciously program complex movements	Poor handwriting, requiring inordinate effort, often with overly tight pencil grasp; special difficulty with timed tasks
Phonologic processing	Ability to perceive differences between similar sounding words and to break down words into constituent sounds	Delayed receptive language skills; attention and behavior problems secondary to not understanding directions; delayed acquisition of letter-sound correlations (phonetics)
Cognitive		
Long-term memory, both storage and recall	Ability to acquire skills that are "automatic" (i.e., accessible without conscious thought)	Delayed mastery of the alphabet (reading and writing letters); slow handwriting; inability to progress beyond basic mathematics
Selective attention	Ability to attend to important stimuli and ignore distractions	Difficulty following multistep instructions, completing assignments, and behaving well; peer interaction problems
Sequencing	Ability to remember things in order; facility with time concepts	Difficulty organizing assignments, planning, spelling, and telling time
Language		
Receptive language	Ability to comprehend complex constructions, function words (e.g., if, when, only, except), nuances of speech, and extended blocks of language (e.g., paragraphs)	Difficulty following directions; wandering attention during lessons and stories; problems with reading comprehension; problems with peer relationships
Expressive language	Ability to recall required words effortlessly (word finding), to control meanings by varying position and word endings, to construct meaningful paragraphs and stories	Difficulty expressing feelings and using words for self-defense, with resulting frustration and physical acting out; struggling during "circle time" and in language-based subjects (e.g., English)

■ TABLE 15–2 Classification of Sex Maturity Stages in Girls

SMR Stage	Pubic Hair	Breasts
1	Preadolescent	Preadolescent
2	Sparse, lightly pigmented, straight, medial border of labia	Breast and papilla elevated as small mound; areolar diameter increased
3	Darker, beginning to curl, increased amount	Breast and areola enlarged, no contour separation
4	Coarse, curly, abundant but amount less than in adult	Areola and papilla form secondary mound
5	Adult feminine triangle, spread to medial surface of thighs	Mature; nipple projects, areola part of general breast contour

SMR = sexual maturity rating.
From Tanner JM: Growth at Adolescence, 2nd ed. Oxford, England, Blackwell Scientific Publications, 1962.

sign in boys, testicular enlargement, begins as early as 9.5 yr. In girls, under the influence of follicle-stimulating hormone and estrogen, the ovaries, uterus, and clitoris enlarge; the endometrium and the vaginal mucosa thicken; and increased vaginal glycogen encourages acid-forming bacteria, predisposing to yeast infections. The labia majora become more vascular and more sensitive. Menarche occurs in approximately 10% of girls in SMR2. In boys, under the influence of luteinizing hormone and testosterone, the seminiferous tubules, epididymis, seminal vesicles, and prostate enlarge. The left testis normally is lower than the right; the opposite may be true in situs inversus.

Growth acceleration begins in early adolescence, although peak growth velocities are not reached until SMR3 or 4. The growth spurt occurs early in girls and later in boys (see Fig. 15–5 for gender-related growth velocities). It begins distally, with early enlargement of hands and feet followed by the arms and legs and finally by the trunk and chest. This asymmetric growth gives the young adolescent a gawky look.

Some degree of breast hypertrophy occurs in 40–65% of pubertal boys as a result of a relative excess of estrogenic stimulation. Gynecomastia sufficient to cause embarrassment and social disability occurs in fewer than 10%. Small swellings (<4 cm in diameter) resolve within 3 yr without therapy in 90%. For greater degrees of enlargement, hormonal or surgical treatment may be indicated.

In both sexes, adrenal androgens stimulate the sebaceous glands, promoting the development of acne. Elongation of the optic globe often results in nearsightedness. Changes occur in vocal quality, reflecting laryngeal and thoracic growth, as well as cultural norms. Dental changes include jaw growth, loss of the final deciduous teeth, and eruption of the permanent cuspids, premolars, and finally molars (see Table 11–6). Orthodontic appliances may be needed.

SEXUALITY. Sexuality includes not only sexual behaviors but also interest and fantasies, sexual orientation, attitudes toward

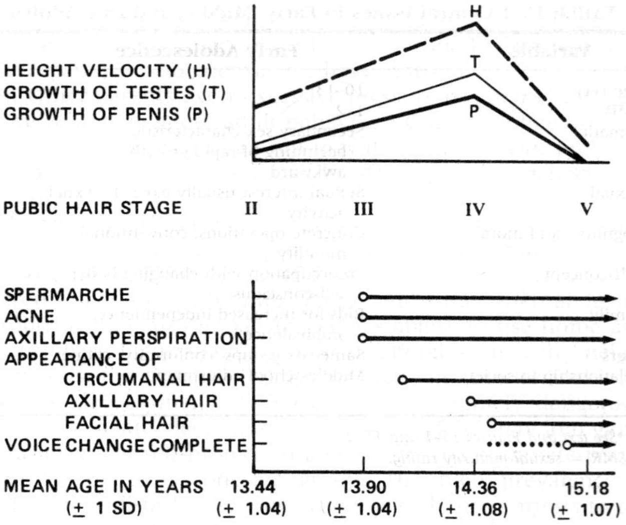

Figure 15–3. Sequence of maturational events in males. (Adapted from Marshall WA, Tanner JM: Variations in the pattern of pubertal changes in boys. Arch Dis Child 45:13, 1970.)

sex and its relationship to emotions, and awareness of socially defined roles and mores.

Interest in sex increases in early puberty. Ejaculation occurs for the first time, usually during masturbation, and later spontaneously in sleep. Some boys worry that these emissions are signs of infection. Early adolescents sometimes masturbate socially; mutual sexual exploration is not necessarily a sign of homosexuality. Sexual behavior, other than masturbation, is less common. At age 13 yr, some 5% of girls and 20% of boys report having had sexual intercourse.

The relationship between hormonal changes and sexual interest and activity is controversial; no consistent links between hormones and sexual arousal, age of first intercourse, or frequency of intercourse have been found.

COGNITIVE AND MORAL DEVELOPMENT. In Piagetian theory, adolescence marks the transition from the concrete operational thinking characteristic of school-age children (Chapter 14) to formal logical operations. Formal operations include the ability to manipulate abstractions such as algebraic expressions, to reason from known principles, to weigh multiple points of view according to varying criteria, and to think about the process of thinking itself. Formal operational thought, which implies an ability to treat possibilities as real entities, may be related to critical decisions, such as whether or not to have unprotected intercourse or engage in other risk-taking behavior.

Some early adolescents demonstrate formal thinking, others acquire the capability later, and others do not acquire it at all. Young adolescents may be able to apply formal operations to

■ TABLE 15–3 Classification of Sex Maturity Stages in Boys

SMR Stage	Pubic Hair	Penis	Testes
1	None	Preadolescent	Preadolescent
2	Scanty, long, slightly pigmented	Slight enlargement	Enlarged scrotum, pink texture altered
3	Darker, starts to curl, small amount	Longer	Larger
4	Resembles adult type, but less in quantity; coarse, curly	Larger; glans and breadth increase in size	Larger, scrotum dark
5	Adult distribution, spread to medial surface of thighs	Adult size	Adult size

SMR = sexual maturity rating.
Adapted from Tanner JM: Growth at Adolescence, 2nd ed. Oxford, England, Blackwell Scientific Publications, 1962.

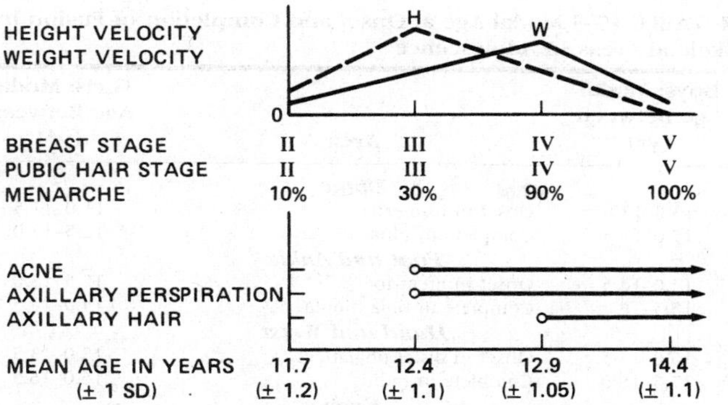

Figure 15–4. Sequence of maturational events in females. (Adapted from Marshall WA, Tanner JM: Variations in pattern of pubertal changes in girls. Arch Dis Child 44:291, 1969.)

schoolwork but not to personal dilemmas. When the emotional stakes are high, magical thinking, such as the conviction of invulnerability, may interfere with higher order cognition.

Some theorists argue that the transition from concrete to formal operations follows from quantitative increases in knowledge, experience, and cognitive efficiency rather than a qualitative reorganization of thinking. Consistent with this view are data showing a steady rise in cognitive processing speed from late childhood through early adulthood. The brain, unlike many other body parts, shows little structural change during puberty, although there is progressive maturation of the electroencephalogram. It is unclear whether or not the hormonal changes of puberty directly affect cognitive development.

The development of moral thinking roughly parallels general cognitive development. Most preadolescents perceive right and wrong as absolute and unquestionable. Taking a loaf of bread to feed a starving child is wrong because it is "stealing." Adolescents often question this received morality, embracing the behavior standards of the peer group. Group membership may allow them to displace guilt feelings for perceived moral infractions from themselves to the group.

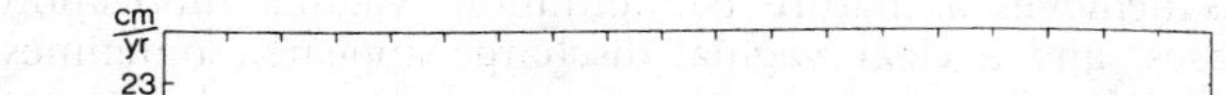

Figure 15–5. Height velocity curves for U.S. boys *(solid line)* and girls *(dashed line)* who have their peak height velocity at the average age (i.e., average growth tempo). (From Tanner JM, Davies PSW: Clinical longitudinal standards for height and height velocity for North American children. J Pediatr 107:317, 1985.)

■ **TABLE 15–4 Variability in Timing of Sexual Maturation**

SMR	*Early (mean −2 SD Early)*	*Average (median)*	*Late (mean +2 SD Late)*
Timing of SMR Stages in Girls			
Pubic Hair			
SMR2	9.0	11.2	13.5
SMR3	9.6	11.9	14.1
SMR4	10.3	12.6	14.8
Breast Development			
SMR2	8.9	10.9	12.9
SMR3	9.8	11.9	13.9
SMR4	10.5	12.9	15.3
Timing of SMR Stages in Boys			
Pubic Hair			
SMR2	9.9	12.0	14.1
SMR3	11.2	13.1	14.9
SMR4	12.0	13.9	15.7
Penis Development			
SMR2	9.2	10.5	13.7
SMR3	10.1	12.4	14.6
SMR4	11.2	13.2	15.4

SMR = sexual maturity rating.
Data from Tanner JM, Davies PSW: Clinical longitudinal standards for height and height velocity for North American children. J Pediatr 107:317, 1985.

SELF-CONCEPT. Self-consciousness increases exponentially in response to the somatic transformations of puberty. Self-awareness at this age tends to center on external characteristics in contrast to the introspection of later adolescence. It is normal for early adolescents to scrutinize their appearance and to feel that everyone else is staring at them too. A mild degree of distortion of body image is probably universal. Serious body image distortions, such as anorexia nervosa, also tend to appear at this age. Puberty may increase self-esteem in boys but undermine it in girls as both sexes assume gender roles that incorporate gross inequalities in power and prestige.

RELATIONSHIPS WITH FAMILY, PEERS, AND SOCIETY. In early adolescence, the trend toward separation from family and increasing involvement in peer activities accelerates. A symbolic expression of this shift is the renunciation of the family code of dress and grooming in favor of the peer group "uniform." Such stylistic changes frequently spark conflicts that are truly about power or difficulty accepting separation. Not all adolescents rebel and not all parents reject such assertions of separateness as signs of insurrection. Most adolescents continue to strive to please their parents even while they disagree on certain points.

Separation from family often involves selecting adults outside of the family as role models and developing close relationships with particular teachers or the parents of other children. Organizations such as the Boy Scouts and Girl Scouts provide an important sense of extrafamilial belonging.

Early adolescents often socialize in same-sex peer groups. Scatologic jokes, teasing directed against the other gender, and rumor mongering about who "likes" whom attest to burgeoning sexual interest. Belonging is all-important. In one-to-one friendships, boys and girls may differ in important ways. Female friendships may center on the sharing of confidences, whereas male relationships may focus more on shared activities and competition.

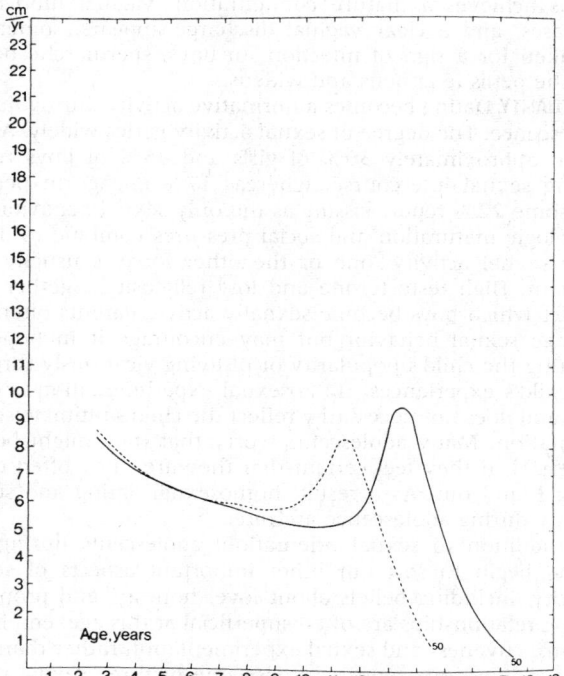

The early adolescent's relationship to society centers on school. The shift from elementary to junior high school entails giving up the protection of the homeroom in exchange for the additional stimulation and responsibility involved in moving from class to class. This change in school structure mirrors and reinforces the changes involved in separating from the family.

Implications for Parents and Pediatricians. Physical growth, body preoccupation, and sexual interest correlate with sexual maturity, whereas cognitive advancement, separation, and changes in social behavior may correlate more closely with chronologic age or grade in school. Discordance between chronologic age and sexual maturation may increase the stress of early adolescence. As a group, early-maturing boys enjoy greater social success and higher self-esteem than do later maturers. For girls, by contrast, early maturation is associated with poorer school performance and lower self-esteem.

Early adolescents often have questions about the somatic and sexual changes they are experiencing. In a multicultural sample of rural and urban adolescents, questions ranged from sophisticated to "poignantly ignorant." During the physical examination, the pediatrician can anticipate concerns and volunteer information that the adolescent may have been too uncomfortable to request. Parents, too, may have concerns that they are hesitant to discuss. If the parent is interviewed alone, it is important that this be done first, before the interview with the child, to avoid undermining the adolescent's trust.

The child's level of cognitive sophistication has implications for the sort of explanations that will be most helpful. Open-ended questions about common dilemmas facing young adolescents, whether or not to join a clique or gang or to abide by family rules that seem unjustified, can provide information about cognitive level and help detect the likelihood of risky behavior.

Parents and children often need help differentiating between the normal discomforts of the period and truly concerning behaviors. Discomfort with one's body is normal; the conviction that one is overweight and needs to diet despite objective evidence to the contrary is concerning. Bids for autonomy in the form of avoidance of family activities, demands for privacy, and increased argumentativeness are normal; extreme withdrawal or antagonism may be a sign of dysfunction. Interest in sex, sometimes heralded by the appearance of pornographic magazines, is normal; sexual intercourse in early adolescence, although fairly common, is usually a sign of developmental dysfunction. Bewilderment and dysphoria at the start of junior high school are normal; continued failure to adapt several weeks later suggests a more serious problem.

MIDDLE ADOLESCENCE

BIOLOGIC DEVELOPMENT. In middle adolescence, growth accelerates above the prepubertal rate of 6–7 cm (3 in) per year. In the average girl, the growth spurt peaks at 11.5 yr at a top velocity of 8.3 cm (3.8 in) per year and then slows to a stop at 16 yr (see Fig. 15–4). In the average boy, the growth spurt starts later, peaks at 13.5 yr at 9.5 cm (4.3 in) per year, and then slows to a stop at 18 yr. Weight gain parallels linear growth, with a delay of several months, so that adolescents seem first to stretch and then fill out. Pubertal weight gains account for approximately 40% of adult weight. Muscle mass also increases, followed several months later by an increase in strength; boys show greater gains in both. Lean body mass, approximately 80% in the average prepubertal child, increases in boys to 90% and decreases in girls to 75% as subcutaneous fat accumulates.

Bone maturation correlates closely with SMR because epiphyseal closure is under androgenic control (Table 15–5). Boys with SMR3 pubic hair and SMR4 genitalia normally have their peak growth spurt ahead of bone maturation; girls at the same SMR are usually past their peaks (see Figs. 15–3 and 15–4). Widening of the shoulders in boys and of the hips in girls is also hormonally determined. Other physiologic changes include a doubling in heart size and lung vital capacity. Blood pressure, blood volume, and hematocrit rise, particularly in boys. Androgenic stimulation of sebaceous and apocrine glands results in acne and body odor. A physiologic increase in sleepiness may be mistaken for laziness.

■ **TABLE 15–5 Modal Age at Onset and Completion of Fusion in Skeletal Areas in Adolescence**

Boys: Modal Age Between (yr)	Area	Girls: Modal Age Between (yr)
	Elbow	
13.0–13.5	Onset in humerus	11.0–11.5
15.0–15.5	Complete in ulna	12.5–13.0
	Foot and Ankle	
14.0–14.5	Onset in great toe	12.5–13.0
15.5–16	Complete in tibia, fibula	14.0–14.5
	Hand and Wrist	
15.0–15.5	Onset in distal phalanges	13.0–13.5
17.5–18.0	Complete in radius	16.0–16.5
	Knee	
15.0–15.5	Onset in tibial tuberosity	13.5–14.0
17.5–18.0	Complete in fibula	16.0–16.5
	Hip and Pelvis	
15.5–16.0	Onset in greater trochanter	14.0–14.5
after 18.0	Complete in symphysis	17.5–18.0
	Shoulder and Clavicle	
15.5–16.0	Onset in greater tubercle of humerus	14.0–14.5
after 18.0	Complete in clavicle	17.5–18.0

Sexual maturation in middle adolescence is dramatic, with the achievement of menarche in 30% of girls by SMR3 and in 90% by SMR4. Menarche usually follows approximately 1 yr after the growth spurt. The timing of menarche, not completely understood, appears to be determined by genetics as well as such factors as adiposity, chronic illness, and exercise. In developed countries, the average age at menarche has decreased over the last century, perhaps in response to better nutrition and less physical activity. Before menarche, the uterus achieves a mature configuration, vaginal lubrication increases, and a clear vaginal discharge appears, sometimes mistaken for a sign of infection. In boys, spermarche occurs and the penis lengthens and widens.

SEXUALITY. Dating becomes a normative activity during middle adolescence. The degree of sexual activity varies widely. At age 16 yr, approximately 30% of girls and 45% of boys report having sexual intercourse, whereas 17% engage in petting, and some 22% report kissing as the only sexual behavior.

Biologic maturation and social pressures combine to determine sexual activity; one or the other force is usually preeminent. High testosterone and low religiosity together may predict which boys become sexually active. Parents often discourage sexual behavior but may encourage it in hopes of boosting the child's popularity or of living vicariously through the child's experiences. Homosexual experimentation is common and does not necessarily reflect the child's ultimate sexual orientation. Many adolescents worry that they might be homosexual. If they feel certain that they are, they often dread being found out. As a result, homosexual dating and sexual activity during adolescence are rare.

In addition to sexual orientation, adolescents during this period begin to sort out other important aspects of sexual identity, including beliefs about love, honesty, and propriety. Dating relationships are often superficial at this age, emphasizing attractiveness and sexual experimentation rather than intimacy. Adolescents tend to choose one of three sexual paths: celibacy, monogamy, or polygamous experimentation. Most have some knowledge of the risks of pregnancy, acquired immunodeficiency syndrome, and other sexually transmitted diseases, but knowledge does not consistently control behavior. A minority use any contraception at first intercourse, and fewer than 75% consistently use condoms or other effective methods.

COGNITIVE AND MORAL DEVELOPMENT. With the transition to formal operational thought, middle adolescents question and analyze extensively. Questioning of moral conventions fosters the development of personal codes of ethics. Often such codes appear designed to sanction the adolescent's sexual appetite: "Anything I want is right." In other cases, the adolescent may embrace a code that is more strict than that of the parents, perhaps in response to the anxiety engendered by the weakening of the conventional limits. The adolescent's new flexibility of thought has pervasive effects on relationships with self and others.

SELF-CONCEPT. The peer group exerts less influence over dress, activities, and behavior. Middle adolescents often experiment with different personae, changing styles of dress, groups of friends, and interests from month to month. Many philosophize about the meaning of their lives and wonder, "Who am I?" and "Why am I here?" Intense feelings of inner turmoil and misery are common and may be difficult to differentiate from psychiatric illness. Girls may tend to characterize themselves and their peers according to interpersonal relationships ("I am a girl with close friends."), whereas boys as a group may focus on abilities ("I am good at sports.").

RELATIONSHIPS WITH FAMILY, PEERS, AND SOCIETY. Puberty commonly results in strained relationships between adolescents and their parents. As part of separation, adolescents may become distant from parents, redirecting emotional and sexual energies toward peer relationships. Dating can become a lightning rod for parent-child battles, in which the real issue may be the fact of separation rather than the particulars of "with whom" or "how late."

As dating increases, the need to belong to same-sex groups declines. Physical attractiveness and popularity remain critical factors both in peer relationships and in self-esteem. Children with visible differences, such as cleft lip, are at risk for problems developing social skills and confidence and may have more difficulty establishing satisfying relationships.

Middle adolescents often begin thinking seriously about what they want to do as adults, a question that formerly had been comfortably hypothetical. The process involves self-assessment and assessment of the opportunities available. The presence or absence of realistic role models, as opposed to the idealized ones of earlier periods, can be crucial.

Implications for Parents and Pediatricians. Physical and sexual maturation, changes in sexual behavior and identity, further emotional distance from parents, waning of peer group influence, introspection, and growing cognizance of life after childhood all combine to make middle adolescence a time when the opportunity to talk confidentially with a nonjudgmatic, informed adult can be particularly appreciated and helpful.

Adolescents vary greatly in the rate of physical and social progress and in the resolution of central conflicts about autonomy and self-esteem. Questions about family and peer relationships can help locate the child along the developmental continuum and facilitate individualized counseling. In asking about dating and sex, it is important not to convey the assumption of heterosexuality because that will reduce the likelihood that concerns about sexual orientation will surface.

LATE ADOLESCENCE

BIOLOGIC DEVELOPMENT. The somatic changes in this period are modest by comparison. The final stages of breast, penile, and pubic hair development occur by age 17–18 yr in 95% of males and females. Minor changes in hair distribution often continue for several years in males, including the growth of facial and chest hair and the onset of male-pattern baldness in a few.

PSYCHOSOCIAL DEVELOPMENT. Sexual experimentation decreases as adolescents adopt more stable sexual identities. Cognition tends to be less self-centered, with increasing thoughts about concepts such as justice, patriotism, and history. The older adolescent is often idealistic but also may be absolutist and intolerant of opposing views. Religious or political groups that promise answers to complex questions may hold great appeal.

Slowing physical changes permit the emergence of a more stable body image. Intimate relationships are also an important component of identity for many older adolescents. In contrast to the often superficial dating relationships of middle adolescence, these relationships increasingly involve love and commitment. Career decisions become pressing because the adolescent's self-concept is increasingly bound up in the emerging role in society (as student, worker, or parent).

Implications for Parents and Pediatricians. Erikson identified the crucial task of adolescence as that of establishing a stable sense of identity, including separation from family of origin, initiation of intimacy, and realistic planning for economic independence. To achieve these milestones, developmental progress is required of both the adolescent and the parents. Continued difficulty in any of these areas may constitute an indication for referral for counseling.

Davis SM, Harris MB: Adolescents' questions about sex. J Adolesc Health Care *4*:225, 1983.

Felice ME: Adolescence. *In:* Levine MD, Carey WB, Crocker AC (eds): Developmental-Behavioral Pediatrics. Philadelphia, WB Saunders, 1992, pp 65–73.

Halpern CT, Udry JR, Campbell B, et al: Testosterone and religiosity as predictors of sexual attitudes and activity among adolescent males: A biosocial model. J Biosoc Sci *26*:217, 1994.

Litt IF, Martin JA: Development of sexuality and its problems. *In* Levine MD, Carey WB, Crocker AC (Eds): Developmental-Behavioral Pediatrics. Philadelphia, WB Saunders, 1992, pp 428–442.

Mahoney CP: Adolescent gynecomastia: Differential diagnosis and management. Pediatr Clin North Am *37*:1389, 1990.

Marshall WA, Tanner JM: Variations in the pattern of pubertal change in girls. Arch Dis Child *44*:291, 1969.

Marshall WA, Tanner JM: Variations in the pattern of pubertal change in boys. Arch Dis Child *45*:13, 1970.

Rutter M, Graham P, Chadwick OFD, et al: Adolescent turmoil: Fact or fiction? J Child Psychol Psychiatr *17*:35, 1976.

Slap GB: Normal physiological and psychosocial growth in the adolescent. J Adolesc Health Care 7:13S, 1986.

Tanner JM, Davies PSW: Clinical longitudinal standards for height and height velocity for North American children. J Pediatr *107*:317, 1985.

CHAPTER 16
Assessment of Growth

Growth assessment is an essential component of pediatric health surveillance because almost any problem within the physiologic, interpersonal, and social domains can adversely affect growth. The most powerful tool in growth assessment is the growth chart (see Figs. 12–1 and 12–2). Combined with an accurate scale, a measuring board, stadiometer, and tape measure, the growth chart provides most of the information needed in routine practice.

GROWTH CHART DERIVATION AND INTERPRETATION

The standard growth chart is based on data collected from 1963 to 1975 by the National Center for Health Statistics (NCHS), an office of the U.S. Bureau of Vital Statistics. A sample of more than 20,000 children was selected to represent the noninstitutionalized U.S. population from birth to 18 yrs.

Children were weighed undressed. The data for the younger

children (0–36 mo) were collected separately from those for the older children (3–18 yr) and were plotted on separate charts (see Figs. 12–1 and 12–2). For infants, the measure of linear growth was *length,* taken by two examiners (one to position the child) with the child supine on a measuring board. For the older children, the measure was *stature,* taken with the child standing on a stadiometer. This technical difference results in children appearing to shift down in length as they change from the younger to the older chart. The data are presented in four standard charts: (1) weight for age, (2) height for age, (3) head circumference for age, and (4) weight for height. Separate charts are provided for boys and girls (see Figs. 12–1 and 12–2).

Each chart is composed of seven percentile curves, representing the distribution of weight, length, stature, or head circumference values at each age. The percentile curve indicates the percentage of children at a given age on the x axis whose measured value falls *below* the corresponding value on the y axis. For example, on the weight chart for boys 0–36 mo of age (see Fig. 12–1*A*), the 9-mo age line intersects the 25th percentile curve at 8.5 kg, indicating that 25% of the 9-mo-old boys in the NCHS sample weigh less than 8.5 kg (75% weigh more). Similarly, a 9-mo-old boy weighing more than 11 kg is heavier than 95% of his peers.

By definition, the 50th percentile is the *median,* the value above (and below) which 50% of the observed values fall. It is also termed the *standard value* in the sense that the *standard height* for a 7-mo-girl is 120 cm (see Fig. 12–1*B*). The weight-for-height charts (see Fig. 12–2) are constructed in an analogous fashion, with length or stature in place of age on the x axis. According to the chart, the median or standard weight for a girl measuring 125 cm is 24 kg.

It is important to appreciate both the strengths and limitations of these charts. The NCHS data are representative of a population of well-nourished and healthy children in the United States. Although this population is dissimilar to much of the rest of the world, the NCHS charts have been accepted by the World Health Organization as the international standard of growth for the first 5 yr of life. Disparities in growth between developed and developing countries reflect nutritional rather than genetic differences. It is recommended to use the NCHS standards for first-generation American children whose immigrant parents may be short. Such children may have better nutrition and grow taller than their parents.

The NCHS curves may be less applicable to adolescents. Growth during adolescence is linked temporally to the onset of puberty, which varies widely (Chapter 15). The NCHS cross-sectional sample, based solely on chronological age, lumps together subjects who are at different stages of maturation. The data for 12-yr-old boys include both early-maturing boys who are at the peak of their growth spurts and later-maturing ones who are still growing at their prepubertal rate. The net result is to artifactually level off the growth peak, making it seem as though adolescent children grow more gradually and over a longer period than they do. The NCHS curves may indicate poor or excessive growth when the child is growing normally but happens to be a late or early maturer.

The numerical data on which the charts are based are presented in Tables 13–1 and 13–2. The charts are more useful because they facilitate assessment of growth over time. Specialized charts have also been developed for U.S. children with various conditions, including Down, Turner, and Klinefelter syndromes and achondroplasia.

ANALYSIS OF GROWTH PATTERNS

Growth is a process rather than a static quality. An infant at the 5th percentile of weight for age may be growing normally, may be failing to grow, or may be recovering from growth failure, depending on the *trajectory* of the growth curve. Typically, infants and children stay within one or two growth channels. This *canalization* attests to the robust control that genes exert over body size.

A normal exception commonly occurs during the 1st 2 yr of life. For full-term infants, size at birth reflects the influence of the uterine environment; size at age 2 yr correlates with mean parental height, reflecting the influence of genes. Between birth and 18 mo, small infants often shift percentiles upward toward their parents' mean percentile. Large neonates with smaller parents often shift downward, with decelerating growth beginning at 3–6 mo and ending as the infant achieves a new growth channel at approximately 13–18 mo.

It is important to correct for various factors in plotting and interpreting growth charts. For premature infants, overdiagnosis of growth failure can be avoided by subtracting the weeks of prematurity from the postnatal age when plotting growth parameters. This correction should continue until 18 mo of age for head circumference, 24 mo for weight, and 40 mo for length, by which times catch-up growth for the various parameters should be complete. Special growth charts based on gestational, rather than chronologic, age have been developed for infants beginning at 26 wk gestational age. These charts are based on a relatively small, possibly nonrepresentative sample, which may limit their general applicability.

For adolescents, normal variations in the timing of the growth spurt can lead to misdiagnosis of growth abnormalities. In general practice, cognizance of the relationship between sexual maturity and growth suffices (see Chapter 15). Special growth charts have been developed for early-, average-, and late-maturing adolescents that can be used when additional precision is needed. For children with particularly tall or short parents, there is a risk of overdiagnosing growth disorders if parental height is not taken into account or, conversely, of underdiagnosing growth disorders if parental height is accepted uncritically as the explanation. Standards have been developed to allow adjustments on the adolescent height curve based on mean parental height. These charts are based on a small, possibly nonrepresentative sample, which limits the generalizability of these standards.

The analysis of growth patterns provides critical information for the diagnosis of failure to thrive (FTT) (see Chapter 39). There is no universally agreed-on criterion for FTT, or growth failure; most consider the diagnosis if the child's weight is below the 5th percentile or drops down more than two major percentile lines. Calculation of weight gain in grams per day, with comparison to Table 11–5, allows more precise estimation of growth rate.

Acute undernutrition results in decreases on the weight-for-age and weight-for-height curves (wasting). After several months of caloric deprivation, the height-for-age curve drops (stunting), whereas the weight-for-height curve may return toward normal, reflecting the fact that chronically undernourished children are often stunted but not necessarily wasted. In infants, chronic, severe undernutrition also depresses head growth, an ominous predictor of later cognitive disability.

When growth parameters fall below the 5th percentile, it becomes necessary to express the values as *percentages* of the median or *standard* value. A 12-mo-old girl weighing 7.3 kg is at 75% of the median weight (9.7 kg) for her age. Using the calculated percentage of standard rather than the percentile, growth failure can be graded from mild to severe according to Table 16–1. These designations correlate with risk of mortality in developing countries; their correlation with short- and long-term sequelae of growth failure in the United States is less well documented. Another way to describe extremes of height is the *height age,* the age at which the standard (median) height equals the child's present height. A 30-mo-old child who is as tall as an average 13-mo-old has a height age of 13 mo. The *weight age* is defined analogously.

■ TABLE 16–1 Severity of Malnutrition: Stunting and Wasting

Grade of Malnutrition	Weight for Age* (Wasting)	Height for Age† (Stunting)	Weight for Height‡
0, normal	>90	>95	>90
1, mild	75–90	90–95	81–90
2, moderate	60–74	85–89	70–80
3, severe	<60	<85	<70

Values represent percentage of median for age.

**Data from Gomez F, Galvan RR, Frank S, et al: Mortality in second- and third-degree malnutrition. J Trop Pediatr 2:77, 1956.*

†Data from Waterlow JC: Evolution of kwashiorkor and marasmus. Lancet 2:712, 1974.

‡Data from Waterlow JC. Classification and definition of protein-calorie malnutrition. Br Med J 3:566, 1972.

Nutritional insufficiency must be differentiated from congenital, constitutional, familial, and endocrine causes of decreased linear growth (see also Chapter 45.1). In the latter cases, the length declines first or at the same time as the weight; weight for height is normal or elevated. In nutritional insufficiency, the weight declines before the length and the weight for height is low (unless there has been chronic stunting). Figure 16–1 depicts typical growth curves for four classes of decreased linear growth. In congenital pathologic short stature, the infant is born small and growth gradually tapers off throughout infancy. Causes include chromosomal abnormalities (Turner syndrome, trisomy 21), infection (TORCH [toxoplasmosis, other infections, rubella, cytomegalovirus infection, and herpes simplex] infections), teratogens (phenytoin [Dilantin], alcohol), and extreme prematurity. In constitutional growth delay, weight and height decrease near the end of infancy, parallel the norm through middle childhood, and accelerate toward the end of adolescence. Adult size is normal. In familial short stature, both the infant and parents are small; growth runs parallel to and just below the normal curves.

Growth charts can confirm an impression of obesity if the weight for height exceeds 120% of the standard (median) weight for height. The body mass index (BMI) can be calculated as weight per height^2 when weight is in kilograms and height is in meters. Standards for BMI have been developed for white children, age 1–19 yr, on the basis of the 1971–1974 National Health and Nutrition Examination Survey (Fig. 16–2). The BMI has a normal nadir between 4 and 8 yr. Children whose BMI begins to rise before 5.5 yr may be at increased risk for adult obesity. BMI may overestimate adiposity for children with high lean muscle mass. Reference standards have also been published to allow estimation of adiposity from caliper measurement of triceps and subscapular skinfold thickness (Fig. 16–3). Considerable experience is needed for accuracy; variability in fat distribution may confound the measurement. Measurement of electrical impedance may offer more precise estimation of body composition for research purposes.

Accurate measurement of weight and length is of obvious importance. Scales should be calibrated regularly. Supine length should be measured on a board; length measurements using a tape are inaccurate. Stature is best measured using a stadiometer; swing-arm measuring sticks attached to office scales are inaccurate. Head circumference is measured from the supraorbital ridge in front to the farthest point of the occiput in back. Cloth tapes stretch and should be avoided.

OTHER INDEXES OF GROWTH

BODY PROPORTIONS. Body proportions follow a sequence of regular changes with development. The head and trunk are relatively large at birth, with progressive lengthening of the limbs throughout development, particularly during puberty (Chapter 15). Proportionality can be assessed by measuring the lower body segment, defined as the length from the symphysis pubis to the floor, and the upper body segment, defined as the height minus the lower body segment. The ratio of upper body segment divided by lower body segment (U/L ratio) equals approximately 1.7 at birth, 1.3 at 3 yr, and 1.0 after age 7 yr. Higher U/L ratios are characteristic of short-limb dwarfism or bone disorders such as rickets.

SKELETAL MATURATION. Reference standards for bone maturation facilitate estimation of bone age (see Tables 11–7 and 15–5). Bone age correlates well with stage of pubertal development and can be helpful in predicting adult height in early- or late-maturing adolescents. In familial short stature, the bone age is normal (comparable to chronologic age). In constitutional delay, endocrinologic short stature, and undernutrition, the bone age is low and comparable to the height age. The most commonly used standards are those of Gruelich and Pyle, which require radiographs of the left hand and wrist; knee films are sometimes added for younger children. Sontag's method

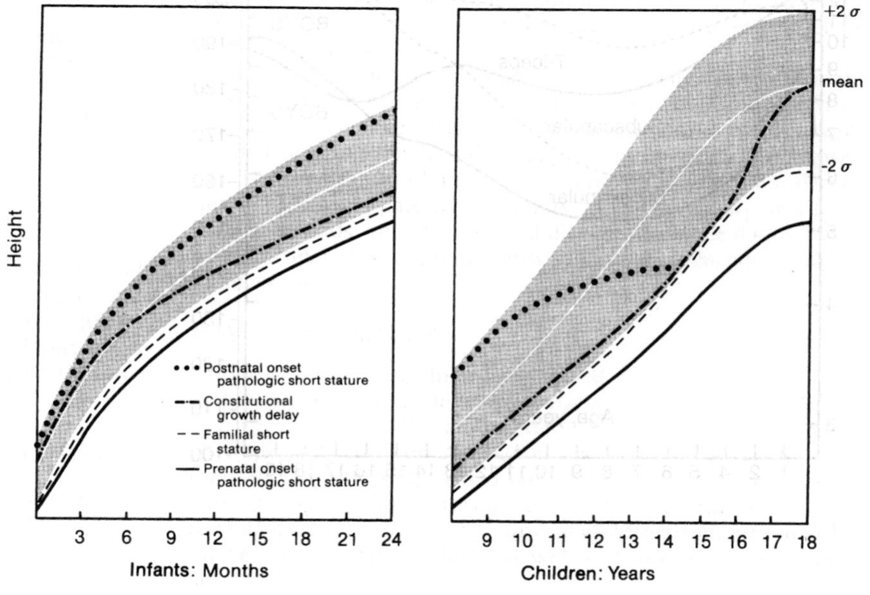

Figure 16–1. Height for age curves of the four general causes of proportional short stature: postnatal onset pathologic short stature, constitutional growth delay, familial short stature, and prenatal onset short stature. (From Mahoney CP: Evaluating the child with short stature. Pediatr Clin North Am 34:825, 1987.)

Pediatricians should play a central role in early identification. In practice, this is not always true. In one large, multicity study, the mean ages at which physicians detected mental retardation, speech, and hearing problems were 34, 38, and 39 mo, respectively; Down syndrome and cerebral palsy were detected earlier, at 0.6 and 10.3 mo. Physicians identified only 23% of emotional problems and 19% of hyperactivity before other professionals. Attempts to improve pediatricians' performance include screening tests and developmental surveillance.

SCREENING TESTS. An acceptable screening test must be highly sensitive (detect nearly all children with problems) and reasonably specific (not identify too many children without problems) (see Chapter 2). It should also measure what it purports to measure (content validity), give similar results on repeat administration and administration by different examiners (test-retest and inter-rater reliability), and be relatively quick and inexpensive. Table 17–1 lists several of the most widely used screening tests and their strengths and limitations. None of these screening tests is entirely satisfactory. Many take too long to administer during a routine health supervision visit. Three screening tests that deserve special discussion are the Denver Developmental Screening Test (DDST), the Early Language Milestone (ELM) Scale, and the Clinical (Capute) Linguistic and Auditory Milestone Scale (CLAMS).

The most widely used developmental screening test is the DDST. Originally published in 1969, the DDST provides pass-fail ratings in four domains of development—personal-social, fine motor-adaptive, language, and gross motor—for children from birth to 6 yr. It can be administered in 20–30 min without extensive training or expensive equipment.

The DDST has been criticized for underidentification of children with developmental disabilities, particularly in the area of language. Predictive validity, the ability of the test to predict cognitive delays at a later age, is limited, except for children in whom severe delays are detected. The test was never intended to predict, only to detect, subnormal performance in comparison with age-matched peers. This caveat, however, leaves the question of need for services unanswered, inasmuch as developmental services would not be indicated for children likely to recover without them. The test was reissued as the DDST-II, with a greatly expanded language section, elimination of difficult-to-administer items, and restandardization on a large normative sample. The DDST-II has been reported to have greater sensitivity, particularly for language delays.

To increase the efficiency of screening, a series of brief parent questionnaires based on the DDST milestones has been recommended as a prescreen: the Prescreening Developmental Questionnaire. Agreement with the full DDST is good, although the questionnaires require a high school reading level and may be subject to the same limitations as the DDST itself. As part of a package of office-based screening assessments, the Denver group has also developed a parent questionnaire, the Home Screening Questionnaire, to provide information on the child-rearing environment analogous to that provided by the HOME Scale (Home Observation for Measurement of the Environment), a well-validated research instrument.

Screening for language delays is particularly important because of the strong link between language and cognitive development. The ELM Scale provides pass-fail ratings in expressive, receptive, and visual language, using a format similar to that of the DDST. The ELM Scale was normed on a racially mixed sample of middle-class children and has been well validated in both low- and high-risk samples. Administration takes 2–3 min; most items can be completed by parental reporting. Sensitivity for language and cognitive delays is high compared with gold standard diagnostic tests; the test identifies many children even before their parents report being concerned. A modified scoring method can be used to generate a numerical score or age equivalent for diagnostic and research purposes.

The CLAMS is a sequence of language milestones that can be quickly administered, has been validated in infants and toddlers suspected of language delay and in those with known motor delays, and correlates well with standard diagnostic language tests. Paired with a similar series of nonverbal adaptive (problem solving) milestones, the test correlated well with a gold standard test of mental retardation. The ELM Scale and CLAMS share many of the same items (see Table 17–1).

Concerns have been raised about the utility of community-wide programs of developmental screening. Screening tests are subject to a number of abuses, including failure to follow the instructions for administration and scoring; overinterpretation of the results (essentially confusing screening with diagnosis, exemplified by the practice of deriving a developmental quotient from the DDST); focus on the screening test to the exclusion of other sources of information; overreliance on measures of child performance at an early age, when they are relatively unreliable; screening too infrequently; using tests that are culturally biased; and failing to follow up with further assess-

■ **TABLE 17–1 Instruments and Questionnaires for Brief Developmental Assessment**

Instrument	Age Range	Time (min)	Notes	Source
DDST	0–6 yr	20–30	Gives well-normed ranges for milestones in multiple domains; most widely used and studied; underidentifies delays, especially language	Denver Developmental Materials, PO Box 6169, Denver, CO 80206
DDST II	0–6 yr	30–45	Like DDST but better sensitivity; may overidentify delays	Same as DDST
Early Screening Inventory	3–6 yr	15–20	A quick, multidomain screen with good sensitivity and specificity compared with McCarthy Scales (a well-accepted test)	Teachers College Press, 1234 Amsterdam Ave, New York, NY 10027
ELM	0–3 yr	5–10	Well-normed, quick screen for expressive, receptive, and visual language; very useful in infancy; does not assess other domains	Pro-Ed, 8700 Shoal Creek Boulevard, Austin, TX 78757-6897
CAT/CLAMS	0–3 yr	10–20	CLAMS alone gives quick language quotient; CAT/CLAMS correlates well with Bayley (traditional gold standard); not yet normed, validated, or sold commercially	Contact Dr AJ Capute, The Kennedy Institute for Handicapped Children, 707 North Broadway St, Baltimore, MD 21205
Peabody Picture Vocabulary Test	2.5–4.0 yr	10–20	Quick, validated test of receptive language alone; correlates well with verbal IQ; easy to administer; beware of limited scope—not an IQ test!	American Guidance Service, PO Box 190, Circle Pines, MN 55014-1796
Infant Monitoring System	4–36 mo	15–20	Series of self-administered questionnaires; multiple domains; good sensitivity and specificity; designed for ages that fall *between* usual pediatric schedule (e.g., 4, 8, 16 mo)	Center on Human Development, 901 East 18th St, University of Oregon, Eugene, OR 97403

DDST = Denver Developmental Screening Test; ELM = Early Language Milestone Scale; CAT = Clinical Adaptive Test; CLAMS = Clinical Linguistic and Auditory Milestone Scale. Adapted from Blackman JA: Developmental screening: Infants, toddlers, and preschoolers. In: *Levine MD, Carey WB, Crocker AC (eds): Developmental-Behavioral Pediatrics. Philadelphia, WB Saunders, 1992, pp 617–623.*

The Pediatric Symptom Checklist[a]

Please mark under the heading that best fits your child:

	Never	Sometimes	Often
1. Complains of aches or pains	____	____	____
2. Spends more time alone	____	____	____
3. Tires easily, little energy	____	____	____
4. Fidgety, unable to sit still	____	____	____
5. Has trouble with a teacher	____	____	____
6. Less interested in school	____	____	____
7. Acts as if driven by a motor	____	____	____
8. Daydreams too much	____	____	____
9. Distracted easily	____	____	____
10. Is afraid of new situations	____	____	____
11. Feels sad, unhappy	____	____	____
12. Is irritable, angry	____	____	____
13. Feels hopeless	____	____	____
14. Has trouble concentrating	____	____	____
15. Less interest in friends	____	____	____
16. Fights with other children	____	____	____
17. Absent from school	____	____	____
18. School grades dropping	____	____	____
19. Is down on him or herself	____	____	____
20. Visits doctor with doctor finding nothing wrong	____	____	____
21. Has trouble sleeping	____	____	____
22. Worries a lot	____	____	____
23. Wants to be with you more than before	____	____	____
24. Feels he or she is bad	____	____	____
25. Takes unnecessary risks	____	____	____
26. Gets hurt frequently	____	____	____
27. Seems to be having less fun	____	____	____
28. Acts younger than children his or her age	____	____	____
29. Does not listen to rules	____	____	____
30. Does not show feelings	____	____	____
31. Does not understand other people's feelings	____	____	____
32. Teases others	____	____	____
33. Blames others for his or her troubles	____	____	____
34. Takes things that do not belong to him or her	____	____	____
35. Refuses to share	____	____	____

[a]School items are in bold. These items were not counted for the 4–5 year old sample.

Figure 17–1. The Pediatric Symptom Checklist. (From Little M, Murphy JM, Jellinek MS, et al: Screening 4- and 5-year-old children for psychosocial dysfunction: A preliminary study with the pediatric symptom checklist. J Dev Behav Pediatr 15:191, 1994.)

ments and treatment when indicated. In a community-based study from Canada, children identified as delayed in the preschool period were no less likely to have academic and behavioral problems during school than children whose parents were not told of the screening results, although parents in the former group reported being more worried. One explanation may have been poor compliance with recommendations for follow-up assessment on the part of both parents and professionals.

DEVELOPMENTAL SURVEILLANCE. Surveillance has been put forward as an antidote to the shortcomings of developmental screening. The transactional nature of development ensures that the child's status at any single point in time can never entirely predict later development; for younger children, particularly, the strongest single predictor of later development is an assessment of the child-rearing environment. Prediction is more accurate when it makes use of multiple sources of information, including the medical and social histories. In many cases, referral for further evaluation and services may be indicated on the strength of family or social risk factors alone in the absence of documented delays. The benefits of early intervention have been demonstrated more convincingly for such cases than in cases of established disability. As with physical growth, a series of observations made over time provides much more information than an assessment at a single time point, allowing for estimation of developmental rate. These considerations underlie the concept of developmental surveillance, a process that includes regular elicitation of the developmental history, attention to parental concerns, careful developmental observations, and promotion of development.

Critics of surveillance have pointed out that it is essentially what pediatricians do now, with qualified success, and that the pediatrician's judgment is subject to a host of biases that undermine its accuracy. Pediatricians may overestimate IQ in children they know well or in children who are physically attractive or socially adept.

COMBINED APPROACHES. An approach combining ongoing surveillance with periodic use of screening tests such as the ELM Scale or CLAMS may be the most effective and practical solution. A multidomain battery of milestones, such as the DDST-II, can be used as a framework for regular observations rather than as a stand-alone test. Parent questionnaires can streamline data collection and may encourage parents to voice their questions and concerns. Questionnaires, such as the Pediatric Symptom Questionnaire, may be particularly useful in eliciting concerns about behavioral problems (Fig. 17–1).

Early identification of developmental and emotional problems will be maximized by keeping the following five principles in mind:

1. Parents, as a rule, are accurate observers of their children's behaviors; parental concerns about possible developmental delays are often appropriate and need to be taken seriously; conversely, a lack of parental concern should not be relied on as the sole indicator of normal development.

2. No child is too young for formal audiologic testing. In-office audiologic screening cannot rule out clinically significant hearing loss. Hearing-impaired children often use visual cues to "pass" hearing tests. Audiologic testing is indicated by the presence of any of the historic and physical findings listed in Table 17–2.

3. Risk factors are additive. Biologic impairments that may be relatively minor on their own (recurrent otitis) may have major impacts in the face of environmental risk factors (maternal depression). The suspicion of problems in one area should trigger increased vigilance in other areas. Emotional problems are common causes and consequences of cognitive and language disorders; environmental risk factors, such as maternal

■ TABLE 17–2 Indications for Audiologic Evaluation

Neonatal intensive care
Birth wt <2,500 g: All cases
Birth wt >2,500 g: If medical complications (asphyxia, seizures, persistent fetal circulation, intracranial hemorrhage, assisted ventilation, hyperbilirubinemia, ototoxic drugs)
Proven or suspected intrauterine infection
Bacterial meningitis
Anomalies of 1st or 2nd brachial arch (microtia, auricular dysplasia, micrognathia)
Anomalies of neural crest/ectoderm (widely spaced eyes; pigmentary defects)
Family history of hereditary or unexplained deafness
Parental concern regarding hearing loss
Delayed speech or language development
Other developmental disabilities (mental retardation, cerebral palsy, autism, blindness)

From Coplan J: Deafness: Ever heard of it? Delayed recognition of permanent hearing loss. Pediatrics 79:206, 1987.

■ TABLE 17–3 Prevalence of Developmental Disabilities*

Condition	Prevalence per 1,000
Cerebral palsy	2–3
Visual impairment	0.3–0.6
Hearing impairment	0.8–2
Mental retardation	25
Learning disability	75
ADHD	150
Behavioral disorders	6–13%

ADHD = Attention deficit hyperactivity disorder

**Adapted from Levy SE, Hyman SL: Pediatric assessment of the child with developmental delay. Pediatr Clin North Am 40:465, 1993.*

depression, frequently coexist with biologic risks, such as prematurity or lead toxicity.

4. Discomfort, fatigue, shyness, and oppositionality may adversely affect a child's performance on developmental testing. Rescreening is appropriate when these factors are suspected but should not be unduly delayed. Caution should be exercised before proclaiming that a child will "grow out of" a problem.

5. Pediatricians and parents may worry about the adverse effects of labeling a child. Screening test results are not diagnoses. Follow-up assessment and intervention are critical. It is the child's progress over time that is important rather than any labels given along the way. In all but the most severe cases, the child's progress cannot be accurately predicted at the outset; an attitude of realistic optimism is appropriate.

DIAGNOSTIC ASSESSMENT

Once a child has been "screened in" as having a potential problem, the next step is diagnostic assessment. The form and content of the assessment depend on the age of the child, the nature of the problem, and the available medical and community resources. The pediatrician functions as part of a team that may also include psychologists, educators, social workers, and other professionals. Central to the pediatrician's role is the medical evaluation of the developmentally disabled child.

MEDICAL EVALUATION OF DEVELOPMENTAL DELAYS. The prevalence of more common developmental disabilities is listed in Table 17–3. The medical evaluation includes history, physical examination, and laboratory testing. A thorough family history, including neurologic, psychiatric, and social difficulties (e.g., legal problems), is indispensable and may also shed light on parents' beliefs about the causes of the child's problem and the intergenerational patterns of parenting within the family. The prenatal history should include a search for potential teratogenic exposures, including radiation or medications, infectious illnesses, fever, addictive substances, and trauma. The perinatal history includes birthweight, gestational age, Apgar scores, and any medical complications. Postnatal medical factors that are sometimes overlooked include chronic respiratory or allergic illness, recurrent otitis, head trauma, and sleep problems (particularly signs of obstructive sleep apnea [Chapter 330]).

In the physical examination, points of particular importance include growth parameters and head circumference, facial and other dysmorphology, thorough eye examination, and signs of neurocutaneous disorders (café au lait spots in neurofibromatosis, hypopigmented macules in tuberous sclerosis).

No specific laboratory tests are indicated in all cases. Screening at birth for phenylketonuria, hypothyroidism, and other metabolic conditions varies from state to state. Iron deficiency and lead toxicity are common contributors to developmental delays and are easily detected. Electroencephalograms and neuroimaging are not routinely indicated but should be used if there is clinical suspicion of seizure or encephalopathy or in cases of microcephaly or of rapidly expanding head circumference.

The medical evaluation for mental retardation and autism should include chromosomal and molecular biologic testing for Fragile X, the most common inherited cause for mental retardation. Classic physical findings in Fragile X such as long facies, large ears, and large testes may be absent in infancy. Milder forms of cognitive and behavioral disturbance have been associated with partial mutations and heterozygosity for Fragile X in girls as well as boys. A diagnosis of Fragile X does not change therapy, but has implications for genetic counseling. Ammonia and organic and amino acids may be included to screen for metabolic disease. With progressive loss of milestones, and particularly if there is associated growth delay, human immunodeficiency virus must be considered.

DEVELOPMENTAL DIAGNOSIS FOR PRESCHOOL-AGE CHILDREN. For infants and preschool-age children, the diagnostic process may include formal developmental testing, playroom observations, parent and family interviews, home observations, and team meetings and often involves a multidisciplinary team of educators, psychologists, parents, social workers, therapists, and pediatricians. The pediatrician contributes medical expertise and knowledge of the child and family accumulated over time. Diagnostic and therapeutic services are provided through the federal- and state-mandated early intervention programs and through multidisciplinary child development teams.

The diagnostic evaluation should include assessments in each domain of development as well as assessments of the parental, family, and social environments. Developmental tests are commonly used as part of multidisciplinary assessments.

For young children, intervention requires parental participation. The importance of family involvement at all stages of the process of assessment, construction of a service plan, and monitoring of the child's progress has been recognized in the federal Early Intervention law (PL 99-457), which mandates the creation of an individualized family service plan for each child. The pediatrician can help parents understand their rights and responsibilities under this legislation, can review the process of diagnosis and service planning to see that the assessment has been complete and that the parents are comfortable with the plan, and can advocate with the early intervention system on behalf of the child.

To monitor the child's progress and advise the parents, the pediatrician needs to have realistic expectations about the effectiveness of early intervention. There is strong evidence for short-term benefits in IQ and long-term benefits in school completion, job satisfaction, and social adjustment for children at environmental risk. For children at biologic risk because of prematurity, interventions combining direct therapy for the child with family support (home visiting, parent education) have resulted in significant gains in cognitive and emotional development. For children with established disabilities, the findings are more complex and controversial. Gains in IQ are generally "modest" and appear greatest for the least severely affected children; improvements in family adjustment and alleviation of parental stress are more consistent findings. For children with autism-spectrum disorders, intensive language and interpersonal therapy may result in significant gains.

DIAGNOSTIC ASSESSMENT FOR SCHOOL-AGE CHILDREN. Pediatricians are often called on to diagnose specific learning disabilities or attention deficit disorder in school-age children with academic or behavioral problems or both (Chapters 18, 27, and 31). The medical evaluation includes the factors discussed in the prior sections. Vision and hearing deficits, although seldom the sole causes of school problems, must be checked. The interview should assess functioning in the home, the school, and the neighborhood and with peers (Chapters 14 and 15).

Definitive diagnosis usually requires a team effort. Educational testing is indicated to define areas of academic strength and weakness. Psychological evaluation is indicated to assess emotional problems, such as depression or anxiety, that may

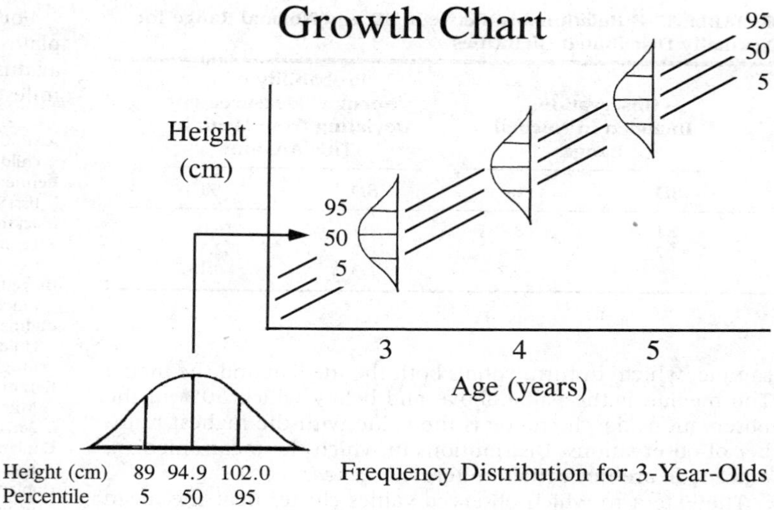

Figure 17–2. Relationship between percentile lines on the growth curve and frequency distributions of height at different ages.

be either causes or consequences of the school problems and to assess family functioning. Neuropsychological testing may be indicated to assess specific functional deficits (short-term memory, verbal processing) that may cause a child to be "lost" and, therefore, inattentive (Chapter 14). The pediatrician can facilitate these referrals and synthesize the information for parents and the school. Pediatricians with special interest in assessment of learning problems may also choose to use one of a series of neurodevelopmental test batteries—Pediatric Early Elementary Examination (PEEX)—to obtain a better sense of the child's functioning in a variety of school-related cognitive areas.

Referrals to psychological and educational specialists may be expensive and may not be covered by insurance. An alternative is assessment in the school. Under PL 94-142, each child is entitled to comprehensive educational assessment and the establishment of an individualized educational plan (IEP) as part of free public education. The assessment must be completed within approximately 2–3 mo (depending on the state), and parents must approve the IEP before it can be instituted. The quality of the assessments varies greatly depending on the skills of the school psychologist, the workload, and the educational resources available within the school system. If the assessment is inadequate, the parents have the right to demand a better one at the school's expense, if necessary. The following questions can aid the pediatrician in the important task of assessing the assessment:

1. Was sufficient time taken for the child to feel comfortable with the examiner and setting? The anxiety of confronting a stranger in a strange room may lower a child's score considerably.

2. Were a psychological interview and projective testing as well as the more standard educational tests performed? Many school psychologists ignore the emotional aspects of learning, focusing solely on the cognitive.

3. Was IQ testing done? Were individual or group tests done?

4. Did the testing address all major areas of functioning (e.g., receptive and expressive language, visuomotor skills, short- and long-term memory?

5. Was an attempt made to synthesize the findings in the report, or were the scores simply reported?

BIOLOGIC VARIATION

STATISTICS USED IN DESCRIBING GROWTH AND DEVELOPMENT (see also Chapters 2 and 5). "Normal" has two potential meanings: that a person or process is healthy or that a measured value falls within the normal range. Quantitative normality must be considered in the context of growth and development. Anthropometric quantities such as height and weight are normally distributed within a population. Given a sufficiently large sample, a graph with the quantity (height) on the x axis and the frequency (the number of children of that height) on the y axis will generate a bell-shaped curve, indicating a normal or Gaussian distribution. In an ideal bell-shaped curve, the peak of the curve corresponds to the arithmetical mean of the

Figure 17–3. Method of presenting percentiles for developmental milestones.

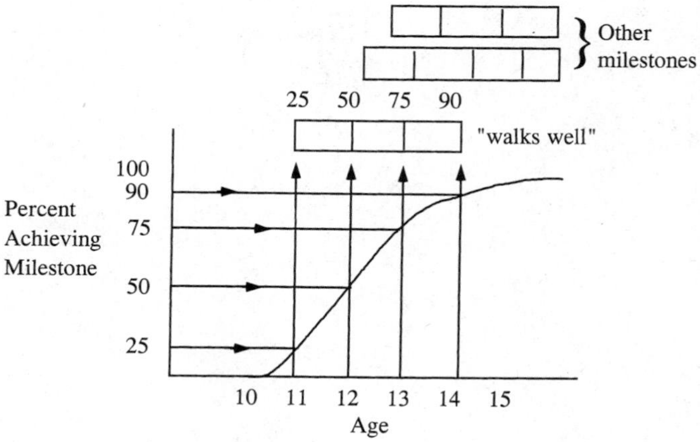

■ **TABLE 17–4 Relationship Between SD and Normal Range for Normally Distributed Quantities**

Observations Included in Normal Range		Probability of a "Normal" Measurement Deviating from Mean by This Amount	
SD	**%**	**SD**	**%**
±1	68.3	≥1	16.0
±2	95.4	≥2	2.3
±3	99.7	≥3	0.13

sample, which, in turn, equals both the median and the mode. The median is the value above and below which 50% of the observations lie; the mode is the value with the highest number of observations. Distributions in which the mean, median, and mode are not equal are termed *skewed.*

The extent to which observed values cluster near the mean determines the width of the bell and is described mathematically by the SD. The SD is tied to the concept of the normal range. For quantities that are normally distributed, a range of values extending from 1 SD below the mean to 1 SD above the mean includes approximately 68% of the subjects; a range encompassing ±2 SD includes 95% of the subjects, and so on (Table 17–4). For any single measurement, the degree of deviation from the mean, expressed in terms of number of SDs, gives the probability that the individual being measured is truly a member of the same population for which the mean was calculated (see Table 17–4). For example, if the population measured is healthy boys, and an individual boy's height falls more than 2 SD above the mean, then the probability that this boy belongs to the population of healthy boys is less than 2.3%. He may belong, instead, to the population of "boys with precocious puberty."

Another way of relating an individual to a group uses percentiles. The percentile is the percentage of individuals in the group who have achieved a certain measured quantity (a height of 95 cm) or developmental milestone. For anthropometric data, the percentile cutoffs can be calculated from the mean and SD. The 5th, 10th, and 25th percentiles correspond to −1.65 SD, −1.3 SD, and −.7 SD, respectively. Figure 17–2 shows how frequency distributions of a particular parameter (height) at different ages translate into percentile lines on the growth curve.

For developmental milestones, the percentiles are often displayed in boxes, derived from graphs plotting age (x axis) against the percentage of subjects achieving the particular milestone (y axis), as shown in Figure 17–3.

AAP Committee on Children with Disabilities: Screening infants and young children for developmental disabilities. Pediatrics *5*:863, 1994.

Bennett FC, Guralnick MJ: Effectiveness of developmental intervention in the first five years of life. Pediatr Clin North Am *38*:1513, 1991.

Blackman JA: Developmental screening: Infants, toddlers, and preschoolers. *In* Levine MD, Carey WB, Crocker AC (eds): Developmental-Behavioral Pediatrics. Philadelphia, WB Saunders, 1992, pp 617–623

Brazelton TB: The Neonatal Behavioral Assessment Scale. Philadelphia, JB Lippincott, 1973.

Cadman D, Chambers LW, Walter SD, et al: Evaluation of public health preschool child developmental screening: The process and outcomes of a community program. Am J Public Health *77*:45, 1987.

Capute AJ, Palmer FB, Shapiro BK, et al: Clinical Linguistic and Auditory Milestone Scale: Predication of cognition in infancy. Dev Med Child Neurol *28*:762, 1986.

Coplan J: Deafness: Ever heard of it? Delayed recognition of permanent hearing loss. Pediatrics *79*:206, 1987.

Coplan J, Gleason JR: Quantifying language development for birth to 3 years using the Early Language Milestone scale. Pediatrics *86*:963, 1990.

Dworkin PH: Developmental screening: (Still) expecting the impossible? Pediatrics *89*:1253, 1992.

First LR, Palfrey JS: The infant or young child with developmental delay. N Engl J Med *330*:478, 1994.

Frankenburg WK, Dodds J, Archer P, et al: The Denver II: A major revision and restandardization of the Denver Developmental Screening Test. Pediatrics *89*:91, 1992.

Glascoe FP, Byrne KE, Ashford LG, et al: Accuracy of Denver-II in developmental screening. Pediatrics *89*:1221, 1992.

Glascoe FP, Dworkin PH: Obstacles to effective developmental surveillance: Errors in clinical reasoning. J Dev Behav Pediatr *14*:344, 1993.

Glascoe FP, Martin ED, Humphrey S: A comparative review of developmental screening tests. Pediatrics *86*:547, 1990.

Hoon AH, Pulsifer MB, Gopalan R, et al: Clinical Adaptive Test/Clinical Linguistic Auditory Milestone Scale in early cognitive assessment. J Pediatr *123*:S1, 1993.

Kemper K: Self-administered questionnaire for structured psychosocial screening in pediatrics. Pediatrics *89*:433, 1992.

Levine M: Middle childhood. *In:* Levine MD, Carey WB, Crocker AC (eds): Developmental-Behavioral Pediatrics. Philadelphia, WB Saunders, 1992, pp 48–64.

Levy SE, Hyman SL: Pediatric assessment of the child with developmental delay. Pediatr Clin North Am *40*:465, 1993.

Little M, Murphy JM, Jellinek MS, et al: Screening 4- and 5-year-old children for psychosocial dysfunction: A preliminary study with the pediatric symptom checklist. J Dev Behav Pediatr *15*:191, 1994.

Meisels SJ, Provence S: Screening and Assessment: Guidelines for Identifying Young Disabled and Developmentally Vulnerable Children and Their Families. Washington, DC, National Center for Clinical Infant Programs, 1989.

Palfrey JS, Singer JD, Walker DK, et al: Early identification of children's special needs: A study in five metropolitan communities. J Pediatr *111*:651, 1987.

Zuckerman BS: Family history: A special opportunity for psychosocial intervention. Pediatrics *87*:740, 1991.

PART III

Psychologic Disorders

CHAPTER 18

Assessment and Interviewing

18.1 The Clinical Interview

(History)

William H. Hetznecker and Marc A. Forman

The clinical interview is the most common procedure in medicine, but the nature of the process is often poorly defined. The interview is not simply history-taking; still less is it a cross-examination of the patient that attempts to fulfill the requirements of a review of systems. It is basically a working alliance between the patient and the physician, aimed at the orderly exchange of any and all clinically relevant information between them (see also Chapter 7). The patient is seeking reassurance or help, and the physician possesses knowledge, skills, and the social sanction to be helpful. *The most useful perspective in which to view the clinical interview is as a major means of engaging the patient in the active management of his or her own care.*

One well-practiced aspect of the clinical interview in most pediatric and general medical settings is the simple collection of those historical medical data that disclose and review the signs and symptoms of a presenting illness, the nature and course of past medical illnesses, the family history, and a review of systems. Other aspects of the patient's life, such as the psychosocial aspects, often get less or scant attention in interviewing. Physicians need to find ways to use clinical interviews to assess the emotional states of their patients, their usual reactions to stress, their levels of self-concept, their systems of values, the natures of their personal relationships, something of their personalities, the quality of their coping abilities, and clues that might point to psychosocial distress or disturbance.

To become an effective interviewer requires motivation, skill, and continuous attentive practice. The skills required develop throughout the course of one's professional life. They are frequently overlooked in medical school, poorly taught, seen as related only to psychiatric patients, or taken for granted once medical school is completed. The development of effective interviewing skills is facilitated when the student has the opportunity to practice with simulated patients, to make and watch recordings of his or her work with simulators or with actual patients, and to have these activities supervised by competent teachers or consultants.

TIME. An interview that attempts comprehensively to explore both psychosocial and biomedical aspects of the condition of a stranger who has just become a new patient needs at least 30–40 min for significant exchange of the most basic relevant information. Physician and patient must have time to become comfortable with each other and to establish the rapport that facilitates the exploration of psychologic and social information. When patient and physician have had an adequate earlier initial interview, and the physician therefore knows some of the major aspects of the patient's psychosocial status, it is possible to focus on particular issues in periods as brief as 10 min, but an initial interview of 10 min is ineffective, and it may communicate to the family a lack of respect for the sensitivity and importance of material given such casual attention.

SETTING. Privacy is essential, but the need for privacy is most likely to be overlooked with children, who are frequently managed with less respect and sensitivity than are given adults. It is difficult to carry on an interview in a relatively unsheltered cubicle in an outpatient department or at bedside, even with curtains drawn to shield the child or family from visual intrusion or distractions. If possible, it is often more productive to seat the hospitalized child in a chair next to the bed rather than to converse with the child while he or she lies in bed. Adverse physical conditions negatively affect the quality and the effectiveness of the clinical interview. Though it may be difficult, it is worth considerable effort to find a private place; in hospitals, this may be a treatment room, an empty conference room, or even an unoccupied office or patient's room. Privacy is more easily arranged in the office of the practicing physician, where closed doors and reasonable comfort are ordinarily routine.

GOALS. The most common deficiency within an interview is the failure of the clinician to define clearly the goals of that particular encounter. No single interview can accomplish everything that needs to be done to complete a clinical assessment. *The clinician must set, define, and state priorities.* These will depend on the nature of the patient's condition, whether the interview is an initial visit or a follow-up one, and whether the physician has to elicit sensitive material or to transmit unpleasant or unhappy diagnostic or prognostic information to patient or family. Physicians must become sufficiently familiar with their own styles and learn enough from past experiences to be able to judge accurately what can be accomplished in each interview. For example, if the work of the first interview is to establish a working alliance with a child and family and to identify the primary problems or concerns, then it may be a mistake to attempt a total developmental, family, or school survey on such an occasion.

COMMUNICATION. The major purpose and process of the clinical interview is the exchange of information. When the patients are children, this exchange occurs between parents and physician, between child and parents, and between parents, as well as between child and physician. In any social interaction, communication has two major features: one is the *content* or *message*; the other is the *process*, or the manner in which content is exchanged within the relationship. (See also Chapter 4.)

The notion of *content* refers to the literal meaning of the words exchanged between communicating parties; content is the message or the *what* of communication. The notion of *process* refers to the relational or nonverbal aspects of communication. The tone of voice, the rate of speech, the inflection of words and phrases, facial expressions, head movements, hand gestures, and body postures and movement all communicate meaning, often more accurately than the words exchanged. The words usually capture the major conscious attention, but the process may frequently determine the success of the venture. The nonverbal features of communication are continually monitored by each sender and receiver, often preconsciously or subconsciously. The nonverbal expression conveys the cognitive, emotional, social, or global state of the sender with respect to what he or she is saying and indicates to the receiver *how the content is to be interpreted.*

Children attend to and interpret nonverbal communication before they understand the meanings of words. Reciprocal communication of basic feelings and emotions between parent and infant takes place through sounds, gestures, and body contacts long before the infant or the toddler can identify feelings or know what words appropriately express them. Physicians should be aware of how their own facial expressions, tones of voice, or gestures influence children's reactions and determine how messages are interpreted; this knowledge contributes greatly to skill in interviewing. The complementary skill required of the physician is to recognize and interpret the child's emotional state correctly through careful observation of facial expression, tone and inflection of voice, body posture, gestures, and other responses. Children may be unresponsive to questions because they are upset by the loudness of the physician's voice, by the suddenness with which he or she initiates an examination, or even by the closeness of the physician's body. Some children have temperamental characteristics predisposing them to anxiety in new or unfamiliar situations, and the physician has the responsibility for recognizing the signs and knowing how anxiety may be dealt with. Many children are frightened of unfamiliar office or hospital settings, of physical pain, of separation, of uncertainty, of persons or figures to whom they may attribute awesome authority and power, and of all else that goes with the word "doctor."

Children need continually to know what is happening and what is going to happen to them in the immediate future. Their anxiety will be significantly reduced when physicians take time to explain what they are doing and what they are going to do, and when they engage the child as an active participant as much as the clinical situation and good judgment will allow. Making life predictable, within the framework of a short or even a 50-min encounter in the office or hospital, can have a profound effect on the likelihood of obtaining the cooperation of children.

Some children as young as 3–4 yr and most children by the age of 8 yr can participate verbally as well as physically in their own health care. All too frequently, conversation involves only the clinician and the parent, with the interaction between clinician and child being limited to the physical examination and some pleasantries. Children can and will respond relevantly to seriously posed questions about themselves.

By about the age of 13 yr, the young person is to be considered the primary informant and should be dealt with directly in his or her own right. If parents are at hand, they may be interviewed with the adolescent or separately, but at this age all explanations of diagnostic and treatment procedures should be directed first to the young person rather than to the parents. This procedure does not imply that the patient has veto power over the recommendations of the physician. The patient is still dependent on his or her parents, and the parents are still the major decision makers. Physical examinations of adolescents should be conducted with their parents not present, unless the patient requests otherwise.

TALKING WITH CHILDREN. Professional conversations with children have certain rules:

1. Don't talk to children in a condescending manner but as a physician talks with any patient.
2. Don't convey to the child your thought that his or her feelings, concerns, or ideas are "childish."
3. Don't laugh at what a child says unless you are quite sure the child intends to be humorous.
4. Don't try always to be funny or amusing to children. Such efforts are best saved for few occasions only and for children you know and who know you very well. Children know the difference between doctors and funny people.
5. Never tease a child unless you know him or her *very* well and the child knows that he or she has permission to tease you in return.
6. Initial or casual encounters with young children are often made easier when introduced in a whisper, which young children may find more personal, private, and reassuring than jollity; they commonly whisper in response.
7. When children are old enough, at 4–5 yr, form the habit of discussing with them their symptoms, diagnoses, and treatments in terms they can understand. The use of drawings to illustrate and explain medical problems can be very useful.
8. Never discuss the illness or treatment of a hospitalized child who has acquired receptive language functions in the child's presence unless you are discussing it with him or her as well.
9. When a child fails to cooperate in his or her care in office or hospital, the first assumption should be that negativism or struggling means that he or she is frightened and reacting to fear in a customary personal manner; such behavior is often erroneously perceived as immature and irritating, embarrassing, provocative, or frightening by parents and other adults.

OTHER ASPECTS OF THE INTERVIEW. Certain signs indicate that the progress of an interview or examination should be assessed or reassessed for the effectiveness of communication.

1. When parents do not appear readily reassured by the diagnostic and treatment procedures, look for hidden anxiety from unanswered questions that they may have difficulty recognizing or stating. Latent anger may have the same result. The physician should make it comfortable and easy for parents to ask "stupid" questions or to admit "shameful" thoughts or "ungrateful" or angry feelings.
2. When a child is giving evidence of feeling pain, it is a psychologic impossibility that nothing hurts. When parents scold a child with "That doesn't hurt," they must be helped to understand that pain is a purely subjective experience and needs to be respected. Their acceptance of this may help greatly to clear the air.
3. Parents will sometimes be heard denigrating or shaming a child by using such terms as "baby," which is almost as bad as being intentionally cruel or frightening. Such behavior should be dealt with by the physician promptly and its inappropriateness discussed, with as much empathy for the parents' position as possible. "I can see that it's upsetting to you to have your child behaving this way, but I don't think that this approach is going to help us. Let's look at it from her (his) point of view. . . ."
4. Exhortation and other emotional appeals to reason are frequently used by parents and are among the weakest methods of attempting to alter behavior or attitudes. Again, ". . . Let's look at it from the child's point of view. . . ."
5. When only one parent accompanies the child, it is almost always the mother. In many families, including those with working mothers, issues of health care are considered as maternal responsibilities. Physicians should feel increasingly uncomfortable as time passes and they have not yet met the fathers of children for whom they have assumed the responsibility of continuing care. Many fathers will be found eager to

see a physician who extends a specific invitation, has clearly stated expectations, and will accommodate his time and schedules.

6. The physician will often, if he or she adequately explores the matter, find that parents have not complied with recommendations made for the care of their children. *Compliance* is not simply a matter of hearing, understanding, and doing what the doctor says, nor is noncompliance to be explained simply as ignorance, neglect, or a personality clash. The parent who fails to comply with recommendations may do so for a number of reasons, and these must be accurately identified.

Did the parent really understand what was prescribed or recommended? Does noncompliance express the parent's reservations as to the appropriateness of the recommendations or were the recommendations beyond the capacity of these parents to execute them, for technical, emotional, or financial reasons? Had the parents enough opportunity to ask questions and to discuss the details and ramifications of the child's condition and treatment? Is a noncompliant parent being influenced or torn by information or advice contrary to that of the physician, which may come from the other parent, a grandmother, a friend, a newspaper or magazine article, or television programs?

Does the parent or do the parents have personal or marital problems which so upset and distract them that they cannot be effective, or does the child's illness itself have them so emotionally upset that they cannot accept the initiative and responsibility that has been thrust on them? Depressed mothers can be so psychologically depleted as to be unavailable to the child even though they may consciously want or intend to carry out recommendations. Is the parent expressing anger at the physician through noncompliance? Is the parent of an anxious and resistant child unable to execute a prescribed regimen that may be difficult or uncomfortable because he or she fears that the child may become hurt, resentful, or angry if the required firmness is exercised?

OTHER SOURCES FOR ASSESSMENT

INSTITUTIONS OR AGENCIES. Besides the clinical interview, other data can greatly help in psychosocial assessment. Birth records, for example, may help in questions of injury during pregnancy or at birth. Such records are often deficient, but they may provide the only objective view of events of the patient's birth and early days. Other health records, including those from other physicians or agencies who have cared for the patient, may provide essential information concerning acute or chronic illness, show a pattern of unusually frequent visits to the physician's office for relatively minor problems, or reveal an obsessive focus on certain areas of the body.

School reports are important to the psychosocial assessment, especially if they include both an academic assessment and a description of the child's relationships with schoolmates and teachers. Requests for school reports should be made only with the written permission of the child's parents or legal guardians.

Reports from child care agencies may also be helpful, especially in the case of adopted children or children in foster care. Such agencies often have extensive background material and may have reports of earlier psychologic examinations.

PSYCHOLOGIC TESTING. Relatively simple screening tests such as the Peabody Picture Vocabulary Test, the Denver Developmental Screening Test, the Thorpe Developmental Inventory, and others may be administered by the trained pediatrician or by his or her assistant. They may indicate areas of possible or patent intellectual or perceptual dysfunction that need further study. The major danger of these tests is that they may be relied on too heavily as giving definitive assessments, whereas they should be regarded purely as screening tests.

Some psychologic tests should be administered and interpreted only by or under the supervision of trained psychologists; others can be used by trained school personnel. They are generally of four types. The first type is concerned with *perceptual-motor* integrity. This type is felt to be especially sensitive to "organicity" or to reflect structural or physiologic abnormalities in the central nervous system. The Bender-Gestalt test is probably the best known test in this category. The second category is that of *intelligence* (IQ) tests such as the Stanford-Binet or the Wechsler Intelligence Scale for Children-Revised (WISC-R). The WISC-R is a 10-category test that gives both verbal and performance IQ scores. The third type of test includes the *achievement* tests that are usually administered in schools. Tests such as the Wide Range Achievement Test report the grade level of achievement in such subject areas as reading, spelling, and mathematics. The fourth type includes the *projective* tests such as the Rorschach test (ink blot) or the Thematic Apperception Test. These give some indication of the fantasy life of the child as well as the reality testing and personality characteristics. When tests have already been done by the school, the results should be examined before new tests that may prove redundant or unnecessary are requested.

Other assessment instruments include various rating scales, questionnaires, checklists, and specific parent-child interactive measures. For example, the *Achenbach Child Behavior Checklist* provides a profile of the child's behavior problems. Ainsworth and associates have developed a structured mother-child paradigm that assesses attachment and affective and cognitive development in infancy. *The Nursing Child Assessment Feeding and Teaching Scales* (Barnard and Eyres) may be used by pediatricians and nurses to evaluate parent-child interaction according to sensitivity to cues and distress, responsiveness, and whether or not the interaction fosters cognitive growth. The *Child Assessment Schedule* developed by Hodges and associates is used in a structured interview setting with the child and correlates with the standard classification system for psychiatric disorders.

The tests to be used should be chosen by the psychologist after the physician and psychologist have discussed the nature of the problem and the reason for consultation. As much as possible, tests should be chosen to assess specific problems rather than as an exhaustive battery, some of which may have only a vague relationship to any clearly defined problems or goals. When the physician is at all uncertain of the nature of the tests or the implications conveyed in their interpretation, a joint meeting should be arranged with the psychologist and parents for an interpretive review; otherwise, costly tests may be ordered, the results of which are never fully exploited.

Occasionally, genetic, endocrine, or neurologic studies will be required to determine whether organic problems may contribute to or be responsible for psychologic disorders.

PSYCHIATRIC CONSULTATION. A psychiatric consultation may be a valuable part of the assessment of children in whom vague or unexplained physical symptoms may have substantial psychogenic determinants; it will often be most acceptable and useful when the child has been hospitalized for study. Other indications include the evaluation of depression in children with major acute or chronic illness, of chronic anxiety problems, of underachievement, and of serious aggressive difficulties. The physician should inform both parent and child of the reasons for the psychiatric consultation, obtain their consent, and prepare them for what to expect.

CORRELATION OF DATA. The physician must avoid early diagnostic closure even when the parents' initial description of their problem gives a reasonably clear idea of what is going on. So long as the physician remains a receptive and perceptive listener, new and important information will emerge, as parents and perhaps patient begin to feel more trusting and as they are educated by the physician's questions. Furthermore, the weighing of data must be done in the context of the family's sociocultural pattern. (See Chapter 4.) It is important that the physician not use his or her personal value system or style of living as a yardstick against which to measure the family's behavior or their success or failure in coping with their life situation. Their own feelings of anger, frustration, anxiety, failure, or depression are more valid indicators of where they need help.

It is important that the principal item of concern be accurately identified. Parents may present as the prime concern, for example, a problem such as bedwetting of many years' duration. Why then have they come for help now? It is important to determine whether there may, in fact, be more important hidden issues the parents do not recognize or acknowledge, or cannot face. By the same token, it must be understood that the parents' assessment of the problem is critical for the child. Sometimes a physician, having collected and assessed appropriate data, can conclude only that a child presented by his or her parents as having a problem is functioning within normal limits. In such a case, it must be determined what personal, familial, social, or cultural considerations compel the parents to see the child's behavior as a major problem. It must then be determined what re-education they may need to feel reassured and not be left with the impression that their anxiety has been casually dismissed.

REFERRAL. When problems have not been internalized by the child, it may be sufficient simply to counsel the parents, school personnel, or both. If this has been done and a maladaptive child or situation continues to present problems, the child and family will probably require more intensive or extensive help and should be referred to a child psychiatrist or to a psychiatric clinic. It is important that physicians avoid the position that psychiatric referral is a last resort. The need for a psychiatric consultation or referral can perhaps best be expressed in terms of the joint need of the family and physician for help in areas where the psychiatrist has special expertise, with the understanding that the collaboration of physician and family in management of the other health care needs of the child remains intact.

Achenbach TM, Edelbrock CS: Manual for child behavior checklist and revised child behavior profile. Burlington, University of Vermont, Dept. of Psychiatry, 1993.

Ainsworth MDS, Bell SM: Attachment, exploration, and separation illustrated by the behavior of one-year-olds in a strange situation. Child Dev 41:49, 1970.

Barnard KE, Eyres SJ: Child health assessment, part 2: *In*: The First Year of Life. Washington, DC, US Government Printing Office, 1979. Publication number DHEW HRA 79–25.

Cohen DJ: The diagnostic process in child psychiatry. Psychiatry Annu 6:29, 1976.

Goodall J: Opening windows into a child's mind. Dev Med Child Neurol 18:1976.

Hodges K, McKnew D, Cytryn L, et al: The Child Assessment Schedule (CAS) diagnostic interview: a report on reliability and validity. J Am Acad Child Adolesc Psychiatry 21:468, 1982.

Kestenbaum CJ: The clinical interview of the child. *In*: Wiener JM (ed): Textbook of Child and Adolescent Psychiatry. Washington, DC, American Psychiatric Press, 1991.

Rich J: Interviewing Children and Adolescents. London, Macmillan, 1968.

Schowalter JE, King RA: The clinical interview of the adolescent. *In*: Wiener JM (ed): Textbook of Child and Adolescent Psychiatry. Washington, DC, American Psychiatric Press, 1991.

Simmons JE: Psychiatric Examination of Children, 4th ed. Philadelphia, Lea & Febiger, 1987.

Wood DJ: Talking to young children. Dev Med Child Neurol 24:856, 1982.

18.2 Psychosocial Problems

Richard Dalton and Marc A. Forman

A psychosocial disorder in a child may become manifest as a disturbance in feelings (e.g., depression, anxiety), in bodily functions (e.g., psychosomatic disorders), in behavior (e.g., conduct disturbances, passive-aggressive behavior), or in performance (e.g., learning problems). Dysfunction may involve any or all of these areas. Psychosocial problems may be produced by such physical or emotional stresses as birth defects, physical injury, inconsistent and contradictory child-rearing practices, marital conflict, child abuse and neglect, overindulgence, chronic illness, and so on. Particular agents do not, however, produce specific symptoms or disorders; rather, children's psychosocial problems are multifactorial in origin, their expression depending on many variables, including temperament, developmental level, the nature and duration of stress, past experiences, and the coping and adaptive abilities of the family. In general, chronic stresses, or a series of stressful events, are much more difficult for the child and family to manage than a single acute stressful episode. Children may react immediately to traumatic events or may keep their feelings dormant until maladaptive reactions become apparent during later periods of vulnerability.

Anticipatory guidance during periods of stress may considerably help children and their families to achieve more positive outcomes. Parents should be encouraged to prepare their children in advance for potentially traumatic events that can be anticipated (e.g., elective surgery, separation, or divorce). Children should be allowed or encouraged to express their feelings of dismay, fear, or anger rather than being told to be a "good girl" or "brave boy."

Infants and toddlers tend to react to stressful situations with impairment of physiologic functions, such as disturbances of feeding and sleep, with relatively global expressions of anger or fear, as in temper tantrums, or with withdrawal and avoidance behavior. School-aged children demonstrate their difficulties through altered interpersonal relationships with peers and family members, through impairment of school performance, by the development of specific psychologic syndromes, such as phobias or psychosomatic disorders, or by "regressing" to earlier, more "childish" modes of functioning.

Parents are frequently concerned whether the particular behaviors of their children are "normal" or whether they represent problems that require intervention. Some "symptomatic" actions of children may be part of normal development. For example, a temper tantrum may express the normal negativism of a toddler; on the other hand, temper tantrums on slight provocation in a 6-yr-old child may indicate psychosocial disturbance. Whether behavior is judged to be a developmental variation or evidence of a more serious problem depends on the age of the child; on the frequency, intensity, and number of symptoms; and especially, on the degree of functional impairment. The decision of parents to seek help is determined, in turn, by the characteristics of their children's behavior; by the amount of distress it causes the children, parents, teachers, and others; and by their past experiences in discussing psychosocial matters with their physicians.

CHAPTER 19
Psychiatric Considerations of Central Nervous System Injury

Richard Dalton and Marc A. Forman

Psychiatric difficulties may follow infection; injury; intoxication; or genetic, metabolic, or idiopathic illness involving the central nervous system. These are not to be confused with the manifestations of "minimal cerebral dysfunction" (also known as minimal brain dysfunction, dysfunctional child, attention deficit disorder, or, in behavioral terms, the hyperactive or hyperkinetic child. For the last condition, see Chapters 27 and 31.).

Brain injury increases the risk of both intellectual impairment and psychiatric disorder, especially when the injury is severe. Social disinhibition appears to be a specific sequela of brain injury, but no typical psychiatric syndrome is associated. The particular expression of disturbance depends as much on the child's developmental level, past history, temperament, and family relationships as on the nature of the insult. Psychosis is not a typical result of brain injury or illness in childhood. Chess has reported an autism-like syndrome in children who have had congenital rubella, but autistic psychosis is probably the result primarily of unspecified genetic, physiologic, and organic factors (see Chapter 29).

Psychiatric disorder accompanies or follows brain injury, illness, or epilepsy in a significant percentage of affected children. The epidemiologic survey of the Isle of Wight found brain-injured or epileptic children 5–15 yr old to have five times the normal risk of psychiatric disorders. Mentally retarded children also are at increased risk of psychiatric disorders.

Prenatal factors have long been suspected of causing brain damage and psychiatric or behavioral disorders. Prematurity and neonatal complications involving hypoxia have been seen as causing such conditions as hyperactivity, impulsivity, difficulties in socialization, and poor control of emotions, especially anger.

Substance abuse during pregnancy may affect both prenatal and early childhood development. Although placental problems, premature labor, intrauterine growth retardation, and low weight have all been reported in infants and fetuses, it is the effect of cocaine and other substances on brain development that has been most closely studied. Reported fetal and infant CNS problems from cocaine include cerebral infarction, microcephaly, developmental delays, and behavioral and learning problems. Although cocaine usage during pregnancy is associated with various learning and behavioral deficits subsequently in some exposed children, a significant percentage of substance-exposed children are not adversely affected by the prenatal exposure (see Chapter 92).

Children under the age of 3 yr who survive encephalitis or meningitis seem to show more lasting effects on personality and behavior than those who have these illnesses later. The result contradicts the notion that the brain might, in the earlier years, have greater potential for recovery without significant residual dysfunction.

Children with hydrocephalus and motor deficits have a seven times greater than average incidence of psychiatric disorder. The additional findings of low intelligence, language disorder, or bilaterality of the motor handicap increase the incidence of psychiatric disturbance significantly, but again there is no specificity in the type of disturbance encountered.

When children with brain damage or injury have problems with impulse or anger control, aggressiveness, hyperactivity, or other emotional reactions, these do not differ in quality from those of children with intact nervous systems who have the same disturbances.

The most significant factor in the child's adjustment to a chronic handicapping organic condition is the capacity of parents to adjust and cope.

In some affected children, stimulant drugs improve the ability to perform in school, smooth out emotional reactivity, and facilitate social interactions with peers and adults. Such medication, taken for extended periods, may produce growth retardation, which must be weighed against possible beneficial effects. Neuroleptics may lessen anxiety and improve emotional control and behavior, but they tend also to produce obtundation and somnolence, which may interfere with learning. In addition, they may have serious side effects (see Chapter 30).

Most children with psychologic disturbances related to central nervous system injuries and their families benefit from understanding psychosocial support. A frequently beneficial approach is to help the child to identify his or her ineffective reaction patterns, along with more successful patterns. The approach combines "coaching" and education with an opportunity to discuss depression, isolation, and anger and those feelings of being different, rejected, or exploited that so much affect self-esteem. The parents have their own needs and will need advice, counseling, and emotional support in dealing with their child's emotional and behavioral problems, both in family matters and in his or her life at school and with friends. Fair, firm discipline is always useful. Behavior modification techniques can help children in whom specific target behaviors can be identified; the technique may be used at home or at school. Both aberrant psychosocial behaviors and learning difficulties may respond to these techniques (see Chapters 30.3 and 31).

Caplan R, Guthrie D, Shields W, Mori L: Formal thought disorder in pediatric complex partial seizure disorder. J Child Psychol Psychiatry 33:1399, 1992.
Cousens P, Waters B, Said J, Stevens M: Cognitive effects of cranial irradiation in leukaemia: a survey and meta-analysis. J Child Psychol Psychiatry 29:839, 1988.
Deonna TH: Annotation: cognitive and behavioural correlates of epileptic activity in children. J Child Psychol Psychiatry 34:611, 1993.
Gonzales N, Campbell M: Cocaine babies: does prenatal exposure to cocaine affect development? J Am Acad Child Adolesc Psychiatry 33:16, 1994.
Griffith D, Azuma S, Chasnoff I: Three-year outcome of children exposed prenatally to drugs. J Am Acad Child Adolesc Psychiatry 33:20, 1994.
Kim WJ: Psychiatric aspects of epileptic children and adolescents. J Am Acad Child Adolesc Psychiatry 30:874, 1991.
Middleton J: Thinking about head injuries in children. J Child Psychol Psychiatry 30:663, 1989.
Richardson G, Day N: Detrimental effects of prenatal cocaine exposure: illusion or reality? J Am Acad Child Adolesc Psychiatry 33:28, 1994.
Rutter M: Psychological sequelae of brain damage in children. Am J Psychiatry 138:1533, 1981.

CHAPTER 20
Psychosomatic Illness

Richard Dalton, Nuria Sabaté, and Marc A. Forman

Psychologic conflict that significantly alters somatic function is the hallmark of the psychosomatic disorders. Any kind of emotional distress may be associated with any type of psychosomatic disorder in a child or adolescent; particular types of feeling or conflict do not produce specific kinds of psychosomatic illness. There appear to be both innate, constitutional vulnerabilities and environmental factors, neither of which are well understood, that determine why one organ or system becomes dysfunctional rather than another.

There are three categories of psychosomatic disorders. The first, psychological factors that affect the physical condition (psychophysiologic disorders), occurs when psychological reactions to either external or internal stimuli affect the development or recurrence of a physical condition with demonstrable organic pathologic aspects (e.g., diabetes mellitus, rheumatoid arthritis, or asthma). The second, somatoform disorder, presents with somatic complaints and/or dysfunctions that are not under conscious control and for which there is no demonstrable organic cause. These disorders include body dysmorphic disorder, conversion disorder, hypochondriasis, somatization disorder, and somatoform pain disorder. The third, factitious disorder, presents with somatic and psychological complaints and/or dysfunctions that are consciously controlled and self-induced for the purpose of secondary gain. Munchausen by proxy syndrome is an example of a chronic factitious disorder.

Although there are multiple theories regarding cause, Engel's biopsychosocial approach to development and psychopathology offers the most cogent understanding. Underlying temperamental factors, environmental stress, family issues, and individual psychodynamics all contribute, some more than others, depending on the situation. The antiquated notion of specific personality types leading to particular disorders has not been substantiated.

Conversion disorder, the loss or alteration of physical functioning without a demonstrable organic illness, is a type of somatoform disorder that usually presents in adolescence or adulthood. However, numerous childhood cases have occurred. Conversion reactions usually start suddenly, can often be traced to a precipitating environmental event, and end abruptly after a period of short duration. Voluntary musculature and organs of special sense are the most frequent target sites for the "hysterical" expressions of psychologic conflict. Such reactions may take many forms, including hysterical blindness, paralysis, diplopia, gait disturbances, seizures, and the like. Physical examination often fails to reveal objective abnormalities. Histories usually reveal a close relationship with a person who exhibited similar symptoms or a recent episode of actual illness. Deep tendon reflexes can be elicited in a paralyzed leg, and pupillary responses to light are noted in patients with hysterical blindness. Affected children and their families tend to be rather dramatic and hypochondriacal and often give a past history of previous conversion episodes. The few follow-up studies that do exist suggest that more than one third of children and adolescents who are initially diagnosed with a conversion disorder ultimately are found to have a not readily apparent organic disorder.

Hypochondriasis, preoccupation with the fear of having a serious illness, and *somatization disorder,* the use of multiple somatic complaints as a means of assuaging inner tension, are also somatoform disorders. As with conversion hysteria, these disorders provide alternative routes and mechanisms for the discharge of physiologic and emotional tension. Adolescence and early adulthood are the most common times for the presentation of each, although both can be seen in some anxious, usually dependent, school-aged children who often have an adult role model with a similar symptom picture.

Munchausen by proxy syndrome is a factitious disorder in which parents induce physical symptoms in their children. It is considered a form of child abuse, sometimes ending in death. Warning observations include (1) a persistent or recurrent illness that cannot be explained; (2) investigation results at variance with the general health of the child; (3) symptoms and signs that lead experienced doctors to say they have never seen such a case; (4) symptoms that do not occur when the parent is away; (5) a particularly attentive primary caregiver who refuses to leave the child alone in the hospital for even a short time; (6) poorly tolerated treatments; (7) a very rare disorder; (8) a primary caregiver who does not seem as worried about his or her child as the staff; and (9) clinical syndromes that do not respond to appropriate treatment.

The signs and symptoms can be varied, including fractures, poisonings, persistent complaints of apnea, and unusual injuries. Therapy includes separation of the child from the abusing parent and further investigation, as in cases of child abuse. The treatment team usually consists of the pediatrician, child psychiatrist, nurse, and social worker. (Also see Chapter 38.3.)

Psychophysiologic disorders have a more insidious onset than somatoform disorders. Chronic anxiety produces functional abnormalities within the autonomic nervous system that lead to structural changes within organ systems. Eczema, bronchial asthma, ulcerative colitis, and peptic ulcer are considered to be psychophysiologic disorders or at least to have significant psychophysiologic components in some children. Although these children have been reported to be obsessive and inhibited, there is no compelling evidence for specific personality characteristics.

Several general principles guide the management of children with psychosomatic disorders:

1. The symptoms of affected children are not within their conscious control; they are not acting or malingering, and their pain and their problems are real.
2. It is essential for a psychiatric assessment to be arranged early in the management of these disorders; otherwise, after elaborate and expensive tests have been done, the child and family will often be convinced that the patient has a very serious illness for which a "real" cause exists that cannot be found.
3. An explanation of the role of the emotions and the genesis of these disorders must be accepted by the parents before truly effective intervention can be accomplished.
4. Psychotherapy for the child and counseling for the family are often indicated, as well as pediatric management. The psychiatrist and pediatrician must be in close communication with each other in a therapeutic alliance. Modest amounts of minor tranquilizing medication may be a useful adjunct.
5. Child and family should be helped to live as normally as possible to avoid crippling psychologic invalidism. Stress should be placed on early return to school after acute illness, participation in recreational activities, and normal peer interactions. Parents should know that some children unconsciously use their symptoms to maintain dependency, and that firm, gentle insistence on the fullest possible range of activities for the child is indicated.
6. The physician should be alert for indications of psychosomatic or physical illness in parents, with which children may unconsciously identify; successful treatment of parental illness may be necessary to ensure a favorable outcome in the child.

Bools CN, Neale BA, Meadow SR: Follow up of victims of fabricated illness (Munchausen syndrome by proxy). Arch Dis Child 69:625, 1993.

Engel G: The clinical application of the biopsychosocial model. Am J Psychiatry 137:535, 1980.

Engstrom I: Mental health and psychological functioning in children and adolescents with inflammatory bowel disease. J Child Psychol Psychiatry 35:568, 1992.

Folks DG, Freeman AM III: Munchausen's syndrome and other factitious illness. Psychiatr Clin North Am 8:263, 1985.

Forman MA: Psychosomatic illness: *In*: Gellis S, Kagan B (eds): Current Pediatric Therapy 12. Philadelphia, WB Saunders, 1986.

Liang S, Boyce WT: The psychobiology of childhood stress. Curr Opin Pediatr 5:545, 1993.

Mitchell I, Brummett J, DeForest J, Fisher G: Apnea and factitious illness (Munchausen syndrome) by proxy. Pediatrics 92:810, 1993.

Nemzer E: Psychosomatic illnesses in children and adolescents. *In*: Garfinkel B, Carlson G, Weller E (eds): Psychiatric Disorders in Children and Adolescents. Philadelphia, WB Saunders, 1990.

Shaffer D, Ehrhardt AA, Greenhill LL: The Clinical Guide to Child Psychiatry. New York, The Free Press, 1985.

Steinhausen HC, von Aster M, Pfeiffer E, et al: Comparative studies of conversion disorders in childhood and adolescence. J Child Psychol Psychiatry 30:615, 1989.

Sugar JA, Belfer M, Israel E, Herzog D: A 3-year-old boy's diarrhea and unexplained death. J Am Acad Child Adolesc Psychiatry 30:1015, 1991.

Taylor DC: Hysteria, belief, and magic. Br J Psychiatry 155:391, 1989.

Taylor DC: Outlandish factitious illness. *In*: David TJ (ed): Recent Advances in Pediatrics No. 10. Edinburgh, Churchill Livingstone, 1992.

Wiener JM: AACAP Textbook of Child and Adolescent Psychiatry. Washington, DC, American Psychiatric Press, 1991.

CHAPTER 21
Vegetative Disorders

Richard Dalton

The five disorders included under this appellation have been reorganized in the *Diagnostic and Statistical Manual of Mental Disorders,* fourth edition, under Eating Disorders (rumination disorder and pica, along with bulimia and anorexia nervosa, which are discussed in Chapter 107), Elimination Disorders (encopresis and enuresis), and Sleep Disorders (dyssomnias and parasomnias of adolescence are also discussed in Chapter 106).

21.1 Rumination Disorder

The hallmark of this disorder is a weight loss or failure to gain at the expected level because of repeated regurgitation of food without nausea or associated gastrointestinal illness. This rare disorder occurs more commonly in males and usually appears between 3 and 14 mo of age. It is potentially fatal; some reports indicate that up to one fourth of affected children die. There are psychogenic and self-stimulating ruminators. The former type occurs in infants with otherwise normal development, although there is often a disturbed parent-child relationship. The self-stimulating variety is usually seen in mentally retarded individuals of any age and often occurs even in the presence of nurturing parents. The differential diagnosis should include congenital anomalies that affect the development of the gastrointestinal system and pyloric valve.

Behavioral *treatment* is directed toward positively reinforcing correct eating behavior and negatively reinforcing rumination. Adverse conditioning is often used. Parent counseling and family therapy are often necessary to discern underlying conflicts and to help educate the parents about appropriate approaches to be taken toward the child and the problem.

21.2 Pica

This eating disorder involves repeated or chronic ingestion of non-nutrient substances, which may include plaster, charcoal, clay, wool, ashes, paint, and earth. The age of onset is usually 1–2 yr of age but may be earlier. Pica usually remits in childhood but can continue into adolescence and adulthood. Mental retardation and lack of parental nurturing (psychologic and nutritional) are predisposing factors. Although tasting or mouthing of objects is normal in infants and toddlers, pica after the 2nd yr of life needs investigation. It is often a symptom of family disorganization, poor supervision, and affectional neglect. Pica appears to be more prevalent in the lower socioeconomic classes. Children with pica are at an increased risk for lead poisoning (see Chapter 665) and parasitic infections (see Part XVII, Section 7). Differential diagnoses include autism, schizophrenia, and certain physical disorders such as Kleine-Levin syndrome.

21.3 Enuresis

(Bedwetting)

The involuntary discharge of urine after the age at which bladder control should have been established is one of the most common and perplexing problems brought to the attention of the pediatrician. The prevalence at age 5 yr is 7% for males and 3% for females. At age 10, it is 3% for males and 2% for females, and at age 18, it is 1% for males and extremely rare in females. Twin studies show that there is a marked familial pattern: a 68% concordance rate in monozygotic twins and a 36% concordance rate in dizygotic twins. (Also see Chapter 497.)

CLINICAL MANIFESTATIONS. Bedwetting may be divided into the persistent (or primary) type, in which the child has never been dry at night, and the regressive (secondary) type, in which a child who has been continent for at least 1 yr begins to wet the bed again. About 75% of all enuretic children have primary enuresis. However, more than 50% of late school-aged enuretic children have secondary enuresis. Persistent nocturnal enuresis is often the result of inadequate or inappropriate toilet training. Nocturnal enuresis has been shown to occur throughout the sleep cycle. Parents who demand coercively that the child become toilet trained promptly may generate an angry response, with the child unconsciously defying them by wetting the bed. On the other hand, parents who are not sufficiently close to the needs of the child to support toilet training appropriately, may undermine his or her attempts at bladder mastery. Chronic psychologic stress, unrelated to toilet training experiences but occurring during the toddler period, can also impair the child's ability to achieve bladder control. Social stress such as overcrowding is sometimes associated with bedwetting. Enuresis is also associated with immigration, socioeconomic disadvantage, and family psychopathologic conditions.

The regressive type of bedwetting is precipitated by stressful environmental events, such as a move to a new home, marital conflict, birth of a sibling, or death in the family. Such bedwetting is intermittent and transitory; the prognosis is better, and management is less difficult than in a child with primary enuresis.

Recent studies suggest that enuresis reflects immature development. Many enuretic children have been found to have reduced bladder capacity, perhaps through inadequate training and genetic predisposition. Environmental factors provide additional stress.

In both types of bedwetting, organic pathologic conditions can be found in only a very small number of cases. However, there is a marked increase in urinary tract infections in enuretic children. Physical examination and urinalysis are indicated, but procedures such as urography and cytoscopy are usually not warranted and should not be pursued unless there is some indication of an organic lesion.

TREATMENT. Management of the child with enuresis depends on an understanding of the possible specific causative factors suggested by an adequate psychosocial evaluation and physical examination. For example, a child can be helped to deal with feelings about a younger sibling, or the parent may be helped to establish the proper attitudes and climate for a child's success in toilet training. Some general suggestions are as follows:

1. It is important to enlist the cooperation of the child to deal with the problem. Rewarding the child for being dry at night is a useful step. The child or parent can chart the dry nights, and with one or two dry nights, a small reward can be given. More substantial rewards should be give for increasing success.

2. Older children should be expected to launder their own soiled bed clothes and pajamas.
3. Children should be given no liquids after dinner time.
4. The child should void before retiring.
5. Waking the child repeatedly to take him or her to the bathroom is useful in only a few children and may further engender or aggravate anger in child or parent.
6. Punishment or humiliation of the child by parents or others should be strongly discouraged.

The use of conditioning devices (e.g., an alarm that rings when the child wets a special sheet) is usually not necessary and should be reserved for persistent and refractory cases in which the child's self-esteem has been seriously eroded. Consent of the child should be a prerequisite for use of such a device. A positive reinforcement system that charts the child's progress is successful in 80–85% of cases. Conditioning devices have been shown to be successful in more than 90% of cases. Imipramine (Tofranil) administration (25 mg/24 hr before bedtime) is also generally effective. Studies suggest that it is only slightly less effective than the alarm system. It usually works within the first 2 wk of initiating the treatment. Enuresis usually returns after brief treatment. Recent studies suggest that therapy for at least 5 mo is necessary to avoid relapse.

Desmopressin acetate nasal spray (DDAVP) has recently been introduced as a treatment for enuresis. Its positive effect, however, is usually temporary, and the medication is also expensive.

21.4 Encopresis

This term refers to the passage of feces into inappropriate places at any age after bowel control should have been established. This predominantly male disorder affects slightly more than 1% of school-aged children. It is more commonly seen in children from low socioeconomic backgrounds. Organic defects are rarely found. Encopresis indicates a more serious emotional disturbance than enuresis and is often associated with anger.

CLINICAL MANIFESTATIONS. Chronic soiling may persist from infancy onward (primary) or may appear as a regressive (secondary) phenomenon. It is often associated with chronic constipation, fecal impaction, and overflow incontinence (in about two thirds of cases) and may progress to psychogenic megacolon. Encopresis usually represents unconscious anger and defiance in the child, and the parents may respond with retaliatory, punitive measures. School performance and attendance may be affected as the child becomes the target of scorn and derision from schoolmates because of the offensive odor.

TREATMENT. Measures similar to those used for the supportive treatment of enuresis may be useful, but the fixed and disabling nature of the symptom frequently requires psychotherapeutic intervention with the child and family. Treatment of secondary encopresis can be facilitated by the judicious use of mineral oil and a high-fiber diet. Relieving constipation and removing impactions leads to significant improvement in about three fourths of all cases. Sitting on the toilet 10–15 min after each meal is often necessary. Rewards for compliance should be offered. Power and autonomy struggles should be avoided, if possible, and records of the child's elimination should be kept. Primary encopresis is more difficult to treat. Initially, enemas may be needed to evacuate the colon. However, chronic use of enemas and laxatives should be avoided. Biofeedback, which is used to train the anal sphincter muscle, has been helpful. The child is encouraged to use the bathroom at specific times and is rewarded accordingly. If the child does not produce a reasonable amount of fecal material, glycerine suppositories may be necessary. A nonhumiliating examination of the child's clothing at the end of the day is necessary. Rewards are offered for nonsoiling, and mild, nonjudgmental consequences are used for soiling. The therapeutic response rate is said to be 80–90%.

21.5 Sleep Disorders

These are common in childhood and may be temporary, intermittent, or chronic in nature. The prevalence rate is said to be 0.2–10%.

CLINICAL MANIFESTATIONS. A substantial portion of children have struggles around bedtime. Many use a special toy or a nightlight to help them fall asleep. Infants who show difficulty in establishing regular night-time sleep patterns may also show general fussiness and irritability as a temperamental characteristic. Sleep disorders in infancy may be a result of parental anxiety or strife. Older children may experience transient night-time fears (of burglars, noises, thunder and lightning, being kidnapped, and so on) that interfere with sleep. Children may express their fears overtly, or they may disguise them, often by invoking tactics designed to delay bedtime. The fearful child may also seek to sleep in the parents' bedroom or may attempt to come into their bedroom after they are asleep. The inability to get to sleep or to maintain sleep is rare in childhood, but is more common in adolescence.

Separation anxiety often contributes to this problem. Children may unconsciously and symbolically consider sleep as a time when they are removed from parental love and concern. If there is conflict within the family or if separation or divorce has occurred, such anxiety will be exacerbated. Bedtime fears are often related to normal separations such as occur with the child's first attendance in nursery school or kindergarten. As growing children become more aware of death, they may be unwilling to go to sleep at night for fear that they may die. This fear will be heightened if a family member has recently died. Anxiety related to any other areas of the child's life—family, peers, and school performance—may be expressed as a sleep disorder. Depression also causes sleep disturbances.

Narcolepsy is a disorder causing frequent daytime naps and cataplexy, sleep paralysis, and/or hypnogogic hallucinations. A genetic predisposition has been noted. Although it usually starts in adolescence, prepubertal cases have been reported. Sleep laboratory studies are required for a definitive diagnosis. Conservative treatment is usually suggested. Stimulants have been used for daytime naps and antidepressants for cataplexy.

About 7–15% of children report current problems with *nightmares.* Anxiety dreams occur during rapid eye movement (REM) sleep; the child awakens, becomes lucid quickly, and usually remembers the content of the dream. Nightmares occur more often in girls than in boys and usually begin before the age of 10. They are especially common in children with anxiety and affective disorders.

Night terrors usually begin in the preschool years and occur with arousal from stage 4 (non-REM) sleep, usually at the beginning of the sleep cycle. The child is confused and disoriented, shows signs of intense autonomic activity (labored breathing, dilated pupils, sweating, tachypnea, and tachycardia), may complain of peculiar visual phenomena, and appears to be frightened. A period of *somnambulism* (sleepwalking) may occur, during which the child may be at risk for injury. Some minutes may pass before the child seems to be oriented. Usually, the child cannot recall the content of the dream that caused the night terror. Night terrors are often self-limited and may be related to a specific developmental conflict or to a precipitating traumatic event. The incidence in children is said to be 2–5%, and it is more common in boys than in girls. There is a familial pattern in the development of night terrors, and febrile illness may be a predisposing factor.

Sleepwalking occurs during stage 3 or 4 in up to 10–15% of school-aged children. Episodes normally remit by early adolescence. Sleepwalking is more likely to be associated with nocturnal enuresis and a family history of somnambulism. Unlike the disorder in adults, childhood sleepwalking is usually benign in regard to psychopathologic conditions. Temporal lobe epilepsy should be ruled out. Therapy is usually supportive, i.e., ensuring that the child is safe and that the parents understand that the course is usually time limited.

TREATMENT. Parental support, reassurance, and encouragement are vital for alleviating sleep disorders. Angry threats and punitive measures should be avoided. Parents should adopt calm and understanding but firm attitudes. Bedtime should be set for a regular, stated time, with variations being kept to a minimum. The parents should discourage the child from sleeping in their room but may temporarily allow a fearful child to sleep in a sibling's room. A night light and permission to leave the child's door open are often reassuring. The interval before bedtime should be quiet and restful; stimulating television programs should be avoided. A warm bath, a light snack, and a quiet affectionate moment with parents are conducive to sleep. Some children may become drowsy if they are allowed to read a favorite book for a few minutes after they are settled in bed. Diphenhydramine (Benadryl) may serve as a mild sedative.

The treatment of persistent nightmares involves an understanding of the underlying anxiety and the provision of reasonable support for the child. Night terrors are treated in the same fashion. Benzodiazepines and tricyclic antidepressants have been used because they suppress stages 3 and 4 of the sleep cycle. There are no studies to confirm their efficacy for night terrors. Sleep laboratory studies and medical examinations are useful in assessing all sleep disorders.

For sleep disorders in adolescents, see Chapter 106.

Benoit D, Zeanah CH, Boucher C, et al: Sleep disorders in early childhood: association with insecure maternal attachment. J Am Acad Child Adolesc Psychiatry 31:86, 1992.

Berg I: Day wetting in children. J Child Psychol Psychiatry 16:289, 1975.

Gandhi KK: Diagnosis and management of nocturnal enuresis. Curr Opin Pediatr 6:194, 1994.

Garfinkel B: The elimination disorders. *In*: Garfinkel B, Carlson G, Weller E (eds): Psychiatric Disorders in Children and Adolescents. Philadelphia, WB Saunders, 1990.

Horne J: Annotation: sleep and its disorders in children. J Child Psychol Psychiatry 33:473, 1992.

Keith PR: Night terrors. J Am Acad Child Adolesc Psychiatry 14:147, 1975.

Levine MD: Encopresis: its potentiation, evaluation and alleviation. Pediatr Clin North Am 29:315, 1982.

Lincheid T, Rasnake L: Sleep disorders in children and adolescents. *In*: Garfinkel B, Carlson G, Weller E (eds): Psychiatric Disorders in Children and Adolescents. Philadelphia, WB Saunders, 1990.

Mayes SD, Humphrey E, Handford A, et al: Rumination disorder: differential diagnosis. J Am Acad Child Adolesc Psychiatry 27:300, 1980.

Minde K, Popiel K, Leos N, et al: The evaluation and treatment of sleep disturbances in young children. J Child Psychol Psychiatry 34:521, 1993.

Moffatt MEK, Harlos MD, Kirshen AI, et al: Desmopressin acetate and nocturnal enuresis: how much do we know? Pediatrics 92:420, 1993.

Taylor DC: Real life soilers—holding on and giving up encopresis. Eur Child Adolesc Psychiatry 1:100, 1992.

CHAPTER 22
Habit Disorders

Richard Dalton

Habit disorders include tension-discharging phenomena, such as head banging, body rocking, thumbsucking, nail biting, hair pulling (trichotillomania), teeth grinding (bruxism), hitting or biting parts of one's own body, body manipulations, repetitive vocalizations, breath holding, and swallowing air (aerophagia). Tics, which involve the involuntary movement of various muscle groups of the body, are also included. Stuttering is discussed with the habit disorders, although it is not generally regarded as a tension-relieving activity.

All children at various developmental points show repetitive patterns of movement that can be described as habits. Whether they are considered disorders depends on the degree to which they interfere with the child's physical, emotional, or social functioning. Some habit patterns may be learned by imitation of adults. Many begin as a purposeful movement that, for some reason, becomes repetitive, with the habit losing its original significance and becoming a means of discharging tension. For example, a child who has an eye irritation or is attempting not to shed tears might try closing the eyelids several times in rapid succession. This activity may become repetitive and incorporated into the child's behavior as an outlet for tension. Such symptoms are often reinforced by attention from parents or others. Other movements, such as rhythmic head banging and rocking in early life, can persist without parental reinforcement, occurring when the child is put to bed or is alone; these movements seem to provide a kind of sensory solace for the child who is feeling otherwise uncared for or understimulated by human touch or interaction. These movements represent a kind of internal stroking. Such patterns are often seen in the mentally retarded or in children suffering from maternal or emotional deprivation. Equivalent movements are evident in children who twist their hair or touch or play with parts of their bodies in repetitive ways. As involved children become older, they learn to inhibit some of their rhythmic habit patterns, particularly in social situations. The prevalence of habit disorders is not known. The natural course can vary, depending on whether the behavior is part of a chronic problem (e.g., mental retardation) or results from an episodic disorder.

Teeth grinding, bruxism, seems to result from tension originating in unexpressed anger or resentment. It may create problems in dental occlusion. Helping the child to find ways to express resentment may relieve the problem. Bedtime can be made more enjoyable and relaxed by reading or talking with the child, permitting re-experience and review of some of the fears or angers experienced during the day. Praise and other emotional support are useful at these times.

Thumbsucking is normal in early infancy. It makes the older child appear immature and may interfere with normal alignment of the teeth. Like other rhythmic patterns, it can be seen as a way of securing extra self-nurturance. The best strategy for dealing with thumbsucking is to provide the child with evidence of interest in his or her well-being and other forms of satisfaction. Parents should ignore the symptom if possible, while giving attention to more positive aspects of the child's behavior. The child who actively tries to restrain thumbsucking should be given praise and encouragement.

Tics involve repetitive movements of muscle groups and represent discharges of tension originating in emotional and physical states that have no apparent useful function. They may have been initially intentional, sometimes becoming nonintentional very quickly. Parts of the body most frequently involved are the muscles of the face, neck, shoulders, trunk, and hands. There may be lip smacking and grimacing, tongue thrusting, eye blinking, throat clearing, and so on. It is very difficult for a person with a tic to inhibit it. Tics can be distinguished from variants of minor seizures in that the child does not experience a transient loss of consciousness or amnesia. They can be distinguished from dyskinetic movements and dystonias by their discontinuation during sleep and by virtue of the conscious control that can be achieved for short periods of time. Tics usually accompany other psychiatric syndromes or follow encephalitis. In most cases, they seem to have had no physical antecedents and are transient. Undue parental attention can reinforce tics, whereas ignoring them may diminish their occurrence. Electroencephalographic (EEG) findings and cognitive testing do not differentiate patients with tics from controls.

Gilles de la Tourette syndrome, which has a lifetime prevalence rate of 0.5/1,000 individuals, is a rare condition in children. It appears prior to 7 yr of age in one half of all cases. It is characterized by multiple tics, compulsive barking and grunting, or shouting obscene words. It is more common in the 1st-degree relatives of patients with Tourette syndrome than in the general population and affects boys 3–4 times more often than girls. It is more common in whites than among other races. Children with Gilles de la Tourette syndrome often suffer from secondary behavioral, emotional, and academic problems. Although the etiology is uncertain, research has shown that it probably results from an interplay among genetic, neurobiologic, psychologic, and environmental factors. Drugs that increase dopaminergic action precipitate or worsen tics and Gilles de la Tourette syndrome. Many environmental precipitants have been noted to serve as emotional stressors, which also precipitate or increase tics and Gilles de la Tourette syndrome. Laboratory studies are nonspecific; up to 80% of patients with Tourette syndrome have nonspecific abnormal EEG findings. Abnormal amounts of various neurotransmitter metabolites have been reported. Lower scores on verbal subscales of psychometric tests have also been reported. Gilles de la Tourette syndrome can be fairly well managed with haloperidol (Haldol), a dopamine antagonist, or pimozide (Orap), a more powerful dopamine antagonist. Clonidine (Catapres), clonazepam (Klonopin), and carbamazepine (Tegretol) have also been used to treat tics and associated behaviors. The disorder usually persists throughout life, but studies have shown a significant diminution in symptoms in one half to two thirds of cases 10–15 yr after the initial evaluation and treatment.

Primary *stuttering* usually begins as an atypical development during the learning of speech. It starts gradually, initially with the repetition of consonants, often followed by a repetition of words and phrases. As the child becomes aware of the dysfluency, anxiety and behavioral responses may occur. As the condition becomes fixed, secondary compulsive and repetitive movements of various muscle systems occur as the child attempts to "force" out the words and release the built-up tension. About 5% of children stutter. Most cases resolve spontaneously, although about 20% continue to suffer the disability in adulthood. A strong family incidence has been noted, and the disorder seems to remit more readily in girls than in boys.

The physician can help parents accept the child's early patterns of dysfluent speech; a decreased emphasis on these early patterns portends a better outcome. The child should be made to feel successful and cared for in other ways. If the pattern persists, a speech therapist should be consulted. Approaches to treatment include breath-control exercises and the use of a miniaturized metronome that "paces" the rhythm of speech.

Cohen D, Leckman J: Sensory phenomena associated with Gilles de la Tourette syndrome. J Clin Psychiatry 53:319, 1992.

Cohen D, Leckman J: Developmental psychopathology and neurobiology of Tourette's syndrome. J Am Acad Child Adolesc Psychiatry 33:2, 1994.

Hetznecker W, Forman MA: Developmental issues and psychosocial problems in children: I. Normal development and minor behavioral problems. II. More serious behavioral and performance disorders. *In*: Smith DWS (ed): Introduction to Clinical Pediatrics, 2nd ed. Philadelphia, WB Saunders, 1977.

Lang A: Patient perception of tics and other movement disorders. Neurology 41:223, 1991.

Lehane MC, Swedo SE, Rapoport JL: Rates of obsessive-compulsive disorder in first degree relatives of patients with trichotillomania. J Child Psychol Psychiatry 33:925, 1992.

Shapiro E, Shapiro AK, Fulop G, et al: Controlled study of haloperidol, pimozide and placebo for the treatment of Gilles de la Tourette's syndrome. Arch Gen Psychiatry 46:722, 1989.

CHAPTER 23 Anxiety Disorders

Richard Dalton

Anxiety, fearfulness, and worrying are regularly experienced as part of normal development. When they become disattached from specific situations or events or when they become disabling to the point that they negatively affect social interactions and development, they are pathologic and warrant intervention. Separation anxiety disorder, avoidant disorder, overanxious disorder, obsessive-compulsive disorder, phobias, and post-traumatic stress disorder are all defined by the occurrence of either diffuse or specific anxiety related to predictable situations. The Isle of Wight study reported by Rutter and associates noted the prevalence of anxiety disorders to be 6.8%. About one third of these children were overanxious, and another third had specific fears or phobias that were disabling. Other studies estimate the prevalence of phobias as 7%, of which 2% are clinically disabling.

The antecedents of developmentally normal anxiety initially present at 7–8 mo of age. As infants begin to differentiate from their primary caregivers they often develop wariness and mood changes that previously did not exist when in the company of strangers. This *stranger reaction* is to be differentiated from *stranger anxiety,* which is a more intense discomfort that includes obvious psychologic and physiologic distress. Although stranger reaction is typically seen in early development, stranger anxiety often heralds later problems related to attachment and separation. Preschoolers typically develop specific fears related to the dark, animals, and imaginary situations. Parental reassurance is usually sufficient to help the child through this period. School-aged children slowly give up imaginary fears and replace them with fears of bodily harm as well as with other potentially real worries. Social anxieties often develop during the teenage years.

There are a number of theories about the origin of fears and phobias. The psychoanalytic view postulates that internal conflict that is not expressed leads to the development of neurotic symptoms. Social learning theory proposes that fears and anxieties are learned within the context of the child's environment. Others think that excessive worrying is related to maternal anxiety. Several studies suggest a genetic cause; 50% of monozygotic twins show concurrent anxiety disorders compared with a much smaller percentage of dizygotic twins. Studies also suggest that anxiety disorders are related genetically to depressive disorders. Finally, recent research has related persistent childhood anxiety to motor (neurologic) "soft" signs.

Children with *phobias* are anxious only under specific conditions. They try to avoid specific objects or situations that will automatically lead to anxiety. As with other forms of anxiety, phobias become pathologic when they interfere with social, professional, and interpersonal functioning. The parents of phobic children should remain calm in the face of the child's anxiety or panic. If they become upset, the child will conclude that there is, in fact, something to fear. Behavioral therapy is indicated, including systematic desensitization, the process of exposing the patient to the fear-inducing situation or object. Anxiety is managed through relaxation techniques. A thorough interpretive session with the parents and child designed to convey an understanding of what is happening is important to the development of a trusting therapeutic relationship. Parent training designed to help the family be supportive during stressful periods is also important.

School phobia, a syndrome in which a child will not attend school because of various reasons, occurs in about 1–2% of children. The literature has underscored the hostile-dependent nature of the relationship between mother and child that often contributes to this disorder. Bernstein and Garfinkel have shown that 70% of these children suffer with depression; 60% with an anxiety disorder, especially *separation anxiety disorder* (SAD); and 50% with both depression and anxiety. Management of the disorder involves treatment of the underlying psychiatric problems, family therapy, parent management training, and liaison work with the child's school.

SAD is characterized by unrealistic and persistent worries of possible harm befalling primary caregivers, reluctance to go to school or to sleep without being near the parents, persistent avoidance of being alone, nightmares involving themes of separation, and numerous somatic symptoms and complaints of subjective distress. These are children who come from the middle to lower socioeconomic classes. Often the first clinical sign of this disorder does not appear until 3rd or 4th grade, typically after the Christmas holidays or after a period in which the child has been absent from school because of an illness. Parents frequently encourage the disability in conscious and unconscious ways.

Children are referred for psychiatric therapy when the usual supportive approaches have failed to return the child to school or to reduce the symptoms. After a thorough assessment, the therapist clearly states to the child the expectations of the family regarding the child's return to school. A program involving the school, the parents, and the child is coordinated by the therapist to minimize the child's use of splitting and manipulation. Parent training as well as family therapy is often necessary to delineate underlying motivations and to teach appropriate ways to help the child fulfill reasonable expectations regarding school attendance. A large percentage of children with SAD develop feelings of panic when they are coerced to separate from their parents. A judicious use of either antidepressant or antianxiety medicines is often necessary to facilitate treatment goals. Young children with affective symptoms have the best prognosis. SAD with school refusal presenting insidiously in adolescence has a more guarded prognosis.

Avoidant disorder is characterized by an excessive fear of contact with unfamiliar people that leads to social isolation. These children and adolescents maintain the desire for involvement with family and familiar peers. Some clinicians think that this diagnosis does not really exist but is part of a generalized anxiety picture. The long-term course is variable.

Children who suffer from *overanxious disorder* have unrealistic worries about future events, the appropriateness of past behavior, and concerns about competence. They frequently present with somatic complaints, are markedly self-conscious, need large amounts of reassurance, and have trouble relaxing. Onset may be gradual or sudden. The disorder is usually seen in white children who are the eldest in their families. The families are usually of a higher socioeconomic status than the families of children with other anxiety disorders and are often overconcerned about issues of competence of their own. Boys and girls are equally affected. Overanxious children are more likely than children with separation anxiety to be diagnosed as having a simple phobia or panic disorder as well. Frequently, overanxious disorder does not become manifest until puberty.

Many children present with repetitive thoughts that invade consciousness or repetitive rituals or movements that do not obviously contribute to a high level of adaptation in any given situation (an *obsessive-compulsive disorder*). In times of stress (e.g., bedtime, preparing for school), some children touch certain objects, verbalize certain words, or wash their hands continually. The most common *obsessions* are concerned with bodily wastes and secretions, the fear that something calamitous will happen, or the need for sameness. The most common *compulsions* are hand washing, continual checking of locks, and touching. These thoughts and acts occur consciously, often causing great distress in the child. Some children externalize the ritualized behavior, attempting to involve their parents in their compulsions.

These behaviors become part of a disorder when they cause distress, consume time, or interfere with usual occupational or social functioning. The National Institute of Mental Health Global Rating Scale and the Yale-Brown Obsessive-Compulsive Scale are very useful in distinguishing individuals with obsessive-compulsive disorder from those without the disorder. The lifetime prevalence rate is about 1%. This disorder may be associated with anorexia nervosa, Gilles de la Tourette syndrome, and epilepsy. Recent positron-emission tomography studies have demonstrated increased metabolic activity in the frontal lobes and the basal ganglia in affected children. Treatment consists of behavioral therapy and pharmacotherapy. Overexposure of the patient to the situations that lead to the symptoms and anxiety is a major therapeutic technique, used especially for rituals. Clomipramine (Anafranil), fluoxetine (Prozac), and fluvoxamine have all shown promise in ameliorating obsessive-compulsive symptoms. Because each blocks the neuronal reuptake of serotonin, some have hypothesized that excessive serotonergic activity may be the basis for the disorder. However, other neurotransmitters, particularly dopamine, are also probably involved.

POST-TRAUMATIC STRESS DISORDER (PTSD). This anxiety disorder has received considerable attention during the past decade as investigators have explored the long- and short-term effects of trauma on children, adolescents, and adults. Many adolescent and adult psychopathologic conditions such as conduct disorder and various character pathologic findings, which were previously thought to be a product of internal psychologic conflict, have been shown to be related to previous trauma.

Etiology. PTSD results from external trauma perceived by the child or adolescent as dangerous. Life-threatening situations that produce considerable stress predispose the child to PTSD. Many investigators have noted the importance of the victim's feelings of helplessness in response to the trauma. Witnessing the traumatic death of a family member or close friend also places the child at risk for PTSD. In addition to the trauma itself, predisposing factors include the level of trait anxiety within the individual prior to the trauma. For example, the children with the greatest PTSD reactions after Hurricane Hugo were those with the greatest tendency to experience anxiety or negative emotionality, as measured on the Revised Children's Manifest Anxiety Scale. Younger children and females are also more likely to suffer with PTSD symptoms after significant trauma.

Epidemiology. About 1% of adults suffer with PTSD symptoms sufficient to satisfy complete *Diagnostic and Statistical Manual of Mental Disorders*, 3rd edition, revised criteria for the disorder. In addition, 15% of adults suffer with symptoms and produce behavior indicative of past trauma. Statistics for children and adolescents are not available.

Clinical Manifestations. PTSD is characterized by recurrent and intrusive recollections and dreams of noxious events in addition to intermittently intense psychologic and physiologic distress in situations that symbolize the original trauma. Individuals with this disorder typically try to avoid stimuli associated with the original trauma. Symptoms and behaviors indicative of this disorder include re-experiencing the trauma through intrusive recollections and dreams and re-enactment through play and other behaviors; psychologic numbing by way of amnesia, isolation, avoidance, and reduced interest in activities; and increased states of arousal, as exemplified by sleep problems, agitated emotions, hypervigilance, extreme startle responses, and difficulty concentrating.

Terr suggests that four long-term symptom complexes are related to childhood traumas. These are visualized or otherwise repeatedly perceived memories of the traumatic event; repetitive behaviors; trauma-specific fears; and changed attitudes about people, life, and the future. Terr further divides childhood trauma into two basic types. Type I trauma is usually a product of an unanticipated, single event and includes subsequently developed detailed memories, omens, and misperceptions. Type II is usually the product of long-standing or repeated exposures to extreme external events and is associated with later developing denial and numbing; self-hypnosis; and dissociation, sadness, and rage. Type II is often associated with repetitive physical and sexual abuse. Some overlap exists between these two types.

Treatment. Initial interventions should be directed toward determining the severity of the trauma, the child's vulnerability to the trauma, and the child's reactions to the trauma. Interviews designed to help children explore their understanding of the trauma are very important. This sort of triage helps to determine which children require brief versus extensive treatment and which therapeutic modalities are necessary (e.g., individual versus group psychotherapy or pharmacotherapy). Treatment goals include the bolstering of ego and reality testing functions; helping children to anticipate, understand, and manage everyday reminders; and assisting the child in making distinctions between current life stresses and past trauma. Both early intervention and psychotherapy provide the child with an opportunity to talk about the trauma and to express feelings of sadness, rage, and helplessness, among others. Family therapy and school consultations are often helpful. Pharmacotherapy designed to modify arousal behavior can be an important adjunctive treatment.

Bernstein GA: Anxiety disorders. *In*: Garfinkel B, Carlson G, Weller E (eds): Psychiatric Disorders on Children and Adolescents. Philadelphia, WB Saunders, 1990.

Bernstein GA, Garfinkel B: School phobia: the overlap of affective and anxiety disorders. J Am Acad Child Adolesc Psychiatry 25:235, 1986.

Famularo R, Fenton T, Kinscherff R: Child maltreatment and the development of post-traumatic stress disorder. Am J Dis Child 147:755, 1993.

Flament MF, Koby E, Rapoport JL, et al: Childhood obsessive-compulsive disorder: a prospective follow-up study. J Child Psychol Psychiatry 31:363, 1990.

Klein RG, Koplewicz HS, Kanner A: Imipramine treatment of children with separation anxiety disorder. J Am Acad Child Adolesc Psychiatry 31:21, 1992.

Leonard HL, Swedo SE, Rapoport JL, et al: Treatment of obsessive-compulsive disorder with clomipramine and desipramine in children and adolescents. Arch Gen Psychiatry 46:1088, 1989.

Lonigan C, Shannon M, Taylor C, et al: Children exposed to disaster: II. Risk factors for the development of post-traumatic symptomatology. J Am Acad Child Adolesc Psychiatry 33:94, 1994.

Moreau D, Weissman MM: Panic disorder in children and adolescents: a review. Am J Psychiatry 149:1306, 1992.

Pine D, Shaffer D, Schonfeld I: Persistent emotional disorder in children with neurological soft signs. J Am Acad Child Adolesc Psychiatry 32:1229, 1993.

Pynoos R: Post-traumatic stress disorder in children and adolescents. *In*: Garfinkel B, Carlson G, Weller E (eds): Psychiatric Disorders in Children and Adolescents. Philadelphia, WB Saunders, 1990.

Riddle MA, Scahill L, King RA, et al: Double-blind crossover trial of fluoxetine and placebo in children and adolescents with obsessive-compulsive disorder. J Am Acad Child Adolesc Psychiatry 31:1062, 1992.

Rutter M, Tizard J, Yule W, et al: Research Report: Isle of Wight studies, 1964–1974. Psychol Med 6:313, 1976.

Shannon M, Lonigan C, Finch A, Taylor C: Children exposed to disaster: I. Epidemiology of post-traumatic symptoms and symptom profiles. J Am Acad Child Adolesc Psychiatry 33:80, 1994.

Simeon JG, Ferguson HG, Knott V, et al: Clinical, cognitive and neurophysiological effects of alprazolam in children and adolescents with overanxious and avoidant disorders. J Am Acad Child Adolesc Psychiatry 31:29, 1992.

Terr LC: Childhood traumas: an outline and overview. Am J Psychiatry 148:1, 1991.

Udwin O: Annotation: children's reactions to traumatic events. J Child Psychol Psychiatry 34:115, 1993.

Yule W: Post-traumatic stress disorder in children. Curr Opin Pediatr 4:623, 1992.

CHAPTER 24 *Mood Disorders*

Richard Dalton and Marc A. Forman

Major depressive disorder, dysthymic disorder, and bipolar disorder with alternating mania and depression are the three major types of affective disorder seen in children and adolescents. *Major depression* is characterized by dysphoria and an obvious loss of interest and pleasure in usual activities but also includes a significant weight change secondary to decreased or increased food intake, insomnia or hypersomnia, psychomotor agitation or retardation, fatigue or loss of energy almost every day, feelings of worthlessness and excessive guilt, diminished ability to think and concentrate, and recurrent thoughts of death. In addition, the melancholic subtype of depression also includes marked anhedonia and greater feelings of depression in the morning with early morning awakening. *Dysthymic disorder* is a less severe but more protracted syndrome involving depressed mood for at least 1 yr. In addition poor appetite, sleep problems, decreased energy and self-esteem, and feelings of hopelessness are present. *Bipolar disorder* involves both mania and depression or mania alone.

24.1 Major Depression

The concept of the existence of depression in children has been controversial. Many have argued that because depression has a component replete with feelings of hopelessness and helplessness about the future, an individual can become depressed only after achieving the ability to string together hypothetical thoughts about the future. Because this ability develops during adolescence, the preponderant belief has been that depression cannot develop until then. However, researchers have now abundantly shown by using structured interviews and other psychologic scales that prepubertal children do manifest mood disturbance, anhedonia, and vegetative symptoms associated with depression. Although some still argue that children assign different values and importance to questions of mood, thus leading to a number of false-positive responses, it has become fairly well accepted that both prepubertal children and adolescents suffer mood disturbances not unlike those affecting adults.

EPIDEMIOLOGY. The prevalence of depressive disorders in childhood has been estimated to be 0.15–2%. In a population that has clinical problems it has been estimated to be 10–20%. The prevalence of major depression in prepubertal children has been reported as 1.8% and in adolescents, 3.5–5%. Girls report significantly more depressive symptoms than boys.

ETIOLOGY. Although the causes of depression have not been established, there is ample evidence of a genetic basis for major depressive disorders. Twin studies have shown a 76% concordance for depression among monozygotic twins reared together and 67% for monozygotic twins reared apart compared with 19% for dizygotic twins reared together. Many studies have demonstrated an increased rate of depression (3–6 times greater) in 1st-degree relatives of patients suffering from a major affective disorder. In attempting to assess exactly what it is that is genetically transmitted, researchers have focused on biogenic amines and neurotransmitters. Because of the low urinary levels of 3-methoxyhydroxyphenylglycol and 5-hydroxyindoleacetic acid in depressed patients, low functional levels of norepinephrine and serotonin are thought to be important genetic markers. These views are reinforced by the therapeutic responses to antidepressants that block their presynaptic reuptake. Cognitive theories have attributed the development of depression to feelings of hopelessness and helplessness secondary to an actual loss or the perception of loss by the individual. Learning theory has postulated that depression is learned within the environment because of a lack of reasonable reinforcers. Others postulate that social skills deficits, learned helplessness, problems with self-control, and life stress play a role in the development and maintenance of depression.

CLINICAL MANIFESTATIONS. Depressive symptoms vary according to age and developmental level. Spitz described the *anaclitic depression of infancy.* Bowlby reported that separation from a primary caregiver after 6–7 mo of age leads to protest (crying, searching, panic-like behavior, and hypermotility of both arms and legs). This is followed by the infant's close scrutiny of each approaching adult, looking for the caregiver. The child turns away from everyone else. The final phase involves apathy in which the infant becomes hypotonic and inactive, exhibiting an obviously sad facial expression. These babies cry silently and stare into space. When picked up, they search again for the familiar face; they cling to the stranger and cry but are not consoled.

Depressed school-aged children present with a variety of symptoms. Sad facial expressions, easy tears, irritability, withdrawal from usually pleasurable interests, and vegetative symptoms involving eating and sleeping disturbances are common. One half of depressed children also present with obvious anxiety symptoms, and 20–30% have behavioral disturbances. Adolescents typically present with impulsivity, fatigue, depression, and suicidal ideation. Psychotically depressed adolescents frequently present with both hallucinations and delusions, whereas psychotically depressed children usually do not have delusions. Hopelessness is much more frequently seen in depressed adolescents than in children.

The symptoms of a major depressive episode usually develop over a period of days or weeks. Sometimes they may develop suddenly secondary to a severe precipitant. The duration of the symptoms is quite variable. Untreated, symptoms often persist for 6 mo. Sometimes, however, they continue for 2–3 yr before they remit. Although the natural history of major depression has not been fully elucidated, several longitudinal studies clearly show that children and adolescents who are depressed are at risk for the development of later episodes of depression. Children who have depression at age 9 have been shown to have numerous depressive symptoms at 11–13 yr of age. Other studies have shown that, within 2 yr of the first depressive episode, 40% of children who have had a major depressive disorder experience a relapse. As many as 20% of teen-agers hospitalized because of major depressive disorders develop a manic episode within 3–4 yr of discharge. Three predictors of such an outcome are (1) a depressive symptom cluster characterized by rapid onset, psychomotor retardation, and mood-congruent psychotic features; (2) a family history of either bipolar illness or other affective illness; and (3) induction of hypomania by antidepressant medication.

DIAGNOSIS. Two measures have been developed that are somewhat useful in diagnosing depression: structured interviews or questionnaires and biologic methods that measure physiologic and neuroendocrine dysfunctions. The Children's Depression Inventory, Children's Depression Scale, Depression Self-Rating Scale, and the Center for Epidemiological Studies Depression Scale for Children have all been shown to be useful in diagnosing depression in children and adolescents, although some researchers have questioned the validity of some scales. There are no biologic tests specific for depression. During major depressive episodes, some children have been shown to hyposecrete growth hormone in response to insulin-induced hypoglycemia. Some preliminary reports have also suggested that depressed prepubertal children produce higher growth hormone peaks during sleep. Dexamethasone (Decadron) suppression tests (DST) have been shown to be inconclusive in children and adolescents, although they show some efficacy in diagnosing depressed adults. About one half of depressed children produce a negative DST result. Current research suggests that those with false-negative results are more likely to relapse but are also more likely to respond to pharmacotherapy. Sleep electroencephalographic (EEG) reports in depressed children and adolescents are inconclusive. Although psychologic and biologic tests show promise in their ability to differentiate depression from other psychopathologic syndromes as well as from a normal state, additional research is needed.

TREATMENT. Major depression in childhood and adolescence is treated with antidepressant medications and various psychologic therapies. Tricyclic antidepressants (imipramine [Tofranil], desipramine [Norpramin]) may be useful in ameliorating symptoms. It is particularly important that these medicines in children and adolescents be followed by adequate determination of blood levels of the drug; children treated with subtherapeutic levels are much less likely to respond efficaciously than those whose drug levels are in the therapeutic range. Six recent sudden deaths of prepubertal boys who were taking desipramine have caused considerable uncertainty about using tricyclic antidepressants in children. These deaths are discussed in Chapter 30.2. The more recently developed serotonin reuptake blockers (trazodone [Desyrel], fluoxetine [Prozac]) are efficacious and have fewer side effects.

Nonpharmacologic treatment, including psychotherapy, is indicated and is especially important for those children who have dual disorders; anxiety disorders and conduct disorders frequently coexist with depression. Play therapies and various talking therapies are important in ameliorating symptoms secondary to these diagnoses in combination with mood disorders.

24.2 Dysthymic Disorder

In this disorder, the dysphoria is generally more intermittent, with periods of normal mood lasting several days to several weeks, than in a major depression. The dysphoria is less intense but more chronic, lasting up to several years.

ETIOLOGY. Although the genetic basis of major depression has been demonstrated, it is questionable whether there is also a genetic basis for dysthymic disorder. Dysthymia may be a partial phenotypic expression of an underlying genetic disorder or a different syndrome altogether that has certain symptom clusters in common with major depression.

Ten per cent of latency-aged children give positive answers to questions pertaining to depression and dysphoria. Other studies have shown a prevalence rate of 3.3% for dysthymia in adolescence.

CLINICAL MANIFESTATIONS. With the exception of hallucinations and delusions, the other symptoms of major depression may be present. Dysthymia frequently is the consequence of preexisting, chronic disorders such as anorexia nervosa, somatization disorder, or anxiety disorder. Children who have dysthymia have had frequent disruptions of important relationships, often beginning as early as infancy. There is often a history of depressive illness in both parents. Affected children show more general emotional and social maladjustment. They often present the picture of helpless, passive, clinging, dependent, and lonely children. Others relate in a more hardened, aloof, negativistic manner. They are reluctant to invest emotion or trust in relationships and frequently develop rather manipulative or expedient approaches to human affairs. They are less likely than acutely depressed children to show episodes of crying. These children attempt to hide their depressed affect. They frequently experience problems in school achievement and in their relationships with family and peers. They are at risk for the development of conduct disorders or substance abuse. Studies show that untreated dysthymic disorder lasts approximately 3 yr. The recovery rate for dysthymic disorder is significantly worse than that for a major affective disorder. The younger the child when dysthymia emerges, the longer it takes to recover.

TREATMENT. Antidepressant pharmacotherapy may be useful in the treatment of dysthymic patients. It is especially helpful for dysthymic patients who display vegetative symptoms of depression. Because the occurrence of dysthymic disorder predisposes the individual to major depression, therapies necessary in the treatment of major depression are often also indicated for the treatment of dysthymic disorder. However, when the dysthymic symptoms are a secondary reaction to an underlying disorder (anorexia, somatization disorder, substance abuse disorder, physical illness, personality disorder), the issues leading to the underlying disorder should be addressed as well. This often requires a full spectrum of therapies, including alliance building and dynamic psychotherapy, family therapy, parent management training, and community liaison work.

24.3 Bipolar Disorder

Bipolar illness is defined as either alternating depression and mania or as mania alone. This illness typically presents in the 3rd or 4th decade of life, but there are descriptions of cases beginning before puberty. Initially, patients may present with either a depressive episode or mania. During the first few years of the illness, manic episodes are more common than depressive episodes. Many adolescents misdiagnosed as schizophrenic on the one hand or adjustment reaction on the other are correctly diagnosed in their adult years as suffering with bipolar illness. The life-time prevalence for the development of bipolar illness is 0.6%. This disorder has been shown to have genetic roots: a concordance rate of 65% in monozygotic twins and less than 20% in dizygotic twins. First-degree relatives of individuals with bipolar disorder are much more likely than the general population to develop various mood disorders. Twenty per cent of adolescents presenting with major depressive symptoms have been shown to develop manic episodes later.

Clinical manifestations in adolescents are similar to those in adults. Overactivity, loquaciousness, insomnia, a grandiose sense of self, expansive mood, paranoid delusions, and overspending are all seen in both populations. The earlier the onset of bipolar symptoms, the more susceptible the patient is to later suicide, increased frequency of episodes, and rapid cycling. Early onset is also associated with an increased frequency of both bipolar disorder and major depression in 1st-degree relatives. (See also Chapter 103.)

Lithium carbonate has proved to be very effective in the *treatment* of bipolar illness and manic symptoms. This is administered orally and is followed by blood levels. The ideal therapeutic range for the initial treatment of acute symptoms is 1.0–1.2 mEq/L, and the recommended level for maintenance therapy is 0.5–0.8 mEq/L. During the acute manic phase, neuroleptic medication may also be required because of the psychotic nature of the symptoms. Carbamazepine (Tegretol), a tricyclic compound used as an antiseizure medicine, has also been effective in controlling manic symptoms in adults. Alliance-building psychotherapy and parent work designed to help manage the behavioral sequelae of mania are also important.

Ambrosini PJ, Bianchi MD, Rabinovich H, et al: Antidepressant treatments in children and adolescents. I. Affective disorders. J Am Acad Child Adolesc Psychiatry 32:1, 1993.
Biederma J: Sudden death in children treated with a tricyclic antidepressant. J Am Acad Child Adolesc Psychiatry 30:3, 1991.
Bowlby J: Attachment and Loss, Vol 2. Separation. New York, Basic Books, 1973.
Bowring MA, Kovacs M: Difficulties in diagnosing manic disorders among children and adolescents. J Am Acad Child Adolesc Psychiatry 31:611, 1992.
Carlson GA: Child and adolescent mania—diagnostic considerations. J Child Psychol Psychiatry 31:331, 1990.
Dwyer JT, Delong GR. A family history of twenty probands with childhood manic-depressive illness. J Am Acad Child Adolesc Psychiatry 26:173, 1987.
Harrington R: Annotation: the natural history of child and adolescent affective disorders. J Child Psychol Psychiatry 33:1287, 1992.
Jones P, Berney T: Early onset rapid cycling bipolar affective disorder. J Child Psychol Psychiatry 28:731, 1987.
Kazdin AE: Childhood depression. J Child Psychol Psychiatry 31:121, 1990.
Riddle MA, Geller B, Ryan N: Another sudden death in a child treated with desipramine. J Am Acad Child Adolesc Psychiatry 32:4, 792. 1993.
Riddle MA, Nelson J, Kleinman C, et al: Sudden death in children receiving Norpramin: a review of three reported cases and commentary. J Am Acad Child Adolesc Psychiatry 30:104, 1991.
Schou M: Lithium prophylaxis: myths and realities. Am J Psychiatry 146:5, 1989.
Spitz R: The First Year of Life. New York, International University Press, 1965.
Steinberg D: The use of lithium carbonate in adolescence. J Child Psychol Psychiatry 21:263, 1980.

CHAPTER 25
Suicide and Attempted Suicide

Richard Dalton

See also Chapter 104.

Adolescents may turn to suicide as a solution to psychologic and environmental problems. It is now the second leading cause of adolescent death. In addition, although few pre-pubertal children kill themselves, many in this age group consider suicide as a means of handling problems and conflicts.

EPIDEMIOLOGY. Nine to 18% of nonpsychiatrically disturbed preadolescents entertain suicidal ideas, whereas 1.5% actually make suicidal threats. The incidence of suicide in children and youth has been rising since 1950. Furthermore, it is estimated that there are 5–45 attempts for each completed act. The suicide rate in males is about threefold that in females, but the opposite sex ratio occurs for attempted suicide. By 1986, suicide was the third leading cause of fatal injuries among those younger than 20 yr of age; 80% of these suicides (2,151) were males, and firearms were associated with 60% of their deaths. The rate is significantly higher in the 15–19 yr olds (8.5/100,000 in 1980) than in those younger than 15 years of age. In 1991, there were 266 suicides among children younger than 15 yr old; the 1990 rate was 0.8/100,000 for this population. Because of undercounting, the rates are estimated to be 1.2 to 3.8 times the reported rates. Brent et al. suggest that this increased incidence of suicide, especially in the 15–19-yr-old age group, is due to increased abuse of alcohol, increased rates of depression and divorce, increased availability of firearms, and an increase in mobility.

The individual and family variables associated with suicidal ideation are different from those associated with suicide. Studies suggest that up to 25% of children and adolescents think about killing themselves. Factors influencing suicidal thoughts include depression, preoccupation with death, and general psychopathologic factors. No particular diagnosis has been associated with suicidal threats. However, a wide range of psychosocial variables were found not to be associated with suicidal ideation: age, sex, social status, race, family size, intelligence, academic achievement, impulse control, reality testing, parental separation and divorce, parental medical and psychiatric problems, and drug or alcohol abuse. Variables associated with completed suicides are different. The preponderance of white, older adolescent males among child and adolescent suicide victims readily points to age, sex, and race as important factors. Alcohol intoxication is a prominent factor in adolescent suicide.

CLINICAL MANIFESTATIONS. Fifteen to 40% of completed suicides are preceded by other suicide attempts. Depression and general psychopathologic factors are related to completed suicides. In one third of suicides, a parent, a sibling, or other 1st-degree relative had previously shown overt suicidal behavior. Just as with suicidal ideation, children and adolescents who kill themselves show an especially prominent preoccupation with death and dying, a wish to die, and feelings of hopelessness or worthlessness prior to the act. In adolescents, the notion of revenge or hostility is particularly prominent, directed either outwardly or against the self; it is present in at least one half of those who succeed in killing themselves. Family studies have shown that fathers of suicidal youngsters have more often been noted to be depressed themselves and to have low self-esteem, whereas mothers have experienced greater anxiety or suicidal ideation. Marital difficulties and child abuse are more likely in families of adolescent suicide victims. Both parents have tended to consume more alcohol than usual. Drug use is a common family problem. Some reports suggest that gender dysphoria is related to adolescent suicide.

Firearms serve as the major method of death in adolescent suicide. Death from carbon monoxide poisoning and medication overdoses are also prominent. Males are more likely to use violent methods than females. Among preadolescents, jumping from heights is the most common method, followed by self-poisoning, hanging, stabbing, and running into traffic. Episodes of self-poisoning that occur after age 6 yr are less likely to be accidental and should be treated as if the behavior had suicidal potential or as a possible case of child abuse and neglect.

School-aged children in general are surprisingly knowledgeable about the subject of suicide. The major difference between children and adolescents lies in the congruence among knowledge, fantasy, and method. Among adolescents, there is a very high correspondence among knowledge about the kinds of acts that will lead to death, fantasies about what will happen to them if they commit one of these acts, and the particular method chosen for suicide. Prepubertal children, on the other hand, show discrepancies between what they know to be a suicidal act and their fantasies of what will kill and what will not. This may, in part, be why so few prepubertal children kill themselves compared with adolescents.

TREATMENT OF THREATS AND ATTEMPTS AT SUICIDE. Threats of suicide should be seen as acts communicating desperation, and all such threats or attempts should be taken seriously. Physicians, parents, and others must scrupulously avoid sarcasm, kidding, daring, or belittling the individual making such threats. If a suicidal threat is labeled "manipulative," power or control becomes a major issue influencing behavior, and the risk of suicide may increase.

The physician assessing suicidal behavior of a child or adolescent should carefully explore, in detail, the child's life during the 48–72 hr prior to either the threat or the suicide attempt. The precipitating events should be identified. The degree of premeditation or impulsivity should be assessed. It is important to understand whether the patient intended to stop or to be discovered and whether the behavior prior to or subsequent to the attempt promoted or impeded the patient's being discovered before or after the attempt. The physician should judge the margin of error allowed by the patient in terms of the method used or proposed, the closeness or remoteness of available help, whether the patient actually called for help after the attempt if it was not immediately discovered, and whether the patient calculated correctly whether the family would return in time to discover the attempt. The most significant factor in assessing intent is the possibility and probability of rescue, as foreseen by the child or adolescent.

When the patient is able, the physician should investigate the child's frame of mind; the degree of hopelessness, helplessness, or overwhelming shame or guilt; and the presence or absence of anger (directed toward others or toward the self). The degree of depression should be evaluated carefully in terms of both the seriousness of the attempt and whether or not the patient presents a continuing risk. It is important to determine whether the child acted out a psychotic delusion or paranoid ideation or whether the act was the result of hallucinatory experiences that produce intolerable anxiety or panic. After recovery, it is important to assess the patient's frame of mind, to determine whether the suicide intent persists, and to assess whether there is now a more optimistic sense of being able to solve or to seek help for problems in a more constructive manner.

When suicidal patients have been seen in the physician's office, the physician should enter into a no-suicide contract with the patient. The parents should be notified, and a psychiatric consultation should be obtained. Because 50% of suicide attempters do not attend even one outpatient psychiatric session, the physician should procure a specifically arranged appointment within 1 or 2 days. If possible, the patient and family should meet the therapist immediately after the examination by the physician. Suicide attempters who are seen in the emergency room should be admitted for 1 day or more to the hospital so that a more adequate evaluation can be made of the patient's frame of mind and of the circumstances of the family or environment. Such admissions usually require 2–3 days, unless medical needs require a longer stay or unless serious psychiatric disorders such as depression or psychosis are found. If social service and psychiatric assessments are adequate and arrangements for appropriate follow-up care can be made, disposition can be made fairly rapidly. The physician must give careful attention to how the family and friends have responded to the patient's act. A hostile and angry family, such as occurs frequently, will necessitate a different disposition or resolution than a family that is supportive, sympathetic, and understanding. The latter supports a decision for the patient to return home. Some families may completely deny the seriousness of the behavior; this can be discouraging and provocative to the patient, whose act has been a desperate attempt to compel a different response. The family members should be helped to examine their roles in the interactions that preceded the attempt, without being made to feel overly guilty.

In planning care of patients after suicidal threats or attempts the physician should consider the following factors:

1. Has the patient been restored physiologically? The patient's state of consciousness, orientation, memory, attention, and concentration should be evaluated. Drugs taken during the suicide attempt may produce an acute brain syndrome or delirium that persists after the coma or stupor phase is no longer present. It is important to determine whether the effects of the drugs have cleared the system.
2. Is the patient less depressed, or is the depression masked? This is difficult to determine quickly and may require a pediatric psychiatric consultation. The family can sometimes help determine if or when the patient seems to be returning to his or her usual self.

3. Does the patient appreciate the seriousness of the act, or does he or she still want to die? Answers to these questions are important in deciding about future psychiatric hospitalization as well as in determining the appropriate time to discharge the patient home.
4. Are the precipitating events or other reasons that provoked the suicidal behavior still actively influential? The answer requires assessment of the family and environment by a health care worker.
5. Have the family, friends, teachers, and other persons significant to the patient responded in a relatively positive manner? It is important to determine whether the parents or other significant adults have recovered from their anger or excessive guilt because the child will need their support after discharge. Have the parents and child been able to identify for themselves some changes that they can make to improve things at home, school, or in the neighborhood?
6. Does the child show evidence of a future orientation after the return home?
7. Have the child's anger, disappointment, shame, guilt, depression, grief, and other strong feelings moderated to the point at which he or she does not feel at the mercy of impulses and feelings? It is particularly important to assess whether hopelessness and helplessness have declined and whether a sense of control over one's life or one's situation has reappeared.

Psychiatric hospitalization is indicated when the individual continues to be actively suicidal, when major psychiatric disorders are found within the attempter, or when major family problems complicate ongoing protection of the attempter.

Brent DA, Kolko DJ, Allan MJ, et al: Suicidality in affectively disordered adolescent inpatients. J Am Acad Child Adolesc Psychiatry 29:586, 1990.
Brent DA, Perper JA, Goldstein CE, et al: Risk factors for adolescent suicide. Arch Gen Psychiatry 45:581, 1988.
Carlson G, Asarnow J, Orbach I: Developmental aspects of suicidal behavior in children. J Am Acad Child Adolesc Psychiatry 26:186, 1987.
deWilde EJ, Kienhorst ICWM, Diekstra FW, et al: The relationship between adolescent suicidal behavior and life events in childhood and adolescence. Am J Psychiatry 149:45, 1992.
Hoberman H, Garfinkel B: Completed suicide in children and adolescents. J Am Acad Child Adolesc Psychiatry 27:689, 1988.
Pfeffer CR, Klerman GL, Hurt SW, et al: Suicidal children grow up: rates and psychosocial risk factors for suicide attempts during follow-up. J Am Acad Child Adolesc Psychiatry 32:106, 1993.

CHAPTER 26
Disruptive Behavioral Disorders

Richard Dalton

Numerous behaviors considered appropriate at certain developmental levels are obviously pathologic when they present at later ages. Lying, impulsiveness, breath holding, defiance, and temper tantrums are frequently noted around the ages of 2–4 yr when children begin to need autonomy but do not have the motor and social skills necessary for successful independence. These behaviors are probably the result of frustration and anger. About one half of preschoolers in the United States are brought to the attention of physicians at some time because of destructive and disobedient behaviors. Moreover, some studies suggest that disruptive, antisocial behaviors are intermittently committed by one half of this country's adolescents.

Breath holding is not unusual during the first years of life. It is frequently used by infants and toddlers in an attempt to control their environment and their caregivers. Whereas some children hold their breath until they lose consciousness, sometimes leading to a seizure, there is no increased risk of their later developing a seizure disorder. Parents are best advised to ignore the behavior and leave the room in response. Without sufficient reinforcement, the behavior soon disappears.

Defiance, oppositionalism, and *temper tantrums* are often used by children 18 mo to 3 yr of age who feel frustrated by their conflicting desires to be in control of their environment on the one hand, and, on the other, to be taken care of and pampered in a developmentally regressed way. Parental and caregiver response to this behavior is very important. Caregivers who respond to toddler defiance with punitive anger run the risk of reinforcing the defiance and teaching the child that out-of-control emotions are a reasonable response to frustration. In response to tantrums and oppositionalism, parents are advised to acknowledge verbally to the child that the reasons for frustration are understandable but that the particular response is not acceptable. The child should be given time and space to recover. If the child is unable to give up this behavior but instead presents with escalating oppositionalism, parents should nonemotionally place the child on time out or a room restriction until he or she is able to adjust more reasonably.

Children are often frightened by the strength and intensity of their own angry feelings as well as by the intensity of the angry feelings they arouse in their parents. It is therefore of prime importance that parents provide models for control of their own anger and aggressive feelings that they wish their children to follow. Many parents who are horrified at their children's loss of control of anger are unable to see that they have often lost control themselves; they are not, therefore, helping their children to internalize controls. Physicians must learn from the parents how they handle anger before making recommendations about how the child's problems are to be helped. One way to help the toddler develop a sense of autonomy and to feel more in control is to allow the child to have simple choices of activities that the parents can accept. This helps to provide the child with options, thus reducing his or her potential feelings of being powerless, overwhelmed, or engulfed. Such negative, internalized feelings may later have adverse effects on developing interpersonal relationships, intimacy, and personality development.

Lying is often used by 2–4 yr olds as a method of playing with the language. By observing the reactions of parents and caregivers, preschoolers learn cognitively and affectively about expectations for honesty in communication. In another sense, lying is a form of fantasy for children who describe things as they wish them to be rather than as they are. For instance, a child who has not done something that a parent wanted may say that it has been done to avoid an unpleasant confrontation. The child's sense of time and reason does not permit the realization that this only postpones an even angrier confrontation.

In school-aged children, lying most often represents the child's attempt to avoid the pain of a relative loss of self-esteem. That is, most lying is an effort to cover up something that the child does not want to accept in his or her own behavior. The lie is invented, therefore, to achieve temporary good feeling. Lying can be the result of parental modeling, in which case the child's interpretations of reality are often conflicting, confusing, or unclear. For instance, when mothers and fathers accuse each other frequently of lying, the child may become hopelessly unsure of how the word lying is to be interpreted; moreover, a loyalty conflict is added to the already distorted process of reality testing.

Many adolescents lie because they fear that their parents would disapprove of what they are doing. Chronic lying, however, often occurs in combination with several other antisocial behaviors and is a sign of an underlying psychopathologic condition. As with other antisocial behaviors, lying is often used as a method of rebellion.

Regardless of the age or developmental level, when lying becomes a frequent way of managing conflict and anxiety, intervention is warranted. Initially, the parents should confront the child to give a clear message of what is acceptable. Sensitivity and support are necessary for a successful intervention because children and adolescents are so developmentally vulnerable to shame and embarrassment. If the situation cannot be equitably resolved (i.e., parental understanding of the situation and the child's understanding that lying is not a reasonable alternative), professional intervention is indicated.

Almost all children *steal* something at some point in their lives. It becomes a problem when it happens more than once or twice. Some preschoolers and school-aged children steal as a response to a sense of internal loss. They frequently feel neglected and are in fact emotionally deprived. Their stealing is impulsive, but the gratification derived does not satisfy the underlying need. In children and adolescents stealing can sometimes be an expression of anger or revenge for real or imagined frustrations by the parents. In many instances of children's stealing, there is a strong wish by the child to be caught. Stealing becomes one way in which the child or adolescent can manipulate and attempt to control interactions with parents. Like lying, stealing can be learned from parents. Parents who boast about outwitting tax laws or exceeding speed limits are implicitly condoning stealing as an acceptable behavior.

It is important for parents to help the child undo the theft by returning the stolen articles or by rendering their equivalent either in money that the child can earn or in services. When it is apparent that children are not able to control temptation, money and valuable objects should not be left where they can reach them, to decrease the chances of stealing. It is also important that the act not be overemphasized, lest the behavior or the response to it becomes so exciting that it is reproduced in future periods of discontent.

Unlike the previous behaviors, *truancy* and *run-away behavior* are never developmentally appropriate. Some children skip school because they are afraid of peers or teachers or because of the sense of humiliation secondary to learning difficulties. Others are truant because of separation anxiety symptoms. Most often, truancy represents disorganization within the home, developing personality problems, or both. Whereas younger children often threaten to run away out of frustration or a desire to get back at parents, children who run away with nowhere to go are almost always expressing a serious underlying problem (see Chapter 42). During the latency years, the most common causes are related to abuse and neglect within the home. In adolescence, disagreements with the parents, developing personality problems, and abuse and neglect all must be considered as possible precipitants.

Although the interest in fire is ubiquitous in early childhood, unsupervised *fire setting* is always inappropriate. Early school-aged children tend to set fires because of both curiosity and latent hostility secondary to deprivation within a disorganized and neglectful family. These young children set fires by themselves within their homes. In adolescence, fire setting is a more delinquent sign. Teenagers usually set fires in small groups, seeking revenge from school and community authorities.

At the very least, fire setting requires intervention by the parents but most often also intervention by mental health professionals. A combination of family therapy, alliance-building individual therapy, parent management training, and community involvement is often necessary to effect a reasonable change. The recidivistic young fire setter is very difficult to manage, however. Many adult arsonists were childhood fire setters.

Although there is no totally satisfactory theory about the nature and cause of *antisocial behavior,* risk factors within the individual and family have been identified. Adoption twin studies strongly suggest that both genetic factors and child-rearing practices contribute to later developing aggressive behaviors. In well-controlled studies, adopted children with antisocial biologic fathers presented later in life with more antisocial behaviors than did those with antisocial adoptive fathers. However, children with both biologic and adoptive antisocial fathers were the most antisocial in later life. Sociocultural factors, temperament, some psychiatric conditions, and cognitive limitations can also predispose individuals to antisocial acting out.

Aggression is an additional behavior, and possibly the most serious, included within this group of disorders. Many theories have attempted to explain human aggression. The drive theory proposes that aggressive responses are biologically programmed within the human species. The phenomenologic approach suggests that everyday life is sufficiently depriving and frustrating that aggression is to be expected. Social learning theory proposes that aggression is learned and successively reinforced throughout young childhood and adolescence. In addition, social theorists suggest that modern crowding, the breakdown of commonly shared values, the demise of traditional family patterns of child rearing in kinship systems, and social alienation both in individuals and in large groups are leading to increased aggression in children, adolescents, and adults. Aggression in childhood has also been correlated with family unemployment, discord, criminality, and psychiatric disorders.

Several factors contribute to aggression. Boys are almost universally reported to be more aggressive than girls. In many animals, administration of male sex hormones to females produces more aggressive behavior. Large children are often more aggressive than smaller ones. More active and intrusive children are perceived as more aggressive. Difficult temperament and later aggressiveness have been shown to be related. Children from larger families are often more aggressive than those from smaller families. Marital discord between parents and aggression within the home certainly contribute to aggression within children.

Clinically, it is important to differentiate the causes and motives for childhood aggression. Many hyperactive, clumsy children are called aggressive because of the accidental results of their behavior. Intentional aggression may be primarily instrumental, to achieve an end, or primarily hostile, to inflict physical or psychologic pain. There is also a relationship between individual aggression and emotional disturbance, school failure, brain damage, overactivity, and character pathologic conditions. Psychopathologic conditions are also associated with conduct-disordered behavior; attention deficit disorder and borderline personality traits have been correlated with aggression. Of particular importance is the relationship between severe reading retardation (as well as cognitive deficits, in general) and the development of symptoms of aggressive conduct disorder, especially in boys.

The child of 2–5 yr may show aggressive outbursts ranging from temper tantrums and screaming to hurting others or destroying toys and furniture. This behavior is frequently the product of particular frustrations and the toddler's inability to manage them. In toddlerhood, aggression is usually directed toward parents; during the preschool years, it is more likely to be directed toward siblings or peers. Verbal aggression increases between 2 and 4 yr, and after 3 yr of age, revenge and retaliation become more prominent as determinants of aggression.

Aggressive behavior in boys is relatively consistent from the preschool period through adolescence; a boy with a high level of aggressive behavior from 3–6 yr of age has a high probability of carrying this behavior into adolescence. On the other hand, girls younger than 6 yr who are aggressive toward peers are less likely to demonstrate that behavior at older ages.

Children exposed to aggressive models on television or in play display more aggressive behavior compared with children not exposed to these models (see Chapter 37). Parents' anger and aggressive or harsh punishment model behavior that children may imitate when they are physically or psychologically hurt. As Lewis has noted, parental abuse may be transmitted to the next generation by several modes: children imitate aggression that they have witnessed, abuse can cause brain injury (which itself predisposes the child toward violence), and internalized rage more often than not results from abuse.

Passive-aggressive behaviors are common in childhood and adolescence. Prevalence rates of 16–22% have been noted. Children with passive-aggressive behavior express hostility indirectly as procrastination, stubbornness, or resistance. Parents often complain that such children do not hear them and that they fail to respond to repeated requests. Academic underachievement is common. Early histories may reveal excessive negativism during infancy and toddlerhood with feeding disturbances and problems in bladder and bowel training.

Children may unconsciously adopt passive-aggressive strategies for a variety of motives: to gain independence while maintaining dependency; to counter underlying low self-esteem; to maintain control and autonomy when threatened by anxiety; and to get revenge. These children are fearful of direct expression of assertiveness, aggression, and hostility. The child-rearing styles of their parents are often intimidating, critical, and inconsistent or, on the other hand, indulgent and permissive. Both children and parents often find it difficult to deal directly with anger.

Parents should be encouraged to handle passive-aggressive behavior by setting firm limits and expectations for the child. Parents and child should reach agreement on what they consider to be the child's important tasks and responsibilities. The most important issues need to be managed first. Age-appropriate assertiveness and independence should be promoted and rewarded. More refractory cases often require psychiatric intervention.

Conduct disorder is a distinct clinical entity manifested by several different antisocial behaviors: stealing, lying, fire setting, truancy, property destruction, cruelty to animals, rape, use of a weapon while fighting, armed robbery, physical cruelty to others, and repeated attempts to run away from home. A pattern of such behaviors that has existed for at least 6 mo warrants the diagnosis of a conduct disorder. One third to one half of adolescent psychiatric clinic patients present with conduct-disordered behavior. *Oppositional defiant disorder* is defined by less severe behavior than a conduct disorder: temper tantrums, continuous arguing, defiance of rules, continual blaming of others, angry and resentful affect, spiteful and vindictive behavior, and frequent use of obscene language. Studies have significantly differentiated oppositionalism seen in patients with oppositional defiant disorder from delinquent behaviors noted in children with conduct disorder. One third of children and adolescents seen in community-based clinics with psychiatric diagnoses are considered oppositional.

Many argue that conduct disorder is not a unitary illness but instead contains three different syndromes characterized primarily by *aggression, intermittent antisocial behaviors,* and *delinquency.* The latter two types of behavior are differentiated by the number and frequency of antisocial behaviors committed by the child. The antecedents and outcome of patients suffering from each of these subtypes, as they relate specifically to conduct disorder, have not been studied.

The risk factors (from child, parent, and environment) associated with the development of conduct disorders are very similar to those previously mentioned in association with the development of specific antisocial and aggressive behaviors. Specific antisocial symptoms in children have been related to similar behavior in their parents. Aggressive behavior is stable across generations within families. Inconsistent parenting practices as well as overly punitive disciplinary measures have been associated with conduct disordered children. Parents of conduct-disordered children are less accepting of their children and show less warmth and support for their children. However, not all children showing antisocial behavior continue that behavior into adulthood. An early age of onset of disordered behavior, an increased number of episodes and varieties of antisocial behaviors, the seriousness of the behavior, as well as the types of symptoms, parental criminality, and marital discord are associated with continuation of antisocial behavior into the adult years.

Many different approaches have been used in the *treatment* of children and adolescents with aggressive behavior, conduct disorder, and oppositional disorder. Individual therapy focusing on alliance building and conflict resolution is sometimes useful in establishing the basic trust necessary for a positive therapeutic outcome; however, this has not been shown to be especially effective in ameliorating behavioral problems. Group therapy has shown some promise in treating adolescents with behavioral difficulties but has been relatively ineffective with latency-aged children. Training in problem-solving skills involves modeling, role play, and practicing to help children deal more successfully with interpersonal relations and is somewhat effective in modifying maladaptive styles of relating and behaving. The most effective results have been obtained with parent management training in which parents are trained directly to promote prosocial behaviors within the home and to place reasonable limits on unwanted, destructive behaviors. Family therapy designed to improve communication among family members and to elicit underlying conflicts to allow them to be more equitably resolved is also somewhat effective. Pharmacotherapy is, by and large, not indicated for this problem. However, children with underlying biologic vulnerability (intermittent psychotic disorders, attention deficit problems) may benefit from judicious use of appropriate medication. There are no medicines specifically intended for treatment of antisocial behaviors. Although lithium and haloperidol (Haldol) have some usefulness in the treatment of aggression, it is not clear whether they are helpful in conduct-disordered children or in patients with psychotic and affective symptoms. Physicians are sometimes pressured by caregivers to use both major and minor tranquilizers to help control specific behavior problems. This pressure should be resisted. Some children present with such severe behavioral problems that residential treatment and psychiatric hospitalization are necessary for a successful outcome.

Dalton R, Haslett N, Daul G: Alternative therapy with a recalcitrant fire-setter. J Am Acad Child Adolesc Psychiatry 25:713, 1986.

Lahey BB, Piacentini JC, McBurnett K, et al: Psychopathology in the parents of children with conduct disorder and hyperactivity. J Am Acad Child Adolesc Psychiatry 27:163, 1988.

Lewis DO: Conduct disorders. *In*: Garfinkel B, Carlson G, Weller E (eds): Psychiatric Disorders in Children and Adolescents. Philadelphia, WB Saunders, 1990.

Marriage K, Fine S, Moretti M, et al: Relationship between depression and conduct disorder in children and adolescents. J Am Acad Child Adolesc Psychiatry 25:687, 1986.

Nunn K: The episodic dyscontrol syndrome in childhood. J Child Psychol Psychiatry 27:439, 1986.

Rey JM: Oppositional defiant disorder. Am J Psychiatry 150:1769, 1993.

Schachar R, Wachsmuth R: Oppositional disorder in children: a validation study comparing conduct disorder, oppositional disorder and normal control children. J Child Psychol Psychiatry 31:1089, 1990.

Stewart JT, Myers WC, Burket RC, et al: A review of the pharmacotherapy of aggression in children and adolescents. J Am Acad Child Adolesc Psychiatry 29:269, 1990.

Wallander JL: The relationship between attention problems in childhood and antisocial behavior eight years later. J Child Psychol Psychiatry 29:53, 1988.

Webster-Stratton C: Annotation: strategies for helping families with conduct disordered children. J Child Psychol Psychiatry 32:1047, 1991.

CHAPTER 27

Attention Deficit Hyperactivity Disorder (ADHD)

Richard Dalton and Marc A. Forman

See also Chapter 31.

This disorder is characterized by poor ability to attend to a task, motoric overactivity, and impulsivity. These children are fidgety, have a difficult time remaining in their seats in school, are easily distracted, have difficulty awaiting their turn, impulsively blurt out answers to questions, have difficulty following instructions and sustaining attention, shift rapidly from one uncompleted activity to another, talk excessively, intrude on others, often seem not to listen to what is being said, lose items regularly, and often engage in physically dangerous activities without considering possible consequences. It is difficult to distinguish adequately between ADHD and conduct disorder, on the one hand, and between ADHD and learning disabilities on the other. Restlessness, inattentiveness, distractibility, and vigilance deficits are commonly seen in conduct-disordered children. In several studies, learning-disabled children could not be differentiated from children with ADHD on the basis of attention or distractibility. Hyperactive behaviors often cannot be shown to be separate from aggressive and antisocial behaviors.

ETIOLOGY. Dopaminergic, noradrenergic, and serotonergic mechanisms have been postulated, but a unitary biologic model has not been established. Children with ADHD differ from normal children in terms of cognitive style, levels and types of arousal, and response to rewards. Zametkin and Rapoport have demonstrated abnormal positron-emission tomographic scans with reduced glucose metabolism in premotor and superior prefrontal cortex in adults having ADHD. These areas involve control of attention and motor activities. Genetic factors have also been postulated as major contributors to the development of ADHD. Despite the plethora of investigations into the cause of ADHD, the cause is still poorly understood.

EPIDEMIOLOGY. Some studies differentiate ADHD from both conduct and anxiety disorders because the former overwhelmingly occurs in males and is primarily a disorder of cognitive impairment, in contrast to the other disorders. European and American investigators differ in their estimates of the prevalence of ADHD. Studies in the United States have suggested a prevalence rate of 1.5–4%. A recent Canadian report found an overall prevalence of 9.0% in boys and 3.3% in girls. The syndrome is 4–6 times more likely to occur in males than in females. In about half the cases, the age of onset occurs before 4 yr. Central nervous system and neurologic disorders serve as predisposing factors for this syndrome. ADHD, developmental disorders, alcohol abuse, conduct disorder, and antisocial personality disorder have all been shown to be more common in 1st-degree relatives of children with ADHD than in the general population.

CLINICAL MANIFESTATIONS. A description of the problem behaviors in specific situations and environments is elicited. A *history* of aggression and fears, poor relationships with peers, academic difficulty, behavioral problems at school, and reaction to authority define the breadth of the problem and provide useful information about the concurrent presence of conduct disorder, anxiety disorders, and learning disabilities. The history should include events of the birth and delivery, a description of the child's temperament, examples of early separation reactions and separation anxiety, a description of the child's behavior between 18 and 30 mo when the child was psychologically separating from the primary caregiver, and the child's activity level between 2 and 5 yr. ADHD is associated with neurologic problems, and some parents of hyperactive children report problems during pregnancy and delivery as well as during infancy. Some children are also described as "colicky," temperamentally difficult, and overactive from a very early age, with sleep and feeding abnormalities. Many parents report excessive temper tantrums and oppositionalism during the preschool years, suggesting a conduct disorder.

The initial identification of many children with this problem commonly occurs when they enter nursery or elementary school. They are often reported as being uncontrollable, refusing to sit still, intruding into the space and activities of other children, being boisterous and inattentive, and refusing to follow instructions. They often provoke others to anger and rarely learn from their mistakes.

During the *examination* of a child who is said to be hyperactive, it is not uncommon for signs and symptoms to be absent. Many hyperactive children are able to suppress characteristic behavior in a structured situation. Although some children have neurologic "soft signs" (mixed hand preference, impaired balance, astereognosis, dysdiadochokinesia), these findings are very inconsistent and do not contribute to the final assessment. Many of these neurologic signs occur in normal children and in various other syndromes.

DIAGNOSIS AND DIFFERENTIAL DIAGNOSES. Laboratory studies do not establish the diagnosis of ADHD. Slow wave activity on electroencephalograms is not relevant unless the child also suffers from a neurologic disorder or epilepsy. It is uncertain whether hyperactive children have significantly lower intelligent (IQ) scores than children appropriately matched for age, school grade level, and socioeconomic status who do not have the syndrome. Some studies have suggested that hyperactive children have higher verbal scores than performance scores on the Wechsler Intelligence Scale for Children-Revised and lower scores on the Attention-Concentration Subset. Psychometric tests should cover four essential areas: language skills, visuospatial skills, sequential-analytic skills, and motor planning and execution skills. Educational levels, as measured on the Peabody Individual Achievement Test and the Wide Range Achievement Test, may be lower than expected for age and IQ, especially for children who also have learning disabilities. Specific tests for learning disabilities (Woodcock Reading Mastery Test, Key Math Diagnostic Test) should be administered to pinpoint areas of difficulty. Projective psychologic tests are not useful in establishing the diagnosis.

Children in whom attention deficit problems are suspected should be evaluated for conduct disorder problems and learning disabilities. Sensory impairment, particularly auditory impairment, should be investigated in children who present with difficulty in concentrating. Petit mal epilepsy should be considered because it can mimic the concentration and attention problems seen in children with ADHD. Various medications (antipsychotics, anticonvulsants) may cause overactivity and attention problems. Overanxious children and those suffering with dysthymic and depressive disorders also may show increased activity and social disturbances similar to those seen in ADHD. Gilles de la Tourette syndrome may coexist with ADHD.

TREATMENT. Stimulant medications should be used only as a part of an ongoing treatment plan of behavioral and psychosocial therapy involving the child, parents, and school. This approach is most likely to be efficacious.

A program that gives *structure to the child's environment* decreases the effects of the handicap and helps in academic and social learning. Children should have a regular daily routine, which they are expected to follow promptly and for which they are rewarded with praise. Rules should be simple, clear, and as few in number as possible, and they should be coupled with firm limits, enforced fairly and sympathetically through restrictions and deprivation for transgressions. Overstimulation and excessive fatigue should be avoided. There should be time for relaxation after play, particularly after vigorous physical activity. The period before bedtime should be quiet, with avoidance of exciting television programs and rough and tumble games. Children with obvious hyperactivity problems should not be taken on long trips in automobiles or on extensive shopping trips. The home should be arranged so that all valuable, dangerous, or breakable objects are out of reach of young hyperactive children. Parents should reward even partially successful efforts to control behavior or to perform academic responsibilities with recognition, affection, and regular praise. More formal operant conditioning techniques that reward the child with stars or tokens contingent on improved behavior are often helpful.

Close communication between the physician and school personnel is essential. Depending on the level of the disability, some children may require special classes in which contingency or operant conditioning is used. Such approaches can be very helpful when carefully planned and implemented. Behavior therapy is a more efficacious treatment than pharmacotherapy for aggression and physical acting out in children with ADHD. Decisions about medication should be made in consultation with school personnel as well as with parents.

When severe psychosocial difficulties have produced serious family distress or when the child has internalized the obvious disapproval rendered by others so that low self-esteem results, *referral* to a mental health professional is indicated. There is no evidence that psychotherapy is primarily beneficial in ADHD, but individual and family therapy are indicated when hyperactivity is complicated by depression, social withdrawal, conduct disorder, eroded self-esteem, or family conflict.

Several *controversial therapies* are not efficacious. There is no evidence to support the use of dietary management. Megavitamins, restriction of sugar, and supplementary trace minerals are not effective. Diets low in food additives or coloring are not effective.

Methylphenidate (Ritalin), dextroamphetamine (Dexedrine), magnesium pemoline (Cylert), and various tricyclic antidepressants are efficacious in reducing overactivity, increasing attention span, improving interaction between the child and the mother and between the child and other family members. Despite short-term improvements with stimulant medication, there is little evidence that stimulants improve retention, retrieval of information, or control of anger. There is marginal evidence that stimulants significantly enhance academic performance. Peer interaction is not favorably altered with long-term drug treatment. The increased likelihood of developing delinquency later is also unaffected by stimulant medication usage. The long-term benefits of these medicines have not yet been established.

Methylphenidate is the most commonly used stimulant; it is efficacious in 75–80% of patients when administered in a dose ranging from 0.3–1.0 mg/kg. It generally has an effect for 2–4 hr, although the sustained-release form, available only in 20-mg tablets, lasts considerably longer. Studies of plasma levels suggest that a dose of 0.3 mg/kg helps to improve attention, whereas amelioration of behavioral problems requires 0.7 mg/kg. Methylphenidate should usually be given for at least 2–3 wk so that efficacy can be adequately determined.

Dextroamphetamine is efficacious in approximately 70–75% of patients. Its optimal dose range is 0.2–0.5 mg/kg. It has a longer half-life than methylphenidate, although the therapeutic effect of amphetamine preparations is reported to be no longer than 4 hr. Both dextroamphetamine and methylphenidate should be given about 20–30 min before meals to avoid their deactivation. They should not be given after 4:00 P.M. to avoid insomnia. The response to both medications should be noticeable soon after they are started. Children who do not respond will show little or no change in behavior with increasing doses.

Magnesium pemoline is effective in 65–70% of children. Its effect develops more slowly, and it may take 2–3 wk to evaluate its efficacy fully. An initial dose of 18.75 mg should be given and increased by one half tablet per week as needed (see Table 30–1, maximum 112.5 mg/24 hr). About 1–2% of children treated with this medicine may show changes in liver function; accordingly, pretreatment studies and monitoring of liver function are required.

Clonidine (Catapres), an α-adrenergic agonist, typically used as an antihypertensive, has been shown to be efficacious in treating ADHD symptoms but may produce hypotension.

Tricyclic antidepressants are efficacious in 60–70% of children. When used for hyperactivity, it is not necessary to determine blood levels in these patients. Many clinicians think that patients who respond best with a diminution of overactivity are those who also suffer from an underlying dysthymic or depressive disorder. Because of possible side effects, these medications should not be used initially.

Stimulant drugs can cause complications such as increased nervousness and jitteriness. Major short-term side effects include anorexia, upper abdominal pain, and difficulty with sleeping. The abdominal discomfort usually remits spontaneously. Tics have been reported with stimulant usage. Although this may not be an absolute contraindication, it is wise to continue stimulant usage if tics develop only with caution and close vigilance. Because the use of desipramine (Norpramin) for children with ADHD and a chronic tic disorder has been shown to be efficacious without increasing tic or Tourette symptoms, it should be considered in these situations. However, the incidence of sudden deaths associated with desipramine usage must be kept in mind (see Chapter 30). Long-term stimulant side effects may include increased heart rate and growth suppression. The effects of increased heart rate are not known. Some think that the decreased growth rate is a short-term problem, but others have reported a drop in height of 2% in children who receive an average of 40 mg/24 hr of a stimulant medicine for 2–4 yr. The growth of children receiving stimulants should be monitored, and drug-free holidays (weekends, holidays, summer vacations) should be used when practical. Stopping the medication each summer permits the parents and child to reassess the need for continued medication. At the very least, a drug-free period of 2–3 wk/yr should be tried routinely for this purpose.

It is difficult to predict which children will respond most favorably to stimulants. Up to 25% of children with ADHD do not respond positively to stimulant medication for poorly understood reasons. The action of these drugs is the same in both hyperactive and nonhyperactive, conduct-disordered children. Some studies suggest that nonanxious children with the poorest levels of concentration respond best to pharmacotherapy.

PROGNOSIS. Although hyperactivity may be short-lived, other symptoms of ADHD may persist into later life. Some anecdotal studies suggest that these other ADHD symptoms continue into adolescence and adulthood and are associated with adult alcoholism, sociopathy, and hysteria. Other studies strongly suggest that hyperactive children do well in adulthood if they are successfully employed. It is likely that the most consistent, predictive symptom of later psychopathologic conditions is the presence of aggression in childhood. Recent research indicates that children with ADHD who are treated with multiple therapies (i.e., medications, psychotherapy, parent counseling) were less likely to present with delinquency in adolescence.

Biederman J, Faraone SV, Keenan K, et al: Family-genetic and psychosocial risk factors in DSMIII attention deficit disorder. J Am Acad Child Adolesc Psychiatry 29:526, 1990.
Elia J, Welsh PA, Gullotta CS, Rapoport JL: Classroom academic performance: improvement with both methylphenidate and dextroamphetamine in ADHD boys. J Child Psychol Psychiatry 34:785, 1993.
Fisher M, Barkley R, Fletcher K, et al: The adolescent outcome of hyperactive children: Predictors of psychiatric, academic, social and emotional adjustment. J Am Acad Child Adolesc Psychiatry 32:324, 1993.
Ialongo NS, Horn WF, Pascoe JM, et al: The effects of a multimodal intervention with attention deficit hyperactivity disorder in children: A 9-month follow-up. J Am Acad Child Adolesc Psychiatry 32:182, 1993.
Spencer T, Biederman J, Kernan K, et al: Desipramine treatment of children with attention-deficit hyperactivity disorder and tic disorder or Tourette's syndrome. J Am Acad Child Adolesc Psychiatry 32:354, 1993.
Szatmari P, Offord DR, Boyle H: Ontario Child Health Study: Prevalence of attention deficit disorder with hyperactivity. J Child Psychol Psychiatry 30:219, 1989.
Werry J, Reeves J, Elkind G, et al: Attention deficit, conduct, oppositional, and anxiety disorders in children: I. A review of research on differentiating characteristics. J Am Acad Child Adolesc Psychiatry 26:133, 1987.
Zametkin A, Rapoport J: Neurobiology of attention deficit disorder with hyperactivity: Where have we come in 50 years? J Am Acad Child Adolesc Phychiatry 26:676, 1987.

CHAPTER 28

Sexual Behavior and Its Variations

Richard Dalton

See also Chapter 516.

Gender identity refers to the individual's sense of self as a male or a female. *Gender role,* on the other hand, refers to those behaviors within a culture commonly thought to be associated with maleness or femaleness. Thus, one's gender identity is intact when a biologic male identifies himself as a man and a biologic female identifies herself as a woman. If the male performs the sort of behavior associated with being a man within his culture, he is said to fit comfortably within his gender role. However, if a man is uncomfortable with those behaviors identified with men within his culture, the implication is that he has trouble with his gender role. The same is true for women. However, as society has changed, gender roles have changed. In the past, gender roles were shaped by traditionally defined masculine and feminine roles. As the economics of family life have changed—and both sexes have become potentially self-sufficient economically—gender roles, as they relate to job choices and performance, have changed dramatically or, in some cases, have simply disappeared. Fewer behaviors are specific solely to one gender.

Children identify themselves as boys or girls by about 18 mo of age (i.e., establish a gender identity). Between 18 and 30 mo of age, children establish *gender stability,* the concept that boys become men and girls become women. By 30 mo, gender constancy, the immutability of one's gender, is firmly established and resistant to change. Although there are numerous theories suggesting which environmental and biologic factors are most important to the establishment of a firm gender identity, at this point, we still do not understand, in a way that has treatment implications, which factors are most important in any given child.

Children are naturally curious about their bodies. The 2-yr-old child ought to be taught the proper names for the parts of the body, including the genitals. Parents should react calmly when their children explore and manipulate their own bodies with enjoyment, although open masturbation by older children suggests poor awareness of social reality or lack of parental censorship. Parents should inform their children that *masturbation* is not a social activity and should be limited to the bedroom when the child is alone. An overly excited or overly punitive reaction will only serve to excite the child. It is important that masturbation be accepted as a normal aspect of the child's sexual life and that guilt be avoided. By puberty, children should be given explanations of its normality. This can be done in conjunction with explanations of ejaculation, orgasm, and menstruation so that children can understand them, too, as normal bodily functions.

It is quite common for preschool children to hug and kiss each other. More explicit sexual behavior, such as oral contact, attempts at simulated intercourse, or anal stimulation are probably learned through observation or direct involvement with older children or adults. Intervention designed to uncover the source of the child's knowledge and appropriate subsequent action is indicated in these situations.

Especially between the ages of 10 and 12 yr, boys and girls typically explore sexual issues with best friends (same-sex friends) as a means of gathering information. This should not be viewed as a prelude for homosexuality but as a developmental stage in most children. At any age, the compulsive need for sex serves as a defense against underlying dependency, separation, and autonomy issues. It is usually during adolescence that gender object interests are realized. The teenager's actual or perceived sexual experiences and their reinforcements are important in shaping ultimate gender role behaviors.

Transsexualism, the conviction by a person biologically of one gender that he or she is a member of the other gender, is the most obvious example of gender identity confusion. Transsexual adolescents feel discomfort and a sense of inappropriateness about their assigned sex. They spend years trying to figure out how to get rid of the primary and secondary sexual characteristics that define them biologically. Gender roles of the opposite biologic sex are usually adopted.

The prevalence of transsexualism is 1/30,000 for males and 1/100,000 for females. Individuals with this disorder usually have a difficult time with social and occupational functioning. Concurrent psychopathologic conditions and depression are part of the reason; societal consternation is the other part. The natural history of transsexualism is not well understood. A preponderance of adult transsexuals had gender identity disorders as children and adolescents. Extreme femininity in boys is a predisposing factor. Some say that they remember being confused about gender identity as early as 2 yr of age. Which particular effeminate boys will later show transsexual behavior cannot be accurately predicted.

Treatment of transsexualism has taken two directions. Many transsexual adults have opted for hormonal and surgical therapies to produce primary and secondary sexual characteristics of the gender with which they identify. Follow-up studies consistently show continued distress after these treatments. Long-term dynamic and behavioral therapies also have been tried. Although there are anecdotal reports of successful reidentification with the given biologic sex, without statistical controls, it is impossible to know whether this represents a response to therapy or a spontaneous change that would have occurred otherwise. Spontaneous remissions have been shown to occur.

Transvestism, cross-dressing, may occur transiently, in preschool boys who dress up in their mothers' clothing, or it may occur chronically in preschool and school-aged boys who feel genuinely excited when dressed in women's clothing. Cross-dressing in girls is rarely an identified problem. Chronic cross-dressing might represent underlying transsexualism, although that is generally not the case. Transvestism usually indicates that other gender roles might also be problematic for the individual. Physicians consulted by parents should investigate other areas of gender identification and gender behavior. Does the child verbalize a preference to be the opposite sex? Does the child deny or disparage his or her own sexual anatomy or assert that opposite anatomic structures will develop? Three to 6% of school-aged boys and 10–12% of school-aged girls often behave like the opposite sex, but fewer than 2% of boys and 2–4% of girls actually wish to be the opposite sex.

28.1 Gender Identity Disorder (GID)

A recent study indicates that 22.8% of school-aged boys and 38.6% of girls exhibit 10 or more gender-atypical behaviors (GABs). Most children exhibit one or more GABs. These behaviors are to be expected in most children and are most often not indicative of GID. However, persistent distress about being a particular gender while being preoccupied with cross-gender roles or repudiation of given anatomic genital structures is the hallmark of GID. It encompasses transsexualism, transvestism, and effeminacy in boys. The etiology of GID is similar to that postulated for homosexuality.

CLINICAL MANIFESTATIONS. Many GID children develop the disorder prior to 4 yr of age. They are often ostracized by peers and have a difficult social adjustment, sometimes with subsequent depression. One half or more of the boys develop a homosexual orientation during adolescence and adulthood. GID is associated with numerous other childhood and adolescent disorders. Using the Child Behavior Checklist, it has been shown that 84% of feminine boys display behavioral disturbances similar to those seen within a psychiatric clinic population. Sixty per cent endorsed items related to peer difficulties and met the criteria for the diagnosis of separation anxiety disorder. Others have found that GID is unrelated to ethnic background, religion, or educational level.

TREATMENT. The relationship between GID and separation anxiety disorder and other disturbances supports the importance of psychotherapy and possibly pharmacotherapy if behaviors satisfy criteria for separation anxiety disorder or other Axis I disorders. Other approaches are often employed and have been shown to be helpful. Parenting techniques that specify which behaviors are appropriate and what is expected of the child regarding gender role behaviors have shown promise in managing a significant percentage of children with GID. The physician needs to help the parents control their own frustration and disappointment to minimize judgmental, rejecting behavior. Punishment, castigation, or shaming will not support the child's attempts to struggle with whatever intrapsychic, interpersonal, or cultural conflicts exist. Underlying family conflicts and parent-child conflicts need to be managed therapeutically.

28.2 Homosexuality

Homosexuality, the romantic and physical attraction to someone of the same gender, has occurred throughout the ages in about 5% of men and women. Historically, acceptance of homosexuality has waxed and waned within societies. The view is currently held by some that homosexuality is best regarded as an alternative lifestyle. The American Psychiatric Association no longer lists it among mental disorders.

The *etiology* is uncertain. Many view its development as a normal variant of sexual development; others point to problematic parent-child relationships. Numerous psychologic theories have been proffered to explain homosexual development. They include problems of sexual identification with parents; problematic relationships between either parent and the child, abuse, overly eroticized attachment, and underlying anxiety and affective proclivities in the individual who will later present with homosexual behavior. Although each theory has been accompanied by anecdotal reports and case studies, none has been substantiated in well-controlled studies.

Biologic causes have also been proposed. Focusing on the perceived homology between homosexual behavior in humans and lower animals, researchers have proposed the "dual mating center" theory, stating that there are hypothalamic areas that regulate male and female sexual behavior. It is hypothesized that too little androgen production in males during a critical prenatal period causes the female center to overdevelop; conversely, excessive androgen production in females leads to the overdevelopment of the male center. Proponents point to the fact that some homosexual men demonstrate "estrogen feedback responses," in which, because of decreased androgen levels, administration of estrogen causes increased production of lutenizing hormone. Many other investigators dispute this theory because of the lack of consistent findings (e.g., XY males with testicular feminization syndrome do not exhibit this response).

LeVay's recent finding that heterosexual and homosexual men have differences in hypothalamic structure and size also suggests a biologic substrate for sexual orientation, although the possibility of acquired immodeficiency syndrome in his postmortem specimens may have biased these findings. Other researchers have recently noted that the anterior commissure in homosexual men is significantly larger than that in heterosexual men. This anatomic difference correlates with both sexual orientation and gender; i.e., the anterior commissure is also larger in heterosexual women than in heterosexual men. Furthermore, Hamer and associates discovered a possible genetic marker for male homosexuality in a small group of individuals and are searching for a gene. Many researchers are skeptical of these biologic findings. Some note that the current evidence that postulates biologic factors in the development of sexual orientation is no more compelling than the current evidence linked to psychologic theories.

There are probably multiple mechanisms leading to homosexuality in adolescence and adulthood, just as there are probably multiple mechanisms leading to heterosexuality; many complex factors contribute to sexual development. At this point, it appears probable that cultural, biologic, and psychologic factors contribute to sexual orientation development.

If a child is found to be engaging in homosexual behavior, parents should not immediately conclude that this means that the child is already homosexual. Sexual behavior during adolescence does not necessarily predict future sexual orientation. It is estimated that 6% of females and 17% of males have had at least one homosexual experience during adolescence. Children sexually explore in the same way that they explore other parts of their environment. The first task of the physician of parents after discovering that a child has engaged in homosexual activity is to help the younger child feel safe and less guilty. Parents should avoid suspicious, scolding, threatening, shaming, or guilt-inducing attitudes or behaviors toward the child. The physician can serve as a model for the parent through his or her own calm, sensitive, careful exploration of feelings and behavior with the child. The physician should expect denials on the part of the child and avoidance of and embarrassment with the subject, but discussion helps the child to understand that sexual behavior is comprehensible and that sexual feelings and curiosity are normal. It is important to know whether the child's information and understanding of sexual matters are appropriate for his or her age.

If the same-sex behavior involves another child in the family, he or she should be treated in the same manner. If an older child is the initiator or seducer, he or she should be told clearly and firmly that such behavior will not be tolerated and that he or she will be expected to act with responsibility and control. The older child should talk with a physician or mental health professional; if concerns about emotional and social adjustment become evident, referral for a psychiatric evaluation is indicated. Physicians must not let their own negative feelings aggravate the negative feelings that parents might have for an older child seen as a perpetrator, especially if the older child is not a member of the younger child's family. The physician may need to help the parents of exploited children refrain from ill-considered acts of revenge against the offenders. On the other hand, if there has been physical violence or psychologic coercion, both psychiatric and legal interventions are indicated.

In taking a history of sexual behavior, the pediatrician should not presume exclusive heterosexual behavior. Confidentiality must be maintained, except in sexual abuse cases. Depending on the patient's prior experience, the physical examination should include an assessment of possible sexually transmitted diseases (STDs). The American Academy of Pediatrics recommends that all sexually active males should have appropriate laboratory testing for STDs. Immunization for hepatitis B is recommended and should be provided for all males who anticipate having sex with another male. Human immunodeficiency virus (HIV) testing with the necessary consent is appropriate in these situations. Counseling before and after HIV testing is also necessary. Homosexual activity between adolescent girls is associated with a far lower risk of STDs. However both HIV and other STDs can be transmitted during lesbian sexual activity, especially if one of the partners has also had sex with a man.

When the social opprobrium is considered, it is not surprising that homosexual feelings and wishes create psychologic conflicts in adolescents. Recent studies suggest that 3–30% of adolescent suicides are attributed to conflicts regarding sexual orientation. Troiden's model of homosexual identity development helps to elucidate the stages associated with sexual orientation acceptance. They include sensitization, i.e., the awareness of being different because of same gender attraction; sexual identity confusion, i.e., turmoil often related to trying to reconcile one's feelings with negative societal stigmatization; sexual identity assumption, i.e., acknowledgment of one's own gay identity; and integration and commitment, i.e., incorporation of sexual identity into a positive self-acceptance.

In spite of some anecdotal reports, very little can be done to change one's sexual orientation. Even in cases in which individuals have expressed the desire to change, significantly fewer than one half of those who have tried have been able to change sexual orientation with various behavioral and dynamic therapies. Often, attempts to change sexual orientation only lead to additional guilt and further stigmatization. Psychotherapy is more appropriately used for concurrent disorders (separation anxiety disorder, conduct disorder, dysthymic disorder, depression) and to help with the conflict that often ensues as one moves toward sexual orientation acceptance. Families usually need assistance in coping with this knowledge and their attendant anger and disappointment. Children need help in understanding how to cope with the reactions of others.

Allen L, Gorski R: Sexual orientation and the size of the anterior commissure in the human brain. Proc Natl Acad Sci U S A 89:7199, 1992.

Bailey J, Michael J, Neale M, et al: Heritable factors influencing sexual orientation in women. Arch Gen Psychiatry 50:217, 1993.

Byrne W, Parsons B: Human sexual orientation: The biologic theories reappraised. Arch Gen Psychiatry 50:228, 1993.

Coates S, Person E: Extreme boyhood femininity: Isolated behavior or pervasive disorder? J Am Acad Child Adolesc Psychiatry 24:702, 1985.

Committee on Adolescence (American Academy of Pediatrics): Homosexuality and adolescence. Pediatrics 92:631, 1993.

Hamer D, Magnuson V, Pattatucci A: A linkage between DNA markers on the X chromosome and male sexual orientation. Science 261:321, 1993.

LeVay S: The Sexual Brain. Cambridge, The M.I.T. Press, 1993.

Sandberg D, Meyer-Bahlburg H, Ehrhardt A, et al: The prevalence of gender-atypical behavior in elementary school children. J Am Acad Child Adolesc Psychiatry 32:306, 1993.

Sreenivasan V: Effeminate boys in a child psychiatric clinic: prevalence and associated factors. J Am Acad Child Adolesc Psychiatry 24:689, 1985.

Troiden R: Homosexual identity development. J Adolesc Health Care 9:105, 1989.

CHAPTER 29
Psychosis in Childhood

Richard Dalton and Marc A. Forman

29.1 Infantile Autism

This psychosis develops before 30 mo of age. It is characterized by a qualitative impairment in verbal and nonverbal communication, in imaginative activity, and in reciprocal social interactions.

CLINICAL MANIFESTATIONS. Among the most notable symptoms and signs are nondeveloped or poorly developed verbal and nonverbal communication skills, abnormalities in speech patterns, impaired ability to sustain a conversation, abnormal social play, lack of empathy, and an inability to make friends. Stereotypic body movements, a marked need for sameness, very narrow interests, and a preoccupation with parts of the body are also frequent. The autistic child is withdrawn and often spends hours in solitary play. Ritualistic behavior prevails, reflecting the child's need to maintain a consistent, predictable environment. Tantrum-like rages may accompany disruptions of routine. Eye contact is minimal or absent. Visual scanning of hand and finger movements, mouthing of objects, and rubbing of surfaces may indicate a heightened awareness and sensitivity to some stimuli, whereas diminished responses to pain and lack of startle responses to sudden loud noises reflect lowered sensitivity to other stimuli. If speech is present, echolalia, pronomial reversal, nonsense rhyming, and other idiosyncratic language forms may predominate.

Intelligence by conventional psychologic testing usually falls in the functionally retarded range; however, the deficits in language and socialization make it difficult to obtain an accurate estimate of the autistic child's intellectual potential. Some autistic children perform adequately in nonverbal tests, and those with developed speech may demonstrate adequate intellectual capacity. Occasionally, an autistic child may have an isolated, remarkable talent, analogous to that of the adult idiot savant.

Although first described as a social illness, most research studies have focused on the communicative and cognitive deficits of autism and, particularly, on the types of cognitive processing deficits most apparent in emotional situations. Deficits in verbal sequencing, abstraction, rote memory, and reciprocal verbal exchange are typical in autistic children. Autistic children also show deficits in their understanding of what the other person might be feeling or thinking, a so-called lack of a "theory of mind."

EPIDEMIOLOGY. The prevalence is generally thought to be 3–4/10,000 children. The disorder is much more common in males than in females (3–4:1). Several systemic, infectious, and neurologic illnesses produce autistic-like symptoms or predispose patients to the development of autistic symptoms. An increased association with seizures also has been noted.

ETIOLOGY. The cause of autism is speculative. Genetic causes have been implicated. There is an 80% concordance rate for monozygotic twins and a 20% concordance rate for dizygotic twins. What is actually inherited is not entirely clear; language and cognitive abnormalities are more common in relatives of autistic children than in the general population. Chromosomal abnormalities, especially fragile X syndrome, are also more common in families with autism.

Abnormal neurochemical findings have been associated with autism. Although dopamine functioning has been thought to be normal in autism, abnormalities have recently been suggested in a number of catecholamine pathways. Increased levels of serotonin have also been noted.

Theories of causation have also centered on a variety of other possibilities, including brain injury, constitutional vulnerability, developmental aphasia, deficits in the reticular activating system, an unfortunate interplay between psychogenic and neurodevelopmental factors, structural cerebellar changes, and forebrain hippocampal lesions. Contrary to notions in vogue in the past, autism is not induced by parents.

TREATMENT. Different therapeutic approaches have been advocated to treat and manage autistic children, but success has been limited. Gains in speech acquisition have been reported with behavior therapy utilizing operant conditioning. Destructive behavior and aggression can often be modified by behavior management. Neuroleptics have shown promise in reducing self-injurious behavior, outwardly directed aggression, stereotypic behavior, and social withdrawal. Potent opiate antagonists have recently been shown to alter behavioral problems, withdrawal, and stereotypies. Day treatment models using play, language therapy, and structured interpersonal exercises have also shown promise.

PROGNOSIS. This is guarded. Some children, especially those with speech, may grow up to live marginal, self-sufficient, albeit isolated, lives in the community, but for some, chronic placement in institutions is the ultimate outcome. The relationship between autism and schizophrenia is uncertain. Cases in which autistic children have later developed schizophrenia have been reported but are not common. A better prognosis is associated with higher intelligence, functional speech, and less bizarre symptoms and behavior. The symptoms often change as children grow older. Seizures and self-injurious behavior becomes more common with advancing age.

29.2 Pervasive Developmental Disorder

Some children have a qualitative impairment in the development of reciprocal social interaction and verbal and nonverbal communication but do not have the quantity of symptoms necessary for a diagnosis of autism. Though somewhat socially aware, these children appear to others to be peculiar and eccentric. The prevalence is said to be 2.0/10,000 children. These patients may be diagnosed as having a schizoid personality disorder or Asperger syndrome, which generally refers to a higher-functioning form of autism, although this distinction remains somewhat controversial.

29.3 Late-Onset Psychosis

Psychotic reactions in older children tend more closely to resemble the psychoses of adulthood, and the same diagnostic criteria apply. Affective psychoses have been described earlier.

In *childhood schizophrenia,* prominent symptoms include thought disorder, delusions, and hallucinations. The latter two symptoms, in addition to later onset, higher intelligence scores, and fewer perinatal complications, differentiate schizophrenia from autism. As the symptoms imply, schizophrenic children often appear to be chaotic. They may have paranoid delusions, aggressive behavior, hebephrenic silliness, social withdrawal, and alternating moods not apparently related to environmental stimuli, among other possibilities.

The prevalence of adult schizophrenia is 1% of the population. Because the typical age of onset is late adolescence to early adulthood, a very small percentage of preschool and latency-aged children actually shows symptoms that meet the criteria for a diagnosis of schizophrenia. Most prepubertal children diagnosed with schizophrenia are later rediagnosed, usually with an affective disorder. The prognosis is poor. The symptoms in childhood that most predict psychotic adult psychopathology are affective blunting and disturbed interpersonal relationships, as opposed to delusions and hallucinations.

A multimodal therapeutic approach is necessary to manage this illness. Parent training is necessary to teach effective techniques to modify the schizophrenic child's behavior to a reasonable extent. Individual therapy designed to build a positive alliance is also very important. Neuroleptic therapy is often effective in managing hallucinations and psychotic delusions. School and community liaison work can establish and maintain a day-to-day schedule for the patient.

29.4 Borderline Personality Disorder

The majority of children with late-onset psychosis suffer from this disorder, also called interactive psychosis or symbiotic psychosis. These children present with a marked instability of mood, interpersonal relationships, and sense of self. They make suicidal threats and gestures, often abuse themselves and others physically, and are very impulsive. Behavioral disorders are almost always present, and unpredictability is frequent, as are rage reactions and manipulativeness. They rarely hallucinate, although they may be suspicious and have paranoid-like thinking.

Although underlying biologic vulnerabilities may be present, most of these children experience a great deal of difficulty with attachment and separation issues. Their behavior often seems to be a product of the child's underlying desire to maintain a self-image of being the center of his or her own environment. Rage reactions result when this desire is frustrated. These children require very consistently applied limits in addition to alliance-building dynamic psychotherapy designed to improve object relations.

Most nonorganically induced psychotic reactions and behaviors in children are a product of either autism, pervasive developmental disorder, affective disorder, schizophrenia, or borderline personality disorder. Some children may present with intermittent psychotic-like behavior (withdrawal, hysterical acting out) in response to a traumatic situation or an ongoing series of psychologic and physical insults. These are either post-traumatic or adjustment reactions.

Baron-Cohen S: The autistic child's theory of mind: A case of specific developmental delay. J Child Psychol Psychiatry 30:285, 1989.

Burd L, Fisher W, Kerbeshian J: Childhood onset pervasive developmental disorder. J Child Psychol Psychiatry 29:155, 1988.

Gillberg C: Outcome in autism and autistic-like conditions. J Am Acad Child Adolesc Psychiatry 30:375, 1991.

Gillberg IC, Hellgren L, Gillberg C: Psychotic disorders diagnosed in adolescence: outcome at age 30 years. J Child Psychol Psychiatry 34:1173, 1993.

Green WH, Padron-Gayol M, Hardesty AS, et al: Schizophrenia with childhood

onset: a phenomenological study of 38 cases. J Am Acad Child Adolesc Psychiatry 31:968, 1992.
Kanner L: Early infantile autism. Am J Orthopsychiatry 19:416, 1949.
Lofgren DP, Bemporad J, King J, et al: A prospective follow-up of so-called borderline children. Am J Psychiatry 148:1541, 1991.
Petti TA, Vela RM: Borderline disorders of childhood: An overview. J Am Acad Child Adolesc Psychiatry 29:327, 1990.
Piven J, Gayle J, Landa R, et al: The prevalence of fragile X in a sample of autistic individuals diagnosed using a standardized interview. J Am Acad Child Adolesc Psychiatry 30:825, 1991.
Pomeroy J: Infantile autism and childhood psychosis. *In*: Garfinkel B, Carlson G, Weller E (eds): Psychiatry Disorders in Childhood and Adolescence. Philadelphia, WB Saunders, 1990.
Ritvo ER, Mason-Brothers A, Freeman BJ, et al: The UCLA-University of Utah epidemiologic survey of autism: The etiologic role of rare diseases. Am J Psychiatry 147:1614, 1990.
Treffert DA: The idiot savant: A review of the syndrome. Am J Psychiatry 145:563, 1988.
Ventner A, Lord C, Schopler E: A follow-up study of high-functioning autistic children. J Child Psychol Psychiatry 33:489, 1992.
Volkmar FR, Cohen DJ: Comorbid association of autism and schizophrenia. Am J Psychiatry 148:1705, 1991.
Werry JS, McClellan JM, Chard L: Childhood and adolescent schizophrenic, bipolar and schizoaffective disorders: A clinical and outcome study. J Am Acad Child Adolesc Psychiatry 30:457, 1991.

CHAPTER 30

Psychologic Treatment of Children and Adolescents

Richard Dalton

30.1 Illness and Death

All clinical phenomena relate to a variety of organizational levels: molecular, anatomic, physiologic, intrapsychic, interpersonal, familial, and social. Accordingly, the physician should focus on the patient's discomfort rather than on a categorization of clinical manifestations as either organically or psychologically determined. The psychologic aspects of illness should be evaluated from the outset, and the physician should act as a model for the parents and the child by showing interest in the child's feelings and demonstrating that it is possible and appropriate to communicate discomfort in verbal, symbolic language.

For *the hospitalized child,* potential challenges include coping with separation, adapting to a new environment; adjusting to multiple caregivers; often associating with very sick children; and sometimes experiencing the disorientation of intensive care, anesthesia, and surgery. To help mitigate potential problems, a preadmission visit to the hospital is often important to meet the people who will be offering care and to ask questions about what will happen. For children younger than 5–6 yr of age, parents should room with the child if feasible. Creative and active recreational or socialization programs, with liberal visiting hours (including visits from siblings), and chances to act out feared procedures in play with dolls or mannequins are all helpful. Sensitive, sympathetic, and accepting attitudes toward the child and parents by the hospital staff are very important. There is often an underlying tension between the hospital caregivers and the parents. Hospital routines and schedules often serve to complicate the relationship between parents and hospital workers. Guilt and anger can result, unnecessarily complicating an already difficult situation.

Ambulatory care in clinics or offices where patients receive discontinuous care from a series of physicians whose intercommunication is often limited may create a problem. Parents often become confused and unable to verbalize major concerns about their children. Recommendations for care may become inappropriate or irrelevant, and compliance with advice or directions becomes poor. At the end of any initial diagnostic or management activity, the physician should habitually inquire whether there are other things parents or children may wish to talk about during this visit. In busy emergency rooms of hospitals and urban centers, conflicting expectations between how the professional staff expects the emergency room to be used and what patients actually need can lead to confusion. When these different expectations are critically examined, ways may be found to deal more effectively with the patterns of use of emergency services.

With *chronically or fatally ill children,* every symptom is experienced by the patient and parent as a threat to physical integrity and life. The more serious the clinical state, the greater the intensity of the emotions aroused. By 9 yr of age, children begin to conceive of death as meaning more than just going away. By adolescence, they think of death in philosophic terms much as adults do, albeit with limited experience.

In dealing with chronic illness that shortens life, such as cystic fibrosis, parents need the physician's early support in developing a relatively guilt-free understanding of the disease and how to manage it. They need guidance to help them comfortably answer the child's questions about the disease. The young child will take most cues from the parents. With the older child, and especially the adolescent, parents must be prepared to deal with the anger of the child because of his or her fate. The child needs both the parents' psychologic strengths and resources and the physician's availability and objectivity.

The role of the physician is difficult. He or she must stand for hope and for relief of discomfort, ready to help parents and child avoid emotionally crippling psychologic handicaps. For example, parents must be encouraged to meet their own needs, even when this requires temporary and perhaps recurrent separation from the child; at times, this may help the child to learn to tolerate frustration. Parents of critically or fatally ill children may creatively support each other in group meetings under the professional guidance of physicians, psychologists, or social workers.

In *potentially fulminant lethal processes,* the intensity of parental anxiety, guilt, and despair may be greater than it is with more chronic illnesses. With most children older than 9–10 yr of age, it is most supportive to treat fatal illness factually with the child, so far as diagnosis and prognosis are concerned, but always offering realistic hope. Children do not usually ask the physician if and when they are going to die, though they may reveal their fears to others in the hospital. Young children primarily want to be reassured that their parents will not desert them and that they are loved. A hospital team approach representing medical, nursing, psychologic, and social work disciplines, among others, should provide support. The primary physician needs to stay involved and close to the child and to the clinical situation.

Organ transplants in children have most often involved the kidney. Dialysis may precede renal transplant for varying lengths of time and begins in the hospital, but parents may be expected to learn to carry out this procedure at home. They may be ambivalent about being given control of a life-threatening process. The child receiving dialysis becomes psychologically dependent and often withdrawn. Bone marrow, heart, lung, and liver transplants also involve many psychologic considerations, such as donor relationships and the stress of isolation and complications.

Family problems multiply with the question of who will donate an organ. If relatives are available as donors, there may be tension about who can and should "make the sacrifice." In some cases, guilt may be relieved if the physician arbitrarily (but thoughtfully) makes this decision. A medical support team of carefully chosen staff is essential to facilitate decision making and continuing care. Although there is a high suicide rate among adults undergoing hemodialysis, this procedure appears to be less traumatic in children, probably owing to the child's greater capacities for denial and acceptance of a support system. Adolescents are concerned with distortions of body image, which they cannot always express verbally.

After *the death of a child,* the parents will need opportunities to talk out their feelings with the physician, one of whose goals should be to help them avoid psychologically encapsulating the lost child in an unmourned state. Many parents can be helped and comforted by being with and holding the dying infant or child or seeing and touching him or her after death. The physician needs the patience to listen (both to the stated and to the implied questions and misconceptions), to answer questions, and to help families with funeral arrangements (see Chapter 41).

30.2 Psychopharmacology (Table 30–1)

Using drugs to modify children's behavior is controversial. Their effects on behavior are influenced by the maturity of the central nervous system, by intrapsychic and psychosocial factors, by the personality or charisma of the physician prescribing them, by the problem itself, and by the milieu (e.g., patient, parents, time of day given).

Neuroleptics are appropriately used for hallucinations, delusions, thought disorders, and severe agitation. They are primarily indicated for children and adolescents suffering with schizophrenic disorders, mood-congruent and mood-incongruent psychotic reactions secondary to major affective disorders, autism presenting with stereotypic and withdrawal symptoms and self-abuse, and Gilles de la Tourette syndrome. Some advocate the use of haloperidol for aggressive behavior in children and adolescents, but this usage remains controversial. Serious questions have been raised about the efficacy of neuroleptics in childhood schizophrenia. This class of medicine is inappropriately used for anxiety, conduct disorder without extreme aggression, and attention deficit disorder.

Neuroleptics can be subdivided into low-potency, midpotency, and high-potency types. Chlorpromazine and thioridazine are both low-potency medicines and usually require a higher dose than the other neuroleptics for symptom remission. They are both rather sedative, producing numerous anticholinergic side effects but causing comparatively fewer extrapyramidal symptoms. Mesoridazine, a midpotency medicine, produces more extrapyramidal symptoms than the low-potency drugs. Thiothixene and haloperidol are high-potency medicines that produce, comparatively, the greatest number of extrapyramidal symptoms.

The most worrisome side effect of the neuroleptics is the development of **tardive dyskinesia.** This is characterized by choreoathetoid movements of trunk, limbs, and facial musculature; these movements develop in approximately 20–30% of children treated long-term with neuroleptics. Dyskinesia can occur during the treatment with the drug or after it has been discontinued, in which case it is referred to as withdrawal dyskinesia. This latter type of dyskinesia, the symptoms of which can include nausea, vomiting, diaphoresis, ataxia, oral dyskinesia, and various dystonic movements, is reversible in most cases, whereas the dyskinesia developing during drug use may not be reversible. The treatment of tardive dyskinesia involves decreasing or discontinuing the medication if possible, despite the fact that it has been noted that increasing the neuroleptic causes a temporary diminution of dyskinetic symptoms. Prophylactic measures involving drug-free holidays and periodic discontinuation of neuroleptics are also advisable to help mitigate the development of tardive dyskinesia.

Extrapyramidal symptoms, a Parkinson-like syndrome (akithesia, bradykinesis, torticollis, drooling, and involuntary hand movements, among others), develop in at least one fourth of children treated with neuroleptics. The imbalance created by the dopaminergic blocking action of the antipsychotic medication disrupts a needed balance between that system and the cholinergic system within the basal ganglia. The high-potency neuroleptics, which contain few anticholinergic properties, are the most likely to produce extrapyramidal symptoms. This syndrome can be treated by decreasing the neuroleptic or adding an anticholinergic agent (trihexyphenidyl HCl [Artane], benztropine mesylate [Cogentin]).

Neuroleptic malignant syndrome, a rare side effect of neuroleptic usage, can be fatal. Its development is heralded by a high fever and a "lead pipe" stiffness of the extremities. The creatinine phosphokinase level is also markedly elevated. Immediate discontinuation of the medicine and supportive care are necessary during the early part of the syndrome.

Stimulant medications are used to treat the signs and symptoms of attention deficit hyperactivity disorder. Although the mechanism of action is not entirely clear, these medications have been shown to increase children's ability to attend, to improve classroom behavior, and to increase social acceptance in various situations. These stimulants should be used concurrently with individual, family, and community therapy, but often this is not done.

Antidepressants and *lithium carbonate* are useful in the treatment of patients with affective disorders. Antidepressants generally are effective for depression, whereas lithium has shown efficacy with mania. Bipolar and unipolar adult patients are often treated with long-term pharmacotherapy, and this is becoming more common in childhood and adolescence. Because of the propensity of tricyclic antidepressants to cause heart block, a pretreatment electrocardiogram (ECG) and follow-up ECGs are necessary. Children and adolescents who receive tricyclic antidepressants should be followed by serial blood levels until an adequate dose is determined. This usually takes at least a few weeks. Although deaths in school-aged children taking desipramine have been reported, sudden deaths have not been reported in conjunction with the use of other tricyclics or with other nontricyclic antidepressants. Prior to prescribing tricyclics in general and desipramine in particular, clinicians must procure a detailed medical history, including examination of the patient's cardiovascular system and family history of cardiac disease (including unexplained syncope and sudden death). A child with a suspicious history or with an abnormal ECG should have a pediatric or cardiologic assessment before these medicines are used. A pretreatment lithium evaluation includes thyroid studies, renal function tests, and electrolyte levels. Lithium blood levels should also be determined while the patient is taking the medication. Prolonged use of lithium may cause hypothyroidism.

Serotonin reuptake blockers, especially fluoxetine (Prozac), sertraline (Zoloft), and paroxetine (Paxil), have been shown to be effective with patients with mild depressive symptoms, anxiety, and compulsions. Paroxetine is especially useful because of its relatively short half-life and lack of side effects. Clonidine has been partially successful in treating children with attention deficit hyperactivity disorder and in those who have a personal history of tics (including Gilles de la Tourette syn-

■ **TABLE 30–1 Psychopharmacology**

Medication Class	Indications	Dosage	Side Effects/Toxicity/Cautions	Pretreatment Workup
Antipsychotics	**All Classes**	**Low Potency**	**All Classes**	CBC with differential, blood chemical panel (including hepatic enzymes)
Low Potency/High Dosage	Severe agitation; childhood and adolescent schizophrenia; mania; stereotypic symptoms of pervasive developmental disorder and autism; self-abuse, extreme aggressiveness.	30–150 mg/24 hr in divided doses; available in concentrated form	Sedation, weight gain; anticholinergic effects (dry mouth, blurred vision, constipation); hypersensitive reactions (hepatic, skin); blood dyscrasias; parkinsonism	
Thioridazine (Mellaril)				
Chlorpromazine (Thorazine)				
Midpotency/Mid-Dosage		**Midpotency**		
Mesoridazine (Serentil)		10–75 mg/24 hr in divided doses		
High-Potency/Low Dosage	**High-Potency Class**	**High-Potency**	**Long-Term Effects**	
Trifluoperazine (Stelazine)	Gilles de la Tourette syndrome; other tic disorders (haloperidol)	1–6 mg/24 hr in divided doses	Risk of tardive dyskinesia and "withdrawal-emergent" syndrome (see text)	
Thiothixene (Navane)				
Haloperidol (Haldol)				
Stimulants (6 yr and older)			Insomnia, decreased appetite, possible weight loss; irritability and tearfulness; abdominal pain, headache; elevated systolic blood pressure; development and worsening of tics. A long-term effect may be height and weight reduction (Chapter 27). Pemoline is associated with hypersensitivity reactions, especially hepatic.	History (medical) Heart rate, blood pressure Hepatic enzymes with pemoline usage
Methylphenidate (Ritalin)	Attention deficit disorder	0.3–1.0 mg/kg/24 hr		
Dextroamphetamine (Dexedrine)	Attention deficit disorder	0.2–0.5 mg/kg/24 hr		
Pemoline (Cylert)	Attention deficit disorder	37.5–112.5 mg/kg/24 hr		
Antidepressants				
Desipramine (Norpramin)	Major depressive disorder; separation anxiety; attention deficit disorder unresponsive to stimulants (12 yr and older)	For major depressive disorder and separation anxiety; 2–3 mg/kg/24 hr in divided doses (blood levels; therapeutic, 100–250 ng/ml)	ECG and blood pressure should be monitored for hypertension, orthostatic hypotension, cardiac arrhythmia, or lengthening of PR or QRS interval (see Chapter 30). Monitor plasma levels for therapeutic range.	Thorough individual and family medical and cardiologic histories; 12-lead ECG; cardiology consultation if necessary.
Fluoxetine (Prozac)	Mild depression and anxiety	10–30 mg/24 hr	Agitation, headaches, anxiety, insomnia, weight loss; binds tenaciously to proteins and has a long half-life.	
Paroxetine (Paxil)	Mild depression and anxiety	10–30 mg/24 hr	Agitation, insomnia, weight loss	
Mood Stabilizers				
Lithium carbonate	Mania, some cases of unipolar illness, extreme aggression	600–1200 mg/24 hr (blood levels: therapeutic—0.6–1.2 mEq/L)	Gastrointestinal disturbance, tremor, ataxia, confusion, coma, death; hypothyroidism	Creatinine clearance, thyroid studies, electrolytes, ECG
Carbamazepine (Tegretol)	Mania, aggression, self-injurious behavior in organically impaired patients	400–1000 mg/24 hr (blood levels: therapeutic 8–12 μg/mL)	Fever, sore throat, hematologic problems (white cell decrease), dizziness, drowsiness, neuromuscular disturbance	Physical examination and medical history; CBC with differential, BUN, hepatic enzymes
Antihypertensives				
Clonidine (Catapres)	ADHD not responding to stimulants ADHD with aggression	0.1–0.25 mg/24 hr	Bradycardia, hypotension	Physical examination and medical history; ECG

ADHD, attention deficit hyperactivity disorder; ECG, electrocardiogram; CBC, complete blood count; BUN, blood urea nitrogen.

drome). Pimozide (Orap) reduces vocal and motor tics effectively in both tic disorder and Gilles de la Tourette syndrome. Carbamazepine, an antiepileptic medicine, is effective in the treatment of mania and episodic dyscontrol syndrome. β-Blocking agents (nadolol [Corgard]) appear to decrease aggressiveness in the mentally retarded. Opiate antagonists significantly change some behaviors in autistic children and have promise in the treatment of self-injurious behavior in severely and profoundly mentally retarded individuals. Clomipramine (Anafranil) is efficacious in the treatment of obsessive-compulsive disorder. Seizures have been reported secondary to its use, however.

Some parents are adamantly opposed to the use of psychotropic medications. If drugs are used, it should be for as short a time as possible. As with any clinical disorder, the physician should avoid using multiple medications and should not shift back and forth from one medication to another when no immediate response occurs. Because psychotropic medications have significant biochemical effects on the developing child, it is important for the physician to give an appropriate explanation to the parents and child about the rationale for medication. The parents and child must have an opportunity to discuss their feelings and thoughts about psychotropic medication usage in general and the specific drug that is ordered. Even with thought disorders, in which pharmacotherapy has a firmly established place, medication is rarely, if ever, the sole treatment indicated. The complexity of emotional conditions demands an integrated approach involving various therapies: psychodynamic (individual, family, or group), behavioral, milieu, medication, and the use of resources in the family, school,

Stimulants (6 yr and older)		
Methylphenidate (Ritalin)	Attention deficit disorder	0.3-1.0 mg/kg/24 hr
Dextroamphetamine (Dexedrine)	Attention deficit disorder	0.2-0.5 mg/kg/24 hr
Pemoline (Cylert)	Attention deficit disorder	37.5-112.5 mg/24 hr

and community. These factors must be knowledgeably selected, judiciously coordinated, and skillfully applied to ensure that maximal benefit for the child results.

30.3 Psychotherapy

When it has been determined that psychopathology exists in a child or within a family that requires intervention, the pediatrician may develop and implement the therapeutic plan or may refer to a more specialized level of care within the community. The choice of treatment should be left to the consultant, with the referring physician reassuring the family and patient that close communication with the consultant will be maintained. The primary physician should continue to evaluate the child's progress throughout the treatment process and to provide medical care for the patient.

There are many types of individual psychotherapy. Most involve the development of an alliance with the patient that provides an opportunity to look at the problems precipitating therapy. Younger children often express their concerns and developmental issues in play therapy, a specific modality designed to foster symbolic and metaphoric individual expression. Older children and adolescents are more likely to participate in talking during therapy. *Dynamic therapy* is designed to understand the psychologic motivations for the child's problems and to develop a therapeutic process based on that understanding. *Behavior therapy* is used to modify specific behaviors through consistently applied positive and negative reinforcements.

There are several types of *family therapy*: directive, structural, strategic, and object-relations. In each, the therapist works primarily with the family to impart understanding or to help organize change. A particular directive approach, *parent management training,* is very useful in the treatment of conduct disorders. This approach involves training parents to respond in specific and consistent ways to the child's behavior.

Group therapy is especially useful for children suffering from poorly developed social skills. Group therapy for preadolescents tends to emphasize structured activities through which therapist and children alike can discover how they relate to each other and find ways to change. It is an especially profitable approach for treating the social problems of adolescents.

Barriers to involving the generalist or pediatrician in psychotherapeutic activities with children include a presumed lack of time and lack of adequate conceptual background. Although psychotherapy primarily emphasizes listening and interviewing, two skills important to all fields of medicine, experience is an important and necessary asset for the psychotherapist.

30.4 Psychiatric Hospitalization

At times psychiatric hospitalization of the disturbed or emotionally ill child in a general, pediatric, or psychiatric hospital is helpful or necessary, and it may serve a number of functions. In children with many psychosomatic disorders or in a suicidal or drugged adolescent, indications may be medical as well as psychiatric. If treatment of a child in a psychiatric hospital is thought necessary, consultation with a child psychiatrist is essential for decision making and planning. The indications for admission include thought, behavior, and affect that is so irrational that it will not respond to less restrictive therapy; complex psychiatric problems that require skilled medical and nursing care; extremely disturbed family interactions that contribute to problematic behavior or interfere with needed care; and dangerous behavior that cannot otherwise be managed. Admission to residential treatment reflects the family's decompensation as often as the child's.

Campbell M, Spencer EK: Psychopharmacology in child and adolescent psychiatry: a review of the past five years. J Am Acad Child Adolesc Psychiatry 27:269, 1988.

Dalton R: Psychiatry on the burn unit. *In:* Salisbury R, Dingeldein P, Newman N (eds): A Guide to Burn Unit Therapies. Boston, Little, Brown, 1984.

Dalton R, Forman MA: Psychiatry Hospitalization of School-Age Children. Washington, DC, American Psychiatric Press, 1992.

Gadow KD: Pediatric psychopharmacology: a review of recent research. J Child Psychol Psychiatry 33:153, 1992.

Krener P, Miller FB: Psychiatric response to HIV spectrum disease in children and adolescents. J Am Acad Child Adolesc Psychiatry 28:596, 1989.

Schowalter JE: Psychodynamics and medication. J Am Acad Child Adolesc Psychiatry 28:681, 1989.

Spinetta JJ: The dying child's awareness of death. Psychol Bull 81:256, 1974.

Van Dongen-Melman JEWM, Sanders-Woudstra JAR: The chronically ill child and his family. *In:* Solnit AJ, Cohen DJ, Schowalter J (eds): Child Psychiatry (Psychiatry, Vol 6). Philadelphia, JB Lippincott, 1986, pp 531–540.

Werry JS, Wollersheim JP: Behavior therapy with children and adolescents: a twenty-year overview. J Am Acad Child Adolesc Psychiatry 28:1, 1989.

CHAPTER 31

Neurodevelopmental Dysfunction in the School-Aged Child

Melvin D. Levine

Neurodevelopmental dysfunctions are central nervous system impairments that generate frustration and anxiety for school-aged children who are struggling to feel effective. These so-called low-severity handicaps of development are commonly associated with academic underachievement, behavioral difficulties, and problems with social adjustment. It is estimated that 5–15% of school children harbor these insidious handicaps. The prevalence may be higher if one includes discrete dysfunctions that lead to a transient self-limited disorder in learning a particular subject area. (Also see Chapter 27.)

ETIOLOGY. Diverse causes underlie these neurodevelopmental dysfunctions. Some reading and spelling disabilities have genetic causes. Many studies have uncovered etiologic associations between disorders of learning and/or attention and abnormal chromosome patterns, low-level lead intoxication, recurrent otitis media, meningitis, acquired immunodeficiency syndrome, intraventricular hemorrhage, serious head trauma, and low birthweight. Abnormalities of thyroid function have also been documented in a group of children with attentional dysfunction. Environmental and sociocultural deprivation have also been implicated as etiologic factors, or at least potentiators, of neurodevelopmental dysfunction. In individual cases, a definite cause usually cannot be ascertained.

CLINICAL MANIFESTATIONS. School-aged children with neurodevelopmental dysfunctions vary widely with regard to clinical symptoms. Their specific patterns of academic performance and behavior represent final common pathways, the convergence of multiple forces, including interacting cognitive strengths and deficits, environmental or cultural factors, temperament, educational experience, and intrinsic resiliency. Consequently, a memory dysfunction has different manifestations in a child with strong language skills, well-controlled attention, and a supportive home environment from those evident in an economically deprived youngster whose memory problems are accompanied by weaknesses of attention and difficulties with language. Eight areas of neurodevelopmental function are especially germane to understand an academically delayed child.

Attention. Attention subsumes a series of control mechanisms through which the central nervous system regulates behavior and learning. Children with attentional dysfunction show varying patterns of impairment of these controls. The resulting symptoms may affect learning, behavior, and/or social interactions. Located in different parts of the brain, these controls are responsible for regulating the following:

1. Central nervous system arousal, levels of alertness, and the mobilization and distribution of mental effort: Children with diminished alertness and arousal are likely to exhibit signs of mental fatigue in a classroom. They often yawn, stretch, fidget, and daydream. Sometimes they become overactive or hyperkinetic in an effort to attain a higher level of arousal. There may be difficulties falling asleep or awakening on time. They are apt to have difficulty sustaining their concentration and they may display a reduced ability to mobilize, allocate (to the appropriate functions), and maintain the mental effort required to initiate and complete many academic tasks. Efforts may be erratic and unpredictable. Those affected by this form of weak control may manifest extreme *performance inconsistency*.
2. The processing of incoming stimuli: These children show evidence of superficial concentration. As a result, directions and explanations may have to be repeated. Furthermore, the child is likely to show weaknesses of *selective attention*, often focusing on the wrong stimuli at home and in school. The resultant distractibility may take the form of listening to extraneous noises instead of a teacher, staring out the window, or constantly thinking about the future rather than current salient inputs. In addition, it takes inordinate incoming stimulation to enable many of these children to feel satisfied. They tend therefore to be restless, to feel bored easily, to require constant high levels of stimulation or excitement, and to want things all the time and not feel satisfied until they receive what they desire.
3. Output or the production of work, behavior, and social activity: There is a tendency for these children to perform without predicting an outcome or thinking through what they are about to do. The consequent *impulsivity* can lead to careless mistakes in academic work and unintended misbehavior. There may be hyperactivity. Such children have difficulty knowing how they are doing during and right after an academic endeavor or a behavior. As a result, they can get into trouble without realizing it. Finally, these children commonly are under-responsive to punishment and reward.

It is important to appreciate that most children with attentional dysfunction also harbor other forms of neurodevelopmental dysfunction. The latter can have a significant impact on the symptoms exhibited by the child. There is also considerable confusion and disagreement about the appropriate terminology to be applied to children with attentional difficulties. The *Diagnostic and Statistical Manual of Mental Disorders,* fourth edition, uses the term attention deficit disorder (ADD) and makes a distinction between individuals who have trouble with inattention and those who exhibit substantial hyperactivity and impulsivity. Over the years, such terms as attention deficit disorder, hyperactivity, hyperkinetic impulse disorder, and minimal brain dysfunction have been used. In part, the taxonomic flux stems from the marked heterogeneity of groups of affected children. The clinical symptoms summarized above are variably present and are of different degrees of severity from case to case. In addition, children with attention deficits show diverse patterns of developmental, academic, or behavioral difficulties. It is likely, therefore, that there are multiple subtypes of attention deficits (see Chapter 27).

Dysfunctions of Memory. As children proceed through school, there is a progressively increasing demand for the efficient use of memory. Students are expected to be selective, systematic, and strategic in entering new procedures and factual data in memory. They must become proficient in their use of both long- and short-term memory to retrieve stored rules, facts, concepts, and skills. By secondary school, rapid and precise recall is heavily stressed. Not surprisingly, some students experience tremendous frustration when memory dysfunctions prevent them from satisfying academic demands.

There are children who experience difficulty with the initial *registration of information in short-term memory.* They have trouble keeping pace with the data flow in a classroom. In some cases, children with attentional dysfunction have problems being selective and sufficiently alert to register salient information in memory. Other students have highly specific registration weaknesses. Some may have trouble with registering visuospatial data in memory, whereas others may be deficient in the registration of verbal material. Still others have a problem putting *linear chunks* of data in short-term memory; they can only enter small amounts of material that comes arranged in a linear configuration or sequence. Finally, some children can register data in short-term memory, but they cannot do so quickly enough to keep pace with classroom demands.

Many children experience problems with *active working memory.* They are ineffective at suspending information in memory temporarily while they are working on it. Normally active working memory enables a student to keep in mind all of the different components of a task, such as a mathematics problem, while completing it. A student with an active memory dysfunction, for example, might carry a number and then forget what it was that he or she intended to do after he or she had carried that number. Active working memory also enables children to remember the beginning of a paragraph when they arrive at the end of it. It lets them remember what they intend to express in writing while they are attempting to remember where to place a comma or how to spell a particular word. Thus, children with active working memory disorders can have trouble performing computations in mathematics, problems with writing, and difficulty in remembering and retelling what they have read.

There are other youngsters who experience frustration in their efforts at *consolidating information in long-term memory.* They are ineffective when filing data for later access. Ordinarily, consolidation in long-term memory is accomplished in one or more of four ways: (1) pairing two bits of information together (such as a group of letters and the English sound it represents), (2) classifying data in categories (e.g., filing all the insects together in memory), (3) linking new information to established rules (so-called rule-based learning), and (4) arranging knowledge in logical chains (such as the months of the year, the alphabet, the steps in a procedure, or the events in a story). Some students struggle unsuccessfully with specific kinds of paired association learning, categories, rules, or chains.

Some children can register and consolidate facts and procedures in memory but seem to have inordinate *difficulty recalling* these when they need them. Their recall may be painfully slow or imprecise. They are prone to encounter difficulty with *simultaneous recall,* the frequent need to retrieve several facts or procedures at once. This can be especially disabling when it comes to writing, a task requiring the simultaneous recall of spelling, punctuation, capitalization, letter formation, ideas, vocabulary, and the directions given for the assignment. Consequently, many children with simultaneous recall problems have their greatest difficulty with written output. When they try to write, they contend with a memory overload, often manifested in illegibility (due to a crowding out of memory for letter formation), poor use of punctuation and capitalization, deficient spelling in context, and surprisingly primitive ideation. Some of these children also do poorly in mathematics.

Finally, some students exhibit *delayed automatization*. Not enough of what they have learned in the past is accessible to them instantaneously and with no expenditure of effort. Such skills as letter formation, the mastery of mathematical facts, and word decoding must ultimately become automatic if students are to make good academic progress.

Language. Linguistically proficient children have a distinct advantage in school because much of what is taught is delivered in literate language. All of the basic academic skills are conveyed largely through language. Therefore, it is not surprising that children with language dysfunctions usually have troubled educational careers.

There are many forms of language disorder. Some children have particular problems with *phonology*. They experience unclear reception of English language sounds. They may have trouble discriminating between and forming associations with the sounds of their native language. Commonly, a weak phonologic sense has a negative effect on reading. A student with a poor appreciation of language sounds is likely to form unstable associative linkages between those sounds and visual symbols (i.e., letter combinations). They may also have problems manipulating language sounds in their minds. Consequently, while analyzing the last sound in a word, they may forget the first two and thus be unable to blend the sounds to form a word.

Semantic deficits are also common. Affected children have trouble learning and using new words. It is especially hard for them to develop a rich *semantic network*, a strong enough sense of how words relate to each other in their meanings. Other common language deficiencies include difficulty with syntax (word order), problems with discourse (paragraphs and passages), an underdeveloped sense of how language works (weak metalinguistics), and trouble with drawing appropriate inferences (i.e., supplying missing information) from language. As children with language dysfunctions progress through school, they are apt to encounter problems dealing with abstract and symbolic language, highly technical vocabulary, verbal concepts, and figures of speech (including metaphors and similes).

It is common to distinguish between *receptive language dysfunctions* (those affecting understanding) and *expressive language dysfunctions* (those impeding production or communication). Children with primarily receptive language problems may have serious difficulty following instructions in the classroom, understanding verbal explanations, and interpreting what they have read. Expressive weaknesses include oromotor problems affecting articulation and verbal fluency. In addition, some children display weaknesses of *word retrieval*; despite an adequate vocabulary, they have problems in finding exact words when they need them (as in a class discussion). Still others with expressive impediments have trouble formulating sentences, using grammar acceptably, and organizing spoken (and possibly written) narrative. Some children with expressive language problems are hesitant when they speak, so that their verbal communication is unduly laborious. They may become passive, taciturn, and nonelaborative in communication. Some studies have linked expressive language dysfunction to delinquent behavior. This is especially true when an expressive language disorder occurs in a context of environmental deprivation or turmoil.

Language dysfunctions may be subtle and diagnostically elusive. For example, some children with mild language difficulties function reasonably well in school until they are required to master a second language or become proficient with abstract verbal material.

Students with strong language function may make use of their linguistic facility to overcome other learning problems. For example, it may be possible to verbalize one's way through a mathematics curriculum, thereby overcoming a tendency to be confused by predominantly nonverbal concepts (such as ratio, equation, and diameter).

Visuospatial Ordering. Visual perceptual abilities entail the appreciation of spatial attributes. Shape, position, relative size, foreground and background relationships, and form constancy (the notion that a shape retains its identity regardless of its position in space) are among the constituents of visuospatial ordering. Children with visuospatial deficiencies may encounter some initial problems with letter and word recognition. Spelling may emerge as a weakness because these children commonly experience trouble recalling the precise visual configurations of words. In general, however, children who are confused about spatial attributes are unlikely to have longstanding or serious academic problems unless their visuospatial weaknesses are complicated by additional academically relevant neurodevelopmental dysfunctions. At one time, it was thought that visuospatial processing dysfunctions were a common cause of chronic reading disabilities; recent research for the most part has refuted this opinion.

Children with visuospatial dysfunctions may be late in discriminating between left and right. They may show signs of fine or gross motor clumsiness because they may be poor at making use of visuospatial data to program motor responses.

Temporal-Sequential Ordering. Awareness of time and sequence is an important neurodevelopmental function. Students in school need to be able to manage time, to process and produce multistep explanations and procedures, and to develop memory capacity for extended sequences. The latter includes the preservation of serial order in spelling, in narrative, and in various mathematical algorithms.

Children who have difficulties with temporal-sequential ordering may be delayed in learning to tell time. They may have great difficulty in following multistep commands, performing acts that necessitate a sequence of steps in the proper order, mastering the months of the year, or organizing narrative. Affected children may also have trouble in managing time. They may be frustrated in adhering to schedules, in learning the order of their classes in school, or in meeting deadlines.

Neuromotor Function. There are three distinct yet related forms of neuromotor ability relating to function in school: *graphomotor fluency, gross motor coordination,* and *fine motor dexterity.* Although these competencies ordinarily develop rapidly throughout childhood, some children experience considerable humiliation related to their insufficiently developed motor abilities.

Graphomotor fluency refers to the specific motor aspects of written output. Several subtypes of graphomotor dysfunction significantly impede the writing of certain children. Some of them exhibit signs of *finger agnosia*; they have trouble localizing their fingers while they write. As a result, they need to keep their eyes very close to the page. Ultimately, their writing becomes agonizingly slow and laborious. Others struggle with *graphomotor production deficits*. Such students have trouble planning the highly coordinated motor sequences needed for writing. Although they may understand and be able to visualize what it is they need to write, they have difficulty assigning writing roles to specific muscle groups in their hands. Some of these students also display oromotor production problems, resulting in speech articulation gaps. Some students harbor *weaknesses of visualization* during writing. They have trouble picturing the configurations of letters and words as they write. Their written output tends to be poorly legible, and their problems with visualization frequently also result in poor spelling. Commonly, these are students who much prefer printing (manuscript) to cursive writing. It is important to stress that a child may show excellent fine motor dexterity (as revealed in mechanical or artistic domains) but very poor graphomotor fluency (with labored or poorly legible writing).

Some children exhibit generalized gross motor delays, weaknesses, or highly specific deficits with or without fine motor or graphomotor problems. Examples of the latter include problems in using visuospatial information to guide their gross motor actions; affected children are inept at catching or throwing a ball because they cannot form accurate judgments about trajectories in space. Others are unable to satisfy the motor praxis demands of certain gross motor activities. It is hard for them to recall or plan complex motor procedures (such as those needed for dancing, gymnastics, and swimming). Still others demonstrate diminished *body position sense.* They do not receive or interpret feedback from peripheral joints and muscles. They are likely to be impaired when activities demand balance and the ongoing tracking of body movement.

Children with gross motor problems may suffer a significant loss of self-esteem. They may incur considerable embarrassment in physical education classes. Gross motor weaknesses can lead to social rejection, withdrawal, and generalized feelings of inadequacy.

Problems with fine motor dexterity can affect a child's ability to excel in artistic and crafts activities. They may also interfere with learning a musical instrument or mastering a computer keyboard. *Eye-hand incoordination* may be prominent because the child has trouble with the rapid and precise use of visual inputs to govern hand movements.

Higher-Order Cognition. This series of functions consists of various sophisticated thinking skills. Included are the formation of concepts, problem-solving skills, critical thinking, brainstorming (and creativity), and metacognition.

Children vary considerably in their capacities to *understand the conceptual bases of skills and content areas.* Some of them acquire only a *tenuous grasp of concepts.* As students progress through their education, concepts become increasingly abstract and complex. New concepts are likely to contain previously encountered concepts. Those youngsters who have chronically tenuous grasps of concepts often underachieve. Some of them have a pervasive weak grasp of concepts, whereas others have difficulty only with concepts in highly specific domains (e.g., mathematics, social studies, or science). There are some students who prefer to conceptualize verbally, whereas others are more comfortable in forming concepts without the interposition of language (perhaps using visual imagery). Many of the best students try to solidify concepts both linguistically and nonverbally.

Problem-solving skills are an important part of mathematics and virtually every other subject in school. Children with good problem-solving skills are good strategists. They are excellent at previewing or estimating answers, coming up with multiple alternative techniques to meet challenges, selecting the best techniques, and monitoring what they are doing so that they can deploy alternative strategies as needed. Poor problem solvers, on the other hand, tend to be rigid or impulsive. They do not come up with the best strategic approaches. Instead, they become committed irreversibly to a particular technique whether or not it works. They may then encounter significant difficulties in course work that requires methodical strategy deployment and flexible problem solving.

Brainstorming skills are needed to develop a topic for a report, to think about the best way to undertake a project, and to deal with a variety of other open-ended academic challenges. Some students cannot generate original ideas. They prefer to be told exactly what to do. They balk at having to devise a topic, deploy imagination, develop an argument, or think freely and independently.

Critical thinking skills represent another higher cognitive ability acquired during childhood. Successful students often display a keen ability to evaluate statements, products, and people using objective criteria. They are able to tease out their own personal biases and appreciate the viewpoints of others. They are effective in comparing and contrasting their own values and views with those of an author. They can think and talk about the qualities of a person. They become adept at assembling qualitative criteria to judge the products they see on television or in stores.

A child's *metacognitive abilities* refer to his or her capacity to think about thinking. Children with good metacognition are able to observe themselves thinking or studying. They can develop thereby an understanding of thought processes, enabling them to enhance their personal learning strategies and become more efficient and active learners. Those youngsters who lack metacognition tend to perform intellectual tasks the hard way. They are unlikely to appropriate effective techniques to study for a test, to write a report, or to meet other complex academic challenges.

Social Cognition. A student's social abilities are stringently tested throughout the school day and in the neighborhood after school. There is increasing evidence that social cognition exists as a discrete area of neurodevelopmental function. Some children are extremely adept in social abilities, whereas others exhibit debilitating social skill deficits. There are multiple subskills within social cognition. These include the ability to enter smoothly into new relationships, the capacity to time and stage interactions effectively, the appropriate degree of sensitivity to social feedback cues, the knowledge of how to resolve social conflict without aggression, the adaptive use of language in social contexts (*verbal pragmatics*), the ability to establish truly reciprocal (sharing) relationships with others (especially peers), and the inclination to overcome one's innate egocentricity to praise or nurture others. In addition to these skills, students need to be conscious of their own "image development" and to be adept at marketing themselves to peers. Regrettably, there are some children who have no idea of how adversely they are affecting others. As a result, they experience agonizing isolation with little or no insight into the reasons for their rejection.

The plight of a socially unskilled child can be tragic. He or she may sustain verbal abuse, bullying, and outright rejection, with various subtle forms of repudiation. Such students may seek refuge in the company of younger children, animals, a fantasy world, or adults. Social skill deficits can exert an enduring negative effect on behavioral adjustment, mental health, and, ultimately, success in a career.

Academic Effects. Neurodevelopmental dysfunctions are likely to occur in varying clusters within individual children. Combinations of dysfunctions commonly result in academic delays, frequently affecting the acquisition of basic skills and subskills in reading, spelling, writing, and mathematics.

Reading. Reading disabilities may stem from multiple neurodevelopmental factors. Most commonly, subtle or blatant language dysfunctions are present in children with significant reading delays. Initially, such children are likely to reveal *poor phonological awareness,* as seen in their difficulty appreciating and manipulating language sounds. They may then have debilitating problems in forming associations in memory between English language sounds and combinations of letters. This gap results in deficiencies at the level of decoding individual words. An affected child may be slow to acquire a *sight vocabulary* (a repertoire of words he or she can identify instantly). When decoding skills are delayed or overly laborious, reading comprehension is subsequently seriously compromised.

Students with visuospatial dysfunctions may also have trouble learning to read, but this is a relatively rare cause of reading difficulty. Children with weaknesses of temporal-sequential ordering or active working memory may experience difficulty in breaking down words into their component sounds (phonemes) and reblending them into correct sequences. Memory difficulties can cause problems with reading recall and summarization skill, with associative memory for sounds and symbols, and with the acquisition of vocabulary. Some youngsters with higher-order cognitive deficiencies experience trouble in understanding what they read because they lack a strong grasp of the concepts in a text.

Commonly, children with reading difficulties avoid reading. Thus, it is not unusual for a child whose reading is deficient to superimpose on this problem a lack of reading practice. Consequently, a delay in reading proficiency becomes increasingly pronounced over time.

Spelling. Impairments in spelling ability take various forms. Those with language disorders may have difficulty in applying a knowledge of phonology to spelling. They may overuse their visual (configurational) sense of words, so that their attempts at spelling are phonetically poor approximations yet visually comparable to the actual word (e.g., faght for fight). Other youngsters seem to have the opposite problem, trouble with revisualization or the recall of word configurations. When their phonologic abilities are adequate, their spelling efforts are often phonetically correct but visually far afield (e.g., fite for fight).

Children with certain memory disorders can spell words adequately during a spelling bee or on a spelling list, but they misspell the same words when writing a paragraph. They appear to have a memory problem that leads to difficulty in sustaining several different operations simultaneously. As a result, spelling becomes "eclipsed" by other task components.

Children who have difficulty preserving *linear chunks* of data tend to omit critical letters in the middle of words. Some students commit *mixed spelling errors,* many of which are orthographically illegal (i.e., they deploy letter combinations never found in English). Such children have the worst prognoses with regard to spelling proficiency.

Writing. Writing is an anathema to many youngsters with learning and attention problems. As children proceed through school, there are growing demands for large amounts of well-organized written output. In many cases, writing is laborious because of an underlying graphomotor dysfunction. In such instances, a child's graphomotor fluency does not keep pace with ideation and language production. Thoughts are literally forgotten or underdeveloped during writing because the mechanical effort is so taxing.

Just as students with simultaneous memory deficiencies experience difficulty with spelling in paragraphs, they are also prone to serious problems with writing in general. Their written output is often inconsistent in its legibility, ideation, and use of rules (of punctuation, capitalization, and grammar). Children with sequential ordering problems may have difficulty in organizing their ideas effectively when they write. Those with language disabilities may not be able to use language effectively on paper. Students with active working memory dysfunctions have difficulty getting the ideas in a paragraph to cohere because they keep forgetting what they wish to express. Finally, students with attentional dysfunction may find it hard to mobilize and sustain the mental effort, the pacing, and the self-monitoring demands of writing. In fact, writing difficulties are the most frequently encountered academic problems among children with weak attention controls.

Mathematics. Delays in mathematical ability can be especially refractory to correction. In one school-based study, it was found that no student who was delayed more than 6 mo in mathematics in 6th grade ever caught up. Thus, significant mathematical weaknesses can become virtually insurmountable, as the subject is so highly cumulative in its structure. Various forms of mathematical disability plague students.

- Some children experience mathematics failure because of discrete higher-order cognitive weaknesses. They cannot grasp arithmetical concepts. Good mathematicians are able to deploy both verbal and nonverbal conceptual abilities to understand such concepts as fractions, percentages, equations, and proportion. Impaired student mathematicians may have serious difficulty in moving back and forth from abstract to concrete thinking. It may also be hard for them to apply concepts effectively or be systematic in solving word problems or when confronted with practical situations.
- There are youngsters who show circumscribed memory weaknesses that compromise mathematical ability. Some have trouble in automatizing mathematical facts (such as the multiplication tables). Others have difficulty in recalling appropriate procedural sequences or *algorithms* (such as the steps involved in solving a long division problem). Still others have weak active working memory, so that, when they focus on one portion of a mathematical problem, they are likely to forget other components of the same problem.
- Some students with language dysfunctions have difficulty in mathematics because they have trouble understanding their teachers' verbal explanations of quantitative concepts and operations. Such students are likely to experience frustration in solving word problems and in processing the vast network of technical vocabulary in this subject area.
- Many students with attention deficits falter in mathematics classes because they are poor at focusing on fine detail (such as operational signs). Consequently, they commit frequent careless errors.
- Mathematics involves a degree of visualization. Children who have difficulty forming and recalling visual imagery to enhance learning may be at a disadvantage in acquiring mathematical skills. It may be hard, for example, for them to picture geometric shapes or to think about fractions.

It is not unusual for individuals with mathematical disabilities to develop superimposed mathematical phobias. Anxiety over mathematics can be especially disheartening and can aggravate an underlying skill delay.

Content Area Subjects. Children with neurodevelopmental dysfunctions may experience difficulty in a wide range of academic content areas. The sciences may be a special problem, especially because they necessitate the processing of dense verbal material in textbooks and the rapid convergent recall of facts. Social studies courses often entail use of sophisticated language and a mastery of verbal abstract concepts (e.g., democracy, liberalism, and taxation with representation). Students with higher cognitive weaknesses may not grasp such concepts.

Foreign language learning can be a serious problem for students with language disorders or memory gaps. Some adolescents require foreign language waivers to graduate from high school and enter college.

Many students with attention deficits can succeed only in content areas that they find romantically attractive. They are likely to exhibit poor performance in courses that contain a great deal of not very exciting detail. They may have trouble distinguishing important data from trivia in a text because their selective attention is too diffuse.

Some students harbor incapacitating *organizational problems* that adversely affect performance in content area subjects. They often lack effective learning strategies. Some are too impulsive to make use of techniques to facilitate studying and work output. Others struggle because they are unable to maintain a systematized notebook, keep track of assignments, get to places on time, meet deadlines, find things, organize a locker, and remember what books to take home from school. Many disorganized students also have trouble studying for tests. They do not seem to know how and what to study and for how long. They frequently lack self-testing skills.

Nonacademic Impacts. Neurodevelopmental dysfunctions commonly exert impacts that extend far beyond school. Some nonacademic impacts are closely related to the dysfunctions themselves, whereas other sequelae are secondary to persistent failure and frustration. The impulsivity and lack of effective self-monitoring of children with attention deficits may lead to unacceptable actions that were unintentional. A child affected by attentional dysfunction may be aggressive or disruptive in the classroom and at home. He or she may have serious difficulty in accepting behavioral limits, assuming responsibilities, and delaying gratification. Insatiability may lead to highly provocative behaviors, as he or she perpetually seeks intense experience (be it ever so negative). These negative behaviors often subvert the function of an entire family. Adolescents with attentional dysfunction have also been shown to be predisposed to serious automobile accidents.

In some cases, children with neurodevelopmental dysfunctions have excessive performance anxiety or clinical depression. Sadness, self-deprecatory comments, declining self-esteem, chronic fatigue, loss of interests, and even suicidal ideation may ensue. Some children lose motivation. They tend to give up and exhibit *learned helplessness*, a sense that they have no personal control over their destinies. Therefore, they feel no need to exert effort. This perspective ultimately can promote depression, pessimism, and a loss of ambition.

DIAGNOSIS (ASSESSMENT). A child who is functioning poorly during the school years requires a careful multidisciplinary evaluation because of the diverse sources and broad effects of underachievement. An optimal evaluation team should consist of a pediatrician, a psychologist or psychiatrist, and a psychoeducational specialist. The latter is a clinician (usually a special educator or educational psychologist) who can undertake a detailed analysis of academic skills and subskills. Other professionals should become involved, as needed, in individual cases, such as a speech and language pathologist, an occupational therapist, a neurologist, and a social worker.

Many children undergo evaluations in school. Such assessments are guaranteed in the United States under Public Law 94-142. In addition, children found to have attentional dysfunction may qualify for educational accommodations under Section 501 of the Individuals with Disabilities Education Act.

Multidisciplinary evaluations conducted in schools are usually very helpful, but they are susceptible to biases and conflicts of interest. For example, if a school does not have a language therapist, that school's evaluation team might tend to be reluctant to recommend language therapy. School budgeting constraints may also affect the quality of evaluations and the extent of recommended services. Because of such limitations, there has been a growing demand for independent evaluations and for second opinions outside of the school setting. Many pediatricians become involved in such outside assessments.

The evaluation of a child with suspected neurodevelopmental dysfunctions should include complete physical, neurologic, and sensory examinations. A physician may also perform an extended neurologic and developmental assessment. Available pediatric neurodevelopmental examination instruments that facilitate direct sampling of various neurodevelopmental functions, such as attention, memory, and so on, include the Pediatric Examination at Three (PEET), the Pediatric Examination of Educational Readiness (PEER), the Pediatric Early Elementary Examination (PEEX II), and the Pediatric Examination of Educational Readiness at Middle Childhood (PEERAMID II). Examinations of this type also include direct behavioral observations and assessment of minor neurologic indicators (sometimes called "soft signs"). The latter include various associated movements and other phenomena frequently associated with neurodevelopmental dysfunction (see also Chapter 541).

The pediatrician can be helpful in gathering and organizing data relating to a child with neurodevelopmental dysfunctions. He or she can obtain such data through the use of questionnaires completed by the parents, the school, and (if old enough) the child. These questionnaires can provide up-to-date information about behavioral adjustment, patterns of academic performance, and traits associated with specific developmental dysfunctions. In addition, questionnaires can elicit relevant data concerning the child's health history, family background, and demographic variables relevant to a child's learning difficulty. The ANSER System Questionnaires have been developed for this purpose. There also exist standardized behavioral checklists that can aid in evaluation. Among these are the Yale Child Behavioral Inventory, the Connors Questionnaire (for hyperactivity), and the Achenbach Child Behavioral Checklist.

Commonly, an evaluation includes *intelligence testing*. Although an overall intelligence quotient (IQ) is seldom helpful, it can be useful in relating specific subtest scores to other diagnostic data. Such comparisons can uncover revealing patterns suggestive of specific neurodevelopmental dysfunctions.

Psychoeducational tests yield relevant data, especially when such assessments include careful analyses that pinpoint where breakdowns are occurring in the processes of reading, spelling, writing, and mathematics. The psychoeducational specialist, making use of input from multiple sources, can help the pediatrician formulate specific recommendations for regular and special educational teachers.

A mental health specialist can be valuable in identifying family-based issues that may be complicating or aggravating neurodevelopmental dysfunctions. Specific psychiatric disorders also may be a part of the clinical picture.

TREATMENT. The management of children with neurodevelopmental dysfunctions often also needs to be multidisciplinary. Most children require several of the following forms of intervention.

Demystification. Many children with neurodevelopmental dysfunctions have little or no understanding of the nature or sources of their difficulties. Once an appropriate descriptive assessment has been performed, it is especially important to explain to the child the nature of the dysfunction and his or her strengths. This explanation should be provided in nontechnical, optimistic, and nonaccusatory language. The Concentration Cockpit is an example of a device that can be used to help children understand attentional dysfunction.

Bypass Strategies. Numerous techniques can enable a child to circumvent neurodevelopmental dysfunctions. Ordinarily, such bypass strategies are used in the regular classroom; individual forms of intervention in other settings are aimed at strengthening deficient functions. Examples of bypass strategies include using a calculator while solving mathematical problems, writing essays with a word processor, presenting oral instead of written reports, solving fewer mathematical problems, seating a child with attention deficits closer to the teacher to minimize distraction, offering visually presented demonstration models of correctly solved mathematical problems, and granting permission for a student to take scholastic aptitude tests untimed. These bypass strategies do not "cure" neurodevelopmental dysfunctions but minimize their academic and nonacademic impacts.

Remediation of Skills. Tutorial programs are commonly used to bolster deficient academic skills. Reading specialists, mathematical tutors, and other such professionals can make use of diagnostic data to select techniques that make use of a student's neurodevelopmental strengths in an effort to improve decoding skills, writing ability, or mathematical computation. Remediation need not focus exclusively on specific academic areas. Many students need assistance in acquiring study skills, cognitive strategies, and productive organizational habits.

Remediation may take place in a resource room or learning center at school. To qualify for these services in school, students may need to be labeled or classified as "learning disabled." To be so designated, testing must document a substantial discrepancy between the child's IQ and his or her academic skill. Unfortunately, some needy students with significant neurodevelopmental dysfunctions do not display such a discrepancy. They commonly "fall between the cracks" and so may require tutoring outside of school.

Increasingly, students with neurodevelopmental dysfunctions are being served within regular classrooms. This approach, known as the *inclusionary model,* places an emphasis on bypass strategies and other accommodations rather than resource rooms or other "pullout" services in schools. The success of inclusionary models is highly dependent on the training and orientation of regular classroom teachers.

Developmental Therapies. Considerable controversy exists about the efficacy of treatments to enhance weak developmental functions. It has not been demonstrated convincingly that it is possible to improve substantially a child's fine motor skills, memory, problem-solving proficiency, or temporal-sequential ordering abilities. Nevertheless, some forms of developmental therapy are widely accepted. *Speech and language pathologists* commonly offer intervention for youngsters with various forms of language disability. *Occupational therapists* strive to improve the motor skills of certain students with writing problems or gross motor clumsiness. Recently, there has been considerable interest in *social skills training* that usually takes the form of small group sessions in which school children are helped to become more aware of the dynamics of social interaction. *Cognitive-behavioral therapy* is another recently introduced intervention. In this modality of treatment, children learn about their neurodevelopmental dysfunctions and are given specific exercises aimed at enhancing the weak areas. For example, a child with attentional dysfunction may be taught about his or her impulsivity and then provided with exercises that encourage reflection, planning, and a less frenetic tempo.

Curriculum Modifications. Many children with neurodevelopmental dysfunctions require alterations in the school curriculum to succeed. This is particularly true as students progress through secondary school. For example, students with memory weaknesses may need to have their courses selected for them so that they do not have an inordinate cumulative memory load in any one semester. The timing of a foreign language, the selection of a mathematical curriculum, and the choice of science courses are critical issues for many of these struggling adolescents.

Strengthening of Strengths. These children need to have their affinities, potentials, and talents identified clearly and exploited widely. It is as important to strengthen strengths as it is to attempt to remedy deficiencies. Athletic skills, artistic inclinations, creative talents, and mechanical aptitudes are among the potential assets of certain students who are underachieving academically. Parents and school personnel need to create opportunities for such students to build on these proclivities and to achieve respect and praise for their efforts. The strengthening of strengths is essential for sustaining self-esteem and motivation. Ultimately, these well-developed personal assets can have implications for transitions into young adulthood, including career and/or college selection.

Individual and Family Counseling. When learning difficulties are complicated by family problems or identifiable psychiatric disorders, psychotherapy may be indicated. Clinical psychologists or child psychiatrists may offer long- or short-term therapy. Such intervention may involve the child alone or the entire family. It is essential, however, that the therapist have a firm understanding of the nature of a child's neurodevelopmental dysfunctions. Both parents and child can become confused if a psychotherapist attributes a child's learning difficulties exclusively to environmental factors, thus ignoring the potent influence of an underlying language disability, attention deficit, or memory problem. Most families do not require a heavily psychoanalytic or psychodynamic approach but instead can benefit from a counseling program that offers them practical advice on behavioral management. Increasingly, there is a recognition of the role of short-term problem-oriented counseling (see Chapter 30).

Advocacy. Children with neurodevelopmental dysfunctions require informed advocacy. They need to have their rights upheld in school and in the community. A physician can be especially helpful in advocating for a child in school. Some children, for example, are devastated by being held back in a grade, and the likelihood of benefit is minimal. A physician may need to represent the rights of the child in opposing such grade retention and other sources of public humiliation. A physician may also need to argue strongly for a child to receive services in school or to benefit from modifications in the curriculum. Physicians can also perform advocacy by becoming vocal citizens of their communities. In serving on a school board, for example, a physician can exert a major influence on local policy and on the allocation of resources to school children with special educational needs. Physicians can also be helpful in offering to conduct inservice educational programs for teachers.

Medication. Certain psychopharmacologic agents may be especially helpful in lessening the toll of neurodevelopmental dysfunctions. Most commonly, stimulant medications are used in the management of children with attention deficits. They are never a panacea because most youngsters with attention deficits have other associated dysfunctions (such as language disorders, memory problems, motor weaknesses, or social skill deficits). Nevertheless, medications such as methylphenidate (Ritalin), dextroamphetamine (Dexedrine), and pemoline (Cylert), can be important adjuncts to treatment because they seem to help some youngsters focus more selectively and control their impulsivity. Stimulant medication, its indications, administration, and complications are described in Chapter 30. When depression or excessive anxiety is a significant component of the clinical picture, antidepressants may be helpful (see Chapter 30). Other drugs may improve behavioral control (see Chapter 30). Children receiving medication need regular follow-up visits that include a review of current behavioral checklists, a physical examination, and appropriate modifications of medication dose, including intervals when they are off the drug so that they can strive to be in control of themselves.

Longitudinal Case Management. All children with neurodevelopmental dysfunctions can benefit from the support and guidance of a case manager, a professional who can offer advice in a continuing manner and be available to monitor function over the years. The pediatrician may be an ideal professional to assume this responsibility. With time, new questions inevitably emerge as a child's neurodevelopmental dysfunctions evolve and academic expectations undergo progressive changes. Because children with neurodevelopmental dysfunctions represent an extremely heterogeneous group, no two children require the same management plan, nor is it possible to predict with certainty at age 7 the needs of a youngster when he or she is 14 yr of age. Consequently, affected children and their families require vigilant follow-up and individualized objective advice throughout their academic careers.

Barkley RA, Guevremont DC, Anastopoulos AD, et al: Driving-related risks and outcomes of attention deficit hyperactivity disorder in adolescents and young adults: A 3- to 5-year follow-up survey. Pediatrics 92:212, 1993.

Gerber A: Language-Related Learning Disabilities. Baltimore, Paul H. Brookes, 1993.

Hauser P, Zametkin AJ, Martinez P, et al: Attention deficit–hyperactivity disorder in people with generalized resistance to thyroid hormone. N Engl J Med 328:997, 1993.

Levine MD: Developmental Variation and Learning Disorders. Cambridge, MA, Educators Publishing Service, 1987.

Levine MD: Keeping a Head in School: A Student's Book About Learning Abilities and Learning Disorders. Cambridge, MA, Educators Publishing Service, 1990.

Levine MD: Attention and memory: Progression and variation during the elementary school years. Pediatr Ann 18:366, 1989.

Levine MD: All Kinds of Minds: A Young Student's Book About Learning Abilities and Learning Disorders. Cambridge, MA, Educators Publishing Service, 1993.

Levine MD: Educational Care. Cambridge, MA, Educators Publishing Service, 1994.

Levine MD: The Pediatric Assessment System for Learning Disorders. (Questionnaires and Neurodevelopmental Examinations.) Cambridge, MA, Educators Publishing Service, 1982.

Lyon R (ed): Frames of Reference for the Assessment of Learning Disability. Baltimore, Paul H. Brookes, 1994.

Lyon R, Gray DB, Kavanaugh JF (eds): Better Understanding Learning Disabilities. Baltimore, Paul H. Brookes, 1993.

Part IV

Social Issues

Chapter 32

Adoption

Marc A. Forman and Richard Dalton

Most adopted children and their families handle this issue with considerable common sense and sensitivity, but some problems of adoption require comment.

Adoptions are accomplished through licensed public or private agencies or independent adoption intermediaries (lawyers, physicians, and other nonagency adoption services). The former have become primarily involved with older or special needs children, who have been neglected or abused; two thirds of newborn adoptions are handled independently. Both agency and independent adoption should include objective counseling of birth parents, professional assessment of prospective adoptive parents, preplacement home evaluation, and postplacement social and legal services. Adoptive placement should be made as soon after birth as possible in order to foster attachment and bonding between infant and adoptive parents. Adoptions of older children, or across religious and ethnic lines, or by single parents are, in appropriate instances, reasonable alternatives to having adoptable children languish in institutions or temporary foster homes, but adoptions of older children present some increased risks. For example, a family seeking to adopt a 4- to 5-yr-old child with a history of severe emotional deprivation and multiple foster home placements may find that the child has been severely traumatized and will later display major psychologic disturbances, even in the best of adoptive homes. Genetic risks and early biologic factors related to pregnancy and perinatal events may have further compounded the disadvantages for such a child. However, most late-adopted children have a relatively good outcome if placed in a nurturing family environment.

Adopted children should be told of their adoption as soon as they have achieved reasonably good verbal facility and comprehension, by the age of 3 or at the latest 4 yr. The explanation can be repeated when circumstances are appropriate, such as during a family discussion about the birth of a neighbor's baby, but should not become ritual. Children's books on adoption can be read to young children; later they can read them themselves.

Controversy continues about whether adopted children are at increased risk for development of emotional problems. Although psychologic, behavioral, and adjustment problems do occur, there is a remarkable degree of consistency in favorable outcome in such widely differing types of adoption as special needs, international, transracial, and transethnic. Adoption need not be perceived by the child as a threat to self-esteem, but in the case of individual and family problems, the child's adoptive status may reinforce otherwise existing doubts about his or her competence and worth. Not infrequently, a natural child is born following an adoption to previously "infertile" parents. For the adopted child, the event may initiate a competitive struggle requiring both understanding and firmness on the part of the parents.

Occasionally, foster parents wish to adopt a child who has been in their care for a number of years but has not been legally relinquished by the natural parents. Historically, the courts have upheld the claim of biologic parents for the child, even in those instances in which the natural parents abandoned the child and the foster parents had been essentially the child's only long-standing, nurturant, and consistent (psychologic) parents. Recent decisions, however, show the courts' growing appreciation of the child's need for continuity of care, although considerable variation exists from state to state in these rulings.

In some states, adopted persons who have attained their majority are entitled to have access to their adoption records and to information about their biologic parents. On the whole, this is a commendable development; this right to know must be weighed, however, against the rights of biologic parents to privacy if they desire it. Increasingly infants are adopted under circumstances in which adoptive parents meet, exchange identifying information, and commonly agree on some degree of continuing contact and communication with the birth parents.

Brodzinsky D, Schechter MD (eds): The Psychology of Adoption. New York, Oxford University Press, 1990.

Hersov L: The seventh Jack Tizard memorial lecture: Aspects of adoption. J Child Psychol Psychiatry 31:483, 1989.

Schulman I (ed): Adoption. The Future of Children Vol. 3(1), 1993.

Chapter 33

Foster Care

Dorothy Bolding and Marc A. Forman

Placement in foster care is typically provided by local welfare authorities for abandoned, severally neglected, or abused children. For many children, foster care offers a life-saving environment that gives them the opportunity to be physically safe and replenished, to grow, and to develop innate potential. For others, however, foster care represents yet another episode in a lifelong history of deprivation. (See also Chapter 42.)

The number of children in foster care in June 1992 was 429,000, a 3% increase from the previous June but a 68% increase from June 1982. Some of this increase was due to placement with relatives, where children tend to stay longer than in placement with nonrelatives. In recent years, the infants of many substance-abusing women have been placed in foster care. It has been estimated that 80–125,000 children will have lost their mothers to acquired immunodeficiency syndrome by the year 2000, and a number of these children will need to be accommodated in the foster care system. In addition, children with serious developmental problems and major emotional disturbances are disproportionately represented in all forms of out-of-home care, including foster care.

Unfortunately, the United States does not have a comprehensive and well-supervised system of foster care. Understaffed and underbudgeted departments of public welfare are often unable adequately to prepare, supervise, and support foster parents who may have to deal with difficult, traumatized children. Children may be transferred from one foster home to another because foster parents move, the child doesn't "adjust," or unsupervised foster parents are deemed to be inadequate. Some children move in and out of placement according to the desires of natural parents who can neither care for them or let them be permanently placed in the care of others.

Only recently have trends in state and federal legislation emphasized "permanency planning," using adoptive placement or permanent foster care. This involves earlier termination of the rights of parents who are unwilling or unable to care for their own children. The United States lags far behind other developed countries in providing economic and social support to all families of young children and thus reducing the number of children going into foster care. Until the needs of children receive high priority in social planning and legislation, children in foster care will continue to be vulnerable to disturbance in personality development, serious retardation in reading, apathetic states, and defects in socialization.

Children's Defense Fund: The State of America's Children, Yearbook 1994. Washington, DC, Children's Defense Fund, 1994.

Eisenberg L: The sins of the fathers: Urban decay and social pathology. Am J Orthopsychiatry 32:5, 1962.

Kemmerman S, Kahn A: Child Care, Parental Leave, and the Under 3's: Policy Innovations in Europe. New York, Auburn House, 1991.

CHAPTER 34

Effects of a Mobile Society

Richard Dalton and Nuria Sabaté

A significant proportion of the population of the United States changes residence each year. The effects of this movement on children and families are frequently overlooked. For children, the move is essentially involuntary; they move because a parent has obtained employment elsewhere, because the birth of a sibling has made a larger home desirable, or for other reasons. When such changes in family structure as divorce or death precipitate moves, children face the stresses created by both the precipitating events and moving itself. When parents are sad because of the circumstances surrounding the move, this unhappiness will be transmitted to their children. Children who move lose their old friends, the comfort of a familiar bedroom and house, and their ties to school and community. Not only must they sever old relationships, they are also faced with developing new ones in new neighborhoods and new schools. Because movement upward in social standing often accompanies a geographic move, children may enter neighborhoods with new and different customs and values, and since academic standards and curricula vary from community to community, children who have performed well in one school may find themselves struggling in a new one. Frequent moves during the school years are likely to have adverse consequences on social and academic performance.

Migrant children and families present as a special population (See Chapter 42). Migrant children not only need to adjust to a new community, school, and house, they also need to adjust to a new culture, and, in many cases, to a new language. Because children have faster language acquisition, they may function as translators for the adults in their families. This powerful position may lead to role reversal and potential conflict within the family. There is controversy in the current literature as to whether or not migrant status per se poses a higher risk to the development of psychopathologic conditions in children. However, there is agreement that migrant children are more likely to come from low socioeconomic status families, live in overcrowded conditions, and have poorly educated parents. All of this, plus the above-mentioned factors, can increase the risk for psychopathologic disorders. In the evaluation of migrant children and families, it is also important to ask about the circumstances of the migration; legal status; conflict of loyalties; and moral, ethical, and religious differences.

Parents should prepare children well in advance of any move and allow them to express any unhappy feelings or misgivings. Parents should acknowledge their own mixed feelings and agree that they will miss their old home while looking forward to a new one. Visits to the new home in advance are often useful preludes to the actual move. Transient periods of regressive behavior may be noted in preschool children after moving, and these should be understood and accepted. Parents should assist the entry of their children into the new community, and exchanges of letters with old friends and visits, whenever possible, should be encouraged.

Jensen PS, Lewis RL, Xenakis SN: The military family in review: Context, risk and prevention. J Am Acad Child Adolesc Psychiatry 25:225, 1986.

Monroe-Blum H, Boyle M, Offord D, Kates N: Immigrant children: Psychiatric disorder, school performance and service utilization. Am J Orthopsychiatry 59:510, 1989.

Puskar KR, Dvorsak KG: Relocation stress in adolescents: Helping teenagers cope with a moving dilemma. Pediatr Nursing 17:295, 1991.

Vernberg EM: Experiences with peers following relocation during early adolescence. Am J Orthopsychiatry 60:466, 1990.

Westermeyer J: Psychiatric Care of Migrants: A Clinical Guide. Washington, DC, American Psychiatric Press, 1989.

CHAPTER 35

Child Care

Paul H. Dworkin

Profound social and demographic changes have resulted in an increasing number of children receiving a portion of their care from someone other than their parents. In the United States, most mothers of children older than age 1 yr are in the labor force, with most employed mothers working full time. A high divorce rate and rise in births to single women have contributed to approximately one child in four living within a single-parent household headed by the mother. Women work for the same reasons as men—economic necessity and personal choice. The economic climate and changes in family structure have necessitated the availability of child care services for working parents.

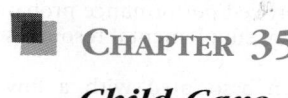

"Child care" is defined as care provided by an individual outside the nuclear family or in a setting separate from the child's home and is inclusive of such services as "babysitting," "day care," "preschool," "early childhood program," and "nursery school." Options for families generally include in-home care, family child care, and center child care. It is used for children of all ages. Less than 5% of children of working parents receive in-home care, in which a relative or nonrelative (such as a nanny, housekeeper, or regular sitter) comes to the child's home to provide care. Approximately 20% of all preschool children who receive supplemental care are in regulated or nonregulated family child care, in which a small group of children, typically six or fewer, receive care in the private home of a caregiver. Nearly one half of employed mothers of 3- and 4-yr-old children report center care as their primary supplemental arrangement. Child care centers provide care for more than 6–10 children at a time and include for-profit centers, which may be independent or operated by large chains, and nonprofit centers, which may be independent or sponsored by the government (e.g., Head Start), religious organizations, public schools, community agencies, or employers. Child care centers are licensed, although standards vary from state to state. Different types of child care have advantages and disadvantages, including cost, familiarity of care provider and environment, convenience, availability, flexibility in scheduling, and reliability. From a developmental perspective, the progression from care in the child's own home to care in another home with a few other children to large-group care may be appropriate. Yet for most families, decisions about child care are based largely on considerations of cost and distance from home.

The effect of child care on children's development depends on a number of interrelated factors, including characteristics of the child, the care setting, and the family. Although some studies have suggested that infants in child care may be at greater risk of insecure attachments to their mothers, most such infants are securely attached and display no long-term emotional insecurity. Children with child care experience have been found to be more sociable, more self-confident, more involved in activities with peers, and less timid. However, such children have also been described as more aggressive (especially boys) and less compliant with adults.

High-quality child care can favorably influence the intellectual development of children, especially those from disadvantaged populations. Such children perform better on school entry on standardized tests of intelligence, academic achievement, and measures of accomplishment such as grades and teacher ratings. Sustaining such improved performance probably requires the continued provision of supplemental resources throughout the school years.

Good quality child care has been associated with a low adult-to-child ratio, small group size, and caregiver training in child development. Other important determinants include staff stability and consistency; a developmentally appropriate curriculum; and a physical setting that affords protection from environmental hazards, cleanliness, sanitation, and adequate space for activities and rest. The lack of national standards for child care and uneven regulation from state to state contribute to the variable quality of child care in the United States. The American Academy of Pediatrics and the American Public Health Association have recently published standards for health and safety in child care programs. See Chapter 250 for discussion of communicable diseases and child care. Some believe that efforts to upgrade the quality of child care should also include the establishment of federal standards that address such characteristics as staff-to-child ratios, group size, and caregiver training and improved salaries for child care providers. Additional critical policy issues include parental leave, tax credits for child care (currently available), flexible work time, and on-site child care provided by employers.

Pediatric providers may assume a number of important roles in promoting successful child care experiences. Pediatricians can help parents become informed consumers by discussing the advantages and disadvantages of various child care options, providing accurate information regarding implications for children's health and development, and directing parents to sources of information about child care in the community. The pediatrician can provide guidance to parents regarding a sick child's participation in child care and serve as health consultant to child care programs. Pediatric advocacy for the availability of high-quality care for all children includes encouraging the implementation of national child care standards, paid parental infant care leaves, and improved salaries and training for child care providers.

American Academy of Pediatrics and American Public Health Association: Caring for Our Children. National Health and Safety Performance Standards: Guidelines for Out-of-Home Child Care Programs. Elk Grove Village, IL, American Academy of Pediatrics, 1993.

Aronson SS: Child care and the pediatrician. Pediatr Rev 10:277, 1989.

Dilks SA: Developmental aspects of child care. Pediatr Clin North Am 38:1529, 1991.

Willer B, Hafferth SL, Kisker EE, et al: The Demand and Supply of Child Care in 1990. Washington, DC, National Association for the Education of Young Children, 1991.

Zigler E, Hall NW: Day care and its effect on children: An overview for pediatric health professionals. J Dev Behav Pediatr 9:38, 1988.

CHAPTER 36

Separation and Death

Marc A. Forman and Richard Dalton

Relatively brief separations of children from their parents, such as vacations, usually produce minor transient effects, but more enduring and frequent separations may cause significant sequelae. The potential impact of each event must be considered in the light of the age and stage of development of the child and the particular relationship with the absent person as well as the nature of the separation. For example, it is more frightening for children to be separated from a parent in a hospital than within the familiar surroundings of home. In a marital separation, the child is faced with a relative loss of one parent who may be vilified by the other.

In young children, the initial reaction to separation may involve crying, either of a tantrum-like, protesting type or of a quieter, sadder type. After a few hours or a day or so of separation, the child may appear more subdued, withdrawn, and quiet or irritable, fussy, moody, and resistant to authority. Disturbance of appetite may occur, and there may be special difficulties at bedtime, such as reluctance in going to bed and problems in getting to sleep, with a resurgence of old fears, and, in younger children, perhaps such regressive behavior as bedwetting. Children may repeatedly ask where the absent parent is and when he or she will return home; some children may not refer to parental absence at all. The child may go to the window or door or out into the neighborhood looking for the absent parent; a few may even leave home or their places of temporary placement to try to find where their parents are. This last rather unusual response needs to be considered when a child cannot be found for a while shortly after the separation or departure of a parent.

The child's response to reunion may surprise or alarm the parent who is not prepared. The parent who joyfully returns to the family may be met by wary or cautious children, who, after a brief interchange of affection, may move away from the parent and seem indifferent to his or her return. The interpretation of this response will depend on the child and his or her style; it may indicate anger at being left and wariness that the event will happen again, or, because children tend to personalize, the child may have felt that he or she caused the parent's departure. For instance, if the mother who frequently says, "Stop it, or you'll give me a headache," is hospitalized, the child may unrealistically feel at fault and guilty. As a result of these feelings, children may seem to be more closely attached to the other parent than to the absent one, or even to the grandparent or babysitter who cared for them during their parent's absence. Immediately after the reunion or after a few days, some children, particularly younger ones, may become more clinging and dependent than they were prior to separation, while continuing any regressive behavior that had occurred during separation. Such behavior may engage the returned parent more closely and help to re-establish the bond that the child felt was broken. Usually such reactions are transient; within 1–2 wk, the child will have recovered his or her usual behavior and equilibrium. Recurrent separations may tend to make the child more wary and guarded about re-establishing the relationship with the repeatedly absent parent, and these traits may affect other personal relationships. Parents should not try to ameliorate a child's behavior by threatening to leave.

Experiences of loss such as divorce or placement in foster care can give rise to the same kinds of reactions listed earlier, but they are more intense and possibly more lasting. School-aged children may respond with evident depression, seem indifferent, or be markedly angry. Other children appear to deny or avoid the issue, behaviorally or verbally. Most children may cling to the hope or fantasy that the actual placement or separation is not real. Guilt may be generated by the child's feeling that this loss, separation, or placement represents rejection and perhaps punishment for misbehavior. The child may protect the parents at his or her own expense, believing and asserting that one's own badness caused the parent to depart or to place him or her with relatives or strangers rather than that the parent has been bad or irresponsible. Besides having their own feelings of guilt, children cannot blame their parents because they sense it may be fairly risky. The parent who discovers that the child harbors resentment might punish further for these thoughts or feelings. Children who feel that their misbehavior caused their parents to separate or become divorced have the fantasy that their own trivial or recurrent behavioral patterns have caused their parents to become angry with each other. Some children develop behavioral or psychosomatic symptoms and unwittingly adopt a "sick" role as a strategy for reuniting the parents.

In response to separation and divorce of parents, *older children and adolescents* commonly show more intense anger. Almost all children cling to the magical belief that their parents will reunite. Wallerstein and Kelly found that, 5 yr after the break-up, about one third of the children studied were "consciously and intensely unhappy and dissatisfied with their life in the post-divorce family." Another third showed clear evidence of a quite satisfactory adjustment, and the remaining third demonstrated "a mixed picture with good achievement in some areas and faltering achievement in others." After 10 yr, 45% were doing well, but 41% were poorly adjusted with academic, social, and emotional problems. As they entered adulthood, many were reluctant to form intimate relationships, fearful of repeating their parents' experience. Good adjustment in children after a divorce is related to ongoing involvement with two psychologically healthy parents who minimize conflict and to the support system offered by siblings and other relatives. Joint custody arrangements may reduce ongoing parental conflict, but a study by Steinman revealed that one third of children in joint custody "felt overburdened by the demands and requirements of maintaining a strong presence in 2 homes."

As to the ultimate separation—*death of a parent*—most preadolescent children do not seem to go through a typical mourning process as psychoanalytically defined. The child's mourning may be masked by behavior not typically seen in adults. Among school-aged to adolescent children who had lost a parent through death, Wolfenstein found that, immediately after the loss, sad feelings were not markedly evident, nor was there much crying. Children continued in daily activities, the major mechanism in dealing with catastrophe being denial, both overt and unconscious, and maintained by the magical wish and hope for reunion and reappearance. Some children seemed to maintain remarkably good moods; some were more active than usual. Wolfenstein saw these good moods as an effective accompaniment of denial, "If one does not feel bad, then nothing bad has happened." Some children show hostile and angry feelings toward the surviving parent and tend to identify with and idealize the lost parent, sometimes with reunion fantasies accompanying denial. Guilt may be present, reflecting the child's egocentric tendency. Alternatively, some children show considerable sorrow at the time of the parent's death or after a delay when the defense of denial is no longer effective.

Children under the age of 5 yr view death as reversible, possibly with belief in the dead coming back to life and in ghosts. In the next stage, up to 8–9 yr, death is personified, for example, as the "grim reaper" who punishes and avenges. Only after this age does the child realistically understand death as a universal and final biologic process.

The physician can help children and surviving caretakers through a period of separation or adjustment to death of parent or sibling, first by helping them recognize that the adults themselves are going through a period of grief and mourning. It is not unhealthy for children to see their surviving or remaining parent mourn the loss of a mate or grieve for a divorced or separated spouse. In the case of a dead parent, the child needs the support and reassurance of having the remaining parent or other important caretakers available. Close physical contact and emotional exchange, with verbal explanations and reassurance for those children who can understand, are important aspects of support. Children should not be expected or forced to discuss all their feelings or to put into words their reactions to a parent's death. They should not be expected to interrupt usual social or recreational activities for weeks or months after the death of a parent, either out of respect for that parent or in recognition of the remaining parent's sorrow or grief. Continuance of usual activities should not be interpreted by adults or older children as callousness or indifference but rather as the child's way of dealing, at his or her stage of development, with what is as much a catastrophe for him or her as it is for the adult. Further, the child should not be expected to serve as a primary support to the remaining parent or others in their grief.

In most cases, it seems helpful for the child to participate appropriately in the rituals that generally surround the death and burial of a parent. A young child can attend a funeral, viewing, or wake so long as there is no morbid preoccupation or demand that the child remain a long time or be involved in prolonged religious ceremonies. To keep the young child away from some participation in the burial rituals, whatever they are, will be a misguided effort to protect and ultimately will be more confusing and isolating than helpful.

Derdeyn AP, Scott E: Joint custody: A critical analysis and appraisal. Am J Orthopsychiatry 54:199, 1984.

Gardner R: The Boys' and Girls' Book about Divorce. New York, Science House, 1970.

Nagy M: The child's meaning of death. *In*: Feifel H (ed): The Meaning of Death. New York, McGraw-Hill, 1959.
Quinn LS, Behrman RE (eds): Children and divorce. The Future of Children, Vol 4(1), 1994.
Steinmann S: The experience of children in a joint custody arrangement: a report of a study. Am J Orthopsychiatry 53:220, 1981.
Wallerstein JS: Children of divorce: the psychological tasks of the child. Am J Orthopsychiatry 53:230, 1983.
Wallerstein JS: The long-term effects of divorce on children: a review. J Am Acad Child Adolesc Psychiatry 30:349, 1991.
Wallerstein JS, Blakeslee S: Second Chances: Men, Women and Children a Decade After Divorce. London, Ticknor & Fields, 1989.
Wolfenstein M: How is mourning possible? *In*: The Psychoanalytic Study of the Child. New York, International Universities Press, 1966.

CHAPTER 37

Impact of Violence

Dorothy Bolding and Marc A. Forman

Anxiety about violence has spread to children of all social classes. A recent poll in the United States revealed that one half of the children questioned said that their most important worry was that someone they loved would become the victim of a violent crime. Another study reported that 25% of the children in a midwestern inner-city grade school described at least one violent event that involved either the child, a family member, or a friend. Many of these children described two or more violent events, and they were nearly twice as likely as their classmates to report low self-esteem, excessive crying, and worries about dying or being injured.

Firearms are now the leading cause of death among 10–24-yr-old black males, the second leading cause of death among all 10–14-yr-old children, and the third major cause of death among children in the 5–14-yr-old age range. In 1993, 48% of American households reported owning at least one gun. Every day, 1.2 million latchkey children go home to a house in which there is a gun.

Acts of violence are invading schools, disrupting learning, and undermining the child's trust and reliance on adults. Nondelinquent adolescent students join gangs and arm themselves for "protection," placing themselves even more at risk. Almost 1.5 million children are reported to have been physically and/or sexually abused. Parents who abuse their children not only injure their child physically and psychologically but also "teach" the child to use force to resolve conflicts. Often, these same parents permit their children to be abusive to their siblings and others.

Concern regarding the impact of television violence on children also seems warranted. Although earlier research indicated that violence on television affected children who were already at risk for aggressive behavior, more recent research has shown that one of the single best predictors of future adolescent violence is the amount of violent television programs watched during childhood. Furthermore, when television watching is substituted for parental affection and guidance, particularly in the preschool years, a child's cognitive and affective resources for coping and adaptation and his or her capacity for imaginative play are likely to be affected. A recent study showed that such overstimulated and undernurtured preschoolers were less happy and more aggressive in their free play in childcare centers and nursery schools. Alternatively, educational television programs specifically designed for preschool children may enhance cognitive development in reading readiness and acquisition of vocabulary. Television may inform older children of current events, politics, history, and science. Such programs can supplement rather than substitute for the activities of parents; can convey knowledge, skills, and information; and may motivate learning. All parents should know what their children are watching on television, should decide whether certain programs are appropriate, and should feel in no way reluctant to set their own standards and impose restrictions on the time and content of television viewing.

Abbott MW: Television violence: A proactive prevention campaign. *In*: Albee GW, Bond LA, Cook Monsey TV (eds): Improving Children's Lives: Global Perspectives on Prevention. Newbury Park, CA, Sage Publications, 1992.
Children's Defense Fund: The State of America's Children: Yearbook 1994. Washington, DC, Children's Defense Fund, 1994.
Friedlander BZ: Community violence, children's development, and mass media: In pursuit of new insights, new goals, new strategies. Psychiatry 56:66, 1993.
Lande RG: The video violence debate. Hosp Community Psychiatry 44:347, 1993.
Lefkowitz MM, Eron LD, Walden LO, et al: Growing Up to Be Violent. New York, Pergamon Press, 1977.
Prothrow-Stith D, Weissman M: Deadly Consequences: How Violence Is Destroying Our Teen-Age Population and a Plan to Begin Solving the Problem. New York, Harper Collins, 1991.
Rothenberg MB: The role of television in shaping the attitudes of children. J Am Acad Child Adolesc Psychiatry 22:86, 1983.
Strasburger VC, Comstock GA (eds): Adolescents and the media. State of The Art Reviews, Vol 4, No 3. Philadelphia, Hanley & Belfus, 1993.
Surger JL, Surger DE: Television, Imagination and Aggression: A Study of Preschoolers. Hillsdale, NJ, Laurence Erlbaum Associates, 1981.

CHAPTER 38

*Abuse and Neglect of Children**

Charles F. Johnson

Child maltreatment encompasses a spectrum of abusive actions, or acts of commission, and lack of actions, or acts of omission, that result in morbidity or death (Fig. 38–1). Acts of omission and commission before birth may also have adverse effects on the child, such as maternal drug abuse and failure to seek appropriate health care during pregnancy. Physical abuse may be narrowly defined as intentional injuries to a child by a caretaker that result in bruises, burns, fractures, lacerations, punctures, and organ damage. A broader definition would include short- and long-term emotional consequences, which can be more debilitating than the physical effects. Physical neglect, and other acts of omission, may result in failure to thrive, develop, and learn. Nutritional neglect is the most common cause of underweight in infancy and may account for more than one half of the cases of failure to thrive (see Chapter 39). Physicians are most likely to identify medical neglect that results from the failure of a parent to provide appropriate medical care, whereas failure to provide heat, schooling, adequate clothing, and protection from environmental hazards tends to be observed by neighbors, relatives, teachers, and social workers. Medical neglect of a child with an acute or chronic disease may result in deteriorization in the condition and death. Neglect accounts for more deaths than physical abuse.

Parents may refuse to allow recommended medical treatments because of personal or religious beliefs. A determination of whether this constitutes neglect and, if it does, the appropriate action a physician should take are difficult decisions. Neglect of appropriate precautions by caretakers to ensure a

*Some parts adapted from previous sections by B. D. Schmitt and R. D. Krugman.

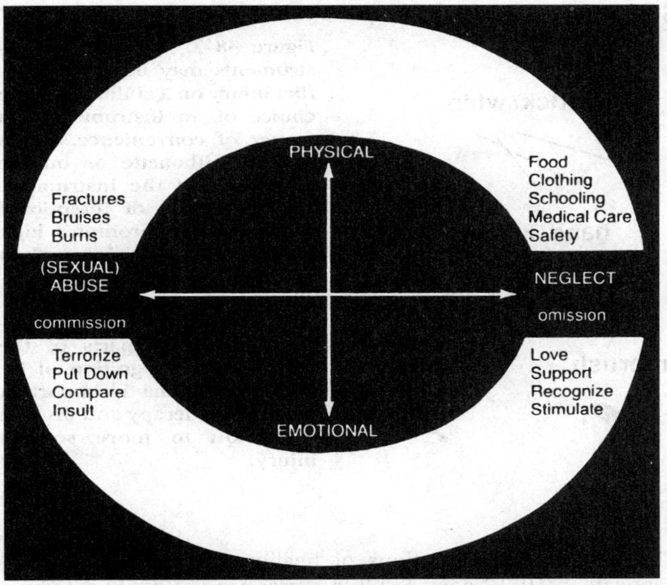

Figure 38–1. The spectrum of child maltreatment. Child maltreatment encompasses acts of commission, or abuse, and acts of omission, or neglect by a caretaker that adversely affect children. The act can be physical or emotional. The boundaries between these areas are indistinct and emotional; physical abuse and neglect overlap and may exist at the same or various times in the child's life. Sexual abuse may be considered a specific type of physical abuse that has emotional components. Physical abuse and neglect invariably have short- and long-term emotional consequences. Emotional consequences may persist long after the physical wounds heal.

child's safety similarly may involve difficult matters of judgment. Children may be injured despite a variety of actions by well-meaning parents to protect them.

Emotional abuse includes intentional verbal or behavioral acts that result in adverse emotional consequences; emotional neglect occurs when a caretaker intentionally does not provide nurturing verbal and behavioral actions that are necessary for healthy development. Emotional abuse can include rejection, scapegoat assignment, isolation, criticism, or terrorizing of a child by caretakers. Emotional neglect, especially by a mother, may have devastating consequences. Emotional abuse and neglect are often difficult to document. It may also be hard to establish that psychopathologic conditions or emotional consequences in the child are the direct result of acts or omissions by caretakers.

Sexual abuse, or involving a child in any act that is intended for the sexual gratification of an adult, has received increased media attention in recent years and accounts for a major proportion of the increase in abuse reports. Sexual abuse may be perpetrated by family members (incest), acquaintances, or least often, by strangers.

Medications and toxins may be given to intentionally poison a child. When this or any other deceptive action is undertaken to stimulate a disorder, it is referred to as Munchausen syndrome by proxy. The induced symptoms and signs may lead to unnecessary medical investigation, hospital admissions, or treatment; in 10% of these cases death occurs.

Legal definitions of abuse and neglect vary from state to state; however, physicians and other providers of child care are required by law in all 50 states, to report suspected child abuse or neglect. These laws provide protection to mandated reporters who report in good faith; also they allow for clinical and laboratory evaluations and documentation without the parent's or guardian's permission. Failure to report suspected child abuse may result in a penalty. It may also result in a malpractice claim for damages incurred as a result of failure to report and thereby protect the child from further injury.

EPIDEMIOLOGY. The number of reports to children's protective services (CPS) and law enforcement agencies in the county in which the alleged abuse or neglect occurred have steadily increased since mandated reporting began in the 1960s. Reports of all types of abuse increased 50%, from 30 per 1,000 children to 45 per 1,000, between 1985 and 1992. In 1992, 2.9 million CPS reports were filed, and 1,261 children died of maltreatment. Of reported children, 85% were younger than 5 yr of age, and 45% were younger than 1 yr of age. Sixty percent of these reports were "substantiated" by CPS. This increase in reports is attributed primarily to improved case finding and reporting. With the advent of child death review teams, it is expected that more child abuse deaths will be revealed. The actual incidence of abuse is unknown. A survey of families with children aged 3–18 yr indicated that 140 of 1,000 (14%) were kicked, bitten, punched, hit with an object, beaten up, or threatened with a knife or gun in 1 yr. Approximately 10% of injuries to children younger than 5 yr of age who are seen in emergency departments are due to abuse; 15% of children admitted for burns and 50% of children younger than 1 yr of age with fractures are abused. In 1991, the National Child Abuse and Neglect Data System indicated that 24% of 838,232 reports were for physical abuse; 7% of children were younger than 1 yr of age, 27% were younger than 4 yr of age, and 28% were 4–8 yr of age. The rate of reports decreases in older children. Of the 1,229 assessments done in a pediatric hospital during that same period, 223 (28%) of 797 reports were for physical abuse and the death rate was 6%. Immediate family members were the perpetrators in 55% of abuse cases. The most common perpetrators were the father (21%), mother (21%), boyfriend of the mother (9%), baby sitter (8%), and stepfather (5%). The average age of the abuser was 25 years.

Although varying definitions and reporting requirements prevent detailed comparisons, parents who abuse their children have been reported from most ethnic, geographic, religious, educational, occupational, and socioeconomic groups. Groups living in poverty may have increased reports of child abuse because (1) of the increased number of crises in their lives (e.g., unemployment or overcrowding); (2) they have limited access to economic or social resources for support during times of stress; (3) of the increased violence in the communities where they live; (4) of an association of poverty with other risk factors, such as teen-age and single parenthood and substance abuse; and (5) there may be more scrutiny by community agencies and neighbors. An increased incidence of physical abuse also has been noted on military bases. The presence of spouse abuse increases the likelihood of child abuse. Substance abuse is a common finding in families with abused children. More than 90% of abusing parents have neither psychotic nor criminal personalities. Rather they tend to be lonely, unhappy, angry, young, and single parents who do not plan their pregnancies, have little or no knowledge of child development, and have unrealistic expectations for child behavior. Mentally retarded children are more at risk for abuse and neglect. Without support, their parents may injure and physically handicap them in anger after being provoked by what they consider a misbehavior that is actually related to the handicap. From 10–40% of abusive parents have experienced physical abuse as children.

Physical abuse is most likely to occur when a high-risk parent is responsible for the care of a high-risk child. High-risk children include premature infants, infants with chronic medical conditions, colicky babies, and children with behavior problems. The child may be normal but misperceived by an unsophisticated parent as difficult, unusual, or abnormal. Nor-

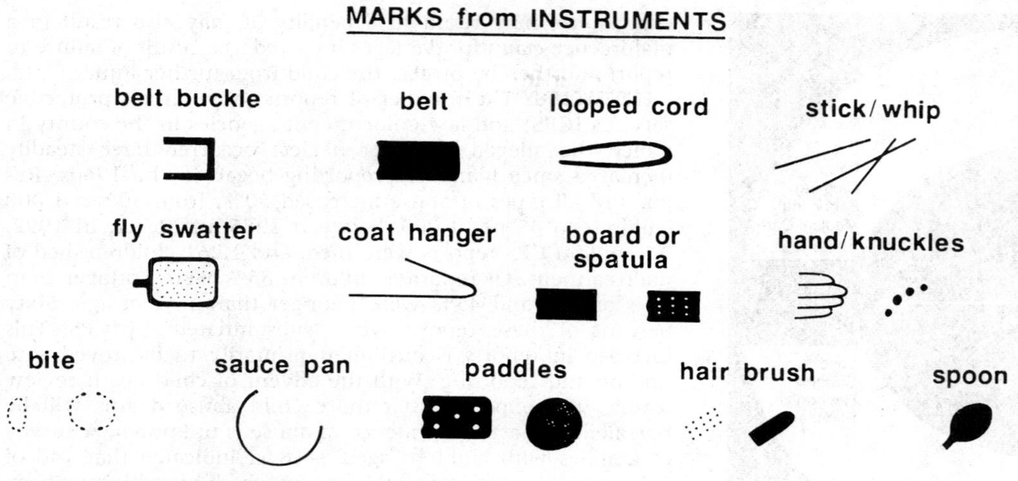

Figure 38–2. A variety of instruments may be used to inflict injury on a child. Often the choice of an instrument is a matter of convenience. Marks tend to silhouette or outline the shape of the instrument. The possibility of intentional trauma should prompt a high degree of suspicion when injuries to a child are geometric, paired, mirrored, of various ages or types, or on relatively protected parts of the body. Early recognition of intentional trauma is important to provide therapy and prevent escalation to more serious injury.

mal behavior, such as crying, wetting, soiling, and spilling may cause the parent to lose control and injure a child. The occasion precipitating the abuse may be associated with a family crisis, such as loss of a job or home, marital strife, death of a sibling, physical exhaustion, or development of an acute or chronic physical or mental illness in the parent or child. Determining risk factors for abuse and neglect should be part of the medical history in all cases of childhood injury. Although not diagnostic, the presence of risk factors increases the suspicion of abuse and, even if no abuse is documented, may necessitate referral for preventive services.

CLINICAL MANIFESTATIONS. Physical abuse is suspected when an injury is unexplained, unexplainable, or implausible. If an injury is incompatible with the history given or the child's development, suspected abuse should be reported. It is expected when children are hurt that parents will bring them immediately for examination. With abused children, there is often delay in seeking medical help. A delay may also be due to a lack of transportation or ignorance about the significance of an injury. Before reporting suspected medical neglect, the physician should determine whether the parents have an understanding of disease processes and have the intellectual, emotional, and physical resources to provide for their children.

Bruises are the most common manifestation of child abuse and may be found on any body surface. Accidental bruises, from impact trauma, are most likely to be found on leading surfaces overlying superficial bone edges, such as the shins, forearms, hips, and brows. Bruises to the buttocks, genitalia, back, and back of the hands are less likely to be due to an accident. In addition to being struck or thrown, children may also be intentionally burned, lacerated, or punctured. The shape of the injury may suggest the object used. Paddles, belts, hands, and other instruments leave specific marks (Fig. 38–2). Bilateral, symmetrical, and geometric injuries should raise suspicion of child abuse. Bruises change color over time; bruise color may be used to estimate the time of injury in order to determine the accuracy of the history of the injury (Fig. 38–3). Bruises of different colors are not compatible with a single event.

Most inflicted *fractures* are due to wrenching or pulling injuries that damage the metaphysis. A classic finding in child abuse is a chip fracture in which a corner of the metaphysis of a long bone is torn off with damage to the epiphysis and periosteum. Inflicted fractures of the shaft are more likely to be spiral rather than transverse; spiral fractures of the femur before the age of walking are usually inflicted. Cardiopulmonary resuscitation rarely causes rib fractures or retinal hemorrhages in children. As with bruises, fractures may be dated. The earliest manifestations of healing, by callus formation, appears in 10–12 days. Skull fractures are not easily dated.

Hair that is pulled causes alopecia in which the hairs are broken at various lengths. Neglected infants, left to lay on their backs, may have an area of missing hair at the back of the head. The existence of bruises, scars, and fractures at various stages of healing is highly suggestive of abuse.

Conditions that suggested abuse, but were not reportable, constituted 25% of cases of physical abuse evaluated at a Children's hospital. Petechiae of the face and shoulders from intense retching, coughing, or crying and a variety of other conditions, such as mongolian spots, capillary hemangiomas, pigmented nevi, and other congenital, allergic, self-inflicted, and infectious skin conditions may be mistaken for abuse. A single 1-cm, round lesion of impetigo may be difficult to differentiate from a fresh cigarette burn. Blood dyscrasias and coagulopathies result in more ready bruising. Old and new fractures may be seen in chromosomal disorders, Wilson disease, Schmid-like metaphyseal chondrodysplasia, and osteogenesis imperfecta. Severe monilia of the diaper area may suggest a burn.

Approximately 10% of cases of physical abuse involve *burns.* The shape or pattern of a burn may be diagnostic when it reflects the geometric pattern of an object or method of injury. Cigarette burns produce circular, punched-out lesions of uniform size and are often found on the hands or feet (Fig. 38–4). An immersion burn occurs when a parent holds the thighs against the abdomen and places the buttocks and perineum in scalding water as punishment for enuresis or resistance to toilet training. This results in a well-demarcated and circular burn restricted to the buttocks. With deeper, forced immersions, the scald line extends to a clear-cut water level on the thighs and waist. Depending on how the child is immersed, the hands and feet may be spared, and there are no splash

DAY	1	2	3	4	5	6	7	8	9	10	13	21	28
	Red-blue			Blue-purple		Green			Yellow-brown			Resolved	

Figure 38–3. Determination of age of bruise or contusion. Bruises change color with time. It is not possible to date a bruise narrowly within hours; however, bruises of varying colors are not in keeping with a single instance of injury. The time of the injury, in days, can be roughly determined from the color of the bruise; however, the depth of the injury; the existence of underlying, unyielding tissue, especially bone; and the child's skin color may influence the time of the appearance of a bruise and its rate of resolution.

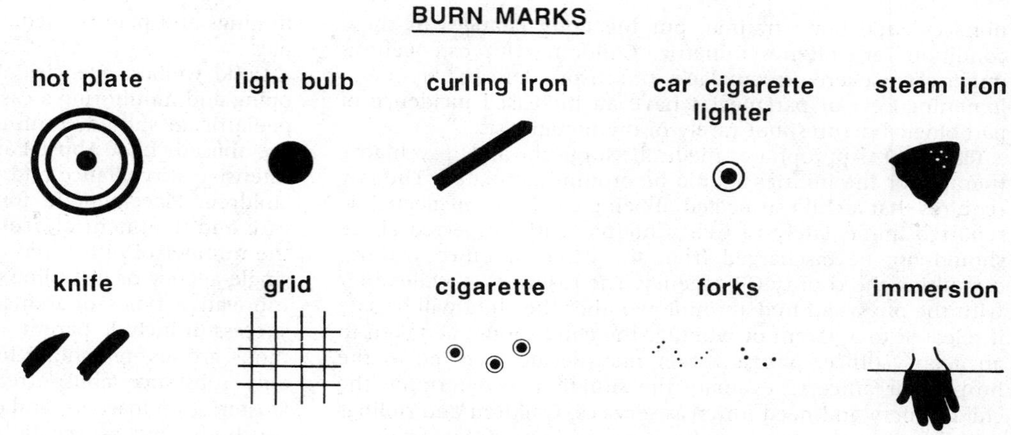

Figure 38–4. Marks from heated objects cause burns in a pattern that duplicates that of the object. Familiarity with the common heated objects that are used to traumatize children facilitates recognition of possible intentional injuries. The location of the burn is important in determining its cause. Children tend to explore surfaces with the palmar surface of the hand and rarely touch a heated object repeatedly.

marks. The burn pattern is incompatible with falling into a tub or turning on the hot water while in the bathtub. It is important to ascertain the developmental level of the child, water temperature, and tub and knob type in the investigation of scald burns. Children younger than 24 mo of age may not be able to enter a tub and may be developmentally unable to turn a rotary knob. Immersion of a hand or foot causes a burn pattern that resembles a stocking or glove. Immersion burns are most common in infants.

The most common cause of death from physical abuse is from *head trauma*. The head, face, or cranial contents were injured in 29% of child abuse reports from a children's hospital. More than 95% of serious intracranial injuries during the 1st yr of life are the result of abuse. Injured infants may present with coma, convulsions, apnea, and increased intracranial pressure. A bloody spinal tap may not be iatrogenic. Subdural hematomas may result from a blow from a hand in which there are no scalp marks or skull fractures. Although grab marks or metaphyseal fractures and rib fractures have been described in association with shaking injuries and slamming the head against a mattress or wall, there may be no external marks. Retinal hemorrhages, which may occur in association with normal birth, coagulopathies, blood dyscrasias, and more rarely in meningitis, endocarditis, and severe hypertension, are also considered markers for acceleration/deceleration injuries. Retinal hemorrhages rarely result from cardiopulmonary resuscitation.

Intra-abdominal injuries are the second most common cause of death in battered children. Affected children may present with recurrent vomiting, abdominal distention, absent bowel sounds, localized tenderness, or shock. Because the abdominal wall is flexible, the force of the blow is usually absorbed by the internal organs, and the overlying skin is free of bruises. If a fist is used, however, a row of three to four 1-cm round bruises in a slight curve may be seen. The most common finding is a ruptured liver or spleen. Much rarer are tears or other injuries of the small intestine at sites of ligamental support such as the duodenum and proximal jejunum. Intramural hematomas at these sites can lead to temporary obstruction. Chylous ascites and pseudocyst of the pancreas have been reported.

LABORATORY DATA. Screening tests for a bleeding diathesis should be obtained in all cases of bruising to rule out a bleeding diathesis. These tests should include a prothrombin time, partial thromboplastin time, and platelet count. Children with a hematologic condition, or any chronic condition, may also be abused.

When physical abuse is suspected in a child younger than 2 yr of age, a roentgenologic bone survey consisting of films of the skull, thorax, and long bones should be ordered; in addition, pelvis, finger, toe, and spine films may be indicated. Bone scans may be of value in detecting new fractures of the hands, feet, or ribs. They are not valuable in detecting skull fractures. For children 2–4 yr of age, a bone survey is indicated unless the child is adequately verbal, has very minor injuries, or has been in a witnessed and supervised setting (e.g., preschool). For verbal children older than 4 or 5 yr of age, roentgenograms need be obtained only if there is bone tenderness or a limited range of motion on physical examination. If films of a tender site are initially negative, they should be repeated in 2 wk to detect any calcification, subperiosteal bleeding, or nondisplaced epiphyseal separations that may have occurred. Bone trauma is found in 10–20% of physically abused children. Fractures considered highly specific of child abuse include metaphyseal, rib, scapular, outer end of clavicle, vertebral, and finger in preambulating children; fractures of different ages; bilateral fractures; and complex skull fractures. Midclavicular, simple linear, and single diaphyseal fractures have a low specificity for abuse. Despite an absence of central nervous system abnormalities, a head computed tomographic (CT) scan and, if indicated, magnetic resonance imaging should be obtained when an infant has been severely injured because the fractures, burns, or bruises may be associated with head injury. Liver and pancreatic enzyme studies or an abdominal CT scan may uncover damage to these organs. Urine and stool should be screened for blood if abdominal trauma is suspected.

DIAGNOSIS. A tentative diagnosis of physical abuse or neglect is usually based on the history and physical findings. All information should be carefully recorded and, when appropriate, photographed with color charts and measuring scales in the field. An analysis of the circumstances of the injury is critical. For example, the consequences of a fall depend on (1) child variables, such as surface contacted, age, size, motor skills, motor tone, clothing, and momentum; and (2) environmental variables, such as distance and physical qualities of contact surfaces. Data from studies of witnessed falls from hospital beds, bunk beds, windows, and school yard equipment have been used to estimate the force required to cause brain damage and fractures. A fall from 3 ft may rarely result in a simple linear fracture of the skull or clavicle. Falls from 6 ft may rarely result in concussions, subdural hemorrhages, or lacerations. There are no reports of death or severe brain injury from witnessed falls of less than 10 ft.

A child older than age 3 yr may be able to tell a sensitive and skillful interviewer that a particular adult hurt him or her. However, verbal children may not give a history of intentional injury if they are concerned about retribution from the perpetrator or separation from even a pathologic home environment.

The differential diagnosis depends on the particular injuries. For example, roentgenograms of bones in scurvy and syphilis and normally growing bone shafts of infants may resemble nonaccidental bone trauma, but the bony changes in these conditions are often symmetric. Children with osteogenesis imperfecta, severe osteomalacia, or sensory deficits (e.g., myelomeningocele or paraplegia) have an increased incidence of pathologic fractures, but rarely of the metaphysis.

TREATMENT. Appropriate medical, surgical, and psychiatric therapy for the injuries should be promptly initiated. The law requires that a child suspected of being abused or neglected be reported immediately to CPS. Children with suspected abuse should not be discharged from the clinic or office without consulting the county CPS agency. The caseworker will confer with the physician to determine whether the child will be safe if released to a parent or whether the child should be taken to an agency office. A caseworker may decide to come to the hospital or office to evaluate the situation to determine the child's safety and need for crisis services. Children and siblings at risk for serious abuse can be placed in homes of appropriate relatives or emergency receiving homes. Some communities offer intensive support that provides for the immediate and safe return of the child to the home. The CPS should complete their investigation within a reasonable stipulated time and contact law enforcement. The role of law enforcement is to perform site investigations, interview suspects, and if a criminal act has taken place, to contact the prosecutor's office. In most states, 48 hr after the initial report by telephone or facsimile communication, an official *written* medical report is required.

Hospital admission is indicated for children (1) whose medical or surgical condition requires inpatient management; (2) in whom the diagnosis is unclear; and (3) when no alternative safe place for custody is available. If in doubt, the physician, agency, or court should err on the side of protecting the child through hospitalization. If parents refuse hospitalization, an emergency court order must be obtained. The parents should be told by the physician why an inflicted injury is suspected; that the physician is legally obligated to report the circumstance; that the referral is being made to protect the child; that the family will be provided with services; and that a CPS social worker will be involved. Siblings should have full examinations within 24 hr of the recognition of child abuse in the family. Approximately 20% of them will be found to have signs of physical abuse.

Experiencing anger with abusing or neglectful parents is to be expected, but expressing the anger to them damages rapport, increases defensiveness, and makes their cooperation less likely. Repeated interrogations, confrontations, and accusations may be avoided by involving CPS workers and law enforcement early in the investigation. If the child is hospitalized, the parents should be encouraged to visit their children, and the hospital staff must be counseled to be courteous, helpful, and observant. The primary physician should maintain contact with the parents. An evaluation by hospital social services should be obtained to determine existing problems and strengths in the family. An agency caseworker and, when needed, a police officer should visit the home. A psychiatric evaluation of the parents may be indicated.

Hospitals caring for these children should designate a team of professionals who are trained and skilled in child abuse recognition and reporting and responsive to the needs of abused or neglected children and their families. This team should include a pediatrician, a hospital social worker, a pediatric nurse, a psychologist or psychiatrist, and a coordinator. The roles of all the members as well as public agencies should be clear and formalized. Legal and medical specialty consultants should be available. When evaluations are completed, the team should meet with the child's primary care physician, ward nurse, the CPS representative, and, as appropriate, a law enforcement officer, prosecutor, or any other community agencies involved with the family to clarify medical and social findings and plan immediate and long-range goals and therapies.

Child welfare agencies are primarily responsible for developing and monitoring a case plan for the child and family. The pediatrician should continue to coordinate the health care of the abused child. Abused and neglected children require more intensive surveillance and well-child care than do nonabused children. Placement in foster care may interrupt preventive care and treatment of acute and chronic illnesses. Because of the number of difficulties experienced by abusive families, no single agency or discipline can provide all the needed services. Innovative types of individualized therapies that have been successful include parent aides, homemakers, Parents Anonymous groups, telephone hot lines, environmental crisis therapy, substance abuse treatment, Big Brothers and Sisters, "foster" grandparents, and child-rearing counseling. Traditional psychotherapy, especially in isolation, may be ineffective.

PREVENTION. A major role of the pediatrician in primary abuse prevention is to identify parents at high risk for being unable to accept, love, and care properly for their offspring. The history obtained from all parents should include information about pregnancy planning and attitudes about the child and child-rearing techniques. Parental risks include a history of family violence, drug addiction, depression, lack of support, socioeconomic problems, serious psychiatric illness, mental retardation, young parental age, closely spaced pregnancies, single parent status of the mother, negative parental comments about the newborn infant, lack of evidence of maternal attachment, infrequent visits to a new baby whose discharge is delayed because of prematurity or illness, anger toward or spanking of a young infant, and severe neglect of infant hygiene. Mentally or physically handicapped and chronically ill children should also be recognized as being at increased risk for abuse and neglect. Abuse and serious neglect may be prevented when at-risk families receive intensive training and support during pregnancy and after delivery. Prevention efforts should include early and frequent contact between mother and baby in the delivery room, rooming-in, increased parental contact with premature infants, extra help calming the crying or "difficult" infant, more frequent office visits for at-risk infants, ongoing counseling regarding discipline and the use of nonphysical responses to annoying behaviors, public health nurse visits or trained home visitors, parenting classes, close follow-up of acute and chronic illnesses, telephone lifelines, arrangement for day care or preschool, and assistance in family planning.

PROGNOSIS. Early studies of abused children returned to their parents without any intervention indicated that about 5% were killed and that 25% were seriously reinjured. With comprehensive, intensive treatment of the entire family, 80–90% of families involved in child abuse or neglect can be rehabilitated to provide adequate care for their children. Approximately 10–15% of such families, especially those with a history of substance abuse, can only be stabilized and will require an indefinite continuation of supporting services, which may include drug monitoring, until their children are old enough to leave home. Termination of parental rights or continued foster placement is required in 2–3% of cases. If a parent is unable to respond to a treatment plan, this should be documented as soon as possible to afford the child the opportunity to develop in a healthy and permanent home.

Children with repeated injuries to the central nervous system may develop mental retardation, organic brain syndrome, seizures, hydrocephalus, and ataxia. Common emotional traits of abused children include fearfulness, aggression, hypervigilance, denial, projection, a lack of trust, low self-esteem, juvenile delinquency, substance abuse, and hyperactivity. Unsuccessfully treated families tend to produce children who become juvenile delinquents, violent and antisocial adults, and the next generation of child abusers.

38.1 Sexual Abuse

Sexual abuse includes any activity with a child, before the age of legal consent, that is for the sexual gratification of an adult or a significantly older child. Sexual abuse includes oral-genital, genital-genital, genital-rectal, hand-genital, hand-rectal or hand-breast contact; exposure of sexual anatomy, forced viewing of sexual anatomy; and showing pornography to a child or using a child in the production of pornography. Sexual intercourse includes vaginal, oral, or rectal penetration. Penetration is entry into an orifice with or without tissue injury. In studies of juvenile offenders, younger perpetrators tend to have younger victims, but are more likely to have intercourse with older victims. Without detection and intervention, sexual abuse may progress from touching to intercourse. Sexual play may be defined as viewing or touching of the genitalia, buttocks, or chest by pre-adolescent children separated by not more than 4 yr, in which there has been no force or coercion. Sex acts perpetrated by young children are learned behaviors and are associated with sexual abuse or exposure to adult sex or pornography.

Sexual mistreatment of children by family members (incest) and non-relatives known to the child are the most common types of sexual abuse. The least common offender is a stranger. Intrafamilial sexual abuse is difficult to document and manage because the child must be protected from additional abuse and coercion to not reveal or deny the abuse, while attempts are made to preserve the family unit. Children also may be coerced to recant accusations of abuse by relatives or they may decide to recant the abuse for fear of ridicule or teasing, retaliation, attending court, or losing contact with a needed or loved relative.

EPIDEMIOLOGY. Most of the increase in child abuse reports is due to increased reporting of sexual abuse. The rate of sexual abuse, estimated by the American Association for Protecting Children, went from 1.4 per 10,000 to 17 per 10,000 children between 1976 and 1984. In a children's hospital, the number of total assessments of sexual abuse increased by a factor of 4 between 1981 and 1991. Of 838,232 cases of child abuse reported to the National Child Abuse and Neglect Data System in 1991, 15% were of sexual abuse. Surveys of adult women indicate that from 12–38% were sexually abused by 18 years of age. The results of one study indicated that the likelihood of extrafamilial and intrafamilial sexual abuse being reported was only 8% and 2%, respectively. The incidence of sexual abuse of males ranges from 3–9% of the population; males constitute up to 20% of reports. Because fixed pedophiles show a predilection for boys, it is theorized that the number of males who are sexually abused is higher. Furthermore, boys may refrain from reporting what might be interpreted as a homosexual action. In addition, in a society that expects males to be able to protect themselves from assault, boys may feel guilty if they are victimized.

Increased recognition of sexual abuse manifestations is responsible for increased reporting; however, as many as 50% of reported cases may not be substantiated. This may be due to the child's young age and an associated inability to give a detailed history or a lack of physical findings or caretaker appreciation of the significance of nonspecific symptoms, such as genital erythema, enuresis, or unusual behaviors. Approximately one third of sexual abuse victims are younger than 6 yr of age, one third are 6–12 yr of age, and one third are 12–18 yr of age. Reported offenders are 97% male. Females are more often perpetrators in child-care settings, including babysitting. The number of female perpetrators may be higher because younger children may confuse sexual abuse by a female with normal hygiene care and adolescent males may not be trained to recognize sexual activity with an older female as a form of abuse. Sexual abuse by stepfathers is nearly 5 times higher than among natural fathers. Incest is described in most cultures and is seen among all socioeconomic levels to a greater degree than physical abuse and neglect.

ETIOLOGY. The abuse of daughters by fathers and stepfathers is the most common form of reported incest, although brother-sister incest is considered to be the most common type. Studies of incarcerated adult perpetrators indicated that sexual relationships begin gradually through selection of vulnerable and available victims with innocent physical contact and seduction. The propensity for pedophiles to become sexually involved with children often begins in their adolescence. Pedophiles indicated that they seek positions and opportunities where they can be in contact with potential victims. The vulnerable children they described included those with mental and physical handicaps, unloved and unwanted children, previously abused children, children in single-parent families, children of drug abusers, and children with low self-esteem and poor achievement. Pornography may be used to initiate sexual activity with a child. Threats and bribes may be used to entice children and keep them from telling. Boys and girls may be convinced that they are guilty because they did not protect themselves. Children's trust in adults make them more vulnerable to abuse. This obedience and trust, coupled with a need to maintain family unity are factors associated with incest. A father's need for sexual gratification and a daughter's need for affection and nurturance may lead to incest when the mother is unavailable and there is a desire to maintain the family unit. These incestuous fathers have been described as rigid, patriarchal, and emotionally immature. They are unlikely to engage in extramarital relationships, and there is a high reported incidence of alcoholism. The characteristics of abusing fathers who are not revealed or confessed may be different from revealed, confessed, or incarcerated fathers. The mothers have been described as chronically depressed, unavailable to their husbands because of work or illness, and often the victims of childhood sexual abuse. The child victim tends to be pseudomature and may have taken on many of the adult roles, including housekeeping. The tendency for some of these families to be closely knit and socially isolated prevents detection.

Violence is not common in sexual abuse; however, its incidence increases with the age and size of the victim and specific traits in the perpetrator. Violence is more likely to occur in association with a single incident by a stranger. In cases of violent incest, the father has been described as sociopathic, with sexual abuse extending outside the family circle.

CLINICAL MANIFESTATIONS. A child may disclose an incestuous relationship to his or her mother and be brought to a physician at that time. If the mother does not believe the child, the child may delay further comment indefinitely or later tell a friend, relative, friend's mother, teacher, or school counselor. Children, given the opportunity, may disclose their abuse to a physician in a private interview. The possibility of sexual abuse should be entertained as the result of associated physical symptoms or behaviors. Symptoms associated with sexual abuse include (1) vaginal, penile, or rectal pain, erythema, discharge, or bleeding; (2) chronic dysuria, enuresis, constipation, or encopresis; and (3) premature puberty in a female. Specific behaviors associated with sexual abuse include sexualized activity with peers, animals, or objects; seductive behavior; and age-inappropriate sexual knowledge and curiosity. Nonspecific behaviors include suicide gestures, fear of an individual or place, nightmares, sleep disorders, regression, aggression, withdrawn behavior, post-traumatic stress disorder (see Chapter 23), low self-esteem, depression, poor school performance, running away, self-mutilation, anxiety, fire setting, multiple personalities, somatization, phobias, trauma, prostitution, drug abuse, eating disorders, dysmenorrhea, and dyspareunia. Because of secrecy or threats by the abuser, the cause of these symptoms or behaviors may be denied by the child. When the perpetrator is a breadwinner or violent, they may also be denied by the nonoffending and dependent parent.

Determining the possibility of sexual abuse requires supportive, sensitive, and detailed *history* taking. Because the type of abuse, the age of the victim and perpetrator, and the time since the abuse vary, fewer than 25% of the victims will have physical or laboratory findings. Ideally, the forensic interview, with open-ended, nonleading questions, should be conducted by an experienced interviewer in the presence of law enforcement and social service workers on videotape to avoid repeated interviews and possible further trauma to the child from the process. After an initial interview, children who gain trust and comfort may experience a decrease in guilt and fear of reprisal or loss of love and give consistent and more detailed information in subsequent interviews. Interviewing should proceed at the child's pace and level of development, beginning with discussion of general topics and naming of body parts, including "private" parts, and proceeding to details about each incident. The sophistication of the information that can be obtained from the child will vary with the development of the child and skill of the interviewer. Experienced interviewers, especially of preadolescent children, may use anatomic pictures or dolls to clarify the names of body parts and aid the child in describing the abuse. If a social worker or law enforcement officer has carried out the initial interview, the physician should review this material and decide whether it is necessary to repeat the interview before performing a physical examination. Questions about the abusive actions, including symptoms of trauma, may be asked during the examination. Familiarity with the child through participation in the interview or a previous examination facilitate a cooperative and nontraumatic physical examination. Both female and male victims may prefer that a physician of the same sex examine them; when possible, their desires should be respected.

A thorough *examination* of the skin should be carried out for any signs of associated trauma, with special attention to the neck and mouth. If present, bite marks should be measured, and wax impressions and wiping for saliva should be obtained to aid in identification of the perpetrator. The abdominal examination should assess the possibility of pregnancy. The mouth should be examined for redness, abrasions, or purpura that may be due to recent trauma. The rectum should be examined for signs of trauma and laxity. The external genitals should be examined for signs of trauma and discharge. Acute injuries to the hymen occur between the 4–8-o'clock positions. Depending on the age of the girl, penetration may injure the labia minora and posterior fourchette first; tears of the posterior hymenal ring occur with deeper penetration. With the child in the frog-leg position, the hymenal orifice is measured in horizontal and vertical directions while separation or lateral traction is applied to the labia with the gloved fingers of the examiner or assistant. Hymenal diameter varies with the child's age and examination technique. The horizontal diameter of the hymen increases with lateral traction and age. If the child is resistant, the parent may provide assistance; occasionally, the child will be able to separate the labia or buttocks themselves. A speculum examination of the vagina is indicated when the victim is postpubertal or when nonmenstrual vaginal bleeding or major trauma of the external genital is present. General anesthesia may be required for this examination. Magnification, using a colposcope or a hand-held magnifier with bright illumination ensures a detailed examination that can reveal abnormalities in the fourchette and rim of the hymen. The tears from penetration may heal with scarring or a permanent notch. Trauma may cause attenuation or narrowing of the lateral or inferior (dorsal) hymenal rim. Photographs with the colposcope or a hand-held 35-mm camera provide useful records that can be used for consultation. Normal values for the hymenal opening of nonsexually abused girls of different ages are available and should be referred to when evaluating the hymen. An opening more than two standard deviations above the norm should be considered suspicious for abnormal enlargement. A hymenal opening greater than 1 cm is considered suggestive of sexual abuse by some experts. Findings such as (1) a hymen with new or healed lacerations and transections, remnants, and attenuations; (2) posterior fourchette lacerations; (3) vaginal wall granulation, tears, or scarring; and (4) perianal lacerations are also considered "suggestive findings" of sexual abuse. The presence of sperm and semen is "clear evidence" of sexual abuse. Other findings suggestive of sexual abuse include genital molluscum contagiosum, bite marks of the genitalia or inner thigh, or scarring or tears of the labia minora. Straddle injuries usually result in trauma to the labia and clitoris and do not involve the relatively protected hymen. Accidental penetration of the hymen is rare and is associated with penetration of underclothing and the wall of the vagina.

LABORATORY DATA. Laboratory investigation depends on the history and the time from injury. Victims of sexual intercourse seen within 72 hr of the event should have tests for sperm and acid phosphatase. In addition, specimens of possible offender blood and hair and the victim's nail clippings and clothing should be collected. Tests for rectal blood may be indicated. Gonorrhea and Chlamydia cultures should be obtained from the mouth, anus, and genitalia. In the vagina, motile sperm can be found for 6 hr; nonmotile sperm exist for 72 hr or longer. Acid phosphatase is present for 24 hr. Sperm and semen may also be recovered from the mouth, rectum, and clothing. Although the presence of semen substantiates the victim's history, the absence of semen does not contradict the history of vaginal intercourse. Fewer than 5% of victims have positive cultures for gonorrhea or Chlamydia. Symptomatic victims, or those with positive cultures for other venereal diseases, should also undergo tests for syphilis. When epidemiologically indicated, or requested, HIV and hepatitis B tests should be performed. All specimens should be transferred to the forensic laboratory in sealed, signed, and dated envelopes to ensure an official chain of evidence.

DIAGNOSIS. It is most common for the diagnosis of sexual abuse to depend on the history offered by the victim. False accusations are rare, except in unusual cases that involve emotionally disturbed patients or in custody disputes. These latter instances generally involve adolescents. Abuse may be revealed during a custody dispute because the child has been separated from an offender, is able to communicate without retaliation and fear, and desires protection from further abuse. The physical examination may corroborate a child's history, but normal physical and laboratory examination findings are compatible with sexual abuse. The genitalia and rectum may heal completely after extensive trauma, and minor trauma, such as abrasions, may heal within 3–4 days. In one study of 18 victims whose abusers confessed to vaginal penetration, 7 children had normal genital examination findings. Abnormal physical findings should be reported if no history is available.

Laboratory findings of pregnancy, sperm, semen, and nonpregnancy or delivery-related syphilis, gonorrhea, *Chlamydia*, herpes type II (genital) and human immunodeficiency virus (HIV) may be considered diagnostic of sexual abuse and reported. Although the following diseases also should be reported as suspect abuse, condylomata acuminata and *Trichomonas vaginalis* are considered "probably diagnostic." Herpes type I may be autoinoculated to the genitorectal area and is considered "possibly diagnostic." The significance of bacterial vaginosis and genital *Mycoplasma* infection, is uncertain. New techniques, such as DNA typing of blood, semen, sperm, or tissue, may positively identify the perpetrator.

TREATMENT. Evaluation and management of sexual abuse is similar to, but more complex than, that of physical abuse. Sexual abuse is considered a criminal offense and is investigated by the police. All victims of sexual abuse require psychologic support. Parents, relatives, and siblings may deny the child's accusation and rebuke or punish the child for reporting the incident. The consequences and appropriate therapy of sexual abuse vary, depending on the type of abuse, the age and other physical and emotional factors in the victim, the frequency of abuse, and the identity of abuser. Victims of a single, nonviolent episode of touching or exposure by a stranger may need only reassurance and a chance to express their feelings about the event in one or two therapy sessions. They may be less distressed by the incident than are their parents. In contrast, a single episode of family-related sexual abuse may cause serious, long-term emotional distress and require individual and group treatment by a child psychiatrist, child psychologist, clinical social worker, arts therapist, or rape victim advocate. The therapist may recommend that the victim of incest be returned home if the perpetrator is out of the home or has confessed and is in therapy. The child victim should be placed in foster care if this is his or her desire, if the mother does not believe the child's story or is likely to encourage the child to recant, if family life is chaotic, or if collection of evidence is not yet complete. Medication to prevent pregnancy may be given to postmenarcheal girls in midcycle who have experienced vaginal intercourse within the previous 72 hr. Treatment with antibiotics is initiated to prevent sexually transmitted disease if the perpetrator is known to be infected, if the victim has signs of infection, or the likelihood of follow-up is poor. All victims should revisit their primary care physicians within 2 wk for evaluation of their psychologic functioning and to ensure that recommended services have been implemented.

Incest offenders may respond to treatment, but success requires a coordinated, multidisciplinary approach. The offending parent should be referred for psychiatric or psychologic evaluation, and the spouse should be evaluated by a social worker. Offenders should be investigated by the police, and criminal prosecution should be supported. There is evidence, especially in pedophilia, that incarceration may ensure access to and efficacy of associated treatment. Sentencing varies with the type and chronicity of offenses and potential or favorable outcome for therapy. The behavior of chronic sexual offenders may be resistant to a variety of therapies. All juvenile and prejuvenile offenders should receive therapy to prevent recurrences. In one diagnostic center, 17% of offenders were younger than 17 yr of age.

PREVENTION. The primary prevention of sexual abuse begins with teaching children the proper names of all body parts, including the names, function, and significance of "private parts" (nipples, genitalia, and rectum). The training should begin in the home and pediatrician's office by 3 yr of age and continue in school. Children should be taught to say "No" to touches by anyone to these areas and to report all the actions that make them uncomfortable to a trusted adult. Caretakers, including baby sitters and their companions, should be carefully screened by parents and agencies. Victim therapy should decrease the potential for reactive abuse. Monthly family and classroom discussions of uncomfortable events in the lives of children may reveal unsuspected abuse. To improve diagnosis and prevent reabuse, physicians should examine the genitalia and rectum routinely, become familiar with normal rectal and genital anatomy and the consequences of trauma, listen to and believe children, and be willing to report and testify.

PROGNOSIS. With early and adequate intervention, victims may lead normal adult lives. However, even with intervention, some victims may run away from home, falling prey to adolescent prostitution, violence, drug addiction, and unprepared parenthood. Others who remain at home may manifest a variety of emotional problems, including depression, suicidal gestures, decrease in school performance, and conversion reactions. As adults, victims may have difficulties with close relationships; enter abusive relationships with men; have a variety of somatic complaints of the genitourinary and other systems; and need psychiatric help for depression, anxiety, substance abuse, disassociation, and eating disorders. The risk of untoward effects are greatest for incest victims.

38.2 Nonorganic Failure to Thrive (NOFTT)

See Chapter 39 for a full discussion of organic and nonorganic failure to thrive. NOFTT mainly occurs when a child, usually an infant, is not fed adequate calories. The mother may neglect proper feeding because she is involved with external demands and the care of others, preoccupied with inner problems, ignorant about appropriate feeding, abusing substances, or does not like the infant. Emotional or maternal deprivation is inevitably concurrent with nutritional deprivation. These mothers often feel deprived and unloved themselves and may be acutely or chronically depressed. Multiple and continuing crises, frequently compounded by the physical absence of the father, may overwhelm a mother, who reacts by neglecting her infant. Poverty may also prevent a caretaker from obtaining adequate food for a child. Retarded and emotionally disturbed parents may not have the ability to provide proper care.

CLINICAL MANIFESTATIONS. The dietary history in infants with nutritional neglect may not be accurate because the parent misinforms the physician that the baby is receiving adequate calories. Depending on severity, the infant with NOFTT may exhibit thin extremities, a narrow face, prominent ribs, and wasted buttocks. Neglect of hygiene is evidenced by diaper rash, unwashed skin, untreated impetigo, uncut and dirty fingernails, or unwashed clothing. A flattened occiput with hair loss may indicate that the child has been on its back and unattended for prolonged periods. Delays in social and speech development are common. Other findings include an avoidance of eye contact, an expressionless face, and the absence of a cuddling response. The amount of time the mother spends holding, playing with, and talking to her baby is usually reduced or inappropriate. A rejecting mother often feeds her baby with anger and unnecessary force. This may result in a torn frenulum and aversion to feeding.

LABORATORY DATA. Extensive laboratory evaluation should be delayed until dietary management has been attempted for at least 1 wk and has failed. A skeletal survey is indicated in those infants who have a rejecting parent or evidence of associated physical abuse.

DIAGNOSIS. Most children with NOFTT should be hospitalized and given unlimited feedings for a minimum of 1 wk of a diet appropriate for age, that approaches 150 kcal/kg (ideal weight)/24 hr. Infants with NOFTT usually gain more than 2 oz every 24 hr for 1 wk (approximately 1 lb/wk) or have a gain that is strikingly greater than that achieved during a similar period at home. These infants may display a ravenous appetite. A nursing plan should include careful charting of intake, weight, and observations of the mother's feeding style and relationship to the child. Deprivational behaviors may improve or resolve in the hospital setting with attention from staff.

TREATMENT. All cases of NOFTT caused by underfeeding from maternal neglect should be reported to CPS. After appropriate hospital management, approximately 75% of infants are discharged home with added services for the family, 20% go into temporary foster care while the parents receive therapy, and 5% enter long-term foster care with plans for voluntary relinquishment or termination of parental rights. This decision should be based mainly on the responsiveness of the mother to treatment. Those infants who are discharged to their natural home require intensive and long-term intervention. The parents should be provided with clear, written dietary instructions at discharge and trained to hold the infant closely during feedings and to provide frequent and appropriate stimulation. Families may require homemaker, public health nurse, health visitor, and other types of outreach services. Weekly medical follow-up is needed to monitor progress.

PROGNOSIS. Without detection and intervention, a small percentage of infants with nutritional neglect die of starvation. Approximately 5–15% of these infants suffer from physical abuse. Weight loss and understature from malnutrition are reversible, but normal head circumference and brain growth may not be achieved if the infant has suffered from NOFTT beyond 6 mo of age. Emotional and educational problems occur in more than one half of these children.

38.3 Munchausen Syndrome by Proxy

The term "Munchausen syndrome" was used initially to describe situations in which patients falsified their own symptoms. In Munchausen syndrome by proxy, first described in 1977, a parent, invariably the mother, simulates or causes disease in a child. The parent may (1) fabricate a medical history; (2) cause symptoms by repeatedly exposing the child to a toxin, medication, infectious agent, or physical trauma; or (3) alter laboratory samples or temperature measurements. Depending on the parent's sophistication and secrecy, a variety of convincing, novel, and exotic diseases may be simulated or created. The parent may deny any involvement and, in instances of intentional poisoning, smothering, or trauma, may continue the action while the child is hospitalized. This syndrome is inflicted on children who are either unable or unwilling to identify the true offense and offender. The abusing caregiver gains attention from the relationships formed with health caregivers or with his or her family as a result of the problems created.

CLINICAL MANIFESTATIONS. The child's symptoms, their pattern, or the response to treatment may not be compatible with a recognized disease. They may involve any organ system and suggest a panoply of disease processes. Although generally reported in preverbal children, cases have been recognized up to 16 yr of age. There may be an associated actual disease. Symptoms are always associated with the proximity of the mother to the child. The mother usually has a background in health care, is supported by the father who may be unavailable, and presents as a devoted and "model" parent, who forms close relationships with members of the health care team. She may have a history of Munchausen syndrome and seem relatively unconcerned about the child's illness.

Apnea and seizures, two common manifestations, the observation of which may be falsified, may also be created by partial suffocation. Symptoms created by toxins, medications, water, and salts require familiarity with those substances available to families and the wide array of consequences from misuse of these substances. The clinical pattern is variable, depending on the agent, and includes forced ingestion of medications such as ipecac to cause chronic vomiting, laxatives to cause diarrhea, or injection of insulin with consequent seizures. The skin, which is more easily accessible to the perpetrator, may be burned, dyed, tattooed, lacerated, or punctured to simulate acute or chronic skin conditions. Infectious or toxic agents may be administered by any available orifice. Provision of intravenous lines during hospitalization may provide an opportunity for injection of infectious agents from feces, toxins, and pharmacologic agents. Urine and blood samples may be contaminated with foreign blood or stool.

Investigations should be based on a high index of suspicion so that unpleasant, dangerous, or unnecessary tests are not undertaken. Specimens should be analyzed for potentially harmful agents and for "foreign" blood. All steps in the diagnosis should be carefully documented. Records from other hospitals should be obtained and carefully reviewed. Hospitalized children should be under constant surveillance. This may include hidden television monitoring. Careful coordination of all individuals involved in working with the child is necessary to ensure that all information is gathered in a planned and reliable manner. Frequent staff meetings are necessary.

TREATMENT. After all laboratory information is collected and the diagnosis is established, the offending parent should be confronted by a nonaccusatory physician who offers help. Even the most sensitive approach may be met with resistance, denial, and threats. These cases should be reported promptly and with careful documentation to children's services and legal authorities. The consequences of Munchausen syndrome by proxy include persistence of abuse, emotional problems, chronic disability in 8% of cases, and death. Other siblings may be or may have been at risk; there is an association of this syndrome with unexplained infant deaths.

GENERAL

Belsey MA: Child abuse: Measuring a global problem. World Health Stat Q 46:69, 1993.

Department of Health and Human Services: National Child Abuse and Neglect Data System Working Paper 2, 1991. Summary Data Component. National Center on Child Abuse and Neglect, Washington, DC, 1993.

Reece RM: Child Abuse: Medical Diagnosis and Management. Philadelphia, Lea & Febiger, 1994.

PHYSICAL ABUSE

Carty HM: Fractures caused by child abuse. J Bone Joint Surg 75B:849, 1993.

Chadwick DL, Chin S, Salerno C, et al: Deaths from falls in children: How far is fatal? J Trauma 31:1353, 1991.

Duhaime AC, Gennarellia TA, Thibault LE, et al: The shaken baby syndrome: A clinical, pathological, and biomechanical study. J Neurosurg 66:409, 1987.

Duhaime AC, Lewander WJ, Schut L, et al: Head injury in very young children: Mechanisms, injury types, and ophthalmologic findings in 100 hospitalized patients younger than 2 years of age. Pediatrics 9:179, 1992.

Johnson CF: Inflicted injury vs accidental injury: The diagnosis of inflicted injury. Pediatr Clin North Am 37:791, 1990.

Kempe CH: The battered child syndrome. JAMA 181:17, 1962.

McClain PW, Sacks JJ, Froehlke RG, et al: Estimates of fatal child abuse and neglect, United States 1979 through 1988. Pediatrics 91:338, 1993.

Paez A, Shugerman RP, Grossman DC, et al: Epidural hemorrhage: Is it abusive? Am J Dis Child 147:421, 1993.

Williams RA: Injuries in infants and small children resulting from witnessed and corroborated free falls. J Trauma 31:1350, 1991.

Wilson EF: Estimation of the age of cutaneous contusions in child abuse. Pediatrics 60:751, 1977.

SEXUAL ABUSE

Adams JA: Significance of medical findings in suspected sexual abuse: Moving toward consensus. J Child Sexual Abuse 1:91, 1993.

Bays J, Chadwick D: Medical diagnosis of the sexually abused child. Child Abuse Negl 17:91, 1993.

Bays J, Jenny C: Genital and anal conditions confused with child sexual abuse. Am J Dis Child 144:1319, 1990.

Faller KC: Child sexual abuse allegations: How to decide when they are true. Violence Update 4:1, 1994.

French GM, Johnson CF: Genital bleeding: Two uncommon causes in patients referred to a sexual abuse clinic. Clin Pediatr 33:38, 1994.

Gibbons M, Vincent EC: Childhood sexual abuse. Am Fam Physician 49:125, 1994.

McCann J, Voris J, Simon M: Genital injuries resulting from sexual abuse: A longitudinal study. Pediatrics 89:307, 1992.

McCann J, Voris J, Simon M, et al: Perianal findings in prepubertal children selected for nonabuse: A descriptive study. Child Abuse Negl 13:179, 1989.

NONORGANIC FAILURE TO THRIVE

Rosenn DW, Loeb LS, Jura MB: Differentiation of organic from non-organic failure to thrive in infancy. Pediatrics 66:698, 1980.

Schmitt BD, Mauro RD: Nonorganic failure to thrive: An outpatient approach. Child Abuse Neglect 13:235, 1989.

MUNCHAUSEN SYNDROME BY PROXY

Rosenberg DD: Web of deceit: a literature review of Munchausen syndrome by proxy. Child Abuse Neglect 11:547, 1987.

Schreier HA, Libow JA: Munchausen syndrome by proxy: Diagnosis and prevalence. Am J Orthopsychiatry 63:318, 1993.

OTHER TYPES OF CHILD MALTREATMENT

Dine MS, McGovern ME: Intentional poisoning of children—an overlooked category of child abuse: Report of seven cases and review of the literature. Pediatrics 70:32, 1982.

Garbarino J: The psychologically battered child: Toward a definition. Pediatr Ann 18:502, 1989.

Garbarino J: Psychological child maltreatment—a developmental view. Primary Care 20:6, 1993.

Johnson CF: Physicians and medical neglect: Variables which affect reporting. Child Abuse Neglect 17:605, 1993.

PART V

Children with Special Health Needs

CHAPTER 39

Failure to Thrive

Howard Bauchner

Failure to thrive (FTT) refers to an infant or child whose physical growth is significantly less than that of his or her peers, and it often leads to poor developmental and socioemotional functioning. Although there is no clear consensus regarding the definition, FTT usually refers to a child growing below the 3rd or 5th percentile or a child whose decreased growth has crossed two major growth percentiles (i.e., from above the 75th percentile to below the 25th) in a short time. Traditionally, the diagnosis has been divided into two categories. Organic FTT refers to a child with an underlying medical condition; nonorganic or psychosocial FTT refers to a child who is younger than age 5 yr and has no known medical condition that causes poor growth (also see Chapter 38.2).

EPIDEMIOLOGY AND ETIOLOGY. The prevalence of FTT depends on the population sampled. From 5–10% of low birthweight children and children living in poverty may have FTT. Family discord, neonatal problems other than low birthweight, and maternal depression are also associated with FTT. In the United States, psychosocial FTT is far more common than organic FTT.

The causes of organic FTT are numerous (Table 39–1). Every organ system is represented. Psychosocial FTT is most often due to poor child-parent interaction. Organic and nonorganic etiologic factors may also occur together, for example, in child abuse and neglect or a temperamentally difficult premature infant.

CLINICAL MANIFESTATIONS. The clinical presentation of FTT ranges from failure to meet expected age norms for height and weight, to alopecia, loss of subcutaneous fat, reduced muscle mass, dermatitis, recurrent infections, marasmus, and kwashiorkor. In developed countries, the most common presentation is poor growth detected in the ambulatory setting; in developing countries, recurrent infections, marasmus, and kwashiorkor are more common presentations.

The degree of failure to thrive is usually measured by calculating each growth parameter (weight, height, and weight/height ratio) as a percentage of the median value for age based on appropriate growth charts. Appropriate growth charts are often not available for children with specific medical problems; serial measurements are especially important for these children. For premature infants, correction must be made for the extent of prematurity. Corrected age, rather than chronologic age, should be used in calculations of their growth until 1–2 yr of corrected age.

For weight, mild, moderate, and severe FTT is equivalent to 75–90%, 60–74%, and less than 60% of standard, respectively. For height, the corresponding values are 90–95%, 85–89%, and less than 85%. For the weight/height ratio, the values are 81–90%, 70–80%, and less than 70%. Traditionally, the weight for age percent of the standard value decreases early in the course of failure to thrive, followed by a decrement of height for age. Children with chronic malnutrition often have a normal weight for height because both their weight and height are reduced.

The laboratory evaluation of children with FTT is often not helpful and, therefore, should be used judiciously. A complete blood count, lead level, urinalysis, and set of electrolyte values represent a reasonable initial screen. Other tests, such as thyroid function studies, tests for gastroesophageal reflux and malabsorption, organic and amino acids, or a sweat test, should be performed if indicated by the history and/or physical examination.

DIAGNOSIS. The history, physical examination, and observation of the parent-child interaction usually suggests the diagnosis. The latter observation, especially with feeding, is often critical to the diagnosis of psychosocial FTT.

The causes of insufficient growth include (1) failure of a parent to offer adequate calories, (2) failure of the children to take sufficient calories, and (3) failure of the child to retain sufficient calories. Reasons why a parent or their substitute may not offer appropriate or sufficient foods include lack of knowledge, parental depression, unusual dietary beliefs, or lack of food. With young infants, it is particularly important to

TABLE 39–1 Major Organic Causes of Failure To Thrive

System	Cause
Gastrointestinal	Gastroesophageal reflux, celiac disease, pyloric stenosis, cleft palate/cleft lip, lactose intolerance, Hirschsprung disease, milk protein intolerance, hepatitis, cirrhosis, pancreatic insufficiency, biliary disease, inflammatory bowel disease, malabsorption
Renal	Urinary tract infection, renal tubular acidosis, diabetes insipidus, chronic renal insufficiency
Cardiopulmonary	Cardiac diseases leading to congestive heart failure, asthma, bronchopulmonary dysplasia, cystic fibrosis, anatomic abnormalities of the upper airway
Endocrine	Hypothyroidism, diabetes mellitus, adrenal insufficiency or excess, parathyroid disorders, pituitary disorders, growth hormone deficiency
Neurologic	Mental retardation, cerebral hemorrhages, degenerative disorders
Infectious	Parasitic or bacterial infections of the gastrointestinal tract, tuberculosis, human immunodeficiency virus disease
Metabolic	Inborn errors of metabolism
Congenital	Chromosomal abnormalities, congenital syndromes (fetal alcohol syndrome), perinatal infections
Miscellaneous	Lead poisoning, malignancy, collagen vascular disease, recurrently infected adenoids and tonsils

■ TABLE 39–2 Approach to Failure to Thrive Based on Age

Age of Onset	Major Diagnostic Consideration
Birth to 3 mo	Psychosocial failure to thrive, perinatal infections, gastroesophageal reflux, inborn errors of metabolism, cystic fibrosis
3–6 mo	Psychosocial failure to thrive, human immunodeficiency virus infection, gastroesophageal reflux, inborn errors of metabolism, milk-protein intolerance, cystic fibrosis, renal tubular acidosis
7–12 mo	Psychosocial failure to thrive (autonomy struggles), delayed introduction of solids, gastroesophageal reflux, intestinal parasites, renal tubular acidosis
12+ mo	Psychosocial failure to thrive (coercive feeding, new psychologic stressor), gastroesophageal reflux

Adapted from Frank D, Silva M, Needlman R: Failure to thrive: Mystery, myth and method. Contemp Pediatr 10:114, 1993.

■ TABLE 39–3 Approach to Failure to Thrive Based on Signs and Symptoms

History/Physical Examination	Diagnostic Consideration
Spitting, vomiting, food refusal	Gastroesophageal reflux
Diarrhea, fatty stools	Malabsorption, intestinal parasite, milk-protein intolerance
Snoring, mouth breathing, enlarged tonsils	Adenoid hypertrophy
Recurrent wheezing, pulmonary infections	Asthma, aspiration
Recurrent infections	Human immunodeficiency virus disease
Travel to/from developing countries	Parasitic or bacterial infections of the gastrointestinal tract

Adapted from Frank D, Silva M, Needlman R: Failure to thrive: Mystery, myth and method. Contemp Pediatr 10:114, 1993.

obtain a detailed dietary history, including how often the infant is fed and how the parent responds when the child cries or sleeps for prolonged periods. A child may have difficulty swallowing if he or she has oral-motor dysfunction, anatomic abnormalities, cardiopulmonary dysfunction, or enlarged and recurrently infected tonsils and adenoids. Vomiting, diarrhea, and malabsorption are general causes of inadequate caloric absorption. It may be helpful to approach the diagnosis in terms of age (Table 39–2) or signs and symptoms (Table 39–3).

TREATMENT. The treatment of FTT requires an understanding of all the elements that contribute to a child's growth: the child's health and nutritional status, family issues, and the parent-child interaction. Regardless of cause, an appropriate feeding atmosphere at home is important. Children with severe malnutrition must be refed carefully.

For children with organic FTT, the underlying medical condition should be treated. The type of caloric supplementation must be based on the severity of FTT and the underlying medical condition. For example, in children with renal failure, the amount of protein in the diet must be carefully monitored. The response to caloric supplementation depends on the specific diagnosis, medical treatment, and severity of FTT.

For older infants and young children with psychosocial FTT, meal times should be approximately 20–30 min, solid foods should be offered before liquids, environmental distractions should be minimized, and the child should eat with other people and not be force fed. The intake of water, juice, and low-calorie beverages should be limited. High-calorie foods, such as peanut butter, whole milk, cheese, and dried fruits, should be emphasized. Sometimes high-calorie supplementation, such as Polycose, or high-calorie liquids, such as Carnation Instant Breakfast with whole milk, or formulas containing more than 20 calories per ounce (Pediasure and Ensure) are necessary. Weight gain in response to adequate caloric feedings usually establishes the diagnosis of psychosocial FTT.

Indications for hospitalization include severe malnutrition, further diagnostic and laboratory evaluation, lack of catch-up growth, and evaluation of the parent-child feeding interaction. Parents of children with organic FTT should be comfortable with the diagnosis and treatment before discharge. The treatment in the hospital should be similar to the treatment at home. For psychosocial FTT, the hospitalization often lasts 10 days to 2 wk. Caloric intake should be monitored, and the parent-child feeding interaction should be observed (Chapter 38.2). The goals of the hospitalization are to obtain sustained catch-up growth and educate parents about appropriate foods and feeding styles.

PROGNOSIS. FTT in the 1st yr of life, regardless of cause, is particularly ominous. Maximal postnatal brain growth occurs during the first 6 mo of life. The brain grows as much during the 1st yr of life, as during the rest of a child's life. Approximately one third of children with psychosocial FTT are developmentally delayed with social and emotional problems. The prognosis of children with organic FTT is more variable, depending on the specific diagnosis and severity of FTT. Ongoing assessment and monitoring of cognitive and emotional development, with appropriate intervention, is necessary for all children with FTT.

Berwick DM, Levey JC, Kleinerman R: Failure to thrive: diagnostic yield of hospitalization. Arch Dis Child 57:347, 1982.
Bithoney WG, Dubowitz H, Egan H: Failure to thrive/growth deficiency. Pediatr Rev 13:453, 1992.
Drotar D, Sturm L: Prediction of intellectual development in young children with early histories of nonorganic failure-to-thrive. J Pediatr Psychol 13:281, 1988.
Frank D, Silva M, Needlman R: Failure to thrive: Mystery, myth and method. Contemp Pediatr 10:114, 1993.
Kelleher KJ, Casey PH, Bradley RH, et al: Risk factors and outcomes for failure to thrive in low birth weight preterm infants. Pediatrics 91:941, 1993.
Wilcox WD, Neiburg P, Miller DS: Failure to thrive—a continuing problem of definition. Clin Pediatr 28:391, 1989.
Wright CM, Waterston A, Aynsley-Green A: Effect of deprivation on weight gain in infancy. Acta Paediatr 83:357, 1994.

CHAPTER 40

Developmental Disabilities and Chronic Illness: An Overview

James M. Perrin and Jack P. Shonkoff

Children with special health needs constitute a heterogeneous population that includes youngsters with a wide variety of developmental disabilities and chronic illnesses. In some cases, persistent problems may overlap, such as when a child with bronchopulmonary dysplasia also has delayed development, or when a child with mental retardation develops diabetes mellitus. Other children fit more clearly into one group or another, such as a youngster with cystic fibrosis who has no cognitive or developmental problems, or a physically healthy child with a complex learning disorder. Nevertheless, a core of basic considerations is applicable to most children with special health needs, and these issues are discussed first in this section.

Most children receive the majority of their health care from a single provider and are educated in regular school settings that require no modifications to meet special developmental or health concerns. Children with special health needs, on the other hand, may see a variety of health care specialists (e.g., neurologists, orthopedists, and cardiologists), interact with multiple professionals (e.g., occupational therapists, respiratory therapists, nutritionists, and psychologists), and need major adaptive modifications in their school setting (e.g., barrier-free facilities, special education services, and specialized nursing care).

Some chronic conditions that are determined genetically are wholly preventable through utilization of new measures for determining carrier states prior to conception and through techniques for prenatal diagnosis. Although emerging advances in molecular genetics are likely to diminish further the incidence of inherited disease, the wide range of conditions that lead to special health needs during childhood and the continued lack of understanding of the causes of many of these disorders make it likely that large numbers of youngsters will continue to manifest chronic impairments of health or development.

An appreciation of the multiple levels at which prevention or treatment efforts can be implemented for children with special health needs requires an understanding of the differences inherent among the concepts of disease, functional limitation, and disability. *Disease* refers to a specific health condition affecting a child, such as arthritis or congenital cytomegalovirus (CMV) infection. *Functional limitation* refers to the problem brought about as a result of the symptoms of the disease, such as a poorly functioning knee or a hearing impairment. *Disability,* on the other hand, refers to the social implications or consequences of having the disease or disability, such as the inability to participate competitively in sports or the social isolation that results from difficulty in communicating orally.

Physicians can play a key role in preventing the occurrence of many special health needs and in diminishing their impact on a child's growth and development. Intervention may be targeted at any level—that of the disease, the functional limitation, or the disability. For the child with arthritis, efforts are directed both toward reducing joint inflammation and toward removing barriers to participation in age-appropriate physical activities. For the child with congenital CMV and deafness, successful management focuses on both audiologic habilitation and social integration. Both types of children have a chronic health condition, although neither may necessarily be perceived as "chronically ill." The two terms (condition and illness) are used interchangeably in the following discussion.

Early detection of persistent conditions, amelioration of the functional consequences of specific disabilities, and prevention of secondary psychosocial handicaps are central to the provision of care for children with special health needs. However, health care providers occasionally and inappropriately refer to such children by the name of their condition, such as "asthmatics," "sicklers," "leukemics," or "Down's babies." This tendency to characterize children by their disease or disability influences both parental and professional attitudes as well as their assessments of the child's current abilities and their expectations for his or her future. In general, parents and professionals should work together on behalf of a child who has a disease rather than allowing the disease to define the child.

The importance of early intervention programs as a mechanism for decreasing the impact of special health or developmental needs on children and their families is increasingly recognized. Because of their strategic relationship with young children and their parents, physicians have an important responsibility with regard to early identification of children at risk and referral to the appropriate services. This includes the need to maintain accurate and updated information on all available resources within a community to ensure that families have access to a full range of needed services. Programs that incorporate the best practices provide individualized services designed to strengthen the inherent adaptiveness of participating children and families. Furthermore, because the best predictors of the well-being of children with special health needs include factors that relate to family functioning, effective pediatric management should embody a comprehensive approach to the child within the context of the family, addressing the needs of all of its members. This will enhance the prospects for a positive outcome.

Several public programs in the United States assist families with children having special health needs. Title V Maternal and Child Health Programs for Children with Special Health Needs provides a variety of coordinating and multidisciplinary clinical services for children who have many chronic illnesses and developmental disabilities. The Individuals with Disability Education Act (IDEA) supports state-sponsored early intervention and special education programs and mandates an appropriate education in the least restrictive environment for children having disabilities. The Supplemental Security Income Program provides cash benefits for families whose children have severe physical, mental, or developmental disabilities, as well as public health insurance coverage (i.e., Medicaid) in almost every state.

In summary, children with special health needs and their families are a diverse group who share common experiences. Those who have symptoms of illness for more than 3 mo or who require hospitalization or extensive home- or community-based health services for more than 1 mo in a 12-mo period are said to have a chronic disease. Children with developmental disabilities, on the other hand, have been defined by the Federal Developmental Disabilities Assistance and Bill of Rights Act Amendments of 1987 as individuals with impairments in physical or mental abilities that are manifested before 22 yr of age, are likely to persist indefinitely, and result in functional limitations in major life activities. Mental retardation is the prototypic developmental disability; others include cerebral palsy, specific learning disabilities, pervasive developmental disorder, autism, visual or hearing impairments, and disorders of communication.

40.1 Chronic Illness in Childhood

James M. Perrin

EPIDEMIOLOGY, SEVERITY, AND OUTCOME

The epidemiology of chronic illness in childhood differs in important ways from the epidemiology of long-term illness in adults. Adults face a relatively small number of common chronic conditions (e.g., diabetes, osteoarthritis, and coronary artery disease) and few rare diseases. Children, in contrast, face a wide variety of mainly quite rare diseases. Only two groups of chronic physical conditions in childhood are common: allergic disorders (mainly asthma, eczema, and hayfever) and neurologic disorders (mainly seizure disorders and neuromuscular conditions such as cerebral palsy). Other conditions often thought to be common, such as childhood diabetes, occur only in about 1 in 1,000 children younger than 16 yr of age, a much lower rate than that seen in adults. Many of the conditions described in this textbook occur with a frequency of much less than 1 in 1,000. Table 40–1 indicates prevalence rates for representative childhood conditions.

These epidemiologic distinctions have implications for both physicians and families. The adult epidemiologic pattern means that health care providers for adults have frequent daily experience with the common chronic illnesses of adults, remaining current and knowledgeable about such conditions as hypertension. Similarly, an adult who has been newly diagnosed with high blood pressure probably knows something about the disease and has friends or family members with hypertension.

■ **TABLE 40–1 Estimated Prevalence of Representative Childhood Chronic Conditions, Ages 0–20, United States, 1980**

Chronic Conditions	Rates/1,000
Asthma (moderate and severe)	10.00
Congenital heart disease	7.00
Seizure disorder	3.50
Arthritis	2.20
Diabetes mellitus	1.80
Cleft lip/palate	1.50
Down syndrome	1.10
Spina bifida	0.40
Sickle cell anemia	0.28
Cystic fibrosis	0.20
Hemophilia	0.15
Acute lymphocytic leukemia	0.11
Chronic renal failure	0.08
Muscular dystrophy	0.06

Adapted from Gortmaker SL, Sappenfield W: Chronic childhood disorders: Prevalence and impact. Pediatr Clin North Am 31:3, 1984.

The practicing pediatrician, however, may see a new case of a malignancy only once a decade and will make the diagnosis of cystic fibrosis or even diabetes infrequently. A family whose child has been newly diagnosed with a rare condition may never even have heard the name of the disease prior to its onset in their child. These epidemiologic facts mean that child health care providers have a difficult task in identifying children with rare conditions and in staying current with the new technologies applicable to rare diseases.

The aggregate number of children with all types of chronic health conditions is high, despite the rarity of individual conditions, mainly because the number of different conditions that affect children is very large. At least 10–20% of American and British children have some chronic condition, and some studies indicate that the number may be even higher. This percentage translates into at least 10 million or more children in the United States with some kind of chronic health condition. Most chronic conditions are mild, such as acne, hayfever, or mild congenital deformity causing a slight limp. Only about 2–4% of children (1–2 million children) have diseases of such physiologic severity that they interfere with a child's usual daily activities on a regular basis.

Severity, a notion simple in concept, is difficult to measure in most chronic illnesses. Few illnesses have a clear biologic marker that is independent of environmental influences and treatment (the factor VIII level in hemophilia is an exception to this rule). Physiologic measures of severity (e.g., asthma rating scales or hemoglobin A_{1c} in diabetes) reflect the interaction of biologic susceptibility, treatment, and other environmental factors. The impact of the condition on the child's functioning with friends or in school or on his or her psychologic status are other aspects of severity. Although this chapter focuses on health conditions that are relatively severe in physiologic terms, many of the issues discussed affect children with milder conditions. Further, one type of severity (e.g., physiologic) may correlate poorly with others (e.g., psychologic or functional).

The percentage of children with severe long-term illnesses has more than doubled in the past 2 decades (Fig. 40–1). This change partly reflects major advances in the technology of medical and surgical care. Current estimates are that, even among severely ill children, at least 90% survive to young adulthood, although often with significant physical morbidity and psychologic disturbance. Most adolescents with chronic conditions, however, make the transition to adulthood well, with little interference in their finishing education, becoming employed, and entering into significant interpersonal relationships. Conditions that may show major changes in incidence, thereby affecting the size of the total population of children with severe illnesses, include AIDS, the aftereffects of fetal substance exposure, and major pulmonary or neurologic disease in children leaving neonatal intensive care units. Alternatively, new genetic techniques allow the prenatal and preconception diagnosis of increasing numbers of health conditions, and genetic counseling and other interventions may diminish the incidence of several diseases.

ISSUES COMMON TO DIVERSE CHRONIC CONDITIONS

Health care providers typically view each chronic illness as a distinct and separate entity that has its own etiology, natural history, treatment, complications, and physiologic impact. However, families whose children have a variety of long-term illnesses face several issues in common, reflecting chronicity itself rather than aspects of the specific disease (Table 40–2).

First, many chronic childhood illnesses are high-cost health conditions. A small percentage of children with major chronic illnesses utilize a large proportion of the child health dollar; 2–4% of children with severe long-term illnesses account for at least 35% of all child health expenditures. These figures reflect only what is paid by public or private insurance. Families face many other costs, such as the costs of transportation, long-distance phone calls, and special diets, few of which may be reimbursed. Furthermore, chronic illness in a child makes

Figure 40–1. Estimated percentage of American children, aged birth through 16 yr, with any limitation of activity due to chronic conditions (1960–1989). (From unpublished analyses by Newacheck of data from the National Center for Health Statistics, Current Estimates from the National Health Interview Survey, Series 10, Annual Reports.)

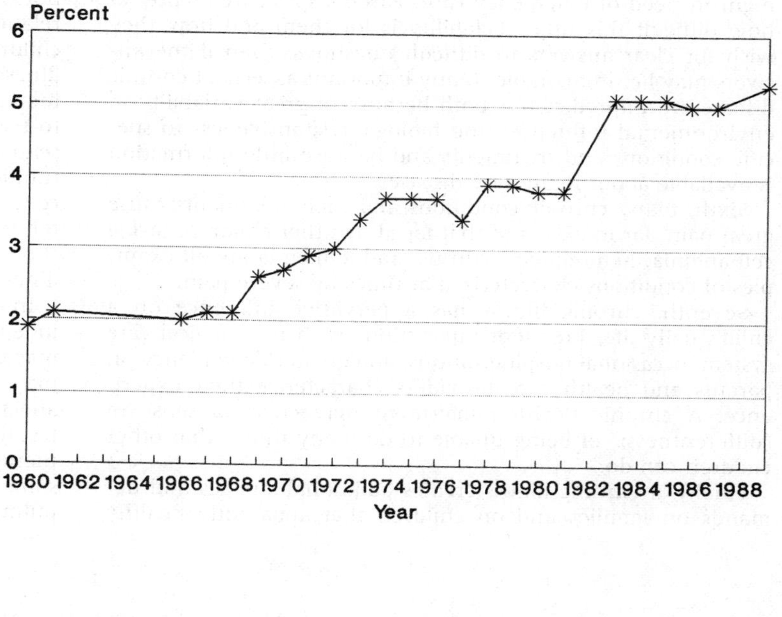

■ **TABLE 40–2 Common Issues for Children with Chronic Illnesses and Their Families**

Costly treatments	Unpredictability
Burden of care on families	Pain
Multiple providers and treatments	Effects on child's daily life
Rarity and isolation	Stress and psychologic impact

it more difficult for both parents to work outside the home, thereby diminishing families' financial resources.

Second, the daily burden of care rests mainly on the families, and that burden can be extensive, as with a family with two teenagers with muscular dystrophy, both wheelchair bound and requiring transportation from place to place, or with a youngster with cystic fibrosis who needs extensive pulmonary care prior to leaving for school each day. These daily burdens greatly extend the work of families.

Third, whereas most children require only a single health care provider for most of their health care and supervision, children with long-term health conditions frequently have multiple providers and multiple treatments. A child with hemophilia may have contact with a hematologist, a pediatrician, a specialized dentist, an orthopedist, a hematology nurse, a physical therapist, a psychologist, and a social worker, among others. The recommendations of any one member of this group may vary from those of another, and families must often choose among conflicting advice. Clinically, there usually are trade-offs among the choices, such as the optimal time to do a surgical procedure or the trade-off between seizure control and alertness. Pediatricians can help families make informed choices.

Fourth, the comparative rarity of most childhood chronic conditions makes families feel isolated. They often wonder why they have been singled out by an unusual condition and feel that no other families have had similar experiences. Several programs in specialty centers (e.g., cystic fibrosis or arthritis centers) and several parent advocacy programs have worked to break this sense of isolation through groups that help parents learn from each other how to raise children with chronic illnesses.

Fifth, many of these conditions are unpredictable in their implications, longevity, complications, and developmental impact on the individual child. The parent whose child has leukemia wonders whether new bleeding signals a relapse that will have a fatal outcome or will be followed by a permanent remission. The parent whose child has mild wheezing at bedtime does not know whether the child will sleep well through the night or awaken severely dyspneic in the middle of the night in need of emergency care. Parents speak frequently of how difficult this unpredictability is for them and how they wish for clear answers to difficult questions, even if the answers may be unfavorable. Many important aspects of chronic disease are unpredictable, both because of great variability in environmental influences and biologic responsiveness to specific conditions and treatments and because little information is available about many rare diseases.

Sixth, many chronic conditions and their treatments cause great pain, far in excess of that faced by other children. Sickle cell anemia, hemophilia, arthritis, and leukemia are all examples of conditions characterized at times by severe pain.

Seventh, chronic illness has a pervasive influence on a child's daily life. Frequent interactions with the medical care system, occasional hospitalizations, and greater dependency on parents and health care providers characterize their experience. A chronic health impairment may create a sense of "differentness," of being unable to do many things that other children can do.

Finally, a chronic illness creates additional stresses and demands on families and on children that apparently healthy children do not face. Perhaps as a result, chronically ill children have about twice the frequency of psychologic or behavioral problems found in healthy controls; children with significant neurologic handicaps or sensory deficits have as much as a 5 times greater risk for these problems. The level of severity correlates poorly with psychologic status. Despite this greater risk of psychologic maladjustment, most children with chronic health conditions are psychologically healthy.

DEVELOPMENTAL ASPECTS OF LONG-TERM ILLNESS

Two issues are central to an understanding of the developmental implications of long-term childhood illness: the development of children's understanding of illness mechanisms and the impact of illness at different stages of child development.

Clinicians working with children who have long-term illnesses should understand the developmental stage of their patients' understanding of illness in order to explain illness and its mechanisms in age-appropriate terms. Because children's understanding follows a typical pattern of growth in cognitive abilities, children need different explanations of their continuing disease as they mature. Young children of preschool or early school age tend to have a concrete and relatively superficial understanding of illness. They view illness as a response to their bad behavior or not following the rules (such as wearing a coat when you go outside in the cold). Children at this age believe that getting well occurs by adhering to another set of rules. By about the 4th–6th grade, children begin to differentiate themselves from external events that may cause illness. For this age group, germ theory seems very important; with the notion that germs cause almost all illnesses, illness can be prevented by avoiding germs, and better results will be gained from taking medicines, which are seen as fighting germs. This notion of germs can cause confusion or isolation for children of this age who have conditions such as leukemia or diabetes. By 8th grade or even later, children begin to understand the physiologic mechanisms for illness, appreciating the many interrelated causes of illness and the several symptoms of illness. At this age, children usually begin to understand the interaction of body parts, for example, that lungs and hearts are not only near each other but actually work together to maintain body functions.

Physical illness has different impacts on children based on their stage of development. In infancy, the illness may affect the parameters of growth and development by influencing feeding, sleeping, motor abilities (and therefore exploration of the environment), or sensory functions. Physical deformity or fatigue may affect a child's responsiveness to parents, who may in turn react differently to this child. Frequent hospitalizations may interfere with the normal development of trusting relationships within a family. In later preschool years, when children are developing autonomy, mobility, and self-control, illness may again interfere with these important developmental functions. Early school-aged children may be subject to teasing from classmates; they may need to be absent from school for illness or its treatment and thus miss normal opportunities for early socialization. Middle childhood and adolescence are periods when children expand their areas of competence; responsibility for the care of the child's health condition should shift gradually from the parents to the child. Chronic illness may interfere with this process.

In adolescence, illness may affect the individual's developing independence, greater responsibility for self-care, growing intimacy, and planning for the future. The disease or its treatment may be particularly embarrassing for adolescents and may affect their body image. Adolescence is frequently a time to test the limits of the illness and compliance with recommended therapies. Health conditions that require another person for some care, such as the teenager with cystic fibrosis who needs pulmonary physical therapy before each day of high school, may hinder growth toward independence. Sensitivity to the developmental impact of chronic illness will help clinicians provide their patients with appropriate planning and anticipatory guidance and help children and their families find acceptable ways of fulfilling the normal developmental tasks of childhood and adolescence.

Children should take increasing responsibility for the management of their own health condition commensurate with their level of maturity, developmental stage, and understanding of their illness. Areas of responsibility include monitoring the condition, assessing indicators of change and exacerbation, asking for help, and self-medication (both at home and at school). Families may need help in learning ways to foster responsibility, and children need education and advice in learning how to become independent in appropriate ways.

INTEGRATING CHILDREN WITH CHRONIC CONDITIONS INTO COMMUNITIES

Changing interests of families and changing notions of the civil rights of people with disabilities have fostered an increasing emphasis on family-centered services for children with chronic conditions. Parents increasingly take responsibility for monitoring and managing the care of their child, and more care is provided in or near the child's home and less in hospitals. Families want most care to be community based, both in the sense of receiving as many services as close to home as possible and in the sense of integrating their chronically ill child into the usual community activities, not limiting him or her to services provided for children with special health needs. The Iowa model of providing most care for children with malignancies through community-based physicians, with supervision and coordination of specialty care provided at the university health center, illustrates that complex health services can be delivered close to home.

Community-based services also strengthen early socialization of the child, mainly through participation in community services such as child care, and later social and educational development through participation in regular school programs. Chronic illness accounts for a sizable number of school absences by children. Part of that time away from classes reflects the direct effects of illness, such as increased fatigue or necessary hospitalization; however, some represents the need to travel great distances for treatments that are often available only during regular school hours.

Some children with chronic illnesses, especially those with cognitive impairments, need special education services. However, most children with long-term illnesses have no intrinsic cognitive impairment and should be in regular education programs. They may need specialized health services (e.g., access to medicines or planning for emergencies) in order to participate in school, and children who must miss classes frequently need home-bound and hospital-bound instruction to allow them to keep up with their classmates.

Families whose children have long-term health conditions should have access to a wide range of coordinated and comprehensive services. The specific services needed by any one family will vary considerably from those needed by another and will change over time as the child grows and the family changes. The main groups of services that should be available for families include primary and specialized medical and surgical care; nursing services, especially those that will help to strengthen a family's own skills in caring for their child; preventive and therapeutic mental health services; social services; educational planning; and certain special therapies, such as physical therapy, occupational therapy, or nutritional services. Preventive mental health services help to diminish the risk of psychologic problems related to the chronicity of the child's condition.

Partly because of the emphasis on specialized medical services, children with chronic health conditions lack regular pediatric health supervision more than other children. Chronically ill children have lower rates of immunization and screening for common health problems and often lack anticipatory guidance in key areas of growth and development, such as behavior and discipline in the preschool years, preparation for entry to school, and preparation for adolescence, with developing sexuality, growth of independence, and opportunity for substance abuse. All children need primary care services, and each of these areas has special significance for children who have chronic conditions.

Teamwork among the multiple professionals and the family and coordination of care are important to serve families of chronically ill children effectively. For some families, especially in the first months or years after the initial diagnosis of a long-term condition, care coordination by another person is an essential service. Most parents prefer to coordinate the care for their children themselves, especially after they become knowledgeable about their child's condition and its management. Therefore, the education of both parents and child about the disease process, its management, its complications, and its developmental implications is a central part of the therapeutic effort.

PEDIATRIC CARE IN THE COMMUNITY

Community pediatricians have a central role in the care of children with chronic illnesses and in supporting their families. Although the pediatrician's involvement may begin with diagnosis and referral to specialty services, the pediatrician should also assume responsibility as a continuing advocate for the child and family. This includes continuing communication with specialty providers and helping families make informed choices, especially when advice is conflicting. Other responsibilities include continued support to children and family members, helping families find appropriate community resources to meet their needs, and, especially, collaboration with schools and other community agencies to integrate the child into the community. Tasks with agencies include referral to early intervention services, when appropriate; providing information that may help determine whether a child needs special or regular education services; and helping the child obtain the school services that enhance school attendance. Needed school services typically include appropriate nursing and related services and access to medications or emergency care, although a few children require more extensive services, including personal attendants.

Communication with families is particularly important. Families want clear information, with details that they can understand and information about both positive and negative aspects of the child's condition. They particularly appreciate receiving information and support from a professional familiar to them who provides compassionate and caring services. The child should also participate in developmentally appropriate ways in information sharing.

American Academy of Pediatrics: Screening infants and young children for developmental disabilities. Pediatrics 93:863, 1994.

Gortmaker SL, Sappenfield W: Chronic childhood disorders: prevalence and impact. Pediatr Clin North Am 31:3, 1984.

Institute of Medicine: Disability in America: Toward a National Agenda for Prevention. Washington, DC, National Academy Press, 1991.

Kisker CT, Strayer F, Wong K, et al: Health outcomes of a community-based therapy program for children with cancer. Pediatrics 66:900, 1980.

Newacheck PW, Stoddard JJ: Prevalence and impact of multiple childhood chronic illness. J Pediatr 124:40, 1994.

Perrin EC, Gerrity PS: There's a demon in your belly: children's understanding of illness. Pediatrics 67:841, 1981.

Perrin EC, Gerrity PS: Development of children with chronic illness. Pediatr Clin North Am 31:19, 1984.

Perrin EC, Newacheck P, Pless IB, et al: Issues involved in the definition and classification of chronic health conditions. Pediatrics 91:787, 1993.

Perrin JM, Shayne MW, Bloom SR: Home and Community Care for Chronically Ill Children. New York, Oxford University Press, 1993.
Pless IB, Power C, Peckham CS: Long-term sequelae of chronic physical disorders in childhood. Pediatrics 91:1131, 1993.
Stein REK (ed): Caring for Children with Chronic Illness. New York, Springer, 1989.
Stein REK, Perrin EC, Pless IB, et al: Severity of illness: concepts and measurements. Lancet 2:1506, 1987.

40.2 Mental Retardation

Jack P. Shonkoff

Mental retardation is a condition of both clinical and social importance. It is characterized by limitations in performance that result from significant impairments in measured intelligence and adaptive behavior. It also confers a social status that can be more handicapping than the specific disability itself. Because the boundaries between "normality" and "retardation" frequently are difficult to delineate, the pediatric identification, evaluation, and care of children with cognitive difficulties and their families require a considerable level of both technical sophistication and interpersonal sensitivity.

Dramatic changes in social and political attitudes toward persons with developmental disabilities during the last 2 decades have revolutionized the pediatric approach to children with mental retardation. Previous practices of withholding life-saving measures from neonates with congenital abnormalities have been modified by legally sanctioned treatments for children with profound and irreversible disorders. The practice of almost automatically placing young children with disabilities in residential institutions has been replaced by extensive efforts to develop community-based service systems that coordinate resources for both children and their families. The pediatric responsibility has shifted from helping to "put the child away" to "normalizing" the life of the child and his or her family.

Concurrent with this shift in sociopolitical values, our theoretical and empirical understanding of the phenomenon of mental retardation has also changed. The expanding knowledge base has led to a rejection of the simplistic debate over "organic" versus "environmental" causes of retardation and to a growing recognition of the mutually interactive contributions of both nature and nurture to the development of all children. Consequently, the traditional medical focus on neuropathology has been expanded to an assessment of the interplay among the biologic factors in the child, the adaptive characteristics of the family, and the social context in which they live.

In 1992, the American Association on Mental Retardation revised its official definition to formalize the paradigm shift from viewing mental retardation as an individual trait to thinking of it as an expression of the interaction between a person with limited intellectual functioning and the environment. Consequently, categories of mild, moderate, severe, and profound retardation have been replaced by a classification system that specifies four levels of support systems needed for daily functioning (i.e., intermittent, limited, extensive, and pervasive). Four assumptions were articulated as essential to the appropriate application of the new definition as follows: (1) valid assessment considers cultural and linguistic diversities; (2) limitations in adaptive skills occur within the context of community environments typical of age peers and indexed to individualized needs for supports; (3) adaptive limitations coexist with strengths; and (4) with appropriate and sustained supports, the life functioning of individuals with mental retardation will generally improve.

ETIOLOGY AND PATHOGENESIS. The determinants of competence in any individual are complex and multifactorial. Regardless of his or her level of performance, each child's abilities are influenced by both the integrity and maturational status of the nervous system and by the nature and quality of his or her life experience. Some children sustain significant neurologic insults and develop normal skills. Others manifest severe cognitive impairment despite the absence of recognizable focal neurologic findings or historical evidence of significant risk factors for central nervous system dysfunction. The neurobiologic roots of mental retardation may be found among such diverse factors as structural malformations of the brain, metabolic abnormalities, and central nervous system deficits related to infection, malnutrition, or hypoxic-ischemic injury. The experiential precursors of retardation may be identified in histories of dysfunctional caregiving related to parental psychopathology, extreme family disorganization, or economic hardship. Children who live in poverty are particularly susceptible to the cumulative burdens of both social stress and the greater biologic vulnerability related to a higher prevalence of such risk factors as perinatal complications and nutritional deficiencies.

Table 40–3 lists potential contributing factors in the pathogenesis of mental retardation from preconception through the early childhood years. Few of the etiologic factors included in this table, however, provide a complete explanation for the phenomenon of retardation in any single individual. Rather, a developmental disability reflects the complex interplay among multiple risk and protective factors.

EPIDEMIOLOGY. Approximately 3% of the general population has an intelligence quotient (IQ) less than two standard deviations below the mean. It has been estimated that 80–90% of persons with mental retardation function within the mild range, whereas only 5% of the population with mental retardation is severely to profoundly impaired. The prevalence of mild retardation varies inversely with socioeconomic status,

■ TABLE 40–3 Potential Contributing Factors in the Pathogenesis of Mental Retardation

Preconceptual Disorders
Single gene abnormalities (e.g., inborn errors of metabolism, neurocutaneous disorders)
Chromosomal abnormalities (e.g., X-linked disorders, translocations, fragile X)
Polygenic familial syndromes
Early Embryonic Disruptions
Chromosomal disorders (e.g., trisomies, mosaics)
Infections (e.g., cytomegalovirus, rubella, toxoplasmosis, human immunodeficiency virus)
Teratogens (e.g., alcohol, radiation)
Placental dysfunction
Congenital central nervous system malformations (idiopathic)
Fetal Brain Insults
Infections (e.g., human immunodeficiency virus, toxoplasmosis, cytomegalovirus, herpes simplex)
Toxins (e.g., alcohol, cocaine, lead, maternal phenylketonuria)
Placental insufficiency/intrauterine malnutrition
Perinatal Difficulties
Extreme prematurity
Hypoxic-ischemic injury
Intracranial hemorrhage
Metabolic disorders (e.g., hypoglycemia, hyperbilirubinemia)
Infections (e.g., herpes simplex, bacterial meningitis)
Postnatal Brain Insults
Infections (e.g., encephalitis, meningitis)
Trauma (e.g., severe head injury)
Asphyxia (e.g., near drowning, prolonged apnea, suffocation)
Metabolic disorders (e.g., hypoglycemia, hypernatremia)
Toxins (e.g., lead)
Intracranial hemorrhage
Malnutrition
Postnatal Experiential Disruptions
Poverty and family disorganization
Dysfunctional infant-caregiver interaction
Parental psychopathology
Parental substance abuse
Unknown Influences

whereas moderate to severe disability occurs with equal frequency across all income groups. Because a diagnosis of mental retardation relies on an assessment of adaptive behavior and not solely on IQ, the epidemiology varies with the life cycle. The reported incidence of retardation increases initially with age, the numbers rising sharply in the early school years and then declining in late adolescence as individuals with mild impairments leave the formal education setting and are assimilated into the "normal" adult world. Identification of children with mild retardation in the preschool period is most commonly precipitated by concerns about the development of language.

CLINICAL MANIFESTATIONS. Children with physical findings suggestive of recognizable syndromes that are associated with mental retardation should be identified at birth or during early infancy. Down syndrome and primary microcephaly are examples of such conditions. These disorders, however, represent a small percentage of the population of youngsters with intellectual impairment. The overwhelming majority are identified because of their failure to meet age-appropriate expectations.

Delayed achievement of developmental milestones is the cardinal symptom of mental retardation. Although youngsters with severe impairment show marked delays in psychomotor skills in the first year of life, children with moderate retardation typically exhibit normal motor development and present with delayed speech and language abilities in the toddler years. Mild retardation, on the other hand, may not be suspected until after entry to school, although participation in a nursery school or child care program can highlight discrepancies in the performance of a preschooler with significantly subaverage abilities.

The natural history of mental retardation is highly variable and dependent on the availability of appropriate educational and therapeutic experiences as well as on neuromaturation and the presence of associated disabilities. Although many youngsters may experience transient "plateau periods" during which measurable progress may be minimal, most individuals with mental retardation acquire new skills and continue to learn throughout their lifetimes. The ability to formulate specific prognoses, except for children who manifest severe to profound retardation, is quite limited, especially during the preschool years. Generally speaking, children within the relatively mild range of retardation who receive appropriate education can achieve 4th to 6th grade reading levels and may be able to function relatively independently as adults. Individuals with more significant intellectual limitations require greater degrees of supervision, depending on their range of adaptive abilities. Children with histories that suggest a loss of previously acquired skills represent an important subgroup for whom the diagnosis of a progressive rather than a static neurologic disorder must be investigated. In such cases, developmental deterioration is rarely reversible, yet a precise diagnosis is important for genetic counseling and informed family support.

A thorough pediatric history is essential to identify relevant contributing factors as well as to document the evolving pattern of the child's developmental skills over time. The product of the history should be a comprehensive inventory of risk factors (both within the child and within his or her environment) that increase the likelihood of developmental dysfunction (see Table 40–3) as well as protective factors that may contribute to more adaptive functioning. Common protective factors include good physical health, a normal rate of growth, healthy parent-child attachment, and a cohesive family unit within a supportive social network.

A systematic physical examination may reveal findings that help to explain the etiology of the child's disability or that identify particular treatment needs. Table 40–4 lists a number of atypical physical features that have been associated with a higher incidence of mental retardation. In some cases, a particular cluster of phenotypic characteristics may suggest a specific syndrome related to a chromosomal abnormality or known teratogenic effect. It should be emphasized, however, that many of these features are found in children without developmental disabilities, some tend to be familial, and several appear with greater prevalence among specific ethnic groups.

■ TABLE 40–4 Atypical Physical Features That May Be Associated with Increased Incidence of Mental Retardation

Hair
- Double whorl
- Fine, friable, prematurely gray or white locks
- Sparse or absent hair

Eyes
- Microphthalmia
- Hypertelorism
- Hypotelorism
- Upward-and-outward or downward-and-outward slant
- Inner or outer epicanthal folds
- Coloboma of iris or retina
- Brushfield spots
- Eccentrically placed pupil
- Nystagmus

Ears
- Low-set pinna
- Simple or abnormal helix formation

Nose
- Flattened bridge
- Small size
- Upturned nares

Face
- Increased length of philtrum
- Hypoplasia of maxilla or mandible

Mouth
- Inverted V shape of upper lip
- Wide or high-arched palate

Head
- Microcrania
- Macrocrania

Hands
- Short 4th or 5th metacarpals
- Short, stubby fingers
- Long, thin tapered fingers
- Broad thumbs
- Clinodactyly
- Abnormal dermatoglyphics (e.g., distal triradius)
- Transverse palmar crease
- Abnormal nails

Feet
- Short 4th or 5th metatarsals
- Overlap of toes
- Short, stubby toes
- Broad, large big toes
- Deep crease leading from angle of 1st and 2nd toes
- Abnormal dermatoglyphics

Genitalia
- Ambiguous genitalia
- Micropenis
- Large testicles

Skin
- Café-au-lait spots
- Depigmented nevi

Teeth
- Evidence of abnormal enamelogenesis
- Abnormal odontogenesis

DIAGNOSIS. The primary care pediatrician is strategically situated to identify young children with possible mental retardation through routine developmental surveillance in the context of general pediatric care. Parental report of a child's typical skills and behaviors in conjunction with the use of in-office screening procedures are important complementary sources of information. For young children involved in a program outside of the home (e.g., child care or preschool), the impressions of the caregiver or teacher also are valuable. Concerns raised by parents, nonparental caregivers, or teachers or by direct observation of the child require systematic investigation. The extent to which a comprehensive developmental assessment can be performed within the primary care setting depends on the expertise of the physician and his or her office staff.

Ultimately, the diagnosis of mental retardation requires confirmation of significantly subaverage general intellectual functioning (i.e., an IQ standard score of 70–75 or below) in association with deficits in two or more of the following 10 adaptive skill areas: communication, self-care, home living, social skills, community use, self-direction, health and safety, functional academics, leisure, and work. Screening instruments (e.g., the Denver Developmental Screening Test) and nonstandardized developmental scales are unacceptable substitutes for validated and reliable diagnostic measures (e.g., the Bayley Scales of Infant Development, the Stanford-Binet Intelligence Scale, or the Wechsler Scales). After the psychometric diagnosis of mental retardation has been confirmed, a comprehensive medical evaluation is necessary to complete the assessment process.

A range of laboratory studies must be considered in the medical evaluation of a youngster with mental retardation. Table 40–5 lists important studies and the indications for their

one lives from day to day and that it is usually possible to avoid undue suffering or pain. When the illness may endure for months or years, it may not be inappropriate to hold out hope that medical research may provide methods of control or cure that are not currently available.

Parents are often reluctant to ask whether the diagnosis may be in doubt, or whether some other physicians or the resources of some other medical center may offer more hope. They should be helped to express such concerns and should be encouraged and helped to seek one or two additional expert medical opinions if they wish. These matters should be discussed in such a way that the family feels no embarrassment, and they should be assured that they are causing none. They can be told that medical communication is good enough so that there will be prompt dissemination of any real breakthrough in the management of the illness of their child. It is also reasonable to advise them that they may do the ill child and the rest of the family a disservice if they dissipate the family's emotional and other resources in a frantic search for something that is not available.

MANAGEMENT. What to tell children who have a fatal illness varies with the developmental status of the child, the nature of the illness, and the circumstances. Initially, they can often be told that their illness may last for some time and may have ups and downs and that it is important for them to get adequate rest and to be active when they feel up to it.

The parents of a child who has a probably fatal illness should be encouraged to handle the life situation of the child as normally as possible. This may be difficult for guilt-ridden or grieving parents who may think that their usual disciplinary activities may make the child's pain or illness worse. The parents should be encouraged to maintain the child in his or her normal place in the family hierarchy. Special arrangements, such as Christmas in the summertime or public dramatizations of the child's illness, may be more anxiety provoking for the child than a fulfillment of any need.

The young child knows from the reactions and behavior of his or her parents to the news of a potentially fatal illness that something is perhaps terribly wrong, but the very young child has only a fragmentary conception of death. Before the age of 2 yr, the concept of death is absent (Piaget); after that the notion develops of a state that is potentially reversible, or temporary, like sleep. The preadolescent child may believe that death is irreversible, but capricious, with internal and external explanations. The adolescent views death as irreversible, but distant, with physiologic and possibly theologic explanations. When magical or irrational thoughts lead the child or adolescent to irrational explanations for the death of self or another, such thoughts may be the root of much guilt.

As an illness that will be fatal progresses, Bluebond-Langner found that the perceptions of the patient evolve through several stages; first, the illness is regarded as simply a change from a prior state of health. Then, the illness is regarded as serious but temporary; later, with a relapse and continuing disability, the illness is seen as persistent but which some day may resolve. The next phase, after further relapses, is a conviction that the illness will continue and the child will not get better; and finally, often after the death of a friend or fellow patient, the conclusion is reached, "I am dying."

Young children do not often ask if they are dying. When they do, they do not so much need a yes or no answer as recognition that the question has arisen from some new perception of their illness. They can be asked why the question comes up at this time, and whether it does not mean that being ill is no fun and having it go on for so long is discouraging. Unrealistic assurances that they look well and are doing fine are counterproductive. It is likely that the child knows the answer at some level and is reaching out to a trusted person for reassurance that he or she will not be abandoned. The person approached for this reassurance may not be a family member or a physician or nurse but some other member of the therapeutic team. Whoever it may be should understand that reassurances of commitment and love are being asked for, rather than denial or efforts at "cheering up."

It is appropriate to keep hope alive for the patient and the parents. This means maintaining a positive attitude toward the needs of the patient and meeting them appropriately. The focus of hope will change as the illness progresses. First there is hope for a cure, then for a longer remission, then for care to be given at home, and finally for death to come without pain.

In the case of temporary hospitalization, the patient can be reassured that school and normal activity will begin again as soon as possible; meanwhile, it is supportive, when appropriate, for the patient to receive attention from schoolteachers and play therapists in the hospital, who will help blunt the sense of inevitability of worsening illness. The child often reveals his or her feelings through art or music.

In the case of preadolescent or adolescent children with chronic and fatal illnesses, the plan for care may often include a decision to share the diagnosis with the child. In this case, the physician examines with parents and child together the implications of diagnosis and prognosis, answering their questions and laying out with them a program of action. The explicit goal is to keep the patient as comfortable as possible and to forestall any end to the effort as long as possible. In this atmosphere of frankness, trust, and cooperation, free of secrets or evasions, many families and patients may find an unexpectedly healthy climate for the expression of tenderness and love toward each other, and the physician may find his or her own work easier. In any case, the decision as to whether, when, or how the diagnosis of a potentially fatal illness is to be shared with the child or adolescent must have the prior full understanding, consent, and cooperation of the parents.

An important consideration at this time is how information about the nature of the child's illness will be shared with other family members, such as siblings or grandparents, or with schoolmates, friends, or neighbors. The status of siblings may need particular attention. They will know from the behavior of their parents that something is gravely amiss. But here, as in the case of the patient, it is important as much as possible to maintain normal family dynamics. The illness of the patient threatens the siblings ("Me, too?"), and they may become resentful of the undue attention or privileges given the sick family member. They, like the parents, may have irrational feelings of responsibility for the patient's condition. Parents can support siblings by staying in contact with them during the hospitalization of the patient, being attentive to their needs, and spending some time alone with each sibling to hear his or her concerns.

Schoolmates may share the anxieties of the patient or develop their own. It may be important that the patient's teacher and school nurse know the condition of the patient and whether or how the course of the school day may need to be modified. In the case of some conditions, such as human immunodeficiency virus positivity, there may be a need for education of classmates in the implications for them of the illness of the patient.

The needs of the patient and family will evolve with the phase of the illness and their understanding of the course of the illness and of each other's needs. The need of the patient for physical comfort and emotional support is universal. Attention to the needs of the family addresses their understanding of the current condition of the patient, their emotional status, their emotional and financial resources, the nature of their support system (family, friends, and community), and their possible need for respite from their immediate investment in the care of the patient. In all of these concerns, the needs of the patient are central.

Management of Pain (also see Chapter 62). Children and adolescents with chronic illness may suffer pain both from the illness and from therapeutic interventions. The prevention or relief of pain calls for sensitivity on the part of the physician or others to the indications given by each patient that he or she is in distress or in fear of pain. Children, especially very young children, do not always or readily complain vocally of discomfort but may give other signs, such as immobility, a facial expression of depression, or physiologic indicators. In the case of chronic or persistent pain, it is not sufficient for the medication for the relief of pain to be given only on indication or request ("prn"); such a procedure makes it inevitable that the child will suffer some pain before relief comes. Rather, medication should be given at regular intervals or continuously in suitable dosage.

Older children and adolescents can be given some responsibility for and control of their own medication. Devices exist that permit continuous intravenous administration of analgesics at designated rates and doses, with the patient able to increase the dose if necessary by calling on an additional pulse of injection. The interval between such injections can be controlled. There is no evidence that the administration of opiates in this manner is addictive for children or adolescents who need relief from pain; the total amount of medication required is often less than if it were given prn.

When diagnostic or therapeutic interventions cause acute discomfort, some relief can be obtained from premedication with analgesic or anxiolytic medication. Some children can readily learn techniques of self-hypnosis, through relaxation imagery; the achievement of this can contribute to self-esteem.

Other Resources. In dealing with the problems of the patient and family in regard to a fatal illness, the physician often calls on other professionals for help. The spiritual advisor of the family can be of immense comfort. When family problems can be ameliorated by counseling or by the use of community resources, the help of social work services may be important. When the family is not intact, owing to the death or previous separation of a parent, the likelihood of emotional difficulties complicating the management of the illness is sufficiently great that social service should probably be involved from the time the diagnosis is first known.

Fatal chronic illnesses of children tend to cluster around certain diagnoses, such as leukemia or other malignancies, cystic fibrosis, and metabolic or degenerative disorders (e.g., Tay-Sachs disease). When groups of families who share a common problem can be formed to discuss aspects of the care of their children, under the guidance of a skillful professional person (physician, social worker, or nurse), they can often help one another in the management of the illness, both medically and socially, and in coping with the feelings that go with the inevitability of ultimate loss.

Terminal Care. As a chronic illness becomes terminal, the patient needs a sense of not being abandoned, assurances of the continuing love and affection of those around him or her, and reasonably prompt responses to his or her needs for care. In the management of terminal illness, the physician should not leave to parents decisions about what is to be done but should give positive advice as to what he or she deems appropriate or plans to do. Such plans should be responsive, however, to the wishes or suggestions of the parents when these represent helpful and realistic appraisals of their children's needs. In cases of disagreement or conflict between family and physicians as to procedure, consultation with others may be indicated (e.g., psychologists, psychiatrists, social workers, ethicists, or the clergy [see also Chapter 3]).

Parents should be encouraged to participate in the care of the child in the hospital so long as their responsibilities to other children at home are adequately met. Parents may also need encouragement to take adequate respite from the care of the ill child.

As the physician follows the evolution of a fatal illness in a child, the manner in which the parents are coping with the situation should be observed. Some parents may turn their attention increasingly to other sick children in the hospital. This is a healthy sign if it is not premature; if it comes too early, it may represent the parents' unresolved burden of guilt or their pain in facing their own ill child. This turning to help other children is healthy so long as the parents still have adequate resources and strength for the needs of their own child.

As death approaches, the child or adolescent may not uncommonly convey his or her knowledge of the imminent end of illness. At this time, the need for relief of any sense of abandonment may be paramount, along with measures to ensure comfort. The sensitive physician sees that the occasion is accorded appropriate dignity and not rendered more frustrating and agonizing by invasive efforts to prolong vital functions in a climate of fruitless hyperactivity.

It may often be easier to achieve death with dignity in a climate of loving parting if the terminal illness is permitted to run its course at home or in a hospice, rather than in a hospital. This can occur when the family, and often also the child or adolescent patient, accept the premise that high technology no longer has anything useful to offer or that the need for intimacy or togetherness has become an overriding concern. The responsibilities of the physician, as discussed below for the hospitalized patient, are not abridged when plans for home or hospice care are adopted.

The hospitalized patient whose illness is terminal should be in a room where he or she can be alone, with parents or loved ones at the bedside or nearby. The physician should be available to both the parents and the patient. The physician's control of his or her own feelings is important; if the physician's personal distress is allowed to increase the distance from or decrease involvement with the patient, the anger of the child or parents with what may be perceived by them as abandonment may make terminal care more difficult. The continued interest and concern of the physician are important in preventing the emotional situation from deteriorating at this time.

When death has occurred, the patient, bed, and room should be made neat, and the paraphernalia of illness removed. If the parents of a hospitalized child are not at hand, they should be asked to come to the hospital and be informed of the circumstances. Parents should be given the opportunity to be with the child for a little while in the relatively peaceful and uncluttered setting that has been created. A brief and tender parting may help the parents in the adjustments they must ultimately make.

Postmortem Examination. A request for postmortem examination should be made by the responsible physician who knows the family best, often not the house officer, but the attending or referring physician. The need for postmortem examination should be urged as strongly as conviction permits. Parents can be assured that such examinations are always helpful and that information is gathered and saved that may be useful in solving similar problems in other children or in providing definitive answers to future questions of other children in the family or of their relatives or descendants concerning the patient's illness. Later, the physician should describe the important and relevant findings for the parents in simple terms, and they should have a chance to discuss them as freely as they wish.

Family Support. There are wide personal and cultural differences in the manner in which families adjust to the death of family members. A period of grief and mourning is inevitable, and elements of these may last a lifetime—for example, in periods of depression on birthdays or holidays. Most families find a new equilibrium within a few months; before that occurs, however, there may be troubling experiences for parents, such as the fear of loss of touch with reality that comes with having set a place at the table for the dead child or finding oneself listening for or hearing his or her footsteps or voice. Parents may experience guilt at earlier wishes that the ordeal be over soon or at an unexpected sense of relief or release at the terminal event itself. The skillful physician watches for signs of these reactions and finds the right words of reassurance or encouragement, saying that such feelings are normal and that the parents have given everything that could have been expected of them in a situation that they have found very trying and toward which they will forever have sensitive and tender feelings.

After the death of an infant or child, the opportunity for groups of parents to share their experiences may be as important and as supportive as before the death, so long as professional guidance is adequate. Members of such groups can help each other with mourning and can foster the reassurance that comes with sharing such experiences as those described. The physician, in any case, should plan a number of visits with the parents in the weeks after a child's death to review such matters with them, to answer their continuing questions, and to assess their status.

DEATH OF THE NEWBORN INFANT. The management of the death of the newborn infant serves as a model for the management of the *acute* and often unanticipated death of an infant, child, or adolescent. Acute fatal illnesses have a major cluster in the neonatal period, and the physicians, nurses, and other personnel of nurseries and neonatal intensive care units must be responsive to the needs of parents who have had no preparation for a catastrophic loss.

The mother and infant are usually apart at the moment of death. When death can be anticipated by minutes or a few hours, it may be possible to involve the mother in the care of the infant so that she may know with certainty what her infant was like. The thought is often expressed that this might make the mother's loss more difficult to adjust to; there is no substantial support for this notion. Many mothers feel that, if the infant were to die in their arms, that would be the preferred form of leave taking.

When mother and infant are apart in the hospital at the time of death, the body of the infant can be taken to the mother or to both parents at her bedside or at some other point in the hospital where the chance to hold and examine the infant may be the mother's only opportunity to establish for herself the reality of the birth and death of her infant and to adjust toward reality her current or future fantasies as to what the baby might *really* have been like or what might *really* have happened. For the mother of the malformed infant, this may be especially important. The defects can be examined by her in reality rather than in fantasy and their implications gently discussed, with the observation perhaps that the baby was in every other way perfectly formed.

Mothers who have lost newborn infants are in critical need of help in mourning. They should have as much opportunity as they may wish, or as circumstances afford, for participation in rituals that follow death, such as funerals or other ceremonies. Words of sympathy and understanding are helpful. It is naive, on the other hand, of health personnel, family, or friends to try to cheer up such a mother with the encouragement that she can soon have another child. The mother has been deeply bonded to *this* infant during pregnancy, and a host of hopes, expectations, and wonderments have perished with the baby. Physicians should make sure that parents understand that the mourning process for a dead infant or older child ought to be reasonably complete and a stable state reached before they decide to have another child. This generally requires 9 mo or 1 yr or more. A new infant conceived too soon is likely to be too closely identified with the dead child and to be surrounded by inordinate anxiety or inappropriate expectations.

Nurseries and neonatal intensive care units find it helpful to create and maintain small discussion groups of mothers, within which, during the first few weeks of mourning, mothers who have lost their infants can share their experiences with others. Unexpected experiences may include the illusion of hearing the baby (even the stillborn baby) cry in the night. Sharing of such normal but distressing experiences may allay anxiety. The quality of guidance of such groups is crucial to their success.

Bluebond-Langner M: The Private Worlds of Dying Children. Princeton, Princeton University Press, 1978.

Davidson GW: Death of the wished-for child: A case study. Death Educ 1:265, 1977.

Doyle D, Hanks GWC, McDonald N (eds): Oxford Textbook of Palliative Medicine. Oxford, Oxford University Press, 1994.

Fleischman AR (ed): Caring for gravely ill children. Pediatrics (in press).

McGrath PJ, Unruh AM: Pain in Children and Adolescents. Amsterdam, Elsevier, 1987.

Olness K, Gardner GG: Hypnosis and Hypnotherapy with Children. Philadelphia, Grune & Stratton, 1988.

Sahler OJZ, van Eys J, Wessel MA: Children: Death and Dying. American Academy of Pediatrics Pediatric Update, Vol 13. Port Washington, NY, Medical Information Systems, 1992.

Schechter NL, Altman AJ, Weisman SJ (eds): Report of the Consensus Conference on the Management of Pain in Childhood Cancer. Pediatrics 86(Suppl.):813, 1990.

Shapiro BS, Cohen DE, Covelman KW, et al: Experience of an interdisciplinary pediatric pain service. Pediatrics 88:1226, 1991.

CHAPTER 42
Children at Special Risk

*Richard E. Behrman**

In this chapter, the health issues faced by some of the most socioculturally and economically disadvantaged children in the United States are discussed: Native Americans, migrants, immigrants, homeless children and runaways, and children in foster care. The role of poverty in the lives of these and other children has a special significance. The biologic causes of special risk are covered elsewhere. The nonbiologic and biologic causes of special risk often overlap and may confound the risks.

Most children in the United States today grow up loved and supported, although many have problems that disturb their parents and blight their future. However, for a small but significant number of children, their circumstances are so dismal that one wonders how many survive. Examples of children with even more dismal futures than these also exist elsewhere in the world, such as children growing up in the midst of the Israel-Palestine conflict or in Northern Ireland, Bosnia, or Rwanda. Many of the children growing up in these environments will be damaged and their futures will be compromised, unless effective interventions are mounted. However, in all of these situations, a few children are so resilient that they survive and actually thrive. Werner has characterized these children as "vulnerable but invincible." The fact that a few defy the odds does not absolve society from attempting to help the majority of those who do not, although these resilient ones can teach us what it takes to survive.

The majority of children at special risk need a nurturant environment but have had their futures compromised by actions or policies arising from their families, schools, communi-

*Modified from the original version in the 14th edition written by Robert J. Haggerty.

ties, and nation. The challenge is to improve the environment of these children so that most can achieve their full potential. Many of their problems are due to multiple causes, and many of these causes are similar, whether the end result is homeless children, runaways, children in foster care, or other disadvantaged groups. From a preventive point of view, the most effective approach involves alleviation of poverty, poor housing, and lack of jobs. From a medical point of view, optimal care of these children requires specially organized programs, multidiscipline teams, and special financing.

CHILDREN IN POVERTY

Poverty and economic loss diminish the capacity of parents to be supportive, consistent, and involved with their children. Clinicians need to be especially alert to the development and behavior of children whose parents have lost their jobs or who live in permanent poverty. Fathers who become unemployed frequently develop psychosomatic symptoms, and their children often develop similar symptoms. Young children who grew up in the Great Depression and whose parents were subject to acute poverty suffered more than older children, especially if the older ones were able to take on responsibilities for helping the family economically. Such responsibilities during adolescence seem to give purpose and direction to an adolescent's life. But the younger children, faced with parental depression and unable to do anything to help, suffered a higher frequency of illness and a diminished capacity to lead productive lives even as adults. Children who are poor have higher than average rates of death and illness from almost all causes (exceptions being suicide and motor vehicle accidents, which are most common among white, nonpoor children) (Table 42–1).

Although physicians cannot cure poverty, they have an obligation to ask parents about their economic resources, adverse changes in their financial situation, and the family's attempts to cope. Encouraging concrete methods of coping, suggesting ways to reduce stressful social circumstances while increasing social networks that are supportive, and referring patients and their families to appropriate welfare, job training, and family agencies can significantly improve the health and functioning of children at risk when their families live in poverty. In many cases, special services, especially social services, need to be added to the traditional medical services, and outreach is required to find and encourage parents to use health services and bring their children into the health care system.

■ **TABLE 42–1 Relative Frequency of Health Problems in Low-Income Children Compared with Other Children**

Health Problem	Relative Frequency in Low-Income Children
Low birthweight	Double
Delayed immunization	Triple
Asthma	Higher
Bacterial meningitis	Double
Rheumatic fever	Double to triple
Lead poisoning	Triple
Neonatal death	1.5 times
Postneonatal death	Double to triple
Child deaths due to accidents	Double to triple
Child deaths due to disease	Triple to quadruple
Complications of appendicitis	Double to triple
Diabetic ketoacidosis	Double
Complications of bacterial meningitis	Double to triple
Percent with conditions limiting school activity	Double to triple
Lost school days	40% more
Severely impaired vision	Double to triple
Severe iron-deficiency anemia	Double

From: Starfield B: Effectiveness of Medical Care: Validating Clinical Wisdom. Baltimore, Johns Hopkins University Press, 1985. In: Starfield B: Child and adolescent health status measures. The Future of Children 2(2):25, 1992.

■ **TABLE 42–2 Observed and Adjusted Poverty Rates for Children, by Ethnicity, 1980 and 1991**

Ethnicity	Percentage of Children below Poverty Thresholds	
	1980	*1991*
All Children		
Observed	17.9%	21.1%
Adjusted using 1980 family composition	17.9%	19.4%
White		
Observed	13.3%	16.1%
Adjusted using 1980 family composition	13.3%	15.0%
Black		
Observed	42.1%	45.6%
Adjusted using 1980 family composition	42.1%	42.2%
Hispanic*		
Observed	33.0%	39.8%
Adjusted using 1980 family composition	33.0%	38.5%

Population poverty rates for children depend on both the poverty rates of specific subgroups of children (e.g., black children in two-parent households) and the proportion of children in the different subgroups. Poverty is more common among children who live in single-parent families, especially those headed by single women. Poverty rates of children can change over time as can the rates for children in different subgroups of the population and the proportion of children in the different subgroups. One way to analyze the impact of changes in the proportion of children in the different subgroups on child poverty rates is to standardize poverty rates by holding the proportion of children in the various groups constant while allowing the subgroup poverty rates to change over time.

The adjusted rates in the table show what child poverty rates would have been in 1991 if children were distributed across different family subgroups (e.g., female-headed, no-spouse-present households, vs all other households, primarily two-parent families) in the same proportion as they were in 1980. For all children and for each ethnic subgroup, adjusted poverty rates are below actual 1991 poverty rates. This suggests that child poverty rates in 1991 would have been lower if children were distributed across single-parent female-headed and all other families in 1991 in the same proportions as they were in 1980.

**May be of any race.*

The calculations were based on data from the following sources: US Bureau of the Census: Poverty in the United States: 1991. Current Population Reports, Series P-60, No 181. Washington, DC, US Government Printing Office, 1992, pp 11, 14; US Bureau of the Census: Characteristics of the Population below the Poverty Level: 1982. Washington DC, US Government Printing Office, 1982, pp 8–9. From Lewit EM: Why is poverty increasing among children? The Future of Children 3(2):198, 1993.

Poverty among children in the United States has increased during the last 25 yr (Fig. 42–1). One in five children lives in poverty, a higher percentage than in any other developed country. The rates vary substantially among ethnic groups, are higher for children than adults, are highest for infants and toddlers, and are usually higher for single-parent female-headed families than for two-parent families (Table 42–2). Many factors associated with poverty are responsible for the illnesses seen in these children—crowding, poor hygiene and health care, poor diet, environmental pollution, poor education, and stress. The basic support for poor families in the United States comes from the Aid to Families with Dependent Children program (AFDC). Support for these families is the foundation on which specially organized health care programs for children at special risk must be built. Unfortunately, AFDC has not kept up with inflation, has been subject to fraud, and varies greatly from one state to another.

NATIVE AMERICANS, INCLUDING ALASKAN ESKIMOS AND ALEUTS

Children of Native Americans have higher than average rates of many physical and psychologic disorders. They are one group in the United States for whom a separately organized health service has long been in place, the Indian Health Service. There are approximately 2.1 million Native Americans, 40% of whom are younger than 20 yr of age, a much higher proportion of children than for the remainder of the United States. More than 50% of Native Americans live in urban areas, not on or near native lands. The unemployment and

Annual Poverty Rates for Children Under 18 in Families and Annual Unemployment Rates, 1959–1991

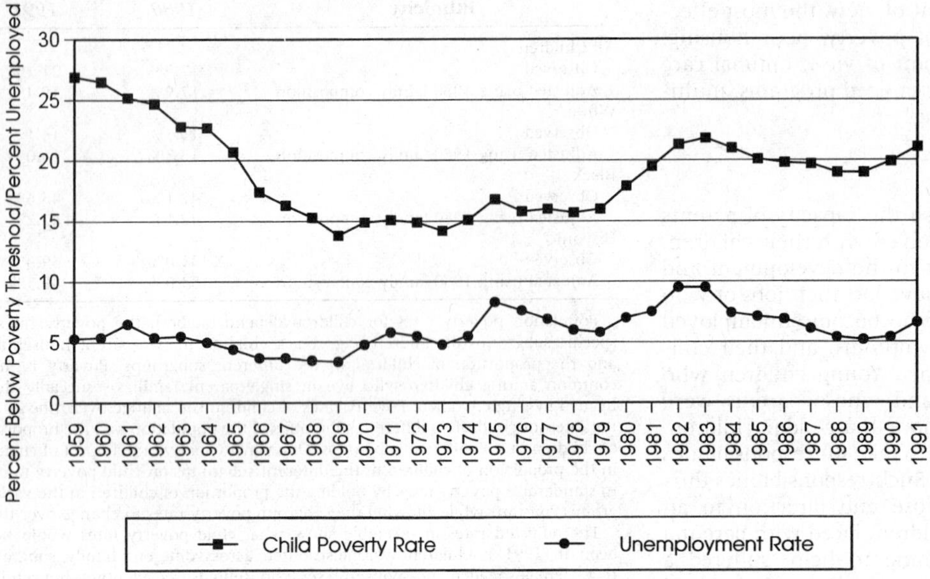

In the period prior to 1969, child poverty rates dropped precipitously. Although official poverty rates have been calculated only for the period since 1959, data from the 1950 census have been used with the official poverty thresholds to estimate that the child poverty rate was 47.6% in 1949.* Thus, between 1949 and 1969, the child poverty rate declined by 33.8 percentage points. As can be seen in the figure, most of this decline, 25.1 percentage points, predated the war on poverty which began in 1964. Since the late 1960s, child poverty rates have fluctuated in tandem with the unemployment rate but have drifted higher with each fluctuation.

Sources: U.S. Bureau of the Census. *Poverty in the United States: 1991*. Current Population Reports, Series P-60, No. 181. Washington, DC: USGPO, 1992, p. 4; U.S. Department of Labor, Bureau of Labor Statistics. *Employment and Earnings*. Washington, DC: USGPO, October 1992, p. 7; * Danziger, S.K., and Danziger, S. Child Poverty and Public Policy, *Daedelus* (Winter 1993) 122,1:57–84.

Figure 42–1.

poverty levels of Native Americans are three- and fourfold that of the white population, respectively, and far fewer Native Americans graduate from high school or go on to college.

The rate of *low birthweight* is more than the white rate and less than the black rate. The *neonatal mortality* rate and the *postneonatal mortality* rate are higher for Native Americans living in urban areas than for urban white Americans. Deaths during the 1st yr of life from sudden infant death syndrome and pneumonia and influenza are higher than the average in the United States, whereas deaths from congenital anomalies, respiratory distress syndrome, and disorders relating to short gestation and low birthweight are similar.

After the newborn period, *accidental deaths* are the most common cause of death in all childhood populations (with the exception that, in New York City in 1988, acquired immunodeficiency syndrome [AIDS] was the most common cause of death in children from 1–4 yr of age). But accidental death among Native Americans occurs at twice the rate for other United States populations, whereas deaths from malignant neoplasms are lower. During adolescence and young adulthood, *suicide* and *homicide* are the second and third causes of death in this population and also occur at about twice the rates of the rest of the population.

Recurrent otitis media is an especially frequent problem among Native American children. As many as three quarters of these children have recurrent otitis media and high rates of hearing loss. This results in learning problems for many children. Other infectious disorders, such as tuberculosis and gastroenteritis, which were so much more common among Native Americans in the past, now occur at about the national average.

Psychosocial problems are more prevalent in these populations than in the general population: depression, alcoholism, drug abuse, out-of-wedlock teenage pregnancy, school failure and dropout, and child abuse and neglect. The reasons for these differences are not clear, but the cultural disruption of Native American populations is probably, in part, responsible.

INDIAN HEALTH SERVICE. Since 1954, the Indian Health Service has been the responsibility of the Public Health Service; since the 1975 Indian Self-Determination Act, tribes have been given the option of managing Native American health services in their communities. Thus, today, the Indian Health Service is managed through local administrative units, and some tribes contract outside of the Indian Health Service for health care. The asthma-related hospitalization patterns of Native American children are similar to those seen in white children despite having socioeconomic characteristics more similar to those of black children. A great deal of emphasis is, however, on adult services: treatment for alcoholism, nutrition and dietetic counseling, and public health nursing services. In addition to programs on Native American reservations, there are currently more than 40 urban programs for Native Americans, with an emphasis on increasing access of this population to existing health services, providing special social services, and developing self-help groups. In an effort to accommodate traditional Western medical, psychologic, and social services to the Native American cultures, such programs increasingly include the

"Talking Circle," the "Sweat Lodge," and other interventions based on Native American culture. The efficacy of any of these programs, especially those to prevent and treat the sociopsychologic problems peculiar to Native Americans, has not been assessed.

The United States has played a long and ambivalent role in dealing with its Native American population. Health services have been among its more socially responsible activities, and today there is increased recognition of the need to maintain cultural sensitivity and to utilize traditional healing models, while at the same time bringing the benefits of modern medicine and social services to this group at special risk. See Chapter 4.

CHILDREN OF MIGRANT FARM WORKERS

There are estimated to be 2.5–4.4 million migratory farm workers and their families in the United States. The eastern stream of workers winters primarily in Florida, while the western stream comes from Texas and the border states, as well as from Mexico. Many children travel with their parents in the migrant streams. The circumstances of migrants often include poor housing, frequent moves, and a socioeconomic system controlled by a crew boss who arranges the jobs, provides transportation, and often, together with the farm owners, provides food, alcohol, and drugs under a "company store" system that leaves the migrant family with little money, or even in debt at the end of the year. Children often go without schooling because of the moves, and medical care is usually limited.

The medical problems of children of migrant farm workers are similar to those of children of homeless families: increased frequency of infections (including human immunodeficiency virus [HIV] and AIDS), trauma, poor nutrition, poor dental care, low immunization rates, exposures to toxic chemicals, anemia, and developmental delays.

In 1964, the Public Health Service initiated a special program to provide funds for local groups to organize medical care for migrant families. This program has continued to grow. In addition, many migrant health projects, which were staffed initially by part-time providers and were open for only part of the year, have been transformed into community health care centers that provide services not only for migrants but also for other residents in the area. However, health services for migrant farm workers often need to be organized separately from existing primary care programs because the families are migratory. Special record-keeping systems that link the health care provided during winter months in the south with the care provided during the migratory season in the north are difficult to maintain in ordinary group practices or individual physicians' offices. Outreach programs that take medical care to the often remote farm sites are necessary, and specially organized Head Start, early education, and remedial education programs should also be provided. Similar to other groups discussed in this section, children of migrant farm workers require health care that is more extensive than physicians' services; and this sort of health care often requires separate organizations to deliver it.

CHILDREN OF IMMIGRANTS

The United States has always been a country of immigrants, and in the last 10 yr immigration has once again increased, especially from Southeast Asia, South America, and the Soviet Union. About 240,000 children legally immigrate each year, and an estimated 50,000/yr enter the country illegally. There may be 850,000 to 1 million illegal immigrant children currently in residence. Families of different origins obviously bring different health problems and different cultural backgrounds, which influence health practices and use of medical care and need to be understood to provide appropriate services (see Chapter 4). Children from Southeast Asia and South America have growth patterns that are generally below the norms established for children of Western European origin, and high rates of hepatitis, parasitic diseases, and nutritional deficiencies are prevalent, as well as high degrees of psychosocial stress. The high prevalence of hepatitis among women from Southeast Asia makes use of hepatitis B vaccine necessary for newborns in this group. While special health care programs have been developed for many of these children (e.g., children of immigrant migrant workers), children of legally immigrant families have usually been more readily incorporated into traditional medical practice in the United States than some of the other groups of children at special risk.

HOMELESS CHILDREN

Estimates are that, in 1992, children constituted about 20–25% of the estimated 1–2 million people who were homeless at some time during the year in the United States. The population of homeless children has been increasing as a consequence of more families with children living in poverty, fewer available affordable dwellings for these families, decreasing public assistance programs for the nonelderly poor, and the rising prevalence of substance abuse.

Homeless children have an increased frequency of illness, including intestinal infections, anemia, neurologic disorders, seizures, behavior disorders, mental illness, and dental problems, as well as increased frequency of trauma and substance abuse. Homeless children are admitted to hospitals at a much higher rate than the national average, have higher school failure rates, and the likelihood of their being victims of abuse and neglect is much higher. In one study, 50% of such children were found to have psychosocial problems, such as developmental delays, severe depression, or learning disorders.

Because families tend to break apart under the strain of poverty and homelessness, many homeless children end up in foster care. And even if their families remain intact, frequent moves make it very difficult for them to receive continuity of medical care. Even in the United Kingdom, which offers the easiest access to primary care of all Western democracies, studies have shown that homeless persons rarely have a family physician, and therefore special programs generally need to be developed to provide health services for this population. Mobile vans, with a team consisting of a physician, nurse, social worker, and welfare worker, have been shown to provide effective comprehensive care, ensure delivery of immunizations, link the children to school health services, and bring the children and their families into a stable relation with the traditional medical system. A special record-keeping system is necessary to enhance continuity and to provide a record of care once the family has moved to a permanent location. Because of the high frequency of developmental delays in this group, linkage of preschool homeless children to Head Start programs is an especially important service. Medical and social services for the parents of homeless children are also essential for preservation of these families.

The basic problem of homeless families cannot, of course, be solved by physicians. Provision of adequate housing, job retraining for the parents, and mental health and social services are necessary to prevent homelessness from occurring. But physicians can play an important role in motivating society to adopt the social policies that will prevent homelessness from occurring by pointing out the likelihood that these homeless children will become burdens both to themselves and to society if their special health needs are not met.

RUNAWAY AND THROWNAWAY CHILDREN

The number of runaway and thrownaway children and youth in 1988 was 577,800 and at least 192,700 of these children had no familiar and secure place to stay. Teenagers make up most of both groups. The usual definition of a runaway is a youth younger than 18 yr of age who is gone for at least one night from his or her home without parental permission. Most runaways leave home only once, stay overnight with friends, and have no contact with the police or other agencies. This group is no different from their "healthy" peers in psychologic status. A smaller but unknown number become multiple or permanent "runners" and are significantly different from the one-time "runners." Thrownaways include children directly told to leave the household, children who have been away from home and are not allowed to return, abandoned or deserted children, and children who run away but their caretaker makes no effort to recover the child or does not care if the child returns.

The same constellation of causes common to many of the other special-risk groups is characteristic of permanent runaways. These causes include environmental problems (family dysfunction, abuse, poverty), as well as personal problems of the young person (poor impulse control, psychopathology, or school failure). Thrownaways experience more violence and conflicts within their families. The reason why one child enters the group of runaways while another child enters foster care, the juvenile justice system, or mental health systems is not clear.

The minority of runaway youths who become homeless street people have a high frequency of problem behaviors. Three quarters engage in some type of criminal activity and half engage in prostitution as a means of support. A majority of permanent runaways have serious mental problems; more than one third are the product of families who engage in repeated physical and sexual abuse. These children also have a high frequency of medical problems, including traditional infections, hepatitis, sexually transmitted diseases, and drug abuse. Although runaways usually distrust most social agencies, they will come to and use medical services. Thus, medical care may become the point of re-entry into mainstream society and to needed services.

Services for the permanent runaways and thrownaways need to be comprehensive and should include social, psychiatric, foster home, drug detoxification, as well as more traditional medical services. The only approach that has been successful has been long-term team efforts by people who develop the trust of runaway youths and then can help them to work out a better solution to their problems than by running away, drug use, and prostitution.

Although there may be significant legal considerations involved in the treatment of homeless minor adolescents, most states, through their "good Samaritan" laws and definitions of "emancipated minors," authorize treatment of homeless youths. Physician liability is based on the usual malpractice standards. Legal barriers should not be used as an excuse to refuse medical care to runaway or thrownaway youths.

The Runaway Youth Act, Title III of the Juvenile Justice and Delinquency Prevention Act of 1974 (Public Law 93–414), and its amended version (Public Law 95–509) have supported shelters and provide a toll-free 24-hr telephone number (1-800-621-4000) for youth who wish to contact their parents or request help after having run away.

Parents who seek a physician's advice about a runaway child should be asked about the child's history of running away, the presence of family dysfunction, and personal aspects of the child's development. If the youth contacts the physician, he or she should be examined and the youth's health status should be assessed, as well as his or her willingness to return home. If it is not feasible for the youth to return home, foster care, a group home, or an independent living arrangement should be sought by referral to a social worker or a social agency.

FOSTER CHILDREN

In the United States, the placement of children, who cannot remain with their families, in out-of-home alternative residential settings (foster family homes [about 70%], group homes or facilities [about 17%], special shelters, medical facilities, or nonfinalized adoptive homes) is commonly referred to as the foster or substitute care system. It is part of the very complex child welfare system, which varies greatly from state to state. The welfare system offers a variety of preventive and rehabilitative services to try to help keep families together when this does not involve unreasonable risks to the children.

Most children placed in foster care have a higher than average number of physical and mental health problems, as well as social problems. The frequency of placement of children in foster care is greater among most of the populations of children at special risk and children from broken families and single-parent families than in the general population. Although extended families (especially grandparents) are frequently the initial source of continuing care, their abilities to cope may be overtaxed and their wards end up receiving foster care from strangers. However, in the past 2 decades, there has been an increase in formal foster placement of children with relatives (kinship care), some of whom are not licensed, approved, or paid.

The total number of children and youth of all ages in foster or substitute care has been increasing in recent years (Fig. 42–2). Substance abuse (especially crack cocaine) and the related increase in child abuse and neglect, and poverty have contributed significantly to this trend. The increase in very young infants and, in some cities, adolescents has been substantial.

Infants who have a positive test result for HIV infection and children whose mothers are substance abusers present special problems. They are especially difficult to place in foster care or adoption and often cannot be returned to their biologic homes. Parental drug abuse is a factor in 35–40% of all foster care placements and is increasing. It contributes significantly to child abuse, both physical and sexual, and to neglect and abandonment of children.

Adolescents have always been difficult to place for adoption, and most who are in foster care have such severe emotional and physical problems that adoption is impossible. They often end up permanently in foster care, revolving in and out of different foster homes. More than 80% have experienced sexual or physical abuse or neglect. There is need to prepare adolescents in foster care for independent living when they reach maturity. The Federal Foster Care Independent Living Initiative (Section 477, Title IV E of the SSA) of 1980 permits payment for such discharge planning, without which many of these youths would end up chronically on welfare.

General considerations concerning foster care and adoption are discussed in Chapters 32 and 33, but children at special risk present the social service and medical systems with especially difficult problems. Every child entering foster care should have a complete health assessment and provision of a medical record. However, it is difficult to provide standard health care to many of these children because frequent moves from one foster home to another obstruct continuity of medical care. Successful medical care programs usually involve special organizations to provide continuity of care.

Foster children are also more likely to have chronic health problems, especially psychoeducational ones. They are often depressed and insecure, and they may have lifelong difficulty in developing intimate relationships. These complex sociomedical problems are another reason why there is a need for specially organized health care programs for children in foster care. Because most foster children are eligible for Medicaid, it

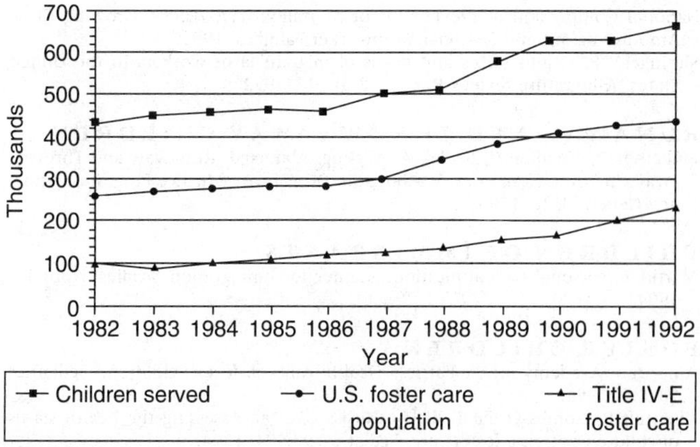

Figure 42–2. There is no uniformly defined, complete source of national data on foster care. Most national data come from the Voluntary Cooperative Information System (VCIS), a voluntary annual survey conducted by the American Public Welfare Association with support from the Department of Health and Human Services. VCIS foster care data should be interpreted cautiously because the number of jurisdictions reporting has fluctuated from year to year, not all reporting states answered all the questions in the survey, and the definitions of terms and reporting periods varied among the states.

- The number of children in foster care in the United States increased by 69% between 1982 and 1992. As a result, the proportion of all children in foster care increased from four per thousand in 1982 to six per thousand in 1992.
- Figure 42–2 presents data on the foster care population, the total number of children in care at a specific point in time (typically the end of the fiscal year), and the total number of children served by the nation's substitute care system during a year. For any year, the number of children served will be greater than the population at a point in time so long as some children leave the system during the year.
- Data on foster children receiving support via the federal AFDC/Title IV-E programs are tied to the flow of matching funds from the federal government to the states to support the services provided and the administration of the program at the state level. Between 1982 and 1990, the population of children eligible for Title IV-E assistance increased by 73%. During this period, the population of foster children eligible for federal reimbursement under Title IV-E grew more than twice as rapidly as the population of foster children not in the federal program and supported largely by state funds. This has led to some concern that, as an open-ended entitlement, the Title IV-E program may provide strong incentives to place children in foster care without strong efforts at family preservation, which are not reimbursed under the program.

Sources: U.S. House of Representatives, Ways and Means Committee: *Overview of entitlement programs. Washington, DC, US Government Printing Office, May 15, 1992, pp 102–44;* Tatara T: *Characteristics of children in substitute and adoptive care: A statistical summary of the VCIS National Child Welfare data base.* Washington, DC, VCIS/APWA, May 1993; Tatara T: U.S. Child Substitute Care Flow Data for FY 1992 and Current Trends in the State Child Substitute Care Populations. *VCIS Research Notes* (August 1993). From Lewit EM: Children in foster care. The Future of Children 3(3): 192, 1993.

is also important to enroll them in this source of medical services.

INHERENT STRENGTHS IN VULNERABLE CHILDREN AND INTERVENTIONS

By 20–30 yr of age, many children who were at special risk will have made moderate successes of their lives. Furstenberg's study of teenage mothers and Werner's study of children in Kauai, most of whom were born prematurely or in poverty, demonstrate that, by this age, the majority in each study had defied the odds and made the transition to stable marriages and jobs and were accepted by their communities as responsible citizens.

Certain biologic characteristics are associated with success over the long term, such as being born with an accepting temperament. Avoidance of additional social risks is even more important. Premature infants or preadolescent boys with conduct disorders and poor reading skills, who must also face a broken family, poverty, frequent moves, and family violence, are at much greater risk than children with only one of these handicaps. But perhaps most important are the protective buffers that have been found to enhance children's resilience because these can be aided by an effective health care system and community. Children generally do better if they can gain social support, either from family members or from a nonjudgmental adult outside the family, especially an older mentor or peer. Providers of medical services should develop ways to "prescribe" supportive "other" persons for children who are at risk and isolated. Promotion of self-esteem and self-efficacy seems to be a very central factor in protecting against risks. It is essential to promote competence in some area of these children's lives.

Providers of medical services need the patience to work over a long time frame and the willingness to accept limited improvement. In addition, prediction of the consequences of risk is never 100% accurate. Health professionals as well as families should have hope. However, the confidence that, even without aid, many such children will achieve a good outcome by age 30 does not justify ignoring or withholding services from them in early life. It should teach us how to focus our resources on those most in need and provide a basis for hope in individual cases.

Programs that seem to work for high-risk children have a similar group of characteristics. A *team* is needed, because it is rare for one individual to be able to provide the multiple services needed for high-risk children. At the same time, successful programs are characterized by at least *one caring person* who can make personal contact with these children and their families. Most successful programs are relatively *small* (or are large programs divided up into small units) and nonbureaucratic but are *intensive, comprehensive,* and *flexible.* They work not only with the individual but also with the *family, school, community,* and even at broader societal levels. In addition, generally the *earlier* the programs are started, in terms of the age of children involved, the better is the chance of success. It is also important for services to be continued over a long period.

GENERAL

Lewit G (ed): Health Care Reform. The Future of Children. 3(2):5, 1993.
Children's Defense Fund: Kids Count Data Book, 1994. The Annie F. Casey Foundation.
Starfield B: Effectiveness of Medical Care: Validating Clinical Wisdom. Baltimore, Johns Hopkins University Press, 1985.
Starfield B: Child and adolescent health status measures. The Future of Children 2(2): 25, 1992.
The State of America's Children. Chicago, Year Book, 1994.
Lewit G (ed): U.S. health care for children. The Future of Children 2(2):4, 1992.
Werner EE: Vulnerable but Invincible: A Longitudinal Study of Resilient Children and Youth. New York, McGraw-Hill, 1982.
Wilson WJ: The Truly Disadvantaged: The Inner City, the Underclass and Public Policy. Chicago, Chicago University Press, 1987.
Zuckerman B, Weitzman M, Alpert JJ (eds): Children at risk: Current social and medical challenges. Pediatr Clin North Am 35:1169, 1988.
Children in Poverty National Center for Children in Poverty: Five Million Children: 1993 Update. New York, National Center for Children in Poverty.
Danziger SK, Danziger S: Child poverty and public policy. Daedalus 122(1): 57, 1993.
Lewit EM: Why is poverty increasing among children? The Future of Children 3(2): 198, 1993.

General Accounting Office: Infants and Toddlers: Dramatic Increases in Numbers Living in Poverty. Washington, DC, US Government Printing Office, 1994.

United States Bureau of the Census: Characteristics of the Population Below the Poverty Level: 1982. Washington, DC, US Government Printing Office, 1982, pp 8–9.

United States Bureau of the Census: Poverty in the United States: 1991: Current Population Reports, Series P-60, No. 181. Washington DC, US Government Printing Office, 1992, p 7.

United States Department of Labor, Bureau of Labor Statistics: Employment and Earnings. Washington, DC, US Government Printing Office, 1992, p 7.

NATIVE AMERICAN, ALASKAN ESKIMO, AND ALEUT CHILDREN

Grossman DC, Krieger JW, Sugarman JR, et al: Health status of urban American Indians and Alaska Natives. JAMA 271:845, 1994.

Hismanick JJ, Coddington DA, Gergen PJ: Trends in asthma-related admissions among American Indian and Alaskan Native children from 1979 to 1989. Arch Pediatr Adolesc Med 148:357, 1994.

The State of Native American Youth Health. University of Minnesota Health Center, 1994.

HOMELESS CHILDREN

Lissauer T, Richman S, Tempia M, et al: Influence of homelessness on acute admissions to hospital. Arch Dis Child 69:423, 1993.

Wood DL, Valdez RB, Hayashi T, et al: Health of homeless children and housed, poor children. Pediatrics 86:858, 1990.

CHILDREN OF MIGRANT FARM WORKERS

Dever GEA: Migrant Health Status: Profile of a Population with Complex Health Problems. Monograph Series. Migrant Clinicians Network. National Migrant Resource Program, 1991.

National Commission to Prevent Infant Mortality:HIV/AIDS: A Growing Crisis Among Migrant and Seasonal Farmworker Families, 1993.

Slesinger DP: Health status and needs of migrant farm workers in the United States: A literature review. Res Rev 8(3):227, 1992.

RUNAWAY AND THROWNAWAY CHILDREN

Finkelhor D, Hotaling G, Sedlak A: Missing, Abducted, Runaway, and Thrownaway Children in America. Washington, DC, Office of Justice Programs. Attorney General U.S., 1990.

CHILDREN OF IMMIGRANTS

Martin J (personal communication). Center for Immigration Studies, April 11, 1994.

FOSTER CHILDREN

American Academy of Pediatrics: Health care of foster children. Pediatrics 93:335, 1994.

Chernoff R, Combs-Orme T, Risley-Curtiss C, et al: Assessing the health status of children entering foster care. Pediatrics 93:594, 1994.

Levine C, Stein GL: Orphans of the HIV Epidemic. The Orphan Project. New York, NY 1994.

Lewit EM: Children in foster care. The Future of Children 3(3):192, 1993.

Tatara T: Characteristics of Children in Substitute and Adoptive Care: A Statistical Summary of the UCIS National Child Welfare Data Base. Washington, DC, VSIS/APWA, 1993.

Tatara T: U.S. Child Substitute Care Flow Data for FY 1992 and Current Trends in the State Child Substitute Care Populations, No. 9. Washington, DC, VSIS Research Notes, August 1993.

United States General Accounting Office: Foster Care. Washington, DC, US Government Printing Office, April 1994.

US House of Representatives, Ways and Means Committee: Overview of Entitlement Programs. Washington, DC, US Government Printing Office, May 15, 1992, pp 102–144.

Part VI

Nutrition

Lewis A. Barness ■ John S. Curran

Chapter 43
Nutritional Requirements

Individual nutritional requirements vary with genetic and metabolic differences. For infants and children, however, the basic goals are satisfactory growth and the avoidance of deficiency states. Good nutrition helps to prevent acute and chronic illness and to develop physical and mental potential; it should also provide reserves for stress.

The Food and Nutrition Board (NAS-NRC, 1989) has identified appropriate dietary allowances for a number of substances that prevent deficiency states in most persons (Table 43–1). Because some essential substances remain unidentifiable, a varied diet may be the only prudent way of providing them after early infancy. Only human milk appears to supply all essentials for a prolonged time. Although some food essentials should be included in the daily diet, others are stored by the body and may be supplied periodically.

Although any diet producing good nutrition varies considerably, mild excesses of nutrients or calories may be as undesirable as mild deficiencies. Because dietary influence on aspects of the aging process, for example, atherosclerosis and longevity, remains incompletely understood, avoidance of excessive caloric and fat intake appears to be wise at all ages.

43.1 Water

Water (see also Chapter 46) is essential for existence; a lack of it results in death in a matter of days. The water content of infants is relatively higher (75–80% of the body weight) than that of adults (55–60%). Although dietary fluids provide the principal source of water, some water is obtained from the oxidation of foods (mixed diets yield about 12 g of H_2O/100kcal) and, when needed, body tissues.

Human needs for water are related to caloric consumption, to insensible loss, and to the specific gravity of the urine. The infant must consume much larger amounts of water per unit of body weight compared with the adult, but when calculated per unit of caloric intake, the amounts required are almost identical (Tables 43–2 and 43–3). The daily consumption of fluid by the healthy infant is equivalent to 10–15% of body weight compared with 2–4% in the adult. The usual food of infants and children is high in water content; most of the solid food in the child's diet contains 60–70% water, with fruits and vegetables containing 90%.

Water is absorbed throughout the intestinal tract. The quantity of water in the interstitial compartment is readily changed to maintain homeostatic balance between the intracellular and vascular compartments. The interchange of water among these compartments depends on their respective protein and electrolyte concentrations. Depending on the rate of growth, about 0.5–3% of the fluid intake will be retained. Retention of water is in the range of 9–13 mL/24 hr for the "male reference infant" in the first year of life.

Water balance depends on variables, such as the protein and mineral content of diet, that determine solute load presented for renal excretion, metabolic and respiratory rates, and body temperature. Water requirements for low-birthweight infants are estimated at 85–170 mL/kg/24 hr. Fecal losses are small (3–10% of intake). Evaporation from lungs and skin accounts for 40–50% of intake (sometimes more) and renal excretion for 40–50% or more. The kidney preserves the fluid and electrolyte equilibrium of the body by varying the osmolar content and volume of urine. Urine usually has a greater osmotic pressure (300–1,000 mOsm/L) than the internal environment (293 mOsm/L); maximum normal urinary concentration is approximately 600–700 mOsm/L.

43.2 Energy

The unit of heat in metabolism is the large calorie or kilocalorie (1 Cal = 1kcal); it is used to refer to the energy content of food. A kilocalorie is defined as the amount of heat necessary to raise the temperature of 1 kg of water from 14.5–15.5° C. The production of heat varies in the oxidation of different foods, so that measuring the amount of oxygen consumed or measuring the end products of oxidation, carbon dioxide, and water approximates the values obtained by direct calorimetry.

Energy needs of children at different ages and under various conditions (Fig. 43–1) vary greatly. The approximate average expenditures of energy by the child 6–12 yr of age are basal metabolism, 50%; growth, 12%; physical activity, 25%; and fecal loss, about 8%, mainly as unabsorbed fat.

Basal metabolism is measured at room temperature (20° C) 10–14 hr after a meal, with the patient physically and emotionally quiet. For each centigrade degree of fever, basal metabolism increases approximately 10%. The basal requirement in infants is about 55 kcal/kg/24 hr; it decreases to 25–30 kcal/kg/24 hr at maturity. The term *thermic effect of food* (TEF) refers to the increase in metabolism over the basal rate by the ingestion and assimilation of food. Protein digestion may increase metabolism as much as 30% above the basal level, except when it is being deposited in tissues, whereas fat and carbohydrate, which have a "sparing" effect on the TEF of protein and upon each other, cause increases of only 4 and 6%, respectively. In infants, about 7–8% of the total caloric

■ **TABLE 43–1 Food and Nutrition Board, National Academy of Sciences–National Research Council Recommended Dietary Allowances (Revised 1989)*†**

							Fat-Soluble Vitamins				Water-Soluble Vitamins							Minerals						
Category	Age (yr) or Condition	Weight‡ (kg)	Weight‡ (lb)	Height‡ (cm)	Height‡ (in)	Protein (g)	Vitamin A (μg RE)§	Vitamin D (μg)‖	Vitamine E (mg α-TE)¶	Vitamin K (μg)	Vitamin C (mg)	Thiamine (mg)	Riboflavin (mg)	Niacin (mg NE)**	Vitamin B_6 (mg)	Folate (μg)	Vitamin B_{12} (μg)	Calcium (mg)	Phosphorus (mg)	Magnesium (mg)	Iron (mg)	Zinc (mg)	Iodine (μg)	Selenium (μg)
Infants	0.0–0.5	6	13	60	24	13	375	7.5	3	5	30	0.3	0.4	5	0.3	25	0.3	400	300	40	6	5	40	10
	0.5–1.0	9	20	71	28	14	375	10	4	10	35	0.4	0.5	6	0.6	35	0.5	600	500	60	10	5	50	15
Children	1–3	13	29	90	35	16	400	10	6	15	40	0.7	0.8	9	1.0	50	0.7	800	800	80	10	10	70	20
	4–6	20	44	112	44	24	500	10	7	20	45	0.9	1.1	12	1.1	75	1.0	800	800	120	10	10	90	20
	7–10	28	62	132	52	28	700	10	7	30	45	1.0	1.2	13	1.4	100	1.4	800	800	170	10	10	120	30
Males	11–14	45	99	157	62	45	1,000	10	10	45	50	1.3	1.5	17	1.7	150	2.0	1,200	1,200	270	12	15	150	40
	15–18	66	145	176	69	59	1,000	10	10	65	60	1.5	1.8	20	2.0	200	2.0	1,200	1,200	400	12	15	150	50
	19–24	72	160	177	70	58	1,000	10	10	70	60	1.5	1.7	19	2.0	200	2.0	1,200	1,200	350	10	15	150	70
	25–50	79	174	176	70	63	1,000	5	10	80	60	1.5	1.7	19	2.0	200	2.0	800	800	350	10	15	150	70
	51+	77	170	173	68	63	1,000	5	10	80	60	1.2	1.4	15	2.0	200	2.0	800	800	350	10	15	150	70
Females	11–14	46	101	157	62	46	800	10	8	45	50	1.1	1.3	15	1.4	150	2.0	1,200	1,200	280	15	12	150	45
	15–18	55	120	163	64	44	800	10	8	55	60	1.1	1.3	15	1.5	180	2.0	1,200	1,200	300	15	12	150	50
	19–24	58	128	164	65	46	800	10	8	60	60	1.1	1.3	15	1.6	180	2.0	1,200	1,200	280	15	12	150	55
	25–50	63	138	163	64	50	800	5	8	65	60	1.1	1.3	15	1.6	180	2.0	800	800	280	15	12	150	55
	51+	65	143	160	63	50	800	5	8	65	60	1.0	1.2	13	1.6	180	2.0	800	800	280	10	12	150	55
Pregnant						60	800	10	10	65	70	1.5	1.6	17	2.2	400	2.2	1,200	1,200	320	30	15	175	65
Lactating	1st 6 mo					65	1,300	10	12	65	95	1.6	1.8	20	2.1	280	2.6	1,200	1,200	355	15	19	200	75
	2nd 6 mo					62	1,200	10	11	65	90	1.6	1.7	20	2.1	260	2.6	1,200	1,200	340	15	16	200	75

*The allowances, expressed as average daily intakes over time, are intended to provide for individual variations among most normal persons as they live in the United States under usual environmental stresses. Diets should be based on a variety of common foods in order to provide other nutrients for which human requirements have been less well defined. See text for detailed discussion of allowances and of nutrients not tabulated.

†Designed for the maintenance of good nutrition of practically all healthy people in the United States.

‡Weights and heights of Reference Adults are actual medians for the population in the United States of the designated age, as reported by National Health and Nutrition Examination Survey (NHANES II). The median weights and heights of those younger than 19 yr of age were taken from Hamill H, et al: Physical growth: National Center for Health Statistics Percentiles. Am J Clin Nutr 32:607, 1979. The use of these figures does not imply that the height-to-weight ratios are ideal.

§Retinol equivalents. 1 retinol equivalent (RE) = 1 μg retinol or 6 μg β-carotene. See text for calculation of vitamin A activity of diets as retinol equivalents.

‖As cholecalciferol. 10 μg cholecalciferol = 400 IU of vitamin D.

¶α-Tocopherol equivalents. 1 mg d-α-tocopherol = 1 mg α-TE. See text for variation in allowances and calculation of vitamin E activity of the diet as α-tocopherol equivalent.

**1 NE (niacin equivalent) is equal to 1 mg of niacin or 60 mg of dietary tryptophan.

■ TABLE 43–2 Water Requirements

Urine Specific Gravity	Infant–3 kg 300 Calories* Intake — Water Intake mL	g/100 kcal	g/kg	Adult–70 kg 3,000 Calories* Intake — Water Intake mL	g/100 kcal	g/kg
1.005	650	217	220	6300	210	90
1.015	339	113	116	3180	106	45
1.020	300	100	100	2790	93	40
1.030	264	88	91	2430	81	35

In this sense Calorie = large calorie = 1 kcal = 1 Cal (see text).

intake goes to the TEF, whereas, in older children on an ordinary mixed diet, it is unlikely to constitute more than about 5% of total intake. The estimated energy necessary to build body tissue (*growth*) is the difference between the calories ingested and those expended for other purposes. The average requirement for *physical activity* is 15–25 kcal/kg/24 hr, with peak utilizations as high as 50–80 kcal/kg/24 hr, for short periods. The amount of energy-producing food lost in the stools, except when absorption is impaired, is not more than 10% of the intake.

Although caloric requirements can best be predicted from the surface area rather than from age or weight, the final criteria for evaluating the child's needs depend on the growth pattern, the sense of well-being, and satiety. The daily requirement is approximately 80–120 kcal/kg for the 1st yr of life, with subsequent decreases of about 10 kcal/kg for each succeeding 3-yr period. Periods of rapid growth and development near puberty require increased caloric consumption. The distribution of calories in human milk, in most formulas, and in a well-balanced diet is similar. Approximately 9–15% of the calories are derived from protein, 45–55% are derived from carbohydrate, and 35–45% are derived from fat.

Each gram of ingested protein or carbohydrate provides 4 kcal. One gram of short-chain fatty acids provides 5.3 kcal; 1 g of medium-chain fatty acid gives 8.3 kcal; and 1 g of long-chain fatty acids provides 9 kcal. A continued caloric intake greater or less than the body expenditure will increase or decrease body fat. In general, a consistent caloric imbalance of 500 kcal/24 hr changes body weight by about 450 g (1 lb)/wk.

43.3 Proteins

Protein constitutes about 20% of adult body weight. Its amino acids are essential nutrients in forming cell protoplasm.

■ TABLE 43–3 Range of Average Water Requirements of Children at Different Ages Under Ordinary Conditions

Age	Average Body Weight (kg)	Total Water in 24 hr (mL)	Water per Kilogram of Body Weight in 24 hr (mL)
3 days	3.0	250–300	80–100
10 days	3.2	400–500	125–150
3 mo	5.4	750–850	140–160
6 mo	7.3	950–1100	130–155
9 mo	8.6	1,100–1,250	125–145
1 yr	9.5	1,150–1,300	120–135
2 yr	11.8	1,350–1,500	115–125
4 yr	16.2	1,600–1,800	100–110
6 yr	20.0	1,800–2,000	90–100
10 yr	28.7	2,000–2,500	70–85
14 yr	45.0	2,200–2,700	50–60
18 yr	54.0	2,200–2,700	40–50

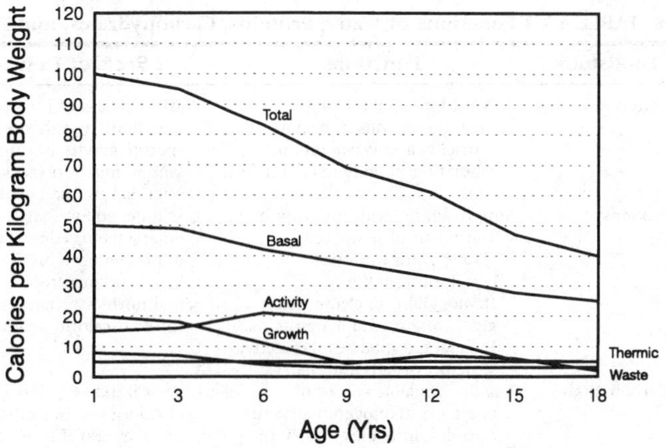

Figure 43–1. Changing energy expenditure with age.

The kind, number, and arrangement of amino acids in a protein molecule determine its characteristics. Twenty-four amino acids have been identified; nine were found to be essential for infants (threonine, valine, leucine, isoleucine, lysine, tryptophan, phenylalanine, methionine, and histidine). Arginine, cystine, and taurine are essential for low-birthweight infants. Nonessential amino acids can be synthesized and need not be supplied in the diet. New tissue cannot be formed without all of the essential amino acids simultaneously present in the diet; the absence or deficiency of only one essential amino acid results in a negative nitrogen balance.

Proteins are broken down in the digestive process to oligopeptides and α-amino acids. The hydrochloric acid of the stomach provides the optimal pH for peptide cleavage by pepsin. Chymosin changes casein of milk to paracasein, which pepsin hydrolyzes along with other proteins. The various proteases show preference for splitting specific peptide linkages; some cleave linkages in the interior of the peptide chain, and others act at more terminal junctures. In the alkaline medium of the intestine, trypsin, chymotrypsin, and carboxypeptidase from the pancreas hydrolyze these proteins and peptones to peptides and to some amino acids; other peptidases from the intestinal juices carry digestion to the amino acid stage.

Minute amounts of certain proteins may be absorbed unchanged, as shown by immunologic reactions, but the hydrolytic products, the amino acids, and some peptides are normally absorbed through the intestinal mucosa. Large oligopeptides may be absorbed in the first few months of life or after episodes of gastroenteritis. The amino acids are carried to the liver by the portal circulation, and from there they are distributed to other tissues. Amino acids are reconstituted to functional human proteins (e.g., albumin, hemoglobin, hormones). Excess amino acids undergo deamination, and the nitrogenous portions are converted to urea in the liver and excreted by the kidneys. The carbon from amino acids is oxidized much like that of carbohydrate or fat; some amino acids are glycogenic; others are ketogenic. Proteins cannot be effectively stored. In protein depletion states, proteins from muscle may be broken down to supply amino acids for more essential sites, such as the brain and for enzyme synthesis.

Aberrations in the metabolism of protein and the amino acids constitute a significant portion of the disease entities known as inborn errors of metabolism (see Part X).

Protein requirements at various ages are listed in Table 43–1. "Biologic value" of proteins indicates effectiveness of utilization; proteins of high biologic value have the quantity and distribution of essential amino acids appropriate for resynthesis of body tissues and provide little waste, as determined by nitrogen balance studies (Table 43–4). Abundant protein is

■ TABLE 43–4 Functions of Water, Proteins, Carbohydrates, and Fats

Foodstuffs	Functions	Effects of Deficiency	Effects of Excess	Sources
Water	Solvent for cellular changes, medium for ions, transport of nutrients and waste products, regulation of body temperature	Thirst, dryness of tongue, dehydration, anhydremia, high specific gravity of urine, loss of kidney function (acidosis, oliguria, uremia, death)	Abdominal discomfort, headache, cramps (water without salt), intoxication, convulsions, edema, and circulatory failure	Water as such, all foods
Proteins	Supply amino acids for growth and repair of tissue cells, solutions for osmotic equilibrium, buffer. Hemoglobin, nucleoproteins, glycoprotein, and lipoproteins. Enzymes, antibodies. Protective structures (nails and hair)	Lassitude, abdominal enlargement, edema, depletion of plasma proteins, kwashiorkor (protein malnutrition); marasmus (protein-calorie malnutrition)	Prolonged high protein intake. May aggravate renal insufficiency	Milk, eggs, meat, fish, poultry, cheese, soybeans, peas, beans, cereals, nuts, lentils
Carbohydrates	Readily available source of energy, antiketogenic, structure of cells, antibodies, source of stored calories (glycogen and fat), resynthesis of amino acids, roughage	Ketosis if intake is less than 15% of calories or in starvation; underweight if total calories are low	Overweight if total calories are high. Various syndromes due to inborn errors of sugar metabolism.	Milk, cereals, fruits, sucrose, syrups, starches, vegetables
Fats	Concentrated source of energy; physical protection for vessels, nerves, organs; insulation against changes in temperature; cell membranes and nuclei; vehicle for absorption of vitamins (A, D, E, and K); essential fatty acids, appetite appeal; aid satiety (delay emptying time of stomach)	Lack of satiety (craving for fat), underweight, skin changes with intakes very low in linoleic acid	Overweight, abdominal symptoms in familial hyperlipidemia, high cholesterol intakes may be harmful to selected populations	Milk, butter, egg yolk, lard, bacon, meat, fish, cheese, nuts, vegetable oils. Breast milk usually supplies 4–5% of calories as linoleic acid; vegetable oils vary greatly, with safflower, corn, soy, and others being especially rich

available for children in the United States, but the supply in many countries is limited.

43.4 Carbohydrates

Carbohydrates, while supplying the necessary bulk of the diet, also supply most of the body's energy needs. In their absence, the body uses proteins and fats for energy. Stored chiefly as glycogen in the liver and muscles, carbohydrates probably constitute no more than 1% of the body weight. Because the size of the infant's liver is 10% of that of the adult's liver and the muscle mass is 2%, the infant's glycogen reserve is a fraction (approximately 3.5%) of that of the adult's.

Carbohydrates are oxidized as glucose (dextrose) but are consumed in various forms: the monosaccharides (glucose, fructose, galactose), the disaccharides (lactose, sucrose, maltose, isomaltose), and the polysaccharides (starches, dextrins, glycogen, gums, cellulose). Pentoses are poorly absorbed.

Through a series of enzymatic and chemical reactions in the digestive tract, complex carbohydrates are split into simpler structures. Salivary and pancreatic amylases are principally involved in the breakdown of starch to oligosaccharides (dextrins) and disaccharides (primarily maltose). Intestinal amylase may be decreased during the first 4 mo of life. The disaccharides are absorbed intact into the intestinal brush border cells, where disaccharidases in the microvilli complete the hydrolysis to the monosaccharides: one molecule of maltose to two molecules of glucose; sucrose to glucose and fructose; lactose to glucose and galactose. The monosaccharides are absorbed rapidly; glucose and galactose are actively taken up against concentration gradients, whereas fructose absorption is passive. During absorption, phosphoric acid "carrier" radicals combine with hexose sugars in the intestinal mucosa for transport across the cell membrane. Sodium must be present for absorption to continue when the intraintestinal sugar concentration is low. These hexose phosphates separate again into their component parts, permitting the sugar to diffuse into the portal bloodstream.

Some glucose may be oxidized directly, such as in the brain and heart. Most of the absorbed sugar is converted to glycogen in the liver, although glycogenesis also occurs in other tissues. Up to 15% of the weight of the liver and 3% of the muscle may be glycogen; small amounts are also found in practically all other organs. Glycogenolysis in the liver yields glucose as the chief product, whereas glycogen breakdown in the muscle yields lactic acid. The overall oxidation of glucose has two phases, the anaerobic (glycolysis) and the aerobic (tricarboxylic acid cycle). In the former, glucose is broken down to pyruvic acid; in the aerobic cycle, pyruvic acid is completely oxidized to carbon dioxide and water. Insulin and the pituitary and adrenal hormones are involved in these processes, and nicotinic acid, thiamine, riboflavin, and pantothenic acid take part in the enzymatic reactions. Carbohydrate that is not oxidized or stored as glycogen is converted to fat.

The principal carbohydrate metabolic disorders are diabetes mellitus, glycogen storage disease, galactosemia, fructose intolerance, and glucose intolerance; deficiencies of sugar-splitting enzymes in the intestines (lactase, sucrase, maltase) are associated with diarrhea and malabsorption resulting from the osmotic effect of the unabsorbed sugar and from fermentation of the carbohydrate by intestinal bacteria.

43.5 Fats

Fats or their metabolic products form an integral part of cellular membranes and are efficient stores of energy. They impart palatability to food and serve as vehicles for fat-soluble vitamins A, D, E, and K. Approximately 98% of natural fats are triglycerides, three fatty acids combined with glycerol. The remaining 2% include free fatty acids, monoglycerides, diglycerides, cholesterol, and phospholipids (including lecithin, cephalin, sphingomyelin, and cerebrosides).

Naturally occurring fats contain straight-chain fatty acids, both saturated and unsaturated, varying in length from 4 to 24 carbon atoms. The degree of absorption generally varies with the melting point, the degree of unsaturation, and the positions of the fatty acids on the glycerol molecule.

Ingested triglycerides are partially hydrolyzed by lingual lipase and emulsified in the stomach. In the duodenum, pancreatic lipase hydrolyzes the triglycerides to monoglycerides and fatty acids and, with bile salts, forms micelles, which increase fat solubility. Unsplit diglycerides and triglycerides are insoluble. Low-birthweight infants have decreased amounts of bile and decreased absorption of fat.

Long-chain fatty acids and monoglycerides (those with more than 10 carbon atoms) in micelles are presumably absorbed into the mucosal cell by diffusion. Transport across the cell involves re-esterification of these fatty acids and monoglycerides to triglycerides, which are then "coated" with lipoprotein to form the chylomicron, in which the fat is transported in the lymph system to the venous circulation via the thoracic duct. Transport proteins include very low-density, low-density, and high-density lipoproteins synthesized in the liver.

Short- and medium-chain triglycerides are handled differently; they are readily hydrolyzed by pancreatic lipase to free fatty acids, which are transported through the cell. Even when intraluminal hydrolysis is inadequate because of deficiency of pancreatic lipase or of bile salts, these fats will be absorbed and hydrolyzed to free fatty acids within the cell by mucosal lipase. With neither esterification to triglycerides nor subsequent chylomicron formation, these free fatty acids directly enter the intestinal veins and pass to the liver via the portal system. This alternative pathway for short- and medium-chain triglycerides is utilized in nutritional formulations for children with severe absorptive problems.

ESSENTIAL FATTY ACIDS. Humans do not synthesize linoleic or linolenic acid. Both must be supplied in the diet and are, therefore, "essential." Linoleic acid is the precursor of arachidonic acid, the prostaglandins, and the leukotrienes. Linolenic acid modulates the rate of production of arachidonic acid metabolites and forms longer chain unsaturated fatty acids, which may be essential for central nervous system structure and function. Essential fatty acids are necessary for growth, skin and hair integrity, regulation of cholesterol metabolism, lipotropic activity, decreased platelet adhesiveness, and reproduction. Diets containing less than 1–2% of the calories as linoleic acid require greater caloric consumption for comparable growth. In children with essential fatty acid deficiency, serum levels of trienoic acid increase relative to tetraenoic acids. Excess unsaturated acids increase peroxidation and may cause membrane destruction. Rapidly growing young infants maintained on diets very low in linoleic acid develop intertrigo and dryness, thickening, and desquamation of the skin.

The relation of dietary fat intake to intimal fat streaking in the major arterial vessels in early life and atheromatous changes in adults remains to be clarified (see Chapter 72.4).

43.6 Minerals

The physiologic roles and dietary sources of the principal minerals with nutritional significance are summarized in Table 43–5. Requirements are shown in Table 43–1, except for several of the trace elements.

The ash content of the fetus is about 3% of the body weight at birth. It increases continuously throughout childhood. Adult ash content is 4.35% of body weight; 83% is in the skeleton, and 10% is in the muscle. For each gram of protein retained, 0.3 g of mineral matter is deposited. The principal cations are calcium, magnesium, potassium, and sodium; the comparable anions are phosphorus, sulfur, and chloride. Iron, iodine, and cobalt appear in important organic complexes. The trace elements fluorine, copper, zinc, chromium, manganese, selenium, and molybdenum have known metabolic roles; silicon, boron, nickel, aluminum, arsenic, bromine, and strontium are also present in the diet and in the body.

43.7 Vitamins

The word "vitamin" refers to organic compounds required in minute amounts to catalyze cellular metabolism essential for growth or maintenance of the organism. Vitamin requirements for infants and children are listed in Table 43–1. For vitamin functions and disorders, see Table 43–6 and Chapter 45.3.

43.8 Miscellaneous Factors

FIBER. The quantity of undigestible vegetable fiber consumed in acceptable diets may be as much as 170–300 mg/kg/24 hr. Most children who receive well-balanced diets obtain sufficient amounts of fiber. Highly refined foods contain little fiber and may be associated with increased incidence of constipation, appendicitis, diverticulitis, and other intestinal disorders. High-fiber intake may result in decreased absorption of cholesterol as well as zinc and other essential nutrients.

DIGESTIBILITY. The relative amount of a given nutrient available for assimilation is high in most of the common food classes: carbohydrate, 97%; fat, 95%; protein, 92%. Cooking is a factor in digestibility. For example, the boiling of milk reduces the size of the curd and renders it more digestible; on the other hand, heating destroys the activity of vitamin C.

SATIETY. The ingestion of a meal should provide a sense of well-being. Whole milk, cream, eggs, and fatty foods have high satiety values; sugar increases the flow of gastric juice and delays emptying of the stomach, thus increasing satiety. Bread and potatoes have relatively low satiety values, as do lean meat, fish, vegetables, and many fruits.

AVAILABILITY. Poverty, ignorance, and lack of practical education in buying and preparing food are the main causes of malnutrition in children. Diets of lower-income families are often deficient in milk, fruits, fresh vegetables, and meats. A suggested method for planning low-cost meals is to divide the money available for food into fifths: one fifth each for vegetables and fruits; for milk and cheese; for meats, fish, and eggs; for bread and cereals; and for fats, sugar, and other food adjuncts.

Geographic location may influence the availability of foods and the development of deficiency disorders, especially among low socioeconomic populations, for example, the relation of dental caries to lack of fluoride in communal water supplies.

BACTERIAL SYNTHESIS OF VITAMINS. Certain vitamins are synthesized in the human gastrointestinal tract; however, the extent to which they can meet the body's needs is uncertain. Once the bacterial flora of the intestinal tract have been established, vitamin K is produced and is available to the body. Pantothenic acid and biotin, essential to human metabolism, can be supplied by bacterial synthesis alone. Thiamine, riboflavin, niacin, vitamin B_6, vitamin B_{12}, and folic acid are synthesized in some species, but synthesis is limited or does not exist in humans. The kind of food or the nature of intestinal flora may affect vitamin production or availability. For instance, 3% of the

Text continued on page 150

■ **TABLE 43–5 Physiology and Sources of Nutritionally Important Minerals**

Mineral	Function and Metabolism	Effects of Deficiency	Effects of Excess	Sources
Calcium	Structure of bone and teeth, muscle contraction, nerve irritability, coagulation of blood, cardiac action, production of milk Absorbed from upper small intestine: aided by vitamin D, ascorbic acid, lactose, acid medium; hindered by excesses of dietary oxalic acid, phytic acid, fat, fiber, phosphate. Deposited in bone trabeculas and maintained in dynamic equilibrium with body tissue through action of parathyroid hormone and thyrocalcitonin About 70% excreted in feces, 10% in urine, 15–25% retained, depending on growth rate. Serum level 9–11 mg/dL, 60% ionized	Poor mineralization of bones and teeth; osteomalacia; osteoporosis; tetany; rickets; impairment of growth	Unknown (dietary) Heart block and renal stones (parenteral)	Milk, cheese, green leafy vegetables, canned salmon, clams, oysters
Chloride	Osmotic pressure; acid-base balance; HCl in gastric juice. Readily absorbed; about 92% of intake is excreted, mainly in the urine, some in feces and sweat; comprises about ⅔ of the blood plasma anions; blood serum level, 99–106 mEq/L; in intracellular and extracellular fluids; parallels sodium intake and output	Hypochloremic alkalosis may occur with prolonged vomiting or excessive sweating, with parenteral administration of glucose without saline, with excessive ACTH therapy, and with congenital alkalosis	Unknown	Table salt, meat, milk, eggs
Chromium	Glycemia regulation and insulin metabolism	Diabetes in animals	None known	Yeast
Cobalt	Component of vitamin B_{12} (cyanocobalamin) molecule and of erythropoietin	None known ? Hypothyroidism	Cardiomyopathy; medicinally, it may be goitrogenic or may produce cardiomyopathy	Widely distributed
Copper	Essential for production of red blood cells; transferrin, hemoglobin formation; absorption of iron, activities of tyrosinase, catalase, uricase, cytochrome C oxidase, 8-aminolevulinic acid dehydrase, lysyl oxidase. Absorbed with sulfur-rich proteins; transported bound to α-2-globulin as ceruloplasmin; present in erythrocytes in a labile form and the more stable hemocuprein; highest concentration in liver and central nervous system (cerebrocuprein); excreted mainly via the intestinal wall and the bile; deranged metabolism in Wilson disease (hepatolenticular degeneration), and Menkes syndrome	May be cause of refractory anemia, osteoporosis, neutropenia, depigmentation and delayed bone age, bone infractions, pseudoparalysis, ataxia. Increase of serum cholesterol	Cirrhosis, gastritis, hemolysis	Liver, oysters, meats, fish, whole grains, nuts, legumes
Fluorine	Tooth and bone structure. Retained when intake is above 0.6 mg/day; excreted in urine and sweat; deposited in bones as fluorapatite (dynamic equilibrium)	Tendency to dental caries	Fluorosis: mottling of teeth with intake of more than 4–8 mg/24 hr	Water, sea foods, plant and animal foods (dependent on content in soil and water)
Iodine	Constituent of thyroxine (T4) and triiodothyronine (T3) Readily absorbed from intestine; circulates as inorganic and organic iodide; selectively concentrated about 25:1 in the thyroid gland, quickly iodized and incorporated into thyroglobulin; proteolytic enzymes release thyroxine and triiodothyronine into the blood. Excretion mainly in urine. Antithyroid compounds: goitrins and brassicae; certain drugs interfere with iodine metabolism	Simple goiter, endemic cretinism	Not harmful (less than 1 mg/24 hr); medicinally, may cause goiter	Iodized salt, sea food, food grown in nongoitrous areas
Iron	Structure of hemoglobin and myoglobin for O_2 and CO_2 transport; oxidative enzymes; cytochrome C and catalase. Absorbed in ferrous form according to body need, aided by gastric juice and ascorbic acid; hindered by fiber, phytic acid, steatorrhea. Transported in plasma in ferric state bound to transferrin; stored in liver, spleen, bone marrow, and kidney as ferritin and hemosiderin; conserved and reused; minimal losses in urine and sweat; about 90% of intake excreted in the stool	Anemia; hypochromic, microcytic, growth failure; hyperactivity (?)	Hemosiderosis in Bantu people of Africa due to low phosphorus and high iron contents of diet. Poisoning by medicinal iron	Liver, meat, egg yolk, green vegetables, whole grains, legumes, nuts

■ TABLE 43–5 Physiology and Sources of Nutritionally Important Minerals *Continued*

Mineral	Function and Metabolism	Effects of Deficiency	Effects of Excess	Sources
Magnesium	Structure of bones and teeth; activation of enzymes in carbohydrate metabolism; muscle and nerve irritability, important intracellular cation, essential to metabolic processes. Principal cation of soft tissue; absorption from small intestine varies with intake; some urinary excretion, but excellent renal conservation; antagonist to calcium action	Occurs in malabsorption and deficiency states; diabetes, may be expressed clinically as tetany; associated frequently with hypocalcemia; hypokalemia	None (dietary); toxicity from intravenous medication	Cereals, legumes, nuts, meat, milk
Manganese	Enzyme activation, especially superoxide dismutase; normal bone structure, carbohydrate metabolism. Poor absorption from intestine; transported in plasma; particularly high turnover rate in mitochondria; excretion mainly via the intestine in bile; competes with iron	Not known	None (dietary); toxicity from chronic inhalation (encephalopathy)	Legumes, nuts, whole grain cereals, green leafy vegetables
Molybdenum	Component of enzymes; xanthine oxidase for conversion to uric acid and mobilization of territin iron in liver, liver aldehyde oxidase. Readily absorbed from intestine; excreted chiefly in urine, some in bile	Not observed in humans	Not established	Legumes, grains, dark green leafy vegetables, animal organs
Phosphorus	Constituent of bones and teeth; structure of nucleus and cytoplasm of all cells; acid-base balance; energy transformations and transmission of nerve impulses; metabolism of carbohydrate, protein, and fat. About 70% of intake absorbed as free phosphates; vitamin D and parathormone implicated in intestinal absorption and kidney retention; excreted in urine and feces; occurs in blood as phospholipids, organic esters, and inorganic phosphates; inorganic phosphates in blood serum of infants and children, 4–7 mg/dL; ratio of inorganic to organic phosphates in whole blood is about 1:20	Rickets may develop in rapidly growing, very low-birthweight babies with low intakes of both P and Ca; muscle weakness	Possibility of tetany during recovery from rickets or in newborn on formula with low Ca:P (1:1) ratio	Milk, milk products, egg yolk, fresh foods, legumes, nuts, whole grains
Potassium	Muscle contraction; nerve impulse conduction; intracellular osmotic pressure and fluid balance; heart rhythm. Primarily intracellular; excretion 80% in urine, some in sweat and feces; about 8% retained by growing child; blood serum level 4.0–5.6 mEq/L	In starvation or in such pathologic conditions as diarrhea, diabetic acidosis, ACTH excess; muscle weakness, anorexia, nausea, abdominal distention, nervous irritability, drowsiness, confusion, tachycardia; deficiency exaggerates effects of sodium	Heart block at serum levels of 10 mEq/L; important in Addison disease, renal failure, or administration of potassium-containing salts	All foods
Selenium	Cofactor of glutathione peroxidase in tissue respiration	Kashin cardiomyopathy, arthritis (?), Kashin cardiovascular disease, myositis	Alopecia, nail abnormalities, garlic odor to breath	Vegetables, meat
Sodium	Osmotic pressure; acid-base balance; water balance; muscle and nerve irritability. Readily absorbed from intestine; excreted chiefly in urine (98%); parallels chloride intake; renal excretion controlled by ACTH; extracellular cation, but small amount in muscle and cartilage; blood serum level, 135–145 mEq/L	Nausea; diarrhea, muscle cramps, dehydration, hypotension	Edema if inadequate excretion or excessive parenteral fluids	Table salt, fresh foods, milk, eggs, sodium compounds as baking soda and powder, glutamate, seasonings, and preservatives
Sulfur	Constituent of cellular protein; cocarboxylase; melanin; mucopolysaccharides, vitreous humor, synovial fluid, connective tissues, cartilage, heparin, insulin; metabolism of nerve tissue; detoxification mechanisms; SH group in coenzyme A, cystathionine, and glutathione. Only sources utilized are cystine and methionine; inorganic forms unavailable to body; excreted as inorganic sulfate or ethereal sulfate via urine and bile	Not known; growth failure from protein deficiency may be due in part to deficiency of sulfur-containing amino acids	Not harmful; excreted in urine as sulfates	Protein foods contain about 1%
Zinc	Constituent of several enzymes; carbonic anhydrase (in erythrocytes) essential for CO_2 exchange; carboxypeptidase of intestine for hydrolysis of protein; dehydrogenase of liver. Found in liver and organs, muscles, bones, red and white blood cells; higher tissue concentration in young subjects; excreted chiefly from intestine, competes with copper	Dwarfism, iron-deficiency anemia, hepatosplenomegaly, hyperpigmentation and hypogonadism, acrodermatitis enteropathica, depression of immunocompetence, poor wound healing	Gastrointestinal upsets (from galvanized iron cooking utensils); copper deficiency; decreased high-density lipoprotein	Meat, grain, nuts, cheese

■ TABLE 43–6 Physical and Metabolic Properties and Food Sources of the Vitamins

Names and Synonyms	Characteristics	Biochemical Action	Effects of Deficiency	Effects of Excess	Sources
Vitamin A: retinol (vitamin A1) is an alcohol of high molecular weight; 1 μg of retinol = 3.3 IU vitamin A Provitamin A: the plant pigments α-, β-, and γ-carotenes and cryptoxanthin; ⅙ activity of retinol	Fat soluble; heat stable; destroyed by oxidation, drying; bile necessary for absorption; stored in liver, protected by vitamin E	Component of retinal pigments, rhodopsin and iodopsin, for vision in dim light; bone and tooth development; formation and maturation of epithelia	Nyctalopia, photophobia, xerophthalmia, conjunctivitis, keratomalacia leading to blindness; faulty epiphyseal bone formation; defective tooth enamel; keratinization of mucous membranes and skin; retarded growth; impaired resistance to infection	Anorexia, slow growth, drying and cracking of skin, enlargement of liver and spleen, swelling and pain of long bones, bone fragility, increased intracranial pressure, alopecia, carotenemia	Liver, fish liver oils, whole milk, milk fat products, egg yolk, fortified margarines Carotenoids from plants: green vegetables, yellow fruits and vegetables
Vitamin B Complex: thiamine: vitamin B_1; antiberiberi vitamin; aneurin	Water and alcohol soluble; fat insoluble; stable in slightly acid solution; labile to heat, alkali, sulfites	Component of thiamine pyrophosphate carboxylases, which act in various oxidative decarboxylations, including that of pyruvic acid	Beriberi, fatigue, irritability, anorexia, constipation, headache, insomnia, tachycardia, polyneuritis, cardiac failure, edema, elevated pyruvic acid in the blood, aphonia	None from oral intake	Liver, meat, especially pork, milk, whole grain or enriched cereals, wheat germ, legumes, nuts
Riboflavin: vitamin B_2	Sparingly soluble in water; sensitive to light and alkali; stable to heat, oxidation, acid	Constituent of flavoprotein enzymes important in hydrogen transfer reactions; amino acid, fatty acid, and carbohydrate metabolism and cellular respiration. Retinal pigment for light adaptation	Ariboflavinosis; photophobia, blurred vision, burning and itching of eyes, corneal vascularization, poor growth, cheilosis	Not harmful	Milk, cheese, liver and other organs, meat, eggs, fish, green leafy vegetables, whole or enriched grains
Niacin: nicotinamide; nicotinic acid; antipellagra vitamin	Water and alcohol soluble; stable to acid, alkali, light, heat, oxidation	Constituent of coenzymes I and II. NAD, NADP cofactors in a number of dehydrogenase systems	Pellagra, multiple B-vitamin deficiency syndrome, diarrhea, dementia, dermatitis	Nicotinic acid (not the amide) is vasodilator; skin flushing and itching, hepatopathy	Meat, fish, poultry, liver, whole grain and enriched cereals, green vegetables, peanuts
Folacin: group of related compounds containing pteridine ring, para-amino benzoic acid, and glutamic acid. Pteroylglutamic acid (PGA)	Slightly soluble in water: labile to heat, light, acid	Concerned with formation and metabolism of one-carbon units; participates in synthesis of purines, pyrimidines, nucleoproteins, and methyl groups	Megaloblastic anemia (infancy pregnancy): usually is secondary to malabsorption disease glossitis, pharyngeal ulcers, impaired immunity	Unknown	Liver, green vegetables, nuts, cereals, cheese, fruits, yeast, beans, peas
Cyanocobalamin: vitamin B_{12}	Slightly soluble in water; stable to heat in neutral solution; labile in acid or alkaline ones; destroyed by light. Castle intrinsic factor of the stomach required for absorption	Transfer of one-carbon units in purine and labile methyl group metabolism; essential for maturation of red blood cells in bone marrow; metabolism of nervous tissue; adenosylcobalamin is the coenzyme for methylmalonyl CoA mutase	Juvenile pernicious anemia, due to defect in absorption rather than to dietary lack; also secondary to gastrectomy, celiac disease, inflammatory lesions of small bowel, long-term drug therapy (PAS, neomycin); methylmalonic aciduria; homocystinuria	Unknown	Muscle and organ meats, fish, eggs, milk, cheese

■ **TABLE 43–6 Physical and Metabolic Properties and Food Sources of the Vitamins** *Continued*

Names and Synonyms	Characteristics	Biochemical Action	Effects of Deficiency	Effects of Excess	Sources
Biotin	Crystallized from yeast; soluble in water	Coenzyme carboxylases; involved in CO_2 transfer	Dermatitis, seborrhea; inactivated by avidin in raw egg white	None known	Yeast, animal products; synthesized in intestine
Vitamin B_6 active forms: pyridoxine, pyridoxal, pyridoxamine	Water soluble; destroyed by ultraviolet light and by heat	Constituent of coenzymes for decarboxylation, transamination, transsulfuration; fatty acid metabolism	Irritability, convulsions, hypochromic anemia; peripheral neuritis in patients receiving isoniazid; oxaluria (see Chapter 45.3)	Sensory neuropathy	Meat, liver, kidney, whole grains, soybeans, nuts, fish, poultry, green vegetables
Vitamin C: ascorbic acid; vitamin C; antiscorbutic vitamin	Water soluble; easily oxidized, accelerated by heat, light, alkali oxidative enzymes, traces of copper or iron	Integrity and maintenance of intercellular material, facilitates absorption of iron and conversion of folic acid to folinic acid; metabolism of tyrosine and phenylalanine, activity of succinic dehydrogenase and serum phosphatase in infants, not in adults	Scurvy and poor wound healing	Oxaluria (see also Chapter 45.3 and discussion of hyperoxaluria oxalosis)	Citrus fruits, tomatoes, berries, cantaloupe, cabbage, green vegetables. Cooking has destructive effect.
Vitamin D: group of sterols having similar physiologic activity, D_2-calciferol is activated ergosterol. D_3 is activated 7-dehydrocholesterol in skin 1 μg = 40 IU vitamin D	Fat soluble, stable to heat, acid alkali, and oxidation; bile necessary for absorption. Prohormone for 25-OH cholecalciferol	Regulates absorption and deposition of calcium and phosphorus, by affecting permeability of intestinal membrane; regulates level of serum alkaline phosphatase, which is believed to be concerned with calcium phosphate deposition in bones and teeth	Rickets (high serum phosphatase level appears before bone deformities); infantile tetany, poor growth, osteomalacia	Wide variation in tolerance; over 500 μg/24 hr toxic when continued for weeks; prolonged administration of 45 μg/24 hr may be toxic (Chapter 45.3); nausea, diarrhea, weight loss, polyuria, nocturia, calcification of soft tissues, including heart, renal tubules, blood vessels, bronchi, stomach	Vitamin D-fortified milk and margarine, fish liver oils, exposure to sunlight or other ultraviolet sources
Vitamin E: group of related chemical compounds—tocopherols with similar biologic activities	Fat soluble; unstable to ultraviolet light, alkali, readily oxidized by oxygen, iron, rancid fats Antioxidant; bile necessary for absorption	Minimizes oxidation of carotene, vitamin A, and linoleic acid; stabilizes membranes	Requirements related to polyunsaturated fat intake; red blood cell hemolysis in premature infants, loss of neural integrity	Unknown	Germ oils of various seeds, green leafy vegetables, nuts, legumes
Vitamin K: group of naphthoquinones with similar biologic activities; K_1 is phytoquinone	Natural compounds are fat soluble; stable to heat and reducing agents; labile to oxidizing agent, strong acids, alkali, light; bile salts necessary for intestinal absorption	Prothrombin formation, coagulation factors II, VII, IX, and X and osteocalcin are vitamin K dependent, proteins C, S, Z	Hemorrhagic manifestations; bone metabolism	Not established; analogs may produce hyperbilirubinemia in premature infants	Green leafy vegetables, pork, liver. Widely distributed

NAD(P), nicotinamide adenine dinucleotide (phosphate); CoA, coenzyme A; PAS, para-aminosalicylic acid.

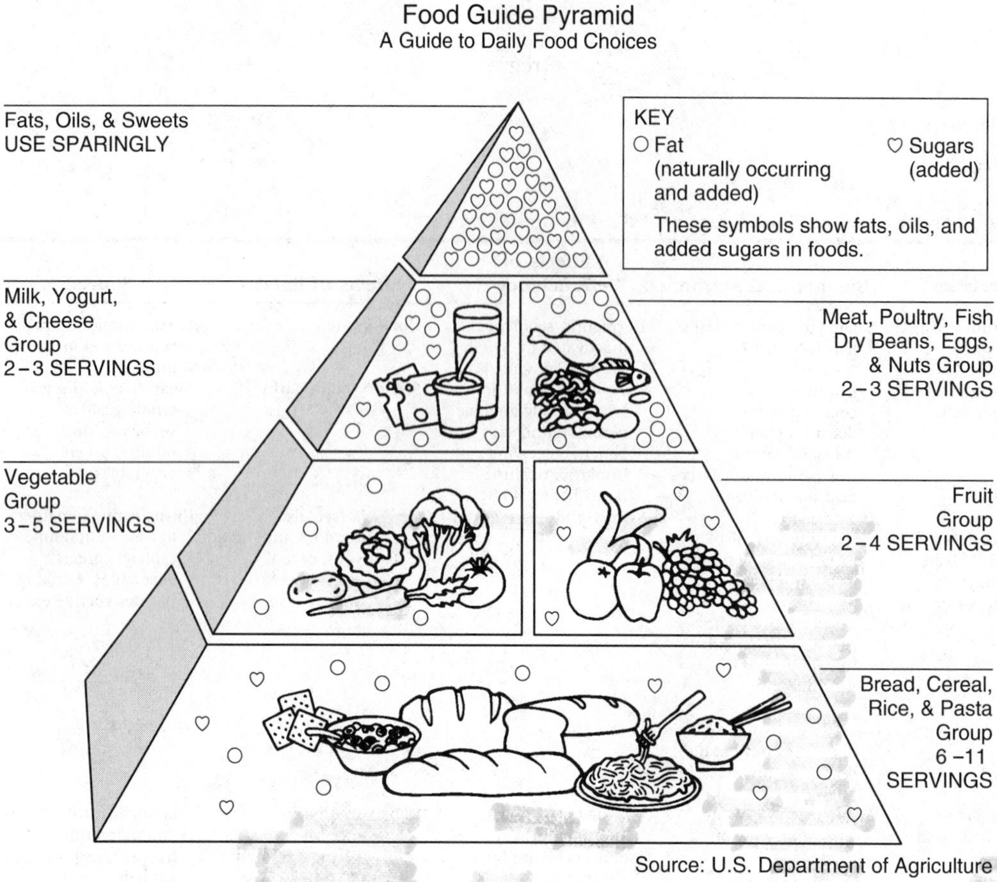

Figure 43–2. Food guide pyramid: a guide to daily food choices.

population in Kobe, Japan, harbored intestinal bacteria that split thiamine; evidence of beriberi appeared in these persons.

ANTIMICROBIAL FACTORS. Administration of antimicrobial agents may affect nutritional status. Appetite is sometimes impaired or bacterial flora producing vitamin K are sufficiently altered to precipitate borderline deficiency. Several antibiotics are known to produce steatorrhea. Orally administered broad-spectrum antibiotics decrease nitrogen balance. Isoniazid combines with pyridoxal phosphate and may produce symptoms of vitamin B_6 deficiency. Antimicrobial compounds may be transmitted in breast milk or in foods from animals that are fed these compounds.

ENDOCRINE FACTORS. Antithyroid substances that increase the requirement for iodine (goitrogens) have been found in turnips, rutabagas, cabbage, soybeans, cobalt-containing foods, food additives, and medications. Administering adrenocorticotropic hormone (ACTH) or corticosteroids necessitates an increase in protein and calcium and a decrease in sodium intake. Transient hypoparathyroidism with tetany has been observed in the neonatal period after excessive intake of vitamin D or of phosphates.

RADIOACTIVITY. Apparently, little danger results from ^{14}C, because of its low activity. ^{131}I is removed from milk by aeration or storage. ^{137}Cs, which may be found in meat and milk products, can be counteracted by a high potassium intake or by acetazolamide. Only 10% of ^{90}Sr ingested by the cow is found in cow's milk.

EMOTIONAL FACTORS. Along with increased knowledge of the significance of various nutrients, excessive parental and professional concern has developed with regard to the food that the individual infant or child eats. The mother, developing a sense of fear or guilt about her child's eating habits, may create a battle of wits between her and her child that may have far-reaching effects. For example, misdirected efforts to control obesity and hypercholesterolemia have led to severe malnutrition in young children.

■ **TABLE 43–7 Recommended Food Intake for Good Nutrition According to Food Groups**

Food Group	Serving Size	Servings/d	1 y	2–3 y	4+ y
Bread, cereal, rice, pasta	1 slice 1 oz (cereal)	6–11	1–2	2–4	3–11
Vegetables	½ cup	3–5	1/2	1	3–5
Fruit	1 apple, banana	2–4	1/2	1	2–4
Milk, cheese	1 cup 1½ oz cheese	2–3	1/2	1	1–3
Meat, poultry, etc	2–3 oz	2–3	1/2–1	1/2–1	1–3

After age 2 yr, fats, oils, and sweets should be consumed sparingly.
C = 1 cup or 8 oz or 240 mL.
Tbsp = tablespoon (1 Tbsp = 15 mL = ½ oz).

43.9 Evaluation of Diet

See Tables 43–7, 670–10, and 670–11 and Figure 43–2.

The recall interview for determining children's food habits is usually satisfactory, but for a more accurate accounting the mother should observe and record the actual food intake and convert to "servings" appropriate to the child's age. It is important to include items that may not be consumed daily.

The 1992 United States Department of Agriculture dietary guide according to food groups provides flexibility (Fig. 43–2). A food intake record can indicate possible nutritional imbalances. An excessive intake of foods of one group may result in a high caloric level, producing an overweight child while at the same time leading to a dangerously low intake of some essential nutrients, such as the overconsumption of milk and the underconsumption of other foods, the resultant danger of which is iron-deficiency anemia. When key foods, such as milk, eggs, and citrus fruits, are eliminated for personal or medical reasons, the deficiencies may be compensated for by judicious substitutions. A list of the principal food groups' nutrients follows:

Milk: high-quality protein, calcium, and phosphorus; riboflavin; vitamin A; vitamin D (if fortified)
Meat and eggs: high-quality protein, iron, B vitamins; vitamin A from liver and eggs
Fruits and vegetables: vitamin C; provitamin A from green and yellow ones; trace elements; fiber
Cereals: less expensive and supplementary amounts of protein, minerals, fiber, B vitamins

Hamil H, et al: Physical growth; National Center for Health Statistics Percentiles. Am J Clin Nutr 32:607, 1979.

CHAPTER 44

The Feeding of Infants and Children

Successful infant feeding requires cooperation between the mother and her baby, beginning with the initial feeding experience and continuing throughout the child's period of dependency. Promptly establishing comfortable, satisfying feeding practices contributes greatly to the infant's and mother's emotional well-being (see Chapter 79). Feeding time should be pleasurable for both mother and child. Because maternal feelings are readily transmitted to the baby and largely determine the emotional setting in which feeding takes place, tense, anxious, irritable, easily upset, or emotionally labile mothers are more likely to experience a difficult feeding relationship, but they frequently become more comfortable and confident with appropriate guidance and support from an empathetic and experienced relative, friend, or physician.

As soon after birth as an infant can safely tolerate enteral nutrition, as judged by normal activity, alertness, suck, and cry, feedings should be initiated to maintain normal metabolism and growth during the transition from fetal to extrauterine life; to promote maternal-infant bonding; and to decrease the risks of hypoglycemia, hyperkalemia, hyperbilirubinemia, and azotemia. Mistakes are made by feeding the infant too much or too little. Inadequate fluid intake, particularly in hot weather, may result in "dehydration fever." Most infants may start breast-feeding shortly after birth and others, within 4–6 hr. When any question about the tolerance of feeding arises because of physical or neurologic status, feeding should be withheld, and parenteral fluids should be substituted. The schedule of initial feeding in a hospital is less important than the principle of the unhurried beginning and patient assistance and support for the mother. Mothers who wish to initiate breast-feeding in the delivery room and continue on a demand basis thereafter should be supported. However, when rooming-in is unavailable or not desired and demand feeding is impractical, the infant can be taken to the mother for the first feeding at 10:00 A.M. or 6:00 P.M., whichever is nearer the end of a 6-hr postpartum rest. Subsequent formula or breast-feedings are given every 3–4 hr/day and night by the mother. Artificially fed infants should receive sterile water for the first feeding because regurgitation and aspiration of this liquid are less likely to cause significant irritation of the respiratory tract.

The feeding of infants requires practical interpretation of specific nutritional needs and of the widely varying limits of the normal baby's appetite and behavior regarding food. The time that it takes the infant's stomach to empty may vary from 1–4 hr or more; thus, considerable difference in the infant's desire for food is expected at different times of the day. Ideally, the feeding schedule should be based on this reasonable "self-regulation." Variation in the time between feedings and in the amount taken per feeding is to be expected in the first few weeks during the establishment of the self-regulation plan. By the end of the first month, more than 90% of infants will have established a suitable and reasonably regular schedule.

Most healthy, bottle-fed infants will want 6–9 feedings/24 hr by the end of the first week of life. Some will take enough at one feeding to satisfy themselves for approximately 4 hr; others who are smaller or whose gastric emptying time is more rapid will want formula about every 2–3 hr; breast-fed infants often prefer shorter intervals. Most term infants will rapidly increase their intake from 30 mL to 80–90 mL every 3–4 hr at 4–5 days of life. Feeding should be considered as having progressed satisfactorily if the infant is no longer losing weight by 5–7 days and is gaining weight by 12–14 days. Some infants will not awaken for a middle-of-the-night feeding after 3–6 wk of age; some may never want it. Many will not want a late evening feeding between 4 and 8 mo of age and will be satisfied with 3 meals/day by 9–12 mo. However, individual feeding needs are quite variable, and one infant should not be expected to fit the pattern of another infant.

It is important to appreciate that infants cry for other reasons besides hunger, and *they need not be fed every time they cry*; some infants are placid, some are unusually active, and some are irritable. Sick infants are often uninterested in food. Infants who awaken and cry consistently at short intervals may not be receiving enough milk at each feeding or may have discomfort from some cause other than hunger, such as too much clothing; colic; soiled, wet, or uncomfortable diapers and clothing; swallowed air ("gas"); uncomfortably hot or cold environment; or illness. Some infants cry to gain sufficient or additional attention, whereas others deprived of adequate mothering become indifferent. Some infants simply need to be held. Those who stop crying when they are picked up or held do not usually need food, but those who continue to cry when held and when food is offered should be carefully evaluated for other causes of distress. The habit of offering frequent, small feedings or of holding and feeding to pacify all crying should not be cultivated.

However, the advantages in satisfying the infant's true hunger needs as they are expressed are several: physiologic requirements are met promptly; the infant does not learn to associate prolonged crying and discomfort with feeding; and the infant is less likely to develop poor eating practices such as gulping the feedings or taking small amounts too frequently. Infants soon establish a regular schedule that permits the family to resume normal function. If this does not occur, individual feedings or the whole day's schedule can be moved ahead or delayed sufficiently to avoid conflicts with necessary family activities.

Some mothers will not understand the goals of infant "self-regulation"; some will misinterpret the physician's instructions; and others may be unable to adjust themselves to the regimen of the infant. *The orderly, overanxious, and compulsive parent may do better with a more specific outline for the infant's activities.*

The postpartum period is often a time of great anxiety and insecurity for the first-time mother, who may be temporarily overwhelmed by the responsibilities of motherhood. The hospital setting and the attitude of the hospital personnel should be comforting and supporting while the mother finds and develops confidence in her maternal abilities. Short hospital stay can interfere with adequate guidance. *Time should be set aside to consider the questions of inexperienced or uncertain mothers at the hospital or in the home.* Fathers and other household members should be included by physicians in these anticipatory guidance sessions. Knowing the personalities and expectations of both parents is invaluable in helping to avert physical and psychologic problems centered on feeding. Parental misconceptions and confusion about the dietary and satiety needs of infants and children are often the bases for abnormal parent-child relations that can be avoided by appropriate counseling.

44.1 Breast-Feeding

Breast-feeding continues to have practical and psychologic advantages that should be considered when the mother selects the method for feeding. Human milk is the most appropriate of all available milks for the human infant because it is uniquely adapted to his or her needs.

ADVANTAGES. *Breast milk is the natural food for full-term infants during the first months of life.* It is always readily available at the proper temperature and needs no time for preparation. The milk is fresh and free of contaminating bacteria, which reduces the chances of gastrointestinal disturbances. Although little if any difference exists in mortality rates in formula-fed and breast-fed infants receiving good care, among the lower socioeconomic groups and those living in unsanitary conditions, the breast-fed infant is more likely to survive. The potential life-saving and protective effects of breast milk against enteric pathogens associated with severe diarrhea are most strongly demonstrated in developing countries or where there is not a safe supply of potable water and effective disposal of human waste.

Allergy and intolerance to cow's milk create significant disturbances and feeding difficulties that are not seen in breast-fed infants. The symptoms include diarrhea, intestinal bleeding, and occult melena. "Spitting up," colic, and atopic eczema are less common in infants receiving human milk. A decreased incidence of otitis media in the first year of life has been reported in infants breast-fed exclusively for at least 4 mo. Similarly, reduction in the incidence of pneumonia, bacteremia, meningitis, and a reduced frequency of certain chronic diseases in later life has been reported.

Human milk contains bacterial and viral antibodies, including relatively high concentrations of secretory IgA antibodies, which prevent microorganisms from adhering to the intestinal mucosa. Breast-fed infants of mothers with high antipoliomyelitis titers are relatively resistant to infection by the attenuated live poliomyelitis vaccine viruses, an effect that may be pronounced in the neonatal period but does not seem to interfere with active immunization. Growth of the mumps, influenza, vaccinia, rotavirus and Japanese B encephalitis viruses can be inhibited by substances in human milk. These ingested antibodies from human colostrum and milk may provide local gastrointestinal immunity against organisms entering the body via this route.

Macrophages normally present in human colostrum and milk may be able to synthesize complement, lysozyme, and lactoferrin. Breast milk is also a source of lactoferrin, the iron-binding whey protein that is normally about one third saturated with iron, which has an inhibitory effect on the growth of *Escherichia coli* in the intestine. The stool of the breast-fed infant has a pH lower than that of the infant fed cow's milk. The intestinal flora of infants fed human milk may protect them against infections caused by some species of *E. coli.* Bile salt–stimulated lipase kills *Giardia lamblia* and *Entamoeba histolytica.* Transfer of tuberculin responsiveness by breast milk also suggests passive transfer of T-cell immunity.

Milk from the mother whose diet is sufficient and properly balanced will supply the necessary nutrients, except, perhaps, fluoride and, after several months, vitamin D. If the water supply is inadequately fluoridated (less than 0.3 ppm), then the infant should receive 0.25 mg of fluoride daily. If the maternal vitamin D intake is inadequate and the infant's exposure to sunlight is rare (especially in dark-skinned infants), 10 μg of vitamin D is recommended. Iron stores are sufficient for the first 6 mo in term infants. Human milk iron is well absorbed by the infant, but the diet should be supplemented by 4–6 mo of age with the addition of iron-fortified cereals and baby foods or by one of the ferrous iron preparations. Human milk contains sufficient vitamin C for the infant's needs, provided the mother's intake is adequate.

The psychologic advantages of breast-feeding for both mother and infant are well recognized, and successful breast-feeding is a satisfying experience for both. The mother is personally involved in the nurturing of her baby, gaining both a feeling of being essential and a sense of accomplishment. The infant is provided with a close and comfortable physical relationship with the mother. Breast-feeding offers increased opportunity for close sensual contact between the mother and the infant (see Chapter 79).

The mother who is unable or does not wish to nurse her infant, however, need have no less sense of accomplishment or of affection for her baby. The quality of attachment and mothering and the degree of security and affection provided can be identical. Reported associations of women who are less likely to either initiate breast-feeding or to be nursing at 6 mo include younger mothers, black race, those enrolled in the Supplemental Food Program for Women, Infants, and Children (WIC), those with a high school education or less, and those with low-birthweight infants.

The resumption of menstruation should not deter continued nursing, although temporary behavior changes of mother or baby may call for reassurance. Pregnancy does not necessitate immediate cessation of nursing, but the combined demands of supplying milk to the infant and nutrients to the fetus are formidable and require special attention to maternal nutrition.

Prematurely born infants weighing 2,000 g (4½ lb) or more usually thrive on breast milk. Infants of lesser birthweights, however, may have such rapid rates of growth that human milk alone may not supply sufficient essential nutrients for normal growth (see Chapter 82). Low-birthweight infants too weak to suck or those tiring before ingesting an adequate volume may be given human milk by gavage. Occasionally, breast milk fortifier preparations may be indicated as a supplement to the breast milk feeding of very low-birthweight infants (less than 1,500 g).

The low vitamin K content of human milk may contribute to hemorrhagic disease of the newborn. *Administration of 1 mg of vitamin K_1 parenterally at birth is recommended for all infants, especially for those who will be breast-fed.*

Unconjugated hyperbilirubinemia in breast-fed infants is discussed in Chapter 88.3.

Hemolytic disease of the newborn (erythroblastosis fetalis) is not a contraindication to breast-feeding if the infant's general condition warrants it because antibodies in the mother's milk are inactivated in the intestinal tract and do not contribute to further hemolysis of the infant's blood cells.

Transmission of human immunodeficiency virus (HIV) by breast-feeding has been well documented in multiple studies and currently contraindicates breast-feeding when there are safe alternatives and there is a low rate of endemic infection.

The risk of HIV acquisition by this route is a contraindication to the use of pooled donor milk in this country. However, in developing countries, breast-feeding may be crucial to infant survival; thus, the risk of HIV transmission must be accepted even though there may be a high endemic infection rate. The World Health Organization currently recommends that, unless safe infant formula is readily available, breast-feeding should continue in areas of high HIV endemicity. Regardless of the risk of transmission of HIV, breast-feeding benefits are significantly greater than the risks of bottle feeding in the developing countries.

Other viruses that have been demonstrated in breast milk include cytomegalovirus (CMV), human T-cell lymphotropic virus type 1, rubella, hepatitis B, and herpes simplex. A study of infants seronegative at birth who were breast-fed by mothers shedding CMV only in their milk demonstrated infection in 63%. Although CMV-specific antibodies may be demonstrated in colostrum and milk, the antibody does not appear to be protective. Transmission to term infants appears to be without symptoms or sequelae; however, the risks to preterm infants may be substantially greater, and the use of fresh donor milk is relatively contraindicated unless it is known to be CMV seronegative.

Although hepatitis B has been isolated from maternal milk, the predominant route of transmission appears to be at delivery. Active immunization of the infant within the first 24 hr of life, together with the use of specific high-titer hepatitis B immune globulin and follow-up active vaccination, should permit the mother to nurse if desired with minimal risk. If a nursing mother acquires hepatitis B, then the infant should receive the accelerated protocol of immunization with doses at birth and 1 and 2 mo.

Herpes simplex virus has been described in breast milk with vesicles in the mouth of one infant. Although evidence of breast milk transmission is rare, it appears prudent that women with active lesions who are nursing should observe scrupulous handwashing technique and should avoid nursing if there are active lesions on or near the nipple while activity is present.

Similarly, rubella virus has been isolated from breast milk, both from maternal acute infection and associated with active immunization of the mother with attenuated virus. Breast-feeding need not be interrupted, because neither virus appears to be associated with significant risk to the infant.

Prematurely born infants who weigh 2,000 g (4½ lb) or more usually thrive on breast milk. Infants of lesser birthweights, however, may have such rapid rates of growth that human milk alone may not supply sufficient essential nutrients for normal growth (see Chapter 82.2). Low-birthweight infants too weak to suck or those tiring before ingesting an adequate volume may require gavage.

PREPARATION OF THE PROSPECTIVE MOTHER. Most women are physically capable of breast-feeding, provided they receive sufficient encouragement and are protected from discouraging experiences and comments while the secretion of breast milk is becoming established. The physician interested in aiding the prospective mother to breast-feed should discuss its advantages during the midtrimester of pregnancy or whenever the mother begins planning for her baby. Many mothers ambivalent toward breast-feeding will be able to nurse successfully if they are reassured and supported. If the mother rejects the suggestion that she should nurse her infant, overpersuasion may be detrimental to mother-infant relationships.

Physical factors conducive to a good breast-feeding experience include establishing and maintaining a state of good health, proper balance of rest and exercise, freedom from worry, early and sufficient treatment of any intercurrent disease, and adequate nutrition.

Retracted nipples usually benefit from daily manual breast-pump traction during the latter weeks of pregnancy; truly inverted nipples may be helped by the use of milk cups, starting as early as the 3rd mo of pregnancy.

The mother may be confidently told that she need not gain or lose weight if her diet is adequate. Nursing will help the uterus return to its normal size sooner and may help the mother return to her prepregnancy weight sooner. She should be reassured that breast tone will be preserved by the use of a properly fitted brassiere to support the breasts, especially before delivery and during the nursing period. During the latter part of pregnancy, the mother gains weight and stores fat, which is utilized in lactation. Nutritional requirements for lactation are listed in Table 43–1.

ESTABLISHING AND MAINTAINING THE MILK SUPPLY

The most satisfactory stimulus to the secretion of human milk is regular and complete emptying of the breasts; milk production is reduced when the secreted milk is not drained. Once lactation is well established, mothers are capable of producing more milk than their infants need. There are many reasons for incomplete nursing, but the principal ones are lack of support, weakness of the infant, and failure to initiate the natural hunger cycle. Efforts should be directed toward the early establishment of normal, vigorous nursing by letting the infant empty the breast frequently during the time when only colostrum is being formed. The infant should be allowed to nurse when hungry, whether or not there appears to be any milk.

Breast-feeding should be begun as soon after delivery as the condition of the mother and of the baby permits, preferably within several hours. Infants who cannot be fed on demand should be brought to the mother for feeding about every 3 hr during the day and every 4 hr during the night. Many infants are hungry within 2 hr of a satisfying nursing episode, and about 75% of the breast's milk has been replenished by this time.

Appropriate care for tender or sore nipples should be instituted before severe pain from abrasions and cracking develops. Exposing the nipples to air; applying pure lanolin; avoiding soap, alcohol, and tincture of benzoin; frequently changing disposable nursing pads lining the brassiere cups; nursing more frequently; manually expressing milk; nursing in different positions; and keeping the breast dry between feedings are recommended. When the tenderness causes the mother apprehension the *milk-ejection reflex* may be delayed, leading to frustration in the infant and to increasingly vigorous nursing, which further injures the nipple and areolar area. Occasionally, nipple shields may be helpful.

The first 2 wk of the neonatal period are crucial for establishing breast-feeding. Lactogenic hormones are ineffective in stimulating human breast secretion. Daily weight gains are overly emphasized, and early supplemental bottle feedings given to achieve this goal compromise attempts at breast-feeding.

Although the difference between breast and bottle nipples may confuse the infant, this is usually not the case. It may be perfectly satisfactory to have the mother pump her breasts and feed the infant breast milk via a bottle for the 1st wk or 2. She can then attempt breast-feeding 1 or 2 times daily when she is relaxed and less anxious until infant and mother have achieved a successful nursing experience. The additional pumping will usually increase milk production, ensuring an adequate supply. Even after nursing is well established, it is acceptable for the mother to pump extra milk to store (in a deep freezer up to 1 mo or refrigerator up to 24 hr) for use when the mother is not available. This will also allow the mother a bit of freedom and allow the father or other caretaker more involvement in the infant's feeding and care.

On the day that the mother is discharged from the hospital, lactation may not be well established, and the excitement of going home may impede an initially successful nursing experience there. A wise physician anticipates this experience and discusses it with the mother. In rare cases, providing her with enough isocaloric formula for 1–2 complementary feedings may prevent discouragement that might prejudice further nursing.

PSYCHOLOGIC FACTORS. No factor is more important than a happy, relaxed state of mind. Worry and unhappiness are the most effective means for decreasing or abolishing breast secretions.

Mothers may worry that their infants are abnormal when they cry or are drowsy, sneeze, or regurgitate milk. Mothers are upset by any suggestion that their milk may be lacking in quantity or quality. They may be disturbed at the scanty supply of colostrum, at tenderness of the nipples, and at the fullness of the breast on the 4th or 5th day. Many mothers do not feel comfortable when trying to nurse in an open ward or with another person in the room. Mothers may worry about what is going on at home while they are in the hospital or about what is going to happen when they arrive home. An alert physician recognizes and appreciates these worries, particularly if the baby is a first born, and by tactful reassurance and explanation can help prevent or minimize worry, thus contributing to successful breast-feeding. Attention should be given to social and cultural factors to provide a support plan for the individual mother.

FATIGUE. Avoiding fatigue is important, but the mother should exercise sufficiently to promote her sense of physical well-being.

HYGIENE. Once a day, the breasts should be washed. If soap is drying to the nipple and areolar area, it should be discontinued. The nipple area should be kept dry. *Boric acid must not be used.* Care should be taken to prevent irritation and infection of the nipples caused by prolonged initial nursing, maceration from wetness of the nipple, or rubbing of clothing.

Some mothers may be more comfortable if they wear a properly fitted brassiere day and night. Plastic liners should be removed. An absorbent pad (commercially available) or a clean cloth or handkerchief may be placed inside the brassiere to absorb any milk that leaks out.

DIET. The diet should contain enough calories to compensate for those secreted in the milk as well as for those required to produce it. The nursing mother needs a varied diet, sufficient to maintain her weight and high in fluid, vitamins, and minerals. She should avoid weight-reducing diets. Milk is important but should not replace other essential foods. If the mother is allergic to or dislikes milk, 1 g of calcium may be added to her daily diet. The fluid intake should approximate 3 qt daily; urinary output is a good measure of the adequacy of fluid in the daily diet.

The idea that substances such as milk, beer, oatmeal, and tea are galactogenic is mistaken. Singular foods in the mother's diet seldom disturb the breast-fed infant. Occasionally, however, eating certain berries, tomatoes, onions, members of the cabbage family, chocolate, spices, and condiments may cause gastric distress or loose stools in the infant. No food need be withheld from the mother unless it causes distress to the infant. Whenever possible, nursing mothers should not take drugs, because many preparations are harmful to the neonate and many have not been evaluated (see Table 79–4). Antithyroid medications, lithium, anticancer agents, isoniazid, all recreationally abused drugs, and phenindione are contraindicated. Temporary cessation of nursing is recommended if the mother requires diagnostic radiopharmaceuticals, chloramphenicol, metronidazole, sulfonamides, or anthroquinone-derivative laxatives. Lactating women should not eat sport fish from waters contaminated with polychlorinated biphenyls. It is better to control maternal constipation by inclusion in her diet of raw and cooked fruits and vegetables, whole wheat bread, and an adequate amount of water than by use of laxatives. Smoking cigarettes and drinking alcoholic beverages should be discouraged. Substances such as arsenicals, barbiturates, bromides, iodides, lead, mercurials, salicylates, opium, atropine, most antimicrobial agents, and cascara may be transmitted through the milk and exert an effect on the infant.

TECHNIQUE OF BREAST-FEEDING

The technical aspects of breast-feeding require careful consideration. Breast-feeding sometimes becomes impossible simply because the attending physician fails to recognize that the difficulties are in the feeding technique.

At feeding time, the infant should be hungry, dry, neither too cold nor too warm, and held in a comfortable, semisitting position for his or her enjoyment and for ease of eructation without vomiting. The mother, too, must be comfortable and completely at ease. When she is able to be out of bed, a moderately low chair with an armrest is preferable, and a low stool is advantageous for resting her foot and raising her knee on the nursing side. The baby is supported comfortably with the face held close to the mother's breast by one arm and hand while the other hand supports the breast so that the nipple is easily accessible to the infant's mouth and yet does not obstruct the infant's nasal breathing. The baby's lips should engage considerable areola as well as nipple.

Success in infant feeding depends greatly on the adjustments made during the first few days of life. Difficulties often result from attempts to adapt the infant to a nursing procedure rather than designing a procedure that satisfies the infant's natural desires. Rigidly adhering to clock schedules may make adjustment difficult. Most problems can be avoided by conforming to the infant's spontaneous pattern. If the infant is breast-fed when he or she normally cries in hunger and feeding ends when the baby's appetite is satisfied, the fundamental requirements are met.

At birth, the normal infant is equipped with several reflexes, or behavior patterns, that facilitate breast-feeding. These reflexes are concerned with obtaining food—rooting, sucking, swallowing, and satiety reflexes. The *rooting reflex* is the first to come into play. When infants smell milk, they move their heads around, attempting to find its source. If their cheek is touched by a smooth object (the mother's breast), they will turn toward that object, opening their mouths in anticipation of grasping the nipple (rooting with their mouths for the nipple).

The infant's rooting reflex brings the entire areolar area into the mouth; the contact of the nipple against the palate and posterior tongue elicits sucking or "milking," and the buccal fat pads help to keep the nipple in place. This *sucking reflex* is a process of squeezing the sinuses of the areola rather than simply suction on the nipple. The infant's sucking results in afferent impulses to the mother's hypothalamus and then to both anterior and posterior pituitary. Prolactin from the anterior pituitary stimulates milk secretion in the cuboidal cells in the acini or alveoli of the breast. Finally, milk in the infant's mouth triggers the *swallowing reflex.* In contrast, bottle-feeding requires the infant to compress the nipple to avoid choking.

Mothers should know that if the infant is not hungry, he or she will not search for the nipple or suck. Infants are usually sleepy for several days, and most, initially, are not avid suckers. On the 3rd day, when there has been some weight loss, mothers become anxious about infants who seem uninterested in nursing. It reassures them to learn that most healthy babies "wake up" and become good nursers on the 4th day. Infants whose mothers received obstetric sedation during labor suck at lower rates and pressures and consume less milk than comparable infants of mothers given no sedation.

Some infants will empty a breast in 5 min; others nurse more leisurely for 20 min. Most of the milk is obtained early in the feeding: 50% in the first 2 min and 80–90% in the first 4 min. The infant should be permitted to suck until satisfied unless the mother has sore nipples. If the infant does not "unlatch" from the breast, a finger inserted into the corner of the infant's mouth decreases suction and facilitates removal. The infant should not be pulled from the breast. Waking a sleepy infant to nurse by slapping feet, pinching, or shaking is usually unsuccessful and inappropriate.

At the end of the nursing period, the infant should be held erect over the mother's shoulder or on her lap with or without gently rubbing or patting the back to assist in expelling swallowed air; often this "burping" procedure is necessary one or more times during the feeding as well as 5–10 min after the infant has been put into the crib. It is an essential procedure during the early months but should not be overdone. When nursing is completed, the infant should be placed in the crib on the back or on the right side to facilitate emptying of the stomach into the intestines and to reduce the chances of regurgitation or aspiration.

ONE OR BOTH BREASTS PER FEEDING. The infant should empty at least one breast at each feeding; otherwise, it will not be stimulated to refill. Both breasts should be used at each feeding in the early weeks to encourage maximal production of milk. After the milk supply has been established, the breasts may be alternated at successive feedings, and the infant will usually be satisfied with the amount obtained from one. If the secretion of milk becomes too great, both breasts may again be offered at each feeding and incompletely emptied with the intent of securing a partial decrease in lactation.

DETERMINING ADEQUACY OF MILK SUPPLY. If the infant is satisfied after each nursing period, sleeps 2–4 hr, and gains weight adequately, the milk supply is sufficient. Infants who are "light sleepers" require a lot of body contact with the mother during the first months. Mothers of these wakeful and alert infants should not be thought to have a poor milk supply. However, if the infant nurses avidly and completely empties both breasts but appears unsatisfied afterward, does not go to sleep, or sleeps fitfully and awakens after 1–2 hr, and fails to gain weight satisfactorily, the milk supply is probably inadequate. The program of La Leche League,* which establishes close relationships between successful nursing mothers and mothers needing assistance, is often helpful in such circumstances.

The "let-down" or *milk-ejection reflex* in the mother is an important sign of successful nursing. Sucking or psychologic stimuli associated with nursing lead to secretion of oxytocin by the posterior pituitary. As a result, the myoepithelial cells surrounding the alveoli deep in the breast contract, squeezing milk into the larger ducts, where it is more easily available to the sucking infant. When this reflex functions well, milk flows from the opposite breast as the infant begins to nurse. This reflex is frequently absent or erratic during periods of pain, fatigue, or emotional distress, and its malfunction is thought to be responsible for milk retention in women unsuccessful in breast-feeding.

In general, a mother's weighing her infant before and after nursing is neither necessary nor desirable in judging milk supply adequacy. The amount of milk an infant takes at a time is usually unimportant (the amount ingested at each feeding ranges from one to several ounces throughout a 24-hr period), and the results obtained are readily misinterpreted. Small gains may worry the mother and in turn may diminish her milk supply. She may give the infant a bottle to reassure herself that the infant is getting enough to eat. The better result with the "test bottle" may be so discouraging that subsequent breast-feeding becomes impossible, even when she has an adequate supply of milk. Before assuming that the mother produces insufficient milk, three possibilities should be excluded: (1) errors in feeding technique responsible for the infant's inadequate progress; (2) remediable maternal factors related to diet, rest, or emotional distress; or (3) physical disturbances in the infant that interfere with eating or with gain in weight. Infrequently, infants who seem to be nursing well may not thrive because of insufficiency of milk; increased frequency of feeding may be indicated. Nursing more than every 2 hr, however, may inhibit prolactin secretion of the anterior pituitary, decreasing production; this is usually corrected by delaying feedings to 2½-hr intervals. Other aids include stimulation of prolactin secretion by administering small doses of chlorpromazine for a few days or by devices such as the Lact-aid, which supplement the infant's intake.

*La Leche League International, 9616 Minneapolis Avenue, Franklin Park, Illinois 60131, has many local affiliates composed of successfully nursing mothers willing to assist other mothers desiring to nurse.

EXPRESSION OF BREAST MILK. Although manual expression of breast milk is useful to relieve engorgement of the breasts in an emergency, the cost and availability of battery-operated and electric breast pumps usually makes this unnecessary. Pumping can increase milk production and relieve sore nipples for a few feedings because it does not cause the same nipple irritation that suckling may. Again, breast milk can be safely stored in the freezer or refrigerator and used at a later time for the father or caretaker to feed the infant. Although the infant may balk at anyone else attempting to feed him or her, perseverance will win out.

SUPPLEMENTARY FEEDINGS. The best-intentioned mother who is returning to work plans on pumping while at work and supplying enough milk to feed her infant in her absence. This is often not possible because of stress and time constraints at work. It is acceptable to feed the infant a commercial formula during the day and to continue nursing in the evening and throughout the night. The breast milk production will gradually decrease so the mother is not plagued by engorged, leaking breasts. She will usually continue to produce enough milk to supply 2 or 3 feedings a day for several months. If formula is to be given after the infant has completed a breast-feeding, the warmed bottle should be available so it can be offered immediately after the infant has been burped. The holes in the nipples should not be so large that the infant gets this portion of food without any effort, or the infant may quickly abandon any efforts to suck adequately at the mother's breast. Some employers are developing day care at the work place that enables mothers to continue nursing successfully. Such efforts by employers should be commended and encouraged.

WEANING. Most infants gradually reduce the volume and frequency of their demand for breast-feedings at 6–12 mo of age, and they become accustomed to increasing amounts of solid foods and liquids by bottle and cup. As they demand less breast milk, the mother's supply gradually diminishes, causing the mother no discomfort from engorgement. Weaning should be initiated by substituting formula or cow's milk by bottle or cup for part of a breast-feeding and subsequently for all of a breast-feeding. Over several days, one of the breast-feedings is replaced and then subsequently another, and so on, until the infant is weaned completely. Occasionally, the infant takes the cup as readily as the bottle, avoiding the intermediate transfer from bottle to cup. These changes should be made gradually, for they should provide a pleasant experience, not a conflict, for the mother and infant. Praise, loving attention, and cuddling are vital to successful weaning.

When cessation of nursing is necessary at an earlier age, a tight breast binder may be used and ice bags may be applied for a few days to decrease milk production. Restriction of the mother's fluid intake is also helpful. Hormones, such as small doses of estrogen for 1–2 days, also may help decrease milk production at the termination of nursing.

CONTRAINDICATIONS. For the average, healthy, full-term infant there are no disadvantages to breast-feeding, provided that the mother's milk supply is ample and that her diet contains sufficient amounts of protein and vitamins. Infrequently, allergens to which the infant is sensitized may be conveyed in the milk. In such cases, an attempt should be made to find the specific allergen and to remove it from the mother's diet; its presence rarely is a valid reason for weaning the baby.

From the mother's standpoint, there are few contraindications to breast-feeding. Markedly inverted nipples may be troublesome. Fissuring or cracking of the nipples can usually be avoided if engorgement is prevented. Mastitis may be alleviated by continued and frequent nursing on the affected breast to keep it from becoming engorged, by local heat applications, and by antibiotics. Acute infection in the mother may contraindicate breast-feeding if the infant does not have the same infection; otherwise, there is no need to stop nursing unless the condition of either necessitates it. When the infant is unaffected and the mother's condition permits, the breast may be emptied and the milk given to the infant. Septicemia, nephritis, eclampsia, profuse hemorrhage, active tuberculosis, typhoid fever, breast cancer, and malaria are contraindications to nursing, as are chronic poor nutrition, substance abuse, debility, severe neuroses, and postpartum psychoses.

44.2 Formula Feeding

Whole cow's milk or its modified form is the basis for most formulas, although other milks and milk substitutes are available for infants who cannot tolerate it. Sterilization and refrigeration of the formula greatly reduce morbidity and mortality from gastrointestinal infections. Milk processing (ranging from simple home boiling to commercial pasteurization, homogenization, and evaporation) alters the casein so that small and readily digestible curds form in the stomach, eliminating the principal cause for undigestibility of cow's milk protein.

Although breast-feeding is considered superior to formula feeding for normal infants, many infants receive formula from birth. Changing social and cultural patterns may encourage formula feeding. Because they are employed outside the home, many mothers are reluctant to nurse their infants. Others believe that nursing will limit their activities or they fear failure at nursing. Some regard weight gain and loss of breast tone as unattractive and some consider breast-feeding as socially unacceptable. Whatever the reasons, the present popularity of artificial feeding could not have been reached without prior improvements in the safety and quality of the substitute milks.

Objective nutritional studies of growing infants (e.g., rate of growth in weight and length, normality of various constituents in blood, performance in metabolic studies, body composition) show relatively small differences between infants fed human milk and those fed cow's milk. Although such techniques may not record small but important variations, these investigations attest to the normal infant's ability to thrive by making satisfactory physiologic adjustments to wide ranges of ingested protein, fat, carbohydrate, and minerals.

Conventional formulas of whole and evaporated cow's milk provide approximately 3–4 g of protein/kg/24 hr ("high-protein" intake largely exceeding the basic need), whereas breast milk and many commercially prepared feedings simulating the composition of breast milk supply 1.5–2.5 g/kg/24 hr ("low-protein" intake supplying a smaller degree of excess).

Fomon has calculated the rate of increase in total body protein mass in the "male reference" term infant to average approximately 3.5 g/24 hr in the first 4 mo of life. Assuming 0.5 g/24 hr of nitrogen loss from the skin, total protein need is estimated to be about 4 g/24 hr during the first 4 mo and slightly less during the remainder of the first year.

Commercial formulas are modified from a cow's milk base, and their protein and ash levels are reduced nearer to those of human milk, thus decreasing osmolality and renal excretory load. The saturated fat of cow's milk is replaced with some unsaturated vegetable fatty acids, and vitamins are added. The concentration of lactose is lower in cow's milk than in human milk. Some formulas include higher whey protein and lower casein, such as in breast milk. Low-birthweight infants in particular may benefit from the increased cystine of whey proteins. Until more information is available, breast-feeding for all infants appears prudent, but if this is impossible, then a formula as compositionally close to breast milk as possible is desirable.

TECHNIQUE OF ARTIFICIAL FEEDING

The setting should be similar to that for breast-feeding, with the mother and infant in a comfortable position, unhurried, and free from distractions. The infant should be hungry, fully awake, warm, and dry and be held as though being breast-fed. The bottle should be held so that milk, not air, channels through the nipple. Bottle propping, even with a "safe" holder, should be avoided because it not only deprives the infant of the physical contact, comfort, and security of being held but may also be dangerous to small infants, who may aspirate if unattended. Otitis media is more common in infants fed with the propped bottle.

The bottle of milk is customarily warmed to body temperature, although no harmful effects have been demonstrated from feedings at room temperature or cooler. The temperature may be tested by dropping milk onto the wrist. The nipple holes should be of the size so that milk will drop slowly.

Especially during the first 6–7 mo of life, the eructation of air swallowed during feeding is important for avoiding regurgitation and abdominal discomfort. This technique is similar to that described after breast-feeding. A few infants relieve themselves best after being replaced in the crib. All infants will, at times, regurgitate or "spit up" a small amount of milk after feeding, a fact that the mother should know. Spitting up occurs more often in the artificially fed than in the breast-fed infant.

A feeding may last from 5–25 min, depending on the vigor and the age of the infant. Because the appetite varies from one feeding to another, each bottle should contain more than the average amount taken per feeding. In no case should the infant be urged to take more than desired, and excess milk should be discarded.

COMPARISON OF HUMAN MILK AND COW'S MILK

Average values for the various constituents of human milk and whole fresh cow's milk are listed in Table 44–1. Both differ during the various stages of lactation and among individuals, although the differences in human milk from women with adequate diets are insignificant. Milk late in pregnancy and early after birth contains more protein, calcium, and other minerals than later during lactation. Cells are also present in colostrum and human milk.

COLOSTRUM. The secretion of the breasts during the latter part of pregnancy and for the 2–4 days after delivery is called "colostrum." It has a deep lemon yellow color, its reaction is alkaline, and its specific gravity is 1.040–1.060, in contrast to the average specific gravity of 1.030 for mature breast milk. The total amount of colostrum secreted daily is 10–40 mL. Human or cow colostrum contains several times the protein of mature breast milk, more minerals, but less carbohydrate and fat. Human colostrum also contains some unique immunologic factors. After the first few days of lactation, colostrum is replaced by secretion of a transitional form of milk that gradually assumes the characteristics of mature breast milk by the 3rd or 4th wk.

WATER. The relative amounts of water and solids in human and cow's milks are about the same.

CALORIES. The energy value of each milk may vary slightly and is approximately 20 kcal/oz or 0.67 kcal/mL.

PROTEIN. There are quantitative differences between the proteins of the two milks. Human milk contains only 1–1.5% protein compared with approximately 3.3% in cow's milk. The increased protein of cow's milk results almost entirely from its 6-fold higher content of casein. Human milk protein consists of approximately 65% whey proteins, largely lactalbumins, and 35% casein; the cow's milk ratio is reversed to 22:78.

CARBOHYDRATE. Human milk contains 6.5–7%, and cow's milk contains about 4.5% lactose. About 10% of the carbohydrate in human milk consists of polysaccharides and glycoproteins.

FAT. The fat content of milks is about 3.5%. In human milk, fat content varies somewhat with maternal diet; during a single nursing, it is higher in the latter portion of the feeding, which may help satiate the infant at the conclusion of nursing.

The milks of different breeds of cattle vary in fat content. Most market milk in urban areas, however, is pooled, and the fat content is adjusted to a standard level, generally from 3.25–4%.

Qualitative differences exist in the fats of human milk and cow's milk. The fats of each consist principally of the triglycerides olein, palmitin, and stearin, but human milk contains twice as much of the more absorbable olein. The volatile fatty acids (butyric, capric, caproic, and caprylic) constitute only about 1.3% of human milk fat but about 9% of cow's milk fat. The small amount of linoleic acid in cow's milk is usually sufficient to prevent deficiency. The premature or debilitated infant may have steatorrhea after ingesting cow's milk fat. For such infants, it is wise to substitute a more readily assimilated vegetable fat or human milk.

MINERALS. Cow's milk contains much more of all the minerals except iron and copper than human milk; total mineral content of cow's milk is 0.7–0.75%; that of human milk is 0.15–0.25%. Cow's milk contains inadequate iron; breast-milk iron, although low, may be sufficient for the infant because it is better absorbed, and during the first 4 mo or so of life iron stored during fetal life compensates for the milk's deficiency. Although the need for calcium and phosphorus is great during periods of rapid growth, adequate balances are maintained on breast milk despite its low content of these minerals.

VITAMINS. The vitamin content of each milk varies with the maternal intake. Cow's milk is low in vitamins C and D. Breast milk usually contains adequate vitamin C, if the mother eats appropriate foods, and adequate vitamin D unless she is insufficiently exposed to sunlight or is darkly pigmented. Cow's milk contains more vitamin K than human milk. Both types of milk seem to contain adequate amounts of vitamin A and the B-complex vitamins for the nutritional needs of infants in the first months of life.

BACTERIAL CONTENT. Although human milk is essentially uncontaminated by bacteria, pathogenic organisms in significant numbers may enter the milk from mastitis. Tubercle and typhoid bacilli and herpes, hepatitis B, rubella, mumps, HIV, and CMV may be found at times in the milk of women infected with these organisms. Cow's milk is regularly contaminated, but in most cases by bacteria that are not harmful to humans. Milk, however, is a good culture medium for pathogenic bacteria, and many infections are milk borne, including streptococcal diseases; diphtheria; typhoid fever; salmonellosis; tuberculosis; and brucellosis. Furthermore, certain bacteria that may not affect older children or adults may cause diarrhea in infants. In most cities, pasteurization of all marketed whole milk is required. In addition, terminal sterilization or boiling the milk immediately before mixing the infant's formula is advisable.

DIGESTIBILITY. The stomach empties more rapidly after human milk than after whole cow's milk; however, no appreciable difference in gastrointestinal passage time exists between human milk and processed milk formulas during the first 45 days of life. The curd of cow's milk is reduced in size by boiling; it is made considerably less tough and much smaller by the heating required in evaporation, by the addition of acid or alkali, and by homogenization. In contrast, the curd of breast milk is fine and flocculent and readily broken down in the stomach. The fat of cow's milk is less readily digested than that of breast milk.

MILK USED IN FORMULAS

RAW MILK. This is not advised for infant feeding; it forms large curds in the stomach, is slowly digested, and is easily contaminated with pathogenic organisms. Its sale is forbidden in most urban communities in the United States.

PASTEURIZED MILK. Pasteurization destroys pathogenic bacteria and modifies casein so that smaller, less tough curds are produced in the stomach. Raw milk is heated at 63° C (145° F) for 30 min or, more commonly, at 72° C (161° F) for 15 sec, then rapidly cooled. Standards for the bacterial content of pasteurized milk vary in different cities and countries, tolerable counts ranging as high as 50,000 nonpathogenic bacteria/mL; average counts in many cities, however, are as low as 5,000–10,000. Pasteurized milk should be boiled when used for infant feeding. If it is allowed to stand in the refrigerator for as long as 48 hr, its bacterial count may increase significantly.

HOMOGENIZED MILK. During the process of homogenization, the fat globules are broken into minute particles and remain dispersed. The principal advantage of homogenized milk is the smaller, less tough curd produced in the stomach.

EVAPORATED MILK. This milk has many advantages, including almost universal availability. The unopened can will keep for months without refrigeration. The casein curd produced in the stomach is softer and smaller than that of boiled whole milk; homogenization of the fat also contributes to smaller curd formation. The whey protein or lactoglobulin appears to be less allergenic than that of fresh milk. Evaporated milk can be fed in higher concentrations than whole milk formulas. The standard can contains 13 fluid oz* (384 mL). Each fluid ounce equals about 44 kcal; in practice, the value is generally considered to be 40 kcal. Vitamin D is usually added in the processing so that each reconstituted quart contains 10 μg.

PREPARED MILKS. Many commercially prepared modified milks (Tables 44–2 and 44–3) are derived from cow's milk, and many are available in powder, concentrated liquid requiring 1:1 dilution with water, and ready-to-feed forms. The composition of the majority simulates breast milk in various ways. All are fortified with vitamin D and other vitamins, and some have added iron.

These milks are nutritionally adequate for normal infants. They cost more than evaporated milk–water formulas.

Other prepared milks that may have virtue for special circumstances are now available. Milks prepared from hydrolyzed whey or casein may be useful for infants having malabsorption or milk allergy. Special formulas with specific amino acid elimination are useful for infants and children having inborn metabolic errors.

CONDENSED MILK. About 45% cane sugar has been added in sweetened condensed milk, making the carbohydrate content approximately 60% in the evaporated form before dilution. Although readily digestible, it has no use in infant feeding for more than short periods when a high-calorie diet is desired.

*One fluid ounce is equivalent to approximately 29.57 mL.

■ **TABLE 44–1 Compositions of Breast Milk and Cow's Milk**

	Breast Milk							
	Mature Milk (15 days–15 mo Postpartum)		*Transitional Milk (6–10 days Postpartum)*		*Colostrum (First 5 days Postpartum)*		Cow's Milk	
	Mean	**Experimental Range**	**Mean**	**Experimental Range**	**Mean**	**Experimental Range**	**Mean**	**Experimental Range**
Calories								
(kcal/L)	747	446–1192	735	678–830	671	588–730	701	587–876
(mJ/L)	3.127	1.867–4.989	3.076	2.838–3.474	2.808	2.461–3.055	2.9344	2.457–3.666
Specific gravity	1.031	1.026–1.037	1.035	1.034–1.036	1.034	—	1.031	1.028–1.033
pH	7.01	6.4–7.6	—	—	—	—	6.6	—
Solids, total (g/L)	129	103–175	133	105–156	128	100–167	124	119–142
Ash, total (g/L)	2.02	1.6–2.66	2.67	2.31–3.38	3.08	2.47–3.50	7.15	6.81–7.71
Minerals								
Electropositive elements (mEq/L)	41	—	55		68	—	149	—
Sodium (g/L)	0.172	0.064–0.436	0.294	0.192–0.539	0.501	0.265–1.37	0.768	0.392–1.39
	0.189	0.080–0.350	0.536	0.170–1.21	0.956	0.330–2.24	—	—
Potassium (g/L)	0.512	0.373–0.635	0.636	0.528–0.769	0.745	0.658–0.870	1.43	0.38–2.87
	0.553	0.425–0.735	0.692	0.450–0.910	0.581	0.220–0.790	—	—
Calcium (g/L)	0.344	0.173–0.609	0.464	0.23–0.628	0.481	0.242–0.656	1.37	0.56–3.81
	0.271	0.207–0.372	0.320	0.166–0.420	0.261	0.180–0.364	—	—
Magnesium (g/L)	0.035	0.018–0.057	0.035	0.026–0.054	0.042	0.031–0.082	0.13	0.07–0.22
Electronegative elements (mEq/L)	28	—	37	—	40	—	108	—
Phosphorus (g/L)	0.141	0.068–0.268	0.198	0.097–0.317	0.157	0.085–0.251	0.91	0.56–1.12
Sulfur (g/L)	0.14	0.05–0.30	0.20	0.15–0.23	0.23	0.20–0.26	0.30	0.24–0.36
Chlorine (g/L)	0.375	0.088–0.734	0.457	0.305–0.721	0.586	0.435–1.01	1.08	0.93–1.41
Excess electropositive elements (mEq/L)	13	—	18	—	28	—	41	—
Trace elements								
Cobalt (μg/L)	Trace	—	—	—	—	—	0.6	—
Iron (mg/L)	0.50	0.20–0.80	0.59	0.29–1.45	1.0	—	0.45	0.25–0.75
Copper (mg/L)	0.51	—	1.04	—	1.34	—	0.102	—
Manganese (mg/L)	Trace	—	Trace	—	Trace	—	0.02	0.005–0.067
Zinc (mg/L)	1.18	0.17–3.02	3.82	0.39–5.88	5.59	0.72–9.81	3.9	1.7–6.6
Fluorine (mg/L)	0.107	0.0–0.24	—	—	0.131	0.0–0.35	—	0.10–0.28
Iodine (mg/L)	0.061	0.044–0.093	—	—	—	0.045–0.450	0.116	0.036–1.05
Selenium (mg/L)	0.021	—	—	—	—	—	0.04	0.005–0.067
Protein (g/L)								
Total	10.6	7.3–20	15.9	12.7–18.9	22.9	14.6–68.0	32.46	28.16–36.76
	—	—	—		55	14–215	—	—
Casein	3.7	1.4–6.8	5.1	4.2–5.9	21	7.3–52	24.9	21.9–28.0
Whey protein	7	4–10	—		—	—	7	6–10
Lactalbumin	3.6	1.4–6.0	7.8	6.9–8.6	—	—	2.4	1.4–3.3
Lactoglobulin	—	—	5.0	2.1–13.6	35	4.2–133	1.7	0.7–3.7
Blood-serum albumin	0.32	0.20–0.47	0.37	0.26–0.65	2.5	—	0.4	—
Blood-serum immunoglobulin	0.09	0.02–0.27	0.36	0.01–0.96	1.0	—	0.8	—
Amino acids (g/L)								
Total	12.8	9.0–16.0	9.4	6.0–10.0	12.0	7.0–40.0	33.0	27.0–41.0
Alanine	—	0.36–0.42	—	—	—	—	0.75	—
Arginine	0.43	0.28–0.64	0.63	0.48–0.73	0.74	0.62–0.96	1.4	1.2–1.6
Aspartic acid	—	0.89–0.98	—	—	—	—	1.7	—
Cystine	—	0.23–0.25	—	—	—	—	—	—
Glutamic acid	—	1.89–2.00	—	—	—	—	6.8	—
Glycine	—	0.23–0.24	—	—	—	—	0.11	—
Histidine	0.24	0.12–0.30	0.38	0.29–0.45	0.41	0.35–0.46	1.2	1.1–1.3
Isoleucine	0.61	0.41–0.92	0.97	0.73–1.21	1.01	0.88–1.15	2.5	2.1–2.9
Leucine	0.97	0.65–1.47	1.51	1.13–1.97	1.66	1.33–2.14	3.6	3.2–3.9

DRIED WHOLE MILK. The fat content of fluid milk is adjusted to 3.5%, and the milk is rapidly evaporated to powder form by spray-, freeze-, or roller-drying. Reconstituted dried milk has most of the advantages of evaporated milk but does not keep well when exposed to air.

DRIED SKIM MILK. Both nonfat skim milk (fat content 0.5%) and half-skim milk (fat content 1.5%) are available for infants with fat intolerance or for children consuming diets with lowered fat content. Skim milk should not be used in the first 2 yr of life. Its high protein and mineral content in proportion to calories may cause severe dehydration. Many of these products do not contain added vitamin D.

ACID AND FERMENTED MILK. So-called acid milks are prepared by adding acid to previously boiled and cooled cow's milk formulas, or these milks are fermented by adding lactic acid–producing organisms. These milks require less hydrochloric acid for gastric digestion. The casein is altered so that smaller, less tough curds form in the stomach. Acidified milks are now rarely used in infant feedings because they are likely to cause acidosis.

GOAT'S MILK. In many countries, goat's milk is used extensively for infant feeding; in the United States, its use is limited to managing cow's milk allergies.

Although similar in composition to cow's milk, goat's milk contains less sodium, more potassium and chloride, and more linoleic and arachidonic acids. Its fat may be more digestible and its curd tension lower than that found in cow's milk. It is low in vitamin D, iron, and folic acid; infants fed exclusively on goat's milk are susceptible to megaloblastic anemia due to folate deficiency. Because the goat is especially susceptible to brucellosis, its milk should be boiled before use. It is commercially available in evaporated and powdered forms.

MILK PROTEIN. Powdered protein is used chiefly for increasing protein content of some formulas fed to premature or debili-

■ **TABLE 44–1 Compositions of Breast Milk and Cow's Milk** *Continued*

	Breast Milk: *Mature Milk (15 days–15 mo Postpartum)*		*Transitional Milk (6–10 days Postpartum)*		*Colostrum (First 5 days Postpartum)*		Cow's Milk	
	Mean	**Experimental Range**	**Mean**	**Experimental Range**	**Mean**	**Experimental Range**	**Mean**	**Experimental Range**
Amino acids (g/L) *Continued*								
Lysine	0.70	0.36–0.93	1.13	0.88–1.48	1.18	0.95–1.41	2.6	2.3–3.1
Methionine	0.12	0.07–0.16	0.24	0.16–0.34	0.25	0.19–0.36	0.8	0.6–0.9
Phenylalanine	0.40	0.24–0.58	0.62	0.48–0.71	0.70	0.60–0.84	1.8	1.5–2.2
Proline	—	0.84–0.94	—	—	—	—	2.5	—
Serine	—	0.47–0.51	—	—	—	—	1.6	—
Threonine	0.52	0.30–0.66	0.78	0.61–0.91	0.85	0.75–1.04	1.7	1.3–2.2
Tryptophan	0.19	0.14–0.26	0.28	0.23–0.32	0.32	0.25–0.42	0.6	0.4–0.8
Tyrosine	—	0.46–0.52	—	—	—	—	—	—
Valine	0.73	0.45–1.14	1.05	0.77–1.36	1.17	0.98–1.49	2.6	2.4–2.8
Nonprotein nitrogen (mg/L)								
Total	324	173–604	479	425–533	910	510–1270	252	181–323
Urea nitrogen	180	127–235	111	—	—	—	132.7	61.3–204
Uric acid nitrogen	22	13–41	—	—	—	—	24.1	11.3–36.9
Creatinine nitrogen	11	8–19	—	—	—	—	7.05	1.9–12.2
Creatine nitrogen	11	2–41	—	—	—	—	40.35	24.5–56.2
Amino acid nitrogen	50	28–113	44	—	—	40–120	6.8	1.7–11.9
Choline nitrogen	10.3	6.2–16.8	—	—	—	—	12	5–19
Enzymes								
Lysozyme (mg/L)	390	30–3000	—	—	460	90–1020	0.13	0.00–2.6
Carbohydrates								
Lactose								
Directly estimated (g/L)	71	49–95	64	61–67	57	11–79	47	45–50
As difference	68	50–92	64	60–68	—	—	—	—
Fucose (g/L)	1.3	—	—	—	—	—	—	—
Glucosamine (g/L)	—	0.7–0.8	—	—	—	1.4–4.3	0	—
Galactosamine (g/L)	—	0.0–0.4	—	—	—	0.04–0.7	0	—
Inositol (g/L)	0.45	0.39–0.56	—	—	—	—	0.08	0.06–0.12
Citric acid (g/L)	—	0.35–1.25	—	—	—	—	2.54	2.15–2.90
Fats, total (g/L)	45.4	13.4–82.9	35.2	27.3–51.8	29.5	24.7–31.8	38.0	34.0–61.0
Cholesterol (mg/L)	139	88–202	241	126–320	280	180–345	110	70–170
Free cholesterol (as percent of total)	76.1	—	76.5	—	79.5	—	—	90–95
Lipid phosphorus (mg/L)	10.5	7–14	15.5	11–20	12	6–17	—	53–70
Vitamins								
Vitamin A (mg/L)	0.61	0.15–2.26	0.88	0.58–1.83	1.61	0.75–3.05	0.27	0.17–0.38
Carotenes (mg/L)	0.25	0.02–0.77	0.38	0.23–0.63	1.37	0.41–3.85	0.37	0.12–0.79
Vitamin D (IU/L)	—	4–100	—	—	—	—	—	5–40
Tocopherol (mg/L)	2.4	1.0–4.8	8.9	4.0–18.5	14.8	2.8–30.0	0.6	0.2–1.0
Thiamine (mg/L)	0.142	0.081–0.227	0.059	0.023–0.105	0.019	0.009–0.034	0.43	0.28–0.90
Riboflavin (mg/L)	0.373	0.198–0.790	0.369	0.275–0.490	0.302	0.120–0.453	1.56	1.16–2.02
Vitamin B_6 (mg/L)	0.18	0.10–0.22	—	—	—	—	0.51	0.40–0.63
Nicotinic acid (mg/L)	1.83	0.66–3.30	1.75	0.60–3.60	0.75	0.50–14.5	0.74	0.50–0.86
Vitamin B_{12} (μg/L)	—	Trace	0.36	0.03–0.70	0.45	0.10–1.5	6.6	3.2–12.4
Folic acid (μg/L)								
(a)	1.4	0.9–1.8	0.2	0.15–0.25	0.5	0.10–1.5	1.3	0.2–4.0
(b)	24.0	7.4–61.0	—	—	—	—	37.7	16.8–63.2
(c)	7.3	2.3–17.6	—	—	—	—	12.6	2.8–43.6
Biotin (μg/L)	2	1–3	—	—	—	—	22	14–29
Pantothenic acid (mg/L)	2.46	0.86–5.84	2.88	1.35–4.12	1.83	0.29–3.02	3.4	2.2–5.5
Ascorbic acid (mg/L)	52	0–112	71	45–90	72	47–104	11	3–23

From Geigy Scientific Tables, 7th ed. Basel, Switzerland, Ciba-Geigy, Ltd.

tated infants or to infants with diarrhea. Because of the increased metabolic products and the easy conversion from a balanced to an unbalanced diet, such products should be used carefully and for short durations.

MILK SUBSTITUTES AND HYPOALLERGENIC MILKS. A number of milks and milk substitutes are available for infants allergic to cow's milk. These include evaporated goat's milk, a preparation in which nutrient nitrogen is supplied as an amino acid mixture (casein or whey hydrolysate), and nonmilk foods in which the protein is derived from soybeans. All appear to be nutritionally satisfactory and have a place in the management of infants who cannot tolerate cow's milk; those not containing lactose are useful for infants with galactosemia. Powdered casein (Casec) and medium-chain triglycerides (MCT oil) are available for special purposes.

FILLED AND IMITATION MILKS. Imitation milk products and nondairy "white" beverages in which vegetable fat is substituted for cow (butter) fat are being tested for use in countries where milk and other high-quality protein sources are in short supply. Many of these products lack the full nutritional benefits of fluid milk; they are not intended as formula for infants or as a substitute for breast milk. When they are used for older children, the physician should be aware of the composition and limitations of the product.

ELEMENTAL DIETARY SUBSTITUTES FOR MILK. A number of specialty products have been developed to meet complicated dietary

■ TABLE 44–2 Natural Milks, Prepared Milks, and Milk Substitutes Used in Infant Feeding

	Normal Dilution (kcal/oz)	Approximate Percentage Composition in Normal Dilution (g/100 mL)					Approximate Electrolyte Composition in Normal Dilution					
							(mEq/L)			(mg/L)		
		Protein	*Carbohydrate*	*Fat*	*PUFA*	*Minerals*	*Na*	*K*	*Cl*	*Ca*	*P*	*Fe*
Human milk, mature, average	22	1.1	7.0	3.8	—	0.21	6.5	14	12	340	150	1.5
Cow's milk, market, average	20	3.3	4.8	3.7	—	0.72	25	35	29	1.170	920	1.0
Cow's milk, evaporated	22	3.8	5.4	4.0	—	0.80	28	39	32	1.300	1.100	1.0
Prepared formulas, cow's milk based												
Aptamil Milupa	20	1.5	7.2	3.6	0.43	0.30	7.8	21.2	11.2	580	350	8.0
Bebelac No. 1, LYEMPF	20	1.5	8.0	3.5	0.55	0.30	9.1	15.9	12.7	550	280	5.5
Benamil, Wyeth Ayerst	20	1.5	7.1	3.6	0.36	0.22	7.8	15.5	11.8	460	360	12.0
Dumex Infant Formula, Dumex	20	2.0	7.3	3.2	0.40	0.37	8.6	15.0	13.0	594	396	7.9
Dutch Baby Food, Friesland	20	1.5	7.8	3.3	0.40	0.33	4.6	23.8	14.9	590	400	4.0
Enfamil, Mead Johnson	20	1.5	7.0	3.8	0.68	0.30	8.0	18.7	12.0	530	360	3.4
Frisolac, Friesland	20	1.4	7.4	3.5	0.48	0.31	4.6	25.4	13.9	560	300	6.2
Gerber Baby Formula	20	1.5	7.2	3.7	0.67	0.37	8.7	18.7	13.2	510	390	3.4
Good Start, Carnation	20	1.6	7.4	3.5	0.80	0.28	7.0	16.5	11.3	430	240	10.0
Lactogen, Nestlē	20	1.7	7.4	3.4	0.46	0.34	9.1	18.5	13.8	530	440	8.0
Latogen FP, Nestlē	20	3.1	7.5	2.7	0.35	0.69	20.0	35.0	29.2	1110	860	12.0
Mamex, Dumex	20	1.6	7.3	3.5	0.45	0.26	6.0	14.0	10.0	500	333	7.7
Nan, Nestlē	20	1.6	7.6	3.4	0.44	0.25	7.0	16.9	12.4	420	210	8.1
Nativa, Nestlē	20	1.8	6.9	3.6	0.60	0.26	7.4	17.4	13.0	410	210	8.1
Nutricia	20	1.8	7.1	3.4	0.28	0.23	8.3	17.2	12.0	600	370	8.0
Pertargon, Nestlē	20	1.9	8.0	3.0	0.39	0.43	13.9	23.1	19.4	700	580	8.0
Similac, Ross (also 13, 24, 27 kcal/oz)	20	1.5	7.2	3.7	0.87	0.23	7.9	18.1	12.9	490	380	12.0
Similac PM 60/40, Ross	20	1.6	6.9	3.8	1.2	0.22	7.1	14.9	11.0	380	190	1.5
SMA, Wyeth-Ayerst (also 13, 24, 27 kcal/oz)	20	1.5	7.2	3.6	0.35	0.25	6.5	14.0	11.0	420	290	12.0
Soy based												
Alsoy, Nestlē	20	1.9	7.4	3.3	0.8	0.35	10.0	20.5	13.8	600	430	8.0
Frisosoy, Friesland	20	1.7	7.1	3.5	0.5	0.29	5.7	28.9	13.9	460	270	7.0
Gerber Soy	20	2.0	6.8	3.6	0.7	0.4	13.9	20.0	16.6	640	500	12.2
Isomil (soy), Mead Johnson	20	1.7	7.0	3.7	1.4	—	13.0	18.0	15.0	710	510	12.0
Isomil/DF	20	1.7	6.8	3.7	0.9	—	13.0	18.0	15.0	693	495	12.0
Nursoy (soy), Wyeth-Ayerst	20	1.8	6.9	3.6	0.34	0.35	8.7	18.9	10.6	634	443	12.7
ProSobee (soy), Mead Johnson	20	2.0	6.8	3.6	0.67	0.4	10.4	21.0	15.2	710	560	12.2
Soyalac (soy), Loma Linda	20	2.1	6.8	3.7	1.9	0.4	13.0	20.0	13.0	635	370	1.3

and nutritional problems in children and adults with malabsorption due to primary disease or extensive surgical resection of the small bowel. These include diets prepared with known quantities of purified chemical elements (free glucose, amino acids, and essential fatty acids). All are low residue, chemically defined, and nutritionally adequate, at least for short-term use. They have been most useful in treating severely ill infants with intractable diarrhea, in reducing stooling or "resting" the colon in inflammatory bowel disease, in making maximum use of short bowel segments after surgery, and in maintaining very ill patients in positive nitrogen balance while decreasing the bulk and bacterial content of the colon prior to and after major bowel surgery (see Table 44–2).

MILK FORMULAS

The formulas combine milk, sugar, and water, and some modification for a more desirable, smaller curd formation. They should contain about 20 kcal/oz.

CALORIC REQUIREMENTS (Chapter 43). The average caloric requirements of full-term infants are about 45–55 kcal/lb or 80–120 kcal/kg during the first few months of life and about 45 kcal/lb or 100 kcal/kg by 1 yr of age; individual variations are significant, and for many infants intakes of this order exceed caloric need.

FLUID REQUIREMENTS (see Table 43–3). Fluid requirements are high during infancy. During the first 6 mo of life, they range from 2–3 oz/lb/24 hr or 130–190 mL/kg/24 hr and may increase during hot weather. As a rule, the infant regulates his or her own fluid intake, provided adequate amounts are offered. Most of the fluid required is in the formula, but some is supplied in juice and other foods and by water between feedings.

NUMBER OF FEEDINGS DAILY. The number of feedings required per day decreases throughout the first year; by 1 yr of age, most infants are satisfied with 3 meals/day (Table 44–4). The interval between feedings differs considerably among infants but, in general, ranges from 3–5 hr during the first year of life, averaging 4 hr for full-term, healthy infants. Small or weak infants may prefer feedings at 2- to 3-hr intervals. For the 1st mo or 2, feedings are taken throughout the 24-hr period, but thereafter, as the quantity of milk consumed at each feeding increases and the infant adjusts his or her demand to the family pattern of daytime activity, the infant usually sleeps for longer periods at night. As the infant develops psychologically and the loving relationship between the parent and infant evolves, demand feeding should gradually progress to a feeding regimen that accounts for the needs of both the infant and the parents.

QUANTITY OF FORMULA. Although the quantity taken at a feeding varies with different infants of the same age and with the same infant at different feedings, it is important to know the average amounts taken at various ages.

Each infant must be primarily responsible for determining the quantity of intake (Table 44–5). Rarely will an infant want to take more than 7–8 oz of milk at one feeding, if caloric and nutritional needs are adequately supplemented by other foods. The relative requirement for milk is somewhat less in the first 2 wk than in the succeeding 5–6 mo. After this time milk, although still of value, has diminishing importance in meeting total nutritional requirements.

It is rarely necessary to use more than 1 can (13 fluid oz) of

	Normal Dilution (kcal/oz)	Approximate Percentage Composition in Normal Dilution (g/100 mL) Protein	Carbohydrate	Fat	Notes	mOsm	Approximate Electrolyte Composition in Normal Dilution (mEq/L) Na	K	(mg/L) Ca	P
Specialty products										
Accupep, Sherwood	30	4.0	19.0	1.0	1	490	30	30	625	625
Alfare, Nestlē	20	2.2	7.0	3.3	—	—	17	21	540	340
Alimentum, Ross	20	1.9	6.9	3.8	2	370	13	20	710	510
Alitra, Q, Ross	30	5.2	16.5	1.5	3.5	575	43	31	733	733
Babelac FL, LYEMPF	20	1.7	7.5	3.7	—	—	9.1	16	550	280
Compleat Mod, Sandoz	32	4.3	14.0	3.7	—	300	43	36	670	870
Comply, Sherwood	45	6.0	18.0	6.0	—	410	48	47	1,000	1,000
Criticare H, Mead Johnson	31	3.8	22.0	0.5	2	650	27	34	530	530
Deliver, Mead Johnson	59	7.5	20	10.2	—	—	35	43	1,010	1,010
Enfamil Human Milk Fortifier, Mead Johnson	14	0.7	2.7	0.04	—	—	7	15	60	3
Enrich, Ross	33	4.0	16.2	3.7	—	480	37	43	720	720
Ensure, Ross	31	3.7	14.5	3.7	6	470	37	40	530	530
Ensure HN, Ross	31	4.4	14.1	3.5	—	470	35	40	750	750
Ensure Plus, Ross	45	5.5	19.2	5.3	—	690	46	50	700	700
Ensure Plus HN, Ross	45	6.3	20.0	5.0	—	650	51	47	1,050	1,050
Entera, Fresenius	32	4.0	14.6	3.6	—	420	35	34	800	640
Entralife, Corpak	30	3.5	13.6	3.5	—	300	26	25	500	500
Entralife HN30, Corpak	4.2	13.3	3.4	—	—	300	40	32	800	800
Follow-up, Carnation	20	1.7	8.8	2.7	—	—	11.3	22.5	900	600
Frisopep 1, Friesland	20	1.5	7.2	3.5	—	—	51	254	500	300
Isocal, Mead Johnson	31	4.4	12.4	4.4	—	230	41	41	850	850
Isocal HN, Mead Johnson	31	4.4	12.4	4.4	—	230	41	41	850	850
Isoservice, Sandoz	36	4.3	17.0	4.1	6	360	52	43	670	670
Jevity, Ross	32	4.4	15.2	3.7	—	300	40	40	912	759
Lactofree, Mead Johnson	20	1.5	7.0	3.7	—	—	8.7	19	530	360
Magnacal, Sherwood	60	7.0	25.0	8.0	—	590	43	32	1,000	1,000
Meritene, Sandoz	32	6.9	12.0	3.4	—	690	48	32	2,200	1,900
Newtrition, Knight	32	3.6	41.0	4.0	—	450	42	?	600	600
Newtrition Isotonic, Knight	32	3.6	14.8	3.6	—	300	26	26	600	600
Newtrition Isofiber, Knight	36	5.0	16.0	3.7	—	310	36	32	847	847
Nutrapak, Corpak	32	3.7	14.5	3.7	—	450	37	40	530	530
Nutren 1.0, Clintec	30	4.0	12.7	3.8	—	340	22	32	500	500
Nutren 1.5, Clintec	45	6.0	17.0	6.7	—	600	33	48	750	750
Nutren 2.0, Clintec	60	8.0	19.6	10.6	—	800	43	64	1,000	1,000
Nutramigen, Mead Johnson	20	1.9	9.1	2.6	2	290	14	18	630	420
Osmolite, Ross	31	3.7	14.5	3.8	—	300	28	26	530	530
Pediasure, Ross	30	3.0	10.9	4.9	6	325	16	33	970	800
Peptamen, Clinitec	30	4.0	12.7	3.9	1	260	22	32	600	500
Perative, Ross	38	6.7	17.7	3.7	3.5	385	45	44	867	867
Portagen, Mead Johnson	20	2.4	7.8	3.2	—	220	16	22	635	470
Pregestimil PO, Mead Johnson	20	1.9	7.0	3.8	2	290	14	19	630	420
Profiber, Sherwood	30	4.0	14.7	3.5	—	300	32	32	800	800
Promil, Wyeth-Ayerst	20	2.5	8.0	2.8	—	360	14	26	1,150	650
Pulmocre, Ross	45	6.3	10.5	9.2	—	465	57	49	1,050	1,050
RCF, Ross	40	2.0	0	3.6	—	74	13	19	700	500
Resource, Sandoz	32	3.7	14.5	3.7	—	430	39	41	525	525
Resource Plus	45	5.5	20.0	5.3	—	600	57	54	700	700
S14, Wyeth-Ayerst	20	1.1	7.1	3.7	—	280	7	12	420	320
S-29, Wyeth-Ayerst	20	1.7	10.1	2.3	—	360	0.4	8	140	170
S-44, Wyeth-Ayerst	20	1.7	10.1	2.3	—	360	0.4	8	140	170
Sustacal, Mead Johnson	30	6.1	14.0	2.3	—	620	41	54	1,010	930
Sustacal Plus	45	6.1	19.0	5.8	6	520	36	38	850	850
Tolerex, Sandoz	30	2.1	22.8	0.15	3	550	20	30	550	550
Traumacal, Mead Johnson	45	8.3	14.3	6.8	—	440	51	36	750	750
Vital HN, Ross	30	4.1	18.0	1.1	3, 4.5	500	25	36	670	670
Vitaneed, Sherwood	30	4.0	13.5	3.5	—	300	27	32	670	670
Vivonex Ten, Sandoz	30	3.8	20.6	0.3	3	630	20	20	500	500

(1) Hydrolyzed whey, (2) hydrolyzed casein, (3) amino acids, (4) partially hydrolyzed whey, and (5) others. Other speciality formulas are available from various manufacturers, low (or free of) carbohydrate, protein, sodium, phenylalanine, branched chain amino acids, histidine, homocystine, lysine, tyrosine, and methionine.

	Normal Dilution (kcal/oz)	Approximate Percentage Composition in Normal Dilution (g/100 mL) Protein	Carbohydrate	Fat	PUFA	Minerals	Approximate Electrolyte Composition in Normal Dilution (mEq/L) Na	K	Cl	(mg/L) Ca	P	Fe
Formulas for low-birthweight infants												
Alprem, Prenan, Nestlē	21	2.1	8.0	3.4	0.5	0.4	11	19	11.3	700	460	11
Enfamil, Premature Formula, Mead Johnson	24	2.4	8.9	4.1	0.8	0.5	14	23	19.4	950	480	1.3
Similac, 24 LBW, Ross	24	2.2	8.5	4.5	0.6	0.5	13	31	23	730	560	3
Similac Special Care, Ross	24	2.2	8.6	4.4	0.6	0.5	15	27	19	1440	720	1.5
SMA Preemie, Wyeth-Ayerst	24	2.0	8.6	4.4	0.4	0.4	13.9	19	15	750	400	3

Table continued on following page

■ **TABLE 44–2 Natural Milks, Prepared Milks, and Milk Substitutes Used in Infant Feeding** *Continued*

	kcal/g	kcal/mL
Carbohydrate supplements		
LC, Corpak	—	2.5
Moducal, Mead Johnson	3.8	—
PC, Corpak	4.0	—
Pollycose, Ross	3.8	2.0
Sumacal, Sherwood	3.8	—
Fat supplements		
Liposyn, Abbott 10%	1.1	1.1
Liposyn, Abbott 20%	2.0	2.0
Intralipid, Cutter 10%	1.1	1.1
Intralipid, Cutter 20%	2.0	2.0
MCT Oil, Mead Johnson	7.7	7.1
MCT Supplement, Corpak	6.1	—
Microlipid, Sherwood	4.5	2.2
Protein supplements		
Casec, Mead Johnson	3.7	—
Electrodialyzed Whey, Wyeth-Ayerst	1.4	—
Pro-Mix, Corpak	1.4	—
Pro-Mod, Ross	4.2	—
Propac, Sherwood	4.0	—

evaporated milk or 1 qt of whole milk/day. By the time the infant is taking these quantities, other foods will be added to the diet in increasing amounts. Ingesting more milk has no advantage, but the disadvantage is that other essential foods may be displaced. Some of the milk may be incorporated in the cereal and in the preparation of foods such as custards, soups, and sauces.

During the first few months, the high quantity of protein and minerals in undiluted cow's milk makes such unmodified milk unsuitable for most infants. Diluting the milk supplies free water, and adding carbohydrate modifies the caloric content (Table 44–6).

Whereas lactose is the milk sugar of most mammals, other carbohydrates are usually used in home-prepared formulas. Cane sugar, dextrin-maltose preparations, or other easily digestible sugars can be added. Ingested lactose produces a lower pH in the intestine than formulas containing other sugars. The acid pH improves calcium absorption.

Representative evaporated or whole milk formulas are given in Table 44–7. Subsequent adjustments of milk and water should be made in accordance with the infant's satiety and the growth curve.

PREPARATION OF FORMULA. Several more bottles than the number required for feedings are needed for holding water and orange juice. Bottles should be smooth inside; and they should be marked in ounces or milliliters. A wide-mouthed bottle is preferable because it is cleaned more easily, and those with an adequate cover for the nipple are preferable if the baby is to be fed away from home. There should be several more nipples than the number required for feedings. Alternatively, disposable bottles and commercially prepared presterilized formula are now widely used.

All utensils required for the mixing and storing of the formula should be purchased sterilized or sterilized by boiling for 5–10 min. The rubber nipples and caps should not be boiled more than 5 min. After each feeding, the nondisposable bottle and nipple should be flushed thoroughly, and the bottle should be filled with water until washed with water and a detergent.

The hands should be scrubbed thoroughly, and the sterilized bottles and utensils should be arranged on a clean table. If whole milk is used, the bottle is shaken so that its contents are mixed, and the top is washed with hot water before the cap is removed. The water for the formula (it is necessary to allow for a slight loss in boiling) is brought to the boiling point in a saucepan; the amount of whole milk is added; and the

■ **TABLE 44–3 Recommended Ranges of Nutrient Levels in Infant Formulas***

Nutrient (per 100 kcal)	Adequate	Not to Exceed
Protein (g)	1.8†	4.5
Fat (g)	3.3 (30% of kcal)	6 (54% of kcal)
Including essential fatty acid (linoleate) (mg)	300 (2.7% of kcal)	
Vitamins		
A (IU)	250 (75 μg)‡	750 (225 μg)‡
D (μg) cholecalciferol§	1	2.5
K (μg)	4	—
E (tocopherol equivalents)‖	0.5 (at least 0.5/g linoleic acid)	
C (ascorbic acid) (mg)	8	—
B_1 (thiamine) (μg)	40	—
B_2 (riboflavin) (μg)	60	—
B_6 (pyridoxine) (μg)	35 μg/g protein	—
B_{12} (μg)	0.15	
Niacin (μg)	250 (or 0.8 niacin equivalent)	—
Folic acid (μg)	4	—
Pantothenic acid (μg)	300	—
Biotin (μg)	1.4	—
Choline (mg)	7¶	—
Inositol (mg)	4¶	—
Minerals**		
Calcium (mg)	60††	—
Phosphorus (mg)	30††	—
Magnesium (mg)	6	—
Iron (mg)	0.15	2.5‡‡
Iodine (μg)	5	25
Zinc (mg)	0.5	—
Copper (μg)	60	—
Manganese (μg)	5	100
Selenium (μg)	3	—
Sodium (mg)	20 (5.8 mEq/L)	60 (17.5 mEq/L)
Potassium (mg)	80 (13.7 mEq/L)	200 (34.3 mEq/L)
Chloride (mg)	55 (10.4 mEq/L)	150 (28.3 mEq/L)

**American Academy of Pediatrics Committee on Nutrition, 1976 recommendations with 1987 modifications.*

†Nutritionally equivalent to casein. For use of other proteins, refer to the commentary on breast feeding and infant formulas, including proposed standards for formulas. Pediatrics 57:278, 1976.

‡Retinol equivalents.

§1 μg cholecalciferol = 40 IU vitamin D.

‖1.49 IU = 1 mg d-α-tocopherol equivalent. The β and γ isomers have less activity.

¶Average present in milk-based formulas; should be included in this amount in other formulas.

***Formula should be made with water low in fluoride and in all cases contain less than 45 μg/100 kcal. For explanation, see statement on fluoride supplementation: revised dosage schedule. American Academy of Pediatrics Committee on Nutrition. Fluoride supplementation: revised dosage schedule. Pediatrics 63:150, 1979.*

††Calcium to phosphorus ratio should not be less than 1.1 or more than 2.

‡‡Prudence indicates there should be an upper limit for iron. If formula is labeled "infant formula with iron," it must not contain less than 1 mg/100 kcal.

■ **TABLE 44–4 Average Daily Number of Feedings**

Age	Average No. of Feedings in 24 hr
Birth–1 wk	6–10
1 wk–1 mo	6–8
1–3 mo	5–6
3–7 mo	4–5
4–9 mo	3–4
8–12 mo	3

■ **TABLE 44–5 Average Quantity of Feedings**

Age	Average Quantity Taken in Individual Feedings
1st and 2nd wk	2–3 oz (60–90 mL)
3 wk–2 mo	4–5 oz (120–150 mL)
2–3 mo	5–6 oz (150–180 mL)
3–4 mo	6–7 oz (180–210 mL)
5–12 mo	7–8 oz (210–240 mL)

■ **TABLE 44–6 Household Measures of Some Commonly Used Sugars***

	Tablespoonfuls per Ounce
Lactose	3
Sucrose (cane)	2
Dextrin-maltose preparations	
Mead's Dextri-Maltose	4
Karo	2
Cartose	2
Dexin	6
Polycose fluid	2

**Caloric value of each is 120 kcal/oz, except Dexin, 115, and Polycose, 60.*

mixture is boiled for 5 min. Constant stirring is necessary. The sugar is added while the milk is still warm.

If evaporated milk is used, the top of the can is washed with soap and hot water and rinsed with hot water; two holes are punctured in it. The water for the formula is boiled for 5 min, and the evaporated milk and sugar are added to it. No further boiling is necessary.

The freshly prepared and sterile formula is poured in appropriate amounts into sterilized nursing bottles. The bottles are capped by aseptic technique and stored in the refrigerator until time for the feedings.

TERMINAL HEATING. This method has practical advantages and does not require presterilization of bottles or utensils. The formula is poured into clean nursing bottles, and the nipples are applied. The nipples are then covered loosely with glass, metal, or paper caps and the bottles are placed in a rack in a container tall enough to prevent the bottles from touching the lid. The container is filled with water to about the midpoint of the bottles, covered, and placed over a moderate flame. The water is allowed to boil gently for 25 min. The bottles are then removed with tongs and placed in a container of cold water for 10 min. The caps are then tightened, and the bottles are stored in a refrigerator. Bottles containing formula should not be warmed in a microwave oven because uneven heating may cause the formula to burn the infant.

44.3 Other Foods

VITAMINS. Most marketed whole and artificial milks are fortified with 10 μg of vitamin D per reconstituted quart, and commercially prepared milks vary in the content of other vitamins. Therefore, knowing the vitamin content of the milk is essential before prescribing additional vitamins for the bottle-fed baby.

Orange and other citrus fruit juices are natural sources of *vitamin C,* but because many young infants do not seem to tolerate them in amounts large enough to supply an adequate vitamin intake, it is preferable to give 35 mg of ascorbic acid. When at least 2 oz of fresh, frozen, or canned orange juice (or equivalent amounts of other sources of vitamin C) is taken daily, the ascorbic acid may be discontinued.

Vitamin D should be started early in the neonatal period with a daily intake of approximately 10 μg only if the infant is taking a formula that does not contain vitamin D or is receiving an insufficient volume of milk to meet the daily requirement. Low-birthweight infants require supplementation (Chapter 82). Vitamin D supplement is not necessary during the first few months of breast-feeding of white infants but may be for black infants and those not exposed to adequate sunlight. Concentrates in water-miscible vehicles are desirable to avoid aspiration of oil.

IRON. Foods rich in iron are less available in the diet of poor families. The most effective way to prevent iron deficiency is to provide iron supplementation in the form of an iron-fortified milk formula or medicinal iron (2 mg/kg up to a total of 15 mg/24 hr) beginning at 6 wk of age. It is doubtful whether iron-supplemented cereals provide sufficient supplementation for infants with reduced iron stores.

"SOLID" FOODS. The caloric contents of the various prepared baby foods differ widely (see Table 670–11). Egg yolk, cereals with added milk, meats, and puddings have greater caloric density than milk, whereas vegetables and fruits have an energy value similar to or lower than milk. Without appropriate advice, many mothers select foods with high caloric values that result in obesity. The inclusion of solid foods to the diet before 4–6 mo of age does not contribute significantly to the health of the normal infant nor does it increase the likelihood of the infant sleeping through the night, providing hunger is avoided with adequate breast-feeding or formula feeding.

Any new food should be initially offered once a day in small amounts (1–2 teaspoonfuls). Any small spoon that easily fits the baby's mouth may be used. New foods are generally best accepted if fairly thin or dilute. Food is frequently pushed out by the tongue rather than back because the baby cannot yet swallow efficiently. This should be mentioned to the mother, who might otherwise interpret the "spitting out" of new foods as dislike. It is usually wise to offer the same food daily until the baby becomes accustomed to it and not to introduce new foods more often than every 1–2 wk.

The feeding at which these foods are offered is not particularly important. They should be given when the baby's hunger is no longer satisfied by milk alone and when they fit into the daily schedule. There is no reason for persisting with or forcing a particular food that is definitely disliked. The family's dislikes and prejudices for particular foods are contagious and should not be displayed before the infant. The physician should avoid prescribing a definite amount of a given food lest the mother interpret the suggestion too literally. *Many infants are overfed by overzealous parents who mistake acceptance of food for appetite.* The infant's appetite is the best index of the proper amount, and respect for the infant's wishes will avoid many problems.

Cereal. The various precooked cereals on the market provide in a convenient form a variety of grains excellent for infants. Most contain iron and factors of the vitamin B complex.

Fruits. Strained or puŕeed cooked fruits furnish minerals and some water-soluble vitamins and usually have a mildly laxative effect. Raw ripe mashed banana is readily digested and enjoyed by most infants. Many infants who are slow in accepting new foods seem to prefer fruits.

Vegetables. Vegetables are moderately good sources of iron and other minerals and of the B-complex vitamins. They should be freshly cooked and strained or commercially prepared. Vegetables are usually added to the infant's diet by about 7 mo of age.

■ **TABLE 44–7 Representative Formulas***

	1–3 Days	kcal	4–10 Days	kcal	>10 Days	kcal
Evaporated milk	6 oz	240	7 oz	280	13 oz	520
Sugar	1 tbsp	60	1 tbsp	60	3 tbsp	180
Water	14 oz		14 oz		17 oz	
	20 oz	300	21 oz	340	30 oz	700
kcal/oz		14		16		22
kcal/100 ml		47		56		70
Whole milk	12 oz	240	14 oz	280	26 oz	520
Sugar	1 tbsp	60	1 tbsp	60	3 tbsp	180
Water	8 oz		7 oz		6 oz	
	20 oz	300	21 oz	340	32 oz	700

**Total volume is divided into six bottles, and the total intake is regulated by the infant.*

Meats, Eggs, and Starchy Foods. Eggs and starchy foods are usually introduced during the second 6 mo of life, although some physicians offer egg yolk at an earlier age. The yolk of the egg is used initially and is preferably hard-cooked. As with all new foods, a small amount is offered at first, with gradual increases up to a whole yolk 1–3 times a week. Egg white should be introduced with equal caution to minimize any possible allergic manifestations.

Potatoes, rice, spaghetti, bread, and similar starchy foods have principally a caloric value. As a rule, they are not included in the infant's diet until the more essential foods mentioned earlier are being taken regularly. Zwieback, toast, or graham crackers may be offered to the infant when he or she shows an interest in "gumming" on coarser foods (usually 6–8 mo of age). It is with such foods that infants learn to chew and to feed themselves.

Meat is an excellent source of protein as well as of iron and vitamins. Ground fresh beef or liver or the strained canned meats may be used initially by about 6 mo of age. Meats may be more readily accepted when mixed with another food.

The commercial soups and meat and vegetable mixtures are relatively high in carbohydrate and are not considered optimal sources of iron or protein. Many home-prepared soups are bulky out of proportion to their food value, and much of the vitamin content is lost by overcooking.

Desserts. Puddings, junkets, and custard are good foods for older infants, particularly if they temporarily prefer milk in that form. If, however, such foods are given as a bribe or reward or only after other foods have been finished, poor eating habits are likely to be established. Sweet foods should be offered as casually as the rest of the meal and at any place in the meal that the child desires.

SALT INTAKE. To increase their palatability, particularly for the parent, excessive salt used to be added to baby foods. This practice has been discontinued. The significance of large intakes of sodium, which are in the ranges seen in populations with a high incidence of hypertension, is not clear, but the possibility that they might contribute to the development of hypertension later in life cannot be ignored.

FOOD ADDITIVES. Naturally occurring chemicals and food additives, particularly the artificial flavors and colors, have been implicated in health problems. It has been estimated that more than 3,000 flavors are currently being used, and few children are spared exposure to them in their daily diet. Artificial flavors and colors have been associated with respiratory allergic disorders, with urticaria and angioedema, with lesions of the tongue and buccal mucosa, with digestive disturbances, with arthralgia and hydrarthroses, and with headache and behavioral disturbances, including hyperkinesis in childhood.

44.4 First-Year Feeding Problems

UNDERFEEDING. Underfeeding is suggested by restlessness and crying and by failure to gain weight adequately, despite complete emptying of the breast or bottle. Underfeeding may also result from the infant's failure to take a sufficient quantity of food even when offered. In these cases, the frequency of feedings, the mechanics of feeding, the size of the holes in the nipple, the adequacy of eructation of air, the possibility of abnormal mother-infant "bonding," and possible systemic disease in the baby should be investigated (see Chapters 38 and 39). The extent and duration of underfeeding determine the clinical manifestations. Constipation, failure to sleep, irritability, and excessive crying are to be expected. There may be poor gain in weight or an actual loss. In the latter case, the skin becomes dry and wrinkled, subcutaneous tissue disappears, and the infant assumes the appearance of an "old man." Deficiencies of vitamins A, B, C, and D and of iron and protein may be responsible for characteristic clinical manifestations.

Treatment consists of increasing the fluid and caloric intake, correcting deficiencies in vitamin and mineral intake, and instructing the mother in the art of infant feeding. If some underlying systemic disease or psychologic problem is responsible, specific management of these disorders is necessary.

OVERFEEDING. Overfeeding may be quantitative or qualitative. Regurgitation and vomiting are frequent symptoms of overfeeding. As a rule, infants can be depended on not to take excessive quantities, but occasionally an infant who has postprandial discomfort from eating too much may nonetheless gain weight excessively. Diets too high in fat delay gastric emptying, cause distention and abdominal discomfort, and may cause excessive gain in weight. Diets too high in carbohydrate are likely to cause undue fermentation in the intestine, resulting in distention and flatulence and in too rapid gain in weight. Such diets may be deficient in essential protein, vitamins, and minerals. Formulas too high in caloric content in the first 1–2 wk of life are likely to result in loose or diarrheal stools. Obesity is undesirable at any time in life; often the excessively fed infant becomes the obese child and adult.

REGURGITATION AND VOMITING. The return of small amounts of swallowed food during or shortly after eating is called "regurgitation" or "spitting up." More complete emptying of the stomach, especially occurring some time after feeding, is called "vomiting." Within limits, regurgitation is a natural occurrence, especially during the first 6 mo or so of life. It can be reduced to a negligible amount, however, by adequate eructation of swallowed air during and after eating, by gentle handling, by avoiding emotional conflicts, and by placing the infant on the right side for a nap immediately after eating. The head should not be lower than the rest of the body during the rest period because gastroesophageal reflux is common during the first 4–6 mo.

Vomiting, one of the most common symptoms in infancy, may be associated with a variety of disturbances, both trivial and serious. It should be distinguished from rumination; its cause should always be investigated (see Chapters 251, 252, and 275).

LOOSE OR DIARRHEAL STOOLS. Acute infectious diarrhea and chronic diarrheal conditions are discussed in Chapters 171, 283, and 287; only mild disturbances of dietary origin are considered here.

The stool of the breast-fed infant is naturally softer than that of the infant fed cow's milk. From about the 4th to the 6th day of life, the stools go through a transitional stage in which they are rather loose and greenish yellow and contain mucus; within a few days, the typical "milk stool" appears. Subsequently, the use of laxatives or the ingestion of certain foods by the mother may be temporarily responsible for an infant's loose stools. Excessive intake of breast milk may also increase the frequency and the water content of the stool. Actual diarrhea in a breast-fed infant is unusual and should be considered infectious until proved otherwise.

Although the stools of artificially fed infants tend to be firmer than those of breast-fed infants, loose stools may result from artificial feeding. In the first 2 wk or so of life, overfeeding is likely to cause loose, frequent stools. Later, formulas too concentrated or too high in sugar content, especially in lactose, may produce loose, frequent stools. Many temporary diarrhea disturbances in artificially fed infants result from food contaminations that would not disturb an older child and are not serious enough to cause prolonged difficulty for the infant. The ease with which artificially fed infants acquire diarrheal disturbances and their potential seriousness are strong arguments for extreme care in providing food free of pathogenic bacteria.

Mild diarrheal disturbances due to overfeeding respond quickly to temporary decrease or cessation of feeding. Withholding all solid food and one or several milk feedings, substituting boiled water or a balanced electrolyte solution, are usually all that is required.

CONSTIPATION (see Chapter 252). Constipation is practically unknown in breast-fed infants receiving an adequate amount of milk and is rare in artificially fed infants receiving an adequate diet. The nature of the stool, not its frequency, is the mark of constipation. Although most infants have one or more stools daily, an infant will occasionally have a stool of normal consistency only at intervals of 36–48 hr. Whenever constipation or obstipation is present from birth or shortly thereafter, a rectal examination should be performed. Tight or spastic anal sphincters may be responsible occasionally for obstipation, and correction usually follows finger dilatation. Anal fissures or cracks may also cause constipation. If irritation is alleviated, healing usually occurs quickly. Aganglionic megacolon may be manifested by constipation in early infancy; the absence of stool in the rectum on digital examination suggests this possibility.

Constipation in the artificially fed infant may be caused by an insufficient amount of food or fluid. In other cases, it may result from diets too high in fat or protein or deficient in bulk. Simply increasing the amount of fluid or sugar in the formula may be corrective in the first few months of life. After this age, better results are obtained by adding or increasing the amounts of cereal, vegetables, and fruits. Prune juice (1/2–1 oz) may be given as a temporary measure, but it is better to add foods with some bulk. Enemas and suppositories should never be more than temporary measures. Milk of magnesia may be given in doses of 1–2 teaspoonfuls but should be reserved for unresponsive or severe constipation.

COLIC. The term "colic" describes a frequent symptom complex of paroxysmal abdominal pain, presumably of intestinal origin, and of severe crying. It occurs usually in infants younger than 3 mo of age.

The clinical pattern is characteristic: the attack usually begins suddenly; the cry is loud and more or less continuous; so-called paroxysms may persist for several hours; the face may be flushed, or there may be circumoral pallor; the abdomen is distended and tense; the legs are drawn up on the abdomen, though they may be momentarily extended; the feet are often cold; the hands are clenched. The attack may terminate only when the infant is completely exhausted, but often there is apparent relief with the passage of feces or flatus.

Certain infants seem to be peculiarly susceptible to colic. The cause of recurrent attacks is usually not apparent, although they may be associated with hunger and with swallowed air that has passed into the intestine. Overfeeding may also cause discomfort and distention. Certain foods, especially those of high carbohydrate content, may be responsible for excessive fermentation in the intestines, but a change in diet only occasionally prevents further colic attacks. Crying from intestinal discomfort is seen in infants with intestinal allergy, but colic is not limited to this group. Intestinal obstruction or peritoneal infection may mimic an attack of colic. Recurrent attacks commonly occur late in the afternoon or evening, suggesting that events in the household routine may possibly cause them. Worry, fear, anger, or excitement may cause vomiting in an older child and may cause colic in an infant. No single factor consistently accounts for colic, nor does any treatment consistently provide satisfactory relief. Careful physical examination is important to eliminate the possibility of intussusception, strangulated hernia, hair in the infant's eye, otitis, pyelonephritis, or other disorders.

Holding the baby upright or permitting the baby to lie prone across the lap or on a hot water bottle or heating pad helps occasionally. Passage of flatus or fecal material spontaneously or with expulsion of a suppository or enema sometimes affords relief. Carminatives before feedings are ineffective in preventing the attacks. Sedation is occasionally indicated for a prolonged attack and is sometimes given to the parent or child for a period of time if other measures fail. Temporary hospitalization of the infant, often without more than a change in the infant's feeding routine and providing a period of rest for the mother, may help in extreme cases. Prevention of attacks should be sought by improving feeding techniques, including burping, providing a stable emotional environment, identifying possibly allergenic foods in the infant's or nursing mother's diet, and avoiding underfeeding or overfeeding. Colic rarely persists after 3 mo of age. A supportive, sympathetic physician is important in successfully resolving the problem.

44.5 Feeding During the Second Year of Life

Most infants naturally adapt themselves to a schedule of three meals a day by about the end of the 1st yr of life. Although considerable latitude in the diet of each infant should be permitted to allow for personal idiosyncrasies and family habits, the mother should be given an outline of the daily basic dietary needs (see Table 43–7 and Fig. 43–2). When malnutrition, either as dietary deficiency or excess, or failure to thrive exists despite an apparently satisfactory food intake, the infant or child's family relationships must be evaluated, not only for organic causes but especially for psychosocial ones (see Chapters 38 and 39).

REDUCED CALORIC INTAKE. Toward the end of the 1st yr of life and during the 2nd yr, because of the constantly decelerating rate of growth, there is a gradual reduction in the infant's caloric intake per unit of body weight. In addition, it is not unusual to have temporary periods of lack of interest in certain foods or even in food in general. Failure to recognize these features, especially the decreasing caloric needs, results in attempts to force feed. The child naturally rebels and feeding problems ensue. Because preventing problems is more effective than correcting them, the changing pattern of the infant's food habits during the 2nd yr of life should be explained to the mother before it appears.

SELF-SELECTION OF DIET. Children's strong likes or dislikes of particular foods should be respected whenever possible and practicable. Spinach is an example of a nonessential food whose virtues have been overemphasized. When consistently rejected foods include basic staples such as milk and cereal, food allergy should be considered.

Children, including infants, tend to select diets that, over several days, assume a balanced nature. Thus, the child may be permitted a wide choice of foods, as long as he or she eats adequately over the longer period. Normally, the child determines the quantity to be eaten of a given food and of the entire meal. At this age, eating habits may be strongly influenced by older children in the family, particularly in respect to food likes and dislikes. Eating patterns and habits developed in the first 2 yr of life usually persist for several years.

SELF-FEEDING BY INFANTS. Before 1 yr of age, the infant should be permitted to participate in the act of feeding. By approximately 6 mo, the infant can hold a bottle; within another 2–3 mo, a cup. Zwieback, graham crackers, or other hand-held foods can be introduced by the age of 7–8 mo. A spoon may be used as soon as it can be held and directed to the mouth, possibly by 10–12 mo of age. Mothers often inhibit this learning process because they object to its messiness.

Acquiring the ability to feed oneself is an important step in developing self-reliance and responsibility. By the end of the

2nd yr of life, infants should be largely responsible for feeding themselves.

Permitting infants and children to go to sleep while sucking intermittently from a bottle of formula, whole milk, sweet fruit juice, or water should be discouraged. Pedodontists emphasize the correlation between this habit and enamel erosion in deciduous teeth, calling it the "baby bottle syndrome."

Although nutritional requirements per unit of body weight constantly decrease with increasing age (110 kcal/kg in infancy; 50 kcal/kg at 15 yr), the need for calories as well as for protein, vitamins, and minerals is relatively greater in children than it is in adults.

DAILY BASIC DIET. Parents should be given a daily basic diet for the child from which the family menu can be prepared. Daily selection from each of the food groups (Fig. 43–2) provides a balanced diet with sufficient macronutrients and micronutrients. The quantity of intake after the basic requirements have been met can be determined usually by the healthy growing child. The child's history of dietary habits is essential for evaluating the nutritive intake, but such histories are often unreliable unless an accurate dietary diary is kept for several days. From such information, correcting the diet may be more effective.

The older child should learn the content of a basic diet and its importance to proper growth and good health, but this information should never be presented as a threat to enforce rigid feeding practices.

EATING HABITS. Eating habits formed in the 1st yr or 2 of life distinctly affect those of the subsequent years. Feeding difficulties between the ages of 2–5 yr frequently result from excessive parental insistence on eating and subsequent anxiety when the child does not conform to some arbitrary standard. The child's negative reactions naturally result from undue mealtime stress, and correction requires improvement in parent-child relations. Other factors that disturb eating are too much confusion at mealtime, insufficient time for eating, either on the part of the adult or of the child, food dislikes of other members of the family, and poorly prepared and unattractively served food. A comfortable chair of proper height with a foot-rest is important for a child's ease at the table. Mealtimes should be happy, and the conversation should be on subjects of interest to the entire family. The child's appetite should be respected; if his or her desire for food at times is below average, there should be no persuasion to eat more. Adults should realize that eating habits are taught better by example than by formal explanation.

SNACKS BETWEEN MEALS. During the 2nd yr and even for several years thereafter, orange juice or other fruit juice or fruit, together with a cracker, may be given in either or both of the between-meal periods. Snacks served in nursery schools and kindergartens should be nutritious. Older children should avoid between-meal snacking if it reduces their appetite for the next meal. After-school snacks, especially of fruit, should be encouraged if they produce greater enthusiasm and energy for play and do not reduce the appetite for the evening meal.

VEGETARIAN DIET

All-vegetable diets supply all necessary nutrients when vegetables are selected from different classes. Vegetables are high in fiber content, vitamins, and minerals. Vegetarians usually have faster gastrointestinal transit time, bulkier stools, and low serum cholesterol levels and are said to have less diverticulitis and appendicitis than meat eaters. Those who consume eggs are ovovegetarians. Those who consume milk are lactovegetarians. Those who consume neither are vegans. Vegans may develop vitamin B_{12} deficiency and, because of high-fiber intake, may develop trace mineral deficiency. Nursing vegan mothers must be given added vitamin B_{12} to prevent methylmalonic acidemia in their infants. Vegetarian infants may not grow as rapidly as omnivores in the first 2 yr.

44.6 Later Childhood and Adolescence

As the child reaches age 2 yr, diet is similar to that of the family. All the known nutrients are supplied by a varied diet and should include selections from each of the food groups: cereals, fruits, vegetables, proteins, and dairy. The relative amounts are described by the food pyramid (see Fig. 43–2) as designed by the United States Department of Agriculture. Emphasis on cereal, fruits, and vegetables supports the recommendations of the National Cholesterol Education Program. Those recommendations include restriction of total fat in the diet to approximately 30% of the total daily calories, of which 10% is saturated fatty acids, 7–8% polyunsaturated, and 12–13% monounsaturated fatty acids. Dietary cholesterol should not exceed 100 mg/1,000 calories. This diet, the American Heart Association Step One Diet, is recommended to decrease atherosclerotic heart disease and may also be effective in limiting the development of obesity. The food selections of the pyramid may be made as the infant begins to take supplemental foods, but fat in the diet should not be restricted until the child is past 2 yr. Some children given a more restricted diet in infancy fail to thrive.

DIET FOR ATHLETIC ACTIVITIES

Adequate caloric intake is necessary for growth and activity. A varied diet supplies all necessary nutrients. Special food supplements are unnecessary and may be harmful. Water intake should be scheduled regularly before and during athletic events.

American Academy of Pediatrics: Pediatric Nutrition Handbook. Committee on Nutrition, 3rd ed. Elk Grove Village, IL, American Academy of Pediatrics, 1993.

Barr RG, Kramer MS, Pless B, et al: Feeding and temperament as determinants of early infant crying/fussing behavior. Pediatrics 84:514, 1989.

Baumgartner TG: Trace elements in clinical nutrition. Nutr Clin Pract 8:251, 1993.

Forman SJ: Infant Nutrition, 2nd ed. Philadelphia, WB Saunders, 1974, pp 68–73.

George DR, De Francesca BA: Human milk in comparison to cow milk. *In*: Labenthal E (ed): Textbook of Gastroenterology and Nutrition in Infancy and Childhood, 2nd ed. New York, Raven Press, 1989, pp 242–243.

Lawrence RA: Breast Feeding, A Guide For the Medical Profession, 4th ed. St. Louis, CV Mosby, 1994.

Lebenthal E (ed): Textbook of Gastroenterology and Nutrition in Infants, 2nd ed. New York, Raven Press, 1989.

La Leche League International: The Womanly Art of Breast Feeding. Franklin Park, IL, La Leche League International, 1976.

Lozoff B: Behavioral alterations in iron deficiency. Adv Pediatr 35:331, 1988.

National Academy of Sciences: Recommended Dietary Allowances, 10th ed. Washington, DC, National Academy Press, 1989.

National Cholesterol Education Program (NCEP): Reports of the Expert Panel on Blood Cholesterol in Children and Adolescents. Pediatrics 89(Suppl):525, 1992.

Oski FA: Iron deficiency in infancy and childhood. N Engl J Med 329:190, 1993.

United States Department of Agriculture: Food Guide Pyramid. A Guide to Daily Food Choices. Home and Garden Bulletin, No. 252. Washington, DC, Human Nutrition Information Services, 1992.

Wright JA, Ashenberg CA, Whitaker RC: Comparison of methods to categorize undernutrition in children. J Pediatr 124:944, 1994.

CHAPTER 45
Nutritional Disorders

45.1 Malnutrition

Worldwide, malnutrition is one of the leading causes of morbidity and mortality in childhood. See Chapter 6.

Malnutrition may be due to improper or inadequate food intake or may result from inadequate absorption of food. Insufficient food supply, poor dietary habits, food faddism, and emotional factors may limit intake. Certain metabolic abnormalities may also cause malnutrition. Requirements for essential nutrients may be increased during stress and disease and during the administration of antibiotics or of catabolic or anabolic drugs. Malnutrition may be acute or chronic, reversible or irreversible.

Precise evaluation of nutritional status is difficult. Severe disturbances are readily apparent, but mild disturbances may be overlooked, even after careful physical and laboratory examinations. The diagnosis of malnutrition rests on an accurate dietary history; on evaluation of present deviations from average height, weight, head circumference, and past rates of growth; on comparative measurements of midarm circumference and skinfold thickness; and on chemical and other tests. Decreased skinfold thickness suggests protein-calorie malnutrition; excessive thickness indicates obesity. Muscle mass is calculated by subtracting skinfold measurements from arm circumference. For older children and adults midarm muscle circumference (cm) = arm circumference (cm) − (skinfold thickness [cm] × 3.14). Lean body mass can be estimated from 24-hr creatinine excretion. Deficiencies of some nutrients may be revealed by finding low blood levels of them or their metabolites, by observing biochemical or clinical effects of administration of the nutrients or their products, or by giving the patient substantial amounts of appropriate nutrients and noting the rate at which they are excreted. Protein reserves are assessed from serum albumin and rapid turnover proteins. The levels of rapid turnover proteins, transthyretin with a half-life of 12 hr, prealbumin with a half-life of 1.9 days, and transferrin with a half-life of 8 days, decrease due to inadequate visceral protein synthesis or depletion of protein stores. Serum levels of essential amino acids may be lower than those of nonessential amino acids. Excretion of hydroxyproline is decreased and of 3-methylhistidine increased, and hair is easily plucked out in the severely malnourished child.

The most acute nutritional disturbances are those which involve water and electrolytes, especially sodium, potassium, chloride, and hydrogen ions (see Part VII). Chronic malnutrition usually involves deficits of more than a single nutrient. Immunologic insufficiency is common in malnutrition and is demonstrated by total lymphocyte counts less than 1,500/mm^3 and anergy to skin test antigens, such as streptokinase-streptodornase, *Candida,* mumps, or tuberculin in exposed persons (see Chapters 39 and 286.5).

MARASMUS

(Infantile Atrophy, Inanition, Athrepsia)

Severe malnutrition in infants is common in areas with insufficient food, inadequate knowledge of feeding techniques, or poor hygiene. The synonyms of marasmus apply to patterns of clinical illness emphasizing one or more features of protein and calorie deficiency.

ETIOLOGY. The clinical picture of marasmus originates from an inadequate caloric intake due to insufficient diet, to improper feeding habits such as those of disturbed parent-child relations, or to metabolic abnormalities or congenital malformations. Severe impairment of any body system may result in malnutrition.

CLINICAL MANIFESTATIONS. Initially, there is failure to gain weight, followed by loss of weight until emaciation results, with loss of turgor in skin that becomes wrinkled and loose as subcutaneous fat disappears. Because fat is lost last from the sucking pads of the cheeks, the infant's face may retain a relatively normal appearance for some time before becoming shrunken and wizened. The abdomen may be distended or flat, and the intestinal pattern may be readily visible. Atrophy of muscle occurs, with resultant hypotonia.

The temperature is usually subnormal, the pulse may be slow, and the basal metabolic rate tends to be reduced. At first, the infant may be fretful but later becomes listless, and the appetite diminishes. The infant is usually constipated, but the so-called starvation type of diarrhea may appear, with frequent, small stools containing mucus.

PROTEIN MALNUTRITION

(Protein-Calorie Malnutrition [PCM], Kwashiorkor)

Because they are growing, children must consume enough nitrogenous food to maintain a positive nitrogen balance, whereas adults need only maintain nitrogen equilibrium.

ETIOLOGY. Although deficiencies of calories and other nutrients complicate the clinical and chemical patterns, the principal symptoms of protein malnutrition are due to insufficient intake of protein of good biologic value. There may also be impaired absorption of protein, such as in chronic diarrheal states, abnormal losses of protein in proteinuria (nephrosis), infection, hemorrhage or burns, and failure of protein synthesis, such as in chronic liver disease.

Kwashiorkor is a clinical syndrome that results from a severe deficiency of protein and an inadequate caloric intake. Either from lack of intake or from excessive losses or increases in metabolic rate caused by chronic infections, secondary vitamin and mineral deficiency may contribute to the signs and symptoms. It is the most serious and prevalent form of malnutrition in the world today, especially in industrially underdeveloped areas. Kwashiorkor means "deposed child," that is, the child no longer suckled; it may become evident from early infancy to about 5 yr of age, usually after weaning from the breast. Although gains in height and weight are accelerated with treatment, these measurements never equal those of consistently well-nourished children.

CLINICAL MANIFESTATIONS (Fig. 45–1). Early clinical evidence of protein malnutrition is vague but does include lethargy, apathy, or irritability. When well advanced, it results in inadequate growth, lack of stamina, loss of muscular tissue, increased susceptibility to infections, and edema. Secondary immunodeficiency is one of the most serious and constant manifestations. For example, measles, a relatively benign disease of the well nourished, can be devastating and fatal in malnourished children. The child may develop anorexia, flabbiness of subcutaneous tissues, and loss of muscle tone. The liver may enlarge early or late; fatty infiltration is common. Edema usually develops early; failure to gain weight may be masked by edema, which is often present in internal organs before it can be recognized in the face and limbs. Renal plasma flow, glomerular filtration rate, and renal tubular function are decreased. The heart may be small in the early stages of the disease but is usually enlarged later.

Dermatitis is common. Darkening of the skin appears in irritated areas but not in those exposed to sunlight, a contrast to the situation in pellagra (see Chapter 45.3). Dyspigmentation may occur in these areas after desquamation or may be generalized. The hair is often sparse and thin and loses its elasticity. In dark-haired children, dyspigmentation may result in streaky red or gray hair color (hypochromotrichia). Hair texture becomes coarse in chronic disease.

Infections and parasitic infestations are common, as are anorexia, vomiting, and continued diarrhea. The muscles are weak, thin, and atrophic, but occasionally there may be an excess of subcutaneous fat. Mental changes, especially irritability and apathy, are common. Stupor, coma, and death may follow.

LABORATORY DATA. Decrease in the concentration of serum albumin is the most characteristic change. Ketonuria is common in the early stage of inanition but frequently disappears in the later stages. Blood glucose values are low, but glucose tolerance

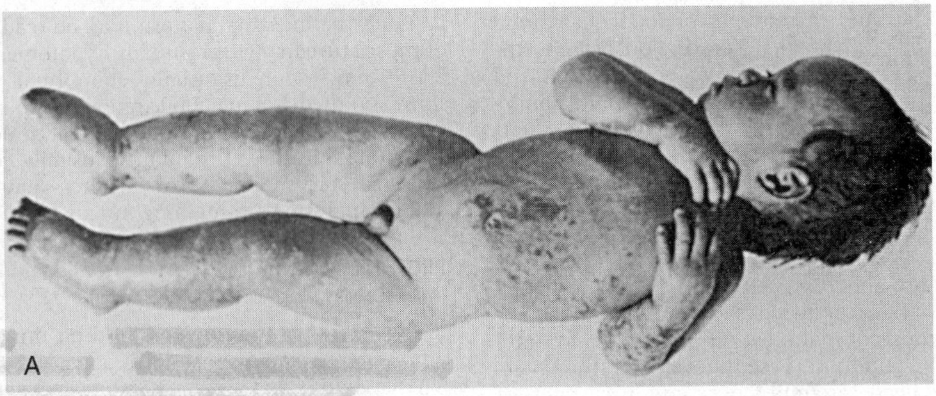

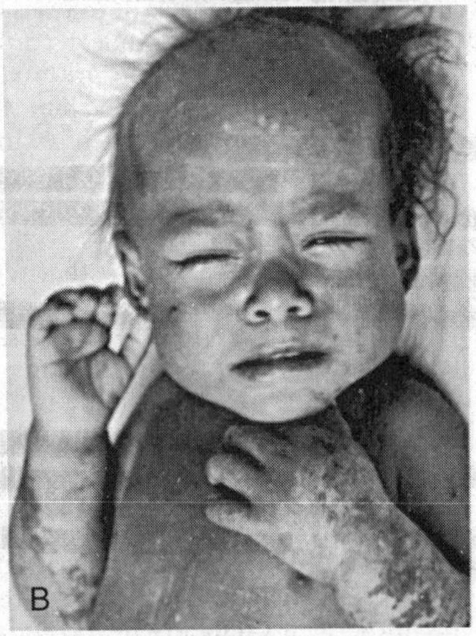

Figure 45–1. *A*, Kwashiorkor in a 2-yr-old boy. Note the generalized edema, the typical skin lesions, and the state of prostration. *B*, Close-up of the same child showing the hair changes and psychic alterations (apathy and misery); the edema of the face and the skin lesions can be seen more clearly. (Photographs made available by the Institute of Nutrition of Central America and Panama, Guatemala, courtesy of Moišes Ɓehar, M.D.)

curves may be diabetic in type. Urinary excretion of hydroxyproline relative to creatinine may be decreased. Plasma values of essential amino acids may be decreased relative to nonessential ones, and there may be increased aminoaciduria. Potassium and magnesium deficiencies are frequent. The serum cholesterol level is low, but it returns to normal after a few days of treatment. The serum values of amylase, esterase, cholinesterase, transaminase, lipase, and alkaline phosphatase are decreased. There is diminished activity of the pancreatic enzymes and of xanthine oxidase, but these values return to normal shortly after the onset of treatment. Anemia may be normocytic, microcytic, or macrocytic. Signs of vitamin and mineral deficiencies are usually evident. Bone growth is usually delayed. Growth hormone secretion may be increased.

DIFFERENTIAL DIAGNOSIS. Differential diagnosis of protein deprivation includes chronic infections, diseases in which there is an excessive loss of protein through urine or stools, and conditions with a metabolic inability to synthesize protein.

PREVENTION. This requires a diet containing an adequate quantity of protein of good biologic quality. Because kwashiorkor has not only a serious and often fatal course but often permanent and devastating aftereffects in recovered children and their offspring, adequate dietary instruction and food distribution are urgently needed in endemic areas.

TREATMENT. Immediate management of any acute problems such as those of severe diarrhea, renal failure, and shock (see Chapter 60) and, ultimately, the replacement of missing nutrients is essential. Moderate or severe dehydration, manifest or suspected infection, eye signs of severe vitamin A deficiency, severe anemia, hypoglycemia, continuing or recurrent diarrhea, skin and mucous membrane lesions, anorexia, and hypothermia all must be treated. For mild to moderate dehydration, fluids are administered orally or by nasogastric tube (see Chapter 54). A breast-fed infant should be nursed as often as he or she wants. For severe dehydration, intravenous fluids are necessary (see Chapter 56). If intravenous fluids cannot be given, a intraosseous (marrow) or intraperitoneal infusion of 70 mL/kg of half-strength Ringer lactate solution may be life saving. Effective antibiotics should be given parenterally for 5–10 days.

When dehydration is corrected, oral feeding starts with small, frequent feeds of dilute milk; strength and volume are gradually increased and frequency decreased over the next 5 days. By days 6–8, the child should receive 150 mL/kg/24 hr in 6 feeds. Cow's milk, or yogurt for the lactose-intolerant child, should be made with 50 g of sugar/L. Special feeds are available from UNICEF. In the recovery period, high-energy feeds made with milk, oil, and sugar are needed. Skim milk, casein hydrolysates, or synthetic amino acid mixtures may be used to supplement the basic fluid and nutritional regimen.

When high-calorie and high-protein diets are given too early and rapidly, the liver may become enlarged, the abdomen becomes markedly distended, and the child improves more slowly. Vegetable fat is better absorbed than cow's milk fat. Impaired glucose tolerance may be improved in some affected children by the daily administration of 250 μg of chromium chloride. Vitamins and minerals, especially vitamin A, potassium, and magnesium, are necessary from the outset of treatment. Iron and folic acid usually correct the anemia.

Bacterial infections must be treated concomitantly with the dietary therapy, whereas treatment of parasitic infestations, if they are not severe, may be postponed until recovery is under way.

After treatment has been initiated, the patient may lose

weight for a few weeks, owing to loss of apparent or inapparent edema. Serum and intestinal enzymes return to normal, and intestinal absorption of fat and protein improves.

If growth and development have been extensively impaired, mental and physical retardation may be permanent. The younger the infant at the time of deprivation, the more devastating are the long-term effects. Deficits in perceptual and abstract abilities are especially long lasting.

MALNUTRITION IN CHILDREN BEYOND INFANCY

ETIOLOGY. Malnutrition in children may be a continuation of an undernourished state begun in infancy, or it may arise from factors that become operative during childhood. In general, the causes are the same as those responsible for malnutrition in infants. The problem may be complex. Poor dietary habits may be associated with a generally poor hygienic situation, with chronic disease, with finicky eating habits of other members of the family, or with disturbed parent-child relations (see Chapter 38).

Poor eating habits in children under the age of 5 or 6 yr can often be traced directly to parental factors, of which overconcern about the quantity or quality of the diet is a common one. In children of all ages, insufficient sleep and too much emotional excitement, such as that associated with the movies and television, are important factors. School-aged children often develop irregular or inappropriate eating habits, especially at breakfast and lunch, because sufficient time is not allotted or because the meals may be inadequate. Some children as young as 5–8 yr eat little because of fear of obesity. These children respond readily to dietary advice and explanation, in contrast to children who have anorexia nervosa. Eating between meals, especially of items such as candy and snack foods, usually reduces the mealtime appetite.

CLINICAL MANIFESTATIONS. Malnutrition does not invariably result in underweight. Fatigue, lassitude, restlessness, and irritability are frequent manifestations. Restlessness and overactivity are frequently misinterpreted by parents as evidences of lack of fatigue. Anorexia, easily induced digestive disturbances, and constipation are common complaints, and even in older children the starvation type of mucoid diarrheal stool may be observed. Malnourished children often have a limited span of attention and do poorly in school. They have increased susceptibility to infections. Muscular development is inadequate, and the flabby muscles result in a posture of fatigue, with rounded shoulders, flat chest, and protuberant abdomen. Such children often look tired; the face is pale, the complexion is "muddy," and the eyes lack luster. Hypochromic anemia is common. In protracted cases, there may be delayed epiphyseal development, irregularities in dentition, and delayed puberty.

Evaluation should always include a careful history of dietary habits, psychosocial maladjustments, physical hygiene, and illness in addition to a thorough physical examination. Laboratory examinations are usually unnecessary.

TREATMENT. Individualized treatment is aimed at correcting underlying psychologic and physical disturbances. An adequate diet (see Chapter 44) should be outlined; vitamin concentrates may be added and continued for a time after the dietary intake has become adequate. When anorexia is a problem, the essential items of the diet should be provided in as concentrated a form as possible, and the fat content should be low. Between-meal snacks need not be prohibited if they do not interfere with the appetite for the next meal; milk or candy should not be given at such times; fruit or fruit juices are appropriate. Re-educating the entire family about eating habits may be necessary.

Committee on Agriculture, House of Representatives: Hunger in America, its effects on children and families, and implications for the future. Committee on Agriculture, House of Representatives: Hearings, Serial No. 102–13, 1991.
Graham GG, Lembeke J, Lancho E, et al: Quality protein maize: digestibility and utilization by recovering malnourished infants. Pediatrics 83:416, 1989.
Hegsted DM: Protein-calorie malnutrition. Am Scientist 66:61, 1978.
Karp RJ (ed): Malnourished Children in the United States. New York, Springer, 1993.
Katz M, Stiehm ER: Host defense in malnutrition. Pediatrics 59:490, 1977.
Robinson H, Picou D: A comparison of fasting plasma insulin and growth hormone concentrations in marasmic, kwashiorkor, marasmic-kwashiorkor and underweight children. Pediatr Res 11:637, 1977.
Select Committee on Hunger, House of Representatives: Hearings, Serial No. 102–28, 36, 38, 1992.
Sleisenger MH, Kim YS: Protein digestion and absorption. N Engl J Med 300:659, 1979.

PROTEIN EXCESS

Excessive protein intake, especially in the absence of sufficient water, may lead to signs of dehydration–protein fever. Signs of protein excess are rare, but premature infants fed a high-protein diet may have an increased morbidity. Marasmic infants fed high-protein diets during the recovery phase may develop hyperammonemia; protein intoxication has also been noted in children with other liver disease. Some weight-reducing diets with high-protein content may be responsible for protein intoxication.

Barness LA, Omans WB, Rose CS, et al: Progress of premature infants fed a formula containing demineralized whey. Pediatrics 32:52, 1963.

45.2 Obesity

The identification of obesity and overweight in childhood may be an important aspect of preventive pediatrics with implications for the promotion of physical, social, and emotional health for children that may have effects in adulthood. Obesity is not a disease in itself but rather a symptom complex with a weak association to adult obesity with its correlates of increased mortality, cardiovascular disease, atherosclerosis, and diabetes rates. Studies have shown that childhood obesity occurred in a minority (10–30%) of obese adults. Thus, it is not a direct predictor of adult obesity; the probability of an obese child becoming an obese adult decreases with greater time intervals between onset of obesity and adulthood but increases with severity of childhood obesity, onset in adolescence, and a pre-existing pattern of family obesity.

Interpretation of studies assessing the impact and management of childhood obesity has been difficult because there has not been a uniform standard to differentiate obesity (defined as an excess accumulation of body fat) from "overweight" in which body size may be increased without increased accumulation of body fat but with increased lean body mass. Excess weight and body fat in adolescents have been associated with increased plasma insulin levels, elevated blood lipid and lipoprotein levels, and elevated blood pressure, which are factors known to be associated with obesity-related adult morbidity.

No exact line separates optimal nutrition from overnutrition; practically, the diagnosis is made from the child's appearance rather than from an arbitrary weight excess. Stocky children may have relatively large skeletal frames and more than the average amount of muscular tissue so that their weight and height and their "bigness" exceed those of the average child of their age, but they should not be considered obese. Obesity or overnutrition is a generalized and excessive accumulation of fat in subcutaneous and other tissues.

Measures used to differentiate obese and overweight adolescents have included relative weight, weight-stature indices, body circumferences, and skinfold thickness, usually triceps. Weight-for-age percentiles are unsatisfactory because they do

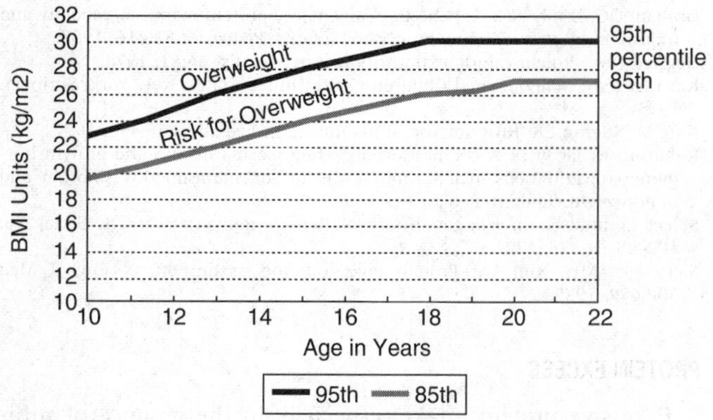

Figure 45–2. Male body mass index, 85th and 95th percentiles. (Adapted from data of Must et al. Am J Clin Nutr 53:839, 1991.)

not allow for variation in lean body mass. The use of adult reference data such as life tables is inappropriate, as children and adolescents differ greatly in the rate of growth and distribution of weight. The body mass index (BMI), defined as weight/stature squared (in kilograms per meter squared), is the most useful index used for screening populations of adolescents for obesity because it correlates significantly with both subcutaneous and total body fat in adolescents, particularly those with the greatest proportion of body fat. In addition, BMI elevations correlate with blood pressure, blood lipid levels, and lipoprotein concentrations in adolescence and predict elevated BMI, lipid levels, and blood pressure in young adults. In adults, elevated BMI is predictive for adult obesity-related morbidity and mortality (Figs. 45–2 and 45–3).

ETIOLOGY. Obesity is usually due to an excessive intake of food rather than from massive overeating. Body fat stores increase when energy intake exceeds expenditure, and this usually occurs when there are small positive energy balances over extended periods. Obese children do not eat differently or eat more "junk" food or starch than their peers. The total energy expenditure during exercise of obese children during controlled exercise is increased but, when corrected for increased body mass, is equivalent to that of the nonobese child. The resting metabolic rate is also equal when adjusted for metabolically active body mass.

Appetite may be influenced by a variety of factors that include psychologic disturbances; hypothalamic, pituitary, or other brain lesions; and hyperinsulinism. Genetic predisposition to obesity occurs in certain animals and may occur in humans, although environmental effects are thought to be more prominent. Obesity may result from increases in the number or in the size of fat cells, *adipocytes*. These appear to

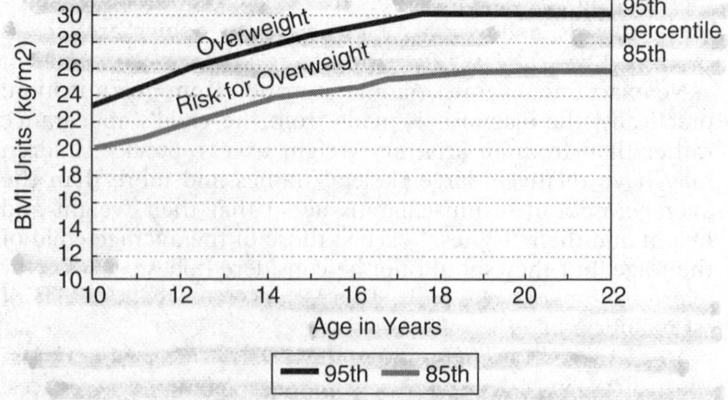

Figure 45–3. Female body mass index, 85th and 95th percentiles. (Adapted from data of Must et al. Am J Clin Nutr 53:839, 1991.)

increase in number when caloric intake is increased, especially in the gestational months and during the 1st yr of life. This stimulus to increase in number continues, although at a reduced rate, throughout puberty, so that during periods of adolescent weight reduction, the size, but not the number of adipocytes decreases.

The obese may become resistant to insulin, resulting in an increase in levels of circulating insulin. Insulin decreases lipolysis and increases fat synthesis and uptake. The obese person responds to a carbohydrate meal with increased insulin and a decreased utilization of free fatty acids. During weight-reduction regimens, the obese person delivers less food to his or her cells than the lean person, owing to decreased mobilization of free fatty acids. In starvation after obesity, fat is mobilized as the serum insulin level decreases. Protein conservation is facilitated as the brain utilizes ketones for energy. During starvation, serum alanine levels decrease, and glycine levels rise. Purified sugars and high-protein diets may cause greater secretion of insulin than do complex carbohydrates.

The chronic and uncritical offering of a bottle as a method of dealing with a fretful or crying infant may establish a habit that leads the infant to expect or seek food whenever experiencing frustration. If obesity is initiated early, it may persist. Similarly, the uncritical early introduction of high-calorie solid foods may lead to rapid weight gain and to obesity.

EPIDEMIOLOGY. Longitudinal studies in industrialized societies over the last century have shown growth in height and weight compared with previous generations. Individual studies have described a prevalence of childhood obesity from 7–43% (Canada), 7.3% (United Kingdom), and 27.1% at ages 6–11 and 21.9% at ages 12–17 (United States). The incidence of childhood obesity in the United States has been estimated to be 10–15%; there are regional differences in incidence, with the highest prevalence in the Northeast and the incidence decreasing in the Midwest, South, and West, respectively. This may relate to decreased seasonal availability of low-caloric density foods and/or decreased access to facilities for play and/or exercise in the winter season. Obesity is more prevalent in urban than rural areas.

The incidence of childhood obesity relates strongly to family variables, including parental obesity, higher socioeconomic status, increased parental education, small family size, and family patterns of inactivity. Children of parents with high activity levels tend to be leaner than their peers. An increased amount of time spent viewing television appears to correlate with an increased incidence of childhood obesity and may relate not only to the sedentary nature of the pastime but also to effects on food consumption related to advertisement of food products.

CLINICAL MANIFESTATIONS. Obesity may become evident at any age, but it appears most frequently in the 1st yr of life, at 5–6 yr of age, and during adolescence. The child whose obesity is due to excessively high caloric intake is usually not only heavier than others in his or her own cohort but also taller, and bone age is advanced. The facial features often appear disproportionately fine. The adiposity in the mammary regions of boys is often suggestive of breast development and, therefore, may be an embarrassing feature. The abdomen tends to be pendulous, and white or purple striae are often present. The external genitalia of boys appear disproportionately small but actually are most often of average size; the penis is often imbedded in the pubic fat. Puberty may occur early, with the result that the ultimate height of the obese may be less than that of their slower maturing peers. The development of the external genitalia is normal in most girls, and menarche is usually not delayed and may be advanced. Obesity of the extremities is usually greater in the upper arm and thigh and is sometimes limited to them. The hands may be relatively small and the fingers tapering. Genu valgum is common.

Children with obesity or overweight experience significant social and psychologic stresses and difficulties. Urban Western society has a strong cultural prejudice against obesity. Social stigmatization in school, the work place, and social environments is common. School children are frequently harassed, intimidated, and excluded from other activities; teachers may treat the obese child differently. Negative social attitudes toward obesity have been demonstrated in children as early as 7 yr of age. Psychologic disturbances are common in obese children. Even in the apparently well-adjusted child, adequate psychologic evaluation often discloses significant underlying emotional problems, which may have initially contributed to the causes of obesity and usually are an additive factor in its maintenance.

DIAGNOSIS. The Expert Committee on Clinical Guidelines for Overweight in Adolescent Preventive Services (an advisory group to the Maternal Child Health Bureau, the American Academy of Pediatrics, and the American Medical Association) has recommended use of the BMI for definition of obesity and overweight populations. Two categories have been defined: (1) adolescents with BMIs at the 95th percentile or more for age and sex or whose BMIs are more than 30 (whichever is smaller) should be considered overweight and be referred for definitive medical evaluation, and (2) adolescents whose BMIs are at the 85th percentile or more but less than the 95th percentile or equal to 30 (whichever is smaller) should be referred to a second level of screening.

The proposed second level of screening includes five areas of health risk as follows: (1) family history, i.e., positive family history of cardiovascular disease, parental elevated total cholesterol level (or an unknown history), positive family history of diabetes mellitus, or positive family history of parental obesity; (2) blood pressure, i.e., elevated blood pressure using methods and criteria of the Second Task Force on Blood Pressure Control in Children; (3) total cholesterol level, i.e., elevation more than 5.2 mmol/L or 200 mg/dL; (4) large annual incremental increase in BMI, i.e., an increase over the previous year of two BMI units; and (5) concern about weight, i.e., assessment of personal concerns, emotional or psychologic, related to overweight or the perception of overweight. If any one or more of the five areas are positive, then the patient should receive careful medical evaluation to consider primary medical pathologic conditions as listed under differential diagnosis.

The use of BMIs for identification of both the population at risk and to serve as a means to define patients requiring definitive evaluation appears to have clinical utility. Recommended cutoff values for both the risk and obese populations by age and sex are shown in Figures 45–2 and 45–3. Supplemental consideration of triceps skinfold thickness measurements more than 85th percentile for age and sex may also be helpful.

DIFFERENTIAL DIAGNOSIS. Children with obesity defined by elevated BMI of 95th percentile or more and/or 30 or more for age should receive careful medical evaluation for disorders that may have a primary medical association with obesity. Most of these disorders are rare. They are usually differentiated from childhood obesity by short stature, delayed bone age, and delayed development of secondary sexual characteristics. The differential diagnoses listed in Table 45–1 relate to less than 1% of all cases of childhood obesity.

COMPLICATIONS. Obese infants and children are at moderately increased risk of becoming obese adults. This increased risk is associated with greater severity of childhood obesity, decreased time interval to adult age, and greater number of obese family members. There is an association between childhood obesity and cardiovascular risk factors. In the Muscatine study, obese children had significantly lower high-density lipoprotein cholesterol levels, higher triglyceride levels, and higher systolic

■ **TABLE 45–1 Differential Diagnosis of Childhood Obesity**

Endocrine Causes
Cushing's syndrome
Hypothyroidism
Hyperinsulinemia
Growth hormone deficiency
Hypothalamic dysfunction
Prader-Willi syndrome
Stein-Leventhal syndrome (polycystic ovary)
Pseudohypoparathyroidism type I
Genetic Syndromes
Turner syndrome
Laurence-Moon-Biedl syndrome
Alstrom-Hallgren syndrome
Other Syndromes
Cohen syndrome
Carpenter syndrome

Adapted from Dietz, W. H. and Robinson, T. N., Assessment and Treatment of Childhood Obesity. Pediatr Rev 14:337, 1993.

blood pressure, although there was no difference from normal ranges for total cholesterol, low-density lipoprotein cholesterol, apolipoprotein A_1, apolipoprotein B, or diastolic blood pressure. Other studies have provided conflicting results and do not prove that childhood obesity increases the risk of cardiovascular disease, nor is there evidence that treatment of childhood obesity decreases the risk of adult coronary artery disease. Table 45–2 provides a list of the complications of obesity described in children, although some of those included have not been firmly established.

The *pickwickian syndrome* (for the fat boy, Joe, in Dickens's *Pickwick Papers*) is a rare complication of extreme exogenous obesity, in which there is severe cardiorespiratory distress with alveolar hypoventilation and a decrease in pulmonary, tidal, and expiratory reserve volumes. The manifestations include polycythemia, hypoxemia, cyanosis, cardiac enlargement, congestive cardiac failure, and somnolence. High concentrations of oxygen may be dangerous in treating the cyanosis because respiration may depend solely on the chemoreceptor stimulation of hypoxemia. Weight reduction is extremely important and should be accomplished as rapidly as feasible.

PREVENTION AND TREATMENT. Because obesity may be self-perpetuating for psychologic or physiologic reasons, obese children, children of obese parents, or those with obese siblings should be encouraged to adhere to a systematic program of energetic exercise and a balanced diet appropriate to their energy expenditure level. Idealized weight is desirable not only for aesthetic reasons but also potentially to prevent complications of obesity such as diabetes, shortness of breath, and early death. Untreated overweight infants may remain overweight as adults. Early attempts to modify behavior commencing in the infant period, such as feeding the infant on demand shortly after birth, providing food only at signs of hunger in the 1st yr, avoiding cueing by showing attractive foods or regimenting

■ **TABLE 45–2 Reported Complications of Childhood Obesity**

Cardiovascular
Increased blood pressure
Increased total cholesterol
Increased serum triglycerides
Increased LDL (low density lipoprotein)
Increased VLDL (very low density lipoprotein)
Decreased HDL (high density lipoprotein)
Hyperinsulinism
Cholelithiasis
Blount disease and slipped capital femoral epiphysis
Pseudotumor cerebri
Pulmonary
Pickwickian syndrome
Abnormal pulmonary function tests

feeding times by the clock, and by teaching the child to eat only when hungry, may effectively prevent overeating and obesity.

After childhood obesity is established, it is extremely difficult to implement an effective plan for weight reduction and maintenance without active participation and motivation of both the child and the family. Techniques used for fat reduction in adults, including surgery, pharmacotherapy, and gastric balloons, are contraindicated in children. Very low-calorie diets are inappropriate because they may impair growth and development at critical points during childhood. Alternatively, however, maintenance of weight during the growth spurt of adolescence leads to an effective weight reduction for age as growth occurs and may be preferable to drastic weight reduction and exercise protocols. Successful treatment of childhood obesity requires attention to at least the following components: (1) modification of diet and caloric content; (2) definition and utilization of appropriate exercise programs; (3) behavior modification for the child; and (4) involvement of the family in therapy. There has been modest success in behavior modification programs; however, results for individuals have been highly variable. Programs which include simultaneous family therapy seem to be effective in preventing progression to severe obesity as measured by reduction in triceps skinfold thickness during adolescence, if the therapy starts at 10–11 yr of age. Such programs also include self-monitoring, stimulus control, reduction in the rate of eating, cognitive restructuring, and increased physical activity. Involvement of the family is most effective if a parent is simultaneously involved in the therapeutic plan and makes efforts to change the family lifestyle. Although these programs have shown some success, the patients did not reach nonobese status (less than 20% overweight).

If the practitioner chooses to implement a diet, the basic nutritional needs must be met. All the essential dietary needs may be included in an 1,100–1,300-calorie diet for children 10–14 yr of age for several months (Table 45–3). Some children avoid excessive eating after they have been allowed to return to a free choice of diet. The diet should contain as much bulk as possible. At times, greater cooperation is secured if small portions of the diet are permitted between meals, especially in the afternoon. If there is doubt that the daily vitamin intake is adequate, vitamin concentrates may be prescribed. Vitamin D should be included, as for all growing children. Rapid decreases in weight should not be attempted, and medical supervision should be maintained. During the growing years, maintenance of weight while the child increases in height is often a sufficient goal. At best, there is a limited place for drug therapy. Psychologic support is often an essential element in management, and both dietary and psychologic treatment should involve the entire family.

PROGNOSIS. Results with dietary and/or exercise modification have been successful only for the short term; follow-up studies of adequate duration show a high rate of relapse at 4–10 yr, with successful maintenance of reduced (but not normal) weight in only slightly less than 50% of patients.

A Canadian meta-analysis that evaluated obesity in children, utilized in the development of practice guidelines, supported the need for sequential weight and height measurements of children principally to rule out failure to thrive, but the analysis was unable to demonstrate sufficient evidence of the success of therapeutic intervention to support screening for childhood obesity. No harm was associated with screening, however. In addition, there was insufficient evidence to either include or exclude counseling about nutrition and exercise for the initial therapy of obese children, although very low-calorie diets should be excluded from the management of preadolescent children. Finally, there was conflicting evidence with regard to the inclusion or exclusion of exercise in the routine management of obese children.

Although data do not support massive screening programs for the identification of childhood obesity as a preventive program of pediatrics, it appears prudent for the practitioner to initiate, on behalf of the individual motivated patient, judicious dietary and exercise management combined with behavior modification and family therapy. The goal should be to facilitate growth and provide substantial social and psychologic support, even if the direct medical preventive aspects are not well substantiated.

■ TABLE 45–3 1,100–1,300 Calorie Diet

Breakfast	*Dinner*
½ cup orange juice	2 oz lean ground beef
¾ cup ready-to-eat cereal	1 oz cheese
6 oz 1% milk	½ tomato
1 tsp sugar	1 cup 1% milk
	2 taco shells, taco sauce
Lunch	1 nectarine
2 oz turkey or lean meat	Lettuce
½ cup noodles or bread	
½ cup carrots	*Snack*
1 tsp margarine	6 Saltines
1 cup 1% milk	1 apple

Total "exchanges": 3 fruit, 2 vegetables, 4 starch, 2¾ milk, 3 medium-fat meat, 2 low-fat meat, 2 fat. Try to incorporate egg, high-fiber sources (e.g., beans, some combination foods).

Canadian Task Force on the Periodic Health Examination: Periodic health examination, 1994 update: 1. obesity in childhood. Can Med Assoc J 150:871, 1994.

Dietz WH, Robinson TN: Assessment and treatment of childhood obesity. Pediatr Rev 14:337, 1993.

Flodmark C, Ohlsson T, Ryden O, et al: Prevention of progression to severe obesity in a group of obese schoolchildren treated with family therapy. Pediatrics 91:880, 1993.

Himes JH, Dietz WH: Guidelines for overweight in adolescent preventive services: recommendations from an expert committee. Am J Clin Nutr 59:307, 1994.

Mossberg H: 40-year followup of overweight children. Lancet 2:491, 1989.

Schlicker SA, Borra ST, Regan C: The weight and fitness status of United States children. Nutr Rev 52:11, 1994.

Williams CL, Kimm SYS (eds): Prevention and treatment of childhood obesity (monograph). Ann N Y Acad Sci 699:310, 1993.

45.3 Vitamin Deficiencies and Excesses

Vitamins are essential nutrients that must be supplied exogenously. Functions of vitamins are summarized in Table 43–6, and recommended daily allowances in Table 43–1. Toxicity is seen more commonly with excesses of the fat-soluble vitamins A and D than with those of the water-soluble vitamins. The vitamin-dependent states are summarized in Table 45–4.

VITAMIN A DEFICIENCY

The term vitamin A is a generic label for all β-ionone derivatives other than provitamin A carotenoids. Retinol signifies vitamin A alcohol, retinyl ester, vitamin A ester; retinal, vitamin A aldehyde; and retinoic acid, vitamin A acid.

"Provitamin A carotenoids" is the generic term for all carotenoids that have the biologic activity of β-carotene. They or their derivatives with vitamin A activity are required in the diets of infants and children.

β-Carotene is partly absorbed by the intestinal lymphatics; the remainder is cleaved into two molecules of retinol. Dietary retinyl ester is hydrolyzed to retinol in the intestine. Retinol is esterified inside the mucosal cell with palmitic acid and is stored in the liver as retinyl palmitate; this in turn is hydrolyzed to free retinol for transport to its site of action. Zinc is required for this mobilization. Normal plasma values of

■ TABLE 45–4 Vitamin Dependency States

Vitamin	Disease	Untreated State	Daily Dosage
A	Darier	Hyperkeratosis follicularis	7,500 μg
B_1	Leigh—pyruvic-lactic acidosis	Ataxia, retardation	600 mg
	Thiamine responsive anemia	Megaloblastic anemia	20 mg
	Maple syrup urine disease	Hypotonia, seizures	10 mg
Riboflavin	Pyruvate kinase deficiency	Hemolysis	10 mg
	Glutaric acidemia (II)	Hypoglycemia	100–300 mg
Niacin	Hartnup	Ataxia, eczema	200 mg
B_6	Cystathioninuria	No symptoms	200 mg
	Homocystinuria	Retardation	200 mg
	B_6-anemia	Hypochromic microcytic anemia	10 mg
	B_6-seizures	Seizures	25 mg
	Xanthurenic aciduria	Retardation	10 mg
	Gyrate atrophy of choroid	Blindness	100 mg
	Oxaluria	Oxalate crystals	100 mg
Folic acid	Formiminotransferase deficiency	Retardation	5 mg
	Folate reductase deficiency	Megaloblastic anemia	5 mg
	Homocystinuria	Retardation	10 mg
B_{12}	Methylmalonic acidemia	Retardation	1 mg
Biotin	Propionic acidemia	Retardation	10 mg
	β-Methylcrotonyl glycinuria	Coma	10 mg
	Biotinidase deficiency	Seizures	5–20 mg
	Holocarboxylase deficiency	Hypotonia	10 mg
C	Chédiak-Higashi	Infections	50 mg
D	Dependency	Rickets	100 μg
	Familial hypophosphatemia	Rickets	2,500 μg

retinol in infants are 20–50 μg/dL; in children and adults, 30–225 μg/dL.

Ingested carotenoids are nontoxic and may result in yellow discoloration of the skin but not of the sclera. This disorder, *carotenemia,* is especially likely to occur in children with liver disease, diabetes mellitus, or hypothyroidism and in those who have congenital absence of enzymes that convert provitamin A carotenoids.

ETIOLOGY. The liver at birth has a low vitamin A content that is rapidly augmented because colostrum and breast milk furnish large amounts of the vitamin. Breast milk and whole cow's milk are satisfactory sources of vitamin A. Other foods (vegetables, fruits, eggs, butter, liver) or vitamin supplements also provide vitamin A. Loss of it in cooking, canning, and freezing of foodstuffs is small; oxidizing agents, however, destroy it.

The risk of vitamin A deficiency is small in healthy children with balanced diets. Deficient diets commonly cause disease by 2–3 yr of age. Vitamin A deficiency also results from inadequate intestinal absorption, such as, for example, with chronic intestinal disorders, celiac disease, hepatic and pancreatic diseases, iron-deficiency anemia, chronic infectious diseases, or chronic ingestion of mineral oil. Low intake of dietary fat results in low vitamin A absorption. Vitamin A excretion is increased in cancer, urinary tract disease, and chronic infectious diseases. Low protein intake results in deficient carrier protein and in decreases in plasma concentration of vitamin A.

PATHOLOGY. The human retina contains two distinct photoreceptor systems: the rods are sensitive to light of low intensity, the cones to colors and to light of high intensity. Retinal is the prosthetic group of the photosensitive pigment in both rods and cones. The major difference between the visual pigments in rods (rhodopsin) and in cones (iodopsin) is the nature of the protein bound to retinal. All-*trans* retinal isomerizes in the dark to 11-*cis* form. This combines with opsin to form rhodopsin. Energy from light quanta reconverts 11-*cis* retinal back to the all-*trans* form; this energy exchange, transmitted via the optic nerves to the brain, results in visual sensation. β-Carotene has been effective in ameliorating photosensitivity in patients with erythropoietic protoporphyria. It has also been suggested that retinitis pigmentosa may be related to a defect in retinol-binding protein.

Retinoids are essential for cell differentiation, in the activation of retinoic acid responsive genes, and in membrane stability. Both excess and deficiency of vitamin A lead to rupture of lysosomal membranes with release of hydrolases.

The vitamin plays a role in keratinization, cornification, bone metabolism, placental development, growth, spermatogenesis, and mucus formation. Characteristic changes in epithelium include proliferation of basal cells, hyperkeratosis, and the formation of stratified, cornified, squamous epithelium. Epithelial changes in the respiratory system may result in bronchiolar obstruction. Squamous metaplasia of the renal pelves, ureters, urinary bladder, enamel organs, and pancreatic and salivary ducts may lead to an increase in infections in these areas.

CLINICAL MANIFESTATIONS. Ocular lesions develop insidiously. Initially, the posterior segment of the eye is affected, with impairment of dark adaptation resulting in night blindness. Later, drying of the conjunctiva (xerosis conjunctivae) and of the cornea (xerosis corneae) is followed by wrinkling and cloudiness of the cornea (keratomalacia) (Fig. 45–4). Dry, silver-gray plaques may appear on the bulbar conjunctiva (Bitot spots), with follicular hyperkeratosis and photophobia.

Vitamin A deficiency may result in retardation of mental and physical growth and in apathy. Anemia with or without hepatosplenomegaly is usually present.

The skin is dry and scaly, and at times follicular hyperkeratosis may be found on the shoulders, buttocks, and extensor surfaces of the extremities. The vaginal epithelium may become cornified, and epithelial metaplasia of the urinary tract may contribute to pyuria and hematuria. Increased intracranial pressure with wide separation of cranial bones at the sutures may occur. Hydrocephalus, with or without paralyses of the cranial nerves, is an infrequent manifestation.

DIAGNOSIS. Dark adaptation tests may be helpful. Xerosis conjunctivae can be detected by biomicroscopic examination of the conjunctiva. Examination of the scrapings from the eye and vagina is recommended as a diagnostic aid. The plasma carotene concentration falls quickly, but that of vitamin A decreases more slowly.

PREVENTION. Infants should receive at least 500 μg daily; older children and adults, 600–1500 μg of vitamin A or carotene. The average diets of infants and children in this country supply enough vitamin A to prevent symptoms of deficiency. One microgram of retinol equals 3.3 IU of vitamin A.

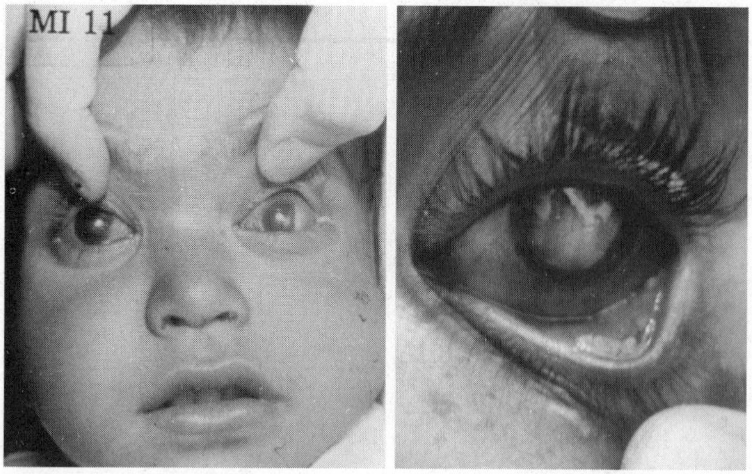

Figure 45–4. Recovery from xerophthalmia, showing permanent eye lesion. (From Bloch CE: Blindness and other diseases arising from deficient nutrition [lack of fat-soluble A factor]. Am J Dis Child 27:139, 1924.)

For therapeutic reasons, low-fat diets should be supplemented with vitamin A. In disorders with poor absorption of fat or increased excretion of vitamin A, water-miscible preparations should be administered in amounts several times the usual daily requirement. Premature infants, who absorb fats and vitamin A less efficiently than do full-term infants, should also receive water-miscible preparations. In areas of the world where vitamin A deficiency occurs, 30,000 μg of vitamin A should be given orally in a water-miscible base 4 times yearly; the same dose should be given postpartum to the mothers of breast-fed infants in these regions.

TREATMENT. In cases of latent vitamin A deficiency, a daily supplement of 1,500 μg of vitamin A is sufficient. For xerophthalmia, 1,500 μg/kg/24 hr is given orally for 5 days and then continued with intramuscular injection of 7,500 μg of vitamin A in oil daily until recovery occurs. Morbidity and mortality rates may decrease in nondeficient children who acquire certain viral infections such as measles when given 1,500–3,000 μg of vitamin A.

HYPERVITAMINOSIS A. Acute hypervitaminosis A may occur in infants after ingesting 100,000 μg or more. The symptoms are nausea, vomiting, drowsiness, and bulging of the fontanel. Diplopia, papilledema, cranial nerve palsies, and other symptoms suggestive of brain tumor (*pseudotumor cerebri*) may also occur. Toxicity has occurred with supplementation during vaccine administration in developing countries.

Chronic hypervitaminosis A appears after ingestion of excessive doses for several weeks or months. The child has anorexia, pruritus, and a lack of weight gain. There is increased irritability, limitation of motion, and tender swelling of the bones. Alopecia, seborrheic cutaneous lesions, fissuring of the corners of the mouth, increased intracranial pressure, and hepatomegaly may develop. Craniotabes and desquamation of the palms and soles are common. Roentgenograms reveal hyperostosis affecting several long bones; it is most notable at the middle of the shafts (Fig. 45–5).

Severe congenital malformations may occur in infants of mothers consuming large amounts of oral retinoids used in treating acne.

A history of excessive ingestion of vitamin A helps to differentiate it from cortical hyperostosis (see Chapter 628). Besides a history of excess, the serum vitamin A level is elevated, and hypercalcemia or liver cirrhosis occurs occasionally.

Caffey J: Pediatric X-Ray Diagnosis, 5th ed. Chicago, Year Book, 1967, p 994.
de Francisco A, Chakrabory J, Chowdhury HR, et al: Acute toxicity of vitamin A given with vaccines in infancy. Lancet 392:526, 1993.
Fisher KD, Carr CJ, Huff JE, et al: Dark adaptation and night vision. Fed Proc 29:1605, 1970.
Goodman DS: Vitamin A metabolism. Fed Proc 39:2716, 1980.
Hussey GD, Klein M.: A randomized controlled trial of vitamin A in children with severe measles. N Engl J Med 323:160, 1990.
Leung AKC: Carotenemia. Adv Pediatr 34:223, 1987.
Mahoney CP, Margolis T, Knauss TA, et al: Chronic vitamin A intoxication in infants fed chicken liver. Pediatrics 65:893, 1980.
McLaren DS, Shirajain E, Tchallian M, et al: Xerophthalmia in Jordan. Am J Clin Nutr 17:117, 1965.
Moon RC: Comparative aspects of carotenoids and retinoids as chemopreventive agents for cancer. J Nutr 119:127, 1989.
Neuzil KM, Gruber WC, Chytil F, et al: Serum vitamin A levels in respiratory syncytial virus infection. J Pediatr 124:433, 1994.
Peck GL: Prolonged remissions of cystic and conglobate acne with 13-*cis*-retinoic acid. N Engl J Med 300:299, 1979.

VITAMIN B COMPLEX DEFICIENCY

Vitamin B complex includes several factors whose chemical composition and function vary widely (see Table 43–6). All are

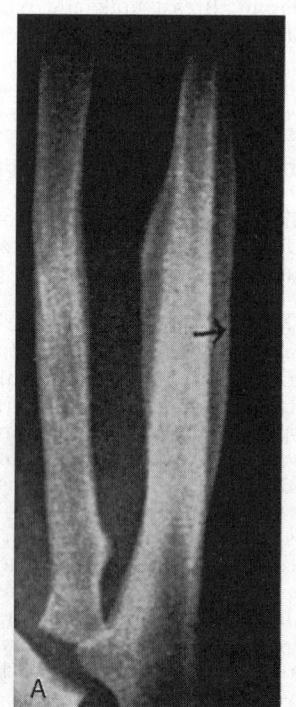

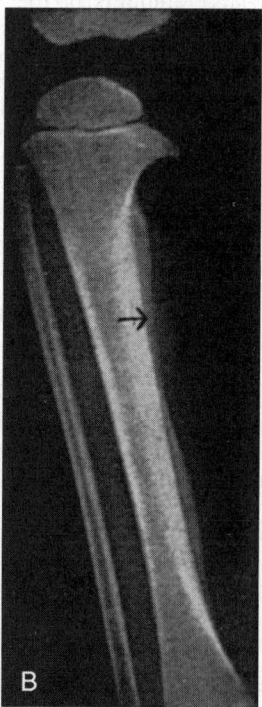

Figure 45–5. Hyperostosis of the ulna and the tibia in an infant 21 mo of age, resulting from vitamin A poisoning. *A*, Long, wavy cortical hyperostosis of the ulna. *B*, Long, wavy cortical hyperostosis of the right tibia; striking absence of metaphyseal changes. (From Caffey J: Pediatric X-ray Diagnosis, 5th ed. Chicago, Year Book, 1967, p 994.)

important constituents of enzyme systems. Because many of these enzymes are closely related functionally, lack of a single factor can interrupt an entire chain of chemical processes, producing diverse clinical manifestations.

Diets deficient in any one factor of the B complex are frequently poor sources of other B vitamins. Because manifestations of several B deficiencies can usually be found in the same patient, it is generally practical to treat the patient with the entire B complex.

Factors such as pantothenic acid, choline, and inositol are important for the normal functioning of the human organism, but at present no specific deficiency syndromes can be ascribed to their lack in the diets of children.

THIAMINE DEFICIENCY

(Beriberi)

ETIOLOGY. Vitamin B_1 (thiamine) is water soluble and, as thiamine pyrophosphate or cocarboxylase, functions as a coenzyme in carbohydrate metabolism. Thiamine is required for the synthesis of acetylcholine, and deficiency results in impaired nerve conduction. It is the coenzyme in transketolation and in decarboxylation of α-keto acids. Transketolase participates in the hexose monophosphate shunt that generates nicotinamide adenine dinucleotide phosphate and pentose.

Breast milk or cow's milk, vegetables, cereals, fruits, and eggs are sources of thiamine. Infants whose source of food is the milk of thiamine-deficient mothers may develop beriberi. Older children whose diet contains good sources of thiamine such as meats and legumes do not require thiamine supplements.

Thiamine is easily destroyed by heat in neutral or alkaline media and is readily extracted from foodstuffs by cooking water. An enzyme factor destructive to thiamine is present in some fish. Because the covering of grains of cereals contains most of the vitamin, polishing reduces its availability.

Thiamine absorption decreases with gastrointestinal or liver disease. Requirements increase with fever, surgery, or stress. Thiamine dependency has been described in a child with megaloblastic anemia and in an infant with otherwise typical maple syrup urine disease. The urine of children with *Leigh encephalomyelopathy* and of their parents inhibits the formation of thiamine pyrophosphate. Large doses of thiamine improve some of the physical abnormalities associated with the disease.

PATHOLOGY. In fatal cases of beriberi, lesions are located principally in the heart, peripheral nerves, subcutaneous tissue, and serous cavities. The heart is dilated, and fatty degeneration of the myocardium is common. Generalized edema or edema of the legs, serous effusions, and venous engorgement may be present. The peripheral nerves undergo varying degrees of degeneration of myelin and axon cylinders, with wallerian degeneration, beginning in the distal locations. The nerves of the lower extremities are affected first. Lesions in the brain include vascular dilatation and hemorrhage.

CLINICAL MANIFESTATIONS. Early manifestations of deficiency include fatigue, apathy, irritability, depression, drowsiness, poor mental concentration, anorexia, nausea, and abdominal discomfort. Signs of progression include peripheral neuritis with tingling, burning, and paresthesias of the toes and feet; decreased tendon reflexes; loss of vibration sense; tenderness and cramping of leg muscles; congestive heart failure; and psychic disturbances. There may be ptosis of the eyelids and atrophy of the optic nerve. Hoarseness or aphonia due to paralysis of the laryngeal nerve is a characteristic sign. Muscle atrophy and tenderness of nerve trunks are followed by ataxia, loss of coordination, and loss of deep sensation. Paralytic symptoms are more common in adults than in children. Later, signs of increased intracranial pressure, meningismus, and coma occur.

In *dry* beriberi, the child may appear plump but is pale, flabby, listless, and dyspneic; the heart rate is rapid and the liver enlarged. In *wet* beriberi, the child is undernourished, pale, and edematous and has dyspnea, vomiting, and tachycardia. The skin appears waxy. The urine may contain albumin and casts.

The cardiac signs at first are slight cyanosis and dyspnea. Tachycardia, enlargement of the liver, loss of consciousness, and convulsions may develop rapidly. The heart is enlarged, especially to the right. The electrocardiogram shows increased Q-T interval, inversion of T waves, and low voltage, changes that rapidly revert to normal with treatment. Cardiac failure may lead to death in either chronic or acute beriberi.

Wernicke Encephalopathy. This is characterized by irritability, somnolence, and ocular signs, and less commonly by mental confusion and ataxias, infrequently occurring in malnourished infants and children. Associated conditions include malignancy, infection, gastrointestinal disorders, and prematurity.

DIAGNOSIS. Since the early symptoms are encountered in many types of nutritional disturbances besides thiamine deficiency, demonstrations of lowered red blood cell transketolase and high blood or urinary glyoxylate values have been proposed as diagnostic tests. Excretion after an oral loading dose of thiamine or its metabolites, thiazole or pyrimidine, may help to identify the deficiency state. Clinical response to administration of thiamine remains the best test for thiamine deficiency.

PREVENTION. A maternal diet containing sufficient amounts of thiamine prevents this deficiency in breast-fed infants (see Table 43–1). Thiamine requirements increase with a high-carbohydrate content of the diet.

TREATMENT. If beriberi occurs in a breast-fed infant, both the mother and child should be treated with thiamine. The daily dose for adults is 50 mg and for children 10 mg or more. Oral administration is effective unless gastrointestinal disturbances prevent absorption. Thiamine should be given intramuscularly or intravenously to children with cardiac failure. Such treatment is followed by dramatic improvement, although complete cure requires several weeks. The heart is not permanently damaged. Because patients with beriberi often have other B complex deficiencies, all other vitamins of the B complex should be administered, in addition to large doses of thiamine chloride.

RIBOFLAVIN DEFICIENCY

(Ariboflavinosis)

Riboflavin deficiency without deficiencies of other members of the B complex is rare. Riboflavin, a yellow, fluorescent, water-soluble substance, is stable to heat and acids but is destroyed by light and alkalis. The coenzymes flavin mononucleotide and flavin adenine dinucleotide (FAD) are synthesized from riboflavin, forming the prosthetic groups of several enzymes important in electron transport. Riboflavin is essential for growth and tissue respiration; it may have a role in light adaptation and is required for conversion of pyridoxine to pyridoxal phosphate. Large amounts of riboflavin occur in liver, kidney, brewer's yeast, milk, cheese, eggs, and leafy vegetables; cow's milk contains about five times as much riboflavin as human milk.

Riboflavin deficiency is usually caused by inadequate intake. Faulty absorption may contribute in patients with biliary atresia or hepatitis or in those receiving probenecid, phenothiazine, or oral contraceptives. Phototherapy destroys riboflavin.

CLINICAL MANIFESTATIONS. Evidences of riboflavin deficiency include cheilosis (perlèche), glossitis, keratitis, conjunctivitis, photophobia, lacrimation, marked corneal vascularization, and seborrheic dermatitis. Cheilosis begins with pallor at the angles of the mouth, followed by thinning and maceration of the epithelium. Superficial fissures often covered by yellow crusts develop in the angles of the mouth and extend radially into the skin for distances of 1–2 cm. With glossitis, the tongue is smooth, and loss of papillary structure occurs. A normocytic, normochromic anemia with bone marrow hypoplasia is common.

DIAGNOSIS. Urinary excretion of riboflavin below 30 μg/24 hr is abnormally low. Levels of erythrocyte glutathionine reductase, a flavoprotein requiring FAD, may reflect the stores of riboflavin. A patient with hemolysis due to pyruvate kinase deficiency and reduced erythrocyte glutathionine reductase had both enzyme activities restored to normal on administration of riboflavin.

PREVENTION. Recommended daily allowances are presented in Table 43–1. Riboflavin deficiency is usually prevented by a diet that contains adequate amounts of milk, eggs, leafy vegetables, and lean meats.

TREATMENT. Treatment consists in the oral administration of 3–10 mg of riboflavin daily. If no response occurs within a few days, intramuscular injections of 2 mg of riboflavin in saline solution may be made three times daily. The child should also be given a well-balanced diet and, at least temporarily, more than the usual requirements of the B complex.

NIACIN DEFICIENCY
(Pellagra)

ETIOLOGY. Pellagra (*pellis,* skin; *agra,* rough), a deficiency disease caused mainly by a lack of niacin (nicotinic acid), affects all tissues of the body. Niacin forms part of two enzymes important in electron transfer and glycolysis: nicotinamide adenine dinucleotide and nicotinamide adenine dinucleotide phosphate. Although dietary tryptophan can partially substitute for niacin, other sources of niacin are necessary. Liver, lean pork, salmon, poultry, and red meat are good sources, but most cereals contain only small amounts of it. Pellagra occurs chiefly in countries where corn (maize), a poor source of tryptophan, is a basic foodstuff. Milk and eggs, which contain little niacin, are good pellagra-preventive foods because of their high content of tryptophan. Because niacin is a stable compound, there are only small losses in cooking.

PATHOLOGY. Histologically, edema and degeneration of the superficial collagen of the dermis occur. The papillary vessels are engorged, and there is perivascular lymphocytic infiltration in the dermis. The epidermis is hyperkeratotic and later becomes atrophic.

Changes comparable with those in the skin are present in the tongue, buccal mucous membranes, and vagina. These changes may be associated with secondary infection and ulceration. The walls of the colon are thickened and inflamed with patches of pseudomembrane; later the mucosa atrophies. Changes in the nervous system occur relatively late in the disease and consist of patchy areas of demyelinization and degeneration of ganglion cells; demyelinization in the spinal cord may involve the posterior and lateral columns.

CLINICAL MANIFESTATIONS. The early symptoms of pellagra are vague. Anorexia, lassitude, weakness, burning sensations, numbness, and dizziness may be prodromal symptoms. After a long period of niacin deficiency, the characteristic symptoms appear. The classic triad consists of dermatitis, diarrhea, and dementia. Manifestations in children who have parasites or chronic disorders may be especially severe.

The most characteristic manifestations are the cutaneous ones, which may develop suddenly or insidiously and may be elicited by irritants, particularly by intense sunlight. They first appear as symmetric erythema of the exposed surfaces that may resemble sunburn and in mild cases may escape recognition. The lesions are usually sharply demarcated from the healthy skin around them, and their distribution may change frequently. The lesions on the hands sometimes have the appearance of a glove (pellagrous glove), and similar demarcations are occasionally seen on the foot and leg (pellagrous boot) or around the neck (Casal necklace) (Fig. 45–6). In some cases, vesicles and bullae develop (wet type), or there may be suppuration beneath the scaly, crusted epidermis; in others, the swelling disappears after a short time and desquamation begins. The healed parts of the skin may remain pigmented.

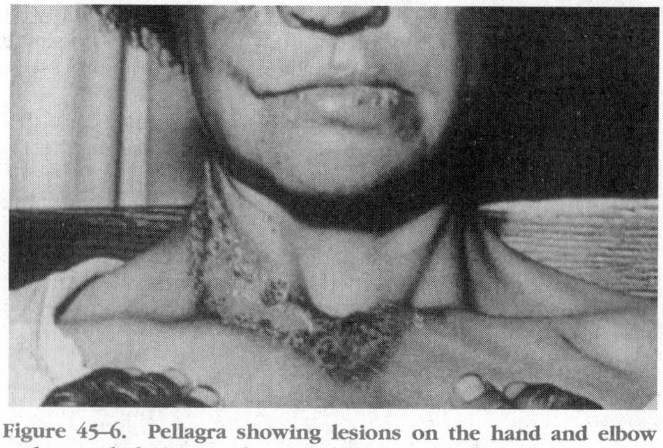

Figure 45–6. Pellagra showing lesions on the hand and elbow and an early lesion on the neck (Casal necklace).

The cutaneous lesions are sometimes preceded by stomatitis, glossitis, vomiting, or diarrhea. Swelling and redness of the tip of the tongue and its lateral margins may be followed by intense redness of the entire tongue and of the papillae and even ulceration.

Nervous symptoms include depression, disorientation, insomnia, and delirium.

The classic symptoms of pellagra are usually not well developed in infants and children. Anorexia, irritability, anxiety, and apathy are common in "pellagra families." They may also have sore tongues and lips, and the skin is usually dry and scaly. Diarrhea and constipation may alternate, and a moderate secondary anemia may occur. Children who have pellagra often have evidence of other nutritional deficiency diseases.

DIAGNOSIS. Diagnosis is usually made from the physical signs of glossitis, gastrointestinal symptoms, and a symmetric dermatitis. Rapid clinical response to niacin is an important confirming test. N-methylnicotinamide, a normal metabolite of niacin, is almost undetectable in urine during niacin deficiency.

PREVENTION. A well-balanced diet containing meat, vegetables, eggs, and milk meets the recommended daily allowances (see Table 43–1); thus supplements of niacin are necessary only in breast-fed infants whose mothers have pellagra or in children on restricted diets.

TREATMENT. Children respond rapidly to antipellagral therapy. A liberal and well-balanced diet should be supplemented with 50–300 mg/day of niacin; 100 mg may be given intravenously in severe cases or in cases of poor intestinal absorption. Administering large doses of niacin is often followed within a half hour by a sensation of increased local heat and flushing and burning of the skin, unpleasant effects that are not produced by niacinamide. Large doses of niacin may cause cholestatic jaundice or hepatotoxicity.

The diet should be supplemented with other vitamins, especially with other members of the B complex. Sun exposure should be avoided during the active phase; the skin lesions may be covered with soothing applications. Hypochromic anemia should be treated with iron. The diet of the cured patient with pellagra should be supervised continuously to prevent recurrence.

THIAMINE DEFICIENCY

Borgna-Pignatti C, Marradi P, Pinelli L, et al: Thiamine-responsive anemia in DIDMOAD syndrome. J Pediatr 114:405, 1989.
Brin M: Erythrocyte as a biopsy tissue for functional evaluation of thiamin adequacy. JAMA 187:762, 1964.

McCandless DW, Schenker S: Neurologic disorders of thiamine deficiency. Nutr Rev 27:213, 1969.
Pihko H, Soarinen U, Paetau A: Wernicke encephalopathy: A preventable cause of death: Report of 2 children with malignant disease. Pediatr Neurol 5:237, 1989.
Vrochota K, Oberg CN, Harris KN: Beriberi in a southeast Asian adolescent. Am J Dis Child 143:270, 1989.

RIBOFLAVIN DEFICIENCY

Rillotson JA, Baker EM: An enzymatic measurement of the riboflavin status in man. Am J Clin Nutr 25:425, 1972.
Rivlin RS: Hormones, drugs and riboflavin. Nutr Rev 37:241, 1979.
Staal GEJ, Van Berkel TJC, Nijessen JG, et al: Normalization of red blood cell pyruvate kinase in pyruvate kinase deficiency by riboflavin treatment. Clin Chim Acta 60:323, 1975.

NIACIN DEFICIENCY

Darby WJ, McNutt KW, Todhunter EN: Niacin. Nutr Rev 33:289, 1975.

PYRIDOXINE (VITAMIN B_6) DEFICIENCY

Vitamin B_6 includes pyridoxal, pyridoxine, and pyridoxamine. These are converted to pyridoxal-5-phosphate (or pyridoxamine-5-phosphate), which acts as a coenzyme in decarboxylation and transamination of amino acids, such as in the decarboxylation of 5-hydroxytryptophan in the formation of serotonin and in the metabolism of glycogen and fatty acids. Vitamin B_6 is also essential for the breakdown of kynurenine. When this does not occur, xanthurenic acid appears in the urine. Adequate functioning of the nervous system depends on pyridoxine, deficiency of which leads to seizures and to peripheral neuropathy. Pyridoxal phosphate is the coenzyme for both glutamic decarboxylase and γ-aminobutyric acid transaminase; each is necessary for normal brain metabolism. It participates in active transport of amino acids across cell membranes, chelates metals, and participates in the synthesis of arachidonic acid from linoleic acid. If it is lacking, glycine metabolism may lead to oxaluria. It is excreted largely as 4-pyridoxic acid.

ETIOLOGY. Pyridoxine is adequately available in human and cow's milk and in cereals, but prolonged heat processing of the latter two destroys it. Diseases with malabsorption, such as celiac syndrome, may contribute to vitamin B_6 deficiency.

There are several types of *vitamin B_6 dependency syndromes,* presumably the result of errors in enzyme structure or function, in which the patient responds to very large amounts of pyridoxine. These syndromes include B_6-dependent convulsions, a B_6-responsive anemia, xanthurenic aciduria, cystathioninuria, and homocystinuria.

Pyridoxine antagonists, such as isoniazid used in the treatment of tuberculosis, increase the requirements for pyridoxine, as do pregnancy and drugs such as penicillamine, hydralazine, and the oral progesterone-estrogen contraceptives.

CLINICAL MANIFESTATIONS. Deficiency symptoms are not as common in children as in adults. Four clinical disturbances caused by vitamin B_6 deficiency have been described in humans: convulsions in infants, peripheral neuritis, dermatitis, and anemia.

Infants fed a formula deficient in vitamin B_6 for 1–6 mo exhibit irritability and generalized seizures. Gastrointestinal distress and an aggravated startle response are common.

Peripheral neuropathy may occur during treatment of tuberculosis with isonicotinic acid hydrazide. The neuropathy responds to administration of pyridoxine or to a decrease in the dose of the drug. Administration of isonicotinic acid may also be followed by manifestations of pellagra.

Skin lesions include cheilosis, glossitis, and seborrhea around the eyes, nose, and mouth. Microcytic anemia, oxaluria, oxalic acid bladder stones, hyperglycinemia, lymphopenia, decreased antibody formation, and infections also occur.

Convulsions from B_6 dependency may occur several hours to as long as 6 mo after birth. Seizures are typically myoclonic with hypsarrhythmic patterns on the electroencephalogram. In several cases, the mother had received large doses of pyridoxine during pregnancy for control of emesis.

In *B_6-dependent anemia,* the red blood cells are microcytic and hypochromic. There are increased serum iron concentrations, saturation of iron-binding protein, hemosiderin deposits in bone marrow and liver, and failure of iron utilization for hemoglobin synthesis.

Xanthurenic aciduria following tryptophan load tests is an apparently benign occurrence in some families. Xanthurenic acid excretion becomes normal following large doses of vitamin B_6. *Cystathioninuria* is similarly not accompanied by any clear clinical disturbance. Cystathioninase is vitamin B_6 dependent (see Chapter 71.4).

In some patients with *homocystinuria,* serum levels of homocysteine will fall following B_6 administration. Cystathionine synthetase is B_6 dependent (see Chapter 71.4 and 71.5).

LABORATORY DATA. Anemia is not common in affected infants. After administration of 100 mg/kg of tryptophan, large amounts of xanthurenic acid will be found in the urine of patients with pyridoxine deficiency; in normal persons, none is detected. The result of this test may be normal in patients with "pyridoxine dependency."

DIAGNOSIS. Infants with seizures should be suspected of having vitamin B_6 deficiency or dependency. If more common causes of infantile seizures, such as hypocalcemia, hypoglycemia, and infection, can be eliminated, 100 mg of pyridoxine should be injected. If the seizure stops, B_6 deficiency should be suspected, and a tryptophan loading test is indicated. Similarly, in older children with seizure disorders, 100 mg of pyridoxine may be injected intramuscularly while the electroencephalogram (EEG) is being recorded; a favorable response of the EEG suggests pyridoxine deficiency.

Erythrocyte glutamic pyruvic transaminase is reduced in pyridoxine deficiency; its concentration may be used as an indicator of vitamin B_6 status.

PREVENTION. Balanced diets usually contain enough pyridoxine so that deficiency is rare. Children receiving high-protein diets should have vitamin B_6 added. Infants whose mothers have received large doses of pyridoxine during pregnancy are at increased risk of seizures due to pyridoxine dependency. Any child receiving a pyridoxine antagonist such as isoniazid should be carefully observed for neurologic manifestations. If these develop, either pyridoxine should be administered or the dose of the antagonist decreased. Daily intake of 0.3–0.5 mg of pyridoxine in the infant, 0.5–1.5 mg in the child, or 1.5–2.0 mg in the adult prevents deficiency states.

TREATMENT. For convulsions possibly due to pyridoxine deficiency, 100 mg of the vitamin should be given intramuscularly. One dose should suffice if the diet is adequate. For "pyridoxine-dependent" children, 2–10 mg intramuscularly or 10–100 mg orally may be necessary daily.

TOXICITY. Excessive intake may cause neuropathy.

Cinnamon AD, Beaton JR: Biochemical assessment of vitamin B_6 status in man. Am J Clin Nutr 26:96, 1970.
Frimpter GW, Andelman RJ, George WF: Vitamin B_6-dependency syndromes. Am J Clin Nutr 22:794, 1959.
Hansson O, Hagberg B: Effect of pyridoxine treatment in children with epilepsy. Acta Soc Med Upsal 73:35, 1968.
Schaumburg H, Kaplan J, Windebank, A, et al: Sensory neuropathy from pyridoxine abuse. N Engl J Med 309:445, 1983.
Scriver CR: Vitamin B_6 deficiency and dependency in man. Am J Dis Child 113:109, 1967.

BIOTIN

Biotin deficiency is rare. It is found in those consuming the biotin antagonist, avidin, found in raw egg white. Many microorganisms produce biotin.

ETIOLOGY. Biotin is discussed in Chapter 71.6. Avidin ingestion causes symptoms of deficiency. Deficiencies have appeared in those receiving all their nutrition parenterally and occasionally in infants whose mothers are deficient in biotin.

CLINICAL MANIFESTATIONS. Brawny dermatitis, somnolence, hallucinations, and hyperesthesia with accumulation of organic acids are common. Other neurologic signs and defective immunity may occur.

DIAGNOSIS. Elevated organic aciduria, particularly propionic and hydroxy short chain acids, with response to clinical and biochemical abnormalities following treatment, suggests biotin deficiency.

PREVENTION AND TREATMENT. Parenteral solutions should contain biotin. Deficient patients respond to oral administration of 10 mg.

VITAMIN B_{12} DEFICIENCY (see Chapter 412).

VITAMIN C (ASCORBIC ACID) DEFICIENCY

(Scurvy)

Ascorbic acid is essential for the formation of normal collagen; the defects in collagen structure arising from deficiency of the vitamin produce many of the metabolic and clinical manifestations of scurvy. Alterations in collagen formation are partly due to failure to incorporate hydroxyproline and proline.

Vitamin C is a potent reducing agent that is easily oxidized and destroyed by heating. The adrenals and lenses have particularly high contents of vitamin C.

Ascorbic acid functions in a number of enzymatic activities (Table 43–6 and Chapter 71.2). Transient tyrosinemia in the neonatal period, relatively common among low-birthweight infants and occasionally seen in full-term ones fed high-protein diets, is corrected by administering ascorbic acid (see Chapter 82).

Ascorbic acid deficiency may also be a factor in some cases of megaloblastic anemia by interfering in the conversion of folic acid or other conjugates (Table 43–6 and Chapter 412.3).

ETIOLOGY. The infant is born with adequate stores of vitamin C if the mother's intake has been adequate; the vitamin C content of cord blood plasma is 2–4 times greater than that of maternal plasma. Under these circumstances breast milk contains about 4–7 mg/dL of ascorbic acid and is an adequate source of vitamin C. Deficiency of vitamin C in the mother's diet may result in scurvy in her breast-fed infant. Infants fed with evaporated milk formula must receive vitamin C supplements; such supplements will provide additional protection for the breast-fed infant.

The need for vitamin C is increased by febrile illnesses, particularly infectious and diarrheal diseases, and by iron deficiency, cold exposure, protein depletion, or smoking.

PATHOLOGY. During vitamin C deficiency formation of collagen and of chondroitin sulfate is impaired. The tendencies to hemorrhage, defective tooth dentin, and loosening of the teeth are caused by deficient collagen. Because osteoblasts no longer form their normal intercellular substance (osteoid), endochondral bone formation ceases. The bony trabeculae that have been formed become brittle and fracture easily. The periosteum becomes loosened, and subperiosteal hemorrhages occur, especially at the ends of the femur and tibia. In severe scurvy, there may be degeneration in skeletal muscles, cardiac hypertrophy, bone marrow depression, and adrenal atrophy.

CLINICAL MANIFESTATIONS. Scurvy may occur at any age but is rare in the newborn infant. The majority of cases occur in infants 6–24 mo of age. Clinical manifestations require time to develop; after a variable period of vitamin C depletion, vague symptoms of irritability, tachypnea, digestive disturbances, and loss of appetite appear. There is evidence of general tenderness, especially noticeable in the legs when the infant is picked up or when the diaper is changed. The pain results in pseudoparalysis, and the legs assume the typical "frog position," in which the hips and knees are semiflexed with the feet rotated outward. Edematous swelling along the shafts of the legs may be present. In some cases, a subperiosteal hemorrhage can be palpated at the end of the femur. The facial expression is apprehensive. Changes in the gums, most noticeable when the teeth are erupted, are characterized by bluish purple, spongy swellings of the mucous membrane, usually over the upper incisors. There may be a "rosary" at the costochondral junctions and a depression of the sternum (Fig. 45–7). The angulation of the "scorbutic beads" is usually sharper than that of the rachitic rosary.

Petechial hemorrhages may occur in the skin and mucous membranes. Hematuria, melena, and orbital or subdural hemorrhages may be found. Low-grade fever is usually present. Anemia may reflect inability to utilize iron or impaired folic acid metabolism (see Chapters 409 and 412). Wound healing is delayed, and apparently healed wounds may break down. Swollen joints and follicular hyperkeratosis may develop, as well as the "sicca" syndrome of Sjögren, which is usually associated with collagen disorders and includes xerostomia, keratoconjunctivitis sicca, and enlargement of the salivary glands (see Chapter 162).

ROENTGENOGRAPHIC MANIFESTATIONS. The diagnosis of scurvy is usually based on roentgenographic changes in the long bones, especially at their distal ends. Changes are greatest, as a rule, in the area of the knee. In the early stages, the appearance resembles that of simple atrophy of bone. The trabeculae of the shaft cannot be discerned, and the bone assumes a

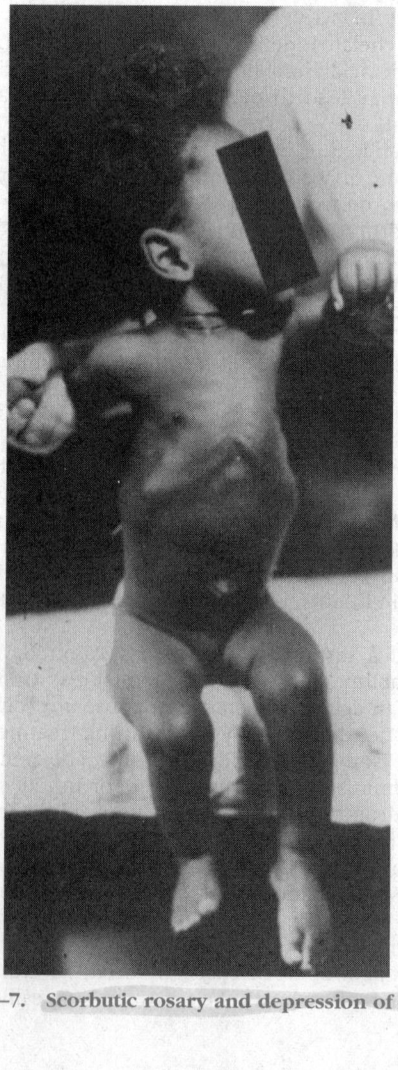

Figure 45–7. Scorbutic rosary and depression of sternum.

"ground-glass" appearance. The cortex is reduced to "pencil-point thinness," and the epiphyseal ends are sharply outlined. The white line of Fraenkel, which represents the zone of well-calcified cartilage, can be clearly discerned as an irregular but thickened white line at the metaphysis. The epiphyseal centers of ossification also have a ground-glass appearance and are surrounded by a white ring (Fig. 45–8).

At this stage, scurvy cannot be diagnosed with certainty from the roentgenogram unless the zone of rarefaction under the white line at the metaphysis becomes apparent. The zone of rarefaction is a linear break in the bone proximal and parallel to the white line. Often, it does not traverse the shaft in its entire width and may be seen only in its lateral parts as a triangular defect (see Fig. 45–8*B*). A spur, as a lateral prolongation of the white line, may be present. Epiphyseal separation may occur along the line of destruction, with linear displacement or compression of the epiphysis against the shaft. Subperiosteal hemorrhages are not visible roentgenographically in active scurvy. During healing, however, the elevated periosteum becomes calcified, and the affected bone assumes a dumbbell or club shape.

DIAGNOSIS. Diagnosis is based mainly on the characteristic clinical picture, the roentgenographic appearance of the long bones, and history of poor intake of vitamin C. Occasionally, a mother may have been boiling the infant's fruit juices.

Laboratory tests for scurvy are unsatisfactory. A fasting vitamin C level of the blood plasma of over 0.6 mg/dL aids in the exclusion of scurvy, but a lower vitamin C level does not prove its presence. Evidence of vitamin C deficiency is better furnished by the ascorbic acid concentration in the white cell-platelet layer (buffy layer) of centrifuged oxalated blood. A level of zero in this layer indicates latent scurvy, even in the absence of clinical signs of deficiency. The saturation of the tissues with vitamin C can be estimated from the amount of urinary excretion of the vitamin after a test dose of ascorbic acid. During the 3–5 hr after parenteral administration of the test dose, 80% of it can be found in the urine of normal children. A generalized, nonspecific aminoaciduria occurs in scurvy, while blood values of amino acids remain normal. After a tyrosine load, the scorbutic infant excretes metabolites similar to those of the premature infant. Prothrombin time may be greatly increased.

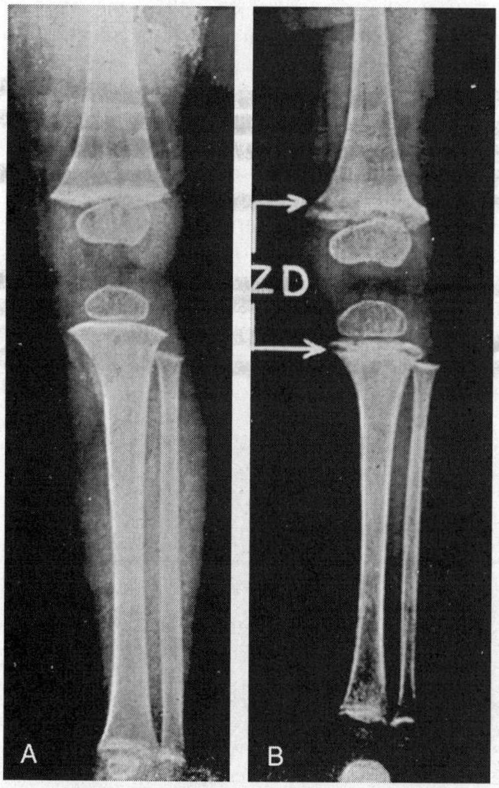

Figure 45–8. Roentgenograms of a leg. *A*, Early scurvy: "white line" is visible on the ends of the shafts of the tibia and fibula; rings around the epiphyses of the femur and tibia. *B*, More advanced scorbutic changes; zones of destruction (ZD) in the femur and tibia.

DIFFERENTIAL DIAGNOSIS. The tenderness of the limbs and the pain elicited by movement have often led to a false diagnosis of arthritis or acrodynia. The patient's age aids in differentiating scurvy from rheumatic fever because rheumatic fever is rare in children under 2 yr of age. Suppurative arthritis and osteomyelitis should be considered in the differential diagnosis. The pseudoparalysis of syphilis occurs usually at an earlier age than does that of scurvy and is often accompanied by other signs of syphilis; a roentgenogram may aid in the diagnosis. Poliomyelitis causes a true flaccid paralysis, and, in infants, the exquisite tenderness present in the limbs in scurvy is absent. Henoch-Schönlein purpura, thrombocytopenic purpura, leukemia, meningitis, or nephritis may be suspected.

PROGNOSIS. With proper treatment, recovery occurs rapidly in infants, but the swelling of subperiosteal hemorrhage may require months to disappear. Body growth usually is quickly resumed.

PREVENTION. Scurvy is prevented by a diet adequate in vitamin C; citrus fruits and juices are excellent sources. Formula-fed infants should receive 35 mg of ascorbic acid daily. Lactating mothers should take 100 mg; 45–60 mg/24 hr is needed by children or adults (see Table 43–1).

TREATMENT. The administration of 3–4 oz of orange juice or tomato juice daily will quickly produce healing, but ascorbic acid is preferable. The daily therapeutic dose is 100–200 mg or more, orally or parenterally.

Irwin MI, Hutchins BK: A conspectus of research on vitamin C requirements in man. J Nutr 106:823, 1976.
Levine M: New concepts in the biology and biochemistry of ascorbic acid. N Engl J Med 314:892, 1986.

RICKETS OF VITAMIN D DEFICIENCY*

Rickets is the term signifying a failure in mineralization of growing bone or osteoid tissue. The characteristic early changes are seen roentgenographically at the ends of long bones; evidence of demineralization also exists in the shafts. Subsequently, if healing is not initiated, clinical manifestations appear (see later). Failure of mature bone to mineralize is called osteomalacia.

ETIOLOGY. During the first third of this century, the predominant cause of rickets was nutritional deficiency of vitamin D due either to inadequate direct exposure to ultraviolet rays in sunlight (296–310 nm; these rays do not pass through ordinary window glass) or to inadequate intake of vitamin D, or both. Vitamin D deficiency rickets is rare among infants and children in the industrialized countries. Deficiency may occur in unsupplemented dark-skinned infants or in breast-fed infants of mothers unexposed to sunlight.

Currently in industrialized countries, it appears that conditions besides inadequate nutritional prophylaxis with vitamin D collectively produce most of the observed rachitic lesions (see Chapters 483 and 648–653). These conditions include clinical entities that interfere with the metabolic conversion

*For a review of the rachitic lesions reference should be made to Table 43–6 and Chapters 50 and 52 for calcium and phosphorus metabolism; Chapter 56.9 for hypocalcemic tetany; Part XXVI, Section 3 for parathormone, vitamin D, and calcitonin activities; and Chapter 647 for additional discussion of vitamin D metabolism and its activities.

and activation of vitamin D, such as hepatic and renal lesions, or that disrupt calcium and phosphorus homeostasis in other ways.

Two forms of vitamin D are of practical importance. Vitamin D_2, or calciferol, available as irradiated ergosterol, largely replaced the fish liver oils (cod and percomorph) as a source of dietary and therapeutic vitamin D. Vitamin D_3, available synthetically, is naturally present in human skin in the provitamin stage as 7-dehydrocholesterol. It is activated photochemically to cholecalciferol and transferred to the liver. Each of these irradiated sterols is hydroxylated in the liver to 25-OH-cholecalciferol and, subsequently, in the renal cortical cells to 1,25-dihydroxycholecalciferol, which functions as a hormone. Receptors of the hormone are found in the kidney, intestine, osteoblasts of bone, parathyroid, islet cells of the pancreas, cells in the brain, mammary epithelium, and elsewhere. Its antirachitic functions include facilitation of intestinal absorption of calcium and phosphorus and of reabsorption of phosphorus in the kidney and a direct effect on mineral metabolism of bone (deposition and reabsorption). In conjunction with parathormone and calcitonin, it has a major role in homeostasis of calcium and phosphorus in the body's fluids and tissues.

The diet of infants may contain only small amounts of vitamin D; cow's milk contains only 0.1–1 μg/qt.* Cereals, vegetables, and fruits contain only negligible amounts. Egg yolk contains 3–10 μg/g. Most marketed cow's milk is fortified with 10 μg/qt of vitamin D, and most commercially prepared milks for infant formulas are also fortified.

Besides lack of dietary vitamin D and the skin's lack of exposure to ultraviolet irradiation, several factors may predispose to vitamin D deficiency. Rickets or epiphyseal dysplasia is particularly likely to develop during rapid growth, such as in low-birthweight infants and in adolescents. Black children are singularly susceptible to rickets, owing to either the pigmentation of their skin or inadequate penetration of sunlight.

Children with disorders of absorption, such as celiac disease, steatorrhea, pancreatitis, or cystic fibrosis, may acquire rickets because of deficient absorption of vitamin D and calcium or of both. Anticonvulsant therapy, as with the phenytoins or phenobarbital, may interfere in the metabolism of vitamin D. Glucocorticoids appear to be antagonistic to vitamin D in calcium transport.

PATHOLOGY. New bone formation is initiated by the osteoblast, which is responsible for matrix deposition and its subsequent mineralization. Osteoblasts secrete collagen, and changes in polysaccharides, phospholipids, alkaline phosphatase, and pyrophosphatase follow until mineralization occurs in the presence of adequate calcium and phosphorus. Resorption of bone occurs when osteoclasts secrete enzymes on the bone surface, dissolving and removing matrix and mineral. Osteocytes covered by bone both resorb and redeposit bone. Factors affecting bone growth are poorly understood, but phosphorus, calcium, fluoride, and growth hormone all have some influence.

In rickets, defective growth of bone results from retardation or suppression of normal growth of epiphyseal cartilage and of normal calcification. These changes depend on a deficiency in serum of calcium and phosphorus salts for mineralization. Cartilage cells fail to complete their normal cycle of proliferation and degeneration, and subsequent failure of capillary penetration occurs in a patchy manner. The result is a frayed, irregular epiphyseal line at the end of the shaft. Failure of osseous and cartilaginous matrix to mineralize in the zone of preparatory calcification, followed by deposition of newly formed uncalcified osteoid, results in a wide, irregular, frayed zone of nonrigid tissue (the rachitic metaphysis) (Fig. 45–9). This zone, responsible for many of the skeletal deformities, becomes compressed and bulges laterally, producing flaring of the ends of the bones and the rachitic rosary (Fig. 45–10). Mineralization is also lacking in subperiosteal bone; pre-existing cortical bone is resorbed in a normal manner but is replaced by osteoid tissues over the entire shaft, which fails to mineralize. If this process continues, the shaft loses its rigidity, and the resultant softened and rarefied cortical bone is readily distorted by stress; deformities and fractures result.

Healing Rickets. With healing, degeneration of cartilage cells occurs along the metaphyseal-diaphyseal border, capillary penetration of the resultant spaces is resumed, and calcification takes place in the zone of preparatory calcification. This calcification, occurring approximately at the line at which normal calcification would have occurred had the rachitic process not supervened, produces a line clearly demonstrable in roentgenograms (Figs. 45–11*A* and *B*). As healing progresses, the osteoid tissue between this line of preparatory calcification and the diaphysis also becomes mineralized (see Fig. 45–9). Osteoid tissue in the cortex and about the trabeculae in the shaft rapidly becomes mineralized.

Chemical Pathology. In healthy infants the inorganic serum phosphorus concentration is 4.5–6.5 mg/dL, whereas in rachitic infants it is usually reduced to 1.5–3.5 mg/dL. The serum calcium level is usually normal, but under certain conditions it too is reduced, and tetany may develop.

Vitamin D deficient rickets can be conceptualized to be the body's attempt to maintain normal serum calcium levels. In the absence of vitamin D, less calcium is absorbed from the intestine. With slightly lowered serum calcium, parathormone is secreted, leading to mobilization of calcium and phosphorus from the bone. The serum calcium concentration is thus main-

*1 μg = 40 IU.

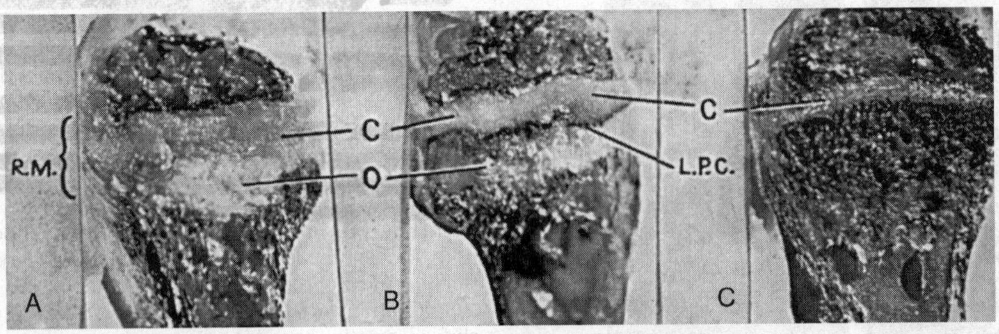

Figure 45–9. Line tests in rats (proximal end of the tibia) (calcified tissue stained with silver appears black). *A,* Active rickets. The light broad zone between the epiphysis and the shaft represents the rachitic metaphysis (R.M.) (C = cartilage; O = osteoid). *B,* Healing rickets. The line of preparatory calcification (L.P.C.) between the zone of cartilage (C) and the osteoid (O). *C,* Healed rickets. Cartilaginous disc (C) between the epiphysis and the normal shaft.

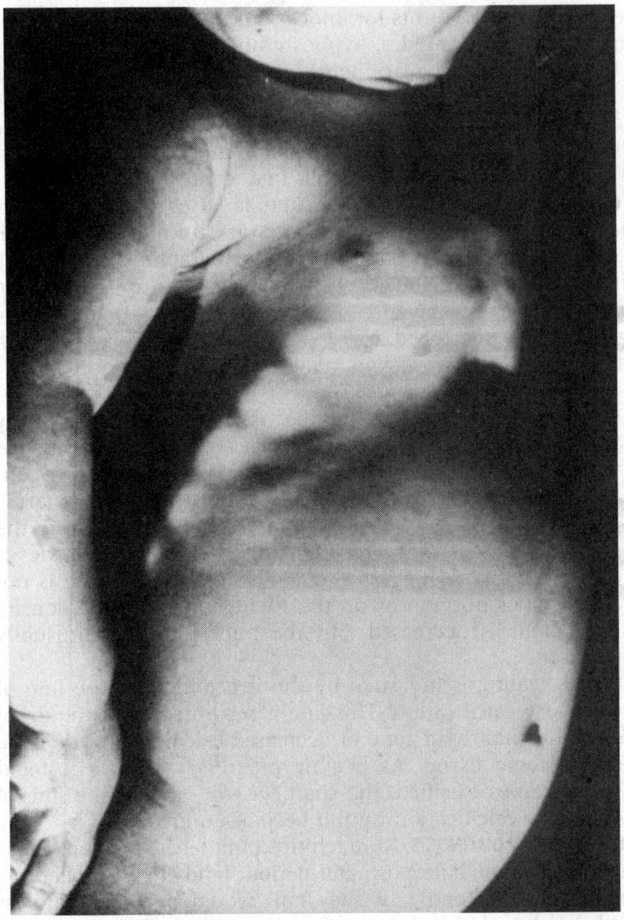

Figure 45–10. Rachitic rosary in a young infant.

tained, but secondary effects occur, including the changes of rickets in bone, the lowered serum phosphorus concentration (because parathormone decreases phosphorus reabsorption in the kidney), and elevated serum phosphatase (due to increased osteoblastic activity).

The alkaline phosphatase of serum, which in normal children is less than 200 IU/dL, is elevated in mild rickets to more than 500 IU/dL. As rickets heals, the phosphatase value returns slowly to the normal range. Serum alkaline phosphatase levels may be normal in infants with rickets who are protein or zinc depleted.

Calcium and phosphorus homeostasis depends on the intestinal absorption of dietary calcium and phosphorus. Maximum calcium absorption occurs in humans when the ratio of calcium to phosphorus in the diet is about 2:1; increase in phosphate decreases absorption of calcium. Acidity of intestinal contents increases absorption of calcium. An increase in calcium absorption also occurs when lactose is the dietary sugar. Chelating agents such as ethylenediaminetetraacetic acid or the phytates of cereals may decrease calcium absorption, and dietary iron may decrease absorption of phosphate. High dietary levels of stearic and palmitic acids, which are poorly absorbed, also decrease calcium absorption.

Calcium absorption is facilitated by 1,25-dihydroxycholecalciferol or similar hydroxylated forms of vitamin D. Calcium deficiency alone rarely leads to the failure of calcification as seen in rickets and osteomalacia; it results in a diminished amount of bone.

Vitamin D deficiency is also accompanied by generalized aminoaciduria, a decrease of citrate in bone and its increased urinary excretion, decreased ability of the kidneys to make an acid urine, phosphaturia, and, occasionally, mellituria. The parathyroid glands hypertrophy in rickets, and urinary cyclic adenosine monophosphate (AMP) level is increased.

CLINICAL MANIFESTATIONS. Osseous changes of rickets can be recognized after several months of vitamin D deficiency. In breast-fed infants whose mothers have osteomalacia, rickets may develop within 2 mo. Florid rickets appears toward the end of the 1st and during the 2nd yr of life. Later in childhood, manifest vitamin D deficient rickets is rare.

One of the early signs of rickets, craniotabes, is due to thinning of the outer table of the skull and detected by pressing firmly over the occiput or posterior parietal bones. A Ping-Pong-ball sensation will be felt. Craniotabes near the suture lines is a normal variant. Low-birthweight infants are particularly susceptible to the early development of rickets and to craniotabes. Palpable enlargement of the costochondral junctions (the "rachitic rosary") (see Fig. 45–10) and thick-

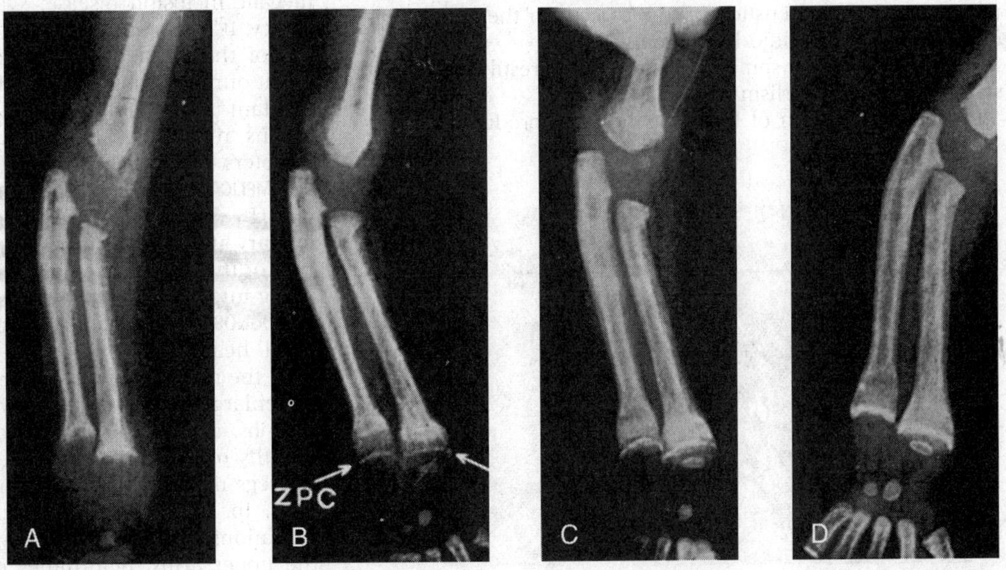

Figure 45–11. *A,* Active rickets; cupping and fraying of the distal ends of the radius and ulna; double contour along the lateral outline of the radius (periosteal osteoid). The two dense zones in the shaft of the ulna are calluses of greenstick fractures. *B,* Healing rickets after 12 days of treatment with vitamin D. Zones of preparatory calcification (ZPC); above them in the rachitic metaphyses there is beginning calcification. *C,* Healing rickets after 18 days of treatment. The zones of preparatory calcification are well defined, and the rachitic metaphyses appear well calcified. The epiphysis of the radius has become visible. *D,* Healing rickets after 29 days of treatment. Zones of preparatory calcification, rachitic metaphyses, and shafts have become united.

ening of the wrists and ankles (see Fig. 45–11) are other early evidences of osseous changes. Increased sweating, particularly around the head, may also be present.

Head. Craniotabes may disappear before the end of the 1st yr, although the rachitic process continues. The softness of the skull may result in flattening and, at times, permanent asymmetry of the head. The anterior fontanel is larger than normal; its closure may be delayed until after the 2nd yr of life. The central parts of the parietal and frontal bones are often thickened, forming prominences or bosses, which give the head a boxlike appearance (caput quadratum). The head may be larger than normal and may remain so throughout life. Eruption of the temporary teeth may be delayed, and there may be defects of the enamel and extensive caries. The permanent teeth that are calcifying may also be affected; the permanent incisors, canines, and first molars usually show enamel defects.

Thorax. Enlargement of the costochondral junctions may become prominent; the beading of the ribs is not only palpable but also visible (see Fig. 45–10). The sides of the thorax become flattened, and the longitudinal grooves develop posterior to the rosary. The sternum with its adjacent cartilage appears to be projected forward, producing the so-called pigeon breast deformity. Along the lower border of the chest develops a horizontal depression, Harrison groove (Fig. 45–12), which corresponds with the costal insertions of the diaphragm. There may be a variety of other thoracic deformities, including those of the shoulder girdle.

Spinal Column. Slight to moderate degrees of lateral curvature (scoliosis) are common, and a kyphosis may appear in the dorsolumbar region of rachitic children when sitting. Lordosis of the lumbar region may be seen in the erect position.

Pelvis. In children with lordosis, there is frequently a concomitant deformity of the pelvis, which is also retarded in growth. The pelvic entrance is narrowed by a forward projection of the promontory; the exit, by a forward displacement of the caudal part of the sacrum and the coccyx. In the female, these changes, if they become permanent, add to the hazards of childbirth and may necessitate cesarean section.

Extremities. As the rachitic process continues, the epiphyseal enlargement at the wrists and ankles becomes more noticeable. The enlarged epiphyses can be seen (see Fig. 45–11) or palpated but are not distinct in roentgenograms because they consist of cartilage and uncalcified osteoid tissue. Bending of the softened shafts of the femur, tibia, and fibula results in bowlegs or knock-knees; the femur and the tibia may also acquire an anterior convexity. Coxa vara is sometimes the result of rickets. Greenstick fractures occur in the long bones; often there are no clinical symptoms.

Deformities of the spine, pelvis, and legs result in reduced stature, rachitic dwarfism.

Ligaments. Relaxation of ligaments helps to produce deformities and partly accounts for knock-knees, overextension of the knee joints, weak ankles, kyphosis, and scoliosis.

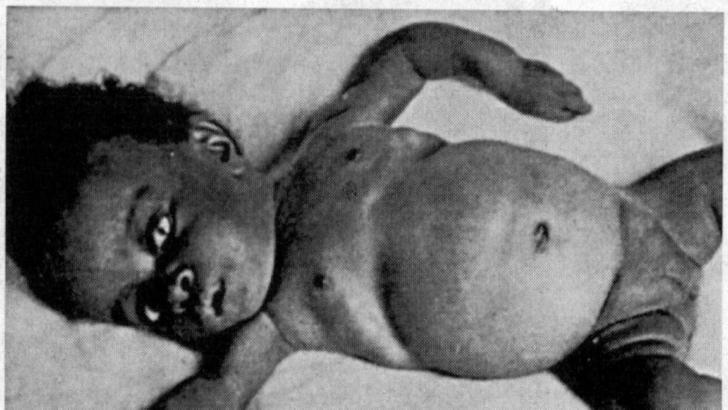

Figure 45–12. Deformities in rickets, showing the curvature of the limbs, potbelly, and Harrison groove.

Muscles. The muscles are poorly developed and lack tone. As a result, children with moderately severe rickets are late in standing and walking. Potbelly (see Fig. 45–12) depends to a large extent on weakness of the abdominal muscles; weakness of the gastric and intestinal walls may contribute.

DIAGNOSIS. The diagnosis of rickets is based on a history of inadequate intake of vitamin D and on clinical observation; it is confirmed chemically and by roentgenographic examination. The serum calcium level may be normal or low, the serum phosphorus level is below 4 mg/dL, and the serum alkaline phosphatase is elevated. Urinary cyclic AMP level is elevated, and serum 25-hydroxycholecalciferol level is decreased.

ROENTGENOGRAPHIC CHANGES (see Fig. 45–11).

Active Rickets. A roentgenogram of the wrist is best for early diagnosis because characteristic changes of the ulna and radius occur at an early stage. The distal ends appear widened, concave (cupping), and frayed, in contrast to the normally sharply demarcated and slightly convex ends. The distance from the distal ends of the ulna and radius to the metacarpal bones is increased because the large rachitic metaphysis, which is not calcified, does not appear on the roentgenogram. The density of the shafts is decreased, but the trabeculae are unusually prominent.

Initial healing is indicated by the appearance of the line of preparatory calcification. This line is separated from the distal end of the shaft by a zone of decreased calcification, the zone of the osteoid tissue. As healing progresses and the osteoid tissue becomes calcified, the shaft "grows" toward the line of preparatory calcification until it becomes united with it.

DIFFERENTIAL DIAGNOSIS. Nonrachitic craniotabes, at times present in the immediate postnatal period, tends to disappear before rachitic softening of the skull would become manifest (2nd–4th mo of life). Craniotabes also occurs in hydrocephalus and osteogenesis imperfecta, but it is not difficult to differentiate these conditions from rickets.

Enlargement of the costochondral junctions occurs in rickets, scurvy, and chondrodystrophy. The enlargements in rickets are rounded knobs, but in scurvy a ledgelike depression with the chondral or sternal portion is displaced below the osseous ribs. In chondrodystrophy, there may be irregular, concave outlines of the distal ends of the bones, but no roentgenographic evidence of fraying. Other epiphyseal lesions that may require differentiation include congenital epiphyseal dysplasia, cytomegalic inclusion disease, syphilis, rubella, and copper deficiency. It is sometimes difficult to distinguish rachitic deformities of the chest from congenital ones. Bowlegs can be the result of rickets but may be a familial characteristic. Vitamin D resistant rickets and other metabolic disturbances with osseous lesions resembling rickets must also be differentiated (see Chapters 483 and 647–656).

COMPLICATIONS. Respiratory infections such as bronchitis and bronchopneumonia are common in rachitic infants, and pulmonary atelectasis is frequently associated with severe deformities of the chest. Anemia due to iron deficiency or accompanying infections often develops in severe rickets.

PROGNOSIS. If sufficient amounts of vitamin D are administered, healing begins within a few days and progresses slowly until the normal bony structure is restored. In many instances, the enlargement of the epiphyses of the long bones, including the ribs, and the deformities of the skull disappear only after months or years of treatment. Even rather severe bowing of the legs may disappear within several years without osteotomies. In advanced cases, there may be permanent osseous alterations in the form of bowlegs, knock-knees, curvature of the upper arms, deformities of the chest and spine, rachitic pelvis and coxa vara, and dwarfism.

Rickets in itself is not a fatal disease, but complications and intercurrent infections such as pneumonia, tuberculosis, and enteritis are more likely to cause death in rachitic children than in normal children.

PREVENTION. Rickets can be prevented by exposure to ultraviolet light or by oral administration of vitamin D. Sunlight, as a prophylactic agent, may be effective in the temperate zones only during the sum [illegible] in haze-free areas.

The daily requirem [illegible] in D is 10 μg or 400 IU. Much of the whole milk av [illegible] an areas and evaporated milk is fortified with vita [illegible] entrate so that 1 qt of fresh, whole milk or 1 can [illegible] d milk contains this amount. Prematurely born inf [illegible] st-fed infants whose mothers are not exposed to a [illegible] light should receive supplemental vitamin D dail [illegible]

Vitamin D should [illegible] ministered to pregnant and lactating mothers.

TREATMENT. Natural an [illegible] light are effective therapeutically, but oral adminis [illegible] vitamin D is preferred. The daily administration of [illegible] of vitamin D_3 or 0.5–2 μg of 1,25-dihydroxychole [illegible] will produce healing demonstrable on roentgenogra [illegible] 2–4 wk except in the unusual cases of vitamin D [illegible] rickets.

Administering 15,000 [illegible] min D in a single dose without further therapy for s [illegible] nths may be advantageous. More rapid healing will f [illegible] sibly with earlier differential diagnosis from genetic [illegible] resistant rickets and less dependence on parents fo [illegible] ministration of the vitamin. If no healing occurs, the r [illegible] robably resistant to vitamin D (see Chapters 647 to 6 [illegible] r healing is complete, the dose of vitamin D should [illegible] d to 10 μg/day.

Argao EA, Heubi JE: Fat-soluble vi [illegible] ency in infants and children. Curr Opin Pediatr 5:562, 1993.
DeLuca HF: New concepts of vit [illegible] ctions. Ann N Y Acad Science 669:59, 1992.
Rasmussen H: Cell communication, calcium ion, and cyclic adenosine monophosphate. Science 170:404, 1970.
Reichel H, Koeffler HP, Norman AW: The role of the vitamin D endocrine system in health and disease. N Engl J Med 320:980, 1989.
Root AW, Harrison HE: Recent advances in calcium metabolism. I. Mechanisms of calcium homeostasis. II. Disorders of calcium homeostasis. J Pediatr 88:1, 177, 1976.
Yetgin S, Ozsoylu S, Raucan S, et al: Vitamin D-deficiency rickets and myelofibrosis. J Pediatr 114:213, 1989.

TETANY OF VITAMIN D DEFICIENCY

(Infantile Tetany)

See also Chapter 56.9.

Tetany due to deficiency of vitamin D occasionally accompanies rickets. Relatively common in former times, this type of tetany is rare today owing to the widespread prophylactic use of vitamin D. Occasionally, tetany is associated with celiac disease, probably as a result of deficient absorption of both vitamin D and calcium. Tetany of vitamin D deficiency occurs most frequently between the ages of 4 mo and 3 yr.

CHEMICAL PATHOLOGY. When the serum calcium concentration falls below 7–7.5 mg/dL, muscular irritability occurs, apparently owing to the loss of the inhibitory control that serum ionized calcium exerts on the neuromuscular junctions. It remains unclear why serum calcium level is occasionally decreased in association with rickets; failure of the parathyroids to compensate for the low serum calcium level may be a factor.

CLINICAL MANIFESTATIONS. The symptoms and signs of tetany are manifested, and rickets usually occurs concurrently. Vitamin D deficient tetany may exist in either a latent or a clinically manifest stage.

Latent Tetany. Symptoms are not evident, but they can be elicited by means of the Chvostek, Trousseau, and Erb procedures. The serum calcium level is less than 7–7.5 mg/dL.

Manifest Tetany. Spontaneous clinical manifestations include carpopedal spasm, laryngospasm, and convulsions. The serum calcium level is often well under 7 mg/dL.

DIAGNOSIS. The diagnosis is based on the combined presence of rickets, low serum calcium level, and symptoms of tetany. The serum phosphorus level is usually low; the serum alkaline phosphatase level is increased. In the differential diagnosis, causes of tetany such as hypoparathyroidism, hypomagnesemia, and ingestion of phenothiazine must be eliminated.

PROGNOSIS. The prognosis is good unless treatment is delayed. Death rarely occurs, though it may result from laryngospasm and possibly from cardiac dilatation, so-called cardiac tetany.

PREVENTION. Prophylactic treatment is identical to that for rickets.

TREATMENT. Active treatment raises the serum calcium above the tetany level. This level may be attained by administration of calcium chloride in 1–2% solution in milk. For the first 1–2 days, 4–6 g/day may be given in 1-g doses, the initial dose being 2–3 g; smaller doses of 1–3 g/day should then be continued for 1–2 wk. Calcium chloride in more concentrated solution may cause severe gastric ulceration, and large doses may cause acidosis. Calcium lactate may be added to milk in doses of 10–12 g/day for 10 days. When oral medication is impractical, calcium gluconate (5–10 mL of a 10% solution) can be administered intravenously but not subcutaneously or intramuscularly owing to the dangers of local necrosis.

Oxygen inhalation is indicated during convulsive seizures. When intravenously administered calcium gluconate does not quickly control the attacks, sodium phenobarbital may be given intramuscularly. Prolonged attacks of laryngospasm are usually controlled by sedation and by administering calcium salts. Intubation is only occasionally necessary. After the acute manifestations have been controlled, vitamin D in daily doses of 50–100 μg should be started and the oral administration of calcium continued (see earlier). When the rickets is healed, the dose of vitamin D should be decreased to the usual prophylactic one.

Fraser D, Kook SW, Scriver CR: Hyperparathyroidism as the cause of hyperaminoaciduria and phosphaturia in human vitamin D deficiency. Pediatr Res 1:425, 1967.

HYPERVITAMINOSIS D

Ingesting excessive amounts of vitamin D results in signs and symptoms similar to those of idiopathic hypercalcemia (see Chapter 655), which may be due to hypersensitivity to vitamin D. Symptoms develop after 1–3 mo of large intakes of vitamin D; they include hypotonia, anorexia, irritability, constipation, polydipsia, polyuria, and pallor. Hypercalcemia and hypercalciuria are notable. Evidence of dehydration is usually present. Aortic valvular stenosis, vomiting, hypertension, retinopathy, and clouding of the cornea and conjunctiva may occur.

The urine may show proteinuria. With continued excessive intake, renal damage and metastatic calcification occur. Roentgenograms of the long bones reveal metastatic calcification and generalized osteoporosis.

Excessive intake of vitamin D may result from inadvertently substituting its concentrated form for one more dilute, from the parents' increasing their child's prescribed dose, and from inadequately controlling dosages for children receiving large amounts of vitamin D for chronic hyperphosphatemic states (see Chapters 483 and 489).

DIFFERENTIAL DIAGNOSIS. Metastatic calcification occurs in chronic nephritis, hyperparathyroidism, and idiopathic hypercalcemia. The latter two are accompanied by hypercalcemia.

PREVENTION. Prevention requires careful evaluation of vitamin D dosage.

TREATMENT. This includes discontinuing vitamin D intake and decreasing intake of calcium. For severely involved infants, aluminum hydroxide by mouth, cortisone, or sodium versenate may be used.

Forbes GB, Cafarelli C, Manning J: Vitamin D and infantile hypercalcemia. Pediatrics 42:203, 1968.

VITAMIN E DEFICIENCY

The effects of vitamin E deficiency vary in different animal species. Vitamin E (α-tocopherol) is a fat-soluble antioxidant that may be involved in nucleic acid metabolism, but its precise biochemical action is unclear. Vitamin E is present in many foods (see Table 43–6).

Deficiency may occur in malabsorption states such as cystic fibrosis and acanthocytosis. Diets high in unsaturated fatty acid increase the vitamin E requirement in premature infants who absorb vitamin E poorly. Excess iron administration exaggerates signs of vitamin E deficiency.

CLINICAL MANIFESTATIONS. Some patients deficient in vitamin E have creatinuria, ceroid deposition in smooth muscle, focal necrosis of striated muscle, and muscle weakness. Some improvement may occur after administration of vitamin E. Vitamin E deficiency has been suggested as a causative factor in the anemia of kwashiorkor. Premature infants may have low serum levels of tocopherol, with development of a hemolytic anemia at 6–10 wk of age, correctable by administration of vitamin E. In deficiency states, platelet adhesiveness increases, as do blood platelet levels. The role of vitamin E in retinopathy of prematurity is discussed in Chapters 82 and 581. Patients with malabsorption and vitamin E deficiency due to biliary atresia develop a degenerative, potentially reversible, neurologic syndrome consisting of cerebellar ataxia, peripheral neuropathy, and posterior column abnormalities.

DIAGNOSIS. If vitamin E has recently been administered, 3 days should elapse before determination of blood levels because oral vitamin E may circulate for 1–2 days.

PREVENTION. Minimal daily requirements of vitamin E are not known; 0.7 mg/g of unsaturated fat in the diet appears adequate. Children with deficient fat absorption should take more. Premature infants may be given 15–25 IU/24 hr. Large oral or parenteral doses of vitamin E may prevent permanent neurologic abnormalities in children with biliary atresia or abetalipoproteinemia.

Argo EA, Heubi JE: Fat soluble vitamin deficiency in infants and children. Curr Opin Pediatr 5:562, 1993.
Gross S: Hemolytic anemia in premature infants: relationship to vitamin E, selenium, glutathione peroxidase, and erythrocyte lipids. Semin Hematol 13:187, 1976.
Sokol RJ: Vitamin E and neurologic deficits. Adv Pediatr 37:119, 1990.

VITAMIN K DEFICIENCY

Vitamin K is a naphthoquinone that participates in oxidative phosphorylation. Its absence or its failure to be absorbed from the intestinal tract results in hypoprothrombinemia and decreased hepatic synthesis of proconvertin. Prothrombin (factor II) and proconvertin (factor VII) are important to the second stage of coagulation (see Chapter 433). The second stage of coagulation is studied by the one-stage prothrombin time (Quick). Administering vitamin K to the newborn infant increases concentrations of prothrombin, proconvertin, plasma thromboplastin component (factor IX), and Stuart-Prower factor (factor X). Four vitamin K dependent proteins contain γ-carboxyglutamate. All require calcium for activity. Factors C and S are anticoagulants. Factors Z and M stimulate platelet activity. Vitamin K dependent calcium binding proteins such as osteocalcin promote phospholipid interactions in coagulation and in calcium metabolism.

SOURCES OF VITAMIN K. Naturally occurring vitamin K is fat soluble; it is found in high concentrations of hog's liver, soybeans, and alfalfa and in smaller amounts in some vegetables, such as spinach, tomatoes, and kale. The natural vitamin (2-methyl-3-phytyl-1,4-naphthoquinone) has been labeled vitamin K_1 to distinguish it from vitamin K_2 of bacterial origin and from synthetic naphthoquinones with vitamin K activity.

Suppression of intestinal bacteria by various antibiotics may be responsible for vitamin K deficiency, which results in diminution of prothrombin. Irradiated foods have produced vitamin K deficiency in animals. Cow's milk has more vitamin K than human milk.

CLINICAL MANIFESTATIONS. Deficiency of vitamin K or hypoprothrombinemia should be considered in all patients with a hemorrhagic disturbance. The incidence of hemorrhagic disease of the newborn (see Chapter 89) has been sharply decreased by the prophylactic administration of vitamin K. In childhood, the deficiency is usually due to factors affecting absorption or utilization of fat or to factors limiting its synthesis in the intestine, such as prolonged use of antibiotics. Diarrhea in infants, particularly breast-fed ones, may cause vitamin K deficiency. Diseases of the liver may lead to hypoprothrombinemia, which usually does not respond to administration of vitamin K.

Hypoprothrombinemia may also result from administering certain drugs. Dicumarol (or bishydroxycoumarin), obtained from spoiled sweet clover, is used specifically for the production of hypoprothrombinemia in the prevention and treatment of venous thrombosis. Dicumarol is thought to prevent the liver from utilizing vitamin K without exerting an effect on prothrombin. Blood prothrombin is continually destroyed in the body; since dicumarol prevents its replacement, a fall in prothrombin occurs. If a dangerously low level results, massive doses of vitamin K_1 may be necessary to restore prothrombin, and whole blood transfusions may also be necessary.

Salicylic acid, a degradation product of dicumarol, produces hypoprothrombinemia by similar action. The fall in prothrombin resulting from salicylates, however, is mild compared with that of dicumarol. The hemorrhagic manifestations in acute rheumatic fever may be due in some cases to large doses of salicylates; vitamin K is effective in neutralizing this action. Its use in children receiving large doses of salicylates would appear justified.

TREATMENT. Oral administration of vitamin K may correct mild prothrombin deficiency. One to 2 mg/day for an infant will usually suffice. If prothrombin deficiency is severe and hemorrhagic manifestations have appeared, 5 mg/day of vitamin K_1 should be given parenterally. Large doses of synthetic vitamin K analogs, but not of vitamin K_1, may result in hyperbilirubinemia and kernicterus in the G-6-PD–deficient newborn and in the premature infant. In hypoprothrombinemia owing to liver damage, vitamin K_1 may be given, but whole blood is usually also necessary.

Corrigan JJ: The vitamin K dependent proteins. Adv Pediatr 28:57, 1981.
Peters C, Casella JF, Marlar RA, et al: Homozygous protein C deficiency. Pediatrics 81:272, 1988.

PART VII

*Pathophysiology of Body Fluids and Fluid Therapy**

Raymond D. Adelman ■ *Michael J. Solhung*

It is important to understand the normal physiology of body fluids to manage the abnormalities that alter the normal condition. The discussion of normal body fluid physiology includes three main topics.

First, *the total amounts of water and solutes in the body as a whole* result from carefully regulated balances of intake and output. Many controlling mechanisms, especially for substances having physiologic significance, are extremely complex. Those especially important to the clinician are discussed in some detail in this section.

Second, *the distribution of water and the concentration of solutes in the various compartments of the body* are critically important, because considerable energy is required to maintain steady-state equilibria for most substances. The concentration of solutes depends on the relative amounts of solute and solvent (i.e., water) in that compartment.

Third, the *regulation of the fluid compartments* that maintain physiologic balance by preventing large changes in solute concentrations that could disturb function is addressed in this section. Alterations of normal body fluid physiology by diseases or other processes are best dealt with when the expected physiologic responses are known and the physiologic impact of the corrective therapies are fully understood. ■

CHAPTER 46
Water

TOTAL BODY WATER. Water is the most important solvent in the fluid composition of living systems. Total body metabolism of water is maintained by several mechanisms that control water intake and output, but is balanced principally through excretion of water by the kidney.

Total body water (TBW) as a percentage of body weight changes with age, decreasing rapidly in early life (Fig. 46–1). Prenatally, TBW decreases during gestation. At birth, TBW is 78% of body weight. In the first few months of life, TBW drops dramatically to approximate the adult level of 55–60% of body weight at 1 yr of age. At puberty, a further change in TBW takes place. Because fat has a low water content, TBW as a percentage of body weight is lower in mature women, who have greater amounts of body fat (55%), than men, who have less fat (60%). Increased body fat in obese children at any age has a similar effect on TBW. In the nonobese child, a close linear relationship is maintained between TBW and body weight, and TBW can be calculated using body weight alone: TBW (L) = 0.61 × weight (kg) + 0.251.

FLUID COMPARTMENTS. TBW consists of intracellular (ICF) and extracellular fluid (ECF) components (Fig. 46–2). In the fetus, the ECF volume is larger than the ICF volume, and the ECF decreases with age. The ECF volume drops precipitously after birth, in large part because of postnatal diuresis. As the ECF volume continues to fall in the first year of life, the ICF volume increases to achieve a ratio of ICF to ECF close to adult levels after 1 yr of age. The relative loss of extracellular fluid beyond the immediate postnatal diuresis results from the increasing growth of cellular tissue and the decreasing rate of growth of collagen relative to muscle during the early months of life.

In older children, the ECF volume bears a fairly straight-line

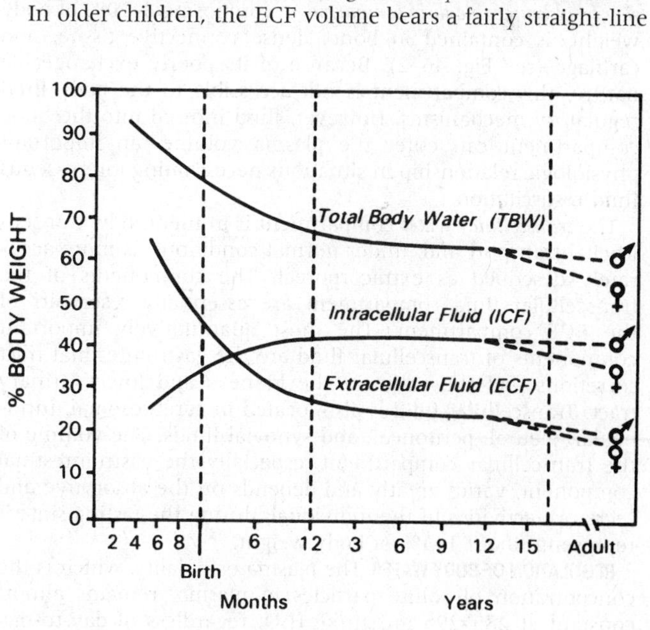

Figure 46–1. Total body water, intracellular fluid, and extracellular fluid as a percentage of body weight and a function of age. (From Winters RW: Water and electrolyte regulation. (*In*: Winters RW [ed]: The Body Fluids in Pediatrics. Boston, Little, Brown & Company, 1973.)

*Modified from the 14th edition written by Alan Robson.

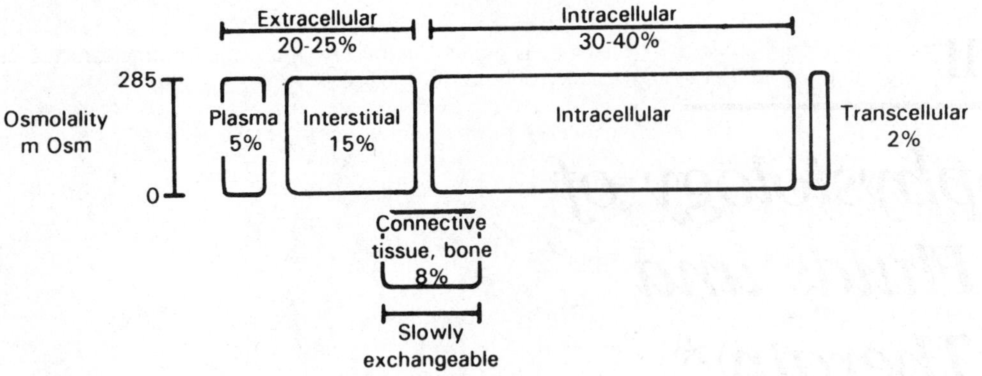

Figure 46–2. Total body water distribution as a percentage of body weight in an older child. (Adapted from Edelman IS, Leidman J: Am J Med 27:256, 1959.)

relation to weight and to total body water in normal infants and children (ECF [L] = 0.239 × weight [kg] + 0.325). Under conditions of normal hydration in the older child, exchangeable ECF constitutes 20–25% of body weight and is composed of plasma water (5% of body weight) and interstitial water (15% of body weight) (see Fig. 46–2). At puberty, the ECF volume differs little between males and females. However, because of decreased TBW at this age, girls have a lower ICF volume than boys.

The ICF volume is bounded by the membranes of the cells of the soft tissues. The ICF volume, representing the difference between total body water and extracellular water, is approximately 30–40% of body weight. Although frequently considered a homogeneous fluid, the ICF represents the sum of fluids from the cells in different locations that have various functions and different intracellular compositions.

The remaining two body water compartments are the *transcellular* and the *slowly exchangeable compartments*. Although actually extracellular because of their unique characteristics, these compartments are less important under normal conditions than the ICF and ECF. However, some clinical conditions, especially in the gastrointestinal tract, render the transcellular compartment an important repository of body water. The *slowly exchangeable fluid compartment*, composing 8–10% of body weight, is contained in bone, dense connective tissue, and cartilage (see Fig. 46–2). Because of its poorly exchangeable nature, this compartment is not accessible to the body fluid regulatory mechanisms. However, fluid infused into the bone compartment can enter the plasma volume, an important physiologic relationship in situations necessitating interosseous fluid resuscitation.

The *transcellular water* compartment is influenced by transepithelial transport and, under normal conditions, is more accurately described as extracorporeal. The components of the transcellular fluid compartment are essentially reservoirs of the ECF compartment. The most quantitatively important components of transcellular fluid are the gastrointestinal tract secretions and the urine in the kidneys and lower urinary tract. Transcellular fluid is also located in cerebrospinal, intraocular, pleural, peritoneal, and synovial fluids. The volume of the transcellular compartment, especially the gastrointestinal component, varies greatly and depends on the absorptive and secretory activities of the individual; during the fasting state it represents about 1–3% of body weight.

REGULATION OF BODY WATER. The plasma osmolality, which is the concentration of solute particles in plasma, remains almost constant at 285–295 mOsm/kg H_2O, regardless of day-to-day fluctuations in solute and water intake (see Fig. 46–2). This stasis is largely a result of precise control of the amount of water in the body through a finely regulated feedback system. To maintain a constant state, the amount of body water derived from intake and from oxidation of carbohydrate, fat, and protein of exogenous and endogenous origin must equal losses from the kidneys, lungs, skin, and gastrointestinal tract. Water balance is controlled by regulating intake and excretion, but excretion is the more important regulatory mechanism.

Intake. Intake of water is normally stimulated by a sensation of *thirst;* although only partially understood, this mechanism is a major defense against fluid depletion and hypertonicity. Thirst sensation, defined as the conscious desire to drink water, is regulated by a center in the midhypothalamus. Many factors induce or depress thirst. The major stimuli are plasma osmolality increases of as little as 1–2% or depletion of ECF volume by 10% or more, as occurs with hemorrhage or sodium depletion. The changes in plasma osmolality are monitored by osmoreceptors located in the hypothalamus and possibly located in the pancreas and hepatic portal vein. The mechanisms by which volume depletion induces thirst are less well understood, but depletion may be monitored by baroreceptors in the atria and elsewhere in the vascular bed. Considerable circumstantial evidence suggests that elevated plasma levels of angiotensin II stimulate drinking and may mediate thirst in hypovolemic and hypotensive states.

In clinical situations of conflicting conditions such as decreased plasma osmolality and decreased intravascular volume, the ECF volume changes dominate, and the resultant stimulated thirst causes increased water intake, restoring volume at the expense of tonicity.

The thirst mechanism and the release of antidiuretic hormone (ADH, i.e., arginine vasopressin) may be interrelated. However, at least some of the thirst centers are separated functionally and physically from those involved in release of ADH.

Disorders of the thirst mechanism may be seen in psychologic disorders, diseases of the central nervous system, potassium deficiency, malnutrition, and alterations in the renin-angiotensin system. These may lead to increased drinking, even though the content of body water is greater than usual and plasma osmolality is decreased, or to a decrease in drinking, as in adipsia.

Excretion. Body water losses can occur from the lungs, skin, gastrointestinal tract, and kidneys. *Obligatory water losses* represent the minimum volume of fluid a person must ingest every day to maintain fluid balance. After the expenditure of energy, obligatory water losses include *insensible water losses,* which are mainly evaporative water loss from the lungs and skin; *urinary water excretion,* which represents the amount of water necessary to excrete a solute load by the kidneys; and *stool water losses,* which under normal conditions are small but can account for significant water losses during intestinal diseases.

Unlike the excretion of water by the kidneys, which responds to the content of water and solute in the body, insensible water losses are regulated by factors generally independent of body water. Because they are evaporative water losses, they are proportionate to the surface area of the body and are influenced by body and environmental temperatures, by the rate of respiration, and by the partial pressure of water vapor in the environment. Evaporative water losses cannot be used to regulate water losses that occur because of changes in the body's water content. The rate of sweating varies with the body temperature and is controlled in part by the autonomic nervous system. It may be reduced in heat stress by *severe* deficits in volume of body fluids or in the concentration of electrolytes, but this does not represent a major mechanism for regulating body water. Because of their proportionately high body surface area, premature newborns have much larger evaporative water losses than term newborns and older infants and children. This increased insensible water loss must be taken into account when formulating a fluid management plan for these infants (see Chapter 82).

Urinary water excretion is obligatory, and because an important function of the kidney is to maintain body homeostasis, urinary water excretion closely regulates the composition and volume of ECF. On a daily basis, the accumulation of an excess amount of urea, as the end product of protein breakdown, and mineral salts, chiefly dietary sodium, are excreted in the urine. The resulting urinary solute load requires a necessary volume of urine for excretion. Alterations in ECF osmolality also require regulation through urinary water excretion. A fall in plasma osmolality, indicating relative excess of water, is corrected by the excretion of an increased volume of dilute urine that has an osmolality below that of plasma. This loss of free water restores plasma osmolality to normal. Conversely, when plasma osmolality rises above normal, the volume of urine falls, and its osmolality rises above that of plasma. This regulation of urine volume and concentration depends principally on the neurohypophyseal-renal axis, the effector of which is ADH. However, because urine volume can be reduced to only that necessary to excrete the solute load, it is also influenced by diet. Other factors that influence urine water output include the glomerular filtration rate (GFR), the state of the renal tubular epithelium, and plasma concentrations of adrenal steroids.

Urinary water excretion is regulated by two complementary mechanisms: the production, storage, and release into the circulation of *ADH*, and by the *renal epithelial tubular cell response to ADH*, determined principally by ADH receptor activity of the collecting duct cells and the maintenance of a medullary concentration gradient to provide the passive reabsorption of water. Human ADH, a cyclic octapeptide, is synthesized in the supraoptic nuclei. This neurosecretory substance is transported down axons that descend through the infundibular stem to be stored in the terminal arborizations in the pars nervosa of the posterior pituitary. Release of ADH into the bloodstream occurs by exocytosis in response to stimuli from the hypothalamus. Depletion of ADH in the posterior pituitary occurs in animals deprived of water; storage occurs when water loads are administered (Chapter 56).

Secretion of ADH is regulated by the effective osmotic pressure of the ECF. Pressure is produced by solutes (primarily sodium and chloride) that do not readily penetrate cell membranes. This process is monitored by vesicles in the supraoptic nuclei that act as osmoreceptors. They swell when the osmolality of ECF is less than that of the ICF and shrink when the osmolality of ECF exceeds that of the ICF. Administering urea, which readily diffuses across cell membranes to increase the osmolality of the ECF and ICF, produces little shift of water between cells and interstitial fluids and does not evoke consistent antidiuresis. However, intravenous hypertonic saline solution evokes intense antidiuresis; the sodium remains predominantly in the ECF, increasing its osmolality in relation to that of the ICF. Conversely, administering water inhibits the release of ADH.

Normally, the threshold for release of ADH is 280 mOsm/kg of H_2O. Release of vasopressin may be initiated or inhibited with changes in plasma osmolality of as little as 1–2%. The response is graded, permitting the urine volume and the osmolality of the ECF to be continuously regulated, preventing the fluctuations in osmolality that would occur as a consequence of normal variations in intake of fluid and solutes. Levels of ADH also increase significantly after 8% or greater dehydration, and the rise is exponential with more marked dehydration.

The primary action of ADH is to increase the permeability of the renal collecting ducts to water. Under conditions of antidiuresis, the interstitium of the renal medulla has an osmolality of as much as 1,200 mOsm/kg H_2O at the level of the papilla. This level of osmolality is achieved by the actions of the countercurrent multiplier (i.e., loops of Henle) and the exchange (i.e., medullary vasa recta blood vessels) systems. ADH activation of specific receptors on the collecting duct cell membrane triggers a series of intracellular events that result in the increase in the cell membrane permeability to water. In the presence of ADH, luminal urine entering the collecting duct has an osmolality of about 285 mOsm/kg H_2O and becomes progressively more concentrated along the course of the collecting duct as water diffuses out of the urine into the hypertonic medullary interstitium by passive osmotic diffusion. By the time the urine enters the calyces, it has achieved the same concentration as the fluid in the hypertonic medullary papillas. Continued reabsorption of sodium in the distal tubule and collecting duct further dilutes the urine. In the absence of ADH, these segments of the nephron are impermeable to water, diffusion into the hypertonic medulla does not occur, and dilute urine is formed.

PATHOPHYSIOLOGIC CONDITIONS. *Diabetes insipidus* is a specific disease state caused by an inability to effectively conserve urinary water. The clinical result of excessive urinary water loss is increased concentration of ECF solute (mainly sodium) or hypernatremia. The two types of diabetes insipidus are named according to the site of abnormal function: central and nephrogenic. Central diabetes insipidus occurs if ADH is not released into the circulation. This abnormality is produced by an interruption of the supraoptic-osmoreceptor-hypophyseal axis, preventing the release of ADH in the circulation despite appropriate physiologic stimuli, such as increases in plasma osmolality. In nephrogenic diabetes insipidus, ADH is normally released in response to plasma osmolality changes, but the renal collecting ducts fail to respond to the ADH, often because of a defect in the epithelial cell membrane receptor for ADH.

Factors altering ADH release disrupt the normal mechanisms that regulate ADH release. ADH release may be stimulated or inhibited by emotional factors. Stressful stimuli such as pain or the mass discharge of peripheral receptors resulting from trauma, burns, or surgery increase ADH output and are important considerations in devising appropriate fluid therapy. Nicotine, prostaglandins, and cholinergic and β-adrenergic drugs are potent stimulators of ADH output. Demerol, morphine, and barbiturates are probably antidiuretic in this way, although their reduction of the GFR may also contribute to their effects in reducing urine flow. Alcohol is a potent inhibitor of ADH release, with a consistent dose-response relationship. Diphenylhydantoin and possibly glucocorticoids also inhibit ADH release.

Factors altering the renal response to ADH produce increased urinary excretion of water despite appropriate ADH levels. Anesthesia reduces urinary flow, probably by altering renal hemodynamics. The presence of nonabsorbable, osmotically active solutes in the renal tubular lumen (e.g., glucose in diabetes mellitus) reduces the amount of water than can diffuse into the hypertonic medulla and limits the ability of ADH to conserve water. Intrinsic renal conditions, such as urinary tract obstruction, particularly if it occurs in utero, tubular damage from nephrotoxins or tubular necrosis, and advanced renal disease, can reduce renal responsiveness to ADH.

MECHANISMS FOR DISTRIBUTING FLUID WITHIN THE BODY. The distribution of water between the ICF and ECF is determined by physical factors. The *maintenance of the ICF volume* is effected by factors that regulate the concentration of solute within the cell and by the ECF. The ICF volume is maintained relatively constant by osmotic forces operating across cell membranes freely permeable to water. The maintenance of these forces depends on the active transport of potassium into and sodium out of cells by energy-requiring processes, although no evidence exists for active transport or secretion of water. A rise in extracellular osmolality (e.g., with a sodium load) results in a decrease in cell water. Conversely, water intoxication decreases extracellular osmolality and leads to an increase in cell volume. Disturbances in cellular function may also result in an increase in the fluid content of cells.

Maintenance of the ECF volume is critical for the preservation of a normal plasma volume. The amount of fluid in the *plasma volume* (i.e., plasma water) is maintained in a steady state by a balance between renal regulation of solute and water excretion and oncotic forces at the capillary level. Oncotic pressure (i.e., colloid osmotic pressure) represents only a small fraction of the total osmotic pressure,* but its osmotic pressure is exerted by molecules, primarily albumin, that do not readily pass through the capillary pores. The colloid osmotic pressure produces an effective osmotic gradient across capillary walls.

At the arteriolar end of the capillaries, the dominant effect of intracapillary hydrostatic pressure results in a net loss of plasma ultrafiltrate. Normally, at the venous end of the capillary, oncotic pressure causes the net return of a somewhat smaller amount of fluid and electrolytes, with the difference returned to the vascular space through the lymphatic system.

Decreases in protein concentration, as in the nephrotic syndrome, may lead to reductions in plasma volume and equivalent increases in *interstitial volume*. These changes may compromise the intravascular volume enough to reduce the GFR and blood flow to other vital organs. Because the volume of plasma is only one third that of interstitial fluid, plasma volume reduction achieved by shifting water into the interstitial space may not be observed clinically as *edema*. An increase in capillary permeability to protein, as in angioneurotic edema and diffuse capillary leak syndromes, produces a rise in protein concentration of the interstitial fluid. This rise reduces plasma oncotic pressure, causing a net shift of fluid to the interstitium. The increase may be generalized or localized, appearing as a wheal or urticaria.

Interstitial fluid volume may also be increased by an increase in the hydrostatic pressure at the venous end of the capillary, as occurs with increased venous pressure associated with heart failure or with retention of sodium and resultant hypervolemia in glomerulonephritis.

The *transcellular fluid* space may increase markedly in inflammatory bowel disease, in early severe diarrhea, or in ileus with multiple fluid levels.

OSMOLALITY OF BODY FLUIDS. Individual solute concentrations in the ECF and ICF vary (Fig. 46–3), but the total ionic concentration in the compartments is balanced between cations and anions. The osmolality in the ECF and ICF compartments is balanced as well (see Fig. 46–2). Except for transient changes, the ECF and ICF compartments are in osmotic equilibrium. Because the cell membranes are highly permeable to water, a change in the osmolality of either fluid compartment results in the rapid movement of water to achieve an equilibration of osmolality. Because of its abundance in plasma and interstitial fluids (see Fig. 46–3), sodium is the most important cation contributing to extracellular osmolality. Because sodium and its accompanying anions, chloride and bicarbonate, account for 90% or more of plasma osmolality, a rough estimate of extracellular fluid osmolality can be obtained by doubling the plasma sodium concentration. For example, if the normal sodium concentration of plasma is 140 mEq/L, the estimated plasma osmolality is 280 mOsm/L. There are two important exceptions to this rule: hyperglycemia and hyperlipidemia.

Of the nonelectrolytes in plasma, the most important contributor to osmolality is glucose, which does not freely penetrate the cells. At normal plasma glucose concentrations, glucose provides 3–5 mOsm/L to plasma osmolality. However, the high plasma glucose concentrations occurring in diabetic

*The principal colloids in the plasma are the plasma proteins, which exert an osmotic pressure of approximately 28 mm Hg, compared with the 5,100 mm Hg exerted by the plasma's crystalloid solutes. However, the capillary walls are very permeable to the crystalloid solutes, which exert no osmotic force across the capillary walls. Albumin, the most abundant plasma protein and the one having the lowest molecular weight, is the principal solute responsible for colloid osmotic pressure and for regulating net water movement across capillary walls.

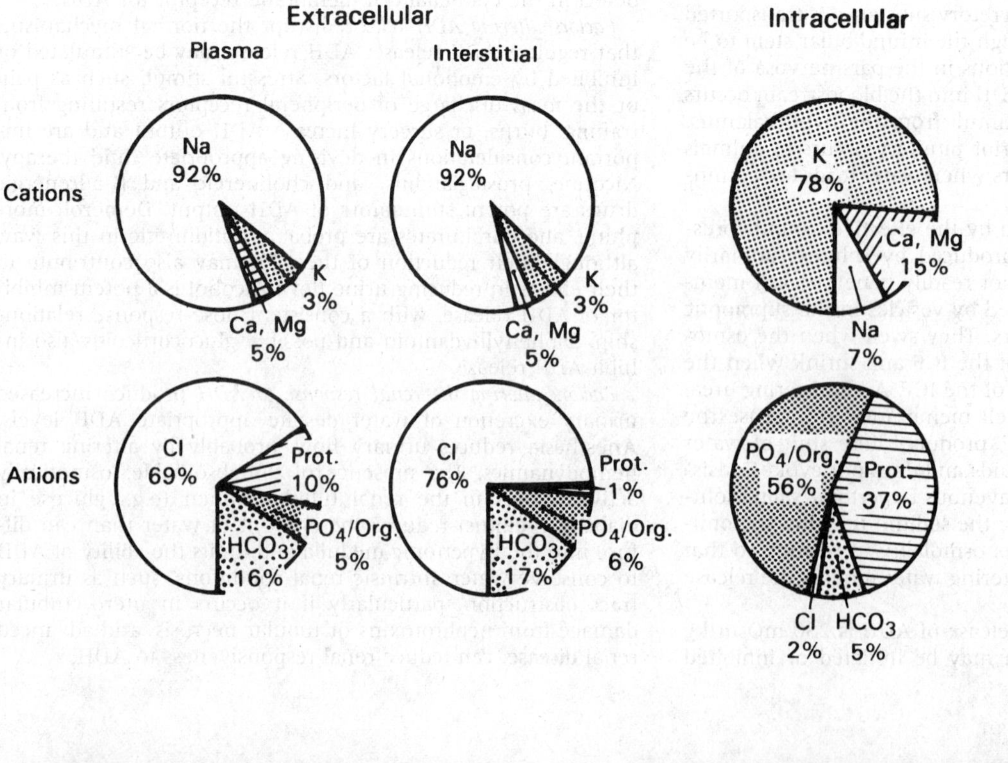

Figure 46–3. The concentrations of the major cations and anions in the extracellular fluids (i.e., plasma and interstitial fluids) and intracellular fluids as a percentage of total electrolyte composition. Na = sodium; K = potassium; Ca = calcium; Mg = magnesium; HCO_3 = bicarbonate; PO_4/Org. = phosphorus and organic anions; Prot. = proteins.

ketoacidosis can increase plasma osmolality, shifting water from the ICF to ECF compartments. The reduced plasma sodium concentration caused by the influx of water into the extracellular fluid volume produces an invalid measure of plasma osmolality. In treating diabetic patients, it is essential to recognize the impact of the changes in plasma glucose concentration on ECF osmolality and on water shifts between the fluid compartments.

The second condition, which does not allow use of plasma sodium to estimate plasma osmolality, occurs with increases in serum solids. For example, when serum solids such as the proteins and lipids are increased, the water content in the serum is markedly decreased (expressed per liter of serum) because of volume displacement of water by lipids. Because electrolytes are dissolved in the aqueous phase of serum, electrolyte concentrations such as that of sodium determined by flame photometry and expressed as milliequivalents per liter of serum appear decreased even though the concentration per liter of serum water is normal. Treatment of such *pseudohyponatremia* is unnecessary and may be detrimental to the patient. Its occurrence can be recognized by measuring serum osmolality by freezing point depression, a method that measures solute concentration of the water fraction of serum and more accurately reflects serum sodium concentration. The problem of pseudohyponatremia is avoided by methods measuring sodium concentration with ion-specific electrodes.

CHAPTER 47
Sodium

BODY CONTENT AND DISTRIBUTION OF SODIUM. Sodium, the bulk cation of the extracellular fluids, is the principal osmotically active solute responsible for the maintenance of intravascular and interstitial volumes. Of the total quantity of sodium in the body, more than 30% is nonexchangeable or only slowly exchangeable, bound in poorly mobilizable tissues (Fig. 47–1). Of total body sodium, 11% is in the plasma sodium pool, 29% is in the interstitial lymph fluid, and 2.5% is in the intracellular fluid. About 43% of total body sodium is in bone, but only one third of the sodium in bone is exchangeable. Dense connective tissue and cartilage contains 12% of body sodium, of which about two thirds is exchangeable (see Fig. 47–1). The *exchangeable sodium content of the fetus* averages 85 mEq/kg, compared with the adult value of 40 mEq/kg, because the fetus has relatively large amounts of cartilage, connective tissue, and extracellular fluid, all of which contain considerable amounts of sodium, and has a relatively small mass of muscle cells, which have a low sodium content.

Although cell membranes are relatively permeable to it, sodium is predominantly distributed in the extracellular compartment. Intracellular concentrations are maintained at levels of approximately 10 mEq/L and extracellular concentrations of approximately 140 mEq/L. The low intracellular concentration is achieved by active extrusion of sodium from cells by the sodium-potassium–activated and magnesium-activated ATPase systems. Calcium inhibits ATPase, as do ouabain and related cardiac glycosides.

Although intracellular concentrations of sodium are low and represent a small part of total body sodium, they may be critical in modifying certain intracellular enzyme activities. The intracellular sodium content usually remains relatively constant, and changes in total body sodium reflect mostly

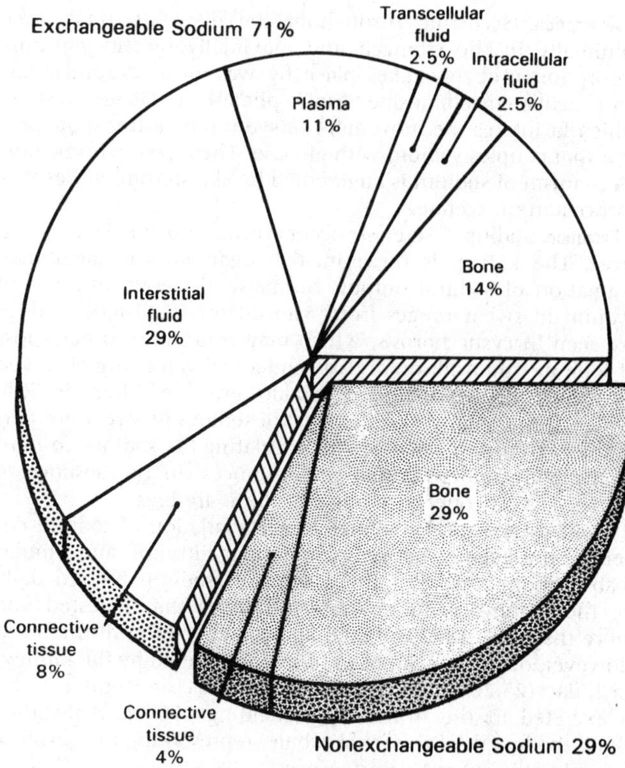

Figure 47–1. Distribution of body sodium as a percentage of the total. Exchangable sodium *(clear)* and nonexchangeable sodium *(stippled)* are indicated. (From Frohnert PP: Body composition. *In*: Knox FG (ed): Textbook of Renal Pathophysiology. Hagerstown, MD, Harper & Row, 1978.)

changes in extracellular sodium. However, redistribution of sodium between the intracellular and extracellular compartments may occur in the absence of significant changes in total body sodium. Such a change (e.g., increased intracellular sodium) may be observed in the severely ill patient, in whom it usually is referred to as the "sick cell syndrome." Intracellular sodium may also be increased in some forms of hypertension.

Because of the Donnan distribution of anionic proteins, the concentration of sodium in interstitial fluid is approximately 97% of that of the serum sodium value; changes in concentration of sodium in the serum are reflected by proportional changes in the concentration of sodium in the interstitial fluid. Concentrations of sodium in transcellular fluids vary considerably because such fluids are not in simple diffusion equilibrium with plasma. Unexpected changes in the composition of these fluids may occur and may necessitate changing the therapeutic regimens designed to replace their abnormal loss.

REGULATION OF SODIUM. Intake. The amount of sodium in the body is determined by the balance between intake and excretion. Compared with the thirst mechanism for water, the regulatory mechanism of sodium *intake* is poorly developed but may respond to large changes; for example, salt craving may occur in some patients with salt-wasting syndromes. However, sodium intake normally depends on cultural customs. In the United States, the average adult usually takes in about 170 mEq/24 hr, equivalent to 10 g of salt. Children take in less, proportionate to their smaller food intake, but still well in excess of maintenance needs. Infants generally have a relatively high sodium intake because of the high sodium content of cow's milk (21 mEq/L). The sodium content of many infant formulas is also high compared with breast milk (7 mEq/L). The sodium dietary intake of older children and adolescents varies but usually is relatively high because of ingestion of fast foods and junk foods.

Absorption. Occurring throughout the gastrointestinal tract, minimally in the stomach and maximally in the jejunum, absorption probably takes place by way of a sodium-potassium–activated adenosine triphosphatase (ATPase) system, which facilitates the movement of sodium by a transport protein that couples sodium with glucose. The intestinal transport mechanism of sodium is augmented by aldosterone or desoxycorticosterone acetate.

Excretion. Sodium excretion occurs through urine, sweat, and feces. The kidney is the principal organ for the facultative regulation of sodium output. Normally, the concentration of sodium in sweat ranges from 5 to 40 mEq/L. Higher values are seen in cystic fibrosis, which may contribute to body loss of sodium, and Addison disease, and lower values are observed in sodium depletion and hyperaldosteronism. There is little evidence that changes in the level of sodium in sweat are part of the excretory mechanism for regulating the sodium content of the body under normal circumstances. In the absence of diarrhea, fecal concentrations of sodium are low.

RENAL REGULATION OF SODIUM EXCRETION. Renal regulation of sodium depends on a balance between glomerular filtration and tubular reabsorption. Normally, the amount of sodium filtered daily by the kidneys is more than 100 times that ingested and more than five times the total amount of sodium in the body. However, of the total amount of sodium filtered by the kidneys each day (25,200 mEq/24 hr), less than 1% or 50 mEq/24 hr, is excreted in the urine; the remaining 99% is reabsorbed along the length of the renal tubule, representing the result of a highly efficient regulatory process.

Glomerular Filtration of Sodium. Under normal conditions, changes in glomerular filtration rate (GFR) do not affect sodium homeostasis. A constant fraction of the filtered load of sodium is reabsorbed in the proximal tubule despite transient, spontaneous variations in the GFR. This balance of filtration and reabsorption, called glomerular-tubular balance, reduces the impact of spontaneous changes in GFR on the amount of renal sodium excretion. Moreover, sodium balance can be achieved when the GFR remains stable even though sodium intake varies. However, the GFR may play a role in sodium excretion during conditions that also stimulate sodium regulatory mechanisms through changes in extracellular volume. The factors that affect the GFR and promote sodium reabsorption in response to a decrease in extracellular volume, such as hemorrhage or dehydration, are activation of sympathetic renal nervous system and stimulation of the renin-angiotensin system. When extracellular volume expansion occurs, atrial natriuretic peptide (ANP) is released into the circulation from the cardiac atria and causes increased urinary losses of sodium, in part as a response to increased GFR.

Tubular Reabsorption of Sodium. The integrated action of all the nephron segments results in the regulation of renal sodium excretion (Fig. 47–2). Renal sodium handling is characterized by two coordinated tubular processes. First, reabsorption of sodium in the proximal tubule and loop of Henle delivers a constant proportion of the filtered load of sodium to the distal nephron. Second, reabsorption of sodium in the distal tubule and collecting duct is the fine regulator of the final amount of sodium excreted, which closely matches the amount of sodium ingested. Under normal circumstances, approximately two thirds of the filtered sodium is reabsorbed by the proximal convoluted tubule (see Fig. 47–2).

Because the percentages of filtered sodium and water reabsorbed in the proximal tubule are proportional, the fluid remaining at the end of the proximal convoluted tubule has a sodium concentration comparable to that in the plasma. Net movement of sodium out of the proximal tubule represents the balance between sodium reabsorbed from the luminal fluid (i.e., transcellular and paracellular) and that returned through intercellular spaces. The movement of transcellularly reabsorbed sodium across the proximal tubule cell membrane is coupled with the reabsorption of organic solutes and anions, such as glucose and chloride, and facilitated by specific membrane transport proteins. Reabsorbed sodium is actively transported out of the cells across their basolateral membranes, producing an osmotic gradient that causes the movement of an equivalent amount of water. The resulting hydrostatic force in the intercellular spaces and interstitial fluid, as well as the exertion of oncotic pressure by the plasma protein in the peritubular capillary, is responsible for returning the reabsorbed sodium and water into the peritubular capillary and, ultimately, into the systemic circulation.

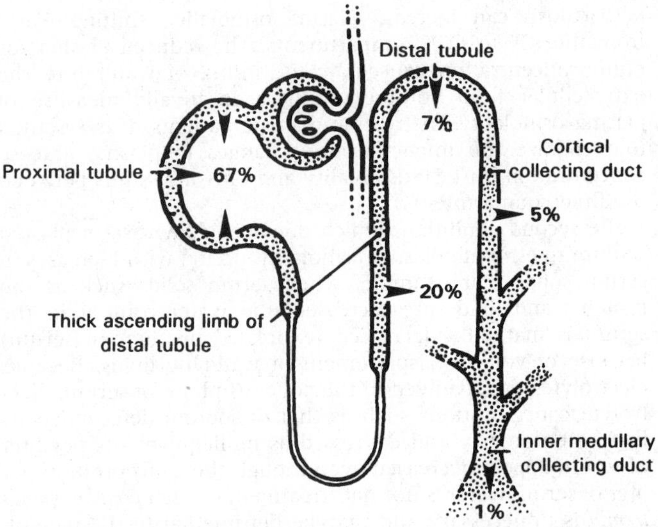

Figure 47–2. Segmental sodium reabsorption along the nephron as a percentage of the filtered load of sodium. (From Koeppen BM, Stanton BA: Renal Physiology. St. Louis, Mosby Year Book, 1992.)

Significant sodium reabsorption (approximately 20%) occurs in the *loop of Henle* (see Fig. 47–2) and is central to the countercurrent multiplier system essential for water balance and the concentration of urine. Water reabsorption occurs in the descending limb of the loop of Henle, and sodium reabsorption occurs in the ascending limb. Sodium transport at the thick ascending limb is active, and it may be secondary to the active transport of chloride rather than primary, as it is at most other sites. Although the loop of Henle is important in the overall control of sodium reabsorption, no precise regulating mechanism has been delineated, nor has a maximal rate for sodium transport at this site been demonstrated. When the load of sodium delivered to the loop is increased by changes in the GFR or in sodium reabsorption in the proximal tubule, most of the excess load is reabsorbed in the loop, providing a further protective mechanism and limiting the magnitude of changes of sodium delivery to the distal convoluted tubule.

The fine regulation of sodium balance probably occurs throughout the distal nephron in the *distal convoluted tubules* and the *collecting ducts*. The distal convoluted tubule reabsorbs 7% and the collecting duct 5% of the filtered load of sodium (see Fig. 47–2). With the proximal tubule and loop of Henle reabsorption of sodium producing a regulated, proportioned delivery of sodium to these sections of the nephron, only small adjustments in distal convoluted tubule and collecting duct reabsorption are required to balance urinary sodium excretion with intake to maintain homeostasis.

Sodium reabsorption at these sites is regulated by aldosterone, whose secretion is governed by the renin-angiotensin system and, to some degree, by potassium balance (Fig. 47–3).

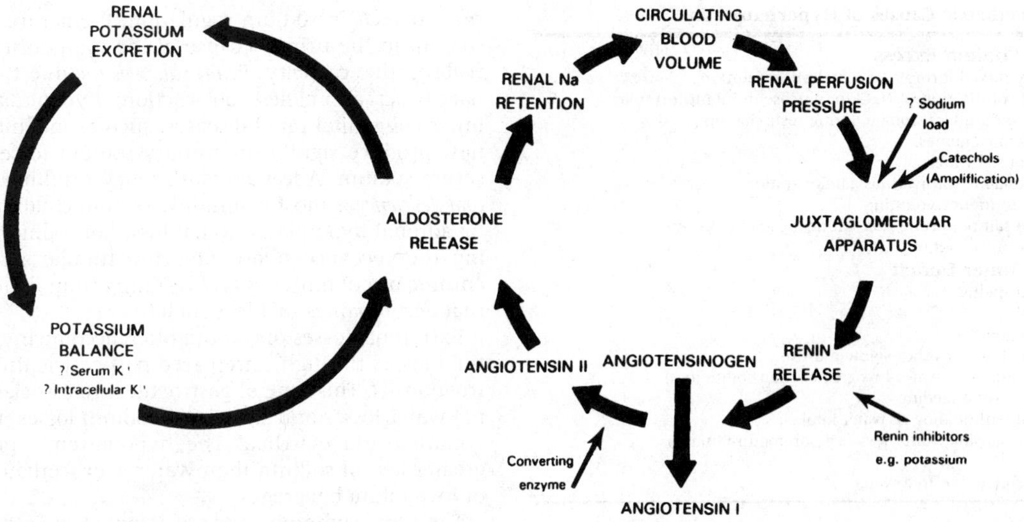

Figure 47–3. Correlations of the volume and potassium feedback loops with aldosterone secretion. Integration of the signals from each loop determines the level of aldosterone secretion. (From Williams GH, Dluhy RG: Aldosterone biosynthesis: interrelationship of regulating factors. Am J Med 53:595, 1972.)

Throughout the distal tubule and collecting duct, sodium is reabsorbed against a large concentration gradient from lumen to plasma. However, compared with the proximal convoluted tubule and the loop of Henle, the total capacity for sodium reabsorption is more limited. If the load of sodium reaching the distal tubule increases significantly, reabsorption does not increase proportionately, and the added load is excreted in the urine.

In health, less than 1% of filtered sodium is normally excreted in the urine. However, to maintain sodium balance, this amount may increase to 10% or higher in response to a high sodium intake and can decrease to very low levels in response to reduced dietary sodium. The considerable flexibility prevents a significantly positive or negative sodium balance when dietary sodium intake fluctuates. However, it takes about 3 days for a new steady state to be achieved after the dietary intake of sodium has been markedly altered.

FACTORS REGULATING SODIUM EXCRETION. An important factor regulating the renal handling of sodium is the *renin-angiotensin system* (see Fig. 47–3). The proteolytic enzyme renin is released from the juxtaglomerular apparatus, which is anatomically composed of the specialized cells in the afferent arteriole and in the segment of the distal tubule that contacts the glomerular vascular pole, the macula densa. Stimuli for the release of renin include decreases in renal perfusion pressure detected in the afferent arteriole and a decrease in sodium chloride concentration or delivery to the macula densa.

Angiotensin I is formed by cleavage of the substrate angiotensinogen by renin. Angiotensin I is converted to angiotensin II by a specific converting enzyme. Angiotensin II, by inhibiting renin secretion, acts as a negative-feedback regulator of renin release. The renin-angiotensin system regulates tubular sodium reabsorption by the direct stimulation of sodium reabsorption in the proximal tubule by angiotensin II and by the stimulation of *aldosterone* secretion by angiotensin II. Aldosterone, a mineralocorticoid produced in the adrenal gland, is an important promoter of sodium reabsorption in the late distal convoluted tubule and collecting duct. While increasing sodium reabsorption, aldosterone also increases potassium secretion and the loss of potassium in the urine. In general, activation of the renin-angiotensin system enhances tubular reabsorption of sodium and results in decreased urinary sodium excretion. Under conditions of extracellular volume expansion or plasma sodium excess, the renin-angiotensin system is suppressed and urinary sodium excretion is increased.

Atrial natriuretic peptide (ANP) is a potent natriuretic and diuretic peptide hormone produced and stored in the atrial myocytes. The target organ of ANP is the kidney, in which it increases sodium and water excretion. ANP is released into the circulation from its cardiac location in response to expansion of the extracellular fluid volume and the resulting stretch of the cardiac atria. The urinary sodium and water excretory actions of ANP generally antagonize the sodium-retaining mechanisms of the renin-angiotensin system. ANP is an important regulator of acute or short-term changes in extracellular fluid volume. However, the role for ANP as a long-term regulator of sodium homeostasis is less certain.

Starling forces in the intercellular space of the proximal tubule cells and the interstitial space between the tubular cells and the peritubular capillaries influence the movement of reabsorbed solute and water into the peritubular capillaries. Normally, the sum of Starling forces favors the movement of solute and water from the intercellular and interstitial spaces into the peritubular capillary. Reabsorbed solute and water are returned to the tubular lumen through paracellular pathways when the normal balance of these forces is altered. Rapid expansion of the extracellular fluid volume increases the interstitial hydrostatic pressure, preventing sodium reabsorption and producing increased urinary sodium excretion.

PATHOPHYSIOLOGIC CONDITIONS. Pathophysiologic changes in serum sodium concentration in the absence of serum solids excess, such as hyperlipidemia or hyperglycemia, usually result from changes in body water, sodium, or a combination of the two. The serum sodium concentration does not necessarily reflect the status of total body sodium content, as previously described. A particular abnormality of serum sodium concentration must be understood in the context of sodium and water regulation.

Hypernatremia. Hypernatremia (serum sodium >150 mEq/L) is caused by conditions that produce an excessive gain of sodium or result in an excessive loss of body water that is greater than the loss of sodium. Hypernatremia due to an excessive gain of sodium, primary sodium excess (Table 47–1), is usually associated with iatrogenic causes: the substitution of NaCl for glucose in infant formulas prepared on site from basic ingredients, the overuse of saline enemas, inappropriate intravenous adminis-

■ **TABLE 47–1 Pediatric Causes of Hypernatremia**

Primary Sodium Excess
Improperly mixed formula or rehydration solution
Accidental substitution of NaCl for glucose in infant formulas
Excessive sodium bicarbonate during resuscitation
Hypernatremic enemas
Ingestion of sea water
Hypertonic saline intravenous administration
NaCl used to induce vomiting
Intentional salt poisoning (i.e., Münchausen by proxy)
High breast milk sodium
Primary Water Deficit
Diabetes insipidus
Central
Nephrogenic
Diabetes mellitus or other solute diuresis
Gastroenteritis (i.e., water loss greater than solute loss)
Inadequate breast feeding
Intentional withholding of water intake
Increased insensible water loss (e.g., premature infant)
Adipsia
Inadequate access to free water

tration of hypertonic saline solutions, and NaCl used to induce vomiting. The more commonly encountered causes of hypernatremia are those caused by a primary water deficit (see Table 47–1), in which the loss of total body water exceeds any loss of sodium.

Diabetes insipidus (see Chapter 46) is caused by one of two fundamental defects in renal water regulation. *Central diabetes insipidus* is caused by a defect in the release of antidiuretic hormone (ADH) into the circulation. The abnormality in central diabetes insipidus can occur in the production, transport, storage, or release of ADH. Any condition, such as trauma, neoplasms, or congenital central nervous system defects, that disrupts the osmoreceptor-hypothalamus-hypophyseal axis results in defective ADH release and excessive urinary water loss. *Nephrogenic diabetes insipidus* is a sex-linked recessive disorder caused by a defective ADH receptor on the tubular cell membrane. The release of ADH in these patients is normal, but the tubular cell is not able to respond to ADH. This condition is present at birth, and if unrecognized, it can be life threatening or result in serious complications. Repeated episodes of extreme hypernatremia may produce permanent central nervous system damage.

Gastroenteritis, usually predominately diarrhea that causes large amounts of stool water loss that is greater than the amount of solute lost, is the most common cause of hypernatremia in childhood.

Inadequate breast feeding must be considered in a newborn with hypernatremia. In most of these cases, the breast milk sodium concentration is not elevated, but there have been case reports of hypernatremia associated with elevated breast milk sodium concentration. In an otherwise normal infant, decreased water intake from an inadequate breast milk supply cannot match the obligatory water losses, and hypernatremia ensues.

Withholding of water intake may produce hypernatremia if the water intake is withheld to such a degree that it is exceeded by obligatory water losses. Two groups of children are vulnerable to developing this type of hypernatremia: neurologically compromised individuals who cannot express thirst or obtain water and severely abused children. Lack of access to water occurs in children who, because of age or a handicapping condition, cannot provide themselves with water intake.

Hyponatremia. Hyponatremia (serum sodium <130 mEq/L) is caused by conditions that create primary sodium deficits resulting in the depletion of sodium; produce a gain in total body water; combine sodium and water abnormalities (Table 47–2).

Primary sodium deficits involve a disruption in renal sodium handling. *Renal sodium losses* occur in conditions with intrinsic renal defects in sodium regulation. Premature infants can lose sodium in the urine because of the immaturity of the sodium reabsorptive capacity. *Renal salt wasting* due to congenital urinary tract anomalies, obstruction, hypoplasia, dysplasia, or other congenital renal diseases, such as medullary sponge kidney, produce significant urinary sodium losses despite a low serum sodium. Adrenal insufficiency resulting in *mineralocorticoid deficiency* is most commonly seen in children with congenital adrenal hyperplasia. Renal losses of sodium also occur during the recovery phase of acute tubular necrosis with the chronic use of diuretics and resulting from the osmotic diuresis that accompanies diabetes mellitus.

Extrarenal losses of sodium often accompany gastrointestinal fluid losses through unreplaced nasogastric fluid losses or gastroenteritis. This type of gastroenteritis, associated with intestinal water losses and significant sodium losses, usually includes vomiting and diarrhea. The hyponatremia produced by the greater loss of sodium than water is exacerbated by the intake of low-solute beverages.

The most common cause of hyponatremia due to decreased *nutritional* sodium intake is the WIC syndrome. This form of water intoxication is seen in small infants who receive large amounts of very-low-sodium–containing fluids, usually to the exclusion of normally concentrated formulas. These infants present with profound hyponatremia and serious central nervous system symptoms, such as seizures.

Of the disorders resulting in a primary water excess, the most common is the *syndrome of inappropriate ADH secretion (SIADH)*. This disorder, which has many potential causes, is marked by the secretion of ADH in the absence of a physiologic stimulus for its secretion. The increased ADH secretion increases collecting duct water reabsorption and dilutes the extracellular fluid, producing hyponatremia. In children, of the many conditions associated with SIADH, the most common occurs as a complication of acute meningitis.

The hyponatremia of water excess involves the addition of

■ **TABLE 47–2 Pediatric Causes of Hyponatremia**

Sodium Deficit with Sodium Depletion
Renal Losses
Prematurity
Acute tubular necrosis, recovery phase
Diuretics
Renal salt wasting
Mineralocorticoid deficiency
Expanded extracellular fluid
Osmotic diuresis
Renal tubular acidosis
Extrarenal Losses
Vomiting and diarrhea
Third spacing
Burns
Nasogastric drainage
Cystic fibrosis
Excess sweating
Nutritional Deficits
WIC syndrome (i.e., inadequate oral sodium intake)
Inadequate sodium in parenteral fluids
Cerebrospinal fluid drainage
Burns
Paracentesis
Water Excess with Water Gain
Syndrome of inappropriate antidiuretic hormone secretion
Glucocorticoid deficiency
Hypothyroidism
Drugs
Excess parenteral fluid administration
Psychogenic polydipsia
Tap water enemas
Excess of Sodium and Water
Nephrotic syndrome
Cirrhosis
Cardiac failure
Acute and chronic renal failure

excess water from an exogenous source, such as the use of dilute or sodium-poor intravenous fluids for the treatment of dehydration. Conditions producing hyponatremia combining abnormal retention of sodium and water usually involve the edema-forming diseases of *nephrotic syndrome and cirrhosis.* In these conditions, water shifts from plasma to the interstitial spaces, which stimulates thirst and releases ADH, causing water and sodium retention. The resulting water retention is greater than the sodium retention, producing hyponatremia. *Cardiac failure* activates similar water- and sodium-retaining mechanisms, but the plasma oncotic pressure remains normal.

CHAPTER 48
Potassium

BODY CONTENT AND DISTRIBUTION OF POTASSIUM. The body content of potassium, the major intracellular cation, correlates well with the lean body mass. Because potassium is predominantly intracellular (see Fig. 46–3), the change in body potassium content that occurs with growth is an excellent index of cellular mass at different ages. In the adult, 90% of total body potassium is exchangeable. The exchangeable components are intracellular potassium (89.6%) and extracellular potassium: plasma (0.4%) and interstitial lymph (1.0%). The remainder (10%) of total body potassium is nonexchangeable and is contained in dense connective tissue and cartilage (0.4%), bone (7.6%) and as a small amount of intracellular potassium (2%).

Intracellular concentrations of potassium approximate 150 mEq/L of cell water. The extracellular concentration of potassium (4 mEq/L) creates a large concentration difference across the cell membranes. The difference between intracellular and extracellular potassium, sustained by the action of Na, K-ATPase, is important for maintaining the resting membrane potential difference across the cell membrane. Potassium is critical for the excitability of nerve and muscle cells and for the contractility of cardiac, skeletal, and smooth muscle. Because of its intracellular osmotic contribution, potassium is also important for the maintenance of cell volume.

REGULATION OF POTASSIUM. Potassium exists in remarkably constant quantities in almost all animal and vegetable tissues. A daily intake of 1–2 mEq/kg body weight is recommended, but intakes vary widely. Absorption of potassium is reasonably complete in the upper gastrointestinal tract. More distally, body potassium is exchanged for sodium in the lumen of the lower bowel.

Two sets of mechanisms participate in potassium homeostasis. These mechanisms maintain an intracellular potassium concentration differential and match potassium dietary intake, mainly through regulating renal potassium excretion. Acute potassium loads require well-developed extrarenal mechanisms to prevent severe hyperkalemia and to avoid potassium toxicity. In the first 4–6 hr after a potassium load, only one half of the potassium is excreted by the kidneys. Some potassium is secreted into the intestinal tract. More than 40% is translocated into cells, primarily in the liver and muscle. This process is an important protective mechanism and is regulated by insulin and epinephrine, which enhance potassium uptake. The catecholamine effect appears to be mediated through β-receptors. Stimulation of α-adrenergic receptors impairs extrarenal disposal of an acute potassium load.

Aldosterone plays a key role in the renal and extrarenal handling of potassium. Its primary extrarenal site of action may be the gastrointestinal tract, although it also affects muscle transport of potassium. Glucocorticoids may also be important in extrarenal potassium homeostasis. Glucagon infusion causes a transient hyperkalemia, but its role in potassium regulation is not clear.

The acid-base balance affects intracellular shifts of potassium. Systemic acidosis results in the movement of potassium out of cells; alkalosis produces the opposite effect. For every 0.1 unit change in blood pH, the plasma potassium concentration changes 0.3–1.3 mEq/L in the opposite direction. The changes depend on numerous factors. For example, the increase in serum potassium accompanying respiratory acidosis is much less than that with metabolic acidosis.

Chronic potassium balance is primarily regulated by the kidneys, which can adjust the amount of potassium excreted over a wide range. Normally, the rate of potassium excretion in the urine approximates 10–15% of that filtered. With the administration of large amounts of potassium, urinary excretion may be more than twice the amount filtered at the glomerulus. Conversely, urinary concentrations can be reduced to very low levels if potassium conservation is required. In the adult, rates of urinary potassium excretion may range from less than 5 mEq to 1,000 mEq/24 hr, depending on the amount of potassium intake.

Potassium is freely filtered in the glomerulus. Its concentration along the length of the proximal convoluted tubule is similar to that of plasma, indicating that reabsorption of potassium in this segment of the nephron is proportionate to that of water, with 60% or more of the filtered potassium absorbed. Concentrations of potassium are increased in the loop of Henle. However, by the time tubular fluid reaches the early distal convoluted tubule, its potassium concentration is below that of plasma, and the amount of potassium delivered to more distal segments of the nephron is less than 10% of the filtered load. The distal tubule and collecting duct have the dual capabilities of potassium reabsorption and secretion.

Under conditions of maximal potassium conservation, continued reabsorption occurs in the distal tubule; when dietary intake is normal or when excretion is increased for other reasons, potassium secretion takes place in the distal tubule and possibly in the collecting duct. The primary mechanism regulating renal control of potassium homeostasis is potassium secretion in these segments of the nephron. The cellular mechanisms of potassium secretion in the distal nephron are regulated by several clinically relevant factors. Increases in plasma potassium stimulate the tubular cell secretion of potassium, and decreases of plasma potassium inhibit tubular secretion.

Aldosterone promotes potassium secretion in the tubule through a series of intracellular events in the tubular cell, including increased luminal membrane permeability to potassium. Aldosterone secretion is stimulated by increased plasma potassium and angiotensin II (see Fig. 47–3). Atrial natriuretic peptide (ANP) and low plasma potassium inhibit aldosterone secretion. Increased tubular flow rate through the potassium-secreting nephron segments due to diuretics or extracellular volume expansion stimulates potassium secretion.

Acid-base status, which affects the cellular potassium concentration, also regulates tubular potassium handling. Alkalosis stimulates and acidosis inhibits secretion. A rise of tubular fluid sodium concentration, such as that produced by diuretics, stimulates potassium secretion. Diuretics can promote renal potassium secretion and urinary potassium loss by increasing tubular fluid flow rate and by increasing tubular sodium concentration. Most of the potassium in the final urine probably results from tubular secretion rather than glomerular filtration.

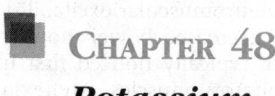

Potassium is also lost in the feces and in sweat. The exchange of plasma potassium for sodium in the colonic contents contributes to sodium conservation and permits the colon to participate in potassium homeostasis. However, even under conditions of chronic potassium loading, fecal potassium constitutes only a small percentage of the total amount of potassium excreted. The human colon responds to mineralocorticoids by decreasing sodium and increasing the potassium content of the stool. Glucocorticoids have a similar effect.

The potassium content of sweat, normally 10–25 mEq/L, is increased by mineralocorticoids and may be elevated in cases of hyperaldosteronism and in cystic fibrosis. Losses of potassium by this route, however, usually are insignificant, even in disease states.

PATHOPHYSIOLOGIC CONDITIONS. Consequences of Hyperkalemia. The major consequences of hyperkalemia result from its neuromuscular effects. Hyperkalemia reduces transmembrane potential toward threshold levels, producing delayed depolarization, faster repolarization, and a slower conduction velocity. Paresthesias are followed by weakness and eventually by flaccid paralysis if treatment is not instituted. The heart is particularly vulnerable to hyperkalemia. The electrocardiogram typically shows peaking of the T waves. Lengthening of the P-R interval and widening of the QRS complex develop later and are particularly ominous, because they often herald the development of ventricular fibrillation. Because the sequence of cardiotoxic events often progresses rapidly, hyperkalemia should be treated as a medical emergency (Chapter 388).

Causes of Hyperkalemia. *Hyperkalemia* with serum potassium levels of 5.5 mEq/L or greater (normal values of serum potassium vary with age) may result from surprisingly small increases in total body potassium. Acute increases in potassium intake, usually through parenteral administration, may result in hyperkalemia, although it is typically transient in duration. Because the kidney has a large capacity to excrete excess potassium and to prevent hyperkalemia, this electrolyte abnormality is most often seen when renal excretory mechanisms are impaired. It may occur in acute or chronic renal failure, in adrenal insufficiency, in hyporeninemic hypoaldosteronism, and with the use of potassium-sparing diuretics.

Sources of potassium include the use of potassium salts of penicillin (1.7 mEq/1 million units) and of salt substitutes by patients on a salt-restricted diet. Acute tissue breakdown, such as from trauma, major surgery, burns, and cell lysis from chemotherapeutic agents, can release sufficient potassium into the extracellular fluid to cause hyperkalemia. An elevated serum potassium may occur with transcellular redistribution of potassium, which is seen typically in metabolic acidosis and shortly before death or in severely ill patients. Certain drugs may increase the serum potassium level by similar mechanisms. Succinylcholine inhibits membrane repolarization, which requires cellular uptake of potassium. Severe digitalis overdose may cause severe hyperkalemia, presumably by inhibiting sodium-potassium exchange by cell membranes.

Because intracellular levels of potassium are 30 times as high as those in the extracellular fluid, lysis of red cells during the collection or handling of a blood sample or release of potassium from platelets during clotting may result in pseudohyperkalemia, in which apparent elevations of serum potassium levels are recorded by the laboratory.

Consequences of Hypokalemia. Although it is impossible to predict the degree of potassium loss from the body accurately by measuring serum potassium, a 1-mEq/L decrease in serum potassium concentration secondary to potassium loss generally corresponds to a loss of approximately 10–30% of body potassium. Many patients tolerate this degree of loss without symptoms. The rate of change in potassium levels and the magnitude of losses probably affects the severity of symptoms.

The relation of extracellular to intracellular potassium concentration is vital to cell function. Membrane depolarization, the process responsible for initiating muscle contraction, requires the abrupt influx of sodium into cells and a comparable efflux of potassium. The process is reversed with repolarization. With hypokalemia, the ratio of intracellular to extracellular potassium concentrations is increased. The transmembrane electrical potential gradient increases so that a wider differential between the resting and excitation potentials exists, which interferes with impulse formation, propagation, and muscle contraction. Hypokalemia produces functional alterations in skeletal muscle, smooth muscle, and the heart. The most observable cardiac manifestations of hypokalemia are electrocardiographic changes, including a prolonged QT interval and flattened T waves.

Hypokalemia also can produce serious neurologic symptoms, including autonomic insufficiency, manifested by orthostatic hypotension, tetany, and decreased neuromuscular excitability. The latter results in weakness and decreased bowel motility. Weakness is an early manifestation, typically noticed first in limb muscles before trunk and respiratory muscles. Areflexia, paralysis, and death from respiratory muscle failure can develop.

Paralytic ileus and gastric dilation reflect smooth muscle dysfunction. Hypokalemia affects protein metabolism and diminishes growth hormone release, contributing to the failure to thrive of children with chronic hypokalemia, most notably Bartter syndrome. Rhabdomyolysis is a dramatic complication of hypokalemia.

In the kidney, potassium deficiency results in vacuolar changes in the tubular epithelium. If sustained for a long time, it leads to nephrosclerosis and interstitial fibrosis, pathologic lesions indistinguishable from those of chronic pyelonephritis. The kidney has a reduced ability to concentrate or dilute the urine, with polyuria and polydipsia developing. An increase in bicarbonate reabsorption and hydrogen ion secretion results in systemic alkalosis. External losses of potassium also result in a shift of potassium from the intracellular to the extracellular fluid. Intracellular potassium is replaced in part by sodium, hydrogen ions, and dibasic amino acids. If these changes become severe, intracellular acidosis in the renal tubular cells may result in excessive exchange of intracellular hydrogen for sodium in the distal tubular fluid, leading to aciduria, with the increased urinary excretion of ammonia, and to systemic alkalosis.

Causes of Hypokalemia. Abnormally low amounts of total body potassium occur in various disease states, such as muscular dystrophy, which are characterized by a decrease in muscle mass. These disorders are not necessarily accompanied by *hypokalemia.* A low serum potassium level may result from a prolonged decreased intake, from increased renal excretion, or from increased extrarenal losses. Renal losses may be increased by the use of diuretics, including osmotic diuretics and carbonic anhydrase inhibitors; by tubular defects such as renal tubular acidosis; by acid-base disturbances; in endocrinopathies such as Cushing syndrome, primary aldosteronism, and thyrotoxicosis; and in diabetic ketoacidosis, Bartter syndrome, and magnesium deficiency.

Extrarenal losses may occur from the bowel (e.g., diarrhea, chronic catharsis, frequent enemas, protracted vomiting, biliary drainage, enterocutaneous fistulas) or from the skin if there is profuse sweating. Movement of potassium into cells during correction of a metabolic acidosis, for example, may also result in hypokalemia, as may *familial hypokalemic periodic paralysis,* a rare disorder in which episodes of paralysis are usually accompanied by an abrupt and marked hypokalemia caused by movement of potassium into an extravascular body compartment (see Chapter 562.1).

When the source of potassium loss is not apparent, measuring urinary potassium may help. A urine concentration of 15 mEq/L or less indicates renal conservation of potassium and suggests that the loss occurred from a nonrenal source.

CHAPTER 49
Chloride

BODY CONTENT AND DISTRIBUTION OF CHLORIDE. Chloride is the major anion of extracellular fluid (Fig. 46–3). Most of total body chloride is extracellular, occurring in plasma chloride (13.6%); interstitial lymph (37.3%); dense connective tissue and cartilage (17%); bone (15.2%); and transcellular fluids (4.5%). Small quantities (12.4%) are present intracellularly. Exchangeable chloride remains relatively constant per unit of body weight at different ages. The low chloride concentration in cells is regulated by two active cell membrane mechanisms. A reciprocal bicarbonate-chloride exchange is sensitive to changes in intracellular pH. When intracellular pH increases, bicarbonate in the cell is exchanged for extracellular chloride, restoring cellular pH to normal. The extrusion of chloride from the cell is mainly accomplished by the large potassium gradient across the cell membrane. The membrane potential, created by the large intracellular potassium concentration, also drives chloride out of the cell passively through anion-selective transport channels or actively by potassium-chloride cotransport.

REGULATION OF CHLORIDE. The intake and output of chloride usually parallel those of sodium, but chloride intake, abnormal extrarenal losses, and renal excretion can occur independently of sodium. The daily turnover of chloride is high, and the renal conservation of chloride is excellent because of efficient renal regulation. In the proximal tubule, a proportional amount (60–70%) of the chloride filtered load is reabsorbed, closely linked to sodium reabsorption (see Fig. 47–2). Chloride reabsorption in the proximal tubule is coupled to sodium, and in the latter portion, chloride is the preferred anion for sodium cotransport. Because of this cotransport mechanism, any change in sodium reabsorption in the proximal tubule influences proximal tubule handling of chloride.

In the thick ascending limb of the loop of Henle, 20–30% of the chloride load is reabsorbed, closely linked to sodium by a special mechanism. Sodium and chloride movement out of the lumen into the tubular cell is driven by active transport. The reabsorption in this segment is mediated by a unique membrane transport symport protein that couples the movement of one sodium, two chlorides, and one potassium ion. Loop diuretics, such as furosemide, inhibit the symport protein, abolishing the reabsorption of sodium and chloride in the thick ascending limb.

Virtually all of the remaining filtered load of chloride is reabsorbed in the distal tubule and collecting duct. Chloride plays a special role in the tubular handling of sodium, potassium, and hydrogen ions in these segments, because it is the only anion available for reabsorption under normal conditions. Chloride reabsorption in this portion of the nephron involves a complex combination of sodium-chloride coupling by a symporter protein, an antiporter protein that facilitates chloride-bicarbonate exchange and a significant amount of chloride transcellular transport by mechanisms not completely understood. The clinically relevant feature of chloride handling in the distal tubule and collecting duct involves the requirement that sodium reabsorption is electroneutral, dictating that sodium is exchanged for potassium or hydrogen ions or cotransported with chloride.

The important participation of chloride handling after the proximal tubule is demonstrated during conditions of chloride deficiency, which are most commonly caused by diets severely restricted in sodium chloride and extended diuretic use. A lower than normal amount of chloride arrives out of the proximal tubule to the thick ascending limb. Because of the special properties of the cotransport protein, less tubular chloride in this segment results in less reabsorption of sodium. More sodium delivered to the distal tubule and collecting duct enhances sodium reabsorption, which increases the exchange of potassium and hydrogen ions, resulting in increased urinary losses and producing hypokalemia and alkalosis with the hypochloremia.

PATHOPHYSIOLOGIC CONDITIONS. Under most clinical circumstances, alterations in chloride concentration in the blood parallel those of sodium. Hypochloremia and hyperchloremia are usually associated with comparable degrees of hyponatremia and hypernatremia, respectively, and are seen most often in patients with dehydration secondary to diarrhea. Occasionally, changes in chloride concentration are not accompanied by equivalent changes in sodium concentration.

Hypochloremia. Hypochloremia is typically seen in metabolic alkalosis. Although chloride is not directly involved in regulating the concentration of free hydrogen ions, it is crucial to the genesis and maintenance of metabolic alkalosis. Chloride depletion as a cause of metabolic alkalosis occurs when chloride is lost from the body in excess of sodium losses. Examples include a loss from the bowel with vomiting or gastric drainage or in chloride diarrhea, a rare congenital disorder in which there is a defect in bowel transport of chloride, and cystic fibrosis. Urinary losses of chloride may exceed those of sodium during the correction of metabolic acidosis and in potassium deficiency.

A decrease in the filtered load of chloride increases bicarbonate reabsorption in the proximal tubule, because it becomes the predominantly available anion for sodium reabsorption. Less chloride available in the thick ascending limb reduces the amount of sodium reabsorbed, and the increased sodium delivered to the distal nephron enhances potassium and hydrogen ion exchange. These same mechanisms allow chloride to maintain a condition of metabolic alkalosis.

Administering chloride is necessary to correct most cases of metabolic alkalosis whether or not it is associated with potassium deficiency. In cases of potassium deficiency, both potassium and chloride must be given before the potassium deficits can be corrected. Treating patients with metabolic alkalosis with potassium or sodium chloride, as appropriate, results in the prompt excretion of bicarbonate into the urine and correction of the alkalosis.

Hypochloremia also results from a protracted, inadequate intake of chloride. Infants fed a chloride-deficient milk formula for several months have developed chronic depletion of body chloride, severe hypochloremia (serum sodium levels usually remained normal), severe hypokalemic metabolic alkalosis, loss of appetite, failure to thrive, muscle weakness, and lethargy. Although adding chloride to the diet quickly reverses the electrolyte abnormalities, long-term sequelae may develop, including disturbed behavioral patterns.

Hyperchloremia. Hyperchloremia may result when chloride is conserved by the kidney in excess of sodium and potassium or when alkaline urine is formed during the renal correction of alkalosis. An increased fractional reabsorption of chloride in the renal proximal tubule in distal renal tubular acidosis also results in hyperchloremia. Early amino acid solutions used in parenteral alimentation contained excessive amounts of chloride, and their administration resulted in hyperchloremic acidosis. Substituting acetate has largely solved this problem. Hyperchloremia also may occur when large amounts of parenteral fluids containing chloride, such as normal saline and lactated Ringer solution, are administered during acute fluid resuscitation.

Anion Gap. Measurements of the serum chloride level are necessary to determine a patient's *anion gap*. The concentration of the most abundant serum cation (i.e., sodium) is greater than the sum of the two most abundant serum anions (i.e., chloride and bicarbonate). The difference is referred to as the anion gap; *anion gap* = [Na] − ([HCO_3] + [Cl]). It is normally about 12 mEq/L (range, 8–16 mEq/L). The anion gap results from the effect of the combined concentrations of the unmeasured anions, such as phosphate, sulfate, proteins, and organic acids, which exceed those of the unmeasured cations, primarily potassium, calcium, and magnesium. Calculating the anion gap permits the detection of an abnormal concentration of an unmeasured anion or cation.

An abnormal condition in which a *normal anion gap* exists is the metabolic acidosis due to renal tubular acidosis or stool losses of bicarbonate. The fractional reabsorption of chloride is increased, because it becomes the predominantly available anion to accompany sodium tubular reabsorption when the plasma bicarbonate concentration is decreased. In the plasma, as bicarbonate falls with this type of acidosis, the chloride rises, and the sum of anions in plasma remains normal.

An *increased anion gap* in renal failure is a result of increased concentrations of phosphate and sulfate; in diabetic ketoacidosis, to β-hydroxybutyrate and acetoacetate; in lactic acidosis, to lactate; in hyperglycemic nonketotic coma, to unidentified organic acids; and in disorders of amino acid metabolism, to various organic acids. Increased anion gap also follows the administration of large amounts of penicillin. After ethylene glycol ingestion, it is caused by glycolate production; after methanol ingestion, by formate production; and after salicylate poisoning, by the salicylate anion and various organic anions secondary to the uncoupling of oxidative phosphorylation.

A *decreased anion gap* occurs less frequently. It may be found in nephrotic syndrome, in which it is caused by a decreased serum concentration of albumin, which is anionic at pH 7.4; after lithium ingestion, with lithium as an unmeasured cation; and in multiple myeloma, because of the presence of cationic proteins.

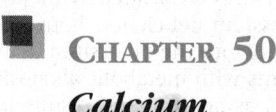

CHAPTER 50
Calcium

BODY CALCIUM. At all stages of life, 99% of the body's calcium is in bone. Because the bones of infants are less densely mineralized than are those of adults, the body contents of calcium in infants and adults are significantly different, about 400 and 950 mEq/kg of body weight, respectively (see Chapters 43, 44, and 45).

Under normal conditions, the extracellular pool of calcium remains remarkably constant despite fairly free exchange with the enormous reservoir in bone. The calcium concentration in serum is also maintained within narrow limits, averaging 2.5 mM/L (10 mg/dL). Approximately 40% is protein bound, and the remaining 60% is ultrafilterable (Table 50–1). Because 1 g of albumin binds 0.8 mg of calcium, but 1 g of globulin binds only 0.16 mg, 80–90% of the bound calcium is bound to albumin, and decreases in serum albumin concentration result in decreases in total serum calcium levels. Of the ultrafilterable calcium, 14% is complexed with anions such as phosphate and citrate, and the remaining 46% (1.2 mM/L or 4.8 mg/dL) is present as free ionic calcium (see Table 50–1).

Ionized calcium exists in equilibrium with the protein-bound form. Changes in hydrogen ion activity in the plasma modify the percentage of calcium that is ionized; for example,

■ **TABLE 50–1 Levels of Plasma, Calcium, Magnesium, and Phosphorus**

Chemical Status	Calcium	Magnesium	Phosphorus
Ionized (diffusible)	46%	55%	85%*
Complexed (ultrafilterable)	14%	25%	5%
Protein-bound (nondiffusible)	40%	20%	10%

**At pH 7.40 = 68% as HPO_4^{2-}, 17% as HPO_4^-.*

a change of 0.1 pH unit alters the concentration of ionized calcium by 10%. Acidosis increases and alkalosis decreases the proportion ionized. The ionized form of calcium is of greatest physiologic importance. The calcium ion plays a major role in many fundamental biologic processes, including bone formation, cell division and growth, coagulation, hormone-response coupling, and electrical stimulus-response coupling in muscle contraction and neurotransmitter release. Although ionized calcium concentrations can be measured, a useful approximation can be made for clinical purposes if the patient's acid-base status is known and by assuming that each 1 g/dL decrease in serum albumin concentration decreases bound and therefore total serum calcium by 1 mg/dL.

REGULATION OF CALCIUM. Overall regulation of calcium homeostasis is provided by a complex system involving intestinal absorption, renal excretion, and hormonal regulation of these processes. Two important variables operate to maintain calcium homeostasis: the total body calcium, mainly determined by the amount of calcium absorbed in the intestinal tract and the amount of calcium excreted by the kidneys, and the distribution of calcium between bone and the extracellular compartment, mainly determined by a balance of hormonal regulation.

Body calcium content is regulated primarily through *intestinal tract absorption of calcium.* The recommended daily dietary intake is 360 mg in the first 6 mo of life, 540 mg in the second 6 mo, 800 mg for 1–10 yr of age, and 1,200 mg for 11–18 yr of age. Dairy products constitute the most important single source. Dietary calcium is absorbed along the small intestine, primarily in the duodenum and early jejunum by an active, carrier-mediated transport mechanism that is stimulated by 1,25-dihydroxyvitamin D_3. It is postulated that hypocalcemia stimulates release of parathyroid hormone (PTH), which increases the renal conversion of 25-hydroxyvitamin D_3 to its more biologically active 1,25-derivative.

The efficiency of intestinal absorption of dietary calcium is increased by low calcium intake in the growing child, in pregnancy, and during depletion of body calcium stores. The mechanisms responsible for this adaptation are unknown. Administering vitamin D and PTH also increases calcium absorption; PTH probably acts by its effect on vitamin D metabolism.

Increases in absorption leading to hypercalcemia occur in sarcoidosis, carcinomatosis, and multiple myeloma. Decreased absorption of calcium results from the presence in the gastrointestinal tract of phytate, oxalate, and citrate, all of which complex the dietary calcium; from increased gastric motility; from reduction of bowel length; and from protein depletion, which may cause a deficiency of the calcium-binding protein in the intestinal mucosa. Some calcium is secreted into the intestinal lumen by the bowel, but this process probably does not represent a regulatory mechanism.

Renal calcium excretion matches the amount of intestinal absorption to maintain the overall calcium balance. Plasma non–protein-bound calcium (i.e., diffusible and ultrafilterable calcium) is filtered at the glomerulus. Normally, about 99% of this filtered calcium is reabsorbed by the tubules, with ionized calcium transported more easily than the complexed form. Reabsorption occurs throughout the nephron. Reabsorption that occurs in the proximal tubule (50–55%) and loop of Henle (20–30%) appears to parallel sodium reabsorption; factors influencing the transport of one of these cations also affect the other. Calcium transport in the distal convoluted tubule (10–15%) and the collecting duct (2–8%) can be dissociated from sodium transport; these sites probably represent the mechanisms that are specifically calciuric. For example, thiazide diuretics decrease tubular sodium reabsorption, producing a natriuresis, but when administered on a chronic basis, they increase calcium reabsorption and reduce urinary calcium excretion. Calcium reabsorption is stimulated specifically by 1,25-dihydroxyvitamin D_3 in the distal tubule.

The most important hormone regulating renal calcium excretion is PTH. PTH dramatically stimulates calcium reabsorption in the thick ascending limb of the loop of Henle and the distal tubule. When PTH is increased, urinary calcium is reduced, and the opposite effect occurs with decreased PTH levels. Contraction of extracellular volume and metabolic alkalosis also stimulates tubular calcium reabsorption and decreases urinary calcium excretion.

Urinary excretion of calcium is also increased by many nonspecific mechanisms. These include expansion of extracellular fluid volume; the administration of osmotic diuretics, furosemide, growth hormone, thyroid hormone, or glucagon; metabolic acidosis; prolonged fasting; and an increase in the serum phosphate level.

There is a diurnal variation in the excretion of calcium, which peaks at the middle of the day. Alterations in dietary calcium result in only small changes in the urinary excretion of calcium, probably reflecting adaptive changes in the intestinal absorption of calcium. Physical inactivity is associated with increased urinary excretion of calcium and, if prolonged, may result in the formation of renal stones.

The balance between deposition and mobilization of calcium in bone largely determines the concentration of ionized calcium in the blood. The *distribution of calcium between bone and the extracellular fluid* is determined by hormonal regulation. PTH and 1,25-dihydroxyvitamin D_3 act to increase plasma calcium. PTH release is stimulated by hypocalcemia or an increase in plasma phosphorus. PTH increases plasma calcium by stimulating release of calcium from bone and by stimulating the production of 1,25-dihydroxyvitamin D_3, which increases intestinal calcium absorption and stimulates bone release of calcium. PTH also increases renal calcium reabsorption.

Thyrocalcitonin, produced in the parafollicular cells of the thyroid gland, is released in response to hypercalcemia. The major effect of thyrocalcitonin is to lower plasma calcium by inhibiting bone resorption. This hormone also increases urinary calcium excretion.

Plasma pH modifies concentrations of plasma-ionized calcium, as do the amounts of calcium absorbed from the renal tubular fluid and from the bowel, although to a lesser extent. Because the serum concentrations of sodium and potassium may play some role in the balance between deposition and mobilization of bone calcium, treating hypernatremia with fluids low in potassium content may result in hypocalcemia.

PATHOPHYSIOLOGIC CONDITIONS. Symptomatic *hypocalcemia* may be caused by a low concentration of ionized calcium resulting from vitamin D deficiency, which is caused by nutritional deficiency, malabsorption, or abnormal metabolism of vitamin D. Hypocalcemia may also be a result of hypoparathyroidism, pseudohypoparathyroidism, hyperphosphatemia, magnesium deficiency, and acute pancreatitis. Because acidosis increases and alkalosis decreases the proportion of calcium that is ionized, symptomatic hypocalcemia may occur during rapid correction or overcorrection of acidosis or with alkalosis.

The neonate is particularly susceptible to hypocalcemia associated with hypoparathyroidism, abnormal vitamin D metabolism, a low calcium intake, or a high phosphate intake (see Chapters 82.2, 92, and 527). Bone mineralization [illegible] inadequate in very-low-birthweight infants durin[illegible] tal period, increasing the incidence of radiologic [illegible] fractures. These lesions probably result from an [illegible] intake of calcium and phosphorus at the time of ra[illegible] tal growth and may not respond to vitamin D metab[illegible]

The causes of *hypercalcemia* include primary or te[illegible] perparathyroidism, hyperthyroidism, vitamin D into[illegible] immobilization, malignancies (especially those that me[illegible] to bone), use of thiazide diuretics, excessive calcium [illegible] parenteral nutrition fluid, milk-alkali syndrome, and sa[illegible] sis. An idiopathic form may occur in infancy associated [illegible] typical "elfin" facies and supravalvular aortic stenosis; this [illegible] drome may be caused by hypersensitivity to vitamin D. If [illegible] dietary intake of phosphorus is inadequate, low-birthwe[illegible] infants may develop hypercalcemia as a result of resorption [illegible] phosphorus and calcium from bone.

Calcium loading increases renal excretion of sodium an[d] potassium and profoundly reduces the ability to concentrat[e] the urine. This effect may explain the polyuria and polydipsia of patients with hypercalcemia resulting from hypervitaminosis D, which may be associated with tubulointerstitial nephropathy. Concentrated calcium solutions should always be administered cautiously, using electrocardiographic monitoring if possible to minimize cardiac arrhythmias (see Chapter 388).

CHAPTER 51
Magnesium

Magnesium is the fourth most abundant cation in the body and second most common intracellular electrolyte (see Fig. 46–3). Because of its relative intracellular abundance, magnesium plays a major role in cellular enzymatic activity, especially in glycolysis and the stimulation of the ATPases.

BODY CONTENT AND DISTRIBUTION OF MAGNESIUM. Body magnesium concentration is approximately 22 mEq/kg in the infant. The concentration increases in adults to 28 mEq/kg. Bone and muscle cells are the major intracellular pools of magnesium. Sixty percent of body magnesium is in bone, of which about one third is freely exchangeable. Most of the remaining 40% is intracellular; more than 50% is in muscle and much of the remainder in liver. Only 20–30% of the intracellular magnesium is exchangeable, and the remainder is bound to proteins, RNA, and adenosine triphosphate.

Extracellular magnesium accounts for only 1% of body magnesium. Although freely exchangeable with the large exchangeable pools in bone and cells, extracellular concentrations are maintained at low levels within a relatively narrow normal range. The range of serum magnesium normally is 1.5–1.8 mEq/L, although wider normal ranges have been reported. Approximately 80% is ultrafilterable; this consists of 55% ionized and 25% complexed magnesium. The remaining 20% is protein bound (see Table 50–1).

REGULATION OF MAGNESIUM. Intake. The intake range of magnesium in children is 10–25 mEq/24 hr, depending on age; the highest intakes are required during periods of rapid growth. Green vegetables and many other foods contain high concentrations of magnesium; the intake of most individuals exceeds the minimum requirement of 3.6 mg/kg/24 hr (i.e., 12 mg of magnesium is equivalent to 1 mEq or 0.5 mM). Absorption of dietary magnesium occurs primarily in the upper gastrointestinal tract by mechanisms that are not fully delineated. Vitamin

, parathyroid hormone (PTH), and increased sodium absorp- on enhance magnesium absorption; calcium, phosphorus, nd increased intestinal motility decrease it. Absorption is far rom complete; an amount of magnesium equal to about two thirds of intake is excreted in the feces. A small portion of this magnesium is secreted by the bowel.

Renal Excretion. Maintenance of magnesium balance depends primarily on urinary excretion. Normally, less than 5% of the filtered load of magnesium appears in the urine, and 20–30% is reabsorbed in the proximal tubule and most of the remainder in the loop of Henle, especially the thick ascending limb, which is the primary site of renal magnesium modification. Under various conditions, magnesium reabsorption parallels that of calcium and sodium. Magnesium competes with calcium for transport. Urinary excretion of magnesium efficiently matches the net intestinal absorption. Renal magnesium reabsorption is inhibited, increasing urinary magnesium, by expansion of the extracellular fluid volume; osmotic, thiazide, mercurial, and loop diuretics; glucagon; calcium loading; and decreased PTH levels. Conversely, volume contraction, magnesium deficiency, thyrocalcitonin, and increased PTH levels increase the renal reabsorption of magnesium, decreasing urinary excretion. Acidosis increases urinary excretion of magnesium, but alkalosis decreases urinary magnesium.

The maintenance of magnesium balance and serum magnesium concentrations requires a complex interaction of renal and nonrenal factors. For example, a low-magnesium diet results in reduced urinary magnesium. This reduction may be the consequence of modest reductions in the serum concentration of magnesium, which have been shown to increase the release of PTH. The release of PTH decreases the urinary loss of magnesium and also causes the release of magnesium and calcium into the extracellular fluid, increasing the concentrations of both cations. Tubular reabsorption of filtered magnesium can be almost complete. However, the gastrointestinal tract continues to secrete small amounts of magnesium, and depletion may result. The concentration of magnesium in serum depends on intake and output and on the mobilization of magnesium from bone and soft tissue. The serum level is not always a reliable indicator of magnesium balance and may remain normal even with marked magnesium depletion. In severe nutritional deficiency states such as kwashiorkor, serum levels of magnesium may be normal even though the content of magnesium in the muscle is decreased. Conversely, reduced levels may be seen without appreciable losses.

PATHOPHYSIOLOGIC CONDITIONS. Hypomagnesemia. *Hypomagnesemia* occurs in various clinical states, including malabsorption syndromes, hypoparathyroidism, diuretic therapy, hypercalcemia, renal tubular acidosis, primary aldosteronism, alcoholism, and prolonged intravenous fluid therapy with magnesium-free fluids. At special risk are infants who undergo surgery and receive such fluids for protracted periods of time. Nephrotoxic agents may produce hypomagnesemia through increased urinary losses. Infants with early or late neonatal tetany often also have hypomagnesemia (see Chapter 56). When associated with early neonatal tetany, hypomagnesemia tends to be mild and transient and may not require treatment with magnesium. In late neonatal tetany, hypocalcemia may fail to respond to treatment until magnesium levels have been returned to normal.

The symptoms of hypomagnesemia are primarily those of increased neuromuscular irritability and include tetany, severe seizures, and tremors. Personality changes, nausea, anorexia, abnormal cardiac rhythms, and electrocardiographic changes may also be seen. Symptoms do not always correlate with serum magnesium levels, perhaps because serum levels do not always reflect the body content of magnesium, a predominantly intracellular cation. Alternatively, the symptoms of hypomagnesemia may be minor compared with the symptoms of the primary disease causing the magnesium depletion. A third possibility is that the symptoms may reflect hypomagnesemia complicated by hypocalcemia. Severe hypomagnesemia interferes with the release of PTH and induces skeletal resistance to the action of PTH. Hypomagnesemia and hypocalcemia often coexist.

Hypermagnesemia. *Hypermagnesemia,* which is an increase in total body magnesium, rarely occurs in the absence of decreased renal function. Normally, the kidney prevents elevations of serum magnesium to dangerous levels even when large magnesium loads are administered. However, hypermagnesemia with serum levels exceeding 5 mEq/L can occur. The usual sources of a magnesium load include magnesium-containing laxatives, enemas, intravenous fluids, and magnesium-containing antacids used as phosphate binders in patients with chronic renal failure. Severe hypermagnesemia may occur in neonates born of mothers who were treated with intramuscular injections of magnesium sulfate for the hypertension of pre-eclampsia. Neonates born prematurely with asphyxia or hypotonia are at special risk, although it remains to be determined whether the elevated magnesium is the cause or consequence of these abnormalities. Serum magnesium levels tend to spontaneously return to normal within 72 hr. There is also an increased incidence of hypermagnesemia in patients with Addison disease.

The symptoms of hypermagnesemia occur when magnesium levels exceed 5 mg/dL. Hyporeflexia antedates respiratory depression, drowsiness, and coma. Manifestations are rapidly reversed by intravenous administration of calcium. Coma and death usually occur when the serum magnesium level increases above 15 mg/dL.

CHAPTER 52
Phosphorus

Confusion may exist in understanding the physiology of phosphorus, because the terms "phosphorus" and "phosphate" have frequently and erroneously been used interchangeably. Measurements of phosphate in biologic samples are usually performed as and expressed in terms of total elemental phosphorus concentration. Because the atomic weight of phosphorus is 30.98, a concentration of 3.1 mg/dL (31 mg/L) of phosphorus is equivalent to 1 mM of phosphorus/L. Most of the measured plasma phosphorus exists as monovalent or divalent orthophosphate and behaves as though it has a valence of 1.8 at pH 7.40 (see Table 50–1). Consequently, at pH 7.40, 1 mM of phosphate is equivalent to 1.8 mEq of phosphate (mM × valence = mEq).

BODY CONTENT AND DISTRIBUTION OF PHOSPHORUS. Infants retain phosphorus avidly. A 3-kg infant may retain 40–80 mg/24 hr, which is more than 50% of usual intake. Consequently, total body phosphorus per unit of fat-free body weight (FFBW) increases throughout childhood; it doubles from birth to adulthood, at which time its value is approximately 12 g/kg FFBW. This doubling is primarily the result of an increase in skeletal phosphorus content; more than 80% of body phosphorus is intracellular (see Fig. 46–3), principally in bone, and the remainder is distributed throughout all soft tissues.

In plasma, two thirds of phosphorus occurs as phospholipids. These compounds are insoluble in acid and are not measured in routine plasma phosphorus determinations. The measured portion of plasma phosphorus is acid soluble and is composed of inorganic phosphorus, primarily orthophosphate, 10% of which is bound to protein (see Table 50–1). The remaining 90% is ultrafilterable, 5% of which is complexed as calcium, magnesium, and sodium phosphates and 85% of which is free phosphate. Of the latter, 80% is the divalent anion (HPO_4^{2-}) and 20% the monovalent anion ($H_2PO_4^-$) (see Table 50–1). Concentrations of phosphorus are low in interstitial fluids.

Cellular phosphorus exists in cell membranes and subcellular organelles as organic phosphoglycerides and sphingolipids. Acid-soluble moieties of intracellular phosphorus include adenosine triphosphate (ATP) and other nucleotides, various glucose-phosphate compounds, creatinine phosphate, and a small amount of cytosolic inorganic phosphate. Intracellular phosphate plays an essential role in forming and releasing energy, as well as in intracellular enzyme activity. Inorganic phosphorus is the principal urinary buffer filtered at the glomerulus and plays a critical function in the regulation of free hydrogen ions (see Chapter 53).

REGULATION OF PHOSPHORUS. Intake and Absorption. The principal sources of *dietary phosphorus* are milk, milk products, and meat. The recommended daily intake is 880 mg/24 hr for children 1–10 yr of age and 1,200 mg for older children. Breast-fed infants ingest 25–30 mg of phosphorus/kg/24 hr. As much as two thirds of the dietary phosphate is absorbed from the bowel, primarily in the jejunum. This absorption is stimulated by vitamin D and its metabolites and by parathyroid hormone (PTH). Absorption is decreased by thyrocalcitonin, by binders such as aluminum hydroxide and carbonate in the bowel, and at least in animals, by a high dietary calcium intake.

Renal Excretion. Even though phosphate is actively transported across the bowel wall, it is the kidney that plays a major role in regulating body phosphate. Renal handling of phosphate consists of glomerular filtration with facultative reabsorption by the tubule. Ultrafilterable phosphate is freely filtered at the glomerulus, with an average of 90% of this filtered load normally reabsorbed. Eighty percent of the filtered load reabsorption occurs in the proximal tubule, and the remainder occurs in more distal segments. Under certain circumstances, phosphate may also be secreted by the distal tubules. A maximal rate for tubular reabsorption of phosphorus (T_m) exists in the proximal tubule. Because this transport maximum is only slightly above the normal filtered load, small increases in plasma phosphorus increase the filtered load above the transport maximum and increase urinary phosphorus excretion. Urinary excretion of phosphate shows a circadian rhythm, with the lowest levels in the morning and highest levels in the early evening.

Tubular reabsorption of phosphate is regulated by *PTH,* the effects of which are mediated by the adenylate cyclase system. This hormone reduces tubular reabsorption of phosphorus mainly in the proximal tubule and is associated with phosphaturia. Conversely, large doses of vitamin D stimulate reabsorption of phosphate in the proximal tubule, as does growth hormone. Under many circumstances, renal tubular transport of phosphate parallels that of sodium. Expansion of extracellular fluid results in phosphaturia, as does the administration of diuretics, especially those that inhibit carbonic anhydrase. Phosphate transport is also linked to that of glucose and to changes in pH; hyperglycemia therefore results in phosphaturia and a reduced T_m for phosphorus. Conditions that result in an alkaline urine also decrease reabsorption of phosphate.

Plasma Phosphate. In addition to the factors already discussed, plasma phosphate concentration is affected by the continuous exchange of phosphate between the large stores in the bone and those in the extracellular fluid. The release of phosphorus from bone stores is stimulated by the same regulating hormones that promote calcium release. Net reabsorption of phosphate from bone is promoted by 1,25-dihydroxyvitamin D_3 and PTH but is opposed by thyrocalcitonin. Phosphate is also readily transported across all cell membranes. Administering glucose or insulin decreases plasma phosphate concentration, probably because of an intracellular flux of phosphate secondary to the phosphorylation of glucose. Hyperventilation, alkalosis, and administration of epinephrine also decrease plasma phosphate concentration. Marked, acute increases in plasma phosphate concentration result in hypocalcemia. Changes in calcium concentration, however, do not necessarily reciprocally alter plasma phosphate concentration.

Plasma phosphorus concentrations are high during infancy and childhood. The range of values at birth is 1.4–2.8 mM/L, which increases progressively in the first week of life to 2.0–3.3 mM/L before declining slowly during childhood. Levels fall to those of the adult (1.0–1.3 mM/L) on completion of growth. Premature infants also have high plasma phosphorus values of 2.5–3.0 mM/L if their intake of phosphorus is adequate.

PATHOPHYSIOLOGIC CONDITIONS. Hyperphosphatemia. *Hyperphosphatemia* is characteristic of hypoparathyroidism but rarely occurs in the absence of renal insufficiency. Although small changes in the glomerular filtration rate (GFR) have little effect on phosphate excretion in health, *reduction of the GFR* to below 25% of normal leads to an elevation of the serum inorganic phosphate level and to reciprocal changes in the serum calcium level, resulting in secondary hyperparathyroidism. This process begins with small decreases in the GFR but usually does not clinically appear until the GFR has fallen to low levels. *In the young infant,* the GFR is low in relation to active cell mass, and the dietary phosphorus intake is high; consequently, the serum inorganic phosphorus level is high. A reduction in the GFR or relative hypoparathyroidism in infants rapidly leads to very high serum values of phosphate, with consequent depression of the calcium concentration and latent or manifest tetany (see Chapters 45 and 56).

Hyperphosphatemia may also result from the excessive administration of phosphate by oral or intravenous routes or of phosphate-containing enemas. Using cytotoxic drugs to treat malignancies, especially lymphomas or leukemias, results in cytolysis, with hyperphosphatemia caused by the release of phosphate into the circulation. The major clinical consequences of hyperphosphatemia are symptoms of the resulting hypocalcemia.

Hypophosphatemia. *Hypophosphatemia* may result from the phosphate deficiency associated with starvation, protein-calorie malnutrition, and malabsorption syndromes. It may result from intracellular shifts of phosphate, such as those that occur with respiratory or metabolic alkalosis, during the treatment of diabetic ketoacidosis (typically during the first 24 hr), and after the administration of corticosteroids. Increased urinary losses of phosphate may be sufficiently severe to reduce the plasma concentration; this reduction is observed in primary and tertiary hyperparathyroidism, in renal tubular defects, after extracellular fluid volume expansion, or after the administration of diuretics. A combination of pathophysiologic mechanisms often is responsible for the hypophosphatemia. Examples include vitamin D–deficient (see Chapter 45) and vitamin D–resistant rickets (see Chapter 649).

The very-low-birthweight infant requires a high phosphorus intake at the time of rapid postnatal growth. Inadequate intake results in phosphorus depletion and hypophosphatemia. Insufficient phosphorus intake occurs particularly in patients receiving total parenteral nutrition when the physician fails to recognize the need to achieve relatively higher levels of serum phosphorus in premature infants. Bone demineralization, hypercalcemia, and calciuria may occur, probably as a result of mobilization of phosphorus and calcium from the bone.

In most instances, hypophosphatemia is mild or moderate in degree and is asymptomatic. Occasionally, plasma phosphate concentration may fall to very low levels (≤0.3 mM/L [≤1.0 mg/dL]). Such low levels have been observed with the *pro-*

longed use of intravenous alimentation without phosphate supplements and may produce a very severe, well-defined syndrome. Red cell concentrations of 2,3-diphosphoglycerate and ATP are decreased. The resulting decreased release of oxygen by the red cells produces tissue anoxia. Increased hemolysis may occur, as may leukocyte and platelet dysfunction. Some patients display the symptoms of a metabolic encephalopathy, including irritability, paresthesias, confusion, seizures, and coma, and some may develop abnormalities revealed by the electroencephalogram. Hypercalcemia, thought to result from the increased release of calcium from bone; rhabdomyolysis; cardiopathy; and possibly hepatocellular dysfunction also have been reported. Renal tubular defects may occur, and the kidney's ability to excrete hydrogen ions is impaired. Promptly recognizing and treating this syndrome, preferably by orally administering phosphate salts, is beneficial, but permanent defects may result. Prevention of severe hypophosphatemia should always be the goal.

CHAPTER 53

Hydrogen Ion

(Acid-Base Balance)

TERMINOLOGY. Acid-base balance has been complicated historically by a confusion of terminologies. The current approach emphasizes the *hydrogen ion* or proton, which is a hydrogen atom with its neutralizing electron removed. The *pH* is the negative logarithm of the concentration of free hydrogen ions.

An *acid* is a proton (i.e., hydrogen ion) donor. Hydrochloric, sulfuric, phosphoric, and carbonic acids are conventional acids, each dissociating to liberate protons. A strong acid is one that is highly dissociated and therefore produces a high concentration of hydrogen ions; a weak acid is one that is poorly dissociated. A *base* is a hydrogen ion acceptor. Bases bind free hydrogen ions, reducing their concentration. Examples include hydroxyl ions, ammonia, and the anions of weak acids.

A *buffer* is defined as a substance that reduces the change in free hydrogen ion concentration of a solution on the addition of an acid or base. The presence of a buffer in a solution increases the amount of acid or alkali that must be added to cause a change in pH. The addition of a strong acid to any of these buffer systems produces a neutral salt and a weak acid. By generating a poorly dissociated acid, the buffer significantly reduces the increment in free hydrogen ion concentration when the reaction is compared with one that is not buffered.

Aprotes are cations such as sodium, potassium, calcium, and magnesium that carry one or more positive charges, depending on valence, or anions such as chloride and sulfate that carry negative charges. Because aprotes can neither donate nor accept protons, they are not acids, bases, or buffers.

NORMAL ACID-BASE REGULATION. The number of potential hydrogen ions in the body is huge. Most are buffered and therefore are not in free form. At the usual pH of 7.4, the concentration of free hydrogen ions in the blood is only 0.0000398 mEq/L or 3.98×10^{-8} Eq/L (often expressed as 40 nEq/L; Fig. 53–1):

$$pH = -\log(H^+) = -\log(3.98 \times 10^{-8}) \quad (1)$$
$$= -(0.60 - 8.0) = 7.4$$

Normally, the hydrogen ion concentrations of body fluids are maintained in relatively narrow ranges by buffers. Buffers represent the first line of defense against changes in pH, but

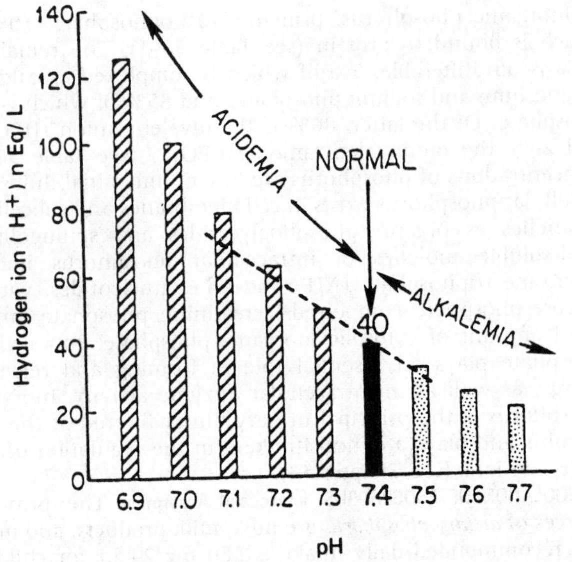

Figure 53–1. Relationship of pH to hydrogen ion concentration. (From Narins RG, Emmett M: Simple and mixed acid-base disorders: a practical approach. Medicine (Baltimore) 59:161, 1980.)

they cannot maintain the acid-base balance. In disease states or abrupt alterations of hydrogen ion production, buffer systems may not be able to maintain a normal pH for a prolonged period, and their action must be supplemented by compensatory and corrective physiologic changes in the lungs and kidneys.

Compensation of a primary acid-base disorder is a slower process than buffering, but it is more effective in returning the pH to normal. In a primary metabolic disorder, the respiratory system provides the compensating mechanism; the kidneys compensate in a primary respiratory disorder by increasing base or by acid excretion. Compensation reduces pH changes but must be followed by *correction*, which returns all acid-base measurements to normal. This stabilization occurs when the primary disorder is cured. The kidneys correct a metabolic disorder, and the lungs correct a respiratory one. Although discussed separately, the buffering, pulmonary, and renal systems are interdependent and act in concert with one another.

BUFFER SYSTEMS. The principal buffer in the extracellular fluid is the bicarbonate-carbonic acid system; intracellular buffers include various proteins and organic phosphates. In the urine, phosphate in its monohydrogen and dihydrogen forms is the major buffer. Only the extracellular fluid buffer mechanisms are considered in detail in this chapter.

Hydrogen ions, when added to the plasma, are buffered in large part by bicarbonate, with the generation of a neutral salt and carbonic acid:

$$HA + NaHCO_3 \rightarrow NaA + H_2CO_3 \quad (2)$$

Carbonic acid is a weak acid with a relatively low solubility coefficient and is in equilibrium with dissolved carbon dioxide, as follows:

$$[H^+]\cdot[HCO_3^-] \leftrightarrows H_2CO_3 \leftrightarrows CO_2 + H_2O \quad (3)$$

The addition of hydrogen ions drives this equation to the right, generating CO_2 and H_2O. Despite the addition of hydrogen ions, the buffering mechanisms result in relatively little change in free hydrogen ion concentration and in pH. However, buffering is accomplished at the expense of a decrease in bicarbonate concentration, which has been referred to as representing a *base deficit*, and an increase in carbon dioxide

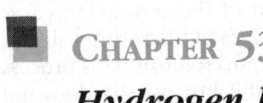

P_{CO_2} levels. The Henderson-Hasselbalch equation indicates that these changes must result in some change in pH:

$$pH = pK + \log \frac{[A^-]}{[HA]} \quad (4)$$

In the bicarbonate-carbonic acid system, pH (a constant derived from the dissociation of the acid-base pair) is 6.1. Thus,

$$pH = 6.1 + \log \frac{[\text{bicarbonate}]}{[\text{carbonic acid}]} \quad (5)$$

Because carbonic acid is in equilibrium with dissolved carbon dioxide, measurement of the partial pressure of carbon dioxide (P_{CO_2}) can be used as a clinical estimate of carbonic acid concentration. By decreasing bicarbonate concentration and increasing P_{CO_2}, the addition of hydrogen ion to the plasma still results in some decrease in pH despite the presence of buffers. However, the changes are of lesser magnitude than would occur in the absence of the buffering mechanism.

CLINICAL ACID-BASE RELATIONSHIPS. The three major components of clinical acid-base balance are *pH*, as determined by the hydrogen ion concentration; the partial pressure of CO_2, P_{CO_2}, regulated by pulmonary ventilation; and plasma bicarbonate concentration, HCO_3, initially an extracellular buffer and then regulated primarily and to a much greater degree by the kidneys. The clinically cumbersome Henderson-Hasselbalch equation has been rearranged by Kasirer and Bleich to an equation that has clinical utility for these three components:

$$[H^+] = 24 + \frac{P_{CO_2}}{HCO_3} \quad (6)$$

This expression emphasizes the important point that *hydrogen ion concentration, and therefore pH, is defined by the ratio of* P_{CO_2} *and plasma bicarbonate*, not the absolute values of the individual components. Defining acid-base balance in terms of this important ratio allows the physician to understand how the acid-base balance operates in clinical settings. The interdependence of the three critical acid-base factors—pH, P_{CO_2}, and HCO_3—is vital for understanding the individual effect on acid-base status of *primary alterations* of P_{CO_2} or HCO_3 produced by clinical abnormalities and for understanding the resultant *compensation* of the counterbalancing factor, P_{CO_2} or HCO_3, to return the acid-base balance toward normal.

Pulmonary Mechanisms. The aforementioned equation indicates that pH depends not on absolute levels of bicarbonate and P_{CO_2} but on the *ratio* of the two concentrations. A decrease or increase in concentration of bicarbonate does not modify pH if the P_{CO_2} is lowered or increased in proportion. By altering the rate at which carbon dioxide is excreted, the lungs can regulate P_{CO_2} and modify pH. Although enormous quantities of carbon dioxide are produced from normal metabolic activity, little change in pH results because of the unique properties of the bicarbonate–carbonic acid buffer system and a highly developed respiratory control mechanism. An increased respiratory rate, stimulated by increased levels of carbon dioxide, increases the excretion of carbon dioxide, decreases P_{CO_2}, and increases pH. Conversely, a decreased respiratory rate increases P_{CO_2} and decreases pH.

Even though the lungs can modify pH by changing the P_{CO_2} and altering the ratio of carbonic acid to bicarbonate, this process cannot cause any loss or gain in hydrogen ions. The lungs are incapable of regenerating bicarbonate to replace that lost when the hydrogen ion concentration was buffered. The generation of new bicarbonate and, when required, the excretion of bicarbonate are the responsibilities of the kidneys.

Renal Mechanisms. The kidneys are the most important regulators of acid-base balance on a daily basis under normal conditions. Renal regulation of acid-base balance fulfills two requirements. First, the kidneys must prevent the loss of bicarbonate in the urine. Second, to maintain acid-base balance, the kidneys must excrete an amount of acid equal to the daily production of nonvolatile acids. Renal regulation to perform these two major requirements is accomplished by two important processes. First, reclamation of most filtered bicarbonate occurs in the proximal tubule. No net hydrogen ion excretion results, but in the adult, this process is responsible for reclaiming up to 5,000 mEq of bicarbonate, which is filtered through the glomeruli each day. If this bicarbonate were not reclaimed, its loss would be equivalent to the retention of an equal amount of hydrogen ions, which would result in severe systemic acidosis. Second, net acid excretion takes place in the distal segments of the nephron through the secretion of hydrogen ion into the tubular lumen and its subsequent excretion in combination with filtered buffers, such as phosphate or ammonia.

The mechanisms for these steps are highly developed, energy-requiring, active transport processes, in contrast to the pulmonary excretion of carbon dioxide, which results from simple passive diffusion. Both processes, the reabsorption of filtered bicarbonate in the proximal tubule and the net excretion of acid in the distal tubules, are accomplished through the secretion of hydrogen ions from the tubular cell into the tubular lumen. For each hydrogen ion secreted into the tubular lumen, a bicarbonate ion moves from the cell into the peritubular capillary and the circulation (see Fig. 53–2). Increased hydrogen ion secretion increases the movement of bicarbonate into plasma, increasing plasma bicarbonate levels. A decrease in tubular hydrogen ion secretion decreases the amount of bicarbonate entering the plasma.

As shown in Figure 53–2, the *reabsorption of bicarbonate in the proximal tubule* depends on the secretion of hydrogen ion from the cell into the tubular lumen in exchange for sodium through an antiporter membrane transport protein. In the proximal tubule cell, hydrogen and bicarbonate ions are produced from the dissolution of carbonic acid catalyzed by carbonic anhydrase. As the hydrogen ion is secreted into the tubular lumen, the bicarbonate exits the cell across the basolateral membrane and into the peritubular capillary. Within the tubular lumen, the secreted hydrogen ion combines with filtered bicarbonate to form carbonic acid (H_2CO_3). The newly formed carbonic acid is rapidly converted to CO_2 and H_2O by the enzyme carbonic anhydrase present on the proximal tubule cell membrane and exposed to the luminal contents. The

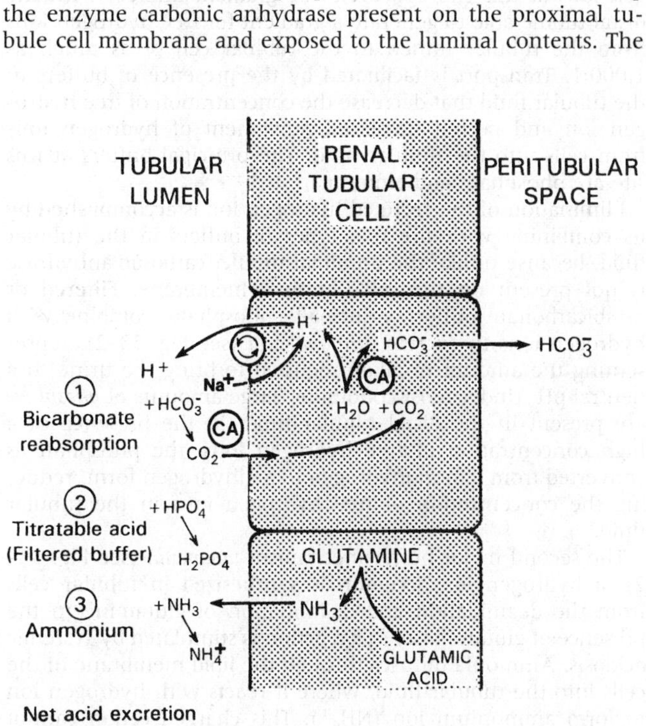

Figure 53–2. The three major renal acidification mechanisms.

carbonic acid conversion products, CO_2 and H_2O, rapidly diffuse into the cell, where they are substrate for the reformation of carbonic acid within the cell, mediated by intracellular carbonic anhydrase. These mechanisms ensure that virtually no bicarbonate passes to more distal segments of the nephron and that an amount of bicarbonate equal to the amount filtered is returned to the peritubular capillaries.

Several factors influence bicarbonate reabsorption in the proximal tubule by regulating hydrogen ion secretion. Some factors increase the rate of hydrogen ion secretion in the proximal tubules and lead to increased bicarbonate reabsorption, with consequent elevation of the serum bicarbonate level. These factors include an increase in the filtered load of bicarbonate (by increasing plasma bicarbonate levels or glomerular filtration rate [GFR]), elevation of plasma Pco_2, hypokalemia, reduction in the extracellular fluid volume (e.g., after vomiting or hemorrhage), and activation of the renin-angiotensin system, mainly through angiotensin II. Conversely, the process of hydrogen ion secretion and bicarbonate reabsorption is decreased by decreases in the filtered load, a decreased plasma Pco_2, by expansion of the extracellular fluid volume, by inhibition of carbonic anhydrase (e.g., by drugs such as acetazolamide), and inhibition of angiotensin II production. Parathyroid hormone (PTH) inhibits proximal tubule bicarbonate reabsorption by reducing the activity of the special transport protein on the cell luminal membrane. Reduction in the plasma bicarbonate level may occur in these situations. Similarly, disease states, such as primary proximal renal tubular acidosis, cystinosis, and heavy metal poisoning, or nephrotoxins associated with structural or functional damage to the proximal tubule may limit bicarbonate reabsorption at this site and result in systemic acidosis.

Renal acid-base regulation in the distal segments of the nephron is accomplished by *net excretion of acid in the distal convoluted tubule and collecting duct*. Hydrogen ions are generated within these tubular cells by the same process as described for the proximal tubular cells, and in the process, bicarbonate is added to the blood (see Fig. 53–2). These nephron segments have a proton-translocating ATPase that actively secretes hydrogen ions under normal conditions. The transport of hydrogen ions at this site appears to be gradient limited, with the distal tubule able to generate a gradient for free hydrogen ions from the tubular lumen to the tubular cell of as much as 1,000:1. Transport is facilitated by the presence of buffers in the tubular fluid that decrease the concentration of free hydrogen ion and permit increased movement of hydrogen ions from cells into the tubular fluid. The principal buffers at this site are phosphate and ammonia.

Elimination of the secreted hydrogen ion is accomplished by its combining with the two types of buffers in the tubular fluid, because unlike the proximal tubule, carbonic anhydrase is not present on the cell's luminal membrane. Filtered or nonbicarbonate buffers, principally phosphate, combine with hydrogen ions to excrete *titratable acid* (see Fig. 53–2), representing the amount of alkali required to bring the urine to a neutral pH. Under most conditions, large amounts of *phosphate* are present in the distal tubular fluid. In the presence of a high concentration of free hydrogen ions, the phosphate is converted from a monohydrogen to a dihydrogen form, reducing the concentration of free hydrogen ions in the tubular fluid.

The second major buffer mechanism, *ammonia* (see Fig. 53–2), a hydrogen ion acceptor, is synthesized in tubular cells from the deamidation and deamination of glutamine in the presence of glutaminase; this reaction is stimulated by systemic acidosis. Ammonia diffuses through the lipid membrane of the cells into the tubular fluid, where it reacts with hydrogen ion to form ammonium ion (NH_4^+). This charged cation cannot readily diffuse back from the luminal fluid.

These two processes, by reducing free hydrogen ion concentration in the tubular fluid, enable an increased rate of transport of hydrogen ions into the distal renal tubule fluid and allow the generation of new bicarbonate, which can enter the plasma and replenish depleted levels of plasma bicarbonate (see Fig. 53–2).

The absolute net rate of excretion of hydrogen ions by the kidney is calculated as the sum of the excretion rates in the urine of titratable acid and ammonium ion minus urine bicarbonate. Living on an average mixed diet, an adult in the United States must excrete about 70 mEq of hydrogen ions each day to maintain pH balance. Approximately one third is excreted as titratable acid, and the remaining two thirds are excreted as ammonium.

Aldosterone is a major regulatory factor of hydrogen ion secretion and therefore of the generation of new bicarbonate in the distal nephron. Aldosterone stimulates hydrogen ion secretion. Other factors influencing distal hydrogen ion secretion include the prevailing Pco_2 and the amount of sodium delivered to these segments. The distal acidification mechanisms may be impaired by intrinsic defects in the tubule, which cause primary distal renal tubular acidosis, or by various insults such as nephrocalcinosis, vitamin D intoxication, or amphotericin B administration, which produce secondary forms of distal renal tubular acidosis.

NORMAL ACID-BASE BALANCE. Most mixed diets produce a net amount of hydrogen ions; true vegetarians ingest a neutral ash diet. Protein is the largest source of hydrogen ions; its metabolism accounts for approximately 65% of the total, generated primarily from the oxidation of sulfur-containing amino acids to yield sulfuric acid and from the oxidation and hydrolysis of phosphoproteins to yield phosphoric acid. The remainder of the hydrogen ions comes from the incomplete catabolism of carbohydrates, fats, and organic acids, such as pyruvic, lactic, acetoacetic, and citric acids. Complete oxidation of these compounds does not produce excess hydrogen ions, because water and carbon dioxide are the final reaction products; incomplete metabolism results in the formation of organic acids and adds hydrogen ions. Milk and meat diets generate about 70 mEq of hydrogen ions/24 hr in the adult and require the kidney to excrete an equal amount daily to maintain a normal blood pH of 7.35–7.45. The infant and child must excrete proportionally similar amounts of hydrogen ions. As a consequence, the daily turnover of hydrogen ions is large, amounting to more than 50% of the hydrogen ions usually in the body buffers and 10% of the maximum storage capacity of the buffers. This hydrogen ion concentration is initially buffered by the intracellular and extracellular fluid buffers and then by respiratory compensation before the kidneys excrete the hydrogen ions to maintain balance.

DISTURBANCES OF ACID-BASE BALANCE. Definitions. Abnormalities in blood pH occur when the hydrogen ion concentration increases above normal, called *acidemia*, or decreases below normal, called *alkalemia* (see Fig. 53–1). The suffix *emia* refers to changes in blood pH. The abnormal clinical processes that cause acid or alkali to accumulate are called *acidosis* and *alkalosis*, respectively. The suffix *osis* is applied to clinical conditions that may or may not imply that a change in blood pH has occurred. For example, metabolic acidosis need not necessarily be associated with acidemia, because the accumulation of acid might have been handled by the buffer defense mechanisms or respiratory compensation might have occurred to bring the blood pH toward normal.

The simple acid-base disorders are shown in Figure 53–3. The *primary alteration* refers to the initiating disturbance that produces, at least transiently, a change in the blood pH by altering Pco_2 or plasma HCO_3. Acidosis is caused by conditions that result in a primary decrease in plasma HCO_3 or an increase in Pco_2 that decreases blood pH below normal (defined as

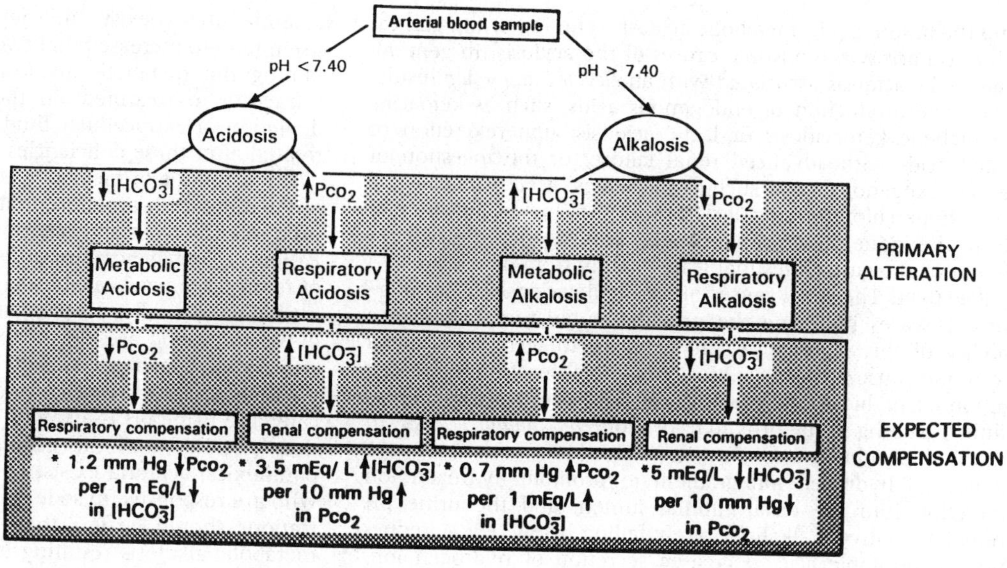

Figure 53–3. Approach for the analysis of simple acid-base disorders. (From Koeppen BM, Stanton BA: Renal Physiology. St. Louis, Mosby Year Book, 1992.)

<7.40 in Fig. 53–3) by increasing the hydrogen ion concentration. Alkalosis is caused when the primary disturbance increases plasma HCO_3 or decreases Pco_2, which increases blood pH above normal (>7.40 in Fig. 53–3) by decreasing hydrogen ion concentration.

When a primary acid-base disturbance in plasma HCO_3 or Pco_2 occurs, a compensatory response restores blood pH toward normal. Referring to Equation 53–6, acid-base balance (i.e., normal blood pH) is defined as the ratio of Pco_2 to plasma HCO_3. The changes of blood pH produced by the primary respiratory and metabolic alterations are determined by the ratio of Pco_2 to HCO_3. The offsetting compensatory response necessarily moves in a direction that attempts to restore the ratio, and therefore the blood pH to normal. Figure 53–3 gives the *expected compensation* for each primary acid-base disturbance. Primary metabolic disorders elicit respiratory compensation, and primary respiratory disorders elicit metabolic compensation. For example, a primary decrease in the plasma HCO_3 concentration increases blood hydrogen ion concentration, and blood pH falls below normal. This primary metabolic acidosis with a lowered blood pH stimulates the respiratory center to increase alveolar ventilation, which reduces Pco_2 and returns the blood pH toward normal. The primary event of metabolic acidosis is a decrease in plasma HCO_3 concentration, lowering blood pH, and the compensatory event is a decrease in Pco_2, accomplished by enhanced ventilation to return the Pco_2/HCO_3 ratio and blood pH toward normal.

A *simple acid-base disorder* is defined as a single primary unidirectional alteration in the respiratory (Pco_2) or metabolic (plasma HCO_3) parameter, with a compensatory response by the remaining parameter. Figure 53–3 provides methods to determine if the expected compensation is appropriate during steady-state conditions. If the actual compensatory response falls outside the expected value, a *mixed acid-base disorder* is likely. Systemic acidosis or alkalosis may result from primary metabolic or respiratory abnormalities. Recovery is unlikely to occur if the blood pH falls below 6.80 or increases above 7.80. The rate of response by the respiratory and renal mechanisms differs. Respiratory responses occur more rapidly: 50% in 6 hrs and 100% in 14–16 hr. Renal mechanisms are slower, with renal base excretion more rapid than acid excretion. Renal base excretion is 50% at 8 hr and 100% at 24 hr. Renal acid excretion is 50% at approximately 36 hr and is 100% at 72 hr.

Metabolic Acidosis. Metabolic acidosis results from an alteration in the balance between production and excretion of acid. Systemic acidosis may result from increased blood hydrogen ion concentration due to accumulation caused by increased intake from an exogenous source or increased endogenous production or by inadequate excretion of hydrogen ions or excessive loss of bicarbonate in the urine or stools. Rapid expansion of the extracellular fluid space by a bicarbonate-free solution may also produce metabolic acidosis by diluting the bicarbonate in the extracellular fluid. The hydrogen ion load is buffered initially by bicarbonate in the extracellular fluid and by intracellular buffers such as hemoglobin and phosphate. Bone may be another source of buffer. The serum bicarbonate level and pH fall (to a lesser extent than if no buffering mechanism were available) and Pco_2 rises.

The resulting systemic acidosis and increased Pco_2 stimulate the respiratory center (and possibly peripheral chemoreceptors in the carotid artery and aorta) to increase the respiratory rate, which increases the rate of excretion of carbon dioxide. Plasma Pco_2 and carbonic acid levels fall, partially or almost totally correcting the acidosis but at the expense of lowering both plasma bicarbonate and Pco_2. The blood pH is decreased but rarely drops as low as might be predicted from the low level of plasma bicarbonate.

The acidosis also stimulates the kidney to increase ammonia production and hydrogen ion excretion into the urine. In the distal nephron, the secretion of hydrogen ion is accompanied by the return of a bicarbonate to the circulation (see Fig. 53–2), increasing the generation of bicarbonate and returning the plasma bicarbonate level to normal if the primary disease process has been alleviated. The respiratory rate subsequently decreases, with the Pco_2 returning to normal. At this point, the patient's acid-base status has returned to the normal state that existed before the hydrogen ion load was administered.

The *clinical manifestations* of metabolic acidosis are often nonspecific. The most important physical sign is hyperventilation, the extreme of which is the deep, rapid respirations (i.e., *Kussmaul breathing*) needed for respiratory compensation. However, severe acidosis itself may cause a decrease in peripheral vascular resistance and cardiac ventricular function, resulting in hypotension, pulmonary edema, and tissue hypoxia. The laboratory findings are decreased serum pH and decreased levels of HCO_3 and Pco_2 (see Fig. 53–3).

The *anion gap* is an important tool in evaluating metabolic acidosis. As described in Chapter 49, the anion gap represents the unmeasured anions, which along with bicarbonate and chloride, counterbalance the positive charge of sodium. The normal anion gap, calculated as $[Na] + [K] - ([Cl] + [HCO_3])$, is 12 mEq/L, with a range of 8–16 mEq/L. Determining the anion gap in metabolic acidosis is an important clinical clue to narrow the possible causes of the acidosis. In general, metabolic acidosis associated with an *elevated anion gap* results from overproduction of endogenous acids, such as ketoacids in diabetic ketoacidosis or lactic acidosis; underexcretion of fixed acids with advanced renal failure; or the ingestion of excess exogenous acids, such as salicylates. A *normal anion gap* (i.e., hyperchloremic) results from the net loss of bicarbonate from the kidney (e.g., renal tubular acidosis, nephrotoxin related) or the gastrointestinal tract, mainly from diarrhea.

Renal Causes. The renal causes of metabolic acidosis are numerous. Diseases involving the proximal tubules may limit the ability of this segment of the nephron to secrete hydrogen ions and cause incomplete bicarbonate reabsorption. Increased amounts of bicarbonate are presented to the distal tubular fluid, resulting in the proximal form of *renal tubular acidosis.* In distal renal tubular acidosis, the distal tubule cannot maintain a normal hydrogen ion gradient to promote hydrogen ion secretion into the distal tubular lumen, and the urine pH remains relatively alkaline, rarely falling below 5.5. A reduction of titratable acid, decreased secretion of hydrogen ion, and systemic acidosis result. With *chronic renal insufficiency,* acidification mechanisms work normally or at supranormal rates. However, the reduced tubular mass limits the ability of the kidney to generate sufficient ammonia and to excrete adequate amounts of hydrogen ions. A *low* GFR, such as in the newborn, also limits the renal capacity to excrete hydrogen ion. The filtered load of phosphate also is reduced, with the bulk reabsorbed in the proximal tubule; little is left for buffering added hydrogen ions in the distal tubule. Hydrogen ion transport is reduced by rapid attainment of a maximal concentration gradient in the absence of buffer. Rarely, *reduction in ammonia synthesis,* as in the cerebro-oculorenal syndrome of Lowe, limits the ability to excrete hydrogens ions.

Other Causes. Metabolic acidosis may also develop in *diabetic ketoacidosis* from incomplete metabolism of body lipids and catabolism of body protein, accompanied by the production of large amounts of acetoacetic, β-hydroxybutyric, phosphoric, and sulfuric acids. In *salicylism,* metabolic acidosis results from hydrogen ions derived from salicylic acid and from the uncoupling of oxidative phosphorylation by salicylate. In severe *diarrhea,* the increased losses of bicarbonate in diarrheal fluid and possibly the formation of organic acids from the incomplete breakdown of carbohydrate in the stools result in metabolic acidosis. *Hyperalimentation, lactic acidosis, starvation,* and *poisoning with either methyl alcohol or ethylene glycol* cause systemic acidosis by increasing the production of various strong acids. Metabolic acidosis is seen also in certain *inherited aminoacidurias* (e.g., methylmalonicaciduria), in hypoxemia, and in shock.

Metabolic Alkalosis. Three basic mechanisms may produce alkalosis: excessive loss of hydrogen ion, as in prolonged gastric aspiration or persistent vomiting associated with pyloric stenosis; increased addition of bicarbonate to the extracellular fluid, which may result from excessive administration by the parenteral route or by oral intake, as in the milk-alkali syndrome, or from increased renal reabsorption of bicarbonate caused by profound potassium depletion, primary hyperaldosteronism, Cushing syndrome, Bartter syndrome, or excessive intake of licorice; and contraction of the extracellular fluid volume, which increases bicarbonate concentration in this fluid space and increases bicarbonate reabsorption in the proximal tubule.

The buffer systems minimize pH change, but the plasma bicarbonate level and pH are increased. Respiration may be depressed with some increase in plasma Pco_2, but this response is limited by increasing hypoxia so that respiratory compensation is always incomplete and never restores the pH to normal. The renal threshold for bicarbonate is exceeded, and bicarbonate appears in the urine, which may have a pH as high as 8.5–9.0. However, factors such as volume depletion and hypokalemia often coexist, and they, along with the increased Pco_2 itself, tend to increase renal reabsorption of bicarbonate, maintaining the metabolic alkalosis. Metabolic alkalosis may be refractory to treatment in the presence of hypokalemia or depletion of extracellular fluid volume and often can only be treated after these deficiencies have been corrected.

The diagnosis of metabolic alkalosis should be considered in any patient with an appropriate history; there are no pathognomonic clinical manifestations of this electrolyte disturbance. Patients may have cramps or feel weak and may have the signs of tetany if ionized calcium has been reduced by the alkalosis.

Characteristically, the pH, plasma bicarbonate level, and Pco_2 of arterial blood are elevated (see Fig. 53–3). Hypochloremia and hypokalemia are usually present, the latter principally resulting from increased urinary losses of potassium. Classically, the urine pH is alkaline, but in the case of severe depletion of potassium, the urinary potassium level is low and paradoxical aciduria exists. In patients with volume depletion who are responsive to sodium chloride, urine chloride concentrations should be less than 10 mEq/L. Patients who have metabolic alkalosis resulting from excessive mineralocorticoid activity or potassium depletion have a urine chloride level exceeding 20 mEq/L and are resistant to sodium chloride treatment.

Respiratory Acidosis. Inadequate pulmonary excretion of carbon dioxide in the case of normal production of this gas produces acidosis. It may occur acutely in neuromuscular disorders, such as brain stem injury, Guillain-Barré syndrome, or sedative overdose; in airway obstruction, such as that caused by a foreign body, severe bronchospasm, or laryngeal edema; in vascular diseases, such as massive pulmonary embolism; and in other conditions, such as pneumothorax, pulmonary edema, or severe pneumonia. Chronic respiratory acidosis may accompany the pickwickian syndrome, poliomyelitis, chronic obstructive airway disease, kyphoscoliosis, or chronic administration of sedatives.

In health, increased production of carbon dioxide stimulates its own respiratory excretion, which maintains a normal Pco_2 and acid-base status. In any of the disease states causing respiratory acidosis, the level of Pco_2 increases until it is elevated sufficiently to cause pulmonary excretion of carbon dioxide equal to its production. Although a new steady state is reached, the increase in Pco_2 (i.e., hypercapnia) causes a systemic acidosis by increasing serum concentrations of carbonic acid and, therefore, of hydrogen ions.

Because carbon dioxide is a major component of the principal buffer system of the extracellular fluid, the rise in Pco_2 must be buffered initially by the nonbicarbonate buffers—the proteins in the extracellular fluid and phosphate, hemoglobin, other proteins, and lactate in the cells. The acidosis and increased Pco_2 stimulate the kidney to increase hydrogen ion excretion as ammonium and titratable acid and to generate and reabsorb more bicarbonate; the plasma bicarbonate levels may be increased somewhat above normal. At this stage, the increase in the plasma bicarbonate level compensates for the primary increase in Pco_2 so that the pH returns toward normal and the respiratory acidosis has been "compensated" by renal mechanisms. The only way to *correct* the abnormality is to reverse the primary disorder.

The causes of acute respiratory acidosis are often associated with hypoxemia, which usually dominates the *clinical manifestations,* along with the signs of respiratory distress. Hypercapnia results in vasodilatation, in increased cerebral blood flow, and may be responsible for the headaches and raised intracranial pressure sometimes found in these patients. Severe hypercapnia may be a cerebral depressant; arterial pH is low, Pco_2 elevated, and plasma bicarbonate level elevated moderately (see Fig. 53–3).

Respiratory Alkalosis. Excessive pulmonary losses of carbon dioxide in the presence of normal production results in a fall in P_{CO_2} and produces respiratory alkalosis. This process may be observed with hyperventilation of psychogenic origin, with overventilation from mechanically assisted ventilation, and in the early stages of salicylate overdosage as a result of stimulation of the respiratory center by salicylate or of increased sensitivity of the respiratory center to P_{CO_2}. Plasma P_{CO_2} falls, and pH rises. A rapid buffering of this pH change occurs, with hydrogen ions released from body buffers to decrease plasma bicarbonate. Approximately 99% of the hydrogen ions are released from intracellular buffers, with the remaining 1% from extracellular buffers. The renal excretion of bicarbonate, slowly increasing by mechanisms that are incompletely understood, reduces plasma bicarbonate levels and compensates for the excessive loss of carbon dioxide, returning the pH toward normal. However, correction cannot occur until the causative disorder has been removed.

The *clinical manifestations* are usually those of the underlying disease process. However, acute hypercapnia may result in neuromuscular irritability and paresthesias in the extremities and periorally because of a decrease in the concentration of ionized calcium. Arterial pH is elevated, and the P_{CO_2} and plasma bicarbonate levels are decreased (see Fig. 53–3). Despite systemic alkalosis, the urine usually remains acid.

Mixed Disorders. Under certain circumstances, mixed disturbances may occur in which more than a single primary cause is responsible for the abnormal acid-base balance. A mixed acid-base disorder should be suspected when the compensatory response falls outside the expected range (see Fig. 53–3). For example, in respiratory distress syndrome, metabolic and respiratory acidoses often coexist. The respiratory disease prevents the compensatory fall in P_{CO_2}, and the metabolic component limits the ability to increase the plasma bicarbonate level, which would normally buffer a respiratory acidosis. In this situation, the decrease in pH is often profound, of greater magnitude than that of a single disturbance.

Other types of mixed disturbances may be seen. Patients with congestive heart failure and chronic respiratory acidosis may develop a component of metabolic alkalosis if they use diuretics excessively. The plasma bicarbonate level and pH are higher than in a simple chronic respiratory acidosis. The pH may be normal or even slightly elevated. Patients with hepatic failure may have metabolic acidosis and respiratory alkalosis. The plasma bicarbonate level and P_{CO_2} may be lower than expected with a simple disorder, although the pH may be little changed from normal. Respiratory and metabolic alkaloses also may coexist in some circumstances.

CLINICAL ASSESSMENT OF ACID-BASE DISORDERS. For clinical purposes, acid-base status is determined from serum pH, P_{CO_2}, and bicarbonate levels.

Measurements. Blood pH can be measured accurately in small blood samples; normal values are 7.35 to 7.45. The concentration of carbonic acid (H_2CO_3) in biologic fluids is quantitatively negligible compared with dissolved carbon dioxide. The latter is measured as the partial pressure of carbon dioxide (P_{CO_2}) in a gas phase in equilibrium with the biologic fluid; the normal value is approximately 40 mm Hg.

The concentration of bicarbonate ion in plasma can be measured directly, but the precision of this determination is not required for clinical purposes. It is customary to determine total carbon dioxide concentration of the serum as an estimate of bicarbonate level. This value is 1–2 mEq/L higher than that of true bicarbonate. It is obtained by titration or by generation of carbon dioxide from serum with a strong acid. The carbon dioxide is derived principally from bicarbonate but also from dissolved carbon dioxide, carbonic acid, carbonate ion, and carbamino compounds. The normal value is 25–28 mM/L, except in the first year of life, when values are 20–23 mM/L, probably because of the low renal threshold for bicarbonate.

If only two of these values are known, the third can be derived from one of the nomograms developed for this purpose, or it can be calculated by one of the several methods based on the Henderson-Hasselbalch equation (see Equation 53–6). If all three measurements have been made, the same formulas can be used to check the validity of the values.

Interpretation. It is relatively easy to diagnose a simple acid-base disorder correctly, based on the blood pH, P_{CO_2}, and bicarbonate levels and using an acid-base nomogram such as that shown in Figure 53–4 or the summary of laboratory findings shown in Figure 53–3. Understanding that blood pH is maintained by the ratio of P_{CO_2} to HCO_3, the patient's acid-base status can be readily ascertained. The following steps provide a useful guide for determining an acid-base abnormality. First, is the condition acidosis or alkalosis? Second, is the primary cause metabolic or respiratory? Third, if it is metabolic acidosis, is the anion gap normal or high? Fourth, is the compensation (respiratory or metabolic) appropriate?

Diagnosing a mixed disorder is more difficult. In simple disorders, P_{CO_2} and bicarbonate levels always change in the same direction to stabilize the blood pH by maintaining the P_{CO_2}/HCO_3 ratio. If any patient's values do not show this relationship or the expected response falls outside the appropriate value (see Fig. 53–3), a mixed disorder should be considered. Similarly, results that plot outside any of the shaded areas shown in Figure 53–4 indicate a 95% chance of a mixed disorder, which can be diagnosed from the clinical setting, as discussed previously.

There are significant arteriovenous differences in acid-base values. In patients with normal cardiac output, central venous pH is lower than arterial pH by an average of 0.03 unit, and the venous P_{CO_2} is higher by about 6 mm Hg. These differences increase with moderate heart failure and are substantial in patients with severe circulatory failure (i.e., pH difference averages 0.1 unit; P_{CO_2} differences average 24 mm Hg). Large arteriovenous differences (i.e., up to 0.35 pH unit and up to 56 mm Hg for P_{CO_2}) occur in patients during cardiac arrest

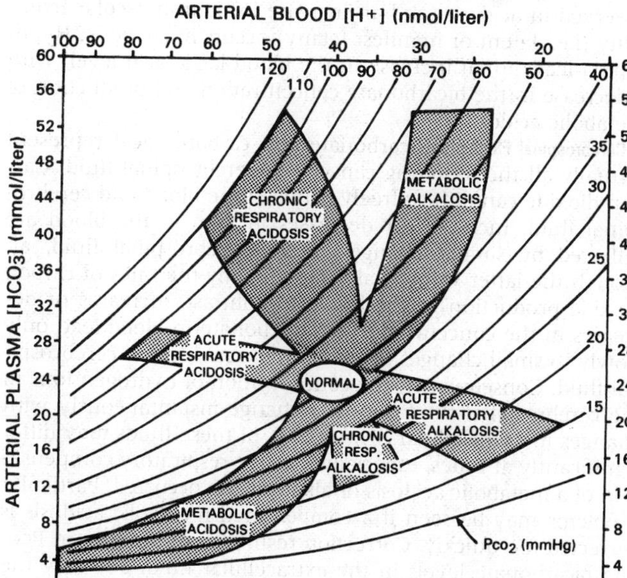

Figure 53–4. The acid-base nomogram shows the 95% confidence limits of metabolic and respiratory compensations for the primary acid-base disturbances. (From Cogan MG, Rector FC: Acid-base disorders. *In*: Brenner BM, Rector FC (eds): The Kidney. Philadelphia, WB Saunders, 1991.)

with mechanical maintenance of ventilation and during cardiorespiratory arrest after sodium bicarbonate administration.

Arterial and central venous blood samples are required to assess acid-base status optimally in patients with critical hemodynamic compromise. Arterial samples provide information about pulmonary gas exchange, and central venous samples provide more accurate information on the acid-base status of tissues during conditions of severe hypoperfusion.

Intracellular pH. Normal intracellular pH has been estimated to be 6.8; values as low as 6.0 have been obtained using microelectrodes. Mitochondrial pH may be even lower because intracellular pH is probably inhomogeneous.

Because carbon dioxide diffuses readily across cell membranes, intracellular and extracellular values for P_{CO_2} are similar. The intracellular changes in hydrogen ion concentration may occur as a result of primary respiratory disorders that cause hypocapnia or hypercapnia. With *hypocapnia,* intracellular alkalosis is proportional to the degree of extracellular alkalosis. With *hypercapnia,* because intracellular bicarbonate concentrations cannot be adjusted as rapidly as those in the extracellular fluid, intracellular acidosis may be proportionally greater than that seen in the extracellular fluid. In contrast to the situation in respiratory acidosis, intracellular pH may be maintained in the face of severe metabolic acidosis until extracellular pH drops below 7.0.

The effects of extracellular acidosis and alkalosis on cellular functions are not fully understood. A low pH produces a slight change in the Donnan distribution across the capillary membrane, and some decrease in oncotic pressure results in a reduced plasma volume. Low pH also seems to reduce myocardial contractility and impair catecholamine action, and it increases the likelihood of arrhythmia, particularly with hypoxia. Moreover, if the hydrogen ion concentration rises rapidly, it may inhibit further transport of the ion in the kidney. Metabolic disturbances also alter the exchange of sodium and potassium ions for hydrogen ions; a potassium deficiency may decrease the intracellular pH at the same time that the extracellular pH is elevated.

Changes in intracellular pH probably affect the activities of many enzymes. A decrease in carbohydrate tolerance has been observed in acidosis, and an increase in neuromuscular irritability (i.e., latent or manifest tetany) occurs in alkalosis. Hypocapnia leads to an increase in the blood lactic acid level, with a decrease in the bicarbonate concentration and production of metabolic acidosis.

Cerebrospinal Fluid pH. Bicarbonate and carbonic acid represent virtually all the buffering capacity in cerebrospinal fluid. Carbon dioxide can diffuse freely between the blood and cerebrospinal fluid. Increases or decreases in P_{CO_2} in the blood are reflected by similar changes in the cerebrospinal fluid, although the latter value is also modified by the rates of carbon dioxide production in the brain. In contrast, increases or decreases in the concentration of bicarbonate in blood lead only slowly to small changes in the bicarbonate level in cerebrospinal fluid. Consequently, the concentration of hydrogen ions in the cerebrospinal fluid does not change instantaneously with changes in extracellular pH; the pHs of these fluids may differ significantly at times, especially if active respiratory compensation of a metabolic acidosis or alkalosis has occurred. Particular problems may be seen if a compensated metabolic acidosis is corrected too quickly. Correction results in an increase in P_{CO_2} and bicarbonate levels in the extracellular fluid, but only the P_{CO_2} rises in the cerebrospinal fluid. The pH of the extracellular fluid returns to normal, but that of the cerebrospinal fluid falls even further, and continuing neurologic symptoms and abnormalities in respiration may result.

Ad Hoc Committee on Acid-Base Terminology: Report. Ann NY Acad Sci 133:25, 1966.

Adrogué HJ, Rashad N, Gorin AB, et al: Assessing acid-base status circulatory failure. N Engl J Med 320:1312, 1989.

Bronner F, Coburn JW (eds): Disorders of Mineral Metabolism, Vol II: Calcium Physiology. Vol III: Pathophysiology of Calcium, Phosphorus and Magnesium. New York, Academic Press, 1981.

Chan JCM, Gill JR Jr (eds): Kidney Electrolyte Disorders. New York, Churchill Livingstone, 1990.

Cogan MG, Rector FC Jr: Acid-base disorders. *In*: Brenner BM, Rector FC Jr, (eds): The Kidney. Philadelphia, WB Saunders, 1991.

Cooke RE (ed): The Biologic Basis of Pediatric Practice. New York, McGraw-Hill, 1969.

Edelman CM Jr (ed): Pediatric Kidney Disease, 2nd ed. Boston, Little, Brown & Company, 1992.

Emmett M, Narins RG: Clinical use of the anion gap. Medicine (Baltimore) 56:38, 1977.

Hicks JM, Boeckx RL (eds): Pediatric Clinical Chemistry. Philadelphia, WB Saunders, 1984.

Holliday MA, Barratt TM, Avner ED (eds): Pediatric Nephrology, 3d ed. Baltimore, Williams & Wilkins, 1994.

Klahr S (ed): The Kidney and Body Fluids in Health and Disease, 2nd ed. New York, Plenum Press 1984.

Koeppen BM, Stanton BA: Renal Physiology. St. Louis, Mosby Year Book, 1992.

Narins RG, Emmett M: Simple and mixed acid-base disorders: a practical approach. Medicine (Baltimore) 59:161, 1980.

Plum F, Price RW: Acid-base balance of cisternal and lumbar cerebrospinal fluid in hospital patients. N Engl J Med 289:1346, 1973.

Schrier RW (ed): Renal and Electrolyte Disorders, 3d ed. Boston, Little, Brown & Company, 1992.

CHAPTER 54
Fluid Therapy

Parenteral or oral fluid therapy is employed to maintain or restore the normal volume and composition of body fluids. It should be administered in a safe and efficient manner, which maximizes the corrective capability of normal physiologic mechanisms within the body, primarily through the circulatory, respiratory, and renal systems. The goal is to normalize the intracellular and extracellular chemical environments that optimize cell and organ function. Although parenteral fluid therapy was first initiated experimentally in the 19th century by Latta, it emerged as a scientific and therapeutic entity in this century with the discovery of methods to measure electrolytes such as sodium, potassium, and chloride and to perform balance studies that documented the net losses of electrolytes and fluid in children being repleted for diarrheal dehydration.

Although parenteral fluid therapy is taken for granted in developed countries as an effective and simple means of treating a child with dehydration from gastroenteritis, it is not widely available in developing countries, where 4 to 5 million youngsters die yearly of dehydration, which is often superimposed on infection and malnutrition. In the United States, about 15–30 million cases of diarrhea in children result annually in 2–3 billion dollars in health care costs, approximately 10% of admissions to pediatric facilities (roughly 200,000 admissions/yr), and approximately 500 deaths. Dehydration from fluid loss, most commonly vomiting and diarrhea, can be particularly devastating in infants because of limited access to fluids and a turnover of total body water of 15–20% per 24 hr, compared with only 5% per 24 hr in adults. Diarrheal losses may not be as evident as in adults but may be much more profound. In a newborn, diarrhea of only 3 Tb every 3 hr results in almost a 50% reduction in extracellular fluid volume in a 36-hr period, which is equivalent in an adult to a loss of 8 L of extracellular fluid. The problem of diarrheal dehydration is magnified in the malnourished infant in whom there may be chronic deficits of electrolytes and limited caloric reserves.

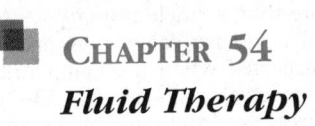

DETERMINATION OF REQUIREMENTS. Fluid therapy consists of three categories: *maintenance, deficit* replacement, and *supplemental* replacement of ongoing losses. Any attempt to lump these categories for the purpose of simplification can lead to serious miscalculations. Maintenance fluid expenditures are a function of metabolic rate, and maintenance therapy is designed to replace usual body losses of fluid and electrolytes. Deficit is described as losses per kilogram of body weight, and deficit therapy is designed to replace abnormal losses of fluid and electrolytes, usually as a result of an illness. Supplemental replacement is based on measured or estimated continuing abnormal losses; supplemental therapy, when indicated, is given in addition to maintenance and deficit fluids.

Each component of therapy must be calculated independently and carefully. A fasting preoperatively stable youngster awaiting surgery may only need maintenance fluid and electrolytes before restoration of oral intake postoperatively, but a child with diarrheal dehydration probably needs maintenance, deficit, and supplemental therapy. Although several modified and simple approaches to parenteral therapy have been described, it is essential that the physician understand the pathophysiology of body fluids, recognize the specific needs in each of the three areas of fluid therapy, and avoid a "cookbook" approach to patient care. Equally important is the recognition that fluid therapy is based on gross estimates of maintenance requirements, deficit, and ongoing losses. The patient is always the final common pathway of therapeutic interventions and must be clinically assessed carefully each step of the way.

If the patient is underhydrated or overhydrated after parenteral therapy, the therapy must be readjusted and individualized to address this reality. Monitoring is usually easily done at the bedside with physical examination and assessment of changes in intake, output, and body weight. Serum chemistries may be followed as indicated, but evaluating their results does not replace close bedside monitoring of the patient.

MAINTENANCE THERAPY. Fluid and electrolyte requirements are directly related to metabolic rate. Changes in metabolic rate affect endogenous water production through the oxidation of carbohydrate, fats, and protein; urinary solute excretion, which influences urinary fluid losses; and heat production, 25% of which must be dissipated through the mechanism of insensible water loss. Although several systems have been used to estimate maintenance fluid and electrolyte requirements, the simplified scheme by Holliday and Segar (Table 54–1) that relates caloric expenditure to body weight for a resting, hospitalized patient is simple to use, physiologic, and applicable over the range of pediatric and adult weights. It compares favorably with other approaches and focuses attention on the caloric needs of patients, not just the fluid and electrolyte needs. This is a critical factor in the highly catabolic patient or the child requiring long-term parenteral management. Estimated caloric requirements, if not provided by oral or parenteral intake, are derived through depletion of fat, glycogen, and protein stores.

Because fecal water losses usually are negligible, fluid requirements of 100 mL/100 calories primarily address insensible and renal water losses. Approximately one third of this water requirement is for insensible water loss, and two thirds are for renal water loss. Insensible water loss occurs through pulmonary and cutaneous routes, with the latter accounting for two thirds and the former for one third of insensible water loss. Conditions that may increase or decrease insensible water loss requirements are associated with changes in caloric expenditure, heat production, and the need for changes in insensible water loss to modulate dissipation of body heat. Insensible water loss increases with increased activity (⩾30%), with fever (i.e., 12% increase for each 1° C rise in body temperature), and with reduced vapor tension in the environment. Conversely, insensible water loss decreases with decreased activity, as in comatose states and with hypothermia, by 12% for every 1° C fall in body temperature. Pulmonary insensible water loss increases with hyperventilation, as in asthma or diabetic ketoacidosis, and decreases with exposure to highly humidified atmospheres or humidified ventilator systems. Cutaneous losses may be especially high in the low-birthweight and very-low-birthweight infant with a large surface area and decreased skin thickness. In this population, insensible water losses of 100–200 mL/kg/24 hr may occur. Insensible water loss is further increased with the use of overhead lights for the treatment of hyperbilirubinemia.

Urinary water requirements may be increased when renal concentrating ability is diminished by an increased solute load or by diminished secretion of or response to antidiuretic hormone (ADH). The solute load may be increased in diabetes mellitus, after the infusion of mannitol or radiocontrast agents, in electrolyte wasting, or by high-protein diets. ADH deficiency is usually associated with central nervous system conditions such as craniopharyngioma or other neoplasms, septo-optic dysplasia, head trauma, granulomas, or infections. A diminished response to ADH by the renal tubules occurs in the condition known as nephrogenic diabetes insipidus (NDI). Primary NDI is uncommon and readily diagnosed by family history and clinical presentation. However, secondary NDI may occur in common conditions such as sickle cell disease, chronic pyelonephritis, renal cystic disease, obstructive uropathy, reflux nephropathy, psychogenic polydipsia, hypokalemia, hypercalcemia, or in response to certain medications.

Urinary water losses are diminished in conditions associated with oligoanuria such as syndrome of inappropriate antidiuretic hormone, acute or chronic renal failure, or genitourinary tract obstruction. If urinary water loss is abnormally high or low, maintenance fluid therapy should include replacing the usual insensible water loss plus urinary output on a milliliter for milliliter basis with free water.

Maintenance requirements for sodium and potassium may also be modified for certain patients. Sodium requirements may be higher in patients with increased cutaneous losses from cystic fibrosis; in patients with increased urinary losses from salt-losing nephritis, obstructive uropathy, chronic pyelonephritis, or diuretic therapy; and in patients with increased gastrointestinal losses from fistulas, diversions, nasogastric drainage, or inflammatory bowel disease. Losses from gastric or intestinal drainage are usually replaced by isotonic or half normal sodium chloride. In some situations, it may be necessary to measure the electrolyte composition of gastrointestinal fluid to aid estimates for electrolyte replacement. Sodium requirements are diminished in edematous states due to hepatic, cardiac, or renal disease, because edema indicates excess body sodium. Patients who have chronic renal failure may require less sodium, especially if they are hypertensive; those with acute anuric renal failure, if euvolemic, should receive no sodium.

Potassium requirements may also be higher in patients with ongoing abnormal gastrointestinal or genitourinary losses. Potassium-losing states generally parallel sodium-losing states and may occur with chronic renal disease associated with renal

■ **TABLE 54–1 Simplified Method for Calculating Caloric Expenditure From Body Weight**

Body Weight (kg)	Caloric Expenditure/Day*
Up to 10	100 kcal/kg
11–20	1,000 kcal + 50 kcal/kg for each kg above 10 kg
Above 20	1,500 kcal + 20 kcal/kg for each kg above 20 kg

**Maintenance fluid and electrolytes: 100 mL water [35 mL insensible water loss, 65 mL urinary water loss] and 2–4 mEq of Na and K for every 100 calories expended.*

medullary injury, with gastric or intestinal drainage, and with chronic laxative or diuretic abuse. Increased renal potassium loss accompanies the alkalosis associated with gastric drainage and loss of hydrochloric acid. In conditions having diminished potassium-excreting ability, such as chronic renal failure and adrenal insufficiency, potassium intake may have to be modified. In cases of acute anuric renal failure, adrenal insufficiency, or severe acidosis with hyperkalemia, no potassium should be administered.

In certain clinical situations, third spacing, which is a shift of extracellular fluid from the plasma compartment elsewhere, such as interstitial or transcellular spaces, may necessitate provision of additional fluid and electrolytes. The volume of third-space fluid is difficult to assess, but the electrolyte composition usually approximates extracellular fluid. Replacement fluid should be based on clinical assessment, including the impact of third spacing on the effective plasma volume and on circulatory status. Massive increases in extracellular fluid due to third spacing may necessitate adjustment of drug dosages for medications that are distributed in the extracellular fluid compartment.

Maintenance fluid and electrolytes may be given orally or parenterally. Although water, sodium, and potassium needs are easily met by this regimen, the provision of calories is insufficient to sustain a positive nitrogen balance. A 5% dextrose solution usually provides enough calories to have some sparing effect on catabolism of protein, but for patients with diminished glycogen and fat storage or those in highly catabolic states, this amount of dextrose may be calorically insufficient. In these patients and those on parenteral therapy for more than a few days, additional nutrition is provided by parenteral alimentation with 5% or higher dextrose solutions, with or without the addition of amino acids, or by the use of total parenteral nutrition (TPN) delivered through a deep central venous catheter, an arterial line, or an arteriovenous fistula. Such lines are at risk for infection and thrombosis and should be inserted, maintained, or changed only by skilled individuals. Of equal importance is the recognition that TPN represents an important and potentially toxic "medication." The careless use of TPN may result in excess sodium, potassium, magnesium, or osmols given to patients with compromised renal function; inadequate provision of intracellular cations and anions such as potassium, magnesium, and phosphate for highly anabolic patients; or excessive amounts of sodium for patients with renal artery thrombosis or renal failure who are at risk for hypertension. Hyperglycemia, hypophosphatemia, and severe metabolic acidosis may also complicate this therapy and even be life threatening. The ratio of calcium to phosphorus in TPN provided to very low birthweight infants is very important in promoting calcium and phosphorus retention and improving bone mineralization. The physician should pay careful attention on a daily basis to the volume and composition of TPN fluid in terms of the patient's nutrient requirements, which may vary significantly from day to day. Careful attention also should be given to serum electrolytes, calcium, phosphorous, magnesium, glucose, and serum urea nitrogen and to fluid intake, output, and body weight.

DEFICIT THERAPY. Deficits in fluid and electrolytes (Table 54–2) represent the cumulative net impact of oral or parenteral dietary intake; pathologic body losses, resulting from disease processes; or physiologic body losses, including corrective attempts to modify the volume and composition of losses through normal excretory routes. The net effect produces deficits that are often similar in their magnitude and composition and often, despite different causes, may be treated in a similar fashion. The severity of the deficit reflects the magnitude and rapidity of change, but the type of deficit reflects the relative loss of water and electrolytes, primarily sodium.

Severity of Deficit. The severity of fluid deficit is represented as the percentage of body weight lost (Table 54–3). Acute losses of body weight reflect losses of fluid and electrolytes rather than of lean body mass. Although the physician may have a recently recorded baseline weight for the patient, in most clinical situations, the percentage of body weight lost is an estimate based on the history and physical examination. Infants with a history of fluid loss and no clinical signs of dehydration are considered to have mild dehydration, representing 3–5% of body weight or 30–50 mL/kg of body weight lost. Infants with signs of moderate dehydration are estimated to have 7–10% of body weight lost, and those with marked clinical signs of dehydration have 10–15% of body weight lost or 100–150 mL/kg. In older children and adults, total body water is a smaller percentage of body weight, and mild, moderate, and severe dehydration represent 5%, 7%, and 10% of body weight lost, respectively.

■ TABLE 54–2 Estimated Deficits of Water and Electrolytes in Infants with Moderately Severe Dehydration

Condition	H_2O (mL)	Na (mEq)	K (mEq)†	Cl (mEq)
Fasting and thirsting	100–120*	5–7	1–2	4–6
Diarrhea				
Isonatremic	100–120	8–10	8–10	8–10
Hypernatremic	100–120	2–4	0–4	−2 to −6‡
Hyponatremic	100–120	10–12	8–10	10–12
Pyloric stenosis	100–120	8–10	10–12	10–12
Diabetic acidosis	100–120	8–10	5–7	6–8

**All estimated deficits are per kilogram of body weight.*
†Converted for breakdown of tissue cells: −1 g N = 3 mEq of K.
‡Negative balance of chloride indicates an excess at the beginning of therapy.

The type of dehydration (Table 54–4) is a reflection of the relative net losses of water and electrolytes and is based on serum sodium concentration or plasma osmolality. These types are often used interchangeably, because extracellular osmolality is largely determined by the concentration of sodium, the dominant extracellular cation, and chloride, the dominant extracellular anion that is closely linked to sodium. Hypotonic or hyponatremic dehydration occurs when serum sodium levels are less than 130 mEq/L, isonatremic or isotonic dehydration occurs when serum sodium levels are 130–150 mEq/L, and hypertonic or hypernatremic dehydration occurs when serum sodium levels are greater than 150 mEq/L. Hypertonic dehydration may occur with serum sodium levels less than 150 mEq/L in the presence of other abnormal osmol levels, such as glucose in diabetic ketoacidosis or mannitol. In uremia, increased urea raises extracellular osmolality, but because urea diffuses well across cell membranes into the intracellular space, it has little to no net effect on extracellular osmolality.

The type of dehydration has important ramifications from the standpoint of pathophysiology, therapy, and prognosis. Intracellular and extracellular osmolality are maintained at equal levels in the body. Changes in the osmolality in one compartment lead to compensatory shifts in water, which is freely diffusible across cell membranes, from one compartment to the other to restore equality of osmolality between body water compartments. In isotonic or isonatremic dehydration, no osmotic gradient across cell walls exists, and intracellular fluid volume remains unchanged. In hypotonic or hyponatremic dehydration, the extracellular fluid is hypotonic relative to the intracellular fluid, and water shifts from the extracellular to the intracellular compartments. Volume depletion through external losses in this form of dehydration is further exacerbated by a shift of extracellular fluid to the intracellular compartment. The resultant marked decrease in extracellular volume may be manifested clinically as profound dehydration leading to circulatory collapse. In patients with hypertonic or hypernatremic dehydration, the converse occurs; water shifts from the

■ **TABLE 54–3 Clinical Assessment of Severity of Dehydration**

Signs and Symptoms	Mild Dehydration	Moderate Dehydration	Severe Dehydration
Body weight loss (%)	3–5	6–9	10 or more
General appearance and condition; infants and young children	Thirsty; alert; restless	Thirsty; restless or lethargic but irritable to touch or drowsy	Drowsy; limp, cold, sweaty, cyanotic extremities; may be comatose
Older children and adults	Thirsty; alert; restless	Thirsty; alert; postural hypotension	Usually conscious; apprehensive; cold, sweaty, cyanotic extremities; wrinkled skin of fingers and toes; muscle cramps
Radial pulse	Normal rate and strength	Rapid and weak	Rapid, feeble, sometimes impalpable
Respiration	Normal	Deep, may be rapid	Deep and rapid
Anterior fontanel	Normal	Sunken	Very sunken
Systolic blood pressure	Normal	Normal or low; orthostatic hypotension	Low, may be unrecordable
Skin elasticity	Pinch retracts immediately	Pinch retracts slowly	Pinch retracts very slowly
Eyes	Normal	Sunken	Grossly sunken
Tears	Present	Absent to reduced	Absent
Mucous membranes	Moist	Dry	Very dry
Urine flow	Normal	Reduced amount and dark	Anuria/severe oliguria
Capillary refill	Normal	± 2 sec	>3 sec
Estimated fluid deficit (mL/kg)	30–50	60–90	100 or more

intracellular space to the extracellular space to restore equality of osmolality between compartments. This is the only form of dehydration that significantly decreases intracellular volume. Signs of extracellular depletion are modified because of this compartmental "steal" syndrome.

A careful history can prove provide information for estimating the magnitude and type of deficit. Careful attention must be paid to the type and quantities of fluid intake and output, to any documented changes in body weight or in the frequency and appearance of urine, and to the general appearance and behavior of the child. A child with diarrhea for several days who has ingested adequate water but little sodium may present with hyponatremia. An infant with a high fever for several days and little access to water may have hypernatremia, as may a child with an inaccurately prepared, highly concentrated formula or home-made electrolyte solution. Infants on diuretics or with renal salt losing conditions may, in the absence of adequate oral intake, develop hyponatremia, but infants with primary or secondary NDI, in the absence of access to free water, are likely to develop hypernatremic dehydration.

Hypernatremic and hyponatremic dehydration each occur in 10–15% of the population, but approximately 70% of pediatric dehydration is isotonic, with hypotonic stool losses being replaced, albeit inadequately, with hypotonic oral fluids. Most infants with severe dehydration have a history of lethargy, listlessness, and decreased responsiveness; those with hypernatremic dehydration tend to be irritable and fussy. Decreased urinary frequency and volume is common in severe dehydration, but this sign may be deceptively absent in children with defective renal concentrating ability, who continue to excrete sizable quantities of urine despite severe volume depletion, and in some low-birthweight infants.

Clinical Manifestations. Table 54–3 summarizes the physical findings in children with mild, moderate, and severe dehydration. Children with mild dehydration have a history compatible with dehydration but few physical findings, while those with severe dehydration have marked physical signs. Patients with moderate dehydration fall somewhere in between.

The clinical signs of dehydration largely represent the depletion of extracellular fluid volume and, therefore, changes in plasma volume, interstitial fluid, and transcellular fluid. Transcellular fluids include fluids of the salivary glands, pancreas, liver, and biliary tracts; mucosal fluids of the respiratory and gastrointestinal tracts; the vitreous humor of the eyes; cerebrospinal fluid; and intraluminal contents of the gastrointestinal tract. Other extracellular-like fluids that may contribute to signs of volume depletion include peritoneal, pleural, and pericardial effusions.

■ **TABLE 54–4 Dehydration and Serum Sodium Concentration**

Type of Dehydration	Electrolyte Status
Hypotonic or hyponatremic	Serum Na <130 mEq/L
Isotonic or isonatremic	Serum Na 130–150 mEq/L
Hypertonic or hypernatremic	Serum Na >150 mEq/L

Mild dehydration may be manifested only by thirst and occasionally by changes in behavior. With moderate to severe dehydration, the anterior fontanel is sunken, reflecting the depletion in cerebrospinal fluid; mucous membranes are dry from depletion of transcellular fluids; skin demonstrates tenting due to decreased interstitial fluid; and eyes are sunken because of the decreased vitreous humor. The appearance of sunken eyes is often obvious to a parent but not necessarily to the physician; it is frequently, however, one of the earliest clinical signs that improves after rehydration. Tenting of the skin, often improperly evaluated, should be tested by pinching and gently twisting the skin of the abdominal or thoracic wall. Tented skin remains in a pinched position rather than springing quickly back to normal. Skin tenting may be difficult to ascertain in the severely malnourished child and in the premature infant. In these patients, dehydration may be overestimated. Tear production may be lacking in severe dehydration, although some tearing still may be observed. With hypovolemia due to contraction of plasma volume, the patient may have hypotension, cool extremities, and activation of the sympathetic nervous system, accompanied by tachycardia and sweating. Postural changes in blood pressure and heart rate occur but are not commonly evaluated. This is unfortunate, because oscillometry and Doppler techniques are usually successful in measuring systolic blood pressure in the infant in whom blood pressure may be difficult to obtain by auscultation.

With very severe dehydration, circulatory collapse occurs, with cool, cyanotic, sweating extremities; a rapid, thready pulse; mottled skin; and severe lethargy or coma. Delayed capillary refill often occurs in patients with severe dehydration. Capillary refill, measured by compressing the ball of the thumb or large toe and estimating or measuring the time for return of blood flow or a blush, is greater than 3 sec with profound volume depletion. Capillary refill may also be delayed in a cool ambient environment.

Different types of dehydration may have different clinical manifestations. Patients with hypotonic dehydration, because of external losses and internal fluid shifts, may present with signs of profound volume depletion and shock. Patients with hypernatremic dehydration tend to have fewer signs of dehydration, even with a similar volume loss. Their skin is warm and has a doughy feel. Patients with hypernatremic dehydration tend to be lethargic, but very irritable when touched, and to be hypertonic and hyperreflexic. Patients with systemic acidosis from diarrhea and excessive stool bicarbonate losses may show Kussmaul breathing; those with hypokalemia may have weakness, abdominal distention, ileus, and cardiac arrhythmias. Patients with hypocalcemia and hypomagnesemia may have associated tetany, muscle twitching, and abnormal electrocardiographic findings.

Laboratory Evaluation. Laboratory tests can be useful in evaluating the nature and extent of dehydration and in guiding therapy, but they cannot substitute for careful bedside observation of the patient. Management of dehydration requires the clinical skills of the physician. In cases of serious dehydration, therapy should always be initiated promptly, even before receipt of the laboratory test results.

Identifying hemoconcentration, indicated by elevated hemoglobin, hematocrit, and plasma proteins, may help in estimating the severity of dehydration and in monitoring the response to rehydration. However, when hemoglobin and hematocrit appear normal despite severe dehydration, the physician should suspect that hemoconcentration exists and that the patient has an underlying anemia, often due to iron deficiency.

Serum or plasma electrolyte values are often helpful. Serum sodium concentration defines the type of dehydration and reflects the relative losses of water and electrolytes, not of total body sodium stores. Hypernatremia usually is not caused by sodium excess but is often associated with a mild to moderate deficiency of total body sodium.

Serum potassium values are usually normal or elevated in diarrheal dehydration. Hyperkalemia may be related to acidosis or diminished renal function. Hypokalemia may occur with significant stool losses; with gastric losses associated with alkalosis, as in pyloric stenosis; or with acute intracellular shifts in potassium with the administration of glucose or alkali. Profound depletion of total body potassium usually occurs before extracellular plasma potassium values fall below normal. Hyperkalemia and hypokalemia must be monitored carefully with serial serum sampling and with electrocardiograms or on-line cardiac monitors. Hyperkalemia of whatever cause is a contraindication to parenteral administration of potassium, but hypokalemia is usually addressed with careful and conservative repletion of this cation.

Serum bicarbonate concentrations are helpful in detecting metabolic acidosis or alkalosis. Acidosis is most commonly associated with diarrheal disease because of stool bicarbonate losses and because of retention of anions from tissue catabolism and diminished renal function. Alkalosis occurs in the setting of protracted vomiting or nasogastric drainage. Acute blood gas determinations may be helpful in defining the extent of changes in blood pH and the relative contribution of metabolic and respiratory disorders to the net acid changes.

Because chloride values usually parallel those of sodium, hyperchloremia accompanies hypernatremia, and hypochloremia accompanies hyponatremia. The difference in the sum of the measured cations (i.e., sodium and potassium) and anions (i.e., chloride and bicarbonate), normally about 12 ± 4 mEq/L, is called the anion gap. The anion gap is elevated in cases of decreased renal function and retention of sulfate, phosphate, and other unmeasured anions and in cases of ketosis and lactic acidosis resulting from tissue breakdown and diminished muscle perfusion. A diminished anion gap may be seen with hypoalbuminemia, but no anion gap often indicates a laboratory error.

Blood urea nitrogen and serum creatinine levels may be elevated in severe dehydration because of a decreased glomerular filtration rate (GFR). Increased back diffusion of urea from the proximal tubule due to decreased urinary flow may produce azotemia in the oliguric child in the absence of elevation in serum creatinine values. Serum urea nitrogen levels may be low in the highly anabolic infant, while actual elevations in serum creatinine values may be overlooked by a physician unaware that normal serum creatinine values in the infant and young child are usually much lower than in the older child and adolescent. A serum creatinine value of 1 mg/dL in an adolescent may represent a normal GFR, but the same value in a 2-mo-old infant could represent a GFR that was 25% of normal. A child may have severe dehydration despite normal values for serum urea nitrogen and creatinine, because accumulation of these waste products owing to a decline in renal function occurs over a protracted period.

Urinalysis is most helpful in the measurement of urine specific gravity, which is usually elevated in cases of significant dehydration but which returns to normal after rehydration. Although infants have a reduced ability to concentrate the urine, even those who are a few weeks of age can show a clear elevation in specific gravity with significant dehydration. A specific gravity less than 1.020 indicates mild or no dehydration or indicates a urinary concentrating defect, as in chronic renal disease or in primary or secondary diabetes insipidus. With dehydration, urinalysis may show hyaline and granular casts, a few white cells and red cells, and 30–100 mg/dL of proteinuria. These findings usually are not associated with significant renal pathology, and they remit with therapy.

CHAPTER 55
Principles of Therapy

In some dehydrated patients, especially those with profound dehydration, circulatory collapse, and shock, intravenous fluid should be administered on an emergent basis, even before a complete evaluation of the patient is undertaken (see Chapter 60). In the less urgent situations, before administration of fluids, the patient must be carefully evaluated clinically and the type and quantity of fluids carefully calculated. Consideration should be given to the magnitude of water and sodium deficits, the projected changes in body composition resulting from the illness, and the impact on potassium and hydrogen ion balance. Similar therapeutic approaches are often used for patients with dehydration of different causes.

Oral rehydration (Table 55–1) may be successful in patients with mild to moderate dehydration. Such therapy requires the close and consistent attention of a qualified caregiver, knowledge of appropriate rehydration formulas, and patient compliance. Parenteral therapy is indicated for patients with severe dehydration and those who refuse oral intake or have

■ **TABLE 55–1 Comparison of Oral Solutions**

Solution	Glucose (g/dL)	Na (mEq/L)	K (mEq/L)	Cl (mEq/L)	Base (mEq/L)
WHO solution	2.0	90	20	80	30 Bicarbonate
Rehydralyte	2.5	75	20	65	30 Citrate
Pedialyte	2.5	45	20	35	30 Citrate
Lytren	2.0	50	25	45	30 Citrate
Ricelyte	3.0	50	25	45	34 Citrate
Naturalyte	2.5	45	20	35	48 Citrate

■ TABLE 55–2 Composition of External Abnormal Fluid Losses

Fluid	Sodium (mEq/L)	Potassium (mEq/L)	Chloride (mEq/L)	Protein (g/dL)
Gastric	20–80	5–20	100–150	
Pancreatic	120–140	5–15	90–120	
Small intestine	100–140	5–15	90–130	
Bile	120–140	5–15	80–120	
Ileostomy	45–135	3–15	20–115	
Diarrheal	10–90	10–80	10–110	
Sweat*				
Normal	10–30	3–10	10–35	
Cystic fibrosis	50–130	5–25	50–110	
Burns	140	5	110	3–5

**Sweat sodium concentrations progressively increase with increasing sweat flow rates.*

persistent vomiting. Although the intravenous route is preferable for parenteral therapy, fluids may be given in unusual situations intraperitoneally or intraosseously. Parenteral therapy has three phases. *Initial* therapy is designed to expand extracellular fluid volume rapidly and improve circulatory and renal function. *Subsequent* therapy is aimed at replacing deficits while providing for maintenance water, electrolyte requirements, and ongoing losses (Table 55–2). During this phase, sodium and water losses are usually almost fully corrected. The *final* phase consists of returning the patient to normal composition, which is usually associated with a return to oral feedings and with the more gradual correction of total body potassium deficits.

INITIAL THERAPY. The goal of initial therapy is to expand extracellular fluid volume rapidly, especially plasma volume, to prevent or treat shock (Table 55–3). An isotonic electrolyte solution, similar to plasma in composition, should be used. Isotonic saline (i.e., 0.9%; sodium and chloride, both 154 mEq/L) containing glucose (5 g/dL) is useful, especially in dehydrated patients with metabolic alkalosis. In patients with severe metabolic acidosis, the acidosis may be worsened with the additional chloride load and by dilution of serum bicarbonate levels. In this situation, an isotonic solution in which some chloride is replaced by bicarbonate (e.g., containing 140 mEq/L of sodium, 115 mEq/L of chloride, 25 mEq/L of bicarbonate) may be used. Lactated Ringer also provides additional buffer but should be used cautiously in patients with lactic acidosis or impaired ability to convert lactate to bicarbonate.

In the initial phase, 20–30 mL/kg of body weight of isotonic solution should be given by bolus and repeated a second or, occasionally, a third time, until the patient is hemodynamically stable. At this time, laboratory values are usually available, and the physician can proceed with a logical and well-planned approach. This initial therapy applies to hypernatremic, hyponatremic, or isotonic dehydration. In cases of hypernatremia, some excess in sodium may be provided, but the impact is usually minimal on sodium levels. In hyponatremia, it is not uncommon to require more than one bolus; this reflects the profound intravascular depletion in this condition and the need for additional sodium to restore normal plasma osmolality.

The physician must *never* initially rehydrate a patient with a hypotonic solution. This approach fails to "capture" rehydration fluid within the extracellular compartment, and perhaps more seriously, it can cause a rapid fall in serum sodium values in patients with hypernatremia, precipitating cerebral edema, a devastating consequence of inappropriate use of initial solutions that are not isotonic.

Potassium should be withheld from intravenous fluids unless the patient is very hypokalemic or renal function is well established. Ringer lactate does contain potassium, but the amount is minimal and usually not a concern when used as an initial hydrating solution. In desperate situations in which electrolyte solutions are unavailable, pure plasma expansion is needed, and a severe coexisting anemia complicates the patient's clinical condition, blood may be used in the amount of 10 mL/kg. It must be used cautiously, because blood may be associated with potential delays in availability, problems of cross-matching, a risk of thrombosis, and the risk of transmission of undetected infectious diseases. A 5% albumin infusion is useful in re-expanding plasma volume but should not replace efforts at restoring the total extracellular volume deficit and may offer only temporary benefit in patients with diffuse capillary leak syndrome.

SUBSEQUENT THERAPY. The subsequent phase of therapy is devoted to continued replacement of existing deficit, provision of maintenance fluid and electrolytes, and replacement of ongoing losses. It is possible to calculate over 8-hr intervals (see Table 55–3) the water and sodium requirements for deficit, maintenance, and ongoing losses and arrive at a volume and composition of replacement fluid to be used. For example, with 10% isotonic dehydration, the final composition of rehydrating fluid for the first 8 hr after the initial boluses have been given is one-third to one-half isotonic, and for the next 16 hr, the composition is one-third isotonic. Physicians should familiarize themselves with this process, because oversimplification of fluid and electrolyte therapy can lead to serious complications in the difficult or unpredictable patient.

Potassium losses usually are replaced gradually, and total body potassium deficits are not fully restored to normal until the patient is on oral feeds or, in cases of protracted parenteral therapy, on total parenteral nutrition. This order is necessary because potassium must move through the extracellular fluid compartment to reach the intracellular compartment in which most potassium is stored. Large amounts of parenterally provided potassium can lead to hyperkalemia, which may have serious cardiac sequelae. Potassium is usually not provided unless the patient has voided and demonstrated acceptable renal function. Some physicians even delay provision of potassium for the first 8–16 hr; however, there are situations,

■ TABLE 55–3 Treatment for 10% Isotonic Dehydration in a 10-kg Infant During the First 24 Hours

	First 8 Hours*		Second 8 Hours		Third 8 Hours	
Hours	Water (mL)	Sodium (mEq/L)	Water (mL)	Sodium (mEq/L)	Water (mL)	Sodium (mEq/L)
Deficit	500	70 (50)†	250	35 (25)	250	35 (25)
Isotonic boluses	−250	−35				
Maintenance	333	10	333	10	333	10
Ongoing losses	150	7	150	7	150	7
Total loss‡	733	52 (32)	733	52 (42)	733	52 (42)
Electrolyte solution	1000	70 (43)	1000	62 (50)	1000	62 (50)

**Approximate electrolyte solutions: for the first 8 hr are 1/2 to 1/3 isotonic, and for the subsequent 16 hr, 1/3 isotonic.*
†Values in parentheses represent net sodium deficits with the assumption of release of intracellular sodium stores during rehydration.
‡After initial boluses have been given, values in parentheses indicate sodium deficits.

tion. To reduce vomiting, the ORS should be given slowly, in small amounts, at short intervals. If sustained, severe vomiting occurs, intravenous therapy should be instituted. The patient's progress should be assessed frequently and changes in body weight monitored, if possible, to determine the degree of rehydration.

When rehydration is complete, maintenance therapy should be started. Patients with mild diarrhea usually can then be treated at home using 100 mL of ORS/kg/24 hr until the diarrhea stops. Breast-feeding or supplemental water intake should be maintained. Patients with more severe diarrhea require continued supervision. The volume of ORS ingested should equal the volume of stool losses. If stool volume cannot be measured, an intake of 10–15 mL of ORS/kg/hr is appropriate.

This regimen has not been universally accepted. The sodium concentration of ORS (90 mM/L) is two to three times that of other fluids (see Table 55–1) that have traditionally been recommended for oral therapy in patients with diarrhea. Low-sodium solutions were advocated because hypernatremia was seen frequently in the United States when oral electrolyte solutions with sodium concentrations of 50 mEq/L or more were used to treat infantile diarrhea. However, extensive use of ORS in many developing countries has documented hypernatremia to be a rare complication, probably because ORS has been used primarily for rehydration (the major previous role for oral therapy was to prevent dehydration or for maintenance); because large amounts of water are ingested in addition to ORS, often a 2:1 ratio of ORS to H_2O; and because ORS has been administered under close supervision by trained personnel. Oral rehydration also has been effective in treating acute diarrheal illnesses in well-nourished children in developed countries. Hypernatremia did not occur even when solutions containing 90 mEq/L of sodium were used. Several commercially available electrolyte solutions for oral use have been reformulated with a sodium concentration increased to 50 mEq/L or higher. Solutions such as Pedialyte with lower sodium concentrations may be used for treatment of diarrhea without dehydration but are not adequate as rehydration solutions.

Occasionally, an infant receiving 2–3 L/24 hr of carbohydrate and electrolyte mixtures orally may have an apparently related increase in the volume of stools, but such instances are sufficiently rare that they do not contraindicate an initial trial of oral therapy.

It has been traditional to omit oral feedings initially when treating infants having more severe diarrhea. However, even during acute diarrhea, the small intestine can absorb various nutrients and may absorb up to 60% of the food eaten. In developing countries, regimens for treating acute diarrhea have encouraged continuing the oral intake of nutrients because better weight gain has been documented in infants given a liberal dietary intake during diarrhea compared with others on a more restricted intake, because fasting has been shown to further reduce the ability of the small intestine to absorb nutrients, and because no physiologic basis exists for giving the bowel a "rest" during acute diarrhea. This approach may cause an increase in the volume of stool in most recipients, resulting in continuing large losses of fluid and electrolytes (see Table 55–2). This loss must be replaced and may require instituting or extending parenteral therapy for several days. Despite this unusual complication, studies have shown that rehydration occurs as rapidly with oral as with parenteral therapy in most patients.

Typically, the frequency and volume of stools lessen within 48 hr in fasted patients treated with intravenous therapy. When stooling subsides, oral feeding of one of the carbohydrate and electrolyte mixtures may be initiated if gastric distention and vomiting are absent. As soon as oral feeding is tolerated without exacerbating the diarrhea, the caloric intake may be increased gradually by substituting mixtures that also contain fat and protein until the usual dietary intake is attained, which usually occurs within 7–8 days. Prematurely administering large quantities of calories in the form of milk may exacerbate the diarrhea. In the young infant with a family history of allergy, a hypoallergenic feeding mixture is recommended for the recovery phase because permeability of the gastrointestinal tract to whole protein may be increased during this time. The routine use of lactose-free formulas in children with diarrhea does not lessen the recovery time.

In addition to replacing the deficits of water and electrolytes, efforts should be made to obtain an etiologic diagnosis so that specific antimicrobial therapy may be given if indicated. Such treatment does not modify fluid therapy. Drugs such as opiates, which inhibit peristaltic activity of the bowel, or absorbents such as kaolin or pectin have relatively little or no effect on the course of infantile diarrhea and are not recommended.

56.2 Diarrhea in Chronically Malnourished Children

Severe malnutrition complicated by diarrheal dehydration is common in tropical and subtropical countries and occurs occasionally in the temperate zones. Therapy should be adapted to meet the specific disturbances in body composition characteristic of the dehydrated *and* malnourished infant, in whom there appears to be an overexpansion of the extracellular space, accompanied by extracellular and presumably intracellular hypo-osmolality. Serum sodium, potassium, and magnesium levels tend to be low, and tetany occasionally may result from a magnesium or calcium deficiency. Serum protein levels are frequently below 3.6 g/dL. The sodium content of muscle is high; potassium and magnesium contents are low. The electrocardiogram frequently shows tachycardia, low amplitude, and flat or inverted T waves. Cardiac reserve seems lowered and heart failure is a common complication.

Despite clinical signs of dehydration and reduced body water, urinary osmolality may be low in the chronically malnourished child. This defect in renal concentration may result from the relative absence of urea to contribute to a hypertonic fluid in the renal papillas, a defect associated with a low dietary protein intake and resulting in a failure of tubular conservation of water. However, the glomerular filtration rate (GFR) is low, resulting in a smaller loss of water than would otherwise be expected, and renal concentrating ability returns after several days of high-protein feedings. The renal acidifying ability is also limited in patients with malnutrition.

Survival of the malnourished infant with diarrhea is limited by caloric deficit to a greater extent than by water and electrolyte deficit. Reparative calories can be given by slow drip through an indwelling nasogastric tube while electrolytes and water are given parenterally. If appetite is poor and vomiting and gastric distention are absent, feeding is begun early (30–40 cal/kg/24 hr), given by slow intragastric drip. Increases to 50–100 cal/kg/24 hr and 1–2 g of protein/kg/24 hr are made in a few days. Ad libitum intake should be permitted in the succeeding days and weeks, up to 250–300 cal/kg/24 hr, and the diet should include an adequate supply of iron and copper.

Initial parenteral therapy is designed to improve the circulation and to expand extracellular volume. The repair solutions resemble those recommended for hyponatremic dehydration. For patients with edema, the quantity of fluid and rate of administration should be reduced from recommended levels to avoid pulmonary edema. Blood should be given if the patient is in shock, severely ill, or anemic. Potassium salts can be given early if the urine output is good. Clinical and electrocardiographic improvement may be more rapid with magnesium therapy, and seizures occurring during recovery from diarrhea complicating severe malnutrition may respond to magnesium.

56.3 Congenital Alkalosis of Gastrointestinal Origin

Rarely, chronic diarrhea may result from a congenital defect in the transport of chloride in the small and large bowels. The watery stools of these patients have a high content of chloride and alkalosis results from the ensuing volume depletion. Potassium is lost in the stools and in the urine; the latter losses are a consequence of the alkalosis. Treatment of fluid and electrolyte deficits is similar to that for pyloric stenosis. Long-term therapy must provide an adequate dietary intake of potassium and chloride. A rare, acute, chloride-losing diarrhea may also occur.

56.4 Pyloric Stenosis

(Also see Chapter 275.1)

This condition exemplifies the correction of deficits associated with alkalosis. The therapy differs little from that for other causes of dehydration, except that potassium replacement should begin early, as soon as the child has urinated. In addition, relatively more sodium and potassium should be given as the chloride salt than is usual in treating dehydration, partly because of the larger deficit of chloride in pyloric stenosis and partly because this results in some correction of the alkalosis as the volume is expanded. Correction of the hypochloremia and alkalosis by administering ammonium chloride without correcting the potassium deficit is not recommended because it results in continued dysfunction of renal tubular and other cells.

Severe depletion of intracellular potassium results in the increased exchange of hydrogen ion for sodium in the distal tubules of the kidney. The paradoxical presence of an acid urine with systemic alkalosis should be interpreted as signifying a marked potassium deficit and a need to increase the amount of potassium used for repletion.

It is not uncommon for deficits to be replaced and serum levels of electrolytes returned to normal within 12 hr. However, except in the mildly ill infant without signs of dehydration, it is preferable to delay surgery for at least 36–48 hr to achieve optimal readjustment of body functions. During this preparation period, adequate fluid therapy prevents dehydration, and the stomach may be decompressed by gentle suction.

56.5 Fasting and Thirsting

Parenteral fluid therapy is usually required in initially treating the infant or child who has taken little or no water and food for 1–5 days. Such infants are deficient in water from insensible water loss and in electrolytes, particularly sodium and chloride, which have been excreted in the urine. If fasting and thirsting continue beyond 4–5 days, urinary output falls to such low levels that there is reduced continued loss of electrolytes. Further severe water deficiency associated with continued evaporative losses may result in hypernatremia.

Therapy is begun with an isotonic solution to produce rapid and safe expansion of extracellular volume and to improve renal function. Subsequent therapy is described in Chapter 55. Sodium and water depletion per kilogram of body weight for a given degree of clinical dehydration is generally greater in infants than in children, but potassium deficits are relatively equal in infants, children, and adults. Water, carbohydrate, and electrolytes may be administered orally to the mildly ill patient. Because infants may vomit when they are dehydrated, they may require parenteral therapy.

For a detailed discussion of the fluid therapy of children with diabetic ketoacidosis and burns, see Part XXVI, Section 6 and Chapter 60.

56.6 Electrolyte Disturbances Associated with Central Nervous System Disorders

Diseases of the central nervous system are frequently associated with disturbances in sodium concentration. Patients with diverse lesions, such as surgical or traumatic damage to the brain, encephalitis, brain abscess, brain tumors, Guillain-Barré syndrome, bulbar poliomyelitis, cerebrovascular accidents, tumors of the fourth ventricle, subdural hematomas, and meningitis, may present with hyponatremia. Most hyponatremia in this setting is associated with normal total body sodium, with minimal or no negative sodium balance. A decrease in serum sodium is almost entirely the result of retention of water.

The diagnosis of a *syndrome of inappropriate antidiuretic hormone* (SIADH) is considered in the absence of hypovolemia, edema, endocrine dysfunction (including primary and secondary adrenal insufficiency and hypothyroidism), renal failure, and drugs impairing water excretion. Along with central nervous system disorders such as those mentioned and neonatal hypoxia or hydrocephalus, this syndrome is also found in patients with pulmonary disorders, including pneumonia, tuberculosis, and asthma; those on positive-pressure ventilation; and in those with certain carcinomas. The diagnosis is established by measuring inappropriate secretion of ADH under hypotonic conditions and represents a defect in osmoregulation of vasopressin. Patients with this syndrome generally have a concentrated urine despite the presence of hyponatremia and a urinary sodium concentration greater than 20 mEq/L.

Treatment of acute symptomatic hyponatremia should be prompt and use hypertonic saline in combination with furosemide to enhance free water excretion. Chronic, asymptomatic hyponatremia is best managed conservatively by water restriction to allow a gradual increase of serum sodium over 24–48 hr. Occasionally, an individual with a central nervous system lesion has hyponatremia associated with true salt wasting. In this situation, there are signs of volume depletion, including weight loss, signs of dehydration, hypotension, and a diminished GFR with azotemia. This situation requires the appropriate administration of salt to restore volume status.

56.7 Perioperative Fluids

Preoperatively, preparing a patient having no pre-existing deficit or in whom the deficit has been repaired consists mainly of supplying adequate carbohydrate for sustenance and sparing of protein breakdown. The usual maintenance requirements of water and electrolytes are appropriate. Young infants who are not vomiting should receive carbohydrate and sodium chloride mixtures by mouth until 3 hr before the operation. Such fluids are readily absorbed from the gastrointestinal tract. Preparing the newborn involves certain unique hazards. Deficits of water and electrolytes from vomiting or from stasis caused by intestinal obstruction should be replaced before operating. In cases of intestinal obstruction, conjugated bilirubin may be deglucuronidated by intestinal enzymes; enterohepatic circulation of unconjugated bilirubin can then lead to high serum levels and kernicterus. Hypoprothrombinemia also should be prevented by administering 1 mg of vitamin K_1 oxide.

During surgery, blood, plasma, saline, or other volume expanders may be given if blood loss, tissue trauma, third spacing, or excessive evaporative loss occurs. The magnitude of such losses is best judged by the experienced surgeon as he or she operates. *The most common error in administering parenteral fluid during and after surgery is excessive administration,* particularly of dextrose in water. Under most circumstances, little to no potassium need be administered during this time, because extensive tissue trauma or anoxia may result in the release of large amounts of intracellular potassium, with the potential of causing hyperkalemia. If shock occurs, acute renal failure may ensue, impairing the ability to eliminate through the renal route large amounts of released potassium.

Postoperatively, intake should be limited for 24 hr. Thereafter, the usual maintenance therapy is gradually resumed. The water intake should not exceed 85 mL/100 kcal metabolized because of antidiuresis resulting from trauma, circulatory readjustment, or anesthesia unless renal ability to concentrate the urine is limited, as in patients with sickle cell disease, chronic pyelonephritis, or obstructive uropathy. If the intake of water is not limited, whether given parenterally or orally, water intoxication may occur. Maintenance sodium intake may also be low because of the low caloric expenditure during anesthesia and postoperatively. Fluid therapy in the postoperative period largely depends on the complex but anticipated response of the body to trauma through modification of water and sodium excretion and the concomitant occurrence of common or unanticipated complications from surgery. The patient's clinical condition dictates the final fluid and electrolyte requirements that occur as a net effect of these processes.

Some postoperative children have elevated blood ADH levels due to SIADH or to an appropriate response to fluid restriction and resultant volume contraction. If decreasing urine output after surgery is the result of SIADH, the patient is euvolemic, has a normal circulatory status, has stable to slightly increased weight, and has an elevated urinary sodium excretion. If a child has oliguria related to third spacing and true depletion of intravascular volume, there is decreased urinary sodium excretion associated with clinical signs of hypovolemia, such as weight loss, tachycardia, changes in skin turgor and peripheral perfusion, and hypotension.

56.8 Isolated Disturbances in Blood pH and Concentrations of Electrolytes

ACIDOSIS. *Respiratory acidosis,* in which the pH may be markedly lowered, primarily as a result of retention of carbon dioxide, may be seen with severe respiratory insufficiency, with respiratory distress syndrome in the newborn infant, and in patients receiving assisted ventilation for any reason who may be inadequately ventilated or have airway blockage. Acute respiratory acidosis may also be a manifestation of child abuse and be associated with strangulation. Mild metabolic acidosis may coexist because hypoxia leads to the accumulation of lactic and other organic acids in the extracellular fluid (see chapter 53).

Measurements of blood pH and gases should guide the correction of acidosis. The appropriate treatment is to improve ventilation by assisting respiration rather than by administering sodium bicarbonate, which may produce hyperosmolality and cardiac failure.

Metabolic acidosis, which can result from renal tubular acidosis, renal insufficiency, or from accumulation of organic acids, may require the administration of alkali, especially if symptoms are evident. In lactic acidosis, in glycogen disorders, or in circulatory insufficiency and hypoxia, sodium lactate may not be adequately metabolized; in these situations, sodium bicarbonate is the preferred agent. The usual initial dose is 1–2 mEq/kg. However, a more precise estimate of the dosage required is given by the general formula,

$$(C_d - C_a) \times k \times \text{body weight [in kg]} = \text{mEq required}$$

in which C_d and C_a represent, respectively, the serum bicarbonate concentration desired and the one measured, expressed in units of mEq/L; k represents that fraction of the total body weight in which the administered material is apparently (not actually) distributed. The k for bicarbonate or potential bicarbonate approximates 0.5–0.6. Such calculations indicate that 0.5 mL/kg of a molar solution of sodium bicarbonate would raise the serum bicarbonate concentration approximately 1 mEq/L. However, responses to administered bicarbonate vary widely because it may be sequestered in bone or muscle, lost in urine, or undergoing accelerated systemic consumption.

With renal insufficiency, acidosis should be corrected cautiously, because the sodium administered with bicarbonate may result in further expansion of the extracellular fluid volume and lead to hypertension or pulmonary edema. Patients are frequently asymptomatic and have "adjusted" to the acidemic state. Overcorrecting acidosis may lead to tetany if there is an associated hypocalcemia from vitamin D deficiency or phosphate retention. It is rarely necessary to increase serum bicarbonate levels acutely above 15 mEq/L unless the patient is symptomatic. If hyperphosphatemia coexists with acidosis, it should be treated simultaneously with low-phosphate diets and oral calcium carbonate.

Treating acidosis with sodium bicarbonate should always be considered a temporizing measure. Every attempt should be made to treat the underlying cause, such as using glucose and insulin in diabetic ketoacidosis; improving circulation in shock; eliminating salicylates, methanol, or other toxins; and treating underlying sepsis.

Severe metabolic acidosis is a part of cardiovascular shock of various causes (see Chapter 60). Because of differences in pH and P_{CO_2} between arterial and central venous values in this situation, it is often useful to sample from arterial and central venous lines.

ALKALOSIS. Normally, the kidney has an enormous capacity to excrete bicarbonate, and increased amounts of blood bicarbonate are promptly excreted. However, under certain circumstances, *metabolic alkalosis* may develop and be maintained. Typically, it is caused by the administration of excess amounts of alkali, intravenously or orally as in milk alkali syndrome; by the loss of hydrogen ion through emesis from pyloric stenosis or nasogastric drainage; or by acute volume contraction with disproportionate losses of chloride. Severe hypokalemia can result in alkalosis or may perpetuate it (see Chapter 53).

When the plasma bicarbonate level is elevated, respiratory compensation may result in hypoventilation and an increase in P_{CO_2}. Rarely, respiration may be so depressed in infants with severe hypochloremic alkalosis that blood oxygenation is diminished. Severe alkalotic tetany may also occur. In such instances, administering ammonium chloride may effect symptomatic improvement; the dose may be calculated from the general formula presented, with a probable k of 0.2–0.3. Such therapy only relieves symptoms and should not be used in place of correcting the contracted volume of body fluids or administering potassium chloride to repair intracellular deficits.

Metabolic alkalosis associated with volume contraction responds to measures designed to expand volume and replace the chloride and potassium deficits. It occurs in patients with acid-base disorders caused by vomiting, gastric suction, congenital chloride diarrhea, dietary chloride deficiency, or administration of diuretics. In this setting of chloride depletion, urinary chloride concentration is low (≤10 mM/L). A minority of patients are chloride resistant, with urinary chloride concentrations of 15 mM/L or greater because of hyperadrenalism, Bartter syndrome, severe potassium depletion, or licorice ingestion. Potassium repletion, using potassium chloride, not potassium phosphate, and specific therapy directed to the underlying condition are indicated.

Respiratory alkalosis occurs in salicylate intoxication; in various central nervous system diseases, such as severe hypoxic insult, trauma, infection, or tumors; with anxiety or fever; with overventilation on a respirator; and in congestive heart failure, hepatic insufficiency, and gram-negative septicemia. Treatment should be directed at removing the underlying cause, although measures designed to return the P_{CO_2} to normal may be indicated. Acidifying agents such as ammonium chloride are not indicated.

HYPONATREMIA. The serum sodium level is most commonly reduced as a result of true sodium depletion, water intoxication, or a combination of both (see Table 47–2). A low serum sodium level, thought to be a result of redistribution of total body sodium, may be associated with severe illnesses or occur in the terminally ill patient. *Apparent* hyponatremia, an artifact, may be seen in diabetic ketoacidosis when the water content of plasma is reduced by the presence of increased quantities of lipids. This error is avoided by laboratory methods that determine sodium activity rather than concentration.

Patients with a serum sodium level below 120 mEq/L are often symptomatic (e.g., convulsions, shock, lethargy), although this depends in part on the rate of change in serum sodium. Some patients with serum sodium values below 120 mEq/L, achieved over a period of several months, may be relatively asymptomatic.

The treatment of *asymptomatic hyponatremia* depends on its cause. With water overload, fluid restriction is the appropriate measure; the serum sodium level may return rapidly to normal if there is good renal function, but this may take several days or weeks for patients with SIADH. Adding extra salt to the diet or increasing the sodium concentration of parenterally administered fluid often corrects a sodium deficit.

Measuring urinary sodium concentration helps determine the cause of hyponatremia. Patients who have hyponatremia with a true deficit in total body sodium due to renal losses from diuretic excess, salt-losing nephritis, metabolic ketoacidosis, osmotic diuresis, or obstructive uropathy or to extrarenal losses from vomiting, diarrhea, third spacing, burns, or fistulas have clinical signs and symptoms of extracellular fluid volume depletion. Urinary sodium concentration is often greater than 20 mmol/L in renal salt-losing conditions and less than 10 mmol/L in other situations. Correction requires administration of isotonic saline. In patients in whom hyponatremia is caused by an excess of total body water (e.g., hypothyroidism, pain, use of certain drugs, SIADH), urinary sodium concentration usually exceeds 20 mmol/L, and therapy employs water restriction.

In patients who have excesses of sodium and water, edematous states such as nephrotic syndrome, cirrhosis, or cardiac failure, the urinary sodium level is usually less than 10 mmol/L; however, in edematous patients with acute and chronic renal failure, the urinary sodium level may be in excess of 20 mmol/L. Treatment for hyponatremia associated with edema due to excess water and salt retention is usually water intake and salt restriction. Inappropriate treatment may not correct an underlying defect and may be detrimental. In some patients, for example, although there is an excess of total body sodium and water, the effective plasma volume is reduced and may be further compromised by aggressive therapy directed toward correction of the edema. In other patients, administering sodium may result in further expansion of extracellular fluid volume without correcting the serum sodium level or, in the patient with renal insufficiency, may produce or exacerbate hypertension.

In the pediatric population, hyponatremia related to sodium deficiency most commonly occurs in conditions with excess gastrointestinal loss from emesis or diarrhea, excess renal loss through salt-losing nephritis and use of diuretics, or excess cutaneous salt losses with cystic fibrosis. Sodium deficiency may also occur in infants receiving inadequate parenteral sodium, such as very-low-birthweight infants who may have excessive urinary sodium losses. Perhaps the most common cause of hyponatremia due to insufficient dietary intake of sodium in an otherwise well population in the United States occurs with the *WIC syndrome,* named for the government aid program for poor women, infants, and children. These infants are fed diluted formula or water when eligible parents do not receive adequate infant formulas through the WIC food supplementation program. Providing adequate oral salt and water intake corrects this common problem, which should be readily identified by the physician through a careful history. Social service involvement is indicated. Water intoxication conditions not associated with true depletion of total body sodium are most commonly seen with SIADH occurring during central nervous system infections, asthma, the use of ventilatory machines, and in the postoperative period. Psychogenic polydipsia, reported even in toddlers, can mimic hyponatremia.

Treatment of *symptomatic hyponatremia* consists of administering a hypertonic saline solution, calculated according to the formula in the preceding section on acidosis, with k representing serum sodium rather than bicarbonate. Because there is osmotic equilibrium between cells and extracellular water, changes in osmolality are distributed over total body water so that the value for k should be 0.6–0.7 for the child and adolescent and 0.7–0.8 for the newborn or premature infant. A dose of 12 mL/kg of body weight of 3% sodium chloride solution (6 mEq sodium/kg) usually raises the serum sodium level by approximately 10 mEq/L. Rapid correction of hyponatremia may be associated with myelinolysis of the central nervous system in adults; there are few data regarding the occurrence and prevalence of this problem in children. The initial rapid therapeutic increase in the serum sodium level should only be to a value of about 125 mEq/L and only in the symptomatic individual. Subsequent elevation of serum sodium concentration should be effected in small increments over several hours. Hypernatremia should be avoided.

HYPERNATREMIA. Hypernatremia (see Table 47–1) may result from faulty preparation of infant formulas, as with the use of condensed instead of evaporated milk or heaped rather than level measures of milk powder. These errors increase the solute load excreted by the kidney relative to the amount of water provided and result in an osmotic diuresis and negative water balance.

Salt poisoning may occur through the accidental ingestion of excessive amounts of sodium chloride (e.g., table salt, sea water) by a child or the ingestion of accidental substitution of salt for sugar. This occurs with sufficient frequency in private homes and institutions to justify the routine use of liquid sugars in infant feeding. Hypernatremia may also result from the intentional salt poisoning of a child or withholding water and may be a manifestation of Münchausen by proxy syndrome (Chapter 38).

The excessive intake of sodium is accompanied by increases in total body sodium and in the volume of extracellular water. Severe acidosis results from a shift of organic acids and free hydrogen ions to extracellular fluid. With the shift of water from brain cells, distention of cerebral vessels occurs, leading to subdural, subarachnoid, and intracerebral hemorrhage. The complications and residual injury of salt poisoning are similar to, but may be more severe than, those seen with hypernatremic dehydration. Hypernatremia may also be seen in infants with high fever, without access to water, with excessive administration of sodium in parenteral fluids, and with inadequate availability of free water. The latter is not uncommon in the very-low-birthweight infant with large free water needs because of huge insensible water losses.

Hypernatremia is associated with a high mortality rate, especially if the serum sodium concentration exceeds 158 mEq/L. Treatment is directed toward the rapid removal of excess sodium from the body. Intravenous fluids should consist of glucose in water, potassium acetate, and calcium as needed. In patients with salt poisoning, *peritoneal dialysis* with glucose solutions can remove large quantities of sodium and correct hyperosmolality without the danger of pulmonary edema and heart failure. Approximately 30–45 mL/kg of a commercial dialysis solution containing 4.25% glucose can be injected intraperitoneally for severe hypernatremia (i.e., serum sodium concentration >200 mEq/L) and withdrawn 1 hr later. As the concentration of sodium in the serum falls, subsequent dialysis may be carried out using a solution with 1.5% glucose to prevent removing too much water and dehydrating the patient. Exchange transfusion is not a substitute for dialysis, because enormous quantities of blood are required to effect a change in the osmolality of total body water. Phenobarbital should be administered to prevent or control seizures. Digitalization may be necessary to treat heart failure.

HYPOKALEMIA. Disturbances in the potassium concentration occurring without changes in volume of body fluids have been described in primary hyperaldosteronism and in Bartter and Gitelman syndromes. Large amounts of potassium are lost in the urine, resulting in low serum potassium and high serum bicarbonate concentrations. In congenital alkalosis of gastrointestinal origin, large amounts of potassium and chloride are lost in the stools. Using thiazide and loop diuretics (e.g., ethacrynic acid, furosemide) causes kaliuresis and natriuresis; prolonged use may result in significant potassium loss and hypokalemia. Several drugs, including penicillin, aminoglycosides, amphotericin, and antitumor drugs such as cisplatin, have been associated with a significant renal potassium loss and hypokalemia.

Severe hypokalemia may result in weakness of skeletal muscles, decreased peristalsis, ileus, and an inability of the kidney to concentrate urine. Patients may present with frank paralysis and significant respiratory difficulty (see Chapter 388 for electrocardiographic changes). Prolonged hypokalemia results in characteristic pathologic changes in the kidney and decreased function, which may persist even after potassium repletion.

Treatment consists of administration of adequate amounts of potassium (usually up to 3 mEq/kg/24 hr); in Bartter syndrome or other causes of hypokalemia associated with massive urinary losses, 10 mEq/kg or more may have to be given orally. Indomethacin has proved helpful in Bartter syndrome. Gitelman's syndrome is treated with $MgCl_2$ alone.

HYPERKALEMIA. Marked elevation of the serum potassium level results in ventricular fibrillation and death. Levels above 6.5 mEq/L should be treated promptly, although such levels are often reasonably well tolerated by newborns. The presence or absence of electrocardiographic changes may be helpful in deciding when to initiate therapy (see Chapter 388). The possibility of oral or parenterally administered excessive amounts of potassium should be considered and all potassium intake discontinued. Occult sources of potassium such as antibiotics and total parenteral nutrition may go unrecognized.

Rapid intravenous administration of sodium bicarbonate (1–3 mEq/kg) or glucose and insulin (0.5–1 g of glucose/kg with 1 unit crystalline insulin/3 g of glucose) results in the movement of potassium into cells and lowers the serum potassium level. Intravenous calcium gluconate (up to 0.5 mL of a 10% solution/kg given slowly over several minutes) counters the cardiac toxicity of potassium, but the electrocardiogram should be monitored while it is being administered. None of these measures removes significant quantities of potassium from the patient. They are temporizing measures until a negative potassium balance can be established by the use of ion exchange resins, such as Kayexalate (1 g/kg/24 hr, divided into oral or rectal doses every 6–12 hr) or by hemodialysis or peritoneal dialysis.

HYPOCALCEMIA AND HYPERCALCEMIA. These topics are discussed in Chapters 43, 50, 56, and 92.

HYPOMAGNESEMIA. The importance of magnesium in intravenous therapy is reviewed in Chapters 51 and 56. The only definitive symptom complex associated with hypomagnesemia (i.e., serum magnesium level <1.3 mEq/L) is that of latent or manifest tetany. Convulsions, muscular twitching, disorientation, athetoid movements, carpopedal spasm, and hyper-reactivity to mechanical and auditory stimulation have been observed. Lowered serum concentrations and whole body deficits of magnesium are found in cases of chronic diarrhea or vomiting, sprue, celiac disease, prolonged parenteral fluid therapy with low magnesium composition, hyperaldosteronism, Gitelman syndrome, and increased urinary losses of magnesium from nephrotoxic medications. Low serum magnesium levels have been observed in infantile tetany, presumably because of transient hypoparathyroidism.

The intramuscular injection of 0.1 mL of a 24% solution of $MgSO_4 \cdot 7\ H_2O$ (0.2 mEq/kg) repeated every 6 hr for three or four doses produces symptomatic and biochemical improvement. Adding 3 mEq/L of magnesium to maintenance fluids for patients requiring long-term therapy may decrease the chance of serious deficiency (see Chapters 51 and 56). *Gitelman syndrome,* frequently confused with Bartter syndrome, is seen in older children and young adults. The characteristic features are hypokalemia, occasional tetany, hypomagnesemia, hypocalciuria, and normal growth.

HYPERMAGNESEMIA. Levels of serum magnesium higher than 10 mEq/L are accompanied by drowsiness and occasionally produce coma. Such levels rarely occur in the absence of renal failure. Deep tendon reflexes may also be abolished, and respiratory depression may occur at higher concentrations. Disturbances in atrioventricular and intraventricular conduction may be detected at a level of 5 mEq/L. Acute renal failure and Addison disease are accompanied by significantly elevated serum magnesium levels. Iatrogenic poisoning can result from using magnesium in treating hypertension or toxemia of pregnancy; deaths have been reported from using magnesium sulfate enemas in megacolon and from orally administering it for purging.

Intravenously administering calcium gluconate rapidly reverses the depressant effects of hypermagnesemia and the associated cardiac abnormalities.

AAP Committee on Nutrition: Use of oral fluid therapy and posttreatment feeding following enteritis in children in a developed country. Pediatrics 75:358, 1985.

Brenner BM, Rector FC Jr (eds): The Kidney. Philadelphia, WB Saunders, 1991.

Darrow DC, Pratt EL: Fluid therapy: relation to tissue composition and expenditure of water and electrolyte. JAMA 154:365, 1950.
European Society of Paediatric Gastroenterology and Nutrition Working Group: Recommendation for composition of oral rehydration for the children of Europe. J Pediatr Gastroenterol Nutr 14:113, 1992.
Finberg L, Kravath R, Hellerstein S, Saenger P (eds): Water and Electrolytes in Pediatrics. Philadelphia, WB Saunders, 1993.
Furth S, Oski FA: Hyponatremia and water intoxication. Am J Dis Child 147:932, 1993.
Gore SM, Fontaine O, Pierce NF: Impact of rice based oral rehydration solution on stool output and duration of diarrhea: meta-analysis of 13 clinical trials. Br Med J 304:287, 1992.
Hellerstein S: Fluid and electrolytes: clinical aspects. Pediatr Rev 14:103, 1993.
Holliday MA, Segar WE. The maintenance need for water in parenteral fluid therapy. Pediatrics 19:823, 1957.
Keating JP, Schears GH, Dodge PR: Oral water intoxication in infants: an American epidemic. Am J Dis Child 145:985, 1991.
Levine MM, Pizarro D: Advances in therapy of diarrhea dehydration: oral rehydration. Adv Pediatr 31:207, 1984.
Lipschitz CH, Carrazza F: Effect of formula carbohydrate concentration on tolerance and macronutrient absorption in infants with severe chronic diarrhea. J Pediatr 117:378, 1990.
Maxwell MH, Kleeman CR, Narins RG (eds): Clinical Disorders of Fluid and Electrolyte Metabolism. New York, McGraw-Hill, 1987.
Meyers A: Fluid and electrolyte therapy for children. Curr Opinion Pediatr 6:303, 1994.
Pizarro D, Posada G, Sandi L, et al: Rice-based oral electrolyte solutions for the management of infantile diarrhea. N Engl J Med 324:517, 1991.
Prestridge LL, Schanler RJ, Shulman RJ, et al: Effect of parenteral calcium and phosphorous therapy on mineral retention and bone mineral content in very low birthweight infants. J Pediatr 122:761, 1993.
Santosham M, Daum RS, Dillman L, et al: Oral rehydration therapy of infantile diarrhea: a controlled study of well-nourished children hospitalized in the United States and Panama. N Engl J Med 306:1070, 1982.
Sharifi J, Ghavami F, Nowrouzi Z, et al: Oral versus intravenous rehydration therapy in severe gastroenteritis. Arch Dis Child 60:856, 1985.
Schrier RW (ed): Renal and Electrolyte Disorders. Boston, Little, Brown & Company, 1992.
Stefano JL, Norman ME, Morales MC, et al: Decreased erythrocyte NA^+, K^+ ATPase activity associated with cellular potassium loss in extremely low birthweight infants with nonoliguric hyperkalemia. J Pediatr 122:276, 1993.
Vesikari T, Isolauri E, Baer M: A comparative trial of rapid oral and intravenous rehydration in acute diarrhoea. Acta Paediatr Scand 76:300, 1987.

56.9 Tetany

Tetany, the state of hyperexcitability of the central and peripheral nervous systems, results from abnormal concentrations of ions in the fluid bathing nerve cells. These abnormalities may include decreases of H^+ (alkalosis), Ca^{2+}, or Mg^{2+}. A decrease in H^+ may precipitate tetany when concentrations of Ca^{2+} or Mg^{2+} may otherwise lie above the threshold for manifest tetany. A decreased K^+ can prevent tetany despite low Ca^{2+} concentrations; a rising K^+ can precipitate tetany in a patient with low Ca^{2+}. Hypomagnesemic tetany can occur despite a reduction of K^+ concentration. A range of ionic concentrations exists at which tetany can be latent or manifest.

The serum calcium level, as usually measured, includes ionized calcium (Ca^{2+}) and undissociated calcium proteinate; albumin is the chief serum protein to complex with calcium. Ionized calcium can be measured, but the procedure is not available in all clinical laboratories. At normal concentrations of serum albumin, about 40–50% of the total calcium is ionized (4.0–5.2 mg/dL). When the serum albumin level is reduced, total serum calcium is decreased without necessarily a decrease in Ca^{2+}; a rule of thumb states that with each decrease of 1 g/dL of albumin, a decrease of 0.8 mg/dL of calcium results. A nephrotic child with a serum albumin level of 1 g/dL may be expected to have a total serum calcium concentration of 7.5–8.0 mg/dL without a reduction of Ca^{2+}.

At physiologic concentrations of H^+ and K^+, tetany may develop at Ca^{2+} concentrations of less than 3.0 mg/dL. Tetany usually is manifested at Ca^{2+} concentrations less than 2.5 mg/dL. At normal concentrations of serum albumin, these levels correspond to total serum calcium concentrations of approximately 7 mg/dL and 5 mg/dL, respectively.

The normal range of magnesium in serum is 1.6–2.6 mg/dL, of which about 75% is Mg^{2+}. Total serum magnesium reduced to less than 1.0 mg/dL may be associated with hyperexcitability of the nervous system.

MANIFEST TETANY. The classic signs of peripheral hyperexcitability of motor nerves are spasms of the muscles of the wrists and ankles (i.e., carpopedal spasm) and of the vocal cords (i.e., laryngospasm). In *carpopedal spasm* the wrists are flexed, the fingers extended, the thumbs adducted over the palms, and the feet extended and adducted. These muscular spasms can be quite painful. *Laryngospasm* causes inspiratory obstruction accompanied by a high-pitched inspiratory crow, which may be confused with asthma or infectious laryngotracheitis; apnea may result. Recurrent croup in an afebrile child without an upper respiratory infection should alert the clinician to the possibility of tetany. The sensory manifestations are paresthesias, particularly numbness and tingling of the hands and feet. Motor excitability of the central nervous system may be manifested by brief but recurrent convulsions, which are usually generalized but may be localized to one side of the body. Between seizures, the patient may be apparently conscious, but after a prolonged series of convulsions, a postictal state may result. In young infants, convulsions are frequently the only evidence of hyperexcitability of the nervous system.

LATENT TETANY. This is the condition in which ischemia or mechanical or electrical stimulation of motor nerves is required to produce the motor response characteristic of tetany. Carpopedal spasm may be induced in latent tetany through the production of ischemia of the motor nerves by reducing the arterial blood supply with a tourniquet (i.e., *Trousseau sign*); a blood pressure cuff on the arm is inflated above the systolic blood pressure for 3 min. Motor nerve impulses can be elicited by mechanical tapping, but under normal physiologic conditions, this is not possible. The facial nerve can be stimulated by tapping anterior to the external auditory meatus. Contraction of the orbicularis oris occurs with a twitch of the upper lip or entire mouth (i.e., *Chvostek sign*). The peroneal nerve can be stimulated by tapping the place where it passes over the head of the fibula; a positive *peroneal sign* is dorsiflexion and abduction of the foot.

The motor nerves can also be stimulated electrically. The *Erb sign* is a positive response of motor nerves to electrical stimulation by galvanic currents of amperage less than that required for their stimulation under normal physiologic conditions.

Another manifestation of reduced Ca^{2+} concentration is a prolonged Q-T interval for a given heart rate on the electrocardiogram. The normal Q-T interval, calculated as

$$QT_c = \frac{\text{Measured QT (sec)}}{\sqrt{\text{R-R interval (sec)}}}$$

is <0.45 in infants and <0.425 in adolescents. QT_c is the corrected Q-T interval.

ALKALOTIC TETANY. Although rare in infants and young children, alkalotic tetany can be induced through spontaneous overventilation, producing respiratory alkalosis; such hyperventilation is most often of psychogenic origin. The treatment of alkalotic tetany resulting from spontaneous hyperventilation is to have the patient rebreathe into a bag or a balloon to increase the P_{CO_2}. In patients with low Ca^{2+} concentrations, tetany may be precipitated by overventilation or by a metabolic alkalosis after the administration of sodium bicarbonate. The metabolic alkalosis resulting from a loss of gastric juice caused by pyloric obstruction is rarely associated with tetany. Alkalotic tetany has occurred in patients with renal disease who have been protected by concurrent metabolic acidosis or hypokalemia from the consequences of a low Ca^{2+} concentration. Correcting acidosis can cause tetany and convulsions; this may occur quite accidentally when the noncompliant patient is given in-hospital medications presumed to be taken at home and well tolerated.

HYPOCALCEMIC TETANY. Disorders of Parathyroid Function. The most common disorder of parathyroid function is transient physiologic hypoparathyroidism of the newborn infant, sometimes referred to as *neonatal hypocalcemia*. Clinically, these infants can be separated into two groups, one group with hypocalcemia during the first 72 hr of life, usually before achieving a significant oral intake of milk, and a second group in which hypocalcemia results from high phosphate load, which develops only after receiving cow's milk for several days. The onset of symptoms in the second group occurs most commonly during the first 5–10 days of life; clinical manifestations have occasionally appeared as late as 6 wk of age. Both forms presumably result from physiologically underactive parathyroid glands that fail to respond normally to low calcium concentrations. Serum calcium values correlate directly with gestational age, and less-mature infants have a greater chance of developing hypocalcemia.

In addition to a relative lack of parathyroid hormone output in the newborn period, a partial refractoriness of the target cells to parathyroid hormone may exist. Moreover, excessive secretion of thyrocalcitonin may be a major contributing factor in persistent hypocalcemia of premature infants, particularly those stressed by anoxia. The low-birthweight infant whose mother has had an inadequate intake of vitamin D and little exposure to sunshine also has a low plasma concentration of 25-hydroxyvitamin D, the deficiency of which is associated with relative refractoriness to parathyroid hormone.

The relative hypoparathyroidism of the newborn has been attributed to the increased serum calcium level of the fetus, which reflects a calcium gradient across the placenta. This inhibition of the fetal parathyroids by calcium ions may be augmented by mild maternal hyperparathyroidism. Physiologic hyperparathyroidism, indicated by increased parathyroid hormone levels during pregnancy, may occur more intensely in diabetic women. Occasional cases of infant transient hypoparathyroidism have been associated with maternal clinical hyperparathyroidism.

EARLY HYPOCALCEMIA. The infants at greatest risk are low-birthweight infants, especially those with intrauterine growth retardation, infants born of diabetic mothers, and infants who have been subjected to prolonged, difficult deliveries (see Chapters 92 and 93). Early hypocalcemia occasionally may be seen in infants of mothers with adenomas or in infants with familial hypoparathyroidism. Calcium intake may be decreased because of the infant's small size or illness, and endogenous phosphate levels may be increased from catabolism. The incidence of hypocalcemia in prematurely born infants is extremely high, particularly in those with respiratory distress and those who have received intravenous sodium bicarbonate. Evaluating the role of hypocalcemia in the morbidity and mortality of such infants is difficult. Although hypocalcemia should be suspected as a possible cause of convulsions, it can be diagnosed only by determining serum concentrations of calcium ions.

Asymptomatic hypocalcemia of premature infants usually resolves spontaneously. However, when possible, oral calcium gluconate should be given, because it usually obviates the subsequent need for intravenous therapy and its attendant complications.

Treatment of clinical manifestations requires the intravenous injection of a 10% solution of calcium gluconate in a dose of about 2 mL/kg (18 mg Ca/kg), which must be given slowly while monitoring the cardiac rate for bradycardia; blood containing excessive calcium concentration that reaches the right atrium may inhibit the rhythmic electrical activity of the sinus node, causing cardiac arrest. Tissue necrosis and calcification may occur if this solution extravasates or is given intramuscularly. Intravenous sites should be carefully watched. The intravenous dose of calcium gluconate can be repeated at 6- to 8-hr intervals until calcium homeostasis becomes stable, or the calcium gluconate (50–75 mg elemental Ca/kg/24 hr) can be added to a constant intravenous infusion. Parenteral calcium should be administered carefully, while monitoring serum ionized calcium levels and urinary calcium levels. Because of decreased protein-bound calcium in hypoalbuminemic infants, parenteral calcium may cause elevations in Ca^{2+} and hypercalciuria associated with nephrocalcinosis.

Administering 1,25-dihydroxyvitamin D_3 during the first day of life to prematurely born infants at risk for hypocalcemia has either successfully prevented or reduced the severity and duration of hypocalcemia, but it is not recommended for routine prevention. When hypomagnesemia occurs with early neonatal tetany, it is usually mild and transient; occasionally, it requires treatment before the hypocalcemia responds to therapy. Calcium gluconate or calcium lactate also may be added to the feeding at the same time, as described later. There may be a gradual return to normal calcium levels after 1–3 days. Oral calcium should be continued for about 1 wk.

LATE HYPOCALCEMIA. After a feeding of high-phosphate milk, tetany can occur in full-term and prematurely born infants and in infants whose clinical histories have been benign. The intake of a high-phosphate food, such as cow's milk, in a relatively large volume leads to an elevated serum phosphate level because of relatively high tubular reabsorption of phosphate and the physiologically low GFR of the newborn. The elevated serum phosphate level depresses the serum calcium level through deposition of calcium phosphate in bone and possibly in other tissues. The normal physiologic response is an increased output of parathyroid hormone, which increases the solubilization of bone mineral and urine phosphate excretion. This restores the normal serum levels of calcium and phosphate. If the infant's parathyroid glands are not yet able to respond by increasing parathyroid hormone, the level of serum calcium progressively falls, and symptomatic hypocalcemia may result.

Clinical Manifestations. The most important presentation of hypocalcemia in infants is convulsions, usually generalized, short, and without loss of consciousness. Carpopedal spasm is not usually seen, and because the Chvostek sign is common in newborn infants, it cannot be interpreted as a sign of tetany. Laryngospasm with cyanosis and apneic episodes may occur. Irritability, muscular twitching, jitteriness, and tremors are common clinical manifestations in the newborn. In addition to the characteristic signs from increased excitability of the nervous system, nonspecific symptoms clinically suggestive of sepsis may also occur, such as poor feeding, vomiting, and lethargy rather than irritability. Serum calcium determinations and other diagnostic studies should be made for infants suspected of having sepsis.

Bradycardia with heart block is rarely noted. A prolonged QT interval on the electrocardiogram suggests hypocalcemia. A serum calcium concentration below 7 mg/dL establishes the diagnosis; a level below 7.5 mg/dL is suggestive. The serum phosphate level is increased, sometimes to 10–12 mg/dL. The blood urea nitrogen or serum creatinine levels are not elevated, differentiating this condition from the hyperphosphatemia of severe renal dysfunction. Normal newborns fed cow's milk have serum phosphate concentrations of 6–8 mg/dL; normal premature infants may have concentrations even higher. Hypomagnesemia may also occur.

A favorable response to administering calcium is insufficient in itself to make the diagnosis, because calcium may act nonspecifically during seizures. Symptoms such as irritability and tremors may subside spontaneously, and convulsions resulting from cerebral edema, anoxia, or injury may recur during the neonatal period. Examination of the spinal fluid is indicated because of the possibility of a convulsion caused by infection or hemorrhage in the central nervous system.

Treatment. Initial treatment of the convulsing infant is intravenous injection of a 10% solution of calcium gluconate (2 mL/kg), with the precautions given previously. The response may be dramatic. After this, specific treatment of late hypocalcemia aims at reducing the serum phosphate level. Because human milk is low in phosphorus, breast-fed infants rarely develop hypocalcemia. Some infant formulas prepared from dialyzed whey of cow's milk are considerable higher in phosphate than human milk.

Phosphate absorption from food can be suppressed by adding a great excess of calcium to the formula, which precipitates as calcium phosphate in the lumen of the gut (e.g., adding calcium lactate or gluconate to the milk feeding to achieve a calcium to phosphorus ratio of 4:1). Calcium lactate powder is preferred, and its addition to milk produces no significant gastrointestinal disturbances. Because calcium lactate is 13% calcium, 770 mg of this salt provides 100 mg of calcium; calcium gluconate is 9% calcium, and 1,100 mg of it provides 100 mg of calcium. A soluble preparation of calcium gluconate (e.g., syrup of Neo-Calglucon), containing 92 mg Ca/tsp, is a less desirable method of adding calcium, because the required amounts may cause diarrhea. Calcium chloride may cause gastric irritation and hyperchloremic acidosis. Because the salt must dissolve in the milk, calcium lactate tablets should not be used; compressed tablets are insoluble even if fragmented.

As treatment decreases the serum phosphorus level, the serum calcium level returns to normal, possibly even rising to hypercalcemic levels. At this point, the calcium supplement is reduced in steps, not stopped abruptly, because the serum phosphorus level may rise precipitously, and the calcium concentration may fall again to tetanic levels. In most infants, restoration of normal calcium homeostasis and presumably normal parathyroid responsiveness occurs in 1–2 wk. In infants with accompanying hypomagnesemia, plasma magnesium levels usually return to normal.

Occasionally, a more prolonged calcium supplementation period is needed, in which case the treatment must be individualized by serial measurements of calcium and phosphate concentrations. If the infant responds poorly to treatment, the calculations should be checked to determine if sufficient calcium is being added, and the feeding should be examined to see if the calcium lactate or gluconate has been dissolving completely. If no errors are found and the therapeutic response is inadequate, the diagnosis of congenital hypoparathyroidism or, in older infants, of vitamin D deficiency or an absorptive or metabolic abnormality of vitamin D should be entertained.

The *prognosis* for early hypocalcemia with seizures depends on the primary disease; infants with late tetany have an excellent prognosis.

Congenital Absence of the Parathyroids. Absent parathyroid glands can occur in association with aplasia of the thymus (i.e., *DiGeorge syndrome*), in combination with abnormalities of the great vessels of the heart, or as an isolated parathyroid aplasia (see Chapter 525). Such patients present with the same symptoms as those of infants with transient physiologic hypoparathyroidism but respond incompletely to the simple treatment outlined previously and have relapsing hypocalcemia, which requires more definitive treatment.

In total parathyroid deficiency, substituting pharmacologic amounts of vitamin D, vitamin D metabolites, or vitamin D analogs for parathyroid hormone is required. Dihydrotachysterol is more potent than vitamin D in correcting hypocalcemia. It is more rapidly inactivated in the body, not stored, and is not as cumulatively toxic as vitamin D. In the young infant, 0.05–0.1 mg of dihydrotachysterol should be given daily and the dose adjusted by determining serum calcium concentrations, which should be returned to levels of about 9–10 mg/dL. The highly active vitamin D metabolite, 1,25-dihydroxyvitamin D_3, is also available, and in doses of 0.25–0.5 μg/24 hr, it is effective in treating hypoparathyroidism. Oral calcium supplements such as calcium glubionate syrup (e.g., Neo-Calglucon) or calcium carbonate tablets (e.g., Tums, Rolaids) are also useful adjunctive therapy. As the child grows, the dosage of either steroid must be increased, as indicated by serum calcium concentrations. Urine calcium to creatinine ratios should be monitored to avoid hypercalciuria (ratio >0.2). Hypoparathyroidism in older children is discussed in Chapter 525.

Hypocalcemia and Tetany Caused by Vitamin D Deficiency or Abnormalities of Vitamin D Metabolism. The onset of vitamin D deficiency tetany usually occurs at 3–6 mo of age, because depletion of the infant's vitamin D stores requires this amount of time. However, an infant born of a vitamin D–deficient mother may develop hypocalcemia from vitamin D deficiency within the first week of life. Tetany and nutritional vitamin D deficiency are now rare, but the latter occasionally develops in a breast-fed infant whose mother, unaware of human milk's vitamin D deficiency, does not provide supplementary vitamin D (see Chapter 45).

Hypocalcemia may also be a result of failure of normal metabolism of vitamin D, which undergoes two hydroxylation steps, first in the liver and then in the kidney, before becoming the metabolically active 1,25-dihydroxyvitamin D_3. Infants with liver disease, such as neonatal hepatitis, cytomegalic inclusion disease, or atresia of the bile ducts, may show manifestations of vitamin D deficiency with hypocalcemia because of failure of the liver to metabolize vitamin D. In atresia of the bile ducts, malabsorption of vitamin D may complicate the problem. Vitamin D deficiency can also result from steatorrhea caused by pancreatic lipase deficiency or by intrinsic intestinal mucosal disorders. Rickets and osteomalacia are associated with the treatment of convulsive disorders by large doses of combined anticonvulsant drugs, principally phenobarbital, diphenylhydantoin, and primidone, which alter the liver's metabolism of vitamin D. Diphenylhydantoin also inhibits intestinal transport of calcium, and patients may present with hypocalcemia and skeletal changes. Vitamin D–dependent rickets type I is caused by a deficiency of 1α-hydroxylase, which converts 25-hydroxyvitamin D to 1,25-dihydroxyvitamin D_3. Levels of the latter are low. Vitamin D–dependent rickets type II is an autosomal recessive condition in which there is target organ resistance to 1,25-dihydroxyvitamin D_3 and early onset of rickets and hypocalcemia. It is associated with elevated levels of parathyroid hormone and 1,25-dihydroxyvitamin D_3.

Initially, patients with tetany resulting from vitamin D deficiency or failure of normal metabolism of vitamin D can be symptomatically relieved by intravenous injections of 2 mL/kg of a 10% solution of calcium gluconate, with the usual precautionary monitoring of the heart rate to prevent a too-rapid injection. Treatment of vitamin D deficiency is achieved with vitamin D (2,000–4,000 units or 50–100 μg daily). Vitamin D–dependent rickets type I is treated with 2–8 μg/24 hr of 1α-hydroxyvitamin D_3 or 1–4 μg/24 hr of 1,25-dihydroxyvitamin D_3. The daily dosage is halved after radiologic confirmation of healing. Vitamin D–dependent rickets type II responds to high dosages of vitamin D (0.5–5.0 mg/24 hr) or 1α-hydroxyvitamin D_3 or 1,25-dihydroxyvitamin D_3 (5–50 μg/24 hr). An alternative therapy for true vitamin D deficiency is 10,000 units of vitamin D daily for 3 wk or a highly concentrated vitamin D preparation, given in amounts adequate to achieve a rapid physiologic effect (e.g., 600,000 units of vitamin D in a single dose) or divided into several doses over a 24-hr period. Propylene glycol (Drisdol) is unsuitable for this type of therapy, because the large volume of propylene glycol is a depressant. The hypocalcemia of hepatic disorders responds to larger doses of vitamin D; more precise treatment with 25-hydroxyvitamin D_3 or 1,25-dihydroxyvitamin D is possible. Treatment must be individualized and patients closely monitored to avoid vitamin D intoxication (see Chapter 45).

HYPOMAGNESEMIC TETANY. Hypomagnesemia has reportedly caused tetany associated with low or normal serum calcium concentrations. In transient physiologic hypoparathyroidism of the newborn, low serum magnesium concentrations may accompany the hyperphosphatemia and hypocalcemia. This hypomagnesemia usually responds to treatment directed at reducing the serum phosphate concentration. Occasionally, newborn infants with hypomagnesemia require specific magnesium therapy: intramuscular injection with 0.2 mL/kg of a 50% solution of $MgSO_4 \cdot 7\,H_2O$ (i.e., 25% solution of $MgSO_4$). This treatment raises serum magnesium concentrations into the normal range within 1 hr and should maintain adequate concentrations for several hours. Often, no further therapy is needed. The mechanism of this transient hypomagnesemia is not understood.

Hypomagnesemic tetany and convulsions beyond the newborn period may result from prolonged parenteral nutrition with magnesium-free solutions or congenital disorders of magnesium transport, causing a failure of absorption of dietary magnesium or failure of tubular reabsorption of magnesium with excessive urinary loss. In Bartter and Gitelman syndromes, hypomagnesemia, hypokalemia, and tetany can occur secondary to a renal tubular dysfunction. Intestinal malabsorption of magnesium can result from acquired intestinal injury, such as inflammatory bowel disease or resection of small intestine, and rarely, in male infants, be caused by a specific malabsorption of magnesium. Renal loss of magnesium may be secondary to nephropathy caused by aminoglycosides or cisplatin. Magnesium depletion, whatever the pathogenesis, can be associated with hypocalcemia, because magnesium is needed for the secretion of parathyroid hormone and responsiveness of target tissues to the hormone. Treatment requires magnesium administered intramuscularly (described earlier), intravenously (2–10 mL/kg of 1% magnesium sulfate solution) by slow infusion, or orally in the form of magnesium salts, such as the chloride, gluconate, or citrate forms (24–48 mg/kg/24 hr; see Chapter 51).

Aarskog D, Harrison H: Disorders of calcium, phosphate, PTH and vitamin D. *In:* Kappy M, Blizzard R, Migeon C (eds): The Diagnosis and Treatment of Endocrine Disorders in Childhood and Adolescence. Springfield, IL, Charles C Thomas, 1994.

Booth BE, Johanson A: Hypomagnesemia due to renal tubular defect in reabsorption of magnesium. J Pediatr 84:350, 1974.

Broner CW, Stidham GL, Westenkirchner DF, et al: A prospective, randomized, double blind comparison of calcium chloride and calcium gluconate therapies for hypocalcemia in critically ill children. J Pediatr 117:986, 1990.

Brown DR, Steranka BH, Taylor FH: Treatment of early-onset neonatal hypocalcemia. Am J Dis Child 135:24, 1981.

Colletti RP, Pan MW, Smith EWP, et al: Detection of hypocalcemia in susceptible neonates. The Q-oTc interval. N Engl J Med 290:931, 1974.

David L, Glorieux FM, Salle BL, et al: Human Neonatal Hypocalcemia. *In:* Holick MF, Anast CS, Gray TK (eds): Perinatal Calcium and Phosphorus Metabolism. Amsterdam, Elsevier Science Publishers, 1983, p. 351.

Ezzedeen F, Adelman RD, Ahlfors CE: Renal calcification in preterm infants: pathophysiology and long-term sequelae. J Pediatr 113:532, 1988.

Fraher LJ, Karmali R, Hinde FRJ, et al: Vitamin D–dependent rickets type II: extreme end organ resistance to 1,25-dihydroxyvitamin D_3 in a patient without alopecia. Eur J Pediatr 145:389, 1986.

Harrison HE, Harrison HC: Disorders of Calcium and Phosphate Metabolism in Childhood and Adolescence. Philadelphia, WB Saunders, 1979.

Markestad T, Halvorsen S, Halvorsen K, et al: Plasma concentrations of vitamin D metabolites before and during treatment of vitamin D deficiency rickets in children. Acta Paediatr Scand 73:225, 1984.

Paunier L, Raddle IC, Kooh SW, et al: Primary hypomagnesemia with secondary hypocalcemia in an infant. Pediatrics 41:385, 1968.

Tsang RC, Light IJ, Sutherland JM, et al: Possible pathogenetic factors in neonatal hypocalcemia of prematurity. J Pediatr 82:423, 1973.

PART VIII

The Acutely Ill Child

CHAPTER 57

Evaluation of the Sick Child in the Office and Clinic

Paul L. McCarthy

Many of the approaches to clinical data gathering presented for the well child evaluation in Chapter 7 are also applicable to the sick child evaluation. There are a number of reasons for a sick child visit but most visits are made because of acute intercurrent infections, and often the child is febrile.

When evaluating an acutely ill, febrile child, the pediatrician must be aware of statistics about the occurrence of serious illness, because one of the major goals of the sick child visit is to identify the seriously ill child who requires the most vigorous therapeutic intervention. The risk among children with acute febrile illnesses for serious illnesses and the cause of the serious illness vary depending on the child's age. In the first 3 mo of life, because of an immature immunologic system, the infant is more susceptible to sepsis and meningitis caused by group B streptococcus and gram-negative organisms. Additionally, urinary tract infections are seen more commonly in male infants; these infants more often have an underlying anatomic abnormality of the urinary tract than older children with urinary tract infections. As the infant matures beyond 3 mo, the bacterial pathogens that usually cause sepsis and meningitis are *Haemophilus influenzae* type b, *Neisseria meningitides*, and *Streptococcus pneumoniae*. Urinary tract infections are seen more commonly in females than males. As the child matures, immunity is developed to the bacterial pathogens common during the 1st 3–4 yr of life. At this time, *N. meningitides* becomes the leading cause of bacterial meningitis. In children older than 36 mo, pharyngitis caused by group A streptococcus is a common bacterial infection. *Mycoplasma pneumoniae* assumes increasing importance as a cause for pulmonary infiltrates in children beyond 5 yr of age. The diagnoses of serious illnesses documented in 996 children in the first 3 yr of life who presented consecutively with fever and acute illnesses are shown in Table 57–1. These children were seen in a university hospital and in private practices.

Identifying the acutely ill child with a serious illness is accomplished by careful observation, history, physical examination, appreciation of age and temperature as risk factors, and the judicious use of screening laboratory tests. Based on these data, the physician can make informed decisions about the need for more definitive laboratory tests (e.g., urine culture), therapy, and the advisability of hospital admission. Observation, history, and physical examination are discussed separately, but these components are integrated in the sick child evaluation, e.g., as the child is being observed, historical data are gathered. History taking and observational assessment often continue as the physical examination is performed. If, for example, abdominal tenderness is found on examination, then additional history about blood in the stool, cramping abdominal pain, and vomiting may be sought.

Observation is a key factor in the evaluation of children with acute problems for the possibility of a serious illness. The child should be observed for specific evidence of a serious illness, such as grunting, which might indicate pneumonia or sepsis, or a bulging fontanelle, which might indicate bacterial meningitis. *Most observational data that the pediatrician gathers during an acute illness should focus, however, on assessing the child's response to stimuli.* How does the child's crying respond to parents' comforting? If the child is sleeping, how quickly does the child awaken with a stimulus? Does the child smile when the examiner interacts with the child? As noted in Chapter 7, assessing responses to stimuli—and often providing those stimuli—requires a knowledge of normal responses for different age groups, the manner in which those normal responses are elicited, and to what degree a response might be impaired.

Sometimes the manner in which the child responds to stimuli is readily apparent—for example, the child vocalizes and smiles as the examiner enters the room. At other times, more effort and more stimuli are needed to cause the child to act in a more normal manner. Often, the fussing, irritable child begins to look around and focus on the examiner when held and walked by the parent. This normal visual behavior is an important indicator of well-being. Thus, during observation, the pediatrician must be both clinically and developmentally oriented.

Six observation items and their scales (the Acute Illness Observation Scales) that have reliably and validly identified serious illness in febrile children are shown in Figure 57–1. The normal point is scored as 1, moderate impairment as 3, and severe impairment as 5. The best possible score is 6 items $\times$ 1 = 6; the worst score is 6 items $\times$ 5 = 30. The chance of serious illness is 1–2% if the total score is $\leq$10; if the score is $>$10, the risk of serious illness increases at least 10-fold. It is not clear whether these scales can be used in the first 2–3 mo of life, because infants may not have developed the skills required to score some of these items.

TABLE 57–1 Diagnosis of Serious Illnesses During 996 Episodes of Acute Infectious Illness in Febrile Children Younger than 36 Mo*

Diagnosis	Cases No.	Cases %
Bacterial meningitis	9	0.9
Aseptic meningitis	12	1.2
Pneumonia	30	3.0
Bacteremia	10	1.0
Focal soft-tissue infection	10	1.0
Urinary tract infection	8	0.8
Bacterial diarrhea	1	0.1
Abnormal electrolytes, abnormal blood gases	9	0.9
Total	89	8.9

**From McCarthy PL: Acute infectious illness in children. Comp Ther 14:51, 1988.*

6 OBSERVATION ITEMS AND THEIR SCALES

(PLEASE CHECK BOXES THAT DESCRIBE YOUR CHILD'S APPEARANCE AND BEHAVIOR)

OBSERVATION ITEM	NORMAL	MODERATE IMPAIRMENT	SEVERE IMPAIRMENT
1. **QUALITY OF CRY**	STRONG WITH NORMAL TONE ☐ *OR* CONTENT AND NOT CRYING ☐	WHIMPERING ☐ *OR* SOBBING ☐	WEAK ☐ *OR* MOANING ☐ *OR* HIGH PITCHED ☐
2. **REACTION TO PARENT STIMULATION** (Effect on crying when held, patted on back, jiggled on lap, or carried)	CRIES BRIEFLY, THEN STOPS ☐ *OR* CONTENT AND NOT CRYING ☐	CRIES OFF AND ON ☐	CONTINUAL CRY ☐ *OR* HARDLY RESPONDS ☐
3. **STATE VARIATION** (Going from awake to asleep or asleep to awake)	IF AWAKE, THEN STAYS AWAKE ☐ *OR* IF ASLEEP AND STIMULATED, THEN WAKES UP QUICKLY ☐	EYES CLOSE BRIEFLY, THEN AWAKENS ☐ *OR* AWAKENS WITH PROLONGED STIMULATION ☐	WILL NOT ROUSE ☐ *OR* FALLS TO SLEEP ☐
4. **COLOR**	PINK ☐	PALE HANDS, FEET ☐ *OR* ACROCYANOSIS (BLUE HANDS AND FEET) ☐	PALE ☐ *OR* BLUE ☐ *OR* ASHEN (GRAY) ☐ *OR* MOTTLED ☐
5. **HYDRATION** (Moisture in skin, eyes, mouth)	SKIN NORMAL *AND* EYES, MOUTH MOIST ☐	SKIN, EYES NORMAL *AND* MOUTH SLIGHTLY DRY ☐	SKIN DOUGHY OR TENTED *AND* EYES MAY BE SUNKEN *AND* DRY EYES AND MOUTH ☐
6. **RESPONSE TO SOCIAL OVERTURES** (Being held, kissed, hugged, touched, talked to, comforted)	SMILES ☐ *OR* ALERTS ☐ (2 months or less)	BRIEF SMILE ☐ *OR* ALERTS BRIEFLY ☐ (2 months or less)	NO SMILE, FACE ANXIOUS ☐ *OR* DULL, EXPRESSIONLESS ☐ *OR* NO ALERTING ☐ (2 months or less)

Figure 57–1. Acute Illness Observational Scales. Clinical evaluation of the well and sick child. (From McCarthy PL, Sharpe MR, Spiesel SZ, et al: Observation scales to identify serious illness in febrile children. Pediatrics 70:802, 1982. Reproduced by permission of Pediatrics.)

The complex nature of history taking has been outlined previously. Parents must transmit how a younger child has been "feeling." In addition, they should also provide information on specific symptoms, such as bloody diarrhea or cyanosis when coughing. The older child's perception of his or her symptoms may reflect a less developmentally mature understanding of the cause of the illness. The examiner pursues the historical information provided by the parents or child to define the symptoms precisely. For example, if the complaint is blood in the stool, additional questions can be asked about other evidence of bowel inflammation, such as watery stools, mucus in the stools, or increased frequency of stooling. On the other hand, if the historical information indicates crying with defecation and streaks of blood on the outer portion of a hard stool, without other changes in the character or frequency of the stool, a diagnosis of a rectal fissure is tenable.

Questions should focus on those entities that are seen most commonly in acute febrile childhood illnesses. The more serious diagnoses are outlined in Table 57–1. Because most acute illnesses in children are caused by minor viral infections, specific questions about the epidemiology of the illness can provide important insights. Are there other children in the family with similar symptoms? Has the child had other illness exposures? Finally, it is important to be aware of any underlying chronic problems that might predispose the child to recurring infections and/or a serious acute illness; for example, the child with sickle cell anemia or AIDS is at increased risk for recurrent episodes of bacteremia.

For the sick child, the physical examination follows the same sequence as outlined for the well child in Chapter 7. The examiner should be aware of illnesses that might be present in the acutely ill child and seek evidence of those illnesses. Initially, it is best to seat the child on the parent's lap; the older child may be seated on the examination table. In addition to the child's general level of interaction, color, and hydration, as assessed in the Acute Illness Observation Scales (see Fig. 57–1), the child's respiratory status is evaluated. This evaluation includes determining respiratory rate and noting any evidence of inspiratory stridor, expiratory wheezing, grunting, or coughing. Evidence of increased work of breathing—retractions, nasal flaring, and use of abdominal musculature—is sought. Because acute infections in children are most often caused by viral infections, the presence of nasal discharge is noted. It is possible at this time to assess the skin for rashes. Frequently, viral infections cause an exanthematous eruption and many of these eruptions are diagnostic, for example, the reticulated rash and slapped-cheek appearance caused by parvovirus infections or "hand-foot-and-mouth disease" caused by Coxsackie virus. The skin examination may also yield evidence of more serious infections, such as bacterial cellulitis or petechiae associated with bacteremia. When the child is seated and is least perturbed, an assessment of fontanelle tension can be completed; it can be determined if the fontanelle is depressed, flat, or bulging. It is also important at this time to assess the child's willingness to move and ease of movement. Usually the child with meningitis will hold the neck stiffly and often cry when any attempt is made to move the neck, even during cuddling by the parent. This is termed *paradoxic irritability.* The child with cellulitis, osteomyelitis, or septic arthritis in an extremity will resist movement of that limb. The child with peritoneal inflammation will sit quietly and become irritable during movement. It is reassuring to see the child moving about on the parent's lap with ease and without discomfort.

During this initial portion of the physical examination, when the child is most comfortable, the heart and lungs are auscultated. In the acutely febrile child, because of the relatively high occurrence of respiratory illnesses, it is important to assess adequacy of air entry into the lungs, the equality of breath sounds, and evidence of adventitial breath sounds, especially wheezes, rales, and rhonchi. The coarse sound of air moving through a congested nasal passage will commonly be transmitted to the lungs. The examiner can become attuned to these coarse sounds by placing the stethoscope near the nose of the child and then compensating for this sound as the chest is auscultated. The cardiac exam is next completed; findings such as pericardial friction rub, loud murmurs, or distant heart sounds may indicate an infectious process involving the heart. The eyes are examined to evaluate findings that might indicate an infectious process. Often, viral infections result in a watery discharge or redness of the bulbar conjunctivae. Bacterial infection, if superficial, results in purulent drainage; if the infection is more deep seated, then tenderness, swelling, and redness of tissues surrounding the eye are present, as well as proptosis, reduced acuity, and altered extraocular movement. The extremities may then be evaluated not only for ease of movement, but also for the possibility of swelling, heat, or tenderness; such abnormalities may be indicative of focal infections.

The components of the physical examination that are more bothersome to the child are completed last. This is best done with the child on the examination table. Initially, the neck is examined to assess for areas of swelling, redness, or tenderness, as may be seen in cervical adenitis. The neck is then flexed to evaluate suppleness; resistance to flexion is indicative of meningeal irritation. Kernig and Brudzinski signs may be sought at this time. During examination of the abdomen, the diaper is removed. The abdomen is inspected for distention. Auscultation is then performed to assess adequacy of bowel sounds. Palpation is then done. It is often the case that the child fusses as the abdomen is auscultated and palpated. Every attempt should be made to quiet the child. If this is not possible, then increases in the fussing pattern as the abdomen is palpated may indicate tenderness, especially if this finding is reproducible. Palpation may elicit, in addition to focal tenderness, involuntary guarding or rebound; these findings indicate peritoneal irritation, as is seen in appendicitis. The inguinal area and genitalia are then sequentially examined. The febrile child may, for example, have inguinal adenitis or a strangulated hernia as the cause of fever. The child is then placed in the prone position and abnormalities of the back are sought. The spine and costovertebral angle (CVA) areas are percussed to elicit any tenderness; such findings might be indicative of osteomyelitis or pyelonephritis, respectively.

The physical examination is completed by examining the ears and throat. These are usually the most bothersome parts of the exam for the child, and parents frequently can be helpful in minimizing head movement. The oropharyngeal examination is important to document the presence of enanthemas; these may be seen in many infectious processes, such as "hand-foot-and-mouth" disease caused by Coxsackie virus. This portion of the examination is important as well in documenting inflammation and/or exudates on the tonsils, which may be viral or bacterial.

At times, repeating portions of observational assessment and the physical examination is indicated. For example, the child may have cried continuously during the initial clinical evaluation. The examiner may not be certain if this is due to the high fever or stranger anxiety, or is indicative of a serious illness. Continual crying also makes portions of the physical examination, such as auscultation of the chest, more difficult. Before a repeat assessment is performed, maneuvers to make the child as comfortable as possible are indicated. Such maneuvers would include reducing the fever with antipyretics and allowing the child to take a bottle. Because most children with fever do not have serious illnesses, repeated assessments are more likely to document normal findings. If, on the other hand, the child is persistently irritable, then the possibility of serious illness increases.

The sensitivity of the carefully performed clinical assessment, observation, history, and physical examination for the presence of serious illness is approximately 90%. Careful data gathering is necessary in the observation, history, and physical examination because each component of the evaluation is as effective as the others in identifying serious illness. Other data, however, should be sought to improve this sensitivity level. In the child with an acute febrile illness, the other important supplemental data are age, temperature, and screening laboratory tests. Febrile children in the first 3 mo of life have yet to achieve immunologic maturity, and therefore are more susceptible to severe infections and to infections by unusual organisms. Thus, the febrile infant is at greater risk for serious illness than the child beyond 3 mo of age (see Chapter 167). In febrile children of any age, the higher the fever the greater the risk for serious illnesses. The risk of bacteremia increases as the degree of fever increases; at ≥40° C the risk is 7%. The limit of physiologic thermoregulation is 41.1° C; fevers in this range and higher indicate not only bacteremia but also possible central nervous system infection, pneumonia, or pathologic hyperthermia.

Screening laboratory tests can be helpful in identifying the febrile child at increased risk for common serious illnesses. For example, a white blood cell count (WBC) ≥15,000/μL and/or erythrocyte sedimentation rate (ESR) ≥30 mm/hr in children younger than 24 mo with a temperature ≥40° C places those children at five times the risk of bacteremia (15% vs. 3%) compared with children in whom the WBC is <15,000/μL and the ESR is <30 mm/hr. A similar association with bacteremia has been found with a WBC ≥15,000/μL, a polymorphonuclear neutrophil count >10,000/μL, and a band count ≥500/μL. The risk of any serious illness in all febrile children is approximately twice as great if the WBC is ≥15,000/μL and/or the ESR is ≥30 mm/hr than if neither of these elevations was present.

DIAGNOSTIC APPROACH (See also Chapter 167). If the febrile child is older than 3 mo, appears well, the history or physical examination does not suggest a serious illness, and no age or temperature risk factors are present, the child may be followed expectantly. If otitis media is present, it should be treated. This profile applies to most children with acute infectious illnesses. If, on the other hand, the child appears ill or the history or physical examination suggests a serious illness, definitive laboratory tests appropriate for those findings are indicated (e.g., a chest roentgenogram for a child with grunting). The area of greatest controversy is the necessity of performing laboratory studies on the febrile child who appears well and has no abnormalities on history and physical examination to suggest serious illness but who is less than 3 mo of age or whose temperature is high. Most would agree that a sepsis workup is indicated in the febrile child <3 mo (see Chapter 167); obtaining blood cultures in children older than 3 mo with higher grades of fever is gaining increasing acceptance.

If the physician feels comfortable in following the child in whom no specific diagnosis has been established on an outpatient basis, a follow-up examination often provides a diagnosis. During the initial visit, or from one visit to the next during the acute illness, the change in symptoms or in the physical examination over time may provide important diagnostic clues. For the child in whom a diagnosis has already been established and hospitalization is not required, follow-up by phone or an office visit should be used to monitor the course of the illness and further educate and support the parents.

Baker MD, Bell L, Avner J: Outpatient management without antibiotics of fever in selected infants. N Engl J Med 329:1437, 1993.
Baskin M, O'Rourke E, Fleisher G: Outpatient treatment of fibrile infants 28 to 89 days of age with intramuscular administration of ceftriaxone. J Pediatr 120:22, 1992.
Fleisher G, Rosenberg N, Vinci R, et al: Intramuscular versus oral antibiotic therapy for the prevention of meningitis and other bacterial sequelae in young, febrile children at risk for occult bacteremia. J Pediatr 124:504, 1994.
Margolis P, Ferkol T, Marsocci S, et al: Accuracy of the clinical examination in detecting hypoxemia in infants with respiratory illness. J Pediatr 124:552, 1994.
McCarthy PL: Fever without apparent source on clinical exam. Curr Opin Pediatr 6:105, 1994.

CHAPTER 58
Injury Control

Frederick P. Rivara and Dena R. Brownstein

Injuries are the most common cause of death during childhood beyond the 1st few mo of life and represent one of the most important causes of preventable pediatric morbidity and mortality. Significant advances have been made in understanding the risk factors for injuries as well as in developing successful programs for prevention and control. These principles should be applied daily by the pediatrician, whether in the office, emergency department, or hospital setting.

INJURY CONTROL

The term *accident prevention* has been replaced by *injury control*. *Accident* implies an event occurring by chance, without pattern or predictability. In fact, most injuries occur under fairly predictable circumstances to high-risk children and families. *Accident* connotes a sense of fatalism, that injuries are an "act of God" and thus cannot be prevented. This fatalistic attitude is one of the most important barriers to decreasing mortality and morbidity from injuries, both among individuals and society. Use of the term *injury* avoids these connotations and focuses attention on the damage to the person.

Reduction in morbidity and mortality from injuries can be accomplished not only through primary prevention of the event from occurring in the first place, but also through secondary and tertiary prevention, that is, appropriate emergency medical services for injured children; regionalized trauma care for the multiply injured, severely burned, or head injured child; and specialized pediatric rehabilitation services that attempt to return children to their prior level of functioning. This broadened scope of prevention is more properly described by the term *injury control*.

This expanded definition also allows us to extend our interest to injuries other than "accidents," that is, assaults and self-inflicted injuries. These injuries are increasingly important among adolescents and young adults, and in some populations rank 1st or 2nd as leading causes of death in these age groups. Many of the same principles of injury control can be applied to these problems, for example, limiting access to firearms.

SCOPE OF THE PROBLEM

MORTALITY. Injuries cause almost 40% of the deaths among 1- to 4-yr-old children and three times more deaths than the next leading cause, congenital anomalies. For the rest of childhood and adolescence up to the age of 19 yr, nearly 70% of deaths are due to trauma, more than all other causes combined. In 1990, injuries caused 21,476 deaths among children and adolescents in the United States (Table 58–1). Injuries result in more years of potential life lost than any other cause.

Motor vehicle injuries lead the list of injury deaths at all ages during childhood and adolescence, even in children under 1 yr of age. Motor vehicle occupant injuries account for the majority of these deaths during childhood, and in adults. However, among children in the 5–9 yr age group, pedestrian injuries are the most common cause of death from trauma. During adolescence, occupant injuries are the leading cause of injury death, accounting for more than 50% of the unintentional trauma mortality in this age group.

Drowning ranks 2nd overall as a cause of unintentional trauma deaths, with peaks in the preschool and later teenage years (see Chapter 60.4). In some areas of the United States, drowning is the leading cause of death from trauma for preschool-age children. The causes of drowning deaths vary with age and geographic area. In young children, bathtub and swimming pool drowning predominate, while in older children and adolescents, drownings occur predominantly in natural bodies of water while swimming or boating.

Fire and burn deaths account for nearly 10% of all trauma deaths and more than 20% in those under 5 yr of age (see Chapter 60.5). The vast majority of these (85%) are due to

■ **TABLE 58–1 Incidence of Fatal Injuries—United States, 1990**

Mechanism	0–4 yr	5–9 yr	10–14 yr	15–19 yr	0–19 yr
Motor vehicle	1123	970	1089	5918	9100
Occupant	648	458	672	5152	6930
Pedestrian	456	406	240	339	1441
Bicycle	18	104	149	124	395
Drowning	640	248	260	478	1626
Fire and flames	683	246	107	165	1201
Poisoning	49	7	17	116	189
Homicide	710	156	356	3042	4264
Firearm homicide	69	63	258	2462	2852
Suicide	0	6	258	1979	2243
Firearm suicide	0	2	142	1332	1476
Unintentional firearms	114	56	160	379	709
Other					
Total	4290	1951	2528	12707	21476

From the National Center for Health Statistics 1990 mortality data tapes.

■ **TABLE 58–2 Morbidity (Hospitalizations) from Injuries to Children and Adolescents—United States, 1985**

Mechanism	0–4 yr	5–14 yr	15–24 yr	0–24 yr
Falls	34,944	59,697	52,363	147,004
Motor vehicle	8,853	42,277	164,892	216,022
Drowning	1,993	672	722	3,387
Fire/burns	11,885	4,940	8,937	25,762
Poisoning	24,986	11,132	50,386	86,504
All firearms	199	2684	28,420	31,303
Other	29,576	83,647	158,362	271,585
Total	112,436	205,049	464,082	781,567

From Rice DP, MacKenzie EJ, et al: Cost of Injury in the United States. A Report to Congress, 1989.

house fires, with death due to smoke inhalation and asphyxiation rather than severe burns. Children and the elderly are at greatest risk of these deaths because of difficulty in escaping from burning buildings.

Asphyxiation and choking account for approximately 40% of all unintentional deaths in children under 1 yr of age. The majority of these deaths are due to choking on food items such as hot dogs, candies, grapes, and nuts. Nonfood items include undersized infant pacifiers, small balls, and balloons.

Homicide is the leading cause of injury death for infants under 1 yr, the 4th leading cause of injury death for ages 1–14 yr, and the 2nd leading cause of injury death in adolescents 15–19 yr. Homicide among children falls into two patterns, "infantile" and "adolescent." Infantile homicide involves children under the age of 5 yr and represents child abuse (Chapter 38). The perpetrator is usually a caretaker; death is generally due to blunt trauma to the head and/or abdomen. In contrast, the adolescent pattern of homicide involves peers and acquaintances, and is due to firearms in more than 80%. The majority of these deaths involve handguns. Children between these two ages experience homicides of both types.

Suicide is rare under age 10 yr; only 1% of all suicides occur in children under 15 yr of age. The suicide rate increases markedly after the age of 10, with the result that suicide is now the 3rd leading cause of death for 15–19 yr olds, accounting for more than 100,000 potential years of life lost. Native American teenagers have the highest risk, followed by white males; black females have the lowest rate of suicide in this age group. Approximately 67% of teenage suicides involve firearms.

MORBIDITY. Mortality statistics represent only a small part of the effects of childhood injuries. Approximately 20–25% of children and adolescents receive medical care for an injury each year in hospital emergency departments, and at least an equal number are treated in physician offices. Of these, 2.5% require inpatient care and 55% have at least short-term temporary disability from their injuries.

The distribution of these nonfatal injuries is very different from that of fatal trauma (Table 58–2). Falls and sports are the leading causes of both emergency room visits and hospitalizations. Although motor vehicle occupant injuries represent the leading cause of death, falls and sports injuries constitute the leading causes of emergency department visits. Bicycle-related trauma is the most common type of sports and recreational injury, accounting for more than 300,000 emergency department visits annually.

Nonfatal injuries may be associated with severe morbidity. For example, anoxic encephalopathy due to near drowning, scarring and disfigurement due to burns, and persistent neurologic deficits due to head injury have a great long-term impact on both the injured child and the family.

TRENDS OVER TIME. The death rate for childhood injuries has declined throughout this century, with substantial decreases in deaths from unintentional injuries over the last 15 yr (Fig. 58–1). In contrast, rates of intentional injuries have increased. Suicide rates among male teens have increased by 50% between 1970 and 1988, largely related to firearms. Homicide is the only leading cause of death to increase from 1950 to 1990; handgun homicides have increased fivefold during this period. Homicide is now the leading cause of death for black males 15–19 yr of age.

PRINCIPLES OF INJURY CONTROL

For many years, prevention of injuries centered around attempts to pinpoint the innate characteristics of a child that result in greater frequency of injury. Most researchers have discounted the theory of the "accident-prone" child. While longitudinal studies have demonstrated an association between hyperactivity, impulsivity, and increased rates of injuries, the sensitivity and specificity of these traits for risk of injury are extremely low. The concept of "accident proneness" is in fact counterproductive in that it shifts attention away from potentially more modifiable factors such as the product or the environment. It is more productive to examine the physical and social environment of children with frequent rates of injuries than to try to identify particular personality traits or temperaments. At-risk children are likely to be relatively poorly supervised, have disorganized or stressed families, and live in hazardous environments.

Efforts to control injuries include *education or persuasion, changes in products,* and *modification of the environment,* whether

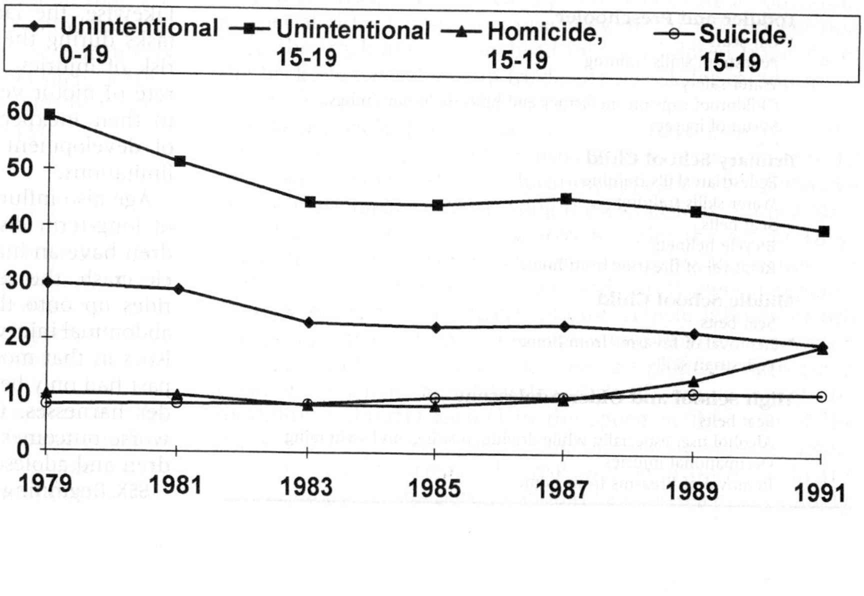

Figure 58–1. Secular changes in mortality from unintentional injuries (0–19, 15–19 yr), homicide and suicide for children and adolescents, 15–19 yr of age in the United States, 1979–1991. (From the National Center for Health Statistics and U.S. Bureau of Census.)

Alcohol use is a major cause of motor vehicle trauma among adolescents. The combination of inexperience in driving and inexperience with alcohol appears to be particularly dangerous. Approximately 50% of all deaths from motor vehicle crashes in this age group involve the use of alcohol, with impairment of driving seen at blood alcohol concentrations as low as 0.05 gm/dL. All adolescent motor vehicle injury victims should have their blood alcohol concentration measured in the emergency department as well as be screened for chronic alcohol use using standard tests such as the CAGE or the Short Michigan Alcohol Screening Test to identify those with alcohol abuse problems. These tests cannot be used for DUI conviction because they do not meet the chain-of-evidence criterion required by the courts. Individuals who have evidence of alcohol abuse should not leave the emergency department or hospital without plans for appropriate alcohol abuse treatment.

BICYCLE INJURIES. Each year in the United States, approximately 400 children and adolescents die due to injuries incurred while riding bicycles; bicycle-related injuries are one of the most common reasons children with trauma visit emergency rooms. The majority of severe and fatal bicycle injuries involve head trauma. A logical step in the prevention of these head injuries is the use of helmets. Rigorous studies indicate that helmets are very effective, reducing the risk of head injury by 85% and brain injury by 88%. Pediatricians can be an effective source of advice to parents and children on the need for bicycle helmets and should incorporate such advice into their anticipatory guidance schedules. Appropriate helmets are those with a firm polystyrene liner and should bear a label indicating that they are either approved by the Snell or American National Standards Institute (ANSI) testing organizations.

Promotion of helmets can and should be extended beyond the office. Community education programs spearheaded by coalitions of physicians, educators, bicycle clubs, and community service organizations have been successful in promoting the use of bicycle helmets, resulting in helmet use rates as high as 60% with concomitant reduction in the rate of head injuries.

Consideration should also be given to other types of activities, although the evidence supporting their effectiveness is limited. Bicycle paths are a logical method for separating bicycles and motor vehicles. Safe bicycling training for children can be provided in the school and community.

PEDESTRIAN INJURIES. Pedestrian injuries are the single most common cause of traumatic death for 5- to 9-yr-old children in the United States and most industrialized countries. While case fatality rates are less than 5%, serious nonfatal injuries constitute a much larger problem. Pedestrian injuries are the most important cause of traumatic coma in children and are a frequent cause of serious lower extremity fractures, particularly in the school-age child.

Most injuries occur during the day, with a peak in the after-school period. Improved lighting or retroreflective clothing would, therefore, be expected to prevent few injuries. Surprisingly, approximately 30% of pedestrian injuries occur while the individual is in a marked crosswalk, perhaps reflecting a false sense of security and decreased vigilance. The risk of pedestrian injury is greater in neighborhoods with high traffic volumes, speeds greater than 40 kph (approx. 25 mph) absence of play space adjacent to the home, household crowding, and low socioeconomic status.

One important risk factor for childhood pedestrian injuries is the developmental level of the child. Children under the age of 5 yr are at risk of being run over in the driveway. Few children under the age of 9 or 10 yr have the developmental skills to successfully negotiate traffic 100% of the time. Young children have poor ability to judge the distance and speed of traffic, and are easily distracted by playmates or other factors in the environment. Many parents, however, are not aware of this potential mismatch between the abilities of the young school-age child and the skills needed to cross streets safely.

Prevention of pedestrian injuries is difficult but should consist of a multifaceted approach. Education of the child in pedestrian safety should be initiated at an early age by the parents and continue into the school-age years. Younger children should be taught not to cross streets at all when alone; older children should be taught and practice how to negotiate quiet streets with little traffic. Major streets should not be crossed alone until the child is age 10 yr or older.

Pedestrian skills training should constitute part of a more comprehensive pedestrian safety program in a community. Legislation and police enforcement are important components of any campaign to reduce pedestrian injuries. Right-turn-on-red laws increase the hazard to pedestrians. In many cities, few drivers stop for pedestrians in crosswalks, a special hazard for young children. Engineering changes in roadway design are extremely important as passive prevention measures. Most important are measures to slow down the speed of traffic and route traffic away from schools and residential areas. Other modifications include one-way street networks, proper placement of transit or school bus stops, sidewalks in urban and suburban areas, edge stripping in rural areas to delineate the edge of the road, and curb parking regulations. Comprehensive traffic "calming" schemes employing these strategies have been very successful in reducing child pedestrian injuries in Sweden, the Netherlands, and Germany.

FIRE- AND BURN-RELATED INJURIES

(see Chapter 60.5)

Fire- and burn-related injuries are the 3rd most common cause of unintentional injury death in the United States; about 6,000 burn injury deaths occur each year in the United States. For both injuries and deaths, the 1st decade of life is the period at highest risk. Burns are 2nd only to motor vehicle crashes in the number of years of life lost *per death,* reflecting the relatively young population involved in serious burn injuries. The likelihood of burn injury is strongly related to low socioeconomic status. Burns are much more frequent among males than females. Among children 10–14 yr of age with burns involving flammable substances, males are burned eight times more frequently than females.

One of the first effective interventions involved flammable fabrics. Flame burns resulting from ignition of clothing were a common, serious burn injury, especially in small children. At least one third of those injuries involved infant sleepwear. Such burns averaged 30% of the body surface, requiring hospitalization for an average of 70 days. In 1967, the Federal Flammable Fabrics Act was passed, requiring children's sleepwear to be flame retardant. As a result of this and similar state legislation, clothing ignition burns in small children now account for only a small fraction of burns in children. Despite the withdrawal of Tris-containing clothing because of potential mutagenicity, federal flammability standards still apply to children's sleepwear. Parents should not circumvent these protective regulations by using cotton tee-shirts for infant and child sleepwear.

Another example of hazard modification resulting in substantial reduction of injury involves scald burns due to tap water. Scalds account for 40% of the burn injuries in children requiring hospitalization, and at least 25% of these scald burns involve tap water. Unlike flame burns, children with scalds generally do not die; however, many children face long hospitalizations, multiple surgical procedures, and severe disfigurement. The risk of full-thickness burns increases geometrically at water temperatures above 130° F. At 150° F, a full thickness burn will be produced in adult skin in 2 sec. A simple and effective preventive maneuver is to turn down the water heater temperature to 125° F. At this setting, dishwashers and washing machines will still operate effectively, but the risk of serious scald injury is greatly reduced. In many cities, the local power company will turn down the temperature without charge. In 1980, Florida became the first state requiring new water heaters to be preset at a temperature of 125° F.

Nearly 70% of all fire deaths in the United States occur in private dwellings. Of these deaths, 60% are caused by smoke asphyxiation and *not* flame burns. Smoke detectors provide an inexpensive but effective method of preventing the majority of these deaths. Physicians can alter parental behavior and increase smoke detector use by offering information on smoke detectors in their offices.

Cigarettes are estimated to cause 45% of all fires and 22–56% of deaths from house fires. The combination of smoking and alcohol use appears to be particularly lethal. Most cigarettes made in this country contain additives in both the paper and tobacco that allow them to burn for as long as 28 min, even if left unattended. If fire-safe or self-extinguishing cigarettes replaced present types, nearly 2,000 deaths and more than 6,000 burns would be prevented annually.

Other common burn risks include scalds from hot tea, coffee, and foods; fireworks injuries; and burns from cigarette lighters. Scalds from hot foods are the most common reason for a burn admission to the hospital for children under the age of 5 yr. Avoiding the use of electric kettles or frying pans with long cords, not using baby walkers, not drinking hot tea or coffee while holding an infant, and keeping children away from pots cooking on the stove will help to prevent many of these injuries. Community restrictions on certain types of fireworks and adult supervision of use of all fireworks have been effective in decreasing burns, amputations, and ocular injuries due to these devices. Change in product modification promises to decrease the hazards associated with certain easy-to-use cigarette lighters commonly found in the home.

Some burns are due to fire setting by children or adolescents. In young children, this usually represents exploratory play. However, such behavior in older children and adolescents may signify a serious conduct disorder and warrants careful psychiatric and family evaluation.

POISONING

(see Chapter 666)

Deaths by poisoning among children have decreased dramatically over the last two decades, particularly for children less than 5 yr of age. In 1970, 226 poisoning deaths of children under 5 yr occurred, compared with only 49 in 1990. Poisoning prevention represents the effectiveness of passive strategies—child-resistant packaging and dose limits per container. The Poison Packaging Prevention Act currently includes 16 categories of household products and nearly all prescription drugs. This law has been remarkably effective in reducing poisoning deaths and hospitalizations. However, compliance with the law by pharmacists is only 70–75% at present, indicating that physicians should always specify that prescriptions be dispensed in child-resistant containers. In addition, difficulty using child-resistant containers is an important cause of poisoning in young children today. A survey by the Centers for Disease Control found that 18.5% of households in which poisoning occurred to children less than 5 yr had replaced the child-resistant closure and 65% of the ones used did not work properly. Nearly 20% of ingestions occur from drugs owned by grandparents, a group that has difficulty using traditional child-resistant containers. There is a need for better child-resistant closures that do not require manual dexterity or strength greater than the capabilities of older adults.

Other poisoning interventions, such as "Mr. Yuk" stickers, are far less effective. They do not deter young children from ingesting labeled medications and may in fact be attractive to children under 3 yr of age. The most important feature of the Mr. Yuk sticker is the phone number of the local or regional poison control center. Parents of toddlers should also be given a bottle of syrup of ipecac to store in the medicine chest. In the case of an ingestion, they should be first instructed to call the poison control center or pediatrician before administering it.

DROWNING

(see Chapter 60.4)

In 1990, 1,626 drownings, primarily associated with recreational activities, occurred in children and adolescents in the United States. For children, drowning ranks 2nd only to motor vehicle injury as a cause of traumatic death. Although no precise data exist on the number of nonfatal water-related injuries, it is estimated that 140,000 occur annually from swimming activities alone. Diving head first into water accounts for the most serious aquatic injuries because of spinal cord damage. Of the estimated 700 spinal cord injuries resulting from aquatic activities each year, the majority result in permanent paralysis.

The proportion of drowning deaths that are pool related varies by region of the country. In Los Angeles, half of all drownings take place in residential pools, similar to those of other areas with large numbers of pools. Children under the age of 5 yr do not understand the consequences of falling into deep water and usually do not call for help. A majority of child victims drown during lapses in adult supervision caused by chores, socializing, and phone calls.

Clearly the most effective way to prevent childhood pool drowning is through fencing. To be most protective, these barriers should restrict entry to the pool from the yard and residence, use self-closing and self-latching gates, be at least 5 ft high, and have no vertical openings more than 4 in wide. Ordinances to require appropriate fencing have been demonstrated to be effective. Many people have advocated "water-babies" and other swimming instruction for young children. The efficacy of such techniques is untested. The potential exists for both parent and child to become less vigilant around water, possibly with tragic consequences.

Among adolescents and young adults, alcohol and drug use have been found to be involved in nearly 50% of all drowning deaths. The restriction of the sale and consumption of alcoholic beverages in boating, pool, harbor, marina, and beach areas may combat this dangerous combination of activities.

More restrictive licensing of boat owners should also be considered. Coast Guard data show that although only 7% of boats involved in mishaps lacked available personal flotation devices, they accounted for 29% of the boating fatalities.

The risk of bathtub drowning is markedly increased in patients with a seizure disorder, including older children and adolescents. These patients should be instructed to shower instead of using a bathtub.

FIREARM INJURIES

Injuries to children and adolescents involving firearms occur in three different situations: non-intentional injury, suicide attempt, and assault. In each case, the injury induced may be fatal or may result in permanent sequelae.

Among children under the age of 18 yr, firearms are the 5th-ranking cause of death from non-intentional trauma in the United States. More than 700 children and adolescents die each year from non-intentional gunshot wounds. An additional 8,000 children and adolescents are left with permanent sequelae, not including emotional and psychological problems.

Non-intentional firearm injuries generally occur in a family dwelling; 85% of firearm deaths occur in the home. In gunshot fatalities to children under 16 yr of age, poverty is more closely related to shooting deaths than race or population density. Urban whites have the lowest death rate, rural whites are intermediate, and urban black children have the highest fatality rate.

Suicide is now the 3rd most common cause of trauma death in teenage males and the 4th for females. During the period from the 1950s to 1982, the suicide rates for children and adolescents have more than doubled; suicide rates have risen by an additional 27% between 1982 and 1991 alone. Firearms have played an important role in this increase and are now the most common means of suicide in males of all ages. The difference in the rate of suicide between males and females is related less to number of attempts than to method. Women die less often in suicide attempts because they use less lethal means, mainly drugs. The use of firearms in a suicidal act usually converts an attempt into a fatality.

Homicides are 2nd only to motor vehicle crashes among causes of death in teenagers over the age of 15 yr. In 1990, 4,264 children and adolescents were homicide victims; nonwhite teenagers accounted for almost 50% of the total, making homicides the most common cause of death among nonwhite teenagers. At present, almost 95% of homicides among males involve firearms, 75% of which are handguns.

In the United States today, there are an estimated 210–220 million firearms. During the last two decades, over 6 million firearms were sold in the United States each year. Handguns account for approximately 20% of the firearms in use today, yet they are involved in 90% of criminal and other firearm misuse. Home ownership of guns increases the risk of adolescent suicide 10-fold and adolescent homicide 4-fold. In homes with guns, the risk to the occupants is far greater than the chance the gun will be used against an intruder; for every death occurring in self-defense, there may be 1.3 unintentional deaths, 4.6 homicides, and 37 suicides.

The data seem to indicate that of all firearms, handguns pose the greatest risk to the health of children and adolescents. Access to handguns by adolescents is surprisingly common and is not restricted to those involved in gang or criminal activity. Regulations and elimination of handguns, rather than all firearms, would appear to be the most appropriate focus of efforts to reduce shooting injuries in children and adolescents.

One approach is information and education campaigns in firearm safety. No data exist to support the effectiveness of such programs in decreasing the number of gunshot wounds in children. Regardless of the merits of safety education, firearms around the home pose a risk to children and adolescents, who have not yet developed adequate judgment for the safe handling of these weapons. Elimination of these weapons from the environment of children and adolescents is the necessary key to reduction in firearm fatalities and injuries. Furthermore, safety education will have no effect on the use of firearms in homicides and suicides. Most homicides are between relatives or acquaintances and are acts of rage. Elimination of handguns would certainly not eliminate arguments, but it would decrease the likelihood of a fatal conclusion. In an assault, the chance of death is five times greater with a firearm than with a knife.

Physicians have a clear responsibility to counsel parents and patients about firearm ownership. This should include information dispelling the myth that families are safer if they own a handgun, the risk of gun injury to all members of the household, and the special risks to adolescent males. Educational information for pediatricians on counseling families and adolescents about guns can be obtained from the American Academy of Pediatrics.

Agran PF, Castillo DN, Winn DG: Comparison of motor vehicle occupant injuries in restrained and unrestrained 4- to 14-year olds. Accid Anal Prev 24:349, 1992.

American Academy of Pediatrics, Committee on Accident and Poison Prevention and Committee on Fetus and Newborn: Safe transportation of premature infants. Pediatrics 87:120, 1991.

Baker S, O'Neill B, Ginsburg MJ, et al: The Injury Fact Book, 2nd ed. New York: Oxford University Press, 1992.

Baker S, Fowler C, Li G, et al: Head injuries incurred by children and young adults during informal recreation. Am J Public Health 84:649, 1994.

Bergman AB, Rivara FP, Richards DD, et al: Anatomy of a children's bicycle helmet campaign. Am J Dis Child 144:727, 1990.

Callahan CM, Rivara FP: Urban high school youth and handguns. A school-based survey. JAMA 267:3038, 1992.

Chiavello C, Christoph R, Bond G: Infant walker related injuries: A prospective study of severity and incidence. Pediatrics 93:974, 1994.

Colletti RB: Longitudinal evaluation of a statewide network of hospital programs to improve child passenger safety. Pediatrics 7:523, 1986.

Davidson L, Durkin M, Kuhn L, et al: The impact of the Safe Kids/Healthy Neighborhood Injury Prevention Project in Harlem, 1988 through 1991. Am J Public Health 84:580, 1994.

Durkin M, Davidson L, Kuhn L, et al: Low income neighborhoods and the risk of severe pediatric injury: A small area analysis in northern Manhattan. Am J Public Health 84:587, 1994.

Fingerhut LA, Ingram D, Feldman J: Firearm and non-firearm homicide among persons 15–19 years of age. JAMA 267:3048, 1992.

Hampson NB, Norkool DM: Carbon monoxide poisoning in children riding in the back of pickup trucks. JAMA 267:538, 1992.

Johnston C, Rivara F, Soderberg R: Children in car crashes: Analysis of data for injury and use of restraints. Pediatrics 93:960, 1994.

Kassirer JP: Guns in the household. N Engl J Med 329:1117, 1993.

Kellermann AL, Rivara FP, Somes G, et al: Suicide in the home in relation to gun ownership. N Engl J Med 327:467, 1992.

Kellermann AL, Rivara FP, Rushforth NB, et al: Gun ownership as a risk factor for homicide in the home. N Engl J Med 329:1084, 1993.

Langley J: The "accident prone child"—the perpetuation of a myth. Austral Paediatr 18:243, 1982.

McLoughlin E, McGuire A: The causes, costs and prevention of childhood burn injuries. Am J Dis Child 144:677, 1990.

National Academy of Sciences: Injury in America: A Continuing Public Health Problem. Washington DC: National Academy Press, 1985.

Quan L, Gore EJ, Wentz K, et al: Ten year study of pediatric drownings and near-drownings in King County Washington. Lessons in injury prevention. Pediatrics 83:1035, 1989.

Rivara FP: Child pedestrian injuries in the United States: Current status of the problem, potential interventions, and future research needs. Am J Dis Child 144:692, 1990.

Rivara FP, Gurney JG, Ries RK, et al: A descriptive study of trauma, alcohol, and alcoholism in young adults. J Adolesc Health 13:663, 1992.

Robertson LS: Injury Epidemiology. New York: Oxford University Press, 1992.

Thompson RS, Rivara FP, Thompson DC: A case-control study of the effectiveness of bicycle safety helmets. N Engl J Med 320:1361, 1989.

Walton W: An evaluation of the Poison Packaging Prevention Act. Pediatrics 69:363, 1982.

Wilson M, Baker SP, Teret S, et al: Saving Children: A Guide to Injury Prevention. New York: Oxford University Press, 1991.

Wintemute GJ: Childhood drowning and near-drowning in the United States. Am J Dis Child 144:6663, 1990.

CHAPTER 59

Emergency Medical Services for Children

Dena R. Brownstein and Frederick P. Rivara

Emergency medical services for children (EMS-C) is a concept rather than a distinct entity, and represents a continuum of care (Fig. 59–1). The primary care physician has an important role in the EMS-C system and is responsible for providing parents and children with education on injury prevention and emergency medical system (EMS) access, participating in the pediatric training of EMS providers in the community and becoming self-educated in appropriate triage and transport of critically ill children. In addition, primary care providers coordinate the care of their sickest patients, from the office to the emergency department, through hospital care to rehabilitation and reintegration into the community.

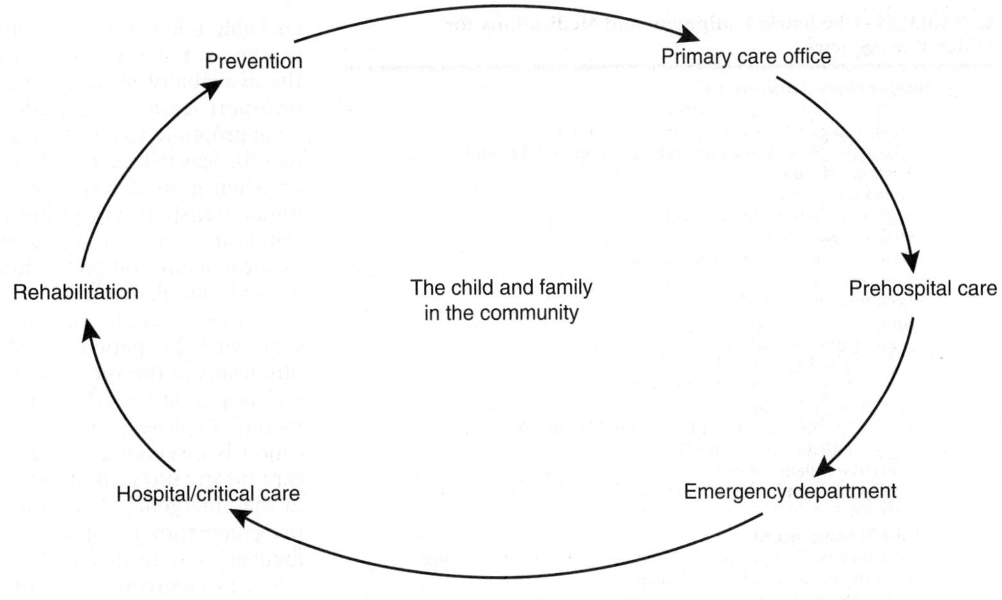

Figure 59–1. The EMS-C Continuum of Care: Seriously ill and injured children will interface with a large number of health care personnel as they move through the EMS-C system. The system both begins and ends in the community.

ANTICIPATORY GUIDANCE. Most injuries are preventable (Chapter 58). Likewise, early recognition and treatment of many illnesses can prevent the need for emergency care. Equally important are education for parents and caregivers on the importance of first aid training, the recognition of signs and symptoms of serious illness or significant injury, and indications for seeking immediate care. Printed handouts, standardized diagnosis-driven discharge instructions, verbal communication during well child or acute care visits, and calendars of first aid/CPR classes are all mechanisms for informing parents of emergency care procedures.

OFFICE PREPAREDNESS. While the need for full cardiopulmonary resuscitation occurs relatively infrequently in the office setting, most practices see children in need of acute intervention or hospitalization on a regular basis. Despite this, primary care providers and their staffs may find themselves ill equipped to treat patients with impending shock, respiratory failure, or a seizure in an exam room, or who deteriorate acutely while waiting to be seen. Emergency preparedness in the office requires training and continuing education for staff members, policies and procedures for emergency intervention, ready availability of appropriate resuscitation equipment, knowledge of local resources for EMS response and transport, and a working relationship with area emergency departments to ensure that children are cared for in facilities with expertise in pediatric emergency care.

STAFF TRAINING AND CONTINUING EDUCATION. Initial recognition by an office staff member that a child requires emergency treatment may occur in the course of a telephone call, in the waiting room, or in an exam room. All office personnel, including those seated at the front desk or answering the phone, must be capable of recognizing the child with altered mental status, shock, or respiratory distress/failure, and be aware of an appropriate action plan for rapid intervention.

It is a reasonable expectation that all office staff, including receptionists and medical assistants, be trained in adult and child CPR and first aid, and that they maintain their certification on an annual basis. In addition to these requirements, nurses and physicians should have training in a systematic approach to pediatric medical and trauma resuscitation. Core knowledge may be obtained through standardized courses in pediatric advanced life support offered by national medical and nursing associations, with frequent recertification important for knowledge and skill maintenance. Examples of such curricula include: the American Heart Association's Pediatric Advanced Life Support (PALS) course, the Advanced Pediatric Life Support (APLS) course sponsored by the American Academy of Pediatrics and the American College of Emergency Physicians, and the Emergency Nurses Pediatric Course (ENPC) and Pediatric Emergency Nursing self-instruction manual sponsored by the Emergency Nurses Association.

To facilitate emergency response when a child needs rapid intervention in the office, all personnel should have a preassigned role. Organizing a "code team" within the office will ensure that necessary equipment is made available to the physician in charge, that an appropriate medical record detailing all interventions and the child's response is generated, and that the call for EMS response or a transport team is made in a timely fashion.

POLICIES AND PROCEDURES. Standardized protocols for telephone triage of seriously ill or injured children are essential, especially if after-hours calls are taken by nonphysician personnel. When a child's status is in question and prehospital care is available, ambulance transport in the care of trained personnel is preferable to transport via private car. This avoids the potentially serious medical consequences of relying on unskilled and worried parents, without the ability to provide even basic life support measures, to transport an unstable child to an emergency department or clinic.

Written policies and procedures for the management of status asthmaticus, upper airway obstruction, seizures, ingestions, shock, sepsis/meningitis, trauma, head injury, anaphylaxis, and cardiopulmonary arrest should be generated and made available to all potentially involved staff members.

RESUSCITATION EQUIPMENT. Availability of necessary equipment is a vital part of a smooth emergency response. Every physician's office should have essential resuscitation equipment and medications packaged in a pediatric resuscitation cart or kit (Table 59–1). This kit should be checked on a routine basis and kept in an accessible location known to all office staff. Outdated medications, a laryngoscope with a failed light source, or an empty oxygen tank represents a catastrophe in a resuscitation setting that can be easily avoided if an equipment checklist and maintenance schedule are implemented. Responsible staff should receive in-service training on a regular basis on equipment location and use, a task that may best be accomplished by a regular schedule of "mock codes" in which all office staff participate. Inclusion in the pediatric kit of posters, laminated cards, or resuscitation tapes specifying emergency drug doses and equipment size by age, weight, or

■ **TABLE 59–1 Pediatric Equipment and Medications for Office Emergencies**

Respiratory Equipment
Oxygen cylinder with flowmeter
Oxygen masks—neonate, infant, child, adult
Bag-valve-mask resuscitator, with reservoir—child, adult
Suction machine
Yankauer suction tip
Suction catheters—8F, 10F, 14F
Oral airways—0–5
Nasal cannulas—infant, child, adult
Nasogastric tubes—8F, 10F, 14F
Feeding tubes—5F, 8F
Intubation equipment*
Laryngoscope handle with
Straight blade 0, 1, 2
Straight or curved blade 2, 3
Endotracheal tubes
Uncuffed 3.0, 3.5, 4.0, 4.5, 5.0, 5.5 mm ID
Cuffed 6.0, 7.0 mm ID
Stylets—infant, adult
Disposable end-tidal CO_2 detector
Nebulizer
Fluid Management
IV catheters, short, over the needle—16, 18, 20, 22, 24 gauge
Butterfly needles—21, 23, 25 gauge
IV boards, tape, povidine iodine and alcohol swabs, tourniquet
Pediatric infusion set/volume control device
Intraosseous needles—15–18 gauge
Isotonic fluids (normal saline or lactated Ringer's solution)
Monitoring
Blood pressure cuffs—infant, child, adult
Sphygmomanometer
Cardiac monitor*
Pulse oximeter with infant and pediatric probe*
ECG monitor/defibrillator with pediatric paddles*
Doppler ultrasound blood pressure monitor*
Cardiac Arrest Board
Medications
Resuscitation
Epinephrine—1:1000, 1:10,000
Atropine
Sodium bicarbonate—4.2%, 8.4%
Glucose—25% solution
Anticonvulsants
Lorazepam or diazepam
Phenobarbital
Antibiotics, parenteral
Poisoning
Ipecac
Activated charcoal
Respiratory/allergic
Albuterol for inhalation
Epinephrine—1:1,000
Methylprednisolone/prednisolone
Diphenhydramine, parenteral
Miscellaneous
Naloxone

**Items are optional.*

height will be invaluable in avoiding critical therapeutic errors during a resuscitation.

TRANSPORT. Every office should be prepared to initiate resuscitation on a child with a life-threatening medical problem. This should include, at a minimum, measures to establish adequate oxygenation, ventilation, and perfusion. A decision must be made on how to transport the child to a facility capable of providing definitive care once the child has been stabilized. If a child has required aggressive airway or cardiovascular support, has altered mental status, continues to have unstable vital signs, or has significant potential to deteriorate en route, it is not appropriate to send the child via private car, regardless of proximity to a hospital. Even when an ambulance is called, it is the primary care provider's responsibility to initiate essential life support measures prior to transport.

In metropolitan centers with multiple public and private ambulance agencies, the primary care provider must be knowledgeable about the level of service that is provided by each. Marked variability will be found between agencies in terms of the availability of basic versus advanced life support services, transport team configuration, and pediatric expertise. It may be appropriate to consider aeromedical transport, when definitive or specialized care is not available within a community, or when ground transport times are prolonged. In that case, initial transport via ground to a local hospital for interval stabilization may be undertaken pending arrival of the aeromedical team. When a child is to be transported by air or ground ambulance, copies of the child's pertinent medical records as well as any radiologic studies or lab results should be sent with the patient (Table 59–2) and a call made to the physicians at the receiving facility to alert them to the referral and any treatments administered. Such prenotification is not merely a courtesy, as direct physician-to-physician communication is essential to ensure adequate transmission of patient care information, to allow mobilization of necessary resources in the emergency department, and to redirect the transport if the emergency physician feels that the child would be better managed at a facility with specialized services.

Not all emergency departments are equally capable of treating an ill or injured child, and it is the responsibility of the referring physician to be aware of the pediatric capabilities of the hospitals in the area. Outcomes for critically ill and injured patients may be improved when cared for in regional referral centers. This is particularly true for neonatal emergencies, major trauma, burns, head injuries, and specific pediatric surgical problems. Thus, while initial stabilization of these patients may take place in a local community hospital, definitive and long-term care may be better delivered in major referral centers especially equipped to provide such care.

PEDIATRIC PREHOSPITAL CARE

Prehospital care refers to emergency assistance rendered by trained emergency medical personnel before a child reaches a fixed medical facility. While most communities in the United States have a formalized EMS system, the nature of the emergency medical response available depends in large part on local demographics and population base. Emergency medical services may be provided by volunteers or paid professionals. There are a number of key points that are important to recognize in considering the interface between the community physician and the local EMS system. These include access to the system, provider capability, response/transport times, and destination.

ACCESS TO THE EMS SYSTEM. Most metropolitan and many rural communities in the United States have a "911" telephone system that provides direct access to a dispatcher who coordinates police, fire, and emergency medical response. Some communities have an "enhanced 911" system, in which the location of the caller is automatically provided to the dispatcher, permitting emergency response even if the caller, such as a young child, cannot give an address. The extent of medical training for these dispatchers varies between communities, as do the protocols by which they assign an emergency response. In some smaller communities, no coordinated dispatch exists

■ **TABLE 59–2 Checklist for Patient Transport**

1. Call appropriate transport agency.
2. Copy patient's current and pertinent past medical records, laboratory reports, and radiologic studies.
3. Obtain written permission for transport from parent/guardian.
4. Call receiving physician and document acceptance of transfer in patient's medical record.
5. Stabilize lines and tubes, splint fractures.
6. Give report to transport team, provide copy of records/studies.
7. Provide parent/guardian with patient's destination in writing.

and emergency medical calls are handled by the local law enforcement agency.

In activating the "911" system, it is important for the physician to make it clear to the dispatcher the nature of the medical emergency and the condition of the child. In many communities, dispatchers will be trained to ask a series of questions per protocol, allowing them to send out emergency medical personnel of an appropriate level of training.

PROVIDER CAPABILITY. There are multiple levels of training for prehospital EMS providers, ranging from individuals capable of providing only first aid to those trained and licensed to provide advanced life support in the field.

First responders may be law enforcement officers, firefighters, or community volunteers who are dispatched to provide emergency medical assistance. They have approximately 40 hr of training in first aid and CPR. Their role is to provide rapid response and stabilization, pending the arrival of more highly trained personnel. In some smaller communities, this will represent the only prehospital emergency medical response.

Emergency medical technicians (EMTs) are volunteers or paid professionals who provide the bulk of emergency medical response in the United States. Basic EMTs may staff an ambulance after undergoing an approximately 100-hr training program. They are licensed to provide basic life support services, but may receive further training to expand their scope of practice to IV placement and fluid administration, endotracheal intubation, and use of an automatic external defibrillator, under the direction of a physician advisor.

Paramedics, or EMT-Ps, represent the highest level of EMT response, with medical training and supervised field experience of approximately 1,000–2,000 hr. They provide advanced life support services in the prehospital setting, functioning out of an ambulance equipped as a mobile intensive care unit. Paramedic skills may include endotracheal intubation; the placement of peripheral, central, or intraosseous lines; IV administration of drugs; administration of nebulized aerosols; needle thoracotomy; and cardioversion/defibrillation. Paramedics work under the supervision of a physician advisor.

Aeromedical transport team configuration can vary widely and may include physicians, nurses, respiratory therapists, or paramedics. The amount of pediatric training of team members will also vary, and it is important to confirm that an appropriate standard of care will be provided during interfacility transport.

The level of training of the prehospital personnel dispatched to the scene of a medical emergency will depend on the acuity of the patient, available resources, and local protocols. It is important to realize that attention has only recently been focused on *pediatric* prehospital care. Only about 10% of all EMS calls are for pediatric emergencies. Training and equipment for pediatric emergency care have historically been given inadequate attention in national certification curricula and by EMS agencies primarily geared toward adult patients. In some communities, the standard of pediatric prehospital care may not match that offered to adult patients of similar acuity. The Emergency Medical Services for Children (EMS-C) initiative sponsored by the Maternal and Child Health Bureau, U.S. Public Health Service, has provided program development grants to improve pediatric emergency services in many states. This has led to increased awareness of the special needs of acutely ill and injured children, and the development of many programs and products to enhance their care.

RESPONSE/TRANSPORT TIMES. Depending on the demographics of a community, the location of the incident, and the nature of the EMS services available, EMS response times after a call for assistance may range from a few minutes to longer than an hour. Unfortunately, even in communities with relatively rapid response times, there may be a reluctance to call for help based on a misperception that 911 should be activated only for full-blown resuscitations. If a child is physiologically unstable (with marked respiratory distress, cyanosis, signs of early shock, or altered mental status) or has significant potential to deteriorate en route to the emergency department, or if a question exists regarding the reliability of the parents to promptly comply with recommendations for emergency department (ED) evaluation, an EMS transport should be initiated. Inherent dangers lie in the attitude that a parent can get to the hospital "faster" by private car. It must be remembered that legal responsibility for the patient lies with the referring physician, until responsibility for care is officially transferred to another medical provider.

DESTINATION. The destination to which an EMT transports a pediatric patient may be defined by parental preference, provider preference, or agency protocol. In communities with an organized trauma system or a system of pediatric designation based on objective capabilities of the area hospitals, seriously ill or injured children may be triaged by protocol to the highest-level center within a reasonable time frame. The Pediatric Trauma Score (PTS) (Table 59–3) or Revised Trauma Score (RTS) can be used to assess the severity of injury. Children with a PTS <8 or an RTS <11 should be treated in a designated trauma center. In communities that do not have a hospital with the equipment and personnel resources to provide definitive inpatient care, interfacility transport of the child to a regional center may be undertaken after initial stabilization. The primary care provider may be involved in this decision-making process, and must make a critical assessment of the local hospital's pediatric intensive care capabilities. When interfacility transport is to be undertaken, indications for transfer, parental consent for transfer, and acceptance of the patient by the receiving physician must all be clearly documented in the medical record.

THE PEDIATRIC PATIENT IN THE HOSPITAL EMERGENCY DEPARTMENT: PRIORITIES IN PEDIATRIC RESUSCITATION

The majority of children who require emergency care will be evaluated in community hospitals by physicians with variable degrees of pediatric training and experience. Children account for approximately 25% of all emergency room visits, but only a fraction of them will represent "true" emergencies. Because the volume of critical pediatrics is low, emergency physicians and nurses often have limited opportunities to reinforce their knowledge and skills in pediatric resuscitation. Pediatricians from the community may be consulted when a seriously ill or injured child presents to the emergency department, and

■ **TABLE 59–3 Pediatric Trauma Score***

Score	+2	+1	−1
Size	≥20 kg	10–20 kg	<10 kg
Airway	Normal	Maintainable	Unmaintainable
Systolic blood pressure	≤90 mm Hg	50–90 mm Hg	<50 mm Hg
Central nervous system	Awake	Obtunded/loss of consciousness	Coma/decerebrate
Open wound	None	Minor	Major/penetrating
Skeletal	None	Closed fracture	Open/multiple fractures

**From Ford EG: Trauma triage.* In: *Ford EG, Andrassy RJ (eds): Pediatric Trauma Initial Assessment and Management. Philadelphia, WB Saunders, 1994, p 112.*

anticonvulsants, and continuous infusion of crystalloid solutions, blood products, and vasopressors, have been successfully used in pediatric resuscitations. Experimental models have demonstrated rapid absorption of resuscitation drugs into the systemic circulation from the tibial marrow space, which serves as a "noncollapsible vein," even in hypotensive subjects or those undergoing CPR.

Although placement of an IOI is easy to learn and rapidly achieved, the technique has some limitations. Flow rates do not approximate those of an IV line of similar caliber, and may be inadequate in cases of severe shock or exsanguinating hemorrhage. However, infusion of an initial crystalloid bolus through an IO line may facilitate subsequent placement of IV lines. More rapid infusion rates may be achieved by placing the bag of IV solution in a pressure bag inflated to 300 torr, or by "pushing" the bolus with a 60 mL syringe. An IOI cannot be placed in a fractured bone.

Concurrent with IV or IO placement, blood for initial laboratory studies should be drawn and sent. In the case of traumatic shock, this should include a type and crossmatch for packed red blood cells as well as a baseline hematocrit.

Initial volume resuscitation of the patient in shock should be with isotonic crystalloid fluids. Unless the patient has cardiogenic shock, an initial bolus of 20 mL/kg administered as rapidly as possible should be given. Further fluid boluses will be administered based on reassessment of the patient's response to therapy, with frequent vital sign checks and attention to signs of end-organ perfusion—skin color and warmth, mental status, and urine output. Placement of an indwelling urinary catheter is helpful in monitoring the effectiveness of shock resuscitation. The production of 1–2 mL/kg/hr of urine is indicative of adequate fluid resuscitation. Transfusion with packed red blood cells may be necessary if an injured child fails to respond to 40 mL/kg of normal saline or Ringer's lactate. Early surgical consultation is imperative in any child who remains hemodynamically unstable after an initial fluid bolus, as emergency operative intervention may be necessary. Pneumatic antishock garments have not been demonstrated to be effective in shock therapy in children.

D: DISABILITY. Rapid assessment of both cortical and brainstem function is an important part of the initial assessment of a seriously ill or injured child. Head injury is the most common cause of death from trauma, accounting for 75% of fatal injuries. The Glasgow Coma Scale or one of the several children's coma scales adapted from that tool may be used to document serial neurologic assessments (Table 59–5). A more abbreviated initial exam consists of an evaluation of pupillary responses, and categorization of mental status based on the acronym AVPU—is the patient **A**lert? Responsive to **V**oice? Responsive to **P**ain? or, **U**nresponsive? Frequent reassessment of neurologic status is of utmost importance.

If signs of elevated intracranial pressure (ICP) are present, immediate stabilizing measures should be undertaken. Elevation of the head of the bed, mild hyperventilation to achieve a $Paco_2$ of 25–30 mm Hg, and the administration of osmotic diuretics may be indicated, depending on the etiology of the ICP elevation. Again, early surgical consultation is imperative. Early attention must also be given to interfacility transport if the hospital does not have CT or neurosurgical capability.

E: EXPOSURE. Undressing and exposing the patient are necessary to perform a thorough exam and to identify all injuries. However, undressed infants and young children are at high risk for excessive heat loss and hypothermia during a resuscitation because of their high surface area–to–volume ratio. Attention must be paid to prevention of heat loss during the emergency evaluation and treatment phase. Blankets, radiant warmers, heat lamps, and warming blankets or chemical heat packs may all have a role in the prevention of hypothermia.

Once the primary survey has been completed and the resuscitation is under way, a thorough head-to-toe physical exam should be performed. A nasogastric or orogastric tube and bladder catheter should be placed unless there are specific contraindications. Radiologic studies, further laboratory evaluation, and consults with specialists may be undertaken at this time. All seriously injured children need lateral neck, chest, and pelvic radiographs. If equipment or personnel resources for optimal definitive care of the patient do not exist, consideration should be given to initiating a patient transfer to a facility with greater capability.

PSYCHOSOCIAL/ETHICAL ISSUES IN PEDIATRIC RESUSCITATION

The resuscitation of a child—and, in particular, a failed resuscitation—is an emotionally draining event for all involved. Aggressive efforts must be undertaken whenever there is hope of saving a child's life. However, with the possible exception of children with profound hypothermia, a child brought in apneic and pulseless from the prehospital setting has essentially no chance of neurologically meaningful survival. Extensive resources may be devoted to such futile efforts, with negative consequences for the child and family. The decision not to start a resuscitation may be just as difficult as the decision to stop (Chapter 3).

Parents, faced with the sudden unexpected loss of their child, may demand that "everything" be done. In reality, when there is good physician-parent communication, most families do not insist on unreasonable measures. In dealing with family members faced with the loss of a child, it is important to remember that the spectrum of normal response may range from apparently unnatural calm, to emotional decompensation, to outrage. The anger of family members is often a reflection of their sense of guilt and helplessness.

Parents need to know that everything reasonably possible has been done to save their child—by bystanders, EMTs, or hospital personnel. At the same time, they need to be told clearly, but compassionately, when there is no hope of survival. By designating one individual to keep the parents informed on the ongoing process of the resuscitation, providing them with realistic information as it evolves, and involving them in the decision-making process when the time comes to stop, parents can be given some sense of empowerment at a time of ultimate helplessness. In some situations, allowing the parents to be present in the treatment room to witness the resuscitation may help them come to terms with the gravity of the situation, and feel that they were with their child in his or her last moments. If this is to be offered, a staff member must be available to stay with the parents. After resuscitation efforts have stopped, parents and family members should be

■ **TABLE 59–5 Glasgow Coma Scale***

Activity	Best Response	Score
Eye opening	Spontaneous	4
	To verbal stimuli	3
	To pain	2
	None	1
Verbal	Oriented	5
	Confused	4
	Inappropriate words	3
	Nonspecific sounds	2
	None	1
Motor	Follows commands	6
	Localizes pain	5
	Withdraws in response to pain	4
	Flexion in response to pain	3
	Extension in response to pain	2
	None	1

**Adapted from Teasdale G, Jennett B: Assessment of coma and impaired consciousness: A practical scale. Lancet 2:81, 1974.*

provided with a private room in which to hold the child and say goodbye.

Death or neurologically poor survival is the rule if asystole persists after administration of two doses of IV epinephrine or after 25 min of CPR. The fact that one can restore a perfusing rhythm with multiple rounds of resuscitation drugs should not be construed as success. We must remember that the goal is survival with good functional neurologic recovery.

At the point at which the code leader wishes to stop CPR and pronounce the child dead, members of the team should be queried to ensure that all personnel involved feel that everything appropriate has been done. An opportunity for staff debriefing should be provided immediately following the code, as emotions tend to run high with the death of a child. Formal code review, looking at process and outcome of each resuscitation, is an important part of the department's quality improvement program.

American Heart Association: Emergency Cardiac Care Committee and Subcommittees. Guidelines for cardiopulmonary resuscitation and emergency cardiac care, VI pediatric advanced life support. JAMA 268:2262, 1992.

Baker MD, Ludwig S: Pediatric emergency transport and the private practitioner. Pediatrics 88:691, 1991.

Cales RH: Trauma mortality in Orange County: The effect of implementation of a regional trauma system. Ann Emerg Med 13:1, 1984.

Chameides L, Hazinski H (eds): Textbook of Advanced Pediatric Life Support. Dallas, TX, American Heart Association, 1994.

Committee on Trauma, American College of Surgeons: Advanced Trauma Life Support. Chicago, IL, American College of Surgeons, 1993.

Day S, McCloskey K, Orr R, et al: Pediatric interhospital critical care transport: Consensus of a national leadership conference. Pediatrics 88:696, 1991.

Doyle CJ, Post H, Burney RE, et al: Family participation during resuscitation: An option. Ann Emerg Med 16:673, 1987.

Durch JS, Lohr KN (eds): Emergency Medical Services for Children. Washington DC, National Academy Press, 1993.

Eichelberger MR, Gotschall CS, Sacco, et al: A comparison of the Trauma Score, the Revised Trauma Score, and the Pediatric Trauma Score. Ann Emerg Med 18:1053, 1989.

Eisenberg M, Berger L, Hallstrom A: Epidemiology of cardiac arrest and resuscitation in children. Ann Emerg Med 12:672, 1983.

Fiser DH: Intraosseous infusion. N Engl J Med 322:1579, 1990.

Fuchs S, Jaffe DM, Christoffel KK: Pediatric emergencies in office practices: Prevalence and office preparedness. Pediatrics 83:931, 1989.

Kaufmann CR, Maier RV, Rivara FP, et al: Evaluation of the Pediatric Trauma Score. JAMA 63:69, 1990.

Lubitz DS, Seidel JS, Chameides L, et al: A rapid method for estimating weight and resuscitation drug dosages from length in the pediatric age group. Ann Emerg Med 17:576, 1988.

Macnab AJ: Optimal escort for interhospital transport of pediatric emergencies. J Trauma 31:205, 1991.

Orlowski JP, Porembka DT, Gallagher JM, et al: Comparison study of intraosseous, central intravenous, and peripheral intravenous infusions of emergency drugs. Am J Dis Child 144:112, 1990.

O'Rourke PP: Outcome of children who are apneic and pulseless in the emergency room. Crit Care Med 14:466, 1986.

Pang D, Wilberger JE: Spinal cord injury without radiographic abnormalities in children. J Neurosurg 57:114, 1982.

Pollack MM, Alexander SR, Clarke N, et al: Improved outcomes from tertiary center pediatric intensive care: A statewide comparison of tertiary and nontertiary care facilities. Crit Care Med 19:150, 1991.

Quan L, Wentz KR, Gore EJ, et al: Outcome and predictors of outcome in pediatric submersion victims receiving prehospital care in King County, Washington. Pediatrics 86:586, 1990.

Schweich PJ, DeAngelis C, Duggan AK: Preparedness of practicing pediatricians to manage emergencies. Pediatrics 88:223, 1991.

Seidel JS: Emergency medical services and the pediatric patient: Are the needs being met? II. Training and equipping emergency medical services providers for pediatric emergencies. Pediatrics 78:808, 1986.

Singer J, Ludwig S (eds): Emergency Medical Services for Children: The Role of the Primary Care Provider. Elk Grove Village, IL, American Academy of Pediatrics, 1992.

Tsai A, Kallsen G: Epidemiology of pediatric prehospital care. Ann Emerg Med 16:284, 1987.

CHAPTER 60

Pediatric Critical Care

George Lister and J. Julio Pérez Fontán

Critical care is defined by the setting where human and technical resources are concentrated to provide sophisticated care, usually in an intensive care unit; by the uniqueness of the knowledge and technical skills required to provide the care; and, most importantly, by the common features of the disease processes that result in critical illness. Although it is unrealistic for every pediatrician to be knowledgeable in all the aspects of critical care, it is essential that those who are involved in the medical management of children be capable of recognizing the sign of potentially life-threatening disease, of evaluating the severity of its manifestations, and of initiating the stabilization of infants or children who suffer these problems. The most common life-threatening problems that afflict infants and children are *respiratory distress, impaired peripheral perfusion,* and *altered consciousness.*

RESPIRATORY DISTRESS

PATHOGENESIS. Significant injuries and diseases of the respiratory system invariably alter the exchange of oxygen and carbon dioxide between air and blood. When the respiratory system is unable to sustain oxygen uptake or carbon dioxide elimination commensurate with metabolic demands, respiratory insufficiency ensues. The means by which this disruption in blood-gas exchange occurs usually involves one or more of three general processes: (1) *abnormalities of mechanical function* of the lungs and chest wall, (2) *neuromuscular abnormalities* affecting the nerves and muscles of respiration, and (3) *disturbances of respiratory control* or drive. Because mechanical abnormalities are the most common type of disturbances, respiratory insufficiency is usually accompanied by *respiratory distress,* the use of excessive effort to sustain breathing.

While the predominant concern with respiratory insufficiency relates to the aberrations in gas exchange, reliance on changes in blood gas tensions alone for detection of problems is not sufficient. Data may be easily subject to misinterpretation because compensatory mechanisms put forth by the patient and the common practice of administering supplemental oxygen maintain blood gas tensions near normal levels until the patient's respiratory muscles cannot sustain the effort any longer. The equipment needed to measure blood gas tensions and pH is not always immediately available, while judgment of oxygenation or ventilation by visual inspection (which is influenced by skin color, perfusion, and ambient lighting) is surprisingly inaccurate and unreliable, even amongst the most skilled physicians. From these disclaimers one might conclude that it is difficult to detect incipient respiratory failure. However, physical signs yield many important clues about the nature of the respiratory dysfunction and how well the patient is tolerating it; these signs often precede abnormalities of blood gas tensions.

Mechanical Dysfunction. Most mechanical dysfunction disease is either restrictive or obstructive in nature. *Restrictive lung disease* occurs when the lungs or the structures that surround the lungs (pleura, rib cage, and abdomen) limit the expansion of the lungs in a volume-dependent fashion. Processes in which the interstitium is infiltrated (pulmonary edema, inflammation), the alveoli are consolidated or collapsed, or the lung is compressed from an external source (tense ascites, pneumothorax) commonly produce this type of problem. The consequences of restrictive disease and the increased elastic recoil are twofold (Fig. 60–1): (1) It takes more force or muscle effort during inspiration to maintain tidal volume (expiration is passive and is not affected), and (2) the alveolar volumes decrease so the lungs operate at a lower end-expiratory volume (functional residual capacity) and average volume. The decreased functional residual capacity causes arterial Po_2 to decrease and the arterial hypoxemia, in turn, causes respiratory drive to increase.

The increased respiratory effort with restrictive disease is manifested by use of accessory inspiratory muscles, such as the scalene and sternocleidomastoid, and, particularly in the infant, by the presence of retractions. Each of these changes raises respiratory work, consumes more energy to breathe, and predisposes the child to fatigue. There is also transient closure of the upper airway at the end of expiration, usually described as grunting (whether or not it is audible), which attempts to increase lung volume and restore functional residual capacity. There is often flaring of the ala nasae, which decreases inspiratory resistance.

As the respiratory muscles become less effective at sustaining their load, respiratory rate increases and tidal volume decreases, a pattern of breathing known as *tachypnea* (to be distinguished from hyperpnea, deep breathing that is slightly increased in frequency). Although depth of breathing is difficult to quantify by physical examination, the respiratory rate is an excellent and reliable guide that can be judged by simple inspection. As restrictive lung disease (whatever the specific etiology) progresses, it should be anticipated that there will be *tachypnea, grunting,* and *signs of increased work,* with the respiratory rate indicating the severity of the mechanical dysfunction. It is very important to recognize that with restrictive disease, whenever there are factors that provoke an increase in minute ventilation, (*fever, acidosis, hypoxemia, exercise*), the tachypnea will be even more apparent. The response to these stresses helps distinguish the child with normal lungs from the one

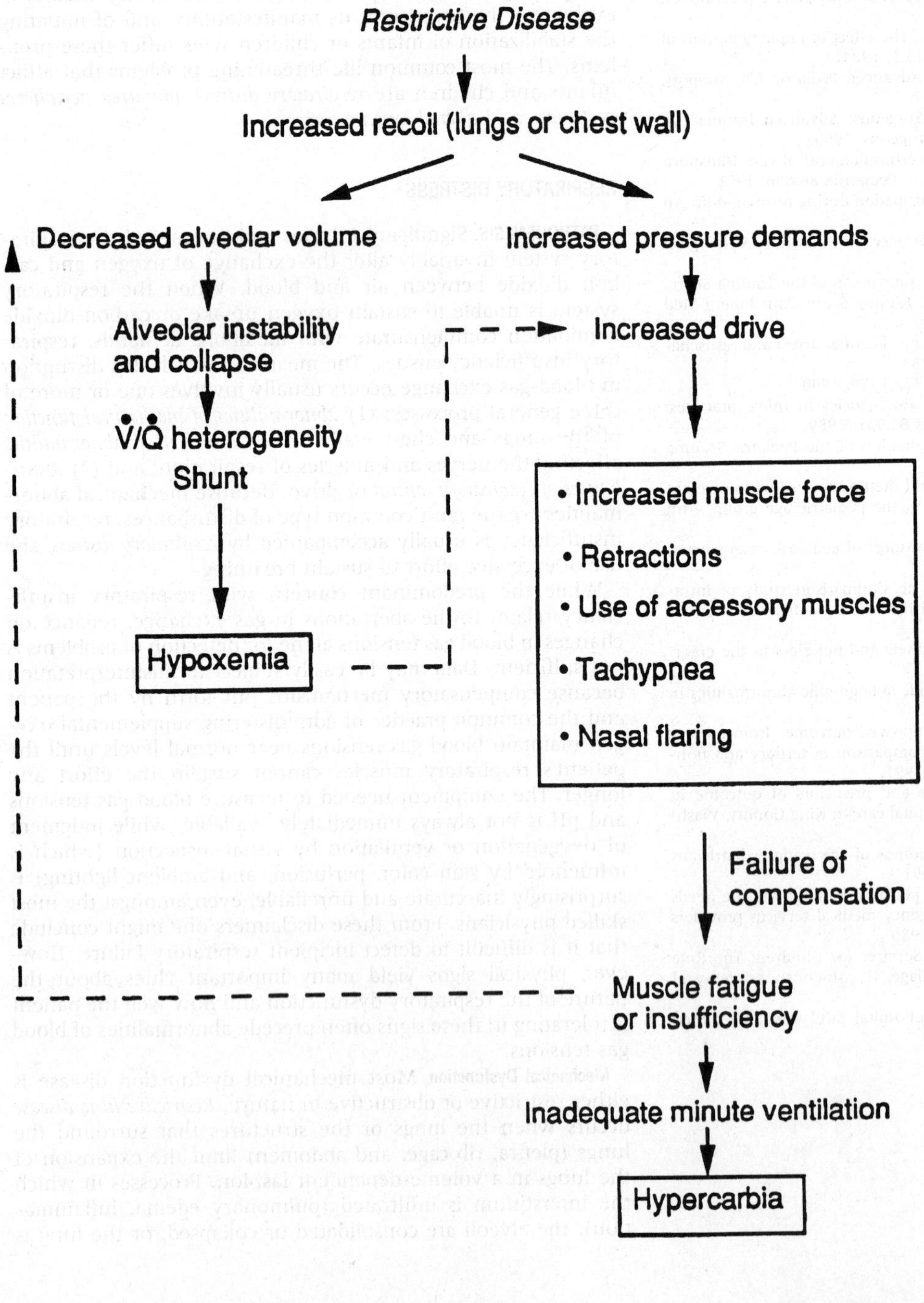

Figure 60–1. The effects of restrictive lung disease on gas exchange and breathing function. As described in the text, restrictive disease causes increased recoil of the lungs or chest wall, either of which causes alveolar volume to decrease and pressure demands to increase. The decreased alveolar volume produces hypoxemia by promoting $\dot{V}/\dot{Q}$ heterogeneity and shunt, and the increased pressure demands provoke responses to overcome the increased work of breathing. When compensation is inadequate, the fatigue causes worsening gas exchange and results in hypercarbia and further hypoxemia.

with restrictive lung disease: the former will become *hyperpneic* and the latter *tachypneic* when minute ventilation is increased.

Obstructive lung disease occurs when the expansion of the lungs is limited in a flow-dependent fashion. It results from narrowing of the intrathoracic or the extrathoracic airways. The consequence is that it will take more effort for gas to flow into or out of the lungs, particularly when the flow rates are high (as during rapid breathing).

With *extrathoracic airway obstruction* (epiglottitis, croup, foreign body, very enlarged tonsils and adenoids, poor hypopharyngeal tone), the time for inspiration relative to expiration increases and inspiratory effort increases, as manifested by the use of accessory inspiratory muscles and retractions, which are often quite severe. Inspiration is specifically affected because of the tendency for the extrathoracic airways to narrow during this phase of respiration. Usually the breathing rate remains low and may decrease below normal. However, the breathing rate also depends on whether there is coexistent restrictive disease (as might occur with croup) and whether there are other factors involved (use of opioids). Regardless of the overall respiratory rate adopted by the patient, inspiration will remain prolonged relative to expiration when there is significant airway obstruction.

There are other important signs that help characterize and localize the pathologic process in a patient with extrathoracic obstruction. For example, stridor is common during inspiration and denotes the presence of extrathoracic obstruction and turbulence to airflow. A hoarse voice or cry strongly suggests that the larynx is affected, as would occur with croup (*laryngotracheobronchitis*). In addition, when changes in the configuration of the airway produced by position or other manipulations alter the degree of inspiratory difficulty, it implies that the obstruction is not fixed and may relate to the hypopharynx or to an unstable cervical spine.

With *intrathoracic airway obstruction,* (bronchiolitis, asthma, foreign body, vascular ring), there is an impediment to airflow out of the lungs. Because of this the emptying of the lungs cannot be completed during expiration and lung volume increases (hyperinflation). Accordingly, breathing effort increases, expiratory or abdominal muscles are used, and the expiratory phase is prolonged. The hyperinflation flattens the diaphragmatic contour and places the diaphragm in a mechanically disadvantageous configuration, which reduces the efficiency of breathing. When there is both obstructive and restrictive disease (bronchiolitis), the respiratory rate may be increased, even though the relative time of expiration also increases. Although the presence of diffuse wheezes usually indicates intrathoracic obstruction, this sign has little value in localizing the precise site of that obstruction. The presence of asymmetric wheezes helps identify a focal problem such as unilateral obstruction of an airway lumen from a foreign body aspiration or an enlarged heart; wheezing that shifts from site to site, or clears and appears abruptly, is often associated with mucus entrapment; and wheezing that is accentuated by changes in position is most likely associated with extrinsic masses.

Adaptation to Increased Work. Both restrictive and obstructive disease increase the work of breathing. Accordingly, they predispose the child to fatigue and eventually to respiratory arrest. The response of the respiratory system to the increased work is analogous to that of other muscular systems during excessive physical labor. Accessory muscles are used to accommodate the increased work load placed on the respiratory system. If, these compensatory mechanisms cannot be sustained, there is muscle fatigue. First, there may be tachypnea, an early sign of respiratory muscle fatigue. Then, some muscles may rest while others are used giving the appearance of a respiratory pattern that is frequently changing. Bobbing of the head as the muscles of the neck and shoulders are rested is one of the clear and late signs of fatigue; unfortunately, this may also interfere with the patency of the upper airway. There may also be brief periods of excessive effort (very rapid respiration with restrictive disease or deep respiration with obstructive disease) preceded and followed by short periods of apnea. This latter pattern is an ominous sign that respiratory arrest is incipient, and the physician should not be comforted by blood gas tensions that are near normal. The patient needs assisted breathing, and skilled assistance should be immediately sought.

Abnormalities of Respiratory Drive or Neuromuscular Function. Even if the mechanical state of the lungs is relatively normal, respiratory insufficiency can occur when the drive to breathe or neuromuscular function is impaired, because either one disrupts the capacity of the respiratory system to respond to chemical signals that control minute ventilation. Impaired neuromuscular function or drive can be relatively insidious and difficult to detect because the patient may not appear distressed. Patients with neuromuscular diseases (Guillain-Barré syndrome, muscular dystrophy, myasthenia gravis) often appear to be relatively apathetic to the disturbances in gas exchange consequent to their weakness. Perhaps this is because the onset in weakness and in respiratory insufficiency is relatively gradual and the signs we use to infer the presence of distress relate to the appearance of excessive muscular effort. With rare exceptions in infants and children, impaired respiratory drive occurs in patients with depressed consciousness from either a global injury (toxic-metabolic injury or drug administration) or injury to the brain stem (trauma, herniation). These patients may fail to increase breathing effort when mechanical dysfunction occurs and therefore have no outward signs of respiratory distress. Thus, it is essential to assess general muscle strength and level of responsiveness when evaluating a patient with disturbed blood gas exchange to ensure that they have the capacity to respond to chemical stimuli that normally provoke an increase in respiratory drive. Moreover, because mechanical, neuromuscular, and respiratory control abnormalities often coexist, one has to make an effort to assess whether the compensatory response for a given mechanical derangement is appropriate.

Disruption of Gas Exchange. Each alveolar-capillary unit functions as a potential site for exchange of oxygen and carbon dioxide in which complete equilibrium of pressure is achieved for each gas between the blood and gas phase, except when the alveolus contains no gas. The pressure for oxygen and carbon dioxide in the capillary blood exiting the lung parenchyma is determined by that equilibrium.

If one envisions that under static conditions inspired alveolar gas mixes with systemic venous blood and reaches equilibrium across a diffusible surface, then it is apparent that the larger the volume of gas relative to blood, the higher will be the equilibrium Po_2 (closer to the Po_2 of inspired gas). Under dynamic conditions when venous blood is flowing into the capillary and gas is entering the alveoli in a tidal fashion, the Po_2 of capillary blood at equilibrium is a function of the respective volume flows of oxygen in inspired gas and mixed venous blood. The flow of oxygen in the gas depends on the Po_2 of inspired gas and the alveolar ventilation; the flow of oxygen in mixed venous blood depends on the oxygen carrying capacity or hemoglobin concentration, the mixed venous Po_2 or hemoglobin-oxygen saturation, and the pulmonary blood flow. If alveolar ventilation (V) is high relative to blood flow (Q), high V/Q, the resultant capillary Po_2 will be relatively high; conversely, if the ventilation is low relative to blood flow, capillary Po_2 will be decreased.

Similar to oxygen, the alveolar-capillary Pco_2 depends on the relationship between ventilation and perfusion; the higher the V/Q, the closer the Pco_2 will be to inspired gas and the lower the V/Q, the closer the Pco_2 will be to mixed venous blood.

release of epinephrine and norepinephrine, while constriction of renal afferent arterioles stimulates an increase in renin production, which initiates an increase in circulating aldosterone, of angiotensin II, and indirectly of antidiuretic hormone. Each of these hormones is a potent vasoconstrictor that raises blood pressure; furthermore, antidiuretic hormone and aldosterone promote water and sodium reabsorption, respectively, which helps restore intravascular volume. Thus, the humoral responses complement the neural reflexes and provide longer range regulation of the circulation.

Regulation of Regional Blood Flow. Even when arterial blood pressure decreases, some organs (brain, heart) maintain blood flow by vasodilation. This *autoregulation* opposes the neural and humoral stimulation by the sympatho-adrenal system and the release of vasoactive peptides that tend to cause vasoconstriction when cardiac output is decreased. How much a given organ responds to the vasodilatory or the vasoconstrictive influences depends on the inherent capacity to autoregulate, the innervation, and the density and nature of the vascular receptors. In addition, local metabolism influences blood flow such that active tissue (working muscle) maintains blood flow even in the presence of neurohumoral stimulation. Therefore, when cardiac output is decreased, organs that are usually metabolically active or have little autonomic innervation (brain, heart) preserve their perfusion, whereas organs that have a low metabolic rate (skin) or have rich autonomic innervation (kidney, gut) have intense vasoconstriction. These responses improve the matching of blood flow to metabolism and, by increasing total vascular resistance, raise blood pressure.

When perfusion to an organ or tissue is reduced there are also local responses, which include opening of previously closed capillaries, that serve to maximize the extraction of oxygen and other nutrients from arterial blood. If oxidative metabolism cannot be sustained, the tissues produce excess H^+ and lactate, metabolic rate declines, and the function of that tissue is reduced. Thus, when there is compromised perfusion to tissue, such as the skin, one would anticipate cooler cutaneous temperature (less perfusion with warm blood, less metabolism), prolonged capillary refill time (less perfusion), bluish or cyanotic discoloration (increased oxygen extraction and lower capillary and venous oxygen saturation), and diminished pulsation of the artery serving that tissue (vasoconstriction).

In addition to redirecting blood flow, the humoral responses serve to augment cardiac output by three mechanisms. Heart rate is increased (response to epinephrine) and a sinus tachycardia should be expected as a compensatory response in any child with compromised perfusion unless there is also a problem in cardiac conduction. Contractility will be enhanced by the catecholamine stimulation, but the effectiveness of this adaptation depends on the capacity of the myocardium to respond and whether there is adequate cardiac filling. Finally, venous return will be increased by the venoconstriction, which decreases venous capacitance and raises the driving pressure for blood to return to the right atrium, and by the renal mechanisms that promote fluid retention.

Causes of Inadequate Cardiac Output. Globally impaired perfusion arises when cardiac output to the tissues cannot keep pace with the demands for blood flow imposed by the body's metabolism. Because cardiac output is the product of stroke volume and heart rate, it can be shown to depend directly on three factors: *end-diastolic* or *filling volume, ejection fraction,* and *heart rate.** If any of these are decreased, a decline in system blood flow would be expected unless adaptive responses compensate. Examples of these physiologic disturbances are shown in Table 60–4.

Reduced filling volume occurs with loss of intravascular volume, increase in vascular capacity, or impedance to venous return. Whereas intravascular volume loss is often apparent from history and measurement of body weight, extravasation of fluid from the vascular space can be subtle and only recognized by careful physical examination, especially when fluid has leaked into the interstitial space, bowel lumen, or peritoneum. Increased vascular (predominantly venous) capacity will reduce venous return and filling volume, and can be a difficult problem to detect because the blood volume remains in the vascular space and there is no sign of vascular congestion nor weight loss. Finally, impedance to venous return, as with pericardial tamponade or tension pneumothorax, can dramatically reduce end-diastolic volume of the heart and will produce signs of increased systemic venous pressure (hepatic enlargement, jugular venous distension, fullness of the fontanel), but it usually is not associated with weight change unless the process has been chronic.

Reduced ejection fraction can result from poor contractile function or impedance to outflow of the heart. With processes that impair contractile function, there is often a gallop rhythm and signs of systemic and pulmonary venous congestion. However, it is very important to recognize that respiratory distress—including tachypnea, wheezing, air trapping, or alveolar collapse—from the congested and edematous lungs may mimic primary pulmonary diseases and obscure the diagnosis of cardiac dysfunction; a useful finding that implicates cardiac rather than respiratory disease is the presence of cardiomegaly. An increased afterload, the pressure against which the ventricle must pump during ejection, can also depress cardiac ejection, especially when the process is abrupt, as in infants with closure of a ductus arteriosus in the presence of aortic stenosis or coarctation. With an increased afterload there are usually signs of systemic or pulmonary venous congestion, depending on which of the ventricle(s) is predominantly affected. Cardiovascular collapse can be the first sign if the load rises abruptly before compensatory responses (hypertrophy) can occur.

Although a *slow heart rate* is uncommon as a primary problem in children, it often occurs in response to asphyxia. Bradycardia can also aggravate other causes of poor perfusion because tachycardia is the expected adaptive response. Peripheral perfusion can be further disturbed by factors that raise the demands for blood flow, such as anemia, hypoxemia, fever, and excessive respiratory work. The importance of recognizing such factors is that they may sometimes be alleviated (fever, anemia) and thus improve the balance between blood flow and metabolic demands.

ASSESSMENT. The first goal in assessment is to determine whether the child's perfusion is adequate to sustain vital functions. This can usually be determined by physical examination. The findings from the physical examination of the child with poor perfusion are a reflection of both the changes that occur primarily from the decrease in blood flow and those that occur in response to the adaptations. Superimposed on this picture may also be factors that relate to the underlying illness or injury that has disturbed the perfusion. The child with severe dehydration can have poor peripheral arterial pulses, cold and cyanotic extremities, and decreased capillary refill, whereas a child with a similar degree of dehydration in combination with systemic infection might have warm rather than cold extremities, even though peripheral pulses are difficult to feel. Table 60–5 gives an overview of the physical examination of the child with reduced systemic perfusion.

Vital signs should be measured and put in perspective with the physical findings. Both systolic and diastolic blood pressure should be measured because with peripheral vasoconstriction

---

*$CO = SV \times HR = (EDV - ESV) \times HR = EDV \times (EDV - ESV)/EDV \times HR = EDV \times EF \times HR$, where EDV and ESV are end-diastolic and end-systolic volumes, respectively, HR is heart rate, and EF is ejection fraction.

■ TABLE 60–4 Causes of Inadequate Cardiac Output

Physiologic Disturbance	Mechanism	Examples
Insufficient cardiac filling	Intravascular volume depletion	
	Fluid loss from body	Hemorrhage, enteric fluid loss, excess insensible H_2O loss (heat stroke), urinary loss (diabetes insipidus or mellitus)
	Extravasation from vascular space	Peritonitis, ileus, intracranial hemorrhage, trauma, sepsis
	Increased vascular capacity	Drug-induced venodilation, spinal trauma, anaphylaxis, sepsis
	Impedance to venous return	Tamponade, tension pneumothorax or pneumomediastinum, positive pressure ventilation, tachyarrhythmia
Impaired ejection	Impedance to ventricular outflow	Coarctation of aorta, aortic stenosis, pulmonary embolus, hypertension
	Decreased myocardial contractility	Asphyxia, myocarditis, myocardial infarction, sepsis
Bradycardia	Disorder of impulse formation	Sick sinus syndrome, hypoxemia
	Disorder of impulse conduction	Hyperkalemia, digitalis or tricyclic antidepressant overdose, complete heart block
Increased demand for blood	Reduced arterial blood concentration of O_2	Anemia, hypoxemia
	Impaired nutrient utilization	Cyanide poisoning, salicylism
	Maldistribution of flow	Arteriovenous fistula, sepsis, acute respiratory distress syndrome
	Increased metabolic rate	Fever, non-neutral thermal environment, excessive work of breathing, thyrotoxicosis, malignant hyperthermia

Adapted with permission from Lister G, Apkon M, Fabry JT: Shock. In: *Emmanouilides GC, Riemenschneider TA, Allen HD, Gutgesell HP (eds): Moss & Adam's Heart Disease in Infants, Children and Adolescents: Including the Fetus and Young Adult, 5th ed. Baltimore, Williams & Wilkins, 1994, pp 1725–1746.*

systolic blood pressure can be normal but pulse pressure will be narrow. Blood pressure should be measured in an upper (preferably right arm) and lower body extremity in an infant because of the possibility of aortic coarctation. During the physical examination, particular attention should be paid to the alertness and interactiveness of the child. Restlessness or apathy are often cause by poor cerebral perfusion. Persistent grunting (which may appear to represent a weak cry) can be a sign of respiratory distress and can be seen with low perfusion states, even when there is no primary or secondary pulmonary involvement.

Once it is determined that perfusion is impaired, data should be sought to determine the primary factors interfering with perfusion, the most rational approach to re-establish adequate circulation, and whether the patient is stable. To determine the cause(s) of the poor perfusion, it is particularly useful to assess whether intravascular volume is expanded or depleted by examining the size of the liver and the fullness of the anterior fontanel or of the jugular veins, and, when possible, weighing the patient (Figure 60–2). Although laboratory data are usually not needed to decide whether perfusion is adequate, they are quite valuable in determining how perfusion has been disturbed. Essential information includes an electrocardiogram (to determine whether there is the expected sinus tachycardia or any dysrhythmia), a radiograph of the chest (to determine whether the circulation is engorged or depleted, and the heart is large or small), and a measure of acid/base status to determine the adequacy of metabolic compensation and whether asphyxia has contributed to myocardial dysfunction. Measurement of hemoglobin concentration and/or hematocrit and blood electrolyte, glucose, creatinine, and urea nitrogen concentration will be helpful in discerning the etiology of the circulatory disturbance and in determining what fluid therapy will be most appropriate after the initial treatment.

When a child is perceived to have poor perfusion, certain monitoring should be initiated to assist with the assessment and to judge the adequacy of the response. At the least, this monitoring should include frequent measurements of blood pressure, continuous display of the heart rate or ECG and arterial O_2 saturation, and measurement of urine output (insertion of a bladder catheter should be considered). Ultrasound imaging and doppler flow velicometry are exceptionally valuable for evaluation and monitoring of myocardial contractile function and cardiac filling volume, and for detection of pericardial effusion.

INITIAL STABILIZATION. If it has been determined that the patient needs restoration of perfusion, vascular access must be established. It is often quite difficult to place a catheter percutaneously in a peripheral vein when the patient's circulating volume is decreased; alternative approaches may be needed, even

■ TABLE 60–5 Signs of Decreased Perfusion

Organ System	↓ Perfusion	↓ ↓ Perfusion	↓ ↓ ↓ Perfusion
CNS	—	Restless, apathetic	Agitated/confused, stuporous
Respiration	—	↑ Ventilation	↑ ↑ Ventilation
Metabolism	—	Compensated metabolic acidemia	Uncompensated metabolic acidemia
Gut	—	↓ Motility	Ileus
Kidney	↓ Urine volume, ↑ Urinary specific gravity	Oliguria	Oliguria/anuria
Skin	Delayed capillary refill	Cool extremities	Mottled, cyanotic, cold extremities
CVS	↑ Heart rate	↑ ↑ Heart rate, ↓ Peripheral pulses	↑ ↑ Heart rate, ↓ blood pressure, central pulses only

CNS, central nervous system; CVS, cardiovascular system; ↑, increased; ↓, decreased.
Adapted with permission from Lister G, Apkon M, Fabry JT: Shock. In: *Emmanouilides GC, Riemenschneider TA, Allen HD, Gutgesell HP (eds): Moss & Adam's Heart Disease in Infants, Children and Adolescents: Including the Fetus and Young Adult, 5th ed. Baltimore, Williams & Wilkins, 1994, pp 1725–1746.*

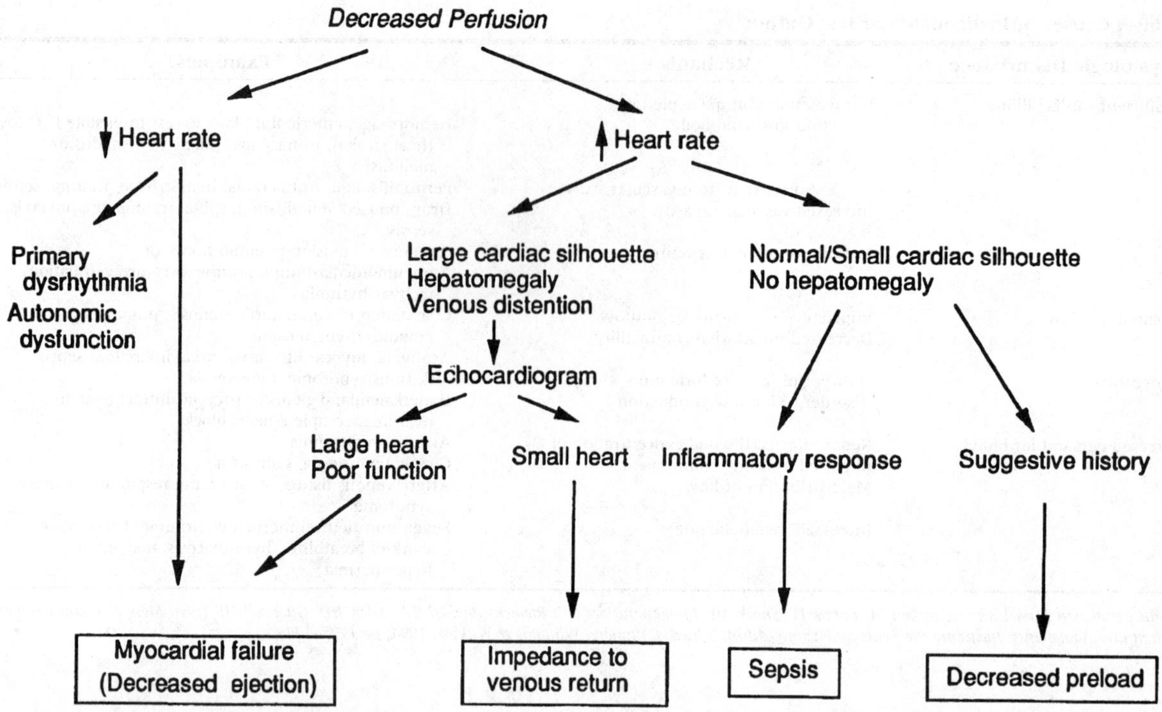

Figure 60–2. Algorithm for discerning the cause of decreased perfusion. Although heart rate is usually increased in response to poor systemic perfusion, the presence of bradycardia should provoke a search for a primary dysrhythmia (e.g., heart block) or autonomic dysfunction (e.g., spinal cord trauma), or raise concern that there is severe myocardial failure. Alternatively, when heart rate is increased, one should attempt to determine whether or not there are signs of systemic venous engorgement. When the heart silhouette is enlarged and there is venous distension, it is important to distinguish whether the heart is well filled and suffering from poor inotropic function, or there is impedance to venous return (e.g., cardiac tamponade, tension pneumothorax); under these circumstances, an echocardiogram is an invaluable tool. When there is tachycardia with no sign of venous distension, inadequate perfusion can be caused by decreased preload and insufficient cardiac filling (e.g., hemorrhage, dehydration) or diminished effective circulation, as in sepsis (with diffuse inflammation, venodilatation, and maldistribution of blood flow). It is also important to recognize that many of the problems that cause decreased perfusion can do so by more than one mechanism. Sepsis is a good example of a process that can diminish preload and produce myocardial failure simultaneously.

in the child who is not necessarily deteriorating but needs therapy. Techniques such as percutaneous cannulation (Seldinger technique) of a large central vein, venisection, or intraosseous cannulation are appropriate when the patient is in shock and there is no means for fluid and medication administration.

Supplemental oxygen should be provided (usually by face mask or face tent, or by head box in the infant) to maximize oxygen delivery and keep the lungs filled with oxygen, even if arterial oxygen saturation is normal. If, however, oxygen administration worsens the patient's perfusion, as can occur in the infant with critical congenital left heart obstruction in whom the ductus arteriosus constricts, then the supplemental oxygen (like any other drug that causes an adverse outcome) should be stopped.

In the course of the physical assessment, it should be determined which of the factors—*heart rate, cardiac ejection,* or *cardiac filling*—is impaired, so that therapy can commence. It is quite possible, depending on how far the underlying process has progressed, that circulatory function is impaired by more than one mechanism. A child with sepsis can have poor contractile function, diminished preload, and increased metabolic demands. However, in any child with poor perfusion, it is essential to start in the repair of the circulation before there is further deterioration. If the circulation is not engorged, perfusion will usually be aided by rapid and repetitive infusion of crystalloid fluid in an isotonic mixture (normal saline, Ringer lactate) in aliquot of 5–10 mL/kg. Volumes as large as 70 mL/kg in 24 hr may be needed in addition to maintenance fluid requirements and replacement of ongoing losses. Following initial attempts at restoration of perfusion with crystalloid, the subsequent choice of fluid should be based on the type of deficits and specific problems identified. For example, if there is anemia and circulating volume depletion, packed red blood cells are needed, whereas fresh plasma may be more appropriate if there is an associated bleeding diathesis.

If there is venous congestion, then it is likely that there is impaired ejection of blood or impedance to filling of the heart. Inotropic support should be provided whenever there is direct evidence of depressed myocardial function (except in obstructive cardiomyopathies), or when it seems likely based on physical findings (venous congestion, cardiomegaly). Depressed function may be apparent on the initial examination or when, after fluid administration, there is a progressive increase in venous engorgement without improvement in perfusion. The inotropic drugs that are most appropriate are given by intravenous route; the dose can be adjusted as conditions change. The most commonly used drugs are the direct and indirect acting β-agonists, including epinephrine, dopamine, and dobutamine, and the phosphodiesterase inhibitor, amrinone (see Chapter 60.2). As these drugs also have peripheral vascular effects, it is worth considering whether some degree of vasoconstriction is needed to increase blood pressure (dopamine, epinephrine) or whether vasodilation would be beneficial (dobutamine, amrinone, isoproterenol). Generally, the former group of drugs is most useful initially until it is clear whether blood pressure is sufficient to support perfusion. More sophisticated approaches to the support of the circulation, such as left-ventricular assist device balloon counterpulsation, are not widely available and are appropriate only in specialized settings. Some of the important and more common causes for impedance to filling are listed in Table 60–4.

If heart rate is not appropriately increased, there should be immediate concern that there is severe hypoxemia or asphyxia, or that the myocardium is intrinsically injured. In this circumstance, oxygen should be given, cardiac rhythm should be checked, and consideration should be given to the use of an inotropic drug with chronotropic properties (isoproterenol).

The response to therapy can be judged by repetitive physical examinations and measurements of vital signs. In particular, one should expect to find a decreasing heart rate, enhanced peripheral perfusion, and possibly increasing blood pressure or pulse pressure as the circulation is improved. If, on the other hand, signs of pulmonary congestion or edema (tachypnea, crackles, wheezing, retractions) develop or worsen, or signs of systemic venous congestion (enlarged liver) develop without appropriate restoration of peripheral perfusion, it is necessary to consider more invasive monitoring. Placement of a central venous catheter can be useful for measuring filling pressure of the right heart and for monitoring oxygen extraction. When there is reason to believe that the right and left ventricles have markedly different filling pressures or disparate functions, a pulmonary artery balloon flotation catheter (Swan Ganz) may be needed to assist in the evaluation of cardiac output and response to therapy.

An important adjunct to therapy can be to use positive pressure ventilation in the patient with shock, even when there are not overt signs of respiratory distress. Supplanting the work of breathing can decrease overall metabolic rate and divert blood flow from respiratory muscles to other vital tissues.

There are some special considerations related to the neonate with left heart obstruction (coarctation or aortic stenosis or atresia) that merit consideration because of the frequency with which these conditions occur and the potential for improvement with infusion of prostaglandin E_1. These conditions commonly produce circulatory shock within the 1st wk after birth; there will be little, if any, improvement in perfusion with conventional approaches, but prostaglandin, by opening a constricted ductus arteriosus, can provide a dramatic increase in distal aortic perfusion until more definitive therapy is initiated.

Once therapy for poor perfusion is started, it is incumbent to search for an underlying etiology to treat, to consider additional strategies for improving circulatory function, and to plan a transfer to a facility equipped to provide extended monitoring and management.

Dantzker DR: Pulmonary gas exchange. *In:* Dantzker DR (ed): Cardiopulmonary Critical Care. Philadelphia, WB Saunders, 1986, pp 25–46.

Lister G, Apkon M, Fahey JT: Shock. *In:* Emmanouilides GC, Riemenschneider TA, Allen HD, Gutgesell HP (eds): *Moss & Adam's Heart Disease in Infants, Children and Adolescents: Including the Fetus and Young Adult,* 5th ed. Baltimore, MD, Williams & Wilkins, 1994, pp 1725–1746.

Matthay MA: Invasive hemodynamic monitoring in critically ill patients. Clin Chest Med 4:233–249, 1983.

Pérez-Fontán JJ: Mechanics of breathing. *In:* Gluckman PD, Heymann MA (eds): *Perinatal and Pediatric Pathophysiology: A Clinical Perspective.* London, Edward Arnold Publishers, 1993, pp 623–632.

Pérez-Fontán JJ, Lister G: Respiratory failure. *In:* Touloukian RJ (ed): *Pediatric Trauma,* 2nd ed. St. Louis, MO, Mosby Year Book, 1990, pp 46–76.

Pontoppidan H, Geffin B, Lowenstein E: Acute respiratory failure in the adult. N Engl J Med 287 part 1:690–698, 1972.

Pontoppidan H, Geffin B, Lowenstein E: Acute respiratory failure in the adult. N Engl J Med 287 part 2:743–752, 1972.

Pontoppidan H, Geffin B, Lowenstein E: Acute respiratory failure in the adult. N Engl J Med 287 part 3:799–806, 1972.

60.1 *States of Altered Consciousness*

George Lister and J. Julio Pérez Fontán

Alterations in the function of the central nervous system (CNS), independent of whether they are caused by a primary disorder in the brain or spinal cord, or occur as part of systemic process, are often life threatening and always serious. The CNS contains the organs responsible for the control of all basic vital functions and coordinates reflex and conscious acts that provide protection against environmental threats. Children, like adults, can present with a wide range of neurologic abnormalities, which are covered in detail in other sections of this textbook. The intent here will be to discuss briefly the diagnosis and management of some common forms of CNS dysfunction that, by virtue of their severity or rapidly progressive nature, require emergent action. Because these forms of CNS dysfunction usually involve alterations in the state of consciousness as their most prominent manifestation, the discussion will focus on the diagnosis and management of the comatose child.

The variability of the physical and behavioral manifestations associated with states of altered consciousness makes their clinical classification difficult. The problem is often solved by judging the severity of the alteration based on scoring systems, like the Glasgow Coma Scale (Chapter 59, Table 59–5). While helpful for descriptive and even prognostic purposes, these systems provide relatively little information on the mechanisms that lead to the alteration of consciousness. Such information needs to be obtained through a thorough neurologic examination and careful evaluation of the clinical history and associated signs and symptoms.

The word *coma* is used to refer to a state in which the infant or child is unable to arouse and is completely unaware of self and surroundings, even in the presence of strong physical stimuli. *Stupor* is characterized by a quiescent attitude that simulates normal sleep. But, in contrast to coma, stupor can be reversed by vigorous stimulation, albeit usually only partially and temporarily. Although, in a strict sense *lethargy* describes what is primarily an attention deficit, the word is often used more loosely to indicate drowsiness or decreased wakefulness. The lethargic patient may be delirious and confused, but retains a minimal ability to communicate, even if it is through cry.

The first concern of the physician confronting a child with an altered state of consciousness should be to assess whether respiration and circulation need to be immediately supported. The next step is to obtain sufficient clinical information to formulate an answer to two essential questions: What is the cause? What is the likely progression? To answer the first question, it is useful to start by considering whether the state of altered consciousness is part of a global or generalized dysfunction of the CNS or results from a more focal structural lesion in the brain.

ACUTE GLOBAL ENCEPHALOPATHY. A global encephalopathy typically occurs when different components of the CNS are affected simultaneously by the disease process. The paradigm is the toxic-metabolic encephalopathy, in which a circulating toxin or an alteration in homeostasis interferes with the function of the brain. The encephalopathies that occur when the brain is acutely deprived of blood flow or oxygen (ischemic-hypoxic encephalopathy), when there is infection of the CNS (encephalitis, meningitis), or during and after generalized seizures are also included. In general, global encephalopathies produce a gradual alteration in the state of consciousness, but they can also be abrupt, as in the case of hypoglycemia and severe ischemic-hypoxic damage. Although motor signs attributable to disruption of individual tracts or organs within the CNS (such as hyperreflexia or a Babinski sign for the corticospinal tract) may be prominent, they are usually symmetric and tend to follow the alteration in consciousness in time. Tremor, asterixis, rapid loss of postural tone, and myoclonus (sudden, nonrhythmic movements of the limbs) are common, especially in the early stages of the encephalopathy. In contrast, basic functions of the brain stem, such as those responsible for the pupillary responses to light, the eye movements, or the control of respiration, are preserved until the alteration of consciousness is severe.

Toxic-Metabolic Encephalopathy. The number of exogenous toxins that can cause acute alterations in the state of consciousness is very large (Part XXXIV). In toddlers and small children, intoxications are usually the result of accidental ingestion, whereas in adolescents they are more frequently deliberate. Toxic ingestion, however, should be suspected at all ages, particularly if the findings of the physical examination and complementary tests cannot be easily reconciled with the history. Often, these findings include alterations that are characteristic (toxidrome) for a toxin or group of toxins. Hypercapneic hypoventilation associated with small pupillary size is typical for opioid intoxication. The coexistence of hyperpnea, respiratory alkalosis, and dehydration should raise the suspicion of salicylate poisoning. The detection of an unexplained gap between calculated and measured osmolarity may be taken as a sign of the presence of high concentrations of small, osmotically active molecules in the blood, as is the case with the ingestion of various alcohols and aromatic compounds available in most households.

Endogenous toxins or compounds that are produced in the course of normal metabolism and have no toxic effects at physiologic concentrations can cause CNS dysfunction if under pathologic conditions they accumulate in the blood. Carbon dioxide, urea, and ammonia are good examples. The presence of endogenous toxins can be suspected by a careful evaluation of the available clinical information. The history is especially important here because it can reveal not only pre-existing illnesses but also genetic disorders like those affecting amino acid or urea metabolism, which may be responsible for unexplained deaths in infant siblings or close relatives. Some endogenous toxins cause specific abnormalities in the physical or laboratory examinations. A few genetic errors of metabolism (maple syrup urine disease, isovaleric acidemia) are associated with a characteristic odor in the urine. Disorders of the amino acid metabolism, the organic acidemia syndromes, and most defects in carbohydrate metabolism result in a prominent anion gap metabolic acidosis. In contrast, urea cycle defects cause hyperammonemia and coma without metabolic acidosis. The encephalopathy of liver failure is associated with hyperpnea and hypocapnia as early manifestations. Metabolic encephalopathies also occur when the homeostatic mechanisms that tightly control the composition of the extracellular fluid malfunction are overwhelmed by disease processes. Examples include alterations in the concentrations of cations such as sodium, calcium, and magnesium, which play important roles in maintaining the normal electrical potentials across the neuronal membranes.

Hypoglycemia can be considered a special case (see Chapter 77). Although, as an isolated homeostatic alteration it is not common outside of the immediate newborn period, hypoglycemia occurs frequently as a manifestation of metabolic and endocrine diseases, in certain intoxications (ethyl alcohol, salicylates), whenever the glycogen stores of the liver are deficient (as in starvation, particularly in small infants, or liver failure), and, of course, in the presence of increased amounts of insulin (hyperinsulinism and excessive insulin administration). Because it can be easily reversed and if left untreated it has ruinous long-term effects for the CNS, hypoglycemia should always be considered in the initial evaluation of a comatose child. For the same reasons, the intravenous administration of dextrose-containing solutions is advisable in practically all cases of unexplained coma until the serum glucose concentrations can be measured.

Ischemic-Hypoxic Encephalopathy. Ischemia and hypoxia start an extremely complex chain of events, which often injures the brain in its entirety. Decreased oxygen supply causes a primary neuronal injury, which is a direct consequence of the dependence of neural tissues on aerobic metabolism for energy production. In addition, hypoxia triggers a secondary injury that amplifies and extends the primary injury. This secondary response involves, among other potential mechanisms, the generation of oxygen free radicals and the activation of cellular receptors (the glutamate receptors), which initiate self-destructive behaviors such as apoptosis (programmed neuronal death) in the surviving neurons. Like other global encephalopathies, the one produced by ischemia or hypoxia can have a variable clinical expression, depending on the severity of the original insult. The latter is not always obvious and therefore ischemic-hypoxic damage needs to be contemplated as a potential diagnosis in children with an altered state of consciousness. Imaging studies using computed tomography, magnetic resonance imaging, and even ultrasound are often helpful by demonstrating the presence of multiple infarcts or global cerebral edema, but these signs take some time to develop. Cranial nerve abnormalities, such as those affecting pupillary size and response to light, are more frequently observed in this than in other global encephalopathies, which tend to preserve brain stem function. Finally, the presence of a lactic acidosis or signs of damage to other hypoxia-sensitive organs (heart, kidney, liver) is highly suggestive of hypoxic-ischemic injury. Poor myocardial function necessitating the continued administration of inotropic medications is frequently associated with severe neurologic injury after water submersion.

Infections of the Central Nervous System. Meningoencephalitis should be considered in the initial differential diagnosis of any acute alteration of consciousness in children, particularly if there are associated infectious manifestations, such as fever or leukocytosis. The presence of signs of meningeal irritation (nuchal rigidity, Kernig and Brudzinski signs) provides a useful clue. These signs, however, are often absent in infancy, when a tense anterior fontanel is more likely to be found and when the infection affects primarily the brain tissue (encephalitis). Uncomplicated meningoencephalitis causes a global encephalopathy; accordingly, localizing signs in a patient with this diagnosis usually indicate the presence of complications such as vascular infarcts, cerebritis, or cranial nerve compression (usually involving cranial nerve VI). Seizures are common in both meningitis and encephalitis. Because early treatment may be critical for the outcome, herpes simplex encephalitis should be suspected when there are signs of depressed levels of consciousness with or without signs of meningeal irritation without a clear etiology, particularly if the computed tomography or the electroencephalogram shows focal temporal lobe abnormalities.

Seizures. Seizures are a frequent cause of altered consciousness in children. Postictal drowsiness or stupor is not always recognized if the seizures were not witnessed or detected (for example, in a patient receiving muscle relaxants). Less often, seizure activity causes a loss of consciousness without abnormal movements (nonconvulsive status epilepticus).

TRAUMA. (See Chapter 551.) Trauma may cause focal or diffuse neurologic injury; both may affect the level of consciousness. Trauma related to diffuse cerebral edema is another mechanism for altered levels of consciousness.

FOCAL ENCEPHALOPATHY. From a clinical point of view, what characterizes most structural lesions of the CNS is the presence of focal manifestations referred to the affected structure or structures. The diagnosis of these lesions, therefore, involves a careful evaluation of the localizing value of each sign and symptom along with imaging studies. Because structural lesions tend to follow a different clinical course depending on whether they are located above or below the tentorium cerebelli (the meningeal fold that separates the anterior and middle fossae from the posterior fossa of the skull), it is useful to divide these lesions into supra- and infratentorial.

Supratentorial lesions can only cause a severe alteration of the state of consciousness if they impair simultaneously the function of the two hemispheres or if they compress the diencephalon or the brain stem. Bilateral hemispheric lesions are common in children. Their symmetric distribution is evident in the case of those pathologic processes, which, like meningitis, encephalitis, or certain cerebrovascular disorders, affect the brain in its entirety, and therefore tend to cause a global encephalopathy. However, a lesion originally restricted to one hemisphere can easily interfere with the function of the contralateral hemisphere by increasing the intracranial pressure (trauma, tumor, abscess, infarct).

Intracranial hypertension is a frequent complication of both global and focal encephalopathies. It usually results from an increase in the volume of the contents of the cranial cavity. Because the cranial vault is a relatively rigid enclosure, even minor expansions of its contents cannot be tolerated without an increase in pressure. This increase in pressure, in turn, decreases the effective perfusion pressure of the brain, which, as intracranial pressure rises above the pressure in the cerebral veins, is defined by the difference between the mean arterial and mean intracranial pressures. Even if the cerebral vessels retain their normal ability to adjust their caliber to maintain cerebral blood flow relatively constant over a wide range of cerebral perfusion pressures (autoregulation), a substantial increase in intracranial pressure inevitably results in a decrease in the perfusion of the brain tissue with the consequent impairment in brain function and neuronal damage. An increase in the volume of any of the contents of the cranial cavity—in tissue (tumor, cerebral edema), blood (hyperemia, hemorrhage), or cerebrospinal fluid (hydrocephalus)—can cause intracranial hypertension. The severity of this hypertension depends on the magnitude of the increase in volume and the ability of the cranial cavity to accommodate the volume increase. The latter is influenced by the state of ossification of the cranial vault and by the speed with which the volume increase occurs. Accordingly, infants develop less intracranial hypertension for a proportionally similar volume expansion because their cranium can undergo some expansion of its own through separation of the sutures and outward deformation of the fontanel (giving rise in the process to valuable clinical signs). Similarly, if the volume increase is slow (with a slow-growing tumor), it may allow enough time for the cranial vault to stretch or for the volume of other cranial contents to be redistributed to spaces outside the cranial cavity (mainly by shifting cerebrospinal fluid to the vertebral space), thereby limiting the increase in intracranial pressure. These adaptations cannot happen when the increase in volume happens over minutes or hours. In the absence of focal manifestations, intracranial hypertension may be indistinguishable from global encephalopathies. The patient is confused and even combative in the early stages, and becomes somnolent and comatose as the intracranial pressure continues to rise. This progression may denote the effects of ischemia on the brain and therefore demands immediate attention. The appearance of focal signs related to the brain stem is particularly ominous in this context, and usually alerts one to the presence of one of the brain herniation syndromes.

Brain herniation occurs when a localized increase in pressure causes the contents of one of the various spaces defined by the meningeal membranes to shift to another space within the intracranial cavity. In transtentorial or central herniation, the diencephalon (thalamus and hypothalamus) is pushed over the tentorium cerebelli into the subtentorial space, compressing in the process the subtentorial portions of the diencephalon and the brain stem. Because the brain stem compression progresses from higher to lower centers in the brain stem, the manifestations of central herniation frequently follow a discernible pattern. In addition to coma, diencephalic compression results in decorticate rigidity (increased extensor tone in the lower extremities and increased flexor tone in the upper extremities). The pupils are small (because sympathetic tone is decreased by the compression of the sympathetic centers in the hypothalamus), but they react normally to light. Occasionally, when the uncus is involved in the herniation, compression of cranial nerve III causes ipsilateral mydriasis without response to light (fixed and dilated). Breathing may be unaltered, but Cheyne-Stokes respiration (a regular pattern consisting of bursts of breaths of increasing-decreasing amplitude alternating with periods of apnea) is not unusual.

As the herniated brain starts to compress the midbrain and pons, the flexor facilitator effects of the corticospinal and rubrospinal pathways become abolished, and decorticate rigidity gives way to decerebrate posturing (increased extensor tone in the upper and lower extremities). In addition, both sympathetic and parasympathetic pupillary pathways become interrupted, causing one or both pupils to be in midposition and unresponsive to light. Ocular movements become disconjugate or altogether absent, even in response to basic reflex mechanisms elicited by movement of the neck (oculo-cephalic or doll's eyes reflex) or by thermal stimulation of the vestibular system (vestibulo-cephalic or caloric reflex). The patient often becomes hyperpneic because of the loss of pontine regulatory influences on the medullary centers of respiration. Finally, medullary compression results in flaccidity, progressive irregularity of the breathing movements, and eventually apnea. The compression of the medullary centers that provide autonomic innervation to the cardiovascular system results in characteristic fluctuations in the blood pressure and heart rate. The association of bradycardia and arterial hypertension, the Cushing reflex, is a particularly ominous sign of medullary involvement in a patient with increased intracranial pressure. Uncal herniation occurs when the medial temporal lobe is pushed medially and caudally, causing it to encroach on the diencephalon. Cranial nerve III is usually compressed in the process, resulting in early ipsilateral anisocoria, loss of the pupillary reflexes, ptosis, and adduction paralysis of the eye. In later stages, the herniated brain goes on to compress the brain stem, producing the same manifestations as central herniation.

INFRATENTORIAL LESIONS. The fact that acute lesions affecting primarily the brain stem are almost always associated with severe alterations of consciousness reflects the importance of the brain stem reticular system in the maintenance of the vigil state. In addition to the reticular system, the brain stem has many structures, which, when disrupted, give rise to a variety of physical findings. In the unconscious child, these findings involve primarily the corticospinal tract and the nuclei and pathways of the cranial nerves. In this regard, the manifestations produced by the infratentorial lesions may not differ from those described earlier for the compression of the brain stem. Infratentorial lesions, however, tend to result in earlier onset of the coma, cranial nerve palsies, and respiratory abnormalities. They also cause early onset of hydrocephalus by compressing the pathways for circulation of the cerebrospinal fluid. Compression and even herniation of the brain stem can occur when expanding lesions in the posterior fossa create sufficient pressure to push the brain stem caudally through the foramen magnum. Infratentorial herniation is characterized by early respiratory and autonomic impairment, sometimes with preservation of the pupillary responses.

MANAGEMENT OF ACUTE NEUROLOGIC DYSFUNCTION

GENERAL THERAPY. The care of a child with an acute neurologic dysfunction must start with an assessment of the circulatory and respiratory functions. Whether caused by ischemia, hypoxemia, or by other mechanisms (carbon monoxide poisoning), cerebral hypoxia will not only cause an acute encephalopathy, it will contribute to the extension of any existing CNS damage. Circulatory deficiencies may result from injuries to other organs (during trauma or as part of a systemic illness) or by primary dysfunction of the premotor and motor autonomic centers located in the brain stem and spinal cord. Arterial hypotension should be treated with fluid and vasoactive medications; bradycardia sufficiently severe to alter perfusion should be treated with chronotropic medications. Respiratory dysfunction is more common than circulatory dysfunction; it usually involves functional or structural abnormalities in either the pontine and medullary centers that control respiratory drive or in the mechanisms that coordinate the contraction of the upper airway and inspiratory muscles. Respiratory drive abnormalities may manifest as alterations in the regularity of the breathing pattern (see herniation syndromes) or as decreased ventilatory amplitude or frequency with a regular pattern. Upper airway control abnormalities cause snoring, stridor, and other signs of inspiratory obstruction because the hypotonic walls of the pharynx and larynx collapse under the negative airway pressures generated during normal inspiration. Although airway obstruction can be relieved temporarily with maneuvers aimed at increasing the anteroposterior diameter of the pharynx (head tilt and jaw thrust), the presence of an unstable airway or of signs of hypoventilation in a child with altered state of consciousness usually constitutes an indication for intubation of the trachea and mechanical ventilation, respectively.

After circulatory and respiratory abnormalities are ruled out or corrected, a more careful neurologic examination can be performed. The initial question that this examination should answer is whether the neurologic dysfunction is global or focal. Answering this question may save valuable time in establishing appropriate therapy. Physical findings indicative of brain stem compression in an unconscious child should prompt immediate measures to reduce intracranial pressure and prevent the progression of herniation.

INITIAL TREATMENT OF INTRACRANIAL HYPERTENSION. The initial treatment of intracranial hypertension should include a number of chiefly supportive measures that carry little or no cost in terms of complications. One of the most important is the prevention of hypoxemia and hypercarbia through the administration of oxygen and, if appropriate, the institution of mechanical ventilation. Cerebral blood vessels dilate if the arterial P_{O_2} decreases below or the arterial P_{CO_2} increases above normal; the resultant increase in the cerebral blood volume raises intracranial pressure. If deemed necessary, intubation of the trachea should be performed by the most experienced person available and with the help of proper sedation to prevent acute hypoxia, hypoventilation, and coughing during laryngoscopy. Continued sedation is often indicated in patients who undergo mechanical ventilation to minimize movement, agitation, and coughing, which tend to increase intracranial pressure by raising cerebral blood flow and impeding cerebral venous outflow. Many sedatives, such as benzodiazepines and barbiturates, and the opioid analgesics have the additional advantage of reducing brain metabolism and blood flow; unfortunately, they also interfere with the ongoing assessment of the patient's neurologic function. Unless otherwise contraindicated (if the arterial pressure is decreased), the patient's head should be elevated with respect to the thorax and placed in midposition to facilitate venous drainage. Maximal effort should be made to keep the surroundings quiet and stimulation to a minimum. Seizures increase cerebral blood flow and may extend the cerebral injury; they should therefore be treated aggressively. Similarly, fever should be suppressed.

MONITORING OF INTRACRANIAL PRESSURE. Additional therapies for intracranial hypertension are not devoid of risk. They should therefore probably be pursued under the guidance of direct monitoring of the intracranial pressure. This is usually accomplished by introducing a measuring device in the intracranial space. The basic design of the intracranial pressure monitors varies from the simple saline-filled catheters introduced into a lateral ventricle and connected to an external pressure transducer to the more sophisticated transducer-tipped fiberoptic systems, which are inserted into the subarachnoid space or directly into the brain parenchyma through a burr hole. Intraventricular catheters permit the withdrawal of cerebrospinal fluid, thereby providing a rapid way to decrease intracranial volume and pressure; however, when the ventricles are reduced in size, they are more difficult to insert and are often unreliable because the catheter often abuts the wall of the ventricle. Perhaps the worst complications of intracranial pressure monitoring derive from actions taken in response to inaccurate measurements caused by faulty calibration, displacement of the measuring device, or, with the fluid-filled systems, obstruction of the catheter. Other possible complications include infection and hemorrhage. The indications for insertion of an intracranial pressure monitor need to be carefully evaluated and the potential benefits for the patient's outcome must be clear. It is interesting, in this regard, that intracranial pressure monitoring has been abandoned for the management of children with ischemic-hypoxic encephalopathy in many institutions after several studies indicated that the practice resulted in no apparent outcome improvement.

SPECIFIC TREATMENT OF INTRACRANIAL HYPERTENSION. The specific measures used to treat intracranial hypertension are aimed primarily at reducing the volume of the cranial contents, starting ideally with the specific content whose volume is increased. For instance, removal of a parenchymal abscess or tumor, aspiration of an intracranial hematoma, or decompression of hydrocephalic ventricles are lifesaving measures, which often require the direct transfer of the patient from the computed tomography scanner to the operating room. Unfortunately, the intracranial pressure is often increased as a result of volume-occupying lesions, which, as in the case of cerebral edema, are diffuse or which, despite being localized, are inoperable or unresponsive to therapy. In such cases, the reduction of intracranial pressure can only be accomplished by decreasing the volume of other intracranial contents. Whether it occurs as part of an inflammatory response to injury or as a result of an isolated alteration in vascular or cell membrane permeability, cerebral edema is a common factor in the genesis of intracranial hypertension. Therapeutic measures directed at controlling edema or, even in the absence of demonstrable edema, directed at reducing the water contained in the brain, have been applied for many years. They include the administration of osmotic agents, which, like mannitol or glycerol, do not cross the blood-brain barrier. By remaining confined to the intravascular space, these agents create an osmotic gradient that favors a net fluid transfer out of the brain. The osmotic agents, which may act also by decreasing blood viscosity and causing reflex cerebral vasoconstriction, are very effective in controlling acute increases in the intracranial pressure. Unfortunately, they become less effective and may even have a negative effect on the resolution of brain edema when the blood-brain barrier is rendered abnormally permeable by disease. The increase in serum osmolarity (which is the basis of their anti-edema effect), the secondary hypernatremia (produced by the osmotic diuresis), and the intravascular volume depletion, limit their long-term use. Complications such as hemolysis, rhabdomyolysis, and renal failure become common when the serum osmolarity is allowed to increase above 320 mOsm/L. Loop diuretics (furosemide) have been used for the treatment of intracranial hypertension alone or combined with osmotic agents. Fluid restriction serves purposes similar to those of the diuretics in the treatment of cerebral edema and intracranial hypertension. It should only be implemented, however, when the patient's circulatory function is stable enough to tolerate a decrease in vascular volume without further impairment of cerebral perfusion. When circulatory function is compromised by diuretics or fluid restriction, it may be facilitated by the administration of inotropic and vasoactive medications.

Another widely used therapeutic modality takes advantage of the vasoconstrictive effects of respiratory alkalosis on the cerebral vessels. Hyperventilation causes a rapid, predictable reduction in cerebral blood flow and cerebral blood volume (the volume of blood contained in the cerebral vessels at any given time), thereby decreasing intracranial pressure. It is easy to apply once the patient is mechanically ventilated and can be adjusted for the desired effect on intracranial pressure, if the latter is being monitored. Unfortunately, the efficacy of hyperventilation tends to decrease with time, as the bicarbonate levels in the cerebrospinal fluid surrounding the cerebral vessels decrease as part of the adaptive response to chronic hypocarbia. Even under these circumstances, however, a short course of increased ventilation is often effective in blunting an acute increase in intracranial pressure. Finally, removal of cerebrospinal fluid from the lateral ventricles or, when appropriate, from other spaces, provides a rapid method to control increased intracranial pressure. Unfortunately, the efficacy of this method is limited almost exclusively to those patients who have a patently open ventricular system. The use of barbiturates and controlled hypothermia, which at one time appeared to be promising treatments for intracranial hypertension, has been widely abandoned after additional studies showed no benefit. Steroids are rarely used for similar reasons, perhaps with the only exception of the treatment of edema related to a tumor or abscess.

Haun SE, Dean JM, Kirsch JR, et al: Theories of brain resuscitation. *In:* Rogers MC (ed): *Textbook of Pediatric Intensive Care,* 2nd ed. Baltimore, MD, Williams & Wilkins, 1992, pp 698–732.

Matthay MA: Invasive hemodynamic monitoring in critically ill patients. Clin Chest Med 4:233–249, 1983.

Plum F, Posner JB: *The Diagnosis of Stupor and Coma,* 3rd ed. Philadelphia, FA Davis, 1982.

60.2 Resuscitation

Jennifer Pratt Cheney

Adults often have primary cardiac disease leading to cardiopulmonary arrest, whereas children are more likely to have a respiratory arrest due to sepsis, infections, aspiration of foreign bodies, trauma including head injury and near-drowning, upper and lower respiratory tract disease, and sudden infant death syndrome. Other less common causes of arrest in children include metabolic abnormalities, cardiac disease and dysrhythmias, and distributive, hypovolemic, and cardiogenic shock (Chapter 60.3). Half of all children who require cardiopulmonary resuscitation (CPR) are infants.

Pediatric patients presenting to an emergency department who are apneic and pulseless have poor survival rates; however, apneic patients generally have excellent survival rates. The potential for a successful outcome in patients with respiratory arrest underlines the importance of competent airway management in the pediatric arrest victim. Because improved outcome following pediatric arrest has been associated with rapid institution of CPR, the current recommendation is that one full minute of CPR be given before a rescuer activates the emergency medical system (EMS).

Recognition of early signs of distress is critical, as appropriate and rapid intervention may prevent a full cardiopulmonary arrest. Signs of respiratory distress include tachypnea, retractions and nasal flaring, stridor, wheezing, and rarely cyanosis. Tachypnea may also indicate metabolic acidosis, as from severe dehydration or diabetic ketoacidosis. Indicators of poor perfusion include delayed (>3 sec) capillary refill, cool skin, diaphoresis, mottling, decreased urine output, and tachycardia. The blood pressure is often maintained early in shock states, progressing to narrowing of the pulse pressure, and finally decreased blood pressure. Altered mental status or seizures may be the result of hypoxia, poor cardiac output, trauma, intoxication, or infection. Attention to these signs, timely intervention, and frequent reassessment may be sufficient to avoid deterioration to cardiopulmonary arrest and result in a good outcome.

BASIC LIFE SUPPORT

AIRWAY AND BREATHING. The airway is opened with the head tilt–chin lift maneuver in the nontraumatized infant or child (Fig. 60–3). If trauma is suspected, the airway is opened with a jaw thrust while the cervical spine is immobilized (Fig. 60–4). Management of the airway in the trauma victim is ideally accomplished by two individuals: One performs the jaw thrust while the other immobilizes the neck. When the airway has been opened, the patient's breathing is assessed by looking for chest rise, listening for exhaled air, and feeling for air flow over the mouth. If there is no spontaneous breathing, ventilation must be provided. Depending on the equipment at hand, this may be delivered by mouth-to-mouth or mouth-to-mask ventilation, or bag-valve-mask ventilation.

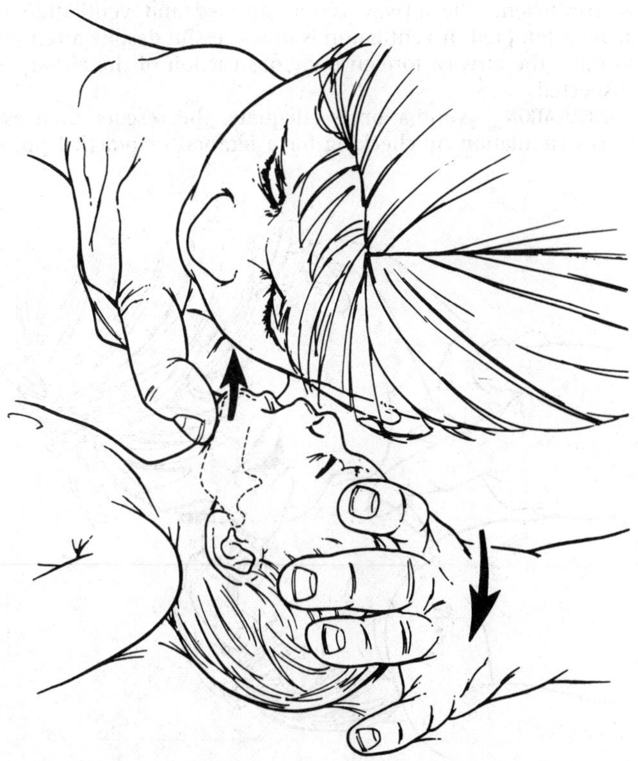

Figure 60–3. Opening the airway with the head tilt–chin lift maneuver. One hand is used to tilt the head, extending the neck. The index finger of the rescuer's other hand lifts the mandible outward by lifting on the chin. Head tilt should not be performed if cervical spine injury is suspected. (From Emergency Cardiac Care Committee and Subcommittees, American Heart Association. Pediatric basic life support, part V. JAMA 268:2251, 1992.)

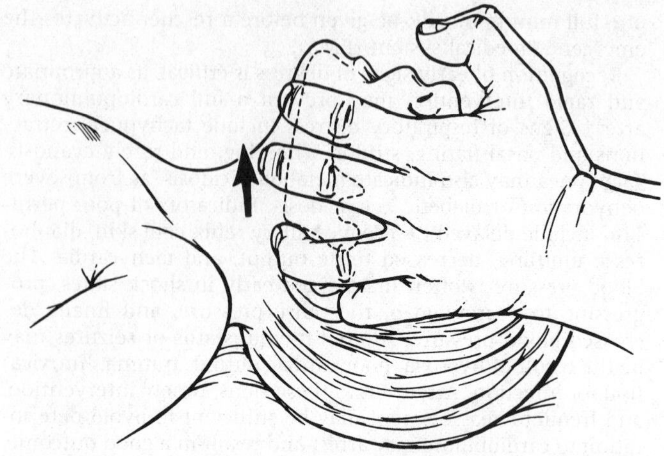

Figure 60–4. Combined jaw thrust–spine stabilization maneuver for the pediatric trauma victim. (From Emergency Cardiac Care Committee and Subcommittees, American Heart Association. Pediatric basic life support, part V. JAMA 268:2251, 1992.)

If mouth-to-mouth ventilation is required, the airway position is maintained while breathing is provided. For an infant under 1 yr of age, the rescuer's mouth forms a seal over the infant's nose and mouth (Fig. 60–5). For the infant over 1 yr of age or a child (up to 8 yr of age), the nose is compressed between the rescuer's thumb and forefinger while the other hand maintains head position (Fig. 60–6). Two slow breaths are delivered, each lasting 1–1½ sec. The rescuer pauses to take a breath before delivering the second breath. The rescuer notes chest rise; if it is adequate rescue breathing may continue at a rate of 20 breaths/min for the infant or child. If chest rise is insufficient, the airway is repositioned and ventilation is again attempted. If ventilation is unsuccessful despite attempts to open the airway, foreign body obstruction of the airway is suspected.

CIRCULATION. If ventilation is adequate, the rescuer then assesses circulation by checking for a femoral or brachial pulse

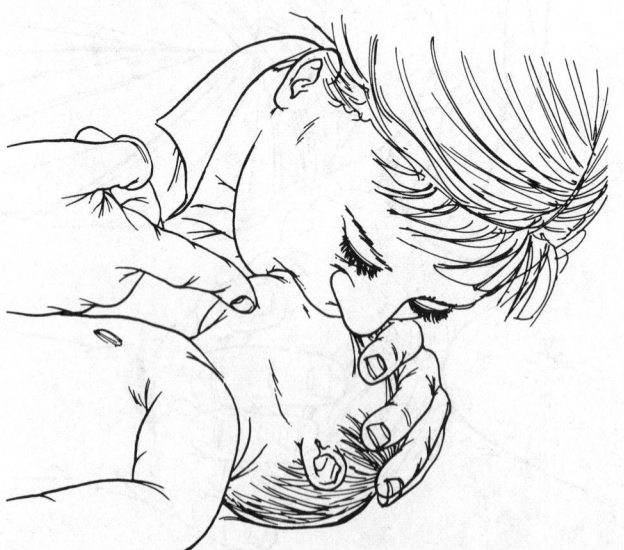

Figure 60–5. Rescue breathing in an infant. The rescuer's mouth covers the infant's nose and mouth, creating a seal. One hand performs head tilt while the other hand lifts the infant's jaw. Avoid head tilt if the infant has sustained head or neck trauma. (From Emergency Cardiac Care Committee and Subcommittees, American Heart Association. Pediatric basic life support, part V. JAMA 268:2251, 1992.)

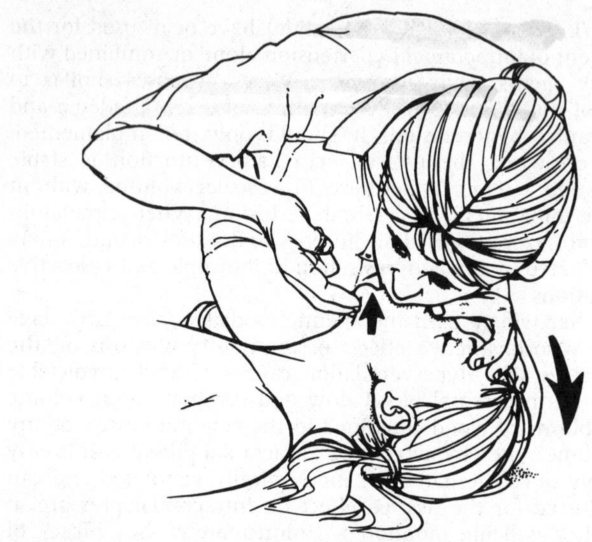

Figure 60–6. Rescue breathing in a child. The rescuer's mouth covers the mouth of the child, creating a mouth-to-mouth seal. One hand maintains the head tilt; the thumb and forefinger of the same hand are used to pinch the child's nose. (From Emergency Cardiac Care Committee and Subcommittees, American Heart Association. Pediatric basic life support, part V. JAMA 268:2251, 1992.)

in the infant under 1 yr of age or the carotid pulse in a child. If the pulse is not palpable, chest compressions are begun. If the pulse is palpable but the child is not breathing, ventilation is provided. The apneic child may also require chest compression, as heart rate and stroke volume are frequently inadequate. The patient should be placed on a hard surface, and in a hospital setting a bedboard, which supports the entire width of the chest from shoulders to waist, may be placed below the patient.

The location for chest compressions for the infant is shown in Figure 60–7. If the infant is being carried, the body may be supported along the rescuer's forearm with the head supported by the rescuer's palm. The head is not allowed to be higher than the body. The rescuer's hand closest to the child's feet is placed with the index finger just below the intermamillary line, the index finger is raised, and the 3rd and 4th fingers are used to deliver compressions to the lower one third of the chest. Alternatively, two hands may be used to encircle the chest and compressions are delivered with both thumbs. The lower one third of the sternum is compressed one-third to one-half the depth of the chest, approximately ½-1 in.

The location for chest compressions in children ages 1–8 yr is shown in Figure 60–8. The hand closest to the child's feet is used to locate the xiphoid notch. The middle finger is placed in the xiphoid notch, and the index finger is placed next to it. The position of the index finger is noted, and the same hand is moved up so that the heel is adjacent and proximal to the line where the index finger rested. The heel of the hand delivers compressions at a depth of 1–1½ in; care is taken to keep the fingers off the chest. Open chest cardiac compression is of little value and is not recommended except under unusual circumstances (cardiac surgery). The role of active compression-decompression CPR for in-hospital or out-of-hospital cardiac arrests in children has not been established.

A rate of 5 compressions to 1 ventilation is appropriate for both infants and children, whether there are one or two rescuers. The chest is compressed at a rate that would result in at least 100 compressions/min, but because compressions are interrupted to deliver ventilation, the effective compression rate is 80+/min. A second rescuer or member of the resuscita-

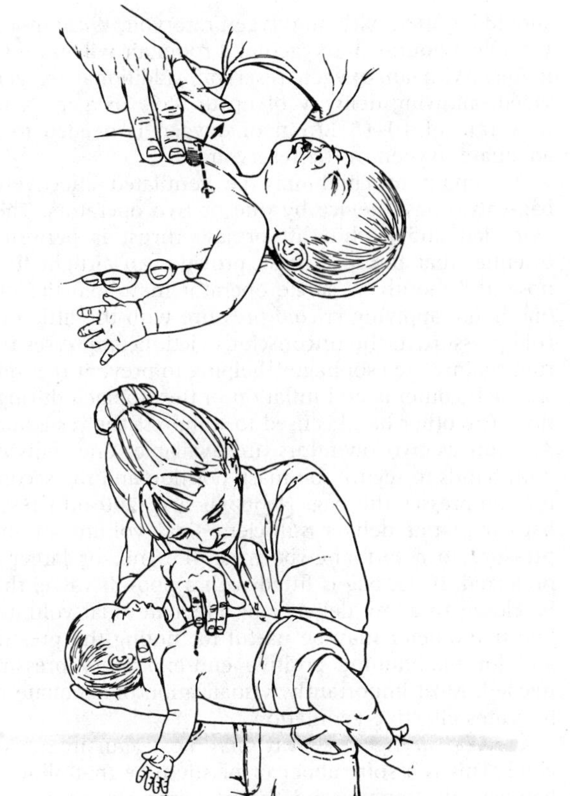

Figure 60–7. Cardiac compressions. *Top*, infant supine on palm of the rescuer's hand. *Bottom*, performing CPR while carrying the infant or small child. Note that the head is kept level with the torso. (From Emergency Cardiac Care Committee and Subcommittees, American Heart Association. Pediatric basic life support, part V. JAMA 268:2251, 1992.)

tion team should frequently reassess adequacy of pulses resulting from chest compressions.

FOREIGN BODY AIRWAY OBSTRUCTION. Foreign-body aspiration should be suspected when there is a sudden onset of respiratory distress, such as cough or stridor, or if the chest does not rise when ventilation is attempted in an unconscious, apneic infant or child. The child should be allowed to cough spontaneously until the cough is no longer effective, there is increased respiratory difficulty associated with stridor, or the child becomes unconscious.

The airway is opened with the head-tilt, chin-lift maneuver and ventilation is attempted. If this is unsuccessful, the airway is repositioned and ventilation is again attempted. If there is still no chest rise, attempts to remove a possible foreign body are indicated. In the infant under 1 yr of age, a combination of 5 back blows and 5 chest thrusts are administered (Fig. 60–9). If the foreign body is then visualized, it is removed. If no foreign body is visualized, ventilation is again attempted. If there is no chest rise, the head is repositioned and ventilation is again attempted. If this is unsuccessful, the series of back blows and chest thrusts is repeated.

A child over 1 yr of age is given a series of 5 abdominal thrusts (the Heimlich maneuver). This may be performed with the victim standing or sitting on the conscious child (Fig. 60–10), or with the victim lying down if unconscious (Fig. 60–11). After the abdominal thrusts, the airway is examined for the presence of a foreign body and it is removed if visualized. If not, the head is repositioned and ventilation is attempted. If the chest does not expand, the head is repositioned and ventilation is again attempted. If unsuccessful, the sequence is repeated.

ADVANCED LIFE SUPPORT

ASSISTED VENTILATION. Mouth-to-mouth ventilation provides only 16–17% oxygen. Mouth-to-mask ventilation may help

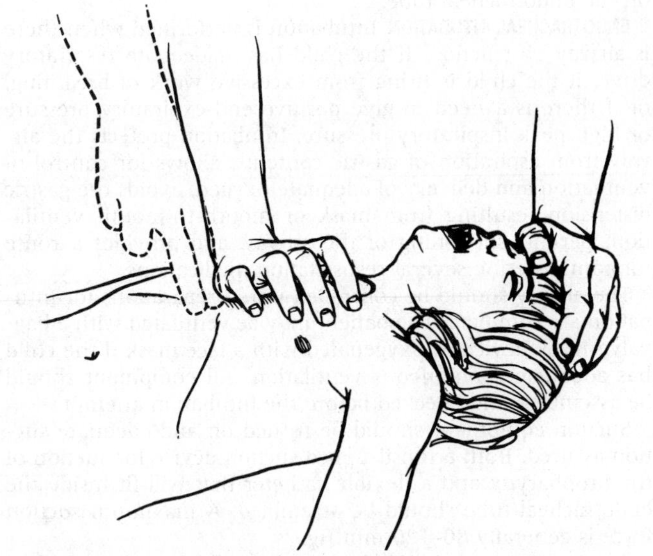

Figure 60–8. Locating hand position for chest compression in a child. Note that the rescuer's other hand is used to maintain head position to facilitate ventilation. (From Emergency Cardiac Care Committee and Subcommittees, American Heart Association. Pediatric basic life support, part V. JAMA 268:2251, 1992.)

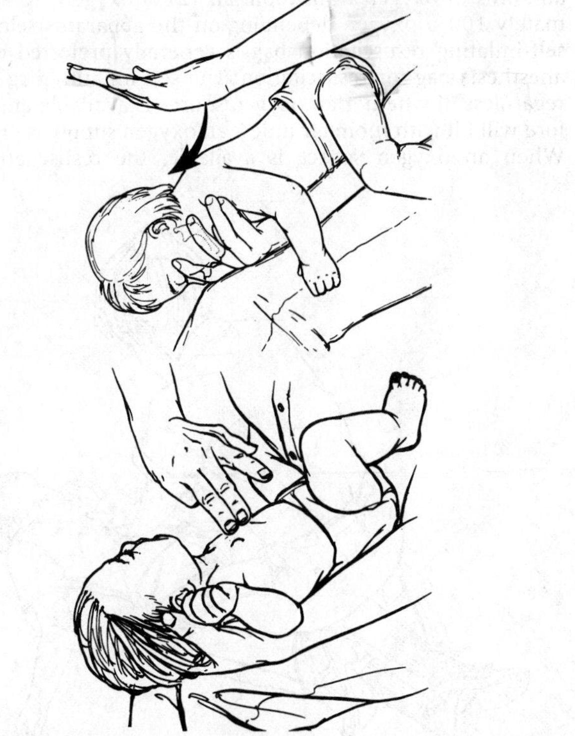

Figure 60–9. Back blows *(top)* and chest thrusts *(bottom)* to relieve foreign-body airway obstruction in the infant. (From Emergency Cardiac Care Committee and Subcommittees, American Heart Association. Pediatric basic life support, part V. JAMA 268:2251, 1992.)

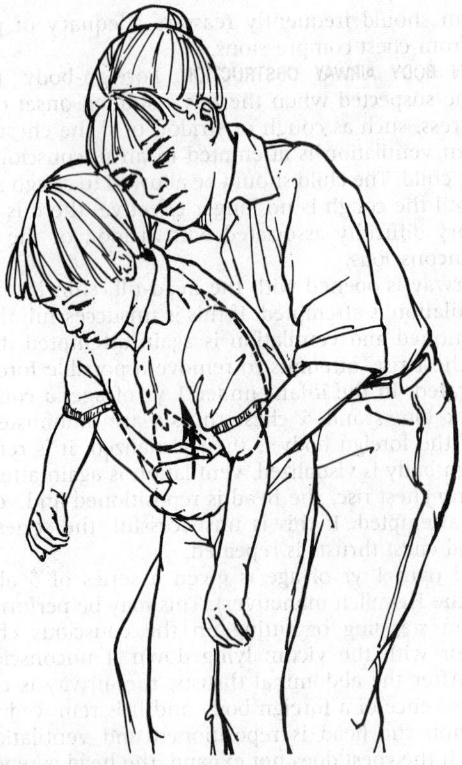

Figure 60–10. Abdominal thrusts with victim standing or sitting (conscious). (From Emergency Cardiac Care Committee and Subcommittees, American Heart Association. Pediatric basic life support, part V. JAMA 268:2251, 1992.)

protect the rescuer from contact with patient secretions or vomitus. Bag-valve-mask ventilation provides variable amounts of oxygen from room air (21% oxygen) to approximately 100% oxygen depending on the apparatus selected. A self-inflating resuscitation bag is generally preferred over an anesthesia bag for resuscitation. The self-inflating bag will fill regardless of whether an oxygen source is available and therefore will fill with room air unless an oxygen supply is provided. When an oxygen source is available, the resuscitation bag

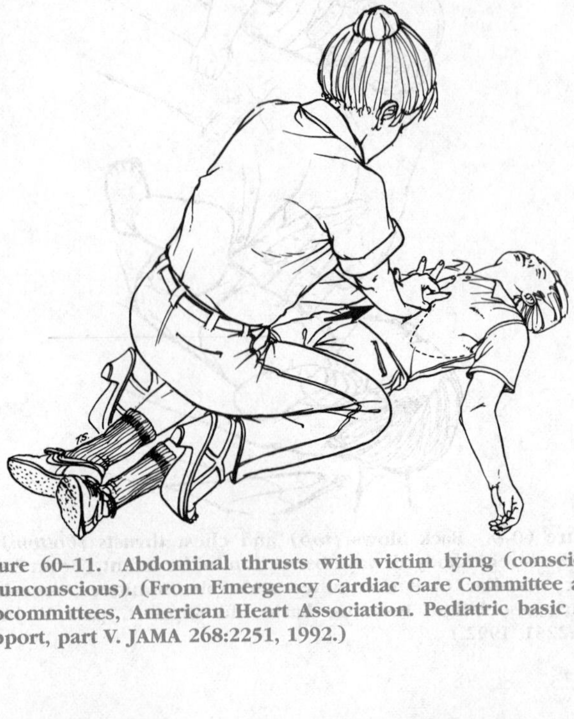

Figure 60–11. Abdominal thrusts with victim lying (conscious or unconscious). (From Emergency Cardiac Care Committee and Subcommittees, American Heart Association. Pediatric basic life support, part V. JAMA 268:2251, 1992.)

should be fitted with an oxygen reservoir. Without a reservoir, variable amounts of oxygen and room air will enter the bag as it fills. With an oxygen reservoir, additional oxygen is provided, allowing delivery of up to 95% oxygen. A minimum flow rate of 10–15 L/min of oxygen is needed to maintain adequate oxygen in the reservoir.

The infant or child may be ventilated effectively with a bag-valve-mask device by one or two operators. The head is extended and a chin lift or jaw thrust is performed. It is essential that the face mask provides an airtight fit over the nose and mouth. A single operator may hold the mask with one hand, applying cricoid pressure with the little finger. Cricoid pressure in the unconscious victim compresses the cricoid ring against the esophagus, helping to prevent regurgitation of stomach contents and inflation of the stomach during ventilation. The other hand is used to compress the resuscitation bag. As soon as two operators are available, one individual uses both hands to secure the mask position and the second operator compresses the bag. Neonatal-size (250 mL) resuscitation bags may not deliver sufficient tidal volume or inspiratory pressure to a term newborn, so 450 mL or larger bags are preferred. If the bag is fitted with a pop-off valve, this should be closed to allow delivery of adequate tidal volume. An in-line manometer may be useful for noting the pressures used and for maintaining positive end-expiratory pressure when needed. Most importantly, visualization of adequate chest rise indicates effective ventilation.

A nasopharyngeal airway may be useful in the conscious child. This is a soft rubber or plastic tube that allows air flow between the tongue and the posterior pharynx. Appropriate airway length is measured from the tip of the nose to the tragus of the ear. The tube is lubricated before gentle insertion, and a mask may then be placed over the face to provide oxygen during spontaneous breathing.

An oropharyngeal airway may be useful in the unconscious child if head tilt–chin lift or jaw thrust is not effective. The airway is generally of hard plastic and moves the tongue from the back of the pharynx. The airway may be held next to the child's face for measurement; the flange is held at the level of the central incisors and the distal tip should reach the angle of the jaw. The oropharyngeal airway cannot be used in a conscious child, as it may cause gagging and vomiting. It may be useful after intubation to prevent the patient from biting down on the endotracheal tube.

ENDOTRACHEAL INTUBATION. Intubation is performed when there is airway obstruction, if the child has inadequate respiratory drive, if the child is tiring from excessive work of breathing, or if there is a need to give positive end-expiratory pressure or high peak inspiratory pressure. Intubation protects the airway from aspiration of gastric contents, allows for control of ventilation and delivery of adequate oxygen, avoids the gastric distension resulting from mask or mouth-to-mouth ventilation, permits suctioning of the airway, and provides a route for administering several resuscitation medications.

The airway should be controlled until preparations for intubation are complete. The patient may be ventilated with a bag-valve-mask device or oxygenated with a face mask if the child has adequate spontaneous ventilation. All equipment should be assembled and checked before the intubation attempt.

Suction equipment should be turned on and adequate suction assured. Both a tonsil-tipped suction device for suction of the oropharynx and a flexible catheter that will fit inside the endotracheal tube should be assembled. A maximum suction force is generally 80–120 mm Hg.

Appropriate endotracheal tube size may be selected by a variety of methods. Resuscitation tapes used to measure the length of the child have been shown to be effective in estimation of weight and appropriate tube sizes. The diameter of the child's little finger can be used to estimate endotracheal tube internal diameter size. Tube size may also be estimated using the formula: internal endotracheal tube diameter (mm) = (age in yr/4) + 4. Endotracheal tubes 0.5 mm larger and 0.5 mm smaller than estimated should also be available.

Cuffed endotracheal tubes are generally reserved for children over 8 yr of age. Before intubation, an appropriate-sized syringe is used to inflate the cuff with air. If the cuff fills properly, it is deflated and not inflated until correct endotracheal positioning has been clinically determined.

Stylets may be used to stiffen the endotracheal tube during intubation, allowing bending of the tube into a hockey-stick shape. If one is used, it must not protrude from the distal end of the tube.

The laryngoscope blade may be curved or straight. The operator should choose a blade with which the operator is most comfortable. A straight blade is preferred by many for children up to age 7 or 8 yr. As a guide, a size 1 blade is generally appropriate for a term newborn, a size 2 for a child age 2–11 yr, and a size 3 for children age 12 or older. It is often wiser to select a larger blade when in doubt, as it may simply be withdrawn slowly from the mouth until the glottis is visualized. The blade is attached to a laryngoscope handle and the light should be checked before intubation to ensure that it is securely in place and that the light is bright. A dim light may indicate a weak bulb or weak batteries in the laryngoscope handle.

The child is preoxygenated with 100% FIO_2 before intubation. Intubation attempts should last no longer than 30 sec. The heart rate and, if available, the oxygen saturation should be monitored. If the child becomes bradycardic, the attempt is interrupted and the child is ventilated by face mask with 100% oxygen. Reflex bradycardia may result from the intubation attempt, and it is also an early indicator of hypoxemia. The spontaneously breathing child may be given atropine before the intubation attempt to avoid reflex bradycardia; however, the bradycardic response warning of early hypoxemia will be blunted. Medications for sedation, pain control, or paralysis may be used before intubation. These techniques require special training and are best performed by an experienced operator.

The head should be placed in the sniffing position to allow optimal alignment for intubation. Infants and children under 2 yr of age have a relatively large occiput, and the airway may be properly positioned with the head resting on a flat surface. A child above age 2 may have a small roll placed under the head to bring the head into a sniffing position. An injured child's head should not be moved, and the cervical spine should remain immobilized during intubation.

Cricoid pressure (Sellick maneuver) should be used during intubation attempts to help prevent aspiration. The trachea is compressed by application of pressure over the cricoid ring, compressing the esophagus and preventing passive regurgitation of stomach contents. An assistant may apply cricoid pressure or the intubator may use the little finger of the left hand.

The mouth should be opened gently and the laryngoscope blade inserted into the right side of the mouth. The blade is held in the left hand and is used to sweep the tongue to the left side of the mouth. The larynx is located more anteriorly and cephalad in the child than in the adult, and the epiglottis is more floppy. Suctioning is used as needed, and the endotracheal tube is inserted into the right side of the mouth. A curved (Macintosh) endotracheal blade is placed into the vallecula, and the glottis is noted below the epiglottis. A straight (Miller) blade is placed below the epiglottis, lifting it out of view, and the glottis becomes visible (Fig. 60–12). Care should be taken to lift the blade upward in the direction of the blade handle. The blade handle should not be used in a prying motion as damage to the teeth may result and visualization of the glottis will be difficult. The endotracheal tube enters the right side of the mouth and is inserted between the vocal cords. Some endotracheal tubes are marked with a black vocal cord line proximal to the tip of the tube; this line may serve as a guide and should be placed at the level of the cords. Cuffed endotracheal tubes are positioned with the cuff just below the vocal cords. The stylet is removed if one was used, and the endotracheal tube adapter is fitted into the resuscitation bag adapter.

The endotracheal tube is held securely in position until it is properly secured with tape. The chest should rise as the bag is compressed. Breath sounds are auscultated in each axilla and over the stomach to ensure proper tube position. If breath sounds are loudest over the stomach, esophageal intubation is suspected and the tube must be removed and endotracheal intubation reattempted. The misplaced tube in the esophagus may be temporarily left in position to indicate the esophageal opening while the trachea is intubated, or may be removed to allow more room for the endotracheal tube and blade. If breath sounds are decreased over the left side of the chest, right mainstem bronchus intubation should be suspected and the endotracheal tube slowly withdrawn until breath sounds are equal. Persistently decreased breath sounds over one area of the chest may indicate pneumothorax, aspiration, or other pulmonary disease. If chest excursion is inadequate despite appropriate compression of the resuscitation bag, there may be an air leak between the trachea and the endotracheal tube. This leak may be audible during auscultation of the neck. In the presence of a significant air leak, the tube should be replaced with a larger tube.

A properly positioned tube is confirmed by symmetric breath sounds, symmetric chest movements, absence of breath sounds over the stomach, and the presence of condensation in the endotracheal tube during exhalation. If the endotracheal tube has a cuff, it is inflated until an audible air leak just disappears. A chest radiograph should be obtained to determine proper midtracheal endotracheal tube position. End-tidal CO_2 monitoring is useful for indicating endotracheal intubation, and pulse oximetry is useful for monitoring adequacy of oxygenation. Tube placement should be frequently reassessed.

Once the child has been intubated, care should be taken to maintain neutral head position, as extension of the neck may result in movement of the tube into the right mainstem bronchus, and flexion of the neck may dislodge the tube.

When intubation is impossible despite measures to clear the airway, it may rarely become necessary to attempt transtracheal catheter ventilation. This technique requires specialized training and little information is available concerning its use in children.

NONINVASIVE RESPIRATORY MONITORING. Pulse oximetry is a noninvasive method of monitoring oxygen saturation. It is an excellent method for indicating improvement or deterioration of respiratory function, such as accidental extubation. The oximeter reading requires a consistent monitoring of the pulse to provide an accurate reading. If the pulse is absent or weak, it may be difficult to obtain a reading, and if the pulse is only occasionally registered because of patient movement, the reported result is likely to be inaccurate. In addition, when interpreting results it is important to remember that oxygen saturation and Po_2 are related but different measurements. End-tidal CO_2 monitoring may be a helpful adjunct in indicating proper endotracheal tube placement or dislodgement, and adequacy of chest compressions.

The presence of CO_2 in expired gas requires the generation of CO_2 by the tissues, transport to the lungs by adequate circulation, and removal from the lungs with adequate ventilation. Esophageal air has low levels of CO_2. For the patient who is not in cardiac arrest, adequacy of ventilation will determine end-tidal CO_2 levels. Esophageal intubation, a significant air leak around the endotracheal tube, or ventilation-perfusion mismatch will result in low levels of CO_2.

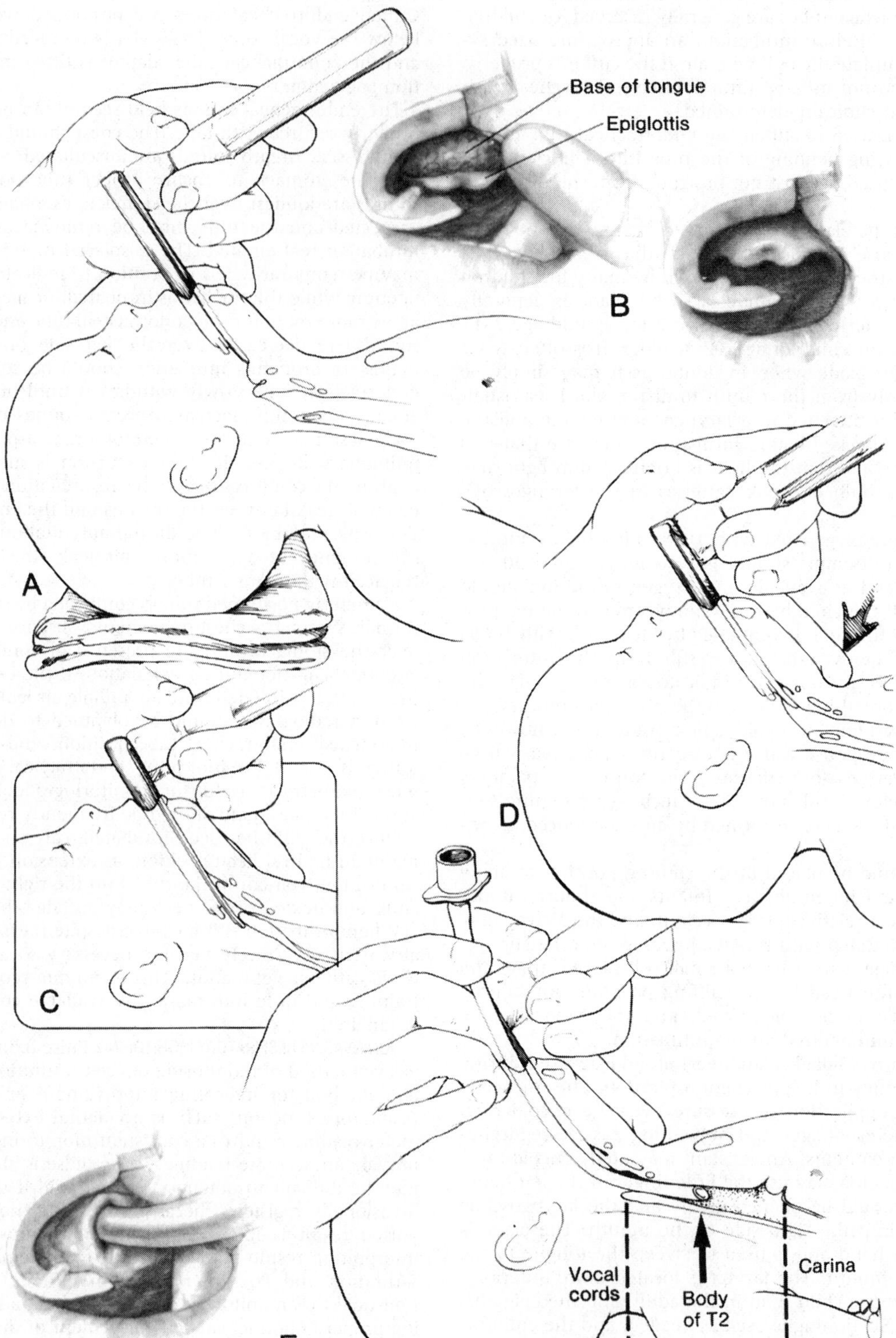

Figure 60–12. Intubation technique. (From Fleisher G, Ludwig S: Textbook of Pediatric Emergency Medicine. Baltimore, Williams & Wilkins, 1983, p 1250.)

In the patient in cardiopulmonary arrest, low end-tidal CO_2 levels may indicate diminished cellular production, the inadequacy of perfusion during resuscitation, or esophageal placement of the endotracheal tube. A drop in end-tidal CO_2 may indicate inadequacy of chest compressions, while a rise in end-tidal CO_2 may indicate spontaneous return of circulation.

VASCULAR ACCESS. Vascular access is often difficult to obtain in infants and children. To ensure timely progression of vascular access attempts, the American Heart Association recommends the following vascular access protocol for children 6 yr of age and younger: If after 90 sec or three attempts venous access attempts are unsuccessful, an intraosseous infusion should be attempted (see Chapter 59, Fig. 59–2). If this is unsuccessful and 3–5 min have elapsed without vascular access, appropriate lipid-soluble resuscitation medications may be given via the endotracheal tube.

The preferred site for vascular access during cardiopulmonary resuscitation should not interfere with resuscitative efforts. A large catheter will allow for volume bolus infusion if needed; therefore, the largest diameter vein accessible and an appropriate catheter should be selected. The skill of the operator determines whether this is obtained most rapidly by a central or peripheral vein. The femoral vein is frequently readily accessed in children; external or internal jugular and subclavian routes may be used by a skilled individual. Medications administered into a peripheral vein should be followed by a saline flush to facilitate entry into the central circulation.

FLUIDS AND MEDICATIONS. The most important therapy in cardiopulmonary resuscitation is careful attention to adequacy of oxygenation, ventilation, and circulation, with frequent reassessment. If these interventions fail to restore cardiopulmonary function, medications and fluids may be indicated.

Correct dosing of fluids and medications during cardiopulmonary resuscitation requires an estimate of the child's weight. Weight may be estimated by a growth chart if the age is known; resuscitation tapes are convenient and have a high degree of accuracy in estimating a weight appropriate for the child's length.

Volume infusion is frequently needed during resuscitation, particularly in patients with hypovolemic shock from trauma, dehydration, or the relative hypovolemic state of septic shock. A fluid bolus of 20 mL/kg of isotonic crystalloid Ringer lactate or normal saline is indicated for the child in shock, and may need to be repeated. Blood products may be needed for the trauma victim with significant blood loss. Recognition and treatment of shock are discussed in Chapter 60.3.

Oxygen is the first and most essential medication to be given during cardiopulmonary resuscitation. The highest concentration of oxygen available should be given during resuscitative efforts, even when measured arterial oxygen tensions or oxygen saturations on pulse oximetry are considered adequate. Delivery of oxygen to the tissues during resuscitative efforts is impaired by poor cardiac output and ventilation-perfusion mismatch in the lungs.

Epinephrine is the drug of choice for cardiac arrest. Epinephrine is indicated for asystole, pulseless arrest (including electromechanical dissociation) (Fig. 60–13), or hemodynamically significant bradycardia (Fig. 60–14). Epinephrine is an endogenous catecholamine with both α- and β-adrenergic effects. α-Mediated vasoconstriction promotes blood flow to the heart

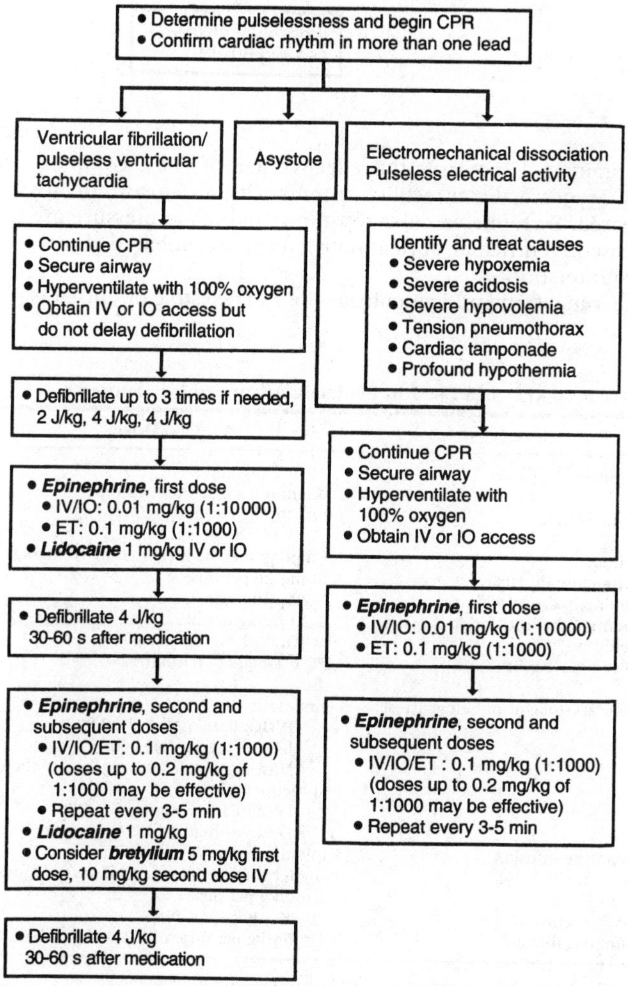

Figure 60–13. Asystole and pulseless arrest decision tree. CPR, cardiopulmonary resuscitation; ET, endotracheal; IO, intraosseous; IV, intravenous. (From Emergency Cardiac Care Committee and Subcommittees, American Heart Association. Pediatric advanced life support, part VI. JAMA 268:2262, 1992.)

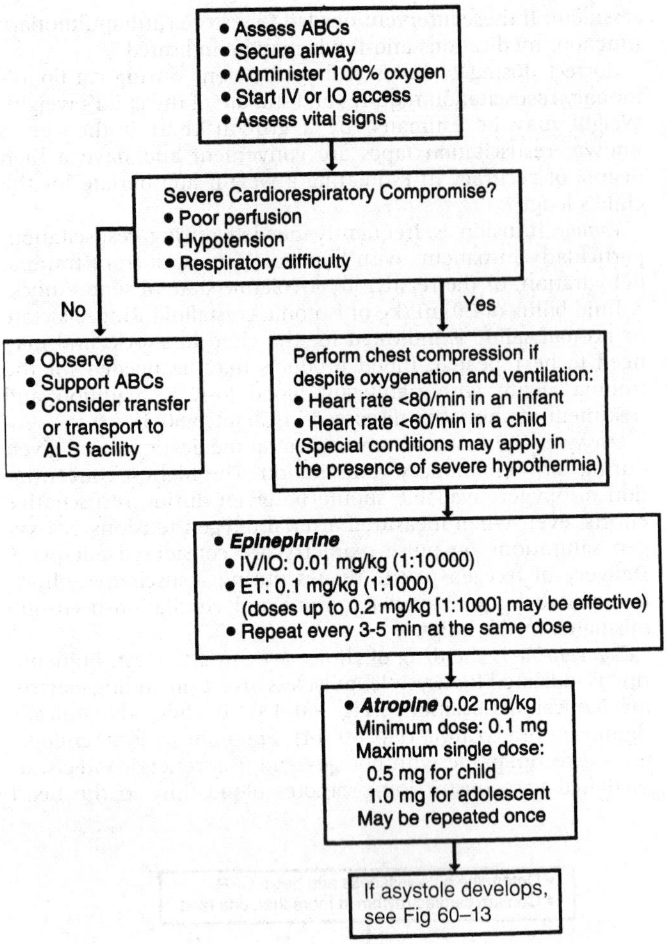

• Assess ABCs
• Secure airway
• Administer 100% oxygen
• Start IV or IO access
• Assess vital signs
Severe Cardiorespiratory Compromise?
• Poor perfusion
• Hypotension
• Respiratory difficulty
No
Yes
• Observe
• Support ABCs
• Consider transfer or transport to ALS facility
Perform chest compression if despite oxygenation and ventilation:
• Heart rate <80/min in an infant
• Heart rate <60/min in a child
(Special conditions may apply in the presence of severe hypothermia)
• Epinephrine
• IV/IO: 0.01 mg/kg (1:10000)
• ET: 0.1 mg/kg (1:1000)
(doses up to 0.2 mg/kg [1:1000] may be effective)
• Repeat every 3-5 min at the same dose
• Atropine 0.02 mg/kg
Minimum dose: 0.1 mg
Maximum single dose:
0.5 mg for child
1.0 mg for adolescent
May be repeated once
If asystole develops, see Fig 60–13

Figure 60–14. Bradycardia decision tree. ABCs, airway, breathing, and circulation; ALS, advanced life support; ET, endotracheal; IO, intraosseous; IV, intravenous. (From Emergency Cardiac Care Committee and Subcommittees, American Heart Association. Pediatric advanced life support, part VI. JAMA 268:2262, 1992.)

and brain and increases the effectiveness of chest compressions. Myocardial contractility, automaticity, and heart rate are increased. Systemic vascular resistance and blood pressure are increased. Ventricular fibrillation is more susceptible to electrical countershock.

The initial standard epinephrine dose for asystole or pulseless arrest is 0.01 mg/kg when administered through an intravenous or intraosseous line (Table 60–6). The value of higher doses of epinephrine in children remains controversial; however, currently the American Heart Association recommends that subsequent epinephrine doses be "high dose," 0.1 mg/kg or 0.2 mg/kg, repeated every 3–5 min as needed. Two

■ **TABLE 60–6 Drugs Used in Pediatric Advanced Life Support**

Drug	Dose	Remarks
Adenosine	0.1–0.2 mg/kg Maximum single dose: 12 mg	Rapid IV bolus
Atropine sulfate	0.02 mg/kg per dose	Minimum dose: 0.1 mg Maximum single dose: 0.5 mg in child, 1.0 mg in adolescent
Bretylium	5 mg/kg; may be increased to 10 mg/kg	Rapid IV
Calcium chloride 10%	20 mg/kg per dose	Give slowly
Dopamine hydrochloride	2–20 μg/kg per min	α-Adrenergic action dominates at ≥15–20 μg/kg per min
Dobutamine hydrochloride	2–20 μg/kg per min	Titrate to desired effect
Epinephrine For bradycardia	IV/IO: 0.01 mg/kg (1:10,000) ET: 0.1 mg/kg (1:1,000)	Be aware of effective dose of preservatives administered (if preservatives are present in epinephrine preparation) when high doses are used
For asystolic or pulseless arrest	First dose IV/IO: 0.01 mg/kg (1:10,000) ET: 0.1 mg/kg (1:1,000) Doses as high as 0.2 mg/kg may be effective Subsequent doses IV/IO/ET: 0.1 mg/kg (1:1,000) Doses as high as 0.2 mg/kg may be effective	Be aware of effective dose of preservatives administered (if preservatives present in epinephrine preparation) when high doses are used
Epinephrine infusion	Initial at 0.1 μg/kg per min Higher infusion dose used if asystole present	Titrate to desired effect (0.1–1.0 μg/kg per min)
Lidocaine	1 mg/kg per dose	
Lidocaine infusion	20–50 μg/kg per min	
Sodium bicarbonate	1 mEq/kg per dose or 0.3 × kg × base deficit	Infuse slowly and only if ventilation is adequate

IV, intravenous route; IO, intraosseous route; ET, endotracheal route.

concentrations of epinephrine are used to provide standard and high-dose epinephrine. Standard-dose epinephrine (0.01 mg/kg) uses 0.1 mL/kg of the 1/10,000 solution, while high-dose epinephrine (0.1 mg/kg) uses 0.1 mL/kg of the more concentrated 1/1,000 solution. Epinephrine should be administered through a secure intravenous or intraosseous line, as inadvertent infiltration into the tissues results in ischemia or necrosis. Endotracheal absorption of medication is inferior to the intravenous or intraosseous routes; therefore, the initial dose of epinephrine given by an endotracheal tube should be 0.1 mg/kg (0.1 mL/kg of the 1/1,000 solution). An epinephrine drip may be given for persistent asystole or pulseless arrest at a dose of 20 μg/kg/min until effective pulses are obtained, when the dose may be lowered.

Epinephrine is extremely useful for hemodynamically significant bradycardia (Fig. 60–14). The initial intravenous or intraosseous dose is 0.01 mg/kg (0.1 mL/kg of 1/10,000 solution) or 0.1 mg/kg (0.1 mL/kg of 1/1,000 solution) when given by endotracheal tube. Epinephrine drips may be used for shock that has not responded to volume infusion; epinephrine is preferred over dopamine in infants and in patients with circulatory instability. In this circumstance it is begun at a dose of 0.1 μg/kg/min and increased up to 1.0 μg/kg/min (Table 60–7).

Atropine is a parasympatholytic medication used for the treatment of bradycardia. It accelerates heart rate by enhancing sinus node automaticity and enhances atrioventricular conduction. Because bradycardia in children is often due to ischemic insult to the myocardium, response to vagolytic treatment is questionable, and epinephrine may be more effective. Atropine is therefore considered only possibly useful for treatment of bradycardia associated with hypotension and poor perfusion. Atropine is indicated for symptomatic bradycardia resulting from atrioventricular blocks. Atropine's role in the treatment of asystole in children is not clear, and it is considered only possibly effective by the American Heart Association. Atropine is also used in the treatment of vagally induced bradycardia during intubation attempts. When atropine is used during intubation, it may block the bradycardic response to hypoxia; pulse oximetry should then be used to monitor oxygenation.

Atropine may be administered through an intravenous or intraosseous line, and if necessary through endotracheal instillation, although absorption through this route is inconsistent. Atropine may produce paradoxical bradycardia when small doses are used. The currently recommended dose is 0.02 mg/kg, with a minimum dose of 0.1 mg. A child should receive a maximum single dose of 0.5 mg, and the adolescent 1.0 mg, which may be repeated in 5 min (see Table 60–6). Maximum total vagolytic doses are 1.0 mg in the child and 2.0 mg in the adolescent.

The use of *sodium bicarbonate* in cardiac arrest is controversial. Cardiopulmonary arrest in infants and children is frequently due to respiratory failure, causing respiratory acidosis and tissue hypoxia. Anaerobic metabolism in the tissues results in metabolic acidosis. Assurance of adequate oxygenation, ventilation, and circulation is therefore recommended before administration of sodium bicarbonate for prolonged cardiac arrest. Sodium bicarbonate is possibly effective in cases of documented metabolic acidosis and shock.

■ TABLE 60–7 Infusion Medications

Drug	Add to 5% Dextrose in Water to Make 100 mL	1 mL/kg/hr/ Delivers
Epinephrine	0.6 mg	0.1 μg/kg min
Dopamine or dobutamine	60 mg	10 μg/kg/min
Lidocaine	120 mg	20 μg/kg/min

Sodium bicarbonate has a number of deleterious side effects. When bicarbonate buffers hydrogen ions, water and CO_2 are produced, potentially worsening respiratory acidosis. Sodium bicarbonate shifts the oxyhemoglobin dissociation curve to the left, impairing delivery of oxygen to the tissues and worsening tissue hypoxia. Large doses may result in hypokalemia, hypocalcemia, hypernatremia, and hyperosmolality, and may decrease the fibrillation threshold.

The dose of sodium bicarbonate is 1 mEq/kg and may be given through an intravenous or intraosseous line (see Table 60–6). Repeated doses of bicarbonate may be considered every 10 min or be based on results of blood gas analysis.

Dopamine is used for hypotension following resuscitation and for the treatment of shock that has not responded to fluid. Dopamine is an endogenous catecholamine with dose-dependent dopaminergic, β-adrenergic, and α-adrenergic effects. Dopaminergic effects occur at low doses, when it enhances flow to renal and mesenteric blood vessels (0.5–2 μg/kg/min). Above 5 μg/kg/min, it has direct cardiac β-adrenergic effects, which increase contractility (inotropy) and heart rate (chronotropy). There is also indirect cardiac stimulation by release of norepinephrine from cardiac sympathetic nerves; however, if norepinephrine stores are depleted, as in chronic congestive heart failure or in infants with immature cardiac innervation, the inotropic effect will be diminished. α-Adrenergic vasoconstriction results in increasing blood pressure as doses are raised from 10 to 20 μg/kg/min. Above 20 μg/kg/min peripheral vascular resistance markedly increases and there is a decline in renal and mesenteric blood flow. As dopamine has a short half-life, it is given by continuous intravenous or intraosseous infusion. Several methods of preparation exist; one commonly used method adds 60 mg of dopamine to 100 mL of 5% dextrose in water; a drip of 1 mL/kg/hr results in an initial dose of 10 μg/kg/min, which is titrated to the desired effect (Table 60–7). Dopamine is inactivated in the presence of sodium bicarbonate and may cause tissue necrosis if infiltration into the tissues occurs.

Dobutamine hydrochloride is a potent synthetic catecholamine that increases contractility and heart rate by relatively selective β-adrenergic effects. Dobutamine is particularly useful for poor cardiac output and inadequate myocardial function. The usual infusion rate is between 2 and 10 μg/kg/min; doses above 20 μg/kg/min are rarely indicated. It is prepared similarly to a dopamine infusion (Table 60–7). Dobutamine is titrated to the desired effect; side effects include ventricular arrhythmias, tachycardia, and hypotension, and it is inactivated by sodium bicarbonate.

Glucose is indicated for documented hypoglycemia, which may be determined at the bedside by rapid reagent strips or in the laboratory. A dose of 2–4 mL/kg of 25% dextrose solution (0.5–1 g/kg) may be administered intravenously; glucose is best provided as a continuous infusion. Hyperglycemia after CPR has been implicated in causing worsened neurologic outcome in some animal studies; however, it may simply reflect prolonged resuscitation and impaired release of insulin during arrest.

Calcium is no longer recommended in the treatment of asystole and electromechanical dissociation, as it has not been associated with improved outcome and may be deleterious. Calcium is indicated when hypocalcemia has been documented, and it may be considered for treatment of hyperkalemia, hypermagnesemia, and calcium channel blocker overdose. Calcium is available in three different salt preparations; calcium chloride is recommended for resuscitation as it does not require hepatic degradation. The recommended dose is 5–7 mg/kg of elemental calcium; a dose of 5.4 mg/kg of elemental calcium (20 mg/kg of salt) is provided by administering 0.2

mL/kg of 10% calcium chloride (see Table 60–6). Several precautions should be noted when calcium is administered: It is highly tissue toxic and should be administered in the largest vein available; it precipitates in the presence of sodium bicarbonate, and it may exacerbate digitalis toxicity.

DEFIBRILLATION AND CARDIOVERSION. Defibrillation is indicated for ventricular fibrillation and pulseless ventricular tachycardia, which are relatively uncommon cardiac rhythms in children (see Fig. 60–13). The diagnosis of ventricular fibrillation should be confirmed in more than one electrocardiographic lead, as loose electrodes, muscle movement, or asystole may initially be difficult to distinguish from fibrillation. Defibrillation is not indicated for asystolic arrest. Defibrillation produces a mass depolarization of myocardial tissue, which may result in a return of sinus rhythm.

Before defibrillation, acidosis and hypoxia should be treated. The airway is secured, ventilation with 100% oxygen provided, and CPR instituted. Vascular access is obtained if it does not delay defibrillation. The largest paddles that provide complete contact with the skin are selected. Larger paddles offer less transthoracic impedance and result in better current flow. Pediatric paddles are recommended for infants under 10 kg, while adult paddles are used for children over 10 kg. The paddles must be prepared with electrode paste or cream, or with saline pads or electrically conductive defibrillation pads. The paddles must never be used bare, or with alcohol, which could result in burns. The electrically conductive material of one electrode must not touch that of the other electrode, as electrical bridging may occur. Bridging results in current passing across the chest; defibrillation will not be effective and a burn to the chest may result. One paddle is placed on the right side of the chest below the clavicle and the other on the left side of the chest lateral to the nipple. Good contact between the electrodes and skin is obtained by applying firm, uniform pressure. The individual attempting defibrillation stands back from the patient's bed and other personnel are instructed to stand clear of the patient and bed.

The initial defibrillation dose is 2 joules (J)/kg; if fibrillation persists the dose is increased to 4 J/kg, and if still unsuccessful a 3rd dose of 4 J/kg is delivered. The rhythm obtained after each defibrillation attempt is quickly noted and the next defibrillation attempt is performed rapidly if needed. If these three attempts are unsuccessful, epinephrine (0.01 mg/kg intravenously or intraosseously, or 0.1 mg/kg endotracheally) and lidocaine 1 mg/kg are administered. Defibrillation at 4 J/kg is again attempted 30–60 sec after medications are given. Persistence of fibrillation or pulseless ventricular tachycardia requires reassessment of adequacy of CPR measures and correction of metabolic derangements and hypothermia.

Lidocaine raises the threshold for ventricular fibrillation and decreases ventricular ectopy. Administration of lidocaine may make electrical defibrillation more likely to succeed; however, defibrillation should not be delayed in order to give lidocaine. Lidocaine may be given by intravenous, intraosseous, and endotracheal routes. The initial dose is 1 mg/kg and may be repeated. A continuous intravenous or intraosseous infusion of 20–50 μg/kg/min is used to suppress ventricular arrhythmias. Excessive doses result in circulatory and myocardial depression and CNS symptoms including seizures; therefore, the recommended dose should remain at 20 μg/kg/min in the patient with cardiac arrest, shock, or congestive heart failure. The infusion may be prepared by a number of different methods; one method uses 120 mg of lidocaine in 100 mL of 5% dextrose in water. When given at a rate of 1 mL/kg/hr, a dose of 20 μg/kg/min is obtained.

Bretylium tosylate may be considered for ventricular fibrillation when the previous measures have failed, and is begun at a dose of 5 mg/kg by rapid intravenous infusion and increased to 10 mg/kg if a 2nd dose is required (see Fig. 60–13). Bretylium has biphasic adrenergic effects, with initial sympathomimetic effects followed by adrenergic blockade. Side effects include nausea and vomiting, and postural hypotension, which may necessitate treatment with Trendelenburg positioning and fluids. Little information exists regarding its usefulness in children.

Synchronized cardioversion is used to convert ventricular tachycardia with a pulse or supraventricular tachycardia associated with hemodynamic compromise (see Chapter 388).

RESUSCITATION MANAGEMENT

Resuscitations are generally unexpected and because of the multitude of simultaneous interventions required and the number of people in attendance, the situation can easily become chaotic. Equipment should be readily available and its location and use familiar to the resuscitation team. The resuscitation team is ideally organized in advance, with assigned roles for individuals. A clear leader should be established, with all team members funneling information through the team leader. The leader will therefore be aware of all interventions and changes in patient status. Attention to documentation is critical; ideally this is the sole responsibility of one of the team members. Whenever possible, a team member should provide updates on the patient's status during resuscitation to the family and private physician.

The decision to terminate resuscitation efforts is frequently difficult. Psychological support of the patient's family is crucial and is often provided by medical personnel, social services, and members of the clergy. Psychologic support of the entire team should not be overlooked; critical incident stress debriefing teams are sometimes useful in helping staff overcome the grief and stress of a difficult or unsuccessful resuscitative effort.

POSTRESUSCITATION STABILIZATION

When resuscitative efforts are successful and the patient adequately stabilized, arrangements will need to be made for admission to an appropriate intensive care department. This may require transfer to another facility. Coordination of efforts with the receiving hospital aids decisions regarding ongoing patient care and mode of transport (helicopter, fixed-wing aircraft, ambulance, or specialized transport team). The patient is frequently reassessed and carefully monitored, and copies of all records, laboratory results, and radiographs are prepared for transport with the patient.

Burke DP, Bowden DF: Modified paediatric resuscitation chart. Br Med J 306:1096, 1993.

Callaham M, Madsen CD, Barton CW, et al: A randomized clinical trial of high-dose epinephrine and norepinephrine vs. standard-dose epinephrine in prehospital cardiac arrest. JAMA 268:2667, 1992.

Cohen TJ, Goldner BG, Maccaro PC, et al: A comparison of active compression-decompression cardiopulmonary resuscitation with standard cardiopulmonary resuscitation for cardiac arrests occurring in the hospital. N Engl J Med 329:1918, 1993.

Goetting MG, Paradis NA: High dose epinephrine in refractory pediatric cardiac arrest. Crit Care Med 17:1258, 1989.

Goetting MG, Paradis NA: High-dose epinephrine improves outcome from pediatric cardiac arrest. Ann Emerg Med 20:22/45, 1991.

Kette F, Weil MH, Gazmuri RJ: Buffer solutions may compromise cardiac resuscitation by reducing coronary perfusion pressure. JAMA 266:2121, 1991.

Lurie KG, Schultz JJ, Callaham ML, et al: Evaluation of active compression-decompression CPR in victims of out-of-hospital cardiac arrest. JAMA 271:1405, 1994.

Madl C, Grimm G, Kramer L, et al: Early prediction of individual outcome after cardiopulmonary resuscitation. Lancet 341:855, 1993.

Neonatal resuscitation, Part VII. JAMA 268:2276, 1992.

Orlowski JP: How much resuscitation is enough resuscitation? Pediatrics 90:995, 1992.

Paediatric Life Support Working Party of the European Resuscitation Council: Guidelines for paediatric life support. Br Med J 308:1349, 1994.

Paradis NA, Martin GB, Rosenberg J, et al: The effect of standard- and high-dose

epinephrine on coronary perfusion pressure during prolonged cardiopulmonary resuscitation. JAMA 265:1139, 1991.
Pediatric advanced life support, Part VI. JAMA 268:2262, 1992.
Schwab T, Callaham M, Madsen C, Utecht T: A randomized clinical trial of active compression-decompression CPR vs standard CPR in out-of-hospital cardiac arrest in two cities. JAMA 273:1261, 1995.
Sheikh A, Brogan T: Outcome and cost of open- and closed-chest cardiopulmonary resuscitation in pediatric cardiac arrests. Pediatrics 93:392, 1994.
Spevak MR, Kleinman PK, Belanger PL, et al: Cardiopulmonary resuscitation and rib fractures in infants. A postmortem radiologic-pathologic study. JAMA 272:617, 1994.

60.3 Shock

P. Pearl O'Rourke

The general definition of shock is the clinical state of inadequate perfusion in which the demands of the body are incompletely met because of massive increases in metabolic demands (oxygen consumption) and/or decreases in metabolic supply (oxygen delivery). The pathophysiology of shock varies with different etiologies, which result in different clinical presentations and require different therapeutic approaches. Initially shock can be divided into two basic categories: intravascular hypovolemia and intravascular hypervolemia or normovolemia.

INTRAVASCULAR HYPOVOLEMIA

Intravascular hypovolemia is caused by a decrease in vascular resistance or, more commonly, by a loss of intravascular volume. The prototypic example for loss of resistance shock is anaphylaxis; other causes include drug ingestion, denervation injuries, and early "warm" sepsis. In loss of resistance shock, the patient is tachycardic and hypotensive with inappropriately vasodilated warm extremities. Postural hypotension can be marked. If measured, the cardiac output is elevated, and the systemic vascular resistance (SVR) and central venous pressure (CVP) are decreased. Treatment is volume resuscitation and administration of a vasoconstrictor. In anaphylaxis in addition to fluid resuscitation and epinephrine administration, attempts also should be made to reverse or block the triggering agent: Benadryl is used to reverse further histamine effect, and steroids are given to decrease the inflammatory response (Chapter 140).

The more common cause of hypovolemic shock is loss of volume, which can be blood (trauma), protein-rich fluid (burns, nephrotic syndrome), or protein-poor fluid (vomiting and diarrhea). These patients are tachycardic with normal or low blood pressure. Children with profound volume loss maintain a normal central arterial pressure much more efficiently than the adult. This is accomplished by extreme vasoconstriction of the peripheral vascular bed, clinically manifested by cool, mottled extremities. The more severe the volume loss, the more proximal the cooling. For example, a child with slight volume depletion will be cool to the wrists and ankles; whereas with more severe depletion, the coolness will extend proximally to the thighs and shoulders. In the child, clinical assessment of peripheral perfusion can be a more reliable indicator of shock than a measured blood pressure. Capillary refill time can be used to assess peripheral perfusion, but care must be given for any interpretation; results are dependent on the ambient temperature. Swan-Ganz catheterization of the pulmonary artery demonstrates a decreased cardiac output or cardiac index, decreased CVP and left atrial pressure (LAP), in concert with a markedly elevated SVR. The treatment is volume replacement. Initially this should be isotonic solutions: Normal saline, lactated Ringer's solution. Five percent albumin, fresh frozen plasma, or whole blood is given for specific etiologies (e.g., blood for hemorrhagic shock). Emergent response with crystalloid is fastest and safest. Fluid should be given in a bolus amount based on weight (usually 10–20 mL/kg). If the patient has had a true blood loss with severe anemia, red blood cells should be part of the resuscitation. The patient's perfusion and vital signs should be carefully reassessed after every fluid bolus. Care should be given to avoid "wide open" volume replacement, which can lead to both overresuscitation as well as inadequate resuscitation.

INTRAVASCULAR NORMOVOLEMIA/HYPERVOLEMIA

This category of shock is caused by cardiac dysfunction, cardiac inflow obstruction, cardiac outflow obstruction, and arrhythmias (also see Chapters 60, 386–388, and 392–394). Inflow obstructions are uncommon: examples include pericardial tamponade and intracardiac tumors. Outflow obstructions presenting as shock include malignant hypertension or, more commonly in pediatrics, congenital heart lesions (critical aortic stenosis, critical aortic coarctation, hypoplastic left heart syndrome). The most common arrhythmia in children causing shock is supraventricular tachycardia (SVT). Because infants and young children cannot describe palpitations or abnormal heart rhythms, the initial presentation of SVT is often profound cardiovascular collapse. The causes of myocardial dysfunction are coronary artery disease, myocarditis, myocardopathy, hypoxemia, and metabolic insults. In the adult patient, myocardial dysfunction is most commonly a result of myocardial infarction, but this is not a common event in the child, who usually has normal coronary arteries. In the rare event of a child developing a myocardial infarction, the diagnoses of Kawasaki syndrome or an anomalous left coronary artery should be entertained.

Patients with normovolemic shock clinically resemble those with intravascular hypovolemia: tachycardia, hypotension, and cool peripheral extremities secondary to profound vasoconstriction, and hypoperfusion. The evaluation of these patients centers around a superb cardiac evaluation. The rhythm should be scrutinized with an electrocardiogram (ECG). A chest radiograph can provide a rapid evaluation of heart size. Echocardiography is used to assess myocardial function, cardiac anatomy, and the status of the pericardium; it also provides information about the filling pressures. Invasive Swan-Ganz catheterization readings demonstrate a decreased cardiac output/cardiac index with normal or increased filling pressures (CVP and LAP) and a markedly increased SVR. The treatment for myocardial failure is careful volume resuscitation and the early administration of antiarrhythmic, inotropic, and possibly afterload-reducing drugs (Chapters 399, 400). Obviously hypoxemia and metabolic abnormalities should be corrected if possible.

EVALUATION. While it is vital to understand the differences between these shock states, they all share a number of common diagnostic and therapeutic features. The diagnosis is based on a combination of history and physical examination with laboratory augmentation. The history should include information about any underlying diseases, any drug history, the duration and symptoms of the acute illness, any extreme volume loss (diarrhea, vomiting), and quantification of fluid intake. Important end-organ perfusion can be rapidly assessed by inquiring about the level of mentation and the amount of urine output.

In all cases, extreme care should be given to guarantee that the patient has adequate oxygenation and ventilation. Monitoring with pulse oximetry should be standard: If the patient is too peripherally vasoconstricted to obtain reliable readings, the probe can be wrapped around the ear lobe, the nose, or the penis. Virtually all patients in shock should have an increase in their ambient oxygen. There should also be a very low threshold for endotracheal intubation and mechanical assistance, particularly in the face of any evidence of increased work of breathing.

Vascular access can be difficult, especially in the small patient with peripheral vasoconstriction. The use of the intraosseous line has facilitated the management of these patients (see Chapters 59 and 60.1). Once the patient is adequately resuscitated, the temporary intraosseous line should be replaced with a standard intravenous catheter (Chapter 59). Central access (femoral, subclavian, internal jugular veins) is helpful for the rapid administration of large volumes of fluid and is mandatory for the infusion of some vasoactive drugs (epinephrine, dopamine) and the assessment of intravascular filling pressures. The initial resuscitation can be started using a sturdy peripheral line.

A number of blood tests are routinely evaluated. Many provide useful information, but in the patient with severe cardiovascular collapse, the initial treatment should proceed—never delay the resuscitation awaiting a laboratory result. The arterial blood gas test is invaluable. In the state of inadequate perfusion, the tissue bed changes to anaerobic metabolism, which results in the accumulation of lactic acid: The degree of metabolic acidosis can be used as an indicator of the severity of the hypoperfusion. A hematocrit reading should be obtained, and if low, packed red blood cells should be included in the resuscitation. Correction of low serum calcium, low serum glucose, or elevated serum potassium levels can be lifesaving. Blood urea nitrogen, creatinine, liver function tests, and a coagulation screen may be helpful after the initial stabilization for further diagnostic and therapeutic decisions. If there is any suspicion of infection and/or septic shock, a complete blood count and blood culture should be obtained prior to the administration of antibiotics if possible.

Antiarrhythmic drugs are discussed in Chapter 388. The clinician should also be knowledgeable about the pharmacology of commonly used positive inotropic agents. There is no perfect inotrope: These drugs often have chronotropic as well as vasomotor effects, which, although not desired, must be tolerated. While many drugs are available, it is prudent to select a few and know them well (Chapter 60.1).

Septic shock deserves specific comment (Chapter 168). Caused by viral, fungal, or more commonly bacterial infections, septic shock is confusing and frustrating because of the continuum of rapidly changing pathophysiology. As the pathophysiology changes, the therapy should change. In warm shock, the primary site of injury is the vascular endothelium. Patients have profound vasodilation (decreased SVR) in the face of a marked increase in the cardiac index: In this stage they present much as patients with loss of resistance from other causes (systemic hypotension and warm vasodilated extremities). The treatment is volume resuscitation and possibly the use of vasoconstrictors. As the vascular endothelium loses its integrity, it begins to leak fluid into the perivascular space. The result is most crucial in the lungs, where the leak contributes to adult respiratory distress syndrome (ARDS) (see Chapter 60.7). As septic shock progresses, myocardial function decreases and the patient enters a phase of decreased cardiac output in concert with secondary profound vasoconstriction (cold shock). At this point, patients are similar to those with myocardial failure (systemic hypotension, cold, vasoconstricted extremities with decreased cardiac index [CI], and increased SVR). Therapy for cold shock is the administration of positive inotropes and afterload reduction. In addition to supporting the cardiovascular effects caused by the infection, it is imperative to eradicate the infection with antibiotics, surgery, or drainage if appropriate. There are a number of controversial therapies for septic shock. Steroids are presently only indicated in the situation of a presumed Waterhouse-Friderichsen syndrome (adrenal necrosis). More general use of high-dose steroids has decreased following the results of a number of clinical studies demonstrating a higher mortality in steroid-treated groups of patients with septic shock.

Alpert JS, Becker RC: Mechanisms and management of cardiogenic shock. Circ Shock 9:205, 1993.

Astiz ME, Rackow EC, Weil MH: Pathophysiology and treatment of circulatory shock. Circ Shock 9:183, 1993.

Rackow EC, Astiz ME: Mechanisms and management of septic shock. Circ Shock 9:219, 1993.

Sáez-Llorens X, McCracken GH: Sepsis syndrome and septic shock in pediatrics: Current concepts of terminology, pathophysiology, and management. J Pediatr 123:497, 1993.

60.4 *Drowning and Near-Drowning*

Harry J. Kallas

Childhood drowning is a common source of injury and fatality. After submersion in a liquid medium, suffocation and asphyxia may occur, with or without pulmonary aspiration. Irreversible pansystemic injury occurs very rapidly, often leading to death. Death within 24 hr of submersion is termed *drowning,* which may be immediate or follow unsuccessful resuscitation. Survival greater than 24 hr is termed *near-drowning,* regardless of whether the victim dies or recovers. While pediatric intensive care has decreased mortality due to the cardiorespiratory consequences of near-drowning, the neurologic injury from hypoxemia and ischemia remains the primary cause of long-term morbidity in survivors.

EPIDEMIOLOGY. Worldwide, approximately 140,000 persons drown each year. In the United States, there are approximately 8,000 drownings/yr, constituting 7% of traumatic deaths in children less than 1 yr of age, 19% of 1–4 yr olds, and 12–14% of older children. From 1986 to 1988, U.S. drowning rates were 2.53/100,000 for children <19 yr old, but 5.80/100,000 for 1–2 yr olds. Drowning is the 4th leading cause of death for U.S. children less than 19 yr old and the single leading cause of injury death for children under 5 yr of age.

Epidemiologic data for near-drowning is scarcer. Estimates of cumulative risk for males from birth to 19 yr of age indicate that 1/1,098 will drown, 1/301 will be hospitalized for near-drowning, and 1/75 will be treated or observed in an emergency room but sent home. Comparable risk estimates for females are 1/3,333, 1/913, and 1/228, respectively. Approximately 80% of pediatric submersion victims survive, and 92% of survivors make a complete recovery; however, in those requiring intensive care, approximately 30% die and 10–30% survive with severe brain damage.

Risk factors for drowning include age, gender, and race. Two age groups are at particular risk: toddlers, who commonly drown in residential swimming pools during brief periods of inadequate supervision; and older adolescent males (15–19 yr old), who often drown in unguarded bodies of water. Children <5 yr old account for 87% of all drownings. Young teenagers (10–14 yr old) actually have the lowest drowning rate in the pediatric age group (1.59/100,000)—half the rate of the older adolescents. Males constitute 85% of drownings. In the United States, black children have almost double the drowning rate of white children (3.8 vs 2.2/100,000, respectively).

The site of drowning also constitutes a major risk factor for various age groups. Residential swimming pools account for half of all U.S. drownings but are the site of almost 90% of immersion events in children <5 yr old. The U.S. Consumer Product Safety Commission (1985) estimated that 3,000 children under 5 yr old are seen annually in emergency rooms after submersion in residential pools; 80% of these children are hospitalized for at least 1 day. Most pool submersion events occur at the child's own home, nearly half occurring within 6 mo of pool exposure. Brief lapses (<5 min) in supervision account for most immersions.

Bathtub drownings are predominately of infants (1.87/100,000 children <2 yr old), with approximately 86% occurring in 7- to 15-mo-old children. Often, these infants have inadequate supervision and parents who overestimate their child's abilities and coordination. Hot tubs and spas pose special hazards as many have suction devices that can entrap hair, clothing, or body parts, preventing children from surfacing. Children <2 yr old are the most frequent victims.

Bucket drownings are common, constituting up to 24% of all toddler drownings in some areas of the United States. Seven- to 15-mo-old children account for 88% of these deaths. Children fall headfirst into the bucket and cannot right themselves due to their relatively cephalad center of gravity and insufficient body mass to tip it over. Bucket drowning has a high mortality, in part because of substances the buckets contain, such as cleaning fluids and other caustic agents.

In older children, adolescents, and young adults, as many as 70% of drownings occur in open bodies of water, such as lakes, ponds, streams, or irrigation ditches, usually when little or no adult supervision exists. One fifth of these drownings involve boats.

The risk of drowning is also increased by the use of alcohol or illicit drugs, which are implicated in approximately 50% of all submersion events. Alcohol clouds judgment, increasing the likelihood of injudicious risk-taking behavior, and retards motor coordination. Vasodilatation from alcohol may also expedite hypothermia, further impairing mental status and motor dysfunction. Intoxicated adults are also incapable of providing adequate supervision for younger children near water.

Concomitant medical conditions may also increase the likelihood of drowning. Children with epilepsy have a 4- to 10-fold increased risk of drowning or near-drowning compared with nonepileptic children. Eighty-six percent of these drownings occur in bathtubs or swimming pools. Other children with mental or motor disabilities may also be at increased risk.

Child abuse and homicide by submersion does occur and requires a careful history, a high index of suspicion, and an understanding of normal childhood developmental capabilities. Overall, 6% of childhood drownings are secondary to abuse or neglect. Approximately 1 in 30 child homicides are by intentional drowning. Most nonaccidental drownings occur in the bathtub, usually to children between 15 and 30 mo of age (compared to the 7–15 mo age range for most accidental bathtub drownings).

PATHOPHYSIOLOGY. Progressive hypoxemia affects all organs and tissues, with the severity of injury dependent on the duration of submersion; if pulmonary aspiration occurs, hypoxemia and respiratory failure are further exacerbated. Additionally, myocardial dysfunction, arrhythmias, or arrest compromise the victim by causing tissue ischemia. Although severe hypothermia may rarely confer some degree of neurologic protection to the submersion victim, its pathologic implications are more commonly catastrophic if not rapidly corrected.

Anoxic-Ischemic Injury. Following submersion, a conscious animal will initially panic, trying to surface. During this stage, small amounts of water enter the hypopharynx, triggering laryngospasm. Most animals struggle violently and swallow copious amounts of water. They eventually lose consciousness from hypoxemia. Vomiting often ensues, accompanied by involuntary aspiration. In about 10% of animals, the initial laryngospasm persists until death without fluid aspiration; similarly, aspiration is absent in a similar percentage of humans who drown. Profound hypoxemia and medullary depression lead to terminal apnea. Cardiovascular changes include an initial tachycardia followed by severe hypertension with reflex bradycardia, presumably from catecholamine release; arrhythmias may be seen. By 3–4 min, the circulation abruptly fails as myocardial hypoxemia supervenes. The heart may continue to have ineffective contractions or electrical activity for a short time, but there is no effective perfusion. The chance of successful resuscitation quickly becomes impossible as hypoxemia and ischemia cause rapid, progressive, and irreversible injury.

The diving reflex may potentially enhance cerebral and myocardial blood flow when the face is submerged in very cold water (less than 20° C) and is felt by some authors to contribute to cerebral protection during prolonged submersion. Although this reflex is prominent in many sea mammals, it is relatively weak in human adults and children. The extent of neurologic protection afforded humans due to the diving reflex is controversial.

The brain is exquisitely sensitive to injury from hypoxia and ischemia. With advances in intensive care, the cardiorespiratory consequences of near-drowning have become increasingly manageable and less often the cause of mortality compared with the central nervous system (CNS) injury, which is now the most frequent cause of mortality and long-term morbidity. Although the duration of hypoxemia before irreversible cerebral injury occurs is uncertain, it is probably on the order of 3–5 min. Different pathophysiologic events during hypoxemia or ischemia may be important. Blood flow during anoxic conditions with ongoing glucose and nutrient delivery results in anaerobic metabolism of these substrates, increasing cellular lactate and other intermediary metabolite concentrations. Neuronal injury may be exacerbated by the release of glutamate and other "excitatory" amino acids. Alteration of calcium channel activity and oxygen free radical generation may further cellular damage. Although blood flow assists the removal of neurotoxic substances, intracellular accumulation can occur as production exceeds removal. Total ischemia halts all nutrient delivery, leading to an abrupt cessation of cellular metabolic activity, less severe lactate and other intermediary product accumulation, and potentially less cerebral injury.

Hyperglycemia has also been implicated in exacerbating ischemic neurologic injury. After near-drowning, children with initial blood glucose concentrations >300 mg/dL are more likely to die or survive in a persistent vegetative state compared with normoglycemic victims. Although the link between hyperglycemia and neuronal injury is tentative, animal studies may suggest a potential mechanism. When subjected to cerebral ischemia, hyperglycemic rats have significantly lower brain production of adenosine and its metabolites compared with normoglycemic controls; this attenuation of adenosine production persists for at least an hour after reperfusion. Adenosine, proposed to be an endogenous neuroprotector, causes cerebral vasodilation, inhibits the release of neuronal excitotoxins, and affects neutrophil-endothelial interactions. Hyperglycemic attenuation of normal adenosine and metabolite production postischemia may make the brain less able to protect itself, worsening injury severity.

Control of hyperglycemia with insulin after near-drowning is not recommended in humans at this time. Although unclear whether treatment of hyperglycemia would mitigate brain injury in human near-drowning victims, it is prudent initially to withhold glucose-containing solutions in patients who are not hypoglycemic to prevent iatrogenic hyperglycemia. Careful monitoring to avoid hypoglycemia is imperative, especially in victims with hypoxic-ischemic injury, to avoid further neuronal injury.

The neurologic consequences of hypoxic-ischemic injury may include the loss of cerebral autoregulation and blood-brain barrier integrity. Generalized neuronal death often follows severe injuries, resulting in cytotoxic cerebral edema and increased intracranial pressure (ICP). It should be emphasized that the extent of cerebral edema in near-drowning probably reflects the severity of the initial cytotoxic injury and, although severe cerebral edema can elevate ICP and cause further ischemia, its very presence is an ominous sign of extensive neuronal death.

Other organs and tissues may also be injured during hypoxia or ischemia. In the lung, hypoxia, ischemia, as well as aspiration can damage pulmonary vascular endothelium, increasing vascular permeability, which can result in noncardiogenic pulmonary edema and the adult respiratory distress syndrome (ARDS) (Chapter 60.7). Myocardial dysfunction, arrhythmias, and infarction may also occur. Acute tubular necrosis and acute cortical necrosis are common renal complications of significant hypoxic-ischemic events. Vascular endothelial injury, exposing basement membrane, can initiate thrombocytopenia and disseminated intravascular coagulation. Factors contributing to gastrointestinal damage include hypoxia, ischemia, hypothermia, the diving reflex, and catecholamine infusions used during resuscitation; a profuse bloody diarrhea with mucosal sloughing may be seen with severe hypoxic-ischemic events and usually portends a fatal injury. Hepatic transaminases and serum pancreatic enzymes are often acutely elevated. Violation of normal mucosal protective barriers predisposes the victim to bacteremia and sepsis.

Pulmonary Aspiration. Pulmonary aspiration occurs in approximately 90% of drowning victims and in 80–90% of the nearly drowned. The amount and composition of the aspirate can affect the patient's clinical course: Water salinity, gastric contents, pathogenic organisms, toxic chemicals, and other foreign matter can injure the lung or cause airway obstruction. A few children may have massive aspiration, increasing the likelihood of fluid shifts or electrolyte abnormalities; however, most submersion victims aspirate only a small volume of water. Nonaspirating victims may still succumb acutely from laryngospasm, hypoxemia, or cardiac arrhythmias.

Although a substantial amount of literature is devoted to the distinction between sea and fresh water aspiration, clinical management is not significantly different. Sea water is hypertonic (approximately 3% normal saline), establishing an osmotic gradient drawing interstitial and intravascular fluid into the alveoli; furthermore, sea water inactivates surfactant, increasing alveolar surface tension, making the alveolus unstable and prone to atelectasis. Hypotonic fresh water aspiration washes out surfactant, also causing alveolar instability and collapse. In either case, hypoxemia and pulmonary insufficiency result from ventilation-perfusion mismatch, increased intrapulmonary shunting, decreased lung compliance, and increased small airway resistance. Profound arterial hypoxemia may result even after the aspiration of as little as 2.2 mL/kg. Pulmonary capillary endothelial injury can lead to ARDS.

Pulmonary infections, caustic aspirations, and barotrauma are still significant causes of morbidity and mortality. Pneumonia may occur primarily from aspirated contaminated water or emesis, or secondary to circumvented normal host respiratory defenses with endotracheal intubation (ventilator-associated, hospital-acquired pneumonia). Gastric acid or caustic agent aspiration can directly injure the lung without infection being present. Patients requiring high airway pressures during mechanical ventilation may develop secondary lung injury, leading to barotrauma, pulmonary interstitial emphysema, pneumothorax, and pneumomediastinum.

Hypothermia. Hypothermia (core temperature <35° C) after submersion is a common event (see Chapter 60.6). Children are at extraordinary risk to develop hypothermia due to their relatively high body surface area–to–mass ratio and decreased subcutaneous fat insulation. Compensatory mechanisms will usually attempt to restore normothermia at body temperatures above 30–32° C; below this core temperature, thermoregulation fails and spontaneous rewarming will not occur. Moderate hypothermia (core temperature 32–35° C) increases oxygen consumption owing to shivering thermogenesis and increased sympathetic tone. Below 32° C (severe hypothermia), shivering ceases and the cellular metabolic rate decreases approximately 7% per degree C in the absence of active thermogenesis.

With moderate to severe hypothermia, progressive bradycardia, impaired myocardial contractility, and loss of vasomotor tone produce hypotension. Below 28° C, extreme bradycardia is most often present and the propensity for spontaneous ventricular fibrillation (VF) or asystole is high. Central respiratory center depression with moderate to severe hypothermia results in hypoventilation and eventual apnea. Deep coma with fixed and dilated pupils and absent reflexes at very low body temperatures (below 25–29° C) may give the false appearance of death.

Depending on the duration and severity of the temperature aberration, other systemic adverse consequences of hypothermia may occur acutely and persist even after rewarming. ARDS secondary to hypothermic pulmonary endothelial injury can be seen even in the absence of submersion or aspiration. Depressed hepatorenal metabolism and perfusion reduce drug clearance. Either hypoglycemia from glycogen store exhaustion or hyperglycemia due to a hypercholinergic state, altered pancreatic insulin release, and depressed peripheral glucose utilization may be observed. Thrombocytopenia, platelet dysfunction, and disseminated intravascular coagulation also occur. Although hypothermia slows bacterial replication, it also renders the host more susceptible to bacterial and fungal invasion and sepsis by impairing neutrophil and reticuloendothelial function. Hypothermia must be expediently corrected to minimize these adverse consequences.

During initial rewarming efforts, core body temperature may actually drop before increasing. This *afterdrop* may occur secondary to the return of cold blood from the extremities to the relatively warmer central core or by the conduction of heat from the warmer core to cooler surface layers. In patients with severe hypothermia, afterdrop may further compromise cardiac, respiratory, or neurologic function or induce arrhythmias. Afterdrop may be less severe if the extremities are not rewarmed during initial resuscitative efforts in moderately hypothermic victims, focusing rather on core rewarming.

Rewarming shock may be observed following rescue. When subjected to the additional metabolic requirements of increasing body temperature, the vasodilatation accompanying surface rewarming, and the removal of external hydrostatic pressure supporting blood pressure, victims with borderline cardiovascular function cannot respond adequately to meet increased physiologic tissue demands. Hypotension, metabolic acidosis, tissue ischemia, and other consequences of shock may be exacerbated (Chapter 60.3).

A few case reports of dramatic neurologic recovery after prolonged (10–150 min) icy water submersions exist; however, in most victims hypothermia is an unfavorable sign. The rare survivor of prolonged submersion typically has been in freezing-temperature water (<5° C) and has a core body temperature less than 28–30° C, or usually much lower. For hypothermia to be protective, core body temperature must fall rapidly, decreasing cellular metabolic rate, *before* significant hypoxemia begins. Submersion in cold water, as opposed to icy water, does not decrease body temperature quickly enough to confer protection unless oxygenation continues (the victim breathing with the head above water) as body temperature rapidly cools. Once cellular death has begun, hypothermia does not confer a protective effect or improve recovery.

Hypothermia is more commonly an unfavorable prognostic sign. In a comprehensive series from King County, Washington, where the water is cold but rarely icy, hypothermic protection has not been observed. Ninety-two percent of good survivors in their series had initial core temperatures of >34° C, whereas 61% of those who died or had severe neurologic injury had core temperatures <34° C.

Fluid and Electrolyte Changes. While submersion victims usually do not aspirate large volumes of fluid, they do swallow copious amounts. Swallowed water, pulmonary aspiration, and intravenous fluids administered during resuscitation can lead to intravascular fluid and electrolyte changes. However, with the exception of pulmonary edema, clinically significant fluid shifts are uncommon in survivors. Only 15% of patients who die in either fresh or sea water are noted to have significant electrolyte changes; children who survive to be seen in the emergency department rarely have electrolyte aberrations requiring therapy.

Massive sea water ingestion and/or aspiration leads to electrolyte changes and fluid shifts because of its high sodium concentration and osmolarity. Hypernatremia occurs to a variable extent. As fluid is osmotically drawn into the lungs and gastrointestinal tract, hemoconcentration from reduced intravascular volume may be observed. Hyposmolar diuresis, hypernatremia, and hemoconcentration can also be observed with diabetes insipidus, usually a sign of brain death after massive cerebral injury.

Water intoxication can occur in fresh water drowning, causing hyponatremia and hemodilution. Rarely, sudden hypoosmolarity results in cellular swelling and hemolysis, leading to hyperkalemia and hemoglobinuria. Hemoglobinuria can cause renal injury; however, plasma-free hemoglobin levels in human near-drowning are usually less than 500 mg/dL, insufficient to cause significant renal dysfunction from tubular plugging alone. Additionally, free water overload may occur from inappropriate antidiuretic hormone secretion, which often accompanies pulmonary and brain injuries. Excess free water can swell cerebral cells, increasing cerebral edema and intracranial pressure.

CLINICAL MANIFESTATIONS AND TREATMENT. A submersion victim's clinical course is primarily determined by the duration of submersion and the resuscitation of the child. Children with brief submersions may arrive at the hospital awake and alert, without obvious clinical injury. Some children may have been apneic at the scene and required assisted ventilation but quickly regain spontaneous respiration; others may develop minimal to severe respiratory insufficiency. Even children who appear "well" after a significant submersion need to be carefully observed for at least 6–12 hr, since delayed respiratory decompensation can occur. At a minimum, vital signs, especially respiratory rate and temperature, careful examination, chest radiography, and assessment of oxygenation by arterial blood gas or oximetry should be performed on all submersion victims.

A smaller subset of children arrive at the hospital in more critical condition. These children have had prolonged hypoxemia and cardiac dysfunction, required more extensive resuscitative efforts, and are at great risk for death or major morbidity. Initial management requires coordinated and experienced prehospital care following the ABCs (Airway, Breathing, and Circulation) of emergency resuscitation, with special attention to correcting hypothermia. Rapid and high-quality out-of-hospital resuscitation has the greatest probability of improving outcome after submersion has occurred. Further in-hospital emergency room and intensive care often requires complex management of multiorgan dysfunction.

Initial Evaluation and Resuscitation (see Chapter 60.1). The initial out-of-hospital resuscitation of submersion victims must focus on rapidly restoring oxygenation, ventilation, and adequate circulation. The airway should be clear of vomitus or foreign material, which may result in obstruction or aspiration. Abdominal thrusts should not be routinely used for removal of lung fluid, as their effectiveness is not established, and they may increase the risk of regurgitation, aspiration, and loss of airway control; interrupt cardiopulmonary resuscitation (CPR); or aggravate spinal trauma. Rather, abdominal thrusts or back blows should be reserved for cases in which airway obstruction by a foreign body is suspected.

The cervical spine should be protected in anyone with potential neck injury, such as victims of child abuse, water-sport accidents, or victims with unknown circumstances surrounding their immersion. The neck should be in a neutral position and protected with a cervical collar.

If the victim has ineffective respiration or apnea, ventilatory support must be initiated immediately. Mouth-to-mouth or mouth-to-nose breathing by trained bystanders often restores spontaneous ventilation. Positive pressure bag-mask ventilation with high inspired oxygen concentration should be substituted as soon as possible. Supplemental oxygen should be administered uniformly regardless of patient condition.

Gastric distension is exacerbated by mouth-to-mouth or bag-mask ventilation. Vomiting is seen in greater than 75% of victims during resuscitation and nearly 25% aspirate their gastric contents. Cricoid pressure during positive pressure breathing and early nasogastric or orogastric decompression may mitigate further gastric distention, decreasing the risk of vomiting and aspiration.

If apnea, cyanosis, hypoventilation, or labored respiration persists after these measures, endotracheal intubation should be performed by trained personnel as soon as possible. Endotracheal intubation is often also indicated to protect the airway in patients with depressed mental status or hemodynamic instability. Hypercapnia and hypoxia must be corrected to minimize secondary injury.

Concurrent with securing oxygenation, ventilation, and airway control, the child's cardiovascular status must be evaluated. Heart rate and rhythm, blood pressure, temperature, and end-organ perfusion require quick assessment; slow capillary refill, cool extremities, and altered mental status are potential indicators of shock. Electrocardiographic (ECG) monitoring assists with the diagnosis and treatment of arrhythmias. Patient core temperature must be evaluated, especially in children, because hypothermia can cause arrhythmias, hypotension, and depressed myocardial function. Rough and excessive stimulation should be avoided in the severely hypothermic victim as this may precipitate ventricular fibrillation (VF). Generally, closed chest cardiac compressions must be instituted immediately in pulseless, bradycardic, or severely hypotensive victims.

Intravenous fluid administration is often required to improve hemodynamic function. Two large-bore intravenous catheters or a central venous line should be established as soon as possible; intraosseous catheter placement is a potentially lifesaving "vascular access" technique that avoids the delay often associated with multiple attempts to establish venous access in critically ill children. Non–dextrose-containing, isotonic fluid is usually employed (lactated Ringer solution or normal saline). Administered fluids should be warmed (40–43° C) in the hypothermic patient; "room temperature" fluids (approximately 21° C) can exacerbate hypothermia. Although patients with cerebral edema are often fluid restricted, cerebral blood flow cannot be restored if cardiac output is insufficient; thus, establishing effective perfusion takes precedence over measures to minimize cerebral edema.

In children with cardiac arrest after submersion, the first recorded rhythm is asystole in 55%, ventricular tachycardia or VF in 29%, and bradycardia in 16%. Electrical defibrillation or cardioversion often is urgently necessary for children with ventricular tachycardia or VF (Chapter 60.2). Catecholamine infusions may be required to support myocardial function and blood pressure (Chapter 60.2). In severely hypothermic patients, the restoration of normal sinus rhythm and adequate perfusion is difficult until core body temperature is at least partially corrected. When VF is present in such victims, up to three defibrillation attempts should be delivered. If defibrillation is unsuccessful, CPR should be reinstituted and further defibrillation attempts generally avoided until the child's core temperature is above 30° C, at which time successful defibrillation may be possible. The dosing of cardioactive medications in hypothermic arrest victims is unchanged, but the frequency of administration should be reduced because of decreased drug metabolism and clearance.

Attention to hypothermia in the field is of great importance, both to initiate rewarming measures and to prevent the consequences of deeper hypothermia. A low recording thermometer and a high index of suspicion are required to diagnose hypothermia. Core temperature is best measured at the tympanic membrane. Adequate rectal temperature determinations require the thermometer be inserted at least 10 cm. Oral and axillary temperature readings are unreliable. Rewarming efforts should be instituted in the field. All hypothermic victims should have damp clothes removed, the skin dried, warm blankets applied, and a warm environmental temperature provided as soon as possible. If available, both warmed intravenous fluids (40–43° C) and humidified oxygen (42–46° C) should be used. For victims not in cardiac arrest with core temperatures <34° C, external rewarming measures should be applied only to truncal areas, attempting to avoid afterdrop. In poorly perfused hypothermic victims, the application of warm packs and other external rewarming devices may cause significant skin burns. Patients with severe hypothermia (core temperatures <30° C) require active internal warming measures provided as soon as possible.

Rapid assessment of blood glucose should be obtained in the field. If hypoglycemic, 0.5–1.0 mL/kg of 50% dextrose or 2–4 mL/kg of 10% dextrose should be administered. Dextrose-containing solutions should be withheld in patients with normal or high blood glucose concentrations, but repeated assessments of glucose must be obtained to avoid unrecognized subsequent hypoglycemia. Insulin should not be used to correct hyperglycemia after submersion injury.

Controversial Issues. The cardiorespiratory management of patients with severe hypothermia (core temperature <28° C) is controversial. Retrospective case reports can be cited of severely hypothermic victims who have ventricular arrhythmias temporally associated with endotracheal intubation or chest compressions. Therefore, some authors advocate withholding artificial ventilation or chest compressions if any respiratory activity or perfusing rhythm is present in order to avoid precipitating VF. In one recent prospective study of severely hypothermic victims, ventricular arrhythmia associated with endotracheal intubation was not observed. Given that the restoration of oxygenation and ventilation are paramount in resuscitating the near-drowning victim, gentle endotracheal tube placement should be performed in most children with hypoxia, apnea, or insufficient respiration.

The provision of chest compressions with CPR in some severely hypothermic victims generates more controversy; no prospective studies are available on this topic to guide the clinician. A few authors would withhold chest compressions if core temperature is <28° C and the ECG shows a perfusing rhythm, regardless of heart rate, pulse, or blood pressure. The logic behind these recommendations follows from observations that effective perfusion often returns with rewarming; rewarming is more effective when any circulation is present; VF or asystole slows rewarming efforts; chest compressions may precipitate VF; and CPR is less effective during severe hypothermia. No one should hesitate to perform full CPR with chest compressions in victims with apparent cardiac arrest if core temperature is unknown or >28° C, no ECG monitor is available, and a pulse cannot be found, or narrow QRS activity is absent on ECG.

Victims with profound hypothermia may appear clinically dead but full neurologic recovery, although unusual, is possible. Attempts at lifesaving resuscitation should not be withheld based on initial clinical presentation, unless the victim is obviously dead (dependent lividity or rigor mortis). Body temperature must be taken into account before terminating resuscitative efforts. Rewarming efforts, in general, probably should be continued until core temperature is at least 32°–34° C; if the victim continues to have no effective cardiac rhythm and remains totally unresponsive to aggressive CPR, resuscitative efforts may be discontinued.

Nonetheless, some children with severe hypothermia and the appearance of death are really dead. Complete core rewarming is not indicated for all victims. The rare profoundly hypothermic near-drowning victim who survives has been in freezing temperature water with the onset of severe hypothermia before significant hypoxia and ischemia are present. In most situations, discontinuing resuscitative efforts in victims of warm water submersions who remain asystolic despite 30–45 min of aggressive advanced CPR is probably warranted. Physicians in hospital settings must use their individual clinical judgment when deciding to stop resuscitative efforts, taking into account the unique circumstances of each incident.

Hospital Management. Emergency room and hospital management of the submersion victim includes and extends the aforementioned resuscitative efforts. Excellent prehospital management gives victims the best possible chance for recovery. Hospitalization allows for ongoing and more sophisticated evaluation, diagnostic testing, and therapy.

RESPIRATORY MANAGEMENT. The level of respiratory support should be appropriate to the patient's condition. Patients may develop atelectasis, pneumonia, pneumothorax, pneumomediastinum, pulmonary edema, or ARDS. Pulmonary edema in the immediate postinjury period may result from increased capillary permeability, massive fluid overload, aspiration, or myocardial failure. A chest radiograph should be obtained. An arterial catheter is also often required for reliable and frequent arterial blood gas assessment and continuous blood pressure monitoring.

Increased inspired oxygen concentration alone contributes minimally to resolving hypoxemia in patients with ventilation-perfusion mismatch. Prolonged use of high inspired oxygen concentration (>70–80%) may also worsen pulmonary injury. Endotracheal intubation and the application of positive end-expiratory pressure (PEEP) are the most effective means of reversing hypoxemia. The routine use of PEEP in near-drowning has made early death from pulmonary insufficiency a rare occurrence. PEEP increases functional residual capacity, decreases intrapulmonary shunting, improves ventilation-perfusion matching, and may improve pulmonary compliance. The level of PEEP and the concentration of inspired oxygen should restore functional residual capacity and reasonable oxygenation, usually to a PaO_2 of 80–120 mm Hg. Excessive PEEP can depress myocardial function and increase intracranial pressure.

Unintubated children who have mild to moderate hypoxemia despite supplemental oxygen and who are alert and adequately self-ventilating may be candidates for mask continuous positive airway pressure (CPAP). CPAP also restores oxygenation and functional residual capacity, possibly averting endotracheal intubation. A nasogastric tube is concomitantly employed to prevent gastric distention. Ongoing hypoxemia, impaired ventilation, labored respiration, depressed mental status, or other intolerance to CPAP requires endotracheal intubation to secure the airway and breathing.

Hypercapnia should be avoided in potentially brain injured children. Mild hyperventilation is usually employed to maintain $PaCO_2$ at 30–35 mm Hg. More excessive hyperventilation is generally not indicated.

ARDS is a serious pulmonary complication of near-drowning (Chapter 60.7). Patients requiring moderate to high pressures during mechanical ventilation are at increased risk for barotrauma. Sedation and neuromuscular blockade are often important adjuncts during respiratory management, increasing thoracic compliance and improving gas exchange on reduced ventilator settings; however, these medications can obscure neurologic evaluation, making prognostication and decision-making more difficult. The use of extracorporeal membrane oxygenation (ECMO) for near-drowning victims with ARDS is extremely controversial. Although a few, uncontrolled, retrospective cases have been reported, the general application of this technology should be limited until good selection criteria and accurate predictors of neurologic disability exist.

Children with bronchospasm after near-drowning may benefit from aerosols of β_2-agonists; however, wheezing may also be caused by pulmonary edema or airway foreign body. Bronchoscopy is usually indicated if a foreign body is suspected. Diuretics may benefit some patients with pulmonary edema and stable cardiovascular status. The routine use of corticosteroids for lung injury after near-drowning is not recommended. Although pneumonia may follow aspiration, prophylactic antibiotics are not generally indicated, except in circumstances in which the aspirate is known to be grossly contaminated.

Cardiovascular Management. Etiologies contributing to myocardial insufficiency include hypoxic-ischemic injury, ongoing hypoxemia, hypothermia, acidosis, high airway pressures during mechanical ventilation, alterations of intravascular volume, and electrolyte disorders. Congestive heart failure, shock, arrhythmias, or cardiac arrest may occur. Continuous ECG monitoring is mandatory to recognize and treat arrhythmias. Fluid resuscitation and inotropic agents are often necessary to improve myocardial function and restore tissue perfusion. Overzealous fluid administration, especially in the presence of depressed myocardial function, can worsen pulmonary edema and hypoxemia. Echocardiography, central venous pressure monitoring, and Swan-Ganz pulmonary artery catheter placement may also aid clinical management in some patients with severe myocardial dysfunction.

Rewarming Measures. Adequate circulation greatly facilitates rewarming. Passive rewarming (warm room, dry blankets) relies upon the patient's ability to self-generate heat and is *not* sufficient for most children with hypothermia. Active external rewarming (warmed blankets, radiant warmers) restores temperature more rapidly, but decreased surface circulation makes this method less effective. Active core rewarming more rapidly improves body temperature and is necessary for moderate to severe hypothermia. Simple active core rewarming measures include the administration of warmed intravenous fluids (36–40° C), heated humidified inspired oxygen (40–44° C), and warmed gastric, bladder, or peritoneal lavage.

More aggressive methods of active core rewarming include hemodialysis, extracorporeal rewarming (venovenous or arteriovenous), and cardiopulmonary bypass. Rewarming rates utilizing extracorporeal rewarming are significantly faster than external active rewarming methods ($2.1 \pm 0.7°$ C/hr vs. $0.8 \pm 0.4°$ C/hr). For profound hypothermia, especially if circulatory collapse is present, cardiopulmonary bypass may be required and has a very rapid rewarming rate ($6.9 \pm 1.9°$ C/hr). The implementation of cardiopulmonary bypass is a difficult decision requiring physician anticipation as well as consultation with and rapid transfer to a tertiary care center. Patients with significant hypothermia, if rapidly rewarmed, may have lower fluid requirements, organ failures, and duration of intensive care unit hospitalization.

Neurologic Management. Near-drowning victims who present to the hospital awake and alert usually have normal neurologic outcomes. For comatose victims, CNS injury is the major consequence of near-drowning. Neurologic management presently relies on preventing secondary injury. The primary injury, cell death from hypoxemia and ischemia, is not currently treatable.

The neurologic management of all patients centers on the rapid restoration and support of oxygenation, ventilation, and perfusion. Hypoxemia, hypercapnia, and vasodilatory medications can exacerbate ICP elevations and should be avoided. Cardiac output, blood pressure, and fluid administration should be adequate for tissue perfusion; excessive fluid administration contributes to pulmonary and cerebral edema. Additionally, the head should be kept in a neutral position and, if the child is not hypotensive, elevated 30 degrees. Hypoglycemia and hyperglycemia should be avoided. Control of seizures (Chapter 543.4) and fever is warranted because they increase cerebral metabolic activity and oxygen utilization. More aggressive neurologic intensive care measures must be critically scrutinized, given that they have not been shown to improve satisfactory patient outcome.

With optimal management, many initially comatose children can have dramatic neurologic improvement, which usually occurs within the first 24–72 hr. Unfortunately, almost half of deeply comatose children admitted to the intensive care unit will die from their brain injury or survive with severe neurologic damage. Some children may become brain dead. Deeply comatose near-drowning victims who do not show substantial improvement in their neurologic examination after 24 hr of aggressive cardiorespiratory support and who do not have other etiologies to explain their altered mental status should seriously be considered for early withdrawal of support.

Other neurointensive care measures do not benefit the usual near-drowning victim. Routine ICP monitoring after near-drowning is no longer employed. Victims with elevated ICP usually have poor outcomes, either death or severe neurologic sequelae, regardless of ICP management. Children with normal ICP can also have poor outcomes, although less frequently. While ICP monitoring and therapy to reduce increased ICP would seem likely to preserve cerebral perfusion and prevent herniation, in fact, they do not improve the near-drowning victim's outcome.

ICP monitoring, "therapeutic" hypothermia, and barbiturate therapy combined with conventional neurointensive therapy (hyperventilation, osmotic agents, diuretics, fluid restriction, muscle relaxants, and steroids), measures often used in victims with different intracranial pathology, also do not benefit the usual near-drowning victim and are not routinely utilized. Indeed, these interventions may only decrease mortality by increasing the number of survivors in a persistent vegetative state; the number of neurologically intact survivors does not increase nor does neurologic morbidity decrease in those who recover consciousness.

Other Management Issues. Some submersion victims may have also incurred traumatic injury, especially if they were participating in water sports such as boating, diving, or surfing. A high index of suspicion is required. Spinal precautions should be maintained in victims with altered mental status suspected to have traumatic injury. Significant anemia should raise suspicion for trauma and internal hemorrhage.

Hypoxic-ischemic injury can result in pansystemic injury, although clinically significant chronic organ dysfunction is uncommon in the absence of significant nervous system injury. Even after initially severe pulmonary injury, lung function returns to normal in most near-drowning victims. Acute renal failure after hypoxic-ischemic injury can result in albuminuria, hemoglobinuria, oliguria, or anuria. Diuretics, fluid restriction, or dialysis may be needed to treat fluid overload or electrolyte disturbances, but renal function also usually normalizes. Profuse, bloody diarrhea and mucosal sloughing usually portend a grim prognosis; conservative management includes bowel rest, nasogastric suction, and gastric pH control. Nutritional support for most near-drowning victims is usually not difficult because the majority of children either die or recover quickly and resume a normal diet within a few days; parenteral nutrition is occasionally indicated.

Severe anoxic encephalopathy is seen in 10–30% of pediatric intensive care unit survivors after near-drowning. Chronic neurologic sequelae after near-drowning include lowered mentation, minimal cerebral dysfunction, spastic quadriplegia, extrapyramidal syndromes, optic and cerebral atrophy, cortical blindness, peripheral neuromuscular damage, or persistent vegetative state. Psychiatric sequelae are also common and counseling for the child and family should be considered.

PROGNOSIS. Accurate neurologic prognostication is important for the child, family, physicians, and society. Victims most likely to have good neurologic outcomes should be offered the most aggressive intensive care measures to prevent death from associated injuries; conversely, children with devastating neurologic injuries can be spared the futility of therapies that will not improve their condition. Ongoing investigation should focus on early and accurate prognostication—not to predict mortality, per se, but rather to identify those children who will die or have devastating neurologic injuries versus survivors with reasonable neurologic outcomes.

Neurologic examination and progression during the first 24–72 hr are probably the best indicators of neurologic outcome. Children who are awake at the rescue scene or regain consciousness within 24 hr, even after prolonged resuscitation, are unlikely to suffer serious neurologic sequelae. In a retrospective series evaluating neurologic outcome of non–icy water, comatose near-drowning victims, many with initial Glasgow Coma Scale scores ≤5, all satisfactory survivors (baseline status or mild to moderate neurologic impairment) were noted to have spontaneous purposeful movements and normal brain-stem function within 24 hr. Good recovery did not occur in any child with abnormal brain-stem function and lack of purposeful movements at 24 hr. The highest cortical function seen in victims with eventual poor outcomes was localization to painful stimuli.

Prehospital predictors of non-icy water immersion events in King County, Washington, have been comprehensively evaluated (1974–1989). Intact survival or mild neurologic impairment occurred in 91% of children with submersion times less than 5 min and in 87% who had successful resuscitation (restoration of cardiovascular function) within 10 min. Children found with normal sinus rhythm, reactive pupils, or neurologic responsiveness at the scene virtually always had good outcomes (≥99%). In children requiring CPR, death or severe neurologic injury resulted in 93% of patients with submersion duration >10 min and in 100% of victims who required more than 25 min of resuscitative efforts. All victims with submersion duration >25 min died.

Several other studies of pediatric non-icy water immersions corroborate these findings. Generally, only a third of victims requiring advanced CPR at the scene survive, but two thirds of survivors have intact recoveries or minimal neurologic injury. However, prolonged CPR after warm water submersion almost invariably leads to death or severe neurologic injury. Therefore, the discontinuation of CPR in the hospital setting is probably warranted for victims of non-icy water submersions who do not respond to aggressive advanced life support within 25–30 min. In a given victim, however, the circumstances surrounding a submersion may not be known, especially during the first 25 min of an ongoing resuscitation; therefore, decisions regarding when to discontinue resuscitative efforts must be individualized, understanding that protracted resuscitation generally does not salvage survivors with good outcomes.

The Glasgow Coma Scale (GCS) has some utility in prognosticating recovery after near-drowning (see Table 59–5). Children with GCS scores ≥6 on admission to the hospital generally have good outcomes, whereas those with GCS scores ≤5 have a higher probability of poor neurologic outcome. Although the initial GCS score fails to adequately distinguish children who will survive intact from those with major neurologic injury, upward trends in GCS during the first several hours of hospitalization may indicate a better prognosis.

PREVENTION. Although therapeutic improvements continue, the best hope for "cure" of drowning lies in preventive efforts. The residential swimming pool is an obvious focus of preventative efforts given the high drowning rate at these sites. In one study of pediatric drowning, approximately 75% of pools were inadequately fenced and only 18% of submersions were witnessed, even though supervising adults could be identified 84% of the time. Additionally, 42% of children who eventually drowned were retrieved by someone who delayed resuscitative efforts until professional medical personnel arrived; only 44% of households had any member who knew basic CPR.

Submersion accidents in young children can be significantly reduced if swimming pools were completely fenced on all four sides with self-latching gates and pool owners were taught basic CPR. Too often, the house serves as one side of the fence, allowing direct access to the pool area. It is estimated that fencing and education could prevent up to 80% of drowning in this age group. Pool alarms are not a reliable preventative measure and pool covers may actually trap the young child underneath them and obscure observation. Drowning will still occur despite optimal barriers—there is no substitute for vigilant adult supervision.

Educating parents about the risks of common household fixtures, such as bathtubs, buckets, toilets, and washing machines, should be every pediatrician's task. For infants and young children, physicians should alert parents that even the briefest periods of absent supervision around standing water poses a risk for drowning.

Swimming lessons in children less than 4 yr old do not "drown-proof" children and may provide a false sense of security. School-age children should be taught to swim, but nonetheless prevented from swimming in unsupervised bodies of water. Water safety education for children, teenagers, and parents, such as wearing floatation devices and never swimming alone, should be reinforced in the school, community, and the physician's office. Teenagers should learn CPR and be counseled about alcohol and drug use, which significantly contribute to submersion and drowning.

Biggart MJ, Bohn DJ: Effect of hypothermia and cardiac arrest on outcome of near-drowning accidents in children. J Pediatr 117:179, 1990.

Bohn DJ, Biggar WD, Smith CR, et al: Influence of hypothermia, barbiturate therapy, and intracranial pressure monitoring on morbidity and mortality after near-drowning. Crit Care Med 14:529, 1986.

Bratton SL, Jardine DS, Morray JP: Serial neurologic examinations after near-drowning and outcome. Arch Pediatr Adolesc Med 148:167, 1994.

Committee on Injury and Poison Prevention: Drowning in infants, children, and adolescents. Pediatrics 92:292, 1993.

Corneli HM: Accidental hypothermia. J Pediatr 120:671, 1992.

Griest KJ, Zumwalt RE: Child abuse by drowning. Pediatrics 83:41, 1989.

Kallas HJ, O'Rourke PP: Drowning and immersion injuries in children. Curr Opin Pediatr 5:295, 1993.

Kyriacou D, Arcinue E, Peek C, et al: Effect of immediate resuscitation on children with submersion injury. Pediatrics 94:137, 1994.

Modell JH: Drowning. N Engl J Med 328:253, 1993.

Quan L, Kinder D: Pediatric submersions: Pre-hospital predictors of outcome. Pediatrics 90:909, 1992.

Peterson B: Morbidity of childhood near-drowning. Pediatrics 29:364, 1977.

Sieber FE, Traystman RJ: Special issues: Glucose and the brain. Crit Care Med 20:104, 1992.

Wintemute GJ: Childhood drowning and near-drowning in the United States. Am J Dis Child 144:663, 1990.

60.5 Burn Injuries

John T. Herrin and Alia Y. Antoon

Burns are a leading cause of accidental death in children, second only to motor vehicular accidents. Although prophylactic measures such as smoke detectors may reduce the likelihood of death in house fires by 85%, a significant number of children continue to suffer fatal burns. Hot water scalding has been reduced by legislation requiring new water heaters to be preset at 120° F, yet scald injury remains the leading cause of hospitalization for burns. Clothing ignition has clearly declined since the Federal Flammable Fabric Act was passed requiring sleepwear to be flame retardant. Despite the most vigorous prophylaxis, some 2 million people in the United States require medical care for burn injuries each year, with 100,000 of these patients requiring hospitalization. Thirty to forty per cent of these patients are under 15 yr of age, with an average childhood age of 32 mo. Scald burns account for 85% of total injuries and is most prevalent in children under 4 yr of age. Flame burns account for 13%; electrical and chemical burns account for the remainder. Approximately 16% of burn injuries occur as a result of child abuse, making it important to assess patterns, site of injury, and its consistency with history.

Burn treatment falls into four major phases: prophylaxis, acute care and resuscitation, reconstruction and rehabilitation, pain relief, and psychosocial adjustment. Children with massive burns require early and appropriate psychologic and social support as well as resuscitation. Surgical debridement, wound closure, and rehabilitative efforts should be concurrently instituted to produce optimal rehabilitation. Aggressive surgical removal of devitalized tissue, early nutrition, and cautious use of intubation and mechanical ventilation are necessary to maximize survival. Children who have sustained burn injuries differ in appearance from their peers, making supportive efforts for re-entry to schooling, social activities, and sporting activities necessary.

PREVENTION. The aim is a continuing reduction in the number of serious burn injuries. Effective first aid and triage can decrease both the extent (area) and severity (depth) of injuries (Table 60–8). Flame-retardant clothing, smoke detectors, and control of hot water temperature (thermostat settings) within buildings and prevention of cigarette smoking have been partially successful in reducing the incidence of burn injuries. Dedicated burn unit treatment of patients with significant burn injuries is to the advantage of the patient in facilitating medically efficient care, improving survival, and leading to greater cost efficiency. Survival of 80% of patients with 90% burns is now usual; overall survival in children with burns of all sizes has been 99%. Deaths are more likely in children with irreversible brain injury sustained at the time of the burn.

Pediatric providers can play a major role in preventing the commonest burns in children by educating parents and children's care providers regarding preventive measures, coordinating such measures with the various stages of child development (Table 60–8). Appropriate clothing, smoke detectors, and planned routes for emergency exit from home are simple, effective, efficient, and cost-effective preventive measures. Child neglect and abuse require serious consideration when the history of the injury and the distribution of the burn do not match.

■ **TABLE 60–8 Burn Prophylaxis**

Prevent Fires
Smoke detectors
Control of hot water thermostat—public buildings (temp. 120° F)
Learn to use fire-matches-lighter to prevent injury
Prevent cigarette smoking
Flame-retardant treated clothing
Prevent Injury
Roll, not run, if clothing catches fire; wrap in blanket
Practice escape procedures
Crawl beneath smoke if indoors
Use of materials for education*

**National Fire Protection Association, pamphlets, and videos.*

■ **TABLE 60–9 Indications for Hospitalization for Burns**

Burns greater than 15% body surface area
High tension electrical burns
Inhalation injury regardless of the size of body surface area burn
Inadequate home situation
Suspected child abuse or neglect
Burns to hands, feet, genitalia

ACUTE CARE AND RESUSCITATION. Careful review of the history of injury will usually reveal a common pattern—scald burn to side of face, neck, and arm if liquid is pulled from a table or stove; a pant leg area burn if clothing ignites; splash areas from cooking; and palm of hand contact with hot stove. However, "glove or stocking" burns of hands and feet; single-area deep burns on the trunk, buttocks, or back; and small-area, full-thickness burns (cigarette burns) in young children should raise a suspicion of child abuse.

Improved resuscitation and survival created multiple new problems: (1) metabolic derangements secondary to topical agents, antibiotics, and parenteral nutrition solutions; (2) translocation of organisms and toxins from the gastrointestinal tract in the presence of hypotensive or shock syndromes; and (3) infective complications that follow necessary monitoring catheters, extensive open wounds, and parenteral nutrition. These infective complications result in a wide spectrum of organisms and produce polymicrobial sepsis, intravascular infections including thrombophlebitis, infected thrombus, aneurysm formation, osteomyelitis, and septic arthritis.

Indications for Admission (Table 60–9). Burns covering greater than 10–15% of total body surface area (BSA); smaller burns of the hands, feet, face, perineum, joint surfaces; burns associated with smoke inhalation; or burns that result from electrical injuries should all be treated as emergencies and the patient should be hospitalized.

Emergency Care (Table 60–10). **First Aid Measures.** These are as follows:

1. Extinguish flames by falling and rolling: Cover the person with blanket or coat.
2. After the airway is checked and found to be patent, smoldering clothing or clothing saturated with hot liquid should be removed. In hot tar burns remove tar with mineral oil. Jewelry, particularly rings or bracelets, should be removed or cut away to prevent constriction and vascular compromise during the edema phase in the first 24–72 hr post burn.
3. In cases of chemical injury—brush off any remaining chemical if a powder or solid; then use copious irrigation or washing of the affected area with water.
4. The burned area should be covered with clean, dry sheeting and cold (not iced) wet compresses applied to small injuries. Significant large burn surface area injury (>15–20% BSA) decreases body temperature control and contraindicates the use of cold compress dressings.
5. Cardiovascular and pulmonary status are rapidly reviewed and pre-existing or physiologic lesions documented (asthma, congenital heart disease, renal or hepatic disease).
6. In patients with greater than 10–15% BSA burns, intravenous access and a nasogastric tube are placed. If genital or perineal burns are present, an indwelling urinary catheter

■ **TABLE 60–10 Acute Treatment of Burns**

First aid
Fluid resuscitation
Supply energy requirements
Pain control
Prevention of infection—early excision and grafting
Control of bacterial wound flora
Biologic and synthetic dressings to close wound

should be placed to allow accurate measurement of urine volume and to protect the area, particularly if transport to a burn center is anticipated.

Life Support Measures. These include the following:

1. Ensure and maintain adequate airway by using humidified oxygen by mask or nasotracheal intubation, if needed (particularly in patients with facial burns or if a burn is sustained in an enclosed space), before facial or laryngeal edema becomes evident. If hypoxia or carbon monoxide poisoning is suspected, 100% oxygen should be used.
2. Intravenous fluid resuscitation: Children with burns greater than 15% of BSA require intravenous fluid resuscitation to maintain adequate perfusion. All patients with inhalation injury, regardless of extent of BSA burn, require venous access to control fluid intake. All high tension and electrical injuries require venous access to ensure forced alkaline diuresis in case of muscle injury and myoglobinuria. Lactated Ringer solution, 10–20 mL/kg/hr (normal saline may be used if Ringer lactate is not available), is infused until proper fluid replacement can be calculated. Consultation with a specialized burn unit should be made to coordinate fluid therapy—type of fluid, preferred formula for calculation, and preferences for use of colloid during treatment, particularly if transfer is anticipated.
3. Evaluate for associated injuries, which are quite common in patients with a history of high tension electrical burn, especially if falling from a height. Injuries to spine, bones, and thoracic or intra-abdominal organs may occur. There is a very high risk of cardiac abnormalities, including ventricular tachycardia or ventricular fibrillation, resulting from conductivity of the high electric voltage. Cardiopulmonary resuscitation should be instituted promptly at the scene, and the patient should be placed on a cardiac monitor on arrival at the emergency room.
4. Patients with burns greater than 15% BSA should not receive oral fluids (initially), as these patients may develop ileus and may need insertion of a nasogastric tube in the emergency room to prevent aspiration.
5. All wounds should be wrapped with sterile towels until a decision is made to treat on an outpatient basis or by referral to an appropriate facility for treatment.

Classification of Burns. Proper triage and treatment of burn injury requires assessment of the extent and depth of the injury. *First degree burns* involve only the epidermis and are characterized by swelling, erythema, and pain (similar to a mild sunburn). Tissue damage is usually minimal and there is no blistering. Pain resolves in 48–72 hr and in a small percentage of patients the damaged epithelium will peel off, leaving no residual scars. A *2nd degree burn* involves injury to the entire epidermis and a variable portion of the dermal layer (vesicles and blister formation are characteristic of 2nd degree burns). A *superficial* 2nd degree burn is extremely painful because a large number of remaining viable nerve endings are exposed. Superficial 2nd degree burns heal in 7–14 days as the epithelium regenerates in the absence of infection. *Mid-level* to *deep* 2nd degree burns also heal spontaneously if wounds are kept clean and infection free. Pain is less than in more superficial burns, because fewer intact nerve endings remain viable. Fluid losses and metabolic effects of deep dermal (2nd degree) burns are essentially the same as those of 3rd degree burns. *Full thickness* or *3rd degree* burns involve destruction of the entire epidermis and dermis, leaving no residual epidermis cells to repopulate the damaged area. The wound cannot epithelialize and can heal only by wound contraction or skin grafting. The lack of painful sensation and capillary filling demonstrates the loss of nerve and capillary elements.

Estimation of Body Surface Area of Burn. It is critical to use appropriate burn charts for different age groups of children to accurately estimate the extent of body surface area burned. The volume of fluid needed in resuscitation is calculated on the estimation of the extent and depth of burn surface. Mortality and morbidity of burn outcome also depend on the extent and depth of the burn. The varying growth of the head and extremities throughout childhood make it necessary to use surface area charts, such as that modified by Lund and Brower or the chart used at the Shriners' Hospital in Boston (Fig. 60–15). The "rule of nines" used in adults may only be used in children over the age of 14 yr or as a very rough estimate to institute therapy before transfer to a definitive therapy center. In small burns under 10%, the "rule of palm" may be used especially in outpatient settings. The area from the wrist crease to finger crease (the palm) in the child equals 1% of the child's body surface area.

OUTPATIENT MANAGEMENT OF MINOR BURNS. First and 2nd degree burns under 10% BSA may be treated on an outpatient basis unless there is inadequate family support or issues of child neglect or abuse. Such patients do not require a tetanus booster or prophylactic penicillin therapy. Children who are not up to date with their immunizations should have their immunizations updated. Blisters should be left intact and dressed with silver sulfadiazine cream (Silvadene). Dressings should be changed twice daily, after the wound is washed with lukewarm water to remove any cream left from the previous application. Very small wounds, especially those on the face, may be treated with Neosporin (neomycin sulfate plus polymyxin B sulfate) or bacitracin ointment and left open. Debridement of the devitalized skin is indicated when the blisters rupture. Burns to the palm with large blisters usually heal beneath the blisters, with close follow-up on an outpatient basis. The great majority of superficial burns heal in 10–20 days. Deep 2nd degree burns take longer to heal. Pain control should be accomplished by using acetaminophen with codeine an hour before dressing changes. Wounds that appear deeper than at initial assessment or that have not healed by 21 days may require a short hospital admission for grafting.

The depth of scald injuries is difficult to assess early; conservative treatment is appropriate to allow maturation and declaration of depth and area before closure is attempted. This obviates the risk of anesthesia and unnecessary grafting and diminishes potential scarring in those patients in whom spontaneous healing is likely to occur.

FLUID RESUSCITATION. For most children the Parkland formula is a good starting guideline for fluid resuscitation (4 mL Ringer lactate/kg body weight/% BSA burned). One half of the calculated fluid is given over the first 8 hr calculated from the time of onset of the injury. The remaining half of the calculated fluid is given at an even rate over the next 16 hr. The rate of infusion is modified to the patient's response to therapy. Pulse and blood pressure should return to normal and an adequate urine output (1 mL/kg body wt/hr) should be accomplished by varying the IV infusion rate. Vital signs, acid-base balance, and mental status reflect the adequacy of the resuscitation. Because of interstitial edema and sequestration of fluid in muscle cells, patients may gain up to 20% over baseline preburn body weight. Patients with burns of 40–60% BSA require a large venous access (central venous line) to deliver the adequate fluid required over the critical 1st hours. Patients with burns greater than 60% BSA may require two central venous lines; these patients are best cared for in a specialized burn unit.

During the second 24 hr after the burn, patients will begin to reabsorb edema fluid and diurese. One half of the 1st day's fluid requirement is infused as lactated Ringer solution in 5% dextrose. Controversies exist over whether colloid should be provided in the early period of burn resuscitation. One preference is to use colloid replacement concurrently, if the burn is greater than 85% total BSA. Colloid is usually instituted 8–24 hr after the burn injury. In children less than 12 mo of age

Moore P, Blackeney P, Broemeling L, Portman S: Psychologic adjustment after childhood burn injuries as predicted by personality traits. J Burn Care Rehab 14:80, 1993.
Remensynder JP: Acute electrical injuries. *In:* Martyn JAJ (ed): Acute Management of the Burned Patient. Philadelphia, WB Saunders, 1990, pp 66–86.
Sheridan RL, Tompkins RG, Burke JF: Management of burn wounds with prompt excision and immediate closure. J Intensive Care Med 9:6, 1994.
Strongin J, Hales CA: Pulmonary disorders in the burn patient. *In:* Martyn JAJ (ed): Acute Management of the Burned Patient. Philadelphia, WB Saunders, 1990, pp 25–45.
Volinsky J, Hanson J, Lustig J: Lightning burns. Arch Pediatr Adolesc Med 148:529, 1994.

60.6 *Cold Injuries*

John T. Herrin and Alia Y. Antoon

The increased involvement of civilians in snowmobiling, mountain climbing, winter hiking, and skiing has increased the risk of problems with cold injury. Cold injury may be either local tissue damage, with the injury pattern depending upon exposure to damp cold—frostnip, immersion or trench-foot—or dry cold, which leads to local frostbite or generalized effects (hypothermia).

PATHOPHYSIOLOGY. Ice crystals may form between or within cells, interfering with the activities of the normal sodium pump and leading to rupture of cell membranes. Further damage may occur from clumping of red cells or platelets, causing microemboli or thrombosis. Blood may be shunted from an affected area by neurovascular impulses secondary to the cold injury; this shunting will often sacrifice an injured part to save the maximal tissue and whole body. The spectrum of injury varies from mild to severe and reflects the result of structural and functional disturbance to small blood vessels, nerves, and skin.

ETIOLOGY. In general, body heat may be lost by conduction (wet clothing, contact with metal or other solid conducting objects), convection (wind chill), and radiation. Susceptibility to cold injury may be increased by dehydration, alcohol or drug excess, substance abuse, impaired consciousness, exhaustion, hunger, anemia, impaired circulation due to cardiovascular disease, sepsis, or in very young or aged persons.

Hypothermia occurs when the body can no longer sustain normal temperature. As shivering ceases, the body is unable to warm itself, and when the body core temperature falls below 35° C, the syndrome of hypothermia occurs. Wind chill, wet, or inadequate clothing or other factors both increase local injury and may cause dangerous hypothermia, even in the presence of an ambient temperature that is not lower than 17–20° C (50–60° F).

CLINICAL MANIFESTATIONS. Frostnip. This results in the presence of firm, cold white areas on the face, ears, or extremities. Blistering and peeling may occur over the next 24–72 hr, occasionally leaving mild increased hypersensitivity to cold for some days or weeks. Treatment is simply to warm with an unaffected hand or warm object before the lesion reaches a stage of stinging or aching, and before numbness supervenes.

Immersion Foot (Trench Foot). This occurs when feet are exposed in the cold to damp or wet, poorly ventilated boots and produce a cold numb extremity, which becomes pale, edematous, and clammy. Tissue maceration and infection are likely and prolonged autonomic disturbance is common. This autonomic disturbance leads to increased sweating, pain, and hypersensitivity to temperature changes, which may persist for years. The treatment is largely prophylactic and consists of using well-fitting, insulated, waterproof, nonconstricting footwear. Once damage has occurred, change in clothing and footwear to more appropriate dry and well-fitting footwear is necessary. The skin integrity is managed by keeping the affected area dry, well ventilated, and preventing or treating infection. Symptomatic measures are all that are possible for control of autonomic symptoms.

Frostbite. Here initial stinging or aching of the skin progresses to cold, hard, white anesthetic and numb areas. On rewarming the area becomes blotchy, itchy, and often red, swollen, and painful. The injury spectrum can be progression to complete normality or to more extensive tissue damage, even with gangrene, if early relief is not obtained.

Treatment consists of warming the damaged area. It is important not to cause further damage by attempting to rub the area with ice or snow; initial warming as in frostnip may be tried. The area may be warmed against an unaffected hand, abdomen, or axilla while in transfer to a facility where more rapid warming with a water bath is possible. If the skin becomes painful and swelling occurs, anti-inflammatory agents are helpful and analgesic is necessary. Freeze and rethaw cycles are much more dangerous for permanent tissue injury, and it may be necessary to delay definitive warming and to apply only mild measures if the patient is required to walk on the damaged feet en route to definitive treatment. In the hospital the affected area can be immersed in warm water (temperature approximately 42° C), being careful not to burn the anesthetic skin area. Vasodilating agents, such as prazosin or phenoxybenzamine, may be helpful. Anticoagulants (heparin, dextran) have provided equivocal results. Oxygen is only of help at high altitudes; results of chemical and surgical sympathectomy have also been equivocal. Meticulous local care, prevention of infection, and keeping the rewarmed area dry, open, and sterile provide optimal results. Recovery can be very good and justifies prolonged observation with conservative therapy before any excision or amputation of tissue is considered. Analgesia and maintenance of good nutrition is necessary throughout the prolonged waiting period.

Hypothermia. Hypothermia may occur in winter sports when injury, equipment failure, or exhaustion decrease the degree of exercise, particularly if there is not sufficient attention to wind chill. Immersion and wet wind chill rapidly produce hypothermia. As the core temperature of the body falls, there is an insidious onset of extreme lethargy, fatigue, incoordination, and apathy, which are followed by mental confusion, clumsiness, irritability, hallucinations, and finally by bradycardia. A number of medical conditions, such as cardiac disease, diabetes mellitus, hyperinsulinemia, and substance abuse, may need to be considered in a differential diagnosis. The decrease in rectal temperature to less than 34° C (93° F) is the most helpful diagnostic feature.

Prevention is a high priority. For those who participate in winter sports, multiple layers of warm clothing, adequate waterproofing, and protection against wind; gloves and socks within insulated boots that do not impede circulation, together with a warm head covering, are all extremely important. Thirty per cent of heat loss occurs from the head. Ample food and fluid need to be provided during the time of exercise. Those who participate in sports should be alert to the presence of cold or numbing of body parts, particularly the nose, ears, or extremities, and should have reviewed methods to produce local warming and know to seek shelter should they detect symptoms of local cold.

Treatment at the scene aims at preventing further heat loss and early removal to adequate shelter (Chapter 60.4). Dry clothing should be provided as soon as practical and transport should be undertaken provided that a pulse is present. If there is no pulse present at the initial review, cardiopulmonary resuscitation is undertaken (Chapter 60.2). During transfer jarring and sudden motion are to be avoided, since these may cause ventricular arrhythmia. It is often difficult to attain a normal sinus rhythm during hypothermia.

If the patient is conscious, mild muscle activity should be encouraged and a warm drink administered. If the patient is unconscious, external warming should be initially undertaken using blankets and a sleeping bag, often with snuggling with a warm companion to increase the efficiency of warming. On arrival at a definitive treatment center, inhalation of warm moist air or oxygen, heating pads, or thermal blankets should be used while a warming bath temperature 45–48° C (113–118° F) is prepared. Monitoring of serum chemistries and electrocardiogram are necessary until the core temperature rises above 35° C and can be stabilized. Control of fluid, pH, blood pressure, and oxygen are all necessary in the early phases of the warming period and resuscitation. In patients with marked abnormalities, warming measures such as gastric or colonic irrigation with warm saline or peritoneal dialysis have limited experience but could be considered.

Chilblain (Pernio). Chilblain (pernio) is a form of cold injury in which erythematous, vesicular, or ulcerative lesions occur. The lesions are presumed to be of a vascular or vasoconstrictive origin. The lesions are often itchy and may be painful and result in swelling and scabbing. The lesions are most often found at the ears, tips of fingers, and toes and on exposed areas of the legs. The lesions last for approximately 1–2 wk but may persist for longer periods. *Treatment* consists of prophylaxis—avoiding prolonged chilling and protecting potentially susceptible areas with caps, gloves, and stockings as a preventive measure. Prazosin and phenoxybenzamine may be helpful in improving circulation if this is a recurrent problem. For significant itching local corticosteroid preparations may be helpful.

Cold-Induced Fat Necrosis (Panniculitis). This common, usually benign, injury occurs on exposure to cold air, snow, or ice and manifests in exposed (less often covered) surfaces as red (less often purple to blue) macular, papular, or nodular lesions. *Treatment* is with nonsteroidal anti-inflammatory agents. The lesions may last 10 days to 3 wk.

Berkow R (ed): Cold injury. The Merck Manual of Diagnosis and Therapy. Rahway, NJ: Merck, Sharp, and Dohme, 1992.
Britt LD, Dascombe WH, Rodriguez A: New horizons in management of hypothermia and frostbite injury. Surg Clin North Am, 71:345, 1991.
Shepard RJ: Metabolic adaptions to exercise in the cold. Sports Med 16:266, 1993.

60.7 Adult Respiratory Distress Syndrome

Thomas B. Rice

Adult respiratory distress syndrome (ARDS) is a syndrome recognized as acute respiratory failure and is characterized by increased permeability pulmonary edema, demonstrated by widespread infiltrates on chest radiograph, impaired oxygenation, and normal cardiac function (noncardiogenic pulmonary edema). This syndrome is more precisely identified as "acute" respiratory distress syndrome because it is acute in onset and has been identified in pediatric patients as young as 1–2 wk of age. The definition of acute respiratory distress syndrome includes: (1) poor oxygenation ($Pao_2/FIO_2 \leq 200$ regardless of the amount of positive end-expiratory pressure [PEEP]), (2) bilateral infiltrates seen on frontal chest radiograph, and (3) pulmonary artery occlusion pressure $\leq$18 mm Hg when measured or no clinical evidence of left atrial hypertension based on clinical data.

ARDS, a diffuse lung injury, is precipitated by a number of triggering agents, including direct and indirect pulmonary events. Shock, sepsis, and near-drowning are the most common causes of ARDS in pediatric patients; ARDS has been associated with trauma, drug overdose, aspiration, inhalation injury, and intravascular coagulation abnormalities. The incidence affecting pediatric patients is unknown; it is estimated that more than 150,000 adults per year develop ARDS. Children with acute respiratory failure compose 8% of total patient days in pediatric intensive care units.

PATHOLOGY. Following the triggering event, diffuse alveolar damage can be identified as the result of structural changes in the alveolar capillary unit. There are three distinct stages in the development of ARDS. In the initial *exudative stage*, there is severe capillary congestion and interstitial pulmonary edema. This is manifested by a protein-rich edema fluid, which develops from increased permeability of the alveolar capillary membrane. The alveoli themselves often contain a nonhomogenous fluid, blood, or aggregated leukocytes. The exudative stage usually begins during the first 6 hr and may last up to 72 hr before resolution or progression. Patients may recover from the exudative phase during the 1st few days; many progress to a chronic or proliferative stage, which occurs between the 1st and 3rd wk after injury. The *proliferative phase* is characterized by an increased density of type II pneumocytes and fibroblasts. Over time the type II pneumocytes are transformed into type I pneumocytes; interstitial edema and inflammatory cells stimulate the fibroblasts to deposit collagen, and eventually the progression from the proliferative stage to the final or *fibrotic stage* takes place. The fibrotic stage is usually present if ARDS has persisted for more than 3 wk. During this time, the lungs are remodeled by collagenous tissue with the development of pulmonary fibrosis. Fibrosis often results in a life-threatening decrease in the surface area available for gas exchange.

PATHOGENESIS. As expected from the severe alterations in lung structure, dysfunction of the cardiorespiratory system is the major physiologic feature of ARDS, with the most salient feature being severe arterial hypoxemia. The precise sequence of events resulting in increased capillary permeability and development of pulmonary edema is not completely understood and appears to be multifactorial. Possible cellular mediators that injure the endothelium include the role of inflammatory cells, neutrophils, mononuclear phagocytes, eosinophils, platelets, fibroblasts, and lymphocytes. Circulating humoral mediators that may cause or amplify the lung injury include complement, endotoxin, cytokines, oxygen free radicals, histamine, serotonin, proteases, free fatty acids, products produced during intravascular coagulopathy, and the products of the arachidonic acid pathway, primarily prostaglandins, thromboxane, and leukotrienes. The role of these various mediators in the development of ARDS is variable and complex. The aggregation of polymorphonuclear leukocytes within the pulmonary circulation appears to play a role through the initiation of a cascade of events for many of the proposed mediators. However, ARDS has been observed in patients with neutropenia; thus the triggering agents may directly affect more distal mechanisms in the cascade that initiates edema formation. Direct toxicity of inhaled substances is also a less common pathophysiologic event.

Abnormalities in the surfactant system have been found in patients with ARDS. This would predispose the lung to develop atelectasis with unstable alveoli and the potential for edema formation, caused in part by inadequate surfactant production, pool size, composition, metabolism, inactivation, or inhibition.

CLINICAL MANIFESTATIONS. Pulmonary symptoms of ARDS may be minimal immediately following the acute injury, because there is often a latent period during which the patient demonstrates mild respiratory distress and possibly hyperventilation. At this stage the lungs are clear to auscultation. During the next 4–24 hr, hypoxemia develops and respiratory distress becomes more evident, with findings of cyanosis, dyspnea, and marked tachypnea with diffuse, moist inspiratory crackles. At this point, a large intrapulmonary shunt can be demonstrated and supplemental oxygen may provide temporary relief. Gradual recovery may ensue, but most patients develop progressive severe hypoxemia and hypercapnia; supplemental oxygen fails to improve the clinical appearance, leading to the need for mechanical ventilation. Many patients in this stage do not survive; those who do often require prolonged respiratory support.

LABORATORY FINDINGS. Arterial blood gas measurements often demonstrate a Pa_{O_2} of <50 mm Hg on a FIO_2 of >0.6%; a Pa_{O_2}/FIO_2 ratio of <200 correlates with a QS/QT (intrapulmonary shunt) of >20%. The radiographic evidence of ARDS is nonspecific. Initially, no significant radiographic abnormalities may exist. Subsequently, over a period of several hours, a fine bilateral reticular infiltrate appears, which can rapidly progress to florid pulmonary edema (whiteout). The development of interstitial and alveolar pulmonary edema, without cardiomegaly, usually becomes apparent within the first 72 hr. Although the chest radiograph on AP film demonstrates diffuse pulmonary infiltrates, CT reveals that the bulk of the infiltrates are in the posterior or dependent regions of the lung. Excessive intravenous fluid therapy may augment the signs of pulmonary edema, while diuretics and PEEP or other ventilator changes that increase mean airway pressure reduces the appearance of edema. With survival, complications such as the development of diffuse interstitial fibrosis and barotrauma (pneumothorax, pneumomediastinum) may become evident. During convalescence the chest radiograph may return to normal. Pulmonary function tests and lung mechanics demonstrate reduced functional residual capacity and diminished lung compliance. Severe increases in pulmonary artery pressure and abnormally high pulmonary artery resistance have been associated with a poor prognosis.

TREATMENT. ARDS must be managed in an intensive care unit where appropriate cardiorespiratory monitoring and therapy can be provided. Clinical management goals are directed towards supportive care, the primary objective of which is to deliver sufficient oxygen to satisfy the metabolic demands of the tissue. Appropriate monitoring includes invasive hemodynamic assessment, including systemic arterial catheterization and often pulmonary artery catheter placement. Measurements of pulmonary function and gas exchange such as arterial blood gases, pulse oximetry, end-tidal CO_2, and lung mechanics are used to adjust inspired oxygen tension and ventilator settings to promote adequate delivery of oxygen to the tissues and minimize complications.

Most patients will require endotracheal intubation and mechanical ventilation with the addition of PEEP when they are unable to maintain a Pa_{O_2} of greater than 50 mm Hg with 60% inspired oxygen. PEEP improves oxygenation and has been the most important contribution to the improvement in early survival in ARDS. PEEP does not restore normal oxygenation in all patients and may adversely affect cardiac function. PEEP settings must be fine-tuned by continued surveillance of clinical and laboratory data. In some instances, extremely high levels of PEEP (10–20 cm H_2O) have been used; however, life-threatening barotrauma may be induced as well as impaired venous return, and thus reduced cardiac output with systemic hypotension. Strict and precise attention must be provided in the maintenance of cardiac function, particularly when high levels of PEEP are used, because stabilization of cardiac output with fluid management is crucial to oxygen delivery. Frequent repositioning (lateral decubitus positioning) is recommended because it may improve oxygenation. Careful evaluation and provision for the child's nutritional needs are essential. Routine use of prophylactic antibiotics is not recommended.

Novel therapies that specifically target underlying pathogenic mechanisms in ARDS have been used and have shown varying degrees of success. Most, however, have not yet been subjected to rigorous, prospective clinical studies, but hold promise as therapies that may impact care. These therapies include pressure-controlled ventilation with permissive hypercapnia; high-frequency ventilation, including high-frequency positive-pressure ventilation, high-frequency oscillation, and high-frequency jet ventilation; negative pressure ventilation, liquid ventilation; extracorporeal membrane oxygenation, including both venoarterial and venovenous methods; exogenous surfactant replacement; inhaled nitric oxide; lung transplant; eicosanoids or their inhibitors; vasodilators; pentoxifylline; and corticosteroids, which have not shown to be effective and may be dangerous in the acute stages, but may be of some value in a selected subset of individuals if used during the later (7–14 days) phases of ARDS.

The primary complications of ARDS include nosocomial infection, severe barotrauma, cardiac output compromise, oxygen toxicity, progressive pulmonary fibrosis, multiple system organ failure (acute tubular necrosis, coagulopathy, myocardopathy, hepatic dysfunction, central nervous system dysfunction, gastrointestinal bleeding, ileus), and death.

PROGNOSIS. Pediatric survival for ARDS varies; most centers report mortality rates of 50–75%. A meta-analysis of four reports of ARDS in children found an overall mortality of 52%. A multicenter study of 41 pediatric intensive care units identified 470 children with acute respiratory failure (defined by mechanical ventilation, PEEP >6 cm H_2O, and a FIO_2 requirement of >0.5 for >12 hr) with a 43% mortality rate. Death is due to the initiating event, multisystem organ dysfunction, or sepsis. For survivors the outlook for functional recovery is good. Most children can return to their pre-illness status within the following year, although minor abnormalities in gas exchange may be identified through pulmonary function testing. The long-term outcome for return of function in those surviving is good and is probably better than in adults.

Bernard GR, Artigas A: European-American Consensus Conference on ARDS. Am J Respir Crit Care Med 149:818, 1994.
Hickling KG: Low volume ventilation with permissive hypercapnia in the adult respiratory distress syndrome. Clin Intensive Care 3:67, 1992.
Hyers TM: Prediction of survival and mortality in patients with ARDS. New Horizons 1:466, 1993.
Kollef MH, Schuster DP: The acute respiratory distress syndrome. N Engl J Med 332:27, 1995.
Lewis JF, Jobe AH: State of the art: Surfactant and the adult respiratory distress syndrome. Am Rev Respir Dis 147:218, 1993.
Lyrene RK, Truog WE: Adult respiratory distress syndrome in a pediatric intensive care unit: Predisposing conditions, clinical course, and outcome. Pediatrics 67:790, 1981.
Marinelli WA, Ingbar DH: Diagnosis and management of acute lung injury. Clin Chest Med 15:517, 1994.
Meduri GU, Chinn AJ, Leeper KV, et al: Corticosteroid rescue treatment of progressive fibroproliferation in late ARDS. Chest 105:1516, 1994.
Moler FW, Palmisano J, Custer JR: Extracorporeal life support for pediatric respiratory failure: Predictors of survival from 220 patients. Crit Care Med 21:1604, 1993.
Ognibene FP, Martin SE, Parker MM, et al: Adult respiratory distress syndrome in patients with severe neutropenia. N Engl J Med 315:547, 1986.
Pfenninger J, Gerber A, Tschaeppeler H, et al: Adult respiratory distress syndrome in children. J Pediatr 101:352, 1982.
Rossaint R, Falke KJ, Lopez F, et al: Inhaled nitric oxide for the adult respiratory distress syndrome. N Engl J Med 328:399, 1993.
Shaffer TH, Wolfson MR, Clark LC: Liquid ventilation. Pediatr Pulmonol 14:102, 1992.
Timmons OD, Dean JM, Vernon DD: Mortality rates and prognostic variables in children with adult respiratory distress syndrome. J Pediatr 119:896, 1991.
Timmons OD, Havens PL, Fackler JC, et al: Predicting death in pediatric patients with acute respiratory failure. Chest (in press).

CHAPTER 61

Anesthesia and Perioperative Care

Charles B. Berde and William S. Schechter

The prospect of surgery and anesthesia provokes anxiety for most children and their parents. Although pediatricians are generally not called upon to direct their patients' perioperative care, they have an essential role in preoperative evaluation and preparation, in counseling patients and families, and in postoperative assessment. Because it is now feasible to provide anesthesia safely for children of all ages, pediatricians should advocate for the rights of infants and children to receive anesthesia and analgesia for both major and minor procedures.

PREOPERATIVE ASSESSMENT

All infants and children scheduled for surgery should be evaluated preoperatively both to screen for conditions that may require specific treatment or optimization (evaluation of anemia, adjustment of asthma medications), and to counsel patients and parents regarding the expected course of anesthesia and surgery. The cornerstone of assessment is a systematic history and detailed physical examination with emphasis on airway anatomy and cardiorespiratory status. A careful history enables the anesthesiologist to plan the management of anesthesia and the postanesthetic period more effectively. The history should include the information listed in Table 61–1.

The physical examination should begin with general observation of the patient and an evaluation of vital signs. The airway is assessed for predictors of difficulty with mask ventilation or intubation, including impaired neck mobility, micrognathia, nasal obstruction, adenotonsillar hypertrophy, impaired mouth opening, macroglossia, and a variety of forms of orofacial dysmorphism. The presence of pectus excavatum in a small child may suggest chronic upper airway obstruction. Determination of hydration status is important because most anesthetics are vasodilators or myocardial depressants, and hypovolemia will predispose the patient to hypotension after induction. Evidence of cardiac failure, such as tachypnea, tachycardia, or hepatomegaly, may alter the choice of induction agents. The presence of wheezing demands further evaluation before proceeding with an elective operation. Venous access must be evaluated with care so that cannulation may proceed rapidly after an inhalation induction. The child's behavior and ability to cooperate can help predict the need for premedication or parental presence at induction.

MATURATION OF ORGAN SYSTEMS: ANESTHETIC IMPLICATIONS. There are major anatomic and physiologic differences between the neonate, infant, child, and adult that influence anesthetic management. These differences are outlined in Table 61–2.

OUTPATIENT SURGERY. Over half of surgery for children is performed on an outpatient basis. This has been made possible in part by advances in anesthetic techniques that involve more rapid recovery and reduced incidence of nausea.

Advantages of day surgery include (1) less time in a threatening hospital environment, (2) reduced health care costs, and (3) reduced exposure to pathogens. Disadvantages include (1) greater difficulty with follow-up care and observation, (2) greater burden for some families, with potential for increased parental anxiety, (3) less continuity of care, and (4) greater difficulty with management of pain and other symptoms.

■ TABLE 61–1 The Preanesthetic History

Child's Previous Anesthetic and Surgical Procedures
- Review anesthetic record for information about mask and endotracheal tube size, type and size of laryngoscope used, difficulties with mask ventilation or intubation

Perinatal Problems (especially for infants)
- Need for prolonged hospitalization
- Need for supplemental oxygen or intubation
- History of apnea and bradycardia

Other Major Illnesses and Hospitalizations

Family History of Anesthetic Complications, Malignant Hyperthermia (MH), or Pseudocholinesterase Deficiency

Respiratory Problems
- Obstructive apnea, breathing irregularities, or cyanosis (especially in infants under age 6 mo)
- History of snoring or obstructive breathing pattern
- Recent upper respiratory tract infection
- Recurrent respiratory infections
- Previous laryngotracheitis (croup)
- Asthma or wheezing during respiratory infections

Cardiac Problems
- Murmurs
- Dysrhythmia
- Exercise intolerance
- Syncope
- Cyanosis

Gastrointestinal Problems
- Reflux and vomiting
- Feeding difficulties
- Failure to thrive
- Liver disease

Exposure to Exanthems or Potentially Infectious Pathogens

Neurologic Problems
- Seizures
- Developmental delay
- Neuromuscular diseases
- Increased intracranial pressure

Hematologic Problems
- Anemia
- Bleeding diathesis
- Tumor
- Immunocompromise
- Prior blood transfusions and reactions

Renal
- Renal insufficiency, oliguria, anuria
- Fluid and electrolyte abnormalities

Psychosocial
- Post-traumatic stress
- Drug abuse, cigarettes, alcohol
- Physical or sexual abuse
- Family dysfunction
- Previous traumatic medical and surgical experiences
- Psychosis, anxiety, depression

Gynecologic
- Sexual history
- Possibility of pregnancy

Current Medications
- Prior administration of corticosteroids

Allergies
- Drugs
- Iodine
- Latex products
- Surgical tapes
- Food allergies (especially soya and egg albumin)

Dental Condition (loose or cracked teeth)

When and What the Child Last Ate (especially in emergency procedures)

Preoperative assessment for "day surgery" patients may vary according to local resources and referral patterns. Patient selection criteria for outpatient surgery are based on three factors: the nature of the operative procedure, parental readiness, and patient status. The most common outpatient procedures are herniorrhaphy, myringotomy, tonsillectomy with or without adenoidectomy, strabismus repair, orchidopexy, and circumcision. In most cases, these procedures cause minor physiologic change and minimal bleeding. Parents must be capable of following specific postoperative instructions. Patients should

■ TABLE 61–2 Anatomic and Physiologic Features of Infancy: Anesthetic Implications

System/Category	Implications
Respiratory	
Airway	
Infant tongue occupies larger proportion of oropharynx	Nasal obstruction may make mask ventilation difficult and require placement of an oral airway; tongue commonly obstructs airway
Cephalad ("anterior") larynx Infant inlet: C_{3-4} Adult inlet: C_{4-5}	Difficult visualization of larynx
Omega-shaped epiglottis	Difficult visualization of larynx
Vocal cords Angled lower anteriorly than posteriorly in infants	Difficult visualization of larynx
Small airway diameter	Poiseille's law Small changes in diameter (e.g., with edema) produce large changes in resistance Greater difficulty with spontaneous ventilation under anesthesia
Cricoid cartilage Narrowest part of pediatric airway	Use uncuffed endotracheal tubes Tubes should have air leak at 20–30 cm H_2O pressure Postanesthetic croup is common in infants
Short tracheal length	Precise endotracheal tube placement required
Lungs	
High ratio of O_2 consumption to FRC	Rapid desaturation with apnea Rapid induction and emergence from inhalation anesthesia
Closing capacity near FRC	Rapid desaturation with apnea Atelectasis
Chest wall compliance high	Atelectasis
Immature ventilatory reflexes	Postoperative apnea Hypoventilation
CNS	Reduced anesthetic requirements at birth, increases to a maximum at 6 mo of age, decreases with age thereafter
Autonomic	Decreased resting sympathetic tone Increased parasympathetic tone
Cardiac	
Noncompliant ventricles	Relatively fixed stroke volume Cardiac output rate dependent
Immature sarcoplasmic reticulum	Greater depression of contractility by inhalation anesthetics
Immature baroreceptors	Less compensatory tachycardia and vasoconstriction with hypotension
Hepatic	
Immature enzyme systems	Slower metabolism of intravenous anesthetics, some muscle relaxants, and opioids
Renal	
Diminished GFR in the first several weeks of life	Delayed elimination of intravenous anesthetics, some muscle relaxants, and opioid metabolites
Thermal regulation	Greater temperature fluctuation with environmental changes

FRC, functional residual capacity; GFR, glomerular filtration rate.

live close to a hospital or emergency medical care facility should the need arise for medical intervention within the first 24 hr after surgery. Children presenting for outpatient surgery should be in good general health or, if they have chronic illness, they should be prepared optimally. Most outpatients are ASA physical status I and II (Table 61–3), although on occasion ASA status III patients may be cared for on an outpatient basis. For example, a suitable ASA III patient may be an oncology patient presenting for a diagnostic or therapeutic procedure or for placement of an indwelling catheter.

LABORATORY TESTING. Preoperative laboratory testing for most children should be extremely parsimonious. The predictive value and cost effectiveness of chest radiography and urinalysis in otherwise healthy children is extremely low. In many centers, even a preoperative hematocrit is no longer required for children undergoing minor surgery who have no specific risk factors for anemia disclosed by history and physical examination. Infants less than 1 yr of age are at increased risk of anemia, and most centers currently require a hematocrit or hemogram for infants less than 6–12 mo of age. If the sickle cell status is unknown, it should be clarified in susceptible populations. Blood typing and cross matching are recommended for children undergoing surgery for which the potential for significant blood loss is high. Coagulation studies are widely obtained for children undergoing diverse procedures from tonsillectomy to craniotomy. In general, their yield is low in patients without a history of bleeding problems.

FASTING GUIDELINES (N.P.O. ORDERS). These guidelines are a frequent source of frustration for patients, parents, and health providers. Preoperative fasting is advised because anesthetic induction involves loss of airway reflexes that prevent aspiration of regurgitated gastric contents. Aspiration involves two

■ TABLE 61–3 American Society of Anesthesiologists Physical Status Classification

ASA PS 1	Healthy patient
ASA PS 2	Mild illness, well controlled
ASA PS 3	Serious illness
ASA PS 4	Life-threatening illness
ASA PS 5	Moribund

problems: airway occlusion from particulates in food and gastric acid–induced chemical pneumonitis.

Although the child's stomach should be free of solids prior to elective anesthesia, it is important not to interrupt fluid intake longer than necessary. Most centers withhold milk or solids for 8 hr prior to elective anesthesia. Several studies have confirmed the safety of preoperative administration of clear liquids (apple juice, glucose-electrolyte solutions) up to 2–4 hr preoperatively in healthy infants and children. Gastric emptying can be delayed in a variety of circumstances, including trauma, gastric outlet obstruction, or severe anxiety. In these circumstances and for most emergency surgery, "full stomach" precautions are recommended.

THE CHILD WITH RHINORRHEA OR COUGHING. Anesthesiologists are frequently faced with the prospect of anesthetizing a child with respiratory signs and symptoms. For convenience, we divide common rhinorrhea and cough into three categories: (1) the child with isolated chronic rhinitis, (2) the child with viral upper respiratory tract infection, and (3) the child with lower respiratory tract disease.

The child with chronic rhinitis may have chronic purulent sinusitis or a noninfectious condition related to allergy, vasomotor rhinitis, or adenotonsillar hypertrophy. In some of these children, signs and symptoms are persistent. One controlled study found no increased risk of pulmonary complications among children with chronic rhinitis undergoing myringotomy and tube placement. Airway management can sometimes be challenging, because many of these children are mouth breathers and may have significant adenotonsillar hypertrophy.

Acute rhinitis or pharyngitis may predispose a child to both intraoperative and postoperative respiratory problems. Because mild airway difficulties are common, but serious adverse events are rare in these patients, anesthesiologists may disagree regarding the safety of proceeding with surgery. The anesthesiologist must judge whether to proceed with an elective anesthetic after the risks and benefits are carefully discussed with the family and surgeon. The presence of fever along with cough, tachypnea, or an abnormal chest examination suggests lower tract disease and argues against proceeding in patients who present for elective surgery.

Children who have had recent viral respiratory tract infection may demonstrate airway hyper-reactivity on pulmonary function tests. These abnormalities may persist for as long as 6–8 wk following resolution of symptoms and are associated with an increased risk of laryngospasm, bronchospasm, and desaturation with anesthesia. Following an upper respiratory infection, children who received endotracheal anesthesia may be at an 11 times higher risk of airway problems than those who were managed by mask alone. Postextubation stridor is more common following a respiratory infection. These complications are more severe in infants and toddlers than in older children or adolescents.

AN ACCEPTABLE HEMATOCRIT. In the past, a hematocrit greater than 30% was widely considered mandatory for patients prior to elective surgery. The rationale for preferring adequate red cell mass lies in providing a safety margin for oxygen delivery and anticipated surgical blood loss. With increasing awareness of the infectious and immunologic consequences of transfusion, and with greater experience in management of hemodilution under anesthesia, this rule has been relaxed. A hematocrit of 28% lies within the normal range for infants at 3 mo of age. In many patients with chronic renal insufficiency or hematologic disorders, it may be appropriate to administer anesthesia with a substantially lower hematocrit. Causes of anemia should be investigated, and purely elective surgery should be delayed pending such assessment.

SURGICAL TIMING AND EVALUATION OF ANESTHETIC RISK. The proper timing of surgery in infants depends both on anesthetic risks and effects of timing on surgical outcome. For example, prostaglandin infusions to maintain patency of the ductus arteriosus permit preoperative stabilization of many infants prior to neonatal cardiac surgery and greatly improves the infant's physiologic stability. Conversely, the newborn exsanguinating from a sacrococcygeal teratoma may need immediate surgery to gain control of bleeding. Many other cases, such as the timing of cleft lip and palate or craniosynostosis repairs, represent a compromise between the benefits of early repair on outcome and the increased risks of anesthesia (or the increased likelihood of transfusion) in younger infants.

Parents and older children often ask for assessment of anesthetic risk. It is useful to place these statistics into a context based on both the patient's disease, age-related risks, and the type of surgery. It should be noted that anesthetic mishap accounts for only a small percentage (less than 5%) of perioperative deaths; the majority of perioperative deaths are related to patient disease–related factors, such as exsanguination following major trauma or inability to remove from cardiopulmonary bypass.

In adults, morbidity and mortality increase as ASA physical status increases; in limited pediatric studies, this trend is less apparent. A study of adverse events in pediatric and adult anesthesia highlights causal differences between pediatric and adult patients. Analyses of critical incidents indicates that two scenarios are most common in infants: (1) inability to manage the airway and deliver oxygen, and (2) overdose of inhalation anesthetics with associated myocardial depression. *Bradycardia and other dysrhythmias under anesthesia are primarily caused by inadequate ventilation and oxygenation until proven otherwise.* A retrospective analysis in one center found statistically reduced mortality among children cared for by pediatric anesthesiologists when compared with nonspecialist anesthesiologists. This difference persisted despite controlling for age, illness, and other factors.

The overall risk of anesthetic death is difficult to estimate because patient age, pre-existing medical condition, type of surgery, and the surgeon's skill all must be considered. Estimates range from 1:10,000 to 1:185,000. Infants remain at greater risk than older children. Emergency surgery is more risky than elective surgery. Perioperative risk appears to have decreased considerably over the past 30 yr. Factors for this improvement include better intraoperative temperature and fluid management, better monitoring equipment (pulse oximetry, capnography), and better training.

THE FORMER PREMATURE INFANT. Physiologic immaturity may complicate anesthetic management of neonates in general and premature infants in particular. Control of airway patency, respiratory drive, temperature, electrolyte balance, and blood pressure is immature. Former preterm infants up to perhaps 60 wk postconception are at risk for periodic breathing, apnea, and bradycardia following general anesthesia or sedation. These risks appear diminished under spinal or caudal epidural anesthesia, provided sedation is avoided. The most common elective procedure in former preterm infants is inguinal hernia repair. It is important to emphasize that general anesthesia may be safely administered in this group of patients if careful monitoring is continued postoperatively and individuals are available to manage respiratory problems. Intravenous caffeine administered after induction of general anesthesia stimulates respiration and reduces, but does not eliminate, the risk of apnea. Other factors may predispose to apnea, including metabolic and electrolyte derangements, sepsis, decreased red cell mass, acidosis, hypocalcemia, and temperature stress. Prudence dictates that nonessential surgery be delayed beyond 60 wk post–conceptual age in former preterm infants. Postoperative apnea rarely occurs in apparently healthy full-term infants. It is our current practice to recommend overnight observation of term infants if they are under 44 wk post–conceptual age.

SPECIFIC DISEASES THAT IMPACT ON ANESTHETIC MANAGEMENT. Table 61–4 outlines a number of disorders that may require anesthetic consultation preoperatively. This listing is not exhaustive.

PREANESTHETIC PREPARATION AND PREMEDICATION

For most children, the primary purpose of premedication is to diminish the fear and anxiety associated with separation from parents and other aspects of anesthetic induction, such as fear of the mask. Terrifying experiences may occur during induction of anesthesia or in the immediate postoperative period, which can contribute to psychologic sequelae such as night terrors, enuresis, and temper tantrums. Certain steps can minimize the psychologic trauma. For children over 3 yr of age, parents should explain the purpose of the proposed operation in simple terms, telling of the probable sequence of events and discomfort involved. Parents' tension and anxiety are readily transmitted to the child. In many locations, preoperative teaching programs are available; the Association for the Care of Children in Hospitals has taken a leadership role in this regard. Teaching films and videotapes are widely available.

Premedication should not substitute for efforts to make the experience of induction as atraumatic as possible. Many healthy children, particularly over the age of 4 yr require no premedication prior to a mask induction, particularly with a supportive and skilled practitioner. Conversely, it is our im-

■ TABLE 61–4 Specific Pediatric Diseases and Their Anesthetic Implications

Disease	Implication
Respiratory System	
Asthma	Intraoperative bronchospasm that may be severe
	Pneumothorax
	Optimal preoperative medical management essential; may require preoperative steroids
Difficult airway	May require special equipment and personnel
	Should be anticipated in children with dysmorphic features or acute airway obstruction as seen in epiglottitis, laryngotracheobronchitis, or airway foreign bodies
	Down syndrome patients may require evaluation of atlanto-occipital joint
	Patients with storage diseases may be at high risk
BPD	Barotrauma with positive pressure ventilation
	Oxygen toxicity, pneumothorax a risk
Cystic fibrosis	Airway reactivity, bronchorrhea
	Risk of pneumothorax, pulmonary hemorrhage
	Atelectasis
	Assess for cor pulmonale
Sleep apnea	Must rule out pulmonary hypertension and cor pulmonale
	Requires careful postoperative observation for obstruction
Cardiac	Need for antibiotic prophylaxis for SBE
	Use of air filters; careful purging of air from intravenous equipment
	Need to understand effects of various anesthetics on the hemodynamics of specific lesions
	Preload optimization and avoidance of hyperviscous states in cyanotic patients
	Possible need for preoperative evaluation of myocardial function and pulmonary vascular resistance
	Provide information concerning pacemaker function
Hematologic	
Sickle cell	Possible need for simple or exchange transfusion based upon preoperative Hgb and percent Hgb S
	Importance of avoiding acidosis, hypoxemia, hyperviscosity states
Oncology	Pulmonary evaluation of patients who have received bleomycin, BCNU, CCNU, MTX, or chest radiation
	Avoidance of high oxygen concentration
	Cardiac evaluation of patients who have received anthracyclines; risk of severe myocardial depression with volatile agents
	Potential for coagulopathy
Rheumatology	Limited mobility of TMJ, C-spine, arytenoid cartilages
	Requires careful preoperative evaluation
	May be difficult airway
Gastrointestinal	
Esophageal, gastric	Potential for reflux and aspiration
Liver	High overall morbidity and mortality in patients with hepatic dysfunction
	Altered metabolism of some drugs
	Potential for coagulopathy
Renal	Altered electrolyte and acid-base status
	Altered clearance of some drugs
	Need for preoperative dialysis in selected cases
	Succinylcholine to be used with extreme caution and only when serum potassium is shown recently to be normal
Neurologic	
Seizure disorder	Avoid anesthetics that may lower threshold
	Ensure optimal control preoperatively
	Preoperative anticonvulsant levels
Increased ICP	Avoid agents that increase cerebral blood flow
	Avoid hypercarbia
Neuromuscular disease	Avoid depolarizing relaxants; at risk of hyperkalemia
	May be at risk of MH
Developmental delay	May be uncooperative at induction
Endocrine	
Diabetes	Greatest risk is unrecognized intraoperative hypoglycemia; if insulin is administered, monitor blood glucose intraoperatively; must provide glucose and insulin with adjustment for fasting condition and surgical stress
Skin	
Burns	Difficult airway
	Risk of rhabdomyolysis and hyperkalemia from succinyl choline
	Fluid shifts
	Bleeding
	Coagulopathy

BPD = bronchopulmonary dysplasia; SBE = subacute bacterial endocarditis; Hgb = hemoglobin; MTX = methotrexate; TMJ = temporomandibular joint; C-spine = cervical; MH = malignant hyperthermia.

pression that many 2 yr olds will be uncooperative unless heavily premedicated. Premedication should be given by a non-noxious route whenever possible. Oral premedications are not intrinsically noxious, but when an uncooperative toddler is forced to drink a bitter-tasting elixir, the result may be heightened distress. Although not FDA approved for oral use, an elixir of midazolam is rapidly becoming the most widely used premedication in the United States. Midazolam is a benzodiazepine anxiolytic with inactive metabolites and considerably more rapid clearance than diazepam or lorazepam. A variety of syrups have been used to mask the bitter taste.

Oral transmucosal fentanyl ("fentanyl lollipop") has the virtue of rapid onset and a pleasant route of administration, but there is potential for significant nausea, chest wall rigidity, and desaturation in preoperative sedation studies. Intranasal medication is commonly disliked by children, although in the uncooperative patient, it may on occasion be a feasible route for administration of midazolam, sufentanil, or ketamine.

Intramuscular injections are painful but have a specific limited role for sedation of the highly distressed or uncooperative child. In the uncooperative child with difficult intravenous access and severe aversion to a mask or oral premedication, a single intramuscular injection of midazolam and ketamine, for example, may be ultimately less distressing than repeated attempts at intravenous cannulation or a forced application of a mask. Rectal administration of the barbiturates methohexital or thiamylal or of benzodiazepines such as midazolam usually produces reliable sedation in less than 10 min.

For patients with pain preoperatively (a child with fractures), it may be helpful to include an opioid as premedication, both to relieve pain and because the risk of dysphoric reactions increases when sedatives are given without analgesics to patients in pain.

Anticholinergics (atropine, scopolamine, glycopyrrolate) were previously routinely given preoperatively, either orally or by intramuscular injection, to patients of all ages to dry secretions, attenuate vagal reflex responses to airway manipulation, and support cardiac output in the face of myocardial depression and relative bradycardia caused by volatile anesthetics. The drying of secretions produced by anticholinergics is generally regarded as unpleasant in awake children. With currently available anesthetic agents, the need for drying of secretions is diminished, and many pediatric anesthesiologists currently limit their use to specific indications such as (1) prolonged surgery in the prone position, (2) airway surgery, and, (3) ophthalmic surgery to block the oculo-cardiac reflex. If pancuronium is used for neuromuscular blockade, it generally provides sufficient vagolysis to obviate the need for anticholinergics.

The effect of premedication is variable. Some children will have inadequate sedation, while others will be deeply sedated with premedication. It is therefore essential that the observation guidelines of the American Academy of Pediatrics be followed with regard to patient observation. In general the patient should be sedated in locations where there is immediate availability of resuscitation equipment and staff skilled in airway management. Along with respiratory observation, constant attention is needed to keep sedated children from falling or injuring themselves.

ANESTHETIC INDUCTION

(Table 61–5)

Before proceeding with an operation, it is important to correct dehydration, decrease excessive fever, correct acid-base balance, and restore a depleted blood volume. Preoperative dehydration can be particularly harmful for children with cyanotic congenital heart disease associated with polycythemia or following Fontan-type procedures. Such patients may at times require that an intravenous catheter be placed preoperatively to avoid the deleterious effects of dehydration.

■ TABLE 61–5 Emotional Responses to Anesthetic Induction

Age	Typical Responses and Implications
0–8 mo	Fewer anticipatory responses Generally calm with strangers Mask induction well tolerated
8 mo to 2 yr	Separation anxiety is high Most difficult for mask induction Premedication, preinduction useful
3–7 yr	Separation anxiety still present Mask induction aided by parental presence
7–11 yr	Generally calm with mask induction Fear of needles Fear of loss of control
12–18 yr	Generally prefers IV to mask induction

Choice of anesthetic induction technique is dictated by specific patient risks and disease status in certain circumstances, such as the requirement for an intravenous "rapid sequence" induction for children at risk of aspiration, but in the majority of cases the primary issue lies in finding a method that is least distressing for the child.

Fear of needles depends on age, developmental factors, and previous experience with noxious procedures. In countries where the local anesthetic lidocaine-prilocaine cream, eutectic mixture of local anesthetics (EMLA), has been used routinely, there is the suggestion that children approach needle procedures with less apprehension. Conversely, a study of EMLA prior to venous cannulation in American children found that apprehension and distress persisted even though the cannulation site was numb. Adolescents, with some notable exceptions, generally prefer intravenous induction to inhalation induction, in part because of the reduced fear of needles and preference for rapid induction of unconsciousness. Intravenous induction is also generally preferred for most children with indwelling intravenous lines prior to surgery.

Intravenous induction is medically indicated for most children coming for emergency surgery, who are generally considered at risk for aspiration of gastric contents. The established method to minimize the risk of aspiration is the "rapid sequence" induction, in which (1) the patient inhales 100% oxygen prior to induction, to prolong the time to arterial desaturation with apnea, (2) anesthesia is induced with a rapid-acting hypnotic along with a muscle relaxant, and (3) cricoid pressure is applied to occlude the esophagus and prevent passive reflux of gastric contents into the pharynx.

Rapid sequence inductions are effective at preventing aspiration in most cases. Nevertheless, they assume certain calculated risks: (1) the ability to intubate the trachea or at least ventilate by mask is assumed but not tested prior to muscle paralysis; (2) a fixed, rather than slowly titrated, dose of hypnotic may produce harmful degrees of hypertension or hypotension in susceptible patients; (3) the younger the infant, the shorter the time to hypoxia following preoxygenation and induction; and (4) cricoid pressure does not protect against aspiration of upper airway contents, such as purulent matter from a retropharyngeal abscess.

Awake intubation, or sedated-awake intubation with topical anesthesia, may be safer than rapid sequence induction in certain emergency cases in which there is potential for airway difficulty, such as the child with severe burns and airway swelling, or certain critically ill neonates. *A cardinal rule is that the risk of loss of airway and hypoventilation takes priority over risks related to aspiration.* A variety of specialized techniques are now available to help in intubation of children with difficult airways, including fiberoptic bronchoscopes, anterior commissure laryngoscopes, and light wands. The laryngeal mask airway is an alternative method for airway maintenance.

Inhalation induction is well accepted by most children ages 4–10 yr, and is the most common induction technique in the United States in this age group. It is aided by (1) calm and quite surroundings, (2) a confident manner on the part of the anesthesiologist, (3) avoidance of delays, (4) use of flavored aromas for the mask, (5) introduction of nitrous oxide (which is odorless) in oxygen for a few minutes prior to introduction of the more aromatic vapor anesthetics, and (6) gradual introduction of the mask.

Inhalation induction may be medically indicated in situations where preservation of spontaneous breathing is important, such as airway foreign bodies. Inhalation induction remains the most widely established technique of induction for children with presumed epiglottitis, although some centers have reported good outcomes with simple intravenous induction. Parental presence at anesthetic induction increasingly is being encouraged in order to diminish the child's distress. Parents should receive specific direction and support from operating room staff.

INTRAOPERATIVE MANAGEMENT

Anesthesia can be maintained by either intravenous agents, inhalation anesthetics, or a combination. In the critically ill infant and child, particularly for whom postoperative ventilation is anticipated, high doses of synthetic opioids, such as fentanyl and sufentanil, provide anesthesia with excellent preservation of hemodynamic stability. Blocking the stress of pain perception has beneficial effects on the newborn's and young infant's metabolic stability by attenuating the stress response, which is characterized by excessive catecholamine release, hyperglycemia, and protein catabolism.

Airway maintenance by mask is useful for many short and elective operations. Tracheal intubation is indicated in the following: (1) operations of the head and neck; (2) thoracic, abdominal, and cranial procedures; (3) operations in the prone position; and (4) most emergency procedures, because there is uncertainty about the contents of the stomach. In younger infants, especially those under 6 mo of age, airway maintenance and adequacy of respiratory effort are more problematic, and there is a widespread preference to use tracheal intubation for all but the most brief of operations. Controlled ventilation (as opposed to spontaneous ventilation) is preferred for intrathoracic and most intra-abdominal operations.

Although most children prefer to be asleep during surgery, there has been rapidly increasing use of regional anesthesia in children, both as a supplement to general anesthesia and as the primary form of anesthesia in selected high-risk infants. Peripheral nerve blocks with bupivacaine can provide prolonged analgesia postoperatively and permit rapid, pain-free emergence that can facilitate early discharge, reduced opioid requirements, and reduced nausea and vomiting. Examples include penile block for circumcision and femoral nerve or fascia iliaca block for femur fractures.

Pediatricians should become familiar with safe dosing guidelines for local anesthetics: 5 mg/kg (7 mg/kg with epinephrine) for lidocaine and 2 mg/kg (2.5–3 mg/kg with epinephrine) for bupivacaine. Thus, for example, if lidocaine 1% is used to infiltrate for chest tube placement in a 2 kg premature infant, then only 1 mL is permitted. Dose calculation and use of more dilute solutions are especially important for young infants. Mucosal application of lidocaine may also produce toxicity. Excessive dosing can produce seizures, arrythmias, and myocardial depression.

For major thoracic, abdominal, and pelvic surgery in children, a useful technique involves epidural analgesia combined with a light general anesthetic intraoperatively, followed by epidural analgesia postoperatively. Both epidural opioids and local anesthetics may be used. Case-control studies of children undergoing esophageal repair, fundoplication, and major urologic reconstructions all suggest a reduced requirement for postoperative ventilation and reduced pulmonary complications in patients receiving epidural analgesia.

FLUID THERAPY. For all but the most superficial operations, children should receive intravenous cannulation, both as a port of access for medications and as a means for replacing fluid deficits and maintenance requirements. Venous cannulation of chronically hospitalized children may be extremely difficult. These difficulties should be anticipated during preoperative assessment, and in appropriate circumstances personnel should be available with expertise in pediatric central venous cannulation or venous access via cutdown. In situations where major bleeding is anticipated, venous access of appropriate gauge is essential.

Hypoglycemia and hyperglycemia are to be avoided. The clinical signs of hypoglycemia are difficult to interpret in anesthetized patients, and the neurologic consequences may be devastating. Studies indicate that hypoglycemia is very rare in anesthetized older children receiving glucose-free solutions, but it may occur more commonly in fasted infants, and in children with medical conditions that prevent an adequate glycemic response to operative stress. In high-risk circumstances, plasma glucose concentrations should be monitored, or the patient should receive maintenance glucose infusions. Rapid infusion of glucose-containing solutions should be avoided, because it can produce hyperglycemia.

BLOOD TRANSFUSION (see Chapter 426). Criteria for perioperative transfusion in children have been modified, in part by improved understanding of the safety of mild hemodilution and because of increased concern regarding blood-borne infections. The decision to transfuse depends not on hematocrit determinations alone (which may not be equilibrated in the setting of ongoing blood loss), but on calculated or estimated blood losses, calculated blood volume, the particular stage of the operation, and patient risk factors. For example, if an infant loses 30% of the blood volume during the initial dissection of a craniotomy or hepatic resection, in which ongoing losses are anticipated and may be rapid, then transfusion should not be delayed. Conversely, if a healthy 45 kg, 12 yr old has lost 30% of a blood volume (roughly 1,200 mL) by the end of a hip osteotomy, has stable hemodynamics, excellent urine output, and a hematocrit of 22% following adequate crystalloid replacement, then transfusion can generally be avoided. Blood component therapy is preferable to whole blood transfusion in most circumstances. Complications of rapid transfusion include hyperkalemia and citrate toxicity (ionized hypocalcemia), which may produce arrhythmias and cardiac arrest. Calcium administration may be lifesaving in this setting. For elective surgery with anticipated bleeding in older children and adolescents, predonation of autologous blood should be encouraged. A variety of techniques are now in use to diminish blood loss, including acute hemodilution, controlled hypotension, and reinfusion of centrifuged, washed erythrocytes from the surgical field.

THERMOREGULATION. Thermoregulation is impaired during general or major regional anesthesia, and the young infant is particularly susceptible to hypothermia or hyperthermia in the operating room. Continuous monitoring of body temperature is essential during general anesthesia. In air-conditioned operating rooms inadvertent hypothermia develops frequently in small infants undergoing laparotomy, thoracotomy, or craniotomy. Deliberate hypothermia is useful for cerebral and myocardial protection in cardiac surgery and other specialized operations. In most other circumstances, hypothermia is to be avoided, because it may detrimentally affect coagulation, ventilatory control, termination of neuromuscular blockade, and metabolic balance. Similarly, hyperthermia increases oxygen consumption and may confuse the differential diagnosis of more serious conditions, such as sepsis and malignant hyperthermia.

Hypothermia can be prevented by the use of overhead radiant heaters, circulating warm water mattresses, heated humidification of inspired gases, and wrapping the head and extremities with heat-retaining, nonabrasive materials. Forced air convective warming is an effective method for treatment of intraoperative hypothermia.

Malignant hyperpyrexia or *malignant hyperthermia* (MH) is a rare life-threatening genetic abnormality of skeletal muscle characterized by tachycardia, tachypnea, hypermetabolism, muscle rigidity, hypercarbia, acidosis, and fever following exposure to the vapor inhalation anesthetics (halothane, isoflurane) or the depolarizing muscle relaxant succinylcholine. Malignant hyperpyrexia is more common among patients with a variety of muscle disorders, including Duchenne muscular dystrophy. Initial management includes (1) cessation of triggering agents, (2) hyperventilation with oxygen, (3) administration of a specific treatment, dantrolene 3 mg/kg, given intravenously mixed in sterile water to a total loading dose of 10 mg/kg if necessary. Along with this, general intensive care measures include: (1) treatment of hyperkalemia and acidosis, (2) circulatory support, (3) active cooling measures, and (4) urinary alkalinization to prevent tubular injury from myoglobinuria. Nontriggering anesthetics that may be used safely include barbiturates, opioids, propofol, nitrous oxide, local anesthetics, benzodiazepines, butyrophenones, and nondepolarizing muscle relaxants (see Chapter 62).

MONITORING. Standard monitors for anesthetized children in the United States undergoing general or major regional anesthesia include an electrocardiogram, a blood pressure cuff, a precordial or esophageal stethoscope, a temperature probe, an oximeter, a capnograph, and in-line oxygen analyzers. Intra-arterial pressure monitoring is indicated for procedures characterized by hemodynamic instability or major blood loss. Other invasive monitoring methods, including central venous or pulmonary artery catheterization or transesophageal echocardiography, may be indicated in specific circumstances.

POSTANESTHETIC RECOVERY

Recovery room facilities and nursing care must be available to provide constant surveillance of airway patency, adequate ventilation, and circulatory stability. Common sequelae of general anesthesia in infants and children include postanesthetic excitement, vomiting, and pain. Vomiting can be relieved in the majority of cases with either butyrophenones (droperidol), phenothiazines (prochlorperazine), metoclopramide, or ondansetron.

The recovery period should be of adequate duration to ensure that the child has adequate relief of pain and is not vomiting. It is neither necessary nor desirable to "force fluids" by mouth because this may exacerbate vomiting, nor is it necessary to delay discharge until the child has voided.

Patients with abnormal upper airways, a history of sleep apnea, or abnormal ventilatory control, or patients who have had airway surgery, require careful and longer observation.

Following tracheal intubation, patients may develop subglottic edema, especially if they have a history of croup or recent upper respiratory tract infection, which can often be relieved by inhaling aerosolized racemic epinephrine. Corticosteroids may be of benefit.

ANESTHESIA AND CONSCIOUS SEDATION AWAY FROM THE OPERATING ROOM

Common diagnostic and therapeutic procedures include bone marrow aspirate and biopsy, radiologic imaging, radiation therapy, and endoscopic procedures. Sedation and anesthesia in these settings can be of great benefit in reducing children's distress and improving ease of conduct of the procedure. The American Academy of Pediatrics has promoted monitoring standards to reduce risk from conscious sedation outside the operating room.

The choice of conscious sedation by pediatric subspecialists (oncologists, gastroenterologists, pediatric radiologists) versus sedation or anesthesia by anesthesiologists depends on several factors, including (1) the patient's medical or psychological condition and risk factors; (2) the duration, painfulness, and degree of immobility or cooperation required for the procedure; and (3) resource availability. A wide range of minor procedures can be managed safely using conscious sedation by nonanesthesiologists. Safe practice of conscious sedation requires (1) standardized protocols regarding monitoring of vital signs; (2) a full-time clinician (nurse, physician, respiratory therapist) who is not occupied with performing the procedure but attends to vital signs, adequacy of airway and breathing efforts, and level of consciousness; and (3) immediate availability of airway equipment, supplemental oxygen, suction, and resuscitative drugs. There should be consensus regarding which procedures are appropriate and maximum doses of sedatives for use by nonanesthesiologists. Pulse oximetry is extremely valuable as a continuous monitor of oxygenation.

There is no perfect combination of medications that provides adequate sedation and cooperation with procedures in all cases with a zero risk of respiratory depression. Dosing should be individualized and titrated slowly enough to gauge the patient's response. For many brief procedures that involve noxious stimulation, a useful combination involves midazolam (a short-acting benzodiazepine to provide anxiolysis and amnesia) along with an opioid (fentanyl) to provide analgesia. This combination of drugs can produce synergistic sedation as well as respiratory depression, so that titrated dosing and monitoring are essential. It is also advisable to have immediate availability of the reversal agents flumazenil and naloxone, respectively, in the event of hypoventilation unresponsive to stimulation, application of supplemental oxygen, and/or ventilatory assistance. For painless procedures that require sleep and immobility, such as magnetic resonance scans, sedatives without analgesic properties, such as pentobarbital or chloral hydrate, are commonly used. There is unresolved debate regarding the toxicology of chloral hydrate's metabolites.

The management of brief anesthetic procedures in remote locations has been greatly facilitated by the design of ultrashort duration intravenous agents such as propofol that permit very rapid and clear-headed emergence and recovery. Propofol has the additional benefit of antiemetic and antipruritic action.

GENERAL REFERENCE

Cote CJ, Ryan JF, Todres ID, Goudsouzian N (eds): The Practice of Anesthesia for Infants and Children, 2nd ed. New York, Grune & Stratton, 1993.
Gregory GA (ed): Pediatric Anesthesia, 3rd ed. New York, Churchill-Livingstone, 1994.
Motoyama E, Davis P (eds): Smith's Anesthesia for Infants and Children, 5th ed. St. Louis, MO, CV Mosby, 1990.
Steward DJ: Manual of Pediatric Anesthesia, 3rd ed. New York, Churchill Livingstone, 1990.

PREOPERATIVE LABORATORY TESTING

O'Connor ME, Drassner K: Pre-operative laboratory testing of children undergoing elective surgery. Anesth Analg 70:176, 1990.

PREOPERATIVE FASTING

Moon R: Fasting before surgery. JAMA 273:1171, 1995.
Schriner MS, Treibwasser A, Koen TP: Ingestion of liquids compared to preoperative fasting in pediatric patients. Anesthesiology 72:593,1990.
Splinter WM, Stewart JA, Muir JG: The effect of pre-operative apple juice on gastric contents, thirst and hunger in children. Can J Anaesth 36:55, 1990.

POSTOPERATIVE APNEA IN THE FORMER PRETERM INFANT

Kurth CD, Spitzer AR, Broennle AM, et al: Post-operative apnea in preterm infants. Anesthesiology 66:483, 1987.

Steward DJ: Preterm infants are more prone to complications following minor surgery than are infants. Anesthesiology 56:304, 1982.

Welborn LG, DeSoto H, Hannallah RS, et al: The use of caffeine in the control of post-anesthetic apnea in former preterm infants. Anesthesiology 68:796, 1988.

CHILD WITH UPPER RESPIRATORY INFECTION

Cohen MM, Cameron CB: Should you cancel the operation when a child has an upper respiratory tract infection? Anesth Analg 72:282, 1991.

Desoto H, Patel RI, Soliman IE, et al: Changes in oxygen saturation following general anesthesia in children with upper respiratory infection signs and symptoms undergoing otolaryngological procedures. Anesthesiology 68:276, 1988.

Tait AR, Knight PR: The effects of general anesthesia on upper respiratory tract infections in children. Anesthesiology 67:930, 1987.

GENERAL ANESTHESIA AND SEDATION

Anand KJS, Sippell WG, Aynsley-Green A: Randomized trial of fentanyl anesthesia in preterm babies undergoing surgery. Effects on the stress response. Lancet 1:243, 1987.

Brustowicz RM, Nelson DA, Betts EK, et al: Efficacy of oral premedication for pediatric outpatient surgery. Anesthesiology 60:475, 1984.

Keenan RL, Boyan CP: Cardiac arrest due to anesthesia. A study of incidence and causes. JAMA 253:2373, 1985.

Nicolson SC, Betts EK, Jobes DR, et al: Comparison of oral and intramuscular preanesthetic medication for pediatric inpatient surgery. Anesthesiology 71:8, 1989.

REGIONAL ANESTHESIA AND PAIN MANAGEMENT

Dalens B: Regional anesthesia in children. Anesth Analg 68:654, 1989.

Schechter N, Berde CB, Yaster M: Pain in Infants, Children, and Adolescents. Baltimore, Williams & Wilkins, 1993.

ANESTHETIC RISK

Holtzman R: Morbidity and mortality in pediatric anesthesia. Pediatr Clin North Am 41:239, 1994.

Morray JP, Geiduschek JM, Caplan RA, et al: A comparison of pediatric and adult anesthesia closed malpractice claims. Anesthesiology 78:461, 1993.

Rosen G, Muckle R, Mahowald M, et al: Postoperative respiratory compromise in children with obstructive sleep apnea syndrome: Can it be anticipated? Pediatrics 93:784, 1994.

MALIGNANT HYPERTHERMIA

Kaus SJ, Rockoff MA: Malignant hyperthermia. Pediatr Clin North Am 41:221, 1994.

CHAPTER 62
Pain Management

Gloria L. Sellman

MISCONCEPTIONS OF PAIN. Pain is a subjective experience comprising both sensory and emotional components. The intensity of the pain experience and the mechanisms for coping with it, therefore, vary among individuals for any given injury. The inability of the pediatric patient, however, to communicate a painful experience clearly has led to the accumulation of complex societal beliefs and medical misjudgments that have resulted in the undertreatment of their pain. Some **misconceptions** about pain in children include (1) children have a higher tolerance to pain, (2) pain perception in children is decreased because of biologic immaturity, (3) children have little or no memory of a painful experience, (4) children are more sensitive to the side effects of analgesics, and (5) children are at special risk for addiction to narcotics. There is no evidence to substantiate these beliefs.

PATHOPHYSIOLOGY. Neurologic immaturity does not render the preterm and term neonate incapable of painful sensation and memory. The neurosensory pathways necessary for nociceptive transmission are anatomically and functionally intact in the newborn infant. Anatomic studies show that peripheral innervation and central nervous system connections at the spinal cord dorsal horn cell level exist early in fetal development. Spinal nerve tracts for pain transmission are myelinated by mid to late gestation and the basic nerve pathways necessary for completing synaptic pain transmission to the level of the neocortex are intact and completely myelinated by the 3rd trimester of gestation. In addition, nociceptive transmitters (substance P) and pain modulator substances (endogenous opioids) function in the fetus, and concentrations of these neuropeptides are significantly increased in the perinatal period.

In the neonate, as in the adult, unmyelinated C fibers transmit nociceptive information peripherally. Nerve pulse transmission in incompletely myelinated A-δ fibers is delayed, not blocked, until myelination has been completed postnatally. The shorter distances necessary for impulse travel offset any delay in conduction velocity. Therefore, lack of well-developed inhibitory control in the newborn may result in exaggerated, hyperalgesic responses to afferent stimuli until postnatal maturation occurs.

Furthermore, evaluation of the neonate undergoing painful procedures (e.g., heel lance, circumcision) without anesthesia indicates a pattern of autonomic response to pain manifested by increases in blood pressure, heart rate, pulmonary vascular resistance, intracranial pressure, palmar sweat, and by a decrease in the transcutaneous partial pressure of oxygen. Behavior responses are diffuse and exaggerated but purposeful, and are characterized by prolonged withdrawal, particularly in the preterm neonate, correlating with increased neuropeptide concentrations at available receptor sites spread diffusely over the cerebral cortex. Pain from such procedures elicits individualized behavioral responses, with some infants actually decreasing activity during painful stimulation. Behavioral changes persist after the pain is over, suggesting memory. Newborns also demonstrate hormonal responses to the pain of surgery with the release of catecholamines, corticosteroids, glucagon, and growth hormone, with simultaneous suppression of insulin release. These metabolic alterations result in marked hyperglycemia, persisting in the postoperative period, and a prolonged state of catabolism, leading to the breakdown of protein substrate. Endocrine responses to the stress of various types of surgical pain can be attenuated or blocked by the use of potent inhaled anesthesia or fentanyl anesthesia, respectively. A lack of attenuation of the neuroendocrine stress response correlates with intraoperative instability and increased postoperative metabolic and circulatory complications, as compared with the course of infants receiving fentanyl anesthesia. The improved surgical outcome of infants given fentanyl has been shown to correlate with shortened stays in the neonatal intensive care unit (NICU) and in the hospital overall, thus resulting in reduced health care costs.

CLINICAL MANIFESTATIONS AND ASSESSMENTS. The assessment of pain in the infant is necessarily indirect and includes the observation of cry, facial expression, autonomic responses, and behavior or motor activity. Facial expression is the most consistently valid indicator of pain in infants. As infants become older, anticipatory behavior also occurs, manifest by posturing and protective limb movement. Preschool children, aged 3–7 yr, have a limited cognitive ability to qualify or quantify their pain. Ladder or linear analog scales using photographed facial expression, serial line-drawn faces, or color schemes may be useful for validating the discomfort of preschool children. Self-reporting methods using numerical rating scales for pain intensity have proven particularly useful for school-aged children and correlate well with simultaneous parent ratings. The psychologic and emotional aspects of the adolescent pain experience are more likely to be factored into self-reporting of their pain. Because behavior is more restrained, and in the absence of a validated pain assessment tool specific to the adolescent's needs, reliance on a more comprehensive self-reporting instrument, such as the McGill Pain Questionnaire, may be helpful. Regardless of age, time must be provided for instruction and practice using self-reporting instruments. Pain assessment should be performed regularly and frequently, and is facilitated by the patients' better understanding of their pain and the reasons it exists.

TREATMENT. The first step in a comprehensive pain management program is the evaluation of each patient's individual needs with the help of a team of pediatric medical and psychosocial specialists, when possible. There should be age-appropriate education and discussion regarding the proposed care plan or any planned procedure, including introducing the patient and family to caregivers, offering hands-on play with benign medical equipment, and encouraging practice sessions with dolls. These techniques may help reveal some of the patient's fears that would otherwise not be easily expressed. By permitting patient participation and incorporating patient preferences in the treatment plan, insofar as possible, patient confidence and cooperation can be improved at almost any age.

The mainstay of the pharmacologic treatment of severe acute or chronic pain is systemic opioid medication. Other analgesic medications given systemically or locally (local anesthetics) can act to provide synergism with opioids or can eliminate the need for systemic opioids (Table 62–1).

Whenever feasible, a child should be offered an appropriate analgesic by a noninvasive route, orally or through an existing intravenous line (Chapter 61). It is important to realize that administering intramuscular injections to children reporting pain sends them the message that to achieve pain relief more pain must be administered. This is a concept that, even if understood, rarely meets with patient acceptance and inevitably leads to the open denial of active pain by fearful children.

Postoperative Pain. Pain control in the perioperative period should be a continuum, beginning with preoperative teaching and medication, and followed by intraoperative analgesia with a regional block or systemic drug, either or both of which can be continued throughout the postoperative period. The concept of pre-emptive analgesia or prophylactic administration of analgesics prior to surgical incision can reduce anesthetic and postoperative pain requirements. In the absence of a regional block (Chapter 61), postoperative pain can be treated effectively by oral preparations of opioids or by their intravenous administration with intermittent or continuous infusion. Continuous infusion is helpful in maintaining uniform plasma drug levels and permits constancy of pain relief, unlike the cycles of alternating pain and analgesia that result from intermittent parenteral administration. The side effects of opioid use can be limited by combination therapy with acetaminophen or nonsteroidal anti-inflammatory drugs (NSAIDs). Moderate to mild postoperative pain may be well controlled with nonopioid analgesics alone but, unlike opioids, nonopioids have ceiling effects for analgesia, and increasing doses may lead to a higher incidence of side effects without improved analgesia. Also, the practice of prn dosing results in inadequate pain relief and is not recommended.

Morphine and fentanyl can be safely administered to infants and children for postoperative pain control. This age group has the same ability as adults for drug clearance and comparable susceptibility to the respiratory side effects of opioids. On the other hand, drug clearance in neonates is highly variable. Therefore, infants younger than 3 mo may safely receive opioid analgesia but must be monitored for apnea until 24 hr after their last dose. This age group, especially preterm infants and those at risk because of underlying disease (e.g., cystic fibrosis), should be intensively observed with immediate access to airway resuscitation available. These patients are at higher risk for apnea after general anesthesia and should be monitored appropriately.

School-aged children benefit greatly from the use of a preprogrammed computerized pump device for the self-administration of intravenous or peridural opioids. This method—patient-controlled analgesia (PCA)—has the advantages of timely drug administration for the maintenance of adequate analgesia, patient participation in self-care, and demonstrated safety in those aged 6–18 yr. It is strongly favored by both patient and caregivers. In addition to improved analgesic efficacy, PCA has been shown to reduce the cost of hospital care and to decrease the nursing work-load. Younger patients may also be acceptable candidates for PCA, but those of all ages must be selected individually according to manual dexterity and conceptual understanding.

Cancer and Other Pain Syndromes. Patients with cancer suffer pain from the disease process, chemotherapy side effects, and repeated diagnostic and therapeutic procedures. It is imperative to establish the precise etiology of all pain to rule out unexpected complications of the underlying disease process. In addition to oral and intravenous opioids, alternative methods of drug administration are sometimes necessary because of patient tolerance, such as when mucositis or nausea preclude the administration of oral medication, or when intravenous access is limited. Options include the following: intermittent, continuous, or PCA subcutaneous infusion of morphine or methadone; subcutaneous, transdermal, or nasal fentanyl; or an opioid agent administered by indwelling epidural or intrathecal catheter. Corticosteroid therapy is also important in the relief of pain resulting from widespread tumor invasion of bone or of the central and peripheral nervous systems, resulting in nerve compression or elevated intracranial pressure.

Adjuvant therapies for potentiating or replacing opioid analgesia (in the case of non–cancer-related pain) include the use of NSAIDs, tricyclic antidepressants, anxiolytic agents, and transcutaneous electrical nerve stimulation (TENS). For example, the most effective pharmacologic therapy for the relief of the neuropathic pain from nerve injury is low-dose tricyclic medication. The pain of sickle cell disease or juvenile rheumatoid arthritis is best treated on a chronic basis by acetaminophen (Tylenol) or NSAIDs. However, in acute vasoocclusive crisis of sickle cell disease, opioid therapy is indicated. In such a case, morphine is the parenteral agent of choice. Generally, meperidine is not recommended because its long-acting metabolite, normeperidine, has poor analgesic properties and is associated with central nervous system excitement and seizures. Also, prolonged administration of meperidine leads to normeperidine accumulation and carries a significant incidence of dysphoria and other toxic effects, particularly in patients with renal dysfunction.

Procedural Pain. Children with chronic illnesses often report that procedural pain related to bone marrow aspirations, lumbar punctures, and intrathecal chemotherapy is their greatest source of anxiety and pain in the hospital setting. Yet these procedures, as well as burn dressing changes and debridements and various intensive care and emergency room procedures, are widely performed without the benefit of a sedative, analgesic, or other coping strategy. Hypnosis and other cognitive-behavioral techniques can be extremely important adjuncts to pharmacologic pain management in this setting. Emphasis should be on maximizing patient participation and control, even for the 18 mo old who might assist with a dressing removal. Older children could have the option of requesting a

■ **TABLE 62–1 Recommended Schedules and Dosages of Analgesic Medication in Infants and Older Children**

Medication	Dosing Schedule: *Infants <3 mo*	Dosing Schedule: *Children >3 mo*	Comments
Morphine	IV: bolus—0.1 mg/kg q3–4 hr; loading—0.05 mg/kg; then infusion—0.01–0.015 mg/kg/hr	Oral: 0.3–0.6 mg/kg q8–12 hr; IV: bolus—0.1 mg/kg q1–2 hr; infusion—0.04–0.06 mg/kg/hr	MS-Contin (oral) Apnea monitoring <3 mo or at risk; bolus over 20 min; beware of hypotension and bronchospasm; naloxone reversal (10 μg/kg) available at all times
		Subcutaneous bolus—0.1–0.15 mg/kg q3–4 hr; infusion—0.05–0.06 mg/kg/hr	>20 mo, syringe pump
Fentanyl	IV: bolus—0.5–2 μg/kg q1–2 hr; loading—1–2 μg/kg; then infusion—1–5 μg/kg/hr	IV: bolus—0.5–2 μg/kg q2–3 hr; increments—0.5 μg/kg q1–2 min; loading—1–2 μg/kg; then infusion—1–5 μg/kg/hr	Intubation or apnea monitoring in infants <3 mo or at risk; beware chest wall rigidity and bradycardia; naloxone standby
Alfentanil		IV increments: 1–2 μg/kg q2–3 min	Potent, ultra–short-acting opioid
Methadone		Oral: 0.1 mg/kg q4 hr × 3; then q6–8 hr IV, bolus: 0.1 mg/kg q2 hr × 2, then 0.04–0.09 mg/kg q 4–8 hr	Full analgesia and toxicity may not be evident until plasma steady state, 3–5 days
Codeine		Oral: 0.5–1 mg/kg q4 hr	Gastric irritation
Tylenol	Oral: 10–15 mg/kg; R: 15–20 mg/kg	Oral: 10–15 mg/kg R: 15–25 mg/kg	Prolonged plasma half-life in neonates; acute hepatotoxicity with excess dosing
Ibuprofen		Oral: 4–10 mg/kg q6–8 hr	Children >2 yr old; can cause gastritis; risk of nephrotoxicity and hepatoxicity with prolonged use
Naprosyn		Oral: 5–7 mg/kg q8–12 hr	
Tolectin		Oral: 5–7 mg/kg q6–8 hr	
Ketorolac		Oral: 1 mg/kg q6 hr × 5–7 days IV: load 1 mg/kg; then 0.5 mg/kg q6hr × 8 doses (60 mg max. dose, all modes)	For mild, moderate pain; no respiratory depression; inhibits platelets; less gastritis; worldwide use supports safety in children; not FDA approved in children
Amitriptyline		Oral: 0.5–1.5 mg/kg q HS	Neuropathic pain; 3–5 days therapy required for pain reduction
Midazolam		Oral: 0.50–0.75 mg/kg IV: 0.05 mg/kg q5 min, titrate to effect R: 0.3–0.7 mg/kg IN: 0.3–0.5 mg/kg	Potent benzodiazepine; 4.5 hr half-life; stable VS; airway resuscitation equipment Time to plasma peak: Oral: 30–60 min; IV, 10 min; R, 45 min; IN, 20–40 min
EMLA		Topical: 2.5 g = 20 cm² (2 in²) Up to 100 cm²—0–10 kg Up to 600 cm²—10–20 kg Up to 2,000 cm²—>20 kg	Topical eutectic mixture 50:50 of lidocaine 2.5%, prilocaine 2.5%; methemaglobinemia: not recommended for <3 mo old; 5 g tube; apply thickly with occlusive dressing
TAC		Topical: 0.05 mL/kg, max. dose	Topical mixture tetracaine, epinephrine, cocaine; highly vasoconstrictive; cardiotoxic in high dose; open wounds only; DO NOT use at end artery sites or on mucous membranes (reported fatality)

R, rectal; HS, at bedtime; IN, intranasal; VS, vital signs.

"time out" during a period of what they perceived to be maximal stress. By optimally controlling pain and anxiety for a 1st procedure, anxiety created by repeated subsequent procedures will be minimized and more easily contained. Children report that the single most helpful factor in coping with any pain experience is for their parent(s) to be present.

Effective topical local anesthetic preparations are available to anesthetize a skin area planned for a procedure. EMLA is a eutectic mixture of local anesthetics consisting of a 50:50 mixture of lidocaine 2.5% and prilocaine 2.5% suspended in an oil and water emulsion. It greatly reduces procedure-related pain in settings varying from IV placement to spinal taps and bone marrow aspirations to burn graft sites. Applied liberally to intact skin and bound by an occlusive dressing, superficial anesthesia is established by 60–90 min. There is a time-dependent increase in the depth of penetration, which peaks at 2 hr and lasts 3–4 hr, providing flexibility for timing procedures in a clinical setting. Infants less than 3 mo of age, and, in particular, preterm infants, may be at increased risk for toxicity. Evidence supports topical 30% lidocaine cream as being safe and beneficial for circumcision in the newborn.

TAC is a topical anesthetic mixture of tetracaine 0.5%, epinephrine 1:2,000, and cocaine 11.8% and is used in pediatric emergency rooms. The solution is applied directly to open lacerations or wounds for which suturing or debridement is indicated. Caution must prevail to avoid contact with mucous membranes, intact or not, due to potentially fatal toxic absorption. TAC **must never** be used in regions supplied by end arteries, such as the digits, penis, and pinna of the ear. Subcutaneous infiltration of a local anesthetic for improved effect can be carried out after topical anesthesia has been applied. Further alteration of the sting of local anesthetic injection can be achieved by the addition of sodium bicarbonate (1 mL per 9 mL of lidocaine or 0.1 mL per 9.9 mL of marcaine) administered via a small-gauge needle.

Pharmacologic sedation plays an important and sometimes essential role in helping patients succeed with their coping strategies during stressful procedures. Fixed combinations of three or more systemic analgesics and tranquilizers are no longer considered safe; they are associated with significantly higher complication rates than more individualized schedules using one or two short-acting medications. By effectively combining the preceding methods, the vast majority of procedures can be performed efficiently without prolonged medication effects.

Patient physical status, the need for an extensive procedure, or any other criteria, such as airway compromise, may require the consultation of a specialty service. For example, with the assistance of a pediatric anesthesiologist in a well-equipped treatment room or in the operating suite, monitored care with profound sedation and analgesia using ultra–short-acting agents or general anesthesia can be provided. Primary care physicians regularly managing procedures of very brief duration should be well acquainted with the pharmacologic and clinical effects of these potent drugs, such as midazolam and alfentanil or fentanyl, and should rely on the anesthesiologist for instruction until they are more experienced. A qualified assistant to the physician should be dedicated to monitoring the patient closely during and after the procedure. Early detection of hypoventilation or airway obstruction is possible with vigilant observation and oxygen saturation monitoring by pulse oximetry. Equipment for airway management and resuscitation should be immediately available at all times.

Agency for Health Care Policy and Research: Acute pain management: Operative or medical procedures and trauma, Part 2. Clin Pharm 11:391, 1992.
Anand KJS, Sippell WG, Aynsley-Green A: Randomized trial of fentanyl anaesthesia in preterm babies undergoing surgery: Effects on the stress response. Lancet 1:243, 1987.
Berde CB: Toxicity of local anesthetics in infants and children. J Pediatr 122:S14, 1993.
Berde CB, Fischel N, Filardi JP: Caudal epidural morphine analgesia for an infant with advanced neuroblastoma: Report of a case. Pain 36:219, 1989.
Berde C, Sethna NF, Masek B, et al: Pediatric pain clinics: Recommendations for their development. Pediatrician 16:94, 1989.
Berman D, Duncan AM, Zeltzer LK: The evaluation and management of pain in the infant and young child with cancer. Br J Cancer 66(Suppl XVIII):S84, 1992.
Ejlersen E, Anderson HB, Eliasen K, et al: A comparison between preincisional and postincisional lidocaine infiltration and postoperative pain. Anesth Analg 74:495, 1992.
Gaukroger PB: Patient-controlled analgesia in children. *In*: Schechter NL, Berde CB, Yaster M (eds): Pain in Infants, Children and Adolescents. Baltimore, MD, Williams and Wilkins, 1993, p 203.
Koren G: Use of eutectic mixture of local anesthetics in young children for procedure-related pain. J Pediatr 122:S30, 1993.
Lynn AM, Slattery JT: Morphine pharmacokinetics in early infancy. Anesthesiology 66:136, 1987.
McGrath PJ, McAlpine L: Psychologic perspectives on pediatric pain. J Pediatr 122:S2, 1993.
Miser AW, Davis DM, Hughes CS, et al: Continuous subcutaneous infusion of morphine in children with cancer. Am J Dis Child 137:383, 1983.
Schechter NL, ed: Acute pain in children. Pediatr Clin North Am 36:781, 1989.
Truog R, Anand KJS: Management of pain in the postoperative neonate. Clin Perinatol 16:61, 1989.
Weatherstone KB, Rasmussen LB, Erenberg A, et al: Safety and efficacy of a topical anesthetic for neonatal circumcision. Pediatrics 92:710, 1993.
Yaster M, Tobin JR, Fisher QA, et al: Local anesthetics in the management of acute pain in children. J Pediatr 124:165, 1994.

CHAPTER 63

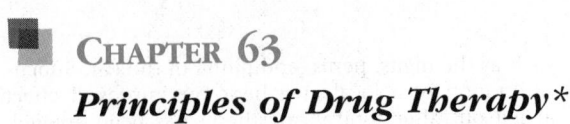

*Principles of Drug Therapy**

Michael D. Reed

Clinical pharmacology is concerned with the integration of a drug's pharmacokinetic and pharmacodynamic profile to optimize drug therapy. *Pharmacokinetics* is the quantitative evaluation of each component of a compound's disposition (absorption, distribution, metabolism, excretion). The ability to estimate a drug's pharmacokinetic parameters depends on the ability to accurately and reproducibly determine the concentration of that drug in a specific body fluid (blood, cerebrospinal fluid, urine, joint fluid). A drug concentration in a specific body fluid is, in theory, a reflection of the drug concentration in tissue, and thus reflects its concentration at its site of action, the receptor. A drug's concentration in blood (or other body fluid), however, is not necessarily equal to the drug's concentration in tissue or at its cellular receptor site. In pediatric practice, it is important to appreciate the factors involved in determining drug concentrations in body fluids, including physical access of that body fluid, available volume that can be safely removed, and the sensitivity and specificity of available laboratory methodology.

Pharmacodynamics is the study of the biochemical and physiologic effects of drugs, that is, their mechanism(s) of action. The pharmacologic or toxicologic effects of most drugs are a result of their interaction with macromolecular components of cells, their receptor. Rational prescribing of drugs depends on a fundamental understanding of a drug's pharmacokinetic and pharmacodynamic profile. Understanding the effect of age is essential to understanding pediatric drug therapy, because age is one of the most important variables that influences the processes responsible for a drug's disposition and action in children. Designing an optimal pharmacologic therapy involves integrating an understanding of the pharmacokinetics and pharmacodynamics of a drug with the patient variables of disease and age.

*This chapter was adapted from previous sections in the 14th edition written by Stanford N. Cohen.

INFLUENCE OF AGE ON DRUG THERAPY

Drugs administered extravascularly must cross physiologic membranes before entering the systemic circulation and being distributed to their site of action.

GASTROINTESTINAL ABSORPTION. Although certain xenobiotics and nutrients are absorbed by active transport or facilitated diffusion, most drugs are absorbed from the gastrointestinal tract by passive diffusion. A number of important patient variables can affect the rate and extent of a drug's gastrointestinal absorption, including pH-dependent diffusion; the presence, absence, and/or type of gastric contents; gastric emptying time; and gastrointestinal motility. These physiologic processes reflect a clear but highly variable dependence on a patient's age. Patient and chemical factors that affect drug absorption are shown in Table 63–1.

Gastric pH. At birth this approaches neutrality but within hours rapidly falls to between 1.5 and 3.0. Postnatally, gastric acid secretion displays a biphasic pattern: The highest gastric acid concentrations occur within the 1st 10 days of life and the lowest between 10 and 30 days of life. Corrected for body weight, the secretion of gastric acid approaches the lower limit of adult values by 3 mo of age. Depending on a drug's pKa, these differences in rate and amount of gastric acid can influence a drug's rate and/or extent of gastrointestinal absorption by influencing the amount of drug present in the ionized or nonionized form. Decreased ionization favors absorption.

Gastric Emptying Time and Intestinal Motility. Most orally administered drugs are absorbed from the small intestine, so the rate of gastric emptying is an important determinant of the rate and possibly overall extent of a drug's absorption. The gastric emptying rate during the neonatal period varies greatly. It is characterized by irregular and unpredictable peristaltic activity, and it is prolonged relative to that in the adult. The rate of gastric emptying is directly related to gestational and postnatal age,

■ **TABLE 63–1 Factors Influencing Drug Absorption**

Physicochemical Factors of the Drug
Molecular weight
Degree of ionization under physiologic conditions
Product formulation characteristics
Disintegration and dissolution rates for solid dosage forms
Drug-release characteristics for time-release preparations
Cosolutes and complex formation
Patient Factors
Surface area available for absorption
Gastric and duodenal pH
Gastric emptying time
Bile salt pool size
Bacterial colonization of the gastrointestinal tract
Presence and extent of underlying diseases
Presence or absence of metabolic pathways or enzymes necessary for biotransformation

and is influenced by the type of feeding (solid or liquid). Gastric emptying time approaches adult values within the 1st 6–8 mo of life. The anatomic location of gastrointestinal feeding tubes (gastric, duodenal) and the dosage form administered can influence markedly the absorption characteristics of the "enterally" administered drug. Small intestinal motility in the perinatal period is also highly variable and is influenced by the presence or absence of food. Contractions of the duodenum in term neonates occur at rates similar to those observed in fasting adults, although the number of contractions/burst is lower. In addition, fasting or interdigestive motor activity is also shorter in children. These physiologic perturbations may influence the time course and extent of drug absorption from the gastrointestinal tract.

Pancreatic Enzyme Activity. The activity of pancreatic enzymes is decreased at birth; it is lower in premature than in full-term neonates. Lipase activity is present by 34–36 wk gestation and increases fivefold during the 1st wk and 20-fold during the first 9 mo of postnatal life. In contrast, amylase activity can be detected as early as the 22nd wk of gestation but remains low even after birth (approximating 10% of adult values). There is decreased duodenal amylase activity in both fasting and fed infants during the 1st yr of life. Trypsin secretion and response to pancreatin and secretin administration are blunted in term infants but develop during the 1st yr of life. Thus, any drug that requires cleavage from its salt by pancreatic enzymes prior to absorption (chloramphenicol palmitate, clindamycin palmitate) may demonstrate highly variable bioavailability during the 1st 1–3 mo of life.

Other Processes. The development of other physiologic processes also may influence the gastrointestinal absorption of drugs and other compounds. Bile salt metabolism during the 1st few months of life is affected by a progressive maturation of gallbladder emptying, intestinal motility and absorption, and hepatic uptake. Also, colonization of the gastrointestinal tract by bacterial flora, a process that influences the metabolism of bile salts and drugs and intestinal motility, varies with respect to age, type of delivery, type of feeding, and concurrent drug therapy. The gastrointestinal tract of a full-term, formula-fed, vaginally delivered infant is colonized with anaerobic bacteria by 4–6 days of postnatal life. The metabolic ability and activity of gastrointestinal bacterial microflora vary greatly. There are differences in the ability of gastrointestinal microflora to metabolize specific substrates among infants, children, and adults. In healthy subjects, complete metabolic activity of gastrointestinal bacterial flora approaches adult values for bile acids and neutral sterols by the age of 4 yr, but the effect of these maturational changes in intestinal flora on drug metabolism is uncertain. For example, although children are colonized with intestinal bacterial flora able to metabolize digoxin by the age of 2 yr, the ability to inactivate the drug develops only gradually, and the metabolic pattern observed in adults is not achieved until adolescence. This finding suggests, at least for digoxin, that intestinal colonization by digoxin-reducing organisms in children approaches adult values. Such variation could influence a drug's absorption profile, which can directly influence a patient's clinical response. Moreover, other drugs the patient is receiving may also influence these processes (broad-spectrum antibiotics and their effect upon gastrointestinal flora).

ALTERNATIVE ROUTES OF DRUG ABSORPTION. The primary means of extravascular drug administration in infants and children, other than the oral route, is the intramuscular route. Similar physiologic and physicochemical factors that affect the rate and extent of drug absorption from the gastrointestinal tract also influence the absorption of drugs from injection sites and through the skin (Table 63–1). Drugs administered intramuscularly should be water soluble at physiologic pH to prevent precipitation and the resultant decreased, delayed, or erratic absorption from the injection site. Lipid solubility of a drug favors diffusion into the capillaries. Blood flow to and from the injection site should be adequate to ensure absorption into the systemic circulation. This physiologic requirement may be compromised in seriously ill infants and children with poor peripheral perfusion resulting from low cardiac output and respiratory disease.

The skin is another important but often overlooked organ for the absorption of various therapeutic agents and environmental chemicals. This is exemplified by the many toxic effects noted in newborn infants exposed to hexachlorophene, aniline-containing disinfectant solutions, and hydrocortisone. The percutaneous absorption of a compound is directly related to the degree of skin hydration and inversely related to the thickness of the stratum corneum. The full-term newborn's integument is a more effective functional barrier than the skin of a premature infant. More importantly, however, the ratio of the newborn's skin surface area to body weight is approximately three times greater than that of an adult. Therefore, the amount of drug absorbed into the systemic circulation (bioavailability) for an identical percutaneous dose of a drug is approximately three times greater in an infant than in an adult. These characteristics of skin make topical creams and patch formulations of drugs important means of drug delivery in infants with adequate perfusion.

The effects of maturational changes on the bioavailability of a drug are unpredictable. A prolonged gastric emptying time and irregular intestinal peristaltic activity can lead to erratic rates of drug absorption, reducing the amount of drug absorbed and/or blunting or delaying the peak serum concentration. Reducing the rate and/or amount of total drug absorbed into the body can be therapeutically important, leading to inadequate dosing, whereas blunting or delaying a drug's peak serum concentration may be of only minor clinical significance. The extent to which maturational changes influence gastrointestinal drug absorption also depends on the specific drug formulation administered. Solid dosage forms (tablets, capsules) must dissolve into solution before the drug can cross cell membranes. Most drugs administered to infants and young children are available in a liquid formulation, some as a suspension. In general, the rate of absorption is faster after administration of a liquid dosing formulation (liquid $>$ suspension) as compared with solid formulations (capsule $\geq$ tablet $>$ sustained/delayed-release tablet).

DRUG DISTRIBUTION. Understanding a drug's distribution characteristics in the body is paramount when selecting the dose to be administered. Although a drug's distribution volume (apparent volume of distribution, V_d) does not denote any real physiologic volume, an estimate of this pharmacokinetic parameter provides insight into the total amount of drug present in the body relative to its concentration in blood. Knowledge of a drug's V_d is important when designing an optimal drug dosage regimen to attain a preselected target concentration. The value of the V_d for a number of drugs differs markedly between newborns (premature vs. full term), infants, and children as compared with adults. These differences are a result of many important age-dependent variables, including the composition and size of body water compartments, protein binding characteristics, and hemodynamic factors, including cardiac output, regional blood flow, and membrane permeability. The absolute amounts and distribution of body water and fat depend on a child's age and are well characterized (Chapter 46). Changes in body water compartment sizes and water distribution account for the differences observed in the V_d in infants and children (Chapter 46).

The extent to which a drug is bound to circulating plasma proteins directly influences the distribution characteristics of the drug. Only the free, unbound drug can be distributed from the vascular space into other body fluids and tissues, where it binds to its receptor and stimulates a response. Drug binding to plasma proteins depends on a number of age-related variables, including the absolute amount of proteins available, their respective number of available binding sites, the affinity constant of the drug for the protein, the influence of pathophysiologic conditions, and/or the presence of endogenous substances, which may compete for protein binding (protein displacement interactions). These and other clinically important variables can affect drug protein binding relative to age. The extent to which a drug is bound to protein markedly influences its V_d and body clearance (Cl).

Albumin, α_1-acid glycoprotein (orosomucoid), and lipoproteins are the most important circulating proteins responsible for drug binding in plasma. The absolute concentration of these proteins are influenced by age, nutrition, and disease. Basic drugs bind mainly to albumin, α_1-acid glycoprotein, and lipoprotein, whereas acidic and neutral compounds bind primarily to albumin. Serum albumin and total protein concentrations are decreased during infancy, approaching adult values by the age of 10–12 mo. A similar pattern of maturation is observed with α_1-acid glycoprotein; concentrations appear to be approximately threefold lower in neonatal plasma compared with those in maternal plasma, achieving values comparable to those of adults by 12 mo of age.

Because the free (unbound) drug can diffuse from the vascular compartment into tissues and bind to its receptor, the developmental perturbations described earlier are of utmost importance when designing optimal dosage regimens. Significantly greater concentrations of free drug in cord blood than in adult plasma has been described for many drugs. Decreased binding of drugs to α_1-acid glycoprotein has also been observed. These differences in the degree of drug protein binding in neonates and young infants may alter target therapeutic drug concentrations compared with those targeted in adult patients.

In addition to drugs, several endogenous substances present in human plasma may bind to plasma proteins and compete for available drug binding sites. During the neonatal period, free fatty acids, bilirubin, and 2-hydroxybenzoylglycine compete for albumin binding sites and influence the resultant balance between free and bound drug concentrations. 2-Hydroxybenzoylglycine is a strong competitor for albumin binding sites in newborn infants and, combined with other endogenous substrates, is a particularly important determinant of drug protein-binding differences between infants and adults.

Bilirubin is noncovalently bound to albumin; the binding affinity of bilirubin for albumin is independent of gestational age at birth and is much lower for the newborn infant than the adult, but by the age of 5 mo it approaches the adult value. This compromised binding affinity of bilirubin for albumin in neonates is a contributing factor in their susceptibility to the development of kernicterus (Chapter 88.4). Clinically significant protein binding displacement reactions occur only when a drug is >80–90% protein bound, the drug's body clearance (Cl) is limited, and its apparent V_d is small, usually <0.15 L/kg. It is prudent to assess a drug's potential for displacement of bilirubin from protein binding sites prior to its administration to premature and newborn infants.

Knowledge of a drug's V_d relative to body weight (L/kg) permits rapid calculation of the dose necessary to achieve a specific target concentration. Imbalances between bound and free drug concentrations caused by changes in protein binding or displacement interactions can influence the intensity of pharmacologic effect and the rate of drug removal from the body (free drug is metabolized and/or excreted from the body).

DRUG METABOLISM. The overall rate of drug removal is described by the pharmacokinetic parameter clearance (Cl) or body Cl. A drug's body Cl is the summation of all clearance mechanisms involved in removing that compound from the body. The primary organ for drug metabolism is the liver, although the kidney, intestine, lung, adrenals, and skin can also biotransform certain compounds. For most drugs (lipophilic weak acids or weak bases), biotransformation to more polar, water-soluble compounds facilitates their elimination from the body through the bile, kidney, or lung. Although the biotransformation of most drugs results in pharmacologically weaker or inactive compounds, parent compounds may be transformed into active metabolites or intermediates (theophylline to caffeine, procainamide to *N*-acetylprocainamide, carbamazepine to 10,11-carbamazepine epoxide). Conversely, pharmacologically inactive parent compounds or prodrugs may be converted to an active moiety (chloramphenicol succinate to active chloramphenicol base, cefuroxime axetil to active cefuroxime) prior to subsequent biotransformation and body elimination.

Drug metabolism within the hepatocyte involves two primary enzymatic processes: phase I, or nonsynthetic, and phase II, or synthetic reactions. Phase I reactions include oxidation, reduction, hydrolysis, and hydroxylation reactions, whereas phase II reactions primarily involve conjugation with glycine, glucuronide, or sulfate. Most drug-metabolizing enzymes are located in the smooth endoplasmic reticulum of cells that are recovered as the microsomal fraction on homogenation. Of these mixed function oxidase systems, the cytochrome P-450 system has been studied in greatest detail. In addition, the extent of fetal hepatic drug metabolism may be influenced by hepatocyte concentrations of ligandin. Ligandin, or Y protein, is a basic protein responsible for substrate uptake by metabolizing cells. Ligandin binds bilirubin and organic anions, including drugs. Although concentrations of ligandin at birth are low, values comparable to those in adults have been observed in the 1st 5–10 days of postnatal life.

At birth, the concentration of drug-oxidizing enzymes in fetal liver (corrected for liver weight) is similar to that in adult liver. The activity of these oxidizing enzyme systems is reduced, however, which is reflected by a prolonged body elimination for drugs that depend on oxidation pathways in newborns (phenytoin, diazepam). Postnatally, the hepatic cytochrome P-450 mono-oxygenase system appears to mature rapidly; metabolic activity similar to or in excess of the adult value is achieved by approximately 6 mo of age. In contrast to mono-oxygenase activity, other phase I enzyme systems have been studied in less detail. Alcohol dehydrogenase activity is detectable by the age of 2 mo at levels ≤3–4% of adult activity. The activity of certain hydrolytic enzymes, including blood esterases, is also reduced during the neonatal period, and appears to account for the highly erratic and variable rates of hydrolysis observed in the conversion of chloramphenicol succinate to the active chloramphenicol base. Blood esterases are also important for the metabolic clearance of cocaine; the reduced activity of these plasma esterases in the newborn may account for the delay often observed in the onset of clinical signs and symptoms of cocaine relative to the infant's time of delivery.

Phase II enzymatic reactions are primarily responsible for the synthesis of more water-soluble compounds, augmenting their renal or biliary elimination. These phase II reactions are also catalyzed by the hepatic microsomal enzyme systems located on the smooth endoplasmic reticulum. Glucuronidation is the most common conjugation reaction because of the relative availability of UDP glucuronic acid and the variety of functional groups with which it can combine. In addition to an altered activity of phase I and II hepatic metabolic pathways, the hepatic metabolism of certain drugs is different in neonates as compared with older children and adults. The *N*-methylation of *theophylline* to caffeine occurs in preterm and full-term infants, whereas adults primarily *N*-demethylate and C-oxidate theophylline to monomethylxanthines and methyluric acid. Caffeine is rarely measured in the serum of older infants, children, or adults receiving theophylline because *N*-methylation represents only a minor pathway in these individuals, and their renal function is active enough to excrete the parent compound effectively (theophylline) and any metabolite (caffeine) that may be formed. The caffeine that accumulates because of the reduced renal excretion of aminophylline or theophylline following their administration in young infants most likely acts additively or synergistically with theophylline, both therapeutically and in the development of adverse effects. A metabolic pattern for theophylline degradation and excretion similar to that of adults is observed by approximately 7–9 mo of age. Similarly, age-related differences in the biotransformation of acetaminophen occur. Numerous attempts have been made to stimulate or induce the activity of phase I and II enzyme systems by either maternal or fetal administration of known enzyme inducers, such as phenobarbital. To date, however, only limited experience is available with such pharmacologic maneuvers, and the erratic and unpredictable nature of enzyme induction raises questions about the overall therapeutic value of this approach.

Understanding the sequence of maturation of processes of drug metabolism is important when developing dosage recommendations for drugs that undergo extensive hepatic metabolism. An example of the consequences of failing to appreciate these processes is the tragedy that occurred following the administration of usual doses of chloramphenicol (100 mg/kg/24 hr) to premature and newborn infants (fatal gray baby syndrome) and the resultant beneficial use of this compound in the same patient population when the dose was appropriately adjusted (15–50 mg/kg/24 hr) to compensate for the decreased hepatic ability for glucuronidation. Chloramphenicol glucuronide is the primary metabolite of chloramphenicol, which is then excreted through the kidneys.

DRUG EXCRETION. The amount of drug that is filtered by the glomerulus/unit of time depends on the functional ability of the glomerulus, on the integrity of renal blood flow, and on the extent of drug-protein binding. The amount of drug filtered is inversely related to the degree of protein binding. Only the free drug is filtered by the glomerulus and excreted. Although highly variable, renal blood flow averages 12 mL/min at birth, approaching the adult value by approximately 5–12 mo of age. The glomerular filtration rate is approximately 2–4 mL/min in full-term infants, increases to approximately 8–20 mL/min by 2–3 days of life, and approaches the adult value by approximately 3–5 mo of age. Before 34 wk of gestation, glomerular filtration is markedly reduced and increases slowly.

PHARMACOKINETICS

Basic Concepts

Pharmacokinetics is the mathematical expression of the time course of drug movement in the body. It is clinically useful only when integrated with the drug's pharmacodynamic characteristics. Because the pharmacologic effects of most drugs are reversible, the time of onset, intensity, and duration of effect of a drug are proportional to the amount of drug in the body at any point in time. Pharmacokinetic-based methods can be used to predict drug concentration at any time after a dose is administered and can facilitate calculation of a drug dose to achieve a desired concentration. The recognition that a drug's pharmacologic and/or toxicologic effects correlate best with its concentration in a biologic fluid rather than the absolute dose administered is the foundation of applied clinical pharmacokinetics.

The biodisposition of most drugs used clinically is best described using the principles of linear or first-order pharmacokinetics; that is, the serum concentration or, more appropriately, the amount of drug in the body, is directly proportional to the dose administered. For example, if the dose of a drug that follows linear pharmacokinetics is doubled, its resultant concentration in blood (at steady state) also doubles. This characteristic of proportionality, combined with appropriate patient monitoring, is often used clinically to make adjustments in drug dosing. In contrast, some drugs, such as phenytoin, salicylate, and alcohol, exhibit saturation kinetics; their elimination pathways become "saturated" and the resultant drug concentration in the blood changes disproportionately to the dose administered. Under usual clinical conditions these drugs exhibit linear (first-order) elimination characteristics at low doses (low serum concentrations) but, as the amount of drug in the body increases with increasing dose, their elimination pathways become saturated. Such drugs are often referred to as drugs that follow the principles of zero-order or Michaelis-Mentin kinetics. The classic principles of elimination half-life ($t_{1/2}$) and clearance (Cl) do not apply to drugs that exhibit zero-order kinetics.

DRUG ABSORPTION AND BIOAVAILABILITY. To be effective, a drug must be absorbed from its site of administration into the systemic circulation, from where it is distributed to its site of action and eliminated from the body. Bioavailability is a measure of the amount of drug absorbed into the systemic circulation over a finite period. With a few exceptions (prodrugs), a drug administered intravenously is 100% bioavailable. A drug's bioavailability is most often described as a fraction of the amount absorbed following extravascular drug administration relative to IV drug administration. Mathematically, bioavailability is ideally calculated as the ratio of the area under the drug concentration time curve (AUC) determined after extravascular drug administration to the drug AUC obtained after intravenous administration, (AUC oral/AUC IV). Drugs administered as prodrug formulations require cleavage of the parent compound from their ester salt-liberating active drug. For example, chloramphenicol succinate and palmitate are inactive prodrug formulations of the antibiotic chloramphenicol that are administered intravenously and orally, respectively. Both require cleavage of the ester salt from the parent compound to liberate (release) antibacterially active chloramphenicol; the succinate ester is hydrolyzed after IV administration in blood by nonspecific plasma and hepatic esterases, whereas the palmitate ester is cleaved from the parent drug by pancreatic enzymes in the duodenum after oral administration.

A drug's absorption profile is a composite that depends on both the bioavailability and rate of absorption into the systemic circulation. A drug's rate and extent of absorption are influenced by a number of physicochemical and patient-related factors, some of which are outlined in Table 63–1. These variables and others (concurrent drug therapy) may interfere with a drug's rate of absorption but not affect its bioavailability. For example, the presence of food in the stomach and duodenum can decrease the rate but generally does not affect the overall extent of absorption of many orally administered drugs. The clinical relevance of this interaction depends on whether the drug's efficacy is related to its peak serum concentration (decreased rate would blunt the peak concentration) or the total amount of drug in the body. Appreciating a drug's rate of absorption can be important in anticipating the onset of toxicologic symptoms in cases of drug overdose. In contrast, a disease or a drug interaction that results in a decrease in drug bioavailability would be expected to influence a patient's response to therapy. The concurrent administration of phenytoin and enteral tube feedings can markedly decrease phenytoin bioavailability.

VOLUME OF DISTRIBUTION. The V_d refers to the hypothetical volume of body fluid in which a drug is distributed; it is a proportionality constant that relates the amount of drug in the body to its serum concentration. The apparent V_d is expressed by the equation $V_d = D/C_{p'}$, where D is the dose of the drug administered and $C_{p'}$ is the peak concentration of drug following administration of the dose D. The V_d may be used to calculate the initial or loading dose (LD) of a drug needed to achieve a desired serum concentration (C_p). If a desired C_p is selected and an age-appropriate "average" V_d is known or obtained from the literature, a dose necessary to obtain that concentration can be easily calculated:

$$LD = C_p \times V_d \times \text{patient's body weight},$$

where C_p is in mg/L, V_d is in L/kg, and the patient's body weight is in kg. Furthermore, it is apparent from this relationship that drug elimination from the body, or drug clearance, does not influence the initial or loading dose of a drug. For example, although a drug may be eliminated from the body only through the kidneys, the initial dose is the same for patients with normal renal function as for those with compromised or no renal function. The 1st dose of drug achieves an equilibrium concentration between body fluids and tissues while undergoing metabolism and elimination from the body to maintain a desired serum concentration without drug accumulation.

ELIMINATION HALF-LIFE. A drug's elimination half-life ($t_{1/2}$) is the time required for any given concentration in blood (or other biologic fluid) to decrease to half of the initial value; that is, the time required for half the amount of drug present in the fluid to be cleared. The $t_{1/2}$ can be determined as $t_{1/2} = 0.693/K_d$, where K_d is equal to the slope of the terminal portion of the natural log of the linear serum concentration versus time curve. The $t_{1/2}$ depends on both the drug's Cl and V_d. A more useful formula for $t_{1/2}$, which reflects these important relationships, would be $t_{1/2} = (0.693\ V_d)/Cl$. Thus, a change in $t_{1/2}$ does not necessarily reflect a change in body elimination (body Cl) of a drug. This dependence of $t_{1/2}$ on V_d is exemplified by the influence of extracorporeal membrane oxygenation (ECMO) on drug disposition. For most drugs, ECMO-induced changes are due to an increase in drug V_d rather than any change in drug Cl. Nevertheless, despite this important distinction, the $t_{1/2}$ is often used clinically to adjust dosing intervals, primarily because it can easily be calculated in the clinic or at the patient's bedside. A drug's $t_{1/2}$ can also be used to determine the time necessary to achieve a steady-state concentration; that is, the point at which the amount of drug administered (dose) is equivalent to the amount of drug cleared from the body. After three half-lives, 87.5% of a drug's steady-state concentration is achieved, after four half-lives it is 93.8%, and after five half-lives it is 100%. When integrated with a target concentration strategy, a drug's $t_{1/2}$ is often used to determine a drug's dosage interval.

CLEARANCE. Clearance (Cl) is the pharmacokinetic parameter that estimates the theoretical volume from which a drug is removed/unit of time. A drug's body clearance reflects the amount of drug removed or eliminated from the body/unit of time, whereas renal Cl reflects the amount of drug cleared by the kidneys/unit of time. Total body Cl is the summation of all Cl mechanisms for a given drug (Cl renal, Cl hepatic, Cl lung). The body Cl can be calculated as $Cl = (0.693\ V_d)t_{1/2}$ with the preferred mathematical method of drug dose/AUC. Knowledge of a drug's Cl is fundamental when determining the need for a drug and how often its dose must be repeated to maintain a given serum concentration. It is the most important pharmacokinetic parameter for determining the steady-state drug concentration for a given dose rate. Changes in organ function responsible for the removal of a drug from the body are reflected as a change in the drug Cl. A drug's body Cl is influenced by the integrity of blood flow and by the functional ability of the organ(s) involved in removing the drug from the body.

INDIVIDUALIZATION OF DRUG DOSE. The clinical response to an average or usual recommended dose of drug can vary considerably, even when the dose is administered relative to a patient's body weight, surface area, and stage of maturation. This variation is a result of interindividual differences in drug pharmacokinetics and pharmacodynamics and a number of biologic variables, including genetic differences in metabolism and concurrent pathophysiology. Individual variability with respect to drug efficacy and possibly toxicity frequently necessitates the adjustment of dosage regimens for specific patients, especially when prescribing drugs with a low therapeutic index. For some drugs, including dopamine, nitroprusside, and furosemide, the drug dose may be adjusted according to the patient's immediate and readily quantifiable clinical response. For other drugs, dosage adjustment may be guided more appropriately by combining clinical response with measuring the concentration of drug in plasma or serum. Such an approach to therapy is often referred to as a *target concentration strategy*, where a drug's pharmacologic or toxicologic response can be directly related to a specific serum concentration range.

Reported therapeutic concentration ranges for drugs (Table 63–2) are usually determined from studies of only a limited number of patients, mostly adults, and these therapeutic ranges represent an average mean value, and therefore 49% of the population is encompassed within the two standard deviations that surround this mean value. Thus, the clinical monitoring of serum drug concentrations serves only as a guide to pharmacologic intervention and dose adjustment. Serum drug concentration values must be interpreted individually for each patient. For example, one patient may have a complete clinical response when the serum concentration of drug X is within the "low" portion of the therapeutic range or window. Conversely, the next patient, with the same disease of similar severity requiring the same drug X, may require a serum drug concentration above or below the reported therapeutic concentration range to achieve the same degree of positive therapeutic response. Toxicity, however, may limit how much above the therapeutic range the serum drug concentration may safely be raised. Therefore, therapeutic ranges for serum drug concentrations serve only as guidelines for therapy. Drug efficacy must be assessed by clinical response. Serum drug concentration–time values or profiles may also be compared with previously determined patient-specific values or literature reports to assess patient compliance with a prescribed drug regimen. More commonly, the determination of a drug concentration in biologic fluid helps to achieve an optimal therapeutic regimen while reducing the likelihood of drug toxicity. Finally, the determination of a drug concentration in a biologic fluid provides a means to assess the influences, if any, of disease process or drug interaction on a drug's disposition profile.

Therapeutic drug monitoring is not appropriate, necessary, or practical for all drugs. Drugs with well-defined and easily recognizable and monitored pharmacodynamic effects do not warrant routine monitoring (diuresis with diuretics, lowering of blood pressure by an antihypertensive). For therapeutic drug monitoring to be of clinical value, a clear concentration-response or -toxicity relationship should be identifiable. Patient age and the extent or severity of disease can influence the relationships among drug concentration, efficacy, and toxicity. A number of variables should be considered when designing strategies to monitor therapy using serum drug concentration. When measuring a drug's concentration in blood, the pharmacokinetic characteristics of that drug must be remembered so that blood samples can be obtained at appropriate times in relation to administration of the drug. This permits proper interpretation of drug concentrations and therapeutic effects, and helps avoid serious therapeutic errors. Peak drug concentrations in blood usually do not refer to the highest concentration achieved in blood with that drug but usually to the postdistribution peak drug concentration. Thus, a lag time

■ **TABLE 63–2 Therapeutic Drug Concentration Ranges for Selected Drugs* in Blood†**

Drug		Usual Therapeutic Range			
		Metric Units		*SI Units*	
Amikacin	Peak	25–40	(μg/mL)	43–68	(mmole/L)
	Trough	<10	(μg/mL)	<17	(mmole/L)
Amitriptyline		120–250	(mg/mL)	430–900	(nmole/L)
Caffeine		5–40	(μg/mL)	26–206	(mmole/L)
Carbamazepine		4–12	(μg/mL)	17–51	(mmole/L)
Chloramphenicol	Peak	25–30	(μg/mL)	77–93	(mmole/L)
	Trough	5–10	(μg/mL)	15–31	(mmole/L)
Cyclosporine‡	Trough	150–300	(ng/mL)	83–250	(nmole/L)
Digoxin		0.8–2	(ng/mL)	1–2.6	(nmole/L)
Ethosuximide		40–100	(μg/mL)	283–708	(mmole/L)
Gentamicin	Peak	5–10	(μg/mL)	10.5–21	(mmole/L)
	Trough	<2	(μg/mL)	4.2	(mmole/L)
Imipramine		125–250	(ng/mL)	446–893	(nmole/L)
Kanamycin	Peak	25–40	(μg/ml)	52–82.4	(mmole/L)
	Trough	<10	(μg/mL)	<20.6	(mmole/L)
Lidocaine		1.5–6	(μg/mL)	6.4–25.6	(mmole/L)
Lithium		0.6–1.4	(mEq/L)	0.6–1.4	(mmole/L)
Methsuximide		10–40	(μg/mL)	53–212	(mmole/L)
Netilmicin	Peak	5–10	(μg/mL)	10.5–21	(mmole/L)
	Trough	<2	(μg/mL)	<4.2	(mmole/L)
Phenobarbital		15–40	(μg/mL)	65–172	(mmole/L)
Phenytoin		10–20	(μg/mL)	40–79	(mmole/L)
Primidone		5–12	(μg/mL)	25–35	(mmole/L)
Procainamide		4–10	(μg/mL)	17–42	(mmole/L)
N-acetylprocainamide		5–30	(μg/mL)	18–108	(mmole/L)
Quinidine		2–6	(μg/mL)	6.2–18.5	(mmole/L)
Salicylic acid					
Analgesia/fever		<100	(μg/mL)	<0.72	(mmole/L)
Anti-inflammatory		150–300	(μg/mL)	1.09–2.17	(mmole/L)
Theophylline		10–20	(μg/mL)	56–111	(μg/mL)
Tobramycin	Peak	5–10	(μg/mL)	10.7–21.4	(mmole/L)
	Trough	<2	(μg/mL)	<4.3	(nmole/L)
Valproic acid		50–100	(μg/mL)	346–693	(mmole/L)
Vancomycin	Peak	30–40	(μg/mL)	21–27.6	(mmole/L)
	Trough	5–10	(μg/mL)	3–7	(mmole/L)
Verapamil		100–500	(ng/mL)	220–1100	(nmole/L)

**Usual therapeutic range shown (see text). Consult a clinical pharmacy/clinical pharmacology service for assistance in the interpretation and appropriate time to obtain a blood sample relative to the specific agent and route of drug administration.*
†Blood, plasma, serum: Consult pathology laboratory for specific matrix for concentration measurement.
‡Whole blood analysis by high pressure liquid chromatography; desired target trough values may differ depending upon the specific organ transplant.
SI Units, Systeme International; μg/mL, micrograms/milliliter; mmole/L, millimoles/liter; ng/mL, nanograms/milliliter.

often exists between the time of drug administration and the time that is recommended to obtain the "peak" blood sample. Also, most clinical determinations of drug concentrations in biologic fluids routinely measure (report) the total drug concentration in that fluid (free drug concentration plus concentration of drug bound to protein equals total drug concentration). This approach assumes a constant ratio of free to bound drug at various concentrations and differing pathophysiologic conditions, which may not always be true, and caution must be exercised in its extrapolation. For example, clinically important imbalances between free and total drug concentrations have been observed with the drug phenytoin in critically ill trauma patients and in patients with severe renal disease. As a result, many laboratories are now beginning to report both free *and* total serum concentrations of drugs or have these results available on request. Despite these differences, it is generally unusual for an imbalance in this ratio to be clinically significant, except for those drugs whose protein binding, under normal circumstances, is greater than 90%.

ADDITIONAL CONSIDERATIONS

METHOD OF DRUG ADMINISTRATION. Although it is often assumed that drugs administered intravenously are administered rapidly and completely, this is not always true. The length of time necessary to infuse the total dose of an intravenously administered drug depends on a number of factors, including the flow rate of the IV fluid, the dead space of the system into which the drug is injected, and the total volume in which the drug is diluted. Because most standard IV fluid delivery systems, including their tubing, are designed for adult use, they contain a large volume/unit of length. This introduces a relatively large dead space factor, which causes substantial infusion delays when operated at the slow flow rates necessary for infants and children. For example, a dose of ceftazidime placed in a volume chamber of an IV system and administered at a flow rate of 1 mL/hr does not begin to infuse into the infant or small child until 1 hr after dosing, and may take up to 3 hr to infuse 90% of the dose. Such a slow infusion rate may profoundly affect the serum concentration and the therapeutic efficacy of the drug. Several steps can be taken to minimize problems with IV drug administration to small infants and children. These include the following: standardization and documentation of the total administration time; documentation of the volume and content of the solution used to "flush" an IV dose; standardization of specific infusion techniques (infusion duration, volumes) for drugs with a narrow therapeutic index; standardization of dilution and infusion volumes for drugs given by intermittent IV injection; avoidance of attaching lines for drug infusion to a central hub with other solutions infused concurrently at widely disparate rates; preferential use of large-gauge cannula; maintenance of the recommended solution at a specific height for use with a gravity-based controller; and the use of low-volume tubing and the most distal sites for access of the drug into an existing IV line.

DRUG-DRUG INTERACTIONS. When two or more drugs are administered to the same patient, the pharmacokinetic and pharmacodynamic properties of each agent may be modified by their

■ **TABLE 63–3 Drug Interactions of Potential Importance in Pediatric Practice (Partial Listing)***

Interacting Drugs	Adverse Effects
Acetaminophen	
Alcohol	Hepatotoxicity
Oral anticoagulants	↑ Anticoagulation
Probenecid	↑ Acetaminophen toxicity
Zidovudine	Granulocytopenia
Acyclovir	
Narcotics	↑ Narcotic toxicity?
Zidovudine	Lethargy
Alcohol	
Antidepressants (tricyclic)	↑ Toxicity
Barbiturates	↑ CNS depression (acute)
Benzodiazepines	↑ CNS depression
Cephalosporins (not all)	Disulfiram effect
Chloral hydrate	↑ CNS depression
Doxycycline	↓ Antibiotic effect
Isoniazid	↑ Hepatotoxicity
Metronidazole	Disulfiram effect
Phenothiazines	Impaired coordination
Phenytoin	↑ Phenytoin toxicity
Allopurinol	
Aluminum hydroxide	↓ Allopurinol absorption
Ampicillin	Rash
Anticoagulants (oral)	↑ Anticoagulant effect
Azathioprine	↑ Azathioprine toxicity
Captopril	↑ Cutaneous hypersensitivity
Cyclophosphamide	↑ Cyclophosphamide toxicity
Theophylline	↑ Theophylline toxicity
Thiazide diuretics	↑ Allopurinol toxicity
Aminoglycoside Antibiotics	
Amphotericin B	↑ Nephrotoxicity
Bumetanide	↑ Ototoxicity
Cisplatin	↑ Nephrotoxicity
Cyclosporine	↑ Nephrotoxicity
Furosemide	↑ Nephrotoxicity and ototoxicity
Magnesium	↑ Neuromuscular blockade
Neuromuscular blocking agents	↑ Blockade
Vancomycin	↑ Nephrotoxicity?
Antacids	
Beta-adrenergic blockers	↓ Absorption
Captopril	↓ Absorption
Cimetidine	↓ Absorption
Corticosteroids	↓ Absorption
Digoxin	↓ Absorption
Iron	↓ Absorption
Isoniazid	↓ Absorption
Ketoconazole	↓ Absorption
Nonsteroidal anti-inflammatory agents	↓ Absorption
Phenytoin	↓ Absorption
Salicylates	↓ Absorption
Tetracycline	↓ Absorption
Theophylline	↑ Toxicity
Aspirin	
Anticoagulants (oral)	↑ Bleeding
Captopril	↓ Antihypertensive effect
Barbiturates	
Anticoagulants (oral)	↓ Anticoagulation
Beta-adrenergic blockers	↓ Beta-blockade
Carbamazepine	↑ Production of carbamazepine expoxide
Chloramphenicol	↑ Barbiturate toxicity
Contraceptives (oral)	↓ Contraception
Corticosteroids	↓ Steroid effect
Influenza vaccine (viral)	↑ Barbiturate toxicity
Rifampin	↓ Barbiturate effect
Theophylline	↓ Theophylline effect
Valproate	↑ Barbiturate toxicity
Bleomycin	
Oxygen	↑ Pulmonary toxicity
Captopril	
Allopurinol	↑ Cutaneous hypersensitivity
Aspirin	↓ Antihypertensive effect
Cimetidine	Neuropathy
Nonsteroidal anti-inflammatory agents	↓ Antihypertensive effect
Potassium	Hyperkalemia
Spironolactone	Hyperkalemia
Carbamazepine	
Anticoagulants (oral)	↓ Anticoagulation
Antidepressants (tricyclic)	↑ Both toxicities
Cimetidine	↑ Carbamazepine toxicity
Contraceptives (oral)	↓ Contraception
Corticosteroids	↓ Steroid effect
Cyclosporine	↓ Cyclosporine effect
Erythromycins	↑ Carbamazepine toxicity
Influenza vaccine (viral)	↑ Carbamazepine toxicity
Isoniazid	↑ Both toxicities
Phenytoin	↓ Carbamazepine effect
Theophylline	↓ Theophylline effect
Valproate	↓ Valproate effect
Cimetidine	
Alcohol	↑ Alcohol effect
Antacids	↓ Cimetidine effect
Anticoagulants (oral)	↑ Anticoagulation
Antidepressants (tricyclic)	↑ Antidepressant toxicity
Benzodiazepines	↑ Benzodiazepine toxicity
Beta-adrenergic blocking agents	↑ Beta-blockade toxicity
Captopril	Neuropathy
Carbamazepine	↑ Carbamazepine toxicity
Digoxin	↑ Digoxin toxicity
Ketoconazole	↓ Ketoconazole absorption
Metoclopramide	↓ Cimetidine effect
Phenytoin	↑ Phenytoin toxicity
Theophylline	↑ Theophylline toxicity
Contraceptives (Oral)	
Anticoagulants (oral)	↓ Anticoagulation
Antidepressants (tricyclic)	↑ Antidepressant toxicity
Barbiturates	↓ Contraception
Carbamazepine	↓ Contraception
Griseofulvin	↓ Contraception
Penicillins (ampicillin, oxacillin)	↓ Contraception?
Phenytoin	↓ Contraception
Rifampin	↓ Contraception
Theophylline	↑ Theophylline toxicity
Cyclosporine	
Alkylating agents	↑ Nephrotoxicity
Aminoglycosides	↑ Nephrotoxicity
Amphotericin B	↑ Nephrotoxicity
Carbamazepine	↓ Cyclosporine effect
Erythromycins	↑ Cyclosporine toxicity
Furosemide	Gout
Ketoconazole	↑ Nephrotoxicity
Metoclopramide	↑ Cyclosporine toxicity
Nafcillin	↓ Cyclosporine effect
Phenytoin	↓ Cyclosporine effect
Rifampin	↓ Cyclosporine effect
Digoxin	
Antacids	↓ Absorption
Anticholinergics	↑ Digoxin toxicity
Cholestyramine	↓ Absorption
Cimetidine	↑ Digoxin toxicity
Diuretics (hypokalemia)	↑ Digoxin toxicity
Phenytoin	↓ Digoxin effect
Quinidine	↑ Digoxin toxicity
Verapamil	↑ Digoxin toxicity
Erythromycins	
Anticoagulants (oral)	↑ Anticoagulation
Astemizole (Hismanal)	↑ Astemizole toxicity: arrhythmias
Carbamazepine	↑ Carbamazepine toxicity
Cyclosporine	↑ Cyclosporine toxicity
Phenytoin	↓ Phenytoin effect
Terfenadine (Seldane)	↑ Terfenadine toxicity: arrhythmias
Theophylline	↑ Theophylline toxicity
Fluoroquinolones	
Antacids	↓ Antibiotic effect
Theophylline	↑ Theophylline toxicity
Griseofulvin	
Anticoagulants (oral)	↓ Anticoagulation
Contraceptive (oral)	↓ Contraception
Isoniazid	
Alcohol	Hepatitis
Antacids	↓ INH absorption
Carbamazepine	↑ Toxicity (both)
Ketoconazole	↓ Ketoconazole effect
Phenytoin	↑ Phenytoin toxicity
Rifampin	↑ Hepatotoxicity
Valproate	↑ Hepatic and CNS toxicity

■ **TABLE 63–3 Drug Interactions of Potential Importance in Pediatric Practice (Partial Listing)*** *Continued*

Interacting Drugs	Adverse Effects
Ketoconazole	
Antacids	↓ Absorption
Anticoagulants (oral)	↑ Anticoagulation
Cimetidine	↓ Ketoconazole effect
Cyclosporine	↑ Nephrotoxicity
Isoniazid	↓ Ketoconazole effect
Phenytoin	Altered metabolism of both drugs
Rifampin	↓ Effects of both drugs
Methotrexate	
Blood transfusion	↑ Toxicity
Cisplatin	↑ Methotrexate toxicity
Etretinate	↑ Hepatotoxicity
Nonsteroidal anti-inflammatory agents	↑ Methotrexate toxicity
Trimethoprim–sulfamethoxazole	Megaloblastic anemia
Metoclopramide	
Carbamazepine	Neurotoxicity
Cimetidine	↓ Cimetidine effect
Cyclosporine	↑ Cyclosporine toxicity
Digoxin	↓ Absorption
Narcotics	↑ Sedation
Nifedipine	
Beta-adrenergic blockers	Heart failure, A-V block
Cyclosporine	↑ Gingival hyperplasia
Phenytoin	↑ Phenytoin toxicity
Prazosin	Hypotension
Quinidine	↓ Quinidine effect
Phenytoin	
Alcohol	↑ Toxicity (acute)
Antacids	↓ Phenytoin effect
Anticoagulants (oral)	↑ Phenytoin toxicity, ↑ ↓ Anticoagulation
Antidepressants (tricyclic)	↑ Phenytoin toxicity
Carbamazepine	↓ Carbamazepine effect
Chloramphenicol	↑ Toxicity (both)
Cimetidine	↑ Phenytoin toxicity
Contraceptives (oral and implant)	↓ Contraception
Corticosteroids	↓ Corticosteroid effect
Cyclosporine	↓ Cyclosporine effect
Digoxin	↓ Digoxin effect
Dopamine	Hypotension
Folic acid	↓ Phenytoin effect
Isoniazid	↑ Phenytoin toxicity
Miconazole	↓ Phenytoin effect
Neuromuscular blocking agents	↓ Blockade
Nifedipine	↑ Phenytoin toxicity
Quinidine	↓ Quinidine effect
Rifampin	↓ Phenytoin effect
Theophylline	↓ Effect (both)
Valproate	↑ Phenytoin toxicity
Quinidine	
Amiodarone	↑ Quinidine toxicity
Anticoagulants (oral)	↑ Anticoagulation
Barbiturates	↓ Quinidine effect
Cimetidine	↑ Quinidine toxicity
Digoxin	↑ Digoxin toxicity
Metoclopramide	↓ Quinidine effect
Phenytoin	↓ Quinidine effect
Procainamide	↑ Procainamide toxicity
Rifampin	↓ Quinidine effect
Verapamil	Hypotension
Rifampin	
Anticoagulants (oral)	↓ Anticoagulation
Barbiturates	↓ Barbiturate effect
Beta-adrenergic blockers	↓ Beta-blockade
Chloramphenicol	↓ Chloramphenicol effect
Contraception (oral)	↓ Contraception
Corticosteroids	↓ Corticosteroid effect
Cyclosporine	↓ Cyclosporine effect
Isoniazid	↑ Hepatotoxicity
Ketoconazole	↓ Effect (both)
Phenytoin	↓ Phenytoin effect
Quinidine	↓ Quinidine effect
Theophylline	↓ Theophylline effect
Verapamil	↓ Verapamil effect
Theophylline	
Barbiturates	↓ Theophylline effect
Beta-adrenergic blockers	↑ Theophylline toxicity
Carbamazepine	↓ Theophylline effect
Cimetidine	↑ Theophylline toxicity
Erythromycins	↑ Theophylline toxicity
Fluoroquinolones	↑ Theophylline toxicity
Influenza vaccine (viral)	↑ Theophylline toxicity
Interferon	↑ Toxicity?
Marijuana smoking	↓ Theophylline effect
Phenytoin	↓ Effect (both)
Rifampin	↓ Theophylline effect
Tobacco smoking	↓ Theophylline effect
Troleandomycin	↑ Theophylline toxicity
Trimethoprim–Sulfamethoxazole	
Anticoagulants (oral)	↑ Anticoagulation
Antidepressants (tricyclic)	Depression
Mercaptopurine	↓ Antileukemia effect
Methotrexate	Megaloblastic anemia
Valproate	
Barbiturates	↑ Phenobarbital toxicity
Benzodiazepines	↑ Diazepam toxicity
Carbamazepine	↓ Valproate effect
Cimetidine	↑ Valproate toxicity?
Ethosuximide	↑ Ethosuximide toxicity?
Phenytoin	↑ Phenytoin toxicity

**When possible, an alternate drug combination should be given. If not possible, drug levels* and *signs of toxicity must be monitored.*
A-V, atrioventricular; CNS, central nervous system; INH, isoniazid; ?, possible effect.
Modified from Rizack M, Hillman C: The Medical Letter Handbook of Adverse Drug Interactions. New Rochelle, NY, The Medical Letter, 1989.

combined interaction. Drugs may interact by a number of different mechanisms; these may be classified on a pharmaceutic, pharmacokinetic, and/or pharmacodynamic basis. These interactions may result in unpredictable clinical effects or toxicologic responses (Table 63–3). Pharmaceutic interactions include those resulting in drug inactivation when compounds are mixed together physically prior to patient administration, as in syringes, infusion tubing, or parenteral fluid preparations. The inactivation of aminoglycosides by certain β-lactam antibiotics when these drugs are mixed together in the same IV solution represents a common, clinically relevant example of this type of interaction.

Pharmacokinetic interactions can occur when the disposition characteristics of one compound (absorption, distribution, metabolism, and/or excretion) are influenced by those of another. This type of interaction may involve one or more aspects of a drug's pharmacokinetic profile. For example, one drug may reduce the rate but not the overall extent of absorption, or a compound may displace a drug from its protein binding sites while concomitantly retarding its elimination from the body. Finally, drugs may interact pharmacodynamically, that is, compete for the same receptor or physiologic system, thus altering a patient's response to drug therapy. The number of known, clinically important drug interactions, combined with the ever-increasing number of available pharmacologic agents, emphasizes the need to make a critical assessment of the possibility or presence of drug-drug interactions in any patient receiving multiple drugs.

DRUGS IN HUMAN MILK. Almost all drugs administered to lactating women are secreted to some extent into their milk and may be ingested by the nursing infant. In general, drug use should be as minimal as possible during lactation; a few drugs have been reported to affect the nursing infant adversely (Chapter 79.5). Obviously, it is not possible nor desirable for lactating women to stop taking needed medications. If a question exists about the amount of drug a breast-feeding infant may be receiving and/or possible drug effects on the infant, a sample of the mother's milk should be analyzed.

PRESCRIBING MEDICATIONS. Factors such as taste, smell, color, consistency, and cost affect the degree to which patients comply with their therapeutic drug regimen. Prescribing generically equivalent medications can sometimes reduce the cost of a drug for a patient. Such prescribing should only be done when it is clearly known that the generic brand affords equivalent bioavailability, bioeffectiveness, and patient acceptability. Unfortunately, complete bioequivalence data are not available for all drugs and, when in doubt, the prescribing physician should consult with the pharmacist.

A prescription issued by the prescribing physician should always direct the dispensing of just enough drug to treat the patient, leaving only a small amount of drug left over after the prescribed course of therapy has been completed. This small residual leaves some drug available for doses accidentally spilled or lost. Parents should be instructed to discard all remaining doses of a prescribed medication after the completed course of therapy to protect against accidental poisoning or improper self-medication at a later date. Patient medication instructions on the prescription should state the specific number of doses the patient should receive each day and the total duration of therapy (number of days of therapy). The number of times the prescribing physician allows the prescription to be refilled should be noted on the prescription label; if no refills are to be permitted, this should also be specified on the written prescription.

COMPLIANCE WITH THE PRESCRIBED REGIMEN. Little is known about the many factors that determine the degree of compliance with a physician's instructions, but it is clear that many patients frequently do not take medication consistently or in the manner intended or prescribed. Moreover, patients frequently take medications not recommended or prescribed by their physician. A child's compliance with a prescribed therapeutic regimen is usually only as good as that of the parents. Compliance can often be maximized by carefully educating the family about the nature of the child's illness, the action of the medications prescribed, and the importance of following the instructions precisely. Often, if the instructions are written down clearly and in detail for the family, and if the regimen results in minimal interference with the daily living schedule (particularly parental sleeping habits), compliance with the therapeutic regimen may be improved.

Besunder JB, Reed MD, Blumer JL: Principles of drug biodisposition in the neonate: A critical evaluation of the pharmacokinetic-pharmacodynamic interface. Clin Pharmacokinet 14:189 (Part I); 14:261 (Part II), 1988.

Brown GR, Miyata M, McCormack JP: Drug concentration monitoring: An approach to rational use. Clin Pharmacokinet 24:187, 1993.

Gilman JT, Gal P: Pharmacokinetic and pharmacodynamic data collection in children and neonates: A quiet frontier. Clin Pharmacokinet 23:1, 1992.

Kalow W: Pharmacogenetics: Its biologic roots and the medical challenge. Clin Pharmacol Ther 54:235, 1993.

Kearns GL, Reed MD: Clinical pharmacokinetics in infants and children. A reappraisal. Clin Pharmacokinet 17(Suppl 1):29, 1989.

May DG: Genetic differences in drug disposition. J Clin Pharmacol 34:881, 1994.

Reidenberg MM: Trends in clinical pharmacokinetics. Clin Pharmacokinet 24:1, 1993.

Tange SM, Grey VL, Senecal PE: Therapeutic drug monitoring in pediatrics: A need for improvement. J Clin Pharmacol 34:200, 1994.

Wilson JT, Kearns GL, Murphy D, Yaffe SJ: Paediatric labelling requirements: Implications for pharmacokinetic studies. Clin Pharmacokinet 26:308, 1994.

PART IX

Human Genetics

CHAPTER 64

*The Molecular Basis of Genetic Disorders**

Larry J. Shapiro

There has been a growing recognition of the influence of genetic factors in human disease. The appreciation of the importance of inherited components of common diseases, congenital malformations, and cancer has increased substantially in recent years. At the same time, revolutionary developments have occurred in the basic science of genetics. Major efforts have focused on the application of molecular genetics to understanding heritable disease, and extraordinary progress has been made to use these advances in the practice of medicine. The approaches to diagnosis, genetic counseling, and screening of individuals at risk for genetic disease have been revolutionized by the application of molecular genetics.

The scope of molecular genetics extends from the structure of genes to the functioning of their products in a cell. This field is dominated by powerful and rapidly changing technology involving the manipulation of DNA, RNA, and protein, resulting in a constant interchange between new insights in basic science and application to medical problems. A fundamental goal of molecular genetics is to identify a heritable disease at the level of the affected gene and to chemically define the precise mutation. Once the mutation has been identified, efforts are made to understand what impact it has on the functioning of the cell, tissue, organ, and organism. The mutation is traced from DNA to the corresponding RNA copies of the gene, to the protein translated from the RNA. Studies at this level of the effects of mutations generally provide novel insights into the biologic design of the normal cellular constituents.

With knowledge of the nature of mutations available at the DNA level, diagnosis of a mutation is aimed at direct examination of an individual's DNA. Diagnosis can now be achieved by examination of the DNA from a single cell, and almost any cell from an individual can suffice. Although our diagnostic possibilities still exceed our therapeutic capabilities, molecular genetics promises the treatment of disease through direct correction of a mutation at the DNA level. In some cases, a gene can be corrected in a somatic cell by replacement with a normal or modified gene and, in a few examples, similar replacement of a gene into the germline of an animal has been accomplished. One portion of this chapter reviews certain essential facts that provide an understanding of how our genetic equipment is organized; another discusses applications that have an impact on this study of human disease.

HUMAN GENOME. Each human somatic cell contains two copies of the entire human genetic program or "genome," amounting to 6 billion base pairs (bp) of DNA. DNA is a double-stranded helix, each "step" of the helix comprising a base from one strand bonded to that from the other (a base pair). DNA is portioned into 46 (23 pairs) large fragments, each contained in a specific autosomal chromosome or the X or Y chromosome. The "gene" is the functional entity of information. Approximately 50,000 genes are thought to be encoded in human DNA, a number similar to what characterizes most mammals. In any one type of cell, only a subset of these genes is actually active and operates to maintain the viability and specialized functions of the cell. The genes within a cell may be expressed at widely varying levels. Some genes are responsible for the specialized function of a cell, like the globin genes of a red blood cell. Other genes are considered to have a "housekeeping" function, that is, genes (the products of which are common to most cells) that are needed for the maintenance of basic cellular functioning. A major question of molecular biology is to explain why certain genes, such as globin in a red blood cell or myosin in the muscle cell, are capable of extraordinary activity in some cells but remain silent in others.

We do not know why genes are located at particular sites in the genome or why they are present on a particular chromosome. Frequently, however, highly related genes are clustered in a particular region of a chromosome. A well-studied example are the genes for globins on chromosome 11. At this location we find a cluster of six related globin genes. In the case of this globin cluster, one gene is turned on in red blood cells during embryonic life, a different gene is turned on during the neonatal period, whereas the β-globin gene is turned on around the time of birth, increases in activity, and remains active into adulthood (see Part XXI). It is believed that precise developmental regulation of the genes within the globin family depends partly on their physical proximity to each other within the cluster.

Many proteins consist of different component proteins, which together are needed for complete function. Often, the genes encoding these component proteins are located on different chromosomes. A well-studied example is the genes for the α- and β-globins, the proteins that assemble into the tetrameric hemoglobin molecule. The genes for α-globin are on chromosome 16, whereas the gene for the β chain is on chromosome 11. The cell carefully regulates the expression of these physically unconnected genes.

It is surprising that only a small fraction of the DNA that makes up the human genome appears to be represented by genes, perhaps only about 10% of the total. Most of the human genome consists of DNA sequences without any clear function. Some of this noncoding DNA may be important in the regulation of gene expression or in aspects of chromosome structure and function. Portions of the noncoding DNA are present as single, unique sequences, while other components are repeated many hundreds or thousands of times in the genome.

Almost all DNA in a human cell is contained in the nucleus, but some genes are also found in the mitochondria. These

*Adapted from sections in the 14th edition by Michael A. Zasloff.

organelles, which serve energy-producing needs of cells, contain their own genome. The mitochondrial genome consists of a circular double-stranded molecule containing about 16,000 base pairs of DNA, which has been completely sequenced. Each mitochondrion may harbor several copies of this circular DNA molecule, and during mitochondrial division the mitochondrial genome is replicated. A cell may contain different mitochondria with distinctly different genomes. What is remarkable about the mitochondrion is that it is constructed of proteins that are encoded on its own genome as well as proteins that are encoded on genes contained in the cell nucleus. Proteins that are encoded in the mitochondrial genome appear to be synthesized within the mitochondrion, whereas those encoded in the nucleus are made in the cell's cytoplasm and transported into the mitochondrion. The design principle on which the mitochondrion is built has an impact on the patterns of inheritance that are observed for mitochondrial characteristics. On fertilization, the sperm does not carry mitochondria into the oocyte. The fertilized egg, therefore, only receives mitochondria from the maternal gamete. Thus, genes expressed on the mitochondrial genome are inherited maternally and, as a consequence, diseases resulting from mutation of mitochondrial genes exhibit a maternal inheritance pattern.

A collaborative international scientific effort of unprecedented scope has been initiated, known as the Human Genome Project. The goal of this undertaking is to determine the entire DNA sequence of the human genome. The spatial location of many human genes and DNA segments have been established and the data base that is being created is having a profound influence on biology and medicine. As a consequence, researchers can now identify and characterize new genes that are important in the pathogenesis of a myriad of inherited *and acquired* human disorders. The diagnostic, investigative, and therapeutic potential of these efforts is reshaping the way in which medicine is practiced.

STRUCTURE OF GENES. A gene is a functional unit of DNA from which RNA is copied (*transcribed*). Most genes implicated in human disease express a class of RNA that is translated by cellular machinery into protein (messenger RNA [mRNA]). Genes range in length from between several hundred base pairs to more than 2 million base pairs of DNA. A specialized nuclear enzyme, *RNA polymerase,* recognizes the beginning or start sequence of a gene, attaches to the double-stranded DNA, and proceeds to copy one strand of the gene's DNA sequence into a single strand of RNA as it travels along the length of the gene. The enzyme recognizes another punctuation signal and falls off the gene, releasing the RNA strand. The RNA strand is then processed. The processing reactions involve additions of certain nucleic acids at both ends and removal of certain internal sequences. The processing reactions are necessary for the RNA to be transported from the nucleus to the cytoplasm and for it to be used effectively by the protein synthetic machinery of the cytoplasm, which must translate this RNA into protein.

The most striking processing reaction involves the splicing out of stretches of the RNA, each splicing event taking place at a very precise point in the precursor. In some cases, the total length of RNA removed exceeds the final length of the mature product. Because of this process, matured RNA differs in sequence from the original DNA template. RNA sequences that are retained are called *exons* of a gene, and those that are excised are called *introns.*

The cellular equipment that splices the RNA precursor accurately is complex and consists of many proteins and small RNA species that are, for the most part, only vaguely characterized. The basic principle underlying splicing is that nuclear splicing machinery somehow recognizes proper splice junctions, cleaves the RNA precisely at these junctions, and rejoins the pieces. The excised piece is destroyed in the nucleus and appears to serve no further function in most cases. Splicing is a very complicated process, fraught with possible opportunities for errors to occur. Mutations have been identified, for example, that prevent normal splicing by altering critical sequences around the splice junction. It is not known why most eukaryotic genes are designed in this manner. However, this splicing mechanism permits a cell to produce different RNA molecules from a single gene by splicing the initial RNA differently. For example, in a muscle cell the initial tropomyosin RNA transcript is spliced into as many as 10 different alternative patterns. Each alternatively spliced RNA actually yields a distinctly different final protein product. From a single gene a family of different proteins, corresponding to RNAs alternatively spliced, can be expressed. This design permits different proteins to be expressed from a single gene. An RNA may be spliced in one way in one cell and in another way in a different cell type, permitting some degree of tissue specificity over the nature of the product expressed from a gene. Splicing permits another level of control and compresses the amount of DNA that we must harbor in our genome.

What causes a particular gene to be expressed in a given cell, and how is the activity of that gene regulated? Certain controls exist that can activate a particular battery of genes in a cell (e.g., the genes activated in response to a hormone). Other specialized controls are necessary for activating genes expressing an abundant product in a specific tissue. Another level of control exists to turn on genes at specific times in development. Many of these controls appear to lie on very small DNA sequences residing in the general neighborhood of the gene, consisting of DNA sequences of about 10–20 base pairs in length. They are commonly found at the front end of the gene (5′ end) outside the DNA sequence that is copied into RNA. The essential control elements of a gene comprise a promoter and, in almost every gene, a group of essential control sequences. Specific proteins bind to these control sequences and make the gene more accessible to productive transcription by RNA polymerase. The precise mechanism by which proteins accomplish this is not known, but it is thought that they permit RNA polymerase to gain access more easily than when they are absent. For example, it appears that steroid hormone-responsive genes are activated by specific proteins that bind to DNA sequences around responsive genes when associated with a specific hormone.

The control elements that are needed for tissue-specific activation are called *enhancers.* These enhancers appear to be special sequences that interact with proteins present only in cells of a specific tissue. The presence of this sequence in the vicinity of a gene may be sufficient to lead to its expression in a tissue-specific fashion.

If DNA were fully extended, the total length of the DNA contained in the nucleus of a cell would stretch to about 1 m. Because DNA is condensed into a considerably smaller volume, it is obvious that DNA must be packaged. Packaging is complicated by the requirement that genes and other sequences must be accessed. In addition, DNA must be replicated during cellular division. Extensive studies have demonstrated that nuclear DNA is packaged with a set of five proteins, *histones,* and some additional nonhistone chromosomal proteins into a DNA-protein assembly called *chromatin.* The histones themselves organize to form spherical particles around which about 200 base pairs of DNA are draped. These "beads on a string" are coiled coaxially to form thicker ropes, which are then draped on proteins that compose the scaffolding of the chromosomes. It is generally believed that when a gene is active the chromatin assembly containing the gene is less condensed, or more "open," and at certain sequences histones may be replaced by specialized proteins.

After a gene sequence has been copied to an RNA and that RNA has subsequently matured, the RNA is transported to the cytoplasm of a cell. In the cytoplasm, the RNA is translated by the ribosome and associated enzymes into a nascent protein. In some cases, the protein remains in the cytoplasm, where it will ultimately function (e.g., glycolytic enzymes). In other cases, the messenger RNA (mRNA) directs its protein product into the internal membrane system of a cell, the endoplasmic reticulum, and the newly made protein is shuttled through the internal membrane compartments of a cell. It can be directed from the endoplasmic reticulum to membrane compartments, such as the Golgi network, where chemical modifications, such as the addition of carbohydrate, occur. Proteins are subsequently delivered into intracellular vesicles, such as lysozomes, secreted constitutively from the cell, or delivered to any of the membranes of the cell, such as plasma membrane. In some cases, proteins synthesized in the cytoplasm are transported into membrane-enclosed organelles, such as the mitochondrion, the peroxisome, or the nucleus. The precise nature of the signals that specify the particular intracellular compartment a protein will ultimately find itself in is unknown.

NATURE OF MUTATIONS. Human genetics deals with the variations between humans. These variations are, in part, reflections of differences that exist at the DNA level. Variations that have an impact on the functioning of a gene are usually referred to as mutations. Other variations that do not have an impact on the health or functioning of an organism are called polymorphisms. Mutations may arise in somatic cells as well as in germ cells, but only those changes present in the germ cells will be heritable. Polymorphisms include single nucleotide substitutions (particularly in introns and extragenic flanking regions of DNA), often creating or abolishing a specific restriction enzyme site and thereby leading to length polymorphisms (restriction fragment length polymorphisms, RFLPs) when restriction endonuclease enzymes are employed to digest or cut DNA. Other neutral variants include variable number of a tandem repeat (VNTRs), the repeating unit consisting of 10–60 nucleotides. The human genome also contains short sequence repeats of dinucleotides or trinucleotides. Many of these polymorphisms are useful in genetic analyses and are exploited either by the use of DNA probes and Southern blotting or increasingly by PCR methodologies (see later).

Mutations result from a change of a single base pair of DNA (substitution), from the loss or addition of DNA (deletions, insertions, duplications, expansions), and from rearrangements (inversions and translocations). The effects of mutations depend on the alteration in the protein that is formed and whether the change occurs in domains of the protein crucial for its normal function, such as the transmembrane spanning domain for membrane-associated proteins. These changes in protein structure can occur during translation, during the extensive post-translational modifications (glycosylation and the like) that many proteins undergo, or by causing silencing of transcription or inappropriate gene expression.

A mutation in which a base is changed within an exon, resulting in change of a corresponding amino acid in the protein, is called a *missense* mutation. Such a mutation may result in a dramatic loss of function or may only mildly affect the protein. In some cases, a single base change can add a new stop signal to an RNA molecule (thereby directing the ribosome to prematurely terminate translation nonsense mutation) and would yield a shortened protein. A classic example of an instructive genotype-phenotype correlation occurs in the dystrophin gene in which the clinical differences between the allelic conditions **Duchenne muscular dystrophy** (DMD; virtually no dystrophin detectable at the muscle level by immunolabeling for the protein) and the much milder **Becker muscular dystrophy** (BMD; variably reduced dystrophin) can usually be attributed to whether the deletion disrupts the translational reading frame. In the case of DMD, the deletion occurs such that translation of dystrophin occurs out of frame, leading to a severely truncated (*nonsense mutation*) or highly unstable protein (*missense mutation*). In contrast, BMD mutations usually tend to maintain the translational reading frame and in consequence merely reduce the amount of dystrophin (see Chapter 560.1).

The human genome is a dynamic apparatus, and rearrangements of DNA sequences occurring as a normal mechanism (evolved perhaps to increase the diversity of gene expression or as divergence from and expansion of a gene family) are susceptible to mutation, and these tracts of DNA are often referred to as unstable. A recently recognized type of mutation involves the expansion of tandemly repeated nucleotide triplets. These trinucleotide repeat arrays are found in normal individuals in certain genes and are capable of occasionally being expanded in size through an increase in trinucleotide repeat number. If the number of repeats exceeds a certain threshold, the repeat array becomes unstable, and additional size increases are likely to occur in succeeding generations. This type of unstable (or dynamic) mutation can result in disease in individuals carrying the expanded repeats. At present these *trinucleotide repeat expansions* fall into three classes, with corresponding classes of phenotypes (Table 64–1). The first class is characterized by large expansions of a CGG trinucleotide (cytosine-guanine-guanine), leading to a *fragile site* in the chromosome. Such a site is so designated because it is associated with chromosome breakage under certain in vitro growth conditions. The prototype for this class is the **fragile X syndrome** (FRAXA), in which an expanded CGG repeat in the 5′ untranslated region of the FMR1 gene leads to underexpression and a clinical phenotype of mental retardation, macro-orchidism, and other somatic changes in affected males (see Chapter 67). The second class of disorder involves the relatively small expansion of an in-frame CAG (cytosine-adenine-guanine) repeat in the coding region of the respective genes, leading to a polyglutamine stretch in the resulting protein. Interestingly, all of the known disorders exhibiting this type of expansion are dominantly inherited, late-onset neurodegenerative diseases, the best known example being **Huntington disease**. The third class of disorder involving triplet repeat expansion is represented by the disorder **myotonic dystrophy** (Chapter 560.3). In this case a CTG (cytosine-thymine-guanine) repeat in the 3′ untranslated region of the relevant gene is greatly expanded in affected individuals. A commonly observed characteristic of this dominantly inherited disease is an increase in disease severity in successive generations, a clinical phenomenon known as *anticipation*. Anticipation results from the successive increases in repeat expansion and is observed to a lesser degree in the other classes of disorders.

Another example of the dynamism within the genome that can lead to either harmless polymorphic variation (and thus usually unrecognized) or to a disease is the insertion of repeated sequences of DNA as they are replicated at meiosis into novel sites in the genome. Although only a single case of this type of mutation in humans (a case of **hemophilia A**) has been attributed to this mechanism to date, *retrotransposons* are likely to become recognized more frequently as detailed investigation of disease at the molecular level continues.

For many conditions a variety of different mutations of the same gene account for individual cases of any single disease. Until recently, the analysis of DNA from patients with hemophilia A revealed point mutations, duplications, and deletions of the factor VIII gene as mutational mechanisms, but did not explain the molecular basis of many cases of more severe disease. Then, it was recognized that a common inversion bought about by aberrant recombination during sperm production (male meiosis) was shown to disrupt the factor VIII gene in these individuals. Similarly, a gene can be disrupted by a translocation, an event that joins a segment of DNA on one

■ TABLE 64–1 Mutations Showing Triplet Repeat Expansion

Condition	Repeat	Repeat Location	Pathologic Repeat Number	
FRAXA	CGG	5′ untranslated	Large	(200–1,000)
FRAXE	CGG	?	Large	(200–1,000)
FRAXF	CGG	?	Large	(300–500)
FRA16A	CGG	?	Very large	(1,000–2,000)
Spinal and bulbar muscular atrophy	CAG	Coding region	Small	(<100)
Huntington disease	CAG	Coding region	Small	(<150)
Spinocerebellar ataxia, type I	CAG	Coding region	Small	(<100)
Dentorubral-pallidoluysian atrophy	CAG	Coding region	Small	(<100)
Machado–Joseph disease	CAG	Coding region	Small	(<100)
Myotonic dystrophy	CTG	3′ untranslated	Very large	(200–4,000)

Adapted from Willems PJ: Nature Genet 8:213, 1994.

chromosome with a segment normally located on another chromosome. In the case of the malignant cells of **chronic myelogenous leukemia** (CML) patients, a balanced translocation between chromosomes 9 and 22 is invariably observed. This translocation brings together two genes (*abl* and *bcr*), allowing expression of an abnormal fusion protein with potent tyrosine kinase activity (it acts to transduce external growth-promoting stimuli to the nucleus), allowing unregulated clonal expansion to occur (see Chapter 449.3).

At the cellular level the effects of mutations in inherited genes responsible for structural proteins can create disease in the heterozygous state and thus be inherited in an autosomal dominant manner. For example, the most common form of **osteogenesis imperfecta (type I)**, or OI, has been associated with a number of mutations in the col α1(I) gene responsible for production of α1 chains of type I procollagen, a triple helical protein composed of α1 and α2 chains that confers tensile and compression strength in those tissues (bone, tendons, skin) that have type I collagen as a major component. The effect of a *knockout* mutation or inactivation in one allele leads to a half-normal amount of αl(I) protein produced and an alteration in the ratio of αI to α2 chains from the normal 2:1 to 1:1. Thus, only half the normal amount of type I collagen is produced, and excess fragility of the bones is seen in cases of OI type I. OI very often has serious consequences, unlike mutations affecting enzymatic proteins, where heterozygotes usually show no clinical abnormalities and inheritance of two mutant alleles is required for expression of the disease phenotype (autosomal recessive inheritance). A related disease mechanism is exemplified by the more severe disorder, **OI type II**; mutation in col α1(I) and col α2 genes reduces the amount of chains available for triple helix formation of type I procollagen, qualitatively altering the assembly, function, or degradation of collagen triple helices. The presence of one mutant allele is sufficient to cause this disruption, and this effect is referred to as a *dominant negative* mutation. This lethal disorder is usually the result of a new dominant mutation in either parent's germline. Comparison of these two OI disease subtypes, caused by different types of mutations in the same gene and having their effects on type I collagen, show that reduced amounts of a normal protein may be less deleterious than normal amounts of an abnormal protein (see Chapter 643).

Mutations also can affect the functioning of a gene by altering the splicing efficiency of the RNA transcribed from the gene. A mutation might lie in an intron and lead to reduced amounts of normally spliced RNA. The classic examples of mutations of this type include several forms of **β-thalassemia** (Chapter 419.9).

Mutations can profoundly disturb a cell by altering the normal regulated function of a gene, rather than through disturbing the quality of the actual protein. An example is the expression of the *myc* gene, a growth-promoting nuclear protein whose gene is translocated into the neighborhood of immunoglobulin heavy chain genes in certain **lymphoid** tumors. The *myc* gene, which is normally regulated when present in its usual chromosomal setting, is activated when it is translocated beside the immunoglobulin gene, which is normally active in the plasma cell. The activation of the *myc* gene in this cell, in an unregulated fashion, results in unrestrained growth and a malignant phenotype (see Chapter 446).

Rearrangements in the human genome occur naturally between generations and are essential for biologic diversity and the evolution of species, including humans. This process, termed *recombination*, occurs during meiosis in germ cells between maternal and paternal homologues, and appears to be exquisitely precise to allow for equal genetic exchange between these homologues. Exchange of DNA even occurs between tiny portions of the short arms of the X and Y chromosomes, and the pseudoautosomal regions of the sex chromosomes. On average there are 52 crossovers per male germ cell examined cytogenetically (obtained by testicular biopsy) and between 0 and 2 crossovers per chromosome arm. Because the chromosomes assort independently during meiosis, there are 2^{23} possible combinations of chromosomes in the germ cells from each parent. The process of pairing and recombination can, however, lead to abnormal exchange of genetic material and mutations, either by insertion or deletion or duplication of DNA sequences, and can prove deleterious to functional genes. **Hereditary sensory and motor neuropathy** (Charcot-Marie-Tooth disease) type IA occurs as a result of acquisition of 1.5 Mb of DNA, including a 3rd copy of the PMP2 gene acquired by abnormal recombination mediated by a 17 kb DNA repeat sequence (Chapter 564.1). This is an example of a *gain of function* mutation. DNA repeat sequences appear to have an important role in the pairing of homologues during meiosis, but this process also can go awry, leading to mutation. Aberrant recombination has been among the many mechanisms elucidated as responsible for familial **hypercholesterolemia** (FH; see Chapter 72.4). In one patient, abnormal pairing occurred between two Alu repetitive elements found within introns of this gene. Unequal exchange and loss of some exons with duplication of other exons occurred in the LDL receptor gene. Deletions can vary in their extent and, even when not visible at the cytogenetic level, can involve several genes and are often termed *microdeletions*. A variety of rearrangement conditions referred to as *contiguous gene syndromes* may be generated, and the clinician may be alerted to this possibility by an unusually diverse array of clinical features in any individual or the presence of additional features to a known condition. For example, due to the close physical proximity of a series of genes, different deletions involving the short arm of the X chromosome can produce patients with various combinations of the following features: icthyosis, Kallmann syndrome, ocular albinism, mental retardation, chondrodysplasia punctata, short stature, and mental retardation. The individual features of each case depend on the involvement of these genes and the loss of DNA sequences in the underlying rearrangement. Many other contagious gene syndromes have been described in humans, including Williams, Prader-Willi, and Angelman syndromes.

Translocations also take place in somatic cells. The most well understood are the rearrangements that occur in lymphoid cells. These rearrangements are required for the formation of functional immunoglobulin in B cells and antigen-recognizing receptors on the T cell. Large segments of DNA, which code for the variable and the constant regions of either immunoglobulin or the T-cell receptor, are physically joined at a specific stage in the development of an immunocompetent lymphocyte. The rearrangements take place during lymphoid cell lineage in humans and result in the extensive diversity of the genes for immunoglobulin and T-cell receptors. It is as a result of this post-germline DNA rearrangement that no two individuals, not even identical twins, are really identical, because mature lymphocytes from each will have undergone random DNA rearrangements at these loci.

During the last decade, as human genes have been cloned and sequenced, and variations in particular sequences have been compared between individuals, certain striking patterns have emerged that characterize DNA variations in humans. We have learned that segments of a gene that play a critical functional role, at any level in the pathway of expression of that gene into a functional product, will exhibit very little variation between individuals. In contrast, segments of our genome that seem to be less "important" (e.g., regions of DNA between genes) exhibit extensive variation between individuals. Indeed, if these less important areas are examined at the level of nucleic acid sequence, the variation in a specific segment of DNA (e.g., an intron in a globin gene) may amount to a different base in every several hundred. As a result of this pattern of variation, a gene and all of the associated sequences that are critical for function may be considered as an "island" lying in a sea of highly variable DNA. The sequences surrounding this "gene island" can exhibit significant sequence difference when these segments, which tolerate variation, are compared between individuals from different pedigrees, while the genes themselves are strikingly similar. We sometimes say that the polymorphic framework that surrounds a gene, and a particular framework, is called a *haplotype*. The variations that characterize the DNA in which the gene is embedded can be used to identify the particular chromosome from an individual and (if the sequence of the framework is known in sufficient detail and number) would provide a **fingerprint**, enabling us to distinguish the particular chromosomal region within a population. If a mutation were to arise in the gene of one individual, that mutation could be followed directly (or by tracking variations in the neighborhood of the gene that distinguish that individual's chromosomes). The linkage concept underlies much of the diagnostic methodology of molecular genetics in use today.

This picture of the genome as consisting of islands of conserved genes embedded in a framework, which tolerates considerably more variation, also helps us to understand the patterns of variation that are observed across evolution. As we compare specific genes between mammals, for example, less variation is noted in the sequences of the genes than in the surrounding genetic environment. When segments of DNA between species are compared by sequence, segments that are conserved in sequence across many species generally mark the presence of genes.

TECHNOLOGY OF MOLECULAR GENETICS. Molecular genetics, as a field, is driven to a large degree by technology, and novel methods are introduced almost monthly that improve and significantly modify experimental approaches to the study of gene structure and function. Both DNA and RNA can be sequenced directly. DNA can be cloned, meaning that a DNA sequence can be amplified to yield unlimited amounts. The procedure involves the insertion of a specific DNA sequence into a *vector* (e.g., a virus or antibiotic-resistant plasmid) that can be propagated indefinitely in bacteria. By simple procedures the vector, containing an inserted DNA sequence, can be purified and the inserted DNA sequence can be cleaved out. RNA can be transcribed into DNA enzymatically and can be cloned and sequenced. Small amounts of DNA (<100 base pairs) can be synthesized efficiently by purely chemical methods. DNA can be manipulated through the use of a variety of enzymes purified from natural sources. Duplex DNA segments can be ligated to each other enzymatically. DNA and RNA can be chemically tagged with radioactive or fluorescent markers. Enzymes (e.g., restriction nucleases, isolated from a variety of microorganisms) cleave specific DNA sequences (between four and eight nucleotides in length) and are used to fragment DNA at specific sites. These tools and others provide an extraordinary ability to manipulate and characterize nucleic acids.

In addition, specific DNA sequences can be detected with high specificity. All methods of detection rely on the double-stranded design of DNA. A single-stranded DNA sequence of sufficient length (a *probe*), corresponding to a segment of DNA in the human genome, will find its complementary sequence when exposed to a preparation of human DNA that has been "melted" into single strands. By several different methods, the formation of such a duplex between a probe and any DNA preparation to which it has been *hybridized* can be readily detected.

Molecular hybridization is used in procedures such as Southern blotting and in situ hybridization. In **in situ hybridization**, a chromosome spread is prepared in the same manner as one would prepare a karyotype (Chapter 67). A DNA sequence, corresponding to a sequence within the human genome, is applied to the chromosome spread after the DNA strands have been separated (or denatured). After a period of time, the probe will hybridize to its complementary sequence at a precise location on a specific chromosome. The method of detecting the location of the probe varies. If the probe is made addictive, an emulsion is laid over the slide and the probe is detected by generation of silver grains overlying the location. Fluorescent-tagged probes have been used more frequently, and their location can be determined by observation of the karyotype under a fluorescent microscope. The precise chromosomal locus can be determined by comparison with karyotypic landmarks. Another technique utilizing molecular hybridization is called **Southern blotting**. In this procedure, DNA is fragmented with a specific restriction nuclease, which is generally chosen empirically. The digestion of DNA with a specific restriction endonuclease permits a preparation of DNA to be fragmented into discrete pieces at cleavage sites dependent on the particular sequence recognized by the nuclease utilized. Thus, the DNA from every cell is fragmented in the same way, and a uniform population of fragments is generated. In the classic procedure, the fragments are separated on the basis of size by electrophoresis in agarose: They are denatured and then transferred (with their position preserved) onto a plastic sheet. The sheet bearing the fragments is exposed to a probe, and the position on the sheet bearing the complement is detected. This procedure tells us the presence of and the size of the fragment bearing the sequence of interest.

RNA can be studied by a similar method called **Northern blotting**. In this procedure RNA is isolated, analyzed by electrophoresis in agarose, and transferred to a nitrocellulose membrane. The presence of a specific RNA and its size is detected by hybridization of the sheet with a probe complementary to the expected RNA sequence.

Southern blotting, along with application of sets of restriction enzymes, permits one to examine the nucleic acid sequence around a gene. Thus, if a sequence necessary for the cutting of a restriction enzyme is missing, that fragment will not be present. A fragment of a different size will result. These differences are called *restriction fragment length polymorphisms* (RFLPs).

Another technique, called **polymerase chain reaction** (PCR), has become increasingly important to molecular genetics. This method permits one to enzymatically amplify a DNA sequence, using short synthetic DNA probes. If a sequence is known, by use of two oligonucleotides one can specifically amplify the DNA sequence bracketed by the probes. From the DNA contained in a single cell, enough DNA corresponding to a specific sequence can be generated to sequence, to probe by hybridization, or to clone. This method permits direct examination of mutations and can be applied to situations in which very limited DNA is available. In practice, the procedure is used to amplify a segment of DNA to be examined. The presence of the mutation is then detected by hybridization methodology or by direct sequencing. In hybridization techniques, the geneticist determines whether or not a probe corresponding to the exact, normal sequence hybridizes to the amplified sequence under conditions in which a perfect match can be distinguished from one that is not perfect.

The power of DNA methodology is that mutations can be studied in essentially every cell. Other very powerful techniques have an impact, not so much on diagnosis as on the search for genes. When a mutation is identified, the dilemma is to prove that the mutation is a gene and not a polymorphism (e.g., that a particular nucleic acid variation observed in an individual is not simply a polymorphism). It is possible to express genes in several systems. A gene can be transcribed directly in RNA and can be translated into protein. The gene can be transferred into a living eukaryotic cell and expression of the gene examined. The gene can be redesigned and expressed in bacterial or yeast cells, and in protein products produced in large quantity. In some cases, it is possible to transfer DNA back into the germline of an animal (e.g., the mouse) and to explore its expression and its effect on development. In the most perfect case, the gene can be returned back to a cell bearing a mutant phenotype and the genetic disease can be corrected.

Perhaps the most important point in this section is that in the past we diagnosed a disease by looking for a specific enzymatic defect or for the presence of an abnormal protein. In the present setting, once a disease is suspected or a carrier is suspected, we can make a diagnosis by examination of the individual's DNA. The gene encoding a liver-specific enzyme or red blood cell's protein can be examined in any available cell from that individual and from every member of the kindred. Any tissue with chemically intact DNA can be studied. With the advent of PCR, it is now possible to perform this study on a single cell's worth of DNA and it need not even be physically intact. The DNA from a single cell of a human blastomere can be defined genetically, or the DNA can be obtained from a single sperm cell or from a few nucleated cells present in a drop of blood.

HUMAN LINKAGE MAP. The chromosomal location of about a thousand human genes is known. In many cases, the precise location on a chromosome, as well as the relative position between individual genes on the same chromosome, are known. This body of data constitutes the *human linkage map*. In some cases, positional information about DNA sequences is available for which there is no known function. These sequences have been mapped to precise locations and help to orient us in a particular region of a chromosome, providing us with further guideposts for mapping.

There are several approaches to mapping genes and other DNA sequences to specific chromosomes. In the classic approach, genes located on the X chromosome were identified on the basis of sex-linked patterns of inheritance (Chapter 66). Other disorders were mapped by virtue of the association of a disease with a visible chromosomal alteration, either a translocation or a deletion (Chapter 67). It was assumed that segments deleted or disrupted when chromosomes break and rejoin represented the positions of the genes lost or altered, and that they were responsible for the disease. By this association, the gene responsible for retinoblastoma was localized to chromosome 13 and that of Wilms tumor was localized to chromosome 11. The precise location of the gene for Duchenne muscular dystrophy (DMD) on the X chromosome was identified by the finding of a deletion encompassing a large enough segment of the X chromosome to be visible by routine cytogenetics.

Another powerful technique for the mapping of genes was the use of human rodent somatic cell hybrids. By this method, cells of a human and rodent are fused in tissue cultures. Through repeated cell cycle passage, human chromosomes are randomly lost, resulting in a variety of hybrid cells containing one or several human chromosomes. Because the chromosomes of humans and rodents are very distinguishable by karyotype analysis, the human chromosomes persisting in the hybrid can be readily identified. By analyzing each of the cell lines for the presence of specific human enzymes or other biochemical markers, it has been possible to assign the genes expressing specific proteins to individual human chromosomes.

The introduction of molecular genetic techniques has dramatically expanded our ability to localize genes to specific chromosome loci. As mentioned earlier in this chapter, through application of in situ hybridization a DNA probe can be physically mapped directly, providing the most powerful and direct approach to this problem.

To construct detailed linkage maps, which relate genes too closely spaced to be visualized as physically distinct on microscopic examination of chromosomes (this amounts to around 1 million base pairs of DNA), Southern hybridization and related methods are used. In this approach, DNA is fragmented, as described previously, into large pieces using restriction endonucleases. To determine if two genes (or DNA sequences) are chromosomal neighbors, one experimentally asks whether or not they lie on the same DNA fragment generated by a restriction nuclease. In addition, once a single gene (or sequence) has been mapped, one can *walk* around the chromosomal region, by cloning segments of DNA that are contiguous with the DNA sequence of interest. By this route, detailed "maps" of many chromosomal loci are assembled and this body of information grows daily.

FINDING A "DISEASE" GENE. The power of modern molecular genetic methodologies is best appreciated in the approach taken to define a gene by positional cloning. When molecular genetics is applied to the study of the cause of disease by the classic approach, the pathophysiology of a disease is determined to a degree or detail that includes our identification of the specific protein that is defective, and we begin a search for the mutation at the genetic level. The protein is purified, and the chemical sequence of that purified protein is determined. A comparison between that sequence and the normal sequence determines the nature of the amino acid error. This was the way that the molecular basis of **sickle cell anemia** was determined, now known to result from a valine to glutamic acid substitution in position 6 of β-globin. In the molecular genetic era, the mRNA for β-globin was isolated, cloned, and sequenced; the gene was subsequently sequenced; and the nature of the mutation was determined at the RNA and DNA level (Chapter 419.1). A similar pathway of discovery characterized the elucidation of the defect in **Tay-Sachs disease**.

After discovering that this degenerative disease of the nervous system resulted from expression of a defective enzyme, *hexosaminidase A*, the enzyme was purified. The protein was partially sequenced, and the corresponding mRNA for the enzyme was cloned and sequenced. Molecular genetic methods revealed heterogeneity to the disease. Those of Ashkenazi Jewish origin exhibited the disease as a result of a frameshift mutation in the coding portion of the hexosaminidase A gene, whereas those from other ethnic backgrounds (e.g., the French Canadian kindred) seemed to be missing a segment of the gene (see Chapter 552).

By the positional cloning approach, it is possible to identify the cause of disease through purely genetic techniques. The defective protein and the biologic processes underlying the disease are studied *after* the gene has been identified by direct genetic analysis. This approach is exemplified by the discovery of the gene that is defective in DMD. It was known for many years that DMD was an X-linked disorder and, although pathophysiology was unclear, the defect was profoundly expressed in muscle tissue. After the discovery of a visible deletion on the X chromosome associated with DMD in a single individual, the chromosomal neighborhood was identified. By use of several techniques, DNA probes were isolated from human DNA, which mapped to the region identified by the deletion. These probes provided a powerful tool. The probes were used to identify genes in the suspected locus that encoded proteins that were expressed in muscle. After one gene was identified successfully, it was later shown that the product of that gene was absent from muscle of many patients with DMD. The protein, dystrophin, was shown to be very large in size and appeared to be associated with certain membrane functions involved in coupling of electrical activity and muscle contractions. At the present time, considerable effort is directed to understanding how defects in dystrophin function result in DMD (Chapter 560.1).

Another example of this "reverse" genetic approach coupled with a linkage approach is the identification of a strong candidate for the gene responsible for cystic fibrosis (CF). Unlike the situation with DMD, no patient has been identified with a visible deletion. Although it was known that the disease was associated with a gene on chromosome 7, the precise location of the gene was not evident. To find this gene required precise mapping of the suspicious region of chromosome 7, narrowing down the neighborhood through careful linkage studies at the molecular genetic level by analysis of many different pedigrees. As the region around chromosome 7 linked to CF narrowed, potential candidate genes were surveyed in the region, using probes to determine if any genes were present that expressed RNA in tissues affected in CF, exocrine tissues. One such candidate gene was identified. After cloning of the RNA product of that gene from the tissues of those with CF and those without, it fortunately appeared that a three-nucleotide deletion occurred in the deduced gene product in about 70% of the common white stock. From the nucleic acid sequence of the putative CF gene product, it was possible to "translate" a protein on paper from the genetic code. The protein sequence deduced appeared to be novel but resembled a group of proteins that were implicated in multidrug resistance, proteins that pump out many different classes of drugs that permeate our cells. Although the biochemical basis of CF is unknown, it appeared that epithelial cells from the respiratory mucosa exhibited a defect in the transport of chloride resulting from aberrant chloride channels. It has now been established that the gene that was isolated by positional cloning is in fact a chloride channel or transporter. Further study has shown that in addition to the most common mutation in the CFTR gene (a three nucleotide deletion), over 300 other discrete alterations of this gene can be found in various patients with cystic fibrosis (see Chapter 363).

CHAPTER 65
Molecular Diagnosis*

Larry J. Shapiro

The most striking advantage of the diagnosis of genetic disease through the molecular genetic approach is that a gene can be identified through examination of the DNA from almost any cell of a patient. The cell can be obtained at any time in the life of the individual. Frequently, whole blood is used as a source of DNA, coming from the nucleated cells present in the circulation. Alternatively, buccal epithelial cells, cells shed from the urinary tract, and even a single sperm can serve as a source for DNA to be examined. In prenatal diagnosis, chorionic villus sampling can be used, or amniocytes can be obtained from amniocentesis. Rare fetal cells in the maternal circulation also can be isolated, providing a noninvasive access to fetal DNA. In combination with in vitro fertilization, a cell can be dissected from the cultured human embryo (without apparent harm!) and used for diagnosis before implantation.

Diagnosis of a genetic disorder can be accomplished by either the direct approach or the indirect approach. In the direct approach, we examine a gene for mutations associated with a disease; in the indirect approach, generally applied before a gene has been characterized, we follow a "disease" gene by its linkage with defined sequences that are inherited with high probability. In general, the direct examination of a gene provides a diagnosis with absolute certainty and represents an essential goal in the advancement of the diagnostic arm of molecular genetics.

If a disease is associated with a single mutation, we can readily determine whether an individual carries the mutant gene. Thus, the diagnosis of sickle cell anemia or the determination of a carrier state involves positive identification of the specific mutation within the β-globin gene (Chapters 419.1 and 419.2). This is accomplished by the application of PCR methodology or by hybridization with DNA, with short DNA probes specific for either normal or mutant DNA sequences, which permit direct examination of the presence of a specific sequence at the DNA level associated with expression of the mutant protein.

In diseases such as Duchenne muscular dystrophy (DMD) or factor VIII deficiency, in which numerous mutations within the corresponding genes have been identified to result in a disease with a common phenotype, the gene is examined for mutations that are observed with highest frequency. If no previously recognized mutation can be localized, the gene itself can be sequenced directly (in some cases, a major research effort), and variations from normal, which appear to be linked to the disease phenotype, can be deduced directly. As data accumulate defining the mutations within a gene responsible for specific diseases, our ability to identify a mutation within a gene directly increases, and catalogues of such data grow more detailed continually at an extraordinary pace.

In many diseases, however, the responsible defective gene has not been identified. Prenatal diagnosis and carrier status must be determined through linkage analysis. An attempt is made to identify DNA sequences that are inherited with the disease phenotype and serve to *mark* the chromosome that has been implicated in carrying the defective allele. In general, these linked sequences lie physically close to the gene and are part of the framework referred to earlier (Chapter 64),

*Adapted from sections in the 14th edition by Michael A. Zasloff.

representing the somewhat polymorphic DNA in which genes are embedded. Molecular genetic methods are used to try to distinguish the DNA neighborhood of the defective gene from the DNA neighborhood or framework surrounding a gene unaffected in a kindred. As stated earlier, sufficient polymorphisms exist in DNA in which our genes are embedded to distinguish nonidentical chromosomal segments (e.g., alleles deriving from either parent). In practice, considerable effort at an investigational level is mounted to determine highly polymorphic DNA sequences that are linked through patterns of inheritance with a disease.

When an individual case is presented for diagnosis, the molecular geneticist must first attempt to *fingerprint* the chromosome associated with the disease gene in the pedigree. If the disorder is recessive, both chromosomal neighborhoods harboring the defective gene must be fingerprinted. The fingerprint amounts to a collection of polymorphic sequences that can distinguish a particular chromosomal framework from another. In the case of a recessive disorder, the chromosomes bearing the defective gene must first be identified by examination of the DNA of the affected child. Then, a determination is made with regard to which of the two maternal and paternal chromosomes is associated with the defective gene. If an unaffected sibling is present, that individual should not have inherited the same set of alleles as that of the affected individual and provides a control for the molecular genetic analysis. Prenatal diagnosis involves a search for the presence of the set of maternal and paternal chromosomes bearing mutations. If only one is inherited, the patient is a *heterozygote* or *carrier.* If neither chromosome is inherited, the patient will not have inherited the defective gene. Carrier detection within the extended family is based on the same general principle that involves tracking of the affected chromosome on which the disease gene is linked.

Prenatal diagnosis or carrier detection through linkage analysis requires an analysis of the DNA of an affected individual. This provides a method of fingerprinting the chromosomes bearing the mutation; DNA from both parents permits the characterization of the chromosome that carries the unaffected gene, and, ideally, DNA of a sibling of the proband who is unaffected provides a "proof" that the chromosomal linkage is correct. The larger the pedigree and the more discriminating the sequence differences characterizing the chromosomal neighborhood in which the gene is embedded, the more accurate will be the diagnosis. It must be appreciated, however, that diagnosis by linkage analysis can never offer 100% certainty about the inheritance of a defective gene. Because by this method we do not actually examine the defective gene, but only track it by association of its immediate chromosomal neighborhood, linkage is never perfect. Significant uncertainty results from a probability that the gene will be separated from the linked DNA sequences during meiosis, and this probability increases as the distance between these linked sequences and the gene increases. In general, however, once the chromosomal neighborhood of a gene has been established, major efforts are directed to characterization of the defective gene itself. If this is accomplished, the diagnosis can be made by direct examination of a gene for the presence of associated mutations.

Molecular genetic diagnosis can be performed on any cell from an individual. Therefore, diseases expressed in highly specialized tissues (e.g., the liver), appearing late in development, can be determined through direct examination of a gene examined from almost any cell of an individual. When a defective gene responsible for human disease is identified and the mutations associated with it are characterized, it will be possible to screen populations for the presence of these mutations. Ethical and societal pressures frequently determine how we apply these techniques in practice (Chapters 3 and 4).

GENETIC ABNORMALITIES. Genetic abnormalities are a common cause of disease, handicap, and death among infants and children. They account for the primary diagnosis of 11–16% of patients admitted to the pediatric units of teaching hospitals. One percent of newborn infants have a hereditary malformation, and an additional 0.5% have an inborn error of metabolism or an abnormality of the sex chromosomes that causes no physical abnormalities and that can be detected only by specific laboratory tests.

The types of biochemical abnormalities that have been identified as causes of genetic disease include: substitution of a single amino acid (e.g., sickle cell disease, Chapter 419.1) or synthesis of extra amino acid residues (e.g., hemoglobin Constant Spring) in a protein molecule; deficient activity of an enzyme located normally in the lysosomes, mitochondria, or extracellular space (e.g., phenylketonuria caused by deficiency of dihydropteridine reductase, Chapter 71.1, and Ehlers-Danlos syndrome, type VII, caused by deficiency of procollagen peptidase); lack of production of a specific protein or protein-sugar complex (e.g., macular corneal dystrophy caused by failure to synthesize keratin sulfate proteoglycan); or defective biosynthesis (e.g., of the C_1 esterase inhibitor in hereditary angioneurotic edema).

Many genes have been localized to specific chromosomes (Table 65–1). Molecular biology technology now makes gene mapping possible so that gene deletions and point mutations, caused by the loss or the substitution of a few base pairs, can be identified (Chapter 64). New methods for straining human chromosomes and identifying subtle duplications and deficiencies of chromosomal material have also enlarged the understanding of human chromosomal abnormalities.

A more complete understanding of the basic defect in many of the genetic diseases has altered current clinical classifications. For example, homocystinuria, once considered a single disease, has been shown to be the manifestation of several different metabolic abnormalities. The lethal type of osteogenesis imperfecta, once considered a single disorder, has been shown to be caused by several different alterations of the collagen gene, including internal deletion in the gene's structure, its failure to properly form the collagen triple helix, and failure to secrete the precursors of collagen from cells (Chapter 64). Furthermore, although lethal osteogenesis imperfecta was once considered to be due to an autosomal recessive gene, spontaneous and presumably autosomal dominant mutations are now known to be the basis for most affected infants. The study of common genetic disorders has shown that for some, such as cystic fibrosis and phenylketonuria (PKU), most affected individuals have the same mutation, whereas others, such as hemophilia, are due to many different mutations. The identification of genetic markers, called *restriction length polymorphisms,* that are close to mutant genes is making it possible to trace mutant genes in diseases, such as Huntington disease, through successive generations.

When clinically appraising and managing the child with an inherited disorder, three phases are critical: (1) recognizing that the condition is inherited, (2) identifying the pattern of inheritance, and (3) clarifying the clinical nature of the disorder, which includes understanding the risk of the disease's occurrence in siblings or other members of the family. Recognition that a condition is hereditary may be difficult when the patient has no affected relatives. The physician should be familiar with the different types of genetic diseases and be able to identify their patterns of inheritance using appropriate references, such as *Mendelian Inheritance in Man* by McKusick, which lists conditions caused by single mutant genes. For those with access to the Internet, this resource is available on line, is heavily annotated, and is frequently updated. No catalog is available for disorders attributed to multifactorial inheritance; their recognition depends on the physician's knowledge of these disorders.

■ **TABLE 65–1 Partial List of Cloned Genes Responsible for Known Hereditary Disorders and Examples of Gross Alterations and Point Mutations in Selected Disorders***

Genes	Chromosome	Disorder	Gross Gene Alterations	Point Mutations (PM)
Antithrombin III	1q	Antithrombin III deficiency	del	
Fucosidase	1p	Fucosidosis		
Protein 4.1	1p	Elliptocytosis-1	del	
Glycocerebrosidase	1q	Gaucher's disease		PM
Uroporphyrinogen decarboxylase	1p	Porphyria cutanea tarda		
Medium-chain acyl-CoA dehydrogenase	1p	Medium-chain acyl-CoA dehydrogenase deficiency		
α-Spectrin	1q	Elliptocytosis-2, spherocytosis		
Carbamylphosphate synthetase deficiency	2p	Carbamylphosphate synthetase deficiency		
Apolipoprotein B	2p	Hypobetalipoproteinemia, premature atherosclerosis?		PM
α_1(III)-Procollagen	2p	Ehlers-Danlos syndrome type IV		
Protein C	2	Thrombophilia due to protein C deficiency		
β-Propionyl-CoA carboxylase	3q	Propionic acidemia type II		
Transferrin	3q	Atransferrinemia		
Fibrinogen α, β, and γ	4q	Dysfibrinogenemias		
β-Hexosaminidase	5q	Sandhoff disease		
Factor XIII	6p	Factor XIII deficiency		
Steroid 21-hydroxylase	6p	Congenital adrenal hyperplasia	del	
Complement factor 2	6p	C2 deficiency		
Complement factor 4	6p	C4 deficiency	del	
Plasminogen	6q	Thrombophilia due to plasminogen variant		
Argininosuccinate lyase	7q	Argininosuccinic aciduria		
β-Glucuronidase	7q	Mucopolysaccharidosis VII		
α_2(1)-Procollagen	7q	Osteogenesis imperfecta, Ehlers–Danlos syndrome type VII A2	del	PM
Plasminogen activator	8p	Thrombophilia due to plasminogen activator deficiency		
Carbonic anhydrase	8q	Renal tubular acidosis with osteopetrosis		
Thyroglobulin	8q	Hereditary congenital hypothyroidism		
Argininosuccinate synthetase	9q	Citrullinemia		
Fructose-1-phosphate aldolase	9q	Fructose intolerance		
Ornithine aminotransferase	10q	Gyrate atrophy		PM
Steroid 17-hydroxylase/17,20-lyase	10	Congenital adrenal hyperplasia		
Insulin	11p	Diabetes mellitus due to abnormal insulins		PM
β-Globin	11p	Sickle cell anemia, β-thalassemia		PM
γ-Globin	11p	Hereditary persistence of fetal hemoglobin	del	PM
Parathyroid hormone	11p	Familial hypoparathyroidism (one form)		
Catalase	11p	Acatalasemia		
Apolipoprotein A1, C3, A4	11q	Premature coronary artery disease	inv	
Muscle glycogen phosphorylase	11q	McArdle disease		
Porphobilinogen deaminase	11q	Acute intermittent porphyria		
Pyruvate carboxylase	11q	Pyruvate carboxylase deficiency		
von Willebrand factor	12p	von Willebrand disease	del	
Triosephosphate isomerase	12p	Triosephosphate isomerase deficiency		
Phenylalanine hydroxylase	12q	Phenylketonuria		PM
Retinoblastoma gene	13q	Retinoblastoma	del	
Factor VII	13q	Factor VII deficiency		
Factor X	13q	Factor X deficiency		
α-Propionyl-CoA carboxylase	13	Propionic acidemia type I		
α-Antitrypsin	14	α_1-Antitrypsin deficiency		PM
Liver phosphorylase	14	Hers disease (glycogen storage disease VI)		
α_1-Hexosaminidase	15q	Tay–Sachs disease	del	PM
P-450 side-chain cleavage enzyme/20,22-desmolase	15	Lipid adrenal hyperplasia		
α-Globin	16p	α-Thalassemia	del	PM
Tyrosine aminotransferase	16q	Tyrosinemia type II		
Lecithin–cholesterol acyltransferase	16q	Lecithin–cholesterol acyltransferase deficiency		
Growth hormone	17q	Isolated familial growth hormone deficiency	del	
α_1(1)-Procollagen	17q	Osteogenesis imperfecta, Ehlers–Danlos syndrome type VII A1	del	PM
Complement factor 3	19p	C3 deficiency		
Apolipoprotein E, C2, and C1	19q	Dyslipoproteinemia		
Low-density-lipoprotein receptor	19q	Familial hypercholesterolemia	del	PM
Adenosine deaminase	20q	Severe combined immunodeficiency due to adenosine deaminase deficiency		
Cystathionine β-synthase	21q	Homocystinuria		
Steroid sulfatase	Xp	X-linked ichthyosis	del	
Ornithine transcarbamylase	Xp	Ornithine transcarbamylase deficiency	del	PM
Chronic granulomatous disease gene	Xp	Chronic granulomatous disease		
Gene for Duchenne muscular dystrophy	Xp	Duchenne muscular dystrophy	del	
α-Galactosidase	Xq	Fabry disease		
Phosphoglycerate kinase	Xq	Phosphoglycerate kinase deficiency		
Hypoxanthine guanine phosphoribosyltransferase	Xq	Lesch–Nyhan syndrome	del	
Factor IX	Xq	Hemophilia B	del	PM
Factor VIII	Xq	Hemophilia A	del ins	PM
Green/red cone pigment	Xq	Color blindness	del	
Glucose-6-phosphate dehydrogenase	Xq	Glucose-6-phosphate dehydrogenase deficiency		

**From Antonarakis SE: Diagnosis of genetic disorders at the DNA level. Reprinted with permission from The New England Journal of Medicine 320:153, 1980.*
del = deletion; inv = inversion; ins = insertion.

ADVANCES IN UNDERSTANDING MORPHOGENESIS. Approximately 3% of all newborns have recognizable congenital malformations. Lethal malformations currently account for 25% of all neonatal deaths in the United States and are responsible for 50% of the neonatal mortality when full-term infants are considered alone. In spite of the major importance of malformations, our understanding of their etiology and prevention is inadequate. Both environmental and genetic factors are operative. Recent experimental work in fruit flies and mice provides some reason for cautious optimism for progress in this area. The genome of the mouse is similar to that of humans in its gross architecture. The rapidly accumulating data base with regard to mouse genetics is yielding profound insights into mammalian development. Specifically, experimenters can introduce any desired cloned or modified gene into a developing mouse, and in principal, control when and where that introduced gene is expressed. Such methods of transgenic technology can be used to create animal models of human disease. A second set of methodologies can be used to ablate virtually any gene within a developing mouse and to construct "knockout" animals in the process. These methods have enabled us to begin to decipher the role of a number of novel genes in molecular detail.

These techniques of experimental mammalian embryology have been augmented by basic discoveries using even simpler organisms, such as flies and worms. This understanding also relates to human morphogenesis and congenital malformations. The fruit fly, *Drosophila melanogaster,* has been the subject of much scrutiny. It is a segmented organism with three head segments, three thoracic segments, and nine abdominal segments. Each segment is destined to give rise to discrete and unique structures. After a finite point in development, the fate of cells in each segment is irreversibly determined and a group of cells will continue to play out this predetermined program, even if transplanted to another location. A number of years ago, a variety of mutations were observed in *Drosophila* that disrupt this otherwise orderly process. The presence of *homeotic* mutations were discovered that have the ability to transform the fate of individual segments such that dramatic phenotypes could be observed. For example, in a fly with the antennapedia mutation, the sensory feelers at the top of the head could be transformed into legs.

Earlier events in *Drosophila* development are also understood. The rostral-caudal axis of the *Drosophila* egg is established by gene products contributed by maternal cells that surround the egg (maternal effect genes). Next, a series of stripes across the axis is established via the action of so-called gap and pair rule genes. Next, the anterior and posterior borders of each segment are directed by the action of segment polarity genes. At this point, while all of the segments are established, their identities and embryonic potential are equal. These **homeobox genes** then act in concert to instruct each segment as to whether it is to become a head segment or an abdominal segment and so on. The homeobox genes are so named because mutations in them cause homeotic transformations in the fate of specific segments and because each homeobox gene contains a relatively similar region encoding 60 amino acids near one end of the gene. The homeobox genes are thought to act as master switches that can regulate the expression of other genes that act downstream in development. Simplistically, they probably do this by actually binding to control regions of DNA of these target genes and regulating their transcription. The homeobox genes of *Drosophila* are organized in a specific order on the 3rd chromosome. This order is identical to the spatial order in which they are expressed in the various segments.

The homeobox genes (as well as some other important developmental genes) are highly conserved through evolution, and very similar genes can be found in most other organisms, including the mouse and human. There are at least 35 human and murine homeobox genes, which are organized into four clusters, each on a different chromosome. At the present time the function of most of these genes is unknown. However, studies of their spatial and temporal expression indicate that they follow a pattern at least grossly reminiscent of that seen in flies. Meticulous studies in the mouse using the methods described earlier are under way, aimed at overexpressing homeobox genes, expressing them in the wrong location, or knocking out their expression in efforts to clarify their function. Early results support the critical role of these genes in development and provide important hints about their role in human malformations. For example, mice in which the Hox 1.6 gene has been knocked out develop defects in neural tube closure. Mice overexpressing Hox 1.1 have vertebral duplications. Mice lacking the Hox 1.5 gene look very similar to human infants with the DiGeorge syndrome. Overexpression of the Hox 1.4 gene produces a phenotype very similar to Hirschsprung disease. There is reason to expect that we will soon have a much more detailed understanding of the genes involved in early development. This will enable us to recognize prenatally (and possibly to treat prenatally) a number of human malformations. For those abnormalities that are the product of environmental triggers, we should be able to specify the genes through which these signals act and are transmitted. This may offer a hope of having better screening procedures to recognize environmental teratogens and to mitigate their effects.

Chapter 66
*Inheritance Patterns**

Larry J. Shapiro

SINGLE MUTANT GENES. Each single mutant gene exhibits one of the four patterns of mendelian inheritance: autosomal recessive, autosomal dominant, X-linked recessive, and X-linked dominant. This method of grouping genetic diseases is often helpful in understanding the clinical presentation of a disorder. Concepts such as the basic structure of the DNA molecule and the transmission of genetic information, initially to messenger RNA and then to the formation of a specific polypeptide, help in understanding the basis of diseases, such as the various disorders of hemoglobin structure in which the primary abnormalities include amino acid substitutions and deletions, elongated globin chains, and fused or "hybrid" globin chains. Other concepts explaining the mechanisms for the occurrence of genetic abnormalities that are apparent in the study of microorganisms, such as defective function of repressor genes and regulator genes, may also be applicable to understanding human genetic diseases (Chapters 64 and 65).

In discussing single mutant genes a number of special terms are used. The 23 chromosomes in the sperm combine with the 23 chromosomes in the egg to form a *zygote* with 23 *pairs* of chromosomes. The *gene locus* is the particular location of a specific gene in a specific chromosome. The coding portions of a gene are interrupted by *intervening sequences* of DNA of variable lengths, *introns.* These *introns* are not represented in the mature messenger RNA that corresponds to the gene (Chapter 64). Errors in splicing out the introns are the basis for the most common types of β-thalassemia. Each gene has an analog

*Adapted from sections in the 14th edition by Lewis B. Holmes.

with similar location in the homologous (other of a pair) chromosome; the identical pair of loci are called *homologous loci.* The genes at the homologous loci are called *alleles.* Allelic genes are analogous (i.e., affect the nature of the same characteristic) but are often not identical; extensive variation may be observed in many of the different types of serum proteins among people of the same as well as different races. Because of the genetic variation that exists at many gene loci, it is arbitrary to consider some genes as mutant; usually the distinction is that the mutant gene has a major, harmful effect. When a person has a mutant gene at a locus in one chromosome but not at the homologous locus of the other, the person is *heterozygous* for the mutant gene. If the mutant gene does not affect the heterozygous individual, it is called a *recessive gene.* If the mutant gene has an effect in the heterozygous state, it is a *dominant gene.* A person having the same mutant gene at both homologous loci is *homozygous* for that gene. Autosomal recessive genes manifest their clinical effect only in the *homozygote.* The distinctions between recessive and dominant genes become arbitrary when identifying the heterozygote by biochemical testing or when the heterozygote only mildly expresses the disorder. Furthermore, molecular genetic studies have demonstrated that many persons considered homozygous for the same autosomal recessive gene actually have two different mutations (Chapter 64).

Each mendelian pattern of inheritance has characteristics that may be useful in establishing a diagnosis or in planning family studies that may be important for a clear explanation to the parents of an affected child.

AUTOSOMAL RECESSIVE INHERITANCE. The pedigree illustrating this pattern of inheritance (Fig. 66–1) shows the following characteristics: The child of two heterozygous parents has a 25% chance of being homozygous (i.e., 1 chance in 2 of inheriting the mutant gene from each parent: $1/2 \times 1/2 = 1/4$); males and females are affected with equal frequency; the affected individuals are almost always born in only one generation of a family; the children of the affected (homozygous) person are all heterozygotes; the children of a homozygote can be affected only if the spouse is heterozygote, which is a rare event because of the low incidence of most adverse recessive genes in the general population.

If the frequency of an autosomal recessive disease is known, the frequency of the heterozygote or carrier state can be calculated from the Hardy-Weinberg formula: $p^2 + 2pq + q^2 = 1$, in which p is the frequency of one of a pair of alleles and q is the frequency of the other. For example, if the frequency of cystic fibrosis among white Americans is 1 in 2,500 (p^2), then the frequency of the heterozygote (2 pq) can be calculated: if $p^2 = 1/2{,}500$, then $p = 1/50$, and $q = 49/50$; $2pq = 2 \times 1/50 \times 49/50$ or approximately 1/25 (or 3.92%).

Every human probably has several rare, harmful, recessive genes. Because these mutant genes are frequently not identifiable by laboratory tests, the heterozygous adult usually learns about his or her harmful recessive genes after the birth of a homozygous (and therefore affected) child. Related parents are much more likely to be heterozygous for the same harmful recessive genes because they have a common ancestor. Consanguineous matings are rare in the United States and in many other countries. Therefore, few genetic studies have been carried out to establish the overall risk for healthy but related parents. Based on the information available, the risk for parents who are first cousins of having a newborn child with a birth defect is about double the 2–3% risk faced by healthy, unrelated parents.

AUTOSOMAL DOMINANT INHERITANCE. The pedigree in Figure 66–2 shows that both males and females are affected, that transmission occurs from one parent to child, and that the responsible mutant gene can arise by a spontaneous mutant gene.

X-LINKED RECESSIVE INHERITANCE. The pedigree in Figure 66–3 shows that only males are clinically affected; that affected males are related through carrier females; that all daughters of affected males are carriers of the mutant gene; and that affected males do not have affected sons but may have affected grandsons born to carrier females. The female carrier has a 50% chance of giving her chromosome that bears the mutant gene to each of her children. In other words, each daughter of a carrier has a 50% chance of being a carrier, and each son has a 50% chance of inheriting the mutant gene and having the disease that it causes. Therefore, in each pregnancy the female carrier has a 25% chance of having an affected son.

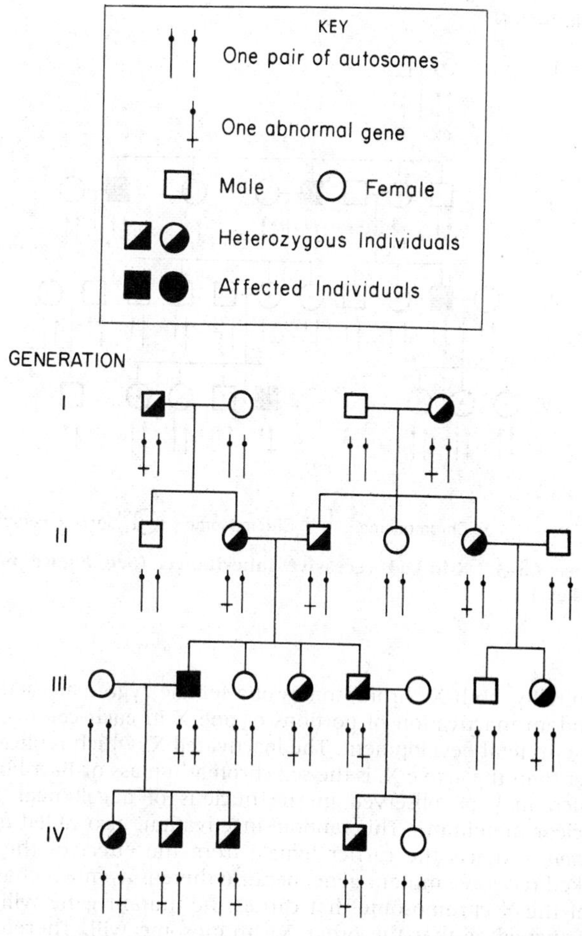

Figure 66–1. Autosomal recessive inheritance.

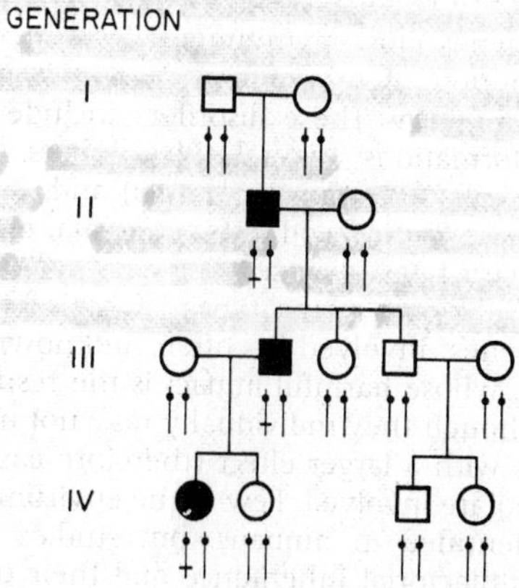

Figure 66–2. Autosomal dominant inheritance. (See Figure 66–1 for key.)

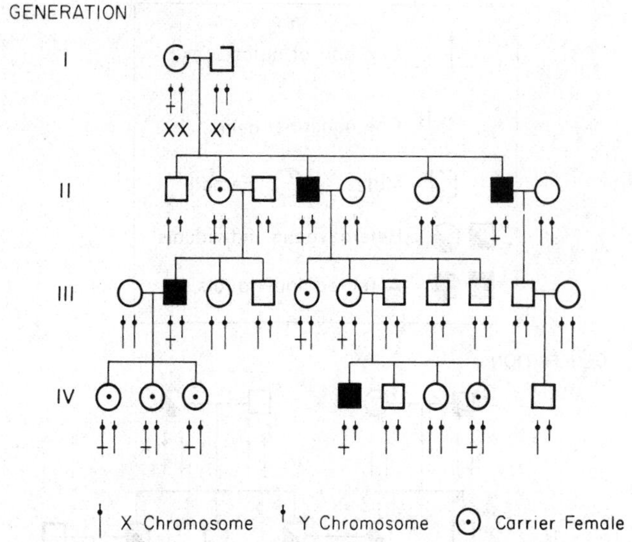

Figure 66–3. X-linked recessive inheritance. (See Figure 66–1 for key.)

Initially, both X chromosomes of a female zygote are active. Random inactivation of portions of one X in each cell occurs early in fetal development. The inactivated X, which replicates later than the active X, is the sex chromatin mass or Barr body, which may be observed in the nucleus of a cell near the nuclear membrane. This random inactivation, also called *lionization,* protects the carrier female from the effect of the X-linked recessive mutant gene, because there is as much chance that the X chromosome that carries the mutant gene will be inactivated as that the other X chromosome will. Therefore, the carrier expresses the effect of the mutant gene in an average of 50% of her cells. For this reason, the female carrier of classic hemophilia will have a reduced level of factor VIII activity, but a level not nearly as low as that in her affected brother.

X-LINKED DOMINANT INHERITANCE. Very few X-linked dominant genes have been identified in humans. Two examples are vitamin D–resistant rickets and the Melnick–Needles syndrome of multiple malformations. The pedigree in Figure 66–4 shows the essential characteristics; both males and females are affected, but males are often more severely affected; the disorder is transmitted from generation to generation; all daughters of an affected father will be affected, but none of his sons.

MULTIFACTORIAL INHERITANCE. The term *multifactorial inheritance* refers to the process in which either continuously variable (quantitative) traits (such as height or blood pressure) or a disease state is the result of additive and interactive effects of one or more genes plus environmental factors. The estimate of the contribution of genes to such a trait or disorder is termed the *heritability.* These disorders include most of the common malformations (neural tube defects, cleft lip and palate, congenital dislocation of the hip) and common multifactorial diseases of adulthood (schizophrenia, essential hypertension, coronary heart disease, diabetes mellitus) and childhood (allergic diseases, some types of hyperlipidemia). The number of genes involved is often unknown and either "minor" genes whose harmful impact is the result of cumulative effect (although they individually may not be harmful) or "major" genes with a larger effect (therefore easier to map in genetic studies) are involved. Few of the environmental factors have been identified in humans, but studies of conditions caused by multifactorial inheritance and their environmental triggers in animals emphasize their relevance. Considerable data must be available on many affected persons and their families before the disease or malformation can be attributed to multifactorial inheritance. More accessible data in studies of mice with such disorders makes mapping of these genes feasible and by locating the syntenic chromosomal region (those conserved blocks of chromosomes that contain very similar DNA sequences between species) in humans, such genes can be identified. As an example, this approach has been used in type I diabetes mellitus.

Some features of multifactorial inheritance are similar to mendelian inheritance of single mutant genes (for example, the incidence of a disorder related to racial background persisting after migration), but some are different. A particularly difficult dilemma can occur in distinguishing between a multifactorial etiology and an autosomal dominant disease gene with reduced penetrance (here "lowered penetrance" refers to the phenomenon of inheriting the mutant gene but not showing the disease phenotype in every instance). Although it may be very difficult to attribute a disease to being of multifactorial etiology in individual instances, most of the features of multifactorial inheritance are quite different and pertinent. Differentiating points are as follows:

1. There is a similar rate of recurrence (typically 2–10%) among all 1st degree relatives (parents, siblings, and offspring of the affected child). It is unusual to find a substantial increase in risk for relatives more distantly related to the index case than 2nd degree.

2. The risk of recurrence is related to the incidence of the disease.

3. Some disorders have a sex predilection, as indicated by an unequal sex incidence. Pyloric stenosis is more common in males, whereas congenital dislocation of the hips is more common in females. Where there is an altered sex ratio, the risk is higher for the relatives of an index case in which the sex is less common. For example, the risk to the son of an affected female with infantile pyloric stenosis is 18% compared with the 5% risk posed to the son of an affected male, the reason being that the female has passed on a greater genetic susceptibility to her offspring.

4. The likelihood that both identical twins will be affected with the same malformation is less than 100%, but much

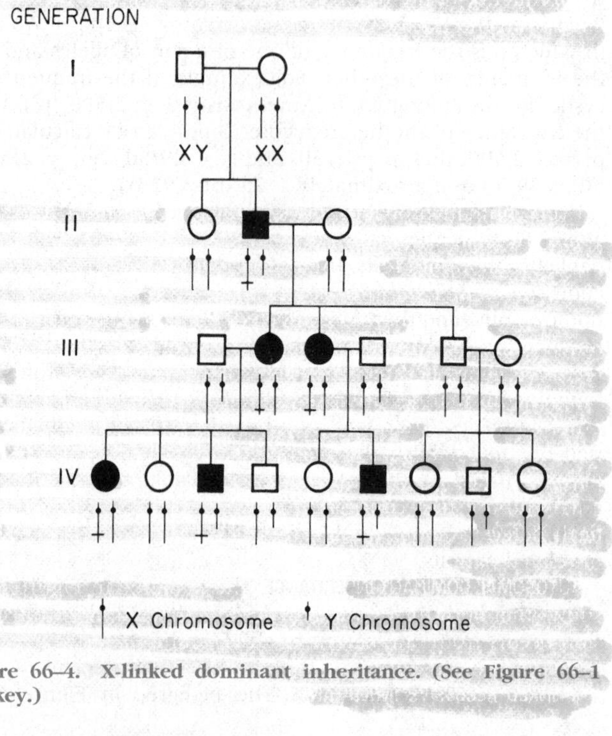

Figure 66–4. X-linked dominant inheritance. (See Figure 66–1 for key.)

greater than the chance that both members of a nonidentical twin pair will be affected. The frequency of concordance for identical twins ranges from 21% to 63%. This distribution contrasts with that of mendelian inheritance, in which identical twins always share a disorder owing to a single mutant gene.

5. The risk of recurrence is increased when multiple family members are affected, and these instances are often the most problematic for distinguishing a multifactorial from a mendelian etiology. A simple example is that the risk of recurrence for unilateral cleft lip and palate is 4% for a couple with one affected child and increases to 9% with two affected children.

6. The risk of recurrence may be greater when the disorder is more severe. For example, the infant who has long-segment Hirschsprung disease has a greater chance of having an affected sibling than the infant who has short-segment Hirschsprung disease.

ATYPICAL PATTERNS OF INHERITANCE. There is a growing appreciation that genetic disorders are sometimes inherited in ways that do not follow the usual patterns of dominant, recessive, X-linked, or multifactorial inheritance. These atypical patterns of inheritance sometimes involve specific diseases, and in other instances can apply to virtually any hereditary disorder. Examples of the latter category are manifested when a de novo mutation occurs at a stage of development of an individual such that the person's gamete population becomes a mixture of normal and mutant alleles. The individual's somatic cells may or may not also constitute a normal/mutant mosaic, but in general, the person is not recognized to be a carrier of a mutant allele, even upon testing for carrier status. An example would be a mother who is not (by routine criteria) a carrier for an X-linked disease such as hemophilia A but who gives birth to more than one affected son. The explanation for this observation is that the mother carries multiple mutant gametes in addition to normal ones. This phenomenon is known as ***gonadal mosaicism*** and is most easily recognized for X-linked, chromosomal, and dominant disorders.

Certain diseases display an atypical mode of inheritance because they result from mutations in mitochondrial DNA. Mitochondria contain small circular chromosomes (as well as ribosomal and transfer RNAs) that encode 13 proteins that function in the respiratory chain of the organelle. Mutations of the mitochondrial genome (which are often deletions) can produce specific diseases. Abnormalities in these disorders are typically seen in one or more specific organs: the brain, the eye, and skeletal muscle. Examples of such disorders are **Kearns-Sayre syndrome** and **Leber hereditary optic neuropathy.** Because mitochondria are inherited virtually exclusively from the mother, the noted diseases are passed from mother to offspring, without regard to the sex of the latter (thus differing from X-linked recessive inheritance). Because the mitochondria of an individual constitute a heterogeneous mixture of genotypes both within and between cells, the mitochondrial complement passed in the egg is often not representative of the total mitochondrial population of the mother. Thus, there is a great variability in symptoms within a family, and the observed inheritance may be more complex than a simple maternal pattern. Nonetheless, the finding of a myopathy or neurologic disease that seems to come from the mother's side should alert the clinician to the possibility of a mitochondrial etiology.

Another type of nontraditional inheritance is the result of a phenomenon known as ***genomic imprinting*** (see Chapter 67). This takes place in the germline and results in certain regions of the genome being inherited differently, depending on the parent of origin. Genes in the relevant region are functionally inactivated (imprinted) during gamete formation and remain inactive in the resulting zygote. The genes imprinted in the two parental germlines are mutually exclusively sets; otherwise, the offspring would have no active copies of the pertinent genes. This imprinting phenomenon leads to clinical consequences in the case of *Prader-Willi syndrome* (PWS). About two thirds of these patients have de novo microdeletions of chromosome 15, and the deletions always occur on the paternally derived chromosome. Similar deletions inherited on the maternal chromosome 15 do not result in PWS but give rise to a different disorder, *Angelman syndrome.* In PWS the relevant gene or genes are silenced on the maternal chromosome 15, so that a deletion on the paternal chromosome leaves the individual with no active alleles (the reverse is true for Angelman patients, where silencing of critical paternal genes with deletion of maternal loci results in the absence of active alleles). Almost all Prader-Willi patients who do not have deletions are found to have inherited two copies of their maternal chromosome 15 and are missing the paternal chromosome. Because both maternal chromosomes are silenced in the critical region, these individuals, like the deletion patients, have no active copies of the critical gene(s). The situation of inheriting both homologous chromosomes from a single parent is called **uniparental disomy**. A number of individuals with abnormal phenotypes have been observed to have uniparental disomy for particular chromosome regions. Thus, at least for certain regions of the genome, it is necessary to have sequences from each parent so that one can express at least one copy of the relevant genes.

GENERAL CLINICAL PRINCIPLES IN GENETIC DISORDERS. Negative Family History (see Chapter 69). A child with a genetic disease or malformation is usually the only known affected member of his or her family. This reflects the fact that the rates of recurrence are very low for common abnormalities of the chromosomes and for conditions attributed to multifactorial inheritance. For example, the recurrence risk for Down syndrome associated with trisomy 21 is 1%; for conditions attributed to multifactorial inheritance it varies from 2% to 10%. The recurrence risk for disorders with a mendelian pattern of inheritance is much higher (e.g., 25% for autosomal recessive disorders), but in small families it is more likely that an autosomal recessive disorder will affect only one of three or four children rather than two. In the case of autosomal dominant disorders, the child may be affected by a spontaneous genetic mutation rather than by inheriting the mutant gene from an affected parent. Generally a negative family history may be misleading.

Environmental Factors. Because the family history is usually negative for the disorder under consideration, the parents often blame themselves and look for environmental factors that might have been the cause. The physician should anticipate their feelings of guilt and should carefully discuss the events, including medications taken, to which congenital disorders may be attributed inappropriately by parents.

Genetic Heterogeneity. A single clinical manifestation may have more than one cause. An elevation in serum phenylalanine may be associated with classic phenylketonuria (either the absence or deficiency of phenylalanine hydroxylase), absence or deficiency of the enzyme pteridin reductase, or deficient biopterin synthesis. Arachnodactyly may be an isolated characteristic of a tall, thin person, or it may be a feature of a number of genetic disorders, including Marfan syndrome and contractual arachnodactyly.

Pleiotropism. Some genetic disorders have many different features, all of which are the pleiotropic effects of a single mutant gene. For example, in classic galactosemia, cataracts, hepatomegaly, malabsorption, neonatal sepsis, and mental deficiency are all related to deficiency of the transferase enzyme, which is the primary effect of the underlying autosomal recessive mutant gene. In neurofibromatosis, café-au-lait spots, subcutaneous nodules, solid tumors, scoliosis, and mental deficiency are caused by a single autosomal dominant gene.

Variable Expression. Publications often present the extreme manifestations of a clinical disorder, but rarely describe its milder forms. The clinician must appreciate that two or three café-au-lait spots may be either innocent birthmarks or the earliest signs of neurofibromatosis in which additional features may become manifest at an older age. This diagnostic dilemma can be resolved only by a careful diagnostic evaluation and sometimes long-term follow-up. In the case of hereditary disorders without progressive changes, such as the Treacher Collins syndrome (mandibulofacial dysostosis), the affected child may have microtia, severe hearing loss, colobomas of the lower eyelids, and marked maxillary hypoplasia, whereas the affected parent may have only mild hearing loss, a downward slant of the palpebral fissures, and a decreased number of lashes on the lower eyelid.

Not Everything Familial Is Genetic. Environmental factors, such as infection and teratogens (see Chapter 81), may simulate genetic conditions; occasionally two or more children of healthy parents may be affected.

Extensive Data. Data from a small number of families cannot establish a pattern of inheritance. For example, when a presumed genetic disorder has occurred in a son and daughter of healthy parents, it is often concluded that each child is homozygous for an autosomal recessive mutant gene. However, a familial chromosomal abnormality and multifactorial inheritance could also cause the same pattern. Similarly, the pattern of occurrence in families with a disorder due to multifactorial inheritance may simulate mendelian inheritance; for example, the parent and child with a cleft lip and palate mimic autosomal dominant inheritance. With the rate of recurrence among parents and siblings only 4% for whites, almost all children with cleft lip and palate are the only affected members of the family. Data on hundreds of families were needed to establish multifactorial inheritance as the basis for the disorder and to exclude the possibility of mendelian inheritance.

Beaudet AL, Scriver CR, Sly WS, et al: Genetics, biochemistry, and molecular bases of variant human phenotypes. *In*: Scriver CR, Beaudet AL, Sly WS, et al (eds): The Metabolic and Molecular Basis of Inherited Disease. New York, McGraw-Hill, 1995.
Lewen B: Genes V. Oxford, Oxford University Press, 1993.
Rosenthal N: Molecular medicine. N Engl J Med 331:39, 331:315, 331:931, 1994.
Sutherland GR, Richards RI: DNA repeats. N Engl J Med 331:191, 1994.

CHAPTER 67

Chromosomal Clinical Abnormalities

Judith G. Hall

The chromosomes are made up of DNA and other protein complexes and contain most of the genetic information that is passed from one generation to the next. Chromosomes are normally only visualized through the microscope when they are in a contracted state as they go through cell division. Chromosome studies are important to the pediatrician because abnormal chromosome number (e.g., trisomy 13) and abnormal chromosomal arrangements (e.g., microdeletion 15q) may lead to multiple congenital anomalies. The first accurate observation and definition of the normal number of chromosomes in a human cell was accomplished by Hsu and Levan in 1956. Improved culture and staining techniques and the use of probes allow the identification of the specific position of gene(s) along the chromosomes and the description of a large number of chromosome abnormalities that are associated with specific disorders and multiple congenital anomalies.

In order to report their findings, cytogeneticists arrange chromosomes by size in pairs—the largest being chromosome 1 and the smallest chromosome 22—and then the sex chromosomes X and Y. The X chromosome is a large submetacentric chromosome, and the Y chromosome is a very small acrocentric chromosome (Fig. 67–1). The position of the centromere in regard to the chromosome arms is another distinguishing feature of each chromosome (Fig. 67–2). The short arm of a chromosome is referred to as p (for petite) and the long arm as q (for the next letter in the alphabet). When the centromere is located in the center between the small and the large arm, the chromosomes are said to be metacentric. In submetacentric chromosomes the centromere is off center. Acrocentric chromosomes have the centromere near the end.

NOMENCLATURE. A karyotype is the designation for the visual display of chromosome studies. This display is obtained after the chromosomes are arrested during cell division in prophase, photographed, and arranged in order according to size. A description of a karyotype consists of three parts: (1) the number of chromosomes, (2) the sex chromosome constitution, and (3) any abnormalities found. The normal karyotype is 46,XX for females and 46,XY for males. If an abnormality is found, it is noted after the sex chromosome constitution. For example, in the case of a female with cri-du-chat syndrome in which a piece of the short arm of the chromosome 5 is missing, the karyotype would be 46,XX,5p−. In a male with Down syndrome in which there is an extra chromosome 21, the karyotype is 47,XY,+21. In the case of translocations, the chromosomes involved are written in brackets preceded by a t, as in 45,XX,t(13q14q), indicating a female carrier of a translocation between the long arms of chromosomes 13 and 14. If the chromosome breaks are along an arm of a chromosome, the band position at which the break occurred is also indicated in the brackets—45,XY, t(13q2.1–14q1.3)—indicating a male carrier of a translocation within the long arms of chromosome 13 and 14.

CELL DIVISION. The process of somatic cell division is called *mitosis*. It is during mitosis, specifically the prophase stage of mitosis, that chromosomes are visible and easy to identify for karyotyping. There is another form of cell division in which the diploid cell (46 chromosomes) becomes haploid (23 chromosomes). This process takes place in the formation of the germ cells and is called *meiosis*.

MITOSIS. This process of cell division occurs in most cells of the body. In mitosis two genetically identical daughter cells are produced from a single parent cell. Prior to cell division DNA replication has occurred so that there is a doubled amount of DNA and the chromosomes contain two identical sister chromatids. Mitosis is divided into stages. *Prophase* is characterized by spiraling of the chromosome threads into coils to form microscopically identifiable chromosomes; the nuclear membrane and the nucleolus disappear and the mitotic spindle forms. In *metaphase*, the chromosomes condense and are clearly visible as distinct structures. The centromeres of the chromosomes attach to the microtubules of the mitotic spindle and the chromosomes align at the middle of the cell along the spindle. *Anaphase* is characterized by division of the chromosomes along their longitudinal axis to form two daughter chromatids and migration of each chromatid of the pair to opposite poles of the cell. *Telophase*, which completes mitosis, is characterized by reconstitution of the nuclear membrane and nucleolus, and duplication of the centriolus as well as cytoplasmic cleavage to form the two daughter cells.

MEIOSIS. This is the form of cell division that occurs to produce germ cells or gametes (sperm and egg). It is divided into two parts: meiosis I and meiosis II. DNA replication occurs before meiosis I, and the cell begins division with two times the

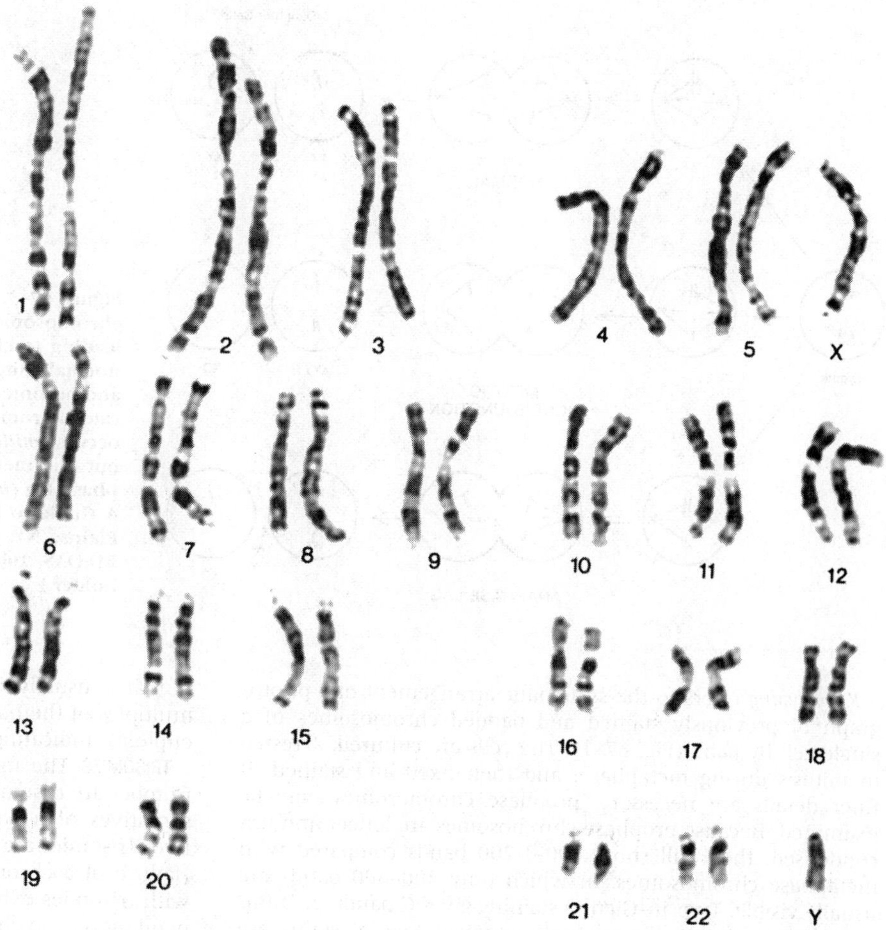

Figure 67–1. Karyotype of normal male with chromosomes in late prophase. The chromosomes are longer, and a greater number of bands are seen than when chromosomes are photographed at metaphase.

normal cellular amount of DNA. In *meiosis I*, each daughter cell gets one of a duplicated chromosome of each pair. At the beginning of *meiosis II*, each cell contains 23 chromosomes, each with a duplicated pair of chromatids. In meiosis II, the duplicated pair separate and each daughter cell ends up with one of each of the 23 chromosomes, that is, there will be four daughter cells, each with a haploid (half the normal number) set of chromosomes.

There is exchange between chromosomes (crossing over of chromosome segments) during meiosis leading to new alignment and combination of genes. Two common errors of cell division occur during meiosis that result in abnormal numbers of chromosomes and chromosomal anomalies. The first is *nondisjunction*, in which two chromosomes fail to separate and migrate together into one of the new cells, producing one cell with two copies of the chromosome and one with no copy. The second is *anaphase lag*, in which a chromatid is lost because it fails to move quickly enough during anaphase to become incorporated into one of the new daughter cells (Fig. 67–3).

METHODOLOGY. Chromosome studies can be obtained from any dividing nucleated cell. The techniques for visualization require condensation of chromatin material that occurs at cell division. Because blood is easy to obtain, cytogenetic studies are usually done on lymphocytes, but fibroblast cytogenetic studies must be considered if there is a suspicion of mosaicism. Chromosome studies for prenatal diagnosis are performed with cells obtained from amniotic fluid, chorionic villi tissue, or fetal blood.

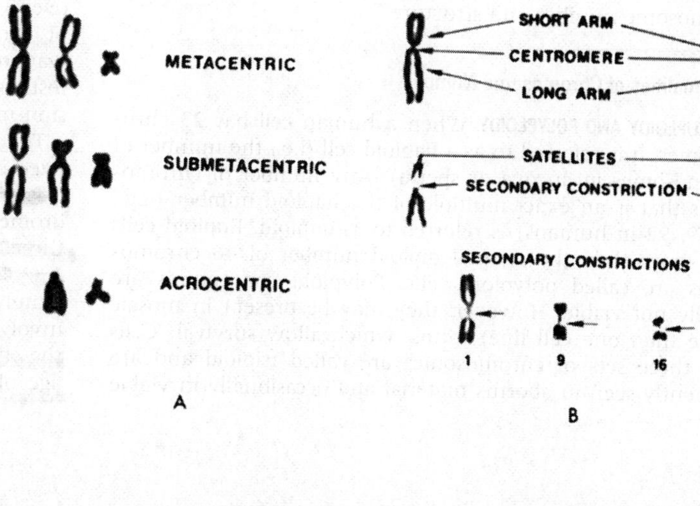

Figure 67–2. *A*, **Centromere position determining the three types of chromosomes seen in the normal human karyotype—metacentric, submetacentric, and acrocentric.** *B*, **Morphologic landmarks useful in chromosome identification.**

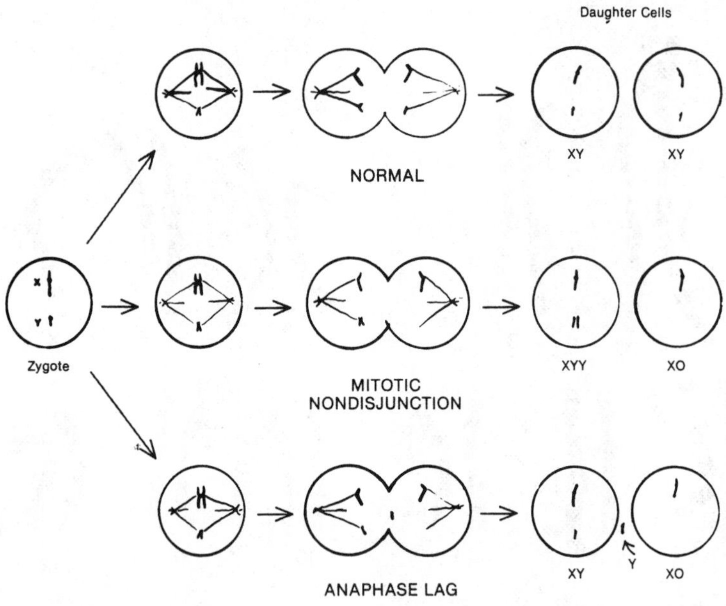

Figure 67–3. The formation of mosaicism. The X and Y chromosomes are used to illustrate two common errors leading to chromosomally abnormal cell populations. In normal mitosis *(top)* duplicated chromosomes separate and become incorporated into daughter cells. If one replicated chromosome fails to separate, mitotic nondisjunction occurs *(middle)*. Occasionally, normal separation occurs, but one member fails to migrate. This is known as anaphase lag *(bottom)*. (From Wisniewski LP, Hirschhorn K: A Guide to Human Chromosome Defects, 2nd ed. White Plains, NY, March of Dimes Birth Defects Foundation, BD:OAS, 16[6], 1980, with permission from the copyright holder.)

Karyotyping refers to the systematic arrangement of a photograph of previously stained and banded chromosomes of a single cell by pairs (Fig. 67–1). The cells are cultured, arrested in mitosis during metaphase, and then fixed and stained. If finer details are necessary, prophase chromosomes may be examined. Because prophase chromosomes are longer and less condensed, they will show 600–1,200 bands compared with metaphase chromosomes, in which only 400–600 bands are usually visible. Trypsin-Giemsa staining gives G banding. Quinacrine gives the Q (fluorescent) banding. Special stains are used to demonstrate centromeres.

In situ hybridization is used to identify the presence or absence of specific DNA sequences on a chromosome spread. The probe recognizes and attaches to homologous DNA sequences on the chromosome spread, identifying a specific chromosome, chromosome segment, or DNA sequence. If fluorescent probes are used, the technique is called fluorescent in situ hybridization (FISH).

CHROMOSOMAL ABNORMALITIES

Chromosomal anomalies occur in 0.4% of live births. They are an important cause of mental retardation and congenital anomalies. Chromosomal anomalies are present in much higher frequencies among spontaneous abortions and still births. The phenotypic anomalies that result from chromosomal aberrations are mainly due to imbalance of genetic information. Chromosomal anomalies include abnormalities of chromosome number and structure.

Abnormalities of Chromosome Number

ANEUPLOIDY AND POLYPLOIDY. When a human cell has 23 chromosomes, it is referred to as a haploid cell (i.e., the number of chromosomes in an ova or sperm). Any number of chromosomes that is an exact multiple of the haploid number (e.g., 46, 69, 92 in humans) is referred to as euploid. Euploid cells with more than the normal diploid number of 46 chromosomes are called polyploid cells. Polyploid conceptions are usually not viable. However, they may be present in mosaic (more than one cell line) forms, which allow survival. Cells with three sets of chromosomes are called triploid and are frequently seen in abortus material and occasionally in viable humans, usually in mosaic forms. Cells deviating from the multiples of the haploid number are called aneuploid (i.e., not euploid), indicating an extra chromosome, as in trisomies.

TRISOMIES. The most common abnormalities of chromosome number are trisomies. These occur when there are three representatives of a particular chromosome instead of the usual two. Trisomies are usually the result of meiotic nondisjunction (failure of a chromosome pair to separate). Most individuals with trisomies exhibit a consistent and specific phenotype depending on the chromosome involved (Table 67–1). The most frequent and best known trisomy in humans is *trisomy 21* or Down syndrome (Fig. 67–4). *Trisomies of chromosome 18* (Fig. 67–5) and 13 (Fig. 67–6) are also relatively common and are associated with a characteristic set of congenital anomalies and mental retardation. *Down syndrome* was first described in 1866, but its cause was not known until 1959, when Lejeune and Turpin showed that these individuals carried 47 chromosomes, the extra chromosome being what was designated at the time as chromosome 21. The incidence is estimated to be more than twice as high among all conceptions than it is among live births. More than half of the trisomic 21 conceptions abort early in pregnancy. The occurrence of trisomy 21 increases with advancing maternal age. In women under 35 yr of age, maternal serum α-fetoprotein concentration is lower, unconjugated estriol decreases, and human chorionic gonadotropin increases in the presence of Down syndrome in the fetus. The combination of these measures are efficacious for prenatal screening. The increased risk of trisomy 21 in women over 35 yr is an indication to offer these women amniocentesis or chorionic-villus sampling and chromosome analysis as a way to detect fetal Down syndrome; the three maternal serum tests can be, when used together, an alternative basis for decision-making in these women.

The clinical manifestations of Down syndrome are summarized in Table 67–1.

Translocation Down Syndrome. All individuals with Down syndrome have three copies of chromosome 21. About 95% have three freestanding copies of chromosome 21. Approximately 1% of individuals are mosaic with some normal cells. Approximately 4% of Down syndrome individuals have a translocation involving chromosome 21. Translocations account for 9% of the children with Down syndrome born to mothers under the age of 30 yr. Half of the translocations arise de novo in the

■ **TABLE 67–1 Chromosomal Trisomies and Their Clinical Findings**

Syndrome	Incidence	Clinical Manifestations
Trisomy 13, Patau syndrome	1/20,000 births	Cleft lip; flexed fingers with polydactyly; hemangiomas of the face, forehead, or neck; broad flat nose; low-set malformed ears; small abnormal skull, cerebral malformation, microphthalmia; cardiac malformations; hypoplastic or absent ribs; visceral and genital anomalies
Trisomy 18, Edwards syndrome	1/8,000 births	Low birthweight; closed fists with index finger overlapping the 3rd digit and the 5th overlapping the 4th; narrow hips with limited abduction; rocker-bottom feet; microcephaly; micrognathia; cardiac and renal malformations and mental retardation; 95% of cases are lethal in the 1st yr
Trisomy 21, Down syndrome	1/600–800 births	Hypotonia, flat face, upward and slanted palpebral fissures and epicanthic folds, speckled irides (Brushfield spots); varying degrees of mental retardation; dysplasia of the pelvis, cardiac malformations, and simian crease; short, broad hands, hypoplasia of middle phalanx of 5th finger, intestinal atresia, and high arched palate; 5% of patients with Down syndrome are the result of a translocation—t(14q21q), t(15q21q), and t(13q21q)—in which the phenotype is the same as trisomy 21 Down syndrome
Trisomy 8, mosaicism		Long face, high prominent forehead, wide upturned nose, thick everted lower lip, microretrognathia, low-set ears, high arched sometimes cleft palate. Osteoarticular anomalies are common; moderate mental retardation.

affected individual, while half are inherited from a translocation carrier parent. Parents who are carriers of a translocation involving chromosome 21 produce three types of viable offspring: normal phenotype and karyotype, a phenotypically normal translocation carrier, and the translocation trisomy 21. The majority of translocations that give rise to Down syndrome are fusions at the centromere between chromosomes 13, 14, 15, or 21 t(21q,21q). The phenotype in translocation Down syndrome is not distinguishable from regular trisomy 21 Down syndrome (Table 67–1). Chromosome studies must be done on every Down syndrome individual. If a translocation is identified, parental studies must be performed to identify normal individuals with a high risk for a chromosomally abnormal child.

MONOSOMIES. Monosomies occur when only one representative of a chromosome is present. They may be complete or partial. Complete monosomies may be the result of nondisjunction or anaphase lag. In nondisjunction during cell division, the two chromosomes in a replicating pair fail to separate; one cell ends up with only one copy (monosomic) and the

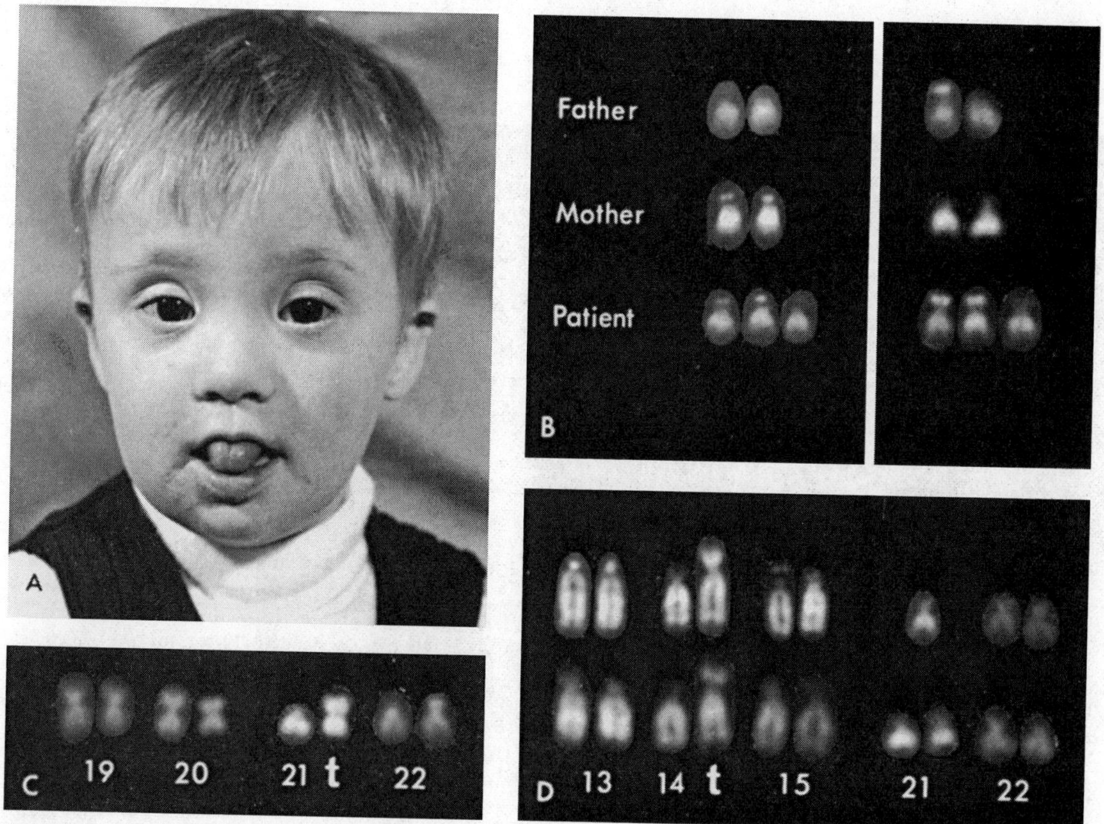

Figure 67–4. Partial karyotypes from patients with Down syndrome. *A*, Patient with trisomy 21. *B*, Chromosome 21 from two patients and their parents. *Left*: Two of a patient's chromosomes with brightly fluorescent satellites were transmitted by the mother. *Right*: Another patient's two chromosomes with bright satellites resulted from paternal nondisjunction at second meiotic division. *C*, 21q21q translocation. *D*, 14q21q translocation in a mother (*above*) and her affected child (*below*).

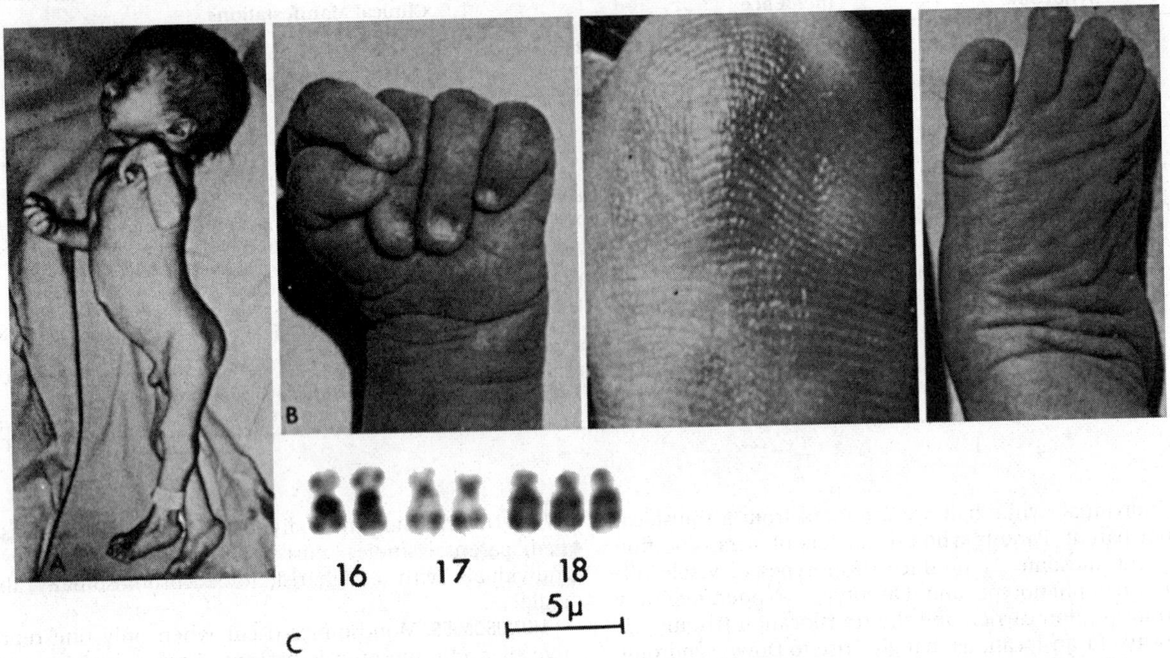

Figure 67–5. *A*, Photograph of male infant with 18-trisomy, age 4 days. Note prominent occiput, micrognathia, low-set ears, short sternum, narrow pelvis, prominent calcaneus, and flexion abnormalities of the fingers. (Courtesy of Robert E. Carrel.) *B*, Several of the common anomalies in the 18-trisomy syndrome, including the unusual position of the fingers with hypoplasia of 5th fingernail; the simple arch pattern of the fingerpads; and the dorsiflexed hallux with hypoplasia of toenails. (From Smith DW: Autosomal abnormalities. Am J Obstet Gynecol 90:1055, 1964.) *C*, Partial karyotype of 18-trisomy prepared with modified Giemsa stain.

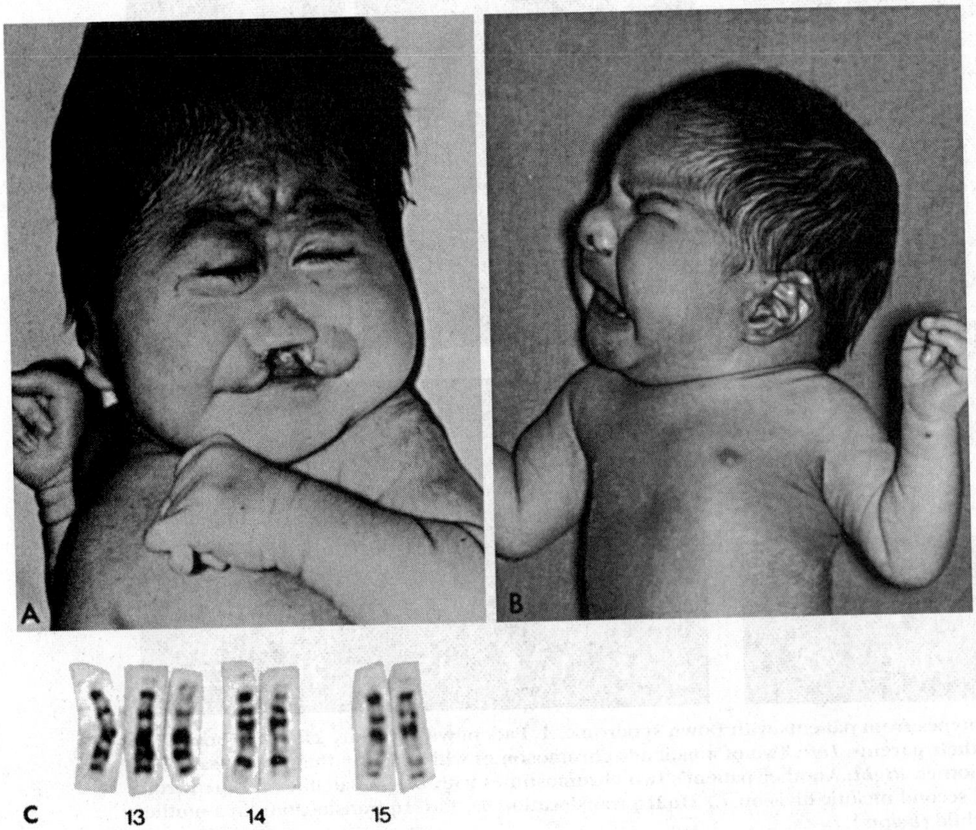

Figure 67–6. *A* and *B*, Female infants with 13-trisomy syndrome. Note the midline cleft of the lip and palate, microcephaly, hypotelorism, microphthalmos, bulbous nose, polydactyly, and overlapping of fingers. Scalp defects (not shown) are also present. (Courtesy of Miriam G. Wilson.) *C*, Partial karyotype showing chromosomes 13, 14, and 15 stained with the trypsin-Giemsa method.

other with three copies (trisomic) of the specific chromosome. In anaphase lag, a chromosome fails to move into the new daughter cell and is lost. All complete autosomal monosomies appear to be lethal early in development in humans and only survive in mosaic forms.

Abnormalities of Chromosome Structure

DELETIONS. Deletions occur when a piece of a chromosome is missing. They may occur as a simple deletion or as a deletion with duplication of another chromosome segment. The latter is usually caused by a crossover in meiosis in a translocation carrier, resulting in an unbalanced reciprocal chromosomal translocation. Deletions may be located at the chromosome ends or in interstitial segments of the chromosome and are usually associated with mental retardation and malformations. The most commonly observed deletions in humans are 4p−, 5p−, 9p−, 11p−, 13q−, 18p−, and 18q−, which are associated with well-described phenotypes (Table 67–2). Deletions may be observed in routine chromosome preparations, but microdeletions are only detectable under the microscope with prophase chromosome studies. In submicroscopic deletions, the missing piece can only be detected by DNA studies.

Microdeletions are defined as small chromosome deletions that are only detectable in high-quality (pro)metaphase preparations. These deletions often involve a gene, and the affected individual is identified by the phenotype of a gene mutation (e.g., Duchenne muscular dystrophy). In addition, the affected individual has other findings not usually seen in the single gene disorder. Prader-Willi, Angelman, Rubinstein-Taybi, Williams, and DiGeorge syndromes have all been found to be associated with microdeletions (Table 67–3). Submicroscopic deletions are not visible by microscopic examination and are detected only with specific probes for a DNA sequence or DNA studies. The deletion is recognized because of the absence of staining or fluorescence.

■ TABLE 67–2 Common Deletions and Their Clinical Manifestations

Deletion	Clinical Abnormalities
4p−	Wolf-Hirschhorn syndrome. The main features are microcephaly, dolichocephaly with frontal bossing, hypoplasia of the eye socket, ptosis, strabismus, nystagmus, bilateral epicanthic folds, cleft lip and palate, large and wide nose bridge, cardiac malformations, and mental retardation.
5p−	Cri-du-chat syndrome. The main features are hypotonia, short stature, characteristic cry, microcephaly with protruding metopic suture, moonlike face, hypertelorism, bilateral epicanthic folds, high arched palate, wide and flat nasal bridge, and mental retardation.
9p−	The main features are craniofacial dysmorphology with trigonocephaly, slanted palpebral fissures, discrete exophthalmos, arched eyebrows, flat and wide nasal bridge, short neck with pterygium colli, genital anomalies, long fingers and toes, cardiac malformations, and mental retardation.
13q−	The main features are low birthweight, failure to thrive, and severe mental retardation. Facial features include microcephaly, flat wide nasal bridge, hypertelorism, ptosis, micrognathia. Ocular malformations are common. The hands have hypoplastic or absent thumbs and syndactyly.
18p−	A few patients (15%) are severely affected and have cephalic and ocular malformations, cleft lip and palate, and varying degrees of mental retardation. Most (80%) have only minor malformations and mild mental retardation.
18q−	The main features are hypotonia with "froglike" position with the legs flexed, externally rotated, and in hyperabduction. The face is characteristic with depressed midface and apparent protrusion of the mandible, deep-set eyes, short upper lip, everted lower lip ("carplike" mouth); the helix and antihelix of the ears are very developed and delimit a deep sulcus. They have varying degrees of mental retardation. Ocular malformations are common.
21q−	The main features are hypertonia, microcephaly, downward-slanting palpebral fissures, high palate, prominent nasal bridge, large low-set ears, micrognathia, and varying degrees of mental retardation. They may have skeletal malformations.

TRANSLOCATIONS. Translocations involve the transfer of chromosomal material from one chromosome to another. Translocations may be Robertsonian or reciprocal. They occur with a frequency of 1 in every 500 liveborn human infants. They may be inherited from a parent or appear de novo, with no other affected family members.

Robertsonian translocations involve two acrocentric (centromere located at the end) chromosomes that fuse near the centromeric region with subsequent loss of the nonfunctional very truncated short arms. The translocation chromosome is made up of the long arms of two fused chromosomes, hence the resulting chromosome count will be only 45 chromosomes. The loss of the short arms of acrocentric chromosomes has no known deleterious effect. Although carriers of a Robertsonian translocation are usually phenotypically normal, they are at increased risk for miscarriages and abnormal offspring. *Reciprocal translocations* are the result of breaks in nonhomologous chromosomes with reciprocal exchange of the broken segments. Carriers of a reciprocal translocation are usually phenotypically normal but also have an increased risk of having chromosomally abnormal offspring and miscarriages due to abnormalities of the segregation of the chromosomes in the germ cells.

INVERSIONS. Inversions require the chromosome to break at two points. The broken piece is then inverted and joined into the same chromosome. Inversions have a frequency of 1 in every 100 liveborns and may be pericentric or paracentric. In *pericentric inversions,* the breaks are in the two opposite arms of the chromosome so that the intervening portion that contains the centromere is reversed. They are usually discovered because they change the position of the centromere. A large number of pericentric inversions have been documented in humans involving every chromosome except 12, 17, and 20. In contrast, *paracentric inversions* involve only chromosomal material from one arm of a chromosome and have been documented for chromosomes 1, 3, 5, 6, 7, 8, 12, 13, 14, and X. Carriers of inversions are usually normal, but they may have an increased risk of miscarriages and chromosomally abnormal offspring.

RING CHROMOSOMES. Ring chromosomes are very rare, but they have been found for all human chromosomes. The formation of a ring involves a deletion at each end of the chromosome. The "sticky" ends then join to form the ring. The phenotype of a ring chromosome ranges from mental retardation and multiple congenital anomalies to normal or nearly normal phenotypes, depending on the amount of chromosomal material that is lost. If the ring replaces a normal chromosome, the result is partial monosomy. The phenotype in these cases often overlaps that seen in comparable deletion syndromes of the same chromosome. If there is a ring in addition to the normal chromosomes, the phenotype reflects the partial trisomy for that chromosome.

DUPLICATIONS. A duplication is the presence of extra genetic material from the same chromosome. Duplications may result from the abnormal segregation in carriers of translocations or inversions.

INSERTIONS. Insertions occur when a piece of chromosome breaks at two points and is incorporated into a break in another part of a chromosome. This requires three breakpoints and may occur between two chromosomes or within one.

Sex Chromosome Anomalies

TURNER SYNDROME. This is one of the most common monosomies in liveborn humans (see Chapter 538). The chromosomal

■ TABLE 67–3 Microdeletions and Their Clinical Manifestations

Deletion	Syndrome	Clinical Manifestations
7q23–	Williams	Round face with full cheeks and lips, stellate patterned in iris, strabismus, supravalvular aortic stenosis and other cardiac malformations, varying degrees of mental retardation, and a very friendly personality
8q24–	Langer-Gideon or tricho-rhino-phalangeal	Sparse hair, multiple cone-shaped epiphyses, multiple cartilaginous exostoses, bulbous nasal tip, thickened alar cartilage, upturned nares, prominent philtrum, large protruding ears, and mild mental retardation
11p13–	WAGR	Hypernephroma (Wilms tumor), aniridia, male genital hypoplasia of varying degrees, gonadoblastoma, long face, upward slanting palpebral fissures, ptosis, beaked nose, low-set poorly formed auricles, and mental redardation
15q11–13–pat	Prader-Willi	Severe hypotonia at birth, obesity, short stature, small hands and feet, hypogonadism, and mental retardation
15q11–13–mat	Angelman	Hypotonia, fair hair, midface hypoplasia, prognathism, seizures, jerky ataxic gait, uncontrollable bouts of laughter, and severe mental retardation
16p13–	Rubinstein-Taybi	Microcephaly, ptosis, beaked nose with low-lying philtrum, broad thumbs and toes, and mental retardation
17p13.3–	Miller-Dieker	Microcephaly, lissencephaly, pachygyria, narrow forehead, hypoplastic male external genitalia, growth retardation, seizures, and profound mental retardation
22q11–	DiGeorge CATCH 22	Hypoplasia or agenesis of the thymus and parathyroid glands, hypoplasia of auricle and external auditory canal, duplication and/or interruption of the aortic arch, cardiac aomalies

finding in Turner syndrome is the loss of part or all of one of the sex chromosomes. Half the affected individuals have 45,X. The other half have a variety of abnormalities of a sex chromosome. The phenotype in Turner syndrome is female. The frequency at birth is 0.4 per 1,000 (i.e., 1/4,000 liveborn females or 1/8,000 livebirths).

Turner syndrome is characterized by short stature and underdeveloped gonads. At least half of the affected individuals have some peripheral edema in the newborn period. One third of affected individuals are recognized at birth because of lymphedema and extra skin or webbing of the neck; one third are recognized during childhood, usually because of short stature; and one third are not recognized until they fail to go through puberty because of gonadal dysplasia. Cardiovascular and renal malformations are common.

Secondary sex characteristics do not appear in 90% of affected girls and hormonal replacement is required. Most individuals with Turner syndrome are infertile. Intelligence is usually normal, but there may be some learning disability. The diagnosis must be made by blood chromosome studies; buccal smear studies are inadequate.

From 5% to 10% of individuals with Turner syndrome have some Y chromosome material in all or some cells and are at risk for developing gonadoblastoma. A careful screening for Y chromosome material should be performed on any individual with Turner syndrome in whom no additional X chromosome (in addition to the one normal X) material has been found.

KLINEFELTER SYNDROME. These children have a male karyotype with an extra X chromosome, 47,XXY, and the phenotype is male (see Chapter 535). Individuals with Klinefelter syndrome are usually relatively tall. They may have gynecomastia and be slow to develop secondary sex development. They usually have azoospermia and small testes, and are infertile.

Many other syndromes occur in which there are extra X chromosomes (i.e., 47,XXX, 48,XXXX, 49,XXXXX, and 48,XXXY, 49,XXXXY). These individuals are often mosaic, having both a normal and an abnormal cell line (46,XX/47,XXX). In all of these syndromes the number of abnormalities increases with the number of X chromosomes and is specific to each syndrome. Abnormalities of chromosome Y also exist. The most common abnormality is the XYY male.

47,XYY MALE. The frequency of XYY males has been estimated to be 1 in every 1,000 livebirths. Because XYY males do not have any striking phenotypical abnormality, this frequency has been estimated from newborn surveys. XYY males are said to be relatively tall and may have some behavioral problems.

Fragile Sites

Fragile sites are defined as regions of chromosomes that show a tendency to separation, breakage, or attenuation under particular growth conditions. Numerous fragile sites have been identified.

FRAGILE X SYNDROME. The fragile site located on the distal long arm of chromosome X at Xq27.3 has been associated with the fragile X syndrome, which is the most common form of mental retardation in males. This fragile site only becomes visible in chromosome studies when it is induced under special culture techniques; regular metaphase studies do not demonstrate the fragile site. The fragile site may not always be visible, even with the appropriate chromosome preparation. The diagnosis of fragile X is now usually made by DNA studies, which demonstrate an expanded segment of DNA from the Xq27.3 region.

The main *clinical manifestations* in affected males are mental retardation, macro-orchidism, and characteristic facial features, including long face, prominent jaw, and large prominent ears. Females affected with fragile X usually only show varying degrees of mental retardation.

The *inheritance of fragile X* is different from the usual single gene inheritance patterns. Three distinct categories of DNA variation occur at the fragile X locus (normal, premutation, and symptomatic). In the normal state the fragment consists of approximately 2,800 trinucleotide repeat base pairs. A person who carries a small increase of trinucleotide repeats without the phenotypic abnormalities is said to be a carrier of a premutation. This usually consists of a 50–600 base pair increase. When inherited, this premutation is unstable and may expand over a few generations, gradually increasing in size when transmitted by females but remaining the same when transmitted by males. As the mutation is transmitted by a female and increases in size, it may become of a size (usually an additional 600–3,000 base pairs) that is clinically significant and leads to the typical fragile X syndrome phenotype with mental retardation.

The fragile X syndrome is due to *allelic expansion.* Allelic expansion refers to a change (increase or decrease) in the size of a particular DNA sequence. The expansion begins as a small increase in the copy number of trinucleotide repeats. The number of repeats may be unstable and may develop different sizes in different cells or tissues. The number of repeats may increase in size from one generation to the next. A change in size of the DNA segment between generations or in tissues means that this type of mutation differs from classical mutations in which the change in DNA sequence usually occurs

■ TABLE 67–4 Allelic Expansion

Gene	Location	Normal	Premutation	Affected	Parent of Origin Effect
Huntington disease	4p16.3	11–24 repeats	30–38	42–82	Male transmission usually increases repeat
Myotonic dystrophy	19q13.3	5–37 repeats	37–50	>50	Male may decrease repeat Female usually increases repeat
Fragile X	Xq23.7	6–54 repeats	52–200	>200	Male constant Female may markedly increase repeat

once and is then passed on from generation to generation. Some of the disorders associated with allelic expansion are fragile X syndrome, myotonic dystrophy (MD), and Huntington disease (HD).

The number of copies seen in disorders associated with allelic expansion may be related to the age of onset and severity of the disease (Table 67–4). For example, the congenital form of myotonic dystrophy is known to occur with the largest number of repeats but only when it is transmitted by the mother. In Huntington disease, the juvenile onset form of the disease is also associated with the largest number of repeats and occurs primarily when inherited from the father.

Chromosomal Breakage Syndromes

There are a number of recessive disorders that are associated with breakage and/or rearrangement of chromosomes. The breaks may be spontaneous or they can be induced by a variety of environmental agents and different techniques. Chromatid breaks are found in Fanconi anemia, Bloom syndrome, incontinentia pigmenti, and Werner syndrome. Breaks and nonrandom rearrangements of chromosomes 7 and 14 have been reported in ataxia-telangiectasia. A special cytogenetic study called sister chromatid exchange can be used in some of these disorders for carrier detection and prenatal diagnosis. These disorders have specific phenotypes, but the growth impairment, malformations, and other dysmorphic features have not been directly attributed to the chromosome breaks.

Mosaicism

Mosaicism is the term used to describe an individual who has two different cell lines derived from a single zygote (fertilized egg) (see Fig. 67–3). Studies of placental tissue from chorionic villus sampling show that at least 2% of all conceptions are mosaic for chromosomal anomalies at or before 10 wk of pregnancy. Compared to complete trisomies, which are usually nonviable for chromosomes other than 13, 18, and 21, the development of a normal cell line may allow a trisomic conception of other chromosomes to come to term and be viable. If a normal cell line develops, the fetus may survive and the original trisomic cell line may even be lost.

Germline mosaicism refers to the presence of mosaicism in the germ cells found in the gonad. This type of mosaicism may be suspected in cases in which there is more than one affected offspring with the same genetic abnormality (usually inherited as a chromosomal or dominant disorder) with phenotypically normal parents.

Depending upon the point at which the new cell line arises during early embryogenesis, a patient may have a variety of clinical presentations. Mosaicism may be present in some tissues and not in others, giving the affected individual a patchy or asymmetric distribution of abnormalities. Cytogenetic studies of fibroblasts must be done to identify mosaicism because blood lymphocyte cells may not tolerate some trisomies and chromosomal rearrangements.

PALLISTER-KILLIAN SYNDROME. This disorder is characterized by coarse facies, pigmentary skin anomalies, localized alopecia, diaphragmatic hernias, cardiovascular anomalies, supernumerary nipples, and profound mental retardation. The syndrome is due to mosaicism for isochromosome 12p. The presence of the isochromosome 12p in cells gives four copies of 12p in the affected cells. The isochromosome 12p is preferentially cultured from fibroblast and is seldom present in lymphocytes. The abnormalities seen in affected individuals probably reflect the presence of abnormal cells during early embryogenesis.

HYPOMELANOSIS OF ITO. This entity is characterized by unilateral or bilateral macular hypopigmented whorls, streaks, and patches. Abnormalities of the eyes, musculoskeletal system, and central nervous system may also be present. Patients with hypomelanosis of Ito appear to have two genetically distinct cell lines. The chromosome anomalies that have been observed involve both autosomes and sex chromosomes and have been demonstrated in about 50% of cases. The mosaicism may not be visible in chromosome studies done on blood but is more likely to be found when the chromosomes are obtained from skin fibroblasts. Sometimes the distinct cell lines may not be due to observable chromosomal anomalies but to single gene mutations or other mechanisms.

UNIPARENTAL DISOMY

Uniparental disomy (UPD) is the term used when both chromosomes of a pair of chromosomes in a person with a normal

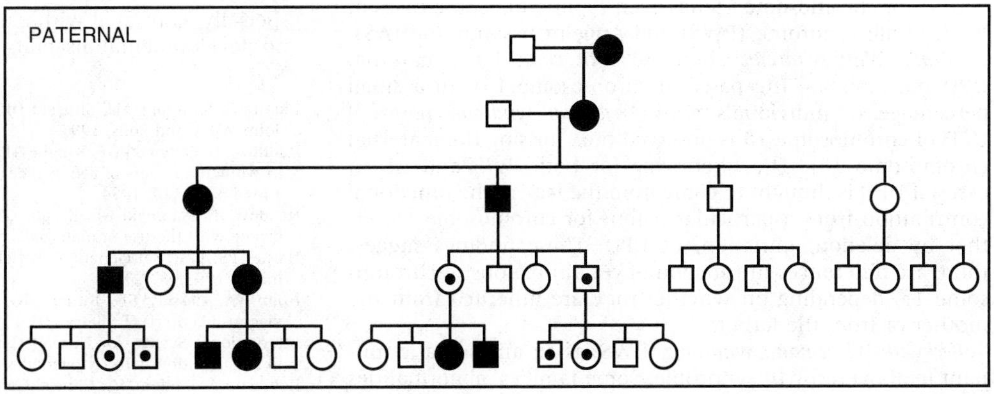

Figure 67–7. In pedigrees suggestive of paternal imprinting, phenotypic effects will occur only when the gene is transmitted from the mother but not when transmitted from the father. There will be an equal number of males and females affected and nonaffected phenotypically in each generation. A nonmanifesting transmitter will give a clue to the sex of the parent who passes the expressed genetic information; in other words, in paternal imprinting there will be "skipped" female nonmanifesting individuals.

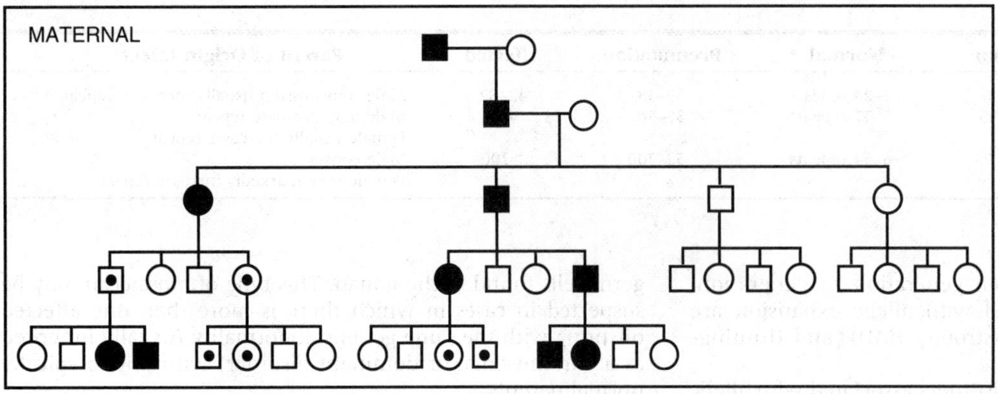

Figure 67–8. In pedigrees suggestive of maternal imprinting, phenotypic effects will occur only when the gene is transmitted from the father but not when transmitted from the mother. There are equal number of males and females affected and nonaffected phenotypically in each generation. A nonmanifesting transmitter will give a clue to the sex of the parent who passes the expressed genetic information; in other words, in paternal imprinting there will be "skipped" female nonmanifesting individuals.

number of chromosomes have been inherited from only one parent. Uniparental isodisomy means that the two chromosomes are identical, while uniparental heterodisomy means that the two chromosomes are different members of a pair. The phenotypical result of UPD may vary according to the specific chromosome involved, the parent who contributed the chromosomes, and whether it is isodisomy or heterodisomy. Two types of phenotypic effects are seen in UPD: (1) those related to imprinted genes (see later), that is, the absence of a gene expressed only when inherited from one parent (these phenotypic effects appear to be primarily on growth, behavior, placenta, and viability) and (2) those related to autosomal recessive disorders.

Because with isodisomy both chromosomes in a pair are identical, consequently the genes in both chromosomes will also be identical. This becomes particularly important for carriers of an autosomal recessive disorder. If the offspring of a carrier parent has isodisomy for a chromosome with an abnormal gene, the abnormal gene will be present in two copies and the phenotype will be one of the autosomal recessive disorder; however, only one parent is actually a carrier of the recessive disorder. This possibility must be kept in mind in situations in which an individual is affected with more than one recessive disorder.

Maternal isodisomy for chromosome 7 has been reported in two patients with cystic fibrosis. Both patients had intrauterine growth retardation and short stature. Another individual reported to have maternal isodisomy for chromosome 7 had intrauterine and postbirth growth retardation and unusual bones. Uniparental disomy, however, is not always associated with phenotypical abnormalities. UPD for chromosomes 21 and 22, for example, is not known to have any deleterious effect. Because maternal uniparental disomy of chromosome 7 has been associated with intrauterine growth retardation, it should be considered in cases of individuals with intrauterine growth retardation and unexplained growth delay.

UPD for chromosome 15 has been reported in some cases of Prader-Willi syndrome (PWS) and Angelman syndrome (AS). In *Prader-Willi syndrome* about 60% of cases have maternal UPD (i.e., missing the paternal chromosome 15). In a small percentage of individuals with *Angelman syndrome* paternal UPD of chromosome 15 is observed (i.e., missing the maternal chromosome 15). The phenotype for both PWS and AS in cases of UPD is thought to come from the lack of the functional contribution from a particular parent for chromosome 15, either by deletion, mutation, or UPD. These findings suggest there are differences in function of certain regions of chromosome 15, depending on whether they are inherited from the mother or from the father.

Beckwith-Wiedemann syndrome (BWS) is an autosomal dominant fetal overgrowth syndrome. Some families' abnormalities have been mapped to the short arm of chromosome 11. Recently sporadic cases of BWS have been associated with a duplication of paternally derived 11p15. A few cases have shown paternal UPD for 11p15 (paternal disomy/maternal deficiency). The gene for insulin growth factor 2 (Igf2) lies in this region, and studies have shown that only the paternal copy of Igf2 is expressed. Igf2 is believed to have a critical role in the growth of undifferentiated cells, and inactivation of the paternal gene in mice causes growth retardation. Overproduction of Igf2 caused by two functioning paternal genes could explain the fetal overgrowth phenotype seen in BWS.

IMPRINTING

Genomic imprinting refers to the observation that phenotypic expression depends on the parent of origin for certain genes and chromosome segments. Whether the genetic material is expressed depends on the sex of the parent from whom it was derived. Genomic imprinting is suspected on the basis of a pedigree (Figs. 67–7 and 67–8). Imprinting probably occurs in many different parts of the human genome and is important in gene expression, development, cancer, evolution, and human disorders.

The classic examples of imprinting in humans are the phenotypic differences seen in Prader-Willi and Angelman syndromes, which are associated with deletion and uniparental disomy of chromosome 15. In Prader-Willi syndrome the deletion, when it occurs, is always of the paternally derived chromosome 15, suggesting that the phenotype of Prader-Willi is due to a lack of paternally derived genetic information carried on that segment of chromosome 15. In contrast, when there is a deleted chromosome 15 in Angelman syndrome, the deleted chromosome is always maternal in origin, that is, there is lack of maternal information and the UPD is always paternal. The clinical manifestations of Prader-Willi syndrome change with age. Hypotonia is prominent in infancy. Obesity, mild mental retardation or learning disability, and behavioral problems, especially associated with eating, result in debilitating physical and developmental disability in adolescence.

Eldon JG, Simmons MJ, Snustad DP: Principles of Genetics, 8th ed. New York, John Wiley and Sons, 1991.

Haddow JE, Palomaki GE, Knight GJ, et al: Reducing the need for amniocentesis in women 35 years of age or older with serum markers for screening. N Engl J Med 330:1114, 1994.

Haddow JE, Palomaki GE, Knight GJ, et al: Prenatal screening for Downs syndrome with the use of maternal serum markers. N Engl J Med 327:588,1992.

Harper PS: Practical Genetic Counselling, 4th ed. Oxford, Butterworth, Heinemann, 1993.

Holm VA, Cassidy SB, Butler MG, et al: Prader-Willi syndrome: Consensus diagnostic criteria. Pediatrics 91:398, 1994.

International System for Human Cytogenetic Nomenclature (ISCN): Published in collaboration with Cytogenetics and Cell Genetics, 1985.

Robinson A, Linden MG: Clinical Genetics Handbook, 2nd ed. Oxford, Blackwell Scientific, 1993.

Stevenson RE, Hall JG, Goodman RM: Human Malformations and Related Anomalies. Oxford, Oxford Monographs on Medical Genetics, 1993.
Thompson M, McInnes R, Willard H: Genetics in Medicine, 5th ed. Philadelphia, WB Saunders, 1991.

CHAPTER 68
Gene Therapy

Gregory A. Grabowski and Jeffrey A. Whitsett

The unprecedented advances in understanding the genetic basis of human diseases are based on the application of molecular biology to clinical medicine. Techniques derived from virology, bacteriology, biochemistry, and cell and molecular biology permit the rapid identification of gene loci that cause or contribute to diseases in humans. Further, the goals of the Human Genome Project are to map, clone, and sequence the 3.3 billion base pairs of DNA that comprise the human genome. The ability to manipulate DNA makes it possible to transfer corrected or correcting genes for therapy of genetic and gene-influenced diseases.

DEFINITION OF GENE THERAPY

Gene therapy is the transfer of recombinant DNA, transiently or permanently, into human cells for correction of disease (Table 68–1). Vectors or gene transfer vehicles transfer plasmid DNA, RNA, or oligonucleotides into target cells, altering expression of specific mRNA that directs the synthesis of a therapeutic protein by the "transfected" cells. The vector is formulated to bind and be internalized by target cells. Vector DNA is transported to the cell nucleus, where the transcriptional machinery of the cell produces a recombinant mRNA. The recombinant RNA is processed and exported from the nucleus to the ribosomes, where translation of the RNA produces the therapeutic protein product. The recombinant protein may correct cellular defects in the target cell or be secreted to alter cellular metabolism at distant sites. Vector DNA may be degraded by lysosomes, maintained within the nucleus as an episomal particle, or integrated permanently into the genome of the host cell. When it is maintained as a nuclear episome, loss of the recombinant DNA will occur with each cell division; expressions depend on the mitotic rate and turnover of the target cells. If recombinant DNA is permanently integrated into the chromosomes of host progenitor cells that are capable of self-renewal, DNA is permanently transferred to all daughter cells. Transfer and integration of genes into germ cells results in a generationally transmitted trait. Germline transfer is routinely achieved in a variety of laboratory mammals, producing transgenic animals. While DNA can be transferred into both somatic and germline cells, only transfer into somatic cells is considered ethical. Intense discussions about the medical, ethical, social, and economic impact of somatic cell or germline gene therapy have accompanied the technical advances that permit gene transfer for human diseases. (See Chapter 3.)

■ TABLE 68–1 Candidate Diseases for Gene Therapy

Single Gene Defects	Gene(s) Involved	Target Organs/ Tissues
Severe combined immunodeficiency	Adenosine deaminase	Lymphoid tissue
α1-Antitrypsin deficiency	α1-Antitrypsin	Lungs (emphysema), liver (cirrhosis)
Cystic fibrosis	Cystic fibrosis transmembrane regulator	Lungs, pancreas
Hemophilia A and B	Factor VIII and IX	Blood clotting
Gaucher disease	Acid β-glucosidase, glucocerebrosidase	Macrophages; liver spleen, lungs
β-Hemoglobinopathies	β-globin	Blood formed elements
Hypercholesterolemia, familial	LDL receptor	Liver; vascular, endothelial; smooth muscle cells
Phenylketonuria	Phenylalanine hydroxylase	Liver
Complex Traits	**Genetic Approach**	**Target Organs/ Tissues**
Cancer	Cytokine, HLA genes, thymidine kinase, p53	Various
HIV-1	Antisence constructs, immunoenhancers	Immune system

Recombinant DNA technology makes it possible to use DNA or genes as therapeutic agents or drugs. Retrovirus, adeno-associated virus, and adenovirus provide delivery vehicles or vectors to transfer the recombinant DNA molecules to a variety of cells and organs. While initial concepts of gene therapy were directed to transfer of genes to somatic cells to correct single gene disorders, that is, inborn errors of metabolism, the field now includes treatment of cancers, infectious diseases, and other acquired disorders. Human disease might also be treated by genes that alter cellular activities or that enhance the properties or activities of existing normal genes. Gene therapy encompasses the broader area of genetic therapeutics, which includes the use of pluripotent stem cell organoids and the use of both prokaryotes and eukaryotes (both plants and animals) as bioreactors for the production of recombinant molecules of therapeutic interest.

SOMATIC VERSUS GERMLINE GENE THERAPY

Germline gene therapy is the permanent introduction of genetic material to germ cells, which allows generational passage of the genes to offspring; transfer of DNA to somatic cells that cannot be transmitted to new generations is called somatic cell gene therapy. Most diseases under consideration for gene therapy result from single genes or interactions among multiple genes, and the affected individual is the target of somatic gene therapy. Treatment is directed to individuals who are affected by or predisposed to the development of significant life-threatening disease. Germline gene therapy would result in the permanent introduction of new or altered traits into the human population. Because it is not possible, or potentially desirable, to "correct" or alter predisposing genes that might be considered as deleterious prior to conception of individuals, germline gene therapy has had no place in the current model of medicine. Germline gene therapy is not being considered or conducted in the United States and is essentially banned worldwide.

VECTORS—DELIVERY SYSTEMS FOR GENES

Design of Transcriptional Unit for Somatic Cell Gene Therapy

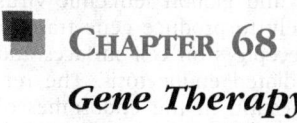

Recombinant complementary DNA (cDNAs) or genes encoding therapeutic proteins, like all eukaryotic or prokaryotic genes, must contain all the elements required to direct the transcription of the gene, including a start site, and the promoters and enhancers that determine the level and cell-specific regulation of the production of mRNA encoding the therapeutic gene product. Transcriptional control of the introduced gene is directed by the nucleotide sequences (*cis*-acting elements) that are recognized by nuclear proteins (*trans*-acting factors)

present in target cells. These *trans*-acting factors direct transcription (the production of RNA from the DNA) of the inserted gene. Transcriptional elements, including enhancers, promoters, silencers, transcriptional start sites, RNA splice-donor sites, termination and polyadenylation signals that can be incorporated to achieve the desired levels of mRNA, and tissue and cell specificity, or other features of gene regulation may be required to achieve the physiologic correction conferred by the recombinant protein. More complex constructs containing cell-specific promoter-enhancers and/or DNA sequences that control mRNA stability can be engineered into the vectors to confer cell specificity and the ability to control the levels of mRNA produced from the inserted gene. A large repertoire of prokaryotic and eukaryotic promoter-enhancer elements has been developed for achieving appropriate levels of gene expression in specific target cells.

Vector Systems

An idealized vector would be capable of direct in vivo administration through a variety of routes, provide for targeted (tropic) delivery to cells of interest, be safely integrated into the genome in somatic cells, and be transferred to all daughter cells. The site of gene integration would be specific and would include the excision of the defective gene and its replacement by the normal gene. Finally, the vector would be integrated in nononcogenic sites in the genome and require a single administration. While significant progress has been made in resolving many technical obstacles, available vectors do not satisfy any of these criteria. Viral, ligand-targeted, and DNA encapsulation vectors are being used to deliver genes (Table 68–2). Each of these methods has distinct limitations and advantages, but none has been fully exploited for therapeutic use.

Viral Vector Systems

Retroviral, adenoviral, and adeno-associated vectors (AAV) are being used in human gene therapy protocols. Viral vectors for gene therapy must be nontoxic, monogenic, and replication defective. The use of viral vectors for human gene therapy requires substantial modification of the genomes of the wild-type viruses prior to their use. For example, retroviruses are oncoviruses, and expression of their unmodified genomes predisposes the infected organism to malignancy. Adenoviruses can cause severe pulmonary infections, stimulate the host immune system, and must be administered repeatedly for correction of genetic disorders because they do not integrate. Although adeno-associated virus (AAV) is nonpathogenic in humans, its small capacity for DNA insertion and its requirement for adenovirus to complement its production have limited its utility. Because of the need to render the vectors nonpathogenic, substantial parts of the viral genome are removed, crippling the replication capacity of the virus in vivo. Cell lines allowing replication and encapsulation of the defective recombinant virus in vitro are required for these vectors.

■ TABLE 68–2 Vectors for Gene Therapy

Plasmid DNA (naked, liposomes, ligand-DNA complexes)
Transient expression
Retrovirus (RNA virus)
Cell division required
Integration into host genome
Adenovirus (DNA virus)
Transient expression
Stable virus
Antigenic
Adeno-Associated Virus (DNA-parvovirus)

The technical details of the "packaging cell lines" are vector specific, but concepts governing their use are similar.

RETROVIRAL VECTORS. Retroviral approaches illustrate the design of packaging cell systems that produce noninfectious virus capable of gene transfer. The genomic structure and life cycle of a recombinant retrovirus is shown in Figure 68–1. Moloney murine leukemic virus (MMLV) and gibbon leukemic virus (GLV) have been used most widely to produce gene transfer vectors. Retroviruses recognize receptors on cell surfaces and are internalized via receptor-mediated endocytosis. The retroviral RNA genome escapes digestion in the endosomes of the transfected cell and is delivered to the nucleus of dividing cells, where preformed viral reverse transcriptase synthesizes a DNA template of the viral genome during mitosis. The viral genome directs the synthetic processes of the host cell to produce its viral RNA genome and capsid proteins. Following encapsidation, the mature viral particles bud off from the plasma membrane of the packaging cell to produce infectious viral particles. The process of incorporation of genomic viral RNA and the use of preformed reverse transcriptase into a complete viral particle is termed *packaging* and requires a specific sequence called the psi (ψ) to signal the packaging events. The ψ sequence is provided in the genome of recombinant viruses used for gene therapy and initiates viral production in the packaging cell lines that complement the genes missing in the disabled retrovirus.

The retroviral genome contains five major elements, which include the long terminal repeats (LTRs) that are powerful promoters, the ψ sequence that signals packaging events, and three genes called GAG, POL, and ENV. These three genes encode encapsidation proteins, reverse transcriptase, and envelope proteins. Preformed reverse transcriptase carried into the cell with the virus is required for the production of the DNA genome from the viral RNA genome prior to viral replication and production of new viruses. Replication and expression of the viral genes can be separated from the packaging and production of infective viral particles. Consequently, most of the retroviral genome, and, in particular, the genes that encode for infectivity and oncogenesis (GAG, POL, ENV), can be removed and the therapeutic genes inserted into the regions of deleted genes. As long as the virus is packaged properly, the genes of the virus are delivered to the appropriate cells and the preformed reverse transcriptase produces the viral DNA for integration into the host genome. Transcription of the therapeutic gene product is directed by gene promoters, such as the retroviral LTRs or other promoter-enhancer sequences that can be engineered into the vector.

To achieve the disassociation between pathogenesis and the reproduction of the viral vector carrying the genes of interest, cell lines are produced containing the appropriate retroviral genes for packaging. The retroviral genome is permanently inserted into the chromosomes of the packaging cell line but lacks the ψ sequence. Consequently, a defective retrovirus, lacking GAG, POL, and ENV but containing the promoter, the ψ sequence, and the therapeutic gene, is transfected into the packaging cell line. The recombinant, defective retrovirus uses the packaging and encapsidation proteins from the genome of the packaging cell line to make infectious viral particles. Resultant viral particles do not contain the genes required for viral pathogenesis but incorporate the encapsulation proteins and the replication-defective recombinant viral RNA genome. High titer infectious viruses are then obtained by multiple passages through the packaging cell line. The "crippled" recombinant virus is used to transfect the recipient cells of interest, integrating the exogenous genes into the genome of the host cell. This single integration event does not produce additional viral particles and is termed *transfection* (Fig. 68–1).

Because intravenously administered retroviruses are rapidly inactivated, recombinant retroviruses must be delivered in

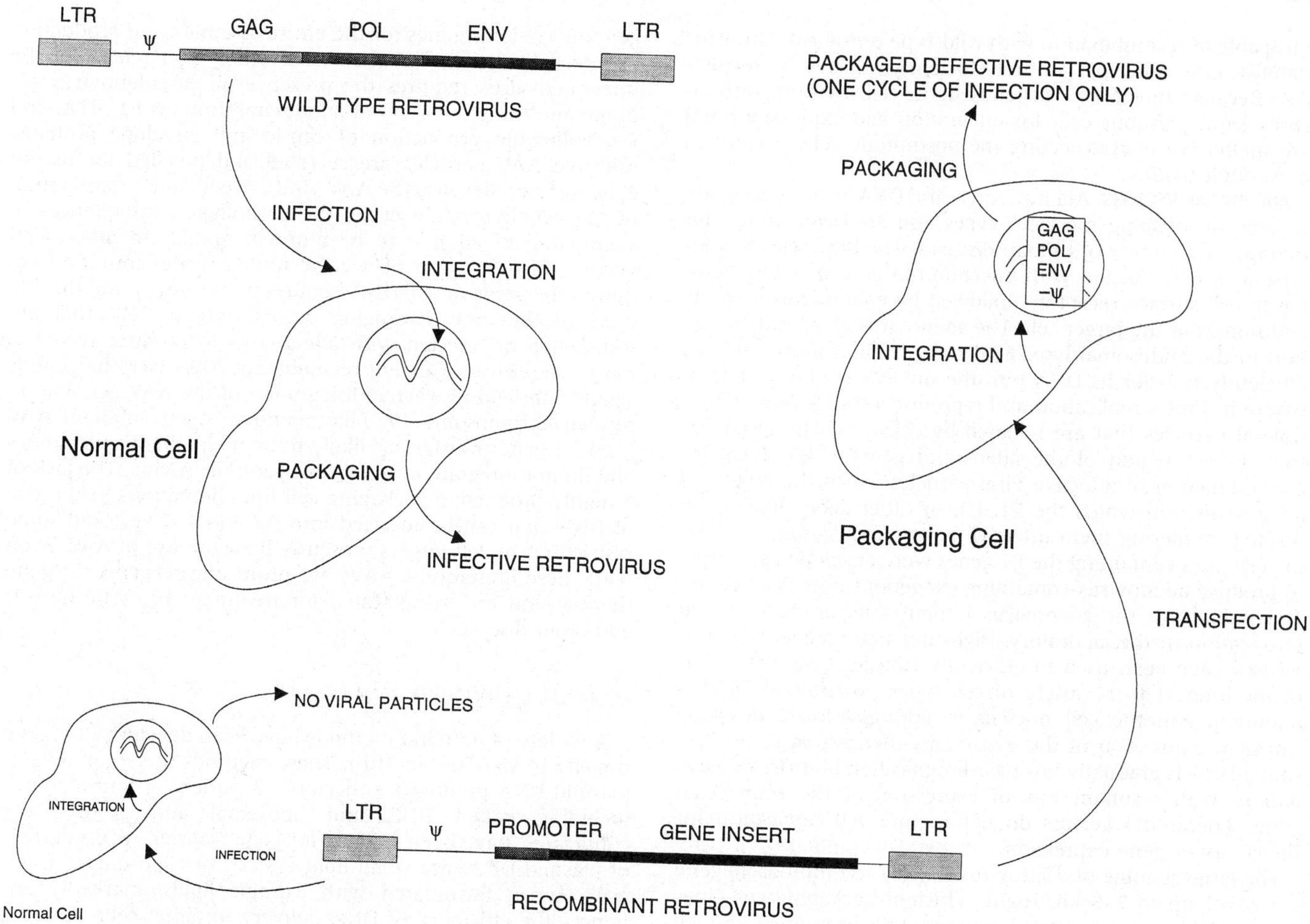

Figure 68–1. Life cycle and organization of wild-type and recombinant retrovirus genomes. Retroviruses bind to specific cellular receptors on the target cell surface and are internalized by receptor-mediated endocytosis. Following entry, the retroviral RNA genome is removed from its capsid coat and is reverse transcribed by viral reverse transcriptase into DNA that is transported to the nucleus, where integration into the host genome occurs. In wild-type virus, the life cycle is completed by the synthesis of viral proteins and RNA by the host cell, packaging the retroviral particle that is released by budding from the cell surface. Recombinant viruses containing the therapeutic gene or cDNA are replication incompetent, with the insert taking the place of the viral genes GAG, POL, and ENV. "Packaging" lines produce these retroviral genes in vitro, allowing encapsulation of virus and production of the infectious virions. The "packaged" recombinant virus contains an RNA copy of the therapeutic gene insert that can be used to infect target cells. The organization of the genome of wild-type and recombinant retroviral vectors is depicted.

high titer to the appropriate target cells, either by direct local application via physical injection, by organ infusion (i.e., portal vein to the liver), or by ex vivo transfection of stem cells that can be transplanted into the patient. Because of these properties and the clinical importance of hematopoietic disorders, pluripotent bone marrow stem cells have been a primary target for retroviral gene therapy (see Part XXI: Section 1). However, pluripotent stem cells make up a very small percentage of bone marrow cells; thus, the isolation of appropriate stem cells remains a major limitation in the development gene therapy. In order to be transfected, pluripotent stem cells must express receptors for retroviruses and undergo mitosis. Once the pluripotent stem cells are transfected with the retroviral vector, they can be returned to the patient so that the genetic abnormality in bone marrow–derived cells can be corrected. Long-term expression of transgenes has occurred in multiply transplanted mice and in humans receiving autologous bone marrow transplants of genetically marked cells, supporting the ability to transfect bone marrow progenitor cells with retroviruses.

Limitations of Retroviruses for Gene Transfer. Retroviral genomes can only incorporate genes of approximately 4 kb. Most cDNAs for human genes are about 2.5–3 kb in length; however, many genes, including hemoglobin, require genomic enhancer sequences on the 5′ and 3′ ends to direct their expression. This effectively limits the use of retroviruses to the transfer of relatively small genes or cDNAs that lack desirable regulatory sequences. The ability to permanently integrate exogenous genes into the human genome is a major advantage of retroviruses. However, integration is predominantly random, making possible integration into normal genes, leading to disrupted expression of essential genes. For example, insertion near a tumor suppressor gene could alter its expression and cause tumors. Although insertional mutagenesis remains an important theoretical and practical concern, such events appear to be rare. A more serious limitation to the safety of retroviruses for gene therapy is the potential recombination of the therapeutic virus with endogenous retroviruses that can complement the defective virus and allow production of infective retroviral particles. Such recombinations are likely to occur in the packaging cell lines, and major efforts have been directed to ensure the production of "minimal" retroviruses that are incapable of recombination with wild-type retrovirus. Unfortunately, many cell types are not efficiently infected by retrovirus. Because integration depends upon cell division, retroviruses require mitotic cells for integration and expression, and are ineffective in transfecting the postmitotic cells present in most adult tissues.

ADENOVIRAL VECTORS. Adenoviruses are DNA viruses that are capable of infecting most cell types and are being tested for therapy of a variety of human diseases. The life cycle of wild-type adenovirus begins with infection of the host cell by binding to cell surface receptors, followed by endocytosis into the endosomes of the target cell. The adenovirus escapes degradation in the endosomal/lysosomal compartment and is able to efficiently transfer its DNA into the nucleus of the host cells, where it directs replication and reproduction of infective adenoviral particles that are released by cell lysis. The discovery that the E1 region of the adenoviral genome is critical for the production of infective viral particles led to the design of adenoviruses in which the E1, E3, or other genes have been deleted, rendering them infective but nonreplicating. Packaging cell lines containing the E1 genes were developed and used to produce adenovirus-containing exogenous cDNAs or genes. The stability of the adenovirus facilitates its production and purification in the laboratory. High-titer noninfectious adenoviruses have been used to efficiently transfer genes of therapeutic interest to a variety of cell types. Adenoviral DNA is maintained in the cell nucleus in episomal form, directing transient expression of the exogenous therapeutic gene. Episomal DNA is gradually lost by cell replication and DNA degradation, with resultant loss of expression of the transfected gene. Adenoviral vectors do not require cell replication for infectivity or gene expression.

The large genome of adenovirus (75 kb) accommodates gene inserts of up to 7–8 kb. Highly efficient packaging cell lines are available, and powerful cell selective promoters can be incorporated into the constructs. In contrast to retroviral vectors, which require substantial ex vivo manipulation for infection of pluripotent stem cells, the adenoviral vectors are highly efficient in vivo for delivery of exogenous genes in a variety of cell types. For example, direct instillation of recombinant adenovirus into the respiratory tract is being studied for gene transfer of the cystic fibrosis transmembrane conductance regulator (CFTR) gene for therapy of cystic fibrosis. Administration of adenovirus into the portal vein in experimental animals directs high levels of gene expression in hepatocytes that could be used to transfer α-1-antitrypsin or blood clotting factors. The transient expression of the adenovirus-delivered genes is a major limitation to permanent gene therapy. Because adenoviruses are highly efficient, they may have advantages in the therapy of some diseases. For example, specific antitumor or highly toxic gene sequences could be used to treat malignancies.

ADENO-ASSOCIATED VECTORS (AAVs). AAV is a small (4.7 kb), parvovirus whose life cycle requires coinfection with adenovirus. AAV is nonpathogenic, infects dividing and nondividing cells, integrates into the human genome, and does not express its own genome following transfection of the target cell. Wild-type AAV is capable of site-specific integration on chromosome 19. Similar to retrovirus and adenovirus, production of AAV requires a packaging cell line for replication of recombinant vectors containing the genes of interest. Adenovirus must be added in vitro to achieve viral replication. The need for the adenovirus derives from the life cycle of the AAV. Infective viral particles enter cells via receptor-mediated endocytosis, and their DNA becomes integrated into the genome of cells. During this phase, the virus is nonreplicative and no additional viral particles are produced. Upon exposure of these cells to adenovirus, AAV replication and protein synthesis is activated and the life cycle of the adenovirus is terminated. The AAV genome contains genes for the entire assembly and production of infective viruses, but their "activation" and release of the integrated virus requires the presence of the adenovirus genome and the production of adenoviral proteins E1, E1A, and E4. Following production of capsid and envelope proteins, infective AAV particles are secreted and purified for use in gene transfer. Because the AAV viral cycle includes termination of the adenovirus life cycle, the pathologic consequences of adenoviral infection may be blunted. Similar to other viral vectors, incorporation of specific human genes into AAV requires the removal of DNA sequences necessary for the life cycle of the AAV. Packaging occurs only in cells that are transfected or infected with adenovirus to produce recombinant AAV viruses. Current recombinant AAVs lack the genetic signals that allow selective integration of the AAV genome on human chromosome 19. Like adenovirus, recombinant AAV used for gene transfer are likely to be maintained as episomes and do not integrate into the host genome in vivo. The lack of a highly productive packaging cell line, limitations in the size of DNA that can be inserted into AAV (<4–5 kb), and some restrictions in cell targets presently limit the use of AAV. Even with these limitations, AAVs are promising reagents for gene therapy and are being tested for treatment of cystic fibrosis and other diseases.

NONVIRAL METHODS OF GENE DELIVERY

A variety of nonviral methods have been developed for gene transfer in vivo and in vitro. These methods use recombinant, plasmid DNA produced in bacteria. A variety of formulations, including naked DNA and liposomal and protein-DNA conjugates, have been utilized for gene transfer. Incorporation of plasmid DNA into small lipid vesicles or "liposomes," especially when formulated with cationic lipids, markedly enhances the efficiency of DNA delivery to target cells. Altering the composition of the liposomes changes the organ distribution and cellular specificity of the expression of the transferred genes. The lipid-DNA complex binds to the plasma membrane of target cells, perhaps via electrostatic interactions, and is internalized into the endosomes and lysosomes of the target cell. Some DNA escapes degradation in the lysosomes, is released to the cytosol, and is transported to the nucleus. The DNA is maintained as an episome in the nucleus of the target cells. Because DNA is not integrated into the genome, gene expression is transient, requiring repeated administration of DNA complexes to correct most genetic disorders. Nevertheless, transient expression may be sufficient for therapeutic effects in some diseases. Plasmid DNA vectors are likely to be applicable for gene therapy of cancer for which toxic genes would be required for relatively short periods of time. The efficiency of gene uptake of plasmid DNA can be further enhanced by linking the recombinant plasmid DNA to proteins (ligands) that bind efficiently to cell surface receptors. The DNA-protein complex may be designed to target specific cellular sites expressing receptors recognized by the ligand. Plasmid DNA is readily produced in large quantities in vitro, and there are no major limitations on the size of plasmid DNA that can be transferred into cells. Thus large cDNAs or genes, including complex regulatory elements, can be incorporated into plasmid-based gene transfer systems. Artificial chromosomes are also being designed for gene transfer.

HOST IMMUNITY AND GENE TRANSFER

Host immune responses, both humoral and cellular, remain a major hurdle in the application of gene transfer technology for therapy of genetic and acquired disease. Immune responses to the vector, as well as to the recombinant therapeutic protein, result in clearance of cells transfected by the vector.

Transfected cells expressing foreign antigens or the recombinant protein can be recognized as non-self. The generation of cytotoxic T cells directed against viral or therapeutic proteins results in the rapid immune cytolysis of transfected cells. Furthermore, neutralizing antibodies will block subsequent transfection by the vectors. Antibodies produced against the therapeutic protein may be recognized as foreign. Protein replacement therapy in hemophilia and Gaucher disease induces antibodies to the administered factor VIII or acid β-glucosidase in 10–15% of patients. The ability to remove genetically corrected cells from the patient may be of practical importance for effective gene therapy.

ALTERNATIVE STRATEGIES FOR GENE THERAPY

Implantation of genetically altered cells that secrete therapeutic gene products systemically or locally is another approach to gene therapy. This approach involves the development of "organoids." Cells that are genetically altered to produce high levels of a secretable gene product are expanded ex vivo. These cells are transplanted back into the recipient so that the gene product is secreted or delivered locally or systemically to a variety of cell types. Organoids have advantages for disorders that can be treated by a secreted protein that functions at distant cellular sites. Examples of this approach include expression of factor VIII for hemophilia, β-glucuronidase for correction of mucopolysaccharidosis (MPS) type VII, and various cytokines for treatment of cancer. The factor VIII cDNA can be permanently transferred to fibroblasts or other cells that are capable of post-translationally modifying and producing factor VIII zymogen for secretion into the circulation. Transfected ex vivo, the cells are placed subdermally, in blood vessels, in the peritoneal cavity, or are attached to synthetic membrane supports and transplanted into the recipient. Following vascularization of the graft, factor VIII is secreted into the circulation. Treatment of mucopolysaccharidosis type VII, a β-glucuronidase deficiency, might be achieved by organoids capable of attaching the specific ligand, mannose-6-phosphate, to the β-glucuronidase polypeptide. The β-glucuronidase–ligand complex may then be delivered to cells expressing mannose-6-phosphate receptors on their surface. The therapeutic enzymes would be delivered to the lysosomes of the target cell via the endosomal pathway, correcting the β-glucuronidase deficiency in cells bearing this receptor. The pathology of the visceral organs in animal models of MPS-type VII is reversible by this approach. Finally, cytokine or cytotoxic genes can be transferred to somatic cells that have been transplanted directly into sites of tumor involvement. The expression of the cytokines, acting as immuno-attractants, stimulates an immune response to the tumor cells. Producer cells containing a retrovirus that expresses herpes thymidine kinase gene have been injected into brain tumors, causing infection of adjacent tumor cells and rendering them susceptible to killing by nucleotide analogs (ganciclovir) that are metabolized to toxic compounds by the viral thymidine kinase (TK) but not by the host cell. Systemic administration of ganciclovir to the patient kills tumor cells expressing retroviral-TK.

DISEASE TARGETS FOR GENE THERAPY

Genetic diseases are invariably lethal targets for gene therapy (Table 68–1). *Adenosine deaminase deficiency* (ADA) is a prototypic genetic disorder that was chosen for initial gene therapy trials. Partial or complete deficiencies of ADA result in severe combined immune deficiency and loss of both T-cell or B-cell function. While bone marrow transplantation corrects ADA deficiency, many patients lack an appropriately matched bone marrow donor. The pathophysiology of the disease derives from the intracellular accumulation of a toxic purine intermediate, deoxyadenosine. Deoxyadenosine is cytotoxic to both T and B cells, resulting in the loss of cellular and humoral immunity, leading to recurrent infections that cause childhood death in patients with ADA deficiency. For gene therapy, autologous bone marrow of ADA patients was transfected ex vivo with a recombinant retrovirus containing the ADA cDNA and returned to cells of the patients. Because autologous marrow is used, the therapy represents a isogenic transplant that avoids graft-versus-host reactions. Correction of the recombinant cells results in their selective growth advantage so that the lymphoid cells expressing recombinant ADA are longer lived than uncorrected cells. Long-term expression of recombinant ADA has been achieved by gene therapy in two patients receiving the retroviral ADA–transfected marrow cells.

Currently, protein therapy with PEG-ADA infusions is used to treat children who lack the matched donors required for bone marrow transplantation (see Chapter 119.6). However, the long-term effects of PEG-ADA treatment have not been assessed, and the therapy leads to partial reconstitution of lymphoid immunity. Although PEG-ADA is now a lifesaving therapy for ADA patients, patients continue to develop serious infections. The early results of gene therapy for ADA deficiency appear promising for reconstitution of lymphoid immunity and represent the first successful application of gene therapy to treat human disease.

Hemoglobinopathies and other hematologic disorders are potential candidates for gene therapy (see Table 68–1). Because hematopoetic stem cells can be permanently transfected by retroviral vectors *ex vivo* and the cells returned to the marrow of the patient, disorders such as sickle cell anemia, thalassemias, Fanconi anemia type C, and other disorders of erythropoiesis and myelopoiesis are potentially amenable to gene therapy.

Gaucher disease and mucopolysaccharidosis VII (MPS-VII) are *lysosomal storage diseases* that are targets for gene therapy. Gaucher disease is caused by mutations in acid β-glucosidase, a protein found in the inner lysosomal membrane of the cell. The lack of MPS-VIII enzyme, β-glucuronidase, causes defects in the soluble lysosomal protein secreted from cells. Transfection of bone marrow progenitor cells with retrovirus containing the cDNAs encoding these proteins should correct the enzymatic defect in the macrophage/monocyte-derived cells. Because acid β-glucosidase is not secreted, correction of Gaucher disease by gene therapy requires transfection of a high percentage of these cells with retrovirus capable of inducing the synthesis of the acid β-glucosidase cDNA. Bone marrow ablation or pretreatment with effective enzyme therapy may be required to provide sufficient space for the growth of transfected bone marrow progenitor cells. Nevertheless, human trials using retroviral gene transfer have been initiated.

The major visceral pathology in MPS-VII derives from involvement of bone marrow monocyte/macrophage–derived cell lines and chondrocytes. Central nervous system involvement also occurs in this disease. Gene therapy for MPS-VII, with retroviral transfection of bone marrow progenitor cells, should provide functional macrophages that are distributed throughout the body and are capable of secreting the recombinant protein. By expressing high levels of β-glucuronidase, macrophages could also act as organoids producing the enzyme that will be taken up by macrophages in various organs. Visceral organ correction of the MPS-VII mouse indicates that both direct cellular correction and uptake of β-glucuronidase by macrophages may repair the metabolic abnormalities in MPS-VII. In the mouse model of MPS-VII, neither enzyme nor transplanted macrophages enter the brain, and pathologic correction was not achieved in that organ, while visceral manifestations of the disease were eradicated by gene transfer.

Mutations in the low density lipoprotein (LDL) receptor gene block LDL uptake in target cells, causing severe, premature atherosclerosis in affected patients (see Chapter 72.4). The normal

LDL receptor was transferred by retroviral vectors into hepatocytes isolated from the livers of patients with LDL receptor gene defects ex vivo. The transfected cells were grown in culture and reinjected into the patient's portal vein and recolonized the liver. To date, two patients have received this therapy, and evidence of decreased serum cholesterol levels was observed after reimplantation with the autologous, genetically corrected hepatocytes. This methodology should be useful for therapy of a variety of metabolic disorders, including phenylketonuria, clotting disorders, α-1 antitrypsin deficiency, and others.

Cystic fibrosis (CF) is the most common lethal genetic disease in whites, affecting approximately 1 in 2,500 infants in North America (see Chapter 363). Cystic fibrosis is caused by mutations in a membrane protein termed the *cystic fibrosis transmembrane conductance regulator* or CFTR. The CFTR is expressed primarily in epithelial cells and acts as a Cl^- transport protein that enhances Cl^- transport across the epithelial surfaces of numerous organs, including the lung, gastrointestinal tract, and pancreas. The most common mutation, a deletion of a phenylalanine codon at position 508 of the polypeptide, produces a CFTR protein that is not properly routed to the apical membrane of the affected cells and therefore fails to transport Cl^- following stimulation with 3′-5′ cyclic adenosine monophosphate (cAMP). Lack of Cl^- and fluid secretion results in the accumulation of mucus in the secretory ducts of many organs, including the liver, pancreas, gastrointestinal tract, reproductive organs, and lung. Strong evidence, in vivo and in vitro, supports the feasibility of transferring the wild-type CFTR to somatic cells of the epithelium of the lung for correction of the lethal pulmonary complications related to mucous plugging and recurrent infection seen in cystic fibrosis. A variety of viral and nonviral strategies for transfer of the CFTR cDNA have been actively studied in the laboratory. Phase I clinical trials, testing the ability to transfer the human CFTR cDNA with liposomes, adenovirus, and adeno-associated viruses have been initiated and more than 40 patients have been studied. Transfer of the CFTR to CF cells and animals with the CF gene defect restores Cl^- ion transport and can correct the intestinal obstruction in CFTR-deficient transgenic mice in the absence of discernible toxicity. The respiratory tract is uniquely accessible via the tracheal-bronchial tree and the systemic and pulmonary vasculatures. Therapeutic strategies using viral and nonviral vectors are being tested in the laboratory. While transfer of the CFTR cDNA to CF epithelial cells can restore normal ion transport properties to the cells, gene therapy for cystic fibrosis will remain a formidable scientific undertaking. Because the vectors fail to integrate into stem cells of the pulmonary epithelium, the present transfer vectors will require repeated administration to patients with cystic fibrosis. Vectors that are neither toxic nor immunologic will be required to correct the CF deficit throughout the life of patients with cystic fibrosis. Unfortunately, retroviruses do not efficiently transfect respiratory epithelial cells in vivo. A number of other genetic and nongenetic diseases of the lung are also being studied as targets for gene therapy, including lethal, hereditary surfactant protein B deficiency, α-1 antitrypsin deficiency, and pulmonary cancer.

RECOMBINANT PROTEIN THERAPIES

The production of recombinant human insulin and human growth hormone in *Escherichia coli* established the value of the application of recombinant DNA technology for the production of medicinal polypeptides. However, bacterial hosts are often incapable of fully processing and secreting many potentially therapeutic polypeptides that can only be produced in eukaryotic cells. The need for mammalian or eukaryotic expression cell systems derives from the specific post-translational processing requirements of many proteins, including proteolytic processing, oligosaccharide addition and modifications, and polypeptide folding required to produce functional, stable recombinant protein. Culture of genetically altered eukaryotic mammalian cells is used to produce many proteins for human therapeutics from recombinant bacteria, for example, DNAse, tissue plasminogen activator (TPA), erythropoetin, GM-CSF, and others. Transgenic animals and plants use the organism to produce human proteins. For example, transgenic goats and cattle have been produced in which the recombinant gene is expressed from promoters that are active only in the mammary gland, with the polypeptide being secreted into the milk. Active recombinant proteins are appropriately processed in the mammary gland and can be obtained in large quantities for therapeutic use. Similarly, domesticated plants, such as tobacco, have been used to express human transgenes in leaves.

PROTEIN MODELING AND ENGINEERING

Progress in structural biology and the use of site-directed mutagenesis to make mutations in polypeptide sequences that can be expressed by recombinant DNA technology makes it feasible to synthesize novel therapeutic proteins. The alteration of amino acids or groups of amino acids that compose functional domains in the polypeptide can improve synthesis rates, processing, stability, or biologic activity. Antigenicity of the proteins can be modified to overcome host cell immunity. Novel proteins can be designed for administration and the improved genes can also be transferred to direct the synthesis of the protein. Combining the approaches of genetic therapeutics and the rational design of proteins may overcome some of the limitations of gene transfer systems. For example, a gene encoding an engineered protein with an increased catalytic rate constant could be incorporated into cells, producing a protein with an enhanced therapeutic effect.

ETHICAL AND REGULATORY CONSIDERATIONS

Gene therapy is considered appropriate for somatic cell therapy of lethal disease but not for cells of the human germline. Extensive procedures have been developed to ensure rigorous scientific assessment of safety and efficacy in gene therapy trials, with final review by the Recombinant DNA Advisory Committee of the National Institutes of Health and required approval by the Food and Drug Agency. More than 200 individuals have been given recombinant cells or recombinant vectors for gene therapy of lethal diseases, including adenosine deaminase deficiency, cancer, cystic fibrosis, and familial hypercholesterolemia. Continued safeguards will be required as application of gene transfer is extended to other nonlethal diseases.

Blaese RM, Culver KW, Anderson WF: The ADA human gene therapy clinical protocol. Hum Gene Ther 1:331, 1990.

Culver KW: Gene Therapy: A Handbook for Physicians. New York, Mary Ann Liebert, Inc., 1994.

Davis BD: Germline gene therapy: evolutionary and moral considerations. Hum Gene Ther 3:336, 1992.

Revised points to consider (document). Hum Gene Ther 1:93, 1990.

Weibel NA, Walters L: Germline gene modification and disease prevention: Some medical and ethical perspectives. Science 262:533, 1993.

CHAPTER 69
Genetic Counseling

Judith G. Hall

When a child is born with multiple congenital anomalies or a family is diagnosed with a genetic disorder, talking with the family is not easy. Giving bad news is always difficult and the information is often somewhat technical. However, it is important to provide the family with as much information as possible in order for them to make informed decisions. Genetic counseling has been defined as "an educational process that seeks to assist affected and/or at risk individuals to understand the nature of a genetic disorder, its transmission and the options available to them in management and family planning."

In recent years the task of providing information about genetic diseases has been done with a team approach using highly trained medical geneticists and genetic counselors, but this information can also be provided by a family physician, pediatrician, or nurse. Genetic counseling must be done based on an understanding of genetic principles, the ability to recognize and diagnose genetic diseases and rare syndromes, and knowledge of the natural history of the disorder and its recurrence risk. Awareness of prenatal diagnosis and screening programs available in a particular region and access to information about new advances in genetic disorders and techniques are also necessary.

TALKING TO FAMILIES. The type of information provided to a family depends on the urgency of the situation, the need to make decisions, or the need to collect additional information. However, in simple terms there are three general situations in which genetic counseling becomes particularly important.

The first is the prenatal diagnosis of a congenital anomaly or genetic disease. This is a very difficult situation, and the need for information is urgent because a family must often decide whether to continue or terminate a pregnancy. The second type of situation occurs when a child is born with a congenital anomaly or genetic disease. This also requires urgent information, and decisions must be made immediately with regard to how much support should be provided for the child and whether certain types of therapy should be attempted. The third situation arises later in life when (1) a diagnosis with a genetic implication is made, (2) a couple is planning a family and there is a family history of the problem (e.g., a couple in which one carries a translocation or is a carrier of cystic fibrosis), or (3) when an adolescent or young adult has a family history of an adult-onset genetic disorder (e.g., Huntington disease or breast cancer). It is often necessary to have several meetings with a family, because all of their questions and concerns cannot be addressed at one time.

GENETIC COUNSELING. Providing accurate information to families requires (1) taking a careful family history and constructing a pedigree that lists the patient's relatives (including abortions, stillbirths, and deceased individuals) with their sex, age, and state of health; (2) gathering information from hospital records about the affected individual (and in some cases, other family members); (3) documenting the prenatal, pregnancy, and delivery history; (4) reviewing the available information concerning the disorder; (5) careful physical examination of the affected individual (with photographs and measurements) and of apparently unaffected individuals; (6) establishing or confirming the diagnosis by the diagnostic tests available; (7) giving the family information about support groups; and (8) providing new information to the family as it becomes available.

In order to provide optimal benefits, the counseling session must include certain information.

Knowledge of the Diagnosis of the Particular Condition. Although not always possible to make an exact diagnosis, having as accurate a diagnosis as possible is important. Estimates of recurrence risk for various family members depend on an accurate diagnosis. When a specific diagnosis cannot be made (as in many cases of multiple congenital anomalies), the various differential diagnoses should be discussed with the family and empirical information provided. If specific diagnostic tests are available, they should be discussed.

Natural History of the Condition. It is very important to discuss the natural history of the specific genetic disorder(s) in the family. Affected individuals and their families will have questions regarding the prognosis and potential therapy that can only be answered with knowledge of the natural history. If there are other possible differential diagnoses, their natural history may also be discussed. If the disorder is associated with a spectrum of clinical outcomes or complications, the worst and best scenario, as well as treatment and referral to the appropriate specialist, should be addressed.

Genetic Aspects of the Condition and Recurrence Risk. This is important information for the family because family members need to be aware of their reproductive choices. The genetics of the disorder can be explained with visual aids (i.e., figures of chromosomes, etc.). It is important to provide accurate occurrence and recurrence risks for various members of the family, including unaffected individuals, cousins, aunts, and so forth. In cases in which a definite diagnosis cannot be made, it will be necessary to use empirical recurrence risks. Counseling should give the individuals the necessary information to understand various options and to make their own informed decisions regarding pregnancies, adoption, artificial insemination, prenatal diagnosis, screening, carrier detection, and termination of pregnancy. In order to complete the educational process, it may be necessary to have more than one counseling session.

Prenatal Diagnosis and Prevention. There are many different methods of prenatal diagnosis available depending on the specific genetic disorder. The use of ultrasound allows prenatal diagnosis of anatomic abnormalities such as neural tube defects. Amniocentesis and chorionic villus sampling (CVS) are used to obtain fetal tissue for analysis of chromosomal abnormalities, biochemical disorders, and DNA studies. Maternal blood or serum sampling is used for some types of screening.

Therapies and Referral. There are a number of genetic disorders that require the care of a specialist. For example, individuals with Turner syndrome usually need to be evaluated by an endocrinologist. Prevention of known complications is a priority. The psychological adjustment of the family may require specific intervention.

Support Groups. Over the last few years a large number of lay support groups have been formed to provide information and fund research on specific genetic and nongenetic conditions. An important part of genetic counseling is to give information about these groups to individuals and to be able to suggest a contact person for the families.

Follow-up. Families should be encouraged to continue to ask questions and keep up with new information about the specific disorder. New developments often influence the diagnosis and therapy of specific genetic disorders. Lay groups are a good source of new information.

Stevenson RE, Hall JG, Goodman RM: Human Malformations and Related Anomalies. Oxford, Oxford Monographs on Medical Genetics, 1993, p 183.

PART X

Metabolic Diseases

CHAPTER 70

An Approach to Inborn Errors of Metabolism

Iraj Rezvani and David S. Rosenblatt

Many disorders originate in mutational events that alter the genetic constitution of an individual, disrupting normal function. Hundreds of human hereditary biochemical disorders, termed *inborn errors of metabolism* by Garrod at the turn of the century, have been discovered, and they are continually being discovered.

Now modern biochemical genetics can describe how genetic information is translated into the synthesis of proteins having specific metabolic or structural properties (see Chapter 64). An inherited mutational event can result in the alteration of either primary protein structure or the amount of the specific protein being synthesized. In either case, the functional ability of the protein, whether it is an enzyme, receptor, transport vehicle, membrane pump, or structural element, may be relatively or seriously compromised.

If the process affected by an inborn error of metabolism is essential for well-being and if the degree of alteration is sufficient to affect the system, clinical consequences may result. Some genetic changes are clinically inconsequential and are responsible only for the many polymorphic differences that set individuals apart. Others produce changes that express themselves only under conditions that may not be encountered during the lifetime of an individual. Still others, however, produce a disease state, which may range from very mild to lethal. Most inborn errors of metabolism exhibiting clinical consequences manifest themselves (or can be detected) in the newborn period or shortly thereafter. It is also now possible to screen and detect many of these disorders in utero (see Chapter 81).

Children with inborn errors of metabolism may present with one or more of a large variety of signs and symptoms. These may include metabolic acidosis, persistent vomiting, failure to thrive, developmental abnormalities, elevated blood or urine levels of a particular metabolite, for example, an amino acid or ammonia, a peculiar odor (Table 70–1), or physical changes such as hepatomegaly. Diagnosis is facilitated by considering those presenting in the neonatal period separately from children presenting later in life.

NEONATAL PERIOD. Inborn errors of metabolism causing *clinical manifestations* in the neonatal period are usually severe and are often lethal if proper therapy is not promptly initiated. Clinical findings are usually nonspecific and similar to those seen in infants with generalized infections. An inborn error of metabolism should be considered in the differential diagnosis of a severely ill neonatal infant, and special studies should be undertaken if the index of suspicion is high (Fig. 70–1).

Neonatal infants with metabolic disorders are usually normal at birth; however, signs and symptoms such as lethargy, poor feeding, convulsions, and vomiting may develop as early as a few hours after birth. A history of clinical deterioration in a previously normal neonate should suggest an inborn error of metabolism. This clinical course contrasts with many other genetic disorders or perinatal insults, which cause abnormalities from the time of birth. Occasionally, vomiting may be severe enough to suggest the diagnosis of pyloric stenosis, which is usually not present, although it has simultaneously occurred in such infants. Lethargy, poor feeding, convulsions, and coma may also be seen in infants with hypoglycemia (see Chapter 77) or hypocalcemia (see Chapter 56.9). Response to intravenous injection of glucose or calcium usually establishes these diagnoses. Because most inborn errors of metabolism are inherited as autosomal recessive traits, a history of consanguinity and/or death in the neonatal period in the immediate family should increase suspicion of this diagnosis. Some of these disorders have a high incidence in specific population groups. For instance, tyrosinemia type 1 is more common among French-Canadians of Quebec than in the general population. Therefore, the knowledge of ethnic background of the patient may be helpful in diagnosis. Physical examination usually reveals nonspecific findings, with most signs related to the central nervous system. Hepatomegaly, however, is a common finding in a variety of inborn errors of metabolism. Occasionally, an unusual odor may offer an invaluable aid to the diagnosis (see Table 70–1). A physician caring for a sick infant should smell the patient and his or her excretions; patients with maple syrup urine disease have the unmistakable odor of maple syrup in their urine and their bodies.

Diagnosis usually requires a variety of specific *laboratory studies*. Measuring serum concentrations of ammonia, bicarbonate, and pH is often very helpful in differentiating major causes of metabolic disorders (see Fig. 70–1). Elevation of blood ammonia is usually due to defects in urea cycle enzymes. These infants with elevated blood ammonia levels commonly have normal serum pH and bicarbonate, and without measurement

TABLE 70–1 Inborn Errors of Amino Acid Metabolism Associated with Abnormal Odor

Inborn Error of Metabolism	Urine Odor
Glutaric acidemia (type II)	Sweaty feet
Hawkinsinuria	Swimming pool
Isovaleric acidemia	Sweaty feet
Maple syrup urine disease	Maple syrup
Methionine malabsorption	Cabbage
Multiple carboxylase deficiency	Tomcat urine
Oasthouse urine disease	Hops-like
Phenylketonuria	Mousy or musty
Trimethylaminuria	Rotting fish
Tyrosinemia	Rancid, fishy, or cabbage-like

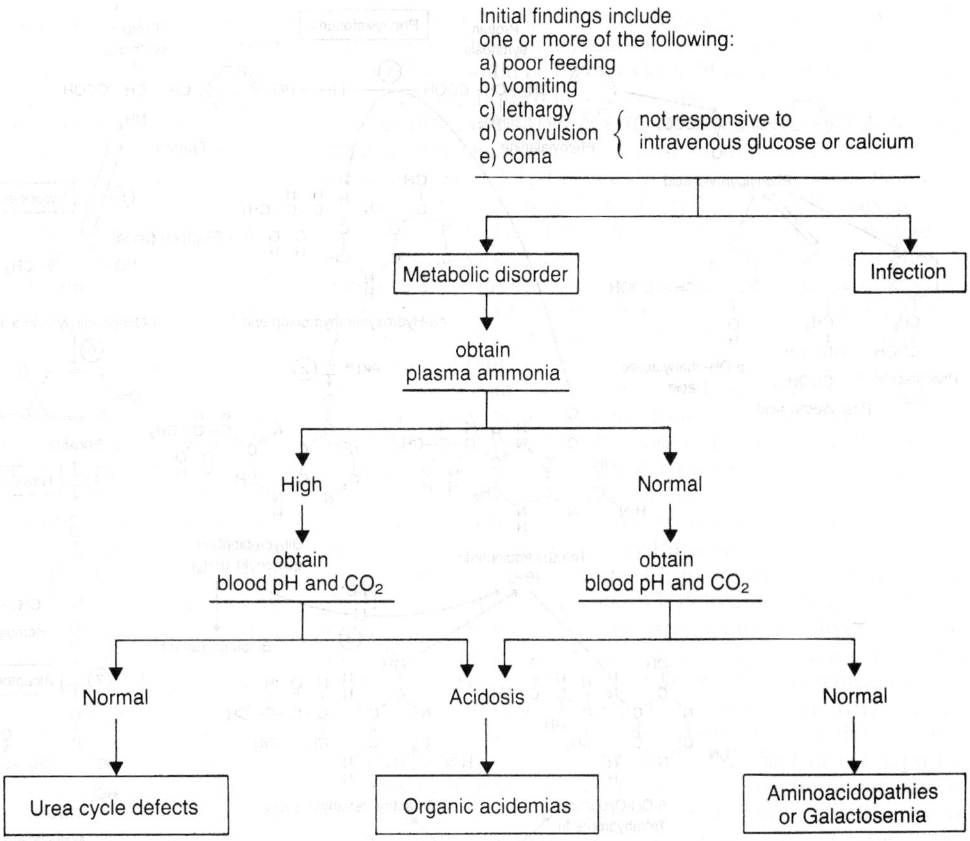

Figure 70–1. Clinical approach to a newborn infant with a suspected metabolic disorder. This schema is a guide to the elucidation of some of the metabolic disorders in newborn infants. Although some exceptions to this schema exist, it is appropriate for most cases.

of blood ammonia they may remain undiagnosed and succumb to their disease. Elevation of serum ammonia, however, has also been observed in some infants with certain organic acidemias. These infants are severely acidotic because of accumulation of organic acids in body fluids.

When blood ammonia, pH, and bicarbonate are normal, other aminoacidopathies, such as hyperglycinemia and galactosemia, should be considered; galactosemic infants may also manifest cataracts, hepatomegaly, ascites, and jaundice.

Most inborn errors of metabolism presenting in the neonatal period are lethal if specific *therapy* is not initiated immediately. Specific diagnosis, even in an infant in whom death seems inevitable, is of great importance for genetic counseling of the family (see Chapter 69). Therefore, every effort should be made to determine the diagnosis while the infant is alive; postmortem examination is usually not helpful.

CHILDREN AFTER THE NEONATAL PERIOD. Most inborn errors of metabolism that cause symptoms in the first few days of life exhibit milder variant forms that have a more insidious onset. These forms may escape detection during the neonatal period, and the diagnosis may be delayed for months or even years. The early clinical manifestations in children with these forms are commonly nonspecific and may be attributed to perinatal insults.

Clinical manifestations, such as mental retardation, motor deficits, and convulsions are the most constant findings in some of these children. There may be an episodic or intermittent pattern with episodes of acute clinical manifestations separated by periods of seemingly disease-free states. The episodes are usually triggered by a stress or a nonspecific insult such as an infection. The child may die during one of these acute attacks. An inborn error of metabolism should be considered in any child with one or more of the following manifestations: (1) unexplained mental retardation, developmental delay, motor deficits, or convulsions; (2) unusual odor, particularly during an acute illness; (3) intermittent episodes of unexplained vomiting, acidosis, mental deterioration, or coma; (4) hepatomegaly; or (5) renal stones.

Inborn errors of metabolism of a given pedigree run true to type. Thus, although symptomatology may vary among siblings, usually if one child in a family, for example, has the form of maple syrup urine disease manifested during the neonatal period, the next affected sibling will have the same defect, not the variant that occurs only intermittently later in childhood.

CHAPTER 71

Defects in Metabolism of Amino Acids

71.1 Phenylalanine

Iraj Rezvani

Phenylalanine is an essential amino acid. Dietary phenylalanine not utilized for protein synthesis is normally degraded via the tyrosine pathway (Fig. 71–1). Deficiency of the enzyme phenylalanine hydroxylase or of its cofactor tetrahydrobiopterin causes accumulation of phenylalanine in body fluids. Several clinically and biochemically distinct forms of hyperphenylalaninemia exist.

CLASSIC PHENYLKETONURIA (PKU). This form of the disorder is caused by the complete or near-complete deficiency of phenyl-

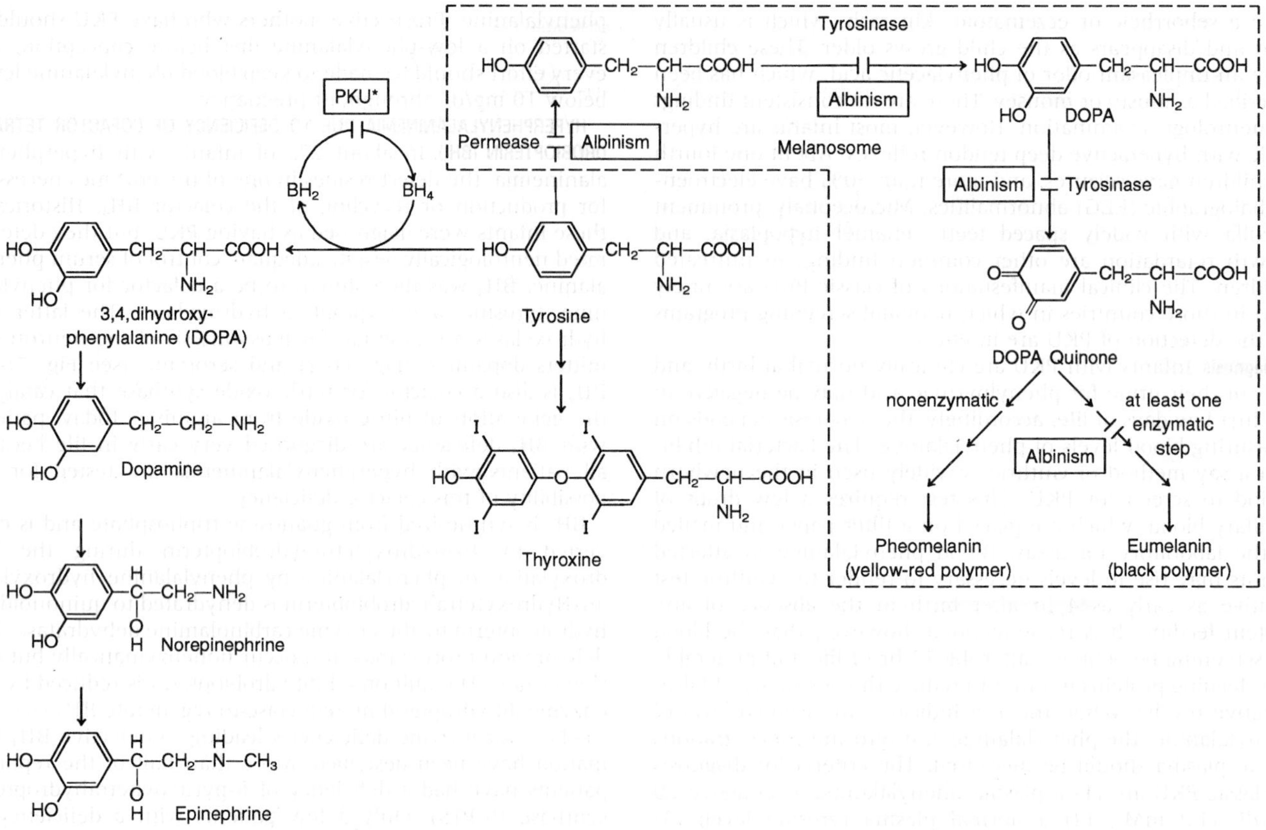

Figure 71–2. Other pathways involving tyrosine metabolism. PKU* = hyperphenylalaninemia due to tetrahydrobiopterin deficiency. (see Fig. 71–1.)

phenylalanine in the diet. Some patients with dihydropteridine reductase deficiency may not respond to this loading test.

3. Enzyme assay. The activity of dihydropteridine reductase can be measured in many tissues, including liver, leukocytes, red blood cells, and cultured fibroblasts. 6-Pyruvoyltetrahydropterin synthase can be measured in liver, kidney, and red blood cells. GTP cyclohydrolase can be measured in liver and in phytohemagglutinin-stimulated lymphocytes (the enzyme activity is normally very low in unstimulated lymphocytes). Measurement of the last two enzymes is technically difficult, and assays are not readily available.

4. Gene study. Genes for dihydropteridine reductase and carbinolamine dehydratase have been identified. Identification of mutations in these gene in affected patients and their families is now possible.

Treatment. The long-term efficacy of various therapies is unknown. The various treatment methods include the following:

1. Low-phenylalanine diet. Although phenylalanine does not prevent neurologic damage, such a diet in conjunction with the following therapies is recommended for at least the first 2 yr of life. High levels of phenylalanine inhibit the synthesis of neurotransmitters.

2. Neurotransmitter precursors. Administration of the L-dopa and 5-hydroxytryptophan seems to be the most effective treatment and may prevent neurologic damage if started early in life. Therefore, *all patients with PKU and hyperphenylalaninemia should be tested for BH_4 deficiency as early as possible.* Treatment started after 6 mo of age, although resulting in some improvement, has not reversed existing neurologic damage.

3. BH_4 replacement. Oral administration of the cofactor in small daily doses normalizes serum levels of phenylalanine. This compound, unless given at high doses (20–40 mg/kg/24 hr), does not readily cross the blood-brain barrier, and neurologic damage may continue to progress.

BENIGN HYPERPHENYLALANINEMIA. Infants with hyperphenylalaninemia are occasionally identified whose blood levels of phenylalanine are only slightly elevated; these concentrations are not enough (less than 20 mg/dL or 1.2 mM) to result in the excretion of phenylpyruvic acid. Like infants with classic PKU, these patients presumably have a deficiency of the phenylalanine hydroxylase enzyme but with some residual enzyme activity; measured activity has ranged from 1% to 35% of normal, in contrast to the nondetectable enzyme activity found in classic PKU. These infants have been detected by screening tests in the neonatal period; they are asymptomatic and may develop normally without special dietary treatment. They should, however, be tested for the presence of the cofactor tetrahydrobiopterin, and if it is deficient they should be treated accordingly (see earlier).

For infants who have serum phenylalanine concentrations in the range of 10–20 mg/dL, with normal tyrosine values and no PKU, a simple reduction of dietary protein intake may be sufficient to control serum concentrations of phenylalanine; if this is not effective, specific restriction of dietary phenylalanine is indicated. All infants who are not treated with dietary restriction should be systematically monitored with repeated determinations of plasma phenylalanine and developmental evaluations to establish the safety of continuing partial treatment or nontreatment. Periodic challenges with natural protein may be helpful in determining the need for continuing dietary restriction.

TRANSIENT HYPERPHENYLALANINEMIA. Moderately elevated levels of phenylalanine occur in transient tyrosinemia of the newborn infant (see Chapter 71.2). When the infant's ability to oxidize tyrosine matures, the elevated levels of tyrosine and phenylalanine return to normal.

Absence of or delayed maturation of phenylalanine transaminase can also produce hyperphenylalaninemia if the patient is fed milk with a high protein content. Such infants cannot produce much phenylpyruvic acid, even when their blood levels of phenylalanine approach 30 mg/dL; they have normal blood levels when fed milk products having the protein content of human milk.

GENETICS AND PREVALENCE. All defects causing persistent hyperphenylalaninemia and PKU are inherited as autosomal recessives. They have a collective prevalence of 1:10,000 to 1:20,000 live births, with classic PKU being the most common and GTP cyclohydrolase the rarest. The gene for phenylalanine hydroxylase is located on the long arm of chromosome 12. Many mutations of the gene have been described in different families. The genes for carbinolamine dehydratase and dihydropteridine reductase are located on the long arm of chromosome 10 and the short arm of chromosome 4, respectively. Prenatal diagnosis and carrier detection are possible using specific genetic probes in cells obtained from chorionic villus biopsy.

71.2 Tyrosine

Iraj Rezvani

Tyrosine, obtained from ingested protein and synthesized endogenously from phenylalanine, is used for protein synthesis and is a precursor of dopamine, norepinephrine, epinephrine, melanin, and thyroxine. Excess tyrosine is metabolized to carbon dioxide and water (see Fig. 71–1). At least two distinct clinical entities are associated with a persistent increase in plasma concentrations of tyrosine, but only in tyrosinemia type II are signs and symptoms attributed to high levels of tyrosine in body fluids. In hereditary tyrosinemia type I the causal relationship with increased tyrosine levels remains unclear. There are also patients who present varied clinical findings and tyrosinemia but do not fit into any specific category, and a transient form of tyrosinemia is seen in newborn infants.

TYROSINEMIA TYPE I (Tyrosinosis, Hereditary Tyrosinemia, Hepatorenal Tyrosinemia). In this condition, caused by a deficiency of the enzyme fumarylacetoacetate hydrolase, a moderate elevation of serum tyrosine is associated with severe involvement of the liver, kidney, and central nervous system. These findings are thought to be due to an accumulation of intermediate metabolites of tyrosine in the body, especially succinylacetone. Decreased activities of 4-hydroxyphenylpyruvate dioxygenase and maleylacetoacetate isomerase observed in this condition are presumed to be secondary phenomena (see Fig. 71–1).

Clinical Manifestations. There are two main forms of the disease: the neonatal or acute form, which comprises most reported cases, and the chronic or latent form. Intermediate forms also occur. Acute and chronic forms have been observed within the same family.

Infants having the *acute form* become symptomatic within the first 6 mo of life. Failure to thrive, developmental delay, irritability, vomiting, diarrhea, and fever are among the early manifestations. Hepatomegaly, jaundice, hypoglycemia, and bleeding tendencies as manifested by melena, hematuria, and ecchymosis are common findings. A cabbage-like odor of some infants is related to metabolites of methionine. Death from hepatic failure usually occurs before the 2nd yr of life.

In the *chronic form,* clinical manifestations may not appear until after the 1st yr of age. Failure to thrive, developmental delay, progressive cirrhosis, renal tubular dysfunction (Fanconi syndrome), and vitamin D–resistant rickets are characteristic. Episodes of acute polyneuropathy resembling acute porphyria have been observed in about 40% of affected infants. These episodes are characterized by severe pains in the legs (occasionally in the abdomen), hypertonia, vomiting, paralytic ileus, and occasionally self-mutilation. Elevation of urinary 5-aminolevulinic acid (presumably due to inhibition of 5-aminolevulinic hydratase by succinylacetone) has been observed in these patients, but the relationship of this abnormality to the polyneuropathic crises is unclear because the urinary excretion of 5-aminolevulinic acid remains elevated between the attacks. Death usually occurs by 10 yr of age from liver failure or hepatoma.

Laboratory findings include normocytic anemia and marked elevations of serum bilirubin (both conjugated and unconjugated), serum transaminases, and α-fetoprotein. An increase in serum levels of α-fetoprotein has been observed in the cord blood of affected infants, indicating intrauterine liver damage. Plasma levels of tyrosine and other amino acids, especially methionine, are moderately increased. Generalized aminoaciduria occurs. Urinary excretion of 5-aminolevulinic acid may be increased. The presence of succinylacetoacetate and succinylacetone in serum and urine is diagnostic (see Fig. 71–1). Liver histology is usually compatible with chronic active hepatitis and nonspecific cirrhosis. Hyperplasia of pancreatic islet cells is also a common finding.

This condition should be differentiated from other causes of hepatitis and hepatic failure in infants, including galactosemia, hereditary fructose intolerance, and giant cell hepatitis. *Diagnosis* is established by measurement of fumarylacetoacetate hydrolyase activity in liver biopsy specimens or fibroblast cultured cells. The degree of residual enzyme activity dictates the severity of the disease.

Treatment. A diet low in tyrosine, phenylalanine, and methionine may result in some clinical improvement in some patients. However, in most patients the progression of the disease cannot be halted by diet alone. Inhibition of the enzyme 4-hydroxyphenylpyruvate dioxygenase by 2-(nitro-4-trifluoromethylbenzoyl)-1-3-cyclohexanedione (NTBC) has been shown to cause significant improvement in clinical and biochemical findings in five patients with this condition. The long-term effect of this treatment, however, has not yet been determined. Liver transplantation, especially if performed early in the course of the disease, remains the most effective therapy.

Tyrosinemia type I is an autosomal recessive trait. The gene for fumarylacetoacetate hydrolase has been mapped to the long arm of chromosome 15. Most reported patients have a French-Canadian ancestry. The prevalence of the condition is estimated to be 1 in 1,846 newborn infants in the French-Canadian population of Quebec. A single mutation in the gene coding for the enzyme has been identified in this population. Prenatal diagnosis has been achieved by measurement of succinylacetone in amniotic fluid and by the enzyme assay in chorionic villus biopsy. Direct gene analysis is now possible in some families.

TYROSINEMIA TYPE II (Richner-Hanhart Syndrome, Oculocutaneous Tyrosinemia). This rare autosomal recessive disorder results in mental retardation, palmar and plantar punctate hyperkeratosis, and herpetiform corneal ulcers. Excessive tearing, redness, pain, and photophobia may occur before skin lesions. Corneal lesions usually occur during the first few months of life and are presumed to be due to tyrosine deposition; skin lesions may develop later in life. Mental retardation is usually mild to moderate and may be associated with self-mutilation.

Significant hypertyrosinemia (20–50 mg/dL) and tyrosinuria are present. The condition is due to the deficiency of the cytosolic fraction of hepatic tyrosine amino transferase (tyrosine transaminase). In contrast to tyrosinemia type I, liver and kidney functions, as well as serum concentrations of other amino acids, are normal.

Treatment with a diet low in tyrosine and phenylalanine has not only corrected the chemical abnormalities but has also resulted in dramatic healing of the skin and eye lesions. Mental retardation may be prevented by early dietary restriction of tyrosine. The gene for tyrosine aminotransferase is located on the long arm of chromosome 16.

TRANSIENT TYROSINEMIA OF THE NEWBORN. In a small number of newborn infants, plasma tyrosine may rise to as high as 60 mg/dL during the first 2 wk of life. Most affected infants are premature and are receiving high-protein diets. Lethargy, poor feeding, and decreased motor activity occur in some of them, but most are asymptomatic and come to medical attention because of a high blood phenylalanine level, rendering the Guthrie test for PKU screening positive. Tyrosinemia usually resolves spontaneously during the 1st mo of life. The condition is presumably due to delayed maturation of 4-hydroxyphenylpyruvate dioxygenase. The condition is often corrected promptly by reducing the amount of protein in the diet (to 2–3 g/kg/24 hr) and by administering vitamin C (200–400 mg/24 hr). Mild intellectual deficits have been reported in some full-term infants with this disorder. Because vitamin C is necessary for optimal functioning of the dioxygenase, it is not surprising that tyrosinemia occurs in patients with scurvy.

HAWKINSINURIA. This rare condition (named after the first affected family) is due to a deficiency of one of the components of the 4-hydroxyphenylpyruvate dioxygenase enzyme complex. This enzyme oxidizes 4-hydroxyphenylpyruvic acid to form an epoxide intermediate first; the epoxide metabolite undergoes a rearrangement to form the final product, homogentisic acid (see Fig. 71–1). A block in the rearrangement step leads to an accumulation of the epoxide intermediate, which either is reduced to form 4-hydroxycyclohexylacetic acid (4-HCAA) or reacts with glutathione (or cysteine) to form the unusual organic acid 2-L-cysteine-S-yl-1-4-dihydroxycyclohex-5-en-1-yl-acetic acid (hawkinsin).

Individuals with this disorder become symptomatic only during infancy. The symptoms usually appear after weaning from breast-feeding with the introduction of a high-protein diet. Severe metabolic acidosis, ketosis, failure to thrive, mild hepatomegaly, and an unusual odor (like that of a swimming pool) are common findings. These infants respond well to a diet low in both phenylalanine and tyrosine, and their clinical manifestations resolve spontaneously by 1 yr of age. Adults with this condition are usually asymptomatic despite metabolic abnormalities. Mental development is usually normal.

Affected children and adults excrete 4-hydroxyphenylpyruvic acid and 4-hydroxyphenylacetic acid as well as the two very unusual organic acids 4-HCAA and hawkinsin in their urine.

Treatment consists of a low-protein diet (such as breast milk) or a diet low in phenylalanine and tyrosine. Large doses of vitamin C (up to 1,000 mg/24 hr) are also recommended. No therapy is needed after 1 yr of age. The condition is inherited as an autosomal dominant trait, and all affected patients reported to date have been presumed to be heterozygous for the trait.

ALBINISM. This condition is due to defects in the biosynthesis and distribution of melanin. Melanin is synthesized by melanocytes from tyrosine in a membrane-bound intracellular organelle called the melanosome. Tyrosine is formed in the skin from phenylalanine by the action of phenylalanine hydroxylase and its cofactor, tetrahydrobiopterin (BH_4). BH_4 seems to be a rate-limiting compound for melanine synthesis because depigmented skin from patients with vitiligo has very low activity of the carbinolamine dehydralase, the enzyme that is necessary for regeneration of BH_4 (see Fig. 71–1). Tyrosine is transported into melanosome, where it is metabolized to dopa and dopaquinolone by the action of a single enzyme, tyrosinase (see Fig. 71–2). Dopaquinone either reacts with cysteine to make pheomelanine, a yellow-red pigment, or undergoes several nonenzymatic steps to form eumelanine, which is brown-black. Albinism (all types) has a world-wide prevalence of 1 in 20,000.

Clinical manifestations common in almost all forms of albinism include depigmentation of the skin, iris, and retina. Nystagmus, strabismus, photophobia, decreased visual acuity, and the presence of red reflex are common eye findings. Binocular vision is absent because of a decussation defect in which all optic nerve fibers from one eye completely cross to the other side at the chiasma. Blindness and skin cancer are the two major late sequelae of albinism in its severe forms.

Many forms of albinism have been identified. However, recent studies of gene mutations in affected patients have indicated that some of the seemingly distinct clinical forms of albinism may be the result of the same gene defect.

OCULOCUTANEOUS (GENERALIZED) ALBINISM. Two major forms of this condition have been identified, tyrosinase negative (type I) and tyrosinase positive (type II). This classification is based on the ability of a plucked hair bulb to form pigment (melanine) when incubated with tyrosine.

Tyrosinase negative (type I) albinism is the most severe and the second most common form (after tyrosinase positive) of generalized albinism. This is an autosomal recessive condition that is caused by deficiency of the tyrosinase enzyme. The gene for this enzyme is mapped to the long arm of chromosome 11. Many different mutations of the gene have been shown to cause this form of albinism. A milder form of the condition, which is seen predominantly in Amish families (type IB), is now known to be caused by mutations in other loci of the same gene. In fact, some of the patients who were thought to have tyrosinase positive albinism have been found to have a mutation in the tyrosinase gene.

Tyrosinase positive (type II) albinism is the most common form of generalized albinism and is inherited as an autosomal recessive trait. The gene is located on the long arm of chromosome 15. About 1% of patients with Prader-Willi and Angelman syndromes who have a deletion of chromosome 15 have this form of albinism. It is speculated that the gene product may be involved in the transport of tyrosine across the melanosome membrane. Several different mutations of the gene have been identified in affected patients. Other clinical forms of albinism that were thought to be different from type II may also be caused by mutation of this gene. For instance, one patient with autosomal recessive ocular albinism was shown to have a mutation in this gene.

Chédiak-Higashi syndrome is a tyrosinase-positive form of partial albinism in which there are abnormal granules in leukocytes and other cells, and a susceptibility to infection (see Chapter 127). Patients who survive childhood may develop a terminal lymphofollicular malignancy. These patients have reduced numbers of melanosomes, which are abnormally large (macromelanosomes).

Hermansky-Pudlak syndrome is a tyrosinase-positive generalized albinism associated with platelet dysfunction owing to the absence of platelet-dense bodies and an accumulation of ceroids in tissues. The degree of albinism is variable in these patients. This is the third most common cause of albinism and is most prevalent in Puerto Rico. Bleeding tendencies and a prolonged bleeding time are seen in all patients. Ceroid storage disease, manifested as restricted fibrotic lung disease and renal failure, occurs during the 4th–5th decades of life.

The gene mutation in other types of oculocutaneous albinism, such as platinum albinism, minimal pigment albinism, rufous albinism, and autosomal dominant albinism has not yet been elucidated.

Ocular Albinism. In these patients albinism is limited to the eyes (iridis and retina). Nystagmus, decreased visual acuity, and photophobia are common findings in all forms. Skin and hair color are within normal limits but are usually lighter than those in nonaffected siblings. Eyes are usually pale blue to light green. Hair bulb tyrosinase is positive in all cases. Four forms of this condition have been identified, differentiated by their mode of inheritance and additional associated anomalies. Ocular albinism of *Nettleship-Falls* and ocular albinism with *sensorineural deafness* are inherited as X-linked traits. In these forms only the hemizygote male has the complete syndrome. Some abnormal pigmentation of the eye may also be seen in heterozygote female carriers. *Autosomal recessive ocular albinism* may be just a mild variant of type II generalized albinism (see earlier). The fourth form of the condition is *autosomal dominant ocular albinism,* with lentigines and deafness.

Partial Albinism (Piebaldism). This disorder is characterized by localized areas of skin and hair devoid of pigment, and is inherited as a dominant trait. In some instances a white forelock or patch of depigmented hair elsewhere may be the sole manifestation.

ALCAPTONURIA. This rare (incidence 1 in 250,000) autosomal recessive disorder is due to a deficiency of homogentisic acid oxidase, which causes large amounts of homogentisic acid to accumulate in the body and then to be excreted in the urine (see Fig. 71–1).

Clinical manifestations of alcaptonuria consist of ochronosis and arthritis. These findings may not become evident until midadult life. The only sign of the disorder in the pediatric age group is a darkening of the urine to almost a black color on standing. This is caused by oxidation and polymerization of the homogentisic acid and is enhanced with an alkaline pH. Therefore, an acid urine may not become dark even after many hours of standing. This is one of the reasons why darkening of the urine may never be noted in an affected person, and the diagnosis may be delayed until adulthood, when arthritis or ochronosis occurs. *Ochronosis,* a term used to describe the darkening of tissue, is due to a slow accumulation of the black polymer of homogentisic acid in cartilage and other mesenchymal tissues. It is manifested clinically as dark, blackened spots in the sclera or as diffuse blackish pigmentation of the conjunctiva, cornea, and ear cartilage. Arthritis is the only disabling effect of this condition, which occurs in almost all affected subjects with advancing age. It involves the large joints (spine, hip, and knee) and is usually more severe in men. The arthritis has the clinical characteristics of rheumatoid arthritis, but the radiologic findings are typical of osteoarthritis. Degenerative changes in the lumbar spine are quite characteristic with narrowing of the joint spaces and fusion of the vertebral bodies. The pathogenesis of arthritic changes remains unclear. High incidences of heart disease (mitral and aortic valvulitis, calcification of the heart valves, and myocardial infarction) have also been noted.

The *diagnosis* is confirmed by measurement of homogentisic acid in urine. Affected subjects may excrete as much as 4–8 g of this compound daily. Homogentisic acid is a strong reducing agent that produces a positive reaction with Fehling or Benedict reagent (but not with glucose oxidase). The dark urine of phenol poisoning and that associated with melanotic tumors do not have these reducing properties. The enzyme is expressed only in the liver and kidneys. The gene for alkaptonuria has been mapped to the long arm of chromosome 3.

There is no effective *treatment* for this disorder.

71.3 Methionine

Iraj Rezvani

The normal pathway for catabolism of methionine, an essential amino acid, produces *S*-adenosylmethionine, which serves as a methyl group donor for methylation of a variety of compounds in the body, and cysteine, which is formed through a series of reactions called trans-sulfuration (Fig. 71–3).

HOMOCYSTINURIA (Homocystinemia). Most homocysteine, an intermediate compound of methionine degradation, is normally remethylated to methionine. This methionine-sparing reaction is catalyzed by the enzyme methionine synthase, which requires a metabolite of folic acid (5-methyltetrahydrofolate) as a substrate and a metabolite of vitamin B_{12} (methylcobalamin) as a cofactor (see Fig. 71–3). Homocysteine (and its dimer homocystine) ordinarily is not detectable in plasma or urine. Three major forms of homocystinemia and homocystinuria have been identified.

Homocystinuria Due to Cystathionine Synthase Deficiency (Homocystinuria Type I, Classic Homocystinuria). This is the most common inborn error of methionine metabolism. The prevalence of this autosomal recessive condition is estimated at 1 in 200,000 live births. The gene for cystathionine synthase is located on the long arm of chromosome 21. Heterozygote carriers are usually asymptomatic. However, thromboembolic disease has been shown to be more common in these individuals than in the normal population. About 40% of affected patients respond to high doses of vitamin B_6 and usually have milder clinical manifestations than those who are unresponsive to vitamin B_6 therapy.

Infants with this disorder are normal at birth. *Clinical manifestations* during infancy are nonspecific and may include failure to thrive and developmental delay. The diagnosis is usually made after 3 yr of age, when subluxation of the ocular lens (ectopia lentis) occurs. This causes severe myopia and iridodonesis (quivering of the iris). Astigmatism, glaucoma, staphyloma, cataracts, retinal detachment, and optic atrophy may develop later in life. Progressive mental retardation is common. Normal intelligence, however, has been reported in about 1/3 of patients. Psychiatric disorders have been observed in more than 50% of affected patients. Convulsions occur in about 20% of patients. Affected individuals with homocystinuria manifest skeletal abnormalities resembling those of Marfan syndrome (see Chapter 646); they are usually tall and thin with elongated limbs and arachnodactyly. Scoliosis, pectus excavatum or carinum, genu valgum, pes cavus, high arched palate, and crowding of the teeth are commonly seen. These children usually have fair complexions, blue eyes, and a peculiar malar flush. Generalized osteoporosis is the main roentgenographic finding. Thromboembolic episodes involving both large and small vessels, especially those of the brain, are common and may occur at any age. Optic atrophy, paralysis, seizure disorders, cor pulmonale, and severe hypertension (due to renal infarcts) are among the serious consequences of thromboembolism, which is due to changes in the vascular walls and increased platelet adhesiveness secondary to elevated homocystine levels. The risk of thromboembolism increases following surgical procedures.

Elevations of both methionine and homocystine (or homocysteine) in body fluids are the diagnostic *laboratory findings.* Freshly voided urine should be tested for homocystine, since this compound is unstable and may disappear as the urine is stored. Cystine is low or absent in plasma. The *diagnosis* may be established by assay of the enzyme in liver biopsy specimens, cultured fibroblasts, or phytohemagglutinin-stimulated lymphocytes. Prenatal diagnosis is feasible by performing an enzyme assay of cultured amniotic cells or chorionic villi. An increasing number of mutations have been recognized in different families.

Treatment with high doses of vitamin B_6 (200–1,000 mg/24 hr) causes dramatic improvement in patients who are responsive to this therapy, but some patients may not respond because of folate depletion; therefore, a patient should not be considered unresponsive to vitamin B_6 until folic acid (1–5 mg/24 hr) has been added to the treatment regimen. Restriction of

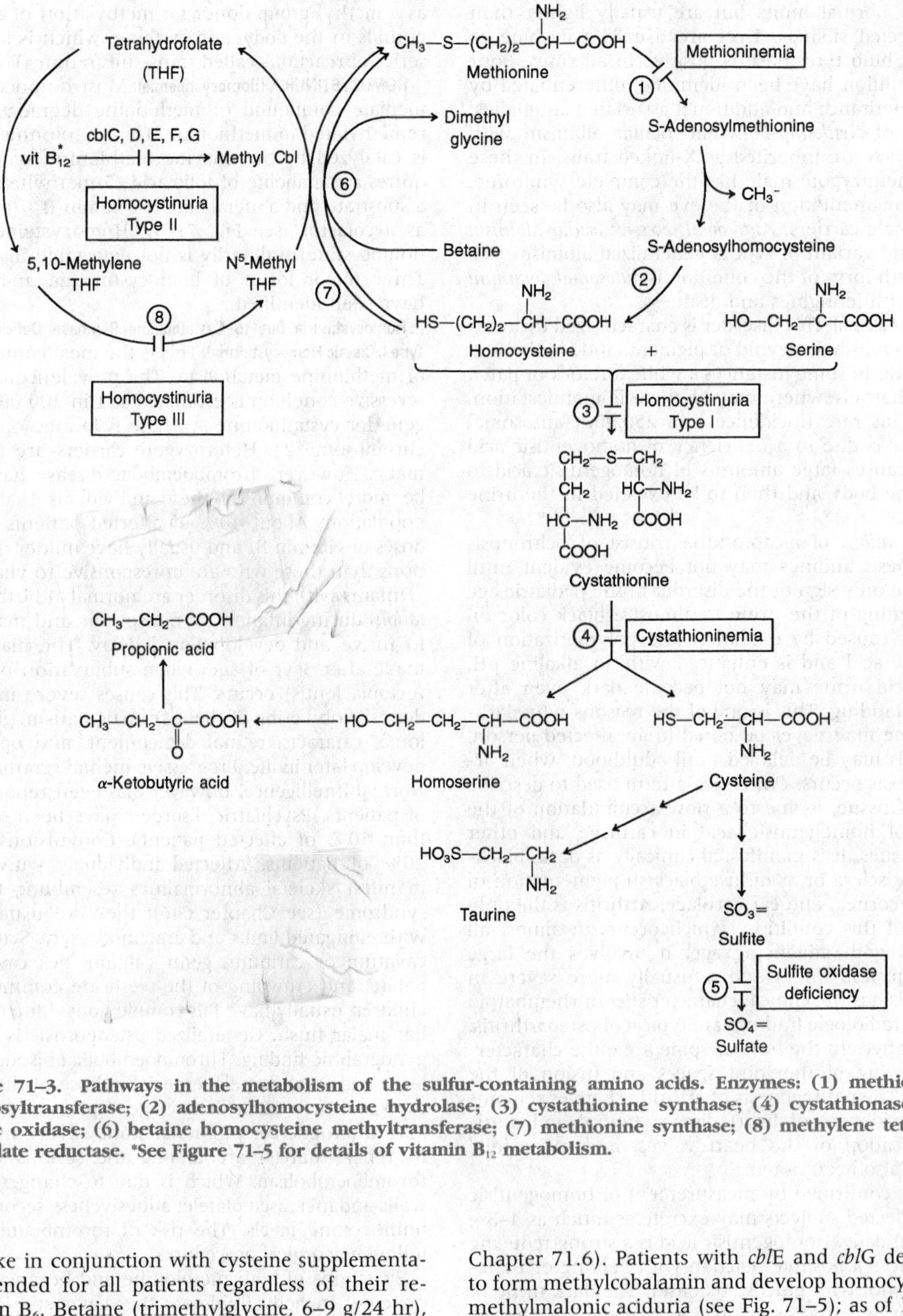

Figure 71–3. Pathways in the metabolism of the sulfur-containing amino acids. Enzymes: (1) methionine adenosyltransferase; (2) adenosylhomocysteine hydrolase; (3) cystathionine synthase; (4) cystathionase; (5) sulfite oxidase; (6) betaine homocysteine methyltransferase; (7) methionine synthase; (8) methylene tetrahydrofolate reductase. *See Figure 71–5 for details of vitamin B_{12} metabolism.

methionine intake in conjunction with cysteine supplementation is recommended for all patients regardless of their response to vitamin B_6. Betaine (trimethylglycine, 6–9 g/24 hr), which also serves as a methyl group donor, lowers homocysteine levels in body fluids by remethylating homocysteine to methionine. This treatment has produced clinical improvement in patients who are unresponsive to vitamin B_6 therapy.

Homocystinuria Due to Defects in Methylcobalamin Formation (Homocystinuria Type II). Methylcobalamin is the cofactor for the enzyme methionine synthase, which catalyzes remethylation of homocysteine to methionine. There are at least five distinct defects in the intracellular metabolism of cobalamin that may interfere with the formation of methylcobalamin. These are designated as *cbl*C, *cbl*D, *cbl*E, *cbl*G, and *cbl*F (see Figs. 71–3 and 71–4). However, the exact nature of these defects is unknown. Patients with *cbl*C, *cbl*D, and *cbl*F defects have methylamalonic aciduria in addition to homocystinuria because formation of both adenosylcobalamin and methylcobalamin is impaired (see Chapter 71.6). Patients with *cbl*E and *cbl*G defects are unable to form methylcobalamin and develop homocystinuria without methylmalonic aciduria (see Fig. 71–5); as of 1994, only a few patients with these two defects have been reported (9 *cbl*E, 14 *cbl*G).

The *clinical manifestations* are similar in patients with all of these defects. Vomiting, poor feeding, lethargy, hypotonia, and developmental delay may occur in the first few months of life. However, one patient with the *cbl*G defect was not symptomatic (except for mild developmental delay) until she was 21 yr old, when she developed difficulty in walking and numbness of the hands. *Laboratory studies* reveal megaloblastic anemia, homocystinuria, and hypomethioninemia. The presence of hypomethioninemia and megaloblastic anemia differentiates these defects from homocystinuria due to either cystathionine synthase deficiency or methylenetetrahydrofolate reductase deficiency.

Diagnosis is established by complementation studies per-

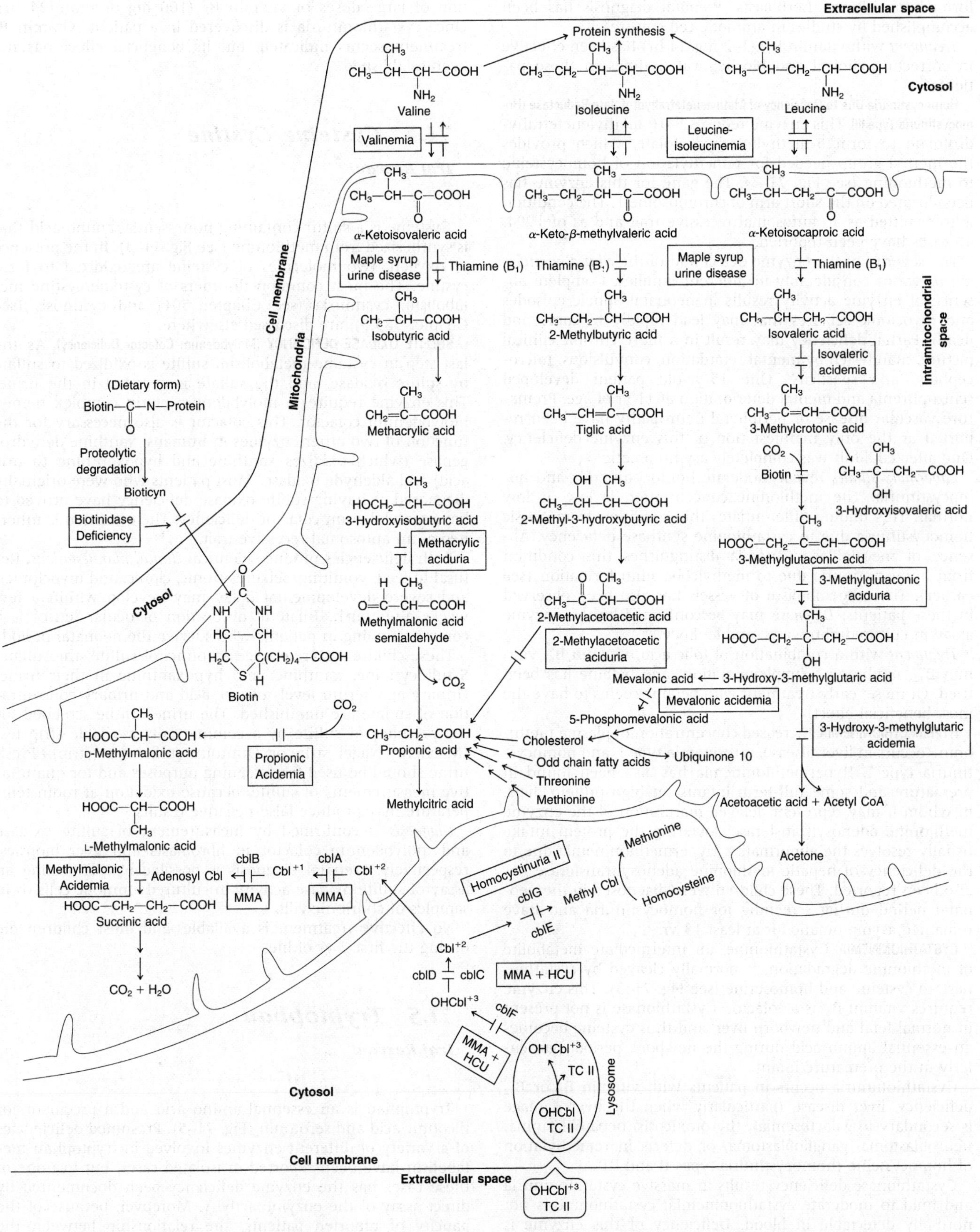

Figure 71–4. Pathways in the metabolism of the branched-chain amino acids, biotin, and vitamin B_{12} (cobalamin). Many of the intermediates (the organic acids) are metabolized via their coenzyme A (CoA) derivatives. For the sake of simplicity, this is not indicated in most of the cases. MMA = methylmalonic acidemia; HCU = homocystinuria; Cbl = cobalamin; OHCbl = hydroxycobalamin; cbl = defect in metabolism of cobalamin; TC = transcobalamin.

formed in cultured fibroblasts. Prenatal diagnosis has been accomplished by studies in amniotic cell cultures.

Treatment with vitamin B_{12} (1–2 mg/24 hr) has been effective in correcting clinical and biochemical findings in these patients.

Homocystinuria Due to Deficiency of Methylenetetrahydrofolate Reductase (Homocystinuria Type III). This enzyme reduces 5–10 methylenetetrahydrofolate to form 5-methyltetrahydrofolate, which provides the methyl group needed for remethylation of homocysteine to methionine (see Fig. 71–3). The gene for this enzyme has been located on the short arm of chromosome 1. The condition is transmitted as an autosomal recessive trait and as of 1994, 40 cases have been reported.

The severity of the enzyme defect and of the *clinical manifestations* varies considerably in different families. Complete absence of enzyme activity results in neonatal apneic episodes and myoclonic seizures that may lead rapidly to coma and death. Partial deficiency may result in a more chronic clinical picture, manifested by mental retardation, convulsions, microcephaly, and spasticity. One 15-yr-old patient developed schizophrenia and mental deterioration at 11 yr of age. Premature vascular disease or peripheral neuropathy have been reported as the only manifestation of this enzyme deficiency. One affected adult was completely asymptomatic.

Laboratory studies reveal moderate homocystinemia and homocystinuria. The methionine concentration is low or low normal. This finding differentiates this condition from classic homocystinuria due to cystathionine synthase deficiency. Absence of megaloblastic anemia distinguishes this condition from homocystinuria due to methylcobalamin formation (see earlier). Thromboembolism of vessels has also been observed in these patients. *Diagnosis* may be confirmed by the enzyme assay in cultured fibroblasts, and leukocytes.

Treatment with a combination of folic acid, vitamin B_6, vitamin B_{12}, methionine supplementation, and betaine has been tried. Of these, early treatment with betaine seems to have the most beneficial effect.

HYPERMETHIONINEMIA. Increased concentration of plasma methionine occurs in liver disease, tyrosinemia type I, and homocystinuria type I. Hypermethioninemia has also been found in premature and some full-term infants on high-protein diets, in whom it may represent delayed maturation of the enzyme methionine adenosyltransferase; lowering the protein intake usually resolves the abnormality. Hypermethioninemia due to the deficiency of hepatic methionine adenosyltransferase has also been reported. These children were diagnosed in the neonatal period during screening for homocystinuria and have remained asymptomatic for at least 13 yr.

CYSTATHIONINEMIA. Cystathionine, an intermediate metabolite of methionine degradation, is normally cleaved by cystathionase to cysteine and homoserine (see Fig. 71–3). This enzyme requires vitamin B_6 as a cofactor. Cystathionase is not present in normal fetal and newborn liver, and thus cysteine becomes an essential amino acid during the newborn period, particularly in the premature infant.

Cystathioninuria occurs in patients with vitamin B_6 or B_{12} deficiency, liver disease (particularly when the liver damage is secondary to galactosemia), thyrotoxicosis, hepatoblastoma, neuroblastoma, ganglioblastoma, or defects in remethylation of homocysteine (homocystinuria types II and III).

Cystathionase deficiency results in massive cystathioninuria and mild to moderate cystathioninemia; cystathionine is not normally detectable in blood. Deficiency of this enzyme is inherited as an autosomal recessive trait. Affected subjects with a wide variety of clinical manifestations have been reported. Lack of a consistent clinical picture and the presence of cystathioninuria in a number of normal persons suggest that cystathionase deficiency perhaps is of no clinical significance. A majority of reported cases are responsive to oral administration of large doses of vitamin B_6 (100 mg or more/24 hr). Once cystathioninuria is discovered in a patient, vitamin B_6 treatment seems indicated, but its beneficial effect has not been established.

71.4 Cysteine/Cystine

Iraj Rezvani

Cysteine is a sulfur-containing nonessential amino acid that is synthesized from methionine (see Fig. 71–3). In the presence of oxygen, two molecules of cysteine are oxidized to form cystine. The most common disorders of cysteine/cystine metabolism, cystinuria (see Chapter 501) and cystinosis (see Chapter 383.3), are discussed elsewhere.

SULFITE OXIDASE DEFICIENCY (Molybdenum Cofactor Deficiency). As the last step in cysteine metabolism, sulfite is oxidized to sulfate by sulfite oxidase, and the sulfate is excreted in the urine. This enzyme requires a molybdenum-pterin complex named molybdenum cofactor. This cofactor is also necessary for the function of two other enzymes in humans, xanthine dehydrogenase (which oxidizes xanthine and hypoxanthine to uric acid) and aldehyde oxidase. Most patients who were originally diagnosed as having sulfite oxidase deficiency have proved to have molybdenum cofactor deficiency. The condition is inherited as an autosomal recessive trait.

Both deficiencies produce identical *clinical manifestations.* Refusal to feed, vomiting, seizures (tonic, clonic, and myoclonic), and severe developmental delay may develop within a few weeks after birth. Bilateral dislocation of ocular lenses is a common finding in patients who survive the neonatal period.

These children excrete large amounts of sulfite, thiosulfate, S-sulfocysteine, xanthine, and hypoxanthine in their urine. Urinary and serum levels of uric acid and urinary concentration of sulfate are diminished. The urine can be screened for the presence of sulfite by a commercially available strip test (Macherey-Nagel strip or Quntofix sulfite test strip). Fresh urine should be used for screening purposes and for quantitative measurements of sulfite, because oxidation at room temperature may produce false-negative results.

Diagnosis is confirmed by measurement of sulfite oxidase and molybdenum cofactor in fibroblasts and liver biopsies, respectively. Prenatal diagnosis is possible by performing an assay of sulfite oxidase activity in cultured amniotic cells or in samples of chorionic villi.

No effective treatment is available, and most children die during the first 2 yr of life.

71.5 Tryptophan

Iraj Rezvani

Tryptophan is an essential amino acid and a precursor for nicotinic acid and serotonin (Fig. 71–5). Presumed deficiencies of a variety of different enzymes involved in tryptophan metabolism have been reported in isolated cases, but in none of these cases has the enzyme deficiency been documented by direct assay of the enzyme activity. Moreover, because of the paucity of reported patients, the relationship between the symptoms and the putative enzyme deficiency has remained uncertain. Therefore, only disorders of tryptophan metabolism that have been well documented are discussed in this section. The most common disorder involving tryptophan metabolism is Hartnup disorder.

HARTNUP DISORDER. In this autosomal recessive disorder, named

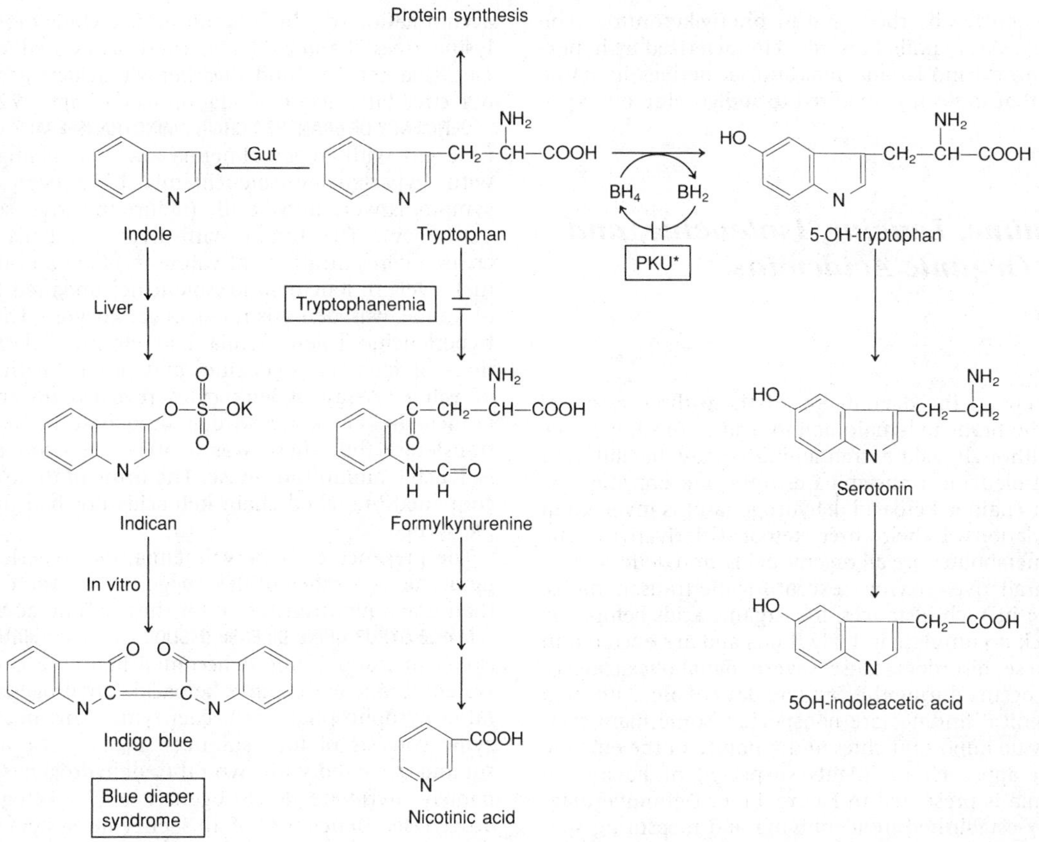

Figure 71–5. Pathways in the metabolism of tryptophan. *Hyperphenylalaninemia due to tetrahydrobiopterin deficiency (see Fig. 71–1).

after the first reported family, there is a single defect in the transport of monoamino-monocarboxylic amino acids (neutral amino acids) by the intestinal mucosa and renal tubules. The condition is thought to be caused by a defect in the amino acid transporter gene located on chromosome 2.

Data from routine urine screening of newborn infants have revealed that most children with Hartnup defect remain asymptomatic. The major *clinical manifestation* in the rare symptomatic patient is cutaneous photosensitivity. The skin becomes rough and red after moderate exposure to the sun, and with greater exposure a pellagra-like rash may develop. The rash may be pruritic, and a chronic eczema may appear. The skin changes have been reported in affected infants as young as 10 days of age. Some patients may have intermittent ataxia with or without the skin rash. Mental deficiency, perhaps an incidental finding in the original kindred, has been reported only in one additional case of a girl who had a severe encephalopathy. Episodic psychologic changes, such as irritability, emotional instability, and suicidal tendencies, have been observed; these changes are usually associated with bouts of ataxia.

Identification of asymptomatic children with Hartnup defect suggests that it can be a benign disorder. The clinical polymorphism may be related to the severity of the defect, especially in the intestinal mucosa. Patients with a severe defect may develop marked amino acid deficiency following minor stress such as diarrhea or a low-protein diet and may then become symptomatic. This theory also explains the episodic nature of the symptoms and the long intervals of spontaneous remission in patients with Hartnup disorder. Hartnup defect, with an overall prevalence of 1 in 24,000 (range 1 in 18,000–42,000) ranks among the most common amino acid disorders in humans. Pregnancy in women with Hartnup disorder has not produced any ill effects in either mother or fetus.

The main *laboratory finding* is aminoaciduria, which is restricted to neutral amino acids (alanine, serine, threonine, valine, leucine, isoleucine, phenylalanine, tyrosine, tryptophan, and histidine). Urinary excretion of proline, hydroxyproline, and arginine remains normal. This is an important diagnostic finding that differentiates Hartnup disorder from other causes of generalized aminoaciduria such as Fanconi syndrome. Plasma concentrations of neutral amino acids are usually within normal limits. This seemingly unexpected finding is due to absorption of the amino acids as dipeptides because the transport system for small peptides remains intact in Hartnup disorder. The indole derivatives (especially indican) are usually excreted in large amounts in this disorder owing to bacterial breakdown of unabsorbed tryptophan in the intestines.

Treatment with nicotinic acid or nicotinamide (50–300 g/24 hr) and a high-protein diet have resulted in a favorable response in symptomatic patients.

SEROTONIN DEFICIENCY. The first step in serotonin synthesis is the hydroxylation of tryptophan by tryptophan hydroxylase. This enzyme requires tetrahydrobiopterin as a cofactor. Defects in biopterin metabolism (see Chapter 71.1) cause a deficiency of serotonin in addition to phenylketonuria (PKU). This fact explains why treatment of patients with PKU due to biopterin defects with the usual low-phenylalanine diet alone does not prevent neurologic manifestations.

INDICANURIA (Tryptophan Malabsorption). This condition occurs when tryptophan, poorly absorbed from the gastrointestinal tract, is converted there by bacterial action to indole. Indole is absorbed, oxidized, sulfated, and excreted as an indican (see Fig. 71–5). Indicanuria is commonly observed whenever stasis in the bowels occurs, such as in constipation or in the *blind loop syndrome*; it also occurs in Hartnup disorder, in which tryptophan is poorly absorbed, and in phenylketonuria. The *blue diaper syndrome,* a familial disorder characterized by hypercalcemia, nephrocalcinosis, and indicanuria, derives its name from the fact that indican is oxidized to indigo blue on exposure to air.

71.6 Valine, Leucine, Isoleucine, and Related Organic Acidemias

Iraj Rezvani

The early steps in the degradation of these three essential amino acids, the branched-chain amino acids, are similar (see Fig. 71–4). Although valine transaminase may be different from leucine-isoleucine transaminase, only one enzyme system (branched-chain α-ketoacid dehydrogenase) is involved in the decarboxylation of their three ketoacid derivatives. The intermediate metabolites are all organic acids, and deficiency of any of the degradative enzymes, except for the transaminases, causes acidosis; in such instances, the organic acids before the enzymatic block accumulate in body fluids and are excreted in the urine. These disorders cause severe metabolic acidosis, which usually occurs during the first few days of life. Although most of the clinical findings are nonspecific, some manifestations may provide important clues to the nature of the enzyme deficiency. An approach to infants suspected of having an organic acidemia is presented in Figure 71–6. Definitive diagnosis is usually established by identifying and measuring specific organic acids in body fluids, especially urine, and by the enzyme assay.

Organic acidemias are not limited to defects in the catabolic pathways of branched-chain amino acids. Disorders causing accumulation of other organic acids include those derived from lysine (see Chapter 71.12), those associated with lactic acid (see Chapter 73), and dicarboxylic acidemia associated with defective fatty acid degradation (see Chapter 72.1).

DEFICIENCY OF BRANCHED-CHAIN AMINOTRANSFERASE. Only one Japanese girl with hypervalinemia and two siblings from France with hyperleucine-isoleucinemia have been reported. The symptoms were nonspecific (failure to thrive, seizures, mental deficiency). The infant with hypervalinemia had only increased concentrations of valine in blood and urine with normal levels of leucine and isoleucine. Impaired transamination of valine was demonstrated in leukocytes. The siblings with hyperleucine-isoleucinemia had elevated plasma concentrations of leucine, isoleucine, and proline with normal levels of valine. Assay of leukocytes revealed no abnormalities of branched-chain ketoacid dehydrogenase or of valine aminotransferase, but there was a 50% reduction in leucine and isoleucine aminotransferase. The urine of these infants neither contained branched-chain ketoacids nor had the odor of maple syrup.

The presence of hypervalinemia and hyperleucine-isoleucinemia as separate entities suggests that there may be more than one aminotransferase for these amino acids.

MAPLE SYRUP URINE DISEASE (MSUD). Decarboxylation of leucine, isoleucine, and valine is accomplished by a complex enzyme system (branched-chain α-ketoacid dehydrogenase) using thiamine pyrophosphate as a coenzyme. This mitochondrial enzyme consists of four subunits: $E_{1\alpha}$, $E_{1\beta}$, E_2, and E_3. The E_3 subunit is shared with two other dehydrogenases in the body, namely, pyruvate dehydrogenase and α-ketoglutarate dehydrogenase. Deficiency of this enzyme system causes MSUD (see Fig. 71–4), named after the sweet odor of maple syrup found in body fluids, especially urine. Several forms of this condition have been reported.

Classic MSUD. This form has the most severe *clinical manifesta-*

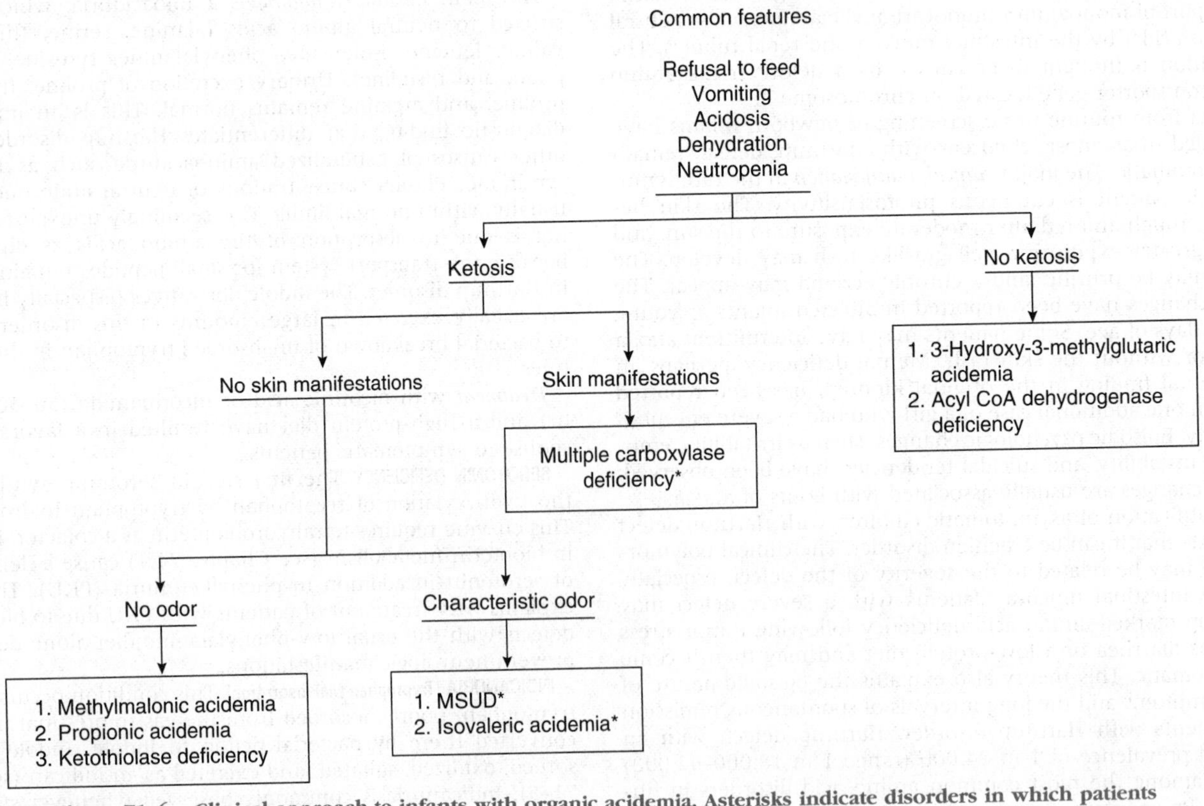

Figure 71–6. Clinical approach to infants with organic acidemia. Asterisks indicate disorders in which patients have a characteristic odor (see text and Table 70–1).

tions. Affected infants who are normal at birth develop poor feeding and vomiting during the 1st wk of life; lethargy and coma ensue within a few days. Physical examination reveals hypertonicity and muscular rigidity with severe opisthotonos. Periods of hypertonicity may alternate with bouts of flaccidity. Neurologic findings are often mistaken for generalized sepsis and meningitis. Convulsions occur in most infants, and hypoglycemia is common. However, in contrast to most hypoglycemic states, correcting the blood glucose concentration does not improve the clinical condition. Routine laboratory studies are usually unremarkable, except for severe metabolic acidosis. Death usually occurs in untreated patients within the first few weeks or months of life.

Diagnosis is often suspected because of the peculiar odor of maple syrup found in urine, sweat, and cerumen (see Fig. 71–6). It is usually confirmed by amino acid analysis showing marked elevations in plasma levels of leucine, isoleucine, valine, and alloisoleucine (a stereoisomer of isoleucine not normally found in blood) and depression of alanine. Leucine levels are usually higher than those of the other three amino acids. Urine contains high levels of leucine, isoleucine, and valine and their respective ketoacids. These ketoacids may be detected qualitatively by adding a few drops of 2,4-dinitrophenylhydrazine reagent (0.1% in 0.1 N HCl) to the urine; a yellow precipitate of 2–4 diphenylhydrazone is formed in a positive test.

Treatment of the acute state is aimed at quick removal of the branched-chain amino acids and their metabolites from the tissues and body fluids. Because renal clearance of these compounds is poor, hydration alone does not produce a rapid improvement. Peritoneal dialysis is the most effective mode of therapy and should be promptly instituted; significant decreases in plasma levels of leucine, isoleucine, and valine are usually seen within 24 hr of institution of treatment. Attempts should also be made to stop the patient's catabolic state by providing sufficient calories intravenously or orally.

Treatment after recovery from the acute state requires a low branched-chain amino acid diet. Synthetic formulas devoid of leucine, isoleucine, and valine are now commercially available.* Because these amino acids cannot be synthesized endogenously, small amounts of them should be added to the diet; the amount should be titrated carefully by performing frequent analyses of the plasma amino acids. A clinical condition resembling acrodermatitis enteropathica occurs in affected infants whose plasma isoleucine concentration becomes very low; addition of isoleucine to the diet causes a rapid and complete recovery. Patients with MSUD should remain on the diet for the rest of their lives.

The long-term *prognosis* of affected children remains guarded. Severe ketoacidosis, cerebral edema, and death may occur during any stressful situation such as infection or surgery. Mental and neurologic deficits are common sequelae.

Intermittent MSUD. In this form of MSUD seemingly normal children develop vomiting, odor of maple syrup, ataxia, lethargy, and coma during stress such as infection or surgery. During these attacks, laboratory findings are indistinguishable from those of the classic form, and death may occur. Treatment of the intermittent variety is similar to that of the classic form. After recovery, although a normal diet is tolerated, a diet low in branched-chain amino acids is recommended. The activity of dehydrogenase in patients with the intermittent form is higher than that in the classic form and may reach 8–16% of the normal activity.

Mild (Intermediate) MSUD. In this form affected children develop milder disease after the neonatal period. They are usually mildly to moderately retarded; have increased plasma levels of leucine, isoleucine, and valine; and excrete ketoacid derivatives of these amino acids in their urine. They usually have the odor of maple syrup. These children are commonly diagnosed during an intercurrent illness when signs and symptoms of classic MSUD occur. The dehydrogenase activity is 2–8% of normal. Since patients with thiamine-responsive MSUD usually have manifestations similar to those seen in the mild form, a trial of thiamine therapy is recommended.

Thiamine-Responsive MSUD. Children with mild or intermittent forms of MSUD have been reported in whom treatment with high doses of thiamine results in dramatic clinical and biochemical improvement. Although some children have responded to treatment with 10 mg/24 hr thiamine, others require as much as 200 mg/24 hr for at least 3 wk before a favorable response is observed.

Other Forms of MSUD. Three patients with combined branched-chain ketoaciduria and lactic acidosis have been reported. These patients were believed to have a deficiency of the E_3 subunit that caused a functional impairment of pyruvate dehydrogenase and α-ketoglutarate dehydrogenase in addition to the branched-chain ketoacid dehydrogenase deficiency. The infants presented with acidosis and hypotonia in the neonatal period that progressed to ataxia, severe neurologic impairment, and death in early childhood. These patients excreted large amounts of lactate, pyruvate, and α-ketoglutarate, and three branched-chain ketoacids in their urine.

Genetics and the Prevalence of MSUD. All forms of this disorder are inherited as an autosomal recessive trait. The deficiency of different subunits of the enzyme may account for the wide clinical and biochemical variability seen in different affected families. Patients with the classic form may have $E_{1\alpha}$, $E_{1\beta}$, or E_2 subunit deficiency. Each subunit of the enzyme resides in different chromosomes. The gene for $E_{1\alpha}$ is mapped to the long arm of chromosome 19, for $E_{1\beta}$ to the short arm of chromosome 6, for E_2 to the short arm of chromosome 1, and for E_3 to the long arm of chromosome 7. Patients with the mild and intermittent forms may also be "double heterozygotes" with two different mutant alleles. The enzyme activity can be measured in leukocytes and fibroblasts, making it possible to diagnose heterozygotes and affected fetuses. The incidence in the United States is about 1 in 200,000; however, the classic form of the disease is more common among Mennonites.

ISOVALERIC ACIDEMIA. This rare condition is due to the deficiency of isovaleryl CoA dehydrogenase, which catalyzes the conversion of isovaleric acid to 3-methylcrotonic acid in the leucine degradative pathway (see Fig. 71–4). Isovaleric acidemia is inherited as an autosomal recessive trait. The gene has been mapped to the long arm of chromosome 15. The gene frequency in the general population is not known.

Clinical manifestations in the acute form include vomiting and severe acidosis in the first few days of life. Lethargy, convulsions, and coma ensue, and death may occur if proper therapy is not initiated. The vomiting may be severe enough to suggest pyloric stenosis. The characteristic odor of "sweaty feet" may be present (see Fig. 71–6). A milder form of the disease also exists in which the first clinical manifestation (vomiting, lethargy, acidosis, or coma) may not appear until the infant is a few months or a few years old (chronic intermittent form).

Laboratory findings reveal severe ketoacidosis, neutropenia, thrombocytopenia, and occasionally pancytopenia. Hypocalcemia and moderate to severe hyperammonemia may be present in some patients. Increases in plasma ammonia may suggest a defect in the urea cycle. However, in the latter conditions the infant is not acidotic. Hyperglycemia may be present in some patients.

Diagnosis is established by demonstrating marked elevations of isovaleric acid and its metabolites (isovalerylglycine, 3-hydroxyisovaleric acid) in body fluids, especially urine. Isovaleric acid is volatile and may disappear from the urine if the specimen is not handled properly; however, isovalerylglycine is a

*MSUD Formula, Mead Johnson Laboratories, Evansville, Indiana.

stable compound that is more reliable for diagnostic purposes. Measuring the enzyme in cultured skin fibroblasts confirms the diagnosis. Intrauterine diagnosis has been accomplished by measuring isovalerylglycine in amniotic fluid.

Treatment of the acute attack is aimed at hydration, correction of metabolic acidosis (by infusing sodium bicarbonate), and removal of the excess isovaleric acid. Because isovalerylglycine has a high urinary clearance, administration of glycine (250 mg/kg/24 hr) is recommended to enhance formation of isovalerylglycine. Carnitine (100 mg/kg/24 hr) also increases removal of isovaleric acid by forming isovalerylcarnitine, which is excreted in the urine. Adequate calories should be provided orally or intravenously to minimize the catabolic state. In patients with significant hyperammonemia (blood ammonia >200 μM) measures that reduce blood ammonia should be employed (Chapter 71.10). Exchange transfusion and peritoneal dialysis may be needed if the above measures fail to induce significant clinical and biochemical improvement. Patients should be kept on a low-protein diet (1.0–1.5 g/kg/24 hr) and should be given glycine and carnitine supplements after recovery from the acute attack. Pancreatitis (acute and recurrent forms) has been reported in survivors. Normal development can be achieved with early and proper treatment.

MULTIPLE CARBOXYLASE DEFICIENCY (Defects in Utilization of Biotin). Biotin is a water-soluble vitamin that acts as a cofactor for all carboxylases in the body: pyruvate carboxylase, acetyl CoA carboxylase, propionyl CoA carboxylase, and 3-methylcrotonyl CoA carboxylase. The latter two of these carboxylases are involved in the metabolic pathways of leucine, isoleucine, and valine (see Fig. 71–4).

Dietary biotin is bound to protein (carboxylases); free biotin is generated in the intestine by the action of digestive enzymes and perhaps biotinidase. The latter enzyme, which is found in serum and most tissues in the body, is also essential for the recycling of biotin in the body by releasing it from a carboxylase (see Fig. 71–4). Free biotin must form a covalent peptide bond with the apoprotein of the above carboxylases in order to render them active. This binding is catalyzed by holocarboxylase synthetase. Deficiencies in this enzyme or in biotinidase result in malfunction of all the carboxylases and in organic acidemia.

Holocarboxylase Synthetase Deficiency (Multiple Carboxylase Deficiency—Infantile or Early Form). Infants with this rare autosomal recessive disorder become symptomatic in the first few weeks of life with breathing difficulties (tachypnea, apnea), hypotonia, seizures, vomiting, and failure to thrive. The urine may have a peculiar odor, which is described as similar to tomcat urine. The clinical finding that may differentiate this disorder from other organic acidemias, especially propionic acidemia, is the skin manifestations, which include generalized erythematous rash with exfoliation and alopecia totalis (see Fig. 71–6).

Laboratory findings include metabolic acidosis, ketosis, and the presence of organic acids such as lactic acid, propionic acid, 3-methylcrotonic acid, 3-methylcrotonylglycine, and 3-hydroxyisovaleric acid in body fluids. Significant hyperammonemia has occurred in some patients. These infants may also have an immunodeficiency manifested by a decrease in the number of T cells.

Treatment with biotin (10 mg/24 hr) results in a dramatic response. Prenatal diagnosis has been accomplished by means of an assay of enzyme activity in cultured amniotic cells and by measurement of intermediate metabolites (3-hydroxyisovalerate and methylcitrate) in amniotic fluid. Prenatal treatment of the mother with biotin has produced normal offspring in two women in whom prenatal diagnosis of holocarboxylase synthetase deficiency was made.

Biotinidase Deficiency (Multiple Carboxylase Deficiency—Juvenile or Late Form). The absence of biotinidase results in biotin deficiency. The prevalence of this autosomal recessive trait is estimated at 1 in 60,000.

Infants with this deficiency may develop *clinical manifestations* similar to those seen in infants with holocarboxylase synthetase deficiency, but, unlike the latter, symptoms may appear later when the child is several months or several years old. The delay is presumably due to the presence of sufficient free biotin derived from the mother or the diet. Atopic or seborrheic dermatitis, alopecia, ataxia, myoclonic seizures, hypotonia, developmental delay, hearing loss, and immunodeficiency may occur. Measurement of biotinidase in 100 Japanese children with intractable seborrheic dermatitis revealed two children with partial (15–30% activity) deficiency of the enzyme; these children were otherwise asymptomatic, and their dermatitis resolved with biotin therapy. Patients with partial deficiency of the enzyme have been identified on neonatal screening and in family members of these infants. Symptoms of biotinidase deficiency were observed only in a few of these individuals. However, the majority of these infants have shown no clinical or biochemical abnormalities.

Laboratory findings and the pattern of organic acids in body fluids resemble those associated with holocarboxylase synthetase deficiency (see earlier). *Diagnosis* can be established by measurement of the enzyme activity in the serum. A simplified method of neonatal screening for biotinidase deficiency is now available that requires a small amount of blood spotted on a filter paper.

Affected children respond dramatically to administration of free biotin (10 mg/24 hr). Treatment with biotin is also suggested for individuals with residual biotinidase activities below 10%.

Multiple Carboxylase Deficiency Due to Dietary Biotin Deficiency. Acquired deficiency of biotin may occur in infants receiving total parenteral nutrition without added biotin, in patients receiving prolonged anticonvulsant drugs, or in children with short gut syndrome or chronic diarrhea who are receiving formulas low in biotin. Excessive ingestion of raw eggs may also cause biotin deficiency because the protein avidin in egg white binds biotin and makes it unavailable for absorption. Infants with biotin deficiency develop dermatitis, alopecia, and moniliasis.

3-METHYLGLUTACONIC ACIDURIA. Clinical manifestations have ranged from mild motor and speech retardation to severe neurologic deficits with self-mutilation. Patients excrete large amounts of 3-methylglutaconic acid, an intermediate metabolite in the catabolism of leucine, in their urine. It is not clear whether the metabolic defect is the cause of the clinical manifestations.

β-KETOTHIOLASE DEFICIENCY (2-Methylacetoacetyl CoA Thiolase Deficiency). 2-Methylacetoacetyl CoA thiolase is one of the three existing ketothiolases in the body. This enzyme cleaves 2-methylacetoacetyl CoA to acetyl CoA and propionyl CoA (see Fig. 71–4). Although deficiencies of the other β-ketothiolases have also been reported (in a total of three patients), the term β-ketothiolase deficiency is traditionally reserved for patients with 2-methylacetoacetyl CoA thiolase deficiency. Fourteen patients with this deficiency have been reported. This condition is inherited as an autosomal recessive trait and may be more prevalent than has been appreciated.

The *clinical manifestations* are quite variable, ranging from an asymptomatic course in an adult to severe episodes of acidosis starting in the 1st yr of life. These children have intermittent episodes of severe acidosis, ketosis, and moderate to severe hyperammonemia that may lead to coma and death. These episodes usually occur following an intercurrent infection and respond quickly to intravenous fluids and bicarbonate therapy. The child may be completely asymptomatic between episodes and may tolerate a normal protein diet well. Mental development is normal in most children. The episodes may be misdiagnosed as salicylate poisoning because of the similarity of clinical findings and the interference of elevated blood levels of acetoacetate with the colorimetric assay for salicylate. In an unreported case of our own, the diagnosis was not made until the child was 3½ yr of age, when a third episode of severe acidosis occurred following an upper respiratory infection. The second episode at 14 mo of age was diagnosed as salicylate ingestion. The child had normal development.

Laboratory findings during the acute attack include acidosis, ketosis, and hyperammonemia. The urine contains large amounts of 2-methylacetoacetate, 2-methyl-3-hydroxybutyrate, and tiglylglycine. Hyperglycinemia may also be present. The clinical and biochemical findings should be differentiated from those seen with propionic and methylmalonic acidemias (see later). *Diagnosis* may be established by assay of the enzyme in cultured fibroblasts.

Treatment of acute episodes includes hydration and infusion of bicarbonate to correct the acidosis; a 10% glucose solution with the appropriate electrolytes and intravenous lipids may be used to minimize the catabolic state. Hyperammonemia should be treated promptly (see Chapter 71.10). Peritoneal dialysis may be required if the above measures do not produce significant clinical improvement. Restriction of protein intake (1–2 g/kg/24 hr) is recommended for long-term therapy. L-Carnitine (50–100 mg/kg/24 hr) may be used to prevent possible secondary carnitine deficiency.

3-HYDROXY-3-METHYLGLUTARIC (HMG) ACIDEMIA. This rare condition is due to a deficiency of hydroxymethylglutaryl (HMG) CoA lyase (see Fig. 71–4). About 60% of these patients become symptomatic between 3 and 11 mo of age, whereas 30% develop symptoms in the first few days of life. One child remained asymptomatic until 2 yr of age. Episodes of vomiting, severe hypoglycemia, hypotonia, acidosis, and dehydration may rapidly lead to lethargy, ataxia, and coma. These episodes often occur during an intercurrent infection. Hepatomegaly is a common physical finding.

Laboratory studies reveal hypoglycemia, moderate to severe hyperammonemia, acidosis, and abnormal liver function test results. There is no ketosis (see Fig. 71–6) because 3-hydroxy-3-methylglutaric acid cannot be converted to acetoacetic acid and β-hydroxybutyric acid. 3-Hydroxy-3-methylglutaryl CoA is also an obligatory intermediate metabolite in the formation of ketone bodies from any other source. Urinary excretion of 3-hydroxy-3-methylglutaric acid and other proximal intermediate metabolites of leucine catabolism (3-methylglutaconic acid and 3-hydroxyisovaleric acid) is markedly increased. This condition should be differentiated from medium-chain acyl CoA dehydrogenase (MCAD) deficiency. The urinary metabolites described earlier are characterisic of 3-hydroxy-3-methylglutaric acidemia and are not found in MCAD deficiency. *Diagnosis* may be confirmed by enzyme assay in cultured fibroblasts, leukocytes, or liver specimens. Prenatal diagnosis has been accomplished by means of an assay of the enzyme in a biopsy specimen of the chorionic villi.

Treatment of acute episodes includes hydration, infusion of glucose to control hypoglycemia, and administration of bicarbonate to correct acidosis. Hyperammonemia should be treated promptly (see Chapter 71.10). Exchange transfusion and peritoneal dialysis may be required in patients with severe hyperammonemia. Restriction of protein and fat intake is recommended for long-term management of these patients. L-Carnitine (50–100 mg/kg/24 hr) may be used to prevent secondary carnitine deficiency. Prolonged fasting should be avoided. One patient died from acute cardiomyopathy at 7 mo of age during a febrile illness. There may be some risk in performing immunization of these children, because one child has died following immunization.

MEVALONIC ACIDURIA. This recently described autosomal recessive condition is due to a deficiency of the enzyme mevalonate kinase (see Fig. 71–5). Eleven patients with this disorder from seven families have been reported. *Clinical manifestations* include mental retardation, failure to thrive, growth retardation, hypotonia, hepatosplenomegaly, cataracts, and facial dysmorphism (dolichocephaly, frontal bossing, low-set ears, down-slanting of the eyes, and long eyelashes). All patients developed recurrent crises characterized by fever, vomiting, diarrhea, arthralgia, subcutaneous edema, and morbilliform skin rash. These episodes last 4–5 days and recur up to 25 times/year. Four patients died during these crises. No metabolic abnormality, such as metabolic acidosis, lactic acidosis, or hypoglycemia, were present. These crises were similar to those seen in capillary leak syndrome and is thought to be related to leukotriene E_4, which is known to cause increased vascular permeability. Increased excretion of leukotriene E_4 has been demonstrated during these episodes. Mevalonic acid production is grossly increased in these patients. Serum cholesterol concentration is normal or mildly decreased. Serum creatine kinase (CK) and sedimentation rate are markedly elevated. Serum levels of ubiquinone-10 (a component of the respiratory chain that is synthesized through steps after mevalonate kinase action) is low. No effective therapy is available. *Treatment* with an HMG CoA reductase inhibitor (lovastatin) has resulted in the development of acute crises. Treatment with high doses of prednisone (2 mg/kg/24 hr) seems to be an effective treatment for recurrent crises. Mevalonate kinase activity is deficient in fibroblasts and lymphocytes. *Prenatal diagnosis* is possible by measurement of enzyme activity in aminocytes or chorionic villus samples.

PROPIONIC ACIDEMIA (Propionyl CoA Carboxylase Deficiency). Propionic acid is an intermediate metabolite of isoleucine, valine, threonine, methionine, odd-chain fatty acids, and cholesterol catabolism. It is normally carboxylated to methylmalonic acid by the mitochondrial enzyme propionyl CoA carboxylase, which requires biotin as a cofactor (see Fig. 71–4). The enzyme is composed of two nonidentical subunits, α and β. Biotin is bound to the α subunit.

The prevalence of propionic acidemia, inherited as an autosomal recessive trait, is not known. The gene for the α subunit is located on chromosome 13 and that of the β subunit is mapped to the long arm of chromosome 3.

Clinical manifestations are nonspecific. The majority of patients develop symptoms in the first few weeks of life. Poor feeding, vomiting, hypotonia, lethargy, dehydration, and clinical signs of acidosis progress rapidly to coma and death. Seizures occur in about 30% of affected infants. If an infant survives the first attack, similar episodes may occur during an intercurrent infection, constipation, or following ingestion of a high-protein diet. Less frequently, the infant may come to medical attention later in life because of mental retardation without acute attacks of ketosis. Some affected children may have episodes of unexplained severe ketoacidosis separated by periods of seemingly normal health. The severity of clinical manifestations may also be variable within a family; in one kindred, a brother was diagnosed at 5 yr of age, whereas his 13-yr-old sister, with the same level of enzyme deficiency, was asymptomatic. The reason for this polymorphism remains unclear.

Laboratory studies during the acute attack reveal severe metabolic acidosis with a large anion gap, ketosis, neutropenia, thrombocytopenia, and hypoglycemia. Moderate to severe hyperammonemia is commonly seen in these infants. Plasma concentration of ammonia usually correlates with the severity of the disease. Measurement of plasma ammonia is especially helpful in planning therapeutic strategy during episodes of exacerbation in a patient whose diagnosis has been established previously. Hyperglycinemia is common in patients with propionic acidemia. Elevations in plasma and urinary levels of glycine have also been observed in patients with methylmalonic acidemia, isovaleric acidemia, and β-ketothiolase deficiency. These disorders formerly were collectively referred to as *ketotic hyperglycinemia* before the specific enzyme deficiencies were elucidated. Hyperglycinemia is presumably due to inhibition of glycine cleavage enzyme by the high levels of accumulated organic acid. Concentrations of propionic acid and methylcitric acid (presumably made by the condensation of propionyl CoA with oxaloacetic acid) are markedly elevated in the plasma and urine of infants with propionic acidemia. Measurement of methylcitric acid is especially helpful in making the diagnosis because, unlike propionic acid, which is volatile, methylcitric acid is a stable compound and does not disappear from the specimen during shipping and handling. 3-Hydroxypropionic acid, propionylglycine, and other intermediate metabolites of isoleucine catabolism, such as tiglic acid, tiglylglycine, and 2-methyloacetoacetic acid, are also found in urine.

The *diagnosis* of propionic acidemia should be differentiated from multiple carboxylase deficiency (see earlier description and Fig. 71–6). Patients with propionic acidemia responsive to biotin in earlier reports were later found to have multiple carboxylase deficiency. The latter infants may have skin manifestations and excrete large amounts of lactic acid, 3-methylcrotonic acid, and 3-hydroxyisovaleric acid in addition to propionic acid. The presence of hyperammonemia may suggest a genetic defect in the urea cycle enzymes. However, infants with defects in the urea cycle are usually not acidotic (see Fig. 70–1). Hyperammonemia is believed to be due to inhibition of carbamylphosphate synthetase (CPS I) by the organic acid. Definitive diagnosis of propionic acidemia can be established by measuring the appropriate enzyme activity in leukocytes or cultured fibroblasts.

Prenatal diagnosis has been accomplished by measuring the enzyme activity in cultured amniotic cells and in samples of uncultured chorionic villi.

Treatment of acute attacks includes rehydration, correction of acidosis, and prevention of the catabolic state by provision of adequate calories through parenteral hyperalimentation. Minimal amounts of protein (0.25 g/kg/24 hr), preferably a protein deficient in propionate precursor, should be provided in the hyperalimentation fluid very early in the course of treatment. To control the possible production of propionic acid by intestinal bacteria, sterilization of the intestinal tract flora by antibiotics (e.g., oral neomycin) should be promptly initiated. Constipation should also be treated. Patients with propionic acidemia may develop carnitine deficiency, presumably as a result of urinary loss of propionylcarnitine formed from the accumulated organic acid. Administration of L-carnitine (50–100 mg/kg/24 hr) normalizes fatty acid oxidation and improves acidosis. In patients with concomitant hyperammonemia measures to reduce blood ammonia should be employed (see Chapter 71.10). Very ill patients with severe acidosis and hyperammonemia require peritoneal dialysis or hemodialysis to remove ammonia and other toxic compounds. Although infants with true propionic acidemia are rarely responsive to biotin, this compound should be administered (10 mg/24 hr) to all infants during the initial attack and should be continued until a definitive diagnosis is established.

Long-term treatment consists of a low-protein diet (1.0–1.5 g/kg/24 hr) and administration of L-carnitine (50–100 mg/kg/24 hr). Synthetic proteins deficient in propionate precursors* (isoleucine, valine, methionine, and threonine) may be used to increase the amount of dietary protein (to 1.5–2.0 g/kg/24 hr) while causing minimal change in propionate production. However, excessive supplementation with these proteins may cause a deficiency of the essential amino acids. To avoid this problem, natural proteins should comprise most of the dietary protein (50–75%). Some patients may require chronic alkaline therapy to correct low-grade chronic acidosis. The concentration of ammonia in blood usually normalizes between attacks, and chronic treatment of hyperammonemia is rarely needed. Stressful situations that may trigger acute attacks (e.g., infections) should be treated promptly and aggressively. Close monitoring of blood pH, amino acids, urinary content of propionate and its metabolites, and growth parameters is necessary to ensure the proper balance of the diet and the success of therapy.

Long-term *prognosis* is guarded. Death may occur during an acute attack. Normal psychomotor development is possible, but most children manifest some degree of permanent neurodevelopmental deficit despite adequate therapy.

METHYLMALONIC ACIDEMIA. Methylmalonic acid, a structural isomer of succinic acid, is normally derived from propionic acid as part of the catabolic pathways of isoleucine, valine, threonine, methionine, cholesterol, and odd-chain fatty acids. Two enzymes are involved in the conversion of D-methylmalonic acid to succinic acid, methylmalonyl CoA racemase (which forms the L-isomer) and methylmalonyl CoA mutase (which converts the L-methylmalonic acid to succinic acid) (see Fig. 71–4). The latter enzyme requires adenosylcobalamin, a metabolite of vitamin B_{12}, as a coenzyme. Deficiency of either the mutase or its coenzyme causes an accumulation of methylmalonic acid and its precursors in body fluids. Deficiency of the racemase has not yet been conclusively identified.

At least two forms of mutase apoenzyme deficiency have been identified. These are designated *mut*^{0}, meaning no detectable enzyme activity, and *mut*$^-$, indicating residual, although abnormal, mutase activity. About half of the reported patients with methylmalonic acidemia have a deficiency of the mutase apoenzyme (*mut*^{0} or *mut*$^-$). These patients are not responsive to vitamin B_{12} therapy. The gene for the mutase has been mapped to the short arm of chromosome 6 and about 20 different mutations have been described. In the remaining patients with methylmalonic acidemia, the defect resides in the formation of adenosylcobalamin.

Defects in Metabolism of Vitamin B_{12} (Cobalamin). Dietary vitamin B_{12} requires intrinsic factor, a glycoprotein secreted by the gastric parietal cells, for absorption in the terminal ileum. It is transported in the blood by three carrier proteins, transcobalamin I, II, and III. The complex of transcobalamin II-cobalamin (CII-Cbl) is recognized by a specific receptor on the cell membrane and enters the cell by endocytosis. The TCII-Cbl complex is hydrolyzed in the lysosome, and free cobalamin is released into the cytosol. The cobalt of the molecule is reduced in the cytosol from three valences (cob[III]alamin) to two (cob[II]alamin) before it enters the mitochondria, where further reduction to cob(I)alamin occurs. The latter compound reacts with adenosine to form adenosyl cobalamin (coenzyme for methylmalonyl CoA mutase). The free cobalamin in the cytosol may also undergo a series of enzymatic steps to form methylcobalamin (coenzyme for methionine synthase, which catalyzes the remethylation of homocysteine to methionine; see Fig. 71–3).

At least seven different defects in the intracellular metabolism of cobalamin have been identified. These are designated *cbl* A through G (*cbl* stands for a defect in any step of cobalamin metabolism). *cbl*A is probably due to a deficiency of mitochondrial cobalamin reductase; *cbl*B is caused by a deficiency of adenosylcobalamin transferase. Both cause methylmalonic acidemia only. The precise enzymatic deficiencies in the remaining defects are not known. In patients with *cbl*C, *cbl*D, and *cbl*F defects, synthesis of both adenosylcobalamin and methylcobalamin is impaired, causing homocystinuria in addition to methylmalonic acidemia. Defects E and G involve only the synthesis of methylcobalamin, resulting in homocystinuria without methylmalonic acidemia. All of the above defects including apoenzyme deficiency (mut^0 and mut$^-$) are inherited as autosomal recessive traits and have an overall prevalence of about 1 in 48,000.

Clinical manifestations of patients with *mut*^{0} and *mut*$^-$ and *cbl*A and *cbl*B are similar to those of patients with propionic

*Milupa OS1. Milupa Corporation, Darien, CT.

acidemia (see earlier). However, fulminating neonatal forms causing severe ketosis, acidosis, hyperammonemia, neutropenia, coma, and death are more common in patients with methylmalonic acidemia than in patients with propionic acidemia. If the infant survives the first attack, similar exacerbations may occur during an intercurrent infection or following ingestion of a high-protein diet. The condition may present later in life with failure to thrive, hypotonia, and developmental delay. Some infants with methylmalonic acidemia have characteristic facial features with a triangular mouth and high forehead. Patients with severe clinical manifestations in the first few days of life tend to have mutase deficiency (*mut*^{0} or *mut*$^-$). However, there are wide variations in the clinical presentation regardless of the nature of the enzyme deficiency. Asymptomatic patients with mutase apoenzyme deficiency have been identified through screening of newborn infants. These patients tolerate a normal protein intake and accumulate high levels of methylmalonate in their body fluids.

Laboratory findings include ketosis, acidosis, anemia, neutropenia, thrombocytopenia, hyperglycinemia, hyperammonemia, hypoglycemia, and the presence of large quantities of methylmalonic acid in body fluids (see Fig. 71–6). Propionic acid and its metabolites 3-hydroxypropionate and methylcitrate are also found in urine. Hyperammonemia may suggest the presence of genetic defects in the urea cycle enzymes. However, patients with defects in urea cycle enzymes are not acidotic (see Fig. 70–1). The increase in ammonia in patients with methylmalonic acidemia is believed to be due to inhibition of CPS I by the organic acid.

Diagnosis can be confirmed by measuring propionate incorporation or mutase activity and by performing complementation studies in cultured fibroblasts. Prenatal diagnosis has been accomplished by performing an assay of propionate incorporation in cultured amniotic cells.

Treatment of acute attacks is similar to that of attacks in patients with propionic acidemia (see earlier) except that large doses (1–2 mg/24 hr) of vitamin B_{12} are used instead of biotin. Long-term treatment consists of a low-protein diet (1.0–1.5 g/kg/24 hr) and administration of L-carnitine (50–100 mg/kg/24 hr) and vitamin B_{12} (1 mg/24 hr for only those patients with defects in vitamin B_{12} metabolism). The protein composition of the diet is similar to that prescribed for patients with propionic acidemia. Chronic alkaline therapy is usually required to correct low-grade chronic acidosis. Blood levels of ammonia usually normalize between the attacks, and chronic treatment of hyperammonemia is rarely needed. Stressful situations that may trigger acute attacks (such as infection) should be treated promptly. Close monitoring of blood pH, amino acid levels, urinary content of methylmalonate, and growth parameters is necessary to ensure proper balance in the diet and the success of therapy.

Prognosis depends largely on the type of enzymatic defect that is present. Patients with mutase apoenzyme deficiency (*mut*^{0}, *mut*$^-$) have a worse prognosis. Acute and recurrent pancreatitis have been reported in survivors as young as 13 mo of age. Two of the five children with this complication died during an acute attack of pancreatitis. Unexplained infarcts of brain and renal dysfunction have been observed in some of these patients.

COMBINED METHYLMALONIC ACIDURIA AND HOMOCYSTINURIA (*cbl*C, *cbl*D, and *cbl*F Defects). About 100 patients with methylmalonic acidemia and homocystinuria due to *cbl*C, *cbl*D, and *cbl*F defects (see Figs. 71–3 and 71–4) have been reported. The majority of the patients (about 90) had the *cbl*C defect; only two brothers with *cbl*D and five patients with *cbl*F defects have been identified.

Neurologic findings were prominent in patients with *cbl*C and *cbl*D defects. Most patients with *cbl*C defect came to medical attention in the first few months of life because of failure to thrive, lethargy, poor feeding, mental retardation, and seizures. However, late-onset defects with sudden development of dementia and myelopathy have been reported. Megaloblastic anemia was a common finding in patients with *cbl*C defect. Mild to moderate increases in concentrations of methylmalonic acid and homocysteine were found in body fluids. However, unlike patients with classic homocystinuria, plasma levels of methionine are low to normal in these defects. Neither hyperammonemia nor hyperglycinemia has been observed in these patients. The first two patients with *cbl*F defect were females in whom poor feeding, growth and developmental delay, and persistent stomatitis became manifest in the first 3 wk of life. The first patient did not have megaloblastic anemia and homocystinuria, but both these signs were present in the second infant. Moderate methylmalonic acidemia was present in both infants. One patient was not diagnosed until age 10 yr. He had findings suggestive of rheumatoid arthritis, a pigmented skin abnormality, and became encephalopathic. Vitamin B_{12} malabsorption is seen in patients with *cbl*F defect.

Experience with *treatment* of patients with *cbl*C, *cbl*D, and *cbl*F defects is very limited. Large doses of hydroxycobalamin (1–2 mg/24 hr) in conjunction with betaine (6–9 g/24 hr) seem to produce biochemical improvement with little clinical effect. Unexplained severe hemolytic anemia, hydrocephalus, and congestive heart failure have been major complications in patients with *cbl*C defect.

Patients with *cbl*E and *cbl*G defects do not have methylmalonic acidemia and are discussed further in the section on homocystinuria (see Chapter 71.3).

71.7 Glycine

Iraj Rezvani

Glycine is a nonessential amino acid synthesized mainly from serine and threonine. The main catabolic pathway requires the complex glycine cleavage enzyme system to cleave the first carbon of glycine and convert it to carbon dioxide. The second carbon is transferred to tetrahydrofolate (THF) to form hydroxymethyltetrahydrofolate, which may either react with another mole of glycine to form serine (Fig. 71–7) or form methyltetrahydrofolate, which serves as a methyl group donor for many reactions in the body (see Fig. 71–3). The glycine cleavage system, a mitochondrial multienzyme system, is composed of four proteins: P protein, H protein, T protein, and L protein. The T protein, also known as aminomethyltransferase, is mapped to the short arm of chromosome 3. More than 80% of patients with nonketotic hypoglycinemia have defects in P protein. Defects in T protein account for nearly the rest of the reported cases.

HYPERGLYCINEMIA. Elevated levels of glycine in body fluids occur in patients having a number of inborn errors of metabolism, including propionic acidemia, methylmalonic acidemia, isovaleric acidemia, and β-ketothiolase deficiency. These disorders have been collectively referred to as *ketotic hyperglycinemia* because episodes of severe acidosis and ketosis occur. The pathogenesis of hyperglycinemia in these disorders is not fully understood, but inhibition of the glycine cleavage enzyme system by the various organic acids has been shown to occur in some of the affected patients. The term *nonketotic hyperglycinemia* is reserved for the clinical condition caused by the genetic deficiency of the glycine cleavage enzyme system (see Fig. 71–7). In this condition hyperglycinemia is present without ketosis.

Nonketotic Hyperglycinemia. The majority of patients with this disorder become ill during the first few days of life. The *clinical*

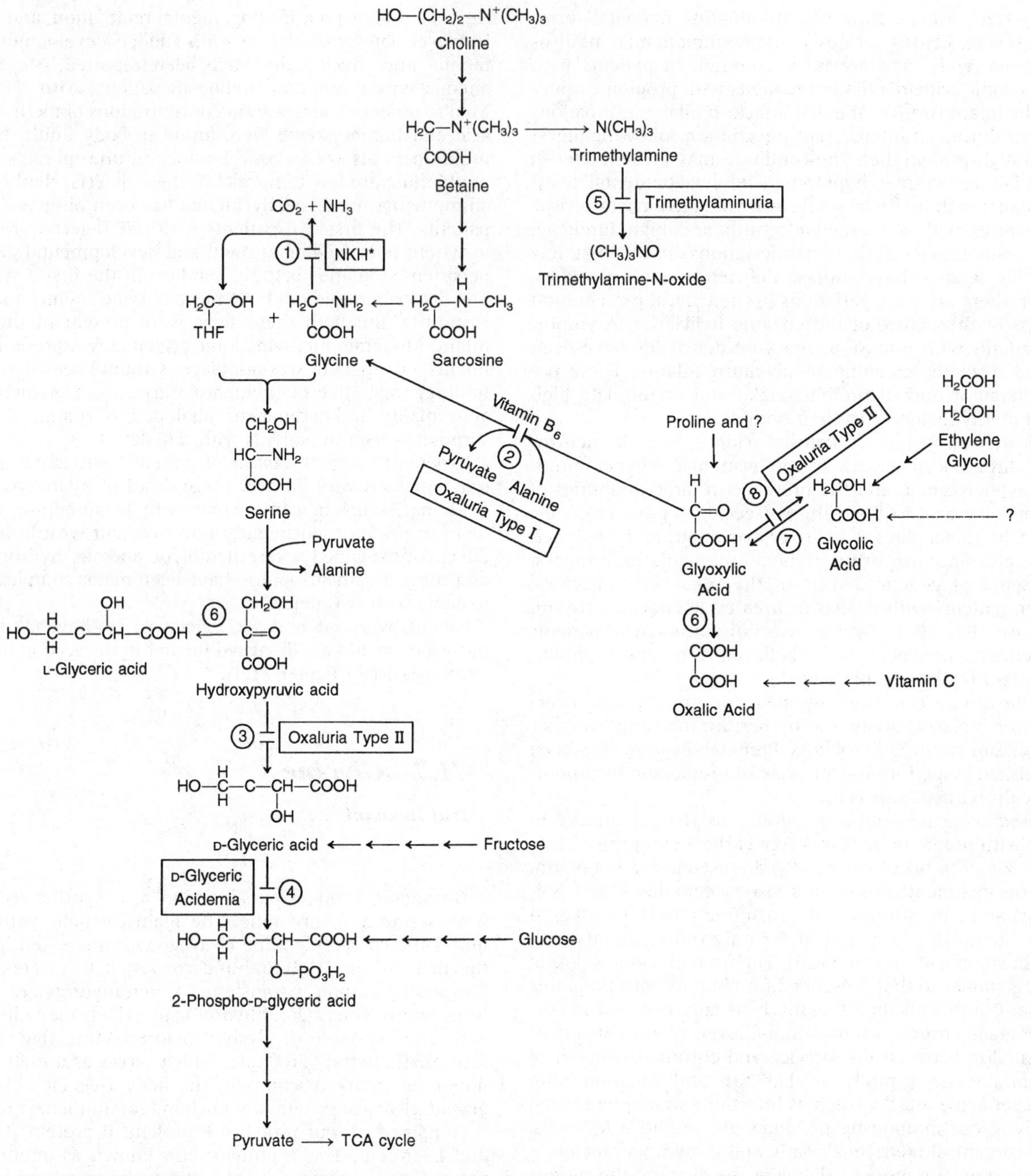

Figure 71–7. Pathways in metabolism of glycine and glyoxylic acid. Enzymes: (1) glycine cleavage enzyme; (2) alanine: glyoxylate aminotransferase; (3) D-glyceric acid dehydrogenase; (4) glycerate kinase; (5) trimethylamine oxidase; (6) lactate dehydrogenase; (7) glycolate oxidase; (8) glyoxylate reductase. NKH* = nonketotic hyperglycinemia; THF = tetrahydrofolate.

manifestations of poor feeding, failure to suck, and lethargy may progress rapidly to a deep coma, apnea, and death. Convulsions, especially myoclonic seizures, and hiccups are common. This disorder is usually fatal; current therapeutic measures may produce only transient improvement. The rare infant who survives this state will have severe mental retardation, repeated myoclonic seizures, and microcephaly. Milder forms of the condition have also been reported; mental retardation, convulsions, and spasticity are frequent findings in these patients. Heterogeneity in clinical severity of the disease has also been observed within a given family.

Laboratory findings reveal moderate to severe hyperglycinemia and hyperglycinuria, and an increased glycine concentration in the spinal fluid. The high ratio of glycine concentration in the spinal fluid to that in blood has been used to differentiate nonketotic hyperglycinemia from other hyperglycinemic states. Plasma serine levels are usually low. Serum pH is usually normal. Organic acidemias that cause hyperglycinemia (propionic and methylmalonic acidemias) should be ruled out by proper urinary assays. *Diagnosis* of nonketotic hyperglycinemia may be suggested in infants who are receiving the anticonvulsant drug valproic acid because this medication is known to cause moderate increases in blood and urinary glycine concentrations. Repeat assays after removal of the drug should establish the diagnosis. The rare condition D-glyceric acidemia, which may cause hyperglycinemia, should also be ruled out (see later).

No effective *treatment* is known. Exchange transfusion, dietary restriction of glycine, and administration of sodium benzoate or folate have not altered the neurologic outcome. Drugs that counteract the effect of glycine on the neuronal cells, such as strychnine and diazepam, have been used; beneficial effects have been observed in some patients with the mild form of the condition.

Nonketotic hyperglycinemia appears to be inherited as an autosomal recessive trait and is more common in Finland than in any other part of the world. The enzyme system may be assayed in specimens obtained from liver or brain. Prenatal diagnosis has been accomplished by performing an assay of enzyme activity in biopsy specimens of chorionic villi.

SARCOSINEMIA. Increased concentrations of sarcosine (*N*-methylglycine) have been observed in both blood and urine, but no consistent clinical picture can be attributed to this metabolic defect. This is probably a recessively inherited inborn error involving sarcosine dehydrogenase, the enzyme that converts sarcosine to glycine (see Fig. 71–7).

D-GLYCERIC ACIDEMIA. D-Glyceric acid is an intermediate metabolite of serine and fructose metabolism (see Fig. 71–7). At least two forms of this rare condition have been identified. In one form (seen in three patients) clinical manifestations of severe encephalopathy (hypotonia, seizures, and mental and motor deficits) and the laboratory findings of hyperglycinemia and hyperglycinuria were suggestive of nonketotic hyperglycinemia. However, these patients excreted large quantities of D-glyceric acid (this compound is not normally detectable in urine). Enzyme studies indicated a deficiency of glycerate kinase in one patient and decreased activity of D-glyceric dehydrogenase in another.

In the other form, the major findings were persistent metabolic acidosis and developmental delay. This infant excreted large amounts of D-glyceric acid without hyperglycinemia. The enzyme defect in this patient was not identified.

TRIMETHYLAMINURIA. Trimethylamine is normally produced in the intestine from the breakdown of dietary choline and trimethylamine oxide by bacteria. Eggs and liver are the main sources of choline, and fish is the major source of trimethylamine oxide. Trimethylamine thus produced is absorbed and oxidized in the liver by trimethylamine oxidase to trimethylamine oxide, which is odorless, and is excreted in the urine. Deficiency of this enzyme results in massive excretion of trimethylamine in urine. Several asymptomatic patients with trimethylaminuria have been reported; there is a foul body odor that resembles that of a rotten fish, which may have significant social and psychosocial ramifications. Restriction of fish, eggs, liver, and other sources of choline (such as nuts and grains) in the diet significantly reduces the odor. The gene for trimethylamine oxidase has been mapped to the long arm of chromosome 1.

HYPEROXALURIA AND OXALOSIS. Normally, oxalic acid is derived mostly from the oxidation of glyoxylic acid and, to a lesser degree, from oxidation of ascorbic acid (see Fig. 71–7). Glyoxylic acid is formed from the oxidation of glycolic acid in the peroxisomes. However, the source of glycolic acid remains unclear. Foods containing oxalic acid, such as spinach and rhubarb, are the main exogenous sources of this compound. Oxalic acid cannot be further metabolized in humans and is excreted in the urine as oxalates. Calcium oxalate is relatively insoluble in water and precipitates in tissues (kidney and joints) if its concentration increases in the body.

Secondary hyperoxaluria has been observed in pyridoxine deficiency (cofactor for alanine-glyoxylate aminotransferase, see Fig. 71–7), following ingestion of ethylene glycol or high doses of vitamin C, after administration of the anesthetic agent methoxyflurane (which oxidizes directly to oxalic acid), and in patients with inflammatory bowel disease or extensive resection of bowel *(enteric hyperoxaluria)*. Acute, fatal hyperoxaluria may develop after ingestion of plants with a high oxalic acid content such as sorrel. Intentional ingestion of oxalic acid was a common suicidal agent at the turn of the century when oxalic acid was easily accessible as a common household cleaning agent. Precipitation of calcium oxalate in tissues causes hypocalcemia, liver necrosis, renal failure, cardiac arrythmia, and death. The lethal dose of oxalic acid is estimated to be between 5 and 30 g.

Primary hyperoxaluria is a rare genetic disorder in which large numbers of oxalates accumulate in the body. Two types of primary hyperoxaluria have been identified. The term *oxalosis* refers to deposition of calcium oxalate in parenchymal tissue.

Primary Hyperoxaluria Type I. This rare condition is the most common form of primary hyperoxaluria. It is due to a deficiency of the peroxisomal enzyme alanine-glyoxylate aminotransferase, which requires pyridoxine (vitamin B_6) as its cofactor. In the absence of this enzyme, glyoxylic acid, which cannot be converted to glycine, is transferred to the cytosol, where it is oxidized to oxalic acid (see Fig. 71–7). It is inherited as an autosomal recessive trait. The gene for this enzyme resides on the long arm of chromosome 2. Several mutations of the gene have been described in patients with this condition. The most common mutation results in the mistargeting of the enzyme to the mitochondria instead of the proxisomes.

There is a wide variation in the age of presentation. The majority of patients become symptomatic before 5 yr of age. In about 10% of cases symptoms develop before 1 yr of age (neonatal oxaluria). The initial *clinical manifestations* are related to renal stones and nephrocalcinosis. Renal colic and asymptomatic hematuria lead to a gradual deterioration of renal function, manifestated by growth retardation and uremia. Most patients die before 20 yr of age from renal failure. Acute arthritis is a rare manifestation and may be misdiagnosed as gout, because uric acid is usually elevated in patients with type I hyperoxaluria. Late forms of the disease presenting during adulthood have also been reported.

A marked increase in urinary excretion of oxalate (normal excretion 10–50 mg/24 hr) is the most important *laboratory finding*. The presence of oxalate crystals in urinary sediment is rarely helpful for diagnosis because such crystals are often seen in normal individuals. Unlike the situation with hyperoxaluria type II, urinary excretion of glycolic acid and glyoxylic acid is increased in patients with type I hyperoxaluria. *Diagnosis* can be confirmed by performing an assay of the enzyme in liver specimens.

Treatment has been largely unsuccessful. In some patients administration of large doses of pyridoxine reduces urinary excretion of oxalate. Renal transplantation in patients with renal failure has not improved the outcome in most cases because oxalosis has recurred in the transplanted kidney. Combined liver and kidney transplants have resulted in a significant decrease in plasma and urinary oxalate in a few patients, and this may be the most effective treatment of this disorder to date.

Primary Hyperoxaluria Type II (L-Glyceric Aciduria). This rare condition is due to the combined deficiencies of L-glyceric acid dehydrogenase and glyoxylic acid reductase enzymes (see Fig. 71–7). In the absence of the former enzyme, hydroxypyruvate (the ketoacid of serine) is reduced to L-glyceric acid by lactate dehydrogenase. Deficiency of glyoxylic acid reductase causes the accumulation of glyoxylic acid, which is converted to oxalic acid by lactate dehydrogenase. It is possible that both glyceric acid dehydrogenase and glyoxylic acid reductase are part of a one-enzyme system. At least 16 patients with the disorder have been reported. Eight patients are from the Saulteaux-Ojibway Indians of Manitoba.

Clinically, these patients are indistinguishable from those with hyperoxaluria type I. Renal stones presenting with renal colic and hematuria may develop before age 2 yr. However, renal failure has not been observed in patients with type II oxaluria;

the urine contains large amounts of L-glyceric acid in addition to high levels of oxalate (L-glyceric acid is not normally present in urine). Urinary excretion of glycolic acid and glyoxylic acid is not increased. The presence of L-glyceric acid without increased levels of glycolic and glyoxylic acids in urine differentiates this type from type I hyperoxaluria. A similar disease has been recently described in cats.

71.8 Proline and Hydroxyproline

Iraj Rezvani

Proline and hydroxyproline are found in high concentrations in collagen. Neither of these amino acids is normally found in urine in the free form except in early infancy. Excretion of "bound" hydroxyproline (dipeptides and tripeptides containing hydroxyproline) reflects collagen turnover and is increased in disorders of accelerated collagen turnover, such as rickets or hyperparathyroidism.

HYPERPROLINEMIA. Two types of this rare autosomal recessive condition have been described. *Type I hyperprolinemia* is due to a deficiency of proline oxidase (dehydrogenase), and *type II* is due to a defect in Δ'-pyrroline-5-carboxylic acid dehydrogenase enzyme (Fig. 71–8). Neither type causes any specific clinical manifestation. Increased blood concentrations of proline (more pronounced in type II) and prolinuria are found in both types. Hydroxyproline and glycine are also excreted in abnormal amounts in the urine because of the saturation of the common tubular reabsorption mechanism by the massive prolinuria. The presence of Δ'-pyrroline-5-carboxylic acid in plasma and urine differentiates type II from type I. No treatment is recommended for the affected individuals.

HYPERHYDROXYPROLINEMIA. This rare autosomal recessive condition is presumably due to a deficiency of hydroxyproline oxidase (see Fig. 71–8). Patients with this disorder are usually asymptomatic. A marked increase in blood concentration of hydroxyproline is diagnostic. These patients also excrete large quantities of proline and glycine in their urine. No treatment is recommended.

PROLIDASE DEFICIENCY. During collagen degradation imidodipeptides (such as glycylproline) are released and are normally cleaved by tissue prolidase. This enzyme requires manganese for its proper activity. Deficiency of prolidase, which is inherited as an autosomal recessive trait, results in the accumulation of imidodipeptides in body fluids. The gene for prolidase has been mapped to the long arm of chromosome 19.

The *clinical manifestations* of this rare condition (only 28 patients are known) and the age of onset are quite variable. Skin lesions (recurrent ulcers, fine purpuric rash, crusting erythematous dermatitis), mental and motor deficits, susceptibility to infections, and joint laxity are major findings. Some patients have characteristic craniofacial features with ptosis, ocular proptosis, and prominent cranial sutures. Asymptomatic cases have also been reported. A marked increase in urinary excretion of imidodipeptides is diagnostic. Enzyme assay may be performed in erythrocytes or cultured skin fibroblasts.

Oral supplementation with proline, ascorbic acid, and manganese and the topical use of proline and glycine result in an improvement in leg ulcers.

FAMILIAL IMINOGLYCINURIA. This asymptomatic defect in renal tubular reabsorption of proline is inherited as an autosomal recessive trait. Because proline, hydroxyproline, and glycine are all transported by a common mechanism, patients with familial iminoglycinuria also excrete proline and hydroxyproline in abnormal amounts. The serum concentrations of these amino acids are normal. Many persons so affected also have impaired intestinal transport of proline, and a few may be coincidentally mentally retarded. In a screening program, iminoglycinuria was found in 1 in 15,000 infants. Iminoglycinuria is also seen in patients with hyperprolinemia, hyperhydroxyprolinemia, and Fanconi syndrome.

71.9 Glutamic Acid

Iraj Rezvani

Glutathione (γ-glutamylcysteinylglycine) is the major product of glutamic acid in the body. This ubiquitous tripeptide is synthesized and degraded through a complex cycle called the γ-glutamyl cycle (Fig. 71–9). Because of its free sulfhydryl (-SH) group and its abundance in the cell, glutathione protects

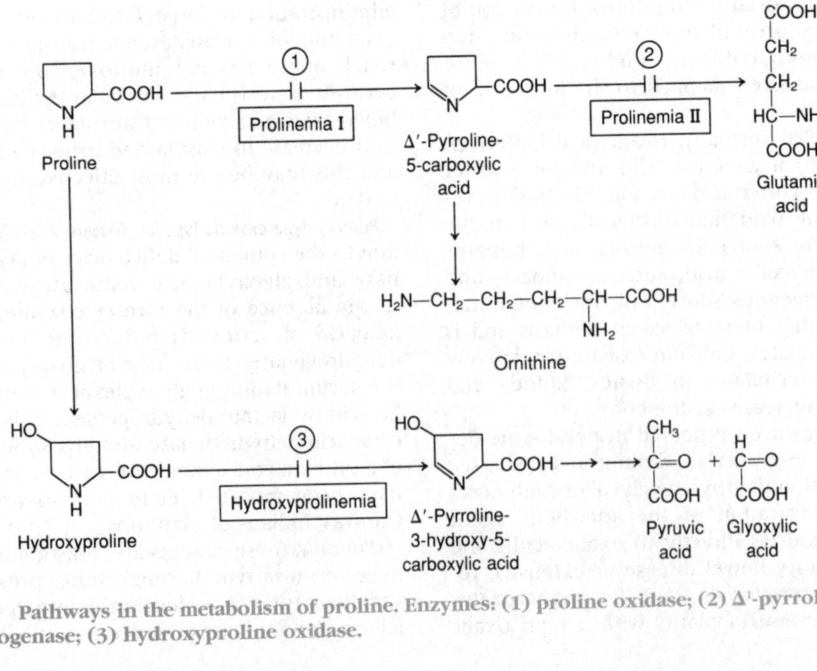

Figure 71–8. Pathways in the metabolism of proline. Enzymes: (1) proline oxidase; (2) Δ'-pyrroline-5-carboxylic acid dehydrogenase; (3) hydroxyproline oxidase.

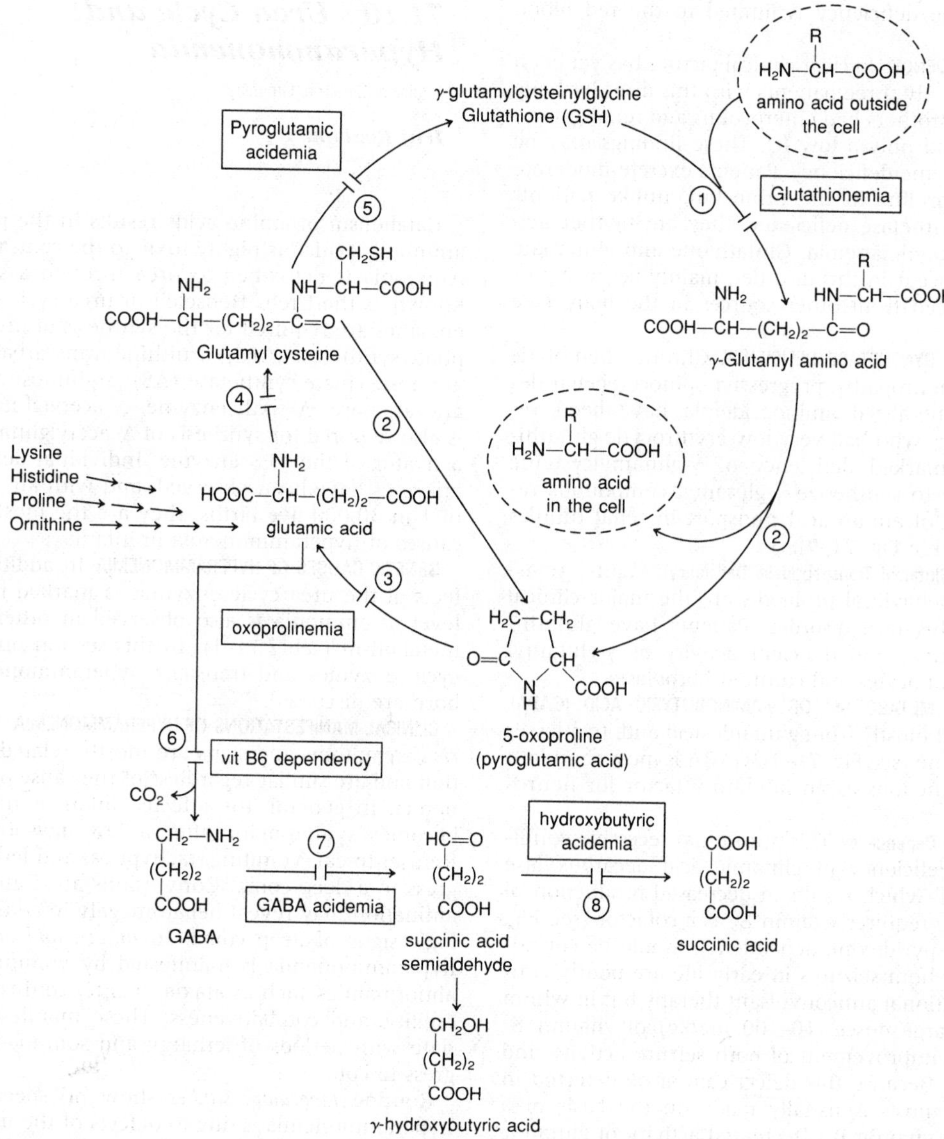

Figure 71–9. The γ-glutamyl cycle. Defects of glutathione synthesis and degradation are noted. Enzymes: (1) γ glutamyl transpeptidase; (2) γ glutamyl cyclotransferase; (3) 5-oxoprolinase; (4) γ glutamylcysteine synthetase; (5) glutathione synthetase; (6) glutamic acid decarboxylase; (7) GABA transaminase; (8) succinic semialdehyde dehydrogenase.

other sulfhydryl-containing compounds (such as enzymes and coenzyme A) from oxidation. It is also involved in the detoxification of peroxides, including hydrogen peroxide, and in keeping the cell content in a reduced state. Glutathione may also participate in amino acid transport across the cell membrane through the γ-glutamyl cycle.

GLUTATHIONE SYNTHETASE DEFICIENCY. Two forms of this condition have been reported. In the *severe form,* which is due to generalized deficiency of the enzyme, severe acidosis and 5-oxoprolinuria are the rule. In the *mild form,* in which the enzyme deficiency is limited to red blood cells only, neither 5-oxoprolinuria nor acidosis has been observed. In both forms, patients have hemolytic anemia secondary to glutathione deficiency.

Glutathione Synthetase Deficiency, Severe Form (Pyroglutamic Acidemia, 5-Oxoprolinuria). Chronic metabolic acidosis and mild to moderate hemolytic anemia, which become manifest in the first few days of life, are cardinal findings in this rare autosomal recessive disorder. Mental and neurologic deficits have been observed in some affected children. Life-threatening metabolic acidosis may occur following a surgical procedure or intercurrent infection. These patients excrete massive amounts (up to 40 g/24 hr) of 5-oxoproline (pyroglutamic acid) in urine. High concentrations of this compound are also found in blood. The glutathione content of erythrocytes is markedly decreased. Increased synthesis of 5-oxoproline in this disorder is believed to be due to the conversion of γ-glutamylcysteine to 5-oxoproline by the enzyme γ-glutamyl cyclotransferase (see Fig. 71–9). γ-Glutamylcysteine production increases greatly because the inhibitory effect of glutathione on the γ-glutamylcysteine synthetase enzyme is removed. A deficiency of glutathione synthetase has been demonstrated in a variety of cells. *Treatment* is mainly directed toward correcting the acidosis, avoiding drugs and oxidants that may cause hemolysis, and preventing stressful states.

Glutathione Synthetase Deficiency, Mild Form. These patients have mild hemolytic anemia and jaundice without 5-oxoprolinuria and acidosis. The enzyme deficiency is limited to the red blood cells.

5-OXOPROLINASE DEFICIENCY. No clear clinical picture has yet been established because only three patients with this disorder have been reported. Two brothers had enterocolitis and renal stones. The other patient had only a low IQ. These findings may be unrelated to the enzyme deficiency. Patients excrete moderate quantities of 5-oxoproline in the urine but, unlike patients with glutathione synthetase deficiency, they are neither acidotic nor have hemolytic anemia. Glutathione and glutamate deficiencies do not occur in this disorder, mainly because glutamic acid is produced from other sources in the body (see Fig. 71–9).

γ-GLUTAMYLCYSTEINE SYNTHETASE DEFICIENCY. Chronic hemolytic anemia, peripheral neuropathy, progressive spinocerebellar degeneration, and generalized aminoacidemia have been reported in two siblings who had very low erythrocytic glutathione levels and a marked deficiency of γ-glutamylcysteine synthetase. Inability to synthesize γ-glutamyl compounds results in impairment of amino acid transport in renal tubules and aminoaciduria (see Fig. 71–9).

GLUTATHIONEMIA (γ-Glutamyl Transpeptidase Deficiency). Mental retardation and severe behavioral problems are the major clinical manifestations of this rare disorder. Patients have glutathionemia, glutathionuria, and deficient activity of γ-glutamyl transpeptidase in leukocytes and cultured fibroblasts.

INBORN ERRORS OF METABOLISM OF γ-AMINOBUTYRIC ACID (GABA). GABA is synthesized mostly from glutamic acid and, to a lesser degree, from ornithine (see Fig. 71–9). GABA is most abundant in the brain and functions as an inhibitory factor for neurotransmitters.

Vitamin B_6 (Pyridoxine) Dependency. This autosomal recessive condition is due to a deficiency of glutamic acid decarboxylase activity in the brain, which results in decreased production of GABA. This enzyme requires vitamin B_6 as a cofactor (see Fig. 71–9). Diagnosis of pyridoxine dependency should be considered in infants in whom seizures in early life are poorly controlled with conventional anticonvulsant therapy but in whom administration of large doses (10–100 mg/kg) of vitamin B_6 results in dramatic improvement of both seizure activity and EEG abnormalities. Because this defect cannot be detected in fibroblasts, the diagnosis is usually made on the basis of a clinical response to vitamin B_6. Decreased activity of glutamic acid decarboxylase, reversible by the addition of pyridoxine, has been demonstrated in renal tissue but not in the brain. These children require high daily doses of vitamin B_6 indefinitely.

γ-Aminobutyric Acidemia (GABA Transaminase Deficiency). This condition is manifest as severe psychomotor retardation, hypotonia, and accelerated linear growth. There is a marked elevation of GABA and β-alanine in cerebrospinal fluid and blood (see Fig. 71–9). Increased linear growth occurs, possibly as a result of hypersecretion of growth hormone induced by GABA. GABA transaminase deficiency has been demonstrated in liver biopsy and lymphocytes. Treatment with high doses of vitamin B_6 is ineffective.

γ-Hydroxybutyric Acidemia. A defect in succinic semialdehyde dehydrogenase, inherited as an autosomal recessive disorder, leads to increased production of γ-hydroxybutyric acid, a normal minor metabolite of GABA, which is abundant in the brain (see Fig. 71–9). Ataxia, hypotonia, and neurologic deficits are the main clinical manifestations, which may occur in early infancy. Ataxia improves with advancement of age. Large amounts of γ-hydroxybutyrate and moderate quantities of succinic semialdehyde are found in the urine. Elevated levels of γ-hydroxybutyrate are also detected in the blood and cerebrospinal fluid. These levels may become normal with advancing age. The enzyme deficiency has been demonstrated in lymphocyte lysates. No effective treatment is yet available.

71.10 Urea Cycle and Hyperammonemia

(Arginine, Citrulline, Ornithine)

Iraj Rezvani

Catabolism of amino acids results in the production of free ammonia, which is highly toxic to the central nervous system. Ammonia is detoxified to urea through a series of reactions known as the Krebs-Henseleit or urea cycle (Fig. 71–10). Five enzymes are required for the synthesis of urea: carbamylphosphate synthetase (CPS), ornithine transcarbamylase (OTC), argininosuccinate synthetase (AS), argininosuccinate lyase (AL), and arginase. A sixth enzyme, *N*-acetylglutamate synthetase, is also required for synthesis of *N*-acetylglutamate, which is an activator of the CPS enzyme. Individual deficiencies of these enzymes have been observed, and with an overall prevalence of 1 in 30,000 live births, they are the most common genetic causes of hyperammonemia in infants.

GENETIC CAUSES OF HYPERAMMONEMIA. In addition to genetic defects of the urea cycle enzymes, a marked increase in plasma level of ammonia is also observed in other inborn errors of metabolism (Table 71–1). In this section only defects of urea cycle enzymes and transient hyperammonemia of the newborn are discussed.

CLINICAL MANIFESTATIONS OF HYPERAMMONEMIA. In the *neonatal period*, symptoms and signs are mostly related to brain dysfunction and are similar regardless of the cause of the hyperammonemia. In general, the affected infant is normal at birth but becomes symptomatic after a few days of protein feeding. Refusal to eat, vomiting, tachypnea, and lethargy quickly progress to a deep coma. Convulsions are common. Physical examination may reveal hepatomegaly in addition to the neurologic signs of deep coma. In *infants and older children*, acute hyperammonemia is manifested by vomiting and neurologic abnormalities such as ataxia, mental confusion, agitation, irritability, and combativeness. These manifestations may alternate with periods of lethargy and somnolence that may progress to coma.

Routine *laboratory studies* show no specific findings when hyperammonemia is due to defects of the urea cycle enzymes. Blood urea nitrogen is usually very low. In infants with organic acidemias, hyperammonemia is commonly associated with severe acidosis. Newborn infants with hyperammonemia are often misdiagnosed as having a generalized infection, and they may succumb to the disease without a correct diagnosis. Au-

■ TABLE 71–1 Inborn Errors of Metabolism Causing Hyperammonemia

Deficiencies of the urea cycle enzymes
Carbamyl phosphate synthetase (CPS)
N-acetylglutamate synthetase
Ornithine transcarbamylase (OTC)
Argininosuccinate synthetase (AS)
Argininosuccinate lyase (AL)
Arginase
Organic acidemias
Propionic acidemia
Methylmalonic acidemia
Isovaleric acidemia
Ketothiolase deficiency
Multiple carboxylase deficiency
Fatty acid acyl CoA dehydrogenase deficiency (glutaric acidemia type II)
3-Hydroxy-3-methylglutaric acidemia
Lysinuric protein intolerance
Hyperornithinemia-hyperammonemia-homocitrullinemia syndrome
Periodic hyperlysinuria with hyperammonemia (?)
Transient hyperammonemia of the newborn

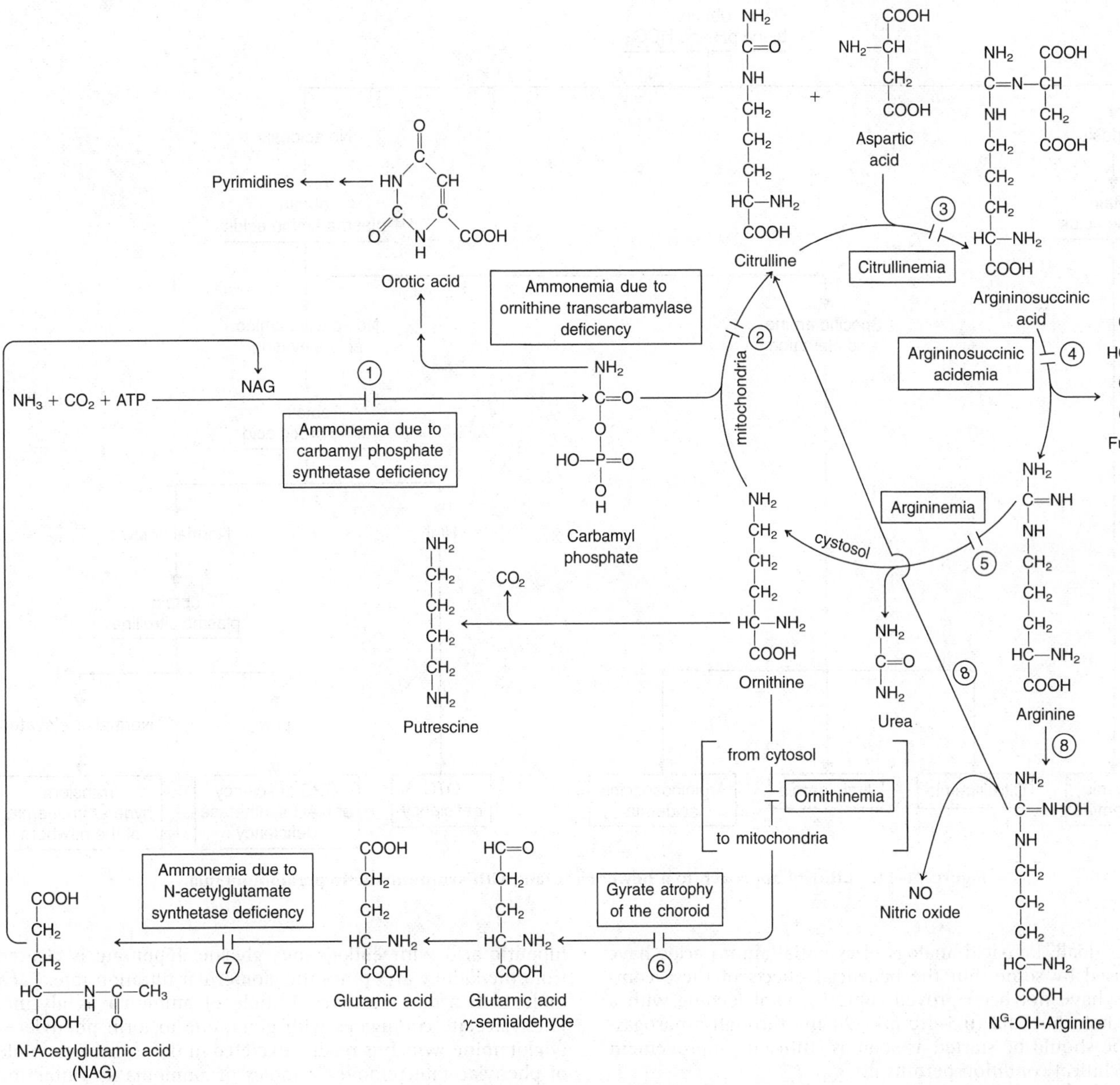

Figure 71–10. Pathways in the metabolism of ammonia and in the urea cycle. Enzymes: (1) carbamyl phosphate synthetase (CPS); (2) ornithine transcarbamylase (OTC); (3) argininosuccinic acid synthetase; (4) argininosuccinic acid lyase; (5) arginase; (6) ornithine 5-aminotransferase; (7) *N*-acetylglutamate synthetase; (8) nitric oxide synthase.

topsy is usually unremarkable. It is therefore imperative to measure plasma ammonia levels in any ill infant whose clinical manifestations cannot be explained by an obvious infection.

DIAGNOSIS. The main criterion for diagnosis is hyperammonemia. The plasma ammonia concentration in the ill infant is usually above 200 μM (normal values <35 μM). An approach to the differential diagnosis of hyperammonemia in the newborn infant is illustrated in Figure 71–11. Patients with a deficiency of carbamylphosphate synthetase or of ornithine transcarbamylase have no specific abnormalities of plasma amino acids except for increased levels of glutamine, aspartic acid, and alanine secondary to hyperammonemia. A marked increase in urinary orotic acid in patients with ornithine transcarbamylase deficiency differentiates this defect from carbamylphosphate synthetase deficiency. Patients with a deficiency of argininosuccinic acid synthetase, argininosuccinic acid lyase, or arginase have a marked increase in the plasma level of citrulline, argininosuccinic acid, or arginine, respectively. Differentiation between the carbamylphosphate synthetase deficiency and the *N*-acetylglutamate synthetase deficiency may require an assay of the respective enzymes. Clinical improvement occurring after oral administration of carbamylglutamate, however, may suggest *N*-acetylglutamate synthetase deficiency.

TREATMENT OF ACUTE HYPERAMMONEMIA. Acute hyperammonemia should be treated promptly and vigorously. The goal of therapy is to remove ammonia from the body and provide adequate calories and essential amino acids to halt further breakdown of endogenous proteins (Table 71–2). Adequate calories, fluid, and electrolytes should be provided intravenously. Lipids for intravenous use (1 g/kg/24 hr) provide an effective source of calories. Minimal amounts of protein (0.25 g/kg/24 hr), preferably in the form of essential amino acids, should be added to the intravenous fluid to prevent a catabolic state. To supply these essential amino acids without increasing the

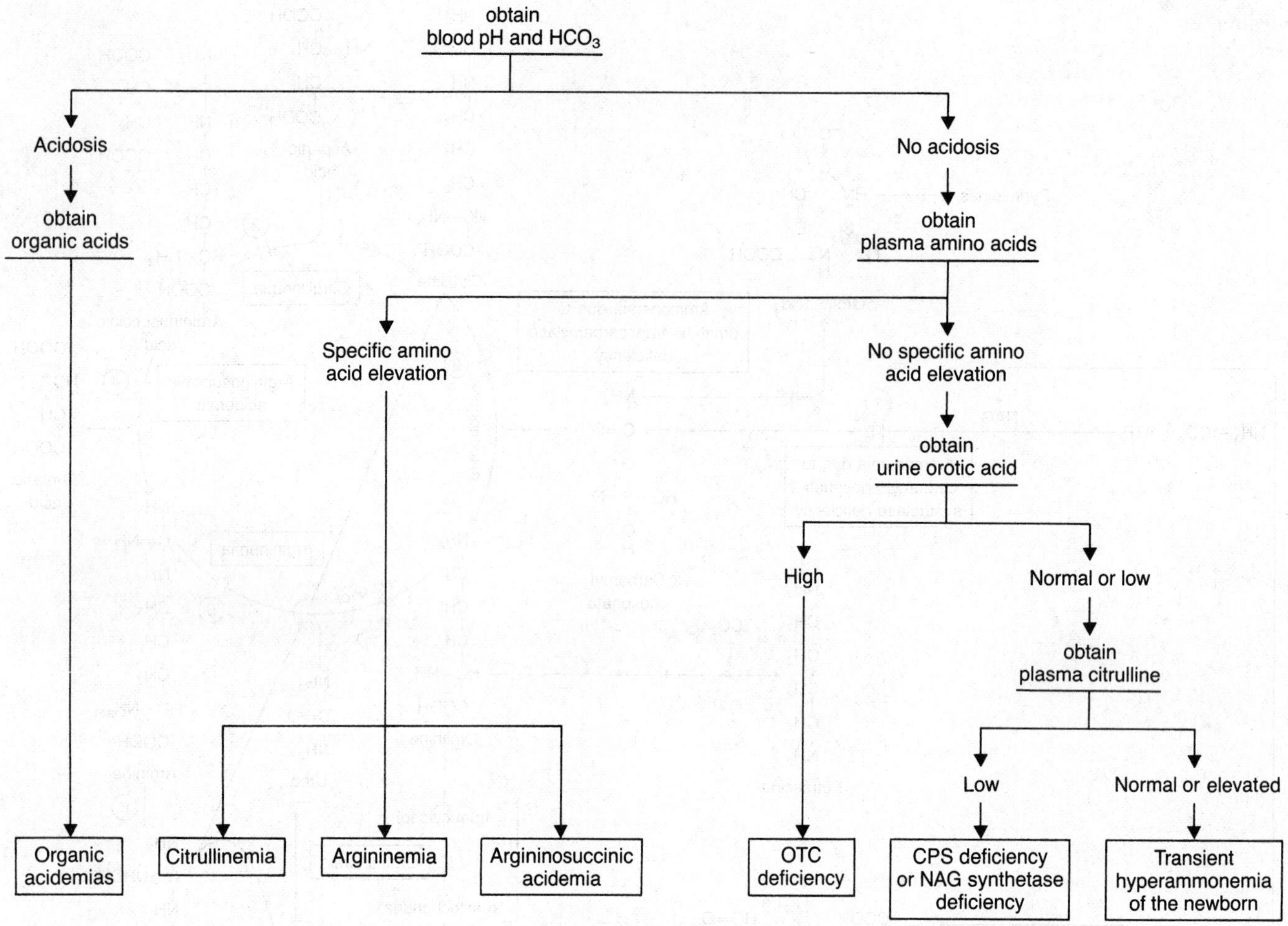

Figure 71–11. Clinical approach to a newborn infant with symptomatic hyperammonemia.

nitrogen load, ketoacid analogs of essential amino acids have been used by some, but the beneficial effects of these compounds have not been proved clinically. Oral feeding with a low-protein formula (0.5–1.0 g/kg/24 hr) through a nasogastric tube should be started as soon as sufficient improvement in the clinical condition permits it.

Because ammonia is poorly cleared by the kidneys, its removal from the body must be expedited by formation of compounds with a high renal clearance. Sodium benzoate forms hippuric acid with endogenous glycine; hippurate is cleared from the kidney at 5 times the glomerular filtration rate. Each mole of benzoate removes 1 mole of ammonia as glycine. Phenylacetate conjugates with glutamine to form phenylacetylglutamine, which is readily excreted in the urine. One mole of phenylacetate removes 2 moles of ammonia as glutamine from the body.

Arginine administration is effective in the treatment of hyperammonemia that is due to defects of the urea cycle (except in patients with arginase deficiency) because it supplies the urea cycle with ornithine and *N*-acetylglumate (see Fig. 71–10). In patients with citrullinemia, 1 mole of arginine reacts with 1 mole of ammonia (as carbamylphosphate) to form citrulline. In patients with argininosuccinic acidemia, 2 moles of ammonia (as carbamylphosphate and aspartate) form argininosuccinic acid with arginine through the urea cycle. Citrulline and argininosuccinic acid are far less toxic and more readily excreted by the kidneys than ammonia. In patients with CPS or ornithine transcarbamylase (OTC) deficiency, arginine administration is indicated because arginine becomes an essential amino acid in these disorders. Patients with OTC deficiency benefit from citrulline supplementation (200 mg/kg/24 hr) because 1 mole of citrulline can accept 1 mole of ammonia (as aspartic acid) to form arginine. In patients whose hyperammonemia is secondary to organic acidemias, treatment with arginine is not indicated because no beneficial effect from such therapy can be expected. However, in a newborn infant with a first attack of hyperammonemia, arginine should be used until the diagnosis is established.

Benzoate, phenylacetate, and arginine may be administered

■ TABLE 71–2 Treatment of Acute Hyperammonemia in an Infant

1. Provide adequate calories, fluid, and electrolytes intravenously (10% glucose and intravenous lipids 1 g/kg/24 hr). Add minimal amounts of protein as a mixture of essential amino acids (0.25 g/kg/24 hr) during the first 24 hr of therapy.
2. Give priming doses of the following compounds:

Sodium benzoate 250 mg/kg* Sodium phenylacetate 250 mg/kg* Arginine hydrochloride 200–800 mg/kg† as a 10% solution	To be added to 20 mL/kg of 10% glucose and infused within 1–2 hr

3. Continue infusion of sodium benzoate* (250–500 mg/kg/24 hr), sodium phenylacetate* (250–500 mg/kg/24 hr), and arginine (200–800 mg/kg/24 hr†) following the above priming doses. These compounds should be added to the daily intravenous fluid.
4. Initiate peritoneal dialysis or hemodialysis if above treatment fails to produce an appreciable decrease in plasma ammonia.

**These compounds are usually prepared as a 5–10% solution for intravenous use. Sodium from these drugs should be included as part of the daily sodium requirement.*

†The higher dose is recommended in the treatment of patients with citrullinemia and argininosuccinic aciduria. Arginine is not recommended in patients with arginase deficiency and in those whose hyperammonemia is secondary to organic acidemia.

together for maximal therapeutic effect. A priming dose of these compounds is followed by continuous infusion until recovery from the acute state occurs (see Table 71–2). It should be noted that both benzoate and phenylacetate are supplied as concentrated solutions and should be properly diluted (1–2% solution) for intravenous use. The recommended therapeutic doses of both compounds deliver a substantial amount of sodium to the patient that should be calculated as part of the daily sodium requirement. Benzoate and phenylacetate should be used with caution in newborn infants with hyperbilirubinemia because they may potentiate the risk of hyperbilirubinemia by displacing bilirubin from albumin. In infants at risk, it is advisable to reduce bilirubin to a safe level by exchange transfusion before administering benzoate or phenylacetate.

If the foregoing therapies fail to produce any appreciable change in the blood ammonia level within a few hours, hemodialysis or peritoneal dialysis should be used. Exchange transfusion has little effect on reducing total body ammonia. It should be used only if dialysis cannot be employed promptly or when the patient is a newborn infant with hyperbilirubinemia (see earlier). Hemodialysis, although the most effective measure for removal of ammonia, is technically difficult to perform and may not be readily available in all centers. Peritoneal dialysis, therefore, is the most practical and expeditious method for treatment of patients with severe hyperammonemia; there is usually a dramatic decrease in the plasma ammonia level within a few hours of dialysis, and in most patients the plasma ammonia returns to normal within 48 hr of initiation of peritoneal dialysis. In a patient whose hyperammonemia is due to an organic acidemia, peritoneal dialysis effectively removes both the offending organic acid and ammonia from the body.

To curtail the possible production of ammonia by intestinal bacteria, oral administration of neomycin and lactulose through a nasogastric tube should be initiated very early in the course of therapy. There may be considerable lag between the normalization of ammonia and an improvement in the neurologic status of the patient. Several days may be needed before the infant becomes fully alert.

Long-Term Therapy. Once the infant is alert, therapy should be tailored to the underlying cause of the hyperammonemia. In general, all patients require some degree of protein restriction (1–2 g/kg/24 hr) regardless of the enzymatic defect. In patients with defects in the urea cycle, chronic administration of benzoate (250–500 mg/kg/24 hr), phenylacetate (250–500 mg/kg/24 hr), and arginine (200–400 mg/kg/24 hr), or citrulline in patients with OTC deficiency (200–400 mg/kg/24 hr), is effective in maintaining blood ammonia levels within the normal range. Phenylacetate may not be accepted by the patient and family because of its offensive odor. Carnitine supplementation has also been recommended for treatment of these patients because benzoate and phenylacetate may cause carnitine depletion, but the clinical benefits of this compound remain to be proved. Catabolic states triggering hyperammonemia should be avoided.

CARBAMYLPHOSPHATE SYNTHETASE (CPS) AND *N*-ACETYLGLUTAMATE SYNTHETASE DEFICIENCIES. Deficiencies of these two enzymes produce similar *clinical and biochemical manifestations*. Affected infants usually become symptomatic in the first few days of life with refusal to eat, vomiting, lethargy, convulsions, and coma. Late forms of the CPS deficiency, characterized by mental retardation with episodes of vomiting and lethargy, have also been reported.

Laboratory findings reveal hyperammonemia without an increase in any specific amino acids in plasma; marked elevations in plasma concentrations of glutamine and alanine seen in these patients are secondary to hyperammonemia. Urinary orotic acid is usually low or may be absent (see Fig. 71–11).

Treatment of patients with CPS deficiency is similar to that outlined above for hyperammonemia. Patients with *N*-acetylglutamate synthetase deficiency were shown to benefit from oral administration of carbamylglutamate. It is therefore important to differentiate between these two enzyme deficiencies by assay of the enzyme activities in biopsies obtained from the liver.

CPS deficiency is inherited as an autosomal recessive trait; the enzyme is normally present in liver and intestine. The gene is mapped to the short arm of chromosome 2. *N*-acetylglutamate synthetase has been assayed only in liver specimens obtained at biopsy.

ORNITHINE TRANSCARBAMYLASE (OTC) DEFICIENCY. In this X-linked dominant disorder the hemizygote males are more severely affected than heterozygote females. More than 20 allelic variants have been documented. The heterozygote female may have either mild disease or no clinical manifestations. This is probably the most common of all the urea cycle disorders.

Clinical manifestations in a male newborn infant are those of severe hyperammonemia. Milder forms of the condition are commonly seen in heterozygote females and in some affected males. These forms characteristically have episodic manifestations. Episodes of hyperammonemia (manifested by vomiting and neurologic abnormalities such as ataxia, mental confusion, agitation, and combativeness) are separated by periods of wellness. Onset may occur in early infancy or early childhood. These episodes usually occur following a high-protein diet or during a situation of stress or infection. Hyperammonemic coma and death may occur during one of these attacks. Some affected children have been diagnosed as having recurrent Reye syndrome. Mental development may proceed normally. However, mild to moderate mental retardation is common. Gallstones have been seen in the survivors; the mechanism remains unclear.

The major *laboratory finding* during the acute attack is hyperammonemia without an increase in any specific amino acid in the blood. As with CPS deficiency, elevation of the plasma concentrations of glutamine and alanine are secondary to hyperammonemia. A marked increase in the urinary excretion of orotic acid differentiates this condition from CPS deficiency (see Fig. 71–11). Orotates may precipitate in urine as gravel or stones. In the mild form, these laboratory abnormalities may revert to normal between attacks. This form should be differentiated from all the episodic conditions of childhood and from poisoning. In particular, lysinuric protein intolerance (Chapter 71.12) mimics the clinical and biochemical characteristics of OTC deficiency. Increased urinary excretion of lysine, ornithine, and arginine and elevated blood concentrations of citrulline, which are salient features of lysinuric protein intolerance, are not seen in patients with OTC deficiency.

The *diagnosis* may be confirmed by performing an assay of enzyme activity that is normally present only in liver. Perinatal diagnosis has been achieved by means of fetal liver biopsy and, more recently, by studying the characteristic DNA polymorphism in chorionic villus samples. Asymptomatic heterozygous female carriers may be identified by using an oral protein load, which increases plasma ammonia and urinary orotic acid levels. A marked increase in urinary excretion of orotidine following an allopurinol loading test has also been used to detect obligate female carriers. Asymptomatic female carriers have mild cerebral dysfunction compared with their unaffected siblings.

Treatment is similar to that given for CPS deficiency except that citrulline may be used in place of arginine. Liver transplantation has been successful as a definite treatment in some patients with OTC deficiency.

ARGININOSUCCINIC ACID SYNTHETASE DEFICIENCY (Citrullinemia). Citrullinemia is inherited as an autosomal recessive trait. The gene is located on the long arm of chromosome 9. The severity of the abnormality of the mutant genes inherited from each parent is different in a given patient, indicating that most affected patients are "double or compound" heterozygotes. This disorder shows considerable clinical and biochemical heterogeneity.

The spectrum of *clinical manifestations* ranges from severe forms to asymptomatic ones. The signs and symptoms in the neonatal form are identical to those seen in the severe forms of CPS and OTC deficiencies (see earlier). Mild forms may have a gradual onset with failure to thrive, frequent vomiting, developmental delay, and dry, brittle hair or, like mild forms of OTC deficiency, may appear episodically (see earlier). In some patients symptoms may not appear until 20 yr of age.

Laboratory findings are similar to those found in patients with OTC deficiency except that the plasma citrulline concentration is markedly elevated in patients with citrullinemia (see Fig. 71–11). Urinary secretion of orotic acid is moderately increased in patients with citrullinemia, and crystalluria due to precipitation of orotates may also occur. Patients with argininosuccinic aciduria also show some increase in the plasma concentration of citrulline in addition to elevated levels of argininosuccinic acid. The *diagnosis* is confirmed by performing an assay of the enzyme activity that is normally present in cultured fibroblasts. Prenatal diagnosis is based on an assay of the enzyme activity in cultured amniotic cells.

Treatment is similar to that for other urea cycle disorders (see earlier). Although *prognosis* is very poor for symptomatic neonates, patients with the mild disease usually do well on a protein-restricted diet. Mild to moderate mental deficiency is a common sequela even in a well-treated patient.

ARGININOSUCCINATE LYASE DEFICIENCY (Argininosuccinic Aciduria). This deficiency is inherited as an autosomal recessive trait with a prevalence of about 1 in 70,000 live births. The gene is located on the long arm of chromosome 7.

The severity of the *clinical and biochemical manifestations* varies considerably. In the neonatal form severe hyperammonemia develops in the first few days of life, and mortality is usually high. In the subacute or late form the major finding is mental retardation, which is associated with episodic vomiting, failure to thrive, and hepatomegaly. Abnormalities of the hair (characterized by dryness and brittleness) are of special diagnostic value. Microscopically, the hair appears similar to that seen in patients with trichorrhexis nodosa. Less severe hair abnormalities are also seen in patients with citrullinemia. Gallstones have been seen in some of the survivors.

Laboratory findings reveal hyperammonemia, moderate elevation in liver enzymes, nonspecific increases in plasma levels of glutamine and alanine, moderate increase in plasma levels of citrulline (less than that seen in citrullinemia), and marked increase in plasma levels of argininosuccinic acid. In most amino acid analyzers, argininosuccinic acid appears within the isoleucine or methionine region, which may cause confusion in the diagnosis. Argininosuccinic acid can also be found in large amounts in urine and spinal fluid. The levels in the spinal fluid are usually higher than those in plasma. The enzyme is normally present in erythrocytes, liver, and cultured fibroblasts. Prenatal diagnosis is based on measuring the enzyme activity in cultured amniotic cells. Argininosuccinic acid is also elevated in the amniotic fluid of affected fetuses.

Treatment is similar to that described for citrullinemia.

ARGINASE DEFICIENCY (Hyperargininemia). This defect is inherited as an autosomal recessive trait. There are two genetically distinct arginases in humans. One is cystosolic and is expressed in liver and erythrocytes, and the other is found in the renal mitochondria. The cytosolic enzyme, which is the one deficient in patients with arginase deficiency, is mapped to the long arm of chromosome 6.

The *clinical manifestations* of this rare condition are quite different from those of other urea cycle enzyme defects. The onset is insidious; the infant usually remains asymptomatic in the first few months or sometimes years of life. A progressive spastic diplegia with scissoring of the lower extremities, choreoathetotic movements, and loss of developmental milestones in a previously normal infant may suggest a degenerative disease of the central nervous system. Two children were followed for several years with the diagnosis of cerebral palsy before the diagnosis of arginase deficiency was confirmed. Mental retardation is progressive; seizures are common, and episodes of severe hyperammonemia are not usually seen in this disorder. Hepatomegaly may be present.

Laboratory findings reveal marked elevation of arginine in plasma and cerebrospinal fluid (see Fig. 71–11). Urinary orotic acid is moderately increased. Plasma ammonia levels may be normal or mildly elevated. Urinary excretion of arginine, lysine, cystine, and ornithine is usually increased, which may suggest a diagnosis of cystinuria. However, urinary excretion of these amino acids may be normal. Therefore, determination of amino acids in plasma is a critical step before the diagnosis of argininemia can be ruled out. The guanidino compounds (α-keto-guanidinovaleric acid, argininic acid) are markedly increased in urine. The *diagnosis* is confirmed by assaying arginase activity in erythrocytes. Prenatal diagnosis has not yet been achieved.

Treatment consists of a low-protein diet devoid of arginine. Administration of a synthetic protein made of essential amino acids usually results in a dramatic decrease in plasma arginine concentration and an improvement in neurologic abnormalities. The composition of the diet and the daily intake of protein should be monitored by frequent plasma amino acid determinations. Sodium benzoate (250–375 mg/kg/24 hr) is also effective in controlling hyperammonemia. One patient developed type I diabetes at age 9 yr while his argininemia was under good control.

TRANSIENT HYPERAMMONEMIA OF THE NEWBORN. Although the plasma levels of ammonia in normal full-term infants are within the normal limits of those seen in older children, a majority of premature infants with low birthweights have a *mild transient hyperammonemia* (40–50 μM), which lasts for about 6–8 wk. These infants are asymptomatic, and follow-up studies up to 18 mo of age have not revealed any significant neurologic deficits.

Severe transient hyperammonemia has been observed in newborn infants. The majority of affected infants have been premature and have had mild respiratory distress syndrome. Hyperammonemic coma may develop within 2–3 days of life, and the infant may succumb to the disease if treatment is not started immediately. Laboratory studies reveal marked hyperammonemia (plasma ammonia as high as 4,000 μM), with moderate increases in plasma levels of glutamine and alanine. Plasma concentrations of urea cycle intermediate amino acids are usually normal except for citrulline, which may be moderately elevated. The cause of the disorder is unknown. Urea cycle enzyme activities are normal. Treatment of hyperammonemia should be initiated promptly and continued vigorously. Recovery without sequelae is common, and hyperammonemia does not recur even with a normal protein diet.

ORNITHINE. Ornithine is one of the intermediate metabolites of the urea cycle that is not incorporated into natural proteins. Rather, it is generated in the cytosol from arginine and must be transported into the mitochondria, where it is used as a substrate for the enzyme OTC to form citrulline. Excess ornithine is catabolized by two enzymes, ornithine 5-aminotransferase, which is a mitochondrial enzyme and converts ornithine to a proline precursor, and ornithine decarboxylase, which resides in the cytosol and converts ornithine to putrescine (see Fig. 71–10). Two genetic disorders result in hyperornithinemia: gyrate atrophy of the retina and ammonemia-hyperornithinemia-homocitrullinemia syndrome.

Gyrate Atrophy of the Retina and Choroid. This is an autosomal recessively inherited disorder due to the deficiency of the enzyme ornithine 5-aminotransferase. About half of the reported cases are from Finland. Clinical manifestations are limited to the eyes and include night blindness, myopia, loss of peripheral vision, and posterior subcapsular cataracts. These eye changes start between 5 and 10 yr of age and progress to complete blindness by the 4th decade of life. Atrophic lesions in the retina resemble cerebral gyri. These patients usually have normal intelligence. There is a 10- to 20-fold increase in plasma levels of ornithine. There is no occurrence of hyperammonemia and no increase in any other amino acids. Some patients respond to high doses of pyridoxine (500–1,000 mg/24 hr) and low dietary arginine. The gene for ornithine 5-aminotransferase is mapped to the short arm of chromosome 10.

Hyperammonemia-Hyperornithinemia-Homocitrullinemia Syndrome (HHH Syndrome). In this rare autosomal recessively inherited disorder the defect is in the transport system of ornithine from the cytosol into the mitochondria, causing an accumulation of ornithine in the cytosol and a deficiency of ornithine inside the mitochondria. The former causes hyperornithinemia and the latter results in disruption of the urea cycle and hyperammonemia. Homocitrulline is formed from the reaction of mitochondrial carbamylphosphate with lysine, which occurs because of the intramitochondrial deficiency of ornithine. Failure to thrive, pyramidal signs (increased deep tendon reflexes, spasticity, clonus), lower limb weakness, mental retardation, and seizures are common findings in these patients. Acute episodes of hyperammonemia in early infancy may result in coma. The onset may be delayed until adulthood in some affected patients. No ocular lesions have been observed in these patients. Marked increases in plasma levels of ornithine and homocitrulline are usually diagnostic. Restriction of protein intake improves hyperammonemia. Ornithine supplementation may produce clinical improvement in some patients. The gene for this disorder is located on the long arm of chromosome 13.

71.11 Histidine

Iraj Rezvani

Histidine is an essential amino acid only during infancy. Its synthetic pathway in older children and adults is poorly understood. Histidine is degraded through the urocanic acid pathway to glutamic acid (Fig. 71–12).

HISTIDINEMIA. This disorder is due to a deficiency of histidase, which normally converts histidine to urocanic acid (see Fig. 71–12). The disorder is inherited as an autosomal recessive trait; its overall prevalence is estimated at 1 in 10,000 worldwide. The gene for histidase is mapped to the long arm of chromosome 12.

Clinical manifestations include impaired speech, growth retardation, or mental retardation. However, the relationship of these findings to histidinemia remains unclear; routine amino acid screening has uncovered a significant number of asymptomatic subjects with histidinemia.

Laboratory studies reveal marked increases in plasma and cerebrospinal fluid concentrations of histidine. There is also an unexplained elevation in the blood level of alanine. Urine contains large amounts of histidine and its transaminated product imidazolepyruvate. The latter compound, like phenylpyruvate, reacts with ferric chloride to produce an intense blue-green color. The *diagnosis* of histidinemia may be confirmed by assay of histidase in liver or skin. Prenatal diagnosis

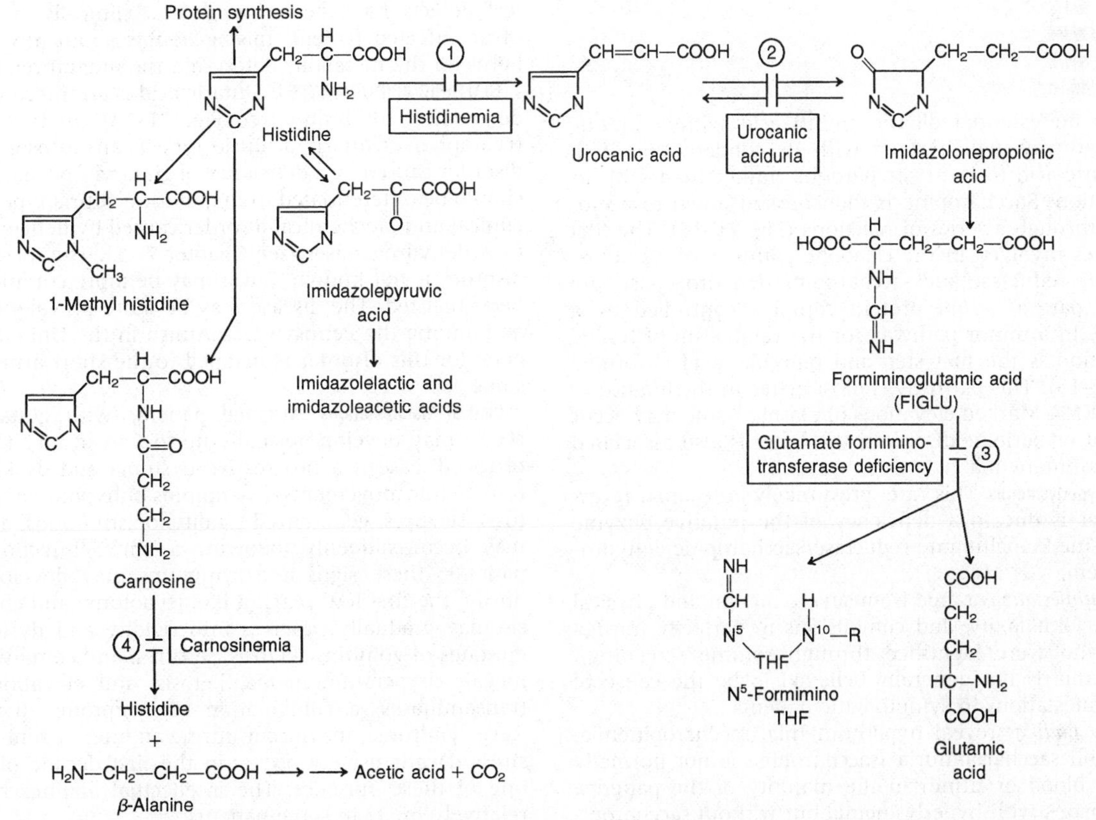

Figure 71–12. Pathways in the metabolism of histidine. THF = tetrahydrofolic acid. Enzymes: (1) histidase; (2) urocanase; (3) glutamate formiminotransferase; (4) carnosinase.

has not yet been achieved because histidase is not present in amniotic cells.

Treatment with a diet low in histidine has produced excellent biochemical control. However, no clinical improvement in symptomatic patients has been observed. Unlike phenylketonuria, maternal histidinemia does not cause any ill effect in the offspring.

UROCANIC ACIDURIA. This disorder is characterized by mental and growth retardation and massive urocanic aciduria (see Fig. 71–12). Urocanase deficiency has been shown in liver biopsies of three of the four reported children. However, the relation of this enzyme deficiency to the clinical findings may be coincidental because normal infants with urocanic aciduria have been identified through routine urine screening of newborns.

GLUTAMATE FORMININOTRANSFERASE DEFICIENCY. This disorder is associated with the excretion of formininoglutamate (FIGLU; see Fig. 71–12). Mildly affected patients have possibly delayed speech. More severely affected patients have mental and physical retardation, abnormal electroencephalogram, and dilatation of the cerebral ventricles with cortical atrophy. Several of the patients had macrocytosis and hyperpigmentation of neutrophils. Only 13 patients have been reported, and the inheritance is autosomal recessive. Although FIGLU excretion may be lowered by folate treatment, it is unclear whether reducing FIGLU excretion is of any value. Glutamate formininotransferase is not expressed in cultured fibroblasts.

HISTIDINURIA. The urinary excretion of histidine normally increases in pregnant women. Histidinuria also occurs as an overflow phenomenon in patients with histidinemia. Isolated histidinuria without histidinemia due to defective renal tubular reabsorption may occur in children whose parents and siblings have been shown to be heterozygotic for the defect.

71.12 Lysine

Iraj Rezvani

Lysine is an essential dibasic amino acid with a unique catabolic pathway, which starts with its condensation with α-ketoglutaric acid to form saccharopine rather than with its transamination. Saccharopine is then broken down to acetoacetic acid through a series of reactions (Fig. 71–13). The first two enzymes involved in the catabolic pathway of lysine, α-ketoglutarate reductase and saccharopine dehydrogenase, are very likely part of a one-protein complex controlled by a single gene. In a minor pathway for the catabolism of lysine, transamination is the first step and pipecolic acid is formed (see Fig. 71–13). This pathway is most active in the brain.

HYPERLYSINEMIA. Marked elevations of plasma lysine may occur as persistent or periodic disorders; the latter is also associated with hyperammonemia.

Persistent Hyperlysinemia. This rare, presumably autosomal recessive disorder is due to a deficiency of the putative enzyme complex lysine ketoglutarate reductase/saccharopine dehydrogenase system.

Clinical manifestations range from severe mental and physical retardation, joint laxity, and convulsions to perfectly normal children (who were identified through routine screening). Hyperlysinemia is not generally believed to be the cause of clinical manifestations in symptomatic patients.

Laboratory findings reveal hyperlysinemia, saccharopinemia, lysinuria, and saccharopinuria (saccharopine is not normally detected in blood or urine) in the majority of the patients. Affected persons with hyperlysinemia but without saccharopinemia have also been reported. In addition, homocitrulline and homoarginine are found in body fluids (see Fig. 71–13). Combined deficiencies of the enzymes lysine ketoglutarate reductase and saccharopine dehydrogenase have been found in all patients having these measurements, except one who had a complete deficiency of saccharopine dehydrogenase with a mild decrease in lysine ketoglutarate reductase activity.

Hyperlysinemia/saccharopinemia is an example of a double deficiency of two sequential enzymes. Another example is the enzyme deficiency causing orotic aciduria (see Chapter 75).

The need for treatment of patients with hyperlysinemia is controversial.

Periodic Hyperlysinemia with Hyperammonemia. Patients with this disorder have episodes of hyperammonemia and hyperlysinemia that may start in the newborn period. They are triggered by a diet high in lysine or in protein. A low-protein diet normalizes plasma concentrations of lysine and ammonia. Patients may have increased levels of plasma arginine or citrulline during the attacks. Enzymes of the urea cycle were within normal limits in patients in the original reports, but subsequently deficiency of the enzyme arginino-succinic synthetase was reported. The basic defect in these patients is obscure but may be a deficiency of one of the urea cycle enzymes because plasma lysine is elevated in some patients with deficiencies of the urea cycle enzymes.

α-AMINOADIPIC ACIDEMIA. Normal children and children with multiple bony anomalies and learning disabilities who excrete large amounts of α-aminoadipic acid have been reported. No relationship could be established between the clinical abnormalities and the biochemical defect. Because lysine loads increased the α-aminoadipic acid excretion, the block is presumed to be an inability to convert α-aminoadipic to α-ketoadipic acid.

α-KETOADIPIC ACIDEMIA. Neonatal seizures, ichthyosis, mild metabolic acidosis, and subsequent marked retardation are associated with elevated α-ketoadipic acid levels in plasma and urine. A defect in the decarboxylation of α-ketoadipic to glutaric acid has been demonstrated. However, the same biochemical defects have been found in a clinically normal sibling of an affected patient, raising doubts about any relationship between the metabolic defect and the mental retardation.

GLUTARIC ACIDURIA TYPE I. Glutaric acid is an intermediate in the degradation of lysine (see Fig. 71–13), hydroxylysine, and tryptophan. Glutaric aciduria type I, an autosomal recessive disorder caused by a deficiency of glutaryl CoA dehydrogenase, should be differentiated from glutaric aciduria type II, a distinct clinical and biochemical disorder caused by deficiencies of acyl CoA dehydrogenases (see Chapter 72.1). The incidence of the disorder is not known, but it may be more common than has been realized. The disease may be more prevalent in Sweden and among the Pennsylvania Amish in the United States. The gene for this disorder is mapped to the short arm of chromosome 19.

Clinical Manifestations. Affected patients with glutaric aciduria type I may develop normally up to 2 yr of life. The hallmark of the disease is a progressive dystonia and dyskinesia (choreoathetoic movements). Symptoms of hypotonia, choreoathetosis, seizures, generalized rigidity, opisthotonos, and dystonia may occur suddenly following a minor infection. In other patients, these signs and symptoms may develop gradually during the first few years of life. Hypotonia and choreoathetosis may gradually progress into rigidity and dystonia. Acute episodes of vomiting, ketosis, seizures, and coma with hepatomegaly, hyperammonemia, ketosis, and elevation of serum transaminases, a combination of symptoms that resembles Reye syndrome, may occur during an intercurrent infection or stress. Death usually occurs in the first decade of life during one of these episodes. The intellectual abilities may remain relatively intact in some patients.

Laboratory Findings. During acute episodes mild to moderate metabolic acidosis and ketosis may occur. Hypoglycemia, hy-

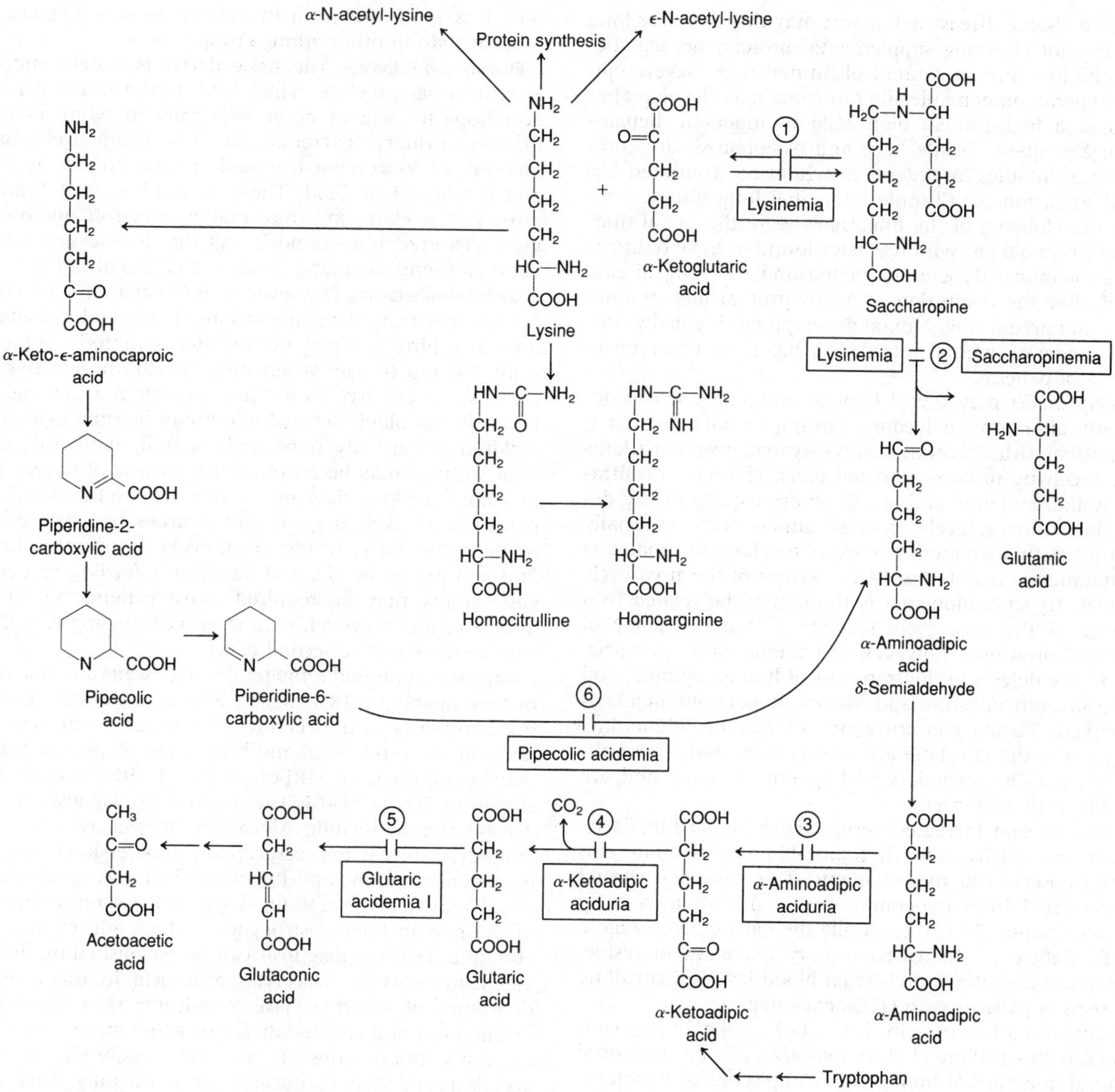

Figure 71–13. Pathways in the metabolism of lysine. Enzymes: (1) lysine ketoglutarate reductase; (2) saccharopine dehydrogenase; (3) α-aminoadipic acid transferase; (4) α-ketoadipic acid dehydrogenase; (5) glutaryl CoA dehydrogenase; (6) α-aminoadipic semialdehyde oxidase.

perammonemia, and elevation of serum transaminases have been seen in some patients. High concentrations of glutaric acid are usually found in urine and blood. 3-Hydroxyglutaric acid may also be present in the urine. This finding differentiated glutaric aciduria type I from type II. In glutaric aciduria type II, 2-hydroxyglutaric rather than 3-hydroxyglutaric acid is elevated. Plasma amino acid concentrations are usually within normal limits. Laboratory findings may be unremarkable between attacks. Severely affected children without glutaric aciduria also have been reported. Therefore, in any child with progressive dystonia and dyskinesia, activity of the enzyme glutaryl CoA dehydrogenase should be measured in leukocytes or cultured fibroblasts.

Treatment. A low-protein diet (especially a diet restricted in lysine and tryptophan) and high doses (200–300 mg/24 hr) of riboflavin (the coenzyme for glutaryl CoA dehydrogenase) and carnitine (50–100 mg/kg/24 hr) have resulted in a dramatic decrease in the levels of glutaric acid in body fluids, but the clinical effect has been variable. The addition of a GABA analog (baclofen) and valproic acid to the therapeutic regimen has produced clinical improvement in some affected children.

PIPECOLATEMIA (Pipecolic Acidemia). Pipecolic acid is one of the intermediate metabolites of the minor pathway of lysine catabolism (see Fig. 71–13). It is oxidized to α-aminoadipic acid within the peroxisomes. Therefore, pipecolic acidemia is a common finding in patients with generalized peroxisomal defects, including Zellweger syndrome, neonatal adrenoleukodystrophy, and infantile Refsum disease (see Chapter 72.2). Previous reported patients with isolated pipecolatemia who all had severe neurologic deficits and hepatomegaly most probably had unrecognized forms of Zellweger syndrome or neonatal adrenoleukodystrophy. The existence of pipecolatemia as a distinct clinical disorder remains doubtful at this time. Pipecolic acidemia is also found in patients with persistent hyperlysinemia.

LYSINURIC PROTEIN INTOLERANCE (Familial Protein Intolerance). This rare autosomal recessive disorder is due to a defect in the transport of lysine, ornithine, and arginine in both kidney and intestine. Unlike patients with cystinuria, urinary excretion of cystine is not increased in these patients. Most reported cases are from Finland, where the prevalence has been estimated to be 1 in 60,000.

Clinical manifestations include refusal to eat, failure to thrive, hypotonia, and repeated episodes of vomiting and diarrhea that may appear anytime after birth. There may be severe multisystem disease. Breast-fed infants may thrive well as long as they are not receiving supplemental protein, perhaps because of the low protein content of human milk. Severe episodes of hyperammonemia leading to coma may develop after ingestion of a high-protein diet. Mild to moderate hepatosplenomegaly; sparse, brittle hair; and osteoporosis are common physical findings in patients in whom the condition has remained undiagnosed. Chronic interstitial lung disease with dyspnea and clubbing of the fingernails were the initial findings in an 11-yr-old girl who was later found to have lysinuric protein intolerance. Hyperammonemia and the lung disease improved after the institution of a low-protein diet, sodium benzoate, and prednisone. Mental development is usually normal, but moderate mental retardation has been observed in about 20% of patients.

Laboratory studies may reveal hyperammonemia, which develops only after protein feeding. Fasting blood ammonia is usually normal. Urinary orotic acid is elevated, even in patients who are receiving protein-restricted diets. Plasma concentrations of lysine, arginine, and ornithine are usually mildly decreased, but urinary levels of these amino acids, especially lysine, are greatly increased. The exact mechanism producing hyperammonemia is not clear. All enzymes of the urea cycle are normal. Hyperammonemia is thought to be related to a disturbance of the urea cycle secondary to a deficiency of arginine and ornithine. However, in patients with cystinuria, who also have defects in the transport of lysine, arginine, and ornithine in both intestine and kidney, hyperammonemia is not observed. Plasma concentrations of alanine, glutamine, serine, glycine, and citrulline are usually increased. These abnormalities may be secondary to hyperammonemia and are not specific to this disorder.

Mild anemia and increased serum levels of ferritin, lactic dehydrogenase (LDH), and thyroxine-binding globulin also have been observed in these patients. This condition should be differentiated from hyperammonemia due to urea cycle defects (see Chapter 71.10), especially the female heterozygote with OTC deficiency. Increased urinary excretion of lysine, ornithine, and arginine and elevated blood levels of citrulline are not seen in patients with OTC deficiency.

Treatment with a low-protein diet (1.0–1.5 g/kg/24 hr), supplemented with citrulline (1–4 mmol/kg/24 hr), has produced biochemical and clinical improvement. Episodes of hyperammonemia should be treated promptly (see Chapter 71.10). Supplementation with lysine is not useful because it is poorly absorbed and tends to produce diarrhea and abdominal pain.

A potential fatal complication in survivors is interstitial pneumonia of unknown etiology. Pathologic examination of the lungs has revealed alveolar proteinosis. One patient has responded to treatment with prednisone.

71.13 Aspartic Acid

(Canavan Disease)

Reuben K. Matalon

N-Acetylaspartic acid is a derivative of aspartic acid that is synthesized in the brain and is found in a high concentration, similar to that of glutamic acid. Its function is unknown, but excessive amounts of *N*-acetylaspartic acid in urine and a deficiency of the enzyme aspartoacylase that cleaves the *N*-acetyl group from *N*-acetylaspartic acid are associated with Canavan disease.

CANAVAN DISEASE. Canavan disease is an autosomal recessive disorder characterized by spongy degeneration of the white matter of the brain, leading to a severe form of leukodystrophy. It is more prevalent in individuals of Ashkenazi Jewish descent than in other ethnic groups.

Etiology and Pathology. The basic defect is a deficiency of the enzyme aspartoacylase, which leads to the accumulation of *N*-acetylaspartic acid in brain, especially in white matter, and massive urinary excretion of this compound. Excessive amounts of *N*-acetylaspartic acid are also present in the blood and cerebrospinal fluid. There is striking vacuolization and astrocytic swelling in white matter. Electron microscopy reveals distorted mitochondria. As the disease progresses, the ventricles tend to enlarge, leading to brain atrophy.

Clinical Manifestations. The severity of Canavan disease comprises a wide spectrum of manifestations. In general, infants appear normal at birth and may not manifest symptoms of the disease until 3–6 mo of age, when they develop progressive macrocephaly, severe hypotonia, and persistent head lag. As the infant grows older, delayed milestones become evident. These children are usually hyper-reflexic and hypotonic, although joint stiffness may be encountered because of disuse. Seizures and optic atrophy develop as they grow older. Feeding difficulties, poor weight gain, and gastroesophageal reflux may occur in the 1st yr of life; swallowing deteriorates during the 2nd and 3rd yr of life, and nasogastric feeding or permanent gastrostomy may be required. Most patients die in the 1st decade of life; however, with improved nursing care they may survive through the second decade.

Diagnosis. Computed tomography (CT) scans and magnetic resonance imaging (MRI) suggest diffuse white matter degeneration, primarily in the cerebral hemispheres with less involvement in the cerebellum and brain stem. Repeated evaluations may be required. An MRI of a 2-yr-old with Canavan disease is shown in Figure 71–14. The differential diagnosis of Canavan disease should include Alexander disease, which is another leukodystrophy with macrocephaly. Progression is usually slow in *Alexander disease,* and hypotonia is not as pronounced as it is in Canavan disease. Brain biopsy shows spongy degeneration of the myelin fibers, astrocytic swelling, and elongated mitochondria. Definite diagnosis can be established by finding elevated amounts of *N*-acetylaspartic acid in the urine and a deficiency of aspartoacylase in cultured skin fibroblasts. The biochemical and enzyme diagnosis is the method of choice for diagnosis; brain biopsy is no longer required. Levels of *N*-acetylaspartic acid in normal urine are only trace amounts (less than 25 μmol/mmol creatinine), whereas in patients with Canavan disease they are in the range of 3,000 ± 1,800 μmol/mmol creatinine. High levels of *N*-acetylaspartic acid in plasma, cerebrospinal fluid (CSF), and brain tissue can also be detected. The activity of aspartoacylase in the fibroblasts of obligate carriers is about half or less of the activity found in normal individuals.

The gene for aspartoacylase has been cloned and mutations leading to Canavan disease have been identified. There are two mutations predominant in the Ashkenazi Jewish population. The first is an amino acid substitution (E285A) in which glutamic acid is substituted to alanine. This mutation is the most frequent and encompasses 83% of 100 mutant alleles examined in Ashkenazi Jewish patients. The second common mutation is a change from tyrosine to a nonsense mutation, leading to a stop in the coding sequence (Y231X). This mutation accounts for 13% of the 100 mutant alleles. In the non-Jewish population more diverse mutations have been observed and the two mutations common in Jewish people are rare. A different mutation (A305E), substitution of alanine for glutamic acid, accounts for 40% of 62 mutant alleles in non-Jewish patients. When the diagnosis of Canavan disease is reached, it is important to obtain a molecular diagnosis because this will lead to accurate counseling and prenatal diagnosis for the family. If the mutations are not known, prenatal diagnosis relies on the level of *N*-acetylaspartic acid in the amniotic

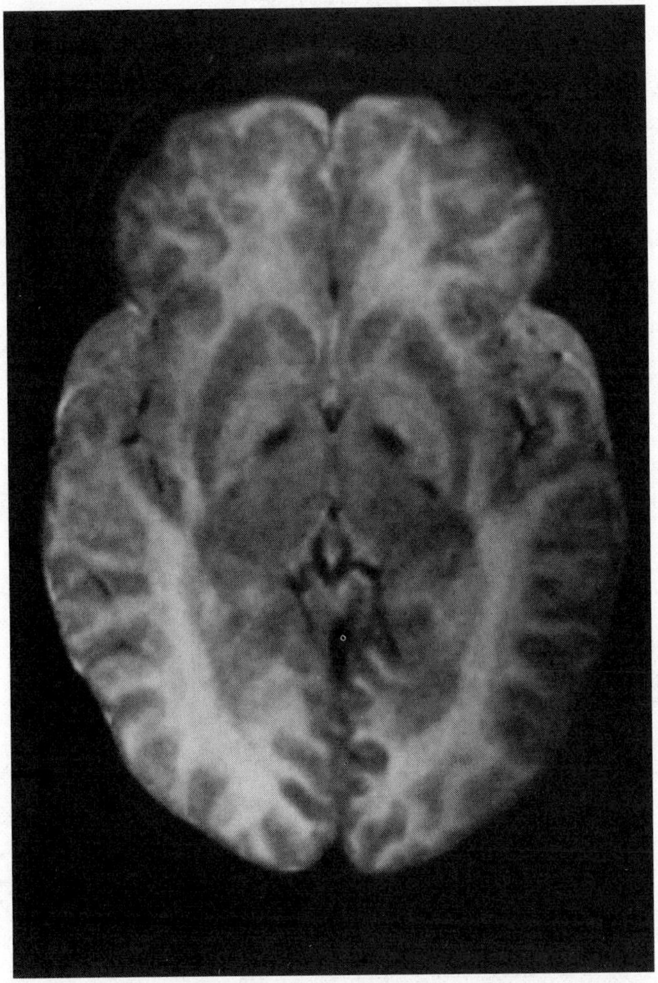

Figure 71–14. Axial T_2-weighted MRI scan taken of a 2-yr-old patient with Canavan disease. Extensive thickening of the white matter radiation is seen.

fluid. In Ashkenazi Jewish patients the carrier frequency may be as high as 1 in 36, which is very close to that of Tay Sachs disease. Ashkenazi Jewish individuals may need to be screened for Canavan disease.

Treatment and Prevention. No specific treatment is available. Feeding problems and seizures should be treated on an individual basis. Genetic counseling, carrier testing, and prenatal diagnosis are the only methods of prevention.

Arn PH, Hauser ER, Thomas GH, et al: Hyperammonemia in women with a mutation at the ornithine carbamyltransferase locus. N Engl J Med 322:1652, 1990.

Arnold GL, Greene CL, Stout JP, et al: Molybdenum cofactor deficiency. J Pediatr 123:595, 1993.

Azen CG, Koch R, Friedman EG, et al: Intellectual development in 12-year-old children treated for phenylketonuria. Am J Dis Child 145:35, 1991.

Citron BA, Kaufman S, Milstein S, et al: Mutation in the 4α-carbinolamine dehydratase gene leads to mild hyperphenylalaninemia with defective cofactor metabolism. Am J Hum Genet 53:768, 1993.

Danpure CJ, Jennings PR, Purdue PE, et al: Primary hyperoxaluria type I: Genotypic and phenotypic heterogeneity. J Inherit Metab Dis 17:487, 1994.

De Raene L, De Meirleir L, Ramet J, et al: Acrodermatitis enteropathica-like cutaneous lesions in organic aciduria. J Pediatr 124:416, 1994.

Dianzani I, Howells D, Ponzone A, et al: Two new mutations in the dihydropteridine reductase gene in patients with tetrahydrobiotern deficiency. J Med Genet 30:465, 1993.

Eisensmith RC, Woo SLC: Molecular basis of phenylketonuria and related hyperphenylalaninemias: Mutations and polymorphisms in human phenylalanine hydroxylase gene. Hum Mutat 1:13, 1992.

Finkelstein JE, Hauser ER, Leonard CO, et al: Late onset ornithine transcarbamylase deficiency in male patients. J Pediatr 117:897, 1990.

Gibson KM, Cassidy SB, Seaver LH, et al: Fatal cardiomyopathy associated with 3-hydroxy-3-methylglutaryl-CoA lyase deficiency. J Inherit Metab Dis 17:291, 1994.

Gibson KM, Lee CF, Hoffman GF: Screening for defects of branched-chain amino acid metabolism. Eur J Pediatr 153:562, 1994.

Goyette P, Sumner JS, Milos R, et al: Human methylenetetrahydrofolate reductase: Isolation of cDNA, mapping and mutation identification. Nature Genet 7:195, 1994.

Grompe M, St Louis M, Demers SI, et al: A single mutation of the fumarylacetoacetate hydroxylase gene in French-Canadians with hereditary tyrosinemia type I. N Engl J Med 331:353, 1994.

Hauser ER, Finkelstein JE, Valle E, et al: Allopurinol-induced orotidinuria. N Engl J Med 322:1641, 1990.

Hayasaka K, Tada K, Fueki N, et al: Prenatal diagnosis of nonketotic hyperglycemia: Enzymatic analysis of the glycine cleavage system in chorionic villi. J Pediatr 116:444, 1990.

Hereditary tyrosinemia (editorial). Lancet 1:1500, 1990.

Hoffmann GF, Charpentier C, Mayatepek E, et al: Clinical and biochemical phenotype in 11 patients with mevalonic aciduria. Pediatrics 91:915, 1993.

Hoffman GF, Gibson KM, Trefz FK, et al: Neurologic manifestations of organic acid disorders. Eur J Pediatr 153:594, 1994.

Jain A, Burst NR, Kennaway NG, et al: Effect of ascorbate or N-acetyl-cysteine treatment in a patient with hereditary glutathione synthetase deficiency. J Pediatr 124:229, 1994.

Janocha S, Wolz W, Srsen S, et al: The human gene for alkaptonuria maps to chromosome 3p. Genomics 19:5, 1994.

Kahler SG, Sherwood G, Woolf D, et al: Pancreatitis in patients with organic acidemias. J Pediatr 124:239, 1994.

Kalayci O, Coskan T, Tokatli A, et al: Infantile spasm as the initial symptoms of biotinidase deficiency. J Pediatr 124:103, 1994.

Kaul R, Balamurugan K, Gao GP, et al: Canavan disease: Genomic organization and localization of human *ASPA* to 17p13-ter; conservation of the *ASPA* gene during evolution. Genomics 21:364, 1994.

Kaul R, Gao GP, Aloya M, et al: Canavan disease: Mutations among Jewish and non-Jewish patients. Am J Hum Genet 55:27, 1994.

Kaul R, Gao GP, Balamurugan K, et al: Cloning of the human aspartoacylase CD gene and a common missense mutation in Canavan disease. Nature Genet 5:118, 1993.

Kelley RI: Prenatal detection of Canavan disease by measurement of N-acetyl-L-aspartate in amniotic fluid. J Inher Metab Dis 16:918, 1993.

Kerem E, Elpeg ON, Shalev RS, et al: Lysinuria protein intolerance with chronic interstitial lung disease and pulmonary cholesterol granulomas at onset. J Pediatr 123:275, 1993.

Koletzko B, Bachmann C, Wendel U: Antibiotic therapy for improvement of metabolic control in methylmalonic aciduria. J Pediatr 117:99, 1990.

Kraus JP: Molecular basis of phenotype expression in homocystinuria. J Inherit Metab Dis 17:383, 1994.

Lamay JF, Lambert MA, Mitchel GA, et al: Hyperammonemia-hyperornithinemia-homocitrullinemia syndrome: Neurologic, ophthalmologic and neuropsychologic examination of six patients. J Pediatr 121:725, 1992.

Lee ST, Nicholas RD, Bundey S, et al: Mutations of the p gene in oculocutaneous albinism, ocular albinism and Prader-Willi syndrome plus albinism. N Engl J Med 330:529, 1994.

Bennett MJ, Gibson KM, Sherwood WG, et al: Reliable Prenatal Diagnosis of Canavan Disease (Aspartoacylase Deficiency): Comparison of Enzymatic and Metabolite Analysis. J Inher Metab Dis 16:831, 1993.

Linstedt S, Holme E, Lock EA, et al: Treatment of hereditary tyrosinemia type I by inhibition of 4-hydroxyphenylpyruvate dioxygenase. Lancet 340:813, 1992.

Maestri NE, Hauser ER, Bartholomew D, et al: Prospective treatment of urea cycle disorders. J Pediatr 119:923, 1991.

Marescau B, DeDeyn PP, Lowenthal A, et al: Guanidino compounds analysis as a complementary diagnostic parameter for hyperargininemia: Follow-up of guanidino compound levels during therapy. Pediatr Res 27:297, 1990.

Matalon R, Kaul R, Casanova J, et al: Aspartoacylase deficiency: The enzyme defect in Canavan disease. J Inherit Metab Dis 12:329, 1989.

Matalon R, Michals K, Azen C, et al: Maternal PKU collaborative study: Pregnancy outcome and postnatal head growth. J Inherit Metab Dis 17:353, 1994.

McKusick V: Mendelian Inheritance in Man, 9th ed. Baltimore, MD, The Johns Hopkins University Press, 1990.

Morton DH, Bennett MJ, Seargeant LE, et al: Glutaric aciduria type I: A common cause of episodic encephalopathy and spastic paralysis in the Amish of Lancaster County, Pennsylvania. Am J Med Genet 41:89, 1991.

Mudd SH, Skovby F, Levy HL, et al: The natural history of homocystinuria due to cystathionine B-synthetase deficiency. Am J Hum Genet 37:1, 1985.

Parenti G, Sebastio G, Strisciuglio A, et al: Lysinuric protein intolerance characterized by bone marrow abnormalities and severe clinical course. J Pediatr 126:246, 1995.

Peinemann F, Danner DJ: Maple syrup urine disease 1954 to 1993. J Inherit Metab Dis 17:3, 1994.

Qureshi AA, Crane AM, Matiaszuk NV, et al: Cloning and expression of mutations demonstrating intragenic complementation in *mut*° methylmalonic aciduria. J Clin Invest 93:1812, 1994.

Rabinowitz LG, Williams LR, Anderson CE, et al: Painful keratoderma and photophobia: Hallmarks of tyrosinemia type II. J Pediatr 126:266, 1995.

Riviello J, Rezvani I, DiGeorge A: Cerebral edema in patients with maple syrup urine disease. J Pediatr 119:42, 1991.

Salt A, Barnes ND, Rolles K, et al: Liver transplantation in tyrosinemia type 1. The dilemma of timing the operation. Acta Paediatr 81:449, 1992.

Schallreuter KU, Wood JM, Pittelkow MR, et al: Regulation of melanin biosynthesis in the human epidermis by tetrahydrobiopterin. Science 263:1444, 1994.
Scheuerle AE, McVie R, Beaudet AL, et al: Arginase deficiency presenting as cerebral palsy. Pediatrics 91:995, 1993.
Scriver CR, Beaudet AL, Sly WS, et al: The Metabolic Basis of Inherited Disease, 7th ed. New York, McGraw-Hill, 1994.
Seargeant LE, de Groot GW, Dilling LA, et al: Primary oxaluria type 2 (L-glyceric aciduria): A rare cause of nephrolithiasis in children. J Pediatr 118:912, 1991.
Secor-McVoy JR, Levy HL, Lawler M, et al: Partial biotinidase deficiency: Clinical and biochemical features. J Pediatr 116:78, 1990.
Shevell MI, Matiaszuk N, Ledley FD, et al: Varying neurological phenotypes among *mut°* and *mut⁻* patients with methylmalomyl CoA mutase deficiency. Am J Med Genet 45:619, 1993.
Spritz RA: Molecular genetics of oculocutaneous albinism. Semin Dermatol 12:167, 1993.
Suormala TM, Baumgartner ER, Wick H, et al: Comparison of patients with complete and partial biotinidase deficiency: Biochemical studies. J Inherit Metab Dis 13:76, 1990.
Vockley J, Parimoo B, Janak K: Molecular characterization of four different classes of mutations in the isovaloyl-CoA dehydrogenase gene responsible for isovaleric aciduria. Am J Hum Genet 49:147, 1991.
Wold B, Heard GS: Screening for biotinidase deficiency in newborns: Worldwide experience. Pediatrics 85:512, 1990.
Zeharia A, Elpeleg ON, Mukamel M, et al: 3-Methylglutaconic aciduria. A new variant. Pediatrics 89:1080, 1992.

CHAPTER 72
Defects in Metabolism of Lipids

72.1 Disorders of Mitochondrial Fatty Acid Oxidation

Charles A. Stanley

Mitochondrial oxidation of fatty acids is an essential energy-producing pathway. It becomes especially important during prolonged periods of starvation when the body switches from using predominantly carbohydrates to using predominantly fat as its major fuel. Fatty acids are also important fuels for exercising skeletal muscle and are the preferred substrate for the heart. In these tissues fatty acids are completely oxidized to carbon dioxide and water. However, in the liver, the end products of fatty acid oxidation are the ketones, β-hydroxybutyrate and acetoacetate. The ketones cannot be oxidized by the liver but are exported to serve as important fuels in peripheral tissues, particularly the brain.

Genetic defects have been recognized in nearly all of the steps in the fatty acid oxidation path. All of these disorders are recessively inherited. *Clinical manifestations* are fairly similar among the disorders. The most common presentation is an acute attack of life-threatening coma and hypoglycemia induced by a period of fasting. Other manifestations frequently include chronic cardiomyopathy and muscle weakness or, more rarely, acute rhabdomyolysis. Because the defects can be asymptomatic except during fasting stress, attacks of illness may be misdiagnosed as Reye syndrome or sudden infant death syndrome. Fatty acid oxidation disorders are easily overlooked because the only specific clue to the diagnosis may be the finding of inappropriately low concentrations of urinary ketones in an infant who has hypoglycemia. In a similar manner, genetic defects in ketone utilization may be overlooked because ketosis is an expected finding with fasting hypoglycemia.

Figure 72–1 outlines the steps involved in mitochondrial oxidation of a typical long-chain fatty acid. In the *carnitine cycle* fatty acids are carried across the barrier of the inner mitochondrial membrane linked to carnitine. Within the mitochondrial matrix, successive turns of the four-step β-*oxidation cycle* convert the fatty acid to acetyl-CoA units. Two to four chain-length specific isoenzymes are needed for each of these β-oxidation steps to accommodate the different-sized fatty acids. The *electron transfer pathway* carries electrons generated in the first β-oxidation step to the electron transport chain for ATP production. In the liver, most of the acetyl-CoA generated

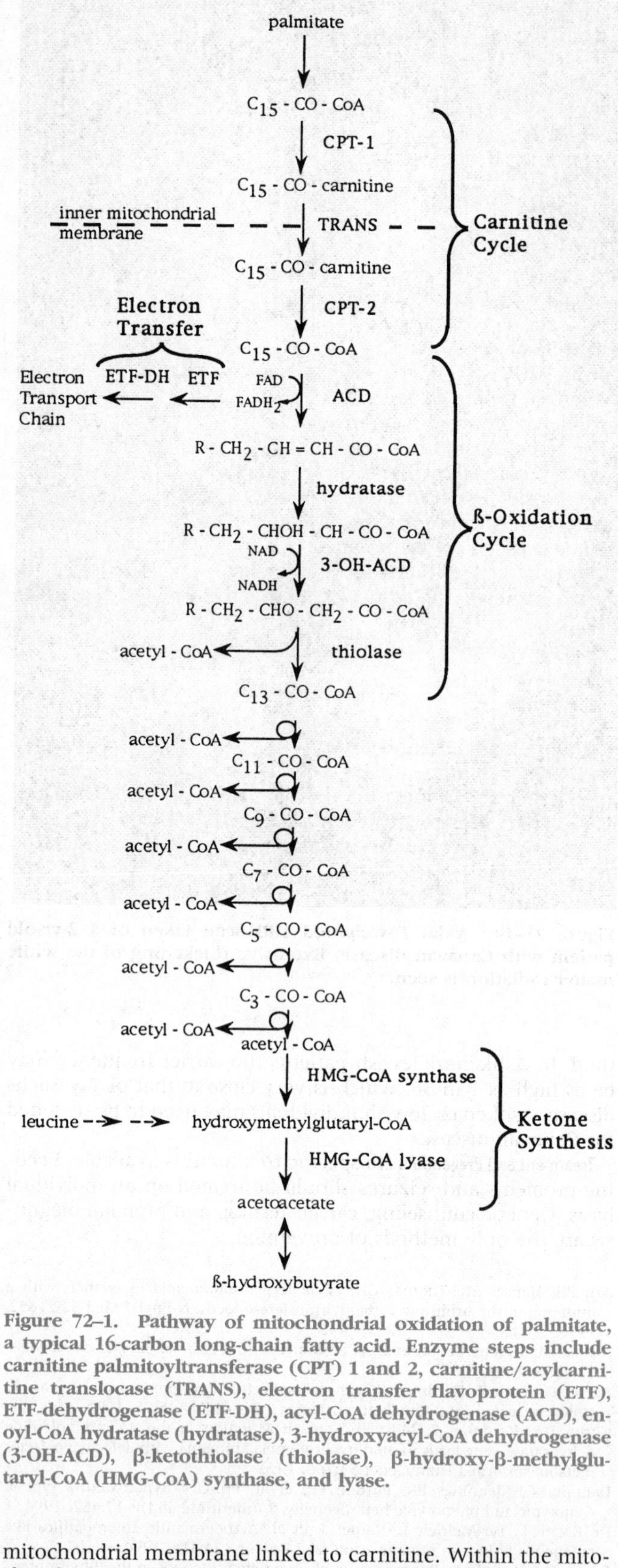

Figure 72–1. Pathway of mitochondrial oxidation of palmitate, a typical 16-carbon long-chain fatty acid. Enzyme steps include carnitine palmitoyltransferase (CPT) 1 and 2, carnitine/acylcarnitine translocase (TRANS), electron transfer flavoprotein (ETF), ETF-dehydrogenase (ETF-DH), acyl-CoA dehydrogenase (ACD), enoyl-CoA hydratase (hydratase), 3-hydroxyacyl-CoA dehydrogenase (3-OH-ACD), β-ketothiolase (thiolase), β-hydroxy-β-methylglutaryl-CoA (HMG-CoA) synthase, and lyase.

from β-oxidation flows through the *ketone synthesis pathway* to β-hydroxybutyrate and acetoacetate.

DEFECTS IN THE β-OXIDATION CYCLE

Medium-Chain Acyl-CoA Dehydrogenase (MCAD) Deficiency

MCAD deficiency is the most common of the fatty acid oxidation disorders. Several hundred cases have been identified since the disease was first reported in 1982–83. The disorder shows a strong founder effect: Most patients have a northwestern European ancestry, and 85–90% are homozygous for a single common mis-sense mutation, an A to G transition at cDNA position 985.

CLINICAL MANIFESTATIONS. Affected patients usually present in the first 2–3 yr of life with episodes of acute illness triggered by prolonged fasting for more than 12–16 hr. Signs and symptoms include vomiting and lethargy, which rapidly progress to coma or seizures and to cardiorespiratory collapse. The liver may be slightly enlarged with fat deposition. Attacks are rare until beyond the first few months of life. Affected infants are at higher risk of illness as they begin to fast through the night or are exposed to fasting stress during intercurrent illnesses. However, presentation in the first days of life has been reported in newborns who were starved inadvertently as they began breast-feeding.

LABORATORY FINDINGS. During acute attacks of illness, hypoglycemia is usually present. Plasma and urinary ketone concentrations are inappropriately low (hypoketotic hypoglycemia). Because of the absence of ketones, there is little or no acidemia. Tests of liver function are abnormal with elevations of transaminases, urate, urea, ammonia, and prolonged thrombin and partial thromboplastin times. Liver biopsies at times of acute illness show increased triglyceride deposition in either a micro- or macrovesicular pattern. During fasting stress or at times of acute illness, urinary organic acid profiles by gas chromatography–mass spectrometry show low concentrations of ketones and elevated levels of medium-chain dicarboxylic acids that derive from microsomal and peroxisomal omega oxidation of fatty acids. Plasma and tissue concentrations of total carnitine are reduced to 25–50% of normal, and the fraction of total carnitine esterified is increased. This pattern of *secondary carnitine deficiency* is seen in almost all of the fatty acid oxidation defects and reflects competition between increased acylcarnitine levels and free carnitine transport at the plasma membrance. Significant exceptions to this rule are the carnitine transporter, CPT-1 and HMG-CoA synthase deficiencies (see below). *Diagnosis* can be made by demonstrating increased octanoylcarnitine in plasma or urine, demonstrating increased glycine conjugates of hexanoate and phyenylpropionate in urine, finding deficient MCAD enzyme activity in cultured fibroblasts or lymphoblasts, or demonstrating the common A985G mutation in homozygous form in, for example, newborn screening filter paper blood spots. A rare mutation G583A is associated with severe MCAD deficiency, hypoglycemia, and sudden neonatal death.

TREATMENT. Acute illnesses should be promptly treated with intravenous fluids containing 10% dextrose in order to suppress lipolysis as rapidly as possible. Chronic therapy consists of ensuring that exposure to starvation stress is eliminated. This usually requires simply adjusting the diet to ensure that overnight fasting periods are limited to less than 10–12 hr. Whether restricting dietary fat or treatment with carnitine is beneficial remains controversial.

PROGNOSIS. Up to 25% of patients may die during their first attack of illness. Some patients may suffer permanent brain injury during an attack. The prognosis for survivors is good because muscle weakness or cardiomyopathy do not occur in MCAD deficiency. With age, fasting tolerance improves and the risk of attacks of illness decreases. It is estimated that as many as 50% of affected patients never have an attack of illness, so testing of sibs of affected patients is important to detect asymptomatic family members.

Long-Chain/Very Long-Chain Acyl-CoA Dehydrogenase (LCAD/VLCAD) Deficiency

This disorder was originally termed *LCAD deficiency* before the existence of an additional VLCAD enzyme specific for longer chain fatty acids was known. Some LCAD patients have been shown to be deficient in the VLCAD enzyme. Patients have usually been more severely affected than those with MCAD deficiency, presenting earlier in infancy and having more chronic problems with muscle weakness or episodes of muscle pain and rhabdomyosis. During acute attacks of fasting illness, evidence of cardiomyopathy may be present. The left ventricle may be hypertrophic or dilated, and show poor contractility on echocardiogram. Other physical and routine laboratory features are similar to MCAD deficiency, including secondary carnitine deficiency. The urinary organic acid profile shows a hypoketotic dicarboxylic aciduria. Increased levels of C_{12-14} dicarboxylic acids may be noted in the urine. *Diagnosis* may be suggested by the demonstration of elevated plasma $C_{14:1}$ fatty acid or acylcarnitine, but the specific diagnosis requires assay of enzyme activities of both LCAD and VLCAD in cultured fibroblasts. *Treatment* is avoidance of fasts more than 10–12 hr. Continuous intragastric feeding has appeared to be useful in some patients.

Short-Chain Acyl-CoA Dehydrogenase (SCAD) Deficiency

The clinical phenotype of this disorder remains somewhat unclear. Most patients have not presented with attacks of fasting coma but instead have had chronic acidosis, failure to thrive, muscle weakness, and developmental delay. Some of these features suggest a toxicity syndrome, perhaps due to accumulation of short-chain fatty acid metabolites. One reported patient had normal ketogenesis, implying that there is no impairment of longer chain fatty acid oxidation. Urinary organic acid profile shows elevations of short-chain fatty acid metabolites, including ethylmalonate and butylrylglycine. Secondary carnitine deficiency is present and butyrylcarnitine may be found in urine. *Diagnosis* may be based on the specific metabolite profile in blood and urine, and confirmed by enzyme assay in cultured cells. *Treatment* is limitation of fasting stress and dietary fat.

Long-Chain 3-Hydroxyacyl-CoA Dehydrogenase (LCHAD) Deficiency

This appears to be the second most common of the fatty acid oxidation disorders. The LCHAD enzyme is actually part of a trifunctional protein, which also contains two other steps in β-oxidation, long-chain enoyl-CoA hydratase and β-keto thiolase. In some patients, only LCHAD is affected, while others have deficiencies of all three enzymes. *Clinical manifestations* include attacks of acute hypoketotic hypoglycemia similar to MCAD deficiency, but patients often show evidence of more severe disease including cardiomyopathy, muscle weakness, and abnormal liver function. Some patients have features implying toxic effects of fatty acid metabolites, such as retinopathy, progressive liver failure, peripheral neuropathy, and rhabdomyolysis. A life-threatening illness, acute fatty liver of pregnancy, has been observed in mothers carrying fetuses affected with LCHAD deficiency. Urinary organic acid profile may show increases in levels of 3-hydroxy dicarboxylic acids. Secondary carnitine deficiency is common and plasma 3-hydroxydicarboxylic acid esters of carnitine may be increased. *Treatment* is similar to that for MCAD or LCAD/VLCAD deficiency.

Short-Chain 3-Hydroxyacyl-CoA Dehydrogenase (SCHAD) Deficiency

One patient has been reported with attacks of fasting hypoglycemia and myoglobinuria associated with deficiency of SCHAD in muscle but not in cultured fibroblasts. The patient died in adolescence with cardiomyopathy and arrhymias. Many questions will remain unanswered about this defect until other affected patients are identified.

DEFECTS IN THE CARNITINE CYCLE

Plasma Membrane Carnitine Transport Defect

(Primary Carnitine Deficiency)

This is the only genetic defect in which carnitine deficiency is the cause, rather than the consequence, of impaired fatty acid oxidation. The most common presentation is progressive cardiomyopathy with or without skeletal muscle weakness that begins at 2–4 yr of age. A smaller number of patients may present with fasting hypoketotic hypoglycemia during the first year of life before the cardiomyopathy becomes symptomatic. The underlying defect involves the plasma membrane sodium-gradient dependent carnitine transporter that is present in heart, muscle, and kidney. This transporter is responsible for maintaining intracellular carnitine 20- to 50-fold higher than plasma concentrations and for renal conservation of carnitine.

Diagnosis of the carnitine transporter defect is aided by the fact that patients have extremely reduced carnitine levels in plasma and muscle to 1–2% of normal. Heterozygote parents have plasma carnitine levels approximately 50% of normal. Fasting ketogenesis may be normal, because liver carnitine transport is normal, but may be impaired if dietary carnitine intake is interrupted. The fasting urinary organic acid profile may show a hypoketotic dicarboxylicaciduria pattern if hepatic fatty acid oxidation is impaired, but is otherwise unremarkable. The defect in carnitine transport can be demonstrated clinically by severe reduction in renal carnitine threshold or in vitro by assay of carnitine uptake using cultured fibroblasts or lymphoblasts. *Treatment* of this disorder with pharmacologic doses of oral carnitine is highly effective in correcting the cardiomyopathy and muscle weakness as well as any impairment in fasting ketogenesis. Muscle total carnitine concentrations remain less than 5% of normal on treatment.

Carnitine Palmitoyltransferase-1 (CPT-1) Deficiency

Several infants and children have been described with a deficiency of the liver isozyme of this enzyme. *Clinical manifestations* include fasting hypoketotic hypoglycemia, occasionally with markedly abnormal liver function tests. The heart and skeletal muscle are not involved because the muscle isozyme is unaffected. Fasting urinary organic acid profile shows a hypoketotic dicarboxylicaciduria but no specific abnormalities. *Diagnosis* is aided by the observation that this is the only fatty acid oxidation disorder in which plasma total carnitine levels are elevated to 150–200% of normal. This may be explained by the fact that the inhibitory effects of long-chain acylcarnitines on the renal tubular carnitine transporter are absent in CPT-1 deficiency. The enzyme defect can be demonstrated in cultured fibroblasts or lymphoblasts. *Treatment* with diet to avoid fasting is similar to MCAD deficiency.

Carnitine/Acylcarnitine Translocase (TRANS) Deficiency

This defect of the inner mitochondrial membrane carrier protein for fatty acylcarnitines blocks the entry of long-chain fatty acids into the mitochondria for oxidation. The few patients identified have had very severe and generalized impairment of fatty acid oxidation. All have presented in the newborn period with attacks of fasting-induced hypoglycemia and cardiorespiratory collapse. All have had evidence of cardiomyopathy and muscle weakness. None have survived beyond 2 yr. No distinctive urinary or plasma organic acids were found. Secondary deficiency of carnitine was noted with unusually increased levels of long-chain acylcarnitines. *Diagnosis* can be made using cultured fibroblasts or lymphoblasts. *Treatment* is similar to other fatty acid oxidation disorders.

Carnitine Palmitoyltransferase-2 (CPT-2) Deficiency

Two forms of this defect have been described. A severe deficiency of enzyme activity is associated with an infantile onset form. This form shares all of the clinical and laboratory features of the TRANS deficiency described earlier. A milder defect is associated with an adult presentation of episodic rhabdomyolysis. The first episode usually does not occur until late childhood or early adulthood. Attacks may be precipitated by prolonged exercise. There is aching muscle pain and myoglobinuria that may be severe enough to cause renal shutdown. Serum levels of creatine kinase are elevated to 5,000–10,000 U/l or more. Fasting hypoglycemia has not been described, but fasting may contribute to attacks of myoglobinuria, and ketogenesis may be impaired. Muscle biopsy shows increased deposition of neutral fat. Diagnosis can be made by demonstrating deficient enzyme activity in muscle or other tissues, and in cultured fibroblasts.

DEFECTS IN ELECTRON TRANSFER PATHWAY

Electron Transfer Flavoprotein (ETF) and ETF Dehydrogenase (ETF-DH) Deficiencies

(Glutaric Aciduria Type 2, Multiple Acyl-CoA Dehydrogenation Deficiencies)

These two enzymes function to transfer electrons into the mitochondrial electron transport chain from dehydrogenation reactions catalyzed by MCAD, SCAD, LCAD, and VLCAD, as well as glutaryl-CoA dehydrogenase and two enzymes involved in branch-chain amino acid oxidation, isovaleryl-CoA dehydrogenase and branch-chain acyl-CoA dehydrogenase. Deficiencies of ETF or ETF-DH, therefore, produce illness that combines the features of impaired fatty acid oxidation and impaired oxidation of several of the amino acids, such as leucine and lysine. Complete deficiencies of either enzyme are associated with severe illness in the newborn period, characterized by acidosis, hypoglycemia, coma, hypotonia, and cardiomyopathy. Some affected neonates have had facial dysmorphia and polycystic kidneys, which suggest that toxic effects of accumulated metabolites may occur in utero. *Diagnosis* can be made from the urinary organic acid profile, which shows abnormalities corresponding to blocks in oxidation of fatty acids (ethylmalonate and dicarboxylic acids), lysine (glutarate), and branch-chain amino acids (isovaleryl-, isobutyryl-, and alpha-methylbutyryl-glycine). Most severely affected infants have not survived the neonatal period.

Partial deficiencies of ETF and ETF-DH produce a disorder that may mimic MCAD deficiency or other milder fatty acid oxidation defects. These patients have attacks of fasting hypoketotic coma. The urinary organic acid profile reveals primarily elevations of dicarboxylic acids and ethylmalonate, derived from short-chain fatty acid intermediates. Secondary carnitine deficiency is present. Some patients with mild forms of ETF/ETF-DH deficiency have been reported to benefit from *treatment* with high doses of riboflavin, the cofactor for these two enzymes as well as for the acyl-CoA dehydrogenases.

DEFECTS IN KETONE SYNTHESIS PATHWAY

β-Hydroxy-β-Methyl Glutaryl-CoA Synthase (HMG-Synthase) Deficiency

This is the rate-limiting step in conversion of acetyl-CoA derived from fatty acid β-oxidation in the liver to ketones.

One patient with this defect has been reported in abstract form, and this may prompt the recognition of other cases. The presentation was one of fasting hypoketotic hypoglycemia without evidence of impaired cardiac or skeletal muscle function. Urinary organic acid profile showed only a hypoketotic dicarboxylic aciduria. Plasma and tissue carnitine levels were normal, in contrast to all of the other disorders of fatty acid oxidation. A separate synthase enzyme present in cytosol for cholesterol biosynthesis was not affected. The HMG-synthase defect is expressed only in the liver and cannot be demonstrated in cultured fibroblasts. Treatment with diet to avoid fasting appears to be successful.

β-Hydroxy-β-Methyl Glutaryl-CoA Lyase (HMG-Lyase) Deficiency (See Chapter 71.6)

DEFECTS IN KETONE UTILIZATION

The ketones, β-hydroxybutyrate and acetoacetate, are the end products of hepatic fatty acid oxidation and serve as important metabolic fuels for the brain during late stages of fasting. Two defects in utilization of ketones in brain and other peripheral tissues that present with episodes of "hyperketotic" hypoglycemia have been described.

Succinyl-CoA Acetoacetyl-CoA Transferase Deficiency

Only one patient with this defect has been reported. He presented with recurrent episodes of severe ketoacidosis beginning in the newborn period and died at 6 mo of age. Treatment of episodes required infusion of glucose and large amounts of bicarbonate for 3–4 days. The enzyme is responsible for activating acetoacetate in peripheral tissues using succinyl-CoA as a donor to form acetoacetyl-CoA. Deficient activity was demonstrated in brain, muscle, and fibroblasts.

β-Ketothiolase Deficiency (See Chapter 71.6)

Brackett JC, Sims HF, Steiner RD, et al: A novel mutation in medium chain acyl-CoA dehydrogenase causes sudden neonatal death. J Clin Invest 94:1477, 1994.
Coates PM, Hale DE, Finocchiaro G, et al: Genetic deficiency of short-chain acyl-coenzyme A dehydrogenase in cultured fibroblasts from a patient with muscle carnitine deficiency and severe skeletal muscle weakness. J Clin Invest 81:171, 1988.
Coates PM, Stanley CA: Inherited disorders of mitochondrial fatty acid oxidation. Prog Liver Dis 10:123, 1992.
Demaugre F, Bonnefont J, Mitchell G, et al: Hepatic and muscular presentations of carnitine palmitoyl transferase deficiency: Two distinct entities. Pediatr Res 24:308, 1988.
Demaugre F, Bonnefont JP, Colonna M, et al: Infantile form of carnitine palmitoyltransferase II deficiency with hepatomuscular symptoms and sudden death. Physiopathological approach to carnitine palmitoyltransferase II deficiencies. J Clin Invest 87:859, 1991.
Frerman FE, Goodman SI: Deficiency of electron transfer flavoprotein or electron transfer flavoprotein:ubiquinone oxidoreductase in glutaric acidemia type II fibroblasts. Proc Natl Acad Sci USA 82:4517, 1985.
Hale DE, Batshaw ML, Coates PM, et al: Long-chain acyl coenzyme A dehydrogenase deficiency: an inherited cause of nonketotic hypoglycemia. Pediatr Res 19:666, 1985.
Hale DE, Bennett MJ: Fatty acid oxidation disorders: a new class of metabolic diseases. J Pediatr 121:1, 1992.
Iafolla AK, Thompson RJ, and Roe CR: Medium-chain acyl-coenzyme A dehydrogenase deficiency: Clinical course in 120 affected children. J Pediatr 124:409, 1994.
Roe CR, Coates PM: Acyl-CoA dehydrogenase deficiencies. In: Scriver CR et al. (eds): The Metabolic Basis of Inherited Disease. New York, McGraw Hill, 1989, pp 889–914.
Stanley CA, Berry GT, Bennett MJ, et al: Renal handling of carnitine in secondary carnitine deficiency disorders. Pediatr Res 34:89, 1993.
Stanley CA, DeLeeuw S, Coates PM, et al: Chronic cardiomyopathy and weakness or acute coma in children with a defect in carnitine uptake. Ann Neurol 30:709, 1991.
Stanley CA, Hale DE: Genetic disorders of mitochondrial fatty oxidation. Curr Opin Pediatr 6:476, 1994.
Stanley CA, Hale DE, Berry GT, et al: A deficiency of carnitine-acylcarnitine translocase in the inner mitochondrial membrane. N Engl J Med 327:19, 1992.
Stanley CA, Sunaryo F, Hale DE, et al: Elevated plasma carnitine in the hepatic form of carnitine palmitoyltransferase-1 deficiency. J Inherit Metab Dis 15:785, 1992.
Tein I, De VDC, Hale DE, et al: Short-chain L-3-hydroxyacyl-CoA dehydrogenase deficiency in muscle: a new cause for recurrent myoglobinuria and encephalopathy. Ann Neurol 30:415, 1991.
Treem WR, Rinaldo P, Hale DE, et al: Acute fatty liver of pregnancy and long-chain 3-hydroxyacyl-coenzyme A dehydrogenase deficiency. Hepatology 19:339, 1994.
Yamaguchi S, Indo Y, Coates PM, et al: Identification of very-long-chain acyl-CoA dehydrogenase deficiency in three patients previously diagnosed with long-chain acyl-CoA dehydrogenase deficiency. Pediatr Res 34:111, 1993.

72.2 Disorders of Very Long Chain Fatty Acids

Hugo W. Moser

PEROXISOMAL DISORDERS

The peroxisomal diseases represent a group of genetically determined disorders in which the major cause of pathology is either the failure to form or maintain the peroxisome or a defect in the function of a single enzyme that normally is located in this organelle. These disorders cause serious disability in childhood and occur more frequently and present a wider range of phenotype than has been recognized in the past.

ETIOLOGY. Table 72–1 shows the current classification of the peroxisomal disorders. The group 1 disorders involve the failure to form normal peroxisomes, and they are therefore referred to as disorders of peroxisome biogenesis. Peroxisomes normally are present in all cells other than mature erythrocytes. The peroxisome is a subcellular organelle surrounded by a single membrane; at least 40 enzymes have been localized to the peroxisome. Some of these enzymes are involved in the production and decomposition of hydrogen peroxide. Other enzymes are concerned with lipid and amino acid metabolism. Most peroxisomal enzymes are first synthesized in their mature form in free polyribosomes and then enter the cytoplasm and are targeted to the peroxisome. It appears that malfunction of the enzyme import mechanisms is the key abnormality in the disorders of peroxisome biogenesis. In the group 2 disorders, peroxisome structure is normal, and there is dysfunction of a single peroxisomal enzyme. The mechanisms of the group 3 disorders are complex and poorly understood.

EPIDEMIOLOGY. Except for X-linked adrenoleukodystrophy, all the peroxisomal disorders listed in Table 72–1 are inherited as autosomal recessive traits. Their combined incidence is estimated to be between 1 in 25,000 and 1 in 50,000. All races are affected.

PATHOLOGY. Absence or reduction in the number of peroxisomes is the pathognomonic feature of disorders of peroxisome biogenesis. In most of these disorders there are membranous sacs that contain peroxisomal integral membrane proteins but lack the normal complement of matrix proteins; these are referred to as peroxisome "ghosts." Pathologic changes are observed in many organs. These include profound and characteristic defects in neuronal migration; micronodular cirrhosis of the liver; renal cysts; chondrodysplasia punctata; corneal clouding, congenital cataracts, glaucoma, and retinopathy; congenital heart disease; and dysmorphic features.

PATHOGENESIS. It is likely that all pathologic changes are secondary to the peroxisome defect. Multiple peroxisomal enzymes fail to function in the group 1 disorders. Table 72–2 lists the defective reactions that are clinically significant. The enzymes that are diminished or absent are synthesized normally but are degraded abnormally fast, presumably because they are unprotected outside of the peroxisome. It is not clear

■ TABLE 72–1 Classification of Peroxisomal Disorders

Group 1 Peroxisomes reduced or absent; multiple enzyme defects	Group 2 Peroxisome normal; single enzyme defect	Group 3 Peroxisomes present, but structure abnormal; more than one defective enzyme
Zellweger syndrome Neonatal adrenoleukodystrophy Infantile Refsum disease Hyperpipecolic acidemia	X-linked adrenoleukodystrophy Acatalasemia Hyperoxaluria type 1 3-oxoacyl-CoA thiolase deficiency "pseudo-Zellweger syndrome" Acyl-CoA oxidase deficiency Bifunctional enzyme deficiency Dihydroxy acetone phosphate acetyl transferase deficiency	Rhizomelic chondrodysplasia punctata Zellweger-like syndrome

how the defective peroxisome functions lead to the widespread pathologic manifestations.

The mechanisms that control the import of peroxisomal enzymes are incompletely understood, but certain of the enzymes have been shown to have specific sequences that are required for appropriate targeting. Complementation studies have subdivided the disorders of biogenesis into 10 separate groups. It is likely that each of these groups represents a distinct genotype, and this suggests that the import of peroxisomal enzymes is controlled by at least six separate mechanisms. A mutation that impairs the formation of a 35 kD peroxisomal membrane protein (peroxisome assembly factor 1) has recently been demonstrated in one of these complementation groups. The patient's parents were heterozygous for this mutation. At this time this is the only group 1 peroxisomal disorder in which carriers can be identified.

CLINICAL MANIFESTATIONS (Disorders of Peroxisome Biogenesis [Group 1]). The three group 1 disorders represent a spectrum of severity. The Zellweger cerebrohepatorenal syndrome is the most severe, infantile Refsum disease the least severe, and neonatal adrenoleukodystrophy intermediate in severity. These distinctions are not definitive. Complementation studies have shown that all three phenotypes are found within a single large complementation group, and the Zellweger phenotype is represented in four of the small complementation groups. However, it seems wisest to retain the current designations until the biochemical basis of the various genotypes is defined.

Newborn infants with *Zellweger syndrome* show striking and consistent abnormalities that are easily recognized. Of central diagnostic importance are the typical facial appearance (high forehead, unslanting palpebral fissures, hypoplastic supraorbital ridges, and epicanthal folds [Fig. 72–2]), severe weakness and hypotonia, neonatal seizures, and eye abnormalities (cataracts, glaucoma, corneal clouding, Brushfield spots, pigmentary retinopathy, and optic nerve dysplasia). Because of the hypotonia and "mongoloid" appearance, Down syndrome is sometimes suspected in these infants. Infants with Zellweger syndrome rarely live more than a few months. More than 90% show postnatal growth failure. Table 72–3 lists the main clinical abnormalities.

Patients with *neonatal adrenoleukodystrophy* show fewer and occasionally no dysmorphic features. Neonatal seizures occur frequently. Some degree of psychomotor development is present, but function remains in the severely or profoundly retarded range and may regress after 3–5 yr of age, probably owing to a progressive leukodystrophy. Several patients are now in a stable, albeit handicapped, state in the 3rd or 4th decade. Enlarged liver and impaired liver function, pigmentary degeneration of the retina, and severely impaired hearing are almost always present. Adrenocortical function is usually impaired, but overt Addison disease is rare. Chondrodysplasia punctata and renal cysts are absent.

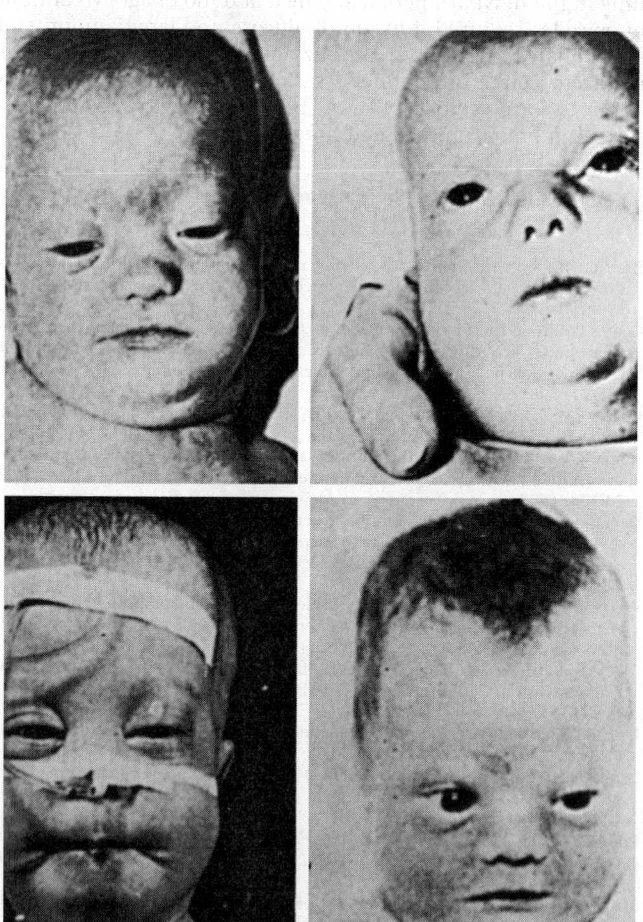

Figure 72–2. Four patients with the Zellweger cerebrohepatorenal syndrome. Note the high forehead, epicanthal folds, and hypoplasia of supraorbital ridges and midface. (Courtesy of Hans Zellweger, M.D. Used by permission.)

■ TABLE 72–2 Abnormal Laboratory Findings Common to Disorders of Peroxisome Biogenesis

Peroxisomes absent or reduced in number
Catalase in cytosol
Deficient synthesis and reduced tissue levels of plasmalogens
Defective oxidation and abnormal accumulation of very long chain fatty acids
Deficient oxidation and age-dependent accumulation of phytanic acid
Defects in certain steps of bile acid formation and accumulation of bile acid intermediates
Defects in oxidation and accumulation of L-pipecolic acid
Increased urinary excretion of dicarboxylic acids

■ TABLE 72–3 Main Clinical Abnormalities in Zellweger Syndrome

Abnormal Feature	Cases in Which Information About the Feature Was Available No.	%	Cases in Which the Feature Was Present No.	%
High forehead	60	53	58	97
Flat occiput	16	14	13	81
Large fontanelle(s), wide sutures	57	50	55	96
Shallow orbital ridges	33	29	33	100
Low/broad nasal bridge	23	20	23	100
Epicanthus	36	32	33	92
High arched palate	37	32	35	95
External ear deformity	40	35	39	97
Micrognathia	18	16	18	100
Redundant skin fold of neck	13	11	13	100
Brushfield spots	6	5	5	83
Cataract/cloudy cornea	35	31	30	86
Glaucoma	12	11	7	58
Abnormal retinal pigmentation	15	13	6	40
Optic disk pallor	23	20	17	74
Severe hypotonia	95	83	94	99
Abnormal Moro response	26	23	26	100
Hyporeflexia or areflexia	57	50	56	98
Poor sucking	77	68	74	96
Gavage feeding	26	23	26	100
Epileptic seizures	61	54	56	92
Psychomotor retardation	45	39	45	100
Impaired hearing	21	18	9	40
Nystagmus	37	32	30	81

From Heymans HSA: Cerebro-hepato-renal (Zellweger) syndrome. Clinical and biochemical consequences of peroxisomal dysfunctions. Thesis, University of Amsterdam, 1984.

Infants with *Refsum disease* have survived to the 2nd decade or longer. They are able to walk, although gait may be ataxic and broad based. Cognitive function is in the severely retarded range. All have sensorineural hearing loss and pigmentary degeneration of the retina. They have moderately dysmorphic features that may include epicanthal folds, flat bridge of the nose, and low-set ears. Early hypotonia and enlarged liver with impaired function are common. Levels of plasma cholesterol and high- and low-density lipoprotein are often moderately reduced. Chondrodysplasia punctata and renal cortical cysts are absent. Postmortem study has been performed in only one child with infantile Refsum disease, who died at 12 yr of age. This revealed micronodular liver cirrhosis and small hypoplastic adrenals. The brain showed no malformations, except for severe hypoplasia of the cerebellar granule layer and ectopic locations of the Purkinje cells in the molecular layer. Although initial reports indicated a preponderance of males, the mode of inheritance is probably autosomal recessive.

The designation of *hyperpipecolic acidemia* was applied to four patients subsequently shown to have diminished or absent peroxisomes, but because of the resemblance of this condition to the Zellweger syndrome or neonatal adrenoleukodystrophy, this disorder is no longer classified as a separate phenotype.

Structurally Abnormal Peroxisomes and Defective Enzymes (Group 3). *Rhizomelic chondrodysplasia punctata (RCDP)* is characterized by the presence of stippled foci of calcification within the hyaline cartilage and is associated with dwarfing, cataracts (72%), and multiple malformations due to contractures. Vertebral bodies have a coronal cleft filled by cartilage that is a result of an embryonic arrest. Disproportionate short stature affects the proximal parts of the extremities (Fig. 72–3*A*). Radiologic abnormalities consist of shortening of the proximal limb bones, metaphyseal cupping, and disturbed ossification (see Fig. 72–3*B*). Height, weight, and head circumference are below the 3rd percentile, and the children are severely retarded mentally. Skin changes such as those observed in ichthyosiform erythroderma are present in about 25% of patients.

Isolated Enzyme Defects of Peroxisomal Fatty Acid Oxidation (Group 2). These rare disorders include oxidase deficiency (pseudoneonatal adrenoleukodystrophy), 3-oxoacyl-CoA thiolase deficiency (pseudo-Zellweger syndrome), and bifunctional enzyme deficiency. Clinically, they resemble the disorders of peroxisome biogenesis and can be distinguished only through laboratory studies.

LABORATORY FINDINGS. The *group 1 disorders* display a spectrum of biochemical abnormalities that are secondary to the defect in peroxisome structure (Table 72–4). The pathognomonic feature is the diminished number or absence of peroxisomes combined with defective function of multiple peroxisomal enzymes.

In the *group 2 disorders* there is a defect in a single peroxisomal enzyme: lignoceroyl-CoA ligase in X-linked adrenoleukodystrophy; alanine:glyoxylate aminotransferase in hyperoxaluria type 1; catalase in acatalasemia; and acyl-CoA oxidase, bifunctional enzyme, or 3-oxoacyl-CoA thiolase, respectively, in the three recently described disorders in which a single peroxisomal β-oxidation enzyme fails to function. In "adult" Refsum disease, there is a defect of phytanic acid oxidase.

The *group 3 disorder (RCDP)* shows three biochemical abnormalities: (1) impaired capacity to oxidize phytanic acid, (2) impaired capacity to synthesize plasmalogens, and (3) failure to process the peroxisomal thiolase enzyme so that it is present in the precursor rather than the mature form. These three defects are also a feature of the group 1 disorders. RCDP differs from them in that the peroxisome structure is intact, and the oxidation of very long chain fatty acids and pipecolic acid is unimpaired.

The *Zellweger-like syndrome,* represented by a single case, has physical findings that resemble those of the Zellweger syndrome and multiple peroxisomal enzyme deficiencies; liver peroxisomes have a normal structure.

DIAGNOSIS. There now are several noninvasive laboratory tests that permit precise and early diagnosis of peroxisomal disorders (see Table 72–4). For the clinician the main decision is when to order these tests. The main challenge in group 1 disorders is to differentiate them from the large variety of other conditions that can cause hypotonia, seizures, failure to thrive, or dysmorphic features. Experienced clinicians can readily recognize classic Zellweger syndrome by its clinical manifestations. However, group 1 patients often do not show the full clinical spectrum of disease and may be identifiable only by laboratory assays. Clinical features that may serve as indications for these diagnostic assays include: severe psychomotor retardation; weakness and hypotonia; dysmorphic features; neonatal seizures; retinopathy, glaucoma, or cataracts; hearing deficits; enlarged liver and impaired liver function; and chondrodysplasia punctata. The combined presence of one or more of these abnormalities increases the likelihood of this diagnosis.

Patients with the isolated defects of peroxisomal fatty acid oxidation (group 2) resemble those with group 1 disorders and can be detected by demonstrating abnormally high levels of very long chain fatty acids.

Patients with RCDP must be distinguished from patients with other causes of chondrodysplasia punctata. In addition to warfarin embryopathy and the Zellweger syndrome, these disorders include the milder autosomal dominant form of chondrodysplasia punctata *(Conradi-Hunermann syndrome)* that is characterized by longer survival, absence of severe limb shortening, and usually intact intellect, an X-linked dominant form, and an X-linked recessive form associated with a deletion of the terminal portion of the short arm of the X chromosome. RCDP is suspected clinically because of the shortness of limbs, psychomotor retardation, and ichthyosis. The most decisive

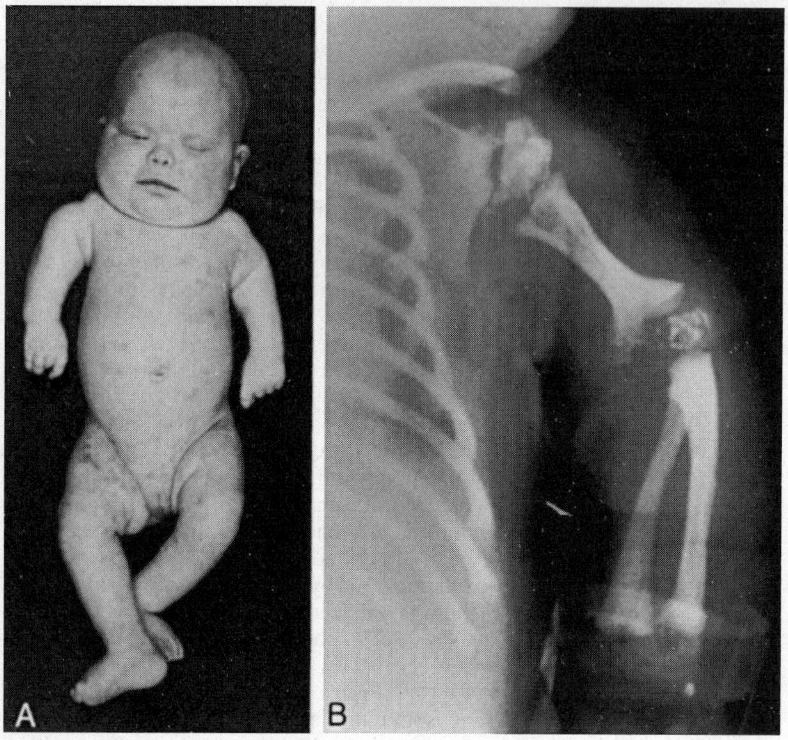

Figure 72–3. *A*, A newborn infant with RCDP. Note the severe shortening of the proximal limbs, the depressed bridge of the nose, hypertelorism, and widespread scaling skin lesions. *B*, Note the marked shortening of the humerus and epiphyseal stippling at the shoulder and the elbow joints. (Courtesy of John P. Dorst, M.D., Johns Hopkins Hospital.)

laboratory test is the demonstration of abnormally low plasmalogen levels in red blood cells and an impaired capacity to synthesize plasmalogens in cultured skin fibroblasts. These biochemical defects are not present in other types of chondrodysplasia punctata.

■ **TABLE 72–4 Peroxisomal Disorders: Biochemical Diagnostic Assays**

Disease	Assay	Findings
Disorders of peroxisome biogenesis: Zellweger syndrome, neonatal adrenoleukodystrophy, infantile Refsum disease, hyperpipecolic acidemia	Plasma	VLCFAs Pipecolic acid Phytanic acid Bile acids
	RBCs	Plasmalogens
	Fibroblasts	Plasmalogen synthesis Catalase subcellular localization
X-linked ALD hemizygote	Plasma/RBCs	VLCFAs
	Fibroblasts	VLCFAs
X-linked ALD heterozygotes	Plasma	VLCFAs
	Fibroblasts	VLCFAs
	DNA probe	
Rhizomelic chondrodysplasia punctata	Plasma	Phytanic acid
	RBCs	Plasmalogens
	Fibroblasts	Plasmalogen synthesis Phytanic acid oxidation
Isolated defects of VLCFA degradation	Plasma	VLCFAs
	Fibroblasts	VLCFAs VLCFA oxidation Immunoblot of peroxisomal fatty acid oxidation enzymes
Hyperoxaluria, type 1	Urine	Organic acids
	Liver	Alanine: Glyoxylate amino transferase in percutaneous liver biopsy
Acatalasemia	RBCs	Catalase

VLCFAs = very long chain fatty acids; RBCs = red blood cells; ALD = adrenoleukodystrophy.

COMPLICATIONS. Patients with the Zellweger cerebrohepatorenal syndrome have multiple disabilities involving muscle tone, swallowing, cardiac abnormalities, liver disease, and seizures. These are treated symptomatically, but the prognosis is poor, and most patients succumb during the first few months of life.

PREVENTION. See later section, Genetic Counseling.

TREATMENT. Because of the multiplicity and severity of deficits, only supportive and symptomatic care is recommended for patients with the classic Zellweger syndrome. For patients with the somewhat milder variants, considerable success has been achieved with multidisciplinary early intervention, including physical and occupational therapy, hearing aids, alternative communication, nutrition, and support for the parents. Although most patients continue to function in the profoundly or severely retarded range, some make significant gains in self-help skills, and several now are in stable condition in their teens or even early twenties.

Several experimental studies are now under way to test strategies that mitigate some of the secondary biochemical abnormalities. These include: (1) the oral administration of cholic acid and chenodeoxycholic acid in a dosage of 100–250 mg/24 hr, with the aim of reducing the levels of presumably toxic bile acid intermediates; (2) administering the ethyl ester of docosahexaenoic acid at 200–250 mg/24 hr by mouth, because the levels of this biologically important polyunsaturated fatty acid are reduced in the plasma and brain of patients with Zellweger syndrome; and (3) the oral administration of plasmalogens in the form of batyl alcohol 5–10 mg/kg/24 hr in 3–5 divided doses. Other measures include the restriction of phytanic acid intake. While these measures do correct, at least in part, some of the biochemical abnormalities associated with the disorders of peroxisomal biogenesis, it is not yet established whether they are of clinical benefit.

GENETIC COUNSELING. All of the peroxisomal disorders can be diagnosed prenatally in the 1st or 2nd trimester, except for hyperoxaluria type 1. The tests used are similar to those described for postnatal diagnosis (see Table 72–4) and utilize chorionic villus samples or amniocytes. More than 300 pregnancies have been monitored, and more than 60 affected fetuses have been identified so far without diagnostic error. Because of the 25% recurrence risk, couples who have previously had an affected child must be advised about the availability of prenatal diagnosis. Except for X-linked adrenoleukodystrophy, there are no techniques for the identification of heterozygotes.

Brul S, Westerveld A, Strijland A, et al: Genetic heterogeneity in the cerebrohepato-renal (Zellweger) syndrome and other inherited disorders with a generalized impairment of peroxisomal functions: A study using complementation analysis. J Clin Invest 81:1710, 1988.

Budden SS, Kennaway NG, Buist NRM, et al: Dysmorphic syndrome with phytanic acid oxidase deficiency, abnormal very long chain fatty acids, and pipecolic acidemia: Studies in four children. J Pediatr 108:33, 1986.

Danpure CJ, Jennings PR, Watts RW: Enzymological diagnosis of primary hyperoxaluria type 1 by measurement of hepatic alanine:glyoxylate amino-transferase activity. Lancet 1:289, 1987.

Hoefler G, Hoefler S, Watkins PA, et al: Biochemical abnormalities in rhizomelic chondrodysplasia punctata. J Pediatr 112:726, 1988.

Kelley RJ, Datta NS, Dobyns WB, et al: Neonatal adrenoleukodystrophy: New cases, biochemical studies and differentiation from Zellweger and related peroxisomal polydystrophy syndromes. Am J Med Genet 23:869, 1986.

Martinez M, Pineda M, Vidal R, et al: Docosahexaenoic acid: A new therapeutic approach to peroxisomal patients. Experience with two cases. Neurology 43:1389, 1993.

Moser AE, Singh I, Brown FR III, et al: The cerebro-hepato-renal (Zellweger) syndrome: Increased levels and impaired degradation of very long chain fatty acids and their use in prenatal diagnosis. N Engl J Med 310:1141, 1984.

Moser HW: Peroxisomal diseases. *In:* LA Barnes (ed): Advances in Pediatrics, Vol. 36. Chicago, Year Book Medical Publishers, 1989, pp 1–38.

Setchell KDR, Bragetti P, Zimmer-Nechemias L, et al: Oral bile acid treatment and the patient with Zellweger syndrome. Hepatology 15:198, 1992.

Shimozawa N, Tsukamoto T, Suzuki Y, et al: A human gene responsible for Zellweger syndrome that affects peroxisome assembly. Science 255:1132, 1992.

ADRENOLEUKODYSTROPHY (X-LINKED)

X-linked adrenoleukodystrophy (ALD) is a genetically determined disorder associated with the accumulation of saturated very long chain fatty acids and a progressive dysfunction of the adrenal cortex and nervous system white matter.

ETIOLOGY. The key biochemical abnormality is the tissue accumulation of saturated very long chain fatty acids. These are unbranched with a carbon chain length of 24 or more. Excess hexacosanoic acid (C26:0) is the most striking and characteristic feature. This accumulation of fatty acids is due to a genetically determined deficient capacity to degrade them, a function that is normally carried out in the peroxisome. The key biochemical defect appears to involve the impaired function of peroxisomal lignoceroyl CoA ligase, the enzyme that catalyzes the formation of the coenzyme A derivative of very long chain fatty acids. The gene defect leads to the defect in the formation of a peroxisomal membrane protein, which is postulated to be required for the import of lignoceroyl CoA ligase into the peroxisome. The gene has been mapped to Xq28.

EPIDEMIOLOGY. X linkage has been confirmed by analysis of more than 900 kindreds. All races are affected. Incidence is estimated to be between 1 in 20,000 and 1 in 50,000. The various phenotypes often occur in members of the same kindred.

PATHOLOGY. Characteristic lamellar cytoplasmic inclusions can be demonstrated with the electron microscope in adrenocortical cells, testicular Leydig cells, and nervous system macrophages. These inclusions probably consist of cholesterol esterified with very long chain fatty acids. They are most prominent in cells of the zona fasciculata of the adrenal cortex, which at first are distended with lipid and later atrophy.

The nervous system of patients with childhood ALD shows acute and relatively symmetric demyelinative lesions that involve the parieto-occipital regions most severely. In addition to the myelin breakdown, there is perivascular infiltration of lymphocytes resembling that seen in multiple sclerosis. Most other tissues are intact. Peroxisomes are normal in number and structure.

PATHOGENESIS. The adrenal dysfunction is probably a direct consequence of the accumulation of very long chain fatty acids. The cells in the zona fasciculata are distended with abnormal lipids. Cholesterol esterified with very long chain fatty acids is relatively resistant to ACTH-stimulated cholesterol ester hydrolases, and this limits the capacity to convert cholesterol to endocrinologically active steroids. In addition, C26:0 excess increases the viscosity of the plasma membrane, and this in turn may interfere with receptor and other cellular functions.

There is no correlation between the severity of the nervous system lesions and the biochemical defect or between the degree of adrenal involvement and that of nervous system involvement. One third or more of patients with adrenoleukodystrophy are free of nervous system involvement or develop a milder disability in adulthood. Thus, nervous system involvement depends on some factor or factors in addition to the very long chain fatty acid excess. These include autoimmune or cytokine-mediated reactions that are triggered in some way by the abnormal accumulation of very long chain fatty acids. Tumor necrosis factor alpha plays a role in the inflammatory response and the severity of the response may be modulated by an autosomal modifier gene.

CLINICAL MANIFESTATIONS. There are seven relatively distinct phenotypes, three of which present in childhood with symptoms and signs. In all of the phenotypes development is usually normal during the first 3–4 yr. Also see Chapter 552.3.

In the *childhood cerebral* form of ALD, symptoms are first noted most commonly between the ages of 4 and 8 yr, 2 yr at the earliest. The most common initial manifestations are hyperactivity, which is often mistaken for an attention deficit disorder, and worsening school performance in a child who had previously been a good student. Auditory discrimination is often impaired, although tone perception is preserved. This may be evidenced by difficulty in using the telephone and greatly impaired performance on intelligence tests in items that are presented verbally. Spatial orientation is often impaired. Other initial symptoms are disturbances of vision, ataxia, poor handwriting, seizures, and strabismus. Visual disturbances often are due to involvement of the cerebral cortex, which leads to variable and seemingly inconsistent visual capacity. Seizures occur in nearly all patients and may represent the first manifestation of the disease. Some patients present with increased intracranial pressure or with unilateral mass lesions. Impaired cortisol response to ACTH stimulation is present in 85% of patients, and mild hyperpigmentation is often noted. However, in most patients with this phenotype adrenal dysfunction is recognized only after the condition is diagnosed because of the cerebral symptoms. Cerebral childhood adrenoleukodystrophy tends to progress rapidly with increasing spasticity and paralysis, visual and hearing loss, and loss of ability to speak or swallow. The mean interval between the first neurologic symptom and an apparently vegetative state is 1.9 ± 2 yr. Patients may continue in this apparently vegetative state for 10 or more yr.

Adolescent ALD designates patients who develop neurologic symptoms between the ages of 10 and 21 yr. The manifestations resemble those of childhood cerebral ALD except that progression is slower.

Adrenomyeloneuropathy first becomes manifest in late adolescence or adulthood as a progressive paraparesis due to long-tract degeneration in the spinal cord. Approximately one half of the patients also have involvement of the cerebral white matter.

The "Addison only" phenotype is an important and underdiagnosed condition. Studies in developed countries, where tuberculosis is no longer a common cause, suggest that as many as 40% of male patients with Addison disease have the biochemical defect of ALD. Many of these patients have intact neurologic systems, whereas others have subtle neurologic signs. Many develop adrenomyeloneuropathy in adulthood.

The term *presymptomatic ALD* is applied to boys up to 10 yr old who have the biochemical defect of ALD but are free of neurologic or endocrine disturbances. Boys in this category who are 10 yr or older are referred to as asymptomatic. A few persons with the biochemical defect of ALD who are relatives of clinically affected patients with ALD have remained asymptomatic even in the 6th or 7th decade.

Approximately 20–30% of female heterozygotes develop a syndrome that resembles adrenomyeloneuropathy but is milder and of later onset. Adrenal insufficiency is very rare.

LABORATORY FINDINGS. Very Long Chain Fatty Acids. The most specific and important laboratory finding is the demonstration of abnormally high levels of very long chain fatty acids in plasma, red blood cells, or cultured skin fibroblasts. The test should be performed in a laboratory that has experience with this specialized procedure. Positive results are obtained in all male patients with X-linked ALD and in approximately 85% of female carriers of X-linked ALD.

Computed Tomography (CT) and Magnetic Resonance Imaging (MRI). Patients with childhood cerebral or adolescent ALD show cerebral white matter lesions that are characteristic with respect to location and attenuation patterns on CT or MRI. In 80% of patients the lesions are symmetric and involve the periventricular white matter in the posterior parietal and occipital lobes. Noncontrast CT scans show bilateral hypodensities in this location. The second characteristic, observed following intravenous injection of contrast material, is the demonstration of a garland of accumulated contrast material adjacent and anterior to the posterior hypodense lesions (Fig. 72–4*A*). This zone corresponds to the zones of intense perivascular lymphocytic infiltration where the blood-brain barrier breaks down. In 12% of patients the initial lesions are frontal. Unilateral lesions that produce a mass effect suggestive of a brain tumor may occur. MRI provides a clearer delineation of normal and abnormal white matter than CT and may demonstrate abnormalities missed by CT (see Fig. 72–4*B*).

Impaired Adrenal Function. More than 85% of patients with the childhood form of ALD have elevated levels of ACTH in plasma and a subnormal rise of cortisol levels in plasma following intravenous injection of 250 μg of $ACTH_{1-24}$ (Cortrosyn).

DIAGNOSIS AND DIFFERENTIAL DIAGNOSIS. The earliest manifestations of childhood cerebral ALD are difficult to distinguish from the much more common attention deficit disorders or learning disabilities. Rapid progression, signs of dementia, or difficulty in auditory discrimination suggests ALD. Even in early stages CT or MRI may show strikingly abnormal changes. Other leukodystrophies or multiple sclerosis may, however, mimic these radiographic findings. Definitive diagnosis depends on demonstration of very long chain fatty acid excess, which occurs only in X-linked ALD and the peroxisomal disorders. The latter may be distinguished from X-linked ALD by their clinical presentation during the neonatal period.

Cerebral forms of ALD may present with increased intracranial pressure and unilateral mass lesions. These have been misdiagnosed as gliomas, even after brain biopsy, and several patients have received radiotherapy before the correct diagnosis was made. Measurement of very long chain fatty acids in plasma or brain biopsy specimens is the most reliable differential test.

Adolescent or adult cerebral ALD can be confused with psychiatric disorders, epilepsy, or dementing disorders. The first clue to the diagnosis of ALD may be the demonstration of

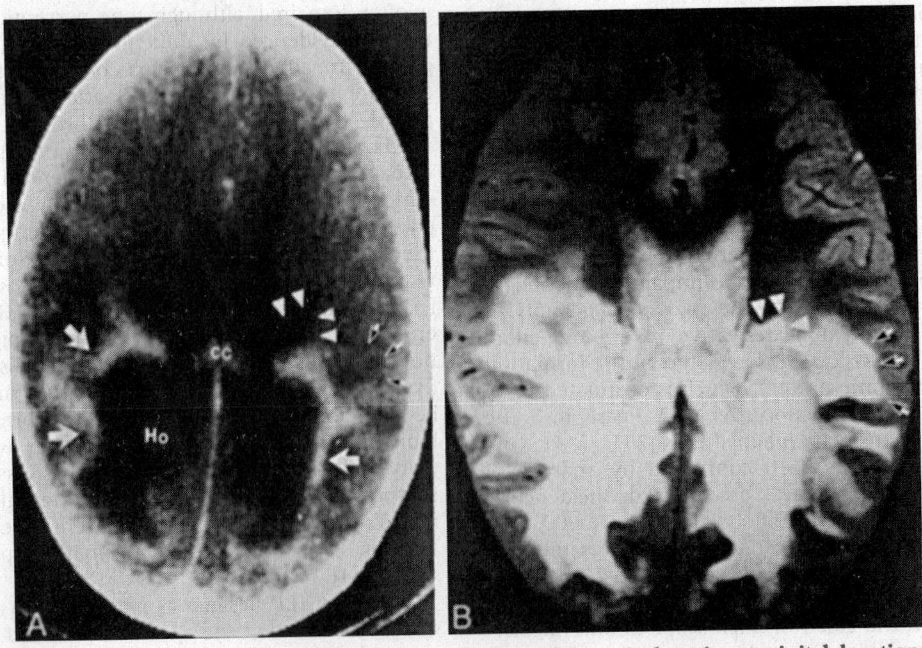

Figure 72–4. *A*, Contrast-enhanced CT abnormalities in ALD with typical parieto-occipital location, showing symmetric bilateral hypodense inactive zones (Ho). The enhancing active periphery zone of hypodensity is demarcated by *arrows*. Compare the anterior zone of hypodensity *(arrowheads)* with the MRI. CC = corpus callosum. (From Kumar et al, 1987, with permission.) *B*, An MRI of the same patient and area shown by CT scanning. MRI-T_2-weighted image shows a high-intensity signal of the abnormally bright parieto-occipital white matter. Subcortical involvement is better identified on MRI. Separation of active zones may be better appreciated by CT scanning, because both inactive and active zones are seen at high-signal areas on MRI. However, it is assumed that such major distinctions afforded by CT will also be demonstrable when IV enhancement (paramagnetic enhancement) becomes readily available. Note the hypodense involvement of CT scanning *(arrowheads* and *arrows)* in *A* compared with the well-resolved lesions on MRI in *B*. (From Kumar et al: Adrenoleukodystrophy: Correlating MR Imaging with CT. Radiology 165:497, 1987.)

white matter lesions by CT or MRI; assays of very long chain fatty acids should be confirmatory.

ALD cannot be distinguished clinically from other forms of Addison disease, and it is recommended that assays of very long chain fatty acid levels be performed in all male patients with Addison disease. ALD patients almost never have antibodies to adrenal tissue in their plasma.

COMPLICATIONS. An avoidable complication is the occurrence of adrenal insufficiency. The most difficult problems are those related to bed rest, contracture, coma, and swallowing disturbances. Other complications involve behavioral disturbances and injuries associated with defects of spatial orientation, impaired vision and hearing, and seizures.

TREATMENT. Steroid replacement for adrenal insufficiency or adrenocortical hypofunction is effective (see Chapter 528). Adrenal function should be tested periodically at minimum intervals of 1 yr.

The progressive behavioral and neurologic disturbances associated with the childhood form of ALD are extremely difficult for the family to cope with. ALD patients require the establishment of a comprehensive management program and partnership between the family, physician, visiting nursing staff, school authorities, and counselors. In addition, parent support groups are often helpful.* Communication with school authorities is important because under the provisions of Public Law 94–142 children with ALD qualify for special services as "other health impaired" or "multihandicapped." Depending on the rate of progression of the disease, special needs might range from relatively low level resource services within a regular school program to home- and hospital-based teaching programs for children who are not mobile.

Management challenges vary with the stage of the illness. The early stages are characterized by subtle changes in affect, behavior, and attention span. Counseling and communication with school authorities are of prime importance. Changes in the sleep-wake cycle can be benefited by the judicious use at night of sedatives such as chloral hydrate (10–50 mg/kg), pentobarbital (5 mg/kg), or diphenhydramine (2–3 mg/kg).

As the leukodystrophy progresses, the modulation of muscle tone and support of bulbar muscular function are major concerns. Baclofen in gradually increasing doses (5 mg twice a day to 25 mg 4 times a day) is the most effective pharmacologic agent for the treatment of acute episodic painful muscle spasms. Other agents may also be used, care being taken to monitor the occurrence of side effects and drug interactions. As the leukodystrophy progresses, bulbar muscular control is lost. Although initially this can be managed by changing the diet to soft and puréed foods, most patients eventually require a nasogastric tube or a surgical procedure such as gastrostomy or lateral esophagostomy. At least one third of patients have focal or generalized seizures, which usually respond readily to standard anticonvulsant medications.

Several specific therapeutic approaches are under investigation. The plasma levels of C26:0 can be normalized within 4 wk by the administration of oils containing certain monounsaturated fatty acids in combination with the dietary restriction of saturated very long chain fatty acids. The most commonly used oil (also referred to as Lorenzo's oil) is a 4:1 mixture of glyceryl trioleate and glyceryl trierucate. Erucic acid (22:1 n-9) is the active component of the latter. These oils appear to act by reducing the rate of endogenous synthesis of the saturated very long chain fatty acids. While the biochemical effect on plasma C26:0 levels is striking, and led to the hope that this could lead to clinical benefit, the general experience has been that this therapy does not alter the rate of neurologic progression in the childhood cerebral or adrenomyeloneuropathy forms of ALD. There is somewhat encouraging, but not yet proven, evidence that administration of the oils prior to the development of neurologic symptoms reduces the frequency and severity of later neurologic disability. While interpretation of the data in the asymptomatic patients requires additional study, it is recommended at this time that neurologically asymptomatic ALD patients be placed on this dietary regimen as part of ongoing therapeutic trials. Moderate reductions in platelet counts are observed in 40% of patients on this dietary regimen and careful medical supervision is required.

Bone marrow transplantation (BMT) is the most effective therapy for X-linked ALD, but its application must be considered with great care. The main indication is in boys with *significant but mild cerebral involvement* for whom a donor with a good HLA match is available. Significant but mild cerebral involvement is judged to be present if an MRI abnormality characteristic of ALD is combined with moderate deficits in visual or auditory processing or memory/learning, which have been shown are known to be associated with ALD, or if there is evidence of mild motor, visual, or auditory dysfunction. Under these circumstances BMT has not only stabilized the course of the disease but in some patients has led to a reversal of the abnormality. It is our impression that severe graft-versus-host disease not only is associated with the expected higher mortality, but also jeopardizes the chance of neurologic benefit. Preliminary, but not yet fully confirmed, data suggest that pretransplant dietary therapy (as described earlier) reduces the risk of transplant-related morbidity and mortality. Because BMT is associated with a 10–20% mortality, even under favorable circumstances, it is not recommended for patients who do not have evidence of cerebral involvement or who have mild cerebral involvement that is nonprogressive (see Chapter 132). Even without therapy, more than half of the patients with the biochemical abnormality of ALD are not "destined" to develop the severe form of the disease. While the majority of these patients will develop adrenomyeloneuropathy in adulthood, and even though this may be a seriously disabling disease, many of these patients have led productive lives and some have survived to the 8th decade. Furthermore, preliminary experience suggests that dietary therapy administered to neurologically asymptomatic patients reduces the frequency and severity of subsequent neurologic disability, and other forms of therapy are under consideration, so that the risk associated with BMT does not appear warranted under these circumstances. BMT is also not recommended for patients with severe cognitive, motor, or visual impairment. Not only has the procedure not been of benefit but it may accelerate the rate of neurologic progression.

It is our current practice to recommend dietary therapy for all persons with the biochemical abnormality of ALD who are asymptomatic or have the "Addison only" phenotype. Neurologic and neuropsychological examinations and MRI are obtained at 6–12 mo in order to ensure that the window of opportunity for BMT is not missed.

Studies are in progress to determine whether the rapid rate of progression of childhood cerebral ALD can be modified by pharmacologic agents such as beta-interferon, immune globulin, or tumor necrosis factor antagonists such as pentoxifylline or thalidomide. Since the ALD gene has been isolated, efforts toward the development of gene therapy have been initiated.

GENETIC COUNSELING AND PREVENTION. The very long chain fatty acid assay can identify 85% of female carriers, and the accuracy of carrier identification can be increased by use of the DXS-52 DNA probe. Prenatal diagnosis of affected male fetuses can be achieved by measurement of very long chain fatty acid levels in cultured amniocytes or chorionic villus cells. Whenever a new patient with X-linked ALD is identified, a detailed pedigree should be constructed, and efforts should be made to identify all at-risk female carriers and affected males.

*United Leukodystrophy Foundation, 2304 Highland Drive, Sycamore, IL 60178.

These investigations should be accompanied by careful and sympathetic attention to social, emotional, and ethical issues during counseling.

Aubourg P, Adamsbaum C, Lavallard-Rousseau MC, et al: A two-year trial of oleic and erucic acids ("Lorenzo's oil") as treatment of adrenomyeloneuropathy. N Engl J Med 329:745, 1993.

Aubourg P, Blanche S, Jambaqué I, et al: Reversal of early neurologic and neuroradiologic manifestations of X-linked adrenoleukodystrophy by bone marrow transplantation. N Engl J Med 332:1860, 1990.

Aubourg PR, Sack GH Jr, Meyers DA, et al: Linkage of adrenoleukodystrophy to a polymorphic DNA probe. Ann Neurol 21:349, 1987.

Kumar AJ, Rosenbaum AE, Naidu S, et al: Role of magnetic resonance imaging in adrenoleukodystrophy. Radiology 165:497, 1987.

Lazo O, Contreras M, Hashmi M, et al: Peroxisomal lignoceroyl-CoA ligase deficiency in childhood adrenoleukodystrophy and adrenomyeloneuropathy. Proc Natl Acad Sci USA 85:7647, 1988.

Moser HW: Lorenzo's oil. Film review. Lancet 341:544, 1993.

Moser HW, Moser AB, Singh I, et al: Adrenoleukodystrophy: Survey of 303 cases: Biochemistry, diagnosis and therapy. Ann Neurol 16:628, 1984.

Moser HW, Moser AB, Smith KD, et al: Adrenoleukodystrophy: Phenotypic variability: Implications for therapy. J Inherit Metab Dis 15:645, 1992.

Moser HW, Moser AB, Trojak JE, et al: Identification of female carriers of adrenoleukodystrophy. J Pediatr 103:54, 1983.

Moser J, Douar AM, Sarde CO, et al: Putative X-linked adrenoleukodystrophy gene shares unexpected homology with ABC transporters. Nature 361:726, 1993.

Powers JM, Liu Y, Moser A, et al: The inflammatory myelinopathy of adrenoleukodystrophy: Cells, effector molecules, and pathogenetic implications. J Neuropathol Exp Neurol 51:630, 1992.

Rizzo WB, Leshner RT, Odone A, et al: Dietary erucic acid therapy for X-linked adrenoleukodystrophy. Neurology 39:1415, 1989.

Wanders RJA, Van Roermund CWT, Van Wijland MJA, et al: Direct demonstration that the deficient oxidation of very long chain fatty acids in X-linked adrenoleukodystrophy is due to an impaired ability of peroxisomes to activate very long chain fatty acids. Biochem Biophys Res Commun 153:618, 1988.

72.3 Lipid Storage Disorders

(Lipidoses)

Reuben K. Matalon

The lipidoses are lysosomal lipid storage diseases, each caused by deficiency of a specific hydrolase. The lipid material stored within the lysosomes, usually a glycosphingolipid, leads to the pathophysiology characteristic of the specific lipid storage disease. For example, if the sphingolipid is stored only in the peripheral tissues, sparing the central nervous system (CNS), then hepatosplenomegaly may be noted and the disease suspected, as in Gaucher disease. On the other hand, if the glycosphingolipid is stored in the CNS only and not in peripheral tissues, there is no hepatosplenomegaly, and the storage disease may not be suspected, as in Tay-Sachs disease. When the CNS is involved, mental retardation and neurologic deterioration are major components of the storage disease. In lipidoses in which storage material accumulates in the periphery and in the CNS, mental retardation together with hepatosplenomegaly is characteristic of the disease, as in Niemann-Pick disease.

The *sphingolipids,* which are components of the cell membrane, are found in every cell of the body. Their basic structure is identical, and all sphingolipids are based on sphingosine (Fig. 72–5). The structure of sphingosine is achieved by the condensation of the amino acid serine with palmitic acid. This compound combines the C_{18} nonpolar region of palmitate and the polar region of serine, which contains an amino group and two hydroxyl groups. Another fatty acid is added to sphingosine through the amino group of serine, forming ceramide. The first hydroxyl group (C_1) of ceramide can become a recipient to sugars, for example, ceramide-glucose, which is also called *glucocerebroside.* Ceramide-galactose is another ceramide-monohexoside, also known as galactocerebroside. Phosphocholine

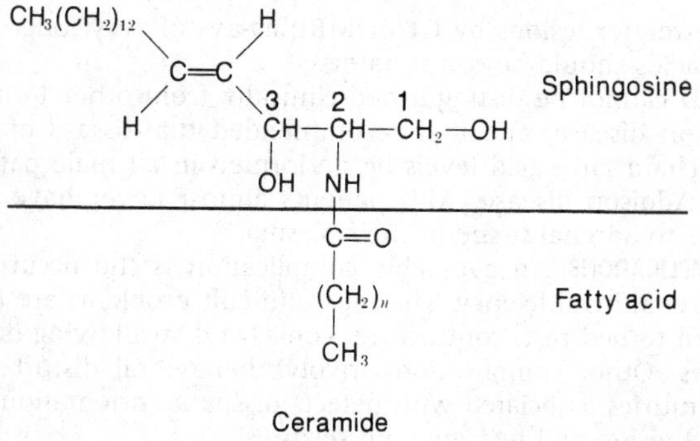

Figure 72–5. **Basic structure of sphingolipids. All additions to ceramide are made through the hydroxyl group of carbon atom 1: Glycosphingolipids = ceramide plus one or more sugars attached to C-1. Gangliosides = glycosphingolipids plus one or more sialic acid residues. Sphingomyelin = ceramide plus phosphorylcholine attached to C-1.**

may substitute for the sugars, forming sphingomyelin. More than one sugar can be added to ceramide, and branches of sialic acid (neuraminic acid [NANA]) may be added, resulting in a rather complex compound (see Fig. 72–5). When neuraminic acid is added to the sphingolipid, the resulting compound is called a *ganglioside.* Despite their complexity, such membrane-associated compounds have similar building blocks and must be degraded or recycled by lysosomal enzymes. A general outline of the stepwise degradation of sphingolipids is shown in Figures 72–6 and 72–7. A defect in any step results in a lysosomal storage disease. The storage of a specific compound in a specific tissue depends on the distribution of that compound in the body.

GM_1 GANGLIOSIDOSIS. This is a group of lysosomal disorders with variable clinical findings. GM_1 ganglioside is a monosialoganglioside found in normal cerebral gray and white matter and in peripheral tissues. There are two major forms of GM_1 gangliosidosis, infantile (type 1) and juvenile (type 2). There is also an adult form, type 3.

Etiology. The biochemical defect of both forms of GM_1 gangliosidosis is a deficiency of the lysosomal enzyme β-galactosidase, which hydrolyzes the terminal galactose from GM_1 ganglioside (see Fig. 72–7). The diagnosis is confirmed by demonstrating deficiency of β-galactosidase in white blood cells or cultured skin fibroblasts.

Clinical Manifestations (see also Chapter 552). The *infantile form* of GM_1 gangliosidosis may be noted at birth by the presence of hepatosplenomegaly, edema of the extremities, and rashes that cannot be explained by the usual newborn skin eruptions. Psychomotor retardation soon becomes evident. A cherry-red spot in the macula is present in 50% of the patients. Umbilical and inguinal hernias with edema of the scrotum are usually present at birth. Because of the coarse facial features and macroglossia these children may be suspected of having Hurler disease. Enlargement of the heart and signs of ventricular hypertrophy occur in most patients with GM_1 gangliosidosis. Lumbar kyphosis and some stiffening of the joints are also characteristic of GM_1 gangliosidosis as well as of Hurler disease. However, rapid mental deterioration, macular cherry-red spot, and early onset of seizures are more characteristic of GM_1 gangliosidosis. The patient becomes dysphagic, deaf, and blind, and death occurs at 3–4 yr of age.

Radiologic changes are those of *dysostosis multiplex.* Vertebral changes occur with anterior beaking, the sella turcica is large, and the calvarium may be thickened. Although these changes are similar to those seen in the mucopolysaccharidoses, they are less severe. CT scans and MRI of the brain show ventricular dilatation and generalized brain atrophy.

Late-onset GM_1 gangliosidosis is clinically distinct. The age

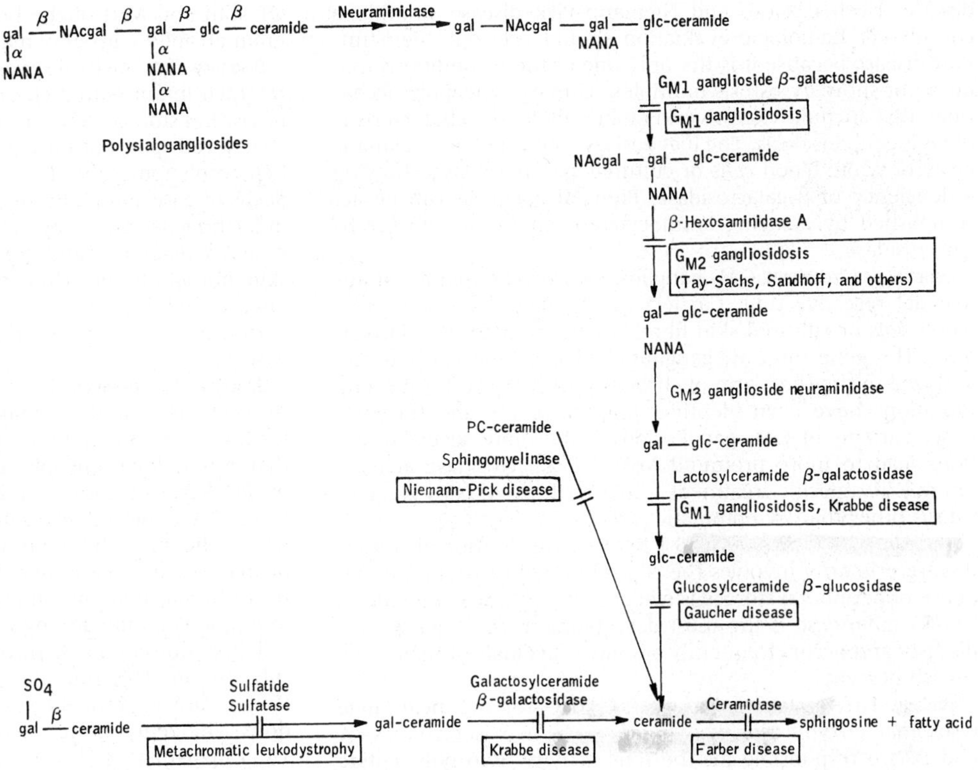

Figure 72–6. Pathways in the metabolism of sphingolipids found in nervous tissues. The name of the enzyme catalyzing each reaction is given with the name of the substrate acted on. Inborn errors are depicted as bars crossing the reaction arrows, and the name of the associated defect or defects is given within the nearest box. The gangliosides are named according to the nomenclature of Svennerholm. Anomeric configurations are given only at the largest starting compound. gal = galactose; glc = glucose; NAcgal = *N*-acetyl-galactosamine; NANA = *N*-acetyl-neuraminic acid; PC = phosphorylcholine.

of onset varies, and such patients may present with ataxia, dysarthria, and cerebral palsy–like spasticity. Deterioration is slow, and patients may survive through the 4th decade of life. These patients lack visceral involvement, do not have coarse facial features, and do not have dysostosis multiplex.

Biochemical and Pathologic Findings. There are foam cells in bone marrow aspirates and in histologic preparations of tissues such as the lungs and liver. GM_1 ganglioside accumulates in the brain and peripheral tissues. In addition, keratan sulfate, a mucopolysaccharide, accumulates in liver and is excreted in the urine of patients with GM_1 gangliosidosis.

Diagnosis. GM_1 gangliosidosis is suspected clinically by developmental delay, coarse facial features, enlarged tongue, hepatosplenomegaly, and a cherry-red spot of the macula. Hurler

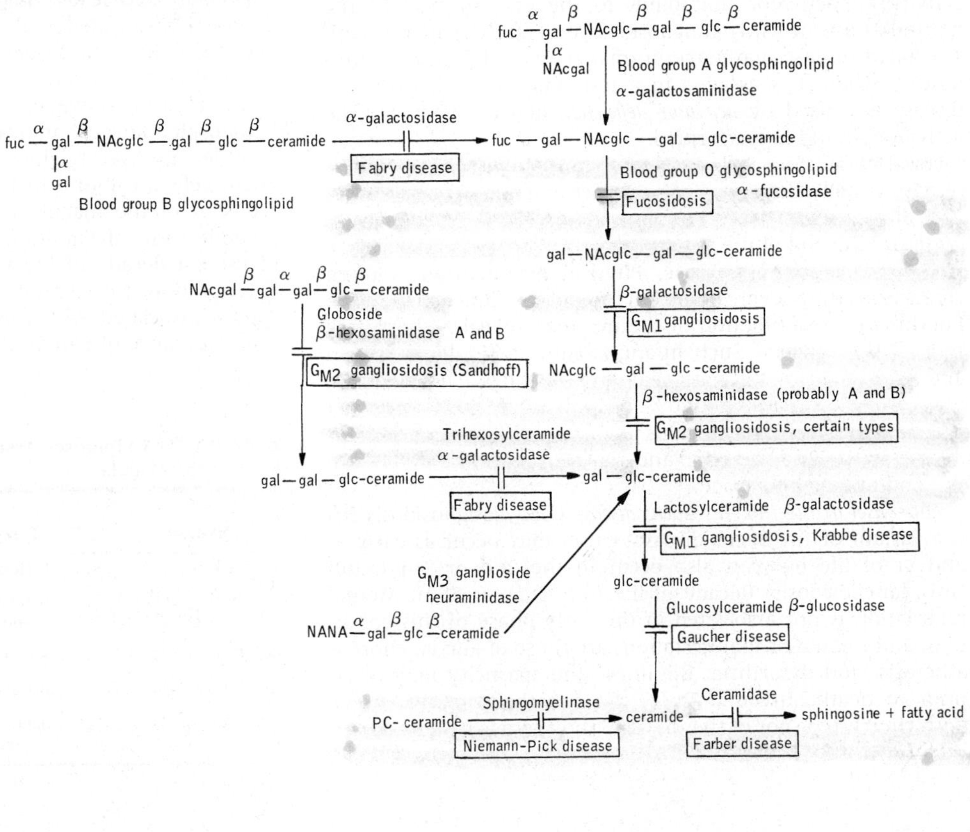

Figure 72–7. Pathways in the degradation of sphingolipids found in visceral organs and red or white blood cells. See also the legend for Figure 72–6. fuc = fucose; NAcglc = *N*-acetylglucosamine.

disease, I-cell disease, and Niemann-Pick disease should be considered. Radiologic evaluation should rule out Niemann-Pick disease because it is the only one of these conditions that does not show dysostosis multiplex. Urinary mucopolysaccharides that include excessive keratan sulfate are characteristic of GM_1 gangliosidosis. The diagnosis is confirmed by enzymatic assay of white blood cells or cultured skin fibroblasts showing a deficiency of β-galactosidase. Prenatal diagnosis can be accomplished by assaying amniocytes or chorionic villi for β-galactosidase.

Genetics and Treatment. GM_1 gangliosidosis is inherited as an autosomal recessive trait. Carriers can be detected using white blood cells or cultured skin fibroblasts to assay for β-galactosidase. The gene for GM_1 gangliosidosis has been isolated and localized to the short arm of chromosome 3 (3p21.33). Several mutations have been identified for the severe and the late-onset variants of GM_1 gangliosidosis. The more severe mutations lead to more profound loss of β-galactosidase activity. There is no specific treatment for either form of GM_1 gangliosidosis other than symptomatic care.

TAY-SACHS (GM_2 GANGLIOSIDOSIS I). Because this lysosomal storage disease primarily involves the central nervous system, no evidence of peripheral storage is evident on physical examination. Tay-Sachs disease is the most devastating of the lipid storage diseases and occurs frequently among individuals of Ashkenazi Jewish descent.

Etiology. The basic defect is a deficiency of the heat-labile lysosomal enzyme β-hexosaminidase A; two isoenzymes, A and B, are responsible for the total activity. Two polypeptide chains, α and β, are required for the formation of β-hexosaminidase A and B. Isoenzyme A is formed with α and β chains, whereas isoenzyme B is composed of β chains only. Therefore, a defect in the α chain results in deficient activity in β-hexosaminidase A, as occurs in both forms of Tay-Sachs disease. Several mutations at the gene locus affecting the production of the α chain of β-hexosaminidase have been identified. A defect in the β chain affects the activity of both isoenzymes A and B, thus causing a deficiency of the total activity of β-hexosaminidase (see later discussion of Sandhoff Disease). The enzyme β-hexosaminidase A requires for its hydrolytic activity an activator that binds to the enzyme and to the natural substrate GM_2 ganglioside. Very rarely, patients with Tay-Sachs disease may have normal activity of β-hexosaminidase A when it is assayed in a test tube. In such cases the disease is caused by *activator deficiency,* and an assay for the activator should be performed.

Clinical Manifestations. Infants develop normally until about 5 mo of age. Usually decreased eye contact and focusing are noted first, along with an exaggerated startle response to noise, *hyperacusis.* By the end of the 1st yr an infant with Tay-Sachs disease becomes severely hypotonic. Physical examination is often characterized by severe hypotonia, blindness, and hyperacusis. Funduscopic examination of the eye may reveal a cherry-red spot of the macula. Such infants assume a froglike position and interact very little with their surroundings. The head size may enlarge more than 50%, but this enlargement is not associated with hydrocephalus. Seizures may complicate the disease in the 2nd yr of life, and death usually occurs between the 2nd and 4th yr of age.

Late-onset or juvenile Tay-Sachs disease (GM_2 gangliosidosis III) is a variant of Tay-Sachs disease. Onset may occur as early as 2nd yr of life but can also occur in the 2nd or 3rd (adult GM_2 gangliosidosis) decade of life (see Chapter 552). Mental retardation is not associated in the early phase of this condition, and the major manifestations are those of ataxia, choreoathetosis, and dysarthria. Blindness and spasticity may occur prior to death. Juvenile Tay-Sachs disease is not associated with cherry-red spot of the macula, and there is no organomegaly. Tay-Sachs disease is not associated with bony changes. CT scan and MRI of the brain reveal enlarged ventricles and brain atrophy with gray matter degeneration.

Diagnosis. Tay-Sachs disease is usually suspected in a severely retarded infant with a cherry-red spot of the macula and lack of visceral storage. Several sphingolipidoses are associated with cherry-red spot, but only patients with Tay-Sachs disease lack hepatosplenomegaly (Table 72–5). The juvenile form of Tay-Sachs disease should be suspected in a child whose ataxia and dysarthria become progressive. The assay for β-hexosaminidase A is diagnostic and can be carried out on plasma, cultured skin fibroblasts, or white blood cells. Carriers for Tay-Sachs disease and juvenile Tay-Sachs disease can be detected by performing an assay for the specific activity of hexosaminidase A.

Genetics and Prevention. There is considerable heterogeneity at the gene level, and the major group of mutations responsible for Tay-Sachs disease in the Jewish population is different from that in non-Jewish people. The mutation for the infantile form of Tay-Sachs disease is different from that for the juvenile form. The gene for hexosaminidase A (Hex A) has been isolated. The most frequent DNA defect in Ashkenazi Jewish people is a four base pair insertion in exon 11. This change results in termination signal and deficiency of mRNA. Another mutation common among Ashkenazi Jews has been located at the first nucleotide of intron 12, where there is a G to C substitution. This mutation also results in loss of activity of Hex A. Other ethnic groups carry a variety of different mutations. The gene for Hex A has been localized to chromosome 15 (15q23–q24).

Both forms of Tay-Sachs disease are inherited as autosomal recessive traits, and both are more frequent among Ashkenazi Jews. The frequency of Tay-Sachs disease is 1 in 3,500–4,000 births, making the carrier rate among Ashkenazi Jews 1 in 30. This high frequency and the availability of carrier testing have led to mass carrier blood screening for β-hexosaminidase A. Carrier testing, counseling, and prenatal diagnosis have markedly decreased the frequency of Tay-Sachs disease among Jewish couples.

Treatment. There is no treatment for either form of Tay-Sachs disease.

SANDHOFF DISEASE (GM_2 Gangliosidosis II). This autosomal recessive disease is associated with total β-hexosaminidase deficiency because both A and B isoenzymes are deficient. *Clinical manifestations* vary but usually mimic those of Tay-Sachs disease in its infantile form. However, Sandhoff disease is associated with hepatosplenomegaly, indicating peripheral storage of GM_2 ganglioside, an *N*-acetylglucosamine containing oligosaccharide. Foam cells are found in bone marrow aspirates. The cherry-red spot of the macula is also seen in Sandhoff disease. A juvenile form of Sandhoff disease presents in the latter half of the 1st decade of life with ataxia, dysarthria, and mental deterioration. No visceral enlargement or macular cherry-red spot is associated with this form of the disease. There is no preponderance of Sandhoff disease among Ashkenazi Jews.

■ **TABLE 72–5 Lipidoses Associated with Cherry-Red Spot of the Macula**

Disease	Enzyme Defect	Visceral Involvement
Tay-Sachs	β-Hexosaminidase A	No organomegaly
Sandhoff	β-Hexosaminidase A and B	Hepatosplenomegaly
Niemann-Pick	Sphingomyelinase	Hepatosplenomegaly
GM_1 gangliosidosis	β-Galactosidase	Hepatosplenomegaly
Mucolipidosis 1	Sialidase (neuraminidase)	Hepatosplenomegaly

The *basic defect* is an abnormal β chain in β-hexosaminidase that affects both the A and B isoenzymes. *Diagnosis* of Sandhoff disease is achieved by demonstrating a total deficiency of β-hexosaminidase on assay of plasma white blood cells or cultured fibroblasts.

Genetics. The β chain for β hexosaminidase (Hex B) gene has been localized to chromosome 5 (5q11). Several mutations have been identified that can be correlated with the clinical severity of the disease.

NIEMANN-PICK DISEASE (Type A). This is an autosomal recessive disorder of sphingomyelin and cholesterol storage within the lysosomes. Niemann-Pick disease is found more frequently among Jewish individuals of Ashkenazi descent.

Etiology. There are increased levels of sphingomyelin and cholesterol in bone marrow cells, liver, spleen, and brain. The enzyme defect is sphingomyelinase deficiency (see Figs. 72–6 and 72–7). Failure to cleave phosphocholine from sphingomyelin results in the storage of sphingomyelin. Storage of cholesterol is not well understood, but there seems to be a close relationship between the metabolism of sphingomyelin and that of cholesterol.

Clinical Manifestations. These begin at 3–4 mo of age with feeding difficulties and failure to thrive. Neurologic deterioration may not be overt because these children are able to sit, stand, and learn other skills, although their development is globally delayed. Physical examination is characterized by hepatosplenomegaly. The liver may be enlarged earlier than the spleen. Bone marrow aspirates show characteristic foam cells containing sphingomyelin and cholesterol. As the disease progresses, children with Niemann-Pick disease begin to look more severely malnourished and have protruding abdomens. Mental retardation becomes more pronounced as new skills are not achieved and existing skills regress. Muscle strength diminishes, and the children become hypotonic. Hearing and vision deteriorate, and blindness occurs in the advanced stages of the disease. Hypoacusis is present. A cherry-red spot on the macula is seen in 50% of cases. Death occurs before the 4th yr of life.

Major bony abnormalities are not associated with Niemann-Pick disease, although some widening of the medullary cavity and thinning of the cortex are observed. CT scan and MRI of the brain show gray matter degeneration, demyelination, and cerebellar atrophy.

Late-onset variants of Niemann-Pick disease are associated with dystonic movements, athetosis, and seizures. Hepatosplenomegaly and sphingomyelinase deficiency are diagnostic.

Diagnosis. Hepatosplenomegaly, mental retardation, foam cells in bone marrow or peripheral blood smears, and a cherry-red spot suggest the diagnosis. Sphingomyelinase deficiency in white blood cells, cultured skin fibroblasts, or other tissues is diagnostic. Carrier detection and prenatal diagnosis are available using a sphingomyelinase assay.

Genetics. The gene for sphingomyelinase has been localized to the short arm of chromosome 11 (11p15) and several mutations have been identified that cause sphingomyelinase deficiency.

Treatment. There is no therapy.

Niemann-Pick Disease (Type B). This is a benign form of sphingomyelinase deficiency that is associated with hepatosplenomegaly and the presence of foam cells in the bone marrow but minor or no neurologic involvement. This disease has an autosomal recessive mode of inheritance but is not associated with any particular ethnic group. It is compatible with a normal life span.

Niemann-Pick Disease (Types C and D). These two autosomal recessive disorders are the same disease with different severity. They *are not caused by sphingomyelinase deficiency,* although the enzyme activity may be reduced. Hepatosplenomegaly exists and foam cells are present in the bone marrow. There are several forms of Niemann-Pick type C. The neonatal form of the disease can be associated with jaundice and hepatosplenomegaly. More commonly type C is associated with normal development until the age of 2–3 yr, when extrapyramidal symptoms develop, with vertical gaze disturbance. Type D is similar to type C but is found more frequently in Nova Scotia. The enzyme defect in these disorders is not known but is related to cholesterol rather than sphingomyelin metabolism.

The *diagnosis* of Niemann Pick type C should be suggested by the triad of gaze paresis, hepatosplenomegaly, and foam cells in the bone marrow. The diagnosis should be confirmed by increased cholesterol in cultured fibroblasts and decreased cholesterol ester synthesis when fibroblasts are incubated with low density lipoprotein (LDL).

GAUCHER DISEASE. In this disorder glucosylceramide (glucocerebroside) is stored in the reticuloendothelial system. The classic form of Gaucher disease, sometimes referred to as the chronic or adult form, is common among Ashkenazi Jews and does not involve the central nervous system. There is an infantile form that is neuropathic and also a juvenile form that is associated with late-onset neurologic deterioration.

Etiology. The enzyme defect is deficiency of beta-glucosidase. Enzyme determination can be performed on white blood cells or cultured skin fibroblasts.

Clinical Manifestations. The chronic form of Gaucher disease is characterized by reticuloendothelial system involvement resulting in splenomegaly. Splenomegaly is usually the first clinical sign of Gaucher disease, but symptoms of hypersplenism and bone marrow failure may occur as early as birth and as late as 80 yr of age. Splenomegaly can be striking, and the spleen may occupy a major portion of the abdomen. In the Ashkenazi Jewish population Gaucher disease may not be identified until the 2nd or 3rd decade of life. The storage of glucocerebroside in the spleen and bone marrow leads to anemia, leukopenia, and thrombocytopenia. In rare cases, thrombocytopenia leads to bleeding. Involvement of the liver is minimal, although moderate hepatomegaly may be encountered. Bone marrow aspirates and cells from the spleen show the characteristic Gaucher cells engorged with glucocerebroside (Fig. 72–8). Radiologic changes include the Erlenmeyer flask shape of the long bones, especially the distal femora.

Diagnosis. Splenomegaly with mild anemia that is unexplained should lead to suspicion of Gaucher disease. Bone marrow aspirates showing Gaucher cells strengthen the suspicion. Gaucher disease is confirmed by the demonstration of a deficiency of β-glucosidase.

Genetics. Gaucher disease is inherited as an autosomal recessive disease. It is very common among Ashkenazi Jews, with a frequency as high as 1 in 500 births, which exceeds the frequency of Tay-Sachs disease. Carrier testing and prenatal

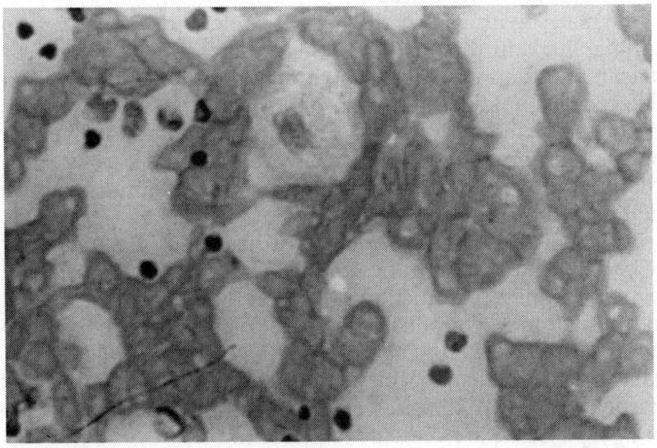

Figure 72–8. Cells from a spleen of a patient with Gaucher disease. A characteristic spleen cell is shown engorged with glucocerebroside.

diagnosis are possible. The gene for glucocerebrosidase has been cloned and localized to chromosome 1 (1q21–q31). The mutation commonly found in the mild form of Gaucher disease is in position 1226, a substitution of A to G. Another common mutation in position 1448 is an insertion of a second guanine in position 84 of the cDNA, referred to as 84GG. The 1226 and the 1448 or 84GG mutations account for 95% of the mutations found in Jewish people. There have been a variety of other mutations described for type II Gaucher and the late-onset form.

Treatment. Splenectomy, which used to be the treatment for Gaucher disease, is now rarely used. Enzyme replacement therapy is the treatment of choice. Glucocerebrosidase isolated from human placenta (Ceredase) or genetically engineered enzyme (Cerezyme) are available. These enzymes are targeted for the lysosomes. The more commonly used therapy is 15–60 units of enzyme per kilogram per 4 wk. The dose is divided and given intravenously every 2 wk. This treatment reduces the size of the spleen dramatically, improves the blood count, and reverses bony changes. Another regimen uses much less enzyme, 1–3 units per kilogram per 4 wk. The dose is divided and given three times weekly. Allergic reactions may occur and patients should be monitored; these are usually not serious.

Ceredase or Cerezyme has not been successful in treating infantile or juvenile Gaucher disease.

Infantile Gaucher Disease. This form of the disease involves the central nervous system. The disease may present with splenomegaly, strabismus, trismus, and dorsiflexion of the head. Seizures are common, and such children usually die around 3–4 yr of age. The diagnosis is made by demonstrating a deficiency of glucocerebrosidase in the tissues.

Juvenile Gaucher Disease. This form of disease has variable age of onset, with neurologic signs occurring in the 1st or 2nd decade of life. Neurologic symptoms include ataxia, peripheral neuropathy, myoclonus, ophthalmoplegia, and dementia. The diagnosis is made by documenting a deficiency of glucocerebrosidase (β-glucosidase). This autosomal recessive disorder is panethnic in distribution.

FABRY DISEASE. This X-linked recessive sphingolipid storage disease results from a deficiency of the enzyme α-galactosidase. Glycosphingolipid with two and three sugar residues with α-galactosyl at the terminal end is deposited and cannot be degraded (see Fig. 72–7).

Clinical Manifestations. Symptoms usually occur in adolescent males and include pain crises of the extremities caused by deposition of sphingolipids in the vascular endothelium supplying the peripheral nerves. Skin eruptions around the naval and over the buttocks and angiokeratomas (tiny dark purple-blue telangiectasias) are characteristic of Fabry disease. Hypohydrosis and corneal lenticular opacities may also be seen early in the course of the disease.

As males with Fabry disease get older, the deposition of sphingolipids in the vascular system increases, leading to cardiac manifestations such as mitral insufficiency, conduction defects, ischemic heart attacks, and thromboses. Fabry disease is not associated with mental retardation. Kidney involvement begins with proteinuria and ends with kidney failure. Corneal changes are the most frequent complication found in female heterozygotes.

Diagnosis. Fabry disease should be considered in a male with pain crises of the extremities, angiokeratomas, proteinuria, and signs of kidney malfunction. A kidney biopsy will show lipid accumulation in epithelial and endothelial cells of the glomeruli and tubules. Confirmation is achieved by documenting α-galactosidase deficiency in white blood cells or cultured skin fibroblasts. Enzymatic tests in females at risk of being carriers of Fabry disease are difficult to perform.

GENETICS. Fabry disease is X-linked. The gene for α-galactosidase has been cloned, and mutations leading to α-galactosidase deficiency have been identified.

Treatment. Pain crises should be treated symptomatically. Renal failure may require renal transplantation.

SCHINDLER DISEASE (α-*N*-Acetylgalactosaminidase Deficiency). This is a newly described autosomal recessive neurodegenerative disorder. Glycolipid with α-*N*-acetylgalactosamine accumulates in brain throughout the cortex, leading to axonal degeneration; other tissues may also contain this lipid. The enzyme defect is α-*N*-acetylgalactosaminidase deficiency, a lysosomal enzyme. This disease should not be confused with α-*N*-acetylglucosaminidase deficiency (Sanfilippo syndrome type B).

These children appear normal until about 1 yr of age. Developmental regression starts in the 2nd yr of life, followed by cortical blindness, myoclonic seizures, spasticity, decerebrate regidity, and profound retardation. Demonstration of α-*N*-acetylgalactosaminidase deficiency in white blood cells or cultured skin fibroblasts confirms the diagnosis.

GENETICS. The disease is inherited as an autosomal recessive trait. The gene of α-*N*-acetylgalactosaminidase has been cloned and mapped to chromosome 22 (22q13-qter).

METACHROMATIC LEUKODYSTROPHY (MLD). This autosomal recessive disorder is caused by a deficiency of arylsulfatase A, which is required for the hydrolysis of sulfated glycosphingolipid. Therefore, sulfatide is stored within lysosomes, especially those of white matter, since sulfatide is a component of myelin. In the infantile, juvenile, and adult forms, the enzyme is defective; however, in the disease form in which the activator protein (SAP-1) is defective, arylsulfatase A is intact, but sulfatide nevertheless cannot be cleaved.

Clinical Manifestations. Metachromatic leukodystrophy represents a spectrum of clinical severity and has variable ages of onset. The *late infantile* form of MLD is the most severe and also the most common. It usually becomes manifest between 12 and 18 mo of life with irritability, inability to walk, and hyperextension of the knee causing genu recurvatum. Deep tendon reflexes are diminished or absent. Muscle wasting, weakness, and hypotonia become gradually evident, and these children eventually become bedridden. Nystagmus, myoclonic seizures, optic atrophy, and quadriparesis are features of the end stage of the disease. Patients with the *late infantile form* usually die in the 1st decade of life. The *juvenile form* of MLD has a slower course, and its onset may occur as late as 20 yr of age. The disease presents with ataxia, mental deterioration, and emotional difficulties. The *adult form* is similar to the juvenile form in its clinical manifestations except that emotional difficulties and psychosis are more prominent and the age of onset is usually after the 2nd or 3rd decade of life. Dementia, seizures, diminished reflexes, and optic atrophy are features of the juvenile and adult forms of MLD. An additional form of MLD is caused by a *deficiency of a sphingolipid activator protein* (SAP-1), a protein required for the formation of substrate-enzyme complex. In this disorder arylsulfatase activity is normal when assayed in the test tube, so an assay for the activator protein is required for the diagnosis.

Pathophysiologic and Pathologic Findings. The undegraded sulfatide is stored primarily in white matter. Therefore, no visceral or bone marrow involvement is encountered. White matter from the brain of patients with MLD undergoes demyelination with deposition of many metachromatic bodies, which stain strongly positive with periodic acid-Schiff (PAS) and Alcian blue. Oligodendroglial cells are markedly reduced in number. Neuronal inclusions are also seen in nerve cells of the midbrain, pons, medulla, retina, and spinal cord, and demyelination occurs in the peripheral nervous system. Biopsies of sural nerve stained with acid cresyl violet show many brown metachromatic deposits containing granules, which accumulate in the perinuclear cytoplasm of Schwann cells and in perivascular histiocytes. All involved areas show a loss of oligodendroglial elements. In patients with MLD excessive amounts of sulfatide are excreted in urine.

Diagnosis. The clinical features of leukodystrophy along with decreased nerve conduction velocities, increased cerebrospinal fluid protein, metachromatic deposits in biopsied segments of sural nerve, and metachromatic granules in urinary sediment suggest MLD. The juvenile and adult forms are more difficult to suspect. In none of the forms of MLD is peripheral storage encountered. Brain CT scan or MRI shows attenuation of white matter. Confirmation of the diagnosis is based on enzymatic studies on leukocytes or on cultured skin fibroblasts, indicating a deficiency of arylsulfatase A activity. Enzymatic studies do not differentiate the various forms of MLD. Measurement of the ability of cultured fibroblasts to metabolize radioactive sulfatide in the culture medium sometimes is required to establish the diagnosis of MLD.

Sphingolipid activator protein–deficient patients can be diagnosed by measuring the concentration of SAP-1 using specific antibodies to leukocytes and cultured skin fibroblasts. A low level of cross-reacting material is found. Carrier detection and prenatal diagnosis can be attained using the specific enzyme assay of arylsulfatase A or an assay for SAP-1. Some carriers of MLD have arylsulfatase A levels near those found in affected children. Therefore, parents of affected children should be checked for their carrier status before prenatal testing is undertaken to avoid abortion of a nonaffected but low-activity child.

Genetics. All forms of MLD are autosomal recessive. The gene for arylsulfatase A has been cloned and assigned to chromosome 22 (22q13.31-qter), which is in the proximity of the gene in Schindler disease. Various mutations have been identified that can explain the clinical forms of MLD. In general, mutations that result in some residual activity lead to a milder phenotype.

Treatment. There is no treatment for any form of MLD—only supportive care can be given. Attempts have been made to treat young patients with MLD with bone marrow transplantation. Although normal enzyme levels can be achieved in peripheral blood, no clear evidence indicates that the treatment decreases the neurologic deterioration.

Prognosis. Patients with the late infantile form usually live 2–4 yr after diagnosis, and those with the juvenile form live 4–6 yr. Some children with the adult form have lived to the 5th decade.

MULTIPLE SULFATASE DEFICIENCY. This is another autosomal recessive disease with deficiencies of arylsulfatases A, B, and C. Sulfatides, mucopolysaccharides, steroid sulfates, and gangliosides accumulate in the cerebral cortex and visceral tissues. The neurologic picture is similar to that of late infantile MLD, but the bony involvement may suggest a mucopolysaccharidosis. Severe ichthyosis occurs in many patients with multiple sulfatase deficiency. Examination of urine for mucopolysaccharides is positive. The urine also contains excess sulfatides. There is a striking abnormality of granulation in the leukocytes. Carrier testing and prenatal diagnosis can be performed. There is no specific treatment for multiple sulfatase deficiency other than supportive care.

KRABBE DISEASE. Krabbe disease, or globoid cell leukodystrophy, is a progressive cerebral degenerative disease affecting the white matter primarily. There is storage of ceramide galactose within lysosomes, leading to degeneration of the white matter. A high incidence of disease occurs in persons of Scandinavian descent. Inheritance is autosomal recessive. The name *globoid cell* comes from the globular distended multinucleated bodies found in the basal ganglia, pontine nuclei, and cerebellar white matter.

Clinical Manifestations. Onset of Krabbe disease may occur very early in life in the *infantile form,* usually around 3 mo of age. These infants are irritable, develop seizures, and are hypertonic. Optic atrophy is evident in the 1st yr of life, and mental development is severely impaired. As the disease progresses, these infants develop opisthotonos and usually die before 3 yr of age. Patients with the *late infantile form* of Krabbe disease become symptomatic after the 2nd yr of life. The clinical course is similar to that of the infantile form but much slower.

Pathophysiologic and Pathologic Findings. The white matter contains large numbers of globoid histiocytes in areas of demyelination. These cells cluster around blood vessels; they have a lacy, pink cytoplasm (on hematoxylin-eosin stain) and prominent staining of intracellular material on PAS stain. The pathologic abnormalities are almost entirely restricted to the white matter. There may, however, be some damage to the cortical gray matter, but the intense intraneuronal deposition usually observed in other cerebral lipidoses is lacking. Visceral organs are usually not involved because of their paucity of galactosylceramide lipids.

Galactosylceramide accumulation is the result of a deficiency of the lysosomal enzyme that cleaves galactosylceramide. This is a specific β-*galactosidase* referred to as *galactocerebrosidase* or galactosylceramide-β-galactosidase. The deficiency can be documented in leukocytes or cultured skin fibroblasts. As a result of this deficiency, galactosylceramide concentration in the brain of patients with Krabbe disease may be 100 times the normal level.

Diagnosis. Diagnosis of Krabbe disease should be suspected in any patient with white matter disease; attenuation of white matter can be found by MRI or CT scan of the brain. Nerve conduction is reduced, and protein is elevated in the CSF (100–500 mg/dL). Elevation of protein in the cerebrospinal fluid is also found in MLD. A definite diagnosis can be made following the demonstration of galactosylceramide-β-galactosidase deficiency in white blood cells or cultured skin fibroblasts. Carriers have lower than normal levels of galactocerebrosidase activity in white blood cells or cultured skin fibroblasts. Prenatal diagnosis can be performed by measuring this activity in chorionic villi or cultured amniocytes.

Genetics. Krabbe disease is inherited as an autosomal recessive trait. The gene for galactocerebrosidase has been cloned and localized on the long arm of chromosome 14 (14q21-q31). Several mutations have been identified at the gene level that lead to galactocerebrosidase deficiency.

Treatment. There is no specific therapy for Krabbe disease.

BATTEN DISEASE. The neuronal storage diseases in this heterogeneous group are sometimes given different labels based on the age of onset: Spielmeyer-Vogt, Jansky-Bielschowsky, and Kufs or amaurotic familial idiocy. Because the storage material, a fluorescent lipopigment, is referred to as lipofuscin, this group of disorders is sometimes called *lipofuscinosis* (see Chapter 552.2).

Clinical Manifestations. In the early form of Batten disease (*late infantile*) a child may develop normally until the age of 2–5 yr. Onset may begin with visual disturbances, intellectual retardation, ataxic gait, or seizures. Patchy macular degeneration and retinitis pigmentosa are also features, especially in the late-onset forms. The *juvenile form* begins at the end of the 1st decade or in the early teens. Visual disturbances may be the first symptom noted. Handwriting becomes unintelligible, and school performance declines. The *adult form* presents in the 2nd decade of life with signs of ataxia, dementia, and choreoathetosis.

Pathologic and Pathophysiologic Findings. There is loss of neuronal perikarya, and neurons contain granules that stain for ceroid and lipofuscin. The neurons also contain cytoplasmic inclusions that resemble fingerprints called *curvilinear bodies.* These inclusions also are found in circulating lymphocytes. The exact biochemical defect is unknown, although *dolichol,* a long-chain lipid containing repeating units of five carbon groups, is excreted in excessive amounts in the urine of many, but not all, patients with Batten disease.

Diagnosis. Young patients with retinitis pigmentosa or other retinal changes, ataxia, or myoclonic seizures should be suspected of having Batten disease. Increased amounts of dolichol in the urine and curvilinear bodies in lymphocytes are diagnostic. Skin, conjunctival, or rectal biopsy may be needed to show lipofuscin storage. No carrier detection is available for this autosomal recessive trait because no enzyme defect has been identified.

Genetics. Batten disease is an autosomal recessive disorder. The basic defect is unknown. Through linkage analysis in large families, the gene for Batten disease has been localized to the short arm of chromosome 16 (16p12.1). The gene itself has not been identified and its function is still not understood.

Treatment. No treatment is available except control of seizures and symptomatic supportive measures.

FARBER DISEASE. This autosomal recessive disease is a result of lysosomal storage of ceramide in various tissues, especially joints.

Clinical Manifestations. Symptoms can begin as early as in the 1st yr of life with painful joint swelling and nodule formation (Fig. 72–9). Sometimes rheumatoid arthritis is suspected in these patients. As the disease progresses these children fail to thrive. Nodule or granulomatous formation affects the vocal cords and leads to hoarseness and breathing difficulties. Children with Farber disease may die from recurrent pneumonias in their teens.

Pathologic and Pathophysiologic Findings. The nodules over the joints are granulomas made of foam cells containing ceramide, the lipid backbone of glycolipids. The kidneys, liver, lungs, and lymph nodes contain an excess of ceramide ranging from 10- to 60-fold. A deficiency of ceramidase leads to a failure to cleave the amino-linked fatty acid attached to sphingosine.

Diagnosis. The diagnosis should be suspected in patients who have nodule formation over the joints but no findings of rheumatoid arthritis. In such patients ceramidase activity should be assayed in cultured skin fibroblasts or white blood cells. Carrier detection is based upon the finding of a lower than normal ceramidase activity. Prenatal diagnosis depends on the presence of ceramidase levels in cultured chorionic villi or amniocytes.

Genetics. Farber disease is inherited as an autosomal recessive trait. The gene has not been cloned or localized to a chromosome.

Treatment. There is no specific therapy.

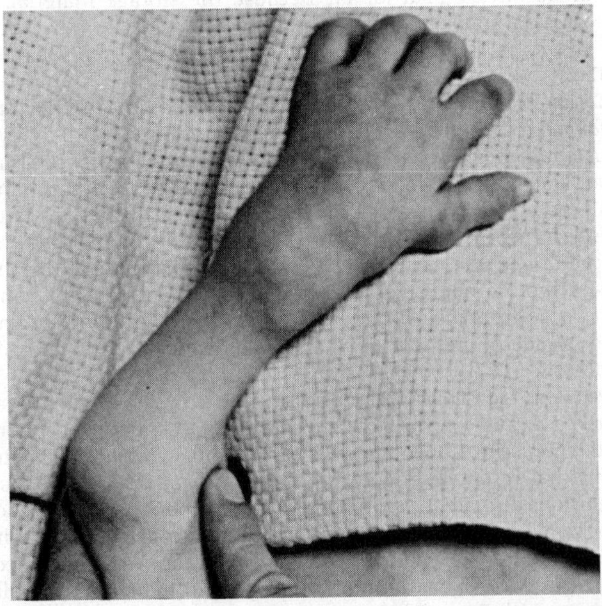

Figure 72–9. A forearm of an 18-mo-old girl with Farber disease. Note the painful joint swelling and the nodule formation. The infant was suspected of having rheumatoid arthritis.

WOLMAN DISEASE. This autosomal recessive lysosomal storage disease of cholesteryl esters is caused by a deficiency of a lysosomal lipase, *acid lipase.* Cholesterol and cholesteryl esters are stored in histiocytic foam cells of visceral organs. The disease is associated with failure to thrive, relentless vomiting, abdominal distention, and hepatosplenomegaly. Calcification of the adrenals is pathognomonic. Usually the disease occurs in the first few weeks of life, and death occurs within 6 mo owing to cachexia and peripheral edema. Diagnosis and carrier identification are based on measuring decreased acid lipase activity in white blood cells or cultured skin fibroblasts. Prenatal diagnosis depends on measuring decreased enzyme levels in cultured chorionic villi or amniocytes. There is a milder form of this acid lipase cholesteryl storage disease that is compatible with long life. The *gene* for lysosomal acid lipase has been cloned and mapped to chromosome 10 (10q23.2-q23.3). Several mutations cause Wolman disease. There is no specific treatment for Wolman disease.

FUCOSIDOSIS. This is an autosomal recessive lysosomal storage disease of fucose-containing glycosphingolipids and glycoproteins.

Pathologic and Pathophysiologic Findings. Lysosomal storage material is found in the liver, brain, and other organs. The hepatocytes and Kupffer cells contain multilamellar structures rich in glycosphingolipid and glycoprotein. The cells in the central nervous system also store this material, and as the disease progresses the features of leukodystrophy become more evident. α-Fucosidase, the enzyme that is deficient in fucosidosis, can be measured in white blood cells, plasma, and cultured skin fibroblasts.

Clinical Manifestations. Children have psychomotor retardation, seizures, hepatosplenomegaly, frontal bossing, coarse facial features, and macroglossia reminiscent of the mucopolysaccharidoses. As they grow older these children develop contractures of the joints and lumbar kyphosis. A *juvenile form* is associated with milder mental involvement and skin lesions over the abdomen and angiokeratomas, similar to those seen in Fabry disease. Fucosidosis is associated with roentgenographic findings of dysostosis multiplex. An MRI or CT scan of the head may suggest the existence of white matter degeneration. Although the radiologic findings of fucosidosis are similar to those of the mucopolysaccharidoses, an enzymatic determination is required to differentiate the former from the latter.

Diagnosis. Visceral storage disease is suggested by hepatosplenomegaly, coarse facial features, and frontal bossing. Urine does not contain mucopolysaccharides but does contain fucose-rich oligosaccharides. In the infantile form, sweat chloride levels are elevated. The diagnosis is confirmed by the demonstration of α-fucosidase deficiency in white blood cells or cultured skin fibroblasts. Carrier detection and prenatal diagnosis can be achieved by performing assays for α-fucosidase. Some ethnic groups, such as Italians and Spanish-Americans, have a high incidence of fucosidosis.

Genetics. Fucosidosis is an autosomal recessive disease. The gene for α-fucosidase has been isolated and localized on the short arm of chromosome 1 (1p34-p36). Several mutations lead to fucosidosis.

Treatment. There is no specific therapy.

Barranger JA, Ginns EL: Glucosylceramide lipidoses: Gaucher disease. *In:* Scriver CR, Beaudet AL, Sly WS, et al (eds): The Metabolic Basis of Inherited Disease, 6th ed. New York, McGraw Hill, 1989, p 1677.

Barton NW, Brady RO, Dambrosia JM, et al: Replacement therapy for inherited enzyme deficiency: macrophage-targeted glucocerebrosidase for Gaucher disease. N Engl J Med 324:1464, 1991.

Beaudet AL, Thomas GH: Acid lipase deficiency: Wolman disease and cholesteryl ester storage disease. *In:* Scriver CR, Beaudet AL, Sly WS, et al (eds): The Metabolic Basis of Inherited Disease, 6th ed. New York, McGraw Hill, 1989, p 1623.

Beutler E: Modern diagnosis and treatment of Gaucher's disease. Am J Dis Child 147:1175, 1993.

Chen YQ, Rafi MA, de Gala G, Wenger DA: Cloning and expression of cDNA

encoding human galactocerebrosidase, the enzyme deficient in globoid cell leukodystrophy. Hum Mol Genet 2:1841, 1993.
Desnick RJ, Bishop DF: Fabry disease: α-galactosidase deficiency; Schindler disease: α-*N*-acetylgalactosaminidase deficiency. *In:* Scriver CW, Beaudet AL, Sly WS, et al (eds): The Metabolic Basis of Inherited Disease, 6th ed. New York, McGraw Hill, 1989, p 1751.
Fujibayashi S, Inui K, Wenger DA: Activator protein deficient metachromatic leukodystrophy: Diagnosis in leukocytes using immunologic methods. J Pediatr 104:739, 1984.
Johnson WG: The clinical spectrum of hexosaminidase deficiency diseases. Neurology 31:1453, 1981.
Kolodny EH: Metachromatic leukodystrophy and multiple sulfatase deficiency: Sulfatide lipidosis. *In:* Scriver CW, Beaudet AL, Sly WS, et al (eds): The Metabolic Basis of Inherited Disease, 6th ed. New York, McGraw Hill, 1989, p 1721.
Kolodny EH, Ullman MD, Mankin HJ, et al: Phenotypic manifestations of Gaucher disease: Clinical features in 48 biochemically verified type 1 patients and comments on type 2 patients. Progr Clin Biol Res 95:33, 1982.
Matthew SW, Callahan WJ: Sphingomyelin-cholesterol lipidoses: The Niemann-Pick group of diseases. *In:* Scriver CW, Beaudet AL, Sly WS, et al (eds): The Metabolic Basis of Inherited Disease, 6th ed. New York, McGraw Hill, 1989, p 1655.
Moser HW, Moser AB, Winston CW, et al: Ceramidase deficiency: Farber lipogranulomatosis. *In:* Scriver CR, Beaudet AL, Sly WS, et al (eds): The Metabolic Basis of Inherited Disease, 6th ed. New York, McGraw Hill, 1989, p 1645.
Moser HW, Moser AB, Trojak JE, et al: Identification of female carriers of adrenoleukodystrophy. J Pediatr 103:54, 1983.
O'Brien JS: β-Galactosidase deficiency (GM_1 gangliosidosis, galactosialidosis and Morquio syndrome type 8); Ganglioside sialidase deficiency (mucolipidosis IV). *In:* Scriver CW, Beaudet AL, Sly WS, et al (eds): The Metabolic Basis of Inherited Disease, 6th ed. New York, McGraw Hill, 1989, p 1787.
Polten A, Fluharty AL, Fluharty CB, et al: Molecular bases of different forms of metachromatic leukodystrophy. N Engl J Med 324:18, 1991.
Rosenberg RN, Prusiner SB, DiMauro S, Barchi RL, Kunkel LM (eds): The Molecular and Genetic Basis of Neurological Disease. Boston, Butterworth-Heinemann, 1993.
Samuel R, Katz K, Papapoulos SE, et al: Aminohydroxy propylidene bisphosphanate (APD) treatment improves the clinical skeletal manifestations of gaucher disease. Pediatrics 94:385, 1994.
Sandhoff K, Conzelmann E, Neufeld EF, et al: The GM_2 gangliosidoses. *In:* Scriver CW, Beaudet AL, Sly WS, et al (eds): The Metabolic Basis of Inherited Disease, 6th ed. New York, McGraw Hill, 1989, p 1807.
Suzuki K, Suzuki Y: Galactosylceramide lipidosis: Globoid cell leukodystrophy (Krabbe disease). *In:* Scriver CW, Beaudet AL, Sly WS, et al (eds): The Metabolic Basis of Inherited Disease, 6th ed. New York, McGraw Hill, 1989, p 1699.
Zimran A, Gross E, West C, et al: Prediction of Gaucher's disease by identification at DNA level. Lancet 2:349, 1989.
Ziyeh S, Harzer K: Bone marrow cytological storage phenomena in lipidosis. Eur J Pediatr 153:224, 1994.

72.4 Disorders of Lipoprotein Metabolism and Transport

Andrew M. Tershakovec, Paul M. Coates, and Jean A. Cortner

Although some children suffer from well-defined familial hyperlipidemia, the majority of individuals with hyperlipidemia do not have such specific syndromes. In addition, although those with hyperlipidemia are at increased risk for heart disease, not all hyperlipidemic individuals develop clinical heart disease. This chapter addresses the basic elements of cholesterol and triglyceride metabolism and the clinical implications of dyslipidemia in order to define a reasonable approach to the evaluation and treatment of children with altered lipoprotein metabolism.

PLASMA LIPOPROTEIN METABOLISM AND TRANSPORT

Cholesterol and triglycerides are transported in the circulation in macromolecular complexes termed *lipoproteins;* the protein components of the complexes are called *apolipoproteins.* Dietary lipoproteins (chylomicrons) are formed in and secreted by the small intestine; other lipoproteins (e.g., very low density lipoproteins, VLDL) are synthesized in the liver; still others (high density lipoproteins, HDL) are secreted as nascent particles by the liver and small intestine, and only reach their mature form in the circulation after exchange of components with other circulating lipoproteins or with tissues.

TRANSPORT OF EXOGENOUS (DIETARY) LIPIDS (Fig. 72–10). After ingestion of a fat-containing meal and hydrolysis by intestinal and pancreatic lipases, free fatty acids and cholesterol are re-esterified in the intestinal epithelium to form triglycerides and cholesteryl esters, respectively. These lipids are then packaged together with phospholipids, free cholesterol, and at least two apolipoproteins, apoA-I and apoB-48, to form chylomicrons. The chylomicrons are then secreted into the intestinal lymph and pass through the thoracic duct into the peripheral circulation. In the circulation, chylomicrons acquire additional apolipoproteins, mainly apoE and several forms of apoC. Triglycerides, which constitute most of the chylomicron mass, are immediately hydrolyzed by lipoprotein lipase at the capillary endothelium. The free fatty acid products of this hydrolysis are transferred primarily to adipose tissue for storage as triglycerides or to muscle tissue for beta oxidation. The lipoprotein particles, now smaller and more dense because they have lost most of their triglyceride content, are called *chylomicron remnants.* They have retained virtually all of their cholesteryl ester content and have transferred some of their apolipoproteins (apoC and apoA-I) primarily to HDL. They also have become enriched with respect to their apoB-48 and apoE content. These remnants are recognized, bound, and internalized

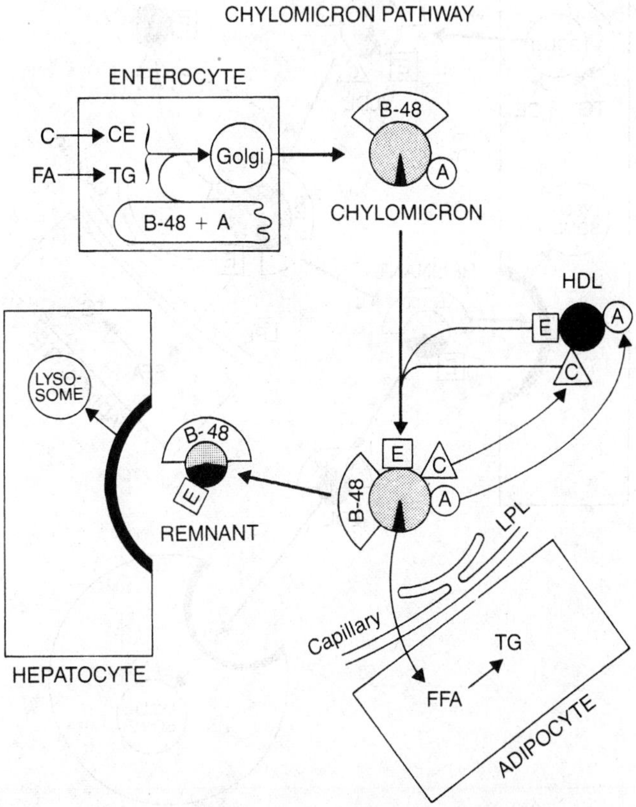

Figure 72–10. Pathway of chylomicron metabolism in human plasma. Fatty acids (FA) and cholesterol (C) are esterified in the intestinal mucosa to form triglycerides (TG) and cholesteryl esters (CE), respectively. They combine with apoA and apoB-48 to form chylomicrons, which are secreted into the circulation: TG *(shaded area)* and CE *(black area)*. Chylomicrons undergo lipolysis in the capillary endothelium near adipose tissue and muscle tissue, losing TG via lipoprotein lipase (LPL), gaining apoE from HDL, and losing apoA and apoC to HDL. The resultant chylomicron remnants are taken up by hepatic apoE receptors for degradation by lysosomes. (Adapted from Havel RJ: Approach to the patient with hyperlipidemia. Med Clin North Am 66:319, 1982.)

in part via hepatic membrane receptors specific for the apoE on the particles. By this mechanism, dietary cholesterol is delivered to the liver, where it plays a role in the regulation of hepatic cholesterol metabolism. Under normal circumstances, chylomicrons and their remnants are very short lived in the circulation; following a 12-hr fast, there are normally no lipoproteins of dietary origin remaining in the plasma.

TRANSPORT OF ENDOGENOUS LIPIDS FROM THE LIVER (Fig. 72–11). The liver secretes a class of lipoproteins called *very low density lipoprotein*, which contain free and esterified cholesterol, triglycerides, phospholipids, and a characteristic set of apolipoproteins, notably apoB-100, apoC, and apoE. Like chylomicrons, VLDL exchange apolipoproteins with other circulating particles and deliver triglycerides to adipose tissue via lipoprotein lipase. In the process, they become smaller and more dense and are termed *VLDL remnants* or intermediate density lipoproteins. Some of these remnant particles are taken up via hepatic cell membrane receptors, while some proportion undergo conversion to low density lipoproteins (LDL); this latter process involves removal of the remaining triglycerides and all apoliproteins except apoB-100 and results in a particle that is almost entirely made up of cholesteryl esters and apoB-100. A specific LDL receptor is present on most cell membranes that recognizes, binds, and internalizes LDL. By this mechanism, LDL particles can deliver cholesterol to extrahepatic tissues to serve their requirements for membrane synthesis; in addition, tissues involved in steroid hormone synthesis can meet their cholesterol needs by receptor-mediated uptake of LDL. LDL particles can circulate in the plasma for several days.

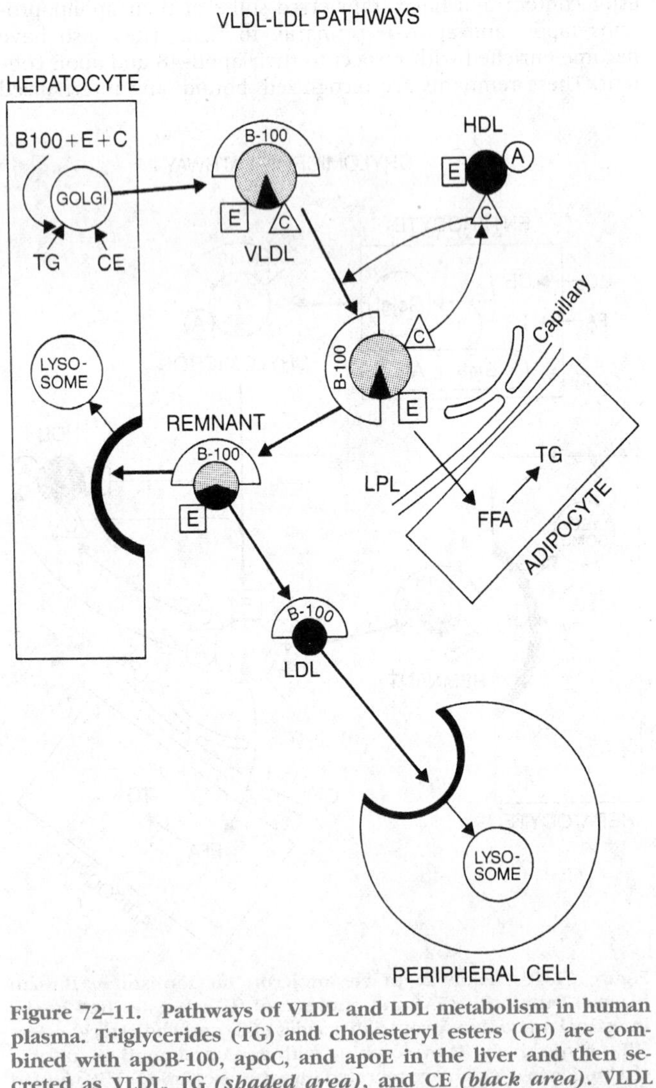

Figure 72–11. Pathways of VLDL and LDL metabolism in human plasma. Triglycerides (TG) and cholesteryl esters (CE) are combined with apoB-100, apoC, and apoE in the liver and then secreted as VLDL, TG *(shaded area)*, and CE *(black area)*. VLDL undergo lipolysis in the capillary endothelium near adipose tissue and muscle tissue, losing TG via lipoprotein lipase (LPL). The resulting VLDL remnants are either converted to low-density lipoproteins (LDL) for transport to peripheral cells via LDL receptor-mediated uptake or are taken up by hepatic receptors. FFA = free fatty acids. (Adapted from Havel RJ: Approach to the patient with hyperlipidemia. Med Clin North Am 66:319, 1982.)

HDL AND REVERSE CHOLESTEROL TRANSPORT. In contrast to chylomicrons and VLDL, which are secreted into the circulation as mature particles, HDL are secreted from the liver and small intestine as nascent discoidal particles composed primarily of phospholipids and proteins. Those secreted by the small intestine are rich in apoA-I and apoA-IV, while those derived from the liver contain predominantly apoA-I, apoA-II, and apoE. The particles accept cholesterol from VLDL and LDL, as well as from tissues; this cholesterol is esterified via the lecithin: cholesterol acyltransferase reaction. Part of the cholesteryl ester is stored in the core of HDL, making it a spherical particle, while part of it is transferred back to VLDL and LDL. Because LDL and remnants of VLDL metabolism can be taken up by the liver, this provides a way for returning tissue-derived cholesterol to the liver (reverse cholesterol transport). HDL itself can also be metabolized by the liver and may provide another vehicle for the return of tissue-derived cholesterol to the liver. The liver can then excrete cholesterol in bile.

PLASMA LIPID AND LIPOPROTEIN LEVELS

NORMAL. Table 72–6 presents normal plasma cholesterol and triglyceride levels from birth through the first 2 decades of life. During the first few months of life, cholesterol levels increase largely because of changes in LDL. Over the next 15–20 yr in both males and females, there is little change in the total cholesterol level; the mean value fluctuates around 150–165 mg/dL. Mean LDL cholesterol levels remain slightly under 100 mg/dL in both males and females during this period. HDL cholesterol levels are comparable in males and females early in life; they remain essentially constant in females but decline markedly in males during the second decade to a level that is maintained through adulthood. Plasma triglyceride levels, on the other hand, tend to rise transiently in both males and females in the first year, fall to a mean of 50–60 mg/dL in the ensuing few years, and then rise to a mean of approximately 75 mg/dL by age 20 yr. In early adulthood, there is a marked rise in plasma cholesterol that is due almost exclusively to an increase in LDL cholesterol. The rate of increase over the next 30 yr is greater in males than in females. When coupled with their lower HDL cholesterol levels and higher triglyceride levels, this puts men at much greater risk than women for atherosclerotic heart disease, at least up to the age of 50–60 yr. Due to the changes in lipid levels with age, it is more appropriate to utilize age- and gender-specific percentile figures when comparing levels between individuals and over long periods of time than it is to consider absolute cholesterol levels.

Cholesterol levels track over time. Thus, children with high cholesterol levels tend to have higher levels as young adults, while those with low levels as children will tend to have lower levels as adults. However, tracking is not perfect. A significant degree of biologic and laboratory variation in cholesterol measurements contributes to this. Lifestyle changes of participants (i.e., weight loss, changes in diet) in longitudinal surveys of cholesterol levels in children and young adults may also have contributed to the lower observed degree of tracking. Recent surveys in adults have described a decline in the prevalence of hypercholesterolemia, presumably related to a decreasing intake of fat in the diet. Assuming similar diet trends in children, a similar shift in the distribution of cholesterol levels may be occurring among children.

■ TABLE 72–6 Plasma Cholesterol and Triglyceride Levels in Childhood and Adolescence: Means and Percentiles

	Total Triglyceride (mg/dL)					Total Cholesterol (mg/dL)					LDL Cholesterol (mg/dL)					HDL Cholesterol (mg/dL)*				
	5th	*Mean*	*75th*	*90th*	*95th*	*5th*	*Mean*	*75th*	*90th*	*95th*	*5th*	*Mean*	*75th*	*90th*	*95th*	*5th*	*10th*	*25th*	*Mean*	*95th*
Cord	14	34	—	—	84	42	68	—	—	103	17	29	—	—	50	13	—	—	35	60
1–4 yr																				
Male	29	56	68	85	99	114	155	170	190	203	—	—	—	—	—	—	—	—	—	—
Female	34	64	74	95	112	112	156	173	188	200	—	—	—	—	—	—	—	—	—	—
5–9 yr																				
Male	28	52	58	70	85	125	155	168	183	189	63	93	103	117	129	38	42	49	56	74
Female	32	64	74	103	126	131	164	176	190	197	68	100	115	125	140	36	38	47	53	73
10–14 yr																				
Male	33	63	74	94	111	124	160	173	188	202	64	97	109	122	132	37	40	46	55	74
Female	39	72	85	104	120	125	160	171	191	205	68	97	110	126	136	37	40	45	52	70
15–19 yr																				
Male	38	78	88	125	143	118	153	168	183	191	62	94	109	123	130	30	34	39	46	63
Female	36	73	85	112	126	118	159	176	198	207	59	96	111	129	137	35	38	43	52	74

**Note that different percentiles are listed for HDL cholesterol.*

Data for cord blood from Strong W: Atherosclerosis: Its pediatric roots. In: *Kaplan N, Stamler J (eds): Prevention of Coronary Heart Disease. Philadelphia, WB Saunders, 1983. Data for children 1–4 yr from Tables 6, 7, 20, and 21, and all other data from Tables 24, 25, 32, 33, 36, and 37 in Lipid Research Clinics Population Studies Data Book, Vol. 1, The prevalence study. NIH Publication No. 80–1527. Washington, DC, National Institutes of Health, 1980.*

SECONDARY HYPERLIPIDEMIA. Much of the hypertriglyceridemia and, to a smaller extent, hypercholesterolemia seen in clinical practice is secondary to exogenous factors or underlying clinical disorders. Obesity, for example, is probably the major cause of mild elevations of plasma triglycerides, and the hypertriglyceridemia is frequently normalized following a return to desirable weight. Weight loss may also reduce cholesterol levels in the overweight.

Pediatric conditions associated with hyperlipidemia include hypothyroidism, nephrotic syndrome, renal failure, storage diseases (e.g., glycogen storage disease, Tay-Sachs disease, Niemann-Pick disease), diabetes mellitus, and occasionally other endocrine and metabolic disorders, such as congenital biliary atresia, other causes of cholestasis, hepatitis, anorexia nervosa, and systemic lupus erythematosus. Excessive alcohol intake is a well-known cause of hypertriglyceridemia in adults and should be considered in teenagers. Oral contraceptives generally increase triglyceride levels, with varying effects on LDL and HDL cholesterol levels. Other drugs that raise triglyceride levels are 13-*cis*-retinoic acid (isotretinoin or Accutane), thiazide diuretics, and some β-adrenergic blocking agents.

Treatment of the underlying condition or removal of the offending drug is usually the first approach to management of the patient with secondary hyperlipidemia. If the elevated lipid level persists, however, consideration must be given to the possibility that the patient has an underlying primary form of hyperlipoproteinemia, and therapy appropriate to that condition should be initiated.

ASSESSMENT AND TREATMENT OF PRIMARY HYPERCHOLESTEROLEMIA

RISK OF ELEVATED CHOLESTEROL LEVELS. A number of studies have described the association between fat intake and cholesterol levels and coronary heart disease mortality. In 1984, the Lipid Research Clinics Coronary Primary Prevention Trial showed that for every 1% drop in plasma cholesterol obtained by cholestyramine therapy in adult males, there was a 2% reduction in the incidence of myocardial infarction.

Several observations have suggested that adult cardiovascular disease has its roots in children and young adults. American casualties in the Korean and Vietnam wars were found to have a significant prevalence of atherosclerosis, despite their young age. The strongest data linking factors in childhood with adult coronary heart disease come from the Bogalusa Heart Study and the Pathobiological Determinants of Atherosclerosis in Youth Research Group. These surveys have found significant correlations between early atherosclerotic changes, identified at autopsy of children and young adults, and both total and LDL cholesterol levels.

Thus, although there are no data directly linking cholesterol levels in children with adult heart disease, most of the evidence suggests that such an association exists. These and other studies suggest that children at risk for developing premature atherosclerosis in adulthood, because they have inherited one or more genes for hypercholesterolemia, should be identified early in life in order to try to reduce the associated risk of premature heart disease. They also suggest the need to intervene to lower even moderately raised cholesterol levels. There is now a consensus that children with cholesterol levels above the 75th percentile should be considered hypercholesterolemic and at risk for adult heart disease. Hypertriglyceridemia, although generally considered to be a lesser risk factor than hypercholesterolemia, is also known to be associated with the early development of atherosclerosis in some individuals.

Children may have moderately raised cholesterol levels for a variety of reasons. Some primary genetic defects (e.g., familial combined hyperlipidemia and hyperapobetalipoproteinemia) may be associated with only mild elevations of cholesterol. In addition, common polymorphic variants of apoE and apoB are known to be associated with moderate elevations of plasma LDL cholesterol. Furthermore, there are secondary causes of hyperlipoproteinemia (e.g., other disease states) that need to be considered. Finally, inappropriate dietary habits, by themselves or by interacting with any of the above, can contribute to moderately raised cholesterol levels.

SCREENING FOR HYPERCHOLESTEROLEMIA. The Expert Panel on Blood Cholesterol Levels in Children and Adolescents of the National Cholesterol Education Program has recommended that children with a parental history of elevated total cholesterol levels (>240 mg/dL) should have their total cholesterol level measured. Children with incomplete or unavailable family histories, or those with other risk factors for coronary heart disease, should be screened at the discretion of the pediatric care provider.

Children with total cholesterol levels below 170 mg/dL require no intervention other than that recommended for the general population, and should be re-evaluated in 5 yr. Those children whose total cholesterol level is above 200 mg/dL should have a lipid profile performed (total and HDL cholesterol, triglycerides, calculated LDL cholesterol; see later). Those with borderline levels (170–199 mg/dL) should have another total cholesterol measurement, and the two values should be averaged; if the average total cholesterol level in these two determinations is >170 mg/dL, then a lipid profile is recommended. The expert panel has likewise recommended that children with a family history of premature coronary heart disease (before the age of 55 in a parent or grandparent) should have a lipid profile completed. Lipid profiles of parents and other first-degree relatives will be necessary to establish whether there is a dominantly inherited defect responsible for the hypercholesterolemia.

A *lipid profile* is obtained after a 24-hr fast. LDL cholesterol can be calculated using the following equation: LDL cholesterol = total cholesterol − [HDL cholesterol + (total triglycerides/5)]. Triglycerides must be less than 400 mg/dL to derive an accurate estimate of LDL cholesterol with this method. The average value from two evaluations is recommended due to the biologic and laboratory variability in lipid values. Children with average LDL cholesterol levels >130 mg/dL are considered to have elevated levels, while LDL cholesterol levels <110 mg/dL are considered acceptable. Levels between 110 and 130 mg/dL are borderline.

These recommendations have been criticized for several reasons. The screening algorithm is complicated to follow for the busy practitioner. Multiple surveys have shown that screening only those with a positive family history will miss half or more of the hypercholesterolemic children. This problem is compounded by the fact that many adults do not know their cholesterol levels, as well as the difficulties in obtaining a complete family history. In addition, many parents who may be at risk for coronary heart disease are too young to have developed clinical heart disease while their children are being evaluated; hence their children may not be identified as being at risk.

Those children with triglyceride levels above the 95th percentile also should be further scrutinized. Although elevated triglyceride levels per se do not represent an independent risk factor for premature cardiovascular disease, levels above the 95th percentile can be a marker for some patients with genetic forms of hyperlipidemia, even with a normal total cholesterol level.

DIETARY MANAGEMENT OF HYPERLIPIDEMIA. For hyperlipidemic children (average LDL cholesterol >110 mg/dL) over the age of 2 yr, dietary modification is the best initial intervention. Their daily food intake should provide 30% of total calories as fat (approximately equally distributed among saturated, monounsaturated, and polyunsaturated fats), and no more than 100 mg cholesterol per 1,000 calories (maximum 300 mg/24 hr) in such a modification program. This has become commonly referred to as the prudent, or Step I, diet. It is recommended that this diet be adopted by all family members above the age of 2 yr in order to encourage optimal compliance and health promotion.

The minimum goal for dietary intervention is to achieve an LDL cholesterol level <130 mg/dL, while the ideal goal is to lower it to <110 mg/dL. If these goals are not reached even after reinforcing the Step I diet, the Step II diet (<7% calories as saturated fat and <66 mg cholesterol/1,000 calories to a maximum of 200 mg/24 hr) should be considered.

When recommending dietary intervention, it is important to explain that the response to dietary management is variable and generally does not lower LDL cholesterol levels by more than 10–15%. People commonly have unrealistic expectations about the cholesterol lowering associated with dietary management, which limits their compliance when the response is modest. Even if the initial response to dietary therapy is limited, the potential for adopting a lifelong healthy style of eating should have long-term benefit.

Dietary modification is safe in the treatment of hyperlipidemia in adults. Several investigators have demonstrated similar effectiveness and safety in children over the age of 2 yr. The results of a large multicenter trial confirming the safety and efficacy of such a program are pending. It must be emphasized that these recommendations are only meant for children over the age of 2 yr. Children under this age placed on a similar or more restrictive diet, and older children placed on more restrictive diets by well-meaning caregivers, have demonstrated poor growth. Children under 2 yr require a relatively large amount of calories to maintain their rapid growth. Due to the higher caloric density of high fat food, it is physically difficult for children less than 2 yr to eat enough low-fat food to ensure normal growth. Furthermore, the higher fat intake may be necessary to help ensure an adequate supply of appropriate nutrients for the rapidly developing central nervous system. There should be proper supervision to ensure the appropriateness of any dietary modification in children. As most pediatricians are unable to provide detailed guidance for such dietary modifications, referral to a trained pediatric dietician is usually indicated. Prior to undertaking a screening program, the physician should assure the availability of such referral for his or her patients. The growth and development of any child undergoing dietary intervention should be monitored and a specific dietary evaluation completed if growth or development is altered. It is also important to explain to the child and family that hypercholesterolemia in childhood is only a risk factor and not an illness and to emphasize the positive changes the child and the family can make to minimize the risk.

OTHER DIETARY FACTORS. Dietary fiber, especially soluble fiber, has a modest cholesterol-lowering effect in hypercholesterolemic individuals. However, high-fiber diets must be used with care in children to ensure adequate delivery of calories and nutrients.

Monounsaturated fats lower LDL cholesterol levels while maintaining or even raising HDL cholesterol levels, in contrast to the lowering of LDL and HDL cholesterol levels commonly observed with a high polyunsaturated fat diet. *Trans*-fatty acids (partially hydrogenated vegetable oils), commonly found in processed foods and margarine, seem to raise LDL cholesterol levels.

Vegetarian diets have a large and significant cholesterol-lowering effect associated with the substitution of vegetable protein for animal protein and the low fat and cholesterol content of the diet. Though many vegetarian groups have demonstrated the safety of vegetarian diets for children, care must be taken to ensure the completeness of the diet for the growing child.

Although fish oil and antioxidants have little if any effect on cholesterol levels, they have been reported to reduce the risk of coronary heart disease by other mechanisms. However, as these compounds are frequently administered in pharmacologic doses, in the absence of additional experience their use in children should be discouraged. Encouraging appropriate fruit and vegetable intake will help optimize natural sources of antioxidants.

DRUG THERAPY. The expert panel recommended that drug therapy be considered in children aged 10 yr and older if, after an adequate trial of diet therapy (6 mo to 1 yr), LDL cholesterol remains above the following levels:

1. Consider drug therapy if LDL cholesterol remains ≥190 mg/dL.
2. Consider drug therapy if LDL cholesterol remains ≥160 mg/dL and
   (a) There is a positive family history of premature coronary heart disease (before 55 yr of age), or
   (b) Two or more other risk factors are present in the child or adolescent after vigorous attempts have been made to control these risk factors (diabetes, hypertension, smoking, low HDL cholesterol, severe obesity, physical inactivity).

Whenever drug therapy is prescribed, diet therapy should be continued to make the treatment regimen as effective as possible. For details of pharmacologic management, see the section on familial hypercholesterolemia (as follows).

OTHER FACTORS. Medical management of hypercholesterolemia should be viewed in the context of other lifestyle factors and conditions associated with risk for premature coronary heart disease, such as lack of exercise, cigarette smoking, hypertension, obesity, and diabetes. These should be evaluated, controlled, minimized, or eliminated as possible and appropriate. Persons already having one risk factor for premature coronary heart disease, hyperlipidemia, should actively strive to minimize any other risk factors. In addition, many of these risk factors are interlinked and, therefore, minimizing one may help to ameliorate others (e.g., increasing exercise may decrease obesity, which helps to lower blood pressure, LDL cholesterol, and triglyceride levels and, potentially, the risk for non-insulin-dependent diabetes mellitus, while also helping raise HDL cholesterol levels).

RISK OF SCREENING AND INTERVENTION. Cholesterol measurements have been shown to be relatively unreliable when undertaken in settings without adequate quality assurance. Thus, screening should only be completed using reliable laboratories and methods in order to avoid inaccurately labeling children as hypercholesterolemic. In addition, the psychosocial influence of screening must be also considered. Identifying children as having sickle cell trait, alpha-1 anti-trypsin deficiency, benign heart murmurs, or hypertension has been found to have a negative psychosocial impact. The potential for a similar effect exists in identifying children as hypercholesterolemic. However, in one cholesterol screening program, the parents of hypercholesterolemic children reported better diets and improved perceptions of the children's health 1 yr after cholesterol screening was completed. This may be an effect of the families' active participation in reducing risk and improving health.

Of some concern are the reports in adults linking low or lowered cholesterol levels with depression, violent tendencies, accidents, and noncardiac illnesses, including some forms of cancer. These reports do not consistently demonstrate the same associations, and other surveys present conflicting data (e.g., those reporting an association between high-fat diets and some forms of cancer). In addition, many of the cholesterol-lowering interventions use diet and/or drugs, and thus negative consequences may be related to the medication. Finally, data from other countries, in which mean cholesterol levels are lower than those in the United States, do not support higher mortality from noncardiac causes. Thus, no clear consensus can be reached from these surveys. However, these issues must continue to be monitored in all age groups and especially in children.

GENETIC DYSLIPIDEMIAS*

One third of patients who have suffered their first myocardial infarction before the age of 50 yr in men and 60 yr in women have hyperlipoproteinemia, and about one half of these are due to a dominantly inherited disorder of lipoprotein metabolism. During a recent 2 yr period at the Lipid-Heart Research Center of The Children's Hospital of Philadelphia, the diagnosis of a dominantly inherited disorder of lipoprotein metabolism was made in 75% of referrals; 21% had familial hypercholesterolemia (FH), 67% familial combined hyperlipidemia (FCHL), 11% hyperapobetalipoproteinemia, and 1% familial hypertriglyceridemia (FHTG).

Familial Hypercholesterolemia (FH)

HETEROZYGOUS FH. This dominantly inherited disease affecting lipoprotein metabolism (and hence plasma lipid levels) occurs with a frequency of at least 1 in 500 in the general population and until recently has been the most common form of inherited hyperlipidemia recognized in childhood. FH results from defects in the LDL receptor, and more than 40 separate allelic mutations in the gene for the LDL receptor, which has been mapped to chromosome 19, have been demonstrated. There are five classes of mutations (null, transport defective, binding defective, internalization defective, and recycling defective) that impair the receptor-mediated uptake of LDL from the circulation (see Fig. 72–11). Most patients with FH are heterozygous for one of these alleles, causing them to produce approximately half normal and half defective receptors, which results in marked elevation of the plasma LDL cholesterol level from birth.

Clinical manifestations of FH, the most important of which is premature coronary atherosclerosis, do not typically develop until the 3rd or 4th decade. The peak incidence of myocardial infarction in affected men is in the 4th–5th decades; by age 60, 85% have suffered a myocardial infarction. In women, the mean age of onset is about 10 yr later. Most adult patients present with a strong family history of premature coronary heart disease and have tendon xanthomas (nodular swellings involving the Achilles and other tendons due to cholesteryl ester deposition in macrophages), as well as deposits in the soft tissues around the eyelid (xanthelasmas) and in the cornea (arcus corneae). These signs are rarely present in pediatric patients with heterozygous FH, except for tendon xanthomas, which are the initial clinical presentation in 10–15% of affected individuals. Therefore, Achilles tendinitis due to xanthomatous deposits in a teenager should suggest the diagnosis of FH because it is very rare in healthy children.

The *diagnosis* of FH is supported by a strong family history of early myocardial infarctions, tendon xanthomas, and total plasma cholesterol levels >300 mg/dL in affected adults. Affected children usually have total cholesterol levels >250 mg/dL, with LDL cholesterol >200 mg/dL.

Treatment by weight control has relatively little impact on the plasma cholesterol level in heterozygous FH. The Step I diet followed by the Step II diet, if needed, is recommended for FH patients and may produce a significant reduction (by as much as 15%) in LDL cholesterol but will rarely return the LDL cholesterol level to normal. Nevertheless, it is important to establish an appropriate diet prior to considering initiating drug therapy. At this point, cholestyramine or colestipol resin is currently recommended to further reduce LDL cholesterol in FH children 10 yr of age or older who continue to have a LDL cholesterol of >160 mg/dL. These nonabsorbable drugs interrupt the enterohepatic cycle through the binding of bile acids in the intestine, enhancing the excretion of cholesterol-containing bile resin complexes in the stool. This has the additional benefit of increasing the number of LDL receptors in the liver, resulting in increased uptake of LDL from the blood and downregulation of cholesterol production by the liver.

One packet or scoop of cholestyramine contains 4 g of active drug. The dose of drug varies with age and with the severity of hypercholesterolemia, ranging from as little as one-half packet or scoop (2 g active drug) twice a day before meals and increasing to two to three packets or scoops twice a day (16–24 g/24 hr). Up to three packets or scoops twice a day (24 g/24 hr) can be well tolerated by some teenagers and may reduce

*Originally, the Fredrickson classification system was used to define hyperlipidemias according to which plasma lipoproteins were elevated. For example, in type I, chylomicrons are increased; type IIa implies elevation of LDL; type IV, elevation of VLDL; type IIb, elevation of both LDL and VLDL; type III, elevation of chylomicron and VLDL remnants; and type V, elevation of VLDL and chylomicrons. These descriptive classifications did not imply specific genetic etiology; furthermore, as knowledge about the molecular basis of specific genetic defects in lipoprotein metabolism has grown, the classification has become much less useful and can contribute to misunderstanding. Therefore, it seems prudent not to continue its use in most cases; however, because it is still quite prevalent in the literature, physicians need to be aware of the classification.

LDL cholesterol by 50–100 mg/dL. Colestipol is available in 5 g packets, all of which is active drug; dosage (in terms of packets or scoops) is similar to that for cholestyramine. In our experience LDL cholesterol was reduced from a mean of 258 ± 35 mg/dL to 190 ± 31 mg/dL in 36 children with FH treated with cholestyramine. Most children tolerate this medication reasonably well for a while; the side effects of constipation and abdominal discomfort usually can be managed effectively. However, we found that 52 of 62 children treated with cholestyramine discontinued the medication after a mean of 21.9 ± 10 mo, 73% of whom complained of its bad taste and texture. Nausea and bloating may also occur. Both drugs may interfere with the absorption of fat-soluble vitamins, suggesting the need for multivitamin supplements. Measurement of a prothrombin time may be indicated after the initial 6 mo period of treatment.

The minimal goal for drug therapy is to achieve an LDL cholesterol level of 130 mg/dL, and <110 mg/dL if possible. If the LDL cholesterol persists above these levels after resin therapy, other drugs should be considered. The practicing pediatrician usually should refer such patients to a lipid center unless he or she has experience with their use. Nicotinic acid is the next drug of choice in adults; however, its side effects (e.g., flushing, gastrointestinal upset, hepatic toxicity) may preclude its effective use in children. Lovastatin and other HMG-CoA reductase inhibitors, which have been successfully used in adults, have not been approved for use in those less than 19 yr of age. Nevertheless, their use in teenage boys with FH and a strong family history of premature coronary heart disease seems to be justified by the risk/benefit ratio, considering what is currently known about their efficacy and safety. They are not indicated for teenage girls at risk of pregnancy because of their unknown potential for teratogenic defects.

HOMOZYGOUS FH. A rare patient (about one per million) with severe FH is either homozygous for one abnormal allele or is a compound heterozygote for two alleles that impair LDL receptor function. They usually have plasma cholesterol levels of 600 mg/dL or higher from birth and have unique planar cutaneous xanthomas over the knees, elbows, and buttocks, which are often evident at birth and always by 6 yr of age. Tendon xanthomas, xanthelasmas, and arcus corneae are virtually always present. Coronary atherosclerosis frequently has its onset before 10 yr of age; most patients die of complications of myocardial infarction before age 30.

Drugs and diet do not have a major impact on the clinical outcome of persons with homozygous FH. Consequently, regular plasmapheresis and aggressive therapies, such as LDL apheresis, ileal bypass surgery and portacaval shunt, have been attempted with some success. Liver transplantation has been successful in several cases and, most recently, ex vivo gene therapy using the patient's hepatocytes transfected with a normal gene for LDL receptors has been tried with promising results.

Familial Defective Apo B-100

This dominantly inherited condition occurs in approximately 1 in 500 people and is associated with moderate to marked elevation of the plasma LDL cholesterol. In some cases, it is clinically instinguishable from FH. As in FH, the high plasma LDL cholesterol level results from defective uptake by LDL receptors; unlike FH, this disorder results from a single missense mutation causing an amino acid substitution in the apoB molecule, which can be identified by molecular genetic techniques. The extent of its expression in childhood has not been fully determined, but some children have been reported with markedly elevated LDL cholesterol levels.

Familial Combined Hyperlipidemia (FCHL)

This familial multiple lipoprotein type of hyperlipoproteinemia is the most frequent inherited disorder of lipoprotein metabolism in adults (1–2 in 100) and is associated with a high risk of myocardial infarction (10% of first episodes). In this dominantly inherited syndrome, approximately one third of the hyperlipidemic family members have hypertriglyceridemia, one third have hypercholesterolemia, and one third have elevations of both cholesterol and triglycerides. The lipid evaluations tend to be modest, often fluctuating between the 90th and 95th percentiles. In addition, the lipoprotein abnormalities can change from time to time in the same affected individual.

This disorder is not usually associated with tendon xanthomas but obesity, hyperinsulinism, and glucose intolerance are frequently found in affected adults. Although adults who inherit this gene(s) will have hyperlipoproteinemia, affected children may not manifest significant hypercholesterolemia and/or hypertriglyceridemia until the 2nd or 3rd decade, presumably due to gradual gene expression. However, in our experience in families with FCHL identified through an affected child, half of the siblings less than 20 yr of age do have hyperlipidemia, compatible with full expression of the gene(s) in those families. We have also observed a correlation between plasma triglyceride level and age and relative weight in affected children, which suggests the gradual expression of hyperlipidemia in some children. Our experience also suggests that at least 0.5% of all children have hyperlipidemia due to FCHL.

Several metabolic defects apparently are associated with the FCHL phenotype. Most commonly, excess hepatic production of VLDL apoB can be demonstrated. In other FCHL families, hyperlipidemia is associated with reduced lipoprotein lipase activity. While a specific genetic defect causing FCHL has not been identified, a variant allele at a locus influencing apoB levels predicts FCHL in a large proportion of families ascertained through affected children; however, the function of this gene is unknown. There is evidence that FCHL is not linked to the apoB structural locus. A restriction fragment length polymorphism near the AI-CIII-AIV gene cluster on chromosome 11 has been reported to be associated with FCHL but has not been confirmed.

The risk of premature heart disease for persons with FCHL is considerable despite the fact that lipid levels in affected individuals may be only moderately elevated. Children in these families, therefore, should be identified and initial *dietary intervention* should be aimed at contolling the hypercholesterolemia and hypertriglyceridemia using the step I or step II diet. We have evaluated the effect of dietary modification in 29 children with FCHL and found a 13.5% reduction in the LDL cholesterol level after dietary modification. Almost all affected children had a reduction of LDL cholesterol levels; however, in only six children did the levels drop to <130 mg/dL and in only one to <110 mg/dL. There were no significant changes in the HDL cholesterol, triglyceride, or apoB levels.

When dietary modification alone does not achieve desired results, *drug therapy* may be recommended. The bile acid sequestrants (cholestyramine and colestipol) have proven efficacy in children with FCHL. We have treated 51 children with FCHL with cholestyramine (8–24 g/24 hr) and obtained reductions in plasma LDL cholesterol from a mean of 207 ± 40 mg/dL to 141 ± 35 mg/dL. HDL cholesterol levels were not significantly changed, but plasma triglyceride levels significantly increased from 81 ± 35 mg/dL to 134 ± 42 mg/dL. Consequently, children who already have elevation of their triglyceride level should be observed carefully for further increases if resin therapy is chosen. Weight loss in the overweight child with FCHL may help lower triglyceride and cholesterol levels. As noted earlier, however, long-term compliance with resin therapy may be poor. If significant elevation of the LDL cholesterol (>160 mg/dL) persists after an adequate trial of the step I diet and resin therapy in the child with FCHL over 10 yr of age, other therapeutic regimens should be considered similar to those described under FH. The general practicing pediatrician should refer these cases to a lipid center for the consultation about therapy.

Hyperapobetalipoproteinemia

In this condition, the plasma apoB level is significantly increased, but the plasma cholesterol and triglyceride levels are within the upper limits of normal. When this occurs in a family with a positive family history of premature coronary heart disease, it may be a variant of FCHL and should be evaluated and managed in a similar fashion. Unfortunately, the measurement of plasma apoB levels is not routinely available and is quite variable among the clinical laboratories that do offer it.

Elevation of Lp(a)

Lp(a) is a large lipoprotein composed of LDL but, in addition to apoB-100, it contains a large glycoprotein called apo(a) which is very similar to plasminogen. The plasma level of Lp(a) is under genetic control and high levels of Lp(a) appear to be a risk factor for coronary heart disease independent of hyperlipidemia.

Familial Dysbetalipoproteinemia

This rare condition, also known as type 3 hyperlipoproteinemia, is characterized by abnormal plasma lipoproteins designated *beta VLDL* or *floating beta lipoproteins.* The presence of planar xanthomas along the palmar creases of the hands (xanthoma striata palmaris) is virtually diagnostic. Other clinical features include tuberoeruptive xanthomas of the trunk, tuberous xanthomas over the elbows and knees, and tendinous xanthomas. Coronary heart disease and peripheral vascular disease are commonly found. The specific genetic abnormality is a mutation that alters the structure of apoE, decreasing the binding of apoE-containing lipoproteins to the liver receptor (Figs. 72–10 and 72–11) and thereby retarding the uptake of chylomicron and VLDL remnants. There are three common alleles at the apoE gene locus, resulting in six phenotypes of apoE, which can be distinguished by isoelectric focusing of VLDL proteins. One of these phenotypes, designated apoE 2/2, occurs in about 1% of the population, but over 90% of patients with familial dysbetalipoproteinemia have this phenotype. Because familial dysbetalipoproteinemia is quite rare (less than 1 in 10,000 adults), the majority of individuals with apoE 2/2 appear to tolerate this clearance disorder well. If they overproduce chylomicrons (e.g., because of dietary indiscretion) or VLDL (e.g., because of a gene for another familial hyperlipidemia), their clinical disease can be fully expressed.

The *diagnosis* can be made on the basis of clinical manifestations or by demonstrating abnormal lipoproteins by electrophoresis. The abnormal chemical composition of the particles also can be demonstrated. The cholesterol content of VLDL in these patients is high; the ratio of their VLDL cholesterol to total triglycerides is greater than 0.3. ApoE phenotyping is not generally available but can be performed in specialized laboratories.

Familial dysbetalipoproteinemia, unlike the other inherited hyperlipidemias, is often exquisitely sensitive to dietary intervention. Weight loss to a level appropriate for height, coupled with institution of the step I diet, can often cause the lipid levels to return to normal. There is little experience with drug treatment of this disorder in children, but adults with familial dysbetalipoproteinemia whose lipid elevations fail to respond to dietary intervention have been treated with fibric acid derivatives.

Sitosterolemia (Phytosterolemia)

This rare inherited disorder is characterized by increased plasma and tissue levels of plant sterols. The clinical presentation includes tendon and tuberous xanthomas; accelerated atherosclerosis, particularly affecting young males; hemolytic episodes; and arthritis and arthralgias. Very low cholesterol synthesis due to reduced HMG-CoA reductase activity along with increased intestinal absorption and slow hepatic removal of sterols are major biochemical features. Bile acid binding resins (cholestyramine, colestipol) are effective treatments for sitosterolemia.

Familial Hypertriglyceridemia (FHTG)

This disorder occurs with a frequency of 2–3 in 1,000 adults but has a considerately lower risk of premature atherosclerosis than either FH or FCHL. It can be diagnosed only by family studies, which commonly show elevation of the fasting plasma triglyceride level in the range of 200–500 mg/dL, not associated with hyperchylomicronemia, and occurring in a dominantly inherited fashion. There are families with endogenous hypertriglyceridemia in which some members have, in addition, hyperchylomicronemia. Only 10–20% of children in families with familial hypertriglyceridemia have elevated triglycerides before the age of 25, while 50% of adults (i.e., those who have inherited the gene) will be affected with hypertriglyceridemia. Obesity, insulin resistance, hyperinsulinemia, glucose intolerance, and hyperuricemia are often associated findings. Although the precise metabolic defect is unknown, some patients appear to have overproduction of VLDL triglycerides, while others appear to have reduced clearance of VLDL.

Children older than 2 yr can usually be managed with weight control and use of the step I diet. Occasionally, further modification of the carbohydrate/fat ratio may be required. The risk/benefit ratio does not ordinarily justify drug intervention.

Hyperchylomicronemia Syndromes

LIPOPROTEIN LIPASE (LPL) DEFICIENCY. This is an extremely rare (<1 in 100,000) autosomal recessive disorder. Although demonstrable shortly after birth, the massive elevation of plasma triglycerides (1,000 mg/dL to >10,000 mg/dL) is often clinically silent and is not discovered until the patient's blood is sampled for another reason; the chylomicronemia is striking. *Clinical manifestations* include eruptive xanthomas over the trunk, lipemia retinalis, mild hepatosplenomegaly, and recurrent bouts of pancreatitis. Rarely, infants present with recurrent "colic," which is probably related to pancreatitis. The hyperchylomicronemia results from failure to hydrolyze chylomicrons due to genetic deficiency of lipoprotein lipase on the endothelial surface of the capillaries. The *diagnosis* of LPL deficiency is made by measuring the enzyme activity in plasma after administration of heparin (postheparin lipolytic activity).

Although patients with this disorder are not at increased risk for early development of atherosclerosis, recurrent bouts of pancreatitis can be life threatening. *Treatment* for these disorders is aimed at making the diet low enough in long-chain fatty acids to keep the patient asymptomatic and free of recurrent bouts of pain. Using medium-chain triglyceride (MCT) oil in food preparation serves both to make the diet more palatable and to provide sufficient calories for growth. MCTs are absorbed directly into the portal vein and are transported to the liver without requiring chylomicron formation and transport through the systemic circulation. None of the presently available hypolipidemic drugs have any sustained effect.

APOC-II DEFICIENCY. The clinical and laboratory manifestations of genetic deficiency of apoC-II, a cofactor of LPL, are similar to those of LPL deficiency. The diagnosis of this autosomal recessive disorder is made by isoelectric focusing of VLDL apolipoproteins.

FAMILIAL TYPE 5 HYPERLIPOPROTEINEMIA. Patients with this rare disorder (<1 in 5,000) have marked elevations of both chylomicron and VLDL triglycerides. Clinical findings include eruptive xanthomas, lipemia retinalis, pancreatitis, and abnormal glucose tolerance associated with hyperinsulinism. The disorder is usually not expressed in childhood, but several families have been found in which the unidentified defect(s) is expressed early in life. The treatment is primarily weight control and dietary modification. Carbohydrate restriction may also be required to reduce endogenous overproduction of VLDL triglycerides. Aggressive dietary measures should be tried before drug therapy is considered to reduce the VLDL triglyceride level.

HDL Deficiency States

Low levels of plasma HDL cholesterol (hypoalphalipoproteinemia) are often associated with an increased risk of atherosclerosis, while high levels of HDL cholesterol appear to protect against its development. Most patients with extremely low levels (<10 mg/dL plasma) have an inherited disorder, such as Tangier disease or lecithin:cholesterol acyltransferase (LCAT) deficiency.

TANGIER DISEASE. Homozygotes for Tangier disease have HDL particles that are structurally abnormal and present in markedly reduced concentrations. Associated lipoprotein abnormalities include low apoA-I and apoA-II levels, low to normal LDL cholesterol levels, and high triglyceride levels. The major clinical manifestations, some of which can be detected in childhood, result from deposition of cholesteryl esters in a number of tissues: enlarged yellowish tonsils, splenomegaly, peripheral neuropathy, hepatomegaly, lymphadenopathy, and diffuse corneal infiltration. Heterozygotes have approximately 50% of normal levels of HDL cholesterol, apoA-I, and apoA-II but none of the clinical manifestations noted above. Premature coronary heart disease, however, is common in both homozygotes and heterozygotes for Tangier disease. The precise molecular defect is unknown, but abnormalities in apoA-I synthesis and metabolism have been identified.

LECITHIN:CHOLESTEROL ACYLTRANSFERASE (LCAT) DEFICIENCY. LCAT normally catalyzes the transfer of fatty acids from phospholipids to cholesterol in plasma. Deficiency of this enzyme, therefore, is associated with markedly reduced levels of cholesteryl esters and results in alterations of virtually all of the plasma lipoproteins. HDL and LDL cholesterol levels are low; triglycerides are generally high; and structural abnormalities result in abnormal electrophoretic mobility of the lipoproteins. Clinically, LCAT deficiency presents early in childhood; corneal opacities, anemia, and proteinuria have been commonly demonstrated, and sea-blue histiocytes in bone marrow and spleen have been reported. In spite of the very low HDL cholesterol levels, LCAT deficiency is not associated with an increased risk of atherosclerosis. This may be explained by the fact that LCAT mutations result in reduced levels and accelerated catabolism of HDL particles containing primarily apoA-II, not those containing exclusively apoA-I; it is the latter particles that are thought to be protective against the development of atherosclerosis. This extremely rare disorder (probably <1 per million) is diagnosed by measuring LCAT activity in plasma. Several different mutations of the LCAT gene have been described. There is no specific treatment, but dietary management generally includes stringent fat restriction.

A related disorder called *Fish-eye disease* results from a partial LCAT deficiency. Clinical features resembling classic LCAT deficiency include corneal opacities and very low levels of HDL cholesterol. Several mutations of the LCAT gene, different from those causing classic LCAT deficiency, have been described, all of which are extremely rare.

OTHER HDL DEFICIENCY DISORDERS. HDL deficiency has been described in several other disorders. Complete absence of HDL (*familial analphalipoproteinemia*), due to a nonsense mutation of the apoA-I gene, is associated with bilateral retinopathy and cataracts, spinocerebellar ataxia, tendon xanthomas, and premature atherosclerosis. Almost complete absence of HDL, with xanthomas and premature atherosclerosis, can be due to one of a series of other mutations of the apoA-I gene; in these cases, the genetic defects result in complex metabolic derangement generally associated with hypercatabolism of apoA-I–containing HDL particles. Other rare inherited HDL deficiency states have been described (apoA-I/apoC-III deficiency, HDL deficiency with planar xanthomas) that share some of the features of Tangier disease. There is no specific treatment for these disorders, but a diet restricted in fat is recommended.

In view of the numerous observations that HDL cholesterol levels tend to be low in patients with premature coronary heart disease, attempts have been made to identify other inherited causes of reduced HDL. Families have been described with low (50% of normal) HDL cholesterol levels apparently segregating in an autosomal dominant fashion, and associated with premature vascular disease. There have been few systematic clinical studies of familial hypoalphalipoproteinemia, and it is not known whether therapies that act on HDL levels in the general population (i.e., exercise, moderate alcohol intake) will influence HDL cholesterol levels in this group of patients.

Abetalipoproteinemia and Hypobetalipoproteinemia

Abetalipoproteinemia is a rare autosomal recessive disorder that is characterized in childhood by fat malabsorption and diarrhea, retinitis pigmentosa, cerebellar ataxia, and acanthocytosis. Homozygotes for abetalipoproteinemia lack all forms of apoB in their plasma and therefore have no detectable chylomicrons, VLDL, or LDL; their plasma cholesterol and triglyceride levels are extremely low (both usually <30 mg/dL). Heterozygotes have no apparent clinical or biochemical abnormalities. The underlying defect generally has been thought to reside in the pathways of lipoprotein assembly or secretion; molecular defects of a protein critical to this process, called microsomal triglyceride transfer protein (MTP), have been recently identified in a few patients with abetalipoproteinemia. MTP catalyzes the transport of triglycerides, as well as cholesteryl esters and phospholipids, between phospholipid surfaces; it is responsible for the assembly of lipoproteins that contain apoB, adding lipid to apoB early in the assembly process in order to protect the apoB from proteolytic degradation. The demonstration of molecular defects in MTP that cause abetalipoproteinemia has stimulated research in the development of therapies to lower plasma cholesterol levels by inhibiting MTP.

The clinical manifestations are directly referable to the failure of transport of lipids and lipid-soluble vitamins. Treatment is symptomatic. Large doses of vitamin E may retard the progress of neurologic and retinal degeneration; water-soluble vitamin A and vitamin K may alleviate symptoms of night blindness and coagulopathy, respectively. Restriction of dietary long-chain fat may lessen the diarrhea. MCT oil may help maintain caloric balance.

Hypobetalipoproteinemia is distinguished from abetalipoproteinemia by its autosomal dominant inheritance, although patients with these two disorders are clinically quite similar. The majority of patients with extremely low plasma cholesterol levels are homozygous for hypobetalipoproteinemia. Heterozygotes have low plasma cholesterol and low-to-normal triglyceride levels but are otherwise usually asymptomatic. Molecular defects of apoB in most cases cause hypobetalipoproteinemia; these usually truncate the apoB molecule, impairing the secretion of fully assembled apoB-containing lipoproteins from the liver.

American Academy of Pediatrics Committee on Nutrition: Indications for cholesterol testing in children. Pediatrics 83:141, 1989.
Breslow JL: Genetic basis of lipoprotein disorders. J Clin Invest 84:373, 1989.
Brunzell JD: Familial lipoprotein lipase deficiency and other causes of the chylomicronemia syndrome. *In:* Scriver CR, Beander AL, Sly WS, Valle D (eds): The Metabolic Basis of Inherited Disease, 6th ed. New York, McGraw-Hill, 1989, p 1165.
Brunzell JD, Schrott HG, Motulsky AG, et al: Myocardial infarction in the familial forms of hypertriglyceridemia. Metabolism 25:313, 1984.
Cortner JA, Coates PM, Liacouras CA, et al: Familial combined hyperlipidemia in children: clinical expression, metabolic defects, and management. J Pediatr 123:177, 1993.
Dennison BA, Kikuchi DA, Srinavasan SR, et al: Parental history of cardiovascular disease as an indication for screening for lipoprotein abnormalities in children. J Pediatr 115:186, 1989.
Framingham Study: An epidemiologic investigation of cardiovascular disease. Washington DC, National Institutes of Health, NIH Publication 1976, No. 76-1083.
Frerichs RR, Srinavasan SR, Webber LS, et al: Serum cholesterol and triglyceride levels in 3,446 children from a biracial community. The Bogalusa Heart Study. Circulation 54:302, 1976.
Goldstein JL, Brown MS: Familial hypercholesterolemia. *In:* Scriver CR, Beaudet AL, Sly WS, Valle D (eds): The Metabolic Basis of Inherited Disease, 6th ed. New York, McGraw-Hill, 1989, p 1215.
Goldstein JL, Schrott HG, Hazzard WR, et al: Hyperlipidemia in coronary heart disease: Genetic analysis of lipid levels in 176 families and delineation of a new inherited disorder, familial combined hyperlipidemia. J Clin Invest 52:1544, 1973.
Granot E, Deckelbaum RJ: Hypocholesterolemia in childhood. J Pediatr 115:171, 1989.
Grundy SM: Hypertriglyceridemia: Mechanisms, clinical significance, and treatment. Med Clin North Am 66:519, 1982.
Grundy SM, Chait A, Brunzell JD: Familial combined hyperlipidemia workshop. Arteriosclerosis 7:203, 1987.
Havel RJ: Approach to the patient with hyperlipidemia. Med Clin North Am 66:319, 1982.
Humphries SE, Mailly F, Gudnason V, et al: The molecular genetics of pediatric lipid disorders: Recent progress and future research directions. Pediatr Res 34:403, 1993.
Linton MF, Farese RV Jr, Young SG: Familial hypobetalipoproteinemia. J Lipid Res 34:521, 1993.
Lipid Research Clinics Population Studies Data Book. Vol. 1, The Prevalence Study. Washington DC, National Institutes of Health, NIH Publication 1980, No. 80-1527.
Lipid Research Clinics Program: The Lipid Research Clinics Coronary Primary Prevention Trial Results. I and II. JAMA 251:351, 365, 1984.
Mahley RW, Rall SC: Type III hyperlipoproteinemia. *In:* Scriver CR, Beaudet AL, Sly, WS, Valle D (eds): The Metabolic Basis of Inherited Disease, 6th ed. New York, McGraw-Hill, 1989, p 1195.
National Cholesterol Education Program: Report of the Expert Panel on Blood Cholesterol Levels in Children and Adolescents. Pediatrics 89(Suppl):525, 1992.
National Institutes of Health Consensus Development Conference: Lowering blood cholesterol to prevent heart disease. JAMA 253:2080, 1985.
Newman WP, Freedman DS, Voors AW, et al: Relation of serum lipoprotein levels and systolic blood pressure to early atherosclerosis: The Bogalusa Heart Study. N Engl J Med 314:138, 1986.
Rader DJ, Brewer HB Jr: Abetalipoproteinemia. New insights into lipoprotein assembly and vitamin E metabolism from a rare genetic disease. JAMA 270:865, 1993.
Rader DJ, Ikewaki K, Duverger N, et al: Markedly accelerated catabolism of apolipoprotein A-II (apoA-II) and high density lipoproteins containing apoA-II in classic lecithin:cholesterol acyltransferase deficiency and Fish-eye disease. J Clin Invest 93:321, 1994.
Salen G, Shefer S, Nguyen L, et al: Sitosterolemia. J Lipid Res 33:945, 1992.
Schaefer EJ: Clinical, biochemical, and genetic features in familial disorders of high density lipoprotein deficiency. Arteriosclerosis 4:303, 1984.
Sharp D, Blinderman L, Combs KA, et al: Cloning and gene defects in microsomal triglyceride transfer protein associated with abetalipoproteinemia. Nature 365:65, 1993.
Weidman W, Kwiterovich PO, Jesse MJ, et al: AHA Committee Report: Diet in the healthy child. Circulation 67:1411A, 1983.
Zwiener RJ, Uany R, Petruska ML, et al: Low density lipoprotein apheresis as a long term treatment for children with homozygous familial hypercholesterolemia. J Pediatr 126:728, 1995.

CHAPTER 73

Defects in Metabolism of Carbohydrates

Robert M. Kliegman*

73.1 Defects in Intermediary Carbohydrate Metabolism

The intracellular conversion of glucose, fructose, and galactose proceeds as shown schematically in Figure 73–1. The demonstration of defective enzyme activity must serve as the basis of diagnosis and therapy in inborn errors of metabolism. However, an enzymatic defect affecting one tissue may not be demonstrable in another tissue for several reasons:

1. The defective enzyme may normally be absent as is glucose-6-phosphatase from muscle. Therefore, the deficiency of this enzyme in liver, kidney, and intestine of glycogen storage disease type I (GSD I) does not affect the skeletal muscle.
2. An enzymatic activity may reflect different enzyme proteins in different tissues. This is the case for glycogen synthetase, phosphorylase, or phosphorylase kinase. Thus, the deficiency of these enzymes in the livers of patients with GSD 0, GSD VI, or GSD IX does not affect their activity in skeletal muscle.
3. There may not have been the opportunity to measure a defective activity in more than one tissue of the patient. Galactokinase deficiency of erythrocytes is likely to affect the liver. However, galactokinase has not been assayed in hepatic tissue of a patient with the defect of this enzyme in erythrocytes.
4. An enzyme may not be effective in vivo, although the usual assay indicates in vitro activity. For example, GSD Ia has clinical and biochemical manifestations similar to those of GSD Ib. Glucose-6-phosphatase activity measured in frozen liver homogenates is deficient in GSD Ia but normal in GSD Ib. Hepatocytes of GSD Ib have a defect in the transport of glucose-6-phosphate to glucose-6-phosphatase across the microsomal membranes that normally separate substrate from enzyme in intact liver cells. In vivo, the result of the transport defect is similar to that of the actual defect of the enzyme. However, in homogenates of frozen liver tissue, normal intracellular topography is destroyed, and membrane barriers are broken down. Substrate added to GSD Ib homogenate can reach the enzyme, although the transport system is defective. Therefore, in GSD Ib, glucose-6-phosphatase is demonstrable in vitro but remains separated from its substrate in vivo.
5. An apparent enzymatic deficiency revealed by tissue analysis may be an artifact of suboptimal tissue handling. For example, liver phosphorylase activity is low or not demonstrable in autopsy liver, and it is altered nonpredictably in hepatic biopsy specimens unless they are frozen at once after removal from the body.

*Dr. George Hug is the author of chapter in 14th edition. Dr. Kliegman is responsible for modifications in this edition.

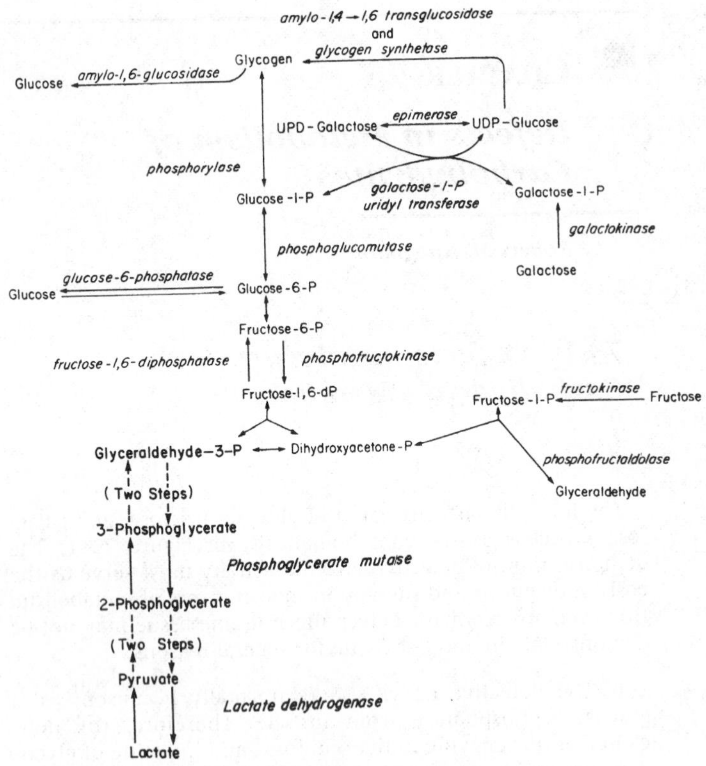

Figure 73–1. Pathway of cytoplasmic glycogen synthesis and degradation.

73.2 *Defects in Galactose Metabolism*

See Figure 73–1.

GALACTOSEMIA: DEFICIENCY OF GALACTOKINASE. This disorder is characterized by galactosemia, galactosuria, and cataracts without mental deficiency or aminoaciduria. Cataracts begin to form after birth when the diet contains galactose derived from the lactose in milk. By the time the diagnosis is made, elimination of dietary galactose may come too late to reverse cataract formation, although younger siblings of the patient may be helped and should be tested at birth.

Galactokinase catalyzes the initial phosphorylation of galactose. If its activity is deficient, the ingestion of galactose leads to increased concentration of galactose in blood and in urine, where it can be found as a reducing substance that is not glucose. Urine specimens tested for galactose should be collected following ingestion of a galactose-containing formula. If an affected infant is receiving a diet without galactose such as glucose water prior to the urine collection, galactose may be absent from the urine and the diagnosis will be missed.

Postnatal institution of a galactose-free diet should prevent cataract formation. Because the children are otherwise normal, the prognosis can be good.

Definitive diagnosis is made by showing that erythrocytes are deficient in galactokinase activity, but the defect is assumed to involve the liver. Some galactose is converted into galactitol, which may be responsible for the cataract formation. Erythrocytic galactokinase activity in affected patients is below the limits of measurement; heterozygous parents and siblings have intermediate activity values. Inheritance is autosomal recessive. The incidence of the condition is about 1 in 40,000.

GALACTOSEMIA: DEFICIENCY OF GALACTOSE-1-PHOSPHATE URIDYL TRANSFERASE. "Classic" galactosemia is a serious disease with early onset of symptoms; the incidence is 1 in 60,000. The newborn infant normally receives up to 20% of caloric intake as lactose, which consists of glucose and galactose. Without the transferase the infant is unable to metabolize galactose-1-phosphate, the accumulation of which results in injury to parenchymal cells of the kidney, liver, and brain. This injury may begin prenatally in the affected fetus by transplacental galactose derived from the diet of the heterozygous mother, who may metabolize dietary galactose with reduced efficiency.

The transferase gene codes for a 379 amino acid peptide. This missence mutation Q188R is one of nine polymorphisms and accounts for 70% of affected Caucasian patients. Severity may not correlate with the genotype in classical galactosemia but may relate to residual enzyme activity in variants (Duarte).

The diagnosis of uridyl transferase deficiency should be considered in newborn infants or older infants or children with any of the following *clinical manifestations:* jaundice, hepatomegaly, vomiting, hypoglycemia, convulsions, lethargy, irritability, feeding difficulties, poor weight gain, aminoaciduria, cataracts, hepatic cirrhosis, ascites, splenomegaly, or mental retardation. Patients with galactosemia are at increased risk for *E. coli* neonatal sepsis; the onset of sepsis often precedes the diagnosis of galactosemia. When the diagnosis is not made at birth, damage to the liver (cirrhosis) and brain (mental retardation) becomes increasingly severe and irreversible. Therefore, galactosemia should be considered for the newborn or young infant who is not thriving or who has any of the above findings.

Because galactose is injurious to persons with galactosemia, diagnostic tests dependent on administering galactose orally or intravenously cannot be used. Galactose administration results in high concentrations of intracellular galactose-1-phosphate, which can function as a competitive inhibitor of phosphoglucomutase. This inhibition transiently impairs the conversion of glycogen to glucose and produces hypoglycemia. Galactose-1-phosphate is responsible for hepatotoxicity and mental retardation, but galactitol causes cataracts. Deficiency of either galactokinase or uridyl transferase produces elevations of galactitol.

Light and electron microscopy of hepatic tissue reveals fatty infiltration, the formation of pseudoacini, and eventual macronodular cirrhosis. These changes are consistent with a metabolic disease but do not indicate the precise enzymatic defect.

The preliminary *diagnosis* of galactosemia is made by demonstrating a reducing substance in several urine specimens collected while the patient is receiving human or cow's milk or another formula containing lactose. The reducing substance found in urine by Clinitest can be identified by chromatography or by an enzymatic test specific for galactose. Clinistix or Testape urine tests are negative because these test materials rely on the action of glucose oxidase, which is specific for glucose and nonreactive with galactose. Deficient activity of galactose-1-phosphate uridyl transferase is demonstrable in hemolysates of erythrocytes, which also exhibit increased concentrations of galactose-1-phosphate. Heterogeneity of the defective enzyme can be shown by electrophoretic techniques using hemolysates. In the complete absence of uridyl transferase activity, very small amounts of galactose may still be metabolized by alternate pathways that are of no clinical significance in most patients.

Primary or secondary amenorrhea was reported in 12 of 18 galactosemic women with transferase deficiency who had laboratory evidence of hypergonadotropic hypogonadism. This condition may result from ovarian toxicity due to galactose and its metabolites, in particular, galactose-1-phosphate, which in patients with galactosemia is present in concentrations toxic to the brain, liver, and kidney. A similar effect is not apparent on the male gonads. This interpretation is consistent with the report of reduced oocytes in offspring of pregnant rats on a high-galactose diet and also with the report that risk factors for ovarian cancer may include increased dietary galactose and decreased transferase activity.

The term *galactosemia*, though adequate for the deficiencies of both galactokinase and uridyl transferase, generally designates the latter for historical reasons.

An occasional infant with galactosemia may tolerate an unexpectedly large amount of food containing lactose, but this is rare. Usually galactose must be excluded from the diet early in life to avoid severe cirrhosis of the liver, mental retardation, cataracts, and recurrent hypoglycemia.

With good dietary control the prognosis is variable. On long-term follow-up, patients may manifest developmental delay and learning disabilities, which increase in severity with age. In addition, most will manifest speech disorders, while a smaller number demonstrate poor growth and impaired motor function and balance (with or without overt ataxia). The relative control of galactose-1-phosphate levels does not always correlate with long-term outcome, leading to the belief that other factors, such as UDP-galactose deficiency (a donor for galactolipids and proteins), may be responsible.

DEFICIENCY OF URIDYL DIPHOSPHOGALACTOSE-4-EPIMERASE. There are two forms of this defect. Depending on the tissue distribution, the condition can be either completely asymptomatic or clinically identical to that of the classic form of galactosemia in which there is a deficiency of transferase activity.

In the benign form the defect is an incidental finding in an otherwise healthy individual without clinical manifestations. The liver is not enlarged, nor are there cataracts or abnormal neurologic findings. Growth and development are normal on an unrestricted normal diet. Patients may be discovered during a newborn screening examination to have an increased concentration of erythrocyte galactose-1-phosphate; galactokinase and uridyl transferase activity is normal. Inheritance is autosomal recessive. The epimerase deficiency affects leukocytes, lymphocytes, and erythrocytes, but its normal activity in tissues other than blood cells may explain the normal tolerance for galactose and the absence of clinical symptoms. No treatment is required.

In patients with generalized epimerase deficiency, the epimerase activity is less than 10% of normal in fibroblasts, in addition to decreased activity in leukocytes and erythrocytes. Parents have about 50% of normal activity in their fibroblasts, consistent with an autosomal recessive mode of inheritance. The clinical manifestations and course are indistinguishable from those of classic galactosemia and include cataracts, hepatomegaly, jaundice, proteinuria, and the presence of a non-glucose-reducing substance in the urine. Treatment is accomplished with a galactose-free diet. Although this form of galactosemia is very rare, it must be considered in a symptomatic patient who has normal transferase activity.

73.3 Defects in Fructose Metabolism

DEFICIENCY OF FRUCTOKINASE (BENIGN FRUCTOSURIA). This condition is not associated with any clinical manifestations. It is an accidental finding usually made because the asymptomatic patient's urine contains a reducing substance. No treatment is necessary. Inheritance is autosomal recessive with an incidence of 1 in 120,000.

Fructokinase deficiency is present in liver, intestine, and kidney. Ingested fructose is not metabolized. Its level is increased in the blood, and it is excreted in urine, there being practically no renal threshold for fructose. Positive Clinitest tests and negative Clinistix tests reveal the urinary-reducing substance to be something other than glucose. It can be identified as fructose by chromatography.

DEFICIENCY OF FRUCTOSE 1,6-BISPHOSPHATE ALDOLASE (ALDOLASE B) (HEREDITARY FRUCTOSE INTOLERANCE). This severe disease of infants appears with the ingestion of fructose-containing food. Either fructose or sucrose (table sugar), the disaccharide of glucose and fructose, may be added as a sweetener to baby foods or formulas. Symptoms may occur quite early in life, soon after birth if foods or formulas containing sucrose or fructose are then introduced into the diet. Early *clinical manifestations* may resemble those of galactosemia and include jaundice, hepatomegaly, vomiting, lethargy, irritability, and convulsions. A urinary-reducing substance that is not glucose can be identified as fructose by chromatography. Acute fructose ingestion produces symptomatic hypoglycemia; chronic ingestion results in hepatic disease.

The deficiency of 1-phosphofructaldolase is practically complete in the liver. Fructose-1-phosphate accumulates in hepatocytes and acts as a competitive inhibitor for phosphorylase in concentrations similar to those of intracellular glucose-1-phosphate. The resulting transient inhibition of the conversion of glycogen to glucose leads to severe hypoglycemia. Some affected children show reduced hepatic conversion of fructose-1,6-diphosphate into the respective trioses in addition to that of fructose-1-phosphate. The concentration of fructose-1-phosphate may be reduced in body tissues by dietary elimination of fructose. However, fructose-1,6-diphosphate is an obligatory metabolite of glycolysis and gluconeogenesis and cannot be eliminated from the body by dietary means.

The severe reduction in the conversion of fructose-1,6-diphosphate in some children may result in *progressive liver disease* despite a fructose-free diet in patients who appear clinically well except for hepatomegaly and elevated levels of serum transaminases. Successive liver biopsies show increasing fatty infiltration and fibrosis, with focal cytoplasmic dissolution, and abnormal appearance of glycogen and mitochondria, and unusual platelike and needle-like crystals in hepatocytes. The prognosis of fructose intolerance must be guarded in some patients, even with good dietary control. Without such control, the disease can result in death during infancy or early childhood. Some infants with hereditary fructose intolerance show fewer and relatively milder symptoms. Owing to dietary avoidance of sucrose, affected patients have few dental caries.

Fructose tolerance tests are contraindicated because they may be followed by hypoglycemia, shock, and death.

Treatment requires completely eliminating fructose from the diet. This may be difficult because fructose is a widely used additive, found even in some aspirin preparations. Inheritance is autosomal recessive, and the incidence (including a mild form in adults) is about 1 in 40,000.

DEFICIENT MUSCLE PHOSPHOGLYCERATE MUTASE. This deficiency has occurred in an otherwise healthy adult exhibiting myoglobinuria and cramps after exercise. The patient was unable to increase blood lactic acid concentration after ischemic exercise, and a muscle biopsy showed normal glycogen concentration and enzyme activities except for low phosphoglycerate mutase activity due to the presence of small normal amounts of B (brain type) isozyme and absence of the M (muscle type) isozyme.

DEFICIENT MUSCLE TYPE LACTATE DEHYDROGENASE. The inability to synthesize the M unit of lactate dehydrogenase (LDH) is inherited as an autosomal recessive disorder and resides on chromosome 11. Affected patients still possess the ability to make the H unit of the enzyme.

The main complaints are fatigue and myoglobinuria after strenuous exercise. There is slightly below normal activity of erythrocyte LDH with a disproportionately high ratio of creatine kinase to LDH activity. Ischemic work results in venous lactate below that of control subjects, and venous pyruvate concentration is at least twice that of normal controls. Patients with deficient M type lactate dehydrogenase can convert muscle glycogen to pyruvate, which is then released into the bloodstream rather than converted to lactate.

73.4 *Defects in Intermediary Carbohydrate Metabolism Associated with Lactic Acidosis*

The defects in carbohydrate metabolism associated with lactic acidosis are discussed here; Figure 73–2 depicts the relevant metabolic pathways.

The normal lactic acid blood concentration is less than 18 mg/dL or 2 mM. Hyperlactic acidemia unrelated to an enzymatic defect occurs in hypoxemia. In this case the serum pyruvic acid concentration may remain normal (<1.0 mg/dL), whereas it is usually increased when hyperlactic acidemia results from an enzymatic defect. It is useful, therefore, to measure lactic and pyruvic acid in the same blood specimen and on multiple blood specimens obtained when the patient is symptomatic because dramatic and ultimately fatal hyperlactic acidemia may be intermittent. Thiamine (vitamin B_1) deficiency (as in alcoholism) also can be associated with life-threatening lactic acidosis that is correctable by thiamine administration. Thiamine participates in the pyruvate dehydrogenase reaction (see Fig. 73–2); this participation and lack of thiamine toxicity are the basis of thiamine treatment that is sometimes used for intractable lactic acidosis.

Deep sighing respirations of the Kussmaul variety should suggest acute metabolic acidosis from hyperlactic acidemia (see Chapter 53). If not corrected, the acidosis can lead to coma, respiratory failure, cardiovascular collapse, renal insufficiency, and death (see Chapter 53).

Hyperlactic acidemia occurs with those defects of carbohydrate metabolism that interfere with the conversion of pyruvate to glucose via the pathway of gluconeogenesis or to CO_2 and water via the mitochondrial enzymes of the citric acid cycle. The concentration of blood lactic acid should be determined in infants and children with unexplained acidosis, especially if the anion gap (see Chapter 53) in blood is greater than 16 mM.

DEFICIENCY OF GLUCOSE-6-PHOSPHATASE. GSD I is the only one of the 12 types of glycogenesis associated with significant lactic acidosis. In most patients the resultant recurrent metabolic acidosis is of minor clinical importance, but in some children it is a life-threatening condition. GSD I is discussed further in Chapter 73.5.

DEFICIENCY OF FRUCTOSE-1,6-DIPHOSPHATASE. These infants are symptom free as long as their diet is limited to human milk. If they receive formulas or food containing fructose or sucrose, they develop intermittent attacks of hypoglycemia, shock, coma, convulsions, and a metabolic acidosis due to hyperlacticacidemia. In symptom-free intervals, physical examination may be normal except for hepatomegaly. If untreated, the disease can lead to psychomotor retardation or death. Inheritance is autosomal recessive.

Fructose-1,6-diphosphatase is one of the four key enzymes of gluconeogenesis. Its activity is markedly reduced or undetectable in hepatic biopsy specimens that show fatty infiltration and reduced glycogen concentration. Other enzymes of fructose metabolism, gluconeogenesis, or glycogen degradation are normal. After glucagon administration, the normal rise in blood glucose concentration may not occur or is abolished after a few hours of fasting. These observations are consistent

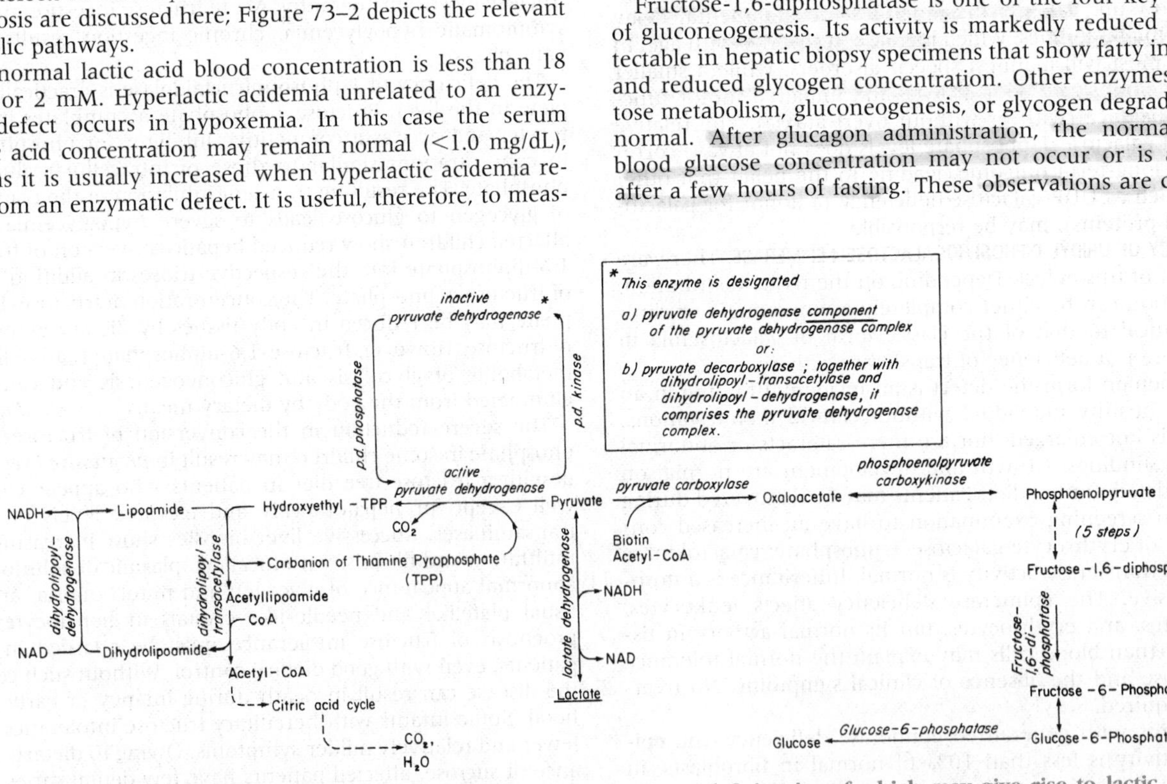

Figure 73–2. Enzymatic reactions of carbohydrate metabolism, deficiencies of which may give rise to lactic acidosis, pyruvate elevations, or hypoglycemia.

with reduced stores of liver glycogen. Biochemical analysis of hepatic biopsy tissue indicates that less than 1.5% of wet liver weight may be glycogen (normal: 2–6%).

Administering galactose produces a normal increase in concentration of blood glucose that is not observed after administering fructose, glycerol, or alanine. The latter substances may produce acute hypoglycemia and lactic acidosis; tolerance tests using them should be avoided. Fasting for more than 10 hr may cause hypoglycemia and lactic acidosis. The clinical presentation may resemble "ketotic hypoglycemia" (see Chapter 77). Untreated fructose-1,6-diphosphatase deficiency is a serious disease with a poor prognosis. Growth and development are normal if the diet is kept free of fructose, sucrose, and sorbitol and is reasonably restricted in fat and protein.

DEFICIENCY OF PYRUVATE DECARBOXYLASE. This enzyme has also been designated the pyruvate dehydrogenase component or the first enzyme (E_1) of the pyruvate dehydrogenase complex. Neonatal onset is associated with lethal lactic acidosis, white matter cystic lesions, agenesis of the corpus callosum, and the most severe enzyme deficiency. Infantile onset may be lethal or associated with psychomotor retardation and chronic lactic acidosis, brain anomalies and cystic lesions, brain stem and basal ganglia pathology typical of Leigh disease, and a greater amount of enzyme activity than that in neonatal disease. Older children, usually boys, may have less acidosis, greater enzyme activity, and manifest ataxia with high carbohydrate diets. Intelligence may be normal. All age patients may have facial dysmorphology similar to fetal alcohol syndrome.

DEFICIENCY OF DIHYDROLIPOYL TRANSACETYLASE. This enzyme is designated the second enzyme (E_2) in the pyruvate dehydrogenase complex, and the only reported patient who might have had this defect was a 9-yr-old boy with profound motor and mental retardation. Blood concentrations of pyruvate and lactate were normal when the patient was fasting but rose to twice the level of controls by 2 hr after a normal meal. A diet high in carbohydrates but not fat (65% and 15%, respectively) precipitated severe lactic acidosis. Dietary thiamine had no effect. Two sisters of the patient had died with severe lactic acidosis; their brains were severely deficient in myelin, but there were no signs of active demyelination. The boy's cultured skin fibroblasts had reduced activity of the pyruvate dehydrogenase complex; activity of the pyruvate decarboxylase was normal. Because the α-ketoglutarate dehydrogenase complex was not defective and because there is evidence that this complex includes an enzyme similar if not identical to E_3 of the pyruvate dehydrogenase complex, it can be inferred that E_2 may have been defective.

DEFICIENCY OF DIHYDROLIPOYL DEHYDROGENASE. The *clinical manifestations* of a deficiency of this third enzyme (E_3) of the pyruvate dehydrogenase complex are severe and include lethargy, hypertonia, irritability, optic atrophy, hyperactive reflexes with muscular hypotonia, lower extremity spasticity, irregular respirations, and laryngeal stridor. Persistent lactic acidosis was not corrected by a diet high in thiamine or fat. Episodes of hypoglycemia may be relieved by alanine. There has been a history of consanguinity.

Laboratory findings include elevations of blood concentrations of pyruvate, lactase, and α-ketoglutarate. Liver function tests may be normal. Dihydrolipoyl dehydrogenase activity in tissues may be as low as 5% of normal. Activities of the pyruvate dehydrogenase complex (but not E_1) and the α-ketoglutarate dehydrogenase complex in liver, muscle, brain, kidney, and skin fibroblasts have also been decreased.

Pathology of the brain in one infant revealed cavitation and lack of myelination in the basal ganglia, thalamus, and brain stem resembling Leigh syndrome.

DEFICIENCY OF PYRUVATE CARBOXYLASE. *Clinical manifestations* of this deficiency have varied from hypoglycemia in infancy to absence of clinical signs and symptoms during the 1st yr of life. Usually psychomotor retardation becomes evident in the 1st yr and may be severe and progressive, culminating in death. Clinical findings have included vomiting, irritability, lethargy, progressive motor and mental retardation, hypotonia, hyporeflexia, abnormal eye movements, optic atrophy, ataxia, and convulsions. There may be a history of psychomotor retardation and death of siblings whose clinical or pathologic findings suggested Leigh syndrome or who were undiagnosed.

Laboratory findings are characterized by elevated concentrations of blood lactate, pyruvate, and alanine. Cerebrospinal fluid protein may be elevated. In one patient, although liver size was normal, glycogen in liver and muscle was increased; there was a normal increase of blood glucose concentration following glucagon administration.

Diagnosis is based upon demonstration of a pyruvate carboxylase deficiency in the liver; a partial defect has been reported in one of two liver pyruvate carboxylases. Activities of the three other gluconeogenic enzymes have been normal.

Treatment with thiamine has prevented episodes of acute metabolic acidosis and controlled the biochemical defect in some patients but has not affected the clinical outcome. Therapy with biotin and lipoic acid is ineffective.

DEFICIENCY OF PYRUVATE CARBOXYLASE SECONDARY TO DEFICIENCY OF HOLOCARBOXYLASE SYNTHETASE OR BIOTINIDASE. See also Chapter 71.6

Deficiency of either of these enzymes of biotin metabolism results in a secondary deficiency of pyruvate carboxylase (and other biotin-requiring carboxylases and metabolic reactions) and in the symptoms associated with the respective deficiencies as well as in skin rash, lactic acidosis, and alopecia. The course of biotinidase deficiency can be protracted, with intermittent exacerbation of chronic lactic acidosis, failure to thrive, and hypotonia leading to spasticity, lethargy, coma, and death. Initial symptoms of this kind in one patient with biotinidase deficiency were reversed by oral biotin, 10 mg/24 hr. In a subsequent sibling the diagnosis was apparent by the finding of less than 5% normal biotinidase activity in serum of cord blood. Biotin therapy prevented the development of discernible symptoms. Because of the curative effect of biotin in an otherwise fatal condition, children with compatible symptomatology, especially children with lactic acidosis and/or unexplained skin rash, should have an assay of serum biotinidase despite the fact that the disease may be rare. The disease can be thought of as biotin dependency. Biotin therapy must be maintained indefinitely.

CARNITINE DEFICIENCY STATES (see also Chapter 72.1). These states may present with recurrent attacks of severe metabolic acidosis (lactic and pyruvic acidemia), hypoglycemia, and hepatomegaly. Cardiomegaly may be present. Untreated, the patient may die during an attack or develop persistent psychomotor retardation, but correction of acidosis and intravenous glucose may terminate the crisis, usually within 12–24 hr. Carnitine concentration may be reduced in serum, liver, muscle, and/or heart. Administration of L-carnitine, the naturally occurring isomer, benefits some but not all patients. Administration of DL-carnitine is without benefit and may be harmful.

L-Carnitine is synthesized in the liver from lysine in four enzymatic steps. The first three steps can also be executed in muscle and heart. The resulting carnitine precursor is transported through blood to the liver, where the synthesis is completed. The finished L-carnitine is returned into cells of muscle and heart. At the outer side of the inner membrane of the mitochondria, the enzyme carnitine palmitoyl transferase I (CPT I) forms fatty acid–carnitine esters. These esters are transferred into the mitochondria, where CPT II cleaves the esters, freeing fatty acid for energy production by β oxidation. Carnitine exits from the mitochondria to begin the next cycle of fatty acid transfer. Carnitine is indispensable in the transport of fatty acids from the cytoplasm into the mitochondria. A newborn girl with CPT II deficiency demonstrated in heart, liver, muscle, and fibroblasts died at age 5 days of encephalocardiomyopathy, hepatomegaly, hypoglycemia, carnitine deficiency, and acidosis. She had appeared normal for the first 2 days of life, probably living off her tissue glycogen stores. However, entry of fatty acids into mitochondria was impaired and energy production could not be sustained once glycogen was depleted. An infant boy with CPT II deficiency demonstrated in fibroblasts appeared healthy until 3 mo of age when he had an episode of lethargy, seizures, hypoglycemia, and respiratory arrest from which he recovered. He died suddenly at age 17 mo.

Carnitine deficiency states can exist either as primary carnitine deficiency, which is the result of a defect within the metabolism of carnitine itself, or more often as secondary carnitine deficiency, which is acquired as the result of some other condition. In primary carnitine deficiency the concentration of carnitine in serum and tissues such as liver, muscle, or heart is usually markedly reduced. Carnitine deficiency can occur with CPT II deficiency, in which acylcarnitine ester is formed normally by CPT I but then is not cleaved by the defective CPT II and is excreted with the loss of the carnitine moiety (see Chapter 72.1).

In secondary carnitine deficiency the concentration of carnitine is reduced in serum and/or tissues because of a carnitine loss that may be associated with many different conditions. These conditions are separable into two groups: (1) those with increased loss or decreased intake of carnitine, and (2) those with an accumulation of carnitine esters that are excreted in the urine, draining the body of carnitine. Group 1 includes renal Fanconi syndrome, type XI glycogenosis, cystinosis, Lowe syndrome, suboptimal diet, and renal dialysis. Group 2 includes defects in β oxidation of fatty acids, various types of organic acidemia, and treatment with the anticonvulsant drug valproic acid, which is excreted in urine as valproylcarnitine ester.

The main danger posed by primary and secondary carnitine deficiencies is the threat to the transfer of fatty acids into the mitochondria and therefore to β oxidation and energy production. The extent to which this threat can be alleviated by carnitine treatment depends on the defective site and mechanism underlying the carnitine reduction. To date, side effects of carnitine treatment are rare and are limited to diarrhea and a fishy body odor. Therefore, after reduced carnitine has been found in serum and/or tissue biopsies, one may consider treatment of children with primary as well as secondary carnitine deficiency with oral L-carnitine in divided doses of up to 200 mg/kg/24 hr.

DEFICIENCY OF PYRUVATE DEHYDROGENASE PHOSPHATASE. This deficiency has been found in a newborn boy who had a metabolic acidosis with high serum concentrations of lactate (up to 7 times normal), pyruvate (2 times normal), and free fatty acids (3 times normal). There was no hypoglycemia or hepatomegaly. The acidosis improved when the intake of glucose was increased and that of fat decreased. Periods of clinical stability and moderate hyperlactic acidemia were interrupted every few days by episodes of severe lactic acidosis. Neurologic damage was evident, with lethargy, convulsions, hypotonia, and irritability. The patient died at 6 mo of age.

The pyruvate dehydrogenase component E_1 of the pyruvate dehydrogenase complex exists in both active and inactive forms. E_1 is inactivated when it is phosphorylated by pyruvate dehydrogenase kinase in the presence of ATP. E_1 is stimulated by calcium. Pyruvate dehydrogenase phosphatase activity was reported deficient in liver and muscle but not in the brain of this child based on the observation that the addition of calcium to a homogenate of liver increased the activity of pyruvate decarboxylase in the patient by 4% and in a control by 50%. Deficiency of this activating phosphatase has been reported in another 7-mo-old boy in whom brain autopsy findings were consistent with Leigh syndrome.

CONGENITAL IDIOPATHIC LACTIC ACIDOSIS. This diagnosis should be considered when there is labored respiration in infancy associated with metabolic acidosis from hyperlactic acidemia. Liver and spleen may be enlarged. Convulsions, hypoglycemia, psychomotor retardation, and neurologic damage usually lead to death in infancy despite dietary administration of thiamine, biotin, steroids, lipoic acid, and other agents. Long-term survival in a few instances is possible.

There are increased serum concentrations of pyruvate, lactate, and alanine, as well as of other amino acids. Cerebral autopsy findings may show severe spongy degeneration and lack of myelination, or there may be only moderate or mild abnormalities.

A variety of deficiencies in enzymatic activities, including those reported and defects in mitochondrial respiratory chain complexes may lead to lactic acidosis. The respiratory chain produces ATP from NADH or $FADH_2$ and includes five specific complexes (I—NADH-coenzyme Q reductase; II—succinate-coenzyme Q reductase; III—coenzyme QH_2 cytochrome C reductase; IV—cytochrome C oxidase; V—ATP synthase). Each complex is composed of 9–25 individual proteins, encoded by nuclear or mitochondrial DNA (inherited only from the mother by mitochondrial inheritance). Such defects produce chronic lactic acidosis in children or adults and are usually diagnosed by muscle biopsy analysis of oxidative mitochondrial function. Some deficiencies resemble Leigh syndrome, while others cause infantile myopathies such as MELAS (mitochondrial encephalopathy, myopathy, lactic acidosis, and strokelike episodes), MERRF (myoclonus epilepsy, with ragged-red fibers), and Kearns-Sayre syndrome (external ophthalmoplegia, acidosis, retinal degeneration, heart block, myopathy, high CSF protein). In patients who have not been examined in a systematic way, excluding the defects described earlier, the diagnosis of congenital idiopathic lactic acidosis should probably not be made.

LEIGH SUBACUTE NECROTIZING ENCEPHALOPATHY (SNE). This condition is characterized by seizures, psychomotor retardation, optic atrophy, hypotonia, vomiting, abnormal movements, lethargy, and lactic acidosis (also see Chapter 548). It is difficult to distinguish this syndrome reliably from many of the enzymatic deficiencies that are associated with lactic acidosis. Gliosis, cavitation, and capillary proliferation in the brain stem, basal ganglia, and thalamus, which are critical criteria for a pathologic diagnosis, may be visible on CT scan. Similar lesions viewed as characteristic have been encountered in patients shown to have pyruvate carboxylase deficiency, or, in one case, defective pyruvate decarboxylase activity in skin fibroblasts. Another boy shown to have SNE by brain autopsy also had a deficiency of pyruvate dehydrogenase phosphatase. The assessment of patients presenting symptoms and signs consistent with Leigh syndrome must include assays of enzymatic activities that result in lactic acidosis. These activities were normal in a 22-mo-old boy who had the cerebral findings of Leigh syndrome associated with increased concentration of endorphin and norepinephrine in cerebrospinal fluid (CSF) and of enkephalins in cerebral cortex.

Thiamine is transiently effective in some patients with Leigh syndrome but not in others. Its use was suggested by the report that extracts of blood, CSF, and urine of patients with SNE inhibited thiamine pyrophosphate–adenosine triphosphate phosphoryl transferase. Thiamine in pharmacologic doses might have over-ridden this inhibitor, which has also been found in the urine of as many as 10% of clinically normal persons.

Attempts to correct hyperlactic acidemia with dichloroacetate, which inhibits the inactivating kinase for pyruvate dehydrogenase (E_1; see Fig. 73–2), thereby maintaining dehydrogenase (E_1) activity, have been ineffective in a child with fatal lactic acidosis of unknown cause.

Acute, life-threatening hyperlactic acidemia can be corrected by the intravenous infusion of *tris-hydroxymethyl aminomethane* (THAM), which avoids the sodium overload of sodium bicarbonate administration. This treatment does not alter the poor prognosis for the majority of conditions that are associated with increased concentrations of lactic and pyruvic acid.

73.5 Glycogen Storage Diseases

These diseases are the result of metabolic errors leading to abnormal concentrations or structure of glycogen. The glycogen storage diseases (GSD) or glycogenosis can be classified according to the identified enzymatic defects or sometimes by the distinctive clinical features (Table 73–1). The separation of

■ **TABLE 73–1 Features of the Glycogen Storage Diseases, Types 0–XI (GSD 0–XI)**

Type, Enzyme Affected	Tissue Distribution of Excessive Glycogen and Enzyme Deficiency	Clinical Symptoms and Signs	Comments *Alternate Names*
GSD 0 Glycogen synthetase	Liver but not muscle (other tissues not analyzed); glycogen depletion in liver; hepatic glycogen synthetase less than 2% of normal, but some hepatic glycogen (1%) demonstrable	Fasting hypoglycemia; prolonged hyperglycemia after a meal or glucose administration; mental retardation follows hypoglycemic convulsions—when these are avoided by frequent protein-rich meals, psychomotor development can be normal	*Aglycogenosis*; defect convincingly demonstrated in two unrelated families; early diagnosis and dietary treatment important for prevention of retardation; some children with "ketotic hypoglycemia" may have GSD 0
GSD Ia Glucose-6-phosphatase	Liver, kidney, intestine; frequent intranuclear glycogen seen in these organs not diagnostic; continuous nighttime feeding by tube and pump may alleviate clinical symptoms; portacaval shunt risky and clinically disappointing; treatment with phenytoin or phenobarbital ineffective	Enlarged liver and kidneys; "doll face," stunted growth, normal mental development; tendency to hypoglycemia, lactic acidosis, hyperlipidemia, hyperuric acidemia, gout, bleeding; IV* galactose or fructose not converted to glucose (caution: these tests may precipitate acidosis); abortive or no rise in blood glucose after SC† epinephrine or IV glucagon; normal urinary catecholamines; prognosis fair to good	*Von Gierke disease, hepatorenal glycogenosis*; no involvement of skeletal or cardiac muscle, or of leukocytes or cultured skin fibroblasts (glucose-6-phosphatase not normally present in these tissues)
GSD Ib In vitro activity of glucose-6-phosphatase is normal, but translocase is deficient	Activity of glucose-6-phosphatase is normal in frozen liver homogenate but is not demonstrable in isotonic homogenate of fresh liver tissue that has never been frozen	Symptoms are as those of GSD Ia; in addition, frequent neutropenia	Transport defect for glucose-6-phosphate at microsomal membrane
GSD Ic In vitro activity of glucose-6-phosphatase can be demonstrated	Activity of glucose-6-phosphatase is normal in frozen liver homogenate but is deficient in isotonic homogenate of fresh liver tissue that has never been frozen	The patient, an 11-yr-old girl, had hepatomegaly, brittle diabetes, frequent hypoglycemia	Transport defect for inorganic phosphate at microsomal membrane
GSD IIa, b Lysosomal acid α-glucosidase (deficient activity of acid α-1,4- and α-1,6-glucosidase; the latter could be considered "lysosomal glycogen debrancher")	In the fatal, infantile, classic form (GSD IIa), glycogen concentration excessive in all organs examined; acid α-glucosidase deficiency was generalized in one patient; in others *normal* renal acid α-glucosidase; amniotic *fluid* (in contrast to cultured amniotic fluid cells) contains acid α-glucosidase activity even if the fetus has the disease	Clinically normal at birth, though minimal cardiomegaly, abnormal ECG,‡ increased tissue glycogen, abnormal lysosomes in liver and skin, and acid α-glucosidase deficiency demonstrable at birth. Within a few months, marked hypotonia, severe cardiomegaly, moderate hepatomegaly; normal mental development; death usually in infancy (GSD IIa). Cases with involvement of muscle and liver but without cardiomegaly described in children and adults (GSD IIb). Normal blood glucose response to glucagon; normal urinary catecholamines	*Pompe disease, generalized glycogenosis, cardiac glycogenosis*; prenatal diagnosis *within* a few days after aminocentesis by the electron microscopic demonstration of abnormal lysosomes in *uncultured* amniotic fluid cells; for prenatal diagnosis by enzyme analysis, *cultured* amniotic fluid cells required, which also show the abnormal lysosomes GSD IIa: *infantile fatal form* GSD IIb: *late juvenile-adult form*
GSD III Amylo-1,6-glucosidase, "debrancher enzyme"	Liver, muscle, heart, etc., in various combinations; designated types IIIA through D; cultured amniotic fluid cells have diagnostic biochemical abnormality	Moderate to marked hepatomegaly; none to moderate hypotonia; none to moderate cardiomegaly, ECG rarely abnormal; no acidosis, hypoglycemia, or hyperlipemia; glucagon produces a normal rise in blood glucose after a meal but not after fasting; normal mental development; failure of liver or heart rare; normal urinary catecholamines; prognosis fair to good	*Limited dextrinosis, debrancher glycogenosis, Cori disease, Forbes disease*; prenatal diagnosis by enzyme assay of cultured amniotic fluid cells feasible but perhaps unnecessary, owing to the usual benign course
GSD IV Amylo-1,4→1,6-transglucosidase, "brancher enzyme"	Generalized (?); low to normal levels of abnormally structured glycogen (amylopectin-like molecules with fewer branch points than normal in animal glycogen)	Hepatosplenomegaly, ascites, cirrhosis, liver failure; normal mental development; death in early childhood	*Amylopectinosis, brancher glycogenosis, Andersen disease*; prenatal diagnosis of this incurable disease may be feasible and indicated by enzyme analysis of cultured amniotic fluid cells
GSD V Muscle phosphorylase deficiency (congenital absence of skeletal muscle phosphorylase; phosphorylase-activating system intact)	Skeletal muscle; liver and myometrium normal	Temporary weakness and cramping of skeletal muscle after exercise; no rise in blood lactate during ischemic exercise; symptoms like those of type VII glycogenosis; normal mental development and urinary catecholamines; myoglobinuria in later life; fair to good prognosis	*McArdle syndrome*; liver and smooth muscle phosphorylase not affected; cardiac muscle phosphorylase not examined; prenatal diagnosis not feasible, does not seem indicated

■ TABLE 73–1 Features of the Glycogen Storage Diseases, Types 0–XI (GSD 0–XI) *Continued*

Type, Enzyme Affected	Tissue Distribution of Excessive Glycogen and Enzyme Deficiency	Clinical Symptoms and Signs	Comments *Alternate Names*
GSD VI Liver phosphorylase deficiency (phosphorylase-activating system intact)	Liver; skeletal muscle normal; leukocytes unsatisfactory for diagnosis	Marked hepatomegaly, no splenomegaly; no hypoglycemia, acidosis, or hyperlipemia; no rise of blood glucose after SC epinephrine or IV glucagon; normal mental development; normal urinary catecholamines; good prognosis	Lack of glucagon-induced hyperglycemia distinguishes GSD VI from GSD IX; the latter shows a normal glucagon response; prenatal diagnosis not feasible, may not be indicated
GSD VII Phosphofructokinase	Skeletal muscle, erythrocytes (in initial report; other tissues not examined); not known whether cultured amniotic fluid cells are affected, but prenatal diagnosis not indicated	Temporary weakness and cramping of skeletal muscle after exercise; no rise in blood lactate during ischemic exercise; normal mental development; symptoms identical to those of type V glycogenosis; good prognosis	*Tarui disease*: reduction of phosphofructokinase activity severe in skeletal muscle, mild in erythrocytes, not established in other tissues; incapacity may be minimal
GSD VIII No enzymatic deficiency yet demonstrated; total liver phosphorylase normal but most is in inactive form (liver phosphorylase activity reduced because control lost over extent of phosphorylase activation)	Liver, brain; skeletal muscle normal; cerebral glycogen increased; electron microscopy shows some cerebral glycogen in the form of α-particles within axon cylinders and synapses	Hepatomegaly; truncal ataxia, nystagmus, "dancing eyes" may be present; neurologic deterioration progressing to hypertonia, spasticity, decerebration, and death; urinary epinephrine and norepinephrine are increased during acute phase of disease, not in stationary end phase	Predominant clinical problem of the three patients with this presumptive diagnosis was progressive degenerative disease of brain
GSD IX a, b, c Liver phosphorylase kinase deficiency (total phosophorylase content normal but in inactive form, owing to the lack of phosphorylase kinase)	Liver; muscle tissue normal biochemically (in IXa and IXb) and microscopically; diagnosis not possible by using leukocytes; D-thyroxine–induced liver phosphorylase kinase activity in one patient, but not in two others of a different family	Marked hepatomegaly, no splenomegaly; no hypoglycemia or acidosis; normal urinary catecholamines; normal rise in blood glucose after IV glucagon or SC epinephrine; prognosis good; treatment may not be necessary ("benign hepatomegaly" may disappear in early adulthood)	Liver phosphorylase can be activated in vitro by addition of exogenous kinase to the homogenate; not the human counterpart of muscle phosphorylase kinase deficiency in mice; normal glucagon response is a distinguishing feature vs GSD VI; GSD IXa, autosomal recessive; GSD IXb, X-linked recessive; prenatal diagnosis not demonstrated
GSD X Loss of activity of cyclic 3′5′-AMP–dependent kinase in muscle and presumably liver (total phosphorylase content of liver and skeletal muscle normal, but the enzyme completely deactivated in both organs; phosphorylase kinase activity 50% of normal, possibly owing to the loss of 3′5′-AMP–dependent kinase activity)	Liver and muscle (other organs not tested); identical biochemical findings were made in two muscle biopsy specimens taken 6 yr apart	Marked hepatomegaly; patient otherwise clinically healthy initially, but 6 yr after diagnosis mild recurrent muscle pain; no cardiomegaly or hypoglycemia; no rise in blood glucose after IV glucagon; the only individual known to have this condition not incapacitated at 12 yr of age	In vitro activation of the patient's phosphorylase occurs (1) under assay conditions not requiring 3′5′-AMP–dependent kinase, or (2) after the patient's muscle homogenate has been fortified with phosphorylase kinase–deficient mouse muscle that supplied 3′5′-AMP–dependent kinase; postulated defect restricted to the activity of the cyclic 3′5′-AMP–dependent kinase that phosphorylates phosphorylase kinase, other cyclic 3′5′-AMP–dependent phosphorylations being intact
GSD XI All enzymatic activities measured to date are normal (adenyl cyclase, 3′5′-AMP–dependent kinase, phosphorylase kinase, phosphorylase, debrancher, brancher, glucose-6-phosphatase)	Liver, or liver and kidney	Tendency for acidosis; markedly stunted growth; vitamin D–resistant rickets (which can be cured with high doses of vitamin D and oral supplementation of phosphate); hyperlipidemia, generalized aminoaciduria, galactosuria, glucosuria, phosphaturia; normal renal size; no rise in blood glucose after IV glucagon or SC epinephrine; urinary excretion of cyclic 3′5′-AMP increases markedly after administration of glucagon	Muscle usually not affected; GSD XI may include patients with glycogenoses with different enzymatic defects; patients exhibit noncystinotic Fanconi syndrome associated with secondary (acquired) carnitine deficiency

**IV = intravenous administration.*
†SC = subcutaneous administration.
‡ECG = electrocardiogram.

a new type of GSD is useful to the clinician if the clinical or biochemical characteristics are sufficiently distinctive to permit their recognition in future patients. Figure 73–3 depicts the relevant metabolic pathways.

DEFICIENCY OF GLYCOGEN SYNTHETASE (GSD 0). Early morning convulsions associated with hypoglycemia are typical symptoms of this condition. There is an associated hyperketonemia but no hepatomegaly. Hypoglycemia appears during periods without food and is not responsive to glucagon administration. After administration of glucose the blood glucose level remains elevated for longer than usual. The diagnosis should be made expeditiously, because hypoglycemic episodes and mental retardation can be avoided if the patient is given frequent meals rich in protein. The clinical picture is similar to that of ketotic hypoglycemia (see Chapter 77), and patients with the latter diagnosis may benefit from an assay of hepatic glycogen synthetase. Persistent hyperglycemia and an increase in serum lactate concentration after administration of glucose should reveal those with a possible deficiency of glycogen synthetase.

Glycogen synthetase activity is deficient in liver but normal in muscle and in white and red blood cells. Glycogen concentration is low (less than 2%) but not absent in liver and normal in muscle. Differential involvement of tissues reflects the fact that different isozymes of glycogen synthetase exist

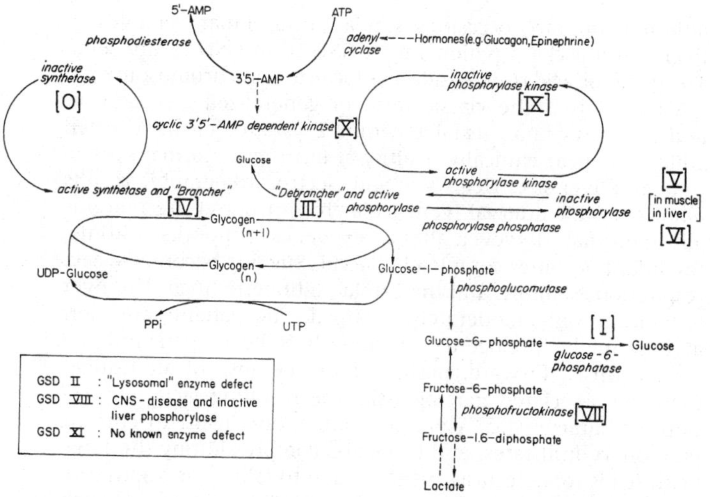

Figure 73–3. Pathway of phosphorylase activation and anaerobic glycolysis. Bracketed numbers refer to the type of glycogenosis in which the activity of the enzyme next to the number is defective. The various types are listed in Table 73–1.

for various tissues. The activation system for glycogen synthetase is normal.

DEFICIENCY OF GLUCOSE-6-PHOSPHATASE (GSD Ia). In GSD Ia, glucose-6-phosphatase activity is defective, and glycogen concentration is increased in liver, kidney, and intestine. *Clinical manifestations* are summarized in Table 73–1. Mild hypotonia is sometimes also reported in GSD Ia, but the disease does not have a primary effect on muscle, because muscle does not normally contain glucose-6-phosphatase. Marked hypoglycemia may be well tolerated; patients with blood glucose levels as low as 10 mg/dL may display normal behavior. Hyperlipidemia (producing xanthomas) and hyperuric acidemia are marked. In adults the latter produces gout, which must be appropriately treated. There is a secondary impairment of platelet function, which may make bleeding a problem when biopsies are done. Young children with GSD Ia have impressive hepatomegaly, but liver involvement may be easily overlooked in the affected adult. In patients with GSD Ia, the kidneys are moderately but consistently enlarged on roentgenographic examination, which helps to differentiate GSD Ia from GSD III, in which renal size is normal.

Administering galactose or fructose does not produce an elevation of blood glucose concentration; tolerance tests with these sugars should not be done because they can lead to severe acidosis. Intravenous administration of glucagon is not followed by a normal rise in blood glucose, regardless of how recently the patient may have eaten. The glucagon tolerance test can, therefore, differentiate between GSD Ia and GSD III; in the latter the concentration of blood glucose will increase if glucagon is given 2 hr after a meal. Subcutaneous administration of epinephrine has no advantage over the glucagon tolerance test and may produce unpleasant side effects.

Acute lactic acidosis may be a recurrent and life-threatening problem. Portacaval shunt has been advocated for its prevention or control, but no patients have benefited from the operation, which has been complicated by closure of the anastomosis and by development of cirrhosis or encephalopathy. Patients in whom this condition is difficult to control can be managed successfully with continuous nighttime feedings by nasopharyngeal or gastrostomy tube. Therapeutic success also has been reported with repeated daily drinking of a solution of uncooked cornstarch. With such dietary regimens, children grow satisfactorily, hepatomegaly and renal disease (hyperfiltration, focal segmental sclerosis, and interstitial fibrosis) recede, and hypoglycemia and lactic acidosis become manageable. However, when the gastric tube feedings are discontinued, the pretreatment tolerance of hypoglycemia may have been lost. Disease-related post-treatment hypoglycemia may result in convulsions. Frequent meals have effects similar to those of gastric tube feedings and may suffice for clinical control. As patients grow older, their metabolic problems become less severe and are more easily manageable.

In GSD Ia, hepatocytes contain many lipid droplets ranging in size from smaller than mitochondria to several times that of the nucleus, and the nuclei themselves frequently contain glycogen. Nuclear glycogenosis can also occur in GSD III, in diabetes mellitus, and in Wilson disease. Patients with GSD Ia have an increased incidence of hepatoma. Abdominal examination by ultrasound or CT scan every 6–12 mo may be indicated. Prenatal diagnosis using amniotic fluid cells is not feasible since glucose-6-phosphatase is not normally present in cultured skin fibroblasts; nor can the enzyme be demonstrated in normal white cells.

GSD Ib (Pseudo-GSD I). Clinically, GSD Ib is indistinguishable from GSD Ia except that children with GSD Ib have an increased incidence of neutropenia, inflammatory bowel disease, and infections. Neutropenia responds to G-CSF. Hepatic glycogen concentration is increased but glucose-6-phosphatase activity is normal in hypotonic homogenates made of frozen liver tissue. The activity is decreased, however, in isotonic homogenates made from fresh liver tissue, which is consistent with a defect in GSD Ib of enzymes that transport glucose-6-phosphate across microsomal membranes. Further evidence that this variant of GSD I is associated with an intracellular transport defect is the finding that when fresh liver homogenates from affected patients are treated with deoxycholate, the activity of glucose-6-phosphatase is normal; deoxycholate is known to break up microsomal membranes.

GSD Ic. Transport of glucose-6-phosphate into microsomes (which is defective in GSD Ib) is normally associated with transport of inorganic phosphates in the opposite direction. A deficiency in this phosphate transfer has been described in an 11-yr-old girl with insulin-dependent diabetes (GSD Ic). Liver glycogen concentration was 9.4%, but because the patient had frequent hypoglycemic attacks, the increased glycogen concentration could have resulted from therapeutic glucose administration. The patient's clinical picture appeared to be similar to that of Mauriac syndrome in diabetic children (see Part XXVI, Section 6).

DEFICIENCY OF LYSOSOMAL ACID α-GLUCOSIDASE (GSD II). This disease, whose clinical manifestations are summarized in Table 73–1, occurs in at least two varieties, one affecting infants (GSD IIa), the other affecting older children and adults (GSD IIb). Both varieties have not occurred in members of the same family. Fibroblast studies indicate that in a patient with GSD IIa, the lysosomal acid α-glucosidase is structurally altered, whereas in a patient with GSD IIb, the amount of the enzyme is reduced. Abnormal lysosomes are the morphologic hallmark of GSD II, although on rare occasions similar intracellular vacuoles in liver and muscle of patients with GSD III or GSD IV are seen. The gene for acid α-glucosidase is localized on chromosome 17.

GSD IIa. This is the classic form of generalized glycogenosis and is always fatal, usually within 2 yr after birth. Affected children appear clinically healthy at birth with normal muscle tone and liver size. Heart size and electrocardiographic results (shortened PR interval, ventricular hypertrophy) are marginally abnormal. However, after a few weeks or months at home, the infant becomes completely flaccid. Sucking becomes weak, respirations shallow, and the cardiac silhouette huge. The liver is typically only moderately enlarged. The patients are alert and normally intelligent. The mouth is kept open and the tongue thrust forward, perhaps more because of air hunger than the associated macroglossia; the resulting facial expression is characteristic. Aspiration pneumonia leads to chronic pulmonary infiltrates, and bronchial compression by the large heart leads to atelectasis. Death is due to failure of respiratory muscles. There is hardly any other condition in which such extreme cardiomegaly and muscular weakness occur in an infant who appears normal at birth. Blood glucose concentrations are normal, as are tolerance tests with glucagon and other carbohydrate test substances.

GSD II is the only lysosomal disease among the glycogenoses; the other types of GSD are associated with defects of enzymes located in the cytoplasm. The deficient acid α-glucosidase is a glycogen-degrading enzyme associated with the lysosomal fraction of tissue homogenates. Fusion of a primary lysosome with an autophagic vacuole normally creates a secondary lysosome. If the primary lysosome is deficient in a lysosomal enzyme (such as α-glucosidase), then the secondary lysosome may become engorged with the material (such as glycogen) that should have been degraded by the defective enzyme. Besides deficiencies of enzymes, other errors in lysosomal mechanisms may be present, such as membrane defects. In GSD IIa the deficiency of lysosomal acid α-glucosidase produces intracellular vesicles (so-called abnormal lysosomes) engorged with glycogen (Fig. 73–4) in cells of liver, muscle, heart and most other tissues of the body. Deficient acid α-glucosidase activity is also associated with the formation of glycogen-filled "abnormal lysosomes" in the cells of placenta and skin of children with I-cell disease (mucolipidosis type II, ML II; see Chapter 72.3).

Increased glycogen concentrations are found in many tissues of affected children. The deficiency of the lysosomal enzyme for glycogen degradation explains the membrane-bound accumulations of glycogen in lysosomes, but it does not explain the excessive accumulation of glycogen in the cytoplasm of heart and muscle cells.

The excessive tissue glycogen as such may not be a cause of death. The normalization of the hepatic ultrastructure is not clinically beneficial for the patient. Bone marrow transplantation in a boy with GSD IIa resulted in engraftment of blood cell lines, but the patient died of GSD IIa 5 mo after the procedure.

The prenatal diagnosis of GSD IIa can be made by electron microscopic examination of cells obtained by chorionic villus biopsy or at amniocentesis (see later).

GSD IIb. Weakness of skeletal muscle begins later in life than in those with GSD IIa. In some the disease is compatible with a normal life span, though it may demand a sedentary lifestyle. In other patients, death from respiratory failure can occur during the 3rd or 4th decade. Cardiomegaly is absent, and the electrocardiogram is normal. The diagnosis is based on electron microscopic examination of skin biopsy showing abnormal lysosomes packed with glycogen particles.

Some cases cannot be explained on the basis of defective activity of lysosomal acid α-glucosidase. For example, a patient who died of unrelated hypertension at 24 yr of age had a deficiency of acid α-glucosidase consistent with GSD IIa. Glycogen concentration was increased in all tissues except heart, though cardiac α-glucosidase activity was deficient. Heart muscle appeared normal on light microscopy; electron microscopy revealed occasional abnormal lysosomes but no excess of glycogen in cytoplasm.

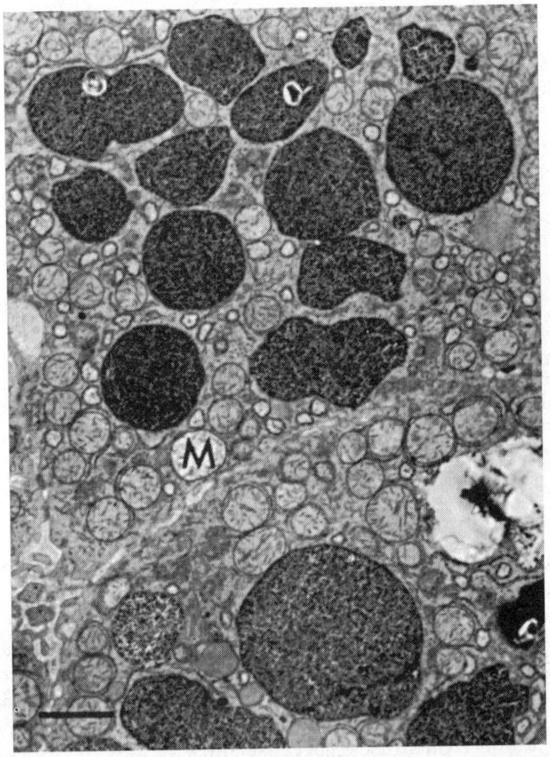

Figure 73–4. Liver autopsy specimen of GSD IIa. "Abnormal lysosomes" with lysosomal glycogen (tightly packed black particles) are ubiquitous, but cytoplasmic glycogen is missing. The absence of cytoplasmic glycogen indicates that this specimen was obtained after starvation or epinephrine treatment, or autopsy. M = mitochondria. (Bar: 2 μm.)

DEFICIENCY OF "DEBRANCHER" ACTIVITY (GSD III). Clinical manifestations are summarized in Table 73–1. In GSD III, hepatomegaly can be as impressive as in GSD I. When generalized, this disorder also affects muscle and heart, but either organ may be clinically involved to a varying degree. Some patients resemble children with muscular dystrophy. Electrocardiographic abnormalities and moderate cardiomegaly are usually found; the size of the kidneys is normal. Patients with GSD III restricted to the liver usually do well. Hypoglycemia is rare and does not present a clinical problem. There may be recurrent pneumonia, but the long-term prognosis is usually good. The serum concentrations of uric acid, lactate, ketones, and lipids are normal. Blood glucose concentration increases if glucagon is given 2 hr after a meal in patients with GSD III but not in those with GSD I, whereas blood glucose levels remain flat in both glycogenoses when glucagon is administered after overnight fasting. These clinical and laboratory findings distinguish GSD III from GSD I.

For "debranching" of the glycogen molecule, two enzymatic reactions need to occur in sequence after phosphorylase activity has reduced the outer chains of the glycogen molecule to within 4 glucose units of the 1,6 branch point. The first reaction is that of a transferase that transfers 3 glucose units of the branched outer chain onto the straight outer chain. The glucose molecule at the branch point becomes exposed and accessible to the subsequent action of α-1,6-glucosidase, which removes it. Both the transferase and the α-1,6-glucosidase activities are deficient in the livers of patients with GSD III. In some patients the activity of transferase in muscle may be low, whereas that of α-1,6-glucosidase remains normal. The overall effect in either liver or muscle is a loss of debrancher activity. Both enzymatic activities may be retained in muscle, the defect being limited to the liver.

Frequently GSD III is a generalized disease, and glycogen concentrations are found to be increased and debranching activity deficient in every (examined) tissue. In generalized GSD III, the concentration of glycogen in muscle may reach the same levels as in GSD II, although patients with the former may be symptom free and those with the latter are markedly hypotonic. In GSD III, starvation induces the degradation of glycogen to within 4 units of the branch point. Glycogen with such short outer chains is called a limit dextrin; hence *limit dextrinosis* is an alternative designation for GSD III. Light microscopic appearance of liver in GSD III is similar to that of GSD I except that GSD III exhibits formation of fibrous septa, more extensive nuclear glycogenosis, and a paucity of intracellular lipid droplets. Hepatic cirrhosis does not usually develop in GSD III; the fibrous septa usually remain stable.

DEFICIENCY OF "BRANCHER" ACTIVITY (GSD IV). This defect is characterized clinically by hepatomegaly and splenomegaly. Progressive portal fibrosis leads to hepatic cirrhosis, ascites, and death in childhood from liver failure. Treatment with corticosteroids may induce temporary remission. Affected children are candidates for liver transplantation.

Hepatic symptoms are associated with reduced rather than increased concentrations of tissue glycogen. The glycogen resembles amylopectin, because it has fewer than the normal number of branch points. This may be the consequence of deficiency of branching enzyme, though one would expect a defect of this enzyme to result in the synthesis of amylose, the glucose polymer with no branch points. The cirrhosis may be the result of the amylopectin-like glycogen, because this glucose polymer is not normally present even transiently in the liver. The limit dextrin of GSD III may not have this effect because it is a transient form normally encountered during synthesis and degradation of glycogen.

DEFICIENCY OF MUSCLE PHOSPHORYLASE (GSD V) (McARDLE SYNDROME). This disorder has a wide clinical spectrum, varying from almost no symptoms to recurrent myoglobinuria, attacks of rhabdomyolysis, and unremitting muscle pain. The muscular pains and cramps after exercise that characterize GSD V can be differentiated from muscle cramps related to more common causes by the ischemic exercise test.

The test requires inflation of a blood pressure cuff on the upper arm to above the arterial pressure. The patient is then asked to squeeze a rubber ball with the hand of the same arm about once every second. The healthy person will easily squeeze 70–110 times, with some discomfort but without cramping of the muscle or residual symptoms after deflation of the blood pressure cuff. In the patient with GSD V, muscle cramps may limit the squeeze to 20–30 movements. When the cuff is released, the cramps persist, with the hand in a tetanic position (wrist bent, fingers extended) that cannot be corrected by the patient or by the examiner. After several minutes there is gradual release of the cramp, but pain may persist for 24–48 hr. In the healthy person, blood samples taken from the antecubital vein of the ischemic arm during exercise show a rise in serum lactate, a rise that does not occur in patients with GSD V because of their inability to produce lactate from glycogen. The diagnosis of GSD V also has been made using magnetic resonance spectroscopy by measuring pH, ATP, and phosphocreatine concentration following both aerobic and ischemic exercise. Molecular diagnosis of DNA from chromosome II reveals characteristic restriction endonuclease mutations; despite genetic heterogeneity, a diagnosis is possible in 90% of cases. A clinical picture consistent with McArdle syndrome, including recurrent rhabdomyolysis, has also occurred in patients with carnitine palmityl transferase deficiency.

Skeletal muscle is without phosphorylase activity. The activity in liver and smooth muscle is normal. The system of phosphorylase activation is intact; patients may have 3 times the normal activity of muscle phosphorylase kinase. Glycogen concentration is increased in muscle but usually not above 4%. Histologically, much of the excessive glycogen is deposited in the cytoplasm beneath the sarcolemma. In patients with phosphorylase deficiency, the energy for muscle contraction can still be provided by glucose entering the myocyte, which may suffice for energy requirements at rest when there are no symptoms. Peak demands for energy, however, which ordinarily are met by supplemental breakdown of muscle glycogen, cannot be satisfied in GSD V because of the phosphorylase defect. The result is pain and cramping during and after exercise, with little or no production of lactic acid. Ischemic exercise tests worsen the situation by interrupting the normal supply of oxygen and glucose.

Treatment includes avoidance of excessive exercise and a high-protein diet.

DEFICIENCY OF LIVER PHOSPHORYLASE (GSD VI). In GSD VI, hepatomegaly may be massive. Otherwise, the affected children are without symptoms and lead normal lives, though there may be some elevation of serum lipids and transaminases (see Table 73–1). Most patients do not have hypoglycemia. The blood glucose concentration does not increase after glucagon administration; this finding can be used to separate GSD VI from GSD IX, in which glucagon tolerance curves are normal. Separation from GSD I also can be made on clinical evidence. The hepatomegaly may recede as the children grow older. Some patients with GSD VI have subtle and unexplained cardiomyopathy.

The low activity of the hepatic phosphorylase system is consistent with but not diagnostic of GSD VI, because low activity may result from a number of defects within the phosphorylase activation system. The diagnosis rests on demonstration of a deficiency in the liver phosphorylase enzyme itself. Leukocyte phosphorylase may also be affected but cannot be relied upon for diagnosis. By light microscopy, formation of fibrous septa is seen in portal areas of the liver. Whether this change remains stationary or progresses to cirrhosis in adulthood is unknown. Phosphorylase activity, glycogen concentration, and histologic appearance are normal in muscle.

DEFICIENCY OF MUSCLE PHOSPHOFRUCTOKINASE (GSD VII). The symptoms of GSD VII resemble those of GSD V, but the muscle pain and cramping after exercise may be more severe. The disease has been tolerated by a young man who plays tennis for pleasure.

Phosphofructokinase is deficient in skeletal muscle but not in the liver; it is only partially defective in erythrocytes. Because this key glycolytic enzyme affects the use of both glycogen and glucose in muscle, it is surprising that the deficiency may cause fewer symptoms than a deficiency in phosphorylase, which affects only the utilization of glycogen. The concentration of glycogen in muscle is moderately elevated, and its distribution is subsarcolemmal, like that observed in GSD V and GSD X.

PROGRESSIVE BRAIN DISEASE AND DEACTIVATED LIVER PHOSPHORYLASE WITHOUT DEMONSTRATED ENZYME DEFECT (GSD VIII). Hepatomegaly without hypoglycemia was apparent soon after birth in one of the four patients in whom the disease has been described. However, the *clinical manifestations,* which are unique for GSD VIII among the glycogenoses and are present in all four patients, are related primarily to the central nervous system (see Table 73–1). The infant may develop nystagmus and rolling of the eyes, ataxia, and truncal tremor. The patient becomes hypotonic and then spastic; spasticity may become severe. Gradually the patient loses rapport with the environment, becomes unresponsive and bedridden, develops swallowing difficulties, and may die of aspiration pneumonia. Urinary excretion of epinephrine and norepinephrine may be increased. The glucagon tolerance test is normal.

Glycogen concentration was increased in hepatic and cerebral biopsies; in muscle, it may be normal or increased. In all patients, electron microscopy of cerebral biopsies revealed increased amounts of glycogen in the form of α particles that are about 10 times wider than the β particles usually found in brain. Liver phosphorylase activity may be low. Cerebral enzymes have not been assayed. The low activity of the hepatic phosphorylase system does not reflect a deficiency of phosphorylase enzyme or of any other enzyme in the hepatic system of phosphorylase activation. This is demonstrated by the normal glucagon tolerance curve and also by the fact that in vivo the phosphorylase activity increases to normal within 2 min after the administration of glucagon or epinephrine to the patient. The low phosphorylase activity observed in a liver specimen obtained before glucagon administration could be increased to normal in vitro by the patient's own liver homogenate. Accordingly, the affected child appears to suffer from impaired control of phosphorylase activation.

DEFICIENCY OF LIVER PHOSPHORYLASE KINASE (GSD IX). This defect occurs in three forms that differ in their pattern of inheritance and tissue distribution. GSD IXa follows an autosomal recessive pattern of inheritance, and GSD IXb is sex-linked recessive. Otherwise, these two forms are indistinguishable. Skeletal muscle is not affected and is normal biochemically (see Table 73–1) and morphologically. In GSD IXc, with autosomal recessive inheritance, the phosphorylase kinase activity of liver and muscle is deficient. Hepatomegaly is massive in early life but recedes as the children grow older; it may disappear completely in teenagers or adults, though the liver can remain somewhat large. Hypoglycemia is unusual. Transaminases are minimally elevated. GSD IX can be classified as a benign hepatomegaly, except in patients who also have defective debrancher activity. Glucagon produces a normal rise in blood glucose concentration that serves to distinguish it from GSD VI, in which the glucagon tolerance curve remains flat. Affected children require no treatment, except perhaps in rare instances of combined deficiencies.

The concentration of liver glycogen is increased and phosphorylase activity is low, as is the case in GSD VI. In GSD IX, however, the low activity of phosphorylase results from a deficiency in phosphorylase kinase. Other enzymes of the activating system, including phosphorylase, are normal. Cultured skin fibroblasts and leukocytes have been reported to be affected but are undependable for diagnosis. The defect persists in adulthood, as demonstrated by rebiopsy of the original patient 25 yr later. In the liver, glycogen remained elevated at 11%, phosphorylase kinase activity was still less than 10% of normal, and some fibrous septa were present.

DEFICIENCY OF CYCLIC 3′5′-AMP-DEPENDENT KINASE (GSD X). The patient with this condition had marked hepatomegaly at 6 yr of age, when the clinical picture was indistinguishable from that of GSD IX except that the blood sugar curve remained flat after intravenous administration of glucagon (see Table 73–1). She had no skeletal muscular symptoms at this time, but 6 yr later she complained of muscular pain, cramping after exercise, and a minimal degree of persistent muscular weakness. The ischemic exercise test was normal, and hepatomegaly was persistent. The patient is doing well without specific therapy.

Liver glycogen concentration was high, and hepatic phosphorylase activity was low. Concentration of glycogen in muscle was increased to 2–4%. Light and electron microscopy showed increased glycogen deposition in liver and skeletal muscle cells. Muscle phosphorylase was present only in the inactive form, whereas normally 60–80% of total phosphorylase is in the active form. GSD X reflects a deficiency in activity of cyclic 3′5′-AMP-dependent kinase. The complete inactivation of muscle phosphorylase in GSD X is clinically well tolerated, whereas the complete lack of muscle phosphorylase in GSD V is characterized by cramps and pains. This difference may be due to the ability of inactive phosphorylase b to degrade glycogen in the presence of adenylic acid (5′-AMP), which is normally found in muscle tissue.

HEPATIC GLYCOGENOSIS WITH STUNTED GROWTH (GSD XI). This disorder is characterized by a greatly enlarged liver and markedly stunted growth (see Table 73–1). Serum transaminase and lipid levels may be elevated. Affected children develop severe hypophosphatemic rickets early in life unless they receive oral phosphate supplementation. Orally administering phosphate alone to the extent necessary for correction of the hypophosphatemia may heal the florid rickets, but adequate growth is not attained through this regimen. The marked rachitic bone changes are due to Fanconi syndrome characterized by urinary loss of phosphate, amino acids, glucose, and galactose that can occur in these children. After puberty the hepatomegaly may recede (although hepatic glycogen concentration remains increased) and the growth rate may increase (although the ultimate body height remains far below normal). However, after puberty the serum phosphate concentration remains normal without supplementation with phosphate.

Glycogen concentration is markedly increased in liver and kidney but normal in muscle. All measured hepatic glycolytic enzyme activities are normal. Administering glucagon does not increase the blood glucose concentration but does increase urinary excretion of cyclic AMP that is usually induced by glucagon administration. Glucose concentration decreases after the oral administration of 1.75 g/kg of galactose, an amount that normally is followed by a significant increase in blood glucose. Conversely, oral administration of an equivalent amount of fructose is followed by the normal increase in blood glucose concentration. On the basis of these findings, it is reasonable to postulate that patients with GSD XI have a functional deficiency of hepatic phosphoglucomutase.

PRENATAL DIAGNOSIS OF GSD

The glycogenoses generally follow an autosomal recessive pattern of inheritance except for GSD IXb, in which inheritance is sex-linked recessive. They should be detectable in the fetus through assay of cultured amniotic fluid cells when these cells normally produce the particular enzyme under study. This criterion is not fulfilled for GSD I because glucose-6-phosphate is not found in normal cultured amniotic fluid cells. Prenatal diagnosis of GSD I is possible by fetal liver biopsy. GSD I, GSD III, GSD VI, GSD IX, and GSD X may not be candidates for prenatal diagnosis because most of the affected children with these conditions lead near-normal lives. In GSD IIa and GSD IV, on the other hand, antenatal diagnosis has been made through assay of cultured amniotic fluid cells. Acid α-glucosidase activity has been present in all amniotic fluid specimens tested, even in GSD IIa. Several weeks may be needed to culture the amniotic fluid cells. Prenatal diagnosis of GSD IIa is feasible within 3 days after amniocentesis through electron microscopic examination of uncultured amniotic fluid cells, which show abnormal intracellular lysosomes that are not present in heterozygous or normal fetuses. These cellular inclusions are also seen by electron microscopy of chorionic villus biopsy specimens in fetal GSD IIa.

73.6 *Deficiency of Xylulose Dehydrogenase*

(Essential Benign Pentosuria)

This benign condition is characterized by a reducing substance in the urine of an otherwise healthy individual. Care should be taken not to mistake the reducing substance for glucose. The pentose in the urine reacts with Clinitest but not with glucose oxidase test papers such as Testape or Clinistix dipsticks.

L-Xylulose dehydrogenase converts L-xylulose (which can arise from D-glucuronate) to xylitol. Xylitol is converted to D-xylulose, which becomes D-xylulose-5-phosphate and enters the pentose phosphate shunt. Deficiency of this enzyme leads to increased concentration of L-xylulose in blood and urine. This rare defect is most common in Jews. No therapy is required.

Pentosuria can be observed in normal individuals if the dietary pentose intake is increased, as with the excessive ingestion of fruit containing pentose. Under these circumstances there may be urinary excretion of xylose and arabinose up to 200 mg/24 hr in normal individuals.

73.7 Deficiency of Acid α-Mannosidase

(Mannosidosis)

The appearance of the patient with mannosidosis is similar to that of a patient with Hurler syndrome (see Chapter 74). The liver and spleen are enlarged in this lysosomal disease; the lymphocytes contain vacuoles. Skeletal roentgenograms reveal structural abnormalities (dysostosis multiplex). Infections are frequent, especially of the middle ear and lungs. There may be corneal or lenticular opacities and psychomotor retardation is usually present. No treatment is available.

Acid α-mannosidase activity is deficient in body fluids and tissues. Mannose-containing macromolecules are stored in the abnormal liver lysosomes, which resemble those characteristic of Hurler syndrome. Mannosidosis exists in heterogeneous forms.

DEFICIENCY OF ACID α-FUCOSIDASE

(Fucosidosis)

See Chapter 72.3.

Baker L, Dahlem S, Goldfarb S, et al: Hyperfiltration and renal disease in glycogen storage disease, type I. Kidney Int 35:1345, 1989.

Beigi B, O'Keefe M, Bowell R, et al: Ophthalmic findings in classical galactosaemia—prospective study. Br J Opthalmol 77:162, 1993.

Bianchi L: Glycogen storage disease I and hepatocellular tumours. Eur J Pediatr 152:S63, 1993.

Carrier H, Maire I, Vial C, et al: Myopathic evolution of an exertional muscle pain syndrome with phosphorylase b kinase deficiency. Acta Neuropathol 81:84, 1990.

Chen Y-T, Cornblath M, Sidbury JB: Cornstarch therapy in type I glycogen storage disease. N Engl J Med 310:171, 1984.

Chen Y-T, Scheinman JI, Coleman RA, et al: Amelioration of proximal renal tubular dysfunction in type I glycogen storage disease with dietary therapy. N Engl J Med 323:590, 1990.

Chen Y-T, Bazzarre CH, Lee MM, et al: Type I glycogen storage disease: Nine years of management with cornstarch. Eur J Pediatr 152:S56, 1993.

Davidson JJ, Ozcelik T, Hamacher C, et al: cDNA cloning of a liver isoform of the phosphorylase kinase α subunit and mapping of the gene to Xp22.2-p22.1, the region of human X-linked liver glycogenosis. Proc Natl Acad Sci USA 89:2096, 1992.

Demaugre F, Bonnefonte J-P, Colonna M, et al: Infantile form of carnitine palmitoyl transferase II deficiency with hepatomuscular symptoms and sudden death. J Clin Invest 87:859, 1991.

DeVivo DC, Haymond MW, Obert KA, et al: Defective activation of the pyruvate dehydrogenase complex in subacute necrotizing encephalomyelopathy (Leigh disease). Ann Neurol 6:483, 1979.

Ding J-A, de Barsy T, Brown BI, et al: Immunoblot analyses of glycogen debranching enzyme in different subtypes of glycogen storage disease type III. J Pediatr 116:95, 1990.

Elleder M, Shin YS, Zuntova A, et al: Fatal infantile hypertrophic cardiomyopathy secondary to deficiency of heart specific phosphorylase b kinase. Virchows Arch A Pathol Anat Histopathol 423:303, 1993.

Garibaldi LR, Canini S, Suporti-Furga A, et al: Galactosemia caused by generalized uridine disphosphate galactose-4-epimerase deficiency. J Pediatr 103:927, 1983.

Gitzelmann R, Steinmann B, Mitchell B, et al: Uridine diphosphate galactose 4'-epimerase deficiency. IV. Report of eight cases in three families. Helv Paediatr Acta 31:441, 1976.

Harris RE, Hannon D, Vogler C, et al: Bone marrow transplantation in type IIa glycogen storage disease. Birth Defects, Original Article Series 22:119, 1986.

Hendrickx J, Coucke P, Bossuyt P, et al: X-linked liver glycogenesis: localization and isolation of a candidate gene. Hum Mol Genet 2:583, 1993.

Hofnaegel D, Worster-Hill D, Child EL: Ovarian failure in galactosaemia. Lancet 2:1197, 1979.

Holton JB, Leonard JV: Clouds still gathering over galactosaemia. Lancet 344:1242, 1994.

Hug G, Chuck G, Walling L, et al: Liver phosphorylase deficiency in glycogenosis type VI: Documentation by biochemical analysis of hepatic biopsy specimens. J Lab Clin Med 84:26, 1974.

Hug G, Soukup S, Ryan M, Chuck G: Rapid prenatal diagnosis of glycogen storage disease type II by electron microscopy of uncultured amniotic-fluid cells. N Engl J Med 310:1018, 1984.

Hug G, Chuck G, Chen Y-T, et al: Chorionic villus ultrastructure in type II glycogen storage disease (Pompe's disease). N Engl J Med 324:342, 1991.

Hug G, Soukup S, Berry H, and Bove K: Carnitine palmitoyl transferase (CPT): Deficiency of CPT II but not of CPT I with reduced total and free carnitine but increased acylcarnitine. Pediatr Res 25:115A, 1989.

Kilimann MW: Molecular genetics of phosphorylase kinase: cDNA cloning, chromosomal mapping and isoform structure. J Inherit Metab Dis 13:435, 1990.

Kornfeld M, LeBaron M: Glycogenosis type VIII. J Neuropathol Exp Neurol 43:568, 1984.

Kristjansson K, Tsujino S, DiMauro S, et al: Myophosphorylase deficiency: An unusually severe form with myoglobinuria. J Pediatr 125:409, 1994.

Lin H-C, Kirby LT, Ng WG, et al: On the molecular nature of the Duarte variant of galactose-1-phosphate uridyl transferase (GALT). Hum Genet 93:167, 1994.

Maire I, Baussan C, Moatti N, et al: Biochemical diagnosis of hepatic glycogen storage diseases: 20 years French experience. Clin Biochem 24:169, 1991.

Malatack JJ, Iwatsuki S, Gartner JC, et al: Liver transplantation for type I glycogen storage disease. Lancet 1:1073, 1983.

Moses SW: Muscle glycogenosis. J Inherit Metab Dis 13:452, 1990.

Moses SW: Pathophysiology and dietary treatment of the glycogen storage diseases. J Pediatr Gastroenterol Nutr 11:155, 1990.

Obara K, Saito T, Sato H, et al: Renal histology in two adult patients with type I glycogen storage disease. Clin Nephrol 39:59, 1993.

Poe R, Snover DC: Adenomas in glycogen storage disease type I. Two cases with unusual histologic features. Am J Surg Pathol 12:477, 1988.

Ratner-Kaufman F, Loro ML, Azen C, et al: Effect of hypogonadism and deficient calcium intake on bone density in patients with galactosemia. J Pediatr 123:365, 1993.

Ratner-Kaufman F, Reichardt JKV, Ng WG, et al: Correlation of cognitive, neurologic, and ovarian outcome with the Q188R mutation of the galactose-1-phosphate uridyltransferase gene. J Pediatr 125:225, 1994.

Reichardt JKV, Levy HL, Woo SLC: Molecular characterization of two galactosemia mutations and one polymorphism: Implications for structure-function analysis of human galactose-1-phosphate uridyltransferase. Biochemistry 31:5430, 1992.

Reitsma-Bierens WCC: Renal complications in glycogen storage disease type I. Eur J Pediatr 152:S60, 1993.

Restaino I, Kaplan BS, Stanley C, et al: Nephrolithiasis, hypocitraturia, and a distal renal tubular acidification defect in type 1 glycogen storage disease. J Pediatr 122:392, 1993.

Schweitzer S, Shin Y, Jakobs C, et al: Long-term outcome in 134 patients with galactosaemia. Eur J Pediatr 152:36, 1993.

Slonim AE, Goans PJ: Myopathy in McArdle's syndrome: Improvement with a high-protein diet. N Engl J Med 312:355, 1985.

Smit GPA, Fernandes J, Leonard JV, et al: The long-term outcome of patients with glycogen storage diseases. J Inherit Metab Dis 13:411, 1990.

Towfighi J, Yoss BS, Wasiewski WW, et al: Cerebral glycogenosis, alpha particle type: Morphologic and biochemical observations in an infant. Hum Pathol 20:1210, 1989.

Treem WR, Stanley CA, Fingeold DN, et al: Primary carnitine deficiency due to a failure of carnitine transport in kidney, muscle, and fibroblasts. N Engl J Med 319:1331, 1989.

Tsujino S, Shanske S, DiMauro S: Molecular genetic heterogeneity of myophosphorylase deficiency (McArdle's disease). N Engl J Med 329:241, 1993.

Verani R, Bernstein J: Renal glomerular and tubular abnormalities in glycogen storage disease type I. Arch Pathol Lab Med 112:271, 1988.

Waggoner DD, Buist NRM, Donnell GN: Long-term prognosis in galactosaemia: Results of a survey of 350 cases. J Inherit Metab Dis 13:802, 1990.

Willems PJ, Gerver WJM, Berger R, et al: The natural history of liver glycogenosis due to phosphorylase kinase deficiency: a longitudinal study of 41 patients. Eur J Pediatr 149:268, 1990.

Willems PJ, Hendrickx J, Van Der Auwera BJ, et al: Mapping of the gene for X-linked liver glycogenosis due to phosphorylase kinase deficiency to human chromosome region Xp22. Genomics 9:565, 1991.

Wolfsdorf JI, Ehrlich S, Landy HS, et al: Optimal daytime feeding regimen to prevent postprandial hypoglycemia in type 1 glycogen storage disease. Am J Clin Nutr 56:587, 1992.

CHAPTER 74
Disorders of Mucopolysaccharide Metabolism

Reuben K. Matalon

The mucopolysaccharidoses are a group of inherited disorders caused by incomplete degradation and storage of acid mucopolysaccharides (glycosaminoglycans). The clinical manifestations result from the accumulation of mucopolysaccharides in various organs. Specific degradative lysosomal enzyme deficiencies have been identified for all the mucopolysaccharidoses.

The mucopolysaccharides are polyanionic polymers, most of which contain alternating carbohydrate residues of *N*-acetylhexosamine and uronic acid. Although the acid mucopolysaccharides are closely related as a group, individual compounds differ in their distribution in body tissues. Dermatan sulfate, heparan sulfate, and keratan sulfate are the major mucopolysaccharides involved in the pathogenesis of the mucopolysaccharidoses. The structural differences of the mucopolysaccharides explain the need for various lysosomal enzymes required for their degradation.

Because the mucopolysaccharides are major components of the intercellular substance of connective tissue, bony changes are characteristic of the mucopolysaccharidoses. The skeletal deformities seen in roentgenograms are referred to as *dysostosis multiplex.* The central nervous system also may be affected, leading to progressive mental retardation. In addition, the cardiovascular system, liver, spleen, tendons, joints, and skin may be involved. The degree of disability and overall prognosis in each of the mucopolysaccharidoses are determined by the extent of the physical and mental involvement.

The mucopolysaccharidoses follow an autosomal recessive mode of inheritance, with the exception of Hunter syndrome, which is inherited as an X-linked recessive trait. They are suspected on the basis of clinical and radiologic manifestations, and the diagnosis is confirmed by the finding of increased urinary excretion of mucopolysaccharides and deficiency of a specific enzyme.

HURLER SYNDROME (MPS IH). This syndrome is the most severe of the mucopolysaccharidoses. Its relentless progression usually results in death by the early teenage years.

Etiology and Pathology. The basic defect in Hurler disease is a deficiency of α-L-iduronidase, which leads to accumulation of the dermatan and heparan sulfates in tissues and their urinary excretion. Almost every tissue in the body is affected, with widespread occurrence of vacuolated, or "gargoyle," cells, which contain lysosomes engorged with mucopolysaccharide. In the brain, lipid storage also occurs with the mucopolysaccharide accumulation. There is unusual hyalinization of collagen and separation of the collagen bundles. These changes lead to joint deformities and stiffness, thickened meninges, hydrocephalus, peripheral nerve compression, and a tendency to develop hernias. As the disease progresses, narrowing of the coronary arteries, thickening of the cardiac valves and endocardium, and stiffening of the myocardium may lead to congestive heart failure. The constricted thorax contributes to the clinical deterioration of these patients.

Clinical Manifestations. Infants with Hurler syndrome appear normal at birth, and during the 1st yr of life only slight developmental delays are noted. Physical examination, however, reveals hepatosplenomegaly, exaggerated kyphosis, persistent nasal discharge, and noisy breathing. The facial features become progressively coarser after the 1st yr of life (Fig. 74–1). The head is large and dolichocephalic, with frontal bossing and prominent sagittal and metopic sutures. The bridge of the nose is depressed, and the nose is broad and flat. Clouding of the corneas becomes evident at about 1 yr of age. Umbilical and inguinal hernias are common. Children afflicted with this disease regress developmentally, and mental retardation becomes obvious. The downhill course continues rapidly after the 2nd or 3rd yr of life. These children become immobile, their joints become progressively stiff and contracted, and they usually die by their early teens.

Roentgenographic Changes. Roentgenograms of patients with Hurler syndrome reveal dysostosis multiplex, which includes a large dolichocephalic skull and thickened calvarium. There may be hyperostosis of the cranium, and the sella turcica may be boot or J shaped. The medial third of the clavicle is thickened. The vertebral bodies are ovoid in the lower thorax and upper lumbar regions. They develop beaklike projections on their lower anterior margins, while their upper portions remain hypoplastic (Fig. 74–2). This results in the gibbus deformity commonly seen in these patients. The ribs are spatulated or oar shaped, and the pelvis shows flaring of the iliac bones, with shallow acetabulae. Roentgenograms of the hips show progressive coxa valga deformity, sometimes resembling the findings of aseptic necrosis. Roentgenograms of the hands show tapering of the terminal phalanges and widening at the distal ends and tapering at the proximal ends of the metacarpals. The 5th metacarpal is the first to show these changes (Fig. 74–3). In the long bones, particularly those of the upper extremities, irregular widenings associated with areas of cortical thinning and expansion of the medullary cavity are seen. Occasionally, there may be cortical thickening. The radius curves toward the ulna, and the articular surfaces of the radius and the ulna face one another, forming a V (see Fig. 74–3). The humerus may be angulated, and the glenoid fossa, like the acetabulum, may be shallow. Severe growth retardation is common in these children.

Diagnosis. The diagnosis of Hurler syndrome is suggested by

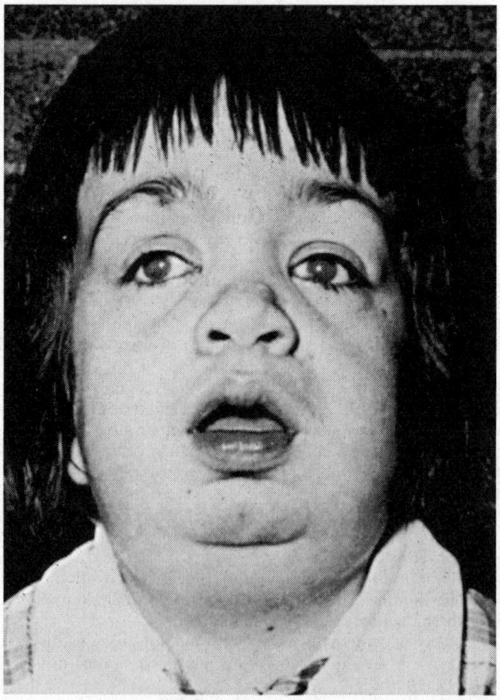

Figure 74–1. Typical appearance of a patient with Hurler syndrome.

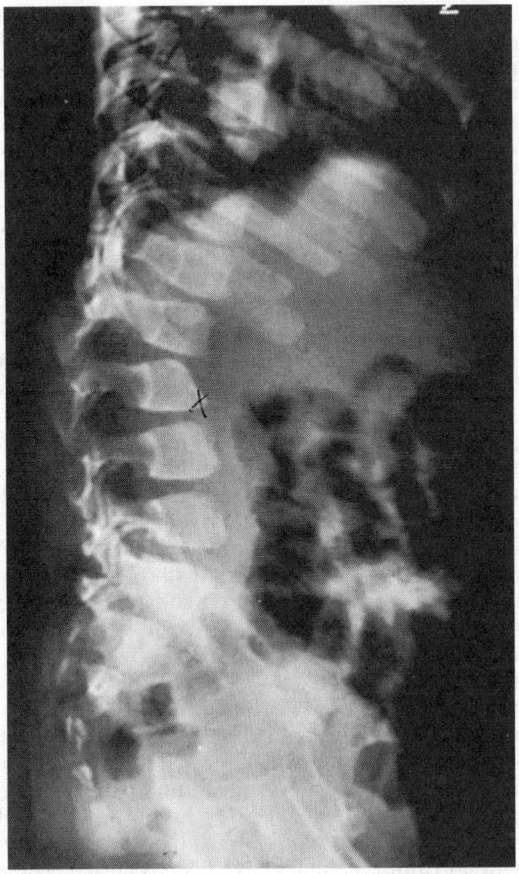

Figure 74–2. Lateral spine roentgenogram of a patient with Hurler syndrome.

the presence of the relevant clinical and roentgenographic findings. Urinary excretion of dermatan and heparan sulfates provides further support. Although there are helpful screening methods for quantifying the mucopolysaccharides in the urine, definitive diagnosis requires detection of α-L-iduronidase deficiency in white blood cells, serum, or cultured skin fibroblasts.

Genetics. Hurler disease is an autosomal recessive disorder. The human α-L-iduronidase cDNA and gene have been isolated, and the genomic organization has been elucidated. The coding sequence for α-L-iduronidase comprises 14 exons. Chromosomal localization of the iduronidase gene has been assigned to the short arm of chromosome 4 (4p16.3), distal to the Huntington disease region. Many mutations of the iduronidase gene have been described. It appears that the phenotypes Hurler-Scheie and Scheie syndromes represent milder mutations on the iduronidase gene. The most frequent mutations associated with Hurler disease, which is the severe phenotype, include substitution of the amino acid tryptophan with a stop codon in position 402. Another stop codon mutation involves the substitution of glutamine in position 70. These are nonsense mutations leading to a nonfunctional enzyme. Other mis-sense, nonsense, insertional deletions, and duplications of coding regions have been described in the severe phenotype of Hurler disease. The multitude of mutations in the iduronidase gene are responsible for the phenotype variability of α-L-iduronidase deficiency.

SCHEIE SYNDROME (MPS IS). This syndrome is the mildest of the mucopolysaccharidoses. It is a distinct clinical and genetic entity; the enzyme deficiency, α-L-iduronidase, is the same as in Hurler syndrome but is specific for dermatan sulfate, which accumulates in tissues and is excreted in excessive amounts in urine.

Clinical Manifestations. Patients with this disease have normal intelligence, mild facial coarsening with striking prognathism, joint stiffness typified by claw hands, and carpal tunnel syndrome. Corneal clouding is a constant feature that leads to loss of visual acuity. Aortic regurgitation is common. The clinical features do not appear until after 5 yr of age, and the disease is compatible with close-to-normal life expectancy. The patient with Scheie syndrome reaches normal height.

Roentgenographic Changes. Findings on roentgenography include mild dysostosis multiplex, without the vertebral changes or the gibbus deformity seen in Hurler disease. There is coxa valga and slight radial and ulnar obliquity with V formation of their articular surfaces.

Diagnosis. Early clinical diagnosis is more difficult in Scheie than in Hurler syndrome because the somatic changes are mild and mental retardation is not present. Detection of urinary dermatan sulfate is helpful, but the diagnosis is confirmed by demonstrating a deficiency of α-L-iduronidase in white blood cells or in cultured skin fibroblasts.

Genetics. Scheie syndrome is the mildest form of iduronidase deficiency diseases. Examples of mutations that lead to a mild form of iduronidase deficiency are substitution of arginine in position 89 for glutamine (R89Q) and an intronic mutation in nucleotide position 678. It is possible, by using molecular tools, to correlate the phenotype of iduronidase deficiency with the genotype.

HURLER-SCHEIE SYNDROME (MPS IH/IS). Few reports exist of patients with this syndrome.

Etiology. The basic defect is α-L-iduronidase deficiency specific for dermatan sulfate, which is excreted in urine and stored in

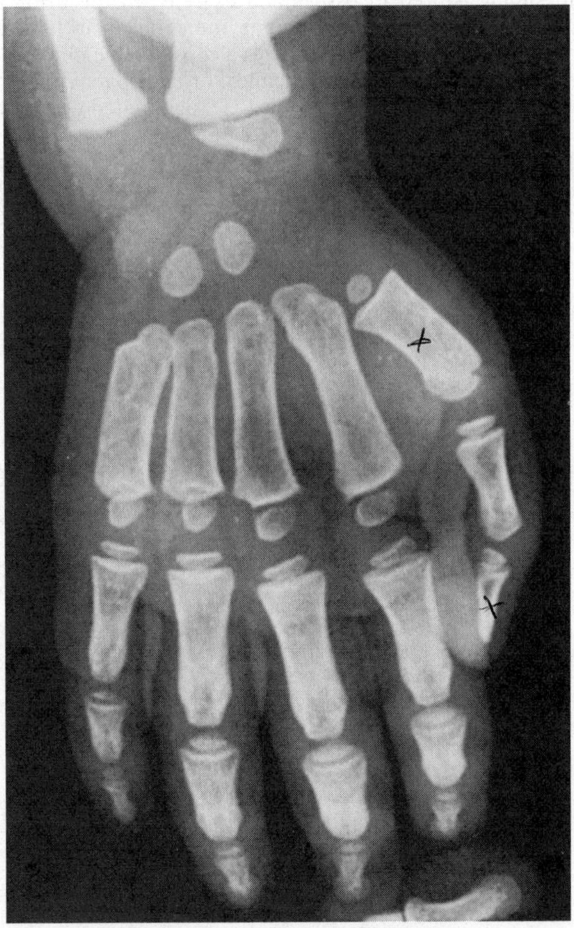

Figure 74–3. Roentgenogram of the hand of a patient with Hurler syndrome.

the liver, spleen, and other tissues. It has been suggested that the Hurler-Scheie syndrome is a genetic compound of two recessive genes, analogous to hemoglobin SC disease, but recent work indicates it is best explained as an allelic mutation of the iduronidase gene.

Clinical Manifestations. Patients develop mild coarseness of facial features, corneal clouding, shortness of stature, joint contractures, hepatosplenomegaly, hernias, and cardiac valvular lesions, primarily mitral insufficiency (Fig. 74–4). Mental development is normal. The clinical features, which usually develop in the first 2 yr of life and in early childhood, are often mistaken for manifestations of a variety of skeletal defects causing growth retardation. The disease is compatible with long life.

Roentgenographic Features. Roentgenograms of patients with this syndrome reveal severe dysostosis multiplex with findings identical to those seen in Hurler syndrome, except that there is no gibbus.

Diagnosis. Diagnosis is based upon the findings of dermatan sulfate in the urine and α-L-iduronidase deficiency. The clinical pattern of onset of joint involvement and the severity of skeletal deformities distinguish Hurler-Scheie from Scheie disease.

Genetics. The cloning and the elucidation of mutations on the iduronidase gene indicate that the Hurler-Scheie form is caused by mutations with moderate phenotype severity. The mutation R89Q, in which arginine is substituted for glutamine, which causes Scheie syndrome, can under certain circumstances lead to the intermediate phenotype, Hurler-Scheie.

HUNTER SYNDROME (MPS II). This syndrome is the only X-linked disorder among the mucopolysaccharidoses. It is milder than Hurler syndrome with respect to the skeletal and mental defects, although the mucopolysaccharides, dermatan and heparan sulfate, stored in tissues and excreted in the urine are similar in the two diseases. The enzyme deficient in tissues is iduronosulfate sulfatase, but there is a considerable phenotypic heterogeneity; there is no biochemical or enzymatic difference between the severe form of the disease, designated *type A*, and the mild disease, *type B*.

Type A. This is the "classic" form of Hunter syndrome. Coarseness of facial features, short stature, joint stiffness, hepatosplenomegaly, and hernias are common clinical manifestations.

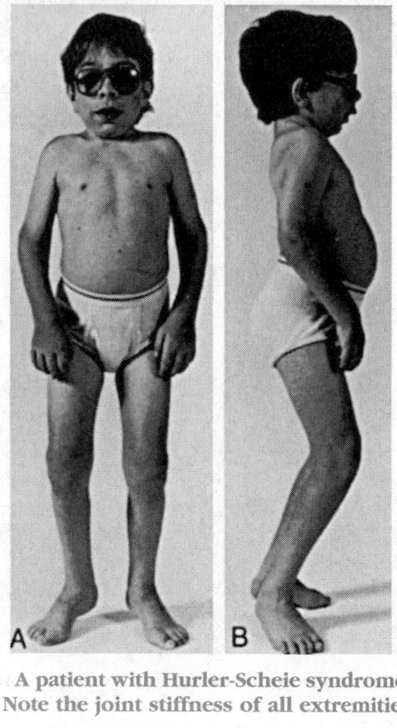

Figure 74–4. A patient with Hurler-Scheie syndrome with normal intelligence. Note the joint stiffness of all extremities.

Mental retardation is severe. Progression of the disease process is slower and the dysostosis multiplex is milder than in Hurler syndrome. Corneal clouding is usually absent, but hearing loss is very common. Skin changes also are frequent, including small raised papules over the skin of the shoulders, the scapulas, and the lower back. Cardiac involvement often occurs. Patients usually do not have gibbus deformity, although mild kyphosis may be present in some. Life expectancy for these patients usually extends into the late teens or early 20s.

Type B. This syndrome is a milder disease than type A, even though the enzyme deficiency and urinary mucopolysaccharides are the same. Retardation is usually lacking or very minimal. The physical features are similar to, but milder than, those in type A, and patients have a longer life expectancy. Airway obstruction caused by mucopolysaccharide accumulation in the trachea and bronchi is a complicating feature of type B.

Diagnosis. The physical features, dysostosis multiplex, and dermatan and heparan sulfaturia suggest either Hurler or Hunter syndrome, but sex-linked inheritance is specific to the latter. Enzyme studies showing iduronosulfate sulfatase deficiency in serum, white blood cells, or cultured fibroblasts confirm the diagnosis of Hunter syndrome. Other sulfatases should be examined, since multiple sulfatase deficiency can be confused with Hunter syndrome.

Genetics. Hunter syndrome is an X-linked disease. The cDNA for iduronosulfatase has been cloned, and the gene has been localized to the Xq28 region close to the fragile X site. The gene for iduronosulfatase is coded for by nine exons. Southern blot analyses of genomic DNA from Hunter patients show that many patients have gross deletions in the iduronosulfatase gene. More than a dozen mutations in the human iduronosulfatase gene in Hunter patients have been reported. These mutations vary from being point mutations to small insertion or deletions in the coding region of the iduronosulfatase gene. There may be a correlation in the nature of mutation and the phenotype observed in patients. For example, patients showing a major change in the gene, such as an insertion of 22 base pairs (nucleotide 1129), are severely affected, type A. Patients with deletions are also severely affected, while patients with point mutations may have a mild phenotype, type B. An example of a mutation causing mild Hunter phenotype is the substitution of lysine for arginine in position 135.

SANFILIPPO SYNDROME (MPS III). This syndrome is a distinct entity and is based on clinical findings and excessive urinary excretion of exclusively heparan sulfate. The coarse facial appearance and skeletal involvement are milder than those seen in the Hurler and Hunter syndromes. There are four enzymatic variants, distinct deficiencies all leading to the same phenotype and mucopolysacchariduria. Heparan sulfate is stored in tissues, and its accumulation is responsible for the neuronal damage and atrophy underlying the profound mental retardation associated with the disease.

Clinical Manifestations. The clinical features of the Sanfilippo syndrome in early life are not very striking. Affected children have delayed developmental milestones and are usually very hyperactive. By the end of the 1st decade there is rapid neurologic deterioration; their gait becomes unsteady, and they become bedridden. Most of the children die in their middle teens. Mental retardation, some joint stiffening, hepatosplenomegaly, hernias, and dysostosis multiplex are common, but dwarfism and corneal clouding are rare.

Patients manifest dysostosis multiplex typical of the mucopolysaccharidoses. The large bones are not as severely involved; the obliquity of the radius and ulna and the tapering of the proximal ends of the metacarpals are very mild.

Diagnosis. Sanfilippo syndrome should be considered in the presence of heparan sulfaturia, hepatosplenomegaly, mental retardation, and dysostosis multiplex. Screening tests for urinary mucopolysaccharides usually give positive results but not as consistently as in the Hurler or Hunter syndrome. The different enzymatic variants can be confirmed by specific enzyme assays provided by special laboratories.

Sanfilippo A Syndrome (MPS III A). Sulfamidase is deficient in this disease and can be assayed using cultured skin fibroblasts or peripheral blood leukocytes. This enzyme is specific for the hydrolysis of the sulfate linked to the amino groups of glucosamine.

Sanfilippo B Syndrome (MPS III B). This form is characterized by α-*N*-acetylhexosaminidase deficiency and can be assayed on serum, white blood cells, or cultured skin fibroblasts. This enzyme is required for the hydrolysis of *N*-acetylglucosamine residues from heparan sulfate.

Sanfilippo C Syndrome (MPS III C). This syndrome is caused by a deficiency of acetyl CoA:α-glucosaminide *N*-acetyltransferase. This enzyme catalyzes the acetylation of the free glucosamine on the polysaccharide terminus. The assay requires cultured fibroblasts or white blood cells.

Sanfilippo D Syndrome (MPS III D). This deficiency of *N*-acetylglucosamine-6-sulfatase is specific for heparan sulfate. The enzyme is assayed using a substrate prepared from heparin.

Genetics. All four Sanfilippo syndromes are autosomal recessive disorders caused by four different enzyme defects. The enzymes are involved in the degradation of heparan sulfate. Therefore, the phenotypes are similar because of the accumulation of heparan sulfate. Cloning of cDNA for glucosamine-6-sulfatase, which is deficient in Sanfilippo D, has been achieved. The sequence analysis of the cDNA has revealed a strong homology with steroid sulfatase as well as with other cloned sulfatases. This gene has been localized to the long arm of chromosome 12 (12q14). The genes for the three other enzymes have not been cloned.

MORQUIO SYNDROME (MPS IV). This disorder is characterized by keratan sulfaturia and skeletal dysplasia. Keratan sulfate is stored in tissues together with chondroitin-6-sulfate. The keratan sulfaturia may decrease with age, but it is always above the normal range. There are two enzyme defects that lead to identical phenotypes in this syndrome.

Clinical Manifestations. The syndrome is associated with severe somatic manifestations and lack of mental involvement. At birth it may not be recognized. Joint laxity and shortness of stature first appear at about 1 yr of age. Skeletal abnormalities include flat vertebrae (platyspondyly universalis), short neck, genu valgum, flat feet, large and unstable knee joints, large elbow joints, and large wrists with ulnar deviation. The platyspondyly leads to short trunk and short stature. The odontoid process is underdeveloped; early on, this may cause atlantoaxial subluxation or translocation, with spinal cord compression. Corneal clouding also may be apparent at an early age. There is midface hypoplasia with a depressed nasal bridge and protrusion of the mandible, which give these patients a permanent grin. Hepatosplenomegaly is not as pronounced as in the other mucopolysaccharidoses, but it is usually present. Cardiac manifestations are secondary to respiratory failure caused by kyphoscoliosis and restricted chest movements, although aortic regurgitation may complicate the Morquio syndrome. Teeth are severely affected and have very thin enamel. Hearing loss may result from recurrent otitis media. Variation in the clinical manifestations is common, and very mild cases may be encountered. Patients usually die in their 3rd or 4th decade of life from cor pulmonale caused by the severe abnormalities of the chest and spine.

Roentgenographic Changes. In the 1st yr of life, roentgenograms may reveal only mild changes in patients with Morquio syndrome. The vertebral bodies show height loss and anterior tonguelike projections. At 2 yr the platyspondyly becomes evident. The hypoplasia of the odontoid process can be clearly seen in tomographic studies. The skull and sella turcica are mildly involved. The long bones are shortened, and the metaphyses appear irregular. There is progressive distortion of the epiphyseal metaphyseal plates. The pelvis shows wide acetabulae with progressive subluxation or dislocation of the femoral heads. The metacarpal bones are short and wide with conical tapering of their proximal ends. The distal ends of the radius and ulna face one another, similar to the obliquity seen in other mucopolysaccharidoses. These changes, especially the coxa valga and the changes in the wrists and lumbar spine, should differentiate Morquio syndrome from other skeletal dysplasias.

Diagnosis. The spondyloepiphyseal dysplasias may mimic the signs of Morquio syndrome both clinically and roentgenographically. Screening tests for acid mucopolysaccharides in the urine of these patients can be negative; therefore, quantitative rather than qualitative isolation methods are preferred. The urinary finding of keratan sulfaturia, moreover, is also found in the Kneist syndrome. Therefore, enzyme determinations are essential for differentiating Morquio syndrome from other conditions. There are two enzyme deficiencies:

MORQUIO SYNDROME, TYPE A (MPS IV A). This syndrome is caused by a deficiency of *N*-acetylgalactosamine-6-sulfate sulfatase, an enzyme that also degrades galactose-6-sulfate.

MORQUIO SYNDROME, TYPE B (MPS IV B). In this syndrome β-galactosidase is deficient. An important clinical difference between the two syndromes is the lack of enamel hypoplasia in type B. In other respects, including roentgenograms of the spine, the two forms may be indistinguishable. Morquio syndrome type B should not be confused with GM_1 gangliosidosis, which also is associated with β-galactosidase deficiency but resembles Hurler syndrome clinically.

Genetics. The two forms of Morquio syndrome are autosomal recessive. Galactosamine-6-sulfate sulfatase, the enzyme that hydrolyzes sulfate from galactose-6-sulfate and galactosamine-6-sulfate, has been purified and found to be specific for the galactose-galactosamine configuration. Deficiency of this enzyme leads to Morquio type A and to the accumulation in tissues and excretion in urine of keratan sulfate and chondroitin-6-sulfate. A full-length cDNA clone for *N*-acetylgalactosamine-6-sulfatase has been isolated and expressed in deficient fibroblasts. The gene has been localized to the long arm of chromosome 16 (16q24.3). Two different mutations in the coding sequence have been reported in Morquio type A patients. In one patient with severe clinical phenotype, a 2 bp deletion (1342delCA) was observed that would shift the reading frame. In another instance, two probands with a mild clinical phenotype had a point mutation, creating a missense mutation substituting asparagine for lysine in position 204. Thus there seems to be a correlation of clinical phenotype with the nature of the coding sequence mutation.

β-Galactosidase is also required for the sequential degradation of keratan sulfate. Deficiency of this enzyme leads to Morquio type B. The cDNA clone for β-galactosidase has been isolated and characterized. Several point mutations have been reported in the β-galactosidase gene. The gene has been assigned to the short arm of chromosome 3 (3p21.33). β-Galactosidase deficiency can also be caused by a protective protein. This disease causes deficiency of sialidase and β-galactosidase (mucolipidosis I).

KERATAN AND HEPARAN SULFATURIA (MPS VIII). A single case of this unusual form of mucopolysacchariduria has been described. The patient was a boy who was noted to have developmental delay at 18 mo of age. At 2 1/2 yr he was severely retarded, bedridden, and blind. He had scaphocephaly and mild pectus excavatum but no organomegaly; corneal clouding was not noted. Roentgenographic studies showed dysostosis multiplex without the platyspondyly seen in Morquio syndrome.

Urinary studies showed excessive excretion of both keratan and heparan sulfates. Enzymatic assays revealed normal activ-

acetylgalactosamine-6-sulfate sulfatase (GALNS) gene to chromosome 16q24. Genomics 16:777, 1993.
Matalon R, Arbogast B, Justice P, et al: Morquio's syndrome: Deficiency of a chondroitin sulfate *N*-acetyl-hexosamine sulfate sulfatase. Biochem Biophys Res Commun 61:759, 1974.
Matalon R, Deanching M, Omura K: Hurler, Scheie and Hurler-Scheie 'compound' residual activity of alpha-L-iduronidase toward natural substrates suggesting allelic mutations. J Inherit Metab Dis 6:133, 1983.
Matalon R, Dorfman A: Sanfilippo A syndrome: Sulfamidase deficiency in cultured skin fibroblasts and liver. J Clin Invest 54:907, 1974.
Matalon R, Kaul R, Michals K: The mucopolysaccharidoses and the mucolipidoses. *In:* Rosenberg R, Prusiner S, DiMauro S, Bachi R, Kunkel L (eds) The Molecular and Genetic Basis of Neurological Disease. Boston, MA, Butterworth-Heinemann, 1993, pp 401–419.
McDowell GA, Cowman TM, Blitzer MG, et al: Intrafamilial variability in Hurler syndrome and Sanfilippo syndrome type A: Implications for evaluation of new therapies. Am J Med Genet 47:1092, 1993.
Miller RD, Hoffman JW, Powell PP, et al: Cloning and characterization of beta-glucuronidase gene. Genomics 7:280, 1990.
Neufeld EF, Muenzer J: The mucopolysaccharidoses. *In:* Scriver CR, Beaudet AL, Sly WS, Valle D (eds): The Metabolic Basis of Inherited Disease, Vol II, 6th ed. New York, McGraw-Hill, pp 1565–1587, 1989.
Oshima A, Kyle JW, Miller RD, et al: Cloning, sequencing and expression of cDNA for human beta-glucuronidase. Proc Natl Acad Sci 84:685, 1986.
Oshima A, Tsuji A, Nagao Y, et al: Cloning, sequencing and expression of cDNA for human beta-galactosidase. Biochem Biophys Res Commun 157:238, 1988.
Peters C, Schmidt B, Rommerskirch W, et al: Phylogenetic conservation of arylsulfatases. cDNA cloning and expression of human arylsulfatase B. J Biol Chem 265:3374, 1990.
Powell PP, Kyle JW, Miller RD, et al: Rat liver beta-glucuronidase. cDNA cloning, sequence comparisons and expression of a chimeric protein in COS cells. Biochem J 250:547, 1988.
Schuchman EH, Jackson CE, Desnick RJ: Human arylsulfatase B: MOPAC cloning, nucleotide sequence of a full length cDNA, and regions of amino acid identity with arylsulfatases A and C. Genomics 6:149, 1990.
Suzuki Y, Oshima A: A β-galactosidase gene mutation identified in the Morquio B disease and infantile Gm1 gangliosidosis. Hum Genet 91:407, 1993.
Tieu PT, Menon K, Neufeld EF: A mutant stop codon (TAG) in the IDUA gene is used as an acceptor splice site in a patient with Hurler syndrome (MPS IH). Hum Mutat 3:333, 1994.
Tomatsu SS, Fukuda M, Masue K, et al: Morquio disease: isolation, characterization and expression of full-length cDNA for human N-acetylgalactosamine-6-sulfate sulfatase. Biochem Biophys Res Commun 181:677, 1991.
Wehnert M, Hopwood JJ, Schroder W, et al: Structural gene aberrations in mucopolysaccharidosis II (Hunter). Hum Genet 89:430, 1992.
Wilson PJ, Morris CP, Anson DS, et al: Hunter syndrome: Isolation of an iduronate-2-sulfatase cDNA clone and analysis of patient DNA. Proc Natl Acad Sci 87:8531, 1990.
Yoshida K, Oshima A, Shimmoto M, et al: β-Galactosidase gene mutations in G_{M1}-gangliosidase: a common mutation among Japanese adult/chronic cases. Am J Hum Genet 49:435, 1991.

74.1 Mucolipidoses

Reuben K. Matalon

Patients with mucolipidoses exhibit clinical features of both lipidoses and mucopolysaccharidoses (see Chapter 72.3). Despite their name, there is little evidence of true storage of lipids or mucopolysaccharides in the organs of affected patients. Technically, fucosidosis, GM_1 gangliosidosis, and multiple sulfatase deficiency are mucolipidoses because there is evidence of storage both of lipids (as glycosphingolipids) and of glycosaminoglycans in various organs. All of the mucolipidoses are inherited as autosomal recessive traits. There is no specific treatment for these disorders.

MUCOLIPIDOSIS (ML-I), LIPOMUCOPOLYSACCHARIDOSIS, OR SIALIDOSIS TYPE 2 (INFANTILE ONSET). This disease produces symptoms in the 1st yr of life. There are Hurler-like features, with dysostosis multiplex, moderate mental retardation, visceromegaly, corneal clouding, cherry-red spot, seizures, vacuolated lymphocytes, and coarse fibroblast inclusions, but no mucopolysacchariduria. Some of these children may appear relatively normal at birth, but all patients develop progressive severe clinical manifestations. There is also a congenital type 2 form characterized by hydrops fetalis and neonatal ascites, hepatosplenomegaly, stippling of the epiphyses, periosteal cloaking, and stillbirth or death during infancy. These patients (infantile and congenital) have an isolated neuraminidase deficiency. There is, in addition, a "juvenile" type 2 form of sialidosis (ML-1), sometimes designated *galactosialidosis,* which is characterized by primary β-galactosialidase deficiency as well as neuraminidase deficiency. In these patients clinical manifestations may begin at any time from infancy to adulthood. In early infancy there may be a phenotype similar to that of GM_1 gangliosidosis with edema, ascites, skeletal dysplasia, and cherry-red spot. Later, the main features are dysostosis multiplex, visceromegaly, mental retardation, dysmorphism, corneal clouding, progressive neurologic deterioration, and bilateral cherry-red spots. The storage compounds in this disorder are predominantly sialylated oligosaccharides similar to those excreted by children with other types of sialidoses.

Sialidosis type 1 is distinguished from type 2 by the cherry-red spot–myoclonus phenotype and the absence of somatic features such as coarse facies and dysostosis multiplex. The age of onset is variable, but usually the disorder occurs in the 2nd decade of life.

Sialidosis types 1 and 2 result from inherited deficiencies of neuraminidase, of which there are at least two forms. Sialic acid terminal oligosaccharides and sialylglycopeptides are excreted in large amounts in the urine. Kupffer cells and hepatocytes are vacuolated, and sural nerve biopsy reveals metachromatic myelin degeneration. These patients are deficient in glycoprotein sialidase activity. Ganglioside sialidase is normal. Diagnosis is based on measurement of neuraminidase activity in fibroblasts or white blood cells. Carriers can be identified, and prenatal diagnosis can be made using cultured amniotic cells.

Two genes may be involved in the expression of the glycoprotein-specific α-neuraminidase absent in sialidosis patients. The sialidase deficiency in a type 2 patient was caused by a mutation in a structural gene on chromosome 10. The neuraminidase deficiency in a galactosialidosis patient was caused by a mutation on a gene located on chromosome 20.

ML-II OR I-CELL. This disease is manifest within the first few months of life. The clinical pattern somewhat resembles Hurler syndrome and GM_1 gangliosidosis (type 1). Affected patients may have congenital dislocation of the hips, inguinal hernias, hypertrophy of the gums, restriction of motion in the shoulders, generalized hypotonia, thick and tight skin, and hepatomegaly. The coarse facial features become more conspicuous with age. Progressive, severe psychomotor retardation occurs as well. Characteristic bone changes related to severe dysostosis multiplex occur, leading to a cloaking of the appearance of long tubular bones, to shortening of vertebral bodies, and to other significant changes in the pelvis, hands, ribs, and skull. Death from pneumonia or congestive heart failure usually occurs at 2–8 yr of age.

Urinary mucopolysaccharides are normal, but sialyloligosaccharides are elevated. Fibroblast cultures reveal characteristic inclusions, which initially set this disease apart from the mucopolysaccharidoses. Enzyme studies show greatly increased lysosomal enzymes in serum, whereas values in leukocytes are near the normal range. Activities of almost all lysosomal enzymes are deficient in cultured skin fibroblasts, whereas the culture medium has an excess of these enzymes compared with those of control fibroblast lines. Normally, the targeting of lysosomal enzymes to lysosomes is mediated by receptors that bind mannose-6-phosphate recognition markers on the enzymes. The marker is synthesized in a two-step reaction in the Golgi complex. UDP-*N*-acetylglucosamine: lysosomal enzyme *N*-acetylglucosaminyl-1-phosphotransferase, the enzyme catalyzing the first step in this process, is defective in ML-II and ML-III. Thus, newly formed lysosomal enzymes cannot be phosphorylated. In the absence of these phosphate groups, which serve as part of a recognition marker, the newly synthesized enzymes do not get into the lysosomes but are excreted from the cell. This specific phosphotransferase activity can be measured in fibroblast cultures, providing a specific diagnostic test for patient and carrier identification and for prenatal diagnosis. There is no effective treatment, although one patient has responded favorably to bone marrow transplantation. Supportive medical and orthopedic care is important.

ML-III OR PSEUDO-HURLER POLYDYSTROPHY. This is a milder form of ML-II. After possibly delayed early psychomotor development, affected 3- to 4-yr-old children may present with progressive joint stiffness, short stature, mild dysostosis multiplex, mild gingival hyperplasia, and normal urinary mucopolysaccharide levels. Corneal clouding or nystagmus may be present. The IQ may range from normal to as low as 50. The prognosis is unknown; some patients have attained the 3rd decade of life. Orthopedic treatment may be indicated in some cases. As in I-cell disease, serum lysosomal enzymes are elevated, and cultured skin fibroblasts reveal characteristic inclusions and decreased activities for many lysosomal enzymes. Measurement of UDP-*N*-acetylglucosamine-1-phosphotransferase activity using exogenous substrate shows more residual activity than in ML-II. Prenatal diagnosis is possible through examination of cultured amniotic fluid cells. There is no effective treatment, but supportive medical and orthopedic management may be helpful.

ML-IV. This is a recently described mucolipidosis. Most cases reported so far have occurred in children of Ashkenazi Jewish descent. Usually, soon after birth affected children present with bilateral corneal opacities and strabismus. Corneal clouding may appear after several years. Retinal degeneration may also occur. After 6 mo hypotonia and psychomotor retardation become more evident. Surviving patients are usually retarded to about the 1-yr level. There is no skeletal dysplasia or excess excretion of mucopolysaccharides in the urine. There are grossly abnormal storage bodies in the cells of the liver, brain, conjunctiva, and fibroblasts. The prognosis is uncertain. One patient has reached 24 yr of age. Treatment to correct the corneal opacities may improve the vision, but no other treatment is available.

Diagnosis is based on examining fibroblast cultures for the characteristic lamellated multivesicular membrane bodies. Patients have been found to have a partial deficiency of ganglioside sialidase activity. Although some obligate heterozygotes have less than normal activity, it has still not been proved whether or not this is the primary defect. Prenatal diagnosis is made by examining cultured amniotic fluid cells for the characteristic storage bodies.

Banerjee A, Burg J, Conzelmann E, et al: Enzyme-linked immunosorbent assay for the ganglioside G_{M2}-activator protein. Hoppe-Seyler's Z Physiol Chem 365:347, 1984.

Crandall BF, Philippart M, Brown WJ, et al: Mucolipidosis IV. Am J Med Genet 12:301, 1982.

Gillow JE, Lowden JA, Gaskin MB, et al: Congenital ascites as a presenting sign of lysosomal storage disease. J Pediatr 104:225, 1984.

Lowden JA, O'Brien JS: Sialidosis: A review of human sialidase deficiency. Am J Hum Genet 31:1, 1979.

O'Reilly RJ, Brochstein J, Dinsmore R, et al: Marrow transplantation for congenital disorders. Semin Hematol 21:188, 1984.

Poenaru L, Kaplan L, Dumez J, et al: Evaluation of possible first trimester prenatal diagnosis in lysosomal diseases by trophoblast biopsy. Pediatr Res 18:1032, 1984.

Reitman ML, Varki A, Kornfeld S: Fibroblasts from patients with I-cell disease and pseudo-Hurler polydystrophy are deficient in uridine 5′-diphosphate-N-acetylglucosamine: glycoprotein N-acetylglucosaminylphosphotransferase activity. J Clin Invest 67:1574, 1981.

Scriver CR, Beaudet AL, Sly WS, et al: The Metabolic Basis of Inherited Disease, 6th ed. New York, McGraw-Hill, 1989.

CHAPTER 75

Defects in Metabolism of Purines and Pyrimidines

R. Rodney Howell

Purines and pyrimidines are heterocyclic nitrogen-containing compounds. Combinations of purines and pyrimidines with ribose or deoxyribose and with phosphate create nucleotides. Combined with ribose and phosphate (hence, ribonucleotide), purines and pyrimidines form the elements of ribonucleic acid (RNA); combined with deoxyribose and phosphate (deoxyribonucleotides), they form deoxyribonucleic acid (DNA). The ability to synthesize the purine ring de novo is virtually universal among living organisms. The final product of purine metabolism in man is uric acid.

Other than uric acid, the purine bases recognized to have clinical importance are adenine and guanine. The important pyrimidines are thymine, cytosine, and uracil. The importance of nucleotides as components of DNA rests on the genetic function of this material. RNA is of central importance in the regulation of protein synthesis and as a component of such important energy-producing compounds and nucleotide cofactors as ATP, UDPG, NAD, NADP, and others.

GOUT. The hallmark of gout is the elevation of serum uric acid concentration. This disease primarily affects adults and rarely occurs in children except those with type I glycogen storage disease (GSD I), in whom hyperuricemia routinely occurs and gouty arthritis and tophi appear in adolescence (see Chapter 73). When hyperuricemia and gout occur in childhood, they are almost always secondary to another disorder.

Elevations of uric acid concentration in serum can result from several general metabolic disturbances. Certain patients have an abnormally active production de novo of uric acid; others have reduction in the renal clearance of uric acid; and some represent combinations of these two major factors.

At least 95% of cases of gouty arthritis are seen in postpubertal males. In a very small group of patients the activity of the enzyme hypoxanthine guanine phosphoribosyl transferase (Fig. 75–1) is reduced to only a few per cent of normal (a total deficiency leads to the Lesch-Nyhan syndrome). In another group of patients overproduction of uric acid and hyperuricemia can be traced to an abnormally high activity of the enzyme phosphoribosylpyrophosphate (PRPP) synthetase (Fig. 75–2). In both of these situations, the increased availability of PRPP leads to an increase in the endogenous production of uric acid. Both enzymes are genetically transmitted as X-linked recessives. The increased availability of PRPP is the mechanism that also leads to hyperuricemia in type I glycogen storage disease; some of the reduction in uric acid clearance that occurs in GSD I may also be due to hyperlactic acidemia, which reduces the renal clearance of uric acid.

Whether or not a patient with elevated levels of uric acid in serum develops gouty arthritis largely depends on the severity and duration of hyperuricemia.

LESCH-NYHAN SYNDROME. Boys with this syndrome are usually normal at birth. The first abnormality consistently noted is a delay in motor development in the first few months of life. Later, extrapyramidal choreoathetoid movements appear, and hyper-reflexia, ankle clonus, and spasticity of the legs develop. The most striking clinical abnormality is the dramatic, compulsive self-destructive behavior usually observed. Older children

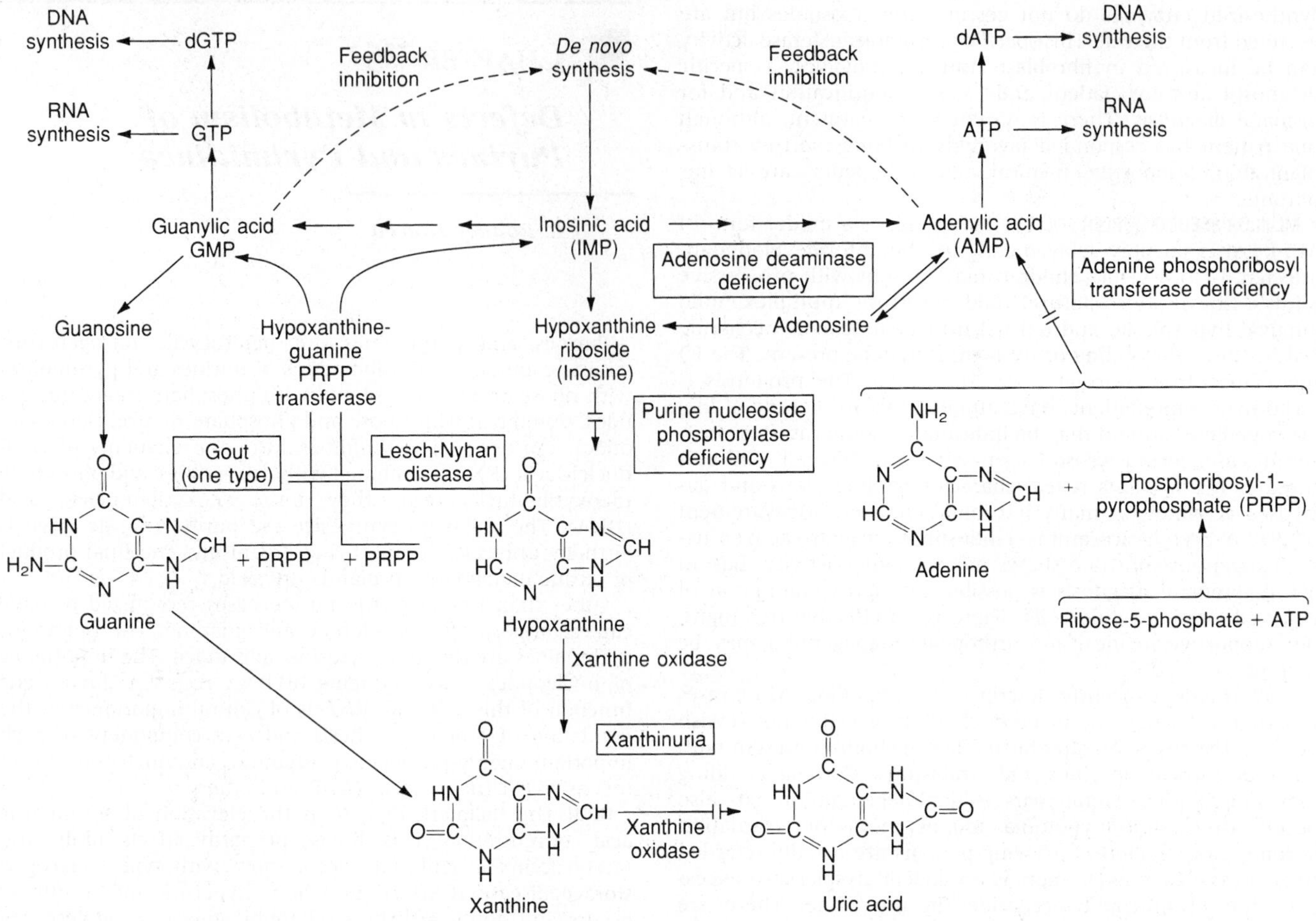

Figure 75–1. Pathways in purine metabolism and salvage.

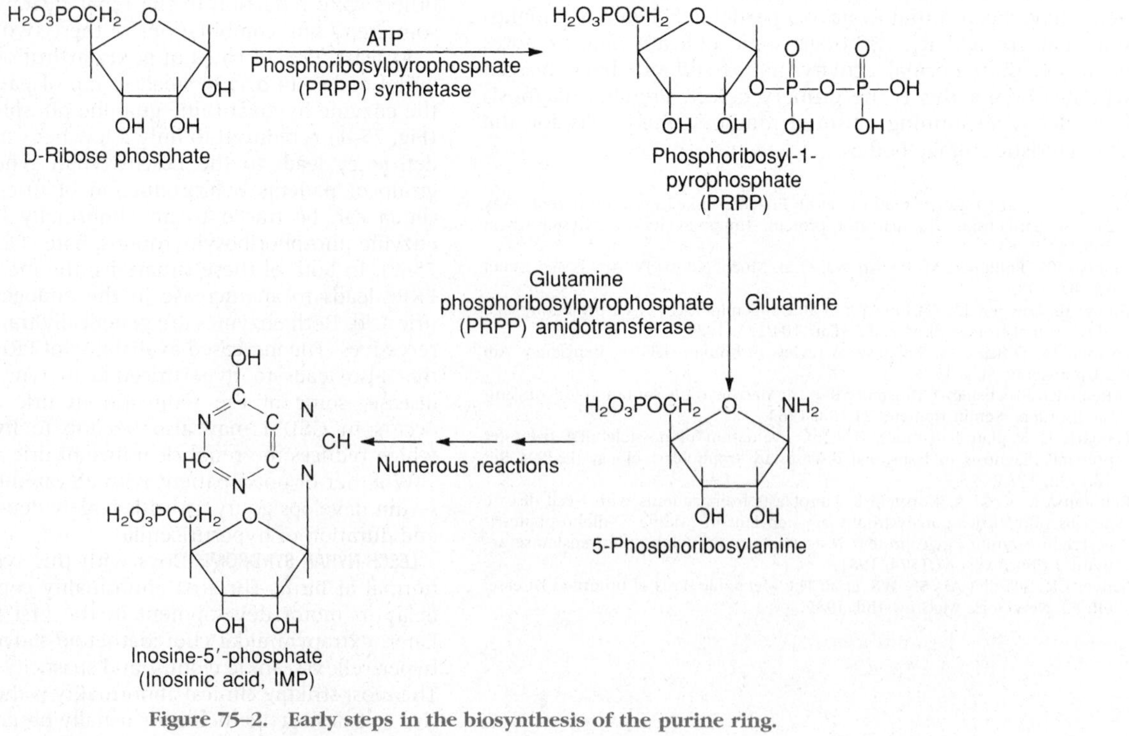

Figure 75–2. Early steps in the biosynthesis of the purine ring.

begin to bite and chew their fingers, lips, and buccal mucosa, leading to mutilation. It is not the result of inability to feel pain but of a compulsive urge that appears so irresistible that it is necessary to restrain the patients. Gouty tophi and gouty arthritis are also sometimes seen in older children with the Lesch-Nyhan syndrome. Tophi result from the accumulation of sodium urate crystals in subcutaneous and other tissues; they occur over the extensor surfaces of the elbows, knees, fingers, and toes.

In the Lesch-Nyhan syndrome, serum uric acid concentrations are commonly in the range seen in the adult with gout (10–12 mg/dL); there are marked increases in the production of uric acid and in its urinary excretion. There is an almost total absence of hypoxanthine guanine phosphoribosyltransferase activity in many tissues, including erythrocytes and fibroblasts. This enzyme is important to the "purine salvage" pathway, through which hypoxanthine and xanthine can be converted to nucleotides, inosinic acid, and guanylic acid (see Fig. 75–1). When this enzymatic pathway is not operative, PRPP synthetase activity increases and PRPP accumulates within the cell, giving rise to accelerated purine production de novo and to excesses of uric acid. The salvage pathway may be important in the synthesis of nucleotides within the brain; when this pathway is inactive, the brain may be unable to synthesize required nucleotides.

This syndrome is transmitted as an X-linked condition. Fibroblasts cultured from biopsies of skin of mothers of patients with Lesch-Nyhan syndrome consist of two cell populations, one normal and one deficient in the crucial enzyme, lending support to the Lyon hypothesis.

The gene for hypoxanthine-guanine phosphoryltransferase is located on the x chromosome in the region q26–q27 and consists of nine exons and eight introns totaling 57 kD. Many different mutations throughout the coding region have been described. Because a loss of central dopaminergic neurons has been demonstrated, D1-dopamine antagonists have been proposed as the cause of the self-destructive behavior. The introduction of this gene into patients with Lesch-Nyhan syndrome is currently being considered as an experimental, potentially curative treatment.

OTHER ABNORMALITIES OF URIC ACID METABOLISM. Hyperuricemia is commonly encountered in situations of a marked increase in cell number and cell destruction, as in myeloproliferative disease. The excessive amount of uric acid results from an increased intensity of degradation of nucleotides to purine end products (uric acid). In the treatment of acute leukemia or lymphoma masses, the sudden lysis of cells may provoke hyperuricemia and hyperuricosuria with clinical consequences (see Chapter 448.1 and 449).

Hyperuricemia may occur in any condition in which renal clearance is reduced. When the serum concentrations of β-hydroxybutyrate and acetoacetate are increased, as in starvation and diabetic ketoacidosis, there are elevations of serum uric acid concentrations related to reduction in renal clearance. Commonly used drugs, such as salicylates, in low doses may reduce renal clearance and produce hyperuricemia. Patients with Down syndrome regularly display modest hyperuricemia. All of these variables must be weighed in the interpretation of serum uric acid concentrations in children.

Hypouricemia due to an increase in renal clearance of uric acid occurs in proximal renal tubular diseases (e.g., Fanconi syndrome). In a clinically normal patient, hypouricemia has been caused by an isolated defect of renal tubular reabsorption of uric acid; the same situation exists in Dalmatian dogs. Hypouricemia is also a prominent feature of xanthinuria and nucleoside phosphorylase deficiency (see later).

Treatment of Hyperuricemia. Several approaches are used. Avoidance of foods high in purines (such as sweetbreads) is of modest benefit. Probenecid is effective in increasing uric acid clearance and may be used to treat hyperuricemia in patients with normal renal function. Allopurinol, an inhibitor of xanthine oxidase, is also widely used. In persons with no known enzymatic defect in purine biosynthesis, this drug reduces total purine production, increases the excretion of the oxypurines (xanthine and hypoxanthine), and reduces the excretion of uric acid. In Lesch-Nyhan syndrome, allopurinol treatment reduces uric acid concentrations (and ameliorates gouty arthritis and tophi); there is no effect on the severe neurologic problems.

For any patient with hyperuricosuria, whether as a result of increased synthesis de novo or of drug therapy, it is essential that high urine volumes be maintained and that urine pH be kept near neutral (7.0). This can ordinarily be done effectively with a balanced mixture of salts, such as Polycitra, which is usually more effective than bicarbonate. The importance of adjusting the urine pH to 7.0 is illustrated by the fact that at pH 5.0 the solubility of uric acid is 15 mg/dL, whereas at pH 7.0 the solubility is 200 mg/dL.

The hyperuricemia associated with type I glycogen storage disease, like other significant hyperuricemia, should be treated; it does not respond to probenecid but does respond appropriately to allopurinol.

XANTHINURIA. Xanthine is the immediate precursor of uric acid. It is formed directly from certain purines, whereas hypoxanthine is an intermediary formed from others. The oxidations of hypoxanthine to xanthine and of xanthine to uric acid are mediated by xanthine oxidase, which is found in liver and intestinal mucosa (see Fig. 75–1).

Xanthinuria is uncommon. Serum uric acid levels in affected persons are virtually undetectable (0.1–0.8 mg/dL). There are low levels of hypoxanthine and uric acid in both plasma and urine; the amount of uric acid in urine falls almost to 0 with a purine-free diet. Xanthine is even less soluble than uric acid in urine; accordingly, some patients with xanthinuria have had *urinary calculi* composed of pure xanthine. The stones are radiolucent, except that slight radiopacity was reported in one instance when the stone contained 5% calcium phosphate. Some patients with muscular pain after exertion were shown to have deposits of xanthine crystals in muscles. Jejunal biopsies of affected patients show no activity of xanthine oxidase toward xanthine and only about 5% of normal activity toward hypoxanthine. (Xanthine stones have also been reported as a rare consequence of allopurinol administration.) There is genetic heterogeneity; some, but not all, xanthenuric patients lack aldehyde oxidase activity (which converts the drug allopurinol to oxypurinol). The enzymes xanthine oxidase and sulfite oxidase require molybdenum as a cofactor. Patients have been recognized to have *molybdenum deficiency* and simultaneous deficiencies of xanthine oxidase and sulfite oxidase activities. All patients with xanthinuria should maintain a high fluid intake, dietary restriction of purines, and alkalinization of the urine. The solubility of xanthine in urine at pH 5.0 is 5 mg/dL, and at pH 7.0 it is 13 mg/dL. The prognosis is excellent.

ADENOSINE DEAMINASE DEFICIENCY. In nearly half of patients with severe combined immunodeficiency (SCID), a deficiency of adenosine deaminase activity has been demonstrated (see Chapter 119).

NUCLEOSIDE PHOSPHORYLASE DEFICIENCY. Deficiencies of this enzyme, whose gene is located on the long arm of chromosome 14, are associated with marked deficiencies of cellular immunity but normal humoral immunity (see Chapter 118). Central nervous system dysfunction has been a prominent clinical feature in six infants with nucleoside phosphorylase deficiency.

ADENINE PHOSPHORIBOSYLTRANSFERASE DEFICIENCY. Twenty Caucasian patients have been described with adenine phosphoribosyltransferase deficiency. The prominent clinical feature was urinary calculi composed of 2,8-dihydroxyadenine and calcium oxalate.

OROTIC ACIDURIA. Orotic acid is an intermediate metabolite in the synthesis of pyrimidines. Orotic aciduria is a rare disorder of children, resulting from a block in the further metabolism of orotic acid. Affected children have megaloblastic anemia that is unresponsive to therapy with vitamin C, folic acid, or vitamin B_{12}; they excrete up to 1.5 g/24 hr of orotic acid and form orotic acid crystals in urine. Although these patients are retarded in growth and development, the hematologic manifestations are more dramatic clinical features because vigorous synthesis of RNA and DNA is so necessary for normal hematopoiesis. Corticosteroid treatment may result in general improvement, but disappearance of abnormalities in the marrow or of the excretion of orotic acid occurs only when pyrimidine compounds found beyond the metabolic block are administered.

In most patients with orotic aciduria, orotidylic acid pyrophosphorylase and orotidylic acid decarboxylase activities are deficient (Fig. 75–3). The enzyme uridine 5′-monophosphate (UMP) synthase is a bifunctional enzyme with these two activities. In orotic aciduria, normal amounts of mRNA are produced that appear to code for a mutant enzyme with either reduced stability or altered kinetic properties. These enzyme deficiencies have been demonstrated in liver, leukocytes, erythrocytes, and fibroblasts grown in culture. Heterozygotes have approximately half the normal level of activities of both enzymes. A single patient has been described who lacks only OMP decarboxylase activity.

The administration of pyrimidine derivatives lowers the urinary excretion of orotic acid. This effect indicates that enzymes in the pathway leading to orotic acid synthesis are under feedback inhibition control. The hematologic response is due directly to the provision for DNA and RNA synthesis of essential material that cannot be made de novo. A patient treated with uridine since infancy was reported to be a normal young adult.

Orotic acid excretion is increased in the urine of children who have primary genetic defects in the urea cycle. These defects result from additional carbamyl phosphate (usually utilized in urea synthesis) that is shunted into de novo pyrimidine synthesis, leading to an apparent overproduction of orotic acid. Orotic aciduria is also seen in nucleoside phosphorylase deficiency.

Unrelated patients with cerebral dysfunction and an increased urinary excretion of uracil, thymine, and 5-hydroxymethyluracil have been reported. These patients are probably deficient in dihydropyrimidine dehydrogenase activity. Such a deficiency has been shown in patients who experienced severe toxicity when receiving 5-flurouracil, which requires this enzyme for its metabolism.

Davidson BL, Tarle SA, Van Antwerp M, et al: Identification of 17 independent mutations responsible for human hypoxanthine-guanine phosphoribosyltransferase (H PRT) deficiency. Am J Hum Genet 48:951, 1991.

Van Acker KJ, Eyskens FJ, Verkerk RM, et al: Urinary excretion of purine and pyrimidine metabolites in the neonate. Pediatr Res 34:762, 1993.

Willis R, Jolly DJ, Miller AD, et al: Partial phenotypic correction of human Lesch-Nyhan (hypoxanthine-guanine phosphoribosyltransferase-deficient) lymphoblasts with a transmissible retroviral vector. J Biol Chem 259:7842, 1984.

Winkler JK, Suttle DP: Analysis of UMP synthase gene and mRNA structure in hereditary orotic aciduria fibroblasts. Am J Hum Genet 43:86, 1988.

OTHER DEFECTS OF ENZYMES AND PROTEINS

Some inborn errors of metabolism cannot be assigned naturally to systems, such as those involved in amino acid, carbohydrate, lipid, pigment, purine, or pyrimidine metabolism. These other defects involving the soluble proteins and formed elements of blood and certain proteins and enzymes of other organs or tissues will be discussed in the following sections.

The absence of any given protein in a specific individual or the presence of a protein that migrates abnormally by electrophoretic and chromatographic techniques is prima facie evidence of the existence of an inborn error of metabolism. Also, immunologic recognition systems depend upon the presence of a variety of cell-surface macromolecules under genetic control, for example, HLA, and the association of various markers with different diseases. Further, a large array of receptor proteins are found in and on cells that mediate hormonal action. Inborn errors of such protein moieties also occur.

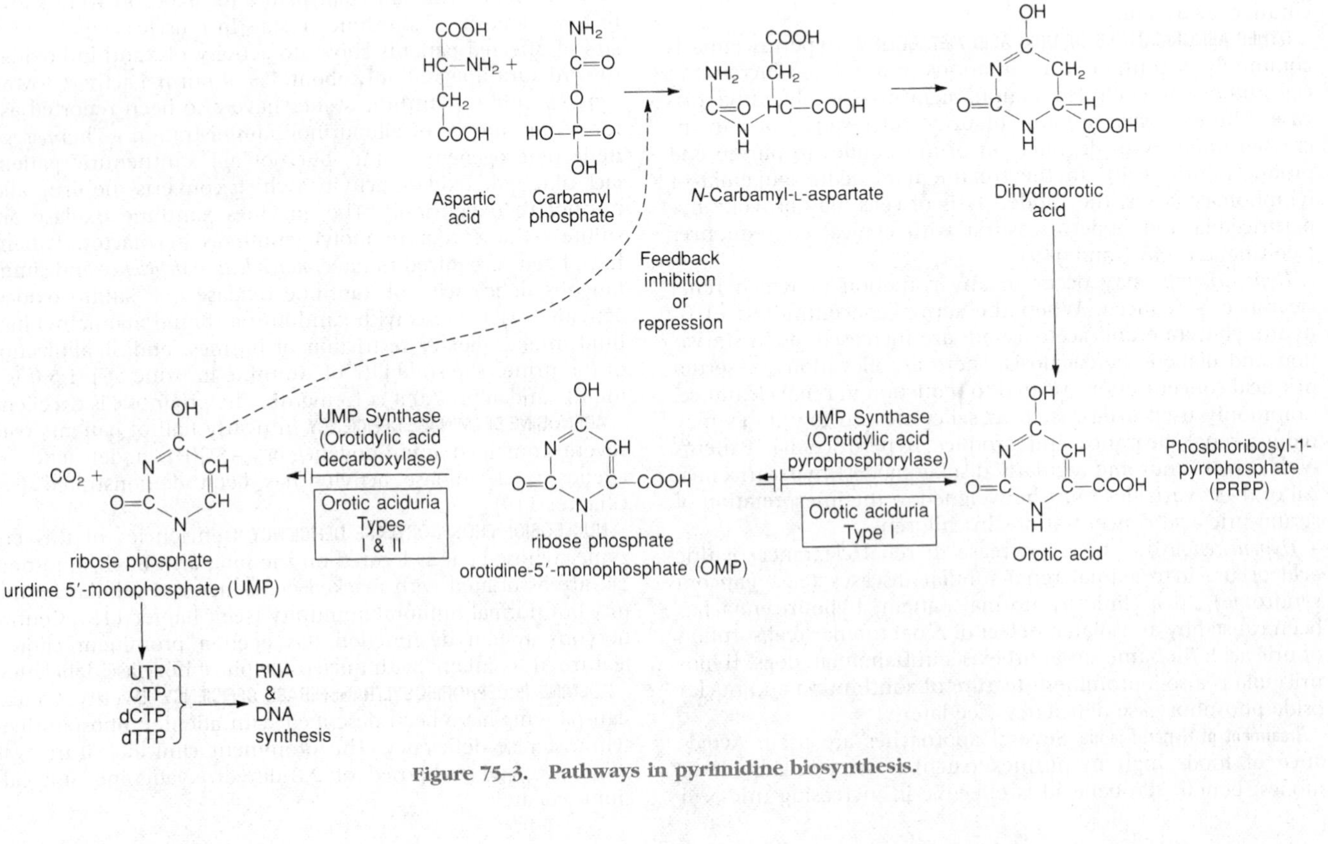

Figure 75–3. Pathways in pyrimidine biosynthesis.

Defects in Plasma Proteins

ANALBUMINEMIA. Plasma albumin maintains the oncotic pressure of blood and serves as a vehicle for the transport of many normal blood constituents. Analbuminemia is a very rare, recessively inherited trait. Molecular cloning studies have shown that three analbuminec individuals had different mutations. Homozygotes have strikingly few symptoms that can be attributed to the lack of albumin. Some heterozygotes have intermediate levels of albumin. Usually no treatment is necessary. The lack of symptoms in analbuminemia may be the result of lifelong compensations in fluid dynamics or to a compensatory increase in other plasma proteins.

HAPTOGLOBIN DEFICIENCY. Haptoglobin is an α_2-globulin that binds proteins. There are numerous phenotypic variations (polymorphisms) in the types of haptoglobins among normal persons, which are under genetic control. With severe hemolytic anemia, haptoglobin levels may be greatly decreased or absent. Healthy persons have been found who have no demonstrable circulating haptoglobin without apparent ill effect.

ABETALIPOPROTEINEMIA. See Chapter 72.4.

ANALPHALIPOPROTEINEMIA (TANGIER DISEASE). See Chapter 72.4.

ABSENCE OF TRANSFERRIN. Transferrin, or siderophilin (a β_2-globulin), is a plasma protein that has a prominent role in the transport of iron. Eighteen or more polymorphisms have been identified. The only recorded instance of a congenital absence of transferrin at birth involved a physically retarded girl with hepatomegaly, splenomegaly, and anemia sufficiently severe to require multiple transfusions. The anemia did not respond to any treatment. Iron was absorbed from the intestinal tract and transported to the tissues. Erythrocytes were hypochromic, and the marrow contained many immature erythroblasts. Liver biopsy revealed cirrhosis and siderosis. Antibodies to transferrin developed after multiple transfusions. Sudden death at 7 yr of age was attributed to hemosiderosis. Both parents had lower than normal amounts of transferrin, suggesting autosomal recessive transmission.

CARBOHYDRATE-DEFICIENT GLYCOPROTEIN (CDG) SYNDROME. Although the basic biochemical defect is unknown, abnormalities of the structure of numerous glycoproteins, including increased amounts of carbohydrate-deficient serum transferrin, are present and diagnostically helpful. Psychomotor or mental retardation is the most consistent clinical manifestation; other common features include growth failure, dysmorphic facies, liver dysfunction, lipocutaneous abnormalities, ataxia and cerebellar hypoplasia, peripheral neuropathy, lower limb atrophy, strabismus and retinal degeneration, hypotonia, and skeletal abnormalities related to neurologic involvement. Strokelike episodes, coma, and cerebral infarctions have been related to coagulopathies. A broad spectrum of additional clinical findings and biochemical abnormalities have been observed. Only supportive treatment is available.

C1 ESTERASE INHIBITOR. See Chapter 121.

COMPLEMENT DEFICIENCIES. See Chapter 121.

α-ANTITRYPSIN PROTEIN DEFICIENCY. See Chapter 354.4.

TRANSCOBALAMIN II DEFICIENCY. Two different serum proteins bind vitamin B_{12}. One of these, transcobalamin I (an α-globulin), has been reported deficient in two siblings without clinical or hematologic sequelae. Deficiency of the other protein, transcobalamin II (a β-globulin), believed to be the primary B_{12} transport protein, was associated with severe megaloblastic anemia and neurologic manifestations in several infants. Partial deficiency in both parents indicated autosomal recessive inheritance. No abnormalities were found in reactions involving the coenzyme forms of vitamin B_{12}, homocysteine methyltransferase and methylmalonyl CoA mutase (see Chapter 71). Treatment consists of parenteral administration of large doses of vitamin B_{12}. Prenatal diagnosis using cultured amniocytes is possible.

Defects in Plasma Enzymes

PSEUDOCHOLINESTERASE. Pseudocholinesterase is found in plasma, liver, and neural tissue; its physiologic function is poorly understood.

Numerous presumably allelic forms of the altered enzyme are known, in some of which enzyme activity is reduced or absent. Homozygotes for each form and mixed heterozygotes are known. About 1 in 25 persons is heterozygous for one or another of these defects. Among whites heterozygote males are more common than females.

The one person in 3,000 who is homozygous for one of these genes is ordinarily asymptomatic. However, the enzyme participates in the destruction of a commonly used muscle relaxant, succinylcholine. Normally this drug is rapidly destroyed by pseudocholinesterase and therefore has a transient effect. Persons homozygous for mutant pseudocholinesterase degrade the drug very slowly or not at all, and apnea results, lasting for hours. Artificial respiration with endotracheal intubation is required. The period of apnea can be shortened by transfusion with normal plasma.

Another genetic alteration of pseudocholinesterase has been described that leads to increased enzyme activity and hence to resistance to the pharmacologic effects of succinylcholine. The human gene has been cloned and mapped to chromosome 3q21–q26.

LECITHIN-CHOLESTEROL ACYLTRANSFERASE DEFICIENCY. See Chapter 72.4.

CARNOSINASE DEFICIENCY. See Chapter 71.11.

γ-GLUTAMYL TRANSPEPTIDASE DEFICIENCY. A moderately retarded adult male with increased levels of glutathione in blood and urine has been shown to have a deficiency of serum γ-glutamyl transpeptidase, which catalyzes the first step in the degradation of glutathione. There was no other abnormality in amino acid excretion. This serum enzyme produced in the liver appears to be under different genetic control from that synthesized in the renal tubule and intestine.

HYPOPHOSPHATASIA. A variety of genetic abnormalities of alkaline phosphatase have been described that lead to a clinical spectrum of bony disorders, sometimes associated with a grave and fatal disorder in infancy (see Chapter 653).

ELEVATED ALKALINE PHOSPHATASE. Elevated serum alkaline phosphatase concentrations (2–10 times normal) usually indicate either liver or bone disease. However, increases (2–4 times normal) also occur in otherwise normal families owing to a genetic alteration, transmitted as an autosomal dominant trait.

Defects of Proteins in Other Tissues

MENKES KINKY HAIR SYNDROME. See Chapter 552.5.

MOLYBDENUM COFACTOR DEFICIENCY. Sulfite oxidase deficiency (see Chapter 71.4) and xanthinuria have been associated with ocular abnormalities (dislocated lenses, Brushfield spots, and nystagmus), neurologic findings (tonic-clonic seizures), and mental retardation. The defect is an inability to form the molybdenum-containing cofactor whose presence is required for the activity of sulfite oxidase, xanthine dehydrogenase, and aldehyde oxidase. Treatment consists of restricting sulfur-containing amino acids and administering allopurinol.

MYOGLOBIN. Myoglobin, a heme protein found in muscle, is responsible for the intracellular transport of oxygen. Two variants of myoglobin have been identified, and the changes in amino acid sequence producing myoglobinopathies are analogous to the changes responsible for the hemoglobinopathies. Patients have been heterozygous for the normal and for the aberrant molecules. Neuromuscular diseases have not been found in these families.

Autosomal dominant myoglobinuria has been reported in three successive generations. Myoglobinuria was precipitated by prolonged exercise, fever, viral illnesses, and alcohol use. There was mild weakness, increased creatine kinase, and enlarged calf muscles. Acute renal failure and death occurred in one such patient.

Myoglobinuria may also occur in a number of disorders of muscle metabolism such as deficient phosphorylase activity (Chapter 73), deficient phosphofructokinase activity (Chapter 73), deficient lactate dehydrogenase activity (Chapter 73.4), and absent carnitine palmityl transferase activity (Chapter 72).

X-LINKED ICHTHYOSIS. See Chapter 608 for discussion of steroid sulfatase deficiency.

XERODERMA PIGMENTOSUM. See Chapter 606.

DYNEIN ARM DEFICIENCY. The absence of this specific ATPase is discussed in Chapter 364.

RECEPTOR PROTEINS. Most if not all communications between cells within the same organ or across organ systems are mediated by specific proteins found on the surface of the cell receiving the message. An increasing number of inborn errors involving receptor proteins have been described. The receptor for LDL is an example (see Chapter 72.4). Another example is the absence of a functional receptor for the hormone vitamin D_3, which leads to vitamin D–dependent rickets type II (see Chapter 649). One form of diabetes mellitus is due to a defect in the specific receptor for insulin (see Part XXVI, Section 6).

PANCREATIC ENZYME DEFICIENCIES. A number of patients have been described in whom malabsorption appears to result from a specific defect involving a pancreatic enzyme or proenzyme (see Chapter 296). They have none of the pulmonary or electrolyte abnormalities of cystic fibrosis.

A syndrome with inability to produce trypsin, lipase, and amylase in conjunction with hematologic evidence of bone marrow dysfunction has also been described (see Chapter 296).

Lipase Deficiency. Congenital absence of active pancreatic lipase leads to malabsorption of lipids and fatty (and sometimes malodorous) stools. It appears to be inherited in an autosomal recessive fashion. Treatment with pancreatin is effective.

Trypsinogen Deficiency. Severe malnutrition, growth failure, and hypoproteinemic edema resembling kwashiorkor are associated with lack of the ability to synthesize pancreatic trypsinogen. As a result, chymotrypsin and carboxypeptidase activities are also low because these enzymes need to be formed from the corresponding proenzymes by trypsin activity. Treatment with a protein hydrolysate diet and exogenous pancreatic enzymes is recommended. Human trypsin-1 gene has been assigned to chromosome 7q22–7qter.

Amylase Deficiency. Less-defined deficiencies of pancreatic amylase activity have been described in at least two children with malabsorption who did not have cystic fibrosis. One of the children also had reduced trypsin activity.

INTESTINAL ENTEROKINASE DEFICIENCY. Enterokinase, an enzyme secreted by the small intestine, initiates the reactions for the conversion of the pancreatic proenzymes to their active forms. Both the clinical findings in and recommended treatment for deficient enterokinase activity in children are identical to those described above for trypsinogen deficiency. Many if not all of the cases originally described as trypsinogen deficiency may be instances of enterokinase deficiency, with the lack of trypsin activity secondary to inability to form trypsin from trypsinogen. Almost all of the infants presented at birth with failure to thrive and diarrhea. Hypoproteinemia and edema are present in 50% of patients.

COLLAGEN METABOLISM. Collagen refers to a group of fibrous proteins that hold the body together and constitute about one fourth of its total protein. Collagens are the major structural proteins of skin, tendons, cartilage, and bone. Collagen contains large amounts of glycine, hydroxylysine, and hydroxyproline. Although the primary structure of the various collagens is under genetic control, the formation of collagen from procollagen and post-translation hydroxylation of lysine and proline, as well as the addition of various carbohydrate side chains, is controlled by a number of specific enzymes. A growing number of disorders involve collagen metabolism at one stage or another; among these are the numerous variants of both osteogenesis imperfecta (see Chapter 643) and Ehlers-Danlos syndrome (see Chapter 609), and Marfan syndrome (see Chapter 646).

MYOADENYLATE DEAMINASE DEFICIENCY. Approximately 2% of all Caucasians and African-Americans are homogyzous for a mutation (nonsense) in exon 2 of the myoadenylate deaminase (AMPD1-AMP deaminase) gene. Although more than 100 patients with AMP-1 deficiency have been reported to have myopathic symptoms, most AMP1 deficient patients are asymptomatic. Symptoms of muscle cramps, easy fatigability, and muscle pain may first occur at any time from infancy to adulthood. The enzyme normally converts AMP to IMP (inosine-monophosphate) with the liberation of ammonia. The IMP formed is then normally recycled back to AMP. In the absence of AMP deaminase activity this cycle is broken, and nucleotides are lost from the muscle cell, leading to impaired activity. No blood ammonia is produced upon ischemic forearm exercise, which distinguishes these patients from those with either McArdle disease (see Chapter 73) or deficient muscle phosphoglycerate mutase or muscle lactic acid dehydrogenase (see Chapter 73) who cannot produce lactic acid upon ischemic forearm exercise. Deficiency of myoadenylate deaminase may be the most common metabolic myopathy, but its exact role is yet to be defined.

MITOCHONDRIAL MYOPATHIES. See also Chapter 562.4. Many patients with muscle weakness and lactic acidosis brought on by mild exercise do not have any of the disorders described either in Chapter 73 or immediately above. Land and colleagues have prepared a very useful resumé of the defects that exist in mitochondrial myopathies: (1) defects in substrate utilization, as in carnitine deficiency, carnitine palmityl transferase deficiency, and defects in various components of the pyruvate dehydrogenase complex; (2) defects in coupling of mitochondrial respiration to phosphorylation, as in Luft disease and mitochondrial ATPase deficiency; and (3) deficiencies of components of the mitochondrial respiratory chain, such as nonheme iron, protein, cytochrome oxidase, cytochrome b deficiency, and NADH-CoQ reductase. The range of clinical manifestations, even within a given biochemical variant, is wide. Some patients go for many years without any signs or symptoms, others become sick at an early age, and still others have been described with a form that is rapidly fatal in the neonatal period. The patients with mitochondrial myopathies may have partial or complete deficiencies limited to muscle or deficiencies with wide tissue distribution.

It is now recognized that the drug zidovudine (AZT), which is widely used to treat acquired immune deficiency syndrome (AIDS), induces a DNA-depleting mitochondrial myopathy. The constitutional features observed in these patients suggest that the drug might well affect cellular function in other tissues.

ACATALASIA. Catalase is found in most tissues, including the erythrocytes. Persons with a decrease of catalase activity in all tissues, to less than 1% of normal, can be detected through the demonstration that blood placed in contact with hydrogen peroxide turns brown and does not produce the oxygen bubbles usually seen. The disorder is heterogeneous; some instances appear to be mutations of the controller gene. In all instances the mode of inheritance is autosomal recessive; the heterozygote can be detected by quantitative catalase assays. Of the two main types, the Japanese variants have oral gangrene *(Takahara disease)*, whereas the Swiss variants are asymptomatic. A genetic strain of mice with acatalasia is known; catalase encapsulated in semipermeable membranes has been used successfully in their treatment.

STORAGE OF GLUTAMYL RIBOSE-5-PHOSPHATE. A mentally and physically retarded boy with seizures and progressive neurologic deterioration who died of renal failure at 8 yr of age had glutamyl ribose-5-phosphate stored in brain and kidney lysosomes. This compound is normally part of the linkage between histones and poly(ADP-ribose) and is thought to accumulate because of an X-linked deficiency of the enzyme ADP-ribose protein hydrolase.

ASPARTYLGLYCOSAMINURIA. The compound 2-acetamido-1(β-L-aspartamido)-1,2-dideoxyglucose (AADG) is a substituted hexose that forms one of the linkage points between the carbohydrate moiety and the amino acid groups of many glycoproteins. Large quantities of urinary AADG (as well as other compounds containing AADG) have been found in some patients with mental retardation, petit mal seizures, or manic-depressive psychosis. Other patients have had vacuolated lymphocytes, facial and osseous features similar to those of the mucopolysaccharidoses, hepatomegaly, and lenticular opacities. The defect is in the lack of the enzyme, glycoasparinase, which hydrolyzes AADG to glucosamine and aspartic acid. The lysosomal enzyme is deficient in liver, brain, and spleen. The structural gene for aspartylglucosaminidase has been assigned to chromosome 4q21–4qter. The gene has been extensively characterized and specific mutations have been demonstrated in patients.

ACID PHOSPHATASE DEFICIENCIES. Two groups of patients have been reported with either decreased or absent activity of lysosomal acid phosphatase. Patients with partial activity of this phospholipid-degrading enzyme have a clinical picture characterized by intermittent vomiting, hypotonia, lethargy, opisthotonos, terminal bleeding, and death within the 1st yr of life. Patients with total deficiency exhibit the same symptoms and die in infancy. Some investigators doubt the existence of this disorder. The enzyme involved is distinct from the normal acid phosphatase found in semen or elaborated by prostatic carcinoma.

TRUE CHOLINESTERASE. True cholinesterase, an enzyme essential for neural and muscular function, is also found in erythrocytes, where its function is unknown. There are no clinical manifestations associated with decreased erythrocyte cholinesterase activities.

Dalakas MC, Leon-Monzon ME, Bernardini I, et al: Zidovudine-induced mitochondrial myopathy is associated with carnitine deficiency and lipid storage. Ann Neurol 35:482, 1994.

Frater-Shroder M: Genetic patterns of transcobalamin II and the relationships with congenital defects. Mol Cell Biochem 56:5, 1983.

Land JM, Morgan-Hughes JA, Clark JB: Mitochondrial myopathy: Biochemical studies revealing a deficiency of NADH-cytochrome B reductase activity. J Neurol Sci 50:13, 1981.

McKusick VA: Mendelian Inheritance in Man. Catalogs of Autosomal Dominant, Autosomal Recessive and X-Linked Phenotypes, 9th ed. Baltimore, MD, Johns Hopkins, 1990.

Monanen I, Fisher KJ, Kaartinen V, et al: Aspartylglycosaminuria: protein chemistry and molecular biology of the most common lysosomal storage disorder of glycoprotein degradation. FASEB J 7:1247, 1993.

Morisaki H, Morisaki T, Newby LK, et al: Alternative splicing: A mechanism for phenotypic rescue of a common inherited defect. J Clin Invest 91:2275, 1993.

Murray JC, Demopulos CM, Lawn RM, et al: Molecular genetics of human serum albumin; restriction enzyme fragment length polymorphisms and analbuminemia. Proc Natl Acad Sci USA 80:5951, 1983.

Park H, Vettese MB, Fensom AH, et al: Characterization of three alleles causing aspartylglycosaminuria; two from a British family and one from an American patient. Biochem J 290:735, 1993.

Pike JW, Dokoh S, Haussler MR, et al: Vitamin D_3-resistant fibroblasts have immunoassayable 1,25-dihydroxyvitamin D_3-receptors. Science 224:879, 1984.

Prockop DJ, Kivirikko KI: Heritable diseases of collagen. N Engl J Med 311:376, 1984.

Prody CA, Zevin-Sonkin D, Gnatt A, et al: Isolation and characterization of full length cDNA clones coding for cholinesterase from fetal human tissues. Proc Natl Acad Sci USA 84:3555, 1987.

Rhead WJ, Amendt BA, Fritchman KS, et al: Dicarboxylic aciduria: Deficient [1-14C] octanoate oxidation and medium-chain acyl-CoA dehydrogenase in fibroblasts. Science 221:73, 1983.

Roesel RA, Bowyer F, Blankenship PR, et al: Combined xanthine and sulfite oxidase defect due to a deficiency of molybdenum cofactor. J Inher Metab Dis 9:343, 1986.

Trijbels JM, Scholte HR, Ruitenbeck W, et al: Problems with the biochemical diagnosis in mitochondrial (encephalo-)myopathies. Eur J Pediat 152:178, 1993.

CHAPTER 76

The Porphyrias

Shigeru Sassa

The porphyrias are inherited and acquired disorders in which the activities of the enzymes of the heme biosynthetic pathway are partially or almost completely deficient. As a result, abnormally elevated levels of porphyrins and/or their precursors are produced, accumulate in tissues, and are excreted in urine and stool. Heme is composed of ferrous iron and protoporphyrin IX (Fig. 76–1) and is an essential molecule for life as the prosthetic group of hemeproteins, such as hemoglobin, myoglobin, mitochondrial and microsomal cytochromes, catalase, peroxidases, and tryptophan pyrrolase. Patients with porphyrias suffer from either cutaneous photosensitivity due to accumulation of porphyrins in the skin, or neurologic disturbances due to accumulation of their precursors, or both.

HEME BIOSYNTHETIC PATHWAY

The steps involved in the heme biosynthetic pathway are illustrated in Figure 76–2. In animal cells, the first step and the last three steps occur in mitochondria; the intermediate steps take place in the cytosol. The two major organs that are active in heme synthesis are the liver and the erythroid bone marrow, and inherited enzymatic defects in the porphyrias are mainly expressed in these tissues. In erythroid cells, hemoglobin is made in erythroblasts or reticulocytes, which still contain mitochondria, while circulating erythrocytes lack the ability to form heme.

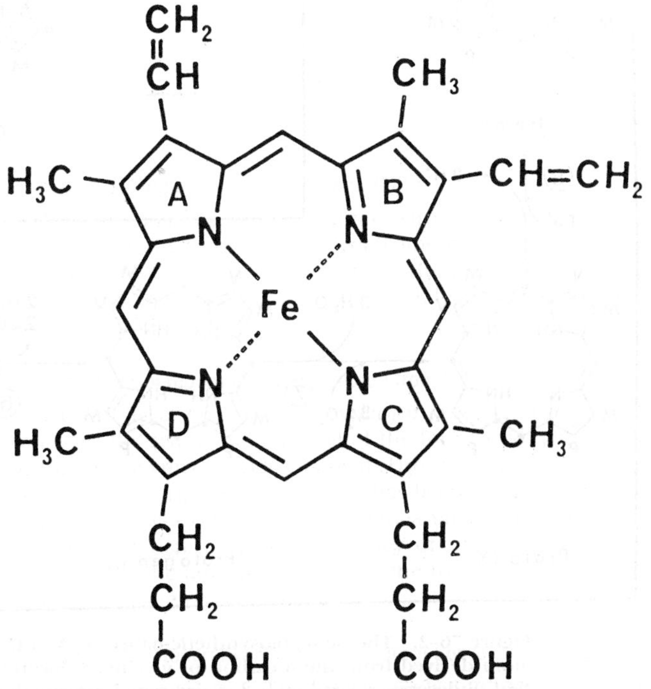

Figure 76–1. Structure of heme.

two hydrogens from the propionic groups of pyrrole rings A and B of Copro′ to form vinyl groups at these positions (Fig. 76–2, Step 6). The gene for human Copro′Ox is localized to chromosome 9. Hereditary coproporphyria (HCP) is due to a partial (or heterozygous) deficiency of Copro′Ox (Fig. 76–3).

Formation of Protoporphyrin from Protoporphyrinogen (Proto′)

The oxidation of Proto′ to protoporphyrin is mediated by *protoporphyrinogen oxidase* (Proto′Ox), which catalyzes the removal of six hydrogen atoms from the porphyrinogen nucleus (Fig. 76–2, Step 7). Variegate porphyria (VP) is due to a partial (or heterozygous) deficiency of Proto′Ox (Fig. 76–3). This is the only enzyme in the heme biosynthetic pathway for which cDNA cloning has not been reported.

Formation of Heme from Protoporphyrin

The final step of heme biosynthesis is the insertion of iron into protoporphyrin (Fig. 76–2, Step 8). This reaction is catalyzed by the enzyme *ferrochelatase* (FeC). Unlike other steps in the heme biosynthetic pathway, this enzyme uses protoporphyrin IX as a substrate, rather than its reduced form. However, the enzyme specifically requires ferrous, not ferric, iron. The gene for human FeC has been assigned to chromosome 18q21.3. Erythropoietic protoporphyria (EPP) is due to a partial (or heterozygous) FeC deficiency (Fig. 76–3).

REGULATION OF HEME SYNTHESIS

Biosynthesis of heme in the liver is controlled largely by the rate of formation of ALAS, that is ALAS-N. The enzyme activity in normal liver cells is very low, while its level increases dramatically when the liver needs to make more heme in response to various chemical treatments. The synthesis of the enzyme is also regulated in a feedback fashion by heme, that is, the end product of the biosynthetic pathway. At higher heme concentrations than those that repress the synthesis of ALAS-N, heme induces microsomal heme oxygenase, resulting in enhancement of its own catabolism. Thus heme concentration is maintained by a balance between the synthesis of ALAS-N and heme oxygenase, both of which are under the regulatory influence of heme. In contrast, ALAS-E synthesis in erythroid cells is either refractory to heme treatment or often stimulated by such treatment.

PATHOPHYSIOLOGIC CONSEQUENCES OF PORPHYRINS AND THEIR PRECURSORS

Photosensitivity

Free porphyrins occur only in small amounts in normal tissues, but their levels may become markedly elevated in porphyrias. Upon illumination at wavelengths ≈400 nm (Soret band) and in the presence of oxygen, porphyrins cause photodynamic damage to tissues, cells, subcellular elements, and biomolecules via the formation of singlet oxygen.

Neurologic Disturbances

Acute hepatic porphyrias, that is ADP, AIP, HCP, and VP, are characterized by neurologic disturbances. Most common symptoms are abdominal pain, disturbances in intestinal motility (e.g., diarrhea and constipation), dysesthesia, muscular paralysis, and respiratory failure, which can often be fatal. The exact nature of the neurologic disturbances in the porphyrias remains unclear, despite the fact that various theories have been proposed, including the involvement of excessive porphyrin precursors, deficient heme synthesis, or increased tryptophan in the central nervous system due to decreased hepatic tryptophan pyrrolase activity.

CLASSIFICATION OF PORPHYRIAS

In this chapter, each porphyria will be described according to the order of the enzymes in the heme biosynthetic sequence (Fig. 76–3). There are eight enzymes involved in the synthesis of heme and, with the exception of the first enzyme, that is, ALAS, an enzymatic defect at each step of heme synthesis is associated with each form of porphyria (Fig. 76–3 and Table 76–1). Porphyrias are classified as either hepatic or erythropoietic, depending on the principal site of expression of the specific enzymatic defect (Table 76–1). They can also be classified as acute hepatic or cutaneous porphyrias. Acute hepatic porphyrias are characterized clinically by neurologic disturbances and biochemically by an overproduction of porphyrin precursors, while cutaneous porphyrias are characterized clinically by cutaneous photosensitivity and biochemically by an excessive production of porphyrins. Cardinal symptoms and laboratory findings of each porphyria are summarized in Table 76–2.

ALAD Deficiency Porphyria (ADP)

ADP is an autosomal recessive disorder resulting from a homozygous ALAD deficiency (Fig. 76–3 and Table 76–1). This is the rarest form of the porphyrias; only four cases have been reported to date. The symptomatology is similar to that seen in AIP.

CLINICAL MANIFESTATIONS. Patients with ADP show vomiting, pain in the arms and legs, and neuropathy, exacerbated following stress, alcohol use, or decreased food intake. A rare infant with ADP has been reported who has a clinical course from birth onward which includes general muscle hypotonia and respiratory insufficiency.

LABORATORY FINDINGS. Urinary ALA excretion is markedly elevated, whereas urinary PBG excretion is within the normal range. Urinary and erythrocyte porphyrins are also markedly elevated (100-fold); no satisfactory explanation has yet been advanced to account for this observation. Fecal porphyrin excretion is normal or marginally elevated. Patients with ADP display markedly decreased activities of ALAD in erythrocytes, as well as in nonerythroid cells (≤2% of normal), and their parents show approximately 50% decreases in enzyme activities.

GENETICS. A patient with adult-onset disease was found to have separate point mutations, one occurring in each ALAD allele. One was a base transition, $G^{820} \rightarrow A$, resulting in an amino acid change, $Ala^{274} \rightarrow Thr$, while the other was a base transition, $C^{718} \rightarrow T$, which resulted in an amino acid change, $Arg^{240} \rightarrow Trp$. The former mutation accompanied markedly reduced enzyme activity, while the latter accompanied instability of the enzyme. These findings demonstrated that the proband was a compound heterozygote for two separate point mutations and accounted for the almost complete lack of enzymatic activity in the proband's cells, and the half-normal activity in cells from his family members. Another compound heterozygosity with point mutations distinct from the above-mentioned proband was also demonstrated in a child with ADP. The four distinct point mutations in two pedigrees suggest a marked heterogeneity in the mutations in this disorder.

DIAGNOSIS. Definitive diagnosis is dependent upon the demonstration of impaired ALAD activity and deficiency of enzyme protein in erythrocytes. Supporting evidence includes massive elevations in urinary ALA, substantial elevations of porphyrins in urine and erythrocytes, and perhaps modest elevations in fecal porphyrins. Clinical symptoms of ADP occur only in homozygous patients, while heterozygous subjects, that is, parents and certain siblings of the proband, remain clinically unaffected.

■ TABLE 76–1 The Porphyrias and Their Enzymatic Defects

Enzyme Deficiency	Porphyria	Prinicipal Site of Expression	Mode of Transmission	Remarks
ALAD	ADP	Liver	Recessive	
PBGD	AIP	Liver	Dominant	
	Type I			CRIM (−)
	Type II			Normal erythrocyte PBGD
	Type III			CRIM (+)
Uro'CoS	CEP	Bone marrow	Recessive	
Uro'D	PCT	Liver		
	Type I		Dominant	Acquired
	Type II			
	Type III		Dominant	
	HEP	Liver and bone marrow	Recessive	
Copro'Ox	HCP	Liver	Dominant	
Proto'Ox	VP	Liver	Dominant	
FeC	EPP	Bone marrow	Dominant	

From Sassa S, Kappas A: The porphyrias. In: *Nathan DG, Oski FA (eds): Hematology in Infancy and Childhood, 4th ed. Philadelphia, WB Saunders, 1993, pp 451–471.*

TREATMENT. The similarities in ptoms between ADP and AIP suggest that prudent management of ADP should probably be directed along the same lines as the management of AIP.

Acute Intermittent Porphyria (AIP)

AIP, which may also be termed Swedish porphyria, pyrroloporphyria, or intermittent acute porphyria, is an autosomal dominant disorder resulting from a partial PBGD deficiency (Fig. 76–3 and Table 76–1). The deficient enzyme activity (≅50% of normal) is found in all tissues, including erythrocytes, in the majority of patients (≥85%). This is consistent with the heterozygous state of affected individuals. However, a subset of patients (≤15%) show deficient enzyme activity only in nonerythroid cells. The majority (≅90%) of individuals with this genetic enzyme deficiency remain biochemically and clinically normal. Clinical expression of the disease is usually linked to environmental or acquired factors, for example, nutritional status, drugs, steroids, other chemicals of endogenous or exogenous origin, etc. The cardinal pathobiology of the disease is a neurologic dysfunction that may affect the peripheral, autonomic, or central nervous systems (Table 76–2).

EPIDEMIOLOGY. AIP is probably the most common of all the genetic porphyrias. The highest incidence occurs in Lapland, Scandinavia, and the United Kingdom, although it has been reported in many population groups. The prevalence of AIP was estimated to be 1–2 in 100,000 in Europe and 2.4 in 100,000 in Finland. The frequency of low PBGD activity, which includes both patients with AIP and latent gene carriers, is, however, as high as 1 in 500 in the general population of Finland. The disorder is expressed clinically after puberty, and more commonly in women than in men.

CLINICAL MANIFESTATIONS. Abdominal pain, which may be generalized or localized, is the most common symptom and is often the initial sign of an acute attack. Other gastroenterologic features may include nausea, vomiting, constipation or diarrhea, abdominal distention, and ileus. Urinary retention, incontinence, and dysuria may frequently be observed. In severe cases, the urine develops a port-wine color due to a high content of porphobilin, an auto-oxidation product of PBG.

■ TABLE 76–2 Clinical and Laboratory Features of the Porphyrias

Porphyria	Clinical Features	Laboratory Features			
		Erythrocytes	*Plasma*	*Urine*	*Stool*
ADP	Neurologic (as in AIP)	ZnPP	—	ALA	—
AIP	Neurologic: nausea, vomiting, abdominal pain, diarrhea, constipation, ileus, dysuria muscle hypotonia, respiratory failure, sensory neuropathy, seizures	—	—	ALA, PBG	—
CEP	Photosensitivity: bullae, crusts, scar formation, sclerodermoid change, hyper- and hypopigmentation, hypertrichosis, erythrodontia, hemolytic anemia, spolenomegaly	Uro I, Copro I	Uro I, Copro I	Uro, 7-carboxyl	—
PCT	Photosensitivity: skin fragility, bullae, crusts, scar formation, sclerodermoid change, hyper- and hypopigmentation, hypertrichosis	—	Uro, 7-carboxyl	Uro, 7-carboxyl	Uro, 7-carboxyl, Isocopro
HEP	Photosensitivity (as in CEP)	ZnPP	Uro, 7-carboxyl	Uro, 7-carboxyl	Uro, 7-carboxyl, Isocopro
HCP	Neurologic (as in ADP, AIP, and VP) and photosensitive (as in VP)	—	Copro	Copro, ALA, PBG	Copro
VP	Neurologic (as in ADP, AIP, and HCP) and photosensitive (as in HCP)	—	Proto	ALA, PBG	Proto
EPP	Photosensitivity: burning sensation, edema, erythema, itching, scarring vesicles	Proto	Proto	—	Proto

7-Carboxyl, 7-carboxylporphyrin; Copro, coproporphyrin; Isocopro, isocoproporphyrin; Uro, uroporphyrin; ZnPP, zinc protoporphyrin. From Sassa S, Kappas A: The porphyrias. In: *Nathan DG, Oski FA (eds): Hematology in Infancy and Childhood, 4th ed. Philadelphia, WB Saunders, 1993, pp 451–471.*

Tachycardia and hypertension, and less frequently fever, sweating, restlessness, and tremor, are also observed. In up to 40% of patients, hypertension may become sustained between acute attacks.

Neuropathy is a common feature of AIP. Muscle weakness often begins proximally in the legs but may involve the arms or the distal extremities. Motor neuropathy may also involve the cranial nerves, or lead to bulbar paralysis, respiratory deficiency, and death. Sensory patchy neuropathy may also occur. Acute attacks of AIP may be accompanied by seizures, especially in patients with hyponatremia due to vomiting, inappropriate fluid therapy, or the syndrome of inappropriate antidiuretic hormone release. The course of an acute attack of AIP is highly variable, both in individuals and among patients, with attacks lasting from a few days to several months. There are no cutaneous manifestations associated with this enzyme deficiency.

Asymptomatic heterozygotes (≅90% of subjects with documented PBGD deficiency) may display neither abnormalities in concentrations of porphyrin precursors nor clinical symptoms. Individuals with both latent or previously clinically expressed AIP may be precipitated into an acute attack by endogenous or exogenous environmental factors. There are at least five different classes of *precipitating factors* in this disease. (1) *ALAS-N inducers:* Most precipitating factors can be related to an associated increase in the activity of ALAS-N in the liver. An overproduction of ALA then makes the partially deficient PBGD activity rate limiting. (2) *Endocrine factors:* The clinical disease is more common in women, especially at the time of menses. (3) *Calorie intake:* Reduced calorie intake often leads to exacerbations of AIP. Additional calories on a diet may reduce PBG excretion and suppress clinical symptoms. (4) *Drugs and foreign chemicals:* Many chemicals, for example, barbiturates, sex steroids, and other foreign chemicals, that exacerbate porphyria have the potential to induce cytochrome P450. The resultant enhanced demand for heme synthesis may lead to induction of hepatic ALAS-N. (5) *Stress:* Stress is known to upregulate the heme oxygenase gene and leads to exacerbations of AIP. Similarly, other forms of stress, including intercurrent illnesses, infections, alcoholic excess, and surgery, are all known to contribute to the genesis of an acute attack of this disorder.

LABORATORY FINDINGS. Patients with clinically expressed AIP, as well as a few individuals with latent AIP, excrete variably increased amounts of ALA and PBG in the urine between attacks. In the majority of cases, the onset of an acute attack is accompanied by further marked increases in excretion of these precursors. Acute attacks may also be associated with elevations in the serum concentrations of ALA, PBG, and porphyrins, which are normally undetectable. Stool porphyrins are usually normal or only slightly elevated. The Watson-Schwartz test is widely used as a screening test for urinary PBG. It is, however, neither specific nor quantitative, and its results need to be confirmed and quantified by the column method of Mauzerall and Granick. Hemoglobin and bilirubin production are normal in AIP.

GENETICS. Patients with AIP can be classified into three subsets (Table 76–1). Patients with *type I* mutations are characterized by cross-reactive immunologic material (CRIM)-negative PBGD mutation; they exhibit both intermediately reduced enzyme activity and protein content (≅50% of normal). *Type II* mutations are observed in <15% of all AIP and are characterized by a decreased PBGD activity in nonerythroid cells, but with normal erythroid PBGD activity. Patients with *type III* mutations are characterized by CRIM-positive mutations, that is, decreased enzyme activity with the presence of structurally abnormal enzyme protein. Various mutations of the human PBGD gene have been described in patients with AIP and are summarized in Table 76–2. Mutations found in type I AIP are single base substitutions or deletions that result in a single amino acid change or in truncated proteins. The mutations found in type II AIP are single base substitutions that occur in the exon/intron boundary of exon 1, resulting in a splicing defect that affects only the nonspecific form of PBGD, but not the erythroid-specific PBGD, because the transcription of the gene in erythroid cells starts downstream of the site of mutation. Mutations characterizing type III AIP are observed in the region that is thought to be essential for catalytic activity.

DIAGNOSIS. Diagnosis of type I and III AIP can be made by demonstrating decreased PBGD activity in erythrocytes in the majority of patients (≥85%), while the distinction between carrier or latent status and clinically expressed AIP requires demonstration of elevated urinary excretion of PBG and ALA. Elevated levels of both ALA and PBG may also be seen in HCP and VP; measurement of urinary and stool porphyrins will usually differentiate these conditions from AIP. The diagnosis of type II AIP requires either the demonstration of PBGD deficiency in nonerythroid cells or DNA hybridization using allele-specific oligonucleotide specific for the mutation.

TREATMENT. The treatment of AIP as well as ADP, HCP, and VP is essentially identical. Treatment between attacks comprises adequate nutritional intake, avoidance of drugs known to exacerbate porphyria, and prompt treatment of other intercurrent diseases or infections. Unresponsive severe cases should be treated with intravenous administration of the carbohydrate dextrose to provide a minimum of 300 g of carbohydrate/24 hr. Intravenous hematin (4 mg/kg, every 12 hr) is also effective in reducing ALA and PBG excretion as well as in curtailing acute attacks. Nasal or subcutaneous administration of long-acting agonistic analogs of LHRH have been shown to inhibit ovulation and greatly reduce the incidence of perimenstrual attacks of AIP in some women with cyclic exacerbations of the disease. Synthetic heme analogs, for example, Sn-mesoporphyrin, have also been shown to diminish the output of ALA, PBG, and/or porphyrins in AIP and VP patients.

Congenital Erythropoietic Porphyria (CEP)

CEP, which may also be referred to as Günther's disease, is an autosomal recessive disorder (Fig. 76–3 and Table 76–1). The primary abnormality is a decreased activity of Uro'CoS activity, which results in accumulation and hyperexcretion of predominantly type I porphyrins (Table 76–2). Clinically, this enzymatic defect is expressed in utero as brownish amniotic fluid due to excessive amounts of porphyrins and results in cutaneous photosensitivity, hemolysis, and a decreased life expectancy after birth.

EPIDEMIOLOGY. Fewer than 200 cases have been reported and some of these cases may really have had PCT or HEP. There is no clear racial or sexual predominance.

CLINICAL MANIFESTATIONS. The diagnosis of CEP is suggested at birth by pink to dark brown staining of the diapers in infants, due to large amounts of porphyrins in urine. Early onset of cutaneous photosensitivity is characteristic and is exacerbated by exposure to sunlight. Subepidermal bullous lesions progress to crusted erosions, which heal with scarring and either hyperpigmentation or, less commonly, hypopigmentation. Hypertrichosis and alopecia are frequent, and erythrodontia (with red fluorescence under ultraviolet light) is virtually pathognomonic of CEP. Patients may display symptoms and signs of hemolytic anemia with splenomegaly and porphyrin-rich gallstones. Bone marrow shows erythroid hyperplasia, which may result in pathologic fractures or vertebral compression-collapse and shortness of stature. Although the onset of symptoms of CEP is most often observed in early infancy, a few patients may first present the syndrome as adults.

PATHOGENESIS. The primary site of expression of the enzymatic defect is the bone marrow; fluorescence secondary to porphyrin accumulation is variably distributed but invariably present.

Most marrow normoblasts display fluorescence, principally localized in the nuclei of the cells. Massive elevations of systemic porphyrins in CEP are derived from porphyrin-laden erythrocytes, which accounts for the multiple pathologies of the integument.

LABORATORY FINDINGS. Urinary porphyrins are always elevated (20- to 60-fold) above normal levels. Uroporphyrin and coproporphyrin are mostly type I isomers. Occasionally anemia may be severe and require transfusion.

GENETICS. There is heterogeneity of mutations in the Uro'CoS gene in patients having CEP. The first molecular analysis in a patient with CEP revealed the compound heterozygosity: a T→C transition resulting in an amino acid change of Cys^{73}→ Arg, and a C→T transition resulting in Pro^{53}→Leu[44]. The second case was, however, homozygous for the same mutation, Cys^{73}→Arg[44]. Subsequently other mutations were also found, indicating that the nature of the enzymatic defect in CEP is heterogenous, as is the case in other porphyrias.

DIAGNOSIS. Pink urine and/or the onset of severe cutaneous photosensitivity in infancy (or rarely in adults) suggests the diagnosis of CEP. Demonstration of elevated urinary, fecal, and erythrocyte porphyrins, with elevated type I isomers of uro- and coproporphyrin, establishes the diagnosis. Demonstration of a deficiency of Uro'CoS activity is definitive.

TREATMENT. The avoidance of sunlight, trauma to the skin, and infections are the most important preventive measures in CEP. Topical sunscreens may be of some help as may oral treatment with β-carotene. Transfusions with packed erythrocytes transiently decrease hemolysis and its attendant drive to increased erythropoiesis, and also decrease porphyrin excretion. Splenectomy has been used fairly frequently and has produced short-term reductions in hemolysis, porphyrin excretion, and skin manifestations but not all cases respond. Treatment with charcoal in a man with CEP was reported to have lowered porphyrin levels and induced complete clinical remission during therapy.

Porphyria Cutanea Tarda (PCT) and Hepatoerythropoietic Porphyria (HEP)

PCT is due to a heterozygous deficiency, and HEP is due to a homozygous deficiency, of Uro'D, respectively (Fig. 76–3 and Table 76–1).

PCT. PCT refers to a heterogeneous group of cutaneous porphyria diseases due to Uro'D deficiency, which may be either inherited or more commonly acquired. Both forms of the disease display reductions in hepatic Uro'D activity, but erythrocyte Uro'D activity may or may not be decreased, depending on their types. *Type I* PCT is an acquired disease that typically presents in adults, with decreased hepatic but not erythrocyte Uro'D activity. The disease may occur spontaneously but more commonly occurs in conjunction with precipitating environmental factors such as alcohol, estrogen, or drug use, or in association with other disorders. *Type II* PCT is, in contrast, inherited in an autosomal dominant fashion and is associated with decreased Uro'D activity in all tissues. *Type III* PCT is also inherited, but the defect is confined to the liver and erythrocyte Uro'D activity and concentrations are normal.

Epidemiology. PCT is probably the most common of all the porphyrias, but its exact incidence is not clear. The disease is recognized worldwide and there is no racial predilection except among the Bantus in South Africa, secondary to their high incidence of hemosiderosis. Type I PCT is generally more common than type II PCT in Europe, South Africa, and South America, although the trend may be less obvious in North America. Previously PCT was thought to be more common in men, perhaps secondary to their higher alcohol intake than women; the incidence in females has recently increased to the level seen in males, perhaps due to increased use of contraceptive steroids, postmenopausal estrogens, and alcohol.

Clinical Manifestations. The pathognomonic clinical feature of PCT is the formation of vesicles on sun-exposed areas of the skin, particularly the dorsa of the hands. The vesicles are superseded by crusting, superficial scar, or milia formation, and residual pigmentation. Facial hypertrichosis may be present and is conspicuous in women. Hypopigmented indurated plaques of skin may develop and resemble those seen in scleroderma. Photo-onycholysis is occasionally present. Neurologic dysfunction does not occur in PCT.

Pathogenesis. Phototoxic porphyrins in the skin may be largely derived from the liver and, to some extent, formed locally in the skin. Activation of the complement system after irradiation has been demonstrated in PCT patients and is presumed to result from the generation of reactive oxygen species, most likely singlet oxygen. Bullous fluid is known to contain prostaglandin E_2 and photoactivation of uroporphyrin damages lysosomes. Liver from patients with PCT almost invariably display siderosis with fatty changes, necrosis, chronic inflammatory changes, and granuloma formation. Iron, estrogens, alcohol, and chlorinated hydrocarbons, which are all potential hepatotoxins, may also aggravate PCT. The incidence of hepatitis B and C infection may also be higher than normal in PCT patients. The incidence of hepatocellular carcinoma in PCT is known to be greater than in the general population. Recently several HIV-infected patients with PCT have been reported.

Laboratory Findings. Increased concentrations of uroporphyrin (mainly isomer I) and 7-carboxylic porphyrins (isomer III) are found in the urine in PCT, with lesser increases of coproporphyrin and 5- and 6-carboxylic porphyrins. Small quantities of isocoproporphyrin may be detected in serum or in urine, but in feces this is often the dominant porphyrin excreted and represents the most important diagnostic criterion for PCT. Total daily fecal porphyrin excretion exceeds total urinary porphyrin excretion. Skin porphyrins are increased, especially in areas that are protected from photoactivation. Serum iron and ferritin concentrations are frequently elevated.

Diagnosis. The clinical picture in PCT is fairly specific but can be confused with other porphyric (e.g., VP) and nonporphyric (e.g., systemic lupus erythematosus or scleroderma) diseases. Urinary fluorescence under ultraviolet light illumination and quantification of porphyrins and separation and identification of porphyrins by TLC and HPLC will assist the diagnosis. Plasma porphyrins are elevated in PCT and in other photosensitizing porphyrias. Fecal porphyrins are often elevated; isocoproporphyrin (or an isocoproporphyrin:coproporphyrin ratio $\geq$0.1) is virtually diagnostic of PCT.

Treatment. In type I PCT, the identification and avoidance of precipitating factors is the first line of treatment. The clinical response to cessation of alcohol ingestion is highly variable; nonetheless, abstinence should be recommended. Phlebotomy is usually effective in reducing urinary porphyrin concentrations and in induction of clinical remissions. There is strong evidence that the beneficial effects of phlebotomy result from a diminution in the stores of body iron. If phlebotomy is ineffective or contraindicated due to the presence of other diseases such as anemia, low-dose chloroquine therapy may be effective. Efficacy of chloroquine therapy and phlebotomy is probably similar and a combined approach may diminish the incidence of side effects. The mechanism of action of chloroquine therapy is thought to be related to its ability to chelate porphyrins in a water-soluble and hence more easily excretable form.

HEP. HEP is a rare form of porphyria probably resulting from a homozygous defect of Uro'D. Clinically, HEP is characterized by the childhood onset of severe photosensitivity and skin fragility, and is indistinguishable from CEP. Fewer than 20 cases have been reported worldwide to date.

Clinical Manifestations. These findings are very similar to those seen in CEP. Pink urine, severe photosensitivity leading to scarring and mutilation of sun-exposed areas of skin, sclerodermoid changes, hypertrichosis, erythrodontia, anemia (often hemolytic), and hepatosplenomegaly characterize HEP. Onset is usually in early infancy or childhood, but adult onset has also been described. In contrast to PCT, serum iron concentrations are usually normal, and phlebotomy has no beneficial effects in HEP patients.

Laboratory Findings. Elevations in urinary porphyrins, predominantly uroporphyrin of isomer type I with lesser quantities of 7-carboxylic porphyrins, mainly type III, are commonly found. Isocoproporphyrin concentrations equal to or greater than coproporphyrin are also found in urine and feces. Elevated erythrocyte Zn-protoporphyrin is commonly observed (Table 76–2). Anemia and biochemical evidence of impaired hepatic function is highly variable.

Genetics. Cloning and sequencing of a cDNA of the mutated gene in a patient with HEP revealed that the enzymatic defect is due to a base transition of $G^{860} \rightarrow A$, resulting in an amino acid change of $Gly^{281} \rightarrow Glu$. This point mutation resulted in an unstable protein. Several other mutations were also reported. None of the mutations found in HEP have not been found in familial PCT, suggesting that HEP may not be a homozygous form of PCT.

Diagnosis. The diagnosis must be suspected in patients with severe photosensitivity and especially considered in the differential diagnosis of CEP. Diagnostic criteria include elevated levels of fecal or urinary isocoproporphyrin and erythrocyte Zn-protoporphyrin. Differential diagnosis of HEP includes EPP in which erythrocyte protoporphyrin is also elevated but in which, in contrast to HEP, urinary porphyrins are normal. EPP is also clinically milder than HEP. Measurement of erythrocyte or fibroblast Uro'D activities typically shows reductions to 2–10% of normal control values with intermediate reductions of Uro'D activities in family members.

Treatment. Avoidance of the sun and the use of topical sun screens is essentially all that can be offered to these patients at present. The response to phlebotomy has not been observed, although this is perhaps not surprising as serum iron levels, in contrast to those in PCT patients, are invariably normal.

Hereditary Coproporphyria (HCP)

HCP is a disease caused by a heterozygous deficiency of Copro'Ox activity, which is inherited in an autosomal dominant manner (Fig. 76–3 and Table 76–1). Clinically, the disease is similar to ADP or AIP, although it is often milder; additionally, HCP may be associated with photosensitivity. Expression of the disease is variable and influenced by the same precipitating factors responsible for the exacerbation of AIP. Very rarely, homozygous deficiency of this enzyme may occur and is associated with a more severe form of the disease.

EPIDEMIOLOGY. Clinically expressed HCP is much less common than is clinically expressed AIP, but, as with the latter disease, latent HCP or HCP gene carriers are being recognized with greater frequency since the advent of improved laboratory techniques for their detection.

CLINICAL MANIFESTATIONS. Neurovisceral symptomatology is essentially indistinguishable from that of ADP or AIP. Abdominal pain, vomiting, constipation, neuropathies, and psychiatric manifestations are common. Cutaneous photosensitivity is a feature in about 30% of cases. Attacks can be precipitated by pregnancy, the menstrual cycle, and contraceptive steroids, but the most common precipitating factor is drug administration, most notably of phenobarbital.

LABORATORY FINDINGS. The biochemical hallmark of HCP is hyperexcretion of coproporphyrin (predominantly type III) into the urine and feces. Fecal coproporphyrin may be chelated with copper, and fecal protoporphyrin may be modestly elevated. Hyperexcretion of ALA, PBG, and uroporphyrin into the urine may accompany exacerbations of the disease, but, in contrast to AIP, these findings generally normalize between attacks. Copro'Ox activity is typically reduced by about 50% in heterozygotes and by about 90–98% in homozygotes.

GENETICS. Recently, molecular analysis of HCP has been reported in two patients. In the first patient, who was homozygous for the CPO deficiency, a $C^{691} \rightarrow T$ transition in CPO cDNA was found that resulted in an $Arg^{231} \rightarrow Trp$ substitution. In the second patient with a heterozygous CPO defect, a single base substitution of $G^{265} \rightarrow A$, resulting in an amino acid substitution of $Gly^{89} \rightarrow Ser$ was detected.

DIAGNOSIS. The diagnosis of HCP should be suspected in patients with the signs, symptoms, and clinical course characteristic of the acute hepatic porphyrias (ADP, AIP, HCP, and VP) but in whom PBGD activity is normal. Urinary excretion of heme precursors is similar in HCP and VP, but the predominant or exclusive presence of fecal coproporphyrin is highly suggestive of HCP. Fecal or urinary predominance of harderoporphyrin, with greatly reduced Copro'Ox activity, was reported in a case of harderoporphyria, a variant form of HCP.

TREATMENT. The identification and avoidance of precipitating factors is essential. Treatment of acute attacks is similar to the treatment of AIP.

Variegate Porphyria (VP)

VP, which may also be termed porphyria variegata, protocoproporphyria, South African genetic porphyria, or Royal malady, is caused by a heterozygous deficiency in Proto'Ox activity and is inherited in an autosomal dominant manner (Fig. 76–3 and Table 76–1). Patients with this disorder may show neurovisceral symptoms, photosensitivity, or both (Table 76–3). Very rare forms of VP are seen with homozygous deficiencies in Proto'Ox activity.

EPIDEMIOLOGY. The incidence of VP of 3 in 1000 in South Africa is substantially higher than elsewhere. In 1980 it was estimated that there were 10,000 affected individuals in South Africa, and there is good evidence to suggest that they are all descendants of a single union between two Dutch settlers in 1680. However, the disease is recognized worldwide, and, with the exception of South Africa, there is probably no racial or geographical predilection. The incidence in Finland is reported at 1.3 in 100,000. Outside of South Africa, VP is probably less common than AIP.

CLINICAL MANIFESTATIONS. The neurovisceral symptomatology is identical to that observed in ADP, AIP, and HCP. Photosensitivity is more common, and the resulting lesions tend to be more chronic in VP than in HCP. Cutaneous manifestations comprise vesicles, bullae, hyperpigmentation, milia, hypertrichosis, and increased skin fragility. Lesions are clinically and histologically indistinguishable from PCT. Skin manifestations are less frequently observed in cold climates than in hot climates. The same spectrum of factors that leads to activation of ADP, AIP, and HCP may also exacerbate VP. Thus, barbiturates, dapsone, lead from "moonshine" whiskey, contraceptive steroids, pregnancy, and decreased carbohydrate intake have all been reported to induce or exacerbate VP.

PATHOGENESIS. Proto'Ox activity in most patients with VP is decreased ≈50%. In very rare cases of homozygous VP, however, there is a virtual absence of Proto'Ox activity. Symptoms were severe photosensitivity, growth and mental retardation, and marked neurologic abnormalities in some cases; onset of homozygous VP was in childhood in all cases.

LABORATORY FINDINGS. The biochemical hallmark of VP is elevated fecal porphyrin, usually with protoporphyrin IX exceeding coproporphyrin (mostly isomer III). Fecal X-porphyrins (ether-acetic acid-insoluble, extracted with urea-Triton), a heterogeneous group of porphyrin-peptide conjugates, are elevated in VP more than in any other type of porphyria. Urinary coproporphyrin (type III), ALA, and PBG are often normal between attacks but may become markedly elevated during acute attacks. Plasma invariably shows a fluorescence emission that probably represents a protoporphyrin-peptide conjugate.

DIAGNOSIS. VP should be considered in the differential diagnosis of acute porphyria, especially if PBGD activity is normal. Characteristic plasma porphyrin fluorescence, having a different fluorescence emission maximum from PCT, is seen in VP. The differentiation of VP from HCP is usually possible following fecal porphyrin analysis and in patients with only cutaneous manifestations. The demonstration of urinary 8- and 7-carboxylic porphyrins and isocoproporphyrin in PCT is usually sufficient for differentiation from VP. Proto'ox deficiency can be demonstrated in fibroblasts or lymphocytes.

TREATMENT. Identification and avoidance of precipitating factors are essential. Photosensitivity can be minimized by protective clothing, and canthaxanthin (a β-carotene analog) may be of some help. The treatment of neurovisceral symptoms is identical to that described for AIP.

Erythropoietic Protoporphyria (EPP)

EPP, which may also be referred to as protoporphyria, or erythrohepatic protoporphyria, is associated with a partial deficiency of FeC and is inherited in an autosomal dominant fashion (Fig. 76–3 and Table 76–1). Biochemically, this defect results in massive accumulations of protoporphyrin in erythrocytes, plasma, and feces. Clinically, the disease is characterized by the childhood onset of cutaneous photosensitivity in light-exposed areas, but skin lesions are milder and less disfiguring than those seen in CEP.

EPIDEMIOLOGY. EPP is the most common form of erythropoietic porphyria. Three hundred case reports were published as of 1976. There is no racial or sexual predilection, and onset is typically in childhood.

CLINICAL MANIFESTATIONS. Cutaneous photosensitivity of EPP is quite different from that seen in CEP or PCT. Stinging or painful burning sensations in the skin occur within 1 hr of exposure to the sun and are followed several hours later by erythema and edema. Some patients experience burning sensations in the absence of such objective signs of cutaneous phototoxicity, resulting in the erroneous diagnosis of a psychiatric illness. Petechiae, or more rarely, purpura, vesicles, and crusting, may develop and persist for several days after sun exposure. Artificial lights may also cause photosensitivity, especially operating theater lights. Symptoms are usually worse during spring and summer and occur in light-exposed areas, especially on the face and hands. Intense and repeated exposure to the sun may result in onycholysis, leathery hyperkeratotic skin over the dorsa of the hands, and mild scarring. Gallstones, sometimes presenting at an unusually early age, are fairly common, and hepatic disease, although unusual, may be severe and associated with significant morbidity. Anemia is uncommon. There are no known precipitating factors and no neurovisceral manifestations.

PATHOGENESIS. The peak light absorption range for porphyrins corresponds well to the wavelength of light (circa 400 nm) known to trigger photosensitivity reactions in the skin of EPP patients. Light-excited porphyrins generate free radicals and singlet oxygen. Thus, such radicals, notably singlet oxygen, may lead to peroxidation of lipids and cross-linking of membrane proteins, which, in erythrocytes, may result in reduced deformability and thus hemolysis. Interestingly, protoporphyrin, but not Zn-protoporphyrin, is released from erythrocytes following irradiation, which may explain why, unlike EPP, lead intoxication and iron deficiency are not associated with photosensitivity. Forearm irradiation in EPP patients leads to complement activation and polymorphonuclear chemotaxis. Similar results have been obtained in vitro, and these events may also contribute to the pathogenesis of skin lesions in EPP.

LABORATORY FINDINGS. The biochemical hallmark of EPP is excessive concentrations of protoporphyrin in erythrocytes, plasma, bile, and feces; this is due to its poor solubility in water, not in urine. The bone marrow and the newly released erythrocytes appear to be the major source of elevated protoporphyrin concentrations, although the liver may contribute in certain cases.

GENETICS. The first molecular analysis of the FeC defect was made in a patient with EPP who had ≈50% enzyme activity, its protein, and its mRNA. The patient's cells contained an unstable transcript encoding an abnormally short protein that completely lacked exon 2. Subsequently, five different mutations were found in other families. Thus far, skipping of exon 2, exon 7, exon 9, and exon 10, and three point mutations have been reported. One patient had a heteroallelic mutation, while five others had a single point mutation in one allele.

DIAGNOSIS. Photosensitivity should suggest the diagnosis, which can be confirmed by the demonstration of elevated concentrations of free protoporphyrin in erythrocytes, plasma, and stools with normal urinary porphyrins. The presence of protoporphyrin in both plasma and erythrocytes is specific for EPP. Fluorescent reticulocytes on examination of a peripheral blood smear may also suggest the diagnosis.

TREATMENT. Avoidance of the sun and use of topical sunscreen agents may be helpful. Oral administration of β carotene may afford systemic photoprotection, resulting in improved, though highly variable, tolerance to the sun. The recommended serum β-carotene level of 600–800 μg/dL is usually achieved with oral doses of 120–180 mg daily, and beneficial effects are typically seen 1–3 mo after the onset of therapy. The mechanism probably involves quenching of activated oxygen radicals.

Bishop DF, Astrin KH, Ioannou YA: Human δ-aminolevulinate synthase: Isolation, characterization, and mapping of house-keeping and erythroid-specific genes. Am J Hum Genet 45:A176, 1989.

Blauvelt A, Harris HR, Hogan DJ, et al: Porphyria cutanea tarda and human immunodeficiency virus infection. Int J Dermatol 31:474, 1992.

Brenner DA, Didier JM, Frasier F, et al: A molecular defect in human protoporphyria. Am J Hum Genet 50:1203, 1992.

Chretien S, Dubart A, Beaupain D, et al: Alternative transcription and splicing of the human porphobilinogen deaminase gene result either in tissue-specific or in housekeeping expression. Proc Natl Acad Sci 85:6, 1988.

Cotter PD, Baumann M, Bishop DF: Enzymatic defect in "X-linked" sideroblastic anemia: Molecular evidence for erythroid δ-aminolevulinate synthase deficiency. Proc Natl Acad Sci 89:4028, 1992.

Deybach JC, de Verneuil H, Boulechfar S, et al: Point mutations in the uroporphyrinogen III synthase gene in congenital erythropoietic porphyria (Gunther's disease). Blood 75:1763, 1990.

Eales L, Day RS, Blekkenhorst GH: The clinical and biochemical features of variegate porphyria: An analysis of 300 cases studied at Groote Schuur Hospital, Cape Town. Int J Biochem 12:837, 1980.

Fujita H, Kondo M, Takatani S, et al: Characterization of cDNA encoding coproporphyrinogen oxidase from a patient with heriditary coproporphyria. Hum Mol Genet 3:1807, 1994.

Goldberg A, Moore MR, McColl KEL, et al: Porphyrin metabolism and the porphyrias. *In:* Ledingham JGG, Warrell DA, Weatherall DJ (eds): Oxford Textbook of Medicine, 2nd ed. Oxford, Oxford University Press, 1987, pp 9136–9145.

Grandchamp B, Weil D, Nordmann Y, et al: Assignment of the human coproporphyrinogen oxidase to chromosome 9. Hum Genet 64:180, 1983.

Held JL, Sassa S, Kappas A, et al: Erythrocyte uroporphyrinogen decarboxylase activity in porphyria cutanea tarda: a study of 40 consecutive patients. J Invest Dermatol 93:332, 1989.

Herrero C, Vicente A, Bruguera M, et al: Is hepatitis C virus infection a trigger of porphyria cutanea tarda? Lancet 341:788, 1993.

Ishida N, Fujita H, Fukuda Y, et al: Cloning and expression of the defective genes from a patient with δ-aminolevulinate dehydratase porphyria. J Clin Invest 89:1431, 1992.

Kappas A, Sassa S, Galbraith RA, et al: The porphyrias. *In:* Scriver CR, Beaudet AL, Sly WS, Valle D (eds): The Metabolic Basis of Inherited Disease, 6th ed. New York, McGraw-Hill, 1989, pp 1305–1365.

Lim HW, Sassa S: The porphyrias. *In:* Lim HW, Soter NA (eds): Photomedicine for Clinical Dermatologists. New York, Marcel Dekker, 1993, pp 241–267.

Mantasek P, Nordmann Y, Grandchamp B: Homozygous hereditary coproporphyria caused by an arginine to tryptophan substitution in coproporphyrinogen oxidase and common introgenic polymorphisms. Hum Mol Genet 3:477, 1994.

Mathews-Roth MM: Systemic photoprotection. Dermatol Clin 4:335, 1986.

Mathews-Roth MM, Pathak MA, Fitzpatrick TB, et al: Beta carotene therapy for erythropoietic protoporphyria and other photosensitivity diseases. Arch Dermatol 113:1229, 1977.

Meguro K, Fujita H, Ishida N, et al: Molecular defects of uroporphyrinogen decarboxylase in a patient with mild hepatoerythropoietic porphyria. J Invest Dermatol 98:128, 1994.
McKay R, Druyan R, Getz GS, et al: Intramitochondrial localization of δ-aminolevulinate synthase and ferrochelatase in rat liver. Biochem J 114:455, 1969.
McLellan T, Pryor MA, Kushner JP, et al: Assignment of uroporphyrinogen decarboxylase (UROD) to the pter-p21 region of human chromosome 1. Cytogenet Cell Genet 39:224, 1985.
Mustajoki P, Tenhunen R, Niemi KM, et al: Homozygous variegate porphyria. A severe skin disease of infancy. Clin Genet 32:300, 1987.
Mustajoki P, Tenhunen R, Pierach C, et al: Heme in the treatment of porphyrias and hematological disorders. Semin Hematol 26:1, 1989.
Mustajoki P, Kauppinen R, Lannfelt L, et al: Frequency of low porphobilinogen deaminase activity in Finland. J Intern Med 231:389, 1992.
Nakahashi Y, Fujita H, Taketani S, et al: The molecular defect of ferrochelatase in a patient with erythropoietic protoporphyria. Proc Natl Acad Sci USA 89:281, 1992.
Nakahashi Y, Miyazaki H, Kadota Y, et al: Human erythropoietic protoporphyria: Identification of a mutation at the splice donor site of intron 7 causing exon 7 skipping of the ferrochelatase gene. Hum Mol Genet 2:1069, 1993.
Nakahashi Y, Miyazaki H, Kadota Y, et al: Molecular defect in human erythropoietic protoporphyria with fatal liver failure. Hum Genet 91:303, 1993.
Pimstone NR, Gandhi SN, Mukerji SK: Therapeutic efficacy of oral charcoal in congenital erythropoietic porphyria. N Engl J Med 316:390, 1987.
Plewinska M, Thunell S, Holmberg L, et al: δ-Aminolevulinate dehydratase deficient porphyria: Identification of the molecular lesions in a severely affected homozygote. Am J Hum Genet 49:167, 1991.
Potluri VR, Astrin KH, Wetmur JG, et al: Human 5-aminolevulinate dehydratase: Chromosomal localization to 9q34 by in situ hybridization. Hum Genet 76:236, 1987.
Romana M, Grandchamp B, Dubart A, et al: Identification of a new mutation responsible for hepatoerythropoietic porphyria. Eur J Clin Invest 21:225, 1991.
Sassa S, Kappas A: Hereditary tyrosinemia and the heme biosynthetic pathway. Profound inhibition of δ-aminolevulinic acid dehydratase activity by succinylacetone. J Clin Invest 71:625, 1983.
Taketani S, Kohno H, Furukawa T, et al: Molecular cloning, sequencing and expression of cDNA encoding human coproporphyrinogen oxidase. Biochim Biophys Acta 1183:547, 1994.
Thunell S, Holmberg L, Lundgreen J: Aminolevulinate dehydratase porphyria in infancy. A clinical and biochemical study. J Clin Chem Clin Biochem 25:5, 1987.
Toback AC, Sassa S, Poh Fitzpatrick MB, et al: Hepatoerythropoietic porphyria: clinical, biochemical, and enzymatic studies in a three-generation family lineage. N Engl J Med 316:645, 1987.
de Verneuil H, Aitken G, Nordmann Y: Familial and sporadic porphyria cutanea: Two different diseases. Hum Genet 44:145, 1978.
Welland FH, Hellman ES, Gaddis EM, et al: Factors affecting the excretion of porphyrin precursors by patients with acute intermittent porphyria. I. The effects of diet. Metabolism 13:232, 1964.
Wetmur JG, Bishop DF, Ostasiewicz L, et al: Molecular cloning of a cDNA for human δ-aminolevulinate dehydratase. Gene 43:123, 1986.

CHAPTER 77
Hypoglycemia

Mark A. Sperling

Glucose plays a central role in mammalian fuel economy and is a source of energy storage in the form of glycogen, fat, and protein (see Chapter 73). Glucose is an immediate source of energy because it provides 38 moles of ATP/mole of glucose oxidized. It is important for cerebral energy metabolism in that it usually is the preferred substrate whose utilization accounts for nearly all of the O_2 consumption in brain (see later). Cerebral glucose uptake occurs through a carrier-mediated, facilitated diffusion process that is dependent on blood glucose concentration. Deficiency of brain glucose transport can result in seizures due to low cerebrospinal fluid glucose concentration while blood glucose is normal. Neither glucose entry into brain cells nor its subsequent metabolism is dependent on insulin. To maintain the blood glucose concentration and prevent it from precipitously falling to levels that impair brain function, an elaborate regulatory system has evolved.

The defense against hypoglycemia is integrated by the autonomic nervous system and by hormones that act in concert to enhance glucose production through enzymatic modulation of glycogenolysis and gluconeogenesis while simultaneously limiting peripheral glucose utilization. In this context, hypoglycemia represents a defect in one or several of the complex interactions that normally integrate glucose homeostasis during feeding and fasting. This process is particularly important for neonates, in whom there is an abrupt transition from intrauterine life, characterized by dependence on transplacental glucose supply, to extrauterine life, characterized ultimately by the autonomous ability to maintain precise glucose balance. Because prematurity or placental factors may limit tissue nutrient deposits, and genetic abnormalities in enzymes or hormones may become evident in the neonate, hypoglycemia is an important cause of neonatal morbidity.

DEFINITION. In neonates, there is not always an obvious correlation between blood glucose concentration and the classic clinical manifestations of hypoglycemia. The absence of symptoms does not indicate that glucose concentration is normal and has not fallen below some optimal level for maintaining brain metabolism. In addition, there is evidence that hypoxemia and ischemia potentiate the role of hypoglycemia in causing brain damage that may permanently impair neurologic development. Consequently, the lower limit of accepted normality of the blood glucose level in newborn infants with associated illness that already impairs cerebral metabolism has not been determined (see Chapter 93). Out of concern for possible neurologic, intellectual, or psychologic sequelae in later life, many authorities now urge that in neonates any value of blood glucose below 40 mg/dL (2.2 mM) be viewed with suspicion and vigorously treated. This is particularly applicable after the initial 2–3 hr of life, when glucose normally has reached its nadir; subsequently, blood glucose levels begin to rise and achieve values of 50 mg/dL (2.8 mM) or higher after 12–24 hr. In older infants and children, a blood glucose concentration of less than 40 mg/dL (10–15% higher for serum or plasma) represents significant hypoglycemia.

SIGNIFICANCE AND SEQUELAE. Metabolism by the adult brain accounts for some 80% of total basal glucose turnover. Studies of in vivo cerebral metabolism indicate that the brain in infants and children can utilize glucose at a rate in excess of 4–5 mg/100 g of brain weight/min. Thus, the brain of a full-term neonate, weighing about 420 g in a 3.5-kg infant, would require glucose at a rate of approximately 20 mg/min, representing glucose production of some 5–7 mg/kg body weight/min. Measurements of the endogenous glucose production rate in infants and children, using stable isotopes, demonstrate values of 5–8 mg/kg/min. Thus, most of the endogenous glucose production in infants and young children can be accounted for by brain metabolism. Furthermore, there is a correlation between glucose production and estimated brain weight at all ages. The correlation between glucose production and body weight demonstrates a marked change in slope beyond 40 kg of body weight, corresponding to the time when brain growth is completed.

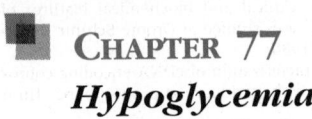

Because the brain grows most rapidly during the 1st yr of life and because the larger proportion of glucose turnover is utilized for brain metabolism, sustained or repetitive hypoglycemia in infants and children has a major impact on retarding brain development and function. In the rapidly growing brain, glucose may also be a source of membrane lipids and protein synthesis, that is, structural proteins and myelination that are important for normal brain maturation. Under conditions of severe and sustained hypoglycemia, these cerebral structural substrates may be broken down to a variety of energy-usable intermediates such as lactate, pyruvate, amino acids, and ketoacids, which can support brain metabolism at the expense of brain growth. The capacity of the newborn brain to take up and oxidize ketone bodies is about five-fold greater than that in the adult brain. However, the liver's capacity to produce ketone bodies may be limited in the newborn period, especially in the presence of hyperinsulinemia, which acutely inhibits hepatic glucose output, lipolysis, and ketogenesis, thereby depriving the brain of alternate fuel sources. The deprivation of the brain's major energy source during hypoglycemia and the limited availability of alternate fuel sources during hyperinsulinemia have predictable consequences on brain metabolism and growth: decreased brain oxygen consumption, increased breakdown of endogenous structural components to release amino acids and free fatty acid, and destruction of functional membrane integrity. All of these factors may combine and lead to permanent impairment of brain growth and function. The potentiating effects of hypoxia may exacerbate brain damage, or indeed be responsible for it, when blood glucose values are not in the classic hypoglycemic range.

The major long-term sequelae of severe, prolonged hypoglycemia are neurologic damage resulting in mental retardation, recurrent seizure activity, or both. Subtle effects on personality are also possible but have not been clearly defined. Permanent neurologic sequelae are present in more than half of patients with severe recurrent hypoglycemia under the age of 6 mo, the period of most rapid brain growth. In the long term, these sequelae are reflected in pathologic changes characterized by atrophic gyri, reduced myelination in cerebral white matter, and atrophy in the cerebral cortex. As indicated, these neurologic sequelae are more likely to occur when alternative fuel sources are limited, as occurs with hyperinsulinemia, when the episodes of hypoglycemia are repetitive or prolonged, or when they are compounded by hypoxia. There is no precise knowledge relating the duration or severity of hypoglycemia to subsequent neurologic development in children in a predictable manner. Although less common, hypoglycemia in older children may also produce long-term neurologic defects.

SUBSTRATE, ENZYME, AND HORMONAL INTEGRATION OF GLUCOSE HOMEOSTASIS

IN THE NEWBORN (see also Chapter 93). Under nonstressed conditions fetal glucose is derived virtually entirely from the mother through placental transfer. Therefore, fetal glucose concentration usually reflects maternal glucose levels. Catecholamine release, which occurs with fetal stress such as hypoxia, mobilizes fetal glucose and free fatty acids through β-adrenergic mechanisms, reflecting the existence of functionally linked β-adrenergic receptors in fetal liver and adipose tissues. In high doses, catecholamines can exert appropriate modulation of fetal pancreatic hormone secretion by inhibiting insulin and stimulating glucagon release.

The acute interruption of maternal glucose transfer to the fetus at delivery imposes an immediate need to mobilize endogenous glucose. Three related events facilitate this transition: changes in hormones, changes in their receptors, and changes in key enzyme activity. In all mammalian species, there is a three- to fivefold abrupt increase in glucagon concentration within minutes to hours of birth. Insulin, on the other hand, usually falls initially and remains in the basal range for several days without demonstrating the usual brisk response to physiologic stimuli such as glucose. A dramatic surge in spontaneous catecholamine secretion also is characteristic of several mammalian species. These changes in epinephrine, glucagon, and insulin may be interrelated because epinephrine is capable of stimulating glucagon and suppressing insulin release. In addition, epinephrine can augment growth hormone secretion by α-adrenergic mechanisms, and growth hormone levels are considerably elevated at birth. Acting in unison, these hormonal changes at birth mobilize glucose via glycogenolysis and gluconeogenesis, activate lipolysis, and promote ketogenesis. As a result of this process, plasma glucose concentration stabilizes after a transient decrease immediately after birth, liver glycogen stores become rapidly depleted within hours of birth, and gluconeogenesis from alanine, a major gluconeogenic amino acid, can account for approximately 10% of glucose turnover in the human newborn infant by several hours of age. Free fatty acid concentrations also rise sharply in concert with the surges in glucagon and epinephrine and are followed by rises in ketone bodies. In this way, glucose is spared for brain utilization while free fatty acids and ketones provide alternative fuel sources for muscle as well as essential gluconeogenic factors such as acetyl-CoA and NADH from hepatic fatty acid oxidation, which is required to drive gluconeogenesis.

In the early postnatal period, responses of the endocrine pancreas favor glucagon secretion at the relative expense of insulin secretion so that blood glucose concentration can be maintained. These adaptive changes in hormone secretion are paralleled by similarly striking adaptive changes in hormone receptors. The surge in epinephrine and glucagon secretion and their coupling to appropriate receptors augment glucose production and lipolysis. Key enzymes involved in glucose production also change dramatically in the perinatal period. Thus, there is a rapid fall in glycogen synthase activity and a sharp rise in phosphorylase after delivery. Similarly, the rate-limiting enzyme for gluconeogenesis, phosphoenol pyruvate carboxykinase (PEPCK), rises dramatically after birth, activated in part by the surge in glucagon and the fall in insulin. This framework permits an interpretation of the normal mechanisms underlying the transition from intrauterine dependence on maternal glucose to extrauterine autonomy of newborn glucose metabolism. This framework can also explain several causes of neonatal hypoglycemia based on inappropriate changes in hormone secretion, unavailability of adequate reserves of substrates in the form of hepatic glycogen, muscle as a source of amino acids for gluconeogenesis, and lipid stores for the release of fatty acids. In addition, appropriate activities of key enzymes governing glucose homeostasis as outlined in Figure 73–2 are required.

IN OLDER INFANTS AND CHILDREN. Hypoglycemia in older infants and children is analogous to that of adults, in whom glucose homeostasis is maintained by glycogenolysis in the immediate postfeeding period and by gluconeogenesis several hours after meals. The liver of a 10-kg child contains 20–25 g of glycogen, which is sufficient to meet glucose requirements of 4–6 mg/kg/min for only 6–12 hr. Beyond this period, hepatic gluconeogenesis must be activated. Both glycogenolysis and gluconeogenesis depend upon the metabolic pathway summarized in Figures 73–1 and 73–3. Defects in gluconeogenesis may not become manifest in infants until the practice of frequent feeding at 3- to 4-hr intervals ceases and infants sleep through the night, a situation usually present by 3–6 mo of age. The source of gluconeogenic precursors is derived primarily from muscle protein. The muscle bulk of infants and small children is substantially smaller relative to body mass than that in adults, whereas glucose requirements per unit of body mass are greater in children, so the ability to compensate for glucose deprivation by gluconeogenesis is more limited in infants and children, as is the ability to withstand fasting for prolonged periods. The ability of muscle to generate alanine, the principal gluconeogenic amino acid, may also be limited, particularly in children with inborn errors of amino acid metabolism. Thus, in young children, the blood glucose level falls after 24 hr of fasting, insulin concentrations fall appropriately to levels of less than 5–10 μU/mL, lipolysis and ketogenesis are activated, and ketones may appear in the urine.

The switch from glycogen synthesis during and immediately after meals to glycogen breakdown and later gluconeogenesis is governed by hormones, of which insulin is of central importance (see Chapter 73). Plasma insulin concentrations increase to peak levels of 50–100 μU/mL after meals, which serves to lower blood glucose through the activation of glycogen synthesis, enhancement of peripheral glucose uptake, and inhibition of gluconeogenesis. In addition, lipogenesis is stimulated, whereas lipolysis and ketogenesis are curtailed. During fasting, plasma insulin concentrations fall to 5–10 μU/mL, and, together with other hormonal changes, this fall results in activation of gluconeogenic pathways (see Fig. 73–2). Fasting glucose concentrations are maintained through the activation of glycogenolysis and gluconeogenesis, inhibition of glycogen synthesis, and activation of lipolysis and ketogenesis. It should be emphasized that a plasma insulin concentration of greater than 10 μU/mL, in association with a blood glucose concentration of 40 mg/dL (2.2 mM) or less, is clearly abnormal, indicating a hyperinsulinemic state and failure of the mechanisms that normally result in suppression of insulin secretion during fasting or hypoglycemia.

The hypoglycemic effects of insulin are opposed by the actions of several hormones whose concentration in plasma increases as blood glucose falls. These counterregulatory hormones are glucagon, growth hormone, cortisol, and epinephrine. Acting in concert, they increase blood glucose concentration by activating glycogenolytic enzymes (glucagon and epinephrine); inducing gluconeogenic enzymes (glucagon and cortisol); inhibiting glucose uptake by muscle (epinephrine, growth hormone, cortisol); mobilizing amino acids from muscle for gluconeogenesis (cortisol); activating lipolysis providing glycerol for gluconeogenesis and fatty acids for ketogenesis (epinephrine, cortisol, growth hormone, glucagon); and inhibiting insulin release and promotion of growth hormone and glucagon secretion (epinephrine).

Congenital or acquired deficiencies in these hormones may therefore result in hypoglycemia, which will occur when endogenous glucose production cannot be mobilized to meet energy needs in the postabsorptive state, that is, 8–12 hr after meals or during fasting. Concurrent deficiency of several hormones such as occurs in hypopituitarism may result in hypoglycemia that is more severe or appears earlier than that seen with isolated hormone deficiencies.

CLINICAL MANIFESTATIONS OF HYPOGLYCEMIA

See also Chapter 93.

Clinical features generally fall into two categories. The first includes symptoms associated with the activation of the autonomic nervous system and epinephrine release, usually associated with a rapid decline in blood glucose (Table 77–1). The second category includes symptoms due to decreased cerebral glucose utilization, usually associated with a slow decline in blood glucose or prolonged hypoglycemia (see Table 77–1). Although these classic symptoms occur in older children, the symptoms of hypoglycemia in infants may be more subtle and include cyanosis, apnea, hypothermia, hypotonia, poor feeding, lethargy, and seizures. Some of these symptoms may be so mild that they are missed clinically. Occasionally hypoglycemia may be asymptomatic in the immediate newborn period. In childhood, hypoglycemia may present as behavior problems, inattention, ravenous appetite, or seizures. It may be misdiagnosed as epilepsy, inebriation, personality disorders, hysteria, and retardation. A blood glucose determination should always be performed in sick neonates, who should be vigorously treated if concentrations are below 40 mg/dL (2.2 mM). At any pediatric age level, hypoglycemia should always be considered a cause of an initial episode of convulsions or a sudden deterioration in psychobehavioral functioning.

■ TABLE 77–1 Manifestations of Hypoglycemia in Childhood

Features Associated with Activation of Autonomic Nervous System and Epinephrine Release*	Features Associated with Cerebral Glucopenia
Anxiety†	Headache†
Perspiration†	Mental confusion†
Palpitation (tachycardia)†	Visual disturbances (↓ acuity, diplopia)†
Pallor	Organic personality changes†
Tremulousness	Inability to concentrate†
Weakness	Dysarthria
Hunger	Staring
Nausea	Seizures
Emesis	Ataxia, incoordination
Angina (with normal coronary arteries)	Somnolence, lethargy
	Coma
	Stroke, hemiplegia, aphasia
	Paresthesias
	Dizziness
	Amnesia
	Decerebrate or decorticate posture

*Some of these features will be attenuated if the patient is receiving β-adrenergic blocking agents.

† Common.

CLASSIFICATION OF HYPOGLYCEMIA IN INFANTS AND CHILDREN

The classification outlined in Table 77–2 is based on knowledge of the control of glucose homeostasis in infants and children discussed earlier.

NEONATAL. Transient. SMALL FOR GESTATIONAL AGE AND PREMATURE INFANTS (see Chapter 93). The overall incidence of symptomatic hypoglycemia in newborns varies between 1.3 and 3.0 per 1,000 live births. This incidence is increased several-fold in certain high-risk neonatal groups (see Table 77–2). The premature, small for gestational age (SGA) infant is especially vulnerable to developing hypoglycemia. The factors responsible for the high frequency of hypoglycemia in this group as well as in other groups outlined in Table 77–2 are related to the inadequate stores of liver glycogen, muscle protein, and body fat needed to sustain the substrates required to meet energy needs. These infants are small by virtue of prematurity or impaired placental transfer of nutrients. In addition, their enzyme systems for gluconeogenesis may not be fully developed.

In contrast to deficiency of substrates and enzymes, the hormonal system appears to be functioning normally at birth in most neonates. Thus, the newborn surge in glucagon secretion occurs normally, low plasma insulin concentrations are usually documented, and plasma concentrations of cortisol and growth hormone are usually normal. Despite the hypoglycemia, plasma concentrations of alanine, lactate, and pyruvate are higher, implying their diminished rate of utilization as substrates for gluconeogenesis. Infusion of alanine elicits further glucagon secretion but causes no significant rise in glucose. During the initial 24 hr of life, plasma concentrations of acetoacetate and β-hydroxybutyrate are lower in SGA infants than in full-term infants, implying diminished lipid stores, diminished fatty acid mobilization, and/or impaired ketogenesis. Diminished lipid stores are most likely, since triglyceride feeding of newborns results in a rise in the plasma levels of glucose, free fatty acids (FFA), and ketones.

The role of FFA and their oxidation in stimulating neonatal gluconeogenesis is essential. The provision of FFA as triglyceride feedings together with gluconeogenic precursors may prevent the hypoglycemia that usually ensues after fasting. For these and other reasons, the practice of delaying feeding of newborns for 12–24 hr has been abandoned, and milk feedings are introduced early (within 4–6 hr) after delivery. In the hospital setting, when feeding is precluded by virtue of respiratory distress or when feedings alone cannot maintain blood glucose concentrations above 40 mg/dL (2.2 mM), intravenous glucose at a rate that supplies approximately 4–8 mg/kg/min should be begun. Infants usually can maintain their blood glucose level spontaneously after 3–5 days of life.

INFANTS BORN TO DIABETIC MOTHERS (see Chapter 93). Of the transient

■ **TABLE 77–2 Classification of Hypoglycemia in Infants and Children**

Neonatal—Transient Hypoglycemia
- Associated with inadequate substrate or enzyme function
  - Prematurity
  - Small for gestational age
  - Smaller of twins
  - Infants with severe respiratory distress
  - Infant of toxemic mother
- Associated with hyperinsulinemia
  - Infants of diabetic mothers
  - Infants with erythroblastosis fetalis

Neonatal—Infantile or Childhood Persistent Hypoglycemia
- Hyperinsulinemic states
  - Nesidioblastosis
  - ß-cell hyperplasia
  - ß-cell adenoma
  - Beckwith-Wiedemann syndrome
  - Leucine sensitivity
  - Falciparum malaria
- Hormone deficiency
  - Panhypopituitarism
  - Isolated growth hormone deficiency
  - ACTH deficiency
  - Addison disease
  - Glucagon deficiency
  - Epinephrine deficiency
- Substrate limited
  - Ketotic hypoglycemia
  - Branched-chain ketonuria (maple syrup urine disease)
- Glycogen storage disease
  - Glucose-6-phosphatase deficiency
  - Amylo-1,6-glucosidase deficiency
  - Liver phosphorylase deficiency
  - Glycogen synthetase deficiency
- Disorders of gluconeogenesis
  - Acute alcohol intoxication
  - Hyperglycinemia, carnitine deficiency
  - Salicylate intoxication
  - Fructose-1,6-diphosphatase deficiency
  - Pyruvate carboxylase deficiency
  - Phosphoenol pyruvate carboxykinase (PEPCK deficiency)
- Other enzyme defects
  - Galactosemia: galactose-1-phosphate uridyl transferase deficiency
  - Fructose intolerance: fructose-1-phosphate aldolase deficiency

Disorders of fat (alternate fuel) metabolism
- Primary carnitine deficiency
- Secondary carnitine deficiency
- Carnitine palmitoyl transferase deficiency
- Long-, medium-, short-chain fatty acid acyl-CoA dehydrogenase deficiency

Other Etiologies
- Poisoning—drugs
  - Salicylates
  - Alcohol
  - Oral hypoglycemic agents
  - Insulin
  - Propranolol
  - Pentamidine
  - Quinine
  - Disopyramide
  - Ackee fruit (unripe)–hypoglycin
  - Vacor (rat poison)
- Liver disease
  - Reye syndrome
  - Hepatitis
  - Cirrhosis
  - Hepatoma
- Amino acid and organic acid disorders
  - Maple syrup urine disease
  - Propionic acidemia
  - Methylmalonic acidemia
  - Tyrosinosis
  - Glutaric aciduria
  - 3-Hydroxy-3-methylglutaric aciduria
- Systemic disorders
  - Sepsis
  - Carcinoma/sarcoma (secreting IGFII—insulin-like growth factor II)
  - Heart failure
  - Malnutrition
  - Malabsorption
  - Anti-insulin receptor antibodies
  - Anti-insulin antibodies
  - Neonatal hyperviscosity
  - Renal failure
  - Diarrhea
  - Burns
  - Shock
  - Postsurgical
  - Pseudohypoglycemia (leukocytosis, polycythemia)
  - Excessive insulin therapy of IDDM—insulin-dependent diabetes mellitus

From Sperling M, Chernausek S: Nelson's Essentials of Pediatrics. Philadelphia, WB Saunders, 1990, p 617.

hyperinsulinemic states, infants born to diabetic mothers are most common. Gestational diabetes affects some 2% of pregnant women, and approximately 1 in 1,000 pregnant women has insulin-dependent diabetes. At birth, infants born to these mothers may be large and plethoric, and their body stores of glycogen, protein, and fat are replete. Thus, in contrast to the transient hypoglycemia of the SGA infant whose body size and tissue nutrient content reflect diminished placental transfer, infants born to diabetic mothers are examples of nutrient surfeit and represent the opposite extreme of the spectrum.

Hypoglycemia in infants of diabetic mothers is related mostly to hyperinsulinemia and partly to diminished glucagon secretion. Hypertrophy and hyperplasia of their islets have been documented, as has their brisk, biphasic, and typically adult insulin response to glucose; this insulin response is absent in normal infants. Infants born to diabetic mothers also have a subnormal surge in plasma glucagon immediately after birth, subnormal glucagon secretion in response to stimuli, and, initially, excessive sympathetic activity that may lead to adrenomedullary exhaustion because urinary excretion of epinephrine is diminished. Thus, despite their abundance of tissue stores of available substrate, the normal plasma hormonal pattern of low insulin, high glucagon, and catecholamines is reversed, and their endogenous glucose production is significantly inhibited compared to that in normal infants, thus predisposing to hypoglycemia.

Infants born with *erythroblastosis fetalis* also have hyperinsulinemia and share many physical features, such as large body size, with infants born to diabetic mothers. The cause of the hyperinsulinemia in infants with erythroblastosis is not entirely clear but may be related to compensatory hypersecretion as a result of the hemolysis that provides increased glutathione, which splits the disulfide bonds of insulin.

Mothers whose diabetes has been well controlled during pregnancy generally have babies near normal size who are less likely to develop neonatal hypoglycemia and other complications formerly considered typical of such infants. Nevertheless, treatment of infants born to mothers with diabetes commonly requires provision of intravenous glucose for several days until the hyperinsulinemia abates. In supplying glucose to these infants, it is important to avoid hyperglycemia that evokes prompt insulin release, which may result in rebound hypoglycemia. Usually glucose should be provided at rates of 4–8 mg/kg/min, but the appropriate dose for each patient should be individually adjusted. During labor and delivery, maternal hyperglycemia should be avoided because it results in fetal hyperglycemia, which predisposes to hypoglycemia when the glucose supply is interrupted at birth. Hypoglycemia persisting or occurring after 1 wk of life requires an evaluation for the causes listed in Table 77–2.

HYPOGLYCEMIA IN INFANTS AND CHILDREN. **HYPERINSULINEMIA.** Most children with hyperinsulinemia causing hypoglycemia present in infancy. Like infants born to diabetic mothers, they may be macrosomic at birth, reflecting the anabolic effects of insulin in utero. There is, however, no history and no biochemical evidence of maternal diabetes. The onset is from birth to 18 mo. Insulin concentrations are inappropriately elevated at the time of documented hypoglycemia. Thus, when blood glucose concentration is less than 40 mg/dL (2.2 mM), plasma insulin concentration should be less than 5 and no higher than 10 μU/mL. In affected infants, however, plasma insulin concentrations at the time of hypoglycemia are commonly greater than 10 μU/mL. The insulin (μU/mL)-glucose (mg/dL) ratio is 0.4 or greater, and plasma ketones and FFA levels are low during hyperinsulinemia. Macrosomic infants may present with hypoglycemia from the first days of life. Infants with lesser degrees of hyperinsulinemia, however, may manifest hypoglycemia after the first few weeks to months, when the frequency of feedings has been decreased to permit the infant to sleep through the night and hyperinsulinemia prevents the mobilization of endogenous glucose. Increasing demands for feeding, wilting spells, jitteriness, and frank seizures are the most common presenting features. Additional clues include the rapid development of fasting hypoglycemia, the need for high rates of exogenous glucose infusion to prevent hypoglycemia, absence of ketonemia or acidosis, and elevated C-peptide or proinsulin levels at the time of hypoglycemia. The latter insulin-related products are absent in factitious hypoglycemia from exogenous administration of insulin. Provocative tests with tolbutamide or leucine are not necessary in infants; hypoglycemia is invariably provoked by withholding feedings for several hours, permitting simultaneous measurement of glucose, insulin, ketones, and FFA in the same sample at the time of clinically manifest hypoglycemia. The glycemic response to glucagon at the time of hypoglycemia reveals a brisk rise in glucose of at least 40 mg/dL and implies that glucose mobilization has been restrained by insulin and that glycogenolytic mechanisms are intact (Table 77–3).

Once organic endogenous hyperinsulinism has been established through concurrent measurement of glucose and insulin, the *differential diagnosis* should include ***nesidioblastosis, β cell hyperplasia,*** and ***β cell adenoma***. These three entities cannot be distinguished by the plasma levels of insulin alone. Although they represent diffuse or localized abnormalities in the pancreas, each is characterized by autonomous insulin secretion that is not appropriately reduced when blood glucose declines spontaneously or in response to provocative maneuvers such as fasting. Celiac angiography, which reportedly has a success rate of 60–75% in localizing pancreatic endocrine tumors (adenoma or carcinoma) in adults, has shown only limited success in infants, in whom the nodules may be small and obscured by the normal rich vascular supply. The chances of detecting a tumor "blush" during arteriography must therefore be balanced by the potential risk of causing vascular trauma in infants under 2 yr. When present, however, a tumor blush may be helpful in localizing the tumor prior to surgery. Computed tomography, high-resolution ultrasonography, and MRI may be helpful in localizing a pancreatic adenoma, but most patients have hyperplasia rather than a discrete tumor.

■ TABLE 77–3 Analysis of Blood Sample Before and 30 Min After Glucagon*

Substrates	Hormones
Glucose	Insulin
Free fatty acids	Cortisol
Ketones	Growth hormone
Lactate	T_4, TSH†
Uric acid	

**Glucagon 30 μg/kg IV or IM.*
†Measure once only before or after glucagon administration.

The term ***islet cell dysmaturation syndrome*** has been used to encompass the spectrum of localized or diffuse (nesidioblastosis) disease, and islet cell histology is highly variable. Rather than a histologically distinct syndrome, the lesions of nesidioblastosis may represent a developmental variant that is present in some normal infants who have hypoglycemia. Islet cell dysmaturity syndrome may produce hyperinsulinism because of an associated deficiency or dysregulation by δ cells, which normally produce somatostatin, a paracrine inhibitor of β insulin-secreting cells.

Because the definitive diagnosis can only be made by histologic examination of removed pancreatic tissue, surgical exploration is usually undertaken in severely affected neonates who are unresponsive to glucose and somatostatin therapy. Near-total resection of 85–90% of the pancreas is recommended. Intraoperative ultrasonography may identify a small unpalpable adenoma, permitting local resection. Further resection of the remaining pancreas may occasionally be necessary if hypoglycemia recurs and cannot be controlled by medical measures, such as the use of somatostatin or diazoxide with cortisone. Surgery should be performed by experienced pediatric surgeons in medical centers equipped to provide the necessary preoperative and postoperative care, diagnostic evaluation, and management.

When the diagnosis is established before 3 mo of life, surgery is usually needed. Frequent feedings coupled with pharmacologic agents such as somatostatin or diazoxide may not consistently maintain blood glucose concentrations or adequately inhibit insulin release. If hypoglycemia first becomes manifest between 3 and 6 mo of life or later, a therapeutic trial using medical approaches with somatostatin, diazoxide, steroids, and frequent feedings can be attempted for up to 2–4 wk. Failure to maintain euglycemia without undesirable side effects from the drugs prompts the need for surgery. Some success in suppressing insulin release and correcting hypoglycemia in patients with nesidioblastosis has been reported with the use of the long-acting somatostatin analog (see later section on treatment). Most cases of neonatal nesidioblastosis are sporadic; familial forms appear to be inherited in an autosomal recessive manner, and the responsible gene has been mapped to chromosome 11. Also, hyperinsulinism, usually transient (weeks–months), may occur in asphyxiated or small for gestational age infants in whom hypoglycemia usually is attributed to asphyxia-induced catecholamine secretion that depletes glycogen stores.

Hypoglycemia associated with hyperinsulinemia is also seen in approximately 50% of patients with the ***Beckwith-Wiedemann syndrome*** (see Chapter 93). This syndrome is characterized by macrosomia, microcephaly, macroglossia, visceromegaly, and omphalocele. Distinctive lateral earlobe fissures are present. Diffuse islet cell hyperplasia and nesidioblastosis both occur in those infants with hypoglycemia. The diagnostic and therapeutic approaches are, therefore, the same as those discussed above, although microcephaly and retarded brain development may occur independently of hypoglycemia. In addition, patients with the Beckwith-Wiedemann syndrome have a predilection for the eventual development of tumors, including Wilms tumor, hepatoblastoma, and retinoblastoma.

Leucine-sensitive hypoglycemia is not being diagnosed as often as it was in previous years. Originally it was considered to occur in a subclass of children with "idiopathic hypoglycemia," in whom protein feeding, specifically leucine, triggered hypoglycemic attacks. Leucine-sensitive hypoglycemia is associated with excessive insulin secretion following leucine administration; and β-cell hyperplasia, adenoma, and nesidioblastosis may also demonstrate hyperinsulinemia in response to leucine, tolbutamide, and other provocative tests. Because nesidioblastosis may not be diagnosed by a routine histologic examination of islets without employing insulin-specific staining techniques, including immunofluorescent techniques for islet hormones, many of the cases previously diagnosed as leucine-sensitive might now be categorized as nesidioblastosis. Occasionally the diagnosis remains in doubt because histologic examination of pancreatic tissue is not undertaken owing to a satisfactory response to a low-leucine diet and diazoxide with or without additional glucocorticoids. In such cases, a functional hyperinsulinemia with leucine sensitivity serves as a descriptive term for patients who eventually outgrow their propensity for hypoglycemia at 5–7 yr of age. Nevertheless, in view of the similarity of excessive insulin response and documented islet cell hyperplasia in previous patients, it is likely that leucine-sensitive hypoglycemia is a variant of the islet cell dysmaturity syndrome.

After the first 12 mo of life, hyperinsulinemic states are uncommon until islet cell adenomas again reappear after several years of age. Hyperinsulinemia due to ***islet cell adenoma*** should be considered in any child 5 yr or older presenting with hypoglycemia. The diagnostic approach is outlined in Table 77–3. Fasting for 24–36 hr usually provokes hypoglycemia; coexisting hyperinsulinemia confirms the diagnosis, providing that factitious administration of insulin by the parents, a form of *Munchausen syndrome by proxy,* has been excluded. Occasionally, provocative tests may be required. Exogenously administered insulin can be distinguished from endogenous insulin by simultaneous measurement of C-peptide concentration. If C-peptide levels are elevated, endogenous insulin secretion is responsible for the hypoglycemia; if C-peptide levels are low but insulin values are high, exogenous insulin has been administered, perhaps as a form of child abuse. Islet cell adenomas at this age are treated by surgical excision; familial multiple endocrine adenomatosis type I (Wermer syndrome) or type II should be considered in the differential diagnosis. Antibodies to insulin or the insulin receptor (insulinomimetic action) are also rarely associated with hypoglycemia.

Endocrine Deficiency. Hypoglycemia associated with endocrine deficiency is usually due to adrenal insufficiency with or without associated growth hormone deficiency (see Chapters 512 and 528). In patients with panhypopituitarism, isolated ACTH or growth hormone deficiency, or combined ACTH deficiency plus growth hormone deficiency, the incidence of hypoglycemia is as high as 20%. In the newborn period, hypoglycemia may be the presenting feature of hypopituitarism; in males, a microphallus may provide a clue to a coexistent deficiency of gonadotropin. Newborns with hypopituitarism often have a form of "hepatitis" and the syndrome of ***septo-optic dysplasia***. When adrenal disease is severe, as in congenital adrenal hyperplasia due to cortisol synthetic enzyme defects, adrenal hemorrhage, or congenital absence of the adrenals, disturbances in serum electrolytes with hyponatremia and hyperkalemia or ambiguous genitalia may provide diagnostic clues (Chapter 529). In older children, failure of growth should suggest growth hormone deficiency. Hyperpigmentation may provide the clue to Addison disease with increased ACTH levels or adrenal unresponsiveness to ACTH due to a defect in the adrenal receptor for ACTH. The frequent association of Addison disease in childhood with hypoparathyroidism (hypocalcemia), chronic mucocutaneous moniliasis, and other endocrinopathies should be considered. Adrenoleukodystrophy should also be considered in the differential diagnosis of primary Addison disease in older children (see Chapter 72.2).

The etiology of hypoglycemia in cortisol–growth hormone deficiency may be due to decreased gluconeogenic enzymes with cortisol deficiency, increased glucose utilization due to lack of the antagonistic effects of growth hormone on insulin action, or failure to supply endogenous gluconeogenic substrate in the form of alanine and lactate with compensatory breakdown of fat and generation of ketones. Thus, deficiency of these hormones results in reduced gluconeogenic substrate, which resembles the syndrome of ketotic hypoglycemia (see later). Investigation of a child with hypoglycemia, therefore, requires exclusion of ACTH-cortisol or growth hormone deficiency, and if diagnosed, its appropriate replacement with cortisol or growth hormone.

Epinephrine deficiency could theoretically be responsible for hypoglycemia. Urinary excretion of epinephrine has been diminished in some patients with spontaneous or insulin-induced hypoglycemia in whom absence of pallor and tachycardia was also noted, suggesting that failure of catecholamine release, due to a defect anywhere along the hypothalamic-autonomic-adrenomedullary axis, might be responsible for the hypoglycemia. However, this possibility has been challenged owing to the rarity of hypoglycemia in patients with bilateral adrenalectomy providing they receive adequate glucocorticoid replacement and because diminished epinephrine excretion is found in normal patients with repeated insulin-induced hypoglycemia. In addition, many of the patients described as having hypoglycemia with failure of epinephrine excretion fit the criteria for ketotic hypoglycemia.

Glucagon deficiency in infants or children may rarely be associated with hypoglycemia.

Substrate Limited. KETOTIC HYPOGLYCEMIA. This is the most common form of childhood hypoglycemia. Usually this condition presents between the ages of 18 mo and 5 yr, and remits spontaneously by the age of 8–9 yr. Hypoglycemic episodes typically occur during periods of intercurrent illness when food intake is limited. The classic history is of a child who eats poorly or completely avoids the evening meal, is difficult to arouse from sleep the following morning, and may have a seizure or be comatose by midmorning. Another common presentation occurs when parents sleep late and the affected child is unable to eat breakfast, thus prolonging the overnight fast.

At the time of documented hypoglycemia, there is associated ketonuria and ketonemia, and plasma insulin concentrations are appropriately low, 5–10 μU/mL, thus excluding hyperinsulinemia. A ketogenic provocative diet, formerly used as a diagnostic test, is not essential to establish the diagnosis because fasting alone will provoke a hypoglycemic episode with ketonemia and ketonuria within 12–18 hr in susceptible individuals. Normal children of similar age can withstand fasting without developing hypoglycemia during the same time period, although even normal children may develop these features by 36 hr of fasting. Thus, the provocative nature of a ketogenic diet appears to be more dependent on its hypocaloric nature than its fat content; its use as a diagnostic tool has been largely replaced by complete caloric restriction.

Children with ketotic hypoglycemia have plasma alanine concentrations that are markedly reduced in the basal state after an overnight fast and decline even further with prolonged fasting. Alanine is the only amino acid that is significantly lower in these children, and infusions of alanine (250 mg/kg) produce a rapid rise in plasma glucose without causing significant changes in blood lactate or pyruvate level, indicating that the entire gluconeogenic pathway from the level of pyruvate is intact but that there is a deficiency of substrate. There is also a normal glycemic response to infusion of fructose and glycerol. Plasma glycerol levels are normal in these children in both the fed and fasted states. Glycogenolytic pathways are also intact because glucagon induces a normal glycemic response in affected children during the fed state. The metabolic response to infusion of β-hydroxybutyrate does not differ from that in normal children. Finally, the levels of hormones that counter hypoglycemia are appropriately elevated, and insulin is appropriately low.

Alanine is quantitatively the major gluconeogenic amino acid precursor whose formation and release from muscle during periods of caloric restriction are enhanced by the presence of a glucose-alanine cycle and by de novo formation from other substrates within muscle, principally branched-chain amino acid catabolism. Thus, the release of alanine (and glutamine) for gluconeogenesis exceeds the content of these amino acids in muscle tissue protein.

The *etiology* of ketotic hypoglycemia, which is characterized by hypoalaninemia, may be a defect in any of the complex steps involved in protein catabolism, oxidative deamination of amino acids, transamination, alanine synthesis, or alanine efflux from muscle. Children with ketotic hypoglycemia frequently are smaller than age-matched controls and often have a history of transient neonatal hypoglycemia. Thus, any decrease in muscle mass may compromise the supply of gluconeogenic substrate at a time when glucose demands per unit of body weight are already relatively high, thus predisposing to the rapid development of hypoglycemia, with ketosis representing the attempt to switch to an alternative fuel supply. Children with ketotic hypoglycemia may represent the low end of the spectrum of children's capacity to tolerate fasting. Similar relative intolerance to fasting is present in normal children, who cannot maintain blood glucose after 30–36 hr of fasting, compared with the adult's capacity for prolonged fasting. Although the defect may be present at birth, it may not become manifest until the child is stressed by more prolonged periods of caloric restriction. Moreover, the spontaneous remission observed in children at age 8–9 yr might be explained by the increase in muscle bulk with its resultant increase in supply of endogenous substrate and the relative decrease in glucose requirement per unit of body mass with increasing age. There is also some evidence to support the contention that impaired epinephrine secretion due to immaturity of autonomic innervation contributes to ketotic hypoglycemia.

In anticipation of spontaneous resolution of this syndrome, *treatment* of ketotic hypoglycemia consists of frequent feedings of a high-protein, high-carbohydrate diet. During intercurrent illnesses, parents should test the child's urine for the presence of ketones, the appearance of which precedes hypoglycemia by several hours. In the presence of ketonuria, liquids of high carbohydrate content should be offered to the child. If these cannot be tolerated, the child should be offered a short course of steroids or admitted to the hospital for intravenous glucose administration.

Branched-Chain Ketonuria (Maple Syrup Urine Disease) (see Chapter 71.6). The hypoglycemic episodes had previously been attributed to high levels of leucine, but evidence now indicates that interference with the production of alanine and its availability as a gluconeogenic substrate during caloric deprivation is responsible for hypoglycemia.

Glycogen Storage Disease. See Chapter 73. Glycogen storage diseases associated with hypoglycemia are summarized in the following sections.

Glucose-6-Phosphatase Deficiency (Type I Glycogen Storage Disease) (see Chapter 73.5). Typically affected children display a remarkable tolerance to their chronic hypoglycemia; blood glucose values in the range of 20–50 mg/dL (1.1–2.7 mM) are not associated with the classic symptoms of hypoglycemia, possibly reflecting the adaptation of the central nervous system to ketone bodies as an alternative fuel. The gene for glucose-6-phosphatase has been identified, and this should permit a better understanding of the variable clinical manifestations of this disorder.

Affected untreated children manifest growth failure, mental retardation, and a shortened life span unless they are treated. Continuous intragastric feeding or total parenteral nutrition improves the metabolic and clinical findings by reducing the frequency and severity of hypoglycemia, thereby avoiding the secondary hormonal changes that appear to be responsible for the metabolic derangements. Continuous intragastric feeding at night, combined with frequent daytime feedings, produces equally effective amelioration of the biochemical disturbances and avoids the inconvenience of 24-hr continuous gastric feeding and the problems associated with long-term parenteral nutrition. The daytime feedings are given every 3–4 hr: 60–70% of the calories as carbohydrate low in fructose and galactose, 12–15% of the calories as protein, and 15–25% of the calories as fat. At night, a small nasogastric tube is passed by the patient (or a parent, for younger children), and approximately one third of the daily caloric requirements is continuously infused over 8–12 hr using a small continuous infusion pump. One commercially available formula for nocturnal infusion contains 89% of the calories as glucose and glucose oligosaccharides, 1.8% as safflower oil, and 9.2% as crystalline amino acids.* Corn starch nocturnal therapy also has been used successfully, and liver transplantation offers promise of long-term cure.

Amylo-1,6-Glucosidase Deficiency (Debrancher Enzyme Deficiency; Type III Glycogen Storage Disease). See Chapter 73.

Liver Phosphorylase Deficiency (Type VI Glycogen Storage Disease). See also Chapter 73. Normal liver phosphorylase activity involves a complex cascade of events that degrades liver glycogen both before and after the debranching step. Consequently, low hepatic phosphorylase activity may result from a defect in any of the steps of activation, and a variety of defects have been described. Hepatomegaly, excessive deposition of glycogen in liver, growth retardation, and occasional symptomatic hypoglycemia occur. A diet high in protein and reduced in carbohydrate usually prevents hypoglycemia.

Glycogen Synthetase Deficiency (see also Chapter 73). The inability to synthesize glycogen is an extremely rare occurrence. There is fasting hypoglycemia and hyperketonemia, but hyperglycemia occurs with glucosuria after meals. During fasting hypoglycemia, levels of the counterregulatory hormones, including catecholamines, are appropriately elevated or normal, and insulin levels are appropriately low. Gluconeogenic capacity appears to be intact. The liver is not enlarged. Glycogen synthetase activity is markedly reduced in the liver but is normal in muscle. Protein-rich feedings at frequent intervals result in dramatic clinical improvement, including growth velocity. This condition mimics the syndrome of ketotic hypoglycemia and should be considered in the differential diagnosis of that syndrome.

Disorders of Gluconeogenesis. Acute Alcohol Intoxication. The liver metabolizes alcohol as a preferred fuel, and generation of reducing equivalents during the oxidation of ethanol alters the NADH-NAD ratio, which is essential for certain gluconeogenic steps. As a result, gluconeogenesis is impaired, and hypoglycemia may ensue if glycogen stores are depleted by starvation or by pre-existing abnormalities in glycogen metabolism. In toddlers who have been unfed for some time, even the consumption of small quantities of alcohol can precipitate these events. The hypoglycemia responds promptly to intravenous glucose, which should always be given to a child who presents initially with coma or seizure, after taking a blood sample to determine glucose concentration. The possibility of the child's ingesting alcoholic drinks must also be considered if there was a preceding evening party. A careful history allows the diagnosis to be made and may avoid needless and expensive hospitalization and investigation.

Defects in Fatty Acid Oxidation (see also Chapter 72.1). The important role of fatty acid oxidation in maintaining gluconeogenesis is underscored by examples of congenital or drug-induced defects in fatty acid metabolism that may be associated with fasting hypoglycemia.

Various congenital enzymatic deficiencies causing defective carnitine or fatty acid metabolism also occur. A severe form of fasting hypoglycemia with hepatomegaly, cardiomyopathy, and hypotonia occurs with long- and medium-chain fatty acid coenzyme-A dehydrogenase deficiency. Plasma carnitine levels

*Vivonex, Eaton Laboratories.

are low, ketones are not present in urine, but dicarboxylic aciduria is present. Clinically, patients with acyl ***CoA dehydrogenase deficiency*** present with a Reye-like syndrome, recurrent episodes of severe fasting hypoglycemic coma, and cardiorespiratory arrest (SIDS-like events). Severe hypoglycemia and metabolic acidosis without ketosis also occur in patients with multiple acyl CoA dehydrogenase disorders. Hypotonia, seizures, and acrid odor are other clinical clues. Survival depends on whether the defects are severe or mild; diagnosis is established from studies of enzyme activity in liver biopsy tissue or in cultured fibroblasts from affected patients. The frequency of this disorder, about one in 15,000 births, suggests that screening for medium chain acyl CoA-dehydrogenase deficiency is indicated; molecular diagnostic methods are being developed. Avoidance of fasting and supplementation with carnitine may be life saving in these patients who generally present in infancy.

Interference with fatty acid metabolism also underlies the fasting hypoglycemia associated with Jamaican vomiting sickness, with atractyloside, and with the drug valproate. In ***Jamaican vomiting sickness***, the unripe ackee fruit contains a water-soluble toxin, hypoglycin, which produces vomiting, central nervous system depression, and severe hypoglycemia. The hypoglycemic activity of hypoglycin derives from its inhibition of gluconeogenesis secondary to its interference with the acyl CoA and carnitine metabolism essential for the oxidation of long-chain fatty acids. The disease is almost totally confined to Jamaica, where ackee forms a staple of the diet for the poor. The ripe ackee fruit no longer contains this toxic principle. ***Atractyloside*** is a reagent that inhibits oxidative phosphorylation in mitochondria by preventing the translocation of adenine nucleotides, such as ATP, across the mitochondrial membrane. Atractyloside is a perhydrophenanthrenic glycoside derived from *Atractylis gummifera*. This plant is found in the Mediterranean basin; ingestion of this "thistle" is associated with hypoglycemia and a syndrome similar to Jamaican vomiting sickness. More commonly, the drug ***valproate***, now used for the treatment of epilepsy, is associated with side effects, predominantly in young infants, which include a Reye-like syndrome, low serum carnitine levels, and the potential for fasting hypoglycemia. In all of these conditions hypoglycemia *is not associated with ketonuria*.

Salicylate Intoxication (see also Chapter 666.3). Both hyperglycemia and hypoglycemia occur in children with salicylate intoxication. Accelerated utilization of glucose, due to augmentation of insulin secretion by salicylates, and possible interference with gluconeogenesis may contribute to hypoglycemia. Infants are more susceptible than older children. Monitoring of blood glucose levels with appropriate glucose infusion in the event of hypoglycemia should form part of the therapeutic approach to salicylate intoxication in childhood. Ketosis may occur.

Fructose-1,6-Diphosphatase Deficiency (see Chapter 73). A deficiency of this enzyme results in a block of gluconeogenesis from all possible precursors below the level of fructose-1,6-diphosphate. Infusion of these gluconeogenic precursors results in lactic acidosis without a rise in glucose, and acute hypoglycemia may be provoked by inhibition of glycogenolysis. Normally, however, glycogenolysis remains intact, and glucagon elicits a normal glycemic response in the fed but not in the fasted state. Accordingly, affected individuals have hypoglycemia only during caloric deprivation as in fasting or during intercurrent illness. While glycogen stores remain normal, hypoglycemia does not develop. In affected families there may be a history of siblings with known hepatomegaly who died in infancy with unexplained metabolic acidosis.

Clinical features simulate those of type I glycogen storage disease. However, hepatomegaly in individuals with fructose-1,6-diphosphatase deficiency is due to lipid storage rather than glycogen storage. Lactic acidosis, ketosis, hyperlipidemia, and hyperuricemia occur; their pathogenesis is related to the severity and duration of hypoglycemia and the resultant low levels of insulin and high levels of counterregulatory hormones. Therapy of these infants, consisting of a diet high in carbohydrates (56%, excluding fructose, which cannot be utilized), low in protein (12%), and normal in fat composition (32%), has permitted normal growth and development. Continuous nocturnal provision of calories through the intragastric infusion system described above for type I glycogen storage disease is also applicable to children with fructose-1,6-diphosphatase deficiency. During intercurrent illnesses with vomiting, intravenous glucose infusion is necessary to prevent severe hypoglycemia.

Pyruvate Carboxylase Deficiency (see Chapter 73). This is predominantly a disease of the central nervous system characterized by a subacute necrotizing encephalomyelopathy and high levels of blood lactate and pyruvate. Hypoglycemia is not a prominent feature of this syndrome, presumably because gluconeogenesis from precursors other than alanine remains intact and these precursors bypass the pyruvate carboxylase step. The utilization of alanine as well as lactate through pyruvate cannot proceed, however, so that these substrates accumulate in blood, and modest hypoglycemia may result during fasting. Affected patients have usually died from progressive central nervous system disease.

Phosphoenol Pyruvate Carboxykinase (PEPCK) Deficiency. Deficiency of this rate-limiting enzyme, which occupies a key step in gluconeogenesis, is associated with severe fasting hypoglycemia and variable onset after birth. Hypoglycemia may occur within 24 hr after birth, and defective gluconeogenesis from alanine can be documented in vivo. At postmortem, liver, kidney, and myocardium demonstrate fatty infiltration, and atrophy of the optic nerve and visual cortex may occur. Although total hepatic PEPCK activity may be normal, the extramitochondrial (cytosolic) fraction is absent, in contrast to the normal situation, in which one third of enzyme activity is in cytosol. This cytosolic fraction is believed to be physiologically important for gluconeogenesis. Extensive fatty deposition in liver, kidney, and other tissues also occurs in PEPCK deficiency. Hypoglycemia may be profound. Lactate and pyruvate levels in plasma have been normal, but a mild metabolic acidosis may be present. The fatty infiltration of various organs is due to increased formation of acetyl CoA, which becomes available for fatty acid synthesis. Diagnosis of this rare entity can be made with certainty only through appropriate enzymatic determinations in liver biopsy material. Avoidance of periods of fasting through frequent feedings rich in carbohydrate should be helpful because glycogen synthesis and breakdown are intact.

Other Enzyme Defects. Galactosemia (Galactose-1-Phosphate Uridyl Transferase Deficiency) (see Chapter 73).

Fructose Intolerance. (Fructose-1-Phosphate Aldolase Deficiency). See Chapter 73. Acute hypoglycemia is due to the inhibition by fructose-1-phosphate of glycogenolysis via the phosphorylase system and of gluconeogenesis at the level of fructose-1,6-diphosphate aldolase. Affected individuals usually learn spontaneously to eliminate fructose from their diet.

DIAGNOSTIC EVALUATION

Table 77–4 lists the pertinent clinical and biochemical findings in the common childhood disorders associated with hypoglycemia. A careful and detailed history is essential in every suspected or documented case of hypoglycemia. Specific points to be noted include age of onset, temporal relation to meals or caloric deprivation, and a family history of prior infants known to have hypoglycemia or to have unexplained infant deaths. In the 1st wk of life the majority of infants have the transient form of neonatal hypoglycemia as a result of either prematurity/intrauterine growth retardation or by virtue of being born to diabetic mothers. In the absence of a history of maternal

■ **TABLE 77–4 Clinical Manifestations and Differential Diagnosis in Childhood Hypoglycemia**

				Serum		Effect of 24- to 36-hr Fast on Plasma					Glycemic Response or Glucagon		Glycemic Response to Infusion of	
Condition	**Hypoglycemia**	**Urinary Ketones (K) or Reducing* Sugars**	**Hepato-megaly**	***Lipids***	***Uric Acid***	***Glucose***	***Insulin***	***Ketones***	***Alanine***	***Lactate***	***Fed***	***Fasted***	***Alanine***	***Glycerol***
Normal	0	0	0	Normal	Normal	↓	↓	↑	↓	Normal	↑	↓	↑	↑
Hyperinsulinemia	Recurrent severe	0	0	Normal or ↑	Normal	↓↓	↑↑	↓↓	Normal	Normal	↑	↑	↑	↑
Ketotic hypoglycemia	Severe with missed meals	Ketonuria + + +	0	Normal	Normal	↓↓	↓	↑↑	↓↓	Normal	↑	↓↓	↑	↑
Hypopituitarism	Moderate with missed meals	Ketonuria + +	0	Normal	Normal	↓↓	↓	↑↑	↓↓	Normal	↑	↓↓	↑	↑
Adrenal insufficiency	Severe with missed meals	Ketonuria + +	0	Normal	Normal	↓↓	↓	↑↑	↓↓	Normal	↑	↓↓	↑	↑
Enzyme deficiencies														
Glucose-6-phosphatase	Severe–constant	Ketonuria + + +	+ + +	↑↑	↑↑	↓↓	↓	↑↑	↑↑	↑↑	0	0–↓↓	0	0
Debrancher	Moderate with fasting	Ketonuria + +	+ +	Normal	Normal	↓↓	↓	↑↑	↓↓	Normal	↑	0–↓↓	↑	↑
Phosphorylase	Mild–moderate	Ketonuria + +	+	Normal	Normal	↓	↓	↑↑	↓↓	Normal	0–↑	0–↓↓	↑	↑
Fructose-1,6-diphosphatase	Severe with fasting	Ketonuria + + +	+ + +	↑↑	↑↑	↓↓	↓	↑↑	↑↑	↑↑	↑	0–↓↓	↓	↓
Galactosemia	After milk or milk products	0 Ketones;(s) +	+ + +	Normal	Normal	↓	↓	↑	↓	Normal	↑	0–↓↓	↑	↑
Fructose intolerance	After fructose	0 Ketones;(s) +	+ + +	Normal	Normal	↓	↓	↑	↓	Normal	↑	0–↓↓	↑	↑

0 = absence.
↑ or ↓ indicates respectively small increase or decrease.
↑↑ or ↓↓ indicates respectively large increase or decrease.
Details of each condition are discussed in the text.

diabetes, the characteristic large plethoric appearance of an "infant of a diabetic mother" should arouse suspicion of the islet cell dysmaturation syndrome; plasma insulin concentrations above 10–15 μU/mL in the presence of documented hypoglycemia confirm this diagnosis. The presence of hepatomegaly should arouse suspicion of an enzyme deficiency; if nonglucose-reducing sugar is present in the urine, galactosemia is most likely. In males, the presence of a microphallus suggests the possibility of hypopituitarism, which may be also associated with a hepatic jaundice in both sexes.

Past the newborn period clues to the cause of persistent or recurrent hypoglycemia can be obtained through a careful history, physical examination, and initial laboratory findings (see Table 77–3), which permit a systematic approach using selective and appropriate investigations. The temporal relation of the hypoglycemia to food intake may suggest that the defect is one of gluconeogenesis if symptoms occur 6 hr or more after meals. If hypoglycemia occurs shortly after meals, leucine sensitivity, galactosemia, or fructose intolerance is most likely, and the presence of reducing substances in the urine will rapidly distinguish these possibilities. The presence of hepatomegaly suggests one of the enzyme deficiencies in glycogen synthesis or breakdown or of gluconeogenesis, as outlined in Table 77–4. The absence of ketonemia or ketonuria at the time of initial presentation strongly suggests hyperinsulinemia or a defect in fatty acid oxidation. In all other causes of hypoglycemia, with the exception of galactosemia and fructose intolerance, ketonemia and ketonuria are present at the time of fasting hypoglycemia. At the time of the hypoglycemia, serum should be obtained for determination of hormones and substrates, followed by repeated measurement after an intramuscular or intravenous injection of glucagon as outlined in Table 77–3. Interpretation of the findings is summarized in Table 77–5. Hypoglycemia with ketonuria in children between the ages of 18 mo and 5 yr is most likely to be ketotic hypoglycemia, especially if hepatomegaly is absent. The ingestion of a toxin, including alcohol or salicylate, can usually be excluded rapidly by the history.

When the history is suggestive but acute symptoms are not present, a 24- to 36-hr fast can usually provoke hypoglycemia and resolve the question of hyperinsulinemia or other conditions (see Table 77–5). Because adrenal insufficiency may mimic ketotic hypoglycemia, plasma cortisol levels should be determined at the time of documented hypoglycemia; increased buccal or skin pigmentation may provide the clue to primary adrenal insufficiency with elevated ACTH (melanocyte stimulating hormone, MSH) activity. Short stature or a decrease in the growth rate may provide the clue to pituitary insufficiency involving growth hormone as well as ACTH. Tests of pituitary-adrenal function such as the arginine-insulin stimulation test for growth hormone and cortisol release may be necessary.

In the presence of hepatomegaly and hypoglycemia, a presumptive diagnosis of the enzyme defect can often be made through the clinical manifestations, presence of hyperlipidemia, acidosis, hyperuricemia, response to glucagon in the fed and fasted states, and the response to infusion of various appropriate precursors (see Tables 77–3 and 77–4). These clinical findings and investigative approaches are summarized in Table 77–4. Definitive diagnosis of the glycogen storage disease may require an open liver biopsy (see Chapter 73). Occasional patients with all the manifestations of glycogen storage disease are found to have normal enzyme activity. These definitive studies require special expertise available only in certain institutions.

THERAPEUTIC CONSIDERATIONS

The prevention of hypoglycemia and its resultant effects on central nervous system development is very important in the newborn period. For neonates with hyperinsulinemia not associated with maternal diabetes, subtotal pancreatectomy may be needed, unless hypoglycemia can be readily controlled with somatostatin analogs or diazoxide. The therapeutic approach to specific causes is discussed with the description of each condition. As knowledge and understanding of glucose homeostasis have increased, fewer children are labeled as having idiopathic hypoglycemia, and precise rational therapy is possible more often.

Treatment of acute neonatal or infant hypoglycemia includes intravenous administration of 2 mL/kg of $D_{10}W$, followed by a continuous infusion of glucose at 6–8 mg/kg/min, adjusting the rate to maintain blood glucose levels in the normal range.

The management of persistent neonatal or infantile hypoglycemia includes increasing the rate of intravenous glucose infusion to 8–15 mg/kg/min. This may require a central venous catheter to administer a hypertonic 15–20% glucose solution. In addition, intramuscular hydrocortisone, 5 mg/kg/24 hr given in divided doses every 8 hr, or oral prednisone, 1–2 mg/kg/24 hr given in divided doses every 6–12 hr, and intramuscular growth hormone, 1 mg/24 hr, may be added if hypoglycemia is unresponsive to intravenous glucose.

Oral diazoxide, 10–25 mg/kg/24 hr given in divided doses every 6 hr, may reverse hyperinsulinemic hypoglycemia but also produces hirsutism, edema, nausea, hyperuricemia, electrolyte disturbances, advanced bone age, IgG deficiency, and, rarely, hypertension with prolonged use. A long-acting somatostatin analog (octreotide, formerly SMS 201–995) has been effective in controlling hyperinsulinemic hypoglycemia in a small number of patients with islet cell dysmaturity syn-

■ **TABLE 77–5 Diagnosis of Acute Hypoglycemia in Infants and Children**

Acute Symptoms Present	History Suggestive: Acute Symptoms Not Present
1. Obtain blood sample before and 30 min after glucagon administration 2. Obtain urine as soon as possible. Examine for ketones; if not present and hypoglycemia confirmed, suspect hyperinsulinemia or carnitine deficiency; if present, suspect ketotic, hormone deficiency, inborn error of glycogen metabolism, or gluconeogenesis 3. Measure glucose in the original blood sample. If hypoglycemia is confirmed, proceed with substrate-hormone measurement as in Table 77–3 4. If glycemic increment after glucagon exceeds 40 mg/dL above basal, suspect hyperinsulinemia 5. If insulin level at time of confirmed hypoglycemia is greater than 10 μU/mL, suspect endogenous hyperinsulinemia; if greater than 100 μUmL, suspect factitious hyperinsulinemia (exogenous insulin injection). Admit to hospital for provocative testing 6. If cortisol less than 10 μg/dL and/or growth hormone less than 5 ng/mL, suspect adrenal insufficiency and/or pituitary disease. Admit to hospital for provocative testing	1. Careful history for relation of symptoms to time and type of food intake, bearing in mind age of patient (see Table 77–2). Exclude possibility of alcohol or drug ingestion. Assess possibility of insulin injection, salt craving, growth velocity, intracranial pathology 2. Careful examination for hepatomegaly (glycogen storage disease; defect in gluconeogenesis); pigmentation (adrenal failure); stature and neurologic status (pituitary disease) 3. Admit to hospital for provocative testing: a. 24-hr fast under careful observation; when symptoms provoked proceed with steps 1–4 as when acute symptoms present b. Pituitary-adrenal function using arginine-insulin stimulation test if indicated 4. Liver biopsy for histology and enzyme determination if indicated 5. Oral glucose tolerance test (1.75 g/kg; max 75 g) if reactive hypoglycemia suspected in an adolescent

drome and islet cell adenoma. Octreotide is administered subcutaneously every 6–12 hr in doses of 20–50 μg in neonates and young infants. Potential but unusual complications include poor growth due to inhibition of growth hormone release, pain at the injection site, vomiting, diarrhea, and hepatic dysfunction (hepatitis, cholelithiasis). Octreotide is usually employed as a temporizing agent for various periods prior to subtotal pancreactomy for nesidioblastosis. It may be particularly useful for the treatment of refractory hypoglycemia despite subtotal pancreatectomy. Total pancreatectomy is not optimal therapy owing to the risks of surgery, permanent diabetes mellitus, and exocrine pancreatic insufficiency.

Amiel SA, Tamborlane WV, Simonson DC, et al: Defective glucose counterregulation after strict glycemic control of insulin-dependent diabetes mellitus. N Engl J Med 316:1376, 1987.

Antunes JD, Geffner ME, Lippe BM, et al: Childhood hypoglycemia: Differentiating hyperinsulinemic from nonhyperinsulinemic causes. J Pediatr 116:105, 1990.

Arky RA: Hypoglycemia associated with liver disease and ethanol. Endocrinol Metab Clin North Am 18:75, 1989.

Aynsley-Green A, Polak JM, Bloom SR, et al: Nesidioblastosis of the pancreas: Definition of the syndrome and the management of the severe neonatal hyperinsulinemic hypoglycemia. Arch Dis Child 56:496, 1981.

Bennish M, Kalam Azad A, Rahman O, et al: Hypoglycemia during diarrhea in childhood. Prevalence, pathophysiology and outcome. N Engl J Med 322:1357, 1990.

Bergada I, Suissa S, Dufresne J, et al: Severe hypoglycemia in IDDM children. Diabetes Care 12:239, 1989.

Bhowmick SK, Lewandowski C: Prolonged hyperinsulinism and hypoglycemia in an asphyxiated, small for gestation infant. Clin Pediatr 28:575, 1990.

Burchell A, Bell JE, Busuttil A: Hepatic microsomal glucose-6-phosphatase system and sudden infant death syndrome. Lancet 2:291, 1989.

Chaussain JL: Glycemic response to 24 hour fast in normal children and children with ketotic hypoglycemia. J Pediatr 82:438, 1973.

Chaussain JL, Georges P, Olive G, Job JC: Glycemic response to 24-hour fast in normal children and children with ketotic hypoglycemia: II. Hormonal and metabolic changes. J Pediatr 85:776, 1974.

Corkey BE, Hale DE, Glennon MC, et al: Relationship between unusual hepatic acyl coenzyme A profiles and the pathogenesis of Reye syndrome. J Clin Invest 82:782, 1988.

Cornblath M, Schwartz R: Disorders of Carbohydrate Metabolism in Infancy, 3rd ed. Boston, Blackwell, 1991.

Cross NCP, DeFranchis R, Sebastio G, et al: Molecular analysis of aldolase B genes in hereditary fructose intolerance. Lancet 1:306, 1990.

Cryer PE: Glucose homeostasis and hypoglycemia. *In*: Wilson JD, Foster DW (eds): Williams Textbook of Endocrinology, 8th ed. Philadelphia, WB Saunders, 1992, pp 1223–1253.

Devaskar SU, Mueckler MM: The mammalian glucose transporters. Pediatr Res 31:1, 1992.

DeVivo DC, Trifiletti RR, Jacobson RI, et al: Defective glucose transport across the blood-brain barrier as a cause of persistent hypoglycorrhachia, seizures, and developmental delay. N Engl J Med 325:703, 1991.

Fischer KF, Lees JA, Newman JH: Hypoglycemia in hospitalized patients: Causes and outcomes. N Engl J Med 315:1245, 1986.

Frakjer DL, Norton JA: Localization on resection of insulinomas and gastroinomas. JAMA 259:3601, 1988.

Hanse IL, Levy MM, Kerr DS: The 2-deoxyglucose test as a supplement to fasting for detection of childhood hypoglycemia. Pediatr Res 18:490, 1984.

Haymond NW: Hypoglycemia in infants and children. Endocrinol Metab Clin North Am 18:211, 1989.

Haymond NW, Ben-Glim E, Strobel KE: Glucose and alanine metabolism in children with maple syrup urine disease. J Clin Invest 62:398, 1978.

Hirsch HJ, Loo SW, Gabbay KH: The development and regulation of the endocrine pancreas. J Pediatr 91:518, 1977.

Kaufman FR, Costin G, Thomas DW, et al: Neonatal cholestasis and hypopituitarism. Arch Dis Child 59:787, 1984.

Kelly RI: The role of carnitine supplementation in valproic acid therapy. Pediatrics 97:892, 1994.

Koh TH, Aynsley-Green A, Tarbit M, et al: Neural dysfunction during hypoglycemia. Arch Dis Child 63:1353, 1988.

Lei KJ, Shelly LL, Pan CJ, et al: Mutations in the glucose-6-phosphatase gene that cause glycogen storage disease type 1a. Science 262:580, 1993.

Lucas A, Morley R, Cole TJ: Adverse neurodevelopmental outcome of moderate neonatal hypoglycemia. Br Med J 297:1304, 1988.

Martin LW, Rychman FC, Sheldon CA: Experience with 95 percent pancreatectomy and splenic salvage for neonatal nesidioblastosis. Ann Surg 200:355, 1984.

Matsubara Y, Narisawa K, Tada K, et al: Prevalence of K329E mutation in medium-chain acyl-CoA dehydrogenase gene determined from Guthrie cards. Lancet 338:552, 1991.

Mayefsky JH, Sarnaik AP, Postellon DC: Factitious hypoglycemia. Pediatrics 69:804, 1982.

Mock DM, Perman JA, Thaler JJ, et al: Chronic fructose intoxication after infancy in children with hereditary fructose intolerance: A cause of growth retardation. N Engl J Med 309:764, 1983.

Pagliara AS, Karl IE, Haymond M, et al: Hypoglycemia in infancy and childhood. J Pediatr 82:365 (part 1), 558 (part 2), 1973.

Palardy J, Havrankova J, Lepage R, et al: Blood glucose measurements during symptomatic episodes in patients with suspected postprandial hypoglycemia. N Engl J Med 321:1421, 1989.

Phillip M, Bashan N, Smith CPA, et al: An algorithmic approach to diagnosis of hypoglycemia. J Pediatr 110:387, 1987.

Rahier J: Relevance of endocrine pancreas nesidioblastosis to hyperinsulinemic hypoglycemia. Diabetes Care 12:164, 1989.

Schwartz SS, Rich BH, Lucky AW, et al: Familial nesidioblastosis: Severe neonatal hypoglycemia in two families. J Pediatr 95:44, 1979.

Schwenk WF, Haymond MW: Optimal rate of enteral glucose administration in children with glycogen storage disease type I. N Engl J Med 314:682, 1986.

Settergren G, Linglbad BS, Persson B: Cerebral blood flow and exchange of oxygen glucose, ketone bodies, lactate, pyruvate and amino acids in infants. Acta Paediatr Scand 65:343, 1976.

Sperling MA, Ganguli S, Leslie N, et al: Fetal-perinatal catecholamine secretion: Role in perinatal glucose homeostasis. Am J Physiol 247:E69, 1984.

Stanley CA, Baker L: Hyperinsulinism in infants and children: Diagnosis and therapy. Adv Pediatr 23:315, 1976.

Stanley CA, Hale DE, Berry GT, et al: A deficiency of carnitine-acylcarnitine translocase in the inner mitochondrial membrane. N Engl J Med 327:19, 1992.

Tauber MT, Harris AG, Rochiccioli P: Clinical use of long acting somatostatin analogue actreotide in pediatrics. Eur J Pediatr 153:304, 1994.

Taylor SI, Barbetti F, Accili D, et al: Syndromes of autoimmunity and hypoglycemia: Autoantibodies directed against insulin and its receptor. Endocrinol Metab Clin North Am 18:123, 1989.

Tyrala EE, Chen X, Boden G: Glucose metabolism in the infant weighing less than 1100 grams. J Pediatr 125:283, 1994.

Thornton PS, Alter CA, Katz LE, et al: Short and long-term use of octreotide in the treatment of congenital hyperinsulinism. J Pediatr 123:637, 1993.

Vidnes J, Oyasaeter S: Glucagon deficiency causing severe neonatal hypoglycemia in a patient with normal insulin secretion. Pediatr Res 11:943, 1977.

Volpe JJ: Hypoglycemia and brain injury. *In*: Volpe II (ed): Neurology of the Newborn. WB Saunders, Philadelphia, 1987, pp 364–385.

Ware AJ, Burton WC, McGarry JD, et al: Systemic carnitine deficiency. Report of a fatal case with multisystemic manifestations. J Pediatr 93:959, 1978.

White NJ, Marsh K, Turner RC, et al: Hypoglycemia in African children with severe malaria. Lancet 1:708, 1987.

Wolfsdorf JI, Keller RJ, Landy H, et al: Glucose therapy for glycogenosis type 1 in infants: comparison of intermittent uncooked cornstarch and continuous overnight glucose feedings. J Pediatr 117:384, 1990.

PART XI

The Fetus and the Neonatal Infant

Robert M. Kliegman

CHAPTER 78

Overview of Mortality and Morbidity

Although the "neonatal period" defines the first 4 wk of life after birth, both fetal and neonatal life form a continuum during which human growth and development are affected by genetic and by intrauterine and extrauterine environmental factors. For example, maternal toxemia may decrease the rate of fetal growth and cause an increased incidence of neonatal hypoglycemia. Social, economic, and cultural influences also affect this continuum. Low economic status is frequently associated with prematurity, which is correlated with high rates of morbidity and mortality, not only in the neonatal period but also throughout infancy. In the United States, the significantly higher black neonatal and infant mortality rate over that of white infants (Figs. 78–1 and 78–2) reflects cultural and socioeconomic factors. Although social influences, such as physician shortages in poor underserved areas, affect the availability of medical care to those most needing it, the failure of many mothers in these areas to use available prenatal and preventive medical care effectively also contributes to fetal and infant morbidity and mortality. Their failure results in part from inadequate public health education, from lack of money to pay for the care, and from limited access to health facilities and providers. Social factors leading to unwed pregnancies and cultural practices, such as the use of illicit drugs, also increase the incidence of fetal and neonatal disease.

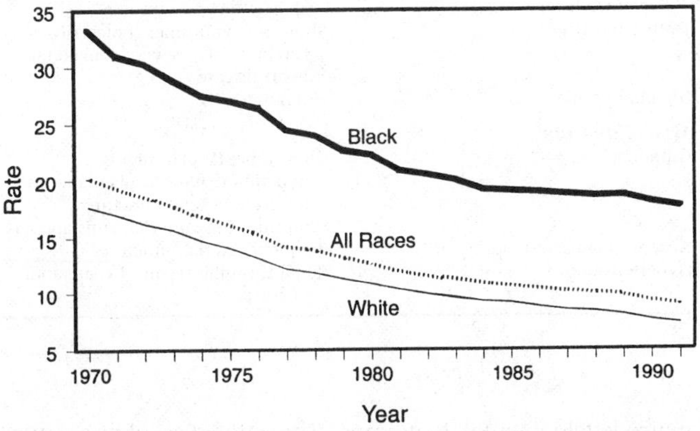

Figure 78–1. Infant mortality rates by race of mother. Deaths at <1 yr of age per 1,000 live births in specified group. Includes Hispanic and non-Hispanic infants; rates are presented only for black and white infants because the Linked Birth/Infant Death Data Set (used to more accurately estimate infant mortality rates for other racial groups) was not available for 1990 and 1991. (From Infant mortality—United States, 1991. MMWR 42:926, 1993.)

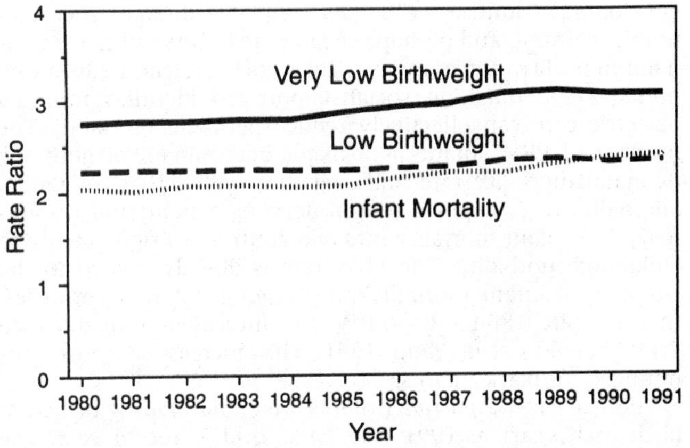

Figure 78–2. Black–white ratios in infant mortality (deaths at age <1 yr) and in low birthweight (LBW) (weight <2500 g [<5 lb, 8 oz] at birth) and very low birthweight (VLBW) (weight <1500 g [<3 lb, 4 oz] at birth) rates (per 1,000 live births)—United States, 1980–1991. (From Differences in infant mortality between blacks and whites—United States, 1980–1991. MMWR 43:288, 1994.)

Neonatal mortality has progressively decreased; it is highest during the first 24 hr of life, and overall accounts for about 65% of deaths under 1 yr of age. Further reduction of mortality and related morbidity depends primarily on preventing the birth of low-birthweight (LBW) infants, prenatal diagnosis, and early treatment of diseases that result from factors acting during gestation and at delivery (Table 78–1 and Fig. 78–3). *Perinatal mortality* designates fetal and neonatal deaths influenced by prenatal conditions and circumstances surrounding delivery. It is often defined as deaths of fetuses and infants from the 20th wk of gestational life through the 28th day after birth.

In the United States each year there are approximately 6 million pregnancies, 4 million live births, and 35,000 infant deaths within the first 12 mo of life. Twelve per cent of births are to women between 15 and 19 yr, and 30% are to unmarried women. Fetal deaths are associated with intrauterine growth retardation and conditions such as placental insufficiency that predispose the fetus to asphyxia. Neonatal deaths are due to diseases associated with low birthweight and to lethal congenital anomalies (see Table 78–1).

■ **TABLE 78–1 Major Causes of Perinatal Mortality**

Fetal	Preterm	Full Term
Placental insufficiency	Respiratory distress syndrome	Congenital abnormalities
Intrauterine infection	Bronchopulmonary dysplasia	Birth asphyxia, trauma
Severe congenital malformations	Severe immaturity	Infection
Umbilical cord accident	Intraventricular hemorrhage	Meconium aspiration pneumonia
Abruptio placentae	Congenital anomalies	Persistent fetal circulation
Hydrops fetalis	Infection	
	Necrotizing enterocolitis	

Infant mortality rates (deaths occurring from birth–12 mo/1,000 live births) vary by country; in 1991 they were lowest in Japan (4.4/1,000 births) and Scandinavia (5.6–6.2/1,000); moderate in the United States (8.9/1,000); and highest in developing countries (30–150/1,000). Although socioeconomic, cultural, and perhaps geographic factors influence perinatal mortality, preventive variables such as health education, prenatal care, nutrition, social support, risk identification, and obstetric care can effectively reduce perinatal mortality. The number of LBW infants is a major determinant of both the neonatal mortality rate and, together with lethal congenital anomalies (e.g., cardiac, central nervous system, and respiratory), the infant mortality rate and contributes significantly to childhood morbidity. The LBW rate is directly related to the variance of infant mortality rates among different countries. In the United States the LBW rate increased from 6.6% to 7.1% between 1981 and 1991. This increase is most pronounced for black infants.

The *low-birthweight rate* (infants weighing 2,500 g or less at birth each year) in 1991 was 7.1%, and in recent years the very low birthweight (VLBW) rate (infants weighing 1,500 g or less at birth) has been 1.1–1.2% of all births. The LBW and VLBW rates and the infant mortality rates are 2 times higher in black infants than in whites (see Fig. 78–2). Despite advances in perinatal care, these data suggest a major need for preventive programs.

The predominant cause of LBW infants in the United States is premature birth, while in developing countries and those nations with higher LBW rates the cause is often intrauterine growth retardation. VLBW infants are most often premature (<37 wks of gestation), although intrauterine growth retardation may complicate their early delivery. VLBW infants represent a larger proportion of infant deaths and infants with neurodevelopmental handicaps. The etiologies of premature birth include amniotic membrane (fluid) infections with genitourinary tract bacteria (*Chlamydia trachomatis, Ureaplasma ureolyticum, Mycoplasma hominis,* group B streptococcus, *Gardnerella vaginalis*), premature rupture of the membranes, uterine abnormalities, placental bleeding (abruptio, previa), multifetal gestation, drug misuse, maternal chronic illnesses, fetal dis-

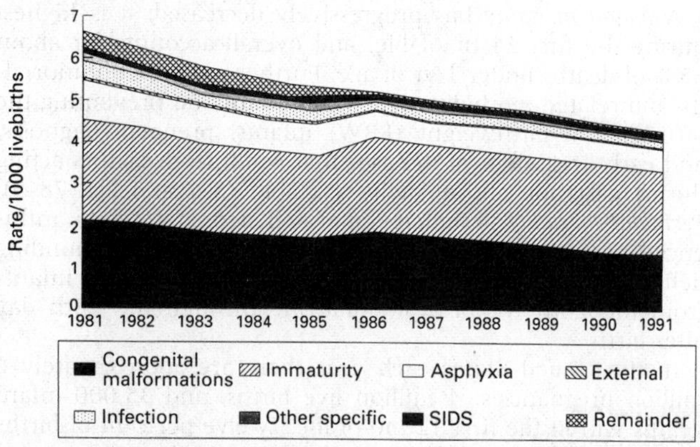

Figure 78–3. Trends in cause groups of neonatal deaths in England and Wales, 1981–1991. External refers to malnutrition, aspiration, pneumonia, hypothermia, injury, or poisoning. (From Alberman E, Botting B, Blatchley N, et al: A new hierarchical classification of causes of infant deaths in England and Wales. Arch Dis Child 70:403, 1994.)

■ **TABLE 78–2 Morbidities and Sequelae of Perinatal and Neonatal Illness**

Morbidities	Examples
Central Nervous System	
Spastic diplegic-quadriplegic cerebral palsy	Hypoxic-ischemic encephalopathy, periventricular leukomalacia, undetermined antenatal factors
Choreoathetotic cerebral palsy	Bilirubin encephalopathy (kernicterus)
Microcephaly	Hypoxic-ischemic encephalopathy, intrauterine infection (rubella, CMV)
Communicating hydrocephalus	Intraventricular hemorrhage, meningitis
Seizures	Hypoxic-ischemic encephalopathy, hypoglycemia
Encephalopathy	Congenital infections (rubella, CMV, HIV, toxoplasmosis)
Educational failure	Immaturity, hypoxia, low socioeconomic status
Mental retardation	Hypoxia, hypoglycemia, cerebral palsy, intraventricular hemorrhage
Sensation-Peripheral Nerves	
Reduced visual acuity (blindness)	Retinopathy of prematurity–ROP (oxygen toxicity)
Strabismus	Undetermined
Hearing impairment (deafness)	Drug toxicity (furosemide, aminoglycosides), bilirubin encephalopathy, hypoxia ± hyperventilation
Poor speech	Immaturity, chronic illness, hypoxia, prolonged endotracheal intubation, hearing deficit
Paralysis-paresis	Birth trauma—brachial plexus, phrenic nerve, spinal cord
Respiratory	
Bronchopulmonary dysplasia (BPD)	Oxygen toxicity, barotrauma
Subglottic stenosis	Endotracheal tube injury
Sudden infant death syndrome	Prematurity, BPD, infant of illicit drug user
Choanal stenosis, nasal septum destruction	Nasotracheal intubation
Cardiovascular	
Cyanosis	Precorrective palliative care of congenital cyanotic heart disease, cor pulmonale from BPD, reactive airway disease
Heart failure	Precorrective palliative care of complex congenital heart disease, BPD, VSD
Gastrointestinal	
Short gut syndrome	NEC, gastroschisis, malrotation-volvulus, cystic fibrosis, intestinal atresias
Cholestatic liver disease (cirrhosis, hepatic failure)	Hyperalimentation toxicity, sepsis, short gut syndrome
Failure to thrive	Short gut syndrome, cholestasis, BPD, cerebral palsy, severe congenital heart disease
Inguinal hernia	Unknown
Miscellaneous	
Cutaneous scars	Chest tube, IV placement; hyperalimentation subcutaneous infiltration; fetal puncture; intrauterine varicella; cutis aplasia
Absent radial artery pulse	Frequent arterial punctures
Hypertension	Renal thrombi; repair of coarctation of aorta

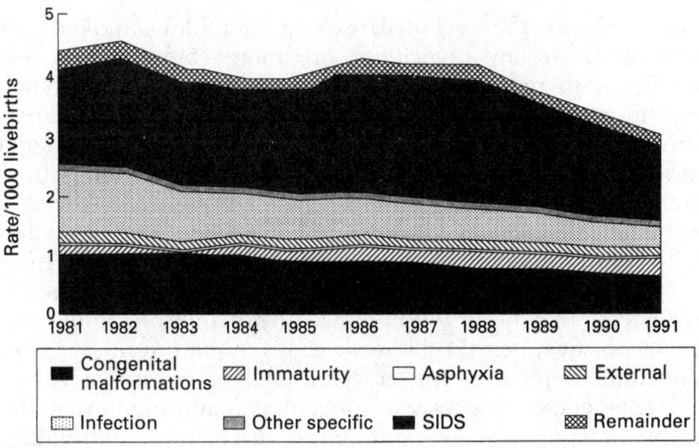

Figure 78–4. Trends in cause groups of postneonatal deaths in England and Wales, 1981–1991. External refers to malnutrition, aspiration, pneumonia, hypothermia, injury, or poisoning. (From Alberman E, Botting B, Blatchley N, et al: A new hierarchical classification of causes of infant deaths in England and Wales. Arch Dis Child 70:403, 1994.)

tress, and maternal pyelonephritis. Nonetheless, in many cases the cause of preterm delivery is unknown.

Although 99% of births occur in hospitals, only 75% of pregnant women receive *prenatal care* in the 1st trimester. Many women who receive inadequate prenatal care are at risk for perinatal complications. The content of prenatal care is critical, as women receiving health behavior advice have a lower incidence of LBW births. Barriers to prenatal care include absent or insufficient money or insurance to pay for care, poor coordination of services, and inadequate effective education about the importance of prenatal care. Successful and adequate provision of high-quality prenatal and perinatal care requires competent health care professionals and coordination of services among physicians' offices, clinics, community hospitals, special regionalized programs for high-risk mothers and infants, and tertiary care centers. Regional perinatal programs should provide continuing education and consultation in both the community and the referral center and transportation for pregnant women and newborn infants to appropriate hospitals; they should also include a regional hospital with facilities, equipment, and personnel for obstetric and neonatal intensive care.

Fetal deaths slightly exceed neonatal deaths in their contribution to perinatal mortality. The obstetrician has a central role in reducing perinatal mortality and morbidity. Recently, intrapartum fetal deaths have declined more than antepartum fetal deaths, which may reflect an increase in the use of fetal monitoring during labor and a more liberal use of cesarean section for fetal distress and other obstetric complications. It also emphasizes the need to be able to predict the maturity and functional reserve of the fetus prior to labor. In order to identify as early as possible those fetuses and infants at greatest risk, the obstetrician and pediatrician must effectively interact to anticipate perinatal problems and to take prompt preventive and therapeutic measures.

Postneonatal mortality refers to deaths between 28 days and 1 yr of life. Historically, these infant deaths were due to causes outside the neonatal period, such as sudden infant death, infections (respiratory, enteric), and trauma. With the advent of modern neonatal care, many VLBW infants who would have died in the 1st mo of life now survive the neonatal period only to succumb to the sequelae noted in Table 78–2 and Figure 78–4. This delayed neonatal mortality is an important contributor to postneonatal mortality.

Along with the need to lower perinatal mortality rates is the need to reduce the incidence of handicaps among high-risk infants (Table 78–2). Because both mortality and permanent neurologic sequelae are largely caused by the same or similar disturbances, research and public health measures directed at reducing perinatal mortality should also reduce the conditions contributing to the incidence of handicaps. For example, reducing the high incidence of mental retardation among infants whose births required vigorous and prolonged resuscitation mandates the early diagnosis of fetal asphyxia, appropriate obstetric management, and optimal resuscitation. However, some injury may be unavoidable; retinal damage may occur among those who had prolonged exposure to high concentrations of oxygen in the immediate postnatal period during which attempts were made to reduce the risk of hypoxic brain damage.

Alo CJ, Howe HL, Nelson MR: Birth-weight-specific infant mortality risks and leading causes of death. Illinois, 1980–1989. Am J Dis Child 147:1085, 1993.
Alberman E, Botting B, Blatchley N, et al: A new hierarchical classification of causes of infant deaths in England and Wales. Arch Dis Child 70:403, 1994.
Div of Nutrition, Nat Ctr for Chronic Disease Prevention and Health Promotion; Div of Vital Statistics, Nat Ctr for Health Statistics, CDC: Increasing incidence of low birthweight—United States, 1981–1991. MMWR 43:335, 1994.
Div of Reproductive Health, Nat Ctr for Chronic Disease Prevention and Health Promotion, CDC: Differences in infant mortality between blacks and whites—United States, 1980–1991. MMWR 43:288, 1994.
Kogan MD, Alexander GR, Kotelchuck M, et al: Relation of the content of prenatal care to the risk of low birth weight. Maternal reports of health behavior advice and initial prenatal care procedures. JAMA 271:1340, 1994.
Lettieri L, Vintzileos AM, Rodis JF, et al: Does "idiopathic" preterm labor resulting in preterm birth exist? Am J Obstet Gynecol 168:1480, 1993.
Mittendorf R, Herschel M, Williams MA, et al: Reducing the frequency of low birth weight in the United States. Obstet Gynecol 83:1056, 1994.
Wegman ME: Annual summary of vital statistics—1992. Pediatrics 92:743, 1993.

CHAPTER 79

The Newborn Infant

See also Chapter 10.

The neonatal period is a highly vulnerable time for the infant, who is completing many of the physiologic adjustments required for extrauterine existence. The high neonatal morbidity and mortality rates attest to the fragility of life during this period; in the United States, of all deaths occurring in the 1st yr, two thirds are of newborn infants. Deaths during the 1st yr mark an annual rate unequaled until the 7th decade.

The infant's intrauterine to extrauterine transition requires many biochemical and physiologic changes. No longer dependent on maternal circulation via the placenta, the newborn's pulmonary function is activated for the self-sufficient respiratory exchange of oxygen and carbon dioxide. The newborn infant also becomes dependent upon gastrointestinal tract function for absorbing food, renal function for excreting wastes and maintaining chemical homeostasis, hepatic function for neutralizing and excreting toxic substances, and the function of the immunologic system for protecting against infection. Unsupported by the maternal placental system, the neonatal cardiovascular and endocrine systems also adapt for self-sufficient functioning. Many of the newborn's special problems are related to poor adaptation due to asphyxia, premature birth, life-threatening congenital anomalies, or adverse effects of delivery.

79.1 History in Neonatal Pediatrics

The neonatal history should (1) identify disabling diseases that are amendable by prompt preventive action or treatment (e.g., asphyxia); (2) anticipate conditions that may be of later importance (e.g., gonococcal conjunctivitis); and (3) uncover possible causative factors that may explain pathologic conditions regardless of their immediate or future significance (e.g., screening for inborn errors of metabolism). The perinatal history should include demographic and social data (socioeconomic status, age, race), past medical illnesses in the child and family (cardiopulmonary disorders, infectious diseases, genetic disorders, diabetes mellitus), prior maternal reproductive problems (stillbirth, prematurity, blood group sensitization), events occurring in the present pregnancy (vaginal bleeding, medications, acute illness, duration of rupture of membranes), and a description of the labor (duration, fetal presentation, fetal distress, fever) and delivery (cesarean section, anesthesia or sedation, use of forceps, Apgar score, need for resuscitation).

79.2 Physical Examination of the Newborn Infant

Many physical and behavioral characteristics of the normal newborn infant are described in Chapter 10, which should be reviewed before reading this section.

The initial examination of the newborn infant should be performed as soon as possible after delivery to detect abnormalities and to establish a baseline for subsequent examinations. For high-risk deliveries this examination should take place in the delivery room and focus on congenital anomalies and pathophysiologic problems that may interfere with a normal cardiopulmonary and metabolic adaptation to extrauterine life. Congenital anomalies may be present in 3–5% of infants. Following a stable delivery room course, a second and more detailed examination should be performed within 24 hr of birth. With healthy infants the mother should be present during this examination; even minor, seemingly insignificant anatomic variations should be explained, since she may become disturbed at her or other relatives' later discovery of them, or she may think the physician is not giving them adequate consideration. However, explaining any problem has the potential for unduly alarming otherwise unworried parents unless it is carefully and skillfully done. No infant should be discharged from the hospital without a final examination, since certain abnormalities, particularly heart murmurs, often appear or disappear in the immediate neonatal period, or there may be evidence of disease that has just been acquired. Pulse (normal 120–160 beats/min), respiratory rate (normal 30–60 breaths/min), temperature, weight, length, head circumference, and dimensions of any visible or palpable structural abnormality should be recorded. Blood pressure is determined if the neonate appears ill.

Examining the newborn requires patience, gentleness, and procedural flexibility. Thus, if the infant is quiet and relaxed at the beginning of the examination, palpation of the abdomen or auscultation of the heart should be performed first before other, more disturbing manipulations are done.

GENERAL APPEARANCE. Physical activity may be absent during the relaxation of normal sleep or decreased by the effects of illness or drugs; the infant may be either lying with extremities motionless, to conserve energy for the effort of difficult breathing, or vigorously crying with accompanying activity of arms and legs. Both active and passive muscle tone and any unusual posture should be recorded. Coarse, tremulous movements with ankle or jaw myoclonus are more common and less significant in newborn infants than at any other age. Such movements tend to occur when the infant is active, whereas convulsive twitching usually occurs in a quiet state. Edema may produce a superficial appearance of good nutrition. Pitting after applied pressure may or may not be present, but the skin of the fingers and toes will lack the normal fine wrinkles when puffed with fluid. Edema of the eyelids commonly results from irritation caused by administration of silver nitrate. Generalized edema may occur with prematurity, hypoproteinemia secondary to severe erythroblastosis fetalis, nonimmune hydrops, congenital nephrosis, Hurler syndrome, or unknown cause. Localized edema suggests a congenital malformation of the lymphatic system; when confined to one or more extremities of a female infant, it may be the presenting sign of Turner syndrome (Chapters 67 and 538.1).

SKIN. Vasomotor instability and peripheral circulatory sluggishness are revealed by deep redness or purple lividity in the crying infant, whose color may darken profoundly with closure of the glottis preceding a vigorous cry, and by harmless cyanosis (acrocyanosis) of the hands and feet, especially when these are cool. Mottling, another example of general circulatory instability, may be associated with serious illness or related to a transient fluctuation in skin temperature. An extraordinary division of the body from forehead to pubis into red and pale halves is **harlequin color change**, a transient and harmless condition. Significant *cyanosis* may be masked by the pallor of circulatory failure or anemia; alternatively, the relatively high hemoglobin content of the first few days and the thin skin may combine to produce an appearance of cyanosis at a higher PaO_2 than in older children. Localized cyanosis is differentiated from ecchymosis by the momentary blanching pallor (with cyanosis) that occurs following pressure. The same maneuver also helps in demonstrating *icterus*, possibly significant but unnoticed if the skin is suffused with blood. *Pallor* may represent asphyxia, anemia, shock, or edema. Early recognition of anemia may lead to a diagnosis of erythroblastosis fetalis, subcapsular hematoma of the liver or spleen, subdural hemorrhage, or fetal-maternal or twin-twin transfusion. Without being anemic, postmature infants tend to have paler and thicker skin than do term or premature infants. The ruddy red appearance of *plethora* is seen with polycythemia.

The vernix and common transitory macular capillary hemangiomas of the eyelids and neck are described in Chapter 597. Cavernous hemangiomas are deeper, blue masses, which, if large, may trap platelets and produce disseminated intravascular coagulation or may interfere with local organ function. Scattered petechial may be present in the scalp or face after a difficult delivery. Slate blue, well-demarcated areas of pigmentation are seen over the buttocks, back, and sometimes other parts of the body in more than 50% of black Native American, or Asian infants and occasionally in white ones. These have no known anthropologic significance despite their name, **mongolian spots**; they tend to disappear within the first year. The vernix, skin, and especially the cord may be stained a brownish yellow if the amniotic fluid has been colored by passage of meconium during or before birth, often because of intrauterine anoxia.

The skin of the premature infant is thin and delicate and tends to be deep red; in extremely premature infants, the skin appears almost gelatinous and bleeds and bruises easily. Fine, soft, immature hair—**lanugo hair**—frequently covers the scalp and brow and may also cover the face in the premature infant. Lanugo hair has usually been lost or replaced by vellus hair in the term infant. Tufts of hair over the lumbosacral spines suggest an underlying abnormality such as an occult spina bifida, sinus tract, or tumor. The nails are rudimentary in the very premature infant, but they may protrude beyond the fingertips in infants born past term. Post-term infants may have a peeling, parchment-like skin (Fig. 79–1), a severe degree of which suggests ichthyosis congenita (Chapter 607).

Many neonates develop small, white, occasionally vesiculopustular papules on an erythematous base 1–3 days after birth. This benign rash, *erythema toxicum*, persists for as long as 1 wk, contains eosinophils, and is usually distributed on the face, trunk, and extremities (Chapter 597). *Pustular melanosis*, a benign lesion seen predominantly in black neonates, contains neutrophils and is present at birth as a vesiculopustular eruption around the chin, neck, back, extremities, and palms or soles; it lasts 2–3 days. Both lesions need to be distinguished from more dangerous vesicular eruptions such as herpes simplex (Chapter 97.2) and staphylococcal disease of the skin (Chapter 174.1).

Amniotic bands may disrupt the skin, extremities (amputation, ring constriction, syndactyly), face (clefts), or trunk (abdominal or thoracic wall defects). Their etiology is uncertain but may be related to amniotic membrane rupture or vascular compromise with fibrous band formation. Excessive skin fragility and extensibility with joint hypermobility suggest Ehlers-Danlos syndrome, Marfan syndrome, congenital contractural arachnodactyly, or other disorders of collagen synthesis.

SKULL. The skull may be molded, particularly if the infant is the first-born and if the head has been engaged for a considerable time. The parietal bones tend to override the occipital and frontal bones. The head of an infant born by cesarean section or from a breech presentation is characterized by its roundness. The suture lines and the size and tension of the anterior and posterior fontanels should be determined digitally. Premature fusion of sutures (cranial synostosis) demonstrates a hard nonmovable ridge over the suture and an abnormally shaped skull. Great variation in the size of the fontanels exists at birth; if small, the anterior fontanel usually tends to enlarge during the first few months of life. Persistence of excessively large anterior (normal: 20 ± 10 mm) and posterior fontanels has been associated with several disorders (Table 79–1). Soft areas **(craniotabes)** are occasionally found in the parietal bones at the vertex near the sagittal suture; they are more common in premature infants and in infants who have been exposed to uterine compression. Although usually insignificant, their possible pathologic cause should be investigated if they persist. Soft areas in the occipital region suggest the irregular calcification and wormian bone formation associated with osteogenesis imperfecta, cleidocranial dysostosis, lacunar skull, cretinism, and occasionally Down syndrome. Transillumination of the abnormal skull in a dark room or examination by ultrasound or computed tomography (CT) scan will rule out hydranencephaly or hydrocephaly (Chapter 542.11). An excessively large head (megalencephaly) suggests hydrocephaly, storage disease, achondroplasia, cerebral gigantism, neurocutaneous syndromes, or inborn errors of metabolism, or it may be familial. The skull of the premature infant may suggest hydrocephaly because of the relatively larger brain growth compared with that of other organs. Depression of the skull (indentation, fracture, ping-pong ball deformity) is usually of prenatal onset from prolonged focal pressure of the bony pelvis.

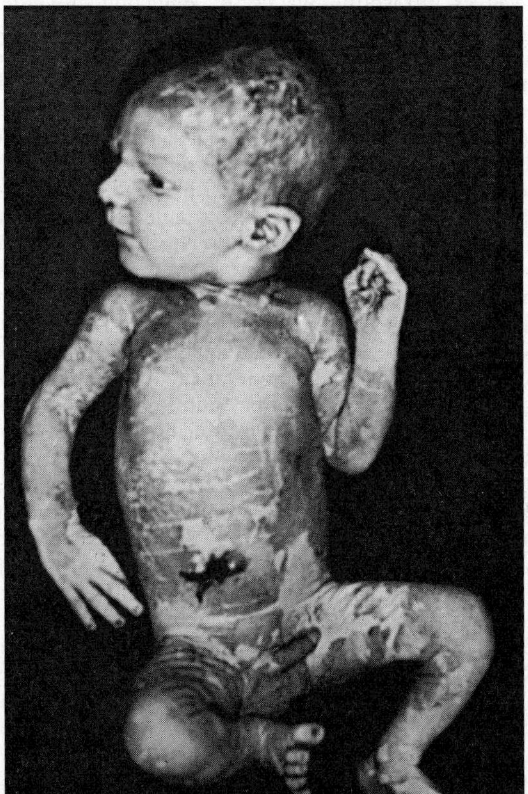

Figure 79–1. Infant with intrauterine growth retardation due to placental insufficiency. Note the long, thin appearance with peeling parchment-like dry skin, alert expression, meconium staining of the skin, and long nails. (From Clifford S: Advances in Pediatrics, Vol 9. Chicago, Year Book Medical Publishers, 1962.)

FACE. The general appearance should be noted with regard to dysmorphic features, such as epicanthal folds, widely spaced eyes, microphthalmia, long philtrum, and low-set ears, often associated with congenital syndromes. The face may be asymmetric from a 7th nerve palsy, from hypoplasia of the depressor muscle at the angle of the mouth, or from an abnormal fetal posture (Chapter 86); when the jaw has been held against a shoulder or an extremity during the intrauterine period, the mandible may deviate strikingly from the midline. Symmetric facial palsy suggests absence or hypoplasia of the 7th nerve nucleus (Möbius syndrome).

EYES. The eyes often open spontaneously if the infant is held up and tipped gently forward and backward. This maneuver, a result of labyrinthine and neck reflexes, is more successful for inspecting the eyes than forcing the lids apart. *Conjunctival and retinal hemorrhages* are not by themselves seriously significant. The pupillary reflexes are present after 28–30 wk of gestation. The iris should be inspected for colobomas and heterochromia. A cornea greater than 1 cm in diameter in a term infant suggests congenital glaucoma and requires prompt ophthalmologic consultation. The presence of bilateral *red reflexes* suggests the absence of cataracts or of intraocular pathology (Chapters 578 to 581). Leukocoria (white pupillary reflex) suggests cataracts, tumor, chorioretinitis, retinopathy of prematurity, or a persistent hyperplastic primary vitreous and warrants an ophthalmologic consultation.

EARS. Deformities of the pinnae are occasionally seen. Unilateral or bilateral preauricular skin tags occur frequently; if pedunculated, they can be ligated tightly at the base; dry gangrene and slough will result. The tympanic membrane, easily seen otoscopically through the short, straight external auditory canal, normally appears dull gray.

■ TABLE 79–1 Disorders Associated With a Large Anterior Fontanel

Achondroplasia	Osteogenesis imperfecta
Apert syndrome	Prematurity
Athyrotic hypothyroidism	Pyknodysostosis
Cleidocranial dysostosis	Rubella syndrome
Hallermann-Streiff syndrome	Russell-Silver syndrome
Hydrocephaly	13-, 18-, 21-Trisomies
Hypophosphatasia	Vitamin D deficiency rickets
Intrauterine growth retardation	

NOSE. The nose may be slightly obstructed by mucus accumulated in the narrow nostrils. The nares should be symmetric.

MOUTH. The normal mouth rarely shows precocious dentition, with natal or neonatal *teeth* in the lower incisor position or aberrantly placed; these teeth are shed before the deciduous ones erupt. Alternatively, neonatal teeth occur in Ellis-van Creveld, Hallermann-Streiff, and other syndromes. Extraction is usually not indicated. Premature eruption of deciduous teeth is even more unusual. The **soft** and **hard palate** should be inspected for a complete or submucosal cleft and the contour noted if the arch is excessively high or the uvula bifid. On the hard palate on either side of the raphe may be temporary accumulations of epithelial cells called **Epstein pearls**. Retention cysts of similar appearance may also be seen on the gums. Both disappear spontaneously, usually within a few weeks of birth. Clusters of small white or yellow follicles or ulcers on an erythematous base may be found on the anterior tonsillar pillars, most frequently on the 2nd–3rd day of life. Of unknown cause, they clear without treatment in 2–4 days.

There is no active salivation. The **tongue** appears relatively large; the **frenulum** may be short, but rarely, if ever, is this a reason for cutting it. Occasionally, the sublingual mucous membrane forms a prominent fold. The **cheeks** have a fullness on both the buccal and the external aspects owing to the accumulation of fat making up the **sucking pads**. These pads, as well as the labial tubercle on the upper lip (sucking callus) disappear when suckling ceases. A marble-sized buccal mass is usually due to fat necrosis.

The **throat** of the newborn infant is hard to see because of the arch of the palate; however, it should be clearly viewed because it is easily possible to miss posterior palatal or uvular clefts. The tonsils are small.

NECK. The neck appears relatively short. Abnormalities are not common; they include goiter, cystic hygroma, branchial cleft rests, and lesions of the sternocleidomastoid muscle that are presumably traumatic or are due to fixed positioning in utero that produces either a hematoma or fibrosis, respectively. *Congenital torticollis* causes the head to turn toward and the face to turn away from the affected side. Plagiocephaly, facial asymmetry, and hemihypoplasia may develop if it is untreated (see Chapter 629.1). Redundant skin or webbing in a female infant suggests Turner syndrome (Chapter 67). Both clavicles should be palpated for fractures.

CHEST. Breast hypertrophy is common, and milk may be present. Asymmetry, erythema, induration, and tenderness should suggest a breast abscess. Look for supernumerary nipples or widely spaced nipples with a shield-shaped chest; the latter suggests Turner syndrome.

LUNGS. Much can be learned by observing breathing. Variations in rate and rhythm are characteristic, fluctuating according to physical activity, state of wakefulness, or presence of crying. Because fluctuations are rapid, the respiratory rate should be counted for a full minute with the infant in the resting state, preferably asleep. Under these circumstances the usual rate for normal term infants is 30–40/min; for premature infants the rate is higher and fluctuates more widely. A rate consistently over 60/min during periods of regular breathing usually indicates cardiac or pulmonary disease. The premature infant may breathe with a Cheyne-Stokes rhythm, known as periodic respiration, or with complete irregularity. Periodic respiration is rare in the first 24 hr of life. Irregular gasping, sometimes accompanied by spasmodic movements of the mouth and chin, strongly indicates serious impairment of respiratory centers.

The breathing of newborn infants is almost entirely diaphragmatic, so that during inspiration the soft front of the thorax usually is drawn inward while the abdomen protrudes. If the baby is quiet, relaxed, and of good color, this "paradoxic movement" does not necessarily signify insufficient ventilation. On the other hand, labored respiration is important evidence of respiratory distress syndrome, pneumonia, anomalies, or mechanical disturbance of the lungs. A weak groaning, whining cry, or **grunting** during expiration signifies a potentially serious cardiopulmonary disease. Flaring of the alae nasi and retractions of the intercostal muscles and sternum are common signs of pulmonary pathology.

Normally, the breath sounds are bronchovesicular. Suspected pulmonary pathology due to diminished breath sounds, rales, or percussion dullness should always be followed up with a chest roentgenogram.

HEART. The size is difficult to estimate owing to normal variations in the size and shape of the chest. The location of the heart should be determined to detect dextrocardia. There may be transitory murmurs. Congenital heart disease may not initially produce the murmur that will be present later; only a 1:12 chance exists that a murmur heard at birth represents congenital heart disease. Evaluating the heart by roentgenography, echocardiography, and electrocardiography is essential when the possibility of significant lesions exists. The pulse may vary normally from 90/min in relaxed sleep to 180/min during activity. The still higher rate of supraventricular tachycardia may be counted better on an electrocardiogram than by ear. Premature infants, whose resting heart rate is usually 140–150/min, may have a sudden onset of **sinus bradycardia**. Pulses should be palpated in the upper and lower extremities to detect coarctation of the aorta on both admission and discharge from the nursery.

Blood pressure measurements may be a valuable diagnostic aid in ill infants (Chapter 380). The *auscultatory method* is often satisfactory, provided the stethoscope head is small enough. The *Doppler method*, using a transducer in the cuff, transmits and receives ultrasound waves. By detecting movements of the arterial wall, it more accurately measures systolic and diastolic pressures. The *oscillometric method* is currently the easiest and most accurate noninvasive method available. In the *palpatory method*, the systolic blood pressure is understood to be the point at which the pulse distal to the cuff becomes palpable during deflation; in the *flush method* the extremity is first compressed, rendering the area below the cuff relatively bloodless, and then, while the cuff is deflated, the mean pressure is recorded at the point where flushing appears in the arm or hand below the cuff. Each of these latter two methods is disadvantageous in that the pulse pressure is not obtained and the reading lies between the systolic and diastolic pressures obtained by the auscultatory method. Continuous or intermittent direct measurement of blood pressure using an umbilical artery catheter may be indicated in special circumstances for infants who are under close observation in an intensive care unit (Fig. 79–2).

ABDOMEN. The liver is usually palpable, sometimes as much as 2 cm below the rib margin. Less commonly, the spleen tip may be felt. The approximate size and location of each kidney can usually be determined on deep palpation. At no other period of life does the amount of air in the gastrointestinal tract vary so greatly, nor is it usually so great under normal circumstances. Gas should normally be present in the rectum on roentgenogram by 24 hr of age. The abdominal wall is normally weak (especially in premature infants), and **diastasis recti** and umbilical hernias are common, particularly among black infants.

Unusual masses should be investigated immediately by ultrasonography. Cystic abdominal masses include hydronephrosis, multicystic-dysplastic kidneys, adrenal hemorrhage, hydrometrocolpos, intestinal duplication, and choledochal, ovarian, omental, or pancreatic cysts. Solid masses include neuroblastoma, congenital mesoblastic nephroma, hepatoblastoma, and teratoma. A solid flank mass may be due to renal vein thrombosis, which becomes manifest with hematuria, hyper-

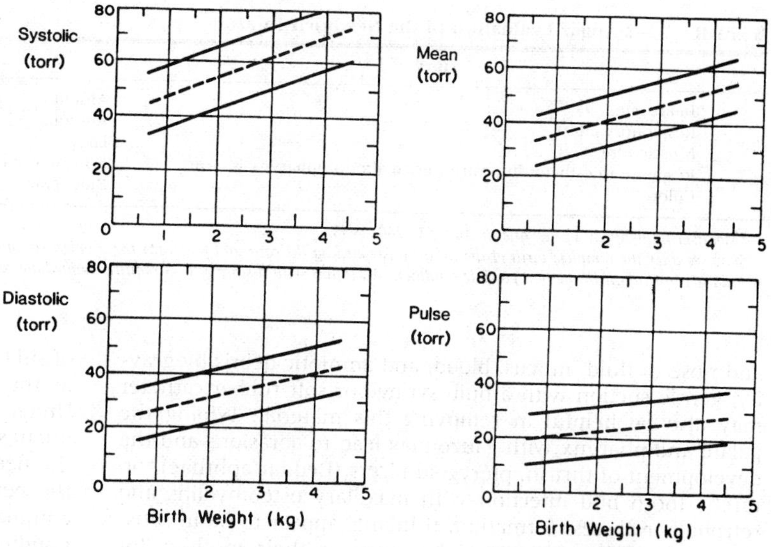

Figure 79–2. Linear regressions *(broken lines)* and 95% confidence limits *(solid lines)* of systolic *(top)* and diastolic *(bottom)* aortic blood pressures on birth weight in 61 healthy newborn infants during the first 12 hr after birth. Linear regressions *(broken lines)* and 95% confidence limits *(solid lines)* of mean pressure *(top)* and pulse pressure (systolic-diastolic pressure amplitude) *(bottom)* on birth weight in 61 healthy newborn infants during the first 12 hr after birth. (From Versmold HT, Kitterman JA, Phibbs RH, et al: Aortic blood pressure during the first 12 hours of life in infants with birth weight 610 to 4,220 grams. Pediatrics 67:607–613, 1981.)

tension, and thrombocytopenia. Renal vein thrombosis in infants is associated with polycythemia, dehydration, diabetic mothers, asphyxia, sepsis, and coagulopathies such as antithrombin III or protein C deficiencies.

Abdominal distention at or shortly after birth suggests either obstruction or perforation of the gastrointestinal tract, often due to meconium ileus; later distention suggests lower bowel obstruction, sepsis, or peritonitis. A scaphoid abdomen in the newborn suggests diaphragmatic hernia. **Abdominal wall defects** produce an omphalocele (Chapter 91) when they occur through the umbilicus and a gastroschisis when they occur lateral to the midline. Omphaloceles are associated with other anomalies and syndromes such as Beckwith-Wiedemann syndrome, conjoined twins, 18-trisomy, meningomyelocele, and imperforate anus. **Omphalitis** is an acute inflammation of the periumbilical tissue that may extend into the portal vein, producing acute pyophlebitis and later chronic portal hypertension.

GENITALIA. The **genitalia** and **mammary glands** normally respond to transplacentally obtained maternal hormones to produce enlargement and secretion of the breasts in both sexes and prominence of the female genitalia, often with considerable nonpurulent discharge. These transitory manifestations require observation but no interference.

Imperforate hymen may result in **hydrometrocolpos** and a lower abdominal mass. The normal scrotum is relatively large; its size may be increased by the trauma of breech delivery or by a **transitory hydrocele**, which is distinguished from a hernia by palpation and transillumination. The testes should be in the scrotum or palpable in the canals. The male black infant usually has dark pigmentation of the scrotum before the rest of the skin assumes its permanent color.

The **prepuce** of the newborn infant is normally tight and adherent. Severe hypospadias or epispadias should always lead one to suspect either that abnormal sex chromosomes are present (Chapter 67) or that the infant is actually a masculinized female with an enlarged clitoris, because this may be the first evidence of the adrenogenital syndrome (Chapter 529). Erection of the penis is common and has no significance. Urine is usually passed during or immediately after birth; a period without voiding may normally follow. However, about 95% of preterm and term infants void within 24 hr.

ANUS. Some passage of **meconium** usually occurs within the first 12 hr after birth; 99% of term infants and 95% of premature infants pass meconium within 48 hr of birth. **Imperforate anus** is not always visible and may require evidence obtained by the gentle insertion of the little finger or a rectal tube. Roentgenographic study is required. The dimple or irregularity of skinfold often normally present in the sacrococcygeal midline may be mistaken for an actual or potential neurocutaneous sinus.

EXTREMITIES. In examining the extremities the effects of fetal posture (Chapter 624) should be noted so that their cause and usual transitory nature can be explained to the mother. This is particularly important after breech presentations. The suspicion of a fracture or nerve injury associated with delivery is more commonly aroused by observing the extremities in spontaneous or stimulated activity than by any other means. The hands and feet should be examined for polydactyly, syndactyly, and abnormal dermatoglyphic patterns such as a simian crease.

The hips of all infants should be examined to rule out a congenital dislocation (Chapter 627.1).

NEUROLOGIC EXAMINATION. See Chapters 7 and 541. In utero neuromuscular diseases associated with limited fetal motion produce a constellation of signs and symptoms that are independent of the specific disease. Severe positional deformation and contractures produce arthrogryposis. Other manifestations of fetal neuromuscular disease include breech presentation, failure to breath at birth, pulmonary hypoplasia, dislocated hips, undescended testes, thin ribs, and clubfoot.

Ordinary Care of the Newborn Infant

The basic requirements of the newborn infant are immediate assistance at birth when needed, primarily to *establish respiration*; and subsequent assistance in obtaining *adequate nutrition*, in maintaining a *normal body temperature*, and in *avoiding contact with infection*. The environment meeting these requirements should also provide constant care by a nursing and medical staff alert to any signs of specific illness and should keep to a minimum the time the mother and infant are separated. The care of full-term and premature infants differs only in the degree of emphasis placed on each of these requirements. Problems to be anticipated after the delivery of a normal fetus include hypoventilation-apnea, hemorrhage, hypoxia, bradycardia, hypothermia, hypoglycemia, hypovolemia, hypotension, and unexpected anomalies.

79.3 Routine Delivery Room Care

The low-risk infant should be placed head downward immediately after delivery in order to clear the mouth, pharynx,

■ TABLE 79–2 Apgar Evaluation of the Newborn Infant*

Sign	0	1	2
Heart rate	Absent	Below 100	Over 100
Respiratory effort	Absent	Slow, irregular	Good, crying
Muscle tone	Limp	Some flexion of extremities	Active motion
Response to catheter in nostril (tested after oropharynx is clear)	No response	Grimace	Cough or sneeze
Color	Blue, pale	Body pink, extremities blue	Completely pink

Modified from Apgar V: Res Anesth Analg 32:260, 1953.
Sixty sec after the complete birth of the infant (disregarding the cord and placenta) the 5 objective signs above are evaluated, and each is given a score of 0, 1, or 2. A total score of 10 indicates an infant in the best possible condition. An infant with a score of 0–3 requires immediate resuscitation.

and nose of fluid, mucus, blood, and amniotic debris by gravity; gentle suction with a bulb syringe or soft rubber catheter may also be helpful in removing this material. Wiping the palate and pharynx with gauze may lead to abrasions and the development of thrush, pterygoid ulcers (Bednar aphthae), or, rarely, tooth bud infection with maxillary osteomyelitis and retrobulbar abscess formation. If infants appear to be in satisfactory condition, they may be given to their mothers for immediate bonding and nursing. If there is any concern about respiratory distress, they should be placed under a warmer, with the head dependent.

The **Apgar score** is a practical method of systematically assessing the newborn infant immediately after birth to help identify infants requiring resuscitation for hypoxic acidosis (Table 79–2). A low score does not necessarily signify fetal hypoxia-acidosis; additional factors may reduce the score (Table 79–3). The Apgar score also does not predict neonatal mortality or subsequent cerebral palsy. Indeed, the score is normal in most patients who subsequently develop cerebral palsy, and the incidence of cerebral palsy is very low among infants with Apgar scores of 0–3 at 5 min. The 1-min Apgar score signals the need for immediate resuscitation, and the 5-, 10-, 15-, and 20-min scores indicate the probability of successfully resuscitating the infant. Apgar scores of 0–3 at 20 min predict high mortality and morbidity.

Infants with a prolapsed cord or delayed delivery and evidence of intrauterine asphyxia should receive prompt resuscitation and close observation subsequently (Chapter 84). The stomachs of infants delivered by cesarean section may contain more fluid than those of infants delivered vaginally. Their stomachs should be emptied by gastric tube to prevent aspiration of gastric contents.

MAINTENANCE OF BODY HEAT. Relative to body weight, the body surface of the newborn infant is approximately 3 times that of the adult, and in low birthweight infants the insulating layer of subcutaneous fat is thinner. The estimated rate of heat loss in the newborn is approximately 4 times that of an adult. Under the usual delivery room conditions (20–25° C), an infant's skin temperature falls approximately 0.3° C/min, and the deep body temperature approximately 0.1° C/min during the period immediately after delivery, resulting usually in a cumulative loss of 2–3° C in deep body temperature (corresponding to a heat loss of approximately 200 kcal/kg). The heat loss occurs by *convection* of heat energy to the cooler surrounding air, by *conduction* of heat to colder materials on which the infant is resting, by heat *radiation* from the infant to other nearby solid objects, and by *evaporation* from moist skin and lungs (a function of alveolar ventilation).

Term infants exposed to cold after birth may develop metabolic acidosis, hypoxemia, hypoglycemia, and increased renal excretion of water and solutes owing to their efforts to compensate for heat loss. They augment heat production by increasing the metabolic rate and oxygen consumption and by releasing norepinephrine, which results in nonshivering thermogenesis through oxidation of fat, particularly of brown fat. In addition, muscular activity may increase. Hypoglycemic or hypoxic infants cannot increase their oxygen consumption when exposed to a cold environment, and their central temperature decreases. After labor and vaginal delivery, many newborn infants have a mild to moderate metabolic acidosis for which they may compensate by hyperventilating, which is more difficult for depressed infants and infants exposed to cold stress in the delivery room. Therefore, it is desirable to ensure that the infant is dried and either wrapped in blankets or placed under a warmer while having skin to skin contact with the mother. Since carrying out resuscitative measures on a covered infant or one enclosed in an incubator is difficult, a radiant heat source should be used to receive the baby immediately.

ANTISEPTIC SKIN AND CORD CARE. To reduce the incidence of skin and periumbilical infections (omphalitis), the entire skin and cord should be cleansed in the delivery room or upon admission to the nursery with sterile cotton soaked in warm water or a mild soap solution. The infant may be rinsed with water at body temperature if care is taken to avoid chilling. The baby is then dried and wrapped in sterile blankets and taken to the nursery. To lessen the chance of carrying pathogenic organisms into the nursery, the outer blanket can be discarded at the nursery door. To reduce colonization with *Staphylococcus aureus* and other pathogenic bacteria the umbilical cord is treated daily with triple dye, a bactericidal agent. Alternatively, chlorhexidine washing or, on rare occasions during *S. aureus* epidemics, a single hexachlorophene bath may be employed. Repeated total body exposure to hexachlorophene may be neurotoxic, particularly in low-birthweight infants, and is not recommended. Nursery personnel should use chlorhexidine or iodophor-containing antiseptic soaps for routine handwashing before caring for each infant. Rigidly enforcing hand-to-elbow washing for 2 min in the initial wash and 15–30 sec in the second wash is recommended for staff and visitors entering the nursery. Shorter but equally thorough washes between handling infants should also be required.

■ TABLE 79–3 Factors Affecting the Apgar Score

False-Positve (No Fetal Acidosis or Hypoxia; Low Apgar)	False-Negative (Acidosis; Normal Apgar)
Immaturity	Maternal acidosis
Analgesics, narcotics, sedatives	High fetal catecholamine levels
Magnesium sulfate	Some full-term infants
Acute cerebral trauma	
Precipitous delivery	
Congenital myopathy	
Congenital neuropathy	
Spinal cord trauma	
CNS anomaly	
Lung anomaly (diaphragmatic hernia)	
Airway obstruction (choanal atresia)	
Congenital pneumonia	
Prior episodes of fetal asphyxia (recovered)	

Regardless of the etiology, a low Apgar score due to fetal asphyxia, immaturity, central nervous depression, or airway obstruction identifies an infant needing immediate resuscitation.

OTHER MEASURES. The **eyes** of all infants must be protected against gonorrheal infection by instilling 1% *silver nitrate* drops, the best-proven therapy; erythromycin (0.5%) and tetracycline (1.0%) sterile ophthalmic ointments are alternative measures that may be effective against chlamydial conjunctivitis. Povidone-iodine (2.5% solution) may also be effective as a one-time prophylactic agent. This procedure may be delayed during the initial short alert period following birth to promote bonding, but once applied, drops should not be rinsed out. Also see Chapters 179 and 197.

Although hemorrhage in the newborn infant can be due to factors other than *vitamin K deficiency*, an intramuscular injection of 1 mg of water-soluble vitamin K_1 (phytonadione) is recommended for all infants immediately after birth to prevent hemorrhagic disease of the newborn (see Chapter 89.4). Higher dose, repeated administration of oral vitamin K may also be useful, but this treatment is not yet established. Larger intravenous doses predispose to the development of hyperbilirubinemia and kernicterus and should be avoided. Administration of vitamin K to the mother during labor is not recommended owing to unpredictable placental transfer.

Neonatal screening is available for various genetic, metabolic, hematologic, and endocrine diseases. Common screening tests performed on infant heel puncture blood samples include those for hypothyroidism, sickle cell anemia, phenylketonuria, homocystinuria, galactosemia, adrenogenital syndrome, cystic fibrosis, possible HIV infection, maple syrup urine disease, and other organic or amino acidopathies. Screening may be cost effective when timely identification and prompt therapy lessen the morbidity of a disease. See Chapter 5.

79.4 Nursery Care

Non-high-risk infants may be taken after the delivery room examination to the "regular" newborn nursery or placed in the mother's room if the hospital has rooming-in.

The bassinet, preferably of clear plastic to allow for easy visibility and care, should be cleaned frequently. All professional care should be given in the bassinet, including the physical examination, clothing changes, temperature taking, skin cleansing, and other procedures that, if performed elsewhere, would establish a common contact point and possibly provide a channel for cross infection. The clothing and bedding should be minimal, only those needed for the infant's comfort; the nursery temperature should be kept at approximately 24° C (75° F). The infant's temperature should be taken once by rectum and thereafter in the axilla; although the interval between temperature taking depends on many circumstances, it need not be shorter than 4 hr during the first 2–3 days and 8 hr thereafter. Axillary temperatures of 36.4–37.0° C (97.0–98.5° F) are within normal limits. Weighing at birth and daily thereafter is sufficient.

Vernix is spontaneously shed within 2–3 days, much of it adhering to the clothing, which should be completely changed daily. The diaper should be checked before and after feeding and when the baby cries; it should be changed when wet or soiled. Meconium or feces should be cleansed from the buttocks with sterile cotton moistened with sterile water. The foreskin of the male infant should not be retracted.

79.5 Parent-Infant Bonding

See also Chapter 10.

Normal infant development depends partly on a series of affectionate responses exchanged between a mother and her newborn infant, binding them together psychologically and physiologically. This bonding is facilitated and reinforced by the emotional support of a loving husband and family. The attachment process may be important in enabling some mothers to provide loving care during the neonatal period and subsequently during childhood. It is initiated before birth with the planning and confirmation of the pregnancy and with the growing acceptance of the fetus as an individual. After delivery and during the ensuing weeks, visual and physical contact between mother and baby triggers a variety of mutually rewarding and pleasurable interactions such as the mother's touching the infant's extremities and face with her fingertips and encompassing and gently massaging the infant's trunk with her hands. Touching the infant's cheek elicits responsive turning toward the mother's face or toward the breast with nuzzling and licking of the nipple, a powerful stimulus for prolactin secretion. The infant's initial quiet alert state provides the opportunity for eye-to-eye contact, which is particularly important in stimulating the loving and possessive feelings of many parents for their babies. The infant's crying elicits the maternal response of touching the infant and speaking in a soft, soothing, higher toned voice. Initial contact between mother and infant should take place in the delivery room, and opportunities for extended intimate contact should be provided within the first hours after birth. Delayed or abnormal maternal-infant bonding, occurring because of prematurity, infant or maternal illness, birth defects, or family stress, may harm infant development and maternal caretaking ability. Hospital routines should be designed to encourage parent-infant contact.

NURSERIES AND BREAST-FEEDING. See Chapter 44 for full discussions of breast- and formula feeding. Many hospital practices contribute to difficulties in breast-feeding by enforcing 4-hr feeding schedules, limiting nursing time, using only one breast at a feeding, washing nipples with substances other than water, delaying the first feeding, providing formula supplements, and using heavy intrapartum sedation.

■ TABLE 79–4 Drugs and Breast-Feeding

Contraindicated	Avoid or Give with Great Caution	Probably Safe But Give with Caution
Antineoplastic agents	Anthroquinones (laxatives)	Anesthetics
Amphetamines	Aspirin (salicylates)	Acetaminophen
Bromocriptine	Atropine	Aldomet
Clemastine	Birth control pills	Antibiotics (not tetracycline)
Cimetidine	Bromides	Antithyroid (not methimazole)
Chloramphenicol	Calciferol	Antiepileptics
Cocaine	Cascara	Antihistamines*
Cyclophosphamide	Danthron	Antihypertensive/cardiovascular
Cyclosporine	Dihydrotachysterol	Bishydroxycoumarin
Diethylstilbestrol	Estrogens	Chlorpromazine*
Doxorubicin	Ethanol	Codine*
Ergots	Metoclopramide	Digoxin
Gold salts	Metronidazole	Dilantin
Heroin	Narcotics	Diuretics
Immunosuppressants	Phenobarbital*	Furosemide
Iodides	Primidone	Haloperidol*
Lithium	Psychotropic drugs	Hydralazine
Meprobamate	Reserpine	Indomethacin
Methimazole	Salicylazosulfapyridine (sulfasalazine)	Methadone*
Methylamphetamine		Muscle relaxants
Nicotine (smoking)		Prednisone
Phencyclidine (PCP)		Propranolol
Phenindione		Propylthiouracil
Radiopharmaceuticals		Sedatives*
Tetracycline		Theophylline
Thiouracil		Vitamins
		Warfarin

Watch for sedation.

Hospital practices that encourage successful breast-feeding include immediate postpartum mother-infant contact with suckling, rooming-in, demand feeding, inclusion of fathers in prenatal breast-feeding education, and support from experienced women. Nursing at least 5 min at each breast is reasonable and allows the baby to obtain most of the available breast contents and to provide effective stimulation for increasing milk supply. Nursing episodes should then be extended according to the comfort and desire of the mother and infant. A confident and relaxed mother, supported by an encouraging home and hospital environment, is likely to nurse well.

DRUGS AND BREAST-FEEDING. Maternal medications may affect the production and safety of breast milk (Table 79–4). Most commonly used medications, such as antihypertensive agents, are safe, but each should be investigated if used during breast-feeding. Maternal sedatives may result in the infant's sedation. Maternal drugs that are weak acids, composed of large molecules, plasma bound, or poorly absorbed from the maternal or neonatal intestine are less likely to affect the neonate. When fresh breast milk is fed by tube or bottle, bacteriologic evaluation of stored milk should be performed within 24 hr.

Medical contraindications to breast-feeding include infection with HIV (except in developing nations), primary CMV, and hepatitis B virus (until infant receives hepatitis immune globulin and vaccine) (see Table 79–4).

American Academy of Pediatrics, American College of Obstetricians and Gynecologists: Guidelines for Perinatal Care, 3rd ed. American Academy of Pediatrics, Elk Grove Village, IL, 1992.

Catlin EA, Carpenter MW, Brann BS IV, et al: The Apgar score revisited: Influence of gestational age. J Pediatr 109:865, 1986.

Cheng TL, Patridge JC: Effect of bundling and high environmental temperature on neonatal body temperature. Pediatrics 92:238, 1993.

Committee on Drugs: The transfer of drugs and other chemicals into human milk. Pediatrics 93:137, 1994.

Committee on Fetus and Newborn: Use and abuse of the Apgar score. Pediatrics 78:1148, 1986.

Committee on Fetus and Newborn: Routine evaluation of blood pressure, hematocrit, and glucose in newborns. Pediatrics 92:474, 1993.

Fenichel GM: Neurological examination of the newborn. Int Pediatr 9:77, 1994.

Isenberg S, Apt L, Wood M: A controlled trial of povidone-iodine as prophylaxis against ophthalmia neonatorum. N Engl J Med 332:562, 1995.

Ito S, Blajchman A, Stephenson M, et al: Prospective follow-up of adverse reactions in breast-fed infants exposed to maternal medication. Am J Obstet Gynecol 168:1393, 1993.

Lawrence R: Breastfeeding and medical disease. Med Clin North Am 73:583, 1989.

CHAPTER 80
High-Risk Pregnancies

Pregnancies in which factors exist that increase the likelihood of abortion, fetal death, premature delivery, intrauterine growth retardation, fetal or neonatal disease, congenital malformations, mental retardation, or other handicaps are called high-risk pregnancies (Table 80–1; see also Chapter 81). Some factors, such as ingestion of a teratogenic drug in the 1st trimester, are causally related to the risk; others, such as hydramnios, are associations that alert the physician to the existence of the risk or risks. Based on their history, 10–20% of pregnant patients can be identified as "high risk"; less than half of all perinatal mortality and morbidity is associated with these pregnancies. Although assessing antepartum risk is important in reducing perinatal mortality and morbidity, some women become at high risk only during labor and delivery; therefore, careful monitoring is critical throughout the intrapartum course.

■ TABLE 80–1 Factors Associated With High-Risk Pregnancy

Economic	**Reproductive**
Poverty	Prior cesarean section
Unemployment	Prior infertility
Uninsured, underinsured health insurance	Prolonged gestation
Poor access to prenatal care	Prolonged labor
Cultural-Behavioral	Prior infant with cerebral palsy, mental retardation, birth trauma, congenital anomalies
Low educational status	Abnormal lie (breech)
Poor health care attitudes	Multiple gestation
No care or inadequate prenatal care	Premature rupture of membranes
Cigarette, alcohol, drug abuse	Infections (systemic, amniotic, extra-amniotic, cervical)
Age less than 16 or over 35 yr	Pre-eclampsia or eclampsia
Unmarried	Uterine bleeding (abruptio placentae, placenta previa)
Short interpregnancy interval	Parity (0 or more than 5)
Lack of support group (husband, family, church)	Uterine or cervical anomalies
Stress (physical, psychologic)	Fetal disease
Black race	Abnormal fetal growth
Biologic-Genetic	Idiopathic premature labor
Previous low-birthweight infant	Iatrogenic prematurity
Low maternal weight at her birth	High or low levels of maternal serum α-fetoprotein
Low weight for height	**Medical**
Poor weight gain during pregnancy	Diabetes mellitus
Short stature	Hypertension
Poor nutrition	Congenital heart disease
Inbreeding (autosomal recessive?)	Autoimmune disease
Intergenerational effects	Sickle cell anemia
Hereditary diseases (inborn error of metabolism)	TORCH infection
	Intercurrent surgery or trauma
	Sexually transmitted diseases

Identifying high-risk pregnancies is important not only because it is the first step toward prevention but also because therapeutic steps may often be taken to reduce the risks to the fetus or neonate if the physician knows of the potential for difficulty. Good prenatal care reduces the incidence of low-birthweight infants.

GENETIC FACTORS. The occurrence of chromosomal abnormalities, congenital anomalies, inborn errors of metabolism, mental retardation, or any familial disease in blood relatives increases the risk of the same condition in the infant. Because many parents recognize only obvious clinical manifestations of genetically determined diseases, specific inquiry should be made about any disease affecting one or more blood relative(s).

MATERNAL FACTORS. The lowest neonatal mortality rate occurs in infants of mothers who receive adequate prenatal care and who are 20–30 yr of age. Both teenage pregnancies and those among women over 35 yr of age, particularly primiparous women, carry an increased risk for intrauterine growth retardation, fetal distress, and intrauterine death.

Maternal illness (Table 80–2); multiple pregnancies, particularly those involving monochorionic twinning; infections (Table 80–3), and certain drugs (Chapter 81) increase the risk for the fetus.

Polyhydramnios and *oligohydramnios* indicate high-risk pregnancies. Although there is a rapid turnover rate, during normal pregnancy the amniotic fluid volume gradually increases at a rate of less than 10 ml/day until about the 34th wk of pregnancy, after which it slowly diminishes. The volumes vary widely in normal pregnancy; term volume may be 500–2000 mL. A volume estimated at greater than 2,000 ml in the 3rd trimester constitutes polyhydramnios, and a volume estimated at less than 500 ml indicates oligohydramnios. Polyhydramnios complicates 1–3%, while oligohydramnios complicates 1–5% of pregnancies. The ultrasonographic criteria for these diagnoses are based on the *amniotic fluid index*, which is determined by measuring the vertical diameter of amniotic fluid pockets

■ TABLE 80–2 Maternal Disease Affecting the Fetus or Neonate

Disorder	Effects	Mechanism
Cholestasis	Preterm delivery	Unknown; possible hepatitis E
Cyanotic heart disease	Intrauterine growth retardation	Low fetal oxygen delivery
Diabetes mellitus		
Mild	Large for gestational age, hypoglycemia	Fetal hyperglycemia—produces hyperinsulinemia; insulin promotes growth
Severe	Growth retardation	Vascular disease, placental insufficiency
Drug addiction	Intrauterine growth retardation, neonatal withdrawal	Direct drug effect, plus poor diet
Endemic goiter	Hypothyroidism	Iodine deficiency
Graves' disease	Transient neonatal thyrotoxicosis	Placental immunoglobin passage of thyroid-stimulating antibody
Herpes gestationalis	Bullous rash	Unknown
Hyperparathyroidism	Neonatal hypocalcemia	Maternal calcium crosses to fetus and suppresses fetal parathyroid gland
Hypertension	Intrauterine growth retardation, intrauterine fetal demise	Placental insufficiency, fetal hypoxia
Idiopathic thrombocytopenic purpura	Thrombocytopenia	Nonspecific maternal platelet antibodies cross placenta
Isoimmune neutropenia or thrombocytopenia	Neutropenia or thrombocytopenia	Specific antifetal neutrophil or platelet antibody crosses placenta following sensitization of mother
Malignant melanoma	Placental or fetal tumor	Metastasis
Myasthenia gravis	Transient neonatal myasthenia	Immunoglobin to acetylcholine receptor crosses placenta
Myotonic dystrophy	Neonatal myotonic dystrophy, congenital contractures, respiratory insufficiency	Genetic anticipation
Obesity	Macrosomia, hypoglycemia	Unknown
Phenylketonuria	Microcephaly, retardation	Elevated fetal phenylalanine levels
Pre-eclampsia, eclampsia	Intrauterine growth retardation, thrombocytopenia, neutropenia, fetal demise	Uteroplacental insufficiency, fetal hypoxia, vasoconstriction
Renal transplant	Intrauterine growth retardation	Uteroplacental insufficiency
Rhesus or other blood group sensitization	Fetal anemia, hypoalbuminemia, hydrops, neonatal jaundice	Antibody crosses placenta directed to fetal cells with antigen
Sickle cell anemia	Preterm birth, intrauterine growth retardation	Maternal sickling producing fetal hypoxia
Systemic lupus erythematosus	Congenital heart block, rash, anemia, thrombocytopenia, neutropenia	Antibody directed to fetal heart, red and white blood cells and platelets

■ TABLE 80–3 Maternal Infections Affecting the Fetus or Newborn

Infection	Mode of Transmission	Outcome
Bacteria		
Group B streptococcus	Ascending cervical	Sepsis, pneumonia
Escherichia coli	Ascending cervical	Sepsis, pneumonia
Listeria monocytogenes	Transplacental	Sepsis, pneumonia
Ureaplasma urealyticum	Ascending cervical	Pneumonia, meningitis
Mycoplasma hominis	Ascending cervical	Pneumonia
Chlamydia trachomatis	Vaginal passage	Conjunctivitis, pneumonia
Syphilis	Transplacental	Congenital syphilis
Borrelia burgdorferi	Transplacental	Prematurity, fetal demise
Neisseria gonorrhoeae	Vaginal passage	Ophthalmia (conjunctivitis)
Mycobacterium tuberculosis	Transplacental	Prematurity, fetal demise, congenital TB
Virus		
Rubella	Transplacental	Congenital rubella
Cytomegalovirus	Transplacental, breast milk (rare)	Congenital CMV, or asymptomatic
Human immunodeficiency virus	Transplacental, vaginal passage, breast milk	Congenital AIDS
Hepatitis B	Vaginal passage, transplacental, breast milk	Neonatal hepatitis, chronic HBsAg carrier
Hepatitis C	Transplacental	Uncommon but neonatal hepatitis, chronic carrier possible
Lymphocytic choriomeningitis	Transplacental	Fetal, neonatal death; hydrocephalus, chorioretinitis
Herpes simplex II	Transplacental	Congenital HSV
	Vaginal passage, ascending	Neonatal encephalitis, disseminated viremia
Varicella-zoster	Transplacental, early	Congenital anomalies
	Transplacental, late	Neonatal varicella
Parvovirus	Transplacental	Fetal anemia, hydrops
Coxsackie virus B	Fecal-oral	Myocarditis, meningitis, hepatitis
Poliomyelitis	Transplacental	Congenital poliomyelitis
Epstein-Barr	Transplacental	Anomalies (?)
Rubeola	Transplacental	Abortion, fetal measles
Parasites		
Toxoplasmosis	Transplacental	Congenital toxoplasmosis or asymptomatic
Malaria	Transplacental	Abortion, prematurity, intrauterine growth retardation
Trypanosomiasis	Transplacental	Congenital Chagas' disease
Fungi		
Candida	Ascending, cervical	Sepsis, pneumonia, rash
Prion		
Creutzfeld-Jakob disease	Transplacental, colostrum	Hypothetical route, no long-term data

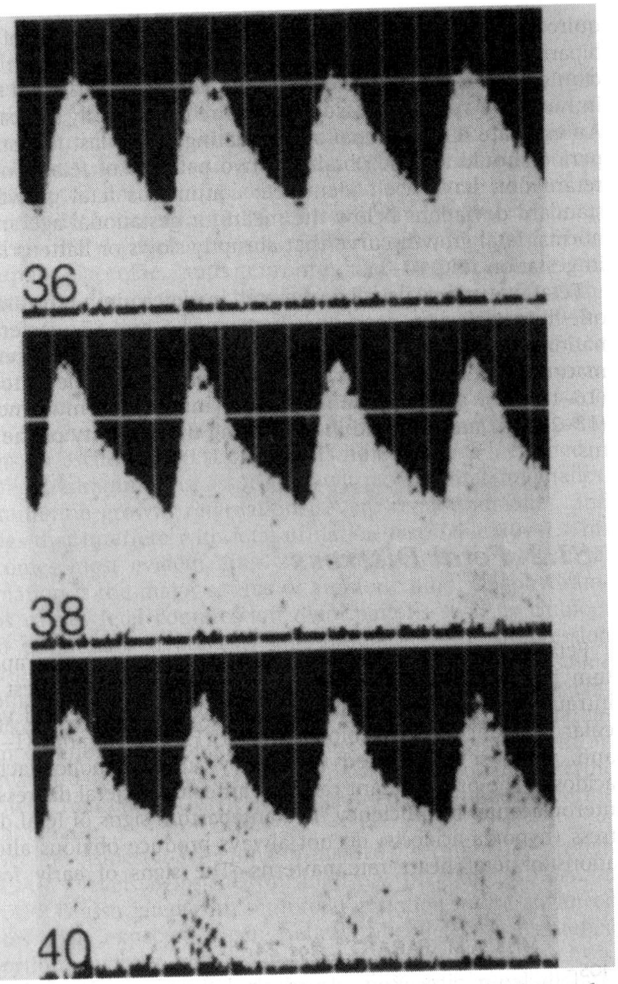

Figure 81–2. Normal Doppler velocimetry. Sequential Doppler studies, from one normal pregnancy, of fetal umbilical artery flow velocity waveforms. Note systolic peak flow with lower but constant flow during diastole. The systolic diastolic ratio can be determined and in normal pregnancies is <3 after the 30th wk gestation. The numbers indicate the week of gestation. (From Trudinger B: Doppler ultrasound assessment of blood flow. *In*: Creasy RK, Resnik R [eds]: Maternal-Fetal Medicine: Principles and Practice, 3rd ed. Philadelphia, WB Saunders, 1994.)

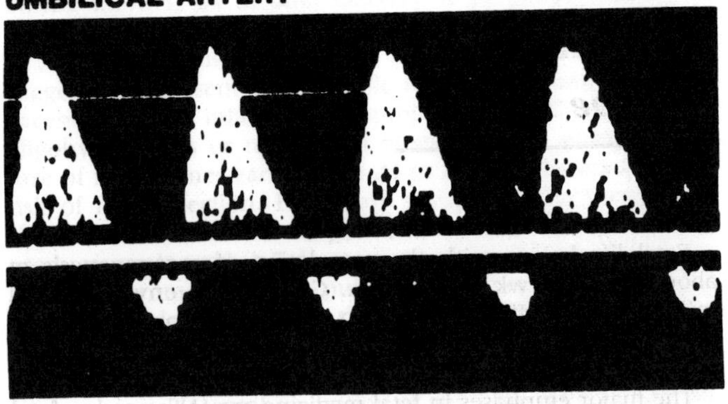

Figure 81–3. Abnormal Doppler velocimetry. An umbilical artery Doppler flow velocity waveform in which umbilical placental impedance is so high that the diastolic component shows flow in a reverse direction. This is an indication of severe intrauterine hypoxia and intrauterine growth retardation. (From Trudinger B: Doppler ultrasound assessment of blood flow. *In*: Creasy RK, Resnik R [eds]: Maternal-Fetal Medicine: Principles and Practice, 3rd ed. Philadelphia, WB Saunders, 1994.)

compromise may be assessed with percutaneous umbilical venous blood sampling (PUBS) to detect hypoxia and acidosis (Table 81–1) and with Doppler ultrasound to detect a reduced, absent, or reversed diastolic blood flow wave-form velocity in the fetal aorta or umbilical artery (Fig. 81–3; see Table 81–1).

The *nonstress test (NST)* monitors the presence of fetal heart rate accelerations that follow fetal movement. A reactive (normal) NST result demonstrates fetal heart rate accelerations of at least 15 beats/min lasting 15 sec. A nonreactive NST result suggests fetal compromise and requires further assessment with a *contraction stress test* (CST) or the *biophysical profile* (BPP). A CST observes the fetal heart rate response to spontaneous, nipple-, or oxytocin-stimulated uterine contractions. Fetal compromise is suggested when 3 contractions in 10 min are followed by late decelerations. CST is contraindicated in women in preterm labor and in those with multiple gestations, an incompetent cervix, polyhydramnios, or placenta previa. The goals of fetal monitoring are to prevent intrauterine fetal demise and hypoxic brain injury. Although the CST and NST have low false-negative rates, both have high false-positive rates. Additional methods of assessing fetal well-being have been combined into the biophysical profile to improve the accurate and safe identification of fetal compromise (Table 81–2). Indications for BPP include intrauterine growth retardation, postdate gestation, maternal diabetes mellitus, rhesus-sensitized pregnancy, previous history of stillbirths, and maternal hypertension. High-risk fetuses often demonstrate combinations of abnormalities such as oligohydramnios, reversed diastolic Doppler umbilical artery blood flow velocity, and a low biophysical profile.

Fetal distress during labor may be detected by monitoring fetal heart rate, uterine pressure, and fetal scalp blood pH (Fig. 81–4).

Continuous fetal heart rate monitoring detects abnormal cardiac patterns by instruments that compute the beat-to-beat fetal heart rate from a fetal electrocardiographic signal. Signals are derived from an electrode attached to the fetal presenting part; from an ultrasonic transducer placed on the maternal abdominal wall to detect continuous ultrasonic waves reflected from the contractions of the heart; or from a phonotransducer placed on the mother's abdomen. Uterine contractions are simultaneously recorded from an amniotic fluid catheter and pressure transducer or from a tocotransducer applied to the maternal abdominal wall overlying the uterus.

Fetal heart rate patterns show various characteristics, some of which suggest fetal distress. Baseline fetal heart rate is the average rate between uterine contractions, which gradually decreases from about 155 beats/min in early pregnancy to about 135 beats/min at term; the normal range at term is 120–160 beats/min. **Tachycardia** (over 160 beats/min) is associated with early fetal hypoxia, maternal fever, maternal hyperthyroidism, maternal β-sympathomimetic or atropine therapy, fetal anemia, and some fetal arrhythmias. The latter do not generally occur with congenital heart disease and tend to resolve spontaneously at birth. **Fetal bradycardia** (<120 beats/min) occurs with fetal hypoxia, the placental transfer of local anesthetic agents and β-adrenergic blocking agents, and, occasionally, heart block with or without congenital heart disease.

Normally, the baseline fetal heart rate is variable, with long-term changes of 3–6 cycles/min as well as short-term beat-to-beat variation. This variability may be decreased or lost with fetal hypoxemia or the placental transfer of drugs such as atropine, diazepam, promethazine, magnesium sulfate, and most sedative and narcotic agents. Prematurity, sleep state, and fetal tachycardia may also diminish beat-to-beat variability.

Periodic accelerations or decelerations of fetal heart rate in

■ TABLE 81–1 Fetal Diagnosis and Assessment

Method	Comment and Indications
Imaging	
Ultrasound (real-time)	Biometry (growth), anomaly (morphology) detection. Biophysical profile. Amniotic fluid volume, hydrops, determine gestational age and IUGR*
Ultrasound (Doppler)	Velocimetry (blood flow velocity). Detection of increased vascular resistance secondary to fetal hypoxia, IUGR*
Embryoscopy	Early diagnosis of limb anomaly
Fetoscopy	Detection of facial, limb, cutaneous anomalies
Fluid Analysis	
Amniocentesis	Fetal maturity (L/S ratio), karyotype (cytogenetics), biochemical enzyme analysis, molecular genetic DNA diagnosis, bilirubin or α-fetoprotein determination. Bacterial culture, pathogen antigen or genome detection
Fetal urine	Prognosis of obstructive uropathy?
Cordocentesis (percutaneous umbilical blood sampling [PUBS])	Detection of blood type, anemia, hemoglobinopathies, thrombocytopenia, acidosis, hypoxia, polycythemia, IgM antibody response to infection. Rapid karyotyping an molecular DNA genetic diagnosis. Fetal therapy (see Table 81–5)
Fetal Tissue Analysis	
Chorionic villus biopsy	Karyotype, molecular DNA genetic analysis, enzyme assays
Skin biopsy	Hereditary skin disease†
Liver biopsy	Enzyme assay†
Maternal Serum α-Fetoprotein	
Elevated	Twins, neural tube defects (anencephaly, spina bifida), intestinal atresia, hepatitis, nephrosis, fetal demise, incorrected gestational age
Reduced	Trisomies, aneuploidy
Maternal Cervix	
Fetal fibronectin	Indicates risk of preterm birth
Bacterial culture	Identifies risk of fetal infection (group B streptococcus, *N. gonorrhoeae*)
Fluid	Determination of premature rupture of the membranes
Antepartum Biophysical (Electrical) Monitoring	
Nonstress test	Fetal distress; hypoxia
Contraction stress test	Fetal distress; hypoxia
Vibroacoustic stimulation	Fetal distress; hypoxia
Intrapartum Fetal Heart Rate Monitoring	(See Fig. 81–4)

**IUGR = intrauterine growth retardation.*

†DNA genetic analysis on chorionic villus samples, amniocytes from amniocentesis, or fetal cells recovered from the maternal circulation may obviate the need for direct fetal tissue biopsy if the gene or genetic marker is available (e.g., the gene for Duchenne muscular dystrophy).

response to uterine contractions may also be monitored (see Fig. 81–4). **Early deceleration** (type I dips), associated with head compression, is a repetitive pattern of slowing, synchronous with and proportional to, the amplitude of the uterine contraction. **Variable deceleration** (associated with cord compression) is characterized by variable shape, abrupt onset and occurrence with consecutive contractions, and return to baseline at or after the conclusion of the contraction. **Late deceleration** (type II dips), associated with fetal hypoxemia, occurs repetitively after a uterine contraction is well established, is proportional to its amplitude, and persists into the interval following contractions. The late deceleration pattern is usually associated with maternal hypotension or excessive uterine activity but may be a response to any maternal, placental, umbilical cord, or fetal factor that limits effective oxygenation of the fetus. Reflex late decelerations with normal beat-to-beat variability are associated with chronic compensated fetal hypoxia and occur during uterine contractions that temporarily impede oxygen transport to the heart. Nonreflex late decelerations are more ominous and indicate severe hypoxic depression of myocardial function. The latter, together with decreased beat-to-beat variability or spontaneous decelerations in the absence of uterine contractions, either warrants further assessment by fetal blood sampling or is an indication for delivery.

Fetal scalp blood sampling during labor through a slightly dilated cervix may aid in confirming fetal distress suspected on the basis of variations in fetal heart rate or the presence of meconium in the amniotic fluid. The proper use of this technique may result in earlier delivery of depressed infants who thus have a better chance of successful resuscitation, increased survival, and less morbidity. Alternatively, when continuous fetal heart rate monitoring or general clinical evaluation suggests that a fetus is at risk, a normal fetal scalp blood sample may help avert obstetric intervention.

Women who are reasonably comfortable and pain-relieved during labor and delivery usually exhibit an early mild respiratory alkalosis due to hyperventilation and, just before delivery, a mild metabolic acidosis due to a lactic acid accumulation that occurs toward the end of labor. However, pain or stress may produce severe hyperventilation, which markedly reduces maternal and subsequent fetal P_{CO_2}; such a reduction may mask fetal acidosis. Fetal scalp blood pH and P_{CO_2} levels fall between values measured in the umbilical vein and artery, in most instances giving a reasonable estimate of systemic fetal acid-base values. Fetal scalp blood pH in normal labor decreases from about 7.33 early in labor to approximately 7.25 at the time of vaginal delivery; the base deficit is about 4–6 mEq/L. Changes in the buffer base may be particularly helpful in assessing fetal status, since they correspond to fetal lactic acid accumulation and do not occur as rapidly as changes in fetal P_{CO_2}, which may be influenced by maternal ventilation as well as by placental diffusion.

Fetal hypoxia and circulatory insufficiency result in a mixed placental respiratory and metabolic acidosis that often, but not invariably, can be detected by the determination of pH, base deficit, and carbon dioxide tension in blood obtained from the fetal scalp. A pH of less than 7.25 strongly suggests fetal distress, and a pH of less than 7.20 is an indication for early delivery.

Normal scalp blood pH values are associated with normal continuous fetal heart rate patterns and accurately indicate the absence of recent moderate to severe hypoxia. In contrast, low scalp blood pH values frequently correlate with severe variable deceleration or late deceleration alone and with loss of beat-to-beat variability or baseline tachycardia associated with these deceleration patterns. However, a wide range of pH is found

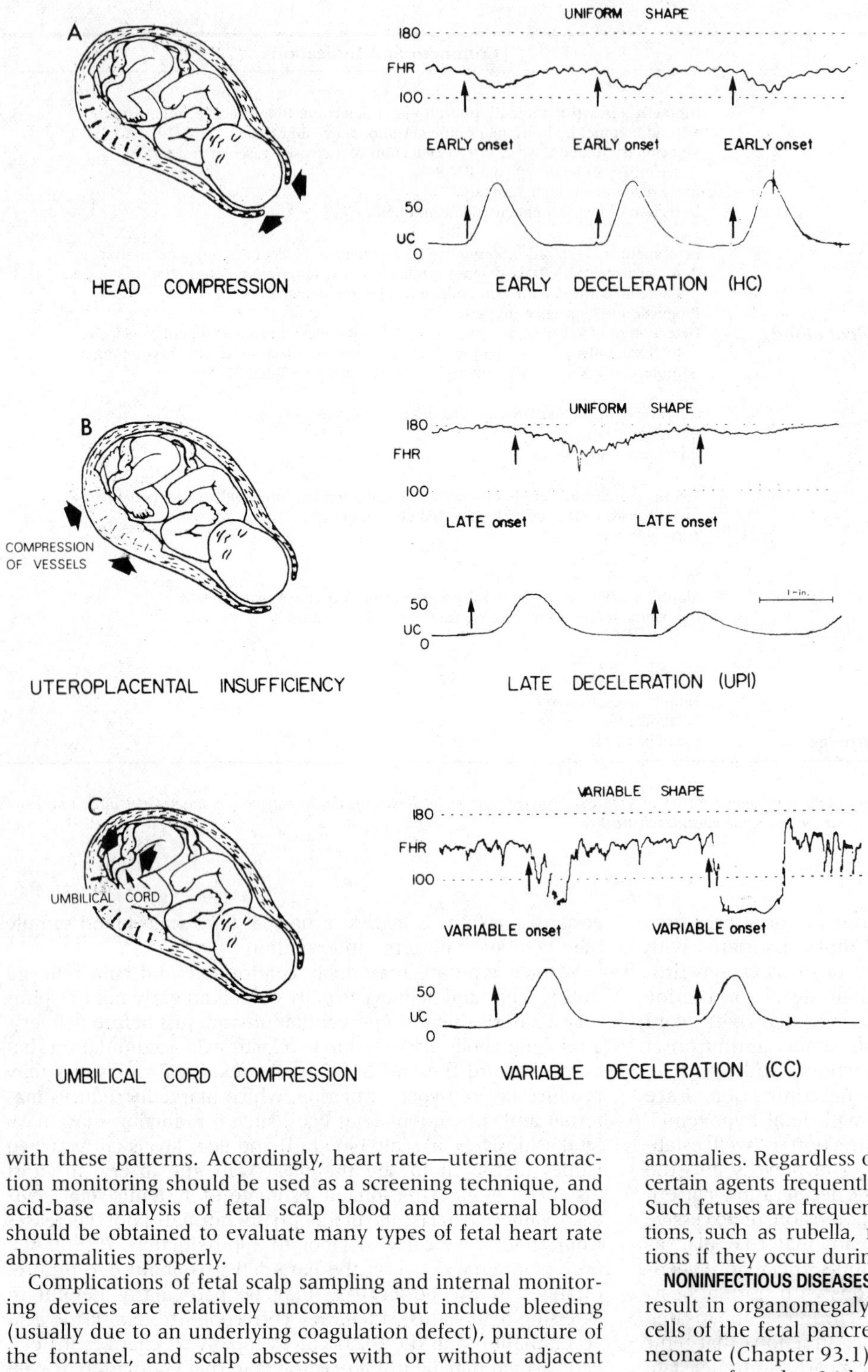

Figure 81–4. Patterns of periodic fetal heart rate decelerations. Tracing in *A* shows early deceleration that occurs during the peak of uterine contractions and is due to pressure on the fetal head. *B*, Late deceleration due to uteroplacental insufficiency. *C*, Variable deceleration due to umbilical cord compression. Arrows denote time relation between the onset of FHR changes and uterine contractions. (From Hon EH: An Atlas of Fetal Heart Rate Patterns. New Haven, CT, Harty Press, 1968.)

with these patterns. Accordingly, heart rate—uterine contraction monitoring should be used as a screening technique, and acid-base analysis of fetal scalp blood and maternal blood should be obtained to evaluate many types of fetal heart rate abnormalities properly.

Complications of fetal scalp sampling and internal monitoring devices are relatively uncommon but include bleeding (usually due to an underlying coagulation defect), puncture of the fontanel, and scalp abscesses with or without adjacent osteomyelitis. Abscesses may be due to *Staphylococcus aureus* or gram-negative rods; more often they are sterile.

81.3 Maternal Disease and the Fetus

INFECTIOUS DISEASES (see Table 80–3). Almost any maternal infection with severe systemic manifestations may result in miscarriage, stillbirth, or premature labor. Whether these results are due to infection of the fetus or are secondary to stress is not always clear. Maternal hyperthermia during infections may be associated with an increased incidence of congenital anomalies. Regardless of the severity of the maternal infection, certain agents frequently infect the fetus, with serious sequelae. Such fetuses are frequently small for gestational age. Some infections, such as rubella, may also produce congenital malformations if they occur during the period of organogenesis.

NONINFECTIOUS DISEASES (see Table 80–2). *Maternal diabetes* may result in organomegaly, hypertrophy and hyperplasia of the β cells of the fetal pancreas, and metabolic derangements in the neonate (Chapter 93.1). A high incidence of intrauterine death occurs after the 36th wk of gestation in unmonitored and poorly controlled mothers. *Toxemia* of pregnancy, chronic hypertension, and renal disease result in small fetal size for gestational age, prematurity, and intrauterine death, all probably due to diminished uteroplacental perfusion. Uncontrolled maternal *hypothyroidism* or *hyperthyroidism* is responsible for relative infertility, a tendency to abort, premature labor, and fetal death. Maternal *immunologic diseases*, such as idiopathic thrombocytopenic purpura, systemic lupus, myasthenia gravis, and Graves disease, all of which are mediated by IgG autoantibodies that cross the placenta, frequently result in a transient illness in the newborn. Untreated maternal *phenylketonuria* results in miscarriage, congenital malformations, and injury to the brain of the nonphenylketonuric fetus.

■ **TABLE 81–2 Biophysical Profile Scoring: Technique and Interpretation***

Biophysical Variable	Normal Score	Abnormal (Score = 0)
Fetal breathing movements	At least 1 episode of FBM of at least 30 sec duration in 30 min observation	Absent FBM or no episode of ≥30 sec in 30 minutes
Gross body movement	At least 3 discrete body/limb movements in 30 min (episodes of active continuous movement considered as single movement)	2 or fewer episodes of body/limb movements in 30 min
Fetal tone	At least 1 episode of active extension with return to flexion of fetal limb(s) or trunk. Opening and closing of hand considered normal tone	Either slow extension with return to partial flexion or movement of limb in full extension or absent fetal movement with fetal hand held in complete or partial deflection
Reactive FHR	At least 2 episodes of FHR acceleration of ≥15 beat/min and of at least 15 sec duration associated with fetal movement in 30 min	Less than 2 episodes of acceleration of FHR or acceleration of <15 beats/min in 30 min
Qualitative AFV†	At least 1 pocket of AF that measures at least 2 cm in 2 perpendicular planes	Either no AF pockets or a pocket <2 cm in two perpendicular planes

**FBM = fetal breathing movement; FHR = fetal heart rate; AFV = amniotic fluid volume; AF = amniotic fluid.*

†Modification of the criteria for reduced amniotic fluid from <1 cm to <2 cm would seem reasonable. Fetal biophysical assessment by ultrasound. (From Creasy RK, Resnik R [eds]: Maternal-Fetal Medicine: Principles and Practice, 3rd ed. Philadelphia, WB Saunders, 1994.)

81.4 Maternal Medication and the Fetus

The effects of drugs taken by the mother vary considerably, especially in relation to the time in pregnancy when they are taken. Miscarriage or congenital malformations result from maternal ingestion of teratogenic drugs during the period of organogenesis. Maternal medications taken later, particularly during the last few weeks of gestation or during labor, tend to affect the function of specific organs or enzyme systems, adversely affecting the neonate rather than the fetus (Tables 81–3 and 81–4). Individual genetic makeup may determine susceptibility to some drugs. For example, phenytoin teratogenesis may be mediated by enzymatic production of epoxide metabolites determined by inheritance. In addition, the effects of drugs may be evident immediately in the delivery room or may be delayed, such as with the development of vaginal adenocarcinoma and genital lesions in adolescent female offspring of women exposed to diethylstilbestrol during pregnancy or childhood tumors following fetal alcohol or phenytoin exposure. Consumption of drugs in pregnancy is frequent; surveys indicate that 90% of pregnant patients have taken at least one drug. The average mother has taken four drugs other than vitamins or iron during pregnancy; 4% have taken 10 drugs or more. In view of the limits of current knowledge of the fetal effects of maternal medication, no drugs should be prescribed during pregnancy without weighing the maternal need against the risk of fetal damage.

81.5 Identification of Fetal Disease

(Intrauterine Diagnosis) (see Table 81–1)

See 81.2 for a discussion of fetal distress.

Diagnostic procedures are used to identify fetal diseases when abortion is being considered, when direct fetal treatment is possible, or when a decision is made to deliver a viable but premature infant to avoid intrauterine fetal demise. Fetal assessment is also indicated in a broader context when the family, medical, or reproductive history of the mother suggests the presence of a high-risk pregnancy or a high-risk fetus (Chapters 80 and 81).

There are various methods of identifying fetal disease (see Table 81–1). Fetal ultrasonographic imaging may detect fetal growth abnormalities (by biometric measurements of biparietal diameter, femur length, or head or abdominal circumference) or fetal malformations. Although 95% of fetuses whose biparietal diameter is 9.5 cm or more are at least 37 wk of gestation, the lungs of these fetuses may not be mature. Serial determination of growth velocity and the head-to-abdominal circumference ratio enhances the ability to detect intrauterine growth retardation. Real-time ultrasound may identify placental abnormalities (abruptio placentae, placenta previa) and fetal anomalies such as hydrocephalus, anencephalus, spina bifida, duodenal atresia, diaphragmatic hernia, renal agenesis, bladder outlet obstruction, congenital heart disease, limb abnormalities, sacrococcygeal teratoma, cystic hygroma, omphalocele, gastroschisis, and hydrops.

Real-time ultrasonography also facilitates performance of *cordocentesis* (PUBS) and the biophysical profile by imaging fetal breathing, body movements, tone, and amniotic fluid volume (see Table 81–2). *Doppler velocimetry* assesses fetal arterial blood flow (vascular resistance) (see Figs. 81–2 and 81–3). Roentgenographic examination of the fetus has been replaced by real-time ultrasound and fetoscopy.

Amniocentesis, the transabdominal withdrawal of amniotic fluid during pregnancy for diagnostic purposes (see Table 81–1), is frequently done to determine the timing of the delivery of fetuses with erythroblastosis fetalis or the need for a fetal transfusion. It is also done for genetic indications, usually between the 16th and 18th gestational weeks. The amniotic fluid may be directly analyzed for amino acids, enzymes, hormones, and abnormal metabolic products; and amniotic fluid cells may be cultivated to permit detailed cytologic analysis for the prenatal detection of chromosomal abnormalities and DNA-gene or enzymatic analysis for the detection of inborn metabolic errors. Analysis of amniotic fluid may also help in identifying neural tube defects (elevation of α-fetoprotein), adrenogenital syndrome (elevation of 17-ketosteroids and pregnanetriol), and thyroid dysfunction. Chorionic villus biopsy (transvaginal or transabdominal) performed in the 1st trimester also provides fetal cells but has a slightly increased risk for fetal loss, limb reduction defects, and oromandibular hypogenesis.

The best available chemical indices of fetal maturity are provided by determinations of amniotic fluid creatinine and lecithin, which reflect the maturity of the fetal kidney and lung, respectively. Lecithin (L) is produced in the lung by type II alveolar cells and eventually reaches the amniotic fluid via the effluent from the trachea. Until the middle of the 3rd trimester, its concentration nearly equals that of sphingomyelin (S); thereafter, S remains constant in amniotic fluid while L increases. By 35 wk, on the average, the L/S ratio is about 2:1, indicating lung maturity.

Earlier lung maturation may occur when there is severe premature separation of the placenta, premature rupture of the fetal membranes, narcotic addiction, or maternal hypertensive and renal vascular disease. A delay in pulmonary maturation may be associated with hydrops fetalis or maternal diabetes without vascular disease. The likelihood of hyaline membrane disease is greatly reduced with L/S ratios of 2:1 or more, although hypoxia, acidosis, and hypothermia may increase the risk despite this "mature" L/S ratio. However,

■ **TABLE 81–3 Agents Acting on Pregnant Women That May Adversely Affect the Fetus**

Drug	Effect on Fetus	Dependability of Evidence
Accutane (isotretinoin)	Facial-ear anomalies, heart disease	Conclusive
Alcohol	Congenital anomalies, IUGR*	Conclusive
Aminopterin	Abortion, malformations	Conclusive
Amphetamines	Congenital heart disease, IUGR	Suggestive
Angiotensin converting enzyme inhibitors (ACE)	Renal failure, oligohydramnios	Suggestive
Azathioprine	Abortion	Suggestive
Busulfan (Myleran)	Stunted growth, corneal opacities, cleft palate, hypoplasia of ovaries, thyroid, and parathyroids	Doubtful
Caffeine	Spontaneous abortion, stillbirth, or LBW birth	Suggestive
Carbamazepine	Spina bifida	Suggestive
Cocaine/crack	Abnormal brain development, microcephaly, LBW, IUGR	Conclusive
Chloroquine	Deafness	Suggestive
Cigarette smoking	Low birthweight for gestational age	Conclusive
Cyclophosphamide	Multiple malformations	Suggestive
Dicumarol	Fetal bleeding and death, hypoplastic nasal structures	Conclusive
Hyperthermia	Spina bifida	Suggestive
Indomethacin	Reducing urination	Suggestive
Lithium	Ebstein anomaly	Suggestive
Meclizine (Bonine)	Congenital malformations	Doubtful
Mepivacaine	Bradycardia, death	Conclusive
6-Mercaptopurine	Abortion	Suggestive
Methimazole	Goiter	Conclusive
Methyl mercury	Minamata disease, microcephaly, deaf, blind, mental retardation	Conclusive
Methyltestosterone	Masculinization of female fetus	Conclusive
17-α-ethinyl-19-nortestosterone (Norlutin)	Masculinization of female fetus	Conclusive
Penicillamine	Cutis laxa syndrome	Suggestive
Phenytoin (Dilantin)	Congenital anomalies, IUGR, neuroblastoma	Conclusive
Progesterone	Masculinization of female fetus	Suggestive
Propranolol	Hypoglycemia, bradycardia, respiratory depression	Suggestive
Propylthiouracil	Goiter	Conclusive
Quinine	Abortion, thrombocytopenia, deafness	Suggestive
Radioactive iodine (^{131}I)	Destruction of fetal thyroid	Conclusive
17-α-ethinyl testosterone (Progestoral)	Masculinization of female fetus	Conclusive
Stilbestrol (diethylstilbestrol [DES])	Vaginal adenocarcinoma in adolescence	Conclusive
Streptomycin	Deafness	Suggestive
Sympathomimetic (tocolytic) agents	Tachycardia, heart failure	Suggestive
Tetracycline	Retarded skeletal growth	Suggestive
	Pigmentation of teeth, hypoplasia of enamel	Conclusive
	Cataract, limb malformations	Doubtful
Thalidomide	Phocomelia, other malformations	Conclusive
Toluene	Craniofacial abnormalities	Suggestive
Trimethadione and paramethadione	Abortion, multiple malformations, mental retardation	Conclusive
Valproate	Spina bifida	Conclusive
Vitamin D	Supravalvular aortic stenosis, hypercalcemia	Doubtful

IUGR = intrauterine growth retardation.

20–25% of infants with L/S ratios less than 2:1 do not have hyaline membrane disease. Maternal and fetal blood have an L/S ratio of about 1:4; thus, contamination will not alter the significance of a ratio of 2:1 or more. Meconium contamination, storage, and centrifugation all may reduce the reliability of the L/S ratio.

A determination of saturated phosphatidylcholine (L), osmophilic bodies, or phosphatidylglycerol (PG) concentrations in amniotic fluid may be more specific and sensitive predictors of pulmonary maturity, especially in high-risk pregnancies such as those occurring in women with diabetes (see Chapter 87).

Although amniocentesis can be carried out with little discomfort to the mother, there is, even in experienced hands, a small risk of direct damage to the fetus, of placental puncture and bleeding with secondary damage to the fetus, of stimulating uterine contraction and premature labor, of amnionitis, and of maternal sensitization to fetal blood. The earlier in gestation amniotic puncture is done, the greater the risk to the fetus. The risks can be reduced by using ultrasound for placental localization. The procedure should be limited to those cases in which the potential benefits of the findings will outweigh the risk.

Cordocentesis, or percutaneous umbilical blood sampling (PUBS), is used to diagnose fetal hematologic abnormalities, genetic disorders, infections, and fetal hypoxia (see Table 81–1). Under direct ultrasonographic visualization, a long needle is passed into the umbilical vein at its entrance to the placenta or fetal abdominal wall. Blood may be withdrawn to determine fetal hemoglobin, platelet concentration, lymphocyte DNA, or $Pa{O_2}$, pH, $P{CO_2}$, and lactate levels. Transfusion or administration of drugs can be given through the umbilical vein (Table 81–5).

81.6 Treatment and Prevention of Fetal Disease

Management of fetal diseases continues to depend on coordinated advances in accuracy of diagnosis; understanding of fetal nutrition, pharmacology, immunology, and pathophysiology; availability of antimicrobial and antiviral drugs; and therapeutic procedures. Progress in providing specific treatments for accurately diagnosed diseases has improved with the advent of real-time ultrasonography and cordocentesis (see Tables 81–1 and 81–5).

The incidence of sensitization of Rh negative women by Rh positive fetuses has been reduced by the prophylactic adminis-

■ **TABLE 81–4 Agents Acting on Pregnant Women That May Adversely Affect the Newborn Infant**

Alcohol—Developmental abnormalities in childhood
Anesthetic agents (volatile)—central nervous system depression
Adrenal corticosteroids—adrenocortical failure (rare)
Ammonium chloride—acidosis (clinically inapparent)
Aspirin—neonatal bleeding, prolonged gestation
Bromides—rash, CNS depression
Cigarettes—possible neurodevelopmental impairment in childhood
Captopril—cardiovascular instability, transient renal failure
Carbamazepine—neurodevelopmental abnormalities
Caudal anesthesia with mepivacaine (accidental introduction of anesthetic into scalp of baby)—bradypnea, apnea, bradycardia, convulsions
CNS depressants (narcotics, barbiturates, tranquilizers) during labor—central nervous system depression
Cephalothin—positive direct Coombs test reaction
Cocaine/crack—microcephaly, growth retardation, behavioral disturbances
Coumarin derivatives—high perinatal mortality, anomalies
Dilantin—bleeding diathesis (vitamin K deficiency), neurodevelopmental abnormalities
Fluoxitine—possible transient neonatal withdrawal, hypertonicity
Hexamethonium bromide—paralytic ileus
Intravenous fluids during labor (e.g., salt-free solutions)—electrolyte disturbances, hyponatremia, hypoglycemia
Iodides—neonatal goiter
Indomethacin—oliguria, necrotizing enterocolitis, bronchopulmonary dysplasia (?)
Isoxsuprine—ileus, hypocalcemia, hypoglycemia, hypotension
Lead—reduced intellectual function
Magnesium sulfate—respiratory depression, meconium plug, hypotonia
Morphine and its derivatives (addiction)—withdrawal symptoms (poor feeding, vomiting, diarrhea, restlessness, yawning and stretching, dyspnea and cyanosis, fever and sweating, pallor, tremors, convulsions)
Naphthalene—hemolytic anemia (in glucose-6-phosphate dehydrogenase [G-6-PD]-deficient infants)
Nitrofurantoin—hemolytic anemia (in G-6-PD–deficient infants)
Oxytocin—hyperbilirubinemia, hyponatremia
Phenobarbital—bleeding diathesis (vitamin K deficiency)
Polychlorinated biphenyls—poor neurologic development
Primaquine—hemolytic anemia (in G-6-PD–deficient infants)
Propranolol—hypoglycemia, bradycardia, apnea
Reserpine—drowsiness, nasal congestion, poor temperature stability
Sulfonamides (long-acting)—interfere with protein binding of bilirubin; kernicterus at low levels of serum bilirubin
Sulfonylurea—refractory hypoglycemia
Thiazides—neonatal thrombocytopenia (rare)
Toluene (solvent abuse)—preterm labor, fetal alcohol–like syndrome, dysmorphology
Vitamin K (excessive amounts)—hyperbilirubinemia

tration of Rh(D) immunoglobulin to mothers early in pregnancy and after each delivery or abortion, thus reducing the frequency of hemolytic disease in their subsequent offspring. Fetal erythroblastosis (Chapter 89) may now be accurately diagnosed by amniotic fluid analysis and treated with intrauterine intraperitoneal or intravenous transfusions of packed Rh negative blood cells to maintain the fetus until it is mature enough to have a reasonable chance of survival.

Fetal hypoxia or distress may now be diagnosed with moderate success. Treatment, however, remains limited to supplying the mother with high concentrations of oxygen, positioning the uterus to avoid vascular compression, and initiating operative delivery before severe fetal injury occurs.

Pharmacologic approaches to fetal immaturity (e.g., administration of steroids to the mother to accelerate fetal lung maturation and to decrease the incidence of respiratory distress syndrome [Chapter 87] in prematurely delivered infants) are promising. Inhibiting labor with β-sympathomimetic tocolytic agents is unfortunately not successful in most patients with premature labor. Treatment of definitively diagnosed fetal genetic disease or congenital anomalies consists of parental counseling or abortion; rarely, high-dose vitamin therapy for a responsive inborn error of metabolism (e.g., biotin-dependent disorders) or fetal transfusion (with red blood cells or platelets) may be indicated. Fetal surgery (see Table 81–5) remains an experimental approach to therapy and is available only in a few highly specialized perinatal centers. The nature of the defect and its consequences as well as the ethical implications for the fetus and the parents must be considered.

Adzick NS, Harrison MR: Fetal surgical therapy. Lancet 343:897, 1994.

Arduini D, Rizzo G, Romanini C: The development of abnormal heart rate patterns after absent end-diastolic velocity in umbilical artery: Analysis of risk factors. Am J Obstet Gynecol 168:43, 1993.

Berrebi A, Kobuch WE, Bessieres MH, et al: Termination of pregnancy for maternal toxoplasmosis. Lancet 344:36, 1994.

CLASP Collaborative Group. CLASP: a randomised trial of low-dose aspirin for the prevention and treatment of pre-eclampsia among 9364 pregnant women. Lancet 343:619, 1994.

Committee on Genetics: Folic acid for the prevention of neural tube defects. Pediatrics 92:493, 1993.

Creasy RK: Preterm birth prevention: Where are we? Am J Obstet Gynecol 168:1223, 1993.

D'Alton ME: Prenatal diagnostic procedures. Semin Perinatol 18:140, 1994.

Elias S, Emerson DS, Simpson JL, et al: Ultrasound-guided fetal skin sampling for prenatal diagnosis of genodermatoses. Obstet Gynecol 83:337, 1994.

Ewigman BG, Crane JP, Frigoletto FD, et al: Effect of prenatal ultrasound screening on perinatal outcome. N Engl J Med 329:821, 1993.

Firth HV, Boyd PA, Chamberlain PF, et al: Analysis of limb reduction defects in babies exposed to chorionic villus sampling. Lancet 343:1069, 1994.

Garmel SH, D'Alton ME: Diagnostic ultrasound in pregnancy: An overview. Semin Perinatol 18:117, 1994.

Ghidini A, Sepulveda W, Lockwood CJ, et al: Complications of fetal blood sampling. Am J Obstet Gynecol 168:1339, 1993.

Guinn DA, Wigton TR, James JA, et al: Mammary stimulation test predicts preterm birth in nulliparous women. Am J Obstet Gynecol 170:1809, 1994.

Heffner LJ, Sherman CB, Speizer FE, et al: Clinical and environmental predictors of preterm labor. Obstet Gynecol 81:750, 1993.

Lockwood CJ, Wein R, Lapinski R, et al: The presence of cervical and vaginal fetal fibronectin predicts preterm delivery in an inner-city obstetric population. Am J Obstet Gynecol 169:798, 1993.

Lynch A, Marlar R, Murphy J, et al: Antiphospholipid antibodies in predicting adverse pregnancy outcome. A prospective study. Ann Intern Med 120:470, 1994.

Manning FA, Snijders R, Harman CR, et al: Fetal biophysical profile score. VI. Correlation with antepartum umbilical venous fetal pH. Am J Obstet Gynecol 169:755, 1993.

McDonnell M, Serra-Serra V, Gaffney G, et al: Neonatal outcome after pregnancy complicated by abnormal velocity waveforms in the umbilical artery. Arch Dis Child 70:F84, 1994.

Morrow R, Ritchie K: Doppler ultrasound fetal velocimetry and its role in obstetrics. Clin Perinatol 16:771, 1989.

Pearson MA, Hoyme HE, Seaver LH, et al: Toluene embryopathy: Delineation of the phenotype and comparison with fetal alcohol syndrome. Pediatrics 93:211, 1994.

Pleet H, Graham J, Smith D: Central nervous system and facial defects associated with maternal hyperthermia at 4–14 wk gestation. Pediatrics 67:785, 1981.

Reece EA, Copel JA, Scioscia AL, et al: Diagnostic fetal umbilical blood sampling in the management of isoimmunization. Am J Obstet Gynecol 159:1057, 1988.

Sharony R, Browne C, Lachman RS, et al: Prenatal diagnosis of the skeletal dysplasias. Am J Obstet Gynecol 169:668, 1993.

Simpson JL, Elias S: Isolating fetal cells from maternal blood. Advances in prenatal diagnosis through molecular technology. JAMA 270:2357, 1993.

Simpson LL, Marx GR: Diagnosis and treatment of structural fetal cardiac abnormality and dysrhythmia. Semin Perinatol 18:215, 1994.

Tejani N, Maran LI, Bhakthavathsalan A, et al: Correlation of fetal heart rate-uterine contraction patterns with fetal scalp blood pH. Obstet Gynecol 46:392, 1975.

Tyrrell S, Obaid AH, Lilford RJ: Umbilical artery Doppler velocimetry as a predictor of fetal hypoxia and acidosis at birth. Obstet Gynecol 74:332, 1989.

Weiner CP, Williamson RA: Evaluation of severe growth retardation using cordocentesis-hematologic and metabolic alterations by etiology. Obstet Gynecol 73:225, 1989.

Workshop on Chorionic Villus Sampling. Report of national institute of child health and human development workshop on chorionic villus sampling and limb and other defects, October 20, 1992. Am J Obstet Gynecol 169:1, 1993.

*81.7 Teratogens**

When an infant or child is malformed or mentally retarded, the parents often wrongly blame themselves and attribute the child's problems to events that occurred during pregnancy.

*Modified in part from original by L. B. Holmes in the 14th Edition.

■ TABLE 81–5 Fetal Therapy

Disorder	Treatment
Hematology	
Anemia with hydrops (erythroblastosis fetalis)	Umbilical vein packed red blood cell transfusion
Thrombocytopenia	
Isoimmune	Umbilical vein platelet transfusion, intravenous immunoglobulin
Autoimmune (ITP)	Maternal steroids, intravenous immunoglobulin
Metabolic-Endocrine	
Maternal PKU	Phenylalanine restriction
Fetal galactosemia	Galactose-free diet (?)
Multiple carboxylase deficiency	Biotin
Methylmalonic acidemia	Vitamin B_{12}
21-Hydroxylase deficiency	Dexamethasone
Hypothyroidism	Thyroid hormone (?)
Maternal diabetes mellitus	Tight insulin control
Fetal Distress	
Hypoxia	Maternal oxygen, position
Intrauterine growth retardation	Maternal oxygen, position
Oligohydramnios, premature rupture of membranes with variable deceleration	Amnioinfusion
Supraventricular tachycardia	Maternal digoxin,* procainamide, amiodarone, propranolol, flecainide
Lupus anticoagulant	Maternal aspirin, prednisone ± heparin
Pre-eclampsia	Maternal aspirin
Premature labor	Sympathomimetics, indomethacin, magnesium sulfate
Respiratory	
Pulmonary immaturity	Dexamethasone(?), thyrotropin releasing hormone
Congenital Anomalies	
Neural tube defects	Folate, vitamins (prevention)
Diaphragmatic hernia	Surgery (?)
Hydrocephalus	Ventricular shunt (unproved)
Hydronephrosis (bladder obstruction)	Vesicostomy tube (unproved), bladder marsupialization (vesicostomy)
Cystic adenomatoid malformation (with hydrops)	Thoracentesis, shunt, or resection
Infectious Disease	
Group B streptococcus	Ampicillin
Chorioamnionitis	Erythromycin (?)
Toxoplasmosis	Spiramycin, pyrimethamine, sulfonamide, and folinic acid
Syphilis	Penicillin
Tuberculosis	Antituberculosis drugs
Lyme disease	Penicillin, ceftriaxone
Parvovirus	Intrauterine red blood cell transfusion
Chlamydia trachomatis	Erythromycin
HIV-AIDS	Zidovudine (AZT)
Other	
Nonimmune hydrops (anemia)	Intrauterine red blood cell transfusion
Narcotic abstinence (withdrawal)	Maternal low-dose methadone
Intraventricular hemorrhage	Vitamin K (?)
Severe combined immunodeficiency disease	Fetal stem cell transfusion
Sacrococcygeal teratoma	In utero resection
Twin-twin transfusion syndrome	Repeated amniocentesis, YAG-laser photocoagulation of shared vessels
Multifetal gestation	Selective reduction
Bilateral chylothorax	Tube, needle drainage
Meconium stained fluid	Amnioinfusion
Congenital heart block	Dexamethasone

(?) *Denotes possible but not proved efficacy.*
**Drug of choice (may require PUBs and umbilical vein administration if hydrops is present).*

Because infections occur and several drugs are often taken during many pregnancies, the pediatrician must evaluate the presumed viral infections and the drugs ingested to help parents understand their child's birth defect. The causes of approximately 40% of congenital malformations are unknown. While only a relatively few agents teratogenic in humans are recognized (see Tables 80–2, 80–3, 81–3, and 81–4), new agents continue to be identified. Overall, only 10% of anomalies are due to recognizable teratogens. The time of exposure is usually <60 days of gestation during organogenesis. Specific agents produce predictable lesions. In some there is a dose or threshold effect; below the threshold there are no alterations of growth, function, or structure. The agent's effects may be species specific. Genetic variables such as the presence of specific enzymes may metabolize a benign agent into a more toxic-teratogenic form (phenytoin conversion to its epoxide). In many circumstances the same agent and dose may not consistently produce the lesion.

Mechanisms of teratogenesis include cell death without reparative regeneration; mitotic delay; delayed differentiation; physical or vascular constraining; reduced histogenesis secondary to cell depletion, necrosis, calcification, or scarring; inhibited cellular migration; and inflammation. Many mechanisms occur secondary to chromosomal or DNA damage and poor molecular repair.

The FDA classifies drugs in five pregnancy risk categories: *Category A* suggests no risk based on evidence from controlled human trials. *Category B* suggests either no risk from animal studies but no adequate studies in humans or some risk in animal studies that are not confirmed by human studies. *Category C* is either definite risk from animal studies but no adequate human studies or no available data for animals or humans. *Category D* includes drugs with some risk but with a benefit that may exceed that risk for the treated life-threatening condition, such as streptomycin for tuberculosis. *Category X* is for drugs that are contraindicated in pregnancy based on animal and human evidence and whose risk exceeds the benefits.

The specific mechanism of action is known or postulated for very few teratogens. Warfarin, an anticoagulant because it is a

■ **TABLE 81–6 Radiation Exposure of the Fetus***

Type of Study	Millirad†
Roentgenogram of:	
Chest	1
Thoracic spine	11
Abdomen	221
Pelvis	210
Hips	124
Roentgenographic contrast studies	
Upper gastrointestinal series	171
Barium enema	903
Cholangiogram	78
Intravenous pyelogram	588

**From US DHEW: Gonad Doses and Genetically Significant Dose from Diagnostic Radiology; US, 1964 and 1970. Washington, DC, US Government Printing Office, 1976.*
†Owing to variation in techniques these estimates may be exceeded.

vitamin K antagonist, prevents carboxylation of γ-carboxyglutamic acid (GLA), which is a component of osteocalcin and other vitamin K–dependent bone proteins. The teratogenic effect on developing cartilage, especially nasal cartilage, appears to be avoided if the pregnant woman's treatment between weeks 6 and 12 of gestation is switched from warfarin to heparin. Hypothyroidism in the fetus may be caused by maternal ingestion of an excessive amount of iodides or of propylthiouracil; each interferes with the conversion of inorganic to organic iodides. Phenytoin may be teratogenic because of the accumulation of a metabolite as a result of deficiency of epoxide hydrolase.

Recognition of teratogens offers the opportunity for prevention of related birth defects. For example, if a pregnant woman is informed of the potentially harmful effects of alcohol on her unborn infant, she may be motivated to control this problem during pregnancy. The woman with insulin-dependent diabetes mellitus may significantly decrease her risk for having a child with birth defects by achieving good control of her disease *before* conception.

Ardinger HH, Atkin JF, Blackston RD, et al: Verification of the fetal valproate syndrome phenotype. Am J Med Genet 29:171, 1988.

Beckman DA, Brent RL: Mechanism of known environmental teratogens: Drugs and chemicals. Clin Perinatol 13:649, 1986.

Brent RL: Evaluating the alleged teratogenicity of environmental agents. Clin Perinatol 13:609, 1986.

Brent RL: The complexities of solving the problem of human malformations. Clin Perinatol 13:491, 1986.

Chervenak FA, Isaacson G: Diagnosing congenital malformation in utero: Ultrasound. Clin Perinatol 13:593, 1986.

Czeizel AE, Elek C, Gundy S, et al: Environmental trichlorfon and cluster of congenital abnormalities. Lancet 341:539, 1993.

Czeizel AE, Intody Z, Modell B: What proportion of congenital abnormalities can be prevented? Br Med J 306:499, 1993.

Jacobson SJ, Jones K, Johnson K, et al: Prospective multicentre study of pregnancy outcome after lithium exposure during first trimester. Lancet 339:530, 1992.

Jones KJ, Lacro RV, Johnson KA, et al: Pattern of malformations in the children of women treated with carbamazepine during pregnancy. N Engl J Med 320:1661, 1989.

Lammer EJ, Chen CT, Hoar RM, et al: Retinoic acid embryopathy. N Engl J Med 313:837, 1985.

Litsey SE, Noonan JA, O'Connor WN, et al: Maternal connective tissue disease and congenital heart block. N Engl J Med 312:98, 1985.

Newman CGH: The thalidomide syndrome: Risks of exposure and spectrum of malformations. Clin Perinatol 13:555, 1986.

Oakley GP: Frequency of human congenital malformations. Clin Perinatol 13:545, 1986.

Olds DL, Henderson CR, Tatelbaum R: Intellectual impairment in children of women who smoke cigarettes during pregnancy. Pediatrics 93:221, 1994.

Pauli RM, Lian JB, Mosher DF, et al: Association of congenital deficiency of multiple vitamin K-dependent coagulation factors and the phenotype of the warfarin embryopathy: Clues to the mechanism of teratogenicity of coumarin derivatives. Am J Hum Genet 41:566, 1987.

Shepard TH: Catalog of Teratogenic Agents, 6th ed. Baltimore, The Johns Hopkins University Press, 1989.

Stickler SM, Dansky LV, Miller MA, et al: Genetic predisposition to phenytoin-induced birth defects. Lancet ii:746, 1985.

81.8 Radiation

Accidental exposure of pregnant women to radiation is a common cause for anxiety among women, their families, and their physicians, usually about whether the fetus will have birth defects or genetic abnormalities. It is unlikely that exposure to diagnostic radiation will cause gene mutations; no increase in genetic abnormalities has been identified in the offspring exposed as unborn fetuses to the atomic bomb explosions in Japan in 1945.

A more realistic concern is whether the exposed human fetus will show birth defects or a higher incidence of malignancy. The recommended occupational limit of maternal exposure to radiation from all sources is 500 millirads (mrad) for the entire 40 wk of a pregnancy. Estimates of the gonadal exposure for the mother and the whole body exposure of the fetus from several common roentgenographic examinations are shown in Table 81–6. The limited data on human fetuses show that large doses of radiation (20,000–50,000 mrad) are harmful to the central nervous system, as evidenced by microcephaly, mental retardation, and intrauterine growth retardation.

Therapeutic abortion is often recommended when exposure exceeds 10,000 mrad. It is more likely that a human fetus will be exposed to 1,000–3,000 mrad, an amount not shown to cause malformations. There is controversy with regard to whether this level of fetal exposure is associated with an increased risk of developing childhood cancer or leukemia.

Brent R: The effects of embryonic and fetal exposure to x-ray, microwaves and ultrasound. Clin Perinatol 13:615, 1986.

The Effects on Populations of Exposure to Low Levels of Ionizing Radiation (BEIR Report). Washington DC, National Academy of Sciences. National Research Council, November, 1972.

Griem ML, Meier P, Dobben GD: Analysis of the morbidity and mortality of children irradiated in fetal life. Radiology 88:347, 1967.

US Department of Health, Education, and Welfare: Gonad Doses and Genetically Significant Dose from Diagnostic Radiology: US., 1964 and 1970. Washington, DC, US Government Printing Office, 1976.

Webster EW: On the question of cancer induction by small X-ray doses. Am J Roentgenol 137:647, 1981.

CHAPTER 82
The High-Risk Infant

Infants particularly at risk during the neonatal period should be identified as early as possible in order to decrease neonatal morbidity and mortality (see also Chapter 79). The term *high-risk infant* designates infants who should be under close observation by experienced physicians and nurses. Approximately 9% of all births require special or neonatal intensive care. Usually needed for only a few days, such observations may last from a few hours to several weeks. Some institutions find it advantageous to provide a special or transitional care nursery for high-risk infants, often within the labor and delivery suite. This facility should be equipped and staffed similarly to a neonatal intensive care area, where well but high-risk term infants can be observed and cared for immediately after birth without being separated from their mothers. Infants in the high-risk category are listed in Table 82–1.

Examination of a fresh *placenta, cord,* and *membranes* may alert the physician to a newborn infant at high risk. Fetal

■ **TABLE 82–1 High-Risk Infants**

Demographic Social Factors
Maternal age < 16 or > 40 yr
Illicit drug, alcohol, cigarette use
Poverty
Unmarried
Emotional or physical stress
Past Medical History
Diabetes mellitus
Hypertension
Asymptomatic bacteriuria
Rheumatologic illness (SLE)*
Chronic medication (see Tables 81–3 and 81–4)
Prior Pregnancy
Intrauterine fetal demise
Neonatal death
Prematurity
Intrauterine growth retardation
Congenital malformation
Incompetent cervix
Blood group sensitization, neonatal jaundice
Neonatal thrombocytopenia
Hydrops
Inborn errors of metabolism
Present Pregnancy
Vaginal bleeding (abruptio placentae, placenta previa)
Sexually transmitted diseases (colonization: herpes simplex, group B streptococcus)
Multiple gestation
Pre-eclampsia
Premature rupture of membranes
Short interpregnancy time
Poly-oligohydramnios
Acute medical or surgical illness
Inadequate prenatal care
Lupus anticoagulant
Labor and Delivery
Premature labor (< 37 wk)
Postdates (> 42 wk)
Fetal distress
Immature L/S ratio: absent phosphatidylglycerol
Breech presentation
Meconium-stained fluid
Nuchal cord
Cesarean section
Forceps delivery
Apgar score < 4 at 1 min
Neonate
Birthweight < 2,500 or > 4,000 g
Birth before 37 or after 42 wk of gestation
SGA†, LGA growth status‡
Tachypnea, cyanosis
Congenital malformation
Pallor, plethora, petechiae

*SLE = Systemic lupus erythematosus.
†SGA = Small for gestational age.
‡LGA = Large for gestational age.

blood loss may be indicated by placental pallor, **retroplacental hematoma**, and tears of a velamentous cord or of chorionic blood vessels supplying succenturiate lobes. **Placental edema** and subsequent deficiency of immunoglobulin G in the newborn may be associated with fetofetal transfusion syndrome, hydrops fetalis, congenital nephrosis, or hepatic disease. **Amnion nodosum** (granules on the amnion) and **oligohydramnios** are associated with pulmonary hypoplasia and renal agenesis, while small whitish **nodules** on the cord suggest a candidal infection. **Short cords** and noncoiled cords occur with chromosome abnormalities and omphalocele. **Chorioangiomas** are associated with prematurity, abruptio, polyhydramnios, and intrauterine growth retardation (IUGR). **Meconium staining** suggests asphyxia and the risk of pneumonia, and opacity of the fetal placental surface suggests infection. **Single umbilical arteries** are associated with an increased incidence of congenital abnormalities.

Many high-risk infants are born prematurely, are breech deliveries, have low weight for gestational age, have significant perinatal asphyxia, or are born with life-threatening congenital anomalies without exhibiting previously identified risk factors. Generally speaking, for any given duration of gestation, the lower the birthweight, the higher the neonatal mortality, and, for any given weight, the shorter the gestational duration, the higher the neonatal mortality (Fig. 82–1). The highest risk of neonatal mortality occurs among infants who weigh less than 1,000 g at birth and whose gestation was less than 30 wk. The lowest risk of neonatal mortality occurs among infants with birthweights of 3,000–4,000 g whose gestational age was 38–42 wk. As birthweight increases from 500 to 3,000 g, a logarithmic decrease in neonatal mortality occurs; for every week increase in gestational age from the 25th to 37th wk, the neonatal mortality rate decreases by approximately one half. Nevertheless, approximately 40% of all *perinatal deaths* occur after 37 wk of gestation in infants weighing 2,500 g or more; many of these deaths occur in the period immediately before birth and are more readily preventable than those of smaller and more immature infants. In addition, neonatal mortality rates rise sharply for infants weighing over 4,000 g at birth and for those whose gestational period is 42 wk or longer. Since neonatal mortality largely depends on birthweight and gestational age, Figure 82–1 helps to identify high-risk infants quickly. However, this analysis is based on total live births and therefore describes the mortality risk only *at birth*. Because most neonatal mortality occurs within the first hours and days after birth, the outlook improves dramatically with increasing postnatal survival.

Amini SB, Catalano PM, Hirsch V, et al: An analysis of birth weight by gestational age using a computerized perinatal data base, 1975–1992. Obstet Gynecol 83:342, 1994.

Bateman DA, O'Bryan L, Nicholas SW, et al: Outcome of unattended out-of-hospital births in Harlem. Arch Pediatr Adolesc Med 148:147, 1994.

Behrman RE: Prevention of low birthweight: A pediatric perspective. J Pediatr 107:842, 1985.

Brett KM, Schoendorf KC, Kiely JL: Differences between black and white women in the use of prenatal care technologies. Am J Obstet Gynecol 170:41, 1994.

Howell EM, Vert P: Neonatal intensive care and birth weight–specific perinatal mortality in Michigan and Lorraine. Pediatrics 91:464, 1993.

Nelson MD: Socioeconomic status and childhood mortality in North Carolina. Am J Public Health 82:1131, 1992.

Strong TH, Finberg HJ, Mattox JH: Antepartum diagnosis of noncoiled umbilical cords. Am J Obstet Gynecol 170:1729, 1994.

Wariyar U, Richmond S, Hey E: Pregnancy outcome at 24–31 weeks' gestation: Mortality. Arch Dis Child 64:670, 1989.

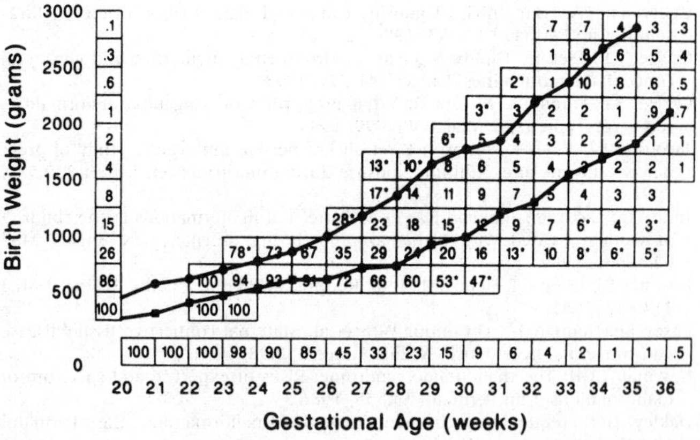

Figure 82–1. Predicted per cent neonatal mortality by 250 g birthweight intervals (y axis), by 1 wk gestational age intervals (x axis), and by combined 250 g birthweight and weekly gestational age intervals *(center cells)* derived from multiple regression model. (●), 90th percentile; (■), 10th percentile; asterisk, fewer than five infants in cell. (From Copper RL, Goldenberg RL, Creasy RK, et al: A multicenter study of preterm birth weight and gestational age-specific neonatal mortality. Am J Obstet Gynecol 168:78, 1993.)

Whitby C, DeCates C, Robertson N: Infants weighing 1.8–2.5 kg: Should they be cared for in neonatal units or postnatal wards? Lancet 1:322, 1982.
Wigton TR, Tamura RK, Wickstrom E, et al: Neonatal morbidity after preterm delivery in the presence of documented lung maturity. Am J Obstet Gynecol 169:951, 1993.
Wolf EJ, Vintzileos AM, Rosenkrantz TS, et al: Do survival and morbidity of very-low-birth-weight infants vary according to the primary pregnancy complication that results in preterm delivery? Am J Obstet Gynecol 169:1233, 1993.

82.1 Multiple Pregnancies

INCIDENCE. The reported incidence of twins is highest among blacks and East Indians, followed by North European whites, and is lowest among the Asian races. Specific rates include: Belgium, 1:56, American blacks, 1:70; Italy, 1:86; American whites, 1:88; Greece, 1:130; Japan, 1:150; China, 1:300. Differences in the incidence of twins mainly involve fraternal (polyovular) dizygotic twins. Triplets are estimated to occur in 1 of 86^2 pregnancies and quadruplets in 1 of 86^3 pregnancies in the United States. The incidence of monozygotic twins is unaffected by racial or familial factors (3–5:1,000). The incidence of twins detected by ultrasonography at 12 wk of gestation (3–5%) is much higher than that occurring later in pregnancy; the vanishing twin syndrome results in a singleton fetus. Although the incidence of spontaneous multifetal gestation is stable, the overall incidence is increasing owing to the treatment of infertility with ovarian stimulants (clomiphene, gonadotropins) and in vitro fertilization.

ETIOLOGY. The occurrence of monovular twins appears to be independent of genetic influences. Polyovular pregnancies are more frequent beyond the second pregnancy, in older women, and in families with a history of polyovular twins. They may result from simultaneous maturation of multiple ovarian follicles, but follicles containing two ova have been described as a genetic trait leading to twin pregnancies. Twin-prone women have higher levels of gonadotropins. Polyovular pregnancies occur in many women treated for infertility.

Conjoined twins (Siamese twins—incidence 1:50000) probably result from relatively late monovular separation, as does the presence of two separate embryos in one amniotic sac. The latter condition has a high fatality rate that is due to obstruction of the circulation secondary to intertwining of the umbilical cords. The prognosis for conjoined twins depends on the possibility of surgical separation. Most conjoined twins are female.

Superfecundation, the fertilization of an ovum by an insemination that takes place after one ovum has already been fertilized, and *superfetation*, the fertilization and subsequent development of an ovum when a fetus is already present in the uterus, have been proposed as uncommon explanations for differences in size and appearance of certain twins at birth.

The *prenatal diagnoses of twins* is suggested by a uterine size that is greater than that expected for gestational age, auscultation of 2 fetal hearts, and elevated maternal serum α-fetoprotein or human chorionic gonadotropin (HCG) level and is confirmed by ultrasound. Ninety per cent of twins are detected prior to delivery.

MONOZYGOTIC VERSUS DIZYGOTIC TWINS. Identifying twins as monozygotic or dizygotic (monovular or polyovular) is important because studying monozygotic twins is useful in determining the relative influence of heredity and environment on human development and disease. Twins not of the same sex are dizygotic. In twins of the same sex, zygosity should be determined and recorded at birth through careful examination of the placenta or later through comparison of physical characteristics, detailed blood typing, DNA fingerprinting, or tissue (HL-A) typing.

Examination of the Placenta. If the placentas are separate, they are always dichorionic (present in 75%), but the twins are not necessarily dizygotic, since initiation of monovular twinning at the first cell division or during the morula state may result in two amnions, two chorions, and even two placentas. One third of monozygotic twins are dichorionic and diamniotic.

An apparently single placenta may be present with either monovular or polyovular twins. Yet inspecting the polyovular placenta usually reveals a separate chorion for each fetus that crosses the placenta between the attachments of the cords and two amnions. Separate or fused dichorionic placentas may be disproportionate in size. The fetus attached to the smaller placenta or portion of placenta is usually smaller than its twin or is malformed. Monochorionic twins may be presumed to be monovular. They are usually diamnionic, and, almost invariably, the placenta is a single mass.

Problems of the twin gestation include polyhydramnios, hyperemesis gravidarum, pre-eclampsia, prolonged rupture of membranes, vasa previa, velamentous insertion of the umbilical cord, abnormal presentations (breech), and premature labor. Compared with the first-born twin, the second or B twin is at increased risk for respiratory distress syndrome and asphyxia. Twins are at risk for IUGR, twin-twin transfusion, and congenital anomalies that occur predominantly in monozygotic twins. Anomalies are due to uterine compression deformations from crowding (hip dislocation); vascular communication with embolization (ileal atresia, porencephaly, cutis aplasia) or without embolization (acardiac twin); and unknown factors that cause twinning (conjoined twins, anencephaly, meningomyelocele).

Placental vascular anastomoses occur with high frequency only in monochorionic twins. In monochorionic placentas, the fetal vasculature is usually joined, sometimes in a very complex manner. The vascular anastomoses in monochorionic placentas may be artery-to-artery, vein-to-vein, or artery-to-vein. They are usually well enough balanced so that neither twin suffers. Artery-to-artery communications cross over placental veins, and when anastomoses are present, blood can readily be stroked from one fetal vascular bed to the other. Vein-to-vein communications are similarly recognized and are less common. A combination of artery-to-artery and vein-to-vein anastomoses is associated with *acardiac fetus.* This rare lethal anomaly (1:35,000) is secondary to the TRAP sequence—Twin Reversed Arterial Perfusion. Neodymium:YAG laser ablation of the anastomosis, in utero, can treat heart failure of the surviving twin. In rare cases one umbilical cord may arise from the other after leaving the placenta. In such cases the twin attached to the secondary cord is usually malformed or dies in utero. Table 82–2 lists the more frequent changes associated with a large uncompensated arteriovenous shunt from the placenta of one twin to that of the other; twins of widely discrepant size are usually monochorionic.

In the **fetal transfusion syndrome**, an artery from one twin delivers blood that is drained into the vein of the other.

■ TABLE 82–2 Characteristic Changes in Monochorionic Twins With Uncompensated Placental Arteriovenous Shunts

Twin on Arterial Side—Donor	Twin on Venous Side—Recipient
Oligohydramnios	Polyhydramnios
Small premature	Large premature
Malnourished	Well nourished
Pale	Plethoric
Anemic	Polycythemic
Hypovolemia	Hypervolemic
Hypoglycemia	Cardiac failure
Microcardia	Cardiac hypertrophy
Glomeruli small or normal	Glomeruli large
Arterioles thin-walled	Arterioles thick-walled

The latter becomes plethoric and large while the former is anemic and small. By definition, there is a 5 g/dl hemoglobin and 20% body weight difference in this syndrome. Maternal hydramnios in a twin pregnancy suggests the fetal transfusion syndrome. Anticipating this possibility by preparing to transfuse the donor twin or to bleed the recipient twin may be lifesaving. Death of the donor twin in utero may result in generalized fibrin thrombi in the smaller arterioles of the recipient twin, possibly as the result of transfusion of thromboplastin-rich blood from the macerating donor fetus. The surviving twin may develop disseminated intravascular coagulation. Treatment of this highly lethal problem includes maternal digoxin, selective twin termination, or Nd:YAG laser ablation of the anastomosis.

Postnatal Identification. *Physical criteria* for determining monovular twins are as follows: (1) Both must be of the same sex; (2) their features, including ears and teeth, must be obviously alike (but they need not resemble one another more than the lateral halves of one individual); (3) their hair must be identical in color, texture, natural curl, and distribution; (4) their eyes must be of the same color and shade; (5) their skin must be of the same texture and color (nevi may be differently apportioned and distributed); (6) their hands and feet must be of the same conformation and of similar size; and (7) their anthropometric values must show close agreement.

PROGNOSIS. Most twins are born prematurely, and maternal complications of pregnancy are more common than with single pregnancies. Although there is a significant increase in perinatal mortality among monochorionic twins, there is no significant difference between the neonatal mortality rates of twin and single births in comparable weight groups. Yet, since most twins are premature by weight, their overall mortality is higher than that of single births. The perinatal mortality of twins is about 4 times that of singletons. Monoamniotic twins have an increased likelihood of entangling their cords, which may lead to asphyxia. If one of the fetuses is macerated, the live twin is usually delivered first. Theoretically, the second twin is more subject to anoxia than the first because the placenta may separate after the birth of the first twin and before the birth of the second. In addition, the delivery of the second twin may be difficult because it may be in an abnormal presentation (breech, entangled), uterine tone may be decreased, or the cervix may begin to close following the first twin's birth. A growth-retarded twin is at high risk for hypoglycemia. Notable differences in size at birth of monovular twins usually disappear by the time the infants are 6 mo of age. The mortality for multiple gestations with 4–5 fetuses is excessively high for each fetus. Because of this poor prognosis, selective fetal reduction to 2–3 fetuses has been proposed.

TREATMENT. Prenatal diagnosis enables the obstetrician and the pediatrician to anticipate the birth of infants who are at high risk because of twinning. Close observation is indicated during labor and in the immediate neonatal period so that prompt treatment of asphyxia or fetal transfusion syndrome can be initiated. The decision to perform an immediate blood transfusion in a severely anemic "donor twin" or to perform a partial exchange transfusion of a "recipient twin" must be based on clinical judgment.

Bruner JP, Rosemond RL: Twin-to-twin transfusion syndrome: A subset of the twin oligohydramnios-polyhydramnios sequence. Am J Obstet Gynecol 169:925, 1993.

Cragan JD, Martin ML, Waters GD, et al: Increased risk of small intestinal atresia among twins in the United States. Arch Pediatr Adolesc Med 148:733, 1994.

Evans MI, Dommergues M, Wapner RJ, et al: Efficacy of transabdominal multifetal pregnancy reduction: Collaborative experience among the world's largest centers. Obstet Gynecol 82:61, 1993.

Luke B: The changing pattern of multiple births in the United States: Maternal and infant characteristics, 1973 and 1990. Obstet Gynecol 84:101, 1994.

Powers WF, Kiely JL: The risks confronting twins: A national perspective. Am J Obstet Gynecol 170:456, 1994.

Prins RP: The second-born twin: Can we improve outcomes? Am J Obstet Gynecol 170:1649, 1994.

82.2 Prematurity and Intrauterine Growth Retardation

DEFINITIONS. Liveborn* infants delivered before 37 wk from the first day of the last menstrual period are termed *premature* by the World Health Organization. "Premature" is also often used to denote immaturity. Infants of extremely low birthweight (ELBW), i.e., less than 1,000 g, are also referred to as immature neonates. Historically, prematurity was defined by a birthweight of 2,500 g or less, but today infants who weigh 2,500 g or less at birth, "low-birthweight (LBW) infants," are considered to be premature with a shortened gestational period, to be intrauterine growth retarded for their gestational age (also referred to as small for gestational age [SGA]), or both. Prematurity and *intrauterine growth retardation* (IUGR) are associated with increased neonatal morbidity and mortality. Ideally, the definitions of low birthweight for individual populations should be based on data that are as genetically and environmentally homogeneous as possible. Figure 82–1 presents variations in neonatal mortality based on birthweight with respect to gestational age.

INCIDENCE. During 1991, 7.1% of live births in the United States weighed less than 2,500 g; the rate for blacks was more than twice that for whites. Since 1981 the LBW rate has increased primarily because of an increased number of preterm births. Approximately 30% of LBW infants in the United States have IUGR and are born after 37 wk. At LBW rates greater than 10%, the contribution of IUGR increases and that of prematurity decreases. In developing countries approximately 70% of LBW infants are IUGR. Infants with IUGR have a greater morbidity and mortality than appropriately grown gestational age-matched infants (see Fig. 82–1).

THE VERY LOW BIRTHWEIGHT (VLBW) INFANT. VLBW infants weigh less than 1,500 g and are predominantly premature. In the United States in 1991 the VLBW rate was approximately 1.2%: 2.6% among blacks and 0.9% among whites. The VLBW rate is an accurate predictor of the infant mortality rate (relative risk of 93). VLBW infants account for over 50% of neonatal deaths and 50% of handicapped infants; their survival is directly related to birthweight, with approximately 20% of those between 500 and 600 g surviving and 85–90% of those between 1,250 and 1,500 g. The VLBW rate has declined minimally in whites and increased in blacks. Perinatal care has improved the rate of survival of LBW infants. Compared with term infants, VLBW neonates have a higher incidence of rehospitalization during the 1st yr of life for sequelae of prematurity, infections, neurologic sequalae, and psychosocial disorders (see later discussion in this section on prognosis).

FACTORS RELATED TO PREMATURE BIRTH AND LOW BIRTHWEIGHT. It is difficult to completely separate factors associated with prematurity from those associated with IUGR. (See also Chapters 79 and 80.) A strong positive correlation exists between both premature birth and IUGR and low socioeconomic status. In families of low socioeconomic status there are relatively high incidences of maternal undernutrition, anemia, and illness; inadequate prenatal care; drug addiction; obstetric compli-

*Live birth is defined by the World Health Assembly (1950) as "the complete expulsion or extraction from its mother of a product of conception . . . which, after such separation, breathes or shows any other evidence of life such as beating of the heart, pulsation of the umbilical cord, or definite movement of the voluntary muscles, whether or not the umbilical cord has been cut or the placenta is attached." This definition is approved by the American Public Health Association.

cations; and maternal histories of reproductive inefficiency (relative infertility, abortions, stillbirths, premature or low birthweight infants). Other associated factors such as single-parent families, teenage pregnancies, close spacing of pregnancies, and mothers who have borne more than 4 previous children are also encountered more frequently. Systematic differences in fetal growth have also been described in association with maternal size, birth order, sibling weight, social class, maternal smoking habit, and other factors. The degree to which the variance in birthweights among various populations is due to environmental (extrafetal) rather than to genetic differences in growth potential is difficult to determine.

The *premature birth* of infants whose LBW is appropriate for their preterm gestational age is generally associated with medical conditions in which there is inability of the uterus to retain the fetus, interference with the course of the pregnancy, premature separation of the placenta, or an undetermined stimulus to effective uterine contractions prior to term (Table 82–3).

Overt (group B streptococcus, *Listeria monocytogenes*) or asymptomatic *(Ureaplasma ureolyticum, Mycoplasma hominis, Chlamydia, Gardnerella vaginalis)* bacterial infection of the amniotic fluid and membranes (chorioamnionitis) may initiate preterm labor. Bacterial products may stimulate local cytokine production (interleukin-6, prostaglandins), which may induce premature uterine contractions or a local inflammatory response with focal membrane rupture. Appropriate antibiotic therapy reduces the risk of fetal infection and may prolong gestation. The use of β-sympathomimetic receptor agonists (ritodrine, terbutaline) has not prevented premature birth. Other agents (indomethacin) have significant neonatal complications (necrotizing enterocolitis), while new oxytocin antagonists remain in the experimental stage of development.

IUGR is associated with medical conditions that interfere with the circulation and efficiency of the placenta, with the development or growth of the fetus, or with the general health and nutrition of the mother (Table 82–4). Many factors are common to both prematurely born and low-birthweight infants with IUGR.

IUGR may be a normal fetal response to nutritional or oxygen deprivation. Therefore, the issue is not the IUGR but rather the ongoing risk of malnutrition or hypoxia. Similarly, some preterm births signify a need for early delivery from a potentially disadvantageous intrauterine environment. IUGR is often classified as reduced growth that is symmetric (head circumference, length, and weight equally affected) or asymmetric (with relative head growth sparing) (see Fig. 81–1). Symmetric IUGR often has an earlier onset and is associated with diseases that seriously affect fetal cell number, such as conditions with chromosomal, genetic, malformation, teratogenic, or severe maternal hypertensive etiologies. Asymmetric IUGR is often of late onset, demonstrates preservation of Doppler waveform velocity to the carotid vessels, and is associated with poor maternal nutrition or late onset or exacerbation of maternal vascular disease (pre-eclampsia, chronic hypertension). Problems of IUGR infants are noted in Table 82–5.

ASSESSMENT OF GESTATIONAL AGE AT BIRTH. Compared with the premature infant of appropriate weight, the infant with retarded intrauterine growth has a reduced birthweight and may appear to have a *disproportionately larger head relative to body size*; infants in both groups lack subcutaneous fat. In general, neurologic maturity (e.g., nerve conduction velocity) correlates with gestational age despite reduced fetal weight.

Physical signs may be useful in estimating gestational age at birth. Commonly used, the Dubowitz scoring system is accurate to ±2 wk (Figs. 82–2 to 82–4). An infant should be presumed to be at high risk of mortality or morbidity if a discrepancy exists between the estimation of gestational age

■ **TABLE 82–3 Identifiable Causes of Preterm Birth**

Fetal
- Fetal distress
- Multiple gestation
- Erythroblastosis
- Nonimmune hydrops

Placental
- Placenta previa
- Abruptio placentae

Uterine
- Bicornate uterus
- Incompetent cervix (premature dilation)

Maternal
- Pre-eclampsia
- Chronic medical illness (e.g., cyanotic heart disease, renal disease)
- Infection (e.g., *Listeria monocytogenes*, group B streptococcus, urinary tract infection, chorioamnionitis)
- Drug abuse (e.g., cocaine)

Other
- Premature rupture of membranes
- Polyhydramnios
- Iatrogenic

■ **TABLE 82–4 Factors Often Associated With Intrauterine Growth Retardation**

Fetal
- Chromosomal disorders (e.g., autosomal trisomies)
- Chronic fetal infections (e.g., cytomegalic inclusion disease, congenital rubella, syphilis)
- Congenital anomalies—syndrome complexes
- Radiation injury
- Multiple gestation
- Pancreatic aplasia

Placental
- Decreased placental weight or cellularity or both
- Decrease in surface area
- Villous placentitis (bacterial, viral, parasitic)
- Infarction
- Tumor (chorioangioma, hydatidiform mole)
- Placental separation
- Twin transfusion syndrome (parabiotic syndrome)

Maternal
- Toxemia
- Hypertensive or renal disease or both
- Hypoxemia (high altitude, cyanotic cardiac or pulmonary disease)
- Malnutrition or chronic illness
- Sickle cell anemia
- Drugs (narcotics, alcohol, cigarettes, cocaine, antimetabolites)

■ **TABLE 82–5 Problems of IUGR (SGA) Infants**

Problem	Pathogenesis
Intrauterine fetal demise	Hypoxia, acidosis, infection, lethal anomaly
Perinatal asphyxia	↓ Uteroplacental perfusion during labor ± chronic fetal hypoxia-acidosis; meconium aspiration syndrome
Hypoglycemia	↓ Tissue glycogen stores, ↓ gluconeogenesis, hyperinsulinism, ↑ glucose needs of hypoxia, hypothermia, large brain
Polycythemia-hyperviscosity	Fetal hypoxia with ↑ erythropoietin production
Reduced oxygen consumption/hypothermia	Hypoxia, hypoglycemia, starvation affect, poor subcutaneous fat stores
Dysmorphology	Syndrome anomalads, chromosomal-genetic disorders, oligohydramnios-induced deformations, TORCH infection

Other problems include pulmonary hemorrhage and those common to the gestational age–related risks of prematurity if born <37 wk (see Table 82–6).
IUGR, intrauterine growth retardation.
SGA, small for gestational age.

EXTERNAL SIGN	SCORE 0	1	2	3	4
Edema	Obvious edema of hands and feet; pitting over tibia	No obvious edema of hands and feet; pitting over tibia	No edema		
Skin texture	Very thin, gelatinous	Thin and smooth	Smooth; medium thickness; rash or superficial peeling	Slight thickening; superficial cracking and peeling, especially on hands and feet	Thick and parchmentlike; superficial or deep cracking
Skin color (infant not crying)	Dark red	Uniformly pink	Pale pink; variable over body	Pale; only pink over ears, lips, palms, or soles	
Skin opacity (trunk)	Numerous veins and venules clearly seen, especially over abdomen	Veins and tributaries seen	A few large vessels clearly seen over abdomen	A few large vessels seen indistinctly over abdomen	No blood vessels seen
Lanugo (over back)	No lanugo	Abundant; long and thick over whole back	Hair thinning, especially over lower back	Small amount of lanugo and bald areas	At least half of back devoid of lanugo
Plantar creases	No skin creases	Faint red marks over anterior half of sole	Definite red marks over more than anterior half; indentations over less than anterior third	Indentations over more than anterior third	Definite deep indentations over more than anterior third
Nipple formation	Nipple barely visible; no areola	Nipple well defined; areola smooth and flat; diameter <0.75 cm	Areola stippled, edge not raised; diameter <0.75 cm	Areola stippled, edge raised; diameter >0.75 cm	
Breast size	No breast tissue palpable	Breast tissue on one or both sides <0.5 cm diameter	Breast tissue both sides; one or both 0.5 to 1.0 cm	Breast tissue both sides; one or both >1 cm	
Ear form	Pinna flat and shapeless, little or no incurving of edge	Incurving of part of edge of pinna	Partial incurving whole of upper pinna	Well-defined incurving whole of upper pinna	
Ear firmness	Pinna soft, easily folded, no recoil	Pinna soft, easily folded, slow recoil	Cartilage to edge of pinna, but soft in places, ready recoil	Pinna firm, cartilage to edge; instant recoil	
Genitalia Male	Neither testis in scrotum	At least one testis high in scrotum	At least one testis down in scrotum		
Female (with hips half abducted)	Labia majora widely separated; labia minora protruding	Labia majora almost cover labia minora	Labia majora completely cover labia minora		

Figure 82–2. External characteristics of the Dubowitz examination. Physical criteria are recorded and a final score is obtained following the addition of each category's score. (From Dubowitz L, Dubowitz V: Gestational Age of the Newborn. Reading, MA, Addison-Wesley, 1977.)

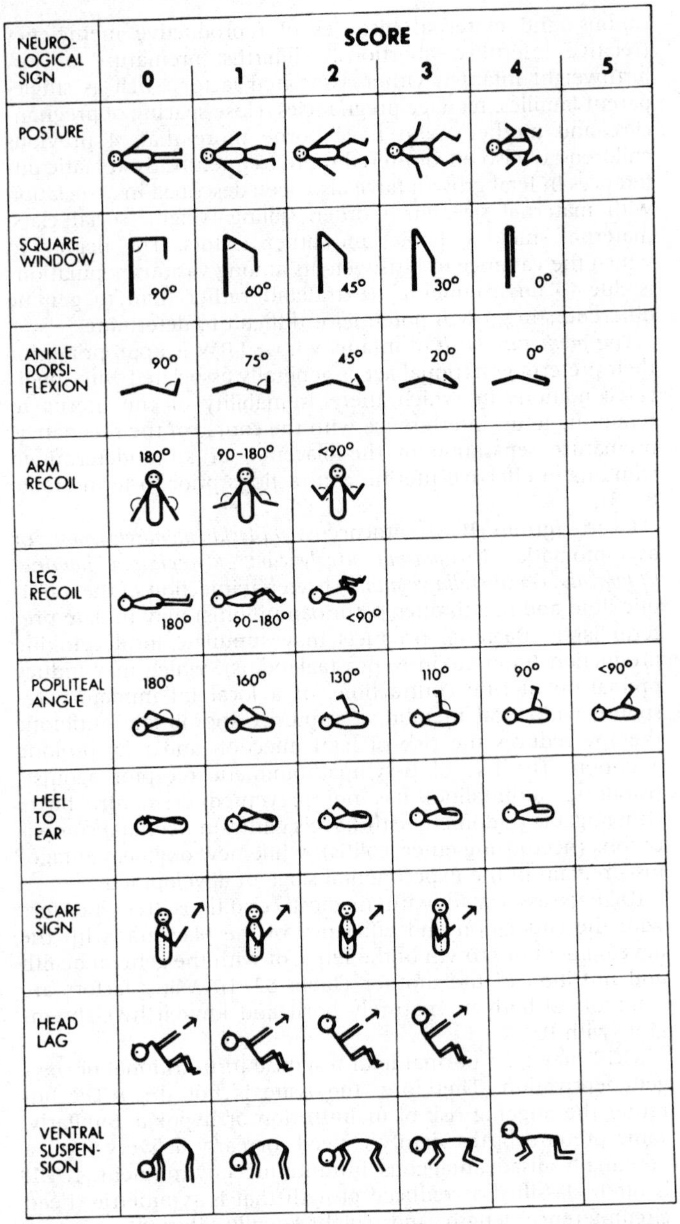

Figure 82–3. Neurologic characteristics of the Dubowitz examination. Neurologic criteria are recorded and added to a final score as performed for the physical assessment. (From Dubowitz L, Dubowitz V: Gestational Age of the Newborn. Reading, MA, Addison-Wesley, 1977.)

by physical examination, the mother's estimated date of last menstrual period, and fetal ultrasonic evaluation.

SPECTRUM OF DISEASE IN LOW-BIRTHWEIGHT INFANTS. Immaturity tends to increase the severity but reduce the distinctiveness of the clinical manifestations of most neonatal diseases. Immature organ function, complications of therapy, and the specific disorders that caused the premature onset of labor contribute to neonatal morbidity and mortality associated with premature, LBW infants (Table 82–6). Problems associated with IUGR LBW infants are noted in Table 82–5; those added problems are often superimposed on those noted in Table 82–6 if the IUGR infant is also premature.

NURSERY CARE. At birth the measures needed for clearing the airway, initiating breathing, caring for the cord and eyes, and administering vitamin K are the same in immature infants as in those of normal weight and maturity (Chapter 79). Special care is required to maintain a patent airway and avoid potential aspiration of gastric contents. Additional considerations are (1) need for incubator care and heart rate and respiration monitoring, (2) need for increased oxygen, and (3) need for special attention to the details of feeding. Safeguards against infection can never be relaxed. Everyone involved must be aware that routine procedures that disturb these infants may result in hypoxia. Finally, the need for regular and active participation by the parents in the infant's care in the nursery, the need to instruct the mother in the at-home care of the infant, and the question of prognosis for later growth and development require special consideration.

Incubator Care. Modern incubators conserve body heat through provision of a warm atmospheric environment and standard conditions of humidity. They also may reduce atmospheric contamination if they are scrupulously cleaned. The survival of LBW and sick infants is greater when they are cared for at or near their *neutral thermal environment*. This is a set of thermal conditions, including air and radiating surface temperatures, relative humidity, and air flow, at which heat production (measured as oxygen consumption) is minimal and the infant's core temperature is within the normal range. It is a function of the size and postnatal age of infants; larger, older infants require lower environmental temperatures than smaller, younger infants. The optimal incubator temperature for minimal heat loss and oxygen consumption for the unclothed in-

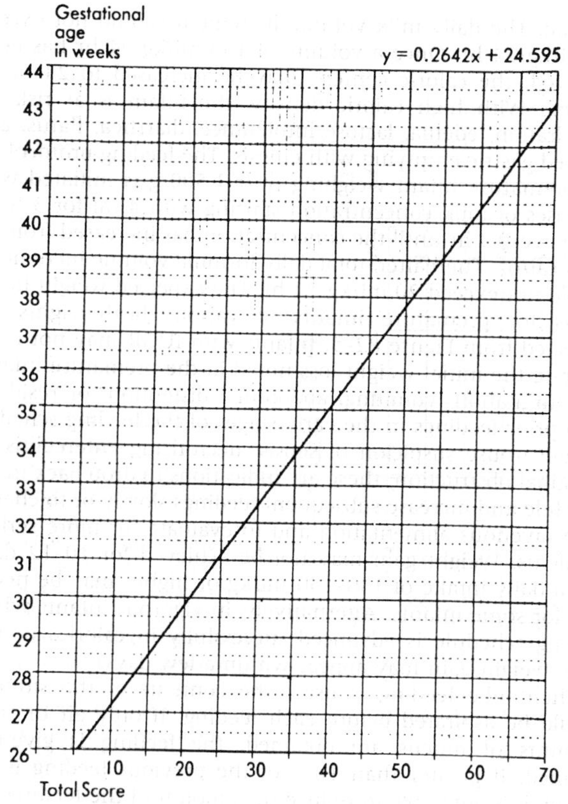

Figure 82–4. Both the external physical criteria score and that for the neurologic criteria are added together and gestational age (± 2 wk) may be read off this graph. (From Dubowitz L, Dubowitz V: Gestational Age of the Newborn. Reading, MA, Addison-Wesley, 1977.)

fant is that which will maintain the infant's core temperature at 36.5–37.0° C. This depends on an infant's size and maturity; the smaller and more immature the infant, the higher the environmental temperature required. A plexiglass heat shield or head caps and body clothing may be required when incubator care alone is insufficient to keep a small premature infant warm. Radiant warmers are alternatives to incubators, especially in seriously ill neonates.

Maintaining a relative *humidity* of 40–60% aids in stabilizing body temperature by reducing heat loss at lower environmental temperatures; by preventing drying and irritation of the lining of respiratory passages, especially during the administration of oxygen and following or during endotracheal or nasotracheal intubation; and by thinning viscid secretions and reducing insensible water loss from the lungs.

Administering *oxygen* to reduce the risk of injury from hypoxia and circulatory insufficiency must be balanced against the risks of hyperoxia to the eyes (retinopathy of prematurity) and oxygen injury to the lungs. When possible, oxygen should be administered by a head hood, continuous positive airway pressure apparatus, or endotracheal tube to maintain stable and safe inspired oxygen concentration. Although cyanosis, tachypnea, and apnea are definite clinical indications whose treatment should include only the amount of oxygen needed to eliminate these signs, the potential harm resulting from hypoxia or hyperoxia cannot be minimized without monitoring the oxygen tension (Po_2) of arterial blood and, based on laboratory analysis, continuously readjusting the concentration of oxygen administered. The development of the transcutaneous oxygen electrode and pulse oximetry for routine clinical management of these infants has significantly improved the

■ **TABLE 82–6 Problems Associated with Premature Infants**

Respiratory
Respiratory distress syndrome—RDS (hyaline membrane disease—HMD)*
Bronchopulmonary dysplasia—BPD*
Pneumothorax, pneumomediastinum; interstitial emphysema
Congenital pneumonia
Pulmonary hypoplasia
Pulmonary hemorrhage
Apnea*
Cardiovascular
Patent ductus arteriosus—PDA*
Hypotension
Hypertension
Bradycardia (with apnea)*
Congenital malformations
Hematologic
Anemia (early or late onset)
Hyperbilirubinemia—indirect*
Hyperbilirubinemia—direct
Subcutaneous, organ (liver, adrenal) hemorrhage*
Disseminated intravascular coagulopathy
Vitamin K deficiency
Hydrops—immune or nonimmune
Gastrointestinal
Poor gastrointestinal function—poor motility*
Necrotizing enterocolitis
Congenital anomalies producing polyhydramnios
Metabolic-Endocrine
Hypocalcemia*
Hypoglycemia*
Hyperglycemia*
Late metabolic acidosis
Hypothermia*
Euthyroid but low T_4 status
Central Nervous System
Intraventricular hemorrhage*
Periventricular leukomalacia
Hypoxic-ischemic encephalopathy
Seizures
Retinopathy of prematurity
Deafness
Hypotonia*
Congenital malformations
Kernicterus (bilirubin encephalopathy)
Drug (narcotic) withdrawal
Renal
Hyponatremia*
Hypernatremia*
Hyperkalemia*
Renal tubular acidosis
Renal glycosuria
Edema
Other
Infections* (congenital, perinatal, nosocomial: bacterial, viral, fungal, protozoal)

**Common*

effectiveness of oxygen monitoring. Capillary blood gases are inadequate for estimating arterial oxygen levels.

If an incubator is not available, the general conditions of temperature and humidity control outlined above can be attained by making intelligent use of radiant warmers, blankets, heating lamps, heating pads, and warm water bottles and by controlling the temperature and humidity of the room. It may be necessary to administer oxygen temporarily by face mask or through an intubation tube.

The infant should be weaned and then removed from the incubator only when the gradual change to the atmosphere of the nursery does not result in a significant change in the infant's temperature, color, activity, or vital signs.

Feeding. The method of feeding each LBW infant should be individualized. It is important to avoid fatigue and the aspiration of food by regurgitation or by the feeding process. No feeding method will avoid these problems unless the person feeding the infant has been well trained in the method. Oral feedings (nipple) should not be initiated or should be discontinued in infants with respiratory distress, hypoxia, circulatory

kg on day 1 and increased to 100–120 mL/kg by day 2–3. Smaller, more premature infants may need to be started with 70–100 mL/kg on day 1 and advanced to 150 mL/kg or more by day 3–4. Fluid volumes should be titrated individually, although it is unusual to exceed 150 mL/kg/24 hr. Daily weights, urine output and specific gravity, and serum urea nitrogen with electrolytes should be monitored carefully to detect abnormal states of hydration, since clinical observations and physical examinations are poor indicators of the state of hydration of premature infants. Conditions that increase fluid losses, such as glycosuria, the polyuric phase of acute tubular necrosis, and diarrhea, may place additional strain on kidneys that have not yet developed their maximum capacity to conserve water and electrolytes, the results of which may be severe dehydration. Alternatively, fluid overload may lead to edema, congestive heart failure, a patent ductus arteriosus, and bronchopulmonary dysplasia.

TOTAL PARENTERAL NUTRITION. When oral feeding is impossible for prolonged periods of time, total intravenous alimentation may provide sufficient fluid, calories, amino acids, electrolytes, and vitamins to sustain growth of LBW infants. This technique has been lifesaving for infants who have had intractable diarrheal syndromes or extensive resection of bowel. Infusions may be administered through an indwelling central vein catheter or through a peripheral vein.

The goal of parenteral alimentation is to deliver enough nonprotein calories to allow the infant to use most of the protein for growth. The infusate should contain synthetic amino acids of 2.5–3 g/dL and hypertonic glucose in the range of 10–25 g/dL in addition to appropriate quantities of electrolytes, trace minerals, and vitamins. The initial daily infusion should deliver 10–15 g/kg/24 hr of glucose and increase gradually to 25–30 g/kg/24 hr when glucose alone is used to meet the full requirements of 100–120 nonprotein kcal/kg/24 hr. If a peripheral vein is used, it is advisable to keep the glucose concentration below 12.5 g/dL. Intravenous fat emulsions such as 20% Intralipid (2.2 kcal/mL) may be used to provide calories without an appreciable osmotic load, thereby decreasing the need for infusion of the higher concentrations of glucose by central or peripheral vein and usually preventing the development of essential fatty acid deficiency. Intralipid may be initiated at 0.5 g/kg/24 hr and advanced to 3 g/kg/24 hr, if triglyceride levels remain normal; 0.5 g/kg/24 hr is sufficient to prevent essential fatty acid deficiency. Electrolytes, trace minerals, and vitamin additives are included in amounts approximating established intravenous maintenance requirements. The content of each day's infusate should be determined after carefully assessing the infant's clinical and biochemical status. Slow and continuous infusion is advisable. A well-trained pharmacist using a laminar flow hood should mix all solutions.

After a caloric intake of greater than 100 kcal/kg/24 hr is established by total parenteral intravenous nutrition, LBW infants can be expected to gain about 15 g/kg/24 hr, with positive nitrogen balances of 150–200 mg/kg/24 hr, if there are no multiple operative procedures, episodes of sepsis, or other severe stress. This goal usually can be achieved and the catabolic tendency during the 1st wk of life reversed with subsequent weight gains by peripheral vein infusions of 2.5 g/kg/24 hr of an amino acid mixture, 10 g/dL of glucose, and 2–3 g/kg/24 hr of Intralipid.

The complications of intravenous alimentation are related to both the catheter and the metabolism of the infusate. **Sepsis** is the most important problem of central vein infusions and can be minimized only by meticulous catheter care and aseptic preparation of the infusate. *Staphylococcus aureus, S. epidermidis,* and *Candida albicans* are the common infecting organisms. Treatment includes appropriate antibiotics. If an infection persists, the line must be removed. Thrombosis, extravasation of fluid, and accidental dislodgment of catheters have also occurred. Sepsis is rarely attributable to peripheral vein infusions, but phlebitis, cutaneous sloughs, and superficial infection occasionally occur. The **metabolic complications** include hyperglycemia from the high glucose concentration of the infusate, which may lead to an osmotic diuresis and dehydration; azotemia; possible increased risk of nephrocalcinosis; hypoglycemia from a sudden accidental cessation of the infusate; hyperlipidemia and possibly hypoxemia from intravenous lipid infusions; tissue accumulation of aluminum; and hyperammonemia, which may be due to high levels of certain amino acids. Cholestatic jaundice has also been noted. Hyperchloremic acidosis occurs in infants receiving synthetic amino acids unless there is an appropriate balance between cationic and anionic amino acids and salts. Abnormal elevations of blood amino acid levels are an additional potential hazard. If intravenous fat emulsions are not used, essential fatty acid deficiency may also occur. When the infusion is given through a peripheral vein, the osmolality of the solution may limit the length of time an infusion site can be used while, at the same time, it may require greater volumes of fluid than can be tolerated. Continuous chemical and physiologic monitoring of infants receiving intravenous alimentation is indicated because of the frequency and seriousness of complications.

Intravenous Supplementation of Tolerated Oral Feedings. A combination of intravenous and gavage alimentation is the usual method of feeding preterm infants. Once the infant is stable (2nd–3rd day of life), small nasogastric milk feedings are supplemented with peripheral alimentation solutions. Initiation of enteric feeding is possible in the presence of an endotracheal tube and an umbilical artery catheter. Glucose, amino acid mixtures, and lipid emulsions may be infused into peripheral veins when sufficient calories cannot be provided to LBW infants by oral feeding alone. Increases in weight, length, and head circumference approaching those expected in utero have been achieved with mixtures of amino acids, glucose, and Intralipid. Although the complications of both techniques may occur, the combination of nutrient delivery methods allows smaller volumes of enteral feedings, thus decreasing the risk of aspiration. Provision of enteral calories reduces the incidence of cholestatic jaundice and rickets of prematurity.

PREVENTION OF INFECTION. Premature infants have an increased susceptibility to infection, which requires nursery personnel to wash rigorously hand to elbow before and after handling the infant, take measures to reduce contamination of food and objects coming in contact with the infant, prevent air contamination, avoid overcrowding, and limit direct and indirect contacts with themselves and other infants. No one with an infection should be permitted into the nursery. However, the risks of infection must be balanced against the disadvantages of limiting the infant's contacts with the family, which may be detrimental to the infant's ultimate development; early and frequent participation by parents in the nursery care of their infant does not significantly increase the risk when preventive precautions are maintained. Prophylactic administration of gamma globulin to premature infants does not reduce the risks of nosocomial infections.

Preventing transmission of infection from infant to infant is difficult because often neither term nor premature newborn infants manifest clear clinical evidence of an infection early in its course. When epidemics occur within a nursery, cohort nursing and isolation rooms should be employed in addition to routine antiseptic care.

The most important factor in the successful care of premature infants is the skill, experience, and number of the nursing staff. It is the responsibility of the physician to insist on an optimal amount of expert nursing.

IMMATURITY OF DRUG METABOLISM. Renal clearances for almost all substances excreted in the urine are diminished in newborn infants, but more so in premature ones. Intervals between doses may, therefore, need to be extended when administering drugs excreted chiefly by the kidney. For instance, highly satisfactory levels of penicillin, gentamicin, and kanamycin are maintained on doses given at 12-hr intervals. Drugs detoxified in the liver or requiring chemical conjugation before renal excretion should also be given with caution and in doses smaller than usual. When possible, blood levels should be obtained for potentially toxic drugs, especially if renal or hepatic dysfunction is present. Decisions about the choice and dose of antibacterial agents and route of administration should be made on an individual basis rather than routinely, owing to the dangers of (1) development of infections with organisms resistant to antibacterial agents, (2) destruction or inhibition of intestinal bacteria that manufacture significant amounts of essential vitamins (e.g., vitamin K and thiamine), and (3) harmful interference in important metabolic processes.

Many drugs apparently safe for adults on the basis of toxicity studies may be harmful to newborn infants, especially premature ones. Oxygen and a number of drugs have proved toxic to premature infants in amounts not harmful to term infants (Table 82–7). Thus, administering any drug, particularly in large doses, without pharmacologic testing in premature infants, should be carefully undertaken after weighing risk against benefit.

PROGNOSIS. There is now a 95% or greater chance of survival for infants born weighing between 1,501 and 2,500 g, but those weighing less still have a significantly higher mortality (see Fig. 82–1). Intensive care has extended the period during which a VLBW infant is likely to die from complications of perinatal disease, such as bronchopulmonary dysplasia, necrotizing enterocolitis, or secondary infection (Table 82–8). The mortality rate of LBW infants who survive to be discharged from the hospital is higher than that of term infants during the first 2 yr of life. Because many of these deaths are attributable to infection, they are at least theoretically preventable. There is also an increased incidence of failure to thrive, sudden infant death syndrome, child abuse, and inadequate maternal-infant bonding among premature infants. Biologic risks from poor cardiorespiratory regulation due to immaturity or to complications of underlying perinatal disease and social risks associated with poverty also contribute to the high mortality and morbidity of these infants. Congenital anatomic anomalies are present in approximately 3–7% of LBW infants.

■ **TABLE 82–7 Adverse Reactions to Drugs Administered to Premature Infants**

Drug	Reaction
Sulfisoxazole	Kernicterus
Chloramphenicol	Gray baby—shock, bone marrow suppression
Vitamin K analogs	Jaundice
Novobiocin	Jaundice
Hexachlorophene	Encephalopathy
Benzyl alcohol	Acidosis, collapse, intraventricular bleeding
Intravenous vitamin E	Ascites, shock
Phenolic detergents	Jaundice
$NaHCO_3$	Intraventricular hemorrhage
Amphotericin	Anuric renal failure
Reserpine	Nasal stuffiness
Indomethacin	Oliguria, hyponatremia, intestinal perforation
Tetracycline	Enamel hypoplasia
Tolazoline	Hypotension, gastrointestinal bleeding
Calcium salts	Subcutaneous necrosis
Aminoglycosides	Deafness, renal toxicity
Enteric gentamicin	Resistant bacteria
Prostaglandins	Seizures, diarrhea, apnea
Phenobarbital	Altered state, drowsiness
Morphine	Hypotension, urine retention, withdrawal
Pancuronium/vecuronium	Edema, hypovolemia, hypotension, tachycardia, contractions, prolonged hypotonia
Iodine antiseptics	Hypothyroidism
Fentanyl	Seizures, chest wall rigidity, withdrawal
Dexamethasone	Gastrointestinal bleeding, hypertension, infection, hyperglycemia
Lasix	Deafness, hyponatremia, hypokalemia, hypochloremia, nephrocalcinosis, biliary stones
Heparin	Bleeding, intraventricular hemorrhage, thrombocytopenia

■ **TABLE 82–8 Sequelae of Low-Birthweight Infants**

Immediate	Late
Hypoxia, ischemia	Mental retardation, spastic diplegia, microcephaly, seizures, poor school performance
Intraventricular hemorrhage	Mental retardation, spasticity, seizures, hydrocephalus
Sensorineural injury	Hearing, visual impairment, retinopathy of prematurity, strabismus, myopia
Respiratory failure	Bronchopulmonary dysplasia, cor pulmonale, bronchospasm, malnutrition, subglottic stenosis, iatrogenic cleft palate, recurrent pneumonia
Necrotizing enterocolitis	Short bowel syndrome, malabsorption, malnutrition, infectious diarrhea
Cholestatic liver disease	Cirrhosis, hepatic failure, carcinoma, malnutrition
Nutrient deficiency	Osteopenia, fractures, anemia, vitamin E, growth failure
Social stress	Child abuse or neglect, failure to thrive, divorce
Other	Sudden infant death syndrome, infections, inguinal hernia, cutaneous scars (chest tube, PDA ligation, IV infiltration), gastroesophageal reflux, hypertension, craniosynostosis, cholelithiasis, urolithiasis, cutaneous hemangiomas

In the absence of congenital abnormalities, central nervous system injury, VLBW or marked IUGR, physical growth of LBW infants tends to approximate that of term infants during the 2nd yr; this occurs earlier in premature infants of larger birth size. VLBW infants may not catch up, especially if they have severe chronic sequelae (see Table 82–8), insufficient nutritional intake, or an inadequate caretaking environment. Premature birth in itself may prejudice later development. In general, the greater the immaturity and the lower the birthweight, the greater the likelihood of intellectual and neurologic deficit; as many as 50% of 500–750 g infants have a significant neurodevelopmental handicap (blindness, deafness, mental retardation, cerebral palsy). Small head circumference at birth may be similarly related to poor neurobehavioral prognosis. The overall incidence of neurologic and developmental handicap in VLBW infants ranges from 10 to 20%, including cerebral palsy (3–6%), moderate to severe hearing and visual defects (1–4%), and learning difficulties (20%). Mean global IQ is 90–97, and 76% have normal school performance. Many surviving LBW infants have hypotonia prior to 8 mo corrected age, which improves by the time they are 8 mo–1 yr old. This transient hypotonia is not a poor prognostic sign.

Mothers of low socioeconomic status are more apt to have LBW babies who tend to develop less well than do those in better postneonatal environments. Major neurologic defects were found to be uncommon in a prospective study of full-term small-for-dates (IUGR) infants, although compared with appropriate-for-gestation term infants, they had an increased incidence of minimal cerebral dysfunction (hyperactivity, short attention span, learning difficulties), electroencephalographic abnormalities, and speech defects.

PREDICTING NEONATAL MORTALITY. Traditionally, birthweight has been used as a strong indicator for the risk of neonatal death. Indeed survival at 22 wk gestation is close to 0%; survival increases with increasing gestational age to approximately 15% at 23 wk, 56% at 24 wk, and 79% at 25 wk. In addition, birthweight-specific neonatal diseases, such as grade IV intraventricular hemorrhage, severe group B streptococcal pneumonia, and pulmonary hypoplasia, also contribute to a poor outcome. Scoring systems have been developed that take into consideration physiologic abnormalities (hypo-hypertension, acidosis, hypoxia, hypercarbia, anemia, neutropenia) in the Score for Neonatal Acute Physiology (SNAP) or clinical parameters (gestational age, birthweight, anomalies, acidosis, FIO_2) in the Clinical Risk Index for Babies (CRIB). CRIB includes 6 parameters collected in the first 12 hr after birth, while SNAP has 26 variables collected in the first 24 hr. Although these risk scoring systems may provide prognostic information for mortality, they may not be useful for predicting morbidity among survivors. Furthermore, when compared with the clinical judgment of experienced neonatologists (based on birthweight, illness severity, low Apgar score, IUGR, therapeutic requirements), objective risk scores provide similar predictability. Combining a physician's judgment and an objective score may produce a more accurate assessment of the mortality risk.

DISCHARGE FROM HOSPITAL. Before discharge, a premature infant should be taking all nutrition by nipple, either bottle or breast. Growth should be occurring at steady increments of approximately 10–30 g/day. Temperature should be stabilized in an open crib. There should have been no recent apnea or bradycardia, and parenteral drug administration should have been discontinued. Stable infants recovering from bronchopulmonary dysplasia may be discharged on oxygen given by nasal cannula as long as careful follow-up is arranged with frequent pulse oximetry monitoring and outpatient visits. Infants previously treated with oxygen should have an eye examination to determine the presence, stage, or absence of retinopathy of prematurity, while all LBW infants should have a hearing test, and those who had indwelling umbilical arterial catheters should have their blood pressure measured to check for renal vascular hypertension. A hemoglobin level or hematocrit should be determined to evaluate possible anemia. If all major medical problems have resolved and the home setting is adequate, premature infants may then be discharged when their weight approaches 1,800–2,100 g; close follow-up and easy access to health care providers are essential for early discharge protocols. Alternatively, if the medical or social environment is not ideal, high-risk neonates transported to neonatal intensive care units whose major illness has resolved may be returned to their hospital of birth for an additional period of hospitalization. Standard vaccinations with full doses should commence after discharge or if in the hospital, with vaccines that do not contain live viruses.

HOME CARE. While the infant is in the hospital the mother should be instructed in how to care for the baby after discharge. This program should include at least one visit to her home by someone capable of evaluating domestic arrangements and advising about any needed improvements.

82.3 Post-Term Infants

Post-term infants are those born after 42 wk of gestation, calculated from the mother's last menstrual period, regardless of weight at birth. This designation is often used synonymously with the term "postmature" for infants whose gestation exceeds the normal 280 days by 7 days or more. Approximately 25% of all pregnancies end on or after the 287th day of gestation, 12% on or after the 294th day, and 5% on or after the 301st day. The cause of post-term birth or postmaturity is unknown. Large size of the infant correlates poorly with late delivery but does correlate with large size of either parent, multigravidity, or a prediabetic or diabetic state in the mother.

CLINICAL MANIFESTATIONS. Post-term infants may be clinically indistinguishable from term infants, but some have received the designation postmature because their appearance and behavior suggest those of an infant 1–3 wk of age. These post-term, postmature infants are often of increased birthweight and characterized by the absence of lanugo, decreased or absent vernix caseosa, long nails, abundant scalp hair, white parchment-like or desquamating skin, and increased alertness. If *placental insufficiency* occurs, the amniotic fluid and fetus may be meconium stained, and abnormal fetal heart rates may be observed; the infant may have growth retardation. Although this syndrome is frequently confused with postmaturity, *only about 20% of infants with placental insufficiency syndrome are post-term.* The majority of those affected are term and preterm infants, particularly those small for gestational age who are the infants of toxemic mothers, older primigravidas, and women with chronic hypertension. The placentas are often small or poorly attached. This syndrome has been postulated to result from degenerative changes in the placenta that progressively reduce oxygen and nourishment to the fetus.

Those infants born post term in association with presumed placental insufficiency may have a variety of physical signs: desquamation, long nails, abundant hair, pale skin, alert faces, and loose skin, especially around the thighs and buttocks, giving them the appearance of having recently lost weight; meconium-stained nails, skin, vernix, umbilical cord, and placental membranes (see Fig. 79–1).

PROGNOSIS. When delivery is delayed 3 wk or more beyond term, there is a significant increase in mortality, which in some series has approximated 3 times that of a control group of infants born at term. Mortality has been lowered markedly through improved obstetric management.

TREATMENT. Careful obstetric monitoring, including nonstress testing, biophysical profile, or Doppler velocimetry, usually provides a rational basis for choosing a course of nonintervention, induction of labor, or cesarean section. Induction of labor or cesarean section may be indicated in older primigravidas who go more than 2–4 wk beyond term, particularly if there is evidence of fetal distress. Meconium aspiration pneumonia or hypoxic encephalopathy is treated symptomatically.

82.4 Large for Gestational Age (LGA)

See also Chapter 92.

Neonatal mortality rates decrease with increasing birth weight until approximately 4,000 g, after which mortality increases. These oversized infants are usually born at term, but preterm infants with weights high for gestational age also have a significantly higher mortality than infants of the same size born at term; maternal diabetes and obesity are predisposing factors. Infants who are very large, regardless of their gestational age, have a higher incidence of birth injuries, such as cervical and brachial plexus injuries, phrenic nerve damage with paralysis of the diaphragm, fractured clavicles, cephalhematomas, subdural hematomas, and ecchymoses of the head and face. The incidence of congenital anomalies, particularly congenital heart disease, is also higher than in term infants of normal weight. Intellectual and developmental retardation is statistically more common in high-birthweight term and preterm infants than in babies of appropriate weight for gestational age.

INFANT TRANSPORT

With the advent of regionalized care of high-risk neonates, increasing numbers of sick infants are being transported to neonatal intensive care units in hospitals at which they were not born. Ideally, high-risk mothers should be transported to and delivered at centers where these specialized units are located. Neonatal transport should include consultation about the infant's problem and care before transport, ease of access to the transport team, and transport and stabilization by the team before moving the infant. Securing an airway, providing oxygen, assisting with infant ventilation, providing antimicrobial therapy, maintaining the circulation, providing a warmed environment, and placing intravenous or arterial lines or chest tubes should all be initiated, if indicated, prior to transport. Infant and maternal records, laboratory reports, and a tube of clotted maternal blood should also be provided. Before departing, the mother should be briefly reassured and allowed to see the stabilized infant, if practical; the father should follow the transport vehicle to the unit. The transport officer or nurse should also call ahead to inform the receiving unit about the nature of the patient's illness.

The transport vehicle should be equipped with appropriate medicines, fluids, oxygen tanks, catheters, chest tubes, endotracheal tubes, laryngoscopes, and an infant warming device. It should be well illuminated and have ample room for emergency procedures and monitoring equipment. With efficient transport and appropriately educated nursing and medical staff at the referring hospitals, the mortality of "outborn" neonates should be no higher than that of those born within the tertiary care center.

Allen MC, Donohue PK, Dusman AE: The limit of viability—neonatal outcome of infants born at 22 to 25 weeks' gestation. N Engl J Med 329:1597, 1993.
American Academy of Pediatrics: Hospital Care of Newborn Infants. Evanston IL, The Academy, 1993.
Anonymous: Breast not necessarily the best. Lancet 1:624, 1988.
Blaymore Bier J, Ferguson A, Anderson L, et al: Breast-feeding of very low birth weight infants. J Pediatr 123:773, 1993.
Bregman J, Kimberlin LVS: Developmental outcome in extremely premature infants. Impact of surfactant. Pediatr Clin North Am 40:937, 1993.
Chan GM: Growth and bone mineral status of discharged very low birth weight infants fed different formulas or human milk. J Pediatr 123:439, 1993.
Committee on Nutrition: Nutritional needs of low-birth-weight infants. Pediatrics 75:977, 1985.
Davey AM, Wagner CL, Cox C, et al: Feeding premature infants while low umbilical artery catheters are in place: A prospective, randomized trial. J Pediatr 124:795, 1994.
Davis DJ: How aggressive should delivery room cardiopulmonary resuscitation be for extremely low birth weight neonates? Pediatrics 92:447, 1993.
Division of Nutrition, National Center for Chronic Disease Prevention and Health Promotion: Division of Vital Statistics, National Center for Health Statistics, CDC. Increasing incidence of low birthweight—United States, 1981–1991. MMWR 43:335, 1994.
Division of Reproductive Health, National Center for Chronic Disease Prevention and Health Promotion, CDC. Differences in infant mortality between blacks and whites—United States, 1980–1991. MMWR 43:288, 1994.
Dunn L, Hulman S, Weiner J, et al: Beneficial effects of early hypocaloric enteral feeding on neonatal gastrointestinal function: Preliminary report of a randomized trial. J Pediatr 112:622, 1988.
Ens-Dokkum MH, Schreuder AM, Veen S, et al: Evaluation of care for the preterm infant: review of literature on follow-up of preterm and low birthweight infants. Report from the collaborative project on preterm and small for gestational age infants (POPS) in the Netherlands. Paediatr Perinatal Epidemiol 6:434, 1992.
Fanaroff AA, Korones SB, Wright LL, et al: A controlled trial of intravenous immune globulin to reduce nosocomial infections in very-low-birth-weight infants. N Engl J Med 330:1107, 1994.
Hack M, Weissman B, Breslau N, et al: Health of very low birth weight children during their first eight years. J Pediatr 122:887, 1993.
Heird WC, Gomez MR: Total parenteral nutrition in necrotizing enterocolitis. Clin Perinatol 21:389, 1994.
Higby K, Xenakis EM-J, Pauerstein CJ: Do tocolytic agents stop preterm labor? A critical and comprehensive review of efficacy and safety. Am J Obstet Gynecol 168:1247, 1993.
Holtrop PC, Ertzbischoff LM, Roberts CL, et al: Survival and short-term outcome in newborns of 23 to 25 weeks' gestation. Am J Obstet Gynecol 170:1266, 1994.
Kashyap S, Schulze KF, Forsyth M, et al: Growth, nutrient retention, and metabolic response in low birth weight infants fed varying intakes of protein and energy. J Pediatr 113:713, 1988.
La Gamma EF, Browne LE: Feeding practices for infants weighing less than 1500 g at birth and the pathogenesis of necrotizing enterocolitis. Clin Perinatol 21:271, 1994.
Lebenthal E, Leung Y: Feeding the premature and compromised infant: Gastrointestinal considerations. Pediatr Clin North Am 35:215, 1988.
Lucas A, Morley R, Cole TJ, et al: A randomised multicentre study of human milk versus formula and later development in preterm infants. Arch Dis Child 70:F141, 1994.
Major CA, Lewis DF, Harding JA, et al: Tocolysis with indomethacin increases the incidence of necrotizing enterocolitis in the low-birth-weight neonate. Am J Obstet Gynecol 170:102, 1994.
Modi N. Sodium intake and preterm babies: Arch Dis Child 69:87, 1993.
Moreno A, Dominguez C, Ballabriga A: Aluminum in the neonate related to parenteral nutrition. Acta Paediatr 83:25, 1994.
Mortality Statistics Branch, Division of Vital Statistics, National Center for Health Statistics, CDC. Infant mortality—United States, 1991. MMWR 42:926, 1993.
Pereira GR, Baumgart S, Bennett MJ, et al: Use of high-fat formula for premature infants with bronchopulmonary dysplasia: Metabolic, pulmonary, and nutritional studies. J Pediatr 124:605, 1994.
Perez-Escamilla R, Pollitt E, Lonnerdal B, et al: Infant feeding policies in maternity wards and their effect on breast-feeding success: An analytical overview. Am J Public Health 84:89, 1994.
Pharoah POD, Stevenson CJ, Cooke RWI, et al: Clinical and subclinical deficits at 8 years in a geographically defined cohort of low birthweight infants. Arch Dis Child 70:264, 1994.
Prestridge LL, Schanler RJ, Shulman RJ, et al: Effect of parenteral calcium and phosphorus therapy on mineral retention and bone mineral content in very low birth weight infants. J Pediatr 122:761, 1993.
Rautonen J, Makela A, Boyd H, et al: CRIB and SNAP: assessing the risk of death for preterm neonates. Lancet 343:1272, 1994.
Richardson DK, Gray JE, McCormick MC, et al: Score for neonatal acute physiology: A physiologic severity index for neonatal intensive care. Pediatrics 91:617, 1993.
Robertson C, Sauve RS, Christianson HE: Province-based study of neurologic disability among survivors weighing 500 through 1249 grams at birth. Pediatrics 93:636, 1994.
Romero R, Sibai B, Caritis S, et al: Antibiotic treatment of preterm labor with intact membranes: A multicenter, randomized, double-blinded, placebo-controlled trial. Am J Obstet Gynecol 169:764, 1993.
Sauer P, Visser M: The neutral temperature of very low birth weight infants. Pediatrics 74:788, 1984.
Schanler R: Human milk for preterm infants: Nutritional and immune factors. Semin Perinatol 13:69, 1989.
Shiono P, Behrman RE (eds): Low birth weight. The Future of Children 5(1):1–213, 1995.
Stevens SM, Richardson DK, Gray JE, et al: Estimating neonatal mortality risk: An analysis of clinicians' judgments. Pediatrics 93:945, 1994.
The International Neonatal Network: The CRIB (clinical risk index for babies) score: a tool for assessing initial neonatal risk and comparing performance of neonatal intensive care units. Lancet 342:193, 1993.
Whyte HE, Fitzhardinge PM, Shennan AT, et al: Extreme immaturity: Outcome of 568 pregnancies of 23–26 weeks' gestation. Obstet Gynecol 82:1, 1993.
Wright K, Dawson JP, Fallis D, et al: New postnatal growth grids for very low birth weight infants. Pediatrics 91:922, 1993.

CHAPTER 83

Clinical Manifestations of Diseases in the Newborn Period

The infant's physician should appreciate the wide variety of disorders that may originate in utero, during birth, or in the immediate postnatal period and the need to distinguish them according to their time of onset, etiology, and place of origin. The disorders may represent genetic mutations, chromosomal aberrations, or acquired diseases and injuries. Recognizing disease in the newborn infant depends on knowledge about the disorder and evaluation of a limited number of relatively nonspecific clinical signs and symptoms.

Central cyanosis usually indicates respiratory insufficiency, which may be due to pulmonary conditions or may be secondary to central nervous system depression due to drugs, intracranial hemorrhage, or anoxia (Table 83–1). If it is caused by the former, respirations tend to be rapid and may be accompanied by retraction of the thoracic cage. If it is due to the latter, respirations tend to be irregular and weak and are often slow. Cyanosis persisting for several days, unaccompanied by obvious signs of respiratory difficulty, suggests cyanotic congenital heart disease or methemoglobinemia. Cyanosis resulting from congenital heart disease may, however, be difficult to distin-

■ **TABLE 83–1 Differential Diagnosis of Neonatal Cyanosis**

System/Disease	Mechanism
Pulmonary	
Respiratory distress syndrome	Surfactant deficiency
Sepsis, pneumonia	Inflammation, pulmonary hypertension, shunting R → L*
Meconium aspiration pneumonia	Mechanical obstruction, inflammation, pulmonary hypertension, shunting R → L
Persistent fetal circulation	Pulmonary hypertension, shunting R → L
Diaphragmatic hernia	Pulmonary hypoplasia, pulmonary hypertension
Transient tachypnea	Retained lung fluid
Cardiovascular	
Cyanotic heart disease with decreased pulmonary blood flow	Right to left shunt as in pulmonary atresia, tetralogy of Fallot
Cyanotic heart disease with increased pulmonary blood flow	Right to left shunt as in d-transposition, truncus arteriosus
Cyanotic heart disease with congestive heart failure	Right to left shunt with pulmonary edema and poor cardiac output as in hypoplastic left heart and coarctation of aorta
Heart failure alone	Pulmonary edema and poor cardiac contractility as in sepsis, myocarditis, supraventricular tachycardia, or complete heart block. High-output failure as in patent ductus arteriosus or vein of Galen or other arteriovenous malformation
Central Nervous System	
Maternal sedative drugs	Hypoventilation, apnea
Asphyxia	CNS depression
Intracranial hemorrhage	CNS depression, seizure
Neuromuscular disease	Phrenic nerve palsy; hypotonia, hypoventilation, pulmonary hypoplasia
Hematologic	
Acute blood loss	Shock
Chronic blood loss	Congestive heart failure
Polycythemia	Pulmonary hypertension
Methemoglobinemia	Low affinity hemoglobin or red blood cell enzyme defect
Metabolic	
Hypoglycemia	CNS depression, congestive heart failure
Adrenogenital syndrome	Shock (salt-losing)

**R → L, Right-to-left intracardiac (foramen ovale), extracardiac (ductus arteriosus), or intrapulmonary shunting.*

guish clinically from cyanosis caused by respiratory disease. Episodes of cyanosis also may be the presenting sign of hypoglycemia, bacteremia, meningitis, shock, or persistent fetal circulation. Peripheral acrocyanosis is common and usually does not warrant concern.

Pallor, in addition to anemia or acute hemorrhage, should suggest hypoxia, hypoglycemia, sepsis, shock, or adrenal failure.

Convulsions (Chapter 543.5) usually point to a disorder of the central nervous system and suggest hypoxic-ischemic encephalopathy resulting from asphyxia, intracranial hemorrhage, cerebral anomaly, subdural effusion, meningitis, hypocalcemia, hypoglycemia, infarction, and, rarely, pyridoxine dependency, hyponatremia, hypernatremia, inborn errors of metabolism, drug withdrawal, or familial seizures. Seizures beginning in the delivery room or shortly thereafter may be due to unintentional injection of maternal local anesthetic into the fetus. Convulsions may also result from administration of large amounts of hypotonic fluids to the mother shortly before and during delivery, leading to subsequent hyponatremia and water intoxication in the infant.

Convulsions (epileptic seizures) should be distinguished from the jitteriness that may be present in normal newborns, in infants of diabetic mothers, in those who experienced birth asphyxia or drug withdrawal, and in polycythemic neonates. Jitteriness resembling simple tremors may be stopped by holding the infant's extremity; it often depends on sensory stimuli and is not associated with abnormal eye movements. Seizures in premature infants are often subtle and associated with abnormal eye or facial movements; the motor component is often that of tonic extension of the limbs, neck, and trunk. Term infants may have focal or multifocal, clonic or myoclonic movements but may also manifest more subtle seizure activity. *Apnea* may be the first manifestation of seizure activity, particularly in a premature infant.

Following severe birth asphyxia infants may have *motor automatisms* characterized by oral-buccal-lingual movements, rotary limb activities (rowing, pedaling, swimming), tonic posturing, or myoclonus. These motor seizures are not usually accompanied by time-synchronized electroencephalographic (EEG) discharges, may not signify cortical epileptic activity, respond poorly to anticonvulsant therapy, and are associated with a poor prognosis. Such automatisms may represent cortical depression that produces a brain stem release phenomenon or subcortical seizures.

Lethargy may be a manifestation of infection, asphyxia, hypoglycemia, hypercarbia, sedation from maternal analgesia or anesthesia, cerebral defect, and, indeed, of almost any severe disease including inborn errors of metabolism. Lethargy appearing after the 2nd day should, in particular, suggest infection.

Irritability may be a sign of discomfort accompanying intra-abdominal conditions, meningeal irritation, drug withdrawal, infections, congenital glaucoma, or any condition producing pain. As in later infancy, the eardrums should always be examined as a possible source of pain.

Hyperactivity, especially of the premature infant, may be a sign of hypoxia, pneumothorax, emphysema, hypoglycemia, hypocalcemia, central nervous system damage, drug withdrawal, thyrotoxicosis, or discomfort due to a cold environment.

Failure to feed well is seen in most sick newborn infants and should always occasion a careful search for infection, central or peripheral nervous system disorder, and other abnormal conditions.

Fever may be the result of too high an environmental temperature due to weather, overheated nurseries or incubators, or too many clothes or bedclothes. It is also seen in "dehydration fever" of newborn infants. If these causes of fever can be eliminated, then serious infection (pneumonia, bacteremia, viremia, meningitis) must be considered, although such infections often occur without provoking a febrile response in newborn infants (see Chapters 97 and 98). An unexplained *fall in body temperature* may accompany infection or other serious disturbances of the circulation or central nervous system. A sudden servo-controlled increase in incubator temperature to maintain body temperature is often associated with sepsis.

Periods of *apnea,* particularly in the premature infant, may be associated with a variety of disturbances (see Chapter 87.2). When apneas recur or when the intervals are longer than 20 sec or are associated with cyanosis or bradycardia, they warrant an immediate diagnostic evaluation.

Jaundice during the first 24 hr of life should be considered to be due to erythroblastosis fetalis until proved otherwise. Septicemia (especially in the low-birthweight infant), cytomegalic inclusion disease, the congenital rubella syndrome, and toxoplasmosis should also be considered, especially if there is an increase in plasma direct-reacting bilirubin.

Jaundice after the first 24 hr may be "physiologic" or may be due to septicemia, hemolytic anemia, galactosemia, hepatitis, congenital atresia of the bile ducts, inspissated bile syndrome following erythroblastosis fetalis, syphilis, herpes simplex, or congenital infections (see Chapter 88).

Vomiting during the 1st day of life suggests obstruction in the upper digestive tract or increased intracranial pressure. Roentgenographic studies are indicated when obstruction is suspected. Vomiting also may be a nonspecific symptom of an illness such as septicemia. It is a common manifestation of overfeeding or inexperienced feeding technique, pyloric steno-

■ **TABLE 83–2 Common Life-Threatening Congenital Anomalies**

Name	Manifestations
Choanal atresia	Respiratory distress in delivery room, apnea, unable to pass nasogastric tube through nares. Suspect CHARGE syndrome
Pierre Robin syndrome	Migrognathia, cleft palate, airway obstruction
Diaphragmatic hernia	Scaphoid abdomen, bowel sounds present in chest, respiratory distress
Tracheoesophageal fistula	Polyhydramnios, aspiration pneumonia, excessive salivation, unable to place nasogastric tube in stomach. Suspect VATER syndrome
Intestinal obstruction: volvulus, duodenal atresia, ileal atresia	Polyhydramnios, bile-stained emesis, abdominal distention. Suspect 21-trisomy, cystic fibrosis, cocaine
Gastroschisis, omphalocele	Polyhydramnios, intestinal obstruction
Renal agenesis, Potter syndrome	Oligohydramnios, anuria, pulmonary hypoplasia, pneumothorax
Neural tube defects: anencephalus, meningomyelocele	Polydramnios, elevated α-fetoprotein, decreased fetal activity
Ductal dependent congenital heart disease	Cyanosis, hypotension, murmur

sis, milk allergy, duodenal ulcer, stress ulcer, or adrenal insufficiency. Infants placed in body casts for orthopedic treatment often vomit transiently. Vomitus containing dark blood is usually a sign of life-threatening illness; the benign possibility of swallowed maternal blood should also be considered. Bile-stained vomitus strongly suggests obstruction below the ampulla of Vater.

Diarrhea may be a symptom of overfeeding (especially high-caloric density formula), acute gastroenteritis, malabsorption, or a nonspecific symptom of infection. It may be seen in conditions accompanied by compromised circulation of part of the intestinal or genital tract, such as mesenteric thrombosis, necrotizing enterocolitis, strangulated hernia, intussusception, and torsion of the ovary or testis.

Abdominal distention, usually a sign of intestinal obstruction or an intra-abdominal mass, may also be seen in infants with enteritis, necrotizing enterocolitis, ileus accompanying sepsis, respiratory distress, or hypokalemia.

Failure to move an extremity (pseudoparalysis) or part of it suggests fracture, dislocation, or nerve injury. It is also seen in osteomyelitis and other infections that cause pain on movement of the affected part.

CONGENITAL ANOMALIES

Congenital anomalies are a major cause of stillbirths and neonatal deaths but are perhaps even more important as causes of physical defects and metabolic disorders. (Anomalies are discussed in general in Chapter 67 and specifically in the chapters on the various systems of the body.) Early recognition of anomalies is important for planning care; for some, such as tracheoesophageal fistula, diaphragmatic hernia, choanal atresia, and intestinal obstruction, immediate medical and surgical therapy is essential for survival (Table 83–2). Parents are likely to have anxiety and guilt upon learning of the existence of a congenital anomaly and require sensitive counseling.

CHAPTER 84
Birth Injury

The term *birth injury* is used to denote avoidable and unavoidable mechanical and anoxic trauma incurred by the infant during labor and delivery. These injuries may result from inappropriate or deficient medical skill or attention, or they may occur, despite skilled and competent obstetric care, independently of any acts or omissions. In order to avoid later misunderstandings, recriminations, or parental guilt, it is important to counsel parents who have a child with a residuum from birth trauma or anoxia about this broad use of the term "birth injury." The definition does not include injury from amniocentesis, intrauterine transfusion, scalp blood sampling, or resuscitation procedures, all of which are discussed elsewhere.

The incidence of birth injuries has been estimated at 2–7/1,000 live births. Predisposing factors include macrosomia, prematurity, cephalopelvic disproportion, dystocia, prolonged labor, and breech presentation. Overall, 5–8/100,000 infants die of birth trauma, and 25/100,000 die of anoxic injuries; such injuries represent 2–3% of infant deaths. Even transient injuries readily apparent to the parents result in anxiety and questioning that require supportive and informative counseling. Some injuries may be latent initially but later result in severe illness or sequelae.

84.1 Cranial Injuries

Caput succedaneum is a diffuse, sometimes ecchymotic, edematous swelling of the soft tissues of the scalp involving the portion presenting during vertex delivery. It may extend across the midline and across suture lines. The edema disappears within the first few days of life. Analogous swelling, discoloration, and distortion of the face are seen in face presentations. No specific treatment is needed, but if there are extensive ecchymoses, phototherapy for hyperbilirubinemia may be indicated. *Molding* of the head and overriding of the parietal bones are frequently associated with caput succedaneum and become more evident after the caput has receded but disappear during the first weeks of life. Rarely, a hemorrhagic caput may result in shock and require blood transfusion.

Erythema, abrasions, ecchymoses and *subcutaneous fat necrosis* of facial or scalp soft tissues may be seen after forceps deliveries. Their location depends on the area of application of the forceps. Ecchymoses may be seen after manipulative deliveries and occasionally in premature infants for no discernible reason.

Subconjunctival and retinal hemorrhages are frequent, and *petechiae* of the skin of the head and neck are common. All are probably secondary to a sudden increase in intrathoracic pressure during passage of the chest through the birth canal. Parents should be assured that they are temporary and the result of *normal* hazards of delivery.

Cephalohematoma (Fig. 84–1) is a subperiosteal hemorrhage, hence always limited to the surface of 1 cranial bone. There is no discoloration of the overlying scalp, and swelling is usually not visible until several hours after birth, since subperiosteal bleeding is a slow process. An underlying skull fracture, usually linear and not depressed, is occasionally associated with cephalohematoma. Cranial meningocele may be differentiated from cephalohematoma by pulsation, increased pressure on crying, and the roentgenographic evidence of bony defect. Most cephalohematomas are resorbed within 2 wk–3 mo, depending on their size. They may begin to calcify by the end of the 2nd wk. A sensation of central depression suggesting but not indicative of an underlying fracture or bony defect is usually encountered on palpation of the organized rim of a cephalohematoma. A few remain for years as bony protuberances and are detectable roentgenographically as widening of the diploic space; cystlike defects may persist for months or

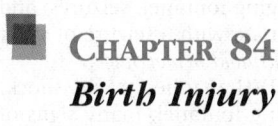

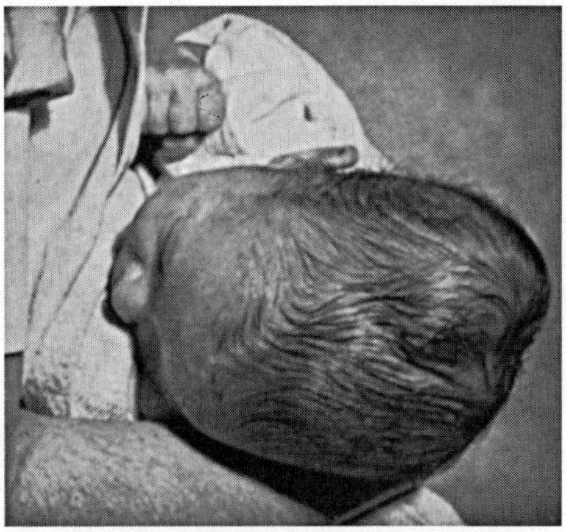

Figure 84–1. Cephalohematoma of the right parietal bone.

years. Despite these residuals, cephalohematomas require no treatment, although phototherapy may be necessary to ameliorate hyperbilirubinemia. Incision and drainage are contraindicated because of the risk of introducing infection in a benign condition. A massive cephalohematoma may rarely result in blood loss severe enough to require transfusion. It may also be associated with a skull fracture, coagulopathy, and intracranial hemorrhage.

Fractures of the skull may occur as a result of pressure from forceps or from the maternal symphysis pubis, sacral promontory, or ischial spines. Linear fractures, the most common, cause no symptoms and require no treatment. Depressed fractures are usually indentations of the calvarium similar to a dent in a ping-pong ball; usually they are a complication of forceps delivery or fetal compression. The infant may be asymptomatic unless there is associated intracranial injury; it is advisable to elevate severe depressions to prevent cortical injury from sustained pressure. Fracture of the occipital bone with separation of the basal and squamous portions almost invariably causes fatal hemorrhage owing to disruption of the underlying sinuses. It may result during breech deliveries from traction on the hyperextended spine of the infant with the head fixed in the maternal pelvis.

84.2 Intracranial (Intraventricular) Hemorrhage

ETIOLOGY AND EPIDEMIOLOGY. Intracranial hemorrhage may result from trauma or asphyxia and, rarely, from a primary hemorrhagic disturbance or congenital vascular anomaly. Traumatic epidural, subdural, or subarachnoid hemorrhage is especially likely when the fetal head is large in proportion to the size of the mother's pelvic outlet; when for other reasons the labor is prolonged; when there are breech or precipitate deliveries; or when there is injudicious mechanical interference with delivery. Massive subdural hemorrhages, often associated with tears in the tentorium cerebelli or, less frequently, in the falx cerebri, are rare but are encountered more often in full-term than in premature infants. Primary hemorrhagic disturbances and vascular malformations are rare and usually give rise to subarachnoid or intracerebral hemorrhage. Intracranial bleeding may be associated with disseminated intravascular coagulopathy, isoimmune thrombocytopenia, and neonatal vitamin K deficiency (especially in infants born to mothers receiving phenobarbital or phenytoin). Intracranial hemorrhages often involve the ventricles **(intraventricular hemorrhage)** of premature infants delivered spontaneously without apparent trauma.

PATHOGENESIS OF INTRAVENTRICULAR HEMORRHAGE (IVH). IVH in the premature infant occurs in the gelatinous subependymal germinal matrix. This periventricular area is the site of embryonal neurons and fetal glial cells, which migrate to the cortex. Immature blood vessels in this highly vascular area may be subjected to various forces that, together with poor tissue vascular support, predispose the premature infant to IVH. By term, the germinal matrix has become attenuated and the tissue's vascular support has strengthened. *Predisposing factors or events* for IVH include prematurity, respiratory distress syndrome, hypoxic ischemic or hypotensive injury, reperfusion of damaged vessels, increased or decreased cerebral blood flow, reduced vascular integrity, increased venous pressure, pneumothorax, hypervolemia, and hypertension. These factors result in rupture of the germinal matrix blood vessels. Similar injurious factors (hypoxic-ischemic-hypotensive) may produce cortical intraparenchymal echodensities (IPE) due to hemorrhagic infarction and later development of *periventricular leukomalacia* (PVL). PVL with or without severe IVH is the result of necrosis of the periventricular white matter and damage to the corticospinal fibers in the internal capsule.

CLINICAL MANIFESTATIONS. The incidence of IVH increases with decreasing birth weight: 60–70% of 500- to 750-g infants and 10–20% of 1,000- to 1,500-g infants. IVH is rarely present at birth; however, 80–90% of cases occur between birth and the 3rd day of life. Twenty to forty per cent of cases progress during the 1st wk of life. Delayed hemorrhage may occur in 10–15% of patients after the 1st wk of life. New-onset IVH is rare after the 1st mo of life regardless of birthweight. The most common symptoms are diminished or absent Moro reflex, poor muscle tone, lethargy, apnea, and somnolence. In premature infants with intraventricular hemorrhage there is often a precipitous deterioration on the 2nd or 3rd day of life. Periods of apnea, pallor, or cyanosis, failure to suck well, abnormal eye signs, a high-pitched shrill cry, muscular twitchings, convulsions, decreased muscle tone, paralyses, metabolic acidosis, shock, and a decreased hematocrit or its failure to increase after transfusion may be the first indications. The fontanel *may* be tense and bulging. Severe neurologic depression progresses to coma after more severe intraventricular hemorrhages, with associated hemorrhage in the cerebral cortex and ventricular dilation. In a small percentage of cases there may be no clinical manifestations.

PVL is usually asymptomatic until the neurologic sequelae of white matter necrosis becomes manifest in later infancy as spastic diplegia. As a result of nonhemorrhagic ischemic injury, PVL often coexists with IVH. PVL may be present at birth but usually occurs later as an early echo-dense phase (3–10 days of life) followed by the typical echo-lucent (cystic) phase (14–20 days of life).

DIAGNOSIS. Intracranial hemorrhage is diagnosed on the basis of the history, clinical manifestations, transfontanel cranial ultrasonography or computed tomography (CT), and knowledge of the birthweight-specific risks of the type of hemorrhage. The diagnosis of *subdural hemorrhage* in a LGA term infant with cephalopelvic disproportion may be delayed 1 mo until the chronic subdural fluid volume expands, producing megalocephaly, frontal bossing, bulging fontanel, seizures, and anemia. Alternatively, the well neonate with a seizure of short duration may have a benign *subarachnoid hemorrhage.*

Although preterm infants with IVH manifest rapid shock, mottling, anemia, coma, or a bulging fontanel, many signs of IVH are nonspecific or absent. Therefore, it is recommended that the premature infant be evaluated with real-time *cerebral ultrasonography* through the anterior fontanel to detect IVH. Infants weighing under 1,000 g are at high risk for IVH and should be examined within the first 3–5 days of life and again the following week. The ultrasound examination will also detect the precystic and cystic symmetric lesions of PVL and the asymmetric intraparenchymal echogenic lesions of cortical hemorrhagic infarction. Furthermore, the delayed development of cortical atrophy, or porencephaly, and the severity, progression, or regression of posthemorrhagic hydrocephalus can be determined with ultrasonography.

Four levels of increasing severity of IVH are defined by ultrasound for LBW infants: Grade I is bleeding confined to the germinal matrix–subependymal region or to less than 10% of the ventricle; grade II is intraventricular bleeding with 10–50% filling of the ventricle; grade III is more than 50% involvement with dilated ventricles; grade IV includes grade III, with corticoperiventricular intraparenchymal lesions that are not necessarily a direct extension of the IVH. Seventy-five per cent of infants with IVH are grade I–II. Severe IVH is independently associated with immaturity and the severity of respiratory distress syndrome (RDS). Immature infants without RDS are at risk for IVH, whereas infants with severe RDS are at greater risk than those with mild or no RDS at the same gestational age.

CT scan is indicated for term infants in whom the diagnosis is suspected, since ultrasound may not reveal intraparenchymal hemorrhage or infarction. Lumbar puncture is indicated in the presence of signs of increased intracranial pressure or deteriorating clinical condition to identify gross subarachnoid hemorrhage or to rule out the possibility of bacterial meningitis; the cerebrospinal fluid usually has elevated protein levels with many red blood cells. Not infrequently there is hypoglycorrhachia and a mild lymphocytosis. Since a small amount of bleeding into the cerebrospinal fluid often occurs in the course of normal and even cesarean deliveries, small numbers of red blood cells or slight xanthochromia in subarachnoid fluid does not necessarily indicate significant intracranial hemorrhage. Conversely, the subarachnoid fluid may be absolutely clear in the presence of severe subdural or intracerebral hemorrhage when there is no communication with the subarachnoid space.

PROGNOSIS. Patients with massive hemorrhage associated with tears of the tentorium or falx cerebri rapidly deteriorate and may die after birth. In utero hemorrhage associated with maternal idiopathic or, more often, fetal alloimmune thrombocytopenia may occur as severe cerebral hemorrhage or a porencephalic cyst after resolution of a fetal cortical hemorrhage.

Most infants with IVH and acute ventricular distention do not develop *posthemorrhagic hydrocephalus*. Ten to fifteen per cent of LBW neonates with IVH have hydrocephalus, which initially may be present without clinical signs such as enlarging head circumference, apnea, bradycardia, lethargy, bulging fontanel, or widely split sutures. In infants who develop symptomatic hydrocephalus, clinical signs may be delayed 2–4 wk despite progressive ventricular distention and compression (thinning) of the cerebral cortex. Posthemorrhagic hydrocephalus is arrested or regresses in 65% of affected infants.

Progressive hydrocephalus requiring ventricular-peritoneal shunting, gestational age of less than 30 wk, prolonged mechanical ventilation (> 28 days), intraparenchymal hemorrhage, and extensive PVL are associated with a poor prognosis. Because PVL and intraparenchymal bleeding represent hypoxic ischemic injury, they are independent risk factors for spastic diplegia and other motor deficits. IVH with intraparenchymal echo-densities greater than 1 cm are associated with a high mortality and a high incidence of motor and cognitive deficits. Grade I–II IVH may be due to factors other than severe hypoxia-ischemia, and in such a case it has a lower risk of long-term neurologic sequelae if it is unassociated with PVL or intraparenchymal hemorrhage.

PREVENTION. The incidence of traumatic intracranial hemorrhage may be reduced by judicious management of cephalopelvic disproportion and operative (forceps, cesarean section) delivery. Fetal or neonatal hemorrhage due to maternal idiopathic thrombocytopenic purpura (ITP) or alloimmune thrombocytopenia may be prevented by maternal treatment with steroids, intravenous immunoglobulin, or fetal platelet transfusion. The incidence of IVH may possibly be reduced by neonatal administration of low-dose indomethacin and vitamin E. Wide fluctuations of blood pressure should be avoided. Vitamin K should be given prior to delivery to all women receiving phenobarbital or phenytoin during the pregnancy.

TREATMENT. IVH associated with hypoxic-ischemic encephalopathy is frequently associated with multiple organ system dysfunction. Seizures are treated with anticonvulsant drugs, anemia-shock requires transfusion with packed red blood cells or fresh frozen plasma, and acidosis is treated with judicious and slow administration of 1–2 mEq/kg sodium bicarbonate. Serial lumbar punctures have no role during the acute hemorrhage; however, repeated lumbar punctures may reduce the symptoms of posthemorrhagic hydrocephalus. Repeat lumbar punctures may increase the risk of nosocomial meningitis. Neurosurgical placement of an external ventriculostomy catheter may be needed in the early stage of uncontrolled symptomatic hydrocephalus. After the protein content of the ventricular fluid declines, a permanent ventricular-peritoneal shunt is put in place.

Symptomatic subdural hemorrhage in large term infants should be treated by removing the subdural fluid collection by means of a spinal needle placed through the lateral margin of the anterior fontanel. In addition to birth trauma, child abuse should be suspected in all infants with subdural effusions.

84.3 Spine and Spinal Cord

Strong traction exerted when the spine is hyperextended or when the direction of pull is lateral, or forceful longitudinal traction on the trunk while the head is still firmly engaged in the pelvis, especially when combined with flexion and torsion of the vertical axis, may produce fracture and separation of the vertebrae. Such injuries, rarely diagnosed clinically, are most likely to occur when difficulty is encountered in delivering the shoulders in cephalic presentations and the head in breech presentations. The injury occurs most commonly at the level of the 4th cervical vertebra with cephalic presentations and the lower cervical–upper thoracic vertebrae with breech presentations. Transection of the cord may occur with or without vertebral fractures; hemorrhage and edema may produce neurologic signs that are indistinguishable from those of transection except that they are not permanent. There is areflexia, loss of sensation, and complete paralysis of voluntary motion below the level of injury, although the persistence of a withdrawal reflex mediated through spinal centers distal to the area of injury is frequently misinterpreted as representing voluntary motion. If the injury is severe, the infant, who from birth may be in poor condition owing to respiratory depression, shock, or hypothermia, may deteriorate rapidly to death within several hours before neurologic signs are obvious. Alternatively, the course may be protracted with symptoms and signs appearing at birth or later in the 1st wk; immobility, flaccidity, and associated brachial plexus injuries may not be recognized for several days. Constipation may also be present. Some infants survive for prolonged periods, their initial flaccidity, immobility, and areflexia being replaced after several weeks or months by rigid flexion of extremities, increased muscle tone, and spasms. Apnea on day 1 and poor motor recovery by 3 mo are poor prognostic signs.

The differential diagnosis includes amyotonia congenita and myelodysplasia associated with spina bifida occulta. The diagnosis is confirmed by ultrasonography or magnetic resonance imaging (MRI). Treatment of the survivors is supportive, and they often remain permanently injured. When there is compression from a fracture or dislocation, the prognosis is related to the time elapsing before the compression is relieved.

84.4 Peripheral Nerve Injuries

BRACHIAL PALSY. Injury to the brachial plexus may cause paralysis of the upper arm with or without paralysis of the forearm or hand or, more commonly, paralysis of the entire arm. These injuries occur in macrosomic infants and when lateral traction is exerted on the head and neck during delivery of the shoulder in a vertex presentation, when the arms are extended over the head in a breech presentation, or when there is excessive traction on the shoulders. Approximately 45% are associated with shoulder dystocia.

In **Erb-Duchenne paralysis** the injury is limited to the 5th and 6th cervical nerves. The infant loses the power to abduct the arm from the shoulder, to rotate the arm externally, and to supinate the forearm. The characteristic position consists of adduction and internal rotation of the arm with pronation of the forearm. The power of extension of the forearm is retained, but the biceps reflex is absent; the Moro reflex is absent on the affected side (Fig. 84–2). There may be some sensory impairment on the outer aspect of the arm. The power in the forearm and the hand grasp are preserved unless the lower part of the plexus is also injured; the presence of the hand grasp is a favorable prognostic sign. When the injury includes the phrenic nerve, alteration of the diaphragmatic excursion may be observed fluoroscopically.

Klumpke paralysis is a rarer form of brachial palsy; injury to the 7th and 8th cervical nerves and the 1st thoracic nerve produces a paralyzed hand, and ipsilateral ptosis and miosis (Horner syndrome) if the sympathetic fibers of the 1st thoracic root are also injured.

The mild cases may not be detected immediately after birth. Differentiation must be made from cerebral injury; from fracture, dislocation, or epiphyseal separation of the humerus; and from fracture of the clavicle. MRI will demonstrate nerve root rupture or avulsion.

The *prognosis* depends on whether the nerve was merely injured or was lacerated. If the paralysis was due to edema and hemorrhage about the nerve fibers, there should be a return of function within a few months; if due to laceration, permanent damage may result. The involvement of the deltoid is usually the most serious problem and may result in a shoulder drop secondary to muscular atrophy. In general, paralysis of the upper arm has a better prognosis than paralysis of the lower arm.

Treatment consists of partial immobilization and appropriate positioning to prevent development of contractures. In upper arm paralysis, the arm should be abducted 90 degrees, with external rotation at the shoulder and with full supination of the forearm and slight extension at the wrist with the palm turned toward the face. This may be done with a brace or splint during the first 1–2 wk. Immobilization should be intermittent through the day while the infant is asleep and between feedings. In lower arm or hand paralysis, the wrist should be splinted in a neutral position and padding placed in the fist. When the entire arm is paralyzed, the same treatment principles should be followed. Gentle massage and range of motion exercises may be started by 7–10 days of age. Infants should be followed closely with active and passive corrective exercises. If the paralysis persists without improvement for 3–6 mo, neuroplasty, neurolysis, end-to-end anastomosis, or nerve grafting offer hope for partial recovery.

PHRENIC NERVE PARALYSIS. Phrenic nerve injury (3rd, 4th, 5th cervical nerves) with diaphragmatic paralysis must be considered when cyanosis and irregular and labored respirations develop. Such injuries, usually unilateral, are associated with ipsilateral upper brachial palsy. Because breathing is thoracic in type, the abdomen does not bulge with inspiration. Breath sounds are diminished on the affected side. The thrust of the diaphragm, which often may be felt just under the costal margin on the normal side, is absent on the affected side. The *diagnosis* is established by ultrasonography or fluoroscopic examination, which reveals the elevation of the diaphragm on the paralyzed side and seesaw movements of the two sides of the diaphragm during respiration.

There is no specific *treatment;* the infant should be placed on the involved side and given oxygen if necessary. Initially, intravenous feedings may be needed; later, progressive gavage or oral feedings may be started depending on the infant's condition. Pulmonary infections are a serious complication. Recovery usually occurs spontaneously by 1–3 mo; rarely, surgical plication of the diaphragm may be indicated.

FACIAL NERVE PALSY. Usually, facial palsy is a peripheral paralysis that results from pressure over the facial nerve in utero, from efforts during labor, or from forceps during delivery. Rarely nonobstetric, it may result from nuclear agenesis of the facial nerve. Peripheral paralysis is flaccid and, when complete, involves the entire side of the face, including the forehead. When the infant cries, there is movement only on the nonparalyzed side of the face, and the mouth is drawn to that side. On the affected side the forehead is smooth, the eye cannot be closed, the nasolabial fold is absent, and the corner of the mouth droops. The forehead will wrinkle on the affected side with central paralysis, since only the lower two thirds of the face is involved. Usually there are also other manifestations of intracranial injury, most commonly a 6th nerve palsy. The *prognosis* depends upon whether the nerve was injured by pressure or whether the nerve fibers were torn. Improvement

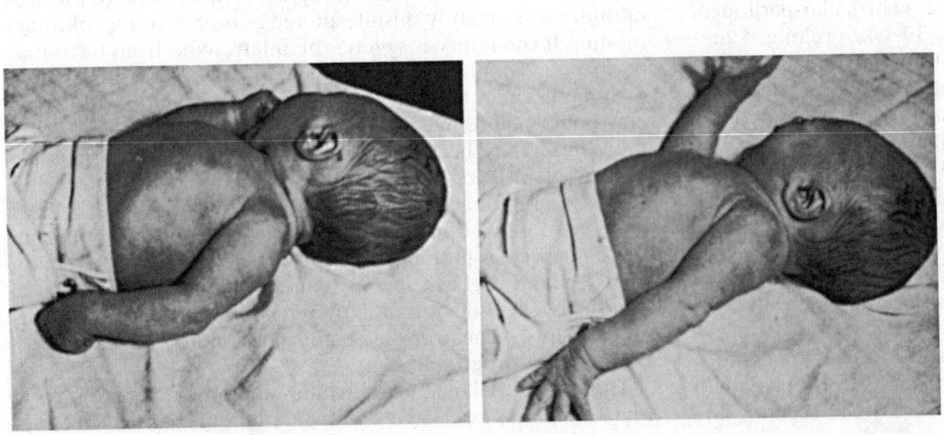

Figure 84–2. Brachial palsy of the left arm (asymmetric Moro reflex).

occurs within a few weeks in the former instance. Care of the exposed eye is essential. Neuroplasty may be indicated when the paralysis is persistent. Facial palsy may be confused with the absence of the depressor muscles of the mouth, which is a benign problem.

Other peripheral nerves are seldom injured in utero or at birth except when they are involved in fractures or hemorrhages.

84.5 Viscera

The **liver** is the only internal organ other than the brain that is injured with any frequency during birth. The damage usually results from pressure on the liver during delivery of the head in breech presentations. Large infant size, intrauterine asphyxia, coagulation disorders, extreme prematurity, and hepatomegaly are contributing factors. Incorrect cardiac massage is a less frequent cause. The liver is ruptured when there is formation of a subcapsular hematoma, which may tamponade further bleeding. The infant usually appears normal for the first 1–3 days. Nonspecific signs related to loss of blood into the hematoma may appear early and include poor feeding, listlessness, pallor, jaundice, tachypnea, and tachycardia. A mass may be palpable in the right upper quadrant; the abdomen may appear blue. The hematoma may be large enough to cause anemia. Shock and death may occur if the hematoma breaks through the capsule into the peritoneal cavity, reducing pressure and allowing fresh hemorrhage. Early suspicion by means of ultrasonographic diagnosis and prompt supportive therapy can decrease the mortality of this disorder. Surgical repair of a laceration may be required.

Rupture of the spleen may occur alone or in association with rupture of the liver. The causes, complications, treatment, and prevention are similar.

Although **adrenal hemorrhage** occurs with some frequency, especially after breech delivery in LGA or infants of diabetic mothers, its cause is undetermined; it may be due to trauma, anoxia, or severe stress, as in overwhelming infections. Ninety per cent are unilateral; 75% are right-sided. Calcified central hematomas of the adrenal have been identified roentgenographically or at autopsy in older infants and children, suggesting that not all adrenal hemorrhages are immediately fatal. In severe cases the diagnosis is usually made at postmortem examination. The symptoms are profound shock and cyanosis. There may be a mass in the flank with overlying skin discoloration; jaundice may also develop. If adrenal hemorrhage is suspected, abdominal ultrasonography may be helpful, and treatment for acute adrenal failure may be indicated (Chapter 528).

84.6 Fractures

CLAVICLE. This bone is fractured during labor and delivery more frequently than any other bone; it is particularly vulnerable when there is difficulty in delivery of the shoulder in vertex presentations and of the extended arms in breech deliveries. The infant characteristically does not move the arm freely on the affected side; crepitus and bony irregularity may be palpated, and occasionally discoloration is visible over the fracture site. The Moro reflex is absent on the affected side, and there is spasm of the sternocleidomastoid muscle with obliteration of the supraclavicular depression at the site of the fracture. In greenstick fractures there may be no limitation of movement, and the Moro reflex may be present. Fracture of the humerus or brachial palsy may also be responsible for limitation of movement of an arm and absence of a Moro reflex on the affected side. The *prognosis* is excellent. *Treatment,* if any, consists of immobilization of the arm and shoulder on the affected side. A remarkable degree of callus develops at the site within a week and may be the first evidence of the fracture.

EXTREMITIES

In fractures of the long bones spontaneous movement of the extremity is usually absent. The Moro reflex is also absent from the involved extremity. There may be associated nerve involvement. Satisfactory results of treatment for a fractured humerus are obtained with 2–4 wk of immobilization during which the arm is strapped to the chest, a triangular splint and a Velpeau bandage are applied, or a cast is applied. For fracture of the femur, good results are obtained with traction-suspension of both lower extremities, even if the fracture is unilateral; the legs, immobilized in a spica cast, are attached to an overhead frame. Splints are effective for treatment of fractures of the forearm or leg. Healing is usually accompanied by excess callus formation.The *prognosis* is excellent for fractures of the extremities. Fractures in preterm infants are related to osteopenia (Chapter 92).

Dislocations and **epiphyseal separations** rarely result from birth trauma. The upper femoral epiphysis may be separated by forcible manipulation of the infant's leg as, for example, in breech extraction or after version. There is swelling, slight shortening, limitation of active motion, painful passive motion, and external rotation of the leg. The diagnosis is established roentgenographically. The prognosis is good for the milder injuries, but coxa vara frequently results from extensive displacement.

NOSE. The most prevalent injury of the nose is a dislocation of the cartilaginous portion of the septum from the vomerine groove and the columella. The infant may have difficulty in nursing and some impairment in nasal respiration. On physical examination, the nares appear asymmetric and the nose flattened. An oral airway rarely is needed, and surgical consultation should be obtained for definitive treatment.

84.7 Hypoxia-Ischemia

(Asphyxia)

Anoxia is a term used to indicate the consequences of a complete lack of oxygen due to a number of primary causes. *Hypoxia* refers to an arterial concentration of oxygen that is less than normal, and *ischemia* refers to blood flow to cells or organs that is insufficient to maintain their normal function. *Hypoxic-ischemic encephalopathy* is an important cause of permanent damage to central nervous system cells, which may result in neonatal death or which may be manifest later as cerebral palsy or mental deficiency. Its prevention and treatment are those of the basic conditions that cause it; death and disability may sometimes be prevented through symptomatic treatment with oxygen or artificial respiration and the correction of associated multiorgan system dysfunction (Table 84–1).

ETIOLOGY. Fetal hypoxia may result from (1) inadequate oxygenation of maternal blood as a result of hypoventilation during anesthesia, cyanotic heart disease, respiratory failure, or carbon monoxide poisoning; (2) low maternal blood pressure as a result of the hypotension that may complicate spinal anesthesia or that may result from compression of the vena cava and aorta by the gravid uterus; (3) inadequate relaxation

■ TABLE 84–1 Effects of Asphyxia

System	Effect
Central nervous system	Hypoxic-ischemic encephalopathy, infarction, intracranial hemorrhage, seizures, cerebral edema, hypotonia, hypertonia
Cardiovascular	Myocardial ischemia, poor contractility, cardiac stun, tricuspid insufficiency, hypotension
Pulmonary	Persistent fetal circulation, pulmonary hemorrhage, respiratory distress syndrome
Renal	Acute tubular or cortical necrosis
Adrenal	Adrenal hemorrhage
Gastrointestinal	Perforation, ulceration, necrosis
Metabolic	Inappropriate secretion of ADH, hyponatremia, hypoglycemia, hypocalcemia, myoglobinuria
Integument	Subcutaneous fat necrosis
Hematology	Disseminated intravascular coagulation

of the uterus to permit placental filling as a result of uterine tetany caused by excessive administration of oxytocin; (4) premature separation of the placenta; (5) impedance to the circulation of blood through the umbilical cord as a result of compression or knotting of the cord; (6) uterine vessel vasoconstriction by cocaine; and (7) placental insufficiency from numerous causes, including toxemia and postmaturity.

Placental insufficiency often remains undetected on clinical assessment. Chronically hypoxic fetuses may develop intrauterine growth retardation without traditional signs of fetal distress (e.g., bradycardia). Doppler umbilical waveform velocimetry (demonstrating increased fetal vascular resistance, Fig. 81–3) and cordocentesis (demonstrating fetal hypoxia) identify the chronically hypoxic infant. Uterine contractions further reduce umbilical oxygenation, depressing the fetal cardiovascular and central nervous systems and resulting in low Apgar scores and postnatal hypoxia in the delivery room.

After birth, hypoxia may result from (1) anemia severe enough to lower the oxygen content of the blood to a critical level due to severe hemorrhage or hemolytic disease; (2) shock severe enough to interfere with the transport of oxygen to vital cells from adrenal hemorrhage, intraventricular hemorrhage, overwhelming infection, or massive blood loss; (3) a deficit in arterial oxygen saturation resulting from failure to breathe adequately postnatally due to a cerebral defect, narcosis, or injury; and (4) failure of oxygenation of an adequate amount of blood resulting from severe forms of cyanotic congenital heart disease or deficient pulmonary function.

PATHOPHYSIOLOGY AND PATHOLOGY. Within minutes of the onset of total fetal hypoxia bradycardia, hypotension, decreased cardiac output, and severe metabolic as well as respiratory acidosis occur. The initial circulatory response of the fetus is increased shunting through the ductus venosus, ductus arteriosus, and foramen ovale with transient maintenance of perfusion of the brain, heart, and adrenals in preference to the lungs (due to pulmonary vasoconstriction), liver, kidneys, and intestine.

The pathology of hypoxia-ischemia is dependent upon the affected organ and the severity of the insult. Early congestion, fluid leak from increased capillary permeability, and endothelial cell swelling may then lead to signs of coagulation necrosis and cell death. Congestion and petechiae are seen in the pericardium, pleura, thymus, heart, adrenals, and meninges. Prolonged intrauterine hypoxia may result in PVL and pulmonary arteriole smooth muscle hyperplasia, which predisposes the infant to pulmonary hypertension (Chapter 87.7). If fetal distress produces gasping, amniotic fluid contents (meconium, squames, lanuga hair) are aspirated into the trachea or lungs.

The combination of chronic fetal hypoxia and acute hypoxic-ischemic injury after birth results in gestational age-specific neuropathology. Term infants demonstrate neuronal necrosis of the cortex (later cortical atrophy) and parasagittal ischemic injury. Preterm infants demonstrate PVL (later spastic diplegia), status marmoratus of the basal ganglia, and IVH. Term, more often than preterm, infants demonstrate focal or multifocal cortical infarcts that produce focal seizures and hemiplegia. Infarctions are best visualized with CT scanning or MRI. In addition to focal lesions, CT scanning may demonstrate diffuse decreases of tissue attenuation. Cerebral edema with resultant increased intracranial pressure occurs in some infants who have severe hypoxic-ischemic encephalopathy. Excitatory amino acids may play an important role in the pathogenesis of asphyxial brain injury.

CLINICAL MANIFESTATIONS. The signs of hypoxia in the *fetus* are usually noted a few minutes to a few days before delivery. IUGR with increased vascular resistance may be the first indication of fetal hypoxia. The fetal heart rate slows, and the beat-to-beat variability declines. Continuous heart rate recording may reveal a variable or late (type II dips) deceleration pattern (see Fig. 81–4), and fetal scalp blood analysis may show a pH less than 7.20. The acidosis is made up of varying degrees of metabolic or respiratory components. Particularly in the infant near term, these signs should lead to the administration of high concentrations of oxygen to the mother and immediate delivery to avoid fetal death or central nervous system damage.

At *delivery* the presence of yellow, meconium-stained amniotic fluid is evidence that there has been fetal distress. At birth these infants are frequently depressed and fail to breathe spontaneously. During the ensuing hours they may remain hypotonic or change from hypotonia to extreme hypertonia, or their tone may appear normal (Table 84–2). Pallor, cyanosis, apnea, slow heart rate, and unresponsiveness to stimulation also are signs of hypoxic-ischemic encephalopathy. Cerebral edema may develop during the next 24 hr and result in profound brain stem depression. During this time seizure activity may occur that may be severe and refractory to the usual doses of anticonvulsants. Lorazepam (0.05–0.1 mg/kg, IV) may be used during the acute seizure, while continuing suppression of seizures may require an IV loading dose of 20–25 mg/kg of phenobarbital or 20 mg/kg of phenytoin. Although most often a result of the hypoxic-ischemic encephalopathy, seizures in asphyxiated newborns may also be due to hypocalcemia and hypoglycemia.

In addition to central nervous system dysfunction, conges-

■ TABLE 84–2 Hypoxic-Ischemic Encephalopathy in Term Infants

Signs	Stage 1	Stage 2	Stage 3
Level of consciousness	Hyperalert	Lethargic	Stuporous, coma
Muscle tone	Normal	Hypotonic	Flaccid
Posture	Normal	Flexion	Decerebrate
Tendon reflexes/clonus	Hyperactive	Hyperactive	Absent
Myoclonus	Present	Present	Absent
Moro reflex	Strong	Weak	Absent
Pupils	Mydriasis	Miosis	Unequal, poor light reflex
Seizures	None	Common	Decerebration
Electroencephalographic	Normal	Low voltage changing to seizure activity	Burst suppression to isoelectric
Duration	<24 hr if progresses, otherwise may remain normal	24 hr to 14 days	Days to weeks
Outcome	Good	Variable	Death, severe deficits

Modified from Sarnat H, Sarnat M: Neonatal encephalopathy following fetal distress: A clinical and electroencephalographic study. Arch Neurol 33:696, 1976. Copyright 1976, American Medical Association.

tive heart failure and cardiogenic shock, persistent pulmonary hypertension (persistent fetal circulation), respiratory distress syndrome, gastrointestinal perforation, hematuria, and acute tubular necrosis are associated with perinatal asphyxia (see Table 84–1).

After delivery hypoxia is due to respiratory failure and circulatory insufficiency (Chapter 87).

PROGNOSIS. The outcome of perinatal asphyxia depends on whether its metabolic and cardiopulmonary complications (hypoxia, hypoglycemia, shock) can be treated, on the infant's gestational age (outcome is poorest if infant is preterm), and on the severity of the hypoxic-ischemic encephalopathy. Severe encephalopathy (stage 3, see Table 84–2), characterized by flaccid coma, apnea, absent oculocephalic reflexes, refractory seizures, and a marked decrease of cortical attenuation on CT, is associated with a poor prognosis. A low Apgar score at 20 min, absence of spontaneous respirations at 20 min of age, and persistence of abnormal neurologic signs at 2 wk of age also predict death or severe cognitive and motor deficits.

Brain death following neonatal hypoxic-ischemic encephalopathy is diagnosed by the clinical findings of coma that is unresponsive to pain, auditory, or visual stimulation; apnea with P_{CO_2} rising from 40 to over 60 mm Hg; and absent brain stem reflexes (pupil, oculocephalic, oculovestibular, corneal, gag, sucking). These must occur in the absence of hypothermia, hypotension, and elevated levels of depressant drugs (e.g., phenobarbital). The absence of cerebral blood flow on radionuclide scan and electrical activity on EEG (electrocerebral silence) is inconsistently observed in clinically brain dead neonatal infants. Persistence of the clinical criteria for 2 days in term and 3 days in preterm infants predicts brain death in most asphyxiated newborns. Nonetheless, there is no universal agreement about the definition of neonatal brain death. Consideration of withdrawal of life support should include discussions with the family, the health care team, and, if there is disagreement, an ethics committee. The best interest of the infant involves judgments about the benefits and harm of continuing therapy and of avoiding continuing futile therapy regardless of the presence of brain death.

Cordes I, Roland EH, Lupton BA, et al: Early prediction of the development of microcephaly after hypoxic-ischemic encephalopathy in the full-term newborn. Pediatrics 93:703, 1994.

Hagberg H, Thornberg E, Blennow M, et al: Excitatory amino acids in the cerebrospinal fluid of asphyxiated infants: Relationship to hypoxic-ischemic encephalopathy. Acta Paediatr 82:925, 1993.

Jongmans M, Henderson S, de Vries L, et al: Duration of periventricular densities in preterm infants and neurological outcome at 6 years of age. Arch Dis Child 69:9, 1993.

Legido A: Perinatal hypoxic ischemic encephalopathy: Recent advances in diagnosis and treatment. Int Pediatr 9:114, 1994.

MacKinnon JA, Perlman M, Kirpalani H, et al: Spinal cord injury at birth: Diagnostic and prognostic data in twenty-two patients. J Pediatr 122:431, 1993.

Ment LR, Oh W, Ehrenkranz RA, et al: Low-dose indomethacin and prevention of intraventricular hemorrhage: A multicenter randomized trial. Pediatrics 93:543, 1994.

Mizrahi EM: Clinical diagnosis and management of neonatal seizures. Int Pediatr 9:94, 1994.

Nocon JJ, McKenzie DK, Thomas LJ, et al: Shoulder dystocia: An analysis of risks and obstetric maneuvers. Am J Obstet Gynecol 168:1732, 1993.

Rehan VK, Seshia MMK: Spinal cord birth injury—diagnostic difficulties. Arch Dis Child 69:92, 1993.

Reynolds EOR: Prevention of periventricular hemorrhage. Pediatrics 93:677, 1994.

Rogers B, Msall M, Owens T, et al: Cystic periventricular leukomalacia and type of cerebral palsy in preterm infants. J Pediatr 125:S1, 1994.

Roth SC, Baudin J, McCormick DC, et al: Relation between ultrasound appearance of the brain of very preterm infants and neurodevelopmental impairment at eight years. Dev Med Child Neurol 35:755, 1993.

Schullinger JN: Birth trauma. Pediatr Clin North Am 40:1351, 1993.

Ventriculomegaly Trial Group: Randomised trial of early tapping in neonatal posthaemorrhagic ventricular dilatation: results at 30 months. Arch Dis Child 70:F129, 1994.

Volpe JJ: Brain injury caused by intraventricular hemorrhage: is indomethacin the silver bullet for prevention? Pediatrics 93:673, 1994.

CHAPTER 85

Delivery Room Emergencies

The most common and important emergency related to the newborn infant in the delivery room is the failure to initiate and maintain respirations. Less frequent, but of major importance, are shock, severe anemia (Chapter 89.1), plethora (Chapter 89.4), convulsions (Chapter 543.5), and management of life-threatening congenital malformations (Chapter 83).

RESPIRATORY DISTRESS AND FAILURE. Disorders of respiration in the newborn infant can be categorized as either *central nervous system failure,* representing depression or failure of the respiratory center, or *peripheral respiratory difficulty,* indicating interference with the alveolar exchange of oxygen and carbon dioxide. Cyanosis occurs in both groups (see Table 83–1). The respiratory problems encountered in the delivery room are most frequently those of airway obstruction and of depression of the central nervous system with the absence of adequate respiratory effort.

Respiratory distress in the presence of good respiratory effort should lead to an immediate consideration of peripheral causes; *it is an indication for a roentgenographic examination of the chest,* if this is at all possible.

If respiratory movements are made with the mouth closed but the infant fails to move air in and out of the lungs, bilateral **choanal atresia** (Chapter 325) or other obstruction of the upper respiratory tract should be suspected. The mouth should be opened, and the mouth and posterior pharynx cleared of secretions by gentle suction. An oropharyngeal airway should be inserted and the source of the obstruction sought immediately. If effective respiratory flow is not produced by opening the infant's mouth and clearing the airway, laryngoscopy is indicated. With obstructive malformations of the epiglottis, larynx, or trachea, an endotracheal tube should be inserted; prolonged endotracheal intubation or tracheostomy may be required. Respiratory failure due to depression or injury of the central nervous system may require continuous artificial ventilation with a face mask and bag or through an endotracheal tube.

Hypoplasia of the mandible (Pierre Robin syndrome) (Chapter 257) with posterior displacement of the tongue may result in symptoms similar to those of choanal atresia, which may be temporarily relieved by pulling the tongue forward. A scaphoid abdomen suggests a **diaphragmatic hernia** or **eventration,** as does asymmetry of contour or movement of the chest or shift of the apical impulse of the heart; these latter manifestations are also compatible with tension pneumothorax.

Causes of peripheral respiratory difficulty are discussed in Chapter 87.

FAILURE TO INITIATE OR SUSTAIN RESPIRATION. This usually originates in the central nervous system as the result of asphyxia; immaturity in itself is seldom a causative factor except in infants weighing less than 1,000 g. Intrapulmonary problems, such as the pulmonary hypoplasia associated with Potter syndrome and severe organized intrauterine pneumonia, may at times result in poorly sustained ventilation. The lungs in these infants are very noncompliant, and efforts to begin respirations may be inadequate to start sufficient ventilation.

Narcosis results from heavy doses of morphine, Demerol, barbiturates, reserpine, or tranquilizers administered to the mother shortly before delivery or from maternal anesthesia, given during the second stage of labor. The infant is cyanotic and hypotonic at birth and slow to cry or breathe; when respiration is established, it is extremely slow.

Narcosis should be avoided by using appropriate analgesic and anesthetic practices. Treatment includes initial physical stimulation and securing a patent airway. If effective ventilation is not initiated, artificial breathing with a mask and bag must be instituted. At the same time, if depression is due to morphine or its derivatives, Narcan (naloxone hydrochloride), 0.1 mg/kg, should be given by intravenous, subcutaneous, intratracheal, or intramuscular routes and repeated q 2–3 min if needed. Ventilation is essential prior to and during the administration of this antidote. If depression is due to other anesthetics or analgesics, artificial respiration should be continued until the infant is able to sustain ventilation. Central nervous system stimulant drugs should not be used because they are ineffective and may be harmful.

Prenatal or **perinatal hypoxia** of whatever cause, if sufficiently severe, will produce brain stem depression and secondary apnea, which is unresponsive to sensory stimulation. Death due to apnea may be prevented by resuscitation, provided the basic cause of the hypoxia can be eliminated within a reasonable time while artificial respiration, if necessary, is being carried out. External cardiac massage, correction of acidosis, and circulatory support with drugs may be important adjuncts to ventilation.

RESUSCITATION. The *goals* of neonatal resuscitation are to prevent the morbidity and mortality associated with hypoxic-ischemic tissue (brain, heart, kidney) injury and to re-establish adequate spontaneous respiration and cardiac output. High-risk situations should be anticipated by the history of the pregnancy, labor, and delivery and by identification of the signs of fetal distress. Although the Apgar score is helpful in evaluating patients in need of attention, infants who are born limp, cyanotic, apneic, or pulseless require immediate resuscitation prior to assignment of the 1-min Apgar score. Rapid and appropriate resuscitative efforts improve the likelihood of preventing brain damage and achieving a successful outcome.

Immediately after birth an asphyxiated neonatal infant should be placed under a radiant heater (to avoid hypothermia), dried, positioned head down and slightly extended, the airway cleared by suctioning, and gentle tactile stimulation provided (slapping the foot, rubbing the back). Simultaneously, the infant's color, heart rate, and respiratory effort should be assessed.

The steps in neonatal resuscitation follow the ABCs: **A,** anticipate and establish a patent *a*irway by suctioning and, if necessary, perform endotracheal intubation; **B,** initiate *b*reathing using tactile stimulation or positive pressure ventilation with a bag and mask or through an endotracheal tube; **C,** maintain the *c*irculation with chest compression and medications, if needed.

If there are no respirations or if the heart rate is below 100/min, *positive pressure ventilation* with 100% oxygen is given through a tightly fitted face mask and bag for 15–30 sec. Although the first breath may require pressures as low as 15–20 cm H_2O, pressures as high as 30–40 cm H_2O may be needed. Subsequent breaths are given at a rate of 40–60 min, with pressures of 15–20 cm H_2O. Noncompliant stiff lungs due to hyaline membrane disease, congenital pneumonia, or meconium aspiration need higher pressures (20–40 cm H_2O). Successful ventilation is determined by good chest rise, symmetric breath sounds, improved pink color, heart rate greater than 100/min, spontaneous respirations, and improved tone.

If there is a history of maternal analgesic narcotic drug administration, *Narcan* (naloxone, 0.1 mg/kg, through the subcutaneous, intramuscular, intravenous, or intratracheal route) is given while adequate ventilation is maintained. Breathing for the depressed infant should be maintained until a response to Narcan is noted. Continuous observation of the infant is important because repeated doses of Narcan may be needed.

If the heart rate does not improve after 15–30 sec with bag and mask (or endotracheal) ventilation and remains below 60/min or if the rate is less than 80/min and not rising, ventilation is continued and *chest compression* with two fingers is initiated over the lower third of the sternum at a rate of 120/min. The ratio of compressions to ventilation is 3:1. Bradycardia in neonatal infants is usually due to hypoxia resulting from respiratory arrest and often responds to ventilation with 100% oxygen. Persistent bradycardia despite ventilation with 100% oxygen suggests more severe cardiac compromise or inadequate ventilation techniques. Poor response to ventilation may be due to a loosely fitted mask, poor positioning of the airway, intraesophageal intubation, airway obstruction, insufficient pressure, pleural effusions, pneumothorax, excessive air in the stomach, asystole, hypovolemia, diaphragmatic hernia, or prolonged intrauterine asphyxia.

Endotracheal intubation should be performed by an experienced person in any infant who does not respond to initial bag and mask ventilation or who was born apneic, pulseless, cyanotic, and limp with signs of fetal distress.

Medications should be administered when the heart rate is less than 80/min following 30 sec of combined ventilation and chest compressions or during asystole. Usually the umbilical vein can be readily cannulated and should be used for immediate administration of medications, glucose, and volume expanders during neonatal resuscitation. Epinephrine (0.1–0.3 mL/kg of a 1:10,000 solution, intravenous or intratracheal) is given for asystole or for failure to respond to 30 sec of combined resuscitation. The dose may be repeated every 5 min. If there is no response, some authorities recommend using 5 to 10 times the standard dose of epinephrine. Ten to 20 ml/kg of volume expanders (normal saline, blood, 5% albumin, Ringer's lactate) should be given for hypovolemia, pallor, electrical-mechanical dissociation (weak pulses with normal heart rate), history of blood loss, suspicion of septic shock, hypotension, or poor response to resuscitation. Sodium bicarbonate (1–2 mEq/kg, 0.5 mEq/mL of a 4.2% solution) should be given slowly (1 mEq/kg/min) if there is a documented metabolic acidosis and the resuscitation is prolonged. Sodium bicarbonate should be given after effective ventilation has been established because such therapy may increase blood CO_2, producing a respiratory acidosis. Restoration of oxygenation and tissue perfusion is the main treatment for the metabolic acidosis associated with asphyxia.

Severe asphyxia also may depress myocardial function, causing cardiogenic shock despite recovery of heart and respiratory rates. Dopamine or dobutamine administered as a continuous infusion (5–20 μg/kg/min) and volume expanders should be started after the initial resuscitation effort to improve cardiac output in an infant with poor peripheral perfusion, weak pulses, hypotension, tachycardia, and poor urine output. Epinephrine (0.1 μg/kg/min) may be indicated for infants in severe shock who do not respond to dopamine or dobutamine.

Less severe degrees of asphyxia can usually be managed by brief periods of bag and mask ventilation of 100% oxygen. Chest compression and medications are not needed for most neonates who have mild to moderate birth depression. Regardless of the severity of asphyxia or the response to resuscitation, asphyxiated infants should be monitored closely for signs of multiorgan hypoxic-ischemic tissue injury (see Table 84–1).

SHOCK. Circulatory insufficiency may present at birth as a result of internal hemorrhage; fetal bleeding during gestation, labor, or delivery (e.g., fetofetal or fetomaternal transfusion syndrome); bleeding from the fetal circulation secondary to a placental tear during amniocentesis; excessive bleeding from a severed or torn umbilical cord; or severe hemolytic anemia. Clinical manifestations include signs of respiratory distress, cyanosis, pallor, flaccidity, cold mottled skin, tachycardia or bradycardia, hepatosplenomegaly, and, rarely, convulsions. **Edema** and hepatosplenomegaly also may suggest hydrops fetalis or congestive heart failure without shock. Shock from overwhelming infection may also be present after birth.

Supportive treatment with type O, Rh negative blood, plasma, or electrolyte solutions is indicated for hypovolemia. Oxygen should be administered and metabolic acidosis corrected with sodium bicarbonate. β-Sympathomimetic agents, such as dopamine or dobutamine, may be needed to support cardiac output and blood pressure. The diagnosis and treatment of erythroblastosis fetalis are discussed in Chapter 89.2. If infection is present, appropriate antibiotics must be started as soon as possible.

After supportive measures have stabilized the infant's condition, a specific diagnosis should be established and appropriate continuing treatment instituted.

Aylward GP, Pfeiffer SI, Wright A, et al: Outcome studies of low birth weight infants published in the last decade: A meta analysis. J Pediatr 115:515, 1989.
Blair E, Stanley FJ: Intrapartum asphyxia: A rare cause of cerebral palsy. J Pediatr 112:515, 1988.
Catlin EA, Carpenter MW, Brann BS IV, et al: The Apgar score revisited: Influence of gestational age. J Pediatr 109:865, 1986.
Davis DJ: How aggressive should delivery room cardiopulmonary resuscitation be for extremely low birth weight neonates? Pediatrics 92:447, 1993.
Emergency Cardiac Care Committee and Subcommittees, American Heart Association: Guidelines for cardiopulmonary resuscitation and emergency cardiac care. Neonatal resuscitation. JAMA 268:2276, 1992.
Lees M, King D: Cyanosis in the newborn. Pediatr Rev 9:36, 1987.
Marrin M, Paes BA: Birth asphyxia: Does the Apgar score have diagnostic value? Obstet Gynecol 72:120, 1988.
Perlman JM, Tack ED, Martin T, et al: Acute systemic organ injury in term infants after asphyxia. Am J Dis Child 143:617, 1989.
Wimmer JE: Neonatal resuscitation. Pediatr Rev 15:255, 1994.

CHAPTER 86
Dysmorphology

Kenneth Lyons Jones

The field of dysmorphology has expanded dramatically as the number of recognizable patterns of malformation has more than tripled during the last 25 yr. New insights have been gained into the pathogenesis of various structural defects; the potential prenatal effect of various drugs, chemicals, and environmental agents has been better appreciated; and the number of defects in which prenatal detection is possible has increased. Because of their vast number, a listing of all known recognizable patterns of malformation will not be presented. Rather, this chapter provides an approach to the child with the prenatal onset of structural defects. The approach is predicated upon the concept that the nature of the structural defects represents a clue to the time of onset, mechanism of injury, and possible etiology of the problem, all of which determine the necessary evaluation. This permits a systematic narrowing of the diagnostic possibilities so that other sections of this textbook or one of the basic compendiums on dysmorphology can be used to make a specific diagnosis.

Structural defects of prenatal onset can be separated into those that represent a *single primary defect* in development and those that represent a multiple malformation syndrome. In most cases, the defect involves only a single structure, the child being otherwise completely normal. The seven most common single primary defects in development are congenital hip dislocation (Chapter 627.1), talipes equinovarus (Chapters 623–624), cleft lip with or without cleft palate (Chapter 256), cleft palate alone (Chapter 256), cardiac septal defects (Chapter 286.5), pyloric stenosis (Chapter 275.1), and defects in neural tube closure (Chapter 542.1). For most, the etiology is unknown, and counseling as to recurrence risk is difficult. However, most single primary defects are explained on the basis of multifactorial inheritance (Chapter 66), which carries a recurrence risk of between 2% and 5% for the next child of unaffected parents with one affected child.

The extent to which multifactorial inheritance contributes to the etiology of some of the less common single defects in development is unclear. The fact that single primary defects are etiologically heterogeneous implies that some have an environmental etiology and others result from dominantly or recessively inherited single altered genes. Craniosynostosis (Chapter 542.12) secondary to in utero constraint is an example of the former, whereas postaxial polydactyly (Chapter 630.7) illustrates the latter. Before multifactorial risk figures are used for counseling when a single primary defect is recognized, references should be consulted to determine whether other risk figures are available.

In contrast to the concept of the single primary defect in development, the designation *multiple malformation syndrome* is used when several observed structural defects all have the same known or presumed etiology. The defects usually include a number of anatomically unrelated errors in morphogenesis. Multiple malformation syndromes are caused by chromosomal abnormalities, by teratogens, and by single gene defects inherited in mendelian patterns. Risks of recurrence range from 0 in cases that represent fresh gene mutations or are caused by teratogens to 100% in the case of a child with the Down syndrome in which the mother is a balanced 21/21 translocation carrier (Chapter 67).

SINGLE PRIMARY DEFECTS IN DEVELOPMENT. These defects are subcategorized according to the nature of the error in morphogenesis that has produced the observed structural defect: malformation, deformation, or disruption of developing structure. A *malformation* is a primary structural defect arising from a localized error in morphogenesis. A *deformation* is an alteration in shape or structure of a part that has differentiated normally. The term *disruption* is used for a structural defect resulting from destruction of a previously normally formed part.

Malformations. Most children with a localized malformation such as cardiac septal defect or pyloric stenosis are otherwise completely normal. After surgical correction, prognosis is excellent. When neither dominant nor recessive inheritance is established, multifactorial recurrence risk factors (2–5%) apply to unaffected parents.

Deformations. Most deformations involve the musculoskeletal system and are probably caused by intrauterine molding. The pressure producing such molding may be intrinsic, due to neuromuscular imbalance within the fetus, or may be extrinsic, secondary to fetal crowding. In either case, the impaired ability of the fetus to kick results in decreased fetal movement, an important factor in development of the normal musculoskeletal system, particularly with respect to normal joint development. In addition, marked positional deformation of any body part can occur when the fetus is unable to change position and thus alter the direction along which potentially deforming forces are being directed.

Intrinsically derived positional deformation of prenatal onset occurs in disorders involving muscle degeneration, such as the Steinert myotonic dystrophy syndrome, and disorders involving motor neurons, such as Werdnig-Hoffmann disease (Chapter 563.2). Early defects in development of the central nervous system are more common causes of positional deformations and should be seriously considered whenever a structural defect is thought to be intrinsically derived.

appropriate grammar and articulation; better reading than mathematics ability; and cognitive dysfunction ranging from learning disabilities to mental retardation. This knowledge of a child's particular strengths and weaknesses may allow educators to develop a curriculum that will give affected children a better chance to reach their potential.

Finally, there are certain nonrandom associations of malformations for which it has not been determined whether the pattern is a sequence or a syndrome. These are designated associations. One important clinical example is the *VATER association*, which includes *v*ertebral defects, *a*nal atresia, *t*racheo-*e*sophageal fistula with atresia, *r*adial upper limb hypoplasia, and *r*enal defects. Single umbilical artery and cardiac and genital anomalies also occur in this association. These defects are likely to occur together in almost any combination of two or more and usually represent a sporadic occurrence in an otherwise normal family.

The ultimate goal in evaluating a child with structural defects is making a specific overall diagnosis. When this is achieved, appropriate recurrence risk counseling for the parents, accurate prognostication about the child's future development, and an appropriate plan to help the child reach his or her potential usually are possible. When an overall diagnosis is lacking, the most that can be expected is a better understanding of the nature and onset of the problem, which often may be helpful to parents and to others dealing with the child.

Breuning MH, Dauwerse HG, Fugazza G, et al: Rubinstein-Taybi syndrome caused by submicroscopic deletions within 16p 13.3. Am J Hum Genet 52:249, 1993.
Briggs GG, Freeman RK, Yaffe SJ: Drugs in Pregnancy and Lactation, 4th ed. Baltimore, Williams & Wilkins, 1994.
Dilts CV, Morris CA, Leonard CO: Hypothesis for development of a behavioral phenotype in Williams syndrome. Am J Med Genet (Suppl)6:126, 1990.
Dunn PM: Congenital postural deformities. Br Med Bull 32:71, 1976.
Ewart AK, Morris CA, Atkinson D, et al: Hemizygosity at the elastin locus in a developmental disorder, Williams syndrome. Nature Genet 5:11, 1993.
Gorlin RJ, Cohen MM, Levin LS: Syndromes of the Head and Neck, 3rd ed. New York, Oxford University Press, 1990.
Higginbottom MC, Jones KL, Hall BD, et al: The amniotic band disruption complex. Timing of amniotic rupture and variable spectra of consequent defects. J Pediatr 95:544, 1979.
Johnson HG, Ekman P, Frieseu W, et al: A behavioral phenotype in the deLange syndrome. Pediatr Res 10:843, 1976.
Jones KL: Smith's Recognizable Patterns of Human Malformation, 4th ed. Philadelphia, WB Saunders, 1988.
Kalter H, Warkany J: Congenital malformation, etiologic factors and their role in prevention. N Engl J Med 308:424, 1983.
Kausseff BG, Newkirk P, Root AW: Brachmann–de Lange syndrome. 1994 update. Arch Pediatr Adolesc Med 148:749, 1994.
Kazazian HH Jr: The nature of mutation. Hosp Pract 20:55, 1985.
Lie RT, Wilcox AJ, and Skjaerven R: A population-based study of the risk of recurrence of birth defects. N Engl J Med 331:1, 1994.
McKusick VA: Mendelian Inheritance in Man. Catalog of Autosomal Dominant, Autosomal Recessive and X-linked Phenotypes, 10th ed. Baltimore, The Johns Hopkins University Press, 1992.
Shepard TH: A Catalog of Teratogenic Agents, 7th ed. Baltimore, The Johns Hopkins University Press, 1992.

CHAPTER 87

Respiratory Tract Disorders

Robert M. Kliegman

Disturbances of respiration in the immediate postnatal period may have originated in utero, in the delivery room, or in the nursery. A wide variety of pathologic lesions may be responsible for one or more of the signs of respiratory distress (see Tables 83–1 and 83–2); cyanosis is common and, if respiratory embarrassment is severe, pallor may also be present. It is occasionally difficult to distinguish cardiovascular from respiratory disturbances on the basis of clinical signs alone. Signs of respiratory distress in the newborn infant may suggest hyaline membrane disease (respiratory distress syndrome), aspiration syndrome, pneumonia, sepsis, congenital heart disease, heart failure, choanal atresia, hypoglycemia, hypoplasia of the mandible with posterior displacement of the tongue, macroglossia, malformation of the epiglottis, malformation or injury of the larynx, cysts or neoplasms of the larynx or chest, pneumothorax, lobar emphysema, pulmonary agenesis or hypoplasia, congenital pulmonary lymphangiectasis, Wilson-Mikity syndrome, tracheoesophageal fistula, avulsion of the phrenic nerve, hernia or eventration of the diaphragm, intracranial lesions, neuromuscular disorders, and metabolic disturbances. *Any sign of postnatal respiratory distress is an indication for a roentgenogram of the chest.*

87.1 Transition to Pulmonary Respiration

The successful establishment of adequate lung function at birth is dependent on unobstructed anatomy and gestational age or maturity. Fluid filling the fetal lung must be removed, gas-containing functional residual capacity (FRC) established and maintained, and a ventilation-perfusion relationship developed that will provide optimal exchange of oxygen and carbon dioxide between alveoli and blood (Chapters 319, 320, and 321).

THE FIRST BREATH. During vaginal delivery, intermittent compression of the thorax facilitates removal of lung fluid. Surfactant in the fluid enhances aeration of the gas-free lung by reducing surface tension, thereby lowering the pressure required to open alveoli. Nevertheless, the pressures required to inflate the airless lung are higher than those needed at any other period of life; they range from 10–50 cm of H_2O for 0.5- to 1.0-sec intervals compared with about 4 cm for normal breathing in term infants and adults. Most infants require the lower range of opening pressures. Higher pressures necessary to initiate respiration are required to overcome the opposing forces of surface tension (particularly in small airways) and the viscosity of liquid remaining in the airways as well as to introduce about 50 mL of air into the lungs, 20–30 ml of which remains after the first breath to establish the FRC. Most of the liquid in the lung is removed by the pulmonary circulation, which increases many fold at birth because all of the right ventricular output perfuses the pulmonary vascular bed. The remainder of the fluid is removed by the pulmonary lymphatics, expelled by the infant, swallowed, or aspirated from the oropharynx; removal may be impaired following cesarean section, endothelial cell damage, or neonatal sedation.

The stimuli responsible for the first breath are multiple, and their relative importance is uncertain. They include a fall in PO_2 and pH and a rise in PCO_2 due to the interruption of the placental circulation, a redistribution of cardiac output after the umbilical cord is clamped, a decrease in body temperature, and a variety of tactile stimuli.

Compared with the term infant, the LBW infant who has a very compliant chest wall may be at a disadvantage in accomplishing the first breath. The FRC is least in the most immature infants, reflecting the presence of atelectasis. Abnormalities in the ventilation-perfusion ratio are greater and persist for longer periods of time, as does gas trapping. There may be a low PaO_2 (50–60 mm Hg) and elevated $PaCO_2$, reflecting atelectasis, intrapulmonary shunting, and hypoventilation. The smallest immature infants have the most profound disturbances, which may resemble respiratory distress syndrome.

BREATHING PATTERNS IN NEWBORNS. During sleep in the first months of life, normal full-term infants may have infrequent episodes when regular breathing is interrupted with short pauses. This **periodic breathing** pattern, shifting from a regular rhythmicity to cyclic brief episodes of intermittent apnea, is more common in the premature infant, who may have apneic pauses of 5–10 sec followed by a burst of rapid respirations at a rate of 50–60/min for 10–15 sec. There is rarely an associated change in color or heart rate, and it often stops without apparent reason. Periodic breathing persists intermittently usually until premature infants are about 36 wk of gestational age. If the infant is hypoxic, an increase in inspired oxygen concentration will often convert periodic to regular breathing. Transfusion of packed red blood cells or external physical stimulation may also reduce the number of apneic episodes. There is no prognostic significance to periodic breathing, a normal characteristic of neonatal respiration.

87.2 Apnea

Periodic breathing must be distinguished from prolonged apneic pauses, since the latter may be associated with serious illnesses. Apnea is due to many primary diseases that affect the neonate (see Table 87–1). Such disorders produce direct depression of the central nervous system's control of respiration (e.g., hypoglycemia, meningitis, drugs, hemorrhage), disturbances of oxygen delivery by perfusion (shock, sepsis, anemia), or ventilation defects (pneumonia, hyaline membrane disease, persistence of fetal circulation, muscle weakness).

Idiopathic apnea of prematurity occurs in the absence of identifiable predisposing diseases and may be due to upper airway obstruction (pharyngeal instability, neck flexion, nasal occlusion) characterized by absent air flow but persistent chest wall movement. Pharyngeal collapse may follow negative airway pressures generated during inspiration, or it may result from incoordination of the tongue and other upper airway muscles involved in maintaining airway patency. Apnea of prematurity may also be due to a decrease of *gestational age dependent reduced* central nervous system stimulus to the respiratory muscles characterized by simultaneous absent air flow and chest wall movement (central apnea). This immaturity of the brain stem respiratory centers is manifest by an attenuated response to carbon dioxide and a paradoxical response to hypoxia, resulting in apnea rather than hyperventilation. The most common pattern of idiopathic apnea among preterm neonates has a mixed etiology, with obstructive apnea preceding (usually) or following central apnea. Short apneas are usually central, whereas apneas of 15 sec or more are often mixed.

■ TABLE 87–1 Potential Causes of Neonatal Apnea and Bradycardia

CNS	IVH, drugs, seizures, hypoxic injury, herniation, neuromuscular disorders
Respiratory	Pneumonia, obstructive airway lesions, atelectasis, extreme prematurity (<1,000 g), laryngeal reflex, phrenic nerve paralysis, severe hyaline membrane distress, pneumothorax
Infectious	Sepsis, necrotizing enterocolitis, meningitis (bacterial, fungal, viral)
Gastrointestinal	Oral feeding, bowel movement, gastroesophageal reflux, esophagitis, intestinal perforation
Metabolic	↓ Glucose, ↓ calcium, ↓ Po_2, ↓ ↑ sodium, ↑ ammonia, ↑ organic acids, ↑ ambient temperature, hypothermia
Cardiovascular	Hypotension, hypertension, heart failure, anemia, hypovolemia, vagal tone
Idiopathic	Immaturity of respiratory center, sleep state, upper airway collapse

Apnea is sleep state dependent; the frequency increases during active (REM) sleep. Paradoxical chest wall movement (inspiratory abdominal expansion and inward chest wall movement) is common during active sleep and may cause a fall in Pao_2 due to ventilation-perfusion defects. Furthermore, increased negative pressure during paradoxical breathing and inhibition of pharyngeal muscle tone during active sleep may contribute to upper airway collapse and obstructive apnea.

CLINICAL MANIFESTATIONS. The incidence of idiopathic apnea of prematurity varies inversely with gestational age. In preterm infants it is rare on the 1st day of life; apnea immediately after birth signifies another illness. The onset of idiopathic apnea occurs on the 2nd–7th day of life. The sudden onset of apnea in a previously well neonate after the 2nd wk of life is a critical event that warrants immediate investigation. In preterm infants serious apnea is defined as cessation of breathing for longer than 15–20 sec or any duration if accompanied by cyanosis and bradycardia. The incidence of associated bradycardia increases with the length of the preceding apnea and correlates with the severity of hypoxia. Short apneas (10 sec) are rarely associated with bradycardia, whereas longer apneas (>20 sec) have a higher incidence of bradycardia. Bradycardia is associated with apnea in more than 95% of cases; vagal responses and, rarely, heart block are causes of bradycardia without apnea.

TREATMENT. Infants at risk for apnea should be monitored with apnea monitors. Gentle *cutaneous stimulation* is often adequate therapy for the neonatal infant having mild and intermittent episodes. Infants having recurrent and prolonged apnea require immediate *bag and mask ventilation. Oxygen* should be administered to treat hypoxia. Apnea of prematurity not due to a precipitating identifiable cause should be treated with *theophylline* or caffeine. Methylxanthines enhance ventilation through a central mechanism or by improving diaphragmatic strength. Loading doses of 5 mg/kg of theophylline should be followed by doses of 1–2 mg/kg given every 8–12 hr using oral or intravenous routes. Loading doses of 10 mg/kg of caffeine are followed 24 hr later by maintenance doses of 2.5 mg/kg/24 hr q.d. PO. These doses should be monitored by observation of vital signs, clinical response, and serum drug levels (therapeutic levels: theophylline, 5–10 μg/ml; caffeine, 8–20 μg/ml). *Transfusion of packed red blood cells* or treatment with erythropoietin (Chapter 89) also may reduce the incidence of idiopathic apnea among anemic infants.

Nasal continuous positive airway pressure (CPAP, 3–5 cm H_2O) is effective therapy for mixed or obstructive apneas. CPAP may splint the upper airway, preventing obstruction. When apnea is due to a precipitating illness, airway stability and oxygenation must be maintained in addition to the therapy of the underlying disease.

PROGNOSIS. Unless severe, recurrent, and refractory to therapy, apnea of prematurity does not alter the infant's prognosis. Associated problems of intraventricular hemorrhage, bronchopulmonary dysplasia, and retinopathy of prematurity are critical in determining the prognosis of apneic infants. Apnea of prematurity usually resolves by 36 wk postconceptional age (gestational age at birth plus postnatal age) and does not predict future episodes of sudden infant death syndrome.

Gerhardt T, Bancalari E: Apnea of prematurity. 1: Lung function and regulation of breathing. Pediatrics 74:58, 1984.
Gerhardt T, Bancalari E: Apnea of prematurity. 2: Respiratory reflexes. Pediatrics 74:63, 1984.
Martin RJ, Miller MJ, Carlo WA: Pathogenesis of apnea in preterm infants. J Pediatr 109:733, 1986.
Miller MJ, Carlo WA, Martin RJ: Continuous positive airway pressure selectively reduces obstructive apnea in preterm infants. J Pediatr 106:91, 1985.

Ruggins NR: Pathophysiology of apnoea in preterm infants. Arch Dis Child 66:70, 1991.
Southall, Richards JM, Rhoden KJ: Prolonged apnea and cardiac arrhythmias in infants discharged from neonatal intensive care units: Failure to predict an increased risk for SIDS. Pediatrics 70:844, 1982.
Upton CJ, Milner AD, Stokes GM: Upper airway patency during apnoea of prematurity. Arch Dis Child 67:419, 1992.
Yazdani M, Kissling GE, Tran TH, et al: Phenobarbital increases the theophylline requirement of premature infants being treated for apnea. Am J Dis Child 141:97, 1987.

87.3 Hyaline Membrane Disease (HMD)

(Respiratory Distress Syndrome, [RDS])

INCIDENCE. This condition is a major cause of death in the newborn. An estimated 30% of all neonatal deaths result from hyaline membrane disease (HMD) or its complications.

HMD occurs primarily in premature infants; incidence is inversely proportional to the gestational age and birthweight. It occurs in 60–80% of infants less than 28 wk of gestational age, in 15–30% of those between 32 and 36 wk, in about 5% beyond 37 wk, and rarely at term. An increased frequency is associated with infants of diabetic mothers, delivery before 37 wk gestation, multifetal pregnancies, cesarean section delivery, precipitous delivery, asphyxia, cold stress, and a history of prior affected infants. The incidence is highest among preterm male or white infants.

ETIOLOGY AND PATHOPHYSIOLOGY. The failure to develop a functional residual capacity (FRC) and the tendency of affected lungs to become atelectatic correlate with high surface tensions and the absence of surfactant. The major constituents of surfactant are dipalmitylphosphatidylcholine (lecithin), phosphatidylglycerol, apoproteins (surfactant proteins: SP-A, B, C, D), and cholesterol (Fig. 87–1). With progressive gestational age, increasing amounts of phospholipids are synthesized and stored in type II alveolar cells (Fig. 87–2). These active agents are released into the alveoli, reducing the surface tension and helping to maintain alveolar stability by preventing the collapse of small air spaces at end-expiration. However, the amounts produced or released may be insufficient to meet postnatal demands because of immaturity. Surfactant is present

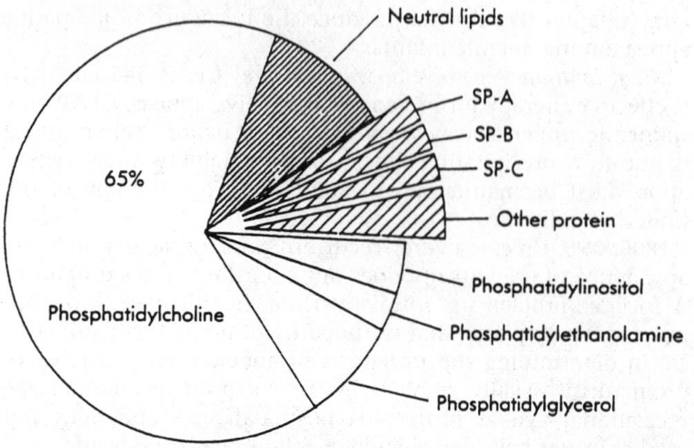

Figure 87–1. Composition of surfactant recovered by alveolar wash. The quantities of the different components are similar for surfactant from mature lungs of mammals. (From Jobe AH: Fetal lung development, tests for maturation, induction of maturation, and treatment. *In*: Creasy RK, Resnik R [eds]: Maternal-Fetal Medicine: Principles and Practice, 3rd ed. Philadelphia, WB Saunders, 1994.)

in high concentrations in fetal lung homogenates by 20 wk of gestation but does not reach the surface of the lung until later. It appears in the amniotic fluid between 28 and 32 wk. Mature levels of pulmonary surfactant are usually present after 35 wk.

Surfactant synthesis depends in part on normal pH, temperature, and perfusion. Asphyxia, hypoxemia, and pulmonary ischemia, particularly in association with hypovolemia, hypotension, and cold stress, may suppress surfactant synthesis. The epithelial lining of the lung may also be injured by high oxygen concentrations and the effects of respirator management, resulting in further reduction in surfactant.

Alveolar atelectasis, hyaline membrane formation, and interstitial edema make the lungs less compliant, requiring greater pressure to expand the small alveoli and airways. In these infants, the lower chest wall is pulled in as the diaphragm descends and the intrathoracic pressure becomes negative, thus limiting the amount of intrathoracic pressure that can be produced; the result is a tendency to atelectasis. The highly compliant chest wall of the preterm infant offers less resistance than that of the mature infant against the natural tendency of the lungs to collapse. Thus, at end-expiration, the volume of the thorax and lungs tends to approach the residual volume, leading to atelectasis.

Deficient synthesis or release of surfactant, together with small respiratory units and compliant chest wall, produces atelectasis, resulting in perfused but not ventilated alveoli, which causes hypoxia. Decreased lung compliance, small tidal volumes, increased physiologic dead space, increased work of breathing, and insufficient alveolar ventilation eventually result in hypercarbia. The combination of hypercarbia, hypoxia, and acidosis produces pulmonary arterial vasoconstriction with increased right-to-left shunting through the foramen ovale, ductus arteriosus, and within the lung itself. Pulmonary blood flow is reduced, and ischemic injury to the cells producing surfactant and to the vascular bed results in an effusion of proteinaceous material into the alveolar spaces (Fig. 87–3).

PATHOLOGY. The lungs appear deep purplish red and are liverlike in consistency. Microscopically, there is extensive atelectasis with engorgement of the interalveolar capillaries and lymphatics. A number of the alveolar ducts, alveoli, and respiratory bronchioles are lined with acidophilic, homogeneous, or granular membranes. Amniotic debris, intra-alveolar hemorrhage, and interstitial emphysema are additional but inconstant findings; interstitial emphysema may be marked when an infant has been ventilated with positive end-expiratory pressure. The characteristic hyaline membranes are rarely seen in infants dying earlier than 6–8 hr after birth.

CLINICAL MANIFESTATIONS. Signs of HMD usually appear within minutes of birth, although they may not be recognized for several hours until rapid, shallow respirations have increased to ≥60/min. The late onset of tachypnea should suggest other conditions. Some patients require resuscitation at birth because of intrapartum asphyxia or initial severe respiratory distress (when birthweight is less than 1,000 g). Characteristically, tachypnea, prominent (often audible) grunting, intercostal and subcostal retractions, nasal flaring, and duskiness are seen. There is increasing cyanosis, which is often relatively unresponsive to oxygen administration. Breath sounds may be normal or diminished with a harsh tubular quality, and, on deep inspiration, fine rales may be heard, especially over the lung bases posteriorly. The natural course is characterized by progressive worsening of cyanosis and dyspnea. If inadequately treated, blood pressure and body temperature may fall; fatigue, cyanosis, and pallor increase, and grunting decreases or disappears as the condition worsens. Apnea and irregular respirations occur as infants tire and are ominous signs requiring immediate intervention. There may also be a mixed respiratory-metabolic acidosis, edema, ileus, and oliguria. Signs of

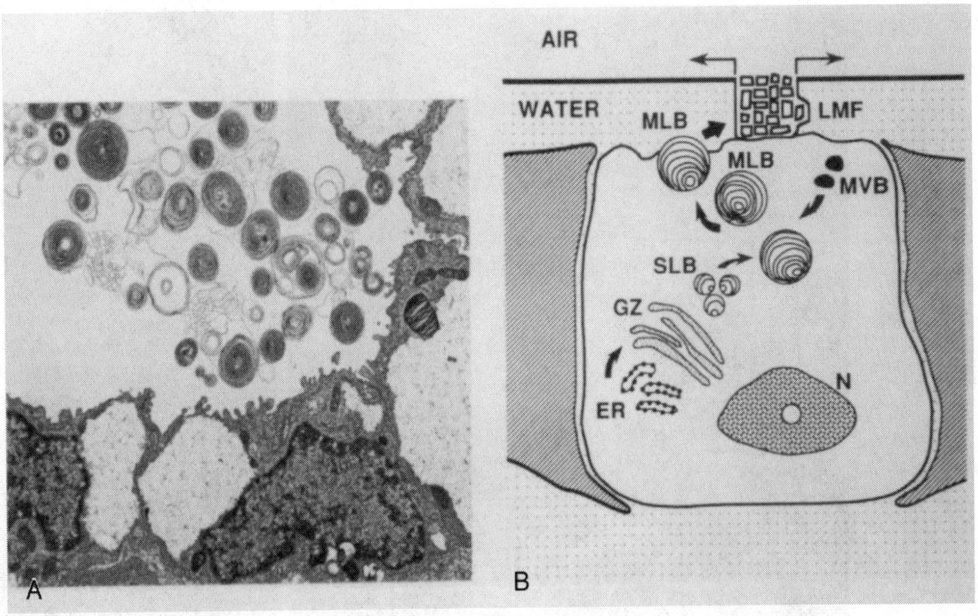

Figure 87–2. *A*, Fetal rat lung (low magnification), day 20 (term day 22), showing developing type II cells, stored glycogen *(pale areas)*, secreted lamellar bodies, and tubular myelin. (Courtesy of Mary Williams, M.D., University of California, San Francisco.) *B*, Possible pathway for transport, secretion, and re-uptake of surfactant. N, nucleus; ER, endoplasmic reticulum; GZ, Golgi zone; SLB, small lamellar body; MLB, mature lamellar body; LMF, lattice (tubular) myelin figure; MVB, multivesicular body. (From Hansen T, Corbet A: Lung development and function. *In*: Taeusch HW, Ballard RA, Avery MA [eds]: Schaffer and Avery's Diseases of the Newborn, 6th ed. Philadelphia, WB Saunders, 1991.)

asphyxia secondary to apnea or partial respiratory failure occur when there is rapid progression of the disease. The condition rarely progresses to death in severely affected infants, but in milder cases the symptoms and signs may reach a peak within 3 days, after which gradual improvement sets in. Improvement is often heralded by a spontaneous diuresis and the ability to oxygenate the infant with lower inspired oxygen levels. Death is rare on the 1st day of illness, usually occurs between days 2 and 7, and is associated with alveolar air leaks (interstitial emphysema, pneumothorax), and pulmonary or intraventricular hemorrhage. Mortality may be delayed weeks or months if bronchopulmonary dysplasia (BPD) develops in mechanically ventilated infants with severe hyaline membrane disease.

DIAGNOSIS. The clinical course, roentgenogram of the chest, and blood gas and acid-base values help to establish the clinical diagnosis. Roentgenographically, the lungs may have a characteristic but not pathognomonic appearance, which includes a fine reticular granularity of the parenchyma and air bronchograms that are often more prominent early in the left lower lobe because of the superimposition of the cardiac shadow (Fig. 87–4). Occasionally, the initial roentgenogram is normal, only to develop the typical pattern at 6–12 hr. There may be considerable variation among films, depending on the phase of respiration and the use of CPAP, often resulting in poor correlation between the roentgenograms and clinical course. The laboratory findings are characterized initially by hypoxemia and later by progressive hypoxemia, hypercarbia, and variable metabolic acidosis.

In the *differential diagnosis,* group B streptococcal sepsis may be indistinguishable from HMD. In pneumonia presenting at birth, the chest roentgenogram may be identical to that for HMD; gram-positive cocci in the gastric or tracheal aspirates and buffy coat smear, a positive test of urine for streptococcal antigen, and the presence of marked neutropenia may suggest this diagnosis. Cyanotic heart disease (e.g., total anomalous pulmonary venous return), persistent fetal circulation, aspiration syndromes, spontaneous pneumothorax, pleural effusions, diaphragmatic eventration, and congenital anomalies such as cystic adenomatoid malformation, pulmonary lymphangiectasia, diaphragmatic hernia, or lobar emphysema must

Figure 87–3. Contributing factors in the pathogenesis of hyaline membrane disease. Potential "vicious circle" perpetuating hypoxia and pulmonary insufficiency. (From Farrell P, Zachman R. *In*: Quilligan EJ, Kretchmer N [eds]: Fetal and Maternal Medicine. © 1980. Reprinted by permission of John Wiley & Sons, Inc.)

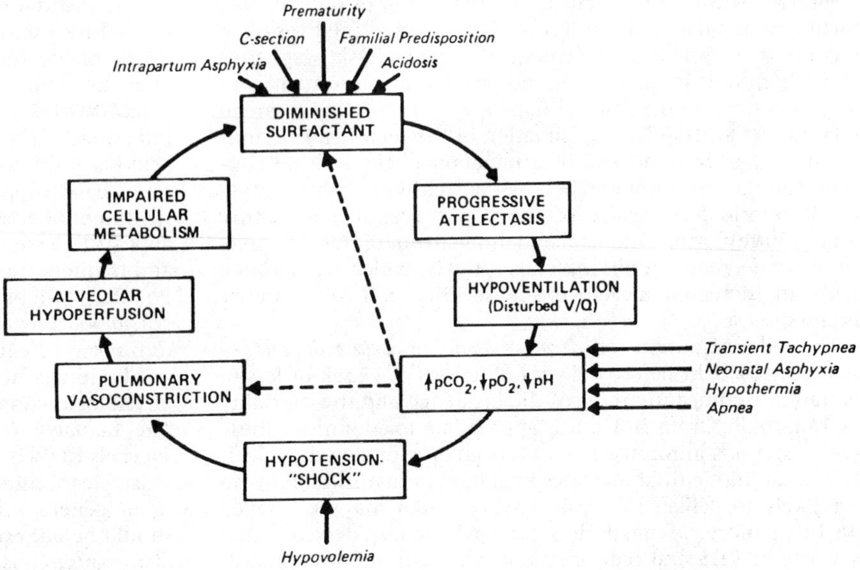

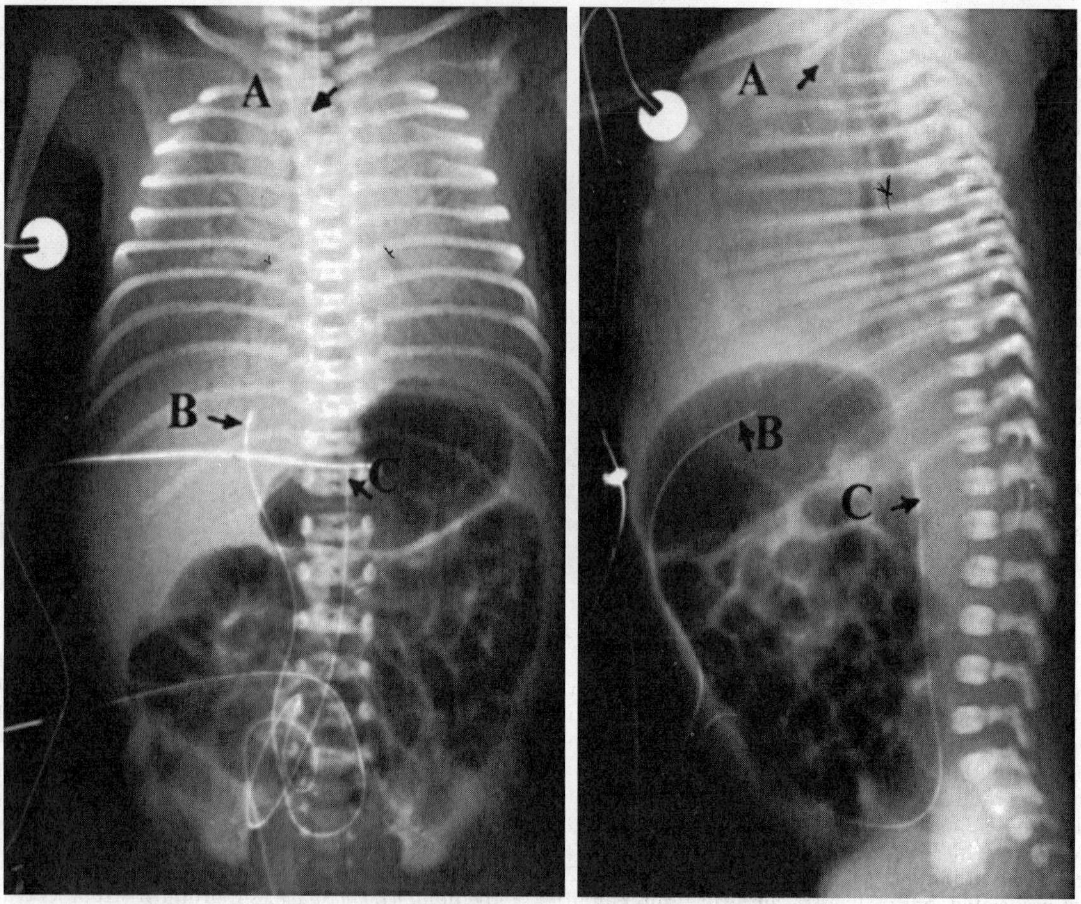

Figure 87–4. Infant with hyaline membrane disease. Note the granular lungs, air bronchogram, and air-filled esophagus. Anteroposterior *(A)* and lateral *(B)* roentgenograms are needed to distinguish umbilical artery from vein catheter and to determine appropriate level of insertion. The lateral view clearly identifies that the catheter has been inserted into an umbilical vein and is lying in the portal system of the liver. *A*, Endotracheal tube; *B*, umbilical venous catheter at the junction of the umbilical vein, ductus venosus, and portal vein; *C*, umbilical artery catheter passed up the aorta to T-12. (Courtesy of Walter E. Berdon, Babies Hospital, New York City.)

be considered and require roentgenographic evaluation. Transient tachypnea may be distinguished by its short and mild clinical course. *Congenital alveolar proteinosis* is a rare familial disease that often presents as severe and lethal RDS (see Chapter 350).

PREVENTION. Most important is the prevention of prematurity, including avoidance of unnecessary or poorly timed cesarean section, appropriate management of the high-risk pregnancy and labor, and the prediction and possible in utero treatment of pulmonary immaturity (Chapter 81). In timing cesarean section or inducing labor, estimation of the fetal head circumference by ultrasound and determination of the lecithin concentration in the amniotic fluid by the lecithin to sphingomyelin (L/S) ratio decrease the likelihood of delivering a premature infant. Intrauterine antenatal and intrapartum monitoring may similarly decrease the risk of fetal asphyxia, which is associated with an increased incidence and severity of hyaline membrane disease.

The administration of *dexamethasone* or *betamethasone* to women 48–72 hr before delivery of fetuses at 32 wk or less of gestation significantly reduces the incidence and the mortality and morbidity from HMD. It is appropriate to administer these corticosteroids intramuscularly to pregnant women whose lecithin in amniotic fluid indicates fetal lung immaturity and who are likely to deliver in 1 wk or whose labor may be delayed 48 hr or more. Prenatal glucocorticoid therapy decreases the severity of RDS and reduces the incidence of other complications of prematurity, such as intraventricular hemorrhage, patent ductus arteriosus, pneumothorax, and necrotizing enterocolitis, without affecting neonatal growth, development, lung mechanics or growth, or the incidence of infection. Prenatal glucocorticoids may act synergistically with postnatal exogenous surfactant therapy.

Administration of one dose of *surfactant* into the trachea of premature infants immediately after birth or during the first 24 hr of life reduces the mortality from HMD but does not alter the incidence of BPD.

TREATMENT. The basic defect requiring treatment is inadequate pulmonary exchange of oxygen and carbon dioxide; metabolic acidosis and circulatory insufficiency are secondary manifestations. Early supportive care of the LBW infant, especially in the treatment of acidosis, hypoxia, hypotension, and hypothermia, appears to lessen the severity of HMD. Therapy requires careful and frequent monitoring of heart and respiratory rates, arterial Po_2, Pco_2, pH, bicarbonate, electrolytes, blood glucose, hematocrit, blood pressure, and temperature. Umbilical artery catheterization is frequently necessary. Since most cases of HMD are self-limiting, the goal of treatment is to minimize abnormal physiologic variations and superimposed iatrogenic problems. The management of these infants is best carried out in a specially staffed and equipped hospital unit, the neonatal intensive care nursery.

The general principles for supportive care of any LBW infant should be adhered to, including gentle handling and minimal disturbance consistent with management. To avoid chilling and to minimize oxygen consumption, infants should be placed in an Isolette and core temperature maintained between 36.5 and 37° C (Chapter 82). Calories and fluids should be provided intravenously. For the first 24 hr, 10% glucose and water should be infused through a peripheral vein at a rate of 65–75 ml/kg/24 hr. Subsequently, electrolytes should be added and fluid volumes increased gradually to 120–150 ml/kg/24 hr. Excessive fluids contribute to the development of a patent ductus arteriosus.

Warm humidified oxygen should be provided at a concentration sufficient initially to keep arterial levels between 55 and 70 mm Hg with stable vital signs to maintain normal tissue oxygenation while minimizing the risk of oxygen toxicity. If the arterial oxygen tension cannot be maintained above 50 mm Hg at inspired oxygen concentrations of 70%, applying CPAP at a pressure of 6–10 cm of H_2O by nasal prongs is indicated, which usually produces a sharp rise in arterial oxygen tension. Although the course may be protracted, the amount of pressure required usually decreases abruptly at about 72 hr of age, and the infant can be weaned from CPAP shortly thereafter. If an infant on CPAP cannot maintain an arterial oxygen tension above 50 mm Hg while breathing 100% oxygen, assisted ventilation is required.

Infants with severe HMD or those who develop complications resulting in persistent apnea require *assisted mechanical ventilation.* Reasonable indications for its use are (1) arterial blood pH of less than 7.20; (2) arterial blood P_{CO_2} of 60 mm Hg or more; (3) arterial blood P_{O_2} of 50 mm Hg or less at oxygen concentrations of 70–100%; or (4) persistent apnea. Assisted ventilation by pressure or flow limited conventional respirators through an endotracheal tube may also include positive end-expiratory pressure (PEEP). (See Chapter 60.)

The goals of mechanical ventilation are to improve oxygenation and carbon dioxide elimination without causing excessive pulmonary barotrauma or oxygen toxicity. Acceptable ranges of blood gas values, balancing the risks of hypoxia and acidosis against those of mechanical ventilation, are Pa_{O_2} of 55–70 mm Hg; P_{CO_2} of 35–55 mm Hg; and pH of 7.25–7.45. During mechanical ventilation, oxygenation is improved by increasing the F_{IO_2} or the mean airway pressure. The latter can be increased by increasing the peak inspiratory pressure, gas flow, inspiratory to expiratory ratio, or PEEP. Excessive PEEP may cause a pneumothorax or impede venous return, reducing cardiac output despite improvement of Pa_{O_2} and thus decreasing oxygen delivery. PEEPs of 4–6 cm H_2O are usually safe and effective. Carbon dioxide elimination is achieved by increasing the peak inspiratory pressure (tidal volume) or the rate of the ventilator.

The rate ranges of conventional ventilators are 10–60 breaths/min; of high-frequency jet ventilation (HFJV), 150–600/min; and of oscillators, 300–1,800/min. HFJV and oscillators may improve carbon dioxide elimination, lower mean airway pressure, and occasionally improve oxygenation in patients not responding to conventional ventilators who have HMD, interstitial emphysema, multiple pneumothoraces, or meconium aspiration pneumonia. HFJV may cause necrotizing tracheal damage, especially in the presence of hypotension or poor humidification; and oscillator therapy has been associated with an increased risk of air leaks, intraventricular hemorrhage, and periventricular leukomalacia. Both methods may cause gas trapping. Complications of endotracheal intubation (plugging of tube, extubation, subglottic granuloma, and stenosis) and mechanical ventilation (pneumothorax, interstitial emphysema, reduced cardiac output) may be minimized by the interventions of specially trained physicians, nurses, and respiratory therapists in neonatal intensive care units.

Multidose endotracheal instillation of *exogenous surfactant* to LBW infants requiring 40% oxygen and mechanical ventilation for the treatment *(rescue therapy)* of RDS has improved survival and reduced the incidence of pulmonary air leaks but has not consistently reduced the incidence of bronchopulmonary dysplasia. The immediate effects include improved alveolar-arterial oxygen gradients, reduced ventilator mean airway pressure, increased pulmonary compliance, and improved appearance of the chest roentgenogram. Survanta is an exogenous surfactant prepared from minced bovine lung with lipid extraction and enriched with phosphatidylcholine, palmitic acid, and triglycerides. Survanta contains SP-B and SP-C but no SP-A. Exosurf is a synthetic surfactant containing dipalmitoylphosphatidylcholine, hexadecanol, and tyloxapol. The latter two organic compounds improve spreading of the surfactant along the alveolus, because dipalmitoylphosphatidylcholine alone has poor surface active properties. Additional surfactants undergoing testing include Curosurf and Infasurf (both natural) and ALEC (artificial lung expanding compound; 7:3 mixture of dipalmitoylphosphatidylcholine and phosphatidylglycerol).

Treatment (rescue) is usually initiated in the first 24 hr of life; therapy is given via the endotracheal tube every 12 hr for a total of 4 doses. Exogenous surfactant should be given by a physician qualified in neonatal resuscitation and respiratory management who is able to care for the infant beyond the 1st hr of stabilization. Additional on-site required staff support includes nurses and respiratory therapists who are experienced in ventilatory management of LBW infants. In addition, appropriate monitoring equipment must be present (radiology, blood gas laboratory, and pulse oximetry). Furthermore, each institution should have an approved protocol for the administration of surfactant. Complications of surfactant therapy include transient hypoxia and hypotension, blockage of the endotracheal tube, and pulmonary hemorrhage.

Respiratory acidosis may require short-term or prolonged assisted ventilation. In severe respiratory acidosis and hypoxia, treatment with sodium bicarbonate may exacerbate hypercarbia.

Metabolic acidosis in HMD may be a result of perinatal asphyxia and hypotension and is often encountered when an infant has required resuscitation (Chapter 85). Sodium bicarbonate, 1–2 mEq/kg, may be administered for treatment over a 10- to 15-min period through a peripheral vein with the acid-base determination repeated within 30 min, or it may be administered over several hours. More often, sodium bicarbonate is administered on an emergency basis through an umbilical venous catheter. Alkali therapy may result in skin sloughs due to infiltration, increased serum osmolarity, hypernatremia, hypocalcemia, hypokalemia, and liver injury when concentrated solutions are administered rapidly through an umbilical vein.

Monitoring of *aortic blood pressure* through an umbilical arterial catheter or by oscillometric technique may be useful in managing the shock-like state that may occur during the 1st hour or so after premature birth of an infant who has been asphyxiated or who has developed respiratory distress (see Fig. 79–2). Hypotension has been associated with an increased risk of IVH and should be treated with dopamine, crystalloid or colloid fluids, or, less often, dobutamine. Occasionally hypotension may be glucocorticoid responsive. Radiopaque catheters should always be used and their position checked roentgenographically after insertion (see Fig. 87–4). The tip of an umbilical artery catheter should lie just above the bifurcation of the aorta (L3–L5) or above the celiac axis (T6–T10). Placement and supervision should be done by skilled and experienced personnel. Catheters should be removed as soon as there is no indication for their continued use, that is, when Pa_{O_2} is stable and the F_{IO_2} is less than 40%.

Periodic monitoring of arterial oxygen and carbon dioxide tension and of pH is an important part of the management; if assisted ventilation is being used, it is essential. Blood should be obtained from the umbilical or peripheral artery. Temporal artery lines are contraindicated because of retrograde cerebral emboli. Tissue Po_2 may also be estimated continuously from transcutaneous electrodes or pulse oximetry (oxygen saturation). Capillary blood samples are of limited value for determining Po_2 but may be useful for evaluating Pco_2 and pH.

Owing to the difficulty of distinguishing some group B streptococcal or other infections from HMD, routinely administering antibacterial agents is indicated until the results of blood cultures are available. Penicillin or ampicillin with kanamycin or gentamicin is suggested, depending on the recent pattern of bacterial sensitivities in the hospital where the infant is being treated (Chapters 94 and 98).

COMPLICATIONS OF HMD AND INTENSIVE CARE. The most serious complications of **tracheal intubation** are asphyxia from obstruction of the tube, cardiac arrest during intubation or suctioning, and the subsequent development of subglottic stenosis. Other complications include bleeding from trauma during intubation, posterior pharyngeal pseudodiverticula, difficult extubation requiring tracheostomy, ulceration of the nares due to pressure from the tube, permanent narrowing of the nostril from tissue damage and scarring from irritation or infection around the tube, erosion of the palate, avulsion of a vocal cord, laryngeal ulcer, papilloma of a vocal cord, and persistent hoarseness, stridor, or edema of the larynx.

Measures to reduce the incidence of these complications include skillfully observing the infant; using polyvinyl endotracheal tubes that do not contain tin, which is toxic to cells; using a tube of the smallest practicable size to reduce local ischemia and pressure necrosis; avoiding frequent changes of the tube; avoiding motion of the tube in situ; avoiding too frequent or vigorous suctioning; and avoiding infection through meticulous cleanliness and frequent sterilization of all apparatus attached to or passed through the tube. The personnel inserting and caring for the endotracheal tube should be experienced and skilled.

The risks of **umbilical arterial catheterization** include vascular embolization, thrombosis, spasm, and perforation; ischemic or chemical necrosis of abdominal viscera; infection; accidental hemorrhage; and impaired circulation to a leg with subsequent gangrene. Although at necropsy the reported incidence of thrombotic complications varies from 1 to 23%, aortography has demonstrated that clots form in or about the tips of 95% of catheters placed in an umbilical artery. Aortic ultrasound can also be used to investigate the presence of thrombosis. The risk of a serious clinical complication resulting from umbilical catheterization is probably between 2 and 5%.

Transient blanching of the leg may occur during catheterization of the umbilical artery. It is usually due to reflex arterial spasm, the incidence of which is lessened by using the smallest available catheters, particularly in very small infants. The catheter should be removed immediately; catheterization of the other artery may then be attempted. Persistent spasm after removal of the catheter may be relieved by topical nitroglycerin applied over the femoral artery or, rarely, by warming the opposite leg. Blood sampling from a radial artery may similarly result in spasm or thrombosis, and the same treatment is indicated. Intermittent severe spasm or unrelieved spasm may respond to the cautious topical nitroglycerin or local infusion of tolazoline (Priscoline), 1–2 mg injected intra-arterially over 5 min. Accidentally lodging the catheter in a smaller artery, either blocking it completely or causing unrecognized local vascular spasm, may result in gangrene of the organ or area supplied by the vessel. To prevent this complication, the catheter should be removed promptly if blood cannot be obtained through it.

Serious hemorrhage on removal of the catheter is rare. Thrombi may form in the artery or in the catheter; their incidence is lowered by using a smooth-tipped catheter with a hole only at its end, by rinsing the catheter with a small amount of saline solution containing heparin, or by continuously infusing a solution containing 1–10 unit/mL of heparin. The risks of thrombus formation with potential vascular occlusion can also be reduced by removing the catheter when there are early signs of thrombosis, such as narrowing of pulse pressure and disappearance of the dicrotic notch. Some prefer to use the umbilical artery for blood sampling only, leaving the catheter filled with heparinized saline between samplings. *Renovascular hypertension* may occur days to weeks following umbilical arterial catheterization in a small number of neonates.

Umbilical vein catheterization is associated with many of the same risks as artery catheterization. In addition, there is an association with subsequent portal hypertension from portal vein thrombosis.

Oxygen is toxic to the lung, particularly if administered by means of a positive-pressure respirator, resulting in **bronchopulmonary dysplasia** (BPD) (see also Chapter 87.9). Additional contributing factors to BPD include alveolar shear stress, volutrauma, hypocapnic saponification, absorption atelectasis, and subsequent inflammation. Instead of showing improvement on the 3rd–4th day, consistent with the natural course in survivors, some infants who have been on prolonged intermittent positive-pressure breathing using increased concentrations of oxygen roentgenographically show a worsening of their pulmonary condition (Fig. 87–5*A*). Respiratory distress persists and is characterized by hypoxia, hypercarbia, oxygen dependency, and the development of right-sided heart failure. The chest roentgenogram is described as gradually changing from a picture of almost complete opacification with air bronchogram and interstitial emphysema to one of small, round, lucent areas alternating with areas of irregular density resembling a sponge (Fig. 87–5*B*). In the histologic picture at this stage (10–20 days after beginning oxygen therapy) there is less evidence of hyaline membrane formation, progressive alveolar coalescence with atelectasis of surrounding alveoli, interstitial edema, coarse focal thickening of the basement membrane, and widespread bronchial and bronchiolar mucosal metaplasia and hyperplasia. This corresponds with a severe maldistribution of ventilation. Oxygen dependency at 1 mo (alternately, at 36 wk gestational age) defines BPD. Most surviving neonates with persistent roentgenographic changes recover by 6–12 mo, but some require prolonged hospitalization and may have respiratory symptoms persisting through infancy. Right-sided heart failure and viral necrotizing bronchiolitis are major causes of death. Pathology reveals cardiac enlargement and pulmonary changes consisting of focal areas of emphysematous alveoli with hypertrophy of the peribronchial smooth muscle of the tributary bronchioles, some perimucosal fibrosis and widespread metaplasia of the bronchiolar mucosa, thickening of basement membranes, and separation of the capillaries from the alveolar epithelial cells.

Infants at risk for BPD have severe respiratory distress requiring prolonged periods of mechanical ventilation and oxygen therapy. Additional associations include the presence of pulmonary interstitial emphysema, lower gestational age, male sex, low Pco_2 at 48 hr, patent ductus arteriosus, high peak inspiratory pressure, increased airway resistance in the 1st wk of life, and possibly a family history of asthma. Some VLBW infants without hyaline membrane disease who require mechanical ventilation for apnea develop chronic lung disease that does not follow the classic pattern for BPD.

Severe BPD requires continued mechanical ventilation until weaning from the respirator becomes possible. Acceptable blood gas concentrations for a patient with BPD include Pco_2 of 50–70 mm Hg (if pH $>$7.30) and Pao_2 of 55–60 mm Hg with oxygen saturation of 90–95%. Lower levels of Pao_2 may exacerbate pulmonary hypertension, produce cor pulmonale and inhibit growth. Airway obstruction in BPD may be due to mucus and edema production, bronchospasm, and collapse of

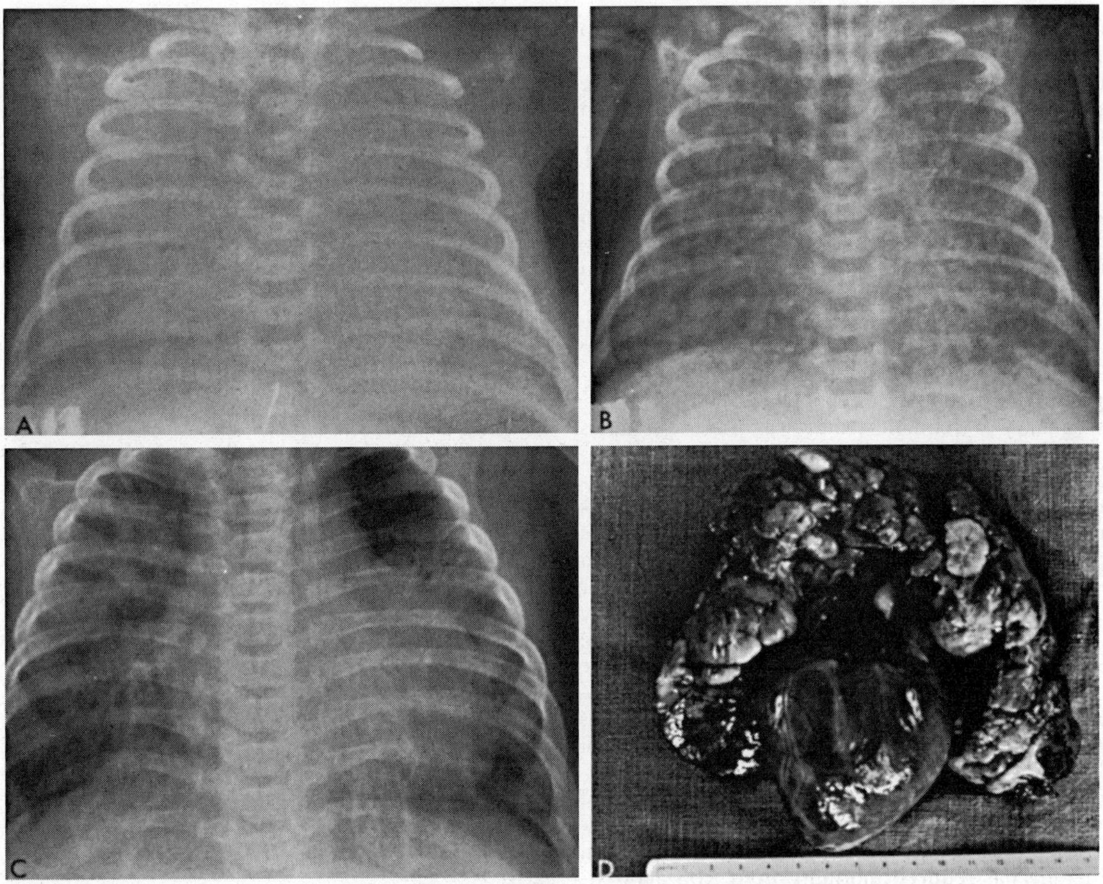

Figure 87–5. Pulmonary changes in infants who were treated in the immediate postnatal period for the clinical syndrome of hyaline membrane disease with prolonged, intermittent positive-pressure breathing with air containing 80 to 100% oxygen. *A*, A 5-day-old infant with nearly complete opacification of lungs. *B*, A 13-day-old infant with "bubbly lungs" simulating the roentgenographic appearance of the Wilson-Mikity syndrome. *C*, A 7-mo-old infant with irregular, dense strands in both lungs, hyperinflation, and cardiomegaly suggestive of BPD. *D*, Large right ventricle and cobbly irregularly aerated lung of an infant who died at 11 mo of age. This infant also had a patent ductus arteriosus. (From Northway WH Jr, Rosan RC, Porter DY: N Engl J Med 276:357, 1967. Reprinted with permission from The New England Journal of Medicine.)

acquired tracheomalacia. These events may contribute to "blue spells." Alternatively, blue spells may be due to acute cor pulmonale or myocardial ischemia.

Treatment of BPD includes use of bronchodilators such as aerosolized β_2-adrenergic agents and theophylline, diuretics, fluid restriction, treatment of infections (*U. urealyticum,* respiratory syncytial virus), high-caloric density formula, CPAP for tracheomalacia, and dexamethasone. Dexamethasone, 0.5 mg/kg/24 hr given in two doses intravenously, is initiated after 2–6 wk of chronic lung disease. This dose is continued for 3 days and then is reduced to 0.3 mg/kg/24 hr for an additional 3 days. Thereafter, the dose is reduced by 10% every 3 days until it reaches 0.1 mg/kg/24 hr. This final dose is given every other day for 1 wk and then is discontinued. Some start dexamethasone after 7–14 days of ventilator dependency. The use of steroids has improved the ability to wean patients from ventilators but increases the risk of hypertension, poor growth, gastrointestinal bleeding, hyperglycemia, infection, and possibly cardiomyopathy. Older infants may respond to vasodilator therapy with reduced pulmonary vascular resistance.

Complications of BPD include growth failure, transient psychomotor retardation, and parental stress as well as such sequelae of therapy as nephrolithiasis (due to diuretics and total intravenous alimentation), osteopenia, and subglottic stenosis, which may require tracheotomy or an anterior cricoid split procedure to relieve upper airway obstruction.

Patients with BPD often go home on oxygen, diuretics, and bronchodilator therapy. The long-term *prognosis* is good for infants who have been weaned off oxygen prior to discharge from the intensive care unit. Prolonged ventilation, interventricular hemorrhage, pulmonary hypertension, cor pulmonale, and oxygen dependence beyond 1 yr of life are poor prognostic signs. Airway obstruction and hyperactivity and hyperinflation may be demonstrated in some adolescents.

Extrapulmonary extravasation of air is another frequent complication of the management of HMD (Chapter 87.8).

There may be clinically significant shunting through a **patent ductus arteriosus** (PDA) in some neonates with HMD, the delayed closure being due to associated hypoxia, acidosis, increased pulmonary pressure secondary to vasoconstriction, systemic hypotension, immaturity, and local release of prostaglandins, which dilate the ductus. This shunting may be bidirectional or right to left through the ductus arteriosus. As HMD resolves, pulmonary vascular resistance decreases, and there may be left-to-right shunting leading to left ventricular volume overload and pulmonary edema. The manifestations of PDA may include (1) persistent apnea for unexplained reasons in an infant recovering from HMD; (2) an active heaving precordium, bounding peripheral pulses, wide pulse pressure, and a systolic or to-and-fro murmur; (3) carbon dioxide retention; (4) increasing oxygen dependency; (5) roentgenographic evidence of cardiomegaly and increased pulmonary vascular markings; and (6) hepatomegaly. The diagnosis is confirmed by echocardiographic visualization of a PDA with Doppler flow evidence of left-to-right shunting. Most infants respond to general supportive measures, including diuretics and fluid restriction. In selected patients in whom spontaneous closure does not occur but in whom there is progressive deterioration despite supportive and cardiotonic treatment, intravenous indomethacin, 0.2 mg/kg at 12- to 24-hr intervals for 3 doses, may induce pharmacologic closure by inhibiting prostaglandin synthesis. An alternative protocol is 0.1 mg/kg/24 hr for 6 days; repeated courses of both protocols may be needed. Contraindications to indomethacin include thrombocytopenia (<50,000/mm^3), bleeding disorders, oliguria (<1ml/kg/hr), necrotizing enterocolitis (NEC), and elevated plasma creatinine level (>1.8 mg/dL). Indications for surgical closure are failure to close the ductus following indomethacin therapy with persistent heart failure and ventilator dependence.

Anemia secondary to frequent withdrawal of blood samples may also occur as a complication of intensive care. The cumulative amount of blood withdrawn should be carefully recorded. Some of its replacement by transfusion may be indicated if more than 10–15% of estimated total blood volume is removed or, more often, if there is a significant decrease in the hematocrit. Oxygen-dependent infants should have their hematocrit maintained close to 40%. Erythropoietin therapy may reduce the need for frequent transfusions (Chapter 89.1).

PROGNOSIS. Early provision of intensive observation and care to high-risk newborn infants can significantly reduce morbidity and mortality due to HMD and other acute neonatal illnesses. However, good results depend on the availability of experienced and skilled personnel, specially designed and organized regional hospital units, proper equipment, and lack of complications such as severe fetal or birth asphyxia, intracranial hemorrhage, or irremediable congenital malformation. Surfactant therapy has reduced mortality from RDS approximately 40%; morbidity has not been measurably affected.

Overall mortality for LBW infants referred to intensive care centers is steadily declining; about 75% of those under 1,000 g survive, and the mortality progressively decreases at higher weights, with over 95% of sick infants weighing more than 2,500 g surviving. Although 85–90% of all infants surviving HMD after requiring ventilatory support with respirators are normal, the outlook is much better for those weighing above 1,500 g; about 80% of those under 1,500 g have no neurologic or mental sequelae. The long-term prognosis for normal pulmonary function in most infants surviving HMD is excellent. However, survivors of severe neonatal respiratory failure may have significant pulmonary and neurodevelopmental impairment.

Archer N: Patent ductus arteriosus in the newborn. Arch Dis Child 69:529, 1993.

Carlo W, Martin R: Principles of neonatal assisted ventilation. Pediatr Clin North Am 33:221, 1986.

Clark RH: High-frequency ventilation. J Pediatr 124:661, 1994.

Cummings JJ, D'Uegenio DB, Gross SJ: A controlled trial of dexamethasone in preterm infants at high risk for bronchopulmonary dysplasia. N Engl J Med 320:1055, 1989.

Durand M, Sardesi S, McEvoy C: Effects of early dexamethasone therapy on pulmonary mechanics and chronic lung disease in very low birth weight infants: A randomized, controlled trial. Pediatrics 95:584, 1995.

Egberts J, de Winter JP, Sedin G, et al: Comparison of prophylaxis and rescue treatment with Curosurf in neonates less than 30 weeks' gestation: A randomized trial. Pediatrics 92:768, 1993.

Fakhoury G, Daikoku NH, Benser J, et al: Lamellar body concentrations and the prediction of fetal pulmonary maturity. Am J Obstet Gynecol 170:72, 1994.

Fiascone J, Rhodes T, Grondgeorge S, et al: Bronchopulmonary dysplasia. A review for pediatricians. Curr Probl Pediatr 29:171, 1989.

Gill AB, Weindling AM: Randomised controlled trial of plasma protein fraction versus dopamine in hypotensive very low birthweight infants. Arch Dis Child 69:284, 1993.

Halliday HL, Tarnow-Mordi WO, Corcoran JD, et al: Multicentre randomised trial comparing high and low dose surfactant regimens for the treatment of respiratory distress syndrome (the Curosurf 4 trial). Arch Dis Child 69:276, 1993.

Helbock HJ, Insoft RM, Conte FA: Glucocorticoid-responsive hypotension in extremely low birth weight newborns. Pediatrics 92:715, 1993.

Horbar JD, Wright EC, Onstad L, et al: Decreasing mortality associated with the introduction of surfactant therapy: An observational study of neonates weighing 601 to 1300 grams at birth. Pediatrics 92:191, 1993.

Hyde I, English RE, Williams JD: The changing pattern of chronic lung disease of prematurity. Arch Dis Child 64:448, 1989.

Jobe AH, Mitchell BR, Gunkel JH: Beneficial effects of the combined use of prenatal corticosteroids and postnatal surfactant on preterm infants. Am J Obstet Gynecol 168:508, 1993.

Kari MA, Hallman M, Eronen M, et al: Prenatal dexamethasone treatment in conjunction with rescue therapy of human surfactant: A randomized placebo-controlled multicenter study. Pediatrics 93:730, 1994.

Klarr JM, Faix RG, Pryce CJE, et al: Randomized, blind trial of dopamine versus dobutamine for treatment of hypotension in preterm infants with respiratory distress syndrome. J Pediatr 125:117, 1994.

Kraybill EN, Runyan DK, Bose CL, et al: Risk factors for chronic lung disease in infants with birth weights of 751 to 1000 grams. J Pediatr 115:115, 1989.

Milner AD, Hoskyns EW: High frequency positive pressure ventilation in neonates. Arch Dis Child 64:1, 1989.

Northway WH Jr, Moss RB, Carlisle KB, et al: Late pulmonary sequelae of bronchopulmonary dysplasia. N Engl J Med 323:1793, 1990.

Ohls RK, Hunter DD, Christensen RD: A randomized, double-blind, placebo-controlled trial of recombinant erythropoietin in treatment of anemia of bronchopulmonary dysplasia. J Pediatr 123:996, 1993.

Parilla BV, Dooley SL, Jansen RD, et al: Iatrogenic respiratory distress syndrome following elective repeat cesarean delivery. Obstet Gynecol 81:392, 1993.

Pramanik AK, Holtzman RB, Merritt TA: Surfactant replacement therapy for pulmonary diseases. Pediatr Clin North Am 40:913, 1993.

Schwartz RM, Luby AM, Scanlon JW, et al: Effect of surfactant on morbidity, mortality, and resource use in newborn infants weighing 500 to 1500 g. N Engl J Med 330:1476, 1994.

Seppänen MP, Kääpä PO, Kero PO, et al: Doppler-derived systolic pulmonary artery pressure in acute neonatal respiratory distress syndrome. Pediatrics 93:769, 1994.

Survanta Multidose Study Group: Two-year follow-up of infants treated for neonatal respiratory distress syndrome with bovine surfactant. J Pediatr 124:962, 1994.

The HIFI Study Group: High-frequency oscillatory ventilation compared with conventional mechanical ventilation in the treatment of respiratory failure in preterm infants. N Engl J Med 320:88, 1989.

Thibeault DW, Emmanoulides GC, Nelson RJ, et al: Patent ductus arteriosus complicating the respiratory distress syndrome in preterm infants. J Pediatr 86:120, 1975.

Walther FJ, Benders MJ, Leighton JO: Early changes in the neonatal circulatory transition. J Pediatr 123:625, 1993.

Walsh-Sukys MC, Bauer RE, Cornell DJ, et al: Severe respiratory failure in neonates: Mortality and morbidity rates and neurodevelopmental outcomes. J Pediatr 125:104, 1994.

87.4 Transient Tachypnea of the Newborn

Transient tachypnea, occasionally called **respiratory distress syndrome type II**, usually follows uneventful normal preterm or term vaginal delivery or cesarean delivery. It may be characterized only by the early onset of tachypnea, sometimes with retractions, or expiratory grunting and, occasionally, cyanosis that is relieved by minimal oxygen. Patients usually recover rapidly within 3 days, although they may rarely appear severely ill and have a more protracted course. The lungs are usually clear without rales or rhonchi, and the chest roentgenogram shows prominent pulmonary vascular markings, fluid lines in the fissures, overaeration, flat diaphragms, and, occasionally, pleural fluid. Hypoxemia, hypercapnia, and acidosis are uncommon. Distinguishing the disease from hyaline membrane disease may be very difficult; the distinctive features of transient tachypnea are the infant's sudden recovery and the absence of a roentgenographic reticulogranular pattern on air bronchography. The syndrome is believed to be secondary to slow absorption of fetal lung fluid resulting in decreased pulmonary compliance and tidal volume and increased dead space.

Avery ME, Gatewood OB, Brumley G: Transient tachypnea of newborn. Possible delayed reabsorption of fluid at birth. Am J Dis Child 111:380, 1966.

Gross TL, Sokol RJ, Kwong MS, et al: Transient tachypnea of the newborn: The relationship to preterm delivery and significant neonatal morbidity. Am J Obstet Gynecol 146:236, 1983.

Sundell H, Garrott J, Blankenship WJ, et al: Studies on infants with type II respiratory distress syndrome. J Pediatr 78:754, 1971.

Goodwin SR, Graves SA, Haberkern CM: Aspiration in intubated premature infants. Pediatrics 75:85, 1985.

87.5 Aspiration of Foreign Material

(Fetal Aspiration Syndrome: Aspiration Pneumonia)

During prolonged labors and difficult deliveries, infants often initiate vigorous respiratory movements in utero because of interference with the supply of oxygen through the placenta. Under such circumstances the infant may aspirate amniotic fluid containing vernix caseosa, epithelial cells, meconium, or material from the birth canal, which may block the smallest airways and interfere with alveolar exchange of oxygen and carbon dioxide. Pathogenic bacteria accompany the aspirated material, and pneumonia may ensue, but even in the noninfected cases respiratory distress accompanied by roentgenographic evidences of aspiration is seen (Fig. 87–6).

Pulmonary aspiration of foreign material may also occur in the newborn infant because of tracheoesophageal fistula, esophageal and duodenal obstructions, gastroesophageal reflux, improper feeding practices, and administration of depressant medicines.

The contents of the stomach should be aspirated through a soft catheter just before operation or other procedures that require anesthesia or significantly disturb an infant. Once aspiration has occurred, treatment consists of general and respiratory support and treatment of pneumonia (Chapters 87 and 99).

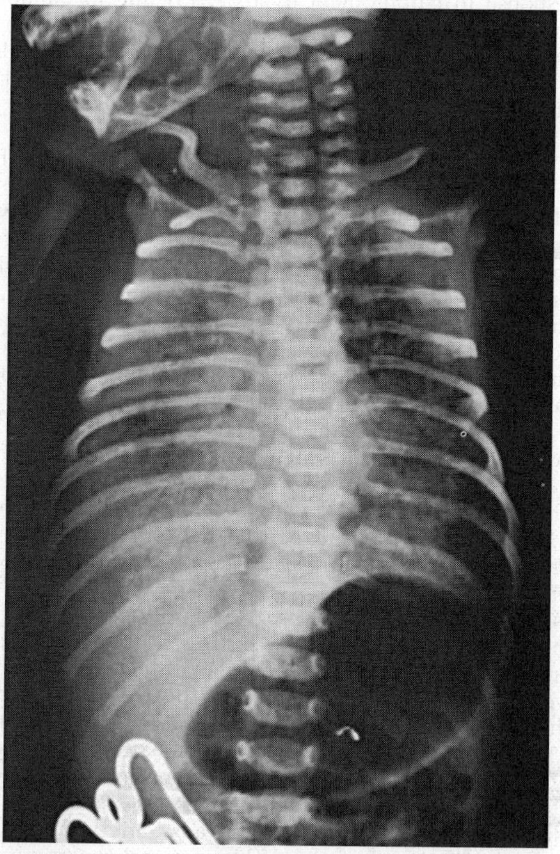

Figure 87–6. Fetal aspiration syndrome (aspiration pneumonia). Note the coarsely granular pattern with irregular aeration typical of fetal distress from aspiration of material, such as vernix caseosa, epithelial cells, and meconium contained in amniotic fluid.

87.6 Meconium Aspiration

Meconium-stained amniotic fluid is seen in 5–15% of births, but this syndrome usually occurs in term or post-term infants. Five per cent of such infants develop meconium aspiration pneumonia, of whom 30% require mechanical ventilation and 5–10% may expire. Usually, but not invariably, fetal distress and hypoxia occur with passage of meconium into the amniotic fluid. These infants are meconium stained and may be depressed and require resuscitation at birth. The pathophysiology is noted in Figure 87–7.

CLINICAL MANIFESTATIONS. Either in utero or more often with the first breath, thick meconium is aspirated into the lungs. The resulting small airway obstruction may produce respiratory distress within the first hours with tachypnea, retraction, grunting, and cyanosis in severely affected infants. Partial obstruction of some airways may lead to pneumothorax or pneumomediastinum, or both. Prompt treatment may delay the onset of respiratory distress, which may consist only of tachypnea without retractions. Overdistention of the chest may be prominent. The condition usually improves within 72 hr, but when its course requires assisted ventilation, it may be severe and its potential for mortality high. Tachypnea may persist for many days or even several weeks. The typical chest roentgenogram is characterized by patchy infiltrates, coarse streaking of both lung fields, increased anteroposterior diameter, and flattening of the diaphragm. A normal chest roentgenogram in an infant with severe hypoxia and no cardiac malformation suggests the diagnosis of persistent fetal circulation (Chapter 87.7). Arterial Po_2 may be low in either disease, and if hypoxia has occurred, metabolic acidosis is usually present.

PREVENTION. The risk of meconium aspiration may be decreased by paying careful attention to fetal distress and initiating prompt delivery in the presence of fetal acidosis, late decelerations, or poor beat-to-beat variability. Amnio-infusion and DeLee suctioning of the oropharynx after the head is delivered reduces the incidence of meconium aspiration.

TREATMENT. In the absence of fetal distress, a vigorous infant (Apgar score of 8 or more) can be born through thin meconium and may not require treatment. Depressed infants (those with hypotonia, bradycardia, or apnea) and those delivered through thick particulate (pea-soup) meconium-stained fluid (particularly those who did not undergo DeLee suctioning) should undergo endotracheal intubation, and suction should be applied directly to the endotracheal tube to remove meconium from the airway. The risks of laryngoscopy with endotracheal intubation (bradycardia, laryngospasm, hypoxia, posterior pharyngeal laceration with pseudodiverticulum formation) are less than the risks of meconium aspiration syndrome in these circumstances.

Treatment of meconium aspiration pneumonia includes supportive care and standard management for respiratory distress. The oxygenation benefit of PEEP must be weighed against the risk of pneumothorax. Severe meconium aspiration resembles persistent fetal circulation and requires similar treatment. Patients who are refractory to conventional mechanical or high frequency ventilation may benefit from surfactant therapy (regardless of gestational age), inhaled nitric oxide, or extracorporeal membrane oxygenation (ECMO) (see Chapter 87.7).

PROGNOSIS. The mortality of meconium-stained infants is considerably higher than that of nonstained infants, and meconium aspiration used to account for a significant proportion of neonatal deaths. Residual lung problems are rare but include

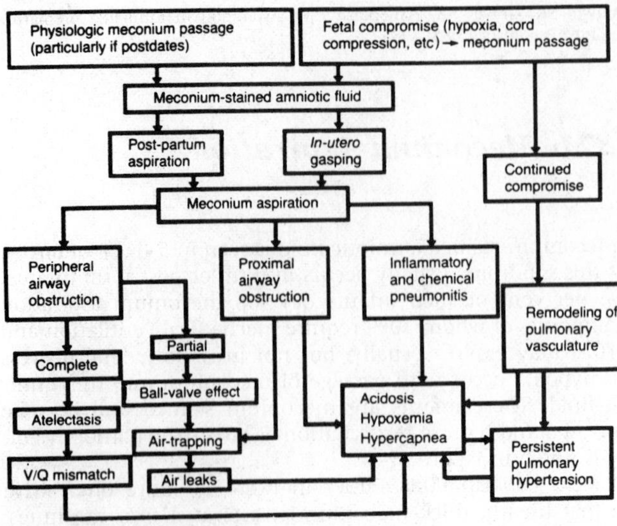

Figure 87–7. Pathophysiology of meconium passage and the meconium aspiration syndrome. (From Wiswell TE, Bent RC: Meconium staining and the meconium aspiration syndrome. Pediatr Clin North Am 40:955, 1993.)

symptomatic cough, wheezing, and persistent hyperinflation for 5–10 yr. Ultimate prognosis depends on the extent of central nervous system injury from asphyxia and the presence of associated problems such as persistence of the fetal circulation.

Anonymous: Lung function in children after neonatal meconium aspiration. Lancet 2:317, 1988.
Cialone PR, Sherer DM, Ryan RM, et al: Amnioinfusion during labor complicated by particulate meconium-stained amniotic fluid decreases neonatal morbidity. Am J Obstet Gynecol 170:842, 1994.
Cunningham A, Lawson E, Martin R, et al: Tracheal suction and meconium: A proposed standard of care. J Pediatr 116:153, 1990.
Gregory GA, Gooding CA, Phibbs RH, et al: Meconium aspiration infants; a prospective study. J Pediatr 85:848, 1974.
Hageman JR: Meconium staining of the amniotic fluid: The need for reassessment of management by obstetricians and pediatricians. Curr Probl Pediatr 23:396, 1993.
Nathan L, Leveno KJ, Carmody TJ, et al: Meconium: A 1990s perspective on an old obstetric hazard. Obstet Gynecol 83:329, 1994.
Sunno C, Kosasa TS, Hale RW: Meconium aspiration syndrome without evidence of fetal distress in early labor before elective cesarean delivery. Obstet Gynecol 73:707, 1989.
Wiswell TE, Bent RC: Meconium staining and the meconium aspiration syndrome. Pediatr Clin North Am 40:955, 1993.
Yoder BA: Meconium-stained amniotic fluid and respiratory complications: Impact of selective tracheal suction. Obstet Gynecol 83:77, 1994.

87.7 *Primary Pulmonary Hypertension—Persistent Fetal Circulation (PFC)*

PFC occurs in term and post-term infants following birth asphyxia, meconium aspiration pneumonia, group B streptococcal sepsis, hyaline membrane disease, hypoglycemia, polycythemia, and pulmonary hypoplasia due to diaphragmatic hernia, amniotic fluid leak, oligohydramnios, or pleural effusions. PFC is often idiopathic. The incidence is 1:500 to 1:700 live births.

PATHOPHYSIOLOGY. Persistence of the fetal circulatory pattern of right-to-left shunting through the patent ductus arteriosus and foramen ovale after birth is due to an excessively high pulmonary vascular resistance. Fetal pulmonary vascular resistance is usually elevated relative to fetal systemic or postnatal pulmonary pressure. This fetal state permits shunting of oxygenated umbilical venous blood to the left atrium (and brain) through the foramen ovale and bypasses the lungs through the ductus arteriosus to the descending aorta. After birth, pulmonary vascular resistance normally declines rapidly as a consequence of vasodilation due to gas filling the lungs, a rise in postnatal PaO_2, a reduction in PCO_2, increased pH, and release of vasoactive substances. Increased neonatal pulmonary vascular resistance may be (1) maladaptive from an acute injury (e.g., not demonstrating normal vasodilation in response to increased oxygen and other changes after birth); (2) the result of increased pulmonary artery medial muscle thickness and extension of smooth muscle layers into the usually nonmuscular, more peripheral pulmonary arterioles in response to chronic fetal hypoxia; (3) due to pulmonary hypoplasia (diaphragmatic hernia, Potter syndrome); (4) obstructive owing to polycythemia or total anomalous pulmonary venous return; or (5) due to alveolar capillary dysplasia, a lethal, possibly familial disorder with thickened alveolar septum and reduced numbers of small pulmonary arteries and capillaries. Apart from the etiology, profound hypoxia from right-to-left shunting and normal or elevated PCO_2 are present.

CLINICAL MANIFESTATIONS. Infants become ill in the delivery room or within the first 12 hr of life. PFC due to polycythemia, idiopathic causes, hypoglycemia, or asphyxia may result in severe cyanosis with tachypnea, although initially there may be minimal signs of respiratory distress. Infants who have PFC associated with meconium aspiration, group B streptococcal pneumonia, diaphragmatic hernia, or pulmonary hypoplasia usually have cyanosis, grunting, flaring, retractions, tachycardia, and shock. Multiorgan involvement may be present (see Table 84–1). Myocardial ischemia, papillary muscle dysfunction with mitral and tricuspid regurgitation, and cardiac stun produce cardiogenic shock with decreased pulmonary blood flow, tissue perfusion, and oxygen delivery. *Hypoxia is quite labile and often out of proportion to the findings on chest roentgenograms.*

DIAGNOSIS. PFC should be suspected in all term infants with cyanosis with or without fetal distress, intrauterine growth retardation, meconium-stained amniotic fluid, hypoglycemia, polycythemia, diaphragmatic hernia, pleural effusions, and birth asphyxia. Hypoxia is universal and is unresponsive to 100% oxygen given by oxygen hood but may respond transiently to hyperoxic hyperventilation administered after endotracheal intubation or application of a bag and mask. A PaO_2 gradient between a preductal (right radial artery) and a postductal (umbilical artery) site of blood sampling greater than 20 mm Hg suggests right to left shunting through the ductus arteriosus and PFC. Real-time echocardiography combined with Doppler flow studies demonstrate right-to-left shunting across a patent foramen ovale and a ductus arteriosus. Deviation of the intra-atrial septum into the left atrium is seen in severe PFC. Tricuspid or mitral insufficiency may be noted on auscultation as a holosystolic murmur and visualized echocardiographically together with poor contractility when PFC is associated with myocardial ischemia. The degree of tricuspid regurgitation can estimate the pulmonary artery pressure. The second heart sound is accentuated and is not split. In asphyxia-associated and idiopathic PFC the chest roentgenogram is normal, whereas in PFC associated with pneumonia and diaphragmatic hernia it shows the specific lesions of parenchymal opacification and bowel in the chest, respectively. The *differential diagnosis* of PFC includes cyanotic heart disease (especially total anomalous pulmonary venous return) and the associated etiologic entities that predispose to PFC (e.g., hypoglycemia, polycythemia, sepsis).

TREATMENT. Therapy is directed toward correcting any predisposing disease (hypoglycemia, polycythemia) and improving poor tissue oxygenation. The response to therapy is often unpredictable, transient, and complicated by adverse effects of drugs or mechanical ventilation. Initial management includes oxygen administration and correction of acidosis, hypotension, and hypercarbia. Persistent hypoxia should be managed with intubation and mechanical ventilation.

One approach to treatment of severe PFC consists of instituting mechanical ventilation without pancuronium paralysis; ventilator settings are selected to achieve a Pa_{O_2} of 50–70 mm Hg and a P_{CO_2} of 50–55 mm Hg. Tolazoline (1 mg/kg), a nonselective α-adrenergic antagonist, is used as an adjunct to vasodilate the pulmonary arterial system but also results in systemic hypotension, which is treated with volume expansion and dopamine. In another approach to treating severe PFC, hyperventilation is used to reduce pulmonary vasoconstriction by lowering P_{CO_2} (20–25 mm Hg) and increasing pH (7.50–7.60). This requires high peak inspiratory pressures and rapid respiratory rates, often necessitating the use of pancuronium paralysis to control ventilation in order to achieve a Pa_{O_2} of between 90 and 100 mm Hg. Complications of hyperventilation include hyperinflation with reduced carbon dioxide elimination, reduced cardiac output, barotrauma, pneumothorax, decreased cerebral blood flow, increased fluid requirements, and edema resulting from pancuronium paralysis. Alkalination with sodium bicarbonate also has been used to elevate the plasma pH to induce pulmonary arterial vasodilation. Both methods of mechanical ventilation may be successful, and specific indications for one or the other have not been defined. Patients not responding to conventional ventilation may later respond to hyperventilation or high-frequency ventilation. Cardiogenic shock should be treated with inotropic agents such as dopamine and dobutamine.

Exogenous surfactant therapy has been beneficial in some patients. Inhaled nitric oxide, a potent and selective pulmonary vasodilator (equivalent to endothelium-derived relaxation factor), when given in 10–20 ppm (occasionally 50) has improved oxygenation in patients with PFC and reduced the need for ECMO.

Extracorporeal Membrane Oxygenation (ECMO). In 5–10% of patients with PFC (approximately 1:4000 births) there is a poor response to 100% oxygen, mechanical ventilation, and drugs. In such patients, the alveolar-arterial oxygen gradient (roughly at sea level [760 − 47] − Pa_{CO_2} − Pa_{O_2}) or the oxygenation index, OI,

$$(\text{mean airway pressure} \times Fi_{O_2} \times 100) \div \text{Postductal } Pa_{O_2}$$

has been used to predict a greater than 80% mortality. AaD_{O_2} gradients of greater than 620 for 8–12 hr and an OI of more than 40 that are unresponsive to nitric oxide inhalation predict a high mortality and are indications for ECMO. ECMO has also been used to treat carefully selected severely ill infants who have hyaline membrane disease, meconium aspiration pneumonia, or group B streptococcal sepsis. ECMO is indicated in hypoxic patients with diaphragmatic hernia, especially when the ventilation index (rate × mean airway pressure) exceeds 1,000 and the P_{CO_2} exceeds 40 mm Hg.

ECMO is a form of cardiopulmonary bypass that augments systemic perfusion and provides gas exchange. Most experience has been with veno-arterial bypass, which requires placement of large catheters in the right internal jugular vein and carotid artery and often necessitates carotid artery ligation. (Venovenous bypass avoids this ligation and provides gas exchange but does not support cardiac output.) Blood is initially pumped through the ECMO circuit at a rate that approximates 80% of the estimated cardiac output of 150–200 ml/kg/min. Venous return passes through a membrane oxygenator, is warmed, and returns into the aortic arch. Venous oxygen saturations are used to monitor tissue oxygen delivery and subsequent extraction. The rate of ECMO flow is adjusted to achieve satisfactory venous oxygen saturation (>65%) and cardiovascular stability. When an infant is started on ECMO the existing ventilator support is weaned to room air at a low rate and pressure to reduce the risk of oxygen toxicity and barotrauma, thus permitting time for the lungs to rest and heal.

Because ECMO requires complete heparinization to prevent clotting in the circuit, patients with or at risk for IVH (weight <2 kg, age <35 wk gestation) are not candidates for this therapy. In addition, infants for whom ECMO is being considered should have reversible lung disease, no signs of systemic bleeding, and an absence of severe asphyxia or lethal malformations, and they should have been ventilated for less than 7–10 days. Complications of ECMO include thromboembolism, air embolization, bleeding, stroke, seizures, atelectasis, cholestatic jaundice, thrombocytopenia, neutropenia, hemolysis, infectious complications of blood transfusions, edema formation, and systemic hypertension.

PROGNOSIS. The outcome for infants with PFC is related to the associated hypoxic-ischemic encephalopathy and the ability to reduce pulmonary vascular resistance. The long-term prognosis for infants with PFC who survive after treatment with hyperventilation is comparable to that for infants who have underlying illnesses of equivalent severity (e.g., birth asphyxia, hypoglycemia, polycythemia). The outcome for infants who have PFC treated with ECMO is also favorable; 85–90% survive, and 70–75% of survivors appear normal at 1 yr of age. Infants who have diaphragmatic hernia associated with severe PFC do poorly if the pre- and postsurgery P_{CO_2} exceeds 40 mm Hg despite mechanical ventilation. Such patients may respond to ECMO; rarely, it is not possible to wean them from bypass, or they expire after ECMO has been discontinued. Lung transplantation may benefit these infants.

Abman SH, Kinsella JP, Schaffer MS, et al: Inhaled nitric oxide in the management of a premature newborn with severe respiratory distress and pulmonary hypertension. Pediatrics 92:606, 1993.

Boggs S, Harris MC, Hoffman DJ, et al: Misalignment of pulmonary veins with alveolar capillary dysplasia: Affected siblings and variable phenotypic expression. J Pediatr 124:125, 1994.

Clark RH, Yoder BA, Sell MS: Prospective, randomized comparison of high-frequency oscillation and conventional ventilation in candidates for extracorporeal membrane oxygenation. J Pediatr 124:447, 1994.

Donn SM: Alternatives to ECMO. Arch Dis Child 70:F81, 1994.

Finer NN, Etches PC, Kamstra B, et al: Inhaled nitric oxide in infants referred for extracorporeal membrane oxygenation: Dose response. J Pediatr 124:302, 1994.

Kanto WP: A decade of experience with neonatal extracorporeal membrane oxygenation. J Pediatr 124:335, 1994.

Roberts JD, Shaul PW: Advances in the treatment of persistent pulmonary hypertension of the newborn. Pediatr Clin North Am 40:983, 1993.

Schumacher RE: Extracorporeal membrane oxygenation. Will this therapy continue to be as efficacious in the future? Pediatr Clin North Am 40:1005, 1993.

Walsh-Sukys MC, Bauer RE, Cornell DJ, et al: Severe respiratory failure in neonates: Mortality and morbidity rates and neurodevelopmental outcomes. J Pediatr 125:104, 1994.

Walsh-Sukys M, Stork EK, Martin RJ: Neonatal ECMO: Iron lung of the 1990s? J Pediatr 124:427, 1994.
Wilcox DT, Glick PL, Karamanoukian H, et al: Pathophysiology of congenital diaphragmatic hernia. V. Effect of exogenous surfactant therapy on gas exchange and lung mechanics in the lamb congenital diaphragmatic hernia model. J Pediatr 124:289, 1994.

87.8 Extrapulmonary Extravasation of Air

(Pneumothorax, Pneumomediastinum, and Pulmonary Interstitial Emphysema)

Asymptomatic pneumothorax, usually unilateral, is estimated to occur in 1–2% of all newborn infants; symptomatic pneumothorax and pneumomediastinum are less common. Pneumothorax is more common in males than in females and in term and post-term infants than in premature ones. The incidence is increased among infants with lung disease, such as meconium aspiration and hyaline membrane disease; in those who have had vigorous resuscitation or are receiving assisted ventilation, especially if high inspiratory pressure or a continuous elevation of end-expiratory pressure is used; and in infants with urinary tract anomalies.

ETIOLOGY AND PATHOPHYSIOLOGY. The most common cause of pneumothorax is overinflation resulting in alveolar rupture. It may be "spontaneous" or idiopathic or secondary to underlying pulmonary disease, such as lobar emphysema or rupture of a congenital or pneumonic cyst; to trauma; or to a "ball-valve" type of bronchial or bronchiolar obstruction resulting from aspiration. Air leaks occur during the first 24–36 hr in infants with meconium aspiration, pneumonia, and hyaline membrane disease when lung compliance is reduced and later during the recovery phase of hyaline membrane disease if inspiratory pressure and PEEP are not reduced simultaneously with improved respiratory function.

Pneumothorax associated with pulmonary hypoplasia is common, occurs in the first day of life, and is due to reduced alveolar surface area and poorly compliant lungs. It is associated with disorders of decreased amniotic fluid volume (Potter syndrome; renal agenesis, renal dysplasia, chronic amniotic fluid leak), decreased fetal breathing movement (oligohydramnios, neuromuscular disease), pulmonary space-occupying lesions (diaphragmatic hernia, pleural effusion, chylothorax), and thoracic abnormalities (asphyxiating thoracic dystrophies).

Air from a ruptured alveolus escapes into the interstitial spaces of the lung, where it may cause *interstitial emphysema* or may dissect along the peribronchial and perivascular connective tissue sheaths to the root of the lung. If the volume of escaped air is great enough, it may follow the vascular sheaths to cause mediastinal emphysema or a rupture with subsequent pneumomediastinum, pneumothorax, and subcutaneous emphysema. Rarely, increased mediastinal pressure may compress pulmonary veins at the hilum, interfering with venous return to the heart and cardiac output. On occasion, air may embolize into the circulation, producing cutaneous blanching, air in intravascular catheters, an air-filled heart on chest roentgenograms, and death.

Tension pneumothorax occurs if an accumulation of air within the pleural space is sufficient to elevate intrapleural pressure above atmospheric pressure. A unilateral tension pneumothorax results in impaired ventilation not only in the collapsed lung but also in the normal lung by a mediastinal shift to the other side. Compression of the vena cava and torsion of the great vessels may interfere with venous return.

CLINICAL MANIFESTATIONS. The physical findings of *asymptomatic pneumothorax* are hyper-resonance and diminished breath sounds over the involved side of the chest with or without tachypnea.

Symptomatic pneumothorax is characterized by respiratory distress, which varies from only an increased respiratory rate to severe dyspnea, tachypnea, and cyanosis. Irritability and restlessness or apnea may be the earliest signs. The onset may be sudden or gradual; an infant may rapidly become critically ill. The chest may appear asymmetric with increased anteroposterior diameter and bulging of the intercostal spaces on the affected side, and there may be hyper-resonance and diminished or absent breath sounds. The heart is displaced toward the unaffected side, and the diaphragm is displaced downward, as is the liver with right-sided pneumothorax. Since both sides are affected in approximately 10% of patients, symmetry of findings does not rule out pneumothorax. In tension pneumothorax there may be signs of shock, and the apex of the heart is pushed away from the affected side.

Pneumomediastinum occurs in at least 25% of patients with pneumothorax and is usually asymptomatic. The degree of respiratory distress depends on the amount of trapped air. If it is great, there is bulging of the midthoracic area, the neck veins are distended, and the blood pressure is low. The last two findings are the result of blockage of the circulation by compression of the systemic and pulmonary veins. Although few clinical signs may exist, subcutaneous emphysema in the newborn infant is almost pathognomonic of pneumomediastinum.

Pulmonary interstitial emphysema (PIE) may precede the development of a pneumothorax or may occur independently, resulting in increasing respiratory distress due to decreased compliance, hypercarbia, and hypoxia. The latter is due to an increased alveolar-arterial oxygen gradient and intrapulmonary shunting. Progressive enlargement of blebs or air may result in cystic dilatations and respiratory deterioration resembling pneumothorax. In severe cases PIE precedes the development of bronchopulmonary dysplasia (BPD). Avoidance of high inspiratory or mean ventilatory pressures may prevent the development of PIE. Treatment may include bronchoscopy if there is evidence of mucus plugging, selective intubation of the uninvolved bronchus, oxygen, general respiratory care, and high-frequency jet ventilation.

DIAGNOSIS. Pneumothorax and pneumomediastinum should be suspected in any newborn infant who shows signs of respiratory distress or who displays restlessness or irritability, or has a sudden change in condition. The diagnosis is established roentgenographically with the edge of the collapsed lung standing out in relief against the pneumothorax (see Fig. 366–1), and in pneumomediastinum with hyperlucency around the heart border and between the sternum and the heart border (Fig. 87–8). Transillumination of the thorax is often helpful in the emergency diagnosis of pneumothorax; the affected side transmits excessive light. Associated renal anomalies are identified by ultrasonography. Pulmonary hypoplasia is suggested by signs of uterine compression (extremity contractures), small thorax on chest roentgenogram, severe hypoxia with hypercarbia, and signs of the primary disease (hypotonia, diaphragmatic hernia, Potter syndrome).

Pneumopericardium may be asymptomatic, requiring only general supportive treatment, but usually presents as sudden shock with tachycardia, muffled heart sounds, and poor pulses suggesting tamponade, which requires prompt evacuation of entrapped air. **Pneumoperitoneum** from air dissecting through the diaphragmatic apertures during mechanical ventilation may also be confused with perforation of an abdominal organ.

TREATMENT. Without a continued air leak, asymptomatic and mildly symptomatic small pneumothoraces require only close observation. Frequent small feedings may prevent gastric dilatation and minimize crying, which can further compromise

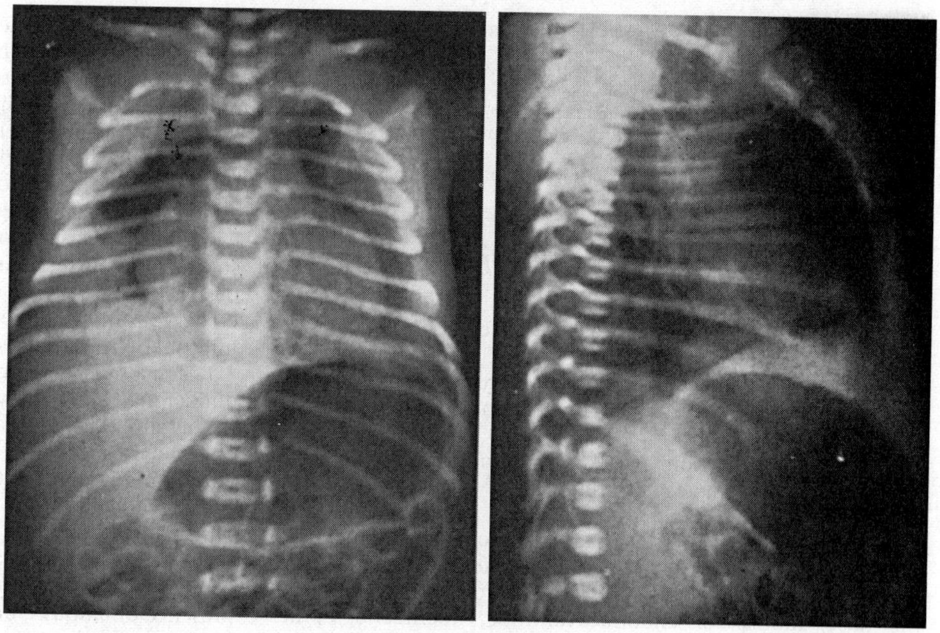

Figure 87–8. Pneumomediastinum in a newborn infant. Anteroposterior view demonstrates compression of lungs and the lateral view shows bulging of the sternum, each resulting from distention of the mediastinum by trapped air.

ventilation and worsen the pneumothorax. Breathing 100% oxygen accelerates the resorption of free pleural air into the blood by reducing the nitrogen tension in blood, producing a resultant nitrogen pressure gradient from the trapped air into the blood, but the benefit must be weighed against the risks of oxygen toxicity. With severe respiratory or circulatory embarrassment, emergency needle aspiration is indicated. If there is adequate time, a chest tube should be inserted and attached to underwaterseal drainage. Severe localized interstitial emphysema may respond to selective bronchial intubation. Judicious use of Pavulon in infants fighting the ventilator may reduce the incidence of pneumothorax.

Gonzalez F, Harris T, Black P, et al: Decreased gas flow through pneumothoraces in neonates receiving high-frequency jet versus conventional ventilation. J Pediatr 110:464, 1987.
Hall RT, Rhodes PG: Pneumothorax and pneumomediastinum in infants with idiopathic respiratory distress syndrome receiving CPAP. Pediatrics 55:493, 1975.
Primhak RA: Factors associated with pulmonary air leak in premature infants receiving mechanical ventilation. J Pediatr 102:764, 1983.
Ryan CA, Barrington KJ, Phillips HJ, et al: Contralateral pneumothoraces in the newborn: Incidence and predisposing factors. Pediatrics 79:417, 1987.

87.9 Interstitial Pulmonary Fibrosis

(Wilson-Mikity Syndrome; Bronchopulmonary Dysplasia; Pulmonary Insufficiency of the Premature)

See also Chapter 87.3 for discussion of bronchopulmonary dysplasia.

Wilson and Mikity described a pulmonary syndrome of premature infants, usually of less than 32 wk gestation and birthweights below 1,500 g, and without a history of hyaline membrane disease; it was characterized by insidious onset of dyspnea, tachypnea, retractions, and cyanosis during the 1st mo of life. Rare cases have been reported in full-term infants, usually those having a history of meconium aspiration or oxygen administration. Viral infections also have been implicated.

Several variations on the clinical presentation have been described with similar roentgenographic findings. Some infants have respiratory distress at birth that is occasionally severe, resembles hyaline membrane disease, and requires oxygen; these may be cases of bronchopulmonary dysplasia (BPD). Others show a more gradual development of dyspnea and cyanosis. Others have no early respiratory symptoms or history of exposure to oxygen, and the onset of symptoms occurs at several weeks of life.

Cough, wheezing, and rales may develop, but fever occurs only with concomitant infection. There may be collapse of a lobe or lung; other complications are right-sided heart failure, osteoporosis, and rib fractures. The symptoms usually increase over 2–6 wk with increasing oxygen dependency persisting for several months, followed by gradual resolution or progressive respiratory and cardiac failure. Infants who recover from the severe form may have an increased number of lower respiratory tract infections in the 1st yr of life. The most characteristic features of this syndrome are roentgenographic. Early, they include bilateral coarse reticular streaky infiltrates and, often, overexpansion of the lungs with small areas of emphysema that develop into multicystic lesions. Subsequently, the cysts enlarge and coalesce to give a hyperlucent, bubbly appearance (see Fig. 87–5*B*). The roentgenograms tend to clear gradually over months to several years. The roentgenographic changes in Wilson-Mikity syndrome may be indistinguishable from those of BPD.

The syndrome must be differentiated from pneumonia due to cytomegalovirus, *Pneumocystis carinii, Ureaplasma urealyticum*, or *Chlamydia* pneumonia, and from cystic fibrosis. *Chronic pulmonary insufficiency of prematurity* is initially different from BPD. Usually a VLBW infant without respiratory distress syndrome develops severe apnea on day 2–5. Atelectasis and a reduced functional residual capacity follow, requiring treatment with CPAP or mechanical ventilation. With prolonged ventilation, a picture of BPD intervenes.

Treatment consists of supportive measures: oxygen for cyanosis, bronchodilators, diuretics for cardiac failure, acid-base correction, correction of anemia with transfusion or erythropoietin, and assisted ventilation when indicated. A trial of erythromycin may be indicated to treat *Chlamydia* or *Ureaplasma* pneumonia.

Abman SH, Wolfe RR, Accurso FJ, et al: Pulmonary vascular response to oxygen in infants with severe bronchopulmonary dysplasia. Pediatrics 75:80, 1985.
Hudak BB, Allen MC, Hudal ML, et al: Home oxygen therapy for chronic lung disease in extremely low-birth-weight infants. Am J Dis Child 143:357, 1989.
Kao LC, Durand DJ, McCrea RC, et al: Randomized trial of long-term diuretic

therapy for infants with oxygen-dependent bronchopulmonary dysplasia. J Pediatr 124:772, 1994.
Ohis RK, Hunter DD, Christensen RD: A randomized, double-blind, placebo-controlled trial of recombinant erythropoietin in treatment of the anemia of bronchopulmonary dysplasia. J Pediatr 123:996, 1993.
Wilson MG, Mikity VG: A new form of respiratory distress in premature infants. Am J Dis Child 99:489, 1960.
Zimmerman JJ, Farrell PM: Advances and issues in bronchopulmonary dysplasia. Curr Probl Pediatr 24:159, 1994.

87.10 Pulmonary Hemorrhage

Massive pulmonary hemorrhage is present in 15% of neonates who come to autopsy in the first 2 wk of life. The reported incidence at autopsy varies from 1–4/1,000 live births. About three fourths of the patients weigh less than 2,500 g at birth.

Most infants in whom pulmonary hemorrhage is demonstrated at autopsy have had symptoms of respiratory distress that are indistinguishable from those of hyaline membrane disease. The onset may occur at birth or may be delayed several days. One fourth to one half of affected infants cough up or regurgitate material containing old or fresh blood from the nose, mouth, or endotracheal tube. Roentgenographic findings are varied and nonspecific, ranging from minor streaking or patchy infiltrates to massive consolidation.

The cause of massive pulmonary hemorrhage is usually not identified; the incidence is increased in association with acute pulmonary infection, severe asphyxia, hyaline membrane disease, surfactant therapy, assisted ventilation, congenital heart disease, erythroblastosis fetalis, hemorrhagic disease of the newborn, kernicterus, inborn errors of ammonia metabolism, and cold injury. Although in the majority of instances bleeding into other organs is observed at autopsy, bleeding other than through the nostrils and mouth and intraventricular bleeding are relatively rare during life and should suggest the possibility of an additional bleeding diathesis such as disseminated intravascular coagulation. Bleeding is predominantly alveolar in about two thirds of cases and interstitial in the rest. In some infants the pulmonary hemorrhage represents hemorrhagic pulmonary edema due to severe left-sided heart failure resulting from hypoxia.

The little information available that describes the prognosis of infants who bleed through the mouth or nostrils suggests that it is extremely poor. Death occurs in the first 48 hr of life in two thirds of the infants who come to autopsy. Treatment includes blood replacement, positive end-expiratory pressure, and epinephrine aerosols.

Acute pulmonary hemorrhage may also rarely occur in postneonatal full-term infants. The etiology is unknown. These infants have acute respiratory distress with bilateral alveolar infiltrates and usually respond to intensive supportive treatment.

Cole VA, Norman ICS, Reynolds EOR, et al: Pathogenesis of hemorrhagic pulmonary edema and massive pulmonary hemorrhage in the newborn. Pediatrics 51:175, 1973.
CDC. Acute pulmonary hemorrhage among infants. MMWR 44:67, 1995.
Pappin A, Shenker N, Hack M, et al: Extensive intraalveolar pulmonary hemorrhage in infants dying after surfactant therapy. J Pediatr 124:621, 1994.

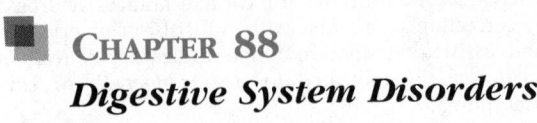

CHAPTER 88
Digestive System Disorders

VOMITING. Infants may vomit mucus, occasionally blood-streaked, in the first few hours after birth. This vomiting rarely persists after the first few feedings; it may be due to irritation of the gastric mucosa by material swallowed during delivery. If the vomiting is protracted, gastric lavage with physiologic saline solution may relieve it.

Vomiting is a relatively frequent symptom during the neonatal period. In the majority of instances it is simply regurgitation from overfeeding or from failure to permit the infant to eructate swallowed air. (See Chapter 269 for discussion of gastric emptying and gastroesophageal reflux.) When vomiting occurs shortly after birth and is persistent, the possibilities of intestinal obstruction and increased intracranial pressure must be considered. A history of maternal hydramnios suggests upper gastrointestinal (esophageal, duodenal, ileal) atresia.

Bile-stained emesis suggests intestinal obstruction beyond the duodenum, but it may also be idiopathic. Abdominal roentgenograms (kidney-ureter-bladder [KUB] and cross-table lateral views) should be performed in neonates with persistent emesis and in all infants with bile-stained emesis to detect air-fluid levels, distended bowel loops, characteristic patterns of obstruction (double bubble: duodenal atresia), and pneumoperitoneum (intestinal perforation). A barium swallow roentgenogram with small bowel follow-through is indicated in the presence of bilious emesis.

Obstructive lesions of the digestive tract occur most frequently in the esophagus and intestines (see Chapters 265, 275, and 276). Vomiting from esophageal obstruction occurs with the first feeding. The diagnosis of esophageal atresia can be suspected if there is unusual drooling from the mouth and if resistance is encountered in the attempt to pass a catheter into the stomach. Diagnosis should be made before the infant chokes on oral feedings and risks aspiration pneumonia. Infantile achalasia (cardiospasm), a rare cause of vomiting in the newborn infant, is demonstrable roentgenographically by obstruction at the cardiac end of the esophagus, without organic stenosis. Regurgitation of feedings due to continuous relaxation of the esophageal-gastric sphincter, chalasia, is a cause of vomiting, which can be controlled by keeping the infant in a semi-upright position.

Vomiting due to *obstruction of the small intestine* usually begins on the 1st day of life and is frequent, persistent, usually nonprojectile, copious, and, unless the obstruction is above the ampulla of Vater, bile-stained; it is associated with abdominal distention, visible deep peristaltic waves, and reduced or absent bowel movements. Malrotation with obstruction from midgut volvulus is an acute emergency that must be considered. Upright roentgenographic films of the abdomen will show the distribution of air in the intestine and often aid in locating the site of the obstruction; malrotation may be identified by contrast studies. Normally, air can be demonstrated roentgenographically in the jejunum by 15–60 min, in the ileum by 2–3 hr, and in the colon by 3 hr after birth. Absence of rectal gas at 24 hr is abnormal. Persistent vomiting may occur with congenital hernia of the diaphragm. The vomiting of pyloric stenosis may begin any time after birth but does not assume its characteristic pattern before the 2nd–3rd wk. Vomiting may occur with many other disturbances that do not obstruct the digestive tract, such as celiac disease, milk allergy, adrenal hyperplasia of the salt-losing variety, galactosemia, hyperammonemias, increased intracranial pressure, septicemia, meningitis, and urinary tract infections.

THRUSH (ORAL CANDIDOSIS). Thrush of the mouth occurs in healthy infants; later, it is rare except in debilitated infants, in those receiving antibiotic or immunosuppressive therapy, and in those with acquired immunodeficiency syndrome (AIDS). Infants with AIDS also manifest failure to thrive, psychomotor retardation, hepatosplenomegaly, diarrhea, lymphadenopathy, and hypergammaglobulinemia (see Chapter 223).

Transmission of the infection from maternal vaginal moniliasis to the infant's oral mucosa is the primary means of infection in healthy newborns. Secondary cases develop in the hospital nursery, presumably owing to contact with infected infants and contaminated supplies or caretakers.

Oral thrush in an otherwise healthy infant is usually a self-limited infection, but treatment is advised, especially in the presence of candidal diaper rash (Chapter 98.6).

DIARRHEA. See Chapters 56.1, 171, 284, and 286.

CONSTIPATION. More than 90% of full-term newborn infants pass meconium within the first 24 hr, and most of the remainder do so within 36 hr; the possibility of intestinal obstruction should be considered in any infant who does not. Intestinal atresia or stenosis, congenital aganglionic megacolon, milk bolus obstruction, meconium ileus, or meconium plugs may present as constipation. About 20% of VLBW infants do not pass meconium within the first 24 hr. Constipation not present from birth but appearing during the 1st mo of life suggests congenital aganglionic megacolon, cretinism, or anal stenosis. It must be kept in mind that infrequent bowel movements do not necessarily mean constipation. A breast-fed infant usually has frequent bowel movements, whereas a formula-fed infant may have 1–2 movements a day or every other day.

MECONIUM PLUGS. Lower colonic or anorectal plugs (Fig. 88–1) with a lower than normal water content may cause intestinal obstruction. Rarely, a firm mass of meconium may form elsewhere in the intestine and cause intrauterine intestinal obstruction and meconium peritonitis unrelated to cystic fibrosis. Anorectal plugs may also cause intestinal ulceration and perforation. Meconium plugs are associated with small left colon syndrome in the infant of a diabetic mother, cystic fibrosis, rectal aganglionosis, maternal drug abuse, and magnesium sulfate therapy for pre-eclampsia. The plug may be evacuated by irrigating it with isotonic sodium chloride solution. Enemas with the iodinated contrast medium Gastrografin usually cause passage of the plug, presumably because the high osmolarity (1,900 mOsm/L) of the medium draws fluid rapidly into the intestinal lumen and loosens inspissated material. Since this rapid loss of fluid into the bowel may result in acute dehydration and shock, it is advisable to dilute the contrast material with an equal amount of water, to correct any existing dehydration and to provide intravenous fluids during and for several hours after the procedure. *After removal of a meconium plug the infant should be observed closely for the possible presence of congenital aganglionic megacolon.*

88.1 Meconium Ileus in Cystic Fibrosis

In the newborn infant impaction of meconium causes intestinal obstructions often associated with cystic fibrosis. The absence of pancreatic enzymes limits normal digestive activities in the intestine, and meconium is left in a viscid, mucilaginous state. It clings to the intestinal wall and is moved with difficulty. The inspissated and impacted meconium fills the intestinal canal but is most concentrated in the lower ileum.

Clinically, the pattern is that of congenital intestinal obstruction with or without intestinal perforation. Abdominal distention is prominent, and persistent vomiting soon occurs. Infrequently, one or more inspissated meconium stools may be passed shortly after birth.

The differential diagnosis involves other causes of intestinal obstruction, including intestinal pseudo-obstruction and pancreatic insufficiency; an exact diagnosis cannot be made except at laparotomy. A presumptive diagnosis can be made on the basis of a history of cystic fibrosis in a sibling, by palpation of doughy or cordlike masses of intestines through the abdominal wall, and by the roentgenographic appearance. Roentgenographically, in contrast to the generally evenly distended intestinal loops above an atresia, the loops may vary in width and are not as evenly filled with gas. At points of heaviest meconium concentration the infiltrated gas may create a bubbly granular appearance (Figs. 88–2 and 88–3). A negative sweat test in the neonatal period may not rule out cystic fibrosis.

The case fatality rate is high, but a number of infants have survived the neonatal period; their subsequent prognosis depends on the basic disturbance, cystic fibrosis (Chapter 363).

Treatment is high Gastrografin enemas as described under Meconium Plugs (see earlier). If they are unsuccessful or if there is reason to suspect a perforation of the bowel wall, laparotomy is performed and the ileum opened at the point of greatest diameter of the impaction. Approximately 50% of infants have associated intestinal atresia, stenosis, or volvulus that does not respond to contrast enema and requires surgery. The inspissated meconium is removed by gentle and patient irrigation with warm isotonic sodium chloride or Mucomyst (acetylcysteine) solution introduced through a fine catheter,

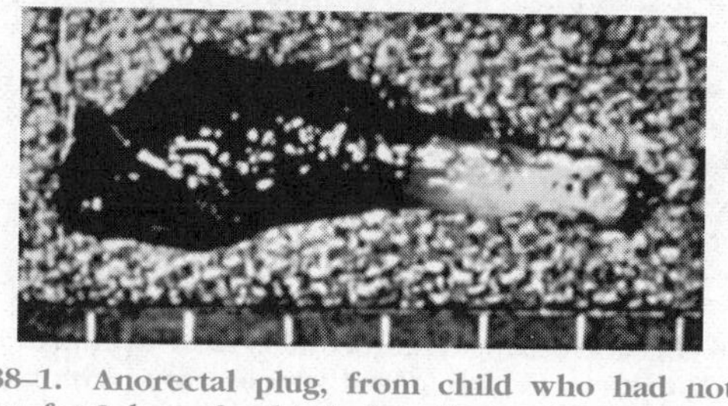

Figure 88–1. Anorectal plug, from child who had not passed meconium for 2 days after birth, is indistinguishable from normal plug. Pale end was adjacent to the anus. (From Emery JL: Arch Dis Child 32:17, 1957.)

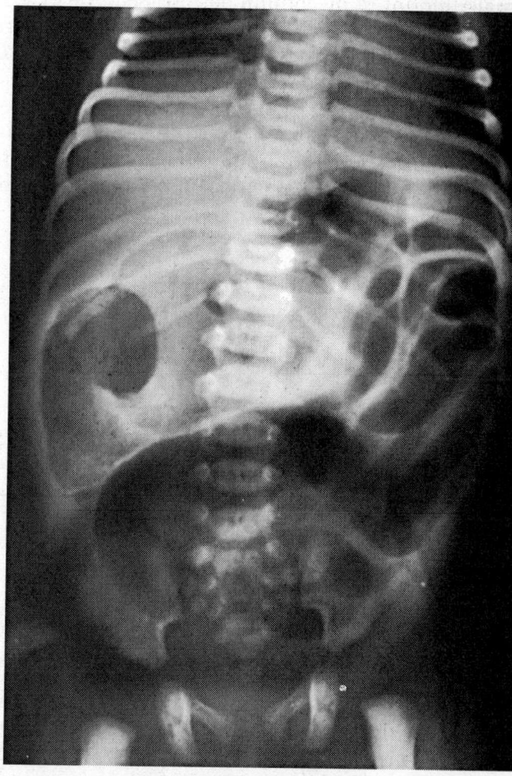

Figure 88–2. Meconium ileus. Impacted meconium with small amounts of air interspersed throughout it in loops of intestine on the right side of abdomen; intestinal loops above this impaction are greatly distended.

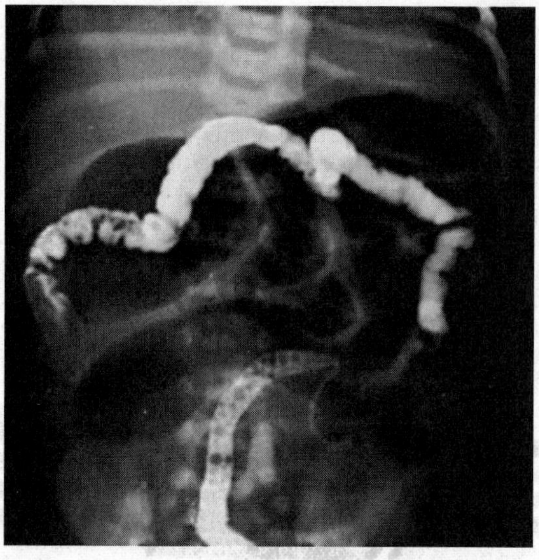

Figure 88–3. Meconium ileus. The colon, outlined by contrast material, is small because meconium has not reached it.

which may be passed between the impaction and the bowel wall.

MECONIUM PERITONITIS. Perforation of the intestine may occur in utero or shortly after birth. Either the tear may be sealed by natural processes relatively quickly with only a small amount of meconium escaping, or the meconial contents may largely be emptied into the peritoneal cavity. Such perforations occur most often as a complication of meconium ileus in infants with cystic fibrosis, but occasionally the perforation is due to a meconium plug or intestinal obstruction of another cause.

When the intestinal perforation is spontaneously sealed and only a small amount of meconium has escaped, the event may never be detected, except when some of the meconial particles become calcified and are later fortuitously discovered on roentgenograms of the abdomen. Alternatively, the clinical picture may be dominated by the signs of intestinal obstruction or peritonitis. Characteristically, there is abdominal distention, vomiting, and absence of stools. Treatment consists primarily of elimination of the intestinal obstruction and drainage of the peritoneal cavity.

88.2 Neonatal Necrotizing Enterocolitis (NEC)

This serious disease of the newborn is of unknown etiology and is characterized by varying degrees of mucosal or transmural necrosis of the intestine. No particular race or sex is unduly susceptible to the disease. Incidence ranges from 1 to 5% of admissions to neonatal intensive care units. Since the very small, ill preterm infant is particularly susceptible to NEC, a rising incidence in recent years may reflect improved survival of this high-risk group of patients. The disease does rarely occur in term infants.

PATHOLOGY AND PATHOGENESIS. Many factors may contribute to the development of a necrotic segment of intestine, the gas accumulation in the submucosa of the bowel wall (pneumatosis, intestinalis), and progression of the necrosis leading to perforation, sepsis, and death. The distal ileum and proximal colon are involved most frequently. A variety of factors such as polycythemia, hypertonic milk or medicines, or too rapid feeding protocols may contribute to mucosal injury and subsequent infection leading to bowel necrosis. NEC also occurs in premature infants without stress, particularly during epidemics. The clustering of cases suggests a primary role for an infectious agent; *Clostridium perfringens, Escherichia coli, Staphylococcus epidermidis,* and rotavirus have commonly been recovered from cultures. Nonetheless, in most situations no identifiable pathogen is recovered.

CLINICAL MANIFESTATIONS. Onset usually occurs in the first 2 wk but can be as late as 2 mo of age in VLBW infants. Meconium is passed normally, and the first signs are abdominal distention with gastric retention. Manifestations usually develop after the onset of enteric feedings. Obvious bloody stools are seen in 25% of patients. The onset is often insidious, and sepsis may be suspected before an intestinal lesion is noted. There is a wide spectrum of illness from mild with only guaiac-positive stools to severe with peritonitis, bowel perforation, shock, and death. Progression may be rapid, but it is unusual for the disease to progress from mild to severe after 72 hr.

DIAGNOSIS. A very high index of suspicion in managing infants at risk is essential. Plain abdominal roentgenograms may demonstrate pneumatosis intestinalis, a finding that is diagnostic of NEC in the newborn infant; 50–75% of patients have pneumatosis when treatment is started (Fig. 88–4). Portal vein gas is a sign of severe disease, and pneumoperitoneum indicates a perforation. (Figs. 88–4 and 88–5).

The differential diagnosis of NEC includes specific infections (systemic or intestinal), obstruction, and volvulus. Indomethacin may produce focal intestinal perforation. Such patients manifest pneumoperitoneum but usually are less ill than those with NEC. Cultures and roentgenograms may be diagnostic. Gastrografin enema may demonstrate pneumatosis intestinalis and should be employed if congenital obstruction or midgut volvulus is a possible diagnosis; hepatic ultrasound may detect portal venous gas despite normal abdominal roentgenograms.

TREATMENT. Intensive therapy is advisable for suspected as well as diagnosed cases. Cessation of feeding, nasogastric decompression, and intravenous fluids with careful attention to acid-base and electrolyte balance are very important. Once cultures are taken of blood, stool, and cerebrospinal fluid, systemic antibiotics (antipseudomonas penicillin [e.g., ticarcillin] and an

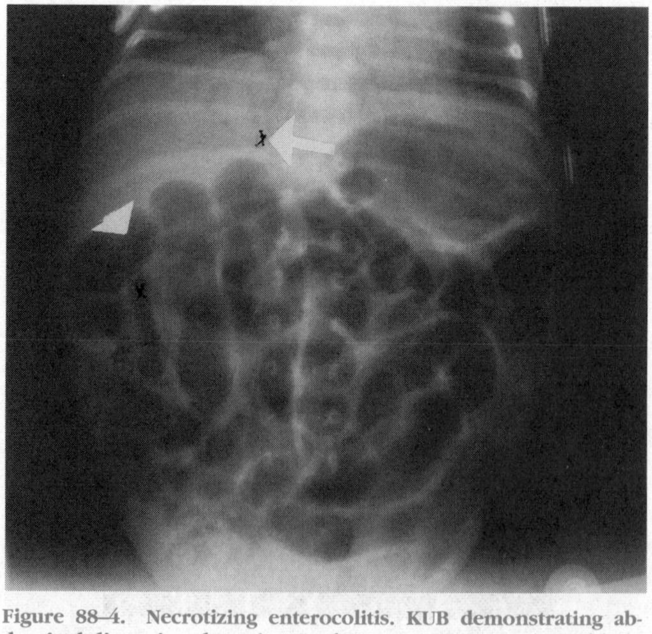

Figure 88–4. Necrotizing enterocolitis. KUB demonstrating abdominal distention, hepatic portal venous gas *(arrow)*, and bubbly appearance of pneumatosis intestinalis *(arrowhead; right lower quadrant)*. The latter two signs are felt to be pathognomonic for NEC.

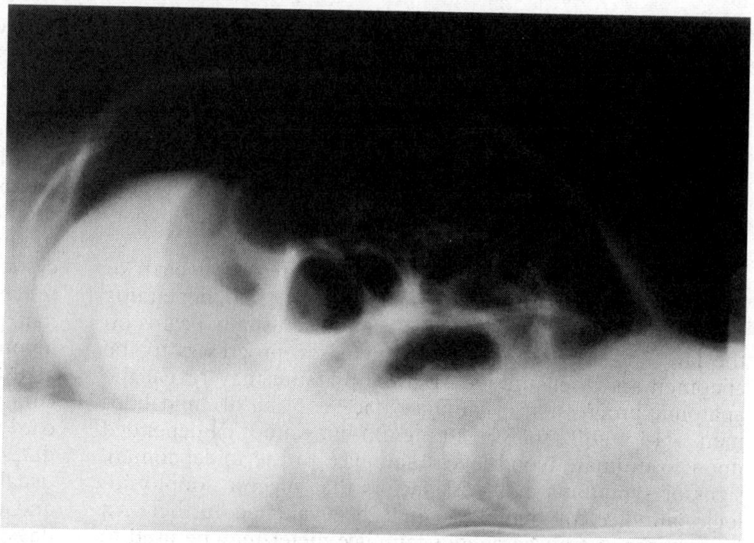

Figure 88–5. Intestinal perforation. Cross-table abdominal roentgenogram in a patient with necrotizing enterocolitis demonstrating marked distention and massive pneumoperitoneum as evident by the free air below the anterior abdominal wall.

aminoglycoside [e.g., gentamicin]) should be started. When present, umbilical catheters should be removed, and ventilation should be assisted if distention is contributing to hypoxia and hypercapnia. If hypotension develops, resuscitation with blood, plasma, crystalloid, and dopamine is essential.

The patient's course should be monitored by frequent cross-table lateral abdominal roentgenograms in search of perforation and by hematocrit, platelet, electrolyte, and acid-base determinations. Gown and glove isolation and grouping infants at similar increased risk into cohorts separate from other infants should be instituted to contain an epidemic.

A surgeon should be consulted early in the course of treatment. Evidence of perforation is usually an indication for resection of necrotic bowel. Pneumoperitoneum and brown paracentesis fluid suggest perforation. Failure to respond to medical management, a single fixed bowel loop, erythema of the abdominal wall, or a mass is an additional indication for exploratory laparotomy, resection of necrotic bowel, and external ostomy diversion. Peritoneal drainage may be helpful for the patient in extremis with peritonitis who is unable to withstand bowel resection.

PROGNOSIS. Medical management fails in about 20% of patients in whom there is pneumatosis intestinalis at diagnosis; of these, at least 25% die. Strictures develop at the site of the necrotizing lesion in about 10% of patients. Resection of the stricture is curative. Complications of NEC following massive intestinal resection include short bowel syndrome (malabsorption, growth failure, malnutrition), complications of total parenteral alimentation due to central venous catheters (sepsis, thrombosis), and cholestatic jaundice that may progress to cirrhosis. *Prevention* may be possible with judicious feeding protocols (slow advancement of no more than 15–20 ml/kg/24 hr) and the use of breast milk.

Buchheit JQ, Stewart DL: Clinical comparison of localized intestinal perforation and necrotizing enterocolitis in neonates. Pediatrics 93:32, 1994.

Kanto WP, Hunter JE, Stoll BJ: Recognition and medical management of necrotizing enterocolitis. Clin Perinatol 21:335, 1994.

Kliegman RM, Walker WA, Yolken RH: Necrotizing enterocolitis: Research agenda for a disease of unknown etiology and pathogenesis. Clin Perinatol 21:437, 1994.

Ricketts RR: Surgical treatment of necrotizing enterocolitis and the short bowel syndrome. Clin Perinatol 21:365, 1994.

Stringer MD, Spitz L: Surgical management of neonatal necrotising enterocolitis. Arch Dis Child 69:269, 1993.

Wang P, Huang F: Time of the first defaecation and urination in very low birth weight infants. Eur J Pediatr 153:279, 1994.

Wilcox DT, Borowitz DS, Stovroff MC, et al: Chronic intestinal pseudo-obstruction with meconium ileus at onset. J Pediatr 123:751, 1993.

88.3 Jaundice and Hyperbilirubinemia in the Newborn

Jaundice is observed during the 1st wk of life in approximately 60% of term infants and 80% of preterm infants. The color usually results from the accumulation in the skin of unconjugated, nonpolar, lipid-soluble bilirubin pigment (indirect-reacting) formed from hemoglobin by the action of heme oxygenase, biliverdin reductase, and nonenzymatic reducing agents in the reticuloendothelial cells; it may also be due in part to the deposition of the pigment after it has been converted in the liver cell microsome by the enzyme uridine diphosphoglucuronic acid (UDPGA) glucuronyl transferase to the polar, water-soluble ester glucuronide of bilirubin (direct-reacting). The unconjugated form is neurotoxic for infants at certain concentrations and under various conditions. Conjugated bilirubin is not neurotoxic but indicates a potentially serious disorder. Mild elevations of bilirubin may have antioxidant properties.

ETIOLOGY. The newborn infant's metabolism of bilirubin is in transition from the fetal stage, during which the placenta is the principal route of elimination of the lipid-soluble bilirubin, to the adult stage, during which the water-soluble conjugated form is excreted from the hepatic cell into the biliary system and then into the gastrointestinal tract. Unconjugated hyperbilirubinemia may be caused or increased by any factor that (1) increases the load of bilirubin to be metabolized by the liver (hemolytic anemias, shortened red cell life due to immaturity or to transfused cells, increased enterohepatic circulation, infection); (2) may damage or reduce the activity of the transferase enzyme (hypoxia, infection, possibly hypothermia and thyroid deficiency); (3) may compete for or block the transferase enzyme (drugs and other substances requiring glucuronic acid conjugation for excretion); or (4) leads to an absence of or decreased amounts of the enzyme or to reduction of bilirubin uptake by the liver cell (genetic defect, prematurity). The risk of toxic effects from elevated levels of unconjugated bilirubin in the serum is increased by factors that reduce the retention of bilirubin in the circulation (hypoproteinemia, displacement of bilirubin from its binding sites on albumin by competitive binding of drugs such as sulfisoxazole and moxalactam, acidosis, increased free fatty acid concentration secondary to hypoglycemia, starvation, or hypothermia), or by factors that increase the permeability of the blood-brain barrier or nerve cell membranes to bilirubin or the susceptibility of brain cells to its toxicity such as asphyxia, prematurity, hyperosmolality, and infection. Early feeding decreases, whereas breast feeding and dehydration increase the serum levels of bilirubin. Meconium has 1 mg bilirubin/dL and may contribute to jaundice by the enterohepatic circulation following deconjugation by intestinal glucuronidase. Drugs such as oxytocin and chemicals employed in the nursery such as phenolic detergents may also produce unconjugated hyperbilirubinemia.

CLINICAL MANIFESTATIONS. Jaundice may be present at birth or may appear at any time during the neonatal period, depending on the condition responsible for it. Jaundice usually begins on the face and, as the serum level increases, progresses to the abdomen and then the feet. Dermal pressure may reveal the anatomic progression of jaundice (face ~ 5 mg/dL, midabdomen ~ 15 mg/dL, soles ~ 20 mg/dL) but cannot be depended upon to estimate blood levels. Jaundice to the midabdomen, signs or symptoms, high risk factors that suggest nonphysiologic jaundice, or hemolysis must be evaluated further. An icterometer or transcutaneous jaundice meter may be used to screen infants, but a serum bilirubin level is indicated for those patients with progressing jaundice, symptoms, or a risk for hemolysis or sepsis. Jaundice resulting from deposition of indirect bilirubin in the skin tends to appear bright yellow or orange; jaundice of the obstructive type (direct bilirubin), a greenish or muddy yellow. This difference is usually apparent only in severe jaundice. The infant may be lethargic and may feed poorly. Signs of kernicterus rarely appear on the first day of jaundice (Chapter 88.4).

DIFFERENTIAL DIAGNOSIS. Jaundice, consisting of indirect or direct bilirubin, that is present at birth or appears within the first 24 hr of life may be due to erythroblastosis fetalis, concealed hemorrhage, sepsis, cytomegalic inclusion disease, rubella, or congenital toxoplasmosis. Jaundice in infants who have received intrauterine transfusions may be characterized by an unusually high proportion of direct-reacting bilirubin. Jaundice that first appears on the 2nd or 3rd day is usually "physiologic" but may represent a more severe form called *hyperbilirubinemia of the newborn.* Familial nonhemolytic icterus (Crigler-Najjar syndrome) is seen initially on the 2nd or 3rd day. *Jaundice appearing after the 3rd day and within the 1st wk should suggest septicemia;* it may be due to other infections, notably syphilis, toxoplasmosis, and cytomegalic inclusion disease. Jaundice secondary to extensive ecchymosis or hematoma may occur during the 1st day or later, especially in premature infants. Polycythemia may lead to early jaundice.

Jaundice that is noted initially after the 1st wk of life suggests breast milk jaundice, septicemia, congenital atresia of the bile ducts, hepatitis, rubella, herpetic hepatitis, galactosemia, hypothyroidism, congenital hemolytic anemia (spherocytosis), or possibly the crises of other hemolytic anemias (such as pyruvate kinase and other glycolytic enzyme deficiencies or hereditary nonspherocytic anemia), or hemolytic anemia due to drugs (as in congenital deficiencies of the enzymes glucose-6-phosphate dehydrogenase, glutathione synthetase, reductase, or peroxidase) (Fig. 88–6).

Persistent jaundice during the 1st mo of life suggests the so-called inspissated bile syndrome (which may follow hemolytic disease of the newborn), hyperalimentation-associated cholestasis, hepatitis, cytomegalic inclusion disease, syphilis, toxoplasmosis, familial nonhemolytic icterus, congenital atresia of the bile ducts, or galactosemia. Rarely, physiologic jaundice may be prolonged for several weeks, as in infants with hypothyroidism or pyloric stenosis.

Low-risk jaundiced infants who are full term and asymptomatic may be evaluated by monitoring serum total bilirubin levels. Regardless of the gestational age or time of appearance of jaundice, significant hyperbilirubinemia and all patients with symptoms or signs require a complete diagnostic evaluation, which should include the determination of the direct and indirect bilirubin fractions, hemoglobin, reticulocyte count, blood type, Coombs test, and an examination of the peripheral blood smear (Table 88–1). Indirect-reacting bilirubinemia, reticulocytosis, and a smear demonstrating evidence of red blood cell destruction suggest hemolysis; in the absence of blood group incompatibility, nonimmunologically induced hemolysis should be considered. If there is direct-reacting hyperbilirubinemia, hepatitis, cholestasis, inborn errors of metabolism, cystic fibrosis, and sepsis are diagnostic possibilities. If the reticulocyte count, Coombs test, and direct bilirubin are normal, physiologic or pathologic indirect hyperbilirubinemia may be present (Fig. 88–6).

PHYSIOLOGIC JAUNDICE (ICTERUS NEONATORUM). Under normal circumstances, the level of indirect-reacting bilirubin in umbilical cord serum is 1–3 mg/dL and rises at a rate of less than 5 mg/dL/24 hr; thus, jaundice becomes visible on the 2nd–3rd day, usually peaking between the 2nd and 4th days at 5–6 mg/dL and decreasing to below 2 mg/dL between the 5th and 7th days of life. Jaundice associated with these changes is designated "physiologic" and is believed to be the result of increased bilirubin production following breakdown of fetal red blood cells combined with transient limitation in the conjugation of bilirubin by the liver.

Overall, 6–7% of full-term infants have indirect bilirubin levels of greater than 12.9 mg/dL and less than 3% have levels greater than 15 mg/dL. Risk factors for indirect hyperbilirubinemia include maternal diabetes, race (Chinese, Japanese, Korean, and Native American), prematurity, drugs (vitamin K_3, novobiocin), altitude, polycythemia, male sex, 21-trisomy, cutaneous bruising, cephalohematoma, oxytocin induction, breast-feeding, weight loss (dehydration or caloric deprivation), delayed stooling, and a sibling who had physiologic jaundice. Infants without these variables rarely develop indirect bilirubin levels above 12 mg/dL, whereas infants with multiple risks are more likely to have higher bilirubin levels. Indirect bilirubin levels in full-term infants decline to adult levels (1 mg/dL) by 10–14 days of life. *Persistent indirect hyperbilirubinemia* beyond 2 wk suggests hemolysis, hereditary glucuronyl transferase deficiency, breast milk jaundice, hypothyroidism, or intestinal obstruction. Jaundice associated with pyloric stenosis may be due to caloric deprivation, deficiency of hepatic UDP-glucuronyl transferase, or ileus-induced increased enterohepatic circulation of bilirubin.

Among premature infants the rise in serum bilirubin tends to be the same or a little slower than that in term infants but is of longer duration, which generally results in higher levels, the peak being reached between the 4th and 7th days; the pattern depends upon the time required for the preterm infant to achieve mature mechanisms for the metabolism and excretion of bilirubin. Usually, peak levels of 8–12 mg/dL are not reached until the 5th–7th day, and jaundice is infrequently observed after the 10th day.

The diagnosis of physiologic jaundice in term or preterm infants can be established only by excluding known causes of jaundice on the basis of the history and clinical and laboratory findings (see Table 88–1). In general, a search to determine the cause of jaundice should be made if (1) it appears in the first 24 hr of life; (2) serum bilirubin is rising at a rate greater than 5 mg/dL/24 hr; (3) serum bilirubin is greater than 12 mg/dL in full-term (especially in the absence of risk factors) or 10–14 mg/dL/24 hr in preterm infants; (4) jaundice persists after the 2nd wk of life; or (5) direct-reacting bilirubin is greater than 1 mg/dL at any time. Among other factors suggesting a nonphysiologic cause of jaundice are family history of hemolytic disease, pallor, hepatomegaly, splenomegaly, failure of phototherapy to lower bilirubin, vomiting, lethargy, poor feeding, excessive weight loss, apnea, bradycardia, abnormal vital signs including hypothermia, light-colored stools,

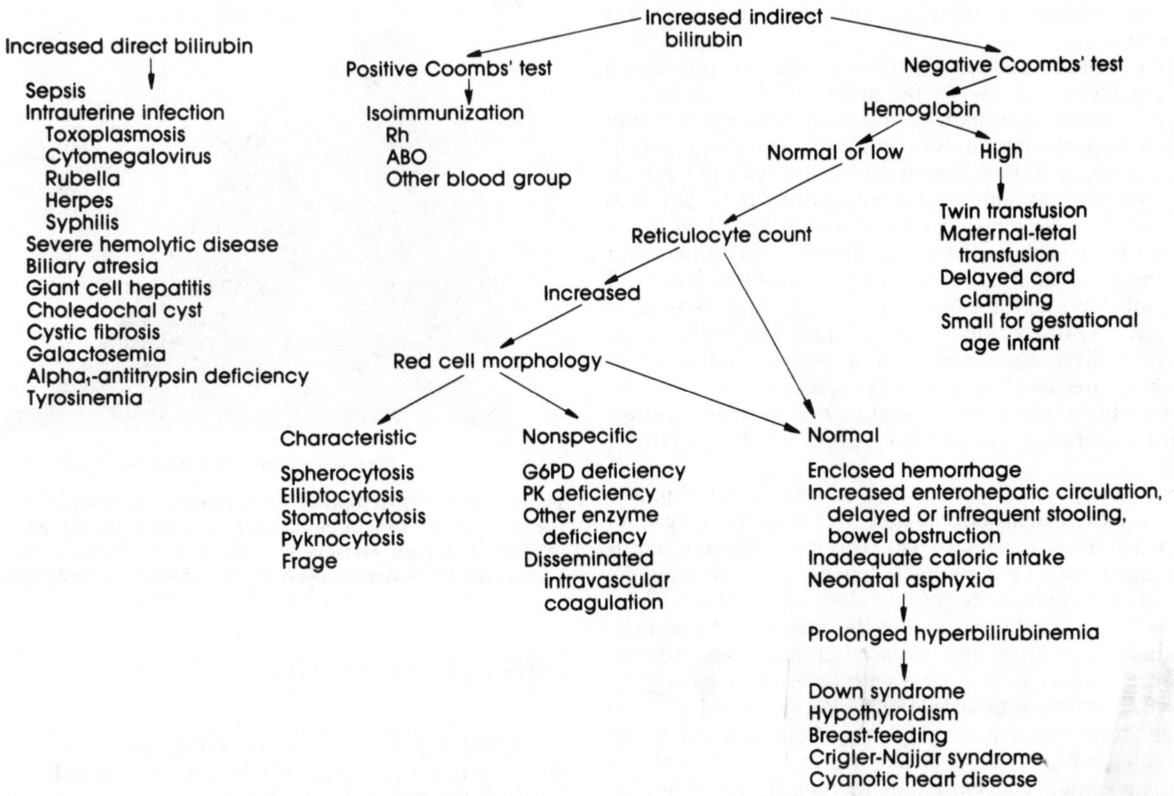

Figure 88–6. Schematic approach to the diagnosis of neonatal jaundice. (From Oski FA: Differential diagnosis of jaundice. *In:* Taeusch HW, Ballard RA, Avery MA [eds]: Schaffer and Avery's Diseases of the Newborn, 6th ed. Philadelphia, WB Saunders, 1991.

■ **TABLE 88–1 Diagnostic Features of the Various Types of Neonatal Jaundice**

Diagnosis	Nature of Van den Bergh Reaction	Jaundice: *Appears*	Jaundice: *Disappears*	Peak Bilirubin Concentration: *mg/dL*	Peak Bilirubin Concentration: *Age in Days*	Bilirubin Rate of Accumulation (mg/dL/day)	Remarks
"Physiologic jaundice":							Usually relates to degree of maturity
Full-term	Indirect	2–3 days	4–5 days	10–12	2–3	<5	
Premature	Indirect	3–4 days	7–9 days	15	6–8	<5	
Hyperbilirubinemia due to metabolic factors							Metabolic factors: hypoxia, respiratory distress, lack of carbohydrate
Full-term	Indirect	2–3 days	Variable	>2	1st wk	<5	Hormonal influences: cretinism, hormones
Premature	Indirect	3–4 days	Variable	>15	1st wk	<5	Genetic factors: Crigler-Najjar syndrome, transient familial hyperbilirubinemia Drugs: vitamin K, novobiocin
Hemolytic states and hematoma	Indirect	May appear in 1st 24 hr	Variable	Unlimited	Variable	Usually >5	Erythroblastosis: Rh, ABO. Congenital hemolytic states: spherocytic, nonspherocytic Infantile pyknocytosis. Drugs: vitamin K. Enclosed hemorrhage—hematoma
Mixed hemolytic and hepatotoxic factors	Indirect and direct	May appear in 1st 24 hr	Variable	Unlimited	Variable	Usually >5	Infection: bacterial sepsis, pyelonephritis, hepatitis, toxoplasmosis, cytomegalic inclusion disease, rubella Drugs: vitamin K
Hepatocellular damage	Indirect and direct	Usually 2–3 days	Variable	Unlimited	Variable	Variable can be >5	Biliary atresia; galactosemia; hepatitis and infection

From Brown AK: Pediatr Clin North Am 9:589, 1962.

dark urine positive for bilirubin, and signs of kernicterus (Chapter 88.4).

PATHOLOGIC HYPERBILIRUBINEMIA. Jaundice and its underlying hyperbilirubinemia are considered pathologic if their time of appearance, duration, or pattern of serially determined serum bilirubin concentrations varies significantly from that of physiologic jaundice; or if the course is compatible with physiologic jaundice but other reasons exist to suspect that the infant is at special risk from the neurotoxicity of unconjugated bilirubin. It may not be possible to determine precisely the etiology for an abnormal elevation of unconjugated bilirubin. Many of these infants have an associated risk factor such as Asian race, prematurity, breast-feeding, or weight loss; hence the terms exaggerated physiologic jaundice and hyperbilirubinemia of the newborn are used for those infants whose primary problem is probably a deficiency or inactivity of bilirubin glucuronyl transferase rather than an excessive load of bilirubin for excretion.

The risk of hyperbilirubinemia is related to the development of kernicterus (bilirubin encephalopathy) at high indirect serum bilirubin levels (Chapter 88.4). The level of serum bilirubin associated with kernicterus is dependent in part on the etiology of the jaundice. Kernicterus develops at lower bilirubin levels in preterm infants and in the presence of asphyxia, IVH, hemolysis, or drugs that displace bilirubin from albumin. Kernicterus is unusual in patients with breast milk jaundice.

JAUNDICE ASSOCIATED WITH BREAST-FEEDING. An estimated 1 of 200 breast-fed term infants develops significant elevations in unconjugated bilirubin between the 4th and 7th days of life, reaching maximum concentrations as high as 10–30 mg/dL during the 2nd–3rd wk. If breast-feeding is continued, the hyperbilirubinemia gradually decreases and then may persist for 3–10 wk at lower levels. If nursing is discontinued, the serum bilirubin level falls rapidly, usually reaching normal levels within a few days. Cessation of breast-feeding for 1–2 days and substitution of formula for breast milk results in a rapid decline in serum bilirubin, after which nursing can be resumed without a return of the hyperbilirubinemia to its previously high levels. If indicated, phototherapy may be of benefit (Chapter 88.4). These infants have no other sign of illness, and kernicterus has not been reported. The milk of some of these mothers contains 5-β-pregnane-3α, 20-β-diol or nonesterified long-chain fatty acids, which competitively inhibit glucuronyl transferase conjugating activity. In others, the milk contains a glucuronidase that may be responsible for jaundice.

This syndrome should be distinguished from an early onset accentuated unconjugated hyperbilirubinemia in the 1st wk of life, when breast-fed infants have higher bilirubin levels than formula-fed infants (Fig. 88–7). This observation may be due to decreased milk intake with dehydration or reduced caloric intake. Giving supplements of glucose water to breast-fed infants is associated with higher bilirubin levels owing in part to reduced intake of the higher caloric density breast milk. Frequent breast feedings (>10/24 hr), rooming-in with night feedings, and discouraging 5% dextrose or water supplementation may reduce the incidence of early breast milk jaundice.

Transient Familial Neonatal Hyperbilirubinemia. Severe unconjugated hyperbilirubinemia leading to kernicterus may occur rarely in the first 2 days of life because of a glucuronyl transferase–inhibiting factor present in the serum of mother and infant.

NEONATAL HEPATITIS. See Chapter 302.1.

CONGENITAL ATRESIA OF THE BILE DUCTS. See Chapter 302.1. Jaundice persisting for more than 2 wk or associated with acholic stools and dark urine suggests biliary atresia. All such infants should have a direct bilirubin determination.

INSPISSATED BILE SYNDROME. See Late Complications in Chapter 89.

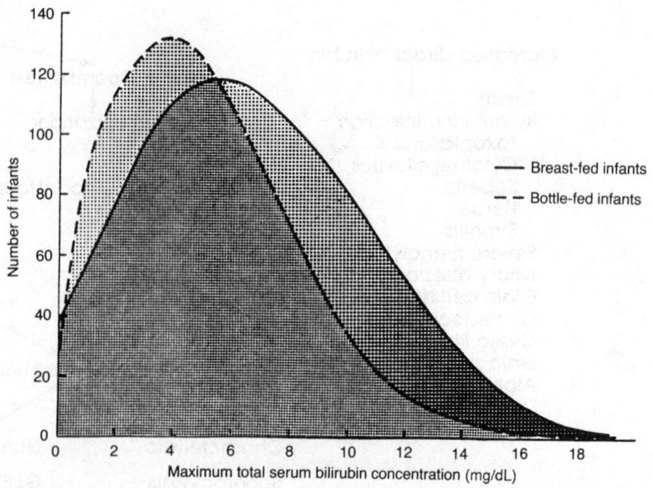

Figure 88–7. Distribution of maximum bilirubin levels during the 1st wk of life in breast-fed and formula-fed white infants >2,500 g. (From Maisels J, Gifford K: Pediatrics 78:837, 1986. Copyright 1986. Reproduced by permission of Pediatrics.)

88.4 Kernicterus

Kernicterus is a neurologic syndrome resulting from the deposition of unconjugated bilirubin in brain cells. The risk in infants with erythroblastosis fetalis is directly related to serum bilirubin levels; the relationship between serum bilirubin level and kernicterus among *healthy term infants* is uncertain. Lipid-soluble indirect bilirubin may cross the blood-brain barrier and enter the brain by diffusion if the bilirubin-binding capacity of albumin and other plasma proteins is exceeded and plasma free bilirubin levels increase. Alternatively, bilirubin may enter the brain following damage to the blood-brain barrier by asphyxia or hyperosmolality.

The precise blood level above which indirect-reacting bilirubin or free bilirubin will be toxic for an individual infant is unpredictable, but kernicterus is rare in healthy term infants and in the absence of hemolysis if the serum level is under 25 mg/dL. The duration of exposure necessary to produce toxic effects is also unknown. There is little evidence to suggest that the level of indirect bilirubin affects the IQ of healthy term infants without hemolytic disease. *Nonetheless the less mature the infant, the greater the susceptibility to kernicterus.* Factors that potentiate the movement of bilirubin into brain cells and its adverse effects on them are discussed in Chapter 88.3. In exceptional circumstances, kernicterus in VLBW infants with serum bilirubin concentrations as low as 8–12 mg/dL has been associated with an apparently cumulative effect of a number of these factors.

CLINICAL MANIFESTATIONS. Signs and symptoms of kernicterus usually appear 2–5 days after birth in term infants and as late as the 7th day in premature ones, but hyperbilirubinemia may lead to the syndrome at any time during the neonatal period. The early signs may be subtle and indistinguishable from those of sepsis, asphyxia, hypoglycemia, intracranial hemorrhage, and other acute systemic illnesses in the neonatal infant. Lethargy, poor feeding, and loss of the Moro reflex are common initial signs. Subsequently, the infant may appear gravely ill and prostrated with diminished tendon reflexes and respiratory distress. Opisthotonos, with bulging fontanel, twitching of face or limbs, and a shrill high-pitched cry may follow. In advanced cases convulsions and spasm occur, with the infant stiffly extending his or her arms in inward rotation with fists clenched. Rigidity is rare at this late stage.

Many infants who progress to these severe neurologic signs die; the survivors are usually seriously damaged but may appear to recover and for 2–3 mo manifest few abnormalities. Later in the 1st yr of life opisthotonos, muscular rigidity, irregular movements, and convulsions tend to recur. In the 2nd yr opisthotonos and seizures abate but irregular, involuntary movements, muscular rigidity, or, in some infants, hypotonia increase steadily. By 3 yr of age the complete neurologic syndrome is often apparent, consisting of bilateral choreoathetosis with involuntary muscle spasm, extrapyramidal signs, seizures, mental deficiency, dysarthric speech, high-frequency hearing loss, squints, and defective upward movement of the eyes. Pyramidal signs, hypotonia, and ataxia occur in a few infants. In mildly affected infants the syndrome may be characterized only by mild to moderate neuromuscular incoordination, partial deafness, or "minimal brain dysfunction," occurring singly or in combination; these problems may be inapparent until the child enters school.

PATHOLOGY. The surface of the brain is usually pale yellow. On cutting, certain regions are characteristically stained yellow by unconjugated bilirubin, particularly the corpus subthalamicum, hippocampus and adjacent olfactory areas, striate bodies, thalamus, globus pallidus, putamen, inferior clivus, cerebellar nuclei, and cranial nerve nuclei. Nonpigmented areas may also be damaged. Loss of neurons, reactive gliosis, and atrophy of involved fiber systems are found in late disease. The pattern of injury has been related to the development of oxidative enzyme systems in various regions of the brain and overlaps with that found in hypoxic brain damage. Evidence favors the hypothesis that bilirubin interferes with oxygen utilization by cerebral tissue, possibly by injuring the cell membrane; antecedent hypoxic injury increases the susceptibility of brain cells to injury. Gross bilirubin staining without hyperbilirubinemia or the specific microscopic changes of kernicterus may not be the same entity.

INCIDENCE AND PROGNOSIS. Using pathologic criteria, one third of infants (all gestational ages) with untreated hemolytic disease and bilirubin levels in excess of 20 mg/dL will develop kernicterus. The incidence at autopsy in hyperbilirubinemic premature infants is 2–16% and is related to the risk factors discussed in Chapter 88.3. Reliable estimates of the frequency of the clinical syndrome are not available because of the wide spectrum of manifestations. Overt neurologic signs have a grave prognosis; 75% or more of such infants die, and 80% of affected survivors have bilateral choreoathetosis with involuntary muscle spasm. Mental retardation, deafness, and spastic quadriplegia are common. Infants at risk should have screening hearing tests.

TREATMENT OF HYPERBILIRUBINEMIA. Regardless of etiology, the goal of therapy is to prevent the concentration of indirect-reacting bilirubin in the blood from reaching levels at which neurotoxicity may occur; it is recommended that phototherapy and, if unsuccessful, exchange transfusion be used to keep the maximum total serum bilirubin below the levels indicated in Tables 88–2 (for preterm) and 88–3 (for healthy term infants). The risk of injury to the central nervous system from bilirubin must be balanced against the risk inherent in the treatment for each infant. The criteria for initiating phototherapy are not generally agreed on. Since phototherapy may require 6–12 hr to have a measurable effect, it must be started at bilirubin levels below those indicated for exchange transfusion. When identified, the underlying cause of the icterus should be treated, for example, antibiotics for septicemia. Physiologic factors that increase the risk of neurologic damage should also be treated (e.g., correction of acidosis).

Exchange Transfusion. This widely accepted treatment should be repeated as frequently as necessary to keep indirect bilirubin levels in the serum under those noted in Tables 88–2 and 88–3. (See Exchange Transfusion in Chapter 89.) A variety of factors may alter this criterion in either direction in an individual patient. Appearance of clinical signs suggesting kernicterus is an indication for exchange transfusion at any level of serum bilirubin. A healthy full-term infant with physiologic or breast milk jaundice may tolerate a concentration slightly higher than 25 mg/dL with no apparent ill effect, whereas a sick premature infant may develop kernicterus at a significantly lower level. A level approaching that considered critical for the individual infant may be an indication for exchange transfusion during the 1st day or two of life when a further rise is anticipated but not on the 4th day in term infants or on the 7th day in premature infants, when an imminent fall may be anticipated as the hepatic conjugating mechanism becomes more effective.

■ **TABLE 88–2 Suggested Maximum Indirect Serum Bilirubin Concentrations (mg/dL) in Preterm Infants**

Birthweight (g)	Uncomplicated	Complicated*
<1000	12–13	10–12
1000–1250	12–14	10–12
1251–1499	14–16	12–14
1500–1999	16–20	15–17
2000–2500	20–22	18–20

**Complications include perinatal asphyxia, acidosis, hypoxia, hypothermia, hypoalbuminemia, meningitis, IVH, hemolysis, hypoglycemia, or signs of kernicterus.*

Phototherapy is usually started at 50–70% of the maximum indirect level. If values greatly exceed this level, if phototherapy is unsuccessful in reducing the maximum bilirubin level, or if there are signs of kernicterus, exchange transfusion is indicated.

Phototherapy. Clinical jaundice and indirect hyperbilirubinemia are reduced on exposure to a high intensity of light in the visible spectrum. Bilirubin absorbs light maximally in the blue range (from 420 to 470 nm). Nonetheless, broad-spectrum white, blue, special narrow spectrum (super) blue, and green lights have been effective in reducing bilirubin levels. Although blue light provides the appropriate wavelengths for photoactivation of free bilirubin, green light may affect photoreactions of albumin-bound bilirubin. Bilirubin in the skin absorbs light energy, which by photoisomerization converts the toxic native unconjugated 4Z,15Z-bilirubin into the unconjugated configurational isomer, 4Z,15E-bilirubin. The latter is the product of a reversible reaction and is excreted in the bile without the need for conjugation. Phototherapy also converts native bilirubin, by an irreversible reaction, to the structural isomer lumirubin, which is excreted by the kidney in the unconjugated state.

The use of phototherapy with fluorescent light bulbs has decreased the need for exchange transfusion in LBW infants without hemolytic disease and in LBW infants with hemolysis as well as for repeated exchange transfusion of infants with hemolytic disease. However, when there are indications for exchange transfusion, phototherapy should not be used as a substitute.

Phototherapy is indicated only after the presence of pathologic hyperbilirubinemia has been established. The basic cause(s) of the jaundice should be treated concomitantly. Phototherapy may be initiated at the bilirubin levels noted in Tables 88–2 and 88–3. Prophylactic phototherapy in VLBW infants may prevent hyperbilirubinemia and may reduce the incidence of exchange transfusions.

Normal infants receiving phototherapy for 1–3 days have peak serum bilirubin concentrations about one-half those of untreated infants. In premature infants without significant hemolysis serum bilirubin usually declines 1–3 mg/dL after 12–24 hr of conventional phototherapy, and peak levels attained may be decreased by 3–6 mg/dL. The therapeutic effect depends on the light energy emitted in the effective range of wavelengths, the distance between the lights and the infant, and the amount

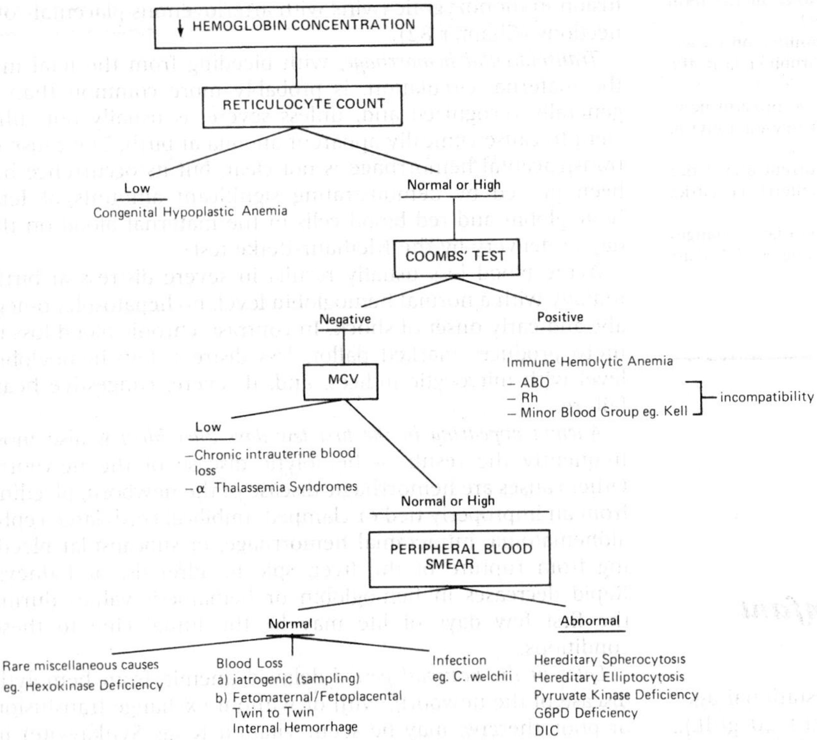

Figure 89–2. Diagnostic approach to anemia in the newborn infant. (From Blanchette V, Zipursky A: Clin Perinatol 11:489, 1984.)

born following an abruptio placentae or with severe hemolytic disease of the newborn warrants immediate transfusion. The preterm infant who has repeated episodes of apnea and bradycardia despite theophylline therapy and a hemoglobin level of less than 10 g/dL may benefit from red blood cell transfusion. In addition, infants with hyaline membrane disease or severe bronchopulmonary dysplasia may need hemoglobin levels of 12–14 g/dL to improve oxygen delivery. Packed red blood cell transfusion (10–15 mL/kg) is given at a rate of 2–3 mL/kg/hr to raise the hemoglobin concentration; 2 mL/kg raises the hemoglobin level 0.5–1 g/dL. Hemorrhage should be treated with whole blood if available; alternatively, fluid resuscitation is initiated and followed by packed red blood cell transfusion.

Recombinant human erythropoietin (rHuEpo) has been used to prevent or treat chronic anemia associated with prematurity and bronchopulmonary dysplasia. The anemia of prematurity is associated with abnormally low endogenous levels of serum erythropoietin but with rHuEpo-responsive erythrocyte progenitor cells. Therapy with rHuEpo is given by intravenous or subcutaneous routes and must be supplemented with oral iron and possibly vitamin E. Doses and regimens vary from 100–200 U/kg/dose 5 d/wk to 400 U/kg/dose 3 d/wk to 150–200 U/kg/dose q 3 d. Transient neutropenia is an inconsistent potential side effect.

89.2 Hemolytic Disease of the Newborn

(Erythroblastosis Fetalis)

Erythroblastosis fetalis results from the transplacental passage of maternal antibody active against red blood cell antigens of the infant, leading to an increased rate of red cell destruction. It continues to be an important cause of anemia and jaundice in newborn infants despite the development of a method of prevention of maternal isoimmunization by Rh antigens. Although more than 60 different red blood cell antigens capable of eliciting an antibody response in a suitable recipient have been identified, significant disease is associated primarily with the D antigen of the Rh group and with incompatibility of ABO factors. Rarely, hemolytic disease may be caused by C or E antigens or by other red blood cell antigens, such as C^w, C^x, D^u, K(Kell), M, Duffy, S, P, MNS, Xg, Lutheran, Diego, and Kidd. Anti-Lewis antibodies do not cause disease.

HEMOLYTIC DISEASE OF THE NEWBORN DUE TO RH INCOMPATIBILITY

The Rh antigenic determinants are genetically transmitted from each parent and determine the Rh type and direct the production of a number of blood group factors (C, c, D, d, E, and e). Each factor can elicit a specific antibody response under suitable conditions; 90% are due to D antigen, the remainder to C or E.

PATHOGENESIS. Isoimmune hemolytic disease from D antigen is approximately three times more frequent in whites than in blacks. When Rh positive blood is infused into an Rh negative woman through error or when small quantities (usually more than 1 mL) of Rh positive fetal blood containing D antigen inherited from an Rh positive father enter the maternal circulation during pregnancy, with spontaneous or induced abortion, or at delivery, antibody formation against D may be induced in the unsensitized Rh negative recipient mother. Once immunization has occurred, considerably smaller doses of antigen can stimulate an increase in antibody titer. Initially, a rise of antibody in the 19S gamma globulin fraction occurs, which later is replaced by 7S (IgG) antibody; the latter readily crosses the placenta, causing hemolytic manifestations.

Hemolytic disease rarely occurs during a first pregnancy, since transfusions of Rh positive fetal blood into an Rh negative mother tend to occur near the time of delivery, too late for the mother to become sensitized and transmit antibody to the infant before delivery. The fact that 55% of Rh positive fathers are heterozygous (D/d) and may have Rh negative offspring and that only 50% of pregnancies have fetal-to-maternal transfusions reduces the chance of sensitization, as does small family size, in which the opportunities for its occurrence are fewer. Finally, the capacity of Rh negative women to form antibodies is variable, some producing low titers even after adequate antigenic challenge. Thus, the overall incidence of isoimmunization of Rh negative mothers at risk is low, with antibody to D detected in less than 10% of those studied, even after five or more pregnancies; only about 5% ever have babies with hemolytic disease.

When mother and fetus are also incompatible with respect to group A or B, the mother is partially protected against sensitization by the rapid removal of Rh positive cells from her circulation by her anti-A or anti-B, which are IgM antibodies and do not cross the placenta. Once the mother has been sensitized, the infant is likely to have hemolytic disease. There is a tendency for the severity of Rh illness to worsen with successive pregnancies. The possibility that the first affected infant after sensitization may represent the end of the mother's childbearing potential for Rh positive infants argues urgently for the prevention of sensitization when this is possible. Such prevention consists of injection into the mother of anti-D gamma globulin (RhoGAM) immediately following the delivery of each Rh positive infant (see below).

CLINICAL MANIFESTATIONS. A wide spectrum of hemolytic disease occurs in affected infants born to sensitized mothers, depending on the nature of the individual immune response. The severity of the disease may range from only laboratory evidence of mild hemolysis (15% of cases) to severe anemia with compensatory hyperplasia of erythropoietic tissue, leading to massive enlargement of the liver and spleen. When the compensatory capacity of the hematopoietic system is exceeded, profound anemia results in pallor, signs of cardiac decompensation (cardiomegaly, respiratory distress), massive anasarca, and circulatory collapse. This clinical picture, termed hydrops fetalis, frequently results in death in utero or shortly after birth; it may also occur from other nonimmune causes (Table 89–1). The severity of hydrops is related to the level of anemia and the degree of reduction in serum albumin (oncotic pressure), which is due in part to hepatic dysfunction. Alternatively, heart failure may increase right heart pressures with the development of edema and ascites. Failure to initiate spontaneous effective ventilation because of pulmonary edema or bilateral pleural effusions results in birth asphyxia; following successful resuscitation, severe respiratory distress may develop. Petechiae, purpura, and thrombocytopenia may also be present in severe cases, reflecting decreased platelet production or the presence of concurrent disseminated intravascular coagulation.

Jaundice is usually absent at birth because of placental clearance of lipid-soluble unconjugated bilirubin, but in severe cases bilirubin pigments stain the amniotic fluid, cord, and vernix caseosa yellow. Icterus is generally evident on the 1st day of life because the infant's bilirubin-conjugating and excretory systems are unable to cope with the load resulting from massive hemolysis. Indirect-reacting bilirubin therefore accumulates postnatally and may rapidly reach extremely high levels, which represent a significant risk of bilirubin encephalopathy. There may be a greater risk of developing kernicterus from hemolytic disease than from comparable nonhemolytic hyperbilirubinemia, although the risk in an individual patient may be a function only of the severity of illness (anoxia, acidosis, and so on). Hypoglycemia occurs frequently in infants with severe isoimmune hemolytic disease and may be related to hyperinsulinism and hypertrophy of the pancreatic islet cells in these infants.

Infants born after intrauterine transfusion for prenatally diagnosed erythroblastosis may be severely affected, since the indications for the transfusion are evidence of already severe disease in utero (e.g., hydrops, fetal anemia). Such infants usually have very high (but extremely variable) cord levels of bilirubin, which reflects the severity of hemolysis and its effects on hepatic function. Infants treated with intraumbilical vein transfusions in utero may have a benign postnatal course, if anemia and hydrops resolve prior to birth. Anemia from continuing hemolysis may be masked by the prior intrauterine transfusion, and the clinical manifestations of erythroblastosis may be superimposed upon various degrees of immaturity resulting from spontaneous or induced premature delivery.

LABORATORY DATA. Prior to treatment, the direct Coombs test is usually positive. Anemia is usual. The cord blood hemoglobin varies, usually proportionally to the severity of the disease; with hydrops fetalis it may be as low as 3–4 g/dL (30–40 g/L). Alternatively, despite hemolysis, it may be within the normal range owing to compensatory bone marrow and extramedullary hematopoiesis. The blood smear usually shows polychromasia and a marked increase in nucleated red blood cells. The reticulocyte count is increased. The white blood cell count is usually normal but may be elevated, and there may be thrombocytopenia in severe cases. The cord bilirubin is usually between 3 and 5 mg/dL (51–86 μmol/L); only rarely is there a substantial elevation of direct-reacting (conjugated) bilirubin. The indirect-reacting bilirubin rises rapidly to high levels in the first 6 hr of life.

After intrauterine transfusions the cord blood may show a normal hemoglobin concentration, negative direct Coombs test, predominantly type O Rh negative adult red cells, and a relatively normal smear. Marked elevation of both indirect- and direct-reacting bilirubin levels has been reported in these infants.

DIAGNOSIS. The definitive diagnosis of erythroblastosis fetalis requires demonstration of blood group incompatibility and of corresponding antibody bound to the infant's red blood cells.

Antenatal Diagnosis. In Rh negative women a history of previous transfusions, abortion, or pregnancy should suggest the possibility of sensitization. Expectant parents' blood types should be tested for potential incompatibility, and the maternal titer of IgG antibodies to D should be assayed at 12–16, 28–32, and 36 wk. The presence of measurable antibody titer at the beginning of pregnancy, a rapid rise in titer, or a titer of 1:64 or greater suggests significant hemolytic disease, although the

■ **TABLE 89–1 Etiologies of Hydrops Fetalis**

Hematologic	Rh and other blood group incompatibilities,* thalassemia, twin-twin transfusion, fetomaternal hemorrhage
Infectious	Parvovirus, syphilis, cytomegalovirus, toxoplasmosis, Chagas' disease, leptospirosis
Cardiovascular	Supraventricular tachycardia, heart failure, arteriovenous malformation, umbilical vein thrombosis, congenital heart block, severe congenital heart disease, rhabdomyoma
Pulmonary	Cystic adenomatoid malformation, diaphragmatic hernia, lymphangiectasia, hypoplasia
Tumor	Congenital neuroblastoma, placental chorioangioma, teratoma, hemangioma
Hepatic	Hepatitis, fibrosis, cirrhosis
Renal	Nephrosis, prune-belly syndrome, urethral valves
Gastrointestinal	Atresias, volvulus, chylous ascites, cystic fibrosis
Metabolic	Gaucher disease, maternal diabetes mellitus, achondroplasia, other macromolecular storage diseases
Malformation Syndromes	Arthrogryposis, thanatophoric dwarf, Noonan syndrome, Meckel syndrome, amniotic bands
Chromosomal Syndromes	XO, 13-, 18-, 21-trisomies, triploidy
Idiopathic	

**The incidence of nonimmune hydrops fetalis is 1:2000–1:3500 births.*

exact titer correlates poorly with the severity of disease. If a mother is found to have antibody against D at a titer of 1:16 or greater at any time during a subsequent pregnancy, the severity of fetal disease should be monitored by amniocentesis, percutaneous umbilical blood sampling (PUBS), and ultrasonography. If there is a history of a previously affected infant or a stillbirth, an Rh positive infant is usually equally or more severely affected than the previous infant, and the severity of disease in the fetus should be followed.

Assessment of the fetus may require information obtained from ultrasound, amniocentesis, and PUBS. Real-time ultrasound is used to detect the progression of hemolysis from mild to severe, with hydrops defined as skin or scalp edema, pleural or pericardial effusions, and ascites. Early ultrasonographic signs of hydrops include organomegaly (liver, spleen, heart), double bowel wall sign (bowel edema), and placental thickening. There may then be progression to polyhydramnios, ascites, pleural or pericardial effusions, and skin or scalp edema. If pleural effusions precede ascites and hydrops by a significant period of time, causes other than fetal anemia should be suspected (see Table 89–1). Extramedullary hematopoiesis and, less so, hepatic congestion compress the intrahepatic vessels, producing venous stasis with portal hypertension, hepatocellular dysfunction, and decreased albumin synthesis.

Hydrops is invariable when fetal hemoglobin is less than 5 g/dL, frequent when under 7 g/dL, and variable between 7 and 9 g/dL. Real-time ultrasound predicts fetal well-being by the biophysical profile (see Table 81–2), whereas Doppler ultrasound assesses fetal distress by demonstrating increased vascular resistance. If there is ultrasonographic evidence of hemolysis (hepatosplenomegaly), early or late hydrops, or fetal distress, an amniocentesis or PUBS should be performed.

Amniocentesis is used to assess fetal hemolysis. Hemolysis of fetal erythrocytes produces hyperbilirubinemia before the onset of severe anemia. Bilirubin is cleared by the placenta, but a significant proportion enters the amniotic fluid and can be measured by spectrophotometry. Amniocentesis is performed if there is evidence of maternal sensitization (titer ≥ 1:16), if the father is Rh positive, or if there are ultrasonographic signs of hemolysis, hydrops, or distress. Ultrasonographic-guided transabdominal aspiration of amniotic fluid may be performed as early as 18–20 wk of gestation. Spectrophotometric scanning of amniotic fluid wavelengths demonstrates a positive optical density (OD) deviation of absorption for bilirubin from normal at 450 nm. The OD 450 is a reflection of fetal bilirubin levels, and thus hemolysis, and indicates the severity of anemia and the risk of intrauterine death. With maturity, the level of amniotic fluid bilirubin normally declines; thus the fetal risk assessed during gestation in terms of three relative but declining zones of OD 450, with zone III representing the highest risk. However, some fetuses in zone III do not have life-threatening fetal anemia and thus do not require intrauterine transfusion. If the OD 450 is in zone III or if hydrops or other signs suggesting fetal anemia are present, PUBS should be performed to determine fetal hemoglobin levels, and packed red blood cells should be transfused if serious anemia (hematocrit of 25–30%) exists.

Postnatal Diagnosis. Immediately after the birth of any infant to an Rh negative woman, blood from the umbilical cord or from the infant should be examined for ABO blood group, Rh type, hematocrit and hemoglobin, and reaction of the direct Coombs test. If the Coombs test is positive, baseline serum bilirubin should be measured, and a commercially available red blood cell panel should be used to identify red blood cell antibodies that are present in the mother's serum, both tests being done not only to establish the diagnosis but also to ensure the selection of the most compatible blood for exchange transfusion should it be necessary. The direct Coombs test is usually strongly positive in clinically affected infants and may remain so for a few days up to several months.

TREATMENT. The main goals of therapy are (1) to prevent intrauterine or extrauterine death from severe anemia and hypoxia and (2) to avoid neurotoxicity from hyperbilirubinemia.

Treatment of the Unborn Infant. The survival of the severely affected fetus has been improved by the use of ultrasonographic and amniotic fluid analysis to identify the need for in utero transfusion. Intrauterine transfusion into the fetal peritoneal cavity is being replaced by direct intravascular transfusion of packed red blood cells. Hydrops or fetal anemia (hematocrit <30%) is an indication for umbilical vein transfusion in infants with pulmonary immaturity (see Fig. 89–1). Intravascular transfusion is facilitated by maternal and hence fetal sedation with diazepam and by fetal paralysis with pancuronium. Packed red blood cells are given by slow-push infusion after cross-matching to the mother's serum. The cells should be obtained from a CMV-negative donor and irradiated to kill lymphocytes in order to avoid graft versus host disease. Transfusions should achieve a post-transfusion hematocrit of 45–55% and can be repeated every 3–5 wk. Indications for delivery include pulmonary maturity, fetal distress, complications of PUBS, or 35–37 wk of gestation.

Treatment of the Liveborn Infant. The birth should be attended by the physician who will care for the affected infant afterward. Fresh, low titer, group O, Rh negative blood, cross-matched against the maternal serum, should be immediately available. If clinical signs of severe hemolytic anemia (pallor, hepatosplenomegaly, edema, petechiae, or ascites) are evident at birth, immediate supportive therapy, temperature stabilization, and monitoring before proceeding with exchange transfusion may save some severely affected infants. Such therapy should include correction of acidosis with 1–2 mEq/kg of sodium bicarbonate; a small transfusion of compatible packed red blood cells to correct anemia; volume expansion for hypotension, especially in those with hydrops; and provision of assisted ventilation for respiratory failure.

Exchange Transfusion. When the infant's clinical condition at birth does not require an immediate full or partial exchange transfusion, the decision to perform one should be based on a judgment that there is a high risk of rapid development of a dangerous degree of anemia or of hyperbilirubinemia. Cord hemoglobin of 10 g/dL or less and bilirubin of 5 mg/dL or more suggest severe hemolysis but inconsistently predict the need for immediate exchange transfusion. Some physicians consider previous kernicterus or severe erythroblastosis in a sibling, reticulocyte counts greater than 15%, and prematurity to be further factors supporting a decision for early exchange transfusion.

The hemoglobin, hematocrit, and serum bilirubin levels should be measured at 4- to 6-hr intervals at first, with extension to longer intervals if and as the rate of change diminishes. The decision to perform an exchange transfusion is based on the likelihood that the trend of bilirubin levels plotted against hours of age indicates that the serum bilirubin will reach the level indicated in Tables 88–2 and 88–3, above which there is an increased risk of kernicterus. Ordinary transfusions of compatible Rh negative red blood cells may be necessary to correct anemia at any stage of the disease up to 6–8 wk of age, when the infant's own blood-forming mechanism may be expected to take over. Weekly determinations of hemoglobin or hematocrit should be done until a spontaneous rise has been demonstrated.

Careful monitoring of the serum bilirubin level is essential until a falling trend has been demonstrated in the absence of phototherapy (Chapter 88.4). Even then, an occasional infant, particularly if premature, may experience an unpredicted significant rise in serum bilirubin as late as the 7th day of life.

Attempts to predict the attainment of dangerously high levels of serum bilirubin, based on observed levels exceeding 6 mg/dL in the first 6 hr or 10 mg/dL in the second 6 hr of life or on rates of rise exceeding 0.5–1.0 mg/dL/hr, can be unreliable. Indices of free bilirubin and bilirubin binding have not been shown to be routinely reliable aids in evaluating the risk associated with hyperbilirubinemia.

Blood for exchange transfusion should be as fresh as possible. Heparin or adenosine-citrate-phosphate-dextrose may be used as an anticoagulant. If the blood is obtained before delivery, it should be taken from a type O, Rh negative donor with a low titer of anti-A and anti-B and should be compatible with the mother's serum by indirect Coombs test. After delivery, blood should be obtained from an Rh negative donor whose cells are compatible with both the infant's and the mother's serum; when possible, type O donor cells are usually employed, but cells of the infant's ABO blood type may be used when the mother has the same type. A complete cross-match, including indirect Coombs test, should be performed prior to the second and subsequent transfusions. Blood should be gradually warmed to and maintained at a temperature between 35° and 37° C throughout the exchange transfusion. It should be kept well mixed by gentle squeezing or agitation of the bag to avoid sedimentation; otherwise, the use of supernatant serum with a low red blood cell count at the end of the exchange will leave the infant anemic. Whole blood or packed red blood cells reconstituted with fresh frozen plasma to a hematocrit of 40% should be used. The infant's stomach should be emptied prior to transfusion to prevent aspiration, and body temperature should be maintained and vital signs monitored. A competent assistant should be present to help monitor, tally the volume of blood exchanged, and perform emergency procedures.

The umbilical vein is cannulated, using strict aseptic technique, with a polyvinyl catheter to a distance no greater than 7 cm in a full-term infant. When free flow of blood is obtained, the catheter is usually in a large hepatic vein or the inferior vena cava. Exchange should be carried out over a 45- to 60-min period, alternating aspirations of 20 ml of infant blood and infusions of 20 ml of donor blood. Smaller aliquots (5–10 ml) may be indicated for sick and premature infants. The goal should be an exchange of approximately 2 blood volumes of the infant (2 × 85 mL/kg). If heparinized blood is used, 0.45 ml (4.5 mg) of a 1% solution of protamine sulfate may be injected intravenously at the conclusion of the transfusion for each deciliter of blood exchanged.

Infants with acidosis and hypoxia from respiratory distress, sepsis, or shock may be further compromised by the significant acute acid load contained in citrated blood, which usually has a pH between 7 and 7.2. The subsequent metabolism of citrate may result in a later metabolic alkalosis if citrated blood is used. Fresh heparinized blood avoids this problem. During the exchange, the blood pH and Pa_{O_2} should be serially monitored, since infants often become acidotic and hypoxic during exchange transfusions. Symptomatic hypoglycemia may occur before or during exchange transfusion in moderately to severely affected infants; it may also occur 1–3 hr after exchange. Acute complications, noted in 5–10% of infants, include transient bradycardia with or without calcium infusion, cyanosis, transient vasospasm, thrombosis, and apnea with bradycardia requiring resuscitation. Infectious risks include CMV, HIV, and hepatitis. Necrotizing enterocolitis is a rare complication of exchange transfusion.

After exchange transfusion the bilirubin level must be determined at frequent intervals (every 4–8 hr), as bilirubin may rebound 40–50% within hours. Repeated exchange transfusions should be carried out to keep the indirect fraction from exceeding the levels indicated in Tables 88–2 and 88–3. Symptoms suggestive of kernicterus are mandatory indications for exchange transfusion at any time.

The risk of death from exchange transfusion performed by experienced physicians is 0.3/100 procedures. However, with the decreasing use of this procedure as a result of the prevalent use of phototherapy and because sensitization is being prevented, the general level of physician competence is decreasing. Thus, it may be best to concentrate this mode of treatment in neonatal referral centers.

Late Complications. The infant who has hemolytic disease or who has had an exchange or an intrauterine transfusion must be observed carefully for the development of anemia and cholestasis. Late anemia may be hemolytic or hyporegenerative. Treatment with supplemental iron, erythropoietin, or blood transfusion may be indicated. A mild graft versus host reaction may be manifested as diarrhea, rash, hepatitis, and eosinophilia.

Inspissated bile syndrome refers to the rare occurrence of persistent icterus in association with significant elevations of direct as well as indirect bilirubin in infants with hemolytic disease. The cause is unclear, but the jaundice clears spontaneously within a few weeks or months.

Portal vein thrombosis may occur among children who have been subjected to exchange transfusion as newborn infants. It is probably associated with prolonged, traumatic, or septic umbilical vein catheterization.

Prevention of Rh Sensitization. The risk of initial sensitization of Rh negative mothers has been reduced from between 10 and 20% to less than 1% by intramuscular injection of 300 μg of human anti-D globulin (1 mL of RhoGAM) within 72 hr of delivery or abortion. This quantity is sufficient to eliminate approximately 10 mL of potentially antigenic fetal cells from the maternal circulation. Large fetal-to-maternal transfers of blood may require proportionately more RhoGAM. RhoGAM, administered at 28–32 wk and again at birth (40 wk), may be more effective than a single dose. The use of this technique, combined with improved methods of detecting maternal sensitization and quantitating the extent of the fetal-to-maternal transfusion, plus the use of fewer obstetric procedures that increase the risk of such fetal-to-maternal bleeding (versions, manual separation of the placenta, and so on), should further reduce the incidence of erythroblastosis fetalis.

HEMOLYTIC DISEASE OF THE NEWBORN DUE TO A AND B INCOMPATIBILITY

Major blood group incompatibility between mother and fetus usually results in milder disease than does Rh incompatibility. Maternal antibody may be formed against B cells if the mother is type A or against A cells if the mother is type B. However, usually the mother is type O and the infant is type A or B. Although ABO incompatibility occurs in 20–25% of pregnancies, hemolytic disease develops in only 10% of such offspring, and usually the infants are of type A_1, which is more antigenic than A_2. Low antigenicity of the ABO factors in the fetus and newborn infant may account for the low incidence of severe ABO hemolytic disease relative to the incidence of incompatibility between the blood groups of mother and child. Although antibodies against A and B factors occur without prior immunization ("natural" antibodies), these are ordinarily present in the 19S (IgM) fraction of gamma globulin, which does not cross the placenta. However, univalent, incomplete (albumin active) antibodies to A antigen may be present in the 7S (IgG) fraction, which does cross the placenta, so that A-O isoimmune hemolytic disease may be seen in first-born infants. Mothers who have become immunized against A or B factors from a previous incompatible pregnancy also exhibit antibody in the 7S gamma globulin fraction. These "immune" antibodies are the primary mediators in ABO isoimmune disease.

CLINICAL MANIFESTATIONS. Most cases are mild, with jaundice as the only clinical manifestation. The infant is not generally affected at birth; pallor is not present and hydrops fetalis is extremely rare. Liver and spleen are not greatly enlarged, if at all. Jaundice usually appears during the first 24 hr. Rarely, it may become severe, and symptoms and signs of kernicterus develop rapidly.

DIAGNOSIS. A presumptive diagnosis is based on the presence of ABO incompatibility, a weakly to moderately positive direct Coombs test, and spherocytes in the blood smear, which may at times suggest the presence of hereditary spherocytosis. Hyperbilirubinemia is often the only other laboratory abnormality. The hemoglobin level is usually normal but may be as low as 10–12 g/dL (100–120 g/L). Reticulocytes may be increased to 10–15%, with extensive polychromasia and increased numbers of nucleated red cells. In 10–20% of affected infants the unconjugated serum bilirubin level may reach 20 mg/dL or more unless phototherapy is employed.

TREATMENT. Phototherapy may be effective in lowering serum bilirubin levels (Chapter 88.4). Otherwise, treatment is directed at correcting dangerous degrees of anemia or hyperbilirubinemia by exchange transfusions with blood of the same group as that of the mother (Rh type should match the infant's). The indications for this procedure are similar to those previously described for hemolytic disease due to Rh incompatibility.

OTHER FORMS OF HEMOLYTIC DISEASE

Blood group incompatibilities other than Rh or ABO (c, E, Kell [K], and so on) account for less than 5% of hemolytic disease of the newborn. The direct Coombs test is invariably positive, and exchange transfusion may be indicated for hyperbilirubinemia and anemia. Hemolytic disease and anemia due to anti-Kell antibodies is not predictable from the previous obstetric history, amniotic fluid OD_{450} bilirubin determinants, or the maternal antibody titer. Erythroid suppression may contribute to the anemia; PUBS is beneficial in actually measuring the fetal hematocrit.

Congenital infections, such as cytomegalic inclusion disease, toxoplasmosis, rubella, and syphilis, may present with hemolytic anemia, jaundice, hepatosplenomegaly, and thrombocytopenia, but the direct Coombs test is negative, and there are usually other distinguishing clinical findings. Homozygous α-thalassemia may present with severe hemolytic anemia and a clinical picture resembling hydrops fetalis; it can be distinguished by a negative direct Coombs test and characteristic clinical and laboratory findings (Chapter 419.9). Anemia and jaundice may occur in infancy from hereditary spherocytosis (Chapter 415) and, if untreated, can result in kernicterus. Hemolytic anemia producing jaundice in the 1st wk of life may also be secondary to congenital deficiencies in red blood cell enzymes, such as pyruvate kinase or G-6-PD.

89.3 Plethora in the Newborn Infant

(Polycythemia)

See also Part XX: Section 4.

Plethora, a ruddy, deep red-purple appearance associated with a high hematocrit, is often due to polycythemia, defined as a central hematocrit of 65% or higher. Peripheral (heelstick) hematocrits are higher than central values, whereas Coulter counter results are lower than hematocrits determined by microcentrifugation. The incidence of neonatal polycythemia is increased at high altitude (Denver 5% vs Texas 1.6%), in postmature (3%) vs term (1–2%) infants, in SGA (8%) vs LGA (3%) vs AGA (1–2%) infants, during the 1st day of life (peak 2–3 hr), in the recipient infant of a twin-twin transfusion, after delayed clamping of the umbilical cord, in infants of diabetic mothers, in 13-, 18-, or 21-trisomy, in adrenogenital syndrome, in neonatal Graves disease, in hypothyroidism, and in Beckwith-Wiedemann syndrome. Infants of diabetic mothers and those with growth retardation may have been exposed to chronic fetal hypoxia, which stimulates erythropoietin production and increases red blood cell production.

Clinical manifestations include anorexia, lethargy, seizures, cyanosis (persistent fetal circulation), tachypnea, respiratory distress, feeding disturbances, necrotizing enterocolitis, hyperbilirubinemia, renal failure, hypoglycemia, and thrombocytopenia. Many affected infants are asymptomatic. Hyperviscosity is present in most infants with central hematocrits of 65% or more and accounts for the symptoms of polycythemia. Hyperviscosity determined at constant shear rates (e.g., 11.5 sec^{-1}) is present when whole blood viscosity is above 18 cycles/sec (18 cps). Hyperviscosity is accentuated because neonatal erythrocytes have decreased deformability and filterability, predisposing to stasis in the microcirculation.

The *treatment* of symptomatic plethora of the newborn is phlebotomy and replacement with saline or albumin. A partial exchange transfusion to reduce the hematocrit to 50% is a technically simpler and therapeutically more effective approach. The volume exchanged is calculated from the formula:

$$\text{Volume of exchange (mL)} = \text{Blood volume} \times \frac{\text{Observed} - \text{desired HCT}}{\text{Observed HCT}}$$

The long-term *prognosis* of polycythemic infants includes speech deficits, abnormal fine motor control, reduced IQ, and other neurologic abnormalities. Partial exchange transfusion may reduce the risk of neurologic problems, poor school performance, and fine motor deficit but is associated with feeding disturbances and may increase the risk of necrotizing enterocolitis.

89.4 Hemorrhage in the Newborn Infant

HEMORRHAGIC DISEASE OF THE NEWBORN. A moderate decrease of factors II, VII, IX, and X normally occurs in all newborn infants by 48–72 hr after birth, with a gradual return to birth levels by 7–10 days of age. This transient deficiency of vitamin K-dependent factors probably is due to lack of free vitamin K in the mother and absence of bacterial intestinal flora normally responsible for synthesis of vitamin K. Rarely, among term infants and more frequently among premature infants there is an accentuation and prolongation of this deficiency between the 2nd and 7th days of life, resulting in spontaneous and prolonged bleeding. Breast milk is a poor source of vitamin K, and hemorrhagic complications have appeared more commonly in breast-fed than in formula-fed infants. This classic form of hemorrhagic disease of the newborn, which is responsive to vitamin K therapy, must be distinguished from disseminated intravascular coagulopathy and from rarer congenital deficiencies of one or more of the other factors that are unresponsive to vitamin K (Chapter 431). Early-onset life-threatening vitamin K deficiency induced bleeding (onset birth–24 hr) is also seen if the mother has been treated with drugs (phenobarbital, phenytoin) that interfere with vitamin K function. Late onset (>1 wk) is often associated with vitamin K malabsorption as noted in neonatal hepatitis or biliary atresia.

Hemorrhagic disease of the newborn resulting from severe transient deficiencies of vitamin K-dependent factors is characterized by bleeding that tends to be gastrointestinal, nasal, subgaleal, intracranial, or a result of circumcision. Prodromal or warning signs (mild bleeding) may occur prior to serious intracranial hemorrhage. The prothrombin time, blood coagulation time, and partial thromboplastin time are prolonged, and the levels of prothrombin (II) and factors VII, IX, and X are significantly decreased. Vitamin K facilitates post-transcriptional carboxylation of factors II, VII, IX, and X. In the absence of carboxylation such factors form PIVKA (protein induced in vitamin K absence), which is a sensitive marker for vitamin K status. Bleeding time, fibrinogen, factors V and VIII, platelets, capillary fragility, and clot retraction are normal for maturity.

Administering 1 mg of natural oil-soluble vitamin K intramuscularly (phylloquinone) at the time of birth prevents the fall in vitamin K-dependent factors in full-term infants but is not uniformly effective in the prophylaxis of hemorrhagic disease of the newborn in premature infants. The disease may be effectively treated with an intravenous infusion of 1–5 mg of vitamin K_1, with improvement of coagulation defects and cessation of bleeding within a few hours. However, serious bleeding, particularly in premature infants or those with liver disease, may require a transfusion of fresh frozen plasma or whole blood. The mortality rate is low among treated patients.

A particularly severe form of deficiency of vitamin K-dependent coagulation factors has been reported in infants born to mothers receiving anticonvulsive medications (phenobarbital and phenytoin) during pregnancy. There may be severe bleeding with onset within the first 24 hr of life, which is usually corrected by vitamin K_1, although in some the response is poor or delayed. A prothrombin time (PT) should be obtained on cord blood and the infant given 1–2 mg of vitamin K intravenously. If the PT is greatly prolonged and fails to improve, 10 mL/kg of fresh frozen plasma should be given.

The recommended drug and dose of vitamin K (IM) in the United States has been safe and not associated with an increased risk of cancer. Although oral vitamin K (birth, discharge, 3–4 wk: 1–2 mg) has been suggested as an alternative, the oral route is not universally accepted and the IM route remains the method of choice.

Other forms of bleeding may be clinically indistinguishable from hemorrhagic disease of the newborn responsive to vitamin K but are neither prevented nor successfully treated with it. A clinical pattern identical to that of hemorrhagic disease of the newborn may also result from any of the congenital defects in blood coagulation (Chapters 432, 433, and 434). Hematomas, melena, and postcircumcision and umbilical cord bleeding may be present; only 5–35% of factors VIII and IX deficiencies become clinically apparent in the newborn period. Treatment of the rare congenital deficiencies of coagulation factors requires fresh frozen plasma or specific factor replacement.

Disseminated intravascular coagulopathy in newborn infants results in consumption of coagulation factors and bleeding. The infants are often premature; the clinical course is frequently characterized by hypoxia, acidosis, shock, hemangiomas, or infection. Treatment is directed at correcting the primary clinical problem, such as infection, and at interrupting consumption and replacing clotting factors. The prognosis is poor regardless of therapy (Chapter 438).

Infants with central nervous system or other bleeding constituting an *immediate threat to life* should receive a small transfusion of fresh, compatible whole blood or plasma, as well as vitamin K, as soon as possible after blood has been drawn for coagulation studies, which should include determination of the number of platelets.

The so-called swallowed blood syndrome, in which blood or bloody stools are passed, usually on the 2nd or 3rd day of life, may be confused with hemorrhage from the gastrointestinal tract. The blood may be swallowed during delivery or from a fissure in the mother's nipple. Differentiation from gastrointestinal hemorrhage is based on the fact that the infant's blood contains mostly fetal hemoglobin, which is alkali-resistant, whereas swallowed blood from a maternal source contains adult hemoglobin, which is promptly changed to alkaline hematin upon the addition of alkali. Apt devised the following test for this differentiation:

> (1) Rinse a bloodstained diaper or some grossly bloody stool with a suitable amount of water to obtain a distinctly pink supernatant hemoglobin solution. (2) Centrifuge the mixture. Decant the supernatant solution. (3) To 5 parts of the supernatant fluid add 1 part of 0.25 normal (1%) sodium hydroxide. Within 1–2 min a color reaction takes place: a yellow-brown color indicates that the blood is maternal in origin; a persistent pink, that it is from the infant. A control test with known adult or infant blood, or both, is advisable.

Widespread subcutaneous ecchymoses in premature infants at or immediately after birth are apparently a result of fragile superficial blood vessels rather than of a coagulation defect. Administering vitamin K_1 to the mother during labor has no effect on their incidence. Occasionally, an infant is born with petechiae or a generalized bluish suffusion limited to the face, head, and neck, which is probably the result of venous obstruction caused by a nuchal cord or sudden increases in intrathoracic pressure during delivery. It may take 2–3 wk for such suffusions to disappear.

NEONATAL THROMBOCYTOPENIC PURPURA. See Chapter 439.

Anonymous: Anaemia in premature infants. Lancet 1:1371, 1987.
Bechensteen AG, Haga P, Halvorsen S, et al: Erythropoietin, protein, and iron supplementation and the prevention of anaemia of prematurity. Arch Dis Child 69:19, 1993.
Burrows RF, Kelton JG: Fetal thrombocytopenia and its relation to maternal thrombocytopenia. N Engl J Med 329:1463, 1993.
Chaou W, Chou M, Eitzman DV: Intracranial hemorrhage and vitamin K deficiency in early infancy. J Pediatr 105:880, 1984.
Delaney-Black V, Camp BW, Lubchenco LO, et al: Neonatal hyperviscosity association with lower achievement and IQ scores at school age. Pediatrics 83:662, 1989.
DeMaio JG, Harris MC, Deuber C, et al: Effect of blood transfusion on apnea frequency in growing premature infants. J Pediatr 114:1039, 1989.
Desjardins L, Blaychman M, Chintu C, et al: The spectrum of ABO hemolytic disease of the newborn infant. J Pediatr 95:447, 1979.
de Almeida V, Bowman JM: Massive fetomaternal hemorrhage: Manitoba experience. Obstet Gynecol 83:323, 1994.
Draper G, McNinch A: Vitamin K for neonates: the controversy. A definitive conclusion is still not possible. Br Med J 308:867, 1994.
Doyle LW, Kelly EA, Rickards AL, et al: Sensorineural outcome at 2 years for survivors of erythroblastosis treated with fetal intravascular transfusions. Obstet Gynecol 81:931, 1993.
Gibson B: Neonatal haemostasis. Arch Dis Child 64:503, 1989.
Liu EA, Mannino FL, Lane TA: Prospective, randomized trial of the safety and efficacy of a limited donor exposure transfusion program for premature neonates. J Pediatr 125:92, 1994.
Lynch L, Bussel JB, McFarland JG, et al: Antenatal treatment of alloimmune thrombocytopenia. Obstet Gynecol 80:67, 1992.
Maier RF, Obladen M, Scigalla P, et al: The effect of epoetin beta (recombinant human erythropoietin) on the need for transfusion in very-low-birth-weight infants. N Engl J Med 330:1173, 1994.
Meyer MP, Meyer JH, Commerford A, et al: Recombinant human erythropoietin in the treatment of the anemia of prematurity: Results of a double-blind, placebo-controlled study. Pediatrics 93:918, 1994.
Reece EA, Cole SW, Romero R, et al: Ultrasonography versus amniotic fluid spectral analysis: Are they sensitive enough to predict neonatal complications associated with isoimmunization? Obstet Gynecol 74:357, 1989.
Rennie JM, Kelsall AWR: Vitamin K prophylaxis in the newborn—again. Arch Dis Child 70:248, 1994.
Stephenson T, Zuccollo J, Mohajer M: Diagnosis and management of non-immune hydrops in the newborn. Arch Dis Child 70:F151, 1994.
Vitamin K Ad Hoc Task Force. Controversies concerning vitamin K and the newborn. Pediatrics 91:1001, 1993.

HYPOCALCEMIA
(Tetany)

See Chapters 50 and 56.9.

OSTEOPENIA OF PREMATURITY. Very small premature infants with chronic illnesses often develop a rickets-like syndrome with pathologic fractures and demineralized bones. There may be associated cholestasis and vitamin D or calcium malabsorption; urine calcium loss due to diuretics; and poor calcium, phosphorus, or vitamin D intake, or aluminum toxicity. The treatment of fractures requires immobilization and administration of calcium, phosphorus, and vitamin D. Appropriate formulas for premature infants should provide a more optimal intake of calcium, phosphorus, and vitamin D and promote bone mineralization. See also Chapters 50, 56.9, 525, and 649.

HYPOMAGNESEMIA

Rarely, hypomagnesemia of unknown etiology may occur in the newborn infant, usually in association with hypocalcemia. It may also be associated with insufficient stores of skeletal magnesium secondary to deficient placental transfer, decreased intestinal absorption, neonatal hypoparathyroidism, hyperphosphatemia, renal loss, a defect in magnesium and calcium homeostasis, or an iatrogenic deficiency due to loss incurred during exchange transfusion or insufficient replacement during total intravenous alimentation. Infants of diabetic mothers may have serum magnesium levels that are lower than normal. The clinical manifestations of hypomagnesemia are indistinguishable from those of hypocalcemia and tetany and may, in fact, contribute to the accompanying hypocalcemia.

Hypomagnesemia occurs when serum magnesium levels fall below 1.5 mg/dL (0.62 mmol/L), although clinical signs usually do not develop until serum magnesium levels fall below 1.2 mg/dL. During exchange transfusion with citrated blood, which is low in magnesium ion because of binding by citrate, the serum magnesium drops about 0.5 mg/dL (0.2 mmol/L); approximately 10 days are required for a return to normal. In noniatrogenic hypomagnesemia the serum magnesium may be less than 0.5 mg/dL. The serum calcium in either instance is usually at levels seen in hypocalcemia tetany, but the serum phosphorus value is normal or high. Since the hypocalcemia accompanying hypomagnesemia is inadequately corrected by administering calcium alone, hypomagnesemia should also be suspected in any patient with tetany not responding to calcium therapy.

Immediate *treatment* consists of the intramuscular injection of magnesium sulfate. For newborn infants 0.25 mL/kg of a 50% solution daily usually suffices. The accompanying hypocalcemia usually corrects itself as the hypomagnesemia is relieved. The same daily dose can be given for oral maintenance therapy. Four to five times higher doses may be required in malabsorptive states. In most cases the metabolic defect is transient, and treatment can be discontinued after 1–2 wk. A few patients appear to have a permanent form of the disease that requires continuous oral supplementation with magnesium to prevent recurrence of hypomagnesemia.* No residual damage to the central nervous system is evident after prompt treatment.

HYPERMAGNESEMIA

Hypermagnesemia may occur in newborn infants of mothers treated with magnesium sulfate for eclampsia. At high serum levels the central nervous system is depressed and totally paralyzed so that artificial respiration is required. Toxicity may also result from magnesium sulfate enemas. Lower levels may result in hypoventilation, hypotension, lethargy, flaccidity, and hyporeflexia. The upper limit of normal magnesium is 2.8 mg/dL (1.15 mmol/L), but serious symptoms occur at levels above 5 mg/dL (2.1 mmol/L). Hypermagnesemia may be associated with failure to pass meconium (meconium plug syndrome). Exchange transfusion has been used as a means of rapid removal of magnesium ion from the blood. Calcium salts and diuresis have also been used. Recovery appears to be complete.

*Four mL/kg/24 hr of the following solution:
Magnesium chloride ($MgCl_2 \times 6\ H_2O$) 4g (39.6 mEq)
Magnesium citrate ($MgHC_6H_5O_7 \times 5\ H_2O$) 6g (39.6 mEq)
Water to 100 mL
Solution provides approximately 0.8 mEq of magnesium/mL.

OTHER METABOLIC DISEASES

A number of inborn errors of metabolism may be manifest during the neonatal period; these include phenylketonuria, galactosemia, the urea cycle defects, methylmalonic acidemia, and maple syrup urine disease (see Chapters 70 and 71). Pyridoxine deficiency and dependency are considered in Chapter 43.7.

SUBSTANCE ABUSE AND WITHDRAWALS

Physiologic addiction to narcotics or toxic effects occur in most infants born to actively addicted mothers, since opiates cross the placenta. Withdrawal may be manifest even before birth by increased activity of the fetus when the mother feels the need for the drug or develops withdrawal symptoms. Heroin and methadone are the drugs most frequently associated with withdrawal syndromes, but these syndromes may also occur with alcohol, phenobarbital, pentazocine, codeine, propoxyphene, and diazepam.

Pregnancy in women who use illegal drugs or alcohol is, by definition, a high risk. Prenatal care is usually inadequate, and there is a higher incidence of sexually transmitted disease including AIDS and hepatitis, toxemia, premature rupture of the membranes, breech presentations, prolapsed cords and limbs, preterm and small for gestational age infants, and prenatal morbidity and mortality. Frequently, more than one drug is being abused in these pregnancies.

Heroin addiction results in a 50% incidence of low birthweight infants, half of whom are small for gestational age. Infections, maternal undernutrition, and a direct fetal growth inhibiting effect are associated abnormalities. The rate of stillbirths is increased, but not the incidence of congenital anomalies. *Clinical manifestations* of withdrawal occur in 50–75% of infants, usually beginning within the first 48 hr, depending on the daily maternal dose (<6 mg/24 hr is associated with no or mild symptoms); duration of addiction (>1 yr has a greater than 70% incidence of withdrawal); and time of last maternal dose (there is a higher incidence if the last dose was taken within 24 hr of birth). Symptoms rarely appear as late as 4–6 wk of age. The incidence of hyaline membrane disease and hyperbilirubinemia may be decreased in low birthweight infants of heroin addicts; hyperventilation leading to respiratory alkalosis or accelerated production of surfactant may explain the former, and enzyme induction of glucuronyl transferase the latter.

Tremors and hyperirritability are the most prominent symptoms. The tremors may be fine or jittery and indistinguishable from those of hypoglycemia but are more often coarse, "flapping," and bilateral; the limbs are often rigid, hyperreflexic, and resistant to flexion and extension. Irritability and hyperactivity are generally marked and may lead to skin abrasions. Other signs include tachypnea, diarrhea, vomiting, high-pitched cry, fist sucking, poor feeding, and fever. Sneezing, yawning, myoclonic jerks, convulsions, abnormal sleep cycles, nasal stuffiness, apnea, flushing alternating rapidly with pallor, and lacrimation are less common. The *diagnosis* is generally established by the history and clinical presentation. Examining the urine for opiates may reveal only low levels during withdrawal, but quinine, which is often mixed with heroin, may be present in higher concentrations. Hypoglycemia and hypocalcemia should be excluded.

Methadone addiction is associated with severe withdrawal symptoms, the incidence varying from 20 to 90%. In general, mothers taking methadone have better prenatal care than those taking heroin; however, there is a high incidence of multiple drug abuse, including alcohol, barbiturates, and tranquilizers, and these mothers are often heavy smokers. There is no increased incidence of congenital anomalies. The average birthweight of infants of mothers taking methadone is higher than that of infants of heroin-addicted mothers; the *clinical manifestations* are similar except that the former group has a higher incidence of seizures (10–20%) and of late onset (2–6 wk of age) of symptoms and signs.

Alcohol withdrawal is uncommon. The infants of women who have been drinking immediately before delivery may have alcohol on their breath for several hours, since it rapidly crosses the placenta, and blood levels in the infant are similar to those in the mother. Hypoglycemia and acidosis may be present. Infants who develop withdrawal symptoms often become agitated and hyperactive with marked tremors lasting for 72 hr, followed by about 48 hr of lethargy before return to normal activity. Seizures may develop.

Phenobarbital withdrawal usually occurs in full-term, appropriate for gestational age infants of addicted mothers. Symptoms begin at a median age of 7 days (range 2–14 days). There may be a brief acute stage consisting of irritability, constant crying, sleeplessness, hiccups, and mouthing movements, followed by a subacute stage that may last 2–4 mo consisting of voracious appetite, frequent regurgitation and gagging, episodic irritability, hyperacusis, sweating, and a disturbed sleep pattern.

Cocaine addiction among pregnant women has increased significantly, but withdrawal in their infants is unusual; pregnancy may be complicated by premature labor, abruptio placentae, and fetal asphyxia. Infants may manifest intrauterine growth retardation, microcephaly, intracranial hemorrhage, possible anomalies of the gastrointestinal and renal tracts, sudden infant death syndrome (SIDS), and neurobehavioral deficits characterized by rigidity, impaired state regulation, developmental delay, and learning disabilities. Child abuse, neglect, and AIDS are common in these families.

Treatment of heroin and methadone withdrawals has been successful using various combinations of narcotics, sedatives, and hypnotics. Therapy is indicated for seizures, for diarrhea, or for such irritability that normal sleep and feeding patterns are disturbed and weight gain is poor. Methadone withdrawal may require larger amounts of medication for longer periods than does heroin withdrawal to control clinical manifestations. Phenobarbital, 8–10 mg/kg/24 hr in 4 divided doses, can effectively reduce irritability and prevent seizures. It is as effective as chlorpromazine, 2.2 mg/kg/24 hr, divided into 3–4 doses. It is usually not necessary to administer either drug for more than 5 days, but on occasion it may be necessary to treat the infant for as long as 6 wk. Patients with severe autonomic symptoms may require gradually diminishing doses of methadone or paregoric for 2–10 wk. Paregoric at a beginning dose of 3–5 drops given every 3–6 hr, increased to 5–10 drops every 4 hr if necessary, depending on the size and response of the infant, will abolish most withdrawal symptoms, especially diarrhea. The dose and duration of therapy may be adjusted according to the clinical response. Parenteral administration of fluids may be necessary to prevent aspiration or dehydration until the symptoms are brought under control. Narcotic and phenobarbital withdrawal requires swaddling, frequent feedings, and protection from noxious external stimuli.

Current mortality from withdrawal is not over 5%, and with early recognition and treatment may be negligible. *Prognosis* for normal development is affected by the adverse circumstances of high-risk pregnancy and delivery and by the environment to which the infant is returned after recovery as well as by the effects of the particular drug on fetal and subsequent neonatal development.

FETAL ALCOHOL SYNDROME. High levels of alcohol ingestion during pregnancy can be damaging to embryonic and fetal development. A specific pattern of malformation identified as the *fetal alcohol syndrome* has been documented, and major and minor components of the syndrome are expressed in 1–2 infants/1,000 live births. Both moderate and high levels of alcohol intake during early pregnancy may result in alterations in growth and morphogenesis of the fetus; the greater the intake, the more severe the signs. Infants born to heavy drinkers have twice the risk of abnormality compared with those born to moderate drinkers; 32% of infants born to heavy drinkers demonstrated congenital anomalies, compared with 9% in the abstinent and 14% in the moderate group.

The characteristics of the fetal alcohol syndrome include (1) prenatal onset and persistence of growth deficiency for length, weight, and head circumference; (2) facial abnormalities, including short palpebral fissures, epicanthal folds, maxillary hypoplasia, micrognathia, and thin upper lip; (3) cardiac defects, primarily septal defects; (4) minor joint and limb abnormalities, including some restriction of movement and altered palmar crease patterns; and (5) delayed development and mental deficiency varying from borderline to severe. Fetal alcohol syndrome is a common cause of mental retardation. The severity of dysmorphogenesis may range from severely affected infants with full manifestations of the fetal alcohol syndrome to those mildly affected with only a few manifestations.

The detrimental effects may be due to the alcohol itself or to one of its breakdown products. Some evidence suggests that alcohol may impair placental transfer of essential amino acids and zinc, both necessary for protein synthesis, which accounts for the intrauterine growth retardation.

The *management* of these infants may be difficult, since no specific therapy exists. The infants may remain hypotonic and tremulous despite sedation, and the prognosis is poor. Counseling with regard to recurrence is important. *Prevention* is achieved by eliminating alcohol intake after conception.

LATE METABOLIC ACIDOSIS

Between 5 and 10% of preterm low birthweight infants develop a metabolic acidosis during the 2nd or 3rd wk of life. Usually there is no history of asphyxia, respiratory distress, or other problems, and the infants are vigorous. However, they often have received cow's milk formulas of high protein and casein content shortly after birth and have had a delayed start of postnatal weight gain. Blood base excess values range from −10 to −16 mEq/L, and P_{CO_2} values are usually less than 40 mm Hg. The condition probably represents an abnormally high rate of endogenous acid formation. Treatment includes administering $NaHCO_3$ and changing to a formula of lower protein content with a whey:casein ratio of 60:40.

Broekhuizen FF, Utrie J, Van Mullem CV: Drug use or inadequate prenatal care? Adverse pregnancy outcome in an urban setting. Am J Obstet Gynecol 166:1747, 1992.

Doberczak TM, Kandall SR, Friedmann P: Relationships between maternal methadone dosage, maternal-neonatal methadone levels, and neonatal withdrawal. Obstet Gynecol 81:936, 1993.

Dreher MC, Nugent K, Hudgins R: Prenatal marijuana exposure and neonatal outcomes in Jamaica: An ethnographic study. Pediatrics 93:254, 1994.

Horsman A, Ryan SW, Congdon PJ, et al: Bone mineral accretion rate and calcium intake in preterm infants. Arch Dis Child 64:910, 1989.

Horsman A, Ryan SW, Congdon PJ, et al: Osteopenia in extremely low birthweight infants. Arch Dis Child 64:485, 1989.

Kildeberg P: Late metabolic acidosis of premature infants. *In* Winters RW (ed): The Body Fluids in Pediatrics. Boston, Little, Brown, 1973.
Kliegman RM, Madura D, Kiwi R, et al: Relation of maternal cocaine use to the risks of prematurity and low birth weight. J Pediatr 124:751, 1994.
Nervez CT, Shott RJ, Bergstrom WH, et al: Prophylaxis against hypocalcemia in low birth weight infants receiving bicarbonate infusion. J Pediatr 87:439, 1975.
Neuman L, Cohen S: The neonatal narcotic withdrawal syndrome. Clin Perinatol 2:99, 1975.
Singer LT, Yamashita TS, Hawkins S, et al: Increased incidence of intraventricular hemorrhage and developmental delay in cocaine-exposed, very low birth weight infants. J Pediatr 124:765, 1994.
Streissguth AP, Herman CS, Smith DW: Intelligence, behavior and dysmorphogenesis in the fetal alcohol syndrome: A report of 20 patients. J Pediatr 92:363, 1978.
Vega WA, Kolody B, Hwang J, et al: Prevalence and magnitude of perinatal substance exposures in California. N Engl J Med 329:850, 1993.

CHAPTER 93

The Endocrine System

The endocrinopathies are discussed in Part XXVI. The purpose of this section is to call attention to those endocrine disturbances that may be identified at birth or during the first month of life.

Pituitary dwarfism is usually not apparent at birth, although panhypopituitary male infants may present with neonatal hypoglycemia and micropenis. Conversely, constitutional dwarfs usually demonstrate length and weight consistent with prematurity when born after a normal gestational period; otherwise their physical appearance is normal.

Thyroid deficiency may be apparent at birth in genetically determined **cretinism** or in infants of mothers treated with thiouracil or its derivatives during pregnancy. Constipation, prolonged jaundice, lethargy, or poor peripheral circulation as shown by persistently mottled skin or cold extremities should suggest cretinism. The early diagnosis and treatment of congenital deficiency of thyroid hormone may be greatly facilitated by screening all newborn infants for this deficiency.

Temporary *hyperthyroidism* may occur at birth in the infants of mothers with hyperthyroidism or of those who have been receiving thyroid medication.

Transient *hypoparathyroidism* may be manifest as tetany of the newborn.

The *adrenal gland* is subject to numerous disturbances, which may become apparent and require lifesaving treatment during the neonatal period. Acute adrenal *hemorrhage* and failure may be seen after breech or other traumatic deliveries or in association with overwhelming infection. *Adrenocortical hyperplasia* is suggested by vomiting, diarrhea, dehydration, hyperkalemia, hyponatremia, shock, or clitoral enlargement. Since the condition is genetically determined, newborn siblings of patients with the salt-losing variety of adrenocortical hyperplasia should be observed closely for manifestations of adrenal insufficiency.

Congenitally hypoplastic adrenal glands may also give rise to adrenal insufficiency during the first few weeks of life.

Female infants with webbing of the neck, lymphangiectatic edema, hypoplasia of the nipples, cutis laxa, low hairline at the nape of the neck, low-set ears, high-arched palate, deformities of the nails, cubitus valgus, and other anomalies should be suspected of having *gonadal dysgenesis*.

Transient *diabetes mellitus* (Part XXVI, Section 6) is rare and is seen only in the newborn. It usually presents as dehydration, loss of weight, or acidosis in small for gestational age infants.

93.1 Infants of Diabetic Mothers

The control of diabetes mellitus with insulin has led to the survival of increasing numbers of diabetic women who bear children. Their infants and the infants of women who later develop diabetes share certain distinctive morphologic characteristics, including large size, macrosomia, and high morbidity risks. Diabetic mothers have a high incidence of polyhydramnios, pre-eclampsia, pyelonephritis, preterm labor, and chronic hypertension; their fetal mortality rate, which is high at all gestational ages, especially so after 32 wk, is greater than that of nondiabetic mothers. Fetal wastage throughout pregnancy is associated with poorly controlled maternal diabetes, especially ketoacidosis and congenital anomalies. Diabetic mothers produce an excess of high-birthweight infants at all gestational ages and, if complicated with vascular disease, of low-birthweight infants at 37- to 40-wk gestations. The neonatal mortality rate is over 5 times that of infants of nondiabetic mothers and is higher at all gestational ages and in every birthweight for gestational age category.

PATHOPHYSIOLOGY. The probable pathogenic sequence is that maternal hyperglycemia causes fetal hyperglycemia, and the fetal pancreatic response leads to fetal hyperinsulinemia; fetal hyperinsulinemia and hyperglycemia then cause increased hepatic glucose uptake and glycogen synthesis, accelerated lipogenesis, and augmented protein synthesis. Related pathologic findings are the hypertrophy and hyperplasia of the pancreatic islets with a disproportionate increase in the number of β cells; increased weights of the placenta and infant organs except for the brain; myocardial hypertrophy; increased amounts of cytoplasm in liver cells; and extramedullary hematopoiesis. Hyperinsulinism produces fetal acidosis, which may result in an increased rate of stillbirth. The separation of the placenta at birth suddenly interrupts glucose infusion into the neonate without a proportional effect on the hyperinsulinism, resulting in hypoglycemia and attenuated lipolysis during the first hours after birth.

Hyperinsulinemia has been documented in infants of gestational diabetic mothers and in those of insulin-dependent diabetic mothers without insulin antibodies. The former group also have significantly higher fasting plasma insulin levels than normal newborns despite similar glucose levels; they respond to glucose with a prompt elevation of plasma insulin and assimilate a glucose load more rapidly. Following arginine administration, they also have an enhanced insulin response and increased disappearance rates of glucose, compared with normal infants. In contrast, fasting glucose utilization rates are diminished. The lower free fatty acid levels in infants of insulin-dependent diabetic mothers probably also reflect their hyperinsulinemia. With good prenatal diabetic control, the incidences of macrosomia and hypoglycemia have decreased.

Although hyperinsulinism is probably the main cause of hypoglycemia, the diminished epinephrine and glucagon responses that occur may be contributing factors. Cortisol and human growth hormone levels are normal. Congenital anomalies correlate with poor metabolic control and may be due to hyperglycemia-induced teratogenesis.

CLINICAL MANIFESTATIONS. The infants of diabetic and gestational diabetic mothers often bear a surprising resemblance to each other (Fig. 93–1). They tend to be large and plump as a result of increased body fat and enlarged viscera, with puffy, plethoric facies resembling those of patients who have been receiving a corticosteroid. These infants may, however, also be of normal or low birthweight, particularly if they are delivered before term or if there is associated maternal vascular disease.

The infants tend to be "jumpy," tremulous, and hyperexcitable during the first 3 days of life, although hypotonia, lethargy, and poor sucking also may occur. They may have any of

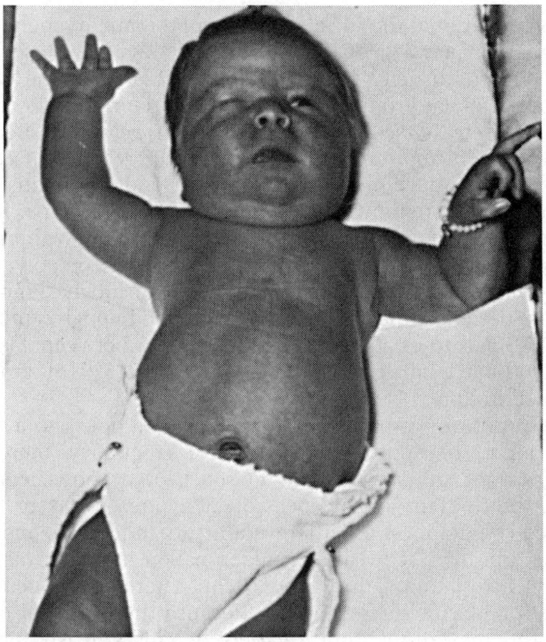

Figure 93–1. Large, plump, plethoric infant of a gestational diabetic mother. Baby was born at 38 wk of gestation but weighed 9 lb 11 oz (4,408 g). Mild respiratory distress was the only symptom other than appearance.

the diverse manifestations of hypoglycemia. Early appearance of these signs is more likely to be related to hypoglycemia and later appearance related to hypocalcemia; these abnormalities also may occur together. Perinatal asphyxia or hyperbilirubinemia may produce similar signs. Rarely, hypomagnesemia may be associated with the hypocalcemia.

About 75% of infants of diabetic mothers and 25% of infants of mothers with gestational diabetes develop hypoglycemia (Chapter 77, but only a small percentage of these infants become symptomatic. The probability of an infant developing hypoglycemia increases and the glucose levels are likely to be lower at higher cord or maternal fasting blood glucose levels. Usually, the nadir in the infant's blood glucose concentration is reached between 1 and 3 hr; spontaneous recovery may begin by 4–6 hr.

Many infants of diabetic mothers develop tachypnea during the first 5 days of life, which may be a transient manifestation of hypoglycemia, hypothermia, polycythemia, cardiac failure, transient tachypnea, or cerebral edema from birth trauma or asphyxia. A greater incidence of respiratory distress syndrome appears in infants of diabetic mothers than in infants of normal mothers born at comparable gestational age; the greater incidence is possibly related to an antagonistic effect between cortisol and insulin on surfactant synthesis.

Cardiomegaly is common (30%), and heart failure occurs in 5–10% of infants of diabetic mothers. Asymmetric septal hypertrophy may occur, becoming manifest similarly to idiopathic hypertrophic subaortic stenosis. Birth trauma is also common due to fetal macrosomia.

Neurologic development and ossification centers tend to be immature and correlate with the brain size (which is not increased) and gestational age rather than with total body weight. There is also an increased incidence of hyperbilirubinemia, polycythemia, and renal vein thrombosis; the latter should be suspected in the presence of a flank mass, hematuria, and thrombocytopenia.

The incidence of congenital anomalies is increased 3-fold in infants of diabetic mothers; cardiac malformations (VSD, ASD, transposition of great vessels, coarctation of the aorta) and lumbosacral agenesis are most common. Additional anomalies include neural tube defects, hydronephrosis, renal agenesis, duodenal or anorectal atresia, and holoprosencephaly. These infants may also develop abdominal distention caused by a transient delay in the development of the left side of the colon, the *small left colon syndrome*.

PROGNOSIS. The subsequent incidence of diabetes mellitus in infants of diabetic mothers is increased compared with that of the general population. Physical development is normal, but oversized infants may be predisposed to obesity in childhood that may extend into adult life. Disagreement persists about whether or not a slightly increased risk of impaired intellectual development exists unrelated to hypoglycemia; symptomatic hypoglycemia probably increases the risk.

TREATMENT. Management of these infants should be initiated before birth by frequent prenatal evaluation of all pregnant women with overt or gestational diabetes, by evaluation of fetal maturity, by biophysical profile, by Doppler velocimetry, and by planning delivery of these infants in hospitals where expert obstetric and pediatric care is continuously available. Regardless of size, all infants of diabetic mothers should initially receive intensive observation and care. Asymptomatic infants should have a blood sugar determination within 1 hr of birth and then every hour for the next 6–8 hr; if clinically well and normoglycemic, oral or gavage feedings initially with 5% glucose water, followed by breast milk or formula, should be started at 2–3 hr of age and continued at 3-hr intervals. If any question arises about an infant's ability to tolerate oral feeding, the feeding should be discontinued and glucose given by peripheral intravenous infusion at a rate of 4–8 mg/kg/min. Hypoglycemia should be treated, even in asymptomatic infants, with intravenous infusions of glucose sufficient to keep the blood levels well above this level. Bolus injections of hypertonic glucose should be avoided because they may cause further hyperinsulinemia and potentially produce rebound hypoglycemia. Managing hypoglycemia in sick or symptomatic infants is discussed in the following section. For treatment of *hypocalcemia* and *hypomagnesemia*, see Chapter 92; for *hyaline membrane disease* treatment, see Chapter 87.3; for treatment of *polycythemia*, see Chapter 89.3.

93.2 Hypoglycemia

See also Chapter 77.

Hypoglycemia is present when serum glucose levels are significantly lower than the range among postnatal age-matched normal infants. Although hypoglycemia may also be defined as the presence of neurologic (lethargy, coma, apnea, seizures) or sympathomimetic (pallor, palpitations, diaphoresis) manifestations that respond to glucose, many neonates with low serum glucose levels are asymptomatic, whereas normoglycemic infants may have nonspecific signs of hypoglycemia.

The *incidence of hypoglycemia* varies with the definition, population, method and timing of feeding, and type of glucose assay (serum levels are higher than whole blood values) (Fig. 93–2). Early feeding decreases the incidence, whereas prematurity, hypothermia, hypoxia, maternal diabetes, maternal glucose infusion in labor, and intrauterine growth retardation increase the incidence of hypoglycemia. Serum glucose levels decline after birth until 1–3 hr of age, when levels spontaneously increase in normal infants. In healthy term infants serum glucose values are rarely less than 35 mg/dL (1.9 mmol/L) between 1 and 3 hr of life, less than 40 mg/dL (2.2 mmol/L) from 3 to 24 hr, and less than 45 mg/dL (2.5 mmol/L) after 24 hr. Although previous studies, performed when premature infants were fasted in the 1st day of life, suggested that prema-

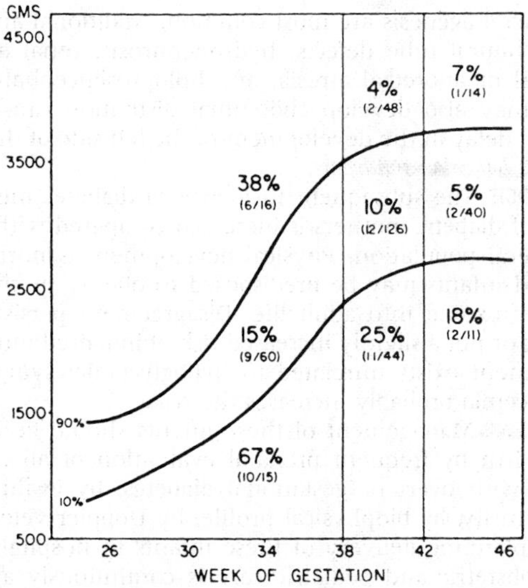

Figure 93–2. Incidence of hypoglycemia by birth weight, gestational age, and intrauterine growth. (From Lubchenco LO [ed]: Incidence of hypoglycemia in newborn infants classified by birth weight and gestational age. Pediatrics 47:832, 1971. Copyright 1971. Reproduced by permission of Pediatrics.)

ture infants have statistically lower glucose levels than term infants and that preterm infants may be unaffected by low glucose values, recent evidence does not support these conclusions. Both premature and full-term infants are at risk for serious neurodevelopmental deficits from equally low glucose levels. This risk is related to the depth and duration of the hypoglycemia.

Four pathophysiologic groups of *neonatal infants are at high risk of developing hypoglycemia*: (1) Infants of mothers with diabetes mellitus or gestational diabetes, infants with severe erythroblastosis fetalis, insulinomas, β cell nesidioblastosis, functional β cell hyperplasia, mutations in the sulfonylurea receptor gene, Beckwith syndrome (see below), and panhypopituitarism seem to have hyperinsulinism. (2) Infants with intrauterine growth retardation or those who are preterm may have experienced intrauterine malnutrition resulting in reduced hepatic glycogen stores and total body fat; the smaller of discordant twins (especially if discordant by 25% or more in weight with a weight of less than 2.0 kg), polycythemic infants, infants of toxemic mothers, and infants with placental abnormalities are particularly vulnerable. (Other factors in the development of hypoglycemia in this group include impaired gluconeogenesis, diminished free fatty acid oxidation, low cortisol production rates, and possibly increased insulin levels and decreased output of epinephrine in response to hypoglycemia.) (3) Very immature or severely ill infants may develop hypoglycemia owing to increased metabolic needs disproportionate to substrate stores and calories supplied; low-birthweight infants with respiratory distress syndrome, perinatal asphyxia, polycythemia, hypothermia, and systemic infections, as well as infants in heart failure with cyanotic congenital heart disease, are at increased risk. The interruption of intravenous infusions, particularly those with high glucose concentrations, may also result in the precipitous onset of hypoglycemia. (4) Rare infants with genetic or primary metabolic defects, such as galactosemia, glycogen storage disease, fructose intolerance, propionic acidemia, methylmalonic acidemia, tyrosinemia, maple syrup urine disease, and long- or medium-chain acyl-CoA dehydrogenase deficiency are also susceptible.

CLINICAL MANIFESTATIONS. In contrast to the frequency of chemical hypoglycemia, the incidence of symptomatic hypoglycemia is highest in small for gestational age infants (see Fig. 93–2). These infants usually fall into category 2 or 3 of the earlier pathophysiologic groupings, and some are referred to as having *transient symptomatic idiopathic neonatal hypoglycemia*. Because many of the symptoms also occur together with other conditions such as infections—especially sepsis and meningitis; central nervous system anomalies, hemorrhage, or edema; hypocalcemia and hypomagnesemia; asphyxia; drug withdrawal; apnea of prematurity; congenital heart disease; or polycythemia—and because some may be seen in normoglycemic well infants, the exact incidence of symptomatic hypoglycemia has been difficult to establish. It probably varies between 1 and 3 per 1,000 live births and affects about 5–15% of growth-retarded infants.

The onset of symptoms varies from a few hours to a week after birth. In approximate order of frequency there are jitteriness or tremors, apathy, episodes of cyanosis, convulsions, intermittent apneic spells or tachypnea, weak or high-pitched cry, limpness or lethargy, difficulty in feeding, and eye-rolling. Episodes of sweating, sudden pallor, hypothermia, and cardiac arrest and failure also occur. There is frequently a clustering of episodic symptoms. Because these clinical manifestations may result from a variety of causes, it is critical to measure serum glucose levels and to determine whether they disappear with the administration of sufficient glucose to raise the blood sugar to normal levels; if they do not, other diagnoses must be considered.

TREATMENT. When seizures are not present, an intravenous bolus of 200 mg/kg (2mL/kg) of 10% glucose is effective in elevating the blood glucose concentration. In the presence of convulsions, 4 mL/kg of 10% glucose as a bolus injection is indicated.

Following initial therapy a glucose infusion should be given at 8 mg/kg/min. If hypoglycemia recurs, the infusion rate should be increased until 15–20% glucose is employed. If intravenous infusions of 20% glucose are inadequate to eliminate symptoms and maintain constant normal serum glucose concentrations, hydrocortisone (2.5 mg/kg/6 hr) or prednisone (1 mg/kg/24 hr) should also be administered. Serum glucose should be measured every 2 hr after initiating therapy until several determinations are above 40 mg/dL. Subsequently, levels should be obtained every 4–6 hr and the treatment gradually reduced and finally discontinued when the serum glucose has been in the normal range and the baby asymptomatic for 24–48 hr. Treatment is usually necessary for a few days to a week, rarely for several weeks. If neonatal hyperinsulinism is present, as in nesidioblastosis, and the infant is unresponsive to steroids and glucose given for a sufficient time, diazoxide or long-acting somatostatin may be employed.

Surgery is the definitive treatment for *nesidioblastosis* and *islet cell adenomas*; glucagon plus somatostatin has been a helpful adjunct in some cases.

Infants who are at increased risk of developing hypoglycemia should have their serum glucose measured within 1 hr of birth and subsequently every 1–2 hr for the first 6–8 hr, then every 4–6 hr until 24 hr of life. Normoglycemic high-risk infants should receive oral or gavage feedings with formula started at 1–3 hr of age and continued at 2- to 3-hr intervals for 24–48 hr. An intravenous infusion of glucose at 4 mg/kg/min should be provided if oral feedings are poorly tolerated or if *asymptomatic transient neonatal hypoglycemia* develops.

PROGNOSIS. Prognosis for life is good. Hypoglycemia recurs in 10–15% of infants after adequate treatment. Some have been reported as late as the age of 8 mo. Recurrences are more common if intravenous fluids are extravasated or are too rapidly discontinued before oral feedings are well tolerated. Children who later develop ketotic hypoglycemia have an increased incidence of neonatal hypoglycemia. Prognosis for normal intellectual function must be guarded, since prolonged and severe hypoglycemia may be associated with neurologic sequelae. Symptomatic infants with hypoglycemia, particularly low-birthweight infants and infants of diabetic mothers, have a poorer prognosis for subsequent normal intellectual development than do asymptomatic infants.

Hypoglycemia with Macroglossia

(Beckwith Syndrome)

Beckwith described a syndrome of intractable neonatal hypoglycemia occurring in infants with macroglossia, large size, visceromegaly, mild microcephaly, omphalocele, facial nevus flammeus, a characteristic earlobe crease, increased risk of tumors (Wilms, hepatoblastoma, gonadoblastoma) and renal medullary dysplasia. The visceromegaly involves chiefly the liver and the kidneys, in which there is a noncystic hyperplasia. Some infants are also polycythemic. Hyperinsulinemia has been demonstrated. Some infants with Beckwith syndrome have a partial duplication of chromosome llp, a region that encodes the insulin-like growth factor II gene. Although usually sporadic, familial inheritance has been noted. Treatment is that of hypoglycemia; in this syndrome hypoglycemia may be severe and persist for several months. The prognosis is poor.

Severe hypoglycemia has also been demonstrated in extremely high-birthweight infants who do not have the anomalies present in Beckwith syndrome. These *infant giants* weigh from 3.8 to 5.3 kg, and, in some, pancreatic hyperplasia has been described.

Anonymous: Brain damage by neonatal hypoglycemia. Lancet 2:882, 1989.

Berk MA, Minouni F, Miodovnik M, et al: Macrosomia in infants of insulin-dependent diabetic mothers. Pediatrics 83:1029, 1989.

Buchanan TA, Kitzmiller JL: Metabolic interactions of diabetes and pregnancy. Annu Rev Med 45:245, 1994.

Daneman D, Ehrlich RM: The enigma of persistent hyperinsulinemic hypoglycemia of infancy. J Pediatr 123:573, 1993.

Demarini S, Mimouni F, Tsang RC, et al: Impact of metabolic control of diabetes during pregnancy on neonatal hypocalcemia: A randomized study. Obstet Gynecol 83:918, 1994.

Koh THHG, Aynsley-Green A, Tarbit M, et al: Neural dysfunction during hypoglycaemia. Arch Dis Child 63:1353, 1988.

Langer O, Rodriguez DA, Xenakis EMJ, et al: Intensified versus conventional management of gestational diabetes. Am J Obstet Gynecol 170:1036, 1994.

Lilien L, Pildes R, Srinivasan G, et al: Treatment of neonatal hypoglycemia with minibolus and intravenous glucose infusion. J Pediatr 97:295, 1980.

Lucas A, Morley R, Cole TJ: Adverse neurodevelopmental outcome of moderate neonatal hypoglycaemia. Br Med J 297:1304, 1989.

Mehta A: Prevention and management of neonatal hypoglycaemia. Arch Dis Child 70:F54, 1994.

Sacks DA: Fetal macrosomia and gestational diabetes: What's the problem? Obstet Gynecol 81:775, 1993.

Sells CJ, Robinson NM, Brown Z, et al: Long-term developmental follow-up of infants of diabetic mothers. J Pediatr 125:S9, 1994.

Swenne I: The fetus of the diabetic mother: Growth and malformations. Arch Dis Child 63:1119, 1988.

Thomas PM, Cate GJ, Wohll KN, et al: Mutations in the sulfonylurea receptor gene in familial persistent hyperinsulinemic hypoglycemia of infancy. Science 268:426, 1995.

Wilcken B, Carpenter KH, Hammond J: Neonatal symptoms in medium chain acyl coenzyme A dehydrogenase deficiency. Arch Dis Child 69:292, 1993.

PART XII

Infections of the Neonatal Infant

SECTION 1

Unique Aspects of Infection

CHAPTER 94

Epidemiology, Immunity, and Pathogenesis

Samuel P. Gotoff

Infections are a frequent and important cause of morbidity and mortality in the neonatal period (see Chapter 1). As many as 2% of fetuses are infected in utero, and up to 10% of infants are infected during delivery or the 1st mo of life. Inflammatory lesions are found in about 25% of newborn infant autopsies; these lesions are second only to hyaline membrane disease in frequency.

The uniqueness of neonatal infections is a result of a number of factors. (1) There are diverse modes of transmission of infectious agents from mother to fetus or newborn infant (Fig. 94–1). Transplacental hematogenous spread may occur at different times during gestation. Manifestations of congenital infections may be present at birth or may be delayed for months or years. Vertical transmission of infection may take place in utero, just prior to delivery, or during the process of delivery. After birth, the newborn infant may be exposed to infectious diseases in the nursery or in the community. With the increasing complexity of neonatal intensive care, gestationally younger and lower birthweight newborns are surviving and remaining for a longer time in an environment with a high risk of infection. (2) The newborn infant may be less capable of responding to infection owing to one or more immunologic deficiencies involving the reticuloendothelial system, complement, polymorphonuclear leukocytes, cytokines, antibody, or cell-mediated immunity. (3) Coexisting diseases of the newborn often complicate the diagnosis and management of neonatal infections. Respiratory disorders such as hyaline membrane disease may coexist with bacterial pneumonia. Acidosis impairs functions of polymorphonuclear leukocytes. (4) The manifestations of infectious diseases in the newborn infant are extremely variable. There may be subclinical infection, congenital malformations, focal disease, and poorly localized systemic infection. The timing of exposure in utero, inoculum size, immune status, and the etiologic agent influence the

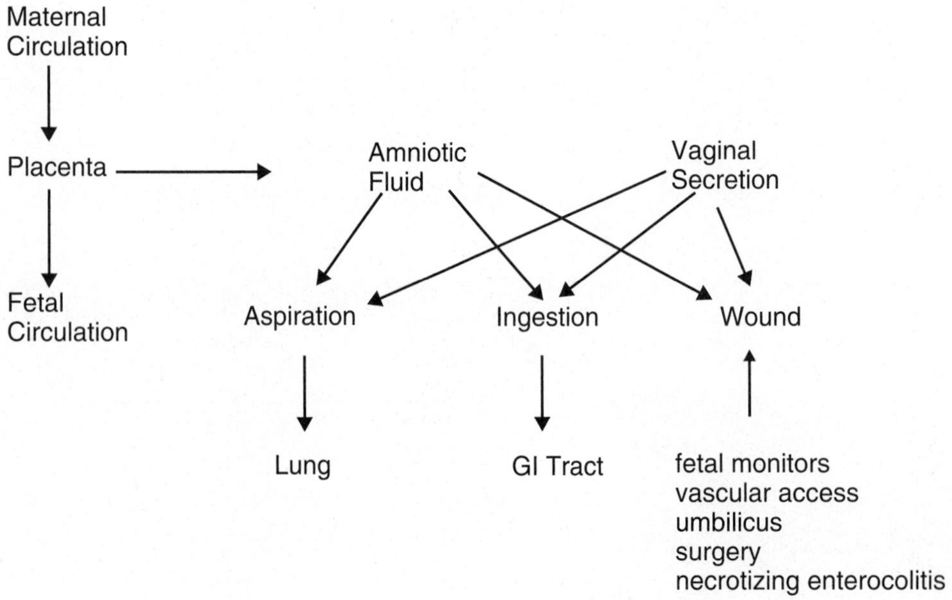

Figure 94–1. The fetus or newborn infant may become infected by the transplacental route, from contamination of amniotic fluid, or by aspiration or ingestion of vaginal secretions. The breakdown of cutaneous or mucous membrane barriers from fetal monitors, vascular catheters, incision of the umbilical cord, surgery, and necrotizing enterocolitis creates additional portals of entry for microorganisms.

expression of disease in the fetus or newborn infant. A variety of organisms, including bacteria, viruses, fungi, protozoa, and mycoplasma, are etiologic agents (Table 94–1).

The status of the mother's immunity, for example, to rubella, and her exposure to various microorganisms, such as *Toxoplasma*, determines whether maternal infection occurs during pregnancy. Maternal infection may be clinical, often with nonspecific symptoms and signs, or subclinical, identified retrospectively by serologic methods, as part of the evaluation of suspected neonatal infection. Transplacental transmission of infection to the fetus is variable. The placenta often functions as an effective barrier. Prenatal infections that are known to be transmitted transplacentally include syphilis, *Borrelia burgdorferi*, rubella, cytomegalovirus (CMV), parvovirus B19, human immunodeficiency virus (HIV), varicella-zoster, *Listeria monocytogenes*, toxoplasmosis, and tuberculosis. Infection acquired in utero may result in resorption of the embryo, abortion, stillbirth, congenital malformation, intrauterine growth retardation, premature birth, acute disease in the neonatal period, or asymptomatic persistent infection with neurologic sequelae later in life.

Perinatal infections are acquired just before or during delivery with vertical transmission of the microorganism from mother to newborn infant. The organisms may be bacteria that colonize the birth canal, such as group B streptococci, gonococci, *L. monocytogenes, Escherichia coli* (particularly the K1 capsular strains), *Chlamydia*, genital *Mycoplasma* and *Ureaplasma*. Other microbial species such as enteroviruses and herpes simplex may also be acquired in a similar fashion. Maternal-to-fetal transfusion at delivery is the usual mechanism of transmission of hepatitis B virus and HIV.

The *amniotic infection syndrome* refers to bacterial invasion of amniotic fluid, usually as a result of prolonged rupture of the chorioamniotic membrane. On occasion, amniotic infection occurs with apparently intact membranes. Amniotic fluid infection may be asymptomatic or may produce maternal fever and local or systemic signs of chorioamnionitis. Microscopic evidence of inflammation of membranes is uniformly present when the duration of rupture exceeds 24 hr. Difficult or traumatic delivery and premature delivery are also associated with an increased frequency of neonatal infections.

Exposure to and aspiration of bacteria in amniotic fluid lead to congenital pneumonia or systemic bacterial infection with manifestations becoming apparent prior to delivery (fetal distress, tachycardia), at delivery (perinatal asphyxia), or after a latent period of a few hours (respiratory distress, shock). Aspiration of bacteria during the birth process may lead to infection after an interval of 1–2 days. Although the term *early-onset neonatal infection* has been used to refer to neonatal infections occurring as late as 1 wk of age, it should be restricted to those infections with a perinatal pathogenesis the usual onset of which occurs within 72 hr (Table 94–2).

The most important neonatal factor predisposing to infection is prematurity or low birthweight; there is a 3- to 10-fold higher incidence of infection and sepsis in these infants than in full-term normal-birthweight infants. Males have an approximately two-fold higher incidence of sepsis than females, suggesting the possibility of a sex-linked factor in host suscepti-

■ **TABLE 94–1 Viral, Parasitic, and Spirochetal Agents Associated with Fetal and Infant Morbidity and Mortality**

Pathogen	Fetus	Neonatal Disease	Congenital Defects	Late Sequelae
Rubella virus	Abortion	Low birthweight, hepatosplenomegaly, petechiae, osteitis	Heart defects, microcephaly, cataracts, microphthalmia	Deafness, mental retardation, thyroid disorders, diabetes, degenerative brain tissue, autism
Cytomegalovirus	—	Anemia, thrombocytopenia, hepatosplenomegaly, jaundice, encephalitis	Microcephaly, microphthalmia, retinopathy	Deafness, psychomotor retardation, cerebral calcification
Varicella-zoster virus	—	Low birthweight, chorioretinitis, congenital chickenpox or disseminated neonatal varicella, possibly zoster	Limb hypoplasia, cortical atrophy, cicatricial skin lesions	Fatal outcome due to secondary infection
Picornaviruses				
Coxsackievirus	Abortion	Mild febrile disease, exanthems, aseptic meningitis, disseminated disease, multiple organ involvement (CNS, liver, heart), gastroenteritis	Possible congenital heart disease, myocarditis	Neurologic deficits
Echovirus	—			
Poliovirus	Abortion	Congenital poliomyelitis		Paralysis
Herpes simplex virus	Abortion	Disseminated disease, multiple organ involvement (lung, liver, CNS), vesicular skin lesions, retinopathy	Possible microcephaly, retinopathy, intracranial calcifications	Neurologic deficits
Hepatitis B virus	—	Asymptomatic HB_sAg positive infection, low birthweight, rarely acute hepatitis	—	Chronic hepatitis, persistent HB_sAg positive
Human immunodeficiency virus	—	AIDS	—	AIDS
Parvovirus B19	Stillbirth Hydrops fetalis	Anemia	—	—
Borrelia burgdorferi	Stillbirth	Rash, prematurity, cortical blindness	?	?
Toxoplasma gondii	Abortion	Low birthweight, hepatosplenomegaly, jaundice, anemia	Hydrocephalus, microcephaly	Chorioretinitis, mental retardation
Treponema pallidum	Stillbirth Hydrops fetalis	Skin lesions, rhinitis, hepatosplenomegaly, jaundice, osteitis, anemia	—	Interstitial keratitis, frontal bossing, saber shins, tooth changes
Malaria	Abortion	Hepatosplenomegaly, jaundice, anemia, poor feeding, vomiting	—	—
Trypanosoma cruzi (Chagas disease)	Abortion	Low birthweight, jaundice, anemia, petechiae, heart failure, hepatosplenomegaly megaesophagus, encephalitis	Cataracts	Myocarditis, achalasia

CNS = central nervous system; HB_sAg = hepatitis B surface antigen; AIDS = acquired immunodeficiency syndrome.

by increased ambient temperature, dehydration, central nervous system disorders, hyperthyroidism, familial dysautonomia, or ectodermal dysplasia. A single temperature elevation is infrequently associated with infection; fever sustained over 1 hr is more likely to be due to infection. Most febrile infected infants have additional signs compatible with infection, although a focus of infection may not be apparent. In premature infants, hypothermia or temperature instability is more likely to be associated with infection, but some degree of temperature instability is not unusual in low-birthweight infants.

Cutaneous manifestations of infection provide useful clues. Impetigo, cellulitis, mastitis, omphalitis, and subcutaneous abscesses should be recognizable. Ecthyma gangrenosum is indicative of pseudomonal infection. The presence of small salmon-pink papules suggests *Listeria monocytogenes* infection. A vesicular rash is consistent with herpesvirus infection. The mucocutaneous lesions of *Candida albicans* are covered later. Petechiae and purpura may have an infectious cause.

Neonatal pneumonia may be difficult to differentiate in premature infants with respiratory distress syndrome or bronchopulmonary dysplasia. Pneumonia should be considered in ventilated infants who have progression of their respiratory failure. Pneumonia is likely in full-term infants with respiratory distress who are not at risk for hyaline membrane disease.

DIAGNOSIS. The maternal history may provide important information about maternal infection, exposure to infection in a sexual partner, maternal immunity (natural or acquired), maternal colonization, and obstetric risk factors (prematurity, prolonged ruptured membranes, maternal chorioamnionitis; Table 95–2). Serologic screening tests may have been performed for *Treponema pallidum,* rubella, and hepatitis B virus. Maternal cultures may have been taken for *Neisseria gonorrhoeae,* GBS, herpes simplex, or *Chlamydia.*

The acronym TORCH refers to toxoplasmosis, other agents, rubella, cytomegalovirus, and herpes simplex. It was modified to STORCH to include syphilis. Although the term may be helpful in remembering some of the etiologic agents of neonatal infections, the TORCH battery of serologic tests has a poor diagnostic yield, and the appropriate diagnostic studies should be selected for each etiologic agent under consideration.

Intrauterine infections due to toxoplasmosis, rubella, cytomegalovirus, herpes simplex, and syphilis present a diagnostic dilemma because (1) their clinical features overlap and may initially be indistinguishable; (2) disease may be inapparent; (3) maternal infection is often asymptomatic; (4) special laboratory studies may be needed; and (5) specific treatment for toxoplasmosis, syphilis, and herpes simplex is predicated on an accurate diagnosis and may reduce significant long-term morbidity. Common shared features that should suggest the diagnosis of an intrauterine infection include prematurity, intrauterine growth retardation, and hematologic involvement (anemia, neutropenia, thrombocytopenia, petechiae, purpura), ocular signs (chorioretinitis, cataracts, keratoconjunctivitis, glaucoma, microphthalmia), central nervous system symptoms (microcephaly, hydrocephaly, intracranial calcifications), and other organ system involvement (pneumonia, myocarditis, nephritis, hepatitis with hepatosplenomegaly, jaundice), or nonimmune hydrops.

The maternal history and physical examination of the newborn add additional diagnostic information; however, neonatal IgG titers are often difficult to interpret because IgG is acquired from the mother by transplacental passage and neonatal IgM titers to specific pathogens are technically difficult to perform and are not universally available. IgM titers to specific pathogens have high specificity but only moderate sensitivity; they should not be employed to exclude infection. Paired maternal and fetal-neonatal IgG titers with higher newborn IgG levels or rising IgG titers during infancy may be used to diagnose some congenital infections. Total cord blood IgM, IgA (both are not actively transported across the placenta to the fetus), or the presence of IgM-rheumatoid factor in neonatal serum may be used as a screening tool to identify infants at risk for any intrauterine infection. Total IgM has a high rate of both false-positive and false-negative results.

Identification of a bacterial or fungal infection may be made by isolating the etiologic agent from a body fluid that is normally sterile (blood, cerebrospinal fluid [CSF], urine, joint fluid), by demonstrating endotoxin or bacterial antigen in a body fluid (CSF, urine, or serum), or by demonstrating bacterial infection at autopsy. It is preferable to obtain two specimens for blood culture by venipuncture from different sites to avoid confusion caused by skin contamination. Samples should be obtained from an umbilical catheter only at the time of initial insertion. A peripheral venous sample should also be obtained when samples for cultures are drawn from central venous catheters. Blood cultures performed by radiometric methods may demonstrate growth within 24–72 hr. Although blood cultures are usually the basis for a diagnosis of bacterial infection, the bacteremic phase of the illness may be missed

■ **TABLE 95–2 Evaluation of a Newborn for Infection or Sepsis**

History (Specific Risk Factors)
Maternal infection during gestation or at parturition (type and duration of antimicrobial therapy)
 Urinary tract infection
 Chorioamnionitis
Maternal colonization with GBS, *N. gonorrhoeae,* herpes simplex
Gestational age/birthweight
Multiple birth
Duration of membrane rupture
Complicated delivery
Fetal tachycardia (distress)
Age at onset (in utero, birth, early postnatal, late)
Location at onset (hospital, community)
Medical intervention
 Vascular access
 Endotracheal intubation
 Parenteral nutrition
 Surgery

Evidence for Other Diseases*
Congenital malformations (heart disease, neural tube defect)
Respiratory tract disease (HMD, aspiration)
Necrotizing enterocolitis
Metabolic disease, e.g., galactosemia

Evidence for Focal or Systemic Disease
General appearance, neurologic status
Abnormal vital signs
Organ system disease
Feeding, stools, urine output

Laboratory Studies

Evidence for Infection
Culture from a normally sterile site (blood, CSF, other)
Demonstration of a microorganism in tissue or fluid
Antigen detection (urine, CSF)
Maternal or neonatal serology (syphilis, toxoplasmosis)
Autopsy

Evidence for Inflammation
Leukocytosis, increased immature/total neutrophil count ratio
Acute-phase reactants: CRP, ESR
Cytokines: IL-6
Pleocytosis in CSF, synovial, or pleural fluid
Disseminated intravascular coagulation: fibrin split products

Evidence for Multiorgan System Disease
Metabolic acidosis: pH, P_{CO_2}
Pulmonary function: P_{O_2}, P_{CO_2}
Renal function: BUN, creatinine
Hepatic injury/function: bilirubin, SGPT, SGOT, ammonia, PT, PTT
Bone marrow function: neutropenia, anemia, thrombocytopenia

**Diseases that increase the risk of infection or may overlap with signs of sepsis.*
GBS = group B streptococci; HMD = hyaline membrane disease; CSF = cerebrospinal fluid; CRP = C-reactive protein; ESR = erythrocyte sedimentation rate; P_{CO_2} = partial pressure of carbon dioxide; P_{O_2} = partial pressure of oxygen; BUN = blood urea nitrogen; SGPT = serum glutamic pyruvic transaminase; SGOT = serum glutamic oxaloacetic transaminase; PT = prothrombin time; PTT = partial thromboplastin time.

by poor timing or blood sample size (sample size may be as little as 0.2 mL, but more than 0.5–1 mL is optimal). Focal infections that produce systemic manifestations such as meningitis, arthritis, and urinary tract infections may be diagnosed by positive culture results from specific sites in the absence of positive blood cultures. Bacterial pneumonia has been reported at autopsy in infants with negative blood cultures before antimicrobial therapy.

Interpretation of tests for bacterial antigen may also be difficult. Latex particle agglutination and counterimmunoelectrophoresis are used for identification of GBS and *E. coli* K1 capsular polysaccharides in biologic fluids. The commercially available antigen detection kits are not as sensitive as blood cultures, and false-positive results may occur, particularly errors from contamination of urine collected in bags. Because urine is an excellent fluid for use in antigen detection, this test should be confirmed with specimens collected by suprapubic aspiration or catheterization.

When the clinical presentation suggests infection and the focus is unclear, additional studies should be performed. This includes, in addition to blood cultures, a lumbar puncture, urine examination and culture, gastric aspirate for Gram stain and culture, and a chest roentgenogram. Urine should be collected by catheterization or suprapubic aspiration; urine culture can be omitted in early-onset infections because urinary tract infection is rare at this time. Demonstration of bacteria and inflammatory cells in Gram-stained gastric aspirates on the 1st day of life may reflect maternal amnionitis, which is a risk factor for early-onset infection. Examination of the buffy coat with Gram or methylene blue stain may demonstrate intracellular pathogens, whereas similar stains of endotracheal secretions in infants with early-onset pneumonia may demonstrate the gram-positive cocci of GBS.

The total white blood cell count and differential and the ratio of immature to total neutrophils provide immediately predictive information when compared to age standards. Neutropenia is more common than neutrophilia in severe neonatal sepsis, but neutropenia also occurs in association with maternal hypertension, neonatal sensitization, NEC, periventricular hemorrhage, seizures, surgery, and possibly hemolysis. An immature neutrophil-total ratio of 0.16 or greater suggests bacterial infection.

Diagnostic evaluations may be indicated for asymptomatic infants because of maternal risk factors. The probability of neonatal infection and subsequent neonatal sepsis correlates with the degree of prematurity and bacterial contamination of amniotic fluid. In an asymptomatic term infant whose mother has chorioamnionitis, two blood cultures and a gastric aspirate should be examined to confirm the maternal diagnosis and identify presumptively the organisms by Gram stain. Presumptive treatment should be initiated. A lumbar puncture is not indicated because infants with meningitis are symptomatic. If the blood culture is positive or if the infant becomes symptomatic, lumbar puncture should be performed. Prolonged rupture of membranes for longer than 18 hr suggests the need for blood cultures in premature infants but not necessarily in asymptomatic term infants without signs of fetal distress.

TREATMENT. Once infection has been suspected and appropriate cultures have been obtained, intravenous or intramuscular antibiotic therapy should be instituted immediately. Initial treatment of suspected neonatal infection is determined by the pattern of disease and the organisms that are common for the age of the infant and the flora of the nursery (see Table 94–2). Initial empiric treatment of early-onset and late-onset community-acquired infections should consist of ampicillin and an aminoglycoside (usually gentamicin). Nosocomial infections acquired in the neonatal intensive care unit (NICU) are more likely to be caused by staphylococci, a variety of Enterobacteriaceae, *Pseudomonas,* or *Candida.* Thus, an antistaphylococcal drug, nafcillin for *S. aureus* or vancomycin for coagulase-negative staphylococci should be substituted for ampicillin. A history of recent antimicrobial therapy or the presence of antibiotic-resistant infections in the NICU suggests the need for a different aminoglycoside agent (amikacin) and vancomycin is used for methicillin-resistant staphylococci. Doses of the commonly used antibiotics are provided in Table 95–3. When the history or the presence of necrotic skin lesions suggests *Pseudomonas* infection, initial therapy should be ticarcillin or carbenicillin and gentamicin.

Once the pathogen has been identified and the antibiotic sensitivities determined, the most appropriate drug(s) should be selected. For most of the gram-negative enteric bacteria, ampicillin and an aminoglycoside, or a third-generation cephalosporin (cefotaxime or ceftazidime) should be used. Enterococci should be treated with both a penicillin (ampicillin or piperacillin) and an aminoglycoside, since synergism has been demonstrated with this combination of antibiotics in many strains. Ampicillin alone is adequate for *L. monocytogenes,* and penicillin will suffice for GBS. Clindamycin or metronidazole is appropriate for anaerobic infections.

Third-generation cephalosporins such as cefotaxime are valuable additions for treating documented neonatal sepsis and meningitis because (1) the minimal inhibitory concentrations needed for treatment of gram-negative enteric bacilli are much lower than those for the aminoglycosides; (2) there is excellent penetration into CSF in the presence of inflamed meninges; and (3) much higher doses can be given. The end result is much higher bactericidal titers in serum and CSF than are achievable with ampicillin-aminoglycoside combinations. However, cephalosporins should not be used alone as empiric therapy or indiscriminantly because they have only modest activity against *S. aureus* and *L. monocytogenes* and enterococci are uniformly resistant. Moreover, rapid emergence of resistant organisms is possible with frequent usage in the NICU.

Therapy for most infections should be continued for a total of 7–10 days or for at least 5–7 days after a clinical response has occurred. The course of treatment for meningitis caused by GBS is usually for 14 days and for a minimum of 14 days after sterilization of the CSF in gram-negative meningitis. A blood culture result taken 24–48 hr after initiation of therapy should be negative. If the culture results are positive, the possibility of an infected indwelling catheter, endocarditis, an infected thrombus, an occult abscess, subtherapeutic antibiotic levels, or resistant organisms should be considered. A change in antibiotics and longer duration of therapy may be indicated.

Management of newborn infants whose mothers received antibiotics during labor should be individualized. If in utero infection is likely, then treatment of the infant should be continued until there is evidence that there was no infection (the infant remains asymptomatic for 24–72 hr) or there is clinical and laboratory evidence of recovery. Antigen detection tests may be helpful in symptomatic infants but are not indicated in asymptomatic infants. The size of the bacterial inoculum needed to produce a positive test in urine should lead to signs of infection.

PREVENTION. Aggressive management of suspected maternal chorioamnionitis with antibiotics before delivery, rapid delivery of the newborn infant, and selective intrapartum chemoprophylaxis appears to have decreased the morbidity and mortality rates of neonatal bacterial infections. (See Chapters 98 and 175.)

Prevention of neonatal nosocomial infection is complex and includes a 2-min scrub before entering the nursery, 15-sec washing between patients, scrub suits for nurses and residents, adequate nursing staff, avoidance of overcrowding, and specific isolation precautions (see Chapter 249 and Tables 249–1 and 249–2). Control of outbreaks depends on the pathogen and epidemiology (see Chapter 249). Commonly used meas-

■ **TABLE 95–3 Dosages of Antibiotics Commonly Used in Newborns***

		Dosages (mg/kg) and Intervals of Administration				
		Weight <1,200g	*Weight 1,200–2,000g*		*Weight >2,000g*	
Antibiotics	**Routes**	**Age 0–4 wk**	**Age 0–7 days**	**>7 days**	**Age 0–7 days**	**>7 days**
Amikacin†	IV, IM	7.5 q12hr	7.5 q12hr	7.5 q8hr	10 q12hr	10 q8hr
Ampicillin,	IV, IM					
Meningitis		50 q12hr	50 q12hr	50 q8hr	50 q8hr	50 q6hr
Other diseases		25 q12hr	25 q12hr	25 q8hr	25 q8hr	25 q6hr
Aztreonam	IV, IM	30 q12hr	30 q12hr	30 q8hr	30 q8hr	30 q6hr
Cefazolin	IV, IM	20 q12hr	20 q12hr	20 q12hr	20 q12hr	20 q8hr
Cefotaxime	IV, IM	50 q12hr	50 q12hr	50 q8hr	50 q12hr	50 q8hr
Ceftazidime	IV, IM	50 q12hr	50 q12hr	50 q8hr	50 q8hr	50 q8hr
Ceftriaxone	IV, IM	50 q24hr	50 q24hr	50 q24hr	50 q24hr	75 q24hr
Cephalothin	IV	20 q12hr	20 q12h	20 q8hr	20 q8hr	20 q6hr
Chloramphenicol‡	IV, PO	22 q24hr	25 q12hr	25 q24hr	25 q24hr	25 q12hr
Clindamycin	IV, IM, PO	5 q12hr	5 q12hr	5 q8hr	5 q8hr	5 q6hr
Erythromycin	PO	10 q12hr	10 q12hr	10 q8hr	10 q12hr	10 q8hr
Gentamicin	IV, IM	2.5 q18–24hr	2.5 q12–18hr	2.5 q8hr	2.5 q12hr	2.5 q8hr
Imipenem	IV, IM	20 q18–24hr	20 q12hr	20 q12hr	20 q12hr	20 q8hr
Kanamycin	IV, IM	7.5 q18–24hr	7.5 q12–18hr	7.5 q8–12hr	10 q12h	10 q8hr
Methicillin	IV, IM					
Meningitis		50 q12hr	50 q12hr	50 q8hr	50 q8hr	50 q6hr
Other diseases		25 q12hr	25 q12hr	25 q8hr	25 q8hr	25 q6hr
Metronidazole	IV, PO	7.5 q48hr	7.5 q12hr	7.5 q12hr	7.5 q12hr	15 q12hr
Mezlocillin	IV, IM	75 q12hr	75 q12hr	75 q8hr	75 q12hr	75 q8hr
Oxacillin	IV, IM	25 q12hr	25 q12hr	30 q8hr	25 q8hr	37.5 q6hr
Nafcillin	IV	25 q12hr	25 q12hr	25 q8hr	25 q8hr	37.5 q6hr
Netilmicin§	IV, IM	2.5 q18–24hr	2.5 q12–18hr	2.5 q8–12hr	2.5 q12hr	2.5 q8hr
Penicillin G	IV					
Meningitis		50,000 U q12hr	50,000 U q12hr	75,000 U q8hr	50,000 U q8hr	50,000 U q6hr
Other diseases		25,000 U q12hr	25,000 U q12hr	25,000 U q8hr	25,000 U q8hr	25,000 U q6hr
Penicillin G	IM					
Benzathine			50,000 U (one dose)	50,000 U (one dose)	50,000 U (one dose)	50,000 U (one dose)
Procaine			50,000 U q24hr	50,000 U q24hr	50,000 U q24hr	50,000 U q24hr
Ticarcillin	IV, IM	75 q12hr	75 q12hr	75 q8hr	75 q8hr	75 q6hr
Tobramycin†	IV, IM	2.5 q18–24hr	2.5 q12–18hr	2.5 q8–12hr	2.5 q12hr	2.5 q8hr
Vancomycin‖	IV	15 q24hr	10 q12–18hr	15 q8–12hr	15 q12hr	15 q8hr

Recommendations for infants weighing <1,000g based on Prober et al: Pediatr Infect Dis J 9:111, 1990.
**Adapted from Nelson JD: Pocketbook of Pediatric Antimicrobial Therapy, 10th ed. Baltimore, Williams & Wilkins, 1993.*
†Aminoglycoside levels should be monitored if therapy continues >3 days. Optimal peak levels 6–8 μg/mL, trough less than 2 μg/mL.
‡Serum levels are highly variable. Chloramphenicol should be given to newborns only if serum levels can be monitored.
§0.5 mg/kg/24 hr can increase to 1 mg/kg/24 hr if needed or give every other day. Treat for cumulative dose of 10–30 mg/kg.
‖Because of variable pharmacokinetics, vancomycin levels should be monitored if therapy continues >3 days. Optimal peak levels 20–30 μg/mL, trough less than 10 μg/mL.

ures include investigation of the extent of colonization in infants and caretakers, a search for a common source or reservoir, cohorting of infants and caretakers, changes in handwashing solutions and protocols, and antimicrobial prophylaxis. Cord care, equipment sterilization, and handwashing are essential, whereas gowns have not consistently been demonstrated to be effective.

Abzug MJ, Levin MJ: Neonatal adenovirus infection: Four patients and review of the literature. Pediatrics 87:890, 1991.

Cantwell MF, Shehab ZM, Costello AM, et al: Brief report: Congenital tuberculosis. N Engl J Med 330:1051, 1994.

Decker MD, Edwards KM: Central venous catheter infections. Pediatr Clin North Am 35:579, 1988.

England JA, Fletcher CV, Balfour HH: Acyclovir therapy in neonates. J Pediatr 119:129, 1991.

Fanaroff AA, Korones SB, Wright LL, et al: A controlled trial of intravenous immune globulin to reduce nosocomial infections in very-low-birth-weight infants. N Engl J Med 330:1107, 1994.

Gladstone IM, Ehrenkranz RA, Edberg SC, et al: A ten-year review of neonatal sepsis and comparison with the previous fifty-year experience. Pediatr Infect Dis J 9:819, 1990.

Grose C, Itani O, Weiner CP: Perinatal diagnosis of fetal infections: Advances from amniocentesis to cordocentesis—congenital toxoplasmosis, rubella, cytomegalovirus, varicella virus, parvovirus, and human immunodeficiency virus. Pediatr Infect Dis J 8:459, 1989.

Heggie AD, Jacobs MR, Butler VT, et al: Frequency and significance of isolation of *Ureaplasma urealyticum* and *Mycoplasma hominis* from cerebrospinal fluid and tracheal aspirate specimens from low birthweight infants. J Pediatr 124:956, 1994.

Ibhanesebhor SE, Okolo AA: Malaria parasitaemia in neonates with predisposing risk factors for neonatal sepsis: Report of six cases. Ann Trop Paediatr 12:297, 1992.

Jacobs RF: Efficacy and safety of cefotaxime in the management of pediatric infections. Infection 19 (suppl.)6:330, 1991.

Jeisser MF, Patterson JE, Kuritza AP, et al: Emergence of resistance to multiple beta-lactams in *Enterobacter cloacae* during treatment for neonatal meningitis with cefotaxime. Pediatr Infect Dis J 9:509, 1990.

Kinney JS, Kumer ML: Should we expand the TORCH complex? A description of clinical and diagnostic aspects of selected old and new agents. Clin Perinatol 15:727, 1988.

Kovatch AL, Wald ER: Evaluation of the febrile neonate. Semin Perinatol 9:12, 1985.

Leland D, Morris MS, French LV, et al: The use of TORCH titers. Pediatrics 72:41, 1983.

Mustafa MM, McCracken GH Jr: Perinatal bacterial diseases. *In:* Feigin RD, Cherry JD (eds): Textbook of Pediatric Infectious Diseases, 3rd ed. Philadelphia, WB Saunders, 1992.

Remington JS, Klein JO: Infectious Diseases of the Fetus and Newborn Infant, 3rd ed. Philadelphia, WB Saunders, 1990.

Singer DB: Infections of fetuses and neonates. *In:* Wigglesworth JS, Singer DB (eds): Textbook of Fetal and Perinatal Pathology. Boston, Blackwell Scientific Publications, 1994.

Spafford PS, Sinkin RA, Cox C, et al: Prevention of central venous catheter-related coagulase-negative staphylococcal sepsis in neonates. J Pediatr 125:259, 1994.

Waites KB, Crouse DT, Cassell GH: Systemic neonatal infection due to *Ureaplasma urealyticum*. Clin Infect Dis 17 (suppl 1):S131, 1993.

Webber S, Wilkinson AR, Lindsell D, et al: Neonatal pneumonia. Arch Dis Child 65:207, 1990.

SECTION 2
Clinical Syndromes

CHAPTER 96
Intrauterine Infection and Prenatal Diagnosis

Charles Grose

Investigations of fetal infection have made enormous advances in the last decade. In particular, the ability to delineate a diagnosis during early gestation is now possible in many situations. Nevertheless, some physicians still elect to use only serologic studies of the mother or, in other cases, await delivery to test the cord blood. This approach is problematic for several reasons. First, the fetus may die in utero, and the correct diagnosis may never be made. Second, the fetal response to viral infection may wane by late gestation so that the infectious agent cannot be identified. Third, the correct prenatal diagnosis may alter the management of both the mother in late gestation and the newborn postpartum. For example, treatment of an infectious agent may be initiated at an earlier period. Alternatively, an accurate diagnosis of fetal infection as the cause of intrauterine growth retardation prevents a preterm delivery based on concerns about uteroplacental insufficiency. Finally, the diagnosis of fetal infection alerts both obstetric and pediatric staffs to follow universal precautions to avoid spread of infection.

The emphasis of this chapter is on the prenatal investigation of fetal infection. The current protocols for fetal diagnosis include both noninvasive and invasive procedures (see Chapter 81). The invasive techniques include amniocentesis, cordocentesis (percutaneous umbilical blood sampling) and chorionic villus sampling. A common noninvasive technique is ultrasound. In many cases, a fetal abnormality detected by ultrasound is the reason for referral of a pregnant woman to a fetal diagnostic center. In the following discussion, an outline is presented for evaluation of suspected fetal infection. Congenital toxoplasmosis is reviewed as an example. Chapter 97 contains the sections on congenital and perinatal viral infections.

TECHNIQUES FOR PRENATAL DIAGNOSIS. *Amniocentesis* is monitored by constant ultrasound visualization (see Chapter 81). The amniotic fluid is aspirated after the percutaneous insertion of a narrow-gauge abdominal needle. As much as 36 mL of amniotic fluid can be safely removed after 15 wk of gestation. When amniocentesis is performed before 15 wk, approximately 1 mL of fluid per week of gestation may be removed. Even the lower quantities of fluid are adequate for diagnosis of infectious agents. The complications are minimal, and the risk of fetal loss is less than 1%.

Fetal blood sampling by percutaneous puncture of the umbilical cord, *cordocentesis,* was developed as a technique for prenatal diagnosis of infection (see Chapter 81). Cordocentesis is usually performed after 15 wk using high-resolution ultrasound. The umbilical vein is punctured, and fetal blood (1–8 mL) is obtained for diagnostic studies. Complications include transient bleeding from the puncture site in the vein or the uterine wall and transient fetal bradycardia. The rate of fetal loss is slightly higher than for amniocentesis but is generally below 2%.

Chorionic villus sampling allows prenatal diagnosis as early as 7 wk of gestation (see Chapter 81). However, because of associated risks of fetal death, subsequent fetal limb anomalies, and cavernous hemangiomas, there is little indication to recommend the procedure for prenatal diagnosis of a suspected infection.

DIRECT EVIDENCE OF INFECTION

MATERNAL SEROLOGY. When a pregnant woman has a febrile illness and concern is raised about fetal infection, maternal serologic testing is the traditional method to evaluate the mother. The acronym TORCH was established to remind the physician of toxoplasmosis, rubella, cytomegalovirus (CMV), and herpes (HSV). Subsequently, S was added because of the resurgence of syphilis as an agent of fetal infection (STORCH). The acronym now also encompasses the known pathogens such as parvovirus and varicella-zoster virus (VZV).

Routine screening of maternal sera for all components of the STORCH profile is now discouraged because of the low yield of useful information. Rather, the physician is encouraged to obtain a thorough history about potential maternal exposures to specific infectious agents and to test the mother for the pathogen in question. In most cases of suspected fetal infection, concern is not raised until the pregnant woman has been ill for several weeks or is only raised in retrospect at parturition. At this time, the maternal immune response to the suspected pathogen may no longer reflect an acute infection, i.e., the specific immunoglobulin (Ig)M response is no longer detectable and the IgG response has already reached a plateau. Also, many of the pathogen-specific IgM serologic assays require considerable skill to perform and tend to be less reliable than the more common IgG assays. For this reason, the results of the IgM assays can be either falsely negative or falsely positive.

FETAL SEROLOGY. If there is a high likelihood of maternal infection with a known teratogenic agent, fetal ultrasound examination is strongly recommended. If the examination demonstrates either delayed growth for gestational age or a physical abnormality, examination of a fetal blood sample may be warranted. Cordocentesis can provide a sufficient sample for both total and pathogen-specific IgM assays. The total IgM value is important because the normal fetal IgM level is less than 5 mg/dL. Any elevation in total IgM may indicate an underlying fetal infection that has stimulated the fetal immune system. For example, a fetus infected by gestational chickenpox at 20 wk had a highly elevated total IgM level of 30 mg/dL at 32 wk. The fetus was delivered at 34 wk and, by 2 wk postpartum, had a low total IgM level. Likewise, fetuses infected in utero with toxoplasmosis may no longer have elevated levels of total IgM at birth. It is also important to remember that cord serum samples with low levels of total IgM (<20 mg/dL) may be unacceptable for detection of pathogen-specific IgM. For these reasons, these IgM tests are only useful when the results are strongly positive. A negative pathogen-specific IgM finding does not necessarily rule out that pathogen as a cause of fetopathy.

CULTURE. If the serologic studies on the mother point to a

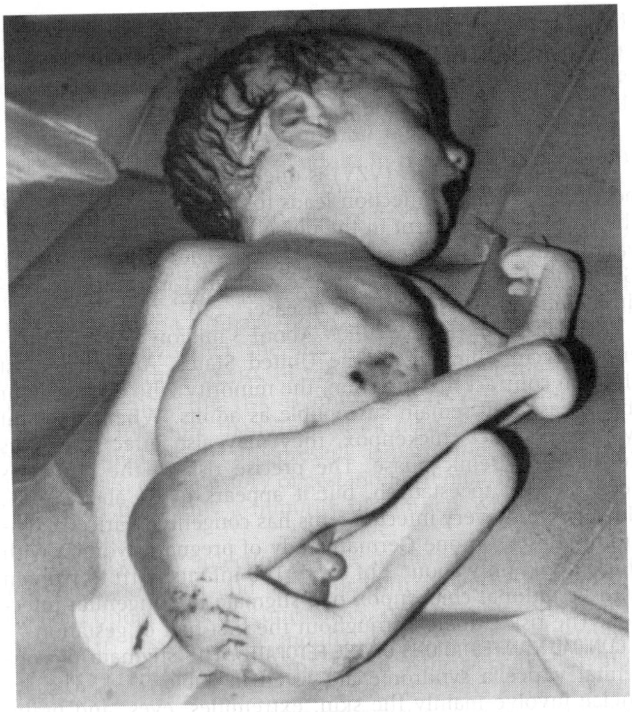

Figure 97–2. Newborn with congenital varicella syndrome. The infant had severe malformations of both lower extremities and cicatricial scarring over his left abdomen. Also see Table 97–1.

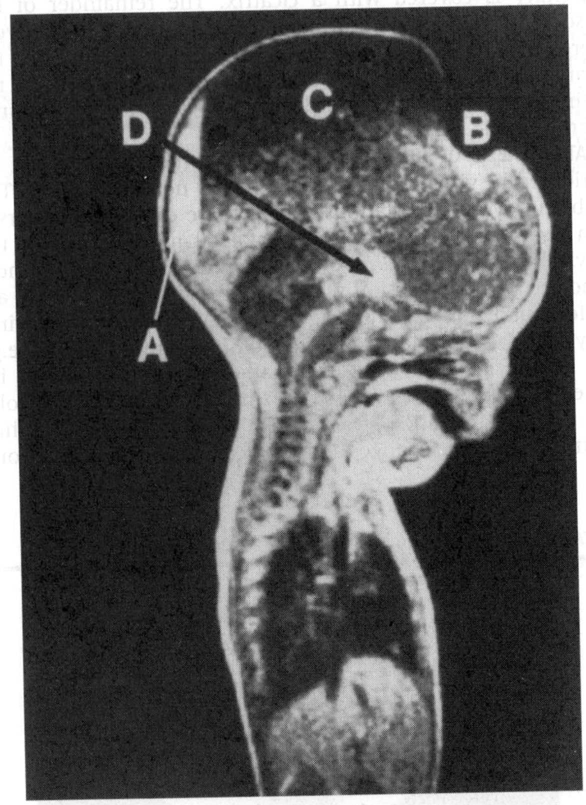

Figure 97–3. Magnetic resonance image of newborn with encephalitis secondary to congenital varicella syndrome. The intrauterine infection occurred about 3 mo antepartum, at which time there was extensive necrosis of the cerebral hemispheres. The image of the newborn head was taken with the patient supine; therefore, there is a fluid/fluid interface in the dependent occiput *(A)*. The hydrocephalus *(C)* and calcifications in the basal ganglia *(D)* are visible; a cranial artifact *(B)* is seen secondary to a scalp vein needle.

and they include shrunken and gliotic posterior horns and lateral columns. The characteristic cicatricial scarring may represent the cutaneous residua of VZV infection of the sensory nerves.

The period of greatest risk to the fetus correlates with the gestational period when there is major development and innervation of the limb buds, and maturation of the eyes. Fetuses infected at 6–12 wk of gestation appear to have maximal interruption with limb development; fetuses infected at 16–20 wk may have eye and brain involvement. In addition, viral damage to the sympathetic fibers in the cervical and lumbosacral cord may lead to divergent effects such as Horner syndrome and dysfunction of the urethral or anal sphincters.

DIAGNOSIS. The diagnosis of VZV fetopathy is based mainly on the history of gestational chickenpox combined with the stigmata seen in the fetus. Virus cannot be cultured from the affected newborn, but viral DNA can be detected in tissue samples by a hybridization technique. Some infants have VZV-specific IgM antibody detectable in the cord blood sample, although the IgM titer drops quickly postpartum. The diagnosis can be made antenatally by obtaining a fetal blood sample for VZV-specific IgM titer. However, VZV has not been cultured from the amniotic fluid.

TREATMENT AND PREVENTION OF FETAL DISEASE. The damage caused by fetal VZV infection does not progress postpartum, an indication that there is no persistent viral replication. Thus, antiviral treatment of infants with congenital VZV syndrome is not indicated. Since the varicella vaccine is now available for general use, VZV fetopathy will be preventable by immunization of VZV-susceptible young women. Vaccination of the same group of women is also indicated because morbidity and mortality rates of gestational chickenpox are considerable.

NEONATAL CHICKENPOX. There is confusion about the terminology of fetal infection when it occurs in the 9th mo of gestation. Although the initial infection is intrauterine, the baby often develops clinical chickenpox postpartum, i.e., after a 10–14-day incubation period. For example, if neonatal chickenpox is first seen on day 5 of life, the infection was contracted about 5 days before delivery. The risk to the newborn under these circumstances reflects the likelihood that the fetus obtained maternal anti-VZV antibody. If there was at least a 1-wk interval between maternal chickenpox and parturition, it is likely that the newborn infant received transplacental antibody to VZV. If the interval was less than 1 wk, the newborn may have no protective VZV antibody. Under the latter circumstances, neonatal chickenpox can be exceptionally severe. Neonatal chickenpox can also follow a postpartum exposure. Chickenpox is a more serious illness throughout the entire 1st yr of life than in later childhood, with more hepatic and CNS involvement. The mortality rate is around 1:13,000; that for older children is less than 1:40,000. The mortality rate is also strikingly increased in pregnant women with chickenpox.

TREATMENT AND PREVENTION IN THE NEONATAL INFANT. The recommendations for varicella-zoster immune globulin (VZIG) reflect the increased risks to the exposed infant. A full-term infant born to a mother who has chickenpox less than 1 wk before parturition should receive one vial of VZIG by intramuscular injection. Every premature infant born to a mother with active chickenpox (even if present longer than 1 wk) should receive VZIG. Because of the higher mortality rate of chickenpox throughout the 1st yr of life, oral acyclovir suspension can be administered as soon as an infant develops chickenpox. The dosage is 80 mg/kg/24 hr, administered as 20 mg/kg every 6 hr. If an infant with chickenpox has signs of pneumonia, hepatitis, or encephalitis, immediate hospitalization and treatment with intravenous acyclovir should be considered.

PROGNOSIS. Many infants with congenital varicella syndrome have severe neurologic deficiencies. However, another group (presumably those infected later in gestation) may have only isolated stigmata, such as cataracts, which can be treated surgically. The latter infants develop normally throughout childhood. Infants with neonatal chickenpox have an excellent prognosis as long as they receive treatment with acyclovir as soon as the diagnosis is made.

Grose C: Congenital infections caused by varicella zoster virus and herpes simplex virus. Semin Pediatr Neurol 1:43, 1994.
Scharf A, Scherr O, Enders G: Virus detection in the fetal tissue of a premature delivery with congenital varicella syndrome. J Perinat Med 18:317, 1990.

97.4 *Parvovirus*

(See Chapter 210)

The human parvoviruses (HPV) are frequently called B19 after the best characterized strain first isolated in 1975.

EPIDEMIOLOGY. Parvovirus infection causes fifth disease, also known as erythema infectiosum. Most children contract the infection by their teenage years, but those who escape infection as children are susceptible as adults. Transmission is presumably by the respiratory route, probably by droplet aerosol. Gestational fifth disease is associated with spontaneous abortions and stillbirths. However, the incidence of maternal parvovirus infection is low. Unless a stillborn fetus has signs of nonimmune hydrops, the diagnosis of parvovirus is unlikely.

CLINICAL MANIFESTATIONS OF FETAL INFECTION. Primary HPV infection in pregnant women is similar to that in children, i.e., the woman may have a subclinical disease or she may complain of sore throat and arthralgia; a skin rash reminiscent of rubella may be seen. During the viremia, maternal HPV infection may be transmitted to the fetus. There are several consequences of fetal infection. The fetus may be infected but have no untoward residua. Alternatively, spontaneous abortion may occur in the first half of pregnancy, or, in the second half, a stillbirth with hydrops fetalis may occur. Live births may also exhibit hydrops, a condition characterized by generalized edema of fetal tissue as a result of fluid extravasation from the intravascular compartment as the result of cardiovascular failure induced by severe fetal anemia. See Chapter 89.

PATHOGENESIS. Transplacental transmission of parvovirus has been proved by detection of viral DNA and viral particles in fetal tissues. Although the virus is found in all tissues, there is a strong predilection for erythroid precursor cells. Parvoviral cytopathic effects are seen in erythroblasts of the bone marrow and sites of extramedullary hematopoiesis in the liver and spleen. Presumably, fetal infection can occur as early as 6 wk of gestation, when erythroblasts are first found in the fetal liver; after the 4th gestational mo, hematopoiesis switches from the liver to the bone marrow.

DIAGNOSIS. Acute parvovirus infection sometimes can be diagnosed in a pregnant woman by detection of virus-specific IgM antibody. Because the disease often occurs in a community-wide outbreak, the diagnosis can be assumed in those with compatible signs and symptoms. Prenatal diagnosis can be accomplished by either detection of viral DNA in fetal blood or visualization of viral particles by immune electron microscopy.

TREATMENT AND PREVENTION. Because HPV usually is spread rapidly through a community, there are few means for prevention. There is neither a vaccine nor a specific antiviral medication to treat HPV infection. Infected fetuses with hydrops can be managed by percutaneous umbilical blood transfusions.

PROGNOSIS. The prognosis of congenital parvovirus infection is difficult to establish because the number of asymptomatic intrauterine infections has not been determined. Once severe hydrops is diagnosed in a fetus, the mother should be referred to a fetal therapy center for further evaluation because of the very high risk for serious complications.

Grose C, Itani O: Pathogenesis of congenital infection with three diverse viruses: varicella-zoster virus, human parvovirus, and human immunodeficiency virus. Semin Perinatol 13:278, 1989.
Naides SJ, Weiner CP: Fetal survival after human parvovirus B19 infection: spectrum of intrauterine response in a twin pregnancy. Am J Perinatol 9:66, 1992.

97.5 *Rubella*

(See Chapter 207)

Rubella is an enveloped RNA virus that causes the disease sometimes called "3-day measles" or "German measles." The disease has almost been eliminated by the production of a live attenuated rubella vaccine. It is the only virus for which a vaccine was made mainly to eliminate the consequences of fetal infection.

EPIDEMIOLOGY OF THE FETOPATHY. Before rubella vaccination, pandemics of rubella occurred every 10–20 yr. In 1964–1965, an epidemic in the United States caused more than 12 million cases of rubella and an additional 20,000 infants with congenital rubella syndrome. After the initiation of a national rubella immunization program in 1969, the number of rubella cases declined by more than 99%. In the early 1990s, there was a modest increase in rubella cases, including congenital rubella syndrome, because of a failure to immunize all children in the United States.

Rubella virus is distinguished by its propensity to infect a fetus. During the first trimester of gestation, a primary maternal rubella infection has an 80% likelihood of transmission to the fetus, and most infected fetuses have rubella fetopathy. Transmission from mother to fetus also occurs in the early second trimester (50%) and persists throughout gestation.

CLINICAL MANIFESTATIONS IN THE FETUS. Rubella involves virtually all organ systems. The most common manifestation is intrauterine growth retardation. Another common finding is cataracts, bilateral or unilateral. Cataracts are frequently associated with microphthalmia. Myocarditis and structural cardiac defects, e.g., patent ductus arteriosus or pulmonary artery stenosis, are common. Blueberry muffin skin lesions, similar to those in CMV infection, may occur. Hearing loss from sensorineural deafness is another common defect. The infants may have active meningoencephalitis at birth; later sequelae include motor and mental retardation. Persistent infection leads to pneumonia, hepatitis, bone lucencies, thrombocytopenic purpura, and anemia in the infant with congenital rubella syndrome.

DIAGNOSIS. Most diagnoses can be made solely on a clinical basis. The diagnosis can be confirmed by finding virus-specific IgM antibody in the neonatal serum or by culturing rubella virus from the infants' urine or tissues. Virus can be shed in the urine for 1 yr or longer. Prenatal diagnosis of fetal rubella infection can be made either by virus isolation from amniotic fluid or by identification of rubella-specific IgM in cord blood.

TREATMENT AND PREVENTION. Congenital rubella syndrome is most easily prevented by universal immunization of all young children with rubella vaccine. When acute rubella infection is documented in a pregnant woman during the first half of gestation, there is a high likelihood of fetal infection with multiple fetal stigmata. Therefore, prenatal diagnosis is recommended so that termination of pregnancy can be considered. There is no effective antiviral medication for treatment of congenital rubella syndrome.

PROGNOSIS. Infants with the complete spectrum of the congenital rubella syndrome have a grim prognosis, especially when the disease continues to progress throughout infancy. The prognosis is obviously better for infants with only a few stigmata of the syndrome, presumably those who were initially infected later in gestation.

Dudgeon JA: Congenital rubella. J Pediatr 87:1078, 1975.
Lee SH, Ewert DP, Frederick PD, et al: Resurgence of congenital rubella syndrome in the 1990s. JAMA 267:2616, 1992.

97.6 Human Immunodeficiency Virus

(See Chapter 223)

Over the past decade, there has been an extraordinary increase in our knowledge of HIV infection and pediatric acquired immunodeficiency syndrome (AIDS). This chapter focuses on intrauterine HIV infection and its consequences.

EPIDEMIOLOGY OF FETAL HIV INFECTION. Pediatric AIDS is nearly always acquired from an infected mother, either by intrauterine or intrapartum transmission. The mother becomes infected by being a member of one of the following risk groups: intravenous drug users who share needles with HIV-infected individuals; prostitutes who contract the disease from one of their partners; or less commonly, recipients of contaminated blood transfusions before 1985; and women married to men who were HIV seropositive, including male hemophiliac patients treated with factor VIII that contained HIV.

The geographic distribution of perinatal AIDS in the United States is heavily concentrated in the coastal metropolitan areas, such as New York/New Jersey, Miami, and Los Angeles, regions that include most women with AIDS. Epidemiologic studies suggest that about 7,000 HIV-seropositive women in the United States will become pregnant annually. The transmission rate to the fetus or newborn depends on maternal factors, such as the severity of her disease and the degree of viremia. For some pregnant women with AIDS, the rate of fetal and perinatal infection may approach 70%. However, a vertical fetal transmission rate for known HIV-seropositive women is around 25%. In the exceptional circumstance in which a woman contracts her primary HIV infection during early gestation, the risk for fetal transmission appears to be higher than 25%.

There are many examples of HIV infection in the second trimester documented by tissue isolation of the virus. There are fewer examples of vertical transplacental transmission during the first trimester, but HIV antigens and nucleic acids have been found in tissues removed from three 8-week-old fetuses. Three mechanisms have been proposed for intrauterine HIV transmission. First, virus in the maternal system is released from decidual cells and subsequently phagocytosed by syncytiotrophoblasts. Second, trophoblasts that are invading decidual tissue come into contact with HIV-infected maternal CD4 lymphocytes. Third, infected maternal macrophages invade the villous stroma. Phagocytosis may be a more important mechanism of intrauterine transmission than the specific CD4-receptor–mediated events because nucleated cells that express the CD4 cell surface molecule have not been observed until 12–14 wk of gestation.

DIAGNOSIS. Both viral culture and HIV-specific PCR assay can be successful in the prenatal diagnosis of HIV infection from fetal blood samples. Amniocentesis and cordocentesis have been carried out successfully in HIV-seropositive pregnant women, but the relative role and timing of these invasive procedures is problematic because the chronology of most intrauterine HIV transmission is uncertain. There is also concern about potential fetal transmission as a result of the procedure itself, especially cordocentesis.

TREATMENT AND PREVENTION. Zidovudine treatment during pregnancy was effective in reducing the risk of fetal infection from HIV-infected women in the 14–34th wk of pregnancy who were not already receiving zidovudine because they had CD4 lymphocyte counts greater than 200 cells/mm^3 without clinical AIDS. The women received oral zidovudine therapy (100 mg five times daily) throughout the remainder of gestation. During labor, the drug was administered intravenously; a loading dose of 2 mg/kg given over 1 hr was followed by continuous infusion of 1 mg/kg/hr until delivery. The newborns received 6 wk of antiviral therapy (zidovudine syrup at 2 mg/kg every 6 hr), beginning 8–12 hr postpartum. This resulted in a 67.5% relative risk reduction.

PROGNOSIS. In 1993, the median age to AIDS diagnosis of all HIV-infected infants was 12 mo, although many children first became symptomatic much later in childhood.

Brandt CD, Rakusan TA, Sison A, et al: Human immunodeficiency virus infection in infants during the first 2 months of life. Arch Pediatr Adolesc Med 148:250, 1994.
Centers for Disease Control: Zidovudine for the prevention of HIV transmission from mother to infant. MMWR Morb Mortal Wkly Rep 43:285, 1994.
Lewis SH, Reynolds-Kohler C, Fox HE, et al: HIV-1 in trophoblastic and villous Hofbauer cells, and haematological precursors in eight-week fetuses. Lancet 335:565, 1990.
Pizzo PA, Wilfert CM: Pediatric AIDS, 2nd ed. Baltimore, Williams & Wilkins, 1994.

CHAPTER 98
Neonatal Sepsis and Meningitis

Samuel P. Gotoff

98.1 Sepsis

Neonatal sepsis, sepsis neonatorum, and neonatal septicemia are terms that have been used to describe the systemic response to infection in the newborn infant. There is little agreement on the proper use of the term, i.e., whether it should be restricted to bacterial infections, positive blood cultures, or severity of illness. Currently, there is considerable discussion of the appropriate definition of sepsis in the critical care literature. This is a result of an explosion of information on the pathogenesis of sepsis and the availability of new potentially therapeutic agents, e.g., monoclonal antibodies to endotoxin and tumor necrosis factor (TNF), which can alter the lethal outcome of sepsis in animal experiments. To evaluate and utilize these new therapeutic modalities appropriately, "sepsis" requires a more rigorous definition. In adults, the term *systemic inflammatory response syndrome* (SIRS) is used to describe a clinical syndrome characterized by two or more of the following: (1) fever or hypothermia, (2) tachycardia, (3) tachypnea, and (4) abnormal white blood cells (WBC) or increase in immature forms. SIRS may be a result of trauma, hemorrhagic shock, other causes of ischemia, pancreatitis, or immunologic injury. When it is a result of infection, it is termed *sepsis.* These criteria have not been established in infants and children and are unlikely to be applicable to the newborn infant. Nevertheless, the concept of sepsis as a syndrome caused by metabolic and hemodynamic consequences of infection is logical and important. In the future, the definition of sepsis in the newborn infant and child will become more precise. At this time, criteria for neonatal sepsis should include documentation of infection in a newborn infant with a serious systemic illness in which noninfectious explanations for the abnormal pathophysiologic state are excluded or unlikely. Serious systemic illness in the newborn infant (Table 98–1) may be caused by perinatal asphyxia, respiratory tract, cardiac, metabolic, neurologic, or hematologic diseases. Sepsis occurs in a small proportion of all neonatal infections. Bacteria and *Candida* are the usual etiologic agents, but viruses and, rarely, protozoa may also cause sepsis. Blood cultures may be negative, increasing the difficulty in establishing infection etiologically. Finally, infection with or without sepsis may be present concurrently with a noninfectious illness in the newborn infant, child, or adult.

EPIDEMIOLOGY. The incidence of neonatal sepsis varies according to definition from 1–4/1,000 live births in developed countries with considerable fluctuation over time and geographic location. Hospital-to-hospital variability in incidence may be related to rates of prematurity, prenatal care, conduct of labor, and environmental conditions in nurseries. Attack rates of neonatal sepsis increase significantly in low-birth-weight infants and in the presence of maternal (obstetric) risk factors or signs of chorioamnionitis such as prolonged rupture of membranes (>18 hr), maternal intrapartum fever (>37.5° C), maternal leukocytosis (>18,000), uterine tenderness, and fetal tachycardia (>180 beats/min).

Host risk factors include male sex, developmental or congenital immune defects, galactosemia (*Escherichia coli*), administration of intramuscular iron (*E. coli*), congenital anomalies (urinary tract, asplenia, myelomeningocele, sinus tracts), omphalitis, and twinning (especially the second twin of an infected twin). Prematurity is a risk factor for both early-onset and late-onset sepsis.

ETIOLOGY. Bacteria, viruses, fungi, and rarely protozoa may produce neonatal sepsis (see Table 98–1). The most common causes of early-onset sepsis are group B streptococci (GBS) and enteric bacteria acquired from the maternal genital tract. Late-onset sepsis may be due to GBS, herpes simplex virus (HSV), enteroviruses, and *E. coli* K1. In very low-birthweight infants, *Candida* and coagulase-negative staphylococci (CONS) are the most common pathogens in late-onset sepsis.

PATHOGENESIS. Rarely, inhalation of infected amniotic fluid may produce pneumonia and sepsis in utero, manifested by fetal distress or neonatal asphyxia. Exposure to pathogens at delivery and in the nursery or community is the mechanism of infection after birth.

The physiologic manifestations of the inflammatory response are mediated by a variety of proinflammatory cytokines, principally TNF, interleukin-1 (IL-1), and IL-6, and by-products of activation of the complement and coagulation systems (see Chapter 168). Studies in the newborn infant are limited, but it appears that some cytokine production may be diminished, which is consistent with an impaired inflammatory response. However, elevated levels of IL-6, TNF, and platelet-activating factor have been reported in newborn infants with neonatal sepsis and necrotizing enterocolitis (NEC). IL-6 appears to be the cytokine most often elevated in neonatal sepsis.

CLINICAL MANIFESTATIONS. Infection is considered in the differential diagnosis of many physical signs in the newborn infant. All of these may have noninfectious explanations. When there is multisystem involvement or when the cardiorespiratory signs are consistent with severe illness, sepsis should be considered. Sepsis may be manifested by the signs listed in Table 95–1. The initial presentation may be limited to only one system, such as apnea, tachypnea with retractions, or tachycardia, but a full clinical and laboratory evaluation will usually reveal other abnormalities (see Table 95–2). Infants with suspected sepsis should be evaluated for multiorgan system disease. Metabolic acidosis is common. Hypoxemia and carbon dioxide retention may be associated with adult and congenital respiratory distress syndrome (RDS) or pneumonia.

Many newborn infants with infections do not have serious systemic physiologic abnormalities. Many infants with pneumonia and infants with stage II NEC (see Chapter 88.2) do not have sepsis. In contrast, stage III NEC is usually accompanied by the systemic manifestations of sepsis, and urinary tract infections (UTIs) secondary to obstructive uropathy may have hematologic and hepatic abnormalities consistent with sepsis. Each infant should be re-evaluated over time to determine whether physiologic changes secondary to infection have reached a moderate to severe level of severity that is consistent with sepsis.

Late manifestations of sepsis include signs of cerebral edema and/or thromboses, respiratory failure as a result of acquired respiratory distress syndrome (ARDS), pulmonary hypertension, cardiac failure, renal failure, hepatocellular disease with hyperbilirubinemia and elevated enzymes, prolonged prothrombin time (PT) and partial thromboplastin time (PTT), septic shock, adrenal hemorrhage with adrenal insufficiency, bone marrow failure (thrombocytopenia, neutropenia, anemia), and disseminated intravascular coagulation (DIC).

DIAGNOSIS. Documentation of infection is the first diagnostic criterion that must be met (see Part XII, Section 1). It is important to note that infants with bacterial sepsis may have negative blood cultures so that other approaches to identification of infection should be taken (see Table 95–2). Tests to demonstrate an inflammatory response include erythrocyte sedimentation rate, C-reactive protein, haptoglobin, fibrinogen, nitroblue tetrazolium dye, and leukocyte alkaline phosphatase. In general, these tests have limited sensitivity and are not helpful. Only the total WBC count with differential and the ratio of immature to total neutrophils provide immediately predictive information compared with age standards. Neutropenia is more common than neutrophilia in severe neonatal sepsis, but it also occurs in association with maternal hypertension, neonatal sensitization, periventricular hemorrhage, seizures, surgery, and possibly hemolysis. An immature neutrophil-total neutrophil ratio of 0.16 or greater suggests bacterial infection.

Criteria for the magnitude of physiologic change in newborn infants with sepsis are not currently defined but should be consistent with the systemic effect of endogenous mediators on one or more organ systems. For example, the effect of

■ **TABLE 98–1 Serious Systemic Illness in the Newborn (Differential Diagnosis of Neonatal Sepsis)**

Infection (Sepsis)	
Bacteria:	Group B streptococci, *E. coli*, *Listeria*, coagulase-negative staphylococcus, *T. pallidum*
Viruses:	Herpes simplex, enterovirus, adenovirus
Fungi:	*Candida*
Protozoa:	Malaria, *Borrelia*
Perinatal Asphyxia	
Respiratory	
Aspiration pneumonia	
Cardiac	
Congenital:	Hypoplastic left heart syndrome
Acquired:	Myocarditis
Metabolic	
Hypoglycemia	
Adrenal insufficiency (congenital adrenal hyperplasia)	
Organic acidoses	
Urea cycle disorders	
Salicylate toxicity	
Neurologic	
Intracranial hemorrhage	
Hematologic	
Neonatal purpura fulminans	
Severe anemia	
Methemoglobinemia	
Malignancies (congenital leukemia)	

life in essentially all infants, at birth or in the nursery. Skin, respiratory tract, and gastrointestinal tract are commonly colonized. CONS are the most common cause of bacteremia in low-birthweight infants. Approximately 50% of bacteremic infants have central venous catheters in place. Central nervous system shunts are also a risk factor for CONS ventriculitis. The mortality rate from CONS infections is lower than that from GBS and gram-negative enteric infections.

The increased prevalence of CONS infections in neonatal intensive care units has been attributed to the increased survival of very low-birthweight infants, which is associated with prolonged hospitalization, heavy exposure to broad-spectrum antibiotics, and the use of invasive procedures for monitoring and treating unstable infants. Recently, the use of intravenous lipid emulsion has been associated with an increased risk of CONS bacteremia.

PATHOGENESIS. Breakdown of the mucocutaneous barrier is the usual initial step. CONS are able to adhere to prosthetic devices, either by contiguous or bacteremic spread. Although there does not appear to be any phenotypic characteristic of CONS responsible for virulence, *S. epidermidis* is the most common species colonizing the newborn and associated with neonatal disease. *S. epidermidis* and *S. hemolyticus* are more virulent in animal models. Colonization and infection are enhanced by production of a slimelike substance, an exopolysaccharide. Slime-producing strains of CONS are often associated with neonatal disease.

Slime enhances adherence to catheters, inhibits neutrophil chemotaxis and phagocytosis, and may affect resistance to glycopeptide antibiotics. Lack of optimal opsonophagocytosis is the most important immunologic defect in the newborn's defense against CONS infection. Opsonic activity for CONS in premature infants is proportional to gestational age. Other possible virulence factors include cytotoxins, hemolysins, and proteinases.

CONS have been associated with NEC in the newborn infant. Like *S. aureus*, strains of CONS produce a delta toxin, which has been found in the stools of infants with NEC. Delta toxin causes lesions resembling NEC in rabbit intestinal loops and may play a role in the pathogenesis of NEC.

CLINICAL MANIFESTATIONS. The manifestations of most CONS neonatal infections are nonspecific. Bacteremia without a focus of tissue damage is associated with a variety of signs, ranging from mild to severe. Respiratory distress, apnea, bradycardia, gastrointestinal abnormalities, thermoregulatory problems, evidence of poor perfusion, and cerebral dysfunction are common. Specific infections caused by CONS include pneumonia, pleural effusions, meningitis, endocarditis, NEC, omphalitis, abscesses, and osteomyelitis.

DIAGNOSIS. Differentiation of CONS in normally sterile biologic fluids from contaminating organisms is a continuing problem for clinicians. Careful collection of specimens for culture and the use of multiple cultures will improve the validity of culture results. Some authors have recommended the use of quantitative cultures; however, low colony counts may occur in infections of the blood and CSF. Specific characteristics of CONS are not helpful in differentiating pathogens from contaminants in any individual case.

TREATMENT. Management of CONS infections involves antimicrobial therapy and, often, a decision regarding the removal of a foreign body. Because most hospital CONS isolates are resistant to penicillin, penicillinase-producing penicillins, and gentamicin and resistance to vancomycin is uncommon, vancomycin is the choice for initial therapy of suspected or proved CONS infections. If the organism is susceptible to penicillin or cephalosporin, these agents should be used to minimize the adverse effects and development of resistance to vancomycin. Vancomycin is nephrotoxic and ototoxic; peak and trough levels should be maintained between 25 and 40 mg/mL and less than 10 mg/mL, respectively. Dosing schedules based on weight and postnatal age have been developed.

Although removal of indwelling catheters or prosthetic devices significantly improves the response to antimicrobial therapy, there is usually a trial of antimicrobial therapy without removal of the foreign body. Infections with slime-producing CONS are less likely to respond, and endocarditis is more difficult to treat without removal of the umbilical venous catheter. If infection persists despite the use of an agent with good in vitro activity, synergistic therapy with rifampin and vancomycin is recommended.

Freeman J, Goldmann DA, Smith NE, et al: Association of intravenous lipid emulsion and coagulase-negative staphylococcal bacteremia in neonatal intensive care units. N Engl J Med 323:301, 1990.

Hall SL: Coagulase-negative staphylococcal infections in neonates. Pediatr Infect Dis 10:51, 1991.

Noel GJ, O'Loughlin JE, Edelson PJ: Neonatal *Staphylococcus epidermidis* right-sided endocarditis: Description of five catheterized infants. Pediatrics 82:234, 1988.

Patrick CC: Coagulase-negative staphylococci: Pathogens with increasing clinical significance. J Pediatr 116:497, 1990.

St. Geme JW III, Harris MC: Coagulase-negative staphylococcal infection in the neonate. Clin Perinatol 18:281, 1991.

Tan TQ, Musser JM, Shulman RJ, et al: Molecular epidemiology of coagulase-negative *Staphylococcus* blood isolates from neonates with persistent bacteremia and children with central venous catheter infections. J Infect Dis 169:1393, 1994.

98.6 Candidiasis

(See Chapter 229.1)

Candida species are a common cause of oral mucous membrane (thrush) and perineal skin infections (diaper dermatitis) in newborn infants. With improved survival of very low-birthweight infants, disseminated fungal infections are occurring more frequently in special care nurseries. The incidence is as high as 5% in very low-birthweight infants.

ETIOLOGY. Candidiasis is caused by members of the genus *Candida*, which includes 80 different species. *C. albicans* accounts for 80–90% of human infections. *C. tropicalis, C. parapsilosis, C. lusitaniae,* and *C. glabrata* are less commonly associated with infection in the newborn infant.

Candida has three predominant morphologic forms. Yeast cells (blastospores) are 1.5–5 μm in diameter, bud asexually, grow on body surfaces and fluids, initiate invasive lesions, and may cause toxic or inflammatory reactions. Chlamydospores are larger (7–17 μm) and are unusual as a form of systemic illness. Hyphae (pseudomycelia) forms are the tissue, rather than the contamination, phase of *Candida* and are filamentous processes that elongate from the yeast cell. *Candida* grows aerobically on routine laboratory media but may take several days of incubation.

EPIDEMIOLOGY. *C. albicans* is commonly isolated from gastrointestinal and vaginal flora of adults. Pregnancy increases the rate of vaginal colonization from less than 20% to about 33%. Approximately 10% of term infants are colonized within the first 5 days of life, but in infants smaller than 1,500 g, fungal colonization rates approach 30%. Early colonization occurs in the gastrointestinal and respiratory tracts. After 2 wk, colonization commonly involves the skin.

Congenital candidiasis has been rarely reported. It occurs as an ascending infection and has been associated with foreign bodies in the genital tract. Postnatal infection most commonly appears as thrush at about 1 wk of age. Monilial diaper dermatitis presents somewhat later with a peak incidence at 3–4 mo.

Systemic candidiasis is predominantly an infection of very low-birthweight infants with an estimated attack rate of 2–5%. Term infants exposed to abdominal surgery or prolonged ventilatory support are also at risk. Prolonged intravenous catheterization, the use of intravenous alimentation, and broad-spectrum antibiotic administration are risk factors.

PATHOGENESIS. Overgrowth of *Candida* on mucocutaneous surfaces and their presence on intravenous catheter tips favor entry and penetration. Clinical infection appears to be related to inoculum size. NEC may provide a mechanism for dissemination. The inability of the newborn infant to localize, control, and eradicate *Candida* infections appears to be related to the relative impairment of specific and nonspecific host defense mechanisms. Hematogenous spread leads to vasculitis and miliary nodules in many organs. The lungs, kidneys, gastrointestinal tract, heart, and meninges are commonly infected. Yeast and filaments are readily identified.

CLINICAL MANIFESTATIONS. Thrush presents with white, curdlike plaques on the oropharyngeal mucosa. The plaques are adherent to the mucosa and scraped off with some difficulty, leaving an erythematous base. *Candida* dermatitis is an erythematous, scaling rash most prominent in the intertriginous areas, with pustules forming along the leading edge and as satellites.

Congenital candidiasis presents as a generalized, intensely erythematous eruption in the first 12 hr of life. The rash may desquamate and become pustular. It contains fungi and is associated with fungal "colonies," which are visible as small yellow-white lesions on the placenta and umbilical cord. Preterm infants frequently have systemic disease characterized by pneumonia, leukocytosis, shock, and a high mortality rate. Full-term infants usually have disease localized to the skin.

The manifestations of systemic infection vary in acuteness and severity. Fungemia may be asymptomatic or may be associated with sepsis and septic shock. Either respiratory tract or gastrointestinal signs may be present. Severe apnea and bradycardia, temperature instability, generalized erythema, and hyperglycemia may be noted.

Vascular disease ranges from vasculitis of the aorta or vena cava to endocarditis. Infected thrombi in vessels and the right atrium are not uncommon. Renal involvement may be subclinical or may present with involvement of the upper or lower urinary tract. Upper tract involvement is manifested as flank mass, hypertension, renal failure, renal abscesses, papillary necrosis, and fungal balls in the collecting system with obstruction and hydronephrosis.

Central nervous system candidiasis may involve the meninges, ventricles, or cerebral cortex with abscess formation. Clinical manifestations of central nervous system disease may be subtle or not apparent. Endophthalmitis may occur in up to 50% of very low-birthweight infants with systemic candidiasis. It begins as chorioretinitis, which may extend to the vitreous. Cotton ball exudates are typical of *Candida* retinal pathologic conditions.

DIAGNOSIS. Isolation of fungi from cultures of normally sterile body fluids is the basis for diagnosis of invasive candidiasis. Occasionally, buffy coat smears of blood may show yeasts, allowing a preliminary diagnosis. Skin scrapings of generalized rashes in very low-birthweight infants with suspected systemic candidiasis should be examined microscopically. Because cultures of blood and CSF are often intermittently positive, multiple samples should be obtained. CSF cultures are positive in 33% of infants with systemic infection. Cultures should be taken from peripheral veins to differentiate true-positive cultures from contaminated catheter. Urine specimens for culture must also be obtained carefully to differentiate perineal colonization. There are no satisfactory antigen detection tests for clinical use. Serologic tests are under investigation but presently unavailable.

It is important to distinguish between catheter-associated transient candidemia and disseminated candidiasis. The former is characterized by positive blood cultures, owing to contamination of in situ intravascular catheters but no evidence of focal or disseminated disease, and may be treated by removing the catheter. Disseminated candidiasis is characterized by involvement of one or more organ systems.

Ultrasonography is useful for localization of *Candida* infection in the cardiovascular, renal, and central nervous systems. Radiographs of the chest may reveal fungal balls. Biochemical analysis of the blood should be performed in patients with suspected sepsis to assess renal and hepatic status.

TREATMENT. Amphotericin B is the drug of choice for systemic candidiasis. The drug is active against both yeast and mycelial forms. The initial dosage ranges from 0.5–1.0 mg/kg/24 hr intravenously. Because of individual variability, determination of serum levels is recommended to avoid drug accumulation. Amphotericin B should be diluted in 5% dextrose in water without electrolytes to a concentration of less than 0.2 mg/mL and administered over 4–6 hr. The duration of therapy varies widely according to clinical response and drug toxicity. The total recommended dose is 20–30 mg/kg. Nephrotoxicity is fairly common in the newborn infant and generally presents with oliguria, azotemia, and hyperkalemia. Some clinicians add flucytosine orally in a dose 100–150 mg/kg/24 hr divided every 6 hr. Flucytosine shows some synergism with amphotericin B and yields good levels in CSF. Fungi develop resistance when flucytosine is used alone. Patients must be observed for bone marrow, gastrointestinal, and hepatotoxicity.

Indwelling catheters should be removed if possible. Infected intracardiac and intravascular thrombi usually must be resected, but resolution without surgery has been described.

Baley JE: Neonatal candidiasis: The current challenge. Clin Perinatol 18:263, 1991.

Butler KM, Baker CJ: *Candida:* An increasingly important pathogen in the nursery. Pediatr Clin North Am 35:543, 1988.

Eppes SC, Troutman JL, Gutman LT: Outcome of treatment of candidemia in children whose central catheters were removed or retained. Pediatr Infect Dis J 8:99, 1989.

Weese-Mayer DE, Fondriest DW, Brouillette RT, et al: Risk factors associated with candidemia in the neonatal intensive care unit: A case-control study. Pediatr Infect Dis J 6:190, 1987.

CHAPTER 99
Pneumonia in the Neonate

Charles G. Prober

ETIOLOGY AND EPIDEMIOLOGY. Pneumonia as a result of infection may be acquired transplacentally, perinatally, or postnatally. When contracted transplacentally, the pulmonary infection usually represents one component of a more generalized congenital process. For example, congenital infection caused by cytomegalovirus (CMV), rubella virus, and *Treponema pallidum* may be associated with pneumonitis, although invariably other manifestations of the congenital process such as prematurity, intrauterine growth retardation, abnormal head size, and/or visceromegaly will also be evident.

Perinatal acquisition of pulmonary infection results from aspiration of infected amniotic fluid or maternal gastrointestinal or genitourinary secretions at delivery. Microorganisms contracted in this fashion include group B streptococci (GBS), gram-negative enteric aerobes, *Listeria monocytogenes,* genital *Mycoplasma, Chlamydia trachomatis,* and viruses including CMV and herpes simplex virus. Factors associated with an increased risk of contracting perinatal pneumonia include prematurity, prolonged rupture of membranes, chorioamnionitis, and fetal distress.

Additional doses of vaccine are administered at 1 and 6 mo of age. The American Academy of Pediatrics and the Centers for Disease Control and Prevention recommend administration of hepatitis B vaccine to all infants at birth. The recommended three-dose schedule of hepatitis B vaccination for infants born to HB_sAg-negative mothers is dose 1 at birth, dose 2 1 mo after dose 1, and dose 3 at 6–18 mo of age. Routine testing of infants to determine the presence of anti-HB_sAg is not recommended.

Lin H-H, Kao J-H, Hsu H-Y, et al: Possible role of high-titer maternal viremia in perinatal transmission of hepatitis C virus. J Infect Dis 169:638, 1994.
Ohto H, Terazawa S, Saski N, et al: Transmission of hepatitis C virus from mothers to infants. N Engl J Med 330:744, 1994.
Pickering LK: Management of the infant of a mother with viral hepatitis. Pediatr Rev 9:315, 1988.
Proceedings of a Symposium: Hepatitis B today. Storch GA, Koff RS, Halsey NA, et al: New guidelines for the pediatrician. Pediatr Infect Dis J 12:427, 1993.
The liver in infancy and childhood. *In:* Sherlock S, Dooley J (eds): Disease of the Liver and Biliary System, 9th ed. London, Blackwell Scientific, 1993, pp 434–459.
Zimmerman HJ, Fang M, Utill R, et al: Clinical conference: jaundice due to bacterial infection. Gastroenterology 77:362, 1979.

CHAPTER 101
*Urinary Tract Infections**

(See Chapter 492)

Ricardo Gonzalez

Urinary tract infections occur in 0.1% of newborn infants, and they differ from infections in children older than 1 yr of age in that they are more frequent in males than in females, the clinical manifestations are vague and nonspecific, and infections in this age group tend to be more severe. Factors predisposing to infection include P blood group secretor status, vesicoureteral reflux, obstructive uropathy, low birthweight, myelomeningocele, bladder catheterization, and, for males, being uncircumcised. The risk of a urinary tract infection for an uncircumcised male in the 1st yr of life is 0.041, and this probability is reduced to 0.002 with neonatal circumcision. Seventy-five per cent of the infections are caused by *Escherichia coli,* but other enterobacteria and gram-positive cocci are not uncommon. The route of infection in most cases is ascending and rarely hematogenous. In addition to renal scarring, newborn infections can cause renal growth retardation, even in the absence of reflux. This renal growth retardation can be reversible after puberty in children without reflux.

*Modified from section in 14th edition by Samuel P. Gotoff.

CLINICAL MANIFESTATIONS AND DIAGNOSIS. The most common manifestations include failure to thrive, weight loss, poor feeding, jaundice, diarrhea, and fever. Fever is usually low grade, but some infants may become septic. A palpable abdominal mass or a weak urinary stream suggests obstructive uropathy. There may be leukocytosis, elevation of the serum creatinine level, and acidosis. The diagnosis is confirmed by a positive bladder urine culture obtained either by catheterization or suprapubic aspiration. Ultrasound guidance for suprapubic aspiration is recommended. Urine cultures collected with an adhesive bag are only useful when negative to exclude infection. Any number of gram-negative bacteria in a suprapubic aspirate of urine indicates infection. A small number of gram-positive cocci may represent skin contaminants. The urinalysis reveals more than 10 leukocytes per high-power field in more than 50% of infants with a urinary tract infection, but the absence of pyuria does not rule out infection. Blood cultures are positive in 33% of infants with a urinary tract infection, and meningitis may develop in some.

EVALUATION. An ultrasound examination of the kidneys and bladder should be obtained soon after the diagnosis in all infected infants. Sepsis is more common in infants with a dilated urinary tract. The ultrasound is also sensitive to rule out pyonephrosis and renal abscess. After resolution of the acute episode, a voiding cystourethrogram is done to exclude reflux. Further evaluation of the newborn with reflux or obstruction is discussed in Chapter 493. In equivocal cases, a dimercaptosuccinic acid (DMSA) renal scan helps to diagnose pyelonephritis.

TREATMENT. Parenteral antibiotics, usually including an aminoglycoside and ampicillin or a cephalosporin, should be initiated even before the sensitivity of the organism is known. If the ultrasonographic examination is suspicious of bladder outlet obstruction (usually posterior urethral valves in males or ectopic ureterocele in females), a bladder catheter is essential for resolution of the obstruction. Likewise, if ureteral obstruction and pyonephrosis are suspected, percutaneous renal drainage (nephrostomy) should be considered.

Although some authors recommend routine newborn circumcision to reduce the risk of urinary tract infection, it is probably more reasonable and effective to evaluate and treat promptly all newborns with a history of renal abnormalities on prenatal ultrasonography.

Alari U, Prey M, Davidai G, et al: Ultrasonography in the evaluation of children with urinary tract infection. Pediatrics 78:58, 1986.
Chessare JB: Circumcision: is the risk of urinary tract infection the pivotal issue? Clin Pediatr 31:100, 1992.
Hellstrom M, Jacobsson B, Jodal U, et al: Renal growth after neonatal urinary tract infection. Pediatr Nephrol 1:269, 1987.

PART XIII

Special Health Problems During Adolescence

Iris F. Litt

CHAPTER 102

Epidemiology of Adolescent Disease

Although adolescents (11–20 yr of age) constituted 17% of the population of the United States during 1980–1990, they were responsible for only 7% of office visits to physicians. Most visits were for acute conditions, compared with all other age groups for whom chronic illness or nonillness health care predominated (see also Chapters 1, 40, and 42). The low rate of utilization of private physicians may reflect the generally good health of adolescents or an inappropriate pattern of physician utilization. Whatever the cause, the result is that physicians, and particularly pediatricians, have relatively less opportunity to evaluate and counsel teenagers than other children.

Younger adolescents had higher rates of office visits than older adolescents. Females in the 15- to 20-yr age group had higher rates than males, primarily because of gynecologic or obstetric care. For the younger adolescents, the leading diagnostic category was respiratory illness (21%), followed by routine examinations, injuries, or poisonings (16%). For older adolescents, after routine examinations, the leading diagnoses included diseases of the skin and subcutaneous tissue (14%), followed by diseases of the respiratory system (13%), injury (13%), and poisoning (13%). In 1985, 35% of office visits of all adolescents were made to general practitioners and family physicians, whereas 23% of office visits were made to pediatricians.

Data from the National Health Examination Survey of 1966–1970 showed that 20% of presumably healthy 12- to 17-yr-olds had previously *undiagnosed health problems*. These problems were primarily related to the rapid growth and maturation that characterizes puberty and included such problems as scoliosis (Chapter 628.1), slipped capital femoral epiphysis (Chapter 627.4), Osgood-Schlatter disease (Chapter 626.4), goiter (Chapter 522), and acne (Chapter 619). In addition, a number of health problems regarded as "adult" problems in the past are actually present during adolescence, albeit in preclinical form (e.g., hypertension, hypercholesterolemia, and carcinoma in situ of the cervix).

Violence, such as accidents, homicides, or suicides, accounts for 70% of all adolescent *deaths*. In the United States, more male adolescents die from gunshot wounds than from any other biologic cause. Neoplasms (7%), infectious diseases, and diseases of a congenital nature (7%) account for a significantly smaller proportion of adolescent deaths. Among the neoplasms, testicular tumors and tumors of bone or lymphatics are most prevalent.

The birth rate has leveled off for all other age groups but continues to rise for young adolescents; they lead the nation in cases of *sexually transmitted disease*, such as gonorrhea, chlamydia, and human papilloma viral infections. Certain non-sexually transmitted infectious diseases now have their peak incidence among adolescents, including rubella, rubeola, infectious mononucleosis, and toxic shock syndrome.

Health-destructive behavior, such as cigarette and marijuana smoking and abuse of alcohol and other drugs (often in combination with driving), continues to present serious problems for adolescents. Eating disorders, such as anorexia nervosa and bulimia, are increasing in prevalence, the former reported to affect 1% of 16- to 18-yr-old females in the United States.

Automobile and motorcycle accidents are the leading causes of adolescent morbidity and mortality. Sixteen- to 19-yr-olds comprise 6% of licensed drivers and account for 13% of vehicular fatalities; 63% of automotive deaths among adolescents involve passengers in cars driven by adolescents. Sports injuries and accidental drowning are additional prominent causes of adolescent morbidity and mortality. See also Chapter 58.

Alcohol is a factor underlying most vehicular fatalities, along with failure to use seat belts in cars or helmets while riding motorcylces. Most of these accidents involve male adolescents and occur between 8:00 P.M. and 4:00 A.M. Lowering the drinking age to 18 yr of age has been associated with a 5% increase in fatal automotive accidents. Driver's education classes have been associated with increased mortality rates because they increase the number of younger drivers on the road. Pediatricians can address this problem among adolescents through anticipatory guidance and legislation aimed at raising the drinking age and enforcing the use of seat belts and helmets (see Chapter 5).

CHAPTER 103

Depression

See also Chapter 24.

Adolescence is a time of increased emotionality, hypothetical thinking, and empathy (Chapter 15). As a result, it is a time for mood swings from the depths of depression to the heights of elation. It is often difficult to decide which sad-looking adolescent is at risk for true depression and even suicide. The hallmarks of the youngster who is at risk are the persistence of the depressed mood, the absence of corresponding periods of elation, the inability to function, and the expression of hopelessness and helplessness. Puig-Antich suggests that the depressed mood should be considered persistent if it lasts for at least 3 consecutive hours for three periods or more each week.

DIAGNOSIS. Assessment of the adolescent's functional status should focus on school performance and on peer and family interactions. Symptoms of depression in the adolescent may include falling school grades, an increase in school absenteeism or truancy, use of alcohol or drugs, accident proneness, and pervasive boredom. Alternatively, persistent euphoria, if combined with acting-out behavior such as promiscuity, may mask depression (see later). Disturbances of eating and sleeping are not as pervasive in adolescents as in depressed adults but may be quite severe when present. Initial insomnia and difficulty in falling asleep, sometimes to the extent of sleeping all day and remaining awake at night without ever feeling rested, are common signs of depression in adolescents. A family history of depressive illness increases the likelihood of depression, particularly if this history includes a suicide attempt.

Suicide (see Chapter 25 and later). When severe depression is suspected, the physician should ask whether the patient has ever felt so sad that death was considered to be a preferable alternative to living. If the patient answers in the affirmative, it is appropriate to inquire about the existence of a plan for self-destruction. The patient who has a suicide plan must be evaluated immediately by a psychiatrist. The adolescent who is not contemplating suicide will not be harmed by such questioning and is often relieved to have an opportunity to discuss his or her concerns with a caring physician. The physician also should not be misled by the adolescent who suddenly appears cheerful after a period of depression, because such a change may accompany the youngster's resolution of ambivalence and the decision to resolve sadness by suicide.

CLINICAL MANIFESTATIONS. Mattsson describes five forms of adolescent depression in order of increasing pathology:

1. **Normal depressive mood swings.**
2. **Acute depressive reactions.** These normally occur after death or separation from a loved one and are the equivalent of a healthy grief response. Although feelings of mourning may preoccupy the adolescent for weeks or months, there is a gradual change toward resolution and restoration of normal functioning. If such an adolescent denies suicidal thoughts and if there is no increase in risk-taking behavior, he or she may be managed by close observation by the primary care physician.
3. **Neurotic depressive disorders.** These disorders may follow lack of resolution of a grief reaction and are characterized by feelings of hopelessness and helplessness, of self-incrimination and guilt in relationship to the lost individual, of difficulty in concentration, of withdrawal from school and social contacts, and of interference with normal sleeping, eating, and activity. A desire to join the deceased may be elicited after careful questioning. This form of depression should be managed by a psychiatrist.
4. **Masked depression.** In this variant of the neurotic depressive disorder, the youngster deals with his or her feelings of despair by denial and somatization. "Acting-out" behavior, such as running away from home, school truancy, multiple accidents, and substance abuse, may be the manifestations of this form of depression, as may the appearance of headaches, abdominal pain, or other physical complaints. Psychiatric management is indicated.
5. **Psychotic depressive disorders.** Impaired reality testing, thought distortion, and delusions of guilt may be present in addition to characteristics already described. Patients should be referred for psychiatric treatment.

CHAPTER 104
Suicide

See Chapter 25.

Suicide is the 3rd leading cause of death among 15- to 19-yr-olds in the United States, accounting for 10% of all deaths among adolescents, and has been increasing in incidence during the last 2 decades. Females lead males in the incidence of suicide attempts, whereas male adolescents outnumber females in completed suicides. Native Americans and Asian Americans have a higher suicide rate than the general population. The chronically ill adolescent is also at increased risk for suicide as a result of feelings of impotence, diminished competence, poor self-image, and vulnerability to loss of a loved one; there is also often increased access to medication that may facilitate suicide.

The *method of suicide* most commonly used by teenagers is ingestion of medication. The medication may be the patient's own or often that of a parent with whom there has been conflict. The drug most often used in suicide attempts is a tricyclic antidepressant. A "bubble-pack" or similar unit-dose form of packaging should be prescribed when there is any concern that medication may be used in a suicide attempt. More violent methods, such as hanging, shooting, or wrist slashing, are used most often by males and by those most intent on completing the act. Nevertheless, it is often difficult to assess the seriousness of the intent by the actual potency of the method. Beck and associates found medical lethality of methods to correlate poorly with seriousness of intent. There was, however, good correlation between the latter and the patient's expectation of lethality, which was often inaccurate.

Other factors to be considered in assessing the seriousness of a suicide attempt are the extent of premeditation and the likelihood of rescue. The adolescent who impulsively grabs a bottle from the medicine cabinet after announcing that he or she plans to kill himself or herself is generally less serious about commiting suicide than is the one who has carefully planned the event, particularly if rescue was unlikely. Leaving a suicide note suggests premeditation and is a sign of seriousness of intent. An attempt by a teenager with a family history of suicide is particularly significant. Any attempt or gesture should be regarded as serious, however, regardless of apparent intent because most successful suicides occur among persons who have made earlier attempts or gestures.

Whenever an adolescent makes a suicide attempt, it is a desperate attempt at conflict resolution. Merely attending to its pharmacologic or surgical sequelae, which is usually the case in hospital emergency rooms, does little to assist in constructive resolution of the conflict. *Short-term hospitalization*, however, effectively accomplishes this latter goal by providing a secure setting for the patient, by impressing parents with the need to attend to the underlying problems, and, most important, by facilitating psychosocial assessment on which to base a recommendation for appropriate therapy or referral. Fewer than one-third of families actually follow up with recommendation for referral made after only emergency room evaluation. Consultation with a skilled psychiatrist is essential in the assessment of every teenager who makes a suicide attempt.

CHAPTER 105
Substance Abuse

The use of mind-altering substances for medicinal, social, and religious purposes has characterized the human race throughout recorded history. The use of such agents by teenagers is also not a new phenomenon. The increased complexity of modern society, as well as the increased availability of a wide variety of drugs, has contributed to increased use by adolescents and an awareness of physical and psychosocial sequelae by health professionals. In our society, drug use may serve a variety of purposes for the adolescent. For the individual aspiring to adult status, the use of drugs may be symbolic of maturity. For those negotiating independence from parental domination, drugs may be viewed as facilitating the process. Peer group acceptance, stress reduction, escapism, and rebellion against the establishment are other functions presumably served by drug use. In addition, the developing teenager, seeking to explore the limits of his or her new cognitive abilities, may attempt to do so through hallucinogenic agents.

Intervention strategies for preventing or stopping drug use by this age group must consider alternatives that meet their developmental needs. Drug use, in the form of alcohol or marijuana, is experienced at some time by more than 90% of teenagers; accordingly, it is no longer useful to think of teenagers as either being drug users or non-drug users. Rather, the clinician should assess the role of drug use in each adolescent's life and the effects of specific drugs on physical and functional parameters in each individual. Because it is much easier to resist pressures to use drugs than to stop once begun, efforts should be focused on prevention (see also Chapter 5).

EPIDEMIOLOGY. Most data on adolescent substance abuse are based on repeated, cross-sectional studies, which makes it difficult to separate effects of maturation from effects caused by changes in the availability of drugs. The use of illicit drugs by high-school seniors in the United States has been declining as a result of a decrease in the use of marijuana. Other drugs exhibiting a marked decline include amphetamines, methaqualone, and lysergic acid diethylamide (LSD). Continuation of a gradual long-term decline also occurred in the use of barbituates, tranquilizers, and phencyclidine (PCP). Heroin use dropped by one-half from 1975 to 1979 and has leveled off at less than 1%; inhalant use has been stable at 4% since 1980. In contrast, the use of *cocaine* doubled between 1975 and 1979, with significant regional differences; rates in West and Northeast sections of the United States were double those in the South and North Central regions. A one-fifth decrease in the use of cocaine was reported in 1987; the rate of use of *crack cocaine* was unchanged from that in 1986 (6%). It is probable, however, that the rate of crack cocaine use among those not in school (and therefore not surveyed) is considerably higher.

Use of *nonprescription stimulants and diet pills* has only been examined in recent years, with the finding of lifetime prevalence of 15–20% for the former and 31% for the latter. Of particular concern is a 45% lifetime prevalence for use of diet pills among adolescent females (Chapter 107). A median of 4% of adolescents surveyed in 1991 reported any lifetime use of *anabolic steroids*.

Alcohol use is reported by 93% of high-school seniors, 69% within the previous month, and 5.5% daily use. The rate of binge drinking (five drinks or more in a row) during the previous 2 wk rose to 41% in 1983 and has declined since then to 37%. Data on adolescent alcohol consumption from four countries for which data are adequate and comparable with those in the United States show a recent decline in three countries and leveling off in one (Australia). In all, however, previously noted male-female differences in usage rates have narrowed.

Smoking on a daily basis by adolescents in the United States decreased from 29% in 1977 to a median of 12% by 1991. Slightly more adolescent females now smoke regularly than males, reversing earlier patterns. Future educational plans correlate significantly with smoking patterns; 8% of college-bound seniors report smoking half a packet or more daily, compared with 21% of those who do not plan to go to college. Use of "smokeless" tobacco by male adolescents is a recent and growing phenomenon (median = 11% for recent use in 1991).

In summary, these cross-sectional studies show that approximately two-thirds of teenagers in the United States try some illicit drug before they finish high-school; 40% have used some illicit drug other than marijuana. Daily cigarette smoking is experienced by one in every 18 high-school seniors; the same percentage drink alcohol on a daily basis.

Cohort longitudinal studies may help separate maturational from historical trends. Kandel and associates evaluated a cohort of New York State adolescents in 1971 and approximately 10 yr later. They found that the time of greatest risk for initiation of cigarette smoking or alcohol and marijuana use was before the age of 20 yr, and for illicit drugs, other than cocaine, before 21 yr of age. A decline in marijuana use began at 22.5 yr of age, whereas the use of cigarettes continued to increase through the end of the period of surveillance, at 25 yr of age. These authors believe that it is unlikely that those who have not experimented with any of these substances by 21 yr of age will do so thereafter. Jessor and Jessor evaluated 7th-, 8th-, and 9th-grade youngsters from a city in the Rocky Mountains, first in 1969, then annually for 4 successive years, and then again in 1979 and 1981. Follow-up data extended to persons who were 25, 26, and 27 yr of age. They defined "problem drinking" as (1) having within the previous year been drunk six times or more or (2) within the same period having on two occasions or more experienced negative consequences of drinking in three or more life areas (difficulty with teachers; difficulties with friends; trouble with parents; criticism from dates; trouble with police; or driving a car while under the influence of alcohol). By this definition, 25% of males and 16% of females in the 1972 sample of 10th, 11th, and 12th graders were problem drinkers. Among the males who were problem drinkers during adolescence, half were no longer in this category by young adulthood. For the females, only 25% of the original problem drinker group remained classified in this way during young adulthood. Among those who were nonproblem drinkers during adolescence, 40% of males and 20% of females became problem drinkers as young adults. Problem drinking during adolescence was correlated with other concurrent problem behaviors, such as smoking marijuana and sexual intercourse. On the other hand, it was not significantly correlated with negative consequences in later life. The authors concluded: "Such findings suggest that post-adolescent development and attainment are not necessarily mortgaged by adolescent problem drinking . . . [and] that premature labeling and social processing of adolescents as problem drinkers might very well set up expectations for chronicity that unnecessarily restrict the developmental options."

Longitudinal studies also provide us with a better picture of the role of marijuana use as a forerunner of later use of hard drugs. Its predictive power is limited to those who begin its use at a young age. The New York study also found that alcohol use was experienced by 20% of children before 10 yr of age and by 50% by 14 yr of age, that marijuana use began to climb at approximately 13 yr of age, and that cigarette use began to rise at about 11 yr of age. The pattern for onset of use of psychedelics parallels that of marijuana, whereas that for cocaine shifts to an older age group (8% by 18 yr of age and 30% by 24 yr of age). Although males outnumber females in the magnitude of illicit drug use, psychoactive substances are prescribed more often for females, beginning in early adolescence and continuing through adulthood. These developmental observations should be used as a basis for preventive strategies.

ETIOLOGY. As indicated earlier, factors that contribute to the adolescent's initial decision to use a substance of abuse include the desire to explore the limits of emotionality; the need to try on new "adult" roles; the wish to expand one's consciousness; the availability of drugs; the desire to escape an unpleasant or stressful experience; and peer pressure. Continued use of a drug after it is first experienced usually suggests that serious problems may underlie usage or may complicate use. For example, drug use is more prevalent among depressed teenagers as well as among those described by the Jessors as being susceptible to problem behavior. No single factor distinguishes "problem" adolescent drug users from those whose drug involvement does not portend major problems, but weighing an aggregate of multiple variables may assist in this process (Table 105–1). The type of drug used (e.g., marijuana versus heroin), the circumstances of use (e.g., alone or in a group setting), the frequency and timing of use (e.g., daily before school versus rarely on a weekend), the premorbid personality (depressed versus happy), as well as the teenager's general functional status should all be considered in evaluating any youngster found to be abusing a drug. In addition, apart from the existence of any high-risk factors, the use of any psychoactive substance in conjunction with operation of a motor vehicle is sufficient reason for immediate intervention to prevent harm to the teenager and to others.

PATHOPHYSIOLOGY. The process of physical growth and development that characterizes puberty may be affected adversely by the use of drugs. For example, one-third of adolescent females who use *heroin* have secondary amenorrhea, even in the absence of weight loss. The higher incidence of menstrual abnormalities in the adolescent heroin user probably results from a greater vulnerability of the hypothalamic-pituitary-ovarian axis in the maturing individual. Experiments with naloxone, the opiate antagonist, suggest that endogenous opiates block the release of gonadotropin-releasing hormone. *Amphetamines* interfere with stage 4 sleep and may impair the intimate relationship between sleep and augmentation of secretion of gonadotropins during early adolescence. To derive calories mainly from *ethanol* during the peak of the pubertal growth spurt deprives the body of the protein necessary for normal muscle growth.

■ **TABLE 105–1 Assessing the Seriousness of Adolescent Drug Abuse**

Variable	0	+1	+2
Age (yr)	>15	<15	
Sex	Male	Female	
Family history of drug abuse		Yes	
Setting of drug use	In group		Alone
Affect before drug use	Happy		Sad
School performance	Good/improving	Always poor	Recently poor
Use before driving	None		Yes
History of accidents	None		Yes
Time of week	Weekend	Weekdays	
Time of day		After school	Before school
Type of drug	Marijuana, beer, wine	Hallucinogens, amphetamines	Whiskey, opiates, cocaine, barbiturates

Total score: 0–3 less worrisome; 3–8 serious; 8–18 very serious.

■ **TABLE 105–2 Interactions Between Alcohol and Prescription Drugs**

Additive	Cross-Tolerant	Antagonistic
Acetaminophen	Anticoagulants (chronic intoxication)	Caffeine
Antihypertensives	Digoxin-digitoxin	Cephalosporins
Anticoagulants (acute intoxication)	Ether	Chloramphenicol
Antihistamines	Fluorinated anesthetics	Griseofulvin
Barbiturates	Imipramine	Ketoconazole
Benzodiazepines	Propranolol	Phenformin
Chloral hydrate	Tetracyclines	
Lithium		
Nonsteroidal anti-inflammatory drugs		
Oral contraceptives		
Phenothiazines		
Propoxyphene		
Salicylates		

The metabolism of certain prescribed drugs may be affected by coincident abuse of illicit drugs or alcohol (Table 105–2). Induction of hepatic smooth endoplasmic reticulum by barbiturates or alcohol may accelerate the metabolism and enhance the excretion of substances requiring glucuronidation. As a result of this mechanism, estrogen-containing oral contraceptives taken by an abuser of these substances may become vulnerable to pregnancy. Conversely, the use of estrogens increases the risk of intoxication from alcohol as a result of decreased ethanol metabolism. The potentiating interaction of alcohol and barbiturates must also be considered when prescribing anticonvulsant medications. Abdominal pain and vomiting occur when metronidazole is ingested by an alcohol-abusing adolescent, because of the antagonistic effect of alcohol on acetaldehyde.

PSYCHOSOCIAL SEQUELAE. Youth may engage in robbery, burglary, drug dealing, or prostitution for the purpose of acquiring the money necessary to buy drugs or alcohol. Regular use of any drug eventually diminishes the ability to function adequately in school, to hold a job, or to operate a motor vehicle. An "amotivational" syndrome has been described in chronic marijuana users who lose interest in age-appropriate behavior.

PREVENTION. The model of prevention relevant to the problem of adolescent drug or alcohol use is one that anticipates experimentation with some agent at some point in the normal development of the adolescent and that attempts to delay that event as long as possible, to make its use as limited in amount and setting as possible, and to prevent entirely any use while operating a motor vehicle. Educational efforts based on scare techniques have not been successful, whereas those that present unemotional, factual information about medical complications of drug use have had some impact. Strategies that teach young adolescents to resist peer pressure to smoke, by the use of trained peer counselors using role-playing techniques, have significantly reduced smoking in a number of studies.

TREATMENT. Acute management is discussed in the following sections on specific agents. A variety of chronic treatment programs are available in inpatient and ambulatory settings. In general, these programs have not been adequately evaluated. Important features of successful long-term management of these adolescents are continuing medical evaluation after detoxification and the provision of developmentally appropriate psychosocial support systems.

105.1 Opiates

Opiate abuse by adolescents decreased considerably during the 1980s, but the magnitude and variety of its medical sequelae warrant continued attention. Moreover, a resurgence of its use in conjunction with "crack" cocaine has occurred.

PHARMACOLOGY. Heroin produces euphoria and analgesia. It is hydrolyzed to morphine, which undergoes hepatic conjugation with glucuronic acid before excretion, usually within 24 hr of administration. It can be detected in urine by thin-layer chromatography up to 48 hr after administration.

The route of administration influences the timing of the onset of action. When the drug is inhaled ("snorting"), it will require almost 30 min until the desired effect is achieved. By the subcutaneous route ("skin-popping"), the effect is achieved within minutes; and when injected intravenously ("mainlining"), it has an immediate effect. A larger dose can be administered intravenously. Tolerance is developed to the euphoric effect and only rarely to the inhibitory effect on smooth muscle, which causes both constipation and miosis.

CLINICAL MANIFESTATIONS. These are determined by the pharmacologic effects of heroin or its adulterants, combined with the conditions and the route of administration.

Neuromuscular. The cerebral effects include euphoria, diminution in pain, and a sleeplike electroencephalogram pattern. An effect on the hypothalamus is suggested by the lowering of body temperature. Transverse myelitis of the thoracic segments has been reported in patients resuming heroin use after a period of abstinence, suggesting a possible hypersensitivity reaction. Rarely, Guillain-Barré syndrome and toxic amblyopia, the latter presumably resulting from the quinine additive, occur in heroin addicts. Brachial and lumbosacral plexitis and polyneuropathies and mononeuropathies, the latter manifested by ankledrop or wristdrop, are the most common peripheral neurologic findings. Acute rhabdomyolysis with myoglobinuria may follow intravenous (IV) injection of heroin and is manifested by generalized muscle tenderness, edema, and marked weakness. Necrotizing fasciitis is a rare complication after inadvertent subfascial injections of heroin. Other rare complications are contractures of the fingers resulting from infection and scarring medial to the proximal interphalangeal joint following injection into the small veins of the hand.

Cardiovascular. Vasodilation is a major cardiovascular manifestation related to the method of administration of the drug. Rare complications of parenteral heroin administration include arteriovenous fistula, arterial and venous thrombosis, embolism, necrotizing arteritis, and mycotic aneurysm.

Respiratory. Respiratory depression is mediated centrally and is characterized by alveolar underventilation. Particles of cotton fibers or nonsoluble adulterants inadvertently injected with the heroin are responsible for granulomatosis and pulmonary fibrosis, which may result in pulmonary hypertension and a decrease in lung volume and in diffusing capacity. Pulmonary edema is common in death from the overdose syndrome, but it may also be seen as an incidental roentgenologic finding in an otherwise asymptomatic adolescent heroin abuser. Pulmonary infections have not been a prominent finding in this age group.

Dermatologic. The most common dermatologic lesions are the "tracks," the hypertrophic linear scars that follow the course of large veins. Smaller, discrete peripheral scars, resembling healed insect bites, may be easily overlooked. The adolescent who injects heroin subcutaneously may have fat necrosis, lipodystrophy, and atrophy over portions of the extremities. Attempts at concealment of these stigmata may include amateur tattoos in unusual sites. Abscesses secondary to unsterile techniques of drug administration are commonly found.

Genitourinary. There is a loss of libido; the mechanism is unknown. The female heroin user may resort to prostitution to support the habit, thus increasing the risks of sexually transmitted disease (including human immunodeficiency virus [HIV]), pregnancy, and other hazards. Urinary retention may result from decreased tone of the detrusor muscles.

Gastrointestinal. Constipation results from decreased smooth-muscle propulsive contractions and increased anal sphincter tone. The practice of concealment of heroin in a swallowed condom or balloon may cause intestinal obstruction or sudden (often fatal) overdosage if the container breaks. Hepatic enzyme activities are frequently elevated in heroin users, the majority of whom have serologic evidence suggesting viral infection with hepatitis B. Elements of chronic aggressive hepatitis on biopsy and persistence of enzyme abnormalities suggest a poor prognosis in some patients.

Infectious. The absence of sterile technique in injection may lead to cerebral microabscesses or endocarditis, usually caused by *Staphylococcus aureus*. Infection with HIV is another complication of needle use.

Immunologic. Elevations in immunoglobulin (Ig) M levels are consistently noted in parenteral heroin users, whereas IgA elevations are reported in those who inhale the drug. Abnormal serologic reactions are also common, including false-positive Venereal Disease Research Laboratory and latex fixation tests. Depression of lymphocyte response to stimulation by mitogens in culture has been reported but may be due to coincident acquired immunodeficiency syndrome (Chapter 223) in parenteral drug users.

Withdrawal. After a period of 8 hr or more without heroin, the addicted individual undergoes, during a period of 24–36 hr, a series of physiologic disturbances referred to collectively as "withdrawal" or the *abstinence syndrome*. The earliest sign is yawning, followed by lacrimation, mydriasis, insomnia, "goose flesh," cramping of the voluntary musculature, hyperactive bowel sounds and diarrhea, tachycardia, and systolic hypertension. The occurrence of grand mal seizures is rare in adolescent addicts. A short course of diazepam is effective and safe treatment for heroin detoxification. An alternative for detoxification is *treatment* with methadone. This synthetic opiate is effective by the oral route and is pharmacologically similar to heroin, with the exception of its lack of euphoric effect. Neither the safety nor the dosage of methadone has been established for children or adolescents.

Overdose Syndrome. Overdose syndrome is an acute reaction after the administration of an opiate. It is the leading cause of death among drug users. The rapidity of onset, the finding of eosinophilia after recovery, and the fact that it occurs only in those who have used the drug previously suggest a hypersensitivity mechanism. The clinical signs include stupor or coma, seizures, miotic pupils (unless severe anoxia has occurred), respiratory depression, cyanosis, and pulmonary edema. The differential diagnosis includes central nervous system (CNS) trauma, diabetic coma, hepatic (and other) encephalopathy, Reye syndrome, as well as overdose of alcohol, barbiturates, PCP, or methadone. Diagnosis of opiate toxicity is facilitated by intravenous administration of the opiate antagonist naloxone, 0.01 mg/kg (a vial of 0.4 mg usually suffices for an adolescent), which causes dilatation of pupils constricted by the opiate. Diagnosis is confirmed by the finding of morphine in the serum. *Treatment* consists of maintaining adequate oxygenation and continued administration of naloxone every 5 min, when necessary, to improve and maintain adequate ventilation. Naloxone may have to be continued for 24 hr if methadone, rather than shorter acting heroin, has been taken.

105.2 Hallucinogens

Several naturally occurring and synthetic substances have been used by adolescents for their hallucinogenic properties. Lysergic acid diethylamide (LSD), which enjoyed popularity in the 1970s, has reappeared recently. LSD flashbacks are terrifying and may be reactivated by fever. Among the other currently popular hallucinogens, PCP, certain mushrooms, and jimsonweed may cause serious toxicity and even death.

Phencyclidine

(PCP, Sternyl, Angel Dust, "Hog," "Peace Pill," "Sheets")

PCP is an arylcyclohexalamine whose popularity is related, in part, to its ease of synthesis in home laboratories. One of the by-products of home synthesis causes cramps, diarrhea, and hematemesis. The drug is thought to potentiate adrenergic effects by inhibiting neuronal reuptake of catecholamines. PCP is available as a tablet, liquid, or powder, which may be used alone or sprinkled on cigarettes ("joints"). The powders and tablets generally contain 2–6 mg of PCP, whereas joints average 1 mg for every 150 mg of tobacco leaves, or approximately 30–50 mg per joint.

CLINICAL MANIFESTATIONS. These are dose related. Euphoria, nystagmus, ataxia, and emotional lability occur within 2–3 min after smoking 1–5 mg and last for hours. Hallucination may involve bizarre distortions of body image that often precipitate panic reactions. With doses of 5–15 mg a toxic psychosis may occur, with disorientation, hypersalivation, and abusive language lasting for more than 1 hr. After oral ingestion of 15 mg or more, the patient usually becomes comatose within 30–60 min, with alternating periods of wakefulness, with dystonic posturing, muscular rigidity, or myoclonic jerks. Hypotension, generalized seizures, and cardiac arrhythmias commonly occur with plasma concentrations from 40–200 μg/dL. Death has been reported during psychotic delirium, from hypertension, hypotension, hypothermia, seizures, and trauma. The coma of PCP may be distinguished from that of the opiates by the absence of respiratory depression; the presence of muscle rigidity, hyper-reflexia, and nystagmus; and lack of response to naloxone. PCP psychosis may be difficult to distinguish from schizophrenia. In the absence of history of use, analysis of urine must be depended on for diagnosis.

TREATMENT. Management of the PCP-intoxicated patient includes placement in a darkened, quiet room on a floor pad, safe from injury. Diazepam, in a dose of 10–20 mg orally or 10 mg intramuscularly every 4 hr, may be helpful if the patient is agitated and not comatose. Ammonium chloride, 500 mg every 6 hr, may be administered orally or by nasogastric tube to maintain urinary pH at 5.5–6, which enhances urinary clearance of PCP. Supportive therapy of the comatose patient is indicated with particular attention to hydration, which may be compromised by PCP-induced diuresis.

Mushrooms

Mushrooms cause both cholinergic and anticholinergic effects, in addition to the sought-after euphoria and hallucinations. Most adverse effects associated with their use are usually self-limited and do not require therapy. Mushrooms containing psilocybin and related antiserotonergic indoles cause LSD-like reactions and agitation and may require treatment with diazepam. Because most hallucination-seeking adolescents are not expert mycologists, mushrooms with other toxic and even fatal effects may be ingested accidentally. Treatment is by induction of vomiting and activated charcoal (see Chapter 666).

Jimsonweed

(*Datura stramonium*)

This is also known as "devil's weed," "locoweed," "stinkweed," and thornapple and grows wild throughout the United States. The seeds, which appear in the autumn, contain alkaloids including hyoscyamine as well as atropine and scopolamine. One hundred seeds, the upper limit of contents of a single pod, contain the equivalent of 6 mg of atropine. Ingestion of the seeds or other plant parts produces dose-related CNS and other anticholinergic effects that range from restlessness, disorientation, and the desired hallucinations at the lower dose range to lethargy and coma and, rarely, convulsions when larger doses are used. The presence of dry mouth, dry hot skin, fever, mydriasis, cycloplegia, urinary retention, and sinus tachycardia, in conjunction with delirium and visual or auditory hallucinations, should alert the physician to the possibility of jimsonweed intoxication.

In addition to supportive care, physostigmine salicylate, an anticholinesterase, is indicated for the treatment of hypertension, convulsions, severe hallucinations, or supraventricular tachyarrhythmias. This agent is administered slowly by the IV route for 2–5 min in an initial dose of 1–2 mg. This dose can be repeated in 20 min. If cholinergic symptoms result from physostigmine administration, atropine sulfate may be given in a dose of 0.5 mg for each milligram of physostigmine.

105.3 Volatile Substances

The practice of inhalation of a variety of euphoriants has enjoyed popularity among adolescents for centuries. The first well-described documentation of this phenomenon related to an "epidemic" of ether sniffing by Irish teenagers in the 19th century. In recent history, the easy availability and low cost of substances such as airplane glue, freons, paint thinners, butane gas lighter refills, and gasoline have provided young adolescents with a wide range of potential hallucinogens. They have been responsible for a similarly wide range of complications, relating to chemical toxicity, to the method of administration (e.g., in plastic bags, with resultant suffocation), and to the often dangerous setting in which the inhalation occurs (e.g., inner-city roof tops).

Airplane glue enjoyed great popularity among young adolescents in the late 1960s and early 1970s and continues to be a problem in some areas of the United States. Toluene, its main ingredient, is excreted rapidly in the urine as hippuric acid, with the residual detectable in the serum by gas chromatography. The glue causes relaxation and pleasant hallucinations for up to 2 hr. Tolerance and physical dependence may occur. Its toxicity is acute as well as chronic. Death in the acute phase may result from cerebral or pulmonary edema or myocardial involvement. Chronic use may cause pulmonary hypertension, restrictive lung defects or reduced diffusion capacity, peripheral neuropathy, acute rhabdomyolysis, hematuria, tubular acidosis, and possibly cerebral and cerebellar atrophy.

Gasoline sniffing is popular among rural adolescents and American Indian youth and may cause ataxia, nausea, and loss of consciousness. Euphoria followed by violent excitement and coma may result from prolonged or rapid inhalation. The long-term effects of chronic exposure include irreversible encephalopathy, bone marrow aplasia (from benzene), and lead encephalopathy when the gasoline contains tetraethyl lead.

Inhalation of *aerosol products*, such as hair sprays, deodorants, frying pan lubricants, and cocktail glass chillers, has also become popular. The method of dispensation involves fluorocarbon propellants (freons) that have been implicated in cardiac sensitization to epinephrine, resulting in arrhythmias and death following inhalation.

A variety of *volatile nitrites*, such as amyl nitrite, butyl nitrite, and related compounds marketed as room deodorizers, are used as euphoriants, enhancers of musical appreciation, and aphrodisiacs among older adolescents and young adults. They may result in headaches, syncope, and lightheadedness; profound hypotension and cutaneous flushing followed by vasoconstriction and tachycardia; transiently inverted T waves and depressed ST segments on electrocardiogram; methemoglobinemia, increased bronchial irritation, and increased intraocular pressure.

105.4 Marijuana

Marijuana and alcohol, the most popular substances of abuse among adolescents, share a number of psychopharmacologic qualities. Both decrease short-term memory and fine coordination, prolong reaction time, and produce "mental clouding." About 300 mg of cannabis is equivalent to 70 g of alcohol.

PHARMACOLOGY. *Marijuana* (THC, "pot," "weed," "hash," "grass") is synthesized from the resin of the *Cannabis sativa* plant, which flourishes in temperate and hot, dry climates. The tetrahydrocannabinol (THC) fraction of the resin is responsible for its hallucinogenic properties and has been synthesized (δ-9-THC). THC is absorbed rapidly by the nasal or oral routes, producing a peak of subjective effect at 10 min and 1 hr, respectively. Marijuana is generally consumed as a "reefer" or joint, made by rolling the crushed plant material in paper. Although there is much variation in content, each cigarette contains approximately 1 g of marijuana or 20 mg of δ-9-THC.

CLINICAL MANIFESTATIONS. In addition to the "desired" effects of elation and euphoria, marijuana may cause impairment of short-term memory, poor performance of tasks requiring divided attention (e.g., those involved in driving), loss of critical judgment, and distortion of time perception. Visual hallucinations and perceived body distortions occur rarely, but there may be "flashbacks" or recall of frightening hallucinations experienced under marijuana's influence that occur usually during stress or with fever.

Temperature may be lowered. Tachycardia is apparent within 20 min of smoking marijuana and is followed ½ hr later by transient systolic and diastolic hypertension, which disappears by 3 hr. Tachypnea is observed only in the experienced user. In placebo-controlled studies of experienced users, smoking marijuana caused hypercapnic ventilation and a decrease in forced expired volume, maximal midexpiratory flow rate, airway conductance, and diffusing capacity. Reduction in bronchospasm has also been demonstrated. Both δ-9-THC and marijuana (smoking a single joint) cause a significant fall in intraocular pressure, lasting for up to 5 hr in normal persons as well as in patients with glaucoma.

Kolodny demonstrated dose-related suppression of plasma testosterone levels and spermatogenesis as a result of smoking marijuana for a minimum of 4 days/wk for 6 mo, prompting concern about the potential deleterious effect of smoking marijuana before completion of pubertal growth and development. Smoking marijuana for 1 wk also decreases glucose tolerance. There is an antiemetic effect of oral THC or smoked marijuana, often followed by appetite stimulation, which is the basis of the drug's use in patients receiving cancer chemotherapy. Although the possibility of teratogenicity and carcinogenesis has been raised because of findings in animals, there is not evidence for such effects in humans at this time. There is no proof of physiologic dependency.

105.5 Cocaine

Cocaine, the most expensive of the inhalants, was not widely used by adolescents before the 1980s. However, its increased availability and decreased cost have now caused its popularity to grow in this age group.

PHARMACOLOGY. The alkaloid extracted from the leaves of the South American *Erythroxylon coca* is supplied as the hydrochloride salt in crystalline form. It is rapidly absorbed from the nasal mucosa, detoxified by the liver, and excreted in the urine as benzoyl ecgonine. Its half-life is slightly more than 1 hr, yet social custom often dictates its repeated administration every 15 min. The perceived effect of "snorting" cocaine may be influenced by some of the many diluents now being added to or actually substituted for the drug (heroin, amphetamines, PCP, or fillers such as mannitol or quinine).

Smoking the cocaine alkaloid ("free basing") in pipes or cigarettes, mixed with tobacco, marijuana, parsley, or as a paste, has become a popular method of use. The effects of smoking in this way appear to be exaggerations of those achieved by other routes. Accidental burns are potential complications of this practice.

CLINICAL MANIFESTATIONS. Cocaine causes euphoria, increased motor activity, decreased fatigability, and occasionally paranoid ideation. Its sympathomimetic properties are responsible for tachycardia, hypertension, and hyperthermia. Binge patterns of use are common. Usage in group settings has been associated with sexual promiscuity and increased risks of sexually transmitted infections. The chronic user may develop tolerance to these physiologic effects, and psychologic dependence may occur. Withdrawal symptoms upon its discontinuation have not, however, been reported, suggesting that physical dependency is not a problem. Pregnant adolescents who use cocaine place their fetus at risk for premature delivery and complications of low birth weight possibly congenital malformations, and developmental disorders.

TREATMENT. Intensive supportive therapy is directed at the clinical manifestations of acute intoxication. See Chapter 105.1 (Treatment) for chronic management.

105.6 Cigarette Smoking

More than 13% of adolescents smoke cigarettes, and the rate among women continues to increase, presumably owing to their appetite-suppressing effect. The severity of atherosclerosis may be correlated with the duration of smoking, increasing its risk among those who begin smoking during adolescence. In addition, adverse health effects of smoking may occur even during adolescence itself. These adverse effects include an increased prevalence of chronic cough, phlegm production, and wheezing. Smoking during pregnancy is associated with an average decrease in fetal weight of 200 g; this, added to the already smaller size of infants born to teenagers, increases perinatal morbidity and mortality. Smoking in combination with use of estrogen-containing oral contraceptives is associated with increased risk of myocardial infarction. Tobacco smoke induces hepatic smooth endoplasmic reticulum and, as a result, may also influence metabolism of drugs and of endogenously produced hormones. Phenacetin, theophylline, and imipramine are examples of drugs affected in this manner. In addition, laboratory test results may be affected by smoking, for example, white blood cell count, hemoglobin, hematocrit, mean corpuscular volume, and platelet aggregation are increased and serum creatinine, albumin, globulin (in females), and uric acid (in males) are decreased. See Chapter 360.

SMOKELESS TOBACCO. Chewing tobacco may result in lesions, primarily in the mandibular mucobuccal fold. With chronic use these may become malignant.

105.7 Alcohol

Alcohol use among adolescents has increased during the past decade and poses a threat to the normal functioning of the teenager as well as to the lives of those potentially jeopardized by drunken drivers. The usual progression is from beer to wine to hard liquor, although regional differences may alter this pattern. Four ounces of hard liquor (86 proof) consumed on an empty stomach produces a plasma ethanol level of approximately 65 mg/dL in an adult male of average weight and 80 mg/dL in a premenstrual female of adult weight. The legal definition of intoxication in most statutes is a blood ethanol level of 100 mg/dL (0.08% or 0.10%).

PHARMACOLOGY AND PATHOPHYSIOLOGY. Alcohol (ethyl alcohol or ethanol) is rapidly absorbed from the stomach, transported to the liver, and metabolized by two pathways. The primary pathway involves removal of two hydrogen atoms to form acetaldehyde, a reaction catalyzed by alcohol dehydrogenase through reduction of a cofactor nicotinamide-adenine dinucleotide. The removed hydrogen atoms supply energy (7.1 kcal/g of alcohol) and contribute to the excess synthesis of triglycerides, a phenomenon that is responsible for producing a fatty liver, even in those who are well nourished. Engorgement of hepatocytes with fat causes necrosis, triggering an inflammatory process (alcoholic hepatitis), which is followed by fibrosis, the hallmark of cirrhosis. Early hepatic involvement may result in elevation in γ-glutamyl transpeptidase and serum glutamic-pyruvic transaminase; cirrhosis has been reported in native American adolescents. The 2nd metabolic pathway, which is utilized at high serum alcohol levels, involves the microsomal system of the liver, in which the cofactor is reduced nicotinamide-adenine dinucleotide phosphate. The net effect of activation of this pathway is to decrease metabolism of drugs that share this system and to allow for their accumulation, enhanced effect, and possible toxicity (e.g., drinking alcohol and ingesting tranquilizers results in potentiation of each [see Table 105–2]).

CLINICAL MANIFESTATIONS. Alcohol acts primarily as a CNS depressant. It produces euphoria, grogginess, talkativeness, and impaired short-term memory, and it increases the pain threshold and the time needed to brake a car under simulated driving conditions. Alcohol's ability to produce vasodilation and hypothermia is also centrally mediated. At very high serum levels, respiratory depression occurs. Its inhibitory effect on pituitary antidiuretic hormone release is responsible for its diuretic effect.

The most common gastrointestinal complication of alcohol use is acute erosive gastritis, which is manifested by epigastric pain, anorexia, vomiting, and guaiac-positive stools. Less commonly, vomiting and midabdominal pain may be caused by acute alcoholic pancreatitis; diagnosis is confirmed by the finding of an elevated serum amylase and lipase activities.

Physiologic dependence upon alcohol may develop in the adolescent who uses it daily over a period of weeks. In such individuals, alcohol deprivation may precipitate a **withdrawal** or **abstinence syndrome** whose manifestations in adolescents are generally mild, occurring within 8 hr of the last dose and lasting no longer than 48 hr in the untreated patient. Anxiety, tremor, insomnia, and irritability are common symptoms. Only rarely are severe reactions found in older adolescents who have been drinking steadily for 1 yr or more; these consist of auditory or visual hallucinations, hyperthermia, delirium, and seizures occurring 48 hr or more after the last drink.

DIAGNOSIS. The *alcohol overdose syndrome* should be suspected in any teenager who appears disoriented, lethargic, or comatose. Whereas the distinctive aroma of alcohol may assist in diagnosis, confirmation by analysis of blood is recommended. There is a high correlation between results obtained by serum and breath analyses so that the latter method may be reliably used. At levels greater than 200 mg/dL, the adolescent is at risk of death, and levels greater than 500 mg/dL (median lethal dose) are usually associated with a fatal outcome. When the level of depression appears excessive for the reported blood level, head trauma or ingestion of other drugs should be considered as possible confounding factors.

TREATMENT. The usual mechanism of death from the alcohol overdose syndrome is respiratory depression, and artificial ventilatory support must be provided until the liver can eliminate sufficient amounts of alcohol from the body. In a patient without alcoholism it generally takes 20 hr to reduce the blood level of alcohol from 400 mg/dL to zero. Dialysis should be considered when the blood level is higher than 400 mg/dL.

Treatment of the alcohol withdrawal or abstinence syndrome uses drugs that are cross-tolerant with alcohol but that have a longer duration of action, such as benzadiazepine derivatives, of which chlordiazepoxide (Librium) is the most popular. The usual regimen consists of an initial oral dose of 25 mg every 6 hr. If a satisfactory effect is not achieved, the dose is repeated at 2-hr intervals. Once symptomatic relief is obtained, the dose is tapered by 25 mg/day.

105.8 Anabolic Steroids

The age-old quest for enhanced athletic performance has led to the phenomenon of abuse of anabolic steroids by competitive athletes of both sexes. It is estimated that 3–5% of all high-school students are users, with a 10% prevalence rate among male adolescent athletes. The perception that these agents increase muscle mass and strength is not supported by objective data, but harmful side effects clearly occur. Among the adverse physical effects are abnormalities of the liver (e.g., hepatocarcinoma, peliosis hepatis, cholestasis); endocrine effects (e.g., in males: gynecomastia, lowered plasma testosterone and gonadotropin levels, testicular atrophy; in females: hirsutism, baldness, deepening of voice, breast atrophy, clitoral enlargement, acne, inhibition of ovulation, menstrual abnormalities, alopecia); effects on cardiovascular risk factors (e.g., increased levels of low-density lipoprotein and decreased levels of high-density lipoprotein cholesterol); and fluid retention. In addition to these effects that occur in individuals of all ages, the adolescent is at risk for growth retardation owing to the possibility of rapid advancement of epiphyseal closure. Serious psychologic effects also have been reported from use of high doses of these agents (often 100 times therapeutic doses), including uncontrollable rage, depression, mania, mood fluctuations, and alterations in libido.

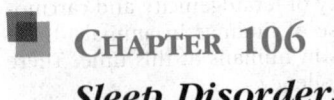

CHAPTER 106
Sleep Disorders

Also see Chapter 21.5.

The maturational changes in sleep patterns during adolescence indicate that between sex maturation stages (SMRs) 3 and 4 there is an increase in daytime sleepiness and a decrease in sleep latency. There is also a secretory spurt of gonadotropins and growth hormone with each completed sleep cycle during early puberty, a pattern not found at any other time of life. This normal pattern of sleep augmentation of gonadotropin secretion is disturbed in anorexia nervosa and possibly in other situations associated with significant weight loss (Chapter 107). The clinical association of sleep disorders with depression has long been appreciated. Shortened rapid eye movement (REM) latency appears to be common in such patients.

Narcolepsy often first becomes symptomatic during adolescence. The syndrome includes (1) attacks of REM sleep during wakefulness, with excessive daytime sleepiness; (2) hypnagogic hallucinations, frightening and recurring visual hallucinations; (3) *cataplexy*, the sudden inhibition of tone of a muscle group, the effects dependent on the muscle group involved; and (4) sleep paralysis, a paralysis of voluntary musculature while falling asleep. The *sleep apnea–hypersomnia syndrome* also may first become symptomatic during adolescence and consists of increased daytime sleepiness after multiple episodes of brief night-time waking after each of the apneic spells, which results from airway obstruction. Also see Chapter 330.

Insomnia affects 10–20% of adolescents. The cause may be depression or the delayed sleep phase syndrome in which the difficulty lies in falling asleep rather than awakening once sleep has begun. According to Anders, "adolescents may be particularly susceptible to this syndrome, because the changing social demands, which result in later bedtimes, interract with the changing neuroendocrine secretion patterns of puberty, which affect sleep state relationships."

CHAPTER 107
Anorexia Nervosa and Bulimia

EPIDEMIOLOGY. The incidence of anorexia nervosa (AN) and bulimia has increased over the last 2 decades. It is estimated that 1 in every 100 females, 16–18 yr old, has anorexia nervosa. A bimodal distribution occurs, with one peak at 14.5 and the other at 18 yr; 25% may be younger than the age of 13. The increased incidence has been documented in all Western countries, with sporadic reports from other nations. Affected females outnumber males by 10 to 1. Initially reported only in middle and upper socioeconomic groups, AN is now occurring in those from the lower socioeconomic levels. It is being diagnosed in a variety of ethnic and racial groups. Bulimia is more common than AN. An increased incidence of eating disorders among primary relatives of those with AN and bulimia suggests a familial basis.

DIAGNOSIS. The *Diagnostic and Statistical Manual of Mental Disorders (DSM-IV)* criteria for the diagnosis of AN include (1) intense fear of becoming obese, which does not diminish as weight loss progresses; (2) disturbance in the way in which one's body weight, size, or shape is experienced (e.g., claiming to "feel fat" even when one is emaciated or believing that one area of the body is "too fat" even when obviously underweight); (3) refusal to maintain body weight over a minimal normal weight for age and height (e.g., weight loss leading to maintenance of body weight 15% below expected, failure to make expected weight gain during period of growth leading to body weight 15% below expected); and (4) in females, absence of at least three consecutive menstrual cycles when otherwise expected to occur (primary or secondary amenorrhea).

AN is characterized further by excessive physical activity in the face of apparent inanition, denial of hunger, preoccupation with food preparation, frequently accompanied by bizarre eating behaviors, and often studiousness and academic success. Most patients are described as having been "model children" before the onset of the illness. Patients who have AN are subdivided into the *restrictor* and *bulimia* subgroups, according to their method of caloric reduction. Restrictors severely limit their intake of carbohydrate and fat-containing foods, whereas bulimics tend to eat in binges and then to purge themselves of food by self-induced vomiting or the use of cathartics. The binge-purge pattern may occur in youngsters who have normal weight or are slightly obese.

DSM-IV separates *bulimia* from AN as a diagnostic entity, defining bulimia as (1) recurrent episodes of binge eating (rapid consumption of a large amount of food in a discrete period of time, usually less than 2 hr); (2) during the eating binges, a fear of not being able to stop eating; (3) regularly engaging in self-induced vomiting, use of laxatives, or rigorous dieting or fasting in order to counteract the effects of binge eating; (4) a minimum average of two binge eating episodes per week for at least 3 mo; and (5) self-evaluation is unduly influenced by body weight and shape, but the disturbance does not occur exclusively during episodes of AN.

ETIOLOGY AND PSYCHODYNAMICS. Eating disorders commonly begin as innocent dieting behavior, not unlike that seen in many other adolescent women, but those with AN gradually progress to profound weight loss with emaciation. Premorbid psychiatric characteristics of patients with AN include excessive dependency, developmental immaturity, and isolation. Their families have been described as having difficulty with problem solving and as being intrusive and overprotective. The onset of these conditions at the time of puberty has prompted psychoanalysts to regard them as defenses against emerging sexuality, an opinion that dominated thinking until the 1950s, when Bruch conceptualized AN as a problem in identity development. Others consider that AN may represent a disorder of mood accompanied by manic or depressive symptomatology. Patients with AN have also been subcategorized on the basis of psychologic characteristics in order to demonstrate that different subgroups are dynamically and prognostically different. Biogenic amine neurotransmitter abnormalities are found in some patients with AN. Their etiologic significance is unclear.

CLINICAL MANIFESTATIONS. AN and bulimia are associated with disturbances in almost every organ system, although it is uncertain which may be primary and which is the result of severe malnutrition. The death rate in AN is approximately 10% and is usually caused by severe electrolyte disturbance, cardiac arrhythmia, or congestive heart failure in the recovery phase. *Bradycardia and postural hypotension* are common, with pulse rates as low as 20/min. Both improve with nutritional therapy. A variety of electrocardiographic abnormalities are common, including low voltage, T-wave inversion and flattening, and ST depression, as well as supraventricular and ventricular dysrhythmias, some preceded by a prolonged QT_c interval. Death from congestive heart failure is a late event and may result from unduly rapid rehydration and refeeding. On a regimen achieving a daily weight gain limited to 0.2–0.4 kg, none of our patients has experienced this complication.

Sleep disturbances occur in some anorexics and include a short rapid eye movement latency time, similar to that often found in depressed patients. Problems of thermal regulation, particularly hypothermia, are very common (15% of our patients had temperatures recorded below 35° C). Hypothermia also occurs in some bulimics of normal weight. Disorders of the hypothalamic-pituitary-ovarian axis are manifested as amenorrhea associated with immature patterns of secretion of luteinizing hormone. These findings may represent a primary hypothalamic defect rather than being secondary to weight loss (which also causes amenorrhea), in as much as amenorrhea antedates weight loss in one-third to one-half of patients with AN, and a similar proportion fail to resume menses when normal weight is restored. One-quarter of patients may be amenorrheic 8 yr later, despite weight rehabilitation. Evidence for hypothalamic-pituitary-adrenal axis dysfunction includes increased secretion of cortisol, loss of diurnal variation in its secretion, and failure of dexamethasone to suppress it. The last may also be found in starvation; however, in 44% of our patients with AN, abnormal results of dexamethasone suppression tests have persisted after weight rehabilitation. Growth hormone secretion is abnormally high in these patients, and somatomedin-C is low. Thyroid-stimulating hormone levels are normal, thyroxine and triiodothyronine (T_3) are low, and reverse T_3 is elevated, presumably in adaptation to a lowered basal metabolic rate as a result of malnutrition and carbohydrate deprivation. Peripheral edema in some patients, in the absence of congestive heart failure or hypoproteinemia, has been attributed to inappropriate secretion of antidiuretic hormone.

Elevations of blood urea nitrogen may occur reflecting dehydration and decreased glomerular filtration rate, but normal levels may be found under these same conditions because of low protein intake even in the dehydrated patient. Mild proteinuria, hematuria, and pyuria, with negative urine cultures, generally resolve with proper rehydration. Pseudoproteinuria is often found because the alkalinity of the urine gives a false-positive reaction to albumin on the dipstick.

Bone marrow hypoplasia is common in AN, with leukopenia, anemia, and (rarely) thrombocytopenia. Low erythrocyte sedimentation rates are common, perhaps reflecting low fibrinogen production secondary to malnutrition.

Constipation is a very common complication of motility problems in AN, as is esophagitis in those who vomit. Decreased gastrointestinal tract motility may be a cause of perforation, which has been reported to occur when a nasogastric tube has been inserted in patients who refuse to eat. Elevations in amylase levels may be associated with bilateral parotid swelling or with pancreatitis.

Electrolyte imbalance results from vomiting, "waterloading" (a practice of surreptitiously drinking large amounts of water in order to achieve an agreed-upon weight gain), or abuse of diuretics or laxatives. Potassium depletion, associated with a hypochloremic alkalosis, is very common. Abnormalities of calcium, magnesium, and phosphorus metabolism may result from laxative abuse, either secondary to malabsorption or to use of preparations containing phosphate.

Patients with AN appear to be remarkably resistant to infection, and the few studies of their immunologic status support this view. The fact that protein intake is relatively good in these otherwise malnourished persons may contribute to this finding. Bone density may be abnormally low, but this osteopenia appears to improve with weight gain. A number of possible mechanisms have been suggested to explain this finding, including low levels of estrogen and calcium and elevated cortisol levels. The skin of patients with AN is dry, and lanugo hair is often seen. Hair loss often occurs in the refeeding phase.

TREATMENT. Systematic, controlled studies of treatment in these disorders are not available. Most of the regimens in current use combine psychotherapy (individual and family), behavior modification techniques, and nutritional rehabilitation. Pharmacologic therapy (primarily of antidepressant medications) appears to be helpful for that subset of depressed patients with eating disorders. The success rate in short-term follow-up studies is about 70%. The frequent occurrence of medical complications and the possibility of death during the acute or rehabilitation phase require the inclusion of a medically and physiologically oriented physician in the management team.

Chapter 108
Pregnancy

For women aged 15–19 the *pregnancy rate* in the United States was 109 per 1000 in 1988, the highest rate among developed countries. The number of births among teenagers has been rising since 1985, despite a decline of teenagers in this age cohort because of an upturn in the birth rate among teenagers. Additional cause for continuing concern arises from the fact that more than two-thirds of the births among teenagers in 1989 involved unmarried mothers. Among those whose pregnancy went to term, there was an increase in teenaged mothers who chose to keep their infants rather than place them for adoption. In addition, there were between 10,200 and 11,800 births to girls younger than 15 yr in each year between 1970 and 1989. This younger group is at increased risk for obstetric and perinatal complications, such as toxemia, postpartum hemorrhage, postpartum infection, infants who are small for gestational age, and stillborn infants.

Adolescent mothers are less likely to marry or to achieve a high-school education, and they are more likely to be unemployed, live in poverty, and have a larger number of children compared with women who postpone childbearing until after 20 yr of age. Children born to teenage mothers have an increased risk of experiencing an accident within the home and of being hospitalized before 5 yr of age.

Because most pregnancies in adolescents are unintended (80%), the challenge to pediatricians, as well as to parents and educators, is to assist in *pregnancy prevention*. Fewer than half of teenagers use any form of contraception at the time of first intercourse. The birth control methods they do use are rarely effective. The lag between becoming sexually active and seeking effective contraception usually exceeds 1 yr. As a result, almost 40% of sexually active teenagers become pregnant within 2 yr of initiating intercourse.

The pediatrician rarely has an opportunity for primary prevention of pregnancy. Discussions of abstinence are usually ignored; on the other hand, stimulating a young girl who has a boyfriend to think about whether she feels ready for intercourse may be helpful if done nonjudgmentally. For the already sexually active adolescent, information, access to, and motivation to use contraception are all necessary for successful pregnancy prevention. The last is most difficult to achieve because many girls who have been sexually active without getting pregnant assume that they are sterile and are not in need of contraception. They are unlikely to use any contraceptive method until they are made to feel vulnerable to an unwanted pregnancy. Those who have become pregnant in the past, and thus have proved their fertility, may shun contraception after vowing that they will be abstinent or out of fear that their fertility has been impaired, as a result of an abortion, infection, or some less well-founded concern. Therefore, it is helpful to inquire about the reason why any sexually active female thinks she has not become pregnant.

Once it is established that the teenager is not pregnant, that intercourse is likely to continue, and that the patient accepts the fact that she is at risk for pregnancy, efforts should be directed toward provision of the most effective and safest contraceptive method. To enhance the likelihood of compliance once the method is prescribed, the physician must learn about the frequency and circumstances of intercourse; past experience and compliance with both contraceptive and non-contraceptive chronic medications; the partner's attitudes about various methods; and parents' knowledge and attitudes about contraception. In the United States, physicians may provide contraception to minors without parental knowledge, but it is helpful in choosing a method to know whether the parents are aware of their daughter's sexual activity.

CHAPTER 109
Contraception

The risk of any contraceptive method should be weighed against the risk of pregnancy, which for young adolescents is a significant one. If contraception is to be successful, however, every effort must be made to individualize the method to the needs of each patient. The risks, benefits, and indications for each of the available methods follow:

Barrier Methods

CONDOM. This method prevents sperm from being deposited in the vagina. There are no major side effects associated with the use of a condom. Its effectiveness in preventing pregnancy is low, however, with 15 pregnancies occurring per 100 woman-years of use by adult women in the United States. No comparative figures are available for adolescents, but acceptance of this method is low in this age group. A 1979 study found that only 23% of 15- to 19-yr-old females reported that their partner ever used a condom. The recent acquired immunodeficiency syndrome (AIDS) scare appears to have increased the use of condoms only among older adolescents. Condoms used in the United States are thicker than those marketed in other countries where they enjoy widespread use. The main advantages of condoms are their low price, availability without prescription, little need for advanced planning, and, most important for this age group, their effectiveness in preventing transmission of sexually transmitted diseases, including human immunodeficiency virus (HIV). A condom to be attached to the vagina, the "female condom," is now available.

DIAPHRAGM. The diaphragm acts by preventing access of sperm to the cervix, while placing spermicidal jelly in a position to be effective. Other than rare cases of contact vaginitis caused by the latex or by the powder used to preserve the diaphragm, there are no adverse side effects associated with its use. Like the condom, the diaphragm is effective in only 85% of women who use it properly. In a study of adolescents who were highly motivated to avoid pregnancy, however, use of a diaphragm was associated with only 2 pregnancies per 100 woman-years. Adolescents may object to the messiness of the jelly or to the fact that the insertion of a diaphragm may interrupt the spontaneity of sex, or they may express discomfort about touching their genitalia. At Stanford University this method is currently used by 21% of sexually active women students, whereas in other studies only 3.5% of 15- to 19-yr-olds chose this method.

A diaphragm must be fitted individually by a trained physician or nurse practitioner. Once fitted, the same diaphragm may be used for 3 yr unless extreme weight gain or loss or pregnancy occurs. After the proper diaphragm is selected, it is important that the teenager be given instructions and ample opportunity to learn to insert and remove it before leaving the office.

CERVICAL CAP. This method is currently being evaluated. The rubber cap, after proper fitting, remains affixed to the cervix by suction for 1–3 intermenstrual days. Like the diaphragm, it must be used in conjunction with spermicidal jelly.

Spermicides

A variety of agents containing the spermicide nonoxynol-9 are available as foams, jellies, creams, or effervescent vaginal suppositories. They must be placed in the vaginal cavity shortly before intercourse and reinserted before each ejaculation in order to be effective. Rare side effects consist of contact vaginitis. Effectiveness is in the range of the barrier methods (approximately 85%), but the finding that nonoxynol-9 is gonococcocidal and spirocheticidal enhances the attractiveness of these agents for adolescents because of the high incidence of sexually transmitted diseases in this group.

Combination Methods

The conjoint use of condom by the male and spermicidal foam by the female adolescent is extremely effective; the failure rate is 2%, without any of the potential side effects and complications associated with the use of other forms of contraception having comparable efficacy. This combination also prevents sexually transmitted diseases, including HIV. The contraceptive sponge, which incorporates the theoretical advantages of barrier and spermicides, has been marketed over the counter, but its efficacy appears to be that of either barrier or spermicide, rather than that found for the combination of foam and condom. Toxic shock syndrome has been reported in users of the sponge, a further reason that caution be used in prescribing this method for teenagers, who are at increased risk for this disease (Chapter 174.3).

Hormonal Methods

These methods currently employ either an estrogenic substance in combination with a progestin or a progestin alone. The action of the estrogen-progestin combination is to prevent the surge of leutinizing hormone and, as a result, to inhibit ovulation. Progestin may prevent ovulation, but this is not reliable. It does, however, affect fallopian tube transport and the composition of cervical mucus in such a way as to make fertilization or implantation less likely.

Combination oral contraceptives are commonly referred to as "the pill" and currently contain either 80, 50, or 35 μg of estrogenic substance, typically either mestranol or ethinyl estradiol, and a progestin. Thrombophlebitis, hepatic adenomas, myocardial infarction, and carbohydrate intolerance are some of the more serious potential complications of use of exogenous estrogens. These disorders are, however, exceedingly rare in adolescents.

Some long-range beneficial effects of estrogen use include decreased risks of benign breast disease, ovarian disease, and anemia. However, adolescents taking estrogen-containing oral contraceptives are reported to have higher levels of high-density lipoproteins than those of controls. Inhibition of ovulation or the suppressant effect of estrogens on prostaglandin production by the endometrium make oral contraceptives effective in preventing dysmenorrhea (Chapter 111).

A potentially untoward effect of estrogens on epiphyseal growth does not occur either because the amount in oral contraceptives is small or because they are taken at a time when most growth has been completed. Post-pill amenorrhea occurs with greater frequency in adolescents than in adults. It may persist for up to 18 mo after the discontinuation of use of the pill. The increased risk may not be due to age alone but may reflect oligomenorrhea or low body weight (less than 47 kg) before the initiation of use of the pill. Acne may be worsened by some and improved by other oral contraceptive preparations. Contraindications to use of estrogen-containing oral contraceptives include hepatocellular disease, migraine headaches, diabetes mellitus, and any condition in which hypercoagulability may be a problem (e.g., replaced cardiac valve, thrombophlebitis, sickle cell anemia) owing to the increased levels of factor VIII and decreased production of antithrombin III.

The pill is one of the most reliable contraceptive methods available, with a pregnancy rate in the range of 0.8% per yr. Some side effects can, without sacrificing their efficacy, be minimized by the use of preparations of low estrogen content. With the use of the 35-μg preparation, however, there may be a higher incidence of breakthrough bleeding, which may lead to noncompliance.

All-progestin contraceptives are available for the adolescent in whom use of estrogen is potentially deleterious, for example, those with liver disease, replaced cardiac valves, or hypercoagulable states. They ("mini-pills") are less reliable in inhibiting ovulation and are associated with a 2.4% per yr pregnancy rate. Acceptance by adolescents is limited by the necessity to take the pill daily, the higher incidence of amenorrhea, and increased bleeding.

An **injectable progestin,** medroxyprogesterone (Depo-Provera), is highly effective in birth control. This substance needs to be administered only once every 3 mo and is completely reversible in its anovulatory action; furthermore, the cessation of menses is conterminous with its use. This agent is particularly attractive for adolescents who have difficulty with compliance or for mentally retarded teenagers.

A *long-acting progestational agent,* levonorgestrel (Norplant) may be contained in a small Silastic tube that is implanted subcutaneously. It can be easily removed, and the contraceptive potency remains for 5 yr. Its use in teenagers is currently under study because it has recently been released for use by the U.S. Food and Drug Administration.

Postcoital Contraception

Unprotected intercourse at midcycle carries a pregnancy risk of 2–30%. The risk may be reduced or eliminated by intervention within 72 hr after unprotected intercourse. Norgestrel (Ovral), a combination oral contraceptive, may be administered in a dose of two pills initially after coitus and two additional pills 12 hr later.

Intrauterine Devices

Intrauterine devices (IUDs) are small, flexible, plastic objects introduced into the uterine cavity through the cervix. They differ in size, shape, and the presence or absence of pharmacologically active substances (e.g., copper or progesterone). The mechanism of action of IUDs is uncertain, although they render the endometrium unsuitable for implantation by inducing a local polymorphonuclear leukocyte response, production of prostaglandins E_2 and $F_{2\alpha}$, and stimulation of uterine contractility. They are effective in preventing pregnancy in 97–99% of women. Women who become pregnant with an IUD in place, however, are at greater risk for having an ectopic pregnancy, especially if the IUD contains progesterone. Additional problems associated with the use of an IUD are increased menstrual bleeding (less so with the newer, smaller versions); increased dysmenorrhea (although those containing progesterone reportedly decrease dysmenorrhea); and of most concern, increased risk of infection, including the risks of septic abortion and death. The highest risk was associated with the use of the Dalkon Shield, which has now been removed from the market. Infection risk varies among the other types of IUDs, being highest with the progesterone-containing IUDs. The small amount of copper that leaches out of the copper-containing IUDs is bactericidal. The risk of infection also varies with characteristics of the patient; young patients and those with multiple sexual partners are at increased risk. The increased risk of infection should limit the prescription of an IUD to teenagers who require passive contraception as a last resort. IUDs were initially proscribed in nulliparous adolescents because of a high rate of expulsion. The newer, smaller types are well tolerated.

CHAPTER 110
Sexually Transmitted Diseases

Adolescents have the highest rate of sexually transmitted disease of any age group. This results from sexual experimentation that characterizes psychosocial development at this time as well as from certain aspects of biologic development. During puberty, increasing levels of estrogen cause the vaginal epithelium to thicken and cornify and cellular glycogen content to rise, the latter causing vaginal pH to fall. These changes increase the resistance of the vaginal epithelium to penetration by certain organisms (including *Gonococcus*) and increase the susceptibility to others (e.g., *Candida albicans* and *Trichomonas*). As a result of these physiologic changes, gonococcal infection becomes primarily cervical, and susceptibility to ascending infection is greatest during menses, when the pH is 6.8–7.0.

Failure to use any contraceptive method or, less frequently, the use of oral contraceptives characterizes most adolescent sexual relationships; both behaviors are conducive to the transmission of venereal organisms. Adolescents are typically reluctant to consider that a sexual partner may have a venereal disease and often lack the communication skills necessary to discuss this issue. Sexually active adolescents should be tested for sexually transmitted diseases, which are often asymptomatic. Minimizing noncompliance with treatment, finding and treating the sexual partner, and making every effort to preserve fertility are additional responsibilities. The latter often requires intensive parenteral therapy for salpingitis or tubo-ovarian abscess.

Diagnosis and therapy are often necessarily carried out within the context of a confidential relationship between the physician and the patient. Therefore, the need to report certain sexually transmitted diseases to health department authorities should be clarified at the outset. Most health departments will not violate confidentiality, if assured that treatment and case finding have been accomplished and that the patient can be expected to follow through in a responsible, mature manner. Gonorrhea, chlamydia, and human papilloma virus are the most common sexually transmitted diseases in adolescents.

GONORRHEA (See also Chapter 179). Infection occurs via the urethral, cervical, anal, pharyngeal, or conjunctival route. An initial inflammatory response is followed either by resolution with a fibrous response, by extension along mucosal planes to adjacent organs (endometrium, fallopian tubes, peritoneum, liver capsule in the female, or urethra, prostate, epididymis in the male), or by hematogenous dissemination to cause arthritis, dermatitis, or rarely meningitis or endocarditis.

Ceftriaxone has replaced penicillin as the drug of choice for the treatment of uncomplicated gonorrhea because of the emergence of strains resistant to the latter and because of the efficacy of a single 125 mg intramuscular dose of ceftriaxone against localized gonococcal infection as well as incubating syphilis in children 45 kg and above and over 9 yr of age. The patient's sexual partner also should be treated. Infection involving higher pelvic structures requires in-patient intravenous administration of cefoxitin, 2 g four times a day, and doxycycline, 100 mg twice a day for 10 days, to ensure compliance and to safeguard future fertility. Disseminated disease (e.g., arthritis, dermatitis) is treated with ceftriaxone 50 mg/kg/24 hr (max 0.2 g) intravenously for 7 days.

SYPHILIS (Chapter 201.1). The incidence of syphilis is rising in adolescents; accordingly, it is advisable to screen high-risk adolescents (e.g., those who are pregnant, sexually promiscuous, homosexual, delinquent, or have evidence of another sexually transmitted disease). The Venereal Disease Research Laboratories (VDRL) is the most sensitive and least specific of the serologic tests for syphilis. False-positive results may occur in intravenous abusers of drugs as well as in those who have liver disease of any cause, collagen-vascular disease, or infectious mononucleosis. A positive result on a test must be confirmed by the use of a more specific test, such as the treponemal immobilization test.

In the infected adolescent, the most common manifestations of syphilis are those of the secondary stage, including condyloma latum or lesions on the palms and soles. Treatment for primary and secondary syphilis is with penicillin benzathine, 2.4 million units intramuscularly (IM). After a rape, prevention of syphilis can be accomplished with the same regimen as for the prevention of gonorrhea (125 mg of ceftriaxone IM).

CHLAMYDIA (Chapter 197). Cases of sexually transmitted infection with *Chlamydia* have increased dramatically in adolescents during the past decade. Most cases of urethritis, previously called "nongonococcal," are now known to be chlamydial in origin, as are approximately one-half of the cases of salpingitis. Moreover, all of the complications of gonococcal infection (e.g., perihepatitis, conjunctivitis, sterility) are potential sequelae of chlamydial infection. Therefore, a laparoscopy, with tubal puncture and culture, is the optimal approach to etiologic diagnosis in salpingitis. If this is not feasible, therapy should address the possibility of either gonococcal or chlamydial cause (cefoxitin, 2 g intravenously [IV] four times a day, and doxycycline, 100 mg IV twice a day for 10 days). Doxycycline is specifically effective against *Chlamydia*, but as with any tetracycline, this drug is contraindicated during pregnancy. *Lymphogranuloma venereum (LGV)* is caused by an agent related to *Chlamydia trachomatis* and should be considered in the differential diagnosis of herpetiform lesions of the genitalia or of inguinal lymphadenopathy, as well as of rectal bleeding, purulent proctitis, or rectal stricture. The sexual history is, therefore, a mandatory part of the evaluation of adolescents thought to have inflammatory bowel disease, as well as a search for more obviously sexually related symptoms.

CHANCROID. Chancroid has increased in incidence recently. The initial lesion is a vesicopustule that rapidly breaks down to form a painful, purulent, sharply delineated ulcer without induration. This latter feature, in addition to its painful nature, helps to distinguish it from the syphilitic chancre with which it shares a similar distribution in the genital region. Autoinoculation may result in multiple lesions, and unilateral painful lymphadenopathy is not uncommon. Biopsy is required for definitive diagnosis. Chancroid is treated with one dose of ceftriaxone, 250 mg IM.

HERPES PROGENITALIS (See also Chapter 211). The characteristic herpetic lesion may be preceded by the less well-recognized symptom of exquisite sensitivity and sharp pain radiating from the perineum along the course of affected nerve roots. Palliation and shortening of the symptomatic and shedding phases in primary infections may be achieved by oral administration of acyclovir, 400 mg three times a day, for 7–10 days. In recurrent cases, acyclovir is less satisfactory; patients with recurrent episodes (>6 per yr) may be given chronic treatment with 200 mg 2–5 times daily. Yearly Papanicolaou (Pap) smears after infection with this premalignant agent are indicated. Cervical cultures may be positive in asymptomatic sexually active adolescents; Pap smears also should be obtained routinely from these adolescents.

HUMAN PAPILLOMA VIRUS (See Chapter 224). This agent is responsible for significant morbidity among adolescents, including genital warts (condylomata acuminata), subclinical infection, and the potential for oncogenic progression. Types 6, 11, and 42 are commonly expressed as warts of the anogenital area and types 16, 18, 31, 33, 35, and 39 as subclinical infections with high risk for dysplasia and cancer of the cervix. Application of a solution of 3–5% acetic acid may reveal mucosal or penile lesions as white plaques; their visualization is further enhanced by use of the colposcope. All patients with genital warts and their sexual partners should have such an examination in addition to Pap smears for females. The latter may reveal a spectrum of cytologic changes from koilocytes (cells with swollen nuclei surrounded by a halo) to cells with nuclear aneuploidy and abnormal mitotic figures (consistent with carcinoma in situ).

Local treatment of *condylomata acuminata* is associated with high failure rates. Application of trichloroacetic acid (85%) three times each week is the best of the chemical treatment methods; liquid nitrogen and podophyllin (20%) is preferred by some. Topical 5-fluorouracil, bleomycin, interferon, and the carbon dioxide laser are now being used for patients with extensive lesions or those who do not respond to other modes of therapy.

TRICHOMONAS. This infection is usually sexually transmitted; it may rarely occur in those who do not engage in sexual intercourse. The symptomatic female patient will have a frothy vaginal discharge. Although males may harbor the organism, they have few clinical manifestations. Diagnosis is based on identification of trichomonads on microscopic examination of a mixture of the discharge with saline. The treatment of both sexual partners with metronidazole (a single dose of 2.0 g orally) is advised unless pregnancy is suspected. The adolescent should be cautioned about the adverse effect (abdominal pain and vomiting) of alcohol ingestion within 24 hr of metronidazole administration.

HEMOPHILUS (GARDNERELLA) VAGINALIS. This is associated with the production of an often foul-smelling vaginal discharge, which gives off a fishy odor when 10% potassium hydroxide is added to a wet preparation, and with the appearance of "clue cells" (epithelial cells ringed with the rod-shaped organisms). The organism is frequently found in vaginal smears from asymptomatic women, but when other etiologic explanations are not found, treatment with metronidazole, 500 mg orally twice a day for 7 days, may bring relief.

HUMAN IMMUNODEFICIENCY VIRUS. (Chapter 223). The risk factors for contraction of infection with human immunodeficiency virus (HIV) include unprotected intercourse and intravenous drug use, both of which occur frequently among adolescents. Therefore, it is anticipated that the numbers of AIDS cases within this age group will increase dramatically. The long incubation period of HIV infection suggests that at least half of the 20- to 24-yr-olds diagnosed as having AIDS in 1988 contracted the infection as adolescents. Pediatricians should take responsibility for educating young people about the transmission of this infection and its prevention and for screening high-risk adolescents to identify those infected so that early treatment can be initiated.

Chapter 111 Menstrual Problems

111.1 Amenorrhea

Amenorrhea, or absence of menses, may be primary or secondary. *Primary amenorrhea* indicates that menarche has never occurred, whereas *secondary amenorrhea* refers to the cessation of menses for more than 3 mo after regular menstrual cycling has been established. The diagnosis of primary amenorrhea assumes that the patient has passed the age at which menarche normally occurs, from 10 to 16 yr. Accordingly, the determination of primary amenorrhea should first be based on an assessment of the patient's stage of pubertal development; 10% of girls have menarche at Sex Maturity Rating (SMR)2, 20% at SMR3, 60% at SMR4, and 10% at SMR5. If the patient has not entered puberty by the expected time or if pubertal development is completed without the onset of menses, she should be thoroughly evaluated, even if her chronologic age is within the normal range. Similarly, the close concordance between the age of menarche between daughters and mothers and among siblings should suggest this diagnosis when the patient is more than 1 yr older than was the mother or sisters when their menarche occurred.

The onset and continuation of normal menstrual cycling depend on the functional and anatomic integrity of (1) the hypothalamus together with higher centers, including possibly the pineal; (2) the anterior pituitary; (3) the ovary; and (4) the uterus. Evaluation of the adolescent with amenorrhea should include consideration of possible abnormalities at each of these levels.

ETIOLOGY. In *primary amenorrhea*, chromosomal or congenital abnormalities, such as gonadal dysgenesis, the triple-x syndrome, isochromosomal abnormalities, testicular feminization syndrome, and, rarely, true hermaphroditism, should be considered in addition to the conditions that cause secondary amenorrhea. Elevated levels of follicle-stimulating hormone (FSH) and leutinizing hormone (LH) suggest primary gonadal failure, and chromosome analysis will elucidate its cause. Once such a diagnosis is made, management includes the use of estrogen and progesterone to produce the development of secondary sex characteristics and cyclic bleeding if a uterus is present to help the patient to feel like her peers as well as to prevent later osteoporosis.

Primary or *secondary* amenorrhea also may be caused by chronic illness, particularly that associated with malnutrition or tissue hypoxia, such as diabetes mellitus, inflammatory bowel disease, cystic fibrosis, or cyanotic congenital heart disease. In most cases, the illness would have been diagnosed previously, but, occasionally, the amenorrhea is its first manifestation.

A central nervous system (CNS) tumor, most commonly a craniopharyngioma, may present with amenorrhea (Chapter 555). In addition to a careful neurologic examination, the finding of a low urine specific gravity, erosion of the clinoids, calcifications in the suprasellar area, or an elevated serum prolactin level (in the case of an adenoma) support the diagnosis of pituitary neoplasm.

Abnormalities of the thyroid gland, typically hyperthyroidism, may first be suspected by delayed sexual maturation or amenorrhea, even in the absence of other signs and symptoms. Hypothyroidism more typically causes precocious puberty and menometrorrhagia. Determination of thyroid-stimulating hormone (TSH), thyroxine (T_4), and triiodothyronine (T_3) assist in establishing this diagnosis. Anorexia nervosa, which may present with either primary or secondary amenorrhea (Chapter 107), is occasionally confused with hyperthyroidism because of weight loss, hyperactivity, and personality changes seen in both entities.

When primary amenorrhea occurs with advanced pubertal development, a structural anomaly of the müllerian duct system should be suspected. **Imperforate hymen** is most common and is associated with recurrent (monthly) abdominal pain and, after some time has passed, a midline lower abdominal mass, the blood-filled vagina, or **hematocolpos**. Diagnosis is made by inspection of the introitus, revealing a bulging hymen with bluish discoloration. If the obstruction is at the level of the cervix, the blood-filled uterus **(hematometrium)** will be apparent on bimanual examination or ultrasonograph. Agenesis of the cervix or uterus is rare but occurs in association with sacral agenesis. Serum levels of gonadotropins are normal in such patients, and diagnosis is made by ultrasonography.

When amenorrhea occurs with signs of virilization, such as clitoromegaly, hirsutism, or excessive acne, adrenal or ovarian disease or abuse of anabolic steroids should be suspected. The adrenal causes are discussed in Chapter 532 and consist of cortical tumors and, very rarely, late-onset congenital adrenal hyperplasia. Determination of the 24-hr urinary 17-ketosteroid and serum testosterone levels will assist in diagnosis. Ovarian causes of virilization include the polycystic ovary syndrome (PCO) and a Sertoli-Leydig cell or lipoid cell tumor, which are both rare. In the young adolescent, PCO may present with amenorrhea or oligomenorrhea and no signs of masculinization; because 17-ketosteroids may be normal or elevated. PCO is diagnosed by the finding of normal serum levels of FSH and marked elevation of the LH level (usually two to three times higher). In adolescence, laparoscopic biopsy may reveal normal ovarian tissue or the histologic findings typical in the adult, consisting of cysts and thickened tunica alburginia. The adolescent may be spared the long-term masculinizing effects of this condition as well as the risk of endometrial carcinoma from continued exposure to estrogens unopposed by progesterone by the administration of combination oral contraceptives (see Chapter 506).

The first diagnosis to be considered in the adolescent with *secondary amenorrhea* is pregnancy. This possibility also exists, albeit rarely, as a cause of primary amenorrhea, if fertilization of the first released ovum occurred before menses. A history of sexual intercourse, nausea, and breast tenderness and physical findings of increased pigmentation of nipples and linea alba, cyanosis and softening of the cervix, and an enlarged uterus form the classic picture. A serum B-subunit human chorionic gonadotropen (HCG) analysis is the most sensitive and specific pregnancy test.

Ingestion of drugs, both legal and illegal, may cause amenorrhea and in the case of phenothiazines, even a false-positive urine pregnancy test. Some drugs, including phenothiazines and certain antihypertensive agents, may cause galactorrhea, further mimicking pregnancy. A thorough drug history is, therefore, necessary.

Psychogenic factors have been implicated in amenorrhea. It is often difficult to separate psychologic factors from nutritional factors because weight loss is a common confounding variable in many of these situations, such as depression, anorexia nervosa, or stress. "Athletic" amenorrhea occurs often in adolescent women engaging in strenuous competitive athletics. Because many patients with anorexia nervosa often use vigorous exercise as a method of weight loss, this possibility must also be considered.

DIAGNOSIS. Evaluation of the adolescent with amenorrhea should include a thorough history and physical examination, a complete blood count, erythrocyte sedimentation rate, pregnancy test, and, if these are negative, serum levels of gonadotropins (LH, FSH), prolactin, TSH, T_4, and T_3; computed tomography (CT) or magnetic resonance imaging (MRI) of the head, if a CNS tumor is suspected; chromosome studies; and determination of urinary 17-ketosteroids. Ultrasonography often can be useful in confirming the presence and size of the uterus and ovaries and identifying tumors and cysts. Ovarian biopsy at the time of exploratory laparoscopy may assist in making a diagnosis.

TREATMENT. Determination of the etiology of amenorrhea may permit the initiation of corrective intervention. When the disorder is not amenable to remediation, consideration should be given to establishing regular pseudomenses to allow the adolescent to feel like her peers. If the result of a vaginal smear is positive for estrogen effect, regular cycling can be accomplished using medroxyprogesterone in a dose of 10 mg orally for 5 days every 6–12 wk. In a patient with gonadal dysgenesis, conjugated estrogens must first be given (Premarin in an oral dose of 0.625 mg for the first 3 wk of each cycle) followed by medroxyprogesterone, 10 mg orally on days 17–21 of the cycle.

111.2 Menometrorrhagia

Excessive menstrual bleeding is one of the few gynecologic emergencies of adolescence. Bleeding may be so severe as to cause death, hypovolemia, and anemia in a frightened young patient. Diagnosis and therapy must be accomplished expeditiously while providing reassurance.

DYSFUNCTIONAL UTERINE BLEEDING. Excessive menstrual bleeding is most often secondary to the anovulatory cycles that normally occur in the 1st year after menarche. Without ovulation, estrogen's effect on the endometrium is unopposed by that of progesterone, resulting in continued endometrial proliferation with eventual massive shedding. The constant estrogen effect also serves to inhibit the LH surge responsible for ovulation, thus perpetuating the problem. Imbalance between FSH and LH, such that the former is higher than the latter, often occurs. Basal body temperature determinations may indicate anovulation.

Treatment is indicated only when there is significant bleeding (i.e., when there is evidence of hypovolemia or anemia). Its goal is to correct the imbalance between estrogen and progesterone, while providing hemostasis. One approach is the immediate oral administration of 25 mg norethynodrel (Enovid). Although this may cause nausea in some patients, the effect is rapid, usually, within 2 hr. Thereafter, the dose is tapered by 5 mg/day until a dose of 5 mg/day is reached. This dose is maintained for the duration of a 21-day cycle, calculated from the day that treatment began. If bleeding recurs at any point in the tapering process, the previous day's dose is resumed, and tapering stopped until there is no further bleeding. A normal menstrual period should begin approximately 2 days after the last pill is taken. On the 5th day of bleeding, a 2-mo course of conventional dose (1/50) oral contraceptive therapy is begun. This may be continued if there is need for contraception, being cognizant of the increased risk of post-pill amenorrhea in adolescents with anovulatory cycles before ingestion of these compounds. An alternative to the use of high-dose norethynodrel consists of oral administration of norethindrone (Ortho-Novum) (2 mg) or norethynodrel (2.5 mg) every 4 hr until the bleeding slows or stops, after which it is administered twice daily until the calendar pack is finished.

In the rare case of a patient whose bleeding cannot be controlled by one of these methods, an endometrial currettage may be indicated. Although this procedure is frequently undertaken in adult women with menometrorrhagia, the rarity of endometrial carcinoma and the usual efficacy of hormonal therapy in adolescence make this procedure unnecessarily invasive in this age group.

CONGENITAL COAGULOPATHIES. Von Willebrand disease should be considered in the adolescent whose first menstrual period is excessive. The finding of a prolonged bleeding time suggests this diagnosis, which is characterized by a defect of platelet adhesiveness and lower levels of factor VIII (Chapter 432.5). The fact that estrogen raises factor VIII levels recommends its use with this condition but underscores the necessity of performing diagnostic studies on blood obtained before the institution of this therapy. Management is the same as for dysfunctional uterine bleeding, with the exception that oral contraceptives will likely be required for the entire menstrual life of the patient.

ASPIRIN. Acquired bleeding diatheses as a result of ingestion of therapeutic doses of aspirin is relatively common and results from disruption of platelet adhesiveness secondary to the effect of the acetyl moiety on the release of adenosine diphosphate. A history of aspirin use within 14 days of menses suggests this possibility and warrants a trial of aspirin avoidance.

THROMBOCYTOPENIA. This may be secondary to toxins, marrow infiltration, hypersplenism, or idiopathic thrombocytopenic purpura and may present with, or be complicated by, menometrorrhagia. Management is the same as that described for dysfunctional uterine bleeding, although platelet transfusions may also be necessary.

EXOGENOUS HORMONES. Improper use of oral contraceptives may cause excessive vaginal bleeding. Careful and sensitive history taking is an important part of evaluation of a patient with this symptom.

THYROID DISORDERS. Hypothyroidism and, rarely, hyperthyroidism may cause excessive vaginal bleeding, occasionally as a presenting symptom. The characteristically low level of T_4 may be altered by the estrogen therapy used to stop the bleeding, but free T_4 should not be affected and TSH remains elevated.

OTHER CAUSES. Rarely, adrenal dysfunction, diabetes mellitus, or estrogen-secreting ovarian tumors may cause increased vaginal bleeding. The bleeding caused by adenocarcinoma of the vagina is typically scant.

In contrast with the conditions described earlier, menometrorrhagia resulting from *trauma, infection,* or *pregnancy* is typically accompanied by pain. Lacerations of the genital tract may result from first or forceful intercourse or athletics, such as water-skiing. The circumstances of the injury may be embarrassing or frightening for the patient, requiring supportive and sensitive history taking. Surgical intervention by a gynecologist is usually needed once the cause of bleeding is identified.

Because approximately 15% of pregnancies in the adolescent age group terminate in *spontaneous abortion,* this possibility should be considered in every case of painful excessive vaginal bleeding. In addition to history and physical examination, performance of a B-subunit HCG pregnancy test should be obtained because this remains positive up to 15 days after an abortion. (Other pregnancy tests revert to negative within 5–8 days.) Involvement of a gynecologist is necessary once the diagnosis is confirmed. Rarely, ectopic pregnancy may present with abnormal vaginal bleeding.

111.3 Dysmenorrhea

Painful menstrual cramps are experienced by nearly two-thirds of postmenarcheal teenagers in the United States, according to the National Health Examination Survey. More than

10% of this group suffer sufficiently to miss school, making dysmenorrhea the leading cause of short-term school absenteeism in female adolescents. Dysmenorrhea may be primary or secondary, the former being the more common. *Secondary dysmenorrhea* results from an underlying **structural abnormality** of the cervix or uterus, a **foreign body** such as an intrauterine device, **endometriosis**, or **endometritis.** Endometriosis, a condition in which implants of endometrial tissue are found at ectopic locations within the peritoneal cavity, is being diagnosed with increasing frequency among adolescents because of the use of ultrasonography and laparoscopy. Characteristically, there is severe pain at the time of menses; its specific location depends on the site of the implants. Some patients respond favorably to treatment with oral contraceptives, whereas the more severe cases are treated with danazol, an antigonadotropin.

A pelvic examination must be performed to exclude the causes of secondary dysmenorrhea, and if none is found a diagnosis of *primary dysmenorrhea* should be considered. Prostaglandins $F_{2\alpha}$ and E_2, produced by the endometrium, stimulate the myometrium to contract, producing pain. Those suffering from dysmenorrhea have high levels of these substances and experience symptomatic relief when prostaglandin-synthetase inhibitors are administered. If given before a menstrual period (or shortly after it begins), administration of a rapidly absorbed prostaglandin-synthetase inhibitor, such as naproxen-sodium, is effective in destroying the prostaglandins before they produce pain (e.g., two tablets of 275 mg each taken with the onset of menses and one tablet taken every 6–8 hr after that for the 1st 24 hr). Medication is rarely needed beyond the 1st day. For the teenager with dysmenorrhea who requires contraception, oral contraceptive therapy may be indicated. It is not certain whether the beneficial effect of their use derives from their ability to inhibit ovulation and thus eliminate progesterone production from the corpus luteum or from their ability to limit endometrial proliferation, and therefore the production of prostaglandins.

111.4 Premenstrual Syndrome

Premenstrual syndrome (PMS), or the late luteal phase syndrome, is a complex of physical signs and behavioral symptoms occurring during the second half of the menstrual cycle, which may resolve with the onset of menses. Clinical manifestations may include breast fullness and tenderness; bloating; fatigue; headache; increased appetite, especially for sweets and salty foods; irritability and mood swings; and depression, inability to concentrate, tearfulness, and violent tendencies. About one-third of women in the reproductive age group may have PMS, but the absence of objective findings makes this difficult to corroborate. It is not common among adolescents, and it does not relate to the presence of dysmenorrhea, which is much more common in this age group. The popular use of vitamin B_6 and progesterone supplementation is not based on evidence of their effectiveness, nor is there a theoretical basis for their use. Use of a gonadotropin-releasing hormone agonist on a short-term basis is supported by carefully controlled studies, but long-term effects and potential complications have not yet been evaluated, making its use in adolescents premature.

CHAPTER 112
The Breast

As one of the most obvious signs of puberty (Chapter 15), breast development is often the focus of attention and a cause of anxiety, particularly when growth is asymmetric or if it occurs in males (gynecomastia). Rarely, the asymmetry is so marked as to create self-consciousness and interfere with self-image. Under those circumstances, consideration may be given to corrective surgery. Although both augmentation and reduction mammoplasty are possible, each has advantages and disadvantages. The former necessitates implantation of a foreign substance, whereas the latter may cause considerable loss of blood and the possibility of later cutaneous hyposensitivity. Surgery is contraindicated before completion of breast growth, which coincides with Sex Maturity Rating 5 (SMR5).

The most common of adolescent breast disorders is the presence of *a mass,* the majority of which are benign cysts or fibroadenomas. Cysts vary in size over the course of a menstrual cycle so that a patient should be re-examined 2 wk after the initial examination. Persistence of the mass or its enlargement over three menstrual cycles is an indication for surgical consultation. Aspiration is usually attempted under local anesthesia, often resulting in curative drainage if it proves to be a cyst. If no fluid is obtained, an excisional biopsy is indicated. This should be done through a circumareolar incision to prevent a disfiguring scar. In one biopsy series, 71% were found to be fibroadenomas, 11% were abscesses, and 2% were cystosarcoma phyllodes, a low-grade malignancy. Carcinoma of the breast in the adolescent is rare, and the efficacy and possible sequelae of mammography are unknown; thus, this procedure is not advised for this age group.

The development of multiple small lumps in the breast is suggestive of **fibrocystic disease,** now considered to be a normal variant. These patients should be taught to examine their breasts regularly and frequently (Chapter 505). The use of combination oral contraceptives of low progesterone potency may be beneficial.

Gynecomastia (Chapter 517) occurs in approximately one-third of normal males during early puberty and often causes concern that may not be openly voiced. The response should be factual information and reassurance of its usual transient nature. Rarely is it of such magnitude or persistence as to warrant surgery.

Nipple discharge in this age group is usually due to local stimulation, use of medications, including oral contraceptives, and pregnancy; rarely, it results from a pituitary or breast neoplasm or infection. Examination of the discharge assists in diagnosis; benign conditions are associated with a milky, sticky, thick discharge, infection with a purulent discharge, and intraductal papilloma and cancer with a serous, serosanguineous, or bloody discharge. Elevation of the serum prolactin level may occur in the **amenorrhea-galactorrhea syndromes,** associated with use of certain antihypertensive medications, oral contraceptives, tranquilizers, or secondary to a pituitary adenoma. The latter is evaluated with a CT scan or MRI of the head. The possibility of a breast neoplasm is an indication for cytologic examination of the discharge and surgical consultation. Infection in the non-breast-feeding adolescent is rare and may be secondary to a human bite or the initial symptom in diabetes mellitus. Culture of the discharge, followed by appropriate antibiotic therapy (usually directed against *Staphylococcus*) is indicated, and surgical drainage is rarely necessary.

CHAPTER 113
Skin Problems

The skin responds as a secondary sex characteristic during puberty, reflecting increased levels of androgens by increased size and secretions of sebaceous follicles and of apocrine glands, the most common manifestation of which is acne. The pathogenesis, clinical picture, and management of acne are discussed in Chapter 619.

As adolescents become preoccupied with their appearance, acne assumes great importance. For that reason, offering treatment even to the youngster whose acne is mild may enhance self-image and is appropriate. Special considerations in the treatment of acne in adolescents include the need to be sure that the patient is not pregnant before instituting therapy with either tetracycline or *cis*-retinoic acid, is alerted to the possibility that chronic tetracycline therapy may cause vaginal infection with *Candida*, and appreciates that acne may be worsened or improved by oral contraceptives, depending on the type of estrogen or progestin.

The skin of the adolescent is influenced not only by the hormones of puberty but also by psychosocial factors occurring at this time. For example, sexual experimentation may result in a sexually transmitted disease with dermatologic manifestations (Chapter 110); stress may be manifested by trichotillomania; contact sports, most notably wrestling, may be associated with herpes simplex infection; and drug abuse may cause skin lesions (Chapter 105).

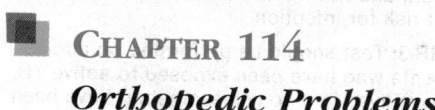

CHAPTER 114
Orthopedic Problems

Puberty is associated with rapid growth of long bones, open epiphyses, and increased traction at sites of insertion of muscles, all of which contribute to the increased rate and unique types of orthopedic problems in this age group. Participation in sports is an additional risk factor, particularly when teams are configured on the basis of chronologic, rather than developmental, age criteria. As a result, such conditions as slipped capital femoral epiphysis, Osgood-Schlatter disease, idiopathic scoliosis (Chapters 626.4, 627.4, and 628.1), and costochondritis of the sternoclavicular junction (Tietze syndrome) are common in adolescents. Certain osseous neoplasms, such as osteogenic sarcoma, are also increased in incidence during adolescence. Infections of bones and joints, although generally less common in adolescents than younger children, may occur as a complication of disseminated gonococcemia or sickle cell anemia. Viral infections, such as rubella and infectious mononucleosis, are more likely to cause arthralgia in adolescents than in younger children.

CHAPTER 115
Delivery of Health Care to Adolescents

The leading causes of death and disability among adolescents are preventable, suggesting that society has failed to address the health needs of this age group adequately. Further, teenagers who require medical treatment also may not receive the care they need. One in seven adolescents in the United States lacks health insurance; others fail to access services because of lack of availability, perceived provider indifference, fear of parental notification, and inadequate information about availability. Even when adolescents access treatment services, the care they receive may not be developmentally appropriate. To address many of these barriers to care, as well as to attempt to optimize the relation between education and health, a number of school-based or school-linked health centers have been developed. To the extent that such centers are accessible, instill trust, provide comprehensive care, and receive support from parents and school personnel, they may be successful.

The complexity and interaction of physical, cognitive, and psychosocial developmental processes during adolescence require sensitivity and skill on the part of the health care provider and a greater number of contacts than is currently appreciated or financed. Health education and promotion and disease prevention should be the focus of every visit with a teenager. To ensure that this is done comprehensively and systematically, guidelines and recommendations have been promulgated by the Department of Adolescent Health of the American Medical Association: Guidelines for Adolescent Preventive Services (GAPS). The frequency of provision of these services is outlined in Figure 115–1. GAPS recommends annual screening for hypertension; eating disorders (based on body mass index), and history; tobacco, alcohol, and drug use by history; sexually transmitted diseases and pregnancy, if sexually active; physical examination, culture and serologic testing, Papanicolaou (Pap) smears, as appropriate; depression; emotional, physical, or sexual abuse; and learning problems by history. Those in high-risk groups should be screened for hypercholesterolemia and hyperlipidemia and for tuberculosis, respectively. Recommendations for immunizations include the following: diphtheria-tetanus 10 years after last diphtheria-pertussis-tetanus vaccine; second trivalent measles-mumps-rubella vaccine unless pregnant; hepatitis B vaccination for those with more than one sexual partner in the previous 6 mo, for those who engaged in paid sex, for male homosexuals, and for intravenous drug users. Also see Chapter 247.

115.1 Legal Issues

In the United States, the right of a minor to *consent* to treatment without parental knowledge is governed by state laws. Usually, the right to self-consent for treatment is granted when there is suspicion of a sexually transmitted disease. Because such diseases are often asymptomatic, this provision is generally interpreted as enabling the physician to perform a pelvic examination on any sexually active adolescent solely upon his or her own consent. In many states, adolescents may consent to receive care for drug abuse or mental health problems.

	Stage of Adolescence: Early (11–14 yrs)	Middle (15–17 yrs)	Late (18–21 yrs)
Health Guidance			
Parenting	●	●	◗
Adolescent Development	■	■	■
Safety Practices	■	■	■
Diet and Fitness	■	■	■
Healthy Lifestyles (sexual behavior, smoking, alcohol and drug use)	■	■	■
Screening			
Hypertension[1]	■	■	■
Hyperlipidemia[2]	HR-1		●
Eating Disorders	■	■	■
Obesity	■	■	■
Tobacco Use	■	■	■
Alcohol & Drug Use	■	■	■
Sexual Behavior	■	■	■
Sexually Transmissible Diseases (STDs)			
Gonorrhea	■*	■*	■*
Chlamydia	■*	■*	■*
Genital Warts	■*	■*	■*
Syphilis	HR-2	HR-2	HR-2
HIV Infection	HR-2	HR-2	HR-2
Cervical Cancer	■*	■*	■**
Depression/Suicide Risk	■	■	■
Physical, Sexual or Emotional Abuse	■	■	■
Learning Problems	■	■	■
Tuberculosis	HR-3	HR-3	HR-3
Immunizations			
Measles, Mumps, & Rubella	HR-4	HR-4	HR-4
Diphtheria & Tetanus		HR-5	
Hepatitis B	HR-6	HR-6	HR-6

1. Recommendation developed by the National Heart, Lung, and Blood Institute Second Task Force on Blood Pressure in Children.

2. Recommendation developed by the National Cholesterol Education Program: Report of the Expert Panel on Blood Cholesterol Levels in Children and Adolescents, 1991.

3. Recommendation developed by the Advisory Committee for Immunization Practices.

*Screening should be performed if the adolescent is currently sexually active.

**Screening should be performed if the adolescent female is sexually active or 18 years of age or older.

HR-1: Test should be performed if there is a family history of cardiovascular disease prior to age 55 or parental history of high cholesterol. Physician may choose to perform test if family history is unknown or if adolescent has multiple risk factors for future cardiovascular disease.

HR-2: Syphilis test should be performed on and HIV test offered to adolescents who are at high risk for infection. This includes having had more than one sexual partner in last six months, having exchanged sex for drugs, being a male who has engaged in sex with other males, having used intravenous drugs (HIV), having had other STDs, having lived in an area endemic for infection, and having had a sexual partner who is at risk for infection.

HR-3: Test should be performed on adolescents who have been exposed to active TB, have lived in a homeless shelter, have been incarcerated, have lived in an area endemic for TB, or currently work in a health care setting.

HR-4: Vaccination should be provided to adolescents who have had only one previous MMR.

HR-5: Vaccination should be given 10 years following previous dT booster.

HR-6: Hepatitis B virus vaccination (HBV) should be given to susceptible adolescents at high risk for infection (see HR-2)

Key and Notations:

- ●: Once per time period
- ■: Yearly
- ◗: Optional

HR: High Risk Category

Figure 115–1. Recommended Frequency of GAPS Preventive Services. (From Elster AB, Kuznets NJ: AMA Guidelines for Adolescent Prevention Services: Recommendations and Rationale. Baltimore, Williams and Wilkins, 1994.)

The minor's right to *contraceptives* has not been reviewed by the Supreme Court, although the right to privacy has been upheld (except in a decision allowing for searches in schools without due process), and accordingly, most states permit the provision of contraceptives to teenagers upon their own consent. Although attempts at restricting Title X–funded programs to provision of contraception only after informing parents has not been legislated, the publicity received by the proposal has left many teenagers with the mistaken notion that their parents will be informed if they seek birth control from any physician. The right of an adolescent to obtain an *abortion* without parental consent or over parental objection varies by state.

With the exception of Delaware, which has an age requirement of 17 yr, all other states require that an individual be 18 yr of age in order to consent to *blood donation. Organ donation* by a consenting minor generally requires parental consent as well as a court order to ensure that there is no alternative adult donor, that the transplant is absolutely necessary in order to save the life of the recipient, and that the adolescent donor will not suffer physically or psychologically as a result of the procedure.

Minors are also exempt from the requirement of parental consent for medical treatment under the following circumstances: (1) *emancipated minors.* These are children who live away from home, are no longer subject to parental control, are economically self-supporting, are married, or are members of the military. (2) *Emergencies.* In a medical emergency, a minor may be treated without consent of parents if, in the physician's judgment, the delay resulting from attempts to contact parents would jeopardize the life or health of the minor. (3) *Mature minor rule.* An emerging trend in the law is the recognition that many minors are sufficiently mature to understand the nature of their illness and the potential risks and benefits of proposed therapy and, therefore, should receive such treatment upon their own consent. In these cases, the physician should document that the adolescent has acted in a responsible manner.

The growing number of cases involving charges of sexual misconduct against male physicians suggests that a chaperone should be present whenever an adolescent female patient is examined. The necessity for chaperoning in the situation of a female physician and a male adolescent patient has not yet become an issue.

115.2 Screening

(See Chapter 5)

Screening tests should be performed only if they are cost effective. This determination for the adolescent involves knowledge of prevalence of the condition in this age group, as well as cost (including possible psychologic and physical sequelae). Screening to detect trivial conditions or those for which there is no immediate intervention should be avoided lest their discovery further the early adolescent's natural tendency to feel flawed or imperfect. During late adolescence, however, it may be appropriate to perform screening tests for genetic disease carrier states in preparation for marriage. Reference standards for adolescents should be available before a screening test is performed to avoid an erroneous diagnosis. Gender and stage of puberty should determine the timing and choice of screening maneuvers.

LABORATORY TESTS. During early adolescence, a screening *urinalysis and culture* are indicated for the female. Polymorphonuclear leukocytes in the urinary sediment suggest the possibility of either cervicitis, vaginitis, urethritis, or an asymptomatic infection of the urinary tract, the last a common finding in adolescent females. The increased incidence of iron-deficiency anemia after menarche also mandates the performance of a *hematocrit* in this group on an annual basis. The reference standard for this test changes with progression of puberty, as estrogen suppresses erythropoietin. Androgens have the opposite effect, causing the hematocrit to rise during male puberty; Sex Maturity Rating 1 (SMR1) males have an average hematocrit of 39%, whereas those who have completed puberty (SMR5) have an average value of 43%. *Tuberculosis testing* on an annual basis is important in adolescents because puberty has been shown to activate this disease in those not previously treated. Sexually active adolescents should undergo screening for *sexually transmitted diseases,* regardless of symptomatology (Chapter 110). *HIV testing* should be included for those at increased risk: bi- and homosexual males, female partners of bisexuals or intravenous (IV) drug abusers, and IV drug users. *Pap smears* are also indicated in sexually active females, regardless of age, because 5–35/1000 have early neoplastic changes. Technique is important; the practice of obtaining two successive cervical scrapes increases the yield by 26% over that obtained by a single cervical specimen. When screening tests for *genetic defect carrier states* are performed, age-appropriate counseling should be immediately available to ensure an opportunity to have questions answered and to have unspoken fears allayed. The use of *spirometry* screening for adolescents who smoke may, over time, serve as a deterrent if deterioration of respiratory status can be demonstrated.

AUDIOMETRY. Highly amplified music of the kind enjoyed by many adolescents may elevate the audiometric threshold, resulting in hearing loss. Therefore, an audiogram should be performed yearly during adolescence, even if earlier tests have been normal.

VISION TESTING. The pubertal growth spurt may involve the optic globe, resulting in its elongation and myopia in genetically predisposed individuals. Vision testing should, therefore, be performed in order to detect this problem before it affects school performance.

BLOOD PRESSURE DETERMINATION. Criteria for a diagnosis of hypertension are based on age-specific norms that increase with pubertal maturation. An individual whose blood pressure exceeds two standard deviations for his or her age is suspect for having hypertension, regardless of the absolute reading. The technique is important; false-positive results may be obtained if the cuff covers less than two thirds of the upper arm. The patient should be seated, and an average should be taken of the 2nd and 3rd consecutive readings, using the change rather than the disappearance as the diastolic pressure. Most adolescents with elevations of blood pressure have labile hypertension (Chapter 404). Half of those with adolescent-onset labile hypertension progress to sustained hypertension in adulthood and require close follow-up. Antihypertensive medication is not indicated, and the effect of reduced salt intake in the adolescent on eventual adult hypertension is unknown. If blood pressure is below two standard deviations for age, anorexia nervosa and Addison disease should be considered.

SCOLIOSIS. Approximately 5% of male and 10–14% of female adolescents have a mild curvature of the spine. This is two to four times the rate in younger children. Scoliosis is typically manifested during the peak of the height velocity curve (Chapter 628.1), at approximately 12 yr in females and 14 yr in males. Curves measuring greater than 10 degrees should be monitored by an orthopedist until growth is completed.

BREAST EXAMINATION. Examination of the female adolescent's breasts is performed to detect masses (Chapters 112 and 505), evaluate progression of sexual maturation, provide reassurance about development, and teach the technique of self-examination with the hope that this practice will continue into the higher risk later years.

SCROTUM EXAMINATION. The peak incidence of germ cell tumors of the testes is in late adolescence and early adulthood. For that reason, palpation of the testes may have an immediate yield and should serve as a model for instruction of self-examination. Because varicoceles often appear during puberty, the examination also provides an opportunity to explain and reassure the patient about this entity (Chapter 499).

PSYCHOSOCIAL. A few questions should be asked directed at detecting the adolescent who is having difficulty with peer relationships (e.g., "Do you have a best friend with whom you can share even the most personal secret?"); with self-image (e.g., "Is there anything you would like to change about yourself?" or "What do you consider to be your best features?"); with depression (e.g., "What do you see yourself doing 5 years from now?" or "Are you ever so sad that you think of dying?"); with school (e.g., "How are your grades this year compared with last year?" and "How many days have you been absent from school this year compared with last year?"); with personal decisions (e.g., "Are you feeling pressured to engage in any behavior for which you do not feel you are ready?" or "Is there anything you would like to change in your relationship with your boyfriend, your father, etc.?"); and with an eating disorder (e.g., "Do you ever feel that food controls you rather than vice versa?"). If the responses to any of these questions suggest a problem, standardized tests are available for more thorough probing or for in-depth interviewing.

Interviewing the Adolescent

It is often difficult to establish open communication with the adolescent patient, unless a prior relationship existed with the physician. Even under that circumstance, the previously comfortable relationship may change with the advent of adolescence, as it often does with parents. The teenager may now wish more privacy than that usually available in the pediatrician's office, and the pediatrician may appear judgmental to a teenager who has some conflict with his or her own parents. Adolescents often imagine that the physician, through the process of physical examination, can detect evidence of behaviors such as smoking, drinking, or masturbation. The physician who takes time to listen, avoids judgmental statements and use of street jargon, and shows respect for the adolescent's emerging maturity will have an easier time communicating with him or her. The use of open-ended questions, rather than closed-ended questions, will further facilitate history-taking (e.g., Question = "Do you get along with your father?" Answer = "Yes." Compare with the question: "What would you like to change in your relationship with your father?" Answer = "I would like to stop him from always putting me down, especially in front of my friends."). The adolescent should be given the opportunity to express concerns and the reasons for seeking medical attention. After the teenager's agenda has been addressed, the physician may wish to define the boundaries of the physician-patient relationship. In such a relationship, the former agrees to provide confidentiality, except if the well-being of the patient or another person may be jeopardized, and the adolescent, in turn, agrees to act maturely and responsibly in terms of medical care.

115.3 Health Enhancement

The health status of adolescents may be enhanced by application of principles of prevention and anticipatory guidance. Prevention of infectious disease should include immunization and counseling. Prevention of sexually transmitted diseases and of pregnancy is an important issue to be addressed in sexually active adolescents of both sexes. Prevention of automotive accidents, the leading killer of adolescents, and of smoking, the leading killer of adults, should also be discussed.

PSYCHOSOCIAL PROBLEMS

Depression/Suicide

Beck AT, Beck R, Kovacs M: Classification of suicidal behaviors. 1: Quantifying intent and medical lethality. Am J Psychol 132:285, 1975.

McAnarney ER: Suicidal behavior of children and youth. Pediatr Clin North Am 22:595, 1975.

Puig-Antich J, Rabinovich H: Major child and adolescent psychiatric disorders. *In*: Levine MD, Carey WB, Crocker AC, Gross RT (eds): Developmental Behavioral Pediatrics. Philadelphia, WB Saunders, 1983, pp 865–890.

Substance Abuse

Centers for Disease Control. Current tobacco, alcohol, marijuana, and cocaine use among high school students, United States. MMWR 41:698, 1991.

Hallagan JB, Hallagan LF, Smyder MB: Anabolic-androgen steroid use by athletes.N Engl J Med 32:1042, 1989.

Henretig FM, Slap GB: A guide to acute medical management of intoxication in adolescents. Adolesc Health Update 6:1, 1994.

Jessor R, Chase JA, Donovan JE: Psychosocial correlates of marijuana use and problem drinking in a national sample of adolescents. Am J Public Health 70:604, 1980.

Jessor R, Jessor SL: Adolescence to young adulthood: A twelve-year prospective study of problem behavior and psychosocial development. *In*: Mednick S, Horway M (eds): Longitudinal Research in the United States. New York, Praeger, 1984.

Johnston LD, O'Malley PM, Bachman JG: Illicit drug use, smoking, and drinking by America's high school students, college students, and young adults, 1975–1987. USDHHS, PHS, Alcohol, Drug Abuse and Mental Health Administration, 1988.

Kandel DB, Logan JA: Patterns of drug use from adolescence to young adulthood. 1: Periods of risk for initiation, continued use, and discontinuation. Am J Public Health 74:660, 1984.

Mott SH, Packer RJ, Soldin SJ: Neurologic manifestations of cocaine exposure in childhood. Pediatrics 93:557, 1994.

Meyer AE, Pottier A, Wright S: Deaths from volatile substance abuse in those under 18 years: Results from a national epidemiological study. Arch Dis Child 69:356, 1993.

Rogol AD: Anabolic steroid hormones for athletes: efficacy or fantasy? Growth, Genetics, and Hormones 4:4, 1988.

Disorders of Sleep

Anders TF, Keener MA: Sleep-wake state development and disorders of sleep in infants, children, and adolescents. *In*: Levine MD, Carey WB, Crocker AC, et al (eds): Developmental-Behavioral Pediatrics. Philadelphia, WB Saunders, 1983.

Anorexia Nervosa

Bruch H: The Golden Cage: The Enigma of Anorexia Nervosa. Cambridge, Harvard University Press, 1978.

Palla B, Litt IF: Medical complications of eating disorders. Pediatrics 81:613, 1988.

Pregnancy and Contraception

Alan Guttmacher Institute: Teenage Pregnancy: The Problem That Hasn't Gone Away. New York, Alan Guttmacher Institute, 1981.

Hatcher RA, Stewart F, Trussell J, et al: Contraceptive Technology, 1990–1992, 15th ed. New York, Irvington Publishers, 1990.

Lewit EM: Teenage childbearing. Future of Children 2:186, 1992.

Sexually Transmitted Diseases

Davis AJ, Emans SJ: Human papilloma virus infection in the pediatric and adolescent patient. J Pediatr 115:1, 1989.

Drugs for sexually transmitted diseases. Med Lett Drugs Ther 36:1, 1994.

Shafer MA: Sexual transmitted diseases in adolescents. Adolesc Health Update, 6:1, 1994.

Menstrual Problems

Litt IF: Menstrual problems during adolescence. Pediatr Rev 4:203, 1983.

Delivery of Health Care to Adolescents

American Medical Association: Guidelines for Adolescent Preventive Services. Chicago, American Medical Association, 1992.

Litt IF: Adolescent health care. *In*: Green M, Haggerty RJ (eds): Ambulatory Pediatrics IV. Philadelphia, WB Saunders, 1990.

U.S. Congress Office of Technology Assessment Adolescent Health: Background and Effectiveness of Selected Preventive and Treatment Services, OTA-H-466: Vol. II. Washington, DC, U.S. Government Printing Office, 1991.

PART XIV

The Immunologic System and Disorders

CHAPTER 116

T-, B-, and NK-Cell Systems

Rebecca H. Buckley

Bodily defense against infectious agents is secured through a combination of physical barriers, including the skin, mucous membranes, mucous blanket, and ciliated epithelial cells, and the various components of the immune system. The latter consists of T, B, and natural killer (NK) cells; phagocytic cells; and the complement proteins. The immune system also serves to protect against autoimmune diseases and malignancy. This chapter reviews T, B, and NK lymphocytes, while the phagocytic cell system is described in Chapter 122 and the complement system in Chapter 120. Genetic defects leading to T-, B-, and/or NK-cell deficiency are discussed in Chapters 117–119.

LYMPHOPOIESIS IN THE FETUS

SOURCE OF LYMPHOID CELLS AND THE PROCESS OF ORGANOGENESIS. The human immune system arises in the embryo from gut-associated tissue. Pluripotential hematopoietic stem cells first appear in the yolk sac at 2.5–3 wk of gestational age and migrate to the fetal liver at 5 wk of gestation; they later reside in the bone marrow, where they remain throughout life. Lymphoid stem cells develop from such precursor cells and differentiate into T, B, or NK cells, depending upon the organs or tissues to which the stem cells traffic. Primary lymphoid organ (thymus, bone marrow) development begins during the middle of the first trimester of gestation and proceeds rapidly; secondary lymphoid organ (spleen, lymph nodes, tonsils, Peyer's patches, lamina propria) development soon follows. These organs continue to serve as sites of differentiation of T, B, and NK lymphocytes from stem cells throughout life. Both the initial organogenesis and the continued cell differentiation occur as a consequence of the interaction of a vast array of lymphocytic and microenvironmental cell surface molecules and proteins secreted by the involved cells. The complexity and number of such cell surface molecules led to the development of an international nomenclature and classification of these differentiation antigens, which are now referred to as *clusters of differentiation* or CDs (Table 116–1).

T and B lymphocytes are the only components of the immune system that have antigen-specific recognition capabilities, that is, they are responsible for adaptive immunity. NK cells are lymphocytes that are also derived from hematopoietic stems cells; they are thought to have a role in host defense against viral infections, in tumor surveillance, and in immune regulation. The proteins synthesized and secreted by T, B, and NK cells, and by the cells with which they interact, are referred to as *cytokines.* Several such proteins have been given an official nomenclature as interleukins or ILs (Table 116–2). Cytokines have the ability to act in an autocrine, paracrine, and/or endocrine manner to promote and facilitate differentiation and proliferation of the cells of the immune system.

T-CELL DEVELOPMENT AND DIFFERENTIATION. The primitive thymic rudiment is formed from the ectoderm of the third branchial cleft and endoderm of the third branchial pouch at 4 wk gestation. Beginning at 7–8 wk, the right and left rudiments move caudally and fuse in the midline. Blood-borne T-cell precursors from the fetal liver then begin to colonize the perithymic mesenchyme at 8 wk gestation. These precursor (pro-T) cells are identified by surface proteins designated as CD7 and CD34. At 8–8.5 wk gestation, CD7+ cells are found intrathymically, and some cells also coexpress CD4, a protein present on the surfaces of mature T-helper cells, and CD8, a protein found on both mature cytotoxic cells and NK cells. In addition, some cells bear single T-cell receptor (TCR) chains (β, δ, or γ) but none bear complete TCRs.

The mature TCR is a heterodimer of two chains, either α and β or γ and δ; it is coexpressed on the cell surface with CD3, a complex of five polypeptide chains (γ, δ, ϵ, ζ, η). TCR gene rearrangement occurs by a process in which large, noncontiguous blocks of DNA are spliced together. These segments, known as V (variable), D (diversity), and J (joining), each have a number of variants. VDJ segments are joined to a constant region of the α gene, and VJ segments are joined to the β gene to complete the receptor polypeptide genes. Random combinations of the segments account for much of the enormous diversity of TCRs that enables humans to recognize millions of different antigens. TCR gene rearrangement requires the presence of recombinase activating genes, referred to as RAG-1 and RAG-2, and possibly other recombinase components. This process is flawed in severe combined immunodeficiency (SCID) mice with and in some humans with SCID. Rearrangement of TCR genes signifies commitment of pro-T cells to T-lineage development, that is, to become pre-T cells. TCR gene rearrangement begins shortly after colonization of the thymus with stem cells, that is, the establishment of the T-cell repertoire begins at 8–10 wk of gestation. By 9.5–10 wk, more than 95% of thymocytes are CD7+, CD2+, CD4+, CD8+, and c(cytoplasmic)CD3+, and approximately 30% bear the CD1 inner cortical thymocyte antigen. By 10 wk, 25% of thymocytes bear αβ TCRs. Tiαβ+ cells gradually increase in number during embryonic life and represent more than 95% of thymocytes postnatally.

As immature cortical thymocytes begin to express TCRs, the processes of positive and negative selection take place. *Positive selection* occurs through the interaction of immature thymocytes (which express low levels of TCR) with major histocom-

■ TABLE 116–1 CD Classification of Some Lymphocyte Surface Molecules

CD Number	Other Names	Tissue/Lineage	Function
CD1	T6	Cortical thymocytes; Langerhans cells	Antigen presentation to TCRγ/δ cells
CD2	SRBC receptor	T and NK cells	Binds LFA-3 (CD58); alternative pathway of T-cell activation
CD3	T3, Leu 4	T cells	TCR-associated; transduces signals from TCR
CD4	T4, Leu3a	Helper T-cell subset	Receptor for HLA class II antigens; associated with p56 *lck* tyrosine kinase
CD7	3A1, Leu 9	T and NK cells and their precursors	Comitogenic for T lymphocytes
CD8	T8, Leu2a	Cytotoxic T-cell subset; also on 30% of NK cells	Receptor for HLA class I antigens; associated with p56 *lck* tyrosine kinase
CD10	cALLA	B-cell progenitors	Peptide cleavage
CD11a	LFA-1a α chain	T, B, and NK cells	With CD 18, ligand for ICAM 1, 2, and 3
CD11b, c	MAC-1, CR3; CR4	NK cells	With CD18, receptors for C3bi
CD16	FcRγIII	NK cells	FcR for IgG
CD19	B4	B cells	Regulates B-cell activation
CD20	B1	B cells	Mediates B-cell activation
CD21	B2	B cells	C3d/EBV receptor; CR2
CD34	My10	Precursor cells	?
CD45	Leukocyte common antigen, T200	All leukocytes	Tyrosine phosphatase that regulates lymphocyte activation; CD45RO isoform on memory T cells, CD45RA isoform on naive T cells
CD56	N-CAM; NKH-1	NK cells	Mediates NK homotypic adhesion

patibility complex (MHC) antigens present on cortical thymic epithelial cells. As a result, thymocytes with TCR capable of interacting with foreign antigens presented on self MHC antigens are activated and develop to maturity. Mature thymocytes that survive the selection process are either CD4+ and restricted to self class II HLA antigens or CD8+ and restricted to self class I HLA antigens when they interact with foreign antigens presented by these MHC molecules. *Negative selection* occurs next and is mediated by interaction of the surviving thymocytes (which have much higher levels of TCR expression) with host peptides presented by HLA class I or II antigens present on bone marrow–derived thymic macrophages, dendritic cells, and possibly B cells. This interaction mediates programmed cell death of such autoreactive thymocytes by a process called *apoptosis.* Fetal cortical thymocytes are among the most rapidly dividing cells in the body; they increase in number by 100,000-fold within 2 wk after stem cells enter the thymus. As these cells mature, the above-mentioned selection process takes place, and, as a consequence, 97% of all cortical thymocytes die. The surviving cells are no longer doubly positive for both CD4 and CD8 but are singly positive for either one or the other and they migrate to the medulla.

T-cell functions are acquired concomitantly with the development of single-positive thymocytes, but they are not fully developed until the cells emigrate from the thymus. It has been estimated that one stem cell gives rise to approximately 3,000 mature medullary thymocytes. Such medullary cells are resistant to the lytic effects of corticosteroids. T cells begin to emigrate from the thymus to the spleen, lymph nodes, and appendix at 11–12 wk of embryonic life and to the tonsils by 14–15 wk. They leave the thymus via the bloodstream and are distributed throughout the body, with heaviest concentrations in the paracortical areas of lymph nodes, the periarteriolar areas of the spleen, and the thoracic duct lymph. The homing of lymphocytes to peripheral lymphoid organs is directed by the interaction of a lymphocyte surface adhesion molecule, L-selectin, with carbohydrate moieties on specialized regions of lymphoid organ blood vessels, called high endothelial venules. By 12 wk gestation, T cells can proliferate in response to plant lectins (phytohemagglutinin and concanavalin A) and to allogeneic cells; antigen-binding T cells have been found by 20 wk gestation. Hassall's bodies (swirls of terminally differentiated medullary epithelial cells) are first seen in the thymic medulla at 16–18 wk of embryonic life.

B-CELL DEVELOPMENT AND DIFFERENTIATION. In parallel with T-cell differention, B-cell development begins in the fetal liver prior to 7 wk gestation. Fetal liver CD34+ stem cells are seeded to the bone marrow of the clavicles by 8 wk of embryonic life and to that of the long bones by 10 wk (Fig. 116–1). ***Antigen-independent*** stages of B-cell development have been defined according to immunoglobulin gene rearrangement patterns and the surface proteins the cells bear. The **pro-B cell** is the first descendent of the pluripotential stem cell committed to B-lineage development and is detected by the presence of both CD34 and CD10 on its surface; in it the immunoglobulin genes remain germline (Fig. 116–2). The next stage is the **pre-pre-B cell** stage, during which immunoglobulin genes are rearranged, but there is no cytoplasmic expression of μ heavy chains or surface IgM (sIgM); these cells are further characterized by the coexpression of membrane CD34, CD10, CD19, and CD40, and (somewhat later) by the additional presence of CD73, CD22, CD24, and CD38. The **pre-B cell** stage is next; these cells are distinguished by the expression of cytoplasmic μ heavy chains but no sIgM, because as yet no immunoglobulin light chains are produced. They also continue to express all CD antigens seen at the pre-pre-B cell stage except CD34 and CD10 (which are lost); in addition, they express CD21. Next is the **immature B-cell** stage, during which sIgM is expressed (because light chain genes have now been rearranged) but not sIgD; CD38 is lost, but all other *pre-B-cell* CD antigens persist. The last stage of antigen-independent B-cell development is the **mature** or **virgin B cell,** which coexpresses both sIgM and sIgD; CD23 is also acquired at this stage, and all of the other CD antigens present on immature B cells persist. Pre-B cells can be found in fetal liver at 7 wk gestation, sIgM+ and sIgG+ B cells at between 7 and 11 wk, and sIgD+ and sIgA+ B cells by 12–13 wk. By 14 wk of embryonic life, the percentage of circulating lymphocytes bearing sIgM and sIgD is the same as in cord blood and slightly higher than in the blood of adults. ***Antigen-dependent*** stages of B-cell development are those that develop after the mature or virgin B cell is stimulated by antigen through its antigen receptor (sIg); the outcome is the differentiation of the cell and its progeny into sIg+ memory B cells (for that particular antigen) and plasma cells, which synthesize and secrete antigen-specific immunoglobulin, that is, antibody. There are five immunoglobulin isotypes (defined by unique heavy chain antigens present on each): IgM, IgG, IgA, IgD, and IgE. IgG and IgM, the only complement-fixing isotypes, are the most important immunoglobulins in the blood and other internal body fluids for protection against infectious agents; IgM is confined primarily to the intravascular compartment because of its large size,

■ **TABLE 116–2 Functional Classification of Cytokines***

Cytokines Involved in Natural Immune Responses

Type I interferons—IFN-α and IFN-β—inhibit viral replication, inhibit cell proliferation, activate NK cells, upregulate class I MHC molecule expression
TNF-α—mediates host response to gram-negative bacteria and other infectious agents
IL-1α and -β—mediate host inflammatory response to infectious agents
IL-1Ra—is a natural antagonist of IL-1, blocks signals delivered by IL-1
IL6—mediates and regulates inflammatory responses
Chemokines (IL-8, monocyte chemotactic protein-1 or MCP-1, RANTES, and others)—mediate leukocyte chemotaxis and activation

Lymphocyte Regulatory Cytokines

Immunostimulatory or Growth-Promoting

IL-1—costimulates activation of T cells
IL-2—growth factor for T, B, NK cells; activates effector cells
IL-4—T and B cell growth factor; stimulates IgE production; upregulates classes I and II MHC molecule and FcRεII expression on macrophages; expansion of T_H2 subset
IL-5—B cell growth and activation
IL-6—growth factor for B cells
IL-7—stromal cell factor; growth factor for precursor B and T cells
IL-10—growth and differentiation factor for B cells
IL-9—growth factor for T cells
IL-12—expansion of T_H1 subset; activates effector cells
IL-13—growth and differentiating factor for B cells; stimulates IgE production; upregulates classes I and II MHC molecule and FcRεII expression on macrophages
TNF-β—stimulates effector cell function
IFN-γ—activates macrophages, NK cells; upregulates classes I and II MHC molecule expression; inhibits IL-4 or IL-13–induced IgE production

Immunosuppressive

IL-1Ra—regulates IL-1 activities
TGF-β—antagonizes lymphocyte responses
IL-10—inhibits activities of T_H1 cells

Hematopoiesis-Regulating Cytokines

GM-CSF, G-CSF, M-CSF—colony stimulating factors
Erythropoietin (EPO)—differentiation of erythroid precursors
IL-3, SCF, *c-kit* receptor—regulate stem cell development
IL-4—mast cell development
IL-5—eosinophil differentiation and proliferation
IL-6—differentiation of B cells
IL-7—differentiation of B and T cells

Proinflammatory Cytokines

IL-1, TNF-α, IL-6—participate in the acute-phase response and synergize to mediate inflammation, shock, and death

Anti-inflammatory Cytokines

IL-4—reduces endotoxin-induced TNF and IL-1 production
IL-6—inhibits TNF production
IL-10—suppresses lymphocyte functions and downregulates production of proinflammatory cytokines
IL-13—downregulates functions of macrophages; suppresses production of proinflammatory cytokines
TGF-β—has immunosuppressive effects, inhibits IL-1 and TNF gene expression
IL-1Ra—competes with the binding of IL-1 to its cell surface receptors and blocks IL-1 effects
TNFsR—soluble TNF receptors; by binding TNF, block interaction of TNF with the target cell

**This is not an exhaustive list. (Modified from Whiteside TL: Cytokine measurements and interpretation of cytokine assays in human disease. J Clin Immunol 14:329, 1994.)*

whereas IgG is present in all internal body fluids. IgA is the major protective immunoglobulin of external secretions, that is, those of the gastrointestinal, respiratory, and urogenital tracts, but it is also present in the circulation as well. IgE, present in both internal and external body fluids, plays a major role in host defense against parasites. However, because of high-affinity IgE receptors on basophils and mast cells, IgE is the principal if not sole mediator of allergic reactions of the immediate type. The significance of IgD is still not clear. There are also immunoglobulin subclasses (again defined by unique heavy chain antigens present on each, in addition to their class-specific heavy chain antigen), including four subclasses of IgG: IgG1, IgG2, IgG3, and IgG4, and two subclasses of IgA: IgA1 and IgA2. These subclasses each have different biologic roles; for example, anti-polysaccharide antibody activity is found predominantly in the IgG2 subclass. Secreted IgM and IgE have been found in abortuses as young as 10 wk, and IgG as early as 11–12 wk. Even though these B-cell developmental stages have been described in the context of B-cell ontogeny, it is important to recognize that the process of B-cell development from pluripotential stem cells goes on throughout postnatal life.

Despite the capacity of fetal B lymphocytes to differentiate into immunoglobulin-synthesizing and secreting cells, plasma cells are not usually found in lymphoid tissues of the fetus until about 20 wk gestation, then only rarely, because of the sterile environment of the uterus. Peyer's patches have been found in significant numbers by the fifth intrauterine month, and plasma cells have been seen in the lamina propria by 25 wk gestation. Prior to birth there may be primary follicles in lymph nodes, but secondary follicles are usually not present.

The human fetus begins to receive significant quantities of maternal IgG transplacentally at around 12 wk gestation, and the quantity steadily increases until at birth cord serum contains a concentration of IgG comparable to or greater than that of maternal serum. IgG is the only class to cross the placenta to any significant degree, and all four subclasses do this but IgG2 does so least well. A small amount of IgM (10% of adult levels) and a few nanograms of IgA, IgD, and IgE are normally found in cord serum; because none of these proteins cross the placenta, they are presumed to be of fetal origin. These observations raise the possibility that certain antigenic stimuli

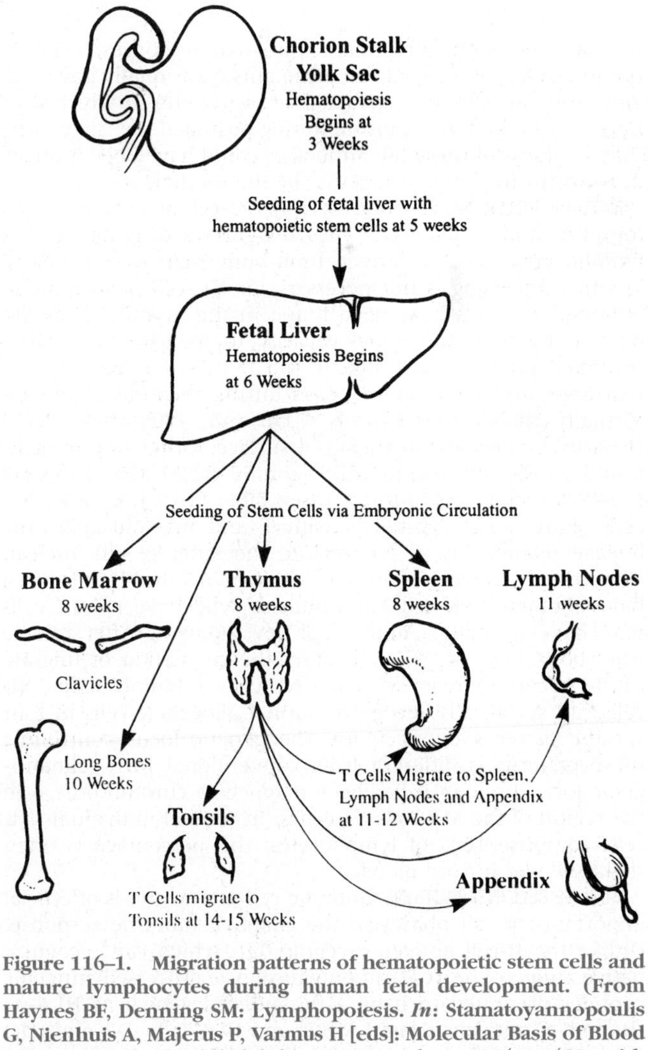

Figure 116–1. Migration patterns of hematopoietic stem cells and mature lymphocytes during human fetal development. (From Haynes BF, Denning SM: Lymphopoiesis. *In*: Stamatoyannopoulis G, Nienhuis A, Majerus P, Varmus H [eds]: Molecular Basis of Blood Diseases, 2nd ed. Philadelphia, WB Saunders, 1994, p 429, with permission.)

Human

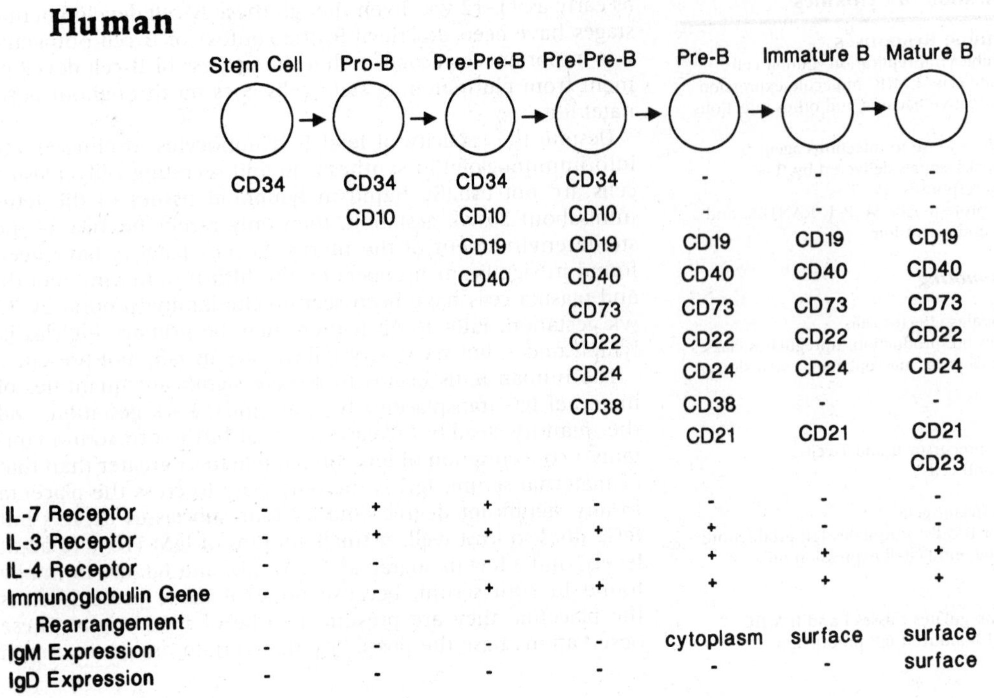

	Stem Cell	Pro-B	Pre-Pre-B	Pre-Pre-B	Pre-B	Immature B	Mature B
	CD34	CD34	CD34	CD34	-	-	-
		CD10	CD10	CD10	-	-	-
			CD19	CD19	CD19	CD19	CD19
			CD40	CD40	CD40	CD40	CD40
				CD73	CD73	CD73	CD73
				CD22	CD22	CD22	CD22
				CD24	CD24	CD24	CD24
				CD38	CD38	-	-
					CD21	CD21	CD21
							CD23
IL-7 Receptor	-	+	+	-	-	-	-
IL-3 Receptor	-	+	+	+	+	-	+
IL-4 Receptor	-	-	-	-	+	+	+
Immunoglobulin Gene Rearrangement	-	-	+	+	+	+	+
IgM Expression	-	-	-	-	cytoplasm	surface	surface
IgD Expression	-	-	-	-	-	-	surface

Figure 116–2. Antigen-independent human B-cell development. (From Haynes BF, Denning SM: Lymphopoiesis. *In*: Stamatoyannopoulis G, Nienhuis A, Majerus P, Varmus H [eds]: Molecular Basis of Blood Diseases, 2nd ed. Philadelphia, WB Saunders, 1994, p 429, with permission.)

normally cross the placenta to provoke responses, even in noninfected fetuses. Some atopic infants occasionally have reaginic antibodies to antigens (such as egg white) to which they have had no known exposure during postnatal life, suggesting that synthesis of these IgE antibodies could have been induced in the fetus by antigens ingested by the mother.

NATURAL KILLER (NK)-CELL DEVELOPMENT. NK-cell activity has been found in human fetal liver cells at 8–11 wk of gestation. NK lymphocytes are also derived from bone marrow precursors. Thymic processing is not necessary for NK-cell development, although NK cells have been found in the thymus. They are defined by their functional capacity to mediate non-MHC–restricted cytotoxicity. Unlike T and B cells, NK cells do not rearrange antigen receptor genes during their development. Virtually all NK cells express CD56 and >90% bear CD16 (FcγRIII) molecules on their cell surface. Other CD antigens found on NK cells include CD57 (on 50–60%), CD7 and CD2 (70–90%), and CD8 (30–40%) (see Table 116–1). Because NK cells share surface antigens with T and myeloid cells, the lineage relationship of NK cells to the latter is still unclear. Humans who have profound deficiencies in T and B cells often have abundant NK cells, and humans who have no NK cells may have normal T- and B-cell development. After release from bone marrow, NK cells enter the circulation or migrate to the spleen; there are very few NK cells in lymph nodes. NK cells can specifically recognize normal allogeneic cells in four specific patterns of reactivity. The genetic locus controlling these patterns is different from conventional MHC alloantigenic loci, although it has been mapped to chromosome 6 in the region of the MHC class I genes. In normal individuals NK cells comprise 10% of lymphocytes; this percentage is often slightly lower in cord blood.

IMMUNE CELL INTERACTIONS. Immune cell interaction is of crucial importance to all phases of the adaptive immune response. Unlike the B-cell antigen receptor (Ig), which can recognize native antigen, the TCR can only recognize processed antigenic peptides presented to it by MHC molecules such as HLA-A, -B, and -C antigens (class I MHC) and HLA-DR, -DP, and -DQ (class II MHC) molecules present on antigen-presenting cells (APCs). The MHC molecules have a groove in their protein structure where peptides fit. Class I MHC molecules are found on most nucleated cells in the body. Class II MHC molecules are found on macrophages and B cells. The peptides found in the groove of class I HLA molecules come from proteins normally made in the cell that are degraded and inserted into the groove. The peptides will include viral peptides if the cell is infected with a virus. The peptides present in the groove of class II molecules come from exogenous native antigens such as vaccine and bacterial proteins. These proteins are taken up by APCs (macrophages and B cells), degraded, and expressed on the cell surface in the groove of class II HLA molecules. The TCR then interacts with the peptide-bearing HLA molecule and, through its functional and physical link to the CD3 complex of signal-transducing molecules, sends a signal to the T cell to produce cytokines that ultimately result in T-cell activation and proliferation.

Two of the main functions of T cells are (1) to signal B cells to make antibody by producing cytokines and membrane molecules that can serve as ligands for B-cell surface molecules and (2) to kill virally infected cells or tumor cells. For the T cell to do either of these functions, it first must bind to an APC or to a target cell. For high-affinity binding of T cells to APCs or target cells, there are several molecules on T cells, in addition to TCRs, that bind to molecules on APCs or target cells. For example, the CD4 molecule present on helper T cells binds directly to MHC class II molecules on APCs. CD8 on killer T cells binds the MHC class I molecule on the target cell. Both CD4 and CD8 molecules are directly involved in the regulation of T-cell activation and are physically linked intracellularly to the p56-lck protein tyrosine kinase. The cytoplasmic tail of CD45 is a tyrosine phosphatase capable of regulating T-cell signal-transduction events by virtue of the fact that p56-lck has been shown to be a substrate for CD45 phosphatase activity. Depending upon which isoform of CD45 is present on the T cell (CD45RO on memory T cells, CD45RA on naive T cells), mechanisms have been proposed whereby CD45 could upregulate or downregulate T-cell triggering. LFA-1 on the T cell binds a protein called ICAM-1 (intracellular adhesion molecule 1), now designated CD54, on APCs. CD2 on T cells binds LFA-3 (CD58) on the APCs. With the adhesion of T cells to antigen presenting cells, helper T cells are stimulated to make interleukins and cell surface molecules, such as the CD40 ligand or gp39, that provide help for B cells, and cytotoxic T cells are stimulated to kill their targets.

In the ***primary antibody response,*** native antigen is carried to a lymph node draining the site, taken up by specialized cells called follicle stimulating cells (FCSs), and expressed on their surfaces. Virgin B cells bearing sIg specific for that antigen then bind to the antigen on the surfaces of the FCSs. If the affinity of the B-cell sIg antibody for the antigen present on the FCSs is high enough, and if other signals are provided by activated T-helper cells, the B cell will develop into an antibody-producing plasma cell. If the affinity is not high enough or if T cell signals are not received, the B cell will die through apoptosis. The signals provided by activated T-helper cells include those from cytokines they secrete (IL-4, IL-5, IL-6, and IL-13; see Table 116–2) and that from a surface T-cell molecule, gp39, which, upon contact of the T cell with the B cell, binds to CD40 on the B-cell surface. CD40 is a type I integral membrane glycoprotein expressed on B cells, monocytes, some carcinomas, and a few other types of cells. It belongs to the tumor necrosis factor (TNF)/nerve growth factor receptor family. Cross-linking of CD40 on B cells by allowing CD40 to interact with gp39 in the presence of certain cytokines causes the B cells to undergo proliferation and to initiate immunoglobulin synthesis. In the primary immune response, usually only IgM antibody is made, and most of it is of relatively low affinity. Some B cells will become memory B cells during the primary immune response. These cells will have switched their immunoglobulin genes so that IgG, IgA, and/or IgE antibodies of higher affinity will be formed upon a secondary exposure to the same antigen. The ***secondary immune response*** occurs when these memory B cells again encounter that antigen. Plasma cells will form, just as in the primary response; however, many more cells are rapidly generated and IgG, IgA, and IgE antibodies will be made. In addition, genetic changes in immunoglobulin genes (somatic mutation) will have led to increased affinity of those antibodies. The exact pattern of isotype response to antigen will vary, depending upon the type of antigen and the cytokines present in the microenvironment.

For NK-mediated lysis, binding to the target is of crucial importance. This is best exemplified by humans with mutations in CD18, or the β chain of three different adhesion molecules, who also lack NK function. Thus, binding of NK cells to their targets is facilitated by LFA-1–ICAM (intracellular adhesion molecule) interactions. CD56 or NCAM (neural cell adhesion molecule) also mediates homotypic adhesion of NK cells. FcγRIII, or the low-affinity IgG receptor, has a higher affinity for IgG when it is present on NK cells than when it is on neutrophils; it permits NK cells to also mediate antibody-dependent cellular cytotoxicity (ADCC). In this reaction, antibody is bound through its Fc region to the FcγRIII. The antibody combining portion of the IgG attaches to the target. The NK cell, now attached to the target by antibody, kills the target cell.

POSTNATAL LYMPHOPOIESIS

T CELLS AND T-CELL SUBSETS. Although the percentage of CD3+ T cells in cord blood is somewhat less than in the peripheral blood of children and adults, T cells are actually present in higher number because of a higher absolute lymphocyte count in all normal infants. An additional distinction is that the ratio of CD4+ to CD8+ T cells is usually higher (3.5–4:1) in cord blood than in blood of children and adults (1.5–2:1). Virtually all T cells in cord blood bear the CD45RA (naive) isoform, and a dominance of CD45RA+ over CD45RO+ T cells persists during the first 2–3 yr of life, after which time there is gradual equalization of the numbers of cells bearing these two isoforms. T-helper (TH) cells can be further subdivided according to the cytokines they produce when activated. TH1 cells produce IL-2 and IFN-γ, thereby promoting cytotoxic T-cell or delayed hypersensitivity types of responses, whereas TH2 cells produce IL-4, IL-5, IL-6, and IL-13 (see Table 116–2), which promote B-cell responses and allergic sensitization. Cord blood T cells have the capacity to respond normally to the two T-cell mitogens, phytohemagglutinin (PHA) and concanavallin A (Con A), and they are capable of mounting a normal mixed leukocyte response. Thus, the absence of these responses in tests of cord blood lymphocytes is evidence of profound primary T-cell dysfunction. The normal newborn infant also has the capacity to develop antigen-specific T cell responses at birth, as evidenced by vigorous tuberculin reactivity a few weeks after BCG vaccination on day 1 of life. Because the level of T-cell function may be depressed in infants with unrecognized severe T-cell defects, most hospitals now routinely irradiate all blood products given young infants.

B CELLS AND IMMUNOGLOBULINS. The newborn infant is quite susceptible to infections with gram-negative organisms, since he or she has not received IgM antibodies (i.e., heat-stable opsonins) to these organisms from the mother. Quantities of the heat-labile opsonin, C3b, are also lower in newborn serum than in adults. These factors probably account for the finding of impaired phagocytosis of some organisms by newborn polymorphonuclear cells. Maternally transmitted IgG antibodies serve quite adequately as heat-stable opsonins for most gram-positive bacteria, and IgG antibodies to viruses afford adequate protection against those agents. However, because there is a relative deficiency of the IgG2 subclass, antibodies to capsular polysaccharide antigens may be deficient. Because premature infants have received less maternal IgG by the time of birth than full-term infants, their serum opsonic activity is low for all types of organisms.

B lymphocytes are present in cord blood in slightly higher percentages but considerably higher numbers than in the blood of children and adults because of higher absolute lymphocyte counts in all normal infants. However, cord-blood B cells do not synthesize the range of immunoglobulin isotypes made by B cells from children and adults when stimulated with either pokeweed mitogen or anti-CD40 plus IL-4 or IL-10, producing primarily IgM and at a much reduced quantity.

The neonatal infant begins to synthesize antibodies of the IgM class at an increased rate very soon after birth, in response to the immense antigenic stimulation of his or her new environment. Premature infants appear to be as capable of doing this as do full-term infants. At about 6 days after birth, the serum concentration of IgM rises sharply. This rise continues until adult levels are achieved by approximately 1 yr of age. Cord serum usually does not contain detectable IgA. Serum IgA is normally first detected at around the 13th day of postnatal life; the level gradually increases during early childhood until adult levels are achieved and preserved between the 6th and 7th yr of life. Cord serum contains an IgG concentration comparable to or greater than that of maternal serum. Maternal IgG gradually disappears during the first 6–8 mo of life, while the rate of infant IgG synthesis increases (IgG1 and IgG3 faster than IgG2 and IgG4 during the 1st year) until adult concentrations of total IgG are reached and maintained by 7–8 yr of age. However, IgG1 and IgG4 reach adult levels first, followed by IgG3 at 10 yr and IgG2 at 12 yr of age. The total immunoglobulin level in the infant usually reaches a low point at approximately 4–5 mo of postnatal life. The rate of development of IgE has generally been found to follow that of IgA. After adult concentrations of each of the three major immunoglobulins are reached, these levels remain remarkably constant for a normal individual. The capacity to produce specific antibodies to protein antigens is intact at the time of birth. However, normal infants cannot produce antibodies to polysaccharide antigens until usually after age 2 yr unless the polysaccharide is conjugated to a protein carrier, as is the case for the *Haemophilus influenzae* type B (HIB) vaccine.

NK CELLS. The percentage of NK cells in cord blood is usually lower than in the blood of children and adults, but the absolute number of NK cells is approximately the same due to the higher lymphocyte count. The capacity of cord-blood NK cells to mediate target lysis in either NK-cell assays or ADCC assays is roughly two-thirds that of adults.

LYMPHOID ORGAN DEVELOPMENT. Lymphoid tissue is proportionally small but rather well developed at birth and matures rapidly in the postnatal period. The thymus is largest relative to body size during fetal life and at birth is ordinarily two thirds of its mature weight, which it attains during the 1st year of life. It reaches its peak mass, however, just before puberty, then gradually involutes thereafter. By 1 yr of age, all lymphoid structures are mature histologically. Absolute lymphocyte counts in the peripheral blood also reach a peak during the 1st yr of life. Peripheral lymphoid tissue increases rapidly in mass during infancy and early childhood. It reaches adult size by approximately 6 yr of age, exceeds those dimensions during the prepubertal years, and then undergoes involution coincident with puberty. The spleen, however, gradually accrues its mass during maturation and does not reach full weight until adulthood. The mean number of Peyer's patches is one half the adult number at birth and gradually increases until the adult mean number is exceeded during adolescent years.

ASSESSMENT OF T-, B-, AND NK-CELL FUNCTION. It is essential that the tests selected for assessing these functions be broadly informative, reliable, and cost effective. The complete blood count and sedimentation rate are among the most cost-effective screening tests. If the sedimentation rate is normal, chronic bacterial infection is unlikely. If the absolute lymphocyte count is normal, the patient is not likely to have a severe T-cell defect. Normal lymphocyte counts are very high in infancy and early childhood. For example, at 9 mo of age—an age when infants affected with severe T-cell immunodeficiency are likely to present—the lower limit of normal is 4,500 lymphocytes/mm^3. Examination of red cells for Howell-Jolly bodies will help exclude congenital asplenia. If the platelet count is normal, Wiskott-Aldrich syndrome is excluded.

B-Cell Function. A simple screening test is used to determine the presence and titer of antibodies to type A and B red blood cell polysaccharide antigens. As assayed in most blood banks, this test measures predominantly IgM antibodies. Measurement of antibodies to diphtheria or tetanus toxoids before and 2 wk after a pediatric or adult D-T booster is helpful in assessing the capacity to form IgG antibodies to protein antigens. To evaluate the ability to respond to polysaccharide antigens, antipneumococcal antibodies can be measured prior to and 3 wk after immunization with Pneumovax. Patients with significant or permanent B-cell defects do not produce either IgM or IgG antibodies normally. However, the finding of normal IgM and IgG antibodies does not exclude IgA deficiency, transient hypogammaglobulinemia of infancy, or protein-losing states. Selective IgA deficiency, the most common B-cell defect, can be excluded by quantifying serum IgA. If the IgA concentration is normal, this also rules out most of the permanent types of hypogammaglobulinemia, as IgA is usually very low or absent in those conditions as well. If the IgA is low, IgG and IgM should also be quantified. Patients who are receiving steroids often have low IgG concentrations but make antibodies normally. If antibody deficiencies are detected despite normal levels of immunoglobulins, IgG subclass measurements may then be helpful. Patients who lack IgG2 are usually unable to make antibodies to polysaccharide antigens; however, this can be true even in those with normal IgG2, and there are healthy people with multiple subclass deficiencies. Thus, antibody measurements are far more cost effective than IgG subclass determinations. Very high serum concentrations of one or more immunoglobulin classes suggest human immunodeficiency virus (HIV) infection or chronic granulomatous disease.

The capacity of blood B lymphocytes to differentiate into plasma cells that synthesize and secrete immunoglobulin can be assessed in in-vitro cultures to which pokeweed mitogen or anti-CD40 plus cytokines is added as a differentiating agent. If all of these tests prove to be normal and the immunoglobulins are still low, trace label studies of serum proteins should be carried out to make certain that the immunoglobulins are not being lost through the urinary or gastrointestinal tract, such as in the nephrotic syndrome, protein-losing enteropathies, or intestinal lymphangiectasia.

T-Cell Function. The *Candida* skin test is the most cost-effective test. Adults and children older than 6 yr should be tested intradermally with 0.1 mL of a 1:1,000 dilution of a known potent *Candida albicans* extract. If the test is negative at 24, 48, and 72 hr, a 1:100 dilution should be tested. The latter concentration can be used in the initial testing of children under 6 yr. If the test is positive, as defined by erythema and induration of 10 mm or more at 48 hr, virtually all primary T-cell defects are excluded, and this will obviate the need for more expensive in vitro tests.

Patients found to have abnormalities on any of the above-mentioned screening tests should be characterized as fully as possible before any type of immunologic treatment is begun, unless there is a life-threatening illness. Some "abnormalities" may prove to be laboratory artifacts, and, conversely, what may appear to be a straightforward diagnosis may prove to be a much more complex disorder. For example, those found to be agammaglobulinemic should have their blood B cells enumerated with dye-conjugated monoclonal antibodies to B-cell–specific CDs (usually CD19 or CD20) in flow cytometry. Usually approximately 10% of circulating lymphocytes are B cells. In X-linked agammaglobulinemia (XLA), such cells are usually missing, whereas in common variable immunodeficiency (CVID), B cells are usually present. This distinction is important, because patients with these two different types of hypogammaglobulinemia can have different clinical problems, and the two defects clearly have different inheritance patterns. As noted in Chapter 117, there are now specific molecular tests for XLA, and these will be needed in cases in which there is no family history and genetic counseling is indicated. XLAs also have a heightened susceptibility to persistent enteroviral infections, whereas those with CVID have more problems with autoimmune diseases and lymphoid hyperplasia.

T-cell numbers and function should also be evaluated because some patients with CVID have such abnormalities. T cells and T-cell subpopulations can be enumerated by reacting them with dye-conjugated monoclonal antibodies recognizing CD antigens present on T cells (i.e., CD2, CD3, CD4, and CD8) and then counting them by flow cytometry. Usually CD3-positive cells make up 70% of the peripheral lymphocytes. T cells express either CD4 or CD8 on their surface; normally there are roughly twice as many CD4-positive (helper) T cells as there are CD8-positive (cytotoxic) T cells. Because there are examples of severe immunodeficiency in which T cells with mature differentiation markers are present, tests of T-cell function are far more informative and cost effective than those just mentioned. T cells are normally stimulated through their TCRs by antigen in the groove of MHC molecules; however, the TCR can also be stimulated directly with mitogens such as phytohemagglutinin, concanavalin A, or pokeweed mitogen. After a 3–5 day period of incubation with the mitogen, the proliferation of T cells is measured by the incorporation of radiolabeled thymidine into DNA. Other stimulants that can be used to assess T-cell function in the same type of assay include antigens (for example, *Candida* or tetanus) and allogeneic cells. Additional assays of T-cell function include determining the ability of allogeneic cells to stimulate the generation of cytotoxic T cells and the measurement of cytokine production by T lymphocytes stimulated with any of the above-mentioned agents (see Table 116–2).

NK cells can be enumerated with monoclonal antibodies to NK-specific CD antigens, usually CD16 or CD56, and flow cytometry. NK function is assessed by a radiolabeled chromium-release assay, using a cell line called K562, which is readily killed by NK cells.

INHERITANCE OF ABNORMALITIES IN T-, B-, AND NK-CELL DEVELOPMENT

More than 50 immunodeficiency syndromes have been described over the past 40 yr. Until recently, there was little insight into the fundamental problems underlying most of these conditions. Several of the primary immunodeficiency diseases involving T, B, and/or NK cells have been mapped to specific chromosomal locations, and the fundamental biologic errors have been identified in a growing number of diseases. Most are recessive traits, some of which are caused by mutations in genes on the X chromosome and others by mutations on autosomal chromosomes. Examples of the latter include (1) combined immunodeficiencies due to abnormalities of purine salvage pathway enzymes, either adenosine deaminase (ADA, encoded by a gene on chromosome 20q13-ter) or purine nucleoside phosphorylase (PNP, encoded by a gene on chromosome 14q13.1) and (2) mutations in the gene encoding ZAP-70 (localized to chromosome 2q12), a non-src family protein tyrosine kinase important in T cell signaling. The molecular bases of four X-linked immunodeficiency disorders affecting T, B, and/or NK cells have been reported: X-linked immunodeficiency with hyper IgM, X-linked agammaglobulinemia, X-linked severe combined immunodeficiency, and the Wiskott-Aldrich syndrome (see Chapters 117–119). The identification and cloning of the genes for several of the primary immunodeficiency diseases have obvious implications for potential future somatic cell gene therapy for these patients.

PRENATAL DIAGNOSIS AND CARRIER DETECTION

Intrauterine diagnosis of ADA and PNP deficiencies can be made by enzyme analyses on amnion cells (fresh or cultured) obtained prior to 20 wk gestation. Diagnosis of several X-linked defects can be made by restriction fragment length polymorphism (RFLP) studies of the X-chromosome in amnion cells from male infants whose mothers have been identified as carriers and who are heterozygous for informative DNA polymorphisms. Diagnosis of enzyme-normal SCID or other severe T-cell deficiencies, MHC class I and/or II antigen deficiencies, CGD, or Wiskott-Aldrich syndrome (by platelet size) can be made by appropriate tests of phenotype and/or function on small samples of blood obtained by fetoscopy at 18–22 wk of gestation, but this procedure carries significant risk. Carriers of ADA and PNP deficiency can be detected by quantitative enzyme analyses of blood samples. Carriers of X-linked agammaglobulinemia, X-linked SCID, or the Wiskott-Aldrich syndrome can be identified by techniques designed to detect nonrandom X-chromosome inactivation in one or more blood cell lineages.

Anonymous: Primary immunodeficiency diseases—report of a WHO Scientific Group meeting. Clin Exp Immunol 99(5):2, 1995.
Buckley RH: Breakthroughs in the understanding and therapy of primary immunodeficiency. Pediatr Clin North Am 41:665, 1994.
Burke F, Naylor MS, Davies B, et al: The cytokine wall chart. Immunol Today 14:165, 1993.
Haynes BF, Denning SM: Lymphopoiesis. *In:* Stamatoyannopoulis G, Nienhuis A, Majerus P, Varmus H (eds): Molecular Basis of Blood Diseases, 2nd ed. Philadelphia, WB Saunders, 1994, pp 425–462.
Noelle RJ, Roy M, Shepherd DM, et al: A 39-kDa protein on activated helper T cells binds CD40 and transduces the signal for cognate activation of B cells. Proc Natl Acad Sci USA 89:6550, 1992.
Puck JM: Molecular and genetic basis of X-linked immunodeficiency disorders. J Clin Immunol 14:81, 1994.
Schlossman SF, Boumsell L, Gilks W, et al (eds): Leucocyte Typing V: White Cell Differentiation Antigens. Oxford, Oxford University Press, 1995.
Zurawski G, de Vries JE: Interleukin 13, an interleukin 4–like cytokine that acts on monocytes and B cells but not on T cells. Immunol Today 15:19, 1994.

CHAPTER 117
Primary B-Cell Diseases

Rebecca H. Buckley

Of all of the primary immunodeficiency diseases, those affecting B-cell function are most frequent. Selective absence of serum and secretory IgA is the most common defect, with reported incidences ranging from 1:333 to 1:16,000 among different races. By contrast, it has been estimated that agammaglobulinemia occurs with a frequency of only 1:50,000. Most B-cell defects are not due to deletions of genes encoding immunoglobulin heavy chains. Patients with antibody deficiency are usually recognized because they have recurrent infections with encapsulated bacteria or a history of failure responding to antibiotic treatment, but some individuals with selective IgA deficiency or infants with transient hypogammaglobulinemia may have few or no infections.

117.1 X-Linked (XLA or Bruton) Agammaglobulinemia

CLINICAL MANIFESTATIONS. Most boys afflicted with XLA remain well during the first 6–9 mo of life by virtue of maternally transmitted IgG antibodies. Thereafter, they repeatedly acquire infections with extracellular pyogenic organisms such as pneumococci, streptococci, and *Haemophilus* unless given prophylactic antibiotics or gammaglobulin therapy. Chronic fungal infections are not usually present, and *Pneumocystis carinii* pneumonia rarely occurs unless there is an associated neutropenia. Viral infections are also usually handled normally, with the exceptions of hepatitis viruses and enteroviruses. Several examples of paralysis after polio vaccine administration have occurred, presumably due to mutation of this vaccine form of enterovirus to a more neurotropic form as it persists. Chronic progressive, eventually fatal, central nervous system infections with various echoviruses have occurred in more than 40 patients. These observations suggest a primary role for antibody, particularly secretory IgA, in host defense against enteroviruses, because normal T-cell function has been present in X-linked agammaglobulinemics with such persistent infections. Infections with mycoplasma are also particularly problematic for these patients.

DIAGNOSIS. The diagnosis of XLA is suspected if serum concentrations of IgG, IgA, IgM, and IgE are far below the 95% confidence limits for appropriate age- and race-matched controls (i.e., usually <100 mg/dL total immunoglobulin). Tests for natural antibodies to blood group substances for antibodies to antigens given during standard courses of immunization, for example, diphtheria, tetanus, or *Haemophilus influenzae,* are useful in distinguishing this disorder from transient hypogammaglobulinemia of infancy. Hypoplasia of adenoids, tonsils, and peripheral lymph nodes is the rule; germinal centers are not found, and plasma cells are rare.

GENETICS. The abnormal gene in X-linked agammaglobulinemia was mapped to q22 on the long arm of the X chromo-

■ **TABLE 117–1 Primary B-Cell Immunodeficiency Diseases**

Disorder	Functional Deficiencies	Molecular Defect
X-linked agammaglobulinemia	Antibody	Mutations in Bruton tyrosine kinase (BTK)
Common variable immunodeficiency (CVID; "acquired" hypogammaglobulinemia)	Antibody	Unknown, ? in MHC class III region
Selective IgA deficiency	IgA antibody	Unknown, ? in MHC class III region
Transient hypogammaglobulinemia of infancy	None; immunoglobulins low, but antibodies present	Unknown
IgG subclass deficiencies	Antibody	Unknown
Immunoglobulin heavy and light chain deficiencies	Antibody	Immunoglobulin heavy or light chain gene deletions
X-linked lymphoproliferative disease	Anti-EBV nuclear antigen antibody; ? also T-cell defect	Unknown

some and was found to encode for a B-cell protein tyrosine kinase, named Bruton tyrosine kinase (or BTK) in honor of the discoverer (Tables 117–1 and 117–2). BTK is a member of the Src-related nonreceptor tyrosine kinase family, which includes Lck, Fyn, and Lyn, and which is thought to be involved in signal transduction in many hematopoietic cells. BTK is expressed at high levels in all B-lineage cells, including pre-B cells; it is not detected in any cells of T lineage but is found in myeloid cells. BTK is hypothesized to have a role in B-cell differentiation at all stages. Pre-B cells are found in the bone marrow; however, blood B lymphocytes are absent or present in very low numbers. Thus far, all males with known XLA (by family history) have low to undetectable BTK mRNA and kinase activity. X-linked inheritance is documented in some agammaglobulinemic boys with no family history who have an abnormal BTK as a new mutation. Determination of the precise mutation, however, requires isolation and sequencing of each patient's BTK gene (Figure 117–1). Carriers are detected by the finding of nonrandom X-chromosome inactivation in B cells in restriction fragment length polymorphism (RFLP) studies of hamster-human B-cell hybrids or by differences in methylation patterns. Prenatal diagnosis of affected male fetuses is possible using closely linked probes and RFLP analysis.

PATHOPHYSIOLOGY. Polymorphonuclear functions are usually normal, but intermittent neutropenia is observed. The fact that BTK is also expressed in cells of myeloid lineage is of interest, because boys with XLA often have neutropenia at the height of an acute infection. It is conceivable that BTK is only one of the signaling molecules participating in myeloid maturation and that neutropenia is observed in XLA only when rapid production of such cells is needed. In most patients, the percentage of T cells is increased, ratios of T-cell subsets are

■ **TABLE 117–2 Chromosomal Map Locations for Faulty Genes in B-Cell Immunodeficiency Diseases**

Chromosome	Disease
2p11	Kappa chain deficiency*
6p21.3	(?) Common variable immunodeficiency and selective IgA deficiency
14q32.3	Immunoglobulin heavy chain deletion*
Xq22	X-linked agammaglobulinemia (Bruton tyrosine kinase or BTK)*
Xq24–26	X-linked lymphoproliferative syndrome

**Gene cloned and sequenced; gene product known.*

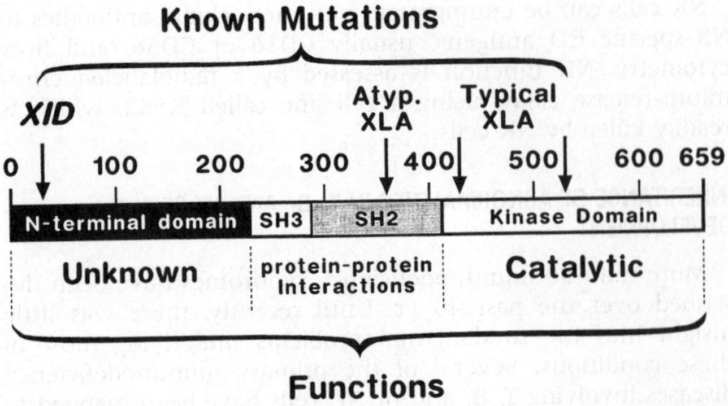

Figure 117–1. Location of mutations in the functional domains of the BTK protein. Deletion and point mutations in BTK identified to date in many boys with classic XLA are in the kinase domain, whereas CBA/N *xid* mice with a less severe B-cell defect have a point mutation causing an amino acid substitution at position 28 in the N-terminal domain. A male with a less severe B-cell defect than in classic XLA has had a point mutation at position 361 in the SH2 domain. However, more recently boys with classic XLA are also reported to have mutations at the *xid* mutation site and in the SH2 domain. (From Buckley RH: Breakthroughs in the understanding and therapy of primary immunodeficiency. Pediatr Clin North Am 41:665–690, 1994, with permission.)

normal, and T-cell function is intact. The thymus appears morphologically normal in autopsied cases. An absence of circulating B cells that resembles XLA phenotypically and functionally is also reported in girls. The molecular basis for this apparently autosomal recessive defect is unknown. XLA is reported in association with growth hormone deficiency.

117.2 Common Variable Immunodeficiency (CVID)

CVID, also known as "acquired" hypogammaglobulinemia, is similar clinically to XLA (see Table 117–1). The infections and bacterial pathogens that occur are generally the same for the two defects. However, echovirus meningoencephalitis is rare in patients with CVID. In contrast to XLA, the sex distribution in CVID is almost equal, the age of onset is later, and infections are less severe.

CLINICAL MANIFESTATIONS. Patients with CVID often have autoantibody formation, normal-sized or enlarged tonsils and lymph nodes, and approximately 25% of cases have splenomegaly. CVID has also been associated with a spruelike syndrome, with or without nodular follicular lymphoid hyperplasia of the intestine; thymoma; alopecia areata; hemolytic anemia; gastric atrophy; achlorhydria; and pernicious anemia. Lymphoid interstitial pneumonia, pseudolymphoma, amyloidosis, and noncaseating granulomata of the lungs, spleen, skin, and liver also occur. There is a 438-fold increase in lymphomas among affected women in the 5th and 6th decades.

PATHOPHYSIOLOGY. The serum immunoglobulin and antibody deficiencies in CVID may be as profound as in XLA. Despite normal numbers of circulating immunoglobulin-bearing B lymphocytes and the presence of lymphoid cortical follicles, blood B lymphocytes from CVID patients do not differentiate normally into immunoglobulin-producing cells when stimulated with pokeweed mitogen in vitro, even when cocultured with normal T cells. However, recent studies have shown that CVID B cells can be stimulated to both switch isotype and to synthesize and secrete immunoglobulin when stimulated with anti-CD40 and IL-4 or IL-10. T cells and T-cell subsets are usually present in normal percentages, although T-cell function is depressed in some patients. Mitogen-activated T cells from some CVID patients are deficient in expression of genes for several lymphokines while retaining a normal capacity to proliferate. Some patients with CVID have significantly depressed (but not absent) expression of CD40 ligand mRNA and surface protein in activated T lymphocytes, suggesting that inefficient signaling by poorly expressed CD40 ligand on T cells could account for failure of B cells to differentiate. CVID is reported to resolve transiently or permanently in patients who acquire human immunodeficiency virus (HIV) infection.

GENETICS. Because this disorder occurs in first-degree relatives of patients with selective IgA deficiency, and some patients with IgA deficiency later become panhypogammaglobulinemic, these diseases may have a common genetic basis. The high incidences of abnormal immunoglobulin concentrations, autoantibodies, autoimmune disease, and malignancy in families of both types of patients also suggest a shared hereditary influence. This concept is supported by the discovery of a high incidence of C4-A gene deletions and C2 rare gene alleles in the class III major histocompatibility complex (MHC) region in individuals with either A Def or CVID, suggesting that the susceptibility gene(s) are in this region on chromosome 6 (see Tables 117–1 and 117–2). A small number of HLA haplotypes are shared by individuals affected with CVID and A Def, with at least one of two particular haplotypes being present in 77% of those affected. In one large family with 13 members, two had A Def and three had CVID. All of the immunodeficient patients in the family had at least one copy of an MHC haplotype that is abnormally frequent in A Def and CVID: HLA-DQB1 *0201, HLA-DR3, C4B-Sf, C4A-deleted, G11-15, Bf-0.4, C2a, HSP70-7.5, TNFα-5, HLA-B8, and HLA-A1. However, four immunologically normal members of the pedigree also possessed this haplotype, indicating that its presence is not sufficient for expression of the defects. Environmental factors, particularly drugs such as phenytoin, D-penicillamine, gold, and sulfasalazine, are suspected to be triggers for disease expression in individuals with the permissive genetic background.

117.3 Selective IGA Deficiency

An isolated absence or near absence (i.e., <10 mg/dL) of serum and secretory IgA is the most common well-defined immunodeficiency disorder, with a frequency of 1:333 being reported among some apparently healthy blood donors. However, this condition is also commonly associated with ill health.

CLINICAL MANIFESTATIONS. Infections occur predominantly in the respiratory, gastrointestinal, and urogenital tracts. Bacterial agents responsible are the same as in other antibody deficiency syndromes. There is no clear evidence that patients with this disorder have an undue susceptibility to viral agents. Children with IgA deficiency vaccinated with killed polio virus intranasally produce local IgM and IgG antibodies. Serum concentrations of other immunoglobulins are usually normal in patients with selective IgA deficiency, although IgG2 (and other) subclass deficiency is reported, and IgM (usually elevated) may be monomeric.

Patients with IgA deficiency often have IgG antibodies against cow milk and ruminant serum proteins. These antiruminant antibodies may cause false-positive results in immunoassays for IgA that use goat (but not rabbit) antisera. A sprue-like syndrome occurs in adults with this defect, which may or may not respond to a gluten-free diet. High incidences of autoantibodies and autoimmune diseases are noted, and the incidence of malignancy is increased. Serum antibodies to IgA are reported in as many as 44% of patients with selective IgA deficiency. If of the IgE isotype, these antibodies can cause severe or fatal anaphylactic reactions after intravenous administration of blood products containing IgA. For this reason, only five times washed (in 200 mL volumes) normal donor erythrocytes or blood products from other IgA absent individuals should be administered to these patients. Immune serum globulin (IVIG; which is >99% IgG) is not indicated because most IgA-deficient patients make IgG antibodies normally. Moreover, many IVIG preparations contain sufficient IgA to cause anaphylactic reactions.

GENETICS AND PATHOPHYSIOLOGY. As is the case for CVID, the basic defect leading to IgA deficiency is unknown (see Tables 117–1 and 117–2). Phenotypically normal blood B cells are present in both conditions. IgA deficiency is known to remit following discontinuation of dilantin therapy or spontaneously. The occurrence of IgA deficiency in both males and females, and in families, suggests autosomal inheritance. In some families, inheritance appears to be dominant with variable expressivity. This defect is commonly seen in pedigrees containing individuals with CVID. Indeed, IgA deficiency has been noted to evolve into CVID, and the recent finding of rare alleles and deletions of MHC class III genes in both conditions suggests that the susceptibility genes for these two defects may reside in the MHC class III region on chromosome 6 (see Tables 117–1 and 117–2). IgA deficiency is noted in patients treated with the same drugs associated with producing CVID, suggesting that environmental factors may also lead to expression of this defect.

117.4 Transient Hypogammaglobulinemia of Infancy (THI)

Unlike patients with X-linked agammaglobulinemia or CVID, patients with THI synthesize antibodies to human type A and B erythrocytes and to diphtheria and tetanus toxoids, usually by 6–11 mo of age, and well before immunoglobulin concentrations become normal (see Table 117–1). IVIG therapy is not indicated in this condition.

117.5 IgG Subclass Deficiencies

Some patients have deficiencies of one or more subclasses of IgG, despite normal or elevated total IgG serum concentrations (see Table 117–1). Most patients with absent or very low concentrations of IgG_2 have A Def. Other patients with IgG_2 deficiency have an evolving pattern of immunodeficiency (such as CVID), suggesting that the presence of IgG subclass deficiency may be a marker for more general immune dysfunction. The biologic significance of the multiple moderate deficiencies of IgG subclasses reported is difficult to assess, particularly because commercial laboratory measurement of IgG subclasses is problematic. The more relevant issue is the capacity of the patient to make specific antibodies to protein and polysaccharide antigens, because profound deficiencies of antipolysaccharide antibodies are noted even in the presence of normal concentrations of IgG_2. IVIG should not be given to IgG subclass–deficient patients unless they are shown to have a deficiency of antibodies to a broad array of antigens.

117.6 Immunoglobulin Heavy and Light Chain Deletions

Some completely asymptomatic individuals have a total absence of IgG_1, IgG_2, IgG_4, and/or IgA_1 due to gene deletions (see Tables 117–1 and 117–2). These abnormalities were discovered fortuitously in 16 individuals, 15 of whom had no history of undue susceptibility to infection. They produced antibodies of all other isotypes in normal quantity. These patients illustrate the importance of assessing specific antibody formation before deciding to initiate IVIG therapy.

117.7 X-Linked Lymphoproliferative Disease (XLP)

X-linked lymphoproliferative disease (XLP), also referred to as Duncan disease (after the original kindred in which it was described), is a recessive trait characterized by an inadequate immune response to infection with Epstein-Barr virus (EBV) (see Table 117–1). The defective gene in XLP has been localized to the Xq25–26 region near DXS42 and DXS37 (see Table 117–2). The affected males are apparently healthy until they acquire EBV infection. Through use of RFLP probes in linkage with XLP, it is possible to identify affected males before they develop primary EBV infection. Immunologic studies demonstrated elevated IgA or IgM and/or variable deficiency of IgG, IgG_1, and IgG_3 in 13/13 RFLP-positive but in none of 14 RFLP-negative, EBV-negative males. Thus, the immunodeficiency in affected males may not all be due to EBV infection, and the preexisting abnormalities found may be related to their inadequate response to EBV. The mean age of presentation is less than 5 yr. The most common form of presentation (75%) is severe fatal (80%) EBV infection, primarily due to extensive liver necrosis caused by polyclonally activated alloreactive cytotoxic T cells that recognize EBV-infected autologous B cells. Most patients surviving the primary infection develop global cellular immune defects involving T, B, and natural killer (NK) cells; lymphomas; and/or hypogammaglobulinemia. There is a marked impairment in production of antibodies to the EBV nuclear antigen (EBNA), whereas titers of antibodies to the viral capsid antigen have ranged from zero to markedly elevated. Antibody-dependent cell-mediated cytotoxicity (ADCC) against EBV-infected cells is low in many patients, and NK function is also depressed. There is also a deficiency in memory T-cell immunity to EBV. The percentage of CD8-positive T cells is often elevated. Immunoglobulin synthesis in response to pokeweed mitogen stimulation in vitro is markedly depressed. Thus, both EBV-specific and nonspecific immunologic abnormalities occur in these patients.

117.8 Treatment of B-Cell Defects

Judicious use of antibiotics and regular administration of antibodies are the only effective treatments for B-cell disorders. The most common form of replacement therapy is with intravenous preparations of IVIG. Broad antibody deficiency should be carefully documented before IVIG therapy is initiated. The rationale for the use of these preparations is to provide missing antibodies, not to raise the serum IgG concentration. The development of safe and effective IVIG is a major advance in the treatment of patients with severe antibody deficiencies, although it is expensive. Seven intravenous preparations of immune globulin are approved by the Food and Drug Administration and are available in the United States; nearly three dozen more are under investigation or marketed abroad. Almost all preparations are isolated initially from normal plasma by the Cohn alcohol fractionation method or a modification of it. Cohn fraction II is then further modified by treatment at low pH or by adding polyethylene glycol, DEAE-Sephadex, or ethanol at low ionic strength to remove aggregated IgG. Additional stabilizing agents, such as sugars, glycine, and albumin, are added to prevent reaggregation and to protect the IgG molecule during lyophilization. HIV is inactivated by the ethanol used in preparation of ISG and IVIG; a detergent is also added to eliminate hepatitis viruses. All commercial lots are produced from plasma pooled from 3,000–6,000 donors and, therefore, contain a broad spectrum of antibodies. Each pool must contain adequate levels of antibody to antigens in various vaccines, such as tetanus and measles. However, there is no standardization based on titers of antibodies to more clinically relevant organisms, such as *Streptococcus pneumoniae* or *Hemophilus influenzae*.

The IVIG preparations currently available in the United States have similar efficacy and safety. There has been no documented transmission of HIV infection by any of these preparations; however, during 1994, hepatitis C virus infections were transmitted by some lots from two of them. The latter problem has been resolved by addition of a detergent. IVIG, 400 mg/kg/mo, achieves trough IgG levels close to the normal range. Systemic reactions to IVIG may occur, but rarely are these true anaphylactic reactions. Anaphylactic reactions caused by patient IgE antibodies to IgA in the IVIG preparation may, however, occur in patients with CVID or IgA deficiency. All newly diagnosed patients with CVID should be screened for anti-IgA antibodies through the American Red Cross before undergoing IVIG therapy. If antibodies are detected, IVIG therapy may still be possible by use of the one available IVIG preparation containing almost no IgA (Gammagard, Baxter-Hyland); carefully screened lots of it can be used safely in patients who have antibodies to IgA.

Buckley RH: Breakthroughs in the understanding and therapy of primary immunodeficiency. Pediatr Clin North Am 41:665, 1994.

Buckley RH, Schiff RI: The use of intravenous immunoglobulin in immunodeficiency diseases. N Engl J Med 325:110, 1991.

Cunningham-Rundles C: Clinical and immunologic analyses of 103 patients with common variable immunodeficiency. J Clin Immunol 9:22, 1989.

Nonoyama S, Farrington M, Ochs HM: Activated B cells from patients with common variable immunodeficiency proliferate and synthesize immunoglobulin. J Clin Invest 92:1281, 1993.

Puck JM: Molecular and genetic basis of x-linked immunodeficiency disorders. J Clin Immunol 14:81, 1994.

Schaffer FM, Palermos J, Zhu ZB, et al: Individuals with IgA deficiency and common variable immunodeficiency share complex polymorphisms of major histocompatibility complex class III genes. Proc Natl Acad Sci 86:8015, 1989.

Spickett GP, Webster ADB, Farrant J: Cellular abnormalities in common variable immunodeficiency. Immunodef Rev 2:199, 1990.

Tsukada S, Saffran DC, Rawlings DJ, et al: Deficient expression of a B cell cytoplasmic tyrosine kinase in human X-linked agammaglobulinemia. Cell 72:279, 1993.

Vetrie D, Vorechovsky I, Sideras P, et al: The gene involved in X-linked agammaglobulinaemia is a member of the src family of protein-tyrosine kinases. Nature 361:226, 1993.

CHAPTER 118

Primary T-Cell Disease

Rebecca H. Buckley

In general, patients with defects in T-cell function have infections or other clinical problems that are more severe than patients with antibody deficiency disorders. These individuals rarely survive beyond infancy or childhood. However, exceptions are being recognized as newer primary T-cell defects are being identified, such as X-linked immunodeficiency with hyper IgM and CD3 deficiency.

118.1 Thymic Hypoplasia (DiGeorge Syndrome)

Thymic hypoplasia results from dysmorphogenesis of the 3rd and 4th pharyngeal pouches during early embryogenesis, leading to hypoplasia or aplasia of the thymus and parathyroid glands. Other structures forming at the same age are also frequently affected, resulting in anomalies of the great vessels (right-sided aortic arch), esophageal atresia, bifid uvula, congenital heart disease (atrial and ventricular septal defects), a short philtrum of the upper lip, hypertelorism, an antimongoloid slant to the eyes, mandibular hypoplasia, and low-set, often notched ears. The diagnosis is often first suggested by hypocalcemic seizures during the neonatal period. Similar facial features and conotruncal heart lesions are seen in the fetal alcohol syndrome.

CLINICAL MANIFESTATIONS. A variable degree of hypoplasia of the thymus and parathyroid glands is more frequent than total aplasia. Patients with variable hypoplasia are referred to as having partial DiGeorge syndrome; they may have little trouble with infections and grow normally. Patients with complete DiGeorge syndrome resemble patients with severe combined immunodeficiency (SCID) in their susceptibility to infections with low-grade or opportunistic pathogens, including fungi, viruses, and *Pneumocystis carinii*, and to graft-versus-host disease (GVHD) from non-irradiated blood transfusions (Table 118–1). Concentrations of serum immunoglobulins are usually near normal for age, but IgA may be diminished and IgE elevated (Table 118–1). Absolute lymphocyte counts are usually only moderately low for age. CD3-positive T cells are variably decreased in number, corresponding to the degree of thymic hypoplasia; as a result, the percentage of B cells is increased. The proportion of CD4- and CD8-positive cells is usually normal. Lymphocyte responses to mitogen stimulation, like intradermal delayed hypersensitivity responses, are absent, reduced, or normal, depending on the degrees of thymic deficiency. Thymic tissue, when found, contains Hassall's corpuscles and a normal density of thymocytes; corticomedullary distinction is present. Lymphoid follicles are usually present, but lymph node paracortical areas and thymus-dependent regions of the spleen show variable degrees of depletion.

GENETICS. DiGeorge syndrome occurs in both males and females. Because familial occurrence is rare, the defect was thought unlikely to be heritable. However, submicroscopic chromosomal deletions at 22q11 are identified in more than 95% of cases (Tables 118–1 and 118–2).

TREATMENT. The immune deficiency in the complete DiGeorge syndrome has been corrected by thymic tissue transplants and by unfractionated HLA-identical bone marrow transplantation.

118.2 X-Linked Immunodeficiency with Hyper IgM (Hyper IgM)

This disorder is characterized by very low serum concentrations of IgG and IgA with a normal or, more frequently, a markedly elevated concentration of polyclonal IgM. Until recently it was classified as a B-cell defect.

CLINICAL MANIFESTATIONS. Like patients with X-linked agammaglobulinemia, affected boys become symptomatic during the 1st or 2nd year of life with recurrent pyogenic infections, including otitis media, sinusitis, pneumonia, and tonsillitis. In contrast to patients with X-linked agammaglobulinemia, the frequent presence of lymphoid hyperplasia often leads away from a diagnosis of immunodeficiency. Thymic-dependent lymphoid tissues and T-cell functions are usually normal, but some affected males have been shown to have decreased T-cell function. High titers of IgM antibodies to blood group substances and to salmonella O antigen are found in some patients, but very low titers or no IgM antibody are noted in others. The frequency of autoimmune disorders is even higher than it is with other antibody-deficiency syndromes. Hemolytic anemia and thrombocytopenia may occur, and transient, persistent, or cyclic neutropenia is a common feature. Normal numbers of B lymphocytes are found in the blood of these patients.

GENETICS. B cells from boys with the X-linked form of this defect are capable of synthesizing not only IgM, but also IgA and IgG when cocultured with a "switch" T-cell line, indicating that the defect is in the T-cell lineage. The abnormal gene is localized to Xq26, and the gene product, gp39 or CD40L, is the ligand for CD40 on B cells; it is upregulated on activated T cells (see Tables 118–1 and 118–2). Mutations in the CD40L on activated T cells from males with X-linked hyper IgM result

■ **TABLE 118–1 Primary T-Cell Immunodeficiency Diseases**

Disorder	Functional Deficiencies	Molecular Defect
DiGeorge syndrome	T cellular; some antibody	Microdeletions in chromosome 22q11
Immunodeficiency with elevated IgM	IgG and IgA antibodies	Mutations in CD40 ligand (gp39) on activated T cells
Defective expression of the T-cell receptor (Ti):CD3 complex	T cellular; antipolysaccharide antibody	Mutation in CD3γ chain or unknown cause
CD8 lymphocytopenia	T cellular; some antibody	Mutations in ZAP-70
Cytokine deficiencies	T cellular; defective IL-2 and other cytokine production	Unknown or due to NF-AT abnormalities
T-cell activation defects	T cellular; some antibody	Defective signal transduction due to various unknown causes

NF-AT, Nuclear factor of activated T cells.

■ **TABLE 118–2 Chromosomal Map Locations for Faulty Genes in T-Cell Immunodeficiency Diseases**

Chromosome	Disease
2q12	CD8 lymphocytopenia (ZAP-70)*
11	CD3 gamma chain deficiency*
22q11.2	DiGeorge syndrome
Xq26	Immunodeficiency with hyper IgM (CD40 ligand—gp39)*

Gene cloned and sequenced, gene product known.

in an inability to signal B cells to undergo isotype switching, so that they produce only IgM. Defective T-cell function may explain the occurrence of *P. carinii* pneumonia and extensive verruca vulgaris lesions in some patients with this condition. At least 16 distinct point mutations or deletions in the gene for CD40L are known, giving rise to frame shifts, premature stop codons, and single amino acid substitutions, all but one of which are clustered in the TNF homology domain located in the carboxy-terminal region. A highly polymorphic microsatellite dinucleotide (CA) repeat region has been identified in the 3′ untranslated end of the gene for the CD40 ligand. Approximately 80% of women are heterozygous for this polymorphism, consisting of eight alleles. This marker can be used to detect carriers of X-linked hyper IgM, and it can be used to make a prenatal diagnosis of this condition. However, not all males with hyper IgM have a mutation in the CD40L; B cells from such patients fail to switch isotype with monoclonal antibodies to CD40, and some patients are females, suggesting that this phenotype has more than one genetic cause.

118.3 Defective Expression of the T-Cell Receptor–CD3 Complex (Ti-CD3)

The first type of this disorder was found in two male siblings in a Spanish family. The proband presented with severe infections and died at 31 mo of age with autoimmune hemolytic anemia and viral pneumonia. His lymphocytes had responded poorly to mitogens and to anti-CD3 in vitro and could not be stimulated to develop cytotoxic T cells. However, his antibody responses to protein antigens had been normal, indicating normal T-helper cell function. His 12-yr-old brother is healthy but has almost no CD3-bearing T cells and has IgG_2 deficiency similar to his sibling. The defect in this family is due to mutations in the CD3γ chain (Tables 118–1 and 118–2). The second type of this disorder was diagnosed in a 4-yr-old French boy who had recurrent *Haemophilus influenzae* pneumonia and otitis media in early life but is now healthy. He has a partial defect in expression of Ti-CD3, and thus the percentage of CD3+ cells is about half-normal but the level of expression is markedly decreased. His T cells do not proliferate in response to anti-CD3 or anti-CD2, nor do they express the IL-2 receptor or have normal calcium influx following these treatments. However, they do respond normally to stimulation with anti-CD28 or antigens, such as tetanus. The defect is attributed to an unstable CD3 protein on the T-cell surface, but its molecular basis is unknown.

118.4 Defective Cytokine Production

Two main defects of cytotokine production are known (see Table 118–1). The first is a selective inability to produce IL-2. In the two reported cases, patients had severe recurrent infections in infancy. The IL-2 gene was present in both, but no IL-2 message or protein was produced. Other T-cell cytokines were produced normally. The second type was seen in a single patient who also presented during infancy with severe recurrent infections and failure to thrive. She had defective transcription of several lymphokine genes, including IL-2, IL-3, IL-4, and IL-5, possibly due to abnormal binding of nuclear factor of activated T cells (NF-AT) to response elements in IL-2 and IL-4 enhancers. She was treated with recombinant IL-2 with some clinical improvement.

118.5 CD8 Lymphocytopenia

Patients with this newly described condition present during infancy with severe, recurrent, often fatal infections. Six cases have been reported, and a majority are Mennonites. They have normal or elevated numbers of blood B cells, and low to elevated serum immunoglobulin concentrations (see Table 118–1). Their blood lymphocytes exhibit normal expression of the T-cell surface antigens CD3 and CD4, but CD8+ cells are almost totally absent. These cells fail to respond to mitogens or to allogeneic cells in vitro or to generate cytotoxic T lymphocytes. By contrast, NK activity is normal. The thymus of one patient exhibited normal architecture with normal numbers of CD4:CD8 double-positive thymocytes, but an absence of CD8 single-positive thymocytes. This condition is due to mutations in the gene encoding ZAP-70, a non-src family protein tyrosine kinase important in T-cell signaling. The gene is localized to chromosome 2q12 (Table 118–2). The hypothesis as to why there are normal numbers of CD4:CD8 double-positive T cells is that thymocytes can use the other member of the same tyrosine kinase family, Syk, to facilitate positive selection. Syk is present at fourfold higher levels in thymocytes than in peripheral T cells, possibly accounting for the lack of normal responses by the CD4+ blood T cells.

118.6 T-Cell Activation Defects

These conditions are characterized by the presence of normal or elevated numbers of blood T cells that appear phenotypically normal but that fail to proliferate or produce cytokines in response to stimulation with mitogens, antigens, or other signals delivered to the T-cell antigen receptor (TCR) due to defective signal transduction from the TCR to intracellular metabolic pathways (see Table 118–1). These patients have problems similar to those of other T-cell–deficient individuals, and some with severe T-cell activation defects may resemble SCID patients clinically.

Allen RC, Armitage RJ, Conley ME, et al: CD40 ligand gene defects responsible for X-linked hyper IgM syndrome. Science 259:990, 1993.

Arnaiz-Villena A, Timon M, Corell A, et al: Brief report: primary immunodeficiency caused by mutations in the gene encoding the CD3-γ subunit of the T lymphocyte receptor. N Engl J Med 327:529, 1992.

Arpaia E, Shahar M, Dadi H, et al: Defective T cell receptor signaling and CD8+ thymic selection in humans lacking zap-70 kinase. Cell 76:947, 1994.

Callard RE, Armitage RJ, Fanslow WC, et al: CD40 ligand and its role in X-linked hyper IgM syndrome. Immunol Today 14:559, 1993.

Chatila T, Wong R, Young M, et al: An immunodeficiency characterized by defective signal transduction in T lymphocytes. N Engl J Med 320:696, 1989.

Disanto JP, Keever CA, Small TN, et al: Absence of interleukin 2 production in a severe combined immunodeficiency disease syndrome with T cells. J Exp Med 171:1697, 1990.

Disanto JP, Markiewicz S, Gauchat J, et al: Brief report: prenatal diagnosis of X-linked hyper IgM syndrome. N Engl J Med 330:969, 1994.

Driscoll DA, Budarf ML, Emanuel BS: A genetic etiology for DiGeorge syndrome: consistent deletions and microdeletions of 22q11. Am J Hum Genet 50:924, 1992.
Elder ME, Lin D, Clever J, et al: Human severe combined immunodeficiency due to a defect in ZAP-70, a T cell tyrosine kinase. Science 264:1596, 1994.
Mayer L, Swan SP, Thompson C: Evidence for a defect in "switch" T cells in patients with immunodeficiency and hyperimmunoglobulinemia M. N Engl J Med 314:409, 1986.
Rijkers GT, Scharenberg JGM, VanDongen JJM, et al: Abnormal signal transduction in a patient with severe combined immunodeficiency disease. Pediatr Res 29:306, 1991.
Weinberg K, Parkman R: Severe combined immunodeficiency due to a specific defect in the production of interleukin-2. N Engl J Med 322:1718, 1990.

CHAPTER 119
Combined B- and T-Cell Diseases

Rebecca H. Buckley

Patients with combined B- and T-cell defects have severe, frequently opportunistic, infections that lead to death in infancy or childhood without bone marrow transplantation early in life. These are rare defects; for example, severe combined deficiency of SCID has been estimated to affect 1:100,000 to 1:500,000 live births.

119.1 Combined Immunodeficiency (CID or Nezelof Syndrome)

Patients with Nezelof syndrome have recurrent or chronic pulmonary infections, failure to thrive, oral or cutaneous candidiasis, chronic diarrhea, recurrent skin infections, gram-negative sepsis, urinary tract infections, and/or severe varicella in infancy. Neutropenia and eosinophilia are common. Serum immunoglobulins may be normal or elevated for all classes, but selective IgA deficiency, marked elevation of IgE, and elevated IgD levels occur in some cases. While antibody-forming capacity is impaired in most patients, it is not absent (Table 119–1). Moreover, plasma cells are usually abundant in the lamina propria and lymph nodes.

Studies of cellular immune function show delayed cutaneous anergy to ubiquitous antigens, lymphopenia, and extremely low but not absent lymphocyte proliferative responses to mitogens, antigens, and allogeneic cells in vitro (Table 119–1). Nezelof syndrome is the primary immunodeficiency disorder most likely to be confused with acquired immunodeficiency syndrome (AIDS) in the pediatric age group. Nezelof patients have profound deficiencies of CD3-positive T cells but usually normal proportions of CD4- and CD8-positive cells. Peripheral lymphoid tissues demonstrate paracortical lymphocyte depletion. The thymuses are very small and have a paucity of thymocytes and usually no Hassall's corpuscles. An autosomal recessive pattern of inheritance is often seen.

119.2 Purine Nucleoside Phosphorylase (PNP) Deficiency

More than 33 patients with Nezelof syndrome have been found to have PNP deficiency (Table 119–1). Point mutations identified in the PNP gene on chromosome 14q13.1 account for these deficiencies (Table 119–2). In contrast to patients with adenosine deaminase (ADA) deficiency, serum and urinary uric acid are usually markedly deficient, and no characteristic physical or skeletal abnormalities have been noted. Deaths occur from generalized vaccinia, varicella, lymphosarcoma, and GVHD mediated by allogeneic T cells in non-irradiated blood or bone marrow. Two thirds of patients have neurologic abnormalities, ranging from spasticity to mental retardation. One third of patients have autoimmune diseases, the most common of which is autoimmune hemolytic anemia. Idiopathic thrombocytopenic purpura and systemic lupus erythematosus are also reported. Lymphopenia is striking due primarily to a marked deficiency of T cells and T-cell subsets; T-cell function is decreased to varying degrees. Cells with the natural killer (NK) phenotype and function are increased. Prenatal diagnosis is possible. Attempts to correct the immunologic and enzymatic deficiencies of PNP-deficient patients by enzyme replacement or deoxycytidine therapy have failed. Gene therapy is a possibility for the future, but thus far bone marrow transplantation has been the only successful form of therapy.

119.3 Cartilage Hair Hypoplasia

In 1965 an unusual form of short-limbed dwarfism with frequent and severe infections was reported among the Pennsylvania Amish; non-Amish cases have since been described.

■ TABLE 119–1 Combined B- and T-Cell Diseases

Disorder	Functional Deficiencies	Molecular Defect
Combined immunodeficiency (CID or Nezelof syndrome)	T cellular; some antibody	PNP deficiency or other unknown defects
Severe combined immunodeficiency syndromes (SCID)	Antibody and T cellular; plus neutropenia in reticular dysgenesis	ADA deficiency; IL2Rγ in x-linked; ? recombinase deficiency in T-B-NK+ type
MHC class I and/or II deficiencies	Antibody; T cellular	Mutation in RFX and C11TA transcription factors that bind to MHC class II gene promoters
Omenn syndrome	Antibody; TH1-like deficiency, TH2-like excess (elevated IgE and eosinophilia)	Unknown
Wiskott-Aldrich syndrome	Antibody; T cellular	Proline-rich protein (WASP)
Ataxia telangiectasia	Antibody; T cellular	Unknown
Hyperimmunoglobulinemia E	Specific immune responses; TH1-like deficiency, TH2-like excess (elevated IgE and eosinophilia)	Unknown

WASP, Wiskott-Aldrich syndrome protein; TH1, T-helper cell type 1; TH2, T-helper cell type 2; PNP, purine nucleoside phosphorylase; ADA, adenosine deaminase.

■ **TABLE 119–2 Chromosomal Map Locations for Faulty Genes in Combined B- and T-Cell Diseases**

Chromosome	Disease
11q22.3	Ataxia-telangiectasia
14q13.1	Purine nucleoside phosphorylase deficiency*
20q13-ter	Adenosine deaminase deficiency*
Xp11.22–11.23	Wiskott-Aldrich syndrome (proline-rich protein, WASP)*
Xq13	Severe combined immunodeficiency (gamma chain of IL-2R, IL-2Rγ)*

**Gene cloned and sequenced, gene product known.*
WASP, Wiskott-Aldrich syndrome protein.

Features include short and pudgy hands; redundant skin; hyperextensible joints of hands and feet but an inability to extend the elbows completely; and fine, sparse, light hair and eyebrows. Radiographically, the bones show scalloping and sclerotic or cystic changes in the metaphyses and flaring of the costochondral junctions of the ribs. Severe and often fatal varicella infections, progressive vaccinia, and vaccine-associated poliomyelitis have been observed.

The severity of the immunodeficiency varies; in one series, 11 of 77 patients died before age 20, but two were still alive at age 76. Three patterns of immune dysfunction have emerged: defective antibody-mediated immunity, Nezelof syndrome (most common form), and severe combined immunodeficiency. In vitro studies have shown decreased numbers of T cells and defective T-cell proliferation due to an intrinsic defect related to the G1 phase, resulting in a longer cell cycle for individual cells. This abnormality also occurs in fibroblasts from these patients. However, NK cells are increased in number and function. Cartilage hair hypoplasia appears to be inherited as an autosomal recessive condition with variable penetrance.

119.4 Severe Combined Immunodeficiency (SCID)

The syndromes of SCID are characterized by (1) absence of T- and B-cell function from birth and (2) great genetic diversity (see Table 119–1). Patients in this group of disorders have the most severe of all of the recognized immunodeficiencies. Unless immunologic reconstitution can be achieved through bone marrow transplantation or enzyme replacement therapy, death usually occurs in the 1st yr of life and almost invariably before the end of the 2nd yr.

CLINICAL MANIFESTATIONS. Affected infants present within the first few months of life with frequent episodes of diarrhea, pneumonia, otitis, sepsis, and cutaneous infections. Growth may appear normal initially, but extreme wasting usually develops after infections and diarrhea begin. Persistent infections with opportunistic organisms such as *Candida albicans, Pneumocystis carinii,* varicella, measles, parainfluenzae 3, cytomegalovirus, Epstein-Barr virus, and bacillus Calmette-Guérin lead to death. These infants also lack the ability to reject foreign tissue and are therefore at risk for graft-versus-host disease from maternal immunocompetent T cells crossing the placenta or from T lymphocytes in non-irradiated blood products or allogeneic bone marrow.

Infants with SCID have profound lymphopenia; an absence of lymphocyte proliferative responses to mitogens, antigens, and allogeneic cells in vitro; and delayed cutaneous anergy. Serum immunoglobulin concentrations are diminished to absent, and no antibody formation occurs following immunization. Analyses of lymphocyte populations and subpopulations demonstrate marked heterogeneity among SCID patients. Patients with ADA deficiency have the lowest absolute lymphocyte counts, usually less than 500/mm^3. Despite the uniformly profound lack of B-cell function, many patients (particularly those with X-linked SCID) have elevated percentages of B cells. T cells and subsets are extremely low or absent in all types; when present, they are in many cases transplacentally derived maternal T cells. All or most of the circulating lymphocytes in some infants with autosomal recessive, non-ADA–deficient SCID are large granular lymphocytes with NK-cell phenotype and function; by contrast, NK cells and function are extremely low in X-linked SCID.

PATHOLOGY. Typically, SCID patients have very small thymuses (less than 1 g) that usually fail to descend from the neck, contain few thymocytes, and lack corticomedullary distinction and Hassall's corpuscles. The thymic epithelium appears histologically normal. Both the follicular and paracortical areas of the peripheral lymph nodes are depleted of lymphocytes; tonsils, adenoids, and Peyer's patches are absent or extremely underdeveloped.

TREATMENT. All forms of human SCID are correctable by bone marrow transplantation. The fact that T cell–depleted haploidentical bone marrow stem cells can correct these defects indicates that the thymi in most human SCIDs have normal T-cell differentiation capacities. This process appears to require 90–120 days whether the stem cells are HLA-identical or haploidentical.

119.5 Autosomal Recessive SCID

This disorder was the first known form of the SCID syndrome identified. Clinically, functionally, and histopathologically, patients with the autosomal recessive form usually resemble those with the X-linked form, except that they have somewhat lower percentages of B cells and higher percentages of NK cells. Those who lack B cells (so-called T-, B-SCID) have abnormal immunoglobulin heavy chain gene rearrangement patterns, reminiscent of abnormalities in SCID mice. The molecular basis of this form of SCID, as well as that of the large subgroup of male SCIDs with no family history, is under intense study (see Table 119–1).

119.6 Adenosine Deaminase (ADA) Deficiency

An absence of the enzyme ADA is observed in approximately 15% of patients with SCID (see Table 119–1), resulting from a variety of point and deletional mutations in the ADA gene (on chromosome 20q13-ter) (see Table 119–2). Marked accumulations of adenosine, 2′-deoxyadenosine, and 2′-*O*-methyladenosine lead directly or indirectly to lymphocyte toxicity, which causes the immunodeficiency. Adenosine and deoxyadenosine are apparent suicide inactivators of the enzyme S-adenosylhomocysteine (SAH) hydrolase, resulting in the accumulation of SAH. SAH is a potent inhibitor of virtually all cellular methylation reactions. These patients usually have profound deficiencies of all types of lymphocytes. Other distinguishing features of ADA-deficient SCIDs include the presence of rib cage abnormalities similar to a rachitic rosary and multiple skeletal abnormalities of chondro-osseous dysplasia, which occur predominantly at the costochondral junctions, at the apophyses of the iliac bones, and in the vertebral bodies.

Enzyme replacement therapy with polyethylene glycol–modified bovine ADA (PEG-ADA) administered subcutaneously once weekly resulted in clinical and immunologic improvement in 29 ADA-deficient patients. However, this therapy should not be initiated if bone marrow transplantation is possible, as it will confer graft-rejection capability. Gene therapy has already been attempted in mature T cells of at least two ADA-deficient patients, as well as in cord blood cells of seven other patients without evidence of striking success.

119.7 X-Linked Severe Combined Immunodeficiency (XSCID)

XSCID is believed to be the most common form of SCID in the United States (Table 119–1). Percentages of blood B cells are usually higher in this defect than in the other forms of SCID, but the number and function of NK cells is as low as in ADA deficiency, and NK junction is low or absent. The abnormal gene in XSCID was mapped by RFLP analysis to Xq13 (see Table 119–2). This gene encodes the gamma chain of the IL-2 receptor (IL-2Rγ) (see Tables 119–1 and 119–2). IL-2, formerly known as T-cell growth factor, plays a key role in intracellular signaling in T cells and, consequently, in the function and regulation of the immune system. However, because humans and genetically engineered mice deficient in IL-2 have T cells and much less severe immunodeficiency than in XSCID, it was initially difficult to see how abnormalities in IL-2Rγ caused such a devastating immunodeficiency. IL-2Rγ has been shown to be a component of the receptors for several other cytokines that regulate the function and development of the immune system, including IL-4, IL-7, and possibly others. IL-2, IL-4, and IL-7 are all facilitators of different stages of the growth and development of both T and B cells. Incapacitation of the receptors for all of these developmentally crucial cytokines by genetic mutations in their common gamma chain explains the severity of the immunodeficiency in XSCID. All XSCID infants reported thus far have point or deletional mutations in IL-2Rγ. Carriers can be detected by demonstration of nonrandom X-chromosome inactivation in their T lymphocytes. Results of X-chromosome inactivation studies in obligate carrier mothers also suggest that the genetic defect affects B- and NK-lineage cells, as well as T cells. This observation is in keeping with the author's observations of very poor B- and NK-cell function in infants with X-linked SCID following nonablated bone marrow cell transplantation, despite excellent reconstitution of T-cell function by donor-derived T cells.

119.8 Reticular Dysgenesis

This condition was first described in 1959 in identical twin male infants who exhibited a total lack of both lymphocytes and granulocytes in their peripheral blood and bone marrow (see Table 119–1). Seven of eight infants with this defect died between 3 and 119 days of age from overwhelming infections; seven infants have been cured by bone marrow transplantation. Mature, normal-appearing granulocytes (although markedly reduced in number) were noted in three patients, arguing against a total failure of stem cell differentiation in this defect. The thymus glands have all weighed less than 1 g, no Hassall's corpuscles have been present, and few or no thymocytes have been seen.

119.9 Defective Expression of Major Histocompatibility Complex (MHC) Antigens

There are three forms of this disorder: (1) class I MHC antigen deficiency (bare lymphocyte syndrome), (2) class II MHC antigen deficiency, and (3) deficiency of both class I and II MHC antigens (see Table 119–1). Sera from infants with class II antigen deficiency contain normal quantities of class I MHC antigens and β_2-microglobulin. Patients (usually of North African descent) present with persistent diarrhea in early infancy and have oral candidiasis, bacterial pneumonia, pneumocystis, septicemia, and undue susceptibility to enteroviruses, herpes, and other viruses. Patients with both class I and II antigen deficiencies also have malabsorption. There is variable hypogammaglobulinemia, with decreased serum IgM and IgA, and poor to absent antibody production. B-cell percentages are usually normal, but plasma cells are absent in tissues. Lymphopenia is only moderate; T-cell functions are decreased in vivo and in vitro but are not absent. The thymus and other lymphoid organs are severely hypoplastic. Most patients die in the first 3 yr of life. The associated defects of both B- and T-cell immunity and of HLA expression emphasize the important biologic role for HLA determinants in effective immune cell cooperation. However, studies of allorecognition and T-cell repertoire selection in patients with MHC class II antigen deficiency demonstrate a normal capacity for self-nonself discrimination by their T cells. This observation suggests that the latter is not absolutely dependent on normal HLA class II expression within the differentiating thymic microenvironment in humans. These conditions are inherited in an autosomal recessive pattern. The defects are not linked to genes encoding MHC antigens on chromosome 6. X-box binding protein abnormalities have been reported (see Table 119–1). Two different molecular defects have been defined. In one, there is a mutation in the gene that encodes a protein called RFX, a transcription factor that binds to MHC class II gene promoters. In the other, there is a mutation in the gene encoding a novel MHC class II transactivator, C11TA, another transcription factor that binds to the MHC class II gene promoter region.

119.10 Omenn Syndrome

Omenn syndrome of combined immunodeficiency with hypereosinophilia is an autosomal recessively inherited, fatal condition characterized by profound susceptibility to infection, with T-cell infiltration of skin, gut, liver, and spleen, leading to an exfoliative erythroderma, lymphadenopathy, hepatosplenomegaly, and intractable diarrhea. Infants so affected have a persistent leukocytosis with marked eosinophilia; elevated serum IgE; low IgG, IgA, and IgM; and impaired T-cell function due to restricted heterogeneity of the host T-cell repertoire. A TH2-like cell dominance was documented in a patient with Omenn syndrome, and the infant was reportedly treated successfully with IFN-γ (see Table 119–1). In another such patient, a clonally expanded Vβ14 positive CD3+CD4-CD8- double-negative T-cell population that spontaneously secreted high levels of IL-5, but had low expression of both IL-4 and IFN-γ mRNA, was found.

119.11 Immunodeficiency with Thrombocytopenia and Eczema (Wiskott-Aldrich Syndrome)

This X-linked recessive syndrome is characterized by atopic dermatitis, thrombocytopenic purpura with normal-appearing megakaryocytes but small defective platelets, and undue susceptibility to infection.

CLINICAL MANIFESTATIONS. Often there is prolonged bleeding from the circumcision site or bloody diarrhea during infancy. The thrombocytopenia appears to be caused by an intrinsic platelet abnormality; survival times of allogeneic but not autologous ^{51}Cr-labeled platelets are normal early on in these patients. Atopic dermatitis and recurrent infections usually develop during the first year of life. Infections are caused by pneumococci and other bacteria having polysaccharide capsules, resulting in otitis media, pneumonia, meningitis, and/or sepsis. Later, infections with agents such as *Pneumocystis carinii* and the herpesviruses become more frequent. Survival beyond the teens is rare; infections or bleeding are major causes of death, but there is also a 12% incidence of fatal malignancy in this condition.

PATHOPHYSIOLOGY AND DIAGNOSIS. Patients with this defect uniformly have an impaired humoral immune response to polysaccharide antigens, as evidenced by absent or markedly diminished isohemagglutinins, and poor or absent antibody responses after immunization with polysaccharide vaccines. Antibody titers to proteins also fall with time, and anamnestic responses are often poor or absent. Studies of immunoglobulin metabolism have shown an accelerated rate of synthesis as well as hypercatabolism of albumin, IgG, IgA, and IgM, resulting in highly variable concentrations of different immunoglobulins, even within the same patient. The predominant pattern is a low serum IgM, elevated IgA and IgE, and a normal or slightly low IgG concentration. IgG_2 subclass concentrations, surprisingly, are normal. Analyses of blood lymphocytes show moderately reduced percentages of T cells reacting with monoclonal antibodies to CD3, CD4, and CD8. Lymphocyte responses to mitogens are moderately depressed, and cutaneous anergy is a frequent finding.

GENETICS. The abnormal gene, on the proximal arm of the X chromosome at Xp11.22–11.23 near the centromere, was recently isolated and found to encode a 501 amino acid proline-rich cytoplasmic protein restricted in its expression to cells of lymphocytic and megakaryocytic lineages (see Table 119–1). This protein, now referred to as the Wiskott-Aldrich syndrome protein (WASP), is suspected of being an important regulator of lymphocyte and platelet function (see Table 119–2). Carriers can be detected by nonrandom X-chromosome inactivation in several hematopoietic cell lineages.

119.12 Ataxia-Telangiectasia

Ataxia-telangiectasia is a complex syndrome with neurologic, immunologic, endocrinologic, hepatic, and cutaneous abnormalities.

CLINICAL MANIFESTATIONS. The most prominent clinical features are progressive cerebellar ataxia, oculocutaneous telangiectasias, chronic sinopulmonary disease, a high incidence of malignancy, and variable humoral and cellular immunodeficiency. Ataxia typically becomes evident soon after the child begins to walk and progresses until he or she is confined to a wheelchair, usually by the age of 10–12 yr. The telangiectasias develop between 3 and 6 yr of age. Recurrent, usually bacterial, sinopulmonary infections occur in roughly 80% of these patients. While common viral infections have not usually resulted in untoward sequelae, fatal varicella occurred in one of the author's patients.

PATHOPHYSIOLOGY AND DIAGNOSIS. Cells from patients as well as those of heterozygous carriers have increased sensitivity to ionizing radiation, defective DNA repair, and frequent chromosomal abnormalities. The sites of chromosomal breakage involve chromosomes 7 and 14 in more than 50% of cases. The breakpoints involve the genes that code for the T-cell receptor and immunoglobulin heavy chains, most likely accounting for the combined T- and B-cell abnormalities seen. The malignancies reported in this condition are usually of the lymphoreticular type, but adenocarcinomas are also seen, and there is an increased incidence of malignancy in unaffected relatives. The most frequent humoral immunologic abnormality is the selective absence of IgA, found in from 50–80% of these patients; hypercatabolism of IgA also occurs (see Table 119–1). IgE concentrations are usually low, and the IgM may be of the low molecular weight variety. IgG_2 or total IgG may be decreased. Specific antibody titers may be decreased or normal. In vitro tests of lymphocyte function have generally shown moderately depressed proliferative responses to T- and B-cell mitogens. There are moderately reduced percentages of CD3- and CD4-positive T cells, with normal or increased percentages of CD8+ and elevated numbers of Tiγ/δ+ T cells. Studies of immunoglobulin synthesis have shown both helper T-cell and intrinsic B-cell defects (see Table 119–1). The thymus is very hypoplastic, exhibits poor organization, and lacks Hassall's corpuscles.

GENETICS. Inheritance follows an autosomal-recessive pattern. The abnormal gene has been mapped to the long arm of chromosome 11 (11q22–23) but has not been identified (see Table 119–2).

119.13 Hyperimmunoglobulinemia E (Hyper IgE) Syndrome

(See Chapter 130)

The hyper IgE syndrome is a relatively rare primary immunodeficiency syndrome characterized by recurrent severe staphylococcal abscesses and markedly elevated levels of serum IgE. The disorder was first reported by the author in two young boys in 1972; since then more than 50 patients with the condition have been evaluated.

CLINICAL MANIFESTATIONS. These patients have histories from infancy of staphylococcal abscesses involving the skin, lungs, joints, and other sites; persistent pneumatocoeles develop as a result of their recurrent pneumonias. The pruritic dermatitis that occurs is not typical atopic eczema, and it does not always persist; respiratory allergic symptoms are usually absent.

The fact that both men and women have been affected, as have members of succeeding generations, suggests an autosomal-dominant form of inheritance with incomplete penetrance.

Laboratory features include exceptionally high serum IgE concentrations; elevated serum IgD concentrations; usually normal concentrations of IgG, IgA, and IgM; pronounced blood and sputum eosinophilia; abnormally low anamnestic antibody responses; and poor antibody and cell-mediated responses to neoantigens (see Table 119–1). In vitro studies have shown normal percentages of CD2-, CD3-, CD4-, and CD8-positive lymphocytes. Paradoxically, however, B cells from these patients demonstrate very low levels of IL-4–stimulated IgE synthesis in vitro, suggesting that they have already been maximally stimulated by a high level of endogenous IL-4. The primary cause of this disorder remains unknown, although it has been speculated to be due to an imbalance of TH1 and TH2 type cells. Most patients have normal T-lymphocyte proliferative responses to mitogens, but very low or absent responses to antigens or allogeneic cells from family members. There is a decreased percentage of T cells with the memory (CD45RO) phenotype in the blood of these patients. Blood, sputum, and histologic sections of lymph nodes, spleen, and lung cysts show striking eosinophilia. Hassall's corpuscles and thymic architecture are normal. Phagocytic cell ingestion, metabolism, and killing and total hemolytic complement activity are normal in all patients. Variable defects of mononuclear and/or polymorphonuclear chemotaxis are present in some but not most patients, and hence are not the basic problem.

TREATMENT. Long-term administration of a penicillinase-resistant penicillin is indicated, with the addition of other antibiotics or antifungal agents as required for specific infections. IVIG should be administered to antibody-deficient patients, and appropriate thoracic surgery should be provided for superinfected pneumatoceles or those persisting beyond 6 mo.

119.14 Treatment of Cellular Immunodeficiency

Transplantation of MHC compatible or haploidentical parental bone marrow is the treatment of choice for patients with fatal T-cell or combined T- and B-cell defects. The major risk to the recipient from transplants of bone marrow is that of graft-versus-host disease. The development of techniques to deplete all post-thymic T cells from donor marrow permits the safe and successful use of haploidentical (half-matched) bone marrow cells for the correction of SCID and other fatal immunodeficiency syndromes. These techniques employ soybean lectin incubation followed by sheep erythrocyte rosette depletion or incubation with monoclonal antibodies to T cells plus complement. Both methods enrich the final cell suspension for stem cells. Patients with less severe forms of cellular immunodeficiency, such as Nezelof syndrome, Wiskott-Aldrich syndrome, cytokine deficiency, or MHC antigen deficiency, reject even HLA-identical marrow grafts unless they are treated with immunosuppressive agents before transplantation. Several patients with Wiskott-Aldrich syndrome, leukocyte adhesion deficiency 1 (LAD1), and other forms of partial cellular immunodeficiency have been treated with HLA-identical bone marrow transplantation after immunosuppression.

From 1968 to 1977 only 14 (or 29%) of 48 infants with SCID worldwide were long-term survivors of successful HLA class II compatible bone marrow transplantation. Possibly due to earlier diagnosis before untreatable opportunistic infections develop, the results of bone marrow transplantation have improved considerably over the last decade. A recent worldwide survey conducted by the author revealed that 195 of 243, or 80%, of patients with primary immunodeficiency transplanted with HLA-identical marrow over the past 26 yr survive. Most encouraging, however, are the results of T-cell–depleted haploidentical (half-matched) marrow transplants in patients with primary immunodeficiency. From the same survey it was ascertained that 535 such transplants have been performed over the past 12 yr and, of these, 291 (or 54%) survive. The significance is even more impressive when it is realized that most of the 535 recipients would have died had not the new T-cell depletion techniques been developed. Enzyme replacement therapy with polyethylene glycol–modified bovine ADA (PEG-ADA) administered subcutaneously once weekly has resulted in clinical and immunologic improvement in approximately 30 ADA-deficient patients. However, bone marrow transplantation remains the treatment of choice, so PEG-ADA therapy should not be initiated first, as it will confer graft-rejection capability. Until somatic cell gene therapy is more fully developed, bone marrow transplantation remains the most important and effective therapy for these inborn errors of the immune system.

Buckley RH, Wray BB, Belmaker EZ: Extreme hyperimmunoglobulinemia E and undue susceptibility to infection. Pediatrics 49:59, 1972.

Buckley RH, Schiff SE, Schiff RI, et al: Haploidentical bone marrow stem cell transplantation in human severe combined immunodeficiency. Semin Hematol 30:92, 1993.

Derry JMJ, Ochs HD, Francke U: Isolation of a novel gene mutated in Wiskott-Aldrich syndrome. Cell 78:635, 1994.

Fischer A, Landais P, Friedrich W: European experience of bone marrow transplantation for severe combined immunodeficiency. Lancet 336:850, 1990.

Hershfield MS, Buckley RH, Greenberg ML, et al: Treatment of adenosine deaminase deficiency with polyethylene glycol-modified adenosine deaminase (PEG-ADA). N Engl J Med 316:589, 1987.

Klein C, Lisowska-Grospierre B, LeDeist F, et al: Major histocompatibility complex class II deficiency: clinical manifestations, immunologic features, and outcome. J Pediatr 123:921, 1993.

Markert ML: Purine nucleoside phosphorylase deficiency. Immunodefic Rev 3:45, 1991.

Noguchi M, Nakamura Y, Russell SM, et al: Interleukin-2 receptor gamma chain: a functional component of the interleukin-7 receptor. Science 262:1977, 1993.

Noguchi M, Yi H, Rosenblatt HM, et al: Interleukin-2 receptor gamma chain mutation results in X-linked severe combined immunodeficiency in humans. Cell 73:147, 1993.

Puck JM, Deschenes SM, Porter JC, et al: The interleukin-2 receptor gamma chain maps to Xq13.1 and is mutated in X-linked severe combined immunodeficiency, SCIDX1. Hum Mol Genet 2:1099, 1993.

Russell SM, Keegan AD, Harada N, et al: Interleukin-2 receptor gamma chain: a functional component of the interleukin-4 receptor. Science 262:1880, 1993.

Voss SD, Hong R, Sondel PM: Severe combined immunodeficiency, interleukin-2 (IL-2), and the IL-2 receptor: experiments of nature continue to point the way. Blood 83:626, 1994.

CHAPTER 120
The Complement System

Richard B. Johnston, Jr.

COMPLEMENT

Complement was originally defined through the study of bacteriolysis, which requires both specific antibody and a nonspecific, heat-labile complementary principle, now termed *complement.* By the 1960s nine complement components were known, one of which had three subcomponents. By the early 1970s a second major pathway of activation of complement, the *alternative pathway,* had been described. The latter system contains two unique factors. In addition, at least seven (perhaps 10) regulators that control activity of either or both pathways exist in serum, and at least five such regulatory proteins exist on the surface of cells. The original system of four components, C1423, is now referred to as the classical pathway. The term *complement system,* as presently broadly conceptualized, refers to both pathways, which interact and depend on each other for their full activity, the *membrane attack complex* (C5b6789), formed from activity of either pathway, the five membrane regulatory proteins, a serosal regulatory protein, and eight cell membrane receptors that bind complement components or fragments (Table 120–1). All of the 20 serum components and regulators are proteins. Together they make up about 10% of the globulin fraction of serum. The normal concentrations of serum complement components in children are given in Reference Ranges for Laboratory Tests, Chapter 670.

■ TABLE 120–1 Constituents of the Complement System*

Serum Components	Membrane Regulatory Proteins
Classical Pathway	CR1
Clq	Membrane cofactor protein
Clr	Decay accelerating factor (DAF)
Cls	Membrane inhibitor of reactive lysis (CD59)
C4	C8 binding protein (C8bp)
C2	
C3	**Serosal Regulatory Protein**
Alternative Pathway	C5a/IL-8 inactivator
Factor B	
Factor D	**Membrane Receptors**
Membrane Attack Complex	CR1
C5	CR2
C6	CR3
C7	CR4
C8	C4a/C3a receptor
C9	C5a receptor
Control Protein, Enhancing	Clq receptors (cClqR, gC1qR)
Properdin	
Control Proteins, Downregulating	
C1 inhibitor (C1 INH)	
C4 binding protein (C4bp)	
Factor H	
Factor I	
S protein (vitronectin)	
Anaphylatoxin inactivator	

* *CR, complement receptor; IL, interleukin.*

NOMENCLATURE. The terminology applied to complement is cryptic but logical and consists of only a few rules: The components have been assigned numbers in the order of their discovery and are preceded by the letter C. Unfortunately, the first four components do not interact in the sequence in which they were discovered but rather in the order C1423. The remaining components react in the appropriate numerical order, C56789. C1 has three subcomponents, Clq, Clr, and Cls. Fragments of components resulting from cleavage by other components acting as enzymes are assigned small letters (a, b, c, d, or e); with the exception of C2 fragments, the smaller piece that is released into surrounding fluids is assigned the lowercase letter a, and the major part of the molecule, bound to other components or to some part of the immune complex, is assigned b, for example, C3a and C3b. When a component is activated (becomes an active enzyme), a bar is placed above the number, for example, $C\overline{1}$.

Components of the alternative pathway have been assigned uppercase letters: B and D, as have the control proteins I and H, which downregulate both pathways. Factor B has an active form denoted $\overline{Bb}$. C3 (in particular, its major fragment, C3b) is a component of both the classical and alternative pathways.

GENERAL CONCEPTS. Complement is a *system* of interacting proteins. The biologic functions of the system depend upon the interaction of individual components, which occurs in sequential fashion. This has been referred to as a cascade, in analogy to the clotting system of blood; activation of each component (except the 1st) depends upon activation of the prior component or components in the sequence.

Interaction occurs along two pathways: the classical pathway, in the order antigen-antibody-C142356789; and the alternative pathway, in the order activator-(antibody)-C3bBD-C356789. Antibody accelerates the rate of activation of the alternative pathway, but activation can occur on appropriate surfaces in the absence of antibody. The classical and the alternative pathways interact with each other through the ability of both to activate C3.

The interaction of the early-acting components of complement (C1423) results in the generation of a series of active enzymes, $C\overline{1}$, $C\overline{42}$, and $C\overline{423}$. Thus, "activation" refers to transformation of the component into part of an active enzyme. In contrast, the interaction among C5b, C6, C7, C8, and C9 is nonenzymatic. In the case of C1, activation is a result of its interaction with antibody. Activation of C4, C2, C3, and C5, as well as factor B of the alternative pathway, is secondary to cleavage by a preceding activated component. Thus, activation of early components generates enzymes that fix to the antigen-antibody complex and catalyze a reaction on the next component, whereas later-acting components (C6–C9) adsorb to the complex or the underlying cell by an interaction that depends on a change in their configuration.

These basic principles can be illustrated by a more detailed analysis of the activation sequence.

SEQUENCE OF ACTIVATION. The sequence in which the components of the classical pathway interact, the interdigitation between classical and alternative pathways, the chemical and some functional by-products of these reactions, and the regulators of the system are summarized in Figure 120–1.

The sequence begins with fixation of C1, by way of C1q, to the Fc non-antigen-binding part of the antibody molecule after antigen-antibody interaction. The C1 tricomplex changes configuration, and the C1s subcomponent becomes an active enzyme, $C\overline{1}$ esterase.

C-reactive protein (CRP), which reacts with C carbohydrate from microorganisms and is elevated in certain inflammatory states, can substitute for antibody in the fixation of C1q and initiate reaction of the entire sequence. Thus, C-reactive protein functions like antibody, although it can combine with only a few specific "antigens" and its size and structure are quite different. This reaction has the potential for initiating inflammation in the absence of antibody. Other agents that can activate C1 directly, without a requirement for antibody, include certain bacteria, mycoplasma, and RNA viruses, uric acid crystals, the lipid A component of bacterial endotoxin, and the membranes of certain intracellular organelles.

In the next two steps of the classical pathway, polypeptide fragments are split from C4 and C2 during their activation and fixation by the enzymatic action of C1. One of these, a kinin-like peptide split from C2, can induce vascular permeability and edema through direct action on postcapillary venules. The peptide C4a has *anaphylatoxin* activity; it reacts with mast cells to release the chemical mediators of immediate hypersensitivity, including histamine. Fixation of C4b to the complex permits it to adhere to a variety of mammalian cells, including neutrophils, monocytes, and erythrocytes.

Cleavage of C3 and generation of C3b is the next step in the sequence and the most crucial in terms of biologic activity. Cleavage of C3 can be achieved through $C\overline{142}$, the C3 convertase of the classical pathway, or through the C3 convertase of the alternative pathway, $\overline{C3bBb}$ (see later). Once fixed to the complex, C3b permits adherence of the antigen-antibody complex to cells with receptors for C3b (complement receptor 1, CR1), including B lymphocytes, erythrocytes, and phagocytic cells (neutrophils, monocytes, and macrophages), leading, in the last case, to phagocytosis. Without C3 bound to them, phagocytosis of most microorganisms in vitro, especially by neutrophils, is very inefficient. The severe pyogenic infections that occur commonly in C3-deficient patients indicate that without C3, phagocytosis is also inefficient in vivo. The biologic activity of C3b is controlled by cleavage by factor I (C3b inactivator) to iC3b, which is further degraded by factor I and serum or tissue enzymes to C3c, which is released, and to C3dg and C3d, which stay bound. iC3b promotes phagocytosis on binding to the iC3b receptor (CR3) on phagocytes. Receptors for C3dg and C3d exist on B lymphocytes (CR2) and phagocytes (CR4). Further cleavage of C3c creates C3e, which induces release of granulocytes from bone marrow.

The peptide C3a, generated when C3 is acted upon by either pathway, has anaphylatoxin activity. The action of $C\overline{423}$ or of the alternative pathway C5 convertase on C5 releases C5a, a powerful anaphylatoxin that can react with neutrophils,

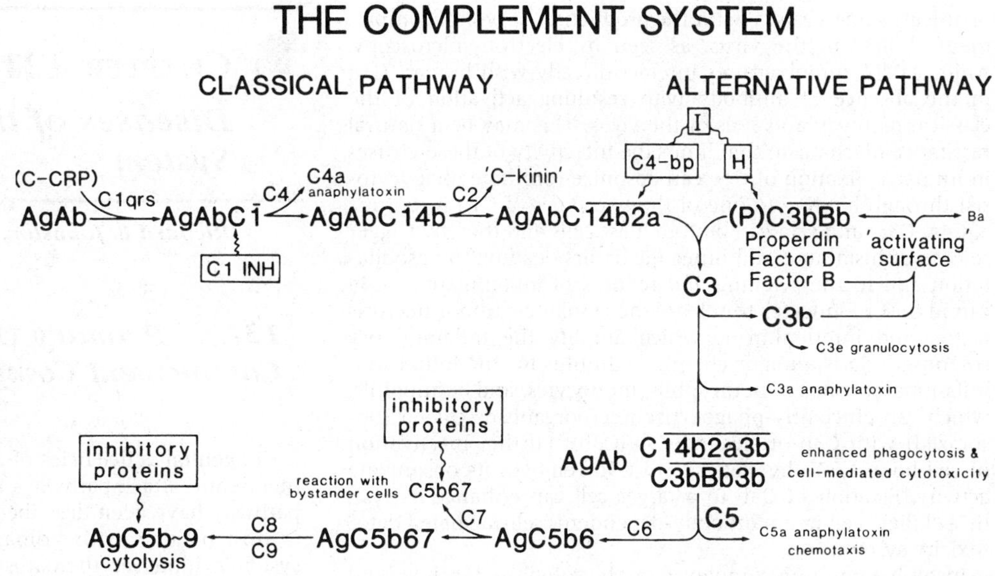

Figure 120–1. Sequence of activation of the components of the classical pathway of complement and interaction with the alternative pathway. (Ag = antigen [bacterium, virus, tumor cell, or erythrocyte]; Ab = antibody [IgG or IgM class only]; C-CRP = C carbohydrate–C-reactive protein; C1 INH = C1 inhibitor; I = factor I; C4-bp = C4-binding protein; H = factor H). Inhibitory regulator proteins are enclosed in a box. S protein is the best defined of the "inhibitory proteins" that act on the membrane attack complex (C5b6789).

macrophages, mast cells, smooth muscle cells, and certain T cells to induce release of a variety of mediators of inflammation. This same peptide serves as a potent chemical attractant for phagocytic cells.

The "membrane-attack" sequence leading to cytolysis begins with the attachment of C5b to the C5-activating enzyme from the classical pathway, C4b2a3b, or from the alternative pathway, C3bBb3b. C6 is bound to C5b without being cleaved, stabilizing the activated C5b fragment. The C5b6 complex then dissociates from C423 and reacts with C7. C5b67 complexes must attach to the cell membrane promptly or lose their activity and remain in the fluid phase. Next, C8 binds, and the C5b678 complex then promotes the addition of multiple C9 molecules. The C9 polymer of at least three to six molecules forms a transmembrane channel, and lysis ensues.

Control mechanisms act at several points to prevent the system's consuming itself in activity that is unnecessary or deleterious to the host. An α_2-globulin, C1 inhibitor (C1 INH), inhibits C1s enzymatic activity and, thus, the cleavage of C4 and C2. Activated C2 has a half-life of about 8 min at 37° C, and this relative instability limits the effective life of C42 and C423. The alternative pathway enzyme that activates C3, C3bBb, also has a short half-life, though it can be prolonged by the binding of properdin (P) to the enzyme complex. Serum contains the protein "anaphylatoxin inactivator," an enzyme that cleaves the carboxy-terminal arginine from C4a, C3a, and C5a, thereby markedly reducing their anaphylatoxic activity and the chemotactic activity of C5a. Factor I inactivates C4b and C3b, thus serving as an important means of controlling both pathways. Factor H accelerates inactivation of C3b by I. An analogous factor, C4 binding protein (C4-bp), accelerates cleavage of C4b by factor I. Three protein constituents of cell membranes, CR1, membrane cofactor protein, and decay-accelerating factor (DAF), promote the disruption of C3 and C5 convertases assembled on those membranes. Other cell membrane–associated proteins (C8 binding protein and CD59) can bind C8 or both C8 and C9, thereby interfering with insertion of the membrane-attack complex (C5b6789). Certain serum proteins (S protein, or vitronectin, being the best studied) can inhibit attachment of the C5b67 complex to cell membranes, bind C8 or C9 in a full membrane-attack complex, or otherwise interfere with the formation or insertion of this complex.

ALTERNATIVE PATHWAY. The alternative pathway can be activated by C3b generated through classical pathway activity, through leukocyte proteases released by degranulation, or perhaps through activation of thrombin or plasmin during blood coagulation. It can also be activated by a form of C3 created by low-grade, spontaneous reaction of native C3 with a molecule of water, which occurs constantly in plasma. Once formed, C3b or this hydrolyzed C3 can bind to any nearby cell or to factor B. Factor B attached to C3b in the plasma or on the surface of a particle can be cleaved to Bb by D, which exists as an active proteolytic enzyme. The complex C3bBb becomes an efficient C3 convertase, which generates more C3b through an "amplification loop" (see Fig. 120–1). P can bind to C3bBb, increasing stability of the enzyme and protecting it from inactivation by factors I and H, which serve to modulate the loop. Cleavage of B releases Ba, which has weak chemotactic activity.

Certain materials promote alternative pathway activation if C3b is fixed to their surface, for example, teichoic acid from bacterial cell wall, endotoxic lipopolysaccharide, or immunoglobulin aggregates, especially of the IgA class. This activation depends on the ability of the C3bBb enzyme complex to escape the efficient control otherwise exercised by factors I and H. The surface of rabbit red blood cells also protects C3bBb from inactivation. This phenomenon serves as the basis for an assay of serum alternative pathway activity. Endotoxin may alter normally "nonactivating" cell surfaces in vivo so that C3bBb is relatively protected from inactivation, which may partially explain the activation of the alternative pathway in patients with gram-negative bacteremia. Sialic acid on the surface of microorganisms or cells prevents formation of an effective alternative pathway C3 convertase by promoting activity of I and H.

Although C3bBb can activate C3 efficiently on only a limited variety of surfaces, significant activation of C3 can occur through this pathway, and the resultant biologic activities are qualitatively the same as those achieved through activation by C142, as illustrated in Figure 120–1.

PARTICIPATION IN HOST DEFENSE. Neutralization of virus by antibody can be enhanced with C1 and C4. When antibody concentrations are low, the additional fixation of C3b to the viral antigen-antibody complex through the classical or alternative pathway improves neutralization; C5 and C6 add little to the effect. Complement may, therefore, be particularly important in the early phases of a viral infection when antibody is limited. Antibody and complement can also eliminate infectivity of at least some viruses, with the production of typical complement "holes" in the virus, as seen by electron microscopy. Animal RNA tumor viruses interact directly with human C1q in the absence of antibody with resulting activation of the classical pathway and lysis of the virus. This may be a natural resistance mechanism that limits the infectivity of these viruses in humans. Fixation of C1q can opsonize (promote phagocytosis) through binding to one of the two types of C1q receptor.

C4a, C3a, and C5a can bind to mast cells and thereby trigger release of histamine and other mediators, leading to vasodilatation and to the swelling and redness of inflammation. C5a can induce monocytes to release the cytokines, tumor necrosis factor, and interleukin 1, which amplify the inflammatory response. C5a is a major chemical stimulus for the influx into inflammatory sites of neutrophils, monocytes, and eosinophils, which can efficiently phagocytize microorganisms coated (opsonized) with C3b or cleaved C3b(iC3b). Further inactivation of cell-bound C3b by cleavage to C3d removes its opsonizing activity. Fixation of C3b to a target cell can enhance its lysis by a "killer" cell in an antibody-dependent, cell-mediated cytotoxicity system.

Insoluble immune complexes can be solubilized if they bind C3b, apparently because C3b disrupts the orderly antigen-antibody lattice. Binding of C3b to a complex also allows it to adhere to C3 receptors (CR1) on red cells, which then transport the complexes to fixed macrophages for removal. These findings offer the best explanation for the immune complex disease found in patients who lack C1, C4, C2, or C3.

The complement system may be involved in certain aspects of B- and T-lymphocyte–mediated specific immunity. C3b- and C3d-coated particles can bind to B lymphocytes, which appears to activate them and to enhance the primary antibody response. C3a may suppress antibody formation, whereas C5a and C1q appear to enhance this response. C3e, a cleavage product generated during the inactivation of C3, induces an increase in circulating granulocytes.

Neutralization of endotoxin in vitro and protection from its lethal effects in experimental animals require later-acting components of complement, at least through C6. Finally, activation of the entire complement sequence can result in lysis of virus-infected cells, tumor cells, and most types of microorganisms. Bactericidal activity of complement has not appeared to be important to host defense, except for the occurrence of infections with *Neisseria* in patients lacking later-acting components of complement (Chapter 121).

Berger M, Frank MM: The serum complement system. *In:* Stiehm ER (ed): Immunologic Disorders in Infants and Children, 4th ed. Philadelphia, WB Saunders, in press.

Johnston RB Jr: The complement system in host defense and inflammation: the cutting edges of a double edged sword. Pediatr Infect Dis J 12:933, 1993.

Kinoshita T, Farries TC, Atkinson JP, et al: The biology of complement. Immunol Today 12:291, 1991.

Müller-Eberhard HJ: Complement: chemistry and pathways. *In:* Gallin JI, Goldstein IM, Snyderman R (eds): Inflammation: Basic Principles and Clinical Correlates, 2nd ed. New York, Raven Press, 1992, p 33.

CHAPTER 121

Diseases of the Complement System

Richard B. Johnston, Jr.

121.1 Primary Deficiencies of Complement Components

Congenital deficiencies of all 11 proteins of the classical and membrane attack pathways and of factor D of the alternative pathway have been described (Table 121–1).

Most patients with primary **deficiency of C1q** have had systemic lupus erythematosus (SLE), an SLE-like syndrome without typical SLE serology, a chronic rash that has shown an underlying vasculitis on biopsy, or membranoproliferative glomerulonephritis (MPGN). Three C1q-deficient children suffered from serious infections; two of these died from meningitis-septicemia. **C1r deficiency** can occur as an isolated defect or in association with C1s deficiency.

Like individuals with C1q deficiency, patients with **C1r, C1r/C1s, C4, C2,** and **C3 deficiencies** have had a high incidence of vasculitis syndromes (see Table 121–1), especially SLE or the SLE-like syndrome in which antinuclear antibody is not elevated. A few patients with **C5, C6, C7,** or **C8 deficiency** have had such a disorder, but recurrent neisserial infections are much more likely to be the major problem in this group. The reason for the concurrence of deficiencies of components of complement and these "autoimmune" diseases is not entirely clear, but deposition of C3 autoimmune complexes facilitates their removal from the circulation through binding to complement receptor (CR) 1 on erythrocytes and transport to the spleen and liver. Inefficiency of this process best explains the particular predisposition to collagen-vascular disease in individuals with a defect in the classical pathway.

Several patients with **C2 deficiency** have had repeated life-threatening septicemic illnesses, most commonly due to pneumococci. Most have not had problems with increased susceptibility to infection, presumably because of the protective function of the alternative pathway. The genes for C2, factor B, and C4 are situated close to each other on chromosome 6, and a depression of factor B levels can occur in conjunction with C2 deficiency. Persons with a deficiency of both proteins might be at particular risk.

Since C3 can be activated by C142 or by the alternative pathway, a defect in the function of either pathway can be compensated, at least to some extent. Without C3, however, the chemotactic fragment from C5 (C5a) is not generated, and opsonization of bacteria is inefficient. Some organisms must be well opsonized in order to be cleared, and **genetic deficiency of C3** has been associated with recurrent, severe pyogenic infections due to pneumococci and meningococci. Some C3-deficient patients have had sluggish neutrophilic responses to infection, in agreement with reports that a cleavage factor of C3 elicits an increase in blood neutrophils.

Over half of the individuals reported to have congenital **C5, C6, C7,** or **C8 deficiency** have had meningococcal meningitis or extragenital gonococcal infection. A few have had a collagen-vascular disease. In seven studies of patients with systemic meningococcal disease, about 15% had a genetic deficiency of C5, C6, C7, C8, or C9. It is not clear why patients with a deficiency of one of the late-acting components suffer a partic-

■ **TABLE 121–1 Genetic Deficiencies of Plasma Complement Components and Associated Clinical Findings**

Deficient Component†	Infection*			Collagen-Vascular Disease*		
	Common	*Less Common*	*Occasional*	*Common*	*Less Common*	*Occasional*
C1q			Pneumococcal B/M, other pyogenic	SLE	GN	DV/DLE
C1r		Other pyogenic	Pneumococcal B/M, DGI	SLE		GN
C1rs		Other pyogenic		SLE		
C4		Other pyogenic		SLE	Other CVD	GN
C2		Other pyogenic, pneumococcal B/M, meningococcal M			SLE, GN, DV/DLE, other CVD	
C3	Other pyogenic	Pneumococcal B/M, meningococcal M			GN, DV/DLE	SLE, other CVD
C5	Meningococcal M	DGI	Other pyogenic			SLE, GN
C6	Meningococcal M	DGI	Other pyogenic			SLE, GN, other CVD
C7	Meningococcal M		DGI, other pyogenic			SLE, other CVD
C8	Meningococcal M	DGI	Other pyogenic			SLE, GN
C9		Meningococcal M				
Factor D			DGI, meningococcal M			

**A finding was reported as "common" if it occurred in 50% or more of reported cases, "less common" if reported in about 5–50% of cases, and "occasional" if present in one or two cases or <5% of the more frequent deficiencies. (Cases are from Figueroa JE, Densen P: Infectious diseases associated with complement deficiencies. Clin Microbiol Rev 4:359, 1991; and from Ross SC, Densen P: Complement deficiency states and infection: Epidemiology, pathogenesis and consequences of neisserial and other infections in an immune deficiency. Medicine 63:243, 1984; table modified from Johnston RB Jr: Disorders of the complement system.* In: *Stiehem ER (ed): Immunologic Disorders in Infants and Children, 4th ed. Philadelphia, WB Saunders, 1985.)*

†No genetic complete deficiency of factor B has been reported to date.

B/M = Bacteremia or meningitis; DGI = disseminated gonococcal infection; DV/DLE = dermal vasculitis or typical discoid lupus erythematosus; GN = glomerulonephritis in various forms, often membranoproliferative; M = meningitis; other CVD = other collagen-vascular diseases (almost all possible diagnoses have been reported); other pyogenic = serious deep or systemic infection due to, or typically caused by, a pyogenic bacterium (abscess, osteomyelitis, pneumonia, bacteremia other than pneumococcal, meningitis other than meningococcal or pneumococcal, cellulitis, myopericarditis, and peritonitis); SLE = typical systemic lupus erythematosus or an SLE-like syndrome without characteristic serologic findings.

ular predisposition to neisserial infections; it may be that serum bacteriolysis is uniquely important in defense against this organism, but some persons with such a deficiency have had no significant illness. Patients with C9 deficiency retain about half-normal hemolytic complement titers; a third of these patients have had neisserial disease.

Three individuals have had **deficiency of factor D** of the alternative pathway. All had recurrent infections. Hemolytic complement activity in their serum was normal, but alternative pathway activity was markedly deficient, or absent.

Deficiencies of C1r, C1rs, C4, C2, C3, C5, C6, C7, C8, and C9 are transmitted as autosomal recessive traits, of the "autosomal codominant" variety; that is, each parent transmits a gene that codes for synthesis of half the serum level of the component. The mode of transmission of deficiency of C1q and factors D, H, and I is probably also autosomal recessive. Properdin deficiency is transmitted as an X-linked trait. A rare form of C4 deficiency may be inherited as an autosomal dominant trait.

121.2 Deficiencies of Plasma, Membrane, or Serosal Complement Control Proteins

Factor I deficiency was originally reported as a deficiency of C3 owing to its hypercatabolism. The first patient described had suffered a series of severe pyogenic infections similar to those seen with agammaglobulinemia or congenital deficiency of C3. Further studies indicated that the primary deficiency was that of factor I, an essential regulator of both pathways. This deficiency permits prolonged existence of C3b in the C3 convertase of the alternative pathway, C3bBb, resulting in constant activation of the alternative pathway and cleavage of more C3 to C3b, in circular fashion. Intravenous infusion of plasma or purified factor I induced a prompt rise in serum C3 concentration in the patient and a return to normal of in vitro C3-dependent functions such as opsonization.

The effects of **factor H deficiency** are like those of factor I deficiency since factor H assists in dismantling the alternative pathway C3 convertase. Levels of C3, factor B, total hemolytic activity, and alternative pathway activity have been low or undetectable in all patients tested. Patients have sustained systemic infections due to pyogenic bacteria, particularly meningococci; and glomerulonephritis has occurred in almost half the cases. The three patients reported to date with **deficiency of C4 binding protein** have had about 25% of the normal levels of the protein and no typical disease presentation.

Persons with **properdin deficiency** have had a predisposition to meningococcal meningitis. All reported patients have been male, and their families have had a striking history of male deaths due to meningitis. The predisposition to infection in these patients indicates a requirement for the alternative pathway in host defense against bacterial infection. Serum hemolytic complement activity is normal in these patients, and the presence of specific antibody should avoid the need for the alternative pathway and properdin. Several patients have had dermal vasculitis or discoid lupus.

Hereditary angioedema occurs in persons born without the ability to synthesize normally functioning C1 inhibitor (C1 INH). In 85% of affected families the affected members have markedly reduced concentrations of inhibitor (5–30% of normal); in the other 15% normal or elevated concentrations of an immunologically cross-reacting but nonfunctional protein occur. Both forms of the disease are transmitted as autosomal dominant traits.

In the absence of C1 INH functions, activation of C1 leads to uncontrolled C1 activity, with breakdown of C4 and C2 and release of a vasoactive peptide (kinin) from C2. Episodic, localized, nonpitting edema results from the vasodilatory effects of the kinin on the postcapillary venule. The mechanism by which C1 is activated in these patients is not known.

Swelling of the affected part accumulates rapidly, without urticaria, itching, discoloration, or redness, and often without severe pain. Swelling of the intestinal wall, however, can lead to intense abdominal cramping, sometimes with vomiting or diarrhea; concurrent subcutaneous edema is often absent, and patients have undergone abdominal surgery or psychiatric examination before the true diagnosis was made. Laryngeal edema can be fatal. Attacks last 2–3 days, then gradually abate. They may occur at sites of trauma, after vigorous exercise, with menses, or with emotional stress. Attacks can begin in the first 2 yr of life but are usually not severe until late childhood or adolescence. The condition can be aquired in association with lymphoid cancer or autoantibody to C1 INH. Systemic lupus erythematosus has been reported in patients with the congenital disease. **Acquired C1 INH deficiency** can occur in association with a B-cell lymphoproliferative disorder or autoantibody to the inhibitor.

Three of the membrane complement control proteins, complement receptor 1 (CR1), membrane cofactor protein, and decay accelerating factor (DAF), prevent the formation of the full C3-cleaving enzyme, C3bBb, that is triggered by C3b deposition. The other two, membrane inhibitor of reactive lysis (CD59) and C8 binding protein (C8bp), prevent the full development of the membrane attack complex that creates the hole. **Paroxysmal nocturnal hemoglobinuria** is a hemolytic anemia that occurs when DAF, CD59, and C8bp are not expressed on the erythrocyte surface. The condition is acquired as a somatic mutation in a hematopoietic stem cell of the PIG-A gene on the X chromosome. The product of this gene is required for the normal synthesis of a glycosylphosphatidylinositol molecule that anchors at least 40 proteins to cell membranes, including DAF, CD59, and C8bp. One case of **genetic isolated CD59 deficiency** had a mild PNH-like disease in spite of normal expression of membrane DAF. In contrast, **genetic isolated DAF deficiency** has not resulted in hemolytic anemia.

Patients with systemic lupus erythrematosus (SLE) and their asymptomatic family members have a partial **deficiency of CR1**, which is possibly inherited. This deficiency could increase the risk of developing immune complex disease, thereby contributing to the pathogenesis of SLE.

There is strong evidence to indicate that serosal fluids contain yet another complement control protein, a protease that normally destroys the chemotactic activity of C5a and interleukin 8 (IL-8), important chemotactic factors for neutrophils. A genetic defect in this protease in peritoneal and synovial fluids results in **familial Mediterranean fever** (FMF). Patients with FMF suffer recurrent episodes of fever in association with painful inflammation of joints and pleural and peritoneal cavities. Thus, it appears that C5a or IL-8, or both, are generated at serosal surfaces under normal conditions and that serosal fluids contain an inhibitor of these chemotactic agents that serves to prevent the inflammatory response that would otherwise ensue.

121.3 Secondary Disorders of Complement

Partial deficiency of C1q has occurred in patients with *severe combined immunodeficiency disease* or *hypogammaglobulinemia*, apparently secondary to the deficiency of IgG, which normally binds reversibly to C1q and prevents its rapid catabolism.

Serum from patients with *chronic membranoproliferative glomerulonephritis* contains a protein termed *nephritic factor* (NeF) that promotes activation of the alternative pathway. Nephritic factor is an IgG antibody to the C3-cleaving enzyme of the alternative pathway, C3bBb, that protects the enzyme from inactivation. The result is increased consumption of C3. Serum C3 concentrations vary widely from patient to patient, however. Pyogenic infections, including meningitis, may occur if the serum C3 level drops below about 10% of normal. This disorder has been found in children and adults with *partial lipodystrophy*. Adipocytes can synthesize C3, factor D, and factor B; exposure to NeF induces their lysis. An IgG nephritic factor that binds to and protects C42, the classical pathway C3 convertase, has been described in *acute postinfectious nephritis* and in *systemic lupus erythematosus*. The consumption of C3 that characterizes poststreptococcal nephritis and lupus could be due to this factor, to activation of complement by immune complexes, or both. A related disorder illustrates the importance of factor H in restraining the uncontrolled conversion of C3. A patient has been described who had a circulating inhibitor of factor H and hypocomplementemic membranoproliferative glomerulonephritis.

Newborn infants are known to have mild to moderate deficiencies of all plasma components of the complement system. Opsonization and generation of chemotactic activity in serum from full-term newborns can be markedly deficient through either the classical or the alternative pathway. Complement activity is even lower in preterm infants than in full-term babies. Patients with *malnutrition* or *anorexia nervosa* may also have significant depletion of components and functional activity of complement. Although synthesis of components is depressed in these conditions, serum from some patients with malnutrition also appears to contain immune complexes that could accelerate depletion. Severe chronic *cirrhosis of the liver* and *hepatic failure* may also result in decreased synthesis of C3.

Patients with *sickle cell disease* have normal activity of the classical pathway, but some have defective function of the alternative pathway in opsonization of pneumococci, in bacteriolysis and opsonization of salmonellae, and in lysis of rabbit erythrocytes. Deoxygenation of erythrocytes from patients with sickle cell disease alters their membranes to increase exposure of phospholipids that can activate the alternative pathway and consume its components. An alternative pathway defect has been described in about 10% of individuals who have undergone *splenectomy* and in some patients with *β-thalassemia major*. The underlying mechanism for this defect in these last two disorders has not been defined. Children with *nephrotic syndrome* may have subnormal serum opsonizing activity in association with decreased serum levels of factor B; factor D also may be low.

Immune complexes, including those initiated by microorganisms or their by-products, may induce consumption of components of complement. Activation occurs primarily through fixation of C1 to antibody thereby initiating the classical pathway. In *systemic lupus erythematosus*, immune complexes activate the classical pathway, and C3 is deposited at sites of tissue damage, including kidneys and skin; depressed synthesis of C3 is also seen. Formation of immune complexes and consumption of complement have been demonstrated in *lepromatous leprosy, subacute bacterial endocarditis, infected ventriculojugular shunts, malaria, infectious mononucleosis, dengue hemorrhagic fever*, and *acute hepatitis B*. Nephritis or arthritis may develop as a result of deposition of immune complexes and activation of complement in these infections. The syndrome of *recurrent urticaria, angioedema, eosinophilia*, and *hypocomplementemia* secondary to activation of the classical pathway may be due to circulating immune complexes. Circulating immune complexes and decreased C3 have been reported in some patients with *dermatitis herpetiformis, celiac disease, primary biliary cirrhosis*, and *Reye syndrome*.

In patients with *bacteremic shock*, bacterial products appear to initiate direct activation of the alternative pathway. *Intravenous injection of iodinated roentgenographic contrast medium* can induce a rapid and significant activation of the alternative pathway, which may explain at least some of the occasional reactions that occur in patients undergoing this procedure.

Burns can induce massive activation of the complement system, especially the alternative pathway, within a few hours after injury. Generation of C3a and C5a occurs, which stimulates neutrophils and induces their sequestration in the lung. These events may play an important part in the development of shock lung after burn injury. Cardiopulmonary bypass, plasma exchange, or hemodialysis using cellophane membranes may be associated with a similar syndrome due to activation of plasma complement, with release of C3a and C5a. In patients with *erythropoietic protoporphyria* or *porphyria cutanea tarda* exposure of the skin to light of certain wavelengths activates complement, generating chemotactic activity. Phototoxicity is associated histologically with lysis of capillary endothelial cells, mast cell degranulation, and the appearance of neutrophils in the dermis.

121.4 Diagnosis of Disorders of the Complement System

Testing for total hemolytic complement activity (CH_{50}) is a useful screening procedure for most of the diseases of the complement system. A normal result in this assay depends on the ability of all 11 component proteins of the classical pathway and membrane attack complex to interact and lyse antibody-coated erythrocytes. The dilution of serum that lyses 50% of the cells determines the end-point. In congenital deficiencies of C1 through C8, the CH_{50} value will be about 0; in C9 deficiency, the value will be approximately half normal. Values in the acquired deficiencies will, of course, vary with the severity of the underlying disorder. This assay will not detect deficiencies of the alternative pathway components B or D, or of properdin. Deficiency of factors I or H (Chapter 120) will permit consumption of C3, with partial reduction in the CH_{50} value.

In *hereditary angioedema*, depression of C4 and C2 during an attack significantly reduces the CH_{50}. Serum concentrations of C4 and C3 can be determined by radial immunodiffusion. In hereditary angioedema, C4 is characteristically low and C3 normal. Concentrations of C1 inhibitor can be determined with antibody, but a normal result can be anticipated in about 15% of cases (Chapter 120). Because C1 acts as an esterase, the specific diagnosis can be made by showing increased capacity of patients' sera to hydrolyze synthetic esters.

Decreased serum concentrations of both C4 and C3 suggest activation of the classical pathway by immune complexes. In contrast, decreased C3 and normal C4 levels suggest activation of the alternative pathway. This difference is particularly useful in distinguishing nephritis secondary to complex deposition from that due to NeF (nephritic factor). In the latter condition and in deficiency of factors I or H, factor B is consumed, and its serum concentration is low as measured by radial immunodiffusion. Alternative pathway activity can be measured with a relatively simple and reproducible hemolytic assay that depends on the capacity of rabbit erythroctyes to serve as both an "activating" (permissive) surface and a target of alternative pathway activity.

A defect of complement function should be suspected in any patient with collagen-vascular disease or chronic nephritis, or with recurrent pyogenic infections, neisserial infections, angioedema, partial lipodystrophy, or a second episode of septicemia at any age. Complement disorders are frequently detected by means of the relatively simple hemolytic complement assay; this procedure should always be available as a screening test.

121.5 Treatment of Disorders of the Complement System

There is no specific therapy presently available for genetic deficiencies of the complement system, but much can be done to protect patients with these disorders from serious complications. Adults with hereditary angioedema respond to danazol, a synthetic androgen with weak virilizing and mild anabolic potential. The drug, given orally, increases the level of C1 inhibitor severalfold and prevents attacks. It can be used for short-term prophylaxis, for example, for oral surgery, by administering it for 1 wk prior to surgery. It has not been recommended for use in children. Purified C1 INH is being investigated for use during acute attacks and for long-term prophylaxis.

Only supportive management is available for other primary diseases of the complement system. It should be emphasized, however, that identification of a specific defect in the complement system may have an important impact on a patient's health. Concern for the associated complications (collagen-vascular disease and infection) should encourage vigorous diagnostic efforts and earlier institution of therapy. With the onset of unexplained fever, cultures should be obtained and antibiotic therapy instituted more quickly and with less stringent indications than in a normal child. The patient and close household contacts should be immunized with vaccines for pneumococci, *Haemophilus influenzae*, and *Neisseria meningitidis*. High titers of specific antibody might opsonize effectively without the full complement system, and immunization of household members could reduce the risk of exposure of the patient to these particularly threatening pathogens.

Ayesh SK, Azar Y, Babior BM, et al: Inactivation of interleukin-8 by C5a-inactivating protease from serosal fluid. Blood 81:1424, 1993.

Colten HR, Rosen FS: Complement deficiencies. Annu Rev Immunol 10:809, 1992.

Davis AE III: C1 inhibitor and hereditary angioneurotic edema. Annu Rev Immunol 6:595, 1988.

Eichenfield LF, Johnston RB Jr: Secondary disorders of the complement system. Am J Dis Child 143:595, 1989.

Figueroa JE, Densen P: Infectious diseases associated with complement deficiencies. Clin Microbiol Rev 4:359, 1991.

Johnston RB Jr: Disorders of the complement system. *In*: Stiehm ER (ed): Immunologic Disorders in Infants and Children, 4th ed. Philadelphia, WB Saunders, 1995.

Kölble K, Reid KBM: Genetic deficiencies of the complement system and association with disease—early components. Int Rev Immunol 10:17, 1993.

Notarangelo LD, Chirico G, Chiara A, et al: Activity of classical and alternative pathways of complement in preterm and small for gestational age infants. Pediatr Res 18:281, 1984.

Ross SC, Densen P: Complement deficiency states and infection: Epidemiology, pathogenesis and consequences of neisserial and other infections in an immune deficiency. Medicine 63:243, 1984.

Tedesco F, Nürnberger W, Perissutti S: Inherited deficiencies of the terminal complement components. Int Rev Immunol 10:51, 1993.

Wang RH, Phillips G Jr, Medof ME, et al: Activation of the alternative complement pathway by exposure of phosphatidylethanolamine and phosphatidylserine on erythrocytes from sickle cell disease patients. J Clin Invest 92:1326, 1993.

Würzner R, Orren A, Lachmann PJ: Inherited deficiencies of the terminal components of human complement. Immunodefic Rev 3:123, 1992.

Yeh ETH, Rosse WF: Perspectives: Paroxysmal nocturnal hemoglobinuria and the glycophosphatidylinositol anchor. J Clin Invest 93:2305, 1994.

CHAPTER 122
The Phagocytic System

Robert L. Baehner

122.1 Normal Physiology of the Phagocytic Inflammatory Response

Understanding the disorders of phagocytic function requires a knowledge of the normal physiology of the inflammatory response of the phagocytic system. The principal phagocytes are neutrophils and monocytes; the former are more heavily involved in acute inflammation and microbial killing and the latter in chronic inflammation. Eosinophils, although capable of phagocytic microbial killing, participate in allergic and certain parasitic responses. Fixed tissue macrophages of liver, spleen, lung, and bone marrow are primed by T lymphocyte cytokines to remove immune complexes, antibody and complement-sensitized blood cells and microbes, and other particulate debris from the circulation.

Neutrophils, eosinophils, and monocytes are derived from a pluripotent stem cell progenitor in the bone marrow, which is further differentiated into specific lineages defined by in vitro culture and influenced by a group of lymphocyte and monocyte cytokines (Fig. 122–1).

Optimal pluripotent stem cell proliferation requires costimulation by multiple cytokines, including stem cell factor, interleukin (IL)-3, IL-1, IL-6, IL-12, and granulocyte-macrophage–colony stimulating factor (GM-CSF). Multipotent myeloid-erythroid progenitors require additional specific hematopoietic regulators, such as erythropoietin for erythrocyte development, IL-5 for eosinophil development, IL-9 and IL-11 for megakaryocyte development, macrophage–colony stimulating factor (M-CSF) for monocyte macrophage development, and granulocyte–colony stimulating factor (G-CSF) for granulocyte development. Neutrophilic granulocytes proliferate and mature in the bone marrow over a 10–12 day period. These cells, in contrast to stem cells, can be recognized on a Wright-Geimsa–stained smear by light microscopy. Proliferation consisting of approximately five divisions takes place only during the 1st three stages of neutrophil maturation (myeloblast, promyelocyte, and myelocyte). After the myelocyte stage, the cells become "end cells," no longer capable of mitosis, and mature further into metamyelocytes, bands, and segmented polymorphonuclear neutrophils (PMNs). They remain in this larger storage pool for about 5 days under normal conditions and then are released into the blood, where they circulate for about 8–10 hr and then migrate to tissues where they may live for 1 or 2 days (Fig. 122–2). PMN maturation is associated with changes in the nucleus and with the production of azurophilic or primary granules, and lighter, less dense specific or secondary granules. The myeloblast is a relatively undifferentiated cell with a large oval nucleus, sizable nuclei, and no granules. Promyelocytes acquire peroxidase-positive azurophilic granules and myelocytes acquire specific granules (see Chapter 125). Chromatin condensation, loss of nucleoli, and shape changes of the nucleus result in the morphometric characteristics of the PMN.

The large store of PMNs in bone marrow moves into the circulation in response to soluble mediators of inflammation such as endotoxin, tumor necrosis factor, interleukin 1, and activated complement by-product C3e. Following intravenous administration of 4 ng/kg endotoxin to humans, after an initial drop in peripheral blood neutrophils by 1 hr, neutrophil counts increase threefold by 6–8 hr with an increase in band forms. Band forms do not increase after a single oral or intravenous dose of glucocorticoids, nor are monoclonal antibody 31D4-positive bone marrow neutrophils seen in the circulation, which calls into question the notion that steroids raise the neutrophil count by causing egress of marrow neutrophils. Steroid neutrophilia may be due to delayed egress into tissues, release of a marginated pool, and increased production. Under normal conditions, neutrophils randomly exit from the circulation at a half-life rate of 4–6 hr, and the marginating pool approximates the circulating pool size. Activation of adenylate cyclase by adrenaline and other adrenergic agonists results in demargination of neutrophils and a doubling of circulating neutrophils associated with a transient elevation in cyclic AMP.

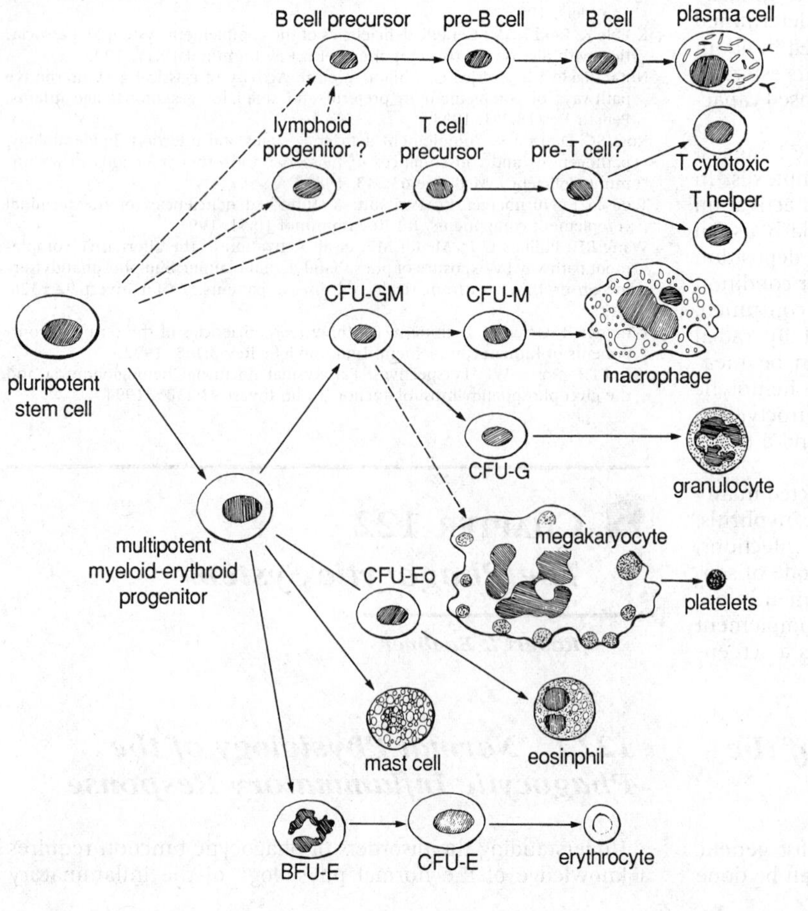

Figure 122–1. Differentiation pathways of hematolymphoid cells. Pluripotent stem cells give rise to multipotent myeloid-erythroid progenitors that commit to restricted precursors of the myeloid and erythroid lineages. Restricted erythroid-myeloid progenitors and precursors are primarily defined through their capacity to give rise to a colony upon stimulation by a defined cytokine and are designated colony forming unit (CFU). The letter(s) after CFU refer to the lineage restriction: E, erythrocytes; M, macrophages; G, granulocytes; Eo, eosinophils. The BFU-E (burst forming unit–erythroid) is an early precursor restricted to the erythroid lineage. Precursors give rise to a colony containing a single mature cell type. Colonies derived from progenitors can be composed of two or more cell types. Lymphoid precursors are believed to separate from myeloid-erythroid progenitors early in the differentiation cascade. Both T- and B-lymphocyte differentiation depend on regulatory stromal cells found in thymus and bone marrow. (From Cooper EL, Nisbet-Brown E [eds]: Developmental Immunology. New York, Oxford University Press, 1993.)

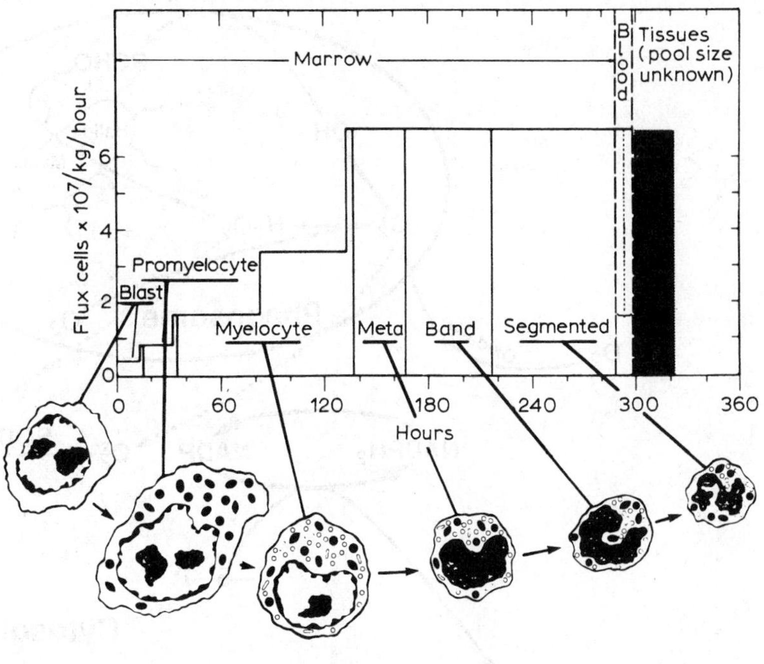

Figure 122–2. Diagrammatic representation of life cycle and stages of maturation of human neutrophilic granulocytes. The myeloblast is a relatively undifferentiated cell with a large oval nucleus, large nucleoli, and cytoplasm lacking granules. It originates from a precursor pool of committed progenitor cells and is followed by two secretory stages: the promyelocyte and the myelocyte. During each of these stages a distinct type of secretory granule is produced—azurophils (solid black) during the promyelocyte stage and specific granules (light forms) during the myelocyte stage. The metamyelocyte and band forms are nonproliferating, nonsecretory cells, which develop into the mature polymorphonuclear neutrophils. The mature form is characterized by a multilobulated nucleus and cytoplasm containing primarily glycogen and granules. The times indicated for the various compartments were obtained by isotope labeling techniques (Cronkite and Vincent, 1969). The ordinate shows the flux through each compartment, and the abscissa shows the time in each compartment. The area of each of the nondividing compartments gives the number of cells in that compartment. The stepwise increase in cell numbers through the dividing compartments represents serial divisions. Note that no mitoses occur after the myelocyte stage. (From Bainton DF: *In*: Weissman G [ed]: Cell Biology of Inflammation. New York, Elsevier, 1980.)

Although the ability of phagocytes to migrate to sites of infection and/or inflammation was recognized more than a century ago, the biologic nature of chemoattractants and their influences on phagocytic cell activities after binding to specific surface receptors have only recently begun to be understood. A variety of chemotactic factors are derived from cells or plasma. The activation of complement generates C5a, clotting generates thrombin, cell membrane phospholipids generate platelet-activating factor, stimulated T lymphocytes provide lymphocyte-derived chemotactic factor, activated macrophages and lymphocytes release IL-8, and activated PMNs generate leukotriene B_4. The ability of the various chemoattractant molecules to activate leukocyte responses is mediated by specific receptors, which, when occupied by a specific chemotactic factor, activate phospholipase C to produce inositol triphosphate (IP3) and diacylglycerol. IP3 in turn increases intracellular calcium-dependent responses associated with phagocyte activation, such as protein kinase C for phosphorylation of several important intracellular proteins required for cell activation and the assembly of actin and associated contractile proteins. The increased expression of a group of adherence proteins, for example, iC3b, and the assembly of actin and associated contractible proteins enable the phagocyte to attach to endothelial surfaces and move in a crawling amoeboid way to the site of infection or inflammation. The pathway is paved by an increasing gradient of chemoattractants that culminate in either a full expression of phagocytic activation or engagement of opsonized microbes.

Microbes are opsonized (prepared for ingestion) by heat-stable and heat-labile factors in human serum that include immunoglobulin G and C3. Human leukocytes have three distinguishable receptors for each of the four immunoglobulin G subclasses (IgG1–4) and four receptors for C3 (CR1–4). CR1 and CR3 are distinct opsonin receptors on neutrophils, monocytes, and macrophages that bind C3b and iC3b, respectively, and facilitate phagocytosis of microbes and other particles or cells opsonized by them. In contrast to the IgG receptors, FcR, and the CR1 receptors (which do not require divalent cation for their ligand binding), CR3 requires 0.5 mM concentrations of calcium and magnesium ions for iC3b binding. The in vivo importance of the CR3 receptor for host defense will be discussed later. The trigger for ingestion by phagocytes of CR1- and CR3-bound microbes or cells appears to involve phosphorylation of the receptor by activated protein kinases. Adhesive proteins found in plasma and tissue matrices (such as fibronectin, laminin, and the protein kinase C stimulant phorbal myristate acetate) have been shown to trigger phagocytic cell ingestion. Ingestion is an active process accompanied by further assembly and disassembly of contractile elements as the pseudopode envelopes its prey as it forms a phagosome. Granules fuse with the phagosomal membrane and discharge their contents into it. In neutrophils, specific granules interact with the phagosome earlier than do azurophilic granules. This process of degranulation occurs in all phagocytic cells and promotes the killing or digestion of microbes. On the other hand, treatment of cells with cytochalasin B disrupts assembled microfilaments, blocks ingestion, and renders the phagocytes secretory. Under such conditions, full activation induces release of the granule contents to the outside of the cell. Soluble chemotactic stimuli at sites of inflammation can induce extensive granule secretion, escalating the inflammatory process. In addition, the microbicidal and cytotoxic system of phagocytes includes the secretory products of the respiratory burst, superoxide anion, hydrogen peroxide, hydroxyl radical, and longer acting hypochlorous acid and chloramines (Fig. 122–3). The azurophilic granule constituent myeloperoxidase participates in the amplification of this system by halides such as iodide and chloride. This system may also inhibit chemotactic factors and lysosomal granule components that may attenuate the inflammatory process. The respiratory burst is discussed in more detail in Chapter 129 in terms of the etiology and pathogenesis of chronic granulomatous disease.

122.2 Other Types of Inflammatory Leukocytes

NEUTROPHILS. As discussed earlier, neutrophils are the predominating type of granulocyte. The nuclei of the cells have three to five segments, and are designated polymorphonuclear leukocytes (PMNs). Qualitatively, neutrophils are the most important phagocytic cells that defend the host against acute bacterial infection. There are several inherited neutrophil

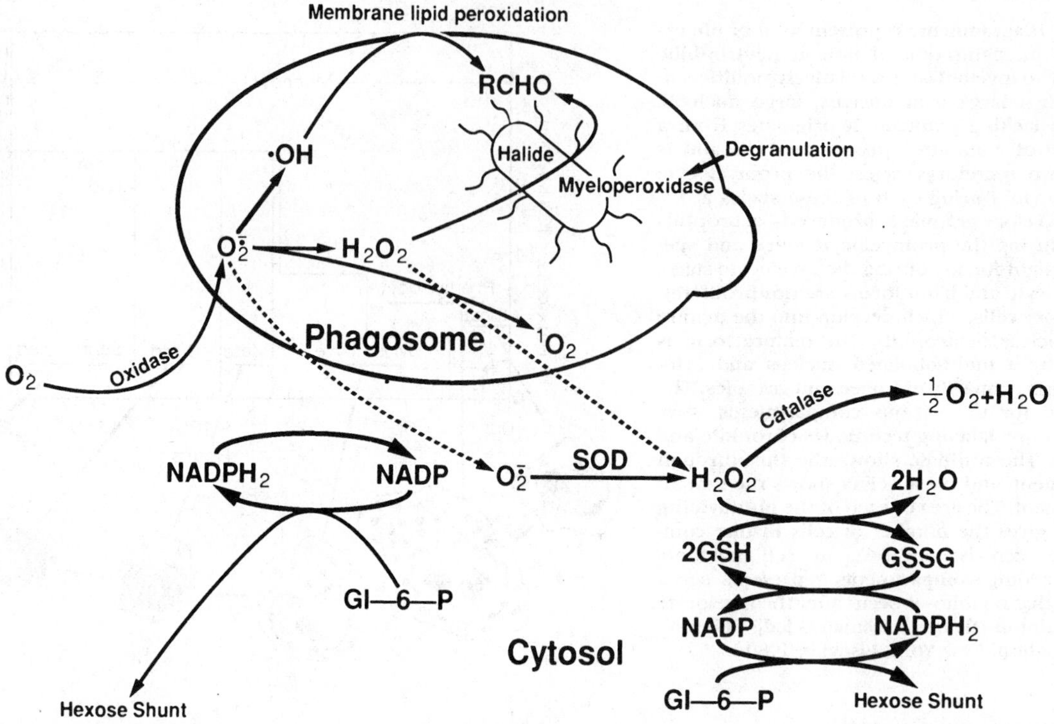

Figure 122–3. **The mechanisms for the production, action, and detoxification of peroxides in neutrophils. Oxygen is reduced to superoxide (O_2^-) by an oxidase. NADPH is regenerated from NADP by the hexose monophosphate shunt. Superoxide may spontaneously decompose to hydrogen peroxide and singlet oxygen ($^1O_2$). Hydrogen peroxide can react with superoxide to form hydroxyl radicals and generate bactericidal aldehydes (RCHO) by oxidizing bacterial constituents in the presence of halide ions and myeloperoxidase that were delivered to the phagosome by degranulation. Hydroxyl radicals (·OH) can peroxidize unsaturated fatty acids of the phagosomal membrane and thus yield the potentially bactericidal aldehydes. Superoxide leaking out of the phagosome may be converted rapidly to hydrogen peroxide by superoxide dismutase (SOD). Hydrogen peroxide in the cytosol is destroyed by catalase or reduced glutathione (GSH). GSH is regenerated by coupled reactions that stimulate the flow of glucose-6-phosphate (G-6-P) into the hexose monophosphate shunt.**

structural abnormalities and these are discussed in Chapter 130.

EOSINOPHILS. Eosinophils are characterized by large coarse granules of prominent red color (with Romanowsky stain) and by a nucleus with one or two segments. They normally account for fewer than 5% of circulating leukocytes. Eosinopenia may be produced by at least two mechanisms: (1) acute stress, with the resultant stimulation of adrenocorticoids or release of epinephrine, or both; and (2) acute inflammatory states. Eosinophil counts are increased in parasitic infections, allergic phenomena, or dermatologic conditions. Other causes of eosinophilia include gastrointestinal disorders, Hodgkin's disease, and immune deficiency diseases, and it can occur during convalescence from viral diseases. The most pronounced eosinophilia encountered in the United States accompanies invasion of the tissues by parasitic helminths, and from such diseases as visceral larva migrans and trichinosis. Hypereosinophilic syndrome refers to a broad continuum of illnesses varying from Löffler syndrome to severe chronic and ultimately fatal eosinophilic leukemia.

BASOPHILS. These leukocytes are distinguished by coarse, deep blue granules that fill the cytoplasm and obscure the nucleus. The granules contain large amounts of heparin and histamine. Basophils account for 0.5% of total leukocytes. Increases occur in those with chronic myelogenous leukemia, ulcerative colitis, juvenile rheumatoid arthritis, iron deficiency, and chronic renal failure, and following radiation therapy.

LYMPHOCYTES. Lymphocytes constitute 30–60% of the blood leukocytes. Most are small cells measuring 9 μm in diameter with a round, dark, blue-black nucleus and thin blue cytoplasm. Lymphocytes are actively motile but not phagocytic. Lymphocytes can be characterized as T or B lymphocytes or natural killer cells on the basis of physical and immunologic properties. Marked absolute lymphocytosis can be seen in certain acute infections such as pertussis, infectious mononucleosis, and acute infectious lymphocytosis. Acute infections with moderate relative lymphocytosis include the common childhood exanthems and other viral illnesses, brucellosis, and typhoid and paratyphoid fevers. Chronic infections, drug and allergic reactions, leukemia, thyrotoxicosis, and Addison disease may also be associated with lymphocytosis. Thymic alymphoplasia is associated with profound lymphopenia.

MONOCYTES. These large phagocytic cells are characterized by a large lobulated nucleus and abundant gray cytoplasm that contains fine azurophilic granules. They normally account for 1–5% of the circulating leukocytes. The blood monocyte is an important component of the body's phagocytic system and is derived from the bone marrow stem cell. There is no substantial bone marrow reserve pool of monocytes, and mature monocytes are released into the bloodstream several days earlier than the bone marrow neutrophils. Consequently, during recovery from bone marrow aplasia or hypoplasia, a relative monocytosis of the peripheral blood may herald the return of neutrophils. This is most commonly noted in patients recovering from the use of chemotherapeutic agents.

In the bloodstream the monocyte functions as a phagocytic cell, similarly to the neutrophil. The half-life of blood monocytes is 8 hr. Unlike the neutrophil, monocytes at inflammatory sites undergo a wide variety of phagocytic functions in response to bacterial products, particularly lipopolysaccharides. Despite its impressive ability to enhance its phagocytic function, the monocyte cannot replace the neutrophil as the primary phagocytic cell, because it moves more slowly than the neutrophil.

After leaving the bloodstream monocytes enter tissues, where they differentiate into tissue macrophages. These long-lived tissue macrophages remain for as long as 2 yr to carry out macrophage functions such as scavenging of debris and ingesting bacteria. In addition to their usually phagocytic functions, tissue macrophages are particularly adept at handling microorganisms and parasites such as *Legionella pneumophila, Listeria monocytogenes,* and *Toxoplasma gondii.* Monocytes are increased in such diseases as tuberculosis, systemic mycosis, bacterial endocarditis, chronic inflammatory bowel disease, and certain protozoan infections. Elevated monocyte counts are also frequently seen in patients with isolated neutropenia.

QUANTITATIVE DISORDERS OF THE NEUTROPHILS

Absolute neutrophil counts vary widely in normal subjects. The relative proportion of neutrophils and lymphocytes in the blood varies with age. Neutrophils predominate at birth but decrease rapidly in the 1st few days of life. During infancy they constitute 20–30% of the circulating leukocytes. Similar proportions of neutrophils and lymphocytes occur by about 5 yr of age, but the approximately 70% predominance of neutrophils characteristic of the adult is not attained until puberty. In normal healthy children, therefore, from 20–70% of the total circulating white blood cells may be neutrophils. In absolute terms they number 1,500–2,500/mm^3. Levels exceeding this range are designated neutrophilia or polymorphonuclear leukocytosis.

Bainton DF: The cells of inflammation: A general view. *In*: Weissman G (ed): The Cell Biology of Inflammation, Vol 2. New York, Elsevier/North Holland, 1980, pp 1–25.
Cooper EL, Møller-Seiburg CE, Spangrude GJ: Stem cells. *In*: Cooper EL, Nisbet-Brown E (eds): Developmental Immunology. Oxford, Oxford University Press, 1993, pp 177–197.
Gallin JI, Goldstein IM, Snyderman R: Inflammation, Basic Principles and Clinical Correlates. New York, Raven Press, 1988.
Shurin SB: Pathologic states associated with activation of eosinophils and with eosinophilia. Hematol Oncol Clin North Am 2:171, 1988.

CHAPTER 123
Neutrophilia

Robert L. Baehner

An increase in circulating neutrophils is the result of a disturbance of the equilibrium involving neutrophil bone marrow production, movement in and out of the bone marrow compartments into the circulation, and neutrophil destruction. Three mechanisms, either alone or in combination, largely account for neutrophilia.

1. Increased numbers of neutrophils may be mobilized from either the bone marrow storage compartment or peripheral marginating pools into the circulating pool.
2. There may be increased blood neutrophil survival because of impaired neutrophil egress into tissue.
3. There may be expansion of the circulating neutrophil pool as a result of increased progenitor cell proliferation and terminal differentiation through the neutrophilic series, increased mitotic activity of neutrophilic cell precursors, or shortening of the cell mitotic cycle of neutrophil precursors.

Acute neutrophilia accompanies physical exercise or an epinephrine-induced reaction, such as a panic response. Epinephrine-induced reactions reflect mobilization of the marginating pool of the neutrophils into the circulating pool. Slower onset of acute neutrophilia can occur following glucocorticosteroid administration or in response to inflammation or infection associated with the generation of endotoxins. Maximal response usually occurs within 4–24 hr and is probably secondary to the release of neutrophils into the circulation from the marrow storage compartments. Glucocorticoids may also impede the release of neutrophils from the circulation into the tissue.

Chronic neutrophilia may be associated with continuous stimulation of neutrophil production, probably through inhibition of marrow feedback mechanisms. Chronic neutrophilia may be associated with prolonged administration of glucocorticoids, chronic inflammatory reactions, or chronic anxiety.

Leukemoid reactions or reactive leukocytosis resembling the blood picture of leukemia has been associated with sepsis, systemic mycotic and protozoan infections, hepatic failure, diabetic acidosis, azotemia, and with disorders associated with malignancy involving the bone marrow. Occasionally, leukemoid reactions may resemble those of chronic myelogenous leukemia. The neutrophils in leukemoid reactions, however, have elevations in alkaline phosphatase activity, whereas this enzyme activity is low in chronic myelogenous leukemia.

Neutrophilia may also accompany various hematologic disorders such as chronic hemolytic anemia, hemorrhage, transfusion reactions, postsplenectomy reactions, and myeloproliferative disorders. Neutrophilia has also been reported in the functional disorder of neutrophils associated with leukocytic adhesion deficiency (see Chapter 125).

CHAPTER 124
Neutropenia

Robert L. Baehner

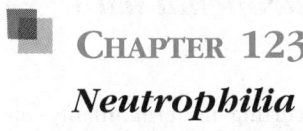

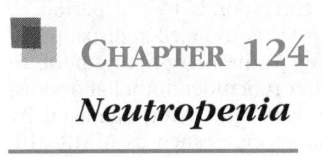

Neutropenia is a deficiency of circulating neutrophils and band forms defined as an absolute neutrophil count (ANC) less than 1,500/μl. The ANC is calculated from the white blood count and differential. Neutropenia is due to either alteration in bone marrow production or exaggerated losses of neutrophils from the circulation. Transient states of neutropenia due to acquired causes last only a few days to weeks, whereas chronic states are usually due to immune, congenital, or genetic causes and may last a few months or be lifelong. In general, the risk for infection in chronic states of neutropenia is roughly proportional to the ANC and to the reserve of neutrophils present in the bone marrow. Normally the bone marrow stores a 10-fold reserve of neutrophils, which are generated from precursor myeloid cells (see Fig. 122–1) regulated by specific bone marrow growth factors and cytokines. The differentiation of uncommitted stem cells into myeloid lineage requires the coordinated action of stem cell factor (SCF), interleukin (IL)-1, IL-3, IL-6, and granulocyte-macrophage colony stimulating factor (GM-CSF) and the further differentiation of mature neutrophils requires granulocyte-colony stimulating factor (G-CSF). Eosinophils require IL-5 and IL-11, and monocytes require monocyte colony stimulating factor. Binding of these growth factors to specific receptors on the surface of the developing myeloid cells initiates a signal intracellularly to promote proliferation and differentiation. Neutrophils are released from the marrow in response to a variety of substances, including endotoxin, corticosteroids, and activated complement components. Neutrophils leave the circulation randomly and upon demand when infection or other inflammatory stimuli provokes them. Neutrophils leave the circulation by rolling against the vascular endothelium, attaching to it, and exiting between endothelial cells into the extracellular space. Chemotactic signals are released by infecting microbes or tissue cells, which activate complement to generate C5a, elaborate leukotrienes, IL-8, and other chemotaxins. The expression of adhesion molecules on neutrophils, including selectins and integrins, is upregulated, leading to margination and attachment of neutrophils to endothelial leukocyte adhesion molecule-1 (ELAM-1, selectin E) on vascular endothelial surfaces. The normal half-life of a circulating neutrophil is about 6–8 hr, but it is shortened by infection, inflammation, or the development of antineutrophil antibody.

Patients with neutropenia may remain asymptomatic or they may experience mild infections of the skin and mucous membranes. However, those with severe forms of neutropenia are at risk for infections that may be life threatening. Table 124–1 lists the causes of neutropenia in infants and children.

124.1 Transient Neutropenia

VIRAL. The most common cause of transient neutropenia in childhood is viral infections. Viruses that commonly cause neutropenia include hepatitis A and B, respiratory syncytial virus, influenza A and B, measles, rubella, and varicella. Neutropenia develops during the first 24–48 hr of illness and may persist for 3–6 days. It usually corresponds to the period of acute viremia and may relate to virus-induced redistribution of neutrophils from the circulating to the marginating pool, to sequestration in the spleen or other reticuloendothelial organs, or to increased uptake into extravascular tissue damaged by viruses. Immunization with viral vaccines such as MMR also may result in transient neutropenia. Mild neutropenia may be associated with transient erythroblastopenia of childhood in approximately half of the cases; it is not associated with a risk of infection and clears when the anemia begins to resolve.

■ TABLE 124–1 Neutropenias of Infants and Children

Transient	
	Viral
	Bacterial
	Drug induced
	Nutritional
	Neonatal with maternal hypertension
	Neonatal with sepsis
Chronic	
Immune Related	
	Benign childhood form (autoimmune)
	Associated with primary immune disease
	Neonatal alloimmune (isoimmune)
	Neonatal maternal autoimmune
Congenital	
	Genetic infantile agranulocytosis (Kostmann disease)
	Cyclic hematopoiesis
	Familial benign
	Chédiak-Higashi syndrome
	Glycogen storage disease type 1b
	Shwachman-Diamond syndrome
	Metaphyseal chondrodysplasia (cartilage-hair hypoplasia)
	Cardioskeletal myopathy (Barth syndrome)
	Dyskeratosis congenita
	Onychotrichodysplasia
Cancer-Related	
	AIDS-related

NUTRITIONAL. Neutropenia may occur with states of nutritional deficiency of vitamin B_{12}, folic acid, or copper. Macrocytic anemia and a megaloblastic bone marrow is present and the hematologic picture responds to folate or vitamin B_{12} therapy. Copper deficiency appears to be linked to production of antineutrophil antibodies. After copper supplementation, antibody titers become negative and ANCs revert to normal.

BACTERIAL. Infection with *Staphylococcus aureus,* brucellosis, tularemia, rickettsia, salmonella typhi, *Shigella sonnei,* and *Mycobacterium tuberculosis* may cause moderate neutropenia. Marked neutropenia often heralds the onset of overwhelming sepsis with high fevers, shaking chills, and shock. A clinical picture of purpura fulminans with diffuse intravascular coagulation may be present.

DRUG INDUCED. Many therapeutic agents cause neutropenia. Most drug-related neutropenias are due to dose-dependent bone marrow suppression or to haptene-associated induction of antineutrophil antibody. Phenothiazines, semisynthetic penicillins, nonsteroidal anti-inflammatory agents, aminopyrine derivatives, and antithyroid medications are most commonly implicated. Recovery usually starts within a few days of stopping the drug and is preceded by the appearance of monocytes and immature neutrophils in the blood. Cytotoxic drugs used in cancer therapy or in attenuation of the immune response regularly cause significant suppression of the bone marrow and result in transient states of neutropenia.

124.2 Neonatal Neutropenia and Maternal Hypertension

Neutropenia is observed in approximately 50% of neonates born to women with severe pregnancy-induced hypertension. It is usually transient, is not associated with a significant risk of infection, and is more common in premature infants. Neutrophil production is inhibited by a placental factor present in cord blood serum.

124.3 Neonatal Neutropenia with Sepsis

Most neutropenic episodes occurring in term infants, although rare, are associated with infections. In contrast, preterm infants experience many more episodes of neutropenia, either associated with infections or from noninfectious causes. Hematologic predictors of sepsis in the neonate include an elevated immature:mature neutrophil ratio in the blood (>0.35) and an ANC less than 500/uL. Those infants with a depleted storage reservoir in the bone marrow (<7% of all nucleated bone marrow cells are polymorphonuclear, band forms, or metamyelocytes) are particularly vulnerable to overwhelming sepsis, meningitis, and death. Granulocyte transfusions are of significant benefit for the newborn with sepsis and neutropenia. High-dose gamma globulin and recombinant G-CSF are currently being evaluated for their efficacy in the treatment of the newborn with suspected or documented sepsis.

124.4 Benign Chronic Neutropenia

AUTOIMMUNE NEUTROPENIA OF INFANCY. This is the most common form of chronic childhood neutropenia. It is a chronic state of mature neutrophil depletion with a compensated increase in immature granulocytes in the bone marrow analogous to erythroid hyperplasia seen in immune hemolytic anemia. The median age of detection is 8 mo and 90% of cases are discovered before 14 mo of age. There is a 3:2 female predominance. Neutropenia is usually not found among other family members. The neutropenia is most often detected as an incidental finding during the workup of a child with fever. Physical examination is normal except for findings related to infection. Pyogenic skin infection, oral ulcerations, abcesses, or cellulitis of the labia majora have been the presenting manifestations in a few patients. Almost all children have a remarkably benign course despite a markedly reduced ANC. The median duration of neutropenia is 20 mo and 95% of the patients recover by 4 yr of age.

The ANC is usually less than 500/μl; moderate eosinophilia or monocytosis is often observed. The bone marrow is cellular with an arrest at the late metamyelocyte or band stage. Antineutrophil antibodies are usually detected, but their absence does not exclude the diagnosis.

Treatment directed at raising the ANC is rarely required, although high-dose gamma globulin as well as recombinant human G-CSF has raised ANC in affected patients. This form of therapy should be reserved for the rare child with significant bacterial infection. Skin infections and upper respiratory tract infections respond to standard antibiotic treatment.

NEUTROPENIA ASSOCIATED WITH PRIMARY IMMUNE DISEASE. Neutropenia is a frequent occurrence in children with congenital and acquired forms of immune deficiencies, including agammaglobulinemia and hypogammaglobulinemia, hypergammaglobulinia, T-cell defects, natural killer cell defects, and autoimmune diseases. Many of these patients have had a positive family history of neutropenia. These patients usually present during infancy or early childhood with recurrent bacterial infections, leading to failure to thrive and life-threatening diseases. Physical examination reveals a child who appears chronically ill with evidence of acute and/or chronic infection, hepatosplenomegaly, and poor growth. The therapy for these disorders is directed at the underlying cause, in addition to aggressive treatment of the infection.

ALLOIMMUNE NEONATAL NEUTROPENIA (ANN). This form of neonatal neutropenia occurs after transplacental transfer of maternal alloantibodies directed against antigens on the infant's neutrophils, analogous to Rh hemolytic disease. Prenatal sensitization induces maternal IgG antibodies to neutrophil antigens on fetal cells. The antibodies are usually complement activating and are frequently directed to the neutrophil-specific NA antigen system (NA1, NA2, NB1). The NA antigens are located in the Fc γ receptor III-1 (FcRIII, CD16), the low-affinity receptor for the Fc domain of IgG. Among the various specificities of antibodies, NA1 is involved 34%, NA2 and NB1 are each involved in 12%, and undefined antigenic sites are likely involved in the remainder. Recently, ANN was reported in two infants whose maternal neutrophils lacked FcγR and were typed as NA-null, a situation that has been noted in 1 in 1,000 blood donors. NA-null individuals are not at risk of infection, presumably because their neutrophils express the other two types of Fc receptors, FcγRI and FcγRII. Antibodies directed to HLA antigens, without NA specificity, have been detected in a few cases of ANN. Among postpartum women, the incidence of granulocyte-specific antibodies is 1.1%, but only 0.4% are directed to known granulocyte antigens. None of the infants of this group of mothers has developed neutropenia, suggesting that the real incidence of ANN is below 0.1%.

The *pathogenesis* of ANN probably involves phagocytosis of antibody-coated neutrophils by macrophages in the liver, spleen, lung, and bone marrow. Most infants with ANN are asymptomatic; symptomatic infants have omphalitis, delayed separation of the umbilical cord, mild skin infections, fever, and pneumonia within the first 2 wk of life, which resolve with antibiotic therapy. Sepsis and death have occurred in a few infants, particularly when the disease was unrecognized. The neutropenia may last a few weeks to as long as 6 mo.

The *diagnosis* is established by demonstrating the presence of maternal neutrophil-specific alloantibodies. Neutrophil-specific antibodies must be demonstrated in maternal serum and parental neutrophils should be typed to determine the antigen specificity.

High-dose gamma globulin improves neutropenia, but it is indicated only for the symptomatic infant. Transfusion of paternal neutrophils that lack the sensitizing antigen is beneficial for infants with suspected sepsis or other serious infection.

NEONATAL MATERNAL AUTOIMMUNE NEUTROPENIA. Mothers with autoimmune diseases may give birth to infants who develop transient neutropenia. The duration of the neutropenia depends upon the time that it takes for the infant to clear the maternally transferred circulating IgG antibody. In most cases this is between a few weeks and a few months. The neonate almost always remains asymptomatic.

124.5 Congenital Neutropenias

GENETIC INFANTILE AGRANULOCYTOSIS (KOSTMANN'S DISEASE). This is a rare autosomal recessive disease characterized by severe neutropenia at birth and frequent bacterial infections, resulting in death in most patients by 3 yr of age. Kostmann collected 19 sibships in Sweden in 1975, and the gene appears to have originated from a small parish in the far north of that country. Since that time other cases of severe congenital agranulocytosis have been described in Asia, North America, and Europe. In addition to persistent neutropenia with less than 200/uL, variable degrees of monocytosis, eosinophilia, hypergammaglobulinemia, and thrombocytosis may be found. Bone marrow morphology suggests maturational arrest of neutrophil precursors at the promyelocyte stage. An association with HLA-B12 has been described, suggesting that a gene controlling neutrophil differentiation is closely linked to the histocompatibility system genes. However, the underlying cause of this disease is unknown and may be heterogeneous. The addition of recombinant human G-CSF (filgrastim) to bone marrow cultures resulted in the development of normal colonies of mature neutrophils.

Administration of G-CSF subcutaneously several times a week to five patients in 1989 resulted in sustained ANC of greater than 1,000/uL for months to over a year during the period of administration. Pre-existing chronic infections resolved and the number of new infectious episodes decreased. Since then most other infants and children with severe congenital neutropenia have achieved normal neutrophil levels when given G-CSF at doses of 3.5–12 μg/kg/24 hr. This form of therapy has dramatically reduced the incidence and duration of infectious complications.

CYCLIC NEUTROPENIA (CYCLIC HEMATOPOIESIS). This is a rare blood disease characterized by regular 18–21 day cyclic fluctuations in the numbers of blood neutrophils, monocytes, eosinophils, lymphocytes, platelets, and reticulocytes. Patients with the disease have recurrent fever, malaise, mucosal ulcers, severe periodontal infections, oral ulcerations, skin infections, and, on rare occasions, life-threatening infection during the nadir of the neutropenia. The disease is usually diagnosed in childhood, often occurs in several generations within the same family, and affects both males and females. A similar disease has been noted in the Grey Collie dog, which is transmitted as autosomal recessive. In both the human and canine forms of the disease, transplantation of the defective bone marrow results in transfer of the cyclic hematopoiesis to the recipient, suggesting that the defect resides in the hematopoietic stem cell. Receptor expression and binding affinity for G-CSF appear to be normal. Neutrophil levels fluctuate between normal and less than 200/μl. Administration of pharmacologic doses of G-CSF raises the ANC nadir, although the cycling pattern of hematopoiesis persists. With G-CSF treatment, most patients also have fewer episodes of fever and mouth and skin infections.

FAMILIAL BENIGN NEUTROPENIA. Both dominant and recessive autosomal forms have been described. A genetic cause is suggested because most cases occur in Jews from Yemen and Ethiopia. In general, African-Americans have lower mean ANCs than Americans of European ancestry, but the differences do not cause any increased susceptibility to infection. Some forms of benign neutropenia seem to be due to intramedullary destruction of the neutrophils associated with morphologic abnormalities of their nuclei. The cells have cytoplasmic vacuoles and thin strands connecting the nuclear lobes, a term called *myelokathexis*.

CHÉDIAK-HIGASHI SYNDROME. This autosomal recessive disorder is characterized by partial albinism, photophobia, nystagmus, decreased pigmentation of the hair and eyes, and increased susceptibility to infection (see Chapter 127).

GLYCOGEN STORAGE DISEASE TYPE 1b. Recurrent infections and neutropenia are a distinctive feature of glycogen storage disease type 1b. Both classical von Gierke glycogen storage disease (GSD1a) and GSD1b cause massive enlargement of the liver and severe growth retardation. In contrast to GSD1a, glucose-6-phosphatase activity is present on in vitro assay but glucose is not liberated from glucose-6-phosphate in vivo in GSD1b. In the liver G6Pase requires two microsomal membrane components, a specific transport system called G6P translocase that shuttles G6P from the cytoplasm to the lumen of the endoplasmic reticulum and another enzyme bound to the lumenal surface of the membrane, called G6P phosphohydrolase. Neutrophils also appear to have a defective transport system, but it may not explain the defects in neutrophil chemotaxis and bactericidal activity noted in these patients. Neutrophil levels improved and recurrent infections ceased after a portocaval shunt operative procedure in one patient, suggesting that sequestration contributed to the neutropenia. Many of the patients have inflammatory bowel disease as well as oral lesions and perianal abscesses. Administration of either G-CSF or GM-CSF has resulted in resolution or significant improvement of neutropenia, recurrent infections, and enteric inflammation. Long-term administration of G-CSF has been associated with fewer side effects, such as local pain at the injection sites, fever, or allergic reactions, compared with GM-CSF.

SHWACHMAN-DIAMOND SYNDROME. This autosomal recessive disorder is characterized by pancreatic insufficiency and neutropenia. The first description of this syndrome in 1964 was in a group of infants referred for steatorrhea suggesting cystic fibrosis but without respiratory symptoms and with normal sweat electrolytes. In contrast to cystic fibrosis patients, these patients usually develop metaphyseal dysostosis during the first several years of life, leading to short stature. Growth failure is also contributed to by malabsorption due to exocrine pancreatic insufficiency with fatty infiltration of the pancreas sparing the islets of Langerhans. The pancreatic abnormality can be seen on computed tomography. Susceptibility to infection and the degree of neutropenia are variable, with the ANC generally between 200 and 400/μL. Anemia and/or thrombocytopenia is sometimes seen. The bone marrow shows myeloid hyperplasia, and peripheral blood neutrophils are defective in their chemotactic response. Cutaneous involvement is frequent and includes various degrees of dry skin, and eczematous and ichthyosiform lesions. The chemotactic defect has been improved in one patient treated with lithium, and it seems likely that G-CSF administration will be effective in improving the neutropenia if clinically indicated. The risk for the development of leukemia is higher among these patients. Two affected sisters, ages 8 and 13, were recently reported to have prominent neurologic abnormalities, including apraxia, diminished motor skills, generalized weakness, and hypotonia.

METAPHYSEAL CHONDRODYSPLASIA (CARTILAGE-HAIR HYPOPLASIA). This form of short-limb dwarfism was first recognized in 1965 in the Amish population in the eastern United States, but the gene has been traced to Finland, where over 100 affected patients from 85 families were identified. The syndrome consists of a variety of skeletal abnormalities, sparse and light-colored hair, and an immunologic defect of T lymphocytes. Affected patients are very susceptible to disseminated varicella infection and death from pneumonia. Macrocytic anemia with reticulocytopenia is frequently observed during infancy, and most affected patients are lymphopenic. About 25% develop neutropenia. The gene has been mapped to chromosome 9 and appears to be transmitted as recessive with reduced penetrance. Bone marrow transplantation has restored cellular immunity and corrected the neutropenia in two patients.

CARDIOSKELETAL MYOPATHY (BARTH SYNDROME). This syndrome was first described in 1981 in a large Dutch family pedigree in males with dilated cardiomyopathy, growth retardation, neutropenia, and skeletal myopathy. The clinical course is characterized by the onset of congestive heart failure during early infancy, recurrent infections associated with neutropenia, and growth retardation. The initial presentation of the syndrome varies from congenital dilated cardiomyopathy to isolated neutropenia without clinical evidence of heart disease. Weakness of skeletal muscles with sparing of extraocular and bulbar muscles has been noted on physical examination. Electron microscopic examination of biopsies from endomyocardium, skeletal muscle, bone marrow granulocyte precursors, liver, and kidneys reveals mitochrondrial abnormalities with concentric tightly packed cristae and occasional inclusion bodies. Neutropenia has been documented in cord blood, and bone marrow reveals arrest at the myelocyte stage. Endocardial fibroelastosis has been documented in several of the affected males. Elevated levels of urinary 3-methylglutaconate, 3-methylglutarate, and 2-ethylhydracrylate was described in 1991 in a group of seven affected boys, some of whom died of sepsis and/or cardiac disease and others of whom seemed to improve in later childhood. Linkage studies of affected families has mapped the gene to Xq2.8. This syndrome may be a relatively common cause of dilated cardiomyopathy and neutropenia in boys during infancy and early childhood.

DYSKERATOSIS CONGENITA. This is a congenital X-linked multisystem disorder in which male infants exhibit skin pigmentation, dystrophic nails, leukoplakia, and neutropenia progressing to bone marrow failure and life-threatening infection during early infancy. A moderate but transient benefit in ANC and infection was reported in an infant treated with GM-CSF. These patients are candidates for bone marrow transplantation.

ONYCHOTRICHODYSPLASIA AND NEUTROPENIA. This autosomal recessive syndrome is characterized by hypoplasia of the fingernails, sparse hair, and neutropenia. Most affected infants and children have moderate degrees of mental retardation. The patients suffer recurrent infections. Head hair is absent at birth, and eyelashes are hypoplastic, causing chronic conjunctivitis. Axillary and pubic hair are absent or sparse in the affected adolescent. Microscopically, hairs show trichorrhexis and, in contrast to other forms of ectodermal dysplasias, sulfur content of the hair is low. The neutropenia is persistent with intermittent episodes of very low ANCs noted during periods of clinical infection of the skin and mucous membranes.

NEUTROPENIA RELATED TO CANCER AND ACQUIRED IMMUNODEFICIENCY SYNDROME (AIDS). Neutropenia may be associated with a primary malignancy such as leukemia, lymphoma, or metastatic tumor from neuroblastoma. In such cases, a bone marrow biopsy will confirm the diagnosis. The peripheral blood may show an erythroblastic response with nucleated erythrocytes, tear drop red cells, and young myelocytes and metamelocytes. Severe neutropenia and its related infections, including both gram-positive and gram-negative bacteria, fungi, and DNA viruses and protozoa, remain a permanent threat for patients receiving intensive chemotherapy. Infants and children with HIV infection also experience neutropenia, either as a direct result of the infection or as a consequence of the antiviral therapy. Because of marked suppression of the immune system in these groups of patients, the risk of overwhelming infection is very high. Aggressive attempts to reduce the risks of neutropenic infection in febrile patients include initiation of broad-spectrum antibiotic and antifungal therapy parenterally immediately after blood and other body fluid cultures have been obtained. Administration of bone marrow growth factors (GM-CSF, G-CSF, IL-3) decrease the duration of chemotherapy-induced neutropenia and may reduce the risk of infection.

Bonilla MA, Gillio AP, Ruggeiro M, et al: Effects of recombinant human granulocyte colony-stimulating factor on neutropenia in patients with congenital agranulocytosis. N Engl J Med 320:1574, 1989.
Boxer LA, Greenberg MS, Boxer GJ, et al: Autoimmune neutropenia. N Engl J Med 293:748, 1975.
Boxer LA, Smolen JE: Neutrophile granule constituents and their release in health and disease. Hematol Oncol Clin North Am 2:101, 1988.
Cairo MS: Neutrophil transfusions in the treatment of neonatal sepsis. Review of G-CSF and GM-CSF effects on neonatal neutrophil kinetics. Am J Pediatr Hematol Oncol 11:227, 1989.
Christenson RD: Neutrophil kinetics in the fetus and neonate. Am J Pediatr Hematol Oncol 11:215, 1989.
Coates T, Baehner R: Leukocytosis and leukopenia. *In*: Benz EJ, Cohen HJ, Furie B, et al (eds): Hematology: Basic Principles and Practice. New York: Churchill Livingstone, 1990, pp 552–566.
Dale DC, Bonilla MA, Davis MW, et al: A randomized controlled phase III trial of recombinant human granulocyte colony stimulating factor (filgrastim) for treatment of severe chronic neutropenia. Blood 81:1496, 1993.
Dale DC, Hammond WP IV: Cyclic neutropenia: A clinical review. Blood Rev 2:178, 1988.
Hutchinson R, Boxer LA: Disorders of granulocyte and monocyte production. *In*: Benz EJ, Cohen HJ, Furie B, et al (eds): Hematology: Basic Principles and Practice. New York, Churchill Livingstone, 1990, pp 193–204.
Jonsson OG, Buchanan GR: Chronic neutropenia in a single institution. Am J Dis Child 145:232, 1991.
Metcalf D: Hematopoietic regulators: Redundancy or subtlety? Blood 82:3515, 1993.

CHAPTER 125
Adhesion Deficiency Disorders

Robert L. Baehner

This inherited syndrome comprises two types of disorders characterized by recurrent or progressive skin, mucous membrane, and subcutaneous infections with diminished pus formation and poor wound healing, including delayed separation of the umbilical cord. The phenotypic expression of type 1 leukocyte adhesion deficiency (LAD) is due to a genetic defect of a group of leukocyte membrane glycoproteins that confer adhesiveness on lymphocyte, monocyte, and neutrophil surfaces. The phenotypic expression of type 2 LAD is due to the absence of the carbohydrate structure sialyl-Lewis X on the cell surface of neutrophils, which serves as a ligand for endothelial cell selectins. Type 1 LAD has been described in over 50 patients, whereas type 2 LAD was first described in 1992 in two unrelated boys, each offspring of consanguineous parents.

ETIOLOGY. Type 1 LAD is defined by the defective expression of three α-β heterodimeric glycoprotein molecules unique to leukocytes called MAC-1, LFA-1, and p150,95. They share a common β subunit (95 kd, also designated CD18) but have distinctive α subunits of varying molecular weights and amino acid sequences, conferring different physicochemical properties and cell distribution. MO-1, or MAC-1 (CD11a), is a physiologically important complement receptor (CR3) that binds the iC3b component of activated complement to granulocytes and monocytes. Another site on MAC-1 is responsible for ensuring the adherence of cells to surfaces and also promotes motility, chemotaxis, and phagocytosis of complement-opsonized microbes. In contrast, LFA-1 (CD11b) is located on all lymphocytes but not on phagocytic cells, and the intercellular adhesion molecule ICAM-1 serves as one of its ligands in promoting cytotoxic T cell activity and other lymphocytic interactions with cells. The third molecule, p150,95 (CD11c), identified by monoclonal antibody LeuM5, is present on phagocytic cells and on cytotoxic and large granular lymphocytes, but its physiologic significance is unclear. The primary genetic lesion affects the common β subunit required for normal α-subunit assemblage of funtionally active α-β molecules. The amino acid sequences of leukocyte adhesion receptor subunits share close homology with other receptors for extracellular matrix proteins called integrins. These include fibronectin, vitronectin, and collagen, suggesting an evolution by gene duplication from single ancestral α and β subunit genes.

Type 2 LAD appears to be related to the lack of expression of sialyl-Lewis X, a carbohydrate ligand on neutrophil surfaces for E-selectin, which, in turn, is present on the surfaces of activated endothelial cells. The synthesis of sialyl-Lewis X requires a fucosyltransferase gene, which could be defective because the red cells in these patients are of the Bombay type, which is due to a deficiency of H antigen, another fucosylated carbohydrate. The blood types of the reported patients were Lewis negative and secretor negative.

EPIDEMIOLOGY. The disease has been observed in North America, Europe, North Africa, Iran, and Japan and is inherited in an autosomal recessive pattern. Family pedigrees from Hispanic, Tunisian, and English families have been described. There often is consanguinity within affected families, and asymptomatic carriers express approximately half the normal amounts of the common β subunit.

PATHOGENESIS. All signs and symptoms observed in affected patients can be related to the absence or diminished expression of adhesive glycoproteins or carbohydrate ligands on leukocyte surfaces. The recruitment of neutrophils to the site of inflammation appears to be initiated by factors that induce rolling of neutrophils on the blood vessel wall, followed by firm adhesion and extravasation into the surrounding infected or inflamed tissue. The initial rolling of neutrophils is mediated by members of the selectin family, including E- and P-selectin, which are expressed on the surface of activated endothelial cells and L-selectin, which is constitutively expressed on neutrophils. The carbohydrate ligands for E- and P-selectin are contained in the structure of sialyl-Lewis X. Thus, in type 2 LAD the affected neutrophil is impaired in its ability to roll, a prerequisite for the upregulated expression of the adhesion molecules LFA-1 and MAC-1, two members of the integrin family present on neutrophils that bind to intracellular adhesion molecule 1 (ICAM-1) on endothelial cells. LFA-1 and MAC-1 are not expressed in type 1 LAD. This interaction is essential to both firm adhesion to the blood vessel wall and to the subsequent chemotactic migration of the neutrophil to extravascular sites of infection and inflammation.

The contrasting clinical picture of high blood granulocyte counts in the presence of necrotic acellular skin and soft tissue ulcers suggests defective migration of inflammatory cells from blood vessels to extravascular sites. In vivo leukocyte migration as monitored by the serial application of glass coverslips to freshly abraded skin (Rebuck skin window test) shows marked impairment of granulocyte and monocyte invasion of tissue sites. However, after granulocyte transfusion of normal cells, the skin window inflammatory response is corrected. In in vitro studies patients' phagocytic cells fail to adhere to endothelial cell monolayers or to protein-coated glass or plastic, and chemotactic stimuli do not promote increases in cellular attachment to surfaces facilitating chemotaxis. Microbes and other particles opsonized with iC3b are not phagocytized. However, LAD phagocytes are capable of both triggering a normal oxidative response that leads to microbial killing and releasing their granule constituents in response to mediators that bypass or do not require MO-1 or CR3.

A variety of in vitro lymphocyte abnormalities dependent on normal LFA-1 expression have been observed in patients with LAD type 1. Cytotoxic T cells, natural killer cells, and antibody-dependent cytotoxic cells are defective. Although total levels of immunoglobulin are normal, the antibody response to protein antigens such as influenza virus is blunted, but the response to polysaccharide antigens is normal. The β subunit gene has been mapped to the distal long arm of chromosome 21 (21q22.3), and studies have suggested a defect in this gene, resulting in abnormal post-translational processing of the molecule.

CLINICAL MANIFESTATIONS. Disease severity correlates with the extent of deficient expression of the leukocyte adherence glycoproteins. The earliest signs occur in the neonatal period with delayed separation or infection of the umbilical cord. Surgical resection of an infected umbilicus has been needed in a few cases. Wound healing is markedly impaired. Skin and subcutaneous infections occur during early childhood. Small (<1 cm) indolent or necrotic abscesses or cellulitis may occur on any area of the body. Perirectal abscesses and lesions on the extremities leading to large ulcers with plaque formation or gangrenous bullous areas measuring between 1 and 10 cm become very difficult management problems. Puncture wounds or skin surface trauma often precipitates cellulitis and abscess formation. Surgical debridement and skin grafting may be required.

Infections of the ears, nose, and mouth are particularly prominent. Recurrent otitis media, pharyngitis, and ulcerative stomatitis are observed in almost all patients. Severe gingivitis often associated with eruption of deciduous teeth in the preschool-aged child usually progresses to generalized alveolar bone loss and severe periodontitis.

Systemic infection with life-threatening sepsis may follow episodes of perirectal abscess or other necrotizing infections of the mouth, pharynx, or intestinal tract. Recurrent bronchopneumonia as well as aseptic meningitis may occur. More than 75% of severely affected patients die before the age of 5 yr, whereas patients with a moderate phenotype are less prone to severe life-threatening infections, although more than half have died between the ages of 12 and 32 yr. Otitis, esophagitis, sinusitis, and pneumonia as well as local soft tissue infections recur in these patients. Biopsy of affected sites reveals a paucity of inflammatory cells and necrosis of tissue. This condition results from a failure of blood leukocytes, especially granulocytes and monocytes, to adhere to the vascular endothelium adjacent to the inflammatory site, inhibiting vascularization of infected tissues. As in agranulocytic patients, severe chronic gingivitis and periodontitis develop during the teenage years, leading to progressive loss of permanent dentition.

The two unrelated boys with type 2 LAD had recurrent episodes of bacterial infection, including pneumonia, periodontitis, otitis media, and localized cellulitis without the formation of pus. In addition, both were severely mentally retarded, short statured, and had distinctive facies. Both were the offspring of consanguineous parents suggestive of an autosomal recessive inheritance.

LABORATORY FINDINGS AND DIAGNOSIS. The laboratory hallmark of the disease is a persistent neutrophilia with white blood cells ranging between 15,000 and 160,000/μL, with 50–90% polymorphonuclear cells. Mild to moderate anemia parallels the extent and chronicity of the infection and inflammation. Inflammatory skin windows fail to show the expected progressive accumulation of inflammatory granulocytes and monocytes over a 24-hr period of study. In vitro studies of leukocyte functions show abnormal chemotaxis, decreased adherence to endothelial monolayers, and abnormal granulocyte aggregation but normal platelet aggregation and adherence, because platelet glycoproteins IIb/IIIa are expressed normally. Complement-coated particles (e.g., serum-treated zymosan or red cells) are not ingested, but oxidative responses (e.g., superoxide release/nitroblue tetrazolium [NBT] reduction) to the for-

■ **TABLE 125–1 Clinical and Laboratory Features of Phagocyte Disorders**

Disorder	Type of Infection	WBC (μL)	Chemotaxis	O_2^- Release	Bacterial Killing
LAD*	Necrotic ulcers, no pus Skin and mucous membranes Mouth affected, gingivitis severe	50,000–100,000 60–90% PMNs‖	Decreased	Decreased—complement opsonized particles Normal—soluble (PMA, fMLP)‡	Normal
Agranulocytosis	Same	<1,000 0–10% PMNs	Normal	Normal	Normal
CGD† Rare severe G-6-PD deficiency	Pustules and abscesses of soft tissue and deep viscera	10,000–20,000 60–80% PMNs	Normal	Decreased	Decreased
Neutrophil granule defects		2,000–15,000			
Myeloperoxidase deficiency	None to mild fungal infections	50–70% PMNs	Normal	Increased	Mildly decreased
Specific granule deficiency	Skin and lung abscesses		Decreased	Normal to increased	Decreased
Chédiak-Higashi syndrome	Skin and mucous membranes		Decreased	Increased	Moderately decreased
Agammaglobulinemia and related disorders	Septicemia, pneumonias	5,000–15,000 50–70% PMNs	Normal	Normal	Normal
Hyperimmunoglobulin E (Job syndrome)	Sinopulmonary Skin and subcutaneous "cold" abscesses Eczema Asthma and allergic rhinitis	5,000–15,000 20–30% eosinophils	Decreased (in some cases)	Normal	Normal

**LAD = leukocyte adhesion deficiency.*
†CGD = chronic granulomatous disease.
‡PMA = phorbal myristate acetate; fMLP = f-met-leu-phe.
‖PMNs = polymorphonuclear leukocytes.

myl-tripeptides, f-met-leu-phe, or phorbal myristate acetate (PMA) are normal. Monoclonal antibodies MO-1 or MAC-1 and LFA-1 to the leukocyte adherence glycoprotein can be employed in a flow cytometer to confirm the diagnosis by demonstrating the absence or reduction of binding of fluorescent-labeled monoclonal antibody to the leukocyte surface. LFA-1-deficient T lymphocytes have reasonably normal responses to normal concentrations of lectins (phytohemagglutinin) or antigens but impaired cytotoxicity as demonstrated by ^{51}Cr release from labeled target cells. Although no humoral deficiency has been described in most patients and serum immunoglobulin concentrations are normal to elevated, a deficiency in synthesis of specific antibody to polypeptide antigens (tetanus, influenza) but not to polysaccharide antigens (pneumococcus, *H. influenzae*) has been noted. Cultures of infected wounds and tissues yield a variety of gram-positive (*Staphylococcus aureus*) and gram-negative (*Escherichia coli, Pseudomonas* species, *Klebsiella*) bacteria or fungi (*Candida* species, *Aspergillus* species).

GENETICS. The common beta subunit of LFA-1, MAC-1, and p150,95, has been mapped to chromosome 21q22.3, and LAD 1 has been shown to be due to a variety of genetic defects of the beta subunit.

DIFFERENTIAL DIAGNOSIS. Patients with significant chronic and recurrent pyogenic and fungal infections usually have a disorder of phagocyte-antibody immunity. Severe forms of agranulocytosis (congenital neutropenia), deficiency of phagocyte NADPH oxidase (chronic granulomatous disease), neutrophil granule defects (specific, azurophilic, and Chédiak-Higashi syndrome [CHS]), agammaglobulinemia or other forms of hypo- and dysgammaglobulinemias, and Job syndrome must be considered. In general, patients with neutrophil disorders associated with chemotactic defects or in vivo inability to mount normal inflammatory responses have skin, soft tissue, mouth, and mucous membrane infections, whereas those with neutrophil bactericidal and fungicidal deficiencies experience abscess formation in subcutaneous sites, lymph nodes, lung, liver, and other abdominal viscera and bone (Table 125–1). Any patient with recurrent documented severe forms of mouth or gum infection, skin abscesses, perianal and perirectal abscesses, poor wound healing, sinopulmonary infections, or deep visceral abscesses must be considered to have a defect of phagocytic function.

The neutrophilia of LAD may be confused with (1) the reactive leukemoid reaction seen at times in collagen-vascular disorders, lung, or deep visceral abscesses, and (2) the chronic myeloproliferative disorders such as the adult form of chronic myelogenous leukemia. Patients with the latter condition usually have moderate to massive splenomegaly, an absence of leukocyte alkaline phosphatase demonstrable by special stain of a blood smear, and the presence of the Philadelphia t(9;22) chromosome. In contrast, leukemoid reactions have elevated leukocyte alkaline phosphatase scores and no leukocyte chromosomal abnormality. A source of infection or inflammation is usually demonstrable by radiologic and bacteriologic studies.

TREATMENT. Aggressive use of antibiotics for treatment of documented infections is indicated. Responses to therapy are much slower than normal. *Candida* and aspergillosis must be considered in any persistent infection not eradicated with antibiotics. Because wound healing is slow, careful attention must be paid to puncture or surgical wounds with proper local treatment and debridement. Selective use of normal granulocyte transfusions may help to eradicate acute infections but are not of value in the long-term management of these patients. Preventive dental hygiene, skin care, and attention to the perianal area often help to alleviate early signs of infection. Bone marrow transplantation has been successful in patients with severe phenotypic LAD. Eight patients have received transplants, five with HLA-identical marrow. LFA-1–deficient patients seem to be able to accept HLA-partially incompatible bone marrow in a manner similar to that seen in patients with severe combined immunodeficiency (SCID) who lack T cells. Transplant candidates should be infection free and in good nutritional condition, and the procedure should be done as soon as possible after diagnosis because the early mortality in severely affected children is high.

GENETIC COUNSELING. Prenatal diagnosis of LAD is possible by obtaining fetal blood samples around 20 wk of gestation. Fetal leukocytes express leukocyte adhesion molecules, although in diminished amounts. The total absence of these adherence glycoproteins indicates the severe phenotype.

Anderson DC: Neonatal neutrophil dysfunction. Am J Pediatr Hematol Oncol 11:224, 1989.

Anderson DC, Schmalsteig FC, Finegold MJ, et al: The severe and moderate phenotypes of heritable MAC-1, LFA-1 deficiency: Their quantitative definition and relation to leukocyte dysfunction and clinical features. J Infect Dis 152:668, 1985.

Etzioni A, Frydman M, Pollack S, et al: Recurrent severe infections caused by a novel leukocyte adhesion deficiency. N Engl J Med 327:1789, 1992.

CHAPTER 126

Neutrophil Granule Defects

Robert L. Baehner

Patients with abnormalities of the neutrophil granules either inherit or acquire them and may remain asymptomatic or experience increased susceptibility to infection. Neutrophils contain two distinct sets of granules. Peroxidase-positive azurophils and peroxidase-negative specific granules form during myeloid cell development in the bone marrow. Azurophilic granules form only during myeloblast and promyelocyte differentiation, whereas specific granules are produced during the later phases of myelocyte proliferation and maturation to the metamyelocyte and band stage. The constituents of the two sets of granules include unique bactericidal proteins, receptors, and enzymes (Table 126–1).

ETIOLOGY. Neutrophil granule defects can be separated into three phenotypic genetic disorders: (1) myeloperoxidase (MPO) deficiency of azurophilic granules, (2) specific granule deficiency (SGD), and (3) Chédiak-Higashi syndrome (CHS); see Chapter 127. Immunohistologic studies reveal the presence of a dysfunctional peroxidase protein in neutrophil and monocyte (but not eosinophil) azurophilic granules from patients

■ **TABLE 126–1 Contents of Neutrophil Granules**

Azurophil	Specific
Bactericidal	
Peroxidase	Lysozyme
Defensins	Lactoferrin
Lysozyme	Cytochrome b
Receptors	
None identified	CR3 (iC3b)
	f-met-leu-phe
	Laminin—adherence
Acid hydrolases and neutral proteinases	
Cathepsins	Collagenase
Elastase	Plasminogen activator
	Vitamin B_{12}–binding protein (transcobalamin I)

with MPO deficiency. The gene, located on chromosome 17q22–23, has been cloned and sequenced. The molecular basis for the defect appears to be a pretranslational defect characterized by diminished amounts of mRNA but no gross alterations of the MPO gene. Specific granules failed to form in developing bone marrow myeloid precursors in the five unrelated patients identified with SGD. On the other hand, azurophilic granules formed normally. The molecular basis for the defect is unknown.

Acquired defects of granules occur in patients with refractory anemia, preleukemia, acute leukemia, and the blastic phase of chronic myelogenous leukemia. MPO and lactoferrin, constituents of azurophilic and specific granules, respectively, are diminished in some patients with acute myeloblastic leukemia and other myelodysplastic syndromes and in newborn neutrophils. Alkaline phosphatase, which is deficient in the neutrophils of patients with SGD, is either absent or diminished in the neutrophils of patients with chronic myelogenous leukemia.

PATHOGENESIS. MPO is essential for the chlorination and iodination of microbes ingested by the neutrophil. Despite a lack of peroxidation in MPO-deficient neutrophils, affected persons are generally asymptomatic, although a few patients with diabetes have experienced recurrent candidal infections. Bactericidal activity is partially compromised during the early phases of in vitro killing, but over a period of several hours effective bacterial killing is accomplished, probably by nonoxidative mechanisms. Patients with neutrophil-specific granule deficiency experience chronic recurrent skin ulcers and abscesses and lung infections, supporting the notion that the specific granule pool is probably more important for normal host defense than the azurophilic granule pool. Defensins, potent bactericidal proteins normally found in azurophilic granules, are almost completely deficient in the neutrophils of patients with SGD. Other azurophilic granule constituents, for example, cathepsin G and elastase, are normal. Conversely, neutrophils of CHS patients lack the latter two cytotoxic proteins but have a normal amount of defensins. These patients also experience recurrent infections due to functional defects of their morphologically abnormal phagocytic blood cells as well as to deficiencies of cytotoxic granule proteins (Chapter 127).

CLINICAL MANIFESTATIONS. Hereditary MPO Deficiency. The overwhelming majority of affected persons have no obvious clinical sequelae from the deficiency. An incidence of 1 in 2,000 was found among asymptomatic persons in the United States, and a similar incidence was recorded in Western Europe. Most patients who experience severe candidiasis also have had diabetes mellitus or other compromises in host defense. Chronic mucocutaneous candidiasis is associated with neutrophils that have a normal MPO content and normal candidacidal activity.

Congenital Specific Granule Deficiency. This rare disorder is described in only five unrelated patients. A history of consanguinity was found in one patient. Clinically, all patients have recurrent infections of the skin and lung, frequently complicated by large indolent skin ulcers and repeated episodes of bronchopneumonia or lung abscesses. Also, lymphadenitis, otitis, and mastoiditis occur. The onset of infections usually occurs within the first few years of life. Both males and females have been affected, suggesting an autosomal recessive mode of inheritance. *Staphylococcus aureus* is the most frequently cultured bacterial species, but a variety of gram-negative microbes as well as *Candida albicans* have been isolated from the lesions. With careful management, these patients may survive into young adulthood.

LABORATORY FINDINGS AND DIAGNOSIS. Routine complete blood count may fail to suggest a neutrophil granule defect unless particular attention is paid to the Wright stained differential. SGD is characterized by bilobed nuclei in more than 80% of the neutrophils, resembling the Pelger-Huet anomaly. The latter defect is not associated with clinical symptoms or significant functional phagocytic defects. Moreover, in SGD there is a striking decrease in cytoplasmic granularity owing to a lack of specific granules. Leukocyte alkaline phosphatase and peroxidase cytochemical stains confirm the absence of alkaline phosphatase and the presence of azurophilic granule peroxidase. Lactoferrin, another constituent of specific granules, is also absent when appropriate immunocytochemistry is employed. On the other hand, patients with hereditary or acquired myeloperoxidase deficiency have either a total or partial deficiency of peroxidase activity, but alkaline phosphatase stains are normal. Occasionally, patients with CHS are discovered because giant granules are noted on routine Wright stained differential counts. The granules are larger and less symmetric than the prominently stained toxic granules or Döhle bodies noted frequently in neutrophils of patients with infection. They result from the progressive coalescence of azurophilic and specific granules formed during myelopoiesis. Moderate neutropenia due to intramedullary destruction of myeloid cells is often noted early in the course of the disease and may contribute to the increased susceptibility to infection.

Phagocytic function is abnormal in all three granule disorders (see Table 125–1). MPO-deficient PMNs show only minor defects in the killing of *S. aureus,* whereas killing of *C. albicans* is much more impaired. The abnormal neutrophil chemotactic response of SGD is associated with impaired upregulation of receptors for the chemoattractant f-met-leu-phe and the adherence receptor iC3b. The absence of the specific granule component cytochrome b may explain the impaired superoxide (O_2^-) release and contribute, along with lack of defensins and lactoferrin, to the impairment in bactericidal killing.

DIFFERENTIAL DIAGNOSIS. The same disorders mentioned in Chapter 125 for any patient with significant chronic and recurrent pyogenic and fungal infections must be considered.

TREATMENT. No therapy is generally required for patients with MPO deficiency. Treatment of patients with SGD is similar to that given to other patients with a functional phagocytic defect (see Chapter 125). With proper use of intravenous antibiotics and drainage of abscesses, these patients may live into adulthood.

GENETIC COUNSELING. Neutrophil granule defects include conditions of clinical diversity ranging from the asymptomatic MPO deficiency to the fatal accelerated phase of CHS. Counseling requires a knowledge of the varied clinical courses of these diseases, all inherited as autosomal recessive traits.

Gallin JI: Neutrophil specific granule deficiency. Annu Rev Med 36:263, 1985.
Ganz T, Metcalf JA, Gallin JI, et al: Microbicidal cytotoxic proteins of neutrophils are deficient in two disorders: Chédiak-Higashi syndrome and "specific" granule deficiency. J Clin Invest 82:552, 1988.
Nauseef WM: Myeloperoxidase deficiency. Hematol Oncol Clin North Am 2:135, 1988.

CHAPTER 127

Chédiak-Higashi Syndrome

Robert L. Baehner

This rare autosomal recessive disorder was initially recognized as one in which leukocytes contained giant cytoplasmic granules (see Chapter 126). It is now recognized as a generalized cellular disease affecting all granule-bearing cells.

ETIOLOGY. The basic abnormalities underlying neutrophil function in the Chédiak-Higashi syndrome are unknown, but altered membrane fusion is probably important. One unifying hypothesis for the functional aberrations of this disorder is that abnormal membrane fluidity leads to uncontrolled granule fusion and to other defects, including the inability of the neutrophils to move normally and to concentrate serotonin into platelets and hydrolytic enzymes into neutrophil lysosomes.

PATHOPHYSIOLOGY. Melanocytes contain giant melanosomes, leading to a failure to dispense pigment. The patients therefore display a partial albinism involving the hair and skin. Schwann cells also contain giant granules, presumably contributing to striking central and peripheral neuropathies that affect many of these patients in later years. Other features of the disease include the presence of giant azurophils and specific granules in circulating neutrophils. These giant granules form in the cytoplasm during myelopoiesis of myeloid precursors, but most of the myeloid precursors die within the bone marrow, producing moderate neutropenia. An increased susceptibility to infection can be explained in part by the neutropenia and in part by defective chemotaxis, degranulation, and bactericidal activity of the remaining neutrophils. The infections usually encountered in those with Chédiak-Higashi syndrome involve the skin, respiratory tract, and mucous membranes and are caused by gram-positive and gram-negative bacteria. Lymphocytes contain giant cytoplasmic granules and function poorly in antibody dependent–cell-mediated cytolysis of tumor cells. Natural killer cell function is also compromised, which may be related to the deranged secretion of the abnormal granules found in these cells, and may explain why some patients develop malignancies.

Patients with Chédiak-Higashi syndrome (CHS) have a prolonged bleeding time in spite of a normal platelet count because of impaired platelet aggregation and associated with a deficiency of granules containing adenosine diphosphate and serotonin. There is also a peculiar propensity for lymphohistiocytic proliferation (known as the *accelerated phase*) to occur in the reticuloendothelial system, which intensifies the already existing neutropenia and leads to pancytopenia. This proliferation is associated with recurrent bacterial and viral infections, fever, and prostation. It usually results in death. The onset of the accelerated phase may relate to the inability of these patients to contain and control Epstein-Barr virus and produces features simulating those of the viral-mediated hemophagocytic syndrome.

CLINICAL MANIFESTATIONS. Patients with this syndrome experience an onset of symptoms in early childhood. Presenting manifestations include photophobia, rotary nystagmus, increased red reflex, partial albinism compared with other family members, recurrent gingivitis, and periodontitis. Hair color varies from blond to dark brown but has a silvery tint that is especially noticeable in bright light. Infections involve the skin, mucous membranes, and respiratory tract and are recurrent. Gram-positive and gram-negative bacteria may be cultured from sites of infection, *Staphylococcus aureus* and β-hemolytic streptococci being the most frequent causes of infection. Affected patients also have prolonged bleeding times with normal platelet counts due to a platelet aggregation defect that is related to storage pool deficiency of ADP and serotonin. If patients survive into adulthood, they develop motor and sensory neurologic defects including cranial and peripheral neuropathy. Ataxia, muscular weakness, decreased motor neuron conduction, diffuse abnormalities in electroencephalograms, and seizures may also occur. Affected patients may die at any age owing to the so-called accelerated phase of the illness, which occurs in 85% of patients. The precipitating event initiating this lethal stage may be related to infection with Epstein-Barr virus or other lymphotrophic viruses, resulting in a lymphoma-like picture with fever, widespread enlargement of lymph nodes, hepatosplenomegaly, and pancytopenia. Sepsis is frequent at this stage of the illness, as is massive bleeding in the brain or gastrointestinal tract. Neutropenia, the result of macrophage sequestration in the bone marrow, liver, and spleen, also may herald the onset of the accelerated phase.

LABORATORY FINDINGS AND DIAGNOSIS. CHS patients have abnormal chemotaxis, and killing is reduced because of delayed fusion of the abnormal granules with phagosomes containing ingested microbes. iC3b receptor expression is markedly reduced, a fact that probably plays an additional role in reduced motility, chemotaxis, and bactericidal activity. The cells have an increased release of superoxide (O_2^-) similar to that seen in myeloperoxidase-deficient neutrophils. In addition, CHS patients have platelet aggregation defects owing to a lack of a storage pool of ADP and a prolonged bleeding time. Lymphocytes contain giant granules and function poorly in tests of antibody-dependent tumor cell lysis and natural killer cell activity. Identification of large lysosomal granules in leukocytes and giant melanosomes in melanocytes and hair roots may confirm the diagnosis.

The accelerated phase of CHS is associated with seroconversion and an abnormal antibody response to *Epstein-Barr virus*. Antibodies to viral capsid antigen and the early antigen reach high levels and persist, supporting the notion of a sustained viral infection.

TREATMENT. Therapy for the stable phase of CHS involves the proper management of infections. Ascorbic acid has improved the clinical status and phagocytic function of some patients. Although antibiotics are valuable during acute infections, their prophylactic use has not been proved effective in patients with CHS. Corticosteroids, vincristine, and cyclophosphamide have been employed for control of the accelerated phase and have partially arrested the infiltrative process but have not been effective in arresting the progression of disease. However, acyclovir 500 mg/m^2 three times daily combined with prednisone 2 mg/kg/24 hr has provided temporary improvement in fever, pancytopenia, and coagulopathy in patients with this fatal disorder. Bone marrow transplantation has been successful in five patients who received HLA-compatible marrow early in their illness before the full-blown accelerated phase occurred. Mismatched transplants have not been successful.

CHAPTER 128
Disorders of Cell Motility and Chemotaxis

Robert L. Baehner

The migration of neutrophils from the circulation to inflammatory sites leads to the accumulation of an exudate responsible for the clinical signs of inflammation and infection. The attraction of cells to chemical substances is known as chemotaxis. For normal chemotaxis to occur, a complex series of events must be carefully coordinated. Chemotactic factors must be generated in sufficient quantities to establish a long-range chemotactic gradient. The neutrophils, in turn, must have receptors for the various chemotactic agents and mechanisms for discerning the direction of the chemotactic gradient. The contractile apparatus, consisting of actin and other actin-associated proteins, enables the cell to deform and crawl from the microvasculature to the site of infection. Because of the complexity of the chemotactic response, it is not surprising that depressed neutrophil chemotaxis is observed in a large

TABLE 128–1 Disorders of Neutrophil Chemotaxis

Defects in the generation of chemotactic factors
Familial deficiency of C1r, C2, C4 (classic complement components)
Familial deficiency of C3, C5, properdin
Acquired C3 deficiency (systemic lupus erythematosus, chronic hemolytic anemia, glomerulonephritis, immunoglobulin deficiency)
Enhanced generation of normal chemotactic inactivators
Hodgkin disease
Sarcoidosis
Malignancy
Lepromatous leprosy
Cirrhosis
Direct inhibitors of the neutrophil itself
Immune complex disease (rheumatoid arthritis)
Bone marrow transplantation
C5a generation in plasma (sepsis, hemodialysis, thermal injury)
Wiskott-Aldrich syndrome
Drugs (corticosteroids, tetracycline, amphotericin B, ethanol, antithymocyte globulin)
Juvenile periodontitis *(Capnocytophaga)*
Hyperimmunoglobulin IgE syndrome
IgA myeloma
Intrinsic defects of neutrophils
Neonatal neutrophils
Leukocyte adhesion defect
Neutrophil-actin dysfunction
Chédiak-Higashi syndrome
Specific granule deficiency
Hypophosphatemia
Shwachman syndrome
Glycogenosis, type 1b
Kartagener syndrome
Hyperimmunoglobulin E
Chromosome 7 abnormalities
Zinc deficiency (acrodermatitis enteropathica)
Alcoholism
Increased microtubule assembly

number of clinical conditions. These disorders are classified according to the presumed derangement of chemotaxis (Table 128–1). However, the chemotactic defects encountered in many of these disorders contribute little to the decreased resistance to bacterial infections.

Patients with chemotactic disorders may be infected by various microorganisms, including gram-positive and gram-negative bacteria and fungi. *Staphylococcus aureus* is the most common bacteria involved. Typically, the skin, gingiva, mucosa, and regional lymph nodes are involved. Respiratory tract infections are frequent, but sepsis is uncommon. Although the cells move slowly in chemotactic chambers, they do accumulate in sufficient numbers to produce pus at inflammatory sites. It is not uncommon to see delayed signs and symptoms of infections, because phagocyte arrival is often delayed. Infections should be appropriately treated.

CHAPTER 129

Chronic Granulomatous Disease

Robert L. Baehner

Chronic granulomatous disease (CGD) is the most common of the inherited disorders of phagocyte function.

ETIOLOGY. The pivotal role of the respiratory burst (which follows within seconds after phagocytes are activated) in the subsequent effective killing of catalase-positive microbes became evident from studies of patients with CGD. The NADPH oxidase that catalyzes the respiratory burst is found exclusively in phagocytes and remains dormant unless activated by a variety of particulate and soluble stimuli, such as opsonized microbes and chemotactic peptides. These stimuli excite a transmembrane electron transport system in which NADPH on the cytoplasmic side of the membrane reduces oxygen through a series of reactions involving flavin adenine dinucleotide (FAD), several soluble cofactors, and membrane-associated cytochrome b. Oxygen is reduced through a univalent reduction to superoxide anion and is rapidly mutated to hydrogen peroxide and hydroxyl radicals. The latter two products are thought to be the principal means by which microbial killing or tissue damage takes place. The components of the phagocyte NADPH oxidase complex are presented in Figure 129–1. The membrane components, a hemoprotein heterodimer with subunits of 91 kD and 22 kD, require at least two cytosolic protein components of 47 kD and 67 kD to achieve maximal oxidase activity. The X-linked and autosomally inherited forms of the disease are associated with missing components or subunits (Table 129–1). The CGD gene is located on the X chromosome proximal to the muscular dystrophy gene and distal to the ornithine transcarbamylase gene on the Xp21 band. The protein encoded by the X-CGD gene is synonymous with the 91-kD subunit of the cytochrome b complex. A reservoir of cytochrome b (~80–90%) is found in neutrophil-specific granules and is translocated to the membrane on activation of the cell. The 22-kD membrane subunit also has been cloned.

PATHOLOGY. Characteristic granulomas, along with phagocytes, giant cells, and occasional pigmented lipid-laden histiocytes, may develop in any organ system. The lung, skin, lymph nodes, liver, spleen, and bone may be affected with abscesses or granulomas. It is likely that the fundamental defect of oxidase activation of phagocytes results in a chronic and persistent inflammatory reaction within tissues owing to seeding with viable microbes.

CLINICAL MANIFESTATIONS. Most patients develop signs and symptoms of chronic and recurrent pyogenic infections during the first 2 yr of life. Milder forms of the disease have been

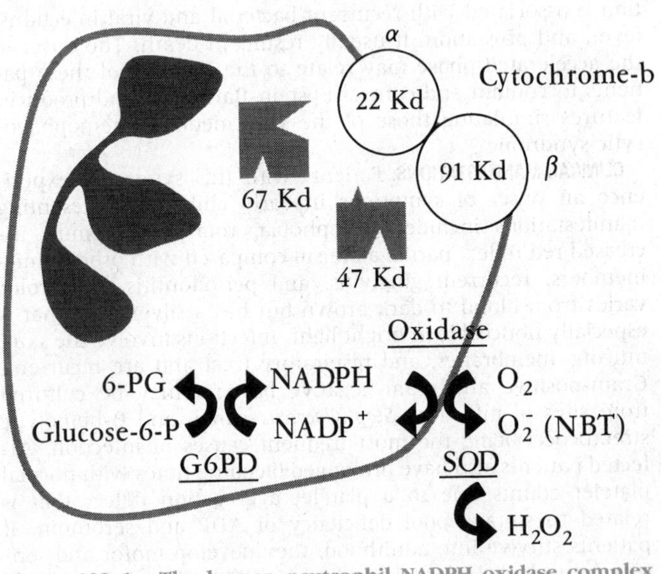

Figure 129–1. The human neutrophil NADPH oxidase complex consists of two cytochrome b membrane subunits, an α (22 kD) subunit and β (91 kD) subunit, and two cytosolic cofactors (67 kD) and (47 kD), required for the respiratory burst. A soluble ras family protein rac-2 (not shown) is also required. NADPH serves as substrate for reduction of oxygen to superoxide O_2, which, in turn, is rapidly dismutated either spontaneously or by superoxide dismutase (SOD) to hydrogen peroxide (H_2O_2). Superoxide is measured by the reduction of nitroblue tetrazolium (NBT). NADPH is generated from glucose-6-phosphate through the hexose monophosphate shunt by glucose-6-phosphate dehydrogenase (G-6-PD).

■ TABLE 129–1 Classification and Incidence of CGD Based on Molecular Defects of Neutrophil

Genetics	Incidence %	Cytochrome b	Defect
X–linked	50–55	Absent	Expression of cytochrome b 91 kD subunit
	5	Present	Function of cytochrome b
Autosomal	30–35	Present	47 kD cytosolic factor absent
	5	Present	67 kD cytosolic factor absent
	5	Absent	?Expression of cytochrome b 22 kD subunit

described with onset occurring in the teenage years or even in adulthood. Lymphadenopathy occurs in almost all cases. A common presentation is recurrent enlargement of the lymph nodes of the neck, which require incision and drainage. Hepatomegaly and splenomegaly occur later and often signify hepatic or perihepatic abscesses or granuloma formation. Chronic or recurrent pneumonia with unusual microbes, for example, *Serratia marcescens,* occurs frequently. Subcutaneous abscesses, recurrent skin furunculosis, eczematoid dermatitis, and impetigo around orifices may be presenting manifestations involving the integumentary system. Granuloma formation may lead to obstruction of the esophageal outlet, pyloris, or urethra. A history of persistent diarrhea may indicate granulomatous colitis. Perianal abscesses or rectal fistulous tracts may occur. Osteomyelitis at multiple sites or in the small bones of the hands and feet are also frequently encountered. Mucous membrane infections are less common than in patients with chemotactic disorders, but conjunctivitis, rhinitis, and stomatitis have occurred in these patients.

LABORATORY FINDINGS AND DIAGNOSIS. The neutrophils of patients with CGD demonstrate normal chemotaxis, phagocytosis, and degranulation, but they do not generate superoxide anion, nor do they kill catalase-positive microbes. Cultures from infected sites will isolate *Staphylococcus aureus, Klebsiella, Aerobacter, Escherichia coli, Shigella, Salmonella, Pseudomonas, Serratia marcescens, Candida albicans,* and *Aspergillus* and other fungi. Common catalase-negative peroxide-producing organisms such as *Streptococcus,* and *Haemophilus influenzae* are not isolated because the fundamental bactericidal defect in CGD is an absence of hydrogen peroxide and related reduced oxygen by-products in the phagocytic vesicle. Bactericidal assays in vitro confirm the selective but significant defect in bacterial killing. The reduction of nitroblue tetrazolium (NBT) remains a convenient method of screening for adequate superoxide anion ($O_2^{\dot{}}$) during phagocytic activation and of detecting CGD. Quantitation of rates of superoxide generation is best carried out by using the ferricytochrome reduction method. Although most patients with CGD fail to generate superoxide, mutations of both X-linked and autosomal forms result in milder forms of the disease in which some superoxide or NBT is formed under appropriate conditions of activation of the cells.

In carriers of the X-linked form of the disease approximately half of the neutrophils are affected, whereas the other half can reduce NBT normally. This is consistent with the Lyon hypothesis. Most female carriers are healthy and do not suffer recurrent infections. A few have had lupus-like skin lesions with photosensitivity, pleuritis, and stomatitis. The parents of children with autosomal recessive forms of CGD have normal results on NBT tests.

CBC shows appropriate neutrophilic leukocytosis during infections. Anemia of chronic infection correlates with the extent of inflammation. Sedimentation rates are usually elevated. Immunoglobulins are normal to increased. Abnormal chest roentgenograms occur in 90% of patients. Liver-spleen scans and bone scans are helpful in documenting the presence of liver abscesses and osteomyelitis, respectively. Ultrasound, endoscopy, and contrast studies usually verify suspected gastric antral obstructions. Cystourethrograms reveal granulomatous involvement of the bladder in some cases.

DIFFERENTIAL DIAGNOSIS. Because of the potential for widespread sites of infection in CGD, this entity must be considered in any child with unexplained recurrent cervical lymphadenitis, bacterial hepatic abscesses, or osteomyelitis as the basis for the primary infection. Lung abscesses or granulomas may at times be confused with tuberculosis or other fungal diseases such as histoplasmosis and coccidioidomycosis. All of the disorders discussed under Differential Diagnosis in Chapter 125 should also be considered. Investigations of the phagocytic functions of chemotaxis, superoxide anion release (NBT test), bacterial killing, quantitative serum immunoglobulins, and complement levels should permit differentiation of this group of disorders.

TREATMENT. Although its results are still not proved, long-term trimethoprim-sulfamethoxasole (TMP-SMZ) prophylaxis appears to increase the duration of infection-free periods. One small series showed significant benefits in reducing clinical manifestations and decreasing the number of isolates causing infection when TMP-SMZ was instituted during early childhood before chronic foci of infection had developed fully. Acute episodes of infection should be managed aggressively by isolating the causative microbe, instituting appropriate intravenous antibiotics, and using short-term (average 1 wk) granulocyte transfusions selectively to achieve control of persistent infections, especially those with gram-negative bacteria. Gastric outlet obstruction and granulomatous cystitis have been successfully managed with prolonged antimicrobial therapy and prednisone.

Based on in vitro studies, which showed the ability of γ-interferon to increase the generation of superoxide anion modestly (between 1 and 10%) in the neutrophils of patients with milder CGD, in vivo treatment of these same patients with γ-interferon was associated with similar improvement in superoxide anion release by neutrophils isolated during treatment. Improved in vivo responses also were observed in a few patients with negative in vitro responses. A large multicenter study showed that γ-interferon administered subcutaneously in a dose of 0.05 mg/m^2 3 times per wk reduced the number of new infections and improved the response to existing infections.

Serious transfusion reactions have occurred in patients with CGD who lack Kell-associated red blood cell antigens, the so-called McLeod phenotype. Prior to transfusion, patients with CGD should be tested for the presence of the Kell antigen.

Bone marrow transplantation has been carried out in several patients with limited success. Graft rejection and partial engraftment have occurred. Attempts to provide somatic gene therapy employing gene transfer of the X-CGD cDNA are in progress.

GENETIC COUNSELING. Cord blood and placental blood obtained by fetoscopy have established the diagnosis of CGD using the NBT slide test. Several molecular DNA probes that are capable of detecting a relatively high proportion of polymorphisms in genomic DNA and are closely linked to the X-CGD gene may be useful in identifying an at-risk male fetus using chorionic villus biopsy. Linkage analysis requires DNA samples from three generations and restriction fragment length polymorphism of maternal DNA and maternal parent DNA. In addition, the carrier status must be identified either by NBT testing or by obtaining a history of affected offspring. Probes recognizing

DNA polymorphisms in the X-CGD gene offer the most promise for improving the results of prenatal diagnosis.

Brown CC, Gallin JI: Chemotactic disorders. Hematol Oncol Clin North Am 2:61, 1988.
Forrest CB, Forehand JR, Axtell RA, et al: Clinical features and current management of chronic granulomatous disease. Hematol Oncol Clin North Am 2:253, 1988.
Hill HR: Biochemical, structural, and functional abnormalities of polymorphonuclear leukocyte in the neonate. Pediatr Res 22:375, 1987.
Orkin SH: Molecular genetics in chronic granulomatous disease. Ann Rev Immunol 7:277, 1989.
Smith RN, Curnutte JT: Molecular basis of chronic granulomatous disease. Blood 77:673, 1991.
The International Chronic Granulomatous Disease Cooperative Study Group: A controlled trial of interferon gamma granulomatous disease. N Engl J Med 324:509, 1991.

CHAPTER 130

Disorders of Neutrophil Oxidative Metabolism and Other Functions

Robert L. Baehner

SEVERE GLUCOSE-6-PHOSPHATE DEHYDROGENASE DEFICIENCY (G-6-PD). Several patients with Caucasian forms of red blood cell G-6-PD deficiency have had neutrophils with less than 5% G-6-PD activity. When activity is approximately 1%, NADPH, the substrate for the oxidase reaction, becomes rate limiting, leading to a clinical phenotype resembling CGD (see Fig. 129–1). Superoxide anion is not generated during neutrophil activation, resulting in a failure of these phagocytes to reduce nitroblue tetrazolium (NBT). G-6-PD activity of 5% results in abnormal results of in vitro tests of NBT and bacterial killing but does not usually cause clinical disease. American blacks with red blood cell G-6-PD deficiency have normal levels of the enzyme in their neutrophils.

GLUTATHIONE REDUCTASE DEFICIENCY. This flavin enzyme catalyzes the reaction of NADPH and oxidized glutathione (GSSG), and deficiencies result in hemolytic anemia. Although these children do not have infections, the respiratory burst in their neutrophils may be abbreviated when activated.

GLUTATHIONE SYNTHETASE DEFICIENCY. The synthesis of glutathione, a potent antioxidant found in high concentrations in most body cells including leukocytes, occurs in two steps: (1) glutamine and cysteine, by the action of γ-glutamyl cysteine synthetase, form glutamyl-cysteine, and (2) glycine is added by the action of glutathione synthetase to form glutathione. Absence of the latter enzyme resulted in hemolytic anemia, recurrent otitis, and an in vitro abnormality in bacterial killing in a child with this very rare defect.

HYPERIMMUNOGLOBULIN E (JOB SYNDROME). This rare disorder is characterized by extremely high serum IgE levels and recurrent serious infections of the skin and sinopulmonary tract and chronic eczema with onset in the first 8 wk of life (see also Chapter 119.13). The infections result in deep-seated abscesses in subcutaneous tissue. Pneumonia, osteomyelitis, arthritis, and visceral abscesses may occur. Associated clinical features include allergic rhinitis, coarse facies, keratoconjunctivitis, asthma, and stunted growth. The most common organisms recovered from the abscesses are *Staphylococcus aureus* and *Candida albicans*, but *Haemophilus influenzae, Streptococcus pneumoniae*, enteric gram-negative bacteria, and herpesvirus also cause infection. Laboratory studies reveal marked eosinophilia, extreme elevation of serum IgE with specificity against *S. aureus* and *C. albicans* and immune complexes containing IgE, variable chemotactic defects of neutrophils and monocytes, and absent delayed hypersensitivity on skin tests to recall antigens in vivo coupled with absent in vitro lymphocyte proliferation in response to the same antigens.

The chemotactic defect may be due to secretion of chemotactic inhibitor substances from mononuclear cells. Recurrent infection may be due to excessive amounts of nonprotective IgE directed against *S. aureus* and other infectious organisms with a concurrent inadequate synthesis of protective IgG antibody against the same organisms.

Treatment should be aggressive. Intravenous gamma globulin prophylaxis may be helpful. Abscesses should be drained surgically, and intravenous antibiotics or antifungal or antiviral agents employed based on results of cultures.

NEWBORN DYSFUNCTION OF NEUTROPHILS. Several clinical observations can be correlated with selective areas of dysfunction of newborn neutrophils: (1) the high incidence of sepsis and meningitis, particularly the poor outcome associated with severe neutropenia and depletion of marrow reserves of neutrophils; (2) the paucity of neutrophils in the alveoli of newborns dying of pneumonia; and (3) the common occurrence of skin infections with *S. aureus* and *C. albicans* in neonatal intensive care units. One of the most consistent abnormalities observed is decreased leukocyte migration, as measured by the Rebuck skin window and response to chemotactic stimuli. Motile responses of phagocytic cells depend in part on the deformability of the cell membrane and the ability of the cell to increase its adherence to endothelial cells and other surfaces in response to chemotactic signals. These are defective in newborns. The impaired movement of lectin receptors or adhesion sites on newborn neutrophil surface membranes and the impaired translocation of C3 receptors from specific granules to surface membranes probably contribute to the newborn neutrophil chemotactic defect. Bactericidal activity in neutrophils from stressed newborns is also diminished, even though the respiratory burst and the ability of those cells to generate superoxide and hydrogen peroxide is preserved. The diminished content of azurophilic myeloperoxidase and specific granule contents such as lactoferrin may contribute to the dysfunction.

The administration of adult donor neutrophil transfusions for treatment of neonatal sepsis is still controversial (see Chapter 98.1). Promising future therapies for the newborn may be forthcoming from the recent observations that recombinant human granulocyte-macrophage–colony-stimulating factor and granulocyte–colony-stimulating factor stimulate neutrophil/monocyte and neutrophil marrow production, respectively; facilitate release of neutrophils from the marrow; prime the chemotactic (C3) receptor expression of the respiratory burst; and stimulate phagocytic responses in adult cells.

CHAPTER 131
Inherited Leukocyte Abnormalities

Robert L. Baehner

Of the neutrophils in the blood of normal persons, 90% have two to four segments. Only about 5% are unsegmented (bands), and fewer than 5% have five or more segments. An increase in unsegmented forms, or a shift to the left, usually indicates infection or inflammation, whereas hypersegmented forms or a shift to the right usually occurs in megaloblastic anemias secondary to folic acid or vitamin B_{12} deficiency.

HEREDITARY HYPERSEGMENTATION OF NEUTROPHILS AND HEREDITARY GIANT NEUTROPHIL LEUKOCYTE. Neutrophil hypersegmentation is inherited as an autosomal dominant trait; no other associated clinical abnormalities have been described. Homozygotes with this condition have a mean nuclear index exceeding four lobes/cell, as opposed to a normal number of slightly less than three.

Giant neutrophils may be inherited as an autosomal dominant trait with no other disorders associated. Giant neutrophils have a volume twice that of normal neutrophils. These cells are also hypersegmented, with six to ten lobes/neutrophil.

HEREDITARY HYPOSEGMENTATION (PELGER-HUËT ANOMALY). This anomaly is characterized by a failure in the normal lobe development of granulocytic cells. Typically, these mature neutrophils have one or two lobes/nucleus and take on a round, dumbbell, or peanut shape. The disorder is inherited as an autosomal dominant trait, is usually not associated with any other congenital abnormality, and does not appear to affect neutrophil function. Patients with specific granule deficiency also demonstrate the Pelger-Huët anomaly, and this disorder is associated with impaired neutrophil function and clinical infections.

ALDER-REILLY ANOMALY. In this condition, which is probably transmitted as an autosomal recessive trait, neutrophil granulations are larger and stain more prominently than normal ones. The granules are distinctly lavender or blue, and are thus easily differentiated from eosinophils. A small proportion of patients with mucopolysaccharidosis may show similar granulations in their neutrophils, although more commonly they have metachromatic granules in their lymphocyte cytoplasm.

MAY-HEGGLIN ANOMALY. This rare, dominantly transmitted anomaly involves neutrophils and platelets. Most of the neutrophils contain irregular blue cytoplasmic inclusions similar to Döhle bodies, which consist of precipitated messenger RNA. Almost all the individuals known to have this disorder have been in good health despite mild leukopenia, thrombocytopenia, and bizarre giant platelets.

CHAPTER 132
Bone Marrow Transplantation

Kent A. Robertson

Bone marrow transplantation (BMT) involves treatment with marrow-ablative chemoradiotherapy followed by an infusion of either the patient's own marrow (autologous BMT) or marrow from a donor (allogeneic BMT) or some other source of marrow stem cells (cord blood, peripheral blood stem cells, fetal liver). BMT is the treatment of choice for some malignant diseases, such as chronic myelogenous leukemia, and for acquired and inherited nonmalignant disorders, such as aplastic anemia and Fanconi's anemia, as well as malignancies that are unresponsive to conventional therapy. The process of stem cell transplantation also encompasses replacing an absent or defective gene with a normal gene in the patient's own cells (gene therapy). Although the use of BMT for malignancies is much more common, relapsed disease continues to be a problem. Because only 25% of patients have human leukocyte antigen (HLA)-matched sibling donors, the use of mismatched related and matched unrelated donors provides an alternate source of marrow, but at the cost of increased graft rejection and graft-versus-host disease (GVHD). As the use of BMT becomes more widespread, the pediatrician will be called upon to take an important role in the evaluation and consideration of patients for possible transplant and the long-term follow-up of BMT patients.

132.1 Clinical Indications

ACQUIRED DISEASES

APLASTIC ANEMIA. Aplastic anemia is a disorder of unknown etiology that results in pancytopenia and bone marrow hypoplasia, and if severe (platelet <20,000; absolute neutrophil count <500; or reticulocyte count <1% when anemic) often results in death within the first 6 mo due to infection or bleeding (Chapter 406). Transfusion should be avoided if at all possible, as sensitization to blood products drastically increases the likelihood of graft rejection should BMT be needed. BMT is the treatment of choice for patients with severe aplastic anemia who have an HLA-matched family donor. The survival rate at 2 yr is 69%, based on data from the International Bone Marrow Transplant Registry. The 10 yr survival rate was 94% among children receiving HLA-matched sibling transplants for aplastic anemia in Seattle. Patients transplanted for aplastic anemia exhibit a higher incidence of graft rejection than other kinds of HLA-matched sibling transplants, but the addition of anti-thymocyte globulin (ATG) to cyclophosphamide for the preparative regimen decreases rejection significantly. Transplants using family donors who are more disparate or the use of matched unrelated donors usually requires more immunosuppressive therapy with the addition of radiation and or chemotherapy, which increases the incidence of secondary cancers from 3.8% to 22% (Fig. 132–1).

ACUTE MYELOGENOUS LEUKEMIA. Acute myelogenous leukemia (AML) is a heterogeneous group of leukemias derived from myeloid progenitor cells (Chapter 449.2). BMT is the accepted therapy for AML in first remission. Disease-free survival rates range from 55% to 83% for matched sibling marrow transplants done in first complete remission (Fig. 132–2).

BMT improves survival of children with acute megakaryocytic (M7) leukemia, an uncommon variant of AML that responds poorly to chemotherapy. BMT is indicated for AML patients who do not enter remission, using marrow from an HLA-identical family donor, mismatched family donors, or matched unrelated donors. In patients who achieve a first remission, BMT is indicated if they have an HLA-identical family donor. One exception to this strategy is M3 or promyelocytic leukemia, which is quite responsive to all-*trans*-retinoic acid and consolidation chemotherapy. Autologous BMT is being explored in clinical trials. Patients who relapse or are in second remission should be considered for BMT using HLA-matched family members, unrelated donors, or previously

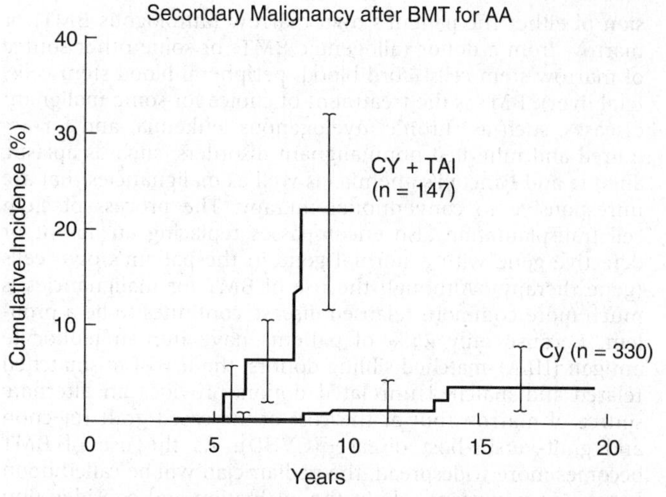

Figure 132–1. Marrow grafts for aplastic anemia (AA). The incidence of secondary malignant tumors in 330 Seattle patients conditioned with cyclophosphamide (Cy) and followed for a period of 20 years after transplant (BMT) versus the incidence in 147 patients reported from Paris who were conditioned with a combination of cyclophosphamide and thoracoabdominal irradiation (TAI) is shown. (From Storb R, Longton G, Anasetti C, et al: Changing trends in marrow transplantation for aplastic anemia. Bone Marrow Transplant 10(Suppl 2):50, 1992.)

stored autologous marrow. In contrast to acute lymphocytic leukemia (ALL), there is no advantage in attempting to induce a second remission. Patients with multiple relapses or resistant disease are candidates for two to three antigen mismatched donor transplants.

ACUTE LYMPHOBLASTIC LEUKEMIA. Acute lymphoblastic leukemia (ALL) is the most common malignancy of childhood, with approximately 70% of children being cured by conventional chemotherapy (Chapter 449.1). A subgroup of these patients have a high risk (75–100%) for relapse with conventional therapy and should be considered for BMT (Table 132–1).

Studies of autologous BMT for ALL involve higher risk patients and a variety of marrow purging techniques and preparative regimens. Disease-free survivals range from 15% to 65% in general, with relapse rates of 30–70%.

Relapsed leukemia is the most common reason for patients to fail marrow transplant for ALL. Purging autologous bone marrow of residual leukemia has theoretical benefit but change in outcome has not been demonstrated with negative purging techniques. Positive selection for stem cells that express surface antigens not expressed on leukemia cells is another possible strategy. Alternative approaches for treating minimal residual leukemia cells include the use of cytokines such as interleukin 2 (IL-2) or immunosuppressants such as cyclosporine post-transplant to simulate a graft-versus-leukemia effect.

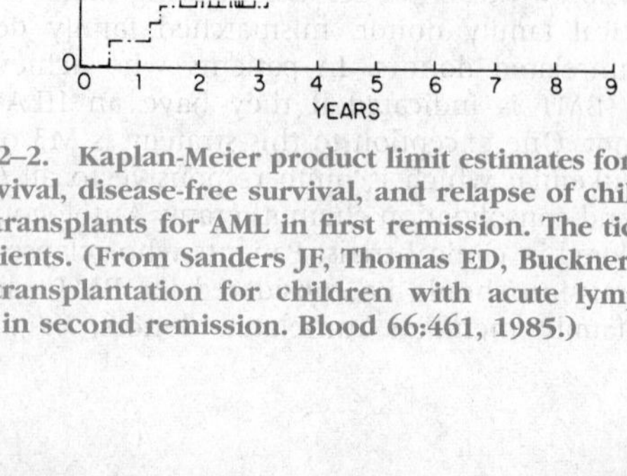

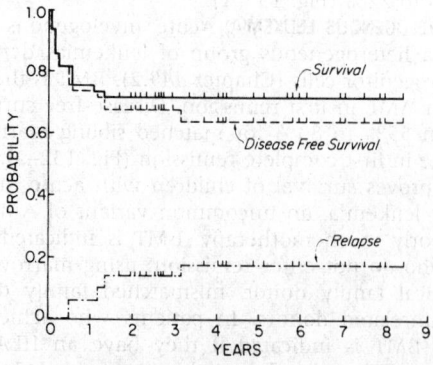

Figure 132–2. Kaplan-Meier product limit estimates for probability of survival, disease-free survival, and relapse of children who received transplants for AML in first remission. The tics indicate living patients. (From Sanders JF, Thomas ED, Buckner CD, et al: Marrow transplantation for children with acute lymphoblastic leukemia in second remission. Blood 66:461, 1985.)

■ TABLE 132–1 High-Risk Acute Lymphoblastic Leukemia

Congenital or infant (<1 yr) ALL
Chromosomal translocations: t(4,11), t(9,22)-Philadelphia, t(8,14)
FAB L-3 morphology (Burkitt)
WBC ≥100,000
More than 1 mo to achieve remission
Failure to achieve a remission
Relapse while on chemotherapy
Second and subsequent remissions
More than one extramedullary site of relapse without a marrow relapse

Patients who have HLA-matched donors may be eligible for allogeneic BMT for high-risk acute lymphoblastic leukemia. Children receiving HLA-matched sibling marrow transplants for high-risk ALL in first complete remission have disease-free survivals of 70–100% with low relapse rates of 0–10%, although the numbers are small. Patients who do not have high-risk features at the time of diagnosis but go on to relapse and have an HLA-identical family donor also benefit from transplantation. Patients have a better outcome if they are transplanted in remission, and earlier remission patients have a higher disease-free survival. Total body irradiation given prior to chemotherapy may be advantageous.

Comparisons of allogeneic and autologous BMT or chemotherapy for ALL relapse support the recommendation that these children should be offered bone marrow transplantation when possible. A review of 376 children receiving HLA-identical sibling marrow transplants compared with 540 children receiving chemotherapy for ALL in second remission revealed disease-free survivals of 40% and 17%, with relapse rates of 45% and 80%, respectively. Other studies comparing allogeneic and autologous marrow transplant for relapsed ALL have shown disease-free survivals of 33–61% for allografts and 21–31% for autografts, illustrating the advantage of allogeneic BMT over autologous transplants despite increased toxicity.

The lower incidence of relapse in allogeneic BMT is related to GVHD/graft-versus-leukemia (GVL) effect. A review of 2,254 pediatric and adult patients from the International Bone Marrow Transplant Registry compared the relapse rate and incidence of GVHD in BMT for ALL, AML, and chronic myelogenous leukemia (CML). The probability of relapse was 25 ± 6%, 22 ± 5%, 10 ± 7%, 7 ± 3%, 46 ± 15%, and 41 ± 8% for allogeneic grafts without GVHD, acute GVHD only, chronic GVHD only, acute and chronic GVHD, syngeneic grafts, and allogeneic T-cell–depleted grafts, respectively. These results were the same for the individual diseases and pointed out the importance of the immune system in eliminating residual leukemia cells.

Infant leukemia (Chapter 449.4) occurring within the first 12 mo of life is a distinct entity, which, although rare, carries a very poor prognosis, with survival rates of 20–30% after 5 yr with conventional chemotherapy. Cytogenetic abnormalities involving the chromosome 11q23 locus occur in as many as 75% of cases with involvement of other loci, including 1p32, 4q21, and 19p13 in ALL, and 1q21, 2p21, 6q27, 9p22, 10p11, 17q25, and 19p13 in AML, with the most common translocation being t(4,11)(q21;q23). Recent screening of infant leukemia for the presence of the rearranged 11q23 locus has demonstrated that infants with a normal 11q23 locus have a very good response to conventional chemotherapy, with a disease-free survival of 80% at a median follow-up of 46 months, while those with a rearranged 11q23 have a very poor response, with a 15% disease-free survival. A total of 29 patients with infant leukemia have received BMT for ALL or AML; disease-free survival is observed in 40–50% of patients transplanted in remission compared with 10–20% if BMT is done after relapse, using various sources of marrow. Children diagnosed with acute leukemia within the first 1–2 yr of life are best treated with intense induction chemotherapy followed by bone marrow transplantation if a suitable donor is available.

MYELODYSPLASTIC AND MYELOPROLIFERATIVE DISORDERS. Myelodysplastic syndrome (MDS) includes a group of disorders with a defects in hematopoietic cell development close to the level of the marrow stem cell, which eventually progresses from a picture of dysplastic ineffective hematopoiesis to aggressive overt myeloid leukemia. These are classified as refractory anemia (RA), refractory anemia with ringed sideroblasts (RARS), refractory anemia with excess blasts (RAEB), refractory anemia with excess blasts in transformation (RAEB-t), and chronic myelomonocytic leukemia (CMMoL). Because of the close relationship to AML, patients with MDS are treated according to AML protocols. The transplant outcome of patients with MDS is similar to AML. In one series of 93 patients, the disease-free survival at 4 yr was 62%. Transplant should be considered early after diagnosis because patients in whom the disease has progressed with increasing blasts have a much poorer outcome and a higher rate of relapse. Conventional chemotherapy and other nontransplant forms of treatment have not made a significant impact of the natural progression of the disease.

The *myeloproliferative disorders* are characterized by a single lineage myeloid proliferation that can progress to an AML-like leukemia. These diseases include CML, essential thrombocythemia (ET), polycythemia vera (PV), agnogenic myeloid metaplasia, and juvenile chronic myelogenous leukemia (JCML). *Chronic myelogenous leukemia* (Chapter 449.3) is characterized by the presence of the t(9,22) or Philadelphia chromosome; it is the most common leukemia in adults but is uncommon in children. BMT is the treatment of choice for CML. HLA-identical sibling transplantation results in an 80% long-term disease-free survival compared with 45–50% for matched unrelated BMT. Transplantation is recommended within 1 yr from diagnosis, as delay results in a significant decrease in the disease-free survival to 40–60%. Patients transplanted in accelerated phase or blast crisis have disease-free survivals of 35–40% and 10–20%, respectively, and a 60% chance of relapse compared with a 10–20% chance of relapse in patients transplanted in the chronic phase.

Successful marrow transplants have also been done for some of the more uncommon myeloproliferative disorders. BMT should be considered in those patients who fail to respond to conservative management or who progress to an AML-like leukemic condition. BMT is a possible approach for childhood *polycythemia vera.* BMT has been attempted for *essential thrombocythemia* in a few patients without success. *Agnogenic myeloid metaplasia* (AMM), or idiopathic myelofibrosis, is characterized by splenomegaly and a progressive fibrosis of the marrow compartment, resulting in anemia. The mean survival for patients with AMM is 5 yr, and the only known curative therapy is BMT; four of 10 patients transplanted for AMM survive.

Juvenile chronic myelogenous leukemia (Chapter 449.3) is an aggressive clonal proliferation of immature myeloid precursors associated with neurofibromatosis type 1 and monosomy 7. The clinical course is rapid, with resistance to conventional chemotherapy and death at an average of 9 mo from the time of diagnosis. The rapid proliferation of JCML blasts appears to be driven by a hypersensitivity to granulocyte-macrophage–colony-stimulating factor (GM-CSF). BMT is curative in these patients and should be pursued aggressively once the diagnosis is confirmed. Among the 10 children transplanted from matched sibling donors in Seattle, three relapsed, four died of transplant complications, and three survive disease free at >5, 7, and 9 yr. Among 17 patients given marrow from mismatched family or matched unrelated donors, 13 died of transplant complications or recurrent leukemia and four have survived >2–5 yr. The Milwaukee transplant group reported six JCML patients given T-cell–depleted matched unrelated marrow transplants; three of the six were alive at 6 mo to 6 yr. Some JCML patients have been found to respond to 13-*cis*-retinoic acid with temporary remissions, which may provide the time needed to identify potential marrow donors for these patients.

LYMPHOMAS. Non-Hodgkin lymphoma (NHL) and Hodgkin disease (HD) are malignant, usually clonal, proliferations arising from the lymphoreticular system (Chapter 450). Childhood lymphomas are quite responsive to conventional chemoradiotherapy, with long-term disease-free survival rates of 60–75% for NHL and 80–90% for HD. A subset of these patients have high-risk disease and relapse, requiring more intensive therapy to achieve a cure. BMT can cure some patients with NHL and HD, and should be offered early after relapse, while the disease is still sensitive to therapy, there is little bulky disease, and there is a greater likelihood of being able to tolerate a transplant regimen. Pretransplant salvage chemotherapy may be of some benefit to reduce the tumor burden. If an HLA-identical sibling is available, allogeneic transplant should be offered to take advantage of the GVL effect, which has reduced the relapse rate by as much as 25–30% in some series. Finally, early results using peripheral blood stem cells for transplantation appear to be as good as or better than autologous transplantation. A French study described BMT for children with relapsed or refractory NHL using either autologous (n = 23) or HLA-identical sibling allogeneic (n = 1) BMT. Eight patients (33%) were alive disease free 1–5.5 yr post-transplant. In a review of 1,060 NHL patients, the European Transplant Registry Group compared allogeneic and autologous BMT in patients matched for age, histology, disease status at transplant, stage at transplant, and conditioning regimen. Children receiving allogeneic BMT had a 38% progression-free survival after 48 mo, and those receiving autologous grafts had a 40% progression-free survival after a median of 30 mo. A lower relapse rate was found in the allogeneic group, but at the cost of a higher transplant-related morbidity/mortality.

The European Transplant Registry Group performed a case-matched comparison of pediatric (age ≤16 yr) and adult autologous BMT for HD. There was no significant difference between the pediatric and adult groups, with the progression-free survival rates being 39% and 48%, while the relapse rates were 52% and 40% for the pediatric and adult groups, respectively.

The Seattle group reviewed their 21 yr experience of allogeneic and autologous BMT for relapsed or refractory HD. The median age was 29 yr (range 10–55 yr). There was no statistical difference in event-free survival between allogeneic and autologous groups, with event-free survivals of 22% and 14% after 5 yr, respectively. Patients with refractory or bulky disease (n = 93) had a survival of 16% compared with 34% in those with less advanced disease (n = 34). HLA-identical sibling transplants had a significantly lower relapse rate (45%) compared with the autologous group (76%). There is one report describing two children who received HLA-identical BMT for aggressive Ki-1 T-cell lymphoma, with both surviving 40–56 mo. Finally, there are several reports of successful BMTs performed in children with Langerhans cell histiocytosis, including histiocytosis-X. Although patients with single-organ involvement histiocytosis do quite well, patients with multiorgan involvement respond poorly to conventional therapy and should be considered for transplant.

NEUROBLASTOMA. The most common extracranial solid tumor of children is neuroblastoma, with about 28 new cases per million children under 4 yr of age each year (Chapter 451).

The 10 yr survival for stage I-II disease is 88–90%, and for stage III disease is 63%, but almost half of all children older than 1 yr have disseminated disease (stage IV), with a 10 yr survival of 21%. Although BMT studies show a trend for improvement over chemotherapy, there have been no randomized trials to compare the two approaches. Disease-free (3 yr) survival rates for patients transplanted after progression of disease are 0–32% compared with 25–56% for those transplanted before progression of disease. Several national and international groups have examined a variety of different preparative regimens for autologous BMT for high-risk neuroblastoma with progression-free survivals of 24–100%, depending on the disease status at transplant. Relapse patterns suggest that minimal residual disease remains in the patient post-transplant as well as in the purged marrow. Whether myeloablative therapy is more effective early before tumor resistance develops and cumulative therapy toxicity becomes a problem, or if extended therapy prior to BMT is more important to eliminate residual disease, is unclear. N-*myc* amplification, histology, age, and ferritin did not correlate with BMT outcome. Current protocols use allogeneic BMT as well as new drug-radiation combinations for intensive consolidation with or without marrow rescue. Biologic agents such as 13-*cis*-retinoic acid that have activity in inducing ganglioneuronal differentiation in neuroblastoma are in clinical trials. Attempts are being directed at inducing a graft-versus-tumor effect with IL-2 or cyclosporine.

BRAIN TUMORS. Tumors of the central nervous system are the most common solid tumors in children, making up 20% of childhood malignancies (Chapter 555). Some forms, such as cerebellar astrocytomas, are amenable to treatment, whereas other forms are resistant because of their biology, for example, glioblastoma multiforme, or location, for example, brain-stem glioma. Phase I-II trials are helping to define the role of BMT in treating brain tumors. The transplant group in Philadelphia treated 10 children with glioblastoma multiforme (9) and anaplastic astrocytoma (1) using a conditioning regimen of thiotepa, etoposide, and bis-chlorethylnitrosourea (BCNU) followed by autologous marrow infusion; the response rate was 60% with two partial remissions and four complete remissions. The French group treated children with recurrent brain tumors using a 7-day course of busulfan and thiotepa followed by autologous bone marrow infusion. The 19 patients transplanted had various brain tumors, including medulloblastoma (5), ependymoma (5), primitive neuroectodermal tumor (2), brain-stem tumor (4), glioblastoma (2), and immature teratoma (1); the response rate was 26%, which is encouraging because all patients had refractory or relapsed disease. A new strategy being tested is the use of sequential rounds of dose-intensified chemotherapy supported with peripheral blood stem cell infusions.

SOLID TUMORS. Many solid tumors are quite responsive to conventional chemoradiotherapy; however, a subset of these have a very poor prognosis (Chapters 452–454). These tumors are high risk by virtue of their histology (alveolar rhabdomyosarcomas, anaplastic Wilms tumor), location (pelvic, trunk, or proximal extremity Ewing sarcoma, axial skeletal osteogenic sarcoma), or widespread metastatic presentation. Phase I-II trials are exploring the use of dose intensification of chemotherapy with or without total body irradiation (TBI) followed by autologous marrow rescue. The European Bone Marrow Transplantation Solid Tumor Registry described 25 children who received autologous BMT for refractory or relapsed Wilms tumor. Eight of 17 children who were transplanted after remission re-induction are disease free 14–90 mo post-transplant; one of eight children transplanted in relapse survives disease free after 3 yr.

The National Cancer Institute reported the results of three protocols to treat high-risk small, round, blue cell tumors, including Ewing sarcoma (n=44; humerus, femur, or trunk), rhabdomyosarcoma (n=25, unresectable), and peripheral primitive neuroectodermal tumors (n=17). The patients were treated with induction regimens, and those achieving complete remission were given consolidation with TBI, vincristine, Adriamycin (doxorubicin), and high-dose cyclophosphamide followed by unpurged autologous marrow infusion. After 6 yr, the event-free survivals for Ewing sarcoma, rhabdomyosarcoma, and primitive neuroectodermal tumors were 30%, 24%, and 24%, respectively, which was not significantly different from conventional chemotherapy. The most important prognostic factor in these patients was the presence of metastatic disease at diagnosis. New protocols will add non-cross-resistant agents such as ifosfamide and etoposide, and TBI may be increased from 8 to 12 Gy. Other groups have reported better success in autologous transplants for Ewing sarcoma using melphalan ± busulfan with 38–40% induction of stable complete remissions. Most reports of autologous BMT to treat osteosarcoma are case reports, but there has been one series of 24 children who were transplanted for relapsed osteosarcoma; after a short follow-up of only 6 mo, half were disease-free survivors.

GENETIC DISEASES

IMMUNODEFICIENCY DISORDERS. The immune deficiency states include a diverse group of disorders with defects in the humoral, cell-mediated, and/or phagocytic immune systems, resulting in life-threatening infections with premature death within the first few years of life. The severe combined immune deficiency (SCID) disorders are the most devastating and include SCID with B cells (45% of all SCID cases), classic SCID with T-B-cell lymphopenia and agammaglobulinemia (25%), adenosine deaminase deficiency (ADA; 15%), SCID with T-cell dysfunction (9%), reticular dysgenesis with lymphopenia and neutropenia (2%), purine nucleoside phosphorylase, and Omenn syndrome with eosinophilia and lymphoid replacement with Langerhans and reticular cells. There are also rare forms of SCID associated with dysostosis (short-limbed dwarfism and ectodermal dysplasia), abnormal T-cell antigen expression (CD-3 and CD-7), and dysfunctional T cells with capping defects.

BMT has been the treatment of choice for SCID since 1968, when the first successful allogeneic bone marrow transplant was performed in an infant with SCID using an HLA-identical unaffected sibling donor. The disease-free survival using matched sibling donors is >90%. Using T-depleted mismatched family member grafts results in disease-free survivals of 69–76%. There is less experience with unrelated donor BMT for SCID, but non-T-depleted marrow was used to treat eight SCID patients by the Minnesota transplant group and six survive 1.5–4 yr post-transplant.

BMT has been performed in other forms of immune deficiency including Wiskott-Aldrich syndrome, Di George syndrome, Kostmann neutropenia, leukocyte adherence deficiency, chronic granulomatous disease, Chédiak-Higashi syndrome, familial erythrophagocytic lymphohistiocytosis, Duncan syndrome, and neutrophil actin deficiencies. Survival rates are 68% when matched sibling donors are used and 35% when mismatched donors are used. Two Wiskott-Aldrich and three Chédiak-Higashi patients have received BMT from unrelated donors, and all five are surviving 1–3 yr post-transplant. If other forms of therapy are available, such as interferon-gamma for chronic granulomatous disease or granulocyte–colony-stimulating factor (G-CSF) for Kostmann's neutropenia, BMT should be reserved for patients who are unresponsive. Patients with ADA SCID may be treated with adenosine deaminase conjugated to polyethylene glycol (PEG-ADA) with variable recovery of immunologic function. Many of these disorders will be amenable to gene therapy to correct the underlying defect. Two patients with ADA SCID have been given T cells with the normal ADA gene inserted by retroviral gene transduction. After several infusions of their transduced T cells, both children have resolution of infections, regrowth of tonsillar tissue, and positive delayed hypersensitivity skin tests.

FANCONI ANEMIA. Fanconi anemia (FA) is an autosomal recessive form of aplastic anemia associated with congenital anomalies, chromosome fragility, pancytopenia, and myelodysplasia/AML (see Chapter 406). Although there is considerable heterogeneity in the phenotype, the diagnosis is made by the observation of increased chromosomal fragility in response to DNA cross-linking agents such as mitomycin-C or diepoxybutane. Patients develop pancytopenia, usually between the ages of 5 and 10 yr, which may respond transiently to low-dose androgens but progresses to fatal complications from bleeding, infection, or leukemia.

The characteristic sensitivity to DNA cross-linking agents makes FA patients quite sensitive to conventional BMT conditioning regimens, requiring dose reduction to avoid excessive toxicity. Transplant-related toxicities include severe oral mucositis, hemorrhagic cystitis, erythroderma, and GVHD. Studies from London (n=23), Paris (n=34), Cincinnati (n=12), and Seattle (n=17) show disease-free survivals of 30–100%, depending on the source of marrow. Patients receiving reduced conditioning regimens and matched sibling transplants have the best outcomes, although mismatched and unrelated donor transplants may be successful. Patients with FA and an HLA-identical family member who has a negative FA screen should be offered BMT at the first sign of pancytopenia. Although the experience with mismatched and unrelated donors is limited, BMT should be considered, given the poor outlook for these patients once leukemic transformation occurs.

STORAGE DISEASES. The metabolic storage diseases are a heterogeneous group of disorders resulting from single gene mutations producing enzyme defects and the subsequent toxic accumulation of metabolites. The end result is progressive neurologic deterioration or visceral infiltration, which is usually fatal. Some disorders, such as adrenoleukodystrophy, respond to dietary measures, while others, such as Gaucher disease type I and III, respond to enzyme supplementation, but in most cases there is no successful supplementation therapy available. BMT provides a source of enzyme through the bone marrow–derived monocyte/phagocytic cell system, which includes the liver (Kupffer cells), brain (microglia), skin (Langerhans cells), marrow (osteoclasts), lung (pulmonary macrophage), and lymph nodes (histiocytes). The results of transplant in several storage disorders are variable, with some showing an excellent response, while others have been more dismal. The risk of transplant-related mortality is about 10% for matched sibling donors and 37% in mismatched and unrelated donors. Transplant before the disease progresses to extensive end-organ damage is necessary. Efforts should be directed toward early diagnosis and BMT before significant neurologic damage occurs.

THALASSEMIA. Homozygous beta-thalassemia (Cooley anemia, thalassemia major) is a hereditary disorder characterized by impaired or absent production of beta globin chains (see also Chapter 419.9). The lack of beta chain production results in the accumulation of alpha globin chains forming unstable tetramers within red cells, resulting in hemolytic anemia and ineffective erythropoiesis. Therapy consists of lifelong transfusions with iron chelation, which allows survival of patients to 30–40 yr. Long-term problems include liver and cardiac failure because of iron deposition, multiple infections, delayed puberty, and diabetes. Although therapy delays their onset, these complications become life threatening.

Three risk factors that influence the outcome of BMT for thalassemia include hepatomegaly, portal fibrosis, and a history of inconsistent iron chelation prior to transplant. Other factors, such as the number of transfusions, ferritin level, degree of hemosiderosis, hepatic iron concentration, and splenomegaly, have no effect. Patients are classified as class 1, no risk factors; class 2, one or two risk factors; and class 3, all three risk factors. In BMT results from Italy, 271 children (≤16 yr) have received HLA-identical family member transplants (Fig. 132–3). Disease-free survivals of up to 94% are obtained in children transplanted before the development of hepatomegaly or portal fibrosis. Hepatic hemosiderosis and portal fibrosis may improve after transplant if the damage is not too extensive.

In the United States, 17 of the 27 children (63%) receiving HLA-matched family donor transplants survived disease free, one of whom required a second transplant. Another five patients survived after graft rejections and lived with recurrent thalassemia for an overall survival of 81%. If an HLA-identical family member is available, BMT should be performed before the patient develops advanced disease.

SICKLE CELL DISEASE. Sickle cell anemia results from a single amino acid substitution of valine for glutamic acid at the 6 position of β-globin (see also Chapter 419.1). With supportive care, more than 90% of children with sickle cell disease live into their 3rd and 4th decades and 60% survive to 50 yr. Disease severity varies among patients with homozygous hemoglobin S (HbS) disease; 5–20% suffer significant morbidity from vaso-occlusive crises and pulmonary, renal, and central nervous system (CNS) damage. New approaches include anti-sickling agents, gene therapy, and induction of increased hemoglobin F by drugs such as hydroxyurea, but BMT is the only curative treatment for sickle cell anemia.

In the United States, five patients (ages 3–10 yr) have been transplanted using HLA-identical sibling donors; two donors had the sickle trait. The first patient receiving a bone marrow transplant for sickle cell disease also had AML. All five patients survive in good health at 8 mo to 9.3 yr.

Forty-two patients (ages 1–23 yr) received HLA-identical family member BMT for SS disease in Belgium and France. After a short follow-up of 1–75 mo, 97.6% survive with a disease-free survival of 90.5%. No vaso-oclusive events have occurred among the 38 patients with successful engraftment, and some have recovered splenic function. Although BMT can cure homozygous HbS disease, the selection of appropriate candidates for transplantation is difficult. Patients with SS disease may survive for decades, but some patients have a poor quality of life, with repeated hospitalizations for painful vaso-occlusive crises and CNS infarcts. SS patients, such as those

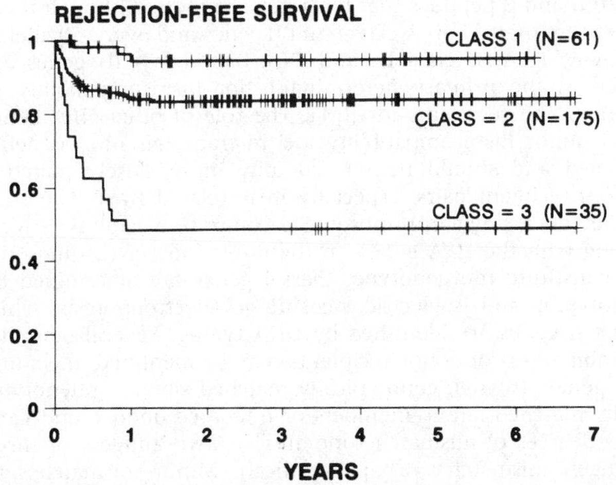

Figure 132–3. The probabilities of rejection-free survival for 271 patients younger than 17 yr with thalassemia who received marrow transplants from human leukocyte antigen identical family members after conditioning with busulfan and cyclophosphamide. (From Forman SJ, Blume KG, Thomas ED: Bone Marrow Transplantation. Boston, Blackwell, 1994, p 835.)

with the Central African Republic haplotype, can be predicted to have serious complications. BMT should be considered in young patients who have recurrent severe vaso-oclusive crises, evidence of developing end-organ damage, CNS infarcts, or a history of strokes, and have an HLA-identical family member donor.

OTHER CONGENITAL ANEMIAS

BMT is successful in some other congenital anemias. *Diamond-Blackfan syndrome* or congenital pure red cell aplasia is characterized by normochromic-macrocytic anemia with a normocellular marrow. The erythroid line is conspicuously decreased or absent with normal megakaryocytes and granulopoiesis. Serum erythropoietin is usually elevated. Patients who fail initial therapies, such as corticosteroids, may benefit from BMT using an HLA-identical sibling donor. Ten of 12 patients who were given BMT for Diamond-Blackfan anemia, are alive disease free 17 mo to 10 yr post transplant. *Congenital sideroblastic anemia* results from a mitochondrial abnormality in erythroblasts. These patients have ineffective erythropoiesis, hypochromic anemia, and elevated serum iron. The disease progresses to transfusion dependency with total body iron overload and secondary hemosiderosis with hepatic and cardiac failure. One 34-mo-old child received a BMT from a phenotypically identical cousin and has some persistent liver enlargement after 3 yr but remains transfusion independent with normal serum iron and ferritin.

132.2 Matching and Rejection

The immunologic goal of BMT is a graft that can respond to foreign antigens without reacting to the host and is not rejected. The most important factor determining tolerance is the histocompatibility between the donor and host. The genes defining histocompatibility are encoded in the major histocompatibility complex (MHC) on the short arm of chromosome 6. The MHC spans approximately 4,000 kilobases of DNA and contains the genes for a series of cell surface glycoproteins termed the *human leukocyte antigens* (HLA). The HLA genes are tightly linked and can be divided into class I glycoproteins that dimerize with β-2-microglobulin and class II glycoproteins with α and β peptides that form heterodimers. Although there are more than 35 HLA class I and II genes and over 250 alleles, HLA-A, HLA-B (class I), and HLA-DRB (class II) genes are used as the primary determinants for histocompatibility of donors and recipients for BMT. The role of other HLA genes and minor histocompatibility loci in transplantation is being studied and should help to identify more closely matched donor-recipient pairs, especially in unrelated BMT. The HLA genes on a single chromosome 6 comprise a haplotype that, along with the HLA genes on the other copy of chromosome 6, constitute the genotype. Class I genes are determined by serotyping and isoelectric focusing gel electrophoresis, while class II genes are identified by DNA typing. Several potential combinations of donor/recipients may be identified, including syngeneic (twins), genotypically matched siblings, phenotypically matched family members or unrelated donors, and various degrees of mismatch (one antigen, two antigen, or three antigen mismatch = haploidentical). Minor mismatches as well as partial matches based on graft-versus-host and rejection vectors may also be identified. Because only 25–30% of patients have an HLA-identical sibling, the identification of phenotypically matched unrelated donors is more feasible using large unrelated donor registries. In the United States, the National Marrow Donor Program has typed more than 600,000 volunteer donors and uses 106 donor centers and 57 transplant centers to add 20,000 potential new donors each month. The chance of identifying an unrelated donor for a given individual is about 20%. Transplants using one-antigen mismatched, unrelated donors may be possible if the mismatch is with cross-reactive or very closely related HLA antigens.

Graft failure and graft rejection are influenced by several factors (Table 132–2); HLA disparity is the most important variable. Failure to engraft may occur in autologous as well as allogeneic BMT and may result from an inadequate stem cell dose or from marrow stromal damage by prior therapy in conjunction with the transplant preparative regimen. Graft rejection may occur immediately, without an increase in cell counts or may follow a brief period of engraftment. Rejection is usually mediated by residual host T cells, cytotoxic antibodies, or lymphokines, and is manifested by a fall in donor cell counts with a persistence of host lymphocytes. BMT using marrow from HLA disparate donors increases the risk for graft rejection/failure significantly. For example, the risk of graft failure in HLA-identical sibling BMT is 1–2%, while in haploidentical BMT the risk is 3–15%. Alloimmunization by exposure to multiple transfusions prior to BMT may sensitize the patient to HLA antigens, increasing the potential for graft rejection; this is observed most often with aplastic anemia. Because adequate immunosuppression of the host prior to marrow infusion is required to ensure engraftment and prevent rejection, the incidence of rejection depends in part on the conditioning regimen. With matched sibling BMT for aplastic anemia, there is a 24% incidence of graft rejection when cyclophosphamide is used alone as a preparative regimen compared with 3% when ATG is added. Post-transplant immunosuppression is useful to prevent GVHD and to minimize the likelihood of graft rejection. One effective approach to GVHD is to eliminate T cells from the donor marrow prior to infusion, but the elimination of T cells allows the persistence of host lymphocytes that are capable of mediating graft rejection in about 10% of cases. Graft rejection may be difficult to differentiate from the effects of drugs or viral infections on the graft.

132.3 Graft-Versus-Host Disease (GVHD)

Engraftment by donor lymphocytes in an immunologically compromised host (congenital, radiation, or chemotherapy-induced immune defects) can result in donor T-cell activation against host MHC antigens, with resultant GVHD. Cell death results from cell-mediated cytotoxic activity (e.g., natural killer cells) and a complex cascade of lymphokines released by activated lymphocytes (e.g., tumor necrosis factor [TNF]). In order for this reaction to occur, the graft must contain immunocompetent cells, the host must be immunocompromised and unable to reject or mount a response to the graft, and there must be histocompatibility differences between the graft and the host. GVHD is classified as the acute form, occurring within

■ TABLE 132–2 Factors Influencing Engraftment and Graft Rejection

HLA disparity
Pretransplant alloimmunization by transfusions
Conditioning regimen
Transplanted marrow cell dose
Marrow stroma/microenvironment
Post-transplant/immunosuppression
Donor T cells
Drug toxicity
Viral infections

■ TABLE 132–3 Clinical Staging and Grading of Graft-Versus-Host Disease

Stage	Skin	Liver	Intestinal Tract
+	Maculopapular rash <25% of body surface	Bilirubin 2–3 mg/100 mL	>500 mL diarrhea/day
+ +	Maculopapular rash <25–50% of body surface	Bilirubin 3–6 mg/100 mL	>1,000 mL diarrhea/day
+ + +	Generalized erythroderma	Bilirubin 6–15 mg/100 mL	>1,500 mL diarrhea/day
+ + + +	Generalized erythroderma with bullous formation and desquamation	Bilirubin >15 mg/100 mL	Severe abdominal pain with or without ileus

GVHD Grade	Skin Stage	Liver Stage	Intestinal Tract Stage	Decrease in Clinical Performance
I	+–+ +	0	0	None
II	+–+ + +	+	+	Mild
III	+ +–+ + +	+ +–+ + + +	+ +–+ + +	Marked
IV	+ +–+ + + +	+ +–+ + + +	+ +–+ + + +	Extreme

Adapted from Thomas ED, N Engl J Med 292:832, 895, 1975.

the first 100 days after bone marrow transplant, and chronic GVHD, occurring after the first 100 days. As discussed earlier, GVHD may have some benefit by producing a graft-versus-leukemia (GVL) effect and a lower relapse rate in patients transplanted for leukemia. The process of GVHD represents a loss of "tolerance" normally maintained by thymic elimination of alloreactive lymphocytes; modulation of the T-cell receptor, rendering alloreactive cells anergic; and active suppressor cells that hold activated T cells in check. Attempts at generating GVHD/GVL effects in autologous BMT patients have been based on altering these tolerance factors with immunomodulatory agents such as cyclosporine.

ACUTE GVHD. The acute form of GVHD (aGVHD) is characterized by erythroderma, cholestatic hepatitis, and enteritis (Table 132–3). Typically aGVHD presents about day 19 (median), when the patient is starting to engraft. It usually starts with a pruritic macular/papular rash on the ears, palms, and soles and may progress to involve the trunk (Fig. 132–4) and extremities, potentially becoming a more confluent erythroderma with bullae formation and exfoliation. Fever may or may not be present. Other diagnostic considerations include toxicity from the immunosuppressive regimen, drug rash, and viral or other infectious exanthems. Hepatic manifestations include cholestatic jaundice with elevated liver function tests.

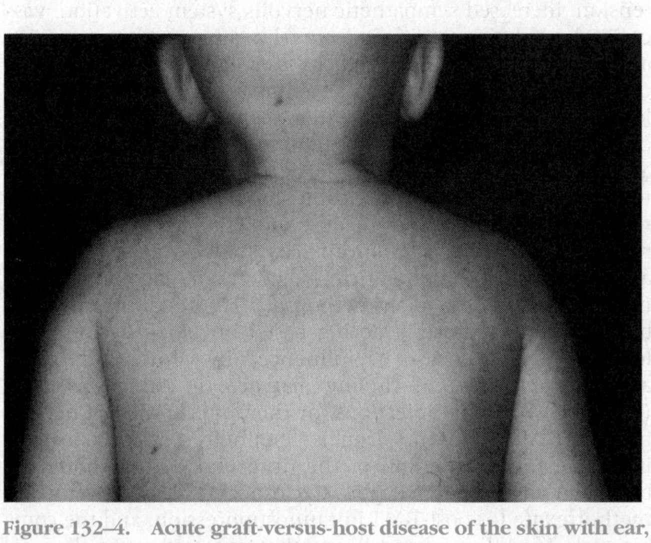

Figure 132–4. Acute graft-versus-host disease of the skin with ear, arm, shoulder, and trunk involvement. (Courtesy of Evan Farmer, MD.) See also color section.

The differential diagnosis includes hepatitis, veno-occlusive disease, or drug effect. The intestinal symptoms of aGVHD include crampy abdominal pain and watery diarrhea, often with blood. The conditioning regimen and infectious agents may produce similar symptoms. Eosinophilia, lymphocytosis, protein-losing enteropathy, bone marrow aplasia (neutropenia, thrombocytopenia, anemia), peripheral edema, and secondary infections may ensue. Factors related to the development of aGVHD include histocompatibility differences between the donor and patient, sex mismatching, donor parity, age, active or relapsed malignancy at the time of BMT, and increasing doses of radiation. The prevention and treatment of GVHD requires a variety of immunosuppressive agents described later.

CHRONIC GVHD. The maturation of the graft may include the development of chronic GVHD, usually after day 100, but as early as day 60–70. Chronic GVHD resembles a multisystem autoimmune process manifesting as Sjögren (sicca) syndrome, systemic lupus erythematosus, and scleroderma (Fig. 132–5), lichen planus, and primary biliary cirrhosis. Recurrent infections (sepsis, sinusitis, pneumonia) with encapsulated bacteria and fungal and viral organisms are common and contribute significantly to transplant-related morbidity and mortality. Prophylaxis with trimethoprim-sulfamethoxazole reduces the incidence of *Pneumocystis carinii* pneumonia. Risks for chronic GVHD include increasing age, prior acute GVHD, buffy coat transfusions, and parity of a female donor. Therapy for cGVHD consists of additional immunosuppression with agents (prednisone and cyclosporine are front-line drugs) described later, again with the disadvantage of putting the patient at risk for infectious complications.

132.4 Principles of Immunosuppression

Immunosuppressive agents are used to prevent and treat allograft rejection and GVHD. Because differences in major or minor histocompatibility antigens induce recipient T lymphocyte activation and subsequent donor allograft rejection, immunosuppression is needed for all tissue transplantation, except from identical twins. Solid organ transplantation requires lifelong immunosuppression to prevent graft rejection, whereas BMT recipients are treated for 6–12 mo until a state of tolerance is attained. New transplant strategies using se-

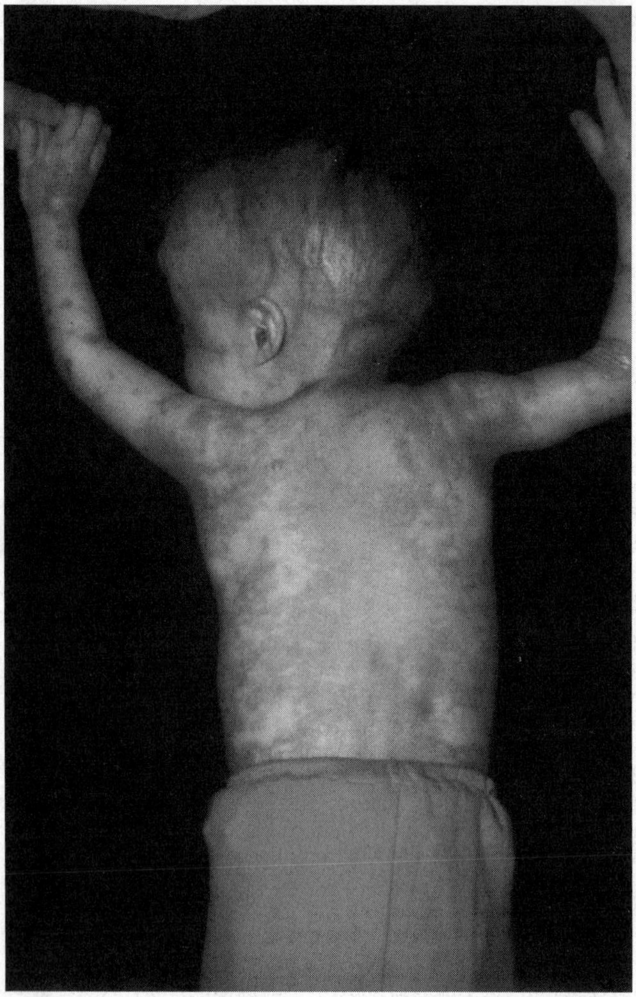

Figure 132–5. Chronic graft-versus-host disease of the skin with sclerodermoid changes. (Courtesy of Evan Farmer, MD.) See also color section.

lected stem and T cells to enhance engraftment but avoid GVHD, as well as newer, more potent immunosuppressive agents, permit successful BMT across greater degrees of mismatched HLA antigens. The ideal immunosuppressive agent inhibits the host lymphocyte subsets that mediate rejection and inhibits donor lymphocytes that mediate GVHD without altering immunity against infection or malignancy (GVL).

PREPARATIVE REGIMEN. Different preparative regimens are used for BMT for different diseases. Most agents have antineoplastic as well as immunosuppressant activity. Cyclophosphamide is a nitrogen mustard derivative that requires metabolic activation to generate a bifunctional alkylating metabolite and is the most widely utilized immunosuppressant in BMT preparative regimens. TBI is also an important therapeutic agent, with excellent antineoplastic activity and immunosuppressive qualities that can effectively treat all parts of the body. Other chemotherapeutic agents that have greater antitumor effects than immunosuppression have been used in combination with TBI and cyclophosphamide and include busulfan, etoposide (VP-16), melphalan, carmustine (BCNU), cytosine arabinoside (ara-C), thiotepa, ifosfamide, and carboplatin. The combinations are designed to achieve adequate immunosuppression allowing rapid engraftment without excessive toxicity and with the capacity to eliminate a malignant clone.

T-CELL DEPLETION. Prevention of graft rejection and GVHD along with treatment of GVHD in the peritransplant period involves several different strategies. Because donor T cells are responsible for GVHD, donor marrows have been depleted of T cells using monoclonal antibodies or physical separation techniques such as soy lectin agglutination. Depletion results in a dramatic reduction in GVHD but can cause problems with graft rejection and relapsed disease. Donor T cells play an important role in eliminating residual host T cells as well as mediating a GVL effect. Alternatives to T-cell depletion are being explored, including adding back-selected T cells that may help engraftment and retain antitumor activity but without GVHD activity.

METHOTREXATE. This competitive inhibitor of dihydrofolate reductase is an excellent immunosuppressive agent, in addition to being a cancer chemotherapeutic drug. A regimen of methotrexate given on days 1, 3, 6, and 11 is quite effective at preventing GVHD, with additional improvement if the drug is given weekly for the first 100 days. Methotrexate may aggravate mucositis resulting from the conditioning regimen and may require rescue with leucovorin if there is renal impairment or a fluid collection such as a pleural effusion. Trimetrexate is an antifolate drug with structural similarity to methotrexate, but it is eliminated by the liver and may be an alternative for patients who have significant renal impairment.

CYCLOSPORINE. This lipophilic (hydrophobic), cyclic, 11-amino acid peptide is a potent and specific immunosuppressive agent that selectively inhibits the translation of IL-2 mRNA by helper T cells. Cyclosporine may also inhibit IL-1, IL-3, and γ-interferon synthesis. T-cell activation is attenuated in the absence of IL-2. Cyclosporine inhibits IL-2 receptor formation at higher doses. Cyclosporine has no myelosuppressive or anti-inflammatory effects, but it is very useful for preventing graft rejection. Cyclosporine is metabolized by the hepatic cytochrome P-450 enzyme system and can be involved in a number of drug interactions. Cyclosporine levels increase in the presence of ketoconazole, erythromycin, methylprednisolone, warfarin, verapamil, ethanol, imipenem-cilastatin, metaclopramide, and fluconazole; cyclosporine levels decrease in the presence of phenytoin, phenobarbital, carbamazepine, valproate, nafcillin, and rifampin.

Cyclosporine has significant nonimmunosuppressant toxic effects, including neurotoxicity (tremors, paresthesias, headache, confusion, somnolence, seizures, coma), hypertrichosis, gingival hyperplasia, anorexia, nausea, vomiting, hepatotoxicity (cholestasis, cholelithiasis, hemorrhagic necrosis), endocrinopathies, (ketosis, hyperprolactinemia, hypertestosteronemia, gynecomastia, impaired spermatogenesis), metabolic disorders (hypomagnesemia, hyperuricemia, hyperglycemia, hyperkalemia, hypocholesterolemia), vascular derangements (hypertension, increased sympathetic nervous system activation, vasculitic-hemolytic uremic syndrome–like illness, atherogenesis), and nephrotoxicity. Renal toxicity is a significant limitation of cyclosporine use and is manifested as an increased creatinine level, oliguria, hypertension, fluid retention, vasoconstriction of the afferent glomerular filtration rate, renal tubular damage, and hemolytic-uremic syndrome–like lesions. Chronic nephrotoxicity (interstitial fibrosis, tubular atrophy) may require a reduction of the cyclosporine dose or a change to other immunosuppressant drugs. Nephrotoxicity may be exacerbated by aminoglycosides, amphotericin B, acyclovir, digoxin, furosemide, indomethacin, or trimethoprim. The renal toxicity may be reduced by adjusting dosing based on blood cyclosporine levels. Levels may also be influenced by clinical conditions affecting absorption, including diarrhea, intestinal disorders (due to GVHD, viral infections, or therapy), or altered hepatic function. Although the drug is lipophilic, obesity does not influence the distribution of the drug and dosing should be based on ideal body weight. Cyclosporine is as effective as methotrexate for post-BMT immunosuppression, and the combination of cyclosporine with methotrexate is better than either drug alone.

FK506. This experimental macrolide immunosuppressive drug produced by the fungus *Streptomyces tsukubaensis* is chemically distinct from cyclosporine but has similar effects on the immune system. Although it binds specific FK506 binding proteins, it has the same effects on the expression of IL-2 and the IL-2 receptor as cyclosporine. FK506 has little advantage over cyclosporine, except possibly for the treatment of GVHD of the liver because it is concentrated in the liver. FK506 has the same toxicities and drug interactions as cyclosporine. The combination of these drugs causes synergistic toxicity.

CORTICOSTEROIDS. Prednisone, usually in combination with other immunosuppressive agents, is often used to treat or prevent GVHD and to prevent rejection. Corticosteroids may interfere with T-lymphocyte proliferation by directly blocking activation of the genes for IL-1 and IL-6. Because IL-2 secretion depends in part on IL-1 and IL-6 release, steroids block IL-2 action indirectly. Corticosteroids also produce a more rapid anti-inflammatory response by inducing the production of lipocortin, an inhibitor of phospholipase A_2, which reduces the synthesis of inflammatory prostaglandins. They may also lyse small populations of activated lymphocytes and reduce the migration of monocytes to sites of inflammation. Nonspecific and pronounced immunosuppressant effects of corticosteroids (and other immunosuppressants) place the patient at risk for serious opportunistic infections. Other long-term complications of steroid use include growth failure, cushingoid appearance, hypertension, cataracts, gastrointestinal bleeding, pancreatitis, psychosis, hyperglycemia, osteoporosis, aseptic necrosis of the femoral head, and suppression of the pituitary-adrenal axis.

ANTITHYMOCYTE GLOBULIN (ATG). Heterologous antibodies against human thymocytes have been generated from horses, rabbits, and other sources. These antibody preparations are potent immunosuppressants and have been useful in preparative regimens as well as for treatment of resistant GVHD. Toxicities include fever, hypotension, rash-urticaria, tachycardia, dyspnea, chills, myalgias, serum sickness, and potential anaphylaxis. All patients should be skin tested for sensitivity prior to treatment. Diphenhydramine, Tylenol (acetaminophen), and hydrocortisone help to minimize side effects.

OKT3. This is a murine monoclonal antibody directed against the T3 (CD3) surface glycoprotein on T cells. Although OKT3 eliminates T cells by binding to CD3 and inducing clearance by the reticuloendothelial system, it also activates T cells with resultant toxicity that includes fever, chills, dyspnea, chest pain, wheezing, nausea, and vomiting. Modified antibodies such as BC3 have been developed that bind CD3 but are unable to interact with the Fc receptors on monocytes and do not activate T cells. These newer antibodies are more effective for treating GVHD and have fewer side effects. Another strategy is to conjugate antibodies to cytologic toxins such as ricin A. Ricin A linked to an anti-CD5 antibody (Xomazyme) that binds T cells and some B cells mediates cytospecific toxicity.

AZATHIOPRINE. This imidazole derivative of 6-mercaptopurine blocks DNA synthesis by inhibiting purine synthesis. Both azathioprine and 6-mercaptopurine inhibit T-cell activation and decrease the number of migrating mononuclear cells. Toxic effects include myelosuppression (neutropenia), hepatic veno-occlusive disease, hepatitis, pancreatitis, and secondary malignancies. It has not been useful for aGVHD because of its toxicities but has been used with some variable benefit for resistant cGVHD.

THALIDOMIDE. Initially used as a sedative but found to have immunosuppressive properties, thalidomide has been studied in phase I-II trials for treating cGVHD. Patients with high risk or refractory cGVHD treated with thalidomide have shown a 59% response rate with a 76% survival for those with refractory cGVHD and 48% for those with high-risk cGVHD. Studies to determine the relative efficacy of thalidomide compared to other regimens for cGVHD are in progress.

132.5 Late Effects of Bone Marrow Transplantation

As more children are undergoing BMT for a widening spectrum of indications and an increasing number of these children become long-term survivors, late effects of the transplant process have a lasting impact on the health and well-being of the individual. The pediatrician should be aware of possible delayed complications, including effects on growth and development, neuroendocrine dysfunction, fertility, second tumors, chronic GVHD, cataracts, leukoencephalopathy, and immune dysfunction.

NEUROLOGIC FUNCTION. Infections, metabolic encephalopathy (resulting from hepatic dysfunction), and drug/radiation therapy may all contribute to neurologic sequelae. Cyclosporine may produce headache (most responsive to propranolol), tremor, confusion, visual disturbance, seizures, and frank encephalopathy. Most of these effects are reversible with discontinuation of the drug. The incidence of cataracts is roughly 80% in patients receiving single-dose TBI, 20–50% with fractionated TBI, and 20% after chemotherapy-only regimens. A dry eye syndrome is often related to chronic GVHD and is treated with artificial tears and lubricants. Leukoencephalopathy is a clinical syndrome characterized by lethargy, slurred speech, ataxia, seizures, confusion, dysphagia, and decerebrate posturing. It may present with minimal symptoms or can result in coma or death in its most severe form. Magnetic resonance imaging (MRI) and computed tomography (CT) scans reveal multifocal areas of white matter degeneration with necrosis. Leukoencephalopathy is almost exclusively observed in patients who have received extensive intrathecal chemotherapy or cranial radiation prior to transplant, with an overall incidence of 7% in patients at risk.

SECONDARY MALIGNANCIES. The overall risk of developing a secondary form of cancer is about 6.7 times that of the general population, with the greatest risk being within the 1st yr. Roughly half of the secondary tumors are non-Hodgkin lymphomas, and two thirds of these are Epstein-Barr virus (EBV) positive. Other malignancies observed include leukemia, brain tumors, melanomas, and a variety of carcinomas of the skin, liver, lung, and thyroid. Risk factors that are associated with second malignancies included the use of ATG, T depletion of the donor marrow, and TBI in the preparative regimen. EBV-related B-cell lymphomas, which are aggressive and resistant to most therapeutic interventions, have been successfully treated with infusions of donor T cells.

GROWTH AND DEVELOPMENT. Long-term follow-up studies of patients who have received TBI-containing regimens reveal significant growth depression and growth hormone deficiency. After 5 yr, TBI-treated patients were more than two standard deviations below the mean height for age and dropped to three to four standard deviations below the mean by 8 yr post-transplant. This decrease in growth velocity is similar for boys and girls, and does not vary with the use of cranial radiation or different regimens of radiation (single vs. fractionated). Children receiving radiation-containing regimens also have no pubertal growth spurt. The pubertal growth spurt depends on the presence of adequate growth hormone and gonadal hormones, both of which may be low post-transplant. A major determinant of final height is the amount of growth done prior to puberty. Children receiving BMT before the age of 11 have a final height below the 10th percentile, while those transplanted after age 11 attain a height close to the average. Chronic GVHD and its treatment with corticosteroids may also contribute to growth impairment post-transplant. In an attempt to avoid TBI-related growth effects in children, chemotherapy-only regimens have been used such as busulfan/cyclophosphamide. Early results of growth studies suggest that busulfan also interferes with growth. Preparative regimens using cyclophosphamide only for aplastic anemia have little effect on normal growth and development, implicating the role of busulfan in affecting growth and development in busulfan/cyclophosphamide regimens. The use of radiation to the long bones and vertebral bodies for neuroblastoma also contributes to decreased growth velocity. Therapy with recombinant growth hormone after age 12 yr prevents a further decrease in growth velocity, but little or no catch-up growth is achieved. Annual growth hormone evaluation is essential in all children post-transplant. Current studies are aimed at identifying children with growth hormone deficiencies at an earlier age and supplementing them with growth hormone to achieve a normal pubertal growth spurt. Gonadal hormones are essential for normal pubertal growth as well as secondary sexual characteristic development. About three quarters of patients receiving TBI-containing regimens show delayed secondary sexual characteristic development, resulting from primary ovarian or testicular failure. Laboratory evaluation reveals elevated follicle stimulating hormone (FSH) and luteinizing hormone (LH) with depressed estradiol and testosterone. These patients require careful follow-up with annual Tanner scores and endocrine evaluation. Supplementation of gonadal hormones is useful for primary gonadal failure, and is given along with growth hormone, to promote normal pubertal growth.

THYROID FUNCTION. Chemotherapy-only preparative regimens have little effect on normal thyroid function. The use of TBI with or without additional conventional radiation involving the thyroid gland may result in compensated or overt hypothyroidism. Some patients, who have received single-dose TBI, develop compensated (28–56%) or overt (9–13%) hypothyroidism. The use of fractionated TBI has reduced the incidence of compensated (10–14%) and overt (<5%) hypothyroidism significantly. Risk factors for the development of hypothyroidism appear to be related only to the use of radiation, with no influence of age, sex, or GVHD. The site of injury by radiation is at the level of the thyroid gland rather than at the pituitary or hypothalamus. Therapy with thyroxine is very effective for overt hypothyroidism, but treatment of compensated hypothyroidism is more controversial. Despite treating hypothyroidism, there remains a risk for thyroid carcinomas. Because the risk of hypothyroidism continues for many years, annual thyroid function studies are important.

IMMUNE RECONSTITUTION. Chemo-radiotherapy for BMT results in complete eradication of host B- and T-cell immunity. After infusion of donor marrow, the recovery of the normal immune functions takes many months or years. The ability of newly engrafting B cells to respond to mitogenic stimulation is intact by 2–3 mo. Because the production of antibodies requires B- and T-cell interaction, normal IgM levels are not observed until 4–6 mo post-transplant; IgG levels take 7–9 mo, and it may take 2 yr before normal IgA levels are achieved. T-cell recovery also takes many months. CD8 T cells recover by about 4 mo but CD4 T cells do not increase until 6–9 mo, resulting in an inverted CD4/CD8 ratio for the first 6–9 mo post-transplant. Factors that prolong this interval include T depletion of the marrow, post-transplant immunosuppression, and chronic GVHD. Patients with cGVHD have a continued decrease in the number of cytotoxic T lymphocytes and helper T cells, along with increased suppressor T cells. Re-immunization of an individual will be successful only after adequate recovery of immune function. For patients without cGVHD, diphtheria and tetanus toxoid (DT) immunizations may be given 3–6 mo post-transplant, inactivated (Salk) polio after 6–12 mo, and measles, mumps, and rubella (MMR) after 1–2 yr. If chronic GVHD is present, re-immunization should be postponed and IgG supplemented until it resolves.

GENERAL REFERENCES

Armitage JO: Bone marrow transplantation. N Engl J Med 330:827, 1994.

Forman SJ, Blume KG, Thomas ED (eds): Bone Marrow Transplantation. Boston, Blackwell Scientific Publications, 1994.

Robertson KA: Pediatric bone marrow transplantation. Curr Opin Pediatr 5:103, 1993.

APLASTIC ANEMIA

Camitta B, Ash R, Menitove J, et al: Bone marrow transplantation for children with severe aplastic anemia: use of donors other than HLA-identical siblings. Blood 74:1852, 1989.

Sanders JE, Storb R, Anasetti C, et al: Marrow transplant experience for children with severe aplastic anemia. Am J Pediatr Hematol Oncol 16:43, 1994.

Storb R, Longton G, Anasetti C, et al: Changing trends in marrow transplantation for aplastic anemia. Bone Marrow Transplant 10(Suppl 2):45, 1992.

ACUTE MYELOGENOUS LEUKEMIA

Appelbaum FR: Indications for bone marrow transplantation in the treatment of acute myeloid leukemia. Leukemia 7:1081, 1993.

Ritter J, Creutzig U, Schellong G: Treatment results of three consecutive German childhood AML trials: BFM-78, -83, -87. Leukemia 6(Suppl 2):59, 1992.

Woods WG, Kobrinsky N, Buckley J, et al: Intensively timed induction therapy followed by bone marrow transplantation for children with acute myeloid leukemia or myelodysplastic syndrome: a Children's Cancer Study Group pilot study. J Clin Oncol 11:1448, 1993.

ACUTE LYMPHOBLASTIC LEUKEMIA

Barrett AJ, Horowitz MM, Pollock BH, et al: Bone marrow transplants from HLA-identical siblings as compared with chemotherapy for children with acute lymphoblastic leukemia in a second remission. N Eng J Med 331:1253, 1994.

Billet AL, Kornmehl E, Tarbell NJ, et al: Autologous bone marrow transplantation after a long first remission for children with recurrent acute lymphoblastic leukemia. Blood 81:1651, 1993.

Bordigoni P, Vernant JP, Souillet G, et al: Allogeneic bone marrow transplantation for children with acute lymphoblastic leukemia in first remission: a cooperative group study of the group d'Etude de la Greffe de Moelle Osseuse. J Clin Oncol 7:747, 1989.

Chen CS, Sorenson PHB, Domer PH, et al: Molecular rearrangements on chromosome 11q23 predominate in infant acute lymphoblastic leukemia and are associated with specific biologic variables and poor outcome. Blood 81:2386, 1993.

Emminger W, Emminger-Schmidmeier W, Haas OA, et al: Treatment of infant leukemia with busulfan, cyclophosphamide, + etoposide and bone marrow transplantation. Bone Marrow Transplant 9:313, 1992.

Lönnerholm G, Simonsson B, Arvidson J, et al: Autologous bone marrow transplantation in children with acute lymphoblastic leukemia. Acta Pædiatr 81:1017, 1992.

Sanders JE, Thomas ED, Buckner CD, et al: Marrow transplantation for children with acute lymphoblastic leukemia in second remission. Blood 70:324, 1987.

Snyder DS, Chao NJ, Amylon MD, et al: Fractionated total body irradiation and high dose etoposide as a preparatory regimen for bone marrow transplantation for 99 patients with acute leukemia in first complete remission. Blood 82:2920, 1993.

Weyman C, Graham-Pole J, Emerson S, et al: Use of cytosine arabinoside and total body irradiation as conditioning for allogeneic marrow transplantation in patients with acute lymphoblastic leukemia: a multicenter survey. Bone Marrow Transplant 11:43, 1993.

MYELODYSPLASTIC AND MYELOPROLIFERATIVE SYNDROMES

Anderson J, Appelbaum FR, Fisher LD, et al: Allogeneic bone marrow transplantation for 93 patients with myelodysplastic syndrome. Blood 82:677, 1993.

Gamis AS, Haake R, McGlave P, et al: Unrelated donor bone marrow transplantation for Philadelphia chromosome positive chronic myelogenous leukemia in children. J Clin Oncol 11:834, 1993.

Sanders JE, Buckner CD, Thomas ED, et al: Allogeneic marrow transplantation for children with juvenile chronic myelogenous leukemia. Blood 71:1144, 1988.

LYMPHOMAS

Anderson JE, Litzow MR, Appelbaum FR, et al: Allogeneic, syngeneic, and autologous marrow transplantation for Hodgkin's disease: the 21 year Seattle experience. J Clin Oncol 11:2342, 1993.

Chopra R, Goldstone AH, Pearce R, et al: Autologous versus allogeneic bone marrow transplantation for non-Hodgkin's lymphoma: a case controlled analysis of the European Bone Marrow Transplant Group Registry data. J Clin Oncol 10:1690, 1992.

Loiseau HA, Hartmann O, Valteau D, et al: High-dose chemotherapy containing busulfan followed by bone marrow transplantation in 24 children with refractory or relapsed non-Hodgkin's lymphoma. Bone Marrow Transplant 8:465, 1991.

Williams CD, Goldatone AH, Pearce R, et al: Autologous bone marrow transplantation for pediatric Hodgkin's disease: a case matched comparison with adult patients by the European Bone Marrow Transplant Group Lymphoma Registry. J Clin Oncol 11:2243, 1993.

NEUROBLASTOMA

Landenstein R, Lasset C, Philip T: Treatment duration before bone marrow transplantation in stage IV neuroblastoma. Lancet 340:916, 1992.

Philip T, Landenstein R, Zucker JM, et al: Double megatherapy and autologous bone marrow transplantation for advanced neuroblastoma: the LMCE2 study. Br J Cancer 67:119, 1993.

BRAIN TUMORS

Kalifa C, Hartmann O, Demeocq F, et al: High-dose busulfan and thiotepa with autologous bone marrow transplantation in childhood malignant brain tumors: a phase I study. Bone Marrow Transplant 9:227, 1992.

SOLID TUMORS

Garaventa A, Hartmann O, Bernard JL, et al: Autologous bone marrow transplantation for pediatric Wilms' tumor: the experience of the European Bone Marrow Transplantation Solid Tumor Registry. Med Pediatr Oncol 22:11, 1994.

Horowitz ME, Kinsella TJ, Wexler LH, et al: Total body irradiation and autologous bone marrow transplant in the treatment of high-risk Ewing's sarcoma and rhabdomyosarcoma. J Clin Oncol 11:1911, 1993.

Seeger RC, Reynolds CP: Treatment of high-risk solid tumors of childhood with intensive therapy and autologous bone marrow transplantation. Pediatr Clin North Am 38:393, 1991.

IMMUNE DEFICIENCY SYNDROMES

Blaese RM: Development of gene therapy for immunodeficiency: adenosine deaminase deficiency. Pediatr Res 33(Suppl 1):S49, 1993.

Blanche S, Caniglia M, Girault D, et al: Treatment of hemophagocytic lymphohistiocytosis with chemotherapy and bone marrow transplantation: a single center study of 22 cases. Blood 78:51, 1991.

Filipovich AH, Shapiro RS, Ramsay NKC, et al: Unrelated donor bone marrow transplantation for correction of lethal congenital immunodeficiencies. Blood 80:270, 1992.

Fischer A, Landais P, Friedrich W, et al: Bone marrow transplantation (BMT) in Europe for primary immunodeficiencies other than severe combined immunodeficiency: a report from the European Group for BMT and the European Group for Immunodeficiency. Blood 83:1149, 1994.

FANCONI ANEMIA

Flowers MED, Doney KC, Storb R, et al: Marrow transplantation for Fanconi anemia with or without leukemic transformation: an update of the Seattle experience. Bone Marrow Transplant 9:167, 1992.

Hows JM, Chapple M, Marsh JCW, et al: Bone marrow transplantation for Fanconi's anemia: the Hammersmith experience 1977–89. Bone Marrow Transplant 4:629, 1989.

METABOLIC STORAGE DISEASES

Krivit W, Shapiro E, Hoogerbrugge PM, et al: State of the art review bone marrow transplantation treatment for storage diseases. Bone Marrow Transplant 10(Suppl 1):87, 1992.

Parkman R: Bone marrow transplantation for immunodeficiency and metabolic diseases. Leukemia 7:1100, 1993.

THALASSEMIA

Giardini C, Angelucci E, Lucarelli G, et al: Bone marrow transplantation for thalassemia, experience in Pesaro, Italy. Am J Pediatr Hematol Oncol 16:6, 1994.

Walters MC, Thomas ED: Bone marrow transplantation for thalassemia, the USA experience. Am J Pediatr Hematol Oncol 16:11, 1994.

SICKLE CELL ANEMIA

Giardini C, Galimberti M, Lucarelli G, et al: Bone marrow transplantation in sickle-cell anemia in Pesaro. Bone Marrow Transplant 12(Suppl 1):122, 1993.

Johnson FL, Mentzer WC, Kalinyak KA, et al: Bone marrow transplantation for sickle cell disease, the United States experience. Am J Pediatr Hematol Oncol 16:22, 1994.

MATCHING AND REJECTION

Quinones RR: Hematopoietic engraftment and graft failure after bone marrow transplantation. Am J Pediatr Hematol Oncol 15:3, 1993.

GRAFT-VERSUS-HOST DISEASE

Atkinson K: Chronic graft-versus-host disease, review. Bone Marrow Transplant 5:69, 1990.

Nash RA, Pepe MS, Storb R, et al: Acute graft-versus-host disease: analysis of risk factors after allogeneic marrow transplantation and prophylaxis with cyclosporine and methotrexate. Blood 80:1838, 1992.

Sullivan KM, Agura E, Anasetti C, et al: Chronic graft-versus-host disease and other late complications of bone marrow transplantation. Semin Hematol 28:250, 1991.

PRINCIPLES OF IMMUNOSUPPRESSION

Martin PJ: Pharmacologic approaches for prevention and treatment of acute graft-versus-host disease. Clin Aspects Autoimmun 4:8, 1990.

Vogelsang GB, Farmer E, Hess A, et al: Thalidomide for the treatment of chronic graft-versus-host disease. N Engl J Med 326:1055, 1992.

LATE EFFECTS

Katsanis E, Shapiro RS, Robison LL, et al: Thyroid dysfunction following bone marrow transplantation: long term follow-up of 80 pediatric patients. Bone Marrow Transplant 5:335, 1990.

Sanders JE: Endocrine problems in children after bone marrow transplant for hematologic malignancies. Bone Marrow Transplant 8:2, 1991.

Thompson CB, Sanders JE, Flournoy N, et al: The risks of central nervous system relapse and leukoencephalopathy in patients receiving marrow transplants for acute leukemia. Blood 67:195, 1986.

Wingard JR, Plotnick LP, Freemer CS, et al: Growth in children after bone marrow transplantation: busulfan plus cyclophosphamide versus cyclophosphamide plus total body irradiation. Blood 79:1068, 1992.

Witherspoon RP, Fisher LD, Schoch G, et al: Secondary cancers after bone marrow transplantation for leukemia or aplastic anemia. N Engl J Med 321:784, 1989.

PART XV

Allergic Disorders*

R. Michael Sly

CHAPTER 133

Allergy and the Immunologic Basis of Atopic Disease

Allergy is a specific, acquired change in host reactivity mediated by an immunologic mechanism and causing an untoward physiologic response. This definition precludes the use of the term *allergy* for disorders in which immunologic mechanisms have not been demonstrated. For example, adverse reactions after food or drug ingestion in some people may resemble typical allergic reactions without any evidence of an immunologic basis. Sometimes there is a biochemical basis for the reaction, as in diarrhea after milk ingestion in people with disaccharidase deficiency. When there is no reason to suspect that allergy is responsible for signs or symptoms, the use of immunologic methods in diagnosis or treatment is irrational.

The terms *antigen* and *allergen* are often used interchangeably, but not all antigens are good allergens and vice versa. For example, tetanus and diphtheria toxoids are highly antigenic but are only rarely responsible for allergic reactions. On the other hand, ragweed pollen protein, one of the most potent allergens, is not a particularly potent antigen by immunologic criteria. Most naturally occurring allergens share several common characteristics. They are protein in part, are acidic with isoelectric points of 2–5.5, and have molecular weights of 10,000–70,000 d. Molecules smaller than 10,000 d would be unable to bridge the gap between adjacent immunoglobulin E (IgE) antibody molecules on the surface of mast cells, a requirement for release of the mediators of the allergic reaction. Molecules larger than 70,000 d would not easily pass through mucosal surfaces to reach IgE-forming plasma cells.

The use of the term *atopy* or *atopic* in designating an allergic reaction implies a hereditary factor expressed as susceptibility to hay fever, asthma, and eczematoid dermatitis in the families of affected individuals. The atopic patient has a predisposition to selective synthesis of IgE antibodies to common environmental antigens. IgE production is under genetic control, and there appears to be an association between human leukocyte antigen (HLA) histocompatibility types and IgE-mediated hypersensitivity responses. In experimental models, the IgE antibody response is regulated by antigen-specific helper and suppressor T cells that secrete IgE-binding factors that potentiate or suppress the reaction. Atopy is often familial and may be localized to chromosome 11q13. Atopic individuals may differ from nonatopic individuals in their ability to regulate IgE antibody production or to dispose of allergens coming in contact with mucosal surfaces. They may also have defective control of mediator release or generation or have impaired mediator inactivation processes.

The formation of IgE antibodies is revealed in atopic persons by "wheal and flare" reactions on skin testing with allergenic extracts. However, the capacity to form IgE antibody is not limited to atopic individuals because IgE is found in the serum and on mast cells of most normal people. Under intense allergen exposure, as in certain occupations, or in response to particular allergens, such as ascaris, nonatopic individuals may form large quantities of allergen-specific IgE antibodies. Atopic people, however, form IgE antibodies on exposure to such common environmental substances as pollens and mites in house dust, and this distinguishes them from the nonatopic. Among patients with asthma, hay fever, or atopic dermatitis, we can identify "highly atopic" subjects and others with lesser atopic tendencies.

It is useful to characterize immunologic reactions in terms of the reactants involved in order to understand the mechanism by which injury occurs. Immunologically mediated tissue injury may occur as a result of the interaction of humoral antibody with antigen or of the interaction of antigen with lymphocytes (cell-mediated or delayed-type hypersensitivity). There are three forms of humoral antibody-antigen reactions, two of which occur on the surface of cells and the third in the extracellular fluids.

Of the two reactions occurring on the surface of the cells, *type I hypersensitivity, mediated by IgE* (immediate type or anaphylactic hypersensitivity), is of greatest interest to the allergist. In this circumstance, circulating basophils and tissue mast cells, the latter strategically located around blood vessels, become "sensitized" through the binding of IgE antibodies to their surface receptors. This is the initial event in the production of immune tissue injury following allergen interaction with cell-bound IgE antibody molecules; the ultimate outcome of the reaction depends on a broad spectrum of secondary events involving various types of lymphoid cells, inflammatory cells, mediator-producing cells, and the soluble products derived not only from all of these cells but from other tissues (platelets, endothelial cells) at the site of the reaction. For example, in particularly intense allergen-induced reactions in the skin, the initial wheal and flare does not entirely disappear but is replaced by an inflammatory lesion that reaches its maximal size at 6–12 hr and disappears in 24–72 hr. This late cutaneous response depends upon recruitment of inflammatory cells (polymorphonuclear leukocytes, eosinophils, and mononuclear cells) by chemotactic factors released in the early response. Late-phase reactions also occur in the lung and nose.

The terms *reaginic IgE, IgE reagins,* and *homocytotropic antibodies* refer to molecules with activities against specific allergens, such as ragweed pollen, whereas "nonspecific" IgE molecules are found in the serum and tissues of all normal individuals. The "normal" role of IgE antibody appears to be to defend the host against tissue-invasive parasites. In humans the ability to

*Adapted from 13th edition sections by Elliot F. Ellis.

induce antigen-specific release of mediators from mast cells and basophils is principally confined to antibodies of the IgE class.

IgE antibodies, like IgA antibodies, are synthesized by plasma cells located predominantly under mucosal surfaces and particularly in the respiratory and gastrointestinal tracts. IgE-forming plasma cells arise following antigen-stimulated differentiation of B cells or their precursors.

Chemical modifications of antigens used in immunotherapy of allergic diseases suppress IgE responses. Although the control of IgE antibody production is better known for animals than for humans, there is good reason to believe that similar mechanisms occur in the human. The association of IgE responses with HLA-linked immune response (IR) genes has been shown for several allergens (ragweed antigen Ra3 and HLA-A2, ragweed antigen Ra5 and HLA-B7, rye grass antigen I and HLA-B8). IgE synthesis in general, and specifically hypersensitivity, is genetically determined by immune cells, probably the specific helper T cells. Bone marrow transplantation from an atopic donor to a nonatopic recipient transfers the allergic diathesis to the recipient. Macrophages and dendritic cells process antigen for presentation to CD_4 (helper T) cells, which are activated by interleukin (IL)-1. As a result, these T cells differentiate into TH2 cells, which after activation by processed antigen can synthesize IL-3, IL-4, IL-5, and granulocyte-macrophage colony-stimulating factor (GM-CSF) as well as other cytokines (Fig 133–1). IL-4 plays an important role in isotype switching of B cells from synthesis of IgM and IgG to synthesis of IgE. For optimal IgE synthesis, IL-5 (a non-isotype B cell growth factor) and IL-6 (a nonisotype B cell differentiation factor) are also needed. IL-5 and GM-CSF also induce eosinophil differentiation. IL-3 and IL-4 are mast cell growth factors. Gamma interferon, produced by another subset of T lymphocytes, can inhibit IL-4–dependent IgE synthesis and IL-4–induced expression of low-affinity IgE receptors (CD_{23}) on B cells.

Once formed, IgE antibody becomes reversibly bound or "fixed" to surface receptors of mast cells and basophils. The binding of IgE to its receptor (F_ER) involves the C4 and C3 domains of the Fc portion of the immunoglobulin molecule. In nonatopic individuals, only 20–50% of the receptors are occupied by IgE molecules. In atopic individuals with high serum IgE concentrations, a larger percentage, up to almost 100%, of their basophil and mast cell receptors is occupied by IgE. Once binding of IgE occurs, the basophils and mast cells are "sensitized." Upon subsequent contact with this specific allergen, and if cell-bound IgE molecules are sufficiently numerous, allergen may bridge adjacent IgE molecules, causing an interaction between the IgE receptors. This causes a series of biochemical reactions (activation of methyltransferases, phospholipid methylation, Ca^{2+} influx, and activation of the phospholipid diacylglycerol cycle). This results in fusion of the mast cell granules with the mast cell plasma membrane, causing release of pharmacologically active substances (such as histamine), known as chemical mediators. The released mediators act on tissue receptors to cause symptoms. The reaction is largely reversible; the mast cells and basophils participating in the reaction are not lysed, and the effects of mediators are only temporary. Although aggregated IgE can fix late components of the complement system through an alternative pathway, participation of the complement system in IgE-mediated hypersensitivity disorders has not been shown. Newly synthesized chemical mediators are released by the mast cell 6–8 hr after antigenic stimulation. Thus, the late-phase reaction may last 12–48 hr.

Interactions of cytokines with endothelial cells are important in localization of eosinophils at the site of the allergic reaction. Activation of endothelial cells by IL-1 causes upregulation of endothelial adhesion molecules, including E-selectin (endothelial leukocyte adhesion molecule-1), intercellular adhesion molecule-1 (ICAM-1), and vascular cell adhesion molecule-1 (VCAM-1). Endothelial activation by IL-4 results in upregulation of VCAM-1. Lectin-binding regions of selectins interact with ligands on leukocytes, causing rolling of leukocytes over endothelial cells. Interactions with the integrins, ICAM-1 and VCAM-1, then arrest the leukocytes, facilitating movement out of the vasculature at the site of the allergic reaction. The ligand for VCAM-1 is very late activation antigen-4; it is found on eosinophils but not neutrophils.

The usual tests for inhalant or food sensitivity make use of the reaction that occurs on the surface of mast cells between antigen and IgE antibody. Small amounts of extracts of pollens, molds, danders, and foods are introduced into the patient's skin by scratch, puncture, or intradermal techniques. If IgE antibody specific for the test antigen is bound to the subject's mast cells, the interaction of injected antigen with cell-bound IgE releases histamine, a potent vasoactive agent that causes increased capillary permeability and dilatation and axon reflex stimulation, leading to the familiar wheal and flare reaction. The prototypic *anaphylactic* or *IgE-mediated* disease is ragweed

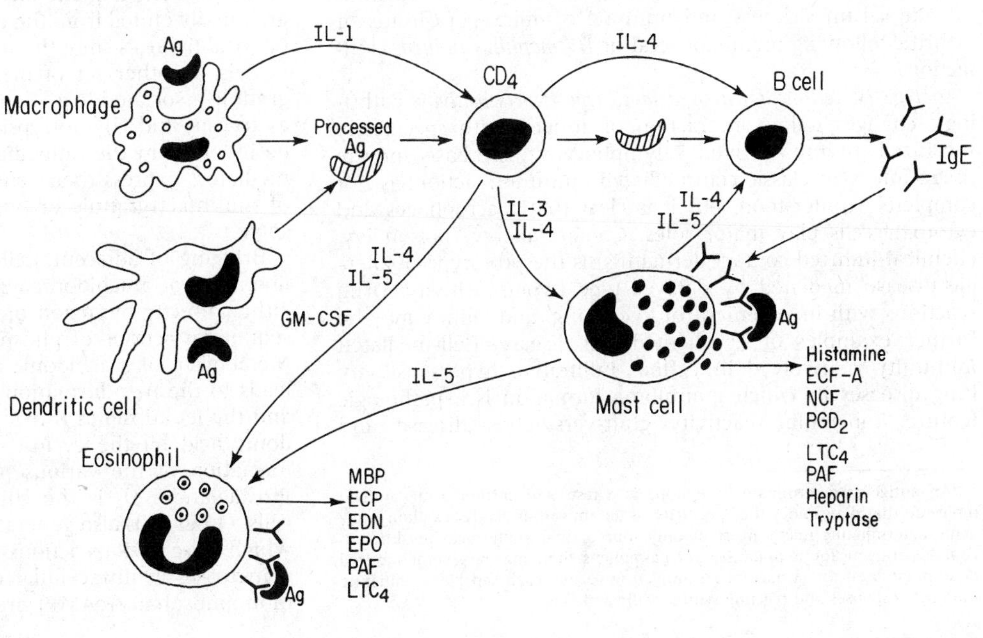

Figure 133–1. Sequential events that lead to allergic sensitization and subsequent allergic reactions after exposure to allergen. (Ag = antigen; IL = interleukin; GM-CSF = granulocyte-macrophage colony-stimulating factor; ECF-A = eosinophil chemotactic factor of anaphylaxis; NCF = neutrophil chemotactic factor; PGD_2 = prostaglandin D_2; LTC_4 = leukotriene C_4; PAF = platelet-activating factor; MBP = major basic protein; ECP = eosinophil cationic protein; IgE = immunoglobulin E; EDN = eosinophil-derived neurotoxin; EPO = eosinophil peroxidase.)

hay fever. Others include anaphylactic reactions to insect venom, food-induced urticaria, and allergic conjunctivitis or rhinitis.

In *type II hypersensitivity (cytotoxic) interactions* between antigen and antibody at cell surfaces, IgG or IgM immunoglobulins react with antigenic determinants* that either are integral parts of the cell membrane or have become adsorbed to or incorporated into the membrane. In contrast to the IgE or anaphylactic type of reaction, this second kind of reaction activates the complement system in most instances, and the involved cell is destroyed. An example of this type of immunologic injury occurs after transfusion of incompatible red cells. The recipient's isohemagglutinins (antibodies directed against determinants on the surface of the red cells) react with the incompatible cells, the complement system is activated, and sequential action of complement proteins leads to lysis of the cell. Analogous immune injury may involve platelets or leukocytes. In the case of drug-induced immune hemolytic anemias, various other mechanisms are also involved ("innocent bystander," drug adsorption).

The *type III immunopathologic mechanism* (Arthus or immune-complex) of tissue injury involving humoral antibody and antigen occurs in the extracellular spaces. At certain ratios of antigen to antibody, antigen-antibody complexes are formed that are "toxic" to tissues in which they are deposited. For example, complexes may lodge in the filtering organs of the body (such as the kidney or lung) or infiltrate the walls of small blood vessels, activating the complement cascade. There is release of biologically active substances, including factors that are chemotactic for polymorphonuclear (PMN) leukocytes, which are attracted to the site. With phagocytosis of the complexes, the PMNs are lysed, and basic proteins and proteolytic enzymes are released that damage tissue. Immune complex disease is responsible for up to 90% of immunologic glomerulonephritis in humans.

Toxic complex injury involves cooperation between different antibodies in the production of tissue injury. The deposition of immune complexes containing IgG_1, IgG_2, IgG_3, and IgM in small blood vessels in the kidney in experimental serum sickness in animals depends on an increase in the permeability of these vessels. This is brought about by histamine liberated in the course of a simultaneous interaction of IgE antibody and antigen, which leads to "leakiness" of the capillaries and prepares them to receive the toxic complexes. Such deposition can be largely prevented by pretreatment with antihistamine drugs in the animal model. Examples of type III reactions include serum sickness and immune complex pericarditis or arthritis following meningococcal or *Haemophilus influenzae* infection.

In *type IV, cell-mediated* or *delayed-type hypersensitivity*, pathologic changes follow interaction of antigen with specifically sensitized, thymus-derived T lymphocytes. The basis for the tissue injury in classic cell-mediated immune reactions is not completely understood, but it is clear that macrophages and cytotoxic cells play major roles. Contact allergy (poison ivy, chemical-induced contact dermatitis) is the prototype of allergic disease mediated by delayed-type hypersensitivity. Drug reactions with involvement of liver, lung, and kidney may be further examples of T cell–mediated disease. Cell-mediated immunity is involved in certain infiltrative hypersensitivity lung diseases in which granuloma formation is a pathologic feature. Tuberculin reactivity, graft-versus-host disease, and tissue transplant reaction are additional type IV hypersensitivity reactions.

*An antigenic determinant or epitope is a restricted portion of an antigen molecule that determines the specificity of an antigen-antibody reaction. Antigenic determinants may consist of only four or five amino acid residues. In complex antigens found in nature, such as pollens, there may be several hundred determinants on the surface of an antigen molecule, each capable of initiating immune responses and reacting with specific antibody.

133.1 Chemical Mediators of Allergic Reactions and Mechanisms of Release

Mast cells play the central role in immediate hypersensitivity responses. Considerable heterogeneity probably exists among populations of mast cells and basophils in humans; differences among these metachromatically staining cells can be measured by morphologic, immunologic, biochemical, and functional criteria. Mast cells and basophils are involved not only in IgE-mediated reactions but also in other chronic inflammatory disorders, for example, inflammatory bowel disease, rheumatoid arthritis, and parasitic infections.

The critical triggering event in mast cell degranulation and release of chemical mediators of allergic injury is the cross-linking of receptor-bound IgE antibodies (which may be viewed as an extension of the receptor) by multivalent specific antigen. Although antigen is usually the principal factor in causing the approximation of IgE receptors, this can be accomplished in the absence of antigen or even of IgE antibody, for example, by the action of purified antibody to the IgE receptor itself. Other stimuli can also cause mast cell activation without involving antigen and cell-bound IgE. These stimuli include products of activation of the complement system (C3a, C5a), kinins, neutrophil-derived lysosomal basic proteins, and lymphokines.

Whatever the nature of the mast cell surface signal that acts as the degranulation stimulus, a series of biochemical reactions takes place that results in granule discharge. Activation of a serine esterase, utilization of intracellular energy stores, calcium influx or remobilization of intracellular calcium, and changes in the mast cell cytoskeleton such as polymerization of microtubules occur during mediator release. Changes in membrane phospholipid metabolism also occur, including methylation and activation of phospholipases and generation of phospholipid by-products, which participate in the fusion of the mast cell granules with the cell membrane, leading to extrusion of the granules. Once discharged from the mast cell, the granules, which are relatively water insoluble, may remain intact for hours. The preformed mediators, such as histamine, eosinophil chemotactic factor, and other chemotactic factors, are rapidly eluted from the granule matrix and act immediately on local tissues—smooth muscles and endothelial cells in blood vessels. Another set of mediators, which are preformed but granule associated (e.g., heparin, arylsulfatase B, enzymes such as trypsin and chymotrypsin, and inflammatory factors) may be involved in the immediate and late-phase reactions; these mediators express their activity either while they are still part of the intact granule or only after the granule begins to dissolve.

Bridging of adjacent, cell-bound IgE molecules also causes liberation of arachidonic acid from membrane phospholipids, either directly by action of phospholipase A_2 or indirectly by sequential actions of phospholipase C and diglyceride lipase. Metabolism of arachidonic acid by the lipoxygenase pathway leads to the new formation of 5-hydroxyeicosatetraenoic acid and the leukotrienes B_4, C_4, D_4, and E_4. Metabolism of arachidonic acid by the cyclo-oxygenase pathway results in new formation of the various prostaglandins and thromboxanes. Prostaglandin D_2 is the chief prostaglandin product of mast cells. Other cells also generate prostaglandins and leukotrienes, which have various actions (Table 133–1).

Increases in intracellular concentrations of cyclic adenosine monophosphate (cAMP) are associated with inhibition of re-

■ TABLE 133–1 Chemical Mediators of Allergic Reactions

Mediator	Structural Characteristics	Actions
Histamine (preformed)	5-β-Imidazolylethylamine MW 111	H_1 receptors: Increase in venular permeability Contraction of smooth muscle Increase in cyclic GMP levels Generation of prostaglandins Increase in nasal mucus production Positive chemokinetic effect on neutrophils and eosinophils* Positive chemotactic effect on neutrophils and eosinophils Bronchial irritant receptor stimulation Pruritus H_2 receptors: Increase in vascular permeability Increase in gastric acid secretion Positive chemokinetic effect on neutrophils and eosinophils Negative chemotactic effect on neutrophils and eosinophils Inhibition of T-cell responses Inhibition of basophil (not mast cell) mediator response Augmentation of gastric acid secretion Stimulation of airway mucus secretion Increase in cyclic AMP Increase in chronotropic and inotropic effects on heart
ECF-A tetrapeptides (preformed)	Val/Ala-Gly-Ser-Glu MW 400–500	Chemotactic attraction and deactivation of eosinophils Increase in eosinophil complement receptors
ECF-oligopeptides (preformed)	Peptides MW 1,500–3,000	Chemotactic attraction and deactivation of eosinophils and mononuclear leukocytes
HMW-NCF (preformed)	Neutral protein MW 600,000	Chemotactic attraction and deactivation of neutrophils
PAF (newly formed)	AGEPC MW 551 (hexadecyl), MW 523 (octadecyl)	Aggregation of platelets and secretion of amines Neutrophil aggregation and enzyme release Production of prostaglandins and thromboxanes by platelets Increase in vascular permeability Mimics physiologic and intravascular sequelae of IgE-mediated human systemic anaphylaxis Potent chemotactic attraction and activation of eosinophils Prolonged increase in bronchial hyper-responsiveness
Heparin (preformed)	Acidic proteoglycan MW 60,000 (human)	Anticoagulation (antithrombin III binding activity) Anticomplementary activity (at several sites) Augments inactivation of histamine
Arachidonic acid (newly formed) Cyclo-oxygenase products: PGD_2 (newly formed)	20-carbon fatty acid	Contraction of smooth muscle Bronchoconstriction Vasodilatation (skin) Chemokinesis of granulocytes Chronotropic effect on heart Increase in vascular permeability Sneezing Rhinorrhea
PGE_2 (newly formed)		Relaxation of smooth muscle Bronchodilatation Vasodilatation
$PGF_{2\alpha}$ (newly formed)		Bronchoconstriction Constriction of microvasculature and pulmonary vasculature
PGI_2 (newly formed)		Relaxation of smooth muscle Pulmonary vasodilation
TXA_2 (newly formed)		Bronchoconstriction Constriction of microvasculature Platelet aggregation
Lipoxygenase products: LTC_4, LTD_4, LTE_4 (newly formed)	MW 400–600	Smooth-muscle contraction and bronchoconstriction, especially of peripheral airway Airway mucus secretion Dilatation and increased permeability of microvasculature Constriction of coronary and cerebral arteries Depression of myocardial contractility
LTB_4 (newly formed)	MW 400	Chemotactic and chemokinetic for neutrophils and eosinophils Increased leukocyte adherence to endothelium Leukocyte activation Suppression of T-lymphocyte function
HETEs (newly formed)		Chemotaxis and chemokinesis of eosinophils and neutrophils

Chemotactic migration requires a concentration gradient from the stimulus side. Movement in the absence of a gradient of the stimulus is termed "positive chemokinesis."
GMP = guanosine monophosphate; AMP = adenosine monophosphate; ECF = eosinophil chemotactic factor; A = anaphylaxis; HMW = high molecular weight; NCF = neutrophil chemotactic factor; PAF = platelet-activating factor; PG = prostaglandin; TXA_2 = thromboxane A_2; MW = molecular weight; Ig = immunoglobulin; HETEs = hydroxyeicosatetraenoic acids; AGEPC = acetyl-glyceryl-ether-phosphorylcholine.

lease of mediators from mast cells. Prostaglandins of the E series and β-adrenergic agonists can cause increases in cAMP.

Factors Not Derived from Mast Cells That Participate in Immediate-Type Hypersensitivity Diseases

Eosinophil-derived molecules of potent biologic activity may contribute to tissue injury in IgE-mediated and other diseases. *Eosinophil major basic protein* (MBP) causes dose-dependent epithelial damage in guinea pig trachea and in human bronchial epithelium. Immunofluorescent staining discloses extracellular deposition of MBP in areas of airway epithelial destruction in patients who have died of status asthmaticus. If MBP causes destruction of airway epithelium, it may play a role in the bronchial hyper-responsiveness characteristic of asthma. Deposition of MBP is also demonstrable in lesions of atopic dermatitis and often in those of chronic urticaria. MBP also stimulates histamine release from human basophils and causes a wheal and flare reaction when injected into human skin. In a variety of in vitro systems (bacteria, parasites, tumor cells), *eosinophil peroxidase* causes injury. Both eosinophil-derived neurotoxin and eosinophil cationic protein cause damage to myelinated cells in animals.

Kinins are another system of proteins activated in inflammatory processes that have amplifier and effector properties. Their activities include chemotaxis, increased vascular permeability, and smooth-muscle contraction. Bradykinin, a nonapeptide, is the most important product of the kinin system. The kinin, complement, and clotting systems are interrelated. Activation of Hageman factor (factor XII) is the initial step in kinin generation and amplification, with positive feedback loops resembling those in the complement pathway. Hageman factor (HF) is activated by tissue injury from a number of agents, including IgG aggregates and immune complexes. HF and complexes of high-molecular-weight kininogen and prekallikrein and high-molecular-weight kininogen and factor XI are bound together. HF appears to autoactivate to form activated HF (HFa), which converts prekallikrein to kallikrein. Kallikrein digests high-molecular-weight kininogen to liberate the vasoactive peptide bradykinin. Bradykinin has potent contractile effects on smooth muscle, causes increased vascular permeability, and dilates peripheral arterioles. It also stimulates pain receptors. At least two other plasma kinins have biologic activities similar to those of bradykinin. The role of bradykinin in allergic disease is uncertain. Several patients with cold urticaria have had increased concentrations of bradykinin in plasma.

Platelet-activating factor (PAF), a phospholipid, is synthesized by a variety of cells, including vascular endothelial cells, monocytes, macrophages, neutrophils, and especially eosinophils, as well as platelets. It is a potent inducer of increased vascular permeability. Its inhalation causes acute transient bronchoconstriction in both normal and asthmatic subjects. Bronchial hyper-responsiveness follows and may persist for weeks in normal subjects but may not occur in patients with asthma, possibly because of hyper-responsiveness already induced by endogenous PAF. Mediators released or formed in response to bridging of cell-bound IgE molecules, such as eosinophil chemotactic factors and LTB_4, may attract eosinophils and other cells that synthesize PAF, which in turn may cause a late-phase reaction several hours after the initial antigen-antibody reaction occurred.

Type I hypersensitivity reactions involve early-phase (10–30 min) and late-phase (4–8 hr) reactions. Early reactions after antigenic stimulation include vasodilation, edema formation from increased vascular permeability, smooth-muscle constriction (bronchoconstriction), and mucus production. This response is due to the release of preformed and newly synthesized mast cell mediators. This response may be treated with antihistamines and mast cell membrane stabilizers such as cromolyn sodium. The late-phase reaction perpetuates the early changes of vascular permeability but includes the recruitment of inflammatory cell types in addition to mast cells. These recruited cells (eosinophils, neutrophils, lymphocytes) are located in the perivascular space. Erythema, edema, and induration are present as is airway hyperirritability to rechallenge with allergens. This late, chronic inflammatory reaction probably contributes to the hyper-responsiveness found in allergic children with asthma, rhinitis, and atopic dermatitis. Late-phase reactions respond poorly to antihistamines or bronchodilator therapy but may respond to corticosteroids.

Serotonin (5-hydroxytryptamine) is a vasoactive amine that, in experimental animals, induces contraction of smooth muscle and increases vascular permeability. Ninety per cent of the body's stores of serotonin are found in the gastrointestinal tract, with the remainder divided between the central nervous system and platelets. Human mast cells lack serotonin. Serotonin has been reported to induce bronchoconstriction in asthmatics but not in normal people, but it has no significant role in immediate hypersensitivity reactions in humans. It is associated distinctively with diarrhea in the carcinoid syndrome.

While not mediators in the same sense as products released from mast cells or basophils, certain components of the *complement system* have activities that may contribute to allergic reactions. (1) Aggregated IgE can initiate complement system activity in vitro through the alternative pathway; this probably does not occur in vivo because of the large quantities of IgE required. (2) Certain "split" or "cleavage" products of the complement cascade, C3a and C5a, can induce mediator (histamine) release from basophils and from mast cells in the skin, producing wheal and flare reactions. C3a and C5a have been termed *anaphylatoxins* because they release histamine and resemble components of serum capable of causing guinea pig anaphylaxis. C5a and, to a much lesser extent, C3a are chemotactic for various leukocytes. Neutrophils attracted to the site of complement activation by C5a may degranulate, releasing basic lysosomal proteins that trigger mediator liberation from mast cells. The result in the skin is urticaria mimicking an antigen-IgE reaction. Small *N*-formylated peptides, derived from bacterial products, also possess potent granulocyte chemotactic activity and may operate in a manner similar to that of C5a to cause urticaria. (3) A kinin-like peptide derived from C2 as a result of reduced functional activity of the inhibitor of C1-esterase (C1s) is thought to mediate the angioedema observed in hereditary angioedema.

From the foregoing considerations it is evident that the signs and symptoms of typical, immediate-type allergic reactions such as anaphylaxis, though most often involving the IgE mechanism, may result from non-IgE immunologic mechanisms or from nonimmunologic mechanisms.

Chung KF, Barnes PJ: Effects of platelet activating factor on airway calibre, airway responsiveness, and circulating cells in asthmatic subjects. Thorax 44:108, 1989.
Gleich GJ, Flavahan NA, Fujisawa T, et al: The eosinophil as a mediator of damage to respiratory epithelium: A model for bronchial hyperreactivity. J Allergy Clin Immunol 81:776, 1988.
Holgate ST: Asthma: past, present and future. Eur Respir J 6:1507, 1993.
Leung D, Kamada M: Developments in allergy. Curr Opin Pediatr 1:27, 1989.

CHAPTER 134
Diagnosis

GENERAL AND SPECIFIC METHODS OF DIAGNOSIS

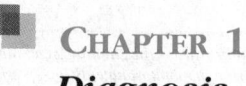

ALLERGY HISTORY. The allergy history differs from the general medical history with respect to the nature of inquiries into possible causes of the symptoms. These inquiries include a detailed history of "exposure" to potential allergens. The frequency, duration, intensity, location, and progression of symptoms are relevant to a determination of their possible causes and to decisions about the types of therapy that may be effective. Seasonal symptoms may correlate with exposure to seasonal allergens such as pollens. Exposure to the highest concentrations of house dust mites, the chief source of allergens in house dust, often occurs at the end of the summer because high humidity favors mite proliferation. Allergy to house dust mites, however, usually causes perennial symptoms. Allergy to pet dogs or cats that have access to the house also usually causes perennial symptoms. Patients may deny an association between exposure to the animal and their symptoms because they fail to recognize that contamination of the house and its furnishings with animal dander results in continual exposure to allergen despite only intermittent exposure to the animal itself. Onset or worsening of symptoms shortly after acquisition of an animal or relief when the child is away from the house should arouse suspicion.

A relationship between symptoms and where they occur may suggest a cause. Exposure to pollens is often more intense outdoors than indoors, especially when windows are closed and air conditioners are operating. Onset of symptoms shortly after moving to a different dwelling should suggest an environmental cause. Changes in symptoms during trips away from home may provide helpful clues to the cause. Worsening of symptoms in a damp, musty basement should suggest allergy to fungi. An increase in symptoms at night may suggest increased exposure to allergen in the bedroom, but asthma commonly worsens at night even without exposure to allergens. Weekend remissions suggest a source of allergen at school or the work place.

An association between symptoms and certain activities may be diagnostically helpful. Respiratory symptoms that follow exposure to freshly cut grass suggest allergy to pollen or fungi. Symptoms provoked by dusting or carpet cleaning are often due to allergy to house dust mites. Coughing or wheezing following strenous exercise may occur in children who have asthma. Provocation of coughing by laughter, crying, or exposure to smoke or specific odors also suggests the bronchial hyper-responsiveness characteristic of asthma.

The nature of the symptoms is important. An intermittent, recurrent, dry cough or a cough productive of clear mucus is consistent with asthma, but a chronic persistent cough productive of purulent sputum suggests bronchiectasis or cystic fibrosis. Aspiration of a foreign body often causes a sudden onset of coughing with choking followed by wheezing. Coughing associated with aphonia or dysphonia may be due to a hypopharyngeal or laryngeal foreign body or laryngeal papilloma. Glottic or subglottic obstruction can cause a harsh, barking cough. Paroxysmal coughing suggests pertussis or a bronchial foreign body.

Allergic rhinitis is the most common cause of a chronic or recurrent, clear nasal discharge, especially when this is associated with sneezing or conjunctival itching and injection with excessive tearing. A purulent nasal discharge suggests infection. A postnasal drip caused by allergic rhinitis or sinusitis may cause frequent clearing of the throat, hoarseness, and nocturnal coughing. Intense conjunctival itching associated with photophobia and a viscid, white conjunctival discharge suggest vernal conjunctivitis.

A history of any beneficial or adverse effects of previous treatment may be helpful in establishing the diagnosis as well as guiding further therapy. Improvement of rhinitis in response to an antihistamine suggests allergy rather than infection. Antihistamines often relieve coughing as a result of postnasal drainage associated with allergic rhinitis, but relief of coughing by a bronchodilator suggests asthma.

The immediate family history is relevant. Atopic allergy manifested by allergic rhinitis, asthma, atopic dermatitis, or urticaria and the specific manifestations of these disorders tend to be familial. Asthma may be familial whether or not it is due to allergy. Nonetheless, any of these conditions can also occur without a positive family history.

PHYSICAL EXAMINATION. Results of the physical examination depend upon the duration and severity of the allergic disorder. *Height and weight* should be compared with normal values for age. Both severe asthma and treatment with adrenal corticosteroids can suppress growth. Poor weight gain may suggest cystic fibrosis, a consideration in the differential diagnosis of asthma.

Pulsus paradoxus, the difference in systemic arterial blood pressure during inspiration and expiration, normally does not exceed 10 mm Hg. During acute asthma it is often increased, and the extent to which it exceeds 10 mm Hg is an index of the severity of the airway obstruction. An increase to more than 20 mm Hg indicates moderate or severe airway obstruction. Other possible causes of increased pulsus paradoxus include cystic fibrosis, heart failure, and cardiac tamponade.

Cyanosis resulting from airway obstruction may be evident if arterial oxygen saturation is less than 85%. Need for a marked reduction in intrapleural (high negative) pressure to initiate inspiration through obstructed airways may cause *supraclavicular and intercostal retractions.* Air trapping during expiration may cause bulging of the intercostal spaces during acute asthma. *Flaring of the alae nasi* may be evident. Bobbing of the head with each inspiration indicates *dyspnea* in infants lying supine.

Mouth breathing and a dark discoloration beneath the lower eyelids *(allergic shiners)* indicate nasal obstruction, usually caused by allergic rhinitis. Frequent wrinkling of the nose and the *allergic salute* (habitual wiping of the running nose) also suggest allergic rhinitis. Frequently repeated salutes for months or years elevate the tip of the nose, causing a transverse nasal crease at the junction of the cartilaginous and bony bridge of the nose. A familial transverse nasal groove, inherited as a mendelian dominant trait, is unrelated to rhinitis. *Dennie lines* (Dennie-Morgan folds), wrinkles beneath the lower eyelids, are associated with allergic rhinitis, asthma, and atopic dermatitis.

Digital clubbing is extremely rare in patients with uncomplicated asthma. Its presence suggests a complication such as bronchiectasis or another disease (Table 134–1). Comparison of the depth of the index finger at the base of the nail with its depth at the distal interphalangeal joint is the best method of recognizing digital clubbing. The depth at the base of the nail is normally smaller. A depth at the base of the nail equal to that at the distal interphalangeal joint is 2.5 standard deviations above normal, indicating mild clubbing.

Inspection of the skin may disclose evidence of *atopic dermatitis:* an erythematous, maculopapular eruption, fine scaling, or weeping and oozing with excoriations caused by frequent scratching (see also Chapters 138 and 596). Crusting may be

■ TABLE 134–1 Diseases Associated with Acquired Digital Clubbing

Cardiac	Gastrointestinal
Cyanotic congenital heart disease	Celiac disease
Subacute bacterial endocarditis	Chronic dysentery
Pulmonary	Chronic ulcerative colitis
Abscess	Multiple polyposis
Bronchiectasis	Regional enteritis
Chronic pneumonia	Hepatic
Cystic fibrosis	Biliary cirrhosis
Empyema	Chronic active hepatitis
Malignant neoplasms	Other
Tuberculosis	Hodgkin disease
Pleural	Thyrotoxicosis
Mesothelioma	

evident if there is superimposed infection. The dermatitis may be generalized, but in infancy there is usually a predilection for the cheeks and extensor surfaces of the extremities. In older children involvement of the antecubital spaces, popliteal spaces, and neck is most frequent. In older children lichenification and either hyperpigmentation or hypopigmentation may be evident.

Urticarial lesions may vary in appearance from multiple, 1- to 3-mm wheals with flares typical of cholinergic urticaria to giant wheals that may be associated with angioedema. Wheals are often evanescent, resolving in minutes or hours, only to appear elsewhere. There is often associated *dermographism. Contact dermatitis* is manifested by an erythematous or papulovesicular eruption in the area exposed to the contactant.

Examination of the eyes may disclose the conjunctival injection, excessive tearing, and periorbital edema of *allergic conjunctivitis.* A tenacious, ropy, mucoid conjunctival discharge associated with giant papillae on the upper palpebral conjunctiva, pseudoptosis, and photophobia should suggest *vernal conjunctivitis.*

The *nasal mucosa* may be pale, blue, or pink in children with allergic rhinitis. A profuse, clear nasal discharge is typical. Nasal turbinates are usually edematous. Hypertrophy of tonsils and adenoids is a common complication of allergic rhinitis.

Examination of the chest may disclose an increase in the *anteroposterior diameter* associated with asthma. Comparison of the depth with the width of the chest, measured with chest or obstetric calipers, permits objective evaluation of the chest configuration. The chest of the normal newborn infant is almost circular in cross-section. With growth, the width increases more than the depth (anteroposterior diameter). By the time the child's height reaches 95 cm at approximately 3 yr of age, the depth-width ratio has decreased to 0.75 and remains between 0.70 and 0.75 thereafter. Abnormal increases in the depth-width ratio occur during acute asthma but return toward normal after response to a bronchodilator. A persistent increase in this ratio may occur in children with frequently recurrent or continual asthma episodes but is more characteristic of chronic conditions associated with persistent airway obstruction, such as cystic fibrosis.

In patients with asthma, auscultation of the lungs may disclose *wheezing,* more pronounced on expiration, and prolongation of the expiratory phase of respiration. Wheezing is usually generalized, but there may be minor differences in intensity from segment to segment as a result of segmental atelectasis.

IN VITRO TESTS. A white cell count and a differential count are useful in establishing whether *eosinophilia* is present. The total eosinophil count is more accurate than estimates from blood smears. Eosinophils are subject to a diurnal rhythm, their numbers being highest in the early morning. Because eosinophilia may be intermittent, two or three normal results should be obtained before concluding that there is no eosinophilia. Eosinophil counts in children usually approximate 250 cells/mm^3, but as many as 700/mm^3 may be normal. Eosinophilia of respiratory tract secretions in a patient with rhinorrhea or cough is important. A smear of nasal secretions or bronchial mucus should be stained on a microscopic slide with an eosin-methylene blue stain (Hansel stain). A finding of more than 5–10% eosinophils in nasal secretions supports the diagnosis of allergic rhinitis. Eosinophils in bronchial mucus strongly suggest asthma. Blood eosinophilia in allergic conditions does not generally exceed 15–20% but may rarely be as high as 35% in allergic children in the absence of other disorders known to cause eosinophilia. Eosinophilia is also noted in drug hypersensitivity, rheumatologic disorders (periarteritis nodosa, rheumatoid arthritis), pemphigus, dermatitis herpetiformis, inherited eosinophilia, allergic bronchopulmonary aspergillosis, various malignancies (leukemias, lymphomas, Hodgkin disease), eosinophilic fasciitis, toxic oil syndrome, and eosinophilic-myalgia syndrome (associated with L-tryptophan). Very high eosinophil counts are also noted in parasitic infections with tissue-invading helminths *(Toxocara,* trichinosis, *Echinococcus, Ascaris)* or malaria, and in hypereosinophilic syndrome (Löffler syndrome, pulmonary infiltrates, cardiomyopathy). Corticosteroids cause eosinopenia for up to 6 hr following a dose; the timing of collection of a blood specimen should be appropriately adjusted.

A number of in vitro immunologic tests are of value in allergy diagnosis, such as measurement of the *total and specific immunoglobulin (Ig) content of serum* and determination of the sensitivity of the patient's leukocytes for antigen-induced histamine release. Table 134–2 shows the serum concentrations of IgE in normal Swedish subjects of different ages. Normal values vary in different populations. Mean concentrations of IgE in atopic people are often higher than normal, although a significant number of allergic individuals have normal or low IgE concentrations. Indeed, very low levels of serum IgE may be more useful in excluding atopic disease than elevated levels are in confirming this diagnosis, although patients with low IgE levels can have atopy. In patients with active atopic dermatitis, however, serum IgE levels are usually greatly elevated. Increased total IgE levels during infancy suggest the likelihood of subsequent development of atopic diseases. Table 134–3 shows some nonatopic disorders associated with increased concentrations of serum IgE.

The *radioallergosorbent test* (RAST) determines antigen-specific IgE concentrations in serum (Fig. 134–1). The correlation among RAST results and medical histories, provocation tests, or leukocyte histamine release tests is good. Correlation with allergy skin testing is also good, but RAST is somewhat less sensitive than skin testing. There has been considerable interlaboratory and intralaboratory variability in RAST results on the same specimen. Selection of a reliable laboratory is essential. More recent modifications of in vitro methods for determining specific IgE incorporate different types of solid supports for binding allergen and different labels for anti-human IgE antibody, resulting in colored, luminescent, or fluorescent detectable products. Few direct comparisons of the results of these newer methods with RAST results have been published, but available data suggest that the newer methods are somewhat less reliable than RAST.

In vitro methods of determining specific IgE to several allergens simultaneously have been marketed as screening tests for allergy. The few published data evaluating such methods indi-

■ **TABLE 134–2 Levels of Serum Immunoglobulin E of Normal Subjects at Different Ages***

Age	Range (IU/mL)	Geometric Mean (± 2 SD) (IU/mL)
0 days	<0.1–1.5	0.22 (0.04–1.28)
6 wk	<0.1–2.8	0.69 (0.08–6.12)
3 mo	0.3–3.1	0.82 (0.18–3.76)
6 mo	0.9–28.0	2.68 (0.44–16.26)
9 mo	0.7–8.1	2.36 (0.76–7.31)
1 yr	1.1–10.2	3.49 (0.80–15.22)
2 yr	1.1–49.0	3.03 (0.31–29.48)
3 yr	0.5–7.7	1.80 (0.19–16.86)
4 yr	2.4–34.8	8.58 (1.07–68.86)
7 yr	1.6–60.0	12.89 (1.03–161.32)
10 yr	0.3–215	23.66 (0.98–570.61)
14 yr	1.9–159	20.07 (2.06–195.18)
18–83 yr	1–178	21.20 (Modal values 10–20 IU/mL)†

Data on ages 0–14 years adapted from Kjellman N-IM, Johansson SGO, Roth A: Clin Allergy 6:51, 1976; data on ages 18–83 years adapted from Nye L, Merrett TG, Landon J, et al: Clin Allergy 1:13, 1975. The method used was a double antibody assay. To convert IU/mL to μg/L, multiply by 2.4.

†Modal values—the most common values observed.

■ **TABLE 134–3 Nonallergic Diseases Associated with Increased Serum IgE Concentrations**

Parasitic Infestations
- Ascariasis
- Capillariasis
- Echinococcosis
- Fascioliasis
- Filariasis
- Hookworm
- Onchocerciasis
- Paragonimiasis
- Schistosomiasis
- Strongyloidiasis
- Trichinosis
- Visceral larva migrans

Infections
- Allergic bronchopulmonary aspergillosis
- Candidiasis, systemic
- Coccidioidomycosis
- Cytomegalovirus mononucleosis
- Infectious mononucleosis (Epstein-Barr virus)
- Leprosy

Immunodeficiency
- Hyperimmunoglobulinemia E syndrome
- IgA deficiency, selective
- Nezelof syndrome
- Thymic hypoplasia (DiGeorge anomaly)
- Wiskott-Aldrich syndrome

Neoplastic Diseases
- Hodgkin disease
- IgE myeloma

Other Diseases and Disorders
- Burns
- Cystic fibrosis
- Dermatitis, chronic acral
- Erythema nodosum, streptococcal
- Guillain-Barré syndrome
- Hemosiderosis, primary pulmonary
- Interstitial nephritis, drug-induced
- Kawasaki disease
- Liver disease
- Pemphigoid, bullous
- Polyarteritis nodosa, infantile
- Rheumatoid arthritis

Ig = immunoglobulin

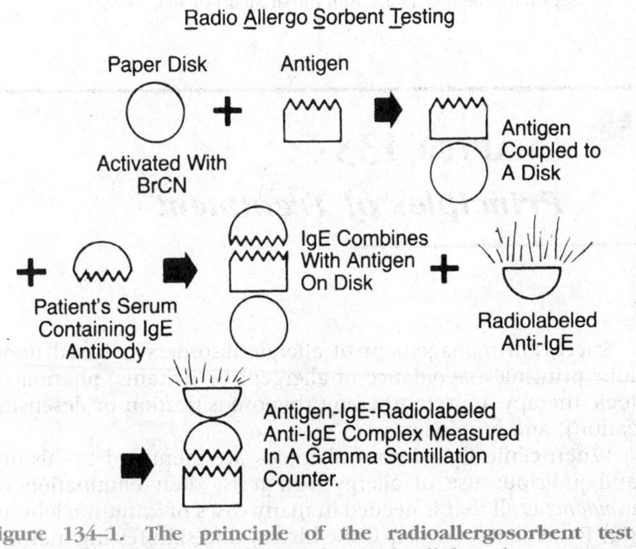

Figure 134–1. The principle of the radioallergosorbent test (RAST). After activation of some form of cellulose (e.g., a paper disk) by cyanogen bromide (BrCN), antigen is coupled covalently to the disk to render the antigen insoluble. Incubation with the patient's serum permits any specific antibodies to bind to the antigen. These antibodies remain bound to antigen after washing. Addition of radiolabeled antihuman immunoglobulin E (IgE) results in labeling of the antigen-IgE complex. The complex is then counted in a gamma scintillation counter. The number of disintegrations per minute is proportional to the amount of specific IgE in the serum sample.

cate that they are relatively insensitive and may fail to identify more than 30% of children with allergy.

Whatever the method for determining specific IgE, results must be correlated with the patient's medical history to establish clinical relevance. In vitro determination of specific IgE has both advantages and disadvantages compared with allergy skin testing (Table 134–4). For experienced clinicians, allergy skin testing remains the method of choice for most patients.

The *leukocyte histamine release test* detects specific IgE antibody attached to the surfaces of peripheral blood basophils by measuring the amount of histamine released in response to challenge with antigen. Incubation of serum with basophils from nonsensitive donors also permits detection of antibody in serum. The amount of histamine release is expressed as a percentage of the total histamine in the cells and varies with the dose of allergen. Small doses of allergen release histamine when cell sensitivity is high. Results generally correlate with allergy skin testing, but skin testing is more sensitive. Approximately 15% of subjects have basophils that do not release histamine in vitro. The complexity of this procedure limits it largely to investigational use.

IN VIVO TESTS. Determination of allergic reactivity through direct *skin testing* of the patient is an important tool in the diagnosis of IgE-mediated sensitivity. A small quantity of allergenic extract is introduced into the skin by prick/puncture (epidermal or epicutaneous method) or by intradermal technique. If the patient's mast cells have IgE antibodies specific for the allergen on their surfaces, an allergen-IgE interaction triggers biochemical events that culminate in release of histamine and other mediators from the mast cell. The histamine acts upon histamine receptors in small vessels, causing increased permeability and dilatation and axon reflex stimulation, which cause a wheal and flare reaction. A positive intradermal reaction is a wheal of at least 5 mm of induration, plus surrounding erythema, occurring 15 min after injection of antigen. The immediate wheal and flare reaction usually peaks within 15–30 min and then resolves. In some patients, however, when the wheal has exceeded 10 mm in diameter, a late-phase reaction may follow. The wheal becomes less distinct, but edema and erythema persist, peak at 6–8 hr, and often resolve by 24 hr. Late-phase reactions are associated with burning, pruritus, and warmth and may become more than double the size of the antecedent immediate reaction. Histologic examination of this late-phase reaction discloses a mixed cellular infiltrate including mononuclear cells, eosinophils, and neutrophils.

The immediate wheal and flare reaction in skin indicates that specific IgE antibody is present also on the mast cells in the tissue of the clinically affected organ. *It does not indicate that*

■ **TABLE 134–4 Determination of Specific IgE by RAST***

Variable	Skin Test	RAST
Risk of allergic reaction	Yes	No
Sensitive†	Very	Less
Affected by antihistamines	Yes	No
Affected by corticosteroids	Usually not	No
Affected by extensive dermatitis or dermographism	Yes	No
Convenience, less patient anxiety	No	Yes
Broad selection of antigens	Yes	No
Immediate results	Yes	No
Expensive	No	Yes
Semiquantitative	No	Yes
Lability of allergens	Yes	No

**RAST as example of other in vitro tests.*

†Because skin tests are more sensitive, they are more reliable than RAST in confirming life-threatening anaphylactic conditions if maximum sensitivity is required (e.g., penicillin, Hymenoptera *hypersensitivity).*

RAST = radioallergosorbent test.

the patient will necessarily have clinical symptoms on exposure to the allergen. Some atopic people have no symptoms following natural exposure to allergens that elicit positive wheal and flare reactions on skin testing. As a general rule, the larger the size of the wheal and flare reaction, the more likely is the test antigen to be clinically relevant. However, one must be cautious not to overinterpret skin test results.

Positive skin tests obtained by the puncture technique correlate better than the more sensitive intradermal tests with measurements of specific IgE antibody and with appearance of clinical symptoms upon exposure to the allergen. With the intradermal technique, only those positive tests obtained with high dilutions (weak concentrations) of extract have as high correlations. If only concentrated solutions of allergenic extract (e.g., 1–100 or 1–10 weight/volume) elicit positive intracutaneous tests, the results will more often than not be of little clinical significance. A histamine control should also be used for comparison. Overinterpretation of such reactions has led to overuse of allergenic extracts in immunotherapy.

Various drugs, extracts that contain irritant materials or substances that are too concentrated, and improper technique can induce nonimmunologic histamine release from tissue mast cells. The resulting wheal and flare reaction cannot be differentiated from that following IgE-allergen interaction, and IgE sensitivity may be mistakenly inferred. Other drugs may inhibit full expression of clinically relevant positive skin tests. Among these are certain adrenergic drugs such as epinephrine and ephedrine and the antihistamines. These drugs should be withheld prior to skin testing (ephedrine for at least 12 hr and most antihistamines for at least 72 hr, hydroxyzine for 5 days, and astemizole for at least 2 mo). To make sure that the skin is capable of reacting to endogenously released histamine, a positive histamine control (histamine phosphate, 1%) should always be used. Corticosteroids administered for only a few days have no appreciable inhibitory effects on IgE-mediated wheal and flare reactions and need not be withheld before skin testing, but administration of systemic corticosteroids daily or on alternate days for as long as 1 yr can suppress cutaneous reactivity to codeine (but not to histamine), suggesting suppression of histamine release from mast cells.

Because the appearance of symptoms on natural exposure may not correlate well with results of skin testing, *provocation testing* by direct exposure of the mucous membrane of the affected organ to the suspected allergen (usually in the form of an extract or aerosol of the material) has received considerable attention. Mucous membrane provocation testing has been used mostly in patients with asthma. As commonly performed, the test requires that increasing concentrations of extracts of various allergens be inhaled by the patient after nebulization with a suitable device. A positive response is manifested by an increase in airway obstruction as monitored with pulmonary function testing. The patient's degree of sensitivity should be determined by skin tests before provocation testing to permit appropriate initial concentrations of allergenic extract to be used. With reasonable precautions the method is safe, and the results of provocation testing correlate well with clinical data. It is time consuming, however, and is not suitable for general use in the office or clinic. Bronchial challenge testing may be most useful in patients who have many positive skin test results, in whom it can guide selection of those allergens that may be most clinically significant for inclusion in an immunotherapy extract mixture. Selection in this way permits a greater concentration of the more clinically significant allergens in the mixture than would be possible if all the allergens possibly implicated by skin testing were to be included. Studies have shown excellent correlations between the results of provocative bronchial challenge testing, RAST, and quantitative intradermal skin tests (end-point dilution method); accordingly, bronchial challenge testing is principally reserved for research purposes. On the other hand, bronchial provocative testing with methacholine or histamine is valuable when the degree of airway reactivity in asthma must be determined and when the diagnosis of asthma is uncertain. Methacholine bronchial challenge testing produces marked bronchoconstriction in patients with asthma compared with normal controls. Atopic children without asthma also have increased hyperresponsiveness to methacholine provocation, suggesting a predisposition to nonspecific bronchial hyperactivity.

Oral provocation should be performed in a facility capable of performing cardiopulmonary resuscitation and is contraindicated if anaphylactic reactions have occurred. Provocation testing with foods has been used to diagnose IgE-mediated food allergy and food-induced atopic dermatitis. Following an elimination diet, food antigens are introduced in a double-blind provocation trial. Skin testing may help to identify the offending food, especially in the presence of an association between ingestion and IgE-mediated events (anaphylaxis, urticaria, angioedema, eczema, abdominal cramps). Oral provocation is indicated if the history is equivocal and symptoms improve during an elimination diet. The specific food is given in gelatin capsules, and the child is evaluated for the immediate recurrence of symptoms or signs. Manifestations of allergy appear within 10–90 min and include pruritus, erythematous macular morbilliform rash, wheezing, sneezing, cough, abdominal pain, nausea, emesis, and increased serum histamine levels.

Aberg N, Engstrom I: Natural history of allergic diseases in children. Acta Pediatr Scand 79:206, 1990.
American College of Physicians: Allergy testing. Ann Intern Med 110:317, 1989.
Bierman CW, Pearlman DS (eds): Allergic Diseases from Infancy to Adulthood, 2nd ed. Philadelphia, WB Saunders, 1988.
Broadbent JB, Sampson H: Food hypersensitivity and atopic dermatitis. Pediatr Clin North Am 35:1115, 1988.
deShazo R, Smith D: Primer on allergic and immunologic diseases. JAMA 268:2785, 1992.
Ownby DR: Allergy testing: In vivo versus in vitro. Pediatr Clin North Am 35:995, 1988.
Pacheco S, Shearer W: Laboratory aspects of immunology. Pediatr Clin North Am 41:623, 1994.
Van Arsdel PP, Larson E: Diagnostic tests for patients with suspected allergic disease: Utility and limitations. Ann Intern Med 110:304, 1989.

CHAPTER 135
Principles of Treatment

Successful management of allergic disorders is based upon four principles: avoidance of allergens or irritants, pharmacologic therapy, immunotherapy (hyposensitization or desensitization), and prophylaxis.

When clinically relevant allergens are identified by history and judicious use of allergy skin tests, their elimination or *avoidance* is all that is needed in many cases of immunoglobulin (Ig) E–mediated disease. If the history and skin testing indicate reactivity to house dust mites or molds, or if dog or cat allergen is contributing to the patient's symptoms, these allergens should be eliminated from the home to the greatest extent possible. The recommendation that a family pet be removed from a home is frequently difficult to implement. When the allergic disorder is a serious one, such as asthma, and when the child has a positive skin test result to the dog or cat allergen, parents can generally be persuaded to remove the animal. When skin tests to danders are negative, the problem may be more difficult; most allergists believe that elimination of potentially sensitizing pets from the household of the allergic child is desirable for prophylaxis.

Allergy to **house dust mites** requires precautions to minimize exposure to mite allergens. Avoidance in the bedroom is often sufficient because children spend more time there than in other rooms of the house. Mattresses, box springs, and pillows should be encased in airtight, allergen-proof covers.* Vacuuming the covered mattress at least weekly is necessary to remove mites. Bedding should be washed at least weekly in hot water (>70° C); cool water does not kill the mites. There should be no carpet or rug in the bedroom because either may be a rich source of mites. A small cotton throw rug may be acceptable if it is washed at least weekly in hot water. There should be no upholstered furniture and no stuffed toys in the bedroom. When removal of carpet from a bedroom is impossible, treatment of the carpet with a solution of tannic acid inactivates mite allergens.* Repeated treatments of the carpet at intervals of 2–3 mo are necessary because the solution does not kill the mites. Benzyl benzoate† kills mites; carpet treatment every few months is necessary to control mite populations.

Household humidity should be kept below 50% to inhibit survival of mites. It is prudent to avoid use of vaporizers. Dehumidifiers may be necessary in damp basements. Air conditioning helps to control humidity and also reduces exposure to atmospheric pollens and molds. If elimination of a cat from a home is impossible, other measures that can reduce allergen exposure include exclusion of the animal from the house, washing the cat more often than weekly, removal of carpets and upholstered furniture, and improvement of ventilation.

Avoidance of irritants is important in the control and prevention of **asthma**. Potential sources of irritants include kerosene heaters and wood-burning stoves. Smoking should not be permitted indoors, and patients with asthma should avoid public facilities where exposure to cigarette smoke is likely.

Pharmacologic therapy is a major element in management of allergic diseases (Chapter 135.1). The drugs used have specific roles in the interruption of pathways leading to tissue damage as a consequence of antigen-antibody interaction. Certain drugs, for example, modulate the antigen-induced release of mediators (histamine, leukotrienes); others affect the tension of smooth muscle; and others prevent the migration to the site of an allergic reaction of inflammatory cells having the potential for producing tissue injury. For patients whose symptoms are not mediated by an immunologic mechanism, avoidance of allergens or attempts to increase the tolerance to allergens by immunotherapy are fruitless. Drug therapy, on the other hand, may be effective whether or not an allergic mechanism is involved. Patients with nonimmunologic or nonallergic asthma may respond to drug treatment as well as do those in whom allergy plays a major role.

Immunotherapy is appropriate for the treatment of allergic rhinitis or asthma mediated by IgE antibody-antigen interactions caused by unavoidable inhalant allergens (Chapter 135.2).

A predisposition to form IgE antibodies to substances of "high" allergenic potential is an important characteristic of the atopic state. Therefore, prevention of exposure of infants and children at risk has a rational basis. It is appropriate to recommend breast-feeding for infants born into families with strong histories of hay fever, asthma, or atopic dermatitis and to delay for at least 6 mo the introduction of solid foods into the diet of such infants, especially foods of highly allergenic potential, such as eggs, cow milk, wheat, fish, citrus fruit, and peanut butter. The nursing mother should avoid highly allergenic foods in her diet because there is evidence that the breast-fed infant can become sensitized to food antigens that are transmitted in breast milk. It is not definitively established whether postponing cow milk feedings in an atopic infant can prevent the development of cow milk allergy, of allergic diseases in general, or of atopic dermatitis in particular, although there is some evidence of such effects.

Environmental exposure to high concentrations of house dust mite allergen is a risk factor for subsequent sensitization and asthma. There are no prospective studies that convincingly indicate that avoidance of environmental exposure of atopic infants and children to other inhalant allergens such as dog and cat allergen lessens the likelihood of their sensitization, although such a result seems reasonable. Cord blood IgE levels greater than 1.3 IU/mL, elevated serum IgE levels, eosinophilia during infancy, and a family history of atopic dermatitis, asthma, or allergic rhinitis may predict a child at risk for future atopic disorders who might benefit from allergic avoidance.

*Allergy Control Products, 89 Danbury Road, PO Box 793, Ridgefield, CT 06877.

†Acarosan, Fisons Corporation, Rochester, NY 14623.

135.1 Pharmacologic Therapy

ADRENERGICS. These agents combine with α- and β-receptors on the surfaces of cells. With several exceptions, drugs that affect α-receptors cause physiologic responses that are excitatory (vasoconstriction), whereas drugs that influence β-receptors produce inhibitory responses (bronchodilation). In a given tissue the response to a drug depends both on the relative numbers of α- and β-receptors and upon whether the drug stimulates predominantly α-receptors, β-receptors, or both.

Variations in sensitivity of β-receptors of different organs to β-agonists (stimulants) and differences in response to β-blocking drugs of diverse chemical structure have led to separation of β-receptors into two subclasses, β_1 and β_2; β_1-receptors have approximately equal affinity for epinephrine and norepinephrine, whereas β_2-receptors have an approximately 10-fold higher affinity for epinephrine than for norepinephrine. Agents with greater β_2-selective activity (isoetharine, metaproterenol, terbutaline, albuterol, fenoterol, bitolterol, pirbuterol, salmeterol) can provide effective bronchodilation in asthma without the significant increase in heart rate that may occur with isoproterenol or epinephrine because the latter drugs stimulate both bronchial β_2-receptors and cardiac β_1-receptors, causing tachycardia. Selectivity for β_2-receptors is relative, however, and some patients experience tachycardia after administration of putative β_2-selective agents. Selective β_2 drugs have essentially no α-adrenergic activity and thus no pressor effect. These agents stimulate skeletal muscle and may induce tremors. They also stimulate glycogenolysis and may produce hypokalemia. Accordingly, such drugs do not cause the pallor that may follow epinephrine administration.

Alpha-adrenergic receptors have been subclassified into α_2 and α_2 subtypes; these have wide distribution and mediate different effects. Stimulation of α_1-receptors contracts vascular and airway smooth muscle.

Although experiments in vitro with human tissues have shown that adrenergic drugs can inhibit allergen-induced mediator release from mast cells and basophils, their use in allergic disorders depends principally upon their effects on smooth muscle in blood vessels and in the bronchial airways. For example, stimulation of α-adrenergic receptors reduces edema of nasal mucous membranes through vasoconstriction and decreases the permeability of venules and capillaries, whereas β-adrenergic stimulation causes smooth-muscle relaxation, which relieves at least one component of obstruction of the airway in asthma.

Adrenergic drugs include catecholamines (epinephrine, isoetharine, isoproterenol, and bitolterol) and noncatecholamines (ephedrine, albuterol, metaproterenol, salmeterol, terbutaline, pirbuterol, procaterol, and fenoterol). Those of the former group are rapidly inactivated by enzymes found in the gastrointestinal tract and liver; accordingly, the use of epinephrine and isoproterenol is limited largely to injection, inhalation, and topical application to mucous membranes. Ephedrine, the oldest of the noncatecholamine sympathomimetics, has relatively weak β-stimulant activity and frequently causes adverse side effects, including increased activity, insomnia, irritability, and headache. Newer noncatecholamine adrenergic agents (metaproterenol, terbutaline, and albuterol), which may also be given orally, have a somewhat longer duration of action (up to 6 hr) than ephedrine (4 hr) and have relatively selective activity on the β_2 receptors in the airways, with less of the cardiovascular effects of isoproterenol and epinephrine, especially when delivered by inhalation. Salmeterol is a very long-acting derivative of albuterol; its long action is due to a long lipophilic side chain that interacts with a binding site near the β_2-receptor, permitting the phenylethanolamine head of the molecule to repeatedly interact with the β_2-receptor. Inhalation of a single dose of salmeterol can elicit bronchodilation for at least 12 hr, inhibit both immediate and late-phase reactions to inhaled allergen, and inhibit allergen-induced bronchial hyper-responsiveness for 34 hr. Because several-fold lower doses of adrenergic drugs are effective when the agents are given by the inhalational rather than the oral route, aerosol administration is preferred wherever possible to minimize adverse side effects.

Autoantibodies against β_2-adrenergic receptors have been identified in small proportions of patients with asthma, a few patients with cystic fibrosis, and a few normal controls. The presence of these autoantibodies has been associated with β-adrenergic hyporesponsiveness. Such autoantibodies may account for some of the abnormalities in autonomic function in some patients with asthma. Tolerance or desensitization to adrenergic agents may occur, but if such agents are used as prescribed, the small decrease in the duration or intensity of drug effect usually has no serious therapeutic implications.

Adverse side effects of adrenergic drugs may include skeletal muscle tremor, cardiac stimulation, worsening of hypoxemia, increased airway obstruction, headache, insomnia, irritability, nausea, vomiting, epigastric pain, flushing, and tolerance (subsensitivity, refractoriness). Benzalkonium chloride, the preservative in most albuterol and metaproterenol nebulization solutions, can cause bronchoconstriction occasionally in asthmatic patients, which may limit the response to the bronchodilator; medications delivered from metered-dose inhalers contain no benzalkonium chloride. Metabisulfite, used as a stabilizing agent in solution for nebulization, may exacerbate bronchoconstriction because of hypersensitivity to this agent. Overreliance on metered-dose adrenergic agents or home-aerosolized sympathomimetic drugs may be responsible for delay in seeking medical attention, increasing the risk of morbidity and even mortality.

THEOPHYLLINE. This is a therapeutic agent for treatment of both acute and chronic asthma. Its mode of action is uncertain. It is no longer held that it inhibits cyclic adenosine monophosphate (cAMP) phosphodiesterase because the concentrations necessary to demonstrate this effect are toxic in vivo. Moreover, other potent phosphodiesterase inhibitors (e.g., papaverine) are ineffective in asthma. Other possible modes of action include adenosine antagonism, an effect on calcium flux across cell membranes, prostaglandin antagonism, release of or synergistic interactions with β-adrenergic agonists, and enhancement of binding of cAMP to a cAMP-binding protein. Theophylline causes bronchodilation by relaxing bronchial smooth muscle, increases concentrations of endogenous catecholamines in the circulation, and enhances the contractility of the fatigued diaphragm. It can inhibit both immediate and late-phase asthmatic responses to allergenic challenge and sometimes reduces bronchial hyperresponsiveness.

Both the therapeutic and toxic effects of theophylline are related to the serum concentration. The incidence of toxic effects increases as the serum levels progressively rise above 20 μg/mL. *Measurement of serum theophylline concentration* is an important element in effective and safe use of the drug. Methods for theophylline analysis are specific, sensitive, rapid, and require only a small serum sample; they should be available in all hospitals. A 15-min method that requires no instrument for determination of theophylline level in finger prick blood (AccuLevel) gives excellent results.

Pharmacokinetics. Both the rapidly absorbed and most (but not all) slow-release (SR) formulations of theophylline are, for all practical purposes, completely bioavailable. Rapidly absorbed preparations may be given with food without significant effect on rate or extent of absorption, but absorption characteristics of SR products may be altered when they are administered with a meal and either accelerated or delayed, depending upon the product. Administration of TheoDur tablets or Slo-bid Gyrocaps with a meal can delay attainment of peak serum concentrations by 1–2 hr usually with little or no effect on bioavailability. On the other hand, administration of TheoDur Sprinkle with a meal can reduce bioavailability by as much as 50%. Administration of Uniphyl with a meal can almost double the amount of drug absorbed. Administration of Theo-24 with meals may be followed by sudden absorption of nearly half the dose within a 4-hr period at variable times after dosing in some patients. Accordingly, unless the physician wishes to take advantage of the fact that food delays absorption of a specific SR product (e.g., Theolair-SR), SR products other than TheoDur tablets and Slo-bid Gyrocaps are best given 60 min before meals. The ultraslow release formulations may be incompletely bioavailable when given to patients with rapid gastrointestinal transit times (especially children). The absorption from an SR product can vary from time to time, even in the same patient, leading to confused interpretation of serum concentration data. Occasionally, a "trough" theophylline level will be higher than that in a specimen drawn at a time thought to represent a "peak" level. Peak serum concentrations usually occur 4–8 hr after administration of most SR products (6–10 hr after TheoDur, Sustaire, or Uniphyl).

The marketed SR products differ in theophylline-release characteristics, and care must be exercised in switching from one product to another. Substitution of a generic for a proprietary preparation without the physician's or patient's knowledge is a potential source of problems. Such unauthorized substitution by the pharmacist is legal in most states unless it is specifically forbidden on the prescription.

Despite these limitations, SR formulations of theophylline represent an advance in dealing with the fluctuations in serum concentrations seen with rapidly absorbed products, particularly in young patients who metabolize the drug rapidly. Even with the SR products, patients who metabolize theophylline rapidly may have unacceptable fluctuations in serum theophylline level if the drug is given at 12-hr intervals rather than 8-hr intervals. Theophylline absorption is slower during nighttime hours; accordingly, administration every 12 hr may produce higher early morning levels than those later in the day. Theophylline salts such as aminophylline (theophylline ethylenediamine) do not improve efficacy and may cause adverse effects because of the development of ethylenediamine hypersensitivity.

After its absorption, about 60% of theophylline is bound to protein (somewhat less in prematures). Free theophylline is distributed rapidly into body fluids, equilibration between serum and tissues being complete within 1 hr following intravenous injection. Salivary concentrations are about 60% of those in serum. Estimates of serum theophylline concentration derived from analysis of *appropriately collected* saliva samples are accurate enough for most clinical purposes. Theophylline distributes freely into umbilical cord blood, breast milk (not clinically significant for the infant), and cerebrospinal fluid.

Theophylline is metabolized by biotransformation in the liver via a cytochrome P450-dependent microsomal mixed-function oxidase. Metabolism occurs via both 1st-order (linear) and nonlinear capacity-dependent processes. Some patients show disproportionate dose-dependent changes in theophylline serum concentration, particularly at the higher doses, owing to the nonlinear elimination. About 10–15% of theophylline is excreted unchanged in urine (50% in prematures). There is substantial intersubject variation in the rate of theophylline body clearance. Intrasubject variations in clearance also occur. As with other drugs eliminated by hepatic metabolism, many environmental and disease factors alter the rate of elimination (Table 135–1). Most of the factors listed tend to decrease clearance, with increased theophylline concentration and risk of adverse effect. The clinical relevance of the factors varies: cigarette smoking, hepatic or heart disease, some drugs (macrolide antibiotics, cimetidine, allopurinol, carbamazepine, phenytoin, rifampin) have substantial effects, whereas others are probably of less clinical relevance (phenobarbital, ranitidine, protein-carbohydrate dietary content, ingestion of charcoal-broiled meats). Average theophylline clearance also varies with age, and dosage is based upon this fact (Table 135–2).

Pharmacodynamics. The logarithmic relationship between the theophylline bronchodilator effect and serum concentration in the 5–20 μg/mL range is well documented. The serum concentration that provides optimal bronchodilator effect probably varies from patient to patient. The physician should use the patient's response rather than the theophylline blood level as a guide to increases in dosage, but dosage should not exceed the average doses for the age group without determination of peak serum theophylline concentrations to ensure safety. Some patients receive good bronchodilator effect with serum concentrations less than 10 μg/mL; in such cases, there is no need to increase the theophylline dose. Regular administration of SR theophylline to maintain trough serum concentrations of 8 to 15 μg/mL can afford symptomatic control of mild to moderate asthma comparable to that achievable with

■ TABLE 135–1 Factors That Affect Theophylline Clearance

Factor	Decreased Clearance: Increased Levels	Increased Clearance: Decreased Levels
Disease	Liver disease (cirrhosis, acute hepatitis)	Hyperthyroidism
	Congestive heart failure	Cystic fibrosis
	Acute pulmonary edema	
	Febrile viral respiratory illness	
	Renal failure	
Drugs	Troleandomycin	Carbamazepine
	Erythromycin	Phenytoin
	Fluoroquinolones	Rifampin
	Cimetidine	Phenobarbital
	Ranitidine (less than cimetidine)	Terbutaline
	Oral contraceptives	Isoproterenol (intravenous)
	Ketoconazole	Sulfinpyrazone
	Mexiletine	
	Pentoxifylline	
	Allopurinol	
	Thiabendazole	
	Propranolol	
	Influenza vaccine	
Habits		
Diet	High carbohydrate, low protein	Smoking (tobacco or marijuana)
	Dietary xanthines	High protein, low carbohydrate
		Charcoal-broiled meats

■ TABLE 135–2 Average Theophylline Dosage Requirements After the Neonatal Period

Age (yr)	Dose (mg/kg/24 hr)
<1	8 + 0.3 × age in weeks
1–9	24
9–12	20
12–16	16–18
>16	12–13

Initial dosage should be one-half to two-thirds the average dose for age. Later changes in dosage should be determined by clinical response and guided by serum theophylline determinations.

inhaled beclomethasone dipropionate, 84 μg four times each day.

Toxicity. Theophylline toxicity is a major clinical problem. Signs and symptoms of acute theophylline intoxication vary from mild nausea, insomnia, irritability, tremors, and headache to severe seizures and death. Gastrointestinal symptoms (nausea, vomiting, hematemesis, cramping) are usually the earliest to appear and generally precede the more serious central nervous system (seizures, coma) manifestations of toxicity. Uncommonly, seizures may appear as the first sign of theophylline intoxication. Disturbances in cardiac rate, most often tachycardia, rhythm disturbances (atrial and ventricular premature contractions or tachycardia), and hypotension are commonly observed with serious toxicity. Additional problems include hypokalemia, hyperglycemia, ataxia, and hallucinations. Signs and symptoms of theophylline intoxication are, by and large, serum concentration dependent, but concentrations associated with symptoms of serious toxicity vary widely. In adults with seizures the mean serum concentration has been reported to be approximately 50 μg/mL with a range of 20–70 μg/mL. Several infants with theophylline-induced seizures have been reported to have very high serum theophylline concentrations (180 μg/mL in one case) with no apparent permanent sequelae. Healthy adolescents who ingest theophylline in suicide attempts may tolerate very high theophylline serum concentrations (over 100 μg/mL) with no permanent sequelae if treated appropriately. On the other hand, children who survive serious theophylline intoxication also may be left with severe brain damage that resembles the sequelae of anoxic encephalopathy.

Treatment of theophylline intoxication should begin with measures designed to induce emesis (e.g., administration of ipecac, if the patient is not already vomiting) or gavage, followed by a slurry of 30 g of activated charcoal to adsorb the theophylline remaining in the gastrointestinal tract. Activated charcoal can also remove serum theophylline that has already been absorbed from the gastrointestinal tract. It may be best to delay administration of charcoal until emesis has occurred when using ipecac to induce emesis, because the charcoal also adsorbs ipecac. After ingestion of SR theophylline, repeated administration of charcoal at 2–3 hr intervals is advisable. The addition of a nonabsorbed saline cathartic is effective for decreasing intestinal transit time when SR products have been ingested. Peritoneal dialysis can remove theophylline from intoxicated patients, but hemoperfusion using a specially prepared charcoal column is the method of choice. The indications for charcoal hemoperfusion are not completely defined; they depend both upon the serum concentration and upon clinical considerations. Diazepam is effective therapy for seizures, propranolol is helpful for treating hypotension or supraventricular or ventricular arryhthmias (lidocaine is also effective for ventricular tachycardia), and ranitidine may be helpful in controlling gastric acid-induced emesis.

Chronic theophylline use may produce or exacerbate subtle behavioral changes, such as hyperactivity and sleep disturbances. These effects are dose dependent. Theophylline has no adverse effect on cognitive function.

ANTIHISTAMINES. These are drugs of diverse chemical structure that compete with histamine for receptors in various tissues. There are at least three histamine receptors: H_1, H_2, and H_3. Initially, only H_1-receptor blockers were used in treatment of allergic disorders. A combination of H_1 and H_2 antagonists, however, may be beneficial in some patients with chronic urticaria and in treatment of anaphylactoid reactions such as those caused by intravenous injections of contrast media for urography. Cimetidine and probably ranitidine, H_2 antagonists, inhibit delayed-type hypersensitivity skin responses, suggesting that H_2-receptor blocking agents may modulate cell-mediated immune injury. The H_1-type antihistamines, as a group, are nitrogenous bases with aliphatic side chains that resemble histamine. The side chains are attached to cyclic or heterocyclic rings of various configurations. The antihistamines may be classified as follows:

Type I—ethylenediamines (tripelennamine [Pyribenzamine], methapyrilene [Histadyl])

Type II—ethanolamines (diphenhydramine [Benadryl], carbinoxamine [Clistin, Rondec])

Type III—alkylamines (chlorpheniramine [Chlor-Trimeton, Teldrin, Novahistine, Demazin], brompheniramine [Dimetane, Bromfed], triprolidine [Actidil, Actifed])

Type IV—piperazines (cyclizine [Manezine], meclizine [Bonine])

Type V—piperidines (cyproheptadine [Periactin], azatadine [Trinalin])

Type VI—phenothiazines (promethazine [Phenergan])

Hydroxyzine (Atarax, Vistaril), which has potent antihistaminic activity and some second-generation H_1 antihistamines do not fit well into any of these types. Second-generation antihistamines such as terfenadine, astemizole, loratadine, and cetirizine (an active metabolite of hydroxyzine) are effective in suppressing the signs and symptoms of allergic rhinitis, do not cross the blood-brain barrier (because they are lipophobic), and have fewer sedative effects than other antihistamines. This is a very important distinction; first-generation antihistamines can cause impairment of function even in patients who perceive no sedation or impairment from the drug. *The antihistamines may be found alone or in combination* with decongestants in the above commercial preparations just mentioned. The chemical classification of antihistamines does not usually have functional significance and, except for cyproheptadine, which also has antiserotonin activity, drugs from each class have equal activity as antihistamines.

In general, the H_1 antagonists are rapidly absorbed after oral administration, with onset of action within 30 min, peak plasma concentration within 1 hr, and complete absorption within 4 hr. Antihistamines are eliminated by biotransformation in the liver; little nonmetabolized drug is found in urine. Some antihistamines (diphenhydramine and chlorcyclizine) stimulate liver microsomal drug-metabolizing enzymes in animals and may accelerate their own metabolism and that of other drugs. There have been relatively few pharmacokinetic studies of the antihistamines; most of the prescribing patterns are empirically based upon clinical experience. Diphenhydramine (Benadryl) has a relatively short serum half-life of 3–4 hr. Yet the drug is effective in suppressing the wheal and flare response to allergy skin testing for over 24 hr. Thus, with this antihistamine there appears to be little correlation between serum concentration and therapeutic effect in the tissue. A study of chlorpheniramine in children showed a mean serum half-life of 13.7 hr (range, 6–34 hr). Significant suppression of clinical symptoms of allergic rhinitis was observed for as long as 30 hr after injection of a single dose, at which time chlorpheniramine was not detectable in the serum. Data indicate that chlorpheniramine, brompheniramine, and hydroxyzine may not need to be given three or four times a day but that twice or even once a day may suffice. In addition to histamine antagonism, the antihistamines have pharmacologic effects on exocrine secretions, the central nervous system, and the cardiovascular system. Some have anticholinergic-like side effects (Benadryl), whereas others are sedatives (hydroxyzine); both groups have the potential to produce drowsiness.

Because antihistamines act as competitive antagonists, they are more effective in preventing than in reversing the action of histamine. To be most effective, they must be administered at doses and intervals that keep tissue histamine receptor sites saturated. Histamine is released explosively at the site of an IgE-mediated reaction; accordingly, antihistamines are less potent in antagonizing the effects of endogenous than of exogenous histamine. Their relative inefficacy in patients with asthma is related not only to this and to the fact that mediators of bronchoconstriction other than histamine are involved in allergic reactions in the lung but also to limitation by sedation to ineffective doses. Second-generation antihistamines may afford protection against bronchoconstriction induced by a variety of stimuli, including allergens, exercise, and histamine. Many antihistamines possess anticholinergic activity, which is valuable in allergic rhinitis for controlling rhinorrhea. Anticholinergic activity may account for some of the response of asthma to some first-generation antihistamines. In children antihistamines usually have neither favorable nor deleterious effects on the course of asthma.

There is little reason to choose one antihistamine over another, except for avoidance of adverse effects, including sedation and impairment of function, which are of great importance for students as well as drivers. Excessive doses of either first-generation or second-generation antihistamines can have adverse cardiac effects. Very large doses of terfenadine or astemizole have elicited cardiac arrest secondary to prolongation of the QT interval and ventricular tachycardia (torsades de pointes) in rare patients. This has occurred in a few patients who denied excessive dosage of their astemizole. There has been no evidence of any similar cardiac arrhythmia with loratadine at daily dosage as high as 40 mg in adults. Patients with prolonged serum elimination of antihistamines may be at increased risk for adverse effects. These patients include those with impaired hepatic function or patients receiving concurrent treatment with an inhibitor of cytochrome P450 enzymes, including erythromycin and other macrolide antibiotics, ketoconazole, and itraconazole.

In general, antihistamines are extraordinarily safe, and most are sold without prescription. They can have other adverse effects, especially in high dosages. Combinations of antihistamines with other central nervous system depressants (e.g., alcohol) should be avoided. In high doses or in certain sensitive patients, the anticholinergic properties of antihistamines cause undesirable adverse reactions. These include excitation, nervousness, tachycardia, palpitations, dryness of the mouth, urinary retention, and constipation. Seizures are common in antihistamine poisoning. Skin eruptions, blood dyscrasias, fever, and neuropathy are rarely observed.

CROMOLYN SODIUM (DISODIUM CROMOGLYCATE). Cromolyn sodium is the disodium salt of 1,3,-*bis* (2-carboxychromon-5-yloxy)-2-hydroxypropane. It is a chemical analog of the drug khellin, which has smooth muscle–relaxing properties. It is soluble in water but insoluble in lipids; only 1% is absorbed from the gastrointestinal tract. The drug is administered as a powder (Intal) with a special turboinhaler, the Spinhaler, or as a 1% (20 mg/2 mL) solution for nebulization, or by metered-dose inhaler (800 μg/actuation). It is used principally in asthma but has some value in allergic rhinitis. It has been used with varying results in patients with aphthous ulcers, food allergy, systemic mastocytosis, ulcerative colitis, and chronic proctitis.

The drug has no bronchodilator properties; it is not, therefore, effective for treatment of actue asthma but is given prophylactically, in a 20-mg dose two to four times each day by Spinhaler or nebulization or 1.6 mg two to four times each day by metered-dose inhaler. Cromolyn has no antimediator or anti-inflammatory properties. It prevents both antibody-mediated and non–antibody-mediated mast cell degranulation and mediator release (from mast cells recoverable by bronchoalveolar lavage). This effect may be due to the ability of cromolyn to block antigen-stimulated calcium transport across the mast cell membrane. Cromolyn inhibition of histamine release may also occur by regulation of phosphorylation of a mast cell protein. The drug also has weak phosphodiesterase inhibitor activity. Cromolyn has no effect on human basophils or human cutaneous mast cells. Cromolyn appears to reduce airway hyperreactivity by a mechanism that is not yet understood, and it can prevent late-phase asthmatic responses when administered before allergen challenge. It inhibits bronchoconstriction produced by nonimmunologic stimuli such as frigid air, exercise, and sulfur dioxide. Some of these stimuli do not cause release of mast cell–derived mediators; accordingly, cromolyn may directly affect neural control of the airway by inhibiting reflex bronchoconstriction through inhibition of the transmission of neural impulses by myelinated afferent nerve fibers.

Cromolyn is of greatest value in allergic or extrinsic asthma, but patients with nonallergic or intrinsic asthma who use it may also improve. Patients with mild degrees of asthma respond more favorably than those with severe disease. About 70% of asthmatic patients receive some benefit from inhalation of the drug. The incidence of toxic reactions to cromolyn is extremely low; dry throat and transient bronchoconstriction have been the most frequently reported side effects. The latter is most likely due to inhalation of the dry powder into irritable airways and is not an intrinsic effect of the drug itself. Rare reports have associated urticaria, angioedema, and pulmonary eosinophilia with the use of cromolyn. There are no known contraindications to its use except that in some patients, during acute asthma, the powder may rarely act as an airway irritant.

Nedocromil sodium is a pyranoquinoline dicarboxylic acid, chemically remote from cromolyn, which has antiallergic and anti-inflammatory activity. Like cromolyn, it inhibits release of mediators from human lung mast cells and suppresses activation of eosinophils, neutrophils, and macrophages. It inhibits both early- and late-phase asthmatic and rhinitic responses and associated increases in airway hyper-responsiveness as well as seasonal increases in nonspecific bronchial responsiveness. It can inhibit bronchoconstrictive effects of exercise; hyperventilation with cold air; inhalation of ultrasonically nebulized distilled water, sulfur dioxide, or adenosine. It can reduce airway hyper-responsiveness in asthmatic patients. Nedocromil, 4 mg four times a day, has a prophylactic effect equivalent to that of inhaled beclomethasone dipropionate at a total daily dose of 400 μg but is less effective than beclomethasone at a total daily dose of 800 μg in asthmatic adults. There are few studies of nedocromil in children; inhalation of 4 mg has been reported to have a protective effect against exercise-induced asthma comparable to that of cromolyn, 10 mg, by metered-dose inhaler in asthmatic children. Such treatment (4 mg four times a day) elicits improvement within 3 to 4 wk. Some adults have complained of unpleasant taste. Less frequent adverse effects have included coughing, sore throat, rhinitis, headache, and nausea; these occasional side effects have been of minor significance.

Lodoxamide tromethamine is a mast cell stabilizer more effective than topical cromolyn sodium in alleviating signs and symptoms of allergic ocular disease. It is used in children older than 2 yr for vernal keratoconjunctivitis, vernal conjunctivitis, and vernal keratitis. Occasional adverse effects have included transient burning or stinging after instillation.

CORTICOSTEROIDS. Corticosteroids are the most potent drugs available for treatment of allergic disorders. Following administration of a well-absorbed tablet of prednisone, peak plasma concentration is attained at 1–2 hr. The systemic availability of the drug is more than 80% of the oral dose. Regardless of the route of administration, there is interconversion of prednisone and prednisolone (the active form), with prednisolone concentrations 4–10 times those of prednisone. There is little effect of liver disease or renal insufficiency on the conversion of prednisone to prednisolone or on prednisolone disposition. The volume of distribution, metabolic clearance, and renal clearance of prednisone increase with increasing doses owing to the partially saturable binding of prednisolone to transcortin in plasma, which provides more unbound drug at higher plasma concentrations of this steroid.

Some effects of prednisolone are evident within 2 hr after oral or intravenous administration (fall in peripheral eosinophils and lymphocytes); others may be delayed 6–8 hr or longer (e.g., hyperglycemia and improvement in pulmonary function in asthmatics). The delayed responses reflect the indirect mechanism of action of glucocorticoids. Steps leading to activity include (1) simple diffusion through the cell membrane, (2) binding to cytosol glucocorticoid receptors (found in most mammalian cells), (3) translocation of the steroid-receptor complex to the nucleus, (4) binding of the complex to chromatin, which affects nuclear gene expression, and (5) subsequent synthesis of messenger ribonucleic acid and proteins with enzyme activity. It is the newly synthesized enzymes that mediate some of the effects of glucocorticoids. The biologic half-life of the steroid is determined by the turnover time of the newly synthesized enzymes, not by steroid plasma concentrations. Plasma half-lives of commonly used steroids vary from 1.5–5 hr, while biologic half-lives vary from 8–54 hr.

Pharmacokinetic studies of prednisolone have shown no differences in distribution, protein binding, plasma clearance, or disposition of unbound drug between males and females or between adults and children. Steroid-dependent asthmatic patients do not differ from normal individuals in prednisolone binding, distribution, or clearance. Clinically significant drug interactions occur with phenobarbital and phenytoin, both of which increase steroid clearance.

The anti-inflammatory actions of glucocorticoids result from (1) alteration in leukocyte number and activity (redistribution, suppression of migration to sites of inflammation, decreased response to mitogens, decreased cytotoxicity, and suppression of delayed hypersensitivity responses in the skin); (2) suppression of mediator release (decreased histamine synthesis and release, decreased synthesis of prostaglandins and other products of arachidonic acid metabolism); (3) enhanced response to agents that increase cAMP (prostaglandin E_2 and histamine via the H_2 receptor); and (4) enhanced response to catecholamines (increased synthesis of β-adrenergic receptors, increased availability of epinephrine as a result of decreased extraneuronal uptake of catecholamines). Humoral antibody synthesis is little affected by glucocorticoids in the dosage usually given for treatment of allergic disorders. Chronic corticosteroid administration may lower total immunoglobulin concentrations.

Topical steroids have direct local effects that include decreased inflammation, edema, mucus production, vascular permeability, and mucosal IgE levels. There is also less local accumulation of neutrophils, eosinophils, basophils, and mast cells and an attenuation of airway hyper-responsiveness. Topical steroids may reduce early- and late-phase reactions, whereas systemic steroids predominantly inhibit late-phase response to antigen. Possible complications of inhaled steroids include oropharyngeal candidiasis, dysphonia, and, at high doses, suppression of the hypothalamic-pituitary-adrenal axis. Total daily dosage of not more than 400 μg probably rarely if ever suppresses linear growth in the majority of asthmatic children;

larger doses may affect growth, but uncontrolled asthma can also impair growth. Growth impairment from inhaled steroids at total daily dosage as high as 800 μg is probably much less than that from oral prednisone, 2.5 mg daily. Suppressive effects of steroids on growth depend on dosage and duration of treatment; attainment of normal height is possible after discontinuation of steroids, but prolonged administration of large doses of systemic steroids can cause permanent short stature.

The short-term use of *systemic corticosteroids* in self-limited allergic conditions such as contact dermatitis due to poison ivy or occasional episodes of severe asthma is not associated with significant adverse effects. Long-term use, on the other hand, especially if daily administration is required, may have substantial undesirable side effects. In children, the most common adverse effect is suppression of linear growth. Posterior subcapsular cataracts develop occasionally in children receiving long-term steroid therapy. Other untoward effects of steroids include osteoporosis (vertebral collapse), hypertension, diabetes mellitus, cushingoid habitus, infections (particularly disseminated varicella or *Pneumocystis carinii*), pancreatitis, gastritis, and myopathy (see also Chapter 137).

Before any decision is made to initiate long-term, systemic corticosteroid therapy, all other modalities of management should be tried. Nevertheless, a small proportion of asthmatic children have severe and continuing symptoms that interfere with normal school attendance, play activities, and sports participation. The judicious use of glucocorticoids can produce substantial improvement in such children with little adverse effect, especially if they are administered as prednisone, prednisolone, or methylprednisolone, in single doses on alternate mornings.

A few considerations in the systemic use of corticosteroids bear emphasis. (1) When given in equivalent anti-inflammatory doses, available drugs do not differ qualitatively in anti-inflammatory effects. Adverse effects are related to dose, dosing interval, and duration of treatment. Prednisone or prednisolone is the preferred drug for oral administration and methylprednisolone or hydrocortisone for intravenous use. Other steroids with longer durations of biologic activity have greater propensities for certain adverse effects, are not suitable for alternate-day therapy, and are more expensive. (2) When corticosteroid therapy is initiated, a sufficient amount should be given daily in three to four divided doses to bring the disease under control. Then an attempt should be made to adjust the dose and the dosing interval to suppress activity of the disease without adverse effects. Whenever possible, alternate-day regimens using prednisone or prednisolone should be tried. In the alternate-day regimen, the drug is given as a single dose every 48 hr between 6:00 and 8:00 A.M.. If daily steroid medication is required, a single dose usually has been given, again between 6:00 and 8:00 A.M.; this regimen mimics endogenous cortisol secretion and causes less suppression of the hypothalamic-pituitary-adrenal axis and fewer other adverse side effects than the same daily dose of drug given in divided doses. Limited data in adults indicate administration of oral prednisone as a single dose at 3:00 P.M. may afford better control of asthma, especially nocturnal asthma, than administration in the morning or evening; the safety of such a regimen remains to be established. Administration of the total daily dose of inhaled triamcinolone acetonide at 3:00 P.M. may be as effective in adults as administration in four divided doses during the day without any increased adverse systemic effect. When exacerbations of asthma occur during low-dose oral maintenance therapy, high-dose suppressive therapy is indicated for a few days, with prompt return to low-dose alternate-day treatment as soon as the acute process is under control. (3) Short-term steroid therapy (<7 days) for exacerbations of asthma or poison ivy suppresses the pituitary-adrenal axis only briefly and can be stopped abruptly without tapering the dose. Patients receiving steroids for longer periods require gradual reduction of the dose to avoid precipitating an acute adrenal crisis.

ADDITIONAL PHARMACOLOGIC AGENTS. *Anticholinergic agents* having antimuscarinic activity may be used as adjuvant aerosol therapy for patients with severe asthma. Atropine sulfate or ipratropium bromide can be added to ongoing therapy with sympathomimetic agents and steroids for patients in status asthmaticus. Atropine methylnitrate may have less systemic effect than atropine sulfate because it is poorly absorbed. The bronchodilation effect of anticholinergic agents is not as great as that of sympathomimetic drugs. Metered dose inhalation therapy has also proved effective in adults with bronchitis.

Ketotifen, a benzocyclohepatathiophene, is an antihistamine with mast cell–stabilizing properties and a leukotriene antagonist. This drug is an antianaphylactic agent, inhibits IgE-dependent mediator release, and attenuates platelet activating factor-induced bronchoconstriction. Ketotifen is a potentially useful drug, but limited experience with it has been recorded in allergic pediatric patients.

Investigational agents that inhibit 5-lipoxygenase enzyme activity or selectively block leukotriene D_4 receptors improve airflow, suggesting that antagonism of these mediators is a potentially new method of treating asthma.

Methotrexate, an immunosuppressant antagonist of folic acid, has anti-inflammatory effects when given in low doses and has been demonstrated to reduce the required doses of steroids among patients with severe chronic asthma. Methotrexate has also been effective in reducing the dose of steroids in patients with severe psoriasis and rheumatoid arthritis. The long-term risks of methotrexate use in children with severe allergic diseases have not been determined. Methotrexate remains an experimental therapy for patients with severe steroid-dependent asthma.

Armenio L, Baldini G, Bardare M, et al: Double-blind, placebo controlled study of nedocromil sodium in asthma. Arch Dis Child 68:193, 1993.
Baker MD: Theophylline toxicity in children. J Pediatr 109:538, 1986.
Barnes PJ, Pedersen S: Efficacy and safety of inhaled corticosteroids in asthma. Am Rev Respir Dis 148:S1, 1993.
Cott G, Cherniack R: Steroids and "steroid sparing" agents in asthma. N Engl J Med 318:634, 1988.
Holgate ST: Asthma: Past, present and future. Eur Respir J 6:1507, 1993.
Rossing TH: Methylxanthines in 1989. Ann Intern Med 110:502, 1989.
Simons FER, Simons KJ: The pharmacology and use of H_1-receptor-antagonist drugs. N Engl J Med 330:1663, 1994.
Sly RM: Aerosol therapy in children. Respir Care 36:994, 1991.
Twentyman OP, Finnerty JP, Harris A, et al: Protection against allergen-induced asthma by salmeterol. Lancet 336:1338, 1990.
Weinberger M: Theophylline: When should it be used? J Pediatr 122:403, 1993.

135.2 Immunotherapy

IMMUNOLOGIC CHANGES. In the early weeks following the institution of regular injections of ragweed pollen extract, IgE antibody against ragweed pollen antigen increases; as treatment continues, however, the titer of antiragweed IgE antibody decreases. In untreated patients with ragweed hay fever, a rise and a fall of antiragweed IgE occur during the year; the rise occurs with the seasonal exposure to ragweed. Injection therapy blunts this anamnestic rise. With continuing treatment, ragweed antibodies of the IgG class ("blocking" or "antigen binding") appear in the serum; the ultimate titer achieved is related to the quantity of ragweed extract injected but does not necessarily correlate with clinical changes, if any occur.

Immunotherapy also can inhibit histamine release from leukocytes (basophils) on challenge in vitro with ragweed antigen E. Leukocytes from treated individuals require exposure to increased amounts of antigen E in order to release the same amount of histamine as they did prior to therapy. Leukocyte preparations from some treated patients behave as if they have been completely desensitized and do not release histamine upon challenge with ragweed antigen E at any concentration. The basis for this change in cell sensitivity is unknown; it does not appear to be related to titers of either antiragweed IgE or IgG. There may be some intrinsic change in receptors for IgE or in the biochemical pathways that cause histamine release. Changes in ratios of helper to suppressor T cells in control of B cells, with an increase in antigen-specific suppressor T cells, have been reported in experimental animals undergoing immunotherapy and to a lesser extent in humans. Immunotherapy inhibits the late-phase asthmatic response to allergenic challenge. In animals it is possible both to suppress IgE antibody production specifically and to induce tolerance to certain chemically modified or conjugated antigens.

STUDIES OF EFFICACY. Critical review of placebo-controlled, double-blind studies of treatment of ragweed hay fever by ragweed extract injections indicates that most patients improve with immunotherapy. Data supporting the efficacy of grass and tree pollen, house dust mite, and *Alternaria* immunotherapy in rhinitis induced by these allergens are less substantial, but the results appear similar to those with ragweed. Controlled, randomized, double-blind studies of treatment of asthmatic patients with extracts of ragweed, mountain cedar, grass pollen, house dust mites, *Cladosporium,* and cat allergen have also shown beneficial effects in most patients. In other studies of asthma, most patients have improved after treatment with extracts of grass pollen and certain molds. Partly because of the multiple factors that can trigger asthma (cold, exercise, smoke, cholinergic agents), immunotherapy does not usually cause complete remission of symptoms. Immunotherapy with Hymenoptera venom in patients having anaphylactic sensitivity to such stinging insect venom protects against anaphylaxis upon subsequent sting.

The cost of immunotherapy, its inconvenience, the possibility of making the disease worse, the risk of inducing anaphylaxis, and other factors must be considered. There is no acceptable evidence for efficacy of injection therapy with allergens other than those just noted. Specifically, the injection of danders (dog, horse), most molds, bacterial vaccines, occupational allergens, synthetic antigens, whole-insect extracts, or food extracts has not been shown to influence favorably the course of rhinitis, anaphylaxis, or asthma.

INDICATIONS, MATERIALS, AND PROCEDURE. Immunotherapy is indicated in patients suffering from allergic rhinitis, IgE-mediated asthma, or allergy to stinging insects. Atopic dermatitis and food allergy are not improved by immunotherapy. A patient is a candidate for a trial of immunotherapy when good correlation exists between symptoms and exposure to an inhalant allergen that cannot be adequately avoided, when the patient has evidence of IgE-mediated allergy by either in vivo (skin testing) or in vitro testing, and when disabling symptoms are not easily controlled with medication. There should also be a reasonable likelihood of good compliance with the regimen because treatment requires injections of allergenic extracts at regular intervals for several years.

Aqueous extracts are used most commonly. Extracts usually contain many different antigens in addition to the specific allergen. In ragweed pollen the allergen, antigen E, represents 8.5% of the protein extract. Pelt or skin proteins constitute the predominant allergens for patients sensitive to a cat or dog, whereas proteins in house dust mite feces are responsible for most dust hypersensitivity. The cat pelt protein, Fel d1, is the most important cat allergen. Alum-precipitated pollen extracts and alum-precipitated pyridine-extracted extracts (Allpyral) do not appear to offer any substantial advantages over aqueous extract therapy. Furthermore, the immunogenicity of one Allpyral extract (ragweed) has been questioned. Allergenic extracts are considered drugs by the U.S. Food and Drug Administration (FDA), but standards of potency exist for only a few. Some extracts sold in the United States for diagnosis and therapy have been totally lacking in allergenic activity when tested by the radioallergosorbent test (RAST) inhibition. Some of the antigens in allergenic extracts (e.g., ragweed antigen E) are quite labile. Methods of extraction, antigen, concentration, and storage temperature are all critical factors in determining the activity and shelf life of an allergenic extract. Pollen extracts are being modified in attempts to reduce their allergenicity without reducing their immunogenicity. Allergens polymerized with glutaraldehyde retain their immunogenicity but are less allergenic. Thus, the initial dose of extract may be substantially increased, the maintenance dose can be reached within 2 mo compared with 5–6 mo with conventional therapy, and there is a greatly reduced incidence of local and systemic reactions. Such modified extracts have not yet been approved in the United States.

In practice, immunotherapy with aqueous extracts involves the repeated injection of increasing amounts of extract until the patient reaches an "optimal" maintenance dose. The dose considered optimal is often arbitrary; clinical trials involving ragweed have reported better results with "high-dose" than with "low-dose" treatment. High-dose therapy is possible only when limited numbers of allergens are included in the extract. No more than 10 and preferably fewer than 6 allergens should be included in a single injection. Children tolerate the same doses as adults.

The injections are given one to three times each week until the patient reaches the maintenance dose, usually after 5–6 mo. In the "rush" method of immunotherapy, the initial injection period is compressed into a few days with apparently satisfactory results. The interval between injections is then extended to 2, 3, and then 4 wk. If more than 1 wk has elapsed since the last dose, the dose is not increased. If more than 6 wk have elapsed between injections, the subsequent dose is reduced to avoid the possibility of a systemic reaction. There is little reason to continue weekly injections for prolonged periods of time after reaching maintenance dosage. During the course of the initial injections, the patient is observed carefully for evidence of excessive local reactions. Large local reactions may sometimes predict systemic reactions, but this is uncertain. If an extensive local reaction or a systemic reaction occurs, the subsequent dose is reduced and then cautiously increased according to the patient's tolerance. Failure to see a local reaction at any time suggests either that the patient is not allergic to the constituents of the extract or that the extract is inactive. Beneficial results often do not become evident until after 6 mo of therapy. Improvement may continue for several years.

Perennial treatment, in which injections are given throughout the year, is preferred to preseasonal treatment, in which the treatment regimen is renewed each year, beginning several months before the pollen season. During the pollen season the maintenance dose of extract is unchanged except for the patient in whom systemic reactions develop presumably because of combined exposure to seasonal and injected allergen. For such patients, the dose may need to be reduced.

The optimal duration of treatment is not known and probably differs from patient to patient. Many allergists believe that if the patient is significantly improved after 3 yr of therapy, it is reasonable to discontinue the injections and observe for recurrence of symptoms. Some children have received "allergy shots" for many years with no evidence that they have been beneficial. Immunotherapy should not be continued if there is no substantial improvement within 2 yr in the condition for which the patient is being treated. Since skin reactivity changes little during the early years of immunotherapy, it is unnecessary to retest the child yearly.

PRECAUTIONS AND ADVERSE REACTIONS. Allergenic extracts should *always* be administered in a physician's office where treatment of a systemic reaction or of anaphylactic shock is readily available. The patient should always remain under observation for at least 20 min after each injection because life-threatening reactions are most likely to occur within this time. Occasionally children will have delayed symptoms; for example, an exacerbation of asthma may occur in the evening of the day on which an injection of extract was given. Rarely, because of distance from a physician's office, it may be necessary to administer allergenic extracts in another setting. Under such circumstances, however, the nonphysician who administers an injection must be prepared to treat a systemic reaction.

Immunotherapy should not be administered during uncontrolled asthma because of diminished pulmonary reserve in the event of a systemic reaction to the allergenic extract. Allergenic extracts are best replaced at intervals of little more than 6 mo because of loss of potency. Dilute extracts lose potency rapidly. Extracts should be kept refrigerated at approximately 4° C. Dilution with .03% human serum albumin minimizes loss of potency. Because of anticipated potency loss, the initial dose of newly prepared allergenic extract should be reduced by at least 50% to minimize the risk of a systemic reaction. Except for the possibility of constitutional reactions, no short- or long-term adverse effects of administration of allergenic extracts to children are known.

Current status of allergen immunotherapy. Lancet 1:259, 1989.

Eggleston P: Immunotherapy for allergic respiratory disease. Pediatr Clin North Am 35:1103, 1988.

Frew A: Injection immunotherapy. Br Med J 307:919, 1993.

Iliopoulis O, Proud D, Adkinson NF Jr, et al: Effects of immunotherapy on the early, late, and rechallenge nasal reaction to provocation with allergen: Changes in inflammatory mediators and cells. J Allergy Clin Immunol 87:855, 1991.

Tinkelman DG, Reed CE, Nelson HS, Offord KP: Aerosol beclomethasone dipropionate compared with theophylline as primary treatment of chronic, mild to moderately severe asthma in children. Pediatrics 92:64, 1993.

CHAPTER 136
Allergic Rhinitis

Seasonal allergic rhinitis, seasonal pollinosis, and hay fever all describe a symptom complex seen in children who have become sensitized to wind-borne pollens of trees, grasses, and weeds. Estimates indicate that 5–9% of children in unselected samples meet diagnostic criteria. Prevalence increases with age; ragweed hay fever is rarely observed before 4–5 yr of age.

In *perennial allergic rhinitis* the patient has symptoms year-round. The causative agents, when they can be identified, are generally allergens to which the patient is exposed more or less continually, though exposure may vary during the year. Indoor inhalant allergens are implicated most often. These include components of house dust, feathers, allergens or danders of household pets, and mold spores. In an occasional patient, foods cause symptoms of allergic rhinitis. Some patients may be able to ingest certain foods with impunity except during a pollen season, when ingestion causes an aggravation of nasal symptoms. The prognosis is not good. Follow-up of children with allergic rhinitis 8–11 yr later disclosed that only 10% were free of symptoms; asthma or wheezing developed in 19%.

PATHOPHYSIOLOGY. Inhaled pollens, mold spores, and animal or mite antigens are deposited on the nasal mucosa. Water-soluble antigens diffuse into the epithelium and, in genetically predisposed atopic individuals, initiate the production of local immunoglobulin (Ig) E. IgE-stimulated release of mast cell mediators, synthesis of new mast cell mediators, and subsequent recruitment of neutrophils, eosinophils, basophils, and lymphocytes are responsible for the early and late-phase reactions to inhalant allergens. These reactions result in mucus, edema, inflammation, pruritus, and vasodilation. Delayed inflammation may contribute to nasal hyper-responsiveness to nonspecific stimuli, a priming effect.

DIAGNOSIS. The symptoms of allergic rhinitis include sneezing, which is frequently paroxysmal; rhinorrhea, which is often watery and profuse; nasal obstruction; and itching of the nose, palate, pharynx, and ears. Itching, redness, and tearing of the eyes may also occur, causing severe discomfort.

The typical patient with allergic rhinitis presents with bilateral nasal obstruction resulting from boggy edema of the mucous membranes. Frequently, redundant mucosa is piled up on the floor of the nose. The mucous membranes are bluish in hue and rather pale, and there is a clear mucoid nasal discharge. The child often has mannerisms caused by itching of the nose or attempts to improve the airway. The child wrinkles the nose (rabbit nose) and may rub it in characteristic ways (allergic salute). Rubbing in an upward direction may lead to a horizontal crease at the junction of the bulbous tip of the nose with the more rigid bridge. Dark circles under the eyes have been attributed to venous stasis resulting from interference with blood flow caused by edematous nasal mucous membranes. Mouth breathing is common. Fever is unusual except when sinusitis or otitis media complicates allergic rhinitis.

The diagnosis of allergic rhinitis is substantiated by the finding of a predominance of eosinophils in a smear made of the nasal secretions. A nasal smear is best prepared by having the child blow the nose into wax paper; the mucous sample is then transferred to a glass slide and stained selectively for eosinophils. There is often a personal or family history of eczema or asthma.

DIFFERENTIAL DIAGNOSIS. *Eosinophilic nonallergic rhinitis* occurs mostly in adults. Symptoms are perennial; the mucous membranes are pale, and there may be associated nasal polyps or sinus disease. Eosinophils are found in the nasal smear, but serum IgE levels are normal and allergy skin tests are generally negative. *Primary nasal mastocytosis,* with onset most often in adulthood, presents with perennial nasal blockage and rhinorrhea. Mast cells are found in the nasal smear, and allergy skin tests are negative. *Neutrophilic (infectious) rhinitis* occurs during the early years of childhood when allergic rhinitis is uncommon; there are complaints of chronic rhinorrhea and nasal blockage, mostly during cold weather. Nasal secretions are commonly mucopurulent, and the nasal smear shows neutrophils, bacteria, and debris. A posterior pharyngeal discharge is often present. Radiographic studies of the maxillary sinuses or computed tomographic scans may show evidence of sinusitis. The condition appears to result from recurrent viral respiratory illnesses complicated by bacterial infections, but the possibility of underlying disease such as humoral antibody deficiency, ciliary dyskinesia, or cystic fibrosis should be considered. *Vasomotor rhinitis* designates a poorly understood disorder presumably resulting from an imbalance of autonomic nervous system control of mucosal vasculature and mucous glands, in which symptoms suggest allergic rhinitis but an allergic cause cannot be identified. Nasal obstruction is the predominant symptom, with minimal itching, sneezing, and rhinorrhea. The obstruction is aggravated by environmental changes in temperature or humidity and by exposure to irritants such as tobacco smoke. The patients do not have eosinophils in their nasal secretions.

Other causes of nasal obstruction include *unilateral choanal atresia* in infants who have a unilateral nasal discharge, *deviated septum, hypertrophy of the adenoids, encephalocele*, and *nasal polyposis*. Nasal polyposis occurs in as many as 20% of children with cystic fibrosis. Fewer than 0.5% of patients in a typical allergy practice have nasal polyps resulting from allergic rhinitis. Nasal polyposis occurs in *ciliary dyskinesia* (immotile cilia syndrome, Chapter 364) and in *immunological deficiencies*. The syndrome of nasal polyps, asthma, and aspirin intolerance is known as *triad asthma*. A foul-smelling, unilateral purulent, or blood-tinged purulent nasal discharge in a child suggests a *foreign body*. A persistent bloody discharge always suggests *malignancy*; nasal obstruction with epistaxis in a male in late childhood or early adolescence suggests *benign nasopharyngeal fibroma*, also known as *angiofibroma*. Nasal obstruction occurs in *hypothyroidism*. Adolescents may suffer from *rhinitis of pregnancy*. A profuse, clear nasal discharge should suggest *cerebrospinal fluid rhinorrhea*, which can be confirmed by measuring the level of glucose in the fluid. Excessive use of vasoconstrictor nose drops or sprays can lead to *rhinitis medicamentosa*, in which nasal obstruction can be severe. Chronic cocaine abuse may produce rhinitis with or without secondary infection or nasal septum perforation. Additional rarer causes of rhinitis-like symptoms include syphilis, diphtheria, Wegener granulomatosis, sarcoidosis, and various malignancies.

Swelling of the mucous membranes of the sinuses frequently occurs with allergic rhinitis in childhood and may be seen in roentgenograms of the involved sinuses, occasionally with fluid levels. The sinuses appear abnormal so often on roentgenography, not only in children with allergic rhinitis but also in those with viral upper respiratory tract infections and in entirely asymptomatic children, that such examination must be carefully interpreted. Sinus infection may complicate allergic rhinitis; the symptoms generally are nocturnal coughing, fetid breath, and persistent mucopurulent nasal and pharyngeal discharge. Headache and facial pain and swelling are prominent symptoms of sinusitis in older children.

TREATMENT. Treatment of either seasonal or perennial allergic rhinitis includes avoidance of exposure to suspected allergens and irritants, immunotherapy for those who cannot avoid inhalant allergens, and drug therapy.

Avoidance. It is difficult or impractical to avoid exposure to seasonal pollens, but much can be done to eliminate exposure to such indoor inhalant factors as house dust, danders, and molds. Control of house dust, with special attention to the child's bedroom, often ameliorates symptoms in the dust-allergic child. Elimination of exposure to danders and feathers is mandatory for a child with perennial allergic rhinitis when these factors contribute to the symptoms. For the child sensitive to indoor molds, avoidance of damp basements and measures to discourage mold growth in the house frequently are beneficial. These measures include dehumidifiers, air conditioners with efficient filters, and air-cleaning devices, either the electronic precipitator type or one containing a high-efficiency particulate air filter. A 1:750 solution of Zephiran Chloride is effective in controlling mold growth. In areas that can be closed off, such as damp cellars, volatilization of paraformaldehyde (25–50 g, depending upon the size of the area to be treated) from several open jars is also frequently effective in inhibiting growth of mold. For infants with persistent rhinorrhea and nasal obstruction, dietary elimination of milk, egg, or wheat is rarely helpful unless allergy skin testing or in vitro testing has confirmed food allergy.

Immunotherapy is discussed in Chapter 135.2.

Drug Therapy. Appropriate drugs usually relieve symptoms of allergic rhinitis. *Antihistamines* are useful, especially in the treatment of seasonal allergic rhinitis (Chapter 135.1). It may be necessary to increase the dosage beyond that routinely recommended until relief of symptoms or side effects occur. Nasal itching, sneezing, and rhinorrhea are usually well controlled by antihistamine therapy, whereas nasal obstruction is relieved to a lesser degree. The major adverse side effect of antihistamine therapy is somnolence, which usually lessens with continued use. Nonsedating antihistamines (astemizole, loratadine, terfenadine) should be used if possible because of evidence that first-generation antihistamines often cause impairment of function even in patients unaware of somnolence.

If nasal obstruction is particularly troublesome, a decongestant such as pseudoephedrine or phenylpropanolamine may be administered alone or in combination with an antihistamine. Nose drops or sprays containing sympathomimetic drugs should be avoided except for short-term use; continued use may lead to progressively severe nasal obstruction due to rebound vasodilatation. Treatment of this latter complication requires complete cessation of use of medicated nose drops and the substitution of nose drops of physiological saline solution.

Cromolyn nasal solution (4%) is useful both in seasonal and in perennial allergic rhinitis. In children with hay fever, use of the nasal spray is best begun before the pollen season. The dose varies from one to two sprays in each nostril three to six times per day. As with the powder, cromolyn nasal solution is used prophylactically (Chapter 135.1).

By far the most effective treatment of allergic rhinitis is topical use of *corticosteroids*. Beclomethasone (Vancenase or Beconase), budesonide (Rhinocort), flunisolide (Nasalide), or fluticasone (Flonase) should be used in children whose nasal symptoms are resistant to antihistamine-decongestant therapy. The initial dosage is usually one to two sprays in each nostril two to three times per day (budesonide, 2 sprays to each nostril twice each day; fluticasone, 2 sprays to each nostril daily). After 3–4 days, as symptoms improve, the dose and frequency of use are reduced until a minimal effective dosage, one to two sprays once or twice each day, is reached and continued as maintenance therapy. Occasionally, temporary use of corticosteroid eye drops is necessary in a child with hay fever and particularly severe eye symptoms. Treatment with 0.1% lodoxamide tromethamine (Alomide) eye drops four times each day is safer and is often effective in preventing symptoms of allergic conjunctivitis. Treatment of allergic conjunctivitis with 0.05% levocabastine hydrochloride eye drops four times each day is also effective, but this H_1 antihistamine is not recommended for use in children younger than 12 yr. Complications of topical nasal steroids include local burning, irritation, and epistaxis. There is no systemic absorption, and nasal or pharyngeal candidiasis and mucosal atrophy are not problems.

For children who suffer from persistent neutrophilic (infectious) rhinitis with or without sinusitis, a 2-wk course of a broad-spectrum antibiotic (such as amoxicillin) frequently is effective. Nasal irrigation with a warm saline solution using a bulb syringe or with an adaptation of the Water Pik device (1 tsp of salt to a full reservoir of warm water) is helpful symptomatically in patients with nonallergic chronic rhinitis.

Abelson MB, George MA, Garofalo C: Differential diagnosis of ocular allergic disorders. Ann Allergy 79:95, 1993.

Fahy GT, Easty DL, Collum LM, et al: Randomised double-masked trial of lodoxamide and sodium cromoglycate in allergic eye disease: A multicentre study. Eur J Ophthalmol 2:144, 1992.

Kaliner M, Lemanske R: Rhinitis and asthma. JAMA 268:2807, 1992.

Linna O, Kokkonen J, Lukin M: A 10-year prognosis for childhood allergic rhinitis. Acta Paediatr 81:100, 1992.

Meltzer EO, Zeiger RS, Schatz M, et al: Chronic rhinitis in infants and children: Etiologic, diagnostic and therapeutic considerations. Pediatr Clin North Am 30:847, 1983.

Simons FE: Allergic rhinitis: Recent advances. Pediatr Clin North Am 35:1053, 1988.

CHAPTER 137
Asthma

Asthma is a leading cause of chronic illness in childhood, responsible for a significant proportion of school days lost because of chronic illness. Asthma is the most frequent admitting diagnosis in children's hospitals and results nationally in 5–7 lost school days/yr/child. As many as 10–15% of boys and 7–10% of girls may have asthma at some time during childhood. Before puberty approximately twice as many boys as girls are affected; thereafter, the sex incidence is equal. Asthma can lead to severe psychosocial disturbances in the family. With proper treatment, however, satisfactory control of symptoms is almost always possible. There is no universally accepted definition of asthma; it may be regarded as a diffuse, obstructive lung disease with (1) hyper-reactivity of the airways to a variety of stimuli and (2) a high degree of reversibility of the obstructive process, which may occur either spontaneously or as a result of treatment. Also known as *reactive airway disease*, the asthma complex probably includes wheezy bronchitis, viral-associated wheezing, and atopic related asthma. In addition to bronchoconstriction, inflammation is an important pathophysiologic factor; it involves eosinophils, monocytes, and immune mediators and has resulted in the alternative designation of *chronic desquamating eosinophilic bronchitis*.

Both large (>2 mm) and small (<2 mm) airways may be involved to varying degrees. Irritability or hyper-reactivity of the airways, while not limited to asthmatic patients, appears to be an intrinsic part of the disease and is present to some degree in almost all asthmatic subjects. This hyper-responsiveness manifests itself as bronchoconstriction following exercise; on natural exposures to strong odors or irritant fumes such as sulfur dioxide, tobacco smoke, or cold air; and upon intentional exposures in the laboratory to inhalations of histamine or parasympathomimetic agents such as methacholine (Mecholyl). This heightened airway irritability is a sensitive objective indicator of asthma and is present to some degree when patients are asymptomatic, free of abnormal physical findings, and capable of normal findings on spirometry. Airway hyper-reactivity relates to the overall severity of the disease. It varies from patient to patient but generally is relatively stable over time in the same patient except for temporary fluctuations; increased reactivity occurs during viral respiratory infections, following exposure to air pollutants and to allergens or to occupational chemicals in sensitized individuals, and following administration of β-receptor antagonists. An acute decrease in airway irritability follows administration of β-receptor agonists, theophylline, and anticholinergics, and decreased irritability follows chronic administration of cromolyn, nedocromil, or systemic or inhaled corticosteroids.

Data on the inheritance of asthma are most compatible with polygenic or multifactorial determinants. A child with one affected parent has about a 25% risk of having asthma; the risk increases to about 50% if both parents are asthmatic. However, asthma is not universally present among monozygotic twins. Lability of bronchoconstriction with exercise is concordant in identical twins but not in dizygotic twins. Bronchial lability in response to exercise testing also has been demonstrated in healthy relatives of asthmatic children. A genetic predisposition combined with environmental factors may explain most cases of childhood asthma.

EPIDEMIOLOGY. Asthma may have its onset at any age; 30% of patients are symptomatic by 1 yr of age, whereas 80–90% of asthmatic children have their first symptoms before 4–5 yr of age. The course and severity of asthma are difficult to predict. The majority of affected children have only occasional attacks of slight to moderate severity, managed with relative ease. A minority experience severe, intractable asthma, usually perennial rather than seasonal; it is incapacitating and interferes with school attendance, play activity, and day-to-day functioning. The relationship of age of onset to prognosis is uncertain; most severely affected children have onset of wheezing during the 1st yr of life and family histories of asthma and other allergic diseases (particularly atopic dermatitis). These children may have growth retardation unrelated to corticosteroid administration, chest deformity secondary to chronic hyperinflation, and persistent abnormalities on pulmonary function testing.

The prognosis for young asthmatic children is generally good. Ultimate remission depends partly upon growth in the cross-sectional diameter of the airways. Longitudinal studies indicate that about 50% of all asthmatic children are virtually free of symptoms within 10–20 yr, but recurrences are common in adulthood. In children who have mild asthma with onset between 2 yr and puberty, the remission rate is about 50%, and only 5% experience severe disease. In contrast, children with severe asthma characterized by chronic steroid-dependent disease with frequent hospitalizations rarely improve, and about 95% become asthmatic adults. Whether the hyperirritability of their airways ever disappears is unknown; abnormal responsiveness to methacholine inhalation in formerly asthmatic patients has been found as long as 20 yr after symptoms have abated.

Both prevalence and mortality from asthma have increased during the last 2 decades. The causes of the increased prevalence are unknown, but some of the factors associated with both onset of asthma and increased mortality have been identified. Risk factors for the occurrence of asthma include poverty, black race, maternal age less than 20 yr at the time of birth, birthweight less than 2,500 gm, maternal smoking (more than one-half pack per day), small home size (<eight rooms), large family size (≥six members), and intense allergenic exposure in infancy (more than 10 μg of house dust mite allergen *Der p* I per gram of dust collected from homes). Additional risk factors may include frequent respiratory infections in early childhood and less than optimal parenting. Sensitization to inhalant allergens can occur in infancy, but it becomes increasingly frequent beyond 2 yr of age and is demonstrable in most children beyond 4 yr of age who require emergency room visits for wheezing. Risk factors for death from asthma include underestimation of severity of asthma, delay in implementation of appropriate treatment, underuse of bronchodilators and corticosteroids, black race, noncompliance with recommendations for management, psychosocial dysfunction and stress that may interfere with compliance or perception of increasing airway obstruction, sedation, and excessive allergenic exposure. Recent emergency treatment or recent admission to a hospital for asthma increases the risk of fatal asthma. Patients subject to sudden, severe airway obstruction and those with chronic, steroid-dependent asthma are at especially high risk for fatal asthma.

PATHOPHYSIOLOGY. Manifestations of the airway obstruction in asthma are due to bronchoconstriction, hypersecretion of mucus, mucosal edema, cellular infiltration, and desquamation of epithelial and inflammatory cells. Various allergic and nonspecific stimuli, in the presence of hyper-reactive airways, initiate the bronchoconstriction and inflammatory response. These stimuli include inhaled allergens (dust mites, pollens, soybean or castor bean proteins), other vegetable proteins, viral infection, cigarette smoke, air pollutants, odors, drugs (nonsteroid anti-inflammatory agents, β-receptor antagonists, metabisulfite), cold air, and exercise.

The pathology of severe asthma includes bronchoconstriction, bronchial smooth muscle hypertrophy, mucous gland hypertrophy, mucosal edema, infiltration of inflammatory cells (eosinophils, neutrophils, basophils, macrophages), and desquamation. Pathognomonic findings include Charcot-Leyden crystals (lysophospholipase from eosinophil membranes), Curschmann spirals (bronchial mucous casts), and Creola bodies (desquamated epithelial cells).

Newly synthesized and stored mediators are released from local mucosal mast cells following nonspecific stimulation or the binding of allergens to specific mast cell-associated immunoglobulin (Ig) E. Mediators such as histamine, leukotrienes C_4, D_4, and E_4, and platelet activating factor initiate bronchoconstriction, mucosal edema, and the immune responses (see Chapter 133). The early immune response results in bronchoconstriction, is treatable with β_2-receptor agonists, and may be prevented by mast cell–stabilizing agents (cromolyn or nedocromil). The late immune response occurs 6–8 hr later, produces a continued state of airway hyper-responsiveness with eosinophilic and neutrophilic infiltration, can be treated and prevented by steroids, and can be prevented by cromolyn or nedocromil.

Obstruction is most severe during expiration because the intrathoracic airways normally become smaller during expiration. Although the airway obstruction is diffuse, it is not entirely uniform throughout the lungs. Segmental or subsegmental atelectasis may occur, aggravating mismatching of ventilation and perfusion (Fig. 137–1). Hyperinflation causes decreased compliance, with consequently increased work of breathing. Increased transpulmonary pressures, necessary for expiration through obstructed airways, may cause further narrowing or complete premature closure of some airways during expiration, thus increasing the risk of pneumothorax. Increased intrathoracic pressure may interfere with venous return and reduce cardiac output, which may be manifested as a pulsus paradoxus.

Mismatching of ventilation with perfusion, alveolar hypoventilation, and increased work of breathing cause changes in blood gases (see Fig. 137–1). Hyperventilation of some regions of the lung compensates initially for the higher carbon dioxide tension in blood that perfuses poorly ventilated regions. However, it cannot compensate for hypoxemia while breathing

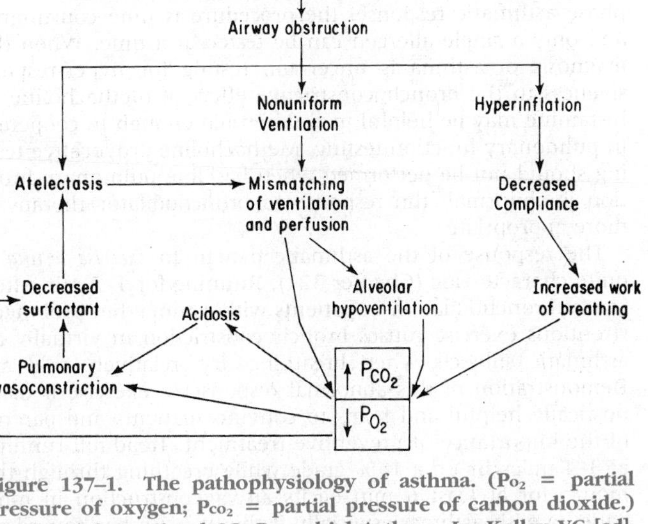

Figure 137–1. The pathophysiology of asthma. (P_{O_2} = partial pressure of oxygen; P_{CO_2} = partial pressure of carbon dioxide.) (Modified from Siegel SC: Bronchial Asthma. *In:* Kelley VC [ed]: Practice of Pediatrics. Chapter 74, Vol 2. Hagerstown, MD, Harper & Row, 1987.)

room air because of the patient's inability to increase the partial pressure of oxygen and oxyhemoglobulin saturation. Further progression of airway obstruction causes more alveolar hypoventilation, and hypercapnia may occur suddenly. Hypoxia interferes with conversion of lactic acid to carbon dioxide and water, causing metabolic acidosis. Hypercapnia increases carbonic acid, which dissociates into hydrogen ions and bicarbonate ions, causing respiratory acidosis.

Hypoxia and acidosis can cause pulmonary vasoconstriction, but cor pulmonale resulting from sustained pulmonary hypertension is not a common complication of asthma. Hypoxia and vasoconstriction may damage type II alveolar cells, diminishing production of surfactant, which normally stabilizes alveoli. Thus, this process may aggravate the tendency toward atelectasis.

ETIOLOGY. Asthma is a complex disorder involving autonomic, immunologic, infectious, endocrine, and psychologic factors in varying degrees in different individuals. The control of the diameter of the airways may be considered a balance of neural and humoral forces. Neural bronchoconstrictor activity is mediated through the cholinergic portion of the autonomic nervous system. Vagal sensory endings in airway epithelium, termed cough or irritant receptors, depending upon their location, initiate the afferent limb of a reflex arc, which at the efferent end stimulates bronchial smooth muscle contraction. Vasoactive intestinal peptide (VIP) neurotransmission initiates bronchial smooth muscle relaxation. VIP may be a dominant neuropeptide involved in maintaining airway patency. Humoral factors favoring bronchodilation include the endogenous catecholamines that act on β-adrenergic receptors to produce relaxation in bronchial smooth muscle. When local humoral substances such as histamine and leukotrienes are released through immunologically mediated reactions, they produce bronchoconstriction, either by direct action on smooth muscle or by stimulation of the vagal sensory receptors. Locally produced adenosine, which binds to a specific receptor, may contribute to bronchoconstriction. Methylxanthines are competitive antagonists of adenosine.

Asthma may be due to abnormal β-adrenergic receptor-adenylate cyclase function, with decreased adrenergic responsiveness. Reports of decreased numbers of β-adrenergic receptors on leukocytes of asthmatic patients may provide a structural basis for hyporesponsiveness to β-agonists. Alternatively, increased cholinergic activity in the airway has been proposed as a defect in asthma, perhaps due to some intrinsic or acquired abnormality in irritant receptors, which seem in asthmatic patients to have lower than normal thresholds for response to stimulation. Neither theory reconciles all the data. In individual patients a number of factors generally contribute in varying degrees to the activity of the asthmatic process.

Immunologic Factors. In some patients with so-called *extrinsic* or *allergic asthma,* exacerbations follow exposure to environmental factors such as dust, pollens, and danders. Often but not always, such patients have increased concentrations both of total IgE and of specific IgE against the allergen implicated. In other patients with clinically similar asthma, there is no evidence of IgE involvement; skin tests are negative and IgE concentrations low. This form of asthma, which is seen most often in the first 2 yr of life and in older adults (late-onset asthma), has been called *intrinsic.* The distinction between intrinsic and extrinsic asthma may be artificial because the basic immune mediator-induced mucosal injury is similar in both groups. Extrinsic asthma may be associated with more easily identified stimuli of mediator release than intrinsic asthma. Patients of all ages with asthma usually have elevated serum IgE levels, suggesting an allergic-extrinsic component in most patients. Although increased IgE levels may be due to atopy, chronic nonspecific stimulation of the mast cell allergen-induced late-phase immune reactions creates a prolonged nonspecific airway hyper-reactivity, which can produce bronchospasm in the absence of identifiable extrinsic factors.

Viral agents are the most important infectious triggers of asthma. Early in life respiratory syncytial virus (RSV) and parainfluenza virus are most often involved; in older children rhinoviruses have also been implicated. Influenza virus infection assumes importance with increasing age. Viral agents may act to initiate asthma through stimulation of afferent vagal receptors of the cholinergic system in the airways. An IgE response to RSV can occur in infants and children with RSV-associated wheezing but not in those whose RSV respiratory disease is without associated wheezing. Wheezing with RSV infection may unmask a predisposition to asthma.

Endocrine Factors. Asthma may worsen in relation to pregnancy and menses, especially premenstrually, or may have its onset in women at the menopause. It improves in some children at puberty. Little else is known about the role of endocrine factors in the etiology or pathogenesis of asthma. Thyrotoxicosis increases the severity of asthma; the mechanism is unknown.

Psychologic Factors. Emotional factors can trigger symptoms in many asthmatic children and adults, but "deviant" emotional or behavioral characteristics are not more common among asthmatic children than among children with other chronic disabling illnesses. On the other hand, the effects of severe chronic illness such as asthma on children's views of themselves, their parents' views of them, or their lives in general can be devastating. Emotional or behavioral disturbances are related more closely to poor control of asthma than to the severity of the attack itself; accordingly, skillful medical intervention can have an important impact.

CLINICAL MANIFESTATIONS. The onset of an asthma exacerbation may be acute or insidious. Acute episodes are most often caused by exposure to irritants such as cold air and noxious fumes (smoke, wet paint) or exposure to allergens or simple chemicals, for example, aspirin or sulfites. When airway obstruction develops rapidly in a few minutes, it is most likely due to smooth muscle spasm in large airways. Exacerbations precipitated by viral respiratory infections are slower in onset, with gradual increases in frequency and severity of cough and wheezing over a few days. Because airway patency decreases at night, many children have acute asthma at this time. The signs and symptoms of asthma include cough, which sounds tight and is nonproductive early in the course of an attack; wheezing, tachypnea, and dyspnea with prolonged expiration and use of accessory muscles of respiration; cyanosis; hyperinflation of the chest; tachycardia and pulsus paradoxus, which may be present to varying degrees depending upon the stage and severity of the attack. Cough may be present without wheezing, or wheezing may be present without cough; tachypnea also may be present without wheezing. Manifestations will vary depending on the severity of the exacerbation (Table 137–1).

When the patient is in extreme respiratory distress, the cardinal sign of asthma, wheezing, may be strikingly absent; in such patients, only after bronchodilator treatment gives partial relief of the airway obstruction can enough movement of air occur to evoke wheezing. Shortness of breath may be so severe that the child has difficulty walking or even talking. The patient with severe obstruction may assume a hunched-over, tripod-like sitting position that makes it easier to breathe. Expiration is typically more difficult because of premature expiratory closure of the airway, but many children complain of inspiratory difficulty as well. Abdominal pain is common, particularly in younger children, and is due presumably to the strenuous use of abdominal muscles and the diaphragm. The liver and spleen may be palpable because of hyperinflation of the lungs. Vomiting is common and may be followed by temporary relief of symptoms.

During severe airway obstruction respiratory effort may be great, and the child may sweat profusely; a low-grade fever may develop simply from the enormous work of breathing; fatigue may become severe. Between exacerbations the child may be entirely free of symptoms and have no evidence of pulmonary disease on physical examination. A barrel chest deformity is a sign of the chronic, unremitting airway obstruction of severe asthma. Harrison sulci, an anterolateral depression of the thorax at the insertion of the diaphragm, may be present in children with recurrent severe retractions. Clubbing of the fingers is rarely observed in uncomplicated asthma, even in severe asthma. Clubbing suggests other causes of chronic obstructive lung disease such as cystic fibrosis.

DIAGNOSIS. Recurrent episodes of coughing and wheezing, especially if aggravated or triggered by exercise, viral infection, or inhaled allergens, are highly suggestive of asthma. However, asthma can also cause persistent coughing in children with no history of wheezing because flow rates are insufficient to generate wheezing, airway obstruction is relatively mild, or caretakers are unable to recognize wheezing. Symptoms may have been ascribed erroneously to "allergic cough," "allergic bronchitis," "wheezy bronchitis," or "chronic bronchitis." Pulmonary function testing before and after administration of methacholine or a bronchodilator or before and after exercise may help establish the diagnosis of asthma. Examination during an episode of severe symptoms may also be helpful if improvement occurs following bronchodilator therapy. Furthermore, when treated by measures that are specific for asthma, affected children show remarkable improvement, strongly suggesting that the cough is a sign of asthma.

Laboratory Evaluation. *Eosinophilia* of the blood and sputum occurs with asthma. Blood eosinophilia of more than 250–400 cells/mm^3 is usual. Asthmatic sputum is grossly tenacious, rubbery, and whitish. An eosin-methylene blue stain usually discloses numerous eosinophils and the granules from disrupted cells. Few diseases in children other than asthma are likely to cause eosinophilia in sputum. Sputum cultures are generally not helpful in asthmatic children because bacterial superinfection is rare and cultures are frequently contaminated with oropharyngeal organisms. Serum protein and immunoglobulin concentrations are generally normal in asthma except that IgE levels may be increased.

Allergy skin testing and *rast* (radioallergosorbent test) or other in vitro determinations of specific IgE are useful in identifying potentially important environmental allergens (Chapter 134).

Inhalation bronchial challenge testing is only rarely done to explore the clinical significance of allergens implicated by skin testing, because the allergenic challenge can provoke a late-phase asthmatic response, the procedure is time consuming, and only a single allergen can be tested at a time. When the diagnosis of asthma is uncertain, testing for hyper-responsiveness to the bronchoconstrictive effect of methacholine or histamine may be helpful in children old enough to cooperate in pulmonary function testing. Methacholine provocative testing should not be performed when baseline pulmonary function is abnormal; the response to bronchodilator therapy is more appropriate.

The response of the asthmatic patient to *exercise testing* is quite characteristic (Chapter 321). Running for 1–2 min often causes bronchodilation in patients with asthma, but prolonged strenuous exercise causes bronchoconstriction in virtually all asthmatic subjects when breathing dry, relatively cold air. Demonstration of this abnormal response to exercise is diagnostically helpful and helps to convince patients and parents of the importance of preventive treatment. Treadmill running at 3–4 miles/hr up a 15% grade while breathing through the mouth for at least 6 min elicits airway obstruction in most patients with asthma, especially if the exercise has caused an increase in pulse rate to at least 180 beats/min. Measurement of pulmonary function immediately before exercise, immedi-

■ **TABLE 137–1 Estimation of Severity of Acute Exacerbation in Children with Asthma**

Sign/Symptom	Mild	Moderate	Severe
Peak expiratory flow rate	70%–90% predicted or baseline	50%–70% predicted or baseline	<50% predicted or baseline
Respiratory rate	Normal to 30% above mean	30%–50% increase above mean	>50% increase above mean
Alertness	Normal	Normal	May be decreased
Dyspnea	Absent or mild, speaks in complete sentences	Moderate, speaks in phrases or partial sentences	Severe, speaks only in single words or short phrases
Accessory muscle use	No intercostal to mild retractions	Moderate intercostal retractions with tracheosternal retractions, use of sternocleidomastoid muscles, chest hyperinflation	Moderate intercostal retractions, tracheosternal retractions with nasal flaring during inspiration, chest hyperinflation
Color	Good	Pale	Possibly cyanotic
Auscultation	End expiratory wheeze only	Inspiratory and expiratory wheezing	Breath sounds inaudible
Oxygen saturation (opt)*	>95%	90%–95%	<90%
$PCO_{2\,(opt)}$	<35	<40	>40

**Oxygen saturation values will have to be adjusted for altitude. These values assume that the patient is at sea level.*
From the Provisional Committee on Quality Improvement: Practice parameter: The office management of acute exacerbations of asthma in children. Pediatrics 93:119, 1994.

ately after exercise, and 5 and 10 min later usually discloses decreases in peak expiratory flow rate (PFR) or forced expiratory volume in 1 sec (FEV_1) of at least 15% without premedication. If exercise causes no airway obstruction, repeat testing on other days when relative humidity is low usually elicits a positive response in patients with asthma. Exercise testing should be deferred whenever significant airway obstruction is already present. If possible, bronchodilators and cromolyn should be withheld for at least 8 hr before testing; slow-release theophylline should not be administered 12–24 hr prior to testing.

Every child suspected of having asthma does not require *roentgenograms of the chest,* but these are often appropriate to exclude other possible diagnoses or complications, such as atelectasis or pneumonia. Lung markings are commonly increased in asthma. Hyperinflation occurs during acute attacks and may become chronic when airway obstruction is persistent. Atelectasis may occur in as many as 6% of children during acute exacerbations and is especially likely to involve the right middle lobe, where it may persist for months. Repeated chest roentgenograms during exacerbations usually are not indicated in the absence of fever, unless there is suspicion of a pneumothorax, or tachypnea greater than 60 beats/min, tachycardia of more than 160 beats/min, localized rales or wheezing, or decreased breath sounds.

Pulmonary function testing (Chapters 321 and 324.8) is valuable in the evaluation of children in whom asthma is suspected. In those known to have asthma, such tests are useful in assessing the degree of airway obstruction and the disturbance in gas exchange, in measuring response of the airways to inhaled allergens and chemicals or exercise (bronchial provocation testing), in assessing the response to therapeutic agents, and in evaluating the long-term course of the disease. Assessments of pulmonary function in asthma are most valuable when made before and after administration of an aerosol bronchodilator, a procedure that indicates the degree of reversibility of the airway obstruction at the time of the testing (Chapters 321 and 324.8). An increase of at least 10% in PFR or FEV_1 after aerosol therapy is strongly suggestive of asthma. Failure to respond does not exclude asthma and may be due to status asthmaticus or to near-maximal pulmonary function.

In mild cases of asthma in remission, no abnormalities may be detected. In others a variety of abnormalities may be found (see Table 137–1). Total lung capacity, functional residual capacity, and residual volume are increased. Vital capacity is usually decreased. Dynamic tests of air flow, forced vital capacity (FVC), FEV_1, PFR, and maximum expiratory flow between 25 and 75% of the vital capacity ($FEF_{25-75\%}$) may also show reduced values, which return toward normal after administration of aerosolized bronchodilators. With the availability of small, relatively inexpensive instruments that measure peak expiratory flow rate (Mini-Wright Peak Flow Meter, Healthscan Assess Plus peak flow meter), it is feasible to monitor expiratory flow rate at home two to three times each day. This provides objective measurements of the degree of airway obstruction between office visits. A fall in peak expiratory flow predicts the onset of an exacerbation and encourages early intervention with additional drug therapy.

Determination of arterial blood gases and pH is important in evaluation of the patient with asthma during an exacerbation requiring hospitalization. During remission, partial pressure of oxygen (PO_2), partial pressure of carbon dioxide (PCO_2), and pH may be normal. In symptomatic periods, low PO_2 is regularly found and may persist days to weeks after an acute episode is over. Determination of oxygen saturation by pulse oximetry is helpful in determining the severity of an acute exacerbation. PCO_2 is generally low during the early stages of acute asthma. As the obstruction worsens, PCO_2 rises; this is an ominous sign. Blood pH remains normal (or sometimes slightly alkalotic owing to hyperventilation) until the buffering capacity of the blood is exhausted, and then acidosis develops. As airway obstruction and hypoxia become more severe, a mixed respiratory and metabolic acidosis develops owing to hypercarbia and lactic acidosis, respectively.

DIFFERENTIAL DIAGNOSIS. Most children who have recurrent episodes of coughing and wheezing have asthma. Other causes of airway obstruction include congenital malformations (of the respiratory, cardiovascular, or gastrointestinal systems), foreign bodies in the airway or esophagus, infectious bronchiolitis, cystic fibrosis, immunologic deficiency disease, hypersensitivity pneumonitis, allergic bronchopulmonary aspergillosis, and a variety of rarer conditions that compromise the airway, including endobronchial tuberculosis, fungal diseases, and bronchial adenoma (Table 137–2). Very rarely in the United States, tropical eosinophilia and other parasitic infections may involve the lung and mimic asthma.

ASTHMA IN EARLY LIFE. Wheezing in the infant merits special mention because it is common and presents substantial diagnostic and therapeutic problems. A significant number of children subsequently shown to have asthma have had symptoms of obstructive airway disease early in life (30% younger than 1 yr and 50–55% younger than 2 yr).

A number of anatomic and physiologic peculiarities of early life predispose to obstructive airway disease: (1) a decreased amount of smooth muscle in the peripheral airways compared to adults may result in less support; (2) mucous gland hyperplasia in the major bronchi compared to adults favors increased intraluminal mucus production; (3) disproportionately narrow peripheral airways up to 5 yr of age result in decreased conductance relative to adults and render the infant and young

■ **Table 137–2 Differential Diagnosis of Childhood Asthma**

Disease	Comment
Infections	
Bronchiolitis (RSV)	Atopic individuals may have predisposition to wheeze with RSV
Pneumonia	Acute febrile illness
Croup	Barking cough, stridor, more than wheezing
Tuberculosis, histoplasmosis	Lymphadenopathy compresses bronchi with wheezing
Bronchiectasis	Congenital, acquired, 1st- or 2nd-degree infections
Bronchiolitis obliterans	Postinfections process (influenza, adenovirus, measles)
Bronchitis	Probably asthma
Anatomic, Congenital	
Cystic fibrosis	Persistent symptoms, clubbing, *Streptococcus aureus, Pseudomonas aeruginosa, P. cepacia*
Vascular rings	Associated esophageal abnomalities
Ciliary dyskinesia	Chronic, recurrent infections, situs inversus
B lymphocyte immune defect	Recurrent sinopulmonary infection
Congestive heart failure	Murmur, large left to right shunt
Laryngotracheomalacia	Stridor, noisy respirations from birth
Tumor, lymphoma	Bronchial obstruction
H-type tracheoesophageal fistula	Rare, difficult to diagnose, recurrent aspiration pneumonia from birth
Repaired tracheoesophageal fistula	Patients have increased risk of reflux and wheezing, possibly asthma
Gastroesophageal reflux	May also exacerbate true asthma
Vasculitis, Hypersensitivity	
Allergic bronchopulmonary aspergillosis	Marked eosinophilia, high serum IgE levels; sputum positive for aspergillosis
Allergic alveolitis, hypersensitivity pneumonitis	Reaction to foreign antigen (fungi, bird protein, plants); occupational
Churg-Strauss syndrome	Allergic angiitis and granulomatosis, eosinophilia
Periarteritis nodosa	Multisystem (kidney, lung, nerves), eosinophilia
Other	
Foreign body aspiration	Sudden cough, gagging, *localized* wheezing and diminished breath sounds
Pulmonary thromboembolism	Acute chest pain, hypoxia
Psychogenic cough	Absent during sleep
Sarcoidosis	Lymphadenopathy-induced bronchial obstruction
Bronchopulmonary dysplasia	History of prematurity, may predispose to asthma

RSV = respiratory syncytial virus; IgE = immunoglobulin E.

child vulnerable to disease affecting the small airways; (4) decreased static elastic recoil of the young lung prediposes to early airway closure during tidal breathing and results in mismatching of ventilation and perfusion and hypoxemia; (5) highly compliant rib cage and mechanically disadvantageous angle of insertion of diaphragm to rib cage (horizontal vs. oblique in the adult) increase diaphragmatic work of breathing; (6) decreased number of fatigue-resistant skeletal muscle fibers in the diaphragm leave the diaphragm poorly equipped to maintain high work output; and (7) deficient collateral ventilation with the pores of Kohn and the Lambert canals deficient in number and size. The infant and young child are therefore predisposed to the development of atelectasis distal to obstructed airways. The combination of these factors with the normal susceptibility of infants and children to viral respiratory infections renders this age group particularly vulnerable to lower respiratory tract obstructive disease.

The clinical, roentgenographic, and blood gas findings in asthma and bronchiolitis are quite similar. It is helpful to remember that the incidence of bronchiolitis caused by RSV peaks during the first 6 mo of life, principally during the cold weather months, and that second and third attacks are uncommon. Some clinicians have proposed using the response to epinephrine or albuterol aerosols to help decide whether an episode is asthma or bronchiolitis, with a favorable response favoring asthma. The validity of this test has not been established; the degree of response may be related more to the severity of the obstructive process than to its underlying nature. Trials of epinephrine or other bronchodilators are worthwhile, however, as discussed later.

The onset of symptoms is rather typical. Previously well infants or young children develop what may seem to be a cold with rhinorrhea, rapidly followed by irritability, cough, tachypnea, and wheezing. The symptoms may progress rapidly and often require hospitalization.

During infancy, respiratory tract infections with viruses or *Chlamydia* may cause symptoms of airway obstruction that can be confused with asthma. Bacterial infections of the lower airway are rare, and the concept that allergic reactions to bacteria cause asthma is unproved. A child with recurrent episodes of coughing and wheezing associated with bacterial infections should be investigated for cystic fibrosis or immunologic deficiency. Chronic aspiration caused by swallowing dysfunction (usually in developmentally delayed children) or gastroesophageal reflux also may cause recurrent cough and wheezing in early life. Symptoms of respiratory distress often occur with or shortly after feeding, and a chest roentgenogram is commonly abnormal. Rarer causes of obstructive airway disease in early life include obliterative bronchiolitis (usually a sequela of a severe viral insult, most often adenovirus) and bronchopulmonary dysplasia (see Table 137–2).

The role of food allergy as a major cause of obstructive airway symptoms during early life is controversial. Positive skin tests for IgE-mediated sensitivity to foods are very unusual in asthmatic infants, but when present, they indicate the need for temporary elimination of the suspected food, usually milk, wheat, or egg from the diet of the asthmatic patient. After elimination from the diet for 3 wk, challenge with the implicated food may be appropriate to confirm the clinical relevance of the positive skin test. Challenge may be necessary two or three times after temporary dietary elimination to ensure clinical relevance. Challenge is contraindicated in patients with a history of anaphylaxis after ingestion of the food. Confirmed food allergy indicates a need for dietary elimination for at least 6 mo (Chapters 135 and 145).

For an infant who has had several episodes of obstructive airway disease, a history of asthma, hay fever, or atopic dermatitis in mother, father, or siblings is an important predictor of subsequent obstructive airway problems. Eczema is also frequently associated with the subsequent appearance of asthma. Eosinophilia >400 cells/mm^3 (and especially >700 cells/mm^3) and high serum IgE concentrations predict continuing respiratory tract problems.

TREATMENT. Asthma therapy includes basic concepts of

avoiding allergens, improving bronchodilation, and reducing mediator-induced inflammation. Systemic or topical inhaled medications are used, depending upon the severity of the episode. The principles of avoidance of allergens outlined under treatment of allergic rhinitis also serve the child with asthma. The hyper-reactivity of the asthmatic airway as an additional factor is dealt with by minimizing exposure to nonspecific irritants such as tobacco smoke, smoke from wood-burning stoves, and fumes from kerosene heaters and to strong odors such as wet paint and disinfectants, and by avoiding ice-cold drinks and rapid changes in temperature and humidity. Maintenance of humidified air is important in dry, cold climates in the winter, but relative humidity should not exceed 50% because house dust mites thrive at higher humidity. If the clinical history suggests IgE-mediated sensitivity to inhalant allergens that cannot be avoided or can be only partially avoided, immunotherapy should be considered; its indications and evidence for its efficacy in asthma are discussed in Chapter 135.

Treatment of acute asthma based on severity and location (home, emergency department, in-patient hospital) is summarized in Figures 137–2 to 137–4.

Pharmacologic therapy is the mainstay of treatment of asthma. Oxygen administered by mask or nasal prongs at 2–3 L/min is indicated in most children during acute asthma. Not only is the Po_2 reduced during an acute episode, but drugs used in therapy (β-adrenergic agonists or intravenous aminophylline) may cause a transient fall in Po_2 secondary to worsening of ventilation-perfusion mismatching, which occurs because these agents cause pulmonary vasodilatation and increased cardiac output. Injection of epinephrine had been the treatment of choice for acute asthma for many years, but bronchodilator aerosols are now preferable.

When epinephrine is used, a dose of 0.01 mL/kg of the 1:1,000 (1.0 mg/mL) concentration of the aqueous preparation may be given. It may be necessary to repeat the same dose once or twice at intervals of 20 min to obtain optimal relief. In infants and small children a dose of 0.05 mL is often effective. The unpleasant side effects of epinephrine (pallor, tremor, anxiety, palpitations, and headache) can frequently be minimized if doses of no more than 0.3 mL are given at any age. Terbutaline, a more selective β_2-agonist (Chapter 135), is available in an injectable form and is an alternative to epinephrine. The usual dose of 0.01 mL/kg of the 1:1,000 (1 mg/mL) concentration does not cause peripheral vasoconstriction and has a longer duration of activity, up to 4 hr. The maximum dose of terbutaline by subcutaneous injection is 0.25 mL; this dose may be repeated once if necessary after 20 min.

Inhalation of bronchodilator aerosols is rapidly effective in relieving the signs and symptoms of asthma. Aerosols have the advantage that substantially less drug is given than would be required by the subcutaneous route; the unpleasant side effects of injected drugs such as epinephrine are avoided. Furthermore, despite airway obstruction, which may limit aerosol delivery to peripheral airways, aerosol therapy is probably more effective than epinephrine in reversing bronchoconstriction. Albuterol (Proventil, Ventolin) solution is safe and effective at a dose of 0.15 mg/kg (maximum 5 mg) followed by 0.05–0.15 mg/kg at intervals of 20–30 min until response is adequate. Albuterol is available as a 0.5% solution (5 mg/mL) to be diluted with 2–3 mL normal saline and as a prediluted 2.5-mg unit dose, 0.083% (0.83 mg/mL). Nebulization with oxygen at 6 L/min prevents hypoxemia that might be related to the treatment. Edetate disodium and benzalkonium chloride, found in some solutions of albuterol and metaproterenol for nebulization, can cause bronchoconstriction in occasional asthmatic patients; Ventolin Nebules contain neither.

If the response to epinephrine or bronchodilator aerosol is not satisfactory, aminophylline may be given intravenously in a dose of 5 mg/kg for 5–15 min at a rate no greater than 25 mg/min. This dose (which will increase the serum theophylline concentration by no more than 10 μg/mL at the peak) is safe in the patient who has had no theophylline in the past few hours. If there is reason to believe that the patient may already have a significant serum theophylline concentration, the intravenous dose should be held until the theophylline level is known. Thereafter, a theophylline dose of 1 mg/kg should increase the serum level by about 2 μg/mL. There is little additional benefit to be gained from adding theophylline to optimal β_2 aerosol therapy, but this combination may be helpful in patients with very severe airway obstruction or those receiving less than maximal treatment with inhaled β_2-adrenergic agonists. Addition of theophylline increases the likelihood of adverse side effects.

Most acute exacerbations of asthma respond to this treatment regimen. Unless the patient either is corticosteroid dependent or has had corticosteroids in the recent past, administration of steroids as part of the emergency room treatment program may be unnecessary. In borderline cases, however, when the decision is made to send the child home rather than to hospitalize him or her, a prescription of prednisone in decreasing doses over 5–7 days may hasten resolution of the exacerbation and causes no harm. The patient should be discharged from the emergency room with sufficient oral medication to continue therapy at home, and appropriate arrangements should be made for follow-up. Good ambulatory management will almost always reduce the need for emergency room visits for acute asthma. Overall, 70% of children treated in the emergency room remain well at home; however, 10–20% experience relapse within 10 days, and 15–20% are hospitalized. Steroid therapy reduces the relapse and hospitalization rates.

Status Asthmaticus

If a patient continues to have significant respiratory distress despite administration of sympathomimetic drugs with or without theophylline, the diagnosis of status asthmaticus should be considered. Status asthmaticus is a clinical diagnosis defined by increasingly severe asthma that is not responsive to drugs that are usually effective. High-risk factors for severe status asthmaticus and for death from asthma are listed in Table 137–3. A patient in whom the diagnosis is made should be admitted to a hospital, preferably to an intensive care unit, where the condition can be carefully monitored. The severity should be determined initially (see Table 137–1) and monitored at regular intervals. An indwelling arterial catheter may be indicated. Baseline complete blood count and serum electrolytes should be measured. Because hypoxemia and acid-base disturbances may predispose to cardiac arrhythmias and potentially cardiotoxic drugs (theophylline, adrenergics) will be used, cardiac monitoring is almost always indicated. Analysis of arterial blood for Po_2, Pco_2, and pH is also indicated. For these determinations well-arterialized capillary blood is adequate but less desirable than arterial blood, particularly if the patient has received epinephrine, which constricts the peripheral vascular bed.

Patients in status asthmaticus are hypoxemic. Oxygen in carefully controlled concentrations is therefore always indicated to maintain tissue oxygenation. It may be administered very effectively by nasal prongs or mask at a flow rate of 2–3 L/min. A concentration of oxygen sufficient to maintain a partial pressure of arterial oxygen of 70–90 mm Hg or oxygen saturation greater than 92% is optimal. A mist tent should not be used; the water does not reach the lower airway to any significant extent, and mists have an irritant effect on the airways of many asthmatic patients, leading to coughing and worsening of the wheezing. Furthermore, it is not possible to observe a patient who is enveloped in a dense fog.

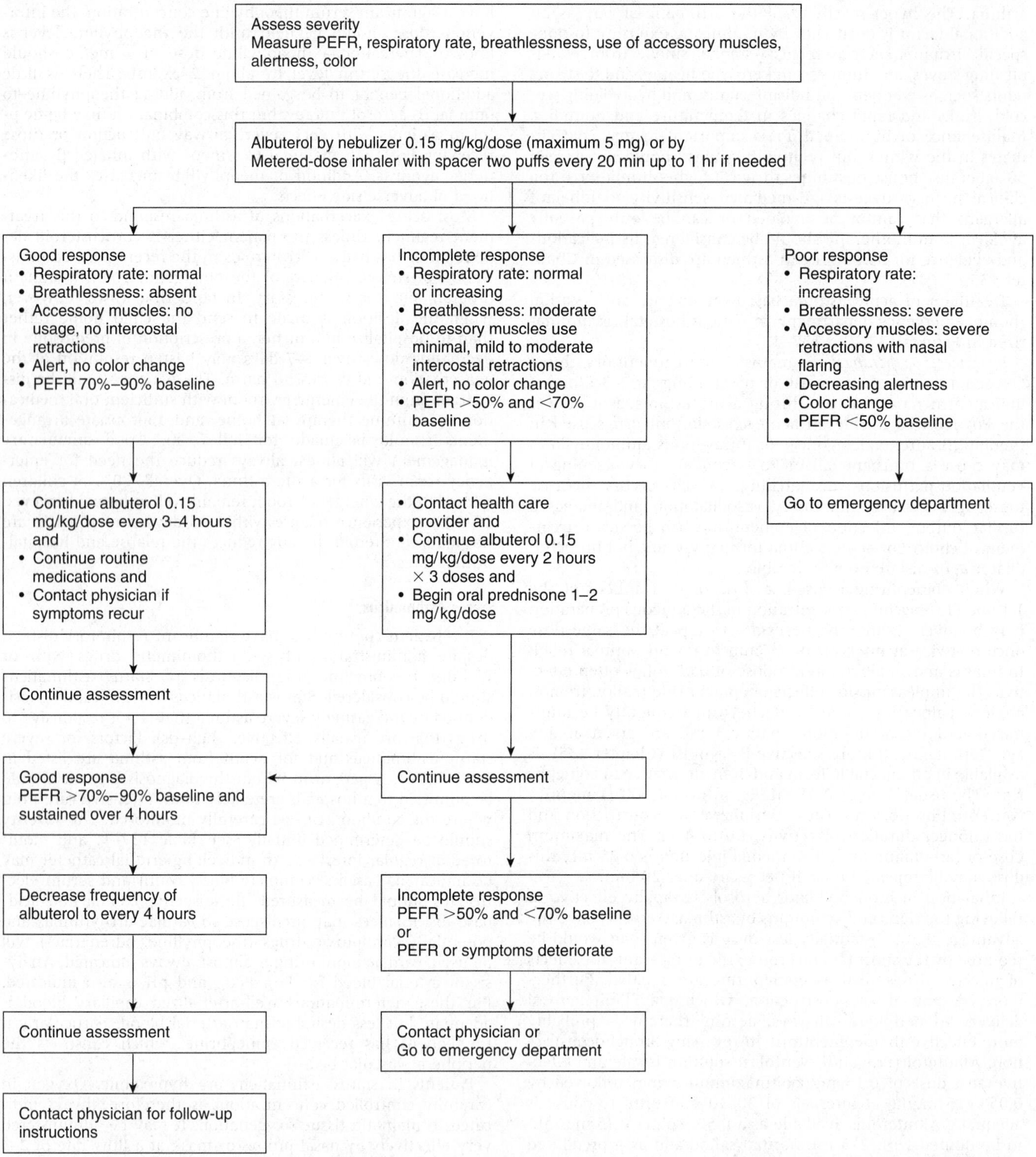

Figure 137–2. Home management of acute asthma. * = Percentage of patient's personal best or percentage predicted on the basis of normal values. PEFR = Peak expiratory flow rate. (Modified from National Asthma Education Program, National Heart, Lung, and Blood Institute, Expert Panel Report: Guidelines for the Diagnosis and Management of Asthma. No. 91-3042. Bethesda, MD, National Institutes of Health, 1991.)

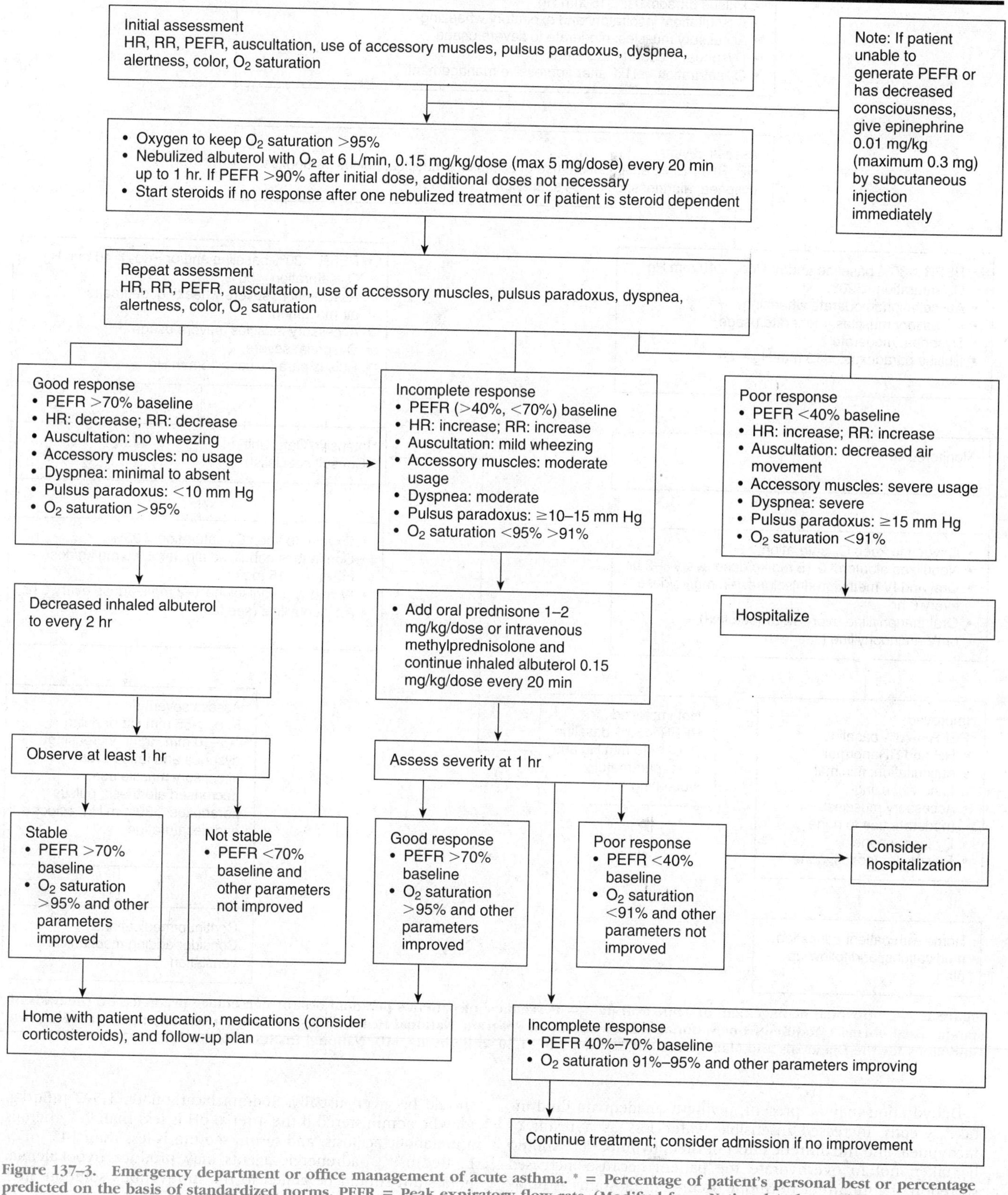

Figure 137–3. Emergency department or office management of acute asthma. * = Percentage of patient's personal best or percentage predicted on the basis of standardized norms. PEFR = Peak expiratory flow rate. (Modified from National Asthma Education Program, National Heart, Lung, and Blood Institute, Expert Panel Report: Guidelines for the Diagnosis and Management of Asthma. No. 91-3042. Bethesda, MD, National Institutes of Health, 1991.)

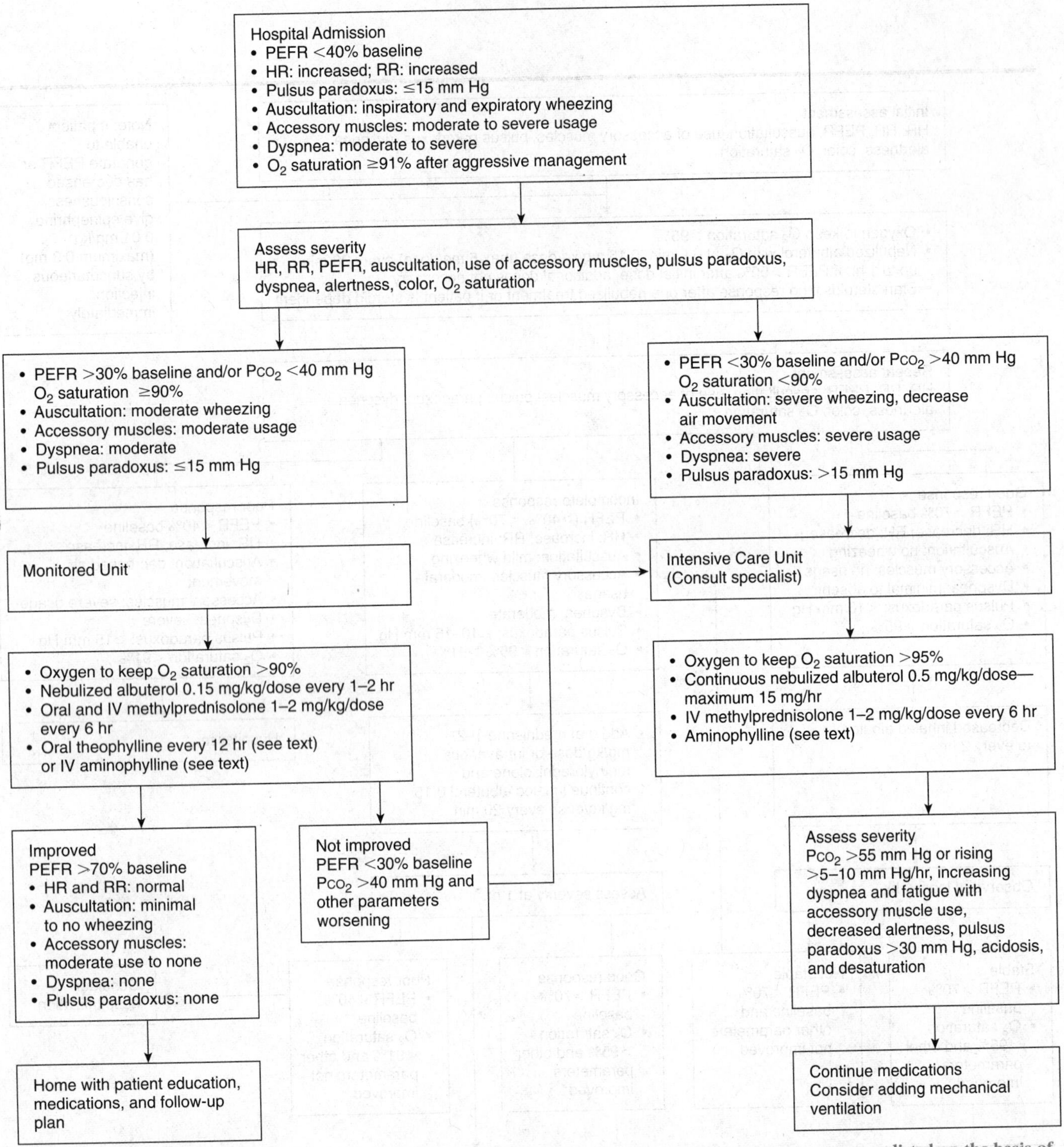

Figure 137–4. Hospital management of acute asthma. * = Percentage of patient's personal best or percentage predicted on the basis of standardized norms. (Modified from National Asthma Education Program, National Heart, Lung, and Blood Institute, Expert Panel Report: Guidelines for the Diagnosis and Management of Asthma. No. 91-3042. Bethesda, MD, National Institutes of Health, 1991.)

Dehydration may be present, owing to inadequate fluid intake, greatly increased insensible water loss as a result of tachypnea, and the diuretic effect of theophylline. Care should be taken not to overhydrate the patient because increased secretion of antidiuretic hormone occurs during status asthmaticus, promoting fluid retention, and because the large negative peak-inspiratory pleural pressures that occur in children favor accumulation of fluid in the interstitial spaces around the small airways. No more than 1–1.5 times maintenance levels of fluid should be given usually. Sodium bicarbonate, 1.5–2 mEq/kg, may be administered if the arterial pH is less than 7.3, there is a metabolic acidosis, and serum sodium is less than 145 mEq/L. Because β_2-adrenergic agents may produce hypokalemia, potassium should be added to the intravenous solution after the patient voids.

Bronchodilator sympathomimetic aerosol therapy initiated in the emergency room should be continued. Aminophylline, 4–5 mg/kg, may be given intravenously over 20 min every 6

■ **TABLE 137–3 Factors Associated with Risk of Severe Status Asthmaticus**

History
Chronic steroid-dependent asthma
Prior intensive care admission
Prior mechanical ventilation for asthma
Recurrent visits to emergency unit in past 48 hr
Sudden onset of severe respiratory distress
Poor compliance with therapy
Poor recognition by patient, family, or physician, of severity of attack
Family dysfunction, crisis
Respiratory arrest
Hypoxic seizures, encephalopathy
Physical Examination
Pulsus paradoxus >20 mm Hg
Hypotension, tachycardia, tachypnea
Cyanosis
1–2 word dyspnea
Lethargy
Agitation
Sternocleidomastoid, intercostal, suprasternal retractions
Poor air exchange (e.g., quiet chest with severe distress)
Laboratory Tests
Hypercarbia
Hypoxia with supplemental oxygen
FEV_1 <30% expected; no improvement 1 hr after aerosol therapy
Chest x-ray (pneumothorax, pneumomediastinum)
Therapy
Over-reliance on aerosol, inhaler therapy
Delayed use of systemic corticosteroids
Sedation
Delayed admission to hospital or intensive care unit

FEV_1 = forced expiratory volume in 1 sec.

hr. Alternatively, a 5-mg/kg loading dose followed by constant infusion in a dose of 0.75–1.25 mg/kg/hr may be administered. If the patient has received aminophylline intravenously in the emergency room, the loading dose should be omitted. It is essential to adjust the aminophylline dose by monitoring serum theophylline concentrations because there are many physiologic derangements that occur during the course of status asthmaticus that may affect the disposition of theophylline. If the every 6-hr regimen is used, serum samples should be obtained 1 hr after the intravenous injection and just before the next dose. During constant infusion, theophylline concentration should be monitored at least at 1, 6, 12, and 24 hr as a basis for dose adjustments and 6 and 12 hr after any change in dosage or every 24 hr while receiving intravenous theophylline. A steady-state serum concentration of approximately 12–15 μg/mL should be sought. Because age affects theophylline kinetics, the starting dose for a continuous infusion of aminophylline varies as follows: 0.5 mg/kg/hr at 1–6 mo, 1.0 mg/kg/hr at 6–11 mo, 1.2–1.5 mg/kg/hr at 1–9 yr, and 0.9 mg/kg/hr over 10 yr of age. Adrenergic drugs are best administered by aerosol as previously described. Administration of β-agonists by inhalation at intervals of 20 min or continually is safer than administration by intravenous infusion and is probably equally effective. Nonetheless, some authorities recommend terbutaline by subcutaneous (0.01 mg/kg; 0.3 mg maximum) or by intravenous (10 μg/kg bolus; 0.4–0.6 μg/kg/min continuous infusion increasing by 0.2 μg/kg/min to 3–6 μg/kg/min) administration for severe status asthmaticus.

Treatment with an antimuscarinic such as atropine sulfate given in combination with a nebulized β-agonist can be more effective than treatment with either alone, although the peak bronchodilation from atropine is reached more slowly than that of the β-agonist. Nebulization of atropine sulfate at doses of 0.05–0.1 mg/kg is safe for most children, but maximal doses of 0.025 mg/kg may be more appropriate for adolescents and adults because of the possible side effects, including tachycardia and mental confusion. Inhalation of nebulized atropine is usually safe at intervals of 4 hr.

Ipratropium bromide causes fewer side effects than atropine. Nebulization at doses of 0.25 mg every 6 hr is safe for children at least 6 yr old, and 0.5 mg every 6 hr is safe for children older than 12 yr.

Corticosteroids, such as methylprednisolone (Solu-Medrol), 1–2 mg/kg every 6 hr, should be administered. Because it has less effect on mineral metabolism when given in high doses and a lower cost for an equivalent anti-inflammatory dose, methylprednisolone is preferable to hydrocortisone. Corticosteroids can sometimes reverse tolerance to β-agonists within 1 hr, but maximal effects of steroids are usually delayed for 6 hr. Steroids improve oxygenation, decrease airway obstruction, and shorten the time needed for recovery.

Treatment is guided by serial measurement of blood gases and pH every few hours, or more often if indicated. If gas and pH analysis both indicate that respiratory failure is impending, an anesthesiologist should be alerted, and facilities and equipment should be available for tracheal intubation and respiratory support.

Mechanical ventilation should be anticipated; elective tracheal intubation with diazepam (Valium), vecuronium, and atropine premedication is safer than emergency intubation. Respiratory care should include patient paralysis on a volume-cycled ventilator with short inspiratory and long expiratory times, a 10- to 15-mL/kg tidal volume, 8–15 breaths/min, and peak pressures of less than 60 cm H_2O. The goals are to improve oxygenation, maintain P_{CO_2} between 40 and 60 mm Hg, and avoid barotrauma. Positive end-expiratory pressure is added in the recovery phase to prevent atelectasis. Sedation during mechanical ventilation may be accomplished with Valium, midazolam (Versed), or ketamine (which at doses of 1–2.5 mg/kg/hr is a sedative-analgesic-anesthetic with bronchodilator activity). Halothane anesthesia produces prompt bronchodilation but is difficult to administer in an intensive care unit. It should be reserved for the most severe cases of status asthmaticus.

Sedation of nonventilated patients with status asthmaticus is hazardous. Tranquilizers, morphine, and other opiates are also contraindicated because of their depressant effects on the respiratory center. The best sedative for the patient is the presence of a competent, compassionate physician and nurse at the bedside and decreased airway obstruction with relief of hypoxia and hypercarbia. Chest roentgenograms should be obtained in all severe cases and repeated as indicated to detect complications such as mediastinal emphysema or pneumothorax. Routine administration of antibiotics has not been shown to alter the course of status asthmaticus in children or to reduce the incidence of infectious complications.

Daily Management of the Asthmatic Child

On the basis of the history, physical examination, laboratory data, pulmonary function testing, and need for medication, patients may be classified as having mild, moderate, or severe asthma. The daily management of these different degrees of illness varies (see Chapter 135; Figs. 137–2 to 137–4).

MILD ASTHMA. Children with mild asthma have exacerbations of varying frequency, up to twice each week, with decreases in peak expiratory flow rate of not more than 20% and respond to bronchodilator treatment within 24–48 hr. Generally, medication is not required between exacerbations for very mild asthma with symptoms less than every 2 wk, when the child is essentially free of symptoms of airway obstruction. Children with mild asthma have good school attendance, good exercise tolerance, and little or no interruption of sleep by asthma. They have no hyperinflation of the chest; their chest roentgenograms are essentially normal. Pulmonary function testing may show mild, reversible airway obstruction, with little or no increase in lung volume.

MODERATE ASTHMA. Children with moderate asthma have symptoms more frequently than those with mild disease and often have cough and mild wheezing between more severe exacerbations. School attendance may be impaired, exercise tolerance will be diminished because of coughing and wheezing, and the child may lose sleep at night, particularly during exacerbations. Such children will generally require continuous rather than intermittent bronchodilator therapy to achieve satisfactory control of symptoms or continuous treatment with cromolyn, nedocromil, or an inhaled corticosteroid to reverse bronchial hyper-responsiveness. Hyperinflation may be evident clinically and roentgenographically. Signs of airway obstruction on physiologic testing are more marked than in the mild group; lung volumes may be increased.

SEVERE ASTHMA. Children with severe asthma have virtually daily wheezing and more frequent and more severe exacerbations; they require recurrent hospitalization, which is rarely required for mild or moderate asthma. Severely affected children may miss significant amounts of school, have their sleep interrupted often by asthma, and have poor exercise tolerance. They have chest deformities as a result of chronic hyperinflation, which is evident on roentgenograms. Bronchodilator medication will be required continuously, and regimens may include the regular systemic or aerosol administration of corticosteroids. Physiologic testing will show more severe airway obstruction than in mild or moderate asthma, less reversibility in response to aerosol bronchodilators, and more severe disturbances of lung volumes.

Tables 137–2 to 137–4 summarize treatment of acute asthma. Children with mild asthma should receive bronchodilator medication only when symptomatic, and most exacerbations may be satisfactorily treated with adrenergic agents, preferably by aerosol (albuterol, metaproterenol, terbutaline, pirbuterol, or bitolterol) or, rarely, by injection (aqueous epinephrine, terbutaline). Use of a chamber such as an AeroChamber or InspirEase enhances delivery of drug to the lower airways when a metered-dose inhaler is used by younger children who are unable to coordinate actuation of the inhaler with inhalation. Such chambers permit effective administration of β-agonists from metered-dose inhalers to children as young as 3 yr of age. Slow inhalation also increases delivery to the lungs because a rapid inhalation causes impaction of drug particles in the pharynx. Breath holding for up to 10 sec after inhalation of the drug also favors deposition in the lungs. When moderate or severe airway obstruction is present, nebulization with an air compressor such as the Proneb with part LC jet or the DeVilbiss No. 561 Pulmo-Aide is often more effective than use of a metered-dose inhaler with a chamber. The apparent advantage of nebulization over metered-dose inhaler is largely due to the different doses administered. Nebulization with such a compressor permits effective delivery of aerosols even to infants. β-Agonist liquids for oral administration are also available for treatment of infants and young children. Theophylline may be added to an oral regimen when indicated. Drug therapy usually can be discontinued after a few days. Exercise-induced asthma is most effectively prevented by inhalation of an adrenergic drug immediately before exercise. Inhaled albuterol usually affords protection for 4 hr; inhaled salmeterol (not labeled for patients younger than 12 yr by the U.S. Food and Drug Administration [FDA]), for 12 hr. Salmeterol should be administered at least 30 min before exercise. Inhalation of cromolyn or nedocromil shortly before exercise is also effective in preventing exercise-induced asthma.

■ TABLE 137–4 Selected Slow-Release Theophylline Preparations

Preparation	Dosage Form	Anhydrous Theophylline Content (mg)
Slo-bid Gyrocaps	Capsule	50, 75, 100, 125, 200, 300
Slo-phyllin Gyrocaps	Capsule	60, 125, 250
Theo-Dur	Tablet	100, 200, 300, 450
Theolair-SR	Tablet	200, 250, 300, 500

Tablets are scored to permit adjustment of dosage.
Capsules may be opened and the contents mixed with moist food for children unable to swallow capsules or tablets.

For children with moderate asthma who require round-the-clock therapy, two inhalations of an adrenergic aerosol every 4–6 hr, or two inhalations of salmeterol every 12 hr, often suffices. Theophylline may be added. Dose and dosing regimen should be individualized. Some experienced allergists reserve monitoring of serum theophylline concentrations for those patients who fail to show a favorable bronchodilator response or who have symptoms of toxicity (gastrointestinal or central nervous system) with average dosages. When slow-release (S-R) formulations of theophylline are used, the peak plasma concentration (assuming that a constant fraction of drug is absorbed, which may not be the case) occurs 4–8 hr after the dose, at which time a blood sample for monitoring should be obtained. Peak concentration may not occur until 12 hr after a bedtime dose of an S-R preparation because of delayed nocturnal absorption. Blood sampling should be delayed until after a day or so of therapy with S-R drugs to ensure that a steady state has been achieved. Some children can be treated successfully on an every-12-hr schedule, but others metabolize theophylline particularly rapidly and experience marked fluctuations in serum concentration. These peaks and troughs of concentration are minimized by dividing the 24-hr dose into equal 8-hr doses.

Younger children (aged 1–9 yr) generally eliminate theophylline more rapidly than older children and adolescents and hence require a higher daily dose on a mg/kg basis. Nonetheless, it is safest to begin with a dose of 14–16 mg/kg/24 hr in most children. If this dose is well tolerated, one may increase by 25% increments at 3- to 4-day intervals to average doses for age as necessary to control symptoms (see Tables 135–2, 137–4). If adequate control of symptoms is not achieved at the maximum doses or if adverse effects become evident, adjustment in the dosing regimen must be guided by determination of the serum theophylline concentration.

Rapidly absorbed liquids and uncoated tablets, while suitable for children with mild asthma who require a few days of therapy for an exacerbation, have no place in the therapeutic regimen of children who require round-the-clock theophylline therapy because wide fluctuations in serum theophylline concentrations are observed when rapidly absorbed products are used. Which of the S-R products to use depends upon the dosage form (tablet vs capsule) and the amount of drug needed (see Table 137–4). Capsule formulations that can be opened are virtually tasteless, should not be chewed, may be mixed with *moist* food, and are particularly suitable for young children. Crushing an S-R tablet destroys its constant-release properties. Exacerbations of asthma in patients receiving round-the-clock theophylline medication should be treated with adrenergic drugs, as described earlier for children with mild asthma (see Fig. 137–2).

Cromolyn powder inhaled four times a day from a Spinhaler or cromolyn aerosol delivered by a metered-dose inhaler or nedocromil (not FDA labeled for patients younger than 12 yr) is useful in children with mild to moderate asthma. A solution of cromolyn is available for home nebulization regimens for young children subject to recurrent attacks of asthma. Cromolyn and albuterol or metaproterenol solutions may be mixed together in the nebulizer for ease of administration if concurrent administration of a bronchodilator is necessary.

In certain children with moderate asthma, significant flare-ups occur from time to time that may require the use of corticosteroids for a few days. Early use of steroids in the child who is known to become severely ill may reduce the need for hospitalization. Early intervention with bronchodilator drugs (with or without steroids, depending upon the clinical setting) is important in the management of all asthmatic children, regardless of the severity of their conditions. Steroids should be given in adequate doses (1–2 mg/kg/24 hr of prednisone or prednisolone in two to three doses) and should be discontinued as quickly as possible, for example, within 5–7 days; a long "weaning" period following acute asthma is unnecessary. In patients who only rarely require steroid administration, return of normal hypothalamic-pituitary-adrenal function is hastened by the *prompt* discontinuation of the drug when the acute episode is over. Inhaled topical steroid preparations are also effective for children with moderately severe asthma.

In a minority of children who have severe asthma despite the management guidelines outlined here, unacceptable degrees of coughing and wheezing persist, severely limiting the child's play activities and school attendance. In such children the judicious administration of oral corticosteroids on an alternate-day basis and as an inhaled aerosol frequently results in significant amelioration of symptoms and allows the child to lead a normal life without suffering the adverse effects of corticosteroids. If alternate-day therapy is indicated because of either chronic disability or the severity or frequency of attacks of status asthmaticus, the patient is given 5–7 days of intensive daily therapy and then switched to an alternate-day regimen with a short-acting steroid (prednisone, prednisolone, or methylprednisolone). A 12-yr-old child might be given 60 mg, 40 mg, 30 mg, 20 mg, and 10 mg of prednisone/24 hr over a 5-day period for an exacerbation of asthma, to be followed by alternate-day therapy at a dose of 20 mg/24 hr given as a single dose at 7.00–8.00 A.M. every 48 hr. If the patient responds well to this regimen, the prednisone may be reduced by 5 mg per dose at 10- to 14-day intervals until the lowest dose compatible with acceptable control of symptoms is reached, usually 5–10 mg on alternate days. Concurrent therapy with aerosol adrenergic drugs, theophylline, or cromolyn should be continued because this reduces the dose of steroid required. Low-dose alternate-day therapy is associated with minimal adverse effects and thus may be justified in a disease that can be life threatening and capable of causing chronic invalidism. Use of steroid therapy should *not,* however, substitute for or delay comprehensive management of the disease.

Inhalational corticosteroids, such as beclomethasone dipropionate (Vanceril, Beclovent), flunisolide (AeroBid), and triamcinolone (Azmacort), may provide an alternative to the use of every-other-day oral corticosteroid medication. Inhalational corticosteroids may be more effective than oral steroids in reversing bronchial hyper-responsiveness and may therefore be indicated even in patients who also require continual treatment with oral steroids. Beclomethasone, which is effective in microgram doses, is rapidly inactivated in the liver into metabolites devoid of glucocorticoid activity. Accordingly, systemic effects in children given less than 14 μg/kg/24 hr (usual dose is two inhalations or 84 μg four times a day) are minimal. Oropharyngeal candidiasis rarely occurs. Its frequency and that of other adverse effects are diminished by rinsing the mouth and expectorating after inhaling the aerosol and inhaling the aerosol through a chamber or spacer. Effective use of inhaled steroid requires a degree of compliance by the patient not often found in children younger than 6–7 yr. Studies of adults who have received beclomethasone for up to 7 yr have shown no evidence of epithelial atrophy or thinning of underlying connective tissue, and there have been no long-term adverse effects of the drug on the pharynx and airways.

Continual treatment with an inhaled corticosteroid or with cromolyn is indicated for any child with symptoms of asthma occurring as frequently as weekly except for exercise-induced asthma preventable by pretreatment with a β-agonist, cromolyn or nedocromil.

Home monitoring of peak expiratory flow rate two to three times a day facilitates early detection of airway obstruction in patients with severe asthma and in patients with infrequent symptoms that may progress to severe airway obstruction. Graphing the results of monitoring will establish the child's diurnal variation and permit the physician to suggest treatment guidelines that anticipate decreases in peak expiratory flow rate. Daily changes in flow rate may also indicate a need for changes in continual treatment regimens. Whatever the degree of severity of the asthma, a personalized, written crisis plan is helpful (Fig. 137–5). This can remind patients and parents about what to do in an emergency.

Emotional tensions surrounding asthma are best handled by unhurried discussion with the parents of the child's difficulty, by avoidance of overdramatization of the child's illness, and by careful examinations with the parents of those areas in which parent and child seem to be in conflict. The use of tranquilizers or sedatives as a substitute for more direct attempts to solve emotional problems should be avoided. As the asthma is brought under control, the emotional climate is often improved.

Various factors may exacerbate asthma or make the disease difficult to treat: gastroesophageal reflux, allergic bronchopulmonary aspergillosis, nonsteroidal anti-inflammatory agents, pregnancy, and sinusitis. Chronic sinusitis may be due to noninfectious immune-mediated inflammation or to bacterial infection. Treatment of sinusitis with antibiotics, intranasal steroids, and oral or topical (3–5 days) decongestants for 3 wk may improve bronchoconstriction as well as sinusitis.

Asthma education programs, for example, ACT (*A*sthma *C*are *T*raining) and Superstuff, are being used in comprehensive asthma management. Their goal is to increase knowledge of asthma and its treatment on the part of both the child and parent, to improve communication within the family and with the physician and nurse, to improve compliance with the treatment plan, and to decrease the need for use of emergency room or hospital.

Prevention of Deaths from Asthma

Death from childhood asthma is rare, but asthma mortality rates have been increasing. In the United States asthma mortality rates increased from 1.2/100,000 general population in 1979 to 2.0 in 1991. Among children 10–14 yr old the asthma mortality rate increased from 0.1 in 1979 to 0.5/100,000 in 1987, the greatest proportional increase for any age group. Rates have been three to nine times as high in black children as in whites. Increases have also occurred in many other countries.

Reasons for these increases in mortality are unknown. Possible causes include increased prevalence of asthma; increased indoor air pollution as a result of tighter construction of homes with emphasis on energy conservation; excessive exposure to allergen; psychosocial dysfunction that may interfere with perception of airway obstruction and with compliance with recommended management; delays in implementation of appropriate treatment for acute asthma; lack of access or utilization of medical care, including preventive care; over-reliance on bronchodilator inhalers leading to delayed treatment with steroids or other therapy until patients are in extremis; unavailability of epinephrine for patients unable to use inhalers effectively; inappropriate use of the metered-dose inhaler; and failure to provide continuity of care or education about what to do for an unusually severe episode of asthma.

Most but not all deaths from asthma are preventable with appropriate care. It is possible to identify many of those at greatest risk for death from their histories, for example, respi-

Guide to Management of Asthma for ______________________________

____

Regular medicines: ______________________________

____

____

____

____

Before exercise: ______________________________

For mild coughing, wheezing, shortness of breath, tightness of chest,
Peak expiratory flow rate (PEFR) reduced by 10 to 30%:
Get away from possible cause (smoke, dust, animal, pollen).
Inhale bronchodilator (______________) every 4 hours.

For more severe symptoms,
PFR reduced by 30 to 50%:
Inhale bronchodilator (______________) every 20 minutes for 1 hour if necessary.
If unimproved, continue bronchodilator (______________) every 2 hours, double your dose of inhaled corticosteroid (______________), contact physician, and start oral prednisone (______________).

For very severe symptoms, struggling to breathe, blue or gray lips or fingernails, difficulty walking or talking, chest and neck sucked in with each breath,
PFR reduced by 50% or more:
Inhale bronchodilator (______________) every 20 minutes *and* go immediately to physician or emergency room.

Figure 137–5. Personalized crisis plan for management of asthma.

ratory failure with hypercapnia, loss of consciousness caused by asthma, or psychosocial dysfunction in the patient or family. These patients require especially close monitoring and psychotherapy when indicated. Each should carry a written emergency protocol indicating current medications and recommended emergency treatment as guidance for emergency personnel who may be unfamiliar with the patient. They should also have a written crisis plan indicating what they should do in an emergency. This should include which medications to use, which doses to use at what intervals, how to reach their physicians, and where to get further assistance. A Medic-Alert emblem can be helpful if such a patient is found unconscious or unable to indicate the nature of the illness. Such patients should be provided with injectable epinephrine in a convenient preparation (e.g., EpiPen or EpiPen Jr.) for use in an emergency when inhalation therapy is ineffective or inappropriate, but use of the EpiPen should not delay transport to an emergency facility.

Adinoff A, Cummings N: Sinusitis and its relationship to asthma. Pediatr Ann 18:785, 1989.

Anto JM, Sunyer J, Reed CE, et al: Preventing asthma epidemics due to soybeans by dust-control measures. N Engl J Med 329:1760, 1993.

Attaway N, Strunk R: Death due to asthma in children: What the pediatrician can do. Pediatr Ann 18:819, 1989.

Burrows B, Martinez F, Halonen M, et al: Association of asthma with serum IgE levels and skin test reactivity to allergens. N Engl J Med 320:271, 1989.

Carter E, Cruz M, Chesrown S, et al: Efficacy of intravenously administered theophylline in children hospitalized with severe asthma. J Pediatr 122:470, 1993.

Cheong B, Reynolds S, Rajan G, et al: Intravenous beta agonist in severe acute asthma. Br Med J 297:448, 1988.

Connett GJ, Warde C, Wooler E, et al: Prednisolone and salbutamol in the hospital treatment of acute asthma. Arch Dis Child 70:170, 1994.

Duff AL, Pomeranz ES, Gelber LE, et al: Risk factors for acute wheezing in infants and children: Viruses, passive smoke, and IgE antibodies to inhalant allergens. Pediatrics 92:535, 1993.

Dworkin G, Kattan M: Mechanical ventilation for status asthmaticus in children. J Pediatr 114:545, 1989.

Editorial: Steroids in acute severe asthma. Lancet 340:1384, 1992.

Fletcher HJ, Ibrahim SA, Speight N: Survey of asthma deaths in the Northern region, 1970–85. Arch Dis Child 65:163, 1990.

Gershel J, Goldman H, Stein R, et al: The usefulness of chest radiographs in first asthma attacks. N Engl J Med 309:336, 1983.

International Paediatric Asthma Consensus Group: Asthma: A follow up statement from an international paediatric asthma consensus group. Arch Dis Child 67:240, 1992.

Katz RW, Kelly HW, Crowley MR, et al: Safety of continuous nebulized albuterol for bronchospasm in infants and children. Pediatrics 92:666, 1993.

Larsen GL: Asthma in children. N Engl J Med 326:1540, 1992.

Lewis CE, Rachelefsky G, Lewis MA, et al: A randomized trial of A. C. T. (Asthma Care Training) for kids. Pediatrics 74:478, 1984.

Martinez FD, Wright AL, Taussig LM, et al: Asthma and wheezing in the first six years of life. N Engl J Med 332:133, 1995.

McFadden ER, Gilbert IA: Exercise-induced asthma. N Engl J Med 330:1362, 1994.

McWilliams B, Kelley H, Murphy S: Management of acute severe asthma. Pediatr Ann 18:774, 1989.

Mrazek DA, Klinnert MD, Mrazek P, et al: Early asthma onset: Consideration of parenting issues. J Am Acad Child Adolesc Psychiatry 30:277, 1991.

National Asthma Education Program, National Heart, Lung, and Blood Institute, Expert Panel Report: Guidelines for the Diagnosis and Management of Asthma (NIH pub no 91-3042). Bethesda, MD, U.S. Department of Health and Human Services, 1991.

Provisional Committee on Quality Improvement: Practice parameters: The office management of acute exacerbations of asthma in children. Pediatrics 93:119, 1994.

Ratto D, Alfaro C, Sipsey J, et al: Are intravenous corticosteroids required in status asthmaticus? JAMA 260:527, 1988.

Rea HH, Scragg R, Jackson R, et al: A case-control study of deaths from asthma. Thorax 41:833, 1986.

Rock M, De LaRocha S, L'Hommedieu S, et al: Use of ketamine in asthmatic children to treat respiratory failure refractory to conventional therapy. Crit Care Med 14:514, 1986.

Scarfone RJ, Fuchs SM, Nager AL, et al: Controlled trial of oral prednisone in the emergency department treatment of children with acute asthma. Pediatrics 92:513, 1993.

Schuh S, Parkin P, Rajan A, et al: High- versus low-dose, frequently administered, nebulized albuterol in children with severe, acute asthma. Pediatrics 83:513, 1989.

Shapiro GG, Furukawa CT, Pierson WE, et al: Double-blind evaluation of nebulized cromolyn, terbutaline, and the combination for childhood asthma. J Allergy Clin Immunol 81:449, 1988.
Sly RM: Mortality from asthma in children 1979–1984. Ann Allergy 60:433, 1988.
Strachan DP: Do chesty children become chesty adults? Arch Dis Child 65:661, 1990.
Strauss RE, Wertheim DL, Bonagura VR, et al: Aminophylline therapy does not improve outcome and increases adverse effects in children hospitalized with acute asthmatic exacerbations. Pediatrics 93:205, 1994.
Volovitz B, Amir J, Malik H, et al: Growth and pituitary-adrenal function in children with severe asthma treated with inhaled budesonide. N Engl J Med 329:1703, 1993.
Weinberger M: Theophylline: When should it be used? J Pediatr 122:403, 1993.
Wiener C: Ventilatory management of respiratory failure in asthma. JAMA 269:2128, 1993.

CHAPTER 138

Atopic Dermatitis

(See Chapter 597)

(Infantile or Atopic Eczema)

Atopic dermatitis is an inflammatory skin disorder characterized by erythema, edema, intense pruritus, exudation, crusting, and scaling. In the acute stages, intraepidermal vesiculation (spongiosis) is present. There appears to be a genetically determined predilection. Infants with atopic dermatitis tend subsequently to experience allergic rhinitis and asthma.

About 80% of patients with atopic dermatitis have serum immunoglobulin (Ig) E concentrations increased 5- to 10-fold above normal. There is conflicting evidence as to whether the level of IgE is related to either the severity or the extent of the dermatitis. The concentration of IgE does, however, fluctuate with the stage of the disease. The level returns to normal when the disease has been quiescent for several years. The high levels of IgE have not been satisfactorily explained. It is not established that atopic dermatitis is primarily an IgE-mediated allergic disorder; it is difficult to demonstrate consistently a role for allergens, whether foods or inhalants, in the pathogenesis of eczema. Moreover, the relationship of atopic dermatitis to allergy or immunology is made more uncertain by reports that IgE is not always increased in affected patients who have neither family history nor clinical evidence of rhinitis or asthma. Children with atopic dermatitis and food hypersensitivity have high rates of spontaneous basophil histamine release. This phenomenon returns to normal following a food elimination diet and is mediated by a monocyte cytokine (histamine-releasing factor), which interacts with a specific subtype of IgE bound to basophils.

The typical dermal manifestation of the interaction of IgE antibody with antigen is the hive (wheal and flare) rather than the erythematous papule of atopic dermatitis; and, although patients with atopic dermatitis frequently possess IgE antibody specific for inhalants or food allergens, it is not generally possible to induce skin lesions of atopic dermatitis by intradermal injection of the suspected allergen. Typical lesions of atopic dermatitis may occur in individuals with X-linked agammaglobulinemia, who have virtually no IgE.

Increased concentrations of IgE in atopic dermatitis may be related to a deficiency of IgE isotype-specific "suppressor" T-cell function. Impairment of cell-mediated immunity in some patients with atopic dermatitis is indicated by (1) absence of the reactions of delayed hypersensitivity upon intradermal skin testing with certain antigens; (2) inability to be sensitized with potent contact sensitizers (e.g., poison ivy, dinitrochlorobenzene); (3) diminished proliferative response of lymphocytes to mitogens such as phytohemagglutinin; and (4) variable phagocytic and chemotactic defects of monocytes and neutrophils.

The hyper-reactive skin of atopic dermatitis differs from normal skin in its response to a variety of physical and pharmacological stimuli. For example, a light mechanical stroke results within 1 min in a white line with a surrounding blanched area. This phenomenon ("white dermographism") is not seen in normal skin, which becomes red. Involved skin has abnormal rates of cooling and warming in response to temperature changes, particularly in flexural areas. Paradoxical responses occur to injections of various pharmacological agents, such as histamine, acetylcholine (blanching rather than erythema), and nicotinic acid ester. Adrenergic responses are decreased in lymphocytes and granulocytes in atopic dermatitis, suggesting that autonomic imbalance may be a basis for the abnormalities in the skin. The abnormal reactivity of the skin has a counterpart in the airway hyper-reactivity of asthma; in both disorders, such hyper-reactivity seems to be intrinsic to the disease, which may, in part, be due to the late-phase immune response (Chapter 133). In addition to its genetic and atopic features, eczema is also characterized by abnormal local essential fatty acid metabolism, disturbed phosphodiesterase activity, cutaneous dysregulation of the autonomic nervous system, expansion of allergen-specific Th2 cells, a reduced threshold for secondary skin infections (*Staphylococcus aureus* molluscum), skin hyperirritability, and exacerbation by stress.

CLINICAL MANIFESTATIONS. Atopic dermatitis affects 2-8% of children and typically occurs in three stages with fairly distinctive features. The disease most often begins in infancy, usually during the first 2-3 mo of life. The onset is sometimes delayed until the 2nd or 3rd yr; 60% of patients are affected by 1 yr of age and 90% by 5 yr of age. The earliest lesions are erythematous, weepy patches on the cheeks, with subsequent extension to the remainder of the face, neck, wrists, hands, abdomen, and extensor aspects of the extremities. Involvement of flexural areas characteristically appears later but may occur as popliteal and antecubital dermatitis in early life (Fig. 138–1).

Pruritus is marked; the affected infant makes incessant efforts to scratch by rubbing the face on bedclothes and against the sides of the crib. This trauma to the skin rapidly leads to weeping and crusting; secondary infection is common and may be extensive.

The onset of dermatitis frequently coincides with the introduction of certain foods into the infant's diet, especially cow's milk, wheat, soy, peanuts, fish, or eggs. Cutaneous symptoms develop after food challenges in 50-90% of infants and children who have dermatitis and high IgE serum concentrations. Overall, about 20-30% of patients with eczema have food hypersensitivity to one or more of the six common allergens. There is unequivocal evidence of reaginic sensitivity in certain infants who have urticaria, colic, and a diffuse erythematous flush following ingestion of the offending food. The erythematous flush appears to be accompanied by intense itching, which results in scratching and then in the appearance of the skin lesions characteristic of eczema. The major role of scratching in the production of skin lesions has been demonstrated when one extremity has been encased in surgical dressings and the other left uncovered; the lesions of atopic dermatitis occur only in the uncovered extremity.

Atopic dermatitis shows a tendency to remission at 3-5 yr of age. In most cases, the disease becomes less prominent by the age of 5 yr; in some, a mild to moderate eczema may persist in the antecubital and popliteal fossae, on the wrists, behind the ears, and on the face and neck. During childhood, antecubital and popliteal involvement becomes common; extensor surfaces of the extremities may still be actively affected. With increasing age, there is a tendency toward drying and thick-

■ TABLE 138–3 Potency of Selected Topical Corticosteroids

Potency	Corticosteroid	Brand
Superpotent	Betamethasone dipropionate	Diprolene ointment, 0.05%
	Clobetasol propionate	Temovate ointment, 0.05%
Very highly potent	Betamethasone dipropionate	Diprosone ointment, 0.05%
	Halcinonide	Halog ointment, 0.1%
	Fluocinonide	Lidex cream, 0.05%
Highly potent	Triamcinolone acetonide	Aristocort cream (HP), 0.5%
	Betamethasone dipropionate	Diprosone cream, 0.05%
	Betamethasone valerate	Valisone ointment, 0.1%
Somewhat less highly potent	Hydrocortisone valerate	Westcort ointment, 0.2%
	Triamcinolone acetonide	Aristocort ointment, 0.1%
	Flurandrenolide	Cordran ointment, 0.05%
Mild potency	Betamethasone valerate	Valisone cream, 0.1%
Milder potency	Mometasone furoate	Elocon cream and ointment, 0.1%
	Alclometasone dipropionate	Aclovate cream and ointment, 0.05%
Low potency	Fluocinolone acetonide	Synalar solution, 0.01%
	Desonide	Tridesilon cream, 0.05%
Lowest potency	Hydrocortisone	Hytone cream and ointment, 1.0%, 2.5%

prescribe the least potent corticosteroid that affords adequate control. Their cost may be a serious problem. Cost can be reduced by purchasing relatively concentrated preparations in bulk, which the pharmacist can dilute to half strength with Aquaphor or a moisturizer (Eucerin), rather than purchasing equivalent material in 15- or 30-g amounts. Small amounts of steroid rubbed in well at frequent intervals give better results than large amounts applied only infrequently. Percutaneous absorption of corticosteroid occurs but is not generally clinically significant. Long-term topical use of steroids leads to an increase in growth of hair in some patients and to atrophy of the skin. The more potent topical steroids should not be applied to the face or to large areas during prolonged periods. Application of 0.5% or 1% hydrocortisone to the face is safe.

Systemic administration of corticosteroids for treatment of atopic dermatitis should be avoided except briefly in the most severely affected patients while awaiting response to other therapies.

Topical treatment with corticosteroids has largely superseded the use of coal tar preparations. Tars stain clothes and skin, and compliance of the patient in their use is often poor. However, newer preparations, such as Estar gel (Westwood) and psoriGel (Owen), are effective and more acceptable cosmetically. Tars are considerably less expensive for long-term topical use than corticosteroids. Coal tar is photosensitizing, and occasionally its use results in a sterile, pustular folliculitis.

In more refractory older patients, experimental therapy has included interferon gamma, cyclosporine, and "Chinese herb." The latter may have untoward effects such as hepatotoxicity or immunosuppression.

PROGNOSIS. With adequate control of factors known to trigger itching, appropriate local treatment, and understanding support for the parents of a child for whom no immediate cure is to be expected, reasonable control of atopic dermatitis is usually possible. Improvement occurs within 5 yr usually.

Bernhisal-Broadbent J, Sampson H: Food hypersensitivity and atopic dermatitis. Pediatr Clin North Am 35:1115, 1988.

Bos JD, Kapsenberg ML, Sillevis Smitt JH: Pathogenesis of atopic eczema. Lancet 343:1338, 1994.

Harper J: Traditional Chinese medicine for eczema: Seemingly effective, but caution must prevail. BMJ 308:489, 1994.

Hoeger PH, Lenz W, Boutonnier A, et al: Staphylococcal skin colonization in children with atopic dermatitis: Prevalence, persistence, and transmission of toxigenic and nontoxigenic strains. J Infect Dis 165:1064, 1992.

Horan RF, Schneider LC, Sheffer AL: Allergic skin disorders and mastocytosis. JAMA 268:2858, 1992.

Przybilla B, Eberlein-Konig B, Rueff F: Practical management of atopic eczema. Lancet 343:1342, 1994.

Sampson HA: Atopic dermatitis. Ann Allergy 69:469, 1992.

Sampson HA, Broadbent K, Bernhisal-Broadbent J: Spontaneous release of histamine from basophils and histamine-releasing factor in patients with atopic dermatitis and food hypersensitivity. N Engl J Med 321:228, 1989.

Sampson HA, Jolie PL: Increased plasma histamine concentration after food challenges in children with atopic dermatitis. N Engl J Med 311:372, 1984.

CHAPTER 139

Urticaria-Angioedema

(Hives)

CLINICAL MANIFESTATIONS. Urticaria, or hives, is a common skin disorder characterized by usually well-circumscribed but sometimes coalescent, localized or generalized, erythematous, raised skin lesions (wheals or welts) of various sizes. The lesions may be intensely pruritic or itch little, if at all. The individual hive usually resolves within 48 hr, but new ones may continue to appear singly or in crops. When urticaria persists for longer than 6 wk, the condition is arbitrarily deemed chronic. Urticaria has been attributed to edema of the upper corium as a result of dilatation and increased permeability of the capillaries.

In angioedema (angioneurotic edema) the deeper layers of skin or submucosa and subcutaneous or other tissues are involved; the upper respiratory tract and the gastrointestinal tract are common target organs. The distinction between urticaria and angioedema is frequently not clear; the lesions appear to differ only in the depth of tissue involvement.

INCIDENCE. As many as 20% of people experience hives at some time during life. Urticaria is somewhat more frequent in females than in males.

PATHOGENESIS. The principal noncytotoxic mechanism for urticaria and angioedema is interaction of antigen with mast cell- or basophil-bound immunoglobulin (Ig) E antibodies. The release of histamine from these cells causes vasodilatation and increased vascular permeability and stimulates an axon reflex, which produces a typical wheal and flare reaction. Leukotrienes may contribute to the edema of the IgE-mediated reaction. A second mediator pathway for urticaria involves the complement system. Two complement component split products, C3a and C5a, act as anaphylatoxins (Chapter 120) and trigger histamine release from mast cells and basophils by direct action on the cell surfaces, independent of antibodies. C3a and C5a can be generated through both the classic and the alternative complement pathways. A third mediator pathway involves the plasma kinin-forming system of the coagulation scheme. Bradykinin is at least as potent as histamine in increasing vascular permeability. Both non-IgE immunological reactions and nonimmunological events can cause urticaria and angioedema when they activate the complement and kinin-forming systems.

ETIOLOGY. A clinical classification of urticaria is given in Table 139–1.

DIFFERENTIAL DIAGNOSIS. With a few exceptions, no laboratory tests establish or exclude the diagnosis of urticaria and angioedema. Allergy skin testing is generally not helpful except when specific drug (penicillin) or food allergies are identified. In the absence of any clue suggesting an ingestant cause, elimination diets are not generally useful. The diagnosis is clinical and requires that the physician be aware of the various forms of urticaria. A careful history usually identifies the type. Except when there are obvious associations with IgE-mediated reactions, naming the "cause" of urticaria may be difficult. Drugs and foods are the most common causes of urticaria. The cause of chronic urticaria is identified in only 10% of cases; some patients demonstrate autoantibodies to the IgE receptor.

Some forms of urticaria need special mention. Papular urticaria usually occurs in small children, generally on the extremities and other exposed parts at the sites of insect bites. Cholinergic urticaria appears as wheals 1–2 mm in diameter surrounded by large areas of erythema (flares) and frequently involves the skin of the neck. It is caused by exercise, hot showers, and occasionally by anxiety. Affected people have increased sensitivity to cholinergic mediators, which can be demonstrated when an intradermal injection of 0.01 mg of methacholine (Mecholyl) in 0.1 ml of saline causes a localized hive surrounded by smaller, satellite lesions. Urticaria is probably due more often to viral infection than is commonly recognized. It is particularly associated with hepatitis, especially during the prodromal stages, and with infectious mononucleosis. Viral infections can also produce erythema multiforme, often confused with urticaria, in which typical iris or target lesions occur and mucosal involvement is common. In some patients, typical hives change spontaneously into lesions of erythema multiforme, which can be a sign of drug allergy (Chapters 63 and 595).

Urticaria pigmentosa typically occurs during the first few years of childhood and has a distinctive presentation. Systemic mastocytosis is a serious form of urticaria pigmentosa in which mast cells infiltrate skeleton, liver, spleen, and lymph nodes. In adults, and rarely in children, urticaria may be associated with malignancy or collagen-vascular disorders.

Cold urticaria is the most common form caused by physical factors. Urticarial lesions, which may be pruritic or painful or burning, appear upon exposure to cold and are confined to the exposed parts of the body. The lesions develop not only on exposure to cold weather but also with local application of cold. The cooling of skin associated with evaporation upon emerging from water can produce urticaria. Swimming in cold water is hazardous; death may occur in patients so exposed. There are two forms: a primary acquired form and a familial form. Cold urticaria can occur in adults with such systemic diseases as cryofibrinogenemia, cryoglobulinemia, cold-agglutinin disease, and secondary syphilis. In some cases of primary acquired urticaria, the phenomenon has been passively transferred using purified IgE and IgM fractions of serum from affected patients. After appropriate cold challenge, there are also increased concentrations of histamine, eosinophil and neutrophil chemotactic factors, and platelet-activating factor in venous blood draining the challenge site. Primary acquired cold urticaria appears and disappears spontaneously; in some cases, its onset occurs with a viral illness.

Hereditary angioedema, a potentially life-threatening form of angioedema (Chapter 121), is the most important familial form of angioedema.

A syndrome of episodic angioedema, urticaria and fever with associated eosinophilia, has been described in both adults and children. In contrast to other hypereosinophilic syndromes, this entity has a benign course.

Exercise-induced anaphylaxis presents with varying combinations of pruritus, urticaria, angioedema, wheezing, laryngeal obstruction, or hypotension after exercise. Cholinergic urticaria is differentiated by positive heat challenge tests and the rare occurrence of anaphylactic shock. The combination of ingestion of various food allergens (shrimp, celery, wheat) and postprandial exercise results in cutaneous mast cell degranulation; food or exercise alone may not produce this reaction.

TREATMENT. In most instances, urticaria is a self-limited illness requiring little treatment other than antihistamines. Hydroxyzine (Atarax), 0.5 mg/kg, is one of the most effective antihistamines for control of urticaria, but diphenhydramine (Benadryl), 1.25 mg/kg, and other antihistamines are also effective. These doses may be repeated at intervals of 4–6 hr if necessary.

Epinephrine 1:1,000, 0.01 mL/kg, max 0.3 mL, usually affords rapid relief of acute, severe urticaria. Hydroxyzine (0.5 mg/kg every 4–6 hr) is the drug of choice for cholinergic and chronic urticaria. The combined use of H_1- and H_2-type antihistamines is sometimes helpful to control chronic urticaria. H_2 antihistamines alone may exacerbate urticaria. Cyproheptadine (Periactin) (2–4 mg every 8–12 hr) is especially useful as a prophylactic agent for cold urticaria. Cyproheptadine can cause appetite stimulation and weight gain in some

■ TABLE 139–1 Types of Urticaria

Caused by ingestants (IgE mechanism in some cases)
Foods, particularly fish, shellfish, nuts, eggs, and peanuts; food additives (tartrazine, azo dyes, benzoates)
Drugs (penicillin, aspirin, sulfonamides, codeine)
Caused by contactants (IgE mechanism in some cases)
Plant substances (e.g., stinging nettle)
Animal–insect (tarantula hairs, Portuguese man-of-war, cat scratch, moth scales)
Drugs applied to the skin
Animal saliva
Caused by injectants (IgE mechanism in some cases)
Drugs (particularly penicillin), transfused blood, therapeutic antisera, insect stings and bites (papular urticaria), allergenic extracts
Caused by inhalants (IgE mechanism)
Pollens, danders, and ? molds
Caused by infectious agents (mechanism unknown)
Parasites
Viruses (e.g., hepatitis, infectious mononucleosis)
Bacteria (*Streptococcus*, mycoplasma)
? Fungi
Caused by physical factors (mechanism mostly unknown)
Dermographism
Cold urticaria
Delayed pressure urticaria
Solar urticaria
Aquagenic urticaria
Local heat urticaria
Exercise induced
Vibratory angioedema
Episodic angioedema with eosinophilia (? a distinct entity)
Cholinergic urticaria (a distinct entity)
Associated with systemic diseases (mechanism mostly unknown)
Collagen-vascular (systemic lupus erythematosus, cryoglobulinuria, Sjögren syndrome)
Cutaneous vasculitis
Serum sickness–like disease
Malignancy (leukemia-lymphoma)
Hyperthyroidism
Urticaria pigmentosa (systemic mastocytosis)
Associated with genetic disorders (various mechanisms)
Familial cold urticaria
Hereditary angioedema
Amyloidosis with deafness and urticaria
C3b inactivator deficiency
Chronic urticaria and angioedema (mechanism unknown)
Psychogenic urticaria (existence as an entity uncertain)

Ig = immunoglobulin.

patients. Sunscreens are the only effective treatment for solar urticaria. Corticosteroids have varying effects on chronic urticaria; the doses required to control the urticaria are often so large that they cause serious side effects. Chronic urticaria does not often respond favorably to dietary manipulation. Unfortunately, chronic urticaria may persist for years. For treatment of hereditary angioedema, see Chapter 121.

Bellanti JA, Kadlec JV, Escobar-Gutiérrez A: Cytokines and the immune response. Pediatr Clin North Am 41:597, 1994.
Casale T, Keahey T, Kaliner M: Exercise-induced anaphylactic syndromes. JAMA 255:2049, 1986.
Coleman R, Trembath RC, Harper JI: Chromosome 11q13 and atopy underlying atopic eczema. Lancet 341:1121, 1993.
Galli SJ: Seminars in medicine of the Beth Israel Hospital, Boston. N Engl J Med 328:257, 1993.
Hide M, Francis DM, Grattan CEH, et al: Autoantibodies against the high-affinity IgE receptor as a cause of histamine release in chronic urticaria. N Engl J Med 328:1599, 1993.
Horan RF, Schneider LC, Sheffer AL: Allergic skin disorders and mastocytosis. JAMA 268:2858, 1992.
Huston DP, Bressler RB: Urticaria and angioedema. Med Clin North Am 76:805, 1992.
Leung DYM: Mechanisms of the human allergic response: Clinical implications. Pediatr Clin North Am 41:727, 1994.
Orfan NA, Kolski GB: Physical urticarias. Ann Allergy 71:205, 1993.
Sandford AJ, Shirakawa T, Moffatt MF, et al: Localisation of atopy and β subunit of high-affinity IgE receptor (FCERI) on chromosome 11q. Lancet 341:332, 1993.
Twarog FJ: Urticaria in childhood: Pathogenesis and management. Pediatr Clin North Am 30:887, 1983.

CHAPTER 140
Anaphylaxis

DEFINITION. Anaphylaxis is an acute, potentially life-threatening reaction caused by rapid release of mediators from mast cells and basophils that follows the interaction of allergen with specific, cell-bound immunoglobulin (Ig) E.

ETIOLOGY. Virtually any foreign substance is capable of eliciting anaphylaxis under appropriate circumstances (Table 140–1). Most anaphylactic reactions are due to drug, food, or Hymenoptera venom allergy. Following IgE production in response to antigen stimulus, re-exposure to the offending antigen may result in a systemic reaction. Exercise can provoke anaphylaxis in occasional patients; in some, it occurs only after antecedent ingestion of a specific food or possibly alcohol or aspirin. Intensive evaluation has failed to identify a cause of recurrent anaphylaxis in occasional patients with idiopathic recurrent anaphylaxis, most of whom have had concomitant allergy or asthma not obviously related to the recurrent anaphylaxis.

■ TABLE 140–1 Etiology of Anaphylaxis

Drugs (penicillin, cephalosporins, chemotherapy, muscle relaxants)
Foods (seafood, nuts, legumes, egg, celery, milk)
Insect Stings (Hymenoptera: kissing bug, deerfly, fire ants)
Biological Agents (L-asparaginase, allergen extracts, blood products, insulin, immunoglobulins)
Food Additives (metabisulfite, monosodium glutamate, aspartame)
Latex
Exercise Induced
Pseudoallergic* (iodinated radiocontrast media, opiates, D-tubocurarine, thiamine, aspirin, captopril)
Idiopathic

**Pseudoallergic or anaphylactoid is not necessarily immunoglobulin E mediated. Substances can produce direct mast cell degranulation.*

Anaphylaxis to latex is a significant problem among patients chronically exposed to this compound (repeated operations or urinary catheterization, e.g., spina bifida).

PATHOGENESIS. In the person in whom IgE-mediated anaphylactic sensitivity to an antigen has developed, subsequent administration of even minute amounts of the antigen may result in an explosive antigen-antibody reaction with massive release of chemical mediators such as histamine. The action of the mediators on various tissue receptors throughout the body produces the symptoms. Histamine plays a central role in the pathogenesis of human anaphylaxis, but other vasoactive substances (arachidonic acid metabolites, kinins, platelet-activating factor) may also have roles. Decreased levels of factor V and factor VIII have been reported, suggesting consumption of coagulation factors as a result of intravascular coagulation. Several patients studied during severe episodes of systemic anaphylaxis have had low levels of high molecular weight kininogen, C3, and C4. When an immunological mechanism cannot be identified (anaphylactoid reactions, see Table 140–1), it is presumed that mediator release occurs as a direct effect of the causative agent on basophils and mast cells or perhaps by activation of the alternative complement pathway, with generation of anaphylatoxins (see prior discussion).

CLINICAL MANIFESTATIONS. Anaphylactic reactions are characteristically explosive, particularly when the antigen is injected. Surviving patients describe a "feeling of impending doom." The more rapidly symptoms appear after administration of the foreign material, the more serious is the reaction. Often the first symptom noted is a tingling sensation around the mouth or face, followed by a feeling of warmth, difficulty in swallowing, and tightness in the throat or chest. There may be apprehension, weakness, and diaphoresis followed by generalized pruritus. The patient becomes flushed; urticaria and angioedema then appear, along with varying degrees of hoarseness, inspiratory stridor, dysphagia, nasal congestion, itching of the eyes, sneezing, and wheezing. Abdominal cramps, diarrhea, and contractions of the uterus and other organs of smooth muscle may also occur. The patient may lose consciousness and, on examination, be hypotensive, with feeble heart sounds, bradycardia, and sometimes an arrhythmia. Cardiorespiratory arrest and death may ensue. In fatal cases, death has most often resulted from acute upper airway obstruction, although profound circulatory collapse may occur without upper airway obstruction.

Most anaphylactic reactions begin within 30 min of exposure to the allergen, especially if by injection. Signs and symptoms usually resolve within a few hours in surviving patients. Some patients experience biphasic reactions with recurrence of signs and symptoms 1 to 8 hr after initial resolution in response to therapy; this may be due to limited durations of action of initially administered pharmacological agents. In a third group of patients, signs and symptoms of anaphylaxis may continue for many hours or days despite aggressive treatment. Protracted anaphylaxis is more likely to follow oral administration of the offending agent than injection. Biphasic or protracted anaphylaxis is more likely when initial manifestations have occurred more than 30 min after exposure.

DIAGNOSIS. Diagnosis depends on recognition of the typical manifestations but sometimes may be uncertain, especially when the victim is found dead. Vasovagal reactions may be confused with anaphylaxis. They are characterized by nausea, pallor, diaphoresis, bradycardia, hypotension, weakness, and occasionally syncope but lack pruritus, urticaria, angioedema, tachycardia, and bronchospasm. Bradycardia can rarely occur with anaphylaxis.

When there has been loss of consciousness and there are no cutaneous manifestations of anaphylaxis, the differential diagnosis also includes pulmonary embolism; cardiac arrhythmia; cerebrovascular hemorrhage, embolism, or thrombosis;

convulsive disorder; foreign body aspiration; and acute poisoning. Systemic mastocytosis can cause symptoms of anaphylaxis occasionally, usually with a history of flushing and maculopapular lesions that urticate with stroking. Hereditary angioneurotic edema can cause laryngeal edema, but associated angioedema is nonpruritic and usually develops gradually over a period of hours. Sudden vascular collapse can occur after exposure to cold in patients with cold urticaria and may be associated with urticaria or airway obstruction; it usually follows swimming in cold water.

Determination of plasma or serum tryptase concentrations can be helpful in the diagnosis of anaphylaxis. Concentrations of 10 ng/ml or more indicate mast cell activation. Increased concentrations may not occur during the first 30 min but tend to peak at 1 to 2 hr and then decline with a half time of 2 hr. Plasma histamine (H) concentrations, on the other hand, peak within 5 to 10 min after a bee sting challenge and return to baseline within 30 min. Therefore, determination of plasma or serum tryptase concentration is usually more helpful in the diagnosis of anaphylaxis. Other causes of increased tryptase concentrations include asthma, provoked, for example, by a nonsteroidal anti-inflammatory drug, and systemic mastocytosis.

Patients with systemic mastocytosis have elevated plasma histamine concentrations when they are asymptomatic. Patients with hereditary angioneurotic edema have absent or dysfunctional C1 inhibitor, and plasma C4 concentrations are usually low both during and between exacerbations.

TREATMENT. Effective treatment depends on prompt diagnosis and rapid implementation of appropriate therapy. The treatment of choice is aqueous epinephrine, 1:1,000, 0.1 mL/kg (maximum 0.3 mL for a child or 0.5 mL for an adult) by subcutaneous injection. If necessary, this dose may be repeated at 15-min intervals. If the reaction is to injection of an allergen extract or to a Hymenoptera sting on an extremity, one half of this dose of epinephrine may be diluted in 2 mL normal saline and infiltrated subcutaneously at the site of the injection or sting to slow absorption. A tourniquet above the site can also slow systemic distribution of the allergen. The tourniquet can be loosened after improvement or briefly at intervals of 3 min.

A persistent, serious reaction can be treated cautiously with careful cardiac monitoring of the intravenous infusion of epinephrine at an initial infusion rate of 0.1 μg/kg/min in a child (or 2 μg/min in an adult) to sustain a systolic blood pressure of 80 mm Hg.

Supplemental oxygen (100%, 4–6 L/min) is indicated. Extension of the neck and use of an oropharyngeal airway may be helpful for upper airway obstruction. Endotracheal intubation may be necessary; if this cannot be accomplished, cricothyrotomy is indicated for laryngeal obstruction. Nebulized albuterol and intravenous aminophylline are effective for treatment of lower airway obstruction as in the treatment of asthma.

If hypotension is unresponsive to administration of epinephrine by subcutaneous injection, rapid intravenous administration of isotonic saline is indicated (up to 100 mL/min to a limit of 3 L for an adult). A supine position with the feet elevated is helpful. Extreme or persistent hypotension may require treatment with norepinephrine by intravenous infusion or dopamine.

An H_1 antagonist such as diphenhydramine, 1 mg/kg, by intramuscular injection or intravenous infusion may be helpful for hypotension as well as urticaria. Combined use of an H_1 antagonist and an H_2 antagonist such as cimetidine, 4 mg/kg (maximum 300 mg), infused intravenously over at least 5 min, may be more helpful than diphenhydramine alone.

Systemic adrenal corticosteroids are appropriate after treatment of the initial manifestations of anaphylaxis, although it is uncertain whether they are helpful in preventing biphasic reactions.

If the only manifestations of anaphylaxis have been urticaria or angioedema and the patient will not be far from medical care, observation is not necessary long after resolution of the cutaneous signs and symptoms; it is prudent for such patients to receive epinephrine initially because of possible progression of involvement to other systems. It is safest to continue observation of patients who have had hypotension or airway obstruction for at least 12 hr because of possible recurrence of the initial life-threatening manifestations.

Serious anaphylactoid reactions to intravenous radiocontrast media are less common in children than in adults but occur occasionally. A prophylactic regimen for patients known to be at risk by virtue of previous reactions consists of prednisone, 50 mg orally every 6 hr for 3 doses, ending 1 hr before the procedure, and diphenhydramine, 50 mg, given by intramuscular injection 1 hr before the procedure. This regimen prevents adverse reactions of any degree in over 90% of high-risk adult patients.

The incidence of drug-induced anaphylaxis would drop substantially if drugs were given only when indicated and only by the oral route unless some compelling reason for injection exists. Not only is anaphylactic sensitivity more easily induced by injection of drugs than by oral administration, but in the sensitized patient anaphylaxis occurs more commonly following parenteral than oral administration. The incidence of anaphylaxis following Hymenoptera stings can be reduced significantly by the appropriate use of venom immunotherapy (Chapters 135 and 142).

Patients with histories of systemic anaphylaxis after eating egg may rarely be at special risk for anaphylaxis after administration of vaccines that contain egg protein, including influenza vaccine and yellow fever vaccine. The Committee on Infectious Diseases of the American Academy of Pediatrics has recommended administration of such vaccines to patients with such histories only after prick and intradermal testing with the vaccine has not elicited a positive reaction or administration with desensitization if a skin test with the vaccine has been positive. Measles, mumps, and measles-mumps-rubella (MMR) vaccines have been included among vaccines with such precautions, but anaphylaxis can follow administration of these vaccines whether or not there is a history of allergy to egg, and the vast majority of egg-allergic children can tolerate MMR vaccine without any significant adverse reaction. It is prudent to skin test such children with influenza vaccine or yellow fever vaccine to evaluate the safety of administration of the vaccine, but skin testing with MMR vaccine may not be necessary. Administration of any of these vaccines in all children should be supervised carefully with preparations for treatment of anaphylaxis if it should occur.

Businco L: Measles, mumps, rubella immunization in egg-allergic children: A long-lasting debate. Ann Allergy 72:1, 1994.

Fasano MB, Wood RA, Cook SK, Sampson HA: Egg hypersensitivity and adverse reactions to measles, mumps, and rubella vaccine. J Pediatr 120:878, 1992.

Herrera AM, deShazo RD: Current concepts in anaphylaxis. Immunol Allergy Clin North Am 12:517, 1992.

Horan RF, Sheffer AL: Exercise-induced anaphylaxis. Immunol Allergy Clin North Am 12:559, 1992.

Kelly KJ, Kurup V, Zacharisen M, et al: Skin and serologic testing in the diagnosis of latex allergy. J Allergy Clin Immunol 91:1140, 1993.

Sampson HA, Mendelson L, Rosen JP: Fatal and near-fatal anaphylactic reactions to food in children and adolescents. N Engl J Med 327:380, 1992.

Schwartz LB, Yunginger JW, Miller J, et al: Time course of appearance and disappearance of human mast cell tryptase in the circulation after anaphylaxis. J Clin Invest 83:1551, 1989.

Stark BJ, Sullivan TJ: Biphasic and protracted anaphylaxis. J Allergy Clin Immunol 78:76, 1986.

Valentine M: Anaphylaxis and stinging insect hypersensitivity. JAMA 268:2830, 1992.

Valentine MD: Insect-sting anaphylaxis. Ann Intern Med 118:225, 1993.

Yunginger JW: Anaphylaxis. Ann Allergy 69:87, 1992.

Yunginger JW: Anaphylaxis to foods. Immunol Allergy Clin North Am 12:543, 1992.

CHAPTER 141
Serum Sickness

The serum sickness syndrome is a characteristic systemic immunologic disorder that follows the administration of foreign antigenic material.

ETIOLOGY. The disorder was first described as a consequence of antitoxin therapy for diseases such as diphtheria and tetanus. The illness was shown to be due to an adverse reaction to the serum proteins of the animal in which the antitoxin was prepared. Therapeutic antisera of animal origin, especially equine, are still occasionally used, but today the major cause of the serum sickness syndrome is drug allergy, particularly that caused by penicillin. Cases have also followed use of other therapeutic agents, including human gamma globulin and even Hymenoptera stings. Preparations of immunoglobulin of human origin are available for treatment of diphtheria and tetanus (and prophylaxis of rabies) in humans, but antitoxins for treatment of crotalid envenomation and clostridial intoxication (botulism, gas gangrene) are still prepared in the horse.

PATHOGENESIS. Serum sickness is the classic example of a type III hypersensitivity, "immune complex" disease in the experimental animal. After a single large dose of isotopically labeled antigen is injected into the rabbit, the symptoms of serum sickness occur coincidentally with the appearance of antibody formed against the injected antigen, at a time when the latter is still present in the circulation. Antigen-antibody complexes formed under conditions of moderate antigen excess lodge in small vessels and in filtering organs throughout the body (deposition being aided in the rabbit by the actions of immunoglobulin [Ig] E antibody, basophils, and platelet-activating factor and by the release of vasoactive amines that increase the permeability of blood vessels); these complexes activate the complement sequence. Complement components bound at the site of immune complex deposition promote accumulation of neutrophils through at least two general processes: adherence of neutrophils to the site of bound complement and chemotactic activity of the C567 complex and C3a and C5a fragments. Tissue injury results from the liberation of toxic molecules from the neutrophils. In this animal model, healing of the lesions occurs following elimination of the complexes from the circulation.

Serum sickness demonstrates how the differing biological activities of the several species of antibodies formed against a complex antigen may be responsible for diverse parts of the clinical picture; the urticaria of serum sickness is thought to be due to IgE antibody molecules reacting with horse serum proteins, whereas the joint symptoms are thought to occur as a result of deposition of antigen-antibody complexes of the IgG and IgM classes. In both rabbits and humans it is suspected that histamine release from basophils and mast cells, mediated by IgE antibodies, facilitates the deposition of immune complexes through increases in vascular permeability.

CLINICAL MANIFESTATIONS. Typically, the symptoms of serum sickness begin 7–12 days following injection of the foreign material but may appear as late as 3 wk afterward. If there has been earlier exposure or previous allergic reaction to the same foreign antigen, symptoms may appear in accelerated fashion, within 1–3 days following injection, or as anaphylaxis. Fever and malaise are almost always present, as are cutaneous eruptions. Urticaria, usually generalized, is a common finding. Faint erythema with a serpiginous border at the margins of palmar or plantar skin of the hands, fingers, feet, and toes may precede the generalized cutaneous eruption. This characteristic cutaneous lesion may become purpuric with time. Edema, particularly around the face and neck, facial flushing, myalgia, lymphadenopathy, arthralgia, or arthritis involving multiple joints (ankle, knee, wrist, fingers, toes), and gastrointestinal complaints (cramping, diarrhea, nausea) also occur. Intense pruritus accompanying the urticaria is the most distressing symptom in many patients. The site of injection of the foreign material generally becomes red and swollen, commonly 1–3 days before systemic symptoms appear. The disease generally runs a self-limited course, and the patient recovers in 7–10 days. Carditis and glomerulonephritis occur rarely; the most serious complications of serum sickness are Guillain-Barré syndrome and peripheral neuritis, especially involving the brachial plexus (C5-6).

LABORATORY MANIFESTATIONS. The blood leukocyte and eosinophil counts are variable; marked thrombocytopenia is often found. Mild proteinuria, hemoglobinuria, and microscopic hematuria may be seen. Plasma cells have been found in blood. The erythrocyte sedimentation rate is often increased. A sheep cell agglutinin titer of the Forssman type is usually elevated. Serum complement levels (C3 and C4) are variably depressed and may fall to low concentrations around the 10th day. C3a anaphylatoxin may be increased. In serum sickness caused by horse serum proteins, antibodies of the IgG, IgA, IgM, and IgE classes may be found directed against various horse serum proteins. Direct immunofluorescence studies of skin lesions often reveal immune deposits of IgM, IgA, IgE, or C3.

TREATMENT. Patients generally respond well to aspirin and antihistamines. When the symptoms are especially severe, corticosteroids have been used with great efficacy. High doses are given and rapidly reduced as the patient improves.

PREVENTION. The use of horse serum or other animal serum in therapy should be limited to cases for which no alternative is available. When only equine antitoxin is available, skin tests should be employed prior to administration of serum, beginning with a puncture test using a 1:10 dilution. If the reaction is negative, one may then begin intradermal testing with 0.02 mL of a 1:10,000 dilution. If there is no reaction, a subsequent skin test should be performed with a 1:1,000 dilution. If a negative result again is obtained, a final intradermal test with a 1:100 dilution of horse serum is done. A negative reaction to the strongest solution indicates that anaphylactic sensitivity to horse serum is very unlikely; skin tests do not predict the likelihood of development of serum sickness.

Occasionally, patients who have evidence of anaphylactic sensitivity to horse serum by virtue of either a previous reaction or a positive immediate wheal and flare skin test require treatment with horse serum. In such a case, the antitoxin can be successfully administered by a process of rapid desensitization. Some allergists medicate the patient with epinephrine and antihistamines before beginning the desensitization procedure. Others prefer not to mask possible evidence of a reaction at an early stage when it still might be of a minor degree and serve as a warning to proceed more slowly with the desensitization. The desensitization process is begun with 0.1-mL amounts of antitoxin, diluted to 1:100,000–1:10,000, depending on an estimate of the degree of the patient's sensitivity, and injected intravenously at 20-min intervals. If the patient tolerates the previous injection without adverse reactions, the amount administered may be doubled every 20 min. Generally, the entire amount of antitoxin can be administered safely over a 4- to 6-hr period. The desensitization, unfortunately, is transient, and the patient often regains the previous anaphylactic sensitivity within a few months. Administration of methylprednisolone in doses of 1–1.5 mg/kg/day has not prevented the development of serum sickness.

Bielory L, Gascon P, Lawley T, et al: Human serum sickness: A prospective analysis of 35 patients treated with equine antithymocyte globulin for bone marrow failure. Medicine 67:40, 1988.
Gilliland BG: Serum sickness and immune complexes. N Engl J Med 311:1435, 1984.
Kunnamo I, Kallio P, Pelkonen P, et al: Serum sickness-like disease is a common cause of acute arthritis in children. Acta Pediatr Scand 75:964, 1986.
Lawley TJ, Bielory L, Gascon P, et al: A prospective clinical and immunologic analysis of patients with serum sickness. N Engl J Med 311:1407, 1984.

CHAPTER 142

Adverse Reactions to Drugs

(See Chapter 63)

DEFINITION. An adverse reaction to a drug may be defined as any unwanted consequence of administration of the agent during or following a course of therapy. Adverse reactions fall into two broad categories: those dependent upon pharmacological mechanisms and those dependent upon immunological mechanisms (Table 142–1). The majority of adverse drug reactions are pharmacological; only 6% have an allergic basis. In a study of hospitalized children who had adverse drug reactions, no more than 15% were thought to be of an allergic nature.

Certain generalities apply to adverse drug reactions. (1) Virtually any organ system may be involved. (2) After the neonatal period, children are less often affected than adults. (3) The incidence of reactions increases almost exponentially with the number of drugs given simultaneously. (4) Certain diseases predispose to adverse drug reactions, especially those in which multiple drug therapy is common (cardiovascular, infectious, and psychiatric illnesses). Diseases that affect organs responsible for absorption (gastrointestinal tract), metabolism (liver), or excretion of drugs (kidney) also increase the likelihood of adverse reactions. (5) The pharmacokinetic properties of a drug (for example, the extent of protein binding) also affect the incidence of adverse reactions.

CLASSIFICATION. Adverse drug reactions can be classified in terms of their underlying mechanisms. Toxicity may result from a high concentration of drug in the body caused by excessive intake—accidental or intentional—or to abnormalities in absorption, metabolism, or excretion of the drug. Various diseases, genetic factors, or drug interactions may permit accumulation of a drug. Some patients for unknown reasons have excessive pharmacological responses (intolerance) to average drug doses. The signs and symptoms are generally intensifications of the expected pharmacologic effects of the agent.

Side effects are undesirable but essentially unavoidable effects of drugs and largely reflect the fact that a given drug rarely affects only one tissue. When theophylline is given as a bronchodilator agent in asthma, for example, central nervous system stimulation is considered a side effect, although this latter effect of theophylline warrants its use in neonatal apnea. Secondary effects of drugs are those not related to their primary pharmacological actions. An example is disturbance of the bacterial flora of the intestine as a consequence of antibiotic therapy. In drug idiosyncrasy, the signs and symptoms of the reaction are unrelated to the known pharmacological properties of the agent, sometimes because of metabolic abnormalities. An example is the hemolytic anemia that follows ingestion of primaquine in patients with G-6-PD deficiency (Chapter 414).

Drug interactions are discussed in Chapter 63, and see also Table 670–3.

Allergic drug reactions occur on the basis of recognized models of immune injury. These include (1) immunoglobulin (Ig) E–mediated reactions; (2) cytotoxic reactions resulting from hapten binding to cell membranes and subsequent reaction with antihapten antibodies; (3) immune complex reactions in which drug-antibody immune complexes with affinity for cell membranes activate the complement system, resulting in cell membrane damage; (4) reactions caused by autoantibody formation; and (5) reactions caused by cell-mediated mechanisms. Most drugs are simple chemicals with molecular weights of less than 1,000 and are rarely immunogenic. Substances with low molecular weights may act as haptens and become immunogenic after covalent chemical binding with tissue proteins to form drug-protein conjugates. Hapten-protein complex formation is necessary for the macrophage–T cell–B cell interaction that leads to formation of hapten-specific humoral antibodies and cellular immunity. In general, only drugs (or their degradative or metabolic products) with sufficient chemical reactivity to bind irreversibly with proteins are capable of inducing hypersensitivity reactions. The major impediment to both study and diagnosis of drug allergy is that the chemically reactive substance is often not the native drug itself but a metabolic or degradative product. Because little is known about the metabolic fate of many drugs in common use, it is often impossible to identify the chemically reactive intermediates necessary for investigative or diagnostic use.

The complexities of understanding allergic reactions to drugs are illustrated by considering the penicillin model. Benzyl penicillin (penicillin G) has produced a wide variety of allergic reactions, including systemic responses such as anaphylaxis, serum sickness, and vasculitis; hematological disorders, including hemolytic anemia, thrombocytopenia, and granulocytopenia; a broad spectrum of cutaneous eruptions; pulmonary disease; and renal disease (see Table 142–1). Under physiologic conditions, both in vivo and in vitro, a number of highly protein-reactive compounds are formed from penicillin. These metabolic products become immunogenic following conjugation with tissue proteins as described earlier. The penicilloyl group, formed by the combination of benzyl penicillenic acid with amino groups of proteins, is the antigenic determinant formed in largest amounts. Ninety-five per cent of all benzyl penicillin that conjugates with tissue proteins in vivo forms benzylpenicilloyl haptenic groups (BPO), and thus benzyl penicillin has been designated the "major" haptenic determinant of penicillin hypersensitivity. A large percentage of people who have been treated with penicillin possess antibodies to the BPO determinant, but most do not experience symptoms of penicillin allergy. BPO-specific IgE antibodies can be detected through a BPO-polylysine skin test reagent in which BPO haptenic groups are attached to a "backbone" of lysine. BPO polylysine is available as a skin test reagent and for coupling to cyanogen bromide-activated disks in the radioallergosorbent test (RAST).

Unfortunately, the most feared consequence of penicillin allergy, anaphylaxis, usually is not due to IgE sensitization to the major BPO haptenic group but to less well defined, so-called minor haptenic determinants. These include penicilloate, penilloate, and penicillenate and its oxidation products. Though only 5% or less of the benzyl penicillin that reacts with proteins forms minor haptenic determinants, these have major clinical significance; unfortunately, antigens with minor determinant specificity are not readily available for testing either in vivo or in vitro.

Allergy to benzyl penicillin is further complicated by the development of related semisynthetic penicillins and cephalopart of a generalized allergic reaction in atopic dermatitis, urticaria, or angioedema, for example, or the eye alone may be affected. Allergic reactions in the eye are known to occur on the basis of immunoglobulin (Ig) E–mediated allergy, as conjunctivitis in a child with ragweed hay fever, for example, or on the basis of a cell-mediated (delayed hypersensitivity) immune reaction, as in contact dermatitis of the eyelids.

EYELIDS. Eyelids are particularly prone to swelling because of their loose areolar connective tissue. Swelling may result from contact dermatitis to a variety of environmental substances. The lids are particularly involved because of the frequency with which offending contact sensitizers are carried to the eyelids with the hands. Occasionally, contact dermatitis appears as a result of sensitization to medication applied to the eyes. Cosmetics and topical ophthalmic medications are common sensitizing agents. Sulfonamides, neomycin, scopolamine, atropine, pilocarpine, contact lens solution, and topical anesthetics cause contact sensitization. The lids become inflamed and indurated, and a scaly, eczematoid reaction is evident. The conjunctiva becomes red, and a follicular conjunctivitis may develop.

Blepharitis. This is an inflammatory eczematous reaction of the eyelid margins that may be caused by infection, allergy, or both. A chronic staphylococcal infection has been implicated as the major cause of chronic eczema of the eyelid margins. The lid margins, particularly of the lower lids, are affected with an itchy, scaly, erythematous eruption with exudate at the base of the lashes. This gives the appearance of "granulated eyelids." The eyelids may be crusted together in the morning. The diagnosis is confirmed by slit-lamp examination.

ALLERGIC CONJUNCTIVITIS. This frequently accompanies allergic rhinitis in patients with hay fever, especially when caused by pollens. In affected children, both eyes itch, the conjunctivae are reddened and edematous, and there may be profuse tearing. Rubbing of the eyes aggravates the condition. There is no photophobia or other signs of corneal involvement. Occasionally, edema of the conjunctiva is so severe that the conjunctiva prolapses over the lower lid in a gelatinous-appearing mass (chemosis) that causes great concern to parents. The secretions are frequently watery but, if persistent, may appear purulent. Even discharges that appear purulent, however, contain predominantly eosinophils; these permit differentiation from infectious conjunctivitis, in which the discharge contains mostly polymorphonuclear leukocytes and bacteria.

Atopic Keratoconjunctivitis. This condition occurs in patients with atopic dermatitis who have extreme ocular itching, red eyes, swollen and thickened eyelids, and, when the cornea is involved, photophobia. Keratoconus, a central corneal ectasia, is thought to be due to repeated eye rubbing, and cataracts are complications.

Vernal Conjunctivitis. This inflammation is more common in children, with a 3:1 male-female predominance, than in adults (80% of patients are under 14 yr old at onset). It appears most often in warm climates and during the spring and summer. The disease affects both eyes and occurs in palpebral and limbal forms. In the palpebral form, which is most common, the tarsal plate of the upper lid presents a characteristic "cobblestone" appearance as a result of hyperplasia and thickening of the conjunctiva. The hyperplasia may cause pseudoptosis. A thick, ropy, whitish discharge may be present over the hypertrophied, giant papillae giving the "cobblestone" appearance. In the limbal form, the junction of the cornea and sclera is involved, with thickening and opacity of the tissue in the area. Whitish Trantas dots, present on the corneoscleral limbus, which represent accumulations of eosinophils, are pathognomonic of the disease. Progression of the limbal form may scar the cornea and lead to blindness in the most severe cases. Symptoms of vernal conjunctivitis include lacrimation, extreme itching, burning, and a particularly distressing photophobia. The seasonal occurrence, the finding of eosinophils, and the frequent coexistence with other atopic diseases such as asthma, hay fever, and eczema suggest that IgE-mediated sensitivity is responsible for the condition; but detailed study of patients with the condition usually fails to identify any cause, and immunotherapy is of little if any value. The symptoms and signs of vernal conjunctivitis are mimicked in a syndrome induced by the wearing of hard or soft contact lenses: giant papillary conjunctivitis.

TREATMENT. Contact dermatitis of the lids is best managed by identification of suspected sensitizers and their elimination. A short course of topical corticosteroids is of value in managing the acute reaction.

Blepharitis is best treated by good lid hygiene, using cotton-tipped applicators and half-strength baby shampoo mixed with water to remove scales and exudate, followed by the use of antistaphylococcal ointments. If an excessive reaction to the treatment results, steroids are applied topically for a few days. Since the disease tends to recur, regular lid care is indicated, often for a lifetime.

Allergic conjunctivitis in the patient with hay fever generally responds well to topical application of sympathomimetics (naphazoline or phenylephrine) in the form of eye drops; 0.05% levocabastine hydrochloride eye drops (not labeled for use by the U.S. Food and Drug Administration [FDA] in patients younger than 12 yr); 0.1% lodoxamide tromethamine eye drops (not FDA labeled for use in patients younger than 2 yr); or, in more severe cases, to eye drops or ointments containing corticosteroids. Lodoxamide is FDA labeled for treatment of only vernal conjunctivitis. As noted later, steroids should be used in the eyes only with caution. Immunotherapy for allergic conjunctivitis in the absence of allergic rhinitis usually gives poor results.

Atopic keratoconjunctivitis requires the use of topical steroids, particularly if the cornea is involved. Referral to an ophthalmologist is indicated.

Vernal conjunctivitis may be treated with topical vasoconstrictors, antihistamines, cold compresses, and 0.1% lodoxamide tromethamine eye drops or, if necessary, with sparing use of corticosteroid eye drops or ointments. Fluorometholone or medrysone, a topically active, poorly absorbed corticosteroid, in a dose of 1–2 drops four times a day, is particularly indicated in allergic conjunctivitis when there is involvement of only the superficial layers of the eye. The drug is less likely to cause increased intraocular pressure than the more readily absorbed preparations such as dexamethasone or methylprednisolone. Whenever topical steroids are used in the eye for more than a few days, intraocular pressure should be monitored. In addition, prolonged topical steroid administration may predispose the patient to cataracts and opportunistic infections.

Abelson MB, George MA, Garofalo C: Differential diagnosis of ocular allergic disorders. Ann Allergy 70:95, 1993.
Fahy GT, Easty DL, Collum LM, et al: Randomised double-masked trial of lodoxamide and sodium cromoglycate in allergic eye disease: A multicentre study. Eur J Ophthalmol 2:144, 1992.
Friedlaender MH: Current concepts in ocular allergy. Ann Allergy 67:5, 1991.
Friedlaender MH: Immunologic aspects of diseases of the eye. JAMA 268:2869, 1992.

CHAPTER 145
Adverse Reactions to Foods

The incidence of adverse reactions to foods is not known and unquestionably varies in different parts of the world.

The average United States diet contains many food antigens, chemical food additives, antibiotics, and other substances; accordingly, a significant frequency of adverse reactions to foods should not be surprising. Food reactions caused by allergic mechanisms are estimated to occur in from 0.3–0.7% of people, but the prevalence of food allergy is a subject of substantial disagreement. Most adverse reactions to food do not have an immunologic basis. In these cases the use of immunologic methods of diagnosis (skin testing or provocative testing [injection or oral administration of food antigen]) is inappropriate. Treatment based on immunologic principles is similarly unwarranted.

ETIOLOGY. Possible mechanisms for adverse reactions to foods include not only allergy but also enzyme deficiencies and nonimmunologic reactions to tyramine, nitrites, and monosodium glutamate (Table 145–1). There is little doubt that intact macromolecules may pass through the epithelium of the gastrointestinal tract and gain access to the systemic circulation, particularly during the first few months of life. Secretory immunoglobulin (Ig) A limits the intestinal absorption of intact macromolecules. Children with IgA deficiency have higher levels of antibodies to cow milk proteins and of immune complexes containing milk antigens than do normal controls. IgE-mediated reactions are characteristically rapid in onset and may present as angioedema of the lips, mouth, uvula, or glottis; as generalized urticaria; as asthma; or occasionally as shock. In such cases, the patient usually recognizes that the symptoms have followed ingestion of a certain food. Persons with such IgE-mediated food allergy are at constant risk of exposure to the offending food hidden in a food mixture. For example, a nut-sensitive individual may have a serious reaction to ingestion of a cookie made with almond extract.

Individuals with IgE-mediated food reactions consistently show positive skin tests to the suspected food. In fact, skin testing itself, particularly if done by the intracutaneous technique, can precipitate the clinical reaction in individuals with anaphylactic allergy to a food. Foods that have the highest potential to cause IgE-mediated sensitivity are fish, shellfish, peanuts (a legume), various nuts and seeds, eggs, cow milk, soy, wheat, and corn.

More difficult to diagnose are reactions that begin a few to 24 hr after ingestion of the offending food. Such reactions have been attributed without much convincing evidence to allergy to a digestive product of the food such as a protease or polypeptide. The roles of antigen-antibody complexes and cell-mediated immunity (delayed hypersensitivity) in the pathogenesis of these late-occurring reactions are unknown.

A variety of reactions have been reported to follow ingestion of cow milk by infants and children. In some cases, an IgE mechanism has been established. In others, however, even with antibodies to milk proteins (particularly α-lactalbumin, β-lactoglobulin, and casein) present in sufficient quantities to be demonstrable by gel diffusion methods, no immunologic mechanism has been established. During the 1st yr of life, vomiting and watery, blood-streaked, mucoid diarrhea may follow cow milk ingestion. An enteropathy with loss of both protein and blood has been found in other young infants fed large volumes of whole pasteurized milk (but not heat-processed formula). In older infants, ingestion of cow milk has been associated with occult fecal blood loss, recurrent roentgenographic pulmonary infiltrates, and multiple precipitating antibodies to cow milk proteins (Chapter 349). Some cases of pulmonary hemosiderosis are said to be responsive to withdrawal of milk from the diet.

Adverse reactions to milk caused by disaccharidase deficiencies are discussed in Chapter 286.11.

A number of enteropathies with varying combinations of malabsorption, steatorrhea, hypoalbuminemia, and fecal blood loss have been reported as a result of cow milk or wheat intolerance. Despite close associations between symptoms or signs and the feeding of these foods, a precise mechanism of immunologic injury has not been identified. It is not known whether wheat-sensitive individuals who have adverse symptoms from the gluten fraction of wheat are reacting to α-gliadin as a toxin or as an antigen in an immune-complex type of injury.

During the first 3 yr of life, rashes and diarrhea following ingestion of fruits and juices are common. There is no evidence of an immunologic mechanism.

Sulfites can cause modest bronchoconstriction in some asthmatic patients and severe, life-threatening airway obstruction in a few, probably in part because of increased airway hyperresponsiveness. Sulfites rarely can cause anaphylactic reactions. In the United States, a ban on the use of sulfiting agents on raw fruit and vegetables has greatly reduced this hazard.

Other nonimmunologic adverse reactions to foods principally in adults include headaches after ingestion of wine and cheese (tyramine), cured meat or "hot dog" headache (sodium nitrite), or the Chinese restaurant syndrome (monosodium glutamate). Affected people apparently have idiosyncratic, but not allergic, reactions to these simple chemicals. In other cases, nonimmunologic adverse reactions may be due to food additives, including the dyes used in foods and drugs. A report of the National Advisory Committee on Hyperkinesis and Food Additives concluded that there was no direct causal connection between artificial food colors and flavors and hyperactivity in children.

DIAGNOSIS. An etiologic diagnosis in a child suspected of an adverse food reaction requires careful objective study. Elimination from the diet for a period of 7–10 days of a food causing difficulty should generally result in improvement in the patient's symptoms. Reintroduction of the food, initially in small quantities and then in increasing amounts, should result in the return of symptoms in a reasonable period of time, within 7 days at most. If symptoms are produced, the food is eliminated from the diet for several months. Reintroduction of the food (except in cases of anaphylactic sensitivity) should be attempted at regular intervals.

The critical testing of foods by the elimination and provocation method is difficult if either patient or parent anticipates an unfavorable reaction because of the emotional bias incident to the ingestion of the suspected food. Food challenges are

■ **TABLE 145–1 Differential Diagnosis of Adverse Reactions to Foods**

Condition	Example
Food allergy	Anaphylaxis, urticaria-angioedema, eosinophilic colitis, eczema, nuts, eggs, seafood, milk, celery, soy
Immune mediated	Celiac disease
Food additives	Dyes (tartrazine), flavoring (MSG), preservatives (metabisulfite)
Food poisoning (toxins)	Botulism, *Bacillus cereus, Clostridium perfringens, Staphylococcus aureus, Scombroid, Ciguatera,* paralytic shellfish
Infections	*Salmonella, Shigella, Escherichia coli, Yersinia, Campylobacter, Giardia,* rotavirus, Norwalk agents, AIDS
Contaminants	Heavy metals, antibiotics (penicillin)
Pharmacologic agents	Caffeine, tyramine, alcohol, histamine
Gastrointestinal disorders	Gastroesophageal reflux, pyloric stenosis, tracheoesophageal fistula, malrotation, peptic ulceration, inflammatory bowel disease
Enzyme deficiencies	Galactosemia, urea cycle defects, phenylketonuria
Malabsorption syndromes	Lactase deficiency, cystic fibrosis, cholestasis
Psychologic	School phobia
Functional	Irritable bowel syndrome, chronic nonspecific diarrhea of infancy

**MSG = monosodium glutamate; AIDS = acquired immunodeficiency syndrome.*

best done in a blind manner, the food being given in a disguised form, for example in opaque capsules or mixed with another food. When symptoms have been continual, dietary elimination of the offending food should cause prompt improvement. On the other hand, when symptoms such as headache have been intermittent, results of elimination and provocation testing are frequently equivocal.

Skin testing with properly prepared food antigens reveals the presence of any IgE antibody to the test antigen. A negative prick skin test with properly prepared potent food extracts virtually excludes the possibility of IgE-mediated allergy to the test food. On the other hand, a positive skin test does not necessarily indicate that the particular food causes symptoms. Positive tests, especially if they do not correlate with the history, should be confirmed by food challenge. In anaphylactic food allergy, skin tests almost invariably show a positive reaction to the offending food, but in this instance the history alone usually establishes the diagnosis, and skin testing is superfluous and may be dangerous. Occasionally, a positive result on a skin test to a food not previously suspected of causing symptoms is clinically corroborated when the history is re-examined in light of the positive test. All too often, undue attention paid to clinically irrelevant skin reactions to food extracts has led to very restricted diets with no attempt made to confirm the clinical importance of suspected foods through elimination and provocative testing. Overdiagnosis of food allergy has sometimes caused malnutrition in infants and children as well as anxiety and depression in mothers who have found it impossible to adhere to severely restrictive diets.

Radioallergosorbent test (RAST) assay has been used to detect IgE antibodies to foods. The correlation among clinical history, puncture skin test, and RAST is excellent for codfish, egg white, nuts, peanuts, and peas. Positive RAST and skin tests to cereals correlate poorly with the results of cereal challenge. RAST for soybeans and white beans is unreliable, apparently because of nonspecific binding of IgE to the RAST disk. RAST does not appear to offer any substantial advantage over skin testing with potent food extracts.

In the provocative-neutralizing method of diagnosis of food allergy, dilutions of food extracts are injected intracutaneously in an attempt to reproduce the patient's symptoms, which are then said to be relieved by successive intracutaneous injections of other dilutions of the same extract. The techniques vary among users of the method. For example, some users both "provoke" and "neutralize" by sublingual administration of the antigen solutions. The validity of all of these methods has not been established, and their use in diagnosis and therapy is unwarranted and experimental at best.

TREATMENT. The treatment of an adverse food reaction is directed at the clinical manifestations, which may be anaphylaxis, urticaria, diarrhea, vomiting, rhinitis, asthma, or atopic dermatitis. Offending foods should be removed from the diet. If elimination diets are prescribed, care must be taken to ensure that they are nutritionally adequate. For reasons that are unclear, some children who are highly reactive to foods become "tolerant" as they grow older; this is especially likely to occur among infants and young children. Foods most likely to become tolerated with the passage of time are cow milk, eggs, and soy. Hypersensitivity to peanuts, nuts, and fish persists for long periods. Cautious periodic attempts to reintroduce offending foods are appropriate. Immunotherapy by injection or sublingual or oral administration of extracts of offending foods is not efficacious.

Atkins FM, Steinberg SS, Metcalfe DD: Evaluation of immediate adverse reactions to foods in adult patients. I: Correlation of demographic, laboratory and prick skin test data with responses to controlled oral food challenge. J Allergy Clin Immunol 75:348, 1985.
Atkins FM, Steinberg SS, Metcalfe DD: Evaluation of immediate adverse reactions to foods in adult patients. II: A detailed analysis of reaction patterns during oral food challenges. J Allergy Clin Immunol 75:356, 1985.
Hill DJ, Ford RPK, Skelton MJ, Hosking CS: A study of 100 infants and young children with cow's milk allergy. Clin Rev Allergy 2:125, 1984.
Sampson HA, Metcalfe DD: Food allergies. JAMA 268:2840, 1992.
Simon RA: Adverse reactions to drug additives. J Allergy Clin Immunol 74:623, 1984.
Weber RW: Food additives and allergy. Ann Allergy 70:183, 1993.

PART XVI

Rheumatic Diseases of Childhood

(Inflammatory Diseases of Connective Tissue, Collagen Vascular Diseases)

Jane Green Schaller

The disorders described in these sections are grouped together because of similarities in symptomatology and pathology; in general, they are associated with inflammatory changes in various connective tissues throughout the body.

The causes of rheumatic diseases of childhood are unknown, and precise diagnostic criteria are often lacking. They usually appear as distinct entities, each presenting characteristic clinical manifestations. For example, rheumatoid arthritis is associated with chronic arthritis, dermatomyositis with inflammation of muscle and skin, and scleroderma with induration of skin. Each of these diseases, however, can affect many organs, and overlapping symptoms and signs may at times make precise diagnosis difficult. ■

CHAPTER 146

Autoimmunity

Marcia J. McDuffie

Although the mammalian immune system can recognize an apparently limitless array of biologic structures, known as antigens, development of an immune response against self-antigens is uncommon. The ability of the immune system to inhibit such reactivity is called self-tolerance, and it is presumed that failure to maintain unresponsiveness to self-antigens results in autoimmunity. Disorders are classified as autoimmune if they lack a direct relationship with infection by a known microbial pathogen and if there is a specific response to self-antigens by B or T lymphocytes. T-lymphocyte infiltration of target tissues is frequently demonstrable histologically, but it is rarely accessible for screening purposes. More frequently, the production of high levels of circulating antibodies against self-antigens is used as a screening and diagnostic tool for organ- or tissue-specific autoimmunity. Despite the importance of antibodies in the diagnosis of autoimmune disease, T lymphocytes appear to control the development of pathologic self-responsiveness as they control the development of normal immune responses.

No syndrome of generalized autoimmunity is recognized clinically, although a model of such a disorder is created through allogeneic bone marrow transplantation when mature T lymphocytes are transferred along with marrow stem cells into immunodeficient or immunosuppressed hosts (see Chapter 132): acute graft-versus-host disease (AGVHD). The target for donor immune activity in this situation appears to be histocompatibility antigens from the major histocompatibility complex (MHC) of the recipient. Because these molecules are expressed on virtually every nucleated mammalian cell, the damaging effects of inappropriate immune system activation in AGVHD are widespread. Unlike AGVHD, naturally occurring autoimmune disease is typically organ or tissue specific, suggesting that it results from an immune response directed against tissue-specific self-antigens.

MECHANISMS OF AUTOIMMUNITY. The development of active autoimmunity appears to require a predisposing genetic background. For example, each well-defined clinical entity studied can be associated with the inheritance of certain haplotypes of the MHC. This large locus has been known for almost 30 yr to contain genes controlling the immune response, and studies of narrowly defined autoimmune disease categories have confirmed that this association can be traced to the structure and expression of the tissue histocompatibility molecules themselves. Using sequence-based typing methods, individual alleles have been shown to determine relative susceptibility to different autoimmune syndromes. However, no published studies of any autoimmune disorder have suggested a simple dominant or recessive mode of inheritance through a single gene. This suggests that multiple genes in addition to MHC genes are involved in determining disease susceptibility, as has been shown for autoimmune or type I diabetes. It also leaves open the possible role of environmental factors, such as diet, infectious agents, and toxins, in regulating or initiating autoimmunity in susceptible individuals.

The mechanisms by which genetic susceptibility is translated into a full-blown immune response against self-antigens are unknown, but disease activity can be modified by interrupting various steps in the immune cascade (Fig. 146–1). An immune response is initiated by antigen uptake by marrow-derived phagocytes. After internalization, the antigen molecules are transported into acidic intracellular vesicles, in which they are enzymatically degraded into small fragments. These fragments associate with MHC molecules during their transport to the cell surface. Cells with a capacity to internalize and re-express antigen fragments bound to MHC molecules are collectively known as antigen-presenting cells (APC). T lymphocytes of the appropriate specificity can form stable attachments to APC through binding of MHC-antigen complexes by clonally unique antigen receptor molecules borne on their surfaces.

When antigen-specific binding occurs before a T lymphocyte has reached complete maturity, the cell is triggered to die or to become nonresponsive. This process eliminates most self-reactive T lymphocytes and results in tolerance to most self-antigens. Failure to develop self-tolerance is postulated to oc-

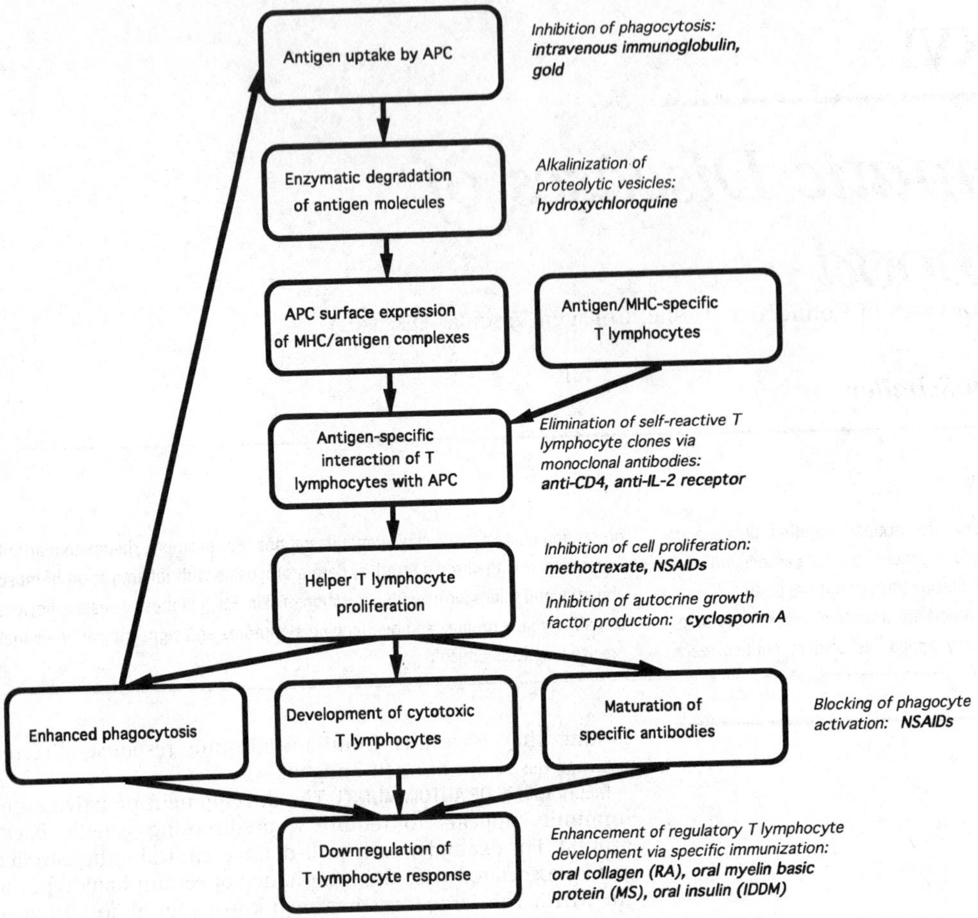

Figure 146–1. Immune response cascade in autoimmunity and therapeutic interventions. APC = antigen-presenting cells; CD4 = cell surface marker for T lymphocytes; IDDM = insulin-dependent diabetes mellitus; IL-2 = interleukin-2; MHC = major histocompatibility complex; MS = multiple sclerosis; NSAIDs = nonsteroidal anti-inflammatory drugs; RA = rheumatoid arthritis.

cur when a self-antigen is delayed in expression or when its structure resembles too closely that of a foreign antigen against which a powerful immune response has been generated. Under these circumstances, self-reactive T lymphocytes proliferate in response to the coordinated secretion of growth factors and expression of growth factor receptors, such as interleukin-2 (IL-2) and its receptor complex. Simultaneously, the responding T cells can activate several mutually exclusive functional programs that direct the progression of the subsequent autoimmune response and the generation of antigen-specific T-lymphocyte subsets with different roles. Among CD4-positive ($CD4^+$) or helper T lymphocytes, one subset interacts specifically with B lymphocytes to promote immunoglobulin class switching and clonal expansion of antigen-specific B cells. A second subset enhances antigen uptake by macrophages and dendritic cells, activates intracellular killing mechanisms, and increases surface expression of antigen-MHC complexes. Activated $CD4^+$ T lymphocytes also trigger the development of a cytotoxic subset among antigen-specific T lymphocytes, primarily those expressing CD8 molecules. Antibody-mediated autoimmune syndromes, such as myasthenia gravis and Graves disease, result from a response that is skewed toward interactions of helper T lymphocytes with antigen-specific B lymphocytes. In T-cell–mediated autoimmunity, typified by autoimmune or type I diabetes, disease appears to result from the predominance of the latter two effector mechanisms. Although active immune responses against foreign pathogens can be terminated by elimination of antigen or by the development of regulatory T lymphocytes with suppressive function, one or both of these mechanisms is deficient in autoimmune disorders, leading to prolonged activation of the responding populations within the immune system.

TREATMENT. Corticosteroids are the most widely used drugs for controlling autoimmune diseases because they inhibit the progression of an immune response at many levels. By enhancing the barrier function of the vascular endothelium, corticosteroids decrease cell migration into sites of active inflammation, preventing continued antigen uptake by APC. They also block the ability of macrophages to interact effectively with T lymphocytes and depress the activation and proliferation of antigen-specific T lymphocytes by inhibiting the expression of growth factors and their receptors.

Other agents are more limited in their effects on the immune response but can be used alone for mild disease or in conjunction with corticosteroids to block disease activity more effectively. As shown in Figure 146–1, colloidal gold and intravenous immunoglobulin preparations decrease phagocytosis, resulting in a nonspecific block to the uptake of antigenic molecules and a decrease in their availability for presentation to T lymphocytes. Further interruption of antigen presentation can be accomplished through alkalinization of proteolytic vesicles in APC with agents such as hydroxychloroquine, which inhibits the enzyme activity required for antigen fragmentation. Agents of this class should be particularly useful in suppressing immune responses against extracellular antigens, such as collagens in rheumatoid arthritis or DNA-histone complexes from necrotic cells in systemic lupus erythematosus.

Proliferation of T lymphocytes can be blocked pharmacologically by drugs such as methotrexate and cyclosporine A. Although use of these drugs is limited by their substantial side effects, they can be employed effectively with agents that block autoimmune reactivity at other points along the pathway. Nonsteroidal anti-inflammatory agents are useful in some autoimmune syndromes involving ongoing recruitment of activated cells because they decrease the level of activation of APC, and they may depress the proliferation of activated T lymphocytes.

Monoclonal antibody therapy directed against lymphocyte surface markers has the theoretical potential for targeting specifically the subpopulation involved in generating a specific immune response. However, this population can only be defined very broadly, because no easily characterized set of antigen-specific T lymphocytes has been identified for any human autoimmune syndrome. The use of CD4 monoclonal antibodies and those targeting only activated T lymphocytes (e.g., antibodies binding the receptor for IL-2) has been proposed as intervention for acute exacerbations of autoimmune disease. Several monoclonal antibody-toxin conjugates that target all T lymphocytes have been selected for therapeutic trials. With the possible exception of CD4 antibodies, these preparations have the undesirable side effect of inducing immune responses against themselves and are therefore useful only for short-term therapy. Modifications of monoclonal antibody molecules that reduce their immunogenicity may increase their utility as therapeutic agents.

Despite the relative efficacy of nonspecific means for controlling pathologic self-reactivity, the therapeutic goal of specific inhibition of autoimmunity without global immunosuppression is not yet possible. As a step in this direction, ongoing clinical trials are attempting to induce specific tolerance to self-antigens by oral or parenteral administration of purified protein targets of autoimmune lymphocyte activation. In preliminary studies, antigen administration has controlled destructive immune activation in animal models of rheumatoid arthritis, multiple sclerosis, and type I diabetes mellitus, suggesting that safe and disease-specific therapy for autoimmune disorders may be available in the future.

Holmdahl R, Malmstrom V, Vuorio E: Autoimmune recognition of cartilage collagens. Ann Med 25:251, 1993.
Nepom GT, Erlich H: MHC class-II molecules and autoimmunity. Annu Rev Immunol 9:493, 1991.
Rashba EJ, Reich EP, Janeway CA, et al: Type I diabetes mellitus: An imbalance between effector and regulatory T cells? Acta Diabetol 30:61, 1993.
Tisch R, McDevitt HD: Antigen-specific immunotherapy: Is it a real possibility to combat T-cell–mediated autoimmunity? Proc Natl Acad Sci USA 91:437, 1994.
Todd JA: Genetic analysis of susceptibility to type I diabetes. Springer Semin Immunopathol 14:33, 1992.
Zinkernagel RM, Pircher H, Ohashi PS, et al: T cells causing autoimmune disease. Springer Semin Immunopathol 14:105, 1992.

CHAPTER 147

Laboratory Evaluation (Table 147–1)

Jane Green Schaller

Although laboratory studies are often helpful, few are diagnostic or specific for rheumatic diseases. These studies include tests for acute-phase phenomena, rheumatoid factors, antinuclear and other autoantibodies, total serum complement and individual complement components, immune complexes, serum proteins and immunoglobulins, and histocompatibility antigens. Other useful tests include blood counts, urinalyses, joint fluid analyses, studies of renal and liver function, and various imaging techniques. Biopsies (skin, kidney) are frequently performed in patients with rheumatic diseases; although tissue histology may provide confirmatory evidence of tissue involvement or aid in classification of disease, it is rarely diagnostic of any specific disease.

TABLE 147–1 Laboratory Tests in the Rheumatic Diseases

- Rheumatoid factors:
  - Classification of JRA
- Antinuclear antibodies:
  - Diagnosis of SLE (DNA, Sm antigen)
  - Diagnosis of MCTD (RNP)
  - Diagnosis of neonatal lupus syndrome (Ro or La antibodies to antigens)
  - Course of SLE (DNA)
  - Classification of JRA
- HLA typing:
  - Chiefly for research interest
  - B27: spondyloarthropathies
- Complement studies:
  - Course of SLE
  - Evidence of immune complex disease
- Acute-phase reactants, serum proteins:
  - Minor role in following disease activity
- Blood counts, bone marrow:
  - Suspicion of malignancy
  - Anemia of chronic disease
  - Autoimmune anemia, thrombocytopenia
- Cultures and serologic studies:
  - Detection of infectious disease
- Radiographs, bone scans, other imaging studies:
  - Detection of underlying bony abnormalities (infection, trauma, malignancy, congenital, or genetic conditions), other anatomic abnormalities, or joint destruction of JRA
- Biopsies:
  - Confirmation of tissue involvement and classification
  - Diagnosis of malignancy or infectious disease
- Organ-specific studies:
  - Detection of specific organ involvement in multisystem disease:
    - Neurologic (spinal fluid, EEG, imaging, angiography)
    - Cardiac (ECG, echo/Doppler)
    - Pulmonary (radiograph, pulmonary function)
    - Hepatic (liver function tests, imaging)
    - Gastrointestinal (barium studies, endoscopy)
    - Renal (urinalysis, renal function)

DNA = deoxyribonucleic acid; ECG = electrocardiogram; Echo = echocardiogram; EEG = electroencephalogram; JRA = juvenile rheumatoid arthritis; MCTD = mixed connective tissue disease; RNP = ribonucleoprotein; SLE = systemic lupus erythematosus.

ACUTE-PHASE REACTANTS. These are plasma constituents that appear or increase during the inflammatory state. They include the erythrocyte sedimentation rate (ESR), C-reactive protein (CRP), serum mucoproteins, various α-globulins, gamma globulins, some complement components, and certain proteins such as transferrin. Because patients with rheumatic diseases have an active inflammatory process, acute-phase phenomena or reactants are usually present during periods of active disease. Such tests are not invariably positive during inflammation, however, and their absence does not exclude the possibility of an active disease process. These tests are of little diagnostic usefulness because they may be positive in a wide variety of conditions associated with inflammation (e.g., malignancy, infection, tissue trauma, tissue necrosis). Acute-phase phenomena are sometimes helpful in following the course of disease in individual patients. The ESR is the most readily available test.

RHEUMATOID FACTORS. These are a group of antibodies that react with the Fc portion of immunoglobulin G (IgG). These antibodies are not specific for host immunoglobulins but may react with immunoglobulin from other individuals or from other species. Rheumatoid factors detected by standard agglutination techniques such as the latex agglutination test or the sheep cell agglutination test are IgM; anti-immunoglobulin antibodies of the IgG, IgA, and IgE classes can also be identified by methods other than agglutination tests. The occurrence of rheumatoid factors in disease states such as chronic infections (e.g., *Toxocara canis*, congenital infections, bacterial endocarditis) or in experimental situations such as hyperimmunization of animals suggests that protracted immune stimulation, chronic infection, or inflammation may underlie their production.

Rheumatoid factors, particularly IgM detected by classic agglutination techniques, are strongly associated with classic adult rheumatoid arthritis; in such patients, rheumatoid factors are present in high titer and on serial tests throughout the course of disease. A small subgroup of patients with juvenile rheumatoid arthritis resembling classic adult rheumatoid arthritis also have rheumatoid factors. However, rheumatoid factors are neither specific for nor diagnostic of rheumatoid arthritis. They also occur in other rheumatic diseases (e.g., lupus erythematosus, scleroderma), chronic active hepatitis, chronic infections, leukemia and lymphoid malignancies, and certain viral infections; in addition, they can be found in patients following immunizations, open heart surgery, or organ transplantation, and in normal aging human beings. Many children with transiently positive low titers on rheumatoid factor tests have probably had antecedent viral illnesses. Rheumatoid factors do not in themselves cause disease nor are they necessary for the occurrence of chronic synovitis; they may play a role in perpetuation of synovial inflammation in people with rheumatoid arthritis by forming immune complexes with immunoglobulins.

ANTINUCLEAR ANTIBODIES. The antinuclear antibodies (ANA) are a group of antibodies that react with various nuclear constituents, including deoxyribonucleoprotein (DNP), DNA, ribonucleoprotein (RNP), ribonucleic acid (RNA), Sm antigen (a soluble nuclear protein antigen), and many others. Stimuli for production of these antibodies remain unknown. ANA are not specific for organs, individuals, or species of cell origin. They usually are detected in the serum of patients by immunofluorescent staining techniques using standard in vitro frozen animal tissue sections or cell culture preparations.

ANA are neither entirely diagnostic of nor specific for any disease. They are found in almost all patients with systemic lupus erythematosus (SLE) but are also found in patients with a number of conditions, including juvenile rheumatoid arthritis (JRA), chronic active hepatitis, and scleroderma. The syndrome called *mixed connective tissue disease* is defined by the presence of antibody to RNP. Nonrheumatic conditions associated with ANA include ingestion of a wide variety of drugs (including anticonvulsants, procainamide, birth control pills); certain infections, notably Epstein-Barr infection; certain malignancies, and the normal aging process. High titers of ANA are most common in SLE and mixed connective tissue disease. Several ANA patterns may be detected on immunofluorescent preparations, including speckled, homogeneous, peripheral, and nucleolar; these distinctions are of limited clinical usefulness. Antibodies to antigens such as DNA, RNP, Sm, Ro, and La are detected by individual tests utilizing specific antigens or substrates. Antibodies reactive with double-stranded DNA are reasonably specific for SLE and are indicative of active disease. Antibodies to antigens called Ro(SSA) and La(SSB) are associated with the neonatal lupus syndrome.

The lupus erythematosus (LE) cell is the result of an ANA that is reactive with DNP. When serum containing this antibody is mixed in vitro with peripheral white blood cells, their nuclei are rendered susceptible to phagocytosis; the LE cell is a granulocyte that has ingested such a nucleus. This test has been largely superseded by the more sensitive tests for ANA.

ANTINEUTROPHIL CYTOPLASMIC ANTIBODIES. Antibodies that react with the granules of neutrophils are called antineutrophil cytoplasmic antibodies (ANCA). They were first found in the serum of patients with Wegener granulomatosis and are detected by immunofluorescence. Two patterns of staining are recognized. One demonstrates diffuse activity of granules (c-ANCA), and the other reveals a perinuclear pattern (p-ANCA). The c-ANCA pattern is associated with Wegener granulomatosis but can also be seen in other forms of vasculitis, including Kawasaki disease. The p-ANCA is less specific and has been found in a number of conditions, including necrotizing or crescentic glomerulonephritis, ulcerative colitis, cholangitis, chronic active hepatitis, and Henoch-Schönlein vasculitis. Both types of ANCA have been noted in patients with HIV infection.

ANTIPHOSPHOLIPID ANTIBODIES. The antiphospholipid antibodies constitute a class of autoantibodies that react with several phospholipid antigens. They include so-called lupus anticoagulants, anticardiolipin antibodies, and antibodies that react with the substrate for the VDRL test for syphilis. Although these antibodies are associated in vitro with prolongation of coagulation, they are associated with thrombosis, not anticoagulation, in vivo. The terminology of lupus anticoagulant is confusing. Several laboratory tests can detect antiphospholipid antibodies, including the partial prothrombin time, the lupus anticoagulant test, the Russell viper venom time, and enzyme-linked immunosorbent assays specific for phospholipid binding. Patients with these antibodies may have false-positive VDRL tests. Laboratory detection remains confusing, awaiting a better understanding of these phenomena.

Antiphospholipid antibodies can be detected in 30–40% of patients with lupus, and, when present, they suggest an increased risk of thrombosis, thrombocytopenia, hemolytic anemia, stroke, chorea, transverse myelitis, and valvular heart disease. Such antibodies also may be found in patients with infections or malignancies. Antiphospholipid antibodies also occur in individuals without apparent underlying disease, a condition called the primary antiphospholipid syndrome. Patients with this syndrome are subject to thrombotic events, thrombocytopenia, recurrent spontaneous abortion, and any of the manifestations cited for SLE. Strokes and thrombotic events have been recognized in children with the primary antiphospholipid syndrome; the antibodies should always be sought in such situations (see Chapter 440). The long-term prognosis for this condition is unknown, and agreement about prophylactic treatment with antiplatelet agents or anticoagulation is lacking.

COMPLEMENT. Complement consists of a group of serum proteins that mediate certain aspects of inflammation and cell injury (see Chapter 120). Serum complement levels can be useful in indicating the activity of SLE and other diseases with an immune complex mechanism; low serum complement levels reflect complement consumption by immune complexes and thus indicate active disease. Measurement of total serum hemolytic complement activity is the most useful test. Measurement of individual complement component C3 or C4 determines only the amount of protein without regard to its biologic activity. Complement studies are not diagnostic of any disease except the rare hereditary deficiencies of complement components.

IMMUNE COMPLEX DETERMINATIONS. Immune complexes of antigen and antibody are responsible for tissue damage in some rheumatic diseases (notably SLE) and in a wide variety of other conditions, including certain infectious diseases. Several assays can measure immune complexes in serum and other fluids; however, these tests are of uncertain clinical value.

SERUM PROTEINS AND IMMUNOGLOBULINS. Increased levels of gamma globulins and α_2-globulins are frequently found in patients with active inflammation; these tests are not specific. Elevated levels of one or more specific immunoglobulins may be found in a number of rheumatic diseases, notably SLE; however, there are no diagnostic patterns. Serum albumin levels may be low in patients with chronic inflammation of various causes. Rarely, patients with immunodeficiency states such as IgA deficiency, hypogammaglobulinemia, or various T-cell or combined immunodeficiency syndromes manifest rheumatic complaints.

HISTOCOMPATIBILITY SYSTEM. Associations of histocompatibility antigens (HLA antigens) with certain diseases provide valuable insights into genetically determined susceptibility to disease and into the immunologic basis of disease. The clinician must remember, however, that HLA typing is not diagnostic of any disease. For example, the finding of HLA-B27 marker in a child with arthritis may suggest, but does not ensure, that the child has spondyloarthropathy. HLA studies are helpful in matching tissue donors to recipients, and they have a limited use in prenatal diagnosis for seeking diseases such as complement component deficiencies. Histocompatibility studies remain of great academic interest in classifying disease, in seeking to identify host factors that predispose to disease, and in unraveling immunologic mechanisms important to the causation of human disease.

HLA antigens are located on the surfaces of most human cells. Loci determining HLA antigens are located on the sixth chromosome. This is a complex system with many loci recognized, including A, B, C, D, DR, DP, and DQ, and with each locus having multiple alleles. The prevalences of various HLA alleles vary in and among different racial groups.

The biologic roles of HLA antigens, other than those determining tissue compatibility, are not fully known. The HLA system is in proximity to genes known to be important to immune reactivity, including loci determining the synthesis of various components of the complement system.

Because the HLA antigens are genetically determined traits that can be accurately identified, they can provide information about disease associations (i.e., occurrence of particular diseases in association with particular HLA antigens) and disease linkages (i.e., passage of a trait along with HLA antigens from generation to generation within the same family, implying that the genes responsible for the trait are close to those of the HLA system on the 6th chromosome).

Other rheumatic diseases with HLA associations include SLE (HLA B8, DR2, DR3) and childhood dermatomyositis (HLA B8, DR3). A group of autoimmune diseases, including insulin-dependent diabetes mellitus, chronic active hepatitis, celiac sprue, thyroiditis, Graves disease, and Addison disease, are associated with the haplotype B8/DR3. Insulin-dependent diabetes mellitus also is associated with DR4. Several human conditions have been linked to the HLA system (transmitted along with HLA antigens from generation to generation); these include deficiencies of the second and fourth components of the complement system and congenital adrenal hyperplasia.

The strongest association of human disease with the HLA system is that of HLA-B27 with ankylosing spondylitis; 95% of patients with ankylosing spondylitis have HLA-B27, compared with only 6% of the unaffected white North American population. An individual carrying HLA-B27 has a 90 times greater relative risk of developing ankylosing spondylitis than one without B27. Only an estimated 8–20% of individuals with HLA-B27 ever actually develop ankylosing spondylitis or a related disease. Reiter syndrome, the spondylitis of inflammatory bowel disease and psoriasis, acute iridocyclitis, pauciarticular arthritis of older children and adult patients, and the "reactive" arthritis following infections with *Salmonella, Shigella, Yersinia enterocolitica,* or *Campylobacter* are also associated with HLA-B27. The mechanism underlying the association between HLA-B27 and susceptibility to these diseases remains unknown. The association of these spondyloarthropathies with HLA-B27 is seen in various racial populations. No corresponding HLA-D or -DR associations have been made.

Three JRA subgroups have distinct HLA associations, suggesting that there are genetic or immunologic factors that influence the occurrence of particular types of disease. Pauciarthritis with onset in older children (pauciarticular JRA type II) is strongly associated with HLA-B27, providing laboratory evidence consistent with clinical observations that many of these children have early spondyloarthropathies. Pauciarthritis of early childhood associated with ANA and chronic iridocyclitis (pauciarticular JRA type I) has an interesting and still incompletely understood set of associations with alleles of HLA-DR8, -DR6, -DR5, DPw2, and DQ. Rheumatoid factor-positive polyarticular disease has a striking association with HLA-DR4, consistent with its clinical resemblance to classic adult-onset rheumatoid arthritis, which is also associated with HLA-DR4. Closer study of DR4-positive children with seropositive arthritis reveals even stronger associations with certain HLA alleles that are detected by the broad test for DR4.

Ansell BM, Rudge S, Schaller JG: A Colour Atlas of Paediatric Rheumatology. London, Wolfe Publishing, 1991.
DeNardo BA, Tucker LB, Miller LC, et al: Demography of a regional pediatric rheumatology patient population. J Rheumatol 21:1553, 1994.
Jacobs JC: Pediatric Rheumatology for the Practitioner, 2nd ed. New York, Springer-Verlag, 1993.
Kelley WN, Harris ED, Ruddy S, Sledge CB (eds): Textbook of Rheumatology, 4th ed. Philadelphia, WB Saunders, 1993.
Schaller JG: Aggressive treatment in childhood rheumatic diseases. Clin Exp Rheumatol 12(Suppl 10):S97, 1994.
Schaller JG: Pediatric and heritable disorders. Curr Opin Rheumatol 6:509, 1994.
Schumacher HR Jr, Klippel JH, Koopman WJ (eds): Primer on the Rheumatic Diseases, 10th ed. Atlanta, Arthritis Foundation, 1993.
Stiehm ER: Immunologic Disorders in Infants and Children. Philadelphia, WB Saunders, 1995.

CHAPTER 148
Juvenile Rheumatoid Arthritis

Jane Green Schaller

Juvenile rheumatoid arthritis (JRA) is a disease or group of diseases characterized by chronic synovitis and associated with a number of extra-articular manifestations. A confusing number of names have been applied, including juvenile arthritis, Still disease, juvenile chronic polyarthritis, and chronic childhood arthritis. JRA encompasses several broad clinical subgroups (Table 148–1). Rheumatoid factor–positive polyarticular disease most closely resembles adult-onset rheumatoid arthritis; rheumatoid factor—negative polyarthritis also occurs in adults. Pauciarticular disease type II is related to the diseases described in adults as "spondyloarthropathies." Systemic-onset disease occurs occasionally in adults. Pauciarticular disease type I with chronic iridocyclitis has not been described in adults. Recognition of these subgroups is useful in the diagnosis, follow-up, and appropriate care of children with chronic arthritis.

ETIOLOGY AND EPIDEMIOLOGY. The cause of rheumatoid arthritis and the mechanisms for perpetuation of chronic synovial inflammation are unknown. Two hypotheses are that the disease results from infection with an unidentified microorganism or that it represents hypersensitivity or an "autoimmune" reaction to unknown stimuli. Attempts to link infectious agents such as rubella virus to JRA remain inconclusive. Infection with *Borrelia burgdorferi,* the spirochete of Lyme disease (see Chapter 198), causes recurrent or chronic pauciarthritis in some children but is not the etiologic agent for pauciarticular JRA. Parvovirus B19 and mycoplasmas have also been associated with arthritis, usually transient, in children. The association of rheumatoid factors (antibodies reactive with IgG) with adult-onset rheumatoid arthritis suggests an immune mechanism. However, these antibodies clearly do not cause the disease, although immune complexes of rheumatoid factor and immunoglobulin may perpetuate synovial inflammation and are responsible for the rheumatoid vasculitis seen in patients with seropositive rheumatoid arthritis. The low levels of complement found in the synovial fluid of some rheumatoid pa-

■ **TABLE 148–1 Subgroups of Juvenile Rheumatoid Arthritis**

Characteristic	Polyarticular Rheumatoid Factor–Negative	Polyarticular Rheumatoid Factor–Positive	Pauciarticular Type I	Pauciarticular Type II	Systemic-Onset
Percentage of JRA patients	20–30	5–10	30–40	10–15	10–20
Sex	90% girls	80% girls	80% girls	90% boys	60% boys
Age at onset	Any	Late childhood	Early childhood	Late childhood	Any
Joints	Any, multiple	Any, multiple	Few large joints: knee, ankle, elbow	Few large joints: hip girdle	Any, multiple
Sacroiliitis	No	Rare	No	Common	No
Iridocyclitis	Rare	No	30% chronic iridocyclitis	10–20% acute iridocyclitis	No
Rheumatoid factor	Negative	100%	Negative	Negative	Negative
Antinuclear antibodies	25%	75%	90%	Negative	Negative
HLA studies	?	HLA DR4	HLA-DR5, -DR6, and -DR8	HLA-B27	?
Ultimate morbidity	Severe arthritis, 10–15%	Severe arthritis, >50%	Ocular damage, 10% Polyarthritis, 20%	Subsequent spondyloarthropathy, ?%	Severe arthritis, 25%

tients and the low serum complement levels observed in patients with rheumatoid vasculitis are consistent with an immune complex mechanism. This mechanism fails, however, to explain most instances of arthritis in children, because most children do not have classic rheumatoid factors. Attempts to link "hidden rheumatoid factors" (antibodies reactive with gamma globulin detected by different methods) to the pathogenesis of JRA have been inconclusive. The occurrence of chronic arthritis in patients with IgA deficiency and hypogammaglobulinemia suggests that immunodeficiency may somehow predispose to chronic arthritis; however, no identifiable immunodeficiency has been detected in children with JRA. The clinical onset of JRA may follow an acute systemic infection or physical trauma to a joint, but no direct relation to such events has been shown. Exacerbations may follow intercurrent illness or psychic stress.

Pauciarticular disease type II is frequently associated with a positive family history for ankylosing spondylitis, Reiter syndrome, acute iridocyclitis, or pauciarticular arthritis. Both pauciarticular JRA type I and rheumatoid factor–positive polyarthritis occasionally occur in one or more 1st-degree relatives of affected children. Each of these subgroups has distinct HLA associations, indicating some genetic predisposition to disease: pauciarticular disease type II with HLA-B27, pauciarticular disease type I with HLA-DR8, -DR5, and -DR6, and rheumatoid factor–positive disease with HLA-DR4. Neither systemic-onset disease nor seronegative polyarthritis has known HLA associations or familial occurrence.

JRA is not rare; there are about a quarter million affected children in the United States. About 5% of all cases of rheumatoid arthritis begin in childhood.

PATHOLOGY. Rheumatoid arthritis is characterized by chronic nonsuppurative inflammation of synovium. Affected synovial tissues are edematous, hyperemic, and infiltrated with lymphocytes and plasma cells. Secretion of increased amounts of joint fluid results in effusions. Projections of thickened synovial membrane form villi that protrude into joint spaces; hyperplastic rheumatoid synovia may spread over and become adherent to articular cartilage (pannus formation). With continuing chronic synovitis and synovial proliferation, articular cartilage and other joint structures may become eroded and progressively destroyed. The duration of synovitis before joint damage becomes permanent varies; in general, lasting articular cartilage damage occurs later in the course of JRA than in adult-onset disease, and many children with JRA never incur permanent joint damage despite prolonged synovitis. Joint destruction occurs more often in children with rheumatoid factor–positive disease or systemic-onset disease. Once joint destruction has commenced, erosions of subchondral bone, narrowing of the "joint space" (loss of articular cartilage), destruction or fusion of bones, and deformity, subluxation, or ankylosis of the joints may result. Tenosynovitis and myositis may be present. Osteoporosis, periostitis, accelerated epiphyseal growth, and premature epiphyseal closure can occur adjacent to affected joints.

Rheumatoid nodules occur less frequently in children than in adults, primarily in rheumatoid factor–positive children, and show fibrinoid material surrounded by chronic inflammatory cells. Pleura, pericardium, and peritoneum may show nonspecific fibrinous serositis; chronic constrictive pericarditis occurs rarely, if ever. The rheumatoid rash appears histologically as a mild vasculitis, with a few inflammatory cells surrounding small vessels in subepithelial tissues.

CLINICAL MANIFESTATIONS. Polyarticular-Onset Disease. Polyarticular disease is characterized by involvement of multiple joints typically including the small joints of the hands (Figs. 148–1 and 148–2) and occurs in 35% of children with JRA. Two subgroups are included: *rheumatoid factor–negative polyarthritis* (20–30% of all patients with JRA) and *rheumatoid factor–positive polyarthritis* (5–10% of all patients with JRA). Rheumatoid factor–positive disease is characterized by onset in late childhood, more severe arthritis, frequent appearance of rheumatoid nodules, and occasional rheumatoid vasculitis. Rheumatoid factor–negative disease may begin at any time during childhood, is frequently mild, and is rarely associated with

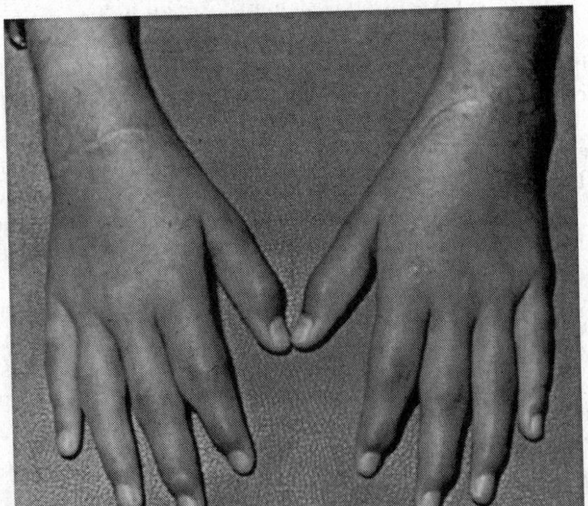

Figure 148–1. Hands and wrists of a girl with rheumatoid factor–negative polyarticular juvenile rheumatoid arthritis. Notice the symmetric involvement of the metacarpophalangeal joints, proximal interphalangeal joints, and distal interphalangeal joints. Both wrists are affected.

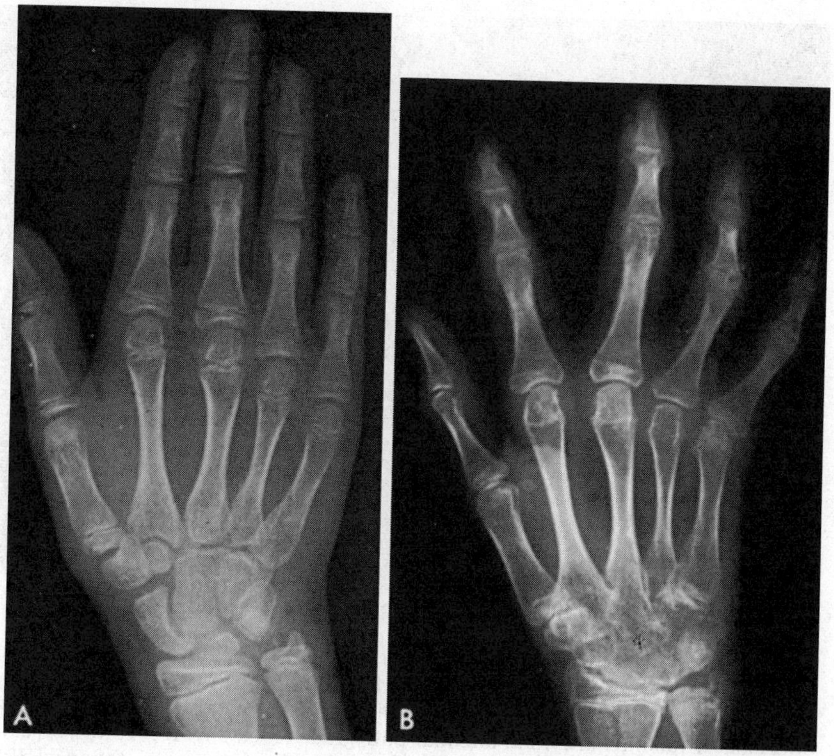

Figure 148–2. Progression of joint destruction in a girl with rheumatoid factor–positive juvenile rheumatoid arthritis despite doses of corticosteroids sufficient to suppress symptoms in the interval between *A* and *B*. *A*, Roentgenogram of the hand at onset. *B*, Roentgenogram 4 yr later, showing a loss of articular cartilage and destructive changes in the distal and proximal interphalangeal and metacarpophalangeal joints and destruction and fusion of wrist bones.

rheumatoid nodules. More girls than boys are affected in both types of disease. Both the polyarticular pattern and the nature of the rheumatoid factor tests are established within the first 6 mo of disease.

Onset of arthritis may be insidious, with gradual development of joint stiffness, swelling, and loss of motion, or fulminant, with sudden appearance of symptomatic arthritis. Affected joints are swollen and warm but rarely red. Swelling results from periarticular edema, joint effusion, and synovial thickening. Some children have "painless" joint stiffness and discomfort before objective changes appear. Affected joints may be tender to touch and painful on motion; however, severe tenderness and pain are unusual, and many children do not complain of pain in obviously inflamed joints. Limited joint motion is related early to muscle spasm, joint effusion, and synovial proliferation and later to joint destruction or soft tissue contracture. Pronounced synovial proliferation may produce cystic swellings about the affected joints; occasionally herniations of synovium and extravasation of synovial fluid affect the neighboring structures, particularly in the popliteal area (popliteal cyst). Morning stiffness and "gelling" following inactivity are characteristic of rheumatoid arthritis in children as in adults. Young children, particularly those with polyarthritis, are often irritable and assume a typical posture of anxious guarding of their joints against movement (Fig. 148–3).

Arthritis, which may affect any synovial joint, often begins in the large joints such as the knees, ankles, wrists, and elbows; initial involvement is often symmetric. Inflammation of proximal interphalangeal joints produces spindling or fusiform changes of the fingers; metacarpophalangeal joint involvement is equally common, and distal interphalangeal joints may also be affected (see Figs. 148–1 and 148–2). Arthritis of the cervical spine, characterized by neck stiffness and pain, occurs in about half of patients. Temporomandibular involvement with limited ability to open the mouth is common; the pain may be referred to as earache. Hip involvement occurs in at least half the children with polyarthritis, usually beginning later in the disease process. Destruction of the femoral heads may ensue; severe hip disease is a major cause of disability in late JRA (Fig. 148–4). Roentgenographic narrowing of the sacroiliac joints occurs in some patients, usually in association with hip disease. Rarely, cricoarytenoid arthritis causes hoarseness and laryngeal stridor. Involvement of the sternoclavicular joints and costochondral junctions may cause chest pain.

Growth disturbances adjacent to the inflamed joints may result in overgrowth or undergrowth of the affected part. Increased leg length may follow chronic arthritis of the knee, and micrognathia after temporomandibular arthritis may be a late hallmark of JRA. Small, deformed feet may result from foot involvement in early childhood and shortened fingers from early hand involvement.

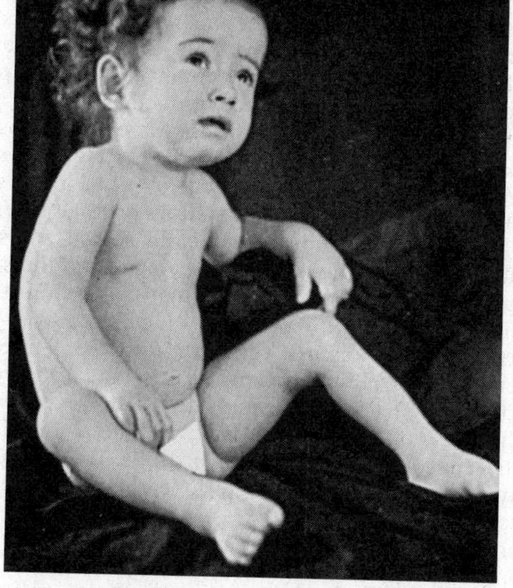

Figure 148–3. Characteristic posture of a child with juvenile rheumatoid arthritis, showing the anxious appearance and guarding of joints.

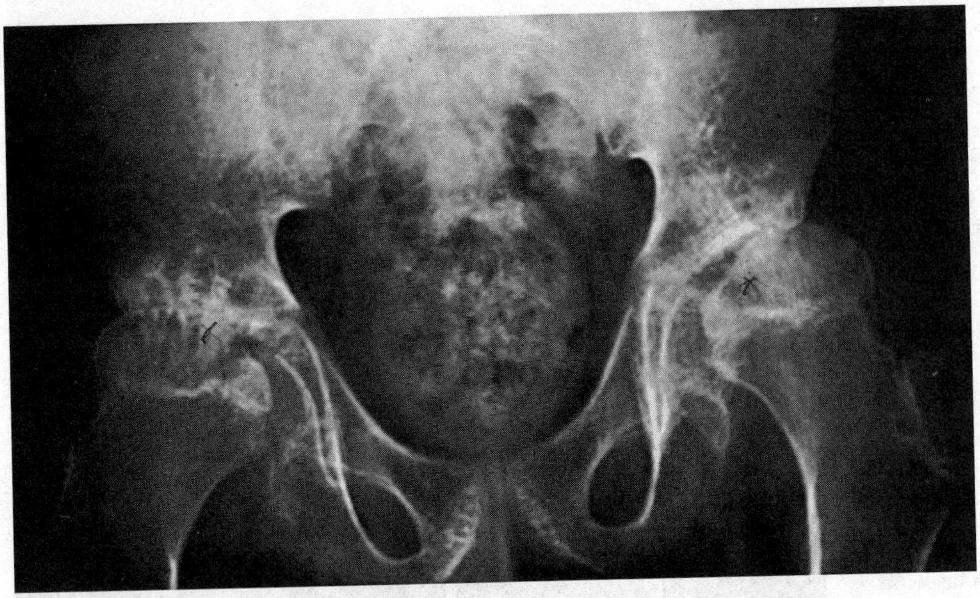

Figure 148–4. Severe hip disease in a 13-yr-old boy with long-active, systemic-onset juvenile rheumatoid arthritis, showing destruction of the femoral heads and acetabula, joint space narrowing, and subluxation of the left hip. The patient had received corticosteroids systemically for 9 yr.

Extra-articular manifestations of polyarticular JRA are not as dramatic as those seen in systemic rheumatoid arthritis. Most patients with active polyarticular disease have malaise, anorexia, irritability, and mild anemia. Low-grade fever, slight hepatosplenomegaly, and lymphadenopathy may be present. Pericarditis is infrequent and iridocyclitis rare. Rheumatoid nodules may occur over pressure points, usually in patients with positive agglutination test results for rheumatoid factor. Rheumatoid vasculitis occurs at times in rheumatoid factor–positive patients, as does Sjögren syndrome. Growth may be retarded during periods of active disease; growth spurts often occur with remission.

Pauciarticular-Onset Disease. This is characterized by arthritis that remains limited to four or fewer joints for the first 6 mo after disease onset. Large joints are primarily affected, and the distribution of arthritis is often asymmetric. There are two distinct subgroups. Type I includes primarily girls who are young at onset and are at risk for chronic iridocyclitis; type II includes primarily boys who are older at onset and who are at risk for subsequent spondyloarthropathy. A few children with pauciarthritis do not fit easily into either type I or type II and remain unclassified.

Pauciarticular disease type I is the most common form of JRA, accounting for 30–40% of all patients. The disease generally begins before the 4th birthday. As many as 90% of patients have positive tests for antinuclear antibodies (ANA). Neither rheumatoid factor nor HLA-B27 is associated. The most commonly affected joints are the knees, ankles, and elbows; occasionally, there is isolated involvement of other joints such as the temporomandibular joints, single toes or fingers, wrists, or neck. The hips and hip girdle are generally spared, and sacroiliitis is not associated. The clinical appearance and the synovial histology of affected joints are indistinguishable from those of polyarticular JRA. Eighty per cent of children with type I pauciarticular-onset disease continue to have limited joint involvement; and although the arthritis may be chronic or recurrent, serious disability or joint destruction is uncommon. The other 20% of children have later additional joint involvement that may result in severe polyarthritis. There is currently no way of identifying either group early in the course of the disease.

Patients with pauciarticular disease type I are at high risk for eye complications; chronic iridocyclitis occurs in 15–30% at some time during the first 10 yr of the disease. *Chronic iridocyclitis* of JRA is characteristically unassociated with early symptoms or signs, activity of arthritis, or elevated ESR. Occasionally, children note early redness, pain, photophobia, or decreased visual acuity. One or both eyes may be affected; if initial involvement is unilateral, the other eye usually remains uninvolved. Iridocyclitis is sometimes the presenting manifestation of JRA, but generally it follows the onset of joint complaints by months to years. Patients with iridocyclitis frequently have positive tests for ANA. The earliest signs of inflammation of the iris and ciliary body are increased numbers of cells and amounts of protein in the anterior chamber of the eye, changes detectable only by slit-lamp examination. The ocular inflammation often remains active for years. Sequelae (Fig. 148–5) include posterior synechiae, complicated cataracts, secondary glaucoma, and phthisis bulbi (degeneration of the globe). Loss of vision may result; in severe cases, permanent blindness occurs. Early detection and therapy before scarring occurs are important for preservation of vision. For this reason all children with pauciarticular disease should have slit-lamp examinations three to four times yearly for at least the first 5 yr of disease regardless of the activity of the joint disease.

Other extra-articular manifestations are usually mild in pauciarticular JRA; low-grade fever, malaise, modest hepatosplenomegaly and lymphadenopathy, and mild anemia may be associated with active joint disease.

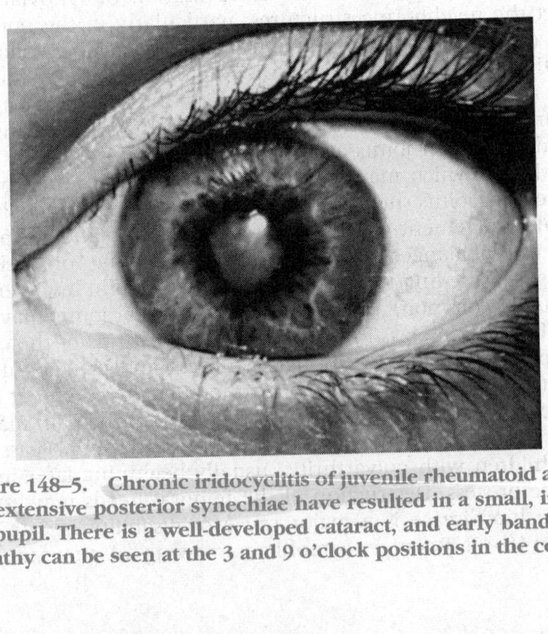

Figure 148–5. Chronic iridocyclitis of juvenile rheumatoid arthritis; extensive posterior synechiae have resulted in a small, irregular pupil. There is a well-developed cataract, and early band keratopathy can be seen at the 3 and 9 o'clock positions in the cornea.

Pauciarticular disease type II affects 10–15% of patients with JRA, predominantly boys older than 8 yr. Family histories often reveal relatives with pauciarticular arthritis, ankylosing spondylitis, Reiter disease, or acute iridocyclitis. Tests for rheumatoid factors and ANA are negative; 75% of patients have HLA-B27. Large joints are affected, particularly those of the lower extremities. Toe joints, temporomandibular joints, and upper extremity joints are involved at times. Heel pain, plantar fasciitis, or Achilles tendinitis is common, and there may be inflammation at the sites of tendon insertion into bone *(enthesopathy)*. Hip girdle involvement is common early in the disease course, and sacroiliitis can often be demonstrated by roentgenography. The peripheral arthritis is generally benign and often transient. Hip and foot pain may be incapacitating at times, although such changes are often reversible with therapy.

With time, some patients with pauciarticular disease type II develop typical ankylosing spondylitis with involvement of the lumbodorsal spine, manifestations of Reiter syndrome (hematuria or pyuria, urethritis, acute iridocyclitis, or mucocutaneous manifestations), or signs of inflammatory bowel disease. The ultimate morbidity for these children lies in the possible occurrence of any of these chronic spondyloarthropathies; the risks for such occurrences are unknown. Physical examination during the follow-up of children with pauciarticular disease type II should include measurements of back flexion and chest expansion. Ten to twenty per cent have self-limited attacks of acute iridocyclitis, which is associated with prominent early symptoms and signs of eye inflammation but few scarring residua.

Systemic-Onset JRA. Systemic-onset disease is characterized by prominent extra-articular manifestations (Table 148–2), particularly high fevers, and rheumatoid rash. This subgroup includes 10 to 20% of patients with JRA. Approximately as many boys as girls are affected.

The disease generally begins with systemic symptoms. Fever is high and intermittent, with daily or twice-daily elevations to 102° F (39° C) or higher and rapid return to normal or subnormal levels (Fig. 148–6). Temperature elevations usually occur in the evening and sometimes in the morning as well. Shaking chills are frequently associated. Patients may seem alarmingly ill during the period of fever and surprisingly well during its remission. Rheumatoid rash (Figs. 148–7 and 148–8) is characterized by its appearance and by its evanescent, recurrent nature. Individual lesions consist of small (several millimeters), pale, red-pink macules, often with central pallor; extensive lesions may coalesce. The rash is most frequently found on the trunk and proximal extremities but may occur anywhere on the body, including the palms and soles. It usually appears during febrile periods but may also be induced by skin trauma (isomorphic response), heat, and embarrassment.

■ TABLE 148–2 Manifestations of Systemic Juvenile Rheumatoid Arthritis

Manifestations	Percentage
High intermittent fever	100
Rheumatoid rash	95
Hepatosplenomegaly or lymphadenopathy	85
Pleuritis or pericarditis	60
Abdominal pain	20
Marked leukocytosis	85
Severe anemia	40
Rheumatoid factors	0
Antinuclear antibodies	0
Arthritis, arthralgia, or myalgia during febrile periods	100
Persistent and chronic*	100
Iridocyclitis	0

**Persistent arthritis (>6 consecutive wk) is necessary for the diagnosis of juvenile rheumatoid arthritis (JRA). Children with only systemic complaints are appropriately considered to have possible systemic JRA.*

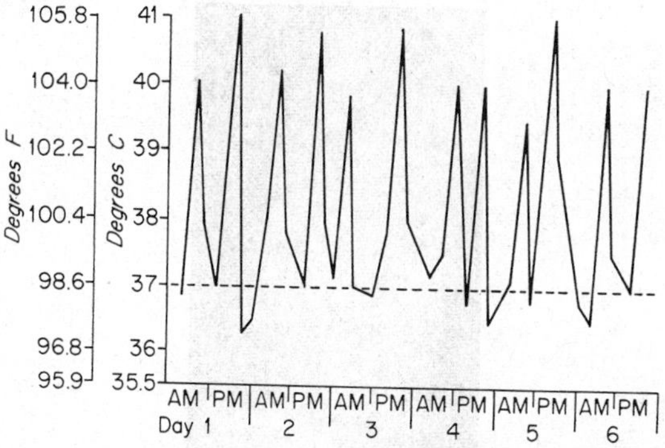

Figure 148–6. Characteristic fever of systemic juvenile rheumatoid arthritis. There are one or two daily temperature elevations to 39° C or greater, with a rapid return of the temperature to normal or subnormal levels.

Hepatosplenomegaly and generalized lymphadenopathy occur in most children with active systemic disease. The degree of organomegaly may be marked. Mild hepatic dysfunction may be present, and lymph node histology may simulate lymphoma. About one third of affected children have pleuritis or pericarditis, often subclinical. Chest roentgenograms may show pleural thickening or small pleural effusions; pericardial effusion may be large and there may be electrocardiographic changes. The pericarditis of JRA is generally benign. Rarely, severe chest pain, dyspnea, or cardiac failure, with or without evidence of myocarditis, demands vigorous therapy. Occasionally, interstitial lung infiltrates occur with active systemic disease (see Chapter 346). A few children have episodes of severe abdominal pain during active disease, probably related to serositis or mesenteric adenopathy.

Leukocytosis and even leukemoid reactions are common. Anemia of chronic disease is also common during active disease and is occasionally profound. Disseminated intravascular coagulation and acute liver failure have been reported; relationships to drug therapies (aspirin, gold) are uncertain.

Most children with systemic JRA have joint manifestations at or within a few months of onset, but the arthritis may initially be overlooked in the presence of the overwhelming

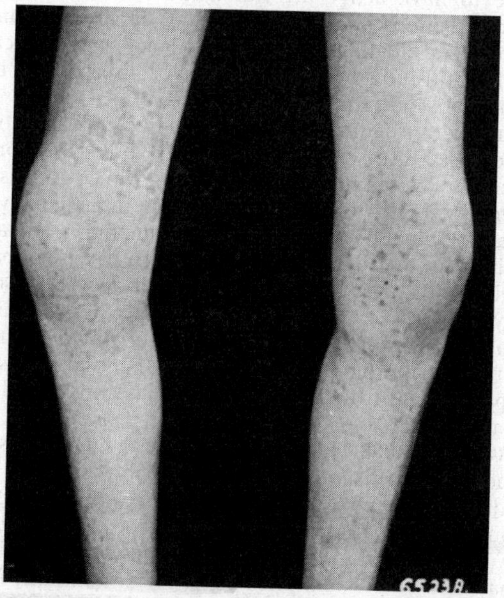

Figure 148–7. The rash of systemic-onset juvenile rheumatoid arthritis.

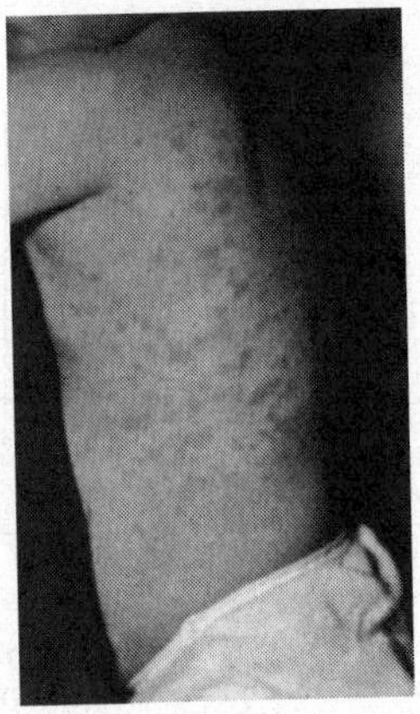
Figure 148–8. Rash of rheumatoid arthritis. See also color section.

systemic symptoms. Some patients initially have only severe myalgia, arthralgia, or transient arthritis. A few patients do not develop arthritis until months or years later. The pattern of joint involvement usually resembles that described for polyarticular disease. Joints of the midcarpus and midtarsus are characteristically affected with corresponding dorsal swellings in the wrists or ankles. The systemic manifestations generally run a self-limited course for several months but may recur. The real morbidity of systemic JRA is arthritis that becomes chronic in some patients and persists after systemic symptoms have remitted. Systemic manifestations rarely recur after patients reach adulthood, even though chronic arthritis may persist.

COURSE AND PROGNOSIS. The ultimate cause of morbidity in polyarticular and systemic JRA is chronic joint disease; in addition, 20% of children with pauciarticular disease type I later develop polyarthritis, which may be severe. In pauciarticular disease, the major morbidity is chronic iridocyclitis in type I patients and subsequent spondyloarthropathy in type II patients. The outcome is unpredictable in any individual patient. Even with severe systemic involvement, the disease is rarely life threatening. There may be exacerbations and remissions, or symptoms may continue for years with mild arthritis causing little disability or, less commonly, with severe arthritis that progresses to joint destruction and permanent deformity. The disease does not always remit at puberty; some patients continue to have active arthritis into adulthood, and some have exacerbations after many years of apparently complete remission. Exacerbations may be associated with intercurrent illness; hepatitis and other forms of liver disease may be followed by transient remission of arthritis.

Patients with rheumatoid factor–positive polyarthritis and systemic-onset disease have the poorest prognosis for joint function. The overall prognosis is good, however. At least 75% of patients with JRA eventually have long remissions without significant residual deformity or loss of function; a few are left with crippling joint deformities. Severe hip disease is particularly debilitating, as is loss of vision from iridocyclitis. Secondary amyloidosis (see Chapter 164), generally heralded by proteinuria and diagnosed by demonstration of amyloid in tissues, may cause late morbidity. In Europe, amyloidosis affects about 5% of patients with JRA; in the United States this complication is very rare.

LABORATORY FINDINGS. There are no specific diagnostic tests. The ESR and CRP are usually but not invariably elevated during active disease. Anemia is common, usually with low reticulocyte counts and a negative Coombs test. Iron deficiency, either dietary or resulting from drug-related gastrointestinal blood loss, may also be present. The white blood cell count is often elevated; leukemoid reactions may occur, particularly in systemic JRA, when counts may be as high as 75,000/mm^3. Thrombocytosis may occur, particularly in systemic-onset disease. Urinalyses are normal; during nonsteroidal therapy a few erythrocytes and renal tubular cells may be seen. There may be an increase in the serum α_2- and gamma globulin fractions and a decrease in albumin. Any or all serum immunoglobulin levels may be elevated.

ANA are found in some children with rheumatoid factor–negative (25%), rheumatoid factor–positive (75%), or pauciarticular type I (90%) disease but are rarely if ever present in those with systemic or pauciarticular type II disease. The finding of ANA does not correlate with disease severity. *Rheumatoid factors* are found in about 5% of children with JRA and correlate with older age at onset. Test results rarely convert from negative to positive despite long-active JRA. Positive test results are most commonly associated with polyarticular disease, late childhood onset, severe destructive arthritis, and rheumatoid nodules; rheumatoid vasculitis is occasionally associated, as is Sjögren syndrome.

Synovial fluid in JRA is cloudy and usually contains increased amounts of protein. The cell count can vary from 5,000–80,000 cells/mm^3; the cells are predominantly neutrophils. Levels of glucose may be low in the joint fluid; levels of complement may be normal or decreased.

Early *roentgenographic changes* consist of soft tissue swelling, osteoporosis, and periostitis about the affected joints (Fig. 148–9). Regional epiphyseal closure may be accelerated and local bone growth increased or decreased. In long-active joint disease, subchondral erosions and narrowing of cartilage spaces may occur, as may varying degrees of bony destruction and fusion. Late roentgenographic changes, for example, in the wrist and hand (see Fig. 148–2), are characteristic. Characteristic changes may occur in the neck, with narrowing and eventual fusion of the neural arch joints (most frequently seen at

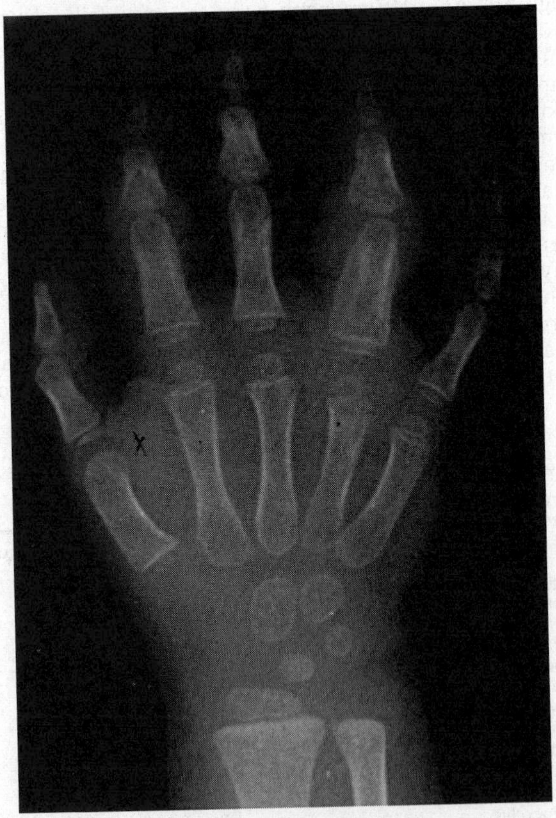
Figure 148–9. Early (6-mo duration) radiographic changes of juvenile rheumatoid arthritis, soft tissue swelling, and periosteal new bone formation appear adjacent to the 2nd and 4th proximal interphalangeal joints.

C2 and C3, Fig. 148–10), erosions of the odontoid process, atlantoaxial subluxation, and underdevelopment of vertebral bodies. Roentgenographic sacroiliitis resembling ankylosing spondylitis is often seen in children with pauciarticular disease type II. Specialized studies utilizing ultrasound, computed tomographic scanning, and magnetic resonance imaging may cast further light on soft tissue and bony abnormalities.

DIAGNOSIS AND DIFFERENTIAL DIAGNOSIS. See Tables 148–3 and 148–4. The diagnosis is clinical and depends on the persistence of arthritis or typical systemic manifestations for 3 consecutive mo or more and on the exclusion of other diseases. Early in the disease pyogenic or tuberculous joint infection, osteomyelitis, sepsis, or arthritis associated with other acute infectious illnesses may be considered. Culture of joint fluid, tuberculin testing, and roentgenograms of affected joints are helpful. Lyme disease should always be considered, particularly in children with pauciarticular disease. Arthritis of limited duration may occur in association with parvovirus and other viral infections and with rubella immunization. Gonococcal infection may result in arthritis. Acute leukemia and other malignancies occasionally present with pain and swelling of one or more joints and should be considered, particularly if there is severe pain, or if severe anemia, thrombocytopenia, or abnormalities of peripheral white blood cells are present.

In acute rheumatic fever the transient, migratory nature of the arthritis and evidence of carditis help in the differentiation. Systemic lupus erythematosus (SLE) and mixed connective tissue disease can cause arthritis indistinguishable from rheumatoid arthritis, but the joint changes are usually milder, and other clinical manifestations of SLE are usually present; however, ANA and occasionally LE cells occur in JRA as well as in SLE. Ankylosing spondylitis may present with arthritis of a few peripheral joints that is indistinguishable from JRA (pauciarticular type II) before the characteristic involvement of the spine becomes manifest; the presence of early roentgenographic sacroiliac joint changes associated with pain in the low back and hip girdle is suggestive. Reiter syndrome (arthritis, urethritis, conjunctivitis) is uncommon in children but should be considered in those with pauciarticular disease type II. The vasculitis syndromes, dermatomyositis, ulcerative colitis, regional enteritis, psoriasis, and sarcoidosis may be associated with arthritis similar to that of JRA but can be differentiated

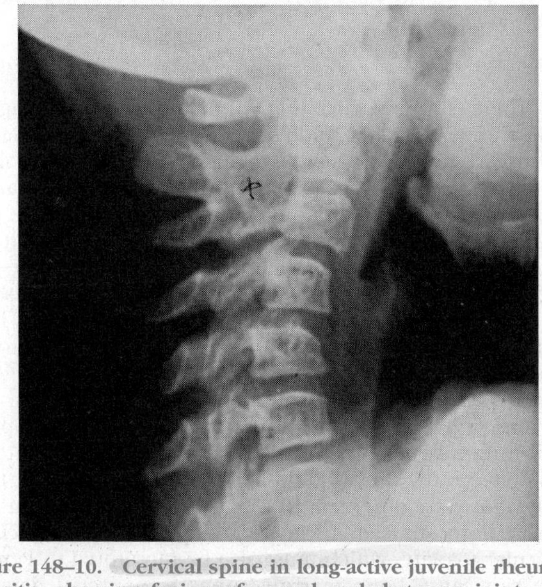

Figure 148–10. Cervical spine in long-active juvenile rheumatoid arthritis, showing fusion of neural arch between joints C2–C3, narrowing and erosions of the remaining neural arch joints, and resultant abnormal curvature.

on clinical grounds. Immunodeficiency diseases may rarely be associated with chronic arthritis resembling JRA.

Various conditions such as joint trauma, Legg-Perthes disease, diskitis, Osgood-Schlatter disease, slipped capital femoral epiphysis, and musculoskeletal pain syndromes may initially mimic JRA. Acute toxic synovitis of the hip is a self-limited condition of uncertain origin; JRA rarely begins in or affects solely the hip. Pigmented villonodular synovitis, an uncommon synovial overgrowth, usually affects only one joint.

Synovial biopsy may be useful, especially to exclude infection in patients with monarticular disease; however, synovial histologic analysis cannot differentiate the various subgroups of JRA, other rheumatic disorders, or even so-called postinfectious states.

TREATMENT. The aims of immediate and long-term treatment are twofold: to preserve joint function and provide adequate care for extra-articular manifestations without causing iatrogenic harm and to support the family and child in achieving an optimal psychosocial adjustment. This requires the devoted attention of a primary physician and may require consultation with a variety of specialists. Although JRA may be of long duration and has no specific cure, the ultimate prognosis is good for most patients, and life is rarely threatened. Management of affected children and their families tests the physician's sympathy, patience, empathy, and clinical skills. Unpredictable exacerbations are discouraging and make evaluation of therapy difficult. There is an understandable tendency for parents to shop for medical help and to grasp for fad or quack cures. The chronic nature of the disease may cause the discouraged family to give up supportive efforts, which may allow unnecessary crippling disability to occur.

There has been a gradual change in the drug therapy for JRA. Salicylates are being less frequently used because of concern about their association with the Reye syndrome, and nonsteroidal anti-inflammatory agents (NSAIDs) are more frequently used. Low-dose methotrexate is increasingly used in patients who have not responded adequately to NSAIDs, and therapies with gold salts, antimalarials, and D-penicillamine are less frequently used.

Acetylsalicylic acid (aspirin) in doses sufficient to maintain blood levels of 20–30 mg/dL often alleviates the arthritic and systemic manifestations of disease. Such blood levels can be achieved by using doses of about 100 mg/kg/24 hr of aspirin for children weighing 25 kg or less and total daily doses of 2.4–3.6 g for older, heavier children. There is considerable individual variation in the doses required, and patients must be watched carefully for toxicity. Hyperventilation or heavy breathing and drowsiness or other central nervous system changes are often the earliest signs of salicylism in children. Tinnitus, a common complaint of adults with salicylism, is rarely reported by children. Salicylates should be given with food because of the possibility of gastric irritation; antacids or buffered salicylate preparations should be added if children complain of stomachaches, and children with persistent gastrointestinal complaints should be investigated for gastritis and ulcer disease. Elevated serum levels of hepatic enzymes may occur; the association of clinically significant liver disease is unusual, but salicylates should be withdrawn if high enzyme levels occur. Hemorrhagic phenomena may occur secondary to effects on platelet function. Epidemiologic studies indicate that aspirin ingestion is associated with the Reye syndrome in children after exposure to chickenpox or influenza. Although this condition has rarely occurred in children with JRA receiving salicylates, it seems prudent to discontinue salicylate use temporarily in children exposed to these infections.

Several NSAIDs are available for therapy of adult arthritis. Of these NSAID agents, tolmetin, naproxen, and ibuprofen are now approved for use in children in the United States; indomethacin, although often used, is still labeled "not to be

■ **TABLE 148–3 Diagnosis of Nonrheumatic Conditions**

Characteristic	Septic Arthritis	Lyme Disease	Osteomyelitis	Viral Arthritis	Childhood Malignancy	Structural, Genetic	Growing Pains, Pain Syndromes
Sex	Any	Any	Any	Any	Any	Any depending on condition	Growing pains, boys > girls
Age at onset	<4 yr: *H. influenzae* Teenage gonococcus Any age: *Staphylococcus*	Over age 2	Any: usually *S. aureus*	More common in older children and adults	Any	Any	Pain syndrome, girls > boys Growing pains, 2–8 yr Pain syndromes, 6 yr or older
Joint manifestations	85% Monoarticular joints swollen, hot, painful, red	Pauciarticular; episodic, recurrent	Sterile joint effusion adjacent to the area of bone infection	Transient arthritis—often polyarticular	Severe bone/joint pain, night pain	Local bone/joint pain or dysfunction	None or bizarre Features of fibromyalgia or reflex sympathetic dystrophy
Extra-articular manifestations	Fever, signs of sepsis, signs of gonococcal disease	Flulike illness, erythema migrans, neurologic, cardiac	Fever, signs of sepsis, bone pain	Those of underlying virus	Those of underlying malignancy	Those of underlying conditions, dysmorphic features, structural abnormalities	Growing pains: none Pain syndromes: bizarre
Laboratory	Cultures: joint fluid, blood, genital	Serologic antibody of *Borrelia burgdorferi*	Culture: blood, bone: bone scan	Viral culture: Serologic rise in antibody titers	Hematologic abnormalities, abnormal radiograph or scan	Demonstration of abnormal structure or metabolic abnormality	Normal
Pathogenesis	Direct bacteremia-synovial infection: occasional immune complex mechanism in gonococcal and meningococcal arthritis	*B. burgdorferi*—synovial and systemic infection	Direct bacteremia-infection of bone, sympathetic joint effusion	Direct viral synovial infection or immune mechanism	Direct primary bone tumor or periarticular or bony infiltrate of malignant cells	Idiopathic or genetic	Unknown, no pathology demonstrable
Diagnosis	Demonstration of organisms in joint fluid, blood culture, or genital culture	Serologic	Demonstration of organisms: blood, bone; bone scan (early), radiograph (late)	Clinical, serologic, or viral culture	Bone marrow or tissue biopsy	Clinical recognition, genetic or metabolic studies	
Natural history	Joint destruction if untreated	Chronic, recurrent; may cause long-term CNS, skin, ocular disease	Bone/joint destruction if untreated	Arthritis, transient	Joint manifestations may wax/wane	Chronic	Growing pains benign, pain syndromes may become chronic and disabling
Therapy	Specific antibiotic	Specific antibiotic	Specific antibiotic	Symptomatic	That of underlying malignancy	That of underlying conditions	Recognition, reassurance, physical therapy, psychosocial attention

CNS = central nervous system.

prescribed for children 14 yr of age and younger unless toxicity or lack of efficacy associated with other drugs warrant the risk." The NSAIDs are of similar potency to aspirin in relieving inflammation, pain, and fever; it is thought that some provide particular relief for patients with spondyloarthropathy. Some of these agents have the advantage of requiring only twice-daily administration. All NSAIDs have side effects similar to those of salicylates: gastric irritation and potential peptic ulcer disease, potential hepatic toxicity, potential renal toxicity, and interference with platelet function. Headache and central nervous system dysfunction may occur in some children. The so-called pseudoporphyria syndrome, with fragile skin subject to scarring lesions, particularly in fair-skinned children exposed to the sun, may be a troubling concomitant of nonsteroidal therapy, particularly with naproxen.

The time for determining efficacy of the NSAIDs is weeks to months. No one of these drugs has been shown superior in efficacy to salicylates in controlled trials, and all have potential toxic hazards. Some patients respond better to one agent than another, and it is reasonable to try two or three in sequence if there is failure to respond adequately to the first agent selected. There is no evidence that combinations of these agents are efficacious, and such combinations may increase toxicity.

The disease-modifying agents include gold salts (oral or intramuscular), antimalarials, D-penicillamine, sulfasalazine, methotrexate, and intravenous immunoglobulin. Oral gold salts, antimalarials, and D-penicillamine have not been shown superior to placebo in controlled studies. Intramuscular gold has never been subject to a controlled study of JRA but is also being used less frequently in children. All of these drugs have significant potential toxicity and must be carefully monitored. The toxicity of gold therapy includes rash, mucosal ulcers, leukopenia, thrombocytopenia, anemia, and proteinuria. Patients receiving gold therapy, either daily oral gold therapy or weekly intramuscular gold therapy, must be closely watched for side effects; the drug should be discontinued, at least temporarily, if any are observed. Hydroxychloroquine, the form of antimalarial most used in rheumatology, can be associated with ocular toxicity, which must also be monitored. D-Penicillamine can cause bone marrow suppression, renal damage, rashes, and myasthenia gravis or various other autoimmune phenomena.

■ **TABLE 148–4 Differential Diagnosis of Rheumatic Disease**

Characteristic	Rheumatic Fever	Juvenile Rheumatoid Arthritis	Systemic Lupus Erythematosus	Kawasaki Disease	Dermatomyositis
Sex	No predilection	Dependent on subgroup	Girls > boys	No predilection	Girls 3:2
Age at onset	3 yr or older	1 yr or older	Usually over age 8 yr	Usually ≤4 yr	2 yr or older
Joint manifestations	Transient migratory arthritis—large joints	Pauciarticular or polyarticular Chronic (6 wk or more)	Arthralgia Transient arthritis Chronic arthritis	Pain and swelling of hands and feet Arthritis occasionally	Joint contractures; arthritis occasionally
Extra-articular manifestations	Fever Cardiac disease Chorea Rash, nodules	Dependent on subgroup: Systemic juvenile rheumatoid arthritis: fever, rash, etc Pauciarticular: iridocyclitis	Occasionally multisystem disease, including nephritis, rash, hematologic and CNS involvement	Fever, conjunctivitis, mucocutaneous lesions, lymphadenopathy, vasculitis of coronary and large vessels	Rash Muscle weakness, pain Gastrointestinal, respiratory
Laboratory	Prior streptococcal infection ECHO or ECG evidence of carditis	May have antinuclear antibodies, rheumatoid factor	Antinuclear antibodies Autoantibodies Low complement Antibody to DNA	Abnormal coronary vessels on ECHO	Abnormal "muscle enzymes," electromyogram, muscle biopsy
Pathogenesis	Poststreptococcal event	Unknown	Immune complex disease	Unknown (question bacterial toxin)	Unknown
Diagnosis	Clinical (Jones criteria)	Clinical (juvenile rheumatoid arthritis criteria)	Clinical plus laboratory (systemic lupus erythematosus criteria)	Clinical (Kawasaki criteria)	Clinical Rash plus myositis Muscle biopsy
Natural history	Arthritis—transient carditis may cause permanent damage	Chronic: arthritis may be destructive	Chronic or recurrent may be fatal	Self-limited Coronary vasculitis May be fatal	Chronic May be fatal
Therapy	Anti-inflammatory group A streptococcus prophylaxis to prevent recurrence	Anti-inflammatory Physical therapy	Anti-inflammatory Corticosteroid Cytotoxic	Intravenous globulin Aspirin	Corticosteroid Cytotoxic

Sulfasalazine, used for years in children with inflammatory bowel disease, is being used to treat JRA and the spondyloarthropathies. There are no controlled trials of this drug in treating childhood rheumatic diseases, but some observers think that this drug may be helpful. Toxicity is the same as that observed in inflammatory bowel disease: gastrointestinal side effects, headache, hypersensitivity reactions, and central nervous system or renal toxicity. Intravenous immunoglobulin has been tested in children with systemic-onset disease and with severe arthritis; no clear-cut demonstration of efficacy has emerged for systemic manifestations or for arthritis.

Methotrexate has now been shown to be an effective agent in many children with severe JRA, and it is being increasingly used in the therapy of children with disease that has not responded to nonsteroidal agents. The doses are low (10–15 mg/m^3/wk, given either orally or intramuscularly). Side effects include gastrointestinal upset after oral methotrexate, potential bone marrow suppression, and hepatotoxicity. Patients should be monitored with periodic blood, liver function, and renal studies. Emerging studies of children who have received this type of therapy for 5 yr or longer do not suggest untoward toxicity over this intermediate period; however, there are no long follow-up studies. A significant proportion of children treated with methotrexate respond within weeks to months with partial or complete clinical remission of disease. Some children who fail low-dose oral methotrexate therapy respond to intramuscular therapy or to higher-dose methotrexate therapy; the latter, however, is still considered experimental and must be very carefully monitored. In those few children with seropositive disease, the potential acceleration of rheumatoid nodule formation during methotrexate therapy should be considered. There is little information concerning whether concomitant nonsteroidal agents should be given with methotrexate; such combinations are commonly used, but their relationship to any drug toxicity observed must be considered. The duration of methotrexate therapy remains a problem; there is accumulating evidence that the drug is suppressive rather than truly remittive, and disease may flare after methotrexate therapy is removed, even after years of apparently successful therapy.

There are few indications for the systemic use of *corticosteroids* in JRA. These agents dramatically suppress symptoms but do not induce permanent remission or prevent the occurrence of joint damage (see Fig. 148–2). In addition, destruction of cartilage and aseptic necrosis of bone, particularly in the femoral heads, may be related to long-term steroid therapy (see Fig. 148–4). Therapeutic doses of corticosteroids also cause adrenal suppression, may suppress growth, and may produce other potentially dangerous side effects. The dose required for suppression of symptoms is unpredictable and may actually increase with prolonged therapy.

Indications for corticosteroid use in JRA include severe systemic disease unresponsive to an adequate trial of salicylates and iridocyclitis uncontrolled by topical steroids. In the former, or in rare instances of vocal cord involvement or of cardiac decompensation due to pericarditis or myocarditis, prednisone in initial doses of 1–2 mg/kg/24 hr is indicated. As soon as symptoms have been suppressed, the dose should be decreased and the drug gradually discontinued under a cover of salicylates. With decreasing doses there is often transient rebound of symptoms, which should be waited out. Because the systemic manifestations of JRA generally run a self-limited course, prednisone can usually be successfully discontinued within weeks or months. In patients with iridocyclitis that does not respond to topical steroid therapy, systemic steroids are indicated in doses sufficient to suppress ocular inflammation as monitored by slit-lamp examination; single doses given daily or on alternate days may be sufficient. Therapy should be managed jointly with an ophthalmologist.

Corticosteroids should rarely be used for relief of joint manifestations alone because they neither cure arthritis nor prevent joint damage, and their chronic side effects may be even less tolerable than the joint disease. Other reasonable therapeutic possibilities should always be exhausted first. If corticosteroids are used, every effort should be made to employ the lowest effective dose, to use alternate-day or single daily doses whenever possible, and to minimize the duration of treatment. Intra-articular injections of corticosteroids may be effective for persistent arthritis in one or a few joints, but many repeated injections should not be made into the same joint.

Physical and occupational therapy are important methods of improving motion and muscular strength about the affected joints and of restoring and maintaining the functional capabilities of the patient. Patients and parents should be instructed in appropriate exercise programs to be carried out at home on a daily basis. Activities such as tricycle riding and swimming are beneficial and should be encouraged. Night splints for knees and wrists may aid in preventing and correcting deformity. Cylindric casts or prolonged immobilization of joints should be avoided. Bed rest has little role in treatment. Children can usually set their own activity levels; in general, they should avoid only those activities that cause overtiring and joint pain. Orthopedic surgery is sometimes required to correct joint deformities. Synovectomy of selected joints is occasionally helpful but not curative. Total replacement of destroyed joints, particularly hips and knees, is now possible when full growth has been attained. Injection of corticosteroids into selected joints may be helpful at times, but repeated injections should not be used. Micrognathia may require orthodontic management and oral surgery. *Functional classification* of JRA includes four classes: I, performs all activities; II, performs adequately with some limitations; III, limited activity, self-care only; and IV, wheelchair-bound or bedridden.

Iridocyclitis requires prompt diagnosis and therapy to preserve vision. The eyes should be examined at each medical visit, and ophthalmologic slit-lamp examinations should be performed at least once each year in children with systemic and polyarticular disease and four times yearly in children with pauciarticular disease. Parents should be cautioned to report at once any eye symptoms or decreased visual acuity. Therapy of iridocyclitis should be supervised by an ophthalmologist. Initially, it consists of topical use of steroids and dilating agents. Systemic steroids or subconjunctival steroid injections should be used if prompt resolution of ocular inflammation is not achieved with topical agents. Frequent and long-term follow-up of eyes is essential. Ophthalmologic surgery may be required for chronic sequelae.

Children with JRA should be encouraged to lead as normal lives as possible. They and their parents need to know what to expect and to be treated optimistically. Affected children should not be led to believe that they are invalids but should be taught to be as self-sufficient as possible. With encouragement most can lead active lives, attend school, and participate in usual activities except strenuous sports. Long hospitalizations should be avoided. Children with residual handicaps need help in vocational planning.

Arthritis Foundation: Arthritis in Children. Atlanta, Arthritis Foundation, 1993.
Arthritis Foundation: Juvenile Dermatomyositis. Atlanta, Arthritis Foundation, 1989.
Arthritis Foundation: When Your Student Has Arthritis. Atlanta, Arthritis Foundation, 1989.
Brewer EJ, Angel KC: Parenting a Child with Arthritis. Los Angeles, Howell House, 1992.
Cassidy JT, Levinson JE, Bass JC, et al: A study of classification criteria for a diagnosis of juvenile rheumatoid arthritis. Arthritis Rheum 29:274, 1986.
DeInocencio J, Giannini EH, Glass DN: Can genetic markers contribute to the classification of juvenile rheumatoid arthritis? J Rheumatol 20(Suppl 40):12, 1993.
Emery HM: Treatment of juvenile rheumatoid arthritis (review). Curr Opin Rheumatol 5:629, 1993.
Fernandez-Vina M, Fink CW, Stastng P: HLA associations in juvenile arthritis. Clin Exp Rheumatol 12:205, 1994.
Giannini EH, Brewer EJ, Kuzmina N, et al: Methotrexate in resistant juvenile rheumatoid arthritis: Results of the USA-USSR double-blind placebo controlled trial. N Engl J Med 326:1043, 1992.
Graham L, Myones B, Rivas-Chacon R, et al: Morbidity associated with long-term methotrexate therapy in juvenile rheumatoid arthritis. J Pediatr 120:468, 1992.
Lindsley CB: Uses of nonsteroidal anti-inflammatory drugs in pediatrics. Am J Dis Child 147:229, 1993.
Malleson PN, Fung MY, Petty RE, et al: Autoantibodies in chronic arthritis of childhood: Relations with each other and with histocompatibility antigens. Ann Rheum Dis 51:1301, 1992.
Prieur AM, Petty RE: Definitions and classification of chronic arthritis in children. Bailleres Clin Pediatr 1:695, 1993.
Pugh MT, Southwood TR, Gaston JSH: The role of infection in juvenile chronic arthritis. Br J Rheumatol 32:838, 1993.
Schaller JG: Juvenile rheumatoid arthritis. Pediatr Rev, in press, 1995.
Sharples AC, Stebulis JA, Weafer-Hodgins M: Just One of the Kids: A Video for Teachers and School Personnel. Boston, Affiliated Children's Arthritis Centers of New England, 1994.
Stebulis JA, DeNardo BA, Tucker LB, Schaller JG: The Pediatric Rheumatology Handbook for Families. Baltimore, Johns Hopkins University Press, in press. [Currently available as Stebulis JA (ed.): The Handbook for Families. Boston, Affiliated Children's Arthritis Centers of New England, 1994].
Stephan JL, Zeller J, Hubert PH, et al: Macrophage activation syndrome and rheumatic disease in childhood: A report of four new cases. Clin Exp Rheumatol 11:451, 1993.
Weatherbee LL, Neil AJ: Educational Rights for Children with Arthritis: A Manual for Parents. Atlanta, Arthritis Foundation, 1989.
Williams RA, Ansell BM: Radiological findings in seropositive juvenile chronic arthritis with particular reference to progression. Ann Rheum Dis 44(10):685, 1985.
Yancey C, Gross RD, et al: Guidelines for ophthalmologic examinations in children with juvenile rheumatoid arthritis. Pediatrics 92:295, 1993.

CHAPTER 149

Ankylosing Spondylitis and Other Spondyloarthropathies

Jane Green Schaller

ANKYLOSING SPONDYLITIS

Ankylosing spondylitis is characterized by stiffness and pain in the back, involvement of the sacroiliac joints, and variable progression to the joints and periarticular tissues of the lumbodorsal and cervical spines. About half the patients have arthritis of the peripheral joints. This is usually a disease of young and middle-aged adults, but it may begin in childhood, usually in males older than 8 yr. There is a striking association between ankylosing spondylitis and HLA-B27. The pathology of synovial tissue from affected joints is similar to that described for rheumatoid arthritis.

Ankylosing spondylitis differs from rheumatoid arthritis by its characteristic involvement of the sacroiliac joints and lumbodorsal spine, predilection for males, lack of association with rheumatoid factor or rheumatoid nodules, association with acute iridocyclitis, occurrence of aortitis with resulting aortic insufficiency, and significant familial incidence.

CLINICAL MANIFESTATIONS. Peripheral arthritis, often transient, may be the first manifestation. Large joints, particularly those of the lower extremities, are affected most frequently. Heel pain is common, as is the occurrence of pain with or without soft tissue swelling at various other sites to which tendons and ligaments attach to bone **(enthesopathy)**. Shoulders, feet, and temporomandibular joints are also involved in a significant number of patients. Affected joints may be warm, swollen, painful, and limited in motion.

Characteristic involvement of the sacroiliac joints and lumbodorsal spine may be present at the onset of disease or may appear months to years later. Pain in the lower back, hip girdles, and thighs is characteristic. The pain is often transient, more severe at night, and relieved by movement. Stiffness in the lower back with loss of normal spinal mobility follows (Fig. 149–1). Spinal involvement characteristically begins in the sacroiliac joints and ascends, involving the lumbar, dorsal, and, finally, cervical spines. In juvenile rheumatoid arthritis (JRA), the neck is involved, but the lumbodorsal spine is spared. Decreased chest wall expansion, related to involvement of the costovertebral joints, may occur early. Low-grade fever, anemia, anorexia, fatigability, and growth retardation may occur. The family history is frequently positive for similar arthritis or for acute iridocyclitis.

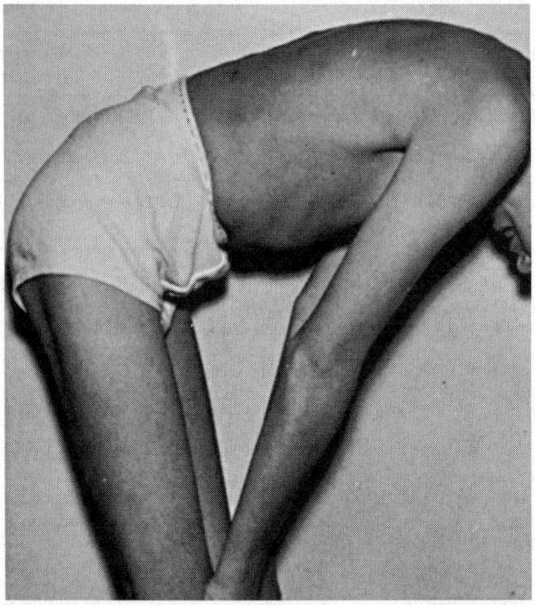

Figure 149–1. Loss of lumbodorsal spine mobility in a boy with ankylosing spondylitis: the lower spine remains straight when the patient bends forward.

Ankylosing spondylitis may arrest at any stage, or the entire spine may become involved over a number of years with loss of virtually all vertebral mobility. Prognosis for functional outcome is usually good if good posture is maintained. Deformity of peripheral joints is uncommon; some patients develop destructive hip disease. Acute iridocyclitis occurs in about 25% of patients at some time; aortitis is rare in children but occurs in a significant number of adults.

LABORATORY FINDINGS. There are no specific laboratory tests. Although HLA-B27 is present in 95% of patients, it is not diagnostic. The erythrocyte sedimentation rate may be elevated. Anemia similar to that of rheumatoid arthritis occurs, but neither rheumatoid factors nor antinuclear antibodies (ANA) are found. Involvement of the sacroiliac joints is demonstrable roentgenographically (Fig. 149–2), usually within the first 3–4 yr; destruction is progressive, with eventual obliteration of the joints. Characteristic roentgenographic changes in the lumbodorsal spine occur some years later.

DIFFERENTIAL DIAGNOSIS. Ankylosing spondylitis should be suspected in any child with persistent pain in the hips, thighs, or

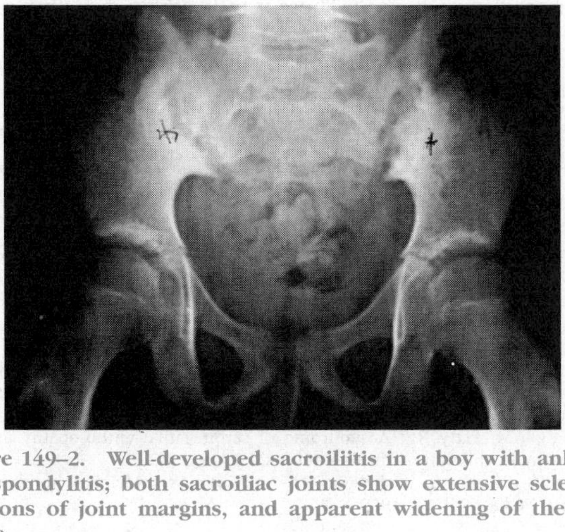

Figure 149–2. Well-developed sacroiliitis in a boy with ankylosing spondylitis; both sacroiliac joints show extensive sclerosis, erosions of joint margins, and apparent widening of the joint space.

lower back, with or without peripheral arthritis. Roentgenographic changes in the sacroiliac joints are necessary for diagnosis, but several years may elapse before they appear. In the differential diagnosis, spinal cord tumors and other childhood malignancies, anatomic defects, infections of the vertebrae or intervertebral disks (diskitis), Scheuermann disease, and other orthopedic conditions of the spine must be considered in any child with persistent back pain. Legg-Perthes disease and slipped capital femoral epiphysis may cause persistent hip and thigh pain. Ulcerative colitis, regional enteritis, psoriasis, and Reiter syndrome may have associated spondylitis resembling ankylosing spondylitis.

TREATMENT. The aims of therapy are to relieve pain and to maintain good posture and function. For relief of pain, salicylates may suffice. Indomethacin or other nonsteroidal anti-inflammatory agents may be helpful. Gold salts are not considered to be effective, and corticosteroid therapy is rarely indicated. Radiation therapy is contraindicated. Maintenance of good posture is essential for preservation of good function; exercises designed to promote posture and strengthen paraspinal muscles should be employed. A firm mattress or bed board should be used for sleeping, and thick pillows should be avoided.

OTHER SPONDYLOARTHROPATHIES

The spondyloarthropathies described in adults include those seronegative types of arthritis associated with sacroilitis and spinal arthritis: ankylosing spondylitis, Reiter disease, psoriatic arthritis, the arthritis of inflammatory bowel disease, and the "reactive arthritis" of yersiniosis and other gastrointestinal infections (Table 149–1). Although these types of arthritis are rarer in children than in adults, some of them, notably ankylosing spondylitis and Reiter disease, may sometimes be mislabeled as JRA. All of the spondyloarthropathies are associated with HLA-B27; none is associated with rheumatoid factors or ANA. The pathology of affected synovial tissues is not distinct from that of rheumatoid arthritis. Some of the spondyloarthropathies, notably Reiter disease and reactive arthritis, may occur after identifiable environmental events such as infections with *Shigella* or *Yersinia*. Spondyloarthropathies may cluster in some families, with several family members having one or another of these types of arthritis; acute iridocyclitis also may be similarly associated. Except for psoriatic arthritis, the spondyloarthropathies affect boys and girls equally or have a male preponderance. Diagnosis rests on clinical grounds.

The pauciarticular disease type II subgroup of JRA probably represents early spondyloarthropathy in most instances. None of the three other seronegative JRA subgroups (seronegative polyarthritis, systemic-onset JRA, and pauciarticular disease type I) is associated with sacroiliitis, HLA-B27, or subsequent spondyloarthropathy.

REITER DISEASE. In its full-blown form, Reiter disease consists of sterile urethritis, arthritis, and ocular inflammation; other manifestations may include gastroenteritis and a variety of rashes. Males are predominantly affected. In children, Reiter disease has been reported after infections with *Shigella, Yersinia enterocolitica, Campylobacter,* and *Chlamydia*; in older children, as in adults, Reiter disease may follow sexual exposure. Reiter disease is strongly associated with HLA-B27. The arthritis is generally pauciarticular, predominantly affecting the large joints. Achilles tendinitis and other enthesopathies are common. Some cases of pauciarticular disease type II may represent "partial" Reiter disease. The long-term prognosis of childhood-onset Reiter disease is unknown. Most children recover within a few months. However, some individuals subsequently have ankylosing spondylitis, some have recurrent or chronic peripheral arthritis, and some have recurrent attacks of ocular or urethral inflammation. The diagnosis is clinical. Infectious

■ TABLE 149–1 The Spondyloarthropathies in Children

Characteristics	Ankylosing Spondylitis	Reiter Syndrome	Inflammatory Bowel Disease	Reactive Arthritis	Psoriatic Arthritis*
Sex	Boys > girls	Boys > girls	No predilection	Boys > girls	Girls > boys
Age at onset	8 yr or older	Occasional in young children, usually over 8 yr	Over age 4	Older children	Over age 2
Joint manifestations	Pauciarticular Lower limb Sacroiliitis Axial arthritis Enthesopathy	Pauciarticular Sacroiliitis Enthesopathy	Pauciarticular Occasional spondylitis	Pauciarticular-transient	Pauciarticular or polyarticular
Extra-articular manifestations	Eye: acute iritis Heart: aortitis	Eye Skin Genitourinary tract Fever, systemic	Those of bowel disease: erythema nodosum, growth failure, etc.	Underlying gastroenteritis: *Yersinia, Shigella, Salmonella, Campylobacter*	Psoriatic rash Nail pitting
Laboratory	HLA-B27 Radiographic sacroiliitis	HLA-B27	HLA-B27 in those with spondylitis	Stool culture positive HLA-B27	None specific
Pathogenesis	Often familial	May follow infectious disease, such as *Shigella, Chlamydia*	Unknown	Reaction to infection	Unknown
Diagnosis	Clinical	Clinical	Clinical, demonstration of bowel disease	Demonstration of gastrointestinal infection	Clinical
Natural history	Chronic May cause spinal fusion and axial joint destruction	Episodic May recur Occasional chronic destructive arthritis	That of underlying bowel disease Peripheral arthritis, benign; spondylitis, chronic	Self-limited arthritis	Arthritis may be chronic
Therapy	NSAIDs Physical therapy	NSAIDs	Bowel disease therapy NSAIDs, physical therapy	That of bowel infection	NSAIDs Remittive agents Physical therapy Skin care

NSAID = nonsteroidal anti-inflammatory drug.
**The inclusion of psoriatic arthritis with spondyloarthropathies may not be appropriate, although it has been traditional.*

urethritis and gonococcal disease must be excluded. Salicylates or one of the other nonsteroidal anti-inflammatory agents is used for treatment. Physical therapy also plays an important role in therapy. Patients should be monitored for subsequent spinal involvement.

ARTHRITIS OF INFLAMMATORY BOWEL DISEASE. Both ulcerative colitis and regional enteritis (see Chapter 283) may be associated with arthritis during childhood; about 10% of children with inflammatory bowel disease will at some time have joint manifestations. Affected children are generally older than 8 yr. The arthritis generally affects a few large joints in a pauciarticular pattern. Arthritis usually begins with or after the onset of active bowel disease; in a few patients arthritis may be the first manifestation of disease. The arthritis of inflammatory bowel disease in children follows two patterns, as it does in adults. Most affected children have peripheral arthritis that waxes and wanes with activity of the bowel disease and causes neither joint destruction nor permanent joint deformity. However, a few children have disease that is inseparable from ankylosing spondylitis and that may progress to disability regardless of control of the underlying bowel disease. For this reason, it is important to follow children with inflammatory bowel disease for evidence of sacroiliitis or spinal arthritis. HLA-B27 is associated with ankylosing spondylitis but not with the peripheral arthritis of inflammatory bowel disease. Therapy for peripheral arthritis includes adequate treatment for the underlying bowel disease with the occasional additional use of salicylates or other nonsteroidal agents. If ankylosing spondylitis occurs, appropriate therapy for that condition is indicated.

REACTIVE ARTHRITIS. Sterile arthritis may follow gastrointestinal infection with *Yersinia enterocolitica, Shigella, Salmonella,* or *Campylobacter.* Generally, only a few joints are affected. The relationship of such arthritis to Reiter disease and other spondyloarthropathies is uncertain. The arthritis usually is transient and the ultimate outcome good. However, some affected patients may subsequently develop chronic spondyloarthropathy. Any child with both gastroenteritis and arthritis should undergo appropriate stool cultures and serologic studies.

PSORIATIC ARTHRITIS. The classification of psoriatic arthritis with the spondyloarthropathies may not be appropriate; there are differences in sex ratios of affected patients and in patterns of arthritis and less strong associations with HLA-B27. Although psoriasis is a relatively common skin condition of children, psoriatic arthritis is uncommon during childhood. Girls are predominantly affected in a 2.5:1 ratio. Psoriatic arthritis in childhood is similar to that seen in adults. Arthritis begins in one or several joints, often in an asymmetric fashion. More than half of patients have involvement of the distal interphalangeal joints; tendinitis is also common. In about half of the patients, psoriasis precedes arthritis by months or years; in others arthritis is the initial manifestation, with psoriasis appearing later. Nail pitting is common. The prognosis of psoriatic arthritis in children appears to be good, although there are few long-term studies. A few patients with psoriatic arthritis develop sacroiliitis and ankylosing spondylitis associated with HLA-B27. Therapy of psoriatic arthritis is similar to that seen in adults; salicylates and other nonsteroidal anti-inflammatory agents are generally used. There is little experience with agents such as methotrexate in children with psoriatic arthritis. As in JRA, physical and occupational therapy play important roles in maintaining good function.

Burgos-Vargas R: Spondyloarthropathies and psoriatic arthritis in children. Curr Opin Rheumatol 5:634, 1993.

Hamilton ML, Gladman DD, Shore A, et al: Juvenile psoriatic arthritis and HLA antigens. Ann Rheum Dis 49:694, 1990.

Jacobs JC, Berdon WE, Johnston AD: HLA-B27 associated spondylarthritis and enthesopathy in childhood: Clinical, pathologic, and radiographic observations in 58 patients. J Pediatr 100:521, 1982.

Lindsley CB, Schaller JG: Arthritis associated with inflammatory bowel disease in children. J Pediatr 84:16, 1974.

Mielants S, Veys EM, Cuvelier C, et al: Gut inflammation in children with late-onset pauciarticular juvenile chronic arthritis and evolution to adult spondyloarthropathy: A prospective study. J Rheumatol 20:1567, 1993.

Rosenberg AM, Petty RE: A syndrome of seronegative enthesopathy and arthropathy in children. Arthritis Rheum 25:1041, 1982.

Schaller JG, Bitnum S, Wedgwood RJ: Ankylosing spondylitis with childhood onset. J Pediatr 74:505, 1969.

CHAPTER 150
Systemic Lupus Erythematosus

Jane Green Schaller

This systemic disease characteristically affects many organ systems and is associated with a variety of immune phenomena. Its natural history is unpredictable; it is often progressive, terminating in death if untreated, but may remit spontaneously or smolder for many years. Systemic lupus erythematosus (SLE) in children is generally more acute and severe than that in adults.

ETIOLOGY AND EPIDEMIOLOGY. The cause is unknown. Many observations support the hypothesis that SLE is a disease of altered immune regulation, perhaps genetically determined. Viruses and other environmental agents may also play a role in pathogenesis. A variety of immune phenomena occur. Serum levels of immunoglobulins are increased. Antibodies are found that react with nuclear constituents (ANA), ribonucleic acid, gamma globulin (rheumatoid factors), red blood cells (positive Coombs test), platelets, white blood cells, antigens used in serologic tests for syphilis (biologic false positive), coagulation factors, and phospholipids (antiphospholipid, lupus anticoagulant, anticardiolipin). There is also an association between inflammation and circulating immune complexes, particularly those consisting of DNA and antibodies reactive with DNA. Such immune complexes are deposited in tissues, fix complement, and initiate an inflammatory response that results in tissue injury such as nephritis. In SLE nephritis immunoglobulins and complement can be demonstrated in renal tissues by immunofluorescence techniques and by direct elution of DNA and anti-DNA antibodies from affected glomeruli; active SLE with nephritis is associated with decreased levels of serum complement and with circulating antibodies reactive with DNA (see Chapter 467).

The onset of exacerbations of disease may appear to be related to intercurrent infections; there may be increased susceptibility to infections, perhaps on the basis of faulty immune mechanisms. Evidence, including studies showing alterations in T- and B-lymphocyte function in patients with SLE, suggests that a state of altered immunologic reactivity underlies the disease. Lupus is sometimes familial and has affected identical twins; hypergammaglobulinemia, other connective tissue diseases, ANA, complement component deficiency, selective IgA deficiency, and other immune abnormalities may be found in patients and 1st-degree relatives of patients.

Lupus-like disease can occur after exposure to a number of drugs, notably hydralazine, sulfonamides, procainamide, and anticonvulsants. Drug-induced disease is generally mild and reversible when the inciting drug is withdrawn. Cutaneous manifestations of SLE and sometimes systemic manifestations may be exacerbated by sunlight.

The incidence is unknown; the disease is not rare. SLE begins in childhood in 20% of patients, usually in children over 8 yr of age. Females are predominantly affected (8:1) in all age groups; however, in prepubertal patients, the ratio is 3:1. All races may be affected, with an apparently higher prevalence in several dark-skinned racial groups, including blacks, Latin Americans, Asians, and some Native American tribes.

PATHOLOGY. Lesions can occur at multiple sites and involve many organ systems. Characteristic masses of amorphous, purple-staining extracellular material are found with hematoxylin staining. These *hematoxylin bodies* probably represent degenerated cell nuclei similar to the inclusions of LE cells. Fibrinoid, an acellular, deeply eosinophilic material, is found in loose connective tissue or in walls of blood vessels of affected tissues. Inflammation of blood vessels (vasculitis) is common. In the spleen, perivascular fibrosis results in characteristic "onion ring" lesions around affected vessels. Granulomas are sometimes found in affected tissues (see Chapter 467) for renal pathology). Deposition of immune complexes, immunoglobulin, and complement can be demonstrated in tissues, including the kidney, skin, and blood vessels.

■ TABLE 150–1 Manifestations of Lupus in Children

Characteristic	% of Patients
Malaise, weight loss, growth retardation	96
Cutaneous abnormalities	96
Hematologic abnormalities	91
Fever	84
Nephritis	84
Musculoskeletal complaints	82
Pleural/pulmonary disease	67
Hepatosplenomegaly or lymphadenopathy	58
Neurologic disease	49
Cardiac abnormalities	38
Hypertension	33
Ocular abnormalities	31
Gastrointestinal symptoms	27
Raynaud phenomenon	13

Reprinted from Arthritis and Rheumatism Journal, copyright 1978. Used by permission of the American College of Rheumatology.

CLINICAL MANIFESTATIONS. SLE may begin insidiously or acutely. Sometimes symptoms antedate the diagnosis of SLE by years. The most frequent early symptoms in children are fever, malaise, arthritis or arthralgia, and rash (Table 150–1). Fever occurs at some time in most affected children; it may be intermittent or sustained. Malaise, anorexia, weight loss, and debility are common.

Cutaneous manifestations occur in most affected children at some time. The "butterfly" rash (Fig. 150–1), consisting of bluish or scaly erythematous patches, involves the malar areas and usually extends over the bridge of the nose. The rash may be photosensitive and may spread to the face, scalp, neck, chest, and extremities; it may become bullous and secondarily infected. Isolated *discoid lupus* (cutaneous manifestations only) is unusual in children. Other skin eruptions include erythematous macules or punctate lesions on the palms, soles, fingertips, extremities, or trunk; vasculitic rashes; livedo reticularis; and nailbed changes. Macular and often painless ulcerative lesions may occur on the palate and mucous membranes of the mouth and nose. Purpura, sometimes associated with thrombocyto-

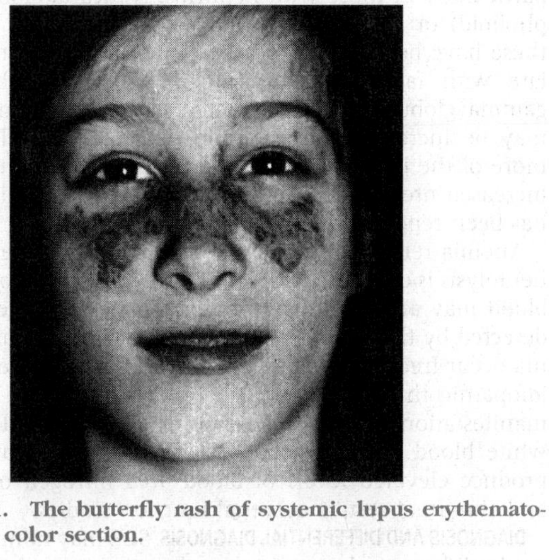

Figure 150–1. The butterfly rash of systemic lupus erythematosus. See also color section.

penia, may appear over dependent or traumatized areas. Erythema nodosum and erythema multiforme are occasionally associated. Alopecia resulting from inflammation about the hair follicles may be patchy or generalized, and the hair may be coarse, dry, and brittle.

Arthralgia and joint stiffness are common and often occur without objective changes. Sometimes affected joints are warm and swollen; pain may be greater than expected for the clinical signs, but persistent deforming arthritis is rare. Aseptic necrosis may affect bone at a number of sites, particularly in the femoral heads. Tenosynovitis and myositis may also occur, as may Raynaud phenomenon. Polyserositis (pleurisy, pericarditis, and peritonitis) is characteristic and produces chest, precordial, or abdominal pain. Hepatosplenomegaly and generalized lymphadenopathy are common. Cardiac involvement may be manifest by variable murmurs, friction rubs, cardiomegaly, electrocardiographic changes, or congestive heart failure, with myocarditis, pericarditis, or verrucous endocarditis (Libman-Sacks endocarditis, recognized by echocardiogram or at postmortem examination). Myocardial infarctions may cause death in relatively young patients, including children. Parenchymal lung infiltrates may occur; infection must be excluded, however, before pneumonia can be ascribed to SLE. Acute pneumonia, pulmonary hemorrhage, or chronic pulmonary fibrosis may occur. Involvement of the nervous system may cause personality changes, seizures, cerebrovascular accidents, chorea, and peripheral neuritis. Gastrointestinal manifestations include abdominal pain, vomiting, diarrhea, melena, and even bowel infarction secondary to vasculitis. Ocular changes may include episcleritis, iritis, or retinal vascular changes with hemorrhages or exudates (cytoid bodies). Thrombotic events affecting either arteries or veins may occur, particularly in patients with antiphospholipid antibodies. Clinical renal involvement is common in children (see Chapter 467).

LABORATORY MANIFESTATIONS. ANA should be demonstrable in all patients with active SLE, and their demonstration provides the best screening test for the disease; however, ANA also occur in many other conditions (see Chapter 147). ANA screening tests are generally done using a fluorescent antibody technique. Tests for specific types of ANA including Ro/SSA, La/SSB, Sm, and DNA should also be performed. Antibodies to Sm are relatively specific for SLE; antibodies to Ro/SSA and La/SSB are associated with the neonatal lupus syndrome. Antibodies to double-stranded DNA are associated with active disease, particularly nephritis; DNA antibodies thus provide a useful index of severity and activity. Serum hemolytic complement and some of its components (C3 is most frequently measured) are decreased in patients with severe active SLE, particularly in those with nephritis. Anticardiolipin (antiphospholipid) or lupus anticoagulant antibodies may be detected; these have been associated with thrombotic events and correlate with false-positive serologic tests for syphilis. Serum gamma globulin levels are often elevated; α_2-globulin levels may be increased and albumin decreased. Levels of one or more of the individual immunoglobulins may be elevated. An increased prevalence of HLA-B8, -DW3/DR3, and -DW2/DR2 has been reported in some series.

Anemia related to chronic inflammatory disease or immune hemolysis is common. Difficulties in typing and cross-matching blood may arise from the presence of erythrocyte antibodies, detected by the Coombs test. Thrombocytopenia and leukopenia occur frequently. Platelet antibodies may be demonstrable; idiopathic thrombocytopenic purpura (ITP) may be the first manifestation of SLE. The urine may contain red blood cells, white blood cells, protein, and casts. Renal insufficiency may produce elevated levels of blood urea nitrogen or creatinine and abnormal results on renal function studies.

DIAGNOSIS AND DIFFERENTIAL DIAGNOSIS. SLE may mimic any rheumatic disease and many other diseases as well. Diagnosis is made on clinical grounds (Table 150–2) and is confirmed by laboratory tests. ANA are usually present; although they are not diagnostic, their absence makes the diagnosis unlikely. Antibodies to double-stranded DNA are virtually diagnostic but may not be present in patients with mild disease. Hypergammaglobulinemia, positive Coombs test, false-positive test for syphilis, anemia, leukopenia or thrombocytopenia, and signs of nephritis may also be diagnostically helpful. Serum levels of hemolytic complement and some of its components are lowered in some patients with active disease; absence of measurable hemolytic complement or failure to achieve normal levels during therapy should suggest a possible congenital complement deficiency. Renal or cutaneous biopsy may confirm the diagnosis of SLE, and renal pathologic studies can indicate the type and severity of renal involvement; however, histologic changes are not entirely specific. Thrombocytopenic purpura and hemolytic anemia may be presenting features; the differential diagnosis of these conditions should include SLE.

Drug-induced lupus or drug-induced ANA may occur in

■ TABLE 150–2 1982 Revised Criteria for Diagnosis of Systemic Lupus Erythematosus

Criterion*	Definition
Malar rash	Fixed erythema, flat or raised, over the malar eminences, tending to spare the nasolabial folds
Discoid rash	Erythematous raised patches with adherent keratotic scaling and follicular plugging; atrophic scarring may occur in older lesions
Photosensitivity	Rash as a result of unusual reaction to sunlight (elicited by patient history or physician observation)
Oral ulcers	Oral or nasopharyngeal ulceration, usually painless, observed by a physician
Arthritis	Nonerosive arthritis involving two or more peripheral joints, characterized by tenderness, swelling, or effusion
Serositis	Pleuritis—convincing history of pleuritic pain or rub heard by a physician or evidence of pleural effusion or Pericarditis—documented by ECG or rub or evidence of pericardial effusion
Renal disorder	Persistent proteinuria greater than 0.5 g/day or greater than 3+ if quantitation not performed or Cellular casts—may be red blood cell, hemoglobin, granular, tubular, or mixed
Neurologic disorder	Seizures—in the absence of offending drugs or known metabolic derangements (e.g., uremia, ketoacidosis, or electrolyte imbalance) or Psychosis—in the absence of offending drugs or known metabolic derangements (e.g., uremia, ketoacidosis, or electrolyte imbalance)
Hematologic disorder	Hemolytic anemia—with reticulocytosis or Leukopenia—less than 4,000/mm^3 total on two or more occasions or Lymphopenia—less than 1,500/mm^3 on two or more occasions or Thrombocytopenia—less than 100,000/mm^3
Immunologic disorder	Positive LE cell preparation or Anti-DNA antibody to native DNA in abnormal titer or Anti-Sm—presence of antibody to Sm nuclear antigen or False-positive serologic test result for syphilis known to be positive for at least 6 mo and confirmed by *Treponema pallidum* immobilization or fluorescent treponemal antibody absorption test
Antinuclear antibody	An abnormal titer of antinuclear antibody by immunofluorescence or an equivalent assay at any point in time and in the absence of drugs known to be associated with "drug-induced lupus syndrome"

From Tan EM, Cohen AS, Fries JF, et al: The 1982 revised criteria for the classification of systemic lupus erythematosus. Anthritis Rheum 25:1271, 1982.

**The proposed classification is based on 11 criteria. For the purpose of identifying patients in clinical studies, a person shall be said to have systemic lupus erythematosus if any 4 or more of the 11 criteria are present, serially or simultaneously, during any interval of observation.*

response to many common pharmaceutical agents, including anticonvulsants, antihypertensive agents, and isoniazid. Most affected individuals have positive ANA tests with no clinical disease. In drug-induced lupus, the clinical features are generally less severe than those of SLE. Fever, arthritis, rash, and serositis are most frequently reported; manifestations of severe lupus, such as nephritis and central nervous system involvement, are unusual. This condition usually responds to symptomatic therapy and discontinuance of the offending agent. Laboratory studies may show cytopenias and autoantibodies such as rheumatoid factors in addition to positive ANA tests. Specific tests frequently reveal antihistone antibodies in drug-induced lupus; however, these antibodies are also found in about one third of patients with SLE. Antibodies to double-stranded DNA and lowered complement levels are rarely associated with drug-induced lupus.

TREATMENT. Therapy should be based on the extent and severity of disease in the individual patient. Patients must be thoroughly evaluated, particularly for involvement of major organ systems such as the kidneys. There is no specific therapy. Drugs used to treat the disease suppress inflammation and immune reactivity. In general, patients should be treated to maintain clinical well-being and serologic (complement and antibody to DNA) normality.

In patients having mild disease without nephritis, nonsteroidal anti-inflammatory agents should be used to provide symptomatic relief of arthritis and other discomfort. Careful follow-up for possible development of nephritis or other major involvement is vital. The antimalarial agent hydroxychloroquine is used for discoid and cutaneous manifestations of systemic lupus, but care must be taken because of potential retinal toxicity. Topical use of corticosteroid preparations may suppress the facial rash.

Systemic use of steroids in doses sufficient to suppress symptoms is required in most patients. In patients with significant systemic involvement but without clinical nephritis and with normal levels of serum complement and DNA antibodies, therapy can also be symptomatic with careful follow-up. Doses of corticosteroid sufficient to suppress symptoms should be given initially (prednisone, 1–2 mg/kg/24 hr may be required) and then tapered to the lowest suppressive doses. Antimalarial agents may be useful adjuncts in therapy of arthritis, sparing steroids. In patients with SLE and nephritis or major systemic involvement, therapy must be geared to maintain the clinical well-being of the patient and to suppress the systemic and renal disease, as reflected by return of serum complement levels to normal and reduction of circulating antibodies to DNA. Large doses of corticosteroids for prolonged periods may be required; initial doses of prednisone of 1–2 mg/kg/24 hr are usual. All the undesirable side effects of steroid therapy may be expected if large doses are required for a significant period of time. Other schedules of steroid administration may be used, including large-dose intravenous pulses or, once symptoms have been controlled, alternate-day doses. Agents such as cyclophosphamide or, less often, azathioprine may be effective adjunctive agents in suppressing severe SLE; however, such therapy must be used with extreme care. Little is known about the long-term effects of such drugs, particularly in children. Side effects include increased susceptibility to severe viral and other infections, gonadal suppression, and possible induction of malignancies. Such agents should never be used in patients with mild SLE or in those whose disease can be satisfactorily controlled with corticosteroids alone. Experience indicates that intravenous pulse therapy with cyclophosphamide (Cytoxan) offers promise in the management of severe childhood lupus; such treatment should be performed only by specialists with experience in its usage.

Seizures and other central nervous system manifestations are generally associated with severe, active disease and demand vigorous control of SLE. Central nervous system disease occurs episodically in patients with SLE and may never recur if the patient is helped over the acute episode and the disease is subsequently controlled. Central nervous system lupus must always be differentiated from infections and steroid psychosis.

Because of the possibility of drug-induced disease, inquiry should be made about possible offending agents; drugs known to be associated with SLE should in general be avoided in patients with the disease.

Patients with *antiphospholipid antibodies* **(lupus anticoagulants)** may manifest venous and arterial thrombosis, recurrent fetal loss, migraine, stroke, transient ischemic attacks, avascular bone necrosis, transverse myelitis, pulmonary hypertension, pulmonary embolism, livedo reticularis, leg ulcers, or thrombocytopenia. Steroid or cytotoxic therapy may lower the levels of the lupus anticoagulant, and antiplatelet agents or anticoagulants may be indicated.

Dialysis and renal transplantation are adjunct therapies for severe lupus nephritis (see Chapters 489 and 490).

Meticulous follow-up is of paramount importance in treating all patients with SLE and includes monitoring the patient's clinical, renal, and serologic status. Any signs of worsening disease should be promptly recognized and appropriately managed. Because there is no cure, the disease is potentially lifelong, and patients must be followed for years. Active lupus should be considered an emergency that demands prompt evaluation and vigorous therapy to bring it under control before irreparable organ system involvement ensues.

PROGNOSIS. SLE was previously considered a potentially or uniformly fatal childhood disease. Children with milder disease are being recognized, and it is apparent that not all children have severe major organ involvement. Although spontaneous exacerbations and remissions occur, prolonged spontaneous remission is unusual in children. Therapy with antibiotics, corticosteroids, and cytotoxic drugs has prolonged survival and brightened the short-term prognosis for many patients with lupus. Although the 5-yr survival rate for children exceeds 90%, a significant number of patients still have ongoing disease and remain at risk of future adverse sequelae. Major causes of death in SLE patients include nephritis, central nervous system complications, infections, pulmonary lupus, and myocardial infarctions. The ultimate prognosis for severe lupus with childhood onset remains to be defined.

Angelini L, Ravelli A, Caporali R, et al: High prevalence of antiphospholipid antibodies in children with idiopathic cerebral ischemia. Pediatrics 94:500, 1994.

Austin HA III, Klippel JH, Balow JE, et al: Therapy of lupus nephritis: Controlled trial of prednisone and cytotoxic drugs. N Engl J Med 314:614, 1986.

Barron KS, Silverman ED, Gonzales J, Reveille JD: Clinical, serologic, and immunogenetic studies in childhood onset systemic lupus erythematosus. Arthritis Rheum 63:348, 1993.

Cameron JS: Lupus nephritis in childhood and adolescence. Pediatr Nephrol 8:230, 1994.

George PM, Tunnessen WW: Childhood discoid lupus erythematosus. Arch Dermatol 129:613, 1993.

Hess E: Drug related lupus. N Engl J Med 318:1460, 1987.

Hughes GRV: The antiphospholipid syndrome: Ten years on. Lancet 342:341, 1993.

Kaufman DB, Laxer RM, Silverman ED, et al: Systemic lupus erythematosus in childhood and adolescence: The problem, epidemiology, incidence, susceptibility, genetics, and prognosis. Curr Probl Pediatr 16:545, 1986.

Lacks S, White P: Morbidity associated with childhood systemic lupus erythematosus. J Rheumatol 17:941, 1990.

Laitman RS, Glicklich D, Sablay LB, et al: Effect of long term normalization of serum complement levels on the course of lupus nephritis. Am J Med 87:132, 1989.

Lang BA, Silverman ED: A clinical overview of systemic lupus erythematosus in childhood. Pediatr Rev 14:194, 1993.

Lehman TJ, McCurdy DK, Bernstein GH, et al: Systemic lupus erythematosus in the first decade of life. Pediatrics 83:235, 1989.

Lehman TJ, Sherry DD, Wagner-Weiner L, et al: Intermittent intravenous cyclophosphamide therapy for lupus nephritis. J Pediatr 114:1055, 1989.

Levy M, Montes de Oca M, Claude-Barron M: Unfavorable outcomes (end-stage renal failure/death) in childhood onset systemic lupus erythematosus. A multicenter study in Paris and its environs. Clin Exp Rheumatol 12(Suppl 10):S63, 1994.

Massengill SF, Richard GA, Donnelly WH: Infantile systemic lupus erythematosus with onset simulating congenital nephrotic syndrome. J Pediatr 124:27, 1994.

Molta C, Meyer O, Dosquet C, et al: Childhood onset systemic lupus erythemato-

sus: Antiphospholipid antibodies in 37 patients and their first degree relatives. Pediatrics 92:849, 1993.
Moore ME, McGrory CH, Rosenthal RS (eds): Learning About Lupus: A User Friendly Guide. Ardmore, PA, Lupus Foundation, 1991.
Ramirez-Seijas F, Cepero-Akselrad A: Systemic lupus erythematosus in children. Int Pediatr 8:334, 1993.
Ravelli A, Caporali R, Bianchi E, et al: Anticardiolipin syndrome in childhood: A report of two cases. Clin Exp Rheumatol 8:95, 1990.
Tucker LB: Antiphospholipid syndrome in childhood: The great unknown. Lupus (in press).

CHAPTER 151

Neonatal Lupus

Jane Green Schaller

Neonatal lupus occurs in infants of mothers who have antibodies to Ro/SSA; most also have antibodies to La/SSB. These mothers are often clinically well. Some show clinical signs of rheumatic disease, most often Sjögren syndrome, occasionally systemic lupus erythematosus (SLE). Affected infants may have a rash, thrombocytopenia, or congenital heart block; liver disease, hemolytic anemia, and leukopenia have been less frequently reported. The neonatal lupus syndrome is assumed to be caused by effects of maternal factors on the fetus, but the exact pathogenesis remains uncertain. The congenital heart block is caused by damage to the conduction system of the fetal heart; this condition is irreversible. The other manifestations of the neonatal lupus syndrome are noticed soon after birth, but they regress within the first year of life. The exact role of the Ro/SSA and La/SSB antibodies has yet to be defined; in one experimental model, heart block was induced in adult rabbits by infusion of Ro/SSA antibody. Only a minority of mothers with these antibodies have infants with neonatal lupus syndrome, and there is striking discordance for this syndrome in infants born to the same mother and even in dizygotic twins of mothers with Ro/SSA or La/SSB antibodies, suggesting that other genetic or environmental factors may be important in the pathogenesis.

The most common abnormality is a rash that is clinically and histologically typical of cutaneous lupus. The rash develops within the first weeks of life and fades over a period of several months. Lesions may occur on the trunk, extremities, or face. They often assume an erythematous, circinate form, closely resembling that of subacute cutaneous lupus in adults, another condition associated with antibodies to Ro/SSA and La/SSB. The thrombocytopenia of neonatal lupus is antibody mediated and also regresses within the first months of life.

Congenital heart block is a permanent condition that usually becomes apparent during fetal life. Most infants with isolated congenital heart block, once considered a rare form of congenital heart disease, have mothers with antibodies to Ro/SSA; many of these mothers do not have overt clinical rheumatic disease. There is little information available about the pathology of the conduction system, but fibrosis, inflammation, and deposition of immunoglobulin have been found in a few instances. Endocardial fibroelastosis has been reported, and fetal myocarditis has been described as part of the syndrome. Congenital heart block should be suspected if the fetal heart rate is low, and antibodies to Ro/SSA and La/SSB should be sought in maternal serum. Therapy for the fetus and mother includes corticosteroids and immunosuppressive agents; plasmapheresis has been proposed and tried in a few instances, but the results are uncertain. The prognosis of congenital heart block is somewhat guarded; more than one half of affected children require pacemakers, sometimes within the first months of life, and follow-up information suggests that as many as 30% of children have died.

Hepatic disease in the form of cholestatic hepatitis has been described in several infants with neonatal lupus. The hepatic disease appears to resolve if infants survive any associated cardiac manifestations.

A few reports have described what appears to be true SLE in infants, particularly in association with the nephrotic syndrome. Several young adults who had the neonatal lupus syndrome developed SLE years later.

Buyon JP, Winchester RJ, Skade SG, et al: Identification of mothers at risk for congenital heart block and other neonatal lupus syndromes in their children. Arthritis Rheum 36:1263, 1993.
Buyon JP: Congenital complete heart block. Lupus 2:291, 1993.
Buyon JP, Ben-Chetrit, Karp S, et al: Acquired congenital heart block: Pattern of maternal antibody response to biochemically defined antigens of the SSA/Ro-SSB/La system in neonatal lupus. J Clin Invest 84:627, 1989.
Buyon JP: Neonatal lupus syndromes. Curr Opin Rheumatol 6:523, 1994.
Jackson R, Gulliver M: Neonatal lupus erythematosus progressing into systemic lupus erythematosus: A 15 year follow up. Br J Dermatol 101:81, 1979.
Julkunen H, Kaaja R, Wallbren E, et al: Isolated congenital heart block: Fetal and infant outcome and familial incidence of heart block. Obstet Gynecol 82:11, 1993.
Julkunen H, Kurki P, Kaaja R, et al: Isolated congenital heart block: Long term outcome of mothers and characterization of the immune response to SS-A/Ro and to SS-B/La. Arthritis Rheum 36:1588, 1993.
Laxer RM, Roberts EA, Gross KR, et al: Liver disease in neonatal lupus erythematosus. J Pediatr 116:238, 1990.
Lee LA, Reichlin M, Ruyle SZ, Weston WL: Neonatal lupus liver disease. Lupus 2:333, 1993.
Watluck J, Buyon JP: Autoantibody associated congenital heart block: Outcome in mothers and children. Ann Intern Med 120:544, 1994.
Watson R, Kang JE, May M, et al: Thrombocytopenia in the neonatal lupus syndrome. Arch Dermatol 124:560, 1988.
Watson RM, Scheel JN, Petri M, et al: Neonatal lupus erythematosus: Report of serological and immunogenetic studies in twins discordant for congenital heart block. Br J Dermatol 130:342, 1994.
Wolach B, Choc L, Pomeranz A, et al: Aplastic anemia in neonatal lupus erythematosus. Am J Dis Child 147:941, 1993.

CHAPTER 152

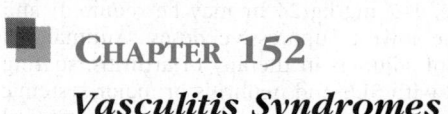

Vasculitis Syndromes

Jane Green Schaller

In these syndromes of blood vessel inflammation, the various patterns of disease depend on the size and location of the affected vessels (Table 152–1). Vasculitis may be a primary disease or may be secondary to a connective tissue disorder, infection, or other process. It may be limited to the skin or exist in multiple organs. When small nonmuscular vessels are involved, the disease takes the form of Henoch-Schönlein vasculitis (anaphylactoid purpura). With involvement of the larger muscular arteries, the disease is called polyarteritis nodosa; variants include Wegener granulomatosis. In Takayasu arteritis, the aorta and other great vessels are sites of inflammation. Some overlap of these syndromes occurs; vessels of various sizes may sometimes be involved in the same patients. Infantile polyarteritis and Kawasaki disease are characterized by vasculitis of the large coronary arteries and to a lesser extent of other large central vessels. Inflammation of blood vessels also occurs in other rheumatic diseases in children, notably lupus erythematosus, dermatomyositis, and scleroderma; in hypertension; and in vessels exposed to local infection, trauma, or thromboemboli.

■ **TABLE 152–1 Vasculitis in Children**

Characteristic	Henoch-Schönlein Syndrome	Kawasaki Disease	Polyarteritis and Variants	Takayasu Disease
Sex	Boys 2:1	No predilection	Boys > girls	Girls > boys
Age at onset	Over 2 yr	Usually before age 5	Any (rare)	Older children (rare)
Clinical characteristics	Purpuric rash Angioedema Arthritis Abdominal pain Nephritis	Fever, conjunctivitis, oral changes, swelling and peeling of hands and feet, rash, cervical adenopathy, coronary vasculitis	Cutaneous or multisystem disease Granulomas of upper airway or lung (Wegener)	Hypertension Absent pulses Various rheumatic complaints
Laboratory characteristics	Elevated serum IgA in half, IgA deposits in tissues	Thrombocytosis Abnormal coronary vessels on echocardiography	None specific except histology or arteriography	None specific except histology or arteriography
Pathogenesis	May follow *Streptococcus* or drug exposure	Unknown	May follow infectious disease Immune complex: Hepatitis B	More common in Asians
Diagnosis	Clinical	Clinical	Clinical: demonstration of vasculitis: biopsy or arteriography	Demonstration of aortic or large central vessel involvement
Natural history	Self-limited Occasionally recurrent Rarely chronic: renal disease	Self-limited Fatal in 1–2% (?)Long-term coronary and large vessel damage	Chronic May be fatal	Chronic, often progressive May be fatal
Therapy	Symptomatic Occasional corticosteroid	Intravenous gamma globulin Aspirin	Corticosteroid Cytotoxic	Corticosteroid Cytotoxic Arterectomy

The causes of these disorders are unknown. Henoch-Schönlein vasculitis and polyarteritis may follow exposure to infectious agents, drugs, or allergens. In serum sickness (see Chapter 141), vasculitis is caused by deposition of immune complexes. Polyarteritis nodosa has been associated with hepatitis B, with vascular damage presumably caused by immune complexes of the viral antigen and its antibody.

In contrast to most other rheumatic diseases, Henoch-Schönlein vasculitis and polyarteritis nodosa affect predominantly males. In childhood, Henoch-Schönlein vasculitis and Kawasaki disease are the most commonly encountered types; polyarteritis and its variants are rare.

152.1 *Henoch-Schönlein Purpura or Vasculitis*

(Anaphylactoid Purpura)

This distinctive syndrome was described by Heberden before 1800; in the 1830s, Schönlein described the typical rash and joint manifestations; and in the 1870s, Henoch recognized the gastrointestinal and renal manifestations. Osler pointed out the similarity between this disease and the hypersensitivity reactions, erythema multiforme, and serum sickness. The skin lesion is the most obvious sign; the visceral lesions are less easily recognized but are more serious. The primary manifestations are due to vasculitis of the small blood vessels.

The cause is unknown. Allergy or drug sensitivity plays a role in some patients. The disease may follow an upper respiratory tract infection, sometimes streptococcal; clustering of cases with no obvious inciting event has been reported. The syndrome may occur at any age; it is more common in children than in adults, with most cases occurring in children 2–8 yr of age. Boys are affected twice as often as girls.

PATHOLOGY. In the skin, small vessels are surrounded by an acute leukocytoclastic inflammatory reaction of polymorphonuclear and round cells; eosinophils and varying numbers of red blood cells may be present. Dermal IgA deposits have been demonstrated. Capillaries are most frequently involved, but small arterioles and venules may be affected also. Scattered nuclear debris, edema, and swelling of collagen fibrils are found adjacent to the affected vessels. Other sites of inflammation or hemorrhage may include the synovium, the gastrointestinal tract, and the central nervous system. Edema and vasculitis of the bowel wall may lead to intussusception and rarely to perforation and may mimic inflammatory bowel disease. In the kidneys, there are focal increases in mesangial cells and matrix, focal glomeralitis, and rarely diffuse changes. Immunofluorescence reveals mesangial deposits of IgA and sometimes of IgG and complement.

CLINICAL MANIFESTATIONS. Onset may be acute, with simultaneous appearance of several manifestations, or gradual, with sequential appearance of different manifestations over a period of weeks. Various combinations of symptoms and signs may occur. Malaise and low-grade fever are present in half the patients.

Skin lesions are present in all identified patients; it is not known whether visceral manifestations occur in the absence of rash. The lesions usually appear on the lower extremities and buttocks but may involve the upper extremities, trunk, and face (Fig. 152–1). Dermatologic manifestations are extremely variable. The classic lesion begins as a small wheal or erythematous maculopapule. Lesions initially blanch on pressure but later lose this feature and generally become petechial or purpuric. Purpuric areas evolve in the usual manner of ecchymoses, changing from red to purple, becoming rusty,

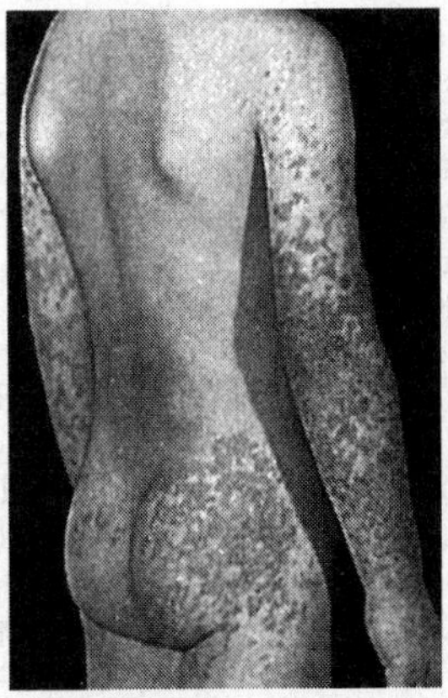

Figure 152–1. Henoch-Schönlein purpura (anaphylactoid purpura). (From Korting GW: Hautkrankheiten bei Kindern und Jugendlichen, 3rd ed. Stuttgart, Germany, FK Schattauer Verlag, 1982.) See also color section.

and eventually fading. The purpura is often palpable. Skin lesions appear in crops, and a variety may be present at any time. In addition to these characteristic lesions, the various patterns of erythema multiforme and erythema nodosum may rarely occur and are rarely pruritic. Angioedema involving the scalp, eyelids, lips, ears, dorsa of the hands and feet, back, scrotum, and perineum is common and may be striking, especially in young children. Rarely, an entire limb segment, such as the forearm, may be transiently swollen and tender.

Arthritis occurs in two thirds of affected children. Large joints, particularly the knees and ankles, are most commonly involved. Affected joints may be swollen, tender, and painful on motion. When present, effusions reveal serous fluid; they are not hemorrhagic. Joint symptoms usually resolve after a few days without residual deformity or articular damage but may recur during periods of active disease.

Gastrointestinal symptoms appear in more than half of affected children. The most common complaint is colicky abdominal pain, which may be severe and is often associated with vomiting. Stools show gross or occult blood in more than 50% of patients, and hematemesis may occur. Failure to recognize this syndrome in children with sudden onset of acute abdominal pain may lead to unnecessary laparotomy. In such cases, peritoneal exudate, enlarged mesenteric lymph nodes, segmental edema, and hemorrhage into the bowel wall may be present. Gastrointestinal roentgenograms may show decreased motility and segmental narrowing, presumably related to submucosal edema and hemorrhage. Rarely, intussusception, obstruction, or infarction with bowel perforation may occur.

Renal involvement occurs in 25–50% of children during the acute phase, the frequency depending in part on the adequacy of examination. It is usually manifest by hematuria with or without casts or proteinuria during the first few weeks of illness; sometimes renal involvement first appears later after other manifestations have become quiescent. The nephrotic syndrome, moderate azotemia, hypertension, oliguria, and hypertensive encephalopathy may occasionally occur. Most children with renal involvement recover, although some continue to have abnormal urinary sediment, with or without abnormal renal function; a few will experience chronic renal disease within a few years of the acute phase of Henoch-Schönlein purpura.

A rare but potentially serious manifestation is central nervous system involvement, with seizures, paresis, and coma. Hepatosplenomegaly and lymphadenopathy may also occur during the acute phase of the disease. Rarely, intramuscular hemorrhage, rheumatoid-like nodules, cardiac involvement, eye involvement, and testicular swelling and hemorrhage have been reported.

The outcome is excellent in the absence of significant renal disease. The course varies. The disease is often mild, lasting for a few days with only transient arthritis and a few purpuric spots. In more seriously affected children, the average duration is 4–6 wk, but subsequent exacerbations and remissions may occur. The illness may occasionally smolder for 1 yr or longer.

LABORATORY FINDINGS. Laboratory test results are not diagnostic. The erythrocyte sedimentation rate (ESR) may be elevated. The white blood cell count is often increased, and eosinophilia may be present. Coagulation studies are normal. With renal involvement, red blood cells, white blood cells, casts, and albumin are present in the urine. There may be gross or occult blood in the stools. Neither rheumatoid factor nor antinuclear antibodies (ANA) are present. Serum complement titers are normal or elevated. Serum levels of IgA are elevated in more than 50% of patients.

DIAGNOSIS AND DIFFERENTIAL DIAGNOSIS. The full-blown picture of rash, arthritis, and gastrointestinal and renal manifestations is characteristic. Diagnostic confusion may result when one symptom predominates or multiple system involvement is not recognized. The rash may suggest a hemorrhagic diathesis or septicemia; platelet counts, blood clotting tests, and cultures can exclude these possibilities. The patient with septicemia usually appears more acutely ill. When gastrointestinal manifestations predominate, the syndrome may suggest a number of intra-abdominal emergencies or inflammatory bowel disease. The possibility of Henoch-Schönlein purpura should be considered in any child with acute abdominal pain, and inquiry made for associated rash, angioedema, arthritis, or nephritis. With prominent renal findings, acute glomerulonephritis may be suggested; other manifestations of Henoch-Schönlein vasculitis should allow differentiation. In children with chronic renal disease, a history of acute Henoch-Schönlein vasculitis should be sought. Differentiation from other rheumatic diseases is rarely difficult. In polyarteritis nodosa, peripheral neurologic changes and cardiac manifestations are more common, but differentiating the clinical manifestations from those of Henoch-Schönlein purpura may be difficult.

TREATMENT. There is no specific therapy. In the rare instance in which a specific allergen can be proved, the patient should avoid the antigen. When the disease follows a bacterial infection, particularly streptococcal illness, the organism should be eliminated and, if the disease recurs, prophylaxis considered. Symptomatic treatment is indicated for arthritis, rash, edema, fever, and malaise. Nonsteroidal anti-inflammatory drugs usually alleviate these self-limited discomforts.

Intestinal hemorrhage, obstruction, intussusception, or perforation may be life-threatening in the acute phase; these complications may be managed by the early use of corticosteroids. Therapy with prednisone, 1–2 mg/kg/24 hr, is often associated with dramatic improvement. Corticosteroid therapy is also indicated for the rare patient with central nervous system manifestations or with the nephrotic syndrome. Acute renal failure should be managed in the same way as acute glomerulonephritis (see Chapter 465). Therapy for severe nephritis with drugs such as corticosteroids, azathioprine, and cyclophosphamide remains experimental and rarely justified.

PROGNOSIS. Rarely, death may occur during the acute phase from gastrointestinal complications (e.g., hemorrhage, intussusception, bowel infarction), acute renal failure, or central nervous system involvement. Chronic renal disease may cause later morbidity in a few patients. About 25% of children with initial renal involvement have persistence of abnormal urine sediment for years; the ultimate prognosis for these patients appears to be good.

152.2 Kawasaki Disease

(Mucocutaneous Lymph Node Syndrome, Infantile Polyarteritis)

Kawasaki disease is a febrile condition affecting children and is notable for its association with vasculitis of the large coronary blood vessels and a constellation of other systemic complaints. First reported in Japanese children after the Second World War, it is similar to a rare condition previously called infantile polyarteritis. Kawasaki disease has surpassed rheumatic fever as the leading cause of acquired heart disease in children in the United States, has been recognized worldwide, and appears to be increasing in frequency. It occurs sporadically or in epidemic form. Children who are 5 yr of age or younger are primarily affected; the condition is recognized only rarely in adults. Although Kawasaki disease has been described in all racial groups, there appears to be a predilection for Japanese, and the condition seems to be rare in some geographic areas such as sub-Saharan Africa. There is no evidence for person-to-person transmission. The cause remains

■ **TABLE 152–2 Diagnostic Criteria for Kawasaki Disease**

A. Fever lasting for at least 5 days*
B. Presence of *four* of the *following five* conditions:
   1. Bilateral nonpurulent conjunctival injection
   2. Changes of the mucosa of the oropharynx, including infected pharynx, infected and/or dry fissured lips, strawberry tongue
   3. Changes of the peripheral extremities, such as edema and/or erythema of the hands or feet, desquamation, usually beginning periungually
   4. Rash, primarily truncal; polymorphous but nonvesicular
   5. Cervical lymphadenopathy
C. Illness not explained by other known disease process

A consensus statement prepared by North American participants of the Third International Kawasaki Disease Symposium, Tokyo, Japan, December, 1988. Pediatr Infect Dis J 8:663, 1989. © by Williams & Wilkins, 1989.

**Many experts believe that, in the presence of classic features, the diagnosis of Kawasaki disease can be made (and treatment instituted) before the 5th day of fever by experienced individuals.*

unknown, but bacterial toxins similar to the staphylococcal toxins of the toxic shock syndrome may be involved in its pathogenesis. Staphylococci and hemolytic streptococci producing such toxins have been cultured from children with Kawasaki disease in a preliminary study. Prior studies seeking a direct role for infectious agents such as retroviruses or rickettsiae in this condition have not been substantiated. There is no evidence that autoimmunity plays a role in pathogenesis; the finding of increased numbers of T-cell subsets (Vβ2-positive T cells) is consistent with toxin superantigen stimulation.

CLINICAL MANIFESTATIONS. Diagnosis rests on the demonstration of characteristic clinical signs (Table 152–2). Atypical cases manifesting few early signs but later characteristic coronary artery lesions have been reported. Atypical patients, often younger than 1 yr of age, may have incorrect admitting diagnoses (gastroenteritis, viral syndrome, sepsis), and a high morbidity rate.

Onset is generally abrupt, heralded by the onset of high sustained fever (generally greater than 104° F) which lasts for 1 wk or longer and is unresponsive to antibiotic therapy. Other characteristic findings include bilateral conjunctivitis without discharge, dry erythematous fissured lips, strawberry tongue (similar to that seen in streptococcal infections), and injected oral pharyngeal mucosa. Lymphadenopathy may affect one or several nodes, generally cervical, or rarely may be generalized; the nodes are nonsuppurative, can be large, and are usually nontender. Erythematous skin eruptions can affect the trunk, face, or extremities; the rash may take maculopapular, morbilliform, or erythema multiforme form. A nonspecific erythematous, desquamating perineal eruption is present in many patients during the 1st wk of illness. After several days of disease, the hands and feet become edematous, swollen, and painful; desquamation of skin from the fingertips, toetips, palms, and soles occurs, generally during the 2nd–3rd wk of illness (Table 152–3). Cutaneous desquamation may also involve other body areas.

Transient arthritis may occur, particularly in old [illegible] children;
painful joint swelling is usually symmetric in [illegible] ion and
may affect both large and small joints. Oth [illegible] ifesta-
tions include diarrhea, vomiting, abdo [illegible] ps of
the gallbladder, myositis, meatitis w [illegible] ni-
tis, ulcerative stomatitis, cough [illegible] with
pulmonary infiltrates), rhino [illegible] seizures,
cranial or peripheral ne [illegible] plenomegaly.
Iridocyclitis may be [illegible] ndergo slit-lamp
examination. Al [illegible] are irritable, and
many may h [illegible] Peripheral large arterial
aneurysm [illegible] evidence of distal vascular
compro [illegible] be noted on physical examination [illegible]

[illegible] s the most important manifestation of
[illegible] en to forty per cent of untreated children
[illegible] coronary vasculitis within the first weeks of
[illegible] ested by dilatation or aneurysm formation in
[illegible] arteries as seen by two-dimensional echocardiogra-
[illegible] is test should be performed in all children with known
[illegible] uspected Kawasaki disease at the time of presentation and again during the first 2 wk of disease. Clinical manifestations of coronary arteritis include signs of myocardial ischemia or rarely overt myocardial infarction or rupture of an aneurysm. Pericarditis, myocarditis, endocarditis, heart failure, and arrhythmias may also occur (see Table 152–3).

LABORATORY FINDINGS. There are no diagnostic tests. Leukocytosis with a predominance of immature forms and thrombocytosis (in the 2nd–3rd wk) can be striking; anemia is also common. Sedimentation rates and C-reactive protein levels are usually greatly elevated. Test results for autoantibodies including ANA and rheumatoid factors are negative, and hemolytic complement levels are normal or high. Mild proteinuria and pyuria may be present, as may cerebrospinal fluid pleocytosis. Serum levels of hepatic transaminases and bilirubin may be slightly elevated.

■ **TABLE 152–3 Kawasaki Disease: Phases, Complications, and Degree of Arteritis in Untreated Patients**

Feature	Acute	Subacute	Convalescent	Chronic
Duration	1–11 days	11–21 days	21–60 days	? yr
Clinical findings	Fever, conjunctivitis, oral changes, extremity changes, irritability, rash, cervical lymphadenopathy, high erythrocyte sedimentation rate	Irritability persists Prolongation of fever may occur Normalization of most clinical findings Palpable aneurysms may develop	Most clinical findings resolve Aneurysmal dilatation of peripheral vessels may persist Conjunctivitis may persist	
Complications	Early arthritis Myocarditis Pericarditis Mitral insufficiency Congestive heart failure Iridocyclitis Meningitis Sterile pyuria	Coronary aneurysms Late-onset arthritis Mitral insufficiency Gallbladder hydrops Fingertip and toe desquamation Thrombocytosis Coronary thrombosis with infarction	Arthritis may persist Coronary and peripheral aneurysms may persist Acute phase reactant normalization	Angina pectoris, coronary stenosis, or myocardial insufficiency may develop
Arterial correlates	Perivasculitis, vasculitis of capillaries, arterioles, venules Inflammation of intima of medium and large arteries	Aneurysms, thrombi, stenosis of medium-sized arteries, panvasculitis, edema of vessel wall Myocarditis less prominent	Vascular inflammation decreases	Scar formation Intimal thickening
Cause of death	Myocarditis	Myocardial infarction Rupture of aneurysm Myocarditis	Myocardial infarction Ischemic heart disease	Myocardial infarction

Modified from Hicks RV, Melish ME: Kawasaki syndrome. Pediatr Clin North Am 33:1151, 1986.

Cardiac studies in the form of chest roentgenograms, electrocardiograms, and echocardiograms are vital for the initial evaluation of all patients; of these, two-dimensional echocardiography is most useful for recognizing coronary vascular disease and revealing coronary vascular dilatation or aneurysm formation. This study should be done initially and in follow-up of all patients. Arteriography of coronary vessels may also reveal lesions in patients with Kawasaki disease, but this invasive procedure is not routinely needed. Occasionally, arteriography of larger central vessels may be warranted by the clinical findings.

Histologic changes at autopsy of patients with fatal lesions include intense inflammatory cell infiltrates of the media and intima of large coronary vessels and other central vessels and arterial obstruction by platelet thrombi. These changes closely resemble those of a rare condition previously called infantile periarteritis nodosa.

DIAGNOSIS. Diagnosis rests on the clinical features. There are no diagnostic laboratory tests, although demonstration of coronary artery involvement revealed by echocardiography is highly suggestive of this condition. The disease manifestations and diagnosis depend on the phase of Kawasaki disease (see Table 152–3). The differential diagnosis includes scarlet fever, toxic shock syndrome, leptospirosis, Epstein-Barr virus infection, juvenile rheumatoid arthritis, measles, acrodynia, Rocky Mountain spotted fever, drug reactions, Stevens-Johnson syndrome, and other vasculitic syndromes.

PROGNOSIS. Recovery is usually complete in patients who do not have detectable coronary vasculitis; second attacks occur only rarely. Most children with demonstrable cardiac involvement also appear to do well, although their long-term prognosis is unknown. In the early Japanese series, 1–2% of all children with Kawasaki disease died of cardiac complications, usually within 1–2 mo of onset. A few reports detail the later occurrence of aneurysms of large vessels other than the coronary arteries.

TREATMENT. Kawasaki disease responds dramatically to therapy with intravenous gamma globulin given during the period of active febrile disease. Fever and other attendant systemic manifestations often abate within 24 hr of initial therapy. Furthermore, controlled studies show that intravenous gamma globulin therapy given early in disease prevents coronary vascular involvement, as demonstrable by echocardiography. The recommended regimen consists of an intravenous infusion of 2 g/kg given as a single dose over 10–12 hr. Therapy given within 10 days of onset appears to be effective in preventing coronary vascular damage; therapy given to symptomatic patients (febrile, high ESR) after 10 days of onset of manifestations may also be effective in providing symptomatic relief. Side effects of intravenous gamma globulin therapy are rare and include anaphylaxis, chills, fever, headache, and myalgia.

Salicylate therapy is also indicated during the febrile phase of the disease; therapeutic serum concentrations of 20–30 mg/dL are desirable but may be difficult to achieve, even with doses of salicylates as high as 100 mg/kg/24 hr. Continuance of low, single-dose (5 mg/kg/24 hr) salicylate therapy for its antithrombotic (antiplatelet) effects has been advocated for 6–8 wk after the period of active disease subsides. Low-dose aspirin with or without dipyridamole should be continued until coronary lesions resolve. Some authorities add heparin or warfarin (Coumadin) therapy for patients with persistent large or multiple nonobstructive or obstructive aneurysms. Careful and repeated follow-up evaluations with stress testing, echocardiography, and at times angiography are warranted for children with significant residual coronary vascular changes. The impact of such coronary vascular changes on the incidence and severity of atherosclerotic coronary artery disease in later life is unknown.

Corticosteroid therapy is rarely used in Kawasaki disease, and some consider it contraindicated.

Thrombolytic therapy with agents such as streptokinase has been used for patients with active coronary thrombosis or peripheral artery ischemia. Arterial bypass surgery may be appropriate for rare patients with severe coronary occlusions.

152.3 Rare Forms of Vasculitis

POLYARTERITIS NODOSA

Medium-sized and small arteries are the sites of inflammation in polyarteritis nodosa. This necrotizing vasculitis is rare in childhood; males are affected more frequently than females. The cause is unknown, but the disease has been reported to follow drug exposure and occur in association with streptococcal infections, serous otitis media, and hepatitis B infection.

Inflammation with polymorphonuclear leukocytes, eosinophils, and round cells may involve the entire vessel wall. Necrosis, thrombosis, or aneurysm formation may occur in affected vessels and result in infarction. Healed vessels become scarred or recanalized.

CLINICAL MANIFESTATIONS. The manifestations are diverse and depend on the sites of vascular involvement. Signs of systemic illness such as fever, anorexia, lethargy, weakness, and weight loss may be prominent. Various cutaneous manifestations are common and include erythematous rashes, nodular lesions, petechiae, purpura, livido reticularis, cutaneous ulcers, and edema. Some children have a limited form of polyarteritis with nodular subcutaneous lesions, fever, malaise, and arthritis or arthralgia, but they have little or no additional systemic involvement. Full-blown polyarteritis nodosa also occurs in children. Arthritis and arthralgia are common and myalgia and myositis also may occur. Rarely, gangrene of the extremities occurs. Peripheral neuropathy (symmetric-distal or mononeuritis multiplex), with pain, numbness, paresthesias, and muscle weakness results from involvement of the peripheral nerves adjacent to affected vessels. Abdominal pain, bleeding, ulcerations, and infarction can follow involvement of the gastrointestinal vessels. Renal involvement may result in renal failure and death. Involvement of large renal vessels results in flank pain and gross hematuria, and that of small vessels and glomeruli results in microscopic hematuria, proteinuria, and cylindruria. Associated hypertension is usual. Inflammation of pulmonary vessels may cause cough, wheezing, pulmonary infiltrates, and pleuritis. Central nervous system manifestations include seizures, encephalitic symptoms, and stroke. Cranial nerve palsies and iridocyclitis may occur. Involvement of coronary vessels may produce tachycardia, heart failure, and myocardial infarction; pericarditis may also be present. Orchitis and epididymitis are common.

LABORATORY FINDINGS. There are no specific laboratory tests. The ESR may be elevated, and acute phase reactants may be present. Anemia is common; eosinophilia and leukocytosis are sometimes found. There may be gross or microscopic hematuria, and renal function studies may be abnormal. ANA and rheumatoid factors are absent.

DIAGNOSIS. Polyarteritis nodosa is readily confused with many other diseases. Differentiation from other rheumatic diseases may be particularly difficult. The diagnosis is based primarily on clinical suspicion and on the presence of histologic changes in involved tissues on biopsy. Muscle, nerve, or skin biopsies may fail to identify vasculitis. Testicular biopsies are said to be helpful but are seldom done. Mesenteric or renal arteriography may reveal arteritis and aneurysms; these are rarely seen in systemic lupus erythematosus.

PROGNOSIS. Full-blown polyarteritis can be a severe, potentially fatal disease, with death resulting from renal failure, heart failure, or severe gastrointestinal or central nervous system involvement. Nodular subcutaneous vasculitis without involvement of major organ systems has a better prognosis.

TREATMENT. Corticosteroids (1–2 mg/kg/24 hr) may suppress acute manifestations and lengthen survival. Cytotoxic agents such as oral or intravenous cyclophosphamide may be effective adjunctive agents.

WEGENER GRANULOMATOSIS

(Lethal Midline Granuloma)

In this rare syndrome, destructive granulomatous lesions of the upper respiratory tract and lungs are associated with a systemic necrotizing vasculitis that is most prominent in the lungs and kidneys. Upper respiratory and pulmonary granulomas may predominate in some cases, antedating recognition of systemic vasculitis by years. Males are predominantly affected (2:1). The cause is unknown; as in other vasculitis syndromes, an association with drug sensitivity, allergy, and parvovirus infection has been suggested.

Respiratory symptoms are prominent *clinical manifestations.* Persistent nasal stuffiness or discharge may be an early symptom, with crusted or pustular lesions in the nares. Lesions are progressively destructive and may result in perforation of the nasal septum, obliteration of the nasal sinuses, and ulcerations of the palate, pharynx, larynx, and trachea. Cough or hemoptysis may occur; fever, weight loss, night sweats, and prostration are common. Other frequently associated manifestations include arthritis, neuropathy, rash, splenomegaly, and severe progressive glomerulitis, often terminating in renal failure. In cases with clinically inapparent systemic involvement, diffuse vasculitis may be found on postmortem examination.

There are no specific laboratory manifestations; eosinophilia may be present. Serum antineutrophil cytoplasmic antibodies (ANCA) are often positive. Roentgenograms may reveal bone destruction in the nose and sinuses and pulmonary infiltrates suggestive of tuberculosis or neoplasm. Urinalyses usually show evidence of nephritis, and renal function studies may be abnormal.

Diagnosis is based on the clinical picture and serologic tests and is confirmed by histologic demonstration of granulomatous lesions of the respiratory tract and systemic vasculitis, particularly nephritis. The differential diagnosis includes other vasculitis syndromes, lymphoma, local or disseminated fungal infections, tuberculosis, allergic alveolitis, and Goodpasture syndrome.

Without therapy, the *prognosis* is poor. Patients with limited forms of the disease may survive for long periods, but the destructive lesions of the upper respiratory tract may be disfiguring.

Treatment with corticosteroids may suppress systemic vasculitis and prevent progression of destructive lesions in the upper respiratory tract. Cyclophosphamide appears to be effective in the management of severe disease. Some patients improve while treated with trimethoprim-sulfamethoxazole.

TAKAYASU ARTERITIS

(Pulseless Disease)

This uncommon condition, an inflammatory process involving the aorta and its major branches, occurs primarily in young women. Some cases have been reported in late childhood, a few in infants. Most reported patients are from Asia or Africa. The cause is unknown; associated congenital defects of the great vessels have been recorded.

The underlying pathology is a segmented panarteritis of the aorta and its major branches. Smaller vessels are generally spared. Aneurysmal dilatation and rupture may occur. Involvement of the great vessels can cause weak or absent pulses in the upper extremities, hence, the term "pulseless disease." Blood pressure in the legs may exceed that in the arms ("reverse coarctation"), in contrast to the situation seen in coarctation of the aorta. Renal arterial involvement may cause renal ischemia, resulting in hypertension. Decreased brain blood flow can result in neurologic disturbances. Visual disturbances are common.

Associated rheumatic complaints include arthritis, myalgia, pleuritis, pericarditis, fever, and rashes, sometimes antedating symptomatic aortitis by years. There are no specific laboratory data. ESR and gamma globulin levels may be elevated. Appropriate angiographic studies will demonstrate changes in affected vessels.

The condition should be considered in any child with obscure hypertension, particularly when fever and an elevated ESR are associated. The prognosis varies. Some adults have survived; most children have died. Therapy with corticosteroids and cytotoxic agents has been tried. Endarterectomy may be warranted.

HENOCH-SCHÖNLEIN VASCULITIS

Allen DM, Dismond LK, Howell DA: Anaphylactoid purpura in children (Schönlein-Henoch syndrome): Review with follow up of renal complications. Am J Dis Child 99:147, 1960.

Farley TA, Gillespie S, Rasoulpour M, et al: Epidemiology of a cluster of Henoch-Schönlein purpura. Am J Dis Child 143:798, 1989.

Ostergaard JR, Storm K: Neurologic manifestations of Schönlein-Henoch purpura. Acta Paediatr 80:339, 1991.

Rosenblum N, Winter H: Steroid effects on the course of abdominal pain in children with Schönlein-Henoch purpura. Pediatrics 79:1018, 1987.

Saulsbury FT: The role of IgA1 rheumatoid factor in the formation of IgA containing immune complexes in Schönlein-Henoch purpura. J Clin Lab Immunol 23:123, 1987.

KAWASAKI DISEASE

American Heart Association Committee on Rheumatic Fever and Kawasaki Disease: Diagnostic guidelines for Kawasaki disease. Am J Dis Child 144:1218, 1990.

Burns JC, Wiggins JW, Toews WH, et al: Clinical spectrum of Kawasaki disease in infants younger than six months of age. J Pediatr 109:759, 1986.

Dajani AS, Taubert KA, Takahashi M, et al: Guidelines for long-term management of patients with Kawasaki disease. Circulation 89:916, 1994.

Kartow H, Ichinose E, Kawasaki T: Myocardial infarction in Kawasaki disease: Clinical analysis of 195 cases. J Pediatr 108:923, 1986.

Kawasaki T, Kosaki F, Okawa S, et al: A new infantile acute febrile mucocutaneous lymph node syndrome (MLNS): Prevalence in Japan. Pediatrics 54:271, 1974.

Klassen TP, Rowe PC, Gafni A: Economic evaluation of intravenous immune globulin therapy for Kawasaki syndrome. J Pediatr 122:538, 1992.

Leung DYM, Meissner HC, Fulton DR, et al: Toxic shock syndrome toxin secreting *Staphylococcus aureus* in Kawasaki syndrome. Lancet 342:1385, 1993.

Levy M, Korean G: Atypical Kawasaki disease: Analysis of clinical presentation and diagnostic clues. Pediatr Infect Dis J 9:122, 1990.

Newburger JW, Takahashi M, Beiser A, et al: A single intravenous infusion of gamma globulin as compared with four infusions in the treatment of acute Kawasaki syndrome. N Engl J Med 324:1633, 1991.

Pelkonen P, Salo E: Epidemiology of Kawasaki disease. Clin Exp Rheumatol 12(Suppl 10):S83, 1994.

Rowley AH, Gonzalez-Crussi F, Gidding SS, et al: Incomplete Kawasaki disease with coronary artery involvement. J Pediatr 110:409, 1987.

Shulman ST, Bass JL, Bierman F, et al: Management of Kawasaki syndrome: A consensus statement prepared by North American participants of the Third International Kawasaki Disease Symposium, Tokyo, Japan, December 1988. Pediatr Infect Dis J 8:663, 1989.

Special Writing Group of the Committee on Rheumatic Fever, Endocarditis, and Kawasaki Disease of the Council on Cardiovascular Disease in the Young of the American Heart Association: Guidelines for the diagnosis of rheumatic fever: Jones criteria [1992 update]. JAMA 268:2069, 1992.

Suzuki A, Kamiya T, Arakaki Y, et al: Fate of coronary arterial aneurysms in Kawasaki disease. Am J Cardiol 74:822, 1994.

POLYARTERITIS NODOSA

David J, Ansell BM, Woo P: Polyarteritis nodosa associated with *Streptococcus.* Arch Dis Child 69:685, 1993.

Fink CW: Vasculitis. Pediatr Clin North Am 33:1203, 1986.

Ozen S, Besbas N, Saatci U, Bakkaloglu A: Diagnostic criteria for polyarteritis nodosa in childhood. J Pediatr 120:206, 1992.

WEGENER GRANULOMATOSIS

Falk RJ, Jennette SC: Antineutrophil cytoplasmic autoantibodies with specificity for myeloperoxidase in patients with systemic vasculitis and idiopathic necrotizing and crescentic glomerulonephritis. N Engl J Med 318:1652, 1988.

Nolle B, Specks U, Ludermann J, et al: Anticytoplasmic autoantibodies: Their immunodiagnostic value in Wegener's granulomatosis. Ann Intern Med 111:28, 1989.

Siberry GK, Cohen BA, Johnson B: Cutaneous polyarteritis nodosa. Report of two cases in children and review of the literature. Arch Dermatol 130:884, 1994.

Rottem M, Fauci AS, Hallahan CW, et al: Wegener's granulomatosis in children and adolescents: Clinical presentation and outcome. J Pediatr 122:26, 1993.

TAKAYASU ARTERITIS

Arend WP, Michel BA, Blaoch DA, et al: The American College of Rheumatology 1990 criteria for the classification of Takayasu arteritis. Arthritis Rheum 33:1129, 1990.

Danaraj TJ, Wong HO, Thomas MA: Primary arteritis of the aorta causing renal artery stenosis and hypertension. Br Heart J 25:153, 1986.

Kerr GS, Hallahan CW, Giordano J, et al: Takayasu arteritis. Ann Intern Med 120:919, 1994.

CHAPTER 153
Dermatomyositis

Jane Green Schaller

This multisystem disease is characterized principally by nonsuppurative inflammation of striated muscle and distinctive cutaneous lesions.

ETIOLOGY AND EPIDEMIOLOGY. The cause of dermatomyositis is unknown. Cellular immune mechanisms may play a basic role in the pathogenesis. Lymphocytes from patients with dermatomyositis release lymphotoxins that kill muscle cells in tissue culture. Immunoglobulin and complement deposition also occur in blood vessels in affected muscle. In adults, but only rarely in children, the disease is associated with malignancies (in 20% of patients). Childhood dermatomyositis is associated with HLA-B8/DR3. Research endeavors continue to seek a link with a viral infection, notably Coxsackie virus.

Dermatomyositis is less common than rheumatoid arthritis, systemic lupus erythematosus (SLE), or Henoch-Schönlein purpura. It rarely begins before the 2nd birthday; the average age at onset is 8–9 yr. Girls are affected more frequently than boys (3:2), and there is no familial or racial predilection.

PATHOLOGY. Lesions in the skin, subcutaneous tissues, gastrointestinal tract, and striated muscles are irregularly distributed; care must be taken to choose an involved site if biopsies are done. The most prominent lesion in children is an occlusive vasculitis involving arterioles, venules, and capillaries in the connective tissues of the skin, nailbed, subcutaneous tissue, and muscle. In muscle, patchy degeneration, atrophy and regeneration of muscle fibers, interstitial edema, and proliferation of connective tissue occur. In affected skin, thinning of the epidermis and edema and vasculitis of the dermis are apparent. Gastrointestinal tract vasculitis may produce mucosal ulcerations and tissue infarction. Mild renal glomerular changes have also been described.

CLINICAL MANIFESTATIONS. The onset is usually insidious, with slowly developing muscle weakness, generally apparent first in the proximal muscles of the extremities and trunk. The child may develop an awkward gait and slowly lose the capacity to perform functions such as climbing stairs, rising from the floor, riding a bicycle, combing hair, and dressing. Weakness can be elicited by observing the child's inability to raise the head when lying supine (weak neck flexors) or to do a sit-up (weak abdominals) or to rise unassisted from the floor (Gower sign; see Chapter 541). Affected muscles tend to be stiff and sore and sometimes brawny, indurated, and tender. Nonpitting edema and thickening of the skin and subcutaneous tissues may be present. Although myositis is generally most pronounced in the proximal muscles, any muscles can be affected, with varying sites and degrees of atrophy or contracture formation. Severe involvement of palatorespiratory muscles may lead to respiratory difficulty, nasal regurgitation, nasal voice, aspiration, and death. Involvement of the respiratory muscles may produce hypoventilation. Cardiac involvement with conduction defects or myocarditis has been reported.

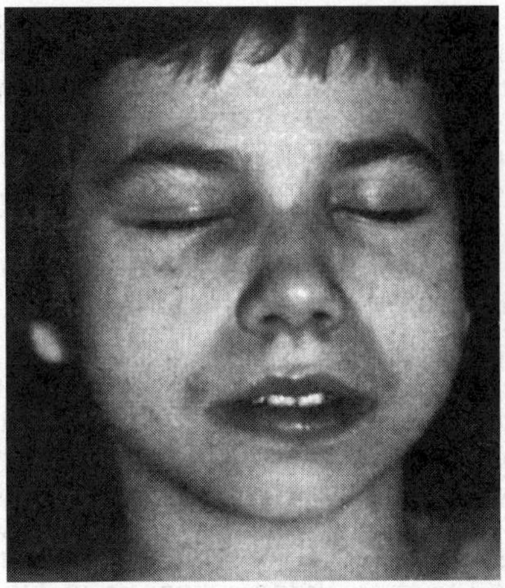

Figure 153–1. The facial rash of dermatomyositis. Notice the faint erythema over the bridge of the nose and malar areas and the heliotropic discoloration of the upper eyelids. See also color section.

The skin lesions are characteristic and often have a distinctive violaceous (heliotrope) erythema. The upper eyelids assume a pathognomonic violaceous discoloration (heliotrope eyelids) (Fig. 153–1 [color plate section]). Periorbital and facial edema may be associated. A butterfly rash similar to that of SLE may be present. Lesions of the palatal and nasal mucous membranes may be associated with the malar rash. The skin over the extensor surfaces of the joints, particularly the knuckles (Gottron papules), knees, elbows, and medial malleoli, becomes erythematous, atrophic, and scaly (Fig. 153–2). These areas later develop pigmentary changes resulting in hyperpigmentation or vitiligo. The capillaries of the nailbed, as seen by capillary microscopy, may become tortuous or occluded. A dusky erythema may cover the upper trunk and proximal extremities. Other nonspecific skin changes also may occur. The skin over the involved extremities may appear tight and glossy; in longstanding disease there may be cutaneous atrophy with binding of the skin to the underlying structures.

Calcium may be deposited in affected subcutaneous tissues, muscles, and fascia; these deposits sometimes break down and are extruded in semisolid or solid form. This calcinosis occurs in 20–50% of children; those with a slowly progressive course

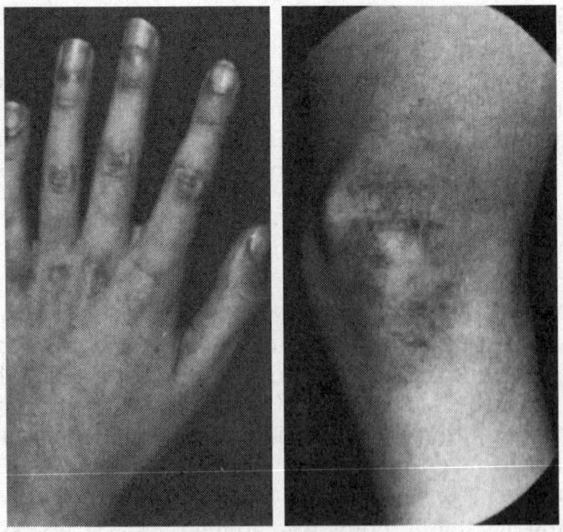

Figure 153–2. Rash of dermatomyositis. Notice the skin changes over the knuckles *(left)* and over the knee *(right)*. See also color section.

are the most susceptible. Calcium deposits may cause contractures, focal atrophy of muscle, and poorly healing ulcers.

Gastrointestinal involvement may occur at any level, heralded by difficulty with swallowing, abdominal pain, perforation, melena, or constipation. Low-grade fever may be present. Arthritis or other evidence of systemic involvement such as lymphadenopathy and hepatosplenomegaly may occur. Pulmonary disease (interstitial, hemorrhagic, or pleuritic), ocular involvement (iritis, retinitis), and central nervous system manifestations (seizures) are rare concomitants of disease.

LABORATORY FINDINGS. Muscle inflammation is usually associated with elevated serum levels of such enzymes as transaminases (SGOT), creatine kinase (CPK), aldolase, and lactate dehydrogenase (LDH). The electromyogram of affected muscles is abnormal, showing a combination of myopathic and neuropathic changes. Motor and sensory nerve conduction is normal. MRI may be useful for visualizing affected muscle groups. The erythrocyte sedimentation rate may be elevated or normal. Tests for rheumatoid factors are generally negative; antinuclear antibodies may be present, usually in low titers. A number of so-called myositis-specific autoantibodies have now been described; these are not very usefulness in clinical medicine but may be of interest in understanding classification of disease. Urinalyses are usually normal. In patients with gastrointestinal involvement, there may be gross or occult blood in the stool. Roentgenograms may reveal calcium deposits in soft tissues.

DIAGNOSIS AND DIFFERENTIAL DIAGNOSIS. In its typical form dermatomyositis should present little diagnostic difficulty. The combination of proximal and axial muscle weakness, characteristic rash, elevated serum levels of enzymes, and abnormal findings on electromyography or MRI is diagnostic; muscle biopsy with evidence of vasculopathy and ischemic myopathy is helpful but is usually unnecessary. In the differential diagnosis, various neuromuscular disorders such as poliomyelitis, Guillain-Barré syndrome, muscular dystrophy, myasthenia gravis, and endocrine or metabolic myopathies should be considered, as should illnesses characterized by predominantly muscular lesions, such as trichinosis or toxoplasmosis. Transient rhabdomyolysis with myoglobinuria should be considered, as well as acute myositis, which has been associated with influenza virus and may occur with other viral infections. SLE, mixed connective tissue disease, juvenile rheumatoid arthritis, and scleroderma are distinguishable clinically and by laboratory tests. When the onset is insidious, a period of observation may be needed to establish the diagnosis.

TREATMENT. During the acute phase, accurate evaluation and management of palatorespiratory function and respiratory muscle status may be lifesaving. If the swallowing mechanism is impaired, soft or liquid diets should be provided under close observation. Patients must be carefully watched for possible deterioration in respiratory function with pulmonary function tests. Constant nursing care is mandatory for any child with palatorespiratory involvement, and equipment for nasopharyngeal suction, endotracheal intubation, and tracheostomy should be available. A respirator may be required. The possibility of serious gastrointestinal manifestations during the acute phase of disease must also be considered.

Functional recovery depends on the preservation of adequate muscle strength and the prevention of crippling contractures. Corticosteroids effectively suppress the inflammatory process in most patients. Serial serum levels of SGOT, CPK, or aldolase provide a helpful gauge of activity and therapeutic response. Prednisone in an initial dosage of 1–2 mg/kg/24 hr (or 60 mg/m^2 of body surface area/24 hr) usually reduces enzyme levels toward normal values within 1–2 wk; clinical improvement with decreased pain and swelling in muscles and increasing muscle strength usually follows. Initial therapy with high-dose intravenous steroid pulses has been advocated by some. When enzyme levels have declined to normal, the steroid dosage should be slowly decreased while maintaining continuous monitoring of the clinical course and serum enzyme levels. If the steroid dosage is reduced too rapidly, rebound in enzyme levels may occur; such rebounds are followed by deterioration in the clinical condition within a few weeks unless the corticosteroid dosage is promptly increased. The lowest dose of steroids sufficient to suppress clinical symptoms and serum enzyme levels should be found and maintained for months. Steroid therapy can generally be discontinued after 2 yr. Steroid preparations such as triamcinolone and dexamethasone, which have been associated with "steroid myopathy," should be avoided. For patients who do not respond to steroids, adjunctive agents such as methotrexate, azathioprine, or cyclosporine may be beneficial. Some success has been reported with intravenous immunoglobulin therapy.

Physical therapy is essential to avoid contractures and to rebuild muscle strength. During the acute phase when muscle weakness is pronounced, passive exercises can be used to maintain range of motion. With clinical improvement active exercises to strengthen muscles should be added. Splints to maintain good limb position may be needed. Bed rest is not necessary, and immobilization without exercise should be avoided at all times. Skin hygiene, especially around the neck, skin creases, and axillae, is important.

PROGNOSIS. The course of dermatomyositis can be favorably modified by early vigorous control of the disease, and the prognosis in adequately treated children is good. For untreated patients, the mortality rate is about 40%. Most deaths are related to palatorespiratory involvement or gastrointestinal complications such as hemorrhage or perforation and occur within 2 yr of onset. Otherwise, the disease usually becomes inactive over a period of several years. Infrequently, the disease may smolder for years. Most surviving patients are able to lead active lives, although they may have residual abnormalities. A few have severe contractures and crippling deformities. Severe calcinosis can be particularly disabling; there is no satisfactory therapy. Surgical excision of calcium lesions may provide some relief. The occurrence of lipodystrophy with insulin resistance and hyperandrogenism has been recognized as a late complication of dermatomyositis.

Bowyer SL, Blane CE, Sullivan DB, Cassidy JT: Childhood dermatomyositis: Factors predicting functional outcome and development of dystrophic calcification. J Pediatr 103:882, 1983.

Dalakas M, Illa I, Dambrosia J, et al: A controlled trial of high dose intravenous immune globulin infusions as treatment for dermatomyositis. N Engl J Med 329:1993, 1993.

Love LA, Leff RL, Fraser DD, et al: A new approach to the classification of idiopathic inflammatory myopathy: myositis-specific antoantibodies define useful homogeneous patient groups. Medicine 70:360, 1991.

Miller LC, Sisson BA, Tucker LB, et al: Methotrexate treatment of recalcitrant childhood dermatomyositis. Arthritis Rheum 35:1143, 1992.

Pachman LM: Inflammatory myopathy in children. Rheum Dis Clin North Am, 919, 1994.

Plotz P: Current concepts in the idiopathic inflammatory myopathies: Polymyositis, dermatomyositis, and related disorders. Ann Intern Med 111:143, 1989.

Reed AM, Pachman LM, Ober C: Molecular genetic studies of major histocompatibility complex genes in children with juvenile dermatomyositis: increased risk associated with HLA-DQA1*0501. Hum Immunol 32:235, 1991.

Tucker LB, Sadeghi-Nejad A, Schaller JG: The association of acquired generalized lipodystrophy with juvenile dermatomyositis. Arthritis Rheum 1994.

CHAPTER 154

Scleroderma

Jane Green Schaller

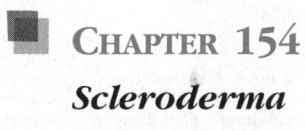

Scleroderma ("hard skin"), a chronic fibrotic disturbance of connective tissue, classically involves skin but may also affect the gastrointestinal tract, heart, lung, kidney, and synovium. Cutaneous involvement may occur in focal patches *(morphea)*, in a linear distribution *(linear scleroderma)*, or in a generalized, symmetric distribution. The latter form is usually associated with systemic involvement *(systemic sclerosis)* and is the usual adult form. Scleroderma in children usually takes the form of morphea or linear scleroderma; systemic sclerosis is uncommon (Table 154–1).

ETIOLOGY AND EPIDEMIOLOGY. The disease is rare, may begin at any time during childhood, and is subject to unpredictable slow progression or remission. Girls are affected more often than boys. There is no known familial predisposition. The etiology is not known. The histopathology of systemic sclerosis is notable for fibrosis of affected tissues, relatively little inflammatory response, and occlusive vasculitis affecting capillaries and small blood vessels.

CLINICAL MANIFESTATIONS. Morphea and Linear Scleroderma. The first signs are patchy lesions of skin and subcutaneous tissues. These often have a linear pattern similar to the distribution of peripheral nerves and may occur primarily on one side of the body. During the early phases, involved areas are slightly erythematous and edematous or have an atrophic, shiny appearance. The child may complain of pain or a prickly sensation. As the disease progresses, the skin lesions become indurated with violaceous, sometimes elevated borders and pale, waxy-appearing centers. Lesions enlarge peripherally and may coalesce to involve an entire extremity or a large portion of the body. Extensive scarring and fibrosis of the involved area can occur with firm binding of cutaneous tissues to underlying structures ("hide-binding"). This may be severe enough to limit growth of the affected part and produce crippling contractures (Fig. 154–1). Chronically involved areas may be hyperpigmented or depigmented. Active disease may be arrested over a period of months to years or may smolder. Prognosis for life is good in the absence of systemic involvement.

Systemic Sclerosis. This systemic form of scleroderma usually is associated with Raynaud phenomenon; Raynaud phenomenon is often the first manifestation of disease (see Chapter 157.2). Cutaneous involvement is symmetric and includes the hands, feet, and sometimes the trunk and face as well. Induration, pigmentary changes, telangiectasia, and hide-binding of involved cutaneous tissues occur as with focal forms of the disease. Cutaneous ulcers may affect the fingertips or other areas on the limbs. Synovitis, particularly about the small hand joints, may mimic rheumatoid arthritis; tenosynovitis and nodules may occur about tendon sheaths. The disease may involve the gastrointestinal tract, heart, lungs, and kidneys. Systemic manifestations, particularly renal, cardiac, and pulmonary lesions, may be fatal. Esophageal dysfunction may result in chronic aspiration pneumonia. Severe hypertension may occur.

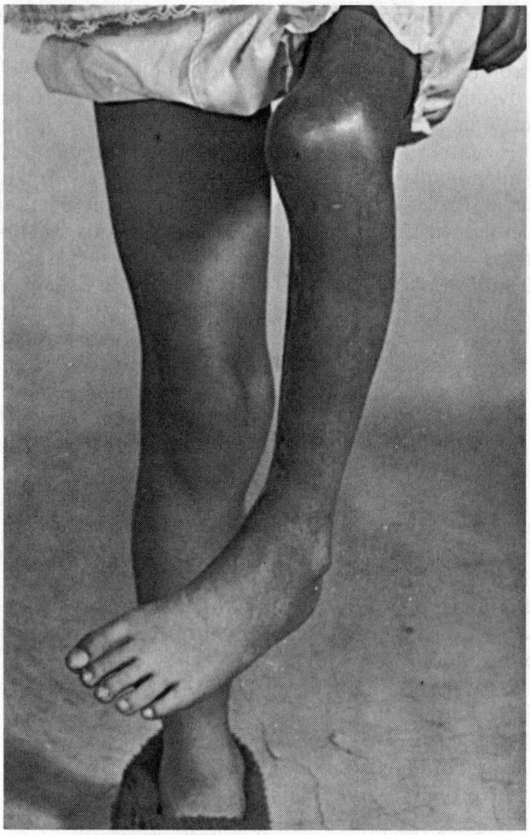

Figure 154–1. Extensive morphea involves the entire left leg, causing scarring, shortening, and flexion contractures. Notice the shiny appearance and patches of hyperpigmentation and vitiligo of affected skin.

LABORATORY FINDINGS. There are no specific laboratory tests. The erythrocyte sedimentation rate is frequently normal. Rheumatoid factors and antinuclear antibodies may be found in both focal and systemic forms of the disease. Roentgenography may show dysfunction of esophageal and bowel motility and erosion of the distal phalanges. Pulmonary function studies, electrocardiograms, and chest roentgenograms may disclose cardiopulmonary involvement. Urinalyses and renal function study results are abnormal in cases of renal involvement.

■ **TABLE 154–1 Scleroderma in Children**

Characteristic	Focal Scleroderma	Systemic Sclerosis	Fasciitis
Sex	Girls > boys	Girls > boys	No prediction
Age at onset	2 yr or older	4 yr or older	4 yr or older
Clinical manifestations	Cutaneous fibrosis; patchy (morphea) or linear (scleroderma); no systemic involvement or Raynaud phenomenon	Raynaud phenomenon Diffuse cutaneous fibrosis: extremities, face, trunk; arthritis; fibrosis of internal organs: heart, lungs, kidneys, gastrointestinal tract; hypertension; cardiopulmonary failure	Pain, inflammation of fascia, particularly in limbs Joint contractures in hands and others; little or no systemic disease
Laboratory characteristics	May have ANA, RF, increased immunoglobulins	May have ANA, RF, increased immunoglobulins; capillary nailbed changes; cutaneous and systemic fibrosis	Negative ANA, RF; eosinophilia: blood or tissue
Diagnosis	Clinical, biopsy	Clinical	Clinical, fascial biopsy
Natural history	May progress or remit; occasionally crippling	May progress or remit May be fatal	May progress or remit; associated with focal scleroderma
Therapy	Uncertain: topical steroid, penicillamine	Uncertain Penicillamine Cytotoxic Control of blood pressure	Corticosteroids, physical therapy

ANA = antinuclear antibody; RF = rheumatoid factor.

DIAGNOSIS AND DIFFERENTIAL DIAGNOSIS. The clinical picture is characteristic in both morphea and progressive systemic sclerosis. Eosinophilic fasciitis may be difficult to distinguish; localization of involvement to the fascial layers with relative sparing of the skin, prominent eosinophilia, and absence of Raynaud phenomenon serves to differentiate the two conditions. However, fasciitis and cutaneous scleroderma are associated in some patients and may represent overlapping conditions.

Scleroderma may bear some superficial resemblance to dermatomyositis, but the absence of severe myositis and the characteristic rash of dermatomyositis should allow differentiation. Subcutaneous fat necrosis and Weber-Christian nonsuppurative panniculitis may suggest morphea, but the course and histology are distinctive. *Scleredema adultorum* (
self-limited benign induration of subcutaneous
acutely, sometimes following streptococcal infe
neous tissues of the neck, upper trunk, and
indurated, but the skin is spared. Several syndrc
environmental events that resemble sclerodern
described, including ingestion of manufacture
(eosinophilia-myalgia syndrome), ingestion of
cooking oil (toxic oil syndrome), exposure to s
graft-versus-host disease following bone marrow
tion (see Table 154–1).

TREATMENT. No specific therapy is known. Many
agents, including corticosteroids, salicylates, chela
chloroquine, radiation, dimethyl sulfoxide, para-ar
acid, penicillamine, and immunosuppressive drugs,
tried without clear-cut benefit. Systemic therapy w
lamine or cytotoxic drugs may be tried for sever
disease. Corticosteroids may be beneficial during acu
tous phases of the disease but are of no benefit for t
manifestations of scleroderma and may complicate t
by exacerbating hypertension. Meticulous control of
sion with agents such as captopril is vital. Topical c
roids may be used for cutaneous lesions. Excision
patches of morphea does not arrest the process. Vigorc
ical therapy is important early in the course of cu
scleroderma to prevent or minimize crippling cont
Avoidance of cold and initiation of therapy for Rayna
nomenon with biofeedback techniques or drugs such a
pine are essential. Good supportive care is needed to
the organ-specific dysfunctions.

Ansell BM, Falcini F, Woo P: Scleroderma in childhood. Clin Dermatol 12:299, 1994.
Black CM: Scleroderma and fasciitis. Curr Opin Rheumatol, in press.
Buckley SL, Skinner S, James P, Ashley RK: Focal scleroderma in children: An orthopaedic perspective. J Pediatr Orthop 13:784, 1993.
Martinez-Cordero E, Fonseca M, Aguilar Leon DE, Padilla A: Juvenile systemic sclerosis. J Rheumatol 20:405, 1993.
Spencer-Green G, Schlesinger M, Bove KE, et al: Nailfold capillary abnormalities in childhood rheumatic diseases. J Pediatr 102:341, 1983.
Suarez-Almazor ME, Cataggio LJ, Maldonado-Cocco JA, Garcia-Morteo O: Juvenile progressive systemic sclerosis: Clinical and serologic findings. Arthritis Rheum 28:699, 1985.

CHAPTER 155

Mixed Connective Tissue Disease

Jane Green Schaller

Mixed connective tissue disease (overlap syndrome) is a syndrome that combines the features of systemic lupus erythematosus (SLE), rheumatoid arthritis, dermatomyositis, and scleroderma. It is characterized by high serum titers of speckled antinuclear antigens (to extractable nuclear antigen) and antibody to ribonucleoprotein (RNP). The syndrome affects girls, usually those older than 6 yr of age. Clinical manifestations include arthritis, scleroderma-like skin changes, Raynaud phenomenon, fever, cardiac involvement (particularly pericarditis), rashes suggestive of SLE or dermatomyositis, myositis, esophageal abnormalities, lymphadenopathy, hepatosplenomegaly, pulmonary disease, and thrombocytopenia. Renal disease occurs in some patients, and neurologic abnormalities and parotitis have also been described.

The diagnosis is made over a period of time by recognizing the overlapping clinical symptoms and by demonstrating serum antibodies to RNP.

Initially, this syndrome was thought to have a better prognosis than SLE and to be responsive to corticosteroid therapy. Although corticosteroid therapy does produce symptomatic improvement in many patients and life-threatening disease manifestations are perhaps not as common as in SLE, mixed connective tissue disease may cause severe morbidity. The ultimate prognosis is unknown. The relationships of this syndrome to other rheumatic diseases are also unclear; many observers consider it a form of SLE. Appropriate therapy consists of symptomatic treatment with corticosteroids, alertness to possible serious complications such as nephritis, physical therapy, and careful attention paid to the function of the musculoskeletal system.

Ioffman RW, Cassidy J, Takeda Y, et al: U1-70-kd autoantibody positive mixed connective tissue disease in children. Arthritis Rheum 36:1599, 1993.
azaro M, Maldonado-Cocco J, Catoggio L, et al: Clinical and serologic characteristics of patients with overlap syndrome: Is mixed connective tissue disease a distinct clinical entity? Medicine (Baltimore) 68:58, 1989.
ngsen BH: Mixed connective tissue disease in childhood. Pediatr Rev 7:309, 1986.
ldens HA, Van Der Net JJ, De Graeff-Meeder ER, et al: Juvenile onset mixed connective tissue disease: Longitudinal follow-up. J Pediatr 122:191, 1993.

CHAPTER 156

Erythema Nodosum

Jane Green Schaller

Erythema nodosum is characterized by the development of painful, indurated, shiny, red, hot, elevated, ovoid nodules 1–3 cm in diameter. They are most frequently distributed symmetrically over the shins (Fig. 156–1) but may also occur on the calves, thighs, buttocks, and upper extremities. Fever, malaise, and arthralgia may precede or accompany the rash, and hilar adenopathy may be seen on chest roentgenograms. The skin lesions have a characteristic progression: Over a period of several days, they become protuberant and violaceous; after 1–2 wk, as induration decreases, a dull purple discoloration predominates and then fades in the manner of a large bruise, leaving a brown residuum without ulceration or scar formation. The lesions come in crops, usually over 3–6 wk. Erythema nodosum is uncommon in children younger than 6 yr, becoming progressively more frequent up to the 3rd decade of life. Females are affected more frequently than males.

The lesions represent a reaction to a variety of stimuli. The eruption has been induced experimentally in patients with the disease by local injection of a single specific bacterial antigen. Epidemiologically, the disease was previously linked to tuberculosis, especially in Europe. In the United States and Europe,

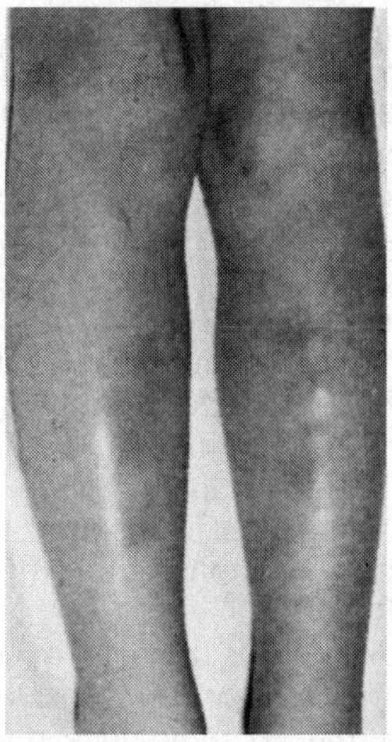

Figure 156–1. Erythema nodosum. See also color section.

streptococcal infections are more frequently implicated as stimuli. The eruption may also accompany sarcoidosis, leptospirosis, cat-scratch disease, Epstein-Barr virus, tularemia, psittacosis, histoplasmosis, coccidioidomycosis, and *Yersinia* infections or the administration of some drugs including sulfonamides and birth control pills. It may also occur with such systemic diseases as systemic lupus erythematosus (SLE), vasculitis, regional enteritis, ulcerative colitis, and Behçet syndrome.

Search for a precipitating infection, drug, or underlying disease should be instituted. The erythrocyte sedimentation rate is usually elevated, and other nonspecific evidences of inflammatory disease, such as acute phase reactants, are found. Suggestive etiologic evidence may include the demonstration of β-hemolytic streptococci in throat cultures or a rising antistreptolysin O titer; conversion of a previously negative tuberculin, histoplasmin, or coccidioidin skin reaction; roentgenographic evidence of pulmonary tuberculosis or fungus disease; or evidence of an underlying disease such as SLE, inflammatory bowel disease, or sarcoidosis.

Salicylates are usually adequate for symptomatic relief of erythema nodosum. The skin lesions and the constitutional manifestations may respond to corticosteroids, but such therapy is usually not warranted in a self-limited disease and may be contraindicated because of underlying active infection.

Aetiology of erythema nodosum in children. Lancet 2:14, 1961.
Kirby JR, Kraft GH: Oral contraceptives and erythema nodosum. Obstet Gynecol 40:409, 1972.

CHAPTER 157

Pain Syndromes

Jane Green Schaller

A significant percentage of children referred to pediatric rheumatology clinics suffer from musculoskeletal pain syndromes that have no demonstrable organic cause. Growing pains, the fibromyalgia syndrome, hypermotility syndromes, and the reflex sympathetic dystrophy syndrome are included. It is important for the clinician to recognize such children and to avoid labeling them as having chronic diseases, such as juvenile rheumatoid arthritis, or prescribing inappropriate and ineffective therapy with anti-inflammatory and immunosuppressive drugs. Children may be disabled by these pain syndromes, and they should receive appropriate management with an accurate diagnosis, appropriate assessment of any psychosocial overlay, and physical therapy to restore function.

Idiopathic limb pains of childhood, commonly called growing pains, affect a significant number of normal children. Diffuse limb pain, usually in the legs, occurs at night and is unassociated with daytime disability or objective physical findings. Therapy includes reassurance and the passage of time.

Fibrositis-fibromyalgia is a poorly defined adult condition that has also been described in children. There is no obvious inflammation associated with this nonarticular form of rheumatism. Little is known about its physiology or pathology; in adults, an association with stress has been suggested. Women are predominantly affected. There are no abnormal laboratory findings. Clinical manifestations consist of poorly defined musculoskeletal pain and discomfort, particularly in the thorax, that can be reproduced by pressure on a number of trigger points. Fatigue, anxiety, insomnia, and headache are common, but this condition is neither progressive nor associated with chronic deformity. Therapy with reassurance, management of stress and sleep disorders, exercise, and perhaps nonsteroidal anti-inflammatory agents may be helpful. The ultimate prognosis is unknown.

In the reflex sympathetic dystrophy syndrome, a limb or a part of a limb is immobilized by severe pain; cutaneous hypersensitivity, osteoporosis, and signs of autonomic nervous dysfunction (temperature changes, sweating) are characteristic. This syndrome may follow what appears to be a minor musculoskeletal injury. Successful therapy involves remobilization of the affected part with physical therapy. Psychosocial intervention may be required, particularly if the condition recurs in the same or another part.

157.1 Fasciitis

(Diffuse Fasciitis, Eosinophilic Fasciitis)

This unusual disorder is characterized by diffuse inflammation of the fascial tissues, usually associated with tissue or blood eosinophilia. No long-term studies have defined the natural history of the disease. It may be a variant of scleroderma. Although most patients have been adults, the disorder does occur in children. Inflammation of fascial tissues occurs primarily in the limbs and trunk; the hands, feet, and face are generally spared. Raynaud phenomenon is not associated. Joint contractures, including contractures of the fingers, may occur. The onset may follow periods of heavy physical exertion. Affected tissues are swollen and tender; however, because the overlying skin is not affected, cutaneous tissues appear puckered. Internal organ involvement has not been described. There are no diagnostic laboratory tests; test results for rheumatoid factors and antinuclear antibodies are generally negative. Some patients have striking eosinophilia, and increased numbers of eosinophils may be found in affected tissues. The diagnosis is clinical and is supported by evidence on biopsy of fascial inflammation. Corticosteroid therapy may be helpful, although results of long-term follow-up studies are not available. The disease appears to be associated with morphea in children, and it overlaps somewhat with scleroderma. Rarely, eosinophilic fasciitis is associated with aplastic anemia, thrombocytopenia, leukemia, or lymphoma.

The *eosinophilia-myalgia syndrome*, which has been reported predominantly in adults, manifests striking similarities to connective tissue disorders such as eosinophilic fasciitis, scleroderma, and eosinophilic myositis. This illness is associated with the ingestion of tryptophan or a manufacturing contaminant. It is characterized by edema, pruritus, paresthesia, myalgia, eosinophilia, perivascular inflammation, and fibrotic or inflamed fascia. Treatment consists of withdrawal of tryptophan. A similar condition has been associated with ingestion of contaminated cooking oil (toxic oil syndrome).

157.2 Raynaud Phenomenon

Raynaud phenomenon is characterized by ischemic blanching of distal phalanges by vasospasm, followed first by cyanosis and then by reactive hyperemia. Hands are more commonly affected than feet; all phalanges may be symmetrically affected, or only a few may be affected asymmetrically. Episodes may be associated with numbness and tingling during the ischemic phase and pain during the recovery phase. Attacks are most often precipitated by cold but can also occur after pressure or stress. Raynaud phenomenon is relatively rare in children.

If it occurs without underlying disease, it is called primary Raynaud phenomenon. Some individuals who present with Raynaud symptoms have an underlying cause, such as scleroderma or less frequently systemic lupus erythematosus (SLE) or mixed connective tissue disease, or rare conditions such as cryogobulinemia. Some individuals with no apparent clinical disease have laboratory abnormalities such as antinuclear antibodies or capillary abnormalities in the nail beds; such individuals are likely to develop rheumatic disease in the future. In cases of scleroderma and in some instances of SLE and mixed connective tissue disease, vasospasm can lead to fingertip ulcers, nail dystrophy, or loss of distal phalangeal mass (sclerodactyly).

Therapy for Raynaud phenomenon includes that for the underlying disease. It is important to maintain central and peripheral body temperatures against environmental cold by dressing warmly and wearing gloves. Individuals can often be taught to control episodes with biofeedback techniques. Vasodilating agents such as nifedipine may be occasionally required.

Farrington ML, Haas JE, Nazar-Stewart V, Mellins ED: Eosinophilic fasciitis in children frequently progresses to scleroderma like cutaneous fibrosis. J Rheumatol 20:128, 1993.
Grisanti MW, Moore TL, Osborn TG, Haber PL: Eosinophilic fasciitis in children. Semin Arthritis Rheum 19:151, 1989.
Miller JJ III: The fasciitis morphea complex in children. Am J Dis Child 146:733, 1992.

CHAPTER 158

Relapsing Nodular Nonsuppurative Panniculitis

(Weber-Christian Syndrome)

Jane Green Schaller

This rare disorder of subcutaneous inflammation is of unknown cause and probably does not represent a single disease. Infection, drug reaction (especially to bromides and iodides), abnormal fat metabolism, and hypersensitivity have all been suggested as etiologic factors. Fat necrosis is associated with several rheumatic diseases, with pancreatic disease, and with corticosteroid withdrawal. Adults are affected predominantly, although the syndrome has been reported in all age groups. Females are affected more frequently than males.

Histologically, there are foci of degeneration and inflammation in subcutaneous fat. Mesenteric, perivisceral, and periarticular adipose tissues may be affected; fatty metamorphosis of the liver and reticuloendothelial hyperplasia may occur. Laboratory findings are not specific. Leukopenia, an elevated erythrocyte sedimentation rate, rheumatoid factor, antinuclear antibodies, and cryoglobulins have been observed.

Clinically, the disease is characterized by the appearance of crops of subcutaneous nodules on any part of the body; thighs, legs, abdomen, breasts, and arms are most frequently involved. Nodules vary in size from a few millimeters to several centimeters and may be painful, with redness and warmth of the overlying skin. Nodules regress in days to weeks, usually leaving a pigmented depression. Fever is common, and a variety of rheumatic complaints may occur, including arthritis, arthralgia, and myalgia. Hepatosplenomegaly, abdominal pain, and episcleritis have been reported. Crops of nodules and systemic symptoms generally recur over long periods of time.

The diagnosis of Weber-Christian syndrome is based on the clinical picture and the histologic changes. The differential diagnosis includes erythema induratum, sarcoidosis, post-injection subcutaneous fat necrosis, and vasculitis. Fat necrosis with subcutaneous nodules, arthritis, and visceral involvement can occur as a manifestation of pancreatic disease, presumably resulting from enzymatic action on fat cells.

No specific therapy is known. Relief may occur after therapy with corticosteroids, chloroquine, or colchicine. Patients with underlying pancreatic involvement may benefit from treatment of the pancreatic disease.

McAdam LP, O'Hanlan MA, Bluestone R, et al: Relapsing polychondritis: Prospective study of 23 patients and a review of the literature. Medicine (Baltimore) 55:193, 1976.
Schuvat SJ, Frances A, Valderrama E, et al: Panniculitis and fever in children. J Pediatr 122:372, 1993.

CHAPTER 159

Relapsing Polychondritis

Jane Green Schaller

Relapsing polychondritis, one of the rarest of rheumatic syndromes, has been described in a few children. It is characterized by pain, swelling, destruction, and deformation of external and internal cartilaginous elements of the ears, nose, eyes, joints, laryngotracheobronchial system, heart, and large blood vessels. Fever, malaise, and myalgia may be associated. Glomerulonephritis has been described. There are no characteristic laboratory tests. The diagnosis rests on the clinical picture and on demonstration of cartilaginous inflammation on biopsy. This condition occasionally occurs in patients who have another established rheumatic disease such as vasculitis, rheumatoid arthritis, systemic lupus erythematosus, or Sjögren syndrome. Death may result from cardiac or respiratory involvement. Therapy with corticosteroid and cytotoxic agents has been advocated, but their long-term benefits are unknown.

CHAPTER 160
Syndrome of Neonatal Fever, Rash, and Arthropathy

Jane Green Schaller

This rare condition is characterized by high intermittent fevers, maculopapular rash, and systemic illness beginning in the first weeks of life. Other features include meningoencephalitis (with pleocytosis and elevated protein levels in cerebrospinal fluid), progressive mental retardation, chronic iridocyclitis, hepatosplenomegaly, and lymphadenopathy. The arthropathy is manifested by swelling, pain, and warmth in one or more joints; joint roentgenograms show periostitis and destruction of the ends of the long bones. Patellar enlargement may be striking. Affected children appear to have a characteristic facies with prominent foreheads.

Nothing is known about the etiology or pathogenesis of this syndrome. Although described in one set of siblings, it has not been familial in other instances. The condition superficially resembles systemic-onset juvenile rheumatoid arthritis, but the neonatal onset and the association of meningoencephalopathy, mental retardation, and chronic iridocyclitis, as well as the nature of the arthropathy, are distinctive. Treatment with nonsteroidal anti-inflammatory agents and physical therapy may assist in improving musculoskeletal function but does not slow progression of the disease. Progressive mental retardation and death in the 1st or 2nd decade of life have been reported, although the true long-term prognosis is unknown.

Prieur A, Griscelli C: Arthropathy with rash, chronic meningitis, eye lesions, and mental retardation. J Pediatr 99:79, 1981.

CHAPTER 161
Behçet Syndrome

Jane Green Schaller

This disorder is characterized by recurrent oral and genital ulcers and ocular inflammation. Arthritis, thrombophlebitis, neurologic abnormalities, skin lesions, fever, and colitis are associated clinical manifestations. The condition is rare in children.

The cause is unknown. Vasculitis of small and medium-sized arteries with cellular infiltrations leads to fibrinoid necrosis and narrowing and obliteration of the vessel lumens.

The clinical course is highly variable, with recurrent exacerbations and disease-free intervals of uncertain duration. The oral ulcers develop in almost all patients, persist for days to weeks, and then heal without scarring. These painful necrotic ulcers (2–10 mm), surrounded by erythema, may occur singly or in crops over the oral-nasal cavity and upper airway. Genital ulcers occur in most patients and follow a parallel course. Ocular manifestations include anterior or posterior uveitis and retinal vasculitis, which may progress to blindness. Arthritis is common and is usually acute, recurrent, asymmetric, and polyarticular, involving the large joints. Central nervous system abnormalities such as meningoencephalitis, cranial nerve palsies, and psychosis usually occur later in the course of the disease and indicate a poor prognosis. Skin manifestations include erythema nodosum, pseudofolliculitis, papulopustular lesions, and acneiform nodules and occur in most patients. Laboratory findings are not diagnostic. Cutaneous pathergy occurs as an erythematous sterile pustule after 24–48 hr at a needle prick skin site.

There is no single effective treatment. Systemic prednisone, colchicine, chlorambucil, azathioprine, and cyclosporine have been effective in some patients.

Ammann AJ, Johnson A, Fyfe GA, et al: Behçet's syndrome. J Pediatr 107:41, 1985.

International Study Group for Behçet's Disease: Criteria for diagnosis of Behçet's disease. Lancet 335:1078, 1990.

CHAPTER 162
Sjögren Syndrome

Jane Green Schaller

This chronic inflammatory, autoimmune disease, rare in children, is characterized by dry eyes (keratoconjunctivitis sicca, xerophthalmia), dry mouth (xerostomia), and associated connective tissue disorders. The salivary and lacrimal glands are infiltrated by lymphocytes and plasma cells; a similar process may reduce secretions in the respiratory tract, vagina, and skin and in the salivary and lacrimal glands.

Clinical manifestations include photophobia, burning and itching eyes, and blurred vision; painless unilateral or bilateral enlargement of the parotid glands, decreased sense of taste, dental caries, dysphagia, fissured tongue, and angular cheilitis; decreased sense of smell and epistaxis; and hoarseness, recurrent bronchitis, pneumonia, and chronic otitis. Sjögren syndrome may occur in the context of rheumatoid arthritis or systemic lupus erythematosus. Lymphoproliferative forms may also occur, with potential lymphoid malignancy. The diagnosis is based on the clinical features supported by biopsy of the lip or glands demonstrating lymphocytic infiltration; hypergammaglobulinemia, cryoglobulinemia, rheumatoid factors, and antibodies to La/SSB and Ro/SSA may be present. Maternal Sjögren syndrome can be antecedent to the neonatal lupus syndrome.

Treatment is symptomatic, with use of artificial tears, lozenges, and fluids to limit the damaging effects of decreased secretions. Corticosteroids may be indicated for severe functional disorders and life-threatening complications.

Fox RI, Saito I: Criteria for diagnosis of Sjögren's syndrome [Review]. Rheum Dis Clin North Am 20:391, 1994.

Hearth-Holmes M, Baethge BA, Abreo F, Wolf RE: Autoimmune exocrinopathy presenting as recurrent parotitis of childhood [Review]. Arch Otolaryngol Head Neck 119:347, 1993.

St. Clair EW: New developments in Sjögren's syndrome [Review]. Curr Opin Rheumatol 5:604, 1993.

CHAPTER 163

Nonrheumatic Conditions Mimicking Rheumatic Diseases of Childhood

Jane Green Schaller

A large number of "nonrheumatic" conditions that can cause musculoskeletal complaints in children, with or without accompanying signs, must be considered in the differential diagnosis of childhood rheumatic diseases (Table 163–1).

Bacterial infections of the bones and joints can cause pain and swelling around one or more joints, generally with accompanying fever and other systemic complaints (see Chapters 148 and 172). Diagnosis may result from appropriate cultures, skin tests, and imaging techniques. Viral and mycoplasmal infections may be associated with transient arthritis, which should not be confused with chronic rheumatic disease. Lyme disease requires differentiation from pauciarticular JRA. Diskitis (see Chapter 628.7) or inflammation of the intravertebral disks and end plates of vertebral bodies may be confused with arthritis, although the pain in diskitis is characteristically spinal; roentgenograms or bone scans may be diagnostic.

A number of childhood malignancies can result in musculoskeletal involvement resembling arthritis, generally through a mechanism of infiltration of malignant cells about the joint capsules and periosteum or destruction of bone. Pain in the affected joints is often severe, and blood studies may reveal abnormal white blood cells (leukopenia or abnormal cellular forms), thrombocytopenia, anemia, hyperuricemia, or elevated LDH. Bone roentgenograms may show metaphyseal rarefaction, periostitis, or lytic lesions. Suspicion of malignancy in a child with "arthritis" demands appropriate investigations, with oncologic consultation and biopsy of the bone marrow or other appropriate tissues.

Costochondral disease *(costochondritis)* is a relatively common disorder characterized by pain localized to the costosternal or costochondral junction. Pain may be of acute onset, sharp, darting, and of short duration, or it may evolve gradually as a dull aching pain lasting hours to days. It may be associated with a feeling of tightness due to muscle spasm and is generally not exacerbated by respiratory or other mild movements. There is often localized tenderness to palpation of one or more costal cartilages and a history of trauma or unaccustomed physical effort. The combination of pain, tenderness, and swelling with or without redness is referred to as the *Tietze syndrome.* Discomfort usually persists for only a few days or responds to mild analgesia and avoidance of strenuous activity.

Several noninflammatory conditions may mimic rheumatic diseases in children. Orthopedic conditions such as bone fractures, soft tissue injuries, avascular necrosis syndromes, and slipped capital femoral epiphysis may mimic arthritis; roentgenograms or bone scans are generally diagnostic. The pain syndromes, growing pains, fibromyalgia, and reflex sympathetic dystrophy (see Chapter 157) must also be considered in the differential diagnosis.

Congenital or genetically determined conditions may superficially resemble rheumatic diseases. For example, congenital myositis ossificans (fibrodysplasia ossificans congenita) is at times confused with dermatomyositis or scleroderma, and conditions such as carpal-tarsal osteolysis or trichorhinophalangeal dysplasia may suggest juvenile rheumatoid arthritis. A positive family history, the presence of associated dysmorphic features (e.g., digital anomalies in congenital myositis ossificans or characteristic facial anomalies in trichorhinophalangeal dysplasia), or the roentgenographic appearance of the affected bones and joints (e.g., lysis of the carpal and tarsal bones in carpal-tarsal osteolysis) can differentiate these entities (see Chapter 634).

Many other miscellaneous conditions may mimic childhood rheumatic diseases. Noteworthy are the hand-foot syndrome of sickle cell anemia and the arthropathy of hemophilia. In general, such conditions can be differentiated on the basis of historical or physical findings that do not appear to be entirely consistent with any of the rheumatic diseases.

■ TABLE 163–1 Conditions Other Than Rheumatic Diseases Associated with Arthritis in Children

- Infectious diseases
  - Pyogenic arthritis
  - Tuberculous arthritis
  - Osteomyelitis with sympathetic joint effusion
  - Virus-related arthritis
  - Reactive arthritis
  - Lyme disease
  - Other (e.g., *Mycoplasma* arthritis)
- Neoplastic diseases
  - Leukemia
  - Neuroblastoma
  - Malignant histiocytosis
  - Lymphoma, Hodgkin disease, reticulum cell sarcoma
  - Rhabdomyosarcoma
  - Osteogenic sarcoma
  - Other primary bone tumors
- "Orthopedic" conditions (noninflammatory conditions of bones and joints)
  - Avascular necrosis syndromes (e.g., Legg-Calvé-Perthes disease, Köhler disease, Osgood-Schlatter disease)
  - Toxic synovitis of the hip
  - Slipped capital femoral epiphysis
  - Trauma (child abuse fractures; joint, ligamentous, and muscle injuries)
  - Chondromalacia patellae
  - Congenital anomalies and genetically determined abnormalities of musculoskeletal system (e.g., muscular dystrophies, congenital subluxation of the hips, other congenital abnormalities of bones, joints, connective tissues)
  - Tenosynovitis
  - Diskitis
- Pain syndromes
  - Idiopathic limb pains (growing pains)
  - Fibromyalgia syndrome
  - Reflex sympathetic dystrophy syndrome
- Hysteria, conversion reactions, "psychogenic rheumatism"*
- Miscellaneous conditions (e.g., sickle cell anemia, hemophilia, hypermobile joint syndrome, immunodeficiency-related arthritis, sarcoidosis, hypertrophic osteoarthropathy)

**These conditions may have associated symptoms suggesting arthritis; they do not produce or represent joint disease.*

Aprin H, Turen C: Pyogenic sacroiliitis in children. Clin Orthop 287:98, 1993.

Cabral D, Petty R, Fung M, Malleson P: Persistent antinuclear antibodies in children without identifiable inflammatory rheumatic or autoimmune disease. Pediatrics 89:441, 1992.

Carr AJ, Cole WG, Roberton DM, Chow CW: Chronic multifocal osteomyelitis. J Bone Joint Surg Br 75:582, 1993.

Cassidy JT: Miscellaneous conditions associated with arthritis in children. Pediatr Clin North Am 33:1033, 1986.

Cassidy JT: Progress in diagnosing and understanding chronic pain syndromes in children. Curr Opin Rheumatol 6:544, 1994.

Cushing AH: Diskitis in children. Clin Infect Dis 17:1, 1993.

Nocton JJ, Miller LC, Tucker LB, Schaller JG: Human parvovirus B19 associated arthritis in children. J Pediatr 122:186, 1993.

Schuval SJ, Bonagura VR, Ilowite NT: Rheumatologic manifestations of pediatric human immunodeficiency virus infection. Rheumatol 20:1578, 1993.

Steere AC, Taylor E, McHugh GL, Logigian EL: The overdiagnosis of Lyme disease. JAMA 269:1812, 1993.

Szer IS, Taylor E, Steere AC: The long-term course of Lyme arthritis in children. N Engl J Med 325:159, 1991.

Tucker LB: Nonrheumatic conditions including infectious diseases and syndromes in children. Curr Opin Rheumatol, in press.

Yunus MB, Masi AT: Juvenile primary fibromyalgia syndrome: A clinical study of 33 patients and matched normal controls. Arthritis Rheum 28:138, 1985.

163.1 Benign Rheumatoid Nodules

Rheumatoid nodule-like lesions unassociated with rheumatic disease occasionally occur in children. Single or multiple lesions may be present over various sites, including the pretibial areas, dorsa of the feet, scalp, hands, and elbows; they may also appear over pressure points or after trauma, as do true rheumatoid nodules. Clinically, the nodules are subcutaneous or fixed to deeper tissues and resemble rheumatoid nodules. Histologically, these lesions show central areas of fibrinoid necrosis with surrounding histiocytes and mononuclear cells; they closely resemble adult-type rheumatoid nodules or the intracutaneous lesions characteristic of granuloma annulare. Indeed, typical granuloma annulare may be associated.

The cause is unknown. Affected children are well and have no associated rheumatic complaints. Laboratory tests are normal; test results for rheumatoid factor and antinuclear antibodies are negative. The nodular lesions wax, wane, and may recur, but recurrences generally cease after months or years. This is a benign condition; affected children are not at increased risk for rheumatic disease, and no therapy other than reassurance is required.

The nodules associated with rheumatic disease (rheumatoid arthritis, acute rheumatic fever, scleroderma, systemic lupus erythematosus) rarely occur as sole manifestations but rather appear with other signs of active rheumatic disease. Rheumatoid nodules in rheumatoid arthritis are generally accompanied by positive test results for rheumatoid factor.

Burrington JD: "Pseudorheumatoid" nodules in children: Report of ten cases. Pediatrics 45:473, 1970.

Simons FE, Schaller JG: Benign rheumatoid nodules. Pediatrics 56:29, 1975.

Chapter 164
Amyloidosis

Jane Green Schaller

Amyloidosis is characterized by the deposition in various body tissues of a homogeneous-appearing eosinophilic material that binds Congo red dye. Amyloid material is composed of microscopic fibrils that are biochemically heterogeneous, with at least 15 different types of protein compositions. The deposition of amyloid material ultimately interferes with the function of organs. Various disease states result from deposition of different types of amyloid material, and different patterns of tissue deposition result in various patterns of organ dysfunction.

Classifications of the amyloid proteins and the various amyloid diseases are complex. The chief types of amyloidosis are those related to multiple myeloma and macroglobulinemia (AL-type amyloid precursors), amyloidosis occurring in individuals with familial Mediterranean fever (AA-type amyloid precursors), and amyloidosis occurring with chronic inflammatory diseases (AA-type amyloid precursors). A group of conditions, including primary amyloidosis, amyloid conditions associated with aging (including Alzheimer disease), and several rare familial types of amyloidosis, are associated with other amyloid precursors. Only the amyloidosis occurring with familial Mediterranean fever and the amyloidosis secondary to chronic inflammatory disease affect children in any appreciable numbers.

Familial Mediterranean fever (FMF) is a genetically determined disorder found most often in North African Jews, Arabs, Turks, and Armenians. Diagnosis rests on clinical grounds of recurrent attacks of fever; serositis, most frequently manifested by abdominal pain; arthritis; and a positive family history. There are no diagnostic tests. Attacks of FMF usually begin during childhood. Transmission of the disease is autosomal recessive. Between one third and one half of individuals with FMF in some populations (Sephardic Jews, Turks) develop secondary amyloidosis, which is independent of the frequency or severity of the attacks of FMF. The genetic locus for FMF is on chromosome 16 and differs from the serum AA gene cluster located on chromosome 11p. The amyloidosis associated with FMF is manifested by proteinuria, which progresses to the nephrotic syndrome and to renal failure over a period of months to several years; death occurs from infection, thromboembolism, or uremia. Attacks of FMF can be prevented by therapy with colchicine. Colchicine therapy also greatly lessens the occurrence of amyloidosis and has resulted in some regression of established amyloidosis. Colchicine taken for FMF during pregnancy is said to harm neither the mother nor the fetus.

Amyloidosis of similar composition (AA fibril precursors) also occurs in some individuals with chronic inflammatory diseases, including juvenile arthritis, cystic fibrosis, inflammatory bowel disease, and chronic infections such as tuberculosis. Because the serum AA protein acts as an acute-phase reactant, increased amounts of this material resulting from chronic inflammation may provide an explanation for the occurrence of this form of secondary amyloidosis. Other inflammatory diseases such as lupus erythematosus or dermatomyositis, which are associated with shorter periods of inflammation, are not associated with secondary amyloidosis. Curiously, secondary amyloidosis in juvenile arthritis affects as many as 10% of children in some European countries but is rarely seen as a complication of seemingly similar disease in children in the United States and Canada; explanations for this difference are unknown. Secondary amyloidosis usually begins some years after the onset of inflammatory disease and is manifested by hepatosplenomegaly or proteinuria, with progression to the nephrotic syndrome and ultimate renal failure.

DIAGNOSIS. The diagnosis of amyloidosis is established by demonstration of amyloid in affected tissues. Renal biopsies are considered hazardous in the presence of amyloidosis because of potential bleeding. The spleen is often affected but is not a suitable site for biopsy. Easier biopsy sites include the rectal mucosa and gingival tissue. A method of scintigraphy using serum amyloid p component has been described as a useful diagnostic tool and as a tool for monitoring the status of amyloidosis. Patients with juvenile arthritis and secondary amyloidosis usually show elevated acute-phase reactants and high levels of immunoglobulins.

TREATMENT. Amyloidosis has been described as being untreatable and irreversible. However, amyloidosis can usually be prevented in FMF by the institution of colchicine therapy, and such therapy may reverse some early amyloidosis, as witnessed by regression of proteinuria. In juvenile arthritis, secondary amyloidosis responds to chlorambucil, which results in a reversal of renal findings and prolongation of life; there is less experience with other cytotoxic agents. Chlorambucil is associated with chromosome breakage and an unknown risk of subsequent malignancy. There is less experience with therapy for the secondary amyloidosis of other conditions.

Castile R, Shwachman H, Travis W, et al: Amyloidosis as a complication of CF. Am J Dis Child 139:728, 1985.

David J, Vouyiouka O, Ansell BM, et al: Amyloidosis in juvenile chronic arthritis: A morbidity and mortality study. Clin Exp Rheumatol 11:85, 1993.

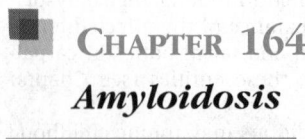

Gedalia A, Adar A, Gorodischer R: Familial Mediterranean fever in children. J Rheumatol 19(Suppl 35):1, 1992.

Hawkins PN, Richardson S, Vigushin DM, et al: Serum amyloid p component scintigraphy and turnover studies for diagnosis and quantitative monitoring of AA amyloidosis in juvenile rheumatoid arthritis. Arthritis Rheum 36:842, 1993.

Pras E, Aksentijevich I, Gruberg L, et al: Mapping of a gene causing familial Mediterranean fever to the short arm of chromosome 16. N Engl J Med 326:1509, 1992.

Saatci U, Bakkaloglu A, Ozen S, Besbas N: Familial Mediterranean fever and amyloidosis in children. Acta Paediatr 81:705, 1993.

Woo P: Amyloidosis in children. Baillieres Clin Rheumatol 8:691, 1994.

Zemer D, Liunch A, Damon YL, et al: Long-term colchicine treatment in children with familial Mediterranean fever. Arth Rheum 34:973, 1991.

Part XVII

Infectious Diseases

Section 1

General Considerations

Chapter 165

Fever

Ann M. Arvin

Fever occurs when various infectious and noninfectious processes interact with the host's defense mechanism. In most children fever is either due to an identifiable microbiologic agent or subsides after a short time. Fever in children may be categorized as (1) fever of short duration with localizing signs for which the diagnosis can be established by clinical history and physical examination, with or without laboratory tests; (2) fever without localizing signs, for which the history and physical examinations do not suggest a diagnosis but laboratory tests may establish an etiology; and (3) fever of unknown origin (FUO).

Fever is an elevation of body temperature mediated by an increase of the hypothalamic heat regulatory set-point. The hypothalamic thermoregulatory center controls body temperature by balancing signals from peripheral cold and warm neuronal receptors. Another regulatory factor is the temperature of blood circulating in the hypothalamus. The integration of these signals maintains normal core body temperature at the set-point of 37° C (98.6° F), within a narrow range of 1–1.5° C. Axillary temperature may be 1° C lower than core temperature, due in part to cutaneous vasoconstriction, and oral temperature may be falsely lowered owing to rapid respirations. Body temperature follows a circadian rhythm: Early morning temperature is low, and the highest level occurs at 4:00–6:00 P.M. Heat generation (increased cell metabolism, muscle activity, involuntary shivering) and heat conservation (vasoconstriction, heat preference behavior) are balanced against heat loss (obligate heat loss [evaporation-radiation-convection-conduction], vasodilation, sweating, and cold preference behavior).

Alterations of the normal homeostatic regulation of temperature by the hypothalamus may be caused by infection, vaccines, biologic agents (granulocyte-macrophage colony–stimulating factor, interferon, interleukins), tissue injury (infarction, pulmonary emboli, trauma, intramuscular injections, burns), malignancy (leukemia, lymphoma, hepatoma, metastatic disease), drugs (drug fever, cocaine, amphotericin B), immunologic-rheumatologic disorders (systemic lupus erythematosus, rheumatoid arthritis), inflammatory diseases (inflammatory bowel disease), granulomatous diseases (sarcoidosis), endocrine disorders (thyrotoxicosis, pheochromocytoma), metabolic disorders (gout, uremia, Fabry disease, type 1 hyperlipidemia), and unknown or poorly understood entities (familial Mediterranean fever). Factitious (self-induced) fever may be due to intentional manipulations of the thermometer or injection of pyrogenic material.

Regardless of the etiology, the final pathway of most common causes of fever is the production of endogenous pyrogens, which then directly alter the hypothalamic temperature set-point, resulting in heat generation and heat conservation (Fig. 165–1). The sequence of cytokine generation in response to exogenous pyrogens, with subsequent hypothalamic prostaglandin E_2 (PGE_2) production, may take 60–90 min. Fever is one manifestation of the inflammatory response produced by cytokine-mediated host defense mechanisms.

Except under unusual circumstances, fever by itself is not beneficial to the host response to infection. Heat production associated with fever increases oxygen consumption, carbon dioxide production, and cardiac output. Thus, it may exacer-

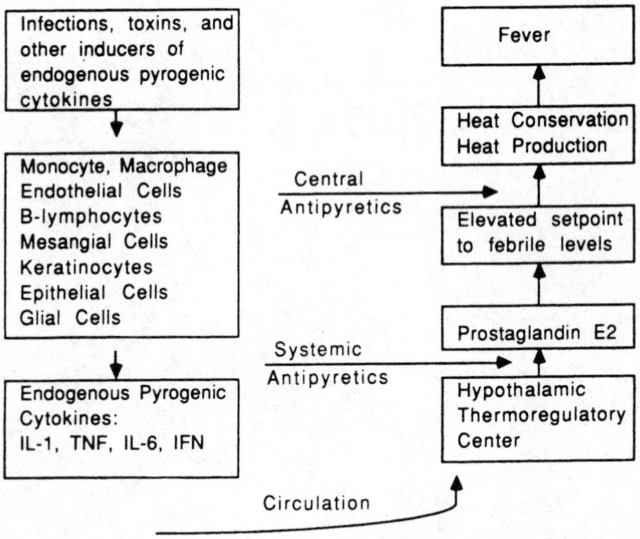

Figure 165–1. ***Pathogenesis of fever.*** **Various infectious, immunologic, or toxin-related agents (exogenous pyrogens) induce the production of endogenous pyrogens by host inflammatory cells. These endogenous pyrogens are cytokines, such as interleukins (IL-1β, IL-1α, IL-6), tumor necrosis factors (TNF-α, TNF-β), and interferon-α (INF). Endogenous pyrogens induce fever within 10–15 min, whereas the febrile response to exogenous pyrogens (e.g., endotoxin) has a delayed onset requiring the synthesis and release of pyrogenic cytokines. Endogenous, pyrogenic cytokines directly stimulate the hypothalamus to produce prostaglandin E_2, which then resets the temperature regulatory set-point; then neuronal transmission to the periphery leads to conservation and generation of heat, thus raising core body temperature. (From Dinarello C, Wolff S: Pathogenesis of fever.** ***In:*** **Mandell G, Douglas R, Bennett J: Principles and Practice of Infectious Diseases, 3rd ed. New York, Churchill Livingstone, 1990.)**

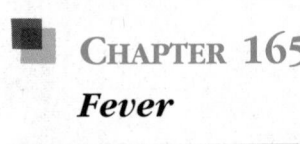

bate cardiac insufficiency in patients with heart disease or chronic anemia (e.g., sickle cell disease), pulmonary insufficiency in those with chronic lung disease, and metabolic instability in children with diabetes mellitus or inborn errors of metabolism. Furthermore, children between the ages of 6 mo and 5 yr are at increased risk of benign febrile seizures, whereas those with idiopathic epilepsy may have increased frequency of seizures as part of a nonspecific febrile illness (Chapter 543.3).

FEVER PATTERNS. The diurnal variation of temperature is usually preserved in patients with febrile illnesses. When this circadian rhythm is associated with tachycardia, chills (rigors), and sweating, a true rather than factitious fever should be suspected. Fever patterns may be *remittent* (daily elevated temperature returning to a baseline but above normal), *intermittent* (daily fever returning to normal), *hectic* (intermittent or remittent with temperature excursion of >1.4° C [2.5° F]), or *sustained* or continuous (fluctuation of elevated temperature of <0.3° C [0.5° F]). In most infectious or inflammatory processes the characteristics of the fever pattern are of little diagnostic importance. The fever associated with malaria, Hodgkin disease (Pel-Ebstein fever), and cyclic neutropenia may indicate the underlying condition.

TREATMENT. Antipyretic therapy is beneficial in high-risk patients who have chronic cardiopulmonary diseases, metabolic disorders, or neurologic diseases and in those who are at risk for febrile seizures. Other than providing symptomatic relief, antipyretic therapy does not alter the course of common infectious diseases in normal children, and thus its use remains controversial in these patients. *Hyperpyrexia* (>41° C) places the patient at higher risk than lower temperature responses, is associated with severe infection, hypothalamic disorders, or central nervous system hemorrhage, and requires therapy (see later). High fever during pregnancy may be teratogenic.

Acetaminophen, aspirin, and nonsteroidal anti-inflammatory agents (e.g., ibuprofen) are inhibitors of hypothalamic cyclo-oxygenase, thus inhibiting PGE_2 synthesis. These drugs are all equally effective antipyretic agents. Because aspirin has been associated with Reye syndrome in children and adolescents, its use is not recommended for the treatment of fever. Acetaminophen, 10–15 mg/kg every 4 hr, is not associated with many adverse effects; however, prolonged use may produce renal injury, and massive overdose may produce hepatic failure. Ibuprofen (suspension 100 mg/5 mL, given in a dose of 5–10 mg/kg every 6–8 hr) may cause dyspepsia, gastrointestinal bleeding, reduced renal blood flow, and, rarely, aseptic meningitis, hepatic toxicity, or aplastic anemia. Serious injury from ibuprofen overdose is unusual. Tepid sponge bathing in warm water (not alcohol) is another recommended method of reducing high body temperature due to infection or hyperthermia resulting from external causes (e.g., heat stroke). The decline of body temperature after antipyretic therapy does not distinguish serious bacterial from less serious viral diseases.

HYPERTHERMIA. High body temperature not caused by hypothalamic thermoregulatory mechanisms may be due to increased endogenous heat production (vigorous exercise, malignant hyperthermia, neuroleptic malignant syndrome, hyperthyroidism), decreased heat loss (wrapping in multiple blanket layers, atropine intoxication), or prolonged exposure to high environmental temperatures (heat stroke) (Chapters 60.8 and 548.3).

Malignant Hyperthermia. This autosomal dominant disorder (which has variable penetrance) may be suggested by a history of drug exposure, previously affected family members, exposure to high environmental temperature, or absence of the hypothalamic-regulated circadian rhythm. It also occurs in patients with various myopathic disorders (Chapter 559).

Neuroleptic malignant syndrome occurs following exposure to phenothiazine-like agents and is indistinguishable from malignant hyperthermia. Therapy with dantrolene and supportive care are similar to the measures described for malignant hyperthermia.

DRUG FEVER. This disorder may be diagnosed when an elevated temperature coincides with drug administration and disappears when the drug is discontinued, and there is no other identified cause of the fever. Drug fever is not associated with a particular fever pattern and is not consistently associated with eosinophilia, rash, pruritus, or drug allergy. Drug fevers may develop at any time after therapy has been initiated (median 8 days, average 21 days); the temperature elevation ranges from 38° to 43° C. Common agents producing drug fever include antibiotics (penicillin, cephalosporins), anticonvulsants (phenytoin, carbamazepine), antineoplastic agents (bleomycin, daunorubicin, cytarabine, L-asparaginase), and cardiovascular drugs (hydralazine, methyldopa [Aldomet], quinidine). *Treatment* includes withdrawal of the drug and, if continued therapy is needed, substitution of another agent. Fever usually resolves within 72 hr of stopping the drug. Subsequent exposure to the drug does not necessarily reproduce a drug fever.

RASHES WITH FEVER. Rashes may be so characteristic of a particular disease that a specific diagnosis can be made without difficulty, but frequently the skin manifestations produced are common to many infections. Skin lesions may be the result of direct inoculation of the skin (anthrax or tularemia); hematogenous dissemination of microorganisms (septicemia due to meningococci, rickettsiae, or other bacteria); or contiguous spread from adjacent foci of infection (impetigo, herpetic lesions). The skin also may reflect the effect of toxins (scarlet fever), antigen-antibody reactions (rheumatic fever), or delayed hypersensitivity to the infecting agent (erythema nodosum). Responses to toxins, pathogens, or inflammation include vasodilation, vaso-occlusion, extravasation of erythrocytes, vasculitis, and necrosis.

Rashes can be classified as macular eruptions, erythematous maculopapular eruptions, papulovesicular or bullous eruptions, petechial or hemorrhagic eruptions, ulcerative eruptions, and nodular eruptions. Many infections produce skin lesions that fall into more than one of these categories. Some infectious diseases and their agents are also associated with erythema multiforme eruptions (Chapter 604) or with erythema nodosum.

The course of the illness and the characteristics of the rash may provide enough information to create a differential diagnosis, establish a specific etiology, or suggest tissue to be obtained for biopsy and culture. Further, the history, physical appearance, and characteristics of the rash help to differentiate acute life-threatening illnesses (meningococcemia, toxic shock syndrome) from more benign diseases (fifth disease, exanthem subitum). Important historical information includes the onset of the rash relative to the onset of the illness, the progression of the rash through various cutaneous stages (macular, papular, purpuric), its distribution and progression through various locations (trunk, face, extremities, palms, and soles), the existence and nature of exposure (drugs, travel, sun, sick contacts, pets, wild animals, season, insect bites, rural vs urban environment, sexual activity), past immunizations, prior illness (congenital heart disease, immunocompromised conditions, allergies), and the severity of the current acute illness. The physical examination should focus on abnormalities of vital signs (tachycardia, hypotension, degree of fever), general appearance, signs of toxicity, characteristics of the rash; the presence of meningismus, lymphadenopathy, mucosal (oral, conjunctival, genital) lesions, hepatosplenomegaly, arthritis, signs of an underlying chronic illness (inflammatory bowel diseases, AIDS, malignancy); and signs suggestive of a noninfectious disease. A rash may be a local cutaneous infection and thus may provide material for diagnostic culture and histologic stain (Gram, immunofluorescent, Tzanck). If hematogenous dissemination produces a distinct rash, as in varicella or Rocky Mountain spotted fever, histologic (Tzanck) or direct immunofluorescent staining (*Rickettsia rickettsii*) or culture, may be diagnostic aids. Skin biopsy may be helpful in differentiating infectious from noninfectious diseases.

Anonymous: Ibuprofen vs acetaminophen in children. Med Lett 31:109, 1989.

Buxton PK: ABC of dermatology. Bacterial infection. Br Med J 296:189, 1988.

Buxton PK: ABC of dermatology. Viral infections. Br Med J 296:257, 1988.

Caspe W, Nucci A, Cho S: Extreme hyperpyrexia in childhood. Presentation similar to hemorrhagic shock and encephalopathy. Clin Pediatr 28:76, 1989.

Cherry JD: Cutaneous manifestations of systemic infections. *In:* Feigin RD, Cherry JD (eds): Textbook of Pediatric Infectious Diseases. Philadelphia, WB Saunders, 1987, p 786.

Dinarello C, Cannon J, Wolff S: New concepts on the pathogenesis of fever. Rev Infect Dis 10:168, 1988.

Guze B, Baxter L: Neuroleptic malignant syndrome. N Engl J Med 313:163, 1985.

Kingston ME, Mackey D: Skin clues to the diagnosis of life threatening infections. Rev Infect Dis 8:1, 1986.

Mackowiak P, LeMaistre C: Drug fever: A critical appraisal of conventional concepts. An analysis of 51 episodes in two Dallas hospitals and 97 episodes reported in the English literature. Ann Intern Med 106:728, 1987.

Musher D, Fainstein V, Young E, et al: Fever patterns. Their lack of clinical significance. Arch Intern Med 139:1225, 1979.

Pleet H, Graham JM, Smith DW: Central nervous system and facial defects associated with maternal hyperthermia at four to 14 weeks' gestation. Pediatrics 67:785, 1981.

Saper CB, Breder CD: The neurologic basis of fever. N Engl J Med 330:1880, 1994.

CHAPTER 166

Clinical Use of the Microbiology Laboratory

Ann M. Arvin

LABORATORY DIAGNOSIS OF BACTERIAL INFECTIONS

GRAM STAIN. The examination of a Gram stain should be carried out on all fluids to be cultured. In addition to giving rapid results, the Gram stain may be useful in interpreting the subsequent cultural data because it allows identification of cellular exudate and the predominant organisms. The identification of cells in respiratory specimens is crucial to the interpretation of the Gram stain because the lack of cells indicates a poor quality specimen.

SPECIAL CULTURES. Most medically important bacteria can be cultivated on blood agar, chocolate agar, and eosin methylene blue or MacConkey agar. New media preparations enhance the recovery of anaerobic organisms. Thioglycollate broth, while an excellent general culture medium, will not foster growth of strict anaerobes. For collection of anaerobic cultures, material should be rapidly transported to the laboratory in a capped syringe, or special swabs supplied in oxygen-free tubes should be used.

BLOOD CULTURE. Culturing the blood is one of the most fruitful procedures in the diagnosis of bacterial disease. It should be done carefully *before* administration of antibiotics, using iodine-alcohol for skin disinfection. A number of different blood culture techniques are now available, most of which use 50- to 100-mL bottles containing broth nutritious for bacteria into which not more than 5–10 mL of blood are introduced. Sodium polyanethanol sulfonate is included in some modern blood culture broth media to prevent coagulation and to inactivate leukocytes; although it may be toxic to certain organisms (e.g., meningococci). Some blood culture bottles also contain an oxygen-free carbon dioxide–enriched atmosphere that allows the recovery of anaerobes. A widely used technique involves lysis of blood cells followed by inoculation of sediment obtained from centrifugation of the lysate. This method provides rapid detection, pathogen identification, and antimicrobial susceptibility data, as well as quantitative blood culture results. Another technique depends on the detection of carbon dioxide released by bacteria from substrates in the medium. The use of media containing resins that adsorb antibiotics that may be present in the patient's blood adds to costs and is usually not necessary. Automated systems have shortened the interval to detection of positive blood cultures and are now used widely in the United States.

Repeating blood cultures may be necessary to determine (1) whether treatment has been successful particularly in high-risk patients who have infections that are difficult to treat and (2) whether the isolate is a contaminant when the organism reported is usually nonpathogenic. Whether an organism isolated from blood is a pathogen or a contaminant should be carefully considered, since "nonpathogens" such as coagulase-negative staphylococci may cause disease.

EXAMINATION OF CEREBROSPINAL FLUID (Table 166–1). Fluid obtained by lumbar puncture or ventricular tap should be collected in sterile, capped containers and transported quickly to the laboratory, where centrifugation is done to concentrate organisms. Gram stains of cerebrospinal fluid (CSF) sediment are helpful; the presence of organisms distinguishes bacterial from viral disease, but stains should not be relied on for the identification of a specific organism. It is better to use broad-spectrum initial therapy in life-threatening disease and to wait for the culture report before ordering specific treatment. Counterimmunoelectrophoresis and agglutination of antibody-coated latex beads are additional rapid, accurate methods for diagnosis. Specific antisera can be used to detect antigens of *Haemophilus influenzae* type b, *Neisseria meningitidis, Staphylococcus pneumoniae*, group B streptococci, and *Escherichia coli* K1.

URINE CULTURE. Urine for culture and colony count can be obtained in midstream (clean-catch), by catheterization, or by suprapubic puncture. The last method is the most reliable; urine so obtained should normally be sterile. Urine collected by catheter is likely to reflect infection if there are 10^3 organisms/mL or more. Clean-catch urine, if obtained after adequate cleansing, can be considered abnormal if 10^5 or more organisms/mL are present, and possibly abnormal if between 10^4 and 10^5 organisms/mL are counted. These limits apply only in uncomplicated urinary tract infection due to enteric gram-negative rods; different criteria may have to be used for gram-positive organisms, for yeasts, for patients in diuresis or with chronic pyelonephritis, or for patients on antibiotics. A Gram stain of unspun urine is helpful in predicting specimens with greater than 10^5 cfu/mL. Clean-catch urine specimens from girls who have inadequately washed, and specimens allowed to sit at room temperature for some time before being transported to the laboratory, may result in unreliable cultures. If delay in transporting specimens is unavoidable, dip-slides coated with bacteriologic media, dipped promptly in the urine specimen as soon as it is passed, give reliable results for urine culture.

CULTURE OF FECES. Rectal swabs or stool specimens are cultured either to identify common bacterial pathogens such as *Salmonella* and *Shigella* or to determine the predominant flora of the intestine in a patient with weakened host defenses whose endogenous flora may become pathogenic. Since feces contain mostly anaerobic bacteria, routine cultures identify only the predominant aerobic organisms among the billions of bacteria contained in each gram of feces.

A number of organisms have recently been added to the list of bacterial pathogens found in feces, including *Helicobacter pylori, Yersinia enterocolitica, Clostridium difficile, Aeromonas* spp.,

TABLE 166–1 Cerebrospinal Fluid Findings in Various Central Nervous System Disorders Associated with Fever

Condition	Pressure (mm H_2O)	Leukocytes mm³	Protein (mg/dL)	Glucose	Comments
Normal	50–80	<5, 75% lymphocytes	20–45	>50 mg/dL or 75% blood glucose	
Acute bacterial meningitis	Usually elevated	100–60,000 +; usually a few thousand; PMNs predominate	Usually 100–500	Depressed compared with blood glucose; usually >40 mg/dL	Organism may be seen on Gram stain and recovered by culture
Partially treated bacterial meningitis	Normal or elevated	1–10,000; PMNs usual but mononuclear cells may predominate if pretreated for extended period of time	100+	Depressed or normal	Organisms may or may not be seen; in disease due to *Haemophilus influenzae*, organism may grow despite pretreatment; pretreatment may render sterile CSF of patients with pneumococcal and meningococcal disease
Tuberculous meningitis	Usually elevated; may be low due to block in advanced stages	10–500; PMNs early but lymphocytes predominate through most of course	100–500; may be higher in presence of block	<50 mg/dL usual in most cases; decreases with time if treatment is not provided	Acid-fast organisms may be seen on smear; organism can be recovered in culture
Fungal meningitis	Usually elevated	25–500; mononuclear cells predominate except PMNs early	25–500	<50 mg/dL, decreases with time if treatment is not provided	Budding yeast may be seen; organism may be recovered in culture; India ink preparation may be positive in cryptococcal disease
Syphilis (acute) and leptospirosis	Usually elevated	200–500, usually lymphocytes	50–200	Generally normal	Positive CSF serology; spirochetes not demonstrable by usual techniques of smear or culture; darkfield examination may be positive
Viral meningitis or meningoencephalitis	Normal or slightly elevated	PMNs early; rarely more than 1,000 cells except in Eastern equine encephalomyelitis, in which counts of up to 20,000 have been recorded; mononuclear cells predominate during most of course	50–200	Generally normal; may be depressed to <40 mg/dL in various viral diseases, particularly mumps (15–20% of cases)	Enteroviruses may be recovered from CSF by appropriate viral cultures
Sarcoidosis	Normal or elevated slightly	0–100; mononuclear	40–100	Normal	No specific findings
Amebiasis	Elevated	500–20,000/+; PMNs predominate	50–100	Normal or slightly depressed	Amebae may be seen rarely in CSF
Chemical (drugs, dermoids, cysts, myelography dye)	Usually elevated	100–1,000/+; PMNs predominate	50–100	20–40 mg/dL	Epithelial cells may be seen within CSF in some children with dermoids by use of polarized light
Subacute bacterial endocarditis with embolism	Normal or slightly elevated	0–100; mixed PMNs and mononuclear cells	50–100	Normal	No organisms on smear or culture
Subdural empyema	Usually elevated	100–5,000; PMNs predominate	100–500	Normal	No organisms on smear or culture of CSF unless meningitis also present; organism found on tap of subdural fluid
Brain abscess	Usually elevated	10–200; fluid rarely acellular; lymphocytes predominate; if abscess ruptures into ventricle, PMNs predominate and cell count may reach >100,000	75–500	Normal unless abscess ruptures into ventricular system	No organisms on smear or culture unless abscess ruptures into ventricular system
Cerebral epidural abscess	Normal to slightly elevated	0–500; lymphocytes predominate	50–200	Normal	No organisms on smear or culture
Spinal epidural abscess	Usually low, with spinal block	10–100; lymphocytes predominate	50–400	Normal	No organisms on smear or culture
Thrombophlebitis (sometimes with subdural empyema)	Normal or elevated	0–500; PMNs and lymphocytes	50–200	Normal	No organisms on smear or culture
Acute hemorrhagic encephalitis	Usually elevated	0–1,000; PMNs predominate	100–500	Normal	No organisms on smear or culture
Collagen-vascular disease	Slightly elevated	0–500; PMNs may predominate; lymphocytes may be present	100	Normal or slightly depressed	No organisms on smear or culture; LE preparation may be positive
Tumor, leukemia	Slightly elevated to very high	0–100+; mononuclear or blast cells	50–1,000	May be depressed to 20–40 mg/dL	Cytology may be positive

PMN = polymorphonuclear leukocyte; CSF = cerebrospinal fluid; LE = lupus erythematosus cell.

Plesiomonas spp., *Vibrio* spp., and *E. coli* 0157:H7. DNA probes, antigen detection methods, and toxin detection have all been applied to the rapid diagnosis of enteric pathogens.

EXUDATES AND TRANSUDATES. Abscesses, pleural fluids, joint fluids, urethral exudates, and other miscellaneous exudates and transudates can be cultured directly on agar. In addition to cultures and stains, glucose and cell count determinations should be done on all transudates for the same reasons they are done on CSF.

NASOPHARYNGEAL, THROAT, AND SKIN SWABS. A dry rayon, Dacron, or calcium alginate swab is most efficient for collecting specimens from the skin and mucous membranes. Since drying rapidly destroys some pathogenic bacteria, swab specimens should be placed promptly in a transport medium.

Interpretation of results of cultures from skin and mucous membranes is difficult because microbial flora are normally recovered from these areas. Some organisms are considered pathogenic wherever found, such as *Corynebacterium diphtheriae, Bordetella pertussis,* and *Neisseria gonorrhoeae*; others, such as *Streptococcus pyogenes, N. meningitidis, H. influenzae,* or staphylococci, may be pathogenic or nonpathogenic, depending on circumstances. Still others, such as *Streptococcus viridans,* are rarely considered pathogenic. In respiratory tract disease there is little correlation between flora of the upper airway and that of the lower airway. Because sputum cultures are seldom reliable in children, bronchoalveolar lavage, tracheal aspirates, and lung punctures are sometimes necessary for accurate diagnosis. If bacteria such as *C. diphtheriae* or *Bordetella* sp. (which grow poorly in ordinary media) are suspected, the laboratory should be informed prior to receipt of the specimen.

ANTIBODY-BASED TECHNIQUES. Fluorescent antibody (FA) techniques have increased the diagnostic scope of direct microscopy. Specific antisera are now available commercially for several common pathogens. In these sera the antibody molecules have been conjugated with a fluorescein dye. The specific dye-labeled serum is added to the smear containing the suspected organism, and the slide is microscopically examined for fluorescence under ultraviolet light. Indirect FA methods are also applicable in the absence of conjugated antibodies. FA is used principally for identifying *B. pertussis, Legionella pneumophila,* and *N. gonorrhoeae*. In the special case of *Mycobacterium tuberculosis* no antibody is used; rather, the smears are stained with auramine-rhodamine, which is taken up by the organisms and fluoresces under ultraviolet light. This acid-fast fluorescent staining procedure is more sensitive but less specific than the Ziehl-Neelsen or Kinyoun acid-fast stain.

Bacteria are often serogrouped or serotyped through agglutination by specific antisera (sometimes attached to latex particles).

ANTIBIOTIC SENSITIVITY TESTS. Most laboratories routinely test bacterial isolates for sensitivity to various antibiotics. The most prevalent technique of antibiotic testing is the agar disk diffusion method, in which a standardized inoculum of the organism is seeded onto a plate. Filter paper disks, each impregnated with an antibiotic, are placed on the agar surface, and after 18–24 hr of incubation, the zone of inhibition of bacterial growth around each disk is measured. Standard zone diameters indicating sensitivity or resistance have been defined according to previous test results correlating zone sizes with sensitivity determined by inhibition of bacteria inoculated into dilutions of antibiotics in culture broth. However, there are some pitfalls in the disk diffusion method. Small differences in zone diameter have large implications, and control of inoculum size, rate of diffusion of antibiotics, and accurate measurement of zones are critical. Automated methods are also now used for antibiotic susceptibility testing.

For more accurate measurement of antibiotic sensitivity, dilutions made in tubes or in wells on microtiter plates have come into wide use. Antibiotic dilutions in growth medium are prepared in steps through the range of attainable blood levels; then each tube or well is inoculated with a standardized suspension of the test organism. After 24 hr the tubes or wells are examined for turbidity; the lowest antibiotic concentration resulting in a clear tube or well indicates the bacteriostatic concentration of the particular antibiotic for the organism (minimal inhibitory concentration, or MIC). In some situations (e.g., endocarditis) it is important to measure the concentration of drug needed to kill bacteria. The tubes or wells are then subcultured to agar plates; the lowest concentration of antibiotic that yields a 99.9% decrease in organism viability is the bactericidal end point (minimal bactericidal concentration, or MBC).

The actual concentrations of certain antibiotics in the blood can be measured by immunochemical assays. These measurements are mandatory when patients with renal disease are treated with aminoglycosides or with vancomycin. Microbiologic assays using susceptible stock strains of bacteria may be useful in special circumstances.

DNA PROBES. The greatest revolution in microbiologic diagnosis to date has occurred through the use of DNA probes. Among those bacteria for which commercial probes are now available, *Mycoplasma pneumoniae, M. tuberculosis, Mycobacterium aviumintracellulare,* and enteric organisms figure prominently.

OFFICE BACTERIOLOGY. Disposable materials have been developed so that rapid, inexpensive bacterial diagnosis can be made in the physician's office. Kits for detecting streptococci, gonococci, and urinary tract infection by culture are most widely used. The only additional purchase required is a small incubator. Unfortunately, quality control by testing of known positive cultures is seldom practiced. Office bacteriology may be inaccurate, unless both positive and negative results are periodically confirmed.

LABORATORY DIAGNOSIS OF VIRUSES

If viral disease is a diagnostic possibility, specimens should be obtained for viral culture and rapid viral detection. Serologic tests are much less useful for viral diagnosis but obtaining an acute phase sample is sometimes indicated for later comparison with convalescent antibody titers.

RAPID VIRAL DETECTION. Fluorescent-antibody techniques or other methods that use antibodies to detect viral antigens in clinical specimens provide rapid identification of viruses. For example, smears of mucosal cells stained by immunologic reagents can identify the antigens of respiratory viruses, such as respiratory syncytial virus or influenza, for which there is a polyclonal or monoclonal antiserum. Rotaviruses, which cause infantile gastroenteritis, and hepatitis B surface antigen can be detected by enzyme-linked immuno-sorbent assay (ELISA) using specific antisera.

Cytologic examination aids in diagnosis when inclusion bodies or syncytia are found but these methods are not sensitive enough to be relied upon for the diagnosis of life-threatening infections, such as neonatal herpes. All rapid detection assays should be done in parallel with and confirmed by viral culture.

ISOLATION. Viruses require living cells for propagation; the cells used most often are human or animal cell tissue cultures. Because some viruses are difficult to isolate and many require a variety of culture systems for their isolation, the clinician should describe the clinical signs, for example, pneumonia or skin lesions, when the specimen is sent to the laboratory. Specimens should be delivered to the laboratory promptly.

Throat and stool or rectal swab specimens should be submitted routinely, along with other site-specific specimens, such as CSF in suspected meningitis. The best throat specimens are taken by vigorous throat swabbing, removing some superficial cells. The swab should be rinsed thoroughly in a transport medium containing antibiotics to inhibit bacterial growth, squeezed against the glass, and discarded. If the laboratory is reasonably close, specimens should be transported at 4° C. Specimens for viral isolation should never be frozen at −20° C (usual temperature of a household freezer).

Rectal swabs should not be heavily covered with feces because the antibiotics present in viral transport media may be insufficient to kill a large inoculum of bacteria. Rectal swabs should be collected even in patients with respiratory and central nervous system syndromes, because many viruses replicate in the intestine as well as in target organs.

Cerebrospinal fluid is often positive during the acute stages of central nervous system inflammation. An extra amount of spinal fluid for viral diagnostic studies should be obtained at the initial lumbar puncture and can be sent for viral culture if the CSF Gram stain is negative and the white cell differential is predominantly lymphocytic.

Urine culture for viruses is most useful for the isolation of cytomegalovirus, but urine is also a good source for isolation of mumps and adenoviruses.

Vesicular fluid can be cultured to distinguish among vaccinia, varicella, herpes simplex, and enteroviruses.

Viremia is part of cytomegalovirus, enterovirus, and other viral infections, and buffy coat cultures are often useful in the diagnosis of febrile syndromes.

VIRAL GENOME AND VIRION DETECTION. New methods for viral diagnosis rely upon the use of probes constructed of sequences complementary to the genome sequences of DNA or RNA viruses. Hybridization of these probes to viral sequences can be detected by Southern blot or in situ methods using fluid or swab specimens or tissue sections. Polymerase chain reaction (PCR) detects viral gene sequences using complementary nucleotides as primers to amplify a conserved region of the genome. These methods are technically complex and difficult to standardize, but reliable commercial assays are available to detect some viruses. For example, the use of PCR makes it possible to prove human immunodeficiency virus (HIV) infection in infants despite the presence of maternal antibodies. However, clinicians should be aware that the reliability of these methods is highly variable and that not all laboratories use adequate quality control measures to assure specificity; false-positive results are common, particularly with PCR methods.

While electron microscopy (EM) provides a tool for direct visualization of virions within infected cells, its use in clinical diagnosis has been replaced for the most part by viral antigen or genome detection methods. Its usefulness is also limited because different viruses in the same family, such as herpes simplex, cytomegalovirus, and other herpesviruses, are indistinguishable by EM morphology.

SEROLOGIC TESTS. Correct diagnosis requires at least two blood specimens: the first should be obtained during the early acute phase of the disease ("acute serum"), and the second ("convalescent serum") 14–21 days later. If the second is taken earlier than 14 days after the first, it is advisable to take a third blood specimen 4–6 wk after the onset, since the rise of antibodies may be delayed, especially in infants. If it is not possible to send blood to the laboratory promptly, serum may be removed for preservation by freezing. Whole blood should never be frozen. To establish the etiologic diagnosis, it is necessary to demonstrate a fourfold rise in titer of antibody to an agent in the convalescent as opposed to the acute phase serum, when all specimens are tested together.

Although the presence of a substantial titer against a suspected agent in a single acute or convalescent specimen of serum will not differentiate between a recent and a past infection, in the following circumstances a study of a single serum specimen can support a clinical diagnosis: (1) Epstein-Barr antibodies; (2) antibody in the young infant not present in the mother; (3) antibody in both infant and mother that remains at the same level as the infant grows older; (4) in patients with suspected mumps, the presence of antibody to the soluble (S) fraction of the mumps virus in the acute serum (this antibody may be found as early as 2–3 days of the disease, when antibodies to the viral [V] antigen may be absent or very low. Pediatricians should be aware that methods for IgM antibody detection are difficult to standardize; false-positive results are especially common. IgM antibody titers should never be relied upon as the only diagnostic test for a serious viral infection. IgG antibody assays are often useful for establishing immune status because viral pathogens usually induce humoral immunity that persists for years after primary infection. Determining immune status will be particularly relevant when newer viral vaccines, such as the varicella or hepatitis A vaccines, become available for clinical use.

Methods of Detecting Antibody. Antibody can be detected by a variety of specific serologic methods; some are more appropriate than others for specific viruses. Complement-fixation (CF) antigens are available for a great range of viruses, and CF antibodies have the advantage of correlating with recent infection but are less useful for showing past infection. Neutralizing antibodies, on the other hand, remain for life; unless one has obtained serum early in the disease, a rise may be difficult to show. Furthermore, neutralization tests have the technical disadvantage of needing to be done in tissue cultures or in whole animals. Hemagglutination-inhibition (HI) antibodies correlate fairly well with neutralizing antibodies. Fortunately, many viruses such as the myxoviruses, rubella, and some enteroviruses can agglutinate erythrocytes. The presence of antibodies can be detected by the extent to which a particular serum specifically inhibits hemagglutination. Many of the viruses that agglutinate red blood cells also cause red blood cells to be adsorbed onto the membranes of infected cell monolayers. Inhibition of adsorption is a particularly useful test for parainfluenza virus antibodies. Antibodies can be detected by the indirect fluorescence technique. ELISA and latex agglutination tests are now used most often to detect antibodies to viral antigens. These depend on the attachment of viral antigens to plastic wells or latex beads.

Balows A (ed): Manual of Clinical Microbiology. Washington, DC, American Society for Microbiology, 1991.

Balows A, Hausler WJ, Ohashi M, Turanol A: Laboratory Diagnosis of Infectious Diseases: Principles and Practice. Vol. I: Bacterial, Mycotic, and Parasitic Diseases. New York, Springer Verlag, 1988.

Lennette EH, Schmidt NJ: Diagnostic Procedures for Viral, Rickettsial and Chlamydial Infections. Washington, DC, American Public Health Association, 1988.

McGowan KL: Infectious diseases: Diagnosis utilizing DNA probes. Understanding a developing clinical technology. Clin Pediatr 28:157, 1989.

Todd JK: Test selection for the pediatric office laboratory. *In*: Aronoff SC, Hughes WT Jr, Kohl S, et al (eds): Advances in Pediatric Infectious Diseases, Vol 3. Chicago, Year Book Medical Publishers, 1988, pp 111–124.

agents. For non-toxic-appearing infants with a rectal temperature of ≥39° C, two options are suggested, either (1) obtain a specimen of blood to culture for bacterial pathogens and give empirical antimicrobial therapy, or (2) obtain a complete blood cell count and if the white blood cell count is ≥15,000 cells/μL obtain a blood culture and give empirical antimicrobial therapy.

A third option, not offered in these guidelines, is to observe selected infants as outpatients without empirical antimicrobial therapy after blood for culture has been obtained. The family should be instructed to return to the office or clinic within 24 hr if there is persistent fever or immediately if the child's condition deteriorates.

If pneumococcus is present in the first blood culture, the child should return to the physician as soon as the culture results have been reported. If the child appears well and is afebrile and the physical examination is normal, a second blood culture should be obtained, and the child may return home without treatment. If the child appears ill and continues to have fever with no identifiable focus of infection, or if *H. influenzae* or *N. meningitidis* is present in the initial blood culture, the child should be evaluated for meningitis, undergo a repeat blood culture, and receive treatment in the hospital with appropriate antimicrobial agents. If the child develops a localized infection, therapy is directed toward the specific pathogen at that particular site.

FEVER WITH PETECHIAE

Independent of age, fever with petechiae with or without localizing signs places the patient at high risk for life-threatening bacterial infections, such as bacteremia, sepsis, and meningitis. Eight to 20% of patients with fever and petechiae have a serious bacterial infection, and 7–10% have meningococcal sepsis or meningitis. *H. influenzae* type b is less common than meningococcus but also produces serious bacterial illness. Management includes prompt hospitalization, culture of blood and cerebrospinal fluid, and administration of appropriate parenteral antimicrobial agents.

FEVER IN PATIENTS WITH SICKLE CELL ANEMIA

Infection is the most common cause of death among children with sickle cell anemia (Chapter 419.1). The incidence of infection is greatest among infants younger than 2 yr old. The increased risk of infection in these children is due in part to functional asplenia and a defect in the properdin (alternate complement) pathway. Fever without a focus is a common presenting sign of sepsis or meningitis due to pneumococcus in patients with sickle cell anemia. *H. influenzae* type b (meningitis), *Salmonella* (osteomyelitis), and *E. coli* (pyelonephritis) are additional pathogens that may present initially as fever without localizing signs.

Treatment of patients with sickle cell hemoglobinopathies requires culture of blood and, if indicated, cerebrospinal fluid, stool, and bone, and administration of antimicrobial agents. Children who appear seriously ill, have a temperature above 40° C, white blood cell counts <5,000/μL or >30,000/μL, and pulmonary infiltrates or complications of sickle cell disease or severe pain should be hospitalized. Other febrile infants with sickle cell disease can be given intramuscular ceftriaxone and managed as outpatients after specimens have been obtained for culture. These children should be seen again in 24 hr or earlier if their condition deteriorates. *Prevention* of pneumococcal sepsis is possible by instituting long-term penicillin therapy continued until adolescence (oral daily or long-acting intramuscular, every 3–4 wk). Alternatively, oral daily amoxicillin has been employed to add coverage against *H. influenzae* type b. Pneumococcal and *H. influenzae* vaccines may provide additional protection, but these vaccines should not be used in place of chronic antimicrobial therapy.

HYPERPYREXIA

Temperatures higher than 41° C are uncommon and are not associated with higher rates of serious bacterial infections than temperatures of 39.1–40.0° C or 40.1–41.0° C. Infants and children with high temperatures should be carefully evaluated, but evaluation and management need not differ from other children with lesser degrees of fever in excess of 39.0° C.

FEVER OF UNKNOWN ORIGIN

Many physicians use the term *fever of unknown origin* (FUO) to describe the condition of any febrile child admitted to the hospital with neither an apparent site of infection nor a noninfectious diagnosis. In most of these children the development of additional clinical manifestations over a relatively short time period makes the infectious nature of the illness apparent. Therefore, the term is better reserved for children with (1) a history of fever of more than 1 wk duration (2–3 wk if an adolescent), (2) documentation of fever by a health care provider, and (3) no apparent diagnosis 1 wk after investigation was begun in either an inpatient or outpatient setting.

The principal causes of FUO in children, using more restrictive criteria, are infections and connective tissue (autoimmune) diseases. Neoplastic disorders should also be seriously considered, although most children with malignancies do not have fever alone. If the patient is receiving drugs, the possibility of drug fever should be considered. Drug fever is not usually associated with other symptoms, and temperature remains elevated at a relatively constant level. Withdrawal of the drug is associated with resolution of the fever, generally within 72 hr (but when drugs, such as iodides, are excreted over a prolonged period of time, fever may persist for up to 1 mo after drug withdrawal).

Most fevers of unknown or unrecognized origin result from atypical presentations of common diseases. In some cases the presentation of a fever of unknown origin is typical of the disease (juvenile rheumatoid arthritis), but a definitive diagnosis can be established only after prolonged observation, because there are no associated findings on physical examination and all laboratory results are negative or normal.

In the United States the systemic infectious diseases most commonly implicated in children with FUO (by the above-mentioned more rigorous definition) are salmonellosis, tuberculosis, rickettsial diseases, syphilis, Lyme disease, cat-scratch disease, atypical prolonged presentations of common viral diseases, infectious mononucleosis, cytomegalovirus infection, hepatitis, coccidioidomycosis, histoplasmosis, malaria, and toxoplasmosis. Less common infectious causes of FUO include tularemia, brucellosis, leptospirosis, and rat-bite fever. Although human immunodeficiency virus type 1 (HIV-1) infection produces fever, acquired immunodeficiency syndrome (AIDS) alone is not usually responsible for FUO. Patients who have AIDS and FUO frequently also have an opportunistic infection with a common or an unusual pathogen.

Table 167–3 lists diseases that have presented as FUO in children with sufficient frequency to merit serious consideration. Specific signs and symptoms of each of these diseases and methods of diagnosis are detailed elsewhere.

Juvenile rheumatoid arthritis and systemic lupus erythematosus are the connective tissue diseases associated most frequently with FUO. Inflammatory bowel disease, rheumatic fever, and Kawasaki disease are also commonly reported as causes of FUO. When factitious fever (inoculation of pyogenic material or manipulation of the thermometer by the patient or parent) is suspected, fever should be documented in the

■ TABLE 167–3 Causes of Fever of Unknown Origin in Children

Infections
Bacterial Diseases
Caused by specific organism
Actinomycosis
Bartonellosis
Brucellosis
Campylobacter
Cat-scratch disease
Listeriosis
Meningococcemia (chronic)
Mycoplasmosis
Salmonellosis
Streptobacillus moniliformis
Tuberculosis
Tularemia
Yersiniosis
Localized infections
Abscesses: abdominal, brain, dental, hepatic, pelvic, perinephric, rectal, subphrenic
Cholangitis
Endocarditis
Mastoiditis
Osteomyelitis
Pneumonia
Pyelonephritis
Sinusitis
Spirochete
Borrelia (borreliosis: *B. recurrentis*)
Leptospirosis
Lyme disease (*B. burgdorferi*)
Spirillium minor
Syphilis
Viral Diseases
Cytomegalovirus
Hepatitis
Human immunodeficiency virus
Infectious mononucleosis (Epstein-Barr virus)
Chlamydial Diseases
Lymphogranuloma venereum
Psittacosis
Rickettsial Diseases
Ehrlichia canis
Q fever
Rocky Mountain spotted fever
Tick-borne typhus
Fungal Diseases
Blastomycosis (nonpulmonary)
Coccidioidomycosis (disseminated)
Histoplasmosis (disseminated)
Parasitic Diseases
Amebiasis
Babesiosis
Giardiasis
Malaria
Toxoplasmosis
Trichinosis
Trypanosomiasis
Visceral larva migrans

Autoimmune Hypersensitivity Diseases
Behçet syndrome
Drug fever
Hypersensitivity pneumonitis
Juvenile rheumatoid arthritis
Pancreatitis
Polyarteritis nodosa
Rheumatic fever
Serum sickness
Systemic lupus erythematosus
Undefined vasculitis
Weber-Christian disease
Neoplasms
Atrial myxoma
Hodgkin disease
Leukemia
Lymphoma
Neuroblastoma
Wilms tumor
Granulomatous Diseases
Granulomatous hepatitis
Sarcoidosis
Crohn disease
Familial-Hereditary Diseases
Anhidrotic ectodermal dysplasia
Fabry disease
Familial dysautonomia
Familial Mediterranean fever
Hypertriglyceridemia
Ichthyosis
Sickle cell crisis
Miscellaneous
Chronic active hepatitis
Diabetes insipidus (non-nephrogenic and nephrogenic)
Factitious fever
Hypothalamic-central fever
Infantile cortical hyperostosis
Inflammatory bowel disease
Kawasaki disease
Pancreatitis
Periodic fever
Poisoning
Pulmonary embolism
Thrombophlebitis
Thyrotoxicosis
Undiagnosed Fever
Persistent
Recurrent
Resolved

hospital by an individual who remains with the patient while the temperature is taken. Prolonged and continuous observation of the patient is imperative. FUO lasting more than 6 mo is uncommon in children and should suggest granulomatosis or autoimmune disease. Repetitive evaluation, including history, physical examination, and roentgenographic studies, may be required.

Diagnostic Clues in the Child with Fever of Unknown Origin

HISTORY. The age of the patient is helpful. Children under 6 yr of age often have a respiratory or genitourinary tract infection, localized infection (abscess, osteomyelitis), juvenile rheumatoid arthritis, or, rarely, leukemia. Adolescent patients are more likely to have tuberculosis, inflammatory bowel disease, autoimmune processes, and lymphoma, in addition to the causes of FUO found in younger children. A history of *exposure to wild or domestic animals* should be solicited. The incidence of zoonotic infections in the United States has been increasing, and they frequently are acquired from pets that are not overtly ill. For example, immunization of dogs against specific disorders such as leptospirosis may prevent canine disease but does not always prevent the animal from carrying and shedding leptospires, which may be transmitted to household contacts. A history of ingestion of rabbit or squirrel meat may provide a clue to the diagnosis of oropharyngeal, glandular, or typhoidal tularemia. A history of tick bite or travel to tick- or parasite-infested areas should be obtained.

A history of *pica* should be sought. Ingestion of dirt is a particularly important clue to infection with *Toxocara* (visceral larva migrans) or *Toxoplasma gondii* (toxoplasmosis).

A history of unusual dietary habits or *travel* reaching back to the birth of the child should be sought. There may be re-emergence of malaria, histoplasmosis, and coccidioidomycosis years after visiting or living in an endemic area. It is important to ask about prophylactic immunizations and precautions taken by the individual against the ingestion of contaminated water or food during foreign travel. Rocks, dirt, and artifacts from geographically distant regions that have been collected and brought into the home as souvenirs may serve as vectors of disease.

A *medication* history should be pursued rigorously. This should include over-the-counter preparations and topical agents, including eye drops (atropine-induced fever).

The *genetic background* of the patient also is important. Descendants of the Ulster Scots may have fever of unknown origin because they are afflicted with nephrogenic diabetes insipidus. Familial dysautonomia (Riley-Day syndrome), a disorder in which hyperthermia is recurrent, is more frequent among Jews than other population groups.

PHYSICAL EXAMINATION. Sweating in a febrile child should be noted. The continuing absence of sweat in the presence of an elevated or changing body temperature suggests dehydration from vomiting, diarrhea, or central or nephrogenic diabetes insipidus. It also should suggest anhidrotic ectodermal dysplasia, familial dysautonomia, or exposure to atropine.

Red, weeping eyes may be a sign of connective tissue disease, particularly polyarteritis nodosa. Palpebral conjunctivitis in the febrile patient may be a clue to measles, coxsackievirus infection, tuberculosis, infectious mononucleosis, lymphogranuloma venereum, cat-scratch disease, or Newcastle disease virus infection. In contrast, bulbar conjunctivitis in a child with FUO suggests Kawasaki syndrome or leptospirosis. Petechial conjunctival hemorrhages suggest endocarditis. Uveitis suggests sarcoidosis, juvenile rheumatoid arthritis, systemic lupus erythematosus, Kawasaki syndrome, Behçet syndrome, and vasculitis. Chorioretinitis suggests cytomegalovirus, toxoplasmosis, and syphilis. Proptosis suggests orbital tumor, thyrotoxicosis, metastasis (neuroblastoma), orbital infection, Wegener granulomatosis, or pseudotumor. A careful ophthalmic examination is important in most patients with FUO.

The ophthalmoscope should also be used to examine for nailfold capillary abnormalities that are associated with connective tissue diseases such as dermatomyositis and systemic scleroderma. Emersion oil or lubricating jelly is placed on the skin adjacent to the nailbed, and the capillary pattern is observed with the ophthalmoscope set on +40. Normal and abnormal nailfold capillary patterns are shown in Figure 167–1 *A* and *B*, respectively.

Fever of unknown origin is sometimes due to hypothalamic dysfunction. A clue to this disorder is failure of pupillary constriction due to absence of the sphincter constrictor muscle of the eye. This muscle develops embryologically when hypothalamic structure and function also are undergoing differentiation.

Lack of tears or an absent corneal reflex may suggest fever resulting from familial dysautonomia. A smooth tongue may reflect absence of fungiform papillae and also suggest this diagnosis. Tenderness to tapping over the sinuses and teeth should be sought, and the sinuses should be transilluminated. Oral candidiasis may be a clue to various disorders of the immune system.

Fever blisters are common findings in patients with pneumococcal, streptococcal, malarial, and rickettsial infection. They also are common in children with meningococcal meningitis (which usually does not present as FUO) but rarely are seen in children with meningococcemia. Fever blisters also are rarely seen with salmonella or staphylococcal infections.

Repetitive chills and temperature spikes are common in children with septicemia (regardless of etiology), particularly when associated with renal disease, liver or biliary disease, endocarditis, malaria, brucellosis, rat-bite fever, or loculated collections of pus.

Hyperemia of the pharynx, with or without exudate, may suggest infectious mononucleosis, cytomegalovirus infection, toxoplasmosis, salmonellosis, tularemia, Kawasaki syndrome, or leptospirosis.

The muscles and bones should be palpated carefully. Point tenderness over a bone may suggest occult osteomyelitis or bone marrow invasion from neoplastic disease. Tenderness over the trapezius muscle may be a clue to subdiaphragmatic abscess. Generalized muscle tenderness suggests dermatomyositis, trichinosis, polyarteritis, Kawasaki syndrome, or mycoplasma or arboviral infection.

Rectal examination may reveal pararectal adenopathy or tenderness, which suggests a deep pelvic abscess, iliac adenitis, or pelvic osteomyelitis. A guaiac test should be obtained on any stool found on the examining finger; occult blood loss may suggest granulomatous colitis or ulcerative colitis as the cause of FUO.

The general activity of the patient and the presence or absence of rashes should be noted. Hyperactive deep tendon reflexes may suggest thyrotoxicosis as the cause of FUO.

LABORATORY STUDIES. Diagnostic tests most likely to provide a prompt definitive diagnosis should be used. Ordering a large number of tests in every child with FUO according to a predetermined sequence may waste time and money. Alternatively, prolonged hospitalization for sequential tests may be more costly. The tempo of diagnostic evaluation should be adjusted to the tempo of the illness; haste may be imperative in a critically ill patient, but if the illness is more chronic, the evaluation can proceed more slowly and deliberately, and, usually, in the ambulatory setting.

A complete blood cell count with a differential cell count and a urinalysis should be part of the initial laboratory evaluation. An absolute neutrophil count $<5,000\ mm^3$ is evidence against nonfulminant bacterial infection other than typhoid. Conversely, patients with >10,000 polymorphonuclear leukocytes or >500 nonsegmented polymorphonuclear leukocytes/mm^3 have a high chance of having a severe bacterial infection. Direct examination of the blood smear treated with Giemsa or Wright stain may reveal malaria, trypanosomiasis, babesiosis, or relapsing fever.

An elevated *erythrocyte sedimentation rate* (ESR; >30 mm/hr, Westergren method) indicates inflammation and the need for further evaluation for infectious, autoimmune, or malignant diseases. A low ESR does not eliminate the possibility of infection or juvenile rheumatoid arthritis, but an ESR of >100 mm/hr suggests tuberculosis, Kawasaki syndrome, malignancy, or autoimmune disease.

Blood cultures should be obtained aerobically. Anaerobic blood cultures have an extremely low yield and should only be obtained if there are specific reasons to suspect an anaerobic infection. Repeated blood cultures may be required to diagnose endocarditis, osteomyelitis, or deep-seated abscesses producing bacteremia. Polymicrobial bacteremia suggests factitious self-induced infection or gastrointestinal pathology. The isolation of leptospires, *Francisella*, or *Yersinia* may require selective media or specific conditions not routinely employed. *Urine culture* should be obtained routinely.

Tuberculin *skin testing* should be performed carefully with polysorbate 80 (Tween) stabilized purified protein derivative (PPD) that has been kept appropriately refrigerated. Other appropriate antigens *should be placed to test for anergy.*

Roentgenographic examination of the chest, sinuses, mastoids, or gastrointestinal tract may be suggested by specific historical or physical findings. Roentgenographic evaluation of the gastrointestinal tract for inflammatory bowel disease may be helpful in evaluating selected children with FUO and no other localizing signs or symptoms.

Examination of the *bone marrow* may reveal leukemia; metastatic neoplasm; mycobacterial, fungal, or parasitic diseases; and histiocytosis, hemophagocytosis, or storage diseases. If a bone marrow aspirate is performed, cultures for bacteria, *Mycobacterium*, and fungi should be obtained.

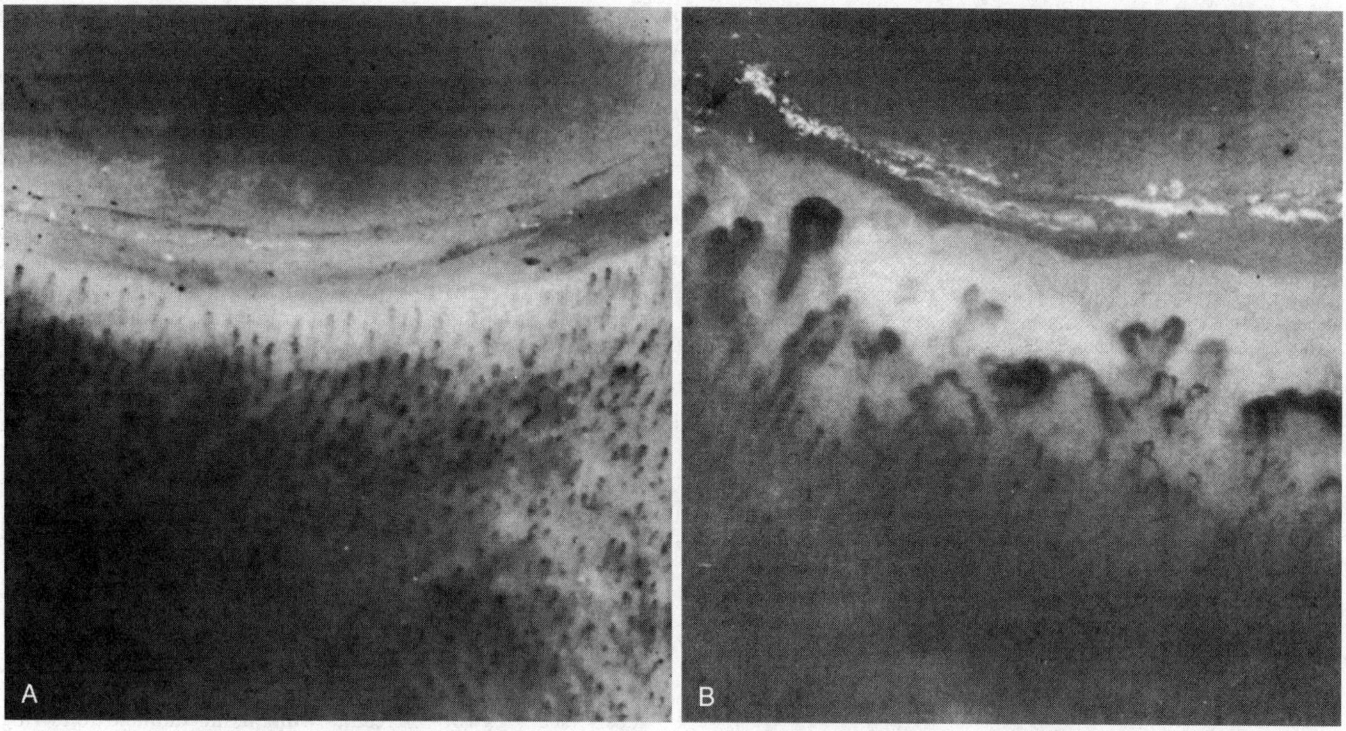

Figure 167–1. *A,* A normal nailfold capillary pattern with a homogeneous distribution and uniform appearance of loops. *B,* Markedly dilated capillary loops next to avascular areas where capillary dropout has occurred (patient with dermatomyositis). (From Spencer-Green G, Schlesinger M, Bove KE, et al: Nailfold capillary abnormalities in childhood rheumatic diseases. J Pediatr 102:341, 1983.)

Serologic tests may aid in the diagnosis of infectious mononucleosis, cytomegaloviral disease, toxoplasmosis, salmonellosis, tularemia, brucellosis, leptospirosis, and, on some occasions, juvenile rheumatoid arthritis. As serologic tests for more diseases become available through commercial laboratories, it is important to ascertain the sensitivity and specificity of each test before relying on these results to make a diagnosis. Serologic tests for Lyme disease are notoriously unreliable.

Radioactive scans may be helpful in detecting osteomyelitis and abdominal abscesses. Gallium citrate (^{67}Ga) localizes in inflammatory tissues (leukocytes) associated with tumors or abscesses. ^{99m}Tc phosphate is useful for detecting osteomyelitis before plain roentgenograms demonstrate bone lesions. Indium-III granulocytes or iodinated IgG may be useful in detecting localized pyogenic processes (see Chapter 304). *Echocardiograms* may suggest the presence of vegetation on the leaflets of heart valves, as in subacute bacterial endocarditis. *Ultrasonography* may identify intra-abdominal abscesses of the liver, subphrenic space, pelvis, or spleen.

Total body computed tomography (CT) or magnetic resonance imaging (MRI) scanning permits the detection of neoplasms and collections of purulent material without the use of surgical exploration or radioisotopes. CT scanning is helpful in identifying lesions of the head, neck, chest, retroperitoneal spaces, liver, spleen, intra-abdominal and intrathoracic lymph nodes, kidneys, pelvis, and mediastinum. CT or ultrasound-guided aspiration or biopsy of suspicious lesions has reduced the need for exploratory laparotomy or thoracotomy. Although scanning procedures can be very helpful in confirming a suspected diagnosis, they rarely lead to an unsuspected one.

Biopsy is occasionally helpful in establishing a diagnosis of FUO. Bronchoscopy, laparoscopy, mediastinoscopy, and gastrointestinal endoscopy may provide direct visualization and biopsy material when organ-specific manifestations are present.

TREATMENT. Fever and infection in children are not synonymous; antimicrobial agents should not be used as antipyretics, and empirical trials of medication should generally be avoided. An exception may be the use of antituberculous treatment in critically ill children with possible disseminated tuberculosis. Empirical trials of other antimicrobial agents may be dangerous and can obscure the diagnosis of endocarditis, meningitis, parameningeal infection, or osteomyelitis. Hospitalization may be required for laboratory or roentgenographic studies that are unavailable or impractical in an ambulatory setting, for more careful observation, or for temporary relief of parental anxiety. After a complete evaluation, antipyretics may be indicated to control fever.

PROGNOSIS. The child with FUO has a better prognosis than that reported for adults. Outcome in the child is dependent on the primary disease process, which is usually an atypical presentation of a common childhood illness. In many cases no diagnosis can be established, but fever abates spontaneously. In as many as 25% of cases in which fever persists, the cause of the fever remains unclear, even after thorough evaluation.

Alpert G, Hibbert E, Fleisher GR: Case-control study of hyperpyrexia in children. Pediatr Infect Dis J 9:161, 1990.

Anonymous: Splenectomy—A long-term risk of infection. Lancet 2:928, 1985.

Baker RC, Sequin JH, Leslie N, et al: Fever and petechiae in children. Pediatrics 84:1051, 1989.

Baraff LJ, Bass JW, Fleisher GR, et al: Practice guidelines for the management of infants and children 0–36 months of age with fever without a source. Pediatrics 92:1, 1993; Ann Emerg Med 22:1198, 1993.

Bass JW, Steele RW, Wittler RR, et al: Antimicrobial treatment of occult bacteremia: a multicenter cooperative study. Pediatr Infect Dis J 12:466, 1993.

Bonadio WA, Hegenbarth M, Zachariason M: Correlating reported fever in young infants with subsequent temperature patterns and rate of serious bacterial infections. Pediatr Infect Dis J 9:158, 1990.

Brusch JL, Weinstein L: Fever of unknown origin. Med Clin North Am 72:1247, 1988.

Dagan R, Hall CB, Powell KR, et al: Epidemiology and laboratory diagnosis of infection with viral and bacterial pathogens in infants hospitalized for suspected sepsis. J Pediatr 115:351, 1989.

Feigin RD, Shearer WT: Fever of unknown origin in children. Curr Probl Pediatr 6:1, 1976.

Fleisher GR, Rosenberg N, Vinci R, et al: Intramuscular versus oral antibiotic

therapy for the prevention of meningitis and other bacterial sequelae in young febrile children at risk for occult bacteremia. J Pediatr 124:504, 1994.
Gartner JC Jr: Fever of unknown origin. Adv Pediatr Infect Dis 7:1, 1992.
Givner LB, Woods CR Jr, Abramson JS: The practice of pediatrics in the era of vaccines effective against *Hemophilus influenzae* type b. Pediatrics 93:680, 1994.
Hayari A, Mahoney DH, Fernbach DJ: Role of bone marrow examination in the child with prolonged fever. J Pediatr 116:919, 1990.
Jaskiewicz JA, McCarthy CA, Richardson AC, et al: Febrile infants at low risk for serious bacterial infection—an appraisal of the Rochester criteria and implications for management. Pediatrics 94:390, 1994.
Larson EB, Featherstone JH, Petersdorf RG: Fever of undetermined origin: Diagnosis and follow up 105 cases, 1970–1980. Medicine 61:269, 1982.
Powell KR: Evaluation and management of febrile infants younger than 60 days of age. Pediatr Infect Dis J 9:153, 1990.
Rogers ZR, Morrison RA, Vedro DA, et al: Outpatient management of febrile illness in infants and young children with sickle cell anemia. J Pediatr 117:736, 1990.
Steele RW, Jones SM, Lowe BA, et al: Usefulness of scanning procedures for diagnosis of fever of unknown origin in children. J Pediatr 119:526, 1991.
Wilimas JA, Flynn PM, Harris S, et al: A randomized study of outpatient treatment with ceftriaxone for selected febrile children with sickle cell disease. N Engl J Med 329:472, 1993.

CHAPTER 168

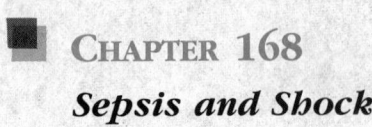

Sepsis and Shock

Keith R. Powell

BACTEREMIA AND SEPTICEMIA

The recovery of bacteria in a blood culture, *bacteremia*, may be a transient phenomenon not associated with disease or the serious extension of an invasive bacterial infection originating in the gastrointestinal *(Salmonella, Pseudomonas, Escherichia coli, Klebsiella-Enterobacter, Enterococcus)*, genitourinary *(E. coli, Klebsiella-Enterobacter, Proteus, Neisseria gonorrhoeae)*, or respiratory *(Pneumococcus, Haemophilus influenzae, Staphylococcus aureus)* tracts or integument *(S. aureus, S. epidermidis, Streptococcus pyogenes)*. Bacteremia may precede or coincide with specific local metastatic foci of infection, such as those occurring with meningitis, osteomyelitis, endocarditis, epiglottitis, and facial cellulitis. Transient or low-grade (<100 colony-forming units [CFU]/mL blood) bacteremia may follow instrumentation of the respiratory, gastrointestinal, or genitourinary tracts. Bacteremia may be asymptomatic or associated with few symptoms. When bacteria are not effectively cleared by host defense mechanisms, a systemic inflammatory response is set into motion that can progress independently of the original infection. Sepsis is a severe systemic response to an infection. Infections with bacteria, viruses, fungi, protozoae, or rickettsiae can result in sepsis. Sepsis is one of the causes of the systemic inflammatory response syndrome (SIRS), but there are noninfectious causes as well. If not recognized and treated early, sepsis can progress to SIRS, septic shock, refractory shock, multiple organ dysfunction, and death. The progression of events from bacteremia to sepsis and subsequent complications is illustrated in Figure 168–1. High-grade bacteremia (>100–1,000 CFU/mL) is commonly noted in patients with sepsis and in those whose condition progresses to septic shock. See Chapter 98.1 for a discussion of neonatal sepsis.

EPIDEMIOLOGY. Patients at high risk for sepsis are noted in Table 167–1. Previously immunocompetent nonhospitalized patients may develop community-acquired bacteremia-sepsis from extension of local tissue infections such as those mentioned earlier. Alternatively, colonization and local mucosal invasion by a particularly virulent pathogen (*N. meningitidis, Streptococcus pneumoniae, H. influenzae* type b) in a previously normal host may produce primary bacteremia and sepsis. Occult pneumococcal bacteremia is discussed in Chapter 167.

Immunocompromised patients, as noted in Table 167–1, are at increased risk for serious nosocomial sepsis. Hospitalized patients develop sepsis due to *S. aureus* or *S. epidermidis* from catheter infection or surgical wounds, whereas serious gram-negative *(E. coli, Pseudomonas, Acinetobacter, Klebsiella-Enterobacter, Serratia)* sepsis is characteristic of the immunocompromised neutropenic patient or the acutely ill patient receiving intensive care. Polymicrobial sepsis also occurs in high-risk patients and is associated with central venous catheterization, gastrointestinal disease, neutropenia, and malignancy. Additional, less frequent causes of bacteremia or sepsis include anaerobic bacilli, *Yersinia pestis* (plague), *Salmonella typhi* (typhoid fever), *Pseudomonas pseudomallei* (melioidosis), *Vibrio vulnificus* (oyster consumption), and DF-2 (dysgonic fermentative organism from cat bites).

Pseudobacteremia may be associated with contaminated solutions such as antimicrobial disinfectants, heparin flush solutions, intravenous infusates, albumin, cryoprecipitate, and contaminated equipment. Unusual water-based organisms such as *Pseudomonas cepacia* are frequently recovered, but true pathogens, such as *P. aeruginosa* or *Serratia*, may also be identified.

PATHOGENESIS OF SEPSIS AND THE SYSTEMIC INFLAMMATORY RESPONSE SYNDROME (SIRS). It is currently thought that SIRS caused by sepsis (see Fig. 168–1) results from tissue damage following the host response to bacterial products such as endotoxin from gram-negative bacteria and the lipoteichoic acid-peptidoglycan complex from gram-positive bacteria. The cardiopulmonary manifestations of gram-negative *(H. influenzae, N. meningitidis, E. coli, Pseudomonas)* sepsis can be mimicked by injection of endotoxin or tumor necrosis factor (TNF). Inhibition of TNF action by monoclonal anti-TNF antibody greatly attenuates the manifestations of septic shock in experimental models. When bacterial cell wall components are released into the bloodstream, cytokines are activated, which in turn can lead to further physiologic derangements (Fig. 168–2). The number of cytokines associated with SIRS continues to increase and currently includes tumor necrosis factor (TNF), interleukin (IL)-1, -6 and -8, platelet-activating factor (PAF), and interferon-γ.

Alone or in combination, bacterial products and proinflammatory cytokines trigger physiologic responses to stop microbial invaders. These responses include: (1) activation of the complement system; (2) activation of Hageman factor (factor XII), which then initiates the coagulation cascade; (3) adrenocorticotrophic hormone and beta-endorphin release, (4) stimulation of polymorphonuclear neutrophils, and (5) stimulation of the kallikrein-kinin system (see Fig. 168–2). TNF and other inflammatory mediators increase vascular permeability, producing diffuse capillary leakage, reduced vascular tone, and an imbalance between perfusion and the increased metabolic requirements of tissues. Inflammatory mediator activity or over-responsiveness contributes to the pathogenesis of sepsis.

Shock is defined by a systolic blood pressure below the 5th percentile for age or by cool extremities. Delayed capillary refill (>2 sec) is no longer considered a reliable indicator of decreased peripheral perfusion. Peripheral vascular resistance is reduced in early (warm) septic shock but becomes greatly elevated in late (cold) shock. Tissue oxygen consumption exceeds oxygen delivery in septic shock. This imbalance is due to early peripheral vasodilation, late vasoconstriction, myocardial depression, hypotension, ventilatory insufficiency, and anemia. Although the cardiac index of children with sepsis is elevated compared with nonseptic patients, the cardiac output is insufficient for the large peripheral tissue oxygen consumption that occurs in septic shock. The resultant tissue hypoxia leads to lactic acidosis.

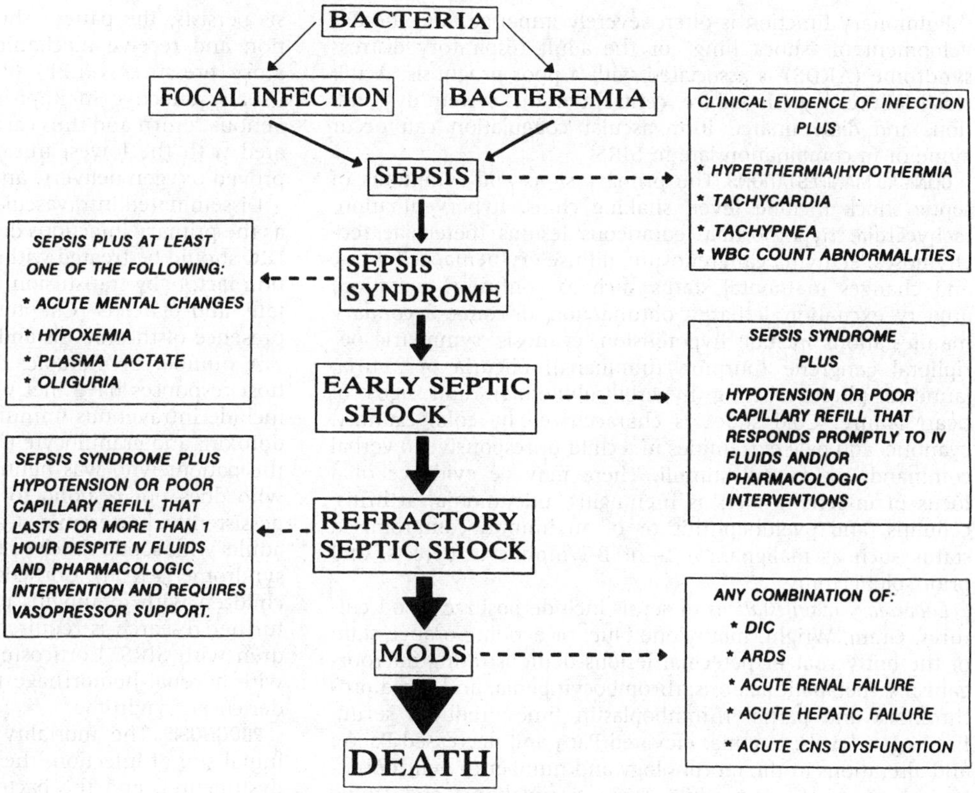

Figure 168–1. Progression from bacteremia to sepsis to the systemic inflammatory response syndrome (SIRS, sepsis syndrome) and its complications. WBC, white blood cell; IV, intravenous; DIC, disseminated intravascular coagulation; ARDS, adult respiratory distress syndrome; CNS, central nervous system; MODS, multiorgan dysfunction syndrome. (From Sáez-Llorens X, McCracken GH Jr: Sepsis syndrome and septic shock in pediatrics: Current concepts of terminology, pathophysiology, and management. J Pediatr 123: 497, 1993.)

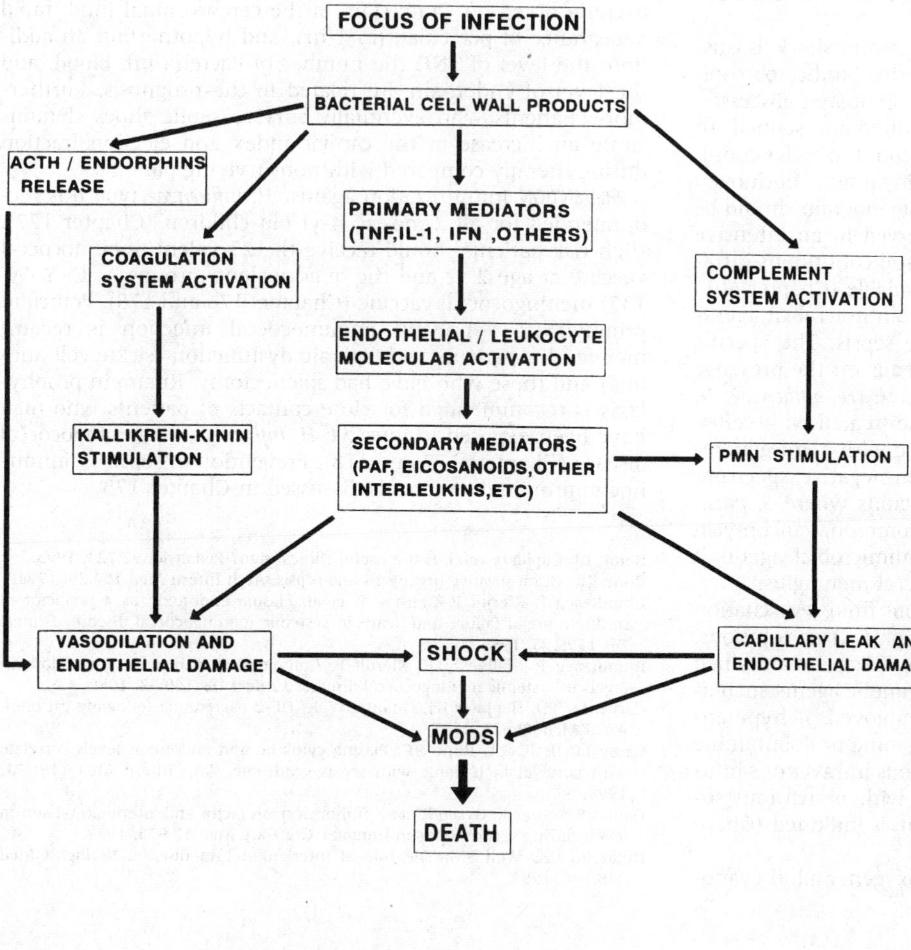

Figure 168–2. Hypothetical pathophysiology of the septic process. ACTH, adrenocorticotrophic hormone; TNF, tumor necrosis factor; IL-1, interleukin-1; PAF, platelet activating factor; PMN, polymorphonuclear lymphocytes; IFN, interferon gamma; MODS, multiorgan dysfunction syndrome. (From Sáez-Llorens X, McCracken GH Jr: Sepsis syndrome and septic shock in pediatrics: Current concepts of terminology, pathophysiology, and management. J Pediatr 123:497, 1993.)

Pulmonary function is often severely impaired, and the development of "shock lung" or the adult respiratory distress syndrome (ARDS) is associated with a poor prognosis. Acute renal failure, hepatic failure, central nervous system dysfunction, and disseminated intravascular coagulation can occur alone or in combination late in SIRS.

CLINICAL MANIFESTATIONS. The primary signs and symptoms of septic shock include fever, shaking chills, hyperventilation, tachycardia, hypothermia, cutaneous lesions (petechiae, ecchymoses, ecthyma gangrenosum, diffuse erythema, cellulitis), and changes in mental status such as confusion, agitation, anxiety, excitation, lethargy, obtundation, or coma. Secondary manifestations include hypotension, cyanosis, symmetric peripheral gangrene (purpura fulminans), oliguria or anuria, jaundice (direct-reacting hyperbilirubinemia), and signs of heart failure. Cold shock is characterized by cold, clammy, cyanotic, and pale extremities in a child unresponsive to verbal commands or painful stimuli. There may be evidence of a focus of infection, such as meningitis, pneumonia, arthritis, cellulitis, and pyelonephritis or of an immunocompromised status such as malignancy, T- or B-lymphocyte defects, and prior splenectomy.

Laboratory manifestations of sepsis include positive blood cultures; Gram, Wright, methylene blue, or acridine orange stain of the buffy coat or petechial lesions demonstrating microorganisms; metabolic acidosis; thrombocytopenia; prolonged prothrombin and partial thromboplastin times; reduced serum fibrinogen levels; anemia; elevated $Pa{O_2}$ and decreased $Pa{CO_2}$; and alterations in the morphology and number of neutrophils. Vacuolization of neutrophils, toxic granulations, and Döhle bodies are also suggestive of bacterial sepsis. Elevated neutrophil and band counts (shift to the left: immature white blood cells) suggest bacterial infection, and neutropenia is an ominous sign of fulminant septic shock. Examination of the cerebrospinal fluid may reveal neutrophils and bacteria, may demonstrate only bacteria in the absence of an inflammatory response, or may be normal.

TREATMENT. Patients in whom sepsis or septic shock is suspected should have specimens of blood, urine, and cerebrospinal fluid cultured for bacterial pathogens. Exudates, abscesses, and cutaneous lesions should also be cultured and stained for organisms. In addition, a complete blood count, platelet count, prothrombin and partial thromboplastin times, fibrinogen level, arterial blood gases, and chest roentgenogram should be obtained. These children should be observed in an intensive care unit where central venous pressure and continuous intra-arterial blood pressure monitoring are available (Chapter 60).

Broad-spectrum bactericidal synergistic antimicrobial agents should be administered for presumptive sepsis. The specific combination of antimicrobial agents depends on the presence of risk factors. Community-acquired disease *(H. influenzae, N. meningitidis, S. pneumoniae)* can initially be treated with ceftriaxone; nosocomial sepsis should be treated with a 3rd-generation cephalosporin or an extended gram-negative spectrum penicillin, plus an aminoglycoside. In regions where *S. pneumoniae* isolates resistant to penicillin are common, vancomycin should be given in addition to other antimicrobial agents if there is a strong possibility of pneumococcal meningitis.

Shock should be managed by intravenous fluid resuscitation using normal saline, albumin, hetastarch, or dextran solutions. If normal blood pressure cannot be achieved and maintained by fluid therapy, intravenous sympathomimetic agents such as dopamine and dobutamine should be employed. If hypotension remains refractory to fluids and dopamine or dobutamine administration, judicious use of a continuous intravenous infusion of epinephrine or norepinephrine, with or without sodium nitroprusside for afterload reduction, is indicated (Chapter 60).

Hypoxia should be treated with nasal oxygen, and, if cyanosis persists, the patient should undergo endotracheal intubation and receive mechanical ventilation. Positive end-expiratory pressures (PEEP) of between 5 and 20 cm H_2O are usually effective in improving oxygenation but may reduce venous return and thus cardiac output. Optimal PEEP is associated with the lowest intrapulmonary right-to-left shunt, improved oxygen delivery, and no impairment of cardiac output.

Disseminated intravascular coagulation (DIC) should resolve as the primary infectious disease is treated. If bleeding is noted, DIC should be treated with replacement of consumed coagulation factors by transfusion of fresh frozen plasma, cryoprecipitate, and platelets (Chapter 60.5). Heparin is indicated in the presence of thrombosis and peripheral gangrene.

A number of therapies aimed at modifying overexuberant host responses have met with limited success. Such therapies include intravenous immunoglobulin, monoclonal IgM to endotoxin, and granulocyte transfusion. The latter is reserved for the patient who was neutropenic prior to the septic episode, who does not respond to antimicrobial therapy, and who is persistently bacteremic. Corticosteroids are not beneficial in adults with septic shock or those with acute respiratory distress syndrome (ARDS). Corticosteroids do improve the outcome of children with meningitis caused by *H. influenzae* type b, and further research is required to determine their effects in children with SIRS. Corticosteroids may be beneficial in patients with adrenal hemorrhage that is part of the Waterhouse-Friderichsen syndrome.

PROGNOSIS. The mortality for septic shock depends on the initial site of infection, the presence of multiple organ system dysfunction, and the bacterial pathogen. It may be 40–60% for patients with gram-negative enteric sepsis. Urosepsis has a much better prognosis than primary sepsis without a focus. Poor prognostic signs in meningococcal sepsis include hypotension, coma, leukopenia (<5,000), thrombocytopenia (<100,000), low fibrinogen level (<150 mg/dL), absence of meningismus, absence of cerebrospinal fluid pleocytosis with bacteria noted on Gram stain of the cerebrospinal fluid, rapid appearance of petechiae (in 1 hr), and hypothermia. In addition, the level of TNF, the number of bacteria/mL blood, and the level of endotoxin are related to the prognosis. Furthermore, patients who eventually survive septic shock demonstrate an increase in the cardiac index and ejection fraction during therapy compared with nonsurviving patients.

PREVENTION. Immunization against *H. influenzae* type b is recommended for all 2-mo- to 4-yr-old children (Chapter 177). High-risk patients should receive the 23-valent pneumococcal vaccine at age 2 yr and the quadrivalent (groups A, C, Y, W-135) meningococcal vaccine (Chapters 176 and 178). Penicillin prophylaxis to prevent pneumococcal infection is recommended for patients with splenic dysfunction (sickle cell anemia) and those who have had splenectomy. Rifampin prophylaxis is recommended for close contacts of patients who may have been exposed to invasive *H. influenzae* or meningococcal disease (Chapters 177 and 178). Prevention of sepsis in immunocompromised patients is discussed in Chapter 173.

Baraff LJ: Capillary refill: Is it a useful clinical sign? Pediatrics 92:723, 1993.
Bone RC: Gram-positive organisms and sepsis. Arch Intern Med 154:26, 1994.
Brandtzaeg P, Kierulf P, Gaustad P, et al: Plasma endotoxin as a predictor of multiple organ failure and death in systemic meningococcal disease. J Infect Dis 159:195, 1989.
Brandtzaeg P, Mollness TE, Kierulf P: Complement activation and endotoxin levels in systemic meningococcal disease. J Infect Dis 160:58, 1989.
Carpenter PD, Heppner BT, Gnann JW Jr: DF-2 bacteremia following cat bites. Am J Med 82:621, 1987.
Casey LC, Balk RA, Bone RC: Plasma cytokine and endotoxin levels correlate with survival in patients with sepsis syndrome. Ann Intern Med 119:771, 1993.
Damas P, Reuter A, Gysen P, et al: Tumor necrosis factor and interleukin-1 serum levels during severe sepsis in humans. Crit Care Med 17:975, 1989.
Dinarello CA, Wolf SM: The role of interleukin-1 in disease. N Engl J Med 328:106, 1993.

Franson TR, Hierholzer WJ Jr, LaBrecque DR: Frequency and characteristics of hyperbilirubinemia associated with bacteremia. Rev Infect Dis 7:1, 1985.
Gullberg RM, Homann SR, Phair JP: Enterococcal bacteremia: Analysis of 75 episodes. Rev Infect Dis 11:74, 1989.
Hilf M, Yu VL, Sharp J, et al: Antibiotic therapy for *Pseudomonas aeruginosa* bacteremia: Outcome correlations in a prospective study of 200 patients. Am J Med 87:540, 1989.
Jacobs RF, Sowell MK, Moss MM, et al: Septic shock in children: Bacterial etiologies and temporal relationships. Pediatr Infect Dis J 9:196, 1990.
Klontz KC, Lieb S, Schreiber M, et al: Syndromes of *Vibrio vulnificus* infections: Clinical and epidemiologic features in Florida cases, 1981–1987. Ann Intern Med 109:318, 1988.
Mercier JC, Beaufils F, Hartmann JF, et al: Hemodynamic patterns of meningococcal shock in children. Crit Care Med 16:27, 1988.
Michie HR, Manogue KR, Spriggs DR, et al: Detection of circulating tumor necrosis factor after endotoxin administration. N Engl J Med 318:1481, 1988.
Reuben AG, Musher DM, Hamill RJ, et al: Polymicrobial bacteremia: Clinical and microbiologic patterns. Rev Infect Dis 11:161, 1989.
Sáez-Llorens X, McCracken GH Jr: Sepsis syndrome and septic shock in pediatrics: Current concepts of terminology, pathophysiology, and management. J Pediatr 123:497, 1993.
Sinclair JF: The management of fulminant meningococcal septicaemia in children. Intensive Care World 5:89, 1988.
Tuchschmidt J, Fried J, Swinney R, et al: Early hemodynamic correlates of survival in patients with septic shock. Crit Care Med 17:719, 1989.
Wong VK, Hitchcock W, Mason WH: Meningococcal infections in children: A review of 100 cases. Pediatr Infect Dis J 8:224, 1989.
Young LS, Glauser MP (eds): Gram negative septicemia and septic shock. Infect Dis Clin North Am 5:739, 1991.

CHAPTER 169

Infections of the Central Nervous System

Charles G. Prober

Acute infection of the central nervous system (CNS) is the most common cause of fever associated with signs and symptoms of central nervous system disease in children. Infection may be caused by virtually any microbe, the specific pathogen being influenced by the age and immune status of the host and the epidemiology of the pathogen. In general, viral infections of the CNS are much more common than bacterial infections, which in turn are more common than fungal and parasitic infections. Infections caused by *Rickettsia* (e.g., Rocky Mountain spotted fever and *Ehrlichia*) are relatively uncommon when the entire country is considered, but, as will be discussed, they assume important roles under certain epidemiologic circumstances. *Mycoplasma* spp. also can cause infections of the CNS, although their precise contribution often is difficult to determine.

Regardless of etiology, most patients with acute CNS infection have similar syndromes. Common symptoms include: headache, nausea, vomiting, anorexia, restlessness, and irritability. Unfortunately, most of these symptoms are quite nonspecific. Common signs of CNS infection, in addition to fever, include: photophobia, neck pain and rigidity, obtundation, stupor, coma, seizures, and focal neurologic deficits. The severity and constellation of signs is determined by the specific pathogen, the host, and the anatomic distribution of the infection. The anatomic distribution of infection may be diffuse or focal. Meningitis and encephalitis are examples of diffuse infection. Meningitis implies primary involvement of the meninges, whereas encephalitis indicates brain parenchymal involvement. Because these anatomic boundaries are often not distinct, many patients have evidence of both meningeal and parenchymal involvement and should be considered to have meningoencephalitis. Brain abscess is the best example of a focal infection of the CNS. The neurologic expression of this infection is determined by the site and extent of the abscess(es).

The diagnosis of diffuse CNS infections depends on careful examination of cerebrospinal fluid (CSF) obtained by lumbar puncture. The usual CSF profile associated with different infections will be detailed in later sections discussing specific syndromes or pathogens. Table 169–1 provides an overview of the expected CSF abnormalities.

■ TABLE 169–1 Cerebrospinal Fluid Findings in Various Central Nervous System Infections

Infection	Pressure (mm H_2O)	Leukocytes Total (m^3)	% PMN	Protein (mg/dL)	Glucose (mg/dL)
No infection (normal)	50–80	<5	<25%	20–45	>50
Viral meningo-encephalitis	100–150	10–1,000	<25%*	50–200	>50
Bacterial meningitis	100–300	100–10,000	>75%	100–500	<40
Brain abscess	100–300	10–200	<25%	75–500	>50

*May be predominance of PMNs in the first several hours of infection.

169.1 Acute Bacterial Meningitis Beyond the Neonatal Period

Bacterial meningitis is one of the most potentially serious infections in infants and older children. This infection is associated with a high rate of acute complications and risk of chronic morbidity. The pattern of bacterial meningitis and its treatment during the neonatal period (0–28 days) are generally distinct from those in older infants and children (see Chapter 98). Nonetheless, the clinical patterns of meningitis in the neonatal and postneonatal periods may overlap, especially in the 1- to 2-mo-old patient in whom group B streptococcus, *H. influenzae* type b, meningococcus, and pneumococcus may all produce meningitis.

The incidence of bacterial meningitis is sufficiently high that it should be included in the differential diagnosis of febrile infants who demonstrate altered mental status, irritability, or evidence of other neurologic dysfunction.

ETIOLOGY. During the first 2 mo of life, the bacteria that cause meningitis in normal infants reflect the maternal flora or the environment of the infant (i.e., group B streptococci, gram-negative enteric bacilli, and *Listeria monocytogenes*). In addition, meningitis in this age group may occasionally be due to *Haemophilus influenzae* (both nontypable and type b strains) and the other pathogens noted in older patients.

Bacterial meningitis in children 2 mo to 12 yr of age is usually due to *H. influenzae* type b, *Streptococcus pneumoniae*, or *Neisseria meningitidis*. Prior to the widespread use of *H. influenzae* type b vaccines, the incidence of disease due to *H. influenzae* type b far exceeded that due to *N. meningitidis* and *S. pneumoniae*. Disease due to *H. influenzae* type b may occur at any age, although historically most episodes occur before 2 yr of age. In children vaccinated against *H. influenzae* type b and in older unvaccinated children and adults, meningitis is usually due to *N. meningitidis* or *S. pneumoniae*. Alterations of host defense due to anatomic defects or immune deficits increase the risk of meningitis from less common pathogens such as *Pseudomonas aeruginosa, Staphylococcus aureus, Staphylococcus epidermidis, Salmonella*, and *L. monocytogenes*.

EPIDEMIOLOGY. A major risk factor for meningitis is the attenuated immunologic response to specific pathogens associated with young age. The risk is greatest among infants between 1 and 12 mo of age; 95% of cases occur between 1 mo and 5 yr of age, but meningitis can occur at any age. Additional risks include recent colonization with pathogenic bacteria, close contact with individuals having invasive disease (home, day-care centers, schools, military barracks), crowding, poverty, black race, male sex, and possibly absence of breast-feeding for infants 2–5 mo of age. The mode of transmission is probably person-to-person contact through respiratory tract secretions or droplets. The risk of meningitis is increased among patients with presumed occult bacteremia; the odds ratio is greater for meningococcus (85 times) than for *H. influenzae* type b (12 times) relative to that for pneumococcus. Other systemic infections also may be associated with an increased risk of meningitis, as exemplified by the association of meningitis with facial cellulitis due to *H. influenzae* type b in children under 4 yr of age. Specific host defense defects due to altered immunoglobulin production in response to encapsulated pathogens may be responsible for the increased risk of bacterial meningitis seen in Native Americans and Eskimos, whereas defects of the complement system (C5–C8) have been associated with recurrent meningococcal infection, and defects of the properdin system have been associated with a significant risk of lethal meningococcal disease. Splenic dysfunction (sickle cell anemia) or asplenia (due to trauma, congenital defect, staging of Hodgkin disease) is associated with an increased risk of pneumococcal, *H. influenzae* type b (to some extent), and, rarely, meningococcal sepsis and meningitis. T-lymphocyte defects (congenital or acquired by chemotherapy, acquired immunodeficiency syndrome [AIDS], or malignancy) are associated with an increased risk of *L. monocytogenes* infections of the CNS. Congenital or acquired CSF communications across the mucocutaneous barrier, such as cranial or midline facial defects (cribriform plate) and middle ear (stapedial foot plate) or inner ear fistulas (oval window, internal auditory canal, cochlear aqueduct), or CSF leakage through a rupture of the meninges due to a basal skull fracture into the cribriform plate or paranasal sinus, is associated with an increased risk of pneumococcal meningitis. Lumbosacral dermal sinus and meningomyelocele are associated with staphylococcal and enteric bacterial meningitis. Penetrating cranial trauma and CSF shunt infections increase the risk of meningitis due to staphylococci (especially coagulase-negative species) and other cutaneous bacteria.

Haemophilus influenzae Type b. Nonencapsulated strains of *H. influenzae* may be found in the throat or nasopharynx of up to 80% of children and adults; 2–5% carry *H. influenzae* type b. Carriage of type b *H. influenzae* occurs predominantly in children 1 mo to 4 yr of age; colonization rates are greatest following close contact with other children who are carriers or have serious *H. influenzae* disease. In unvaccinated children, invasive *H. influenzae* type b infections are most common in infants 2 mo to 2 yr of age; peak incidence occurs in infants 6–9 mo of age, and 50% of cases occur in the first year of life. Rates of infection are highest among Alaskan Eskimos and Navajo Indians. The risk to children is also markedly increased among family or day-care center contacts of patients with *H. influenzae* type b disease. Otitis media due to *H. influenzae* type b, human immunodeficiency virus (HIV) infection, CSF leaks, and occult bacteremia also increase the risk of *H. influenzae* meningitis. The widespread use of vaccines against *H. influenzae* type b, beginning at 2 mo of age, has been associated with marked reduction in the frequency of infection caused by this bacteria.

Streptococcus pneumoniae. The risk of sepsis and meningitis due to *S. pneumoniae* depends, at least in part, on the infecting serotype. Throat or nasopharyngeal carriage of *S. pneumoniae* is acquired from family contacts after birth, is transient (2–4 mo), is often associated with homotype antibody production, and, if recent (<1 mo), is a risk factor for serious infection. The incidence of pneumococcal meningitis is 1–3 per 100,000; infection may occur throughout life. The midwinter months are the peak season. The risk of meningitis is 5- to 36-fold greater among blacks than whites. Among blacks with sickle cell anemia, this incidence increases to more than 300-fold that in white children. Approximately 4% of children with sickle cell anemia will develop pneumococcal meningitis before the age of 5 yr if they are not given prophylactic antibiotics. Additional risk factors for contracting pneumococcal meningitis include an associated otitis media, sinusitis, pneumonia, CSF otorrhea or rhinorrhea, splenectomy, and chronic graft-versus-host disease following bone marrow transplantation.

Neisseria meningitidis. Meningococcal meningitis may be sporadic or cases may occur in epidemics. In the absence of an epidemic, most infections are due to group B. Epidemics usually are caused by groups A and C. Cases occur throughout the year but may be more common in the winter and spring. Nasopharyngeal carriage of *N. meningitidis* occurs in 1–15% of adults. Colonization may last weeks to months; recent colonization places the nonimmune younger child at greatest risk for meningitis. The incidence of simultaneous disease occurring in association with an index case in the family is 1%, a rate that is 1,000-fold the risk in the general population. The risk of secondary cases occurring in contacts at day-care centers is about 1 in 1,000. Most infections of children are acquired from a contact in a day-care facility, a colonized adult family member, or an ill patient with meningococcal disease.

PATHOLOGY. A meningeal exudate of varying thickness may be distributed around the cerebral veins, venous sinuses, convexity of the brain, and cerebellum and in the sulci, sylvian fissures, basal cisterns, and spinal cord. Ventriculitis with bacteria and inflammatory cells in ventricular fluid may be present, as may subdural effusions and, rarely, empyema. Perivascular inflammatory infiltrates may also be present, and the ependymal membrane may be disrupted. Vascular and parenchymal cerebral changes characterized by polymorphonuclear infiltrates extending to the subintimal region of the small arteries and veins, vasospasm, vasculitis, thrombosis of small cortical veins, occlusion of major venous sinuses, necrotizing arteritis producing subarachnoid hemorrhage, and, rarely, cerebral cortical necrosis in the absence of identifiable thrombosis have been described at autopsy. Cerebral infarction is a frequent sequelae of vascular occlusion from inflammation, vasospasm, and thrombosis. Infarct size ranges from microscopic to involvement of an entire hemisphere.

Inflammation of spinal nerves and roots produces meningeal signs, and inflammation of the cranial nerves produces cranial neuropathies of optic, oculomotor, facial, and auditory nerves. Increased intracranial pressure also produces oculomotor nerve palsy due to the presence of temporal lobe compression of the nerve during tentorial herniation. Abducens nerve palsy may be a nonlocalizing sign of raised intracranial pressure.

Increased intracranial pressure is due to cell death (cytotoxic cerebral edema), cytokine-induced increased capillary vascular permeability (vasogenic cerebral edema), and, possibly, increased hydrostatic pressure (interstitial cerebral edema) following obstructed reabsorption of CSF in the arachnoid villus or obstruction of the flow of fluid within or exiting from the ventricles. Intracranial pressure often exceeds 300 mm H_2O; cerebral perfusion may be further compromised if the cerebral perfusion pressure (mean arterial pressure minus intracranial pressure) is less than 50 cm H_2O owing to reduced cerebral blood flow. Inappropriate secretion of antidiuretic hormone may produce excessive water retention, increasing the risk of raised intracranial pressure. Hypotonicity of brain extracellular spaces may cause cytotoxic edema following cell swelling and lysis. Herniation syndromes occur in 5% of infants and children with meningitis, and should suggest markedly raised intracranial pressure, a cerebral abscess, or subdural empyema. Tentorial, falx, or cerebellar herniation does not usually occur because the increased intracranial pressure is transmitted to the entire subarachnoid space and there is little structural displacement. Furthermore, if the fontanelles are still patent, increased intracranial pressure is readily dissipated.

Hydrocephalus is an uncommon acute complication of meningitis occurring after the neonatal period. Most often it takes the form of a communicating hydrocephalus due to adhesive thickening of the arachnoid villi around the cisterns at the base of the brain. Thus, there is interference with the normal resorption of CSF. Less often, obstructive hydrocephalus develops following fibrosis and gliosis of the aqueduct of Sylvius or the foramina of Magendie and Luschka.

Raised CSF protein levels are due in part to increased vascular permeability of the blood-brain barrier and the loss of albumin-rich fluid from the capillaries and veins traversing the subdural space. Continued transudation may result in subdural effusions, noted in the later phase of acute bacterial meningitis. Hypoglycorrhachia (reduced CSF glucose levels) is due to decreased glucose transport by the cerebral tissue. The latter may produce a local lactic acidosis.

Damage to the cerebral cortex may be due to the focal or diffuse effects of vascular occlusion (infarction, necrosis), hypoxia, bacterial invasion (cerebritis), toxic encephalopathy (lactic acidosis), raised intracranial pressure, ventriculitis, and transudation (subdural effusions). The resultant manifestations of impaired consciousness, seizures, hydrocephalus, cranial nerve deficits, motor and sensory deficits, and later psychomotor retardation can be explained by one or more of the pathologic factors described earlier.

PATHOGENESIS. Bacterial meningitis most commonly results from hematogenous dissemination of microorganisms from a distant site of infection; bacteremia usually precedes meningitis or occurs concomitantly. Bacterial colonization of the nasopharynx with a potentially pathogenic microorganism is the usual source of the bacteremia. There may be prolonged carriage of the colonizing organisms without disease or, more likely, rapid invasion following recent colonization. Prior or concurrent viral upper respiratory tract infection may enhance the pathogenicity of bacteria producing meningitis.

H. influenzae type b and meningococci attach to mucosal epithelial cell receptors by pili. Following attachment to epithelial cells, bacteria breach the mucosa and enter the circulation. *N. meningitidis* may be transported across the mucosal surface within a phagocytic vacuole following ingestion by the epithelial cell. Bacterial survival in the bloodstream is enhanced by large bacterial capsules that interfere with opsonophagocytosis and are associated with increased virulence. Host-related developmental defects in bacterial opsonophagocytosis also contribute to the bacteremia. In the young nonimmune host the defect may be due to an absence of preformed IgM or IgG anticapsular antibodies, whereas in immunodeficient patients various deficiencies of components of the complement or properdin system may interfere with effective opsonophagocytosis. Direct activation of the antibody-independent properdin system is one mechanism that counteracts the effects of antibody deficiency and the antiphagocytic properties of the bacterial capsule. Splenic dysfunction also may reduce opsonophagocytosis by the reticuloendothelial system.

Bacteria gain entry to the CSF through the choroid plexus of the lateral ventricles and the meninges. The bacteria then circulate to the extracerebral CSF and subarachnoid space, and rapidly multiply because the CSF concentrations of complement and antibody are inadequate to contain bacterial proliferation. Chemotactic factors then incite a local inflammatory response characterized by polymorphonuclear cell infiltration. The presence of bacterial cell wall lipopolysaccharide (endotoxin) of gram-negative bacteria *(H. influenzae* type b, *N. meningitidis)* and of pneumococcal cell wall components (teichoic acid, peptidoglycan) stimulates a marked inflammatory response with local production of tumor necrosis factor, interleukin-1, prostaglandin E, and other cytokine inflammatory mediators. The subsequent inflammatory response, directly related to the presence of these inflammatory mediators, is characterized by neutrophilic infiltration, increased vascular permeability, alterations of the blood-brain barrier, and vascular thrombosis. Excessive cytokine-induced inflammation continues after the CSF has been sterilized and is thought to be partly responsible for the chronic inflammatory sequelae of pyo[illegible] meningitis.

Meningitis may rarely follow bacterial invasi[illegible] tiguous focus of infection, for example, [illegible] otitis media, mastoiditis, orbital cellu[illegible] cranial or vertebral osteomyeliti[illegible] or meningomyeloceles. Me[illegible] ditis, pneumonia, or t[illegible] associated with severe b[illegible] ntaminated equipment.

CLINICAL MA[illegible] [illegible] te meningitis has two predomi[illegible], with rapidly progressive mani[illegible] pura, disseminated intravascular c[illegible] levels of consciousness, is a dramatic [illegible] itation of meningococcal sepsis with meni[illegible] volve to death with 24 hr. *H. influenzae* type b a[illegible] ococcal meningitis less frequently present as a rapidly [illegible] ogressive infection. More often, meningitis due to *H. influenzae* type b or pneumococcus, and some cases of meningococcal meningitis, is preceded by several days of upper respiratory tract or gastrointestinal symptoms.

The signs and symptoms of meningitis are related to the nonspecific findings associated with a systemic infection or bacteremia and to the specific manifestations of meningeal irritation with CNS inflammation. Nonspecific findings include fever (present in 90–95%), anorexia and poor feeding, symptoms of upper respiratory tract infection, myalgias, arthralgias, tachycardia, hypotension, and various cutaneous signs, such as petechiae, purpura, or an erythematous macular rash. Meningeal irritation is manifest as nuchal rigidity, back pain, *Kernig sign* (flexion of the hip 90 degrees with subsequent pain with extension of the leg), and *Brudzinski sign* (involuntary flexion of the knees and hips following flexion of the neck while supine). In some children, particularly in those less than 12–18 mo of age, these signs may not be evident. Increased intracranial pressure is suggested by headache, emesis, bulging fontanel or diastasis (widening) of the sutures, oculomotor or abducens nerve paralysis, hypertension with bradycardia, apnea or hyperventilation, decorticate or decerebrate posturing, stupor, coma, or signs of herniation. Papilledema is uncommon in uncomplicated meningitis and should suggest a more chronic process, such as the presence of an intracranial abscess, subdural empyema, or occlusion of a dural venous sinus. Focal neurologic signs usually are due to vascular occlusion. Cranial neuropathies of the ocular, oculomotor, abducens, facial, and auditory nerves also may be due to focal inflammation. Overall, about 10–20% of children with bacterial meningitis have focal neurologic signs. This frequency increases to >30% with pneumococcal meningitis, as this bacteria tends to stimulate the most vigorous inflammatory response.

Seizures (focal or generalized) due to cerebritis, infarction, or electrolyte disturbances are noted in 20–30% of patients with meningitis. They are more frequently noted in patients with *H. influenzae* and pneumococcal meningitis than in those with meningococcal infection. Seizures that occur on presentation or within the first 4 days of onset are usually of no prognostic significance. Seizures that persist after the 4th day of illness and those that are difficult to treat are associated with a poor prognosis.

Alterations of mental status and a reduced level of consciousness are common among patients with meningitis and may be due to increased intracranial pressure, cerebritis, or hypotension; manifestations include irritability, lethargy, stupor, obtundation, and coma. Comatose patients have a poor prognosis; this sign is noted more often with pneumococcal or meningococcal infection than with meningitis due to *H. influenzae*. Additional manifestations of meningitis include photophobia and tache cérébrale, which is elicited by stroking the skin with a blunt object and observing a red raised streak within 30–60 sec.

Complications. During the treatment of meningitis complications due to CNS or systemic effects of infection are common. Neurologic complications include seizures, increased intracranial pressure, cranial nerve palsies, stroke, cerebral or cerebellar herniation, transverse myelitis, ataxia, thrombosis of dural venous sinuses, and subdural effusions.

Collections of fluid in the subdural space develop in 10–30% of patients with meningitis and are asymptomatic in 85–90% of patients. Subdural effusions are especially common in infants. Symptomatic subdural effusions may result in a bulging fontanel, diastasis of sutures, enlarging head circumference, emesis, seizures, fever, and abnormal results of cranial transillumination. However, many of these manifestations are also present in patients with meningitis without subdural effusion. Computed tomography (CT) scanning will confirm the diagnosis of a subdural effusion. In the presence of increased intracranial pressure or a depressed level of consciousness, a symptomatic subdural effusion should be treated by aspiration through the open fontanel. Fever alone is not an indication for aspiration.

The syndrome of inappropriate secretion of antidiuretic hormone (SIADH) occurs in the majority of patients with meningitis, resulting in hyponatremia and reduced serum osmolality in 30–50%. This may exacerbate cerebral edema or independently produce hyponatremic seizures. Later in the course of therapy, central diabetes insipidus may develop as a result of hypothalamic or pituitary dysfunction.

Fever usually resolves earlier in patients with meningococcal or pneumococcal disease than in those with *H. influenzae* meningitis. By the 6th day of therapy more than 90% of patients with meningococcal or pneumococcal meningitis are afebrile compared with 70% of patients with *H. influenzae*. *Prolonged fever* (>10 days) is noted in 15% of patients with *H. influenzae* meningitis, 9% of those with pneumococcal, and 6% of those with meningococcal meningitis. Prolonged fever usually is due to an intercurrent viral infection, a nosocomial or secondary bacterial infection, thrombophlebitis, or a drug reaction. Pericarditis or arthritis may occur in patients being treated for meningitis. Involvement of these sites may result either from bacterial dissemination or from immune complex deposition. In general, infectious pericarditis or arthritis occurs earlier in the course of treatment than does immune-mediated disease. Secondary fever refers to the recrudescence of elevated temperature after an afebrile interval. Nosocomial infections are especially important to consider in the evaluation of these patients.

Thrombocytosis, eosinophilia, and anemia may develop during therapy for meningitis. Anemia may be due to hemolysis and is most commonly noted with *H. influenzae* disease. Alternatively, anemia may be due to bone marrow suppression. Disseminated intravascular coagulation (DIC) is most often associated with the rapidly progressive pattern of presentation and is noted most commonly in patients with shock and purpura (purpura fulminans). The combination of endotoxemia and severe hypotension initiates the coagulation cascade; the coexistence of ongoing thrombosis may produce symmetric peripheral gangrene.

Repeated episodes of meningitis are rare but have three distinct patterns. *Recrudescence* is the reappearance of infection during therapy with appropriate antibiotics. CSF culture reveals the growth of bacteria that have developed antibiotic resistance. *Relapse* occurs between 3 days and 3 wk after therapy and represents persistent bacterial infection in the CNS (subdural empyema, ventriculitis, cerebral abscess) or other site (mastoid, cranial osteomyelitis, orbital infection). Relapse is often associated with an inadequate choice, dose, or duration of antibiotic therapy. *Recurrence* is a new episode of meningitis due to reinfection with the same bacterial species or another pyogenic pathogen. Recurrent meningitis suggests the presence of an acquired or congenital anatomic communication between the CSF and a mucocutaneous site. Defects in immune host defense also predispose to recurrent meningitis.

DIFFERENTIAL DIAGNOSIS. In addition to *H. influenzae* type b, *S. pneumoniae*, and *N. meningitidis*, a number of other microorganisms can cause generalized infection of the CNS with similar clinical manifestations. These organisms include: less typical bacteria, such as tuberculosis, *Nocardia*, syphilis, and Lyme disease; fungi, such as those endemic to specific geographic areas *(Coccidioides, Histoplasma*, and *Blastomyces)* and those responsible for infections in compromised hosts *(Candida, Cryptococcus*, and *Aspergillus)*; parasites, such as *Toxoplasma gondii* and *Cysticercus*; and, most frequently, viruses. Noninfectious illnesses also can cause generalized inflammation of the CNS. These disorders are uncommon relative to infections and include: malignancy, collagen vascular syndromes, and exposure to toxins.

Focal infections of the CNS also may be confused with meningitis. Examples of these infections include brain abscesses and parameningeal infections, such as subdural empyema. Determining the specific etiology is facilitated by careful examination of the CSF with specific stains (Kinoyoun carbol fuchin for mycobacteria, India ink for fungi), cytology, antigen detection (partial bacterial treatment, *Cryptococcus*), serology (syphilis), and viral culture (enterovirus, HIV). Other potentially valuable diagnostic tests include CT or magnetic resonance imaging (MRI) of the brain, blood cultures, serologic tests, and possibly brain biopsy. Acute viral meningoencephalitis is the most likely infection to be confused with bacterial meningitis. Although, in general, children with viral meningoencephalitis appear less ill than those with bacterial meningitis, both types of infection have a spectrum of severity. Some children with bacterial meningitis may manifest relatively mild signs and symptoms, whereas some with viral meningoencephalitis may be critically ill. The CSF profiles associated with bacterial versus viral infection tend to be distinct, as summarized on Table 169–1, but, as with clinical manifestations, there may be considerable overlap in neutrophil count and differential and concentrations of glucose and protein.

Another diagnostic conundrum in the evaluation of children with suspected bacterial meningitis is the analysis of CSF obtained from children already receiving antibiotic therapy. This is an important issue as 25–50% of children being evaluated for bacterial meningitis are receiving oral antibiotics when their CSF is obtained. It is imperative to recognize that such *partial treatment* of a patient with acute bacterial meningitis usually will not completely alter the typical bacterial CSF profile. Partially treated meningitis may reduce the incidence of positive CSF Gram stain to less than 60% and the ability to grow the bacteria, especially meningococcus. It does not consistently alter the CSF glucose, protein, or neutrophil profile, nor does it interfere with the detection of bacterial antigens in the CSF.

DIAGNOSIS. The diagnosis of acute pyogenic meningitis is confirmed by analysis of the CSF, which reveals microorganisms on Gram stain and culture, a neutrophilic pleocytosis, an elevated protein, and reduced glucose concentrations (see Table 169–1). Lumbar puncture (LP) should be performed when bacterial meningitis is suspected. *Contraindications for an immediate LP* include (1) evidence of increased intracranial pressure (other than a bulging fontanel), such as 3rd or 6th cranial nerve palsy with a depressed level of consciousness, or hypertension and bradycardia with respiratory abnormalities; (2) severe cardiopulmonary compromise requiring prompt resuscitative measures for shock or in patients in whom positioning for the LP would further compromise cardiopulmonary function; and (3) infection of the skin overlying the site of the LP. Thrombocytopenia is a relative contraindication for immediate LP. Immediate LP is indicated in a child who shows evidence of disseminated intravascular coagulation or petechiae but may be delayed in immunosuppressed patients with chronic thrombocytopenia until platelet transfusion has been given. *If an LP is delayed by any of the above-mentioned factors, immediate empiric therapy should be initiated.* CT scanning for evidence of a brain abscess or increased intracranial pressure also should not delay therapy. Lumbar puncture may be performed after increased intracranial pressure has been treated or a brain abscess has been excluded.

A number of bacterial antigen detection systems have been developed, the most popular and widely used being based upon latex particle agglutination. In the presence of bacterial meningitis, antigen is most consistently detected in the CSF. Antigenuria also is quite common. Serum is not a good specimen for antigen detection as false-positive reactions are common. Tests for antigen are best reserved for patients who were receiving antibiotics when their cultures were obtained, as antigen may remain detectable for several days following the initiation of antibiotics, whereas cultures may be negative. Recent immunization with the *H. influenzae* type b polysaccharide vaccine may produce a false-positive result of the antigen test in serum and urine but not in CSF.

A *blood culture* should be performed in all patients with suspected meningitis, especially those who will be treated empirically prior to examination of CSF. Blood cultures may reveal the responsible bacteria in 80–90% of cases of childhood meningitis.

Lumbar puncture is traditionally performed with the patient in the flexed lateral decubitus position; the styletted needle is passed into the L3–L4 or L4–L5 intervertebral space. After entry into the subarachnoid space, the patient's position is changed to a more extended one to measure the opening CSF pressure. When the pressure is high, only a small volume of CSF should be removed to avoid a precipitous decline in intracranial pressure.

The CSF *leukocyte count* in bacterial meningitis is usually elevated to >1,000 and reveals a neutrophilic predominance (75–95%). Turbid CSF is present when the CSF leukocyte count is >200–400. Normal healthy neonates may have as many as 30 leukocytes and older children without viral or bacterial meningitis may have five to six leukocytes in the CSF; in both age groups there is a predominance of lymphocytes or monocytes.

A low CSF leukocyte count (<250) may be present in as many as 20% of patients with acute bacterial meningitis; absent pleocytosis may be evident in patients with severe overwhelming sepsis, and meningitis and is a poor prognostic sign. Pleocytosis with a lymphocyte predominance may be present in acute bacterial meningitis during the early stage of the illness; conversely, neutrophilic pleocytosis may be present in patients during the early stages of acute viral meningitis. The shift to lymphocytic-monocytic predominance in viral meningitis invariably occurs within 12–24 hr of the initial LP.

The *Gram stain* is positive in most (70–90%) patients with meningitis. Despite the identification of gram-positive or gram-negative diplococci or pleomorphic coccobacilli, treatment should not be modified on the basis of the stain but should remain empiric until a microorganism is identified by culture.

Traumatic lumbar puncture complicates the diagnosis of meningitis. Repeat LP at another interspace may produce less hemorrhagic fluid, but this fluid usually also contains red blood cells. The Gram stain, culture, and glucose level may not be influenced by a traumatic LP. However, interpretation of CSF leukocytes and protein concentration are affected by LPs that are traumatic. Although methods for correcting for the presence of red blood cells have been proposed, it is probably prudent to rely upon the bacteriologic results rather than to attempt to interpret the CSF neutrophil and protein results.

TREATMENT. Initial Antibiotic Therapy. The therapeutic approach to a patient with presumed bacterial meningitis depends on the nature of the initial manifestations of the illness. A child with rapidly progressing disease of less than 24 hr duration, in the absence of increased intracranial pressure, should receive antibiotics immediately after an LP is performed. If there are signs of increased intracranial pressure or focal neurologic findings, antibiotics should be given without performing an LP and before obtaining a CT scan. Increased intracranial pressure should be treated simultaneously. Immediate treatment of associated multiple organ system failure, such as shock and adult respiratory distress syndrome, is also indicated.

Patients who have a more protracted subacute course and become ill over a 1- to 7-day period should also be evaluated for signs of increased intracranial pressure and focal neurologic deficits. Unilateral headache, papilledema, and other signs of increased intracranial pressure suggest a focal lesion such as a brain or epidural abscess, or subdural empyema. Antibiotic therapy should be initiated prior to LP and CT scanning. If no signs of increased intracranial pressure are evident, an LP should be performed.

The initial (empiric) choice of therapy for meningitis in immunocompetent infants and children should be based on the antibiotic susceptibilities of *H. influenzae* type b, *S. pneumoniae*, and *N. meningitidis*. The antibiotic(s) should achieve bactericidal levels in the CSF. Either of the 3rd generation cephalosporins, ceftriaxone or cefotaxime, represents current standard therapy for bacterial meningitis. The dose of *ceftriaxone* is either 100 mg/kg/24 hr administered once per day or 50 mg/kg/dose, given every 12 hr. The dose of *cefotaxime* is 200 mg/kg/24 hr, given every 6 hr. Both drugs achieve high bactericidal levels in the CSF; virtually all patients have sterilization of CSF within 24 hr. Patients allergic to beta lactam antibiotics should be treated with chloramphenicol, 100 mg/kg/24 hr, given every 6 hr. Although chloramphenicol is bacteriostatic against many bacteria, it is bactericidal against *H. influenzae* type b, *S. pneumoniae*, and *N. meningitidis*. Chloramphenicol use currently is reserved for patients unable to tolerate cephalosporins because serum concentrations need to be monitored during therapy and chloramphenicol has the potential adverse effects of aplastic anemia, shocklike gray infant syndrome, and dose-dependent bone marrow suppression.

If *L. monocytogenes* infection is suspected, as in infants 1–2 mo old or patients with a T-lymphocyte deficiency, ampicillin should be given with ceftriaxone or cefotaxime because all cephalosporins are inactive against *L. monocytogenes*. Intravenous trimethoprim-sulfamethoxazole is an alternate treatment for *L. monocytogenes*.

If the patient is immunocompromised and gram-negative bacterial meningitis is suspected, initial therapy might include ceftazidine and an aminoglycoside.

Duration of Antibiotic Therapy. Uncomplicated *H. influenzae* type b meningitis should be treated for a total of 7–10 days. After determining that the organism is sensitive to ampicillin and does not produce a β-lactamase, initial antimicrobial therapy may be changed to ampicillin.

If *S. pneumoniae* is cultured from the CSF, the isolate should be tested for penicillin resistance. Relative resistance to penicillin (MIC 0.1–1.0 μg/mL) is present in 5–25% of *S. pneumoniae* isolates, and highly resistant organisms (MIC >2.0 μg/mL) are found in a small number of patients. Meningitis caused by relatively resistant *S. pneumoniae* isolates can be treated with cefotaxime or ceftriaxone, whereas chloramphenicol is the treatment of choice for highly resistant organisms if the organism is sensitive to the antibiotic. If chloramphenicol resistance also is present, vancomycin is the drug of choice. Therapy for uncomplicated penicillin-sensitive pneumococcal meningitis should be accomplished with intravenous penicillin 300,000 U/kg/24 hr, given every 4–6 hr for 10–14 days.

Intravenous penicillin 300,000 U/kg/24 hr for 5–7 days is the treatment of choice for uncomplicated *N. meningitidis* meningitis. Successful therapy with one to two doses of antibiotics has been demonstrated in underdeveloped countries, but this approach is not recommended in developed countries. Rare meningococcal isolates have demonstrated relative (0.25–0.5 μg/mL) and absolute (>250 μg/mL) resistance to penicillin, and these organisms may require alternate therapy.

Patients who receive intravenous or oral antibiotics prior to LP and do not have an identifiable pathogen (on Gram stain, culture, or antigen detection) but do have evidence of an acute bacterial infection on the basis of their CSF profile should continue to receive therapy with ceftriaxone or cefotaxime for 7–10 days. If focal signs are present or the child does not respond to treatment, a parameningeal focus may be present and a CT scan should be performed.

A routine repeat LP is not indicated in patients with uncomplicated meningitis due to *H. influenzae* type b, *N. meningitidis*, or *S. pneumoniae*. Repeat examination of CSF is indicated in some neonates, in patients with gram-negative bacillary meningitis, and in those who do not respond to conventional antimicrobial therapy within 48–72 hr. Improvement in the CSF profile is indicated by an increase in CSF glucose levels and the appearance of lymphocyte-monocyte cells; although the Gram stain may remain positive at this time, the CSF should be sterile.

Meningitis due to *E. coli* or *P. aeruginosa* requires therapy with a 3rd generation cephalosporin active against the isolate in vitro. Most isolates of *E. coli* will be sensitive to cefotaxime or ceftriaxone, whereas most isolates of *P. aeruginosa* will be sensitive to ceftazidine. Gram-negative bacillary meningitis should be treated for 3 wk or for at least 2 wk after CSF sterilization, which may occur after 2–10 days of treatment.

Side effects of antibiotic therapy of meningitis include phlebitis, drug fever, rash, emesis, oral candidiasis, and diarrhea. Ceftriaxone may cause reversible gallbladder pseudolithiasis, detectable by abdominal ultrasound. This is usually asymptomatic but may produce emesis and right upper quadrant pain.

Supportive Care. Repeated *medical* and *neurologic assessments* of the patient with bacterial meningitis are essential to identify early signs of cardiovascular, CNS, and metabolic complications. Pulse rate, blood pressure, and respiratory rate should be monitored frequently. Neurologic assessment, including pupillary reflexes, level of consciousness, motor strength, cranial nerve signs, and evaluation for seizures, should be made frequently during the first 72 hr, when the risk of neurologic complications is greatest. Thereafter, the neurologic assessment should be performed once a day. Important laboratory studies include an assessment of BUN, serum sodium, chloride, potassium, and bicarbonate levels, urine output and specific gravity, complete blood and platelet counts, and coagulation factors (fibrinogen, prothrombin, and partial thromboplastin times) in the presence of petechiae, purpura, or abnormal bleeding.

Initially, the patient should receive nothing by mouth. If the patient is judged to be normovolemic, with normal blood pressure, intravenous fluid administration should be restricted to one half to two thirds of maintenance, or 800–1,000 mL/m^2/24 hr, until it can be established that increased intracranial pressure or SIADH is not present. Fluid administration may be returned to normal (1,500–1,700 mL/m^2/24 hr) when serum sodium levels are normal. Fluid restriction is not appropriate in the presence of systemic hypotension, because reduced blood pressure may result in a cerebral perfusion pressure of <50 cm H_2O with subsequent CNS ischemia. Therefore, shock, which occurs in the rapidly progressive pattern of meningococcal meningitis, must be treated aggressively to prevent brain and other organ dysfunction (acute tubular necrosis, adult respiratory distress syndrome). Patients with shock, a markedly raised intracranial pressure, coma, and refractory seizures require intensive monitoring with central arterial and venous access, and frequent vital signs, necessitating admission to a pediatric intensive care unit. Patients with septic shock require fluid resuscitation and therapy with vasoactive agents such as dopamine, epinephrine, and sodium nitroprusside. The goal of such therapy in patients with meningitis is avoidance of excessive increases in intracranial pressure without compromising blood flow and oxygen delivery to vital organs (brain, heart, lung, kidney).

Neurologic complications include *increased intracranial pressure* with subsequent herniation, seizures, and an enlarging head circumference due to a subdural effusion or hydrocephalus. Signs of increased intracranial pressure, other than a bulging fontanel or isolated coma, should be treated emergently with endotracheal intubation and hyperventilation (P_{CO_2} approximately 25 mm Hg). In addition, intravenous furosemide (Lasix; 1 mg/kg) and mannitol (0.5–1 g/kg) osmotherapy may reduce intracranial pressure. Furosemide may reduce brain swelling by venodilation and diuresis without increasing intracranial blood volume, whereas mannitol produces an osmolar gradient between the brain and plasma, thus shifting fluid from the CNS to the plasma with subsequent excretion during an osmotic diuresis.

Seizures are common during the course of bacterial meningitis. Immediate therapy for seizures includes intravenous diazepam (0.1–0.2 mg/kg/dose) or lorazepam (0.05 mg/kg/dose), paying careful attention to the risk of respiratory suppression. Serum glucose, calcium, and sodium levels should be monitored to determine if hypoglycemia, hypocalcemia, or hyponatremia is precipitating seizures. After immediate management of seizures, the patient should receive phenytoin (15–20 mg/kg loading dose, 5 mg/kg/24 hr maintenance) to reduce the likelihood of recurrence. Phenytoin is preferred to phenobarbital because it produces less CNS depression and permits assessment of the patient's level of consciousness. Serum phenytoin levels should be monitored to maintain them in the therapeutic range (10–20 μg/mL).

Rapid killing of bacteria in the CSF effectively sterilizes the meningeal infection but releases toxic cell products following cell lysis (cell wall endotoxin), which precipitates the cytokine-mediated inflammatory response. The resultant edema formation and neutrophilic infiltration may produce additional neurologic injury with worsening of CNS signs and symptoms. Therefore, agents that limit production of inflammatory mediators may be of benefit to patients with bacterial meningitis. Recent data support the use of *intravenous dexamethasone* (0.15 mg/kg/dose, given every 6 hr for 4 days) in the management of children with acute bacterial meningitis. Steroid recipients had less fever, lower CSF protein and lactate levels, and a reduction in permanent auditory nerve damage, as manifest by sensorineural hearing loss, than placebo recipients. Most experience with dexamethasone treatment has been gained with *H. influenzae* type b infection, and extrapolation to other bacterial pathogens should be done with caution, balancing potential benefits against risks. It appears that steroids have maximum benefit if given just before antibiotics. Complications of this therapy include gastrointestinal bleeding, hypertension, hyperglycemia, leukocytosis, and rebound fever after the last dose.

PREVENTION. Vaccination and antibiotic prophylaxis of susceptible, at-risk contacts represent the two available means of reducing the likelihood of bacterial meningitis. The availability and application of each of these approaches is different for each of the three major causes of bacterial meningitis in children.

Haemophilus influenzae Type b (see Chapter 177). Rifampin prophylaxis should be given to all *household contacts,* including adults, if there are any close family members less than 4 yr old who have not been immunized fully. A household contact is one who lives in the residence of the index case or who has spent a minimum of 4 hr with the index case for at least 5 of 7 days preceding the patient's hospitalization. Family members should receive rifampin prophylaxis immediately after the diagnosis is confirmed in the index case because more than 50% of secondary family cases occur in the 1st week after the index patient has been hospitalized.

The risk of secondary cases of *H. influenzae* type b infection in *day-care center contacts* is less than that for household contacts and probably greater than that for the general population. The risk is exceedingly low for day-care center children who are nonclassroom contacts and those over 2 yr old. The efficacy of chemoprophylaxis in day-care centers is uncertain, and there are difficulties in ensuring that all at-risk day-care center attendees receive the drug. Chemoprophylaxis for children and adults in day-care centers that resemble households (e.g., >25 hr/wk of close contact) should be provided to all adults and children if two or more cases of *H. influenzae* type b infection occur within 60 days and some of the children are <2 yr of age and not fully immunized. The dose of rifampin is 20 mg/kg/24 hr (maximum 600 mg) given once each day for 4 days. Rifampin discolors the urine and sweat red-orange, stains contact lenses, and reduces the serum concentrations of some drugs, including oral contraceptives. Rifampin is contraindicated during pregnancy. In addition to prophylaxis, day-care center workers and parents should be educated about the signs of serious *H. influenzae* infection and the importance of seeking prompt medical attention for fever or other potential manifestations of *H. influenzae* disease.

The most exciting development in the prevention of childhood bacterial meningitis is the development and licensure of vaccines against *H. influenza* type b. The recently licensed conjugate vaccines have been shown to be safe and immunogenic in infants during the first months of life. Currently, four conjugate vaccines and a combination vaccine that combines one of these conjugates with diphtheria, pertussis, and tetanus toxoid (DPT) are licensed in the United States. Although each of these vaccines elicits different profiles of antibody response in infants immunized at 2–6 mo of age, all result in protective levels of antibody after two to four doses. Prelicensure studies demonstrated that each of the conjugate vaccines was effective, with efficacy rates ranging from 70% to 100%. Efficacy was not as consistent in Native American populations, a group recognized as having an extremely high incidence of disease. Postlicensure surveillance for cases of meningitis caused by *H. influenzae* type b also support a high degree of protection afforded by vaccination. As a result, the Committee on Infectious Diseases of the American Academy of Pediatrics recommends that all children should be immunized with an *H. influenzae* type b conjugate vaccine beginning at about 2 mo of age or as soon as possible thereafter.

H. influenzae type b nasopharyngeal colonization may not be eradicated despite 10 days of appropriate parenteral antibiotic therapy. Prior to discharge from the hospital, *the patient* should receive rifampin (20 mg/kg/dose every day for 4 days) to prevent introduction or reintroduction of the organism into the household or day-care center.

Neisseria meningitidis. Chemoprophylaxis is recommended for all close contacts of patients with meningococcal meningitis regardless of age or immunization status. Close contacts should be treated wtih rifampin 10 mg/kg/dose every 12 hr for 2 days (maximum dose of 600 mg) as soon as possible after identification of a case of meningococcal meningitis or sepsis. Close contacts include household, day-care center, and nursery school contacts, and health care workers who have direct exposure to secretions (e.g., mouth-to-mouth resuscitation, suctioning, intubation). Exposed contacts should be treated immediately upon suspicion of infection in the index patient; bacteriologic confirmation of infection should not be awaited. In addition, all contacts should be educated about the early signs of meningococcal disease and the need to seek prompt medical attention if these signs develop.

Meninogococcal quadrivalent vaccine against serogropus A, C, Y, and W135 is recommended for high-risk children over 2 yr of age. High-risk patients include those with asplenia, functional splenic dysfunction, or deficiencies of terminal complement proteins. The vaccine may also be used as an adjunct with chemoprophylaxis for exposed contacts and during epidemics of meningococcal disease. Unfortunately, most cases of endemic meningococcal meningitis are due to group B, for which there currently is no effective vaccine.

Streptococcus pneumoniae. No chemoprophylaxis or vaccination is required for normal hosts who may be contacts of patients with pneumococcal meningitis, as secondary cases rarely have occurred. High-risk patients should receive the 23-valent pneumococcal vaccine, and patients with sickle cell anemia should also receive chemoprophylaxis with daily oral penicillin, amoxicillin, or trimethoprim-sulfamethoxazole.

PROGNOSIS. Appropriate recognition, prompt antibiotic therapy, and supportive care have reduced the mortality of bacterial meningitis beyond the neonatal period to 1–8%. The highest mortality rates are observed with pneumococcal meningitis. Severe neurodevelopmental sequelae may occur in 10–20% of patients recovering from bacterial meningitis, and as many as 50% have some, albeit subtle, neurobehavioral morbidity. Prognosis is poorest among infants less than 6 mo and in those with more than 10^6 CFU of bacteria/mL in their CSF. Those with seizures occurring more than 4 days into therapy, or with coma or focal neurologic signs on presentation, also tend to have more long-term sequelae. Interestingly, there is not a good correlation between duration of symtpoms prior to diagnosis of meningitis and outcome.

The most common neurologic sequelae include hearing loss, mental retardation, seizures, delay in acquisition of language, visual impairment, and behavioral problems.

Sensorineural hearing loss is the most common sequela of bacterial meningitis. It is due to labyrinthitis following cochlear infection and occurs in as many as 30% of patients with pneumococcal meningitis, 10% with meningococcal, and 5–20% of those with *H. influenzae* type b meningitis. Hearing loss may also be due to direct inflammation of the auditory nerve. Adjunctive therapy with dexamethasone may reduce the incidence of severe hearing loss. Regardless of the bacterial agent, type of antibiotic therapy, or use of dexamethasone, all patients with bacterial meningitis should undergo careful audiologic assessment before or soon after discharge from the hospital. Frequent reassessment on an outpatient basis is indicated for all patients who have a hearing deficit.

169.2 Viral Meningoencephalitis

Viral meningoencephalitis is an acute inflammatory process involving the meninges and, to a variable degree, brain tissue. These infections are relatively common and may be caused by a number of different agents. The CSF is characterized by pleocytosis and the absence of microorganisms on Gram stain and routine culture. In most instances the infections are self-limited; in some cases, however, substantial morbidity and mortality may be observed.

ETIOLOGY. Although the specific etiologic agent is not identified in many instances, clinical and research experience indicate that viruses are usually the responsible pathogens, accounting for the seasonal pattern of disease. Enteroviruses cause more than 80% of all cases. Other frequent causes of infection include arboviruses and herpesviruses. Mumps is a common pathogen in regions where vaccine is not used widely.

EPIDEMIOLOGY. Because most cases are due to enteroviruses, the basic epidemiologic pattern of viral meningoencephalitis reflects their prevalence. Infection with enteroviruses is spread directly from person to person, and the incubation period is usually 4–6 days; most cases in temperate climates occur in the summer and fall. Epidemiologic considerations in aseptic meningitis due to agents other than enteroviruses also include season, geography, climatic conditions, animal exposures, and factors related to the specific pathogen.

COMMON PATHOGENS. Arboviruses are zoonoses in which humans, not being essential in the viral life cycle, are infected accidentally by an arthropod vector. Most commonly, mosquitoes or ticks acquire arboviruses by biting infected birds or small mammals, which often have prolonged viremia without illness. The insect vectors transmit the virus to other vertebrates, including humans and horses. Encephalitis in horses ("blind staggers") may be the first indication of an incipient epidemic. Although rural exposure is most common, urban and suburban outbreaks are also frequent. The most common arboviruses responsible for central nervous infection in the United States are St. Louis and California virus (see Chapter 225).

Enteroviruses are small RNA-containing viruses; 68 specific serotypes have been identified. The severity of disease ranges from mild, self-limited illness with primarily meningeal involvement to severe encephalitis with death or significant sequelae. Epidemics, some devastating, have been observed among newborns in nurseries.

Herpes simplex virus type 1 (HSV-1) is an important cause of severe, sporadic encephalitis in children and adults. Infection may accompany primary or recurrent infection. Brain involvement usually is focal; progression to coma and death occurs in 70% of cases without antiviral therapy. Severe encephalitis with diffuse brain involvement is caused by *herpes simplex virus type 2* (HSV-2) in neonates who have contracted the virus from their mothers at delivery. A mild transient form of meningoencephalitis may accompany genital herpes infection in sexually active adolescents; most of these infections are caused by HSV-2. *Varicella-zoster virus* (VZV) may cause CNS infection in close temporal relationship with chickenpox. The most common manifestation of CNS involvement is cerebellar ataxia, and the most severe is an acute encephalitis. Following primary infection, VZV becomes latent in spinal and cranial nerve roots and ganglia, expressing itself later as herpes zoster, often with accompanying mild meningoencephalitis. *Cytomegalovirus* (CMV) infection of the CNS may be part of congenital infection or disseminated disease in compromised hosts, but it does not cause meningoencephalitis in normal infants and children. *Epstein-Barr virus* (EBV) has been associated with a myriad of CNS syndromes (see Chapter 215).

Meningoencephalitis is caused occasionally by respiratory viruses, rubeola, or rubella. Mumps meningoencephalitis is mild but deafness from damage to the 8th cranial nerve is not uncommon. Encephalitis caused by rabies is discussed in Chapter 227.

PATHOGENESIS AND PATHOLOGY. The sequence of events varies with the infecting agent and host. In general, viruses enter the lymphatic system, either through ingestion of enteroviruses; inoculation of mucous membranes by measles, rubella, VZV, or HSV; or by hematogenous spread from a mosquito or other insect bite. There, multiplication begins, and seeding of the bloodstream leads to infection of several organs. At this stage (the extraneural phase) a systemic, febrile illness is present, but if further viral multiplication takes place in the seeded organs, a secondary propagation of large amounts of virus may occur. Invasion of the CNS is followed by clinical evidence of neurologic disease. HSV-1 probably reaches the brain by direct spread along neuronal axons.

Neurologic damage is caused (1) by a direct invasion and destruction of neural tissues by actively multiplying viruses and/or (2) by a host reaction to viral antigens. Most neuronal destruction is probably due directly to viral invasion, whereas the host's vigorous tissue response induces demyelination and vascular and perivascular destruction.

Tissue sections of the brain generally are characterized by meningeal congestion and mononuclear infiltration, perivascular cuffs of lymphocytes and plasma cells, some perivascular tissue necrosis with myelin breakdown, neuronal disruption in various stages, including ultimately neuronophagia and endothelial proliferation or necrosis. A marked degree of demyelination with preservation of neurons and their axons is considered predominantly to represent "postinfectious" or "allergic" encephalitis. The cerebral cortex, especially the temporal lobe, is often severely affected by herpes simplex virus; the arboviruses tend to affect the entire brain; rabies has a predilection for the basal structures. Involvement of the spinal cord, nerve roots, and peripheral nerves is quite variable.

CLINICAL MANIFESTATIONS. The progression and ultimate severity of the clinical course is very much determined by the relative degree of meningeal and parenchymal involvement, which in turn is determined, at least in part, by the specific infectious agents. However, there is a wide range of severity of clinical manifestations, even with the same etiologic agent. Some children may appear to be mildly affected initially, only to lapse into coma and die suddenly. In others, the illness may be ushered in by high fever, violent convulsions interspersed with bizarre movements, and hallucinations alternating with brief periods of clarity, but then complete recovery.

The onset of illness is generally acute, although CNS signs and symptoms often are preceded by a nonspecific acute febrile illness of a few days' duration. The presenting manifestations in older children are headache and hyperesthesia, and in infants, irritability and lethargy. Headache is most often frontal or generalized; adolescents frequently note retrobulbar pain. Fever, nausea, and vomiting, pain in the neck, back, and legs, and photophobia are common. As the temperature rises, there may be mental dullness, eventuating in stupor in combination with bizarre movements, and convulsions. Focal neurologic signs may be stationary, progressive, or fluctuating. Loss of bowel and bladder control and unprovoked emotional bursts may occur.

Exanthems often precede or accompany the CNS signs, especially with echoviruses, coxsackieviruses, VZV, measles, and rubella. Examination often reveals nuchal rigidity without significant localizing neurologic changes, at least at the onset.

Specific forms or complicating manifestations of CNS viral infection include Guillain-Barré syndrome, acute transverse myelitis, acute hemiplegia, and acute cerebellar ataxia (see Chapter 547.1).

LABORATORY ABNORMALITIES AND DIAGNOSIS. The CSF contains from a few to several thousand cells per cubic millimeter. Early in the disease the cells are often polymorphonuclear; later mononuclear cells predominate. This change in cellular type is often demonstrated in CSF samples obtained 8–12 hr apart. The protein concentration in CSF tends to be normal or slightly elevated, but concentrations may be very high if brain destruction is extensive, as illustrated by HSV encephalitis in later stages. The glucose level is usually normal, although with certain viruses, for example, mumps, a substantial depression of CSF glucose concentrations is often observed. The spinal fluid should be cultured for viruses, bacteria, fungi, and mycobacteria; in some instances special examinations are indicated for protozoa, mycoplasma, and other pathogens. The success of isolating viruses from the CSF of children with viral meningoencephalitis is determined by the time in the clinical course that the specimen is obtained, the specific etiologic agent, whether the infection is a meningitic as opposed to a localized encephalitic process, and the skill of the diagnostic laboratory. Isolating a virus is more likely early in the illness and the enteroviruses tend to be the easiest to isolate, although recovery of these agents from the CSF rarely exceeds 70%. In order to increase the likelihood of identifying the putative viral pathogen, specimens for culture also should be obtained from nasopharyngeal swabs, feces, and urine. Although isolating a virus from one or more of these sites does not prove causality, it is highly suggestive.

A serum specimen should be obtained early in the course of illness and, if viral cultures are not diagnostic, again 2–3 wk later for serologic studies. Serologic methods are not practical for diagnosing CNS infections caused by the enteroviruses because there are too many potential serotypes. This approach may be useful to confirm that a case is caused by a known circulating viral type. Serologic tests also may be of value in determining the etiology of nonenteroviral CNS infection. Newer diagnostic techniques for suspected viral meningoencephalitis that use polymerase chain reaction to detect viral DNA or RNA in CSF appear to be promising but are not yet clinically available.

Other tests of potential value in the evaluation of patients with suspected viral meningoencephalitis include an electroencephalogram and neuroimaging studies.

DIAGNOSIS AND DIFFERENTIAL DIAGNOSIS. A number of clinical conditions that cause CNS inflammation mimic viral meningoencephalitis. The most important group of alternate infectious agents to consider is bacteria. Most children with bacterial infections of the CNS have a more acute onset and appear more critically ill, but this is not always the case. Meningitis caused by the most common bacteria invading the CNS, *H. influenza* type B, *S. pneumoniae,* and *N. meningitidis,* may be insidious in onset. CNS infection caused by other bacteria, such as tuberculosis, *T. pallidum* (syphilis), *Borralia burgdorferi* (Lyme disease), and the bacillus associated with cat-scratch disease, also may have very indolent courses. Analysis of CSF and appropriate serologic tests is necessary to differentiate these bacterial and viral pathogens. Parameningeal bacterial infections, such as brain abscess or subdural or epidural empyema, may have features similar to viral CNS infections. CNS imaging procedures are critical for the diagnosis of these processes.

Nonbacterial infectious agents also need to be considered in the differential diagnosis of CNS infections. These agents include *Rickettsia, Mycoplasma, Protozoa,* and other parasites, and a number of fungi. Consideration of these agents usually arises as a result of accompanying symptoms, geographic distribution of infection, and/or host immune factors.

A variety of noninfectious disorders also may be associated with CNS inflammation and have manifestations overlapping with those associated with viral meningoencephalitis. Some of these disorders include: malignancy, collagen-vascular diseases, intracranial hemorrhage, and exposure to certain drugs or toxins. Attention to history and other organ involvement usually allows early elimination of these diagnostic possibilities. Recent exposure to possibly infected persons, animals, mosquitos and ticks, and any recent travel should be noted. Inquiry should also be made about recent injections of biologic substances and about the possibilities of exposure to heavy metals, pesticides, or noxious substances.

PREVENTION. The widespread use of effective attenuated viral vaccines for polio, measles, mumps, and rubella has almost eliminated CNS complications from these diseases in the United States. The availability of domestic animal vaccine programs against rabies has reduced the frequency of rabies encephalitis. The control of encephalitis due to arboviruses has been less successful because specific vaccines for the arboviral diseases that occur in North America are not available. However, control of insect vectors by suitable spraying methods and eradication of insect breeding sites reduce the incidence of these infections.

TREATMENT. Until a bacterial cause is excluded, parenteral antibiotic therapy should be administered. With the exception of the use of acyclovir for herpes simplex encephalitis, treatment of viral meningoencephalitis is nonspecific. For mild infections, treatment is limited to providing symptomatic relief, whereas for severe infection it is aimed at maintaining life and supporting each organ system.

Headache and hyperesthesia are treated with rest, non-aspirin-containing analgesics, and a reduction in room light, noise, and visitors. Acetaminophen is recommended for fever. Codeine, morphine, and the phenothiazine derivatives may be necessary for pain and vomiting, but, if possible, their use in children should be minimized because they may induce misleading signs and symptoms.

It is crucial to anticipate and be prepared for convulsions, cerebral edema, hyperpyrexia, inadequate respiratory exchange, disturbed fluid and electrolyte balance, aspiration and asphyxia, and cardiac or respiratory arrest of central origin.

Therefore, all patients with severe encephalitis should be monitored carefully. In patients with evidence of increased intracranial pressure, placement of a pressure transducer in the epidural space may be indicated for monitoring intracranial pressure as a guide to therapy aimed at reducing cerebral edema. The risks of cardiac and respiratory failure or arrest are high. All fluids, electrolytes, and medications are initially given parenterally. In prolonged states of coma, parenteral alimentation is indicated. Inappropriate secretion of antidiuretic hormone is quite common in acute CNS disorders, so that constant evaluation is required for its early detection. Normal blood levels of glucose, magnesium, and calcium must be maintained in order to minimize the threat of convulsions. If cerebral edema or seizures become evident, vigorous treatment should be instituted.

Supportive and rehabilitative efforts are very important after the patient recovers. Motor incoordination, convulsive disorders, squint, total or partial deafness, and behavioral disturbances may appear only after an interval of time. Visual disturbances due to chorioretinopathy and perceptual amblyopia may also have a delayed appearance. Special facilities and, at times, institutional placement may become necessary. Some sequelae of infection may be very subtle. Therefore, neurodevelopmental and audiologic evaluations should be part of the routine follow-up of children who have recovered from viral meningoencephalitis, even if they appear to be grossly normal.

PROGNOSIS. Most children completely recover from viral infections of the CNS, although prognosis depends upon the severity of the clinical illness, the specific etiology, and the age of the child. If the clinical illness is severe with evidence of substantial parenchymal involvement, the prognosis is poor, with potential deficits being intellectual, motor, psychiatric, epileptic, visual, or auditory in nature. Severe sequelae also should be anticipated in those with infection caused by HSV. Although some literature suggests that infants who contract viral meningoencephalitis have a poorer long-term outcome than older children, recent data refute this observation. Although about 10% of children younger than 2 yr of age with enteroviral CNS infections manifest an acute complication such as seizures, increased intracranial pressure, or coma, almost all have favorable long-term neurologic outcomes.

Arditi M, Ables L, Yogev R: Cerebrospinal fluid endotoxin levels in children with *H. influenzae* meningitis before and after administration of intravenous ceftriaxone. J Infect Dis 160:1005, 1989.
Baraff LJ, Lee SI, Schriger DL: Outcomes of bacterial meningitis in children: a meta-analysis. Pediatr Infect Dis J 12:389, 1993.
Blazer S, Berant M, Alon U: Bacterial meningitis: Effect of antibiotic treatment on cerebrospinal fluid. J Clin Pathol 80:386, 1983.
Committee on Infectious Diseases: *Haemophilus influenzae* type b conjugate vaccines: Recommendations for immunization with recently and previously licensed vaccines. Pediatrics 92:480, 1993.
Dodge PR, Davis H, Feigin RD, et al: Prospective evaluation of hearing impairment as a sequela of acute bacterial meningitis. N Engl J Med 311:869, 1984.
Epstein F: Bacterial meningitis: Pathogenesis, pathophysiology, and progress. N Engl J Med 327:864, 1992.
Feigin RD, McCracken GH, Klein JO: Diagnosis and management of meningitis. Pediatr Infect Dis J 11:785, 1992.
Fijen C, Hanneman AJ, Kuiper E, et al: Complement deficiencies in patients over ten years old with meningococcal disease due to uncommon serogroups. Lancet 2:585, 1989.
Glimaker M, Kragsbjerg P, Forsgren M, et al: Tumor necrosis factor-α (TNFα) in cerebrospinal fluid from patients with meningitis of different etiologies: High levels of TNFα indicate bacterial meningitis. J Infect Dis 167:882, 1993.
Guerra-Romero L, Tauber MG, Fournier MA, et al: Lactate and glucose concentrations in brain interstitial fluid, cerebrospinal fluid, and serum during experimental pneumococcal meningitis. J Infect Dis 166:546, 1992.
Kilpi T, Anttila M, Kallio MJT, et al: Severity of childhood bacterial meningitis and duration of illness before diagnosis. Lancet 338:406, 1991.
Kilpi T, Anttila M, Kallio MJT, et al: Length of prediagnostic history related to the course and sequelae of childhood bacterial meningitis. Pediatr Infect Dis J 12:184, 1993.
Klass PE, Klein JO: Therapy of bacterial sepsis, meningitis and otitis media in infants and children: 1992 poll of directors of programs in pediatric infectious diseases. Pediatr Infect Dis J 11:702, 1992.
Klein JO, Feigin RD, McCracken GH: Report of the task force on diagnosis and management of meningitis. Pediatrics 78(Suppl):956, 1980.
Mustafa MM, Ramilo O, Saez-Llorens X, et al: Cerebrospinal fluid prostaglandins, interleukin 1β, and tumor necrosis factor in bacterial meningitis. Am J Dis Child 144:883, 1990.
Quagliarello V, Sheld WM: Bacterial meningitis: pathogenesis, pathophysiology, and progress. N Engl J Med 327:864, 1992.
Pomeroy SL, Holmes SJ, Dodge PR, et al: Seizures and other neurologic sequelae of bacterial meningitis in children. N Engl J Med 323:1651, 1990.
Prober CG: Commentary—The role of steroids in managing bacterial meningitis. Pediatrics 95:29, 1995.
Quagliarello V, Scheld WM: New perspectives on bacterial meningitis. Clin Infect Dis 17:603, 1993.
Radetsky M: Duration of treatment in bacterial meningitis: A historical inquiry. Pediatr Infect Dis J 9:2, 1990.
Radetsky M: Duration of symptoms and outcome in bacterial meningitis: an analysis of causation and the implications of a delay in diagnosis. Pediatr Infect Dis J 11:694, 1992.
Rautonen J, Koskiniemi M, Vaheri A: Prognostic factors in childhood encephalitis. Pediatr Infect Dis J 10:441, 1991.
Rodriguez WJ, Khan WN, Cocchetto D, et al: Treatment of *Pseudomonas* meningitis with ceftazidime with or without concurrent therapy. Pediatr Infect Dis J 9:83, 1990.
Rorabaugh ML, Berlin LE, Heldrich F, et al: Aseptic meningitis in infants younger than 2 years of age: acute illness and neurologic complications. Pediatrics 92:206, 1993.
Saez-Llorens X, Ramilo O, Mustafa M, et al: Molecular pathophysiology of bacterial meningitis: Current concepts and therapeutic implications. J Pediatr 116:671, 1990.
Spanos A, Harrell FE, Durack DT: Differential diagnosis of acute meningitis: An analysis of the predictive value of initial observations. JAMA 262:2700, 1989.
Strikas RA, Anderson LJ, Parker RA: Temporal and geographic patterns of isolates of nonpolio enterovirus in the United States, 1970–1983. J Infect Dis 153:346, 1986.
Syrogiannopoulos GA, Nelson JD, McCracken GH: Subdural collections of fluid in acute bacterial meningitis: A review of 136 cases. Pediatr Infect Dis 5:343, 1986.
Talan DA, Guterman JJ, Overturf GD, et al: Analysis of emergency department management of suspected bacterial meningitis. Ann Emerg Med 18:856, 1989.
Talan DA, Hoffman JR, Yoshikawa TT, et al: Role of empiric parenteral antibiotics prior to lumbar puncture in suspected bacterial meningitis: State of the art. Rev Infect Dis 10:365, 1988.
Taylor HG, Mills EL, Ciampi A, et al: The sequelae of *Haemophilus influenzae* meningitis in school-age children. N Engl J Med 323:1657, 1990.
Tzou-Yien L, Nelson JD, McCracken GH: Fever during treatment for bacterial meningitis. Pediatr Infect Dis 3:319, 1984.
Wenger JD, Hightower AW, Facklam RR, et al: Bacterial meningitis in the United States, 1986: Report of a multistate surveillance study. J Infect Dis 162:1316, 1990.
Whitley RJ: Viral encephalitis. N Engl J Med 323:242, 1990.
Wilfert CM, Lehrman SN, Katz SL: Enteroviruses and meningitis. Pediatr Infect Dis 2:333, 1983.

CHAPTER 170
Pneumonia

Charles G. Prober

Pneumonia is an inflammation of the parenchyma of the lungs. Most cases of pneumonia are caused by microorganisms, but there are a number of noninfectious causes that sometimes need to be considered. These noninfectious causes include, but are not limited to, aspiration of food and/or gastric acid, foreign bodies, hydrocarbons, and lipoid substances; hypersensitivity reactions; and drug- or radiation-induced pneumonitis. Infections in neonates and other compromised hosts are distinct from infections occurring in otherwise normal infants and children. This chapter will focus only on the common microbiologic causes of pneumonia in the normal child, including respiratory viruses, *Mycoplasma pneumoniae*, and selected bacteria. Less common causes of infectious pneumonia, such as nonrespiratory viruses, enteric gram-negative bacteria, mycobacteria, *Chlamydia* spp., *Rickettsia* spp., *Coxiella*, *Pneumocystis carinii*, and a number of fungi are discussed elsewhere.

Pneumonia has been classified on an anatomic basis as a lobar or lobular, alveolar, or interstitial process, but classification of infectious pneumonia on the basis of presumed or proven etiology is diagnostically and therapeutically more relevant.

Respiratory viruses are the most common cause of pneumonia during the first several years of life. *Mycoplasma pneumonia* assumes a predominant role in the etiology of pneumonia in the school-aged and older child. Although bacteria are numerically less important as causes of pneumonia, they tend to be responsible for more severe infections than those caused by the nonbacterial agents. The most common bacterial causes of pneumonia in the normal child are *Streptococcus pneumoniae, S. pyogenes*, and *Staphylococcus aureus. Haemophilus influenza* type b also has been responsible for bacterial pneumonia in young children in the past, but likely will become much less common with the widespread, routine use of effective vaccines.

PNEUMONIAS OF VIRAL ORIGIN

ETIOLOGY. The most common viruses causing pneumonia include respiratory syncytial virus (RSV), parainfluenza, influenza, and adenoviruses. In general, lower respiratory tract viral infections are much more common during the winter months and RSV is the most common virus responsible for pneumonia, especially during infancy. Although the seasonality of these viral agents is quite predictable, local epidemics may skew incidence figures for a given year. The type and severity of the illness are influenced by several factors, including age, sex, season of the year, and crowding. Boys are affected slightly more often than girls. Unlike bronchiolitis, for which the peak attack rate is within the 1st year, the peak attack rate for viral pneumonia is between the ages of 2 and 3 yr and decreases slowly thereafter.

CLINICAL MANIFESTATIONS. Most viral pneumonias are preceded by several days of respiratory symptoms, including rhinitis and cough. Often other family members are ill. Although fever usually is present, temperatures are generally lower than in bacterial pneumonia. Tachypnea, accompanied by intercostal, subcostal, and suprasternal retractions; nasal flaring; and use of accessory muscles are common. Severe infection may be accompanied by cyanosis and respiratory fatigue. Chest auscultation may reveal widespread rales and wheezing, but it often is difficult to localize the source of these adventitious sounds in very young children with hyper-resonant chests. The viral pneumonias cannot be definitely differentiated from mycoplasmal disease on purely clinical grounds and may, on occasion, be difficult to distinguish from bacterial pneumonias. Furthermore, evidence of viral infection is present in many patients who have confirmed bacterial pneumonia.

DIAGNOSIS. The chest roentgenogram is characterized by diffuse infiltrates (Fig. 170–1). In some patients, transient lobar infiltrates may also be present or even dominate the picture. Hyperinflation is common. The peripheral white blood cell count of children with viral pneumonia tends to be normal or only slightly elevated (<20,000/mm^3), with a predominance of lymphocytes. Acute phase reactants (e.g., erythrocyte sedimentation rate [ESR] or C-reactive protein [CRP]) usually are normal or only slightly elevated. Definitive diagnosis requires the isolation of a virus from a specimen obtained from the respiratory tract. Growth of a respiratory virus in tissue culture usually takes 5–10 days. However, an immediate diagnosis can be established by demonstrating viral antigens in respiratory secretions. Most tests use labeled viral-specific antibodies to detect viral antigens. Reliable reagents for the rapid detection of RSV, parainfluenzae, influenzae, and adenoviruses are available. Finally, serologic techniques can be used to diagnose a recent respiratory viral infection. Acute and convalescent serum samples are collected, and a rise in antibodies to a specific viral agent is sought. This diagnostic technique is laborious, slow, and not generally clinically useful, as the infection usually is resolved by the time it is confirmed serologically. Nevertheless, serology may be useful as an epidemiologic tool to define the incidence and prevalence of the various respiratory viral pathogens.

TREATMENT. Many patients are given antibiotic agents initially if bacterial pneumonia is suspected. Failure to respond to antibiotic treatment is additional evidence for a viral etiology. Usually, only minimal supportive measures are required, although some patients need hospitalization for intravenous fluids, oxygen, or even assisted ventilation. The only specific agents available for the treatment of respiratory viral infections are oral amantadine (or rimantadine) and aerosolized ribavirin. The former agents are active against influenza A isolates. They have demonstrable efficacy in preventing influenza A infections in exposed, susceptible individuals and in the treatment of patients infected with influenza A virus. Treatment appears to be beneficial only if started within 48 hr of the onset of the infection. Ribavirin is active in vitro against RSV. It appears to be beneficial for certain infants hospitalized with lower respiratory tract infection caused by RSV. It is, however, a very expensive agent that needs to be administered, virtually continuously, by aerosolization. Its precise role in the management of RSV-infected infants remains a subject of debate.

PROGNOSIS. Most children with viral pneumonia recover uneventfully and have no sequelae, although the course may be prolonged, especially in infants. There is increasing evidence, however, that some patients, particularly infants, may develop bronchiolitis obliterans, unilateral hyperlucent lung, or other complications after a single episode of viral pneumonia. Adenovirus, especially types 1, 3, 4, 7, and 21, seems to be the most dangerous agent in this regard, capable of causing fatal acute fulminant pneumonia.

MYCOPLASMAL PNEUMONIA. See Chapter 196.

BACTERIAL PNEUMONIA

GENERAL CONSIDERATIONS. Bacterial pneumonia during childhood is not a common infection, in the absence of an underlying chronic illness, such as cystic fibrosis or immunologic deficiency.

The most common event disturbing the defense mechanisms of the lung is a viral infection that alters the properties of normal secretions, inhibits phagocytosis, modifies the bacterial flora, and may temporarily disrupt the normal epithelial layer of the respiratory passages. A viral respiratory disease often precedes the development of bacterial pneumonia by a few days.

An underlying disorder should be considered if a child experiences recurrent bacterial pneumonias. Defects to consider include: abnormalities of antibody production (e.g., agammaglobulinemia), cystic fibrosis, cleft palate, congenital bronchiectasis, ciliary dyskinesia, tracheoesophageal fistula, abnormalities of polymorphonuclear leukocytes, neutropenia, increased pulmonary blood flow, or deficient gag reflex. Trauma, anesthesia, and aspiration are examples of iatrogenic factors promoting pulmonary infection.

Pneumococcal Pneumonia

Although the incidence of pneumococcal pneumonia has declined over the last several decades, *S. pneumoniae* is still the most common cause of bacterial infection of the lungs.

PATHOLOGY AND PATHOGENESIS. Pneumococcal organisms are probably aspirated into the periphery of the lung from the upper airway or nasopharynx. Initially, a reactive edema occurs that supports proliferation of the organisms and aids in their spread into adjacent portions of the lung. Usually, one or more lobes, or parts of lobes, are involved, leaving the remaining bronchopulmonary system uninvolved. However, this pattern of lobar pneumonia is often not present in infants, who may have a more patchy and diffuse disease that follows a bronchial distribution and that is characterized by many limited areas of consolidation around the smaller airways. Permanent injury is rare.

CLINICAL MANIFESTATIONS. The classic history of a shaking chill followed by a high fever, cough, and chest pain described in adults with pneumococcal pneumonia may be seen in older children, but it is rarely observed in infants and young children, in whom the clinical pattern is considerably more variable.

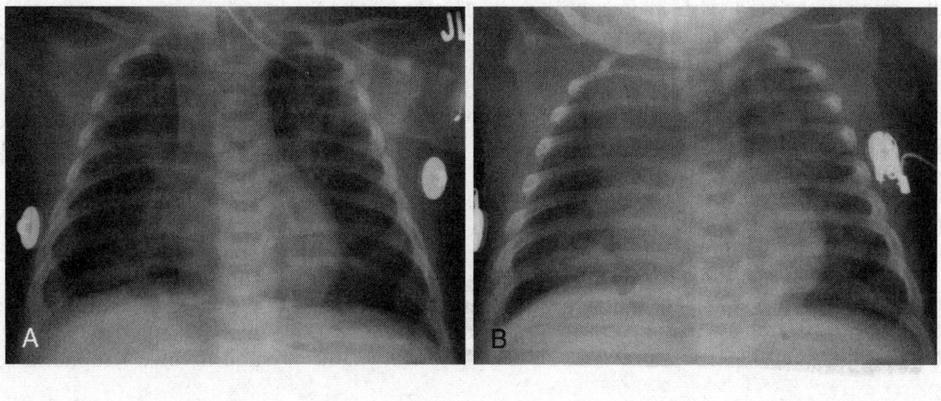

Figure 170–1. *A,* Six-mo-old infant with rapid respirations and fever. An anteroposterior (AP) radiograph of the chest shows hyperexpansion of the lungs with bilateral fine air space disease and streaks of density, indicating the presence of both pneumonia and atelectasis. An endotracheal tube is in place. *B,* One day later the AP radiograph of the chest shows increased bilateral pneumonia.

Infants. A mild upper respiratory tract infection, characterized by stuffy nose, fretfulness, and diminished appetite, usually precedes the onset of pneumococcal pneumonia in infants. This mild illness of several days' duration ends with abrupt onset of fever of 39° C or higher, restlessness, apprehension, and respiratory distress. The patient appears ill with moderate-to-severe air hunger and often cyanosis. The respiratory distress is manifested by grunting; flaring of the alae nasi; retractions of the supraclavicular, intercostal, and subcostal areas; tachypnea; and tachycardia.

A physical examination of the chest is often unrevealing. Auscultation may reveal diminished breath sounds and fine, crackling rales on the affected side, and there may be localized dullness to percussion, but these findings are less common than in older children. On the opposite side, breath sounds may be exaggerated and almost tubular in nature. Abdominal distention may be prominent, reflecting gastric dilation owing to swallowed air or to ileus; it may suggest an acute surgical emergency. The liver may seem enlarged because of downward displacement of the right diaphragm or superimposed congestive heart failure. Nuchal rigidity without meningeal infection may also be prominent, especially with involvement of the right upper lobe. Physical findings in the lung usually change little during the course of illness, although more rales may become audible during resolution.

Children and Adolescents. The signs and symptoms are similar to those of adults. After a brief, mild, upper respiratory infection, there is often onset of a shaking chill followed by fever as high as 40.5° C. This is accompanied by drowsiness with intermittent periods of restlessness; rapid respirations; a dry, hacking, unproductive cough; anxiety; and occasionally delirium. There may be circumoral cyanosis, and many children are noted to be splinting on the affected side to minimize pleuritic pain and improve ventilation; they may lie on their side with knees drawn up to the chest. Abnormal chest findings include retractions, flaring of alae nasi, dullness, diminished tactile and vocal fremitus, diminished breath sounds, and fine and crackling rales on the affected side.

The physical findings undergo change during the course of illness. Classic signs of consolidation are noted on the 2nd to 3rd day of illness and are characterized by dullness to percussion, increased fremitus, tubular breath sounds, and the disappearance of rales. As resolution occurs, moist rales are heard, and the cough loosens and becomes productive of large amounts of blood-tinged mucus.

The development of a pleural effusion or empyema may cause a visible lag in respiration on the affected side, with exaggerated excursion on the opposite side. There usually is dullness to percussion over the area of the effusion, with diminished fremitus and breath sounds. Tubular breathing is often noted immediately above the fluid level and on the unaffected side.

LABORATORY FINDINGS. The white blood cell count is usually elevated to 15,000–40,000 cells/mm^3, with a preponderance of polymorphonuclear cells. White blood cell counts <5,000/mm^3 are often associated with a poor prognosis. The hemoglobin value is usually normal or only slightly diminished. Arterial blood samples usually show hypoxemia without hypercapnia.

In most patients pneumococci can be isolated from the nasopharyngeal secretions, but this finding cannot be considered proof of a causative relation as 10–15% of the population may be uninfected carriers of *S. pneumoniae*. However, isolation of the bacteria from blood in pleural fluid is diagnostic of infection. Bacteremia is found in about 30% of patients having pneumococcal pneumonia.

ROENTGENOGRAPHIC FINDINGS (Figs. 170–1 and 170–2). The roentgenographic changes do not always correspond to the clinical observations. Consolidation may be demonstrated by roentgenography before it can be detected by physical examination. Lobar consolidation is not as common in infants and young children as in the older child. Pleural reaction with the presence of fluid is not uncommon. Radiographic resolution of the infiltrate may not be complete until several weeks after the child is clinically well. Therefore, unless there is evidence of clinical deterioration, it is not prudent to perform serial radiographs early in the illness.

DIFFERENTIAL DIAGNOSIS. Pneumococcal pneumonia cannot be differentiated from other bacterial and viral pneumonias without appropriate microbiologic studies. Conditions possibly confused with pneumonia are bronchiolitis, allergic bronchitis, congestive heart failure, acute exacerbations of bronchiectasis, aspiration of a foreign body, sequestered lobe, atelectasis, and pulmonary abscess.

An older child with right lower lobe pneumonia may have diaphragmatic irritation with pain referred to the right lower quadrant of the abdomen. Because ileus may accompany pneumonia, right lower quadrant pain and absent bowel sounds may be misinterpreted as acute appendicitis.

When meningismus is severe and associated with positive Kernig and Brudzinski signs, it can be differentiated from meningitis only by examining the spinal fluid.

COMPLICATIONS. With the use of antibiotic therapy, complications of bacterial pneumonia have become unusual. Although concomitant pneumococcal infection in other locations may be present prior to the onset of the symptoms of pneumonia, metastatic infection after the initiation of antibiotic treatment is infrequent. Empyema may occur as a result of extension of infection to the pleural surfaces. It is more common in infants than in older children.

PROGNOSIS. In the preantibiotic era, the mortality rate in infants and small children ranged from 20% to 50% and in older children from 3% to 5%. Furthermore, the incidence of chronic empyema with altered pulmonary function was relatively high. With appropriate antibiotic therapy instituted early in the course of the illness, the mortality rate during infancy and childhood is now less than 1%, and long-term morbidity is low.

TREATMENT. The drug of choice is penicillin (100,000 units/kg/24 hr). The majority of older children with pneumococcal pneumonia can be treated at home; the decision to hospitalize depends on the severity of the illness and the ability of the family to supply good nursing care. Pneumonia in the young infant is best treated in the hospital, because fluids and antibiotics may have to be administered intravenously. Furthermore, the course of illness in young infants is more variable and complications are more common. Patients with pneumonia associated with pleural effusion or empyema should also be hospitalized. Oxygen administered promptly to patients with respiratory distress greatly reduces the need for sedatives and analgesics; it should be given before the patient becomes cyanotic.

Streptococcal Pneumonia

Group A streptococci most commonly cause disease limited to the upper respiratory tract, but the organisms may spread to other areas of the body, including the lower respiratory tract. Streptococcal pneumonia and tracheobronchitis are uncommon, but certain viral infections, particularly those causing exanthems and epidemic influenza, predispose to these diseases, which are encountered most frequently in children 3–5 yr of age and very rarely in infants.

PATHOLOGY. Streptococcal infections of the lower respiratory tract result in tracheitis, bronchitis, or interstitial pneumonia. Lobar pneumonia is uncommon. Lesions consist of necrosis of the tracheobronchial mucosa with the formation of ragged ulcers and large amounts of exudate, edema, and localized hemorrhage. The process may extend to the interalveolar septa and involve lymphatic vessels. Pleurisy is relatively common;

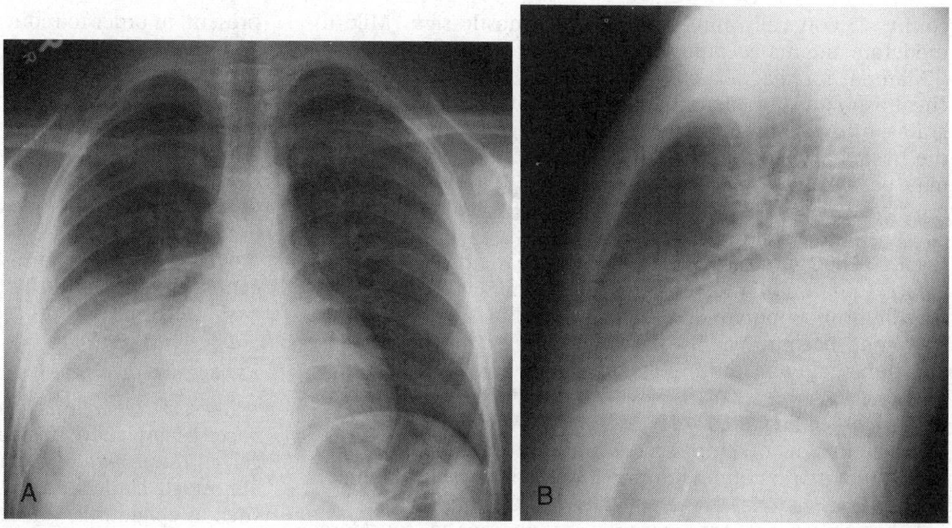

Figure 170–2. Fourteen-year-old male with cough and fever. Posteroanterior *(A)* and lateral *(B)* chest radiographs reveal consolidation in the right lower lobe, strongly suggesting bacterial pneumonia.

the effusion is often large and serous, occasionally serosanguineous, or thinly purulent, with less fibrin than the exudate of pneumococcal pneumonia.

CLINICAL MANIFESTATIONS. The signs and symptoms of streptococcal pneumonia are similar to those of pneumococcal pneumonia. The onset may be sudden, characterized by high fever, chills, signs of respiratory distress, and, at times, extreme prostration. However, it may occasionally be more insidious, and the child will appear only mildly ill, with cough and low-grade fever. If an exanthem or influenza precedes the pneumonia, the onset may be seen only as an increasingly severe clinical course of the viral illness.

LABORATORY MANIFESTATIONS. Leukocytosis occurs as in pneumococcal pneumonia. A rise in serum antistreptolysin titer is supportive diagnostic evidence. The disease may be suspected if large amounts of group A β-hemolytic streptococci are isolated from throat swab, nasopharyngeal secretions, bronchial washings, or sputum, but definitive diagnosis rests on recovery of the organism from pleural fluid, blood, or lung aspirate. Bacteremia occurs in about 10% of patients.

Chest roentgenograms usually show diffuse bronchopneumonia, often with a large pleural effusion. Final roentgenographic resolution may not be complete for up to 10 wk.

DIFFERENTIAL DIAGNOSIS. The clinical course and roentgenographic findings of streptococcal pneumonia with purulent pleurisy are similar to those of staphylococcal pneumonia. Pneumatoceles may occur in both conditions. The roentgenographic changes of uncomplicated streptococcal pneumonia may be indistinguishable from other interstitial pneumonitides, including those caused by *M. pneumoniae*.

COMPLICATIONS. Bacterial complications and long-term morbidity are common in the untreated patient but rare after antibiotic treatment is begun. Empyema occurs in 20% of children, and occasionally septic foci develop in other areas, such as the bones or joints; otherwise extension of the disease is uncommon.

TREATMENT. The drug of choice is penicillin G (100,000 units/kg/24 hr). Parenteral penicillin is used initially, and a 2–3 wk course may be completed orally after clinical improvement has begun in the hospital. If empyema develops, a thoracentesis should be performed for diagnostic purposes and for removal of fluid. On occasion, repeated thoracentesis or closed drainage with indwelling chest tubes may be required if the fluid reaccumulates.

Staphylococcal Pneumonia

Pneumonia caused by *S. aureus* is a serious and rapidly progressive infection that, unless recognized early and treated appropriately, is associated with prolonged morbidity and high mortality. It occurs less frequently than pneumococcal or viral pneumonia, and is more common in infants than in children.

EPIDEMIOLOGY. Most cases occur between October and May. As with other bacterial pneumonias, staphylococcal pneumonia is frequently preceded by a viral upper respiratory tract infection. Although it may occur at any age, 30% of all patients are under 3 mo of age and 70% are under 1 yr. Boys are affected more commonly than girls.

PATHOGENICITY AND PATHOLOGY. Staphylococci cause confluent bronchopneumonia that is often unilateral or more prominent on one side than the other and is characterized by the presence of extensive areas of hemorrhagic necrosis and irregular areas of cavitation. The pleural surface is usually covered by a thick layer of fibrinopurulent exudate. Multiple abscesses occur, containing clusters of staphylococci, leukocytes, erythrocytes, and necrotic debris. Rupture of a small subpleural abscess may result in pyopneumothorax, which in turn may erode into a bronchus, producing a bronchopleural fistula.

CLINICAL MANIFESTATIONS. Most commonly, the patient is an infant under 1 yr of age, often with a history of signs and symptoms of an upper respiratory tract infection for several days to 1 wk. Abruptly, the infant's condition changes, with the onset of high fever, cough, and evidence of respiratory distress. Signs and symptoms include tachypnea, grunting respirations, sternal and subcostal retractions, nasal flaring, cyanosis, and anxiety. If left undisturbed, the infant is lethargic but upon arousal is irritable and appears toxic. Severe dyspnea and a shocklike state may be present. Some infants have associated gastrointestinal disturbances, characterized by vomiting, anorexia, diarrhea, and abdominal distention secondary to a paralytic ileus. A rapid progression of symptoms is characteristic.

Physical findings depend on the stage of pneumonia. Early in the course of illness diminished breath sounds, scattered rales, and rhonchi are commonly heard over the affected lung. With the development of effusion, empyema, or pyopneumothorax, dullness on percussion is noted, and breath sounds and vocal fremitus are markedly diminished. A lag in respiratory excursion often occurs on the affected side. A physical examination may, however, be misleading, particularly in the young infant, with meager findings disproportionate to the degree of tachypnea.

LABORATORY MANIFESTATIONS. In the older infant and child a leukocytosis of ≥20,000 cells/mm^3 usually occurs, with the increase primarily among the polymorphonuclear cells; in the young infant the white blood cell count may remain within the normal range. As in other forms of bacterial infection, a count <5,000 cells/mm³ is a poor prognostic sign. Mild-to-moderate anemia is common.

Material for diagnostic cultures should be obtained by tracheal aspiration or pleural tap; Gram stain frequently reveals gram-positive cocci in clusters. The finding of staphylococci in the nasopharynx is of no diagnostic value, but blood cultures may be positive. Pleural fluid reveals an exudate with polymorphonuclear cell counts of 300–100,000/mm³, protein above 2.5 g/dL, and a low glucose level.

ROENTGENOGRAPHIC MANIFESTATIONS. Most patients with staphylococcal pneumonia have roentgenographic evidence of nonspecific bronchopneumonia early in the illness. The infiltrate may soon become patchy and limited in extent, or be dense and homogeneous and involve an entire lobe or hemithorax. The right lung alone is involved in about 65% of cases; bilateral involvement occurs in fewer than 20% of patients. A pleural effusion or empyema is noted during the course in most patients; pyopneumothorax occurs in approximately 25%. Pneumatoceles of varying sizes are common.

Although no roentgenographic change can be considered diagnostic, rapid progression from bronchopneumonia to effusion or pyopneumothorax with or without pneumatoceles is highly suggestive of staphylococcal pneumonia. Chest films should be obtained at frequent intervals if the diagnosis is suspected. Clinical improvement usually precedes roentgenographic clearing by days or weeks, and pneumatoceles may persist for months.

DIFFERENTIAL DIAGNOSIS. Recognizing early staphylococcal pneumonia in the infant is often difficult. Abrupt onset and rapid progression of symptoms of pneumonia should be considered to be due to staphylococci until proven otherwise. A history of furunculosis, a recent hospital admission, or maternal breast abscess should also alert the physician to the possibility of this diagnosis. Other bacterial pneumonias that cause empyema or pneumatoceles, and thus may be readily confused with staphylococcal disease, include streptococcal, *Klebsiella*, *H. influenzae*, and pneumococcal pneumonias and primary tuberculous pneumonia with cavitation. Occasionally, the aspiration of a nonradiopaque foreign body followed by pulmonary abscesses may lead to a similar clinical and radiologic picture.

COMPLICATIONS. Because empyema, pyopneumothorax, and pneumatoceles are so commonly seen with stapylococcal pneumonia, they are considered part of the natural course of the illness and not complications. Septic lesions outside the respiratory tract occur rarely, except in the young infant, in whom staphylococcal pericarditis, meningitis, osteomyelitis, and multiple metastatic abscesses in soft tissue may occur.

PROGNOSIS. Survival has improved substantially with present-day management, but mortality still ranges from 10% to 30% and varies with the length of illness prior to hospitalization, age of patient, adequacy of therapy, and the presence of other illness or complications. Children who do not have underlying disease have an excellent prognosis for complete recovery, including normal growth and development, normal pulmonary function, and no increased susceptibility to pulmonary infections. The course may be prolonged, with hospitalization for several weeks.

TREATMENT. Therapy consists of appropriate antibiotics and drainage of collections of pus. The infant should be given oxygen and placed in a semireclining position to relieve cyanosis and anxiety. During the acute phase, intravenous hydration and nutrition are indicated. Assisted ventilation may occasionally be needed.

A *semisynthetic, penicillinase-resistant penicillin* should be administered intravenously immediately after cultures are obtained (e.g., nafcillin, 200 mg/kg/24 hr).

Although patients with staphylococcal pneumonia may occasionally recover completely without chest tube drainage, it is recommended, even if only a small effusion or empyema is present, in order to reduce the chance of bronchopleural fistula and the necessity for repeated pleural taps. Generally, pus reaccumulates so rapidly and becomes so viscous or loculated that closed drainage with a chest tube of the largest possible caliber is required. The appearance of pyopneumothorax is another indication for immediate insertion of a catheter into the pleural space. It is often necessary to use several chest tubes when loculation occurs. Once the infant begins to improve and the lung has re-expanded, the tubes may be removed, even if they are still draining small amounts of pus. In general, tubes should not remain in the chest more than 5–7 days. Decortication procedures are rarely needed.

Haemophilus Influenzae Pneumonia

Haemophilus influenzae type b is a frequent cause of serious bacterial infection in infants and children who have not received *Haemophilus* vaccine. Nasopharyngeal infection precedes almost all clinical varieties of localized *H. influenzae* disease, such as epiglottitis, pneumonia, and meningitis. Pneumonia is second in frequency only to meningitis in children with invasive *H. influenzae* disease; most cases occur during winter and spring.

CLINICAL MANIFESTATIONS. *Haemophilus influenzae* pneumonias are usually lobar in distribution, but there is no characteristic chest roentgenogram. Segmental infiltrates, single or multiple lobe involvement, pleural effusion, and pneumatoceles occur. Disseminated pulmonary disease and bronchopneumonia have also been described. Males are affected slightly more often than females. Pathologically, involved areas show a polymorphonuclear or lymphocytic inflammatory reaction with extensive destruction of the epithelium of smaller airways, interstitial inflammation, and marked, often hemorrhagic, edema.

Although the clinical manifestations may be difficult to distinguish from those of pneumococcal pneumonia, *H. influenzae* pneumonia is more often insidious in onset, and the course is usually prolonged over several weeks. Many patients are already receiving treatment for otitis media at the time of diagnosis. Although ceftriaxone or chloramphenicol and ampicillin are recommended for treatment of *H. influenzae* pneumonia, a clinical response to penicillin G is common and does not exclude this diagnosis. Cough is almost always present but may not be productive, and the patient is febrile and often tachypneic with nasal flaring and retractions. There may be localized dullness to percussion and rales and tubular breath sounds; pleural fluid is often present on roentgenogram in the young infant.

DIFFERENTIAL DIAGNOSIS. The diagnosis is established by isolating the organism from the blood, pleural fluid, or lung aspirate. There is usually moderate leukocytosis with a relative lymphopenia. In the absence of a positive culture, a positive urine latex agglutination test supports the diagnosis of this infection. If atelectasis is present, bronchoscopy may be indicated to rule out a foreign body.

COMPLICATIONS. Complications are frequent, particularly in the young infant, and include bacteremia, pericarditis, cellulitis, empyema, meningitis, and pyarthrosis. Meningitis occurred in 15% of the younger patients in one study; examination of cerebrospinal fluid should be strongly considered when pneumonia due to *H. influenzae* is diagnosed.

TREATMENT. Treatment consists of the same symptomatic and supportive measures utilized in pneumococcal and staphylococcal pneumonias. When *H. influenzae* is suspected as the causative agent, ampicillin (100 mg/kg/24 hr) and chloramphenicol (100 mg/kg/24 hr) or ceftriaxone (100 mg/kg/24 hr) should be included in the initial antibiotic therapy until it is known whether the organism produces penicillinase; if the strain is sensitive, ampicillin (100 mg/kg/24 hr) alone may be administered. Appropriate in vitro susceptibility studies are essential. Effusion and pyarthrosis may require drainage. Needle thoracentesis is often adequate for effusion drainage, but the procedure may occasionally have to be repeated. Closed chest drainage may be required if purulent pleural fluid is present, but open drainage is infrequently needed. If the initial response to antibiotics is good, oral treatment can be instituted to complete a 10- to 14-day course. Roentgenographic demonstration of complete resolution may be delayed for several weeks.

Isaacs D: Problems in determining the etiology of community-acquired childhood pneumonia. Pediatr Infect Dis J 8:143, 1989.
Knight GJ, Carmen PG: Primary staphylococcal pneumonia in childhood: A review of 69 cases. J Paediatr Child Health 28:447, 1992.
Peter G: The child with pneumonia: Diagnostic and therapeutic considerations. Pediatr Infect Dis J 7:453, 1988.
Ray CG, Holberg CJ, Minnich LL, et al: Acute lower respiratory illnesses during the first three years of life: Potential roles for various etiologic agents. Pediatr Infect Dis J 12:10, 1993.
Schutze GE, Jacobs RF: Management of community-acquired bacterial pneumonia in hospitalized children. Pediatr Infect Dis J 11:160, 1992.
Turner RB, Lande AE, Chase P, et al: Pneumonia in pediatric outpatients: Cause and clinical manifestations. J Pediatr 111:194, 1987.

CHAPTER 171
Gastroenteritis

Larry K. Pickering and John D. Snyder

Infections of the gastrointestinal tract are caused by a wide variety of enteropathogens, including bacteria, viruses, and parasites (Table 171–1). Clinical manifestations depend on the organism and host, and include asymptomatic infection, watery diarrhea, bloody diarrhea, and chronic diarrhea. A presumptive etiologic diagnosis can be made from epidemiologic clues, clinical manifestations, physical examination, and knowledge of the pathophysiologic mechanism of enteropathogens. The two basic types of acute infectious diarrhea are inflammatory and noninflammatory. Enteropathogens elicit noninflammatory diarrhea through enterotoxin production by some bacteria, destruction of villus (surface) cells by viruses, and adherence and/or translocation by bacteria. Inflammatory diarrhea is usually caused by bacteria that invade the intestine directly or produce cytotoxins. Some enteropathogens possess more than one of these virulence properties.

Laboratory studies to identify the diarrheal pathogen are often not required because most episodes are self-limited. All patients with diarrhea require fluid and electrolyte therapy, a few need other nonspecific support, and some may benefit from antimicrobial therapy. This chapter presents a broad overview of diarrheal diseases due to infectious agents, and illnesses associated with ingestion of contaminated food. Although many aspects of this chapter deal with all children with diarrhea, the focus is on children in developed countries.

EPIDEMIOLOGY. Diarrheal diseases are one of the leading causes of morbidity and mortality in children worldwide, causing one billion episodes of illness and 3–5 million deaths annually. In the United States, 20–35 million episodes of diarrhea occur each year, among the 16.5 million children younger than 5 yr of age, resulting in 2.1–3.7 million physician visits, 220,000 hospitalizations, 924,000 hospital days, and 400–500 deaths. The major mechanism of transmission for diarrheal pathogens is fecal-oral, with food and water being the vehicles for most episodes. Enteropathogens that are infectious in a small inoculum (*Shigella*, enteric viruses, *Giardia lamblia*, *Cryptosporidium*, and perhaps *Escherichia coli* 0157:H7) may be transmitted by person-to-person contact. Factors that increase susceptibility to infection with enteropathogens include young age, immune deficiency, measles, malnutrition, travel to an endemic area, lack of breast-feeding, exposure to unsanitary conditions, ingestion of contaminated food or water, level of maternal education, and day-care center attendance.

CAUSATIVE AGENTS. The relative importance and epidemiologic characteristics of diarrheal pathogens vary by geographic location (see Table 171–1). Children in developing countries become infected with a diverse group of bacterial and parasitic pathogens, whereas all children in developed as well as developing countries will acquire rotavirus, and in many cases the other viral enteropathogens and *G. lamblia* during their first 5 yr of life. Acute diarrhea or diarrhea of short duration may be associated with any of the bacteria, viruses, or parasites listed in Table 171–1. Chronic or persistent diarrhea lasting 14 days or longer may be due to (1) an infectious agent, including *G. lamblia*, *Cryptosporidium*, and enteroaggregative or enteropathogenic *E. coli*; (2) any enteropathogen that infects an immunocompromised host; or (3) residual symptoms due to damage to the intestine by any enteropathogen following an acute infection. There are also many noninfectious causes of diarrhea in children (Table 171–2).

Bacterial Enteropathogens. Bacterial enteropathogens may cause either inflammatory or noninflammatory diarrhea, and specific

■ **TABLE 171–1 Causative Agents of Gastroenteritis**

Bacteria	Viruses	Parasites
Aeromonas sp.	Astrovirus	*Cryptosporidium*
*Bacillus cereus**	Calicivirus	*Cyclospora* spp.
Campylobacter jejuni	Coronavirus	*Entamoeba histolytica*
*Clostridium perfringens**	Enteric adenovirus	*Enterocytozoon bieneusi*
Clostridium difficile	Norwalk virus	*Giardia lamblia*
Escherichia coli	Rotavirus	*Isospora belli*
Plesiomonas shigelloides		*Strongyloides stercoralis*
Salmonella		
Shigella		
*Staphylococcus aureus**		
Vibrio cholerae		
Vibrio parahaemolyticus		
Yersinia enterocolitica		

**Generally associated only with foodborne outbreaks.*

■ **TABLE 171–2 Noninfectious Causes of Diarrhea**

Feeding Difficulty	**Food Poisoning**
Anatomic Defects	Heavy metals
Malrotation	Scombroid
Intestinal duplications	Ciguatera
Hirschsprung disease	Mushrooms
Fecal impaction	**Neoplasms**
Short bowel syndrome	Neuroblastomas
Microvillus atrophy	Ganglioneuromas
Strictures	Pheochromocytomas
Malabsorption	Carcinoid
Disaccharidase deficiencies	Zollinger-Ellison syndrome
Glucose-galactose monosaccharide malabsorption	Vasoactive intestinal peptide syndrome
Pancreatic insufficiency	**Miscellaneous**
Cystic fibrosis	Milk allergy
Shwachman syndrome	Crohn disease (regional enteritis)
Reduced intraluminal bile salts	Familial dysautonomia
Cholestasis	Immune deficiency disease
Hereditary fructose intolerance	Protein-losing enteropathy
Abetalipoproteinemia	Ulcerative colitis
Celiac disease	Acrodermatitis enteropathica
Endocrinopathies	Hartnup disease
Thyrotoxicosis	Laxative abuse
Addison disease	Motility disorders
Adrenogenital syndrome	

■ TABLE 171–3 Antimicrobial Therapy for Bacterial Enteropathogens in Children

Organism	Antimicrobial Agent	Indication for Antimicrobial Therapy
Aeromonas	Trimethoprim/sulfamethoxazole (TMP/SMX)	Dysentery-like illness, prolonged diarrhea
Campylobacter	Erythromycin	Early in the course of illness
Clostridium difficile	Vancomycin or metronidazole	Moderate to severe disease
Escherichia coli		
Enterotoxigenic	TMP/SMX	Severe or prolonged illness
Enteropathogenic	TMP/SMX	Nursery epidemics, life-threatening illness
Enteroinvasive	TMP/SMX	All cases if organism susceptible
Salmonella	Ampicillin or chloramphenicol or TMP/SMX or cefotaxime	Infants <3 mo and immunodeficient patients, typhoid fever, bacteremia, dissemination with localized suppuration
Shigella	TMP/SMX	All cases if organism susceptible
	Cefixime	Resistant strains
	Ciprofloxacin	Resistant strains in persons over 17 yr of age
Vibrio cholerae	Tetracycline or doxycycline or TMP/SMX	All cases

enteropathogens may be associated with either clinical manifestation. Generally, inflammatory diarrhea is associated with *Aeromonas* spp., *Campylobacter jejuni* (Chapter 186), *Clostridium difficile* (Chapter 194), enteroinvasive *E. coli* (Chapter 184), enterohemorrhagic *E. coli* (Chapter 184), *Plesiomonas shigelloides, Salmonella* spp. (Chapter 182), *Shigella* spp. (Chapter 183), *Vibrio parahaemolyticus* (Chapter 185), and *Yersinia enterocolitica* (Chapter 188). Noninflammatory diarrhea may be caused by enteropathogenic *E. coli*, enterotoxigenic *E. coli*, and *Vibrio cholerae*. Antimicrobial therapy is administered to selected patients with diarrhea to shorten the clinical course, to decrease excretion of the causative organism, or to prevent complications. Indications for specific antimicrobial therapy of patients infected with bacterial enteropathogens are shown in Table 171–3. Discussion of *Helicobacter pylori*, which involves the stomach and duodenum, can be found in Chapter 187.

Parasitic Enteropathogens. *Giardia lamblia* is the most common parasitic cause of diarrhea in the United States (Chapter 244.5); other pathogens include *Cryptosporidium* (Chapter 244.4), *Entamoeba histolytica, Strongyloides stercoralis* (Chapter 245.12), *Isospora belli*, and *Enterocytozoon bieneusi*. The latter two agents have been found most often in persons with acquired immune deficiency syndrome (AIDS). The role of *Dientamoeba fragilis, Blastocystis hominis*, and *Cyclospora* spp. as causes of diarrhea has not been fully defined. Patients with diarrhea normally do not need to have their stools examined for ova and parasites unless there is a history of recent travel to an endemic area, stool cultures are negative for other enteropathogens, and diarrhea persists for more than 1 wk; they are part of an outbreak of diarrhea; or they are immunocompromised. Examination of more than one stool specimen may be necessary to establish a diagnosis. Certain medications, antidiarrheal compounds, and barium may interfere with identification of parasitic enteropathogens. Treatment of these organisms depends on the clinical condition and availability of effective therapy (Table 171–4).

■ TABLE 171–4 Antimicrobial Therapy for Enteric Parasites in Children

Organism	Antimicrobial Agent
Giardia lamblia	Quinacrine HCl or metronidazole or furazolidone
Entamoeba histolytica	Metronidazole followed by iodoquinol
Cryptosporidium	None available
Cyclospora spp.	Trimethoprim/sulfamathoxazole (TMP/SMX)
Isospora belli	TMP/SMX
Enterocytozoon bieneusi	None available
Strongyloides	Thiabendazole

■ TABLE 171–5 Immune-Mediated Extraintestinal Manifestations of Enteric Pathogens

Manifestation	Related Enteric Pathogen(s)
Reactive arthritis	*Salmonella, Shigella, Yersinia, Campylobacter, Cryptosporidium*
Reiter syndrome	*Shigella, Salmonella, Campylobacter, Yersinia*
Guillain-Barré syndrome	*Campylobacter*
Glomerulonephritis	*Shigella, Campylobacter, Yersinia*
IgA nephropathy	*Campylobacter*
Erythema nodosum	*Yersinia, Campylobacter, Salmonella*
Hemolytic anemia	*Campylobacter, Yersinia*

Viral Enteropathogens. The four causes of viral gastroenteritis include rotavirus, enteric adenovirus, astrovirus, and calicivirus (Chapters 219 and 222).

GENERAL APPROACH TO CHILDREN WITH ACUTE DIARRHEA. Enteric infections cause signs of gastrointestinal tract involvement as well as systemic manifestations and complications. Gastrointestinal tract involvement may include diarrhea, cramps, and emesis. Systemic manifestations may include fever, malaise, and seizures. Extraintestinal infections related to bacterial enteric pathogens include local spread, causing vulvovaginitis, urinary tract infection, and keratoconjunctivitis. Remote spread can result in endocarditis, osteomyelitis, meningitis, pneumonia, hepatitis, peritonitis, chlorioamionitis, soft tissue infection, and septic thrombophlebitis. Immune-mediated extraintestinal manifestations of enteric pathogens usually occur after diarrhea has resolved (Table 171–5).

The main objectives in the approach to a child with acute diarrhea are to (1) assess the degree of dehydration and provide fluid and electrolyte replacement, (2) prevent spread of the enteropathogen, and (3) in select episodes determine the etiologic agent and provide specific therapy if indicated. Information regarding oral intake, frequency and volume of stool output, general appearance and activity of the child, and frequency of urination must be obtained (Table 171–6). Information should be obtained regarding day-care center attendance, recent travel to a diarrhea endemic area, use of antimicrobial agents, exposure to contacts with similar symptoms, and intake of seafood, unwashed vegetables, unpasteurized milk, contaminated water, or uncooked meats. The duration and severity of diarrhea, stool consistency, presence of mucus and blood, and other associated symptomatology, such as fever, vomiting, and seizures, should be determined. Fever is suggestive of an inflammatory process and also occurs as a result of dehydration. Nausea and emesis are nonspecific symptoms, but vomiting suggests organisms that infect the upper intes-

■ TABLE 171–6 Assessment of Dehydration

	Mild <5%	Moderate 5–9%	Severe ≥10%
Blood pressure	Normal	Normal to ↓	↓ to ↓↓↓
Pulse pressure	Normal	Normal to ↓	↓↓
Heart rate	Normal	Increased	Tachycardia
Skin	Normal	Decreased turgor	Decreased turgor
Fontanel	Normal	Normal	Sunken
Mucous membrane	Slightly dry	Dry	Dry
Extremities	Perfused	Delayed capillary refill	Cool, mottled
Mental status	Normal	Normal to lethargic	Lethargy, coma
Urine output	Slightly decreased	Decreased	Absent
Thirst	↑	↑↑	↑↑↑

tine, such as viruses, enterotoxin-producing bacteria, *Giardia*, and *Cryptosporidium*. Fever is common in patients with inflammatory diarrhea, abdominal pain is more severe, and tenesmus may occur in the lower abdomen and rectum, indicating involvement of the large intestine. Emesis is common in noninflammatory diarrhea; fever usually is absent or low grade; pain is crampy, periumbilical, and not severe; and diarrhea is watery, indicating upper intestinal tract involvement. Because immunocompromised patients require special consideration, information about an underlying immunodeficiency or chronic disease is important. Chronic diarrhea is defined as diarrhea lasting more than 14 days.

Examination of Stool. Stool specimens should be examined for mucus, blood, and leukocytes, the presence of which indicates colitis. Fecal leukocytes are produced in response to bacteria that invade the colonic mucosa diffusely. A positive fecal leukocyte examination indicates the presence of an invasive or cytotoxin-producing organism such as *Shigella, Salmonella, C. jejuni*, invasive *E. coli*, enterohemorrhagic *E. coli, C. difficile, Y. enterocolitica, V. parahaemolyticus*, and possibly an *Aeromonas* species or *Plesiomonas shigelloides*. Not all patients with colitis have a positive leukocyte examination.

Stool cultures should be obtained as early in the course of the disease as possible from patients in whom the diagnosis of hemolytic uremic syndrome (HUS) is suspected, in patients with bloody diarrhea, if stools contain fecal leukocytes, during outbreaks of diarrhea, and in persons with diarrhea who are immunosuppressed. Fecal specimens that cannot immediately be plated for culture can be transported to the laboratory in a non-nutrient-holding medium such as Cary-Blair to prevent drying or overgrowth of specific organisms.

Because certain bacterial agents, such as *Y. enterocolitica, V. cholerae, V. parahaemolyticus, Aeromonas* species, *C. difficile*, and *Campylobacter* species, require modified laboratory procedures for identification, laboratory personnel should be notified when one of these organisms is the suspected etiologic agent. Serotype and toxin assays are available for further characterization of *E. coli*. Detection of *C. difficile* toxins is valuable in the diagnosis of antimicrobial-associated colitis. Proctosigmoidoscopy may be helpful in establishing a diagnosis in patients in whom symptoms of colitis are severe or the etiology of an inflammatory enteritis syndrome remains obscure after initial laboratory evaluation.

Management of Fluids and Electrolytes and Refeeding. Management of dehydration remains the cornerstone of therapy of diarrhea. Children, especially infants, are more susceptible than adults to dehydration because of the greater basal fluid and electrolyte requirements per kilogram and because they are dependent on others to meet these demands. Patients with diarrhea and possible dehydration should be evaluated to assess the degree of dehydration as evident from clinical signs and symptoms, ongoing losses, and daily requirements.

Oral hydration usually is the treatment of choice for all but the most severely dehydrated patients whose caretakers cannot administer fluids. Rapid rehydration with replacement of ongoing losses during the first 4–6 hr should be carried out using an appropriate oral rehydration solution. Once the patient is rehydrated, an orally administered maintenance solution should be used (Table 171–7). Home remedies including decarbonated soda beverages, fruit juices, Jell-O, Kool-aid, and tea, are not suitable for use because they contain inappropriately high osmolalities due to excessive carbohydrate concentrations, which may exacerbate diarrhea; low sodium concentrations, which may cause hyponatremia; and inappropriate carbohydrate to sodium ratios. Once rehydration is complete, food should be reintroduced while the oral electrolyte solution is continued to replace ongoing losses from stools and for maintenance. Breast-feeding in infants should be resumed as soon as possible. Older children should be refed as soon as they can tolerate feeding.

■ **TABLE 171–7 Composition of Representative Glucose Electrolyte Solutions**

GES	Concentration (mmol/L) CHO	Na	CHO:Na	K	Base	Osmolality
Naturalyte	140	45	3.1	20	48	265
Pediatric electrolyte	140	45	3.1	20	30	250
Pedialyte	140	45	3.1	20	30	250
Infalyte	70	50	1.4	25	30	200
Rehydralyte	140	75	1.9	20	30	310
WHO/UNICEF ORS	111	90	1.2	20	30	310

GES = glucose electrolyte solution; CHO = carbohydrate; ORS = oral rehydration salts.

Antidiarrheal compounds are classified by their mechanism of action, which includes alteration of intestinal motility, adsorption of fluid or toxins, alteration of intestinal microflora, and alteration of fluid and electrolyte secretion. Antidiarrheal compounds are generally not recommended for use in children with diarrhea because of their minimal benefit and potential for side effects.

PREVENTION. Patients who are hospitalized should be placed under enteric precautions, including handwashing before and after patient contact, gowns when soiling is likely, and gloves when touching infected material. Patients and their families should be educated about the mode of acquisition of enteropathogens and methods to decrease transmission. Patients who attend day-care centers should be excluded from the center or cared for in a separate area until diarrhea has subsided. Cases of diarrhea caused by *Entamoeba histolytica*, episodes secondary to *E. coli* 0157:H7, *Giardia, Campylobacter, Salmonella, Shigella, V. cholerae*, and *V. parahaemolytica* should be reported to the local health department.

Vaccines are available to prevent or modify infection by *Salmonella typhi* (Chapter 182) and *Vibrio cholerae* (Chapter 185). Both vaccines have limited use in the United States.

ACUTE FOODBORNE AND WATERBORNE DISEASE. Foodborne and waterborne disease is a major cause of morbidity and mortality in all developed countries, including the United States. Changes in food production, flaws in inspection systems, rapid international distribution of food, alterations in dietary habits, and lack of recognition of methods of prevention magnify these problems. Foodborne illness in the United States is estimated to cause 6–81 million cases of gastroenteritis yearly, to cause 500–7,000 annual deaths, and to cost $8–23 billion yearly in medical costs and lost productivity.

The diagnosis of a foodborne or waterborne illness should be considered when two or more persons who have ingested common food or water develop a similar acute illness that usually is characterized by nausea, emesis, diarrhea, or neurologic symptoms. Pathogenesis and severity of bacterial disease depends on whether organisms have preformed toxins *(S. aureus, B. cereus)*, produce toxins, or are invasive, and whether they replicate in the food. The severity of disease due to viral, parasitic, and chemical causes depends on the amount inoculated into the food or water. The epidemiology of outbreaks often suggests specific etiologic agents. Determination of the incubation period and the specific clinical syndrome often lead to the correct diagnosis. Confirmation is established by specific laboratory testing of food, stool, or emesis. As a general rule, when outbreaks are grouped by incubation period of illness, those less than 1 hr are associated with chemical poisoning, toxins from fish or shellfish, or preformed toxins of *S. aureus* or *B. cereus*. Enterotoxin-producing bacteria, invasive bacteria, Norwalk virus, and some forms of mushroom poisoning have longer incubation periods.

Clinical Syndromes. Several clinical syndromes follow the ingestion of contaminated food or water, including nausea and

■ **TABLE 171–8 Characteristics of Foodborne Illness by Symptoms and Incubation Period**

Symptoms	Incubation Period (hr)	Cause
Nausea and vomiting	1–6	*Staphylococcus aureus, Bacillus cereus,* heavy metals
Paresthesia	0–6	Fish and shellfish
Neurologic, gastroenteritis	0–2	Mushroom (early onset)
Watery diarrhea, abdominal cramps	8–16	*B. cereus, C. perfringens*
	16–48	Norwalk virus, enterotoxigenic *E. coli, Vibrio cholerae* 01 and non-01
Diarrhea, fever, abdominal cramps	16–72	*Salmonella, Shigella, C. jejuni, Y. enterocolitica,* enteroinvasive *E. coli*
Bloody diarrhea, abdominal cramps	72–120	Enterohemorrhagic *E. coli*
Neurologic	6–24	Mushroom (late onset)
Paralysis, nausea, vomiting	18–48	*Clostridium botulinum*

vomiting within 6 hr; paresthesia within 6 hr; neurologic and gastrointestinal symptoms within 2 hr; abdominal cramps and watery diarrhea within 16–48 hr; fever, abdominal cramps, and diarrhea within 16–72 hr; abdominal cramps, bloody diarrhea without fever within 72–120 hr; neurologic signs and symptoms within 6–24 hr; and nausea, vomiting, and paralysis within 18–48 hr (Table 171–8).

Short incubation periods with vomiting as the major sign are associated with toxins that produce direct gastric irritation, such as heavy metals, or with preformed toxins of *B. cereus* or *S. aureus*; *B. cereus* also produces an enterotoxin. Paresthesias after a brief incubation period are suggestive of scombroid (histamine fish poisoning), paralytic or neurotoxic shellfish poisoning, Chinese restaurant syndrome (monosodium glutamate poisoning), niacin poisoning, or ciguatera fish poisoning. The early-onset syndrome associated with ingestion of toxic mushrooms ranges from gastroenteritis to neurologic symptoms that include parasympathetic hyperactivity, confusion, visual disturbances, and hallucinations to hepatic or hepatorenal failure, which occurs after a 6–24 hr incubation period.

Watery diarrhea and abdominal cramps after an 8–16 hr incubation period is associated with enterotoxin-producing *Clostridium perfringens* and *B. cereus*. Abdominal cramps and watery diarrhea following a 16–48 hr incubation period can be associated with Norwalk virus and several enterotoxin-producing bacteria. *Salmonella, Shigella, C. jejuni, Y. enterocolitica,* and enteroinvasive *E. coli* are associated with diarrhea, which may contain fecal leukocytes, abdominal cramps, and fever, although these organisms can cause watery diarrhea without fever. Bloody diarrhea and abdominal cramps following a 72–120 hr incubation period is associated with enterohemorrhagic *E. coli,* such as *E. coli* 0157:H7. Hemolytic uremic syndrome (Chapter 184) is a sequelae of infection with enterohemorrhagic *E. coli*. The combination of gastrointestinal tract symptoms followed by blurred vision, dry mouth, dysarthria, diplopia, or descending paralysis should suggest *C. botulinum* as the cause.

Therapy of most persons with foodborne disease is supportive, because the majority of these illnesses are self-limited. The exceptions are botulism, paralytic shellfish poisoning, and long-acting mushroom poisoning, all of which may be fatal in previously healthy persons. If a foodborne or waterborne outbreak is suspected, public health officials should be notified.

Brown KH, Peerson JM, Fontaine O: Use of nonhuman milks in the dietary management of young children with acute diarrhea: A meta-analysis of clinical trials. Pediatrics 93:17,1994.
Cicirello HG, Glass RI: Current concepts of the epidemiology of diarrheal diseases. Semin Pediatr Infect Dis 5:163, 1994.
Guerrant RL: Lessons from diarrheal diseases: Demography to molecular pharmacology. J Infect Dis 169:1206, 1994.
Guerrant RL, Bobak DA: Bacterial and protozoal gastroenteritis. N Engl J Med 325:327, 1991.
Hedberg CW, Osterholm MT: Outbreaks of foodborne and waterborne viral gastroenteritis. Clin Microbiol Rev 6:199, 1993.
Levine MM, Noriega F: Current status of vaccine development for enteric diseases. Semin Pediatr Infect Dis 5:245, 1994.
Pavia AT: Approach to acute foodborne and waterborne disease. Semin Pediatr Infect Dis 5:222, 1994.
Pickering LK, Morrow AL: Factors in human milk that protect against diarrheal disease. Infection 21:355, 1993.
Pickering LK, Obrig TG, Stapleton FB: Hemolytic uremic syndrome and enterohemorrhagic *Escherichia coli*. Pediatr Infect Dis J 13:459, 1994.
Snyder J: The continuing evolution of oral therapy for diarrhea. Semin Pediatr Infect Dis 5:231, 1994.
Velazquez FR, Calva JJ, Guerrero ML, et al: Cohort study of rotavirus serotype patterns in symptomatic and asymptomatic infections in Mexican children. Pediatr Infect Dis J 12:56, 1993.

CHAPTER 172

Osteomyelitis and Septic Arthritis

Nandini Narasimhan and Melvin Marks

OSTEOMYELITIS

Osteomyelitis is an infectious process primarily involving the bone. Hematogenous osteomyelitis is most common in children ≤10 yr of age.

PATHOLOGY AND PATHOGENESIS. Clinical osteomyelitis occurs when sufficient numbers of virulent organisms overcome host defenses to establish a focal infection in bone, with suppuration and ischemic necrosis, followed by fibrosis and bony repair. The entire bone (marrow, cortex, and periosteum) is typically involved.

Acute hematogenous osteomyelitis occurs as a result of localization of bloodborne bacteria in the bone. Bacteria such as *Staphylococcus aureus* possess the ability to adhere to connective tissue elements in bone (collagen, dentin, sialoprotein, and glycoprotein) via the elaboration of extracellular polysaccharide. Thrombosis occurring as a result of local trauma may predispose to localization of infection consequent to bacteremia. The source of bacteremia may be a focal suppurative infection or a clinically inapparent, unidentified colonization or infection.

Infection usually begins in the metaphyseal region of a long bone, probably because this region contains a potentially stagnant network of end arterioles and capillaries and lacks effective phagocytic cells. Bacterial infection typically leads to the production of an inflammatory exudate, which collects under pressure in the marrow and cortex. The resultant septic thrombosis of vessels and compromised vascular supply causes ischemic infarction of the bone with local pain. Sufficient pus may collect in the subperiosteal space to elevate the intact periosteum, causing disruption of the periosteal component of blood supply and infarction of cortical bone. The net result is the formation of an area of necrotic bone, called *sequestrum,* which separates from the underlying viable bone during the later stages to form a free foreign body or undergo gradual resorption. During the reparative phases of acute osteomyelitis, osteogenic precursor cells of the elevated periosteum form new bone (called *involucrum*) in the subperiosteal region, enveloping the infected focus.

The inflammatory response in the overlying soft tissues results in signs of acute inflammation near the site of osteomyelitis. Rupture of the periosteum may allow purulent material to drain into the soft tissues and skin through single or multiple "sinus tracts." The inflammatory process also extends in both directions within the marrow cavity and into the epiphysis in infants, via transphyseal vessels, which present in infants up to about 18 mo of age. These vessels traverse the cartilaginous growth plate. Epiphyseal infection may lead to infection within the joint space, causing *pyarthrosis* or *septic arthritis.* Ischemic necrosis of the growth plate can cause growth disturbance. Infection of the joint space can also occur if the area of metaphysis involved lies within the articular capsule. The proximal ends of the femur, humerus, radius, and the distal lateral end of tibia are intracapsular.

Chronic osteomyelitis is favored by ischemia and lack of effective host defenses, especially in the presence of a foreign body or necrotic bone. Microorganisms remain relatively inaccessible to the action of systemic antibiotics and cellular host defenses.

A subacute or chronic localized abscess walled off by a rim of sclerotic tissue is called a *Brodie abscess* and is seen most commonly in the distal tibia. Often the only clinical manifestations of this are dull pain and local tenderness. Plain radiographs may reveal a lucent area. Spontaneous sterilization may ensue, or it may persist as a chronic nidus of infection, requiring surgical and long-term medical therapy.

Infection of the partly ossified or nonossified flat bones of the foot in children, often due to penetrating injuries, results in suppuration of cartilage (including articular surfaces and growth plate) and adjacent bone, called *osteomyelitis-osteochondritis.* Spread of infection to adjacent joint spaces causes *pyarthrosis.* The latter may also result from direct penetration by puncture wounds.

ETIOLOGY. The most common bacterial pathogen is *Staphylococcus aureus,* accounting for 40–80% of cases. *Haemophilus influenzae* type b has been an important pathogen causing osteomyelitis, especially in children less than 3 yr of age. However, its incidence is likely to be significantly reduced by routine and widespread immunization. In neonates, group B streptococci and coliforms assume greater importance. Less common bacterial pathogens include *Streptococcus pneumoniae*; *Streptococcus pyogenes*; gram-negative bacilli, such as *Salmonella, Brucella, Kingella, Pseudomonas,* and *Serratia*; as well as anaerobes, coagulase-negative *Staphylococcus,* and *Neisseria* spp. The latter two organisms occasionally cause sepsis and osteomyelitis in neonates. In addition, *Neisseria gonorrhoeae* may cause osteomyelitis in sexually active adolescents.

Pseudomonas aeruginosa has a propensity to infect avascular cartilaginous structures of the foot, following puncture wounds. *Pseudomonas* also causes osteomyelitis in intravenous drug users.

Salmonella and *Brucella* tend to cause nonsuppurative osteomyelitis, with a predilection to involve the vertebral bones. Multifocal nonsuppurative osteomyelitis is described elsewhere (see Differential Diagnosis). *Salmonella* osteomyelitis tends to occur more often in children with hemoglobinopathies, although even in this group, *Staphylococcus aureus* remains the predominant pathogen. *Kingella kingae* is an underappreciated cause of osteomyelitis, septic arthritis, and spondylodiskitis in children, especially under 5 yr of age.

Anaerobic osteomyelitis complicates infections following trauma, human bites, and decubitus ulcers. Pathogens causing osteomyelitis associated with sinusitis, mastoiditis, or dental infections are reflective of the microbiologic flora of the adjacent infected mucosal surface (paranasal sinus, mastoid, gingiva). Actinomycetes may cause osteomyelitis of the spine and jaw with insidious onset. Mycobacteria and fungi *(Cryptococcus, Candida, Sporothrix, Blastomyces, Aspergillus)* are less common pathogens causing osteomyelitis. Predisposing factors for fungal osteomyelitis include age (neonates), penetrating wounds, and immunosuppression.

CLINICAL MANIFESTATIONS. The patient may have fever or no symptoms during the bacteremic phase. Local signs of inflammation and pain develop as a result of inflammation and increased intraosseous pressure. Older children can describe and localize the pain; younger children and infants demonstrate decreased voluntary movement (pseudoparalysis) or limp. Periosteal pain and muscle spasm result in limited active range of motion; passive range of motion around the contiguous joint is not affected, except with abscess formation or pyarthrosis. Local warmth, tenderness, and soft tissue swelling occur in direct proportion to dissection of pus through periosteum and deep soft tissues. The physical examination includes an evaluation for any source of primary infection that may have caused bacteremia.

Osteomyelitis in neonates can occur as a result of iatrogenic procedures such as heel punctures and fetal scalp monitoring and often has few or nonspecific clinical signs. Common etiologic agents are staphylococci, group B streptococci, and coliforms. Multifocal disease is seen in up to 50% of cases, and involvement of the joint adjacent to the site of bone involvement is more common.

The diagnosis of osteomyelitis in patients with sickle cell disease is complicated by the fact that similar symptoms can occur with vaso-occlusive (thrombotic) crises. Multiple bone site involvement is also common to osteomyelitis and vaso-occlusive crisis. Common etiologic agents include *Staphylococcus aureus* and gram-negative bacilli, especially *Salmonella.*

Vertebral osteomyelitis occurs mostly in children over the age of 8 yr, typically as a result of hematogenous infection. The diagnosis is difficult because symptoms and signs are poorly localized. Clinical features include fever, back pain, abdominal pain, or referred pain in the thigh and gait disturbances. The condition is often mistaken for primary hip disease and intra-abdominal or intrapelvic disorders. Features that are more diagnostic of vertebral osteomyelitis are point tenderness on percussion of the spinous process or paraspinous muscle spasm with limitation of range of movement. The predominant etiologic agent is *Staphylococcus aureus,* but gram-negative organisms, including *Salmonella, Brucella,* and *Kingella,* account for up to 30% of cases. Destruction of the vertebral body and formation of a paraspinous abscess can result in spinal cord compression, requiring emergency surgical intervention.

Pelvic osteomyelitis is also difficult to localize based on clinical presentation. Common presenting features are pain in the region of hip, buttock, or knee, and gait disturbances; most patients are afebrile. The etiologic agents are usually *Staphylococcus aureus* and *Salmonella.* Some cases are caused by mycobacteria.

Osteomyelitis following puncture wounds of the foot, occurring with osteochondritis/septic arthritis, is usually caused by *Pseudomonas,* especially in children ≥9 yr who suffer puncture wounds of the foot while wearing sneakers. *Staphylococcus aureus,* streptococci, and anaerobes may also be pathogens.

Chronic osteomyelitis presents with localized symptoms and signs of inflammation, often with a sinus tract. Acute exacerbations occur, with signs of acute inflammation and sinus tract drainage.

DIAGNOSIS. Microbiologic Studies. Establishing a definitive diagnosis of osteomyelitis requires isolation of the etiologic agent. Blood cultures yield positive results in up to 50–60% of cases; however, the microbiologic yield is enhanced by culture of material from bone aspiration or biopsy. In those cases where recovery of the pathogen is not possible by culture methods, a positive urine bacterial antigen test for *S. pneumoniae* or *H. influenzae* type b is useful as corroborative evidence. For chronic draining osteomyelitis, needle biopsy of the bone is more accurately predictive of the pathogen involved than are cultures of exudates from the surface of wounds, sinus tracts, or decubitus ulcers, since colonization or secondary infection of these structures can occur independent of the underlying osteomyelitis. Osteomyelitis in these cases is often polymicrobial in etiology. It is therefore important to include cultures for anaerobes.

If tuberculous etiology is suspected, a tuberculin skin test (PPD) and chest roentgenogram should be obtained in addition to mycobacterial cultures. Biopsy from a radiographically evident area of bone involvement showing granulomatous tissue, with or without caseation, is indicative of tuberculosis.

Imaging Studies. Roentgenograms may often be negative in the 1st week of illness or may demonstrate deep soft-tissue swelling with obscuring of fat lines between muscles, suggestive, but not diagnostic, of osteomyelitis. Vertebral osteomyelitis is suggested by plain radiographs demonstrating erosion and collapse of vertebral bodies with disk or without narrowing of the intervening space.

Specific changes of periosteal reaction (periosteal elevation and/or subperiosteal new bone formation) or bony destruction (rarefaction and/or lysis) take about 10–14 days to become radiographically evident (Fig. 172–1). However, institution of treatment early in the course of acute osteomyelitis may halt the progression of radiographic changes by arresting bone mineral loss.

The three-phase bone scan involves use of a ^{99m}Tc isotope–labeled compound, such as ^{99m}Tc methylene diphosphonate (^{99m}Tc-MDP). The uptake of the isotope is affected by the vascularity and osteoblastic activity of bone. Focal increased uptake in the initial phase, with subsequent decline in the later phases (especially the bone phase), is suggestive of cellulitis without osteomyelitis. In osteomyelitis, localized uptake is seen in all three phases, especially in the bone phase. Initial scans, taken within the first 2 days of acute osteomyelitis, may be negative or show areas of reduced uptake ("cold spots") as a result of ischemia or infarction.

The major advantage of technetium bone scanning over plain radiography is its ability to detect multiple sites of involvement earlier in the course of disease than plain radiographs. Neonates have been shown to have false-negative bone scans with osteomyelitis. Yet in this group of patients, bone scans are of value in detecting multiple sites of bony involvement that are frequently missed by the initial clinical exam and plain radiography. In the diagnosis of pelvic osteomyelitis, a delayed image at 24 hr is particularly useful because early images may be inaccurate due to urinary excretion of the isotope overlapping the pelvic bones. When it is difficult to delineate osteomyelitis from overlying cellulitis, septic arthritis, or noninfectious causes of inflammation, combining technetium bone scanning with other radionuclide scanning techniques or tomography may be useful.

Radionuclide scans such as gallium-67 citrate scans and labeled white blood cell scans (using indium-111 oxide or ^{99m}Tc-MDPAO) are useful in detecting acute inflammation. These scans have a role in the diagnosis of pelvic bone osteomyelitis due to its sensitivity over that of plain radiographs in detecting bone inflammation.

An indium-111–tagged white blood cell scan may be more sensitive in detecting acute than chronic inflammation. It is

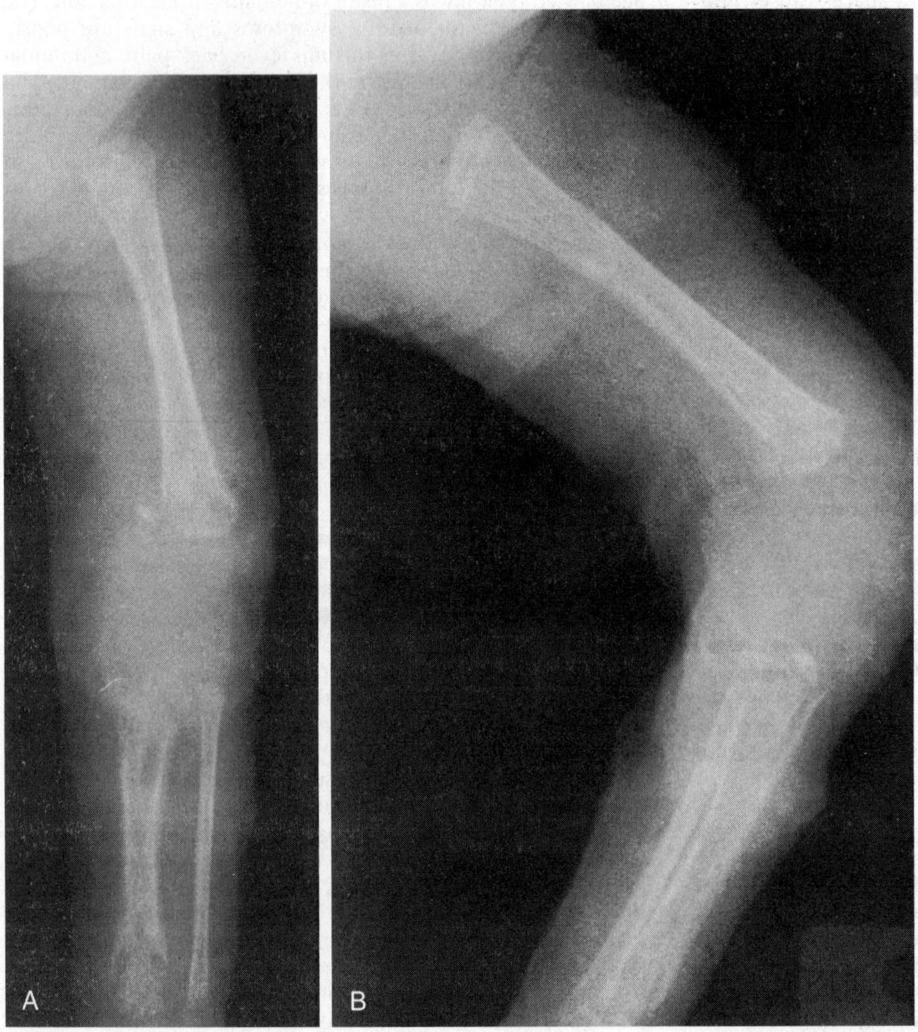

Figure 172–1. Plain radiographs of a neonate with multifocal osteomyelitis involving the left leg, caused by *S. aureus*. *A*, Anteroposterior view showing severe destructive changes in the distal femur, proximal tibia, distal tibia, and distal fibula. A sequestrum may be seen adjacent to the distal femur. The large effusion of the knee joint demonstrates septic arthritis that has arisen as a complication of contiguous osteomyelitis. *B*, Lateral view of the same limb.

considered to be relatively more specific for detecting infection than the gallium-67 scan, which may not distinguish between infection and increased turnover of bone due to inflammation.

In patients with sickle cell disease, the diagnostic value of technetium scans is limited due to residual scintigraphic alterations (foci of increased or decreased uptake) that may result from prior and/or current episodes of infarction, even in the absence of infection. In this context, the combined use of gallium-67 and technetium-99 scintigraphy is helpful in distinguishing osteomyelitis from infarction due to vaso-occlusive crisis.

Computed tomography (CT) is useful in osteomyelitis of the pelvic and vertebral bones and for demonstration of sequestra. Magnetic resonance imaging (MRI) is most sensitive in detecting inflammatory processes in soft tissue or bone and is often useful in providing detailed, precise, anatomic information in a localized area. However, MRI has its limitations, including the limited area surveyed (as opposed to the whole-body survey with radionuclide imaging studies), cost, necess[illegible] of adequate sedation in pediatric patients (to prevent [illegible] artifacts), and the lack of specificity in distinguishing [illegible] from neoplasm in bones of the appendicular skelet[illegible] areas with inflammation (e.g., due to prior trauma).

Markers of Acute Inflammation. Acute-phase reactants, such a[illegible] [illegible]eukocyte count (total and differential), erythrocyte sedimentation rate (ESR), and serum C-reactive protein (CRP), are useful in the diagnosis of acute osteomyelitis, monitoring its course, and response to therapy. At the time of initial diagnosis, leukocyte counts are normal in up to 60% of cases. The ESR may be elevated, but normal values are seen in up to 25% of patients with early acute osteomyelitis. If elevated, the ESR usually returns to normal with treatment in 3–4 wk in uncomplicated cases of acute osteomyelitis. CRP rises rapidly within the first 8 hr, attaining a peak value around 2 days and declining to normal values within 1 wk.

DIFFERENTIAL DIAGNOSIS. Infections of other structures in proximity to bone can mimic osteomyelitis, for example, pyomyositis, cellulitis, bursitis, abscess, septic arthritis, and diskitis. Trauma, primary or secondary bony malignancy (neuroblastoma, osteogenic and Ewing sarcoma, etc.), leukemia, lymphoma, and bone infarction need to be considered in the differential diagnosis of osteomyelitis. Differential diagnosis of pelvic osteomyelitis includes arthritis (toxic and septic), retroperitoneal abscess, and avascular necrosis of the femoral head (Legg-Calvé-Perthes disease).

Chronic Recurrent Multifocal Osteomyelitis

Chronic recurrent multifocal osteomyelitis (CRMO) is a noninfectious, inflammatory condition of children and young adults. Typical features are multiple sites of involvement and a temporal course of remissions and exacerbations, coincident with lack of isolation of etiologic agents or response to empiric antimicrobial therapy. Females are affected approximately twice as often as males. Sites of involvement include the metaphyses of tubular bones, especially the proximal and distal tibia, sternal end of the clavicle, femur, fibula, radius, ulna, as well as vertebrae. Conditions associated with CRMO include palmoplantar pustulosis, Sweet syndrome (neutrophilic dermatosis), vertebral sclerosis, and psoriasis.

Bone biopsy shows acute inflammation, granulation tissue, and noncaseating granulomas with negative cultures for pathogens.

Differential diagnosis of this condition includes multifocal acute or subacute pyogenic osteomyelitis, leukemia, neuroblastoma, and histiocytosis X. Exacerbations respond to therapy with nonsteroidal anti-inflammatory agents and physiotherapy. Steroids may be required for severe cases. Although radiologic changes may persist, the overall prognosis is excellent.

Diskitis

Diskitis refers to an inflammatory condition that primarily involves the intervertebral disk. Most cases occur in children under the age of 5 yr, probably because the vasculature to the cartilaginous end plate at the disk-vertebral interface undergoes involution with age.

The infectious etiology of diskitis is proven in up [illegible] of cases, with the predominant pathogen bein[illegible] *aureus.* Other organisms identified includ[illegible] ganisms, such as *Salmonella* and *Kin*[illegible] tive staphylococci.

Clinical manifestations ar[illegible] [illegible]imp, and refusal to sit, sta[illegible] [illegible]r antecedent trauma m[illegible] examination is usually nor[illegible] [illegible]use spinal tenderness and/o[illegible] [illegible]on of movement. The L4–L5 [illegible] [illegible]ost commonly involved. [illegible] [illegible]evated with a normal leukocyte count. [illegible] features include narrowing of the disk space [illegible]ar erosion of adjacent vertebral surfaces, but these [illegible]ges may be absent within the first 1–2 wk after the onset of symptoms. Technetium bone scans may show increased uptake of the radionuclide in vertebral bodies adjacent to the involved disk(s), and gallium scans demonstrate localization to specific disk(s). For early or atypical cases, MRI is useful.

Antistaphylococcal antibiotics are administered intravenously and orally (sequentially) until clinical resolution. Chronic backache and functional impairment occur infrequently.

TREATMENT (Table 172–1). The goal of antimicrobial therapy in osteomyelitis is to maintain concentrations of an effective antibiotic in infected tissue (bone and pus) at levels that exceed the minimum inhibitory concentration for the pathogen. High serum concentrations of a bactericidal antibiotic must be attained to ensure adequate antibiotic concentration in bone.

In the neonate, initial empirical antibiotics should include an antistaphylococcal agent (e.g., methicillin, nafcillin, oxacillin) to cover *S. aureus* and group B streptococci, in combination with an aminoglycoside (see Tables 172–1 and 172–2) to additionally cover Gram-negative coliforms. If staphylococci that are known or suspected to be resistant to methicillin or oxacillin are involved, vancomycin should be substituted as the antistaphylococcal agent.

Antibiotic therapy in a healthy, immunized child under the age of 5 yr should cover *Staphylococcus aureus* and, possibly, *Haemophilus influenzae* type b. The latter pathogen should be considered when osteomyelitis is associated with septic arthritis in an adjacent joint. Cephalosporins with antistaphylococcal and anti-*Haemophilus* activity, such as cefuroxime or ceftriaxone, can be used. Alternatively, a combination of an antistaphylococcal penicillin and chloramphenicol may be used. In children over the age of 5 yr, an antistaphylococcal penicillin is the drug of choice. Patients with osteomyelitis and sickle cell disease should be given an aminoglycoside or an extended-spectrum cephalosporin along with an antistaphylococcal penicillin. Clindamycin is the preferred antibiotic for anaerobic osteomyelitis.

Treatment for osteomyelitis associated with puncture wounds of the foot should include an antistaphylococcal penicillin and an antipseudomonal penicillin, possibly with an aminoglycoside. However, the mainstay of therapy for ensuing osteomyelitis is surgical.

The initial response to therapy in acute osteomyelitis is judged by the resolution of systemic and local signs of infection; a decline in white blood cell count, CRP, and ESR; and resolution, or at least lack of progression, of plain radiologic changes.

Although the duration of antimicrobial therapy is not well established, 3–6 wk is recommended for most uncomplicated

■ **TABLE 172–1 Antibiotics for Initial Therapy of Osteomyelitis in Children**

Host/Associated Factors	Likely Pathogen	Choice of Empirical Antibiotics	Antibiotic Dosages (IV)
Neonate	Group B streptococci, gram-negative bacilli, *S. aureus*	Nafcillin *and*	100–200 mg/kg/day in 4 div. doses (>7 days old), 3 div. doses (0–7 days old)
		gentamicin *or*	5–7.5 mg/kg/day in 3 div. doses (<7 days old), 2 div. doses (0–7 days old)
		cefotaxime	100–200 mg/kg/day in 3–4 div. doses (>7 days old), 2 div. doses (0–7 days old)
Younger than 5 yr	*S. aureus, H. influenzae* type b	Cefuroxime *or*	100–150 mg/kg/day in 3 div. doses
		cefotaxime *or*	100–150 mg/kg/day in 4 div. doses
		ceftriaxone	50–100 mg/kg/day in 2 div. doses
Older than 5 yr	*S. aureus*	Nafcillin *or*	150 mg/kg/day in 4 div. doses
		oxacillin *or*	100–200 mg/kg/day in 4 div. doses
		clindamycin	40 mg/kg/day in 4 div. doses
After puncture wound of the foot (esp. through sneakers)	*P. aeruginosa, S. aureus*	Ceftazidime *and*	100 mg/kg/day in 3 div. doses
		nafcillin	150 mg/kg/day in 4 div. doses
Chronic granulomatous disease	*S. aureus, Serratia* spp., *Aspergillus* spp.	Nafcillin *and*	150 mg/kg/day in 4 div. doses
		gentamicin *or*	5–7.5 mg/kg/day in 3 div. doses
		cefotaxime	100–150 mg/kg/day in 4 div. doses
Sickle cell disease	*S. aureus, Salmonella* spp.	Nafcillin *and*	150 mg/kg/day in 4 div. doses
		cefotaxime	100–150 mg/kg/day in 4 div. doses

div. = *divided.*

cases. Initial therapy is always given by the intravenous route so as to ensure high concentrations of the antibiotic in serum, and therefore, bone. Besides the initial response to treatment, the duration of parenteral antibiotic therapy depends upon the acute or chronic nature of disease and host status (immune function, sickle cell disease). With a favorable initial response, oral therapy can be considered in selected cases, using high doses of oral antibiotics (often two to three times those used to treat minor infections.

Oral antibiotic therapy should be pursued only when tolerance to oral antibiotics, compliance, availability of a suitable oral agent, and an adequate serum bactericidal activity by measurement of serum bactericidal titer (SBT) are ensured. A trough SBT value, that is, bacteriostatic activity of serum at a time when antibiotic concentration is at its nadir, of at least 1:2 seems to correlate best with cure in acute osteomyelitis. Although peak SBTs are not as directly correlated with clinical outcome, a value of 1:8 is desirable. In the case of orally administered beta-lactams (including penicillin), concomitant use of probenecid may augment achieved serum concentrations. Commonly used oral antibiotics in children are cephalexin, amoxicillin (with or without clavulanic acid), dicloxacillin, and clindamycin. In older children ciprofloxacin is sometimes used.

For cases that fail to show a satisfactory initial response to intravenous therapy, additional therapy (medical and surgical) should be considered in consultation with an infectious disease specialist. Parenteral antibiotics are given for 1–2 mo followed by oral antibiotics for 2–4 mo. For chronic osteomyelitis, a trough SBT level of at least 1:4 is desirable, with a peak level of ≥1:16. Surgical intervention is required for removal of sequestra (sequestrectomy) and sinus tracts, curettage of a Brodie abscess, and irrigation with debridement of osteomyelitis associated with foreign bodies, decubitus ulcers, or open fractures.

Adjunctive therapy for osteomyelitis includes pain relief, nutrition, hydration, and immobilization. The latter seldom requires casting of the limb. Physical therapy is useful after the acute stage when pain has decreased. Weight bearing in lower limb osteomyelitis is usually allowed only after the radiologic changes show improvement.

PROGNOSIS AND COMPLICATIONS. The prognosis for uncomplicated osteomyelitis is good. Septic arthritis may complicate the course of osteomyelitis, necessitating surgical intervention. Sequelae, such as bony deformity and altered growth, may occur as a result of involvement of the bone and cartilaginous growth plate (Fig. 172–2). Pathologic fractures can also occur.

SEPTIC ARTHRITIS

Septic or pyogenic arthritis is an inflammation of the joint caused by pyogenic microorganisms.

PATHOLOGY AND PATHOGENESIS. Septic arthritis can result from hematogenous dissemination of bacteria, contiguous spread of an osteomyelitis, or direct inoculation of microorganisms into the joint cavity as a result of penetrating trauma. Hematogenous seeding of bacteria to the highly vascular synovium triggers a marked inflammatory response. The combination of leukocyte-initiated cytokine mediators and bacterial toxins produces synovial inflammation, with resultant increased vascular permeability and increased fluid production. Turbid fluid collects within the joint space under increased pressure. This may result in compression and/or thrombosis of intra-articular vessels, which, in the case of the hip joint, can rapidly cause avascular necrosis of the femoral head. The lack of a basement membrane allows the inflammatory process to involve the matrix in the superficial zone of the articular surface as early as within 24 hr after infection. Proteolytic enzymes, derived from activated polymorphonuclear cells and, presumably, synovial lining cells and bacteria, cause lysis of the connective tissue matrix of articular cartilage. More prolonged inflammation causes degeneration of chondrocytes and can lead to involvement of the subchondral bone (epiphysis) and cartilaginous growth plate (physis). Furthermore, as a complication of spread of infection across the physis, either by chondrolysis or through patent vascular channels (transphyseal vessels), osteomyelitis can occur.

ETIOLOGY (Table 172–3). *Haemophilus influenzae* type b has been the most common pathogen, accounting for 20–50% of cases occurring in patients between 2 mo and 5 yr of age. Along with the observed decline in the incidence of other invasive diseases caused by *H. influenzae* type b with the practice of routine immunization of infants against this organism, the incidence of septic arthritis is also certain to show a similar trend. As a bacteremic illness, *H. influenzae* septic arthritis is often complicated by concurrent meningitis (10–30%), osteomyelitis (5–10%), otitis media (10%), cellulitis (10–30%), and pneumonia (5%).

Staphylococcus aureus, the most common agent causing neonatal septic arthritis, is also the most common pathogen caus-

■ TABLE 172–2 Epidemiology and Manifestations of Osteomyelitis

Category	Affected Sites	Symptoms and Signs	Expected Organism
Acute Hematogenous Osteomyelitis			
Neonate (0–2 mo)	Femur, humerus; multiple sites may be affected in 20–50%. Associated septic arthritis	Sepsis-like appearance or pseudoparalysis ± fever	Group B streptococci, *Staphylococcus aureus, Escherichia coli*
Infant (2–24 mo)	Metaphysis of long bone; femur affected most commonly, followed by tibia, humerus, fibula, radius, phalanx, in that order. May involve joint space	Fever, limp, pain, tenderness, pseudoparalysis	*S. aureus* (most common), *Streptococus pneumoniae, Haemophilus influenzae* type b, group B streptococci
Child (2–20 yr)	Metaphysis of long bones (as for infant), rarely vertebrae or pelvis	Focal pain with fever for 1–5 days, focal tenderness, swelling, rarely joint effusion	*S. aureus* (most common), streptococci, *E. coli, Salmonella,* anaerobes, rarely fungi
Intravenous drug abuse	Femur, pubis, vertebra, sternum. May be acute or chronic	Indolent, local pain, may be afebrile, swelling	*Pseudomonas aeruginosa,* methicillin-resistant *S. aureus,* streptococci, *Candida,* anaerobes
Sickle cell anemia	Diaphysis and metaphysis, long bones, vertebra, clavicle, calvarium, small bones of hand	Difficult to distinguish from bone vaso-occlusive crises	*S. aureus, Salmonella,* gram-negative bacilli, *S. pneumoniae*
Chronic granulomatous disease	Metaphyseal, chronic; possibly contiguous. Possibly associated or independent septic arthritis	Indolent, local pain, limp, soft tissue swelling	*S. aureus, Aspergillus, Serratia*
Contiguous Osteomyelitis			
Fetal scalp monitoring	Scalp	Open wound, drainage, swelling, may have associated meningitis	*S. aureus, S. epidermidis,* group B streptococci, gram-negative bacilli
Neonatal heel punctures	Calcaneous	Open wound, cellulitis, drainage, tenderness, swelling	*S. aureus, S. epidermidis,* gram-negative bacilli
Decubitus ulcer	Sacrum, bony prominences (chronic)	Tend to occur in patients with paraplegia (spinal cord injury, spina bifida); delayed healing of pressure sores, recurrent drainage. ESR >100, WBC >15,000	Mixed organisms, *S. aureus,* anaerobes, gram-negative bacilli, streptococci
Animal-human bites: paronychia	Hand (fist-fighting), other sites	Open wound, drainage, erythema, cellulitis	*Eikenella corrodens, S. aureus,* streptococci, anaerobes, *Pasteurella multocida* (animals)
Nail puncture through sneaker	In order of frequency—calcaneous, metatarsals, cuboid, navicular, cuneiforms; acute or chronic	Open wound, cellulitis, focal pain and tenderness, swelling, limp	*P. aeruginosa, S. aureus*
Facial-cranial injury	Bone in area contiguous to infected mucosal surface (mastoiditis, sinusitis, periodontal abscess); chronic	Pain, swelling, tenderness. Pott puffy tumor (frontal sinus–associated osteomyelitis)	*Bacteroides fragilis, B. melaninogenicus,* anaerobic cocci
Trauma	Long bone open fracture; surgery (e.g., sternotomy)	Pain, draining sinus tract, wounds fail to heal, fever in 30%	*P. aeruginosa, S. aureus, S. epidermidis* mixed organisms. Sternotomy also may be associated with atypical mycobacteria, *Mycoplasma hominis,* anaerobes

ing septic arthritis in patients more than 5 yr of age and the second most frequent agent in children between the ages of 2 mo and 5 yr. Septic arthritis caused by this organism is often complicated by contiguous osteomyelitis (10–40%).

Neonatal septic arthritis can also be caused by group B streptococci, *Escherichia coli,* or *Candida albicans.* Other pathogens are *S. pneumoniae, Neisseria* spp., and gram-negative bacilli *(Kingella kingae, Salmonella).*

In sexually active adolescents, *N. gonorrhoeae* is an important cause of both polyarticular and monoarticular septic arthritis, occurring almost always in association with infection of the genitourinary tract, rectum, or pharynx.

Streptobacillus moniliformis or *Spirillum minus* (causal agents of rat-bite fever) and *Borrelia burgdorferi* (the causal agent of Lyme disease) are other bacteria that can cause arthritis. *Corynebacterium diphtheriae* is a rare cause of bacterial arthritis in immunocompromised, as well as normal, patients. In up to a third of cases no bacterial pathogen is identified. This observation, at least in part, may be reflective of the fastidious nature of certain bacteria that cause pyogenic arthritis (e.g., *Neisseria, Kingella*) and that require special culture techniques to enhance microbial growth.

Chronic septic arthritis in normal and immunocompromised patients may also be due to *Brucella,* mycobacteria (atypical and tuberculous), and fungi (*Sporothrix schenckii, Coccidioides immitis, Blastomyces dermatitides, Candida albicans, Pseudallescheria boydii, Histoplasma capsulatum,* and dematiaceous fungi).

CLINICAL MANIFESTATIONS. The main feature of septic arthritis is acute inflammation localized to the region of joint(s). This may produce pain, tenderness, swelling, erythema, and decreased range of motion. Early septic arthritis may resemble a bacteremic illness with fever and a toxic appearance. Septic arthritis in the neonate often presents with few systemic signs other than irritability or poor feeding. Pseudoparalysis of the involved extremity and pain when the diaper is changed are common early manifestations of septic arthritis involving the hip in a neonate. Diagnosis in this group of patients is based on a high index of suspicion. Multiple joint involvement and contiguous osteomyelitis are common in infants.

In older patients, pain may be localized to the involved joint, but it may also be referred to a site other than the joint itself. For example, pain from the hip may be referred to the knee, whereas pain from the pelvis may be referred to the back, hip, or anterior thigh.

Muscle spasm reflects the natural tendency to keep the joint in a position that maximizes articular volume, therefore minimizing intra-articular pressure and pain *(antalgic position).* The hip tends to be kept in a position of flexion, abduction, and external rotation, the knee and ankle in partial flexion, the shoulder in adduction and internal rotation, and the elbow in

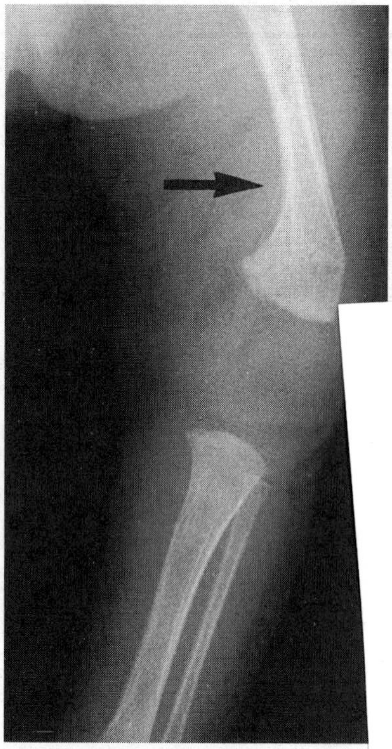

Figure 172–2. Follow-up radiograph 6 wk afte taken showing excellent healing of previousl changes and interval resolution of knee joint eff ment of the region of the growth plate (physis) h residual varus deformity of the distal femur *(arr* of M. T. Gyepes, MD.)

midflexion. Pain may also result in gait disturb denced by limp *(antalgic gait).*

Pyogenic sacroiliitis can present with fever, an region of the hip, thigh, back, or buttock that is a movement. Localized tenderness over the region c iac joint and pain elicited on compression of th gs are important diagnostic signs.

Gonococcal septic arthritis follows disseminate nic infection and is manifested by chills, fever, migratory poly-arthralgias, tenosynovitis, and rash, with eventual development of a monoarticular infection involving the knee, shoulder, wrist, ankle, or interphalangeal joints of the hand. Disseminated gonococcal infection (DGI) is more common in females (4:1) and often occurs during menstruation or the 2nd or 3rd trimester of pregnancy.

Tuberculous arthritis is often chronic, usually involving a single joint. The knee, wrist, hip, interphalangeal-metacarpal joints, spine, and ankle joints may be involved. Concomitant involvement of the synovial sheath is often seen. Pain in the region of the involved joint is a common presenting feature; this may last for weeks to months prior to the onset of other symptoms and signs.

DIAGNOSIS. Initial laboratory studies reveal elevated ESR, CRP, and peripheral white blood cell and neutrophil counts. Blood cultures are positive in 30–40% cases. Diagnostic arthrocentesis should be performed in every patient in whom the diagnosis of septic arthritis is entertained. It is important to try to avoid traversing an overlying superficial cellulitis, because this may introduce organisms into a previously sterile uninvolved joint.

Normal synovial fluid is clear, colorless, or straw colored. The appearance of synovial fluid in patients with septic arthritis may be helpful in distinguishing it from other diseases that produce synovitis (Table 172–4). However, in most cases of septic arthritis grossly purulent synovial fluid with white blood cell counts over 100,000/μL is not obtained. Hence, microbiologic diagnosis is the cornerstone to the establishment of an infectious etiology. If no fluid is obtained on diagnostic aspiration, the joint space can be irrigated with preservative-free saline and the resultant aspirate sent for bacteriologic studies. Culture of synovial fluid is positive in 70–80% of patients. The microbiologic yield may be enhanced by the use of selective or growth-enhancing media. Gram stain is positive in 50%.

Many patients may be partially treated, owing to the use of pecific, nonlocalizing symptoms prior thritis. In such cases, positive antigen detection tests (for *S.* ci, *N. meningitidis,* and *H. in-* hough recoverable from blood recovery of *N. gonorrhoeae* from ult. Hence, culture on selective dditional sites such as blood, cer- asopharynx, should be performed recovering this fastidious organism. from a clinically inapparent primary eristic clinical features can lead to a of gonococcal arthritis.

ding the establishment of a diagnosis of ude plain radiography, ultrasonography, and g. Roentgenograms often reveal swelling with ne joint space and superficial and deep periarticu- ue swelling, with displacement or loss of fat planes ma of fat pads. In the case of the hip joint, effusion esult in lateral displacement of the femoral head or even uxation. If septic arthritis is present for longer than 10–14 ys, roentgenograms may also reveal osteoporosis or subluxa- on. Additionally, in the presence of osteomyelitis, periosteal elevation with or without a characteristic lytic lesion is seen.

Ultrasonography is an important tool in assessing the hip joint for effusions or intra-articular bony disease. For septic arthritis involving the pelvic and vertebral joints, CT or bone scanning may be required. Technetium bone scans demonstrate increased soft tissue uptake in the region of the joint, as do gallium scans.

Synovial biopsy, special stains, and culture may be needed to differentiate chronic arthritis caused by *Mycobacterium tuberculosis* or fungi from other causes of granulomatous inflammation (sarcoidosis, foreign body reaction, or rheumatologic conditions).

DIFFERENTIAL DIAGNOSIS. Suppurative arthritis must be differentiated from infections of contiguous structures: osteomyelitis, deep cellulitis, pyomyositis, psoas or retroperitoneal abscess, synovitis, and septic bursitis (olecranon or prepatellar bursae). It should also be differentiated from other infectious and noninfectious etiologies of arthritis, such as reactive arthritis (rheumatic fever, poststreptococcal reactive arthritis, reactive arthritis following gastrointestinal, or genitourinary infections). Arthritis may occur as a component of systemic vasculitis syndromes, such as lupus erythematosus, serum sickness, Henoch-Schönlein purpura, and Kawasaki disease, as well as metabolic joint diseases (gout, ochronosis, Farber disease). Viral arthritis is often polyarticular and involves the interphalangeal-metacarpal joints most commonly, followed by the knee, wrist, ankle, and elbow joints (see Table 172–3).

Synovitis may also be caused by mycobacterial, gonococcal, and fungal infections. Toxic synovitis refers to a noninfectious inflammatory condition that is common in children less than 5 yr of age, often involving the hip, and following a viral upper respiratory tract infection. Signs include mild fever, limp, or irritability. Unlike bacterial septic arthritis, the extremity has minimal limitation of range of motion; the ESR and white blood cell counts are also usually normal (see Chapter 627).

■ TABLE 172–3 Epidemiology of Infectious Arthritis

Agent	Frequency	Characteristics
Bacterial		
Staphylococcus aureus	Most common pathogen in patients <2 mo, >5 yr of age	Monoarticular; knee most commonly affected, followed by hip, ankle, elbows, in that order
Haemophilus influenzae type b	Most common pathogen in patients <5 yr and particularly <2 yr age, excluding neonates	Monoarticular; may also be reactive
Streptococcus pneumoniae	Common in patients with sickle cell anemia and patients <2 yr of age	Monoarticular, hip affected more often than knee
Neisseria gonorrhoeae	Common in sexually active adolescent females	Monoarticular; follows a bacteremic phase with associated polyarthralgia, fever, chills, rash and tenosynovitis. Onset in 2nd–3rd trimester of pregnancy or during menstruation
N. meningitidis		Monoarticular
Group B streptococci	Common in neonates	Other neonatal pathogens include *S aureus, Escherichia coli, Candida* sp.
Group A streptococci (other streptococci)	Occurs in 10–20% of cases regardless of age	Monoarticular
Borrelia burgdorferi (Lyme arthritis)	Intermittent, migrating, polyarticular. Common in endemic areas. Chronic mono- or pauciarticular disease is uncommon	Knees: Baker cyst formation. Remote history of tick bite and erythema chronicum migrans
Brucella	Uncommon unless patient exposed to animal vector (cattle, swine, goat, sheep) including cheese, milk, carcass; 40% of children with brucellosis have arthritis	Peripheral (hip or knee) ± sacroiliitis. 70% of cases are monoarticular and chronic
Pseudomonas aeruginosa	Common in intravenous drug-abusing adolescents	Other pathogens in intravenous drug-abusing population include methicillin-resistant *S aureus, Serratia, Candida.* Joints include knee, sternoclavicular and sacroiliac joints, hip, or elbow
Mycobacterium tuberculosis	Uncommon	Chronic granulomatous monoarticular disease: knee affected most commonly followed by wrist, hip, and interphalangeal-metacarpal joints
Kingella kingae	Occurs in previously healthy children	Monoarticular; knee, ankle, and spine involved frequently; may also cause osteomyelitis; growth of this pathogen on routine culture media may be slower
Viral		
Rubella	Common (15–30%) in postpubertal susceptible females	Polyarticular; interphalangeal-metacarpal joints affected most commonly, followed by knee, wrist, elbow
Mumps	Affects <1% of postpubertal males	Polyarticular; knees most commonly affected, asymmetric
Parvovirus B19	Common in adults (60% of patients are >20 yr old, 5% are <9 yr old). Rash may be absent	Symmetric peripheral polyarthropathy. Interphalangeal-metacarpal joints affected most commonly, then knees and wrists
Hepatitis B	Variable incidence—0–25%	Interphalangeal-metacarpal joints. Urticaria, angioedema, arthritis, circulating HBsAg immune complexes precede jaundice by days to weeks
Varicella-zoster	Uncommon	Must exclude staphylococcal cellulitis or arthritis. Monoarticular, affecting knee
Human immunodeficiency virus (AIDS)	1. AIDS-related arthritis, common 2. Reiter syndrome, common 3. Septic arthritis, uncommon	1. Etiology unknown 2. Associated with psoriatic arthritis 3. Opportunistic agents, e.g., atypical mycobacteria, *Cryptococcus, Histoplasma*
Fungal		
Sporothrix schenckii	Uncommon	Chronic arthritis, knee affected most commonly, then wrist, then elbow. Occult pulmonary lesion is source, not direct inoculation
Pseudallescheria boydii	Uncommon	Penetrating knee trauma
Blastomyces dermatitides	Uncommon	Associated with adjacent osteomyelitis
Candida albicans	Uncommon	Pathogen in neonates; affects knee, elbow, wrist
Coccidioides immitis	Uncommon	Knee involvement ± disseminated disease in other sites
Histoplasma capsulatum	Uncommon	Migratory polyarthritis, carpal tunnel syndrome, erythema nodosum
Aspergillosis	Uncommon except in chronic granulomatous disease	Other pathogens in chronic granulomatous disease include *S. aureus, Serratia*
Others		
Chronic aseptic arthritis in hypogammaglobulinemic patients	10–20% of cases occur in patients with Bruton agammaglobulinemia: 5–10% occur in patients with common variable immunodeficiency	Arthritis may be rheumatologic or due to *Mycoplasma pneumoniae, M. hominis, Ureaplasma urealyticum,* enterovirus. Aseptic arthritis responds to intravenous immunoglobulin therapy. Acute bacterial arthritis is due to *H. influenzae, S. aureus*

Polyarthritis can be seen with disseminated gonococcal infection and rat-bite fever. Migratory or recurrent polyarthritis can also be associated with rheumatic fever, juvenile rheumatoid arthritis, Lyme disease, and serum sickness. Based on clinical signs, the distinction between gonococcal and reactive arthritis due to nongonococcal genital infection *(Reiter syndrome)* may not be clear cut. The clinical response to initiation of empirical antibiotic therapy is often helpful for clarification. Gonococcal arthritis usually resolves rapidly with antibiotics, whereas continued joint symptoms and development of new joint effusions occur in Reiter syndrome.

TREATMENT. The principles of treatment of septic arthritis are antibiotic therapy, irrigation and drainage of the joint, and immobilization of the joint in a functional position. Choice of empiric antibiotics for therapy for septic arthritis is based on considerations of age, host-specific pathogens, Gram stain, and

■ **TABLE 172–4 Synovial Fluid Analyses in Various Joint Diseases**

Condition	Appearance	Total White Blood Cell Count (/μL)	Polymorphonuclear Cells (%)	Mucin Clot	Synovial Fluid-to-Serum Glucose (mg/dL) Difference	Mutiple Joints	Comments
Normal	Clear-straw colored, yellow	0–200 (200)*	<10	Good	None (<10)	—	—
Trauma	Xanthochromic serosanguineous, sanguineous	50–4,000 (600)	<30	Good	None	No	Hemophilia or rupture of internal ligament, meniscus
Gout	Turbid	10,000–160,000 (20,000)	70	Poor	10–20	No	Synovial fluid urate, long needle-shaped crystals with negative birefringence on polarization microscope
Systemic lupus erythematosus	Clear to slightly turbid	0–9,000 (3,000)	<20	Good to fair	None	Yes	LE cell present: decreased synovial fluid complement
Rheumatoid arthritis	Turbid	250–50,000 (19,000)	50–70	Fair to poor	30	Yes	Decreased synovial fluid complement in 50%
Infectious							
Acute bacterial (septic, pyogenic, suppurative)	Very turbid, white-gray	10,000–250,000 (80,000)	90	Poor	50–90	No	Positive synovial Gram stain culture. Positive blood culture. Prior antibiotic therapy may reduce identification of pathogen
Lyme arthritis	Turbid	500–100,000 (25,000)	>50	Poor	—	Yes	History of tick bite, erythema migrans
Tuberculosis	Turbid rice bodies†	2,500–100,000 (20,000)	60	Poor	40–70	No	Positive PPD test, plus synovial fluid culture and acid-fast stain. May require synovial biopsy and culture
Viral	Clear, serosanguineous	5,000–10,000 (7,000)	<20	Good	None, occasionally 10–20	Yes	Small joints of hands most common sites
Postinfectious, Reactive, Sterile							
Rheumatic fever (streptococcal reactive arthritis)	Cloudy to turbid yellow	10,000–30,000 (20,000)	50	Good to fair	20–30	Yes	Positive serum group A streptococcal antibodies
Reactive arthritis (Reiter, postenteric, or postvenereal); Reiter syndrome includes urethritis, uveitis, conjunctivitis, arthritis, rash	Cloudy to turbid; may be clear	1,000–150,000 (25,000)	65	Fair to poor	30–50	Yes	Postenteric *(Shigella, Salmonella, Campylobacter, Yersinia)*; postvenereal *(Chlamydia)*. Bacterial antigen present in synovial fluid. Association with HLA-B27. Increased synovial fluid complement

**Averages in parentheses.*
†Particulate fibrinous deposits.
Synovial fluid protein content is elevated in many conditions and is nonspecific.

antigen-detection studies of the synovial fluid. Initial antibiotic therapy is given by the intravenous route, with most antibiotics achieving synovial fluid concentrations that equal, or even exceed, serum levels. The duration of antimicrobial therapy is longer in cases caused by pathogens such as *S. aureus* and gram-negative bacilli than with those caused by streptococci, *H. influenzae* type b, and gonococci. Septic arthritis due to *S. aureus* usually requires 4–6 wk of antibiotic therapy. Uncomplicated septic arthritis due to *H. influenzae* type b, *S. pneumoniae*, and group A streptococci should be treated for 14–21 days. Gonococcal arthritis should be treated for 7–10 days. Neonates and immunocompromised hosts may require longer durations of antibiotic therapy.

Fever usually lasts for about 3–5 days in uncomplicated septic arthritis; persistence of fever should raise the suspicion of complications (abscess, loculation, or osteomyelitis). Joint inflammation usually appears to resolve within 5–7 days, although swelling may persist for 10–14 days. Unless concurrent osteomyelitis can be accurately ruled out, septic arthritis of the hip and shoulder joints should be treated for at least 3 wk. Initial intravenous antimicrobial therapy may be changed to high-dose oral therapy with appropriate bactericidal antibiotics after the patient demonstrates signs of improvement, such as remission of fever, a reduction in inflammatory markers, and diminished synovial swelling. Therapy with oral antibiotics (clindamycin, dicloxacillin, amoxicillin) must be rigorously monitored.

Empirical therapy for pyogenic arthritis caused by *S. aureus* should include an antistaphylococcal penicillin (methicillin, oxacillin, or nafcillin) administered through the intravenous route (not intra-articular).

If *H. influenzae* type b is suspected, an extended spectrum cephalosporin (e.g., ceftriaxone or cefuroxime), or a combination of chloramphenicol with an antistaphylococcal penicillin, can be used. Septic arthritis caused by gram-negative enteric bacilli is treated with a combination of an antipseudomonal penicillin and an aminoglycoside until susceptibility results are available. *Kingella kingae* is usually susceptible to penicillins but resistant to vancomycin. For suspected *N. gonorrhoeae* infections, a parenteral 3rd-generation cephalosporin, such as ceftriaxone or cefoxitin, should be used because some strains produce penicillinase. If susceptibility testing subsequently reveals sensitivity to penicillin, oral amoxicillin may be initiated by day 3–5 of therapy. In sexually active adolescents, doxycycline should be included in order to treat concurrent *Chlamydia trachomatis* genital infection.

Fungal arthritis is treated with intravenous amphotericin B; intra-articular amphotericin may be used in certain cases. Given the fact that it attains good levels in synovial fluid, 5-fluorocytosine may also be used in some cases. Experience with the newer triazoles (fluconazole, itraconazole) in the treatment of fungal arthritis is limited. Therapy for tuberculosis is discussed elsewhere.

Prompt, open surgical drainage at the time of presentation is indicated for every case of septic arthritis of the hip, for most infections involving the shoulder, and for cases in which frank pus is obtained on initial diagnostic aspiration. Emergent open drainage of the hip joint is primarily indicated to reduce the intra-articular pressure, thus avoiding septic necrosis of the femoral head and the chances of permanent joint damage. Removal of necrotic bone and inflammatory mediators in this deep joint are also best performed by an initial open drainage.

Open surgical drainage is required for recurrent purulent or culture-positive effusions, or for those lasting longer than 7 days. Arthroscopic drainage is now gaining favor as an effective alternative to open drainage of joints (other than the hip).

Supportive treatment for septic arthritis includes splinting to immobilize the joint in a functional position during the first 72 hr of therapy or until improvement in signs of synovial inflammation are seen. Thereafter, passive range-of-motion exercises may aid in maintaining physiologic circulation of synovial fluid and reduce the risk of contracture. For the lower limb, the hip and knee joints are rested in a position of extension, and the ankle in neutral position (90 degree to the rest of the leg); for the upper limb, the shoulder is kept adducted and internally rotated, and the elbow in midflexion. Active range-of-motion and weight-bearing exercises are permitted after resolution of pain and other signs of acute inflammation. Early institution of passive range-of-motion exercises may improve the functional outcome from joint inflammation.

PROGNOSIS. The most important prognostic factor in predicting a favorable outcome in septic arthritis is early diagnosis and therapy. Delay in the institution of therapy has been correlated with increased morbidity. Poor prognostic features include young age (<6 mo), delayed therapy (especially beyond 5 days after symptoms are apparent), arthritis due to *S. aureus*, gram-negative or fungal pathogens, hip or shoulder joint involvement (with the tendency to associated osteomyelitis), and associated osteomyelitis with epiphyseal damage. Long-term follow-up may reveal effects of epiphyseal damage (angular deformity, limb length shortening), early degenerative changes, and limitation of range of motion.

OSTEOMYELITIS

Asmar BI: Osteomyelitis in the neonate. Infect Dis Clin North Am 6:117, 1992.

Cushing AH: Diskitis in children. Clin Infect Dis 17:1, 1993.

Dagan R: Management of acute hematogenous osteomyelitis and septic arthritis in the pediatric patient. Pediatr Infect Dis J 12:88, 1993.

Demopulos GA, Bleck EE, McDougall IR: Role of radionuclide imaging in the diagnosis of acute osteomyelitis. J Pediatr Orthop 8:558, 1988.

Faden H, Grossi M: Acute osteomyelitis in children. Am J Dis Child 45:65, 1991.

Farley T, Conway J, Shulman ST: Hematogenous pelvic osteomyelitis in children. Am J Dis Child 139:946, 1985.

Frederiksen B, Christiansen P, Knudsen FU: Acute osteomyelitis and septic arthritis in the neonate, risk factors and outcome. Eur J Pediatr 152:S77, 1993.

Fisher MC, Goldsmith JF, Gilligan PH: Sneakers as a source of *Pseudomonas aeruginosa* in children with osteomyelitis following puncture wounds. J Pediatr 106:607, 1985.

Gamble JG, Rinsky LA: Chronic recurrent multifocal osteomyelitis. J Pediatr Orthop 6:579, 1986.

Gold R: Diagnosis of osteomyelitis. Pediatr Rev 12:292, 1991.

Hamdan J, Asha M, Mallouh A, et al: Technetium bone scintigraphy in the diagnosis of osteomyelitis in children. Pediatr Infect Dis J 6:529, 1987.

Jacobs RF, McCarthy RE, Elser JM: *Pseudomonas* osteochondritis complicating puncture wounds of the foot in children: A 10-year evaluation. Infect Dis 160:657, 1989.

Jansen BRH, Hart W, Schreuder O: Discitis in childhood. Acta Orthop Scand 64:33, 1993.

King SM, Laxer RM, Manson D, Gold R: Chronic recurrent multifocal osteomyelitis: A non-infectious inflammatory process. Pediatr Infect Dis J 6:907, 1987.

Lacour M, Duarte M, Beutler A, et al: Osteoarticular infections due to *Kingella kingae* in children. Eur J Pediatr 1991; 150:612.

Nelson JD: Acute osteomyelitis in children. Infect Dis Clin North Am 4:513, 1990.

Prober CG, Yeager AS: Use of the serum bactericidal titer to assess the adequacy of oral antibiotic therapy in the treatment of acute hematogenous osteomyelitis. J Pediatr 95:131, 1979.

Schauwecker DS, Braunstein EM, Wheat LJ: Diagnostic imaging of osteomyelitis. Infect Dis Clin North Am 4:441, 1990.

Syrogiannopoulos GA, McCracken GM, Nelson JD: Osteoarticular infections in children with sickle cell disease. Pediatrics 78:1090, 1986.

Unkila-Kallio L, Kallio MJT, Eskola J, Peltola H: Serum C-reactive protein, erythrocyte sedimentation rate, and white blood cell count in acute hematogenous osteomyelitis of children. Pediatrics 93:59, 1994.

Weinstein MP, Stratton CW, Hawley HB, et al: Multicenter collaborative evaluation of a standardized serum bactericidal test as a predictor of therapeutic efficacy in acute and chronic osteomyelitis. Am J Med 83:218, 1987.

SEPTIC ARTHRITIS

Afghani B, Stutman HR: Bacterial arthritis caused by *Corynebacterium diphtheriae*. Pediatr Infect Dis J 12:881, 1993.

Barton LL, Dunkle LM, Habib FH: Septic arthritis in childhood. Am J Dis Child 141:898, 1987.

Cuellar ML, Silveria LH, Espinoza LR: Fungal arthritis. Ann Rheum Dis 51:690, 1992.

Dagan R: Management of acute hematogenous osteomyelitis and septic arthritis in the pediatric patient. Pediatr Infect Dis J 12:90, 1993.

Goldenberg DL, Reed JI: Bacterial arthritis. N Engl J Med 312:764, 1985.

Jacobs NM: Pneumococcal osteomyelitis and arthritis in children. Am J Dis Child 145:70, 1991.

Nade SML: Acute septic arthritis in infancy and childhood. J Bone Joint Surg [Br] 65:234, 1983.

Rotbart HA, Glode MP: *Haemophilus influenzae* type b septic arthritis in children: Report of 23 cases. Pediatrics 75:254, 1985.

Welkon CJ, Long SS, Fisher MC, et al: Pyogenic arthritis in infants and children: A review of 95 cases. Pediatr Infect Dis J 5:669, 1986.

CHAPTER 173

Infections in the Compromised Host

Walter Hughes

The compromised host is one who has a preexisting condition at the time of microbial exposure, reducing one or more mechanisms for defense against infection. The compromise may be due to a defect or dysfunction of the immune system (compromised host with immunodeficiency) or factors not directly related to the immune system (compromised host without immunodeficiency). While such a categorization allows a conceptual basis for evaluation, compromised patients with infection often do not fall completely in one group or the other. More than one defect in the defense mechanism may be impaired. Especially in the compromised host with immunodeficiency. For example, patients with a specific T-lymphocyte defect caused by the human immunodeficiency virus (HIV) may also have neutropenia caused by drugs used for antiviral therapy; breech of the integrity of the skin and mucous membranes from indwelling central lines, and intravenous drug abuse; secondary malignancy; malnutrition; and increased exposure to infections such as tuberculosis and sexually transmitted diseases, including hepatitis. However, knowledge of the primary defect of the compromised host is useful in predicting the types of infections that might occur and in establishing strategies for the evaluation and management of infectious episodes.

COMPROMISED HOST WITH IMMUNODEFICIENCY (see Part XIV)

Much of our knowledge of how the immune system protects against infectious disease comes from observations of individuals who have congenital or acquired defects in one or more functions of the immune response. The importance of humoral antibody became obvious when infants with Bruton X-linked agammaglobulinemia were observed to have an unusually high rate of serious bacterial infections while susceptibility to viral infections was near normal. Table 173–1 lists the major immunodeficiency disorders and indicates the predominant functional defect(s) in the immune system. Table 173–2 is a compilation of microbial organisms known to cause infection in the immunocompromised host and the defect most frequently associated with risk for infection by the respective organism. Children with one type of immune deficiency disorder may be prone to specific infections, but the defect is not limited solely to these pathogens. The immunocompromised host is at risk for all of the infections that occur in otherwise healthy children.

CLINICAL MANIFESTATIONS. The clinical features of infections in the compromised, as well as the otherwise normal, host are dependent primarily upon the host responses to the invading microbe. The causative organisms are limited by their tissue or cellular tropism in eliciting specific clinical manifestations of disease. The basic clinical responses of the host are fever and the acute inflammatory reaction. The acute inflammatory reaction stems from granulocytic infiltrations, hyperemia, and capillary leakage, evidenced as cellulitis if involving the skin, pneumonitis in the lung and meningitis in the central nervous system. Defects in the normal host response may be reflected in clinical manifestations. For example, extensive bacterial infection may occur in the lung in the severely neutropenic patient without a discernible infiltrate by chest radiography; the swelling and erythema of cellulitis may not be evident, and the anemic and neutropenic patient may have acute otitis media without erythema and congestion of the tympanic membrane. Diagnostic evaluation is complicated when the defect is in the humoral immune function, such as agammaglobulinemia, because serological tests for antibody responses are of the little value. With an impaired cell-mediated immune response, antigenic skin tests are often nonreactive. Some general axioms about clinical features of infection in the immunocompromised host are:

1. Any organism is a potential pathogen in the immunosuppressed host. The microbiologist in the laboratory cannot determine whether or not a microbial isolate is the cause of disease. The physician must assess the individual case to delineate a relationship.
2. Fever is a sensitive and specific sign of an infectious disease, even in the immunocompromised host. Almost all infections of significance will be associated with a febrile response. Immunosuppressive drugs, such as corticosteroids and anticancer drugs, do not mask febrile responses during infections. Thus, fever in the immunocompromised host must be considered of infectious etiology until proven otherwise.
3. Aside from fever, characteristic signs and symptoms of infection may be absent in the compromised host.
4. Microbes of low virulence and components of the normal flora of the skin and mucous membranes may cause severe life-threatening infections. Some organisms may directly evoke signs and symptoms due to specific tropism or toxin production, such as pneumonitis from *Pneumocystis carinii*, diarrhea from *Cryptosporidium* spp. or *Clostridium difficile*, and thrush from *Candida albicans*.
5. Extreme granulocytopenia with absolute neutrophil counts of 0.5×10^9 cells/L or less is predictive of impending infection. With counts between 0.5 and 1.0×10^9 cells/L, the risk of infection is still increased above that of normal individuals but is less than with lower counts. Generally, with counts less than 0.5×10^9 cells/L, the risk for serious infection is inversely proportional to the count. Infections in neutropenic patients are usually caused by bacteria or fungi.
6. The CD_4^+ T lymphocyte count of 200/mm^3 or less (20% or less) in children of 5 yr and older indicates high risk for *P. carinii* pneumonitis in HIV-infected patients. Unfortunately, little information on the relationship between lymphocyte subsets and infection risks in other immune deficiency syndrome patients is available.
7. Multiple infections, either concomitant or sequential, are common.
8. Known and suspected bacterial infections should be treated immediately with antibacterial antibiotics given intravenously in maximum tolerated doses. Often drugs must be given empirically before a diagnosis has been established.
9. Many of the drugs required for the treatment of infections in the immunocompromised host have toxic side effects.

INFECTIONS IN PATIENTS WITH IMMUNODEFICIENCY. Antibody Deficiency. Patients with X-linked agammaglobulinemia and common variable immunodeficiency are unable to generate adequate

■ **TABLE 173–1 Major Immunodeficiency Diseases and the Major Functional Defect**

Antibody Deficiency (Humoral-Lymphocyte Abnormality)
X-linked agammaglobulinemia
IgG subclass deficiencies
Common variable immunodeficiency
Immunodeficiency with increased IgM
Selective IgA deficiency
Hyperimmunoglobulin E syndrome
Selective IgM deficiency
Cell-Mediated Immunodeficiency (T-Lymphocyte Defects)
DiGeorge syndrome
Nezelof syndrome
Lymphocyte activation defects
Acquired immunodeficiency syndrome (AIDS) caused by human immunodeficiency virus
Combined B- and T-Lymphocyte Defects
Severe combined immunodeficiency syndrome
Wiskott-Aldrich syndrome
Ataxia-telangiectasia
Lymphocyte-Phagocyte Defects
Leukocyte adhesion deficiency (CD-11-18 deficiency)
Complement Deficiency
Genetic deficiencies of complement
Phagocyte-Neutrophil Abnormalities
Congenital agranulocytosis
Chronic granulomatous disease
Chédiak-Higashi syndrome
Hereditary specific granule deficiency
Defective Opsonization
Splenic insufficiency

■ TABLE 173–2 Microbial Organisms Common in Patients with Specific Immunodeficiencies

Organism	Granulocytopenia*	Phagocytic Defects†	Antibody Defects‡	Impaired Cell-Mediated Immunity¶	Splenic Dysfunction‖
Escherichia coli	+	+			
Klebsiella pneumoniae	+				
Pseudomonas aeruginosa	+		+		
Serratia marcescens	+	+			
Salmonella spp.		+	+	+	
Haemophilus influenzae	+		+		+
Enterobacter spp.	+				
Aeromonas hydrophilia	+				
Acinetobacter spp.	+				
Bacteroides spp.	+				
Legionella spp.				+	
Staphylococcus aureus	+	+	+		
Coagulase-negative staphylococci	+				
Viridans streptococci	+				
Listeria monocytogenes	+			+	
Corynebacterium spp.	+				
Enterococci	+				
Streptococcus pneumoniae	+	+	+	+	+
Streptococcus pyogenes	+	+			
Bacillus spp.	+				
Clostridium difficile	+	+	+	+	
Nocardia spp.		+		+	
Neisseria spp.			+		+
Mycobacteria spp.				+	
Candida spp.	+	+		+	
Aspergillus spp.	+	+			
Aseptate fungi	+				

Table continued on following page

immunoglobulins. They are especially susceptible to pyogenic bacterial infection from *Staphylococcus aureus, Haemophilus influenzae,* and *Streptococcus pneumoniae* as well as infection from other bacteria (Table 173–2). To a lesser extent, progressive viral and protozoan infections may affect these patients. Infections of the upper and lower respiratory tracts are the most frequent types encountered. Chronic and recurrent pulmonary infections lead to bronchiectasis. Arthritis and pneumonitis may also be caused by mycoplasma species. *Salmonella* and *Campylobacter* species cause enteritis. Pyoderma, sepsis, pneumonia, meningitis, and otitis media are often due to the pyogenic bacteria.

Patients with selective IgA deficiency lack secretory IgA at the mucosal barrier and have recurrent bacterial infections of mild to moderate severity. The causative organisms are included in Table 173–2, although there seems to be no increase in susceptibility to viral infections.

Patients with hyper-IgM syndrome have decreased levels of IgG, IgA, and IgE and often neutropenia. In addition to the bacterial sinopulmonary infectious characteristic of agammaglobulinemia, these children are also at increased risk for *P. carinii* pneumonitis.

The IgG subclass deficiencies are not clearly understood but are associated with mild to severe cases of sinopulmonary diseases, meningitis, bacteremia, osteomyelitis, and pyoderma. In IgG subclass 2 deficiency poor antibody responses follow infections with polysaccharide-encapsulated bacteria, such as *H. influenzae* and pneumococcus, as well as immunization with the polysaccharide bacterial vaccines.

Defects in Cell-Mediated Immunity. Patients with congenital T-lymphocyte or combined T- and B-lymphocyte immunodeficiency states develop infection after birth because T-lymphocyte function is greatly reduced and protection by passive transfer of maternal IgG is transient. Early infectious complications include chronic mucocutaneous candidiasis, chronic rhinitis and otitis media, recurrent pneumonia, and diarrhea. Because of

■ **TABLE 173–2 Microbial Organisms Common in Patients with Specific Immunodeficiencies** *Continued*

Organism	Granulocytopenia*	Phagocytic Defects†	Antibody Defects‡	Impaired Cell-Mediated Immunity¶	Splenic Dysfunction‖
Pseudoallescheria spp.	+				
Fusarium	+				
Histoplasma/Coccidioides				+	
Cryptococcus neoformans				+	
Mycoplasma spp.			+		
Campylobacter spp.			+		
Cytomegalovirus				+	
Herpes simplex				+	
Varicella-zoster virus				+	
Epstein-Barr virus				+	
Enteroviruses			+	+	
Adenoviruses				+	
Measles virus				+	
Rotavirus			+	+	
Polyomavirus BK/JC				+	
Hepatitis viruses			+		
Pneumocystis carinii				+	
Toxoplasma gondii				+	
Cryptosporidium spp.				+	
Babesia spp.					+
Giardia lamblia			+	+	
Plasmodium spp.					+
Chlamydia spp.					
Strongyloides stercoralis				+	

**Granulocytopenia includes aplastic anemia, myelosuppressive agents, congenital neutropenia, bone marrow transplant recipients, malignancy.*
†Phagocytic dysfunction includes chronic granulomatous disease, hyperimmunoglobulin E syndrome, leukocyte adhesion defects, Chédiak-Higashi syndrome.
‡Antibody defects include congenital and acquired immunoglobulin deficiencies, complement deficiencies, properidin deficiencies.
¶Impaired cell-mediated immune defects include AIDS, congenital T-lymphocyte deficiency syndrome, immunosuppression drugs, organ transplantation, Hodgkin's disease, severe malnutrition.
‖Splenic dysfunction includes splenectomy, congenital aspenia, sickle cell anemia, a combined immunoglobulin and reticuloendothelial cell deficiency.

the marked heterogeneity of the immunodeficiency state in DiGeorge syndrome, some children may have minor infections, whereas others who survive after early severe infections may have less frequent or less serious infections as the immune defect spontaneously improves.

The most commonly acquired disorder resulting from a predominantly T-lymphocyte defect is AIDS. Antibody production is also deficient in patients with AIDS due to a defect of helper T-lymphocyte function. Therefore, patients with AIDS are at increased risk for infections with microorganisms that typically infect patients with both T- and B-cell deficiencies (see Chapter 223).

A presumed primary immunodeficiency identified as chronic mucocutaneous candidiasis is uncommon. It is rarely associated with systemic candidiasis. Impaired cell-mediated responses also predispose to other infections, including histoplasmosis.

Combined B- and T-Lymphocyte Defects. Patients with severe combined immunodeficiency syndrome (SCID), Wiskott-Aldrich syndrome, and ataxia-telangiectasia suffer from high frequencies of infections mentioned in Table 173–2. The SCID patient has acute and chronic infections with all classes of microbes. Bacterial infections are less likely in early infancy than later because of maternally acquired IgG. Surface and systemic candidiasis, cytomegalovirus (CMV) infection, bacterial infections, and *P. carinii* pneumonitis may be life threatening. Even live-attenuated vaccines for polio and measles may cause serious disease. The Wiskott-Aldrich syndrome has a pattern of infectious diseases similar to the other combined cell-mediated and humoral immunodeficiencies. Late-onset sinopulmonary infections from streptococcus, enterococcus, *H. influenzae*, and respiratory viruses are found in ataxia-telangiectasia.

Lymphocyte-Phagocyte Defects. Infants with the leukocyte adhesion deficiency have delayed separation of the umbilical cord, cellulitis, gingivitis, and necrotic skin lesions.

Complement Deficiency. Deficiencies of complement components are associated with familial susceptibility to rheumatologic disorders, and increased risk for recurrent pneumococcemia, meningococcemia, and gonococcemia. Fulminant infection due to *N. meningitidis* is also noted in patients with deficiencies of the alternate pathway (Chapter 178).

Phagocyte-Neutrophil Defects. Infants and children with quantitative or qualitative defects in neutrophils and phagocytes (Table 173–2) have increased susceptibility to *S. aureus*, gram-negative bacilli, and *C. albicans* predominantly, but can acquire other infections to a lesser extent. The skin and mucous membranes are frequently the sites of bacterial infections and candidiasis. Systemic bacterial infection with sepsis, pneumonia, and meningitis may occur. Chronic and recurrent pyogenic lymphadenitis, hepatic abscesses, gingivitis, pneumonia, and osteomyelitis are features of patients with impaired neutrophil microbicidal activity.

The risks of infection increase as the neutrophil count decreases to <1,000. Neutropenia may be congenital (cyclic neutropenia, severe infantile agranulocytosis, benign familial neutropenia) or acquired (antineutrophil antibodies, e.g., autoimmune conditions, AIDS; drug reaction, e.g., phenothiazines, sulfonamides, penicillin, chloramphenicol, cancer chemotherapy). The neutropenia associated with common febrile viral illnesses is usually benign. Neutropenia may be isolated, or it may be a sign of more significant bone marrow deficiency (aplastic anemia, leukemia). Patients with chronic granulomatous disease have normal neutrophil counts but deficient mechanisms of bacterial killing. Patients with hyper-IgE syndrome may also have variable leukocyte dysfunction.

The *clinical manifestations* of infection include fever, chills, sore throat, and localizing signs and symptoms, such as local erythema, tenderness, pain, swelling, and limitation of motion. Neutropenia may attenuate but may not eliminate the local manifestations of infection, as noted in cellulitis, pharyngitis, catheter tract infection, and perirectal abscess. It reduces the purulent nature of local infection; pus formation is unusual at sites of cellulitis, and sputum is unusual in neutropenic patients with pneumonia. Patients with severe neutropenia (<500 neutrophils), in the absence of other host defense defects, are at a high risk of fulminant bacterial sepsis, which may be subclinical, associated only with fever, or manifest as fever, chills, disorientation, lethargy, warm-pink or cold-cyanotic extremities, and hypotension. The risk of sepsis and other serious infections in the febrile neutropenic cancer patient is excessively high (see later section on host defense defects associated with malignancy).

The *treatment* of infection in patients with congenital or acquired neutropenia depends on the microorganisms responsible for the infection, the duration and severity of the neutropenia, the possibility of bone marrow recovery, and any associated impairment of host defense. Empiric therapy for bacterial sepsis is necessary for high-risk granulocyte disorders, such as leukocyte adhesions, defects, chronic granulomatous disease, and congenital neutropenia. The antibiotic regimens described for the empiric treatment of febrile neutropenic patients with cancer can usually be applied to other neutrophil disorders and to counts of <500 cells/μL. In addition to antibiotics, corticosteroids may help to resolve granulomas in patients with chronic granulomatous disease. Granulocyte transfusions should be reserved for patients with documented bacterial or fungal infections who are unresponsive to conventional therapy with intravenous bactericidal antibiotics. Although granulocyte transfusions may be beneficial, they are expensive and include the risk of transmission of cytomegalovirus, allosensitization to HLA antigens, graft-versus-host disease in immunosuppressed patients, pulmonary infiltrates and hypoxia if given in conjunction with amphotericin B, and transfusion reactions (especially in patients with X-linked chronic granulomatous disease who lack the X_kKell-related antigen). The role of recombinant colony stimulating factor has been defined.

Prevention of infection in patients with neutrophil functional defects may occasionally be accomplished with the use of prophylactic antibiotics. Intracellular penetration of the broad-spectrum antibiotic combination trimethoprim-sulfamethoxazole improves phagocytic killing in patients with chronic granulomatous disease. Recombinant human interferon-γ in the dose of 50 μg/M^2 subcutaneously three times per week plus oral trimethoprim-sulfamethoxazole has been reported to significantly reduce the infection rate in chronic granulomatous disease.

Defective Opsonization. Splenectomy, congenital asplenia, and splenic dysfunction from sickle cell disease are associated with an increased risk for serious bacterial infections. *Streptococcus pneumoniae*, *H. influenzae*, and *Salmonella* spp. are common causative organisms of sepsis, pneumonia, meningitis, and osteomyelitis. Impaired phagocytic function and defective complement-mediated opsonization are some of the underlying defects. The efficacy of penicillin prophylaxis has been demonstrated for sickle cell disease and is recommended for patients at 6 mo of age and older. In addition to routine immunizations, the pneumococcal vaccine should be given at 2 yr of age, with the expectation that only modest protective efficacy will be attained.

INFECTIONS WITH ORGAN AND TISSUE TRANSPLANTATIONS

Transplantation of bone marrow, liver, kidney, and heart has achieved acceptance as a therapeutic modality for selected diseases and at medical centers with specialized competence. Graft-versus-host disease and infectious complications pose the major barriers to successful outcome. Although the organisms causing infections in transplant recipients are the same as those responsible for infections of other immunocompromised hosts, the relative frequencies of occurrence, magnitude of disease, and response to therapy may vary (Table 173–2). The extent of donor-recipient match, organ or tissue to be transplanted, and the intensity of immunosuppressive preparatory regimens influence infectious complications.

BONE MARROW TRANSPLANTATION. Autologous Bone Marrow Transplantation. Autologous bone marrow transplantation involves using the patient's own bone marrow to re-establish hematopoietic cell function after intensive chemotherapy or irradiation. The risk for infection is relatively small but may occur in 5–10% of patients during the period required for hematologic recovery. These infections most often affect the lung and may be due to the organisms described for allogeneic transplants. Prophylactic precautions used for allogeneic transplantation should also be used with autologous transplant recipients until the functional marrow has been re-established.

Allogeneic Bone Marrow Transplantation. *Allogeneic* transplantation involves the transplantation of bone marrow from one person to another. If the donor and recipient are identical twins, the transplantation is *syngeneic*. Infection and graft-versus-host disease are the major serious complications of allogeneic transplantation. Infection limits the extent of immunosuppression possible for control of graft rejection; infection is less likely in the absence of graft-versus-host disease infection.

Preparative immunosuppressive management for allogeneic transplantation usually consists of radiotherapy plus chemotherapy with the alkylating agents, etoposide and cytarabine. During the pretransplantation period, the type and extent of infections depend in part on the primary underlying disease, the harboring of subclinical or unresolved infection when preparative immunosuppression is started, and the intensity of the preparative regimen. Bacterial infections are common, especially as neutropenia evolves. Cellulitis, mucositis, pneumonia, urinary tract infection, and sepsis may occur (Table 173–

■ TABLE 173–3 Infections with Bone Marrow Transplantation

Stage	Compromised Defense Mechanism	Most Common Infections
Pretransplant days 0–14	Skin and mucous membranes integrity Neutropenia	Mucositis, cellulitis Sepsis, pneumonia UTI
Post-transplant before engraftment days 0–30	Skin and mucous membranes integrity Neutropenia Change in microbial flora Acute GVHD	Oral thrush, herpes Bacterial sepsis; *S. epidermidis, S. aureus*, streptococci, *Corynebacterium* spp.; *Aspergillus* spp. Catheter infections Fungal infections: *Candida* spp., *Aspergillus* spp. Pneumonia: bacterial, fungal, RSV Sinusitis: bacterial fungal
Post-transplant, post-engraftment days 30–100	Impaired cell-mediated immunity Hypogammaglobulinemia Impaired neutrophil and phagocytic function Acute GVHD	CMV infection: pneumonitis, hepatitis, gastroenteritis, esophagitis, retinitis Diffuse interstitial pneumonia: RSV, parainfluenza, adenovirus EBV infection Cystitis: adenovirus, BK papovavirus Systemic candidiasis, aspergillosis *Pneumocystis carinii* pneumonia Toxoplasmosis Viral hepatitis
Post-transplant, post-engraftment days 100–365	Impaired cell-mediated immunity Impaired humoral immunity Reticulo-endothelial tissue abnormalities Chronic GVHD	Varicella (chicken pox) Herpes zoster CMV disease Viral hepatitis *Pneumocystis carinii* pneumonia Toxoplasmosis Common bacterial infection: *Strep. pneumonia, H. influenzae*

GVHD, graft-versus-host disease; UTI, urinary tract infection; CMV, cytomegalovirus; RSV, respiratory syncytial virus; EBV, Epstein-Barr virus.

3). Fatal infections during this time are uncommon. Antibiotic therapy is urgent at the earliest sign of infection because gram-negative bacilli and gram-positive cocci cause most of these infections.

During the month following the transplantation, granulocytopenia is profound and is a major determinant in the type and extent of infections. Damage to mucous membranes resulting in mucositis and breach of the skin barrier by indwelling catheters provides portals of entry for gram-positive cocci, gram-negative bacilli, and opportunistic fungi. Respiratory syncytial virus (RSV) may cause upper and lower respiratory tract infection. RSV pneumonitis has serious consequences during the early post-transplantation period.

Infections occurring between about 30 and 100 days after the transplantation are usually not due to granulocytopenia, but to other derangements in the immune system (Table 173–3); graft rejection adds to the risk of infection. Cytomegalovirus may cause disease in 50–60% of patients if no prophylaxis is used.

Interstitial pneumonia is common in patients with leukemia, occurs about the 60th day post-transplant, and may be due to cytomegalovirus, *P. carinii*, or RSV; in 30% of patients it is idiopathic. Idiopathic interstitial pneumonia may be due to graft-versus-host disease or prior conditioning irradiation or chemotherapy, and has a significant mortality.

The pattern of infection changes after about the 100th post-transplant day, when chronic graft-versus-host-associated antibody deficiency predisposes the recipient to pneumococcal sepsis or meningitis, and sinopulmonary infections. In addition, varicella-zoster virus reactivation occurs with increased frequency in this later period. Additional infections include hemorrhagic cystitis due to reactivation of papovavirus BK, rotavirus enteritis, pseudomembranous colitis due to *C. difficile*, and possibly human herpesvirus virus-6 infection.

The *treatment* of infection after bone marrow transplantation depends on the amount of time elapsed since transplantation and the presence of neutropenia or of acute or chronic graft-versus-host disease. The approach to the febrile neutropenic transplant recipient is similar to management of the febrile neutropenic patient with malignancy and includes prompt institution of empiric bactericidal broad-spectrum antibiotics, which are usually continued until the neutrophil count is >500 cells/mm³.

Acyclovir is effective therapy for herpes simplex and varicella-zoster virus infections, which are usually reactivations of latent virus. Ganciclovir and CMV hyperimmune globulin have improved the survival of patients with serious primary CMV pneumonitis. Foscarnet provides an alternative for patients who fail ganciclovir therapy.

Prevention of early bacterial infection has been attempted by administering intravenous immunoglobulin and fluorinated quinolones, and by preventing acute graft-versus-host disease. Prevention of CMV infection has been attempted by avoiding administration of blood products from CMV-positive donors to a CMV-negative recipient and minimizing the incidence of graft-versus-host disease; the value of acyclovir prophylaxis is unproved. Rowe et al and the Eastern Cooperative Oncology Group recommend weekly blood, urine, and throat cultures for CMV during the first 120 days after allogeneic transplantation; prophylaxis with ganciclovir and intravenous gamma globulin is instituted if the virus is identified.

LIVER TRANSPLANTS. About one half of pediatric liver transplant recipients will have one or more infections from bacteria, fungi, protozoa, and viruses after the transplantation. The highest risk for infection is during the 1st mo post-transplantation, when an average of 2.5 episodes of infection occur per patient. During the 2nd and 3rd mo the rates decrease to about 0.35 and 0.17 episodes per patient, respectively. In addition to immunocompromise from suppressive drugs, the liver transplant recipient has the additional risk of the surgical procedure enhancing access of the microbial flora of the gastrointestinal tract to the biliary tract and liver.

Common early infections include gram-negative enteric bacterial pneumonia, soft tissue and wound infections, intra-abdominal abscesses due to enterococci and anaerobic and gram-negative enteric bacteria, peritonitis, disseminated candidiasis, and cholangitis. The latter characteristically presents with the Charcot triad of fever, abdominal pain, and jaundice; it should be distinguished from liver rejection by microscopic examination of a liver biopsy, Gram stain, and culture. Hepatic abscesses are often due to biliary or vascular obstruction, whereas cholangitis may be related to biliary stricture or the use of endoscopic retrograde cholangiopancreatography. Ischemic injury to the bile ducts from hepatic artery occlusion or bile duct anastomotic breakdown may produce bile leakage and gram-negative bacillary or candidal peritonitis, which will be detected by culture of the abdominal drains.

Cytomegalovirus infections occur in 30–60% of children who receive liver transplants. Most of these are found in the first 3 mo post-transplantation. Up to 15% of transplanted children will have CMV hepatitis. Pneumonitis and gastroenteritis may also be caused by this virus.

Reactivation of Epstein-Barr virus (EBV) may produce a mononucleosis-like syndrome, or it may progress to a late-onset lymphoproliferative syndrome that may improve by reducing the dosage of immunosuppressive therapy.

Evaluation of the febrile liver transplant recipient for infection includes cultures of blood and abdominal drains, chest roentgenogram, abdominal ultrasound and computed tomography imaging, and Doppler assessment of hepatic artery blood flow. Percutaneous liver biopsy is needed to diagnose cholangitis and to exclude the possibility of rejection.

Treatment is directed at the specific infectious complication present and may include broad-spectrum antibiotics and aspiration or drainage of abscesses. *Prevention* of infection has been attempted by using prophylactic antibacterial agents, acyclovir, and trimethoprim-sulfamethoxazole for *P. carinii* infection, avoiding neutropenia due to azathioprine, and maintaining good surgical technique.

RENAL TRANSPLANTS. Recipients of kidney transplants are susceptible to the array of opportunistic infections encountered by other severely immunocompromised patients. Infection is the major cause of death in children with renal transplants. Urinary tract infection is the most common infection, with the highest incidence (10%) during the 1st mo post-transplantation. During this time *P. aeruginosa* is the most common cause, but after the first month *E. coli* is more frequent.

The risk of CMV infection has been reduced by the prophylactic use of antiviral drugs, administration of CMV-antibody negative blood products, and selection of seronegative organ donors. In a recent series of 70 children, the overall incidence of infection was only 10%, and none were fatal. The most common clinical pattern is a syndrome occurring 1–4 mo after transplantation with fever, malaise, myalgia, arthralgia, and leukopenia. Hepatitis and pneumonitis may occur, as well as infrequent involvement of other organs. Infections with other herpesviruses (herpes simplex, varicella-zoster, Epstein-Barr), *P. carinii*, *Aspergillus* spp., *Candida* spp., and viral hepatitis pose additional hazards of low frequency.

Treatment of infection is directed at the specific manifestation (e.g., pneumonia or urinary tract infection) and the responsible microbiologic agent. Urine, blood, and sputum should be cultured prior to antibiotic therapy. Biopsy of the transplanted kidney may be needed to differentiate infection from rejection.

Prevention of infection is similar to that used for other transplant recipients. Prophylactic trimethoprim-sulfamethoxazole may reduce the incidence of pyelonephritis as well as *P. carinii* pneumonitis. Careful evaluation of the urinary tract for abnormalities, such as urethral, ureteral, and vesicoureteral strictures, ureteral reflux, lymphocele, and neurogenic bladder, may identify the cause of recurrent urinary tract infections. Primary CMV infection can be prevented by avoiding the use of CMV-positive blood products as well as transplantation from a CMV-positive donor to a CMV-negative recipient.

HEART TRANSPLANT. Heart transplant recipients are at risk for the same infections as patients with other organ transplants. In addition, mediastinitis caused by *S. areus*, *S. epidermidis*, or gram-negative bacilli may result from an infected surgical wound. Fever, sternal tenderness, erythema, and purulent drainage with bone destruction suggest the diagnosis of mediastinitis. *Treatment* is directed to the specific pathogen and the precautions and prophylaxis used in other organ transplantations are indicated.

INFECTIONS IN PATIENTS WITH CANCER

The child with malignancy may be severely compromised from immunodeficiency caused by the cancer, the therapy, or both. Increased risk for infection is also associated with damage to the skin and mucous membranes, indwelling catheters, malnutrition, prolonged antibiotic usage, and hospitalization.

Because the immunodeficiency is related primarily to anticancer therapy, the risk of infection may be estimated from the type, intensity, and duration of chemotherapy. More than one aspect of the immune system is usually involved. For example, corticosteroid drugs and radiation cause destruction of both T and B lymphocytes; methotrexate and other antifols inhibit DNA synthesis; alkylating agents such as cyclophosphamide block DNA replication; and 6-mercaptopurine interferes with purine synthesis. All of these agents inhibit the inflammatory response to invading microbes. The organisms causing infections in cancer patients are listed in Table 173–2.

The significance of the neutrophil count in predicting the risk and response to infections was clearly elucidated in the 1960s. This parameter serves as the basis for the management of infections in children with malignancies. While CD_4^+ T-lymphocyte counts are dependable predictors of certain infections in AIDS patients, no studies to date have used this measure in cancer patients. Infections in children with cancer are categorized as those occurring in neutropenia and non-neutropenic patients, keeping in mind that exceptions occur with each category.

INFECTIONS IN THE NONGRANULOCYTIC PATIENT. Table 173–2 indicates the organisms that may cause infection in the nongranulocytic patient. These include the viral infections, *P. carinii*, *Toxoplasma gondii*, and certain fungal infections such as histoplasmosis, cryptococcosis, and coccidiomycosis. These patients are also at risk for infections encountered in the otherwise normal host, such as pneumococcal pneumonia, otitis media, streptococcal pharyngitis, and urinary tract infection. Infections from coagulase-negative staphylococci, *P. aeruginosa*, *Serratia marcescens*, *Candida* spp., *Aspergillus* spp., etc. are rare.

Although the need to start specific antimicrobial therapy is urgent, the empirical antibiotic therapy used for neutropenic patients is usually not initiated until after an attempt to establish an etiologic diagnosis has been made.

INFECTION IN THE GRANULOCYTOPENIC CANCER PATIENT. When the granulocyte (neutrophil) count is 500 cells/mm^3 or less, the patient is at high risk for a serious infection, usually of bacterial etiology. The risk is less at counts of 500–1,000 cell/mm^3 but is greater than for normal children. As the count decreases below 500 cells/mm^3, the risk for infection increases proportionately. Because of the granulocytopenia and the poor inflammatory response, fever is often the only manifestation of infection.

Because the etiology of infection in the febrile granulocytopenic patient cannot be predicted from physical signs and symptoms, initial antibiotic treatment requires broad-spectrum antibiotics. The gram-positive cocci have emerged as the most frequent cause of febrile episodes in recent years, but gram-negative bacilli continue to play a significant role in these serious infections (Table 173–2). Coagulase-negative staphylococci, *S. aureus*, and alpha-hemolytic streptococci are the most frequent organisms cultured from the blood of febrile children with neutropenia. In some cases of alpha-hemolytic streptococcal bacteremia, an acute septic shock syndrome may occur, resembling the adult respiratory distress syndrome; this manifestation is most common in children receiving cytarabine. *Pseudomonas aeruginosa*, *E. coli*, and *Klebsiella pneumoniae* are the most common gram-negative bacillary infections. Antibiotic therapy is usually effective in the control of bacterial infections, but the need for prolonged antibiotic therapy predisposes patients to opportunistic fungal infections, especially from species of *Candida* and *Aspergillus*.

Gram-negative sepsis is typically more severe than sepsis due to *S. epidermidis*. *Escherichia coli* or *Pseudomonas* infection results in septic shock in 30–50% of episodes. Oropharyngeal infection manifests as ulcerating stomatitis, gingivitis, and periodontal lesions. Mucositis may be due to anaerobic bacteria, herpes simplex, *Candida* spp., or to a mixed infection. Esophagitis may be due to these same microorganisms or to CMV, and may be associated with mucositis or may occur independently. Cutaneous lesions may occur as perirectal cellulitis at sites of central venous catheter insertion, venipuncture, lumbar puncture, bone marrow biopsy, or abrasions, or as infection of sweat glands and paronychia. Cutaneous signs of disseminated infection include ecthyma gangrenosum (*P. aeruginosa* and other microorganisms), nodules (*Candida* spp., mucormycosis), gangrenous cellulitis (*Aspergillus*, mucormycosis), and thrombotic arterial occlusion with distal ischemia due to *Aspergillus* spp.

Pneumonia in granulocytopenic cancer patients may be subtle and manifest as local rales, tachypnea, chest pain, or the adult respiratory distress syndrome. Pulmonary infiltrates may be absent or faint, only to appear more obvious when the neutrophil count increases above 500 cells/mm^3. Pneumonia is usually due to gram-negative enteric bacteria but may also be due to fungi. *Aspergillus* may produce a characteristic wedge-shaped infiltrate typical of arterial invasion and subsequent thrombotic pulmonary infraction. Pulmonary cavitation is suggestive of aspergillosis, mucormycosis, and, rarely, infection with gram-negative enteric bacteria. Pulmonary infiltrates in neutropenic cancer patients may also represent noninfectious disorders, such as hemorrhage, malignancy, emboli, edema, reactions to granulocyte transfusions, and radiation- or chemotherapy-induced pneumonitis.

Additional infectious complications include sinusitis with possible intracranial extension due to aspergillosis, mucormycosis, or mixed bacteria; hepatic and splenic candidiasis in the absence of candidemia; candidal endophthalmitis; and severe diarrhea due to *C. difficile*.

Blood samples for cultures should be drawn from a peripheral vein and from each lumen of the central venous catheter. Cultures or biopsies should be made of local cutaneous lesions, and a chest roentgenogram should be examined for infiltrates, infarction, or cavitation. Nasal secretions and sputum should be cultured for the presence of *Aspergillus*. Sinus roentgenograms or CT may reveal asymptomatic sinusitis. Esophageal endoscopy may be indicated to identify the cause of odynophagia. If pseudohyphae are demonstrated from esophageal lesions, a presumptive diagnosis of disseminated candidiasis is suggested. Serum C-reactive protein levels of greater than 40 mg/L suggest bacterial infection.

Meningitis is unusual in granulocytopenic febrile cancer patients. Lumbar puncture should be obtained in the presence of significant signs of central venous system infection, following platelet transfusion if needed.

In certain situations fiberoptic bronchoscopy, bronchoalveolar lavage, transbronchial biopsy, or open lung biopsy may be required to identify the microorganism responsible for pneumonia.

Treatment of infections in febrile granulocytopenic cancer patients requires prompt initiation of empiric broad-spectrum, bactericidal antibiotics to decrease the risks of septic shock, the adult respiratory distress syndrome, hypotension, renal and other organ dysfunction, and death. There are several possible choices for initial empiric antibiotics for patients who do not have fulminant septic shock. Monotherapy with ceftazidime or imipenem/cilastatin, with subsequent modification by the addition of vancomycin if *S. epidermidis* or another resistant organism is recovered, is one therapeutic approach. Monotherapy should be limited to patients who have brief episodes of mild neutropenia (500–1,000 neutrophils) when *S. epidermidis* and methicillin-resistant *S. aureus* are not considered likely pathogens. Double β-lactam therapy with an extended gram-negative spectrum carboxy- or ureido-penicillin (ticarcillin with or without clavulanic acid, mezlocillin, piperacillin) and a cephalosporin (ceftazidine, cefoperazone, cefotaxime, ceftriaxone) is another broad-spectrum bactericidal regimen that avoids potentially nephrotoxic drugs such as vancomycin and the aminoglycosides. Its disadvantages include selection of resistant bacteria, possible antibiotic antagonism, and poor antistaphylococcal coverage.

A combination of an anti-*Pseudomonas* β-lactam penicillin or cephalosporin plus aminoglycoside avoids the risk of the emergence of resistant organisms, is synergistic, and includes anaerobic coverage. The disadvantages are the nephrotoxicity, hypokalemia, and ototoxicity resulting from aminoglycoside therapy, and poor coverage of staphylococci. The triple-drug regimen includes a combination of an extended gram-negative spectrum penicillin or a cephalosporin, plus vancomycin, plus an aminoglycoside (gentamicin, tobramycin, amikacin). This regimen is most beneficial if there is a risk of serious staphylococcal, enterococcal, or bacterial multidrug-resistant infection.

If the patient becomes afebrile after 72 hr of empiric antibiotic therapy and a bacterial source of infection is identified, the antimicrobial therapy should be modified based on the antibiotic sensitivity of the isolated bacteria. Antibiotic therapy should be continued for a minimum of 7 days in patients who respond to therapy, are afebrile, have negative repeat cultures, and are free of signs and symptoms of infection. Optimally, the neutrophil count should also exceed 500 when antibiotics are stopped. High-risk patients with profound granulocytopenia, mucositis, signs of persistent infection, central line tract infections, bleeding, impending invasive procedure, or chemotherapy may benefit from continuation of antibiotics until the neutrophil count is >500 cells/mm^3.

Some clinicians recommend that antibiotics be continued until the neutrophil count is >500/mm^3 in all patients who have had fever and neutropenia regardless of defervescence or clinical well-being.

If the patient remains febrile despite broad-spectrum antibiotic therapy and no pathogen is identified, it is important to reassess the patient's condition. The etiology of persistent fever includes a nonbacterial pathogen (*Candida, Aspergillus, Toxoplasma,* herpes simplex, cytomegalovirus, Epstein-Barr virus, enterovirus), emergence of a second resistant species of bacteria, inadequate serum or tissue antibiotic levels, drug fever, deep tissue absess or catheter infection, and fever resulting from the underlying malignancy.

If no identifiable cause of the fever is evident, the fever and granulocytopenia remain after 5–7 days of antibiotic therapy, there is no progression or deterioration in the patient's condition, and the patient appears clinically well, the original antibiotics may be continued. If the patient appears ill or if the manifestations of infection progress, vancomycin or a 3rd generation cephalosporin should be added if the patient was not receiving these antibiotics as part of the initial empiric therapeutic regimen. If the patient remains neutropenic and febrile for 7 days despite modification of antibacterial therapy, intravenous amphotericin B should be started. Approximately 33% of such patients have shown evidence of invasive fungal disease that was either the primary infection or a superinfection that developed after 7 days of broad-spectrum antibiotics. Prior to the initiation of amphotericin B, an evaluation to determine the source of invasive candidiasis, aspergillosis, or mucormycosis should be performed. Biopsies of lesions should be performed, several blood and urine cultures obtained, chest and sinus roentgenogram repeated, abdominal CT performed to identify hepatic or splenic microabscesses, and an ophthalmologic examination carried out to identify candidal ophthalmitis. Amphotericin B is given daily for 2 wk if no fungal infection is identified. Antifungal therapy is then stopped and the patient's condition re-evaluated. Documented fungal infection is treated with prolonged amphotericin B and aspiration or incision and drainage of cutaneous lesions or deep abscesses. New antifungal agents such as fluconazole may be effective, especially if amphotericin is not well tolerated or if severe nephrotoxicity is present. To reduce the risk of renal impairment, concurrent administration of potentially nephrotoxic drugs should be avoided during amphotericin therapy. Third-generation cephalosporins may be substituted for aminoglycosides, and the use of chemotherapeutic agents such as cisplatin should be minimized if possible.

If a documented bacteremia occurs while a central venous catheter or implanted device is in place, antibiotics should be administered through each lumen in an attempt to sterilize the line. Most episodes of catheter-related sepsis respond to systemic antibiotics, and there is no need to remove the catheter. Line infections that are difficult to sterilize include tract infections and sepsis due to *Bacillus* spp., fungi, gram-negative enteric bacteria, and multiple organisms.

Empiric antiviral therapy for the febrile neutropenic patient is not indicated in the absence of typical mucocutaneous lesions suggestive of herpes simplex or varicella-zoster. Intravenous acyclovir is the treatment of choice for these viral infections.

Prevention of infection in neutropenic cancer patients is difficult. Methods include reverse isolation and a total protective environment. Prophylactic oral nonabsorbable antibiotics, such as colistin, nystatin, and polymyxin, and oral absorbable antibiotics such as trimethoprim-sulfamethoxazole (for *P. carinii* and gram-negative enteric bacteria) and the new fluorinated quinolones (norfloxacin, ciprofloxacin) may reduce the risk of infection in severely granulocytopenic (<100 cells/mm^3) patients receiving cancer chemotherapy or bone marrow transplantation. Trimethoprim-sulfamethoxazole may delay bone marrow recovery and produce drug rashes.

Indications for recombinant human granulocyte–colony-stimulating factor (G-CSF) and granulocyte-macrophage–colony stimulating factor (GM-CSF) are not adequately defined. Their use in febrile neutropenic patients appears to reduce the period of granulocytopenia, the incidence of infection, and the number of days for hospitalization and antibiotic therapy, but overall survival from infection has not been affected.

BREECH IN SKIN AND MUCOUS MEMBRANE BARRIERS TO INFECTION (Table 173–4)

In order to establish infection, microbial pathogens must first penetrate the important protective covering of the skin, conjunctivae, and mucous membranes. Commensal organisms colonize these surfaces without invasion. The barrier may be overcome by organisms of very high virulence or by a defect in this host barrier. In addition to being a physical obstacle that few pathogens can penetrate, the skin contains bacteriostatic and bacteriocidal fatty acids secreted by the sebaceous glands. Mucous membrane secretions contain various enzymes (lactoperoxidase, lysozyme, lactoferrin) and secretory IgA, and specific areas have unfavorable acidic environments (stomach, urine, vagina) that reduce bacterial activity. Furthermore, a normal bacterial flora of mucosal surfaces may prevent local colonization by pathogenic microorganisms. This *colonization resistance* is due to the local bacterial production of antimicrobial compounds (bacteriocins), alteration of the redox potential, and competition for nutrients. Additional local defense mechanisms include mucociliary clearance, the cough reflex, unobstructed flow of secretions, and the activity of tissue phagocytic cells. Interference or disruption of any of these local defense mechanisms may predispose to infection. Broad-spectrum antibiotics may alter the normal flora and reduce colonization resistance; therapy intended to increase gastric pH may increase gastric colonization with pathogenic bacteria; obstruction to the flow of urine or lung secretions may cause pyelonephritis or pneumonia, respectively; and surgical incision, burns, or trauma may alter the physical barrier.

■ TABLE 173–4 Some Defects in Nonimmunologic Barriers to Infection

Skin
Traumatic break: treatment or nontreatment related
Blockage of sweat excretion
Change in fatty acid components of sebaceous glands
Change in normal microbial flora
Mucous Membranes
Decrease in tears; lysozyme, normal desquamation; mucus production; acidity of stomach, vagina, and skin; flow of urine; ciliary escalation of respiratory tract; coughing and sneezing; salivation; bile salts, and peristaltic activity
Change in the normal microbial flora
Obstruction to Normal Organ Excretion/Secretion
Impaired Febrile Response
Foreign Body Locus

BURNS. Infections in children with burns (Chapter 60.8) are related to interruption of the skin and mucous membrane barriers and to the presence of necrotic tissue, which serves as a culture medium, to pulmonary injury, to long-term administration of antibiotics, and to prolonged intravenous or urinary catheterization. Septicemia with *P. aeruginosa, S. aureus,* and *S. epidermidis* is frequent. Burn injury has been associated with abnormal immune response to infection, including neutrophil dysfunction, abnormal antibody responses to specific antigens, and delayed rejection of homografts. The risk of infection is directly related to the extent of the burn, the neutrophil chemotactic defect, and an associated hypogammaglobulinemia. The burn site may aid in selection of antibiotics if evidence of infection occurs, such as fever, cellulitis, necrosis, etc. Fever may be due to a metabolic response to injury or to infection. Broad-spectrum antibiotic coverage is recommended if infection is suspected. Sepsis is a major cause of death with extensive burns, and *P. aeruginosa* is the most common cause. Occlusive dressings with silver sulfadiazine may be used prophylactically against infection.

IMPLANTED FOREIGN MATERIALS. Intravascular Devices. Intravascular access devices range from short stainless-steel needles to multilumen implantable catheters. While any may provide a source for local or systemic infection, the long-term indwelling multilumen catheters are a greater risk for infection than the short-term intravenous needles. Infection from the microbial skin flora at the insertion site may extend along the external surface of the catheter and is the most common type of infection with intravascular catheters. Organisms may also gain access to the intraluminal portion of the catheter through contaminated infusion, improper handling of the catheter hub, or hematogenous spread from distant sites.

When prolonged intravenous access is required, a cuffed silicone rubber (silastic) catheter may be inserted into the right atrium through the subclavian, cephalic, or jugular vein. The extravascular proximal segment of the catheter passes through a subcutaneous tunnel before exiting the skin, usually on the superior aspect of the chest. The Broviac or Hickman catheters are the prototype devices used for long-term venous access. The implanted venous access systems (Mediport, Port-a-cath, Infus-port) consist of a reservoir placed in a subcutaneous pocket with a self-sealing silicone septum that permits repeated percutaneous needle insertion and administration of drugs. The reservoir is attached to a distal catheter, which is tunneled in the subcutaneous tissue before it is inserted into the superior vena cava through the same veins as those used for the Hickman or Broviac catheter. The reservoir and catheter are totally intracorporeal and have no exit site or externalized material, such as that needed for the Hickman and Broviac systems. The use of these central venous devices has improved the quality of life of high-risk patients but has also increased the risk of various infections, such as exit site and tunnel infections, as well as catheter-associated bacteremia or fungemia.

The incidence of local (exit site, tunnel, pocket) infection is 0.3–0.6 episodes/1,000 catheter days. The incidence of Broviac or Hickman catheter sepsis is 2–4/1,000 days, whereas that for implantable systems is 0.3–0.7/1,000 catheter days. The risk of catheter infection is increased among premature infants and young children, patients with neutropenia or catheter thrombosis, and those receiving total parenteral nutrition.

The pathogenesis of catheter sepsis is related to local contamination and subsequent colonization of the catheter rather than primary bacteremia seeding the intravascular device. Gram-positive bacteremia accounts for 60–70% of episodes of catheter sepsis *(S. epidermidis, S. aureus, S. pyogenes, S. faecalis)*, gram-negative enteric bacteria occur in 20–30% of episodes (*Klebsiella* spp., *E. coli, Pseudomonas* spp., *Acinetobacter* spp.), and fungi account for 5–10% of catheter sepsis episodes *(Candida* spp., *Malassezia furfur). Mycobacterium fortuitum, Bacillus* spp., and polymicrobial sepsis are rare causes of catheter infections.

The *clinical manifestations* of local infection include erythema, tenderness, and purulent discharge. Catheter sepsis may also present as fever without an identifiable focus, especially in neutropenic patients. All episodes of fever are not due to catheter sepsis, and all episodes of bacteremia are not related to the catheter.

The *diagnosis* of catheter sepsis is confirmed by simultaneously performing blood cultures from the catheter and a peripheral vein. If quantitative blood cultures are obtained, a higher grade of bacteremia will be evident from the catheter than from the peripheral blood sample. A Gram stain of pericatheter drainage may be helpful in the recognition of a bacterial etiology. If no organism is seen, and especially if the discharge has a green tinge, an acid-fast stain is indicated to search for mycobacterial species.

The *treatment* of suspected catheter sepsis in a neutropenic patient includes initiation of broad-spectrum antibiotics such as ceftazidine and vancomycin (see later). Treatment of catheter sepsis in non-neutropenic patients is directed against the specific organism recovered in the blood or exit site culture. If the catheter is no longer needed, it should be removed immediately. If the catheter is required, the catheter does not need to be removed for all exit site or septic episodes; most episodes of *S. epidermidis* infection can be treated with the catheter in place. Repeated negative blood cultures through the catheter ensure that therapy has been successful. However, tunnel infections and episodes of sepsis due to *S. aureus, P. aeruginosa, Bacillus*, spp., *Candida* spp., *Aspergillus* spp., and *Corynebacterium* spp. usually require removal of the catheter.

Prevention of catheter-related infection includes placement using meticulous surgical aseptic technique in an operating room-like environment. Use of antibacterial ointment, avoidance of occlusive or semipermeable dressings, avoidance of bathing or swimming, and careful catheter care may reduce the incidence of catheter infection. The incidence of sepsis with totally implanted devices may be lower than that with external catheters owing to elimination of chronic irritation at the exit site.

Cerebrospinal Fluid Shunts. Cerebrospinal fluid (CSF) shunting is required for the treatment of many children with hydrocephalus. The usual procedure uses a silicone rubber device with a proximal portion inserted into the ventricle, a unidirectional valve, and a distant segment that diverts the CSF to the peritoneal cavity or right atrium. The incidence of shunt infections ranges from 3% to 15% and includes meningitis, purulent perishunt abscesses, septicemia, peritonitis, and nephritis. Many shunt infections are limited to febrile episodes with bacteria cultured from the CSF in the absence of discernible meningitis. *Staphylococcus epidermidis* is the most frequent causative agent. Infection occurred in 8% of cases in a study of 350 shunt procedures. The infecting organisms were gram-positive cocci in 79% and gram-negative bacilli in 7% of the cases. The infection rate was 13.6% for an operation lasting more than 90 min and 5.2% for procedures of less than 30 min duration.

The *clinical manifestations* of infections of ventriculoperitoneal shunts include indolent fever, abdominal pain, signs of peritonitis, and headache due to shunt malfunction. There may be erythema over the shunt tract and meningismus. Patients with infection of a ventriculoatrial shunt may manifest fever, shunt dysfunction, and meningismus; chronic *S. epidermidis* bacteremia may cause hypocomplementemic glomerulonephritis due to antigen-antibody complex deposition in the glomeruli.

The *diagnosis* of shunt infection is confirmed when a shunt CSF culture is positive or the shunt CSF white blood cell count is increased above 10 with a predominance of neutrophils. Bacteremia is present in more than 85% of patients with ventriculoatrial shunt infections. Signs of immune complex glomerulonephritis include hypertension, microscopic hematuria, elevated BUN and serum creatinine levels, and anemia. Infected ventriculoatrial shunts may also produce septic pulmonary emboli, pulmonary hypertension, and endocarditis. If a sample of shunt CSF cannot be obtained and there is meningismus, a lumbar puncture may reveal bacteria and a predominance of neutrophils. Occasionally, no bacterial organism is identified, and presumptive therapy must be initiated.

Treatment of shunt infection includes the use of antibiotics against the specific organism and in some situations removal of the shunt. A combination of systemic vancomycin and intraventricular gentamicin is effective initially. Resistant infections that are difficult to clear may be treated with intraventricular gentamicin plus systemic vancomycin or trimethoprim-sulfamethoxazole and rifampin. The distal end of the ventriculoperitoneal shunt should be externalized; this will usually relieve abdominal complaints within 30–60 min. If abdominal signs continue 4–6 hr after shunt externalization, other intra-abdominal pathology, such as viscus perforation or appendicitis, should be considered. Shunt revision may be performed according to either of two protocols: immediate revision within 24 hr of defervescence or delayed revision after three consecutive negative CSF cultures. This latter protocol is preferred for infections due to *S. aureus* and gram-negative bacteria. In either situation antibiotics should be continued for 10–14 days after shunt revision. Some CSF-shunt infections due to *S. epidermidis* may respond to treatment with systemic and intraventricular antibiotics without performing shunt revision. This approach has been used in patients with ventriculoatrial shunts and in some patients with ventriculoperitoneal shunts (after changing the peritoneal end only).

Prevention of shunt infection includes meticulous cutaneous preparation and surgical technique. Systemic and intraventricular antibiotics and soaking the shunt tubing in antibiotics have been used to reduce the incidence of infection, with varying success. A meta-analysis of 12 clinical trials involving 1,359 randomized patients showed that perioperative use of an antimicrobial agent in CSF shunt placement reduced the risk for infection.

Urethral Catheters. The nosocomial urinary tract infection rate in hospitalized children is about 14 infections per 1,000 admissions; 92% of the infections occur in catheterized patients.

Studies have shown that bacteria adhere to the catheter surface and establish a biofilm composed of bacteria, bacterial glycocalices, Tamm-Horsfall protein, and urinary salts. The biofilm is believed to protect the bacteria from antibiotics. Almost all patients catheterized for more than 30 days develop bacteriuria.

The urinary tract is considered infected if specimens of urine obtained directly from an indwelling catheter yield a level of 100 or greater colony-forming units. *Escherichia coli* and *P. aeruginosa* are the most common causes of catheter-associated infection. Coagulase-negative staphylococci cause about 15% of these infections. Symptomatic infection should be treated with antibiotics as described in Chapter 492. Usually asymptomatic infections are unaffected by antibiotic therapy.

Periodic changes of urethral catheters reduce the likelihood of infection. Some studies suggest that oral antibiotics, such as trimethoprim-sulfamethoxazole, reduce the incidence of infection from intermittent catheterization, but prophylactic antibiotics do not reduce the infection rates for long-term indwelling urethral catheters.

Peritoneal Dialysis. During the 1st year of peritoneal dialysis for end-stage renal disease, 65% of children will have one or more episodes of peritonitis. Bacterial entry comes from luminal or periluminal contamination of the catheter. Hematogenous infection is a rare event. Organisms responsible for peritonitis include *S. epidermidis* (30–40%), *S. aureus* (10–20%), streptococci (10–15%), *E. coli* (5–10%), *Pseudomonas* spp. (5–10%), other gram-negative bacteria (5–15%), enterococci (3–6%), fungi (2–10%) such as *Candida* spp., *Fusarium* spp., *Alternaria* spp., or *Aspergillus* spp., and rare organisms such as *Diphtheroid* spp., *Mycobacterium* spp., and anaerobic bacteria. The culture may be negative in 0–20% of episodes.

The *clinical manifestations* of peritonitis may be subtle and include low-grade fever, mild abdominal pain, and tenderness. Cloudy peritoneal dialysis fluid may be the first or predominant sign. The dialysis fluid will be cloudy when the neutrophil count exceeds 100. The cell count may be influenced by the intraperitoneal volume and the duration of time the dialysate has perfused the peritoneum. Infection is suggested by an increased number and predominance of dialysate neutrophils, a positive Gram stain and culture of peritoneal fluid, and signs of peritoneal inflammation (tenderness, guarding, rebound). Exit site and tunnel infections may occur independent of or precede peritonitis.

Treatment of peritonitis should be initiated prior to identification of the organism and modified after culture and sensitivities are known. Intraperitoneal instillation of a 1st-generation cephalosporin or vancomycin plus an aminoglycoside is reasonable initial antibiotic treatment prior to identification of the pathogen. Antifungal agents usually cannot be given through the dialysis catheter because their peritoneal penetration is poor; these agents must be given by the intravenous (amphotericin B) or oral (5-flucytosine, ketoconazole) route. The catheter may need to be removed in fungal or recurrent bacterial peritonitis. Treatment is continued for 7 days after the last positive culture or for 10 days for gram-positive organisms and 14 days for gram-negative organisms or for culture-negative peritonitis. Recurrent (same organism within 4 wk) peritonitis is treated for 2–4 wk.

SURGICAL PROCEDURES. The surgical incision is an obvious breech in the skin or mucous membrane barrier and introduces an increase in risk for infection, usually bacterial. The risk is proportionate to the number and virulence of microbes entering the wound, the site, and the length of time postincision. A useful classification of surgical procedures based on this risk recognizes four categories:

1. *Clean wounds* are uninfected operative wounds in which no inflammation is noted and the respiratory, alimentary, and genitourinary tracts and the oropharynx are not entered. In addition, the procedure is elective and is performed as primarily closed or drained with closed drainage. Operative incisional wounds following nonpenetrating trauma are included in this category. *In clean wounds prophylactic antimicrobial therapy is not recommended, except in circumstances in which the consequences of infection are potentially life threatening (e.g., implantation of a prosthetic foreign body such as a prosthetic heart valve; open heart surgery for repair of structural defects; surgery in patients who are immunocompromised as a result of an inherited disease or are receiving corticosteroids or chemotherapy for malignancy; and newborn infants).* Systemic antimicrobial agents have been recommended empirically for a clean procedure in patients with infection at another site.

2. *Clean contaminated* wounds are operative wounds in which the respiratory, alimentary, or genitourinary tract is entered under controlled conditions and does not have unusual contamination preoperatively. These include surgery involving the biliary tract, appendix, vagina, and oropharynx in which no evidence of infection or major break in technique is encountered. In clean but potentially contaminated procedures the risk of contamination is variable. *Recommendations for pediatric patients derived from data on adults suggest that prophylaxis be provided for procedures in patients with obstructive jaundice, certain alimentary tract procedures, and urinary tract surgery or instrumentation in the presence of bacteriuria or obstructive uropathy.*

3. *Contaminated wounds* include open, fresh, and accidental wounds; major breaks in otherwise sterile operative technique; gross spillage from the gastrointestinal tract; and incisions in which acute nonpurulent inflammation is encountered.

4. *Dirty and infected wounds* include old traumatic wounds with retained devitalized tissue and those in which clinical infection is apparent or in which the viscera have been perforated. *In contaminated and dirty or infected wound procedures, antimicrobial therapy is indicated.*

In the truest sense antimicrobial prophylaxis refers to the use of antibiotics prior to the attachment of contaminating bacteria to the host tissues, as in the clean and potentially contaminated categories. Antibiotics given after the microbial attachment constitutes therapy, as in the case for contaminated and dirty wounds.

When prophylactic antibiotics are used administration should begin about 30 min before the incision is made, with the intent of having peak concentrations of the drug at this time. In most instances an intravenous dose is preferred for major procedures. The intent is to maintain adequate plasma and tissue concentration of the drugs until the incision is closed. With prolonged procedures lasting longer than 2–3 hr, an additional dose may be required. Drugs administered postoperatively for prophylaxis do not reduce the infection rate. For patients undergoing colonic procedures, additional oral antibiotics may be used and should be given on the day prior to surgery.

The selection of antibiotics for prophylaxis is based upon the procedure, the expected contaminating organisms, and safety of the drugs. Because of the vast array of antibiotics available now, more than one may qualify equally for use. Some suggested regimens for selected *clean-contaminated* procedures are as follows:

Appendectomy	Cefoxitin or clindamycin plus gentamicin
Colorectal surgery	Cefoxitin or clindamycin plus gentamicin
Oropharyngeal surgery	Clindamycin alone or with gentamicin
Compound fracture	Cefazolin, nafcillin, or vancomycin
Biliary tract surgery	Cefazolin, or ampicillin with or without gentamicin

■ TABLE 173–5 Immunizations for Immunocompromised Infants and Children

Vaccine	Routine	HIV/AIDS	Severe Immuno-suppression*	Asplenia	Renal Failure	Diabetes
			Routine Infant Immunizations			
DTP(DT/T/Td)†	Recommended	Recommended	Recommended	Recommended	Recommended	Recommended
OPV	Recommended	Contraindicated	Contraindicated	Recommended	Recommended	Recommended
e/IPV	Use if indicated	Recommended	Recommended	Use as indicated	Use as indicated	Use as indicated
MMR/MR/M/R	Recommended	Recommended/ considered	Contraindicated	Recommended	Recommended	Recommended
Hib	Recommended	Recommended	Recommended	Recommended	Recommended	Recommended
Hepatitis B‡	Recommended	Recommended	Recommended	Recommended	Recommended	Recommended
			Other Childhood Immunizations			
Pneumococcal§	Use if indicated	Recommended	Recommended	Recommended	Recommended	Recommended
Influenza‖	Use if indicated	Recommended	Recommended	Recommended	Recommended	Recommended

**Severe immunosuppression can be the result of congenital immunodeficiency, HIV infection, leukemia, lymphoma, aplastic anemia, or generalized malignancy or from alkylating agents, antimetabolites, radiation, or large amounts of corticosteroids.*
†Including DTaP boosters.
‡HB vaccine is now recommended for all infants.
§Recommended for persons ≥2 yr of age.
‖Not recommended for infants <6 mo of age.
From Centers for Disease Control and Prevention: Immunizing immunocompromised infants and children. MMWR 42:(RR-4)15, 1993.

Antibiotics for *clean* surgical procedures include the following:

Cardiac surgery	Cefazolin, cefuroxime, or vancomycin (See section on cardiology and endocarditis for additional information on antibiotic prophylaxis in children with underlying cardiac disease.)
Orthopedic surgery (e.g., hip surgery, prosthesis, initial fixation)	Cefazolin, vancomycin, or nafcillin

Knowledge of the prevalent bacterial causes of nosocomial infection in one's hospital is especially important in choosing drugs. For example, if methicillin-resistant *S. aureus* or coagulase-negative staphylococci are common contaminants, vancomycin would be chosen over the cephalosporin drugs.

CHRONIC DISEASES

Many chronic diseases and debilitating circumstances render the patient at high risk for infection. Because these diseases, such as sickle cell disease, cystic fibrosis, diabetes mellitis, malnutrition, nephrotic syndrome, uremia, cirrhosis, and AIDS, are discussed elsewhere in this book, no further reference to them will be made here.

IMMUNIZATION IN IMMUNOCOMPROMISED INFANTS AND CHILDREN

Because many immunocompromised children survive into adult life and some may eventually be restored to immunocompetence, immunization with the live-attenuated and killed vaccines in general use deserves consideration. Key factors are adverse effects that might come from use of live-attenuated vaccines, such as the oral poliovirus vaccine, and the inability of the host to muster an adequate immune response. In 1993 the Advisory Committee on Immunization Practices of the U.S. Public Health Service made the recommendations summarized in Table 173–5. Additional details are provided in the Report of the Committee on Infectious Diseases, 1994.

American Academy of Pediatrics: Immunization in special circumstances. *In*: Peter G (ed): 1994 Redbook: Report of the Committee on Infectious Diseases, 23rd ed. Elk Grove Village, IL, American Academy of Pediatrics, 1994, pp 51–71.

Armitage JO: Bone marrow transplantation. N Engl J Med 330:827, 1994.

Ascher NL, Stock PG, Bumgardner GL, et al: Infection and rejection of primary hepatic transplant in 93 consecutive patients treated with triple immunosuppressive therapy. Surg Gynecol Obstet 167:474, 1988.

Ezekowitz RAB, Dinauer MC, Jaffe HS, et al: Partial correction of the phagocyte defect in patients with X-linked chronic granulomatous disease by subcutaneous interferon gamma. N Engl J Med 319:146, 1988.

Hughes WT, Armstrong D, Bodey GP, et al: Guidelines for the use of antimicrobial agents in neutropenic patients with unexplained fever. J Infect Dis 161:381, 1990.

Kontny V, Hofling B, Gutjahr P, et al: CSF shunt infections in children. Infection 21:89, 1993.

Langley JM, LeBlanc JC, Drake J, Milner R: Efficacy of antimicrobial prophylaxis in placement of cerebrospinal fluid shunts: meta-analysis. Clin Infect Dis 17:98, 1993.

Lohr JA, Donowitz LG, Salder JE: Hospital-acquired urinary tract infection. Pediatrics 83:193, 1989.

Morissette I, Gourdeau M, Francoeur J: CSF shunt infections: a fifteen-year experience with emphasis on management and outcome. Can J Neurol Sci 20:118, 1993.

Patrick CC: Infections in Immunocompromised Infants and Children. New York, Churchill Livingstone, 1992.

Pizzo PA: Management of fever in patients with cancer and treatment-induced neutropenia. N Engl J Med 328:1323, 1993.

Raad II, Hohn DC, Gilbreath J, et al: Prevention of central venous catheter-related infections by using maximal sterile barrier precautions during insertion. Infect Control Hosp Epidemiol 15:231, 1994.

Riikonen P, Saarinen UM, Mäkipernaa A, et al: Recombinant human granulocyte-macrophage colony-stimulating factor in the treatment of febrile neutropenia: a double blind placebo-controlled study in children. Pediatr Infect Dis J 13:197, 1994.

Rowe JM, Ciobanu N, Ascesao J, et al: Recommended guidelines for the management of autologous and allogenic bone marrow transplantation: a report from the Eastern Cooperative Oncology Group. Ann Intern Med 120:143, 1994.

Rubin RH, Tokoff-Rubin NE: Antimicrobial strategies in the case of organ transplant recipients. Antimicrob Agents Chemother 37:619, 1993.

Sable CA, Donowitz GR: Infections in bone marrow transplant recipients. Clin Infect Dis 18:272, 1994.

Santolaya ME, Cofre J, Beresi V: C-reactive protein: a valuable aid for the management of febrile children with cancer and neutropenia. Clin Infect Dis 18:589, 1994.

So SKS, Simmons RL: Infections following kidney transplantation in children. *In*: Patrick CC (ed): Infection in Immunosuppressed Infants and Children. New York, Churchill Livingstone, 1992, pp 215–230.

Stamm WE, Hooton TM: Management of urinary tract infections in adults. N Engl J Med, 329:1328, 1993.

Wong W-Y, Overturf GD, Powars DR: Infections caused by *Streptococcus pneumoniae* in children with sickle cell disease: epidemiology, immunologic mechanisms, prophylaxis, and vaccination. Clin Infect Dis 14:1124, 1992.

SECTION 3
Bacterial Infections

CHAPTER 174
Staphylococcal Infections

*James Todd**

Staphylococci are hardy, non–spore-forming, ubiquitous bacteria and are present in air, fomites, and dust or as normal flora of humans and animals. They are resistant to heat and drying and may be recovered from nonphysiologic environments weeks to months after inoculation. These organisms are gram positive and grow in clusters, aerobically or as facultative anaerobes. Strains are classified as *Staphylococcus aureus* if they are coagulase positive or as coagulase-negative staphylococci (e.g., *S. epidermidis, S. saprophyticus, S. haemolyticus*). Generally, *S. aureus* produces a yellow pigment and β-hemolysis on blood organ and *S. epidermidis* produces a white pigment with variable hemolysis results.

174.1 Infections Due to Staphylococcus aureus

S. aureus is the most common cause of pyogenic infection of the skin; it also may cause furuncles, carbuncles, osteomyelitis, septic arthritis, wound infection, abscesses, pneumonia, empyema, endocarditis, pericarditis, meningitis, and toxin-mediated diseases, including food poisoning, scalded skin syndrome, and toxic shock syndrome (TSS).

ETIOLOGY. Disease may be the result of tissue invasion or may reflect injury due to a variety of toxins and enzymes elaborated by these organisms. Strains of *S. aureus* can be identified and classified by means of bacteriophage group typing (groups I–IV, miscellaneous). Strains typing in certain phage groups often have similar pathogenic potential (e.g., phage group I is associated with TSS).

Many strains of *S. aureus* release *exotoxins.* Four immunologically distinct hemolysins have been identified. α-Toxin acts on cell membranes and causes tissue necrosis, injures human leukocytes, and produces aggregation of platelets and spasm of smooth muscle. A β-hemolysin degrades sphingomyelin, causing hemolysis of red blood cells, and a δ-hemolysin disrupts membranes by a detergent-like action. Little is known about γ-hemolysin other than that it also appears to act on cell membranes.

Leukocidin, produced by most strains of *S. aureus,* combines with the phospholipid of the phagocytic cell membrane, producing increased permeability, leakage of protein, and eventual death of the neutrophil and macrophage.

Exfoliative toxins A and B are two serologically distinct proteins that produce localized (e.g., bullous impetigo) or generalized (e.g., scalded skin syndrome, scarlatiniform eruption) dermatologic complications (see Chapter 607). Exfoliative toxin A is a chromosomal gene product, and exfoliative toxin B is a plasmid gene product. Individual strains may produce one or both toxins or neither; no consistent phage type is associated with toxin production, although phage group II has been implicated in some cases. Exfoliative toxin produces skin separation by splitting the desmosome and altering the intracellular matrix in the stratum granulosum.

One or more *Staphylococcal enterotoxins* (types A, B, C_1, C_2, D, E) are elaborated by most strains of *S. aureus.* Ingestion of preformed enterotoxin A or B is associated with vomiting and diarrhea and, in some cases, with the development of profound hypotension. Virtually all individuals by the age of 10 yr have antibodies to at least one enterotoxin.

TSS toxin-1 (TSST-1) is associated with TSS related to menstruation and focal staphylococcal infection. Enterotoxin A and enterotoxin B also may be associated with nonmenstrual TSS. TSST-1 induces production of interleukin 1 and tumor necrosis factor, resulting in hypotension, fever, and multisystem involvement.

A variety of *enzymes* may be released by staphylococci. Production of coagulase differentiates *S. aureus* from *S. epidermidis* and other coagulase-negative staphylococci. Coagulase causes plasma to clot by interacting with fibrinogen. Other enzymes elaborated by staphylococci include catalase (inactivates H_2O_2, promoting intracellular survival), penicillinase or β-lactamase (inactivates penicillin at the molecular level), hyaluronidase (spreading factor), lipase, and phosphodiesterase.

Most strains of *S. aureus* possess an *agglutinogen* (i.e., protein A). This material can react with the Fc fragments of IgG molecules, generates complement-derived chemotactic factors, and has antiphagocytic properties. Capsular antigens 5 and 8 account for up to 70% of strains resistant to phagocytosis by polymorphonuclear leukocytes in vitro. The cell wall peptidoglycan, a polysaccharide polymer, elicits endogenous pyrogen production from monocytes, is chemotactic, activates complement, has endotoxin-like properties, and stimulates opsonic antibody production. Many staphylococci also produce a loose polysaccharide capsule, or slime layer, which may interfere with opsonophagocytosis.

EPIDEMIOLOGY. Most neonates are colonized within the first week of life and 20–30% of normal individuals carry *S. aureus* in the anterior nares at all times.

The organisms may be transmitted from the nose to the skin, where colonization seems to be more transient. Repeated recovery of *S. aureus* from the skin suggests repeated transfer rather than persistent skin colonization. Persistent umbilical and perianal carriage has been described.

Transmission of *S. aureus* generally occurs by direct contact or by spread of heavy particles over a distance of 6 ft or less. Spread by fomites is rare. Heavily colonized individuals and perianal carriers are particularly effective disseminators. Neonates are extremely susceptible to staphylococci; the nasopharynx, skin, perineum, and umbilical stump are the most common sites of colonization. Autoinfection is common, and minor infection (e.g., styes, pustules, paronychia) may be the source of disseminations. Handwashing between contacts with patients decreases the spread of staphylococci from patient to patient. Older children and adults are more resistant than the neonate to colonization.

Infection may follow colonization. Antibiotic therapy with a

*Modified from the 14th edition by Robert M. Kliegman and Ralph D. Feigin.

drug to which *S. aureus* is resistant favors colonization and the development of infection. Other factors that increase the likelihood of infection include wounds, skin disease, ventriculoatrial shunts, intravenous or intrathecal catheterization, corticosteroid treatment, starvation, acidosis, and azotemia. Viral infections of the respiratory tract also may predispose to secondary bacterial infection with staphylococci.

PATHOGENESIS. The development of staphylococcal disease is related to resistance of the host to infection and to virulence of the organism. The intact skin and mucous membranes serve as barriers to invasion by staphylococci. Defects in the mucocutaneous barriers produced by trauma, surgery, foreign surfaces (e.g., sutures, shunts, intravascular catheters), and burns increase the risk of infection. Adhesion of *S. aureus* to mucosal cells is mediated by teichoic acid in the cell wall, and exposure to the submucosa or subcutaneous sites increases adhesion to fibrinogen, fibronectin, laminin, and perhaps collagen IV. The ability of virulent staphylococci to establish disease may be related directly to their capacity to inhibit chemotaxis.

Protein A, present in most strains of *S. aureus* but not in *S. epidermidis,* reacts specifically with IgG1, IgG2, and IgG4. It is located on the outermost coat of the bacterium and can absorb serum immunoglobulin, preventing antibacterial antibodies from acting as opsonins and thus inhibiting phagocytosis. Leukocidin, causing degranulation of leukocytes, and staphylococcal hemolysin that is toxic to erythrocytes and leukocytes also contribute to the virulence of *S. aureus.*

Proliferation of staphylococci in the gastrointestinal tract is also controlled by the prevalence of other bacterial species. If this balance is upset during antibiotic therapy, resistant staphylococci may proliferate and invade the bowel wall. Elaboration of enterotoxin by staphylococci within the gastrointestinal tract or ingestion of preformed enterotoxins may produce disease in the absence of tissue invasion.

The infant may acquire type-specific humoral immunity to staphylococci transplacentally. Older children and adults develop antibodies to staphylococci as a result of intermittent minor infections of the skin and soft tissues; the antistaphylococcal titer of serum generally increases after overt staphylococcal disease. The presence of antibody, however, does not always protect the individual from staphylococcal disease. There is some indication that disseminated *S. aureus* disease in previously healthy children may occur after a viral infection that suppresses neutrophil or respiratory epithelial cell function.

Individuals with congenital or acquired defects in the complement system required for chemotaxis, defective chemotaxis (Job, Chédiak-Higashi, Wiskott-Aldrich, and lazy leukocyte syndromes), defective phagocytosis, and defective humoral immunity (antibodies required for opsonization) as well as those with an impaired intracellular bactericidal capacity are at increased risk of infection with staphylococci. Patients with *chronic granulomatous disease,* in which phagocytosis proceeds normally but killing of ingested catalase-positive bacteria is severely impaired, are particularly susceptible to staphylococcal disease. Impaired mobilization of polymorphonuclear leukocytes has been documented in children with diabetic ketoacidosis and in healthy individuals after ingesting alcohol. Patients with human immunodeficiency virus (HIV) infection have neutrophils that are defective in their ability to kill *S. aureus* in vitro.

CLINICAL MANIFESTATIONS. The signs and symptoms vary with the location of the infection, which, although most commonly located on the skin, may involve any organ, the subcutaneous tissues, and the musculoskeletal system. Disease states of various degrees of severity are generally the result of local suppuration, systemic dissemination with metastatic infection, or systemic effects of toxin production. Although the nasopharynx and skin of many persons may be colonized with *S. aureus,* disease due to this organism is relatively uncommon. Lesions, especially those of the skin, are considerably more prevalent among persons living in low socioeconomic circumstances and particularly among those in tropical climates.

Newborn. Nosocomial infections are discussed in Part XII, Section 1, staphylococcal diseases in general sepsis and meningitis in Chapter 168, pneumonia in Chapter 170, otitis media in Chapter 590, conjunctivitis in Chapter 577, and osteomyelitis and septic arthritis in Chapter 172.

Skin. Pyogenic skin infections may be primary or secondary to wounds or may be a superinfection of other noninfectious skin disease (eczema) or of impetigo contagiosa.

Impetigo contagiosa, ecthyma, bullous impetigo, folliculitis, hydradenitis, furuncles, carbuncles, staphylococcal scalded skin syndrome (i.e., Ritter disease), and a syndrome resembling the rash of scarlet fever are described in Chapter 175. An identical clinical picture may be seen in patients with wounds, especially burns, that are secondarily infected with staphylococci. Folliculitis (i.e., pyodermia of the hair follicle) may extend to a deep-seated furuncle or carbuncle if more than one hair follicle is involved. *Recurrent furunculosis* is a disorder of unknown cause and is associated with repeated episodes of pyoderma over months to years. The patient should be evaluated for immune defects associated with recurrent infection, and the family should be evaluated for nasal colonization with *S. aureus.* Nosocomial skin lesions, including pustules and cellulitis, are discussed in Part XII, Section 1.

Respiratory Tract. Infections of the upper respiratory tract due to *S. aureus* are rare considering the frequency with which this area is colonized. Otitis media (see Chapter 590) and sinusitis (see Chapter 327) due to *S. aureus* may rarely occur. Staphylococcal sinusitis is relatively common in children with cystic fibrosis or defects in white blood cell function. Suppurative parotitis is a rare infection, but *S. aureus* is a common cause. Staphylococcal tonsillopharyngitis is rare except in children whose response to infection has been compromised. **Tracheitis** that clinically complicates viral croup may be caused by *S. aureus.* Patients typically have high fever, leukocytosis, and evidence of severe upper airway obstruction. Direct laryngoscopy or bronchoscopy shows a normal epiglottis with subglottic narrowing and thick purulent secretions within the trachea.

Pneumonia (see Chapter 170) due to *S. aureus* may be primary (hematogenous) or secondary after a viral infection such as influenza. Hematogenous pneumonia may be secondary to septic emboli, right-sided endocarditis, or the presence of intravascular devices. Inhalation pneumonia is caused by alterations of mucociliary clearance, leukocyte dysfunction, or bacterial adherence initiated by a viral infection. In children younger than 1 yr of age, the onset may be heralded by expiratory wheeze, briefly simulating bronchiolitis. More common are high fever, abdominal pain, tachypnea, dyspnea, and localized or diffuse bronchopneumonia or lobar disease. Staphylococci cause a necrotizing pneumonitis; empyema, pneumatoceles, pyopneumothorax, and bronchopleural fistulas develop frequently. Occasionally, staphylococcal pneumonia produces a diffuse interstitial disease characterized by extreme dyspnea, tachypnea, and cyanosis. Cough may be nonproductive. See the discussion of pneumonia in cystic fibrosis in Chapter 363.

Sepsis (see Chapter 168). Staphylococcal bacteremia and sepsis may be associated with any localized infection. The onset may be acute and marked by nausea, vomiting, myalgia, fever, and chills. Organisms may localize subsequently at any site but are found especially in the lung, heart, joints, bones, kidneys, and brain. If appropriate antibiotic therapy is provided, blood cultures may remain positive for 24–48 hr. The fever begins to decrease at a median time of 22 hr (range, 8–90 hr), and the body temperature returns to normal at a median time of 58 hr (range, 12–180 hr) in patients with *S. aureus* septicemia.

Differentiating sepsis from endocarditis may be difficult. Echocardiographic evidence of vegetations, intravenous drug abuse, presence of immune complexes and antistaphylococcal antibodies, and absence of a primary focus of infection suggests endocarditis.

In some instances, especially if treatment of a local infection has been inadequate, disseminated staphylococcal disease occurs, characterized by fever, bone or joint pain, and urticarial, petechial, maculopapular, or pustular rashes. Less frequently, hematuria, jaundice, seizures, nuchal rigidity, and cardiac murmurs are detected. Leukopenia or leukocytosis, proteinuria, and red and white blood cells in the urinary sediment may be noticed.

Muscle. Localized staphylococcal abscesses in muscle associated with elevation of muscle enzymes but without septicemia have been called **tropical pyomyositis.** Although this disorder has been reported most frequently from tropical areas, it also has occurred in the United States in otherwise healthy children. Multiple abscesses occur in 30–40% of cases. Prodromal symptoms may include coryza, pharyngitis, diarrhea, or prior trauma at the site of the abscess. Surgical drainage and appropriate antibiotic therapy are essential.

Bones and Joints. *S. aureus* is the most common cause of osteomyelitis and septic arthritis in children (see Chapter 172).

Central Nervous System. *Meningitis* (see Chapter 169.1) due to *S. aureus* is associated with cranial trauma and neurosurgical procedures (e.g., craniotomy, cerebrospinal fluid [CSF] shunt placement), and less frequently with endocarditis, parameningeal foci (e.g., epidural or brain abscess), diabetes mellitus, or malignancy. The CSF profile in *S. aureus* meningitis is indistinguishable from that of other bacterial causes of meningitis.

Heart. *Acute bacterial endocarditis* (see Chapter 390) may follow staphylococcal bacteremia. *S. aureus* is a common cause of acute virulent endocarditis on native valves. Perforation of heart valves, myocardial abscesses, heart failure, conduction disturbances, acute hemopericardium, purulent pericarditis, and sudden death may ensue.

Kidney. *S. aureus* is a common cause of renal and perinephric abscess (see Chapter 492). Urinary tract infection due to *S. aureus* is unusual.

Toxic Shock Syndrome. See Chapter 174.3.

Intestinal Tract. *Staphylococcal enterocolitis* follows overgrowth of normal bowel flora by staphylococci. This infection most commonly follows use of broad-spectrum oral antibiotic therapy. Diarrhea is associated with blood and mucus.

Peritonitis associated with *S. aureus* in patients receiving chronic ambulatory peritoneal dialysis usually involves the catheter tunnel. Removal of the catheter is required to achieve a bacteriologic cure.

Food poisoning (see Chapter 171) may be caused by ingestion of enterotoxins preformed by staphylococci contaminating foods. Two to 7 hr after ingestion of the toxin, sudden, severe vomiting begins. Watery diarrhea may develop, but fever is absent or low. Symptoms rarely persist longer than 12–24 hr. Rarely, shock and death may occur.

DIAGNOSIS. The diagnosis of staphylococcal infection depends on isolation of the organisms from skin lesions, abscess cavities, blood, cerebrospinal fluid, or other sites of infection. Toxin-producing organisms may be recovered from sites of colonization (e.g., nasopharynx, vagina). The organisms can be grown readily in liquid and on solid media. After isolation, identification is made on the basis of Gram stain and coagulase and mannitol reactivity. Patterns of sensitivity to antibiotics can be assessed and the organism phage-typed if necessary for epidemiologic reasons.

Diagnosis of staphylococcal food poisoning generally is made on the basis of epidemiologic and clinical findings. Food suspected of contamination should be examined by Gram stain, cultured, and tested for enterotoxin. Enterotoxin testing can be done by the Centers for Disease Control and Prevention.

DIFFERENTIAL DIAGNOSIS. Skin lesions due to *S. aureus* and those due to group A β-hemolytic streptococci may be indistinguishable. Staphylococcal pneumonia can be suspected on the basis of chest roentgenograms that may reveal pneumatoceles, pyopneumothorax, or lung abscess. These changes suggesting a necrotizing pneumonitis are not pathognomonic for staphylococcal infection and may be seen in patients with pneumonia due to other bacteria, including *Klebsiella* and many anaerobes. Fluctuant skin and soft tissue lesions also can be caused by many organisms, including *Mycobacterium, Francisella tularensis,* and various fungi and may be seen in patients with cat-scratch disease.

PREVENTION. Staphylococcal infection is transmitted primarily by direct contact. *Strict attention to handwashing techniques* is the most effective measure for preventing the spread of staphylococci from one individual to another (see Chapter 249). Use of a detergent containing an iodophor, chlorhexidine, or hexachlorophene is recommended. In hospitals or other institutional settings, all persons with acute staphylococcal infections should be isolated until they have been treated adequately. There should be constant surveillance for nosocomial staphylococcal infections within hospitals. Infectious disease control measures may reduce the spread of infection (Table 174–1).

Patients in an intensive care unit who received sucralfate instead of H_2-blocking agents for prophylaxis against stress ulceration were shown to have reduced gastric colonization with *S. aureus.* The reduction in colonization is secondary to the maintenance of natural gastric acidity with sucralfate. This difference in therapy was associated with a decrease in the frequency of pneumonia.

Patients with recurrent staphylococcal furunculosis may be treated with hexachlorophene washes and dicloxacillin or clindamycin to prevent recurrences.

Food poisoning may be prevented by excluding individuals with staphylococcal infections of the skin from the preparation and handling of food. Prepared foods should be eaten immediately or refrigerated appropriately to prevent multiplication of staphylococci with which the food may have been contaminated.

TREATMENT. Antibiotic therapy alone is rarely effective in individuals with undrained abscesses or with infected foreign bodies. Loculated collections of purulent material should be relieved by incision and drainage. Foreign bodies should be removed, if possible. Therapy always should be initiated with a penicillinase-resistant antibiotic because more than 90% of all staphylococci isolated, regardless of source, are resistant to penicillin.

For serious infections parenteral treatment is indicated. Although clinically they are equally efficacious, methacillin and nafcillin have a more stable β-lactam ring against β-lactamase

■ TABLE 174–1 Infectious Disease Control Measures Used to Prevent Spread of *Staphylococcus* Epidemics

Reinforcement of regulation for handwashing prior to examining each patient
Hand-to-elbow wash with chlorhexidine or an iodophor
Barrier precautions and/or strict isolation: gowns and/or gloves worn by staff
Isolation of cohort nurses with patients
Identification of nosocomial strain (e.g., antibiotic sensitivity, phage type, DNA profile)
Colonization surveillance of staff
Reassignment of staff with active lesions or colonization
Discharge of colonized patients as soon as possible
Notation on patient chart of colonization status if readmitted to hospital
Monitoring of fomites (e.g., instruments) for colonization
Elimination of nasal colonization with topical bacitracin or mupirocin, and oral rifampin or ciprofloxacin
Topical hexachlorophene (3%) washing during neonatal epidemics*
Triple dye to the umbilical cord

**Excessive use of topical hexachlorophene may be absorbed and may produce neurotoxicity in premature infants or patients with extensive cutaneous lesions.*

than does oxacillin. This stability is most important if there is a large bacterial burden, since the associated inoculum effect may neutralize the antibacterial activity of β-lactam antibiotics. Generally, a dose of 200 mg/kg/24 hr should be employed intravenously in six divided doses. Serious staphylococcal infections, with or without abscesses, tend to persist and recur, necessitating prolonged therapy.

The antibiotic employed as well as the dose, route, and duration of treatment depends on the site of infection, the response of the patient to treatment, and the sensitivity of the organisms recovered from blood or from local sites of infection. In patients with staphylococcal pneumonia, intravenous treatment is recommended until the patient has been afebrile for 72 hr and other signs of infection have disappeared. Oral therapy is continued for a total of 3 wk, longer in selected cases. The treatment of staphylococcal osteomyelitis (see Chapter 172), meningitis (see Chapter 168), and endocarditis (see Chapter 390) are discussed in their respective chapters. In all of these infections, oral treatment should be provided when parenteral therapy has been discontinued; dicloxacillin is penicillinase resistant, absorbed well orally, and quite effective. This drug is administered in a dose of 50–75 mg/kg/24 hr in four divided oral doses. The duration of oral therapy also depends on the response of the patient as determined by the clinical, roentgenographic, and laboratory findings and by culture results.

Skin and soft tissue infection and minor upper respiratory tract infection may be managed by oral therapy alone or by an initial brief course of antibiotics provided parenterally, followed by oral medication. Dicloxacillin (25–50 mg/kg/24 hr), oxacillin (100 mg/kg/24 hr), or nafcillin (100 mg/kg/24 hr), each in four divided oral doses, provides excellent blood and tissue concentrations of these antibiotics. Amoxicillin combined with the β-lactamase inhibitor clavulanic acid also is effective at a dose based on the amoxicillin component of 40 mg/kg/24 hr in three divided doses. In patients with very mild, localized skin infection, repeated cleansing with a mild antiseptic and use of topical antibiotics (e.g., bacitracin, mupirocin) may be effective. Penicillin should not be applied topically.

Penicillin G can be used to treat infections due to *S. aureus* if the organism proves sensitive to this antibiotic in vitro.

Individuals sensitive to penicillin and its derivatives must be treated with other antibiotics or desensitized to the penicillin derivative to be employed. About 5% of penicillin-sensitive children are also sensitive to cephalosporins. Clindamycin and lincomycin have proved effective for the treatment of skin, soft tissue, bone, and joint infections due to *S. aureus*. Clindamycin may be provided in 3–4 divided doses parenterally or orally (total daily dose, 30–40 mg/kg/24 hr). Clindamycin and lincomycin should *not* be used to treat endocarditis, brain abscess, or meningitis due to *S. aureus*. Vancomycin can be used to treat penicillin-sensitive individuals with endocarditis, but serum levels of this antibiotic should be monitored when it is used. Peak serum concentrations should be 25–40 μg/mL. It can be administered in a dose of 10–15 mg/kg/dose given every 6 hr intravenously. Vancomycin or teicoplanin (a vancomycin derivative) should be used to treat bacteremic staphylococcal infections when the organism is resistant to semisynthetic penicillin derivatives. Despite in vitro susceptibility of *S. aureus* to ciprofloxacin and other quinolone antibiotics, these agents should not be used in serious staphylococcal infections, because their use has not consistently been associated with high cure rates.

Staphylococcal infection of the central nervous system can be treated by intravenous methicillin or nafcillin and, in penicillin-allergic children, by vancomycin, trimethoprim-sulfamethoxazole, or imipenem. Rifampin may be added to vancomycin for synergy.

METHICILLIN-RESISTANT *STAPHYLOCOCCUS AUREUS*. Methicillin-resistant *S. aureus* (MRSA) has become a major nosocomial pathogen. Patients at risk for MRSA infection are the seriously ill (e.g., those with burns, surgical wounds, chronic venous access, lengthy hospitalizations, contact with other MRSA-infected patients, and premature infants). Most MRSA strains belong to phage group II (types 77, 83A, 84, and 85); however, outbreaks with nontypable and phage group I strains have been reported.

The resistance to semisynthetic penicillins is thought to be related to a novel penicillin-binding protein that is relatively insensitive to antibiotics containing a β-lactam ring. A low-level resistance related to enhanced production of β-lactamases also may occur. MRSA strains appear to be as virulent as their methicillin-sensitive counterparts. Vancomycin and its derivative, teicoplanin, are highly effective in the treatment of these infections. Vancomycin is the drug of choice if MRSA is considered a possible cause of infection or has been isolated. MRSA is also resistant to cephalosporins and imipenem but often remains sensitive to trimethoprim-sulfamethoxazole and ciprofloxacin.

When MRSA is recovered, strict isolation of affected patients has been shown to be the most effective method for preventing nosocomial spread of infection. Thereafter, control measures should be directed toward identification of new isolates and strict isolation of newly colonized or infected patients. It also may be necessary to identify colonized hospital personnel and eradicate carriage in affected individuals (Table 174–1).

PROGNOSIS. Untreated staphylococcal septicemia is associated with a mortality rate of 80% or greater. Mortality rates have been reduced to 20% by appropriate antibiotic treatment. Staphylococcal pneumonia can be fatal at any age but is more likely to be associated with high morbidity and mortality in young infants or in patients whose therapy has been delayed.

A total white blood cell count below 5,000/mm^3 or a polymorphonuclear leukocyte response of less than 50% is a grave prognostic sign. Prognosis also may be influenced by numerous host factors, including nutrition, immunologic competence, and the presence or absence of other debilitating diseases.

174.2 Infections Due to Coagulase-Negative Staphylococci

S. epidermidis is one of 11 recognized species of coagulase-negative staphylococci (CONS) affecting or colonizing humans. Originally thought to be avirulent commensal bacteria, CONS, particularly *S. epidermidis*, is now known to produce nosocomial infections in patients with indwelling foreign devices (intravenous catheters—sepsis; hemodialysis shunts and grafts—sepsis; cerebrospinal fluid shunts—meningitis; peritoneal dialysis catheters—peritonitis; pacemaker wires and electrodes—pocket infection; prosthetic cardiac valves—endocarditis; urinary catheters—pyelonephritis; prosthetic joints—arthritis), surgical trauma (sternal osteomyelitis, endophthalmitis), immunocompromised states (malignancy, granulocytopenia, neonates), and, rarely, community-acquired disease in patients with no underlying disease (urinary tract infection, osteomyelitis). *S. haemolyticus*, another CONS species, is an important cause of invasive infection and may develop resistance to vancomycin and teicoplanin.

EPIDEMIOLOGY. CONS consist of normal inhabitants of the human skin, throat, mouth, vagina, and urethra. *S. epidermidis* is the most common and persistent species, representing 65–90% of staphylococci present on the skin and mucous membranes. Colonization, usually acquired from hospital staff, precedes infection; alternatively, direct inoculation during surgery may initiate infection through CSF shunts or prosthetic valves. For epidemiologic purposes, CONS can be identified on the basis of phage typing, antibiotic sensitivities, slime layer production, and molecular DNA methods (chromosomal and phage DNA hybridization—restriction enzyme analysis).

PATHOGENESIS. *S. epidermidis* produces an exopolysaccharide protective biofilm (slime) that surrounds the organism and may enhance adhesion to foreign surfaces, resist phagocytosis, and impair penetration of antibiotics.

CLINICAL MANIFESTATIONS. Bacteremia. CONS, specifically *S. epidermidis*, are the most common cause of nosocomial bacteremia. In the neonate *S. epidermidis* bacteremia, with or without a central venous catheter, may manifest as apnea, bradycardia, temperature instability, abdominal distention, hematochezia, meningitis in the absence of CSF pleocytosis, cutaneous abscesses, and persistence of positive blood cultures for as long as 2 wk despite adequate antimicrobial therapy. *S. epidermidis* bacteremia in patients with bone marrow transplantation and malignancy (e.g., leukemia, lymphoma) is associated with neutropenia, central venous access (Hickman or Broviac catheters), and gastrointestinal colonization. In most circumstances *S. epidermidis* bacteremia is indolent and is not usually associated with overwhelming septic shock.

Endocarditis. Infection of native heart valves or the right atrial wall secondary to an infected thrombosis at the end of a central line may produce endocarditis. *S. epidermidis* and other CONS may also produce native valve, subacute indolent endocarditis in previously normal patients without a central venous catheter. *S. epidermidis* is a common cause of prosthetic valve endocarditis, presumably due to inoculation at the time of surgery. Infection of the valve sewing ring, with abscess formation and dissection, produces valve dysfunction, dehiscence, arrhythmias, or valve obstruction. See Chapter 390 for clinical manifestations.

Central Venous Catheter Infection. Central venous catheters become infected through the exit site and subcutaneous tunnel, which provide a direct path to the bloodstream. *S. epidermidis* is the most common CONS, owing in part to its high rate of cutaneous colonization. Line sepsis manifests as fever, leukocytosis, tenderness and erythema at the exit site or along the subcutaneous tunnel, and catheter thrombosis.

Central Nervous System CSF Shunts. *S. epidermidis*, introduced at the time of surgery, is the most common pathogen associated with CSF shunt meningitis. Most (70–80%) infections occur within 2 mo of the operation and are manifest by signs of meningeal irritation, fever, increased intracranial pressure (headache), and peritonitis due to the intra-abdominal position of the distal end of the shunt tubing.

Urinary Tract Infection. *S. epidermidis* causes asymptomatic urinary tract infection in hospitalized patients with urinary catheters and after urinary tract surgery or transplantation. *S. saprophyticus* is a common cause of symptomatic urinary tract infection in previously healthy, sexually active teenage girls after urethral colonization. Manifestations are similar to those characteristic of urinary tract infection due to *Escherichia coli* (see Chapter 492).

S. epidermidis is the most common pathogen producing peritonitis in patients on continuous ambulatory peritoneal dialysis. Manifestations of infection include abdominal pain, fever, more than 100 neutrophils/mm^3, and a positive culture or Gram stain.

DIAGNOSIS. Because *S. epidermidis* is a common skin inhabitant and may contaminate poorly collected blood cultures, it may be difficult to differentiate bacteremia from contamination. Similarly, it may be difficult to differentiate bacteremia due to line sepsis from sepsis not associated with central venous line colonization. Bacteremia should be suspected when blood cultures grow rapidly (within 24 hr), when two or more blood cultures are positive with the same CONS, when the peripheral venous blood culture has a quantitative colony count comparable to that drawn from a central venous catheter, and when clinical and laboratory signs and symptoms compatible with CONS sepsis are present and subsequently resolve with appropriate therapy. No blood culture that is positive for *S. epidermidis* should be considered contaminated without careful assessment of the above criteria and examination of the patient.

TREATMENT. Most *S. epidermidis* are resistant to methicillin. Vancomycin is the drug of choice for methicillin-resistant *S. epidermidis*. The new quinolones and teicoplanin have some activity against CONS, and the addition of rifampin or gentamicin to vancomycin may increase antimicrobial efficacy. In many cases of CONS infection associated with foreign bodies, the catheter, valve, or shunt must be removed to ensure a cure. Prosthetic heart valves and CSF shunts usually have to be removed to treat the infection adequately.

Antibiotic therapy given through an infected central venous catheter (through each lumen) may effectively cure *S. epidermidis* line sepsis. If the catheter or reservoir is no longer needed, it should be removed. Unfortunately, this is not always possible owing to the therapeutic requirements of the underlying disease (nutrition for short bowel syndrome, chemotherapy for malignancy). A trial of intravenous vancomycin is indicated to preserve the use of the central line.

Peritonitis in patients on continuous ambulatory peritoneal dialysis due to *S. epidermidis* is another infection that may be treated with intravenous or intraperitoneal antibiotics without removing the dialysis catheter. If the organism is resistant to methicillin, vancomycin adjusted for renal function is appropriate therapy.

PROGNOSIS. Most episodes of CONS bacteremia respond successfully to antibiotics. Poor prognosis is associated with malignancy, neutropenia, and infected prosthetic or native heart valves. CONS increases morbidity, the duration of hospitalization, and mortality rates among patients with underlying complicated illnesses.

174.3 Toxic Shock Syndrome

TSS is an acute, multisystemic disease characterized by high fever, hypotension, vomiting, abdominal pain, diarrhea, myalgias, nonfocal neurologic abnormalities, and an erythematous rash.

ETIOLOGY AND EPIDEMIOLOGY. Many cases occur in menstruating women between 15 and 25 yr of age who use tampons or other vaginal devices (e.g., diaphragm, contraceptive sponge) in the presence of vaginal colonization or infection with toxin-producing strains of *S. aureus*. TSS, however, also occurs in children, nonmenstruating women, and men. Nonmenstrual TSS has been associated with wounds, nasal packing, sinusitis, tracheitis, pneumonia, empyema, abscesses, burns, osteomyelitis, and primary bacteremia. Without antimicrobial therapy, there is a high recurrence rate (30%) in menstrual TSS, with secondary cases being milder and occurring within 3 mo of the original episode; the overall mortality rate is 3%.

A majority of *S. aureus* strains isolated from confirmed cases are phage group I, are noninvasive, do not adhere to vaginal epithelium, and produce a number of extracellular toxins. The primary toxin associated with TSS is toxic shock syndrome toxin (TSST-1). TSST-1 causes massive loss of fluid from the intravascular space directly or following production of interleukin-1 and tumor necrosis factor. However, TSST-1 negative strains have been isolated from patients with TSS, suggesting that other toxins (including the enterotoxins) play a role in TSS (especially nonmenstrual) and that TSST-1 production is not essential to the pathogenesis of this illness. Epidemiologic and in vitro studies suggest that these toxins are selectively produced in a clinical environment consisting of a neutral pH, a high P_{CO_2}, and an "aerobic" P_{O_2}, which are the conditions found in the vagina with tampon use during menstruation.

CLINICAL MANIFESTATIONS. The diagnosis of TSS is based on clinical manifestations (see Table 174–2). The onset is abrupt with high fever, vomiting, and diarrhea and is accompanied by sore throat, headache, and myalgias. A diffuse erythematous macular rash (sunburn-like) appears within 24 hr and may be associated with hyperemia of pharyngeal, conjunctival, and vaginal mucous membranes. Petechiae may develop on day 3–4. Symptoms often include alterations in the level of consciousness, oliguria, and hypotension, which in severe cases may progress to shock and disseminated intravascular coagulation. The most frequent manifestations include diarrhea (98%), myalgia (96%), emesis (92%), fever of more than 40° C (87%), headache (72%), and sore throat (75%). Recovery occurs within 7–10 days and is associated with desquamation, particularly of palms and soles; hair and nail loss have also been observed after 1–2 mo.

There is no specific laboratory test; appropriate selective tests reveal involvement of multiple organ systems including the hepatic, renal, muscular, gastrointestinal, cardiopulmonary, and central nervous system. The most frequent laboratory signs include increased creatinine (69%), thrombocytopenia (59%), hypocalcemia (58%), azotemia (57%), hyperbilirubinemia (54%), elevated liver enzymes (50%), and leukocytosis of 15,000 or more (48%). Bacterial cultures of the associated focus (e.g., vagina, abscess), prior to administration of antibiotics, usually yield *S. aureus.*

DIFFERENTIAL DIAGNOSIS. Kawasaki disease (mucocutaneous lymph node syndrome) closely resembles TSS clinically but is usually not as severe. Both are associated with fever unresponsive to antibiotics, hyperemia of mucous membranes, and an erythematous rash with subsequent desquamation. Many of the clinical features of TSS, however, are absent or rare in Kawasaki disease, including diffuse myalgia, vomiting, abdominal pain, diarrhea, azotemia, hypotension, adult respiratory distress syndrome (see Chapter 152), and shock. Kawasaki disease typically occurs in children under 5 yr of age, and some cases of "adult Kawasaki disease" may be TSS. Scarlet fever, Rocky Mountain spotted fever, leptospirosis, toxic epidermal necrolysis, sepsis, and measles must also be considered in the differential diagnosis. Group A streptococci can cause a similar toxic shock–like illness.

PREVENTION AND TREATMENT. The low risk of acquiring TSS (6.2 cases/100,000 menstruating women) can be reduced by not using tampons or by using them intermittently during each menstrual period.

Management of adolescents suspected of having TSS includes the careful removal of any retained tampons at the time of taking initial samples for cervical and vaginal cultures. Fluid replacement should be aggressive to prevent or treat cardiovascular collapse. Inotropic agents may be needed to treat shock; corticosteroids and intravenous immune globulin are reserved for severe cases.

Parenteral administration of a β-lactamase–resistant antistaphylococcal antibiotic (e.g., nafcillin, oxacillin, methicillin) is recommended after appropriate cultures have been obtained. Culture of the vagina in menstrual TSS and of infected or colonized sites in nonmenstrual TSS is indicated. Antistaphylococcal therapy with methicillin, nafcillin, or oxacillin (150–200 mg/kg/24 hr, given in four to six divided doses [adult: 8–10 g/24 hr]) for 10–14 days does not affect the immediate outcome but prevents recurrence in menstrual TSS. Antibiotics and drainage are indicated for specific staphylococcal infections such as sinusitis or osteomyelitis. Alternative antibiotics for patients allergic to penicillin include clindamycin, erythromycin, rifampin, and trimethoprim-sulfamethoxazole.

■ TABLE 174–2 Clinical and Laboratory Criteria for Toxic Shock Syndrome

Fever (temperature ≥ 38.9° C)
Rash (diffuse macular erythroderma) with desquamation, 1–2 wk after onset of illness, particularly of palms and soles
Hypotension (systolic blood pressure ≤ 90 mm Hg in adults or <5th percentile for age in children aged <16 years, or orthostatic syncope)
Involvement of three or more of the following organ systems:
Gastrointestinal (vomiting or diarrhea at onset of illness)
Muscular (severe myalgia or creatine kinase level ≥ twice upper limits of normal for laboratory)
Mucous membrane (vaginal, oropharyngeal, or conjunctival hyperemia)
Renal (blood urea nitrogen level or serum creatinine level ≥ twice upper limits of normal for laboratory or ≥5 leukocytes/high-power field, in the absence of urinary tract infection)
Hepatic (total bilirubin, serum aspartate aminotransaminase [AST] or serum alanine aminotransaminase [ALT] activity ≥ twice upper limits of normal for laboratory)
Hematologic (platelet count ≤ 100 × 10^9/L)
Central nervous system (disorientation or alterations in consciousness without focal neurologic signs when fever and hypotension are absent)
Negative results on the serologic tests for Rocky Mountain spotted fever, leptospirosis, and measles

Staphylococcus aureus

Brumfitt W, Hamilton-Miller J: Methicillin-resistant *Staphylococcus aureus.* N Engl J Med 320:1188, 1989.

Eng RHK, Bishburg E, Smith SM, et al: *Staphylococcus aureus* bacteremia during therapy. J Infect Dis 155:1331, 1987.

Hodes DS, Barzilai A: Invasive and toxin mediated *Staphylococcus aureus* diseases in children. Adv Pediatr Infect Dis 5:35, 1990.

Kim JH, van der Horst C, Mulrow CD, et al: *Staphylococcus aureus* meningitis: Review of 28 cases. Rev Infect Dis 2:698, 1989.

Marrack P, Kappler: The staphylococcal enterotoxins and their relatives. Science 248:705, 1990.

Ribner BS: Endemic, multiply resistant *Staphylococcus aureus* in a pediatric population. Am J Dis Child 141:1183, 1987.

Todd JK, Todd BH, Franco-Buff A, Smith C, Lawellin DW: Influence of focal infection conditions on the pathogenesis of toxic shock syndrome. J Infect Dis 155:673, 1987.

Coagulase-Negative Staphylococcus

Boyce MJ, Potter-Bynoe G, Opal SM, et al: A common-source outbreak of *Staphylococcus epidermidis* infections among patients undergoing cardiac surgery. J Infect Dis 161:493, 1990.

Gruskay J, Harris MC, Costarino AT, et al: Neonatal *Staphylococcus epidermidis* meningitis with unremarkable CSF examination results. Am J Dis Child 143:580, 1989.

Latham RH, Running K, Stamm WE: Urinary tract infections in young adult women caused by *Staphylococcus saprophyticus.* JAMA 250:3063, 1983.

Patrick CC: Coagulase-negative staphylococci: Pathogens with increasing clinical significance. J Pediatr 116:497, 1990.

Patrick CC, Kaplan SL, Baker CJ, et al: Persistent bacteremia due to coagulase-negative staphylococci in low birth weight neonates. Pediatrics 84:977, 1989.

Younger JJ, Christensen GD, Bartley DL, et al: Coagulase-negative staphylococci isolated from cerebrospinal fluid shunts: Importance of slime production, species identification, and shunt removal to clinical outcome. J Infect Dis 156:548, 1987.

Toxic Shock Syndrome

Ferguson MA, Todd JK: Toxic shock syndrome associated with *Staphylococcus aureus* sinusitis in children. J Infect Dis 161:953, 1990.

Todd JK: Toxic shock syndrome. Clin Microbiol Rev 1:432, 1988.

Todd JK: Therapy of toxic shock syndrome. Drugs 39:856, 1990.

Todd JK, Todd BH, Franco-Buff A, et al. Influence of focal infection conditions on the pathogenesis of toxic shock syndrome. J Infect Dis 155:673, 1987.

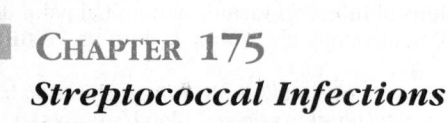

CHAPTER 175
Streptococcal Infections

James Todd

Streptococci are among the most common causes of bacterial infection in infancy and childhood. Group A streptococci, the most common *bacterial* cause of acute pharyngitis, also produce a large variety of other infections and nonsuppurative sequelae such as rheumatic fever (see Chapter 175) and glomerulonephritis (see Chapter 465). Infection during the first 3 mo of life with group B β-hemolytic streptococci is common and may present as bacteremia, meningitis, osteomyelitis, or septic arthritis (see Chapter 98).

ETIOLOGY. Streptococci are gram-positive cocci that grow in pairs or variable length chains, classified on the basis of their ability to hemolyze red blood cells: those with hemolysins producing complete hemolysis (β-*hemolytic*), those producing partial hemolysis (α-*hemolytic*), and those producing no hemolysis (γ-*hemolytic*). α-Hemolysis produces a green color on sheep erythrocytes (viridans group).

Lancefield further separated the streptococci on the basis of differences in carbohydrate components (C-carbohydrate) within the cell wall; streptococcal groups A through H and K through V have been identified so far. The cell wall is composed of three distinct layers. The outer portion contains several antigenic proteins; the most important is M protein. Group A β-hemolytic streptococci can be divided into more than 80 immunologically distinct types that are based on differences in the M protein. M antigen resists phagocytosis and is the major virulence factor. Lipoteichoic acid, another cell wall constituent, is another virulence factor that promotes colonization by binding to fibronectin on the surface of epithelial cells. The hyaluronic acid capsule resists phagocytosis, further facilitating virulence. Acquired immunity is directed at the M protein.

Streptococci elaborate toxins, enzymes, and hemolysins. More than 20 extracellular antigens released by group A hemolytic streptococci growing in human tissues have been identified. The extracellular products of greatest clinical significance are pyrogenic (formerly erythrogenic) exotoxins (A, B, and C), streptolysin O, streptolysin S, NADase, streptokinases, DNase, hyaluronidase, proteinase, amylase, and esterase. Pyogenic exotoxins are responsible for the rash of scarlet fever and for shock in toxic shock–like illness. Generally, the elaboration of pyogenic exotoxins depends on bacteriophage infection (lysogeny) of the streptococcus. Streptolysin S is largely cell bound and damages the membranes of neutrophils and platelets. Streptolysin O is produced by most group A and some group G streptococci. It lyses red blood cells and is toxic to neutrophils, platelets, and mammalian heart muscle. Elaboration of streptolysins S and O produces the clear zone of hemolysis permitting classification of the organisms as β-hemolytic strains. Extracellular digestive enzymes liquefy pus and, together with hyaluronidase, facilitate rapid spreading of streptococci through tissue planes. The proteinase, in particular, is associated with tissue destruction of severe invasive streptococcal disease. Antibodies to streptolysin O (ASO), DNase B, hyaluronidase, NADase, and streptokinase are useful in the serodiagnosis of group A streptococcal disease. M-type specific antibodies are detectable 4–8 wk after infection; antibiotic therapy ablates this response.

Separation by type of hemolysis and Lancefield typing as methods of classifying streptococci are not mutually exclusive. Table 175–1 shows classifications by both methods and outlines the relationship of streptococci to human colonization and disease.

GROUP A STREPTOCOCCI

Sequelae of group A β-hemolytic streptococcal disease (e.g., rheumatic fever, glomerulonephritis) are discussed in Chapters 175.1 and 465.

EPIDEMIOLOGY. The incidence of suppurative and nonsuppurative sequelae from group A streptococci increased in the late 1980s and 1990s. The reason for this resurgence of serious streptococcal disease is unknown but is suspected to be related to an increased prevalence of streptococcal strains that produce more of the aforementioned virulence factors. Group A streptococci are normal inhabitants of the nasopharynx; colonization rates in children vary from 15–20%. The incidence of disease depends on the age of the child, the season of the year, climate and geographic location, and the degree of contact with infected individuals.

Generally, incidence is lowest among infants, who may be protected by transplacental acquisition of type-specific antibodies and a lack of pharyngeal receptors for streptococcal binding. Streptococcal infection of the skin is most common in children younger than 6 yr; streptococcal pharyngitis is most common between 5 and 15 yr of age. Streptococcal disease, including scarlet fever, is uncommon in children less than 3 yr of age, but in families with known streptococcal infection, it may present as nonspecific upper respiratory tract infection, pharyngitis, and otitis media, with or without impetigo. The incidence of streptococcal pharyngitis is higher in temperate climates; incidence and severity appear to increase in cold weather. Streptococcal skin disease is more prevalent in tropical climates and in warmer weather in temperate climates.

Group A β-hemolytic streptococci are spread from person to person. Infection may be spread by droplets; nasal and pharyngeal carriers are effective disseminators. Infection also may be spread by contact with skin lesions or transmitted by food, milk, and water.

Acquisition of streptococci generally is associated with crowding in the home, school, military installation, or other institution. Disruption of the cutaneous epithelium predisposes to streptococcal pyoderma or impetigo. Acquisition from an infected individual is most common during the acute illness (3–5 days) and decreases during the colonization stage. Colonization (nasopharyngeal) may precede or follow (2–6 wk) overt infection. Immunity, which is type specific, may be induced either by carriage of the organism or by overt infection. The risk of streptococcal disease diminishes during adult life as immunity develops to the more prevalent serotypes.

PATHOGENESIS. After inhalation or ingestion, streptococci attach themselves to respiratory epithelial cells by their surface fibrils and cell wall lipoteichoic acid. Fibrils contain antiphagocytic epitopes of type-specific M proteins, which with capsular hyaluronic acid resist phagocytosis. Extracellular digestive enzymes facilitate the spread of infection by interfering with local thrombosis (streptolysins) and pus formation (DNase) and enhancing connective tissue digestion (hyaluronidase, proteinase). Suppurative complications follow local inflammation (peritonsillar abscess, retropharyngeal abscess), direct extension (otitis media, sinusitis), lymphangitic spread (lymphadenitis), or bacteremia (sepsis, osteomyelitis, pneumonia).

Scarlet fever–producing streptococci lead to clinical manifestations that are similar to those produced by nonpyrogenic exotoxin-containing strains except for the scarlatiniform rash. Serologically distinct pyrogenic exotoxins (A–C) produce the rash in nonimmune hosts. Rash production is dependent in part on a host hypersensitivity reaction and is decreased by host synthesis of specific antitoxins. These toxins also exhibit pyrogenicity and cytotoxicity; enhance the effects of endotoxin; and have been associated with toxic shock–like illness. Streptococcal pyrogenic exotoxin A has partial amino acid homology with staphylococcal enterotoxin B, which is associated with staphylococcal toxic shock syndrome.

CLINICAL MANIFESTATIONS. The most common infections caused by group A β-hemolytic streptococci involve the respiratory tract, skin, soft tissues, and blood.

Respiratory Tract Infection. See Chapter 327.

Scarlet Fever. This disease is the result of infection by streptococci that elaborate one of three pyrogenic (erythrogenic) exotoxins. The incubation period ranges from 1–7 days, with an average of 3 days. The onset is acute and is characterized by fever, vomiting, headache, toxicity, pharyngitis, and chills.

■ TABLE 175–1 Relationship of Streptococci Identified by Lancefield Grouping and Hemolytic Reactions to Sites of Colonization and Disease

Lancefield Antigen Group	Streptococcal Species	Hemolysis on Sheep Blood Agar*	Site of Colonization	Common Human Diseases
A	*S. pyogenes*	β	Pharynx, skin, rectum	Pharyngitis, tonsillitis, erysipelas, impetigo, septicemia, wound infections, necrotizing fasciitis, cellulitis, meningitis, pneumonia, scarlet fever, toxic shock–like syndrome, rheumatic fever, acute glomerulonephritis
B	*S. agalactiae*	β	Pharynx, vagina	Puerperal sepsis, chorioamnionitis, endocarditis, neonatal sepsis, meningitis, osteomyelitis, pneumonia
C–H, K–O	Various species	β, α	Mouth, pharynx, vagina, skin	Wound infections, puerperal sepsis, cellulitis, sinusitis, endocarditis, brain abscess, sepsis, nosocomial infections, opportunistic infections
Nontypable	*S. viridans*	α	Pharynx	Endocarditis
Nontypable	*S. mutans*	α	Pharynx	Endocarditis
Nontypable	*Enterococcus faecalis, faecium*	α, β, γ	Colon contents	Endocarditis, urinary tract infections, biliary tract infections, intestinal infections, peritonitis, superinfection bacteremia

*α = *partial hemolysis*; β = *complete hemolysis*; γ = *no hemolysis.*

Abdominal pain may be present; when this is associated with vomiting prior to the appearance of the rash, an abdominal surgical condition may be suggested. Within 12–48 hr the typical rash appears.

Generally, temperature increases abruptly and may peak at 39.6–40° C (103–104° F) on the 2nd day and gradually returns to normal within 5–7 days in the untreated patient; it is usually normal within 12–24 hr after initiation of penicillin therapy. The tonsils are hyperemic and edematous and may be covered with a gray-white exudate. The pharynx is inflamed and covered by a membrane in severe cases. The tongue may be edematous and reddened. During the early days of illness the dorsum of the tongue has a white coat through which the red and edematous papillae project (i.e., *white strawberry tongue*). After several days the white coat desquamates; the red tongue studded with prominent papillae persists (i.e., *red strawberry tongue*, raspberry tongue). The palate and uvula may be edematous, reddened, and covered with petechiae.

The exanthem is red, is punctate or finely papular, and blanches on pressure. In some individuals, it may be palpated more readily than it is seen, having the texture of gooseflesh or coarse sandpaper. The rash appears initially in the axillae, groin, and neck but within 24 hr becomes generalized. Punctate lesions generally are not present on the face. The forehead and cheeks appear flushed, and the area around the mouth is pale (i.e., *circumoral pallor*). The rash is most intense in the axillae and groin and at pressure sites. Petechiae may occur owing to capillary fragility. Areas of hyperpigmentation that do not blanch with pressure may appear in the deep creases, particularly in the antecubital fossae (i.e., *pastia lines*). In severe disease, small vesicular lesions (*miliary sudamina*) may appear over the abdomen, hands, and feet.

Desquamation begins on the face in fine flakes toward the end of the 1st wk and proceeds over the trunk and finally to the hands and feet. The duration and extent of desquamation vary with the intensity of the rash; it may continue for as long as 6 wk.

Scarlet fever may follow infection of wounds (i.e., surgical scarlet fever), burns, or streptococcal skin infection. Clinical manifestations are similar to those just described, but the tonsils and pharynx generally are not involved. A similar picture may be observed with certain strains of staphylococci that produce an exfoliative toxin.

Scarlet fever must be differentiated from other exanthematous diseases, including measles (characterized by its prodrome of conjunctivitis, photophobia, dry cough, and Koplik spots), rubella (disease is mild, postauricular lymphadenopathy usually is present, and throat culture is negative), and other viral exanthems. Patients with infectious mononucleosis, have pharyngitis, rash, lymphadenopathy, and splenomegaly as well as atypical lymphocytes. The exanthems produced by several enteroviruses can be confused with scarlet fever, but differentiation can be established by the course of the disease, the associated symptoms, and the results of culture. Roseola is characterized by the cessation of fever with the onset of rash and the transient nature of the exanthem. Kawasaki disease, drug eruption, and toxic shock syndrome must also be considered.

Septic or severe scarlet fever associated with bacteremia or toxemia may manifest high fever and may be complicated by arthritis, jaundice, and hydrops of the gallbladder. Scarlet fever may be differentiated from Kawasaki disease by an older age at onset, absence of conjunctival involvement, and recovery of group A streptococci. Streptococcal toxic shock–like syndrome, associated with the pyrogenic toxins, produces toxicity, fever, shock, tissue injury (necrotizing fasciitis, myositis), pneumonia, rash (local or diffuse erythema, maculopapular, petechial, desquamation), and multiorgan dysfunction (kidney, lung, central nervous system). The shock, local tissue injury, older age, and nonscarlatiniform rash differentiate this syndrome from scarlet fever. *Arcanobacterium haemolyticum* (formerly *Corynebacterium haemolyticum*) also produces tonsillitis, pharyngitis, and a scarlatiniform rash in adolescents and young adults. Severe sunburn can also be confused with scarlet fever.

Pneumonia. See Chapter 170.

Skin Infections. The most common form of skin infection due to group A β-hemolytic streptococci is superficial pyoderma (impetigo) (see Chapter 605). Colonization of unbroken skin precedes pyoderma by about 10 days. Skin lesions such as impetigo, ecthyma, and cellulitis develop after intradermal inoculation by insect bites, scabies, or minor trauma. Skin colonization or pyoderma may predispose the patient to later nasopharyngeal colonization with the same strain.

Deeper soft tissue infections may occur. Streptococcal cellulitis is a painful, erythematous, indurated infection of the skin and subcutaneous tissues. It more frequently complicates varicella and may develop into a severe necrotizing fasciitis or myositis. Lymphangitis and regional lymphadenitis are common. Streptococcal soft tissue abscesses are rare but have occurred following immunization with contaminated needles. Fever and other systemic manifestations of disease may be noted.

Erysipelas is an acute, well-demarcated infection of the skin with lymphangitis involving the face (associated with pharyngitis) and extremities (wounds). The skin is erythematous and indurated; the advancing margins of the lesions have raised, firm borders. The skin lesion usually is associated with fever, vomiting, and irritability. In some cases streptococci break through the lymphatic barrier, and subcutaneous abscesses, bacteremia, and metastatic foci of infection are observed. Bacteremia and death have been associated with streptococcal cellulitis, and progression may be so rapid that there is no response to treatment with penicillin. Lesions may last from days to weeks.

Bacteremia (see Chapters 167 and 168). Bacteremia may follow a localized cutaneous (wounds, cellulitis, varicella lesions, hemangioma, abscess) or respiratory (pharyngitis, otitis media, sinusitis, pneumonia) infection in previously healthy or immunocompromised (malnutrition, malignancy) patients. It has also occurred in children with no obvious focus of infection. Sepsis may be rapidly progressive, leading to a toxic shock–like illness with hypotension, fever, leukocytosis, disseminated intravascular coagulation, and peripheral gangrene. Metastatic foci may result in meningitis, brain abscess, osteomyelitis, septic arthritis, pneumonia, and peritonitis. Rarely, endocarditis may complicate group A streptococcal bacteremia. The prognosis is poorest for patients with an underlying disease such as malignancy.

Vaginitis. The β-hemolytic streptococcus is a common cause of vaginitis in prepubertal girls. There is usually a serous discharge and marked erythema and irritation of the vulvar area, accompanied by discomfort in walking and in urination. Perianal streptococcal cellulitis produces local itching, pain, blood-streaked stools, erythema, and proctitis.

DIAGNOSIS. Although 30% of children with sore throat have a positive throat culture for group A streptococci, only 50% of these have a positive antibody response indicative of active infection rather than colonization. Streptococcal pharyngitis is suggested by age greater than 5 yr, high fever, exudates, tender anterior cervical lymphadenopathy, scarlatiniform rash, and a history of exposure. However, only 15% of children with pharyngitis and 25% of those with exudates have streptococcal infection; 50% of those with streptococcal pharyngitis do not have tonsillar exudates. Clinical judgment does not predict which children may have streptococcal infection, which must be diagnosed by throat culture or antigen detection.

Throat culture is the most useful laboratory aid in reaching a diagnosis in patients with acute tonsillitis or pharyngitis. Selective media give a higher yield than sheep blood agar plates. A positive result for a throat culture may indicate streptococcal pharyngitis, but hemolytic streptococci are common inhabitants of the nasopharynx in well children. Isolation of a group A streptococcus from the pharynx of a child with pharyngeal infection does not necessarily indicate that the disease is caused by this organism. When streptococci are isolated from children with moderate or severe exudative pharyngitis who have petechiae on the palate and cervical adenitis, the diagnosis is more secure. Rapid antigen detection tests are not sufficiently sensitive to be used without a back-up culture. *Treatment is, however, recommended for all children with pharyngitis and a positive throat culture or rapid antigen test for group A streptococci, even though in some cases the streptococci represent colonization.*

The immunologic response of the host after exposure to streptococcal antigen can be assessed by measuring antistreptolysin O (ASO) titers. An increase in ASO titer to greater than 166 Todd units occurs in more than 80% of untreated children with streptococcal pharyngitis within the first 3–6 wk following infection. This response may be modified or abolished by early and effective antibiotic therapy. ASO titers may be very high in patients with rheumatic fever; in contrast, they are weakly positive or not elevated at all in patients with streptococcal pyoderma; responses in patients with glomerulonephritis are variable. Group A β-hemolytic streptococci also may be recovered from the pharynx of asymptomatic individuals who develop an antibody response to this organism, indicating that subclinical infection has occurred.

Individuals with impetigo may react strongly to stimulation by other streptococcal extracellular products. Anti-DNase (deoxyribonuclease) B provides the best serologic test for streptococcal pyoderma; it begins to rise 6–8 wk after infection. Most patients with streptococcal pharyngitis also develop elevated titers to this enzyme. Patients with pyoderma and pharyngitis also may develop antibody responses to hyaluronidase, but antihyaluronidase (AH) titers are elevated with less regularity than are ASO titers.

A 2-min, inexpensive Streptozyme slide test (Wampole Laboratories, Cranbury, NJ) is designed to detect antibodies against multiple streptococcal extracellular antigens. This test detects more patients with increased antibody titers than any other single test presently available. Nonspecific (false-positive) reactions have been limited in number, and the test is capable of detecting antibody responses within 7–10 days of infection. However, the strength of the Streptozyme reagent varies from lot to lot, and it may not be specific for antibodies to extracellular products of group A streptococci.

The white blood cell count may or may not be elevated. Because leukocytosis may occur in many bacterial and viral diseases, this finding is nonspecific. Similarly, elevations in the erythrocyte sedimentation rate and C-reactive protein do not help to establish a specific diagnosis.

DIFFERENTIAL DIAGNOSIS. Acute pharyngitis that is indistinguishable clinically from that caused by group A β-hemolytic streptococci may be caused by many viruses, including Epstein-Barr virus (infectious mononucleosis). A viral cause may be suggested by failure to isolate streptococci and can be identified specifically by viral culture and serologic studies. Infectious mononucleosis may be suggested by the clinical manifestations, the presence of atypical lymphocytes in the peripheral blood, and a rise in heterophil and Epstein-Barr viral antibody titers. Acute pharyngitis similar to that caused by β-hemolytic streptococci may occur in patients with diphtheria, tularemia, toxoplasmosis, infection with *Mycoplasma* or *A. haemolyticum,* and, rarely, in individuals with tonsillar tuberculosis, salmonellosis, and brucellosis or infections caused by *Neisseria gonorrhoeae, Neisseria meningitidis,* and *Yersinia enterocolitica.* These diseases can be differentiated by appropriate cultures and serologic tests.

Streptococcal pyoderma must be differentiated from staphylococcal skin disease. Often these bacterial species coexist. The lesions produced are clinically indistinguishable; distinction is made only by culture.

Streptococcal septicemia, meningitis, septic arthritis, and pneumonia present signs and symptoms similar to those produced by other bacterial organisms. The offending pathogen can be established only by culture.

COMPLICATIONS. Complications generally reflect extension of streptococcal infection from the nasopharynx. This may result in sinusitis, otitis media, mastoiditis, cervical adenitis, retropharyngeal or parapharyngeal abscess, or bronchopneumonia. Hematogenous dissemination of streptococci may cause meningitis, osteomyelitis, or septic arthritis. Nonsuppurative late complications include rheumatic fever and glomerulonephritis.

PREVENTION. Administration of penicillin will prevent most cases of streptococcal disease if the drug is provided prior to the onset of symptoms. Except for rheumatic fever (see Chapter 175), indications for prophylaxis are not clear. Oral penicillin G or V (400,000 U/dose) is provided four times each day for 10 days. Alternatively, 600,000 U of benzathine penicillin in combination with 600,000 U of aqueous procaine penicillin may be given as a single intramuscular injection. This approach should be used for institutional epidemics. Children exposed to an individual case at school may be observed carefully.

Management of carriers of group A β-hemolytic streptococci is controversial. It has been suggested that treatment of the carrier precludes the development of type-specific immunity, thereby leaving the individual susceptible to reinfection later in life. It is probably unnecessary to re-treat asymptomatic convalescent patients with persistently positive throat cultures for group A streptococci, since they are generally carriers who do not have persistent or recurrent streptococcal infections. Children thought to have recurrent streptococcal infections may be carriers who have frequent viral respiratory infections masquerading as streptococcal infections. Parental anxiety may be high after several such episodes. Treatment with a non-penicillin antibiotic (e.g., cephalosporin, erythromycin, clindamycin) may be useful in eradicating the carrier state but should be reserved for the rare problem case.

No streptococcal vaccines are available for clinical use.

TREATMENT. The goals of therapy are to decrease symptoms and prevent septic, suppurative, and nonsuppurative complications. Penicillin is the drug of choice for the treatment of streptococcal infections. All strains of group A β-hemolytic streptococci isolated to date have been sensitive to concentrations of penicillin achievable in vivo.

Blood and tissue levels of penicillin sufficient to kill streptococci should be maintained for at least 10 days. Children with streptococcal pharyngitis should be treated with penicillin (125–250 mg/dose three times a day) for 10 days. Penicillin G or penicillin V may be employed; the latter is preferable because satisfactory blood levels are achieved even when the stomach is not empty. A single intramuscular injection of a long-acting benzathine penicillin G (600,000 U for children <60 lb and 1,200,000 U for children >60 lb) may be more effective for treatment or prevention of relapse and is indicated for all noncompliant patients or those having nausea, vomiting, or diarrhea.

Erythromycin (40 mg/kg/24 hr), clindamycin (30 mg/kg/24 hr), or cefadroxil monohydrate (15 mg/kg/24 hr) may be used for treating streptococcal pharyngitis in patients who are allergic to penicillin. Generally, relapse rates are lower with regimens other than penicillin. Tetracyclines and sulfonamides should not be used for treatment, although sulfonamides may be used for prophylaxis of rheumatic fever.

Treatment failure, defined as persistence of streptococci after a complete course of penicillin, occurs in 5–20% of children and is more common with oral than with intramuscular therapy. It may be due to poor compliance, reinfection, the presence of β-lactamase–producing oral flora, tolerant streptococci, or presence of a carrier state. Persistent carriage of streptococci predisposes a small number of patients to symptomatic relapse. Repeating the throat culture after a course of penicillin therapy is indicated only in high-risk situations, such as in patients with a history of previous rheumatic fever. If the throat culture is again positive for group A streptococci, some clinicians recommend a second course of treatment. Persistence after a second course of antibiotics probably indicates a carrier state, which has a low risk for the development of rheumatic fever and does not require further therapy.

Patients with severe scarlet fever, streptococcal bacteremia, pneumonia, meningitis, deep soft tissue infections, erysipelas, streptococcal toxic shock syndrome, or complications of streptococcal pharyngitis should be treated parenterally with penicillin, preferably intravenously. The dose and duration of therapy must be tailored to the nature of the disease process, with daily doses as high as 400,000 U/kg/24 hr required in the most severe infections. Severe, necrotizing infections may require the addition of a second antibiotic (e.g., clindamycin) to ensure complete bacterial killing.

PROGNOSIS. The prognosis for adequately treated streptococcal infections is excellent; most suppurative complications are prevented or readily treated. When therapy is provided promptly, nonsuppurative complications are prevented and complete recovery is the rule. In rare instances, particularly in neonates or in children whose response to infection is compromised, fulminant pneumonia, septicemia, and death may occur despite usually adequate therapy.

INFECTIONS DUE TO OTHER STREPTOCOCCI

In many centers, the group B *Streptococcus* has become the leading cause of neonatal septicemia and meningitis (see Chapter 98).

Human infection with streptococci of groups C to H and K to O, as well as with nontypable strains, has been reported in normal infants and children. The classification of these organisms and the infections with which they have been associated are shown in Table 175–1. Penicillin G provides effective therapy for non-group A streptococci, except for selected α-hemolytic strains and the enterococci; these organisms generally are susceptible to ampicillin. When endocarditis or other serious infections are caused by enterococci, therapy with ampicillin plus an aminoglycoside is recommended. Some enterococcal strains may be highly resistant to ampicillin or an aminoglycoside and should be treated with vancomycin.

Bacterial endocarditis in children is commonly caused by infection with *Streptococcus viridans*. A variant of this organism that grows slowly and requires vitamin B_6 or thiol compounds for optimal growth has also caused endocarditis in adults and children. It is important to know that supplemented media are needed for their isolation and sensitivity testing; spuriously low minimal inhibitory concentrations (MIC) may be reported when nonsupplemented media are used. Some of these organisms are relatively tolerant to penicillin; therapy with penicillin and an aminoglycoside is recommended until results of sensitivity studies are available. In several instances, these organisms have been resistant even to this combination of drugs but have been sensitive to clindamycin and vancomycin.

DiNubile MJ: Treatment of endocarditis caused by relatively resistant nonenterococcal streptococci: Is penicillin enough? Rev Infect Dis 12:112, 1990.

Hodge CW, Schwartz B, Talkington DF, et al: The changing epidemiology of invasive group A streptococcal infections and the emergence of streptococcal toxic shock-like syndrome. JAMA 269:384, 1993.

Kokx NP, Comstock JA, Facklam RR: Streptococcal perianal disease in children. Pediatrics 80:659, 1987.

Levin RM, Grossman M, Jordan C, et al: Group A streptococcal infection in children younger than three years of age. Pediatr Infect Dis J 7:581, 1988.

Miller RA, Brancato F, Holmes KK: *Corynebacterium hemolyticum* as a cause of pharyngitis and scarlatiniform rash in young adults. Ann Intern Med 105:867, 1986.

Pichichero ME, Disney FA, Talpey WB, et al: Adverse and beneficial effects of immediate treatment for Group A beta-hemolytic streptococcal pharyngitis with penicillin. Pediatr Infect Dis J 6:635, 1987.

Pichichero ME, Margolis PA: A comparison of cephalosporins and penicillins in the treatment of Group A beta-hemolytic streptococcal pharyngitis: A meta-analysis supporting the concept of microbial copathogenicity. Pediatr Infect Dis J 10:275, 1991.

Radetsky M, Solomon JA, Todd JK: Identification of streptococcal pharyngitis in the office laboratory: Reassessment of new technology. Pediatr Infect Dis J 6:556, 1987.

Shulman ST: Streptococcal pharyngitis: Clinical and epidemiologic factors. Pediatr Infect Dis J 8:816, 1989.

Todd JK: The sore throat: Pharyngitis and epiglottis. Infect Dis Clin North Am 2:149, 1988.

Wheeler MC, Roe MH, Kaplan EL, et al: Clinical epidemiological, and microbiological correlates of an outbreak of group A streptococcal septicemia in children. JAMA 266:533, 1991.

Wittler RR, Yamada SM, Bass JW, et al: Penicillin tolerance and erythromycin resistance of group A β-hemolytic streptococci in Hawaii and the Philippines. Am J Dis Child 144:587, 1990.

The Working Group: Defining the group A streptococcal toxic shock syndrome. JAMA 269:390, 1993.

175.1 Rheumatic Fever

*James Todd**

As recently as the early 1960s, rheumatic fever and its major complication, valvular heart disease, were major problems

*Modified from E. L. Kaplan in 14th edition.

worldwide. During the decades of the late 1960s and 1970s this disease almost disappeared in the United States and Western Europe, although it continues unabated in developing countries. However, the recent resurgence of acute rheumatic fever noted in the United States in the middle and late 1980s has once again emphasized the threat of this nonsuppurative sequel of group A streptococcal pharyngitis. The resurgence of rheumatic fever in the United States has also re-emphasized the need for better understanding of its pathogenesis so that appropriate public health and other preventive measures can be more effective.

ETIOLOGY. Group A β-hemolytic *Streptococcus* is the inciting agent leading to the development of acute rheumatic fever, although the exact pathogenetic mechanisms remain unexplained. Not all of the serotypes of group A streptococci can cause rheumatic fever. When some strains (e.g., M type 4) were present in a very susceptible rheumatic population, no recurrences of rheumatic fever ensued. In contrast, other serotypes prevalent in the same population caused recurrence attack rates of 20–50% of those with pharyngitis. The concept of "rheumatogenicity" is further supported by studies suggesting that those serotypes of group A streptococci that were frequently associated with skin infection, usually the higher serotypes, were frequently isolated from the upper respiratory tract but seldom caused recurrences of rheumatic fever in individuals with a previous history of rheumatic fever. Further, certain serotypes of group A streptococci (e.g., M types 1, 3, 5, 6, 18, 24) are more frequently isolated from patients with acute rheumatic fever than are other serotypes. However, because the serotype is unknown at the time of clinical diagnosis of streptococcal pharyngitis, clinicians must assume that all group A streptococci have the capacity to cause rheumatic fever, and of all episodes of streptococcal pharyngitis should be treated accordingly.

EPIDEMIOLOGY. The epidemiology of acute rheumatic fever is essentially the epidemiology of group A streptococcal pharyngitis. Rheumatic fever is most frequently observed in the age group most susceptible to group A streptococcal infections, children from 5–15 yr of age. However, susceptibility to rheumatic fever is also evident in older age groups, as is noted by the outbreaks of acute rheumatic fever that have occurred in specific closed populations such as military recruits. Increased numbers of cases also occur in socially and economically disadvantaged groups. This has been attributed to crowding, which is more frequent in this segment of the population. Furthermore, the increased incidence of group A streptococcal pharyngitis in fall, winter, and early spring is associated with an increased number of cases of acute rheumatic fever during these same periods of the year.

Group A streptococcal impetigo does not result in acute rheumatic fever, but infection of the upper respiratory tract or the skin may lead to another nonsuppurative complication of streptococcal infection, acute poststreptococcal glomerulonephritis. The reasons for this are not fully understood. Hypotheses relating to differences in rheumatogenic potential of "skin strains" and "throat strains" as well as observed differences in the immunologic response to group A streptococcal impetigo compared to streptococcal upper respiratory tract infection have been proposed to explain the contrast.

The major epidemiologic risk factor for development of acute rheumatic fever is group A streptococcal pharyngitis. The major reservoir for group A streptococci is the upper respiratory tract of humans.

The attack rate of acute rheumatic fever following group A upper respiratory tract infection is approximately 3% of individuals with untreated or inadequately treated infection. This figure has been remarkably constant, and the occasionally reported lower rates probably reflect inclusion of group A streptococcal carriers. Many children who harbor the group A *Streptococcus* are carriers of group A streptococci in the upper respiratory tract. The group A streptococcal carrier is at much reduced risk for development of acute rheumatic fever and for spread of the organism to close family or school contacts.

Of particular epidemiologic interest is the resurgence of acute rheumatic fever that occurred in the United States in the middle and late 1980s. Although the annual incidence of acute rheumatic fever in many communities in the United States was less than 1 in 100,000 in the years through the early 1980s, beginning in the mid-1980s, outbreaks of acute rheumatic fever occurred in numerous areas across the United States. The initial and largest outbreak was reported from Utah, but subsequent reports from eastern states, including Ohio and Pennsylvania, indicated that this resurgence was multifocal. One survey of pediatric cardiologists in large referral medical centers in the United States suggested that an increase in numbers of cases of acute rheumatic fever between 1985 and 1989 occurred in approximately 25 states. There were also at least two outbreaks of acute rheumatic fever in military recruit populations in the United States between 1985 and 1988.

The reasons for this resurgence of acute rheumatic fever in the United States remain unknown. Although rheumatic fever has been associated with socially and economically disadvantaged populations, the 1980s' resurgence has been associated with middle-class, often suburban and rural families. In addition, serotypes of group A streptococci that have been isolated only rarely during the previous 2 or 3 decades have emerged and spread. These serotypes began to be isolated in greater numbers when rheumatic fever cases were being reported. An increased number of isolates from rheumatic fever patients or simultaneously from their household contacts and siblings were shown to be M types 1, 3, 5, 6, and 18. These types have historically been associated with rheumatic fever. Very mucoid strains, especially strains of M type 18 group A streptococci, have appeared in a number of communities prior to the appearance of rheumatic fever. Mucoid strains have historically been associated with virulence.

PATHOGENESIS. Despite remarkable increases in our knowledge of the biology of the group A streptococcus and of the human host and despite important observations about the epidemiologic association between group A streptococci and the human host, the pathogenetic mechanism responsible for the development of acute rheumatic fever remains unknown. There have been two basic theories attempting to explain the development of this sequel to group A streptococcal pharyngitis: a toxic effect produced by an extracellular toxin of group A streptococci on target organs such as myocardium, valves, synovium, and brain; and an abnormal immune response by the human host. The search for the correct hypothesis has been severely hampered by the fact that there is no adequate animal model.

The hypotheses suggesting that rheumatic fever may be related to a direct effect of a streptococcal extracellular toxin have not been proved. For example, although streptolysin O, an extracellular product of group A streptococci, is cardiotoxic in animals, it has not been possible to establish a direct in vivo toxic effect by streptolysin O on the myocardium and valves or an injury of host tissue by streptolysin O resulting in "neoantigen" formation, with a subsequent immunologic response and damage to the host tissues.

The most popular hypotheses are those that postulate an abnormal immune response by the human host to some still, undefined component of the group A streptococcus. The resulting antibodies might then cause the immunologic damage leading to clinical manifestations. The latent period, usually 1–3 wk between the onset of the actual group A streptococcal infection and the onset of symptoms of acute rheumatic fever, lends support to an immunologic mechanism of tissue damage. Although the specific antigen or antigens responsible for inciting such an immune response have still to be identified, several possibilities exist. The group A streptococcus is a complex microorganism producing a large number of somatic and extracellular antigens that evoke brisk immune responses. This theory is further supported by the observation that different humans appear to respond quantitatively differently to streptococcal antigens. For example, in in vitro studies with human lymphocytes, individuals can be divided into high and low responders to streptococcal blastogen A, an extracellular product of the organism. This finding is compatible with the clinical and epidemiologic observations that not all people appear to be susceptible to developing rheumatic fever (see later).

Two streptococcal antigens are excellent examples of how an abnormal immunologic response might cause the clinical manifestations. First, the group-specific polysaccharide of the group A β-hemolytic streptococcal cell wall is antigenically similar to the glycoprotein found in human and bovine cardiac valves. There is prolonged persistence of antibody against the group A polysaccharide in individuals with chronic rheumatic valvular heart disease compared with individuals recovering from uncomplicated streptococcal infection or those with acute nephritis. When rheumatic mitral valves were surgically removed and replaced with prosthetic valves, serum antibody levels against the group A polysaccharide fell, as if the antigenic stimulus had been removed. However, important questions remain about whether this antigen is responsible for the valvulitis of rheumatic heart disease. For example, it has been shown that antibodies to group-specific carbohydrate develop after group A streptococcal skin infection, and rheumatic fever does not follow group A streptococcal skin infection (pyoderma). A second so-called cross-reactive antigen was originally described in the cell wall or cell membrane. Antibodies to this (these) somatic antigen(s) are found in sera of patients with rheumatic fever (i.e., heart-reactive antibodies), and it has been postulated that the myocarditis of acute rheumatic fever is related to an abnormal or autoimmune response against sarcolemma membrane. However, the significance of these observations has been questioned because these serum antibodies also develop after uncomplicated pharyngitis in individuals without evidence of rheumatic carditis.

The possibility of an abnormal immune response is also based on cross-reactivity between group A streptococci M protein and human tissue. The M protein is the virulence factor that is responsible for the organism's ability to resist phagocytosis. In addition, following infections with group A streptococci, type-specific immunity is conferred against the specific M protein type. The group A streptococcal M protein shares certain amino acid sequences with some human tissues, and this has been proposed as a possible source of cross-reactivity between the organism and its human host, leading to the abnormal immune response. One of the two classes of M protein correlates with serotypes of group A streptococci that are frequently isolated from patients with acute rheumatic fever.

In patients with Sydenham chorea, common antibodies to antigens are found in the group A streptococcal cell membrane and the caudate nucleus of brain. This observation further supports the concept of an abnormal autoimmune mechanism for the central nervous system manifestations of rheumatic fever and Sydenham chorea.

An understanding of the pathogenesis of rheumatic fever must encompass the fact that there are differences in human susceptibility to the development of acute rheumatic fever, including an unusual incidence of rheumatic fever and rheumatic heart disease among members of certain family groups. In regard to this genetic influence, there is a specific alloantigen present on the surface of non–T lymphocytes in 70–90% of rheumatic individuals, but fewer than 30% of "control" nonrheumatic individuals have the marker. The marker is more common in family members in which there is an index case of rheumatic fever than in nonaffected members of "control" families.

Although there may be genetic differences in rheumatic susceptibility among humans, the exact mechanism remains unknown. It is unlikely that the recent outbreaks of acute rheumatic fever in the United States are caused by an increasingly susceptible population based only on genetics. It is most likely that the pathogenetic mechanism for the development of rheumatic fever after upper respiratory tract infection with group A β-hemolytic streptococci involves a combination of specific characteristics of the organism and some as yet incompletely defined genetic predisposition in the human host.

CLINICAL MANIFESTATIONS AND DIAGNOSIS. There is no single specific clinical manifestation or specific laboratory test that unequivocally establishes the diagnosis of rheumatic fever. Rather, there are a number of selective clinical findings, called Jones criteria, that make the diagnosis of acute rheumatic fever highly probable and necessitate discussing the clinical manifestations and the diagnosis together. Although the Jones criteria have been changed several times since their original publication, they have remained basically stable and are the accepted method by which the diagnosis of this disease is confirmed. The current recommendations of the American Heart Association for the diagnosis of the initial attack of rheumatic fever are presented in Table 175–2.

Major Criteria. Because the five major criteria are considered to be the most specific findings, more weight is given to major criteria.

CARDITIS (see Chapter 390). This important finding in acute rheumatic fever is a pancarditis that involves the pericardium, epicardium, myocardium, and endocardium. Carditis is the only residual of acute rheumatic fever that results in chronic changes. Common manifestations include evidence of valvular insufficiency, most frequently affecting the mitral valve, but the mitral and the aortic valve may be affected. Isolated involvement of the aortic valve is rare. Tricuspid valve or pulmonary valve involvement is unusual. Valvular insufficiency is present in the acute state of the disease. Later, in the chronic stage, scarring of the valve with either typical "fishmouth" abnormality or even calcified valve tissue may lead to stenosis. Often there is a combination of insufficiency

■ TABLE 175–2 The Jones Criteria for Diagnosis of the Initial Attack of Rheumatic Fever

Major Criteria*	Minor Criteria
Carditis	Fever
Polyarthritis, migratory	Arthralgia
Erythema marginatum	Elevated acute-phase reactants (ESR, CRP)
Chorea	Prolonged P-R interval on an electrocardiogram
Subcutaneous nodules	
Plus	
Evidence of a preceding group A streptococcal infection (culture, rapid antigen, antibody rise/elevation)	

C = C-reactive protein; ESR = erythrocyte sedimentation rate.

**Two major criteria or one major and two minor criteria* plus *evidence of a preceding streptococcal infection indicate a high probability of rheumatic fever. In the three special categories listed below, the diagnosis of rheumatic fever is acceptable without two major or one major and two minor criteria. However, only for a and b can the requirement for evidence of a preceding streptococcal infection be ignored. (From Special Writing Group of the Committee on Rheumatic Fever, Endocarditis, and Kawasaki Disease of the Council on Cardiovascular Disease in the Young of the American Heart Association: Guidelines for the diagnosis of rheumatic fever.* In: *Jones Criteria, 1992 update. JAMA 268:2069, 1992.)*

a. Chorea, *if other causes have been excluded.*
b. Insidious or late-onset carditis *with no other explanation.*
c. Rheumatic recurrence: *In patients with documented rheumatic heart disease or prior rheumatic fever the presence of one major criterion, or of fever, arthralgia, or elevated acute-phase reactants suggests a presumptive diagnosis of recurrence. Evidence of previous steptococcal infection is needed here.*

and stenosis. Carditis occurs in 40–80% of patients with rheumatic fever. In the recent outbreaks in the United States, more than 80% of patients in one of the large series had evidence of carditis.

Other manifestations of carditis include pericarditis, pericardial effusion, and arrhythmias (usually 1st-degree heart block, but 3rd-degree or complete heart block may occur). The carditis of rheumatic fever may be mild or very severe, leading to intractable heart failure; rarely, surgical intervention, even in the acute stage of the disease, may be necessary if medical management cannot control the heart failure. These patients usually have myocardial involvement and significant valvular insufficiency.

Polyarthritis. This is the most confusing of the major criteria and probably leads to more diagnostic errors than any of the other manifestations. The arthritis of acute rheumatic fever is exquisitely tender. It is not uncommon for children with this form of arthritis to refuse to allow even bed sheets or clothing to cover an affected joint. The joints are red, warm, and swollen. The arthritis is migratory and affects several different joints: the elbows, knees, ankles, and wrists. It rarely occurs in the fingers, toes, or spine. It need *not* be symmetric. Effusions may be present. If the joint is aspirated, a leukocytosis is usually found; polymorphonuclear leukocytes are the cells found most frequently. However, there are no specific laboratory findings in the synovial fluid.

The arthritis does *not* result in chronic joint disease. After initiating anti-inflammatory therapy, the arthritis may disappear in 12–24 hr. Untreated, it may persist for a week or more. In many patients with early arthritis of rheumatic fever, because of treatment with anti-inflammatory drugs, the classic migratory polyarthritis does not develop, confusing the diagnosis.

Chorea. Sydenham chorea, a unique part of the rheumatic fever syndrome, occurs much later than other manifestations. These choreoathetoid movements may begin very subtly. The latent period following streptococcal pharyngitis may be as long as several months, and the movements are often very difficult to detect at the onset. However, careful questioning of parents and teachers usually reveals evidence of increased clumsiness. One of the best signs of this in school-aged children is a marked deterioration in their handwriting. Emotional lability is a frequent finding. Sydenham chorea may affect all four extremities or may be unilateral. Although at one time it could be seen in as many as one half of patients with acute rheumatic fever, more recent evidence suggests that it is seen, at least in the United States, in 10% or fewer cases. Sydenham chorea frequently is the only symptom of rheumatic fever. It is for this reason that this symptom alone is adequate to satisfy the Jones criteria. Sydenham chorea usually disappears within weeks to months. It may return, but this has become a rare occurrence.

Erythema Marginatum. The unique rash seen in patients with rheumatic fever is another of the major manifestations that can be very difficult to diagnose. It occurs very infrequently, and therefore few clinicians have had extensive experience in recognizing it. Although early in the disease it may manifest as nonspecific pink macules that are usually seen over the trunk, later in its fully developed form, there is blanching in the middle of the lesions, sometimes with fusing of the borders, resulting in a serpiginous-looking lesion. This rash can be made worse with application of heat, but characteristically it is evanescent. The rash does not itch. It often occurs in patients with chronic carditis. The rash of erythema marginatum can be mistaken for the rash seen with Lyme disease.

Subcutaneous Nodules. These lesions occur infrequently and are most commonly observed in patients with severe carditis. These pea-sized nodules are firm and nontender, and there is no inflammation. They are characteristically seen on the extensor surfaces of the joints, such as the knees and elbows, and also over the spine.

Minor Criteria. The minor manifestations are much less specific but are necessary to confirm a diagnosis of rheumatic fever. They include the clinical findings of fever and arthralgia. Arthralgia is present if the patient feels discomfort in the joint in the absence of objective findings (e.g., pain, redness, warmth) on physical examination. (Arthralgia cannot be counted in satisfying the Jones criteria if arthritis is present.) Fever, usually no higher than 101° or 102° F, may be present. High fever of 103° or 104° F requires careful re-evaluation and consideration of other diagnoses.

Included in the minor criteria are several laboratory tests. Acute-phase reactants, such as the ESR or C-reactive protein, may be elevated. These tests may remain elevated for prolonged periods of time (months) and are used by some clinicians as a guideline for modifying doses of anti-inflammatory drugs (see later). A prolonged PR interval on the electrocardiogram is also included among the minor criteria. This also is a nonspecific finding and should be used only after careful consideration.

Evidence of Group A Streptococcal Infection. This is one of the most important aspects of the Jones criteria. There must be evidence of a preceding group A streptococcal infection documented by a positive throat culture, a history of scarlet fever, or elevated streptococcal antibodies such as antistreptolysin O (ASO), anti-deoxyribonuclease B (anti-DNase B), or antihyaluronidase (AH). The diagnosis of rheumatic fever should *not* be seriously considered in patients without evidence of a recent group A streptococcal infection (see later exceptions for chorea and indolent carditis). Approximately 80% of individuals with rheumatic fever have an elevated ASO titer, but if the titers of two additional streptococcal antibodies are also elevated or rising, an elevation of at least one antibody is found in more than 95% of patients with rheumatic fever.

There are three categories of patients who may be diagnosed as having acute rheumatic fever even in the absence of two major criteria or one major and two minor criteria, as required by the revised Jones criteria (see Table 175–2). These include strongly considering rheumatic fever if chorea or indolent carditis is present with no other likely cause. In addition, a recurrence of rheumatic fever should be considered in patients with prior rheumatic fever or rheumatic heart disease who have evidence of a recent streptococcal infection with one major or two minor criteria.

DIFFERENTIAL DIAGNOSIS. The differential diagnosis is extensive because so many of the clinical and laboratory findings associated with rheumatic fever are not specific and there is no single laboratory test that can confirm the diagnosis. Juvenile rheumatoid arthritis or other connective tissue diseases often need to be considered. Infective endocarditis is frequently confused with rheumatic fever, especially in patients with recurrences of rheumatic fever. Patients with a previous history of rheumatic fever or rheumatic valvular heart disease should be carefully evaluated for infective endocarditis before the diagnosis of recurrent rheumatic fever is made. This may be difficult because such patients may be taking an antibiotic for secondary rheumatic fever prophylaxis in a dose high enough to prevent blood cultures from becoming positive. The typical rash of Lyme disease may be confused with erythema marginatum.

COMPLICATIONS. The major complication of acute rheumatic fever is the development of rheumatic valvular heart disease. None of the other manifestations results in a chronic disease. The mitral valve is most frequently involved, but the aortic and tricuspid valves also may be affected. Usually, the tricuspid valve becomes involved only in patients who have significant mitral or aortic disease resulting in pulmonary hypertension.

LABORATORY FINDINGS. No single specific laboratory test can confirm the diagnosis of acute rheumatic fever. Laboratory evidence of a previous streptococcal infection is confirmed by a search for the organism itself (i.e., culture) or evidence of an immune response to a group A streptococcal antigen. The throat culture remains the gold standard for confirmation of the presence of group A streptococci, although rapid antigen detection tests are available. All patients suspected of having acute rheumatic fever should have at least one throat culture performed before beginning antibiotic therapy. Rapid antigen detection tests may be used if it is recognized that these tests have reduced sensitivity. For small numbers of group A streptococci, the test may be falsely negative. On the other hand, because the specificity of most of these tests is quite good, a positive result of a rapid antigen detection test provides evidence of group A streptococci. If a rapid antigen detection test is negative, a throat culture should be obtained in patients in whom rheumatic fever is suspected.

Streptococcal antibody tests are another method of documenting the presence of a previous group A streptococcal infection. The most commonly used test is the ASO test. Other tests that may be used are the anti-DNase B test and the AH test. A commercially available agglutination screening test is less satisfactory because of its technical difficulties. An elevated streptococcal antibody titer is clear evidence of a previous group A streptococcal infection, but a more reliable way of demonstrating the earlier infection is by showing a rise in titer between acute and convalescent sera. The ASO test reaches its peak 3–6 wk after infection, whereas the anti-DNase B test reaches its peak slightly later (6–8 wk). If acute and convalescent sera are tested, they should be tested simultaneously. Values defining an elevated titer may vary with the age of the patient, the interval since the streptococcal infection, and the population.

Acute-phase reactants such as the ESR or CRP are usually elevated at the onset of acute rheumatic fever. However, these tests are nonspecific. Determination of rheumatoid factor, tests for the presence of antinuclear antibody, and determination of the complement level are rarely helpful in making a diagnosis of acute rheumatic fever. Occasionally, nonspecific elevations of serum gamma globulin may be seen.

The electrocardiogram may indicate a 1st-degree heart block (prolonged PR interval), and on rare occasions, 2nd- or 3rd-degree block may also be present. In first attacks, electrocardiograms are otherwise usually unremarkable. In patients with chronic rheumatic heart disease, electrocardiographic manifestations of resulting cardiac disease, such as left atrial enlargement, may be evident.

No specific findings are revealed by the common, chest roentgenogram, but cardiomegaly is common, especially in individuals with significant carditis.

Some individuals with subclinical evidence of valvular disease may show valvular regurgitation on two-dimensional Doppler echocardiography. This observation may explain why many patients without evidence of carditis at the time of the acute attack present in the 4th or 5th decade of life with evidence of mitral valve disease. An echocardiogram is useful in evaluating patients suspected of having rheumatic fever or rheumatic heart disease.

TREATMENT. Management of acute rheumatic fever can be divided into three approaches: treatment of the group A streptococcal infection that led to the disease, use of anti-inflammatory agents to control the clinical manifestations of the disease, and other supportive therapy, including management of congestive heart failure, if that has occurred.

All patients presenting with acute rheumatic fever should be treated for a group A streptococcal infection at the time the diagnosis is made, whether or not the organism is initially isolated from the patient. It can be difficult to recover the organism from the patient at onset because of the latent period, especially in patients with chorea. A 10 full days of an appropriate oral agent or a single intramuscular injection of 1,200,000 units of benzathine penicillin G is recommended. Treatment for group A B-hemolytic streptococcal infections is discussed in more detail in Chapter 175. Because some patients receiving intramuscular benzathine penicillin G may experience nonspecific rises in the ESR, some clinicians elect to treat patients initially with oral penicillin, especially if they are following the ESR as a measure of the effectiveness of anti-inflammatory therapy given for other rheumatic manifestations. Sulfadiazine is not an appropriate agent for treatment of acute streptococcal pharyngitis.

There are three systemic manifestations of acute rheumatic fever for which therapy is given acutely. These are arthritis, carditis, and Sydenham chorea. Salicylates provide prompt and dramatic relief for the patient with the arthritis of acute rheumatic fever. The exquisitely tender migratory polyarthritis can be relieved in 12–24 hr by the use of salicylates. Early administration of salicylates to a patient suspected of having rheumatic fever before the diagnosis is established with certainty may obscure the diagnosis by interrupting the development of migratory arthritis. Therefore, salicylates or other anti-inflammatory agents should be withheld until the clinical course of the disease has adequately defined itself. For patients with very painful arthritis, comfort can be provided by the use of small doses of codeine or similar drugs, because they do not interfere with the progression of the disease and its subsequent diagnosis. Corticosteroids are seldom indicated for the treatment of arthritis of rheumatic fever. No studies are available documenting the efficacy of other nonsteroidal anti-inflammatory agents in the treatment of rheumatic fever.

For patients with mild carditis without evidence of congestive heart failure, salicylates alone are indicated. However, in patients with congestive heart failure or other significant manifestations of carditis, corticosteroids are required. There is no definitive evidence that the use of salicylates or corticosteroids is beneficial in preventing the subsequent development of rheumatic heart disease. This is in contrast to the clinical impression that corticosteroids may have a beneficial effect in patients with moderate to severe carditis. It is appropriate to restrict the use of corticosteroids to patients who have moderate or severe carditis, especially those with evidence of heart failure.

Administration of steroids should be limited both in amount and in duration to reduce their untoward side effects. For most children, a total dose of 2.5 mg/kg/24 hr of prednisone divided into two doses is appropriate. A short course of steroids over 2–3 wk is usually sufficient, depending on patient response clinically and on laboratory tests (e.g., ESR, CRP). Even with short courses of steroids in these doses, side effects may occur, including some cushingoid changes and hypertension. Alternate-day steroids may reduce the side effects, but controlled studies have not been done. The dose should be tapered rather than abruptly stopped.

Salicylates should be given in a dose that results in blood levels of 20–25 mg/dL. Usually 90–120 mg/kg/24 hr in four divided doses is adequate to reach this level in children. However, serum salicylate levels should be carefully monitored to reduce the possibility of toxicity. Liver function should also be monitored. In patients who are receiving corticosteroids for therapy of carditis, it is advisable to add salicylates to the steroids, especially when the doses are being tapered to prevent the possibility of rheumatic rebound. The salicylates should be given during the last week of corticosteroid therapy and continued for approximately 3–4 wk after the steroids have been discontinued. The duration of salicylate therapy depends on the patient's response and clinical course.

Congestive heart failure should be treated by conventional techniques (see Chapter 403). Diuretics are indicated in patients with severe congestive heart failure. Cardiac glycosides such as digitalis also may be used, although usually in relatively small doses. Long periods of bed rest are not necessary for most patients. In the past, bed rest was used primarily for two groups of patients. The first were patients who had arthritis, but this usually is not a factor after 24 hr of salicylate therapy. Strict bed rest is not needed. The second group of patients are those with carditis, especially those with congestive heart failure. Although bed rest is indicated for the therapy of patients with congestive heart failure, prolonged bed rest is usually unnecessary. It is, however, preferable to keep patients at bed rest until the ESR approaches normal and congestive heart failure has been controlled. Occasionally, steroids, bed rest, and anticongestive measures are not effective in treating the carditis of rheumatic fever. In these rare cases, cardiovascular surgery with replacement of the valve or valvuloplasty may be required.

The treatment of Sydenham chorea has been controversial. Originally, phenobarbital or other sedatives were used; then chlorpromazine became popular. Diazepam, a benzodiazepine derivative, is prescribed for patients with mild chorea. In patients with severe chorea, haloperidol has been used successfully. These children must be closely observed, because severe toxic reactions to this drug have been reported.

There is no specific therapy for erythema marginatum or the subcutaneous nodules of acute rheumatic fever.

PREVENTION. Prevention and treatment of group A streptococcal infection can prevent rheumatic fever. There are two forms of prevention for acute rheumatic fever, primary prophylaxis and secondary prophylaxis.

Primary prophylaxis refers to antibiotic treatment of the streptococcal upper respiratory tract infection to prevent an initial attack of rheumatic fever. Appropriate diagnosis and adequate antibiotic therapy with eradication of group A streptococci from the upper respiratory tract reduce the risk of developing rheumatic fever to near zero. Antibiotic therapy initiated up to approximately 1 wk after onset of the streptococcal sore throat can prevent rheumatic fever. See Chapter 175 for treatment of group A streptococcal infections. However, antibiotic therapy must be adequate. Ten full days of oral therapy are essential if the oral method is used. Suggested doses are shown in Table 175–3.

Secondary prophylaxis refers to the prevention of colonization or infection of the upper respiratory tract with group A β-hemolytic streptococci in people who have already had a previous attack of acute rheumatic fever. Patients who receive antibiotics continuously and do not have group A streptococcal infections do not have recurrences of rheumatic fever. The recommended methods of secondary prevention include regular monthly (every 3–4 wk) injections of intramuscular benzathine penicillin G, daily administration of oral penicillin, daily administration of oral sulfadiazine, or daily oral administration of erythromycin (for individuals who cannot take any of the previously recommended antibiotics). Although sulfadiazine or other sulfa drugs should *never* be used for the treatment of group A streptococcal infections (because a high percentage of organisms are resistant to these antimicrobial agents), sulfadiazine *is* effective in preventing colonization of the upper respiratory tract and is an acceptable form of oral secondary prophylaxis. Regular injections of intramuscular benzathine penicillin G are preferable to oral secondary prophylaxis because of better compliance. Individuals at high risk for rheumatic recurrence should be given 1,200,000 units intramuscularly every 3 wk. Penicillin levels during the 4th wk following injection may be lower than the MIC for group A β-hemolytic streptococci. However, in most instances in the United States 4-wk intervals for injections are sufficient because the risk of recurrence of rheumatic fever is small.

The necessary duration of secondary prophylaxis in individuals with a documented history of rheumatic fever or with rheumatic heart disease is controversial. Recurrences of acute rheumatic fever occur less frequently 5 yr or more after the most recent attack, and for this reason, some clinicians think that patients may not need secondary prophylaxis more than 5 yr after the most recent attack or when they reach their 18th birthday, whichever comes first. Others recommend that, in patients who have significant rheumatic heart disease or who have a significant risk of contracting group A streptococcal upper respiratory tract infection (e.g., medical professionals, school teachers, those living in crowded conditions), the duration of secondary prophylaxis should be longer. Some recommend that treatment be continued for life in patients with rheumatic valvular heart disease. Recommendations for each patient must be individualized, depending on the patient's condition and the environment in which he or she lives and works.

No streptococcal vaccine is available. Physicians and public health authorities must still depend on the accurate and timely diagnosis and therapy of group A streptococcal upper respiratory tract infections and prevention of recurrent infections in known rheumatics to prevent the crippling effects of rheumatic fever and rheumatic heart disease.

■ **TABLE 175–3 Primary and Secondary Prevention of Rheumatic Fever**

Route of Administration	Antibiotic	Dose	Frequency
Primary Prevention: Treatment of Streptococcal Pharyngitis to Prevent a Primary Attack of Rheumatic Fever			
Intramuscular	Benzathine penicillin G	1,200,000 units (600,000 units if <27 kg)	Once
Oral	Penicillin V	250 mg/kg/24 hr	bid for 10 days
	Erythromycin	40 mg/kg/24 hr (not to exceed 1 g/24 hr)	tid or qid for 10 days
	Others, such as clindamycin, nafcillin, ampicillin, amoxicillin, cephalexin	Dosage varies	
Do not use tetracyclines or sulfa drugs			
Secondary Prevention: Prevention of Recurrences of Rheumatic Fever			
Intramuscular	Benzathine penicillin G	1,200,000 units	Every 3–4 wk
Oral	Penicillin V	250 mg	bid
	Sulfadiazine	500 mg	od
	Erythromycin	250 mg	bid
Do not use tetracyclines			

Adapted from Rheumatic fever and heart disease: Report of a WHO Study Group. Geneva, World Health Organization, 1988.

Berrios X, del Campo E, Guzman B, Bisno AL: Discontinuing rheumatic fever prophylaxis in selected adolescents and young adults: A prospective study. Ann Intern Med 118:401, 1993.

Bisno AL: The concept of rheumatogenic and nonrheumatogenic group A streptococci. *In:* Reed SE, Zabriskie JB (eds): Streptococcal Diseases and the Immune Response. New York, Academic Press, 1980, p 789.

Denny FW Jr, Wannamaker LW, Brink WR, et al: Prevention of rheumatic fever: Treatment of the preceding streptococcal infection. JAMA 143:151, 1950.

Dudding BA, Ayoub EM: Persistence of streptococcal group A antibody in patients with rheumatic valvular disease. J Exp Med 128:1081, 1968.

Fischetti VA: Streptococcal M protein: Molecular design and biological behavior. Clin Microbiol Rev 2:285, 1989.

Gerber MA, Wright LL, Randolph MF: Streptozyme test for antibodies to group A streptococcal antigens. Pediatr Infect Dis J 6:36, 1987.

Kaplan EL: The rapid identification of group A beta-hemolytic streptococci in the upper respiratory tract. Pediatr Clin North Am 35:535, 1988.

Kaplan EL, Berrios X, Speth J, et al: Pharmacokinetics of benzathine penicillin G: Serum levels during the 28 days after intramuscular injection of 1,200,000 units. J Pediatr 115:146, 1989.

Kaplan EL, Hill HR: Return of rheumatic fever: Consequences, implications, and needs. J Pediatr 111:244, 1987.

Kaplan EL, Johnson DR, Cleary PP: Group A streptococcal serotypes isolated from patients and sibling contacts during the resurgence of rheumatic fever in the United States in the mid-1980s. J Infect Dis 159:101, 1989.
Kavey RW, Kaplan EL: Resurgence of acute rheumatic fever. Pediatrics 84:585, 1989.
Markowitz M, Kaplan EL: Reappearance of rheumatic fever. Adv Pediatr 36:39, 1989.
Secord E, Emre U, Shah BR, Tunnessen WW Jr: Picture of the month: Erythema marginatum in acute rheumatic fever. Am J Dis Child 146:637, 1992.
Special Writing Group of the Committee on Rheumatic Fever, Endocarditis, and Kawasaki Disease of the Council on Cardiovascular Disease in the Young of the American Heart Association: Guidelines for the diagnosis of rheumatic fever. *In:* Jones Criteria, 1992 update. JAMA 268:2069, 1992.
Swedo SE, Leonard HL, Schapiro MB, et al: Sydenham's chorea: Physical and psychological symptoms of St Vitus dance. Pediatrics 91:706, 1993.
Siegel AC, Johnson EE, Stollerman GH: Controlled studies of streptococcal pharyngitis in a pediatric population: Factors related to the attack rate of rheumatic fever. N Engl J Med 265:559, 1961.
Veasy LG, Tani LY, Hill HR: Persistence of acute rheumatic fever in the intermountain area of the United States. J Pediatr 124:9, 1994.
Veasy LG, Wiedmeier SE, Orsmond GS, et al: Resurgence of acute rheumatic fever in the intermountain area of the United States. N Engl J Med 316:421, 1987.
Wald ER: Acute rheumatic fever. Curr Probl Pediatr 23:264, 1993.
Wannamaker LW, Rammelkamp CH Jr, Denny FW Jr, et al: Prophylaxis of acute rheumatic fever by treatment of the preceding streptococcal infection with various amounts of depo penicillin. Am J Med 10:673, 1951.
Wood HF, Feinstein AR, Taranta A, et al: Rheumatic fever in children and adolescents: III. Comparative effectiveness of three prophylaxis regimens in preventing streptococcal infections and rheumatic recurrences. Ann Intern Med 60 (Suppl 5):31, 1964.
World Health Organization Study Group: Rheumatic Fever and Rheumatic Heart Disease, Technical Report Series No. 764. Geneva, World Health Organization, 1988.

CHAPTER 176
Pneumococcal Infections

James Todd*

The pneumococcus *(Streptococcus pneumoniae)*, a normal inhabitant of the upper respiratory tract, can be an invasive pathogen. *S. pneumoniae* is the most common cause of community-acquired bacterial pneumonia and otitis media and the third most common cause of meningitis. The significance of this agent is accentuated by the emergence of penicillin-resistant and multidrug-resistant strains in many communities.

ETIOLOGY. *S. pneumoniae* is a gram-positive, lancet-shaped, encapsulated diplococcus. In body fluids and culture media, the organisms may be found as individual cocci or as chains. Serotypes (84) are identified by their type-specific capsular polysaccharides. Antisera to some pneumococcal capsular polysaccharides cross-react with other pneumococcal types or with other bacterial species (e.g., *Escherichia coli,* group B streptococci, *Haemophilus influenzae* type b). Only smooth, encapsulated strains are pathogenic for humans. Virulence is related in part to the size of the capsule, but pneumococcal types with capsules of identical size may vary widely in virulence. Fully encapsulated strains (e.g., type 3) are extraordinarily virulent. Capsular material impedes phagocytosis; the mechanism is unclear.

On solid media, the pneumococcus forms unpigmented, umbilicated colonies surrounded by a zone of incomplete (α) hemolysis. Pneumococcal capsules can be seen and the organisms typed by exposing them to homologous type-specific antisera that combine with their respective capsular polysaccharides, rendering the capsules refractile (i.e., quellung reaction).

*Modified from Ralph D. Feigin in the 14th edition.

C substance is a cell-wall antigen that is related to species rather than to specific pneumococcal serotypes. It is a teichoic acid–containing phosphocholine and galactosamine-6-phosphate. C substance precipitates with an acute β-globulin, the C-reactive protein, which may activate complement and stimulate phagocytosis. R antigen is a species-specific protein on or near the cell surface. A *type*-specific protein (M antigen) also has been detected, but it does not confer significant antiphagocytic properties. Antibodies to the C, R, or M antigens produce negligible immunity. Antibodies to pneumococcal surface protein A (PspA) are protective against some pneumococcal strains when tested in mice. The pneumococcus produces a hemolytic toxin called pneumolysin and a toxic neuraminidase. During autolysis, pneumococci release a purpura-producing factor that causes dermal and internal hemorrhages when injected into rabbits. The role of these substances, if any, in the pathogenesis of human disease is unknown. In humans, antibodies to the capsular polysaccharide are protective by promoting opsonization and phagocytosis.

EPIDEMIOLOGY. Many healthy individuals carry *S. pneumoniae* in their upper respiratory tracts. As many as 91% of children between 6 mo and 4.5 yr of age carry *S. pneumoniae* at some time. Serotypes 6, 19, and 23 constitute 50% of all isolates in children. These, plus types 1, 4, 9, 11, 14, 15, and 18, account for 85% of all pneumococcal isolates. Frequently, the same serotype is carried continuously for extended periods (45 days–6 mo). Carriage of a particular serotype does not consistently induce local or systemic immunity sufficient to prevent later reacquisition of the same serotype. Multiple serotypes may coexist in the same nasopharynx. Pneumococcal isolation rates peak during the first 2 yr of life and decline gradually thereafter; carriage rates are highest in institutional settings and from December to April and lowest from July to September.

S. pneumoniae is the most frequent bacterial cause of bacteremia, pneumonia, and otitis media and the third most common cause of meningitis in infants and children. The peak incidence of meningitis occurs among infants 3–5 mo of age, that of otitis media from 6 to 12 mo, and that of hospitalization for pneumonia from 13 to 18 mo of age. The decreased ability to produce antibody to polysaccharide capsule antigens in children less than 2 yr of age may explain, in part, the increased susceptibility to pneumococcal infection and the decreased vaccine effectiveness in this age group. Males are more commonly affected than females, and native Americans and blacks more than whites; the unusual susceptibility of black children is not entirely explained by the increased risk associated with sickle cell disease.

Pneumococcal disease generally occurs sporadically. *S. pneumoniae* is spread from person to person by respiratory droplet transmission. Its frequency and severity are increased in patients with sickle cell disease, asplenia, splenosis, deficiencies in humoral (B cell) immunity, acquired immunodeficiency syndrome, malignancy (e.g., leukemia, lymphoma), and complement deficiencies.

PATHOGENESIS AND PATHOLOGY. Pneumococci must invade to produce disease. Nonspecific host defense mechanisms, including the presence of other bacteria in the nasopharynx, usually limit the multiplication of pneumococci. Aspiration of secretions containing pneumococci is hindered by the epiglottic reflex and by the cilia of the respiratory epithelium, which continuously move infected mucus upward toward the pharynx. Whether disease develops when pneumococci reach the alveoli depends on the outcome of the interaction of the bacteria with the alveolar macrophages. Pneumococci are highly resistant to phagocytosis by alveolar macrophages.

Pneumococcal disease frequently follows a viral respiratory tract infection that may produce mucosal damage, diminish the epithelial ciliary activity, and depress the function of alveolar macrophages. Phagocytosis may be impeded by respiratory secretions and the alveolar exudate. In the tissues, pneumococci multiply and spread through the lymphatics or bloodstream (bacteremia) or by direct extension from a local site of infection.

The severity of disease is related to the virulence and number of organisms causing bacteremia and to the integrity of specific host defenses. Generally, a poor prognosis correlates with very large numbers of pneumococci or significant concentrations of capsular polysaccharide in the circulation; despite effective antibiotic therapy, patients with heavy antigenemia may have severe and protracted illness.

Deficiency of the terminal components of complement (C3–C9) has been associated classically with recurrent pyogenic infection, which includes those caused by *S. pneumoniae.* C2 deficiency also appears to be associated with *S. pneumoniae* infection. The propensity for pneumococcal disease in asplenic persons is presumed to relate to deficient opsonization of the pneumococcus as well as to absence of the filtering function of the spleen on circulating bacteria. Pneumococcal disease is more prevalent in patients with sickle cell disease and other hemoglobinopathies. This risk is greatest in infants less than 2 yr of age when antibody production is attenuated. Patients with sickle cell anemia have a deficit in antibody-independent properdin (alternate) pathway of complement activation. Properdin deficiency and deficient antibody production result in defects in antibody-independent and antibody-dependent opsonophagocytosis of pneumococcus. With advancing age, patients with sickle cell anemia produce anticapsular antibody, augmenting antibody-dependent opsonophagocytosis and reducing but not eliminating the risk of severe pneumococcal disease.

The efficacy of phagocytosis also is diminished in patients with B- and T-cell immunodeficiency syndrome because of a lack of opsonic anticapsular antibody and a failure to produce lysis and agglutination of bacteria. These observations suggest that opsonization of the pneumococcus depends on the classic and the properdin (or alternative) complement pathways and that recovery from pneumococcal disease depends on the development of anticapsular antibodies that act as opsonins, enhancing phagocytosis and ultimately killing the pneumococcus.

In the lung and other body tissues, the spread of infection is enhanced by the antiphagocytic properties of the pneumococcal capsule. The surface fluid of the respiratory tract contains only small amounts of IgG and is deficient in complement. Both are necessary for opsonization of encapsulated microorganisms. After inflammation has been established in the lung, there is an influx of IgG, complement, and polymorphonuclear leukocytes (PMNs). Phagocytosis of bacteria by PMNs may occur, but even normal human serum may not be able to opsonize pneumococci to prepare them for phagocytosis by alveolar macrophages. Macrophages eventually replace the leukocytes in the exudate, and the lesion resolves. The sequence of events evolves over 7–10 days but may be modified by appropriate antibiotic therapy or by the administration of *type*-specific serum.

CLINICAL MANIFESTATIONS. The signs and symptoms are related to the site of infection; see pneumonia (see Chapter 170), otitis media (see Chapter 590), sinusitis and pharyngitis, abscesses of the upper airway (see Chapter 327), laryngotracheobronchitis (see Chapter 332), peritonitis, and bacteremia (see Chapter 167). Local spread of infection may occur, causing empyema, pericarditis, mastoiditis, epidural abscess, or, rarely, meningitis. Colonizing pneumococci may spread through the eustachean tube, producing otitis media, and aspiration of infected pharyngeal secretions may produce pneumonia. Bacteremia may be followed by meningitis (see Chapter 169), septic arthritis, osteomyelitis (see Chapter 172), endocarditis (see Part XX, Section 4), and brain abscess (see Chapter 554).

The incidence of pneumococcal bacteremia, meningitis, endocarditis, and endophthalmitis is increasing in infants under 1 mo of age.

Renal glomerular-capillary and cortical arteriolar thromboses have been associated with pneumococcal bacteremia. Localized gingival lesions, gangrenous areas of skin on the face or extremities, immune complex glomerulonephritis, and disseminated intravascular coagulation also occur as manifestations of pneumococcal disease.

DIAGNOSIS. This may be established by recovery of pneumococci from the site of infection or the blood. However, pneumococci found in the nose or throat of patients with otitis media, pneumonia, septicemia, or meningitis may not be related causally to their disease.

Blood cultures should be obtained for all children with pneumonia, meningitis, arthritis, osteomyelitis, peritonitis, pericarditis, or gangrenous skin lesions. It may also be advisable to obtain blood cultures in children 1–24 mo of age with fever who have no localized signs of infection but are not consolable, are toxic, or have leukocytosis.

Pneumococci can be identified in body fluids as gram-positive, lancet-shaped diplococci. Early in the course of pneumococcal meningitis, many bacteria may be seen in a relatively acellular cerebrospinal fluid. The latex particle agglutination test may be helpful in establishing a diagnosis rapidly; however, it is not necessary if organisms are seen on the Gram stain. The latex test is not as sensitive for the diagnosis of pneumococcal bacteremia. In patients with localized disease (e.g., nonbacteremic pneumonia, otitis media), the latex particle agglutination test is usually negative.

Leukocytosis generally is pronounced, with total white blood cell counts of 30,000/mm^3 a common occurrence. The sedimentation rate may be elevated.

PREVENTION. Polyvalent pneumococcal vaccines have proved to be immunologic and associated with few untoward reactions. However, responsiveness to pneumococcal polysaccharide is unpredictable in children younger than 2 yr of age. A licensed 23-valent pneumococcal vaccine contains purified polysaccharide from 23 pneumococcal serotypes responsible for more than 95% of cases of bacteremia and meningitis and for 85% of cases of otitis media seen in children. The clinical efficacy of the vaccine is controversial, with several large studies producing conflicting results. In children, the mean postimmunization antibody titers after vaccine administration are, on the average, lower than those seen in healthy adults. A minimum titer of 300 ng/mL of antibody nitrogen for each serotype is considered necessary for protection. In addition, antigen 6A, 14, 19F, and 23F are poorly immunogenic in children younger than 6 yr of age. Pneumococcal serotype 6A is one of the strains most likely to produce disease in children. Reimmunization has been shown to increase antibody concentrations; however, routine reimmunization is not recommended currently because of the likelihood of more frequent and severe adverse reactions.

Immunization is recommended for children over 2 yr of age who have sickle cell anemia, functional or anatomic asplenia, nephrotic syndrome, splenectomy after staging laparotomy for Hodgkin disease, cerebrospinal fluid leaks, or human immunodeficiency virus infection. Vaccine is not recommended for prevention of recurrent otitis media or sinusitis. Reimmunization may be given to particular high-risk patients; however, the optimum time interval between initial immunization and booster immunizations is unknown. Immunization does not prevent pneumococcal disease related to serotypes not found in the vaccine and does not invariably prevent infection from a pneumococcal strain that is serotypically identical to one of the vaccine strains. There have been many reports of serious and even fatal infections in vaccinated children.

For this reason, penicillin prophylaxis is still warranted in children at risk of pneumococcal sepsis. Penicillin V potassium (125 mg twice daily for children < 5 yr and 250 mg twice daily for children ≥ 5 yr) substantially decreases the incidence of pneumococcal sepsis in children with sickle cell anemia. In addition, once-monthly intramuscular benzathine penicillin is efficacious in preventing overwhelming sepsis. Erythromycin may be used in children with penicillin allergy. If oral prophylaxis is used, strict compliance must be encouraged.

TREATMENT. Historically, penicillin has been the treatment of choice for pneumococcal infection. The incidences of relative and complete penicillin resistance and multiple drug resistance (e.g., penicillin, tetracycline, chloramphenicol, rifampin, erythromycin, sulfonamides, clindamycin) have increased during the last decade. Intermediate resistance varies but may be as high as 40% in some areas of North America. Multiply-resistant strains have been identified in South Africa, Spain, Great Britain, Australia, and the United States. Resistance to antibiotics is seen most often in the pneumococcal serotypes 6, 14, and 19 and 23, the serotypes that most often cause disease in children.

Problems in treatment may be encountered by organisms that are intermediately resistant to penicillin (minimum inhibitory concentration [MIC] 0.1–1.0 mg/L), organisms that are highly resistant to penicillin (MIC > 1.0 mg/L), and organisms that are resistant to multiple antibiotics. Because of varying patterns of resistance, all isolates should be tested for susceptibility to antibiotics. The use of an oxacillin disk is the preferred method for measuring penicillin susceptibility because it identifies intermediately resistant strains more specifically. Strains identified as intermediately resistant to penicillin should be tested further to establish MICs. Vancomycin resistance has not been reported.

Treatment of pneumococcal disease should be based on knowledge of susceptibility patterns seen in specific communities. Penicillin G is the drug of choice for penicillin-susceptible strains. Oral penicillin V (50–100 mg/kg/24 hr, every 6–8 hr) for minor infections, intravenous penicillin G (200,000–250,000 U/kg/24 hr, every 4–6 hr) for bacteremia or pneumonia, and intravenous penicillin G (300,000 U/kg/24 hr, every 4–6 hr) for meningitis are recommended. For serious infections with strains that are intermediately resistant to penicillin and for all infections with highly penicillin-resistant strains, vancomycin (60 mg/kg/24 hr, every 6 hr) is the treatment of choice. Resistance to the third-generation cephalosporins, such as cefotaxime and ceftriaxone, and treatment failures have been reported.

For susceptible strains and patients without meningitis, erythromycin, cephalosporins, trimethoprim-sulfamethoxazole, and chloramphenicol provide effective, alternative therapy for individuals who are allergic to penicillin. In areas with an increasing incidence of penicillin-resistant pneumococci, vancomycin should be given an initial treatment for suspected pneumococcal meningitis and other severe disease.

PROGNOSIS. This depends on the integrity of host defenses, the virulence of the infecting organism, the age of the host, the site of infection, and the adequacy of treatment. See sections listed under Clinical Manifestations for specific diseases.

Alario AJ, Nelson EW, Shapiro ED: Blood cultures in the management of febrile outpatients later found to have bacteremia. J Pediatr 115:195, 1989.

Bjornson A, Lobel J: Direct evidence that decreased serum opsonization of *Streptococcus pneumoniae* via the alternative complement pathway in sickle cell disease is related to antibody deficiency. J Clin Invest 79:388, 1987.

Davidson M, Schraer CD, Parkinson AJ, et al: Invasive pneumococcal disease in an Alaska native population, 1980 through 1986. JAMA 261:715, 1989.

Friedland IR, Klugman KP: Antibiotic-resistant pneumococcal disease in South African children. Am J Dis Child 146:920, 1992.

Hansman D: Pneumococcal carriage amongst children in Adelaide, South Australia. Epidemiol Infect 101:411, 1988.

Henderson FW, Gilligan PH, Wait K, et al: Nasopharyngeal carriage of antibiotic-resistant pneumococci by children in group day care. J Infect Dis 157:256, 1988.

Jacobs MR: Treatment and diagnosis of infections caused by drug-resistant *Streptococcus pneumoniae.* Clin Infect Dis 15:119, 1992.

Jonsson S, et al: Phagocytosis and killing of common bacterial pathogens of the lung by human alveolar macrophages. J Infect Dis 152:4, 1985.

Johnston RB Jr: Pathogenesis of pneumococcal pneumonia. Rev Infect Dis 13:S509, 1991.

Paton JC, Toogood IR, Cockington RA, et al: Antibody response to pneumococcal vaccine in children aged 5 to 15 years. Am J Dis Child 140:135, 1986.

Tan TQ, Mason EO Jr, Kaplan SL: Penicillin-resistant systemic pneumococcal infection in children: A retrospective case-control study. Pediatrics 92:761, 1993.

Wong WY, Overturf GD, Powars DR: Infection caused by *Streptococcus pneumoniae* in children with sickle cell disease: Epidemiology, immunologic mechanisms, prophylaxis, and vaccination. Clin Infect Dis 14:1124, 1992.

CHAPTER 177

Haemophilus influenzae

Lilly Cheng Immergluck and Robert Daum

The first recognition of *Haemophilus influenzae* occurred during an outbreak of influenza in Europe in 1889–1892, when Richard Pfeiffer identified a bacillus species in the sputum of many patients with influenza during a pandemic. This resulted in the name *Haemophilus influenzae.* The realization that *H. influenzae* was the cause of several important infectious syndromes in childhood and not the cause of influenza came from the work of Margaret Pittman, who, in 1931, also recognized that the serotype b capsule was the major virulence factor among isolates causing invasive disease. Subsequent investigations determined that antibody to polyribosylribitol phosphate (PRP), the serotype b capsular polysaccharide, could protect against invasive disease, an observation that spawned efforts to develop immunity by active immunization.

The vaccine era began in 1985 with the licensure of a purified PRP vaccine for routine use in children 24 mo of age and older. Subsequently, Rachel Schneerson and John Robbins postulated that covalently linking PRP to one of several protein carriers would improve immunogenicity in younger infants, allow immunologic priming, and probably, therefore, prove effective in the prevention of invasive disease. The introduction of such PRP-protein conjugate vaccines into clinical practice has been associated with a dramatic decline in the incidence of invasive infections due to *H. influenzae* type b.

MICROBIOLOGY. *H. influenzae* is a fastidious, gram-negative, pleomorphic coccobacillus that requires factors X (i.e., hematin, heat stable) and V (i.e., phosphopyridine nucleotide, heat labile) for growth. These factors are present within erythrocytes, and the demonstration of their requirement for growth is the basis for speciating *H. influenzae* in the laboratory.

Some *H. influenzae* isolates are surrounded by a polysaccharide capsule. Such isolates can be serotyped into six antigenically and biochemically distinct types, designated a–f. The most virulent isolates belong to serotype b; they are responsible for almost all *H. influenzae* invasive infections in children.

Several schemes have been devised to further classify *H. influenzae* isolates, mainly to subclassify serotype b isolates. None of these methods has consistently identified bacterial factors important in epidemiology or pathogenesis. For example, *H. influenzae* can be classified into eight biotypes based on indole and urea metabolism and the presence of ornithine decarboxylase. Biotype I, the most common isolate from blood and cerebrospinal fluid, accounts for more than 94% of serotype b organisms, and this scheme therefore provided little help in subclassifying serotype b strains. Biotypes II, III, and

IV are isolated mainly from the genitourinary tract, and biotype IV is responsible for most neonatal infections. Biotype V isolates often cause otitis media or may asymptomatically colonize the respiratory tract.

EPIDEMIOLOGY. *H. influenzae* is encountered in many clinical situations. It is a major cause of certain invasive diseases in children; serotype b isolates account for more than 95% of these. Disease caused by other capsular serotypes of *H. influenzae* is rare. Nonecapsulated (nontypable) *H. influenzae* organisms cause invasive disease in the neonate, immunocompromised children, and children in certain developing countries. Nontypable isolates are common etiologic agents in certain mucosal infections such as otitis media and sinusitis. They have also been associated with chronic bronchitis in adults.

Humans are the only natural hosts for *H. influenzae.* This species is a constituent of the normal respiratory flora in 60–90% of healthy children. Most isolates are nontypable. Colonization by serotype b organisms is infrequent. Before the advent of conjugate vaccine immunization, *H. influenzae* type b could be isolated from the pharynx of 2–5% of healthy preschool and school aged children; lower rates occurred among infants younger than 1 yr of age and adults. Such asymptomatic colonization with *H. influenzae* type b probably occurs at lower rates in immunized populations. In the era before *H. influenzae* type b conjugate vaccine availability in the United States, the annual attack rate of invasive disease was estimated to be 64–129 cases per 100,000 children younger than 5 yr of age per year. This incidence decreased by more than 90%.

A striking epidemiologic feature of invasive *H. influenzae* type b infections has been the age distribution. More than 90% of all infections occur in children 5 yr of age or younger in the United States, although a few occur in older children and adults. Moreover, 69–82% of invasive infections occur in children younger than 2 yr of age; about 50% occur in those younger than 12 mo. The peak attack rate occurs at 6–12 mo of age. Most studies also show a predominance among males.

The incidence of invasive disease varies in different countries and certain populations. For example, in the prevaccine era, Finland reported an annual incidence of 41 cases per 100,000 children; 40% occurred in children older than 2 yr of age. Populations identified to have an increased incidence of invasive disease include Alaskan Eskimos, Apaches, Navajos, and blacks. In these populations, the proportion of cases of invasive disease in children younger than 12 mo of age is relatively high. Persons known to be at an increased risk for invasive disease include those with sickle cell disease, asplenia, congenital and acquired immunodeficiencies, and malignancies. Nonvaccinated infants younger than 12 mo of age who had previously documented invasive infection are at increased risk for recurrence.

Socioeconomic risk factors for invasive *H. influenzae* type b disease include day care outside the home, the presence of siblings of elementary school age or younger, short duration of breast feeding, and parental smoking. Previous hospitalization for invasive *H. influenzae* type b disease and a history of otitis media are associated with an increased risk for invasive disease. Much less is known about the epidemiology of *H. influenzae* infections other than serotype b.

The mode of transmission is most commonly by direct contact or inhalation of respiratory tract droplets containing *H. influenzae.* The incubation period for invasive disease is variable, and the exact period of communicability is unknown. Most children with invasive *H. influenzae* type b disease are colonized in the nasopharynx before initiation of antimicrobial therapy; 25–40% may remain colonized during the first 24 hr of therapy.

Among age-susceptible household contacts who have been exposed to a case of invasive *H. influenzae* type b disease, the risk of developing "secondary" invasive disease in the first 30 days is estimated at 0.26%. The attack rate for "secondary" *H. influenzae* type b disease in household contacts is highest in susceptible children younger than 24 mo of age (3.2%) and rare (<0.1%) in contacts older than 47 mo of age. Unlike the case in the general population, asymptomatic carriage of *H. influenzae* type b is frequent in household contacts of patients with disease. More than 75% of families have at least one colonized household member in addition to the index patient.

PATHOGENESIS. The precise mechanisms that facilitate successful colonization of the respiratory epithelium have not been identified. In an organ culture of human nasopharyngeal tissue, type b and non-b strains of *H. influenzae* organisms attach to nonciliated columnar epithelial cells and subsequently can be seen within those cells and in the intercellular spaces.

The events that result in entry into the intravascular compartment by serotype b organisms are unclear. Once there, however, type b strains resist intravascular clearance mechanisms more readily than do strains of other serotypes and nonencapsulated organisms. Whether it is the type b PRP capsule itself that confers the potential for invasive disease or another closely linked virulence factor is not certain. An undeciphered clue may lie in the predilection of genes encoding for PRP to be present in an unusual tandem arrangement on the genome of 98% of clinical isolates.

Once established, *H. influenzae* type b bacteremia is sustained. Data from animal models and patients suggest that the magnitude of bacteremia and its duration are independent variables that determine the likelihood of dissemination of bacteria into sites such as the meninges or joints. The bacterial and host mechanisms that determine the magnitude of bacteremia are poorly understood.

Noninvasive *H. influenzae* infections such as otitis media, sinusitis, and bronchitis, usually caused by nontypable strains, probably gain access to sites such as the middle ear or sinus cavity by direct extension from the pharynx. Serotype b organisms are infrequent causes of these noninvasive infections, probably causing disease by the same mechanism. The factors facilitating spread from the pharynx are not fully understood but include eustachian tube dysfunction and certain antecedent viral infections of the respiratory tract.

ANTIBIOTIC RESISTANCE. Before 1974, all *H. influenzae* isolates were presumed susceptible to ampicillin, and clinical laboratories did not perform routine testing. Isolates that produced β-lactamase were identified in that year for the first time and their incidence increased in the subsequent decade. The most recent multicenter collaborative surveillance study conducted in the United States in 1988 showed that 29.5% of *H. influenzae* type b isolates produced a β-lactamase and were resistant to ampicillin. A few isolates have been identified that are ampicillin resistant but do not produce β-lactamase. The mechanism of resistance in this instance is the production of a penicillin-binding protein with decreased affinity for β-lactam compounds.

When ampicillin resistance was first recognized, chloramphenicol became the agent of choice for therapy against invasive *H. influenzae* type b disease. The advantages of chloramphenicol include low cost and good penetration into cerebrospinal fluid. Chloramphenicol is effective against most isolates of *H. influenzae* type b regardless of β-lactamase production. The disadvantages of chloramphenicol include the necessity for complex monitoring strategies and the rare occurrence of idiosyncratic aplastic anemia.

Isolates of *H. influenzae* type b have been identified that are resistant to chloramphenicol; resistance is usually mediated by the action of chloramphenicol acetyl transferase (CAT), although a few isolates do not produce this enzyme. Chloramphenicol-resistant isolates have remained relatively rare in the United States and throughout the world, although they are more common in a few locales such as Barcelona and Taiwan.

Isolates resistant to both chloramphenicol and ampicillin have been identified rarely. In the United States, fewer than 1% of isolates were resistant to both compounds. Resistance to trimethoprim-sulfamethoxazole (TMP-SMX) or amoxicillin-clavulanate occurred in fewer than 1% of clinical isolates in the most recent national survey conducted in the United States in 1987–1988. That study also reaffirmed the poor activity of erythromycin against *H. influenzae*. Resistance to extended-spectrum cephalosporins, which are commonly used in therapy, and fluoroquinolones, which are seldom used in pediatric populations, has not been documented.

IMMUNITY. In the 1930s, LeRoy Fothergill and Joyce Wright demonstrated that the susceptibility to invasive *H. influenzae* type b disease was related to lack of "bactericidal power" in the blood. They showed that bactericidal power was acquired in an age-related fashion that inversely mirrored the age distribution of *H. influenzae* type b disease. It is now known that bactericidal power of the blood reflects the sum of several elements of host defense. By far the most important is antibody directed against the type b capsular polysaccharide, PRP. Anti-PRP antibody is acquired in an age-related fashion and facilitates clearance of *H. influenzae* type b from blood in experimental animal models; its presence was correlated with protection in several clinical trials that employed active and passive immunization.

The mechanism of action of anti-PRP antibody is related in part to its opsonic activity; other antibodies directed against antigens such as outer membrane proteins or lipopolysaccharides may also play a role in opsonization. Both the classic and alternative complement pathways are important in the opsonization of *H. influenzae* type b. The macrophages of the reticuloendothelial system aid in intravascular clearance of *H. influenzae* type b by affecting intracellular killing after opsonization.

Before the introduction of vaccination and among recipients of unconjugated PRP vaccines, protection from *H. influenzae* type b infection was presumed to correlate with the concentration of circulating anti-PRP antibody at the time of exposure. A serum antibody concentration of 0.15–1.0 μg/mL was considered protective against invasive infection; the higher concentration in PRP vaccinees may predict maintenance of a level of more than 0.15 μg/mL over time. Most infants lack an anti-PRP antibody concentration of this magnitude and are susceptible to disease on encounter with *H. influenzae* type b. This lack of antibody in young infants may reflect a maturational delay in the immunologic response to thymus-independent type 2 (TI-2) antigens such as PRP. Immunization with PRP induces responses markedly influenced by the age at immunization. Infants younger than 6 mo of age produce little if any anti-PRP antibody. A gradual increase in the geometric mean anti-PRP antibody response with increasing age at immunization is consistently observed. Infants 18–24 mo of age and older have a geometric mean anti-PRP response greater than 1 μg/mL, an observation that provided initial enthusiasm for immunizing children of that age group and older. Convalescent sera from unvaccinated children younger than 24 mo of age who develop *H. influenzae* type b disease show inconsistent or negligible anti-PRP antibody responses, but unvaccinated patients older than 24 mo of age have an increased antibody concentration in convalescent sera.

Unlike the PRP unconjugated vaccine, the conjugate vaccines—with the exception of PRP-OMP, which also has thymus independent type 1 (TI-1) properties—act as thymus-dependent (TD) antigens (Table 177–1). They elicit serum antibody responses in young infants, although multiple doses may be required, and prime memory antibody responses on subsequent encounters with PRP. The concentration of circulating anti-PRP antibody in a child primed by a conjugate vaccine may not correlate precisely with protection, because a memory response may occur rapidly on exposure to PRP and provide protection.

■ TABLE 177–1 ***Haemophilus influenzae*** **Type b Conjugate Vaccines**

Manufacturer	Abbreviation	Trade Name	Carrier Protein
Connaught Laboratories	PRP-D*	Prohibit	Diphtheria toxoid
Lederle-Praxis	HbOC†	HIBTITER	CRM_{197} (a nontoxic mutant diphtheria toxin)
Merck, Sharp & Dohme	PRP-OMP	PedvaxHIB	OMP (an outer membrane protein complex of *Neisseria meningitidis*)
Pasteur Merieux Vaccins (distributed by SmithKline Beecham and Connaught Laboratories)	PRP-T‡	ActHIB/OmniHib	Tetanus toxoid

**PRP-D is recommended only for infants 12 months of age or older. HbOC, PRP-OMP, and PRP-T are recommended for infants beginning at about 2 months of age.*
†HbOC is also available as a combination vaccine with DTP (Tetramune).
‡PRP-T may be reconstituted with U.S. Connaught DTP immediately before administration in a single syringe.

The anti-PRP antibody response to natural infection and immunization may be partly under genetic control in that certain individuals have a higher relative risk for invasive *H. influenzae* type b disease and may also respond suboptimally to vaccine administration. More information is required to clarify this interesting possibility.

Less is known about immunity to nontypable *H. influenzae*. Evidence suggests that antibodies directed against one or more outer membrane proteins (OMP) are bactericidal and protect against experimental challenge. For example, P6, a major OMP, is present in all strains of *H. influenzae* and is highly conserved among encapsulated and nontypable strains. In infant rats, antibody to P6 is bactericidal for encapsulated and nontypable *H. influenzae* and is protective against *H. influenzae* type b disease. Another OMP, P2, has substantial interstrain heterogeneity. Antibody elicited to the nonconserved regions of P2 had complement-dependent bactericidal activity to the homologous strain. Monoclonal antibodies directed against a group of surface exposed high molecular weight OMPs have bactericidal activity against certain isolates.

LABORATORY DIAGNOSIS. Presumptive identification of *H. influenzae* is made by direct examination of the collected specimen after Gram staining. Because of its small size, pleomorphism, poor uptake of stain by some isolates, and the tendency for fluids, particularly when proteinaceous, to have a red background, visualization of *H. influenzae* is sometimes difficult; staining with methylene blue may be helpful. With this technique, *H. influenzae* appears as a blue-black coccobacillus against a light blue–gray background. Because identification of microorganisms on smear by either technique requires at least 10^5 bacteria/mL, failure to visualize them does not exclude their presence.

Culture of *H. influenzae* requires prompt transport and processing of specimens, because the organism is fastidious. Specimens should not be exposed to drying or temperature extremes. Primary isolation of *H. influenzae* can be accomplished on chocolate agar, *Haemophilus* isolation agar, or on blood agar plates using the *Staphylococcus* streak technique.

Serotyping of *H. influenzae* is accomplished by slide agglutination with type-specific antisera. In practice, many clinical laboratories identify isolates as serotype b by testing bacterial suspensions or supernatants of broth cultures for the presence of PRP. Isolates from which PRP is not detected are called non-b types.

Detection of PRP in cerebrospinal fluid (CSF) serum, urine, or other relevant body fluids using techniques such as counter-immunoelectrophoresis, latex particle agglutination (LA), staphylococcal protein A coagglutination, and enzyme immunoassay have been employed. LA is perhaps the most sensitive, versatile, and accessible method for direct detection of PRP. Use of immunologic methods for detection of type b PRP capsular antigen is most helpful for diagnosing *H. influenzae* type b infections in patients who received prior antimicrobial therapy when culture results may not be revealing.

CLINICAL MANIFESTATIONS AND TREATMENT. Invasive Disease. Serotype b isolates account for almost all invasive infections. Invasive disease caused by other encapsulated organisms occurs rarely. Nontypable invasive disease is also infrequent and probably constitutes about 5% of all *H. influenzae* invasive infections beyond the neonatal period. Nontypable invasive disease is evidenced more often in isolates obtained from neonates, immunodeficient patients, and children in some developing countries with invasive disease. The clinical manifestations and treatment of all invasive *H. influenzae* disease appear to be similar regardless of serotype.

The initial antibiotic therapy of invasive infections possibly due to *H. influenzae* type b should be a parenterally administered antimicrobial agent effective in sterilizing all foci of infection and against ampicillin-resistant strains. Extended-spectrum cephalosporins, such as cefotaxime or ceftriaxone, have been used as the initial antimicrobial agent when *H. influenzae* type b is considered a likely pathogen, and they have achieved popularity because of their relative lack of serious adverse effects and ease of administration (see Chapter 161 for dosages). Alternatively, chloramphenicol can be used with ampicillin. After the antimicrobial susceptibility of the isolate has been determined, an appropriate agent can be selected to complete the therapy. Ampicillin remains the drug of choice for the therapy of infections caused by susceptible isolates. If the isolate is resistant to ampicillin, extended-spectrum cephalosporins such as cefotaxime or ceftriaxone are useful; the latter can be administered once daily in selected circumstances to outpatients. Chloramphenicol has also received extensive clinical experience.

Oral antimicrobial agents are sometimes used to complete a course of therapy initiated by the parenteral route. If the organism is susceptible to ampicillin, it or amoxicillin is the compound of choice. Cefixime or amoxicillin-clavulanate may be used when the isolate is resistant to ampicillin. Chloramphenicol is another option that continues to enjoy popularity in some countries because of its low cost.

MENINGITIS (see Chapter 169). Before the development of *H. influenzae* type b conjugate vaccines, *H. influenzae* type b was the leading cause of bacterial meningitis in the United States in children. Although its incidence has decreased, it remains an important cause. Clinically, meningitis due to *H. influenzae* type b cannot be differentiated from that due to *Neisseria meningitidis* or *Streptococcus pneumoniae* and may be complicated by other foci of infection, such as the lungs, joints, bones, pericardium, orbit, or globe.

Antimicrobial therapy should be administered parenterally for 7–14 days for uncomplicated cases. Cefotaxime, ceftriaxone, ampicillin, and chloramphenicol are all thought to cross the blood-brain barrier during acute inflammation in concentrations adequate to render them effective. Chloramphenicol has been administered orally to complete a therapeutic regimen for meningitis. It is well absorbed from the gastrointestinal tract and attains high concentrations in the CSF (≈50% of the concentration in serum), independent of meningeal inflammation. However, its use should be reserved for patients who are not vomiting, when there is a compelling reason why parenteral antimicrobials cannot be administered, when serum concentrations of chloramphenicol can be monitored, and when compliance can be ensured.

The prognosis of *H. influenzae* type b meningitis depends on the age of presentation, duration of illness before appropriate antimicrobial therapy, the CSF capsular polysaccharide concentration, and the rapidity with which it is cleared from CSF, blood, and urine. Low intelligence quotients correlate with clinically manifested inappropriate secretion of antidiuretic hormone and evidence of focal neurologic deficits at presentation. About 6% of patients with *H. influenzae* type b meningitis are left with some hearing impairment, probably because of inflammation of the cochlea and the labyrinth. Several studies evaluating the role of dexamethasone (0.6 mg/kg/24 hr divided every 6 hr for 4 days), particularly when given shortly before or concurrent with the initiation of antimicrobial therapy, demonstrated a decrease in the incidence of bilateral hearing loss associated with *H. influenzae* type b meningitis. However, because dexamethasone may not prevent hearing loss from meningitis due to other causes, the likelihood that *H. influenzae* type b is the cause and the risks of steroids must be weighed. Major neurologic sequelae occurring in children who recovered from *H. influenzae* type b meningitis include behavior problems, language disorders, and delayed development of language. Before the use of conjugate vaccination, about 9% of children who recovered from *H. influenzae* type b meningitis had behavioral problems. Other neurologic sequelae seen include impaired vision, mental retardation, motor abnormalities, ataxia, seizures, and hydrocephalus.

CELLULITIS. *H. influenzae* type b is responsible for 5–14% of the cases of cellulitis in young children; more than 85% of children with *H. influenzae* type b cellulitis are 2 yr of age or younger. Frequently, these children have an antecedent upper respiratory tract infection. There is usually no prior history of trauma, and the infection is thought to represent seeding of the organism to the involved soft tissues during bacteremia. The head and neck, particularly the cheek and preseptal region, are the most common sites of involvement. The involved region generally has indistinct margins and is tender and indurated. Buccal cellulitis is classically erythematous with a violaceous hue, although this sign may be absent. *H. influenzae* type b may often be recovered directly from an aspirate with or without prior injection of 0.1 mL of a nonbacteriostatic sterile solution into the area of involvement. The blood culture may reveal the causative organism. Other infectious foci such as meningitis and septic arthritis may complicate cellulitis, particularly if the patient is younger than 18 mo of age or febrile. A diagnostic lumbar puncture should be considered at the time of diagnosis.

Parenteral antimicrobial therapy is indicated until the patient becomes afebrile, usually a prompt occurrence. However, local inflammation at the involved site may not decrease until 24–48 hr later. Prolonged fever may be a sign of distant, concomitant infection (e.g., meningitis, arthritis). After the patient becomes afebrile and the signs of inflammation decrease, an appropriate orally administered antimicrobial agent may be substituted. A 7–10 day course is customary.

ORBITAL AND PRESEPTAL INFECTIONS. The clinical syndrome of the red and swollen eye includes several infectious diseases. Infection involving the superficial tissue layers anterior to the orbital septum is termed preseptal cellulitis. *H. influenzae* type b is an important cause. Infectious processes that involve the orbit and its contents include orbital cellulitis, orbital abscess, or subperiosteal abscess.

Uncomplicated preseptal cellulitis does not imply a risk for visual impairment or direct central nervous system extension. However, concurrent bacteremia may be associated with the development of meningitis. *H. influenzae* type b preseptal cellulitis is characterized by fever, edema, tenderness, warmth of the lid, and, occasionally, purple discoloration. Evidence of interruption of the integument is usually absent. There may be associated conjunctival drainage. *S. pneumoniae, Staphylococcus aureus,* and group A β-hemolytic streptococci cause clinically indistinguishable preseptal cellulitis. The latter two pathogens are more likely when fever is absent and with an interruption of the integument (e.g., an insect bite).

Infections involving the orbit occur rarely. These may also variably have lid edema but have distinguishing features such as proptosis, chemosis, impaired vision, limitation of the extraocular movements, decreased mobility of the globe, or pain on movement of the globe. The distinction between preseptal and orbital cellulitis may be difficult to make. The extent of the infection can often be delineated by computed tomography or ultrasonography.

As for children with cellulitis, those with preseptal cellulitis in whom *H. influenzae* type b or *S. pneumoniae* are etiologic considerations (i.e., young age, high fever, intact integument) should have blood submitted for culture, and a diagnostic lumbar puncture should be considered.

Parenteral antibiotics are indicated for both preseptal and orbital infections. Because *S. aureus, S. pneumoniae,* and group A β-hemolytic streptococci are other causes of these syndromes, empiric therapy should include agents active against these pathogens. Children with uncomplicated preseptal cellulitis older than 5 yr of age may not require therapy directed against *H. influenzae* type b.

Patients with preseptal cellulitis without concurrent meningitis should receive parenteral therapy for about 5 days until fever and erythema have abated. In the case of orbital infections, parenteral therapy is continued for the duration of treatment. For both syndromes, in uncomplicated cases, antimicrobial therapy should be given for a total of 10 days.

Abscesses in the orbit usually require prompt surgical drainage and more prolonged antimicrobial therapy. If no abscess is found at the initial evaluation, the necessity for surgical exploration to drain a subperiosteal or orbital abscess should be reconsidered if the response to therapy is not prompt.

Supraglottitis or Acute Epiglottitis (see Chapter 332). Epiglottitis is a cellulitis of the tissues comprising the laryngeal inlet that include the epiglottis, aryepiglottic folds, and arytenoid cartilage. The cause is almost always *H. influenzae* type b. Epiglottitis caused by other pathogens is exceedingly rare. Direct invasion of the involved tissues by *H. influenzae* type b is probably the initiating pathophysiologic event. This dramatic, potentially lethal condition usually occurs in children 2–7 yr old. Because of the risk of sudden, unpredictable airway obstruction, supraglottitis is a medical emergency. Pneumonia is present by chest radiograph in about 25% of cases. Other foci of infection, such as meningitis, are rare. Antimicrobial therapy directed against *H. influenzae* type b should be administered parenterally but only after the airway is secured, and therapy should be continued until the patient is able to take fluids by mouth. The duration of antimicrobial therapy typically is 7 days.

Uvulitis. *H. influenzae* type b uvulitis is rare; it may occur alone or as a concomitant of pharyngitis, or epiglottitis. Like supraglottitis, infection of the uvula most likely arises by direct invasion by *H. influenzae* type b. Unlike epiglottitis, there is generally no associated respiratory distress. When uvulitis occurs with concomitant epiglottitis, the symptoms and signs are more typical of the latter: high fever, dysphagia, and progressive respiratory distress. A lateral neck radiograph may help to exclude involvement of the supraglottic laryngeal structures. Because group A β-hemolytic streptococci may also cause uvulitis, parenteral antimicrobial therapy targeted against this bacterium and *H. influenzae* type b should be promptly initiated when appropriate cultures are obtained, usually from the blood and the surfaces of the uvula and epiglottis.

Pneumonia (see Chapter 170). The true incidence of *H. influenzae* type b pneumonia in children is unknown because of the invasive procedures required to obtain cultures. It is considered an important cause of pneumonia in unvaccinated children 4 yr of age or younger. The signs and symptoms of pneumonia due to *H. influenzae* type b cannot be differentiated from those of pneumonia caused by many other microorganisms. Associated infectious foci such as meningitis and epiglottitis are common. Antigen detection tests performed on blood or urine may aid in diagnosis.

Children suspected of having *H. influenzae* type b pneumonia who are younger than 12 mo of age should receive parenteral antimicrobial therapy initially because of their increased risk for bacteremia and its complications. Older children who do not appear severely ill may be managed with an orally administered antimicrobial. Therapy is continued for 7–10 days of combined parenteral-oral therapy.

Uncomplicated pleural effusion associated with *H. influenzae* type b pneumonia requires no special intervention. However, if empyema develops, insertion of a chest tube and a more prolonged course of antimicrobial therapy may be necessary.

Septic Arthritis (see Chapter 172). Large joints, such as the knee, hip, ankle, and elbow, are affected most commonly. Associated infections such as meningitis commonly occur; a diagnostic lumbar puncture should be considered. Although single joint involvement is the rule, multiple joint involvement occurs in about 6% of cases. The signs and symptoms of septic arthritis due to *H. influenzae* type b are indistinguishable from those of arthritis caused by other bacteria.

Uncomplicated septic arthritis should be treated with an appropriate antimicrobial administered parenterally for at least 5–7 days. If the clinical response is satisfactory (i.e., absence of fever, decreased signs of inflammation, and a decrease in the C-reactive protein or the erythrocyte sedimentation rate) the remainder of the course of antimicrobial treatment may be given orally (amoxicillin, 100 mg/kg/24 hr, divided three times each day if the isolate is susceptible, or cefixime, 8 mg/kg/24 hr, given as a single dose or divided into two daily doses of 4 mg/kg). Ensuring compliance is an important consideration in the selection of candidates for oral therapy. Some experts think that the dose of the antimicrobial agent should be adjusted so that the serum bactericidal titer is at least 1:8. Therapy is typically given for 3 wk for uncomplicated septic arthritis, but it may be continued beyond 3 wk until the erythrocyte sedimentation rate is normal.

Osteomyelitis (see Chapter 172). *H. influenzae* type b is an uncommon cause of osteomyelitis. However, it should be considered as an etiologic cause in children younger than 3 yr of age with suspected osteomyelitis, particularly when there is concurrent suppurative arthritis. Treatment guidelines are similar to those for septic arthritis except that a 4-wk course is preferred.

Pericarditis (Part XX, Section 7). *H. influenzae* type b is the etiologic agent in about 15% of children with bacterial pericarditis. The children are most commonly 2–4 yr of age and often have had an antecedent upper respiratory tract infection. Fever, respiratory distress, and tachycardia are consistent findings. Other infectious foci are common concomitants.

The diagnosis may be established by recovery of the organism from blood or pericardial fluid. Gram stain or detection of PRP in pericardial fluid, blood, or urine may aid the diagnosis. Antimicrobials should be provided parenterally in a regimen similar to that used for meningitis (see Chapter 169). Pericardiectomy is useful for draining the purulent material effectively and preventing tamponade and constrictive pericarditis.

Bacteremia Without an Associated Focus (see Chapter 167). Bacteremia due to *H. influenzae* type b may be associated with fever without any apparent focus of infection. In this situation, risk factors for "occult" bacteremia include the magnitude of fever (≥ 39° C) and the presence of leukocytosis (≥ 15,000/mm^3).

It is estimated that 26.6% of children with occult *H. influenzae* type b bacteremia develop meningitis if left untreated. All children with *H. influenzae* type b bacteremia in this clinical setting should be re-evaluated for a focus of infection when the blood culture result is obtained. If no source of infection is found but the child remains febrile or appears ill, a follow-up blood culture, diagnostic lumbar puncture, and chest radiograph are recommended. Such children should be hospitalized and given parenteral antimicrobial therapy. If no focus is identified, oral antimicrobial therapy may be substituted after 2–5 days to complete a 7–10-day course.

If no source is found at the time of re-evaluation and the child is afebrile and appears well, a follow-up blood culture should also be obtained. In this instance, further diagnostic evaluation (e.g., lumbar puncture) may not be necessary. However, many experts think that oral antimicrobial therapy may not be adequate because of the risk of serious focal infection. Therefore, a single daily dose of ceftriaxone (50 mg/kg) may be given. The child should be closely monitored until it is apparent that the fever has not recurred, the second blood culture is known to be sterile, and no focus of infection has developed.

MISCELLANEOUS INFECTIONS. Urinary tract infection, epididymo-orchitis, cervical adenitis, acute glossitis, infected thyroglossal duct cysts, endocarditis, endophthalmitis, primary peritonitis, and periappendiceal abscess are rarely caused by *H. influenzae* type b.

INVASIVE DISEASE IN THE NEONATE (see Chapter 98). In the neonate with invasive *H. influenzae* infection, nontypable isolates are more common than serotype b isolates, although both are rare. When illness occurs in the first 24 hr of life, especially in association with maternal chorioamnionitis or prolonged rupture of membranes, transmission of the organism to the infant is likely to have occurred through the maternal genital tract, which may be (< 1%) colonized with nontypable *H. influenzae.* Transmission to the neonate by colonized mothers may occur at a rate of up to 50%. Manifestations of neonatal invasive infection include bacteremia with a septic-like clinical picture, pneumonia, respiratory distress syndrome with shock, conjunctivitis, scalp abscess or cellulitis, or meningitis. Less commonly, mastoiditis, septic arthritis, or a congenital vesicular eruption may occur.

Noninvasive Disease. OTITIS MEDIA (see Chapter 590). Acute otitis media is one of the most common infectious diseases of childhood. It is thought to result from bacteria spreading from the nasopharynx through the eustachian tube into the middle ear cavity. Because of the usually associated upper respiratory tract infection, the mucosa in the area becomes hyperemic and swollen, an event that results in obstruction and an opportunity for bacterial multiplication in the middle ear.

Clinical isolates obtained by needle tympanocentesis from middle ear effusions during acute otitis media indicate that the most common bacterial pathogens are *S. pneumoniae, H. influenzae,* and *Moraxella catarrhalis.* Most *H. influenzae* isolates are nontypable, although a few are serotype b. Amoxicillin (or ampicillin) is a suitable first-line oral antimicrobial agent; the combined probability of an isolate being resistant to amoxicillin and of invasive potential is sufficiently infrequent to justify this approach. Alternatively, a single dose of ceftriaxone may constitute adequate therapy.

In the case of treatment failure or if a β-lactamase–producing isolate is obtained by tympanocentesis or from drainage fluid, cefaclor, amoxicillin-clavulanate, trimethoprim-sulfamethoxazole, or erythromycin-sulfisoxazole are among the available alternatives. The latter two combinations may be useful as first-line agents for patients allergic to β-lactam compounds.

CONJUNCTIVITIS (see Chapter 577). Acute infection of the conjunctiva is the most common eye infection in childhood. In the neonate, *H. influenzae* is an infrequent cause. However, it is an important pathogen in older children, as are *S. pneumoniae* and *S. aureus.* Most *H. influenzae* isolates associated with conjunctivitis are nontypable, although serotype b isolates and other microorganisms are occasionally found. Empiric treatment of conjunctivitis beyond the neonatal period usually consists of topical antimicrobial therapy with sulfacetimide and erythromycin.

SINUSITIS (see Chapter 327). *H. influenzae* is an important cause of acute sinusitis in children, second in frequency only to *S. pneumoniae.* Chronic sinusitis lasting longer than 1 yr or severe sinusitis requiring hospitalization or combined medical and surgical management is often caused by *S. aureus* or anaerobes such as *Peptococcus, Peptostreptococcus,* or *Bacteroides* species. Nontypable *H. influenzae* and viridans group *streptococci* are also frequently recovered.

For uncomplicated sinusitis, amoxicillin is acceptable therapy. However, if clinical improvement does not occur, a broader-spectrum regimen may be appropriate, such as amoxicillin-clavulanate or erythromycin-sulfisoxazole; hospitalization with parenteral therapy is occasionally required. For uncomplicated sinusitis, a 10-day course is sufficient.

PREVENTION OF SEROTYPE B INFECTIONS. Chemoprophylaxis. Unvaccinated close contacts younger than 48 mo of age of patients with invasive *H. influenzae* type b infections are at increased risk of invasive infection when exposed to an index case. The risk of secondary disease is inversely related to age (for children older than 3 mo). About half of the cases of secondary disease among susceptible household contacts occur in the 1st wk after hospitalization of the index patient, and new cases in susceptible household contacts occur 1–11 mo after illness in the index patient. More than 25% of secondary cases are recognized after 30 days. However, many children are now protected against spread of *H. influenzae* type b by prior immunization. With the use of high-efficacy conjugate vaccines, important changes in the recommendations for chemoprophylaxis of household contacts have been made.

The goal of chemoprophylaxis is to prevent a susceptible child from acquiring *H. influenzae* type b from contacts by eliminating colonization in the close contacts. Rifampin prophylaxis is indicated for all members of the close contact group, including the index patient, if one or more children younger than 48 mo are not fully immunized. Fully immunized in this instance is defined as having received at least one dose of a *H. influenzae* type b conjugate vaccine at 15 mo of age or older, two doses at 12–14 mo of age, or two or more doses when younger than 12 mo of age with a booster dose at 12 mo of age or older. An exception is made when the household contact group includes a fully vaccinated immunocompromised child, because the vaccination may have been ineffective. The household contact group is defined as individuals residing with the index patient or a nonresident who has spent 4 or more hr with the index patient for at least 5 of the 7 days preceding the day of hospitalization of the index patient.

Parents of children hospitalized for invasive *H. influenzae* type b disease should be told that there is an increased risk for secondary infection due to this organism in other young children in the same household, if they are partially immunized. The parents should be alerted to any signs or symptoms that might be related to such an infection and should be instructed to seek prompt medical attention when such signs do appear. Although parents of children exposed to a single case of invasive *H. influenzae* type b disease in a child care center or nursery school should be similarly warned, there is disagreement about the use of rifampin for these children. Because the data on the risk of secondary *H. influenzae* type b infection among children who attend group day care are conflicting, some experts think that the risk is too low to justify chemoprophylaxis. It is difficult to institute a uniform policy that would include all the many different caretakers and physicians involved.

A few guidelines for chemoprophylaxis are useful in evaluating a day-care setting for possible rifampin administration. In child care homes resembling households, such as those with children younger than 2 yr of age in which contact is at least 25 hr per week, rifampin prophylaxis may be of benefit. When two or more cases of invasive disease have occurred within 60 days among attendees, regardless of the size of the care facility, administering rifampin to all attendees and supervisory personnel is recommended. If all day-care contacts are older than 2 yr of age, chemoprophylaxis need not be given.

For chemoprophylaxis, children should be given rifampin orally (0–1 mo of age, 10 mg/kg/dose; >1 mo, 20 mg/kg/dose, not to exceed 600 mg/dose), once each a day for 4 consecutive days. The adult dose is 600 mg once daily. It is not recommended for pregnant women, because the effects on the fetus are not established. Because rifampin induces enzymes that metabolize oral contraceptives, other methods of contraception should be implemented during the period of rifampin administration. Rifampin turns body fluids (e.g., urine, saliva, tears) reddish orange and may permanently stain soft contact lenses.

Immunoprophylaxis Vaccines (see Chapter 247). The first-generation unconjugated PRP vaccine has been replaced by four licensed *H. influenzae* type b conjugate vaccines that differ in the carrier protein used, the saccharide molecular size, and the method of conjugating the saccharide to the protein (see Table 177–1): PRP-D (ProHIBit, Connaught Laboratories) employs diphtheria toxoid as the carrier protein; HbOC (HIBTITER, Lederle-Praxis) has an oligosaccharide linked to a nontoxic mutant diphtheria toxin called CRM197; PRP-OMP (Pedvax HIB, Merck, Sharp & Dohme) has an outer membrane protein complex of *N. meningitidis* group B as the carrier; and PRP-T (ActHIB/OmniHib, Pasteur-Merieux-Connaught/SmithKline Beecham) employs a tetanus toxoid carrier. There are two opportunities to combine vaccines which contain *H. influenzae* type b conjugate vaccines with DTP. In one, HbOC is combined with the DTP (TETRAMUNE, Lederle-Praxis) prior to distribution. In the other, PRP-T is reconstituted with U.S. Connaught DTP immediately before administration. The introduction of effective immunization against *H. influenzae* type b with the use of the conjugate vaccines has greatly decreased the occurrence of *H. influenzae* type b infections.

Barenkamp SJ: Outer membrane proteins and lipopolysaccharides of nontypable *Haemophilus influenzae.* J Infect Dis 165 (Suppl):S181, 1992.

Committee on Infectious Diseases: *Haemophilus influenzae* type b conjugate vaccines: Recommendations for immunization with recently and previously licensed vaccines. Pediatrics 92:480, 1993.

Daum RS, Granoff DM: Lessons from the evaluation of the immunogenicity. *In:* Ellis RW, Granoff DM (eds): Development and Clinical Uses of *Haemophilus* b Conjugate Vaccines. New York, Marcel Dekker, 1994, pp 291–312.

Holmes SJ, Granoff DM: The biology of *Haemophilus influenzae* type b vaccination failure. J Infect Dis (Suppl):S121, 1992.

Jorgensen JH, Doern GV, Maher LA, et al: Antimicrobial resistance among respiratory isolates of *Haemophilus influenzae, Moraxella catarrhalis,* and *Streptococcus pneumoniae* in the United States. Antimicrob Agents Chemother Infect 34:2075, 1990.

Jorgenson JH: Update on mechanisms and prevalence of antimicrobial resistance in *Haemophilus influenzae.* Clin Infect Dis 14:1119, 1992.

Liu VC, Smith AL: Molecular mechanism of *H. influenzae* pathogenicity. Antibiot Chemother 45:30, 1992.

Mendelman PM: Targets of β-lactam antibiotics penicillin-binding proteins in ampicillin-resistant, non-β-lactamase-producing *Haemophilus influenzae.* J Infect Dis 165(Suppl):S107, 1992.

Murphy TV, White KE, Pastor P, et al: Declining incidence of *Haemophilus influenzae* type b diseases since introduction of vaccination. JAMA 269:246, 1993.

Takala AK, Clements DA: Socioeconomic risk factors for invasive *Haemophilus influenzae* type b disease. J Infect Dis 165(Suppl):S5, 1992.

Tuomanen E, Powell KR, Laferriere CI, et al: Oral chloramphenicol in the treatment of *Haemophilus influenzae* meningitis. J Pediatr 99:968, 1981.

Vadheim CM, Greenberg DP, Bordenave N, et al: Risk factors for invasive *Haemophilus influenzae* type b in LA County children, 18–60 months of age. Am J Epidemiol 136:221, 1992.

Vadheim CM, Ward JI: Epidemiology in developed countries. *In:* Ellis RW, Granoff DM (eds): Development and Clinical Uses of *Haemophilus* b Conjugate Vaccines. New York, Marcel Dekker, 1994, pp 231–245.

van Alphen L: Epidemiology and prevention of respiratory tract infections due to nonencapsulated *Haemophilus influenzae.* J Infect Dis 165(Suppl):S177, 1992.

CHAPTER 178

Meningococcal Infections

Michele Estabrook

Meningococcal disease, first described by Vieusseaux in 1805 as epidemic cerebrospinal fever, remains a significant health problem, particularly in the developing world. Although nasopharyngeal colonization rarely leads to disseminated disease, the fulminant, rapidly fatal course of a child with meningococcemia is not soon forgotten.

ETIOLOGY. *Neisseria meningitidis* is a gram-negative diplococcus (0.6 × 0.8 μm) that is often described as biscuit shaped. It is a common commensal organism of the human nasopharynx and has not been isolated from animal or environmental sources. The meningococcus is fastidious, and growth is facilitated in a moist environment at 35–37° C in an atmosphere of 5–10% carbon dioxide. It grows well on several enriched media, including supplemented chocolate agar, Mueller-Hinton agar, blood agar base, and trypticase soy agar. On solid media, colonies are transparent, nonpigmented, and nonhemolytic. *N. meningitidis* is identified by its ability to ferment glucose and maltose to acid and its inability to ferment sucrose or lactose. Indole and hydrogen sulfide are not formed. The cell wall contains cytochrome oxidase, which results in the positive oxidase test result.

The meningococci have been divided into serogroups based on antigenic differences in their capsular polysaccharides. At least 13 serogroups have been identified, but groups A, B, C, W, and Y account for most meningococcal disease. The other serogroups often colonize the nasopharynx but rarely disseminate. Lipooligosaccharides (e.g., endotoxin) and proteins found in the outer membrane complex are also used to serotype meningococcal strains.

EPIDEMIOLOGY. Meningococcal dissemination occurs as endemic disease punctuated by outbreaks of cases that are often clustered geographically. True epidemics have become rare in developed countries but remain a significant problem in much of the developing world. Endemic disease appears to be caused by a heterogeneous group of meningococcal serotypes, and epidemics are caused by a single serotype. Analysis with multilocus enzyme genetic methods has confirmed that a meningococcal epidemic is caused by strains derived from a single clonotype.

The Centers for Disease Control (CDC) reported the results of a laboratory-based surveillance for meningococcal disease in a large United States population for the years 1989 through 1991. The average annual rate of invasive disease remained fairly constant at 1.1 per 100,000 members of the population. It was estimated that 2,600 cases of meningococcal disease occurred annually in the United States during this period. The highest attack rates were during the winter and early spring months. Males accounted for 55% of the total cases, and 29% of the cases occurred in children younger than 1 yr of age, with the peak incidence of disease being 26 per 100,000 infants less than 4 mo of age. Forty-six per cent of the cases occurred in children 2 yr of age or younger, and an additional 25% of the cases occurred in persons 30 yr of age or older. Serogroup B and serogroup C meningococci accounted for near-equal proportions of disease (46% and 45%, respectively), but 69%

of group C disease occurred in persons older than 2 yr of age. Fifty-eight per cent of the cases were reported to have meningitis. *N. meningitidis* was isolated from blood in 66% of cases, cerebrospinal fluid (CSF) in 51%, and joint fluid in 1%.

Meningococcal disease, particularly group A, remains a major health problem in much of the developing world. Many areas, such as China and Africa, have an endemic rate of disease of 10–25 per 100,000 persons and major periodic epidemics (100–500 cases/100,000). Epidemic disease typically involves individuals who are older than those with endemic disease.

PATHOGENESIS. *N. meningitidis* is thought to be acquired by a respiratory route. Colonization of the nasopharynx with meningococci usually leads to asymptomatic carriage, and only rarely does dissemination occur. Colonization can persist for weeks to months. Carriage rates vary from 2–30% in a normal population during nonepidemic periods but are higher among children in day-care centers and in conditions of crowding. The carriage rate can approach 100% in a closed population during an epidemic.

For colonization to take place, meningococci must evade mucosal IgA and adhere to epithelial cells in the nasopharynx. This is facilitated by the secretion of proteases that cleave the proline-rich hinge region of IgA and render it nonfunctional. Meningococci and gonococci produce this enzyme, but nonpathogenic *Neisseria* organisms do not. Meningococci then bind selectively to nonciliated epithelial cells. Pili appear to be of major importance in the attachment of meningococci to the human nasopharynx. The bacteria enter nonciliated epithelial cells by a parasite-directed endocytotic process and are carried across the cell in membrane-bound vacuoles.

Meningococci disseminate from the upper respiratory tract through the bloodstream. Serum antibody leading to complement-mediated bacterial lysis has been shown to block this dissemination, and a deficiency of antimeningococcal antibody is associated with the development of meningococcemia. Bactericidal antibody is directed against the capsular polysaccharide, subcapsular protein, and lipooligosaccharide antigens. Newborn infants have protective antibody that is primarily IgG of maternal origin. As this antibody wanes, infants 3–24 mo of age experience the highest incidence of meningococcal disease. By adulthood, most individuals have developed natural immunity against *N. meningitidis.*

The source of this immunity comes from nasopharyngeal colonization with *N. meningitidis* and colonization of the gastrointestinal tract with enteric bacteria that express cross-reactive antigens. Infants have a high carriage rate of an unencapsulated, nonpathogenic neisserial strain, *N. lactamica,* that leads to the development of bactericidal antibody against the meningococcus.

The importance of the complement system in host defense against *N. meningitidis* is underscored by the fact that individuals with primary or acquired complement deficiency have an increased risk of developing meningococcal disease, and 50–60% of individuals with properdin, factor D, or terminal-component deficiencies develop bacterial infections that are caused almost solely by *N. meningitidis.* Recurrent infection is common with terminal component deficiencies but is uncommon with properdin deficiency. Acquired complement deficiency also carries an increased risk and can be seen with systemic diseases that deplete serum complement. Examples are systemic lupus erythematosus, nephrotic syndrome, multiple myeloma, and hepatic failure.

The group B capsule is a homopolymer of sialic acid, which is known to inhibit alternative complement pathway activation. Antibody that activates the classic pathway can overcome this inhibition. The lack of specific antibody coupled with the inhibition of the alternative pathway may explain the prevalence of serogroup B meningococcal disease in young children.

PATHOLOGY. Disseminated meningococcal disease is associated with an acute inflammatory response. Hemorrhage and necrosis may be seen in any organ system and appears to be mediated by intravascular coagulation with deposition of fibrin in small vessels. The major organ systems involved in fatal cases of meningococcemia are the heart, central nervous system, skin, mucous and serous membranes, and adrenals. Myocarditis is found in more than 50% of patients who die of meningococcal disease. Cutaneous hemorrhages, ranging from petechiae to purpura, occur in most fatal infections and are associated with acute vasculitis with fibrin deposition in arterioles and capillaries. Diffuse adrenal hemorrhage may occur in patients with fulminant meningococcemia (i.e., Waterhouse-Friderichsen syndrome). Meningitis is characterized by acute inflammatory cells in the leptomeninges and perivascular spaces. Focal cerebral involvement is uncommon.

The interaction of endotoxin released by *N. meningitidis* and the complement system probably is key in the pathogenesis of the clinical manifestations of meningococcal disease. Complement activation correlates with the concentration of meningococcal lipooligosaccharide in the plasma. The concentration of circulating endotoxin is directly correlated with activation of the fibrinolytic system, development of disseminated intravascular coagulopathy, multiple organ system failure, septic shock, and death. The level of endotoxemia correlates with the concentration of circulating cytokines, which are released from endotoxin-stimulated monocytes and macrophages. The concentrations of tumor necrosis factor-α and interleukins have been directly associated with fatal meningococcal disease.

CLINICAL MANIFESTATIONS. The spectrum of meningococcal disease can vary widely, from fever and occult bacteremia to sepsis, shock, and death. Recognized patterns of disease are bacteremia without sepsis, meningococcemic sepsis without meningitis, meningitis with or without meningococcemia, meningoencephalitis, and infection of specific organs.

A well-recognized entity is occult bacteremia in a febrile child. Upper respiratory or gastrointestinal symptoms or a maculopapular rash can be evident. The child often is sent home on no antibiotics or oral antibiotics for a minor infection. Spontaneous recovery without antibiotics has been reported, but some children have developed meningitis.

Acute meningococcemia can mimic a viral-like illness with pharyngitis, fever, myalgias, weakness, and headache. With widespread hematogenous dissemination, the disease rapidly progresses to septic shock characterized by hypotension, disseminated intravascular coagulation, acidosis, adrenal hemorrhage, renal failure, myocardial failure, and coma. Meningitis may or may not develop. Concomitant pneumonia, myocarditis, purulent pericarditis, and septic arthritis have been described. More often, meningococcal disease manifests as acute meningitis that responds to appropriate antibiotics and supportive therapy. Seizures and focal neurologic signs occur less frequently than in patients with meningitis caused by the pneumococcus or *Haemophilus.* Rarely, meningoencephalitis can occur with diffuse brain involvement.

A review of 100 children with invasive meningococcal disease revealed that 71% presented with fever, 4% with hypothermia, and 42% with shock. Skin lesions occurred in 71% of the cases with petechiae and/or purpura, and in 49% with both. Purpura fulminans developed in 16%. Other rashes described were maculopapular, pustular, and bullous lesions. Additional presenting symptoms and signs were irritability in 21%, lethargy in 30%, and emesis in 34%. Diarrhea, cough, rhinorrhea, seizure, and arthritis occurred much less frequently (6–10%). Leukopenia and low platelet counts affected 21% and 14%, respectively, and the white blood cell counts ranged from 0.9 to $46/mm^3 \times 10^3$. *N. meningitidis* was isolated in blood culture from 48% of the children, and meningitis was diagnosed in 55%. Six children had meningococci isolated from CSF in the absence of CSF pleocytosis, hypoglycorrhachia, or organisms detected by Gram stain. Five of eight children who presented with arthritis had *N. meningitidis* isolated from joint aspiration fluid. Eight per cent of the children had radiographic evidence of pneumonia on presentation.

Uncommon manifestations of meningococcal disease include endocarditis, purulent pericarditis, septic arthritis, endophthalmitis, mesenteric adenitis, and osteomyelitis. Primary purulent conjunctivitis can lead to invasive disease. Sinusitis, otitis media, and periorbital cellulitis also can be caused by the meningococcus. Primary meningococcal pneumonia is a recognized clinical entity that is associated with pleural effusions or empyema in 15% of cases. *N. meningitidis* is a rare isolate of the genitourinary tract in asymptomatic or symptomatic individuals and has been the causal organism in urethritis, cervicitis, vaginitis, and proctitis.

Chronic meningococcemia is a rare manifestation of meningococcal disease that can occur in children and adults. It is characterized by fever, nontoxic appearance, arthralgias, headache, and rash. The rash resembles that of disseminated gonococcal infection. Symptoms are intermittent, with the rash often appearing with fever. The mean duration of illness is 6–8 wk. Blood cultures may initially be sterile. Without specific therapy, complications such as meningitis can result.

DIAGNOSIS. Definitive diagnosis of meningococcal disease is made by the isolation of the organism from a usually sterile body fluid such as blood, CSF, or synovial fluid. Isolation of meningococci from the nasopharynx is not diagnostic for disseminated disease. Blood and CSF are the usual sources of organism isolation. The blood culture yields *N. meningitidis* in about one half of the cases of disseminated disease, and culture or Gram stain usually reveal the organism in those with meningitis. Culture or Gram stain of petechial or papular lesions has been variably successful in identifying meningococci. Occasionally, bacteria can be seen on Gram stain of the buffy coat layer of a spun blood sample.

In meningitis, the morphologic and clinical characteristics of CSF are those of acute bacterial meningitis (see Chapter 169.1). CSF cultures can be positive in patients with meningococcemia but without clinical evidence of meningitis or CSF pleocytosis. CSF cultures may be negative if the lumbar puncture has been performed early in the course of disease or if the patient has received previous antibiotic treatment.

Techniques of counterimmunoelectrophoresis and latex agglutination detect meningococcal capsular polysaccharide in CSF, serum, joint fluid, and urine. False-negative results occur, and specificity may be limited when organisms with cross-reactive antigens are involved, such as *Escherichia coli* K1, which cross reacts with the group B meningococcus. Antisera and monoclonal antibodies can be used to identify different serogroups of meningococci. These studies are useful early in infection and if the patient has received antibiotics, rendering cultures sterile.

Ancillary data may support a systemic bacterial infection and includes elevated sedimentation rate and C-reactive protein, leukocytopenia or leukocytosis, thrombocytopenia, proteinuria, and hematuria. Patients with disseminated intravascular coagulation may have decreased serum concentrations of prothrombin and fibrinogen. Screening for complement deficiency is recommended for individuals diagnosed with meningococcal disease. In one series of 20 patients with a first episode of meningococcal meningitis, meningococcemia, or meningococcal pericarditis, three had a deficiency of a terminal-pathway component and three had deficiencies of multiple complement components associated with underlying systemic diseases.

DIFFERENTIAL DIAGNOSIS. This includes acute bacterial or viral meningitis, mycoplasma infection, leptospirosis, syphilis, acute hemorrhagic encephalitis, encephalopathies, serum sickness, collagen vascular diseases, Henoch-Schönlein purpura, hemolytic uremic syndrome, and ingestion of various poisons. The petechial or purpuric rash of meningococcemia is similar to that noted in any patient with a disease characterized by generalized vasculitis. These diseases include septicemia due to many gram-negative organisms; overwhelming septicemia with gram-positive organisms; bacterial endocarditis; Rocky Mountain spotted fever; epidemic typhus; *Ehrlichia canis* infection; infections with echoviruses, particularly types 6, 9, and 16; coxsackievirus infections, predominantly of types A2, A4, A9, and A16; rubella; rubeola and atypical rubeola; Henoch-Schönlein purpura; Kawasaki disease; idiopathic thrombocytopenia; and erythema multiforme or erythema nodosum due to drugs or infectious or noninfectious disease processes. The morbilliform rash occasionally observed may be confused with any macular or maculopapular viral exanthem.

COMPLICATIONS. Acute complications are related to the inflammatory changes, vasculitis, disseminated intravascular coagulation, and hypotension of invasive meningococcal disease. These can include adrenal hemorrhage, arthritis, myocarditis, pneumonia, lung abscess, peritonitis, and renal infarcts. The vasculitis can lead to skin loss with secondary infection, tissue necrosis, and gangrene. Skin sloughing can necessitate the use of skin grafts. Bone involvement can lead to growth disturbance and late skeletal deformities secondary to epiphyseal avascular necrosis and epiphyseal-metaphyseal defects. Limb amputation has been reported for patients with purpura fulminans.

Meningitis rarely is complicated by subdural effusion or empyema or by brain abscess. Deafness is the most frequent neurologic sequelae, but the reported incidence varies from 0–38%. Other rare sequelae include ataxia, seizures, blindness, cranial nerve palsies, hemiparesis or quadriparesis, and obstructive hydrocephalus.

The late complications of meningococcal disease are thought to be immune complex–mediated and become apparent 4–9 days after the onset of illness. The usual manifestations are arthritis and cutaneous vasculitis. The arthritis is usually monoarticular or oligoarticular. Effusions are usually sterile and respond to nonsteroidal anti-inflammatory agents. Permanent joint deformity is uncommon. Because most patients with meningococcal meningitis are afebrile by the 7th hospital day, the persistence or recrudescence of fever after 5 days of antibiotics warrants an evaluation for immune complex-mediated complications.

PREVENTION. Close contacts of patients with meningococcal disease are at increased risk of infection and should be carefully monitored and brought to medical attention if fever develops. Prophylaxis is indicated as soon as possible for household, day-care, and nursery school contacts. Prophylaxis is also recommended for persons who have had contact with patients' oral secretions. Prophylaxis is not routinely recommended for medical personnel except those with intimate exposure, such as with mouth-to-mouth resuscitation, intubation, or suctioning before antibiotic therapy was begun. Rifampin is given (10 mg/kg; maximum dose, 600 mg) orally every 12 hr for 2 days (total of four doses). The dose is reduced to 5 mg/kg for very young infants. If the isolate is known to be sensitive to sulfonamides, suflisoxazole prophylaxis is preferred. Penicillin does not eradicate nasopharyngeal carriage, and patients with meningococcal disease should receive rifampin before discharge.

A quadrivalent vaccine composed of capsular polysaccharide of meningococcal groups A, C, Y, and W-135 is licensed in the United States. The vaccine is immunogenic in adults but is unreliable in children under 2 yr of age. The group B polysaccharide is poorly immunogenic in children and adults, and no vaccine is available against this serogroup. Routine immunization of the United States population is not recommended at this time, but the vaccine is routinely given to all American military recruits.

Immunization is useful to control outbreaks of meningococcal disease of the serogroups represented in the quadravalent vaccine. It is also recommended for travelers to countries with a high incidence of meningococcal disease. Immunization of close contacts of individuals with A, C, Y, or W disease should be considered, because it has been useful in the prevention of secondary cases. Individuals with anatomic or functional asplenia and those with complement component deficiencies should be immunized.

Polysaccharide-protein conjugate vaccines are being developed for the prevention of meningococcal disease, and subcapsular proteins and detoxified lipooligosaccharides are being investigated as possible vaccines.

TREATMENT. Aqueous penicillin G is the drug of choice and should be given in doses of 250,000 to 300,000 U/kg/24 hr, administered intravenously in six divided doses. Chloramphenicol sodium succinate (75–100 mg/kg/24 hr, intravenously in four divided doses) provides effective treatment for patients who are allergic to penicillin. Cefotaxime (200/mg/24 hr) and ceftriaxone (100 mg/kg/24 hr) are effective empirical therapy for meningococcal disease and may be useful in patients who are allergic to penicillin. Therapy is continued for 7 days.

Isolates of *N. meningitidis* have been reported from Spain, South Africa, and Canada as being relatively resistant to penicillin, defined as having a minimal inhibitory concentration of penicillin of 0.1–1.0 μg/mL. Moderate resistance is caused, at least in part, by altered penicillin-binding protein 2. High-level resistance due to β-lactamase production has been reported from South Africa. The CDC estimated that about 4% of meningococcal disease in 1991 in the United States was caused by *N. meningitidis* strains that were relatively resistant to penicillin. None of the strains isolated produced β-lactamase. The clinical significance of moderate penicillin resistance is unknown. The CDC decided that routine susceptibility testing of clinical meningococcal isolates is probably not indicated in the United States at this time, but continued surveillance is necessary.

Patients with acute meningococcal infections should be monitored carefully. Supportive care and other therapy are discussed in Chapter 60.5.

PROGNOSIS. Despite the use of appropriate antibiotics, the mortality rate for disseminated meningococcal disease remains at 8–12% in the United States. Poor prognostic factors include hypothermia, hypotension, purpura fulminans, seizures or shock on presentation, leukopenia, thrombocytopenia, and high circulating levels of endotoxin and tumor necrosis factor. Some studies have included the development of petechiae within 12 hr of admission, hyperpyrexia, and the absence of meningitis.

Centers for Disease Control: Laboratory-based surveillance for meningococcal disease in selected areas—United States, 1989–1991. MMWR 42:21, 1993.
DeVoe IW: The meningococcus and mechanisms of pathogenicity. Microbiol Rev 46:162, 1982.
Edwards MS, Baker CJ: Complications and sequelae of meningococcal infections in children. J Pediatr 99:540, 1981.
Ellison RT, Kohler PF, Gurd JG, et al: Prevalence of congenital or acquired complement deficiency in patients with sporadic meningococcal disease. N Engl J Med 308:913, 1983.
Figueroa JE, Densen P: Infectious diseases associated with complement deficiencies. Clin Microbiol Rev 4:359, 1991.
Frasch CE: Vaccines for prevention of meningococcal disease. Clin Microbiol Rev 2(Suppl):S134, 1989.
Gedde-Dahl TW, Bjark P, Hoiby EA, et al: Severity of meningococcal disease: assessment by factors and scores and implications for patient management. Rev Infect Dis 12:973, 1990.
Jackson LA, Tenover FC, Baker C, et al: Prevalence of *Neisseria meningitidis* relatively resistant to penicillin in the United States, 1991. J Infect Dis 169:438, 1993.
Leggiadro RJ: Prevalence of complement deficiencies in children with systemic meningococcal infections. Pediatr Infect Dis J 6:75, 1987.
Wong VK, Hitchcock W, Mason WH: Meningococcal infections in children; a review of 100 cases. Pediatr Infect Dis 8:224, 1989.

CHAPTER 179

Gonococcal Infections

Michele Estabrook

Neisseria gonorrhoeae produces various forms of gonorrhea, an infection of the genitourinary tract mucous membranes and rarely of the mucosa of the rectum, oropharynx, and conjunctiva. Gonorrhea transmitted by sexual contact or perinatally is the most frequently reported communicable disease in the United States and affects children of all ages. This high prevalence and the development of antibiotic-resistant strains have produced significant morbidity in adolescents.

ETIOLOGY. *N. gonorrhoeae* is a nonmotile, aerobic, non–spore-forming, gram-negative intracellular diplococcus with flattened adjacent surfaces. Optimal growth occurs at 35–37° C and at pH 7.2–7.6 in an atmosphere of 3–5% CO_2. The specimen should be inoculated immediately into fresh, moist modified Thayer-Martin or specialized transport (Transgrow) media because gonococci do not tolerate drying. Presumptive identification may be based on colony appearance, Gram stain, and production of cytochrome oxidase. Gonococci are differentiated from other *Neisseria* species by the fermentation of glucose but not maltose, sucrose, or lactose. Gram-negative diplococci are seen in infected material, often within polymorphonuclear leukocytes.

The cell surface of the gonococcus is similar to that of other gram-negative bacteria and contains pili, outer membrane proteins, and lipooligosaccharides (endotoxin), which contribute to cell adherence, tissue invasion, and resistance to host defenses. *N. gonorrhoeae* may be subdivided on the basis of the presence of pili, serologic typing, colony appearance, and nutritional requirements. The two systems primarily used to characterize gonococcal strains are auxotyping (i.e., nutritional requirements) and serotyping. The most widely used serotyping system is based on antigenic differences in protein I found in the outer membrane. Protein I can be antigenically classified into two groups: IA and IB. Monoclonal antibodies are used to further subdivide strains as serovars (e.g., IA-1, IB-12).

EPIDEMIOLOGY. *N. gonorrhoeae* infection occurs only in humans. The organism is shed in the exudate and secretions of infected mucosal surfaces and is transmitted through intimate contact, such as sexual contact or parturition and, rarely, by contact with fomites. Gonococcal infections in the newborn period generally are acquired during delivery. Gonococcal infections in children after the newborn period and before puberty are acquired rarely through household exposure to infected caretakers. In such cases, the possibility of sexual abuse should be seriously considered.

Almost 1 million cases of gonorrhea are reported annually in the United States. About 50% of treated cases are reported; the number of undetected asymptomatic cases may be twice the number reported, placing the estimated annual U.S. incidence in excess of 3 million. The highest incidence of gonococcal infection is reported for men 20–24 yr of age, followed by those 15 to 19 yr of age. The highest rates for females are for those who are 15–19 yr of age. Risk factors include nonwhite race, homosexuality, increased number of sexual partners, prostitution, presence of other sexually transmitted diseases, unmarried status, poverty, and failure to use condoms. Peak incidence occurs in July–September, and the nadir is January–April. Techniques of auxotyping and serotyping can be used together to analyze the spread of individual strains of *N. gonorrhoeae* within a community.

Maintenance and subsequent spread of gonococcal infections in a community require a hyperendemic, high-risk core group such as prostitutes or inner city youth. Transmission occurs after intercourse with an asymptomatic patient or one who ignores the signs of infection or has limited access to health care. Frequently, clonal transmission of one strain spreads in waves through communities. Proper education, contact identification, and local treatment clinics may limit transmission.

Gonococcal infection of the neonate usually results from peripartum exposure to infected exudate from the cervix of the mother. An acute infection begins 2 to 5 days after birth. The incidence of neonatal infection depends on the prevalence of gonococcal infection among pregnant women, on whether prenatal screening for gonorrhea is used, and on whether newborns receive ophthalmic prophylaxis. The prevalence of gonorrhea is <1% in most U.S. prenatal populations but may be higher in some areas.

PATHOLOGY. Mucosal invasion by gonococci results in a local inflammatory response that produces a purulent exudate consisting of polymorphonuclear leukocytes, serum, and desquamated epithelium. The gonococcal lipooligosaccharide (endotoxin) exhibits direct cytotoxicity, causing ciliostasis and sloughing of ciliated epithelial cells. Once the gonococcus traverses the mucosal barrier, the lipooligosaccharide binds bactericidal IgM antibody and serum complement, causing an acute inflammatory response in the subepithelial space. Tumor necrosis factor and other cytokines are thought to mediate the cytotoxicity of gonococcal infections.

The purulent discharge produced by urogenital gonococcal infection may block the ducts of paraurethral (Skene) or vaginal (Bartholin) glands, causing cysts or abscesses. In the untreated patient, the inflammatory exudate is replaced by fibroblasts, and fibrous tissue may lead to stricture of the urethra. Gonococci may ascend the urogenital tract, causing acute endometritis, salpingitis, and peritonitis (collectively termed acute pelvic inflammatory disease) in postpubertal females and urethritis or epididymitis in postpubertal males. Perihepatitis (Fitz-Hugh–Curtis syndrome) follows dissemination through the peritoneum from the fallopian tube to the liver capsule. Gonococci that invade the lymphatics and blood vessels may lead to inguinal lymphadenopathy; to perineal, perianal, ischiorectal, and periprostatic abscesses; and to disseminated gonococcal disease.

PATHOGENESIS. A number of gonococcal virulence and host immune factors are involved in the penetration of the mucosal barrier and subsequent manifestations of local and systemic infection. Selective pressure from different mucosal environments probably leads to changes in the outer membrane of the organism, including expression of variants of pili, opacity or Opa proteins (formerly protein II), and lipooligosaccharides. These changes may enhance gonococcal attachment, invasion of human cells, replication, and evasion of the host's immune response.

For infection to occur, the gonococcus must first attach to host cells. A gonococcal IgA protease inactivates IgA1 by cleaving the molecule in the hinge region and may be an important factor in colonization or invasion of host mucosal surfaces. Gonococci adhere to the microvilli of nonciliated epithelial cells by hairlike protein structures (pili) that extend from the cell wall. Pili are thought to protect the gonococcus from phagocytosis and complement-mediated killing. Pili undergo high-frequency antigenic variation that may aid in the organism's escape from the host immune response and may provide specific ligands for different cell receptors. Opacity proteins, most of which confer an opaque appearance to colonies, are also thought to function as ligands to facilitate binding to human cells. Gonococci that express certain Opa proteins adhere and are phagocytosed by human neutrophils in the absence of serum.

Other phenotypic changes that occur in response to environmental stresses allow gonococci to establish infection. Examples include iron-repressible proteins for binding transferrin or lactoferrin, anaerobically expressed proteins, and synthesis of proteins that is mediated by contact with epithelial cells. Gonococci may grow in vivo under anaerobic conditions or in an environment with relative lack of iron.

Approximately 24 hr after attachment, the epithelial cell surface invaginates and surrounds the gonococcus in a phagocytic vacuole. This phenomenon is thought to be mediated by the gonococcal outer membrane protein I inserting into the host cell and causing alterations in membrane permeability. Subsequently, phagocytic vacuoles begin releasing gonococci into the subepithelial space by means of exocytosis. Viable organisms may then cause local disease (i.e., salpingitis) or disseminate through the bloodstream or lymphatics.

Serum IgG and IgM directed against gonococcal proteins and lipooligosaccharides lead to complement-mediated bacterial lysis. Stable serum resistance to this bactericidal antibody probably results from the particular type of porin protein expressed in gonococci, and these strains are often the cause of disseminated disease. Other strains are sensitive when grown in vitro but are not killed in vivo because of blocking antibodies directed against protein III or sialylation of lipooligosaccharide that probably interferes with complement fixation. Gonococcal adaptation also appears to be important in the evasion of killing by neutrophils. Examples include sialylation of lipooligosaccharides, increases in catalase production, and changes in the expression of surface proteins.

N. gonorrhoeae isolates from patients with disseminated gonococcal infection (DGI) share common features that distinguish them from other gonococci. Most gonococci that produce DGI form transparent colonies (Opa−). Most contain outer membrane protein IA. They are resistant to the bactericidal activity of normal human serum. Local infections with these organisms fail to elicit an inflammatory response and are asymptomatic. Human IgG antibodies ("blocking antibodies") that do bind to DGI gonococci may interfere with bactericidal antibody- and complement-mediated lysis. DGI isolates have unique nutritional requirements (58% belong to the Arg−Hyx−Ura− auxotype) and greater sensitivity to penicillin.

Host factors may influence the incidence and manifestations of gonococcal infection. Prepubertal females are susceptible to vulvovaginitis and, rarely, experience salpingitis. *N. gonorrhoeae* infects noncornified epithelium, and the thin noncornified vaginal epithelium and alkaline pH of the vaginal mucin predispose this age group to infection of the lower genital tract. Estrogen-induced cornification of the vaginal epithelium in the neonate and mature female resists infection. Postpubertal females are more susceptible to salpingitis, especially during menses, when diminished bactericidal activity of the cervical mucus and the reflux of blood from the uterine cavity into the fallopian tubes facilitate passage of gonococci into the upper reproductive tract.

Populations at risk for DGI include asymptomatic carriers; neonates; menstruating, pregnant, and postpartum females; homosexuals; and immunocompromised hosts. The asymptomatic carrier state implies failure of the host immune system to recognize the gonococcus as a pathogen, the capacity of the gonococcus to avoid being killed, or both. Pharyngeal colonization has been proposed as a risk factor for DGI. The high rate of asymptomatic infection in pharyngeal gonorrhea may account for this phenomenon. Women are at greater risk for developing DGI during menstruation and pregnancy and postpartum, presumably due to the maximal endocervical shedding and decreased peroxidase bactericidal activity of the cervical mucus during these periods. A lack of neonatal bactericidal IgM antibody is thought to account for the neonate's increased susceptibility to DGI. Persons with terminal complement component deficiencies (C5–C9) are at considerable risk of developing recurrent episodes of DGI.

An increasing number of gonococcal isolates show significant penicillin resistance, which is of two basic types: plasmid-mediated β-lactamase (penicillinase) production, which confers absolute resistance (MIC 10–100 μg/mL), and chromosomally mediated resistance, which does not depend on β-lactamase production and confers relative resistance (MIC 1.0–4.0 μg/mL).

Penicillinase-producing *N. gonorrhoeae* (PPNG) are resistant to all penicillins and first-generation cephalosporins but not to second- and third-generation cephalosporins. An increasing number of gonococcal strains are resistant to tetracycline (TRNG), which can be plasmid-mediated or chromosomally mediated. Many strains are resistant to penicillin and tetracycline. Results of susceptibility data collected by the Centers for Disease Control (CDC) for 1991 indicated that 32% of the strains were resistant to penicillin or tetracycline. Eleven per cent of the isolates were PPNG, 5.7% were TRNG, and 2% were PPNG and TRNG. Almost 14% had chromosomally mediated resistance to one or both of these drugs.

CLINICAL MANIFESTATIONS. Asymptomatic Gonorrhea. The incidence of this form of gonorrhea in children has not been ascertained. Gonococci have been isolated from the oropharynx of young (2–9 yr of age) children who have been abused sexually by male contacts; oropharyngeal symptoms are usually absent. In a study of 12- to 19-yr-old females in a school for delinquents, the incidence of gonorrhea was 12%, and most girls affected were asymptomatic. About 68% of infected United States military men are asymptomatic; 66% of this group remained culture positive but asymptomatic for several months. As many as 80% of sexually mature females with urogenital gonorrhea infections are asymptomatic; asymptomatic rectal carriage of *N. gonorrhoeae* has been documented in 40–60% of females with urogenital infection. At least 20% of rectal infections are asymptomatic and 78% of pharyngeal gonococcal infections are asymptomatic in homosexual men. Individuals with asymptomatic gonorrhea are an important reservoir of infection and may develop disseminated disease.

Uncomplicated Gonorrhea. Genital gonorrhea has an incubation period of 2–5 days in men and 5–10 days in women. Primary infection develops in the urethra of the male, the vulva and vagina of the prepubertal female, and the cervix of the postpubertal female. Neonatal ophthalmitis occurs in both sexes.

Urethritis is usually characterized by a purulent discharge and by burning on urination without urgency or frequency. Untreated urethritis in the male resolves spontaneously in several weeks or may be complicated by epididymitis, penile edema, lymphangitis, prostatitis, or seminal vesiculitis. Gram-negative intracellular diplococci are found in the discharge.

In the prepubertal female, vulvovaginitis usually is characterized by a purulent vaginal discharge with a swollen, erythematous, tender, and excoriated vulva. Dysuria may occur. In the postpubertal female, symptomatic gonococcal cervicitis and urethritis are characterized by purulent discharge, suprapubic pain, dysuria, intermenstrual bleeding, and dyspareunia. The cervix may be inflamed and tender. In urogenital gonorrhea limited to the lower genital tract, pain is not enhanced by moving the cervix, and the adnexae are not tender to palpation. Purulent material may be expressed from the urethra or ducts of the Bartholin gland. Rectal gonorrhea, although often asymptomatic, may cause proctitis with symptoms of anal discharge, pruritus, and bleeding, pain, tenesmus, and constipation. Asymptomatic rectal gonorrhea may not be due to anal intercourse but may represent colonization from vaginal infection.

Gonococcal ophthalmitis may be unilateral or bilateral. It may occur in any age group following inoculation of the eye with infected secretions. Ophthalmia neonatorum due to *N. gonorrhoeae* usually appears from 1–4 days after birth (see Chapter 577). Ocular infection in older patients results from inoculation or autoinoculation from a genital site. The infection begins with mild inflammation and a serosanguineous discharge. Within 24 hr, the discharge becomes thick and purulent, and tense edema of the eyelids with marked chemosis occurs. If the disease is not treated promptly, corneal ulceration, rupture, and blindness may follow.

Disseminated Gonococcal Infection. Hematogenous dissemination occurs in 1–3% of all gonococcal infections, following asymptomatic primary infections more frequently than symptomatic infections. Women account for the majority of cases, with symptoms beginning 7–30 days after infection and within 7 days of menstruation. The most common manifestations are arthritis, tenosynovitis, dermatitis, and, rarely, carditis, meningitis, and osteomyelitis. The most common initial symptoms are acute onset of polyarthralgia with fever. Only 25% of patients complain of skin lesions. Most deny genitourinary symptoms; however, primary mucosal infection is documented by genitourinary cultures. Approximately 80–90% of cervical cultures are positive in women with DGI. In males, urethral cultures are positive in 50–60%, pharyngeal cultures are positive in 10–20%, and rectal cultures are positive in 15% of cases.

DGI has been classified into two clinical syndromes that have some overlapping features. The first and more common is the tenosynovitis-dermatitis syndrome, which is characterized by fever, chills, skin lesions, and polyarthralgias predominantly involving the wrists, hands, and fingers. Blood cultures are positive in approximately 30–40% of cases, and synovial fluid cultures are almost uniformly negative. The second syndrome is the suppurative arthritis syndrome in which systemic symptoms and signs are less prominent and a monoarticular arthritis, often involving the knee, is more common. A polyarthral phase may precede the monoarticular infection. In cases of monoarticular involvement, synovial fluid cultures are positive in approximately 45–55%, whereas blood cultures are usually negative. DGI in neonates usually occurs as a polyarticular septic arthritis.

Dermatologic lesions usually begin as painful discrete, 1- to 20-mm pink or red macules that progress to maculopapular, vesicular, bullous, pustular, or petechial lesions. The typical necrotic pustule on an erythematous base is distributed unevenly over the extremities, including the palmar and plantar surfaces, usually sparing the face and scalp. The lesions number between 5 and 40; 20–30% may contain gonococci. Although immune complexes may be present in DGI, complement levels are normal, and the role of the immune complexes in pathogenesis is uncertain.

Acute endocarditis is an uncommon (1–2%) but often fatal manifestation of DGI that usually leads to rapid destruction of the aortic valve. Acute pericarditis is a rarely described entity in patients with disseminated gonorrhea. Meningitis with *N. gonorrhoeae* has been documented. Signs and symptoms are similar to those of any acute bacterial meningitis.

COMPLICATIONS. Complications of gonorrhea result from the spread of gonococci from a local site of invasion. The time interval between primary infection and development of a complication is usually days to weeks. In postpubertal females, endometritis may occur, especially during menses. This may progress to salpingitis and peritonitis (pelvic inflammatory disease [PID]). Manifestations of PID include signs of lower genital tract infection (e.g., vaginal discharge, suprapubic pain, cervical tenderness) and upper genital tract infection (e.g., fever, leukocytosis, elevated erythrocyte sedimentation rate, and adnexal tenderness or mass). The differential diagnosis includes gynecologic (ovarian cyst, ovarian tumor, ectopic pregnancy) and intra-abdominal (appendicitis, urinary tract infection, inflammatory bowel disease) pathology.

Once inside the peritoneum, gonococci may seed the liver capsule, causing a perihepatitis. The resultant right upper quadrant pain, with or without signs of salpingitis, is known as the Fitz-Hugh–Curtis syndrome. Perihepatitis may also be caused by *Chlamydia trachomatis.* Progression to PID occurs in about 20% of cases of gonococcal cervicitis. *N. gonorrhoeae* is isolated in approximately 40% of cases of PID in the United States. Untreated cases may lead to hydrosalpinx, pyosalpinx, tubo-ovarian abscess, and eventual sterility. Even with adequate treatment of PID, the risk of sterility caused by bilateral tubal occlusion approaches 20% after one episode of salpingitis and exceeds 60% with three or more episodes. The risk of ectopic pregnancy is increased approximately 7-fold after one or more episodes of salpingitis. Additional sequelae of PID include chronic pain, dyspareunia, and increased risk of recurrent PID.

Urogenital gonococcal infection acquired during the 1st trimester of pregnancy carries a high risk of septic abortion. After 16 wk, infection causes chorioamnionitis, a major cause of premature rupture of the membranes and premature delivery.

Because these patients are at high risk for other sexually transmitted diseases, all patients with gonorrhea should have a serologic test for syphilis and be evaluated for recurrent *C. trachomatis* infection at the time of diagnosis. Human immunodeficiency virus (HIV) testing is also indicated. The VDRL should be repeated 3 mo later.

DIAGNOSIS AND DIFFERENTIAL DIAGNOSIS. A definite diagnosis of gonococcal disease depends on isolation of *N. gonorrhoeae.* It is not possible to distinguish gonococcal from nongonococcal urethritis on the basis of symptoms and signs alone. Gonococcal urethritis and vulvovaginitis must be distinguished from other infections that produce a purulent discharge, including β-hemolytic streptococci, *C. trachomatis, Mycoplasma hominis, Trichomonas vaginalis,* and *Candida albicans.* Rarely, infection with human herpesvirus type 2 may produce symptoms similar to those of gonorrhea.

In the male with symptomatic urethritis, a presumptive diagnosis of gonorrhea can be made by identification of gram-negative intracellular diplococci (within leukocytes) in the urethral discharge. A similar finding in females is not sufficient because *Mima polymorpha* and *Moraxella* (normal vaginal flora) have a similar appearance. The sensitivity of the Gram stain for diagnosing gonococcal cervicitis and asymptomatic infections is also low. The presence of commensal *Neisseria* species in the oropharynx prevents the use of the Gram stain for diagnosis of pharyngeal gonorrhea. Although nonpathogenic neisseria are gram-negative diplococci, they are not intracellular or associated with neutrophilia.

Bacteriologic cultures remain the gold standard for the diagnosis of *N. gonorrhoeae.* Male urethral specimens are obtained by placing a small swab 2–3 cm into the urethra. Material for cervical cultures is obtained after wiping the exocervix and placing a swab in the cervical os and rotating it gently for several seconds. For optimal culture results, specimens should be obtained with noncotton swabs, inoculated directly onto culture plates, and incubated immediately. Samples from the urethra should be cultured for heterosexual men, and samples from the endocervix and rectum should be cultured for all females, regardless of the absence of a history of anal intercourse. Symptomatic sites plus the pharynx should be cultured in patients with orogenital exposure. Specimens from sites (e.g., cervix, rectum, pharynx) that normally are colonized by other organisms should be inoculated on a selective culture medium, such as modified Thayer-Martin medium (fortified with vancomycin, colistin, nystatin, and trimethoprim to inhibit growth of indigenous flora). Specimens from sites that are normally sterile or minimally contaminated (i.e., synovial fluid, blood, cerebrospinal fluid [CSF]) should be inoculated on a nonselective chocolate agar medium. If DGI is suspected, blood, pharynx, rectum, urethra, cervix, and synovial fluid (if involved) should be cultured. Cultured specimens should be incubated promptly at 35–37° C in 3–5% CO_2. When specimens must be transported to a central laboratory for culture plating, a reduced, nonnutrient holding medium (i.e., Amies modified Stuart medium) preserves specimens with minimal loss of viability for up to 6 hr. When transport may delay culture plating by more than 6 hr, it is preferable to inoculate the sample directly onto a culture medium and transport it at an ambient temperature in a candle jar. The Transgrow and JEMBEC systems of modified Thayer-Martin medium are alternative transport systems. Colonies of *N. gonorrhoeae* are oxidase positive. Further differentiation from oxidase-positive *M. polymorpha* and *N. lactamica* (both found in normal vaginal and oral secretions) can be made by carbohydrate utilization tests; gonococci ferment glucose but not maltose, lactose, or sucrose. The organism should be tested for β-lactamase production.

When microbiology laboratory facilities are not readily available or when patients may be lost to follow-up, rapid diagnostic techniques may prove efficacious. Care must be taken in selecting and interpreting results because most rapid tests are less specific than cultures. A rapid slide coagglutination test (Phadebact) has a sensitivity of 96–98% for identification of gonococci in anogenital specimens from females and urethral specimens from males. This test cross-reacts with commensal *Neisseria* species. Enzyme immunoassay tests such as Gonozyme are comparable to Gram stain in their sensitivity and specificity for diagnosing gonococcal urethritis in males. Gonozyme is more sensitive than the Gram stain in diagnosing gonococcal cervicitis (80–92% in most studies). This test is limited by a low positive predictive value in populations with a low prevalence of gonorrhea and cannot be used for rectal or pharyngeal infections. On balance, these tests offer a more sensitive means for making a presumptive diagnosis of urogenital gonorrhea in females but has no advantage over the Gram stain for diagnosing gonococcal urethritis in males. They cannot replace bacteriologic cultures for definitive diagnosis of *N. gonorrhoeae* or for antimicrobial susceptibility testing. They may serve as useful adjuvant diagnostic tools in high-prevalence, transient populations (i.e., in adolescent sexually transmitted disease [STD] clinics), in which a rapid and accurate presumptive diagnosis is required for prompt institution of therapy.

Gonococcal arthritis must be distinguished from other forms of septic arthritis as well as from rheumatic fever, rheumatoid arthritis, Reiter syndrome, inflammatory bowel disease, and arthritis secondary to rubella or rubella immunization. Gonococcal conjunctivitis in the newborn period must be differentiated from chemical conjunctivitis caused by silver nitrate drops as well as from conjunctivitis caused by *C. trachomatis, Staphylococcus aureus,* group A or B streptococcus, *Pseudomonas aeruginosa,* or human herpesvirus type 2.

PREVENTION. Efforts to develop a gonococcal pilus vaccine have been unsuccessful thus far. The high degree of inter- and intrastrain antigenic variability of pili poses a formidable deterrent to the development of a single effective pilus vaccine. Other gonococcal surface structures such as the porin protein, stress proteins, and lipooligosaccharides may prove more promising as vaccine candidates. In the absence of a vaccine, prevention of gonorrhea can be achieved through education, use of barrier contraceptives (especially condoms and spermicides), intensive epidemiologic and bacteriologic surveillance (screening sexual contacts), and early identification and treatment of infected contacts.

Gonococcal ophthalmia neonatorum can be prevented by instilling a 1% solution of silver nitrate into the conjunctival sac shortly after birth (see Chapter 577). Erythromycin (0.5%) or tetracycline (1%) ophthalmic ointment may also be used. Infants born to mothers with active gonorrhea are at high risk for developing gonococcal ophthalmitis and should be given a single 125-mg intramuscular injection of ceftriaxone for prophylaxis. For low-birthweight infants, the dosage is 25–50 mg/kg.

TREATMENT. General principles in the treatment of gonorrhea include the need to consider therapy for coexisting sexually transmitted diseases (syphilis, *Chlamydia* infection, HIV) and infection due to PPNG and tetracycline-resistant *N. gonorrhoeae.* The incidence of *Chlamydia* coinfection is 15–25% among males and 35–50% among females. It is recommended that *Chlamydia* infection be treated simultaneously with gonorrhea (see Chapter 197). Sexual partners exposed in the preceding 30 days should be examined, cultures should be taken, and presumptive treatment started.

Because of the increased prevalence of resistance of *N. gonorrhoeae* to penicillin, a third-generation cephalosporin, specifically ceftriaxone, is recommended as initial therapy for all ages. Routine culture and antimicrobial susceptibility testing should be used as guides to therapy. A single intramuscular injection of ceftriaxone, (125 mg) for prepubertal children weighing less than 45 kg and 125 mg for adults is the treatment of choice for uncomplicated urethritis, vulvovaginitis, proctitis, or pharyngitis. Ceftriaxone may also be effective against incubating syphilis but is ineffective against *Chlamydia* infections. In sexually active individuals infected with *N. gonorrhoeae,* simultaneous infection with *C. trachomatis* is common, accounts for most postgonococcal urethritis, and contributes to fallopian tube scarring and infertility. The addition of doxycycline (100 mg orally twice daily for 7 days) is recommended. Children younger than 9 yr and pregnant women should not be given tetracycline drugs, and erythromycin is recommended for them.

Several options exist for treating uncomplicated gonorrhea in penicillin-allergic individuals. A single intramuscular dose of spectinomycin may be given, 40 mg/kg for children weighing less than 45 kg, and 2 g for adults. It is relatively ineffective for pharyngeal gonorrhea, is ineffective against incubating syphilis or *Chlamydia* infections, but is effective against PPNG. Spectinomycin must be followed by a course of doxycycline. Alternatively, ceftriaxone may be used because the incidence of cross-reactivity to cephalosporins is low. Additional therapy for penicillin-allergic patients includes ciprofloxacin (500 mg in a single oral dose). During pregnancy erythromycin should be added to spectinomycin or ceftriaxone. Tetracyclines should not be used as single-drug therapy for gonorrhea.

Although many gonococcal isolates causing disseminated disease are sensitive to penicillin, ceftriaxone is recommended as the initial treatment of choice for DGI. Hospitalization is recommended. A 7-day course of parenteral ceftriaxone (50 mg/kg/24 hr; maximum, given 1g/24 hr) given intravenously or intramuscularly for children and 1g/24 hr given intravenously or intramuscularly for adults is recommended unless the organism is sensitive to penicillin. Endocarditis or meningitis should be treated with 50 mg/kg of ceftriaxone (maximum dose, 2g) twice daily for children and 1–2 g every 12 hr for adults. Endocarditis is treated for at least 4 wk and meningitis is treated for 10–14 days. Children with disseminated gonococcal disease sensitive to penicillin should be hospitalized and treated with intravenous aqueous penicillin G in a dose of 100,000–200,000 U/kg/24 hr in six divided doses for 7–10 days. For gonococcal meningitis and endocarditis, the dosages are 250,000 U/kg/24 hr for 14 days and 4 wk, respectively. Penicillin-allergic patients may be treated with ceftriaxone or spectinomycin in a dose of 2g given intramuscularly every 12 hr. Concurrent therapy with doxycycline is indicated for treatment of genital *Chlamydia* infection in sexually active patients.

Infants born to mothers with known gonococcal infection should be evaluated for sepsis with blood and CSF cultures. Ceftriaxone (50 mg/kg intramuscularly or intravenously given once, 125 mg maximum) is the drug of choice. Topical prophylaxis with this drug is not adequate. Neonates with gonococcal ophthalmitis must be hospitalized and evaluated for DGI. Ceftriaxone (25–50 mg/kg/24 hr intravenously or intramuscularly every day for 7 days) is the treatment of choice. In the absence of systemic infection some specialists treat gonococcal ophthalmia with a single injection of ceftriaxone. Concomitant saline irrigation of the eyes is recommended. Infants with DGI, including meningitis, arthritis, and septicemia are treated for 10–14 days.

PID requires hospitalization for evaluation and initiation of treatment. PID encompasses a spectrum of infectious diseases of the upper genital tract due to *N. gonorrhoeae, C. trachomatis,* and endogenous flora (streptococci, anaerobes, gram-negative bacilli). Therapy must cover a broad spectrum and must be given to adolescents as inpatients. A commonly recommended therapeutic regimen is 2 g of cefoxitin given intravenously every 6 hr or 2 g of cefotetan given intravenously every 12 hr, plus 100 mg of doxycyline administered orally or intravenously every 12 hr. Therapy is continued for at least 48 hr after the patient shows improvement. Thereafter, oral doxycycline is continued for a total of 10–14 days. An alternative recommended regimen is clindamycin (900 mg intravenously every 8 hr) plus a loading dose of gentamicin (2 mg/kg intravenously), followed by maintenance gentamicin (1.5 mg/kg every 8 hr). Therapy is then continued for 48 hr after the patient improves and is followed by oral doxycycline for 10–14 days. If an intrauterine device (IUD) is present, it must be removed and an alternative form of birth control used. Sexual partners should be examined and treated for uncomplicated gonorrhea. Follow-up culture (test of cure) of cephalosporin-doxycycline therapy of gonococcal STD is not recommended owing to the low treatment failure rate. A follow-up examination and culture is recommended in 1–2 mo to evaluate the possibility of reinfection or, rarely, treatment failure.

PROGNOSIS. Prompt diagnosis and correct therapy ensure complete recovery from uncomplicated gonococcal disease. Complications and permanent sequelae may be associated with delayed treatment, recurrent infection, metastatic sites of infection (meninges, aortic valve), and delayed or topical therapy of gonococcal ophthalmia.

Cates W, Wasserheit JN: Gonorrhea, chlamydia, and pelvic inflammatory disease. Curr Opin Infect Dis 3:10, 1990.

Centers for Disease Control: 1993 Sexually transmitted diseases treatment guidelines. MMWR 42:56, 1993.

Centers for Disease Control: Special focus: surveillance for sexually transmitted diseases. MMWR 42:29, 1993.

Cohen MS, Sparling PF: Mucosal infection with *Neisseria gonorrhoeae,* bacterial adaptation and mucosal defenses. J Clin Invest 89:1699, 1992.

Hook EW, Holmes KK: Gonococcal infections. Ann Intern Med 102:229, 1985.

O'Brien JP, Goldenberg DL, Rice PA: Disseminated gonococcal infection: A prospective analysis of 49 patients and a review of pathophysiology and immune mechanisms. Medicine (Baltimore) 62:395, 1983.

Rawstron SA, Hammerschlag MR, Gullans C, et al: Ceftriaxone treatment of penicillinase-producing *Neisseria gonorrhoeae* infections in children. Pediatr Infect Dis J 8:445, 1989.

Treatment of sexually transmitted diseases. Med Lett 32:5, 1990.

Whitington WL, et al: Incorrect identification of *Neisseria gonorrhoeae* from infants and children. Pediatr Infect Dis J 7:34, 1988.

CHAPTER 180

Diphtheria

Sarah S. Long

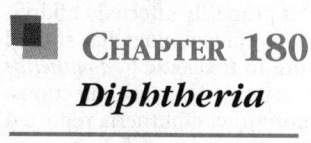

Diphtheria is an acute toxicoinfection caused by *Corynebacterium diphtheriae.* Diphtheria was the first infectious disease to be conquered on the basis of principles of microbiology and public health. Reduced from a major cause of childhood death in the West in the early 20th century to a medical rarity, modern reminders of the fragility of such success underscore the need to assiduously apply those same principles in an era of vaccine dependency and a single global community.

ETIOLOGY. *Corynebacterium* species are aerobic, nonencapsulated, non–spore-forming, mostly nonmotile, pleomorphic, gram-positive bacilli. Not fastidious in growth requirements, their isolation is enhanced by selective media (i.e., cystine-tellurite blood agar) that inhibits growth of competing organisms and, when reduced by *C. diphtheriae,* renders colonies gray-black. Three biotypes (i.e., *mitis, gravis,* and *intermedius*), each capable of causing diphtheria, are differentiated by colonial morphology, hemolysis, and fermentation reactions. A lysogenic bacteriophage carrying the gene that encodes for production of exotoxin confers diphtheria-producing potential to strains of *C. diphtheriae,* but it provides no essential protein to the bacterium. Investigation of outbreaks of diphtheria in England and the United States using a molecular technique suggested that indigenous nontoxigenic *C. diphtheriae* had been rendered toxigenic and disease producing after the importation of toxigenic *C. diphtheriae.* Diphtheritic toxin can be demonstrated in vitro by the agar immunoprecipitin technique (Elek test), an investigational polymerase chain reaction test, or by the in vivo toxin neutralization test in guinea pigs (lethality test). Toxigenic strains are indistinguishable by colony type, microscopy, or biochemical tests.

EPIDEMIOLOGY. Unlike other diphtheroids (coryneform bacteria), which are ubiquitous in nature, *C. diphtheria* is an exclusive inhabitant of human mucous membranes and skin. Spread is primarily by airborne respiratory droplets or direct contact with respiratory secretions of symptomatic individuals or exudate from infected skin lesions. Asymptomatic respiratory carriers are important in transmission. Where diphtheria is endemic, 3–5% of healthy individuals may harbor toxigenic organisms, but carriage is exceedingly rare if diphtheria is rare. Skin infection and skin carriage are silent reservoirs of diphtheria. Viability in dust and on fomites for up to 6 months has less epidemiologic significance. Transmission through contaminated milk and an infected food handler have been proved or suspected.

In the 1920s, more than 125,000 cases and 10,000 deaths due to diphtheria were reported annually in the United States, with highest fatality rate among very young and elderly patients. From 1921–1924, diphtheria was the leading cause of death among Canadian children 2–14 yr of age. The incidence began to fall, and with the widespread use of diphtheria toxoid in the United States after World War II, it declined steadily, with dramatic reductions in the latter 1970s. Since then, there have been zero to five cases per year and no epidemics of respiratory tract diphtheria. Similar decreases have been seen in Europe. Although disease incidence has fallen worldwide, diphtheria remains endemic in many developing countries. The sustained low incidence of diphtheria and high level of childhood vaccination have led authorities to set a goal to eliminate diphtheria among persons 25 yr of age or younger in the United States by the year 2000.

When diphtheria was endemic, it primarily affected children younger than 15 yr of age, but recent epidemiology has shifted to adults who lack natural exposure to toxigenic *C. diphtheriae* in the vaccine era and have low rates of boosting injections. In the 27 sporadic cases of respiratory tract diphtheria reported in the United States in the 1980s, 70% occurred in persons older than 25 yr of age. The largest outbreak of diphtheria in the developed world since the 1960s occurred from 1990–1995 throughout the New Independent States of the former Soviet Union, where more than 47,000 cases and 1,700 deaths occurred in 1994 alone. This outbreak is due to lack of immunization for diphtheria. Most affected individuals were older than 14 yr of age. Smaller epidemiologically similar outbreaks have occurred in Denmark and Sweden.

A survey of antitoxin levels in Sweden is particularly noteworthy, because the childhood immunization rate exceeds 95%, but 19% of persons younger than 20 yr of age and 81% of women and 56% of men older than 60 yr of age lacked the protective antibody. Other broad serosurveys have identified large subgroups of underimmunized individuals in the United States and elsewhere where immunization is "universal" that would be at perilous risk if the organism were introduced. Only 40–60% of 2-yr-old urban and rural poor children are appropriately immunized. Twenty per cent of 396 children younger than 5 yr of age in a Dade County, Florida, serosurvey lacked protective immunity to diphtheria (antitoxin level >0.01 IU/mL). State laws requiring vaccination for school entry have ensured protective immunity for more than 97% of children 5–14 yr of age. In serosurveys in the United States and other developed countries with almost universal immunization during childhood, such as Sweden, Italy, and Denmark, 25% to more than 60% of adults lacked protective antitoxin levels, with particularly low levels found in the elderly.

Cutaneous diphtheria, a curiosity when diphtheria was common, accounted for more than 50% of *C. diphtheriae* isolates reported in the United States by 1975 and features prominently in the changing epidemiology of diphtheria in the 1990s. An indolent local infection with infrequent toxic complications, cutaneous infection, compared with mucosal infection, is associated with more prolonged bacterial shedding, increased contamination of the environment, and increased transmission to pharynx and skin of close contacts. Outbreaks are associated with homelessness, crowding, poverty, alcoholism, poor hygiene, contaminated fomites, underlying dermatosis, and introduction of new strains from exogenous sources. No longer a tropical or subtropical disease, 1,100 *C. diphtheriae* infections were documented in the Skid Row neighborhood in Seattle, Washington, from 1971–1982; 86% were cutaneous, and 40% involved toxigenic strains. Cutaneous diphtheria is the important reservoir for toxigenic *C. diphtheriae* in the United States and a frequent mode of importation of source cases for subsequent sporadic respiratory tract diphtheria. In an attempt to focus attention on respiratory tract diphtheria, which is much more likely to cause acute obstructive complications and toxic manifestations, skin isolates of *C. diphtheriae* were removed from annual diphtheria statistics reported by the Centers for Disease Control (CDC) after 1979.

PATHOGENESIS. Toxigenic and nontoxigenic *C. diphtheriae* organisms cause skin and mucosal infection and some cases of distant infection after bacteremia. The organism usually remains in the superficial layers of skin lesions or respiratory mucosa, inducing local inflammatory reaction. The major virulence of the organism lies in its ability to produce the potent 62–kD polypeptide exotoxin, which inhibits protein synthesis and causes local tissue necrosis. Within the first few days of respiratory tract infection, a dense necrotic coagulum of organisms, epithelial cells, fibrin, leukocytes, and erythrocytes forms, advances, and becomes a gray-brown adherent pseudomembrane. Removal is difficult and reveals a bleeding edematous submucosa. Paralysis of palate and hypopharynx are early local effects of the toxin. Toxin absorption can lead to necrosis of kidney tubules, thrombocytopenia, mycocardiopathy, and demyelination of nerves. Because the latter two complications can occur 2–10 wk after mucocutaneous infection, the pathophysiologic mechanism in some cases may be immunologically mediated.

CLINICAL MANIFESTATIONS. Respiratory Tract Diphtheria. In the classic description of 1,400 cases of diphtheria from California published in 1954, the primary focus of infection was the tonsils or pharynx in 94%, with the nose and larynx the next two most common sites. After an average incubation period of 2–4 days, local signs and symptoms of inflammation develop. Fever is rarely higher than 39° C. Infection of the anterior nares (more common in infants) causes serosanguinous, purulent, erosive rhinitis with membrane formation. Shallow ulceration of the external nares and upper lip are characteristic. In tonsillar and pharyngeal diphtheria, sore throat is a universal early symptom, but only one half of patients have fever, and fewer have dysphagia, hoarseness, malaise, or headache. Mild pharyngeal injection is followed by unilateral or bilateral tonsillar membrane formation, which extends variably to affect the uvula, soft palate, posterior oropharynx, hypopharynx, and glottic areas. Underlying soft tissue edema and enlarged lymph nodes can cause a "bull-neck" appearance. The degree of local extension correlates directly with profound prostration, bull-neck appearance, and fatality from airway compromise or toxin-mediated complications.

The leather-like adherent membrane, extension beyond the faucial area, relative lack of fever, and dysphagia help differentiate diphtheria from exudative pharyngitis due to *Streptococcus pyogenes* and Epstein-Barr virus. Vincent angina, infective phlebitis and thrombosis of the jugular veins, and mucositis in patients undergoing cancer chemotherapy are usually differentiated by the clinical setting. Infection of the larynx, trachea, and bronchi can be primary or a secondary extension from the pharyngeal infection. Hoarseness, stridor, dyspnea, and "croupy" cough are clues. Differentiation from bacterial epiglottitis, severe viral laryngotracheobronchitis, and staphylococcal or streptococcal tracheitis hinges partially on the relative paucity of other signs and symptoms in the patient with diphtheria and primarily on visualization of the adherent pseudomembrane at the time of laryngobronchoscopy and intubation.

The patient with laryngeal diphtheria is highly prone to suffocation because of edema of soft tissues and the obstructing dense cast of respiratory epithelium and necrotic coagulum. Establishment of an artificial airway and resection of the pseudomembrane are lifesaving, but further obstructive complications are common, and systemic toxic complications are inevitable.

Cutaneous Diphtheria. Classic cutaneous diphtheria is an indolent, nonprogressive infection characterized by a superficial, ecthymic, nonhealing ulcer with a gray-brown membrane. Diphtheritic skin infections cannot always be differentiated from streptococcal or staphylococcal impetigo, and they frequently coexist. In most cases, underlying dermatoses, lacerations, burns, bites, or impetigo have become secondarily contaminated. Extremities are more often affected than the trunk or head. Pain, tenderness, erythema, and exudate are typical. Local hyperesthesia or hypesthesia is unusual. Respiratory tract colonization or symptomatic infection and toxic complications occur in the minority of patients with cutaneous diphtheria. Among infected Seattle adults, 3% with cutaneous infections and 21% with symptomatic nasopharyngeal infection, with or without skin involvement, had toxic myocarditis, neuropathy, or obstructive respiratory tract complications. All had received at least 20,000 units of equine antitoxin at the time of hospitalization.

Infection at Other Sites. *C. diphtheriae* occasionally causes mucocutaneous infections at other sites, such as the ear (otitis externa), eye (purulent and ulcerative conjunctivitis), and genital tract (purulent and ulcerative vulvovaginitis). The clinical setting, ulceration, membrane formation, and submucosal bleeding help differentiate diphtheria from other bacterial and viral causes. Rare cases of septicemia are described and are universally fatal. Sporadic cases of endocarditis occur, and clusters among intravenous drug users have been reported in several countries; skin was the probable portal of entry, and almost all strains were nontoxigenic. Sporadic cases of pyogenic arthritis, mainly due to nontoxigenic strains, are reported in adults and children. Diphtheroids isolated from sterile body sites should not be dismissed as contaminants without careful consideration of the clinical setting.

Toxic Myocardiopathy. Toxic myocardiopathy occurs in approximately 10–25% of patients with diphtheria and is responsible for 50–60% of deaths. Subtle signs of myocarditis can be detected in most patients, especially the elderly, but the risk for significant complications correlates directly with the extent and severity of exudative local oropharyngeal disease and delay in administration of antitoxin. Characteristically, the first evidence of cardiac toxicity occurs in the 2nd to 3rd wk of illness as pharyngeal disease improves but can appear acutely as early as the 1st wk when a fatal outcome is likely, or insidiously as late as the 6th wk of illness. Tachycardia out of proportion to fever is common and may be evidence of cardiac toxicity or autonomic nervous system dysfunction. A prolonged PR interval and changes in the ST-T wave in electrocardiographic tracing are relatively frequent findings, and dilated and hypertrophic cardiomyopathy detected by echocardiogram have been described. Single or progressive cardiac dysrhythmias can occur, such as first-, second-, and third-degree heart block, atrioventricular dissociation, and ventricular tachycardia. Clinical congestive heart failure may have an insidious or acute onset. Elevation of the serum aspartate aminotransferase concentration closely parallels the severity of myonecrosis. Severe dysrhythmia portends death. Histologic postmortem findings may show little or diffuse myonecrosis with acute inflammatory response. Survivors of more severe dysrhythmias can have permanent conduction defects; for others, recovery from toxic myocardiopathy is usually complete.

Toxic Neuropathy. Neurologic complications parallel the extent of primary infection and are multiphasic in onset. Acutely or 2–3 wk after onset of oropharyngeal inflammation, hypesthesia, and local paralysis of soft palate occur commonly. Weakness of the posterior pharyngeal, laryngeal, and facial nerves may follow, causing a nasal quality in the voice, difficulty in swallowing, and risk of death from aspiration. Cranial neuropathies characteristically occur in the 5th wk and lead to oculomotor and ciliary paralysis, which manifest as strabismus, blurred vision, or difficulty with accommodation. Symmetric polyneuropathy has its onset 10 days to 3 mo after oropharyngeal infection and causes principally motor deficit with diminished deep tendon reflexes. Proximal muscle weakness of the extremities progressing distally and, more commonly, distal weakness progressing proximally are described. Clinical and cerebrospinal fluid findings in the latter are indistinguishable from those of polyneuropathy of Landry-Guillain-Barré syndrome. Paralysis of the diaphragm can ensue. Complete recovery is likely. Rarely, 2 or 3 wk after onset of illness, dysfunction of the vasomotor centers can cause hypotension or cardiac failure.

MANAGEMENT. The Patient. Diagnostic Tests. Specimens for culture should be obtained from the nose and throat and any other mucocutaneous lesion. A portion of membrane should be removed and submitted with underlying exudate. The laboratory must be notified to use selective medium. *C. diphtheriae* survives drying. In remote areas, a swab specimen can be placed in a silica gel pack and sent to a reference laboratory. Evaluation of a direct smear using Gram stain or specific fluorescent antibody is unreliable. Coryneform organisms should be identified to the species level, and toxigenicity and antimicrobial susceptibility tests should be performed for *C. diphtheriae* isolates.

Antitoxin. Specific antitoxin is the mainstay of therapy and should be administered on the basis of clinical diagnosis, because it neutralizes only free toxin. Efficacy diminishes with elapsing time after the onset of mucocutaneous symptoms. Only an equine preparation is available in the United States, from Connaught Laboratories (Swiftwater, PA) or from the

in humans involve any body site and typically occur in immunocompromised patients or young children with unusual exposure to animals. Protracted coughing can be caused by *Mycoplasma*, parainfluenza or influenza viruses, enteroviruses, respiratory syncytial virus, or adenoviruses. None is an important cause of pertussis.

EPIDEMIOLOGY. Worldwide there are 60 million cases of pertussis a year with more than half a million deaths. During the prevaccine era of 1922–1948, pertussis was the leading cause of death from communicable disease among children under 14 yr of age in the United States. Widespread use of pertussis vaccine is responsible for a dramatic decline in cases. The high incidence of disease in developing and developed countries, such as Italy and certain regions of Germany, where vaccine coverage is low, or Nova Scotia, where a less potent vaccine may have been utilized, and the dramatic resurgence of disease when immunization was halted attest to the pivotal role of vaccination. In the United States, lax implementation of policy is partially responsible for the rise in annual pertussis incidence to 1.2 cases/100,000 population from 1980 through 1989 and epidemic pertussis in many states in 1989–1990 and 1993. The more than 4,500 cases reported to the Centers for Disease Control and Prevention in 1993 is the highest incidence since 1967.

Pertussis is endemic, with superimposed epidemic cycles every 3–4 yr after accumulation of a sizable susceptible cohort. The majority of cases occur from July through October. Pertussis is extremely contagious, with attack rates as high as 100% in susceptible individuals exposed to aerosol droplets at close range. *B. pertussis* does not survive for prolonged periods in the environment. Chronic carriage by humans is not documented. Following intense exposure as in households, the rate of subclinical infection is as high as 50% in fully immunized and naturally immune individuals. When carefully sought, a symptomatic source case can be found for most patients.

Neither natural disease nor vaccination provide complete or lifelong immunity against reinfection or disease. Protection against typical disease begins to wane 3–5 yr after vaccination and is unmeasurable after 12 yr. Subclinical reinfection undoubtedly contributes significantly to immunity against disease ascribed to both vaccine and prior infection. Adults in the United States have inadequate antibody to *B. pertussis*. Despite history of disease or complete immunization, outbreaks of pertussis have occurred in the elderly, in nursing homes, in residential facilities with limited exposures, in highly immunized suburbia, and in adolescents and adults with lapsing time since immunization. Coughing adolescents and adults (usually not recognized as having pertussis) are the major reservoir for *B. pertussis* currently and are the usual sources for "index cases" in infants and children.

In the prevaccine era and in countries such as Germany, Sweden, and Italy with limited immunization, the peak incidence of pertussis is in children 1–5 yr of age; infants younger than 1 yr account for less than 15% of cases. In contrast, of the almost 5,000 cases of pertussis reported in the United States during 1993, 44% were younger than 1 yr of age, 21% were aged 1–4 yr, 11% were aged 5–9 yr, and 24% were 12 yr of age or older. For those younger than 1 yr, 79% were under 6 mo and could benefit little from immunization. Children with pertussis between 7 mo and 4 yr were underimmunized. The proportion of teenagers and adults with pertussis has risen concurrently, from less than 20% in the prevaccine era to 27% in 1992–1993. Partial control by vaccination has led to the current epidemiology of pertussis in the United States and has caused vulnerability of age groups never previously affected. Without natural reinfection with *B. pertussis* or repeated booster vaccinations, older children and adults are susceptible to clinical disease if exposed, and mothers provide little if any passive protection to young infants. The latter observation provides correction to an old tenet that there was little transplacental protection against pertussis.

PATHOGEN AND PATHOPHYSIOLOGY. *Bordetella* are tiny gram-negative coccobacilli that grow aerobically on starch blood agar or completely synthetic media with nicotinamide growth factor, amino acids for energy, and charcoal or cyclodextrin resin to absorb noxious substances. *Bordetella* species share a high degree of DNA homology among virulence genes, and there is controversy whether sufficient diversity exists to warrant classification as distinct species. Only *B. pertussis* expresses pertussis toxin (PT), the major virulence protein. Serotyping is dependent upon heat-labile K agglutinogens. Of 14 agglutinogens, 6 are specific to *B. pertussis*. Serotypes vary geographically and over time.

B. pertussis produces an array of biologically active substances, many of which are postulated to play a role in disease and immunity. Following aerosol acquisition, filamentous hemagglutinin (FHA), some agglutinogens (especially FIM2 and FIM3), and a 69-kD nonfimbrial surface protein called pertactin (PRN) are important for attachment to ciliated respiratory epithelial cells. Tracheal cytotoxin, adenylate cyclase, and PT appear to inhibit clearance of organisms. Tracheal cytotoxin, dermonecrotic factor, and adenylate cyclase are postulated to be predominantly responsible for the local epithelial damage that produces respiratory symptomatology and facilitates absorption of PT. PT has multiple proven biologic activities (e.g., histamine sensitivity, insulin secretion, leukocyte dysfunction), some of which may account for systemic manifestations of disease. PT causes lymphocytosis immediately in experimental animals by rerouting lymphocytes to remain in the circulating blood pool. PT appears to play a central but not a singular role in pathogenesis.

CLINICAL MANIFESTATIONS. Pertussis is a lengthy disease, divided into catarrhal, paroxysmal, and convalescent stages, each lasting 2 wk. Classically, following an incubation period ranging from 3 to 12 days, nondistinctive catarrhal symptoms of congestion and rhinorrhea occur, variably accompanied by low-grade fever, sneezing, lacrimation, and conjunctival suffusion. As symptoms wane, coughing begins first as a dry, intermittent, irritative hack and evolves into the inexorable paroxysms that are the hallmark of pertussis. Following the most insignificant startle from a draught, light, sound, sucking, or stretching, the well-appearing young infant begins to choke, gasp, and flail extremities, eyes watering and bulging, face reddened. Cough (expiratory grunt) may not be present, prominent, or appreciated at this stage and age. Whoop (forceful inspiratory gasp) infrequently occurs in infants under 3 mo who are exhausted or lack muscular strength to create sudden negative intrathoracic pressure. The well-appearing playful toddler with similarly insignificant provocation suddenly expresses an anxious aura and may clutch a parent or comforting adult before beginning a machine-gun burst of uninterrupted coughs, chin and chest held forward, tongue protruding maximally, eyes bulging and watering, face purple, until at the seeming last moment of consciousness, coughing ceases and a loud whoop follows as inspired air traverses the still partially closed airway. The episode may end with expulsion of a thick plug of inspissated tracheal secretions, denuded cilia, and necrotic epithelium. Adults describe a sudden feeling of strangulation followed by uninterrupted coughs, feeling of suffocation, bursting headache, diminished awareness, and then the chest heaves and air rushes into the lungs, usually without a whoop. Post-tussive emesis is common in pertussis at all ages and is a major clue to the diagnosis in adolescents and adults. Post-tussive exhaustion is universal. The number and severity of paroxysms progress over days to a week (more rapidly in young infants) and remain at that plateau for days to weeks (longer in young infants). At the peak of the paroxysmal stage, patients may have more than one episode hourly. As paroxysmal stage fades into convalescence, the number, severity, and duration of episodes diminish. Paradoxically in infants, with growth and increased strength, cough and whoops may become louder and more classic in convalescence.

Immunized children have foreshortening of all stages of pertussis. Adults have no distinct stages. In infants under 3 mo the catarrhal phase is usually a few days or not recognized at all when apnea, choking, or gasping cough herald the onset of disease; convalescence includes intermittent paroxysmal coughing throughout the 1st yr of life including "recurrences" with subsequent respiratory illnesses; these are not due to recurrent infection or reactivation of *B. pertussis.*

The physical examination is generally uninformative. Signs of lower respiratory tract disease are not expected. Conjunctival hemorrhages and petechiae on the upper body are common.

DIAGNOSIS AND DIFFERENTIAL DIAGNOSIS. Pertussis should be suspected in any individual who has pure or predominant complaint of cough, especially if the following are absent: fever, malaise or myalgia, exanthem or enanthem, sore throat, hoarseness, tachypnea, wheezes, and rales. For sporadic cases, a clinical case definition of cough of 14 or more days' duration with at least one associated symptom of paroxysms, whoop, or post-tussive vomiting has sensitivity of 81% and specificity of 58% for culture confirmation. Approximately 25% of university students studied randomly in California and Australia without known contact with pertussis who had coughing illness for 7 days or more had pertussis. Apnea or cyanosis (before appreciation of cough) is a clue in infants under 3 mo. *B. pertussis* is an occasional cause of sudden infant death.

Adenoviral infections are usually distinguishable by associated features, such as fever, sore throat, and conjunctivitis. *Mycoplasma* causes protracted episodic coughing, but there is usually a history of fever, headache, and systemic symptoms at the onset of disease as well as frequent finding of rales on auscultation of the chest. Although pertussis is often included in the laboratory evaluation of young infants with "afebrile pneumonia," *B. pertussis* is associated uncommonly with staccato cough (breath with every cough), purulent conjunctivitis, tachypnea, rales or wheezes that typify infection due to *Chlamydia trachomatis,* or predominant lower respiratory tract signs that typify infection due to respiratory syncytial virus. Unless the infant with pertussis has secondary bacterial pneumonia (and is then ill appearing), the examination between paroxysms is entirely normal, including respiratory rate.

Leukocytosis (15,000–100,000 cells/mm^3) due to absolute lymphocytosis is a characteristic in late catarrhal and paroxysmal stages. Lymphocytes are of T- and B-cell origin and are normal small cells, rather than the large atypical lymphocytes seen with viral infections. Adults and partially immune children have less impressive lymphocytosis. Absolute increase in neutrophils suggests a different diagnosis or secondary bacterial infection. Eosinophilia is not common in pertussis, even in young infants. A severe course and death are correlated with extreme leukocytosis (median peak white cell count fatal vs nonfatal cases, 94 vs 18 $\times$ 10^9 cells/L) and thrombocytosis (median peak platelet count fatal vs nonfatal cases, 782 vs 556 $\times$ 10^9/L). Mild hyperinsulinemia and reduced glycemic response to epinephrine have been demonstrated; hypoglycemia is only reported occasionally. The chest radiograph is mildly abnormal in the majority of hospitalized infants showing perihilar infiltrate or edema (sometimes with a butterfly appearance) and variable atelectasis. Parenchymal consolidation suggests secondary bacterial infection. Pneumothorax, pneumomediastinum, and air in soft tissues can be seen occasionally.

All current methods for confirmation of infection due to *B. pertussis* have limitations in sensitivity, specificity, or practicality. Isolation of *B. pertussis* in culture remains the gold standard and is a more sensitive and specific method of diagnosis than direct fluorescent antibody (DFA) testing of nasopharyngeal secretions if careful attention is paid to specimen collection, transport, and isolation technique. Cultures are positive during the catarrhal stage and escalating paroxysmal stage but are less likely to be positive in partially immune individuals and in those who have received amoxicillin or erythromycin. The specimen is obtained by deep nasopharyngeal aspiration or by use of a flexible swab (Dacron or calcium alginate preferred) held in the posterior nasopharynx for 15–30 sec. (or until coughing). A 1.0% casamino acid liquid is acceptable for holding a specimen up to 2 hr; Stainer-Scholte broth or Regan-Lowe semisolid transport media is used for longer periods, up to 4 days. Regan-Lowe charcoal agar with 10% horse blood and 5–40 μg/mL cephalexin or Stainer-Scholte media with cyclodextrin resins are the preferred isolation media. Cultures are incubated at 35–37° F in humid environment (with or without 5% CO_2) and examined daily for 7 days for slow-growing, tiny glistening colonies. DFA testing of potential isolates using specific antibody for *B. pertussis* and *B. parapertussis* maximizes recovery. Direct testing of nasopharyngeal secretions by DFA is a rapid test, especially helpful in patients who have received antibiotics, but is only reliable in laboratories with continuous experience. Experience with the polymerase chain reaction to test nasopharyngeal specimens is increasing rapidly. Serologic tests for detection of a variety of antibodies to components of the organism in acute and convalescent samples are the most sensitive tests and are useful epidemiologically. They are not generally available, are not helpful during acute illness, and are difficult to interpret in immunized individuals.

COMPLICATIONS AND PROGNOSIS. Rates of complications are difficult to establish because severe outcomes are preferentially reported, but infants under 6 mo of age have excessive mortality and morbidity. Those under 2 mo of age have the highest reported rates of pertussis-associated hospitalization (82%), pneumonia (25%), seizures (4%), encephalopathy (1%), and death (1%).

The principal complications of pertussis are apnea, secondary infections (such as otitis media and pneumonia), and physical sequelae of forceful coughing. The need for intensive care and artificial ventilation is usually limited to infants under 3 mo of age. Apnea, cyanosis, and secondary bacterial pneumonia are events precipitating intubation and ventilation. Bacterial pneumonia and/or adult respiratory distress syndrome are the usual cause of death at any age; pulmonary hemorrhage has occurred in the neonate. Fever, tachypnea or respiratory distress between paroxysms, and absolute neutrophilia are clues to pneumonia. Expected pathogens include *Staphylococcus aureus, S. pneumoniae,* and bacteria of mouth flora. Bronchiectasis has been reported rarely following pertussis. Abnormal pulmonary function may persist for 12 mo after uncomplicated pertussis in children under 2 yr.

Increased intrathoracic and intra-abdominal pressure during coughing can result in conjunctival and scleral hemorrhages, petechiae on the upper body, epistaxis, hemorrhage in the central nervous system and retina, pneumothorax and subcutaneous emphysema, and umbilical and inguinal hernias. Laceration of the lingual frenulum is not uncommon. Rectal prolapse, once reported as a frequent complication of pertussis, was probably due to pertussis in malnourished children or missed diagnosis of cystic fibrosis. It is distinctly unusual and should elicit evaluation for underlying condition. Especially in infants in developing countries, dehydration and malnutrition following post-tussive vomiting can have a severe impact. Tetany has been associated with profound post-tussive alkalosis.

Central nervous system abnormalities occur at a relatively high frequency and are almost always the result of hypoxemia or hemorrhage associated with coughing or apnea in young infants. Apnea or bradycardia or both may occur from apparent laryngospasm or vagal stimulation just before a coughing episode, from obstruction during an episode, or from hypoxemia following an episode. Lack of associated signs in some young infants with apnea raises the possibility of a primary effect of PT on the central nervous system. Seizures are usually the result of hypoxemia, but hyponatremia from inappropriate secretion of antidiuretic hormone during pneumonia can occur. Although hypoglycemia, a direct effect of PT, or secondary infection due to neurotropic virus have been postulated mechanisms for neurologic symptomatology, no animal data support such theories, and the only neuropathology documented in humans is parenchymal hemorrhage and ischemic necrosis.

TREATMENT. Assessment and Supportive Care. Goals of therapy are to limit the number of paroxysms, to observe severity of cough to provide assistance when necessary, and to maximize nutrition, rest and recovery without sequelae (Table 181–1). Infants less than 3 mo of age are admitted to hospital almost without exception, at between 3 and 6 mo unless witnessed paroxysms are not severe, and at any age if complications occur or the family is unable to provide supportive care. Prematurely born young infants and children with underlying cardiac, pulmonary, muscular, or neurologic disorders have a high risk for severe disease.

The specific, limited goals of hospitalization are to (1) assess progression of disease and likelihood of life-threatening events at peak of disease, (2) prevent or treat complications, and (3) educate parents in the natural history of the disease and in care that will be given at home. For most infants without complications, this is accomplished in 48–72 hr. Heart rate, respiratory rate, and pulse oximetry are continuously monitored, with alarm settings so that every paroxysm is witnessed by health care personnel. Detailed cough records and documentation of feeding, vomiting, and weight change provide data to assess severity. Typical paroxysms that are not life threatening have the following features: duration less than 45 sec; red but not blue color change; tachycardia, bradycardia (not <60 beats/min in infants), or oxygen desaturation that spontaneously resolves at the end of the paroxysm; whooping or strength for self-rescue at the end of the paroxysm; self-expectorated mucus plug; and post-tussive exhaustion but not unresponsiveness. Assessing the need to provide oxygen, stimulation, or suctioning requires skilled personnel who can document an infant's ability for self-rescue but who will intervene rapidly and expertly when necessary. Infants whose paroxysms repeatedly lead to life-threatening events despite passive delivery of oxygen require intubation, paralysis, and ventilation.

■ TABLE 181–1 Reminders in Assessment and Care of Infants with Pertussis

Infants with potentially fatal pertussis may appear completely well between episodes.
In making the decision between hospital and home care, a paroxysm must be witnessed.
Only careful compilation and analysis of cough record permits assessment of severity and progression of illness.
Suctioning of nose, oropharynx, or trachea always precipitates coughing, occasionally causes bronchospasm or apnea, and should not be performed on a "preventive" schedule.
If the patient is alert and has retained strength following a coughing episode, feeding is best taken and retained during this brief refractory period for coughing.
Hospital discharge is appropriate if over a 48 hr period disease severity is unchanged or diminished, no intervention is required during paroxysms, nutrition is adequate, no complication has occurred, and parents are adequately prepared for care at home.
Family support begins with empathy for the child's and family's experience to date, transfer of the burden of responsibility for the child's life to the health care team, and delineation of assessments and treatments to be performed.
Family education, recruitment as part of the team, and continued support after discharge are essential.

Subsequent management is difficult, with frequent need to suction the airway and intervene when bradycardia or secondary pulmonary processes occur. Mist by tent, specifically avoided by some experts, can be useful in some infants with thick tenacious secretions and excessively irritable airways. The benefit of a quiet, dimly lighted, undisturbed, comforting environment cannot be overestimated or forfeited in a desire to monitor and intervene. Feeding children with pertussis is challenging. The risk of precipitating cough by nipple feeding does not warrant nasogastric, nasojejunal, or parenteral alimentation in most infants. The composition or thickness of formula does not affect the quality of secretions, cough, or retention. Large-volume feedings are avoided.

Within 48–72 hr, the direction and severity of disease is usually obvious by analysis of recorded information. Many infants have marked improvement following hospitalization and antibiotic therapy, especially if they are early in the course of disease or have been removed from aggravating environmental smoke, excessive stimulation, or a dry or polluted heat source. Apnea and seizures occur in the incremental phase of illness and in those with complicated disease. Portable oxygen, monitoring, or suction apparatus should not be needed at home.

Therapeutic Agents. **ANTIMICROBIAL AGENTS.** An antimicrobial agent is always given when pertussis is suspected or confirmed for potential clinical benefit and to limit the spread of infection. Erythromycin, 40–50 mg/kg/24 hr, orally in four divided doses (maximum 2 g/d 24 hr) for 14 days is standard treatment. Some experts prefer the estolate preparation, but ethylsuccinate and stearate are also efficacious. Small studies of erythromycin ethylsuccinate given at a dosage of 50 mg/kg/24 hr divided into two doses, at a dosage of 60 mg/kg/24 hr divided into three doses, and erythromycin estolate given at a dosage of 40 mg/kg/24 hr divided into two doses showed elimination of organisms in 98% of children. Ampicillin, rifampin, and trimethoprim-sulfamethoxazole are modestly active but 1st and 2nd generation cephalosporins are not. In clinical studies, erythromycin is superior to amoxicillin for eradication of *B. pertussis* and is the only agent with proven efficacy.

SALBUTAMOL. A handful of small clinical trials and reports suggest a modest reduction of symptoms from the β_2-adrenergic stimulant salbutamol (albuterol). No rigorous clinical trial has demonstrated a beneficial effect; one small study showed no effect. Fussing associated with aerosol treatment triggers paroxysms.

CORTICOSTEROIDS. No randomized, blinded clinical trial of sufficient size has been performed to evaluate the usefulness of corticosteroids in the management of pertussis. Studies in animals have shown a salutary effect on disease manifestations that do not have a corollary in respiratory infection in humans. Their clinical use is not warranted.

PERTUSSIS IMMUNE GLOBULIN. Hyperimmune serum, derived from adults convalescing from pertussis, was widely prescribed and regarded as beneficial in the 1930s and 1940s; later studies and the only placebo-controlled trial demonstrated little or no value. In a recent double-blind study in Sweden using large intramuscular doses of hyperimmune serum (raised by immunization of adults), whooping (but not cough or vomiting) was significantly reduced in infants treated in the 1st wk of disease compared with patients given placebo. Use of an immunoglobulin preparation of any sort is not warranted unless further study confirms beneficial effect.

CONTROL MEASURES. Isolation. The patient is placed in respiratory isolation for at least 5 days after initiation of erythromycin therapy.

Care of Household and Other Close Contacts. Erythromycin, 40–50 mg/kg/24 hr, orally in four divided doses (maximum 2 g/24 hr) for 14 days should be given promptly to all household contacts and other close contacts, such as those in day care, regardless of age, history of immunization, or symptomatology. Visitation and movement of coughing family members in the hospital must be assiduously controlled until erythromycin has been taken for 5 days. Close contacts younger than 7 yr who are underimmunized should be given a pertussis-containing vaccine, with further doses to complete recommended series. Children younger than 7 yr who received a 3rd dose 6 mo or more before exposure, or a 4th dose 3 yr or more before exposure, should receive a booster dose. If infection with *B. pertussis* is documented at any age, the individual is exempted from routine pertussis immunization. Antimicrobial prophylaxis is not routinely recommended for exposed health care workers. Coughing health care workers, with or without known exposure to pertussis, should be tested for pertussis promptly. For major hospital outbreaks, multifaceted control procedures including targeted erythromycin treatment of coughing individuals and subsequent mass erythromycin prophylaxis may contain hospital spread.

PREVENTION (see also Chapters 247 and 248). Universal immunization of children with pertussis vaccine, beginning in infancy, is central to the control of pertussis. Despite enormous effort, the critical mechanism(s) of immunity following disease or vaccination, a serologic correlate of protection, and the cause of vaccine-associated adverse events are not known. The only current standards for vaccine usefulness are clinical efficacy and safety. Current goals of immunization are protection of the individual from a significant coughing illness and control of endemic and epidemic disease.

Whole Cell Vaccine. The vaccine currently used for primary immunization series in the United States and recommended by the World Health Organization for use throughout most of the world is a killed whole cell vaccine composed of a suspension of inactivated *B. pertussis,* combined with diphtheria and tetanus (DT) toxoids and aluminum-containing adjuvants (DTP vaccine). Potency of pertussis vaccine is assayed in the mouse by intracerebral challenge–protection test, a standard shown to correlate with protective efficacy of vaccine in humans. Vaccine potency is translated to opacity units (also a safety standard) or protective units. U.S. preparations contain 4–12 protective units and not more than 16 opacity units per 0.5-mL dose. Efficacy of whole cell vaccine varies by case definition from 64% for mild cough, to 81% for paroxysmal cough, and to 95% for severe clinical illness. Composition of the preparation used, degree of match between agglutinogen types in vaccine and challenge strain, type of exposure, time after immunization, and requirement for culture confirmation of cases all impact on estimates of vaccine efficacy. Individuals over 7 yr of age are not routinely given pertussis-containing vaccine. When used in adults to control a hospital outbreak, whole cell vaccine was found to be less reactogenic than reported in children.

A major limitation of whole cell vaccine use has been the associated reactogenicity, reported a decade ago to occur in approximately 75% of vaccinees. Compared to DT, DTP vaccine has significantly more local reactions, such as pain, swelling, erythema, and systemic reactions, such as fever, fretfulness, crying, drowsiness, and vomiting. These manifestations occur within several hours of immunization and subside spontaneously without sequelae. Recent studies report lower rates of common local and systemic reactions, suggesting that modifications of whole cell vaccine have occurred. Severe anaphylaxis or sterile abscess are extremely rare following DTP vaccine. Transient urticaria is uncommon, is probably related to circulating antigen antibody complex, and unless it occurs within minutes of immunization is unlikely to be IgE mediated, serious, or recur on subsequent immunization.

Seizures, occurring within 48 hr of approximately 1:1,750 doses administered, are brief, generalized, and self-limited, occurring in febrile children in almost all instances. They occur more commonly in those with a personal or family history of convulsion and do not result in epilepsy or permanent neurologic sequelae. Persistent inconsolable crying or screaming for 3 or more hours reported after 1% of doses administered, usually in very young infants who have local reactions, is not unique to pertussis immunization and appears to be a manifestation of pain in many instances. Collapse or shocklike state (hypotonic-hyporesponsive episode), usually unrelated to fever or local reactions, has been observed after approximately 1:1,750 pertussis vaccinations, usually in young infants. It appears to be uniquely associated with pertussis vaccine and has no permanent neurologic sequelae. Sixty children were carefully evaluated immediately following serious pertussis vaccine-related adverse events, including seizure, persistent inconsolable crying, extremely high fever, and hypotonic-hyporesponsive episode. Ninety per cent of seizures were typical febrile seizures. No metabolic derangement or measurable pertussis toxin was found in the blood. Infants under 1 yr of age tended to have higher than expected insulin values, suggesting a possible individual age-related susceptibility or vaccine-induced alteration in insulin regulation.

Very rarely (1:140,000 doses administered) pertussis vaccine may be associated with acute neurologic illness in children who were previously normal. Severe adverse events, such as death, encephalopathy, onset of a seizure disorder, developmental delay, or learning or behavioral problems, have occurred in individuals temporally associated with pertussis immunization or alleged to be causally associated. Five major epidemiologic studies have examined neurologic risks related to pertussis immunization. Sudden infant death (SIDS) and infantile spasm were found to be neither temporally nor causally related. Analysis and reanalysis by seven major committees found information insufficient to accept a causal relationship between DTP and chronic neurologic disorders. Consideration of benefits versus risks of whole cell vaccine has repeatedly concluded in favor of its continued use.

Acellular Vaccine. Purified component acellular pertussis (aP) vaccines, originally developed in Japan, are immunogenic and associated with fewer adverse events when compared with DTP. Vaccines provided by six manufacturers have been used exclusively in Japan since 1981, and their use has controlled pertussis. A randomized, placebo-controlled (but not DTP-controlled) efficacy trial of two acellular pertussis vaccines (developed by the Japanese Institute of Health and conducted in Sweden during 1986 and 1987 under sponsorship of the United States) showed slighter lower efficacy of these acellular vaccines compared historically with whole-cell pertussis vaccine used in the United States. Lower reactogenicity of acellular vaccines and good immunogenicity in American toddlers, coupled with evidence of efficacy in household-exposure and population-based studies from Japan, led to U.S. licensure (1991 and 1992) of DTaP for use in children 15 mo of age or older as the 4th and/or 5th doses of the recommended DTP series. These vaccines have been well tolerated, and use is associated with fewer common local reactions and systemic symptoms, fever, and febrile seizures. Whether rare, more serious adverse events associated with DTP will occur less frequently after DTaP is not known.

Immunogenicity and low reactogenicity of 13 candidate acellular vaccines, multinationally manufactured, and containing variably PT, FHA, PRN, FIM2, FIM3 have been documented. Efficacy trials for primary immunization are ongoing in several countries. Experience is accumulating with use of acellular vaccines in adults as well. Licensure of one or more DTaPs in the United States for primary immunization awaits results of these trials. In countries where pertussis has been partially controlled, further reduction of cases will require implementation of booster doses of pertussis vaccine throughout life.

American Academy of Pediatrics: Pertussis. *In:* Peter G (ed): 1994 Red Book: Report of the Committee on Infectious Diseases, 23rd ed. Elk Grove Village, IL, American Academy of Pediatrics, 1994, pp 355–367.

Binkin NJ, Salmaso S, Tozzi AE, et al: Epidemiology of pertussis in a developed country with low vaccination coverage: The Italian experience. Pediatr Infect Dis J 11:653, 1992.
Centers for Disease Control: Diphtheria, tetanus, and pertussis: Recommendations for vaccine use and other preventive measures. MMWR 40:1, 1991.
Centers for Disease Control: Resurgence of pertussis—United States, 1993. MMWR 42:952, 1993.
Cherry JD: Acellular pertussis vaccines—a solution to the pertussis problem. J Infect Dis 168:21, 1993.
Christie CDC, Marx ML, Marchant CD, et al: The 1993 epidemic of pertussis in Cincinnati: Resurgence of disease in a highly immunized population of children. N Engl J Med 331:16, 1994.
Edwards KM: Acellular pertussis vaccines: A solution to the pertussis problem? J Infect Dis 168:15, 1993.
Edwards KM, Decker MD, Graham BS, et al: Adult immunization with acellular pertussis vaccine. JAMA 269:53, 1993.
Farizo KM, Cochi SL, Zell ER, et al: Epidemiologic features of pertussis in the United States, 1980–1989. Clin Infect Dis 14:708, 1992.
Gale JL, Thapa PB, Wassilak SGF, et al: Risk of serious acute neurological illness after immunization with diphtheria-tetanus-pertussis vaccine: A population-based case-control study. JAMA 271:37, 1994.
Halperin SA, Bortolussi R, MacLean D, et al: Persistence of pertussis in an immunized populations: Results of the Nova Scotia Enhanced Pertussis Surveillance Program. J Pediatr 1989; 115:686, 1989.
Hewlett EL: *Bordetella* species. *In:* Mandell GL, Douglas RG Jr, Bennett JE (eds): Principles and Practice of Infectious Diseases, 3rd ed. New York, Churchill Livingstone, 1990, pp 1756–1762.
Howson CP, Fineberg HV: Adverse events following pertussis and rubella vaccines: Summary of a report of the Institute of Medicine. JAMA 267:392, 1992.
Long SS, Welkon CJ, Clark JL: Widespread silent transmission of pertussis in families: Antibody correlates of infection and symptomatology. J Infect Dis 161:480, 1990.
Mink CAM, Sirota NM, Nugent S: Outbreak of pertussis in a fully immunized adolescent and adult population. Arch Pediatr Adolesc Med 148:153, 1994.
Onorato IM, Wassilak SG, Meade B: Efficacy of whole-cell pertussis vaccine in preschool children in the United States. JAMA 267:2745, 1992.
Preston NW: Pertussis vaccination: Neither panic nor complacency. Lancet 344:491, 1994.
Sutter RW, Cochi SL: Pertussis hospitalizations and mortality in the United States, 1985–1988: Evaluation of the completeness of national reporting. JAMA 267:386, 1992.

CHAPTER 182
Salmonella Infections

Shai Ashkenazi and Thomas G. Cleary

Salmonella infections occur worldwide. Acute gastroenteritis, the most frequent presentation, is usually self-limited, although bacteremia and focal extraintestinal infections may develop, especially in immunocompromised patients. The latter group has become more important and complex because of the increasing number of children who are compromised because of acquired immunodeficiency syndrome (AIDS), organ transplant, or chemotherapy. Enteric fever, a severe systemic disease typically caused by *Salmonella typhi,* is found mainly in developing countries, but it is seen elsewhere because of international travel.

ETIOLOGY. *Salmonella* is a genus that belongs to the family Enterobacteriaceae and contains three species: *S. typhi, S. choleraesuis,* and *S. enteritidis.* The former two species have one serotype each, but *S. enteritidis* contains more than 1800 distinct serotypes. For convenience, serotypes are sometimes artificially identified as if they were *Salmonella* species (e.g., *S. typhimurium*).

Salmonellae are motile, nonsporulating, nonencapsulated, gram-negative rods. Most strains ferment glucose, mannose, and mannitol to produce acid and gas, but they do not ferment lactose or sucrose. *S. typhi* does not produce gas. *Salmonella* organisms grow aerobically and are capable of facultative anaerobic growth. They are resistant to many physical agents but can be killed by heating to 130° F (54.4° C) for 1 hr or 140° F (60° C) for 15 min. They remain viable at ambient or reduced temperatures for days and may survive for weeks in sewage, dried foodstuffs, pharmaceutical agents, and fecal material. Like other members of the Enterobacteriaceae, *Salmonella* possesses somatic O antigens and flagellar H antigens. The O antigens are the heat-stable lipopolysaccharide components of cell wall; the H antigens are heat-labile proteins that can be present in phase 1 or 2. The Kauffmann-White scheme commonly used to classify salmonellae serotypes is based on O and H antigens. Serotyping is important clinically because certain serotypes tend to be associated with specific clinical syndromes and because the detection of an unusual serotype is sometimes epidemiologically useful. Another antigen is a virulence (Vi) capsular polysaccharide present on *S. typhi* and rarely found on strains of *S. paratyphi C (S. hirschfeldii).*

These classification schemes are based on biochemical or serologic reactions. Molecular technology has enabled classification at the gene level. DNA hybridizations have proven that all *Salmonella* organisms are closely related genetically as a single species with six subgroups; most isolates causing human or animal disease belong to subgroup 1.

182.1 Nontyphoidal Salmonellosis

EPIDEMIOLOGY. About 50,000 cases of culture-proven salmonellosis, approximately 98% of which are caused by nontyphoidal salmonellae, are reported annually in the United States. Because culturing and reporting are incomplete, the actual number of cases has been estimated as 1–5 million per year. These figures are higher than those of the 1970s and may be related to modern practices of mass food production, which increase the potential for epidemic salmonellosis. About one half of the reported cases occur in persons younger than 20 yr of age and one third occur in children 4 yr of age or younger; the highest isolation rate is for infants younger than 1 yr of age. Nontyphoidal *Salmonella* infections have a worldwide distribution, with an incidence related to water potability, sewage disposal, and food preparation practices.

Salmonella infections occur with highest frequency in the warm months, July through November in the United States. Although most reported cases of nontyphoidal salmonellosis occur sporadically, outbreaks are well documented, usually as foodborne (i.e., "food poisoning"). Each year, about 500 foodborne *Salmonella* outbreaks are reported, representing over 50% of all gastroenteritis outbreaks with a documented bacterial cause. Some of the *Salmonella* outbreaks are widespread—interstate or even international—and affect thousands of individuals. Refinement of outbreak tracing has improved with the development of molecular epidemiology techniques, such as plasmid analysis and endonucleases digestion of chromosomal genes for recognition of small differences in chromosomal structure. These can "fingerprint" a particular clone and are especially useful in tracing outbreaks caused by common serotypes. The *Salmonella* serotypes most often encountered in the United States include *S. typhimurium, S. enteritidis, S. heidelberg,* and *S. newport.*

The major reservoir of nontyphoidal salmonellae is infected animals, which constitute the principal source of human disease. Infected animals are often asymptomatic. *Salmonella* organisms have been isolated from many animals, including poultry (i.e., chickens, turkeys, ducks), sheep, cows, pigs, pets, and birds. Animal-to-animal transmission may occur. Animal feeds containing fish meal or bone meal contaminated with *Salmonella* are an important source of infection for animals. Moreover, subtherapeutic concentrations of antibiotics are often added to animal feed. Such practices promote the emergence of antibiotic-resistant bacteria, including *Salmonella*, in the gut flora of the animals. During slaughtering, these gut organisms may contaminate the meat, which is subsequently consumed by humans. Data suggest that animal antibiotic exposure may be responsible for antibiotic-resistant *Salmonella* infections in man.

Studies of outbreaks have enabled the collection of numeric data regarding the sources of human salmonellosis. Poultry and poultry products (mainly eggs) caused about half of the common-source outbreaks. Foods containing raw or undercooked eggs (e.g., Caesar salad, egg-dipped bread, homemade eggnog) are of special importance. *Salmonella* infections in chickens increase the risk for contamination of eggs. Salmonellae can contaminate the shell surface, penetrate the egg, or be transmitted from an ovarian infection directly to the egg yolk. *Salmonella* serotypes have been isolated in as many as 50% of poultry, 16% of pork, 5% of beef, and 40% of frozen egg products purchased in retail stores. Meats, especially beef and pork, caused about 13% of the outbreaks, and raw or powdered milk and dairy products were the source of about 5% of the outbreaks. Food product–related outbreaks are often caused by contaminated equipment in processing plants or infected food handlers. Pets, especially turtles, caused about 3% of the outbreaks.

The estimated number of bacteria that must be ingested to cause symptomatic disease in healthy adults is 10^6–10^8 *Salmonella* organisms. In infants and in persons with certain underlying conditions, the inoculum size that can produce disease is smaller. Because of the relatively high inoculum size of *Salmonella* infection, ingestion of contaminated food, in which the organisms can multiply, is a major source of human infection. Unlike *S. typhi*, infection with nontyphoidal salmonellae by contaminated water is infrequent. Because of the high infecting dose, person-to-person transmission by direct fecal-oral spread is unusual but can occur, especially in young children who are not yet toilet-trained and do not maintain proper hygiene. Perinatal transmission during vaginal delivery has been reported.

Nosocomial infections have been related to contaminated medical instruments (particularly endoscopes) and diagnostic or pharmacologic preparations, particularly those of animal origin (e.g., pancreatic extracts, pituitary extracts, bile salts, pepsin, gelatin, vitamins, carmine dye). Foodborne nosocomial transmission is also possible. Hospitalized patients are at increased risk of severe and complicated *Salmonella* infections. Intravenous transmission by platelet transfusion has been reported.

After infection, nontyphoidal salmonellae are excreted in feces for a median of 5 wk. In young children and in individuals with symptomatic infections, the excretion period is longer. Prolonged carriage of *Salmonella* organisms is rare in healthy children but has been reported in those with underlying immune deficiency. During the period of *Salmonella* excretion, the individual may infect others, directly by the fecal-oral route or indirectly by contaminating foods. If one household member becomes infected, the probability that another will also become infected is about 60%.

PATHOLOGY. Enterocolitis is the typical disorder caused by nontyphoidal *Salmonella* infection. Findings include diffuse mucosal inflammation and edema, sometimes with erosions and microabscesses. Although *Salmonella* organisms are capable of penetrating the intestinal mucosa, neither destruction of epithelial cells nor production of ulcers is usually seen. Intestinal inflammation, with polymorphonuclear leukocytes and macrophages, usually involves the lamina propria. Underlying intestinal lymphoid tissue and mesenteric lymph nodes enlarge and may develop small areas of necrosis. Such lymphoid hypertrophy may cause interference with the blood supply to the gut mucosa. Hyperplasia of the reticuloendothelial system is seen also within the liver and spleen. If bacteremia develops, it may lead to localized infection and suppuration (with polymorphonuclear leukocyte response) of almost any organ.

PATHOGENESIS. The development of disease after infection with *Salmonella* depends on the number of infecting organisms, on their virulence traits, and on several host defense factors. Ingested *Salmonella* organisms reach the stomach, where acidity is the first protective barrier. The acidity inhibits multiplication of the salmonellae, and when gastric pH reaches 2.0, most organisms are rapidly killed. Achlorhydria, buffering medications, rapid gastric emptying after gastrectomy or gastroenterostomy, and a large inoculum enable viable organisms to reach the small intestine. Neonates and young infants have hypochlorhydria and rapid gastric emptying, which contribute to their increased vulnerability to symptomatic salmonellosis. Because the transit time through the stomach is faster for drinks than for foods, a lower inoculum may cause disease in waterborne infection.

In the small and large intestines, salmonellae have to compete with normal bacterial flora to multiply and cause disease; prior antibiotic therapy disrupts this competitive relationship. Decreased intestinal motility due to anatomic causes or medications increases the contact time of the ingested salmonellae with the mucosa and the likelihood of symptomatic disease. After multiplication within the lumen, the organisms penetrate the mucosa, typically at the distal part of the ileum and the proximal part of the colon, with subsequent localization in the Peyer patches. The penetration process includes specific attachment to the luminal surface of epithelial cells, internalization into the cell by receptor-mediated endocytosis, cytoplasmic translocation of the infected endosome to the basal epithelial membrane, and release of the salmonellae in the lamina propria. The role of cytotoxins, which are produced by most salmonellae, is uncertain. Penetration usually occurs without destroying epithelial cells, and ulcers are not produced.

Heat-labile, cholera-like enterotoxin is produced by many *Salmonella* isolates. This toxin and the prostaglandins that are produced locally increase cyclic adenosine monophosphate levels within intestinal crypts, causing a net efflux of electrolytes and water into the intestinal lumen.

Genes code for adherence to epithelial cells, invasion of epithelial cells, a cholera toxin–like enterotoxin, spread beyond the Peyer patches to mesenteric lymph nodes, intracellular growth in the liver and spleen, survival in macrophages, serum resistance, and complement resistance. Some of these traits are shared by all salmonellae, but others are serotype restricted. These virulence traits have been defined in tissue culture and murine models; it is likely that clinical features of human *Salmonella* infection will eventually be related to specific DNA sequences.

With most diarrhea-associated nontyphoidal salmonelloses, the infection does not extend beyond the lamina propria and the local lymphatics. *S. dublin* and *S. choleraesuis* rapidly invade the bloodstream with little or no intestinal involvement. Specific virulence genes are related to the ability to cause bacteremia. These genes are found significantly more often in strains of *S. typhimurium* isolated from the blood than the feces of humans. Bacteremia, however, is theoretically possible with any *Salmonella* strain, especially in individuals with reduced host defenses. An impaired reticuloendothelial or cellular immune response is important. Children with chronic granulomatous disease, other white cell disorders, and AIDS are at increased risk. Children with sickle cell disease are prone to *Salmonella* septicemia and osteomyelitis. The numerous in-

■ TABLE 182–1 Conditions that Increase the Risk of *Salmonella* Bacteremia During *Salmonella* Gastroenteritis

Neonates and young infants (≤3 mo)
Acquired immunodeficiency syndrome, chronic granulomatous disease, and other immune deficiencies
Malignancies, especially leukemia and lymphoma
Immunosuppressive and steroid therapy
Hemolytic anemia, including sickle cell disease, malaria, and bartonellosis
Collagen vascular disease
Inflammatory bowel disease
Gastrectomy or gastroenterostomy
Achlorhydria or antacid medication
Impaired intestinal motility
Schistosomiasis
Malnutrition

farcted areas in the gastrointestinal tract, bones, and reticuloendothelial system may initially permit organisms greater access to the circulation from the intestine and then furnish an optimal environment for localization. The decreased phagocytic and opsonizing capacity of patients with sickle cell disease also contributes to the high infection rate.

Chronic infection is associated with cholelithiasis, *Schistosoma mansoni* hepatosplenic involvement, and urinary tract *Schistosoma hematobium* infection. Localized infections are more common in areas with impaired local defenses (e.g., effusions, tumors, hematomas).

CLINICAL MANIFESTATIONS. Several distinct clinical syndromes can develop in children infected with nontyphoidal *Salmonella*, depending on host factors and the specific serotype involved.

Acute Gastroenteritis. This is the most common clinical presentation. After an incubation period of 6–72 hr (mean, 24 hr), there is an abrupt onset of nausea, vomiting, and crampy abdominal pain primarily in the periumbilical area and right lower quadrant, followed by mild to severe watery diarrhea and sometimes by dysenteric diarrhea, containing blood and mucus. Moderate fever of 101–102° F (38.5–39° C) affects about 70% of patients. Some children develop severe disease with high fever, headache, drowsiness, confusion, meningismus, seizures, and abdominal distention. Abdominal examination reveals some tenderness. The stool, which is usually not bloody, typically contains a moderate number of polymorphonuclear leukocytes and occult blood. Mild leukocytosis may be detected. Symptoms subside within 2–7 days in healthy children; fatalities are rare.

In certain high-risk groups, the course of *Salmonella* gastroenteritis is distinct. Neonates, young infants, and children with primary or secondary immune deficiency may have symptoms persisting for several weeks. In patients with AIDS, the infection may become widespread and overwhelming, causing multisystem involvement, septic shock, and death. In patients with inflammatory bowel disease, especially active ulcerative colitis, *Salmonella* gastroenteritis may cause invasion of the bowel with rapid development of toxic megacolon, systemic toxicity, and death. Patients with schistosomiasis have increased susceptibility to salmonellosis and exhibit persistence of infection unless the schistosomiasis is also treated. *Salmonella* organisms are able to multiply within the schistosomes, where they are protected from antibiotics.

Bacteremia. Transient bacteremia during nontyphoidal *Salmonella* gastroenteritis is thought to occur in 1–5% of patients. The precise incidence is unclear, because blood cultures often are not obtained from patients with *Salmonella* gastroenteritis, especially those who are not hospitalized, and because most studies are retrospective. *Salmonella* bacteremia is associated with fever, chills, and often with a toxic appearance. Bacteremia has been documented, however, in afebrile, well-looking children, especially neonates. Prolonged or intermittent bacteremia is associated with low-grade fever, anorexia, weight loss, diaphoresis, and myalgias. Children with certain underlying conditions who have *Salmonella* gastroenteritis are at increased risk of bacteremia (Table 182–1), which may lead to extraintestinal infection. Recurrent *Salmonella* septicemia is one of the criteria for diagnosing AIDS according to the Centers for Disease Control and Prevention (CDC) case definition. In these patients, recurrent septicemia appears despite antibiotic therapy, often with a negative stool culture for *Salmonella* and sometimes with no identifiable focus of infection. Prolonged or recurrent bacteremia is also seen in patients with schistosomiasis. Hemolytic anemias, malaria, and bartonellosis are associated with an increased risk of bacteremia, presumably because of reticuloendothelial system dysfunction. In pregnancy, *Salmonella* septicemia and fetal loss have been reported. *S. typhimurium* is the most common serotype causing *Salmonella* bacteremia in the United States.

Extraintestinal Focal Infections. After salmonellae have entered the blood stream, they have a unique capability to metastasize and cause a focal, suppurative infection of almost any organ (Table 182–2). Sites of pre-existing abnormalities are typically involved. The most common focal infections involve the skeletal system, meninges, and intravascular sites. *Salmonella* is a common cause of osteomyelitis in children with sickle cell disease. *Salmonella* osteomyelitis and suppurative arthritis also occur in

■ TABLE 182–2 Extraintestinal Focal *Salmonella* Infections

Infection	Comments
Arteritis	Large arteries; sites with aneurysm, arteriovenous fistula, atherosclerotic plaques; causes persistent bacteremia
Arthritis	
Suppurative	Extension of osteomyelitis or primary; knee, shoulder, hip, sacroiliac; in neonates
Reactive	In HLA-B27–positive patients
Brain abscess	In AIDS; poor prognosis
Endocarditis	In sites of pre-existing heart disease, prosthetic valve; causes persistent bacteremia
Endophthalmitis	In neonates
Hepatic abscess	Usually in pre-existing amebic abscess, echinococcal cyst and hematoma; associated with biliary tract disease; high mortality rate
Infected cyst or tumor	Produces abscess-like disease, also infected cephalohematoma in neonates
Intra-abdominal abscess	Subphrenic, pancreatic; multifocal in patients with AIDS
Mastitis	In neonates
Meningitis	In infants and AIDS patients; complications, high mortality rate
Osteomyelitis	Can develop in normal bone, typically in ischemic bone with sickle cell disease; in systemic lupus erythematosus, hematologic malignancies, after bone surgery or trauma
Pericarditis	In systemic lupus erythematosus; in neonates
Peritonitis	Primary peritonitis in patients with ascites
Pleuropneumonia	In immunocompromised patients, especially with leukemia or lymphoma; secondary empyema of malignant pleural effusion
Soft tissue abscess	After trauma; in neonates; in skin or subcutaneous sites
Splenic abscess	In pre-existing splenic cyst; infected post-traumatic subcapsular hematoma
Genitourinary tract infection	Cystitis, pyelonephritis, renal abscess, testicular and ovarian abscess

AIDS = acquired immunodeficiency syndrome.

sites of previous trauma or skeletal prosthesis. Reactive arthritis may follow *Salmonella* gastroenteritis, usually in children with the HLA-B27 antigen. Meningitis appears mainly in infants. Patients usually present with little or no fever and minimal symptoms, but rapid deterioration, a high mortality rate (~50%), and neurologic sequelae occur despite appropriate antibiotic therapy. *Salmonella* meningitis occurs also in patients with AIDS, for whom the mortality rate is more than 50%, and relapse and brain abscesses can occur. Persistent bacteremia suggests endocarditis, arteritis, or an infected aneurysm. The serotypes causing most extraintestinal focal infections are *S. typhimurium* and *S. choleraesuis.*

Asymptomatic Infection. Asymptomatic fecal excretion of salmonellae after infection with these organisms has been documented, for instance, as part of an outbreak investigation. The precise incidence is unclear. After clinical recovery from *Salmonella* gastroenteritis, asymptomatic fecal excretion of salmonellae occurs for several weeks. A chronic carrier state is defined as asymptomatic excretion of *Salmonella* organisms for more than 1 yr. Although the carrier state does occur after nontyphoidal salmonellosis, it is rare (<1%), and it develops especially in patients with biliary tract disease. The only significance of asymptomatic fecal excretion of nontyphoidal *Salmonella* is the potential transmission of the infection to other individuals.

DIAGNOSIS. Definitive diagnosis of the various clinical syndromes is still based on culturing and subsequent identification of *Salmonella* organisms. In children with gastroenteritis, cultures of stools have higher yields than rectal swabs. In patients with sites of local suppuration, aspirated specimens should be used for Gram staining and culture. *Salmonella* organisms grow well on nonselective or enriched media, such as blood agar, chocolate agar, or nutrient broth. Normally sterile body fluids (e.g., cerebrospinal fluid, joint fluid, urine) can be cultured on any of these. For specimens normally containing bacterial flora (e.g., stools), selective media, such as MacConkey, XLD, bismuth sulfite (BBL) or *Salmonella-Shigella* (SS) agar, which inhibit the growth of normal flora, should be used.

Several methods are being developed to answer the need for rapid diagnosis. Two tests, based on latex agglutination and fluorescence, are commercially available for the rapid diagnosis of *Salmonella* colonies growing in stool culture enrichment broth or culture plates. Clinical experience is limited. Alternatively, chromosomal fragments that are unique to the genus *Salmonella* have been employed as DNA probes to detect *Salmonella* species. The method is still experimental and needs evaluation with clinical specimens. Serologic assay for detecting antibodies against *S. typhimurium* and *S. enteritidis* has been reported, but clinical usefulness is still unclear.

DIFFERENTIAL DIAGNOSIS. *Salmonella* gastroenteritis should be differentiated from other bacterial, viral, and parasitic causes of diarrhea. The presentation of inflammatory diarrhea with moderate fever should be particularly differentiated from *Shigella,* enteroinvasive *Escherichia coli, Yersinia enterocolitica,* and *Clostridium difficile* infections. Rotavirus infections in infants can mimic *Salmonella* enterocolitis. Etiologic diagnosis on the basis of the clinical picture is not possible. Epidemiologic data may be helpful. If abdominal pain and tenderness are severe, appendicitis, perforated viscus, and ulcerative colitis merit consideration in the differential diagnosis.

PREVENTION. Chlorinated water, proper sanitary systems, and adequate food hygiene practices are necessary to prevent nontyphoidal salmonellosis in humans. Handwashing is of paramount importance in controlling person-to-person transmission by means of food. In hospitalized patients, enteric precautions should be used for the duration of illness. Individuals with symptomatic or asymptomatic excretion of *Salmonella* strains should be excluded from activities that involve food preparation or child care until repeated stool cultures are negative. Promotion of breast-feeding may reduce infection, especially in developing communities.

Control of the transmission of *Salmonella* infections to humans requires control of the infection in the animal reservoir, judicious use of antibiotics in dairy and livestock farming, prevention of contamination of foodstuffs prepared from animals, and use of appropriate standards in food processing in commercial and private kitchens. Whenever cooking practices prevent food from reaching a temperature greater than 150° F (65.5° C) for more than 12 min, salmonellosis may be transmitted. Because large outbreaks are often related to mass food production, it should be recognized that contamination of just one piece of machinery used in food processing may cause an outbreak; meticulous cleaning of the equipment is essential. No vaccine against nontyphoidal *Salmonella* infections is available.

TREATMENT. Proper therapy depends on the specific clinical presentation of *Salmonella* infection. Assessment of the hydration status, correction of dehydration and electrolyte disturbances, and supportive care (see Chapter 60) are the most important aspects of managing *Salmonella* gastroenteritis in children. Antimotility agents prolong intestinal transit time and are thought to increase the risk of invasion; they should not be used when salmonellosis is suspected. In patients with gastroenteritis, antimicrobial agents do not shorten the clinical course, nor do they eliminate fecal excretion of *Salmonella.* By suppressing normal intestinal flora, antimicrobial agents may prolong the excretion of *Salmonella* and increase the risk of creating the chronic carrier state. Antibiotics therefore are not indicated routinely in treating *Salmonella* gastroenteritis. They should be used in young infants and other children who are at increased risk of a disseminated disease (see Table 182–1) and in those with a severe or protracted course.

Children with bacteremia or extraintestinal focal *Salmonella* infections should receive antimicrobial therapy. Ampicillin (200 mg/kg/24 hr in four divided doses) is efficacious and used to be the drug of choice; trimethoprim-sulfamethoxazole (TMP-SMX; 10–50 mg/kg/24 hr in two divided doses) and chloramphenicol (75 mg/kg/24 hr in four divided doses) are also effective. Because of the increasing worldwide antibiotic resistance of *Salmonella* strains, it is necessary to perform susceptibility tests on all human isolates. About 20% of *Salmonella* isolates in the United States are resistant to ampicillin. Multiresistance to ampicillin, TMP-SMX, and chloramphenicol has been reported. The third-generation cephalosporins, cefotaxime (150–200 mg/kg/24 hr in three to four divided doses) or ceftriaxone (100 mg/kg/24 hr in one or two doses), are effective in these cases, although clinical experience is still limited. Quinolones are also effective, but they are not approved for use in children because of the potential damage to growing cartilage. In children with severe disease, initial treatment with a third-generation cephalosporin is recommended until antibiotic susceptibility is known. Thereafter, antibiotics should be changed accordingly.

The duration of antimicrobial therapy is 10–14 days in children with bacteremia, 4–6 wks for acute osteomyelitis, and 4 wk for meningitis. In a child with a focal suppurative process, surgical drainage is necessary in addition to antibiotic treatment. Surgical intervention is often necessary in intravascular *Salmonella* infections (e.g., repair of aneurysm, replacement of valve) and in cases of chronic osteomyelitis.

PROGNOSIS. Complete recovery is the rule in healthy children who develop *Salmonella* gastroenteritis. Young infants and immunocompromised patients often have systemic involvement, a prolonged course, and complications. The prognosis is poor for children with *Salmonella* meningitis (~50% mortality rate) or endocarditis.

Centers for Disease Control: *Salmonella* surveillance—annual summary. Atlanta, GA, Public Health Services, 1990.

Cohen JI, Bartlett JA, Corey GP: Extra-intestinal manifestations of *Salmonella* infections. Medicine (Baltimore) 66:349, 1987.
Goldberg MB, Rubin RH: The spectrum of *Salmonella* infection. Infect Dis Clin North Am 2:571, 1988.
Hedberg CW, David MJ, White KE, et al: Role of egg consumption in sporadic *Salmonella enteritis* and *Salmonella typhimurium* infection in Minnesota. J Infect Dis 167:107, 1993.
Isomaki O, Vuento R, Granfors K: Serologic diagnosis of *Salmonella* infections by enzyme immunoassay. Lancet 1:1411, 1989.
Sperber SJ, Schleupner CJ: Salmonellosis during infection with human immunodeficiency virus. Rev Infect Dis 9:925, 1987.
St. Geme JW, Hodes HL, Marcy SM, et al: Consensus: Management of *Salmonella* infection in the first year of life. Pediatr Infect Dis J 7:615, 1988.

182.2 Enteric Fever

Enteric fever is a systemic clinical syndrome produced by certain *Salmonella* organisms. It encompasses the terms typhoid fever, caused by *S. typhi,* and paratyphoid fever, caused by *S. paratyphi A, S. schottmuelleri* (formerly *S. paratyphi B*), *S. hirschfeldii* (formerly *S. paratyphi C*), and occasionally other *Salmonella* serotypes. Typhoid fever, the most frequent and best studied type of enteric fever, tends to be more severe than the other forms.

EPIDEMIOLOGY. The incidence, mode of transmission, and consequences of enteric fever differ significantly in developed and developing countries. The incidence has decreased markedly in developed countries. In the United States, about 400 cases of typhoid fever are reported each year, giving an annual incidence of less than 0.2 per 100,000, which is similar to that in Western Europe and Japan. In Southern Europe, the annual incidence is 4.3–14.5 per 100,000. In developing countries, *S. typhi* is often the most common *Salmonella* isolate, with an incidence than can reach 500 per 100,000 (0.5%) and a high mortality rate. The World Health Organization has estimated that 12.5 million cases occur annually worldwide (excluding China).

Because humans are the only natural reservoir of *S. typhi,* direct or indirect contact with an infected person (sick or chronic carrier) is necessary for infection. Ingestion of foods or water contaminated with human feces is the most common mode of transmission. Waterborne outbreaks due to poor sanitation and direct fecal-oral spread due to poor personal hygiene are seen, mainly in developing countries. Oysters and other shellfish cultivated in water contaminated by sewage are also a source of widespread infection. In the United States, about 65% of the cases result from international travel. Travel to Asia (especially to India) and Central or South America (especially Mexico) is usually implicated. Domestically acquired enteric fever is most frequent in the southern and western United States and is usually caused by consumption of foods contaminated by individuals who are chronic carriers. Congenital transmission of enteric fever can occur by transplacental infection from a bacteremic mother to her fetus. Intrapartum transmission is also possible, occurring by a fecal-oral route from a carrier mother.

PATHOLOGY. In younger children, the morphologic changes of *S. typhi* infection are less prominent than in older children and adults. Hyperplasia of Peyer patches with necrosis and sloughing of overlying epithelium, producing ulcers, is typical. The mucosa and lymphatic tissue of the intestinal tract are severely inflamed and necrotic. Ulceration that heals without scarring is common. Strictures and intestinal obstruction virtually never occur after typhoid fever. Hemorrhages may occur. The inflammatory lesion may occasionally penetrate the muscularis and serosa of the intestine and produce perforation. The mesenteric lymph nodes, liver, and spleen are hyperemic and generally reveal areas of focal necrosis. Hyperplasia of reticuloendothelial tissue with proliferation of mononuclear cells is the predominant finding. A mononuclear response may be seen in the bone marrow associated with areas of focal necrosis. Inflammation of the gallbladder is focal, inconstant, and modest in proportion to the extent of local bacterial multiplication. Bronchitis is common. Inflammation also may be observed in the form of localized abscesses, pneumonia, septic arthritis, osteomyelitis, pyelonephritis, endophthalmitis, and meningitis.

PATHOGENESIS. Bloodstream invasion by *S. typhi* or occasionally by other serotypes is necessary to produce the enteric fever syndrome. The inoculum size required to cause disease in volunteers is 10^5–10^9 *S. typhi* organisms. These estimates may be higher than in naturally acquired infection because the volunteers ingested the organisms in milk; stomach acidity is an important determinant of susceptibility to salmonella. After attachment to the microvilli of the ileal brush borders, the bacteria invade intestinal epithelium, apparently through the Peyer patches. Organisms are transported to intestinal lymph follicles, where multiplication takes place within the mononuclear cells. Monocytes, unable to destroy the bacilli early in the disease process, carry these organisms into the mesenteric lymph nodes. Organisms then reach the bloodstream through the thoracic duct, causing a transient bacteremia. Circulating organisms reach the reticuloendothelial cells in the liver, spleen, and bone marrow and may seed other organs. After proliferation in the reticuloendothelial system, the bacteremia recurs. The gallbladder is particularly susceptible to being infected from the bloodstream or through the biliary system. Local multiplication in the walls of the gallbladder produces large numbers of salmonellae, which secondarily reach the intestine through the bile.

Several virulence factors seem to be important. A surface Vi capsular antigen is found in most *S. typhi* and some other serotypes; it interferes with phagocytosis by preventing the binding of C3 to the surface of the bacterium and correlates with invasion capability. The sequence of the gene *(viaB)* encoding Vi has been defined. The ability of organisms to survive within macrophages after phagocytosis is an important virulence trait encoded by the *phoP* regulon; it may be related to metabolic effects on host cells. Circulating endotoxin, a lipopolysaccharide component of the bacterial cell wall, is thought to cause the prolonged fever and toxic symptoms of enteric fever, although its levels in symptomatic patients are low. Alternatively, endotoxin-induced cytokine production by human macrophages may cause the systemic symptoms. The occasional occurrence of diarrhea may be explained by presence of a toxin related to cholera toxin and *E. coli* heat-labile enterotoxin.

Cell-mediated immunity is important in protecting the human host against typhoid fever. Decreased numbers of T lymphocytes are found in patients who are critically ill with typhoid fever. Carriers show impaired cellular reactivity to *S. typhi* antigens in the leukocyte migration inhibition test. In carriers, a large number of virulent bacilli pass into the intestine daily and are excreted in the stool, without entering the epithelium of the host.

CLINICAL MANIFESTATIONS. The incubation period is usually 7–14 days, but it may range from 3–30 days, depending mainly on the size of the ingested inoculum. The clinical manifestations of enteric fever depend on age.

School-Age Children and Adolescents. The onset of symptoms is insidious. Initial symptoms of fever, malaise, anorexia, myalgia, headache, and abdominal pain develop over 2–3 days. Although diarrhea having a pea soup consistency may be present during the early course of the disease, constipation later becomes a more prominent symptom. Nausea and vomiting are uncommon and suggest a complication, particularly if occurring in the 2nd or 3rd wk. Cough and epistaxis may be seen. Severe lethargy may develop in some children. The fever, which rises in a step-wise fashion, becomes unremittent and high within 1 wk, often reaching 40° C (104° F).

During the 2nd wk of illness, high fever is sustained, and fatigue, anorexia, cough, and abdominal symptoms increase in severity. The patient appears acutely ill, disoriented, and lethargic. Delirium and stupor may be observed. Physical findings include a relative bradycardia, which is disproportionate to the high fever. Hepatomegaly, splenomegaly, and distended abdomen with diffuse tenderness are very common. In about 50% of patients with enteric fever, a macular (i.e., rose spots) or maculopapular rash appears on about the 7th to 10th day. Lesions are usually discrete, erythematous, and 1 to 5 mm in diameter; the lesions are slightly raised, and blanch on pressure. They appear in crops of 10 to 15 lesions on the lower chest and abdomen and last 2 or 3 days. They leave a slight brownish discoloration of the skin on healing. Cultures of the lesions have a 60% yield for *Salmonella* organisms. Rhonchi and scattered rales may be heard on auscultation of the chest. If no complications occur, the symptoms and physical findings gradually resolve within 2–4 wk, but malaise and lethargy may persist for an additional 1–2 mo. The patients may be emaciated by the end of the illness. Enteric fever caused by nontyphoidal *Salmonella* is usually milder, with a shorter duration of fever and a lower rate of complications.

Infants and Young Children (<5 yr). Enteric fever is relatively rare in this age group. Although clinical sepsis can occur, the disease is surprisingly mild at presentation, making the diagnosis difficult and underdiagnosis possible. Mild fever and malaise, misinterpreted as a viral syndrome, are seen in infants with culture-proven typhoid fever. Diarrhea is more common in young children with typhoid fever than in adults, leading to a diagnosis of acute gastroenteritis. Others may present with signs and symptoms of lower respiratory tract infection.

Neonates. In addition to its ability to cause abortion and premature delivery, enteric fever during late pregnancy may be transmitted vertically. The neonatal disease usually begins within 3 days of delivery. Vomiting, diarrhea, and abdominal distention are common. Temperature is variable but may be as high as 40.5° C (105° F). Seizures may occur. Hepatomegaly, jaundice, anorexia, and weight loss can be marked.

LABORATORY FINDINGS. A normochromic, normocytic anemia is often seen after several weeks of illness and is related to intestinal blood loss or bone marrow suppression. Blood leukocyte counts are frequently low in relation to the fever and toxicity, but there is a wide range in counts; leukopenia, usually not below 2500 cells/mm^3, is often seen after the 1st or 2nd wk of illness. When pyogenic abscesses develop, leukocytosis may reach 20,000–25,000/mm^3. Thrombocytopenia may be striking and persist for as long as 1 wk. Liver function test results are often disturbed. Proteinuria is common. Fecal leukocytes and fecal blood are very common.

COMPLICATIONS. Common complications include intestinal perforation, myocarditis, and central nervous system manifestations. Severe intestinal hemorrhage and intestinal perforation occur in 1–10% and 0.5–3% of the patients, respectively. These and most other complications usually occur after the 1st wk of the disease. Hemorrhage, which usually precedes perforation, is manifested by a drop in temperature and blood pressure and an increase in the pulse rate. Perforations, which are usually pinpoint size but may be as large as several centimeters, typically occur in the distal ileum and are accompanied by a marked increase in abdominal pain, tenderness, vomiting, and signs of peritonitis. Sepsis with various enteric aerobic Gram-negative bacilli and anaerobes may develop. Although disturbed liver function test results are found for many patients with enteric fever, overt hepatitis and cholecystitis are considered complications. An increase in serum amylase levels may be seen sometimes with clinically obvious pancreatitis.

Pneumonia often caused by superinfection with organisms other than *Salmonella* is more common in children than in adults. In children, pneumonia or bronchitis is common (approximately 10%). Toxic myocarditis may be manifested by arrhythmias, sinoatrial block, ST-T changes on the electrocardiogram, cardiogenic shock, fatty infiltration, and necrosis of the myocardium. Thrombosis and phlebitis occur rarely. Neurologic complications include increased intracranial pressure, cerebral thrombosis, acute cerebellar ataxia, chorea, aphasia, deafness, psychosis, and transverse myelitis. Peripheral and optic neuritis have been reported. Permanent sequelae are rare. Other reported complications are fatal bone marrow necrosis, pyelonephritis, nephrotic syndrome, meningitis, endocarditis, parotitis, orchitis, and suppurative lymphadenitis. Although osteomyelitis and septic arthritis can occur in a normal host, they are more frequently seen in children with hemoglobinopathies.

DIAGNOSIS. Culturing the *Salmonella* strain involved is usually the basis for the diagnosis. Blood cultures are positive in 40–60% of the patients seen early in the course of the disease, and stool and urine cultures become positive after the 1st wk. The stool culture is also occasionally positive during the incubation period. Because of the intermittent and low-level bacteremia, repeated blood cultures should be obtained. Cultures of bone marrow are often positive during later stages of the disease, when blood cultures may be sterile; although seldom obtained, cultures of mesenteric lymph nodes, liver, and spleen may also be positive at this point. A culture of bone marrow is the single most sensitive method of diagnosis (positive in 85–90%) and is less influenced by prior antimicrobial therapy. Stool and sometimes urine cultures are positive in chronic carriers. In suspected cases with negative stool cultures, a culture of aspirated duodenal fluid or of a duodenal string capsule may be helpful in confirming infection.

Because identification of *S. typhi* from culture usually takes at least 3 days, several methods for earlier diagnosis are being developed. Direct detection of *S. typhi*–specific antigens in the serum or *S. typhi* Vi antigen in the urine has been attempted by immunologic methods, often using monoclonal antibodies. Polymerase chain reaction (PCR) has been used to amplify specific genes of *S. typhi* in the blood of patients, enabling diagnosis within a few hours. This method is specific and more sensitive than blood cultures given the low level of bacteremia in enteric fever. More experience with these new methods is needed before they can be endorsed.

Serology is of little help in establishing the diagnosis, but it may be useful in epidemiologic studies. The classic Widal test measures antibodies against O and H antigens of *S. typhi*. Because many false-positive and false-negative results occur, diagnosis of typhoid fever by Widal test alone is prone to error. Experience is still limited with new serologic assays.

DIFFERENTIAL DIAGNOSIS. During the initial stage of enteric fever, the clinical diagnosis may mistakenly be gastroenteritis, viral syndrome, bronchitis, or bronchopneumonia. Subsequently, the differential diagnosis includes sepsis with other bacterial pathogens; infections caused by intracellular microorganisms, such as tuberculosis, brucellosis, tularemia, leptospirosis, and rickettsial diseases; viral infections, such as infectious mononucleosis and anicteric hepatitis; and malignancies, such as leukemia and lymphoma.

PREVENTION. In endemic areas, improved sanitation and clean, running water are essential to control enteric fever. To minimize person-to-person transmission and food contamination, personal hygiene measures, handwashing, and attention to food preparation practices are necessary. Efforts to eradicate *S. typhi* from carriers are recommended, because humans are the only reservoir of *S. typhi*. When such efforts are unsuccessful, carriers should be prevented from working in food- or water-processing plants, in kitchens, and in occupations related to patient care. These individuals should be made aware of the potential contagiousness of their condition and the importance of handwashing and personal hygiene.

Several vaccines against *S. typhi* are available. A parenteral heat-phenol–inactivated vaccine confers limited protection (51–76% efficacy) and is associated with adverse effects, including fever, local reactions, and headache in at least 25% of recipients. Two doses of 0.5 mL administered subcutaneously 4 wk or more apart have been recommended for children 10 yr or older; 0.25 mL per dose is recommended for younger children. A second newly licensed vaccine (Vivotif) is an oral, live-attenuated preparation of the Ty21a strain of *S. typhi.* Several large studies have shown efficacy (67–82%). Significant adverse effects are rare. Four enteric-coated capsules on alternate days are given. The oral vaccine is not recommended for children younger than 6 yr because of limited experience. Infants and toddlers do not develop immune responses with this preparation. It should not be used in persons with immunodeficiency syndromes. Vaccines against typhoid fever made from the Vi capsular polysaccharide, with or without protein conjugation, are under investigation.

A typhoid vaccine is recommended to travelers to endemic areas, especially Latin America, Southeast Asia, and Africa. Such travelers need to be cautioned that the vaccine is not a substitute for personal hygiene and careful selection of foods and drinks, because neither vaccine has efficacy approaching 100%. Vaccination is also recommended to individuals with intimate exposure to a documented carrier and for control of outbreaks.

TREATMENT. Antimicrobial therapy is essential in treating enteric fever, especially for typhoid fever. Because of increasing antibiotic resistance, however, choosing the appropriate empiric therapy is problematic and sometimes controversial. Most antibiotic regimens are associated with a 5–20% recurrence risk. Chloramphenicol (50 mg/kg/24 hr orally or 75 mg/kg/24 hr, intravenously in four equal doses), ampicillin (200 mg/kg/24 hr, intravenously in four to six doses), amoxicillin (100 mg/kg/24 hr, orally in three doses), and trimethoprim-sulfamethoxazole (10 mg of TMP and 50 mg of SMX/kg/24 hr, orally in two doses) have demonstrated good clinical efficacy. Although chloramphenicol therapy is associated with a more rapid defervescence and sterilization of blood, the rate of relapse is somewhat higher, and this agent can cause potentially serious adverse effects. Most children become afebrile within 7 days; treatment of uncomplicated patients should be continued for at least 14 days or 5–7 days after defervescence. In children with underlying disturbances, including severe malnutrition, extending antibiotic therapy for 21 days may reduce the rate of complications.

Although antibiotic resistance of *S. typhi* isolates in the United States is relatively low (3–4%), most infections are acquired abroad, where resistance occurs. Increasing rates of plasmid-mediated antibiotic resistance of *S. typhi* have been reported from Southeast Asia, Mexico, and certain countries in the Middle East. Reports from India describe multiresistance to chloramphenicol, ampicillin, and TMP-SMX in 49–83% of *S. typhi* isolates. Resistant strains are usually susceptible to third-generation cephalosporins. Cefotaxime (200 mg/kg/24 hr, intravenously in three to four doses) and ceftriaxone (100 mg/kg/24 hr, intravenously in one to two doses) have been successfully used to treat typhoid fever caused by resistant strains, although the response to ceftriaxone was somewhat better. Aztreonam has also been successfully used. Fluoroquinolones are efficacious, but they are not approved for children. In adults, ciprofloxacin at a dose of 500 mg twice daily for 7–10 days is effective and associated with a low relapse rate. In patients with suspected resistant strains, we recommend empirical therapy with ceftriaxone (or cefotaxime) until antibiotic susceptibility patterns are available.

In addition to antibiotic therapy, a short course of dexamethasone, using 3 mg/kg for the initial dose, followed by 1 mg/kg every 6 hr for 48 hr, improves the survival rate of patients with shock, obtundation, stupor, or coma. This does not increase the incidence of complications if antibiotic therapy is adequate. Supportive treatment and maintenance of appropriate fluid and electrolyte balance are essential. When intestinal hemorrhage is severe, blood transfusion is needed. Surgical intervention with broad-spectrum antibiotics is recommended for intestinal perforation. Platelet transfusions have been suggested for the treatment of thrombocytopenia that is sufficiently severe to cause intestinal hemorrhage in patients for whom surgery is contemplated.

Although attempts to eradicate chronic carriage of *S. typhi* are recommended for public health considerations, eradication is difficult despite in vitro susceptibility to the antibiotic used. A course of 4–6 wk of high-dose ampicillin (or amoxicillin) plus probenecid or TMP-SMX results in an approximately 80% cure rate of carriers if no biliary tract disease is present. Ciprofloxacin has been used successfully in adults. In the presence of cholelithiasis or cholecystitis, antibiotics alone are unlikely to be successful; cholecystectomy within 14 days of antibiotic treatment is recommended.

PROGNOSIS. The prognosis for a patient with enteric fever depends on prompt therapy, the age of the patient, previous state of health, the causative *Salmonella* serotype, and the appearance of complications. In developed countries, with appropriate antimicrobial therapy, the mortality rate is below 1%. In developing countries, the mortality rate is higher than 10%, usually because of delays in diagnosis, hospitalization, and treatment. Infants younger than 1 yr of age and children with underlying debilitating disorders are at higher risk. *S. typhi* causes a more severe disease, with higher rates of complications and death, than other serotypes. The appearance of complications, such as gastrointestinal perforation or severe hemorrhage, meningitis, endocarditis, and pneumonia, are associated with high morbidity and mortality rates.

Relapse after the initial clinical response occurs in 4–8% of the patients who are not treated with antibiotics. In patients who have received appropriate antimicrobial therapy, the clinical manifestations of relapse become apparent about 2 wk after stopping antibiotics and resemble the acute illness. The relapse, however, is usually milder and of shorter duration. Multiple relapses may occur. Individuals who excrete *S. typhi* 3 mo or longer after infection are usually excretors at 1 yr and defined as chronic carriers. The risk of becoming a carrier is low in children and increases with age; of all patients with typhoid fever, 1–5% become chronic carriers. The incidence of biliary tract diseases is higher in chronic carriers than in the general population. Although chronic urinary carriage may also occur, it is rare and found mainly in individuals with schistosomiasis.

Butler T, Islam A, Kabir I, Jones PK: Patterns of morbidity and mortality in typhoid fever dependent on age and gender: A review of 552 patients hospitalized with diarrhea. Rev Infect Dis 13:85, 1991.

Centers of Disease Control: Typhoid immunization: recommendations of the Immunization Practices Advisory Committee. MMWR 39:1, 1990.

Edelman R, Levine MM: Summary of an international workshop on typhoid fever. Rev Infect Dis 8:329, 1986.

Mahle WT, Levine MM: *Salmonella typhi* infection in children younger than five years of age. Pediatr Infect Dis J 12:627, 1993.

Mosley JG, Chaudhuri AK: Surgery and *Salmonella:* Complications require prompt diagnosis and treatment. Br Med J 300:552, 1990.

Ryan CA, Hargrett-Bean NT, Blake PA: *Salmonella typhi* infections in the United States, 1975–1984: Increasing role of foreign travel. Rev Infect Dis 11:1, 1989.

Soe GB, Overturf GD: Treatment of typhoid fever and other systemic salmonelloses with cefotaxime, ceftriaxone, cefoperazone and other newer cephalosporins. Rev Infect Dis 9:719, 1987.

Song JH, Cho H, Park MY, et al: Detection of *Salmonella typhi* in the blood of patients with typhoid fever by polymerase chain reaction. J Clin Microbiol 31:1439, 1993.

Thisyakorn U, Mansuwan P, Taylor DN: Typhoid and paratyphoid fever in 192 hospitalized children in Thailand. Am J Dis Child 141:862, 1987.

CHAPTER 183
Shigella

Henry F. Gomez and Thomas G. Cleary

Although dysenteric syndromes have long been recognized as a scourge of man, it is only in the last 90 yr that the bacteriology of the most common form of epidemic dysentery has been appreciated. Four species of *Shigella* are responsible for illness: *S. dysenteriae* (serogroup A), *S. flexneri* (serogroup B), *S. boydii* (serogroup C), and *S. sonnei* (serogroup D). There are 12 serotypes in group A, 6 serotypes and 13 subserotypes in group B, 18 serotypes in group C, and 1 serotype in group D.

PATHOPHYSIOLOGY. The basic virulence trait shared by all shigellae is the ability to invade colonic epithelial cells. This characteristic is encoded on a large (120–140 MD) plasmid that is responsible for synthesis of a group of polypeptides involved in cell invasion and killing. Shigellae that lose the virulence plasmid no longer act as pathogens. *Escherichia coli* that naturally or artificially harbor this plasmid behave like shigellae. In addition to the major plasmid-encoded virulence traits, chromosomally encoded factors are also required for full virulence; some of these chromosomal traits are important for all shigellae (e.g., lipopolysaccharide synthesis), whereas others are important only in some serotypes (e.g., shigatoxin synthesis). Shigatoxin, a potent protein synthesis–inhibiting exotoxin, is produced in significant amounts only by *S. dysenteriae* serotype 1 and certain *E. coli* (enterohemorrhagic *E. coli* or shiga-like toxin–producing *E. coli*). The watery diarrhea phase of shigellosis may be caused by unique enterotoxins: shigella enterotoxin 1 (ShET-1), encoded on the bacterial chromosome, and ShET-2, encoded on the virulence plasmid.

Shigellae require very low inocula to cause illness. Ingestion of as few as 10 *S. dysenteriae* serotype 1 organisms can cause dysentery in some susceptible individuals. This is in contrast to organisms such as *Vibrio cholerae,* which require ingestion of 10^8–10^{10} organisms to cause illness. The inoculum effect explains the ease of person-to-person transmission of shigellae in contrast to *V. cholerae.*

Immune Responses. Secretory IgA and serum antibodies develop within days to weeks after infection with *Shigella.* Although both antilipopolysaccharide and antivirulence plasmid polypeptide antibodies have been described, identification of the major determinant of protection against subsequent infection remains unclear. There is evidence that protection is serotype specific, but there is also the suggestion that a degree of cross-protection against all shigellae follows infection with a given serotype. Cell-mediated immunity may also play some role in protection, although it appears to be minor.

PATHOLOGY. The pathologic changes of shigellosis take place primarily in the colon, the target organ for shigellae. The changes are most intense in the distal colon, although pancolitis may occur. Grossly, localized or diffuse mucosal edema, ulcerations, friable mucosa, bleeding, and exudate may be seen. Microscopically, ulcerations, pseudomembranes, epithelial cell death, infiltration extending from the mucosa to the muscularis mucosae by polymorphonuclear and mononuclear cells, and submucosal edema occur.

EPIDEMIOLOGY. Infection with shigellae occurs most often during the warm months in temperate climates and during the rainy season in tropical climates. The sexes are affected equally. Although infection can occur at any age, it is most common in the 2nd and 3rd yr of life. Infection in the first 6 mo is rare for reasons that are not clear. Breast milk, which in endemic areas contains antibodies to both virulence plasmid-coded antigens and lipopolysaccharides, may partially explain the age-related incidence. Asymptomatic infection of children and adults occurs but is uncommon.

In industrialized societies, *S. sonnei* is the most common cause of bacillary dysentery, with *S. flexneri* second in frequency; in preindustrial societies, *S. flexneri* is most common with *S. sonnei* second in frequency. *S. dysenteriae* serotype 1 tends to occur in massive epidemics, although it is also endemic in Asia.

Contaminated food (often a salad or other item requiring extensive handling of the ingredients) and water are important vectors. However, person-to-person transmission is probably the major mechanism of infection in most areas of the world. Spread within families, custodial institutions, and day-care centers demonstrates the ability of low numbers of organisms to cause disease on a person-to-person basis.

CLINICAL MANIFESTATIONS. Bacillary dysentery is clinically similar regardless of whether the disease is caused by an enteroinvasive *E. coli* (see Chapter 184) or any of the four species of *Shigella;* however, there are some clinical differences, particularly relating to the severity and risk of complications with *S. dysenteriae* serotype 1 infection.

After ingestion of shigellae there is an incubation period of several days before symptoms ensue. Characteristically, severe abdominal pain, high fever, emesis, anorexia, generalized toxicity, urgency, and painful defecation occur. Physical examination at this point may show abdominal distention and tenderness, hyperactive bowel sounds, and a tender rectum on digital examination.

The *diarrhea* may be watery and of large volume initially, evolving into frequent small-volume, bloody mucoid stools; however, some children never progress to the stage of bloody diarrhea, whereas in others the first stools are bloody. Significant dehydration related to the fluid and electrolyte losses in both feces and emesis can occur. Untreated diarrhea may last 1–2 wk; only about 10% of patients have diarrhea persisting for more than 10 days. Chronic diarrhea is uncommon except in malnourished infants.

Neurologic findings are among the most common extraintestinal manifestations of bacillary dysentery, occurring in as many as 40% of hospitalized infected children. Convulsions, headache, lethargy, confusion, nuchal rigidity, or hallucinations may be present before or after the onset of diarrhea. The cause of these neurologic findings is not understood. In the past, these symptoms were attributed to the neurotoxicity of shigatoxin, but it is now clear that that explanation is wrong. Seizures sometimes occur when little fever is present, suggesting that simple febrile convulsions do not explain their appearance. Hypocalcemia or hyponatremia may be associated with seizures in a small number of patients. Although symptoms often suggest central nervous system infection, and cerebrospinal fluid pleocytosis with minimally elevated protein levels can occur, meningitis due to shigellae is rare.

The most common complication of shigellosis is dehydration with its attendant risks of renal failure and death (see Chapter 56.1). Inappropriate secretion of antidiuretic hormone with profound hyponatremia may complicate dysentery, particularly when *S. dysenteriae* is the etiologic agent.

Other major complications, particularly in very young, malnourished children, include sepsis and disseminated intravascular coagulation. Given that these organisms penetrate the intestinal mucosal barrier, these events are surprisingly uncommon. Shigellae and sometimes other gram-negative enterics are recovered from blood cultures in 1–5% of cases in whom blood cultures are taken; because patients selected for blood cultures represent a biased sample, the risk in unselected cases of shigellosis is presumably lower. Bacteremia is more common with *S. dysenteriae* serotype 1 than with other shigellae. The mortality rate is high (20–50%) when sepsis occurs.

In those who have *S. dysenteriae* serotype 1 infection, hemolysis, anemia, and hemolytic uremic syndrome are common complications; these events may occasionally follow *S. flexneri* infection. This syndrome is thought to be related to shigatoxin, because those *E. coli* that produce toxins closely related to shigatoxin (enterohemorrhagic *E. coli*) also cause hemolytic uremic syndrome (see Chapter 184).

Rectal prolapse, toxic megacolon or pseudomembranous colitis (usually associated with *S. dysenteriae*), cholestatic hepatitis, conjunctivitis, iritis, corneal ulcers, pneumonia, arthritis (usually 2–5 wk after enteritis), Reiter syndrome, cystitis, myocarditis, and vaginitis (typically with a blood-tinged discharge associated with *S. flexneri*) are uncommon events. The rare syndrome of extreme toxicity, convulsions, hyperpyrexia, and headache followed by brain edema and a rapidly fatal outcome without sepsis or significant dehydration (Ekiri syndrome or "lethal toxic encephalopathy") is not well understood. Death is a rare outcome in the well-nourished, older child; malnutrition, illness in the 1st yr of life, hypothermia, severe dehydration, thrombocytopenia, hyponatremia, renal failure, and bacteremia are common in children who die during bacillary dysentery.

DIAGNOSIS. Although clinical features suggest shigellosis, they are insufficiently specific to allow confident diagnosis. Infection by *Campylobacter jejuni, Salmonella* sp, enteroinvasive *E. coli,* enterohemorrhagic *E. coli, Yersinia enterocolitica,* and *Entamoeba histolytica* as well as inflammatory bowel disease may cause confusion. Unfortunately, the laboratory is often not able to confirm the clinical suspicion of shigellosis even when it is present. Presumptive data supporting a diagnosis of bacillary dysentery include the finding of fecal leukocytes (confirming the presence of colitis) and demonstration in peripheral blood of leukocytosis with a dramatic left shift (often with more bands than segmented neutrophils). The total peripheral white blood cell count is usually 5,000–15,000 cells/mm^3, although leukopenia and leukemoid reactions occur.

Culture of both stool and rectal swab specimens optimizes the chance of diagnosing *Shigella* infection. Culture media should include MacConkey agar as well as selective media such as xylose-lysine deoxycholate (XLD) and SS agar. Transport media should be used if specimens cannot be cultured promptly. Appropriate media should be used to exclude *Campylobacter* and other agents. Culture is the gold standard for diagnosis, but it is not absolute. Stool cultures of adult volunteers with dysentery after ingestion of shigellae failed to detect the organism in nearly 20% of subjects. Studies of foodborne outbreaks suggest that a single culture allows diagnosis in about half of symptomatic patients with shigellosis. Although additional tools to improve diagnosis (e.g., gene probes) are being developed, the diagnostic inadequacy of cultures makes it incumbent on the clinician to use judgment in the management of clinical syndromes consistent with shigellosis. In children who appear to be toxic, blood cultures should be obtained; this is particularly important in very young or malnourished infants because of their increased risk of bacteremia.

TREATMENT. As with gastroenteritis of other causes, the first concern about a child with suspected shigellosis should be for fluid and electrolyte correction and maintenance (see Chapters 54 and 56.1). Drugs that retard intestinal motility should not be used because of the risk of prolonging the illness.

The next concern is a decision about the use of antibiotics. Although some authorities recommend withholding antibacterial therapy because of the self-limited nature of the infection, the cost of drugs, and the risk of emergence of resistant organisms, there is a persuasive logic in favor of empiric treatment of all children in whom shigellosis is suspected. Even if not fatal, the untreated illness may cause the child to be quite ill for 2 weeks or more; chronic or recurrent diarrhea may ensue. There is a risk of malnutrition developing or worsening during prolonged illness, particularly in children in developing countries. The risk of continued excretion and subsequent infection of family contacts further argues against the strategy of withholding antibiotics.

There are major geographic variations in drug susceptibility. In the United States, shigellae are so frequently resistant to ampicillin that it should not be used for empiric therapy; occasional strains are also resistant to trimethoprim-sulfamethoxazole (TMP-SMX). Cefixime and ceftriaxone are effective alternative drugs in areas where TMP-SMX resistance is common. Nalidixic acid is also an acceptable option in this setting. Resistance to nalidixic acid is uncommon. With the exception of nalidixic acid, the quinolones that have been recommended for use in adults have not been used in children (because of the putative risk of arthropathy). Treatment regimens involve a 5-day course. For strains known to be susceptible to ampicillin, this drug is given at 100 mg/kg/24 hr divided into four doses each day. The usual empiric choice before the availability of susceptibility data is TMP-SMX, given at 5–10 mg/kg/24 hr of the TMP component in two divided doses. For strains known to be resistant to the usual drugs, cefixime (8 mg/kg/24 hr in two divided doses given orally for 5 days), ceftriaxone (50 mg/kg/24 hr as a single daily dose given parenterally for 2–5 days), or nalidixic acid (55 mg/kg/24 hr in four divided doses for 5 days) can be given. Of these agents, given a susceptible organism, TMP-SMX is preferred because of the rapidity with which it causes resolution of symptoms. In patients too ill to take oral medications, intravenous therapy with TMP-SMX is effective if the organism is susceptible. Oral first- and second-generation cephalosporins are inadequate as alternative drugs. Amoxicillin is less effective than ampicillin in therapy of ampicillin-sensitive strains.

Treatment of patients suspected on clinical grounds of having *Shigella* infection should be started when the patient is first examined. Stool culture is obtained to exclude other pathogens and to assist in antibiotic selection should the child fail to respond to empiric therapy. A child who has typical dysentery and who responds to initial empiric antibiotic treatment should be continued on that drug for a full 5-day course even if the stool culture is negative. The logic of this recommendation is based on the difficulty of culturing *Shigella* and on the fact that enteroinvasive *E. coli,* which cause dysentery indistinguishable from that due to shigellae, cannot be diagnosed in routine clinical microbiology laboratories. In a child who fails to respond to therapy of a dysenteric syndrome in the presence of initially negative stool cultures, cultures should be retaken and the child re-evaluated for other possible diagnoses.

PREVENTION. Two simple measures decrease the risk of shigellosis in children. The first is to encourage prolonged breastfeeding in settings in which shigellosis is common. Breastfeeding decreases the risk of symptomatic shigellosis and lessens its severity in infants who acquire infection despite breast-feeding. The second measure is to educate families in handwashing techniques, especially after defecation and before food preparation and consumption. Other public health measures, including water and sewage treatment, are expensive and are unlikely to be universally available in the near future in developing countries.

Ashkenazi S, Amir J, Waisman Y, et al: A randomized, double-blind study comparing cefixime and trimethoprim sulfamethoxazole in the treatment of childhood shigellosis. J Pediatr 123:817, 1993.

Nelson JD, Kusmiesz H, Shelton S: Oral or intravenous trimethoprim-sulfamethoxazole therapy for shigellosis. Rev Infect Dis 4:546, 1982.

Salam MA, Bennish ML: Therapy for shigellosis: I. Randomized, double-blind trial of nalidixic acid in childhood shigellosis. J Pediatr 113:901, 1988.

Varsano I, Eidlitz-Marcus T, Nussinovitch M, Elian I: Comparative efficacy of ceftriaxone and ampicillin for treatment of severe shigellosis in children. J Pediatr 118:627, 1991.

CHAPTER 184

Escherichia coli, Aeromonas, and Plesiomonas

Donald K. Winsor and Thomas G. Cleary

ESCHERICHIA COLI

ETIOLOGY AND PATHOGENESIS. Five classes of *E. coli* are recognized as agents associated with pediatric gastroenteritis. Because *E. coli* organisms are normal fecal flora, demonstration of virulence characteristics is the only way by which the diarrheagenic *E. coli* can be defined. The mechanism by which *E. coli* produces diarrhea typically involves adherence of organisms to a glycoprotein or glycolipid receptor, followed by production of some noxious substance that injures gut cells or disturbs gut function. The genes for virulence properties and for antibiotic resistance are often carried on transferable plasmids or bacteriophages. The current classification is summarized here; the classification changes as new virulence genes are cloned and sequenced.

Enterotoxigenic *E. coli* (ETEC). These *E. coli* serogroups produce a heat-labile enterotoxin (LT) and/or a heat-stable enterotoxin (ST). LT, a large molecule consisting of five receptor-binding subunits and one enzymatically active subunit, is structurally, functionally, and immunologically related to cholera toxin produced by *Vibrio cholerae*. ST is a small molecule (18–19 amino acids) not related to LT or cholera toxin, although it is related to an enterotoxin produced by some strains of *Yersinia enterocolitica*. These toxins do not injure or kill cells; rather, they disturb cyclic nucleotide–regulated fluid and electrolyte absorption. ST stimulates guanylate cyclase, resulting in increased cyclic GMP, but LT (like cholera toxin) stimulates adenylate cyclase, resulting in increased cyclic AMP. The ETEC typically also possess fimbria or colonization factor antigens (CFAs) that allow them to adhere tightly to intestinal epithelium, thereby efficiently colonizing and delivering toxin to the epithelium. Several CFAs have been recognized as important in effecting the adherence of ETEC to gut mucosal cells. These CFAs are called CFA I, CFA II, CFA III, CFA IV, CS7, CS17, 2230, 8786, PCF 09, PCF 0166, PCF 0148, and PCF 0159. After colonization of intestinal epithelium, the ETEC release ST or LT. The genes for both colonization factors and enterotoxins are typically encoded on the same plasmid. Of the more than 170 *E. coli* serogroups only a relatively small number typically are ETEC; these serogroups (06, 08, 015, 020, 025, 027, 063, 078, 080, 085, 0115, 0128ac [but not subgroups 0128ab or 0128ad], 0139, 0148, 0153, 0159, and 0167) are generally different from those found in the other diarrhea-associated *E. coli*.

Enteroinvasive *E. coli* (EIEC). These *E. coli* serogroups behave like shigellae in their capacity to invade gut epithelium and produce a dysentery-like illness. The EIEC adhere to and invade gut epithelium. This *Shigella*-like behavior occurs because these *E. coli* possess a large virulence plasmid closely related to the plasmid that endows *Shigella* with its invasiveness (see Chapter 183). As with *Shigella*, a small group of polypeptides encoded on these plasmids is critical to the invasion of intestinal epithelium. Invasion of epithelium causes cell death and a brisk inflammatory response (clinically recognizable as colitis). The bacterial product that kills intestinal cells is not known. EIEC encompass a small number of serogroups (028ac, 029, 0124, 0136, 0143, 0144, 0152, 0164, 0167, and some untypable strains). These serogroups have lipopolysaccharide (LPS) antigens related to *Shigella* LPS, and, like shigellae, the organisms are nonmotile (they lack H or flagellar antigens) and are usually nonlactose fermenters.

Enteropathogenic *E. coli* (EPEC). These diarrheagenic *E. coli* belong to serogroups (O antigen or lipopolysaccharide antigen) that have been associated with outbreaks of infantile gastroenteritis but do not produce conventional enterotoxins or invade epithelial cells. Low levels of invasion are observed in some assay systems. However, organisms within these serogroups also have been isolated from well individuals. The EPEC adhere to the intestinal mucosa in a distinctive way. This pattern of adherence, seen on transmission electron microscopy, has been called "close attaching and effacing" adherence or "pedestal-forming" adherence. The lesion consists of loss of microvilli with adherence of bacteria to the epithelial cells, which form a cup or pedestal in which the bacteria can be seen. Chronic inflammation with flattened villi may also be seen on small bowel biopsy of affected children. EPEC cause localized or diffuse adherence based on HEp-2 cell assays. EPEC with localized adherence attach loosely to the microvilli of the epithelial cell through ropelike structures called bundle-forming pili, which are encoded on a plasmid (EAF plasmid), followed by attachment to the epithelial cell through the action of the *eae* gene (*E. coli* attaching-effacing). Attachment results in increased intracellular calcium concentration and dense polymerization of actin at the site of attachment. How these cytoskeletal changes cause diarrhea is not clear. EPEC, which are diffusely adherent in the HEp-2 cell assay system, produce an adhesin involved in diffuse adherence (AIDA-I), which has homology to a *S. flexneri* protein associated with intercellular spread (VirG). Some serogroups are associated with localized adherence and are EAF probe positive (055, 086, 0111, 0119, 0125, 0126, 0127, 0128ab, and 0142) whereas others are nonadherent or diffusely adherent to HEp-2 cells and are usually EAF probe negative (018, 044, 0112, and 0114).

Enterohemorrhagic *E. coli* (EHEC). These *E. coli* serogroups produce one or more toxins that kill mammalian cells. They have also been called enterocytotoxic *E. coli*, *Shiga*-like toxin–producing *E. coli* (SLT-EC), and verotoxin-producing *E. coli* (VTEC). Two major toxins are produced by EHEC. One is essentially identical to shigatoxin, the protein synthesis–inhibiting exotoxin of *Shigella dysenteriae* serotype 1. The second is more distantly related to shigatoxin (only 55% amino acid homology). The first toxin is called SLT-I (VT-1) and the second SLT-II (VT-2). Multiple variants of these toxins probably exist. Some EHEC produce only SLT-I, others only SLT-II, but most EHEC produce both toxins. These toxins kill cells by cleaving an adenine residue from ribosomal RNA at the site where elongation factor 1–dependent attachment of aminoacyl t-RNA occurs; the result is protein synthesis inhibition and cell death. EHEC adhere to intestinal cells and produce attaching-effacing lesions that resemble, on electron microscopy, those seen with EPEC, although they are more restricted in their distribution (being found primarily in the colon) compared with EPEC (which infest the entire intestine). The protein product of the *eae* gene of EHEC is closely related but not identical to intimin, the product of the *eae* gene of EPEC, and to invasin, produced by *Yersinia pseudotuberculosis*. The most common serotypes are *E. coli* 0157:H7 and *E. coli* 026:H11, although a number of other serotypes have also been described. *E. coli* 026:H11 was formerly considered an EPEC.

Enteroaggregative *E. coli* (EAggEC). These *E. coli* serogroups have the ability to adhere to HEp-2 cells in tissue culture. They are also referred to as autoagglutinating and enteroadherent-aggregative *E. coli*. It is likely that this group will be further subdivided, and some of these organisms will be shown to be nonpathogens. EAggEC attach to HEp-2 cells and colonic epithelial cells by plasmid-encoded aggregative adherence fimbriae (AAF/I). These organisms do not possess the *eae* genes or produce attaching-effacing lesions. A 4.1-kD heat-stable toxin EAST 1, related to the heat-stable toxin of ETEC, is encoded on a plasmid. A second toxin is a 120-kD heat-labile protein related to the pore-forming cytolytic toxin family, which contains the *Bordetella pertussis* adenylate cyclase hemolysin. This heat-labile toxin increases intracellular levels of calcium. The role of these toxins in EAggEC pathogenesis is unknown. EAggEC appear to colonize the colon.

EPIDEMIOLOGY. In the developing world, the various diarrheagenic serogroups of *E. coli* cause frequent infections in the first few years of life. They occur with increased frequency during the warm months in temperate climates and during rainy season months in tropical climates. Most *E. coli* strains (except EHEC and perhaps some EPEC) require a large inoculum of organisms to induce disease; person-to-person spread is atypical, but foodborne or waterborne illness is common. Infection is most likely when food-handling or sewage-disposal practices are suboptimal. Although infection occurs in children in the United States, it is more often seen in those who live in or have recently visited the developing world. EHEC and EPEC organisms are transmitted person to person as well as by food, suggesting that ingestion of a lower number of these organisms is sufficient to cause disease. Poorly cooked hamburger is the most common cause of foodborne outbreaks of EHEC.

PATHOLOGY. ETEC cause little or no structural alterations in the gut mucosa. EIEC cause colonic lesions like those of bacillary dysentery; ulcerations, hemorrhage, and infiltration of polymorphonuclear leukocytes with mucosal and submucosal edema are typical. EPEC are associated with blunting of villi, inflammatory changes and sloughing of superficial mucosal cells on light microscopy, and attaching and effacing changes on transmission electron microscopy; these lesions are found from the duodenum through the colon. EHEC affect the colon most severely. These organisms cause edema, fibrin deposits, hemorrhage in the submucosa, mucosal ulceration, neutrophil infiltration, and microvascular thrombi. Some of these effects may result from a synergistic action of the *Shiga*-like toxin and the lipid A portion of the LPS. The pathology of EAggEC consists of secretory diarrhea caused by heat-stable or heat-labile toxins.

CLINICAL MANIFESTATIONS. As might be expected from the different mechanisms of disease production, the clinical features of *E. coli*–associated diarrhea vary from group to group. ETEC are a major cause of dehydrating infantile diarrhea in the developing world. The typical signs and symptoms include explosive watery diarrhea, abdominal pain, nausea, vomiting, and little or no fever. Resolution usually occurs in a matter of days. These infections have an untoward effect on infant nutritional status.

EIEC cause an illness that is indistinguishable from classic bacillary dysentery. Fever, systemic toxicity, crampy abdominal pain, tenesmus, and urgency with water or bloody diarrhea are characteristic.

EPEC usually are isolated from infants and children in the first few years of life who have a nonbloody diarrhea with mucus; fever may occur. Unlike ETEC, EIEC, or EHEC, these organisms often cause a prolonged diarrheal disease.

EHEC may cause a nondescript diarrheal illness or an illness characterized by abdominal pain with diarrhea that is initially watery but within a few days becomes grossly bloody (hemorrhagic colitis). Although this pattern resembles that of shigellosis or EIEC disease, it differs in that fever is an uncommon manifestation. The major risk with EHEC is that approximately 10% of symptomatic infections are complicated by development of hemolytic-uremic syndrome.

EAggEC cause significant fluid loss with dehydration, but vomiting and grossly bloody stools are relatively infrequent. These organisms, like the EPEC, are often associated with prolonged diarrhea.

COMPLICATIONS. The major complications are those related to dehydration and electrolyte loss. Some complications are related to specific pathogens. EPEC and EAEC are likely to cause persistent diarrhea. Infection with EHEC is frequently associated with the hemolytic-uremic syndrome.

DIAGNOSIS. The clinical features of illness are seldom distinctive enough to allow confident diagnosis, and routine laboratory studies are of very limited value. Diagnosis currently depends heavily on laboratory studies that are not readily available to the practitioner. Routine stool cultures from which *E. coli* organisms are isolated are interpreted as showing "normal flora." Biochemical criteria (e.g., fermentation patterns) are of minimal value. EHEC serotype O157:H7 is suggested by failure of a suspect colony to ferment sorbitol on MacConkey sorbitol medium; latex agglutination confirms that the organism contains O157 LPS. The other EHEC cannot be detected in routine hospital laboratories, although it is likely that assays based on toxin detection will become available. Culture of duodenal fluid may be helpful in the diagnosis of EPEC because of their tendency to colonize the small intestine. This study is generally indicated only in the child with chronic diarrhea.

Other laboratory data are at best nonspecific indicators of etiology. Fecal leukocyte examination of the stool is usually positive with the EIEC but negative with all other diarrheagenic *E. coli*. Blood counts, especially with EIEC and EHEC, often show an elevated leukocyte count with a left shift. Electrolyte changes are nonspecific, reflecting only fluid loss.

The traditional methods of identification of these organisms require animal or tissue culture models that are unacceptably cumbersome and expensive for routine use by hospital laboratories. Some of these organisms, especially the EPEC, could theoretically be defined serologically. However, the frequency of cross reactions, the unavailability of suitable reagents, and the infrequency with which the serogroup alone is adequate to define a pathogen make these methods unsuitable. DNA probes for genes encoding the various virulence traits hold the greatest promise for the future; they are currently appropriate only in the research laboratory setting. Probes have been developed for ETEC, EIEC, EPEC, EAggEC, and EHEC.

Suspected organisms should be forwarded to reference or research laboratories for definitive evaluation. Such efforts are seldom necessary, but they may be critical for correct diagnosis of the child with severe or life-threatening complications or for the occasional outbreak investigation.

TREATMENT. The cornerstone of proper management is related to fluid and electrolyte therapy. In general, this therapy should include oral replacement and maintenance with rehydrating solutions such as those specified by the World Health Organization. Early refeeding with breast milk or dilute formula should be encouraged as soon as dehydration is corrected. Prolonged withholding of feeding frequently leads to chronic diarrhea and malnutrition.

Specific antimicrobial therapy of diarrheagenic *E. coli* is problematic because of the difficulty of making an accurate diagnosis of these pathogens and the unpredictability of antibiotic susceptibilities. ETEC respond to antimicrobial agents such as trimethoprim-sulfamethoxazole (TMP-SMX) when the *E. coli* strains are susceptible. However, other than for a child recently returning from travel to the developing world, empirical treatment of severe watery diarrhea with antibiotics is seldom appropriate. Although treatment of EPEC infection with TMP-SMX (6.4 mg/kg/24 hr of the trimethoprim component in four divided doses intravenously or orally for 5 days) is effective in speeding resolution, the lack of a rapid diagnostic test makes treatment decisions difficult. EIEC infections are usually treated prior to the availability of culture results because the clinician typically suspects shigellosis and begins empirical therapy. If the organisms are susceptible, TMP-SMX is an appropriate choice. The EHEC represent a particularly difficult therapeutic dilemma. The data suggest that antibiotic treatment, particularly with sulfa-containing regimens, may increase the risk of hemolytic-uremic syndrome; however, the lack of prospective controlled trials makes these observations questionable. It is too early to assess the usefulness of antibiotics in the treatment of EAEC.

Antibiotic resistance is often encoded on the same plasmids that carry virulence properties and continues to make rational decisions about antibiotic therapy difficult. Because emergence of resistance to widely used regimens is typical, new antimicrobial agents must continue to be evaluated.

Prophylactic antibiotic therapy, although effective in adult travelers, has not been studied in children and is not generally recommended. Public health measures, including sewage disposal and food-handling practices, have made pathogens that require large inocula to produce illness relatively uncommon in industrialized countries. Foodborne outbreaks of EHEC are a problem for which no adequate solution has been found. During the occasional hospital outbreak of EPEC disease, attention to enteric isolation precautions and cohorting may be critical.

PREVENTION. In the developing world, prevention of disease caused by diarrheogenic *E. coli* is probably best done by maintaining prolonged breast-feeding, paying careful attention to personal hygiene, and following proper food- and water-handling procedures. Children traveling to these places can be best protected by paying careful attention to diet, in particular consuming only processed water, bottled beverages, breads, fruit juices, fruits that can be peeled, or foods that are served steaming hot.

AEROMONAS

Aeromonas can cause disease in cold-blooded and warm-blooded animals. Species that cause disease in cold-blooded animals are nonmotile and psychrophilic, and species that cause disease in warm-blooded animals are motile and mesophilic. The species associated most often with human disease are *A. hydrophila, A. sobria,* and *A. caviae*.

BACTERIOLOGY. *Aeromonas* organisms are oxidase-positive, facultatively anaerobic, gram-negative rods that belong to the family Vibrionaceae. Their fermentation of lactose is variable. *Aeromonas* are differentiated from Enterobacteriaceae because they are cytochrome oxidase positive. These organisms may not be detected unless oxidase testing is done.

Aeromonas species are easily cultivated on media routinely used in clinical laboratories, such as blood agar and MacConkey agar. *A. hydrophila* and *A. sobria* are hemolytic on blood, and *A. caviae* is not. Selective and enrichment media are available to culture *Aeromonas* from fecal specimens, including alkaline peptone water, blood agar containing ampicillin (to which they are routinely resistent), and cefsulodin-irgasan-novobiocin agar.

EPIDEMIOLOGY. *Aeromonas* is found in fresh and salt water. Gastrointestinal infection is associated with ingestion of well water and pretreatment with antibiotics (particularly ampicillin or other drugs susceptible to β-lactamases), and wound infections are associated with contamination by environmental water. *Aeromonas* species are isolated from raw chicken and produce in grocery stores. Infections are more common in warm weather. Symptomatic and asymptomatic infections occur.

PATHOGENESIS. Some strains of *A. hydrophila* and *A. sobria* produce hemolysins, cytotoxins and enterotoxins. One of the enterotoxins causes water, potassium, and sodium losses in rat intestine and is antigenically related to cholera toxin. A second toxin is a β-hemolysin that produces fluid accumulation in sucking mice and rabbit intestinal loops. A heat-stable cytotoxin of *A. caviae* differs from those made by *A. hydrophila* and *A. sobria*. Several strains of *Aeromonas* adhere to tissue culture cells, but the role of pili in this adherence and in pathogenesis is unclear. *A. hydrophila* and *A. sobria* invade HEp-2 cells; they also invade mucosa and produce bacteremia in animal models. Volunteers given large numbers of organisms thought to be fully virulent do not develop diarrhea. It is likely that, as with *E. coli*, some *Aeromonas* organisms lack virulence genes and are not pathogens.

CLINICAL MANIFESTATIONS. Aeromonads have been associated with gastrointestinal illness, septicemia, and infections of skin, respiratory tract, abdomen, pelvis, and rarely of the eye or bone.

Gastroenteritis is the most common disease caused by *Aeromonas* in humans. *Aeromonas* has been isolated from 2–10% of patients with acute diarrhea and 1–5% of asymptomatic controls in many different locations. *A. caviae* is far more common than *A. hydrophila* or *A. sobria*. Diarrhea is more common in the first 3 yr of life than later. These organisms are probably underdiagnosed because clinical laboratories do not routinely perform oxidase tests on fecal flora. Patients usually present with watery diarrhea that may be cholera-like, but 10–30% of patients have a dysentery-like febrile diarrhea with bloody stools (with *A. caviae* or occasionally *A. sobria*). Fecal leukocytes are unusual. Diarrhea caused by *A. caviae* may last for many months.

Aeromonas septicemia is usually seen in patients with other underlying illnesses. The mortality rate is high (30–70%). Septicemia also occurs in immunocompetent hosts after trauma or respiratory tract infections. *A. hydrophila* and *A. sobria* are the most common species causing septicemia.

Penetrating trauma or open fractures with contamination of the injured extremities by water or fecal material can cause wound infections. Purulent soft tissue infections, cellulitis, fulminating myonecrosis with or without bacteremia, or ecthyma gangrenosum resembling pseudomonal infections can be seen. Mixed infections with other organisms occur in more than 80% of trauma-associated cases.

TREATMENT. Although controlled clinical studies of antibiotic treatment have not been done, clinical observations and susceptibility studies suggest that treatment of gastrointestinal infections shortens the duration of illness. Antimicrobial therapy with trimethoprim-sulfamethoxazole is recommended for patients with dysenteric forms of illness and for those having chronic intestinal complaints associated with *Aeromonas*. Septicemia should be treated parenterally with an aminoglycoside or a third-generation cephalosporin until susceptibility data are available.

PLESIOMONAS SHIGELLOIDES

Plesiomonas shigelloides is reported in sporadic cases and outbreaks of diarrheal disease. There is debate about whether its association with gastroenteritis is causal. Infection is commonly associated with ingestion of foods, such as oysters, likely to be contaminated with other enteropathogens, and virulence factors have been difficult to demonstrate. However, the occurrence of bloody diarrhea and high fever responsive to antibiotics suggest that *P. shigelloides* is a true pathogen.

BACTERIOLOGY. The *P. shigelloides* organisms are gram-negative, non–spore-forming, facultatively anaerobic, indole-producing, slow lactose fermenters that are catalase positive. They ferment glucose but not sucrose or mannitol, and they possess two to seven polar flagella. They are differentiated from the Enterobacteriaceae by being oxidase positive and from other members of the Vibrionaceae (i.e., *Aeromonas* and *Vibrios*) by positive ornithine decarboxylase and fermentation of inositol. Some strains (serotype C27) have a lipopolysaccharide (LPS) that is antigenically identical to that of *Shigella sonnei* phase I LPS. Hospital laboratories often fail to identify these organisms because the colonies look like normal stool flora unless an oxidase test is done.

PATHOGENESIS AND PATHOLOGY. The clinical features suggest that enteroinvasiveness is the mechanism of disease. Virulence traits have been difficult to demonstrate, and volunteer studies have failed to prove pathogenicity, but negative results may reflect inappropriate growth conditions for virulence expression.

EPIDEMIOLOGY. These organisms are cultured from fresh water and sewage, particularly during the warm months. Many cases have a history of recent travel or ingestion of seafood, particularly raw oysters. Persons with occupations that bring them in contact with water are at increased risk of infection. Cold-blooded (e.g., fish, frogs, turtles, snakes, lizards, shellfish) and warm-blooded (e.g., dogs, cats, cows, sheep, pigs, goats, monkeys, chimpanzees) animals are sometimes colonized. Children and adults can be affected, although the risk appears to be increased in the first 5 yr of life. Cases of gastroenteritis are reported from industrialized and developing countries.

CLINICAL MANIFESTATIONS. Diarrhea may be watery, with or without blood in the stools, and fever is common. Abdominal pain and vomiting are frequently present. The illness usually lasts for 1–2 wk. Rarely, bacteremia, cellulitis, meningitis (particularly in neonates), or other extraintestinal infections occur. Usually, these complications occur in immunocompromised hosts (e.g., persons with collagen vascular disease, malignancies, hepatobiliary disease).

DIAGNOSIS. Routine stool culture media support the growth of *P. shigelloides*, but because clinical microbiology laboratories do not routinely perform oxidase tests, the organisms are often undetected. Fecal leukocytes are often detected.

TREATMENT. Because gastroenteritis is usually self-limited, no therapy is recommended routinely. TMP-SMX is used in patients with bloody diarrhea or persistent diarrhea. In the rare patient who develops extraintestinal infection, an aminoglycoside is often chosen, although the organisms are usually susceptible to chloramphenicol and cephalothin as well as 2nd- and 3rd-generation cephalosporins.

Baldwin TJ, Knutton S, Sellers L, et al: Enteroaggregative *Escherichia coli* strains secrete a heat-labile toxin antigenically related to *E. coli* hemolysin. Infect Immun 60:2092, 1992.

Donnenberg MS, Kaper JB: Enteropathogenic *Escherichia coli*. Infect Immun 60:3953, 1992.

Holmberg SD, Farmer JJ: *Aeromonas hydrophila* and *Plesiomonas shigelloides* as causes of intestinal infections. Rev Infect Dis 6:633, 1984.

Kelly J, Oryshak A, Wenesteck M, et al: The colonic pathology of *Escherichia coli* O157:H7 infection. Am J Surg Pathol 14:87, 1990.

Knutton S, Shaw RK, Bhan MK, et al: Ability of enteroaggregative *Escherichia coli* strains to adhere in vitro to human intestinal mucosa. Infect Immun 60:2083, 1992.

Mathewson JJ, Dupont HL: *Aeromonas* species: Role as human pathogens. Curr Clin Top Infect Dis 12:26, 1992.

Tesh VL, O'Brien AD: Adherence and colonization mechanisms of enteropathogenic and enterohemorrhagic *Escherichia coli*. Microb Pathog 12:245, 1992.

184.1 Infections Due To Pseudomonas

*Ann M. Arvin**

Pseudomonas lives abundantly in soil and water and is widespread throughout nature. Most infections are opportunistic and occur among low-birthweight infants and in older infants and children with impaired host defenses, such as those with cystic fibrosis, immunodeficiency disorders, malignancies, extensive burns, or malnutrition (especially in impoverished populations) and in those receiving immunosuppressive therapy (see Chapter 173).

*As modified from the Chapter in the 14th edition by R. D. Feigin.

ETIOLOGY. There are a large number of identified *Pseudomonas* species, but only a few are pathogenic for man; of these, *P. aeruginosa* is by far the most common. Other species occasionally recognized as human pathogens include *P. cepacia*, *P. maltophilia*, *P. fluorescens*, *P. putrefaciens*, and *P. mallei*.

The pseudomonads are gram-negative rods and are strict aerobes. Because they can use any source of carbon, they multiply in most moist environments that contain minimal amounts of organic compounds. Strains from clinical specimens may produce β-hemolysis on blood agar; more than 90% of strains produce a bluish-green phenazine pigment (blue pus) as well as fluorescein, which is yellow-green and fluoresces. These pigments diffuse into and color the medium surrounding the colonies. Strains of *Pseudomonas* can be differentiated for epidemiologic purposes by serologic, phage, and pyocin typing.

EPIDEMIOLOGY. Pseudomonads frequently enter the hospital environment on the clothes, skin, or shoes of patients or hospital personnel, in plants or vegetables brought into the hospital, and in the gastrointestinal tracts of patients. Colonization of any moist or liquid substance may ensue; for example, they may be found growing in distilled water, hospital kitchens and laundries, some antiseptic solutions, and equipment used for respiratory therapy. Colonization of patients' skin, throat, stool, and nasal mucosa is low on admission to the hospital but increases to as high as 50–70% with prolonged hospitalization and the use of broad-spectrum antibiotics, chemotherapy, mechanical ventilation, and urinary catheters.

PATHOGENESIS. The requirement of oxygen for growth may account for the lack of invasiveness of *Pseudomonas* after it has colonized or even infected the skin. It produces endotoxin that is weak compared with that of other gram-negative bacilli and exotoxin A, which produces local necrosis and systemic bacterial invasion. Exoenzyme S is another toxic virulent factor. *Pseudomonas* produces disease by three stages. Bacterial colonization and attachment are facilitated by pili or fimbriae and by opportunistic adhesion to epithelium damaged from prior injury such as ulcerating keratitis or influenzal pneumonia. A mucopolysaccharide may inhibit phagocytosis, whereas extracellular proteins, proteases, elastases, and cytotoxin (formerly leukocidin) digest cell membranes and antibodies produce capillary vascular permeability and inhibit leukocyte function. Dissemination and bloodstream invasion follow extension of local tissue damage and are facilitated by the antiphagocytic properties of the mucosal exopolysaccharide, protease cleavage of IgG, and other characteristics that resist serum phagocytosis. The host responds to infection by producing antibodies to *Pseudomonas* exotoxin (exotoxin A) and lipopolysaccharide. Compromised host defense mechanisms (due to trauma [cutaneous], neutropenia, mucositis, immunosuppression, impaired mucociliary transport) explain the predominant role of this organism in producing opportunistic infections.

CLINICAL MANIFESTATIONS. Although most clinical patterns (Table 184–1) are related to opportunistic infections (see Chapter 173), *P. aeruginosa* introduced into a minor wound of a healthy child may be followed by cellulitis and a localized abscess that exudes green or blue pus. The characteristic skin lesions of *Pseudomonas*, caused by direct inoculation or secondary to septicemia, begin as pink macules and progress to hemorrhagic nodules and eventually to areas of necrosis with eschar formation, surrounded by an intense red areola (ecthyma gangrenosum).

Outbreaks of dermatitis and urinary tract infections caused by *P. aeruginosa* have been reported in healthy children following use of community swimming pools, recreational whirlpools, or family-owned hot tubs. Skin lesions develop several hours to 2 days after contact with these water sources. Skin lesions may be erythematous, macular, papular, or pustular. Illness may vary from a few scattered lesions to extensive

■ TABLE 184–1 *Pseudomonas aeruginosa* Infections

Infection	Characteristics
Endocarditis	Native right-sided (tricuspid) valve disease in intravenous drug addicts
Pneumonia	Compromised local (lung) or systemic host defense mechanisms. Nosocomial (respiratory), bacteremic (malignancy), or abnormal mucociliary clearance (cystic fibrosis) may be pathogenetic. Cystic fibrosis is associated with mucoid *P. aeruginosa* organisms producing capsular slime and *P. cepacia*.
Central nervous system infection	Meningitis, brain abscess; contiguous spread (mastoiditis, dermal sinus tracts, sinusitis); bacteremia or direct inoculation (trauma, surgery)
External otitis	Swimmer's ear; humid warm climates, swimming pool contamination
Malignant otitis externa	Invasive, indolent, febrile toxic, destructive necrotizing lesion in young infants, immunosuppressed neutropenic patients, or diabetics; associated 7th nerve palsy and mastoiditis
Chronic mastoiditis	Ear drainage, swelling, erythema; perforated tympanic membrane
Keratitis	Corneal ulceration; contact lens keratitis
Endophthalmitis	Penetrating trauma, surgery, penetrating corneal ulceration; fulminant progression
Osteomyelitis/septic arthritis	Puncture wounds of foot and osteochondritis; intravenous drug abuse; fibrocartilaginous joints, sternum, vertebrae, pelvis; open fracture osteomyelitis; indolent; pyelonephritis and vertebral osteomyelitis
Urinary tract infection	Iatrogenic, nosocomial; recurrent urinary tract infections in children, instrumented patients, and those with obstruction or stones
Gastrointestinal tract infection	Immunocompromise, neutropenia, typhlitis, rectal abscess, ulceration, rarely diarrhea; peritonitis in peritoneal dialysis
Ecthyma gangrenosum	Metastatic dissemination; hemorrhage, necrosis, erythema, eschar, discrete lesions with bacterial invasion of blood vessels; also subcutaneous nodules, cellulitis, pustules, deep abscesses
Primary and secondary skin infections	Local infection; burns, trauma, decubitus ulcers, toe web infection, green nail (paronychia); whirlpool dermatitis: diffuse, pruritic, folliculitis, vesiculopustular or maculopapular, erythematous lesions

truncal involvement. In some children, malaise, fever, vomiting, sore throat, conjunctivitis, rhinitis, and swollen breasts may be associated with dermal lesions.

Pseudomonads other than *P. aeruginosa* rarely cause disease in healthy children, but pneumonia and abscesses due to *P. cepacia*, otitis media due to *P. putrefaciens* or *P. stutzeri*, abscesses due to *P. fluorescens*, and cellulitis and septicemia due to *P. maltophilia* have been reported. Septicemia and endocarditis due to *P. maltophilia* have also been associated with intravenous abuse of drugs.

Shunts, Catheters, and Equipment (see Chapter 173 and Table 184–1).

Burns and Wound Infection. The surfaces of wounds or burns are frequently populated by *Pseudomonas* and other gram-negative organisms; this does not necessarily imply infection but is a necessary prerequisite to invasive disease. Septicemia with *P. aeruginosa* is a major problem in the burned patient (see Chapters 60 and 173). It may be related to multiplication of organisms in devitalized tissues or associated with prolonged use of intravenous or urinary catheters. Administration of antibiotics may diminish the susceptible microbiologic flora but permit selected strains of *Pseudomonas* to flourish.

Cystic Fibrosis (see Chapter 363).

Malignancy. Children with leukemia or other debilitating malignancies, particularly those who are receiving immunosuppressive therapy and who are neutropenic, are extremely susceptible to septicemia from invasion of the bloodstream by *Pseudomonas* with which the patient is already colonized. Anorexia, malaise, nausea, vomiting, diarrhea, and fever may occur. A generalized vasculitis develops, and hemorrhagic necrotic lesions may be found in all organs, including skin, where they appear as purple nodules or ecchymotic areas that become gangrenous. Hemorrhagic or gangrenous perirectal cellulitis or abscesses may occur, associated with ileus and profound hypotension.

DIAGNOSIS AND DIFFERENTIAL DIAGNOSIS. This diagnosis depends upon recovery of the organism from the blood, cerebrospinal fluid, urine, or needle aspirate of the lung or from purulent material obtained by aspiration of subcutaneous abscesses or areas of cellulitis.

Bluish, nodular skin lesions and ulcers with ecchymotic and gangrenous centers and bright areolae (ecthyma gangrenosum) are virtually pathognomonic of *Pseudomonas* infection of the skin. Rarely, skin lesions clinically indistinguishable from those caused by *P. aeruginosa* may follow septicemia due to *Aeromonas hydrophila*. The differential diagnosis includes local and disseminated diseases due to other gram-negative rods, fungi, or viruses.

PREVENTION. In part, this depends upon continuous surveillance of the hospital environment to identify and subsequently eradicate sources of the organism as quickly as possible. *Pseudomonas* may grow in distilled water, disinfectants, parenteral alimentation solutions, and medications. In newborn nurseries infection generally has been transmitted to the infants by the hands of personnel, from washbasin surfaces, from catheters, and from solutions used to rinse suction catheters.

Strict attention to handwashing, particularly with an iodophor-containing liquid, before and between contacts with neonates may prevent or interdict epidemic disease. Growth of *Pseudomonas* on suction catheters can be prevented by rinsing catheters in a 3% solution of acetic acid. Meticulous care in the preparation of solutions for total parenteral alimentation and in the insertion and care of catheters as well as frequent replacement of all apparatus used for intravenous administration greatly reduces the hazard of extrinsic contamination by *Pseudomonas* and other gram-negative organisms.

Prevention of follicular dermatitis caused by *Pseudomonas* contamination of whirlpools or hot tubs is possible by maintaining pool water at a pH of 7.2–7.8 and free chlorine concentration at 70.5 mg/L.

Burn patients may be actively immunized with a polyvalent *Pseudomonas* vaccine that reduces bacteremia and mortality. The administration of specific hyperimmune globulin also prevents septicemia. Infection also may be minimized by careful protective isolation, by the topical application of sulfadiazine or 10% mafenide acetate cream, and by debridement of devitalized tissue.

Pseudomonas infection of dermal sinuses communicating with the cerebrospinal space can be prevented by early discovery and surgical repair. *Pseudomonas* infection of the urinary tract may be minimized or prevented by early identification and corrective surgery of obstructive lesions.

TREATMENT. Systemic infections with *Pseudomonas* should be treated promptly with an antibiotic to which the organism is sensitive in vitro. Response to treatment may be limited, and prolonged treatment may be necessary for systemic infection in the compromised host.

Septicemia usually should be treated with carbenicillin (200–400 mg/kg/24 hr in six divided doses) or ticarcillin (200 mg/kg/24 hr in six divided doses intravenously). Gentamicin should be used concomitantly for a possible synergistic effect, in a dose of 5–7.5 mg/kg/24 hr in three divided doses. The higher dose may be used after the 1st wk of life. This drug may be given intramuscularly or intravenously (if it is infused slowly over a period of 1 hr. Carbenicillin or ticarcillin alone is not recommended, because strains of the organism rapidly become resistant to these agents. Tobramycin (3–5 mg/kg/24 hr) or amikacin (15–25 mg/kg/24 hr) in three divided doses intramuscularly or intravenously (over 1 hr) may be used to replace gentamicin in the therapeutic regimen.

Of the newer β-lactam antibiotics, ceftazidime is the most active against *P. aeruginosa*, and it has also proved to be extremely effective in patients with cystic fibrosis (150–200 mg/kg/24 hr in three or four divided doses). Azlocillin and piperacillin also have proved to be effective therapy for selected strains of *P. aeruginosa* when combined with an aminoglycoside; they can be given in doses of 300 mg/kg/24 hr intravenously in three or four divided doses. Additional effective antibiotics include imipenem, aztreonam, and ciprofloxacin.

Meningitis should be treated with ceftazidine or carbenicillin or ticarcillin in combination with gentamicin, given intravenously. Concomitant intraventricular or intrathecal treatment with gentamicin (1–2 mg once daily, independent of body weight, until the cerebrospinal fluid is sterile) may be required.

PROGNOSIS. This depends in large part on the nature of the underlying disease; for example, the leading cause of death in childhood leukemia is septicemia, and half of these cases are due to *Pseudomonas*. The outcome for patients with *P. aeruginosa* sepsis is improved by combined antimicrobial therapy, a urinary tract portal of entry, absence of neutropenia or recovery from neutropenia, and drainage of local sites of infection. *Pseudomonas* is recovered from the lungs of most children who die of cystic fibrosis and may be responsible for the slow deterioration of these patients; *P. cepacia*, which is frequently resistant to standard antimicrobial agents, has been associated with a more rapid decline in pulmonary function and lower survival. The prognosis for normal development is poor in the few infants who survive *Pseudomonas* meningitis.

Disease Due to Other Pseudomonads

Glanders

Glanders is a severe infectious disease of horses due to *P. mallei* that is occasionally transmitted to man. It is relatively common in Asia, Africa, and the Middle East. The clinical manifestations include acute or chronic pneumonitis and hemorrhagic necrotic lesions of the skin, nasal mucous membranes, and lymph nodes.

Melioidosis

This important disease of Southeast Asia and northern Australia is seen in the United States mainly in persons from endemic areas. The causative agent is *P. pseudomallei*, an inhabitant of soil and water in the tropics. Infection follows inhalation of dust or direct contamination of abrasions or wounds. Melioidosis may present as a single primary skin lesion (vesicle, bulla, or urticaria). Pulmonary infection may be subacute and mimic tuberculosis. Occasionally, septicemia occurs and multiple abscesses are noted in various organs of the body. Myocarditis, pericarditis, endocarditis, intestinal abscess, cholecystitis, acute gastroenteritis, urinary tract infections, septic arthritis, paraspinal abscess, osteomyelitis, and generalized lymphadenopathy have all been observed. Melioidosis may also present as an encephalitic illness with fever and seizures; generally, antibiotic therapy results in recovery. The disease may remain latent and appear when host resistance is reduced, sometimes years after the initial exposure.

Glanders is treated with tetracycline or chloramphenicol and streptomycin over a period of many months. Melioidosis is treated with ceftazidime or chloramphenicol with doxycycline and TPM-SMX.

Adam D: Use of quinolones in pediatric patients. Rev Infect Dis 11(Suppl 5):S1113, 1989.

Chaowagul W, White NJ, Dance DAB, et al: Melioidosis: A major cause of community-acquired septicemia in northeastern Thailand. J Infect Dis 159:890, 1989.

Feder HM Jr, Grant-Kels JM, Tilton RG: *Pseudomonas* whirlpool dermatitis. Clin Pediatr 22:638, 1983.

Hilf M, Yu VL, Sharp JS, et al: Antibiotic therapy for *Pseudomonas aeruginosa* bacteremia: Outcome correlations in a prospective study of 200 patients. Am J Med 87:540, 1989.

Isles A, Maclusky I, Corey M, et al: *Pseudomonas cepacia* infection in cystic fibrosis: An emerging problem. J Pediatr 104:206, 1984.

Jones RJ, Roe EA, Gupta JL: Controlled trials of a polyvalent *Pseudomonas* vaccine in burns. Lancet 2:977, 1979.

Kerem E, Corey M, Gold R, et al: Pulmonary function and clinical course in patients with cystic fibrosis after pulmonary colonization with *Pseudomonas aeruginosa*. J Pediatr 116:714, 1990.

Kusne S, Eibling DE, Yu VL, et al: Gangrenous cellulitis associated with gram-negative bacilli in pancytopenic patients: Dilemma with respect to effective therapy. Am J Med 85:490, 1988.

McManus AT, Mason AD, McManus WF, et al: Twenty-five year review of *Pseudomonas aeruginosa* bacteremia in a burn center. Eur J Clin Microbiol 4:219, 1985.

Olgle JW, Janda JM, Woods DE, et al: Characterization and use of a DNA probe as an epidemiologic marker for *Pseudomonas aeruginosa*. J Infect Dis 155:119, 1987.

Reed MD, Stern RC, O'Brien CA, et al: Randomized double blind evaluation of ceftazidime dose ranging in hospitalized patients with cystic fibrosis. Antimicrob Ag Chemother 31:698, 1987.

Reed RK, Larter WE, Sieber OF Jr, et al: Peripheral nodular lesions in *Pseudomonas* sepsis: The importance of incision and drainage. J Pediatr 88:977, 1976.

Rodriguez WJ, Khan WN, Cocchetto DM, et al: Treatment of *Pseudomonas* meningitis with or without concurrent therapy. Pediatr Infect Dis J 9:83, 1990.

Salmen T, Dwyer DM, Vorse H, et al: Whirlpool associated *Pseudomonas aeruginosa* urinary tract infections. JAMA 15:2025, 1983.

Whimbey E, Kiehn TE, Brannon P, et al: Bacteremia and fungemia in patients with neoplastic disease. Am J Med 82:723, 1987.

CHAPTER 185
Cholera

Henry F. Gomez and Thomas G. Cleary

The 1990s have seen dramatic changes in the understanding of cholera. The major developments are the spread of epidemic cholera to the Western Hemisphere, the emergence in India of a new and unique strain of *Vibrio cholerae*, and the discovery of new virulence genes in *V. cholerae*. Cholera is acute watery diarrhea caused by a group of enterotoxins produced by *V. cholerae* serotype O1 or serotype O139 (Bengal). The clinical spectrum includes asymptomatic infection, mild watery diarrhea, and severe watery diarrhea with vomiting that rapidly leads to hypovolemic shock, metabolic acidosis, and death.

ETIOLOGY. *V. cholerae* are gram-negative, non–spore-forming, motile, slightly curved rods (1.5–3.0 × 0.5 μm), each with a polar flagellum. They grow in alkaline media with bile salts. The two biogroups (i.e., biotypes) of *V. cholerae* O1 are classified as classic and El Tor based on hemolysin, hemagglutination, susceptibility to polymyxin B, and susceptibility to bacteriophages. They are also subdivided into serogroups (i.e., serovars) based on the somatic or O antigen. *V. cholerae* O1 has two major O antigenic types (Ogawa and Inaba) and unstable intermediate type (Hikojima). The new epidemic strain, *V. cholerae* O139 (Bengal), does not agglutinate with O1 antiserum but is closely related to the El Tor biotype. Non-O1 *V. cholerae* (nonagglutinating *V. cholerae* or NAG) has long been present in the Gulf states of the United States, but unlike the new O139 strain, the NAG *V. cholerae* is not associated with epidemic cholera.

EPIDEMIOLOGY. *V. cholerae* organisms survive in warm, salty water with nutrients and oxygen. They have been found in roots of plants, undercooked shellfish (e.g., shrimp, crabs), and raw bivalves (e.g., clams, oysters, mussels). Direct person-to-person transmission is rare. In endemic areas, cholera primarily affects children 2–15 yr of age. Breast milk may play a role in protecting children from severe cholera during the first 2 yr of life.

In January 1991, epidemic cholera appeared in the Western Hemisphere for the first time in this century. It began on the north coast of Peru and rapidly spread through much of South and Central America. As of 1993, a total of 820,735 cases and 6942 deaths were reported. The low case-fatality rate (0.8%) reflects the success of current therapy rather than decreased virulence of the epidemic strain. This epidemic is characterized by rapid spread, high attack rates (300–900 cases per 100,000 inhabitants), and low mortality rates. Children and adults are affected. Several outbreaks of cholera have occurred in the United States as a result of this epidemic.

In 1992, *V. cholerae* strains of a new serotype, *V. cholerae* O139, were isolated during an outbreak in Madras, India. This outbreak represents the first epidemic cholera due to an organism that is not serotype O1. In the first 3.5 mo of 1993, 13,275 patients were hospitalized and 434 deaths were recorded. Illness due to this pathogen is indistinguishable from typical cholera in its clinical features and potential for epidemic spread. Data suggest that this new strain is more hardy than O1 and may therefore pose a greater risk of transmission. The outbreaks are characterized by high frequency of secondary infection, a high ratio of symptomatic to asymptomatic infection, and high attack rates in adults.

PATHOLOGY AND PHYSIOPATHOLOGY. Vibrios are very acid sensitive; the stomach is a formidable barrier in preventing these organisms from reaching the small bowel. Vibrios must colonize the small bowel to establish infection and cause disease. They attach to small bowel mucosa and proliferate (10^7–10^8/mL of intestinal fluid). The mucous layer contains factors that are chemotactic for vibrios. The vibrios produce proteolytic enzymes, including mucinase. Motility has also been postulated as an important virulence trait. Colonization of the duodenum and jejunum, followed by enterotoxin-mediated fluid secretion, is responsible for the clinical features. The mucosa is not destroyed during this process, although edema fills the interstitial spaces, and the capillaries and lymphatics in the tips of villi become dilated. A few inflammatory cells are present in the lamina propria. The fluid lost is isotonic with plasma and has high concentrations of bicarbonate and potassium. Although there is some impairment of jejunal disaccharidases, including lactase, glucose absorption is usually preserved.

The fluid losses in cholera result from production of enterotoxins encoded on the bacterial chromosome in a virulence cassette. The most important of these toxins is cholera toxin, a large, periplasmic protein whose structural genes (*ctxA* and *ctxB*) encode an enzymatically active A subunit and cell-binding B subunits. Classic strains have two copies of unlinked *ctxAB,* but El Tor strains usually have one copy. The receptor for subunit B is the ganglioside GM1. The A1 portion of A subunit is an ADP-ribosyltransferase that activates the α-subunit of the stimulatory G protein to bind and activate adenylate cyclase, resulting in prolonged elevation of cyclic adenosine monophosphate (cAMP) levels. The high cAMP causes a decrease in active absorption of sodium and chloride by villous cells and an increase in active secretion of chloride by crypt cells.

The role of a second toxin produced by *V. cholerae* is evident from vaccine studies in which genetically engineered strains with a deletion of cholera toxin A subunit still cause diarrhea. This factor alters the intercellular tight junctions by decreasing the strand complexity of the zonula occludens, resulting in fewer strand intersections. The function of intestinal zonula occludens is to restrict or prevent the diffusion of water-soluble molecules through the intercellular space back into the lumen. When this function is altered by the zonula occludens toxin (zot), the intestinal mucosa becomes more permeable, and water and electrolytes leak into the lumen because of hydrostatic pressure and cause diarrhea.

A third potential enterotoxin (accessory cholera enterotoxin [*ace*]) gene shows striking similarity to eukaryotic ion-transporting ATPases, including the product of the cystic fibrosis transmembrane conductance gene (*CFTR*). The *ctx, zot,* and *ace* genes, along with the pilin genes, flanked by a transposable element called *RS1,* represent a "virulence cassette" of *V. cholerae.* The severity of fluid and electrolyte losses in cholera compared with losses due to other enteropathogens that produce enterotoxins closely related to cholera toxin (e.g., enterotoxigenic *Escherichia coli, Campylobacter, Salmonella*) may be the result of other toxins in the *V. cholerae* virulence cassette.

The non-O1, non-O139 *V. cholerae* (NAG) produce an enterotoxin unrelated to cholera toxin. This toxin is heat stable and is related to a heat-stable enterotoxin produced by *Yersinia enterocolitica.*

CLINICAL MANIFESTATIONS. Watery diarrhea and vomiting develop after an incubation period of 6 hr to 5 days (average, 2–3 days). Low-grade fever occurs in some children. In severe cases, there is profuse, painless, watery diarrhea having a "rice water" consistency with a fishy odor, sometimes with flecks of mucus but no blood. The fluid and electrolyte losses lead to thirst and tachycardia, followed by tachypnea, irritability, a sunken anterior fontanel, and poor skin turgor, and progress to circulatory collapse, stupor, and renal failure if untreated. Diarrhea may be so massive that vascular collapse occurs less than 24 hr after onset. Fluid losses may continue for as long as 1 wk.

COMPLICATIONS. Lethargy, seizures, altered consciousness, fever, hypoglycemia, and death occur more frequently in children than adults. Inadequate fluid and electrolyte replacement may lead to acute renal failure due to acute tubular necrosis. In severely ill children with potassium depletion and acidosis, hypokalemic arrhythmia can cause sudden death. Children with low potassium levels can develop paralytic ileus and abdominal distention that may make oral rehydration impossible. In as many as 10% of small children, prolonged drowsiness, coma, or seizures occur. When the seizures are associated with hypoglycemia, they are often followed by coma and death. Studies have found that 14.3% of children with cholera complicated by hypoglycemia died, compared with 0.7% of children without hypoglycemia. Pulmonary edema occurs in some children, probably because of fluid overload during rehydration. Transient tetany may occur during correction of electrolyte imbalances. In children treated with excessive sugar and salt before medical supervision, hypernatremia can be observed. Despite its high sodium content, the World Health Organization Oral Rehydration Solution (WHO-ORS) is not associated with hypernatremia if used properly; it can be used to treat children with hypernatremic dehydration.

DIAGNOSIS. In endemic areas, any child with severe, watery diarrhea should be considered a possible case of cholera pending laboratory investigations. In the United States, the diagnosis should be suspected in any child with severe, watery diarrhea and a history of recent travel to an endemic area.

Two selective media are used for culturing *V. cholerae;* thiosulfate-citrate-bile-sucrose (TCBS) and tellurite-taurocholate-gelatin agar (TTGA). On TCBS, *V. cholerae* organisms stand out as large, yellow, smooth colonies against the bluish-green background of the medium. On TTGA, the colonies are small and opaque, with a zone of cloudiness around them. Colonies of O139 strains grown in TTGA are described as grayish, opaque colonies with dark centers. Biotyping of *V. cholerae* into classic or El Tor can be obtained on the basis of direct hemagglutination with chicken or sheep red blood cells (i.e.,

El Tor strains agglutinate), sensitivity to polymyxin B (i.e., classic strains are sensitive), or susceptibility to cholera-phage group IV (i.e., classic strains are susceptible). Polyclonal- and monoclonal-based antibody tests are used for direct detection of *V. cholerae* O1 in stool samples. Various enzyme-linked immunosorbent assays for toxin detection and DNA methods (e.g., probes, polymerase chain reaction) are being evaluated as tools for rapid diagnosis. Serologic assays can be used for retrospective detection of vibriocidal, agglutinating, or toxin-neutralizing antibodies 7–14 days after the onset of illness.

TREATMENT. The mainstay of treatment for cholera is fluid and electrolyte replacement. Whether the optimal fluid replacement is the WHO-ORS or one of the newer oral solutions, such as rice-based ORS, is still under investigation. Per liter, the WHO-ORS contains 90 mmol of Na^+, 20 mmol of K^+, 80 mmol of Cl^-, 111 mmol of glucose, and 30 mmol of bicarbonate (citrate can be substituted for bicarbonate). Although rice-based ORS may be superior to WHO-ORS, it presents more logistical problems, because it requires boiling rice flour (50 g/L boiled for 7 min) before adding the salts and because it should be discarded and prepared fresh every 8 hr. Oral rehydration given ad libitum is the treatment of choice, unless the child is obtunded, has an ileus, or is in shock; in these cases, intravenous rather than oral rehydration is appropriate. Vomiting is not a contraindication to oral rehydration. Although all patients with cholera should be carefully monitored, attention to intake and output are especially important in the infant who can take orally only those fluids which are offered. Food should be restarted as soon as deficits are replaced to minimize nutritional impact of the illness; refeeding does not affect purging rates or the duration of diarrhea. The success of oral rehydration was well demonstrated when epidemic cholera arrived in Peru in 1991; the mortality rate was less than 1% despite the fact that this massive outbreak was totally unanticipated.

Antibiotics represent therapy of secondary importance, although they are useful in shortening the duration of illness. Antibiotic resistance is common. The antimicrobial agents used are trimethoprim-sulfamethoxazole (10 mg/kg/24 hr of trimethoprim and 50 mg/kg/24 hr of sulfamethoxazole as two divided doses for 3 days) or, in older children, tetracycline (50 mg/kg/24 hr divided in four doses for 2–3 days). Other antidiarrheal compounds usually are not appropriate.

PREVENTION. The most practical method of preventing life-threatening cholera in infants is prolonged breast-feeding. Safe food and water and proper handling of sewage are the long-term solutions to the problem. Cost, ignorance, and politics have kept these basic needs from being met, and for the immediate future, development of an improved vaccine is a high priority. The currently available vaccine uses killed organisms administered parenterally as a two-dose primary series followed by boosters every 6 mo. This vaccine has about 50% efficacy by 3–6 mo after vaccination. Because of its low efficacy and high frequency of reactions (i.e., pain, erythema, local induration, fever, headaches), this vaccine probably should be used only in very-high-risk hosts (e.g., those with achlorhydria) with a very high probability of exposure. It is not recommended for children younger than 6 mo of age.

Progress has been made in development of better *V. cholerae* vaccines. Several different strategies have been used in preparing these new vaccines. These approaches include combinations of killed whole cells with cholera toxin B subunit, live recombinant *V. cholerae* organisms in which the toxin genes have been genetically altered (strain CVD 103-HgR), synthetic peptides that include immunodominant epitopes, and manipulations of the idiotypic network, using a mouse monoclonal antibody specific for the GM1 binding epitope to induce antibodies to cholera toxin epitopes. The three-dose, oral, killed-whole-cell with B subunit vaccine (which has been shown to decrease the severity of symptomatic infection) and the single oral dose of CVD 103-HgR (which has been shown to induce good vibriocidal antibodies and to provide protection during experimental challenge) are the most promising new vaccines, although neither of these is licensed in the United States at the time of this publication. However, vibriocidal antibodies (directed primarily to lipopolysaccharide), rather than anti–cholera toxin antibodies, appear to be of primary importance in protection from severe disease. This fact, coupled with the experience with *V. cholerae* O139 (Bengal), in which adults in cholera endemic areas have developed severe cholera, suggests that current vaccines are unlikely to be effective against this new epidemic strain.

Bhattacharya SK, Bhattacharya MK, Balakrish-Nair G, et al: Clinical profile of acute diarrhoea cases infected with the new epidemic strain of *Vibrio cholerae* O139: Designation of the disease as cholera. J Infect 27:11, 1993.

Calia KE, Murtagh M, Ferraro MJ, et al: Comparison of *Vibrio cholerae* O139 with *V. cholerae* O1 classical and El Tor biotypes. Infect Immun 62:1504, 1994.

Fasano A, Baudry B, Pumplin DW, et al: *Vibrio cholerae* produces a second enterotoxin, which affects intestinal tight junctions. Proc Natl Acad Sci USA 88:5242, 1991.

Trucksis M, Galen JE, Michalski J, et al: Accessory cholera enterotoxin (Ace), the third toxin of a *Vibrio cholerae* virulence cassette. Proc Natl Acad Sci USA 90:5267, 1993.

World Health Organization: WHO guidelines for cholera control. Geneva, World Health Organization, 1993.

CHAPTER 186
Campylobacter

Shai Ashkenazi and Thomas G. Cleary

Initially considered animal pathogens only, *Campylobacter* organisms are now recognized as an important cause of bacterial gastroenteritis and of systemic infections, primarily in neonates and compromised patients.

ETIOLOGY. The genus *Campylobacter* (meaning curved rod) includes 14 species, of which eight are considered pathogenic for humans: *C. jejuni, C. fetus, C. coli, C. hypointestinalis, C. laridis, C. cinaedi, C. fennelliae,* and *C. upsaliensis*. There are more than 90 different serotypes of *C. jejuni*. *Helicobacter pylori* (formerly *C. pylori*) is a new genus, differentiated from *Campylobacter* by RNA sequence differences (see Chapter 187).

The clinical presentation depends on the species (Table 186–1). Intestinal disease is usually associated with *C. jejuni*, and extraintestinal and systemic infections are associated with *C. fetus*. Less frequently, enteritis is caused by *C. coli, C. laridis,* or *C. fetus*; systemic infections may rarely be caused by *C. jejuni* or *C. coli*.

Campylobacter organisms are thin, gram-negative rods; they are short and S-shaped or long, multispiraled, and filamentous. In older cultures, coccal forms may be seen. The organism is

■ **TABLE 186–1 Main *Campylobacter* Species Causing Human Disease**

Species	Clinical Presentation	Source
C. jejuni	Gastroenteritis, bacteremia (rare)	Poultry, raw milk, cats, dogs, cattle
C. coli	Gastroenteritis	Poultry and swine
C. fetus	Bacteremia, meningitis, endocarditis, mycotic aneurysm	Sheep, cattle, birds
C. laridis	Gastroenteritis	Wild birds, mammals

motile, with a flagellum at one or both poles. The organisms appear as small (0.5–1 mm), slightly raised, smooth colonies on solid media. Visible growth in blood culture is often not apparent until 5–14 days after the initial inoculation. *Campylobacter* organisms are microaerophilic, requiring reduced oxygen tension for growth, with optimal growth occurring in 5–6% oxygen. They neither oxidize nor ferment carbohydrates.

EPIDEMIOLOGY. *Campylobacter* infections are among the most frequent causes of bacterial gastroenteritis worldwide. In developed countries, *C. jejuni* gastroenteritis is usually more common than *Salmonella* or *Shigella* infections. *C. coli* also causes gastroenteritis, although the frequency is about 400-fold lower than for *C. jejuni*. Population-based studies in the United States showed isolation rates of *Campylobacter* ranging from 28 to 71 per 100,000 inhabitants annually. *Campylobacter* gastroenteritis occurs most often in summer and fall; in subtropical areas, it peaks in the rainy season.

The age distribution of *Campylobacter* gastroenteritis in developed countries is bimodal, with one peak in children younger than 4 yr of age and a second in adolescents and young adults. The highest incidence occurs in the first year of life. In developing countries, infections occur early in life, usually below the age of 5 yr. Many infections are asymptomatic, especially in older children.

Campylobacter enteritis is a worldwide zoonosis. The gastrointestinal tract of many domestic and wild animals is the main reservoir of infection. *C. jejuni* has been isolated from the feces of 30–100% of chickens, turkeys, and water fowl. Most farm animals, meat sources, and pets can harbor the organisms. Volunteer studies do not show consistent dose-response patterns, some individuals developing diarrhea after ingesting 2×10^2 organisms and others remaining well after ingesting 10^8 organisms. Transmission of *C. jejuni* from animals to persons occurs most often by the fecal-oral route by ingestion of contaminated food, especially undercooked poultry, unpasteurized milk, and untreated water. Perinatal and person-to-person transmission occurs but is much less common. Household transmission from young dogs and cats with diarrhea also occurs. Outbreaks of *Campylobacter* diarrhea are reported in nurseries and day-care centers. Communicability is greatest during the acute phase of the illness and can last as long as 2–3 wk, but appropriate antibiotic treatment can shorten this period to 2–3 days. Chronic carriage is uncommon. Homosexual men are at increased risk for *C. cinaedi* and *C. fennelliae* infections.

Restriction enzyme analysis of bacterial chromosomal DNA or ribosomal RNA can be used to analyze the distribution of *Campylobacter* infections. The polymerase chain reaction (PCR) fingerprinting assay is useful for generating species-specific and isolate-specific DNA fragments.

PATHOLOGY. *C. jejuni* infection involves the terminal ileum and colon, often producing inflammatory diarrhea. Macroscopically, mucus, pus, and blood are present in the lumen of the bowel, with friable, ulcerated mucosa. Microscopically, rectal biopsies of such patients demonstrate colitis with acute inflammatory infiltrates and swelling of the lamina propria and crypt abscesses. These findings are similar to those seen in shigellosis. Damage to the intestinal mucosa may also be minimal.

PATHOGENESIS. Invasion, enterotoxin production, and cytotoxin production have been demonstrated in *C. jejuni* infections. Mucosal invasion, which is mediated by bacterial surface proteins and occurs after specific binding, seems to be the most important virulence trait. Low levels of cytotoxins that damage mammalian cells are produced by some isolates and may help in the invasion process. Some strains of *C. jejuni* produce a cholera-like enterotoxin, which may explain the watery diarrhea seen clinically. It is not clear that all *C. jejuni* possess virulence traits. Asymptomatic infection may reflect this phenomenon. *C. fetus* tends to penetrate the intestinal mucosa without significantly damaging it, reaching the reticuloendothelial system and bloodstream. This organism contains a surface protein capsule that inhibits opsonophagocytosis and enables a systemic infection.

CLINICAL MANIFESTATIONS. Several clinical presentations of *Campylobacter* infections are possible, depending on the species involved and host factors, such as age, immunosuppression, and underlying conditions.

Acute Gastroenteritis. This is the most common presentation of *Campylobacter* infections, usually caused by *C. jejuni* (95–99% of cases); *C. coli* and *C. laridis* are responsible for the remaining 1–5% of cases. The incubation period is 1–7 days. Diarrhea consists of loose, watery stools or blood- and mucus-containing stools (typically dysentery). Blood appears in the stools 2–4 days after the onset of symptoms. Fever, vomiting, malaise, and myalgia are common. Fever may be the only initial manifestation, but 60–90% of older children also complain of abdominal pain. The abdominal pain is periumbilical; cramping may precede other symptoms or persist after the stools return to normal. Abdominal pain mimics appendicitis or intussusception.

Mild infection lasts only 1 to 2 days and resembles viral gastroenteritis. Most patients recover in less than one week, but 20% have a relapse or prolonged or severe illness. Persistent or recurrent *Campylobacter* gastroenteritis and emergence of erythromycin resistance during therapy are reported in patients with hypogammaglobulinemia (congenital or acquired) and acquired immunodeficiency syndrome (AIDS). Persistent infection mimics acute inflammatory bowel disease. Fecal shedding of the organisms in untreated patients usually lasts for 2–3 wk, with a range of a few days to several months. Young children tend to shed the organisms for longer periods.

Bacteremia. Bacteremia without localized infection is the most common systemic infection caused by *Campylobacter*. *C. jejuni* or *C. coli* gastroenteritis rarely (<1%) cause bacteremia. *C. fetus* usually causes bacteremia without diarrheal symptoms; diarrhea caused by this organism is seen in debilitated or immunocompromised patients.

Bacteremia presents with fever, headache, and malaise. Relapsing or intermittent fever is associated with night sweats, chills, and weight loss when the illness is prolonged. Lethargy and confusion are common, but specific neurologic signs are unusual in the absence of cerebrovascular disease or meningitis. Abdominal pain is frequent; diarrhea, jaundice, and hepatomegaly are less common. Cough may occur, but pulmonary parenchymal involvement is unusual. The physical examination is unimpressive except for the ill appearance of the child. There may be a moderate leukocytosis. Transient asymptomatic bacteremia that clears without antibiotic therapy occurs, as does rapidly fatal septicemia. Prolonged bacteremia of 8–13 wk is described with spontaneous remissions and relapses, especially in the immunocompromised host.

Focal Extraintestinal Infections. Focal infections caused by *C. jejuni* such as meningitis, pancreatitis, cholecystitis, urinary tract infection, arthritis, and peritonitis occur mainly in neonates or immunocompromised patients. *C. fetus* bacteremia is more often associated with focal infections. This organism shows a predilection for vascular endothelium, causing endocarditis, pericarditis, thrombophlebitis, and mycotic aneurysms; focal infections include meningitis, septic arthritis, urinary tract infections, lung abscess, and cholangitis.

Perinatal Infections. Severe perinatal infections are usually caused by *C. fetus* and rarely by *C. jejuni*. *C. fetus* tends to colonize the genital tract and infect fetal tissue. Maternal *C. fetus* and *C. jejuni* infections, which may be asymptomatic, cause abortion, stillbirth, premature delivery, or neonatal infection with sepsis and meningitis. Newborn infection with *C. jejuni* is associated with diarrhea that may be bloody; *C. fetus* rarely causes diarrhea.

COMPLICATIONS. Guillain-Barré syndrome has been reported 1–3 wk after culture-proven *C. jejuni* gastroenteritis. Stool cultures obtained from patients with Guillain-Barré syndrome at the onset of neurologic symptoms have yielded *C. jejuni* in more than 25% of the cases. Serologic studies suggest that 20–40% of patients with Guillain-Barré syndrome have evidence of recent *C. jejuni* infection. These patients have antibodies against gangliosides (GM1 and GD1b) that may trigger demyelination.

Reactive arthritis is an immunoreactive complication seen in adolescents and adults; it appears 5–40 days after onset of diarrhea, involves mainly large joints, and resolves in 1–21 wk without any sequelae. Typically, the arthritis is migratory, but the child is afebrile. Synovial fluid is always sterile. Reiter syndrome (i.e., reactive arthritis with conjunctivitis, urethritis, and rash) and erythema nodosum occur less commonly. IgA nephropathy and immune complex glomerulonephritis with *C. jejuni* antigens in the kidneys are reported. Other complications are hemolytic anemia and rectal bleeding.

DIAGNOSIS. The diagnosis of *Campylobacter* is usually confirmed by identification of the organism in culture. Selective media, such as Skirrow's or Batzler's media, microaerophilic conditions (5–10% oxygen), and, for *C. jejuni*, an optimal temperature of 42° C are necessary. For rapid diagnosis of *Campylobacter* enteritis, direct carbolfuchsin stain of fecal smear, indirect fluorescence antibody test, darkfield microscopy, or latex agglutination can be used, but the sensitivity of these methods is generally low (~70%). Species-specific DNA probes and specific gene amplification by PCR have been described, although clinical experience is limited. Serologic diagnoses have been reported, using enzyme-linked immunoassays to measure antibody (IgG, IgM, IgA) levels to *C. jejuni*. This method may help delineate individuals with acute, chronic, or no exposure to *C. jejuni* antigens but is not yet a standard diagnostic approach.

TREATMENT. Fluid replacement, correction of electrolyte imbalance, and supportive care are the mainstays in the management of children with *Campylobacter* gastroenteritis. Antimotility agents may cause prolonged or fatal disease and should not be used. Controversy exists regarding the need for antibiotic therapy in patients with uncomplicated gastroenteritis. Several studies showed no improvement in clinical symptoms or shortening of the course of the disease. When erythromycin ethylsuccinate suspension is initiated early in the course of the disease in patients with the dysenteric form of *Campylobacter* enteritis, the duration of symptoms and shedding is shortened. Antibiotic therapy significantly shortens fecal excretion of *Campylobacter* from 2–3 wk without treatment to about 2 days with treatment.

Erythromycin (50 mg/kg/24 hr in four divided doses for 5 days) is the drug of choice. Late therapy (4 or more days after onset of symptoms) does not cause clinical improvement, although it still decreases shedding. Erythromycin resistance has been reported in Thailand, Spain, Canada, and Sweden, but it is relatively infrequent (1–7%). *C. coli* may be more resistant than *C. jejuni*. Alternative antibiotic agents are tetracycline (useful in children >7 yr), ciprofloxacin (useful in older adolescents >17 yr), and furazolidone. The new macrolides, clarithromycin and azithromycin, show good in vitro activity, but clinical evaluation is needed. Antibiotics are recommended for patients with the dysenteric form of the disease, high fever, or a severe course; children attending childcare centers or other institutions; and children who are immunosuppressed or have underlying disturbances.

Campylobacter bacteremia or extraintestinal infection caused by *C. fetus* requires parenteral antibiotic therapy for 3–4 wk. Gentamicin is the recommended treatment until antibiotic susceptibility of the isolate is known; *C. fetus* isolates resistant to erythromycin are reported.

PROGNOSIS. Although *Campylobacter* gastroenteritis is usually self-limited, immunosuppressed children, including those with AIDS, may experience a protracted, prolonged, or severe course. Septicemia in the newborn and immunocompromised host has a poor prognosis, with an estimated mortality rate of 30–40%.

PREVENTION. As with many enteric infections, prolonged breast-feeding decreases the risk of symptomatic *Campylobacter* infection. Proper food handling, particularly of chicken, decreases the frequency of *C. jejuni* infections.

Ashkenazi S, Danziger Y, Varsano Y, et al: Treatment of *Campylobacter* gastroenteritis. Arch Dis Child 62:84, 1987.

Blaser MJ, Sazie E, Williams LP: The influence of immunity on raw milk-associated *Campylobacter* infection. JAMA 257:43, 1987.

Giesendorf BA, vanBelkum A, Koeken A, et al: Development of species-specific DNA probes for *Campylobacter jejuni, Campylobacter coli* and *Campylobacter laridis* by polymerase chain reaction fingerprinting. J Clin Microbiol 31:1541, 1993.

Mishu B, Blaser MJ: Role of infection due to *Campylobacter jejuni* in the initiation of Guillain-Barré syndrome infect Dis 17:104, 1993.

Reina J, Borrell N, Serra A: Emergence of resistance to erythromycin and fluoroquinolones in thermotolerant *Campylobacter* strains isolated from feces, 1987–1991. Eur J Clin Microbiol Infect Dis 11:1163, 1992.

Ruiz-Palacios GM, Calva JJ, Pickering LK, et al: Protection of breast-fed infants against *Campylobacter* diarrhea by antibodies in human milk. J Pediatr 116:707, 1990.

Salazar-Lindo E, Sack RB, Chea-Woo E, et al: Early treatment with erythromycin of *Campylobacter jejuni*-associated dysentery in children. J Pediatr 109:355, 1986.

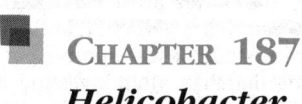

CHAPTER 187
Helicobacter

Jane T. Atkins and Thomas G. Cleary

Although spiral organisms have been seen in the stomach of humans and animals since 1893, it was not until 1983 that Warren and Marshall associated these S-shaped spiral bacilli with chronic gastritis. The organism was first called *Campylobacter pyloridis* but was reclassified as *Helicobacter pylori*. *H. pylori* is now generally accepted as one of the most common causes of acute and chronic antral gastritis. It is also associated with peptic ulcer disease, gastric carcinoma, and lymphoma, although the association with the cancer is still open to debate.

ETIOLOGY. *H. pylori* is a spiral, gram-negative organism with a smooth surface and multiple, sheathed, unipolar flagella. It is fastidious and grows slowly on chocolate agar, producing tiny translucent colonies after incubation for 72–96 hr under microaerophilic conditions at 37° C. Older colonies often assume a coccoid shape. The abundant production of urease is a distinct characteristic of *H. pylori* and is the basis for several diagnostic tests. Although *Helicobacter* and *Campylobacter* species resemble each other in growth requirements and morphology, *H. pylori* has a unique fatty acid composition, 16S ribosomal RNA sequence, and ultrastructural characteristics that differentiate it from *Campylobacter* species.

EPIDEMIOLOGY. *H. pylori* is distributed worldwide. The prevalence of infection varies with age, ethnic background, and socioeconomic status. Factors associated with increased risk of infection include unsanitary and overcrowded living conditions, lack of running water, and sharing a bed. In developing countries, half of the children are infected by 10 yr of age, and by adulthood, more than 80% of the population is infected. In developed countries, infection with *H. pylori* in childhood is uncommon, and only about 40% of adults are infected. Children of lower socioeconomic status have infection rates that parallel those of children from developing countries. Its high prevalence rate caused much confusion about the significance of *H. pylori,* but it is now clear that chronic gastritis in adults is the result of chronic *H. pylori* infection that can be reversed by therapy.

There is no animal or environmental reservoir for *H. pylori.* The mechanism of transmission of *H. pylori* is unknown. The isolation of *H. pylori* from dental plaque and stool suggest that person-to-person transmission occurs. The familial tendency of peptic ulcer disease also supports person-to-person transmission. Whether this transmission occurs by the oral-oral or fecal-oral route is not clear. Nosocomial transmission of *H. pylori* from contaminated endoscope has been reported.

PATHOGENESIS AND PATHOLOGY. *H. pylori* is highly host and tissue specific. It is found predominately in the mucous layer overlying the gastric epithelium in the antrum. Although a few organisms have been found between the tight junctions of adjacent epithelial cells, *H. pylori* does not invade the gastric mucosa. The organism has been isolated from areas of gastric metaplasia in the intestine, but it is not found on intestinal epithelium or in areas of intestinal metaplasia in the stomach.

Virulence factors that allow the organism to adapt to the gastric milieu include urease-mediated ammonia production to neutralize the acidic pH, the spiral morphology and flagella that allow it to penetrate the protective mucous layer and resist peristalsis, and adhesins that allow the organism to attach to the gastric epithelium. In vivo this attachment resembles the attachment of enteropathogenic *Escherichia coli* to intestinal epithelium. Other virulence factors include the production of cytotoxin and mediators of inflammation.

Infection with *H. pylori* virtually always results in gastric inflammation. Although acute infection is associated with neutrophilic infiltration, the histopathologic hallmark of *H. pylori* infection is chronic inflammation. In adults, the characteristic inflammatory response is acute and chronic inflammation with neutrophilic and lymphocytic infiltrates. The inflammatory response in children is lymphocytic and usually associated with lymphonodular hyperplasia.

CLINICAL MANIFESTATIONS. Infection with *H. pylori* is usually clinically silent. The major manufestations of symptomatic infection with *H. pylori* include gastritis, peptic ulcer disease, and possibly gastric carcinoma. *H. pylori* has also been implicated as a cause of nonulcer or functional dyspepsia; however, its role in this disorder is controversial. It appears that gastroesophageal reflux, esophagitis, delayed gastric emptying, and various motility disorders are more important in dyspepsia than *H. pylori.*

Acute infection with *H. pylori* is usually asymptomatic, although a syndrome characterized by abdominal pain, achlorhydria, and neutrophilic gastritis is observed in adults who have experimentally been challenged with *H. pylori* and occasionally seen in the clinical setting. Chronic gastritis is a more common manifestation of infection with *H. pylori;* most patients are asymptomatic. Although the typical clinical presentation of children with chronic gastritis is recurrent abdominal pain and vomiting, most chronic recurrent abdominal pain in childhood is not caused by *H. pylori.* The signs and symptoms associated with chronic active gastritis are nonspecific. Endoscopic findings range from grossly normal-appearing mucosa with microscopic evidence of gastritis to nodular antritis with antral hyperemia.

The term *peptic ulcer disease* is used to encompass gastric and duodenal ulcers. Peptic ulcer disease is uncommon in children; the true incidence in childhood is unknown. Although *H. pylori* is seen in 50–80% of adults with gastric ulcer, its role in gastric ulcers in children is not clear. *H. pylori* plays a significant role in duodenal ulcers in children and adults and is demonstrated in the gastric antrum in 90–100% of these patients. Eradication of *H. pylori* results in recurrence of duodenal ulcer in 0–27% of patients, compared with a recurrence rate of 67–95% if *H. pylori* is not eradicated. The clinical presentation of peptic ulcer disease in children varies. The classic presentation of epigastric pain that is aggravated by fasting and relieved with eating is not common in younger children, although it is seen in older children and adolescents. Fewer than 20% of children with peptic ulcer disease have hematemesis and melena.

The evidence links chronic infection with *H. pylori* with peptic ulcer disease and gastric carcinoma, but, unlike gastritis, a causal relationship has not been established unequivocally. There appears to be an inverse relationship between peptic ulcer disease and gastric cancer. It is estimated that 10–15% of patients with chronic infection with *H. pylori* will develop peptic ulcer disease and another 1–2% will develop gastric carcinoma. Factors that determine which patients develop peptic ulcer disease or gastric cancer probably involve a combination of host, organism, and environmental factors.

DIAGNOSIS. Although other conditions (e.g., anti-inflammatory drugs, Zollinger-Ellison syndrome, eosinophilic gastroentopathy, pernicious anemia) causing gastric inflammation and ulcers are well described, *H. pylori* is among the most common causes. *H. pylori* can be diagnosed by invasive and noninvasive methods. Invasive methods require flexible endoscopy to biopsy the gastric mucosa for culture, histopathology, or rapid urease test. Noninvasive tests include the serology and urea breath test.

H. pylori is a slow-growing organism that is technically difficult to isolate. Culture of biopsied tissue yields growth in approximately 90% of the cases for which the organism is detected by histopathologic analysis. Culture of gastric brushing is less sensitive than culture of tissue. *H. pylori* can be demonstrated in tissue by Gram stain, Giemsa stain, hematoxylin-eosin stain, Warthin-Starry silver stain, acridine-orange stain, and phase-contrast microscopy. None of these techniques are specific for *H. pylori,* but histologic examination of the tissue provides important information on the degree of inflammation. Rapid urease tests such as the CLO test capitalize on the fact that *H. pylori* produces an abundance of urease. A positive result can be obtained within hours of endoscopy. Sensitivity and specificity of these tests appear to be comparable to histology and culture. The polymerase chain reaction has also been employed as a rapid diagnostic test for *H. pylori.*

Serology is helpful in following the response to antimicrobial therapy, but it adds little to the acute diagnosis. If treatment is adequate, serum antibody titers revert to negative or fall to low levels within 6 mo of therapy. Serology also is a reasonable means for estimating prevalence of infection. The urea breath test uses ^{13}C- or ^{14}C-labeled urea and measures the release of radiolabelled CO_2 in the breath after the ingestion of these compounds. This test reportedly has a sensitivity of 97% and a specificity of 100%; it also can be used to follow the response to therapy.

TREATMENT AND PROGNOSIS. The success of treatment is the most important factor in establishing *H. pylori* as a major human pathogen. Antibiotic therapy clears *H. pylori* infection and heals gastritis and peptic ulcer disease. Long-term eradication is associated with continued well-being. Eradication of *H. pylori* infections is difficult, and relapse is common. There is no indication for treatment of patients with asymptomatic or uncomplicated gastritis due to *H. pylori.* When the subpopulation of asymptomatic patients at risk for gastric cancer and duodenal ulcer is better defined, these patients may be treated empirically for *H. pylori.*

Therapy is indicated for patients with symptomatic gastritis or duodenal ulcer. H_2 blockers are dramatically less effective in achieving long-term remission than antibiotic regimens. In vitro, *H. pylori* is susceptible to a wide range of antimicrobial agents, including penicillin G, ampicillin, tetracycline, clindamycin, ciprofloxacin, metronidazole, and erythromycin. In vivo, no single agent effectively eradicates the organism; monotherapy should never be used. Triple therapy with a bismuth compound and ampicillin (or tetracycline) for 4–6 wk plus metronidazole for 3–4 wk eradicates the organism in 75–95% of the patients. A study of a small group of pediatric patients showed that dual therapy with bismuth subsalicylate and amoxicillin for 6 wk was as effective as triple therapy. In adults, the combination with omeprazole (a proton pump inhibitor) and amoxicillin was well tolerated and effective in eliminating *H. pylori.* In an uncontrolled study, amoxicillin and metronidazole in combination with a proton pump inhibitor resulted in elimination of *H. pylori* in children who failed dual therapy with amoxicillin and metronidazole. Further studies are necessary to determine the optimal therapy for symptomatic *H. pylori* infection in children.

Triple therapy of *H. pylori* duodenal ulcer disease has changed the prognosis of this condition dramatically. The high recurrence rates (up to 70%) associated with H_2 blockers, antacids, diet manipulation, and psychotherapy have been replaced by the expectation for cure if the organism is eradicated. There are no data proving that treatment of chronic asymptomatic *H. pylori* infection decreases the frequency of gastric adenocarcinoma. However low-grade gastric B-cell lymphoma was shown to regress with antibiotic treatment of the associated *H. pylori* in a small number of patients.

Blaser MJ: *Helicobacter pylori:* its role in disease. Clin Infect Dis 15:386, 1992.
Drumm B: *Helicobacter pylori* in the pediatric patient. Gastroenterol Clin North Am 22:169, 1993.
Forbes GM, Glaser ME, Cullen DJE, et al: Duodenal ulcer treated with *Helicobacter pylori* eradication: seven-year follow-up. Lancet 343:256, 1994.
Israel DM, Hassall E: Treatment and long-term follow-up of *Helicobacter pylori*-associated duodenal ulcer disease in children. J Pediatr 123:53, 1993.
Raymond J, Bergeret M, Benhamou Ph, et al: A 2-year study of *Helicobacter pylori* in children. J Clin Microbiol 32:461, 1994.
Solnick JV, Tompkins LS: *Helicobacter pylori* and gastrointestinal disease: pathogenesis and host-parasite interaction. Infect Agents Dis 1:294, 1993.
Wotherspoon AC, Doglioni C, Diss TC, et al: Regression of primary low-grade B-cell gastric lymphoma of mucosa-associated lymphoid tissue type after eradication of *Helicobacter pylori.* Lancet 342:575, 1993.

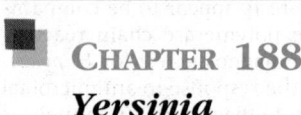

CHAPTER 188
Yersinia

*William Albritton**

Yersinial infections are enzootic in many animal species, including birds, rodents, and wild and domestic mammals. The genus *Yersinia* has 11 named species, but only three species are known to be regularly transmitted to humans: *Yersinia enterocolitica* (enterocolitis), *Y. pseudotuberculosis* (mesenteric adenitis), and *Y. pestis* (plague). Domestic animals, especially swine, and household pets, such as cats and dogs, are major reservoirs for *Y. enterocolitica* and *Y. pseudotuberculosis. Y. pestis* is endemic in wild rodents in the western United States and in many other areas of the world. Humans are accidental hosts for *Y. enterocolitica* and *Y. pseudotuberculosis* and are usually infected by handling contaminated animal tissues or ingesting contaminated meat, water, or milk. *Y. pestis* is transmitted to humans from infected rodents by flea bites.

YERSINIA ENTEROCOLITICA

Infections due to *Y. enterocolitica* far outnumber infections due to *Y. pseudotuberculosis* and *Y. pestis.* Disease is usually manifested as an acute enteritis with fever, diarrhea, abdominal pain, nausea, and vomiting. Stools may be mucoid and bloody or, less commonly, watery.

ETIOLOGY. The genus *Yersinia* was transferred from the family Pasteurellaceae to the family Enterobacteriaceae on the basis of DNA-DNA hybridization studies and the presence of the enterobacterial common antigen. They resemble "atypical" coliforms morphologically and biochemically. *Y. enterocolitica* organisms are oxidase-negative, non–lactose-fermenting, gram-negative bacilli that are motile at 22° C but not at 37° C. Strains resembling *Y. enterocolitica* are isolated from extraintestinal infections and stool from asymptomatic patients or patients with mild gastroenteritis. These strains are considered to be nonenteropathogenic in that they lack the genes required for invasion and have now been assigned to a new species.

EPIDEMIOLOGY. Animals, food, and water are the major reservoirs for *Y. enterocolitica.* Many animal species harbor *Yersinia,* but swine, cattle, goats, dogs, and cats are more commonly involved. *Y. enterocolitica* has been isolated or detected by the polymerase chain reaction in commercial meat products, especially pork. Infections occur primarily in children and young adults, with most occurring in children under 7 yr of age. Infecting serogroups show variable geographic distributions with O:3, O:5, O:8, and O:9 strains predominant. Disease is more common in the colder months and in males than females. Common source outbreaks due to contaminated food or water are reported with incubation periods ranging from 1 to 11 days. Institutional and hospital person-to-person spread, including neonatal transmission from a symptomatic mother and transfusion-related disease from red blood cell–containing products are reported. Extraintestinal infections due to *Y. enterocolitica* are rare.

PATHOLOGY AND PATHOGENESIS. *Y. enterocolitica* pathogenesis is multifactorial, involving chromosomal and plasmid genes. All strains pathogenic for humans carry a related virulence plasmid that encodes several calcium- and thermally regulated virulence factors. The essential mechanisms involved in pathogenesis appear to be adherence, toxin production, and invasion. Adherence and production of a heat-stable enterotoxin appear to be sufficient to produce a watery diarrhea, with elaboration of cytotoxin and one or more invasin genes necessary to produce the classic enteric pathology: a superficial ulcerative ileocolitis with mesenteric adenitis, lymphoid hyperplasia, and abscesses of the Peyer patches. Necrotizing granulomas in the mesenteric nodes seen with *Y. pseudotuberculosis* are absent.

Several features of the organism are important for transfusion-acquired disease. First, pathogenic strains require iron and survive only in red blood cell–containing products. The role of iron is supported by reports of septicemia in patients with hemochromatosis and after accidental overdose of oral iron in previously healthy children. Second, the risk of transfusion-associated disease increases with blood stored for more than 2 wk. *Y. enterocolitica* grows at 4° C, and release of organisms from the phagocytic cell fraction in aging units allows the organism to proliferate under normal storage conditions. This cold-enhanced growth is useful for isolating the organism from mixed sources, such as stool, but increases the bacterial load in stored meat products and blood products.

CLINICAL MANIFESTATIONS. The most common presenting signs and symptoms are fever (occasionally to 40° C), abdominal pain (usually colicky), and diarrhea (watery or mucoid with fecal leucocytes). Illness may be as short as 2 days or persist for 3–4 wk. It is usually self-limiting in older children, but bacteremia develops in 20–30% of infants younger than 3 mo of age. Fever occurs in 40–50% of cases, abdominal pain in 20–80%, and diarrhea in 80–95%. Asymptomatic infections are readily detected in family contacts.

Complications are uncommon in children. Erythema nodo-

*Modified from the section in the 14th edition by R. D. Feigin.

sum, hemolytic anemia, thrombocytopenia, and bacteremic spread to other sites with meningitis, hepatic abscess, and pneumonia have all been reported, but the most frequent complication is reactive arthritis. Joints of the extremities are usually affected, with one to four joints involved. Intact organisms are not detected in synovial specimens known to contain bacterial antigen, suggesting only stable degradation products or immune complexes trapped from the circulation are associated with *Yersinia*-triggered reactive arthritis.

DIAGNOSIS. The history may suggest enterocolitis due to *Y. enterocolitica* based on contact with animals or ingestion of uncooked meat products, especially pork. Direct examination of diarrheal stool for fecal leukocytes is helpful in establishing invasive diarrhea. Culture is the most useful diagnostic test. Because many laboratories do not routinely culture for *Yersinia,* it is important to notify the laboratory of suspected cases. *Yersinia*-selective agar is inoculated with stool and incubated at reduced temperatures of 25° or 32° C. Some laboratories use cold enrichment methods and subculture material held at 4° C for as long as 4 wk. Isolations from nonstool sources and sterile body fluids may be made on routine media. Speciation is important from nonenteric sources. Pathogenic stool strains of *Y. enterocolitica* can be differentiated from nonpathogenic strains using Congo red–magnesium oxalate agar, the pyrazinamidase test, salicin fermentation, and esculin hydrolysis.

Serotyping of isolates and serodiagnosis in culture-negative cases is of value for epidemiologic purposes only.

DIFFERENTIAL DIAGNOSIS. Enterocolitis due to *Y. enterocolitica* is similar in clinical presentation to invasive diarrheal disease due to other enteric pathogens, such as *Shigella* or enteroinvasive *Escherichia coli,* mesenteric adenitis due to *Y. pseudotuberculosis,* inflammatory bowel disease, and reactive arthritis due to other causes.

PREVENTION. Infection is preventable by careful attention to the preparation of meat, especially the slaughter of swine, and by avoiding ingestion of uncooked meat, precooked pork products held at 4° C, potable water of questionable purity, and unpasteurized milk or milk products made from unpasteurized milk. Person-to-person transmission can be reduced by careful personal hygiene, especially handwashing, and institution of enteric precautions in hospitalized patients. Vaccines are not available.

TREATMENT. Uncomplicated enterocolitis due to *Y. enterocolitica* is a self-limited disease, and the benefit of antimicrobial therapy has not been established. Culture-proven septicemia at any age and patients under 3 mo of age who have a high rate of septicemia should be treated. In one retrospective study, aminoglycosides in combination with third-generation cephalosporins, fluoroquinolones, or other agents, such as rifampin and trimethoprim-sulfamethoxazole, were effective, whereas other β-lactams, such as amoxicillin with or without clavulanate and benzylpenicillin were associated with treatment failures.

YERSINIA PSEUDOTUBERCULOSIS

Infection due to *Y. pseudotuberculosis* is most often seen as a pseudoappendicitis syndrome without diarrhea.

ETIOLOGY. *Y. pseudotuberculosis* is differentiated biochemically from *Y. enterocolitica* on the basis of ornithine decarboxylase activity, fermentation of sucrose, sorbitol, cellobiose, and other tests, although some overlap between species may be seen. Antisera to somatic O antigens and sensitivity to yersinial phages may also be used to differentiate the two species. Subspecies-specific DNA sequences have been isolated that allow direct probe- and primer-specific differentiation of *Y. pestis, Y. pseudotuberculosis,* and *Y. enterocolitica.*

EPIDEMIOLOGY. Less is known of the epidemiology of *Y. pseudotuberculosis* infections than for *Y. enterocolitica* or *Y. pestis.* The seasonal incidence in humans parallels that in wild and domestic animals. Transmission from cats and cat-contaminated substances is established. There is a low reported incidence in the 5–12-yr age range.

PATHOLOGY AND PATHOGENESIS. The pathology is similar to that described for *Y. enterocolitica,* with ileal and colonic mucosal ulceration and mesenteric adenitis. Necrotizing, epithelioid granulomas are seen in the mesenteric nodes. The appendix is frequently grossly and microscopically normal. Mesenteric nodes are frequently the only source of positive cultures. *Y. pseudotuberculosis* antigens bind directly to HLA class II molecules and function as superantigens, which may partly explain the clinical syndromes resembling Kawasaki syndrome caused by this organism.

CLINICAL MANIFESTATIONS. Children usually present with fever and abdominal pain that is diffuse or localized to the right lower quadrant. Frequently, there is tenderness over the McBurney point and strong clinical suspicion of appendicitis. At surgery, the terminal ileum is thickened and shiny with enlarged mesenteric nodes, which may appear necrotic. The appendix is normal or only mildy inflammed.

Presentations resembling scarlet fever or Kawasaki syndrome are reported.

DIAGNOSIS. Mesenteric adenitis should be suspected in children with unexplained fever and abdominal pain. A characteristic picture of enlarged mesenteric lymph nodes, thickening of the terminal ileum, and no image of the appendix may appear on ultrasound. *Y. pseudotuberculosis* is rarely isolated. It is almost never isolated from stools, and the best source is an involved mesenteric node. Culture conditions are the same as for *Y. enterocolitica.*

Serologic tests have been described, but commercially available tests or standardized antigens are not available.

DIFFERENTIAL DIAGNOSIS. Appendicitis is the most common diagnosis. Inflammatory bowel disease and nonspecific intra-abdominal infections are also considered.

PREVENTION. Specific preventive measures other than avoiding exposure to potentially infected animals and careful food-handling practices are not apparent. Vaccines for prevention of *Y. pseudotuberculosis* have not been developed.

TREATMENT. Uncomplicated mesenteric adenitis due to *Y. pseudotuberculosis* is a self-limited disease, and antimicrobial therapy is not required. Culture-confirmed bacteremia should be treated with an aminoglycoside in combination with another agent, as for infections due to *Y. enterocolitica.*

YERSINIA PESTIS

The first pandemic of plague (Black Death) was described in 541 A.D. Subsequent pandemics through the Middle Ages devastated portions of Europe, with losses of 30–50% of the population. The psychologic effect of such misunderstood mortality is apparent in the nursery rhyme "Ring around the rosies; A pocket full of posies," describing the signs, and "We all fall down," describing the outcome of plague.

The plague bacillus was introduced into the western United States in the 1800s from infected rats carried by ships returning from Asia. The disease is endemic in the wild rodent population of the western and southwestern United States.

ETIOLOGY. *Yersinia pestis* was first described by Yersin in 1894. Based on DNA-DNA hybridization analysis *Y. pestis* and *Y. pseudotuberculosis* are subspecies of the same species. *Y. pestis* shares with *Y. pseudotuberculosis* characteristic bipolar (safety pin) staining but is differentiated from *Y. pseudotuberculosis* by biochemical reactions, serology, and susceptibility to selected yersinial phage.

EPIDEMIOLOGY. Sylvatic plague occurs as a stable enzootic infection or as epizootic disease with a high mortality rate for the host, usually rodent, population. Hibernating animals are able to maintain the infection over winter, and transmission from animal to animal is achieved by way of a rodent-flea cycle.

Different species of fleas show variable efficiencies of transmission, based on their relative preference for other hosts and whether or not they regurgitate infected material when they feed.

Plague is transmitted to man by the bite of fleas that have fed on infected animals, by direct contact with infected domestic or wild animals, or by direct inhalation of infected droplets from patients or animals with the pneumonic form of the disease.

PATHOLOGY AND PATHOGENESIS. *Y. pestis* ingested by the flea proliferate in the intestine and are regurgitated into the dermal lymphatics of the human host when the flea next feeds. Organisms are initially trapped in the regional lymph nodes, which become enlarged and tender (i.e., buboes). In severe bubonic plague, organisms gain access to the efferent lymphatics and disseminate, causing septicemia, meningitis, and secondary pneumonia. Organisms are readily demonstrated in buboes and on direct smear of peripheral blood in septicemia.

Primary pneumonic plague occurs when infected material is aspirated. The organism is highly transmissible from person to person in this form. Droplets containing large numbers of organisms are expelled and may cause fulminant fatal infections when inhaled.

Y. pestis carries three virulence plasmids, two of which are shared by *Y. enterocolitica* and *Y. pseudotuberculosis* and that promote intracellular survival and suppression of cytokine synthesis. One plasmid unique to *Y. pestis* enhances dissemination and resistance to phagocytosis. The adhesin and invasin genes found in the enteropathogenic species are cryptic in *Y. pestis.*

CLINICAL MANIFESTATIONS. The incubation period of bubonic plague is 2–6 days, and that of pneumonic plague is 1–72 hr. Most cases in children are bubonic plague. Sudden onset of fever and painful lymphadenopathy are common. Femoral, inguinal, axillary, and cervical nodes may be involved, depending on the site of inoculation. Meningitis may present after starting therapy for bubonic plague, particularly when streptomycin is used as a sole agent, and occurs in association with axillary and cervical buboes or septicemia without apparent lymphadenopathy. Undifferentiated septicemia is reported more often in adults. Secondary pneumonia occurs in as many as 25% of patients with bubonic or septicemic plague. Primary pneumonic plague acquired by inhalation of infected droplets from person-to-person or animal-to-human transmission is rare. Pulmonary signs and symptoms may not be apparent until just before death. Gastrointestinal symptoms and signs, including abdominal pain, nausea, vomiting, and bloody diarrhea, occur in more than 50% of patients with plague. Cutaneous manifestations have included nonspecific petechial or purpuric and vesicular or pustular rashes.

DIAGNOSIS. The diagnosis of sporadic plague depends on a high index of suspicion. Outside of endemic areas, a history of travel to an endemic area, especially camping, or contact with ground squirrels and the presence of flea bites are very important clues to the clinical diagnosis. Case-fatality rates are higher in patients diagnosed outside of endemic areas, probably because of missed or delayed diagnosis. Sputum, blood, purulent exudates, and lymph node aspirates should be examined directly with Gram and Giemsa or Wayson stains for bipolar, staining organisms and should be cultured for *Y. pestis.* Commercial identification systems may not identify *Y. pestis.* Suspected isolates of *Y. pestis* should be forwarded to a public health laboratory for confirmation. Serologic tests are not clinically useful in diagnosing the acute disease but may help to establish a retrospective diagnosis in patients inadvertently treated with appropriate antibiotics.

DIFFERENTIAL DIAGNOSIS. Mild and subacute forms of bubonic plague may be confused with other disorders causing localized lymphadenitis and lymphadenopathy. Septicemic plague may be indistinguishable from other forms of bacterial sepsis.

PREVENTION. Primary prevention requires avoidance of exposure to infected animals and their fleas. In endemic areas, the public should be educated to avoid burrows, to refrain from handling sick or dead rodents, to deflea household pets, and to reduce the domestic rat habitat. The prevalence and distribution of plague can be determined in wild rodent populations by surveillance for disease or by using the polymerase chain reaction to detect *Y. pestis* in fleas.

Patients with plague should be quarantined until treated and managed under strict respiratory isolation if they have pulmonary symptoms. Infected material should be handled with extreme caution, and the laboratory should be notified of suspected cases.

A killed whole-cell vaccine is available for laboratory and field personnel working directly with the organism, persons engaged in aerosol experiments, and persons engaged in field operations where enzootic plague is known and preventing exposure to rodents and fleas is not possible. Routine immunization of children in endemic areas is not recommended.

TREATMENT. The treatment of choice has been intramuscular streptomycin (30 mg/kg/24 hr) divided every 12 hr for bubonic plague. Septicemia and meningitis are usually treated with intravenous chloramphenicol (100 mg/kg/24 hr) divided every 6 hr. Mild disease may be treated with oral chloramphenicol or tetracycline in children older than 10 yr of age. Prophylaxis or expectant treatment should be given to close contacts of patients with pneumonic plague. Recommended regimens include tetracycline or trimethoprim-sulfamethoxazole. Contacts of cases of uncomplicated bubonic plague do not require prophylaxis.

PROGNOSIS. Acute bubonic plague progresses to delirium, shock, and death within 3–5 days if untreated. The overall mortality rate for untreated bubonic plague is 60–90%. The progression of pneumonic plague is rapid and almost always fatal within 24–48 hr if untreated.

When bubonic plague is treated early, the mortality rate is less than 10%. The prognosis in primary pneumonic plague remains poor if specific treatment is not provided within 18 hr of onset.

Brubaker RR: Factors promoting acute and chronic diseases caused by yersiniae. Clin Microbiol Rev 4:309, 1991.

Butler T: The black death past and present: I. Plague in the 1980s. Trans R Soc Trop Med Hyg 83:458, 1989.

Gayraud M, Scavizzi MR, Mollaret HH, et al: Antibiotic treatment of *Yersinia enterocolitica* septicemia: A retrospective review of 43 cases. Clin Infect Dis 17:405, 1993.

Gong J, Hogman CF, Hambraeus A, et al: Transfusion-transmitted *Yersinia enterocolitica* infection. Vox Sang 65:42, 1993.

Kane DR, Reuman PD: *Yersinia enterocolitica* causing pneumonia and empyema in a child and a review of the literature. Pediatr Infect Dis J 11:591, 1992.

Krogstad P, Mendelman PM, Miller VL, et al: Clinical and microbiologic characteristics of cutaneous infection with *Yersinia enterocolitica.* J Infect Dis 165:740, 1992.

Naqvi SH, Swierkosz EM, Gerard J, et al: Presentation of *Yersinia enterocolitica* enteritis in children. Pediatr Infect Dis J 12:386, 1993.

Nikkari S, Merilahti-Palo R, Saario R, et al: *Yersinia*-triggered reactive arthritis. Arthitis Rheum 35:682, 1992.

Sato K, Ouchi K, Taki M: *Yersinia pseudotuberculosis* infection in children, resembling Izumi fever and Kawasaki syndrome. Pediatr Infect Dis J 2:123, 1983.

Tertti R, Vuento R, Mikkola P, et al: Clinical manifestations of *Yersinia pseudotuberculosis* infection in children. Eur J Clin Microbiol Infect Dis 8:587, 1989.

Uchiyama T, Miyoshi-Akiyama T, Kato H, et al: Superantigenic properties of a novel mitogenic substance produced by *Yersinia pseudotuberculosis* isolated from patients manifesting acute and systemic symptoms. J Immunol 151:4407, 1993.

Weber J, Finlayson NB, Mark JBD: Mesenteric lymphadenitis and terminal ileitis due to *Yersinia pseudotuberculosis.* N Engl J Med 283:172, 1970.

CHAPTER 189
Tularemia

William Albritton*

Tularemia is a zoonotic infectious disease caused by *Francisella tularensis,* a gram-negative bacterium first isolated from ground squirrels in Tulare County, California, in 1906. Clinical manifestations depend on the infecting biovar and the route of inoculation. In the pediatric population, infection occurs more commonly in the second decade, is usually associated with direct animal contact, and presents as ulceroglandular disease (60–80%). Other clinical presentations, such as typhoidal (5–15%), glandular (10–15%), oropharyngeal (5–10%), and oculoglandular (1%) are less common, and subclinical infections are rare.

ETIOLOGY. *Francisella tularensis* is an aerobic, short, non–spore-forming, nonmotile, gram-negative pleomorphic coccobacillus that possesses a thin capsule and consists of two subspecies. *F. tularensis* subsp. *tularensis* (Jellison type A) is found only in North America, is associated with ticks and lagomorphs (i.e., rabbits, hares), and is highly virulent for humans. *F. tularensis* subsp. *palaeartica* (Jellison type B) occurs in Europe, Asia, and North America; is associated with mosquitoes and rodents; and is less virulent for humans and avirulent for rabbits. Biovar *tularensis* can be differentiated from biovar *palaeartica* by its ability to ferment glycerol and the presence of citrulline ureidase. Genus-specific and type-specific 16S rRNA probes have been described.

EPIDEMIOLOGY. *F. tularensis* is transmitted to humans by direct contact with infected animals, through the bite of infected ticks or other biting insects, by inhalation of dust from contaminated environments, or by consumption of contaminated water. More than 100 wild animal species have been associated with human transmission, including rats, mice, squirrels, muskrats, beavers, moles, and birds, and with nine species of domestic animals, including sheep, cattle, and cats. Common vectors include deerflies, horseflies, fleas, mosquitoes, and lice. Seasonal and geographic associations have also been observed. In the United States, 60% of cases are reported from the Midwest, where rabbits and ticks are the principal reservoir, especially during hunting season. Aerosol transmission is reported after farming activities such as haying or threshing because of rodent contamination and when infected rabbit carcasses are run over with lawnmowers or played with by children. Person-to-person transmission is not documented.

PATHOLOGY AND PATHOGENESIS. The host may be infected by inoculation through broken or intact skin or mucous membranes, ingestion (including penetration of the pharyngeal mucosa by ingested organisms), inhalation, or the bite of infected arthropod vectors. Ten to 50 organisms produce disease if inhaled or injected, but thousands of organisms are needed if they are ingested. Within 48–72 hr after the organisms enter the skin, an erythematous maculopapular lesion may be noticed, followed shortly by ulceration and regional lymphadenopathy. The organisms multiply and produce granulomas within lymph nodes. Subsequently, bacteremia may occur. Although any organ of the body may be involved, infection of the reticuloendothelial system is most prominent and common.

Pneumonia may follow inhalation of *F. tularensis.* An inflammatory reaction develops around the site of bacterial deposition, and necrosis of alveolar walls follows. The organisms that reach the lung are ingested by alveolar macrophages and enter the hilar lymphatics and then the blood.

F. tularensis is resistant to the bactericidal effect of normal serum and polymorphonuclear leukocytes, presumably because of the presence of a capsule. It is an intracellular or facultative intracellular parasite capable of adapting to the intracellular environment of monocytes and may be killed only after activation by specifically committed T lymphocytes. Infection is followed by effective immunospecific protection, with chronic infection or reinfection rarely documented.

CLINICAL MANIFESTATIONS. The incubation period varies from a few hours to several weeks, but is usually 3–5 days. The onset is acute and characterized by myalgia, arthralgia, chills, fever of 40–41° C, nausea, vomiting, and diaphoresis. Headache is prominent and may be associated with photophobia. A generalized maculopapular, papular, or pustular rash occurs in 20% of patients.

In the ulceroglandular form, the primary maculopapular lesion is noticed within 72 hr and ulcerates within 4–5 days. The ulceration is painful, requires about a month to heal, and is located at the site of inoculation, usually the hands when associated with cleaning infected game. Regional lymphadenopathy occurs, usually without lymphangitis. The lymph nodes are tender and become fluctuant in about 25% of untreated cases. Generalized lymphadenopathy, splenomegaly, or both may develop.

Oropharyngeal tularemia is characterized by purulent tonsillitis and pharyngitis and occasionally by ulcerative stomatitis.

Glandular tularemia is similar to the ulceroglandular form, but no local lesion is apparent.

Oculoglandular disease is similar to the ulceroglandular form, except that the primary lesion is a severe, painful conjunctivitis accompanied by preauricular or cervical lymphadenitis.

The typhoidal form resembles typhoid fever. Fever is protracted, and cutaneous or mucous membrane lesions may not be apparent. A dry cough, severe retrosternal chest pain, and hemoptysis are common. Clinical evidence of bronchitis, pneumonitis, or pleuritis may be found in 20% of cases, and roentgenographic evidence of pulmonary involvement and nodular enlargement of the mediastinum is seen in the most cases. Hepatosplenomegaly is common.

Meningitis, encephalitis, pericarditis, endocarditis, peritonitis, thrombophlebitis, and osteomyelitis have been reported in association with infection due to *F. tularensis.*

DIAGNOSIS. The history and physical findings may suggest tularemia, particularly a history of exposure to animals, especially rabbits, or ticks and other biting insects. Hematologic data are not discriminating. Direct Gram-stained smears are usually negative, and routine diagnostic laboratories should not attempt culture because of the danger to laboratory personnel. When cultures are performed, blood-glucose-cystine agar, Müller-Hinton broth, chocolate agar with IsoVitaleX, and modified charcoal-yeast agar have been used. Small, smooth, transparent colonies appear after 24–48 hr with a small zone of α-hemolysis on blood agar media. The organism also grows in chick yolk sac or embryo and in guinea pigs, but these isolation procedures are even more hazardous to laboratory personnel than artificial media and should only be attempted in level 3 animal facilities. Usual sources of cultured material include blood, gastric washings, and drainage from wounds.

The serum agglutination test is the most useful diagnostic test for tularemia. The conventional tube agglutination test is widely used and a four-fold or greater rise in titer is usually found after the 1st wk of illness. A sensitive microagglutination modification appears to be more sensitive, and serum agglutinins were detected on average 9 days earlier. A competitive enzyme immunoassay using a 43-kD outer membrane protein (OMP) has also been reported. The antibody response is spe-

*Modified from the section in the 14th edition by R. D. Feigin.

cific, but cross-reactions in certain tests have been reported with *Brucella, Yersinia, Proteus vulgaris* OX19, and cholera vaccine. IgM antibodies may appear a few days earlier or concomitant with IgG antibodies, depending on the test used. Antibody titers are maximal during the 2nd mo after onset, and IgM and IgG antibodies may persist for years.

Other tests, such as a skin test and lymphocyte stimulation test, have also been described but are not generally available.

DIFFERENTIAL DIAGNOSIS. Ulceroglandular and glandular tularemia may resemble cat-scratch disease, infectious mononucleosis, sporotrichosis, plague, anthrax, meliodosis, glanders, rat-bite fever, or lymphadenitis due to *Mycobacterium tuberculosis,* atypical mycobacteria, or *Staphylococcus aureus.*

Oropharyngeal tularemia must be differentiated from the same diseases and from acquired cytomegalovirus infection, toxoplasmosis, and severe pharyngitis due to adenovirus and herpes simplex.

Pneumonic tularemia must be differentiated from other bacterial and nonbacterial pneumonias, particularly due to *Mycoplasma, Chlamydia,* mycobacteria, fungi, and rickettsia.

Typhoidal tularemia must be differentiated from typhoid and other enteric fevers, brucellosis, and other severe septicemic illnesses.

PREVENTION. Avoidance of exposure is the most important means of preventing transmission. Children should be taught not to handle sick or dead animals, and rubber gloves should be worn in cleaning or handling the flesh of wild animals. Children living in endemic areas should wear protective clothing with tightly fitting cuffs at the ankles and wrists when out of doors and should be checked frequently for the presence of ticks. Ticks should be removed by an instrument or gloved hand and should not be squeezed. The area of attachment should be cleaned with 70% alcohol.

Face masks, rubber gloves, and biologic containment hoods should be used by technologists working with cultures or infective material in the laboratory.

An attenuated, live strain (LVS) of *F. tularensis* has reduced the incidence of typhoidal tularemia and the severity of ulceroglandular tularemia in laboratory-acquired disease. The vaccine efficacy in preventing naturally occurring disease in children is not known.

TREATMENT. Streptomycin 30 mg/kg/24 hr divided in two intramuscular doses for 7–14 days is the treatment of choice. Gentamicin intravenously is an acceptable alternative. Bacteriostatic antibiotics, such as tetracycline and chloramphenicol, have been effective in older children and adults, but clinical relapse may occur unless continued for extended periods. In vitro susceptibility may not correlate with in vivo clinical efficacy because of the intracellular nature of the infection, and β-lactams that show in vitro susceptibility may not be useful. A mixed pattern of macrolide (e.g., erythromycin, clarithromycin) susceptibility but uniform susceptibility to the fluoroquinolones has been reported. Case reports of success with fluroquinolones and imipenem with cilastin have been published. Because of the sporadic nature of tularemia, good controlled treatment trials are not available.

PROGNOSIS. Untreated ulceroglandular tularemia has a reported case-fatality rate of 2–5%, but the case-fatality rates in pneumonic tularemia may reach 30%. Fatalities have been reported to be more common in patients 50 yr of age or older. Untreated patients who survive experience symptoms for 2–4 wk and a subsequent period of disability of 8–12 wk. Recovery usually provides lifelong immunity. Second attacks, if they occur, are mild. If treatment is provided promptly, recovery usually is rapid and fatality exceedingly rare.

Bevanger L, Maeland JA, Naess AI: Competitive enzyme immunoassay for antibodies to a 43,000-molecular-weight *Francisella tularensis* outer membrane protein for the diagnosis of tularemia. J Clin Microbiol 27:922, 1989.
Forsman M, Sandstrom G, Jaurin B: Identification of *Francisella* species and discrimination of type A and type B strains of *F. tularensis* by 16S rRNA analysis. Appl Environ Microbiol 56:949, 1990.
Rohrbach BW, Westerman E, Istre GR: Epidemiology and clinical characteristics of tularemia in Oklahoma, 1979 to 1985. South Med J 84:1091, 1991.
Sato T, Fujita H, Ohara Y, et al: Microagglutination test for early and specific serodiagnosis of tularemia. J Clin Microbiol 28:2372, 1990.
Scheel O, Hoel T, Sandvik T, et al: Susceptibility pattern of Scandinavian *Francisella tularensis* isolates with regard to oral and parenteral antimicrobial agents. APMIS 101:33, 1993.
Tarnvik A: Nature of protective immunity to *Francisella tularensis.* Rev Infect Dis 11:440, 1989.
Taylor JP, Istre GR, McChesney TC, et al: Epidemiologic characteristics of human tularemia in the Southwest-Central states, 1981–1987. Am J Epidemiol 133:1032, 1991.
Uhari M, Syrjala H, Salminen A: Tularemia in children caused by *Francisella tularensis* biovar *palaeartica.* Pediatr Infect Dis J 9:80, 1990.

CHAPTER 190

Brucellosis

*William Albritton**

Brucellosis is a zoonotic infectious disease caused by one of four species or biovars of *Brucella* known to infect humans: *Brucella melitensis* (goats and sheep), *B. abortus* (cattle), *B. suis* (swine), and *B. canis* (dogs). *B. neotomae* (rodents) and *B. ovis* (sheep) cause animal infections but have not been transmitted to humans. In the pediatric population, infection occurs from direct contact, from inhalation of aerosols, and by ingesting raw milk or milk products from infected animals. Efforts to control disease in domestic animals and pasteurization of milk has greatly reduced the incidence of disease in industrialized countries, but sporadic outbreaks occur, and the disease remains endemic in wild animals. The clinical presentation in children is similar to adults. Only about 50% of patients present with acute disease; the remainder have subclinical or subacute infections.

ETIOLOGY. Brucellae, named for Sir David Bruce, who first isolated the organism in 1887 from a patient with Malta fever, constitute a single genospecies, but they have historically been divided into species based on the natural animal host. Species other than *B. ovis* and *B. canis* demonstrate colonial dissociation and the smooth (S) colonial variants are more virulent and cross-react antigenically more than the rough (R) colonial variants. Organisms are small, aerobic, non–spore-forming, nonmotile, gram-negative bacilli and without apparent capsule. Growth requirements are fastidious, and growth in CO_2 is enhanced for some biovars.

EPIDEMIOLOGY. In industrialized countries, occupational or recreational exposure to infected animals is the usual route of infection. Direct contact and aerosol exposure of infected tissue has been well documented in abattoir workers, veterinarians, farmers, hunters, and others who have frequent contact with animals. In the United States, fewer than 10% of reported cases occur in the pediatric population. Endemic brucellosis is usually transmitted by the ingestion of unpasteurized milk, cream, butter, cheese, or ice cream. The organism may also directly invade the eye, nasopharynx, and genital tract. Organisms may remain viable for as long as 3 wk in a refrigerated carcass and can survive the curing of ham. Compulsory pasteurization of milk, immunization of cattle, and other control measures have greatly reduced endemic disease in the United States.

*Modified from the section in the 14th edition by R. D. Feigin.

Endemic disease is maintained in animals through the excretion of large numbers of organisms in genital secretions and milk, with vertical and horizontal transmission. Transmission is through oral or respiratory contact. The presence of growth-enhancing erithritol in placental tissues of some animals has been suggested as a predisposing factor for abortion in these species.

Human-to-human transmission is rare but has been reported in association with blood transfusion, bone marrow transplantation, and transplacental or perinatal exposure. Outbreaks among microbiology laboratory workers are not uncommon, especially when the organism is not suspected or misidentified by commonly used identification systems. Iatrogenic disease due to inadvertent inoculation with the live attenuated vaccine strain used for cattle and swine and produced from *B. abortus* has been reported in adults.

PATHOLOGY AND PATHOGENESIS. Brucellae are facultative intracellular parasites and are capable of surviving and multiplying within phagocytes and many other cell types, including red blood cells. On initial infection nonspecific host factors, such as nonspecific agglutinins, complement, and polymorphonuclear leukocytes, lead to opsonization and phagocytosis, but intracellular killing is less effective than for other organisms, and intracellular organisms in tissue monocytes of the reticuloendothelial system are not killed in the native host.

Multiplication of organisms within the host appears to be essential for the induction of immunity. The host responds by elaborating specific antibodies, including agglutinins, opsonins, precipitins, and complement-fixing antibodies. Specific IgM antibodies appear within 1 wk and decline by 3 mo. Specific IgG antibodies increase by 2–3 wk and persist in untreated or partially treated cases. Cross-reacting antibodies with *Yersinia, Francisella, Vibrio cholerae,* and *Salmonella* are the result of similarities of O-specific side chains of the lipopolysaccharide.

Brucellae do not stimulate effective degranulation or a respiratory burst. The more virulent smooth strains are more resistant to intraleukocyte killing. Intracellular killing of brucellae by fixed-tissue macrophages requires activation by specifically committed T lymphocytes.

All species of *Brucella* produce granulomas in the liver, spleen, lymph nodes, and bone marrow. Granulomatous inflammation of the gallbladder, interstitial orchitis with scattered areas of fibroid atrophy, endocarditis with vegetations of the valves, granulomatous lesions of the myocardium, and involvement of the brain, kidney, and skin have also occurred.

CLINICAL MANIFESTATIONS. In the absence of a history of animal exposure or ingestion of unpasteurized milk, the clinical diagnosis of brucellosis in children is difficult. Nonspecific manifestations of fever, arthralgia, malaise, weakness, and central nervous system manifestations, particularly depression, are most common. Incubation periods of a few days to several months are reported. The interval between onset of symptoms and diagnosis is as long as 150 days, with a mean of 4 wk. Hepatomegaly and splenomegaly are found in 30–40% of cases. Specific organ system localization, such as osteomyelitis, myocarditis, endocarditis, and genitourinary tract infections are uncommon. Bone scintigraphy is more sensitive than radiography in detecting skeletal brucellosis. Neonatal brucellosis cannot be differentiated from other perinatal infections.

DIAGNOSIS. The history may suggest brucellosis, particularly exposure to animals or ingestion of unpasteurized milk or milk products. Anemia, hemolysis, leukopenia, thrombocytopenia or pancytopenia due to hypersplenism, hemophagocytosis, and bone marrow involvement have been reported. Blood cultures are positive for as many as 75% of patients with acute disease before antibiotics. Blood culture isolation is much less frequent in subacute disease. Culture diagnosis may be improved to more than 90% with the use of bone marrow cultures. Common commercial blood culture media may be used with venting and added CO_2. The lysis-centrifugation method may improve isolation rates because of the intracellular location of organisms. It is important to notify the laboratory in suspected cases of brucellosis, because blood cultures should be held for as long as 4 wk, and routine blood cultures are held for only 7–10 days.

In the absence of culture diagnosis, serologic diagnosis is possible. The standard tube agglutination test is used in most public health laboratories. IgM antibodies are measured by a reduction in titer after 2-mercaptoethanol (2-ME) treatment. IgM antibodies appear early in infection, followed within 1–2 wk by IgG antibodies. Because of the delay in considering the diagnosis, high-titered sera may demonstrate a "prozone" inhibition, and it is necessary to dilute the sera to detect antibody. Successful therapy is followed by a rapid decline in IgG antibodies, but IgM antibodies may persist for months or years. High IgG antibodies or a rising titer after treatment suggest persistent infection or relapse. Infection with rough strains of *Brucella,* especially *B. canis,* are not detected with the standard agglutination test, which uses smooth *B. abortus* antigens as the test material. Specific *B. canis* or *B. ovis* antigens may be used to specifically diagnose these infections, but an appropriate exposure history is required. Similar results have been seen with the more sensitive enzyme immunoassay–based test. Differentiation between active and inactive infection has also been reported using lipopolysaccharide–depleted cytoplasmic proteins.

DIFFERENTIAL DIAGNOSIS. Acute brucellosis can mimic many diseases, including tularemia, typhoid fever, rickettsial diseases, influenza, tuberculosis, histoplasmosis, coccidioidomycosis, and infectious mononucleosis. Persistent brucellosis may resemble malignant histiocytosis, lymphoma, or other neoplastic diseases. Appropriate history, radiologic findings, culture, and serology may help to differentiate these disorders. Biopsy of appropriate tissues may be useful.

PREVENTION. Control is best achieved by immunization of domestic herds and pasteurization of milk. Periodic agglutination tests of milk and blood should be used to identify infected animals, and infected herds should be slaughtered. Ingestion of unpasteurized milk and of products derived from unpasteurized milk should be avoided. Hunters should use caution in handling potentially infected animals, such as elk, moose, bison, and caribou.

TREATMENT. Tetracycline in combination therapy is the regimen of choice for the treatment of brucellosis. Doxycycline in a dose of 5 mg/kg/24 hr (maximum, 200 mg/24 hr), given orally in two doses with intramuscular streptomycin (30 mg/kg/24 hr) divided every 12 hours or intravenous gentamicin (5–7.5 mg/kg/24 hr) divided every 8 hr, is a commonly used regimen. Because of the problems with tetracyclines in children under 10 yr of age and the requirement for intramuscular or intravenous administration of aminoglycosides, alternative regimens have been considered. In one prospective trial the combination of two oral agents, trimethoprim-sulfamethoxazole (10–12 mg/kg trimethoprim) and rifampin (15–20 mg/kg) was effective. Treatment failures with β-lactams, including third-generation cephalosporins such as ceftriaxone, may be due to the intracellular nature of the pathogen and the presence of nondividing cells in subacute or persistent infections. The total duration of treatment is usually 3–6 wk.

Initiation of antimicrobial therapy after a delay in diagnosis may be accompanied by a Jarisch-Herxheimer–like reaction described for syphilis, presumably because of the large antigen load. Steroids may be given when this reaction is seen, if necessary.

PROGNOSIS. The case-fatality rate for untreated brucellosis is about 3%. Most deaths are due to specific organ system involvement, such as endocarditis. The prognosis following specific therapy is excellent. A prolonged course is usually due

CHAPTER 192

Botulism*

Stephen S. Arnon

DEFINITION. Botulism is the acute, flaccid paralytic illness caused by the neurotoxin produced by *Clostridium botulinum,* or rarely, an equivalent neurotoxin produced by unique strains of *C. butyricum* and *C. baratii.* Three forms of human botulism are known: infant botulism (the most common), foodborne (classic) botulism, and wound botulism.

ETIOLOGIC AGENTS. Botulinum toxin is the most poisonous substance known, the parenteral human lethal dose being estimated at 10^{-7} mg/kg. The toxin blocks neuromuscular transmission and causes death through airway and respiratory muscle paralysis. Seven antigenic toxin types, assigned the letters A–G, are distinguished by the inability of protective (neutralizing) antibody against one toxin type to protect against a different type. The seven toxin types serve as convenient clinical and epidemiologic markers. Neurotoxigenic *C. butyricum* strains produce a type E–like toxin, while neurotoxigenic *C. baratii* strains produce a type F–like toxin. Toxin types A, B, E, and F are well-established causes of human botulism, while C and D cause illness in other animals. Type G has not been established as a cause of either human or animal disease.

Botulinum toxin is a simple di-chain protein that consists of a 100 kD heavy chain that contains the neuronal attachment site and a 50 kD light chain that is taken into the cell after binding. The phenomenal potency of botulinum toxin is explained by the fact that its seven light chains are Zn^{2+}-endopeptidases, whose substrates are one of three protein components of the docking complex by which synaptic vesicles fuse with the terminal cell membrane and release acetylcholine into the synaptic cleft.

Clostridium botulinum is a gram-positive, spore-forming obligate anaerobe whose natural habitat worldwide is soil, dust, and marine sediments, and is found in a wide variety of fresh and cooked agricultural products. Spores of some *C. botulinum* strains survive boiling for several hours, which enables the organism to survive human efforts at food preservation. In contrast, botulinum toxin is heat labile and easily destroyed by heating at 80° C or above for 5–10 min. Little is known about the ecology of neurotoxigenic strains of *C. butyricum* and *C. baratii.*

PATHOGENESIS. All three forms of botulism produce disease through a final common pathway: Botulinum toxin is carried by the bloodstream to peripheral cholinergic synapses, where it binds irreversibly, blocking acetylcholine release and causing impaired autonomic and neuromuscular transmission. *Infant botulism* is an infectious disease that results from ingesting the spores of any of the three botulinum toxin–producing clostridial strains, with subsequent spore germination, multiplication, and production of botulinum toxin in the large intestine. *Foodborne botulism* is an intoxication that results when preformed botulinum toxin contained in an improperly preserved or cooked food is swallowed. *Wound botulism* results from spore germination and colonization of traumatized tissue by *C. botulinum;* it is the analogue of tetanus, but much more rare.

EPIDEMIOLOGY. *Infant botulism* has been reported from all inhabited continents except Africa. Notably, the infant is the only family member ill. The most striking epidemiologic feature of infant botulism is its age distribution, in which 95% of cases are between 3 wk and 6 mo of age, with a broad peak between 2 and 4 mo of age. This pattern is matched only by one other condition, the sudden infant death syndrome. However, cases as young as 6 days or as old as 363 days at onset have been reported. The male:female ratio of cases is essentially 1:1, and cases have occurred in all major racial and ethnic groups.

Infant botulism is an uncommon and often unrecognized illness. In the United States about 75–100 cases are diagnosed annually; 1,145 cases were reported from 1976 to 1992. Almost half of U.S. cases were reported from California. Reflecting the known asymmetry of the soil distribution of toxin types of *C. botulinum,* most cases west of the Mississippi River have been caused by type A strains, while most cases east of it have been caused by type B strains. One case each in the states of New Mexico and Oregon resulted from *C. baratii* and type F–like toxin, while two cases in Rome, Italy, resulted from *C. butyricum* and type E–like toxin. Identified risk factors for the illness include the ingestion of honey and a slow intestinal transit time (less than one stool per day). Breastfeeding appears to provide protection against fulminant, sudden death from infant botulism. Under rare circumstances of altered intestinal anatomy, physiology, and microflora, older children and adults may contract infant botulism.

Foodborne botulism results from the ingestion of a food in which *C. botulinum* has multiplied and produced its toxin. Recent outbreaks in North America associated with restaurants in which foods such as baked potatoes, sautéed onions, and chopped garlic were implicated have revised the traditional view of foodborne botulism as resulting mainly from home-canned foods. Other United States outbreaks have occurred from commercial foods sealed in plastic pouches that relied solely on refrigeration to prevent outgrowth of *C. botulinum* spores. Noncanned foods responsible for recent foodborne botulism episodes include the hazelnut flavoring added to yogurt, sautéed onions in "patty melt" sandwiches, potato salad, and fresh and dried uneviscerated fish. A recent trend toward a single case per outbreak or of cases presenting separately in different cities or hospitals has meant that the physician cannot rely on the temporal and geographic clustering of illness (often in a family) to suggest the diagnosis.

Most preserved foods have been implicated in foodborne botulism, but the usual offenders in the United States are the "low-acid" (pH 6.0 and above) home-canned foods such as jalapẽno peppers, asparagus, olives, and beans. The potential for foodborne botulism exists throughout the world, but outbreaks occur most commonly in the temperate zones rather than the tropics, where preservation of fruits, vegetables, and other foods is less common.

In the past 10 yr approximately 250 cases of foodborne botulism from about 15 outbreaks per year have occurred in the United States. Most of the continental U.S. outbreaks resulted from either proteolytic type A or type B strains, which produce a strongly putrefactive odor in the food that some people find necessary to verify by tasting. In contrast, in Alaska most foodborne outbreaks have resulted from nonproteolytic type E strains in Native American foods, such as salmon eggs and seal flippers, that do not exhibit signs of spoilage. A further hazard of type E strains is their ability to grow at temperatures as low as 5° C, the temperature of household refrigerators.

Wound botulism is an exceptionally rare disease, with somewhat less than 100 cases reported worldwide, but it is important to pediatrics because about one quarter of cases affect adolescent or younger persons. Most cases have occurred in young, physically active males at greatest risk of traumatic injury, but wound botulism also occurs with crush injuries in which no break in the skin is evident. In the last 10 yr wound botulism has become increasingly common in drug abusers, resulting from self-injection or nasal inhalation of nonsterile street products, not always with evident abscess formation.

PATHOLOGY. Botulinum toxin is a physiologic, not cytotoxic, poison that causes no overt macroscopic or microscopic pathol-

*All material in this chapter is in the public domain, with the exception of any borrowed figures or tables.

ogy. However, secondary pathologic changes (e.g., pneumonia, petechiae on intrathoracic organs) may be found at autopsy. No diagnostic technique is available to identify botulinum toxin bound at the neuromuscular junction. The healing process in botulism consists of sprouting of new terminal unmyelinated motoneurons. Movement resumes when these new twigs locate noncontracting muscle fibers and reinnervate them by inducing formation of a new motor end-plate. Clinically and in experimental animals, this process takes about 4 wk.

CLINICAL MANIFESTATIONS. Botulinum toxin is distributed hematogenously. Because relative blood flow and density of innervation are greatest in the bulbar musculature, all three forms of botulism manifest neurologically as a symmetrical, descending flaccid paralysis of the cranial nerve musculature. *It is not possible to have botulism without having bulbar palsies,* yet in infants such symptoms as poor feeding, weak suck, feeble cry, drooling, and even obstructive apnea are often not recognized as bulbar in origin. Patients with evolving illness may already have generalized weakness and hypotonia in addition to bulbar palsies when first seen.

In older children with foodborne or wound botulism, the onset of neurologic symptoms follows a characteristic pattern of diplopia, blurred vision, ptosis, dry mouth, dysphagia, dysphonia, and dysarthria, with deceased gag and corneal reflexes. Importantly, because the toxin acts only on motor nerves, paresthesias are not seen in botulism, except when a patient hyperventilates from anxiety. The sensorium remains clear, but this may be difficult to ascertain because of the slurred speech.

Foodborne botulism begins with gastrointestinal symptoms of nausea, vomiting, and diarrhea in about one third of cases. These symptoms are thought to result from metabolic byproducts of growth of *C. botulinum* or from the presence of other toxic contaminants in the food, as gastrointestinal distress is not seen in wound botulism. Constipation is common in foodborne botulism once flaccid paralysis becomes evident. Illness usually begins 18–36 hr after ingestion of the contaminated food but can range from as little as 2 hr to as long as 8 days. The incubation period in wound botulism is 4–14 days. Fever may be present in wound botulism but is absent in foodborne botulism unless a secondary infection (e.g., pneumonia) is present. All three forms of botulism display a wide spectrum in their clinical severity, from the very mild with minimal ptosis, flattened facial expression, minor dysphagia, and dysphonia to the fulminant, with rapid onset of extensive paralysis, respiratory distress, and frank apnea. *Fatigability with repetitive muscle activity is the clinical hallmark of botulism.*

Infant botulism differs in apparent initial symptoms of illness only because the infant cannot verbalize them. Almost invariably, the first indication of illness is constipation, defined as 3 or more days without defecation, although this sign is frequently overlooked. Parents usually notice lethargy, listlessness, poor appetite, weak cry, and diminished spontaneous movement. Dysphagia may be evident as secretions drooling from the mouth. Gag, suck, and corneal reflexes diminish as the paralysis advances. Oculomotor palsies may be evident only with sustained observation. Paradoxically, the pupillary light reflex may be unaffected until the child is severely paralyzed, or it may be initially sluggish. Loss of head control is typically a prominent sign. Respiratory arrest may occur suddenly from airway occlusion by unswallowed secretions or from obstructive flaccid pharyngeal musculature. Occasionally, the diagnosis of infant botulism is suggested by a respiratory arrest that occurs after the infant is curled into position for lumbar puncture.

In mild cases or in the early stages of illness, the physical signs of infant botulism may be subtle and easily missed. Eliciting cranial nerve palsies and fatigability of muscular function requires careful examination. Ptosis may not be seen unless the head of the child is kept erect. The presence of decreased anal sphincter tone may suggest a generalized neuromuscular disease.

■ **TABLE 192–1 Diagnoses Considered in Patients with Foodborne and Wound Botulism**

Acute gastroenteritis	Aminoglycoside-induced paralysis
Myasthenia gravis	Tick paralysis
Gullain-Barré syndrome	Hypocalcemia
Organophosphate poisoning	Hypermagnesemia
Meningitis	Carbon monoxide poisoning
Encephalitis	Hyperemesis gravidarum
Psychiatric illness	Laryngeal trauma
Cerebrovascular accident	Diabetic complications
Poliomyelitis	Inflammatory myopathy
Hypothyroidism	Overexertion

DIAGNOSIS AND DIFFERENTIAL DIAGNOSIS. The classic picture of botulism is the acute onset of a flaccid descending paralysis with clear sensorium, no fever, and no paresthesias. The rarity of foodborne and wound botulism makes them easily confused with other diseases (Table 192–1). Routine laboratory studies, including the cerebrospinal fluid (CSF), are normal in botulism unless dehydration or starvation ketosis are present. Electromyography (EMG) may demonstrate a defect in neuromuscular transmission, and the typical EMG finding in foodborne and wound botulism is facilitation (potentiation) of the evoked muscle action potential at high frequency (50 Hz) stimulation. In infant botulism a characteristic pattern, known by the acronym BSAP (*b*rief, *s*mall, *a*bundant motor-unit action *p*otentials), is present only in clinically weak muscles.

Foodborne and wound botulism are often difficult to distinguish from myasthenia gravis and Guillain-Barré syndrome (GBS). The edrophonium (Tensilon) test helps with the former, and a lumbar puncture and EMG help with the latter. In GBS the CSF protein concentration usually has become elevated and nerve conduction velocity has slowed by 4–6 wk after onset. Paresthesias are common in GBS. Possible organophosphate intoxication should be pursued aggressively because a specific antidote (PAM) is available and because the patient may be part of a commonly exposed group, some of whom have yet to develop illness.

Infant botulism requires a high index of suspicion for early diagnosis (Table 192–2). Even today, almost 20 yr after its recognition, "rule-out sepsis" is the most common admission diagnosis. If a previously healthy infant, usually 6 mo of age or less, has a history of constipation and then acutely develops weakness with difficulty in sucking, swallowing, crying, or breathing, infant botulism should be considered the most likely diagnosis. A careful cranial nerve examination is then quite helpful.

The diagnosis of botulism is unequivocally established by demonstrating the presence of botulinum toxin in serum, or

■ **TABLE 192–2 Differential Diagnosis of Infant Botulism**

Admission Diagnosis	Common Subsequent Diagnoses
Suspected sepsis	Guillain-Barré syndrome
Pneumonia	Myasthenia gravis
Dehydration	Disorders of amino acid metabolism
Viral syndrome	Hypothyroidism
Hypotonia of unknown etiology	Drug ingestion
Constipation	Brain stem encephalitis
Failure to thrive	Heavy metal poisoning (Pb, Mg, As)
	Poliomyelitis
	Viral polyneuritis
	Hirschsprung disease
	Werdnig-Hoffmann disease
	Metabolic encephalopathy
	Medium chain acetyl-CoA dehydrogenase (MCAD) deficiency

of *C. botulinum* toxin or organisms in wound material or feces. *C. botulinum* is not part of the normal resident intestinal flora of humans, and its presence in the setting of acute flaccid paralysis is diagnostic. State Health Departments (first call) and the Centers for Disease Control and Prevention (second call; phone: 404-639-3311 workdays and 404-639-2888 at other times) can arrange for specimen testing, epidemiologic investigation, and provision of equine antitoxin. *Suspected botulism represents a medical and public health emergency that is immediately reportable in virtually all United States health jurisdictions.* An epidemiologic diagnosis of foodborne botulism can be made when *C. botulinum* organisms and toxin are found in a food item incriminated by ingestion history.

TREATMENT. Management of botulism rests on three principles: (1) fatiguability with repetitive muscle activity is the clinical hallmark of the disease; (2) complications are best avoided by anticipating them; and (3) meticulous supportive care is a necessity. The first principle applies mainly to feeding and breathing. Correct positioning is imperative to protect the airway and improve respiratory mechanics. The patient is placed face up on a *rigid-bottomed crib* (or bed), the head of which is tilted at 30 degrees. A small cloth roll is placed under the cervical vertebrae to tilt the head back so that secretions drain to the posterior pharynx and away from the airway. In this tilted position the abdominal viscera pull the diaphragm down, thereby improving respiratory mechanics. The patient's head should not be elevated by bending the middle of the bed; if this is done, the hypotonic thorax will slump into the abdomen and breathing will be compromised.

Endotracheal intubation should be done prophylactically to maintain airway patency and avoid aspiration. A rising Pco_2 signals alveolar hypoventilation and irreversible muscle fatigue. About one half of hospitalized patients will need intubation. Tracheostomy is almost never required because with proper positioning patients with global flaccid paralysis can tolerate intubation for weeks or months without permanent sequelae.

Feeding should be done by a nasogastric or nasojejunal tube until sufficient oropharyngeal strength and coordination enables an entire feeding by breast or bottle. Expressed breast milk is the most desirable food, in part because of its immunologic components (sIgA, lactoferrin, leukocytes). Tube feeding also assists in the restoration of peristalsis, a nonspecific but probably essential part of eliminating *C. botulinum* from the intestinal flora. Intravenous feeding (hyperalimentation) is discouraged because of the potential for infection and the advantages of tube feeding.

Antibiotic therapy is not part of the treatment of uncomplicated infant or foodborne botulism because the toxin is primarily an intracellular molecule that is released into the intestinal lumen with vegetative bacterial cell death and lysis. Antibiotics are reserved for the treatment of secondary infections, and in this setting a nonclostridiocidal antibiotic such as trimethoprim/sulfamethoxazole or nalidixic acid is preferred. Aminoglycoside antibiotics should be avoided because they may potentiate the blocking action of botulinum toxin at the neuromuscular junction. However, wound botulism requires aggressive treatment with antibiotics and antitoxin in a manner analogous to tetanus (Chapter 193). The currently available botulinum antitoxin is a horse-serum–derived product that has side effects of serum sickness, anaphylaxis, and potential lifelong sensitization to equine proteins; its use in children requires careful consideration. A clinical trial of botulism immune globulin, a human-derived botulinum antitoxin, for the treatment of infant botulism is now under way in California.

Because sensation remains intact, providing auditory, tactile, and visual stimuli is beneficial. Maintaining strong central respiratory drive is essential, so sedatives or CNS depressants (e.g., Reglan) are contraindicated. Full hydration and stool softeners may mitigate the protracted constipation. Cathartics are not recommended. Patients with foodborne and infant botulism excrete *C. botulinum* toxin and organisms in their feces, often for weeks, and care should be taken in handling their excreta. Bladder atony occurs, and gentle suprapubic pressure with the patient in the sitting position with the head supported may help attain complete voiding and reduce the risk of urinary tract infection.

■ TABLE 192–3 Complications of Infant Botulism

Adult respiratory distress syndrome	Recurrent atelectasis
Aspiration	Seizures secondary to hyponatremia
Fracture of the femur	Sepsis
Inappropriate antidiuretic hormone secretion	Tension pneumothorax
	Transfusion reaction
Misplaced or plugged endotracheal tube	Urinary tract infection
	Subglottic stenosis*
Necrotizing enterocolitis	Tracheal granuloma*
Otitis media	Tracheitis*
Pneumonia	Tracheomalacia*

**A single hospital's experience.*

COMPLICATIONS. Avoidance of complications is best accomplished by noting past experience (Table 192–3). Even so, some critically ill, paralyzed patients who must spend weeks or months on ventilators in intensive care units will inevitably develop complications. All of the complications listed in Table 192–3 are nosocomially acquired; some of them are iatrogenic. Infant botulism does not have a relapsing course, and suspected "relapses" usually reflect premature hospital discharge or an undiscovered underlying complication, such as pneumonia.

PROGNOSIS. In the absence of complications, particularly those related to hypoxia, the prognosis in infant botulism is for full and complete recovery. When the regenerating nerve endings have induced formation of a new motor end-plate, neuromuscular transmission is restored. In the United States, the case-fatality ratio for hospitalized infant botulism is <1%. The case-fatality ratio in foodborne and wound botulism varies by age, with younger patients having the best prognosis. Some adults with botulism have reported chronic weakness and fatigue as sequelae.

Hospital stay in infant botulism averages approximately 1 mo but differs significantly by toxin type, with type B cases being hospitalized a mean of 3.7 wk and type A cases 5.6 wk. Infant botulism is also a costly illness. For all California patients in the years 1984–1993, hospital costs averaged $2,400 per day in constant 1993 dollars. Twenty-five per cent of patients had hospital stays costing $100,000 or more.

PREVENTION. Foodborne botulism is best prevented by adhering to safe methods of home canning (pressure cooker and acidification), by avoiding suspicious foods, and by heating all home-canned foods to 80° C for at least 5 min. Wound botulism is best prevented by thorough cleansing and surgical debridement of contaminated traumatic injuries with provision of appropriate antibiotics and by not abusing illicit drugs. Most infant botulism patients probably inhale and then swallow airborne clostridial spores; these cases are unpreventable. The one identified, avoidable source of botulinum spores for infants is *honey*. Honey is an unsafe food for any child less than 1 yr old. Corn syrups were once thought to be a possible source of botulinum spores, but recent evidence indicates otherwise. Breast-feeding appears to slow the onset of infant botulism and to diminish the risk of respiratory arrest in infants in whom the disease develops. Other preventive measures may emerge from a better understanding of the composition and determinants of the infant intestinal microflora, the pathophysiologic key to this unique infectious disease.

Arnon SS: Infant botulism: anticipating the second decade. J Infect Dis 154:201, 1986.

Arnon SS, Damus K, Chin J: Infant botulism: epidemiology and relation to sudden infant death syndrome. Epidemiol Rev 3:45, 1981.
Arnon SS, Damus K, Thompson B, et al: Protective role of human milk against sudden death from infant botulism. J Pediatr 100:568, 1982.
Arnon SS, Werner SB, Faber HK, Farr WH: Infant botulism in 1931: Discovery of a misclassified case. Am J Dis Child 133:580, 1979.
Aureli P, Fenicia L, Pasolini B, et al: Two cases of type E infant botulism in Italy caused by neurotoxigenic *Clostridium butyricum*. J Infect Dis 54:207, 1986.
Hurst DL, Marsh WW: Early severe infantile botulism. J Pediatr 122:909, 1993.
Long SS: Epidemiologic study of infant botulism in Pennsylvania: report of the infant botulism study group. J Pediatr 75:928, 1985.
Long SS, Gajeweski JL, Brown LW, Gilligan PH: Clinical, laboratory, and environmental features of infant botulism in southeastern Pennsylvania. Pediatrics 75:935, 1985.
MacDonald KL, Cohen ML, Blake PA: The changing epidemiology of adult botulism in the United States. Am J Epidemiol 124:794, 1986.
Montecucco C, Schiavo G: Tetanus and botulism neurotoxins: a new group of zinc proteases. Trends Biochem Sci 18:324, 1993.
Schreiner MS, Field E, Ruddy R: Infant botulism: a review of 12 years' experience at the Children's Hospital of Philadelphia. Pediatrics 87:159, 1991.
Smith LDS, Sugiyama H: *Botulism: The Organism, its Toxins, the Disease*, 2nd ed. Springfield, IL, Charles C. Thomas, 1988.
Thilo EH, Townsend SF, Deacon J: Infant botulism at 1 week of age: report of two cases. Pediatrics 92:151, 1993.
Weber JT, Goodpasture HC, Alexander H, et al: Wound botulism in a patient with a tooth abscess: case report and review. Clin Infect Dis 16:635, 1993.
Woodruff BA, Griffin PM, McCroskey LM, et al: Clinical and laboratory comparison of botulism from toxin types A, B, and E in the United States, 1975–88. J Infect Dis 166:1281, 1992.

CHAPTER 193

*Tetanus**

Stephen S. Arnon

DEFINITION. Tetanus (lockjaw) is an acute, spastic paralytic illness caused by tetanospasmin, the neurotoxin produced by *Clostridium tetani.*

ETIOLOGIC AGENT. *C. tetani* is a motile, gram-positive, spore-forming obligate anaerobe whose natural habitat worldwide is soil, dust, and the alimentary tracts of various animals. It forms spores terminally, thus producing a drumstick or tennis racket appearance microscopically. Tetanus spores can survive boiling but not autoclaving, but the vegetative cells are killed by antibiotics, heat, and standard disinfectants. Unlike many clostridia, *C. tetani* is not a tissue-invasive organism, instead causing illness through the effects of a single toxin, *tetanospasmin,* more commonly referred to as *tetanus toxin.* Tetanus toxin is the second most poisonous substance known, being surpassed in potency only by botulinum toxin; a lethal dose of tetanus toxin is estimated to be 10^{-6} mg/kg.

EPIDEMIOLOGY. Tetanus occurs worldwide and is endemic in 90 developing countries, but its incidence varies considerably. The most common form, neonatal (umbilical) tetanus, kills at least 500,000 infants each year because the mother was not immunized; over 70% of these deaths occur in just 10 tropical Asian and African countries. In addition, an estimated 15,000–30,000 unimmunized women worldwide die each year from maternal tetanus that results from postpartum, postabortal, or postsurgical wound infection with *C. tetani.* Approximately 50 cases of tetanus are reported each year in the United States, mostly in persons 60 years of age or older, but toddler-aged and neonatal cases also occur.

Most non-neonatal cases of tetanus are associated with a traumatic injury, often a penetrating wound inflicted by a dirty object, such as a nail, splinter, fragment of glass, or unsterile injection, but a rare case may have no history of trauma. Tetanus following illicit drug injection is becoming more common, while uncommon settings include animal bites, abscesses (including dental abscesses), ear piercing, chronic skin ulceration, burns, compound fractures, frostbite, gangrene, intestinal surgery, ritual scarification, and female circumcision. The disease also occurs after the use of contaminated suture material or after intramuscular injection of medicines, most notably quinine for chloroquine-resistant falciparum malaria.

PATHOGENESIS. Tetanus occurs after introduced spores germinate, multiply, and produce tetanus toxin in the low oxidation-reduction potential (E_h) of an infected injury site. A plasmid carries the toxin gene; the toxin is released with vegetative bacterial cell death and subsequent lysis. Tetanus toxins (and the botulinum toxins) are 150 kD simple proteins consisting of a heavy (100 kD) and a light (50 kD) chain joined by a single disulfide bond. Tetanus toxin binds at the neuromuscular junction and is then endocytosed by the motor nerve, after which it undergoes retrograde axonal transport to the cytoplasm of the alpha-motoneuron. In the sciatic nerve the transport rate was found to be 3.4 mm/hr. The toxin exits the motoneuron in the spinal cord and next enters adjacent, spinal inhibitory interneurons, where it prevents neurotransmitter release. Tetanus toxin thus blocks the normal inhibition of antagonistic muscles that is the basis of voluntary coordinated movement; in consequence, affected muscles sustain maximal contraction. The autonomic nervous system is also rendered unstable in tetanus.

The phenomenal potency of tetanus toxin is enzymatic in nature. The light chain of tetanus toxin (and of several of the botulinum toxins) is a Zn^{2+} containing endoprotease whose substrate is synaptobrevin, a constituent protein of the docking complex that enables the synaptic vesicle to fuse with the terminal cell membrane. The heavy chain of the toxin contains its binding domain.

PATHOLOGY. *C. tetani* is not an invasive organism and its toxin-producing vegetative cells remain where introduced into the wound, which may or may not display local inflammatory changes and a mixed infectious flora.

CLINICAL MANIFESTATIONS. Tetanus may be either localized or generalized, the latter being more common. The incubation period typically is 2–14 days, but may be as long as months after the injury. In *generalized tetanus* trismus (masseter muscle spasm, or "lockjaw") is the presenting symptom in about half the cases. Headache, restlessness, and irritability are early symptoms, often followed by stiffness, difficulty chewing, dysphagia, and neck muscle spasm. The so-called sardonic smile of tetanus (risus sardonicus) results from intractable spasm of facial and buccal muscles. When the paralysis extends to abdominal, lumbar, hip, and thigh muscles, the patient may assume an arched posture, opisthotonos, in which only the back of the head and the heels touch ground. Opisthotonos is an equilibrium position that results from unrelenting total contraction of opposing muscles, all of which display the typical "boardlike" rigidity of tetanus. Laryngeal and respiratory muscle spasm can lead to airway obstruction and asphyxiation. Because tetanus toxin does not affect sensory nerves or cortical function, the patient unfortunately remains conscious, in extreme pain, and in fearful anticipation of the next tetanic seizure. These seizures are characterized by sudden, severe tonic contractions of the muscles, with fist clenching, flexion, and adduction of the arms and hyperextension of the legs. Without treatment, the seizures range from a few seconds to a few minutes in length with intervening respite periods, but as the illness progresses the spasms become sustained and exhausting. The smallest disturbance by sight, sound, or touch may trigger a tetanic spasm. Dysuria and urinary retention result from bladder sphincter spasm; forced defecation may occur. Fever, occasionally as high as 40° C, is common because of the substantial metabolic energy consumed by spastic muscles. Notable autonomic effects include tachycardia, arrhythmias, labile hypertension, diaphoresis, and cutaneous vasoconstriction. The tetanic paralysis usually becomes more severe in the 1st wk after onset, stabilizes in the 2nd wk, and ameliorates gradually over the ensuing 1–4 wk.

Neonatal tetanus (tetanus neonatorum), the infantile form of generalized tetanus, typically manifests within 3–12 days of birth as progressive difficulty in feeding (i.e., sucking and swallowing), with associated hunger and crying. Paralysis or diminished movement, stiffness to the touch, and spasms, with or without opisthotonos, characterize the disease. The umbilical stump may hold remnants of dirt, dung, clotted blood or serum, or it may appear relatively benign.

Localized tetanus results in painful spasms of the muscles adjacent to the wound site and may precede generalized tetanus. *Cephalic tetanus* is a rare form of localized tetanus involving the bulbar musculature that occurs with wounds or foreign bodies in the head, nostrils, or face. It also occurs in association with chronic otitis media. Cephalic tetanus is characterized by retracted eyelids, deviated gaze, trismus, risus sardonicus, and spastic paralysis of tongue and pharyngeal musculature.

DIAGNOSIS AND DIFFERENTIAL DIAGNOSIS. The picture of tetanus is one of the most dramatic in medicine, and the diagnosis may be made clinically. The typical setting is an unimmunized patient (and/or mother) who was injured or born within the preceding 2 wk and who presents with trismus, other rigid muscles, and a clear sensorium.

Regular laboratory studies are usually normal. A peripheral leukocytosis may result from a secondary bacterial infection of the wound or may be stress induced from the sustained tetanic spasms. The cerebrospinal fluid (CSF) is normal, although the intense muscle contractions may raise its pressure. Neither the electroencephalogram nor the electromyogram show a characteristic pattern. *C. tetani* is not always visible on Gram stain of wound material, and it is isolated in only about one third of cases.

Fully developed, generalized tetanus cannot be mistaken for any other disease. However, trismus may result from parapharyngeal, retropharyngeal, or dental abscesses, or rarely, from acute encephalitis involving the brain stem. Either rabies or tetanus may follow an animal bite, and rabies may present as trismus with seizures. However, rabies may be distinguished from tetanus by its hydrophobia, marked dysphagia, predominantly clonic seizures, and CSF pleocytosis. Although strychnine poisoning may result in tonic muscle spasms and generalized seizure activity, it seldom produces trismus, and unlike tetanus general relaxation usually occurs between spasms. Hypocalcemia may produce *tetany,* characterized by laryngeal and carpopedal spasms, but trismus will be absent. Occasionally, epileptic seizures, narcotic withdrawal, or other drug reactions may suggest tetanus.

TREATMENT. Management of tetanus requires eradication of *C. tetani* and the wound environment conducive to its anaerobic multiplication, neutralization of all accessible tetanus toxin, control of seizures and respiration, palliation and provision of meticulous supportive care, and finally, prevention of recurrences.

Surgical wound excision and debridement is often needed to remove the foreign body or devitalized tissue that created anaerobic growth conditions. Surgery should be done promptly, after the administration of human tetanus immune globulin (TIG) and antibiotics. Excision of the umbilical stump in neonatal tetanus is no longer recommended.

Once tetanus toxin has begun its axonal ascent to the spinal cord, it cannot be neutralized by TIG. Accordingly, TIG is given as soon as possible to neutralize toxin that diffuses from the wound into the circulation before the toxin can bind at distant muscle groups. An optimal dose of TIG has not been determined. A single intramuscular injection of 500 U of TIG is sufficient to neutralize systemic tetanus toxin, but doses as high as 3,000–6,000 U are also recommended. Infiltration of TIG into the wound is now considered unnecessary. If TIG is unavailable, use of human intravenous immune globulin (IVIG), which contains 4–90 U/mL of TIG, or of equine- or bovine-derived tetanus antitoxin (TAT), may be necessary. IGIV may be considered for the treatment of tetanus if TIG is unavailable, but the dosage is not known, and it is not approved for this usage. The usual dose of TAT is 50,000–100,000 U, with half given intramuscularly and half intravenously, but as little as 10,000 U may be sufficient. Approximately 15% of patients given the usual dose of TAT will experience serum sickness. When using TAT, it is essential to check for possible sensitivity to horse serum, and desensitization may be needed. The human-derived immune globulins are much preferred because of their longer half-life (30 days) and the virtual absence of allergic and serum sickness side effects. Intrathecal TIG, given to neutralize tetanus toxin in the spinal cord, is not effective.

Penicillin G remains the antibiotic of choice because of its effective clostridiocidal action and its diffusability, an important consideration because blood flow to injured tissue may be compromised. The dose is 100,000 U/kg/24 hr divided and administered in 4–6 hr intervals for 10–14 days. Metronidazole appears to be equally effective. Erythromycin and tetracycline (in patients ≥9 yr old) are alternatives for penicillin-allergic patients.

All patients with generalized tetanus need muscle relaxants. Diazepam provides both relaxation and seizure control; the initial dose of 0.1–0.2 mg/kg every 3–6 hr given intravenously is then titrated to control the tetanic spasms, after which it is sustained for 2–6 wk before its tapered withdrawal. Magnesium sulfate, other benzodiazepines, chlorpromazine, dantrolene, and baclofen are also used. Intrathecal baclofen produces such complete muscle relaxation that apnea often ensues; like most other agents listed, baclofen should be used only in an intensive care unit setting. The best survival rates in generalized tetanus are achieved with neuromuscular blocking agents such as vecuronium and pancuronium, which produce a general flaccid paralysis that is then managed by mechanical ventilation. Autonomic instability is regulated with standard alpha- and beta- (or both) blocking agents; morphine has also proved useful.

Meticulous supportive care in a quiet, dark, secluded setting is most desirable. Because tetanic spasms may be triggered by minor stimuli, the patient should be sedated and protected from all unnecessary sounds, sights, and touch, and all therapeutic and other manipulations must be carefully scheduled and coordinated. Endotracheal intubation may not be required, but it should be done to prevent aspiration of secretions before laryngospasm develops. A tracheotomy kit should be immediately at hand for unintubated patients. However, endotracheal intubation and suctioning easily provoke reflex tetanic seizures and spasms, and early tracheostomy deserves consideration for severe cases not managed by pharmacologically induced flaccid paralysis. Cardiorespiratory monitoring, frequent suctioning, and maintenance of the substantial fluid, electrolyte, and caloric needs are fundamental. Careful nursing attention to mouth, skin, bladder, and bowel function is needed to avoid ulceration, infection, and obstipation. Prophylactic subcutaneous heparin use is sensible.

COMPLICATIONS. The seizures and the severe, sustained rigid paralysis of tetanus predispose the patient to many complications. Aspiration of secretions and pneumonia may have begun before the first medical attention is received. Maintaining airway patency often mandates endotracheal intubation and mechanical ventilation with their attendant hazards, including pneumothorax and mediastinal emphysema. The seizures may result in lacerations of the mouth or tongue, in intramuscular hematomas or rhabdomyolysis with myoglobinuria and renal failure, or in long bone or spinal fractures. Venous thrombosis, pulmonary embolism, gastric ulceration with or without hemorrhage, paralytic ileus, and decubitus ulceration are constant hazards. Excessive use of muscle relaxants, an integral part of care, may produce iatrogenic apnea. Cardiac arrhythmias, including asystole, unstable blood pressure, and labile temperature regulation reflect disordered autonomic nervous system control that may be aggravated by inattention to maintenance of intravascular volume needs.

PROGNOSIS. Recovery in tetanus occurs through regeneration of synapses within the spinal cord and thereby the restoration of muscle relaxation. However, because an episode of tetanus does not result in the production of toxin-neutralizing antibodies, active immunization with tetanus toxoid at discharge with provision for completion of the primary series is mandatory.

The most important factor influencing outcome is the quality of supportive care. Mortality is highest in the very young and the very old. A favorable prognosis is associated with a long incubation period, with the absence of fever, and with localized disease. An unfavorable prognosis is associated with a week or less between the injury and the onset of trismus and with 3 days or less between trismus and the onset of generalized tetanic spasms. Sequelae of hypoxic brain injury, especially in infants, include cerebral palsy, diminished mental abilities, and behavioral difficulties. Most fatalities occur within the 1st wk of illness. Reported case fatality rates for generalized tetanus range between 5% and 35% and for neonatal tetanus extend from <10% with intensive care treatment to >75% without it. Cephalic tetanus has an especially poor prognosis because of breathing and feeding difficulties.

PREVENTION. Tetanus is an entirely preventable disease; a serum antibody level of ≥0.01 U/mL is considered protective. Active immunization should begin in early infancy with combined diphtheria toxoid–tetanus toxoid–pertussis (DTP) vaccine at 2, 4, and 6 mo of age, with a booster at 4–6 yr of age and at 10 yr intervals thereafter throughout adult life with tetanus-diphtheria (Td) toxoids. Immunization of women with tetanus toxoid prevents neonatal tetanus; a single dose of toxoid that contains 250 Lf units may be safely given in the third trimester of pregnancy and provides enough transplacental antibody to protect the child for at least 4 mo. For unimmunized persons 7 or more yr old, the primary immunization series consists of three doses of Td toxoid given intramuscularly, the second 4–6 wk after the first and the third 6–12 mo after the second.

Tetanus prevention measures following trauma consist of inducing active immunity to tetanus toxin and of passively providing antitoxic antibody. Tetanus prophylaxis is an essential part of all wound management, but specific measures depend on the nature of the injury and the immunization status of the patient. Tetanus toxoid should always be given after a dog or other animal bite, even though *C. tetani* is infrequently found in canine mouth flora. All wounds, except those in a fully immunized patient, require human TIG. In any other circumstances (e.g., patients with an unknown or incomplete immunization history; or crush, puncture, or projectile wounds; wounds contaminated with saliva, soil, or feces; avulsion injuries; compound fractures; or frostbite), 250 U of TIG should be given intramuscularly, and increased to 500 U for highly tetanus-prone wounds (i.e., undebridable, with substantial bacterial contamination, or >24 hr old). If TIG is unavailable, then use of human IGIV may be considered. If neither of these products is available, then 3,000–5,000 U of equine- or bovine-derived tetanus antitoxin (TAT) may be given intramuscularly after testing for hypersensitivity; even at this dose, serum sickness may occur.

The wound itself should have immediate, thorough surgical cleansing and debridement to remove foreign bodies and any necrotic tissue in which anaerobic conditions might develop. Tetanus toxoid should be given to stimulate active immunity and may be administered concurrently with TIG (or TAT) if given in separate syringes at separate sites. A tetanus toxoid booster (preferably Td) is given to all persons with *any* wound if their tetanus immunization status is unknown or incomplete. A booster is given to injured persons who have completed their primary immunization series if (a) the wound is clean and minor but ≥10 yr have passed since the last booster, or (b) the wound is more serious and ≥5 yr have passed since the last booster. With delayed wound care, active immunization should be started at once. Although fluid tetanus toxoid produces a more rapid immune response than the adsorbed or precipitated toxoids, the adsorbed toxoid results in a more durable titer.

Abrutyn E, Berlin JA: Intrathecal therapy in tetanus: a meta-analysis. JAMA 226:2262, 1991.

Dastur FD, Awatramani VP, Chitre SK, et al: A single dose vaccine to prevent neonatal tetanus. J Assoc Phys India 41:97, 1993.

Expanded Program on Immunization: The global elimination of tetanus: progress to date. WHO Wk Epidemiol Rec 68:277, 1993.

Fauveau V, Mamdani M, Steinglass R, et al: Maternal tetanus: magnitude, epidemiology and potential control measures. Int J Gynecol Obstet 40:3, 1993.

Lee DC, Lederman HM: Anti-tetanus antibodies in intravenous gamma globulin: an alternative to tetanus immune globulin. J Infect Dis 166:642, 1992.

Luisto M: Unusual and iatrogenic sources of tetanus. Ann Chir Gynaec Fenn 82:25, 1993.

Luisto M, Iivanainen M: Tetanus of immunized children. Dev Med Child Neurol 35:346, 1993.

Montecucco C, Schiavo G: Tetanus and botulism neurotoxins: a new group of zinc proteases. Trends Biochem Sci 18:324, 1993.

Muguti GI, Dixon MS: Tetanus following human bite. Br J Plastic Surg 45:614, 1992.

Saissy JM, Demaziere J, Vitris M, et al: Treatment of severe tetanus by intrathecal injections of baclofen without artificial ventilation. Intensive Care Med 18:241, 1992.

Sesardic D, Wong MY, Gaines Das RE, et al: The first international standard for antitetanus globulin, human; pharmaceutical evaluation and international collaborative study. Biologicals 21:67, 1993.

Wesley AG, Pather M: Tetanus in children: an 11-year review. Ann Trop Pediatr 7:32, 1987.

Wright DK, Lalloo UG, Nayiger S, et al: Autonomic nervous system dysfunction in severe tetanus: current perspectives. Crit Care Med 17:371, 1989.

Yen LM, Dao LM, Day NPJ, et al: Role of quinine in the high mortality of intramuscular injection tetanus. Lancet 344:786, 1994.

CHAPTER 194

Anaerobic Infections

*Stephen S. Arnon**

OTHER CLOSTRIDIAL INFECTIONS

The genus *Clostridium* encompasses all gram-positive, anaerobic, spore-forming bacilli, which are widely distributed in nature and are responsible for a variety of infectious syndromes, including bacteremia and intra-abdominal, biliary, pulmonary, genital tract, central nervous system, and soft tissue infections, including gas gangrene (myonecrosis).

ETIOLOGY. More than 60 species comprise the clostridia, but only a few are important human pathogens. In the developed world, *C. difficile* is the most commonly isolated species because of its etiologic role in antibiotic-associated colitis (pseudomembranous colitis), which principally affects adults. Elsewhere, with the possible exception of *C. tetani* (see Chapter 193), *C. perfringens* remains the most common human pathogen; it is

*Modified from sections in the 14th edition by R. D. Feigin and K. M. Finta.

immunocompromised status and exposure to potable water are the major risk factors. Infection in a few children with chronic pulmonary disease without immune deficiency has also been reported. Apparently, infection in children lacking any risk factors is very uncommon. The modes of transmission of community-acquired disease in children include exposure to mists, water coolers, and other aerosol-generating apparatuses. Nosocomial *Legionella* infection occurs more frequently than community-acquired disease in children, and the modes of acquisition include microaspiration, frequently associated with nasogastric tubes, and aerosol inhalation. Bronchopulmonary *Legionella* infections occur in patients with cystic fibrosis and has been associated with aerosol therapy or mist tents. Legionnaires' disease is also reported in pediatric patients with asthma and tracheal stenosis.

Pontiac fever in adults and children is characterized by high fever, myalgia, headache, and extreme debilitation, lasting for a few days. Cough, breathlessness, diarrhea, confusion, and chest pain may occur, but there is no evidence for invasive infection. The disease is self-limited without sequelae. Virtually all exposed individuals seroconvert to *Legionella* antigens. A very large outbreak in Scotland that affected 35 children was attributed to *L. micdadei*, which was isolated from a whirlpool spa. The onset of illness was 1–7 days (median, 3 days), and all exposed children developed significant titers of specific antibodies to *L. micdadei*. The pathogenesis of Pontiac fever is not known. In the absence of evidence of true infection, the most likely hypothesis is that this syndrome is caused by a toxic or hypersensitivity reaction to microbial, or protozoan, antigens.

LABORATORY DIAGNOSIS. Culture of *Legionella* from sputum, other respiratory tract specimens, blood, or tissue is the gold standard method against which indirect methods of detection should be compared. Specimens obtained from the respiratory tract that are contaminated with oral flora must be treated and processed to reduce contaminants and plated onto selective media. Since these are costly and time-consuming methods, many laboratories do not process specimens for culture. The microorganisms can be identified presumptively by direct immunofluorescence antibody (DFA) screening, although the sensitivity of the test is generally low in most laboratories, in part because of the lack of antisera directed against other *Legionella* serogroups and species. This method failed to detect the infection in several well-documented pediatric cases. Retrospective diagnosis can be made serologically using the indirect immunofluorescence assay to detect specific antibody production. Seroconversion may not occur for several weeks following onset of infection, and the available serologic assays do not detect all strains of *L. pneumophila* or all species. In view of the low sensitivity of direct detection and the slow growth of the microorganism in culture, the diagnosis of legionellosis should be pursued actively when there is suggestive clinical evidence, including the lack of response to "usual" antibiotics, even when other laboratory studies are negative.

TREATMENT. Erythromycin, with or without rifampin, has been empirically established as effective therapy. The newer macrolides, including azithromycin and clarithromycin, and the fluoroquinolone agents (ciprofloxacin) are more active than erythromycin in experimental models of infection. In serious infections or in high-risk patients, parenteral therapy is recommended initially; a switch to oral therapy can be made when the patient has had a clinical response. The duration of therapy for Legionnaires' disease is 2–3 wk. Treatment of extrapulmonary infections, including prosthetic valve endocarditis and sternal wound infections, may require prolonged therapy. Alternative antibiotics include doxycycline and trimethoprim-sulfamethoxazole (TMP-SMZ). Beta-lactams and aminoglycosides, and other antibiotics that do not penetrate mammalian cells, are not clinically effective. Relapse (recrudescence) may occur following cessation of erythromycin therapy.

PROGNOSIS. The mortality rate of community acquired Legionnaires' disease in adults is approximately 15%. The prognosis depends upon underlying host factors and possibly upon the duration of the illness before appropriate therapy is begun. In spite of appropriate antibiotic therapy, patients may succumb to respiratory complications, such as acute respiratory distress syndrome, associated with artificial ventilation and intubation.

Anderson RD, Lauer BA, Fraser DW, et al: Infections with *Legionella pneumophila* in children. J Infect Dis 143:386, 1981.

Brady MT: Nosocomial Legionnaires' disease in a children's hospital. J Pediatr 115:46, 1989.

Edelstein PH. Legionnaires' disease. Clin Infect Dis 16:741, 1993.

Goldberg DJ, Collier PW, Fallon RJ, et al: Lochgoilhead fever: outbreak of non-pneumonic legionellosis due to *Legionella micdadei*. Lancet 1:316, 1989.

Holmberg RE Jr, Pavia AT: Nosocomial *Legionella* pneumonia in the neonate. Pediatrics 92:450, 1993.

Lowry PW, Tompkins LS: Nosocomial legionellosis: a review of pulmonary and extrapulmonary syndromes. Am J Infect Control 21:21, 1993.

Muder RR, Hu VL, Woo AH: Mode of transmission of *Legionella pneumophila*. A critical review. Arch Intern Med 146:1607, 1986.

CHAPTER 196
Mycoplasmal Infections

Dwight A. Powell

RESPIRATORY MYCOPLASMAS

Among the five mycoplasma species isolated from the human respiratory tract, *Mycoplasma pneumoniae* is the only known human pathogen. It is a major cause of respiratory infections in school-aged children and young adults.

ETIOLOGY. *M. pneumoniae*, originally thought to be a virus and called the Eaton agent, was found to be a mycoplasma in the early 1960s. Mycoplasmas are the smallest self-replicating biologic system and are dependent on attachment to host cells for obtaining essential precursors such as nucleotides, fatty acids, sterols, and amino acids. They contain double-stranded DNA with genome sizes ranging from 577 to 1380 kb. Growth of *M. pneumoniae* in commercially available culture systems is fastidious and generally too slow to be of practical clinical use.

EPIDEMIOLOGY. *M. pneumoniae* infections occur worldwide. In contrast to the acute, short-lived epidemics of some respiratory agents, *M. pneumoniae* infection is endemic in larger communities, with epidemic outbreaks occurring every 4–7 yr. In smaller communities, infections are sporadic with long-lasting and smoldering outbreaks occurring at irregular intervals. Infections occur throughout the year.

The occurrence of mycoplasmal illness is related, in part, to the age and immune status of the patient. Overt illness is unusual before 3–4 yr of age; younger children appear to have frequent mild or subclinical infections, and reinfections appear to be common. The peak incidence of illness occurs in school-aged children: *M. pneumoniae* accounts for 33% and 70% of all pneumonias in children aged 5–9 yr and 9–15 yr, respectively. Recurrent infections occur infrequently but are well documented to occur in adults at intervals of 4–7 yr.

M. pneumoniae infections are not highly communicable, as evidenced by the slow rate at which susceptible family contacts become infected; such periods may extend for weeks or months. Infection occurs through the respiratory route by large droplet spread, and the incubation period is thought to be 1–3 wk. Explosive epidemics have been reported among military recruits and summer camps for children.

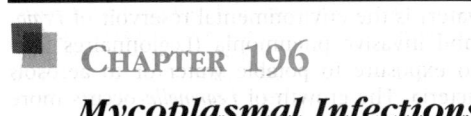

PATHOLOGY, IMMUNOLOGY, AND PATHOGENESIS. Cells of the ciliated respiratory epithelium are the target cells of *M. pneumoniae* infection. The organism is an elongated snakelike structure with an attachment tip characterized by an electron-dense core and a trilaminar outer membrane. Attachment to the ciliary membrane is mediated by a P1 adhesion protein localized to the mycoplasma membrane of the attachment tip.

Restriction fragment length polymorphisms and sequence divergence are observed in the P1 gene, permitting classification of clinical isolates of *M. pneumoniae* into groups I and II. Pretreatment of *M. pneumoniae* with anti-P1 antibody inhibits attachment and subsequent disease in experimental animals. The organisms attach to cell surfaces via sialated glycoprotein receptors and burrow down between cells, resulting in eventual sloughing of the cells. Although the mechanisms of cytopathology have not been determined, intracellular organisms have not been found, and *M. pneumoniae* rarely invade beyond the basement membrane.

A variety of serologic responses occur following *M. pneumoniae* infection. Nonspecific cold hemagglutinins reacting to the I antigen of red blood cell glycoproteins are usually the first antibodies detected. Appearing with titers of at least 1:32 in approximately 50% of patients, cold hemagglutinins develop late in the 1st or 2nd wk of illness, and increase fourfold or more by the 3rd wk. They disappear in about 6 wk. The presence of elevated titers of cold hemagglutinins and the height of the titer correlate with the severity of the illness. Specific immunologic reactions to *M. pneumoniae* can be measured by a variety of techniques and persist for long periods of time.

Although the presence of circulating antibodies in humans can be correlated with protection against *M. pneumoniae* infections, studies in the hamster have shown that circulating antibody alone, in the absence of other forms of immunity, is incompletely protective. In hamsters, most of the peribronchial mononuclear cells are laden with antibody. However, ablation of the T-cell system with antithymocyte serum completely prevents the development of pneumonia. Thus, the disease produced by *M. pneumoniae* is very complex; the immunologic response of the host may be responsible for the disease itself as well as for protection against it, depending on the qualitative and quantitative balance of humoral and cellular immunity. Patients with immunodeficiency states such as hypogammaglobulinemia and sickle cell anemia may have more severe mycoplasma pneumonia than do normal hosts. *M. pneumoniae* is the most common infectious cause of acute chest syndrome in sickle cell patients but is not prevalent in patients with acquired immune deficiency syndrome (AIDS).

CLINICAL MANIFESTATIONS. Bronchopneumonia is the most commonly recognized clinical syndrome following *M. pneumoniae* infections. Although the onset of illness may be abrupt, it is usually characterized by gradual onset of headache, malaise, fever, rhinorrhea, and sore throat with progression of lower respiratory symptoms, including hoarseness and cough. Coryza is unusual in *M. pneumoniae* pneumonia and usually suggests a viral etiology. Although the clinical course in untreated individuals is variable, coughing usually worsens during the first 2 wk of illness, and then all symptoms gradually resolve within 3–4 wk. The cough is initially nonproductive, but older children and adolescents may produce a frothy white sputum. The severity of symptoms is usually greater than the condition suggested by the physical signs, which appear later in the disease. Rales, which are often fine and crackling and resemble those heard in asthma and bronchiolitis, are the most prominent sign. With progression of the disease, the fever intensifies, the cough becomes more troublesome, and the patient may become dyspneic.

Roentgenographic findings are not specific. Pneumonia is usually described as interstitial or bronchopneumonic; involvement is most common in the lower lobes, with unilateral centrally dense infiltrates described in 75% of cases. Lobar pneumonia is seen infrequently. Hilar lymphadenopathy may be described in up to 33% of patients. Significant amounts of pleural fluid are unusual, but patients with large effusions due to *M. pneumoniae* have been described as having more severe and prolonged illness compared with those without pleural involvement. The white blood cell and differential counts are usually normal, while the sedimentation rate is usually elevated.

Additional respiratory illnesses caused infrequently by *M. pneumoniae* include undifferentiated upper respiratory tract infections, pharyngitis, sinusitis, croup, bronchitis, and bronchiolitis. *M. pneumoniae* is a common inducer of wheezing in asthmatic children. Otitis media and bullous myringitis have been described but are rarely seen without associated lower respiratory tract infection.

Despite the rare isolation of *M. pneumoniae* from nonrespiratory sites such as joints, pleurae, and cerebrospinal fluid (CSF), nonrespiratory illness is generally thought to involve autoimmune mechanisms rather than direct organism invasion. Patients with respiratory infections may occasionally manifest illness involving the skin, central nervous system (CNS), blood, heart, gastrointestinal tract, and joints. Skin lesions include a variety of exanthems, most notably maculopapular rashes, erythema multiforme, and the Stevens-Johnson syndrome (SJS). SJS associated with *M. pneumoniae* usually develops 3–21 days after initial respiratory symptoms, lasts less than 14 days, and is rarely associated with severe complications. Meningoencephalitis, transverse myelitis, aseptic meningitis, cerebellar ataxia, and the Guillain-Barré syndrome have been reported. Encephalitis may occur without respiratory symptoms and most commonly manifests as seizures (50%), impaired consciousness (75%), and meningeal signs (85%). CSF is usually normal. Mild degrees of hemolysis with positive Coombs test and minor reticulocytosis occurring 2–3 wk after the onset of illness is common. Severe hemolysis with high titers of cold hemagglutinins ($\geq$1:512) is rare, as are thrombocytopenia and coagulation defects. Mild hepatitis, pancreatitis, and protein-losing hypertrophic gastropathy are reported gastrointestinal complications. Myocarditis, pericarditis, and a rheumatic fever-like syndrome are uncommon manifestations but arrhythmias, ST-, and T-wave changes and cardiac dilation with heart failure may accompany *M. pneumoniae* infection in adults more commonly than children. Transient monoarticular arthritis was described in 1% of patients in one large series.

DIAGNOSIS. No specific clinical, epidemiologic, or laboratory observations permit a definite diagnosis of mycoplasmal infection early in the clinical course. Certain observations, however, are suggestive and can be helpful to the astute physician. For example, pneumonia in school-aged children and young adults, especially if cough is a prominent finding, is always suggestive of *M. pneumoniae* disease. Cultures of the throat or sputum on special media may demonstrate *M. pneumoniae*, but growth is rarely detected earlier than 1 wk. Serum cold hemagglutinins in a titer of 1:64 or greater or a positive IgM *M. pneumoniae* antibody support the diagnosis. A rise or fall in convalescent-phase complement-fixing serum antibody to *M. pneumoniae* obtained after 10 days to 3 wk is diagnostic. Rapid diagnostic tests to detect the presence of *M. pneumoniae* antigens or DNA are not commercially available, but several promising approaches are emerging. When *M. pneumoniae* is confirmed in the community in a few patients, the probability of the existence of other mycoplasmal illnesses is greatly increased.

TREATMENT. In general, *M. pneumoniae* illness is mild, and hospitalization is infrequent. Fatal infections are rare. Complications are unusual, as is bacterial superinfection. *M. pneumoniae* is exceptionally sensitive to erythromycin, clarithromycin, scarring and blindness. Bacterial superinfection may contribute to the scarring. Blindness occurs years after the active disease. Trachoma is caused primarily by the A, B, Ba, and C serotypes of *C. trachomatis*. In areas that are endemic for trachoma, such as Egypt, genital chlamydial infection is caused by the serotypes responsible for oculogenital disease: D, E, F, G, H, I, J, and K.

Trachoma can be diagnosed clinically. The World Health Organization suggests that at least two of the following four criteria be met for diagnosis: lymphoid follicles on the upper tarsal conjunctivae, typical conjunctival scarring, vascular pannus, and limbal follicles. The diagnosis is confirmed by culture or staining methods during the active stage of the disease. Serologic tests are not helpful clinically because of the long duration of the disease and high background prevalence of antibody in many populations where trachoma is endemic. Poverty and lack of sanitation are important factors in the spread of trachoma. As socioeconomic conditions improve, the incidence of the disease decreases substantially. Treatment is discussed within each of the following sections.

Oculogenital Infections in Adults and Adolescents

EPIDEMIOLOGY. The trachoma biovar of *C. trachomatis* causes a large spectrum of diseases that occur in sexually active adults. In men, it is the cause of 30–50% of all cases of nongonococcal urethritis. The Centers for Disease Control estimate that probably one to three cases of chlamydial urethritis occur for every reported case of gonococcal urethritis. The symptoms are less acute than gonorrhea, and the discharge is usually mucoid rather than purulent. As many as 50% of men with gonorrhea may be coinfected with *C. trachomatis*.

C. trachomatis is the major cause of epididymitis in men less than 35 yr of age. It can cause proctitis. Proctocolitis may develop in individuals who have rectal infection with an LGV strain. Asymptomatic urethral infection is frequent in sexually active men. Autoinoculation from the genitals to the eyes can lead to inclusion conjunctivitis.

In women, *C. trachomatis* infects the endocervix; women may have mucopurulent cervicitis but frequently are asymptomatic. The prevalence of cervical chlamydial infection among sexually active women ranges from 2% to 35%. Rates of infection among adolescent girls exceed 20% in many urban populations but can be as high as 15% in suburban populations as well. *C. trachomatis* can infect the urethra, leading to the urethral syndrome of dysuria with "sterile" pyuria. Complications of genital chlamydial infections in women include perihepatitis (Fitz-Hugh-Curtis syndrome) and salpingitis. The latter may cause significant morbidity, leading to infertility and ectopic pregnancy.

Teenagers may be at higher risk for developing complications, especially salpingitis, than older women. Salpingitis in these girls is also more likely to lead to tubal scarring, subsequent obstruction with secondary infertility, and increased risk of ectopic pregnancy.

DIAGNOSIS. The definitive diagnosis of genital chlamydial infection is by isolation of the organism in tissue culture from the urethra in men and the endocervix in women. *C. trachomatis* can be grown in cycloheximide-treated HeLa, McCoy, and HEp-2 cells. *Chlamydia* culture has been further defined by the Centers for Disease Control as isolation of the organism in tissue culture and confirmation by microscopic identification of the characteristic inclusions by fluorescent antibody staining. Care should be taken to obtain cells, not discharge. Alternatively, one of the recently developed nonculture methods can be used. The four types currently available are a direct fluorescent antibody (DFA) test, in which chlamydial EBs are identified directly on a specimen smear stained with a conjugated antichlamydial monoclonal antibody, enzyme immunoassay (EIAs), DNA probe, and a recently approved polymerase chain reaction (PCR) assay. The DFA, EIA, and DNA probes perform best for screening in high-prevalence populations (prevalence of infection >7%). All of these assays perform equivalently when compared with culture, with sensitivities ranging from 80% to over 90% and specificities over 95%. PCR is probably the most sensitive and specific nonculture test available, but data on performance in clinical settings are limited. Nonculture tests can also be used to test for the presence of *C. trachomatis* in concentrated male urine.

TREATMENT. The 1993 STD Treatment Guidelines from the Centers for Disease Control (CDC) recommend either doxycycline, 100 mg bid for 7 days, or azithromycin, 1 g, as a single dose, for the treatment of uncomplicated genital infection in men and nonpregnant women. Neither of these regimens can be used in pregnant women. Another alternative regimen is ofloxacin, 300 mg bid for 7 days. Ofloxacin cannot be used during pregnancy or in persons ≤17 yr of age. In pregnant women, the CDC recommends three different regimens of oral erythromycin base or ethylsuccinate (800 mg qid for 7 days or 400 mg qid for 14 days) or amoxicillin, 500 mg tid for 7–10 days. Experience with any of these regimens is limited. Because *C. trachomatis* may be responsible for 25–50% of all cases of salpingitis, any therapeutic regimen should also contain doxycycline or tetracycline. Sexual partners should always be treated as well.

Perinatally Transmitted Infections

Cervical chlamydial infection is reported in 20–30% of pregnant women. Genital infections, are frequently asymptomatic, especially in women. If a woman has active chlamydial infection during pregnancy, her infant may acquire the infection during parturition. The risk of transmission from mother to infant is about 50%. The infant may become infected at one or more anatomic sites, including the conjunctivae, nasopharynx, rectum, and vagina. Approximately 70% of infected infants are infected in the nasopharynx. Clinically, the infant may develop conjunctivitis or pneumonia.

INCLUSION CONJUNCTIVITIS. *C. trachomatis* is the most frequent identifiable infectious cause of neonatal conjunctivitis, and conjunctivitis is the major *clinical manifestation* of neonatal chlamydial infection. Approximately 30–50% of infants born to chlamydial-positive mothers develop conjunctivitis. The incubation period is 5–14 days after delivery, or earlier with premature rupture of membranes. Infection is rare following cesarean section with intact membranes. At least 50% of infants with chlamydial conjunctivitis also have nasopharyngeal infection. The presentation is extremely variable, ranging from mild conjunctival injection with scant mucoid discharge to severe conjunctivitis with copious purulent discharge, chemosis, and pseudomembrane formation. The conjunctiva may be very friable and bleed when stroked with a swab. Chlamydial conjunctivitis should be differentiated from gonococcal ophthalmia.

PNEUMONIA. Pneumonia due to *C. trachomatis* develops in 10–20% of infants born to women with chlamydial infection. Only about 25% of infants with nasopharyngeal chlamydial infection develop pneumonia. *C. trachomatis* pneumonia of infancy has a very characteristic presentation. The onset is usually between 1 and 3 mo of age and is often insidious, with persistent cough, tachypnea, and lack of fever. Auscultation reveals rales; wheezing is uncommon. The absence of wheezing and lack of fever helps to distinguish *C. trachomatis* from respiratory syncytial virus (RSV) pneumonia. A distinctive laboratory finding is the presence of peripheral eosinophilia (>400 cells per mm^3). The most consistent finding on chest radiograph is hyperinflation accompanied by interstitial or alveolar infiltrates.

INFECTIONS AT OTHER SITES. Infants born to chlamydia-positive mothers may become infected in the rectum and vagina. Although infection at these sites appears to be totally asymptomatic, the infection may cause confusion if detected at a later date. Perinatally acquired rectal, vaginal, and nasopharyngeal infections may persist for at least 3 yr. *C. pneumoniae* can also be confused with *C. trachomatis* in nasopharyngeal cultures if a genus-specific monoclonal antibody is used for culture confirmation.

DIAGNOSIS OF *C. TRACHOMATIS* CONJUNCTIVITIS AND PNEUMONIA. The gold standard remains isolation by culture of *C. trachomatis* from the conjunctiva or nasopharynx. Several nonculture methods have U.S. Food and Drug Administration (FDA) approval for diagnosis of chlamydial conjunctivitis, specifically DFA and EIA. These tests have sensitivities of ≥90% and specificities of ≥95% for conjunctival specimens compared to culture. Their accuracy for nasopharyngeal specimens is not as good. DNA probe and PCR assays are not approved for testing any sites in children, including the conjunctiva. Nonculture tests should never be used to test rectal or vaginal specimens from children. Because all of the available EIAs use genus-specific antibodies, these tests will also detect *C. pneumoniae* if used for respiratory specimens.

PREVENTION AND TREATMENT. An initial study in 1980 suggested that neonatal ocular prophylaxis with erythromycin ointment could prevent chlamydial conjunctivitis, but subsequent studies have not confirmed this observation. The best way to prevent neonatal chlamydial infection is prenatal screening and treatment of pregnant women, as is done for gonococcal infection. Treatment of *C. trachomatis* infection requires 1–2 wk of erythromycin, which causes problems related to compliance and tolerance. The CDC and the American Association of Pediatrics (AAP) recommend an oral erythromycin suspension, 50 mg/kg/24 hr in 2 or 4 divided doses, for 10–14 days, for both conjunctivitis and pneumonia in infants. The rationale for using oral therapy for conjunctivitis is that 50% or more of these infants have nasopharyngeal infection or disease in other sites, and studies have demonstrated the lack of efficacy of topical therapy with sulfonamide drops and erythromycin ointment. The failure rate with oral erythromycin remains 10–20%, and some infants require a second course of treatment. There are no treatment studies of *C. trachomatis* pneumonia but these infants should be treated with erythromycin, in the same dosage for 2 wk.

Infections in Older Children

C. trachomatis is not associated with specific clinical syndromes in older infants and children. Children who have been sexually abused may acquire anogenital infection. These infections usually are asymptomatic. It is not known whether *C. trachomatis* causes vaginitis. Perinatally acquired rectal and vaginal infections may persist for at least 3 yr; the presence of *C. trachomatis* in the vagina or rectum of a prepubertal child is not absolute evidence of sexual abuse. Cultures, rather than DFA or EIA methods, should be obtained from these sites when a prepubertal child is being evaluated, in order to avoid false-positive results.

Lymphogranuloma Venereum

LGV is a systemic, sexually transmitted disease caused by the L_1, L_2, and L_3 serotypes of the LGV biovar. Unlike strains of the trachoma biovar, LGV strains have a predilection for lymphoid tissue. About 20 cases of LGV have been reported in children. Fewer than 1,000 cases are reported in adults in the United States each year.

CLINICAL MANIFESTATIONS. The first stage of LGV is characterized by the appearance of the primary lesion, a painless, usually transient papule on the genitals. The second stage is characterized by lymphadenitis of lymphadenopathy, with enlarging, painful buboes, usually in the groin. The nodes may break down and drain, especially in males. In females, the lymphatic drainage of the vulva is to the retroperitoneal nodes. Fever, myalgia, and headache are common. In the tertiary stage, a full-blown genitoanorectal syndrome is seen, with rectovaginal fistulas, rectal strictures, and urethral destruction.

DIFFERENTIAL DIAGNOSIS. Chancroid and herpes simplex virus (HSV) can readily be distinguished from LGV because of the concurrent presence of painful genital ulcers. The nodes in chancroid may also break down and drain. Syphilis can be readily differentiated by serology and a history of a chancre. However, coinfections can occur. LGV is diagnosed by culture of *C. trachomatis* from a bubo aspirate or serologically. Most patients with LGV have complement-fixing antibody titers above 1:16.

TREATMENT. Doxycycline, 100 mg by mouth for 21 days, is the recommended treatment. Alternative regimens include erythromycin 500 mg qid for 21 days or sulfisoxizole, 500 mg qid for 21 days.

INFECTIONS DUE TO *C. PNEUMONIAE,* STRAIN TWAR

EPIDEMIOLOGY. The first isolates of *C. pneumoniae* were obtained during trachoma studies in the 1960s. Subsequent serologic studies demonstrated that the organism caused an outbreak of mild pneumonia among school children in Finland in 1978. In 1986, the organism was isolated from the respiratory tract of college students with acute respiratory disease. DNA studies show less than 5% relatedness between *C. pneumoniae* and *C. trachomatis* and *C. psittaci*. Ultrastructural studies demonstrate a loose periplasmic membrane, giving the EB a pear-shaped appearance distinct from the other two species. However, some strains of *C. pneumoniae* resemble *C. trachomatis* and *C. trachomatis* and *C. psittaci*. *C. pneumoniae* appears to be a primary human respiratory pathogen, but no zoonotic reservoir has been identified. Transmission is probably from person to person through respiratory droplets. Spread of the infection occurs among members in the same household. *C. pneumoniae* may be responsible for 10–20% of community-acquired "atypical" pneumonia, including acute chest syndrome in children with sickle-cell disease, 10% of bronchitis, and 5–10% of pharyngitis. *C. peumoniae* appears to affect individuals of all ages. A recent multicenter study of community-acquired pneumonia in children, 3–12 yr of age, found evidence of *C. pneumoniae* infection in 16% and *Mycoplasma pneumoniae* in 22%. The prevalence of *C. pneumoniae* infection in the children ≤6 yr of age was 15% and 18% in those >6 yr of age. Almost 20% of the children with *C. pneumoniae* infection were coinfected with *M. pneumoniae*.

C. pneumoniae may serve as an infectious trigger for asthma and for pulmonary exacerbations in patients with cystic fibrosis. *C. pneumoniae* is isolated from middle-ear aspirates of adults and children with acute otitis media. Asymptomatic respiratory infection is documented in 2–5% of adults and children, and may persist for 1 yr or longer.

Serologic surveys document a rising prevalence of *C. pneumoniae* antibody beginning in school-age children and reaching 30–45% by adolescence, suggesting that clinically inapparent infection is common.

CLINICAL MANIFESTATIONS. Clinically, infections caused by *C. pneumoniae* cannot be readily differentiated from thoses caused by other agents, especially *M. pneumoniae*. The pneumonia usually presents as a classic atypical (or nonbacterial) pneumonia, characterized by mild to moderate constitutional symptoms, including fever, malaise, headache, cough, and frequently pharyngitis. The chest radiograph often looks worse than the patient. Auscultation reveals the presence of rales and often wheezing. Chest radiographs reveal lobar infiltrates. Pleural effusions can also be present. *C. pneumoniae* has been isolated from pleural fluid. The complete blood count is often unremarkable.

DIAGNOSIS. Specific diagnosis of *C. pneumoniae* infection is based on isolation of the organism in tissue culture and serology. *C. pneumoniae* grows best in cycloheximide-treated HEp-2 and HL cells. The optimum site for culture is the posterior nasopharynx, collected with wire-shafted swabs in the same manner as for *C. trachomatis*. The organism can also be isolated from sputum, throat cultures, bronchoalveolar lavage fluid, and pleural fluid.

Direct detection of elementary bodies in clinical specimens using fluorescent antibody stains is sometimes possible, but it is not very sensitive or specific. Chlamydial antigen is detected in some clinical specimens by EIA. All the currently available EIAs detect *C. pneumoniae* as well as *C. trachomatis* because they use polyclonal or genus-specific monoclonal antibodies. Initial reports of the use of PCR appear to be promising, but there are no commercially available kits.

Serologic diagnosis can be accomplished using the microimmunofluorescence (MIF) and the CF tests. The CF test is genus specific and is used for diagnosis of lymphogranuloma venereum and psittacosis. Most individuals with oculogenital *C. trachomatis* infections do not have detectable CF antibody. Its sensitivity in hospitalized patients with *C. pneumoniae* infection is variable. Criteria for serologic diagnosis of *C. pneumoniae* infection are for acute infection, the patient should have a fourfold rise in the MIF IgG titer or a single IgM titer $\geq$1:16 or a single IgG titer $\geq$1:512; past or pre-existing infection is defined as an IgG titer $\geq$1:16 and $<$1:512. These criteria are based mainly on data from adults. Studies of *C. pneumoniae* infection in children with pneumonia and asthma show that almost 50% will have no detectable MIF antibody.

TREATMENT. Information about the response of *C. pneumoniae* infection to antibiotic therapy is limited. In vitro susceptibilities indicate that tetracyclines and erythromycin as well as several new macrolides (azithromycin and clarithromycin) and quinolones (ofloxacin) are active in vitro. Like *C. psittaci, C. pneumoniae* is highly resistant to sulfonamides. The optimum dose and duration of therapy remain uncertain. Anecdotal data suggest that prolonged therapy (i.e., at least 2 wk) may be desirable because recrudescent symptoms have been described following 2 wk courses of erythromycin and even after 30 days of tetracycline or doxycycline. The dose and duration of therapy recommended for treating *M. pneumoniae*, 1 g erythromycin per day for 10 days, is probably not adequate. Preliminary data in children with *C. pneumoniae* pneumonia suggest that an erythromycin suspension of 40–50 mg/kg/24 hr day for 10–14 days is effective in eradication of the organism from the nasopharynx in more than 80% of cases.

INFECTIONS DUE TO *C. PSITTACI* (PSITTACOSIS)

EPIDEMIOLOGY. *C. psittaci* is a very diverse species that infects most avian and mammalian species. There is only 10% DNA homology between *C. psittaci* and *C. trachomatis*. *C. psittaci* is differentiated from *C. trachomatis* by lack of glycogen in the inclusions, inclusion morphology, and resistance to sulfonamides. Analysis of strains of *C. psittaci* indicates that there are at least five biovars. The avian biovar contains at least four serovars, as determined by monoclonal antibody staining. Two of these serovars, psittacine and turkey, are of major importance in the avian population of the United States.

Psittacosis caused 1,136 cases and 8 deaths in the United States from 1975 to 1984. Seventy percent of the cases were the result of exposure to pet caged birds. Those at highest risk of acquiring psittacosis included bird owners or fanciers, pet shop employees, or pigeon fanciers. Several major outbreaks of psittacosis have occurred in turkey processing plants. Workers exposed to turkey viscera were at the highest risk of infection. Inhalation of aerosols from feces, fecal dust, and secretions of animals infected with *C. psittaci* is the primary route of infection. Source birds are asymptomatically infected or have anorexia, ruffled feathers, lethargy, and watery green droppings. Psittacosis is uncommon in children. Children may be less likely to be exposed to birds.

CLINICAL MANIFESTATIONS. The mean incubation period is 15 days after exposure, with a range of 5–21 days. The onset is usually abrupt with complaints of fever, cough, and headache. The fever is high and often associated with rigors and sweats. The headache can be so severe that meningitis is considered. The cough is usually nonproductive. Rales may be heard on auscultation. Chest radiographs are usually abnormal with variable infiltrates, and pleural effusions may be present. The white blood cell count is usually not elevated, but there may be a mild leukocytosis. Abnormal liver function tests, including elevated aspartate aminotransferase, alkaline phosphatase, and bilirubin, are common.

DIAGNOSIS AND TREATMENT. The diagnosis of psittacosis can be difficult because of the varying clinical presentations. A history of exposure to birds is very important but as many as 20% of patients with psittacosis have no known contact. Pneumonia due to *C. pneumoniae* should be suspected if there is evidence of person-to-person spread, which is unusual with psittacosis. Other infections that produce the syndrome of pneumonia with high fever, unusually severe headache, and myalgia include *M. pneumoniae*, tularemia, tuberculosis, fungal infections, Legionnaires' disease, and, of course, bacterial infection. The diagnosis of psittacosis in humans is based on clinical presentation, epidemiology, and serology. Culture of *C. psittaci* is not available outside of research laboratories.

Cases of psittacosis are classified based on laboratory findings or exposures: (1) Confirmed case—clinical specimen yielding *C. psittaci* or compatible clinical illness and fourfold rise in CF antibody titer; (2) presumptive case—compatible clinical illness and single serum sample titer of $\geq$1:32 or a stable antibody titer of $\geq$1:32 in two samples; (3) suspect case—a case that does not meet the criteria in one or two but is associated with another case of avian chlamydiosis. The CF test is a genus-specific test, thus infection due to *C. pneumoniae* can give titers $\geq$1:32. Early treatment with tetracycline may suppress the antibody response.

The recommended treatment for psittacosis in humans is 500 mg tetracycline every 6 hr, orally for 7–10 days. Erythromycin, 2 g day for 7–10 days, is an alternative regimen.

Alexander ER, Harrison HR: Role of *Chlamydia trachomatis* in perinatal infection. Rev Infect Dis 5:713, 1983.

Bell TA, Stamm WE, Wang SP, et al: Chronic *Chlamydia trachomatis* infections in infants. JAMA 267:400, 1992.

Centers for Disease Control, 1993: Sexually Transmitted Diseases Treatment Guidelines. MMWR 1993;42 (no. RR-14).

Centers for Disease Control: Recommendations for the prevention and management of *Chlamydia trachomatis* infections, 1993. MMWR 1993; 42 (no. RR-12).

Chirgwin K, Roblin PM, Gelling M, et al: Infection with *Chlamydia pneumoniae* in Brooklyn. J Infect Dis 163:757, 1991.

Eagar RM, Beach RK, Davidson AJ, et al: Epidemiologic and clinical factors of *Chlamydia trachomatis* in black, hispanic and white female adolescents. West J Med 143:37, 1985.

Gaydos CA, Roblin PM, Hammerschlag MR, et al: Diagnostic utility of PCR-enzyme immunoassay, culture and serology for the detection of *Chlamydia pneumoniae* in symptomatic and asymptomatic patients. J Clin Microbiol 32:903, 1994.

Grayston JT, Campbell LA, Kuo CC, et al: A new respiratory pathogen: *Chlamydia pneumoniae* strain TWAR. J Infect Dis 161:618, 1990.

Hammerschlag MR: Chlamydial infections. J Pediatr 114:727, 1989.

Hammerschlag MR, Doraiswamy B, Alexander ER, et al: Are rectogenital chlamydial infections a marker of sexual abuse in children? Pediatr Infect Dis 3:100, 1984.

Hammerschlag MR, Roblin PM, Gelling M, et al: Comparison of two enzyme immunoassays to culture for the diagnosis of chlamydial conjunctivitis and respiratory infections in infants. J Clin Microbiol 28:1725, 1990.

Hammerschlag MR, Golden NH, Oh MK, et al: Single dose azithromycin for the treatment of genital chlamydial infections in adolescents. J Pediatr 122:961, 1993.

Miller ST, Hammerschlag MR, Chirgwin K, et al: Role of *Chlamydia pneumoniae* in acute chest syndrome of sickle cell disease. J Pediatr 118:30, 1991.

Roblin PM, Hammerschlag MR, Cummings C, et al: Comparison of two rapid microscopic methods and culture for detection of *Chlamydia trachomatis* in ocular and nasopharyngeal specimens from infants. J Clin Microbiol 27:968, 1989.
Schachter J, Grossman M, Sweet RL, et al: Prospective study of perinatal transmission of *Chlamydia trachomatis*. JAMA 255:3374, 1986.
Yung AP, Grayson ML: Psittacosis—a review of 135 cases. Med J Austral 148:228, 1988.

CHAPTER 198

Lyme Disease (Lyme Borreliosis)

Eugene D. Shapiro

Lyme disease is the most common vector-borne disease in the United States. Although there is no question that Lyme disease has become a public health problem, extensive publicity as well as a very high frequency of misdiagnoses have resulted in a degree of anxiety about Lyme disease that is out of proportion to the actual morbidity that it causes.

ETIOLOGY. Lyme disease is caused by the spirochete *Borrelia burgdorferi*. This organism is a fastidious, microaerophilic bacterium that replicates very slowly and requires special media for in vitro growth. *B. burgdorferi* is a cylindrically shaped organism, the cell membrane of which is covered by flagella and a loosely associated outer membrane. The three major outer-surface proteins—OspA, OspB, and OspC (which are highly charged basic proteins of molecular weights of about 31, 34, and 23 kD, respectively)—as well as the 41 kD flagellar protein, are important targets for the immune response. Differences in the molecular structure of *B. burgdorferi* strains, especially between isolates from Europe and the United States, are well documented. Clinical manifestations of Lyme borreliosis in Europe and in the United States, such as the greater frequency of radiculoneuritis in Europe, may be explained by these differences.

EPIDEMIOLOGY. Lyme disease has been reported from 49 states and from more than 50 countries. In the United States, most of the cases of Lyme disease occur in southern New England, the eastern parts of the Middle Atlantic states, and the upper midwest (primarily in Wisconsin). There is a smaller endemic focus of Lyme disease along the Pacific coast. In Europe, most cases occur in the Scandinavian countries and in central Europe (especially Germany, Austria, and Switzerland). Estimates of the incidence of Lyme disease are complicated by passive systems for reporting of Lyme disease and the high frequency of misdiagnosis of this illness. In endemic areas, the reported annual incidence ranges from 20 to 100 cases/100,000 people, although this figure may be as high as 1,000 cases/100,000 people in hyperendemic areas such as Lyme, Connecticut. The reported incidence is highest among children 5–10 yr of age, which is almost twice as high as the incidence among older children and adults.

Lyme disease is a zoonosis. It is caused by the transmission of *B. burgdorferi* to humans through the bite of an infected tick of the *Ixodes* species. In the eastern and midwestern United States the vector is *Ixodes scapularis* (formerly known as *Ixodes dammini*), the deer tick. This tiny tick, which is responsible for most cases of Lyme disease in the United States, has a 2 yr three-stage life cycle. The larvae hatch in the early summer and are usually uninfected with *B. burgdorferi*. The tick may become infected at any stage of its life cycle by feeding on a host, usually a small mammal such as the white-footed mouse (*Peromyscus leucopus*), which is a natural reservoir for *B. burgdorferi*. The larvae overwinter and emerge the following spring in the nymphal stage, which is the stage in which the tick is most likely to transmit the infection. The nymphs molt to adults in the fall. The females lay their eggs the following spring before they die and the 2 yr life cycle begins again.

Several factors have been associated with the risk of transmission of *B. burgdorferi* from ticks to humans. First, the proportion of infected ticks varies by geographic area and the stage of the tick in its life cycle. In endemic areas in the northeastern and midwestern United States, approximately 15–20% of nymphal-stage deer ticks and 35–40% of the adult ticks are infected with *B. burgdorferi*. There are small foci in which the rate of infection of adult deer ticks is 60–80% or even higher. By contrast, *Ixodes pacificus* often feeds on lizards, which are not a competent reservoir for *B. burgdorferi*. Only 1–3% of these ticks, even in the nymphal and adult stages, are infected with *B. burgdorferi*. The risk of transmission of *B. burgdorferi* from infected deer ticks is related to the duration of feeding. It takes hours for the mouth parts of ticks to implant fully in the host and much longer (days) for the tick to become fully engorged. Experiments with animals have shown that nymphal ticks must feed for 36–48 hr or longer, and infected adults must feed for 48–72 hr or longer before the risk of transmission of *B. burgdorferi* becomes substantial. Most individuals who recognize that they have been bitten will remove the tick before the transmission of *B. burgdorferi* can occur. People with increased occupational, recreational, or residential exposure to tick-infested woods and fields (the preferred habitat of ticks) in endemic areas are at increased risk of developing Lyme disease. Other risk factors, such as age, race, or gender, have not been adequately studied.

PATHOLOGY. Histologically, Lyme disease is characterized by inflammatory lesions that contain both T and B lymphocytes, macrophages, plasma cells, and some mast cells. The erythema migrans rash consists of a moderately dense infiltrate of lymphocytes, plasma cells, and occasional macrophages, located around the small blood vessels of the upper dermis. Lyme myocarditis is a transmyocarditis with a widespread interstitial lymphocytic and plasma-cell infiltrate. Similar infiltrates have been seen in the meninges and cerebral cortex. There are few reports of the histology of synovial tissue during the acute stages of Lyme arthritis. At this stage of the illness the synovial fluid often has a marked predominance of polymorphonuclear cells, suggesting that the synovial tissue also will have a polymorphonuclear inflammatory infiltrate. By contrast, chronic, recurrent arthritis is characterized by a chronic hypertrophic synovitis. This nonspecific abnormality, also found in other disorders such as rheumatoid arthritis, is marked by hyperplasia of the synovial cells with varying degrees of lymphocytic infiltrates that sometimes form abortive germinal centers and follicles. Plasma cells are present at the periphery of the lymphoid aggregates. In advanced disease, neovascularization (a nonspecific response to chronic inflammation) may be seen.

PATHOGENESIS. The skin is the initial target of infection by *B. burgdorferi*. Inflammation induced by *B. burgdorferi* leads to the development of the characteristic rash. Early disseminated Lyme disease is caused by the spread of spirochetes, via the bloodstream, to tissues throughout the body. The spirochete will adhere to the surfaces of a wide variety of different types of cells, which may explain why it is able to cause clinical manifestations in so many organs. Because the organism may persist in tissues for prolonged periods of time, symptoms may appear very late after infection. The symptoms of early disseminated and of late Lyme disease are due to inflammation, mediated by interleukin 1 and other lymphokines, which is a direct result of the presence of the organism. It is likely that relatively few organisms actually invade the host, but cytokines serve to amplify the inflammatory response and lead to much of the tissue damage. The illness may have an immunogenetic basis in a small subset of patients with refractory symptoms of late Lyme disease, such as chronic recurrent Lyme arthritis. Patients with the HLA-DR2, DR3, and DR4 allotypes may be genetically predisposed to develop chronic recurrent Lyme arthritis. These class II histocompatibility molecules are located on macrophages and B cells that are involved in the presentation of antigens to T-helper cells that initiate the immune response. In genetically susceptible individuals, *B. burgdorferi* may initiate an autoimmune response that causes inflammation and clinical symptoms long after the bacteria have been killed.

CLINICAL MANIFESTATIONS. The clinical manifestations of Lyme disease are divided into early and late stages. Early Lyme disease is further classified as early localized or early disseminated disease. Untreated patients may progressively develop clinical symptoms of each stage of the disease, or they may present with early disseminated or with late disease without apparently having had any symptoms of the earlier stages of Lyme disease.

Early Localized Disease. The first clinical manifestation of Lyme disease is the typical annular rash, which is called erythema migrans. Although it usually occurs 7–14 days after the bite, the onset of the rash has been reported from 3 to 32 days later. The initial lesion occurs at the site of the bite. The rash may be uniformly erythematous, or it may appear as a target lesion with central clearing or central vesicular or necrotic areas. The rash may be itchy or painful. The lesion can occur anywhere on the body, although the most common locations are the axilla, the periumbilical area, the thigh, and the groin. Erythema migrans may be associated systemic symptoms, such as fever, myalgia, headache, or malaise. Without treatment, the rash gradually expands (hence the name *migrans*) to an average diameter of 15 cm and remains present for at least 1–2 wk and usually longer.

Early Disseminated Disease. In the United States a substantial proportion of patients with acute *B. burgdorferi* infection develop secondary erythema migrans lesions, a common manifestation of early disseminated Lyme disease caused by hematogenous spread of the organisms to multiple skin sites. The secondary lesions, which may develop several days or even weeks after the first lesion, usually are smaller than the primary lesion and are often accompanied by fever, myalgia, headache, and malaise; conjunctivitis and lymphadenopathy also may develop. Occasionally, when the erythema migrans rash resolves, new evanescent lesions, which usually are small (1–3 cm), erythematous annular lesions that do not expand, continue to appear over several weeks. Aseptic meningitis, with signs of meningeal irritation, such as nuchal rigidity, uveitis, and rarely, carditis, with varying degrees of heart block, may occur with early disseminated Lyme disease. Focal neurologic findings, especially cranioneuropathies, are a manifestation of this stage of the illness. Paralysis of the facial (seventh) nerve is relatively common in children and may be the initial and the only manifestation of Lyme disease. The paralysis usually lasts from 2 to 8 wk and resolves completely in most cases. There is no evidence that the clinical course of the facial palsy is affected by antimicrobial treatment.

Late Disease. Arthritis, beginning months after the initial infection, is the usual manifestation of late Lyme disease. Arthritis typically involves the large joints, especially the knee, which is affected in more than 90% of the cases, but any joint may be affected. Although the joint is swollen and tender, patients do not experience the exquisite pain that is typical of bacterial arthritides. Although it may last for several weeks, the joint swelling usually resolves within 1–2 wk before recurring, often in other joints. When untreated, the episodes of arthritis often increase in duration, sometimes lasting for months, but in most cases, the disease eventually resolves, even in patients who are untreated and who have had many recurrences of arthritis.

Late manifestations of Lyme disease involving the central nervous system (CNS) (sometimes termed tertiary neuroborreliosis) are rarely reported in children. In adults, chronic demyelinating encephalitis, polyneuritis, and impairment of memory have been attributed to Lyme disease.

Congenital Lyme Disease. Although *B. burgdorferi* has been identified from several abortuses and from a few live-born children with congenital anomalies, the placentas and the abortuses in which the spirochete was identified usually did not show histologic evidence of inflammation. No consistent pattern of fetal damage has been identified, as would be expected in a "syndrome" due to congenital infection. Furthermore, studies conducted in endemic areas have indicated that there is no difference in the prevalence of congenital malformations among the offspring of women with serum antibodies against *B. burgdorferi* and the offspring of those without such antibodies. If it does exist, congenital Lyme disease must be extremely rare.

LABORATORY FINDINGS. Standard laboratory tests rarely are helpful in diagnosing Lyme disease because the associated laboratory abnormalities usually are nonspecific. The peripheral white blood cell count may be either normal or elevated. The erythrocyte sedimentation rate usually is elevated. The white blood cell concentration in joint fluid may range from 25,000 to 125,000/mL, often with a preponderance of polymorphonuclear cells. When the CNS is involved, there usually is a mild pleocytosis with a lymphocytic predominance. The protein may be elevated but the glucose usually is normal in the cerebrospinal fluid.

DIAGNOSIS. The clinical manifestations of Lyme disease, other than erythema migrans, are not specific. The mono- or pauciarticular arthritis may mimic either an acute septic joint or other causes of arthritis in children, such as juvenile rheumatoid arthritis or poststreptococcal arthritis. Clinically, 7th nerve palsy due to Lyme disease is indistinguishable from idiopathic Bell's palsy, and Lyme meningitis may mimic enteroviral meningitis. Even the diagnosis of erythema migrans may be difficult, because the rash initially may be confused with nummular eczema, tinea, granuloma annulare, an insect bite, or cellulitis. However, the relatively rapid expansion of erythema migrans helps to distinguish it from these other conditions.

The isolation of *B. burgdorferi* from a symptomatic patient should be considered diagnostic of Lyme disease. Although *B. burgdorferi* has been isolated from blood, skin biopsies, cerebrospinal fluid (CSF), myocardial biopsies, and the synovium of patients with Lyme disease, the medium in which *B. burgdorferi* is cultured is expensive, it can take as long as 4 wk for the bacteria to grow in culture, and the frequency of isolation of *B. burgdorferi* from patients with active Lyme disease is low. It usually is necessary for patients to undergo an invasive procedure, such as a biopsy or a lumbar puncture, to obtain appropriate tissue or fluid for culture. *B. burgdorferi* has been identified with silver stains (Warthin-Starry or modified Dieterle) and with immunohistochemical stains (with monoclonal or polyclonal antibodies) in skin, synovial, and myocardial biopsies. However, *B. burgdorferi* can be confused with normal tissue structures or it can be missed because it usually is present in low concentrations.

Although attempts have been made to develop antigen-based diagnostic tests, including the polymerase chain reaction, all of these tests are experimental. None of the tests for *B. burgdorferi* antigens that have been adequately evaluated were sufficiently sensitive and specific to be clinically useful. Consequently, the confirmation of Lyme disease usually is based on the demonstration of antibodies to *B. burgdorferi* in the patient's serum.

The normal antibody response to acute infection with *B. burgdorferi* is well described. Specific IgM antibodies appear first, usually 3–4 wk after the infection begins. These antibodies peak after 6–8 wk and subsequently decline. Occasionally, a prolonged elevation of IgM antibodies occurs despite effective antimicrobial treatment. Specific IgG antibodies usually appear 6–8 wk after the onset of the infection. These antibodies peak after 4–6 mo and may remain elevated indefinitely. Once antibodies have developed, antimicrobial treatment may result in a decline in the IgG antibody concentration, but even after the patient is clinically cured, these antibodies usually remain detectable for several years, and often for much longer.

Because the immunofluorescent antibody test requires subjective interpretation and is time consuming to perform, it has been replaced by enzyme-linked immunosorbent assays (ELISA) for the detection of antibodies against *B. burgdorferi.* The ELISA method produces false-positive results because of cross-reactive antibodies in patients with other spirochetal infections (e.g., syphilis, leptospirosis, or relapsing fever), certain viral infections (e.g., varicella), and certain autoimmune diseases (e.g., systemic lupus erythematosus), as well as because antibodies directed against spirochetes that comprise part of the normal oral flora may cross-react with antigens of *B. burgdorferi.*

Immunoblots (Western blots) are also used to detect serum antibodies to *B. burgdorferi* as a diagnostic test for Lyme disease. Although some investigators have suggested that the immunoblot is more sensitive and specific than the ELISA, there is still a great deal of debate about its interpretation. For example, many people who do not have Lyme disease have antibodies against the 41 kD protein (the flagellar protein) of *B. burgdorferi.* Minimum criteria for a "positive" test have not been established. The immunoblot is most useful to validate a positive or equivocal ELISA in a patient with a low clinical likelihood of having Lyme disease.

One reason for the poor sensitivity of serologic tests for Lyme disease is that erythema migrans which is the clinical finding that usually brings patients to medical attention, usually develops within 2–3 wk of the onset of the infection with *B. burgdorferi.* Antibodies to *B. burgdorferi* are often not detected at this early stage of the disease. The antibody response to *B. burgdorferi* also may be abrogated in patients with early Lyme disease who are treated promptly with an effective antimicrobial agent; these patients may never develop antibodies against *B. burgdorferi.*

The currently available serologic tests, especially widely used commercially produced kits, have poor specificity and reproducibility. The estimates of the mean sensitivity of these kits ranges from 26% to 57%, and the mean specificity ranges from 12% to 60%. With these commercial diagnostic test kits, serologic testing for Lyme disease will result in a high rate of misdiagnosis.

The serologic tests for Lyme disease performed by reference laboratories are relatively accurate. Even with these tests, the predictive value still depends primarily on the likelihood that the patient has Lyme disease based on the clinical and epidemiologic history and the physical examination. With few exceptions, the pretest probability that a patient has Lyme disease will be very low in areas in which Lyme disease is rare.

Even in areas with high prevalence, patients with nonspecific signs and symptoms, such as, fatigue, headache, and arthralgia, are not likely to have Lyme disease; most positive serologic tests are false positives. Even when more accurate tests performed by reference laboratories are available, clinicians should order serologic tests for Lyme disease selectively, reserving them for patients from populations with a relatively high prevalence of Lyme disease who have specific clinical findings that are suggestive of Lyme disease so that the predictive value of a positive test is high. Even though a symptomatic patient has antibodies to *B. burgdorferi,* Lyme disease may not be the cause of the patient's symptoms. The test may be falsely positive, or the patient may have been infected previously. Once serum antibodies to *B. burgdorferi* develop, they may persist for many years despite adequate treatment and clinical cure of the disease. Because many people who become infected with *B. burgdorferi* are asymptomatic, the background rate of seropositivity among patients who have never had clinically apparent Lyme disease is significant in endemic areas.

PREVENTION. Children are often bitten by deer ticks in endemic areas, but the overall risk of acquiring Lyme disease is low (approximately 1–2%), even in these areas. Even if the patient is bitten by a nymphal-stage deer tick infected with *B. burgdorferi,* the risk of acquiring Lyme disease is only about 8–10%. If infection develops treatment of the infection is highly effective. The efficacy of routine administration of antimicrobial prophylaxis for persons who have been bitten by a deer tick is not known, and it is not recommended. The routine testing of ticks that have been removed from humans for infection with *B. burgdorferi* is not recommended because the predictive value of a positive test for infection in the human host is unknown. A more reasonable approach to preventing Lyme disease is to wear appropriate protective clothing when entering tick-infested areas and to check for and remove ticks after spending time in such areas. Insect repellants may provide temporary protection, but they may be absorbed from the skin and, if used frequently or in large doses, they may produce significant toxicity, especially in children.

TREATMENT. No clinical trials of treatment for Lyme disease have been conducted in children. Recommendations for the treatment of children that have been extrapolated from studies of adults are shown in the Table 198–1. Children <9 yr of age should not be treated with doxycycline because it may cause permanent discoloration of their teeth. Patients who are treated with doxycycline should be alerted to the risk of developing a sun-induced dermatitis in sun-exposed areas while taking the medication. Some patients may develop a Jarisch-Herxheimer reaction soon after treatment is initiated. The manifestations of this reaction are increased temperature, sweats, and myalgias. These symptoms resolve spontaneously,

■ TABLE 198–1 Antimicrobial Treatment of Lyme Borreliosis

Early Disease

Erythema Migrans and Disseminated Early Disease Without Focal Findings

Doxycycline, 100 mg bid for 21 days (do not use in children <9 yr) or
Amoxicillin, 50 mg/kg/24 hr divided tid (maximum 500 mg/dose) for 21 days
An alternative agent for those who cannot take either amoxicillin or doxycycline is erythromycin, 30–50 mg/kg/24 hr divided qid (maximum 250 mg/dose) for 21 days

Palsy of the Cranial Nerves (Including 7th Nerve Palsy)

Treat as for erythema migrans for 21–30 days. Do not use corticosteroids.

Carditis

Treat as for late neurologic disease. Do not use corticosteroids.

Meningitis

Treat as for late neurologic disease.

Late Disease

Neurologic Disease*

Ceftriaxone 50–80 mg/kg/24 hr in a single dose (max. 2 g) for 14–21 days administered IV or IM, or penicillin G, 200,000–400,000 U/kg/24 hr (max. 20 million units/24 hr) divided q4h administered IV for 14–21 days.

Arthritis

Initial treatment is the same as for erythema migrans except treat for 30 days. If symptoms fail to resolve after 2 mo or there is a recurrence, then give either a 2nd course of orally administered antimicrobials for 30 days or treat as for late neurologic disease.

**For isolated palsy of the facial nerve or of other cranial nerves, see Palsy of the Cranial Nerves above.*

although administration of nonsteroidal anti-inflammatory drugs often is beneficial. Nonsteroidal anti-inflammatory agents also may be useful in treating symptoms of early Lyme disease and of Lyme arthritis.

Other antimicrobial agents, such as cefuroxime, clarithromycin, and azithromycin, may be effective for the treatment of Lyme disease, although none has been either adequately tested or licensed for such use. Preliminary results with azithromycin have been disappointing. There is little need to use new agents because the results of treatment with either amoxicillin or doxycycline have been good.

Fatigue, arthralgia, and myalgia sometimes persist for some time after completion of a course of treatment for Lyme disease. These nonspecific symptoms, which may accompany or follow more specific symptoms and signs of Lyme disease but almost never are the sole presenting manifestations of Lyme disease, generally resolve over a period of weeks to months. There is little evidence that these symptoms are related to persistence of the organism. Likewise, there is no evidence that repeated courses of antimicrobials hasten the resolution of such symptoms. Finally, because antibodies against *B. burgdorferi* persist after successful treatment, there is no reason to obtain follow-up serologic tests.

PROGNOSIS. There is a widespread misconception that Lyme disease is difficult to treat successfully and that chronic symptoms and clinical recurrences are common. In fact, the most common reason for failure of treatment is misdiagnosis in patients who do not have Lyme disease. The impression that Lyme disease requires prolonged treatment, including intravenously administered antimicrobials, and that treatment is often unsuccessful can be attributed to the treatment of patients whose symptoms were not due to Lyme disease.

The prognosis for children treated for Lyme disease is excellent. None of 65 children who were treated for erythema migrans and evaluated at a mean of more than 3 yr later had developed symptoms of late Lyme disease. In a 2nd prospective study, all children with newly diagnosed Lyme disease, most of whom had early localized or early disseminated disease, were cured at a mean of 1.5 yr later. The long-term prognosis for patients who are treated beginning in the late phase of Lyme disease also is excellent. Although recurrences of arthritis do occur rarely, especially among patients with the DR-2, DR-3, or DR-4 HLA-type, most children who are treated for Lyme arthritis are permanently cured. Although there are rare reports of adults who have developed late neuroborreliosis after being treated for Lyme disease, no cases have been diagnosed in children.

American College of Rheumatology and the Council of the Infectious Diseases Society of America: Appropriateness of parenteral antibiotic treatment for patients with presumed Lyme disease. Ann Intern Med 119:518, 1993.

Aronowitz RA: Lyme disease: The social construction of a new disease and its social consequences. Millbank Q 69:79, 1991.

Gerber MA, Shapiro ED: Diagnosis of Lyme disease in children. J Pediatr 121:157, 1992.

Rahn DW, Malawista SE: Lyme disease: Recommendations for diagnosis and treatment. Ann Intern Med 114:472, 1991.

Salazaar JC, Gerber MA, Goff CW: Long-term outcome of Lyme disease in children given early treatment. J Pediatr 122:591, 1993.

Shapiro ED, Gerber MA, Holabird N, et al: A controlled trial of antimicrobial prophylaxis for Lyme disease after deer-tick bites. N Engl J Med 327:1769, 1992.

Steere AC: Lyme disease. N Engl J Med 321:586, 1989.

Steere AC, Taylor E, McHugh GL, et al: The overdiagnosis of Lyme disease. JAMA 269:1812, 1993.

CHAPTER 199
Tuberculosis

Jeffrey R. Starke

After decades of decline in the incidence of tuberculosis, the number of tuberculosis cases has increased dramatically over the past decade. Almost 1.3 million cases and 450,000 deaths occur among children each year. The incidence of childhood tuberculosis increased by 40% in the United States from 1987 to 1993 as a consequence of poverty, immigration from high prevalence countries, the epidemic of human immunodeficiency virus (HIV) infection, and limitations in health care services to high risk populations.

ETIOLOGY. The agents of tuberculosis, *Mycobacterium tuberculosis, Mycobacterium bovis,* and *Mycobacterium africanum,* are members of the order Actinomycetales and the family Mycobacteriaceae. The tubercle bacilli are non–spore forming, nonmotile, pleiomorphic, weakly gram-positive curved rods about 2–4 μm long. They may appear beaded or clumped in stained clinical specimens or culture media. They are obligate aerobes that grow in synthetic media containing glycerol as the carbon source and ammonium salts as the nitrogen source. These mycobacteria grow best at 37–41° C, produce niacin, and lack pigmentation. A lipid-rich cell wall accounts for resistance to the bactericidal actions of antibody and complement. A hallmark of all mycobacteria is acid-fastness—the capacity to form stable mycolate complexes with arylmethane dyes such as crystal violet, carbolfuchsin, auramine, and rhodamine. Once stained, they resist decoloration with ethanol and hydrochloric or other acids.

Mycobacteria grow slowly, their generation time being 12–24 hr. Isolation from clinical specimens on solid synthetic media usually takes 3–6 wk, and drug-susceptibility testing requires an additional 4 wk. However, growth can be detected in 1–3 wk in selective liquid medium using radiolabled nutrients (the BACTEC radiometric system), and drug susceptibilities can be determined in an additional 3–5 days. *M. tuberculosis* has a typical colony morphology, produces niacin but no pigment, is able to reduce nitrates, and produces catalase. Some isoniazid-resistant strains lose the ability to make catalase. The presence of *M. tuberculosis* in clinical specimens can be detected within hours using a polymerase chain reaction (PCR) that employs a DNA probe that is complementary to mycobacterial DNA or RNA. Data from children are limited, but the sensitivity of some PCR techniques is similar to that for culture.

EPIDEMIOLOGY. Infection and Disease. The World Health Organization estimates that one third of the world's population—2 billion people—are infected with *M. tuberculosis.* Infection rates are highest in Southeast Asia, China, India, Africa, and Latin America. Tuberculosis is especially prevalent in populations undergoing the stresses of poor nutrition, overcrowding, inadequate health care, and displacement. Ten to 20 million people living in the United States harbor the tubercle bacillus.

Tuberculosis case rates fell during the first half of the century long before the advent of antituberculosis drugs as a result of improved living conditions. The incidence began to rise in the United States in 1985 (Fig. 199–1). Most people in developed countries remain at low risk for tuberculosis except for certain fairly well-defined groups (Table 199–1). Cities with populations of greater than 250,000 account for 18% of the U.S. population but more than 45% of tuberculosis cases. At every age, tuberculosis case rates are strikingly higher in foreign born and nonwhite individuals. Genetics may play a small role, but

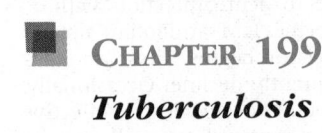

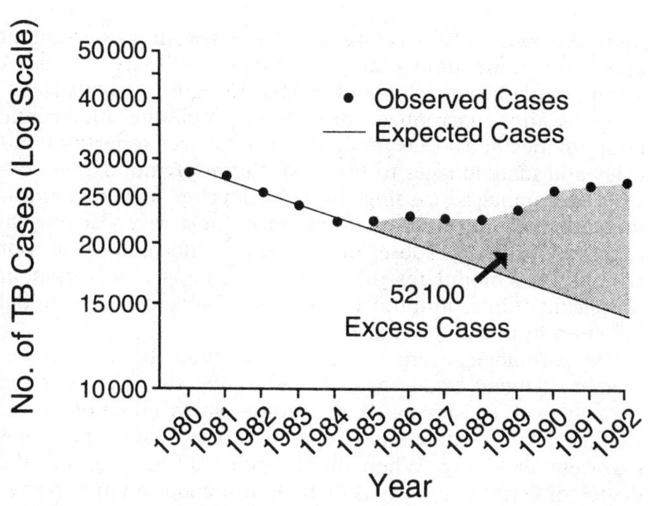

Figure 199–1. Observed cases of tuberculosis in the United States, 1980–1992. Compared with the number of cases expected from the previous decline, 52,100 excess cases were reported from 1985 to 1992. (Data from the Centers for Disease Control and Prevention, 1993.)

environmental factors such as socioeconomic status undoubtedly play the major role in the incidence.

Among adults, two thirds of cases occur in males, but there is a slight predominance of tuberculosis among females in childhood. Tuberculosis rates are highest among the elderly in white populations in the United States; these individuals acquired the infection decades ago. In contrast, among nonwhite populations tuberculosis is most common in young adults and children less than 5 yr of age. The age range of 5–14 yr is often called the "favored age" because in all human populations this group has the lowest rate of tuberculous disease.

In the United States, most children are infected with *M. tuberculosis* in their home by someone close to them, but outbreaks of childhood tuberculosis also occur in elementary and high schools, nursery schools, child-care centers, homes, churches, school buses, and sports teams. Human immunodeficiency virus (HIV)-infected adults with tuberculosis can transmit *M. tuberculosis* to children, some of whom develop tuberculous disease, and children with HIV infection probably are at increased risk of developing tuberculosis after infection.

The incidence of drug-resistant tuberculosis has increased dramatically. In the United States, about 14% of *M. tuberculosis* isolates are resistant to at least one drug, while 3% are resistant to both isoniazid and rifampin. However, in some countries drug resistance rates range from 20% to 50%. The major reasons for the development of drug resistance are poor patient adherence to treatment and prescription of inadequate drug regimens by the physician.

■ TABLE 199–1 Groups at High Risk for Tuberculous Infection and Disease in Developed Countries

Tuberculous Infection
Foreign-born persons from high-incidence countries
Poor and indigent persons, especially in large cities
Present and former residents of correctional institutions
Homeless persons
Injecting drug users
Health care workers caring for high-risk patients
Children exposed to high-risk adults
Tuberculous Disease Once Infected
Coinfection with the human immunodeficiency virus
Other immunocompromising diseases, esp. malignancy
Immunosuppressive medical treatments
Infants and children ≤3 yr of age

Transmission. Transmission of *M. tuberculosis* is person to person, usually by mucus droplet nuclei that become airborne. Transmission rarely occurs by direct contact with an infected discharge or a contaminated fomite. The chance of transmission increases when the patient has an acid-fast smear of sputum, an extensive upper lobe infiltrate or cavity, copious production of thin sputum, and severe and forceful cough. Environmental factors, especially poor air circulation, enhance transmission. Most adults do not transmit the organism within several days to 2 wk after beginning adequate chemotherapy, but some patients remain infectious for many weeks. Young children with tuberculosis rarely, if ever, infect other children or adults. Tubercle bacilli are sparse in the endobronchial secretions of children with pulmonary tuberculosis, and cough is often absent or lacks the tussive force required to suspend infectious particles of the correct size.

PATHOGENESIS AND IMMUNITY. The primary complex of tuberculosis includes local infection at the portal of entry and the regional lymph nodes that drain the area. The lung is the portal of entry in over 98% of cases. The tubercle bacilli multiply initially within alveoli and alveolar ducts. Most of the bacilli are killed but some survive within nonactivated macrophages, which carry them through lymphatic vessels to the regional lymph nodes. When the primary infection is in the lung, the hilar lymph nodes usually are involved, although an upper lobe focus may drain into paratracheal nodes. The tissue reaction in the lung parenchyma and lymph nodes intensifies over the next 2–12 wk as tissue hypersensitivity develops. The parenchymal portion of the primary complex often heals completely by fibrosis or calcification after undergoing caseous necrosis and encapsulation. Occasionally, this portion continues to enlarge, resulting in focal pneumonitis and pleuritis. If caseation is intense the center of the lesion liquefies and empties into the associated bronchus, leaving a residual cavity.

The foci of infection in the regional lymph nodes develop some fibrosis and encapsulation, but healing is usually less complete than in the parenchymal lesion. Viable *M. tuberculosis* can persist for decades within these foci. In most cases of initial tuberculous infection the lymph nodes remain normal in size. However, hilar and paratracheal nodes that enlarge significantly as part of the host inflammatory reaction may encroach upon a regional bronchus or bronchiole. Partial obstruction of the bronchus caused by external compression may cause hyperinflation in the distal lung segment. Inflamed caseous nodes can attach to the bronchial wall and erode through it, causing endobronchial tuberculosis or a fistula tract. The cesium causes complete obstruction of the bronchus. The resulting lesion, a combination of pneumonitis and atelectasis, has been called a collapse-consolidation or segmental lesion (Fig. 199–2).

During the development of the primary complex, tubercle bacilli are carried to most tissues of the body via the blood and lymphatic vessels. Disseminated tuberculosis occurs if the number of circulating bacilli is large and the host response is inadequate. More often the number of bacilli is small, leading to clinically inapparent metastatic foci in many organs. These remote foci usually become encapsulated, but they may be the origin of both extrapulmonary tuberculosis and reactivation tuberculosis in some individuals.

The time between initial infection and clinically apparent disease is quite variable. Disseminated or meningeal tuberculosis are early manifestations, often occurring within 2–6 mo of the infection. Clinically significant lymph node or endobronchial tuberculosis usually appears within 3–9 mo. Lesions of the bones and joints take several years to develop, while renal lesions may become evident decades after infection. Pulmonary tuberculosis that occurs more than a year after the primary infection is usually caused by endogenous regrowth of bacilli persisting in partially encapsulated lesions. This reactiva-

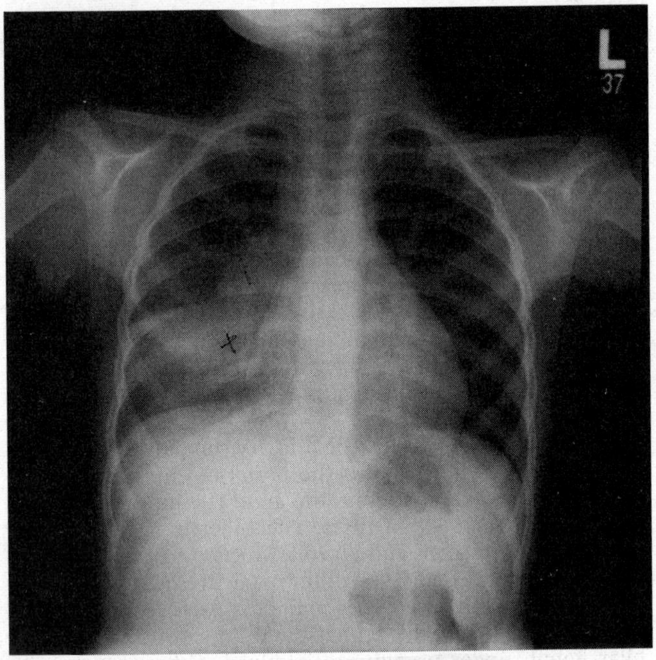

Figure 199–2. Right-sided hilar adenopathy and collapse-consolidation lesions of primary tuberculosis in a 4-yr-old child.

tion tuberculosis is rare in children but is common among adolescents and young adults. The most common form is an infiltrate or cavity in the apex of the upper lobes, where oxygen tension and blood flow are great. Dissemination during reactivation tuberculosis is rare in immunocompetent hosts but is common in adults with the acquired immune deficiency syndrome (AIDS). Only 5–10% of immunocompetent adults who become infected with *M. tuberculosis* ever develop clinical disease. However, approximately 40% of infants with untreated infection develop disease within 1–2 yr. The risk declines throughout childhood. About 25–35% of children with tuberculosis develop extrapulmonary manifestations compared with about 10% of immunocompetent adults.

Pregnancy and the Newborn. Congenital tuberculosis is rare because the most common result of female genital tract tuberculosis is infertility. Congenital transmission occurs most commonly from a lesion in the placenta through the umbilical vein. Primary infection in the mother just before or during pregnancy is more likely to cause congenital infection than is reactivation of a previous infection. The tubercle bacilli first reach the fetal liver, where a primary focus with periportal lymph node involvement may occur. Organisms pass through the liver into the main fetal circulation and infect many organs. The bacilli in the lung usually remain dormant until after birth, when oxygenation and pulmonary circulation increase significantly.

Congenital tuberculosis may also be caused by aspiration or ingestion of infected amniotic fluid. However, the most common route of infection for the neonate is postnatal airborne transmission from an adult with infectious pulmonary tuberculosis.

Immunity. Conditions that adversely affect cell-mediated immunity predispose to progression from tuberculous infection to disease. Tuberculosis is associated with a vast antibody response, but these antibodies appear to play little role in host defense. In the first several weeks after infection, tubercle bacilli undergo a short period of uninhibited growth in both free alveolar spaces and within inactivated alveolar macrophages. Sulfatides in the mycobacteria cell wall inhibit fusion of the macrophage phagosome and lysosomes, allowing the organisms to escape destruction by intracellular enzymes. Cell-mediated immunity develops about 4–8 wk after infection, at about the same time that tissue hypersensitivity begins. A small population of lymphocytes that recognize mycobacterial antigens after macrophage processing proliferate and secrete lymphokines and other mediators that attract other lymphocytes and macrophages to the area. Certain lymphokines activate macrophages, causing them to develop high concentrations of lytic enzymes that enhance their mycobactericidal capacity. A discrete subset of regulator helper and suppressor lymphocytes modulates the immune response. Development of specific cellular immunity prevents progression of the initial infection in most individuals.

The pathologic events in the initial tuberculous infection seem to depend upon the balance among the mycobacterial antigen load; cell-mediated immunity, which enhances intracellular killing; and tissue hypersensitivity, which promotes extracellular killing. When the antigen load is small and the degree of tissue sensitivity is high, granuloma formation results from the organization of lymphocytes, macrophages, and fibroblasts. When both antigen load and the degree of sensitivity are high, granuloma formation is less organized. Tissue necrosis is incomplete, resulting in formation of caseous material. When the degree of tissue sensitivity is low, as is often the case in infants or immunocompromised individuals, the reaction is diffuse and the infection is not well contained, leading to dissemination and local tissue destruction. Tissue necrosis factor and other cytokines released by specific lymphocytes promote cellular destruction and tissue damage in susceptible individuals. Tuberculosis itself may suppress the host immune response, although the exact immunologic mechanisms are poorly understood.

Tuberculin Skin Tests. The development of delayed-type hypersensitivity (DTH) in most individuals infected with the tubercle bacillus makes the tuberculin skin test a useful diagnostic tool. Multipuncture tests (MPTs) are not as accurate as the Mantoux test because the exact dose of tuberculin antigen introduced into the skin cannot be controlled. Since mass tuberculin skin testing of children has been abandoned, MPTs have no role in current pediatric practice.

The Mantoux tuberculin skin test is the intradermal injection of 0.1 mL containing 5 tuberculin units (TU) of purified protein derivative (PPD) stabilized with Tween 80. The amount of induration in response to the test should be measured by a trained person 48–72 hr after administration. Occasional patients will have the onset of induration more than 72 hr after placement of the test; this is a positive result. Host-related factors, including very young age, malnutrition, immunosuppression by disease or drugs, viral infections (measles, mumps, varicella, influenza), live-virus vaccines, and overwhelming tuberculosis, can depress the skin test reaction in a child infected with *M. tuberculosis*. Corticosteroid therapy may decrease the reaction to tuberculin, but the effect is variable. Tuberculin skin testing done at the time of initiating corticosteroid therapy is usually reliable. Approximately 10% of immunocompetent children with tuberculous disease—up to 50% of those with meningitis or disseminated disease—do not react initially to PPD; most become reactive after several months of antituberculosis therapy. Nonreactivity may be specific to tuberculin or more global to a variety of antigens, so positive "control" skin tests with a negative tuberculin test never rules out tuberculosis. The most common reasons for a false-negative skin test are poor technique or misreading the results.

False-positive reactions to tuberculin can be caused by cross-sensitization to antigens of nontuberculous mycobacteria (NTM), which generally are more prevalent in the environment as one approaches the equator. These cross reactions are usually transient over months to years and produce less than 10–12 mm of induration. Previous vaccination with bacille Calmette-Gúerin (BCG) also can cause a reaction to a tuberculin skin test. Approximately one half of infants who receive a BCG vaccine never develop a reactive tuberculin skin test, and the reactivity usually wanes in 2–3 yr in those with initially positive skin tests. Older children and adults who receive a BCG vaccine are more likely to develop tuberculin reactivity, but most lose the reactivity by 5–10 yr after vaccination. When skin test reactivity is present, it usually causes less than 10 mm of induration, although larger reactions occur in some individuals. In general, a tuberculin skin reaction ≥10 mm in a BCG-vaccinated child or adult indicates infection with *M. tuberculosis*, which necessitates further diagnostic evaluation and treatment. Prior vaccination with BCG is never a contraindication to tuberculin testing.

The interpretation of the Mantoux tuberculin skin test should be influenced by the purpose for which the test was given. The appropriate size of induration indicating a positive test varies with related epidemiologic factors. In children with no risk factors for tuberculosis, smaller skin test reactions are usually false-positive results. Possible exposure to an adult with or at high risk for infectious pulmonary tuberculosis is the most crucial factor for determining risk for children. To minimize false results, reaction size limits for determining a positive result vary with the individual's risk of infection. For adults and children at the highest risk of infection—those with recent contact with infectious persons, clinical illnesses consistent with tuberculosis, or HIV infection or other immunosuppression—a reactive area ≥5 mm is classified as a positive result, indicating infection with *M. tuberculosis*. For other high-risk groups (Table 199–1), and all children less than 3 yr of age, a reactive area ≥10 mm is considered positive. For low-risk persons, especially those residing in communities where the prevalence of tuberculosis is low, the cutoff point for a positive reaction may be ≥15 mm. Classifying children with this scheme depends upon the willingness and ability of the clinician and family to develop a thorough exposure history for the child and the adults who care for the child. To interpret the tuberculin skin test correctly, the clinician must clearly understand the epidemiology of tuberculosis in the community and the correct indication for tuberculin testing of the individual.

Purified protein derivative is also available in 1-TU and 250-TU strengths. The 1-TU preparation is used only when it is suspected that the patient may have a severe reaction to the 5-TU test. Use of the 250-TU solution is controversial because interpretation of reactions has not been standardized. Absence of reaction to a 250-TU test does not rule out tuberculous infection, but a reaction is often caused by cross sensitization from NTM. In general, the 250-TU test is of little use in the diagnosis of tuberculous infection or disease.

CLINICAL MANIFESTATIONS. Primary Pulmonary Disease. The primary pulmonary complex includes the parenchymal focus and the regional lymph nodes. About 70% of lung foci are subpleural, and localized pleurisy is common. The initial parenchymal inflammation usually is not visible on chest radiograph, but a localized, nonspecific infiltrate may be seen prior to the development of tissue hypersensitivity. All lobar segments of the lung are at equal risk of initial infection. Two or more primary foci are present in 25% of cases. The hallmark of primary tuberculosis in the lung is the relatively large size of the regional lymphadenitis compared with the relatively small size of the initial lung focus. In most cases, the parenchymal infiltrate and adenitis resolve early. The hilar lymph nodes continue to enlarge in some children, especially infants. Bronchial obstruction begins as the nodes compress the regional bronchus. The common sequence is hilar adenopathy, focal hyperinflation, and then atelectasis. The resulting radiographic shadows have been called collapse-consolidation or segmental tuberculosis (Fig. 199–2). These radiographic findings are similar to those seen with foreign body aspiration but are different from typical cases of bacterial pneumonia in children. Occasionally, extensive lung involvement occurs without obvious adenopathy.

The symptoms and physical signs of primary pulmonary tuberculosis in children are surprisingly meager considering the degree of radiographic changes often seen. More than 50% of infants and children with radiographically moderate to severe pulmonary tuberculosis have no physical findings and are discovered only by contact tracing. Infants are more likely to experience signs and symptoms. Nonproductive cough and mild dyspnea are the most common symptoms. Systemic complaints such as fever, night sweats, anorexia, and decreased activity occur less often. Some infants have difficulty gaining weight or develop a true failure-to-thrive syndrome that often does not improve significantly until several months of effective treatment have been taken. Pulmonary signs are even less common. Some infants and young children with bronchial obstruction have localized wheezing or decreased breath sounds that may be accompanied by tachypnea or, rarely, respiratory distress. These pulmonary symptoms and signs are occasionally alleviated by antibiotics suggesting bacterial superinfection.

Children may have lobar pneumonia without impressive hilar adenopathy. If the primary infection is progressively destructive, liquefaction of the lung parenchyma can lead to formation of a thin-walled primary tuberculosis cavity. Rarely, bullous tuberculous lesions can occur in the lungs and lead to pneumothorax if they rupture. Enlargement of the subcarinal lymph nodes can cause compression of the esophagus and, rarely, a bronchoesophageal fistula.

Most cases of tuberculous bronchial obstruction in children resolve fully with appropriate treatment. Occasionally, there is residual calcification of the primary focus or regional lymph nodes. The appearance of calcification implies that the lesion has been present for at least 6–12 mo. Healing of the segment is rarely complicated by scarring or contraction associated with cylindrical bronchiectasis.

The most specific confirmation of pulmonary tuberculosis is isolation of *M. tuberculosis*. The best culture specimen is usually the early morning gastric acid obtained before the child has arisen and peristalsis has emptied the stomach of the pooled secretions that have been swallowed overnight. Unfortunately, even under optimal conditions, three consecutive morning gastric aspirates yield the organisms in less than 50% of cases. The yield from bronchoscopy is even lower. Negative cultures never exclude the diagnosis of tuberculosis in a child. For most children, the presence of a positive tuberculin skin test, an abnormal chest radiograph consistent with tuberculosis, and history of exposure to an adult with infectious tuberculosis is adequate proof that the disease is present. The drug susceptibility test results from the adult source case's isolate can be used to determine the best therapeutic regimen for the child. Cultures should be obtained from the child whenever the source case is unknown or the source case has possible drug resistant tuberculosis.

Progressive Primary Pulmonary Disease. A rare but serious complication of tuberculous infection in a child occurs when the primary focus enlarges steadily and develops a large caseous center. Liquefaction may cause formation of a primary cavity associated with large numbers of tubercle bacilli. The enlarging focus may slough necrotic debris into the adjacent bronchus, leading to further intrapulmonary dissemination. Significant signs or symptoms are frequent in locally progressive disease in children. High fever, severe cough with sputum production, weight loss, and night sweats are common. Physical signs include diminished breath sounds, rales, and dullness or egophony over the cavity. The prognosis for full but usually slow recovery is excellent with appropriate therapy.

Reactivation Tuberculosis. Pulmonary tuberculosis in adults usually represents endogenous reactivation of a site of tuberculous infection established previously in the body. This form of tuberculosis is rare in childhood but may occur in adolescence. Children with a healed tuberculous infection acquired before age 2 yr rarely develop chronic reactivation pulmonary disease, which is more common in those who acquire the initial infection after 7 yr of age. The most frequent pulmonary sites are the original parenchymal focus, lymph nodes, or the apical seedings (Simon foci) established during the hematogenous phase of the early infection. This form of disease usually remains localized to the lungs because the established immune response prevents further extrapulmonary spread. The most common radiographic presentation of this type of tuberculosis is extensive infiltrates or thick-walled cavities in the upper lobes.

Older children and adolescents with reactivation tuberculosis are more likely to experience fever, anorexia, malaise, weight loss, night sweats, productive cough, and chest pain than children with primary pulmonary tuberculosis. However, physical examination findings usually are minor or absent, even when cavities or large infiltrates are present. Most signs and symptoms improve within several weeks of starting effective treatment, although the cough may last for several months. This form of tuberculosis may be highly contagious if there is significant sputum production and cough. The prognosis for full recovery is excellent when patients are given appropriate therapy.

Pleural Effusion. Tuberculous pleural effusions, which can be local or general, originate in the discharge of bacilli into the pleural space from a subpleural pulmonary focus or caseated lymph node. Asymptomatic local pleural effusion is so frequent in primary tuberculosis that it is basically a component of the primary complex. Larger and clinically significant effusions occur months to years after the primary infection. Tuberculous pleural effusion is infrequent in children younger than 6 yr of age and rare in those below 2 yr of age. Effusions are usually unilateral but can be bilateral. They are virtually never associated with a segmental pulmonary lesion and are rare in disseminated tuberculosis. Often the radiographic abnormality is more extensive than would be suggested by physical findings or symptoms (Fig. 199–3).

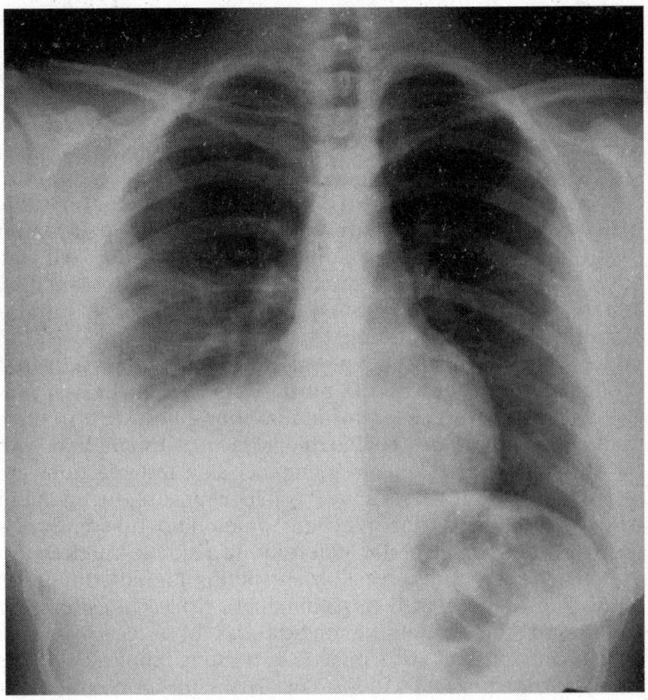

Figure 199–3. Pleural tuberculosis in a 16-yr-old girl.

Clinical onset of tuberculous pleurisy is often sudden, characterized by low to high fever, shortness of breath, chest pain on deep inspiration, and diminished breath sounds. The fever and other symptoms may last for several weeks after the start of antituberculosis chemotherapy. The tuberculin skin test is positive in only 70–80% of cases. The prognosis is excellent but radiographic resolution often takes months. Scoliosis is a rare complication from a long-standing effusion.

Examination of pleural fluid and the pleural membrane is important to establish the diagnosis of tuberculous pleurisy. The pleural fluid is usually yellow and only occasionally tinged with blood. The specific gravity is usually 1.012–1.025, the protein is usually 2–4 g/dL, and the glucose may be low, although it is usually in the low-normal range (20–40 mg/dL). Typically there are several hundred to several thousand white blood cells/mm^3 with an early predominance of polymorphonuclear cells followed by a high percentage of lymphocytes. Acid-fast smears of the pleural fluid are almost never positive. Cultures of the fluid are positive in only 30–70% of cases. Biopsy of the pleural membrane is more likely to yield a positive acid-fast stain or culture and granuloma formation usually can be demonstrated.

Pericardial Disease. The most common form of cardiac tuberculosis is pericarditis. It is rare, occurring in 0.5–4% of tuberculosis cases in children. Pericarditis usually arises from direct invasion or lymphatic drainage from subcarinal lymph nodes. The presenting symptoms are usually nonspecific including low-grade fever, malaise, and weight loss. Chest pain is unusual in children. A pericardial friction rub or distant heart sounds with pulsus paradoxicus may be present. The pericardial fluid is typically serofibrinous or hemorrhagic. Acid-fast smear of the fluid rarely reveals the organism but cultures are positive in 30–70% of cases. The culture yield from pericardial biopsy may be higher and the presence of granulomas often suggests the diagnosis. Partial or complete pericardiectomy may be required when constrictive pericarditis develops.

Lymphohematogenous (Disseminated) Disease. Tubercle bacilli are disseminated to distant sites, including liver, spleen, skin, and lung apices, in all cases of tuberculous infection. The clinical picture produced by lymphohematogenous dissemination depends upon the quantity of organisms released from the primary focus and the adequacy of the host immune response. Lymphohematogenous spread is usually asymptomatic. Rare patients experience protracted hematogenous tuberculosis caused by the intermittent release of tubercle bacilli as a caseous focus erodes through the wall of a blood vessel in the lung. Although the clinical picture may be acute, more often it is indolent and prolonged, with spiking fever accompanying the release of organisms into the bloodstream. Multiple organ involvement is common, leading to hepatomegaly, splenomegaly, lymphadenitis in superficial or deep nodes, and papulonecrotic tuberculids appearing on the skin. Bones and joints or kidneys also may become involved. Meningitis, which occurs only late in the course of the disease, was often the cause of death in the prechemotherapy era. Early pulmonary involvement is surprisingly mild, but diffuse involvement becomes apparent with prolonged infection. Culture confirmation of this form of tuberculosis can be difficult as sputum and gastric aspirate cultures are often unrevealing. Bone marrow examination or liver biopsy with appropriate stains and cultures may be necessary and should be performed if the diagnosis is considered and other tests are not diagnostic. The tuberculin skin test is usually reactive.

The most clinically significant form of disseminated tuberculosis is miliary disease, which occurs when massive numbers of tubercle bacilli are released into the bloodstream, causing disease in two or more organs. Miliary tuberculosis usually complicates the primary infection, occurring within 2–6 mo of the initial infection. Although this form of disease is most common in infants and young children, it is also found in adolescents and older adults, resulting from the breakdown of a previously healed primary pulmonary lesion. The clinical manifestations of miliary tuberculosis are protean, depending on the load of organisms that disseminate and where they lodge. Lesions are often larger and more numerous in the lungs, spleen, liver, and bone marrow than other tissues. Because this form of tuberculosis is most common in infants and malnourished or immunosuppressed patients, the host's immune incompetency probably also plays a role in pathogenesis.

The onset of miliary tuberculosis is sometimes explosive and the patient may become gravely ill in several days. More often, the onset is insidious with early systemic signs, including anorexia, weight loss, and low-grade fever. At this time abnormal physical signs are usually absent. Generalized lymphadenopathy and hepatosplenomegaly develop within several weeks in about 50% of cases. The fever may then become higher and more sustained, although the chest radiograph usually is normal and respiratory symptoms are minor or absent. Within several more weeks, the lungs may become filled with tubercles and dyspnea, cough, rales, or wheezing occur. The lesions of miliary tuberculosis are usually smaller than 2–3 mm in diameter when first visible on chest radiograph (Fig. 199–4). The smaller lesions coalesce to form larger lesions and sometimes extensive infiltrates. As the pulmonary disease progresses an alveolar-airblock syndrome may result in frank respiratory distress, hypoxia, and pneumothorax, or pneumomediastinum. Signs or symptoms of meningitis or peritonitis are found in 20–40% of patients with advanced disease. Chronic or recurrent headache in a patient with miliary tuberculosis usually indicates the presence of meningitis, while the onset of abdominal pain or tenderness is a sign of tuberculous peritonitis. Cutaneous lesions include papulonecrotic tuberculids, nodules, or purpura. Choroid tubercles occur in 13–87% of patients and are highly specific for the diagnosis of miliary tuberculosis. Unfortunately, the tuberculin skin test is nonreactive in up to 40% of patients with disseminated tuberculosis.

Diagnosis can be difficult and a high index of suspicion by the clinician is required. Often the patient presents with fever of unknown origin. Early sputum or gastric aspirate cultures have a low sensitivity. Biopsy of the liver or bone marrow with appropriate bacteriologic and histologic examinations more often yields an early diagnosis. The most important clue is usually history of recent exposure to an adult with infectious tuberculosis.

The resolution of miliary tuberculosis is slow, even with proper therapy. Fever usually declines within 2–3 wk of starting chemotherapy, but the chest radiographic abnormalities may not resolve for many months. Occasionally, corticosteroids hasten symptomatic relief, especially when airblock, peritonitis, or meningitis is present. The *prognosis* is excellent if the diagnosis is made early and adequate chemotherapy is given.

Upper Respiratory Tract Disease. Tuberculosis of the upper respiratory tract is rare in developed countries but is still observed in developing countries. Children with laryngeal tuberculosis have a croupy cough, sore throat, hoarseness, and dysphagia. Most children with laryngeal tuberculosis have extensive upper lobe pulmonary disease, but occasional patients have primary laryngeal disease with a normal chest radiograph. Tuberculosis of the middle ear results from aspiration of infected pulmonary secretions into the middle ear or from hematogenous dissemination in older children. The most common signs and symptoms are painless otorrhea, tinnitus, decreased hearing, facial paralysis, and a perforated tympanic membrane. Enlargement of lymph nodes in the preauricular or anterior cervical chains may accompany this infection. Disease is almost exclusively unilateral, and the most common finding is a single draining ear. Diagnosis is difficult because stains and cultures of ear fluid are frequently negative and histology of the affected tissue often shows a nonspecific acute and chronic inflammation without granuloma formation.

Lymph Node Disease. Tuberculosis of the superficial lymph nodes, often referred to as scrofula, is the most common form of extrapulmonary tuberculosis in children. Historically, scrofula was usually caused by drinking unpasteurized cow's milk laden with *M. bovis*. Most current cases occur within 6–9 mo of initial infection by *M. tuberculosis*, although some cases appear years later. The tonsillar, anterior cervical, submandibular, and supraclavicular nodes become involved secondary to extension of a primary lesion of the upper lung fields or abdomen. Infected nodes in the inguinal, epitrochlear, or axillary regions result from regional lymphadenitis associated with tuberculosis of the skin or skeletal system. The nodes usually enlarge gradually in the early stages of lymph node disease. They are firm but not hard, discrete, and nontender. The nodes often feel fixed to underlying or overlying tissue. Disease is most often unilateral, but bilateral involvement may occur because of the crossover drainage patterns of lymphatic vessels in the chest and lower neck. As infection progresses multiple nodes are infected, resulting in a mass of matted nodes. Systemic signs

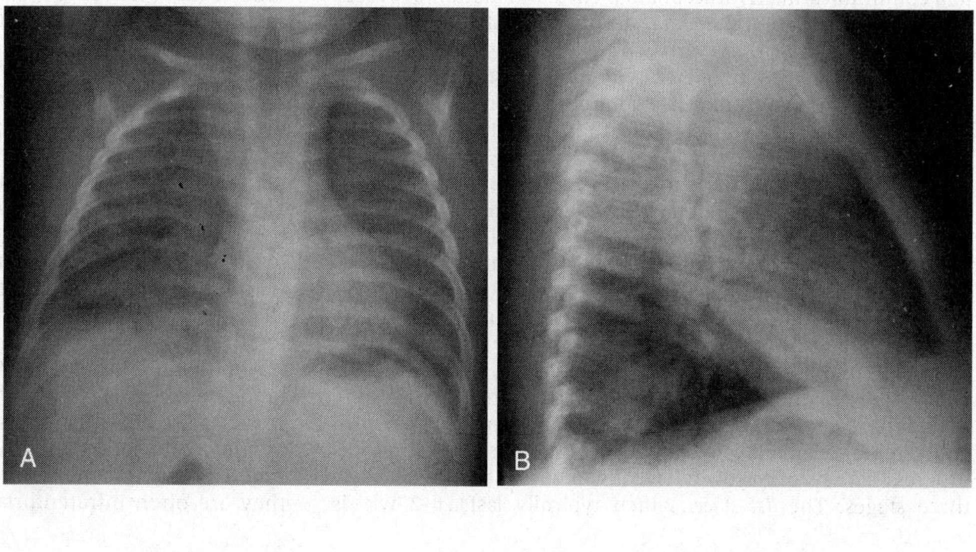

Figure 199–4. Posteroanterior *(A)* and lateral *(B)* chest radiographs of an infant with miliary tuberculosis. The child's mother had failed to complete treatment for pulmonary tuberculosis twice within 3 yr of this child's birth.

and symptoms other than a low-grade fever are usually absent. The tuberculin skin test is usually reactive. The chest radiograph is normal in 70% of cases. The onset of illness is occasionally more acute with rapid enlargement of lymph nodes, high fever, tenderness, and fluctuance. The initial presentation is rarely a fluctuant mass with overlying cellulitis or skin discoloration.

Lymph node tuberculosis may resolve if left untreated but more often progresses to caseation and necrosis. The capsule of the node breaks down, resulting in the spread of infection to adjacent nodes. Rupture of the node usually results in a draining sinus tract that may require surgical removal. Tuberculous lymphadenitis usually responds well to antituberculosis therapy, although the lymph nodes do not return to normal size for months or even years. Surgical removal is not adequate therapy because the lymph node disease is but one part of a systemic infection.

A definitive *diagnosis* of tuberculous adenitis usually requires histologic or bacteriologic confirmation, which is best accomplished by excisional biopsy of the involved node. Culture of lymph node tissue yields the organisms in only about 50% of cases. Many other conditions can be confused with tuberculous adenitis, including infection due to nontuberculous mycobacteria (NTM), cat-scratch disease, tularemia, brucellosis toxoplasmosis, tumor, branchial cleft cyst, cystic hygroma, and pyogenic infection. The most frequent problem is distinguishing infection due to *M. tuberculosis* from lymphadenitis due to NTM in geographic areas where NTM are common. Both conditions are usually associated with a normal chest radiograph and a reactive tuberculin skin test. An important clue to the diagnosis of tuberculous adenitis is an epidemiologic link to an adult with infectious tuberculosis. In areas where both diseases are common, the only way to distinguish them may be culture of the involved tissue.

Central Nervous System Disease. CNS tuberculosis is the most serious complication in children and is fatal without effective treatment. Tuberculous meningitis usually arises from the formation of a metastatic caseous lesion in the cerebral cortex or meninges that develops during the lymphohematogenous dissemination of the primary infection. This initial lesion increases in size and discharges small numbers of tubercle bacilli into the subarachnoid space. The resulting gelatinous exudate may infiltrate the corticomeningeal blood vessels, producing inflammation, obstruction, and subsequent infarction of cerebral cortex. The brain stem is often the site of greatest involvement, which accounts for the frequently associated dysfunction of cranial nerves III, VI, and VII. The exudate also interferes with the normal flow of CSF in and out of the ventricular system at the level of the basilar cisterns, leading to a communicating hydrocephalus. The combination of vasculitis, infarction, cerebral edema, and hydrocephalus results in the severe damage that can occur gradually or rapidly. Profound abnormalities in electrolyte metabolism, due to salt wasting or the syndrome of inappropriate antidiuretic hormone secretion, also contribute to the pathophysiology of tuberculous meningitis.

Tuberculous meningitis complicates about 0.3% of untreated primary infections in children. It is most common in children between 6 mo and 4 yr of age. Occasionally, tuberculous meningitis may occur many years after the primary infection, when rupture of one or more of the subependymal tubercles discharges tubercle bacilli into the subarachnoid space. The clinical progression of tuberculous meningitis may be rapid or gradual. Rapid progression tends to occur more often in infants and young children, who may experience symptoms for only several days before the onset of acute hydrocephalus, seizures, and cerebral edema. More commonly, the signs and symptoms progress slowly over several weeks and can be divided into three stages. The *1st stage*, which typically lasts 1–2 wk, is characterized by nonspecific symptoms, such as fever, headache, irritability, drowsiness, and malaise. Focal neurologic signs are absent, but infants may experience a stagnation or loss of developmental milestones. The *2nd stage* usually begins more abruptly. The most common features are lethargy, nuchal rigidity, seizures, positive Kernig or Brudzinski signs, hypertonia, vomiting, cranial nerve palsies, and other focal neurologic signs. The accelerating clinical illness usually correlates with the development of hydrocephalus, increased intracranial pressure, and vasculitis. Some children have no evidence of meningeal irritation but may have signs of encephalitis, such as disorientation, movement disorders, or speech impairment. The *3rd stage* is marked by coma, hemiplegia or paraplegia, hypertension, decerebrate posturing, deterioration of vital signs, and eventually, death. The prognosis of tuberculous meningitis correlates most closely with the clinical stage of illness at the time treatment is initiated. The majority of patients in stage 1 have an excellent outcome, whereas most patients in stage 3 who survive have permanent disabilities, including blindness, deafness, paraplegia, diabetes insipidus, or mental retardation. The prognosis for young infants is generally worse than for older children. It is imperative that antituberculosis treatment be considered for any child who develops basilar meningitis and hydrocephalus with no other apparent etiology. Often the key to the correct diagnosis is identifying an adult in contact with the child who has infectious tuberculosis. Because of the short incubation period of tuberculous meningitis, the presenting adult has not yet been diagnosed in many cases.

The *diagnosis* of tuberculous meningitis can be difficult early in its course requiring a high degree of suspicion on the part of the clinician. The tuberculin skin test is nonreactive in up to 50% of cases and 20–50% of children have a normal chest radiograph. The most important laboratory test for the diagnosis of tuberculous meningitis is examination and culture of the lumbar CSF. The CSF leukocyte count usually ranges from 10 to 500 cells/mm^3. Polymorphonuclear leukocytes may be present initially, but lymphocytes are predominant in the majority of cases. The CSF glucose is typically less than 40 mg/dL but rarely goes below 20 mg/dL. The protein level is elevated and may be markedly high (400–5,000 mg/dL) secondary to hydrocephalus and spinal block. Although the lumbar CSF is grossly abnormal, ventricular CSF may have normal chemistries and cell counts because this fluid is obtained from a site proximal to the inflammation and obstruction. The success of the microscopic examination of acid-fast stained CSF and mycobacterial culture is related directly to the size of the CSF sample. Examinations or culture of small amounts of CSF are unlikely to demonstrate *M. tuberculosis*. When 5–10 mL of lumbar CSF can be obtained, the acid-fast stain of the CSF sediment is positive in up to 30% of cases and the culture is positive in 50–70% of cases. Cultures of other fluids, such as gastric aspirates or urine, may help confirm the diagnosis. Radiographic studies may aid in the diagnosis of tuberculous meningitis. Computed tomography (CT) or magnetic resonance imaging (MRI) of the brain of patients with tuberculous meningitis may be normal during early stages of the disease. As disease progresses, basilar enhancement and communicating hydrocephalus with signs of cerebral edema or early focal ischemia are the most common findings. Some small children with tuberculous meningitis may have one or several clinically silent tuberculomas, occurring most often in the cerebral cortex or thalamic regions.

Another manifestation of CNS tuberculosis is the tuberculoma, which usually presents clinically as a brain tumor. Tuberculomas account for up to 40% of brain tumors in some areas of the world, but they are rare in North America. In adults tuberculomas are most often supratentorial, but in children they are often infratentorial, located at the base of the brain near the cerebellum. Lesions are most often singular but may be multiple. The most common symptoms are headache, fever, and convulsions. The tuberculin skin test is usually reactive, but the chest radiograph is usually normal. Surgical excision is often necessary to distinguish tuberculoma from other causes of brain tumor. However, surgical removal is not necessary because most tuberculomas resolve with medical management. Corticosteroids are usually administered during the first few weeks of treatment or in the immediate postoperative period to decrease cerebral edema. On CT scan or MRI of the brain, tuberculomas usually appear as discrete lesions with a significant amount of surrounding edema. Contrast enhancement is often impressive and may result in a ringlike lesion. Angiographic studies show that, unlike most types of brain tumors, tuberculomas usually are avascular. Since the advent of CT scanning, the paradoxical development of tuberculomas in patients with tuberculous meningitis who are receiving ultimately effective chemotherapy has been recognized. The cause and nature of these tuberculomas are poorly understood, but they do not represent failure of drug treatment. This phenomenon should be considered whenever a child with tuberculous meningitis deteriorates or develops focal neurologic findings while on treatment. Corticosteroids may help alleviate the occasionally severe clinical signs and symptoms that occur. These lesions may persist for months or even years.

Cutaneous Disease. See Chapter 616.

Bone and Joint Disease. See Chapters 172 and 628. Bone and joint infection complicating tuberculosis is most likely to involve the vertebrae. The classic manifestation of tuberculous spondylitis is progression to Pott disease, in which destruction of the vertebral bodies leads to gibbus deformity and kyphosis. Skeletal tuberculosis is a late complication of tuberculosis and has become a rare entity since antituberculous therapy became available.

Abdominal and Gastrointestinal Disease. Tuberculosis of the oral cavity or pharynx is quite unusual. The most common lesion is a painless ulcer on the mucosa, palate, or tonsil with enlargement of the regional lymph nodes. Tuberculosis of the esophagus is rare in children but may be associated with a tracheoesophageal fistula in infants. These forms of tuberculosis are usually associated with extensive pulmonary disease and swallowing of infectious respiratory secretions. However, they can occur in the absence of pulmonary disease, presumably by spread from mediastinal or peritoneal lymph nodes.

Tuberculous peritonitis, which occurs most often in young men, is uncommon in adolescents and rare in children. Generalized peritonitis may arise from subclinical or miliary hematogenous dissemination. Localized peritonitis is caused by direct extension from an abdominal lymph node infection, intestinal focus, or genitourinary tuberculosis. Pain and tenderness are mild initially. Rarely the lymph nodes, omentum, and peritoneum become matted and can be palpated as a "doughy" irregular nontender mass. Ascites and low-grade fever commonly accompany this complication. The tuberculin skin test is usually reactive. The diagnosis can be confirmed by paracentesis with appropriate stains and cultures, but this procedure must be performed carefully to avoid entering a bowel that is intertwined with the matted omentum.

Tuberculous enteritis is caused by hematogenous dissemination or by swallowing tubercle bacilli discharged from the patient's own lungs. The jejunum and ileum near Peyer's patches and the appendix are the most common sites of involvement. The typical findings are shallow ulcers that cause pain, diarrhea or constipation, and weight loss with low-grade fever. Mesenteric adenitis usually complicates the infection. The enlarged nodes may cause intestinal obstruction or erode through the omentum to cause generalized peritonitis. The clinical presentation of tuberculous enteritis is nonspecific, mimicking other infections and conditions that cause diarrhea. The disease should be suspected in any child with chronic gastrointestinal complaints and a reactive tuberculin skin test. Biopsy, acid-fast stain, and culture of the lesions are usually necessary to confirm the diagnosis.

Genitourinary Disease. Renal tuberculosis is rare in children because the incubation period is several years or longer. Tubercle bacilli usually reach the kidney during lymphohematogenous dissemination. The organisms often can be recovered from the urine in cases of miliary tuberculosis and in some patients with primary pulmonary tuberculosis in the absence of renal parenchymal disease. In true renal tuberculosis, small caseous foci develop in the renal parenchyma and release *M. tuberculosis* into the tubules. A large mass develops near the renal cortex that discharges bacteria through a fistula into the renal pelvis. Infection then spreads locally to the ureters, prostate, or epididymis. Renal tuberculosis is often clinically silent in its early stages, marked only by sterile pyuria and microscopic hematuria. Dysuria, flank or abdominal pain, and gross hematuria develop as the disease progresses. Superinfection by other bacteria, which often causes more acute symptoms, occurs frequently but may also delay recognition of the underlying tuberculosis. Hydronephrosis or ureteral strictures may complicate the disease. Urine cultures for *M. tuberculosis* are positive in about 80–90% of cases, and acid-fast stains of large volumes of urine sediment are positive in 50–70% of cases. The tuberculin skin test is nonreactive in up to 20% of patients. An intravenous pyelogram often reveals mass lesions, dilatation of the proximal ureters, multiple small filling defects, and hydronephrosis if ureteral stricture is present. Disease is most often unilateral.

Tuberculosis of the genital tract is uncommon in both males and females before puberty. This condition usually originates from lymphohematogenous spread, although it can be caused by direct spread from the intestinal tract or bone. Adolescent girls may develop genital tract tuberculosis during the primary infection. The fallopian tubes are most often involved (90–100% of cases) followed by the endometrium (50%), ovaries (25%), and cervix (5%). The most common symptoms are lower abdominal pain and dysmenorrhea or amenorrhea. Systemic manifestations are usually absent and the chest radiograph is normal in the majority of cases. The tuberculin skin test is usually reactive. Genital tuberculosis in adolescent males causes epididymitis or orchitis. The condition usually manifests as a unilateral nodular painless swelling of the scrotum. Involvement of the glans penis is extremely rare. Genital abnormalities and a positive tuberculin skin test in an adolescent male or female should suggest the diagnosis of genital tract tuberculosis.

Disease in HIV-Infected Children. Relatively few cases of children with coexisting tuberculosis and HIV infection have been reported. The diagnosis of tuberculosis can be missed in an HIV-infected child because the skin test reactivity may be absent, culture confirmation is difficult, and the clinical appearance of tuberculosis is similar to many other HIV-related infections and conditions. Tuberculosis in HIV-infected children is often more severe and more likely to be disseminated. Pulmonary symptoms accompanied by fever and weight loss are the most common findings. HIV-infected children may be more likely than other children to develop progressive pulmonary disease with cavitation and extrapulmonary disease.

Perinatal Disease. Symptoms of congenital tuberculosis may be present at birth but more commonly begin by the 2nd or 3rd wk of life. The most common signs and symptoms are respiratory distress, fever, hepatic or splenic enlargement, poor feeding, lethargy or irritability, lymphadenopathy, abdominal distention, failure to thrive, ear drainage, and skin lesions. The clinical manifestations vary in relation to the site and size of the caseous lesions. Many infants have an abnormal chest radiograph, most often a miliary pattern. Some infants with no pulmonary findings early in the course of the disease later develop profound radiographic and clinical abnormalities. Hilar and mediastinal lymphadenopathy and lung infiltrates are common. Generalized lymphadenopathy and meningitis occur in 30–50% of patients.

The clinical presentation of tuberculosis in newborns is similar to that caused by bacterial sepsis and other congenital infections such as syphilis, toxoplasmosis, and cytomegalovirus. The diagnosis should be suspected in an infant with signs and symptoms of bacterial or congenital infection whose response to antibiotic and supportive therapy is poor and evaluation for other infections is unrevealing. The most important clue for rapid diagnosis of congenital tuberculosis is a maternal or family history of tuberculosis. Frequently, the mother's disease is discovered only after the neonate's diagnosis is suspected. The infant's tuberculin skin test is negative initially but may become positive in 1–3 mo. A positive acid-fast stain of an early morning gastric aspirate from a newborn usually indicates tuberculosis. Direct acid-fast stains on middle-ear discharge, bone marrow, tracheal aspirate, or biopsy tissue (especially liver) can be useful and should be performed. The CSF should be examined and cultured, although the yield for isolating *M. tuberculosis* is low. The mortality rate of congenital tuberculosis remains very high because of delayed diagnosis; many children will have a complete recovery if the diagnosis is made promptly and adequate chemotherapy is started.

TREATMENT. Microbiologic Basis for Treatment. Tubercle bacilli can be killed only during replication. Individual organisms that are naturally resistant to each antimycobacterial drug are present within large populations of *M. tuberculosis*. All known drug resistance within *M. tuberculosis* is chromosomal and is not passed from one organism to another. The estimated frequency of these naturally drug-resistant organisms is about 10^{-6} but varies among drugs: with streptomycin it is 10^{-5}, with isoniazid 10^{-6}, and with rifampin 10^{-8}. A cavity containing 10^{9} tubercle bacilli has thousands of drug-resistant organisms, whereas a closed caseous lesion with its much smaller population contains few if any naturally resistant organisms. Fortunately, the natural occurrence of resistance to one drug is independent of resistance to any other drug. The chance that an organism is naturally resistant to both isoniazid and rifampin is on the order of 10^{-14}. Because populations of this size do not occur in patients, organisms naturally resistant to two drugs are essentially nonexistent.

The major biologic determinant of the success of antituberculosis chemotherapy is the size of the bacillary population within the host. For patients with large bacterial populations, such as adults with cavities or extensive infiltrates, many naturally drug-resistant organisms are present and at least two antituberculosis drugs must be used to effect a cure. Conversely for patients with infection (reactive skin test) but no disease, the bacterial population is small, drug-resistant organisms are rare or nonexistent, and a single drug can be used. Children with primary pulmonary tuberculosis and most patients with extrapulmonary tuberculosis have medium-sized populations in which significant numbers of naturally drug-resistant organisms may or may not be present. In general, these patients are treated with at least two drugs. The phenomena of drug resistance mutation and microbial population size explain why poor patient adherence to treatment or an inadequate treatment regimen can lead to the development of drug-resistant tuberculosis. If a patient with extensive pulmonary tuberculosis is given a single medication, the subpopulation of bacilli susceptible to that drug will be eliminated but the subpopulation of bacilli resistant to the drug have the opportunity to multiply and become the predominant strain. The patient will temporarily improve but will suffer a relapse from tuberculosis resistant to that drug. With treatment using two drugs to which the *M. tuberculosis* isolate is susceptible, drug X eliminates the subpopulation of bacilli resistant to drug Y, and drug Y eliminates the subpopulation of bacilli resistant to drug X. If all the organisms have initial resistance to a certain medication (called primary resistance) and the patient is treated with that plus one other medication, only one effective medication is being used and the patient will eventually relapse with tuberculosis that is resistant to both drugs.

The various antituberculosis drugs (Table 199–2) differ in their primary site of activity and their actions. Isoniazid and rifampin are highly bactericidal for *M. tuberculosis*. Streptomycin and several other aminoglycosides are also bactericidal for extracellular tubercle bacilli, but their penetration into macrophages is poor. Pyrazinamide cannot be shown to be bactericidal in the laboratory but clearly contributes to the killing of *M. tuberculosis* within the patient. Other antituberculosis drugs, such as ethambutol at low doses (15 mg/kg/24 hr), ethionamide, and cycloserine, are bacteriostatic for *M. tuberculosis* and their primary purpose in the therapeutic regimen is to prevent emergence of resistance to other drugs. Ethambutol at 25 mg/kg/24 hr has some bactericidal activity, which may be important in treating cases of drug-resistant tuberculosis. Isoniazid and rifampin are also effective in preventing emergence of resistance to other drugs, but pyrazinamide has almost has no similar activity.

Antituberculosis Drugs in Children. ISONIAZID (INH). Isoniazid is inexpensive, diffuses into all tissues and body fluids, and has a very low rate of adverse reactions. It can be administered either orally or intramuscularly. At the usual daily dose of 10 mg/kg, serum concentrations greatly exceed the minimum inhibitory concentration for *M. tuberculosis*. Peak concentrations in blood, sputum, and CSF are reached within a few hours and persist

TABLE 199–2 Most Commonly Used Antituberculosis Drugs

Drug	Daily Dose (mg/kg/24 hr)	Twice-Weekly Dose (mg/kg/dose)	Maximum Dose
Isoniazid*	10–15	20–30	Daily: 300 mg; twice weekly: 900 mg
Rifampin*	10–20	10–20	600 mg
Pyrazinamide*	20–40	40–60	2 g
Streptomycin (IM)	20–40	20–40	1 g
Ethambutol	15–25	25–50	2.5 g
Ethionamide	15–20 (1–3 divided doses)	—	1 g
Cycloserine	10–20 (1–2 divided doses)	—	1 g
Kanamycin or capreomycin (IM)	15–30	15–30	1 g
Amikacin (IV)	15–30	15–30	1 g

IM = intramuscular; IV = intravenous.
**Isoniazid (150 mg) and rifampin (300 mg) are combined in one preparation called Rifamate.*
Isoniazid, rifampin, and pyrazinamide are combined in one preparation called Rifater.

for at least 6–8 hr. Isoniazid is metabolized by acetylation in the liver. Rapid acetylation is more frequent among African-Americans and Asians than among whites. There is no correlation between acetylation rate and either efficacy or adverse reactions in children.

Isoniazid has two principal toxic effects, both which are rare in children. Peripheral neuritis results from competitive inhibition of pyridoxine utilization. Pyridoxine levels are decreased in children taking INH but clinical manifestations are rare and pyridoxine administration is not generally recommended. However, teenagers with inadequate diets, children from groups with low levels of milk and meat intake, and breast-feeding babies often require supplemental pyridoxine. The most common physical manifestation of peripheral neuritis is numbness and tingling in the hands or feet. CNS toxicity from INH is rare, occurring usually when there is a significant overdose. The major toxic effect of INH is hepatotoxicity, which is also rare in children but increases with age. Three to ten percent of children taking INH experience transient elevated serum transaminase levels. Clinically significant hepatotoxicity is very rare, being more likely to occur in adolescents or children with severe forms of tuberculosis. For most children routine biochemical monitoring is not necessary, and toxicity can be monitored using clinical signs and symptoms. Allergic manifestations or hypersensitivity reactions caused by INH are very rare. INH can increase phenytoin levels and lead to toxicity by blocking its metabolism. Occasionally INH interacts with theophylline, requiring modification of the dosage. Rare side effects of INH include pellagra, hemolytic anemia in patients with glucose-6-phosphate dehydrogenase deficiency, and a lupus-like reaction with skin rash and arthritis.

RIFAMPIN (RIF). This is a key drug in the modern management of tuberculosis. It is well absorbed from the gastrointestinal tract during fasting, with peak serum levels achieved within 2 hr. Oral and intravenous forms of RIF are now readily available. Like INH, RIF is distributed widely in tissues and body fluids, including the CSF. While excretion is mainly via the biliary tract, effective levels are reached in the kidneys and urine. Side effects are more common than with INH and include orange discoloration of urine and tears (with permanent staining of contact lenses), gastrointestinal disturbances, and hepatotoxicity, usually manifested as asymptomatic elevations in serum transaminase levels. When RIF is administered with INH, there is an increased risk of hepatotoxicity, which can be minimized by lowering the daily dose of INH to 10 mg/kg/24 hr. Intermittent administration of RIF has been associated with thrombocytopenia and an influenza-like syndrome consisting of fever, headache, and malaise. Rifampin can render oral conceptives ineffective and interacts with several drugs, including quinidine, sodium warfarin, and corticosteroids. Rifampin is generally available in 150 mg and 300 mg capsules that, unfortunately, are inconvenient for many weight ranges of children. A suspension can be made using a variety of carriers but should not be taken with food because of malabsorption. A preparation called Rifamate contains both INH (150 mg) and RIF (300 mg); this preparation helps to ensure that the patient gets both INH and RIF or neither drug so that selective drug resistance is not created.

PYRAZINAMIDE (PZA). In adults, a once-daily dose of PZA, 30 mg/kg/24 hr, produces serum levels of 20 μg/mL and little liver toxicity. The optimal dose in children is unknown, but this same dose causes high CSF levels, is well tolerated by children, and correlates with clinical success in treatment trials of tuberculosis in children. Extensive experience with PZA in children has verified its safety. Approximately 10% of adults treated with PZA develop arthralgias, arthritis, or gout due to hyperuricemia. Although uric acid levels are slightly elevated in children taking PZA, clinical manifestations of the hyperuricemia are extremely rare. Hypersensitivity reactions are rare in children. The only dosage form of PZA is a rather large 500 mg tablet, which produces some dosing problems for children, especially infants. These pills can be crushed and given with food in the same manner as INH, but formal pharmacokinetic studies using this method have not been reported.

STREPTOMYCIN (STM). Streptomycin is used less frequently than in the past for the treatment of childhood tuberculosis but is important for the treatment or prevention of drug-resistant disease. It must be given intramuscularly. Streptomycin penetrates inflamed meninges fairly well but does not cross uninflamed meninges. Its major current use is when initial INH resistance is suspected or when the child has a life-threatening form of tuberculosis. The major toxicity of STM is to the vestibular and auditory portions of the 8th cranial nerve. Renal toxicity is much less frequent. Streptomycin is contraindicated in pregnant women because up to 30% of their infants will suffer severe hearing loss.

ETHAMBUTOL (EMB). Ethambutol has received little attention in children because of its potential toxicity to the eye. At a dose of 15 mg/kg/24 hr it is primarily bacteriostatic, and its historic purpose has been to prevent emergence of resistance to other drugs. However, at 25 mg/kg/24 hr EMB has some bactericidal activity, which may be important in the treatment of drug-resistant disease. It is well tolerated by both adults and children when given orally as a once or twice a day dose. The major potential toxicity is optic neuritis. There have been no reports of optic toxicity in children, but the drug has not been widely used because of the inability to routinely test visual fields and acuity in young children. Ethambutol is not recommended for general use in young children for whom vision cannot be adequately examined but should be considered for children with drug-resistant tuberculosis when other agents are not available or cannot be used.

ETHIONAMIDE (ETH). Ethionamide is a bacteriostatic drug whose major purpose is treatment of drug-resistant tuberculosis. Ethionamide penetrates into CSF very well and may be particularly useful in cases of tuberculous meningitis. It is generally well tolerated by children but often must be given in 2 or 3 divided daily doses because of gastrointestinal disturbance. Ethionamide is chemically similar to INH and can cause significant hepatitis.

OTHER DRUGS. These drugs are used less commonly for tuberculosis because they are significantly less effective or more toxic. Several aminoglycosides, especially kanamycin and amikacin, have significant antituberculosis activity and are used in cases of streptomycin-resistant tuberculosis. A closely related drug, capreomycin, is used more commonly in adults. These drugs can be given either intramuscularly or intravenously, are bactericidal, and usually do not demonstrate cross resistance with STM. Cycloserine is an effective antituberculosis drug in adults but has been used infrequently in children due to its major side effects of impairment with thought processes and tendency to cause depression and other psychiatric abnormalities. The drug is usually given in one or two divided doses, and most experts recommend monitoring serum levels during administration. Pyridoxine supplementation should be given when cycloserine is used. Ciprofloxacin and ofloxacin are fluoroquinolones with significant antituberculosis activity that are used commonly for drug-resistant tuberculosis in adults. These drugs are generally contraindicated in children because they cause destruction of growing cartilage in some animal models. However, they have been used effectively in some cases of multiple drug-resistant tuberculosis in children when few other effective agents were available.

Treatment Regimens for Disease. Historically, recommendations for treating children with tuberculosis have been extrapolated from clinical trials involving adults with pulmonary tuberculosis. The trend over the past several decades has been to develop regimens that are increasingly intense and shorter. It is well established that a 9-mo regimen of INH and RIF cures more than 98% of cases of drug-susceptible pulmonary tuberculosis in adults. After daily administration of medication for the first 1–2 mo, both drugs can be given daily or twice weekly for the remaining 7–8 mo with equivalent results and low rates of adverse reactions. Twice weekly administration is supported by pharmacologic and animal model data and extensive clinical trials. The addition of PZA at the beginning of the regimen reduces the duration of necessary treatment to 6 mo.

Over the past 15 yr, a number of trials of antituberculosis therapy for children with drug-susceptible tuberculosis have demonstrated that a 9-mo regimen of INH and RIF is highly successful. Medication should be given daily initially but may be administered twice weekly during the final months of treatment. The major drawbacks of this two-drug, 9-mo regimen are the necessary length of treatment, the need for good adherence by the patient, and the relative lack of protection against possible initial drug resistance. Several clinical trials have shown that a 6-mo duration of INH and RIF, supplemented during the first 2 mo of treatment with PZA, yields a success rate approaching 100% with an incidence of clinically significant adverse reactions of less than 2%. Based on the reported studies, the American Academy of Pediatrics has endorsed a regimen of 6 mo of INH and RIF supplemented during the first 2 mo by PZA as standard therapy of intrathoracic tuberculosis in children. Most experts recommend that all drug administration be directly observed, meaning that a health care worker is physically present when the medications are administered to the patients. In locales where the community rate of INH resistance is greater than 5–10%, most experts recommend adding a 4th drug—usually STM, EMB, or ETH—to the initial regimen. The reason to add the 4th drug is that PZA is not effective in preventing the emergence of RIF resistance during therapy when INH resistance already exists.

Controlled clinical trials for treating various forms of extrapulmonary tuberculosis are virtually nonexistent. Extrapulmonary tuberculosis is usually caused by small numbers of mycobacteria. In general, the treatment for most forms of extrapulmonary tuberculosis in children is the same as for pulmonary tuberculosis. One exception may be bone and joint tuberculosis, which has been associated with a higher failure rate when only 6 mo of chemotherapy is used, especially if surgical intervention has not been performed. Some experts recommend at least 9–12 mo of effective chemotherapy for bone and joint tuberculosis.

Tuberculous meningitis usually has not been included in trials of tuberculosis therapy because of its serious nature and low incidence. As with other forms of extrapulmonary tuberculosis, the number of mycobacteria causing disease is usually small. Daily treatment with INH and RIF for 12 mo is generally effective. Several recent reports have suggested that 6–9 mo of therapy is effective if INH, RIF, and PZA are administered during the initial phase of treatment. Most experts add a 4th drug at the beginning of treatment to protect against unsuspected initial drug resistance. When drug susceptibility information becomes available, the 4th drug can be discontinued.

The optimal treatment of tuberculosis in HIV-infected children has not been established. Adults with tuberculosis who are HIV seropositive can be treated successfully with standard regimens that include INH, RIF, and PZA. The total duration of therapy should be 6–9 mo or 6 mo after culture of sputum becomes sterile, whichever is longer. Data for children are limited to isolated case reports and small series. It may be difficult to determine whether a pulmonary infiltrate in a HIV-infected child who has a positive tuberculin reaction or history of exposure to an adult with infectious tuberculosis is being caused by *M. tuberculosis*. The radiographic appearance of other pulmonary complications of HIV infection in children, such as lymphoid interstitial pneumonitis and bacterial pneumonia, may be similar to that of tuberculosis. Treatment is often empiric based on epidemiologic and radiographic information. Therapy should be considered when tuberculosis cannot be excluded. Most experts believe that HIV-seropositive children with drug-susceptible tuberculosis should receive at least INH, RIF, and PZA for 2 mo followed by INH and RIF to complete a total treatment duration of 9–12 mo. It is recommended that all children with tuberculosis be evaluated for HIV infection because the presence of HIV may necessitate a longer duration of treatment.

Drug-Resistant Tuberculosis. The incidence of drug-resistant tuberculosis appears to be increasing in many areas of the world, including North America. There are two major types of drug resistance. Primary resistance occurs when an individual is infected with *M. tuberculosis* that is already resistant to a particular drug. Secondary resistance occurs when drug-resistant organisms emerge as the dominant population during treatment. The major causes of secondary drug resistance are poor adherence with the medication by the patient or inadequate treatment regimens prescribed by the physician. Nonadherence with one drug is more likely to lead to secondary resistance than failure to take all drugs. Secondary resistance is rare in children because of the small size of their mycobacterial population. Therefore, most drug resistance in children is primary, and patterns of drug resistance among children tend to mirror those found among adults in the same population. The main predictors of drug-resistant tuberculosis among adults are history of previous antituberculosis treatment or exposure to another adult with infectious drug-resistant tuberculosis.

Treatment for drug-resistant tuberculosis is successful only when at least two bactericidal drugs are given to which the infecting strain of *M. tuberculosis* is susceptible. When a child has possible drug-resistant tuberculosis, at least three and usually four or five drugs should be administered initially until the susceptibility pattern is determined and a more specific regimen can be designed. The specific treatment plan must be individualized for each patient according to the results of susceptibility testing on the isolates from the child or the adult source case. Treatment of 9 mo duration with RIF, PZA, and EMB is usually adequate for INH-resistant tuberculosis in children. When INH and RIF resistance are present, the total duration of therapy often must be extended to 12–18 mo. The prognosis of single or multiple drug-resistant tuberculosis in children is usually good if the drug resistance is identified early in the treatment, appropriate drugs are administered under directly observed therapy, adverse reactions from the drugs do not occur, and the child and family are in a supportive environment. The treatment of drug-resistant tuberculosis in children always should be undertaken by a clinician with specific expertise in the treatment of tuberculosis.

Corticosteroids. These are useful in the treatment of some children with tuberculous disease. They are most beneficial when the host inflammatory reaction contributes significantly to tissue damage or impairment of organ function. There is convincing evidence that corticosteroids decrease mortality rates and long-term neurologic sequelae in some patients with tuberculous meningitis by reducing vasculitis, inflammation, and, ultimately, intracranial pressure. Lowering the intracranial pressure limits tissue damage and favors circulation of antituberculosis drugs through the brain and meninges. Short courses of corticosteroids also may be effective for children with endobronchial tuberculosis that causes respiratory distress, localized emphysema, or segmental pulmonary lesions. Several randomized clinical trials have shown that corticosteroids can help relieve symptoms and constriction associated with acute tuberculous pericardial effusion. Corticosteroids may cause dramatic improvement in symptoms in some patients with tuberculous pleural effusion and shift of the mediastinum. However, the long-term course of disease is probably unaffected. Some children with severe miliary tuberculosis have dramatic improvement with corticosteroid therapy if the inflammatory reaction is so severe that alveolocapillary block is present. There is no convincing evidence that one corticosteroid preparation is better than another. The most commonly prescribed regimen is prednisone 1–2 mg/kg/24 hr in 1–2 divided doses for 4–6 wk with gradual tapering.

Supportive Care. Children receiving treatment should be followed carefully to promote adherence with therapy, to monitor for toxic reactions to medications, and to ensure that the tuberculosis is being adequately treated. Adequate nutrition is important. Patients should be seen at monthly intervals and should be given just enough medication to last until the next visit. Anticipatory guidance with regard to the administration of medications to children is crucial. The physician should foresee difficulties that the family might have in introducing several new medications in inconvenient dosage forms to a young child. The clinician must report all cases of suspected tuberculosis in a child to the local health department to be sure that the child and family receive appropriate care and evaluation.

Nonadherence to treatment is the major problem in tuberculosis therapy. The patient and family must know what is expected of them through verbal and written instructions in their primary language. At least 30–50% of patients taking long-term treatment are significantly nonadherent with medications, and clinicians are usually not able to determine in advance which patients will be nonadherent. If the clinician suspects any chance of nonadherence with daily self-administered medications, directly observed therapy should be instituted with the help of the local health department.

TREATMENT OF TUBERCULOUS INFECTION WITHOUT DISEASE. The treatment of children with asymptomatic tuberculous infection (reactive tuberculin skin test, normal chest radiograph, normal physical examination) to prevent the development of tuberculous disease is an established practice. The effectiveness of INH therapy in children has approached 100% and has lasted for at least 30 yr. INH therapy should be given to any child with a positive tuberculin skin test but no clinical or radiographic evidence of disease. The currently recommended regimen is 9 mo of daily INH therapy. INH can be given twice weekly under direct observation if adherence with daily treatment is likely to be poor. INH therapy also should be started for children less than 6 yr of age with a negative tuberculin skin test who have had recent exposure to an adult with infectious tuberculosis, including infants born to mothers who have tuberculosis. These children may already be infected with *M. tuberculosis* but have not yet developed delayed hypersensitivity. Significant tuberculous disease may develop simultaneously with skin test reactivity in small children and infants, and the illness may develop before the positive skin test is recognized. In exposed children, tuberculin skin testing is repeated 3 mo after contact with the adult source case has been interrupted. If the repeat tuberculin skin test is negative, INH can be discontinued; if the second skin test is reactive, the child has tuberculous infection and a full course of INH therapy can be administered.

Treatment of Drug-Resistant Strains. The optimal treatment for tuberculous infection caused by drug-resistant strains of *M. tuberculosis* has not been established. For infections with strains that are INH resistant only, most experts recommend a 6–9 mo course of RIF. No data from controlled clinical trials support this practice, however. Similarly, no data are available concerning treatment of tuberculous infection caused by organisms that are resistant to both INH and RIF. Some experts have recommended a combination of a fluoroquinolone and PZA for 6–9 mo. An alternative regimen is high-dose EMB and PZA for a similar period of time. For infection with isolates that are resistant to many drugs, the clinician usually administers two drugs to which the organism is susceptible. The efficacy and safety of these regimens in children are not established, and an expert in pediatric tuberculosis should be consulted for treatment of multiple drug-resistant tuberculous infection in children.

PREVENTION. Finding Infected Children. The highest priority of any tuberculosis control program should be case finding and treatment, which interrupts transmission of infection between close contacts. The children and adults in close contact with an adult suspected of having infectious pulmonary tuberculosis should be tuberculin skin tested and examined as soon as possible. On average, 30–50% of household contacts to infectious cases will be tuberculin skin test positive, and 1% of contacts already have overt disease. This scheme relies on effective and adequate public health response and resources. Children, particularly young infants, should receive high priority during contact investigations because their risk of infection is high and they are more likely to rapidly develop severe forms of tuberculosis.

Mass testing of large groups of children for tuberculous infection is an inefficient process. When large groups of children at low risk for tuberculosis are tested, the vast majority of skin test reactions are actually false-positive reactions due to biologic variability or cross sensitization with NTM. However, testing of high-risk groups of adults or children should be encouraged because most of these individuals with positive tuberculin skin tests have tuberculous infection. Testing should take place only if effective mechanisms are in place to assure adequate evaluation and treatment of the individuals who test positive. In many testing programs less than one third of the infected individuals complete effective treatment when adequate resources are not available.

Bacille Calmette-Guérin Vaccination. The only available vaccine against tuberculosis is the bacille Calmette-Guérin (BCG), named for the two French investigators responsible for its development. The original vaccine organism was a strain of *M. bovis* attenuated by subculture every 3 wk for 13 yr. This strain was distributed to dozens of laboratories that continued to subculture the organism on different media under various conditions. The result has been production of many BCG vaccines that differ widely in morphology, growth characteristics, sensitizing potency, and animal virulence. The route of administration and dosing schedule for the BCG vaccines are important variables for efficacy. The preferred route of administration is intradermal injection with a syringe and needle because it is the only method that permits accurate measurement of an individual dose. However, the intradermal route is expensive, and needles and syringes are reused in developing countries, creating a danger of HIV and hepatitis virus transmission. A unit-dose multipuncture technique is the only technique available in the United States and many other parts of the world.

The BCG vaccines are extremely safe in immunocompetent hosts. Local ulceration and regional suppurative adenitis occur in 0.1–1% of vaccine recipients. Local lesions do not suggest underlying host immune defects and do not affect the level of protection afforded by the vaccine. They usually resolve spontaneously but chemotherapy is needed occasionally. Surgical excision of a suppurative draining node is rarely necessary and should be avoided if possible. Osteitis is a rare complication of BCG vaccination that appears to be related to certain strains of the vaccine that are no longer in wide use. Systemic complaints such as fever, convulsions, loss of appetite, and irritability are extraordinarily rare after BCG vaccination. Profoundly immunocompromised patients may develop disseminated BCG infection after vaccination. Children with HIV infection appear to have rates of local adverse reactions to BCG vaccines that are comparable to rates in immunocompetent children. However, the true incidence in these children of disseminated infection months to years after vaccination is currently unknown.

Recommended vaccine schedules vary widely among countries. The official recommendation of the World Health Organization is a single dose administered during infancy. In some countries repeat vaccination is universal. In others it is based on either tuberculin skin testing or the absence of a typical scar. The optimal age for administration and dosing schedule are unknown because adequate comparative trials have not been performed.

Although dozens of BCG trials have been reported in various human populations, the most useful data have come from several controlled trials. The results of these studies have been disparate. Some demonstrated a great deal of protection from BCG vaccines, but others showed no efficacy at all. A recent meta-analysis of published BCG vaccination trials suggested that BCG is 50% effective in preventing pulmonary tuberculosis in adults and children. The protective effect for disseminated and meningeal tuberculosis appears to be slightly higher, with BCG preventing 50–80% of cases. A variety of explanations for the varied responses to BCG vaccines have been proposed, including methodologic and statistical variations within the trials, interaction with NTM that either enhances or decreases the protection afforded by BCG, different potencies among the various BCG vaccines, and genetic factors for BCG response within the study populations. BCG vaccination administered during infancy has little effect on the ultimate incidence of tuberculosis in adults, suggesting that the effect of the vaccine is time limited.

In summary, BCG vaccination has worked well in some situations but poorly in others. Clearly BCG vaccination has had little effect on the ultimate control of tuberculosis throughout the world because over 8 billion doses have been administered but tuberculosis remains common in most regions. BCG vaccination does not substantially influence the chain of transmission because those cases of contagious pulmonary tuberculosis in adults that can be prevented by BCG vaccination constitute a rather small fraction of the sources of infection in a population. The best use of BCG vaccination appears to be prevention of life-threatening forms of tuberculosis in infants and young children.

BCG vaccination has never been adopted as part of the strategy for the control of tuberculosis in the United States. Widespread use of the vaccine would render subsequent tuberculin skin testing less useful. However, BCG vaccination may contribute to tuberculosis control in selected population groups. BCG is recommended for tuberculin skin test negative infants and children who (1) are at high risk of intimate and prolonged exposure to persistently untreated or ineffectively treated adults with infectious pulmonary tuberculosis and cannot be removed from the source of infection or placed on long-term preventive therapy; or (2) are continuously exposed to persons with tuberculosis who have bacilli that are resistant to INH and RIF. Any child receiving BCG vaccination should have a documented negative tuberculin skin test prior to receiving the vaccine. After receiving the vaccine, the child should be separated from the possible sources of infection until it can be demonstrated that the child has had a vaccine response (demonstrated by tuberculin reactivity, which usually develops within 1–3 mo). Occasionally, a second BCG vaccination must be given to children who fail to develop skin test reactivity after the first dose.

PERINATAL TUBERCULOSIS. The most effective way of preventing tuberculous infection and disease in the neonate or young infant is through appropriate testing and treatment of the mother and other family members. High-risk pregnant women should be tested with a tuberculin skin test, and those with a positive test should receive a chest radiograph with appropriate abdominal shielding. If the mother has a negative chest radiograph and is clinically well, no separation of the infant and mother is needed after delivery. The child needs no special evaluation or treatment if he remains asymptomatic. Other household members should receive tuberculin skin testing and further evaluation as indicated.

If the mother has suspected tuberculous disease at the time of delivery, the newborn should be separated from the mother until the chest radiograph is taken. If the mother's chest radiograph is abnormal, separation should be maintained until the mother has been evaluated thoroughly, including examination of the sputum. If the mother's chest radiograph is abnormal but the history, physical examination, sputum examination, and evaluation of the radiograph show no evidence of current active tuberculosis, it is reasonable to assume that the infant is at low risk for infection. The mother should receive appropriate treatment, and she and her infant should receive careful follow-up care. In addition, all household members should be evaluated for tuberculosis.

If the mother's chest radiograph or acid-fast sputum smear shows evidence of current tuberculous disease, additional steps are necessary to protect the infant. INH therapy for newborn infants has been so effective that separation of the mother and infant is no longer considered mandatory. Separation should occur only if the mother is ill enough to require hospitalization, she has been or is expected to become nonadherent with her treatment, or there is strong suspicion that she has drug-resistant tuberculosis. INH treatment for the infant should be continued until the mother has been shown to be sputum culture negative for at least 3 mo. At that time, a Mantoux tuberculin skin test should be placed on the child. If positive, INH is continued for a total duration of 9–12 mo; if negative, INH can be discontinued. Because INH resistance is increasing in the United States, it is not always clear that INH therapy will be effective for the neonate. If INH resistance is suspected or the mother's adherence to medication is in question, separation of the infant from the mother should be considered. The duration of separation must be at least as long as is necessary to render the mother noninfectious. An expert in tuberculosis should be consulted if the young infant has potential exposure to the mother or another adult with tuberculous disease caused by an INH-resistant strain of *M. tuberculosis*.

If the family with tuberculosis cannot be relied upon to receive proper treatment or if the strain of *M. tuberculosis* is resistant to both INH and RIF, then BCG vaccination of the infant should be considered. Previous reports from the United States, Europe, Africa, and Asia have shown that early BCG vaccination of the infant is very effective in preventing disease when a family member has active tuberculosis. Although routine BCG vaccination of newborns is not appropriate in the United States, it should be considered for the neonate whose household is chaotic and cannot be made free from tuberculosis or who is likely to be lost at follow-up.

Although INH is not thought to be teratogenic, the treatment of pregnant women with asymptomatic tuberculous infection is often deferred until after delivery. However, symptomatic pregnant women or those with radiographic evidence of tuberculous disease should be appropriately evaluated. Because pulmonary tuberculosis is harmful to both the mother and the fetus, and it represents a great danger to the infant after delivery, tuberculous disease in pregnant women always should be treated. The most common regimen for drug-susceptible tuberculosis is INH, RIF, and EMB. The aminoglycosides and ethionamide should be avoided because of their teratogenic effect. The safety of PZA in pregnancy has not been established.

American Academy of Pediatrics, Committee on Infectious Diseases: Chemotherapy for tuberculosis in infants and children. Pediatrics 89:161, 1992.

American Academy of Pediatrics, Committee on Infectious Diseases: Screening for tuberculosis in infants and children. Pediatrics 93:131, 1994.

American Thoracic Society: Diagnostic standards and classification of tuberculosis. Am Rev Respir Dis 142:725, 1990.

American Thoracic Society: Treatment of tuberculosis and tuberculous infection in adults and children. Am J Respir Crit Care Med 149:1359, 1994.
Brudney K, Dobkin J: Resurgent tuberculosis in New York City. Human immunodeficiency virus, homelessness, and the decline of tuberculosis control programs. Am Rev Respir Dis 144:745, 1991.
Cantwell MF, Snider DE Jr, Cauthen GM, et al: Epidemiology of tuberculosis in the United States, 1985 through 1992. JAMA 272:535, 1994.
Centers for Disease Control and Prevention: Initial therapy for tuberculosis in the era of multidrug resistance: recommendations of the Advisory Council for the Elimination of Tuberculosis. MMWR 42:1, 1993.
Colditz GA, Brewer TF, Berkey CS, et al: Efficacy of BCG vaccine in the prevention of tuberculosis. Meta-analysis of the published literature. JAMA 271:698, 1994.
Hsu KHK: Thirty years after isoniazid. Its impact on tuberculosis in children and adolescents. JAMA 251:1283, 1984.
Hussery G, Chisholm T, Kibel M: Miliary tuberculosis in children: a review of 94 cases. Pediatr Infect Dis J 10:832, 1991.
Kochi A: The global tuberculosis situation and the new control strategy of the World Health Organization. Tubercle 72:1, 1991.
O'Brien R, Long M, Cross F, et al: Hepatotoxicity from isoniazid and rifampin among children treated for tuberculosis. Pediatrics 72:491, 1983.
Pineda PR, Leung A, Muller NL, et al: Intrathoracic paediatric tuberculosis: a report of 202 cases. Tubercle Lung Dis 74:261, 1993.
Schaaf HS, Gie RP, Beyers N, et al: Tuberculosis in infants less than 3 months of age. Arch Dis Child 69:371, 1993.
Starke JR: Current chemotherapy for tuberculosis in children. Infect Dis Clin North Am 6:215, 1992.
Starke JR, Jacobs RF, Jereb J: Resurgence of tuberculosis in children. J Pediatr 120:839, 1992.
Steiner P, Rao M: Drug-resistant tuberculosis in children. Semin Pediatr Infect Dis 4:275, 1993.
Vallejo JG, Starke JR: Tuberculosis and pregnancy. Clin Chest Med 13:693, 1992.
Vallejo JG, Ong LT, Starke JR: Clinical features, diagnosis and treatment of tuberculosis in infants. Pediatrics 94:1, 1994.
Waecker NJ, Conner JD: Tuberculous meningitis in 30 children. Pediatr Infect Dis J 9:539, 1990.

CHAPTER 200
Nontuberculous Mycobacteria

Dwight A. Powell

Nontuberculous, nonleprous *Mycobacterium* species (NTM), which are also referred to as atypical mycobacteria, mycobacteria other than tuberculosis (MOTT), or potentially pathogenic environmental mycobacteria are members of the family of Mycobacteriaceae. They differ from *M. tuberculosis* in their nutritional requirements, ability to produce pigments, enzymatic activity, and susceptibility patterns to antituberculous drugs. In contrast to *M. tuberculosis,* NTM are generally acquired from contact with the environment rather than by person-to-person spread.

ETIOLOGY. Thirteen strains of NTM are associated with human infections. Phenotypically, they are divided into four groups described by Runyon in 1959 (Table 200–1) based on their colony growth and morphology on solid media. Groups I, II, and III are slow growing (>7 days to detect growth); group IV is rapid growing (<7 days to detect growth). Photochromogens form pigment following exposure to light, scotochromogens form pigment in the dark, and nonchromogens fail to produce pigment. Species and serovars of NTM are now defined by biochemical reactions, antibody specificity, radiolabeled DNA probes, DNA restriction fragment length polymorphism, or ribosomal-RNA sequencing. Biochemically and immunologically related species that are difficult for clinical laboratories to differentiate are referred to as "complexes," for example, the *M. fortuitum* complex *(M. fortuitum* and *M. chelonae)* and the *M. avium* complex *(M. avium* and *M. intracellulare).*

EPIDEMIOLOGY. NTM are distributed worldwide and are ubiquitous in the environment, existing as saprophytes in soil and water; as pathogens in swine, birds, and cattle; and as part of the normal human pharyngeal flora. Some NTM have well-defined ecological niches that help explain transmission patterns. The natural reservoir for *M. marinum* is fish and other cold-blooded animals, so infections follow injury in an aquatic environment. *M. fortuitum* and *M. chelonae* are ubiquitous in the hospital environment and have caused clusters of nosocomial surgical wound and venous catheter-related infections. *M. ulcerans* is recovered only from soils and waters of rain forests and is associated with chronic skin infections in the tropics. *M. avium* complex is found in abundance in the waters, soils, and aerosols of the acid, brown-water swamps of the southeastern United States. In rural counties in this area, asymptomatic infections with *M. avium* complex approach 70% by adulthood.

With the exception of cervical lymphadenitis, illness related to NTM infections is relatively uncommon in children. NTM, particularly *M. avium* complex, are one of the most common terminal infections in patients with the acquired immune deficiency syndrome (AIDS).

PATHOLOGY. The histologic appearances of lesions produced by *M. tuberculosis* and NTM are often indistinguishable. Mycolic acids and other lipids in the cell wall of mycobacteria give them their hallmark trait of acid-fastness with the Ziehl-Neelsen or Kinyoun stains. They may also be identified with the fluorochrome stain auramine-rhodamine. The sensitivity of these stains for detecting NTM in tissue samples is less than with the tubercle bacilli. As with *M. tuberculosis,* the classic pathologic lesion consists of caseating granulomas. However, NTM infections are more likely to result in granulomas that are noncaseating, ill defined (nonpalisading), and irregular or serpiginous. Granulomas may be absent, with only chronic inflammatory changes observed. In patients with AIDS and disseminated NTM infection, the inflammatory reaction is usually scant and tissues are filled with large numbers of histiocytes packed with acid-fast bacilli.

CLINICAL MANIFESTATIONS. Lymphadenitis of the superior anterior cervical or submandibular nodes is the most frequent manifestation of NTM infection in children. Preauricular, posterior cervical, axillary, and inguinal nodes are involved occasionally. This infection is most common in children 1–5 yr of age because of their tendency to put objects contaminated with soil, dust, or standing water into their mouths. Affected children usually lack constitutional symptoms and present with a unilateral subacute and slowly enlarging lymph node or group of closely approximated nodes >1.5 cm that are firm, painless, freely movable, and not erythematous (Fig. 200–1). The involved nodes occasionally resolve without treatment, but most undergo rapid suppuration after several weeks. The center of the node becomes fluctuant, and the overlying skin becomes erythematous and thin. Eventually, the nodes rupture

■ **TABLE 200–1 Nontuberculous Mycobacteria Associated with Human Disease**

Runyon Group	Mycobacteria
I. Photochromogens	*M. kansasii*
	M. marinum
	M. simiae
II. Scotochromogens	*M. scrofulaceum*
	M. xenopi
	M. szulgai
III. Nonchromogens	*M. avium*
	M. intracellulare
	M. malmoense
	M. haemophilum
	M. ulcerans
IV. Rapid growers	*M. chelonei*
	M. fortuitum

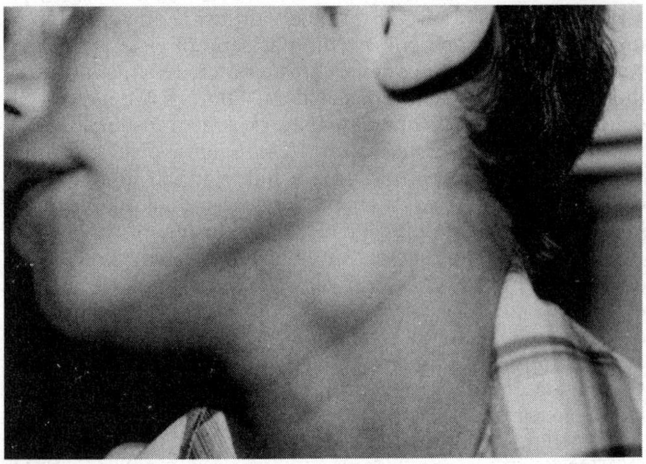

Figure 200–1. Enlarging lymph node, which is firm, painless, freely movable, and not erythematous.

and form cutaneous sinus tracts that drain for months or years, resembling the classic scrofula of tuberculosis (Fig. 200–2). In the United States, *M. avium* complex accounts for approximately 80% of NTM lymphadenitis in children. *M. scrofulaceum* and *M. kansasii* account for most other cases, particularly in the southwestern United States. Rarely, *M. xenopi, M. malmoense, M. haemophilum,* and *M. szulgai* are described.

Cutaneous disease due to NTM is rare in children. Infection usually follows percutaneous inoculation with fresh or salt water contaminated by *M. marinum.* Within several weeks of exposure, a solitary nodule develops at the site of minor abrasions on the elbows, knees, or feet ("swimming pool granuloma"), and on the hands and fingers of fish fanciers ("fish tank granuloma"). The lesions are usually nontender and enlarge over 3–5 wk to ulcerated granuloma or warty lesions, as seen in cutaneous tuberculosis. The lesions sometimes resemble sporotrichosis; satellite lesions near the site of entry extend along the skin following the superficial lymphatics. Lymphadenopathy is usually absent. Although most infections remain localized to skin, penetrating *M. marinum* infections may result in tenosynovitis, bursitis, osteomyelitis, or arthritis.

M. ulcerans also causes cutaneous infection in children living in tropical countries (Africa, Australia, Asia, and South America). Infection follows percutaneous inoculation and presents as a painless erythematous nodule, most frequently

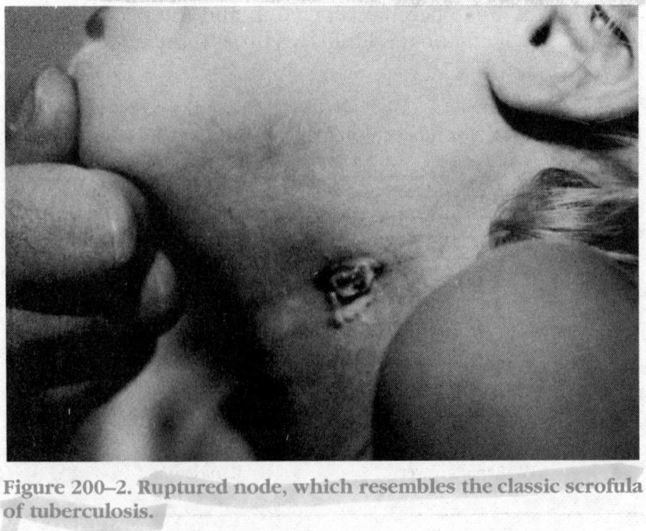

Figure 200–2. Ruptured node, which resembles the classic scrofula of tuberculosis.

on a leg, which undergoes central necrosis and ulceration. The lesion, often called Buruli ulcers after the region in Uganda where most cases are reported, has a characteristic undermined edge, gradually expands, and may result in extensive soft tissue destruction with secondary bacterial infection. The lesion may heal slowly over 6–9 mo or may continue to spread, leading to deformities and contractures.

Skin and soft tissue infections due to *M. fortuitum* and *M. chelonae* are rare in children and usually follow percutaneous inoculation due to puncture wounds and minor abrasions. Clinical disease usually arises after a 4–6 wk incubation period and presents as a localized cellulitis, painful nodules, or a draining abscess. *M. haemophilum* may cause painful subcutaneous nodules, which often ulcerate and suppurate in immunocompromised patients, particularly post renal transplant.

Pulmonary infections, although the most common cause of NTM illness in adults, are uncommon in children. *M. avium* complex is described as a cause of acute pneumonitis, chronic cough, or wheezing associated with paratracheal or parabronchial lymphadenitis and airway compression in normal children. Chronic infections in older cystic fibrosis patients have been caused by *M. avium* complex and *M. fortuitum* complex. *M. kansasii, M. xenopi,* and *M. szulgai* are uncommon in children and usually occur in adults with underlying chronic lung disease. The onset is insidious and consists of low-grade fever, cough, night sweats, and general malaise. Thin-walled cavities with minimal surrounding parenchymal infiltrates are characteristic, but radiographic findings may resemble those of tuberculosis.

In unusual circumstances, NTM cause bone and joint infections that are indistinguishable from those produced by *M. tuberculosis* or bacterial agents. Such infections usually result from operative incision or accidental puncture wounds. *M. fortuitum* infections from puncture wounds of the foot resemble infections caused by *Pseudomonas aeruginosa* and *Staphylococcus aureus*.

Disseminated disease, usually associated with *M. avium* complex infections, occurs occasionally in children without any apparent immunodeficiency. Some of these patients have defective interferon gamma production. The majority of disseminated NTM infections occur in patients with AIDS, usually late in the illness when CD4 cell counts are less than 100 cells/mm^3. Colonization of the respiratory or gastrointestinal tract probably precedes disseminated *M. avium* complex infections, but screening studies of respiratory secretions or stool samples are not useful to predict dissemination. Continuous high-grade bacteremia is usual, and multiple organs are infected, including most commonly lymph nodes, liver, spleen, bone marrow, and gastrointestinal tract; thyroid, pancreas, adrenal gland, kidney, muscle, and brain may be involved. The most common signs and symptoms of disseminated *M. avium* complex infections are fever, night sweats, chills, anorexia, marked weight loss, wasting, weakness, generalized lymphadenopathy, and hepatosplenomegaly. Jaundice, anemia, and neutropenia may occur. Infection with *M. avium* complex appears to shorten the lifespan of AIDS patients by as much as 6 mo.

DIAGNOSIS. The differential diagnosis of NTM lymphadenitis includes tuberculosis, cat-scratch disease, mononucleosis, toxoplasmosis, brucellosis, tularemia, and malignancies, especially lymphomas. An intermediate strength tuberculin skin test is usually weakly positive with 3–15 mm induration. Although the Centers for Disease Control and Prevention have produced skin tests representing the different Runyon groups of NTM, these antigens are no longer available. Differentiation between NTM and *M. tuberculosis* may be difficult, but children with NTM lymphadenitis usually have unilateral anterior cervical node involvement, a normal lung roentgenogram, and no exposure to tuberculosis; children with tuberculous lymphadenitis most often have bilateral posterior cervical node involvement, an abnormal lung roentgenogram, and exposure to adult tuberculosis. Definitive diagnosis requires excision of involved nodes and recovery of the responsible pathogen.

Diagnosis of cutaneous infections depends on isolating the responsible microorganisms from an excised lesion because acid-fast stains are rarely positive. The diagnosis of pulmonary NTM infection in children is also difficult because many species of NTM, including *M. avium* complex, can be isolated from oral and gastric secretions of healthy children. Definitive diagnosis requires invasive procedures such as bronchoscopy and pulmonary or endobronchial biopsy.

Blood cultures are usually diagnostic in AIDS patients with disseminated infection. *M. avium* complex may be detected within 7 days of inoculation in nearly all patients with the BACTEC radiometric blood culture system. Commercially available DNA probes differentiate NTM from *M. tuberculosis*. Identification of histiocytes containing numerous acid-fast bacilli from bone marrow and other biopsy tissues provides a rapid presumptive diagnosis of disseminated mycobacterial infection.

TREATMENT. Therapy of NTM infections involves medical, surgical, or combined treatment. Isolation of the infecting strain with susceptibility testing is ideal because susceptibility patterns vary. *M. kansasii, M. marinum, M. xenopi, M. ulcerans,* and *M. malmoense* are usually susceptible to some standard antituberculous drugs. *M. fortuitum, M. chelonae, M. scrofulaceum,* and *M. avium* complex are often resistant to standard antituberculous drugs but have variable susceptibility to newer antibiotics such as quinolones and macrolides. Multiple drug therapy is essential to avoid development of resistance.

The preferred treatment of NTM lymphadenitis is complete surgical excision. Nodes should be removed while still firm and encapsulated. Excision is more difficult if extensive caseation with extension to surrounding tissue has occurred, and complications of facial nerve damage or recurrent infection are more likely. Incomplete surgical excision is not advised because chronic drainage may develop. Antituberculous medications are not necessary with complete excision, but if there is concern for *M. tuberculosis* infection, therapy with isoniazid, rifampin, and pyrazinamide should be given until cultures confirm the etiology.

Cutaneous NTM lesions usually heal spontaneously following incision and drainage without other therapy. *M. marinum* is susceptible to rifampin, amikacin, ethambutol, sulfonamides, trimethoprim-sulfamethoxazole, and tetracyclines. Therapy with one or a combination of these drugs should be given for 3–4 mo. Corticosteroid injections should not be used. Superficial infections with *M. fortuitum* or *M. chelonae* usually resolve following surgical incision and open drainage, but deep-seated infections require therapy with parenteral amikacin and cefoxitin, or oral clarithromycin. Pulmonary infections should be treated initially with isoniazid, rifampin, and pyrazinamide pending culture identification and susceptibility testing. Chemotherapy for disseminated disease due to *M. avium complex* does not cure the infection but various multiple drug combinations of clarithromycin, azithromycin, clofazimine, rifabutin, rifampin, ciprofloxacin, and ethambutol may limit progression.

Havlik JA Jr., Metchock B, Thompson SE: A prospective evaluation of *Mycobacterium avium* complex colonization of the respiratory and gastrointestinal tracts of persons with human immunodeficiency virus infection. J Infect Dis 168:1045, 1993.

Horsburgh CR Jr: *Mycobacterium avium* complex in the acquired immunodeficiency syndrome. N Engl J Med 324:1332, 1991.

Kilby JM, Gilligan PH, Yankaskas JR, et al: Nontuberculous mycobacteria in adult patients with cystic fibrosis. Chest 102:70, 1992.

Levin RH, Bolinger AM: Treatment of non-tuberculous mycobacterial infections in pediatric patients. Clin Pharm 7:545, 1988.

Lewis LL, Butler KM, Husson RN, et al: Defining the population of human immunodeficiency virus-infected children at risk for *Mycobacterium avium-intracellulare* infection. J Pediatr 121:677, 1992.

Margileth AM, Chandra R, Altman P: Chronic lymphadenopathy due to mycobacterial infection. Am J Dis Child 138:917, 1984.

Peloquin CA: Controversies in the management of *Mycobacterium avium* complex infection in AIDS patients. Ann Pharmacother 27:928, 1993.

Raad II, Vartivarian S, Khan A, et al: Catheter-related infections caused by the *Mycobacterium fortuitum* complex: 15 cases and review. Rev Infect Dis 13:1120, 1991.

Stark JR: Nontuberculous mycobacterial infections in children. Adv Pediatr Infect Dis 7:123, 1992.

Wallace RJ Jr, Tanner D, Brennan PJ, et al: Clinical trial of clarithromycin for cutaneous (disseminated) infection due to *Mycobacterium chelonae*. Ann Intern Med 119:482, 1993.

Wolinsky E: Mycobacterial diseases other than tuberculosis. Clin Infect Dis 15:1, 1992.

200.1 Leprosy

(Hansen Disease)*

Leprosy is a chronic disease produced by infection with *Mycobacterium leprae* and the ensuing host response. The organs most prominently affected are the skin and the peripheral nervous system, but upper respiratory, testicular, and ocular involvement are also relatively common. Humans were long believed to be the sole host of *M. leprae*, but naturally acquired infection has been documented in armadillos in the southeastern United States, and experimental infection has been established in primates, nude mice, and armadillos.

Chronic skin lesions, madarosis, sensory neuropathy resulting in the loss of digits or limbs, and paresis secondary to motor nerve dysfunction are among the sequelae of leprosy. The highly visible nature of these debilities led to the historical stigmatization of the "leper." The psychologic and sociologic sequelae of this stigma can be as debilitating as the disease itself and may result in delays in seeking medical attention. To combat this prejudice, the term *leprosy patient* has replaced the word *leper*, and *Hansen disease* has become an accepted designation.

ETIOLOGY. *M. leprae* is an acid-fast bacillus of the family Mycobacteriaceae. The exceedingly slow multiplication of *M. leprae* observed in animal models may partially explain the long incubation period seen in human disease; a period of 3–5 yr is believed to be typical. The rare occurrence of leprosy in infants as young as 3 mo of age suggests that in utero transmission may occur or that very short incubation periods may be possible in certain situations. Possible modes of transmission include contact with desquamated infected epidermis, ingestion of infected breast milk, and bites of mosquitoes or other vectors. At present, however, transmission via infected nasal secretions appears to be the basis for most infections. Extensive involvement of the nasopharynx manifested as chronic rhinitis is common in lepromatous disease.

EPIDEMIOLOGY. The World Health Organization estimated that worldwide there were 11 million cases of leprosy in 1975. This figure must be considered an underestimate because of inadequate case finding and reporting. The insidious onset of the disease and the social stigma assigned to it delay medical consultation, and the lack of an inexpensive, simple diagnostic test makes confirmation of the diagnosis difficult.

Most of the world's leprosy patients reside in Africa, India, Southeast Asia, and Central and South America. Prevalence rates vary widely between and within countries; the highest rates for entire countries are 25 or more cases per 1,000 population, but rates as high as 200 cases per 1,000 population have been found in small, hyperendemic pockets. Human-to-human transmission accounts for an overwhelming majority of cases; a high percentage of them occur in family members

*Modified from the section in the 14th edition by R. A. Miller.

or in close contacts of known patients. Approximately 200 cases are reported annually in the United States, of which 90% are in immigrants. The remaining 10% develop in localized foci along the Gulf coast, in Hawaii, and in the Micronesian territories.

Leprosy occurs at all ages, but infections in infants are extremely rare; incidence rates peak during childhood and early adulthood in endemic areas. Human immunodeficiency virus infection may alter the risk of leprosy in areas of high prevalence for both pathogens.

PATHOGENESIS AND PATHOLOGY. Damage is mediated through many pathways, some of which are release of humoral mediators of inflammation by activated lymphocytes and macrophages, nerve compression by enlarging granulomata, and deposition of immune complexes. Multiple mechanisms may operate simultaneously or sequentially.

The site of entry of *M. leprae* into the human host is unknown. Primary respiratory or gastrointestinal tract involvement has not been documented prior to the appearance of lesions involving the skin and peripheral nerves. Growth and multiplication of *M. leprae* are maximal at 34–35° C. Nothing is known of the host immune responses in the initial period after infection, but skin testing (Mitsuda reaction, see later) and serologic studies suggest that up to 80–90% of those infected develop immunity without ever manifesting clinical disease. Most of the remaining patients, after a highly variable incubation period, develop typical skin lesions of *indeterminate leprosy.* Studies in endemic areas using the polymerase chain reaction show widespread presence of the organism in nasal secretions from asymptomatic individuals.

Fully developed clinical leprosy is classified into five categories that can be aligned upon a spectrum representing the range of intensity and efficacy of the cellular limb of the host immune response.

One end of the spectrum is *polar tuberculoid leprosy,* in which there is a vigorous and specific cell-mediated immune response. In tissue biopsies there are tightly organized granulomas composed of epithelioid cells and lymphocytes, but bacilli are scant or absent. Macrophages, when present, do not contain intracellular organisms. Caseation is rare. Nerve involvement is usually limited to cutaneous sensory nerve endings and to, at most, a single peripheral nerve trunk.

At the other end of the spectrum is *polar lepromatous leprosy,* in which there is total and specific anergy to *M. leprae* both by skin testing and by in vitro assays of cell-mediated immunity. Large amounts of circulating and tissue-based antibody to mycobacterial antigens are present, but they afford no protective immunity. Bacilli are found in enormous numbers in the skin, nasal mucosa, and peripheral nerves. There is continual bacillemia as well as bacillary invasion of all major organs except the central nervous system. Tissue granulomas are poorly formed and are composed chiefly of loose aggregates of foamy histiocytes. Macrophages teeming with undigested bacilli (globi) are common. There is extensive, symmetric involvement of peripheral nerves, although the cutaneous nerve endings are usually spared.

An *M. leprae*–specific suppressor T-cell population is found in the circulation of patients with lepromatous leprosy, and increased numbers of suppressor T cells are found in their skin granulomas. T cells from lepromatous patients also produce less interleukin 2 and less gamma interferon following stimulation with *M. leprae* antigens than do T cells from tuberculoid patients or normal controls. These findings may relate to the underlying cellular defect that permits development of clinical leprosy in the susceptible individual.

Borderline or *dimorphous leprosy* is subdivided into three subclasses that lie between the tuberculoid and lepromatous poles on the clinical spectrum.

CLINICAL MANIFESTATIONS. Indeterminate Leprosy (I). This is the earliest clinically detectable form of leprosy. Although it is observed in only 10–20% of infected individuals, it is a stage through which most patients with advanced leprosy have passed. Usually there is a single hypopigmented macule, 2–4 cm in diameter, with a poorly defined border but having no erythema or induration. Anesthesia is minimal or absent, particularly if the lesion is on the face. Biopsies of tissue may contain granulomas, but bacilli are rarely demonstrable. The histopathology is not distinctive; the diagnosis is usually made by exclusion, in contacts (especially children) of leprosy patients. In 50–75% of patients with indeterminate leprosy, the lesions heal spontaneously; in the remainder, they progress to one of the classic forms. Thus, only 5–10 of every 100 infected individuals are likely to develop progressive leprosy.

Polar Tuberculoid (TT). There is usually a single, large (often over 10 cm in diameter) lesion with a well-demarcated, elevated erythematous rim. The interior of the lesion is flat, atrophic, hypopigmented, and anesthetic. Rarely, there may be as many as four lesions. The closest superficial nerve is often impressively thickened. The ulnar, posterior tibial, and great auricular nerves are most commonly affected. Periodic examination of all leprosy patients and their contacts should include palpation of these nerves. Without therapy, the lesion tends to enlarge slowly, but documented instances of spontaneous resolution exist. The coloration of the rim slowly fades with therapy, and the induration resolves, resulting in a flat lesion with central hypopigmentation and a ring of postinflammatory hyperpigmentation. Loss of hair follicles, sweat glands, cutaneous nerve receptors, and of sensation in the central portion of the lesion is irreversible. Marked improvement should be apparent within 1–2 mo after initiating therapy, but complete resolution may take up to 8–12 mo. There is an entity of "pure neural" tuberculoid leprosy, which presents as a mononeuropathy with prominent nerve thickening but no cutaneous lesions. Histopathology is mandatory to establish this diagnosis. Nerve trunk size varies widely, and overdiagnosis of "enlarged" nerves is common among inexperienced observers. Nodular or fusiform nerve thickening has greater diagnostic value than a palpable nerve that is smooth and symmetric.

Borderline Leprosy. The clinical and histologic criteria for the three subdivisions of borderline leprosy are less well defined than are those of the two polar categories. In contrast to the tuberculoid and lepromatous patterns, those in the borderline divisions are unstable. For example, host or bacterial factors can result in downgrading the clinical condition toward the lepromatous pattern or upgrading it toward the tuberculoid pattern. Therapy is the most common cause of upgrading reactions; downgrading can be seen in conditions that compromise host immunity, for example, pregnancy. Clinical characteristics of the three generally accepted borderline subclasses are as follows.

In *borderline tuberculoid* (BT) leprosy the lesions are greater in number but smaller in size than in tuberculoid leprosy. There may be small satellite lesions around older lesions, and the margins of the borderline tuberculoid lesions are less distinct and the center is less atrophic and anesthetic. There is usually thickening of two or more superficial nerves.

In the *borderline* (BB) pattern the lesions are more numerous and more heterogeneous in appearance. They may become confluent, and plaques may be present. The borders are poorly defined, and the erythematous rim fades into the surrounding skin. There may be anesthesia, but hypesthesia is more common. Mild to moderate nerve thickening is common, but severe muscle wasting and neuropathy are unusual.

In the *borderline lepromatous* (BL) pattern, there are a large number of asymmetrically distributed lesions that are heterogeneous in appearance. Macules, papules, plaques, and nodules may all coexist. Individual lesions are small unless confluent. Anesthesia is mild and superficial nerve trunks are spared. The initial response to therapy is often dramatic; nodules and plaques flatten within 2–3 mo. With continued therapy the lesions become macular and almost invisible.

Polar Lepromatous Leprosy (LL). The lesions are innumerable, often confluent, and symmetric. Initially there may be only vague macules or even uniform, diffuse skin infiltrations without discernible lesions. As the disease progresses, the lesions become increasingly papular and nodular, so that with the diffuse thickening and infiltration of the skin, the characteristic leonine facies accompanied by loss of the eyebrows and distortion of the earlobes becomes apparent. Anesthesia of the lesions either does not occur or is mild, but a symmetric peripheral sensory neuropathy may develop. Testicular infiltration leading to azoospermia, infertility, and gynecomastia is common in adults but not in children. Bacilli are demonstrable in most internal organs other than the central nervous system, but tissue damage or interference with function is infrequent. Glomerulonephritis, when it occurs, is felt to be secondary to immune complex deposition rather than to infection per se. The initial response to therapy may be encouraging but is often followed by a long (2–5 yr) period of very slow improvement. In true polar lepromatous leprosy, the specific anergy to the leprosy bacillus persists despite therapy, thus making the patient theoretically susceptible to relapse if even a single viable bacillus remains at the end of therapy.

Reactional States. Acute clinical exacerbations are common in leprosy and are believed to reflect abrupt changes in the host-parasite immunologic balance. Although these reactional states do occur in the absence of therapy, they are especially common during the initial years of treatment. Three major variants are recognized.

Erythema nodosum leprosum (ENL) occurs in the majority of patients with polar lepromatous leprosy and in 25–40% of borderline lepromatous cases. Tender dermal nodules, clinically resembling erythema nodosum, are the hallmark of this syndrome. High fever, migrating polyarthralgia, orchitis, and increased activity in pre-existing cutaneous lesions complete the clinical picture. Circulating and tissue-based immune complexes are frequently present and may explain the resemblance to other immune complex disorders, but the underlying mechanism appears to involve the activation of a helper T-cell subset. There is a strong tendency to recurrence, and there is a risk of amyloidosis and renal failure if treatment is inadequate.

Reversal reactions are observed throughout the borderline range. Acute tenderness and inflammation at the site of existing cutaneous and neural lesions and the development of new lesions are the major manifestations. Fever and systemic toxicity are uncommon, but the acute neuritis can lead to irreversible nerve injury if it is not treated immediately. Reversal reactions constitute perhaps the only medical emergency related to leprosy per se. Patients should be instructed to contact their physicians immediately if signs of a reaction appear. A sudden increase in effective cell-mediated immunity with rapid killing of bacilli within nerve sheaths is the initiating event.

Lucio's phenomenon, a severe, necrotizing, cutaneous vasculitis, is uncommon; it occurs predominantly in patients of Mexican origin who have diffuse lepromatous leprosy. Conventional therapy for vasculitis has had only modest success, and fatalities are common. Experimental therapies, including plasmapheresis and cyclophosphamide, have been successful in isolated cases. The pathogenesis is unknown, although immune complexes almost certainly contribute.

DIAGNOSIS. The critical factor in the diagnosis of leprosy is its inclusion in the differential diagnosis of a skin disorder in anyone who has resided in an endemic leprosy region. Anesthetic skin lesions with or without thickened peripheral nerves are virtually pathognomonic of leprosy. A full-thickness skin biopsy from an active lesion (stained with both a standard histologic stain and an acid-fast stain such as Fite-Faraco) is the optimal procedure for confirmation of the diagnosis and accurate disease classification. Acid-fast bacilli are rarely found in patients with indeterminate or tuberculoid disease, so diagnosis in these cases is based on the clinical picture and the presence of typical dermal granulomas. Other routine clinical, microbiologic, and radiologic tests have little or no role in the diagnosis of leprosy, although they may be useful in the exclusion of other diagnoses. Various assays for serum antibodies directed against unique antigens of *M. leprae* have been developed, but current tests lack sufficient sensitivity and specificity for active disease to be useful for clinical diagnostic purposes.

Lepromin is a suspension of killed *M. leprae* obtained from infected human or armadillo tissue. Following intradermal inoculation, early (48 hr, Fernandez reaction) as well as late (3–4 wk, Mitsuda reaction) reactions may be seen. The Mitsuda reaction, a granulomatous response to the antigen, is more consistent. Patients with tuberculoid leprosy have strongly positive (5 mm) responses, whereas patients with lepromatous leprosy do not respond. The test is not useful in the diagnosis of leprosy, because the majority of the population in both endemic and nonendemic leprosy areas will be Mitsuda positive. Lepromin is not available in the United States.

Many diseases endemic in developing countries can mimic the appearance of leprosy; these include secondary syphilis, cutaneous leishmaniasis, yaws, and cutaneous fungal infections. None of these entities involves paresthesia/anesthesia localized to the skin lesions or causes thickening of peripheral nerves. The presence of nerve thickening with skin lesions also differentiates leprosy from primary neurologic disease. Indeterminate leprosy may present with minimal anesthesia, no nerve thickening, and equivocal histopathology suggesting a superficial fungal infection, particularly tinea versicolor. The diagnosis of indeterminate leprosy should be considered one of exclusion and will rarely be made in anyone other than a close contact of a known patient.

TREATMENT. Only three antimycobacterial agents have proven to be consistently effective in the treatment of leprosy.

Since the early 1940s, *dapsone* (diaminodiphenyl sulfone) has remained the cornerstone of therapy because of its low cost, minimal toxicity, and wide availability. Unfortunately, secondary resistance tends to develop when it is used as the sole agent. More worrisome is the increasing incidence of primary resistance, which has been reported in up to 30% of newly diagnosed patients in Malaysia and Ethiopia. Dermatitis, hepatitis, and methemoglobinemia are the most common side effects; granulocytopenia is rare but potentially fatal. Dose-related hemolytic anemia, which can be severe, is seen in patients with glucose-6-phosphate dehydrogenase (G-6-PD) deficiency, methemoglobin reductase deficiency, or hemoglobin M. Pregnancy studies have not shown an increased risk of fetal abnormalities.

Rifampin is the most rapidly mycobactericidal drug for *M. leprae,* achieving excellent levels inside cells, where most leprosy bacilli reside. Resistance has been reported infrequently. The widespread use of rifampin has been limited by cost more than by toxicity. Hepatitis is the most common side effect that necessitates discontinuance.

Clofazimine, a phenazine dye with both antimycobacterial and anti-inflammatory activity, is particularly useful in cases of dapsone resistance or when recurrent reactional states have developed. The pharmacokinetics are poorly understood, but the half-life is several days. The drug is avidly taken up by epithelial cells, a feature that may be important for its activity but also results in cutaneous hyperpigmentation, ichthyosis, xerosis, and enteritis. The intense reddish-brown discoloration of the skin is cosmetically a deterrent to use and often results in discontinuation or poor compliance.

The increasing incidence of drug-resistant *M. leprae* has led to an intensified search for alternative therapeutic agents. Minocycline, certain 2nd-generation quinolones, and some new macrolide derivatives have shown promise in experimental models or preliminary human trials.

Delineation of the optimal therapeutic regimens for leprosy has been hampered by deficient patient compliance, the long durations of therapy required, and inadequacies in the long-term follow-up for late relapses. All patients with leprosy should receive multidrug therapy to reduce the emergence of resistance. The following recommendations reflect the standard of practice among leprologists in the United States; they differ slightly from those of WHO, which largely reflect the economic realities in developing countries. The initial treatment regimen is determined by the number of bacilli in the skin (as estimated by smear or biopsy) and the histology of the skin lesions. The duration of therapy is dependent on both the initial histology and the clinical and microbiologic response.

Paucibacillary patients (bacillary index ≤2+: all indeterminate and polar tuberculoid and most borderline tuberculoid patients) should receive dapsone (2 mg/kg/24 hr up to 100 mg/24 hr) and rifampin (10–20 mg/kg/24 hr up to 600 mg/24 hr) for 6–12 mo (depending on the clinical response), followed by dapsone alone to complete 1 yr of therapy for patients with indeterminate leprosy and 2–3 yr for those with tuberculoid and borderline tuberculoid disease. All patients with lepromatous or borderline lepromatous disease and most patients with borderline disease have large numbers of bacilli present in the skin (multibacillary leprosy). Common practice in the United States is to initiate treatment with dapsone and rifampin (same dosages as above) for a minimum of 2 yr, followed by dapsone alone for at least 10 yr after skin smears or biopsies become negative for morphologically intact bacilli. Patients with lepromatous and borderline lepromatous disease may require therapy for life. WHO and the American Academy of Pediatrics recommend the addition of clofazimine (adult dosage: 50–100 mg/24 hr; pediatric dosage: 1 mg/kg/24 hr). to the dapsone-rifampin regimen in patients with multibacillary disease, particularly in areas in which there is a high prevalence of primary dapsone resistance.

Therapy of reactional states can become very complicated and will generally require expert consultation. Erythema nodosum leprosum usually responds to corticosteroid therapy (1 mg/kg/24 hr of prednisone) but often relapses when the drug is discontinued. Clinical remission of acute and suppression of chronic erythema nodosum can be achieved with thalidomide.* *Thalidomide is absolutely contraindicated in women of child-bearing age*; otherwise it is much safer than corticosteroids for chronic use. The major side effect is fatigue. Pediatric dosages have not been established. Clofazimine is also useful in managing chronic erythema nodosum. Reversal reactions are optimally treated with corticosteroids. Alternate-day regimens may be effective in patients with frequent relapses.

Serial skin smears or repeat biopsies are useful in assessing response to therapy. Bacilli in the skin are quantitated on a logarithmic scale (bacillary index). Four to 8 yr of effective therapy are commonly required in lepromatous patients before the bacillary index becomes zero, but the appearance of the bacilli will gradually change, becoming first beaded and then fragmented. Persistence of intact bacilli in the skin or nerves during therapy suggests poor patient compliance or drug resistance and usually correlates with clinical failure or recrudescence. Serologic monitoring of IgM antibodies to antiphenolic glycolipid-I may provide a new approach for evaluating treatment responses. Drug sensitivity testing of *M. leprae* is difficult and not widely available but may be necessary to confirm suspected drug resistance.

*Thalidomide is available as an investigational agent through the Gillis W. Long Hansen's Disease Center, Carville, Louisiana. The Gillis W. Long Hansen's Disease Center and its Regional Centers are available for consultation and assistance in patient management. The use of this service is strongly encouraged.

PROGNOSIS. The prognosis for arresting progression of tissue and nerve damage is good, but recovery of lost sensory and motor function is variable and generally incomplete; hyperpigmentation, hypopigmentation, and loss of skin organs persist. Intercurrent reactional states, poor compliance, and emergence of dapsone resistance can all lead to clinical exacerbations or relapses necessitating close follow-up of patients. Much of the chronic debility results from repeated trauma to anesthetic digits and limbs. Careful counseling of patients and consultation with physical and occupational therapy services is essential for an optimal outcome.

PREVENTION. Two approaches are advocated for interrupting leprosy transmission in endemic areas. The first is directed at the risk of infection among household contacts of leprosy patients, especially those with multibacillary disease. It is based on regular periodic examination of contacts and early treatment at the first evidence of leprosy. Prophylactic therapy is reserved for special circumstances so that the inappropriate treatment of the 90–95% of contacts not expected to develop leprosy can be avoided.

The second approach to leprosy control has been through vaccination. Results from clinical trials with various vaccines, including bacille Calmette-Guérin, have been disappointing, but the recent cloning of the genes for the major antigens of *M. leprae* has renewed hope for the development of an effective vaccine.

One historical practice that has fortunately been abandoned is the forcing of leprosy patients into leprosariums. Mouse footpad inoculation studies have demonstrated that viability of *M. leprae* in skin biopsies falls sharply within 3 wk of initiating therapy with dapsone and rifampin. This rapid drop in infectivity combined with the high probability that family members have had prolonged exposure to the patient prior to the diagnosis makes physical isolation of leprosy patients unnecessary.

Bloom BR, Godal T: Selective primary health care. Strategies for control of disease in the developing world. V. Leprosy. Rev Infect Dis 5:765, 1983.
Brubaker ML, Meyers WM, Bourland J: Leprosy in children one year of age and under. Int J Lepr 53:517, 1985.
Chemotherapy of leprosy (Editorial). Lancet 2:487, 1988.
Dayal R: Early detection of leprosy in children. J Trop Pediatr 37:310, 1991.
Neill MA, Hightower AL, Broome CV: Leprosy in the United States, 1971–1981. J Infect Dis 152:1064, 1985.
Orege PA, Fine PE, Lucas SB, et al: A case control study on human immunodeficiency virus-1 (HIV-1) infection as a risk factor for tuberculosis and leprosy in western Kenya. Tuber Lung Dis 74:377, 1993.
Ridley DS, Jopling WH: Classification of leprosy according to immunity: A five-group system. Int J Lepr 34:255, 1966.
Roche PW, Britton WJ, Failbus SS, et al: Serological monitoring of the response to chemotherapy in leprosy patients. Int J Lepro Other Mycobact Dis 61:35, 1993.
Sehgal VN, Srivastava G: Leprosy in children. Int J Dermatol 26:557, 1987.
van Beers SM, Izumi S, Madjid B, et al: An epidemiological study of leprosy infection by serology and polymerase chain reaction. Int J Lepr Other Mycobac Dis 62:1, 1994.
Young RA, Mehra V, Sweester D, et al: Genes for the major protein antigens of *Mycobacterium leprae*. Nature 316:450, 1985.

CHAPTER 201
Spirochetal Infections

Parvin Azimi

201.1 Syphilis

ETIOLOGY. Syphilis is a systemic communicable infection caused by *Treponema pallidum*, a long, slender, tightly coiled, motile spirochete with finely tapered ends belonging to the family Spirochaetaceae and the genus *Treponema*. The pathogenic members of this genus include *T. pallidum* (syphilis), *T. pertenue* (yaws), and *T. carateum* (pinta). Because these microorganisms stain poorly, detection in clinical specimens requires dark-field microscopy or immunofluorescent staining techniques. *T. pallidum* cannot be cultured in vitro but has been propagated by intratesticular inoculation in rabbits. Transmission occurs via sexual contact or transplacentally. Other modes of transmission include transfusion of tainted blood or by direct contact with infected tissues.

EPIDEMIOLOGY. Two forms of syphilis are encountered by the pediatrician. *Congenital* syphilis results from transplacental transmission of spirochetes; rarely, infant contact with a maternal chancre leads to postnatal infection. The risk of transplacental transmission varies with the stage of maternal illness. Untreated pregnant women with primary and secondary syphilis and spirochetemia are more likely to transmit infection to the unborn infant than are women with latent infection. Transmission can occur throughout pregnancy. The incidence of congenital infection in the offspring of untreated infected women remains highest during the first 4 yr after acquisition of primary infection, secondary, and early latent disease. *Acquired* syphilis results almost exclusively from sexual contact. Although curative treatment has been available for syphilis for over 4 decades, syphilis remains an important and common health problem. The incidence within the United States increased dramatically during the 1980s, most notably among inner city minority populations in the Northeast, Southwest, and West Coast of the country. Among the risk factors, the use of illegal drugs, especially the epidemic in crack cocaine use, and lack of partner notification and treatment rank high.

CLINICAL MANIFESTATIONS. *Primary syphilis* is characterized by syphilitic chancre and regional adenitis. A painless papule appears at the site of inoculation 2–6 wk after *T. pallidum* has been introduced. The papule soon develops into a clean, painless ulcer with raised borders called a chancre. The chancre is usually on the genitals, contains viable *T. pallidum*, and is highly contagious. Extragenital chancres can also be seen, depending on the site of primary inoculation. Adjacent lymph nodes are generally enlarged. The chancre heals spontaneously within 4–6 wk, leaving a thin scar. Untreated patients develop manifestations of *secondary syphilis* 2–10 wk after the healing of the chancre. Manifestations of secondary syphilis are related to spirochetemia and include a nonpruritic maculopapular rash, which can cover the entire body involving palms and soles; pustular lesions may also develop. Condylomata lata (gray-white to erythematous wartlike plaques) can occur in moist areas around the anus and vagina, and white plaques called mucous patches may be found in mucous membranes.

A flulike illness with low-grade fever, headache, malaise, anorexia, weight loss, sore throat, myalgias, and arthralgias, and generalized lymphadenopathy is often present. Renal, hepatic, and ophthalmologic manifestations may be seen, as well as meningitis. Meningitis occurs in 30% of patients with secondary syphilis, manifested by cerebrospinal fluid (CSF) pleocytosis and elevated protein, but the patient may not show neurologic symptoms. Secondary infection becomes *latent* within 1–2 mo after the onset of the rash. Relapses with secondary manifestations can be seen during the 1st year of latency. This period is referred to as the early latent period. No relapses occur after the 1st year; what follows is late syphilis, which may be either asymptomatic *(late latent)* or symptomatic *(tertiary)*. At this stage, patients may begin showing the manifestations of tertiary disease, which include neurologic, cardiovascular, and gummatous lesions. The latter are granulomas of the skin and musculoskeletal system resulting from the host's delayed hypersensitivity reaction.

CONGENITAL INFECTION. Syphilis during pregnancy has a transmission rate approaching 100%. Fetal or perinatal death occurs in 40% of affected infants. Among survivors, manifestations have traditionally been divided into early and late stages. The former appear during the first 2 yr of life, whereas the latter appear gradually during the first 2 decades. Early congenital syphilis results from transplacental spirochetemia and is analogous to the secondary stage of acquired syphilis. The majority of infants may be asymptomatic at the time of birth; but if they are untreated, symptoms develop within weeks or months. The manifestations of congenital infection are varied and involve multiple organ systems. Hepatosplenomegaly, jaundice, and elevated liver enzymes are common. Histologically, liver involvement includes bile stasis, fibrosis, and extramedullary hematopoiesis.

Lymphadenopathy tends to be diffuse and resolve spontaneously; shotty nodes may persist. Coomb negative hemolytic anemia is characteristic. Thrombocytopenia is often associated with platelet trapping in an enlarged spleen. Characteristic osteochondritis and periostitis (Fig. 201–1) and mucocutaneous rash (Fig. 201–2), presenting with erythematous maculopapular or bullous lesions, followed by desquamation involving hands and feet, are common. Mucous patches, rhinitis (snuffles), and condylomatous lesions are highly characteristic features of mucous membrane involvement in congenital syphilis. Bone involvement occurs frequently. Roentgenographic abnormalities include multiple sites of osteochondritis at the wrists, elbows, ankles, and knees; and periostitis of the long bones, and rarely the skull. The osteochondritis is painful and often results in irritability and refusal to move the involved extremity (pseudoparalysis of Parrot). Central nervous system (CNS) abnormalities, failure to thrive, chorioretinitis, nephritis, and nephrotic syndrome may also be seen. Clinical manifestations of renal involvement include hypertension, hematuria, proteinuria, hypoproteinemia, hypercholesterolemia, and hypocomplementemia. They appear to be related to glomerular deposition of circulating immune complexes. Less common clinical manifestations of early congenital syphilis include gastroenteritis, peritonitis, pancreatitis, pneumonia, eye involvement (glaucoma and chorioretinitis), non-immune hydrops, and testicular masses.

The manifestations of late congenital syphilis result primarily from chronic inflammation of bone, teeth, and the CNS. Skeletal changes due to persistent or recurrent periostitis and associated thickening of bone include frontal bossing, a bony prominence of the forehead ("olympian brow"); unilateral or bilateral thickening of the sternoclavicular portion of the clavicle (Higoumenakis sign); an anterior bowing of the midportion of the tibia (saber shins); and scaphoid scapula, a convexity along its medial border. Dental abnormalities are common and include (1) Hutchinson teeth (Fig. 201–3), which are the peg- or barrel-shaped upper central incisors that erupt during the 6th yr of life; (2) abnormal enamel, which results in a notch along the biting surface; and (3) mulberry molars, abnormal 1st lower (6 yr) molars, characterized by a small biting surface

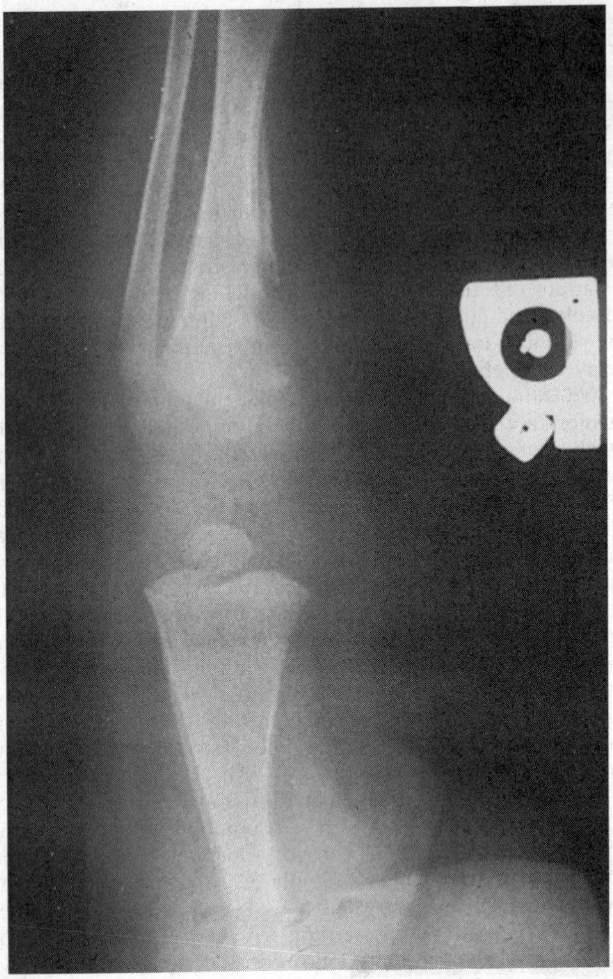

Figure 201–1. Osteochondritis and periostitis in a child with congenital syphilis.

and an excessive number of cusps. Defects in enamel formation lead to repeated caries and eventual tooth destruction.

A saddle nose (Fig. 201–4), a depression of the nasal root is a result of syphilitic rhinitis, which destroys the adjacent bone and cartilage. A perforated nasal septum is an associated abnormality. Rhagades are linear scars that extend in a spokelike pattern from previous mucocutaneous lesions of the mouth, anus, and genitalia. Juvenile paresis, an uncommon latent

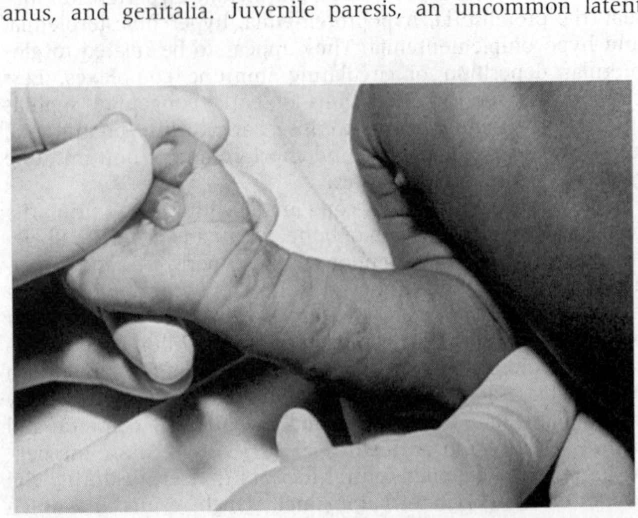

Figure 201–2. The mucocutaneous rash of congenital syphilis. See also color section.

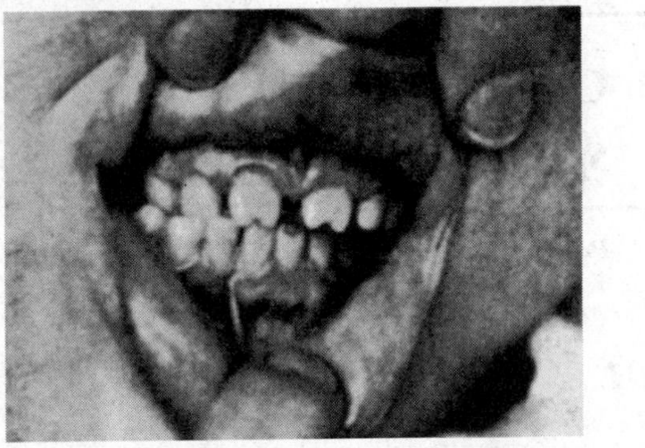

Figure 201–3. Hutchinson teeth in congenital syphilis.

meningovascular infection, typically presents during adolescence with behavioral changes, focal seizures, or loss of intellectual function. Juvenile tabes with spinal cord involvement and cardiovascular involvement with aortitis are extremely rare.

Other clinical manifestations of late congenital syphilis may represent a hypersensitivity phenomenon. These include unilateral or bilateral interstitial keratitis with symptoms such as intense photophobia and lacrimation, followed within weeks or months by corneal opacification and complete blindness. Less common ocular manifestations include choroiditis, retinitis, vascular occlusion, and optic atrophy. Eighth nerve deafness may be unilateral or bilateral, appears at any age, presents initially with vertigo and high-tone hearing loss, and progresses to permanent deafness. The Clutton joint represents a unilateral or bilateral synovitis involving the lower extremities (usually the knee), which presents as painless joint swelling with sterile synovial fluid; spontaneous remission usually occurs after a period of several weeks. Soft tissue gummas (identical to those of acquired disease) and paroxysmal cold hemoglobinuria are rare hypersensitivity phenomena.

DIAGNOSIS. Diagnosis of congenital syphilis is made with certainty when *T. pallidum* is demonstrated by dark-field microscopy or immunofluorescence on specimens from skin lesions, placenta, or umbilicus; or when the mother of an infant has reactive treponemal and nontreponemal serologic tests with characteristic clinical findings of congenital syphilis in the infant. In asymptomatic cases, diagnosis is based on treponemal and nontreponemal serologic tests in mother and infant, as well as maternal history.

Nontreponemal tests, such as Venereal Disease Research Laboratory (VDRL) and rapid plasma reagin (RPR), detect antibodies against a cardiolipin-cholesterol-lecithin complex, not specific for syphilis. The quantitative results of these nontreponemal tests tend to correlate with disease activity and therefore are very helpful in screening. Titers rise when disease is active (including treatment failure or reinfection) and fall when

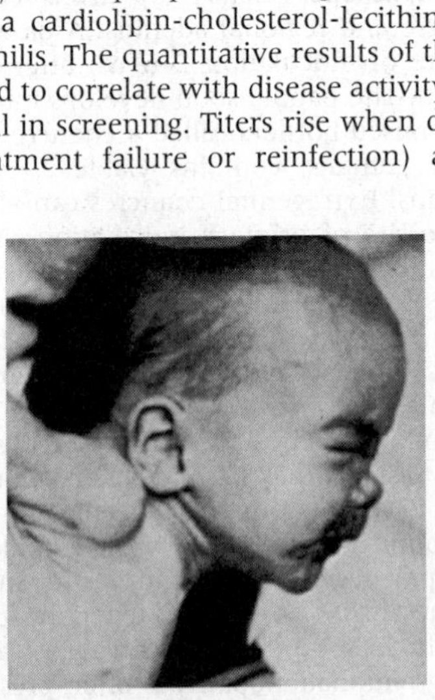

Figure 201–4. Saddle nose in early syphilis.

treatment is adequate. Figure 201–5 depicts the serologic response in untreated syphilis for both treponemal and nontreponemal tests. Serum usually becomes nonreactive in the nontreponemal tests within 1 yr of adequate therapy for primary syphilis and within 2 yr of treatment for secondary disease. In congenital infection, these tests become nonreactive within a few months after adequate treatment.

A major disadvantage of the nontreponemal tests, particularly VDRL, is that they are not specific for active infection and may be falsely positive, particularly in the presence of immunologic stimulation such as infection, immunization, collagen-vascular disease, pregnancy, and drug addiction. Often these "biologic false-positive" tests for syphilis have low titers, and their true nature is verified by demonstration of a negative specific antitreponemal test. Despite their value as screening tests for primary and secondary syphilis, the nontreponemal tests may be used improperly in diagnosing congenital syphilis. Maternal antibody crosses the placenta, and accordingly a false-positive VDRL can occur in an uninfected infant delivered to a VDRL-positive mother.

Passively acquired antibody is suggested when neonatal titers are significantly less (at least four-fold) than maternal titers and can be verified when antibody is no longer demonstrable by 3 mo of age. False-negative nontreponemal test results may occur in patients who acquire infections late in pregnancy; such infants become seropositive in the postnatal period.

Treponemal tests measure antibody specific for *T. pallidum* and include the *T. pallidum* immobilization test (TPI), the fluorescent treponemal antibody absorption test (FTA-ABS), and the microhemagglutination assay for antibodies to *T. pallidum* (MHA-TP). The TPI measures the ability of test serum (antibody) plus complement to immobilize *T. pallidum*; there are few laboratories where this test is available. The MHA-TP and FTA-ABS are the confirmatory tests that are generally used. These tests are not quantitated, because the degree of reactivity does not correlate with disease activity; they are reported only as "reactive" or "nonreactive." Treponemal tests are especially useful for confirming positive results from nontreponemal tests. False-positive reactions are uncommon but occur in a few normal individuals during pregnancy and in patients with diseases such as lymphoproliferative disorders, cirrhosis, collagen-vascular disease, and drug addiction. The major disadvantages of these tests are that their interpretation is subjective, their results cannot be quantitated, and, once positive, they remain so for life, even when therapy is adequate. Therefore, treponemal tests should not be used as a basis for monitoring the effectiveness of treatment. The FTA-ABS and MHA-TP tests are subject to misinterpretation during the neonatal period because seropositivity in an adequately treated mother results in a seropositive, uninfected newborn. Follow-up titers will distinguish passively acquired antibody from disease-specific antibodies, the former becoming negative after the 6th month of life. In congenitally infected infants, similar to their adult counterparts, the treponemal tests can remain reactive even after adequate treatment.

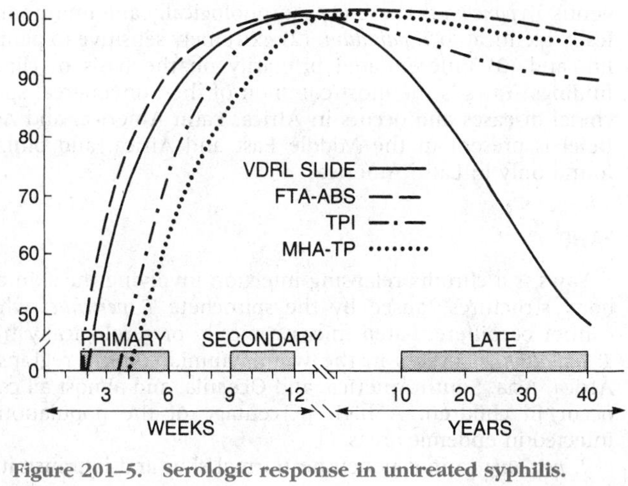

Figure 201–5. Serologic response in untreated syphilis.

IgM-based immunologic tests have been useful in confirming the diagnosis in symptomatic newborns but have not proved sensitive enough for the diagnosis of syphilis in the asymptomatic newborns at risk. At the present time, the asymptomatic infant considered at risk for congenital syphilis because the maternal nontreponemal and treponemal serology is positive should be evaluated if maternal treatment was inadequate, unknown, or undocumented within the 30 days prior to delivery or if the mother was treated with erythromycin; or if the maternal nontreponemal titers did not decrease sufficiently to demonstrate a cure (fourfold or greater). If the maternal treatment was adequate and more than 1 mo before delivery and the infant's positive nontreponemal test represents passively acquired antibody, the infant does not need treatment at delivery, but follow-up serology should be obtained. If the maternal evaluation is unable to be completed, these infants must be assumed to be infected and treated. For this group of asymptomatic infants, an antigen-based test such as polymerase chain reaction specific for *T. pallidum* is needed.

The Centers for Disease Control (CDC) recommend that infants be treated if (1) they were born to mothers who had untreated syphilis at delivery; (2) there is evidence of maternal relapse or reinfection; (3) there is physical evidence of active disease; (4) there is radiologic evidence of syphilis; (5) there is a reactive CSF VDRL or, for infants born to seropositive mothers, an abnormal CSF white blood cell count or protein, regardless of CSF serology; (6) a serum quantitative nontreponemal serologic titer in the infant is at least fourfold greater than the mother's titer; or (7) the infant has specific antitreponemal IgM antibody detected by a testing method that has been given provisional or standard status by the CDC.

The diagnosis of neurosyphilis in acquired disease is made by demonstrating pleocytosis and increased protein in the CSF, and a positive CSF VDRL along with neurologic symptoms. CNS involvement is common and the CSF VDRL is not always reactive. The diagnosis of neurosyphilis in the newborn with syphilitic infection is difficult owing to the poor sensitivity of the CSF VDRL in this age group and the lack of CSF abnormalities. In general, a positive CSF VDRL in a newborn infant warrants treatment for neurosyphilis, even though it might reflect passive transfer of antibodies from serum to CSF. More importantly, it is now accepted that all infants with a presumptive diagnosis of congenital syphilis should be treated with regimens effective for neurosyphilis because this diagnosis cannot be ruled out.

Dark-field microscopy of scrapings from primary lesions or congenital or secondary lesions can reveal *T. pallidum*, often before serology becomes positive, but this technique is usually not available in clinical practice. Placental examination by gross and microscopic techniques can be useful in the diagnosis of congenital syphilis. The disproportionately large placentas are characterized histologically by focal proliferative villitis, endovascular and perivascular arteritis, and focal or diffuse immaturity of placental villi.

TREATMENT. Acquired Syphilis. *T. pallidum* is extremely sensitive to penicillin, and there is no evidence of increasing penicillin resistance. A concentration of 0.018 μg/mL (0.03 U/mL) of penicillin is needed to ensure killing of spirochetes in serum and CSF. Table 201–1 presents the recommended therapeutic regimens for syphilis. Although nonpenicillin regimens are available to the penicillin-allergic patient, desensitization followed by penicillin therapy is the most reliable strategy.

For primary, secondary, and early latent disease, a single

■ TABLE 201–1 Treatment of Syphilis

Stage	Treatment and Dosage	Alternatives
Early: (primary, secondary or latent < yr)	Penicillin G benzathine, 2.4 million U IM, in one dose	Tetracycline (500 mg PO qid for 2 wk) or doxycycline (100 mg PO bid for 2 wk) or erythromycin (500 mg PO qid for 2 wk)
Late: (>1 yr duration)	Penicillin G benzathine, 2.4 million U IM, weekly for 3 doses	Tetracycline (500 mg PO qid for 4 wk) or doxycycline (100 mg PO bid for 4 wk)
Neurosyphilis	Aqueous crystalline penicillin G (12–24 million U/24 hr IV given as 2.4 million U every 4 hr) for 10–14 days	Penicillin G procaine (2.4 million U/day IM) PLUS probenicid (500 mg PO qid). Both for 10–14 days
Congenital syphilis	Aqueous crystalline penicillin G (100,000–150,000 U/kg/24 hr, given as 50,000 U/kg IV every 12 hr for the first 7 days and every 8 hr thereafter) for 10–14 days or Procaine penicillin G (50,000 U/kg IM daily in a single dose) for 10–14 days	

dose of 2.4 million units IM of benzathine penicillin is recommended. Nonpregnant penicillin-allergic patients without neurosyphilis may be treated with either doxycycline (100 mg orally 2 times a day for 2 wk) or tetracycline (500 mg orally 4 times a day for 2 wk). If ceftriaxone is used, treponemicidal serum levels should be provided for 8–10 days; single-dose ceftriaxone therapy is not effective for treating syphilis. Single-dose benzathine penicillin may not result in treponemicidal levels of drug in the CSF and may not be an effective treatment for neurosyphilis, which is especially true in patients who are coinfected with human immunodeficiency virus (HIV), in whom neurosyphilis may be difficult to cure. Although CDC guidelines continue to recommend single-dose benzathine penicillin for early acquired disease, careful follow-up and multiple-dose therapy may be required for some patients, especially those who are HIV infected. These patients are best treated with three injections of benzathine penicillin, a 10-day therapy with aqueous penicillin has been suggested for those known to have neurosyphilis.

Incubating syphilis may be effectively treated with the currently recommended penicillin regimens for gonorrhea, and all patients treated for gonorrhea should have serologic testing for syphilis at the time of treatment and at follow-up 6–8 weeks later. Therapy with ampicillin, amoxicillin, or ceftriaxone is probably also effective. Spectinomycin therapy will not cure incubating syphilis. Because of the high risk of acquiring infection, "prophylactic treatment" should be given to sexual contacts of persons with infectious syphilis within the preceding 3 mo, regardless of serology. Three additional elements of syphilis therapy are obligatory: (1) Follow-up serology should be performed on treated individuals to establish adequacy of therapy; (2) sexual contacts should be identified and treated; and (3) testing for other sexually transmitted diseases (STDs), including HIV, should be performed on all patients.

Syphilis in Pregnancy. Routine serologic tests for syphilis should be performed during the 1st trimester and, for women at high risk, again at the beginning of the 3rd trimester and at delivery. When clinical or serologic findings suggest active infection or when the diagnosis of active syphilis cannot be excluded with certainty, treatment is indicated. Patients should be treated with the penicillin regimen appropriate for the woman's stage of syphilis. Women who have been adequately treated in the past do not require additional therapy unless quantitative serology suggests evidence of reinfection (four-fold rise in titer). Doxycycline and tetracycline should not be administered during pregnancy, and erythromycin does not effectively treat fetal infection.

Congenital Syphilis. Adequate maternal therapy should eliminate the risk of congenital syphilis. All such infants, however, should be followed until nontreponemal serology is negative. The risk of giving penicillin to a newborn infant is minimal; the infant should be treated when there is an uncertainty about the adequacy of the mother's treatment.

Current recommendations for treatment of congenital syphilis include regimens of IV aqueous penicillin G (100,000–150,000 U/kg/24 hr) and IM procaine penicillin (50,000 U/kg/24 hr), given for 10–14 days. Higher concentrations of penicillin are achieved in the CSF of infants treated with IV aqueous penicillin G than in those treated with IM procaine penicillin. Both penicillin regimens are still recognized as adequate therapy for congenital syphilis. Treated infants should be followed serologically to confirm decreasing nontreponemal antibody titers.

An acute systemic febrile reaction, the *Jarisch-Herxheimer reaction*, with exacerbation of lesions, occurs in 15–20% of all patients with acquired or congenital syphilis who are treated with penicillin. It is not an indication for discontinuation of penicillin therapy.

Azimi PH, Janner D, Berne P, et al: Concentrations of procaine and aqueous penicillin in the cerebrospinal fluid of infants treated for congenital syphilis. J Pediatr 124:649, 1994.

Beck-Sague C, Alexander ER: Failure of benzathine penicillin G treatment in early congenital syphilis. Pediatr Infect Dis J 6:1061, 1987.

Centers for Disease Control: 1993 Sexually Transmitted Diseases Treatment Guidelines. MMWR 42:14, 1993.

Centers for Disease Control: Syphilis and congenital syphilis—United States, 1985–1988. MMWR 37:486, 1989.

Musher DM: Syphilis, neurosyphilis, penicillin, and AIDS. J Infect Dis 163:1201, 1991.

Zenker PN, Berman SM: Congenital syphilis: trends and recommendations for evaluation and management. Pediatr Infect Dis J 1:105, 1991.

201.2 Nonvenereal Syphilitic Diseases

Several variants of endemic syphilis are recognized by their geographic distribution. These diseases, which include yaws, bejel, and pinta, are caused by spirochetes belonging to the genus *Treponema* that are (1) morphologically and immunologically identical to *T. pallidum*, (2) extremely sensitive to penicillin, and (3) differentiated primarily on the basis of clinical findings. Yaws is the most common of the nonvenereal spirochetal diseases and occurs in Africa, Latin America, and Asia. Bejel is present in the Middle East and Africa, and pinta is found only in Latin America.

YAWS

Yaws is a chronic relapsing infection involving the skin and bony structures caused by the spirochete *T. pertenue*, which cannot be differentiated microscopically or serologically from *T. pallidum*. It occurs in the warm, humid tropical regions of Africa, Asia, South America, and Oceania, and almost all cases occur in children. A high percentage of the population is infected in endemic areas.

T. pertenue cannot penetrate normal skin and is transmitted via direct contact from an infected lesion through a skin abrasion or laceration. Transmission is facilitated by overcrowding and poor personal hygiene. The initial papular lesion (the "mother yaw") occurs 2–8 wk following inoculation. The papule develops into a raised raspberry-like papilloma, which is often associated with regional lymphadenopathy. Secondary lesions erupt before or after the ulceration and healing of the mother yaw. With the healing of the mother yaw, there is hypopigmented scar formation. Secondary papillomas may appear anywhere and can be associated with lymphadenopathy, anorexia, and malaise. Ulcerated lesions are covered by exudates containing treponemes. Secondary lesions heal without scarring, but relapses are common within 5 yr after the primary lesion.

The lesions and exacerbations are often associated with bone pain and underlying periostitis or osteomyelitis, especially in the fingers, nose, and tibia. Following the initial period of clinical activity, the patient enters a 5–10 yr period of latency. This is followed by the appearance of tertiary lesions at puberty, which are often solitary and destructive. These present as painful papillomas on the hands and feet, gummatous skin ulcerations, or osteitis. Bony destruction and deformity are common, as are juxta-articular nodules, depigmentation, and painful hyperkeratosis ("dry crab yaws") of the palms and soles.

Diagnosis depends on the clinical manifestations of the disease in an endemic area. Dark-field examination of cutaneous lesions and serologic tests for syphilis, both treponemal and nontreponemal, are confirmatory.

Treatment of patients and all contacts consists of a single intramuscular injection of benzathine penicillin (1.2 million U), which cures the lesions of active yaws, renders them noninfectious, and prevents relapse. Eradication of yaws from endemic foci may be accomplished by treating the entire population with penicillin. Patients allergic to penicillin may be treated with erythromycin or tetracycline.

ENDEMIC SYPHILIS

(Bejel, Nonvenereal Childhood Syphilis)

Bejel affects children living in the Saharan regions of Africa and the Middle East. Infection with a strain of *Treponema pallidum* follows penetration of the spirochete through traumatized skin or mucous membranes. In experimental infections, a primary papule forms at the inoculation site after an incubation period of 3 wk; in human infections a primary lesion is almost never visualized. The *clinical manifestations* of the secondary stage of bejel are confined to the skin and mucous membranes and consist of highly infectious mucous patches on the oral mucosa and condyloma-like lesions on the moist areas of the body, especially the axilla and anus. These mucocutaneous lesions resolve spontaneously over a period of several months, but recurrences are common. The secondary stage is followed by a variable latency period before the onset of late or tertiary bejel. The late complications, identical to those of yaws, include gumma formation in skin, subcutaneous tissue, and bone, resulting in painful destructive ulcerations, swelling, and deformity.

Diagnosis is suspected on epidemiologic and clinical grounds and is confirmed either by dark-field examination of the skin and mucous membrane lesions or by serologic testing (positive VDRL, TPI, and FTA-ABS tests). Differentiation from syphilis is extremely difficult in an endemic area. Bejel can be suspected by the absence of a primary chancre and lack of involvement of the CNS and cardiovascular system during the late stage. *Treatment* of early infection consists of a single intramuscular dose of benzathine penicillin (1.2 million U); late infection is treated with three injections, each of the same dose at intervals of 7 days. Patients allergic to penicillin may be treated with erythromycin or tetracycline.

PINTA

Pinta is a chronic, nonvenereally transmitted infection caused by *Treponema carateum,* a spirochete morphologically and serologically indistinguishable from other human treponemes. The disease is endemic in Mexico, Central America, South America, and parts of the West Indies. Infection follows direct inoculation of the treponeme through abraded skin. Following a variable incubation period of days, a primary lesion appears at the inoculation site as a small asymptomatic erythematous papule resembling localized psoriasis or eczema. The regional lymph nodes are often enlarged, and spirochetes can be visualized on dark-field examination of skin scrapings or of the involved lymph nodes. After a period of enlargement, the primary lesion disappears. Secondary lesions follow within 6–8 mo; they consist of small macules and papules on the face, scalp, and other exposed portions of the body. These pigmented lesions are scaly and nonpruritic and may coalesce to form large plaquelike elevations resembling psoriasis. In the late stage, atrophic and depigmented lesions develop on the hands, wrists, ankles, feet, face, and scalp. Hyperkeratosis of palms and soles is uncommon. *Diagnosis* is confirmed by dark-field examination of early lesions and a positive serologic test for syphilis. *Treatment* consists of a single intramuscular injection of benzathine penicillin (1.2 million U). Tetracycline and erythromycin are satisfactory alternatives for patients allergic to penicillin.

LEPTOSPIROSIS

ETIOLOGY. Leptospirosis is a generalized infection of humans and animals caused by spirochetes of the genus *Leptospira.* The pathogenic leptospires belong to a single species, *Leptospira interrogans,* which contains approximately 200 distinct serovars. A single serovar may produce a variety of distinct syndromes, and a single clinical manifestation (e.g., aseptic meningitis) may be caused by multiple serotypes.

EPIDEMIOLOGY. Leptospirosis is a zoonosis of worldwide distribution. Leptospires infect many species of wild and domestic animals and have been isolated from birds, fish, and reptiles. The rat is the principal source of human infection. Other important animal reservoirs include dogs, cats, livestock, and wild animals. Animal infection varies from inapparent to fatal. Once infected, animals excrete spirochetes in urine for an extended period of time. Leptospire survival outside the animal host is dependent upon the moisture content, temperature, and pH of the soil or water into which they are shed. The majority of human cases worldwide result from occupational exposure to rat-contaminated water or soil. Occupational groups with a high incidence of leptospirosis include agricultural workers, persons who live or work in rat-infested environments, individuals involved in animal husbandry or veterinary medicine, and laboratory workers. In the United States, the major animal reservoir is the dog, and contact with spirochetes is often associated with recreational activities that result in contact with contaminated soil or water during the summer months.

PATHOPHYSIOLOGY. Leptospires enter humans through moist and preferably abraded skin or through mucous membranes. Following penetration of the skin or mucus membranes, leptospires circulate in the bloodstream and spread to all organs of the body. The primary lesion caused by leptospires is damage to the endothelial lining of small blood vessels with resultant ischemic damage to the liver, kidneys, meninges, and muscles. After an incubation period of 7–12 days, an initial *septicemic phase* begins in which leptospires can be isolated from the blood, CSF, and other tissues. Initial symptoms, which last approximately 2–7 days, may be followed by a brief period of well-being and a second symptomatic or *immune phase.* The immune phase is associated with the appearance of circulating antibody, the disappearance of organisms from the blood and CSF, and the appearance of additional signs and symptoms. Despite the presence of circulating antibody, leptospires may persist in the kidney, urine, and aqueous humor. The immune or leptospiruric phase may last for several weeks.

CLINICAL MANIFESTATIONS. Most cases of human leptospirosis are subclinical, with inapparent infection particularly common in high-risk occupational groups such as farmers and their families. Symptomatic infection may present as an acute febrile illness with nonspecific signs and symptoms (70%), as meningitis (20%), or as hepatorenal dysfunction (10%). The onset is typically sudden, and the illness tends to follow a biphasic course (Fig. 201–6).

Anicteric Leptospirosis. The onset of the initial or septicemic phase is abrupt, with fever, shaking chills, severe headache, malaise, nausea, vomiting, and severe, often debilitating muscular pain. Circulatory collapse is uncommon, but some patients have bradycardia and hypotension. Typically, the child is lethargic, with mild to moderate dehydration. Additional physical findings include extreme muscle tenderness, which is most prominent in the lower extremities, the lumbosacral spine, and abdomen. Conjunctival suffusion with photophobia and orbital pain (in the absence of chemosis and purulent exudate), generalized lymphadenopathy, and hepatosplenomegaly may also be present. Cutaneous lesions are common (10%), usually consisting of a truncal erythematous maculopapular rash, but they may be urticarial, petechial, purpuric, or desquamating. Less common manifestations include pharyngitis, pneumonitis, arthritis, carditis, cholecystitis, and orchitis. The second or immune phase may follow a brief asymptomatic interlude and is characterized by recurrence of fever. Aseptic meningitis is the hallmark of this phase. Despite abnormal CSF profiles in 80% of infected children, only 50% have meningeal manifestations. Spinal fluid abnormalities include a modest elevation in pressure, a mononuclear pleocytosis rarely exceeding 500 cells/mm^3 (polymorphonuclear leukocytes predominate initially), normal or slightly elevated protein, and normal glucose values. Encephalitis, cranial and peripheral neuropathies, papilledema, and paralysis are uncommon. Symptoms referable to the CNS resolve spontaneously within a week or so. Uveitis may occur during this phase; it can be unilateral or bilateral and is usually self-limited, rarely resulting in permanent visual impairment.

Icteric Leptospirosis (Weil Disease). This severe form of leptospirosis occurs in fewer than 10% of affected children. The initial manifestations are similar to those described for anicteric leptospirosis. The immune phase, however, is distinctive, being characterized by clinical and laboratory evidence of hepatic and renal dysfunction. In fulminating cases, hemorrhagic phenomena and cardiovascular collapse also occur. Hepatic abnormalities include right upper quadrant pain, hepatomegaly, direct and indirect hyperbilirubinemia, and modest elevation of serum liver enzymes. Renal manifestations are common, may dominate the clinical picture, and are the principal cause of death in fatal cases; all patients have abnormal findings on urinalysis (hematuria, proteinuria, and casts), and azotemia is common, often associated with oliguria or anuria. Congestive heart failure is uncommon; however, abnormal electrocardiograms are present in 90% of affected children. Hemorrhagic manifestations are rare but when present may include epistaxis, hemoptysis, and gastrointestinal and adrenal hemorrhage. Thrombocytopenia and hypoprothrombinemia also occur.

DIAGNOSIS. Leptospirosis should be considered in the differential diagnosis of any acute febrile illness when there is a history of direct contact with animals or with soil or water contaminated with animal urine, and especially when the onset is abrupt with chills, fever, severe myalgias, conjunctival suffusion, headache, nausea, and vomiting. Isolation of the infecting organism from clinical specimens or a four-fold rise in antibody titer in the presence of clinical symptoms compatible with leptospirosis establishes the diagnosis. A presumptive diagnosis is made in symptomatic children with stable titers of 1:100 or greater in two or more specimens and in asymptomatic children with evidence of exposure and a seroconversion (i.e., a four-fold rise in antibody titer in specimens obtained 2 or more wk apart).

Silver impregnation and fluorescent antibody techniques permit identification of *leptospires* in infected tissue or body fluids. Spirochetes may also be demonstrated by phase-contrast or dark-field microscopy; however, the skill required and the high frequency of artifacts found with these tests limit their use. Unlike other pathogenic spirochetes, *leptospires* are easily cultured on commercially available media.

Media containing rabbit serum or bovine serum albumin and long-chain fatty acids are suitable. Repeated blood cultures in the 1st wk of infection with very small inocula of blood are recommended. A small inoculum (i.e., one drop in 5 mL of medium) is used to minimize growth inhibitory factors. They can be recovered from the blood or CSF during the first 10 days of illness and from urine after the 2nd wk. The number of *leptospires* in clinical specimens is small and their growth rate is slow; leptospires may be seen in several days, although

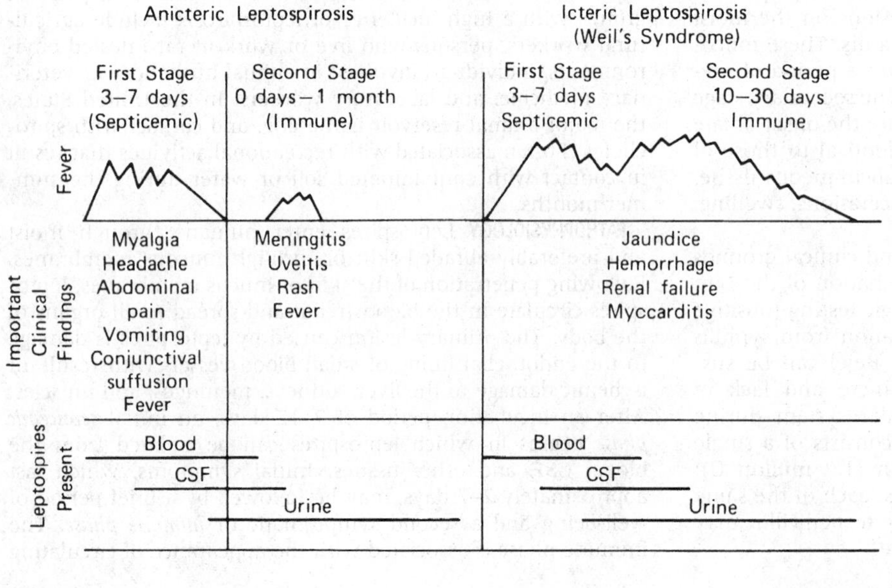

Figure 201–6. Stages of anicteric and icteric leptospirosis. Correlation between clinical findings and presence of leptospires in body fluids. (Reprinted with permission from Feigin RD, Anderson DC: CRC Crit Rev Clin Lab Sci 5:413, 1975. Copyright CRC Press, Inc., Boca Raton, FL.)

cultures may not become positive for 2–4 mo. Prolonged incubation is thus required.

The diagnosis is most often established by serologic testing. A microscopic slide-agglutination test utilizing killed antigen is the most useful screening test. A microscopic slide-agglutination test with a live or formalin-treated antigen may be used to determine antibody titer and tentatively identify the infecting serotype. Agglutinins usually appear by the 12th day of illness and reach a maximum titer by the 3rd wk. Low titers may persist for years. Approximately 10% of infected persons do not have detectable agglutinins, presumably because available antisera do not identify all *Leptospira* serotypes. The indirect hemagglutination test or the highly specific and sensitive enzyme-linked immunosorbent assay (ELISA) and dot ELISA tests have replaced the conventional slide agglutination tests.

TREATMENT AND PREVENTION. Despite the in vitro sensitivity of *Leptospira* to penicillin and tetracycline and the efficacy of these agents in treating experimental infection, their effectiveness in human leptospirosis remains controversial. It does appear that initiation of treatment before the 7th day will probably shorten the clinical course and decrease the severity of the infection. On this basis, treatment with penicillin or tetracycline (in children over 12 yr) should be instituted as soon as the diagnosis is suspected. Parenteral penicillin G, 6–8 million U/m²/24 hr, in 6 divided doses for 7 days is recommended. In patients allergic to penicillin, tetracycyline (10–20 mg/kg/24 hr) should be administered orally or intravenously in 4 divided doses for 7 days.

Prevention of human leptospirosis is possible by instituting rodent control measures and avoiding contaminated water and soil. Immunization of livestock and family pets has been recommended as a means of eliminating animal reservoirs, but these programs have met with limited success. A formalin-killed polyvalent human vaccine has been utilized in "at risk" occupation groups in Europe and Asia; however, there have been no clinical trials to determine its efficacy. Leptospirosis has been prevented in American servicemen stationed in the tropics by administering doxycycline, 200 mg once a week, as prophylaxis. This schedule may be similarly effective for the traveler entering a highly endemic area for a limited period of time.

Edwards GA, Domm BM: Human leptospirosis. Medicine 39:117, 1960.

Feigin RD, Anderson DC: Human leptospirosis. CRC Crit Rev Clin Lab Sci 5:413, 1975.

Heath CW Jr, Alexander AD, Galton MM: Leptospirosis in the United States. Analysis of 483 cases in man, 1949–1961. N Engl J Med 273:857, 1965.

Watt G, Alquiza LM, Padre LP, et al: The rapid diagnosis of leptospirosis: A prospective comparison of the dot enzyme-linked immunosorbent assay and the genus-specific microscopic agglutination test at different stages of illness. J Infect Dis 157:4, 1993.

Wong ML, Kaplan S, Dunide LM, et al: Leptospirosis: A childhood disease. J Pediatr 90:532, 1977.

RAT-BITE FEVERS

Two distinctly different diseases are categorized under the term *rat-bite fever*. These are spirillary and streptobacillary rat-bite fever. Both illnesses usually follow the bite or scratch of a rat; however, cases have been reported in the absence of a history of rodent exposure. Isolated case reports and several epidemics of streptobacillary rat-bite fever have been described following the ingestion of raw milk contaminated by rats *(Haverhill fever)*. The illnesses exist worldwide, with higher incidences reported in urban settings with poor sanitation and large rat populations. Infections are more common in children than adults and occur in approximately 10% of children bitten by wild rats.

Spirillary Rat-Bite Fever
(Sodoku)

The disease is caused by *Spirillum minor*, a short, tightly coiled, gram-negative spirochete that is present in the saliva of about 10% of healthy wild and laboratory rats. It cannot be grown in commercially available media; laboratory isolation requires inoculation of mice and guinea pigs. However, it can be visualized by direct dark-field examination of infected lymph obtained from the inoculation site (preferably during the ulcerative phase) or from regional lymph nodes. Occasionally, the spirochete is visualized on peripheral blood smears.

CLINICAL MANIFESTATIONS. The initial inoculation of spirochetes is followed by an asymptomatic incubation period of 14–18 days. The wound appears to heal but then becomes erythematous and indurated, and eventually undergoes suppuration and eschar formation (Fig. 201–7). During this phase, localized lymphangitis and lymphadenitis are observed in about 50% of affected children. At the onset there are fever, chills, severe myalgia, and a reddish-brown or purple macular rash (80%), typically beginning at the inoculation site and spreading to involve the entire body. Arthralgia may be severe, but there is no joint effusion. In untreated children, the fever persists for 3–4 days, at which time the constitutional symptoms subside, the rash disappears, and the inoculation site heals. This asymptomatic period persists for several days and is followed by a second cycle of fever, rash, and constitutional symptoms. This relapsing pattern of illness may continue for up to a year in untreated patients; however, the disease is eventually self-limiting. Fatalities are uncommon (1%) and are usually associated with meningitis, endocarditis, and myocarditis.

DIAGNOSIS. In patients with a history of rat bite, the major differential diagnosis is etiologic—whether the infectious agent is *Streptobacillus moniliformis* or *Spirillum minor*. The long incubation period, the prompt initial healing of the primary wound followed by induration, ulceration, and eschar formation, and the absence of arthritis suggest *Spirillum minor* infection. The laboratory diagnosis depends on the presence of negative blood and joint fluid cultures for *Streptobacillus moniliformis*, the presence of spirochetes on direct dark-field examination of tissue specimens, and recovery of spirochetes following animal inoculation.

TREATMENT. *Spirillum minor* is extremely sensitive to penicillin; however, because this illness is often confused with rat-bite fever due to *Streptobacillus moniliformis*, which is more resistant to penicillin, and because dual infection has been described, large doses of procaine penicillin G (600,000 U every 12 hr for 10 days) are recommended. In patients allergic to penicillin, tetracycline or an aminoglycoside may be used.

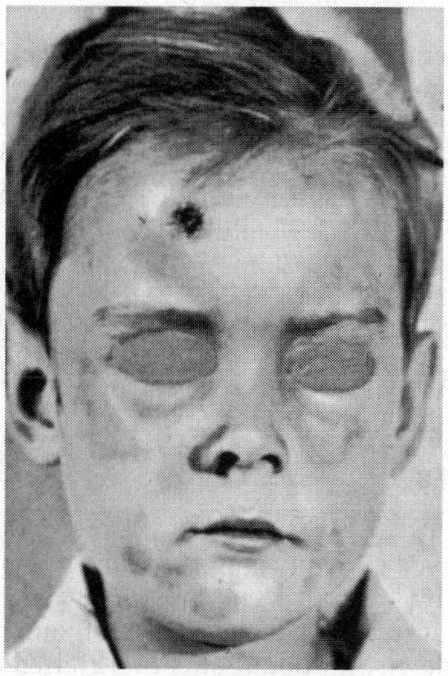

Figure 201–7. Sodoku: chancre-like indurated ulcer at a bite site on the forehead; secondary macular eruption of the face.

Streptobacillary Rat-Bite Fever

(Haverhill Fever)

This form of rat-bite fever is caused by *Streptobacillus moniliformis*, an aerobic, nonmotile, pleomorphic, unencapsulated gram-negative bacillus, which can be isolated from the nasopharynx of about 50% of healthy wild and laboratory rats. The organism has also been isolated from mice, squirrels, dogs, cats, and weasels. *S. moniliformis* can be grown on commercially available artificial media. The morphologic characteristics of the pathogen, including the formation of L-forms devoid of cell walls, and the relative resistance to penicillin vary with the age of the inoculum and the components of the culture medium. Giemsa or Gram stain may reveal short rods, long chains, or long tangled filaments with fusiform swellings.

CLINICAL MANIFESTATIONS. The incubation period is short, rarely exceeding 7 days. The onset is abrupt with fever and chills. Associated symptoms include severe myalgia, weakness, headache, and upper respiratory symptoms, most notably pharyngitis. A generalized rash and joint involvement appear within several days after the onset of fever. The rash may be maculopapular, petechial, or urticarial; most often it appears as a diffuse morbilliform rash involving the hands and feet. Papules, vesicles, pustules, and scabs are also seen. Joint involvement occurs in approximately half the patients and consists of a polyarticular, occasionally migratory arthritis that has a predilection for knees and large joints as well as the small joints of the hands and feet. The initial inoculation site heals without suppuration, and lymphangitis and lymphadenitis are uncommon. In untreated patients the symptoms spontaneously resolve after several days, whereupon the illness assumes a relapsing course of paroxysms of fever, rash, and arthritis occurring at irregular intervals for several months; the illness is eventually self-limiting, and the mortality rarely exceeds 10%. Life-threatening complications include endocarditis and pneumonitis.

DIAGNOSIS. In patients with a history of a rat bite or rodent contact, the major differential diagnosis involves the two forms of rat-bite fever. In the streptobacillary form of infection the incubation period is short, the inoculation site heals without suppuration or eschar formation, lymphangitis and lymphadenitis are uncommon, and the responsible pathogen can be readily cultured from blood and joint fluid. Diagnosis is more difficult when there is no history of rat bites or other direct contact with rodents, such as infection following consumption of contaminated raw milk (Haverhill fever). Other bacterial infections to be considered in the differential diagnosis include disseminated gonococcal infection, chronic meningococcemia, and leptospirosis.

TREATMENT. Penicillin is the treatment of choice. It can be given parenterally, using aqueous penicillin G (100,000–200,000 U/kg/24 hr IV) or procaine penicillin G (600,000–1.2 million U/hr IM), or orally using penicillin V in large doses, all for 7–10 days. Alternative agents include tetracycline for children over 7 yr of age or an aminoglycoside.

Brown R, McPherson J, Nunemaker JC: Rat-bite fever—A review of the American cases with re-evaluation of etiology, report of cases. Bull Johns Hopkins Hosp 70:201, 1942.

Raffin BJ, Freemark M: Streptobacillary rat-bite fever: A pediatric problem. Pediatrics 64:214, 1979.

RELAPSING FEVER

(Recurrent Fever, Louse-Borne Fever, Tick-Borne Fever)

Relapsing fever is an uncommon arthropod-borne infection characterized by recurrent episodes of fever. It is caused by spirochetes of the genus *Borrelia*, a fastidious microorganism with worldwide distribution that is transmitted to man by lice or ticks.

ETIOLOGY AND EPIDEMIOLOGY. *Epidemic relapsing fever* is caused by *B. recurrentis* and is transmitted from person to person by the human body louse *(Pediculus humanus)*. Following ingestion of an infective blood meal by the louse, the spirochetes penetrate its midgut, migrate to and multiply within the hemolymph, and remain viable throughout its lifespan (several weeks). Human infection occurs as a result of crushing lice during scratching, allowing infected hemolymph to enter through the abraded skin. Louse-borne disease tends to occur in epidemics, often in association with typhus. It occurs more commonly during the winter, and the major endemic focus of the disease is the highlands of Ethiopia.

Endemic relapsing fever is caused by several species of *Borrelia* and is transmitted to humans by ticks (genus *Ornithodoros*). Following ingestion of an infective blood meal, spirochetes invade all tissues of their arthropod hosts, including the salivary glands and reproductive tract. The latter permits transovarian passage of infected spirochetes, perpetuating arthropod infection in successive generations. Human infection occurs when saliva, coxal fluid, or excrement is released by the tick during feeding, thereby permitting spirochetes to penetrate the skin and mucous membranes. *Ornithodoros* is distributed worldwide (including the western United States), prefers warm, humid environments and high altitudes, and is found in rodent burrows, caves, and other nesting sites; rodents are the principal reservoirs. Infected ticks gain access to human dwellings on the rodent host. Human contact is often unnoticed, because these ticks are nocturnal feeders, have a painless bite, and detach immediately following a short blood meal.

PATHOPHYSIOLOGY. The cyclic nature of relapsing fever is explained by the ability of *Borrelia* organisms to continually undergo antigenic (phase) variation: Multiple variants evolve simultaneously during the first relapse, with one type becoming predominant, and spirochetes isolated during the primary febrile episode differ antigenetically from those recovered during a subsequent relapse. During febrile episodes, spirochetes enter the bloodstream, promote the development of specific IgM and IgG antibody, and undergo agglutination, immobilization, lysis, and phagocytosis. During remission, *Borrelia* spirochetes may remain in the bloodstream, but spirochetemia is insufficient to produce symptoms. The number of relapses in untreated patients depends upon the number of antigenic variants of the infecting strain.

CLINICAL MANIFESTATIONS. Louse-borne disease has a longer incubation period, longer periods of pyrexia, fewer relapses, and longer remission periods than tick-borne disease. Each illness is associated with sudden onset of high fever, headache, photophobia, nausea, vomiting, myalgia, and arthralgia. Additional symptoms may appear later and include abdominal pain, a productive cough, and mild respiratory distress. Bleeding manifestations are common and include epistaxis, hemoptysis, hematuria, and hematemesis. The child may be lethargic and often has a diffuse, erythematous, macular, or petechial rash over the trunk and shoulders. This rash is more common in louse-borne fever (25%), is of 1–2 days' duration, and occurs almost exclusively during the end of the primary febrile episode. There may also be lymphadenopathy, pneumonia, and splenomegaly. Hepatic tenderness associated with hepatomegaly is a common sign. Jaundice is not uncommon and may occur in half of affected children. CNS manifestations may be the principal feature of late relapses in tick-borne disease; they include lethargy, stupor, meningismus, convulsions, peripheral neuritis, focal neurologic deficits, and cranial nerve paralysis. Myocarditis and hepatitis are not uncommon and may be responsible for death.

The initial symptomatic period characteristically ends with a crisis in 4–10 days, marked by abrupt diaphoresis, hypothermia, hypotension, bradycardia, profound muscle weakness, and prostration. In untreated patients subsequent relapse occurs within 1 wk and is followed by up to five relapses with symptoms during each relapse becoming milder and shorter; the afebrile remission period lengthens. Severe manifestations include myocarditis, hepatic failure, and disseminated intravascular coagulation.

Diagnosis depends on demonstration of spirochetes in thin or thick blood smears stained with Giemsa or Wright stain. During afebrile remissions, spirochetes disappear from the blood.

TREATMENT AND PROGNOSIS. Oral or parenteral tetracycline is the drug of choice for louse-borne and tick-borne relapsing fever. In children under 12 yr of age erythromycin (50 mg/kg/24 hr) for a total of 10 days is recommended. For older children and young adults, tetracycline (500 mg every 6 hr) for 10 days has been effective. Single-dose treatment with erythromycin or tetracycline (a single 500-mg oral dose) is efficacious in adults, but experience in children is limited.

Resolution of each febrile episode either by natural crisis or as a result of antimicrobial treatment is usually accompanied within 2 hr by the Jarisch-Herxheimer reaction, which is associated with clearing of the spirochetemia. Attempts to control this reaction by prior treatment with corticosteroids or antipyretics have met with limited success.

With adequate therapy the *mortality rate* for relapsing fever is below 5%. A majority of patients recover from their illness with or without treatment after the appearance of antiborrelial antibodies, which agglutinate, kill, or opsonize the spirochete.

No vaccine is available, and disease control requires avoidance or elimination of the arthropod vectors. In epidemics of louse-borne disease, dissemination can be prevented by good personal hygiene and delousing of persons, dwellings, and clothing with commercially available insecticides.

Butler T: Relapsing fever: New lessons about antibiotic action. Ann Intern Med 102:397, 1985.
Butler T, Jones PK, Wallace CK: *Borrelia recurrentis* infection. Single dose antibiotic regimens and management of Jarisch-Herxheimer reaction. J Infect Dis 137:573, 1978.
Perine PL, Teklu B: Antibiotic treatment of louse-borne relapsing fever in Ethiopia: A report of 377 cases. Am J Trop Med Hyg 32:1096, 1983.
Stoennerita DT, Larcen C: Antigenic variation in *Borrelia hermsii.* J Exp Med 156:1297, 1982.

CHAPTER 202
Actinomycosis

Richard F. Jacobs

Actinomyces species are slow-growing, gram-positive bacteria that are part of the normal oral flora in humans. Their filamentous structure gives them a fungus-like appearance and infections that are caused by these bacteria are termed *actinomycosis.* The disease actinomycosis is a chronic, granulomatous, suppurative disease characterized by peripheral spread with extension to contiguous tissue in the formation of multiple draining sinus tracts. These infections usually involve the cervicofacial, thoracic, abdominal, or pelvic regions.

ETIOLOGY. *Actinomyces israelii* is the predominant organism causing disease in humans. Other implicated species, in order of importance, include: *Arachnia propionica, Actinomyces odontolyticus, A. meyeri, A. naeslundii, A. viscosus,* and *Bifidobacterium eriksonii.* Additionally, four or five other species of *Actinomyces* have been shown to cause human disease but are rare.

EPIDEMIOLOGY. Actinomycosis occurs worldwide without relation to age, sex, race, season, or occupation. In a classic review published in 1952, Bates and Cruikshank described 85 cases of actinomycosis. Of these patients, 27% were less than 20 yr of age with 7% of the patients being less than 10 yr of age. The youngest patient in this description was 28 days of age. Although actinomycosis is usually not an opportunistic infection, disease has been described in patients on steroids, with leukemia, renal failure, congenital immunodeficiency diseases, and human immunodeficiency virus (HIV)/acquired immune deficiency syndrome (AIDS). Antecedent disease and surgery predisposed 81 of 181 subjects to infection. The source of human infection is almost always endogenous flora.

Actinomycosis, even in closed infections, is usually part of a polymicrobial infection involving mixed bacteria. In a large study of over 650 cases, Holm was unable to identify a single infection in which *Actinomyces* occurred in pure culture; *Actinomyces* was identified with other bacteria, most notably *Actinobacillus actinomycetemcomitans* and *Haemophilus aphrophilus,* as well as other local flora.

PATHOGENESIS. The organism infects the host after introduction into the tissue by trauma or aspiration into the lung. It spreads locally and, rarely, hematogenously. *Actinomyces* are gram-positive, facultative, or strict anaerobes with a variable morphology. The irregular morphology ranges from diphtheroid to mycelial. The organisms are found in clinical specimens, such as sputum, purulent exudates, and tissues obtained surgically or at necropsy. Staining of crushed tissue specimens rinsed with sterile saline or purulent exudate stained by Gram or acid-fast procedures can reveal organisms within the classic sulfur granules. Cultures on brain-heart infusion agar incubated at 37° C anaerobically (95% N and 5% CO_2) and a separate set incubated aerobically will reveal organisms within the lines of streak at 24–48 hr. *Actinomyces israelii* colonies appear as loose masses of delicate branching filaments with a characteristic spider-like growth. Colonies of *A. naeslundii, A. viscosus, A. propionica,* and *Bifidobacterium eriksonii* may have similar growth characteristics. Due to the similarity in growth characteristics from colony morphology, various biochemical tests are performed in order to identify the specific organism.

Actinomycosis is a chronic, suppurative, scarring inflammatory process. Sites of infection show dense cellular infiltrates and suppuration that form multiple interconnecting abscesses and sinus tracts. This may be followed by cicatricial healing from which the organism then spreads by burrowing along fascial planes. This causes deep communicating scarred sinus tracts. Characteristic sulfur granules have an adherent mass of polymorphonuclear neutrophils that are attached to the radially arranged eosinophilic clubs of the granule.

The three important sites of *Actinomyces* infection in order of frequency are cervicofacial, abdominal, and thoracic. Many less common infections occur, involving every organ in the body. Actinomycosis must be differentiated from several other chronic inflammatory diseases, including tuberculosis, mycotic infections, *Yersinia enterocoliticus* "pseudoappendicitis," appendicitis, amebiasis, hepatic abscess, osteomyelitis, nocardiosis, and other chronic bacterial infections. In addition to introduction at wound sites, use of intrauterine devices (IUD) permits the development of pelvic and gastrointestinal actinomycosis. Pulmonary actinomycosis occurs following inhalation or aspiration of organisms, introduction of a colonized foreign body, or spread from an existing cervicofacial or abdominal actinomycotic infection.

CLINICAL MANIFESTATIONS. The three major forms of actinomycosis: cervicofacial, abdominal/pelvic, and pulmonary infections arise by different routes but may predispose to other forms of the disease. The diagnosis of actinomycosis in children should raise suspicion for an underlying immunodeficiency disease state, especially chronic granulomatous disease.

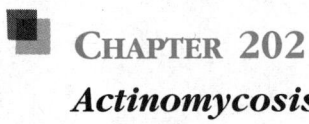

Cervicofacial Actinomycosis. In cervicofacial actinomycosis, the organisms enter the tissue through trauma to the mucous membranes of the mouth or pharynx by way of caries or through tonsillar tissue. Clinical characteristics are pain, trismus, firm swelling, and fistula with drainage containing the characteristic sulfur granules. Cervicofacial actinomycosis is usually painless, slow growing, with a hard mass that can produce cutaneous fistulas, a condition commonly known as lumpy jaw (Fig. 202–1). Less frequently, cervicofacial actinomycosis can present as an acute, tender, fluctuant mass suggestive of an acute pyogenic infection. Bone is not involved early in the disease, but later a periostitis, mandibular osteomyelitis, or perimandibular abscess may develop. Infection may spread via sinus tracts to the cranial bones, which may give rise to meningitis. The ability of the organisms in this disease to burrow through tissue planes, and even bone, is a key differentiating point between actinomycosis and nocardiosis. The cervicofacial type of actinomycosis has the best prognosis, and the disease is usually cured with surgical debridement and excision as an adjunct to proper antibiotic therapy.

Abdominal and Pelvic Actinomycosis. This disease usually develops as a result of an acute, perforative gastrointestinal disease or after trauma to the abdomen. Of all the forms of actinomycosis, a delayed diagnosis is typical for abdominal or pelvic disease. Gastrointestinal disease occurs as appendicitis in 25% of cases, but can manifest as a variety of ulcerative diseases. Infection classically appears after appendectomy as a hard, irregular mass in the ileocecal area that softens and then drains to the outside via a fistula. Hepatic involvement has been described in approximately 15% of abdominal actinomycosis cases as solitary or multiple liver abscesses or in a miliary pattern. The clinical course is indolent with chills, fever, night sweats, and weight loss, and is similar to the presentation of tuberculous peritonitis. Extension from this focus is usually by direct continuity or, rarely, hematogenously to involve any tissue or organ, including muscle, spleen, kidney, fallopian tubes, ovaries, uterus, testes, bladder, or rectum.

Pulmonary Actinomycosis. Neither the clinical or radiographic presentation of pulmonary actinomycosis is specific. Principal symptoms include fever, productive cough, chest pain, and weight loss. Infection frequently dissects along tissue planes and may extend through the chest wall or diaphragm, producing multiple sinuses. These characteristic sinus tracts contain small abscesses and purulent drainage. Other complications include boney destruction of adjacent ribs, sternum, and vertebral bodies. Occasionally, multiple lobe involvement is found in the lung. Associated conditions, such as dental caries, aspiration, inhalation injury, introduction of a colonized foreign body, or pre-existing cervicofacial or abdominal disease, should heighten the index of suspicion. A specific diagnosis can be made by examining purulent sinus tract drainage for sulfur granules and appropriate cultures. The presence of *Actinomyces* in sputum or bronchoscopy is hampered because these organisms are normal oral flora. The differential diagnosis of pulmonary actinomycosis includes lung abscess and tuberculosis.

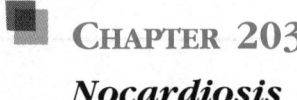

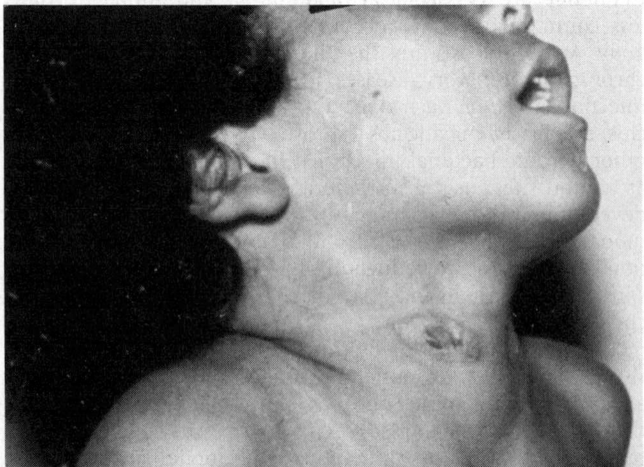

Figure 202–1. A 2-yr-old HIV-infected male with cervicofacial actinomycosis and a chronic draining fistula.

DIAGNOSIS. Microscopic examination with appropriate stains and culture of purulent drainage from fistulae, abscesses, or draining sinus tracts, along with bronchoalveolar lavage and sputum, can reveal one of the three major agents *Actinomyces, Arachnia,* and *Bifidobacterium.* Appropriate anaerobic and aerobic techniques and an index of suspicion for *Actinomyces* will enhance the yield on microbiological cultures.

TREATMENT. The mainstay of treatment for actinomycosis is prolonged antibiotics and an appropriate surgical approach to sinus tracts and abscesses. Prompt use of antibiotics results in a high rate of cure. Actinomycosis is treated with penicillin (250,000 U/kg/24 hr intravenously divided every 4 hr). Other appropriate antibiotics include tetracycline, clindamycin, chloramphenicol, and imipenem, given parenterally. Although controversy still exists over the dosage and duration of therapy, appropriate therapy usually includes parenteral antibiotics for 2–6 wk followed by oral antibiotics for 3–12 mo. The oral antibiotic of choice is penicillin (100 mg/kg/24 hr divided every 6 hr). Although most *Actinomyces israelii* strains are sensitive to penicillin with minimum inhibitory concentrations (MICs) in the 0.03–0.5 μg/ml range, some resistant strains have been identified. Antibiotic susceptibility testing should be performed on all patients with significant disease or with an underlying immunocompromised disease state. Hepatic abscesses or other deep tissue infections need to be treated for 6–12 mo. Large abscesses usually require surgical excision. Removal of chronically infected tonsils and treatment of pyorrhea or caries may eliminate possible sources of infection. Generally, the prognosis is excellent with adequate therapy and early diagnosis.

CHAPTER 203
Nocardiosis

Richard F. Jacobs

Nocardiosis is an acute, subacute, or chronic suppurative infection with a tendency to remissions and exacerbations. Nocardiosis is uncommon in children, presenting primarily as lung disease in immunocompromised hosts. Hematogenous dissemination to other body sites, most notably brain and skin, may also occur. *Nocardia* are classified as Actinomycetales, an order of gram-positive filamentous bacteria that includes *Actinomyces, Streptomyces,* and mycobacteria. Soil and decaying vegetable matter are their natural habitat. Infection in humans occurs by the respiratory route or by direct skin inoculation.

ETIOLOGY. Numerous taxonomic studies have established the heterogeneity of the species, *Nocardia asteroides,* and has led to the description of *N. asteroides* complex. Current methods of recognition of *N. asteroides* in the clinical laboratory include microscopic and colonial morphology, and inability to hydrolize caseine, tyrosine, xanthine, and hypoxanthine with resistance to lysozyme. Unfortunately, the species *N. asteroides, N. farcinica, N. carnia, N. nova,* and *N. transvalensis* share similar features and have contributed to the apparent heterogeneity of *N. asteroides.* In 1988, a susceptibility study of 78 clinical isolates of the *N. asteroides* complex from the United States found that 95% of strains exhibited one of five antibiotic resistance patterns. The first pattern studied (type 5) was seen in approximately 20% of isolates including, essentially, all isolates in the *N. asteroides* complex that were resistant to cefotaxime, ceftriaxone, and cefamandole. Recent studies have established these isolates as *N. farcinica*. The second group studied (Type 3) comprises approximately 20% of the strains and was characterized by susceptibility to ampicillin and erythromycin. Isolates with this susceptibility pattern were determined to be *N. nova*. The remaining groups had susceptibility patterns that included resistance to broad-spectrum cephalosporins, susceptibility to ampicillin and carbenicillin, but intermediate susceptibility to imipenem, and the most common group occurring in 35% of isolates was resistant to ampicillin but susceptible to the broad-spectrum cephalosporins and imipenem. The most active parenteral agents were amikacin (95%), imipenem (88%), ceftriaxone (82%), and cefotaxime (82%). The most active oral agents were the sulfonamides (100%), minocycline (100%), and ampicillin (40%).

Systemic nocardiosis is caused most frequently by the bacteria in the *N. asteroides* complex. *N. brasiliensis* is the principal cause of localized, chronic mycetoma but has recently been described in the United States and worldwide as a form of pulmonary and systemic disease, especially in immunocompromised patients. *Actinomadura madurae* (madura foot), *N. farcinica, N. nova,* and *N. transvalensis* are also causes of human disease. *Nocardia asteroides* complex are the most common agents of systemic nocardiosis in the United States, while *N. brasiliensis* is seen more commonly in Central America, South America, and Asia. These agents are similar morphologically and can be distinguished only by biochemical and serological procedures.

EPIDEMIOLOGY. Nocardiosis was once thought to be a rare cause of human disease but is now being recognized more frequently. It has been diagnosed in individuals ranging from 4 wk to 82 yr of age. Almost all of the patients have one or more severe underlying diseases, usually accompanied by compromised cellular immunity due to steroids, primary immunodeficiency (chronic granulomatous disease), organ transplantation, cytotoxic chemotherapy or human immunodeficiency virus (HIV)/acquired immune deficiency syndrome (AIDS). Although not a surveillance organism for HIV/AIDS, HIV-infected patients may present with nocardiosis. Soil is the natural habitat of *Nocardia* and it has been isolated throughout the world. The organism is inhaled in aerosolized dust and causes pulmonary infection with widespread dissemination in the susceptible host. Although communicability from human to human has not been proven to be common, a recent description of human-to-human transmission of *N. farcinica* resulting in sternal wound infections in open-heart surgery patients has raised concern of *Nocardia* as a nosocomial pathogen.

PATHOGENESIS. *Nocardia asteroides* complex and *N. brasiliensis* organisms are obligate aerobes and grow on ordinary culture media. These organisms are sensitive to a variety of antibiotics, so media containing these specific drugs will not support growth. Many isolates of *Nocardia* are thermophilic and can grow at temperatures up to 50° C; however, best growth is achieved at 37° C. At 25° C, the organisms grow very slowly. Colonies appear within 1–2 wk on brain-heart infusion agar and Lowenstein-Jensen media, usually as waxy, folded, or heaped colonies at the edges. With further incubation, these colonies develop aerial hyphae that tend to give them a white, chalky appearance. Classification of species of *Nocardia* are based on physiologic reactions with various substrates and antibiotic susceptibility testing. A recently isolated 55 kD protein that has apparent specificity for *N. asteroides* complex and an enzyme immunoassay with antibody titers ≥1:256 appear sensitive and specific but will require further clinical testing. On biopsy specimens or clinical body fluids, the appearance of *Nocardia* using the modified Kinyoun acid-fast staining technique would demonstrate fragmented bacilli with stain concentrated in a beaded fashion along portions of the branching filaments.

The primary infection of *Nocardia* is pulmonary, and the disease becomes systemic by hematogenous spread. Direct inoculation from soil into traumatized skin (madura foot) is also a frequent cause of *Nocardia* infection. In patients with impaired cellular immunity, direct spread from lungs or hematogenous spread to brain, skin, and other organs can occur.

CLINICAL MANIFESTATIONS. Nocardiosis is primarily a pulmonary disease in 75% of all cases. Almost all cases occur in immunocompromised patients or patients with underlying pulmonary disease, especially alveolar proteinosis. A demonstration of tissue invasion is important for identifying active infection because the organism can occasionally exist as a respiratory saprophyte. Clinical manifestations include pneumonia, and necrotizing pneumonia with single or multiple abscesses. Diagnosis is established in one third of cases by sputum analysis and culture in adults. Bronchoalveolar lavage or lung biopsy may be required to establish the diagnosis in the remaining two thirds of adults and in children. Generally, the mortality with nocardiosis exceeds 50%, but may be lower when the diagnosis is made early in infection.

Metastatic lesions may occur anywhere in the body, but the brain is the most common secondary site, occurring in 15–40% of cases. Brain lesions may be multiple or single. Brain abscess is the most common presentation, with meningitis the second most common, as manifested by pleocytosis (lymphocytes or neutrophils), elevated cerebrospinal fluid (CSF) protein, and hypoglycorrhachia. Persistent neutrophilic meningitis with sterile cultures is classic for central nervous system (CNS) *Nocardia* infection. The onset of CNS infection may be gradual or sudden and includes manifestations varying from headache to coma. Cranial computed tomography scan (CT) is recommended in all immunocompromised patients with pulmonary nocardiosis, even when asymptomatic, because of the frequency of CNS involvement and should be considered in all patients with pulmonary nocardiosis.

The skin is the 3rd most commonly involved organ. Renal nocardiosis is the 4th most common site, presenting with dysuria, hematuria, or pyuria. Lesions may extend from the cortex into the medulla. Gastrointestinal involvement may also be seen associated with nausea, vomiting, diarrhea, abdominal distension, and melana. Infection may metastasize to skin, pericardium, myocardium, spleen, liver, or adrenal glands; bone involvement is rare. Almost all of the involved organs have multiple abscesses, but, in contrast to actinomycosis, granules are rarely found.

DIAGNOSIS. Laboratory diagnosis of nocardiosis requires the direct examination of clinical material for characteristic gram-positive, acid-fast organisms and isolation by culture methods. Smears of clinical material are Gram stained or stained by the modified Kinyoun acid-fast technique. *Nocardia asteroides* complex and *N. brasiliensis* appear as delicately branched gram-positive structures that tend to fragment and may have a coccoid to bacillary shape. In properly stained and decolorized acid-fast smears, the organisms may appear as fragmented bacilli with the stain concentrated in a beaded fashion along the portions of the filaments.

TREATMENT. Sulfonamides are the treatment of choice in human nocardiosis. Trisulfapyrimidines or sulfasoxazole (120–150 mg/kg/24 hr divided every 6 hr) therapy for 3–6 mo is standard. For severe infections, amikacin (15–30 mg/kg/24 hr divided every 8 hr) as a single agent or in combination with a beta-lactam antibiotic (cefotaxime, ceftriaxone, or imipenem) can be used. In addition, and for specific *N. asteroides* complex isolates with in vitro susceptibility testing, alternative drugs may include combinations of erythromycin, imipenem, streptomycin, minocycline, or 3rd generation cephalosporins. Clinical trials have shown ampicillin or amoxicillin-clavulanate to be effective in *N. brasiliensis* infections. Relapses of *Nocardia* have been demonstrated in patients who were treated for less than 3 mo. Patients with AIDS probably should be treated indefinitely. Surgical drainage of abscesses is important. Despite adequate therapy, the overall mortality is approximately 50%, which may be secondary to a delay in diagnosis or to the debilitated state of the patient with severely compromised host defenses.

Ajello J, Georg LK, Kaplan W, et al: Mycotic infections. *In:* Bodily HL, Updyke GL, Mason JO (eds): Diagnostic Procedures for Bacterial, Mycotic and Parasitic Infections, 5th ed. New York, American Public Health Association, 1970, pp 633–723.
Angeles AM, Sugar AM: Rapid diagnosis of nocardiosis with an enzyme immunoassay. J Infect Dis 155:292, 1987.
Baghdadlian H, Sorger S, Knowles K, et al: *Nocardia transvalensis* pneumonia in a child. Pediatr Infect Dis J 8:470, 1989.
Bates M, Cruikshank G: Thoracic actinomycosis. Thorax 12:99, 1952.
Bodily HL, Updyke GL, Mason JO: Diagnostic Procedures for Bacterial, Mycotic and Parasitic Infections, 5th ed. New York, American Public Health Association, 1970, pp 868–869.
Bronner M: Actinomycosis, 2nd ed. Bristol, John Wright and Sons, 1971.
Brown JR: Human actinomycosis. A study of 181 subjects. Hum Pathol 4:319, 1973.
Feder HM Jr: Actinomycosis manifesting as an acute painless lump of the jaw. Pediatrics 85:858, 1990.
Georg LK: Diagnostic procedures for the isolation of the etiological agents of actinomycosis. Proceedings International Symposium on Mycoses. Pan American Health Organization Pub 205, 1970, pp 71–81.
Gordon KE, Mihm JM: The type species of the genus *Nocardia*. J Gen Microbiol 27:1, 1962.
Holm G: Studies on the etiology of human actinomycosis: I. The other microbes of actinomycosis and their importance. Acta Pathol Microbiol Scand 27:736, 1950.
Law BJ, Marks MI: Pediatric nocardiosis. Pediatrics 70:560, 1982.
McNeil MM, Brown JM, Georghiou PR, et al: Infections due to *Nocardia transvalensis:* Clinical spectrum and antimicrobial therapy. Clin Infect Dis 15:453, 1992.
Pinkhas J, Oliver I, deVries A, et al: Pulmonary nocardiosis complicating malignant lymphomas successfully treated with chemotherapy. Chest 63:367, 1973.
Schaal KP, Lee HJ: Actinomycete infections in humans—a review. Gene 115:201, 1992.
Slack JM: The epidemiology of actinomycosis. *In:* Al Dowry Y (ed): The Epidemiology of Human Mycotic Disease. Springfield, IL, Charles C. Thomas, 1975, pp 13–39.
Waksman SA, Henrici AT: The nomenclature and classification of the actinomycetes. J Bacteriol 46:337, 1942.
Wallace RJ, Septimus EJ, Williams TW, et al: Use of trimethoprim-sulfamethoxazole for treatment of infections due to *Nocardia*. Rev Infect Dis 4:315, 1982.
Wallace RJ, Steele LC, Sumter G, et al: Antimicrobial susceptibility patterns of *Nocardia asteroides*. Antimicrob Agents Chemother 32:1776, 1988.
Wallace RJ, Tsukamura M, Brown BA, et al: Cefotaxime-resistant *Nocardia asteroides* strains are isolates of the controversial species *Nocardia farcinica*. J Clin Microbiol 28:2726, 1990.
Wallace RJ, Brown BA, Tsukamura M, et al: Clinical and laboratory features of *Nocardia nova*. J Clin Microbiol 29:2407, 1991.
Weisse WC, Smith I: A study of 57 cases of actinomycosis over a 36-year period. Arch Intern Med 135:1562, 1975.
Young LS, Armstrong D, Blevins A, et al: *Nocardia asteroides* infection complicating neoplastic disease. Am J Med 50:356, 1971.

CHAPTER 204
Bartonellosis

Barbara W. Stechenberg

Bartonellosis is a geographically distinct disease caused by *Bartonella bacilliformis,* which produces two predominant forms of illness: Oroya fever, a severe, febrile hemolytic anemia; and verruca peruana, an eruption of hemangioma-like lesions. The organism also causes asymptomatic disease. Also called Carrion disease in honor of the medical student who inoculated himself with infectious material and proved the unitary etiology of the two clinical illnesses, it is found only in mountain valleys of the Andes Mountains in Peru, Ecuador, Colombia, Chile, and Bolivia.

ETIOLOGY AND EPIDEMIOLOGY. *B. bacilliformis* is a small, motile gram-negative organism with a brush of 10 or more unipolar flagella, which appear to be important components of its invasiveness. An obligate aerobe, it grows best at 28° C in semisolid nutrient agar containing rabbit serum and hemoglobin. Recent studies have shown genetic similarity with the alpha-2 subgroup of the class Proteobacteria.

The vector of this disease is the sand fly, *Phlebotomus noguchi.* After the bite, the Bartonella organisms enter the endothelial cells of blood vessels, where they proliferate. Found throughout the reticuloendothelial system, they then re-enter the bloodstream and parasitize the erythrocytes. They bind to the cells, induce deformation of the membranes, and then enter intracellular vacuoles. The resultant hemolytic anemia may involve as many as 90% of the erythrocytes. Patients who survive this acute phase may or may not develop the cutaneous manifestations, which are nodular hemangiomatous lesions or verrucae ranging in size from a few millimeters to several centimeters.

CLINICAL MANIFESTATIONS. The incubation period is from 2 to 14 wk. Patients may be totally asymptomatic or manifest nonspecific symptoms such as headache and malaise without anemia. Patients with Oroya fever are febrile with rapid development of anemia. Clouding of the sensorium and delirium are common symptoms and may progress to overt psychosis. Physical examination demonstrates signs of severe anemia, icterus, and pallor, which may be associated with generalized lymphadenopathy.

The anemia is macrocytic and hypochromic with reticulocyte counts as high as 50%. *B. bacilliformis* may be seen on Giemsa stain as red-violet rods in the erythrocytes. In the recovery phase, these organisms change to a more coccoid form and disappear from the blood.

In the pre-eruptive stage, patients may complain of arthralgias, myalgias, and paresthesias. Inflammatory reactions such as phlebitis, pleuritis, erythema nodosum, and encephalitis may develop. The appearance of verrucae is pathognomonic of the eruptive phase. They vary greatly in size and number.

The *diagnosis* is made on clinical grounds in conjunction with a blood smear with typical organisms or via blood cultures. In the absence of anemia, the diagnosis depends on blood cultures. In the eruptive phase, the typical verruca confirms the diagnosis. Recently antibody testing with ELISA has been used to document infection.

TREATMENT. *B. bacilliformis* is sensitive to many antibiotics, including penicillin, tetracycline, and chloramphenicol. Treatment is very effective in rapidly lowering fever and eradicating the organism from the blood. Chloramphenicol is considered the drug of choice, as it also is useful in the treatment of intercurrent infections such as *Salmonella.* Blood transfusions and supportive care are critical in patients with severe anemia. Treatment for verruca peruana is not necessary unless large lesions are disfiguring or interfere with function; then, surgical excision may be needed. Oral tetracycline may aid in healing of lesion.

Prevention depends on avoidance of the vector, particularly at night, and the use of insect repellents.

Gray GC, Johnson AA, Thornton SA, et al: An epidemic of Oroyo fever in the Peruvian Andes. Am J Trop Hyg 42:215, 1990.
Ricketts WE: Clinical manifestations of Carrion's disease. Arch Intern Med 84:751, 1949.

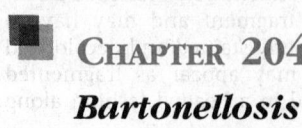

CHAPTER 205
Cat Scratch Disease

Andrew M. Margileth

Cat scratch disease (CSD) is a relatively common, self-limited, benign infectious disease that occurs in persons of all ages. It is the most common cause of chronic (≥3 wk) lymphadenopathy that usually develops following cat contact and/or a cat scratch in children and young adults.

ETIOLOGY. In 1988 English and associates isolated and cultured pleomorphic bacilli from lymph nodes obtained from 10 patients with CSD and fulfilled Koch's postulates. The vegetative form of the bacillus grew best at skin temperature and was found more often in inoculation lesions than in lymph nodes. In contrast, the cell-wall–defective form grew best at both skin and core body temperatures. In 1991, Brenner and colleagues cultured six species and proposed the genus *Afipia* on the basis of phenotypic characterization and DNA determinations. The genus name was derived from the abbreviation AFIP, for Armed Forces Institute of Pathology. All six *Afipia* species are gram negative, mobile, possess a single flagellum, and grow on buffered charcoal-yeast extract (BCYE) agar and in nutrient broth.

Two *Rochalimaea* species (*R. quintana* and *R. henselae*) were isolated from four human immunodeficiency virus (HIV)-infected patients with bacillary angiomatosis, an infectious disease causing proliferation of small blood vessels in the skin and visceral organs of immunocompromised patients. The bacillus is visualized in tissue sections by Warthin-Starry silver stain and is morphologically similar to *A. felis*. *Rochalimaea* infection appears to be another cause of CSD in HIV-infected patients. Two immunocompetent individuals whose involved lymph nodes yielded *R. henselae* on culture have also been reported.

Serologic evidence suggests that CSD is associated with infection caused by *Rochalimaea*, not *A. felis*. *R. henselae* has been isolated from cats and cat fleas and is a relatively common feline infection. Comparable data linking *A. felis* with a feline host are lacking. Samples of cat scratch skin–test antigen used for years in the diagnosis of cat-scratch disease contain *Rochalimaea* antigen (not *A. felis*). *Bartonella* is the new preferred nomenclature replacing the genus *Rochalimaea*. The genera *Bartonella* and *Rochalimaea* have been united.

EPIDEMIOLOGY. Cat scratch disease occurs worldwide and in all races. In temperate climates, 62–88% of cases occur from September through February. In warmer climates, cases occur frequently in July and August. About 55% of cases occur in males. Over 80% of patients are less than 21 yr of age. The incidence of patients discharged from hospitals with a diagnosis of cat scratch disease is 0.77–0.86 per 100,000 population per year. The estimated incidence of disease in ambulatory patients is 9.3 per 100,000 population per year. Family outbreaks, usually involving siblings, were found in 4.8% of 521 families. These families had one or more cats and almost always had a kitten. Cases in family units usually occur within a few weeks of each other, suggesting that the cat or kitten may transmit the organism for a limited period.

TRANSMISSION AND COMMUNICABILITY. Infection follows direct cat or dog contact. In over 2,000 patients, cat contact occurred in 95%, especially with kittens, and dog contact in 4%, whereas no history of animal contact occurred in 1%. Most animals implicated in cases of CSD are healthy and have negative CSD skin tests. The domestic cat is a major persistent reservoir for *R. henselae*. Animal scratches occur less often. About 76% of patients have a cat scratch, 2% a dog scratch or bite, and 22% have no history of an animal scratch. Rarely, CSD follows a scratch from a thorn or wood splinter, insect bites, or chickenpox. There is also an association between mucous membrane lesions, such as canker sores, and regional cervical lymphadenopathy. Human-to-human transmission is not reported.

PATHOLOGY. Biopsied lymph nodes exhibit a broad spectrum of histopathology: arteriolar proliferation with widening of anteriolar walls, reticulum cell hyperplasia, multiple microabscesses, frank abscess formation, and round or stellate granulomas. Except for the vascular changes, similar histopathologic findings are found in tularemia, brucellosis, tuberculosis, lymphogranuloma venereum, and the solid granulomas of sarcoidosis; reticulum cell hyperplasia with granulomas is suggestive of Hodgkin disease. Cat scratch bacilli are demonstrated best by the Warthin-Starry silver impregnation stain of lymph nodes removed during the first 4 wk of illness. In these nodes, bacteria are abundant in clumps or filaments, and are found most readily in vessel walls, collagen fibers, and microabscesses. The bacilli range in size from 0.2 to 0.3 nm to 0.5 to 1.5 nm in length. The bacilli may be seen in areas of necrosis (80%), and less often (40%) in association with giant cell granulomas. Similar bacteria were detected in the inoculation skin lesion of several patients meeting the criteria for CSD. In two of these patients, the same bacilli were identified in regional lymph nodes draining the lesion.

PATHOGENESIS. An atypical presentation occurs in 10–14% of patients with CSD (Table 205–1). Parinaud oculoglandular syndrome is the most common, followed by encephalopathy, severe, chronic systemic disease, and neuroretinitis. *A. felis* and *B. henselae* have low endotoxin potency and lower biologic oxidative metabolism compared with *Escherichia coli*, 0:111. These characteristics may explain the intracellular growth of these bacteria, their survival and eventual reproduction in phagocytic cells, and a possible mechanism for the variable severity of CSD.

CLINICAL MANIFESTATIONS. In spite of extensive lymphadenopathy, patients usually are not ill. Only one third of patients have fever greater than 101° F (38.3° C). Malaise, fever, fatigue, headache, and anorexia may occur in about 50% of patients. Less often, splenomegaly, sore throat, conjunctivitis, blindness, various rashes, and rarely, arthralgias and/or parotid swelling occur (Table 205–2). About 50% of children and adolescents have adenopathy only, whereas nearly 75% of adults develop some systemic signs or symptoms.

Inoculation Lesion. Sixty percent to 93% of patients with CSD develop a 3–5 mm inoculation lesion (vesicle or pustule that

TABLE 205–1 Clinical Features of Cat Scratch Disease

	1957–1993 No.	%
Typical presentation (lymphadenopathy)	1,723	86
Inoculation lesion (skin, eye, mucous membrane)	1,202	60
Unusual major manifestations	283	14
Parinaud oculoglandular syndrome	123	6
Encephalopathy (radiculopathy 14*)	47	2.3
Systemic disease, severe, chronic	43	2
Erythema nodosum	14	0.7
Neuroretinitis	30	1.5
Thrombocytopenic purpura	7	0.4
Hepatosplenomegaly	6	0.3
Primary atypical pneumonia	3	0.2
Breast tumor	3	0.2
Angiomatoid papules	2	0.1
Osteomyelitis	5	0.3
Total	2,006	100

*Complication in 14 with typical cat scratch disease. Mediastinal adenopathy—1.

■ TABLE 205–2 Clinical Features in Cat Scratch Disease

	1975–1993	
Symptoms and Signs	*Percent of Patients**	*Duration (Days)*
Adenopathy	100	14–730
Adenopathy only	49	14–730
Fever (38.3–41.2° C)	28.5	1–60
Malaise/fatigue	30	1–21
Headache	13	1–7
Anorexia, emesis	14	3–30
Splenomegaly	9.5	7–30
Sore throat	7	1–5
Exanthem	4.4	5–17
Blindness	1.7	30–200
Arthralgia	2.5†	3–42
Seizures/coma	2.8	1–5
Conjunctivitis	3.3	1–11

**A total of 1,656 patients were evaluated.*
†Data from 1989 through 1993.

evolves to a papule) 3–10 days after introduction of the organism into the skin. This lesion may persist for several days to several months. Careful examination of the skin, particularly of the upper extremities, head, and scalp, may reveal a lesion that had been overlooked or mistaken for an insect bite. In 5–10% of patients, the inoculation lesion manifests as a nonsuppurative conjunctivitis, an ocular granuloma, or both. Inoculation lesions are nonpruritic and heal without scar formation. Occasionally, a superficial ulcer of the oral mucous membranes precedes or is found at the onset of lymphadenopathy.

Lymphadenopathy. Regional lymphadenopathy with single or multiple nodes is a hallmark of CSD. Within 2 wk of the scratch (range, 7–60 days), enlarged tender lymph nodes appear proximal to the inoculation site. Because the upper extremities, head, and neck are the most likely locations for scratches, over 80% of the involved nodes are in the axillary, epitrochlear, cervical, and/or supraclavicular areas. Submandibular and preauricular lymphadenopathy also occurs and requires careful examination of the mucous membrane and ocular areas for a primary inoculation lesion. In about two thirds of patients, the adenopathy consists of a single or several nodes in one region; the other one third of patients have enlarged nodes in two or more anatomic sites. If adenopathy is detected in more than one area, a search should be made for additional inoculation lesions.

The majority of lymph nodes are 1–5 cm in diameter, but initially edema and swelling may extend 10–12 cm. During the first 2 wk of illness, the nodes are usually tender. Erythema of overlying skin may occur early in the disease and resolve as the node decreases in size. Cellulitis is observed rarely.

The lymphadenopathy usually regresses over 2–4 mo, but it persists for 1–3 yr in 1–2% of patients. Large lymph nodes with erythema and tenderness regress more slowly and tend to be suppurative. Approximately 15% of nodes suppurate.

Atypical CSD. From 9 to 14% of cases present with symptoms other than regional lymphadenopathy (Table 205–1).

Oculoglandular Syndrome. The most frequent of the atypical forms of CSD is Parinaud oculoglandular syndrome, which manifests as a conjunctival granuloma at the inoculation site and preauricular lymphadenopathy. The involved eye may reveal nonsuppurative conjunctivitis. Cat scratch bacilli have been found in the conjunctival granulomas using the Warthin-Starry silver stain. Spontaneous resolution of the lymphadenopathy usually occurs within 2–4 mo.

Neurologic Syndromes. Nervous system manifestations occur in about 2% of patients, including encephalopathy with coma and/or seizures, myelitis, radiculitis, polyneuritis, paraplegia, neuroretinitis, and cerebral arteritis. Neurologic symptoms usually follow the onset of lymphadenopathy by 1–6 wk and are characterized by a sudden change in mental status and seizures. Severe symptoms last 1–2 wk and recovery is complete. Rarely, patients with focal abnormalities noted by electroencephalogram or a computed tomography scan have recurrent seizures or persistent neurologic deficits. Cerebrospinal fluid may show pleocytosis, elevated protein, or both. Electroencephalograms are abnormal in most patients. *Afipia felis* was detected with use of the polymerase chain reaction (PCR) in a submandibular lymph node obtained from a 6-yr-old child with status epilepticus. Of 35 patients with neurologic disease and no encephalopathy, 2 children displayed cranial nerve palsies, 30 had neuroretinitis, and 3 had peripheral neuritis. Of 30 older children and young adults with neuroretinitis, 29 recovered their vision within several weeks to 12 mo. Treatment for encephalopathy includes control of convulsions and supportive measures. Commonly used antibiotics administered to many of the patients appeared to be ineffective.

Systemic Cat Scratch Disease. Systemic illness caused by CSD is associated with a longer duration of fever, malaise, fatigue, skin rashes, myalgias, and arthralgias. Other findings include generalized lymphadenopathy, larger lymph nodes, and weight loss greater than 5 lb. Some patients have pleurisy, arthralgia, or arthritis, splenic or liver abscesses, mediastinal masses, enlarged nodes at the head of the pancreas, and severe systemic disease with prolonged fevers lasting up to 60 days associated with weight loss of up to 40 lb. All patients recovered, although the severity of the disease was variable.

Granulomatous hepatitis is reported in some children with CSD. These patients often have high fever (40° C) for more than 3–4 wk, no peripheral lymphadenopathy, and organisms consistent with CSD bacillus in biopsies of the liver, spleen, mesenteric lymph nodes, and at times, peripheral lymph nodes. Antibiotic therapy may be helpful in these patients.

Hematologic manifestations of CSD include hemolytic anemia with hepatosplenomegaly, thrombocytopenic purpura, nonthrombocytopenic purpura, and eosinophilia. Other atypical and rare manifestations of CSD include osteolytic lesions, atypical pneumonia, recurrent CSD over 3–4 yr, breast tumor, and angiomatoid papules in both immunocompromised and immunocompetent patients.

CSD in Immunocompromised Hosts. CSD may be a severe illness in the immunocompromised patient. CSD may be missed or confused with other clinical manifestations related to human immunodeficiency virus (HIV). Although CSD has not been reported in children with HIV the syndrome in adults is characterized by unusual manifestations and, paradoxically, an excellent response to antibiotic therapy. These patients often present with numerous generalized skin lesions, ranging from pink to deep reddish-purple papules to sessile or pedunculated nodules. The nodules are firm, indurated, and usually nontender and range in size from 1 to 6 cm. Clinically, the lesions are indistinguishable from Kaposi sarcoma, histiocytoid hemangioma, epithelioid hemangioma, and/or pyogenic granuloma. Radiographs of lesions located over bone may show bone loss and periostosis, and a large, soft, tender mass.

DIAGNOSIS. The most important clues for diagnosis are the history of contact with animals, particularly kittens, and identification of an inoculation skin or ocular lesion. Regional lymphadenopathy developing several weeks after cat contact suggests CSD, especially if a primary inoculation papule or pustule occurs following a cat scratch. Criteria for a definitive diagnosis include: (1) contact with a cat, and the presence of a scratch or primary lesion of the dermis, eye, or a mucous membrane; (2) a positive skin test for CSD or positive serologic test for *B. henselae* antibody; (3) negative serologies, including purified protein derivative (PPD-T and PPD-Battey) skin tests and cultures of aspirated pus or lymph nodes performed for other causes of lymphadenopathy; and (4) characteristic histopathologic features in a biopsy specimen of skin, lymph node, or ocular granuloma. In clinical practice, the diagnosis can be made when three of these four criteria are met.

The diagnosis can be confirmed in atypical cases of CSD by a fourfold rise in titer for *B. henselae* or by demonstrating small, pleomorphic bacilli in Warthin-Starry stained sections of lymph nodes, skin, or conjunctiva. Biopsies are recommended only when the disease is atypical. Generally, the diagnosis can be made on the basis of history of cat or kitten exposure, clinical findings, exclusion of the other causes of lymphadenopathy, and observation until resolution. A cat scratch skin test is not always required.

A biopsy must be considered to rule out malignancy if a cat scratch antigen skin test and/or a test for antibodies to *B. henselae* is negative. Ultrasonography may be useful for identifying and aspirating cervical abscesses, and may detect liver or spleen defects in patients with systemic CSD.

Cat Scratch Skin Test. The skin-test antigen (0.1 mL) should be injected intradermally on the flexor (volar) surface of the arm, and the site should be circled. The exact extent of induration is delineated after 72–96 hr by drawing a ballpoint pen held perpendicular with firm pressure toward the area of induration. After several strokes of the pen in each of four quadrants, the maximum amount of induration can be measured accurately. A positive reaction requires induration of 5 mm or more. Rarely, patients with negative skin tests at 48–72 hr may have a positive test 7–10 days post-test. CSD antigen for diagnosis is available from the author on written request.

LABORATORY. A mild to moderate leukocytosis may occur for several days at the onset of the illness; eosinophilia has been reported. The erythrocyte sedimentation rate usually is elevated during the first few weeks of adenopathy. Diagnostic serologic tests for CSD are commercially available, including an indirect immunofluorescent antibody (IFA) test for genus-specific antibodies to *Bartonella* antigens. PCR analysis of cat scratch skin test antigen identified *Bartonella* nucleic acid sequences in samples. Computed tomographic scan or magnetic resonance imaging is useful in patients with atypical CSD and hepatic or splenic granulomatous or nodular microabscesses.

DIFFERENTIAL DIAGNOSIS. Bacterial adenitis commonly is caused by group A B-hemolytic streptococci and *Staphylococcus aureus*, and less often by anaerobic bacteria, atypical and typical mycobacteria, and rarely, *Francisella tularensis* or *Brucella* species. Cytomegalovirus, Epstein-Barr virus, HIV, *Toxoplasma*, or fungi usually produce lymphadenopathy in two or more anatomic sites. A cystic hygroma or bronchogenic cyst should be considered in the differential diagnosis in children and adolescents. Neoplastic disease occurs more often in adolescents and adults.

Parinaud oculoglandular syndrome may be associated with chlamydial infection, tularemia, tuberculosis, or syphilis. The differential diagnosis of persistent skin papules or nodules with regional adenopathy includes sarcoidosis, infection with typical or atypical mycobacteria or fungi, syphilis, and leishmaniasis.

PREVENTION. The patient with CSD does not require isolation or quarantine. The disease cannot be spread directly from one person to another. Because the animals involved are invariable healthy, disposing of the cat or dog is not recommended. About 5% of family members develop CSD within a 2–3 wk period of each other. Because 46% of American households have a cat and there are approximately 65 million cats in the United States, CSD is difficult to prevent. The most common pitfall in the diagnosis of CSD is failure to inquire about animal contact or scratches, especially by a cat or dog.

TREATMENT. No antimicrobial therapy is required in the majority of cases, because the adenopathy subsides spontaneously within 2–4 mo. Bed rest is rarely required, but it may lessen extreme fatigue. The patient should avoid trauma to the involved nodes or enlarged spleen. Local application of moist saline compresses for 3–5 days continuously to the swollen nodes may reduce pain and decrease swelling.

Fever (>38.3° C) occurs in only one third of patients with CSD. Antipyretics and analgesics such as aspirin or acetaminophen are advised for tender adenitis. Incision and drainage is not recommended if suppuration occurs (15%) because a chronic sinus tract may develop and persist for several months. Needle aspiration relieves painful adenopathy and provides material for culture. Surgical excision of nodes usually is not indicated unless a noninfectious etiology, such as a neoplasm or cyst, is suspected. Close follow-up for several months to assess resolution of adenopathy is recommended.

Systemic Antibiotics. *A. felis* is resistant to a broad array of antimicrobials but susceptible in vitro to ceftriaxone, cefotaxime, and cefoxitin as well as amikacin sulfate, gentamicin, tobramycin, ciprofloxacin, and imipenem/cilastatin. Oral trimethoprim (TMP)/sulfamethoxazole 2 or 3 times daily (10–20 mg TMP/kg/24 hr) for 7 days is effective therapy in more than 50% of patients. Rifampin (15–20 mg/kg/24 hr PO 2 or 3 times daily; maximum dose: 600 mg/24 hr) for 7–14 days is very effective. Children over 12 years of age can be treated with ciprofloxacin in two daily doses (20–30 mg/kg/24 hr PO) for 7–14 days. In the rare, severely ill patient, parenteral gentamicin sulfate, 5 mg/kg/24 hr given every 8 hr IM, is quite effective, usually within 72 hr. Paradoxically, *Bartonella* species usually respond to a prolonged course of commonly used antibiotics given for several weeks or months in immunocompromised patients.

PROGNOSIS. The prognosis for CSD is excellent. Lymphadenopathy regresses spontaneously in 2–6 mo in 96% of patients but may take 1–3 yr in 1–2% of patients. Overt disease appears to confer lifelong immunity in most patients, although recurrence of lymphadenopathy 6–13 mo after initial disease may occur.

Fatal complications and irreversible sequelae are not documented. Patients with encephalopathy or encephalitis have recovered completely, and those with radiculopathy, neuroretinitis, or both have recovered completely or with minimal decreased visual acuity during several to 12 mo.

Adal KA, Cockerell CJ, Petri WA: Cat scratch disease, bacillary angiomatosis, and other infections due to *Rochalimaea*. N Engl J Med 330:1509, 1994.

Fumarola D, Guiliani G, Petruzzelli R, et al: Pathogenicity of cat-scratch disease bacilli. Pediatr Infect Dis J 13:162, 1994.

Golden SE: Hepatosplenic cat-scratch disease associated with elevated anti-*Rochalimaea* antibody titers. Pediatr Infect Dis J 12:868, 1993.

Koehler JE, Glaser CA, Tappero JW: *Rochalimaea henselae* infection: A new zoonosis with the domestic cat as a reservoir. JAMA 271:531, 1994.

Margileth AM: Antibiotic therapy for cat-scratch disease: Clinical study of therapeutic outcome in 268 patients and review of literature. Pediatr Infect Dis J 11:474, 1992.

Margileth AM: Cat-scratch disease. Adv Pediatr Infect Dis 8:1, 1993.

Margileth AM, Hayden GF: Cat-scratch disease: From feline affection to human infection. N Engl J Med 329:53, 1993.

Malatack JJ, Jaffe R: Granulomatous hepatitis in three children due to cat-scratch disease without peripheral adenopathy. Am J Dis Child 147:949, 1993.

Regnery RL: Cat-scratch disease: An update of the case for a *Rochalimaea* etiology. Infect Med 10:44, 1993.

Waldvogel K: Disseminated cat-scratch disease: Detection of *Rochalimaea henselae* in affected tissue. Eur J Pediatr 153:23, 1994.

Wong MT, Dolan MJ, Lattwada CP et al: Neuroretinitis, aseptic meningitis, and lymphadenitis in immunocompetent and HIV-infected patients. Clin Infect Dis (in press).

SECTION 4
Viral Infections

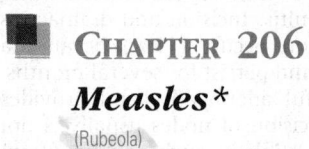

CHAPTER 206
Measles*
(Rubeola)

Yvonne Maldonado

Measles, an acute communicable disease, is characterized by three stages: (1) an incubation stage of approximately 10–12 days with few, if any, signs or symptoms; (2) a prodromal stage with an enanthem (Koplik spots) on the buccal and pharyngeal mucosa, slight to moderate fever, mild conjunctivitis, coryza, and an increasingly severe cough; and (3) a final stage with a maculopapular rash erupting successively over the neck and face, body, arms, and legs and accompanied by high fever.

ETIOLOGY. Measles is an RNA virus of the family Paramyxoviridae, genus *Morbillivirus.* Only one antigenic type is known. During the prodromal period and for a short time after the rash appears, it is found in nasopharyngeal secretions, blood, and urine. It can remain active for at least 34 hr at room temperature.

Measles virus may be isolated in cultures of human embryonic or rhesus monkey kidney tissue. Cytopathic changes, visible in 5–10 days, consist of multinucleated giant cells with intranuclear inclusions. Circulating antibody is detectable when the rash appears.

INFECTIVITY. Maximal dissemination of virus is by droplet spray during the prodromal period (catarrhal stage). Transmission to susceptible contacts often occurs prior to diagnosis of the original case. An infected person becomes contagious by the 9th–10th day after exposure (beginning of prodromal phase), in some instances as early as the 7th day. Isolation precautions, especially in hospitals or other institutions, should be maintained from the 7th day after exposure until 5 days after the rash has appeared.

EPIDEMIOLOGY. Measles is endemic over most of the world. In the past, epidemics tended to occur irregularly, appearing in the spring in large cities at 2- to 4-yr intervals as new groups of susceptible children were exposed. Measles is very contagious; approximately 90% of susceptible family contacts acquire the disease. It is rarely subclinical. Prior to the use of measles vaccine, the age of peak incidence was 5–10 yr; most adults were immune. At present in the United States, measles occurs most often in unimmunized preschool-aged children and in teenagers and young adults who have been immunized. Epidemics have occurred in high schools and colleges where immunization levels were high. These epidemics are thought to be due primarily to vaccine failure. Despite a resurgence of measles in the United States from 1989–1991, reported numbers of measles cases dropped to an all-time low in 1993, probably a result of widespread vaccination. Those older than 30 years are virtually all immune. Because measles is still a common disease in many countries, infective persons entering this country may infect United States citizens, and Americans traveling abroad risk exposure there.

The many similarities among the biologic features of measles and smallpox suggest the possibility that measles may be eradicable. These features are (1) a distinctive rash, (2) no animal reservoir, (3) no vector, (4) seasonal occurrence with disease-free periods, (5) no transmissible latent virus, (6) one serotype, and (7) an effective vaccine. A prevalence of more than 90% immunization of infants has been shown to produce disease-free zones. In 1980, three fourths of all counties in the United States did not report a single case of measles, but by 1988 the number of measles cases was increasing and the disease was more widespread.

Infants transplacentally acquire immunity from mothers who have had measles or measles immunization. This immunity is usually complete for the first 4–6 mo of life and disappears at a variable rate. Although maternal antibody levels are generally undetectable in the infant by the usual tests performed after 9 mo of age, some protection persists, which may interfere with immunization administered prior to 15 mo. Most women of child-bearing age in the United States now have measles immunity by means of immunization rather than disease. Some studies now suggest that infants of mothers with measles vaccine–induced immunity lose passive antibody at a younger age than infants of mothers who had measles infection. Infants of mothers susceptible to measles have no measles immunity and may contract the disease with the mother before or after delivery.

PATHOLOGY. The essential lesion of measles is found in the skin; in the mucous membranes of the nasopharynx, bronchi, and intestinal tract; and in the conjunctivae. Serous exudate and proliferation of mononuclear cells and a few polymorphonuclear cells occur around the capillaries. There is usually hyperplasia of lymphoid tissue, particularly in the appendix, where multinucleated giant cells of up to 100 μm in diameter (Warthin-Finkeldey reticuloendothelial giant cells) may be found. In the skin, the reaction is particularly notable about the sebaceous glands and hair follicles. Koplik spots consist of serous exudate and proliferation of endothelial cells similar to those in the skin lesions. A general inflammatory reaction of the buccal and pharyngeal mucosa extends into the lymphoid tissue and the tracheobronchial mucous membrane. Interstitial pneumonitis resulting from measles virus takes the form of Hecht giant cell pneumonia. Bronchopneumonia may be due to secondary bacterial infection.

In fatal cases of encephalomyelitis, perivascular demyelinization occurs in areas of the brain and spinal cord. In Dawson subacute sclerosing panencephalitis (SSPE), there may be degeneration of the cortex and white matter with intranuclear and intracytoplasmic inclusion bodies (see Chapter 552.5).

CLINICAL MANIFESTATIONS. The *incubation period* is approximately 10–12 days if the first prodromal symptoms are selected as the time of onset, or approximately 14 days if the appearance of the rash is selected; rarely it may be as short as 6–10 days. A slight rise in temperature may occur 9–10 days from the date of infection and then subside for 24 hr or so.

The *prodromal phase,* which follows, usually lasts 3–5 days and is characterized by low-grade to moderate fever, a hacking cough, coryza, and conjunctivitis. These nearly always precede Koplik spots, the pathognomonic sign of measles, by 2–3 days. An enanthem or red mottling is usually present on the hard and soft palates. Koplik spots are grayish white dots, usually as small as grains of sand, with slight, reddish areolae; occa-

*As modified from the section in the 14th edition by C. Phillips.

sionally they are hemorrhagic. They tend to occur opposite the lower molars but may spread irregularly over the rest of the buccal mucosa. Rarely they are found within the midportion of the lower lip, on the palate, and on the lacrimal caruncle. They appear and disappear rapidly, usually within 12–18 hr. As they fade, red, spotty discolorations of the mucosa may remain. The conjunctival inflammation and photophobia may suggest measles before Koplik spots appear. In particular, a transverse line of conjunctival inflammation, sharply demarcated along the eyelid margin, may be of diagnostic assistance in the prodromal stage. As the entire conjunctiva becomes involved, the line disappears.

Occasionally, the prodromal phase may be severe, being ushered in by sudden high fever, at times with convulsions and even pneumonia. Usually the coryza, fever, and cough are increasingly severe up to the time the rash has covered the body.

The temperature rises abruptly *as the rash appears* and often reaches 40–40.5° C (104–105° F). In uncomplicated cases, when the rash appears on the legs and feet, within about 2 days, the symptoms subside rapidly; the subsidence includes a usually abrupt temperature drop. Patients up to this point may appear desperately ill, but within 24 hr after the temperature drop, they appear essentially well.

The rash usually starts as faint macules on the upper lateral parts of the neck, behind the ears, along the hairline, and on the posterior parts of the cheek. The individual lesions become increasingly maculopapular as the rash spreads rapidly over the entire face, neck, upper arms, and upper part of the chest within approximately the first 24 hr (Fig. 206–1 [color plate section]). During the succeeding 24 hr it spreads over the back, abdomen, entire arms, and thighs. As it finally reaches the feet on the 2nd–3rd day, it begins to fade on the face. The fading of the rash proceeds downward in the same sequence in which it appeared. The severity of the disease is directly related to the extent and confluence of the rash. In mild measles the rash tends not to be confluent, and in very mild cases there are few, if any, lesions on the legs. In severe measles the rash is confluent, the skin being completely covered, including the palms and soles, and the face is swollen and disfigured.

The rash is often slightly hemorrhagic; in severe cases with a confluent rash, petechiae may be present in large numbers, and there may be extensive ecchymoses. Itching is generally slight. As the rash fades, branny desquamation and brownish discoloration occur and then disappear within 7–10 days.

The rash may vary markedly. Infrequently a slight urticarial, faint macular, or scarlatiniform rash may appear during the early prodromal stage and disappear in advance of the typical rash. Complete absence of rash is rare except in patients who have received human antibodies during the incubation period, in some patients with human immunodeficiency syndrome (HIV) infection, and possibly in infants younger than 8 mo who have appreciable levels of maternal antibody. In the hemorrhagic type of measles (black measles), bleeding may occur

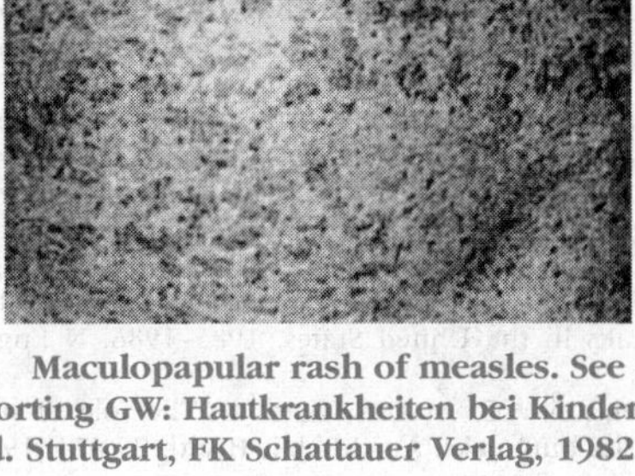

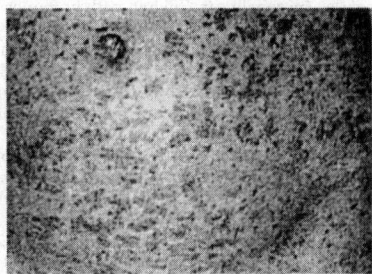

Figure 206–1. Maculopapular rash of measles. See also color section. (From Korting GW: Hautkrankheiten bei Kindern und Jugendlichen, 3rd ed. Stuttgart, FK Schattauer Verlag, 1982.)

from the mouth, nose, or bowel. In mild cases the rash may be less macular and more nearly pinpoint, somewhat resembling that of scarlet fever or rubella.

Lymph nodes at the angle of the jaw and in the posterior cervical region are usually enlarged, and slight splenomegaly may be noted. Mesenteric lymphadenopathy may cause abdominal pain. Characteristic pathologic changes of measles in the mucosa of the appendix may cause obliteration of the lumen and symptoms of appendicitis. Changes of this type tend to subside with the disappearance of Koplik spots. Otitis media, bronchopneumonia, and gastrointestinal symptoms, such as diarrhea and vomiting, are more common in infants and small children (especially malnourished ones) than in older children.

The diagnosis of measles is frequently delayed in adults because practitioners providing health care for adults are not used to encountering the disease and rarely include it in the differential diagnosis. The clinical picture is similar to that seen in children. Liver involvement, with abdominal pain, mild to moderate elevation of aspartate aminotransferase (AST) levels, and occasionally jaundice, is common in adults. In developing countries and in recent outbreaks in the United States, measles frequently occurs in infants younger than 1 yr; possibly because malnutrition is concomitant there, the disease is very severe and has a high mortality.

DIAGNOSIS. This is usually made from the typical clinical picture; laboratory confirmation is rarely needed. During the prodromal stage multinucleated giant cells can be demonstrated in smears of the nasal mucosa. Virus can be isolated in tissue culture, and diagnostic rises in antibody titer can be detected between acute and convalescent sera. The white blood cell count tends to be low with a relative lymphocytosis. Lumbar puncture in patients with measles encephalitis usually shows an increase in protein and a small increase in lymphocytes. The glucose level is normal.

DIFFERENTIAL DIAGNOSIS. The rash of rubeola must be differentiated from exanthem subitum, rubella, infections resulting from echovirus, coxsackie virus, and adenovirus, infectious mononucleosis, toxoplasmosis, meningococcemia, scarlet fever, rickettsial diseases, serum sickness, Kawasaki disease, and drug rashes.

Koplik spots are pathognomonic for rubeola, and the diagnosis of unmodified measles should not be made in the absence of cough.

Roseola infantum (exanthem subitum) is distinguished from measles in that the rash of the former appears as the fever disappears. The rashes of rubella and of enteroviral infections tend to be less striking than that of measles, as do the degree of fever and severity of illness. Although cough is present in many rickettsial infections, the rash usually spares the face, which is characteristically involved in measles. The absence of cough or the history of injection of serum or administration of a drug usually serves to identify serum sickness or drug rashes. Meningococcemia may be accompanied by a rash that is somewhat similar to that of measles, but cough and conjunctivitis are usually absent. In acute meningococcemia the rash is characteristically petechial purpuric. The diffuse, finely papular rash of scarlet fever with a "goose flesh" texture on an erythematous base is relatively easy to differentiate.

The milder rash and clinical picture of measles modified by gamma globulin or by partial immunity induced by measles vaccine, or in infants by maternal antibody, may be difficult to differentiate.

COMPLICATIONS. The chief complications of measles are otitis media, pneumonia, and encephalitis. Noma of the cheeks may occur in rare instances. Gangrene elsewhere appears to be secondary to purpura fulminans or disseminated intravascular coagulation following measles.

Pneumonia (see Chapter 170) may be caused by the measles virus itself; the lesion is interstitial. Measles pneumonia in patients with HIV infection is often fatal and not always accompanied by rash. Bronchopneumonia is more frequent, however; it is due to secondarily invading bacteria, particularly the pneumococcus, streptococcus, staphylococcus, and *Haemophilus influenzae*. Laryngitis, tracheitis, and bronchitis are common and may be due to the virus alone.

One of the potential dangers of measles is exacerbation of an existing *tuberculous process*. There may also be a temporary loss of hypersensitivity to tuberculin.

Myocarditis is an infrequent serious complication; transient electrocardiographic changes are said to be relatively common.

Neurologic complications are more common in measles than in any of the other exanthems. The incidence of *encephalomyelitis* is estimated to be 1-2/1,000 reported cases of measles. There is no correlation between the severity of the measles and that of the neurologic involvement or between the severity of the initial encephalitic process and the prognosis. Rarely, encephalitis has been reported in association with measles modified by gamma globulin or by live attenuated measles virus vaccine. Infrequently, encephalitic involvement is manifest in the preeruptive period, but more often the onset occurs 2–5 days after the appearance of the rash. The cause of measles encephalitis remains controversial. It is suggested that when encephalitis occurs early in the course of the disease, viral invasion plays a large role, although measles virus has rarely been isolated from brain tissue; encephalitis that occurs later is predominantly demyelinating and may reflect an immunologic reaction. In this demyelinating type the symptoms and course do not differ from those of other parainfectious encephalitides. Fatal encephalitis has occurred in children receiving immunosuppressive treatment for malignancies. Other central nervous system complications, such as Guillain-Barré syndrome, hemiplegia, cerebral thrombophlebitis, and retrobulbar neuritis, are rare.

Subacute sclerosing panencephalitis (see Chapter 552.5) is due to measles virus.

PROGNOSIS. Case fatality rates in the United States have decreased in recent years to low levels for all age groups, largely because of improved socioeconomic conditions but also because of effective antibacterial therapy for the treatment of secondary infections.

When measles is introduced into a highly susceptible population, the results may be disastrous. Such an occurrence in the Faroe Islands in 1846 resulted in the deaths of about one fourth, nearly 2,000, of the total population regardless of age. At Ungava Bay, Canada, where 99% of 900 persons had measles, the mortality rate was 7%.

PROPHYLAXIS. Quarantine is of little value because of the contagiousness during its prodromal stage, when measles may not be suspected.

Active Immunization. See also Chapter 247.

The initial measles immunization may be given at 12 to 15 mo but may be given earlier in areas where disease is occurring. Because the seroconversion rate following immunization is not 100% and there may be some waning of immunity with time, a second immunization against measles, usually given as measles-mumps-rubella (MMR), is indicated. This dose can be given when the child enters school or later on entry to middle school. Adolescents entering college should also have received a second measles immunization.

The response to live measles vaccine is unpredictable if immune globulin has been administered in the 3 mo preceding immunization. Anergy to tuberculin may develop and persist for 1 mo or longer after administration of live, attenuated measles vaccine. A child with active tuberculous infection should be receiving antituberculosis treatment when live measles vaccine is administered. A tuberculin test prior to or concurrent with active immunization against measles is desirable.

Use of live measles vaccine is not recommended for pregnant women or for children with untreated tuberculosis. Live vaccine is contraindicated in children with leukemia and in those receiving immunosuppressive drugs because of the risk of persistent, progressive infection such as giant cell pneumonia. After exposure of these susceptible children to measles, measles immune globulin (human) should be given intramuscularly in a dose of 0.25 mL/kg as soon as possible. A larger dose may be advisable in children with acute leukemia, even those in remission. Children with HIV infection should receive measles vaccine because mortality from measles is high in this group and they tolerate the vaccine well. Despite a history of having received measles immunization, these children should receive gamma globulin after exposure to measles in a dose of 0.5 mL/kg (maximum 15 mL). This is twice the usual recommended dose. Measles vaccine can be given following exposure to the disease. Reactions are not increased, and measles may be prevented.

The use of inactivated (killed) virus vaccine is not recommended.

Passive Immunization. Passive immunization with pooled adult serum, pooled convalescent serum, placental globulin, or gamma globulin of pooled plasma is effective for prevention and attenuation of measles. Measles can be prevented by using immune serum globulin (gamma globulin) in a dose of 0.25 mL/kg given intramuscularly within 5 days after exposure but preferably as soon as possible. Complete protection is indicated for infants, for children with chronic illness, and for contacts in hospital wards and children's institutions. Attenuation may be accomplished by the use of gamma globulin in a dosage of 0.05 mL/kg. Gamma globulin is approximately 25 times as potent in antibody titer as pooled adult serum, and it avoids the risk of hepatitis. Attenuation is variable, and the modified clinical patterns may vary from those with few or no symptoms to those with little or no modification. Encephalitis may follow measles modified by gamma globulin.

After the 7th–8th day of incubation the amounts of antibody administered must be increased greatly for any degree of protection. If the injection is delayed until the 9th, 10th, or 11th day, slight fever may already have started and only slight modification of the disease may be expected.

TREATMENT. Sedatives, antipyretics for high fever, bed rest, and an adequate fluid intake may be indicated. Humidification of the room may be necessary for laryngitis or an excessively irritating cough, and it is best to keep the room comfortably warm rather than cool. The patient should be protected from being exposed to strong light during the period of photophobia. The complications of otitis media and pneumonia require appropriate antimicrobial therapy.

With complications such as encephalitis, subacute sclerosing panencephalitis (see Chapter 552.5), giant cell pneumonia, and disseminated intravascular coagulation, each case must be assessed individually. Good supportive care is essential. Gamma globulin, hyperimmune gamma globulin, and steroids are of limited value. Currently available antiviral compounds are not effective. Treatment with oral vitamin A (400,000 IU) reduces morbidity and mortality in children with severe measles in the developing world.

Aicardi J: Acute measles encephalitis in children with immunosuppression. Pediatrics 59:232, 1977.
Brem J: Koplik spots for the record: An illustrated historical note. Clin Pediatr 11:161, 1972.
Centers for Disease Control and Prevention. Reported vaccine - preventable diseases.—United States, 1993, and the Childhood Immunization Intiative. MMWR 43:57, 1994.
Gustafson TL, Brunell PA, Lievens, AW, et al: Measles outbreak in a "fully immunized" secondary school population. N Engl J Med 316:771, 1987.
Hussey G, Klein M: A randomized trial of vitamin A in children with severe measles. N Engl J Med 323:160, 1990.
Jabbour JT, et al: Subacute sclerosing panencephalitis. JAMA 220:959, 1972.
Markowitz LE, Preblud SR, Orenstein WA, et al: Patterns of transmission in measles outbreaks in the United States, 1985–1986. N Engl J Med 320:75, 1989.
Mathias RG, Meeklson WG, Arcand TA, et al: The role of secondary vaccine failures in measles outbreaks. Am J Public Health 79:474, 1989.

McLaughlin M, Thomas P, Onorato I, et al: Live virus vaccines in human immunodeficiency virus-infected children: A retrospective study. Pediatrics 82:229, 1988.
Modlin JF: Epidemiologic studies of measles, measles vaccine, SSPE. Pediatrics 59:505, 1977.
Payne FE, Baublis JV, Itabashi HH: Isolation of measles virus from cell cultures of brain from a patient with subacute sclerosing panencephalitis. N Engl J Med 281:11, 1969.
Ruuskanen O, Salmi TT, Halonen P: Measles vaccination after exposure to natural measles. J Pediatr 98:43, 1978.
Starr S, Berkovich S: The effect of measles, gamma globulin modified measles and attenuated measles vaccine on the course of treated tuberculosis in children. Pediatrics 35:97, 1965.

CHAPTER 207

Rubella*

(German or Three-Day Measles)

Yvonne Maldonado

Rubella is a common communicable disease of childhood characterized ordinarily by mild constitutional symptoms, a rash similar to that of mild rubeola or scarlet fever, and enlargement and tenderness of the postoccipital, retroauricular, and posterior cervical lymph nodes. In older children and adults, especially adult women, the infection may occasionally be severe, with manifestations such as joint involvement and purpura.

Rubella in early pregnancy may cause severe congenital anomalies. The congenital rubella syndrome is an active contagious disease with multisystem involvement, a wide spectrum of clinical expression, and a long postnatal period of active infection with shedding of virus (Chapter 94).

ETIOLOGY. Rubella is caused by a pleomorphic, RNA-containing virus currently listed in the family Togaviridae, genus *Rubivirus.* The virus is usually isolated in tissue culture, and its presence is demonstrated by the ability of rubella-infected African green monkey kidney (AGMK) cells to resist challenge with enterovirus. During clinical illness the virus is present in nasopharyngeal secretions, blood, feces, and urine. Virus has been recovered from the nasopharynx 7 days before exanthem and 7–8 days after its disappearance. Patients with subclinical disease are also infectious.

EPIDEMIOLOGY. Humans are the only natural host of rubella virus, which is spread by oral droplet or transplacentally through congenital infection. Prior to institution of the rubella vaccine program in 1969, the peak incidence of the disease was in children 5–14 yr of age. Now most cases occur in susceptible teenagers and young adults. Large outbreaks have been reported among college students and in unvaccinated populations, such as Amish communities. Hospital epidemics among employees, with transmission to susceptible patients, have prompted hospitals to require that employees having contact with patients be immune to rubella. Health care personnel in physicians' offices should also be screened for rubella antibody and, if necessary, immunized. Maternal antibody is protective for the first 6 mo of life. Boys and girls are equally affected. In closed populations, such as institutions and military barracks, almost 100% of susceptible individuals may become infected. In family settings the spread of the virus is less: 50–60% of susceptible family members acquire the disease. Many infections are subclinical, with a ratio of 2:1 inapparent to overt disease. Rubella usually occurs during the spring. It can be difficult to diagnose clinically because enteroviral and other rashes may produce a similar appearance. A single attack usually confers permanent immunity. Epidemics occurred every 6–9 yr before vaccine was available. Serologic studies prior to the use of rubella vaccine showed that about 80% of adult populations in the United States and other continents had antibody to rubella. In island populations, such as those of Trinidad and Hawaii, only 20% of adults screened had detectable antibody.

The epidemiology of the congenital rubella syndrome is discussed in Chapters 96 and 97. Infants with rubella are a source of infection for older children who are not immune and for nonimmune adults, including pregnant women and nursery personnel.

CLINICAL MANIFESTATIONS. The incubation period is 14–21 days. The prodromal phase of mild catarrhal symptoms is shorter than that of measles and may be so mild as to go unnoticed. The most characteristic sign is retroauricular, posterior cervical, and postoccipital adenopathy. No other disease causes the tender enlargement of these nodes to the extent that rubella does. An enanthem may appear just before the onset of the skin rash. It consists of discrete rose spots on the soft palate that may coalesce into a red blush and extend over the fauces.

Lymphadenopathy is evident at least 24 hr before the *rash* appears and may remain for 1 wk or more. The exanthem is more variable than that of rubeola. It begins on the face (Fig. 207–1 [color plate section]) and spreads quickly. Its evolution is so rapid that the rash may be fading on the face by the time it appears on the trunk. Discrete maculopapules are present in large numbers; there are also large areas of flushing which spread rapidly over the entire body, usually within 24 hr. The rash may be confluent, particularly on the face. During the 2nd day the rash may assume a pinpoint appearance, especially over the trunk, resembling that of scarlet fever. Mild itching may occur. The eruption usually clears by the 3rd day. Desquamation is minimal. Rubella without a rash has been described.

The pharyngeal mucosa and the conjunctivae are slightly inflamed. In contrast to rubeola, there is no photophobia. Fever is slight or absent during the rash and persists for 1, 2, or occasionally 3 days. The temperature seldom exceeds 38.4° C (101° F). Anorexia, headache, and malaise are not common. The spleen is often slightly enlarged. The white blood cell

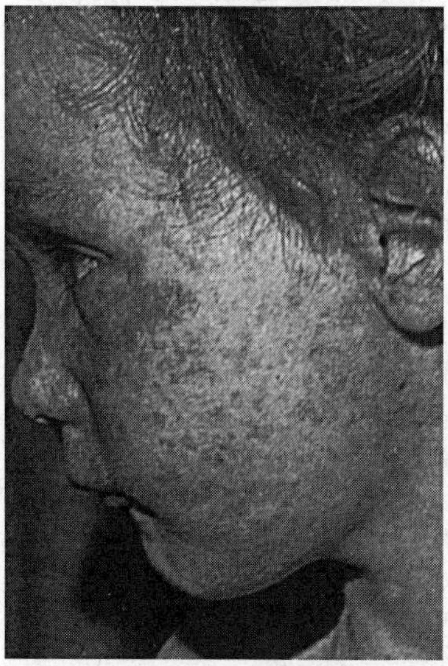

Figure 207–1. Rash of rubella (German measles). See also color section. (From Korting GW. Hautkrankheiten bei Kindern und Jugendlichen, 3rd ed. Stuttgart, Germany, FK Schattauer Verlag, 1982.)

*As modified from the section in the 14th edition by C. Phillips.

count is normal or slightly reduced; thrombocytopenia is rare, with or without purpura. Especially in older girls and women, polyarthritis may occur with arthralgia, swelling, tenderness, and effusion but usually without any residuum. Any joint may be involved, but the small joints of the hands are affected most frequently. The duration is usually several days to 2 wk; rarely it persists for months. Paresthesia also has been reported. In one epidemic, orchidalgia was reported in about 8% of infected college-aged males.

The congenital rubella syndrome is discussed in Chapter 97.5.

DIFFERENTIAL DIAGNOSIS. Because similar symptoms and rashes can occur with many other viral infections, rubella is a difficult disease to diagnose clinically except when the patient is seen during an epidemic. A history of having had rubella or rubella vaccine is unreliable; immunity should be determined by testing for antibodies. Particularly in its more severe forms, rubella may be confused with the mild types of scarlet fever and rubeola. *Roseola infantum* (exanthem subitum) is distinguished from rubella by the severity of the fever and by the appearance of the rash at the end of the febrile episode rather than at the height of the signs and symptoms. *Drug rashes* may be extremely difficult to differentiate from rubella. The characteristic enlargement of the lymph nodes strongly supports a diagnosis of rubella. In *infectious mononucleosis* a rash may occur that resembles that of rubella, and enlargement of the lymph nodes in each disease may lead to confusion. The hematologic findings in infectious mononucleosis should be sufficient to distinguish the two diseases. Enteroviral infections accompanied by a rash can be differentiated in *some* instances by respiratory or gastrointestinal manifestations and the absence of retroauricular adenopathy.

Diagnostic tests include isolation of virus from various tissues and serologic tests. Hemagglutination-inhibition (HI) antibody has been the usual method of determining immunity to rubella. Several newer tests including latex agglutination, enzyme immunoassay, passive hemagglutination, and fluorescent immunoassay appear to be equal or superior to the HI test in sensitivity. Rubella-specific immunoglobulin (Ig) M can be present in the blood of affected newborn infants.

COMPLICATIONS AND PROGNOSIS. Complications are relatively uncommon in childhood. Neuritis and arthritis occur occasionally. Resistance to secondary bacterial infection is not altered significantly. Encephalitis similar to that seen with rubeola occurs in about 1/6,000 cases. The prognosis of childhood rubella is good; that of congenital rubella varies with the severity of the infection (Chapter 97.5). Only about 30% of infants with encephalitis appear to escape residual neuromotor deficits, including an autistic syndrome.

PREVENTION. In a susceptible person, passive protection from or attenuation of the disease may be variably afforded by intramuscular injection of immune serum globulin (ISG) given in large dosage (0.25–0.50 mL/kg or 0.12–0.20 mL/lb) within the first 7–8 days after exposure. The effectiveness of immune globulin is not predictable. It apparently depends upon the antibody content of the product used and upon unknown factors. The value of ISG has been questioned also because in some instances rash was prevented and clinical manifestations were absent or minimal though viable virus was demonstrable in the blood. This form of prevention of rubella is not indicated, except in nonimmune pregnant women.

Since 1979 live-virus vaccine RA 27/3 (human embryonic lung fibroblasts of the WI-38 line) has been used exclusively for active immunization against rubella in the United States. RA 27/3 vaccine has many advantages over other rubella vaccines used in the past because it produces nasopharyngeal antibody and a wide variety of serum antibodies, provides better protection against reinfection, and more closely resembles the protection provided by natural infection. The vaccine virus is heat and light sensitive; therefore, the vaccine should be stored in the refrigerator at 4° C and used as soon as it is reconstituted. Vaccine is administered as a single subcutaneous injection. See Chapter 247 for routine immunization.

Antibody develops in about 98% of those vaccinated. Although virus may persist, especially in the nasopharynx, and shedding occurs from 18–25 days after vaccination, communicability does not appear to be a problem.

The duration of persistence of rubella antibody following vaccination with RA 27/3 is uncertain but is probably lifelong. Preventive measures are of the greatest importance for the protection of the fetus. It is especially important that girls have immunity to rubella before reaching child-bearing age, either by contracting the natural disease or by active immunization. The immune status can be evaluated by appropriate serologic tests.

The rubella vaccine program in the United States calls for immunization of all boys and girls between the ages of 12 and 15 mo and puberty and of nonpregnant postpubertal females. Immunization is effective at 12 mo of age but may be delayed until 15 mo and given as measles-mump-rubella (MMR) vaccine. Rubella immunization should be offered to potentially susceptible postpubertal women at any health care visit. For women who say they might be pregnant immunization should be deferred. Pregnancy testing is not routinely necessary, but counseling about the advisability of avoiding pregnancy for 3 mo after immunization should be provided. The current immunization policy has successfully interrupted the usual epidemic cycle of rubella in the United States and decreased the reported incidence of congenital rubella syndrome to only 20 cases in 1994. However, it has not resulted in a decrease in the percentage of women of child-bearing age who are susceptible to rubella.

Pregnant women should not be given live rubella virus vaccine, but inadvertent immunization should not ordinarily be a reason to interrupt the pregnancy. The infants of more than 200 women immunized during pregnancy with RA 27/3 vaccine have been studied; no cases of clinically evident congenital rubella syndrome were found to occur. Other contraindications include immune deficiency states, severe febrile illness, hypersensitivity to vaccine components, and therapy with antimetabolites, corticosteroids, and steroid-like substances.

Clinical manifestations that may follow rubella immunization include fever, typical lymphadenopathy, rash, and arthritis and arthralgia. The last two occur more frequently in older girls and adult women and may last for weeks. Two unusual syndromes have been reported in association with rubella vaccine: one with paresthesia of the hand or arm that occurs at night lasts for up to 1 hr and may recur frequently during the night; the other is manifested by pain behind the knee and limitation of motion. Symptoms are worst in the morning, diminishing during the day. They may last for up to 5 wk. Both syndromes may recur.

Management of Pregnant Women Exposed to or Acquiring Rubella. Pregnant women, especially early in pregnancy but also during the entire gestational period, should avoid exposure to rubella regardless of history of the disease during childhood or of history of active immunization. Exposure of pregnant women to infants with congenital rubella syndrome should be especially guarded against because of prolonged shedding of virus. Risk of damage to the fetus decreases after the 14th wk of gestation.

Because approximately 80% of women of child-bearing age are immune to rubella as a result of the natural infection or of immunization, the immune status to rubella of women who may become pregnant should be determined.

If a pregnant woman whose immune status is unknown is exposed to rubella, an antibody test should be performed *immediately as an emergency measure.* If determined to be immune, she can be reassured that the pregnancy can be continued without added risk. If she is found to be susceptible and therapeutic abortion is unacceptable or unavailable to her, passive immunization with ISG, 20–30 mL intramuscularly, should be attempted immediately. Active immunization of pregnant women is not advised.

If exposure to rubella occurs in a susceptible pregnant woman to whom abortion is available and desirable because of significant potential hazard to the fetus, it is probably advisable to withhold ISG, observe her carefully, and repeat the rubella antibody test. If rubella then develops at a stage of pregnancy at which she feels the risk is greater than she wants to assume or if serial antibody tests show that subclinical infection has occurred, abortion may be induced.

REINFECTION. The incidence of reinfection on exposure of individuals who are serologically immune to wild virus is 3–10% among those demonstrating serologic immunity without a history of immunization and 14–18% among those immunized with RA 27/3 vaccine. Infection has been demonstrated among the fetuses of reinfected pregnant women as well as among pregnant women who had received rubella vaccine. The relevance of reinfection of serologically immune pregnant women to the production of congenital malformations remains to be determined. Until these questions are answered, *all* pregnant women should make every effort to avoid exposure to rubella.

TREATMENT. Unless bacterial complications occur, treatment is symptomatic. Adamantanamine hydrochloride (amantadine) has been reported to be effective in vitro in inhibiting early stages of rubella infection in cultured cells. An attempt to treat a child having congenital rubella with this drug was unsuccessful. *Because amantadine is not recommended for pregnant women, its usefulness is very limited.* Interferon and isoprinosine have been used with limited success.

Centers for Disease Control and Prevention: Summary of notifiable diseases, United States, 1992. MMWR 41:3, 1992.
Chang TW: Rubella reinfection and intrauterine involvement (Editorial). J. Pediatr 84:617, 1974.
Clark M, et al: Effect of rubella vaccination programme on serological status of young adults in United Kingdom. Lancet 1:1224, 1979.
Howson CP, Katz M, Johnston RB, et al: Chronic arthritis after rubella vaccination. Clin Infect Dis 15:307, 1992.
Immunization practices in colleges—United States. MMWR 36:209, 1987.
Miller E, Cradock-Watson JE, Pollock TM: Consequences of confirmed maternal rubella at successive stages of pregnancy. Lancet 2:781, 1982.
O'Shea S, Best JB, Banatvala JE, et al: Development and persistence of class-specific antibodies in the serum and nasopharyngeal washings of rubella vaccines. J Infect Dis 151:89, 1985.
Plotkin SA, Klaus RM, Whitely JP, et al: Hypogammaglobulinemia in an infant with congenital rubella syndrome: Failure of L-adamantanamine to stop virus excretion. J Pediatr 69:1085, 1966.
Rawls WE, Desmyter J, Melnick JL: Serologic diagnosis and fetal involvement in maternal rubella. JAMA 203:627, 1968.
Rawls WE, Phillips CA, Melnick JL, et al: Persistent virus infection in congenital rubella. Arch Ophthalmol 77:430, 1967.
Rubella and congenital rubella syndrome—United States 1985–1988. MMWR 38:173, 1989.
Rubella vaccination during pregnancy—United States 1971–1986. MMWR 36:458, 1987.
Tardieu M, Grospierre B, Durandy A, et al: Circulating immune complexes containing rubella antigens in late-onset rubella syndrome. J Pediatr 97:370, 1980.
Townsend JJ: Progressive rubella panencephalitis: Late onset after congenital rubella. N Engl J Med 292:990, 1975.

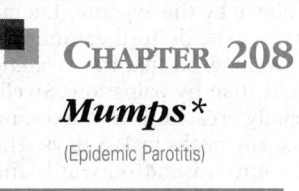

CHAPTER 208
Mumps*
(Epidemic Parotitis)

Yvonne Maldonado

Mumps is an acute, generalized viral disease in which painful enlargement of the salivary glands, chiefly the parotids, is the usual presenting sign.

ETIOLOGY. The virus is a member of the paramyxovirus group, which also includes the parainfluenza, measles, and Newcastle disease viruses. Only one serotype is known. Primary cultures of human or monkey kidney cells are used for viral isolation. Cytopathic effect is occasionally observed, but hemadsorption is the most sensitive indicator of infection. Virus has been isolated from saliva, cerebrospinal fluid, blood, urine, brain, and other infected tissues.

EPIDEMIOLOGY. Mumps is endemic in most urban populations; the virus is spread from a human reservoir by direct contact, airborne droplets, fomites contaminated by saliva, and possibly by urine. It is distributed worldwide and affects both sexes equally; 85% of infections occurred in children younger than 15 yr prior to widespread immunization. Now disease often occurs in young adults, producing epidemics in colleges or in the work place. Epidemics appear to be primarily related to lack of immunization rather than to waning of immunity. Epidemics occur at all seasons but are slightly more frequent in late winter and spring. Sources of infection may be difficult to trace because 30–40% of infections are subclinical. There has been a decrease in the incidence since the introduction of mumps vaccine in 1968.

Virus has been isolated from saliva as long as 6 days before and up to 9 days after appearance of salivary gland swelling. Transmission does not seem to occur longer than 24 hr before appearance of the swelling or later than 3 days after it has subsided. Virus has been isolated from urine from the 1st–14th day after the onset of salivary gland swelling.

Lifelong immunity usually follows clinical or subclinical infection, although second infections have been documented. Transplacental antibodies seem to be effective in protecting infants during their first 6–8 mo. Infants born to mothers who have mumps in the week prior to delivery may have clinically apparent mumps at birth or experience illness in the neonatal period. Severity ranges from mild parotitis to severe pancreatitis. The serum neutralization test is the most reliable method for determining immunity but is cumbersome and expensive. A complement-fixing antibody test is available (see Diagnosis). The presence of V antibodies alone suggests previous mumps infection.

PATHOGENESIS. After entry and initial multiplication in the cells of the respiratory tract, the virus is blood-borne to many tissues, among which the salivary and other glands are the most susceptible.

CLINICAL MANIFESTATIONS. The incubation period ranges from 14–24 days, with a peak at 17–18 days. In children, prodromal manifestations are rare but may be manifest by fever, muscular pain (especially in the neck), headache, and malaise. The onset is usually characterized by pain and swelling in one or both parotid glands. The parotid swells characteristically; it first fills the space between the posterior border of the mandible and the mastoid and then extends in a series of crescents down-

*As modified from the section in the 14th edition by C. Phillips.

ward and forward, being limited above by the zygoma. Edema of the skin and soft tissues usually extends further and obscures the limit of the glandular swelling, so that the swelling is more readily appreciated by sight than by palpation. Swelling may proceed extremely rapidly, reaching a maximum within a few hours, although it usually peaks in 1–3 days. The swollen tissues push the ear lobe upward and outward, and the angle of the mandible is no longer visible. Swelling slowly subsides within 3–7 days but occasionally lasts longer. One parotid gland usually swells a day or two before the other, but swelling limited to one gland is common. The swollen area is tender and painful, pain being elicited especially by tasting sour liquids such as lemon juice or vinegar. Redness and swelling about the opening of the Stensen duct are common. Edema of the homolateral pharynx and soft palate accompanies the parotid swelling and displaces the tonsil medially; acute edema of the larynx has also been described. Edema over the manubrium and upper chest wall may occur probably because of lymphatic obstruction. The parotid swelling is usually accompanied by moderate fever; normal temperatures are common (20%), but temperatures of 40° C (104° F) or more are rare.

Although the parotid glands alone are affected in the majority of patients, swelling of the submandibular glands occurs frequently and usually accompanies or closely follows that of the parotid glands. In 10–15% of patients only the submandibular gland(s) may be swollen. Little pain is associated with the submandibular infection, but the swelling subsides more slowly than that of the parotids. Redness and swelling at the orifice of the Wharton duct frequently accompany swelling of the gland.

Least commonly the sublingual glands are infected, usually bilaterally; the swelling is evident in the submental region and in the floor of the mouth.

A maculopapular erythematous rash, most prominent on the trunk, occurs infrequently; rarely it is urticarial.

COMPLICATIONS. Viremia early in the infection probably accounts for the widespread complications.

Meningoencephalomyelitis. This is the most frequent complication in childhood. The true incidence is hard to estimate because subclinical infection of the central nervous system, as evidenced by cerebrospinal fluid pleocytosis, has been reported in more than 65% of patients with parotitis. Clinical manifestations occur in over 10% of patients. The incidence of mumps meningoencephalitis is approximately 250/100,000 cases; 10% of these cases occurred in patients older than 20 yr. The mortality rate is about 2%. Males are affected three to five times as frequently as females. Mumps is one of the most common causes of aseptic meningitis (see Chapter 169).

The pathogenesis of mumps meningoencephalitis has been described as (1) a primary infection of neurons and (2) a postinfectious encephalitis with demyelination. In the first type, parotitis frequently appears at the same time or following the onset of encephalitis. In the latter type, encephalitis follows parotitis by an average of 10 days. Parotitis may in some cases be absent. Aqueductal stenosis and hydrocephalus have been associated with mumps infection. Injecting mumps virus into suckling hamsters has produced similar lesions.

Mumps meningoencephalitis is clinically indistinguishable from meningoencephalitis of other origins (see Chapter 169). Moderate stiffness of the neck is seen, but the remainder of the neurologic examination is usually normal. The cerebrospinal fluid (CSF) usually contains fewer than 500 cells/mm^3, although occasionally the count may exceed 2,000. The cells are almost exclusively lymphocytes, in contrast to enteroviral aseptic meningitis, in which polymorphonuclear leukocytes often predominate early in the disease. Mumps virus can be isolated from cerebrospinal fluid early in the illness.

Orchitis, Epididymitis. These complications rarely occur in prepubescent boys but are common (14–35%) in adolescents and adults. The testis is most often infected with or without epididymitis; epididymitis may also occur alone. Rarely, there is a hydrocele. The orchitis usually follows parotitis within 8 days or so; it may also occur without evidence of salivary gland infection. In about 30% of patients both testes are affected. The onset is usually abrupt, with a rise in temperature, chills, headache, nausea, and lower abdominal pain; when the right testis is implicated, appendicitis may be suggested as a diagnostic possibility. The affected testis becomes tender and swollen, and the adjacent skin is edematous and red. The average duration is 4 days. Approximately 30–40% of affected testes atrophy. Impairment of fertility is estimated to be about 13%, but absolute infertility is probably rare.

Oophoritis. Pelvic pain and tenderness are noted in about 7% of postpubertal female patients. There is no evidence of impairment of fertility.

Pancreatitis. Severe involvement of the pancreas is rare, but mild or subclinical infection may be more common than is recognized. It may be unassociated with salivary gland manifestations and be misdiagnosed as gastroenteritis. Epigastric pain and tenderness, which are suggestive, may be accompanied by fever, chills, vomiting, and prostration. An elevated serum amylase value is characteristically present with mumps, with or without clinical manifestations of pancreatitis.

Nephritis. Viruria has been reported frequently. In one study of adults, abnormal renal function occurred at some time in every patient, and viruria was detected in 75%. The frequency of renal involvement in children is unknown. Fatal nephritis, occurring 10–14 days after parotitis, has been reported.

Thyroiditis. Although uncommon in children, a diffuse, tender swelling of the thyroid may occur about 1 wk after the onset of parotitis with subsequent development of antithyroid antibodies.

Myocarditis. Serious cardiac manifestations are extremely rare, but mild infection of the myocardium may be more common than is recognized. Electrocardiographic tracings revealed changes, mostly depression of the ST segment, in 13% of adults in one series. Such involvement may explain the precordial pain, bradycardia, and fatigue sometimes noted among adolescents and adults with mumps.

Mastitis. This is uncommon in each sex.

Deafness. Unilateral, rarely bilateral, nerve deafness may occur; although the incidence is low (1:15,000), mumps is a leading cause of unilateral nerve deafness. The hearing loss may be transient or permanent.

Ocular Complications. These include *dacryoadenitis,* painful swelling, usually bilateral, of the lacrimal glands; *optic neuritis (papillitis)* with symptoms varying from loss of vision to mild blurring with recovery in 10–20 days; *uveokeratitis,* usually unilateral, with photophobia, tearing, rapid loss of vision, and recovery within 20 days; *scleritis; tenonitis,* with resultant exophthalmos; and *central vein thrombosis.*

Arthritis. Arthralgia associated with swelling and redness of the joints is an infrequent complication; complete recovery is the rule.

Thrombocytopenic Purpura. This sign is infrequent.

Mumps Embryopathy. There is no firm evidence that maternal infection is damaging to the fetus; a possible relationship to endocardial fibroelastosis has not been established. Mumps in early pregnancy does increase the chance of abortion.

DIAGNOSIS. The diagnosis of mumps parotitis is usually apparent from the symptoms and physical examination. When the clinical manifestations are limited to those of one of the less common lesions, the diagnosis is not so clear but may be suspected, especially during an epidemic. The routine laboratory tests are nonspecific; there is usually leukopenia with relative lymphocytosis, but complications often result in polymorphonuclear leukocytosis of moderate degree. An elevation of serum amylase is common; the rise tends to parallel the parotid swelling and then to return to normal within 2 wk or so. The etiologic diagnosis depends on isolation of the virus from the saliva, urine, spinal fluid, or blood or the demonstration of a significant rise in circulating complement fixation antibodies during convalescence. Serum antibodies to the S antigen reach their peak early in about 75% of patients and are detectable at the time of the presenting symptoms. They gradually disappear within 6–12 mo; antibodies against the V or viral antigen usually reach a peak titer in about 1 mo, remain stationary for about 6 mo, and then slowly decline during the ensuing 2 yr to a low level, at which they persist. The presence of a high anti-S titer and a low anti-V titer during the acute stage of an otherwise undiagnosed meningoencephalitis, for example, strongly suggests a mumps infection, which would be confirmed if a convalescent serum (taken 14–21 days later) revealed a fourfold rise of anti-V antibodies accompanied by little change in the titer of anti-S antibodies.

DIFFERENTIAL DIAGNOSIS. This includes *parotitis* of other origin, as in viral infections including human immunodeficiency virus (HIV) infection, influenza, parainfluenza 1 and 3, cytomegalovirus, or the rare instances of coxsackievirus A and lymphocytic choriomeningitis infections. These infections can be distinguished by specific laboratory tests; *suppurative parotitis,* in which pus can often be expressed from the duct; *recurrent parotitis,* a condition of unknown origin, but possibly allergic in nature, which has frequent recurrences and a characteristic sialogram; *salivary calculus,* obstructing either a parotid or, more commonly, a submandibular duct, in which the swelling is intermittent; *preauricular or anterior cervical lymphadenitis* from any cause; *lymphosarcoma* or other rare *tumors* of the parotid; *orchitis resulting from infections other than mumps,* for example, the rare infections by coxsackievirus A or lymphocytic choriomeningitis viruses; and *parotitis caused by cytomegalovirus* in immunocompromised children.

TREATMENT. Treatment of parotitis is entirely symptomatic. Bed rest should be guided by the patient's needs, but no statistical evidence indicates that it prevents complications. The diet should be adjusted to the patient's ability to chew. Orchitis should be treated with local support and bed rest. Mumps arthritis may respond to a 2-wk course of corticosteroids or a nonsteroidal anti-inflammatory agent. Salicylates do not appear to be effective.

PROPHYLAXIS

Passive. Hyperimmune mumps gamma globulin is not effective in preventing mumps or decreasing complications.

Active. The routine administration of live, attenuated mumps vaccine is discussed in Chapter 247. Vaccinated children usually do not experience fever or other detectable clinical reactions, do not excrete virus, and are not contagious to susceptible contacts. Rarely, parotitis can develop 7–10 days after vaccination. The vaccine induces antibody in about 96% of seronegative recipients and has a protective efficacy of about 97% against natural mumps infection. The protection appears to be long lasting. In one outbreak of mumps, several children who had been immunized with mumps vaccine in the past experienced an illness characterized by fever, malaise, nausea, and a red papular rash involving the trunk and extremities but sparing the palms and soles. The rash lasted about 24 hr. No virus was isolated from these children, but increases in the titer of mumps antibody were demonstrated.

Bistrian B, et al: Fatal mumps meningoencephalitis. JAMA 222:478, 1972.
Cochi SI, Preblud SR, Orenstein WA: Perspectives in the relative resurgence of mumps in the United States. Am J Dis Child 142:499, 1988.
Gordon SC, Lauter CB: Mumps arthritis: A review of the literature. Rev Infect Dis 6:338, 1984.
Quast U, Hennessen W, Widmark RM: Vaccine induced mumps-like disease. Develop Biol Standard 43:269, 1979.

CHAPTER 209

*Enteroviruses**

Abraham Morag and Pearay L. Ogra

Enteroviruses are a large group of viral agents that inhabit the intestinal tract and are responsible for significant and frequent human illnesses with protean clinical manifestations.

ETIOLOGY. Enteroviruses are RNA viruses belonging to the Picornaviridae family. The original enteroviral subgroups—coxsackieviruses, echoviruses, and polioviruses—were differentiated by their effects in tissue culture and animals (Table 209–1). Coxsackieviruses are named after the town of Coxsackie, New York, where they were first isolated in 1948, as nonpoliovirus agents causing paralysis in children. Echo virus, or enteric cytopathogenic human orphan viruses, were not, at first, known to cause any disease in animals or humans. The coxsackieviruses consist of two groups, A and B. Since 1970 new enteroviral types have been classified by enteroviral numbers. Enteroviruses retain activity for several days at room temperature and can be stored indefinitely at ordinary freezer temperatures (−20° C). They are rapidly inactivated by heat (>56° C), formaldehyde, chlorination, and ultraviolet light. Enteroviruses, except for most members of Coxsackie group A, grow well in many cell cultures and cause cytopathic effects (CPE) that are different from those caused by herpesvirus, adenoviruses, and reoviruses. Coxsackieviruses from group A are identified by their pathologic effects in suckling mice.

EPIDEMIOLOGY. Humans are the only known reservoir for the human enteroviruses. Viruses related to human enteroviruses have been isolated from dogs and cats, but there is no evidence of spread from animals to humans. They are spread from person to person by fecal-oral and possibly oral-oral (respiratory) routes. The enteroviruses infect the human gastrointestinal tract, but they do not colonize it. Even during the season of greater prevalence, very few strains circulate, probably as a result of interference among the virus types.

Children are immunologically susceptible, and their unhygienic habits facilitate spread. Transmission occurs from child to child (via feces to skin to mouth) and then within family groups. Even when an enterovirus is spreading through a community, it is often confined to households with young children. Rapid and extensive spread occurs in other similar environments such as summer camps and day-care centers. Recovery of enteroviruses is inversely related to age, and prevalence of specific antibodies is directly related to age. The incidence of infections and the prevalence of antibodies do not differ between boys and girls, but significant disease is more common in boys. Enteroviruses are often isolated from sewage and survive for up to 6 mo in wet soil, but person-to-person spread is the primary mode of transmission. Environmental contamination is probably the result rather than the cause of human infection.

Enteroviruses have a worldwide distribution. In tropical and semitropical areas, they are found year-round. In temperate climates, they are detected during winter and spring but are more common during summer and fall, with peaks from August to October. Winter outbreaks are rare. Infection and acquisition of postinfection immunity occur with greater frequency and at earlier ages among crowded, economically deprived populations. Under such conditions, the incidence of

*Modified from the section in the 14th edition by J. D. Cherry.

■ **TABLE 209–1 Human Enteroviruses**

Polioviruses: types 1–3
Coxsackieviruses A: types A1–A24 (A23 reclassified as echovirus 9)
Coxsackieviruses B: types B1–B6
Echoviruses: types 1–33 (type 10 reclassified as reovirus type 1 and type 28 reclassified as rhinovirus type 1A)
Enteroviruses: types 68–72 (hepatitis A has been provisionally classified as type 72)

infection, with one or more enterovirus serotypes, may exceed 50%; mixed infections are common.

Although there are 68 identified enteroviral types, most illness in the United States is due to about a dozen nonpolio enteroviral types. Recently, the most prevalent types have been echoviruses 4, 6, 9, 11, and 30, coxsackieviruses A9, A16, and B2-B5, and enteroviruses 70 and 71. The universal use of live polio vaccine in the United States has virtually eliminated epidemic poliomyelitis. However, poliomyelitis still occurs in many regions of the developing world. In countries in which vaccines are not available and economic conditions are poor, poliomyelitis remains a disease of infants and young children. A changing epidemiologic pattern is emerging in some underdeveloped countries as economic standards improve. Significant epidemics are being reported in these countries, where paralytic poliomyelitis had been rare.

PATHOGENESIS AND IMMUNE RESPONSES. Figure 209–1 shows a schematic diagram of the events of pathogenesis and target tissues involved. Following initial acquisition of virus by the oral or respiratory route, implantation occurs in the pharynx and the lower alimentary tract. Two or more enteroviruses may invade and replicate at the same time in the gastrointestinal tract, but replication of one type often interferes with the growth of the heterologous type. Interference has been documented between echovirus, coxsackievirus, and poliovirus, including vaccine strains. Within 1 day the infection extends to the regional lymph nodes. On about the 3rd day minor viremia occurs, involving many secondary sites. Multiplication of virus in these sites coincides with the onset of clinical symptoms. Illness can vary from minor to fatal infections. Major viremia occurs during the period of multiplication of virus in the secondary sites, usually lasting from the 3rd–7th day of infection. In many enteroviral infections central nervous system involvement occurs at the same time as other secondary organ involvement, but the occasional delay of central nervous system symptoms suggests that seeding occurred later in association with the major viremia or by another pathway such as autonomic nerve fibers. Cessation of viremia correlates with the appearance of serum antibody. The viral concentration in secondary sites begins to diminish on about the 7th day. However, infection continues in the lower intestinal tract for prolonged periods (Fig. 209–2).

Immunity to Poliovirus. Passive antibodies transferred across the placenta persist for about 6 mo. Active immunity, after natural infection, probably lasts for life. Neutralizing antibodies against enteroviruses form within several days after exposure, often before the onset of illness. This early production of serum antibodies is a result of replication of the virus in the intestinal tract and deep lymphatic tissues, which occurs before the invasion of target organs, such as the central nervous system. Local (mucosal) immunity, conferred mainly by secretory immunoglobulin (Ig)A, is an important defense against enteroviral infection, mediating protection against intestinal reinfection after recovery from natural infection with wild-type poliovirus or after immunization with live polio vaccine. Enhanced potency inactivated polio vaccine (E-IPV) elicits higher serum antibodies but is less effective than oral polio vaccine (OPV) in preventing and limiting intestinal infection. A decrease in resistance to poliovirus has been observed after tonsillectomy and adenoidectomy, which correlates with decreased secretory antibodies in the nasopharynx.

PATHOLOGY AND PATHOPHYSIOLOGY

Polioviruses. The neuropathy of poliomyelitis and other paralytic diseases caused by nonpolio enteroviruses is due to direct cellular destruction. Secondary damage may be due to immunologic mechanisms. Other syndromes caused by viral lysis of

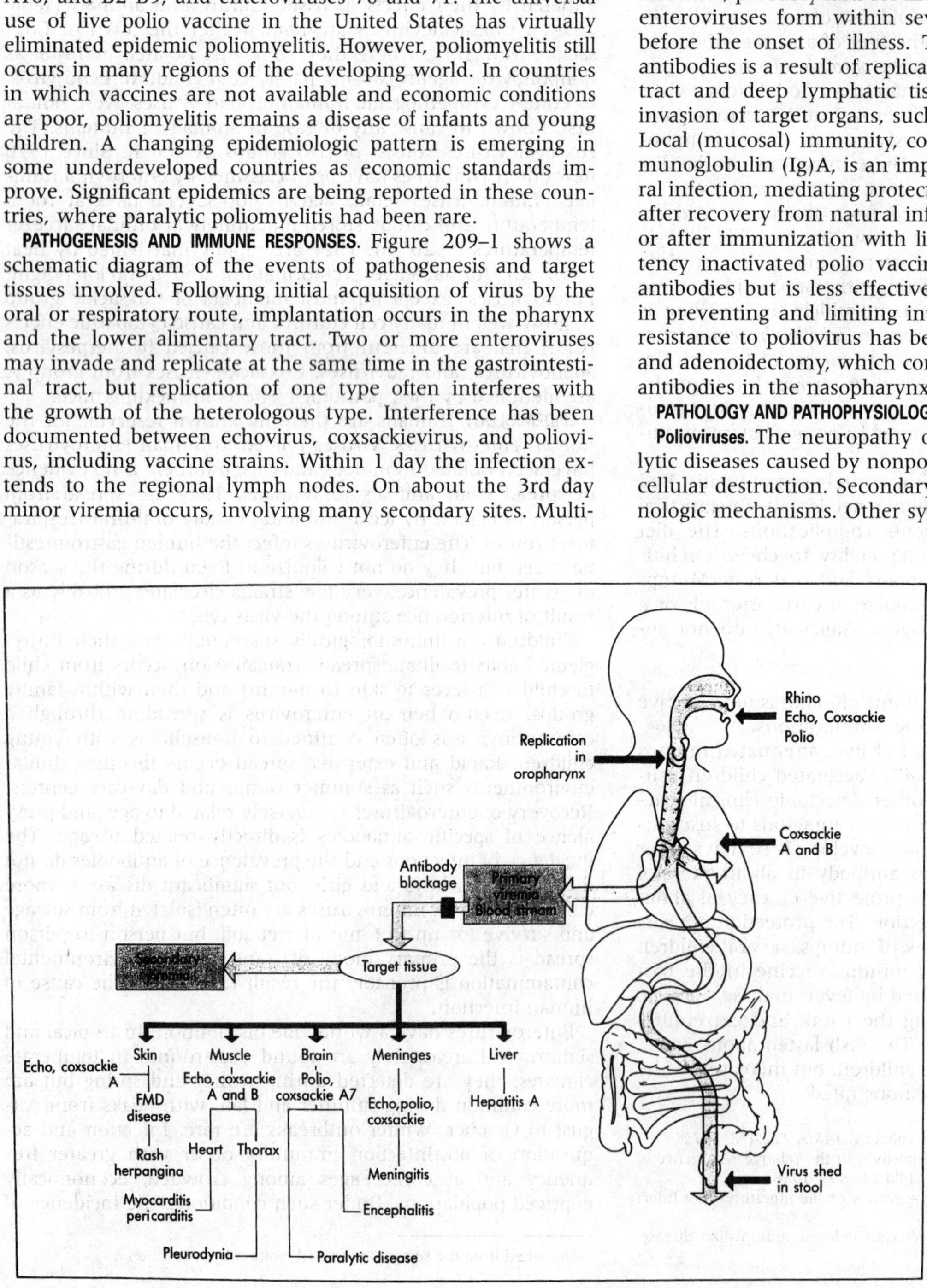

Figure 209–1. The pathogenesis of enteroviral infections. (FMD = foot and mouth disease.)

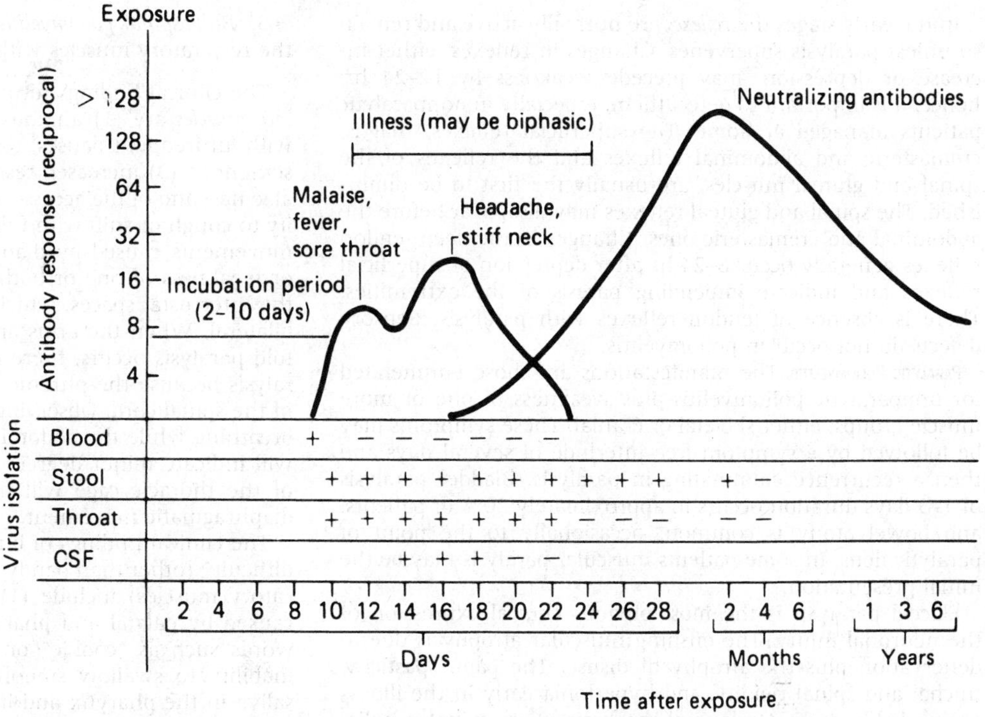

Figure 209–2. Time course of clinical and laboratory manifestations. (CSF = cerebrospinal fluid.)

host cells include disseminated disease of the newborn, aseptic meningitis, encephalitis, and acute respiratory illness. In poliomyelitis, neuronal lesions occur in the (1) spinal cord (anterior-horn cells chiefly and to a lesser degree the intermediate and dorsal horn and dorsal root ganglia); (2) medulla (vestibular nuclei, cranial nerve nuclei, and the reticular formation, which contains the vital centers); (3) cerebellum (nuclei in the roof and vermis only); (4) midbrain (chiefly the gray matter but also the substantia nigra and occasionally the red nucleus); (5) thalamus and hypothalamus; (6) pallidum; and (7) cerebral cortex (motor cortex). The following areas are spared: (1) the entire cerebral cortex except the motor area; (2) the cerebellum except the vermis and deep midline nuclei; and (3) the white matter of the spinal cord.

Enteroviruses have been detected in some cases of myopericarditis. The pathogenesis of enterovirus-associated nephritis, myositis, polyradiculitis, pancreatitis, hepatitis, pneumonitis, and other syndromes is unclear; these disorders may be due to the inflammatory response to viral antigens or virus-induced tissue damage. Enteroviral RNA sequences have been demonstrated in cardiac tissues from patients with cardiomyopathies, but a causal relationship has not been established. Some peptide sequences that constitute viral epitopes are shared by host tissues, which may provide a mechanism for autoimmune reactions in enteroviral infection.

CLINICAL MANIFESTATIONS

Poliovirus Infections. When a susceptible person has been infected with poliovirus, one of the following responses may occur, in this order of frequency: (1) inapparent infection in 90–95% of those infected, (2) abortive poliomyelitis, (3) nonparalytic poliomyelitis, (4) paralytic poliomyelitis.

Abortive Poliomyelitis. A brief febrile illness occurs with one or more of the following symptoms: malaise, anorexia, nausea, vomiting, headache, sore throat, constipation, and unlocalized abdominal pain. Coryza, cough, pharyngeal exudate, diarrhea, and localized abdominal tenderness and rigidity are uncommon. The fever seldom exceeds 39.5° C (103° F), and the pharynx shows usually little change despite the frequent complaint of sore throat.

Nonparalytic Poliomyelitis. The symptoms are those enumerated for abortive poliomyelitis, except that headache, nausea, and vomiting are more intense, and there is soreness and stiffness of the posterior muscles of the neck, trunk, and limbs. Fleeting paralysis of the bladder is not uncommon, and constipation is frequent. Approximately two thirds of the children have a short symptom-free interlude between the first phase (minor illness) and the second phase (central nervous system or major illness). This two-phase course is less common in adults, in whom the evolution of symptoms is more insidious. Nuchal and spinal rigidity should occur as a basis for the diagnosis of nonparalytic poliomyelitis during the second phase.

Physical examination reveals nuchal-spinal signs and changes in superficial and deep reflexes. With cooperative patients the nuchal-spinal signs are first sought by active tests. The child is asked to sit up unassisted. If this causes undue effort and if the knees flex upward and the patient writhes a bit from side to side in sitting up and uses hands on the bed for the tripod supporting position, there is unmistakable spinal rigidity. Still sitting, the patient is asked to flex the chin to the chest and is observed for nuchal rigidity. Alternatively, from the supine position, with knees held down gently, the patient is asked to sit up and kiss his or her knees. If the knees draw up sharply or if the maneuver cannot be adequately completed, there is stiffness of the spine as a result of muscle spasm. If the diagnosis is still uncertain, attempts should be made to elicit Kernig and Brudzinski signs. Gentle forward flexion of the occiput and neck will elicit nuchal rigidity, which may precede spinal rigidity. Head drop may be demonstrated by placing the hands under the patient's shoulders and raising the trunk. Normally the head follows the plane of the trunk, but in poliomyelitis it often falls backward limply. The head-drop sign is not due to true paresis of the neck flexors. In struggling infants it may be difficult to distinguish voluntary resistance from clinically important involuntary nuchal rigidity. One may place the infant's shoulders flush with the edge of the table, support the weight of the occiput in the hand, and then flex the head anteriorly. Nuchal rigidity that persists during this maneuver may be interpreted as involuntary. When not closed, the anterior fontanel may be tense or bulging as in meningitis.

In the early stages the *reflexes* are normally active and remain so unless paralysis supervenes. Changes in reflexes, either increase or depression, may precede weakness by 12–24 hr; hence, it is important to detect them, especially in nonparalytic patients managed at home. The superficial reflexes, that is, cremasteric and abdominal reflexes and the reflexes of the spinal and gluteal muscles, are usually the first to be diminished. The spinal and gluteal reflexes may disappear before the abdominal and cremasteric ones. Changes in the deep tendon reflexes generally occur 8–24 hr after depression of superficial reflexes and indicate impending paresis of the extremities. There is absence of tendon reflexes with paralysis. Sensory defects do not occur in poliomyelitis.

Paralytic Poliomyelitis. The manifestations are those enumerated for nonparalytic poliomyelitis plus weakness of one or more muscle groups, either skeletal or cranial. These symptoms may be followed by a symptom-free interlude of several days and then a recurrence culminating in paralysis. Bladder paralysis of 1–3 days duration occurs in approximately 20% of patients, and bowel atony is common, occasionally to the point of paralytic ileus. In some patients muscular paralysis may be the initial presentation.

Flaccid paralysis is the most obvious clinical expression of the neuronal injury. The ensuing muscular atrophy is due to denervation plus the atrophy of disuse. The pain, spasticity, nuchal and spinal rigidity, and hypertonia early in the illness are probably due to lesions of the brain stem, spinal ganglia, and posterior columns. Respiratory and cardiac arrhythmias, blood pressure and vasomotor changes, and the like are reflections of damage to vital centers in the medulla.

On physical examination the distribution of paralysis is characteristically spotty. To detect mild muscular weakness, it is often necessary to apply gentle resistance in opposition to the muscle group being tested. In the spinal form there is weakness of some of the muscles of the neck, abdomen, trunk, diaphragm, thorax, or extremities. In the bulbar form there is weakness in the motor distribution of one or more cranial nerves with or without dysfunction of the vital centers of respiration and circulation. Components of both the preceding forms occur together in bulbospinal poliomyelitis. In the encephalitic form irritability, disorientation, drowsiness, and coarse tremors not explained by inadequate ventilation are noted; peripheral or cranial nerve paralysis coexists or ensues. Hypoxia and hypercapnia caused by inadequate ventilation from respiratory insufficiency may produce disorientation without true encephalitis.

A number of components acting together may produce insufficiency of ventilation, resulting in hypoxia and hypercapnia, which may produce profound effects on many other systems. Because respiratory insufficiency may develop rapidly, continued clinical evaluation is essential. Despite weakness of the respiratory muscles, the patient may respond with so much respiratory effort (associated with anxiety and fear) that overventilation may occur at the outset, resulting in respiratory alkalosis. Such effort is fatiguing and soon leads to respiratory failure.

Certain characteristic patterns of disease occur:

1. *Pure spinal poliomyelitis with respiratory insufficiency* involves tightness, weakness, or paralysis of respiratory muscles (chiefly the diaphragm and intercostals) without discernible clinical involvement of cranial nerves or vital centers. The cervical and thoracic spinal cord segments are chiefly affected.

2. *Pure bulbar poliomyelitis* involves paralysis of motor cranial nerve nuclei with or without involvement of the vital centers that control respiration, circulation, and body temperature. Involvement of the 9th, 10th, and 12th cranial nerves results in paralysis of the pharynx, tongue, and larynx with consequent airway obstruction.

3. *Bulbospinal poliomyelitis with respiratory insufficiency* affects the respiratory muscles with coexisting bulbar paralysis.

The clinical findings resulting from *involvement of the respiratory muscles* are (1) anxious expression; (2) inability to speak without frequent pauses, resulting in short, jerky, "breathless" sentences; (3) increased respiratory rate; (4) movement of the alae nasi and of the accessory muscles of respiration; (5) inability to cough or sniff with full depth; (6) paradoxical abdominal movements caused by diaphragmatic immobility from spasm or weakness of one or both leaves; (7) relative immobility of the intercostal spaces, which may be segmental, unilateral, or bilateral. When the arms are weak, and especially when deltoid paralysis occurs, there may be impending respiratory paralysis because the phrenic nerve nuclei are in adjacent areas of the spinal cord. Observing the patient's capacity for thoracic breathing while the abdominal muscles are splinted manually will indicate minor degrees of paresis. Light manual splinting of the thoracic cage will help to assess the effectiveness of diaphragmatic movement.

The clinical findings of bulbar poliomyelitis with respiratory difficulty (other than paralysis of extraocular, facial, and masticatory muscles) include (1) nasal twang to the voice or cry caused by palatal and pharyngeal weakness (hard-consonant words such as "cookie" or "candy" bring this out best); (2) inability to swallow smoothly, resulting in accumulation of saliva in the pharynx and indicating partial immobility (holding the larynx lightly and asking the patient to swallow will confirm immobility); (3) accumulated pharyngeal secretions, which may cause irregular respirations because each inspiration must be "planned" to avoid aspirating; the respirations may thus appear interrupted and abnormal even to the point of falsely simulating intercostal or diaphragmatic weakness; (4) the impossibility of effective coughing, with constant fatiguing efforts to clear the throat; (5) nasal regurgitation of saliva and fluids as a result of palatal paralysis, with inability to separate the oropharynx from the nasopharynx during swallowing; (6) deviation of the palate, uvula, or tongue; (7) involvement of vital brain stem centers, manifested by irregularity in rate, depth, and rhythm of respiration; by cardiovascular alterations which include blood pressure changes (especially increased), alternate flushing and mottling of the skin, and cardiac arrhythmias; and by rapid changes in body temperature; (8) paralysis of one or both vocal cords causing hoarseness, aphonia, and ultimately asphyxia unless recognized by laryngoscopy and managed by immediate tracheostomy; (9) the "rope sign," an acute angulation between the chin and larynx caused by weakness of the hyoid muscles (the hyoid bone is pulled posteriorly, narrowing the hypopharyngeal inlet).

Nonpolio Enterovirus Infections. Coxsackie-viral and echoviral infections are exceedingly common, and their spectrum of disease is protean. Because many of the clinical-virologic associations are based upon a limited number of cases and because enteroviruses are frequently carried asymptomatically in the gastrointestinal tract for relatively long periods of time, some of the observed illnesses and coincidentally recovered viruses may not have a cause and effect relationship. However, repeated observations have confirmed many virus-illness associations, even though their occurrence has been sporadic. More than 90% of infections caused by nonpolio enteroviruses are asymptomatic or result in undifferentiated febrile illnesses. Some clinical syndromes are highly but not exclusively associated with certain serotypes.

Asymptomatic Infection. Coxsackieviruses and echoviruses can frequently be recovered from the stools of well children, but there are few data on the rate of asymptomatic infection with nonpolio enteroviruses. The isolation of enteroviruses from the stool cannot be equated with asymptomatic infection because illness, if it occurs, happens shortly after virus acquisition and is of short duration; a particular infection may have been associated with nonspecific illness 1–3 mo prior to collection of a stool specimen. In general, the more carefully clinical symptomatology is sought, the lower is the percentage of truly asymptomatic infections. Clinical expression is also inversely related to age and varies by viral type. Overall, probably fewer than 50% of all infections are asymptomatic.

NONSPECIFIC FEBRILE ILLNESS. This is the most common manifestation of enteroviral infections. All viral types cause this clinical presentation, but the frequency varies considerably among the individual viruses. The onset of illness is usually abrupt and without prodrome. In young children the initial finding is fever and associated malaise. In older children headache and myalgia are usually also noted. The temperature ranges from 38.5–40° C (101–104° F) and has a mean duration of 3 days. In some instances the fever is biphasic; it occurs for 1 day, is absent for 2–3 days, and then recurs for an additional 2–4 days. In many young children the only manifestation of illness is fever, and its presence is discovered by chance by a parent. Malaise and anorexia are often related to the degree of temperature elevation, as is headache in older patients. The complaint of a sore or scratchy feeling in the throat is common, but an inflamed pharynx is not seen. Nausea and vomiting occasionally occur at the onset of illness, as does mild abdominal discomfort. A few mildly loose stools may be noted. Generalized myalgia is also noted. Findings on physical examination are generally benign. There may be minimal conjunctivitis, injection of the pharynx, and cervical lymphadenitis. The duration of illness varies from 24 hr to 6 days with an average of 3–4 days. The white blood cell count is normal.

RESPIRATORY MANIFESTATIONS. *Pharyngitis, tonsillitis, tonsillopharyngitis,* and nasopharyngitis are common clinical manifestations of coxsackieviral and echoviral infections; probably all enteroviruses on occasion cause mild pharyngitis. Pharyngitis is frequently associated with other clinical findings such as meningitis, pleurodynia, and exanthem. Although evidence of pharyngeal involvement may be present at the time of disease onset, the initial complaint is most often fever. Sore throat, coryza, and vomiting or diarrhea, or both, may also be noted. Examination of the tonsils and pharynx reveals varying degrees of erythema; in some, patches of exudate will be seen. The usual duration of uncomplicated pharyngitis is 3–6 days. The total white blood cell count may be normal or slightly elevated with a normal differential count.

Herpangina is usually characterized by the sudden onset of fever, although the initial temperature can be quite variable with a range from normal to 41° C (106° F). In general, the temperature tends to be higher in younger patients. Older children frequently complain of headache and backache. Vomiting occurs in about 25% of children younger than 5 yr. In the majority of children the oropharyngeal lesions are present on the first examination at the time or shortly after fever is observed (Fig. 209–3 [color plate section]). The characteristic lesions are small, 1- to 2-mm vesicles and ulcers. They are usually discrete with an average of 5 per patient; some patients have only 1 or 2 lesions; in others 14 or more may be noted. When seen early, the vesicular lesions enlarge over a 2- to 3-day period to 3–4 mm in size. Each vesicular and ulcerative lesion is surrounded by an erythematous ring that varies in size up to 10 mm in diameter. The major site of the lesions is the anterior tonsillar pillars. They also occur on the soft palate, uvula, tonsils, pharyngeal wall, and occasionally the posterior buccal surfaces. Aside from these lesions, the remainder of the throat appears either normal or minimally erythematous. Although occasionally noted in association with aseptic meningitis or other more severe enteroviral illness, most cases of herpangina are mild and without complication. The usual duration of signs and symptoms is 3–6 days.

Pleurodynia (Bornholm disease) is an epidemic disease, but sporadic cases do occur. Following an incubation period of about 4 days, there is sudden onset of fever and pain. The typical pain is located in the chest or upper abdomen, is muscular in origin, and is of variable intensity. Occasionally, the pain occurs in other areas of the body. It is often excruciatingly severe and sudden and is associated with profuse sweating. The patient may appear pale and shocklike. The pain is spasmodic, with durations varying from a few minutes to several hours. Most commonly, the spasmodic periods last about 15–30 min. During spasms, the respirations are usually rapid, shallow, and grunting, suggesting pneumonia of pleural inflammation. Pleural friction rubs may be noted on auscultation, and they may appear and disappear with the coming and going of the pain episodes. Coughing, sneezing, or deep breathing makes the pain worse. In older children and adults the pain is described as stabbing or knifelike. When pain is localized to the abdomen, it is frequently crampy and suggests colic in the younger child. The child may double over and refuse to walk or move. Occasionally, the abdominal pain in association with a pale, sweaty, shocklike appearance suggests acute intestinal obstruction. Splinting and guarding of the abdomen also suggests appendicitis and peritonitis. Tenderness to some degree is present in areas of pain, but frank myositis with muscle swelling is not observed. Fever and pain usually last 1–2 days. Frequently, however, the illness is biphasic; after the initial febrile period the patient is asymptomatic for several days; then pain and fever recur. Rarely, patients have several recurrent episodes over a period of a few weeks. In these cases fever is less prominent during the recurrences.

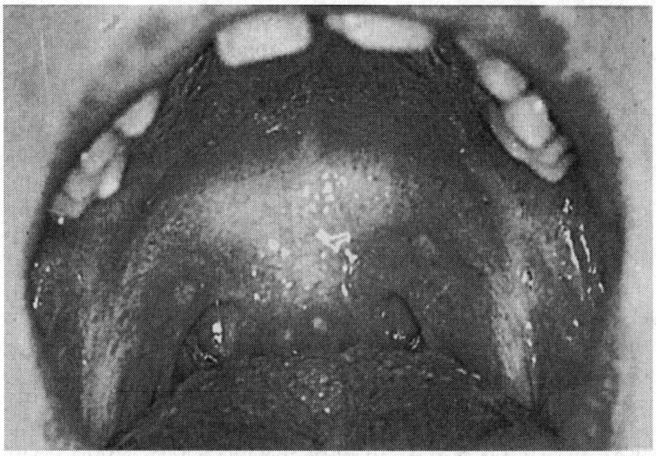

Figure 209–3. Herpangina. This enanthem is predominantly a disease of children and is caused by coxsackieviruses group A. These lesions resemble the ones caused by herpes simplex virus. See also color section. (From Edmond's Color Atlas of Infectious Diseases. Wolfe Medical Publishers, 1990, p 313.)

In epidemics both children and adults are afflicted, with the majority of cases occurring in persons younger than 30 yr. Most children have other signs of enteroviral infection such as anorexia, nausea, vomiting, headache, and sore throat. Routine laboratory studies are not very helpful. The white blood cell count is variable, but an increased percentage of polymorphonuclear neutrophils and band forms is frequent. The erythrocyte sedimentation rate is also inconsistent, with normal to extremely high values observed. The chest roentgenogram is most often normal.

Complications in pleurodynia are uncommon. Aseptic meningitis has been noted, and adult males have experienced orchitis. Myocarditis and pericarditis may also complicate pleurodynia.

The major etiologic agents in epidemic pleurodynia are coxsackieviruses B3 and B5; other associated viruses include coxsackieviruses B1 and B2 and echoviruses 1 and 6.

A variety of nonpolio enteroviruses have been associated

with sporadic instances of parotitis, croup, bronchitis, bronchiolitis, infectious asthma, and pneumonia as well as outbreaks of lymphonodular pharyngitis, stomatitis, and other lesions in the anterior mouth.

GASTROINTESTINAL MANIFESTATIONS. Gastrointestinal manifestations are common (7–30%) in enteroviral infections. Vomiting is a common manifestation of infections with many coxsackieviral and echoviral types, but it is rarely the major complaint of the patient or the parent. Except for the hand, foot, and mouth syndrome (coxsackievirus A16), in which vomiting is uncommon, this manifestation occurs in about 50% of all cases in epidemic enteroviral disease. Vomiting is most common in meningitis and least common in pleurodynia and uncomplicated exanthematous disease.

Diarrhea occurs commonly in coxsackieviral and echoviral infections as one of many manifestations of the systemic illness. It is rarely severe. In most instances loose stools occur for a 2- to 4-day period. The stools are rarely watery and never bloody and number at most 6–8/day.

Abdominal pain is also a common complaint in many enteroviral infections. About 10% of patients with coxsackievirus A16 (hand, foot, and mouth syndrome) complain of abdominal pain. Coxsackieviral and echoviral meningitis is associated with abdominal pain in about 25% of the cases. The severity of pain in enteroviral infections is quite variable and on occasion may suggest a surgical abdomen. The pain is most often periumbilical; it may be either constant or colicky. The associated fever is most often greater than 38.3° C (101° F).

Nonpolio enteroviruses have been associated with a variety of other gastrointestinal and abdominal complaints. In most situations the findings are just one manifestation of a more typical enteroviral illness.

ACUTE HEMORRHAGIC CONJUNCTIVITIS. Conjunctivitis may be the dominant complaint. In the majority of epidemics, enterovirus 70 has been the etiologic agent. Acute hemorrhagic conjunctivitis has a sudden onset that is accompanied by severe eye pain and associated photophobia, blurred vision, lacrimation, erythema and congestion of the eye, and edematous and chemotic lids. There are subconjunctival hemorrhages of varying size and frequently a transient punctate epithelial keratitis, conjunctival follicles, and preauricular lymphadenopathy. Eye discharge is initially serous but becomes mucopurulent with secondary bacterial infection. Systemic symptoms (including fever) are rare. Occasionally, a picture suggestive of pharyngoconjunctival fever has occurred. A small number of patients have had a polyradiculomyeloneuropathy or paralytic poliomyelitis following enterovirus 70 acute hemorrhagic conjunctivitis. Persons 20–50 yr of age have the highest attack rates, and children are less often involved. Initially most epidemics occurred in coastal areas of tropical countries toward the end of hot rainy periods. More recently, outbreaks of disease have occurred in temperate climates, including many areas of the United States. Epidemics are explosive and are spread mainly by the eye-hand-fomite-eye route.

PERICARDITIS AND MYOCARDITIS. These manifestations have been noted in association with 27 different nonpolio enteroviruses. The group B coxsackieviruses have been most frequently implicated, and B5 has been the most common causative agent. Of the echoviruses, type 6 has been most frequently associated with cardiac involvement. Hepatitis, pneumonia, nephritis, meningitis, and orchitis have also been occasional associated findings with coxsackievirus B. The mortality resulting from acute coxsackieviral and echoviral heart disease is significant. In nonfatal cases recovery is usually complete without residual disability; occasionally, constrictive pericarditis occurs as well as other sequelae.

GENITOURINARY MANIFESTATIONS. Group B coxsackieviruses are second only to mumps as causative agents of orchitis; B5 is the most commonly associated virus, but B2 and B4 have also been implicated on many occasions. In almost all instances the orchitis is a secondary event, most commonly associated with pleurodynia. The illness is frequently biphasic; fever and pleurodynia or meningitis are followed by apparent recovery and then by orchitis about 2 wk after onset. Many patients also have epididymitis. In epidemics of disease resulting from group B coxsackieviruses, the occurrence of testicular involvement is quite variable. Generally, orchitis is infrequent, but in one B2 outbreak 17% of the postpubertal males had orchitis and 7% also had epididymitis. Other genitourinary manifestations of nonpolio enteroviral infections include acute glomerulonephritis; mesangiolytic glomerulonephritis in an infant with immune deficiency; hemolytic-uremic syndrome; acute renal failure; pyuria, hematuria, or proteinuria; hemorrhagic cystitis; and vaginal ulcerative lesions.

MYOSITIS AND ARTHRITIS. Myalgia is a common complaint accompanying many coxsackieviral and echoviral illnesses. However, there is almost no direct (demonstration of virus in muscle) or indirect (muscle enzyme elevations) evidence of muscle involvement in routine enteroviral illnesses. Coxsackievirus A2 has been associated with myositis, and coxsackievirus A9 and echovirus 18 have been associated with polymyositis. A dermatomyositis-like syndrome has been associated with immune deficiency and enteroviral infection. Arthritis has occurred rarely in enterovirus infection.

SKIN MANIFESTATIONS. Nonpolio enteroviruses are a common cause of a large variety of skin manifestations. In the summer and fall they are the leading cause of exanthems. There is a marked variation in the rates at which exanthems occur among the various viral types and also among different age groups of the host. In general, the frequency is inversely related to the age of the infected patient, and several different agents can produce similar skin manifestations. The relative importance of enteroviruses as causative agents of exanthems in developed countries is due to immunization programs, which have decreased the classic childhood exanthems, such as measles and rubella.

Echovirus type 9 is the most prevalent nonpolio enterovirus, and exanthem is a common clinical manifestation. Nonspecific febrile illness and aseptic meningitis are the usual major manifestations of echovirus 9 infection. Exanthem occurs in about one third of the cases; 57% of children younger than 5 yr have rash, whereas only 6% of those older than 10 yr have similar cutaneous findings. The rash is most frequently rubelliform, but in addition or as the sole manifestation, petechiae frequently occur. Rash and fever usually appear at about the same time, and frequently the illness closely mimics meningococcemia. The rash usually lasts 3–5 days. The disease may be confused with measles in some patients with lesions of the oral mucosa resembling Koplik spots and patchy rash, but the coryza and conjunctivitis of measles are absent.

Coxsackievirus A16 is the major cause of the hand, foot, and mouth syndrome, which has a typically enteroviral pattern, with a short incubation period (4–6 days) and a summer and fall seasonal pattern. The clinical expression rate of the enanthem-exanthem complex is high, being close to 100% in young children, 38% in school children, and 11% in adults. The intraoral lesions are ulcerative and average about 4–8 mm in size. The tongue and buccal mucosa are most frequently involved. The hands are more commonly involved than the feet. Buttock lesions are also common, but these do not usually progress to vesiculation. The lesions on the hands and feet are usually vesicular and vary in size from 3–7 mm; they are generally more common on the dorsal surfaces but frequently occur on the palms and soles as well. They clear by absorption of the fluid in about 1 wk. Coxsackievirus A16 is frequently associated with subacute, chronic, and recurring skin lesions. Recently, enterovirus 71 has been the etiologic agent in several outbreaks of hand, foot, and mouth syndrome. Illness with this virus is frequently more severe than with coxsackievirus A16; aseptic meningitis, encephalitis, and paralytic disease are common.

Neurologic Manifestations. Aseptic meningitis resulting from enteroviruses occurs in epidemics and as isolated cases (Chapter 169.2). Epidemics have been most common with coxsackievirus B5 and echoviruses 4, 6, 9, and 11. In general, illness is more common in children than in adults. Virtually all patients have fever, and many have mild pharyngitis; other respiratory manifestations are also common. Rash is common but varies with the specific viral agents; 30–50% of all patients with echovirus 9 meningitis have exanthem. Frequently, the rash is petechial, thus suggesting meningococcemia. Except for the occurrence of rash, herpangina, pleurodynia, or myocarditis, there is little clinical evidence that helps in identifying the cause in a sporadic case of aseptic meningitis. Generalized muscle stiffness or spasm is usually observed, although the degree varies considerably; Kernig and Brudzinski signs are positive in fewer than half the cases. Deep tendon reflexes are usually normal.

The duration of illness is variable. In the majority of instances the temperature returns to normal within 4–6 days and disability resulting from neurologic involvement lasts 1–2 wk. Occasionally, a biphasic illness pattern occurs consisting of an initial period with fever, headache, nausea, vomiting, and muscle aches and pains of a few days duration followed by general recovery; then the same symptoms return with more pronounced neurologic involvement.

About 2% of the reported cases of *encephalitis* (Chapter 169.2) in the United States are demonstrated to have an enteroviral etiology. This is probably an underestimate of the number of severe cases, which may total over 1,000/yr. Echovirus type 9 is the most common cause of enteroviral encephalitis; other commonly associated enteroviral types are echoviruses 3, 4, 6, and 11 and coxsackieviruses B2, B4, and B5. In general, the prognosis in encephalitis caused by enteroviral infections is good, but fatalities have occurred in association with coxsackieviruses B3 and B6, echoviruses 2, 9, 17, and 25, and enterovirus 71.

Paralysis on the basis of anterior horn cell disease occasionally results from infection with nonpolio enteroviruses. Many coxsackieviruses and echoviruses have been associated with the *Guillain-Barré syndrome. Cerebellar ataxia* has been noted in association with coxsackieviruses A4, A7, A9, B3, and B4 and with echoviruses 6, 9, and 16. *Peripheral neuritis* has been reported with echovirus 9 infection, and coxsackievirus A9 has been noted in association with a *focal encephalitis and acute hemiplegia*.

Neonatal Infections. Nonpolio enteroviral infections in neonatal infants result in a wide variety of clinical manifestations ranging from asymptomatic infection to fatal encephalitis and myocarditis (see Chapter 97). Coxsackieviruses B1–B5 are associated with neonatal myocarditis. The illness usually begins within the first 2 wk of life. Most often, the mother is the source of infection. Nursery outbreaks also occur. The onset of neonatal myocarditis is sudden and associated with acute respiratory illness. Other symptoms are fever, feeding difficulties, respiratory distress, cyanosis, and lethargy. Later signs include cardiomegaly, hepatomegaly, and electrocardiographic changes. Cardiovascular signs are accompanied by various neurological manifestations in up to one third of cases. The prognosis is poor despite extensive supportive care.

DIAGNOSIS. The clinical differentiation of enteroviral disease from treatable bacterial illnesses is frequently very difficult, although when all the circumstances of a particular illness are considered, enteroviral diseases often can be suspected on clinical grounds. The most important factors in clinical diagnosis are season of the year, geographic location, exposure, incubation period, and clinical symptoms. In temperate climates enteroviral prevalence is distinctly seasonal; therefore, disease is usually seen in the summer and fall and unlikely to be seen in the winter; in the tropics enteroviruses are prevalent throughout the year. A careful history of maternal illness is vitally important in neonatal disease. For example, a mother's nonspecific mild febrile illness that occurs in the summer and fall should suggest the possibility of severe neonatal illness. Certain findings (i.e., aseptic meningitis, paralysis, pleurodynia, herpangina, pericarditis, myocarditis) should alert the clinician to enteroviral illnesses. The short incubation period of enteroviral infections should be taken into consideration. Polioviral infection should be considered in any unimmunized or incompletely immunized child with nonspecific febrile illness, aseptic meningitis, or paralytic disease.

Most viral diagnostic laboratories have facilities for recovering the majority of enteroviruses that cause illness. Tissue culture systems allow the isolation of polioviruses, group B coxsackieviruses, echoviruses, and coxsackieviruses A9 and A16. Enteroviral growth in tissue culture takes only a few days in many cases and less than a week in most; identification of type frequently takes much more time. A complete diagnostic isolation spectrum can be obtained using suckling mouse inoculation. Specimens for virus isolation should be obtained from the throat and rectum (feces) and any other clinically involved site. Virus isolation from all sites except the feces can usually be considered causally related to a specific illness. Molecular biology methods may detect viral RNA. Demonstration of a rise in neutralizing antibody titer to a virus recovered from the feces indicates recent infection and tends to indicate a causal role for the isolated virus. Serum should be collected and stored frozen as soon as possible after the onset of illness and then again 2–4 wk later.

DIFFERENTIAL DIAGNOSIS. The differential diagnosis of enteroviral infections depends upon the clinical manifestations. It is most important to distinguish bacterial diseases such as those commonly associated with pharyngitis, pneumonia, pericarditis, meningitis, and septicemia, although other viral illnesses must also be considered.

Paralytic Poliomyelitis. Conditions causing muscular weakness include the following:

1. *Infectious neuronitis* (Guillain-Barré syndrome) is the most common disease and the most difficult to distinguish from poliomyelitis. Generally, the fever, headache, and meningeal signs are less notable. Paralysis is characteristically symmetric, and sensory changes and pyramidal tract signs are common but are absent in poliomyelitis. Characteristically, there are few cells but elevated globulin content in the cerebrospinal fluid.
2. *Peripheral neuritis*—postinjectional, toxic (lead, avitaminosis), paralytic cranial herpes zoster, postdiphtheritic neuropathy—is excluded by history, sensory examination, and related findings.
3. Arthropod-borne viral *encephalitis, rabies,* and *tetanus* have been confused with bulbar poliomyelitis.
4. *Botulism* may closely simulate bulbar poliomyelitis; nuchal-spinal rigidity and pleocytosis are absent.
5. *Demyelinizing types of encephalomyelitis* are associated with or follow the exanthems and other infections or occur as an untoward sequel of antirabies vaccination.
6. *Tick-bite* paralysis is uncommon; meningeal signs are absent, and removal of the tick is followed by swift recovery.
7. *Neoplasms* originating in and around the spinal cord may rarely have a fairly abrupt onset.
8. *Familial periodic paralysis, myasthenia gravis,* and *acute porphyria* are uncommon causes of weakness.
9. *Hysteria* and *malingering* are rare in children.

Conditions causing pseudoparalysis do not present with nuchal-spinal rigidity or pleocytosis and include the following:

1. *Unrecognized trauma* from contusions, sprains, fractures,

and epiphyseal separation is a common cause of diagnostic confusion.

2. *Nonspecific (toxic) synovitis* produces a limp, usually unilaterally; the hip and the knee are the most common sites. There may be low-grade fever for several days.

3. *Acute osteomyelitis* has a more septic course; there is polymorphonuclear leukocytosis, with localized signs, positive blood culture, and, later, roentgenographic changes.

4. In *acute rheumatic fever* the clinical pattern is usually diagnostic.

5. *Scurvy* is revealed by a history of inadequate intake of vitamin C and by roentgenographic changes in the bones.

6. *Congenital syphilitic osteomyelitis* of the acute painful type is found only in early infancy.

Other Enteroviral Illnesses. The differential diagnoses of other enteroviral syndromes (respiratory, pericarditis and myocarditis, exanthems, meningitis and encephalitis, and so forth) are presented in the respective sections of this book relating to the clinical category.

COMPLICATIONS

Paralytic Poliomyelitis. *Melena* severe enough to require transfusion may result from single or multiple superficial intestinal erosions; perforation is rare. *Acute gastric dilatation* may occur abruptly during the acute or convalescent stage, causing further embarrassment of respiration; immediate gastric aspiration and external application of ice bags are indicated. Mild *hypertension* of a few days or weeks duration is common in the acute stage, probably related to lesions of the vasoregulatory centers in the medulla and especially to underventilation. In the later stages, because of immobilization, hypertension may occur along with hypercalcemia, nephrocalcinosis, and vascular lesions. Dimness of vision, headache, and a lightheaded feeling in association with hypertension should be regarded as premonitory of a frank convulsion. Cardiac irregularities are uncommon, but electrocardiographic abnormalities suggesting myocarditis are not rare. Acute pulmonary edema occurs occasionally, particularly in patients with arterial hypertension. Pulmonary embolism is uncommon despite the immobilization. Skeletal decalcification begins soon after immobilization and results in hypercalciuria, which in turn predisposes to calculi, especially when urinary stasis and infection are present. A high fluid intake is the only effective prophylactic measure. The patient should be mobilized as much and as early as possible.

Complications of enteroviral infections such as those associated with myocarditis or encephalitis are presented in other sections of this text.

PREVENTION. Vaccination is the only effective method of preventing poliomyelitis. Hygienic measures help to limit the spread of the infection among young children, but immunization is necessary to control transmission in older age groups. The efficacy of inactivated polio vaccine (IPV) and live, attenuated, orally administered polio vaccine (OPV) is well established. Both vaccines induce production of antibodies against the three strains of poliovirus. The specific immune response depends on the dose and potency of the vaccine and the age and immune status of the vaccinee. Very young infants may not respond well to either vaccine. The immunogenicity of the enhanced-potency killed vaccine is not affected by the presence of maternal antibodies. IPV has no adverse effects if manufactured properly. Live vaccine may undergo reversion to neurovirulence as it multiplies in the human intestinal tract and may cause vaccine-associated paralytic poliomyelitis (VAPP) in vaccinees or in their contacts. This risk is very low; hundreds of millions of doses have been given without incident.

IPV does not induce intestinal IgA production, whereas OPV induces significant mucosal immunity along the upper and lower alimentary tracts. Intestinal infection with wild-type virus may occur in recipients of IPV and be transmitted to nonimmune individuals. OPV stimulates pharyngeal as well as intestinal secretory IgA production, preventing virus replication at these sites. Transmission of wild-type virus by fecal spread is limited in OPV recipients. Most countries, including the United States, rely on OPV, whereas Sweden, Finland, and Holland use only IPV as the standard vaccine preparation. IPV and OPV are used in a combined regimen in Denmark and Israel.

Attenuated viral vaccines for enteroviruses other than polioviruses are not available. However, passive protection with pooled human immune globulin (0.2 mL/kg intramuscularly) may be useful in preventing disease. This is worthwhile only in sudden and virulent nursery outbreaks. Pooled human immune globulin in most instances can be expected to contain antibodies against coxsackievirus types B1-B5, offering protection to those infants without transplacentally acquired specific antibody who have not yet become infected.

TREATMENT

Poliomyelitis. The broad principles of management are to allay fear, to minimize ensuing skeletal deformities, to anticipate and meet complications in addition to the neuromusculoskeletal ones, and to prepare the child and family for the prolonged treatment that may be required and for permanent disability when this seems likely. Patients with the nonparalytic and mildly paralytic forms of poliomyelitis may be treated at home.

For the *abortive form* simple analgesics, sedatives, an attractive diet, and bed rest until the child's temperature is normal for several days suffice. Avoidance of exertion for the ensuing 2 wk is desirable, and there should be a careful neuromusculoskeletal examination 2 mo later to detect any minor involvement.

Treatment for the *nonparalytic form* is similar to that for the abortive form, relief being indicated in particular for the discomfort of muscle tightness and spasm of the neck, trunk, and extremities. Analgesics are more effective when combined with the application of hot packs for 15–30 min every 2–4 hr. Hot tub baths are sometimes useful. A firm bed is desirable and can be improvised at home by placing table leaves or a sheet of plywood beneath the mattress. A footboard should be used to keep the feet at a right angle with the legs. Muscular discomfort and spasm may continue for some weeks, even in the nonparalytic form, necessitating hot packs and gentle physical therapy. Such patients should also be carefully examined 2 mo after apparent recovery to detect minor residuals that might cause postural problems in later years.

Most patients with the *paralytic form* require hospitalization. A calm atmosphere is desirable. Suitable body alignment is necessary to avoid excessive skeletal deformity. A neutral position with the feet at a right angle, knees slightly flexed, and hips and spine straight is achieved by use of boards, sandbags, and, occasionally, light splint shells. Active and passive motions are indicated as soon as the pain has disappeared. Opiates and sedatives are permissible only if no impairment of ventilation is present or impending. Constipation is common, and fecal impaction should be prevented. When bladder paralysis occurs, a parasympathetic stimulant such as bethanechol (Urecholine), 5–10 mg orally or 2.5–5.0 mg subcutaneously, may induce voiding in 15–30 min; some patients do not respond, and others have nausea, vomiting, and palpitation. Bladder paresis rarely lasts more than a few days. If bethanechol fails, manual compression of the bladder and the psychologic effect of running water should be tried. If catheterization must be performed, strict asepsis is essential. An interesting diet and a relatively high fluid intake should be started at once unless there is vomiting. Additional salt should be provided if the environmental temperature is high or if the application of hot packs induces sweating. Anorexia is common initially. Adequate dietary and fluid intake can be maintained by the placement of a central venous catheter. The orthopedist and the physiatrist should see these patients as early in the course of illness as possible and assume responsibility before fixed deformities develop. The management of *pure bulbar poliomyelitis* consists of maintaining the airway and avoiding all risks of inhalation of saliva, food, or vomitus. Gravity drainage of accumulated secretions is favored by using the head-low (foot of bed elevated 20–25 degrees) prone position with the face to one side. Aspirators with rigid or semirigid tips are preferred for direct oral and pharyngeal use, and soft, flexible catheters may be used for nasopharyngeal aspiration. Fluid and electrolyte equilibrium is best maintained by intravenous infusion because tube or oral feeding in the first few days may incite vomiting. In addition to close observation for respiratory insufficiency, the blood pressure should be taken at least twice daily because hypertension is not uncommon and occasionally leads to hypertensive encephalopathy. Patients with pure bulbar poliomyelitis may require tracheostomy because of vocal cord paralysis or constriction of the hypopharynx; the majority who recover have little residual impairment, although some patients exhibit mild dysphagia and occasional vocal fatigue with slurring of speech.

Impaired ventilation must be recognized early; mounting anxiety, restlessness, and fatigue are early indications for prompt intervention. Tracheostomy is indicated for some patients with pure bulbar poliomyelitis, spinal respiratory muscle paralysis, and bulbospinal paralysis because these patients are generally unable to cough, sometimes for many months. Mechanical respirators are often needed.

Nonpolio Enteroviruses. There is no specific therapy for any enterovirus infection. In severe, catastrophic, and generalized neonatal infection, it is probably advisable to administer immune globulin to the infant, but there is no evidence that this therapy is beneficial. Corticosteroids should not be given during acute severe enteroviral infections, such as neonatal myocarditis or encephalitis, although some authors believe this therapy has been beneficial in patients with coxsackievirus myocarditis. These agents have had deleterious effects in experimental coxsackieviral infections of mice. Because the possibility of bacterial sepsis cannot be ruled out in many instances of enteroviral infections, antibiotics should frequently be administered for the most likely potential bacterial pathogens.

PROGNOSIS. Mortality in large urban epidemics of poliomyelitis in the United States in the prevaccine era was 5–7%. Most deaths occur within the first 2 wk after onset. Mortality and the degree of disability are greater after the age of puberty. In general, the more extensive the paralysis in the first 10 days of illness, the more severe is the ultimate disability. Unexpected improvement may appear soon after defervescence and again about 6 wk after onset, a time that corresponds to functional restoration of temporarily inactive neurons. The degree of functional recovery also depends upon the adequacy and promptness of therapy as related to proper body positioning, active motion, use of assistive devices, and, of great importance, the psychologic motivation of the patient to return to as full and normal a life as possible. A long-term follow-up study of adults with postpoliomyelitis neuromuscular symptoms has shown slowly progressive non–life threatening muscle weakness, with a greater effect occurring in patients in whom poliomyelitis had caused severe disability and muscle weakness.

The prognosis in nonpolio enteroviral infections in the vast majority of instances is excellent. Morbidity and mortality are related almost entirely to cardiac and neurologic disease in older children and these same diseases accompanied by general disseminated infection in neonates.

GENERAL

Cherry JD: Enteroviruses: Polioviruses (poliomyelitis), coxsackieviruses, echoviruses and enteroviruses. *In*: Feigin RD, Cherry JD (eds): Textbook of Pediatric Infectious Diseases, 2nd ed. Philadelphia, WB Saunders, 1992, pp 1705–1753.

Christie AB: Infectious Diseases, Epidemiology and Clinical Practice, 4th ed. London, Longman Group UK, LTD, 1987, p 753.

Melnick JL: Enteroviruses. *In*: Evans AS (ed): Viral Infections of Humans; Epidemiology and Control, 3rd ed. New York, Plenum Medical Book Co, 1989, pp 191–263.

Modlin JF: Poliovirus, coxsackieviruses, echoviruses and newer enteroviruses. *In*: Mandel GL, Gordon DR, Bennet JE (eds): Principles and Practice of Infectious Diseases, 4th ed. New York, Churchill Livingstone, 1995, pp 1606–1636.

Murray PR, Kabayashi GS, Pfaller MA, et al: Medical Microbiology, 2nd ed. London, Mosby-Year Book, 1994, pp 607–619.

SPECIFIC

Dagan R, Hall CB, Powell KR, et al: Epidemiology and laboratory diagnosis of infection with viral and bacterial pathogens in infants hospitalized for suspected sepsis. J Pediatr 115:351, 1989.

Faden H, Modlin JF, Thomas ML, et al: Comparative evaluation of immunization with live attenuated and enhanced-potency inactivated trivalent poliovirus vaccines in childhood: Systemic and local immune responses. J Infect Dis 162:1291, 1990.

Hayward JC, Gillespie SM, Kaplan KM, et al: Outbreak of poliomyelitis-like paralysis associated with enterovirus 71. Pediatr Infect Dis J 8:611, 1989.

Howard RS, Wiles CM, Spencer GT: The late sequelae of poliomyelitis. Q J Med (New Series 66) 251:219, 1988.

Kaplan MH, Klein SW, McPhee J, et al: Group B coxsackievirus infections in infants younger than three months of age: A serious childhood illness. Rev Infect Dis 5:1019, 1983.

Modlin JF: Perinatal echovirus infection: Insights from a literature review of 61 cases of serious infection and 16 outbreaks in nurseries. Rev Infect Dis 8:918, 1986.

Moore M: Enteroviral disease in the United States, 1970–1979. J Infect Dis 146:103, 1982.

Ogra PL, Garofalo R: Secretory antibody response to viral vaccines. Prog Med Virol 37:156, 1990.

Strikas RA, Anderson LJ, Parker RA: Temporal and geographic patterns of isolates of nonpolio enterovirus in the United States, 1970–1983. J Infect Dis 153:346, 1986.

Yin-Murphy M: Acute hemorrhagic conjunctivitis. Prog Med Virol 29:23, 1984.

CHAPTER 210
Parvovirus B19

William C. Koch

Parvoviruses are small, DNA-containing viruses that infect a variety of animal species. Several parvoviruses are recognized as important causes of disease in animals such as canine parvovirus and feline panleukopenia virus, but parvovirus B19 is the only strain that is pathogenic in humans. Parvovirus B19 was discovered by Cossart and coworkers in 1975 as an anomalous precipitin line during counterimmunoelectrophoresis screening of blood for hepatitis B antigen. The new virus was associated with human disease in 1981 when Pattison and colleagues linked it with the aplastic crisis of sickle cell disease. The frequency of B19 infection in the general pediatric population was not understood until 1983 when Anderson and colleagues identified B19 as the cause of erythema infectiosum.

ETIOLOGIC AGENT. Parvovirus B19 is a member of the genus *Parvovirus* in the family Parvoviridae. The mammalian parvoviruses are very species specific. B19 does not infect other animals, and animal parvoviruses do not infect humans.

B19 is composed of an icosahedral protein capsid without an envelope that contains single-stranded DNA approximately 5.5 kb in length. It is relatively heat and solvent resistant. It is antigenically distinct from other mammalian parvoviruses, and there is only one known serotype. Parvoviruses replicate in dividing cells. Because of their limited genome, they require host cell factors present in late S phase to replicate. B19 can be propagated only in erythropoietin-stimulated erythropoietic cells derived from human bone marrow or primary fetal liver culture.

EPIDEMIOLOGY AND TRANSMISSION. Infections with parvovirus B19 are common and worldwide. In outbreak studies, clinically apparent infections (rash illness and aplastic crisis) are most prevalent in school-age children, with 70% of cases occurring among children 5–15 yr old. Although sporadic infections occur year-round, community outbreaks show seasonal peaks in the late winter and spring. Serologic testing demonstrates that many infections are clinically inapparent. Antibody prevalence increases with increasing age. Serologic surveys from many different countries have shown that 40–60% of adults have evidence of prior infection.

Transmission of B19 is by the respiratory route, presumably via large droplet spread. In studies of volunteers infected intranasally, virus could be detected in respiratory secretions 7–11 days after inoculation at a time when they were also viremic. Virus is detected in the respiratory secretions of children immediately before an aplastic crisis. The incubation period for erythema infectiosum ranges from 4–28 days (average, 16–17 days). The incubation period for other clinical manifestations such as aplastic crisis is shorter because viremia precedes the rash.

The transmission rate in households ranges from 15–30% in susceptible contacts; mothers are more commonly infected than fathers. In outbreaks of erythema infectiosum in elementary schools, the secondary attack rates range from 10–60%. Nosocomial outbreaks are described with secondary attack rates of 30% in susceptible health care workers.

Although respiratory spread is the primary mode of transmission, B19 is transmissible in blood and blood products, as shown in hemophiliac children receiving pooled donor clotting factor. Given its resistance to solvents, fomite transmission could be important, but this mode of transmission is not documented.

PATHOGENESIS AND IMMUNITY. The primary target of B19 infection is the erythroid cell line, specifically erythroid precursors near the pronormoblast stage. The virus lyses these cells, leading to a progressive depletion and a transient arrest of erythropoiesis. The virus has no apparent effect on the myeloid cell line. The tropism for erythroid cells is related to the erythrocyte P blood group antigen, which seems to act as a receptor site for B19 on these cells. Endothelial cells and myocardial cells also possess this antigen. Viral suppression of erythropoiesis is reversed *in vitro* by convalescent serum containing B19 antibodies. Humoral immunity is crucial in controlling infection. Thrombocytopenia and neutropenia are often observed, but their pathogenesis is unexplained.

Individuals with conditions of chronic hemolysis and increased red cell turnover are very susceptible to perturbations in erythropoiesis. Infection with B19 leads to a transient arrest in red cell production and a precipitous fall in serum hemoglobin, usually requiring transfusion. The reticulocyte count falls to near zero, reflecting the lysis of infected erythroid precursors. Specific immunoglobulin (Ig) M appears within 1–2 days followed by anti-B19 IgG and the infection is controlled, leading to a reticulocytosis and a rise in serum hemoglobin.

Experimental infection of normal volunteers reveals a biphasic illness. Seven to 11 days after inoculation, the subjects acquired viremia with fever, malaise, and mild upper respiratory infection symptoms. Their reticulocyte counts dropped to less than 0.1% but resulted only in a mild, clinically insignificant fall in serum hemoglobin. Symptoms resolved and hemoglobin returned to normal with the appearance of specific antibodies. Several subjects experienced a rash 17–18 days after inoculation associated with arthralgia. Some manifestations of B19 infection, such as transient aplastic crisis, appear to be a direct result of viral infection, whereas others, including the exanthem and arthritis, appear to be postinfectious phenomena related to the immune response. Skin biopsy results from patients with erythema infectiosum are compatible with an immune process, showing edema in the epidermis and a perivascular mononuclear infiltrate.

Individuals with impaired ability to produce specific antibodies are likely to be at risk for more serious or persistent infection with B19, which usually manifests as chronic red cell aplasia, but neutropenia, thrombocytopenia, and marrow failure are also described. Children with leukemia on chemotherapy or with congenital immunodeficiency states, and patients with AIDS are at risk for chronic B19 infections.

Infections in the fetus and neonate are somewhat analogous to infections in the immunocompromised host. B19 is associated with nonimmune fetal hydrops and stillbirth in women experiencing a primary infection. Like most mammalian parvoviruses, B19 can cross the placenta and gain access to the fetus during primary maternal infection. Most infections during pregnancy result in normal deliveries at term. Some of these asymptomatic infants have been reported to have chronic postnatal infection with B19 of unknown significance. In some cases, fetal infection leads to profound anemia and subsequent high-output cardiac failure. Fetal hydrops ensues and mortality is high. There may also be a direct effect of the virus on myocardial tissue.

CLINICAL MANIFESTATIONS

ERYTHEMA INFECTIOSUM (FIFTH DISEASE). The most common manifestation of parvovirus B19 is erythema infectiosum (EI), also known as fifth disease, which is a benign, self-limited exanthematous illness of childhood. It was the fifth in a classification scheme of childhood exanthems; the others were rubella, measles, scarlet fever, and Filatov-Dukes disease (atypical scarlet fever). The hallmark of fifth disease is the characteristic rash. The prodromal phase is mild and consists of low-grade fever, headache and mild URI symptoms. The typical rash of EI occurs in three stages that are not always distinguishable. The initial stage is an erythematous facial flushing, often described as a "slapped-cheek" appearance. The rash spreads rapidly or concurrently to the trunk and proximal extremities as a diffuse macular erythema in the second stage. Central clearing of macular lesions occurs promptly, giving the rash a lacy, reticulated appearance. Palms and soles are spared, and the rash tends to be more prominent on extensor surfaces. Affected children are afebrile and not ill-appearing. Older children and adults often complain of mild pruritus. The rash resolves spontaneously without desquamation but tends to wax and wane over 1–3 wk. It can recur with exposure to sunlight, heat, exercise, and stress. Lymphadenopathy and atypical papular, purpuric, vesicular rashes are also described.

Transient Aplastic Crisis. Individuals with chronic hemolytic conditions may experience transient red cell aplasia after contact with B19. The transient arrest of erythropoiesis and absolute reticulocytopenia induced by B19 infection leads to a sudden fall in serum hemoglobin. In contrast to children with EI, these patients are ill with fever, malaise, and lethargy and have signs and symptoms of profound anemia, such as pallor, tachycardia, and tachypnea. Rash is rarely present. Children with sickle hemoglobinopathies may also have a concurrent vaso-occlusive pain crisis. B19-induced aplastic crises occur in patients with all types of chronic hemolysis, including sickle cell disease, thalassemia, hereditary spherocytosis, and pyruvate kinase deficiency.

Arthropathy. Arthritis and arthralgia occur as a complication of fifth disease or as the only clinical manifestation of B19 infection. Joint symptoms are much more common in adults and older adolescents. Females are affected more frequently than males. In one outbreak of fifth disease, 60% of adults and 80% of adult women reported joint symptoms. Joint symptoms range from diffuse arthralgias with morning stiffness to frank arthritis. The joints most often affected are the hands, wrists, knees, and ankles, but practically all have been reported. The joint symptoms are self-limited and, in the majority of patients, resolve within 2–4 wk. Some patients have a prolonged course of many months, suggesting rheumatoid arthritis. Transient rheumatoid factor positivity is reported in some of these patients but with no joint destruction.

Infection in the Immunocompromised Host. Patients with impaired humoral immunity are at risk for chronic infections with parvovirus B19. Chronic anemia is the most common manifestation, sometimes accompanied by other cytopenias or complete marrow suppression. Chronic infections are seen in children with cancer receiving cytotoxic chemotherapy, children with congenital acquired immunodeficiency syndrome (AIDS), and patients with defects in IgG class switching who are unable to generate neutralizing antibodies.

Fetal Infections. Primary maternal infection is associated with nonimmune fetal hydrops and intrauterine fetal demise. The incidence of these outcomes after maternal infection is low, estimated at 5% or less. The mechanism of fetal disease appears to be a viral-induced red cell aplasia at a time when the fetal erythroid fraction is rapidly expanding. This can lead to profound anemia, high-output cardiac failure, and hydrops. Viral DNA has been detected in infected abortuses. The second trimester seems to be the most sensitive time, but fetal losses are reported at every stage of gestation. Most infants infected in utero are born normally at term, even when there is evidence of hydrops by ultrasonography. Some of these infants may acquire a chronic or persistent postnatal infection with B19, but its significance is unknown. Fetal infection has not been associated with other birth defects.

COMPLICATIONS. Erythema infectiosum is often accompanied by arthralgias or arthritis in adolescents and adults, which may persist after resolution of the rash. B19 causes thrombocytopenic purpura and rarely aseptic meningitis in normal individuals after EI. B19 is also a cause of virus-associated hemophagocytic syndrome, usually in immunocompromised patients.

DIFFERENTIAL DIAGNOSIS. The rash of erythema infectiosum must be differentiated from rubella, measles, enteroviral infections, and drug reactions. Older children with rash and arthritis should prompt consideration of juvenile rheumatoid arthritis, systemic lupus erythematosus, and other connective tissue disorders.

DIAGNOSIS. Laboratory tests for the diagnosis of B19 infection are not available routinely. Diagnosis of EI is usually based on clinical observation of the typical rash and exclusion of other conditions. The virus cannot be isolated by culture. Determination of anti-B19 IgM is the best marker of recent or acute infection on a single serum sample when B19 serology is available. IgM develops rapidly after infection and persists for up to 6–8 wk. Seroconversion in paired sera can also be used to confirm recent infection. Anti-B19 IgG serves as a marker of past infection or immunity. Serologic diagnosis is unreliable in patients with immunodeficiencies. Methods to detect viral particles or viral DNA such as polymerase chain reaction or DNA hybridization are necessary to make the diagnosis.

TREATMENT AND PREVENTION. There is no specific antiviral therapy. Commercial lots of intravenous immunoglobin (IVIG) have been used with some success to treat B19-related episodes of anemia and bone marrow failure in immunocompromised children. Specific antibody may allow clearance of the virus, but it is not always necessary because cessation of cytotoxic chemotherapy will often suffice. In patients whose immune status is not likely to recover, such as in AIDS, administration of IVIG may give only a temporary remission, and periodic reinfusions may be required.

Anecdotal reports of treating nonimmune fetal hydrops caused by B19 with intrauterine transfusion and IVIG have appeared. This therapy carries its own risks and is not generally recommended. There are no data to support the use of IVIG for postexposure prophylaxis in pregnant care-givers or in immunocompromised children.

Preventive strategies are based on an understanding of the pathophysiology of the particular clinical syndrome. Children with erythema infectiosum are not likely to be infectious at presentation because the rash and arthropathy represent immune-mediated, postinfectious phenomenon. Isolation and exclusion from school or day care are unnecessary and ineffective after diagnosis.

Children with B19-induced red cell aplasia (aplastic crisis) are infectious when they present and experience a more intense viremia. Most of these children require transfusion and supportive care until their hematologic status is stable. They should be isolated in the hospital to prevent spread to susceptible patients and staff. Isolation should continue for at least 1 wk and until the patient is afebrile. Pregnant care-givers should not be assigned to these patients. Exclusion of pregnant women from the workplace where children with EI may be present is not recommended as a general policy because it is unlikely to reduce their risk. No vaccine is available.

Anand A, Gray ES, Brown T, et al: Human parvovirus infection in pregnancy and hydrops fetalis. N Engl J Med 316:183, 1987.
Anderson LJ: Human parvoviruses. J Infect Dis 161:603, 1990.
Anderson MJ, Jones SE, Fisher-Hoch SP, et al: Human parvovirus, the cause of erythema infectiosum (fifth disease)? Lancet 1:1378, 1983.
Cherry JD: Parvovirus. *In*: Feigin RD, Cherry JD (eds): Textbook of Pediatrics Infectious Diseases, 3rd ed. Philadelphia, WB Saunders, 1992, pp 1626–1633.
Chorba T, Coccia R, Holman RC, et al: The role of parvovirus B19 in aplastic crisis and erythema infectiosum (fifth disease). J Infect Dis 154:383, 1986.
Koch WC, Massey G, Russell CE, Adler SP: Manifestations and treatment of human parvovirus B19 infection in immunocompromised patients. J Pediatr 116:355, 1990.
Pattison JR (ed): Parvoviruses and Human Disease. Boca Raton, FL, CRC Press, 1988.
Ware R: Human parvovirus infection. J Pediatr 114:343, 1989.

CHAPTER 211
Herpes Simplex Virus

Steve Kohl

Herpes Simplex Virus (HSV) is common among humans, and has a variety of clinical manifestations involving the skin, mucous membranes, eye, central nervous system, and genital tract. It also causes generalized systemic disease. Disease manifestations are in large part determined by the immune competence of the host. Two strains of the virus are identified: HSV-1 commonly infects skin and mucous membranes above the waist. HSV-2 primarily infects the genitalia and the neonate.

Two types of infection are recognized:

1. *Primary* infection is the susceptible host's first experience with the virus, which in most instances is a subclinical infection; otherwise there are usually local superficial lesions (see later discussion) accompanied by varying degrees of systemic reaction. In newborn infants and severely malnourished infants, a serious systemic infection, often without superficial lesions, may occur. Circulating antibodies and a cell-mediated response develop in nonfatal cases.

2. Recurrent herpetic lesions represent reactivation of a latent infection in an immune host with circulating antibodies. Reactivation follows such nonspecific stimuli as changes in the external milieu (e.g., cold, ultraviolet light) or in the internal milieu (e.g., menstruation, fever, or emotional stress). The lesions tend to be localized and, generally, are not associated with systemic reactions. Viral reactivation may take place in

the absence of clinical recurrence, leading to asymptomatic viral shedding.

ETIOLOGY. HSV is a double-stranded DNA containing enveloped virus. The icosahedral protein core is surrounded by a lipid envelope in which is embedded a number of viral glycoproteins (e.g., glycoproteins B, C, D) responsible for viral–target cell interaction and infection. These glycoproteins are also key targets for the host humoral and cellular immune response. HSV grows rapidly in human and nonhuman cell lines and produces characteristic cytopathic changes. HSV-1 and HSV-2 may be differentiated by DNA analysis (endonuclease restriction analysis) and commercially by reactivity with type-specific monoclonal antibodies in a variety of fluorescent and enzyme-linked immunosorbent (ELISA) assays. Several enzymes important for viral DNA synthesis, such as thymidine kinase and DNA polymerase, are useful targets for antiviral agents.

EPIDEMIOLOGY. The virus develops an extremely compatible relationship with its host. In about 85% of instances the infection is subclinical. Even when clinical manifestations are present, the host is only rarely seriously disabled. Occasionally, the primary or recurrent infection may lead to institutional or family outbreaks of stomatitis. This has been reported in orphanages and day-care center settings. HSV may also be transmitted by infection of digits (whitlows), during contact sports such as rugby or wrestling (herpes gladiatorum), and rarely in the hospital setting. The incubation period is 2–12 days (average, 6 days). The spread of infection appears to be determined by two factors: close bodily contact and trauma such as teething or a break in the skin.

The higher incidence of HSV antibodies in lower socioeconomic groups correlates with crowded living conditions. The epidemiology differs for the two types of HSV. Detailed serologic studies have been done primarily in low-income groups, in which most infants have transplacental antibody for about the first 6 mo of life. From 1–4 yr, there is a sharp rise in antibodies to HSV-1 and then a much slower rate of acquisition up to 14 yr. At this time, there is a second sharp rise in antibodies, mostly to HSV-2. By adult life HSV antibodies are seen in by far the majority of persons in the lower socioeconomic groups. HSV-1 antibodies are found in 30% of university students. HSV-2 antibodies are found in up to 60% of the lower socioeconomic status adults. The incidence of type 2 antibody in higher socioeconomic groups is about 10–30% and in nuns about 3%.

Once infected, the majority of people continue to carry the virus in a latent state and maintain an almost constant level of circulating antibodies. The initial level of antibodies reached after a primary infection may fall, and several subclinical reinfections may occur before a stable antibody level is established. Carriers may distribute the virus without having any manifest lesion. Herpes simplex virus can be isolated from the pharynx of about 5% of asymptomatic adults.

PATHOLOGY. The pathologic changes vary with the tissue infected. In general, a specific lesion is characterized by the presence of intranuclear inclusion bodies, homogeneous masses lying in the midst of a severely disorganized nucleus in which the basic chromatin has marginated to the nuclear membrane. Around the specific lesion there is always evidence of an acute inflammatory reaction. In the skin and mucous membranes the typical lesion is a unilocular vesicle. In the skin the vesicle is tense. Ballooned epithelial cells containing intranuclear inclusions can best be seen at the margins of the vesicle. The vesicular fluid contains infected epithelial cells, including multinucleated giant cells and leukocytes. In the corium there is no necrosis, but capillaries are dilated, and there is infiltration with mononuclear and polymorphonuclear cells. In the mucous membrane, because of maceration, there is early leakage of the vesicular fluid resulting in a collapsed vesicle, mainly filled with fibrin. The edematous roof cells form a gray membrane over the lesion.

In otherwise healthy persons, the lesions are confined to the skin and mucous membranes; viremia has rarely been described. Bloodstream spread of the virus with resultant widely disseminated disease is seen mainly in the newborn, in severely malnourished children, in persons with skin diseases such as eczema, and in those with defects in cell-mediated immunity. In these patients the virus spreads hematogenously from the portal of entry to susceptible organs. Virus increases within these organs, and secondary viremia occurs with evidence of extensive cell destruction. It is probable, however, that most cases of HSV-1 encephalitis other than in the newborn are caused by neurogenic transmission of the virus to the brain. Healing begins with clearing of the viremia and a decrease in the production of virus within the cells.

CLINICAL MANIFESTATIONS. HSV characteristically produces a vesicular lesion. Only rarely is there a viremic distribution that results in widespread systemic disease or neurogenic transmission that leads to meningoencephalitis (see later and Chapter 169.2). Furthermore, although the occurrence of primary and recurrent lesions is an accepted characteristic of herpetic infection, their distinction clinically is often not possible without knowledge of the presence or absence of serum antibodies in the patient.

Lesions of the Skin and Mucous Membranes. On the skin the lesion consists of aggregates of thin-walled vesicles on an erythematous base. These rupture, scab, and heal within 7–10 days without leaving a scar except after repeated attacks or secondary bacterial infections; temporary depigmentation may occur in blacks. The local lesions may be preceded by mild irritation or burning at the local site or by severe neuralgic pain in the region. In children the vesicles often become secondarily infected, introducing impetigo contagiosa into the differential diagnosis. The lesions tend to recur at the same site, particularly at mucocutaneous junctions, but may occur anywhere.

Primary infection, especially in the immunocompromised patient, may, uncommonly, result in a generalized vesicular eruption in which the lesions are small and may continue to appear over a period of 2–3 wk. If the systemic manifestations are mild, the infection must be differentiated from varicella.

Traumatic lesions of the skin can be infected by HSV. Primary lesions can also occur on apparently unbroken skin, as, for example, on the chin of a drooling infant with herpetic stomatitis, in whom scattered isolated vesicles appear, in contrast to the grouped vesicles of recurrent attacks. When the skin of a limb is infected, vesicles appear in 2–3 days at the site of trauma. There is often centripetal spread along lymph channels, causing enlargement of regional lymph nodes and scattered vesicles on the intervening undamaged skin. The final clinical picture may be mistaken for that of *herpes zoster,* especially if accompanied by neuralgic pain, unless the lesions are recognized as not being confined to a dermatome. The lesions heal slowly, often taking 3 wk; recurrences at the site of local trauma are common and may assume a bullous pattern. Wrestlers and medical personnel are prone to herpetic infections of superficial abrasions (herpes gladiatorum and herpetic whitlow). In the latter, infection of minor trauma about the nails leads to extremely painful, deep-seated spreading lesions with vesicles that resolve spontaneously in 2–3 wk. Similar lesions occur on the fingers of thumb suckers who are suffering from herpetic gingivostomatitis. The lesions should not be incised.

Acute Herpetic Gingivostomatitis (Acute Infectious Gingivostomatitis; Catarrhal Stomatitis; Ulcerative Stomatitis; Vincent Stomatitis). This primary infection, probably the most common cause of stomatitis in children 1–3 yr of age, can also occur in older children and adults. The symptoms may appear abruptly, with pain in the mouth, salivation, fetor oris, refusal to eat, and fever, often as high as

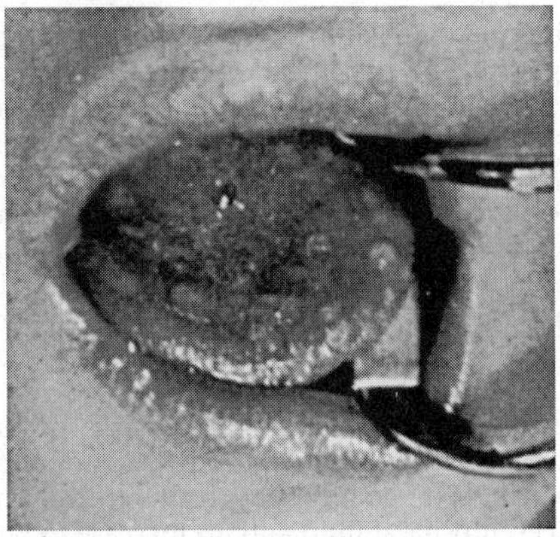

Figure 211–1. Lesions of herpetic stomatitis on the tongue.

40–40.6° C (104–105° F). The onset may be insidious, with fever and irritability preceding the oral lesions by 1–2 days. The initial lesion is a vesicle (Fig. 211–1), which is seldom seen because of its early rupture. The residual lesion is 2–10 mm in diameter and is covered with a yellow-gray membrane (Fig. 211–2). When this membrane sloughs, a true ulcer remains. Although the tongue and cheeks are most commonly involved, no part of the oral lining is exempt. Except in edentulous infants, acute gingivitis is characteristic of the disease and may precede the appearance of mucosal vesicles. Submaxillary lymphadenitis is common. The acute phase lasts 4–9 days and is self-limited. Pain tends to disappear 2–4 days before healing of the ulcers is complete. In some instances the tonsillar regions are involved early and appear exudative, and acute tonsillitis of bacterial origin or enterovirus-induced herpangina may be suspected. Negative cultures for *Streptococcus* and other bacterial pathogens and failure of the lesion to respond to antibiotic therapy differentiate a bacterial infection. The spread of the vesiculation to the buccal mucosa and anterior portion of the mouth is atypical for herpangina.

Recurrent Stomatitis and Herpes Labialis. The typical oral recurrence of HSV is one or a few vesicles grouped at the mucocutaneous junction. Lesions are usually accompanied by local pain, tingling, or itching and lasts 3–7 days. Systemic symptoms are unusual. Less commonly, localized lesions may occur on the palate in association with a febrile illness or on the mucosa adjacent to a lesion on the lip. Recurrent aphthous ulcers, however, are not caused by HSV. In some persons a generalized stomatitis recurs consistently 7–10 days after a recurrent herpetic lesion of the lip or elsewhere and is often accompanied by skin lesions of erythema multiforme. Indeed, recurrent HSV infection is one of the most common causes of recurrent erythema multiforme.

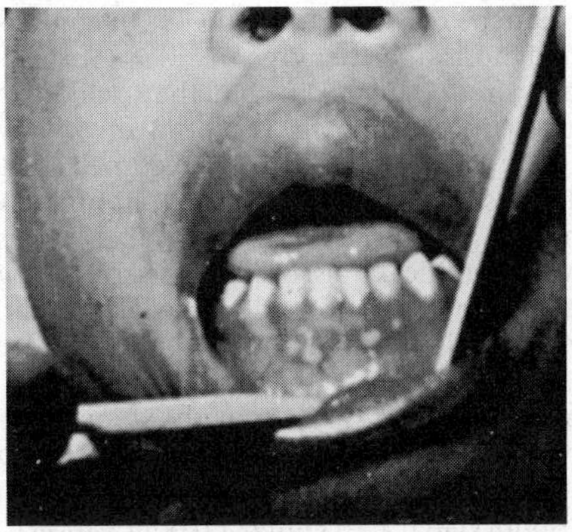

Figure 211–2. Herpetic stomatitis.

Eczema Herpeticum (Kaposi Varicelliform Eruption; Juliusberg Pustulosis Vacciniformis Acuta). This, the most serious manifestation of "traumatic herpes," results from a widespread and usually primary infection of the eczematous skin with HSV. The severity of this complication varies; the lesion may be so mild as to be overlooked, or it may be fatal. In a typical severe primary attack, vesicles develop abruptly in large numbers over the area of eczematous skin. They continue to appear in crops for as long as 7–9 days. Isolated at first, they later become grouped and may occur on adjoining areas of normal skin (Fig. 211–3). Wide denudation of the epidermis may occur. Scabs eventually form, and epithelialization occurs. The systemic reaction varies, but temperatures of 39.4–40.6° C (103–105° F) for 7–10 days are not uncommon. Recurrent attacks develop on chronic atopic skin lesions. Death may result from profound physiologic disturbances from loss of fluid, electrolytes, and protein through the skin, from dissemination of the virus to the brain and other organs, or from secondary bacterial invasion. A differentiation from *eczema vaccinatum* can usually be made by determining with reasonable certainty that the child has not been exposed to vaccinia and by the occurrence of crops of vesicles in herpes. The diagnosis can be accurately established by examination of vesicular fluid with rapid viral diagnostic techniques (see later discussion, Diagnosis).

Ocular Lesions. *Conjunctivitis* and *keratoconjunctivitis* may occur as manifestations of either a primary or recurrent infection. The conjunctiva appears congested and swollen, but there is little, if any, purulent discharge. In primary infection the preauricular node is usually enlarged and tender. Cataracts, uveitis, and chorioretinitis have been described in newborn infants and in the immunocompromised.

Corneal lesions may be superficial, in the form of a dendritic ulcer, or deep, as a disciform keratitis. Dendritic keratitis is unique to HSV eye involvement. The diagnosis is suggested by the presence of herpetic vesicles on the lids; it is established by the isolation of the virus. The highly contagious *epidemic keratoconjunctivitis* (shipyard conjunctivitis) caused by any of several serotypes of adenovirus must be considered in the

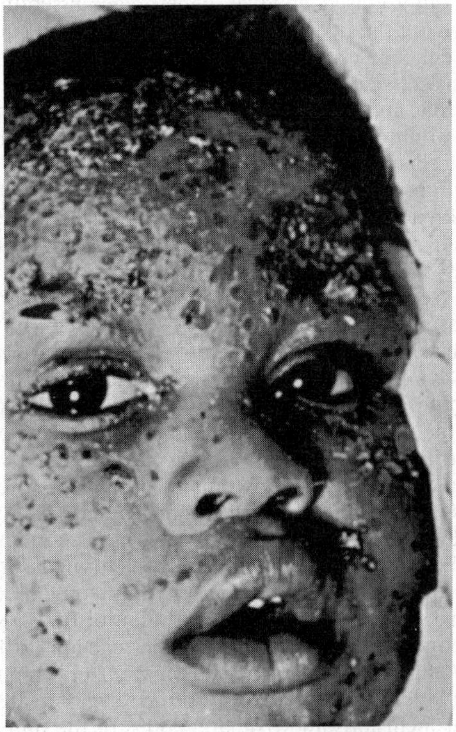

Figure 211–3. Eczema herpeticum.

differential diagnosis. Recurrent herpetic corneal infection may result in scarring of the cornea and vision impairment.

Genital Herpes. Genital infections with herpesvirus occur most commonly in adolescents and young adults, are usually due to HSV-2, and are usually spread by sexual activity. Although hand to genital infection and autoinoculation are possible, genital or rectal herpes in a young child warrants a sensitive and careful appraisal of the possibility of child abuse. Ten to 25% of cases of primary genital herpes are caused by HSV-1. Almost all cases of recurrent genital herpes are due to HSV-2. In primary genital infection, when the patient has no antibody to either type of herpes (approximately 30% of cases), systemic symptoms such as fever, regional adenopathy, and dysuria are more likely to occur. In adult women, the vulva and vagina may be involved with vesicles and ulcers, but the cervix is the primary site of infection. Recurrence is common. Both primary and recurrent disease are frequently subclinical, but virus shed during this time may infect a sex partner or an infant during passage through the birth canal.

In males herpetic vesicles or ulcers are usually seen on the glans penis, prepuce, or shaft of the penis. The scrotum is less frequently involved. Genital HSV is a risk factor for human immunodeficiency virus (HIV) infection.

Systemic Infection

IN THE NEWBORN INFANT. See Chapter 97.2.

IN THE IMMUNOCOMPROMISED HOST. Unusually severe HSV infection may occur in a variety of hosts including the newborn (see Chapter 95); the severely malnourished; and children with malignancies or other conditions necessitating immunosuppressive therapy, with acquired immunodeficiency virus (AIDS), with burns, or with primary immunodeficiency diseases that particularly impair cell-mediated immunity. In children receiving therapy for cancer or organ transplantation, the risk of severe HSV infection coincides with the time of maximum immunosuppression. The most common syndrome is local and chronic mucocutaneous disease. The lesions may resemble typical vesicles and ulcers or progress to large necrotic painful erosions or atypical exophytic, wartlike lesions. Mucositis, esophagitis, proctitis and pneumonitis are less common. The most severe manifestation, usually a result of primary infection in the immunocompromised child, is widespread disseminated disease involving the liver, lungs, adrenal gland, and central nervous system. These patients have a sepsis-like syndrome with leukopenia, disseminated intravascular coagulopathy, fever, or hypothermia and progression to death. Skin lesions may be localized to mucous membranes, widely disseminated, resembling varicella infection, or absent. This form of HSV infection has a high mortality rate even with therapy.

Central Nervous System Infection. (See Chapter 169.2.) HSV has a predilection to infect the nervous system. Both types 1 and 2 may cause a meningoencephalitis as part of neonatal HSV infection (see Chapter 97.2). In patients with primary genital herpes, usually resulting from HSV-2, an aseptic meningitis syndrome may complicate the course. The cerebrospinal fluid reveals a lymphocytic pleocytosis, and the virus may be cultured from it in patients with this self-limited syndrome. HSV-1 is the most common cause of fatal sporadic encephalitis. It has a striking predilection to involve the frontal and parietal areas. Typical signs and symptoms include fever, altered consciousness, headache, personality changes, seizures, dysphasia, and focal neurologic signs. If untreated, the mortality rate is apparently 75%, with severe sequelae in survivors. HSV is the cause of some cases of recurrent aseptic meningitis (Mollaret meningitis), on the basis of demonstration of HSV DNA in the cerebrospinal fluid by polymerase chain reaction (PCR).

LABORATORY DATA. Microscopic examination of scrapings from lesions (Tzanck stain) reveals multinuclear giant cells and intranuclear inclusions approximately 50% of the time. Specific antigen detection methods such as ELISA and immunofluorescent techniques applied to these specimens can be useful in rapidly diagnosing herpes infection and in differentiating the two types of herpes. Virus can be readily isolated from vesicles and from conjunctival swabs in 1–4 days. Cerebrospinal fluid is positive for virus in about one third of infected neonates but is rarely positive in older children with encephalitis. Brain biopsy is required for a definitive diagnosis and exclusion of other treatable entities. PCR permits detection of viral DNA in cerebrospinal fluid and, if positive, will make brain biopsy unnecessary. At this writing, PCR for HSV is available through specialized research laboratories only.

Moderate polymorphonuclear leukocytosis occurs in acute herpetic gingivostomatitis, eczema herpeticum, and meningoencephalitis. In meningoencephalitis there are frequently red cells in the cerebrospinal fluid and an increase in lymphocytes, usually fewer than 100 but occasionally up to 1,000/mm^3; the protein level is elevated, and the sugar is usually within the normal range. Electroencephalogram (EEG) and magnetic resonance imaging (MRI) may demonstrate a temporal lobe lesion in early encephalitis. The computed tomographic (CT) scan may be normal in early encephalitis but becomes abnormal as the disease progresses. Thrombocytopenia and elevated liver function tests often occur with systemic infection.

DIAGNOSIS. The diagnosis is based on any two of the following: (1) a compatible clinical pattern; (2) isolation of the virus; (3) development of specific antibodies; (4) demonstration of characteristic cells, histologic changes, viral antigen, or HSV DNA in scrapings or biopsy material. A rise in cerebrospinal fluid HSV antibody occurs in HSV encephalitis, but it is late in the illness and is useful only for retrospective diagnosis. HSV serologic changes (fourfold rise or seroconversion from negative to positive) usually occur after the critical period for diagnosis and therapy. Illnesses resulting from HSV recurrence may not demonstrate a diagnostic serologic rise, and neonates or severely immunocompromised individuals may fail to produce antibody during primary infection. Reliable antibody tests to differentiate HSV-1 from HSV-2 are not commercially available. HSV-1 and HSV-2 viral isolates may be typed by a variety of readily available antigen (ELISA, fluorescent antibody) and molecular techniques. HSV isolates that are unrelated epidemiologically are all slightly different at the nucleic acid level, as discerned by DNA endonuclease restriction analysis. Using this technique, it is possible to confirm infection of one individual by another and to demonstrate that apparent nosocomial outbreaks or viral transmission represent a chance collection of unrelated cases, which may be extremely important for counseling and medicolegal reasons.

COURSE AND PROGNOSIS. Primary localized infections with HSV in the normal host are self-limited, usually lasting 1–2 wk. Mortality rates are high in newborn infants who also have systemic infection and in older infants who are severely immunocompromised or malnourished. In patients with meningoencephalitis the prognosis for survival or for recovery without serious permanent residuals is guarded. Outcome is improved with early diagnosis and therapy.

Attacks may frequently recur, but they seldom cause more than temporary inconvenience except in the eye, where they may eventually cause scarring of the cornea and blindness. Recurrent herpes lesions can be a significant problem in immunocompromised patients. Recurrent genital disease may be associated with significant discomfort and psychologic morbidity. The major complication of any form of genital HSV infection in a woman is infection of her newborn (see Chapter 97.2).

Treatment. Acyclovir (9-[-2-hydroxyethoxymethyl] guanine, a purine nucleoside analog) is the mainstay of therapy for HSV. Viral thymidine kinase will phosphorylate acyclovir, which is then triphosphorylated by cellular enzymes to act as an HSV DNA polymerase inhibitor and DNA chain terminator. Thymidine kinase–negative HSV isolates are resistant to acyclovir. Topical acyclovir may decrease the period of viral shedding but has little effect on symptoms of oral or genital herpes.

Topical trifluorothymidine, vidarabine, and idoxuridine are all usually effective in treating herpetic keratitis but do not reduce the recurrence rate. Topical corticosteroids may increase ocular involvement, if used alone, and should only be utilized with antiviral therapy.

Patients with primary genital infection who are treated with *oral acyclovir* (200 mg five times daily for 5 days) have significantly less pain, itching, and time to crusting; a shorter duration of viral shedding; and fewer new lesions compared with control patients. A dose of 800 mg twice a day appears to be just as effective and well tolerated and is easier to administer. Those with recurrent genital infections who are treated similarly with oral acyclovir have a shorter duration of viral shedding and heal faster. Therapy of primary attacks does not prevent recurrences. However, daily prophylactic administration of oral acyclovir can diminish the number of recurrences and may be prescribed if recurrences are frequent or severe. In small studies, oral acyclovir has modest effects in children with primary gingivostomatitis by decreasing drooling, gum swelling, pain, and new lesion formation compared with placebo. Therapy of recurrent oral herpes with oral acyclovir has limited effects. Acyclovir has no effect on HSV-associated erythema multiform. Suppression of the HSV infection by prophylactic therapy as for genital disease prevents the erythema multiforme recurrences. Oral acyclovir therapy is useful for treating recurrent herpes whitlow and rectal herpes.

Intravenously administered acyclovir (10 mg/kg/dose given over 1 hr every 8 hr for 14–21 days) is the treatment of choice for herpes encephalitis. The drug is well tolerated. The best results are obtained when treatment is started early. Patients younger than 30 yr and those who are only lethargic compared with those who have progressed to coma have a better prognosis. Supportive care to minimize increased intracranial pressure, seizure activity, and respiratory compromise requires an intensive care setting and a team of experts. Intravenous acyclovir (5–10 mg/kg/dose given over 1 hr every 8 hr [duration depending on clinical response]) is therapeutic for HSV infection in the immunocompromised host. The larger doses are used for severe and systemic infections. The lower dose may be used for localized mucocutaneous disease. As the patient responds, therapy may be switched to the oral route. Oral acyclovir, as used in genital disease, may be used to suppress HSV recurrences in seropositive patients during periods of maximum immunosuppression after organ or marrow transplantation or during induction therapy for leukemia, lymphoma, or solid tumors. Immunosuppressed patients with frequently recurring HSV infection, such as those with AIDS or primary immunodeficiencies, benefit from chronic suppressive oral therapy. In the neonate, all forms of HSV are treated with high doses (10–20 mg/kg/dose every 8 hr) of acyclovir for 14–21 days (see Chapter 97.2).

Acyclovir-resistant HSV is rare in the normal host but occurs in the immunocompromised host treated with multiple, intermittent courses of acyclovir. When immunocompromised patients have unresponsive or worsening HSV infection despite acyclovir therapy, the virus should be forwarded to reference laboratories for drug susceptibility testing. The drug of choice for acyclovir-resistant HSV is intravenous foscarnet (phosphonoformic acid), 40 mg/kg/dose every 8 hr. This drug has serious side effects (azotemia, electrolyte disturbance, anemia, granulocytopenia). Acyclovir and foscarnet dosages must be modified in patients with renal impairment.

Symptomatic and supportive therapy is of great importance. In infants especially, eczema herpeticum and stomatitis may lead to severe dehydration, shock, and hypoproteinemia, requiring replacement of fluids, electrolytes, and proteins.

Oral lavage should be used for mouth care; Ceepryn 1:4,000 or Zephiran 1:1,000 may be useful. Local analgesics, such as viscous lidocaine or benzocaine lozenges, are not advocated because they may cause the child to damage friable and anesthesized parts of the mouth. Genital lesions may be made less painful by using sitz baths. Local drying agents prolong healing and may increase secondary infection. Analgesics should be used systemically as required. Antibiotics are useful only in treating secondary bacterial infections.

Food and fluid intake will be facilitated by acquiescing to the child's whims. Ice-cold fluids, ice slush, or semisolids are often accepted when other food is refused.

The child or adolescent with recurrent oral or genital herpes may have severe psychologic problems and may benefit from anticipatory guidance or formal counseling. Genital disease should be destigmatized and safer sex practices emphasized. Parents of children with most types of HSV infection, such as gingivostomatitis or skin infection, should be reassured that common childhood HSV infections are not related to sexual activity or abuse.

PREVENTION. Acyclovir administered during periods of high risk in immunocompromised hosts and chronically in individuals with frequently recurrent genital or oral disease markedly decreases the rate of recurrence. Acyclovir administered before a known trigger factor, such as intense sunlight, usually prevents recurrences.

HSV spread can be limited by standard methods of infection control. Open lesions on skin, hands, and mucous membranes should be well covered. Wrestlers with possible HSV cutaneous lesions should be excluded from practice and competition until they are healed. Wrestling mats should be cleansed with a bleach solution at least daily. Children with immunodeficiencies or chronic skin diseases that predispose to severe HSV infection should not be cared for by persons with herpetic whitlow or active uncovered fever blisters. Active herpes lesions that can be covered are not a reason to exclude children from day-care or school activities. Prevention of neonatal herpes by cesarean section is discussed in Chapter 97.2.

There is active research to develop a vaccine to prevent HSV infection. HSV may be prevented in some animal models by live, attenuated or subunit viral particle vaccines. Several purified HSV glycoprotein vaccines are antigenic in humans, but whether these vaccines will prevent disease or ameliorate recurrences is not known.

Aurelius E, Johansson B, Skoldenberg B, et al: Rapid diagnosis of herpes simplex encephalitis by nested polymerase chain reaction assay of cerebral spinal fluid. Lancet 337:189, 1991.

Frenck RW, Kohl S: Herpes simplex virus in the immunocompromised child. *In*: Patrick CC (ed): Infections in Immunocompromised Infants and Children. New York, Churchill Livingstone, 1992, pp 603–624.

Kohl S: Postnatal herpes simplex virus infection. *In*: Root RK, Sande MA (eds): Viral Infections, Contemporary Issues in Infectious Diseases, Vol 10. New York, Churchill Livingstone, 1992, pp 331–356.

Leigh IM: Management of non-genital herpes simplex virus infections in immunocompetent patients. Am J Med 85:34, 1988.

Straus SE, Takiff HE, Seidlin M, et al: Suppression of frequently recurring genital herpes. N Engl J Med 310:1545, 1984.

Whitley RJ, Alford CA, Hirsch MS, et al: Vidarbine versus acyclovir therapy in herpes simplex encephalitis. N Engl J Med 314:144, 1986.

Whitley RJ, Cobbs CG, Alford CA, et al: Diseases that mimic herpes simplex encephalitis: Diagnosis, presentation, and outcome. JAMA 262:234, 1989.

Whitley RJ, Guann JW Jr. Acyclovir: A decade later. N Engl J Med 327:782, 1992.

CHAPTER 212
Human Herpesvirus 6
(Roseola Infantum, Exanthem Subitum)

Steve Kohl

In 1986, a new virus was isolated from the peripheral blood mononuclear cells of several patients with acquired immunodeficiency syndrome (AIDS), or lymphoproliferative diseases. Originally named the human B-cell lymphotrophic virus, further characterization revealed it to be a novel herpesvirus, now known as human herpesvirus 6 (HHV-6). In the years since its discovery, primary infection in infants has been associated with roseola infantum (exanthem subitum) or a nonspecific febrile disease.

ETIOLOGY. HHV-6 is one of the seven human herpesviruses. It is a large (185–200 nm), enveloped, double-stranded DNA virus of approximately 170 kilobases. Originally isolated from human peripheral blood cells, it replicates in human T cells (both CD4 and CD8 cells), monocytes, megakaryocytes, natural killer cells, glial cells, and epithelial and salivary cells. The virus produces balloon-like cytopathic effects and cell lysis in mitogen-stimulated mononuclear leukocytes. The A variant is more commonly isolated from adult patients with AIDS or lymphoproliferative disease. The B variant appears to account for most symptomatic primary HHV-6 infections in infants. HHV-6 is most closely related to human cytomegalovirus (CMV). The molecular and antigenic relationships explain some degree of serologic cross-reactivity with CMV.

EPIDEMIOLOGY. The seroepidemiology of HHV-6 infection parallels the clinical epidemiology of roseola. Most (70–95%) newborns are seropositive for HHV-6, reflecting transplacental antibodies. Seropositive rates drop between 4 and 6 mo of age (5–50%), followed by rapid acquisition of antibodies. By age 1–2 yr, more than 90% of infants are seropositive. Almost all young adults are seropositive, although HHV-6 titers may be lower than in children. In late adulthood, the prevalence of antibody to HHV-6 declines to approximately 60%. The pattern of antibody prevalence fits the clinical prevalence of roseola, an uncommon disease in the first 3 mo of life (although rarely documented in the neonate) with a peak incidence at 6–12 mo and 90% occurrence within the first 2 yr of age. Approximately one third of children experience clinical roseola. Infection occurs in both sexes equally and occurs year-round with a somewhat higher incidence in late spring and early summer. Some of the seasonal cases of roseola may be due to enteroviruses, which, in the absence of specific virologic diagnosis, simulate a roseola-like illness. Small outbreaks of HHV-6–mediated roseola are documented in closed populations, such as orphanages. The incubation period suggested from small outbreaks and experimental infections is 5–15 days.

PATHOGENESIS. The mode of acquisition of HHV-6 is not yet known, but the frequent detection of the virus in saliva of healthy humans suggests horizontal spread by oral viral shedding. Primary infection may be associated with clinical signs and symptoms or may be asymptomatic, although the frequency of the latter is unknown. Viremia can be documented in the first 4–5 days of clinical roseola with a mean of 10^3 infected cells per 10^6 peripheral blood mononuclear cells. The amount of virus in blood is associated directly with severity of disease.

There is a complex immune response composed of induction of a variety of cytokines (interferon alpha and gamma, interleukin-1 beta, tumor necrosis factor alpha), antibody responses, and T-cell reactivity. Clearance of primary viremia, fever, and appearance of rash are temporally associated with the appearance of anti–HHV-6 serum-neutralizing antibody and possibly increased natural killer cell activity. Transplacental antibody appears to protect young infants from infection. Infection of bone marrow cells in vitro suppresses progenitor cell differentiation of all cell lines. HHV-6 infection in vitro inhibits the lymphoproliferative response of human peripheral blood mononuclear cells.

High levels of antibody in adults, frequent viral shedding in saliva, and detection of viral nucleic acid in salivary glands and peripheral blood mononuclear cells in seropositive children and adults support a long-lived state of viral latency of HHV-6. The precise cell harboring latent HHV-6 is unknown, but leukocytes (possibly macrophages) and salivary glands cells are likely candidates. The nature of reactivation disease in older children and adults, especially those who are immunocompromised, is just being recognized. Because most of these individuals have antibodies, defects in cell-mediated immunity, as found in transplant patients or those with AIDS, may predispose to symptomatic reactivation.

CLINICAL MANIFESTATIONS

Roseola Infantum (Exanthem Subitum). HHV-6 is the etiologic agent of roseola in at least 80–92% of cases. Some remaining cases are probably due to HHV-6, whereas a few cases are due to enteroviral and other less common pathogens. The onset is sudden, with fever as high as 39.4–41.2° C (103–106° F); a bulging anterior fontanelle or convulsions may occur at this time or later. When seizures occur (5–35% of cases), they do so in the pre-eruptive stage of roseola. Although the pharyngeal mucosa may be slightly inflamed and there may be slight coryza, there are no diagnostic signs. A variety of signs and symptoms have been clearly associated with HHV-6 roseola infection (Table 212–1). The outstanding feature is the absence of physical findings sufficient to explain the fever. Usually the child looks relatively well despite the degree of the fever.

The fever falls by crisis on the 3rd–4th day. As the temperature returns to normal, a macular or maculopapular eruption appears over the body, starting on the trunk, spreading to the arms and neck, and involving the face and legs to some degree. The rash fades within 3 days. Desquamation is rare, and usually no pigmentation remains. Cases without a rash are described. Occasionally, the lymph nodes, especially in the cervical area, are enlarged but not to the extent that they are in rubella. Less commonly, the illness may present without the characteristic fever. Before defervescence and rash appearance, the diagnosis is suggested by excluding other common causes of high fever at this age, such as otitis media, acute pyelonephritis, pneumonia, meningitis, and pneumococcal bacteremia.

Fever in Infants without Characteristic Roseola. Specific diagnostic tests

■ **TABLE 212–1 Human Herpesvirus 6–Associated Roseola**

Fever (98%)	
Maximum level:	39–40° C (range, 37.5–41.2° C)
Duration:	3–4 days (range, 1–7 days)
Rash	
Day of appearance:	3–5 days after onset of fever
Duration:	3–4 days (range, 1–6 days)
Characterization:	Macular, coalescent (measles-like), 40%; Papular (rubella-like), 55%;
Site:	Neck, abdomen, trunk, back, extremities
Associated Signs and Symptoms	
Occipital or cervical adenopathy	30–35%
Respiratory signs or symptoms	50–55%
Mild diarrhea	55–70%
Seizures	5–35%
Edematous eyelids	0–30%
Anterior fontanelle bulging	26–30%
Papular pharyngitis	65%

for HHV-6 have allowed for definition of a number of HHV-6–associated syndromes. In two prospective studies, among 1,792 U.S. children 3 yr old or younger with an acute febrile illness, 10–14% were diagnosed with primary HHV-6 infection. The age range of these children was 9.5–9.9 mo. They were irritable and febrile (mean temperature, 39.7° C), and 47–62% had inflamed tympanic membranes with few other localizing signs. Thirteen per cent had a febrile seizure; fever lasted an average of 4 days. Only 9% had a roseola-like rash, although 17–33% had a rash during or after the period of fever. HHV-6 may account for as much as 50% of the first febrile illness of a child's life.

Disseminated Infection in Infants and Adults. Rare cases of HHV-6 causing severe or fatal disseminated diseases in otherwise healthy infants are reported. These occur as acute febrile illnesses at times resembling an infectious mononucleosis syndrome (lymphadenopathy, hepatosplenomegaly, maculopapular rash) or fulminant hepatitis. HHV-6 is also associated with small numbers of cases of intussusception in infants, with single or recurrent febrile seizures, rare cases of meningoencephalitis or encephalopathy, exacerbation of idiopathic thrombocytopenic purpura, and fatal hemophagocytic syndrome.

In otherwise healthy adults, HHV-6 primary infection is occasionally associated with a severe infectious mononucleosis-like syndrome, fulminant hepatitis, or a milder illness with malaise and cervical lymphadenopathy. HHV-6 may be associated with Kikuchi lymphadenitis (lymphadenitis and remittent fever) and sinus histiocytosis with massive lymphadenopathy (Rosai Dorfman disease).

Infection in the Immunocompromised. HHVs cause reactivation disease in immunocompromised individuals. This appears to be the case with HHV-6 as well, although the full spectrum of these syndromes and their frequencies are just being elucidated. In bone marrow transplantation patients, HHV-6 viremia has been associated with otherwise unexplained fever and marrow suppression. In small series of patients with bone marrow transplantation or AIDS, HHV-6 has been associated with idiopathic interstitial pneumonitis. These findings must be viewed with caution because HHV-6 infection is nearly universal in these patients, and its association with reactivation disease in any given patient is difficult.

HHV-6 infects many of the same cells as the human immunodeficiency virus (HIV), transactivates the HIV promoter in vitro, and under some conditions increases HIV replication. HHV-6 infection of human CD8 T cells and natural killer cells induces CD4 expression and susceptibility to HIV infection in vitro. Nevertheless, there are no data to indicate that HHV-6 hastens the course of HIV infection in patients.

LABORATORY FINDINGS. In roseola, during the first few days of fever, the white blood cell count averages 8,000/mm^3, with an increase in neutrophils. By the 3rd–4th day of fever, the white cell count drops to a mean of 6,000/mm^3, at times with an absolute neutropenia and a lymphocytosis that may be as high as 90%. Occasionally, a large number of monocytes are present. The cerebrospinal fluid is usually normal, although HHV-6 DNA may be detected by polymerase chain reaction (PCR) in the cerebrospinal fluid of some of the rare infants with HHV-6–mediated encephalopathy. These patients may also have a mild cerebrospinal fluid pleocytosis.

DIFFERENTIAL DIAGNOSIS. Children with roseola present with the differential diagnosis of a fever of unknown origin (Chapter 167) until the temperature drops precipitously and the rash appears. Rubella's other prodromal manifestations and the persistence of its fever after a rash appears usually distinguish it from roseola. Rubeola and dengue can be distinguished primarily by the time of appearance of their rash in relation to fever and other clinical findings. In rubeola, although there is usually a fever of variable degree for 3–4 days just before the rash, the temperature is abruptly elevated to 39.4–40° C (103–104° F) at the time the rash appears and remains elevated for the next 2 days, when the rash fades rapidly. The lack of Koplik spots, severe coryza, and conjunctivitis also helps to distinguish roseola from rubeola. Pneumococcal bacteremia may present with high fever and a well-appearing child. The white cell count is frequently elevated, and the blood culture is positive for *Pneumococcus*. Distinguishing roseola from entero- and adenoviral diseases and drug reactions is difficult. Recently, second cases of roseola in the same child have been associated with primary HHV-7 infection.

HHV-6 infection is an uncommon cause of a heterophil-negative infectious mononucleosis syndrome and hepatitis and should be distinguished from the other viruses that cause these syndromes. In the immunocompromised host, it is part of the differential diagnosis of interstitial pneumonitis and bone marrow failure along with cytomegalovirus, *Pneumocystis carinii,* and a host of other less common agents.

DIAGNOSIS. Specific diagnosis of HHV-6 infection depends on viral isolation during primary infection, demonstration of antibody production to HHV-6, or localization of HHV-6 in infected tissue by molecular methods. In the case of roseola, the virus may be recovered from peripheral blood leukocytes in the first 3–4 days of illness by cocultivation with mitogen-treated human umbilical cord blood mononuclear cells or established T-cell lines. The infected cells form a ballooning cytopathic effect, undergo lysis, and produce detectable antigen. Virus is not recovered from blood of normal, healthy, seropositive children or adults but may be recovered from asymptomatic, immunocompromised individuals.

After the 1st wk of primary infection, production of antibody may be demonstrated by a variety of assays including immunofluorescence, neutralization, immunoblot, and enzyme immunoassays. Immunoglobulin (Ig) M antibody appears early and declines as IgG antibody, which lasts well into adulthood, is produced. Although seroconversion (negative to positive antibody response) is indicative of primary infection, a fourfold rise may indicate either primary infection or reactivation of virus. IgM antibody may also reappear during viral reactivation. In the immunocompromised patient, low or falling levels of antibody may be associated with disease but are not reliably diagnostic. Apparent rises in HHV-6 antibodies may be due to CMV infection because there are antigenic cross-reactivities between these related herpes viruses. Definitive diagnosis of HHV-6 infection by serologic methods requires exclusion of primary CMV infection.

HHV-6 antigen or high levels of viral DNA are detected by immunohistochemical techniques or PCR in tissues of immunocompromised hosts, which is the only way to associate particular illnesses with HHV-6, because antibody changes are unreliable and viral recovery from blood leukocytes or saliva is not uncommon, even in the absence of a recognized syndrome. Most seropositive children and adults have viral DNA detected by PCR in their peripheral blood cells, probably indicating a state of viral latency. Almost all HHV-6 diagnostic tests are available only in research laboratories.

PROGNOSIS. The prognosis of roseola is good except in the rare patient who has extreme hyperpyrexia, persistent seizures, severe encephalitis, or fatal hepatitis. Preliminary indications in the immunocompromised host suggest that HHV-6–induced interstitial pneumonia has a better prognosis than that caused by CMV.

PROPHYLAXIS AND TREATMENT. No methods for shortening the course of roseola or for prophylaxis are known. In infants and young children who are prone to convulsions, administering a sedative when the sharp, febrile onset of roseola appears may be effective as prophylaxis against such seizures. An antipyretic may be of help in partially reducing the fever and in allaying restlessness. HHV-6 is susceptible in vitro to ganciclovir and foscarnet and much less so to acyclovir. There are no controlled studies of use of these agents in therapy for the rare severe cases of HHV-6 infection in the otherwise normal or the immunocompromised host.

Asano Y, Yoshikawa T, Suga S, et al: Fatal fulminant hepatitis in an infant with human herpesvirus-6 infection. Lancet 335:862, 1990.

Asano Y, Yoshikawa T, Suga S, et al: Clinical features of infants with primary human herpes virus 6 infection (exanthem subitum, roseola infantum). Pediatrics 93:104, 1994.

Cone RW, Hackman RC, Huang MW, et al: Human herpes virus 6 in lung tissue from patients with pneumonitis after bone marrow transplantation. N Engl J Med 329:156, 1993.

Hall CB, Long CE, Schnabel K, et al: Human herpes virus 6 infection in children: A prospective study of complications and reactivation. N Engl J Med 331:432, 1994.

Levy J, Greenspan D, Ferro F, et al: Frequent isolation of HHV-6 from saliva and high seroprevalence of the virus in the population. Lancet 335:1047, 1990.

Linnavuori K, Peltola H, Tapani H: Serology versus clinical signs or symptoms and main laboratory findings in the diagnosis of exanthema subitum (roseola infantum). Pediatrics 89:103, 1993.

Pruksananonda P, Hall CB, Insel RA, et al: Primary human herpes virus 6 infection in young children. N Engl J Med 326:1445, 1992.

Tanaka K, Kondo T, Torigoe S, et al: Human herpes virus 7: another causal agent for roseola (exanthem subitum). J Pediatr 125:1, 1994.

Yamanishi K, Skiraki K, Kondo T, et al: Identification of human herpesvirus-6 as a causal agent for exanthem subitum. Lancet 1:1065, 1988.

CHAPTER 213

Varicella-Zoster Virus

Ann M. Arvin

Primary infection with varicella-zoster virus (VZV) causes varicella (chickenpox). The virus establishes latent infection in dorsal root ganglia; its reactivation causes herpes zoster (shingles).

ETIOLOGY. VZV is a human herpesvirus; it is classified as an alpha herpesvirus because of its similarities to the prototype for this group, which is herpes simplex virus (HSV). VZV is an enveloped, double-stranded DNA virus; the viral genome encodes more than 70 proteins, including proteins that are targets of immunity and a viral thymidine kinase, which makes the virus sensitive to inhibition by acyclovir and related antiviral agents.

PATHOLOGY. Varicella begins with mucosal inoculation of virus transferred in respiratory secretions or by direct contact with skin lesions of varicella or herpes zoster. Inoculation is followed by an incubation period of 10–21 days, during which subclinical viral spread occurs. Widespread cutaneous lesions result when the infection enters a viremic phase; peripheral blood mononuclear cells carry infectious virus, generating new crops of vesicles for 3–7 days. VZV is also transported back to respiratory mucosal sites during the late incubation period, permitting spread to susceptible contacts before the appearance of rash. The transmission of infectious virus by respiratory droplets distinguishes VZV from other human herpes viruses. Visceral dissemination of the virus follows the failure of host responses to terminate viremia, which results in infection of lungs, liver, brain, and other organs. VZV becomes latent in dorsal root ganglia cells in all individuals who experience primary infection. Its reactivation causes a localized vesicular rash that usually involves the dermatomal distribution of a single sensory nerve; necrotic changes are produced in the associated ganglia, sometimes extending into the posterior horn. The histopathology of varicella and herpes zoster lesions is identical; infectious VZV is present in herpes zoster lesions, as it is in varicella lesions, but is not released into respiratory secretions. Varicella elicits humoral and cell-mediated immunity that is highly protective against symptomatic reinfection. Suppression of cell-mediated immunity to VZV correlates with an increased risk of VZV reactivation as herpes zoster.

EPIDEMIOLOGY. In the United States and other temperate climates, 90–95% of individuals acquire VZV in childhood. Annual varicella epidemics occur in winter and spring. Wild-type VZV strains that cause the annual epidemics of varicella do not exhibit changes in virulence as judged by the clinical severity of primary VZV infections from year to year. Household transmission rates are 80–90%; more casual contact, such as school classroom exposure, is associated with attack rates of 30% or less. Varicella is contagious from 24–48 hr before the rash appears and while uncrusted vesicles are present, which is usually 3–7 days. Susceptible children acquire varicella after close, direct contact with adults who have herpes zoster; this route of transmission maintains the circulation of the virus in the population. For unexplained reasons, varicella is much less common in tropical areas, so that susceptibility rates among adults are as high as 20–30%. Herpes zoster shows no seasonal variation in incidence because it is due to the reactivation of endogenous, latent virus. Despite anecdotal reports, epidemiologic studies demonstrate that exposure to varicella does not cause herpes zoster. Herpes zoster is very rare in children younger than 10 yr except among those given immunosuppressive therapy for malignancy or other diseases, those who have human immunodeficiency virus (HIV) infection, and those who have been infected in utero or during the first year of life. The risk of severe or life-threatening primary or recurrent VZV infection is related primarily to host factors rather than variations in the pathogenicity of VZV strains.

CLINICAL MANIFESTATIONS OF VARICELLA. Although the incubation period of varicella ranges from 10–21 days, the illness usually begins from 14–16 days after exposure. Almost all exposed, susceptible children experience a rash, but it may be limited to fewer than 10 lesions. Prodromal symptoms are common, particularly in older children; fever, malaise, anorexia, headache, and occasionally mild abdominal pain occur 24–48 hr before the rash appears. Temperature elevation is usually moderate, ranging from 100–102° F but may be as high as 106° F; fever and other systemic symptoms persist during the first 2–4 days after the onset of the rash. Varicella lesions appear first on the scalp, face, or trunk. The initial exanthem consists of intensely pruritic erythematous macules that evolve to form clear, fluid-filled vesicles. Clouding and umbilication of the lesions begin in 24–48 hr. While the initial lesions are crusting, new crops form on the trunk and then the extremities; the simultaneous presence of lesions in various stages of evolution is characteristic of varicella (Fig. 213–1 [color plate section]). Ulcerative lesions involving the oropharynx and vagina are common; many children have vesicular lesions on the eyelids and conjunctivae, but serious ocular disease is rare. The average number of varicella lesions is about 300, but healthy

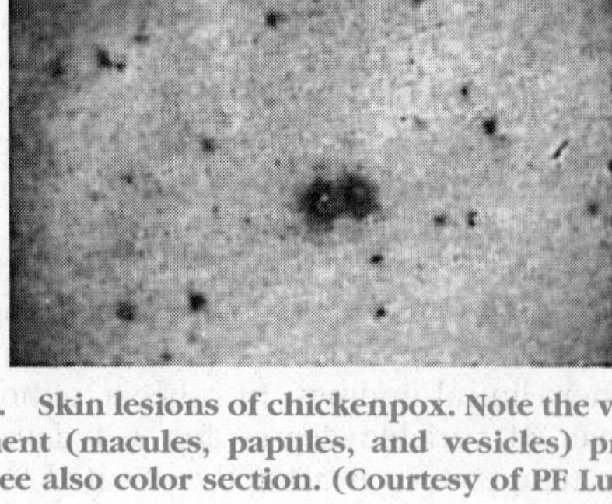

Figure 213–1. Skin lesions of chickenpox. Note the varying stages of development (macules, papules, and vesicles) present at the same time. See also color section. (Courtesy of PF Lucchesi, M.D.)

children may have from fewer than 10 to more than 1,500 lesions. In secondary household cases and cases involving older children, more days of new lesion formation and more lesions are likely. The exanthem is more extensive in children with skin disorders, such as eczema or recent sunburn. Hypopigmentation of lesion sites persists for days to weeks in some children, but scarring is unusual.

The differential diagnosis of varicella includes vesicular rashes caused by other infectious agents, such as enterovirus or *Staphylococcus aureus*, drug reactions, contact dermatitis, and insect bites.

COMPLICATIONS OF VARICELLA. Secondary bacterial infections, usually resulting from *S. aureus* or *Streptococcus pyogenes* (group A β-hemolytic streptococcus), are the most common complication of varicella. Cellulitis, lymphadenitis, and subcutaneous abscesses also occur. Varicella gangrenosa, usually resulting from *S. pyogenes*, is a rare but potentially life-threatening consequence of secondary infection. Acute bacterial sepsis is uncommon, but transient bacteremia may cause focal infections, including staphylococcal or streptococcal pneumonia, arthritis, or osteomyelitis. Encephalitis and cerebellar ataxia are well-described neurologic complications of varicella; the incidence of central nervous system morbidity is highest among patients younger than 5 yr and older than 20 yr. Meningoencephalitis is characterized by seizures, altered consciousness, and nuchal rigidity; patients with cerebellar ataxia have a more gradual onset of gait disturbance, nystagmus, and slurred speech. Neurologic symptoms usually begin from 2–6 days after the onset of the rash but may occur during the incubation period or after resolution of the rash. VZV-related encephalitis and cerebellar ataxia may be immune mediated; the severe hemorrhagic encephalitis caused by HSV is very rare in children with varicella. Clinical recovery is typically rapid, occurring within 24–72 hr, and is usually complete. Before the association of salicylates was documented, some children with varicella had neurologic symptoms caused by the encephalopathy associated with Reye syndrome. Varicella hepatitis is relatively common and is usually subclinical, but some children have severe vomiting, which must be differentiated from that associated with Reye syndrome. Acute thrombocytopenia, accompanied by petechiae, purpura, hemorrhagic vesicles, hematuria, and gastrointestinal bleeding, is a rare complication that is usually self-limited. Other rare complications of varicella include nephritis, nephrotic syndrome, hemolytic-uremic syndrome, arthritis, myocarditis, pericarditis, pancreatitis, and orchitis.

Progressive disease caused by primary VZV infection occurs in otherwise healthy adolescents and adults, immunocompromised children, pregnant women, and newborn infants. Varicella pneumonia is very rare in children, but this complication accounts for most of the increased morbidity and mortality in high-risk populations. Respiratory symptoms, which may include cough, dyspnea, cyanosis, pleuritic chest pain, and hemoptysis, usually begin within 1–6 days (average, 3 days) after the onset of the rash. Hypoxemia is often much more severe than is suggested by the physical findings; the chest radiograph may be normal or may show diffuse bilateral infiltrates. Varicella pneumonia is often transient, resolving completely within 24–72 hr, but in severe cases, the interstitial pneumonitis progresses rapidly to cause respiratory failure. Hemorrhage into the cutaneous lesions is a sign of severe varicella in high-risk patients, as is severe abdominal or back pain, although its pathogenesis is uncertain.

The risk of progressive varicella is highest in children with malignancy if chemotherapy was given during the incubation period and the absolute lymphocyte count is less than 500 cells. In one large series, the mortality rate without antiviral therapy was 7%, and all varicella-related deaths occurred within 3 days after the diagnosis of varicella pneumonia. Hepatitis, encephalitis, and disseminated intravascular coagulopathy are other frequent complications. The syndrome of inappropriate antidiuretic hormone secretion may accompany disseminated varicella with or without clinical encephalitis. Children who acquire varicella after organ transplantation are also at risk for progressive VZV infection. Children on long-term, low-dose steroid therapy usually have no complications, but fatal varicella has occurred in patients receiving high-dose steroids. Untreated varicella is severe or fatal in children with congenital immunodeficiency disorders, especially involving cell-mediated immunity. Unusual clinical findings of varicella, including lesions that develop a unique hyperkeratotic appearance and chronic new lesion formation for weeks or months, have been described in children with HIV infection.

In rare instances, maternal varicella results in the congenital varicella syndrome, associated with unusual cutaneous defects, atrophy of an extremity, microcephaly, ocular defects, and damage to the autonomic nervous system. Infants who are born within 4 days after or 2 days before the onset of maternal varicella may acquire progressive varicella.

CLINICAL MANIFESTATIONS OF HERPES ZOSTER. VZV reactivation is rare in childhood. When it occurs, it causes vesicular lesions clustered unilaterally in the dermatomal distribution of one or more adjacent sensory nerves, which are preceded or accompanied by localized pain, hyperesthesias, pruritus, and low-grade fever (Fig. 213–2). The rash is mild, with new lesions appearing for a few days, symptoms of acute neuritis are minimal, and complete resolution usually occurs within 1–2 wk. Immunocompromised children have more severe dermatomal disease and may experience viremia, causing pneumonia, hepatitis, encephalitis, and disseminated intravascular coagulopathy. Severely immunocompromised children, particularly those with HIV infection, may have unusual, chronic, or relapsing cutaneous disease, retinitis, or central nervous system disease without rash. Transverse myelitis with transient paralysis is a rare complication of herpes zoster. In contrast to adults, postherpetic neuralgia is very unusual in children.

LABORATORY FINDINGS AND DIAGNOSIS. Laboratory evaluation is not necessary for appropriate management of healthy children with varicella or herpes zoster. Abnormal laboratory values are common during varicella. Leukopenia is typical during the first 72 hr; it is followed by a relative and absolute lymphocytosis. Liver function tests are also often moderately elevated. Patients with neurologic complications of varicella or uncomplicated herpes zoster have a mild lymphocytic pleocytosis and a slight to moderate increase in protein; the cerebrospinal fluid glucose is usually normal. Rapid laboratory diagnosis of VZV is often important in high-risk patients and can be accomplished by direct immunohistochemical staining of cells from cutaneous lesions. Multinucleated giant cells can be detected with non-specific stains, but false-negative results are common, and these methods do not differentiate VZV and HSV infections.

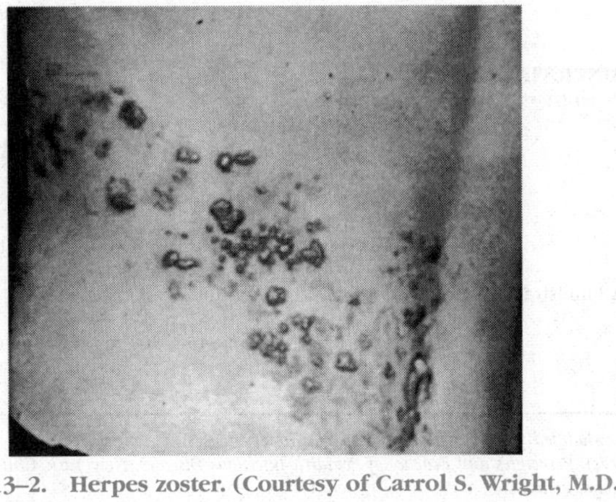

Figure 213–2. Herpes zoster. (Courtesy of Carrol S. Wright, M.D.)

The definitive diagnosis of VZV infection requires the recovery of infectious virus using tissue culture. VZV immunoglobulin G (IgG) antibodies can be detected by several methods, but serologic diagnosis is retrospective; testing for VZV IgM antibodies is not useful for clinical diagnosis because commercially available methods are unreliable. VZV IgG antibody tests are valuable to determine the immune status of individuals whose clinical history of varicella is unknown or equivocal.

TREATMENT. Acyclovir—9-[(2-hydroxyethoxy) methyl] guanine—is the drug of choice for varicella and herpes zoster when specific therapy is indicated (Table 213–1). Any patient who has signs of disseminated VZV including pneumonia, hepatitis, thrombocytopenia, or encephalitis should receive immediate treatment with intravenous acyclovir. Acyclovir therapy given within 72 hr prevents progressive varicella and visceral dissemination in high-risk patients; the dosage is 500 mg/m^2 every 8 hr, administered intravenously for 7 days or until no new lesions have appeared for 48 hr. Delaying antiviral treatment until prolonged new lesion formation is evident is not an option because visceral dissemination occurs during the same time period. Recent large, placebo-controlled clinical studies have shown that oral acyclovir diminishes the clinical symptoms of varicella in otherwise healthy children, adolescents, and adults when it is administered within 24 hr after the appearance of the initial cutaneous lesions. Drug efficacy was established for all groups, but the clinical benefit may be considered more significant in older children and in secondary household cases. Acyclovir therapy does not interfere with the induction of VZV immunity.

Acyclovir is also effective for treatment of herpes zoster in healthy and immunocompromised patients. Patients at high risk for disseminated disease should receive 500 mg/m^2 or 10 mg/kg every 8 hr intravenously. Onset of VZV reactivation reduces the duration of new lesion formation to only about 3 days. Oral acyclovir is an option for immunocompromised patients who are considered at low risk for visceral dissemination. Antiviral drug resistance is rare but has occurred in children with HIV infection; foscarnet is the only drug now available for the treatment of acyclovir-resistant VZV infections.

■ TABLE 213–1 Use of Acyclovir for the Treatment of Varicella

Acyclovir Indicated	
Patients:	Malignancy, bone marrow or organ transplantation, high-dose steroids
	Congenital T-cell immunodeficiency
	Human immunodeficiency virus infection
	Neonatal varicella after maternal varicella beginning within 5 days before or 2 days after delivery
	Associated pneumonia or encephalitis
Administration:	Initiate as soon as possible after initial lesions appear
	Intravenous route
	Dose
	$<$ 1 yr: 10 mg/kg/dose given every 8 hr as 1-hr infusion
	$>$ 1 yr: 500 mg/m^2/dose given every 8 hr as 1-hr infusion
	Duration: 7 days or until no new lesions have appeared for 48 hr
Acyclovir Optional	
Patients:	Chronic cutaneous disorders
	Chronic diseases that may be exacerbated by acute varicella-zoster virus infection such as cystic fibrosis or other pulmonary disorders, diabetes mellitus
	Disorders requiring chronic salicylate therapy or intermittent steroid therapy
	Otherwise healthy children, especially those older than 12 years or secondary household contacts
Administration:	Initiate within 24 hr after initial lesions appear
	Oral route
	Dose: 20 mg/kg/dose (maximum 800 mg/dose) given as four doses a day
	Duration: 5 days

Modified from Arvin AM: Varicella-zoster virus. In: *Long S, Prober C, Pickering L (eds): Principles and Practice of Pediatric Infectious Diseases. New York, Churchill Livingstone, in press.*

PREVENTION. VZV transmission is difficult to prevent because the infection is contagious for 24–48 hr before the rash appears. Infection control practices, including caring for infected patients in isolation rooms with filtered air systems, are essential in hospitals that treat immunocompromised children. Susceptible health care workers who have had a close exposure to varicella should not care for high-risk patients during the incubation period.

Varicella-zoster immune globulin (VZIG) prophylaxis is recommended for immunocompromised children, pregnant women, and newborn infants exposed to maternal varicella. VZIG is distributed by the American Red Cross Blood Services; the dosage is one vial per 10 kg intramuscularly given within 96 hr or, if possible, within 48 hr after exposure. Adults should be tested for VZV IgG antibodies before VZIG administration because many adults with no clinical history of varicella are immune. Because VZIG prophylaxis does not eliminate the possibility of progressive disease, patients should be monitored and treated with acyclovir if necessary. Immunocompromised patients who have received high-dose intravenous immune globulin (100–400 mg/kg) for other indications within 2–3 wk before the exposure can be expected to have serum antibodies to VZV. Close contact between a susceptible high-risk patient and a patient with herpes zoster is also an indication for VZIG prophylaxis. Passive antibody prophylaxis does not reduce the risk of herpes zoster or alter the clinical course of varicella or herpes zoster when given after the onset of symptoms.

Acyclovir should not be given as prophylaxis against varicella. Acyclovir prophylaxis for herpes zoster is not essential because the prompt initiation of acyclovir for the treatment of recurrent VZV infections is very effective in reducing morbidity and mortality among immunocompromised patients. Prolonged low-dose administration of acyclovir should be avoided to minimize the emergence of drug-resistant VZV.

The live, attenuated varicella vaccine, made from the Oka strain, is the first human herpesvirus vaccine. The live, attenuated varicella vaccine (Oka-Merck strain) has been given to more than 8,500 healthy children and adults in clinical trials in the United States. The vaccine induced seroconversion rates of more than 95%, with complete protection against disease in 85–95% of exposures. Persistence of humoral and cell-mediated immunity has been documented in 94–100% of vaccine recipients monitored for 1–6 yr. The Oka-Merck varicella vaccine can be given to children with acute leukemia in remission, with careful attention to the status of their underlying disease and immunosuppressive therapy regimens. VZV reactivation has been described in a few healthy vaccine recipients, but the incidence of herpes zoster resulting from vaccine virus in children with leukemia was significantly lower than reactivation of naturally acquired VZV. Licensure of the Oka-Merck vaccine was approved in 1995 in the United States; live, attenuated varicella vaccines have been approved for clinical use in Japan, Korea, and some European countries.

Arvin AM: Varicella-zoster virus. In: Long S, Prober C, Pickering L (eds): Principles and Practice of Pediatric Infectious Diseases. New York, Churchill Livingston, in press.

Balfour HH Jr: Varicella zoster virus infections in immunocompromised hosts: A review of the natural history and management. Am J Med 85:68, 1988.

Balfour HH Jr, Rotbart HA, Feldman S, et al: Acyclovir treatment of varicella in otherwise healthy adolescents. J Pediatr 120:627, 1992.

Brunell PA: Varicella in pregnancy, the fetus and the newborn: Problems in management. J Infect Dis 166(Suppl 1): S42, 1992.

Dunkle LM, Arvin AM, Whitley RJ, et al: A controlled trial of acyclovir for chickenpox in normal children. N Engl J Med 325:1539, 1991.

Feldman S, Lott L: Varicella in children with cancer: Impact of antiviral therapy and prophylaxis. Pediatrics 80:465, 1987.

Gershon AA, LaRussa P, Hardy I, et al: Varicella vaccine: The American experience. J Infect Dis 166(Suppl 1):S63, 1992.

Gershon AA, Steinberg SP, Schmidt NJ. Varicella-zoster virus. *In:* Balows A, Hauseler WJ, Herrman KL, Isenberg HD, Shadomy HJ (eds): Manual of Clinical Microbiology. Washington, DC, American Society for Microbiology, 1991, pp 838–852.

Grose C. Varicella-zoster virus: Pathogenesis of the human diseases, the virus and viral replication. *In:* Hyman R (ed): The Natural History of Varicella-Zoster Virus. New York, CRC Press, 1987, pp 1–66.
Guess HA, Broughton DD, Melton LJ II, et al: Population-based studies of varicella complications. Pediatrics 78:723, 1987.
Kelley R, Mancao M, Lee F, et al: Varicella in children with perinatally acquired human immunodeficiency virus infection. J Pediatr 124:271, 1994.
Pastuszak AL, Levy M, Shick B, et al: Outcome after maternal varicella in the first trimester of pregnancy. N Engl J Med 330:901, 1994.
Plotkin SA, Starr SE, Connor K, et al: Zoster in normal children after varicella vaccine. J Infect Dis 159:1000, 1989.
Prober CG, Gershon AA, Grose C, et al: Consensus: varicella-zoster infections in pregnancy and the perinatal period. Pediatr Infect Dis J 9:865, 1990.
Report of Committee on Infectious Diseases: Varicella-Zoster Infections, 23rd ed. Elk Grove Village, IL, American Academy of Pediatrics, 1994, pp 510–517.
Starr SE: Varicella in children receiving steroids for asthma: Risks and management. Pediatr Infect Dis J 11:419, 1992.
Takahashi M: Current status and prospects of live varicella vaccine. Vaccine 10:1007, 1992.
White CJ, Kuter BJ, Hildebrand CS, et al: Varicella vaccine (VARIVAX) in healthy children and adolescents: Results from clinical trials, 1987 to 1989. Pediatrics 87:604, 1991.
Whitley RJ: Varicella-zoster virus infections. *In:* Galasso GJ, Whitley RJ, Merigan TC (eds): Antiviral Agents and Viral Diseases of Man. Raven Press, New York, 1990, pp 235–263.

CHAPTER 214
Cytomegalovirus

Sergio Stagno

Cytomegaloviruses (CMVs) are a group of agents within the herpesvirus family known for their wide distribution among humans and other animals. In vivo and in vitro CMV infections are highly species specific. Most CMV infections are inapparent, but the virus can cause a variety of clinical illnesses that range in severity from mild to fatal. CMV is the most common congenital viral infection, which occasionally causes the syndrome of cytomegalic inclusion disease (hepatosplenomegaly, jaundice, petechia, purpura, and microcephaly) (Chapter 96 and 97). In normal, immunocompetent adults, the infection is occasionally characterized by a mononucleosis-like syndrome. Among immunosuppressed individuals, including recipients of transplants and patients with acquired immunodeficiency syndrome (AIDS), CMV pneumonitis, retinitis, and gastrointestinal disease are common and can be fatal. The infection, which occurs in a seronegative, susceptible host, is referred to as primary infection, whereas recurrent infection represents reactivation of latent infection or reinfection in a seropositive immune host. Disease may result from primary or recurrent CMV infection, but the former is a more common cause of severe disease.

ETIOLOGY. CMV is the largest of the herpesviruses, with a diameter of 200 nm. It contains double-stranded DNA in a 64-nm core enclosed by an icosahedral capsid composed of 162 capsomers. The core is assembled in the nucleus of the host cells. The capsid is surrounded by a poorly defined amorphous tegument, which is itself surrounded by a loosely applied, lipid-containing envelope. The envelope is acquired during the budding process through the nuclear membrane into a cytoplasmic vacuole, which contains the protein components of the envelope. Mature viruses exit the cells by reverse pinocytosis. The CMV genome encodes for at least 35 structural proteins, glycoproteins, and an undefined number of nonstructural proteins. Serologic tests do not define specific serotypes. In contrast, restriction endonuclease analysis of CMV DNA shows that, although all known human strains are genetically homologous, none are identical unless they were obtained from epidemiologically related cases.

EPIDEMIOLOGY. Seroepidemiologic surveys demonstrate CMV infection in every population examined. The prevalence of infection, which increases with age, is higher in developing countries and among lower socioeconomic strata of the more developed nations. Sources of CMV include saliva, milk, cervical and vaginal secretions, urine, semen, stools, and blood. The spread of CMV requires very close or intimate contact because it is very labile. Transmission occurs by direct person-to-person contact, but indirect transmission is possible via contaminated fomites such as toys. The incidence of congenital infection ranges from 0.2–2.4% of all live births. The higher rates occur in populations with a lower standard of living. The fetus may become infected as a consequence of both primary and recurrent infections. The latter, which is more common in highly immune populations, is less likely to cause disease in the newborn infant or to lead to developmental sequelae.

Perinatal transmission is common, reaching 10–60% by 6 mo of age. The most important sources of virus are genital tract secretions at delivery and breast milk. Infected infants excrete virus for years in saliva and urine. After the 1st year of life, the prevalence of infection is dependent on child-rearing practices, with day-care centers contributing to the rapid spread of CMV. Infection rates of 50–80% are common. For children who are not exposed to other toddlers, the rate of infection increases very slowly throughout the 1st decade of life. A 2nd peak occurs in adolescence as a result of sexual transmission.

Seronegative child care workers and parents of young children shedding CMV have a 10–20% annual risk of acquiring CMV, which contrasts with 1–3% per year for the general population. Health care providers are not at increased risk for acquiring CMV infection from patients. Nosocomial infection is a hazard of transfusion of blood and blood products. In a population with a 50% prevalence of infection, the risk has been estimated at 2.7% per unit of whole blood. Leukocyte transfusions have a much greater risk. Infection is usually asymptomatic, but, even in well children and adults, there is a risk of disease if the patients are seronegative and receive multiple units. Immunosuppressed patients and seronegative premature infants have a much higher (10–30%) risk of disease. CMV infection is transmitted in transplanted organs (kidney, heart, and bone marrow). After transplantation, many patients excrete CMV as a result of infection acquired from the donor organ or from reactivation of latent infection caused by immunosuppression. Seronegative recipients of organs harvested from seropositive donors are at greatest risk for severe disease.

PATHOLOGY. Strikingly enlarged intranuclear inclusion-bearing cells that also have cytoplasmic inclusions are pathognomonic for CMV infections. The virus induces focal mononuclear cell infiltrates, which may be present with or without cytomegalic cells. The virus may induce focal necrosis in the brain and liver, which may be extensive and accompanied by granulomatous change with calcifications. The lung, liver, kidney, gastrointestinal tract, and salivary and other exocrine glands are the most commonly infected organs, although the virus has been found in most cell types. The extent of abnormal organ function and the quantity of virus that can be recovered from affected organs are not related to the number of cytomegalic inclusion-bearing cells, which may be few or absent in each organ section examined.

CLINICAL MANIFESTATIONS. The signs and symptoms of CMV infection vary with age, route of transmission, and immune competence of the individual. The infection is subclinical in most patients, including those with congenital infection (see Chapters 96 and 97). Infections acquired from the mother and other contacts are almost always asymptomatic and do not cause sequelae. Premature infants with transfusion-acquired infection constitute an exception. If infected, seronegative infants with birthweights of 1,500 g or less have a 40% risk of experiencing hepatosplenomegaly, pneumonitis, gray pallor, jaundice, petechia, thrombocytopenia, atypical lymphocytosis, and hemolytic anemia. In young children, the infection occasionally causes pneumonitis, hepatitis, hepatomegaly, and petechial rashes. In older children, adolescents, and adults, CMV may cause mononucleosis-like syndrome characterized by fatigue, malaise, myalgia, headache, fever, hepatosplenomegaly, abnormal liver function test results, and atypical lymphocytosis.

The course of CMV mononucleosis is generally mild, lasting 2–3 wk. An occasional patient may present with persistent fever, overt hepatitis, or morbilliform rash, or a combination. Recurrent infections are asymptomatic in the normal host. In immunocompromised individuals, the risk of CMV disease is increased with both primary and recurrent infections. Illness with a primary infection ranges from pneumonitis (most common), hepatitis, chorioretinitis, gastrointestinal disease, or fever with leukopenia as isolated entities to generalized disease, which is often fatal. The risk is greatest in patients who underwent bone marrow transplantation and in those with AIDS. Pneumonia, retinitis, and involvement of the central nervous system and gastrointestinal tract are usually severe and progressive. Submucosal ulcerations can occur anywhere in the gastrointestinal tract. Hemorrhage and perforation are known complications, as are pancreatitis and cholecystitis.

DIAGNOSIS. Active CMV infection is best demonstrated by virus isolation from urine, saliva, bronchoalveolar washings, milk, cervical secretions, buffy coat, and tissues obtained by biopsy. Rapid (24-hr) identification is now routine with the centrifugation-enhanced rapid culture system based on the detection of CMV early antigens by monoclonal antibodies. Polymerase chain reaction and DNA hybridization techniques can be used, but their sensitivities and cost effectiveness remain to be established. Virus isolation alone cannot distinguish between primary and recurrent infections. A primary infection is confirmed by seroconversion or the simultaneous detection of immunoglobulin (Ig)G and IgM antibodies. Rising IgG antibody titers may be caused by primary and recurrent infection and must be interpreted with caution. Sensitive and specific serologic tests to measure IgG antibodies are available in diagnostic laboratories.

To define rises in antibody titers complement fixation, neutralization, anticomplement immunofluorescence, and indirect immunofluorescence, assays are preferable because they are quantitative. In contrast, radioimmunoassay (RIA) and enzyme-linked immunosorbent assay (ELISA) are less reliable for demonstrating significant changes in titers because most laboratories establish binding ratio (RIA) and absorbance units (ELISA) at a fixed serum dilution to compare the quantities of antibodies present in two sera. A simple rise in antibody titers in initially seropositive subjects must be interpreted with caution because these are occasionally seen years after primary infection. IgG antibodies persist for life. IgM antibodies can be demonstrated transiently (4–16 wk) during the acute phase of symptomatic as well as asymptomatic primary infection in adults. RIA, ELISA, and an IgM capture RIA have acceptable specificity and sensitivity to detect primary infections. IgM antibodies are rarely found with these assays (0.2–1%) in patients with recurrent infection.

A recurrent infection is defined by the reappearance of viral excretion in a patient known to have been seropositive in the past. The distinction between reactivation of endogenous virus and reinfection with a different strain of CMV requires restriction enzyme analysis of viral DNA to demonstrate homology between viral isolates.

In immunocompromised patients, excretion of CMV, rises in IgG titers, and even the presence of IgM antibodies are common, making the distinction between primary and recurrent infections more difficult. Determining pretransplantation and preimmunosuppressive treatment serologic status of the patients is helpful. Demonstrating viremia by buffy coat culture implies active disease and worse prognosis whether the type of infection is primary, recurrent, or unknown.

The definitive method for diagnosis of congenital CMV infection is virus isolation or demonstration of specific DNA sequences (see Chapters 96 and 97). Urine and saliva are the best specimens to submit to the laboratory. An IgG antibody test is of little diagnostic value because a positive result generally reflects maternal immunity, although a negative result excludes the diagnosis. Demonstration of stable or rising titers in serial specimens during the 1st year of life does not help because perinatal infection is common. In general, IgM tests lack sensitivity and specificity and are technically demanding. No reliable IgM test is commercially available.

PREVENTION

Passive Immunoprophylaxis. The use of hyperimmune plasma or globulin for prophylaxis of infection in transplant recipients reduces the risk of symptomatic disease but does not prevent infection. The efficacy of immunoglobulin is more striking in situations in which the hazard of primary CMV infection is greatest, such as in bone marrow transplantation. One recommended regimen is 1.0 g/kg of immunoglobulin given as a single intravenous dose beginning within 72 hr of transplantation and once weekly thereafter until day 120 after transplantation.

Active Immunization. The beneficial role of immunity is substantial, as illustrated by the fact that most severe disease follows primary infections, especially in congenital infection, transfusion-acquired infection, and infection in transplant recipients. Candidates for a CMV vaccine include seronegative women of childbearing age and seronegative transplant recipients. Live, attenuated vaccines are immunogenic, but immunity wanes quickly. The investigational Towne vaccine produces self-limited asymptomatic infection, which results in the production of humoral and cell-mediated immune responses in most healthy volunteers. Vaccine virus does not seem to be transmissible. Vaccines are protected when challenged with low but not high doses of challenge virus and illness occurs from higher vaccine doses. The vaccine does not protect renal transplant recipients from CMV infection but appears to reduce the virulence of primary infection. In a study of vaccine efficacy in normal adult women, the Towne vaccine did not provide protection against naturally acquired infection. Other types of vaccines, such as subunit and recombinant vaccines, are being developed.

The use of CMV-free blood and blood products and, when possible, the use of organs from CMV-free donors represent important measures to prevent CMV infection and disease in nonimmune patients.

TREATMENT. Ganciclovir has been used to treat life-threatening CMV infections in immunocompromised hosts (such as bone marrow, heart, and kidney transplant recipients and patients with AIDS). A regimen of 10 mg/kg/24 hr, with individual doses administered at 12-hr intervals for 2–3 wk, followed by maintenance dose of 5 mg/kg/24 hr administered until regression of clinical manifestations, has had some efficacy. CMV retinitis and gastrointestinal disease appear to be clinically responsive to therapy but, like viral excretion, often recur on cessation. Toxicity with ganciclovir is extensive, including neutropenia, thrombocytopenia, liver dysfunction, reduction in spermatogenesis, and gastrointestinal and renal abnormalities. No controlled studies of treatment of congenital CMV infection are available. One phase I-II study shows encouraging results at a dose of 12 mg/kg/24 hr for a total of 6 wk. A randomized study of symptomatic congenital CMV infection is in progress.

PROGNOSIS

Congenital Disease. See Chapters 96 and 97.

Acquired Disease. Patients with CMV mononucleosis usually recover fully, although some have a protracted illness. Many whose infections are acquired in association with immunosuppression and transplantation recover, but a significant number have severe pneumonitis, and the fatality rate is high if hypoxemia develops. CMV infection and disease may be terminal events in individuals with increased susceptibility to infections such as those with AIDS.

Alford CA, Britt WJ: Cytomegalovirus. *In:* Fields BN, Knipe DM, et al. (eds): Virology, 2nd edition. New York, Raven Press, 1990, pp 1981–2010.

Ho M: Cytomegalovirus. *In:* Mandell GL, Douglas RG, Bennett JE (eds): Principles and Practice of Infectious Diseases, 3rd ed. New York, Churchill Livingston, 1990, pp 1159–1172.

Plotkin SA: Cytomegalovirus vaccines. *In:* Plotkin SA, Mortimer EA Jr (eds): Vaccines. Philadelphia, WB Saunders, 1988, pp 513–516.

Stagno S: Cytomegalovirus. *In:* Remington JS, Klein JO (eds): Infectious Diseases of the Fetus and Newborn Infant, 4th ed. Philadelphia, WB Saunders, in press.

Stagno S, Pass RF, Britt WJ: Cytomegalovirus. *In:* Schmidt NJ, Emmons RW (eds): Diagnostic Procedures for Viral, Rickettsial and Chlamydial Infections. 6th ed. Washington, DC, The American Public Health Association, 1989, pp 321–378.

Weller TH: The cytomegaloviruses: Ubiquitous agents with protein clinical manifestations. N Engl J Med 285:203, 267, 1971.

CHAPTER 215

Epstein-Barr Virus

Hal B. Jenson

Infectious mononucleosis is the best-known clinical syndrome caused by Epstein-Barr virus (EBV). It is characterized by systemic somatic complaints consisting primarily of fatigue, malaise, fever, sore throat, and generalized lymphadenopathy. Originally described as glandular fever, it derives its name from the mononuclear lymphocytosis with atypical-appearing lymphocytes that accompany the illness. Other less common infections may cause infectious mononucleosis–like illnesses.

ETIOLOGY. EBV, a member of the Herpesviridae, causes more than 90% of infectious mononucleosis cases. Approximately 5–10% of infectious mononucleosis–like illnesses are caused by primary infection with cytomegalovirus, *Toxoplasma gondii*, adenovirus, viral hepatitis, human immunodeficiency virus (HIV), and possibly rubella virus. In the majority of EBV-negative infectious mononucleosis–like illnesses, the exact cause remains unknown.

EPIDEMIOLOGY. The epidemiology of infectious mononucleosis is related to the epidemiology and age of acquisition of EBV infection. EBV infects up to 95% of the world's population. It is transmitted in oral secretions by close contact such as kissing or exchange of saliva from child to child, such as occurs between children in out-of-home child care. Nonintimate contact, environmental sources, or fomites do not contribute to spread of EBV.

EBV is shed in oral secretions for 6 mo or longer after acute infection and then intermittently for life. Healthy individuals with serologic evidence of past EBV infection excrete virus 10–20% of the time. Immunosuppression may permit reactivation of latent EBV; approximately 60% of seropositive, immunosuppressed patients shed the virus. EBV is also found in the genital tract of women and may possibly be spread by sexual contact.

Infection with EBV in developing countries and among socioeconomically disadvantaged populations of developed countries usually occurs during infancy and early childhood. In central Africa, almost all children are infected by 3 yr of age. Primary infection with EBV during childhood is usually inapparent or indistinguishable from other childhood infections; the clinical syndrome of infectious mononucleosis is practically unknown in undeveloped regions of the world. Among more affluent populations in industrialized countries, infection during childhood is still most common, but approximately one third of cases occur during adolescence and young adulthood. Primary EBV infection in adolescents and adults is manifest in 50% or more of cases by the classic triad of fatigue, pharyngitis, and generalized lymphadenopathy, which constitute the major clinical manifestations of infectious mononucleosis. This syndrome may be seen at all ages but is rarely apparent in children younger than 4 yr, when most EBV infections are asymptomatic, or in adults older than 40 yr, when most individuals have already been infected by EBV. The true incidence of the syndrome of infectious mononucleosis is unknown but is estimated to occur in 20–70 of 100,000 persons per year; in young adults the incidence rises to about 1 in 1,000 persons per year. The prevalence of serologic evidence of past EBV infection increases with age; almost all adults in the United States are seropositive.

PATHOGENESIS. After acquisition in the oral cavity, EBV initially infects oral epithelial cells; this may contribute to the symptoms of pharyngitis. After intracellular viral replication and cell lysis with release of new virions, virus spreads to contiguous structures such as the salivary glands with eventual viremia and infection of B lymphocytes in the peripheral blood and the entire lymphoreticular system including the liver and spleen. The atypical lymphocytes that are characteristic of infectious mononucleosis are $CD8^+$ T lymphocytes, which exhibit both suppressor and cytotoxic functions that develop in response to the infected B lymphocytes. This relative as well as absolute increase in $CD8^+$ lymphocytes results in a transient reversal of the normal 2:1 $CD4^+/CD8^+$ (helper-suppressor) T-lymphocyte ratio. Many of the clinical manifestations of infectious mononucleosis may result, at least in part, from the host immune response, which is effective in reducing the number of EBV-infected B lymphocytes to less than one per 10^6 of circulating B lymphocytes.

Epithelial cells of the uterine cervix may become infected by sexual transmission of the virus, although neither local symptoms nor infectious mononucleosis have been described following sexual transmission.

EBV, like the other herpesviruses, establishes lifelong latent infection after the primary illness. The latent virus is carried in oropharyngeal epithelial cells and systemic B lymphocytes as multiple episomes in the nucleus. The viral episomes replicate with cell division and are distributed to both daughter cells. Viral integration into the cell genome is not typical. Only a few viral proteins, including the EBV-determined nuclear antigens (EBNA), are produced during latency. These proteins are important in maintaining the viral episome during the latent state. Progression to viral replication begins with production of EBV early antigens (EA), proceeds to viral DNA replication, followed by production of viral capsid antigen (VCA), and culminates in cell death and release of mature virions. Reactivation with viral replication occurs at a low rate in populations of latently infected cells and is responsible for intermittent viral shedding in oropharyngeal secretions of infected individuals. Reactivation is apparently asymptomatic and not recognized to be accompanied by distinctive clinical symptoms.

Oncogenesis. EBV was the first human virus to be associated with malignancy and, therefore, was the first virus to be identified as a human tumor virus. EBV infection may result in a spectrum of proliferative disorders ranging from self-limited, usually benign disease such as infectious mononucleosis to aggressive, nonmalignant proliferations such as the virus-associated hemophagocytic syndrome to lymphoid and epithelial cell malignancies. Benign EBV-associated proliferations include oral, hairy leukoplakia, primarily in adults with the acquired immunodeficiency syndrome (AIDS), and lymphoid interstitial pneumonitis, primarily in children with AIDS. Malignant EBV-associated proliferations include nasopharyngeal carcinoma, Burkitt lymphoma, Hodgkin disease, and lymphoproliferative disorders and leiomyosarcoma in immunodeficient states including AIDS.

Nasopharyngeal carcinoma occurs worldwide but is 10 times more common in persons in southern China, where it is the most common malignant tumor among adult men. It is also common among whites in North Africa and Inuits in North America. All malignant cells of undifferentiated nasopharyngeal carcinoma contain a high copy number of EBV episomes. Undifferentiated and partially differentiated, nonkeratinizing nasopharyngeal carcinomas have diagnostic and prognostic antibodies to EBV antigens. High levels of immunoglobulin (Ig) A antibody to EA and VCA may be detected in asymptomatic individuals and can be used to follow response to tumor therapy (Table 215–1). Cells of well-differentiated, keratinizing nasopharyngeal carcinoma contain a low or zero copy number of EBV genomes and have EBV serologic patterns similar to those of the general population.

Endemic (African) Burkitt lymphoma, often found in the jaw, is the most common childhood cancer in equatorial East Africa and New Guinea. The median age of onset is 5 yr. These regions are holoendemic for *Plasmodium falciparum* malaria and have a high rate of EBV infection early in life. The constant malarial exposure acts as a B-lymphocyte mitogen that contributes to the polyclonal B-lymphocyte proliferation with EBV infection. It also impairs the T-lymphocyte control of EBV-infected B lymphocytes. Approximately 98% of cases of endemic Burkitt lymphoma contain the EBV genome compared with only 20% of nonendemic (sporadic or American) Burkitt lymphoma cases. Individuals with Burkitt lymphoma have unusually and characteristically high levels of antibody to VCA and EA that correlate with the risk of developing tumor (see Table 215–1).

All cases of Burkitt lymphoma, including those that are EBV negative, are monoclonal and demonstrate chromosomal translocation of the c-*myc* proto-oncogene to the constant region of the immunoglobulin heavy-chain locus, t(8;14), to the kappa constant light-chain locus, t(2;8), or to the lambda constant light-chain locus, t(8;22). This results in the deregulation and constitutive transcription of the c-*myc* gene with overproduction of a normal c-*myc* product that autosuppresses c-*myc* production on the untranslocated chromosome.

The incidence of *Hodgkin disease* peaks in childhood in developing countries and in young adulthood in developed countries. Levels of EBV antibodies are consistently elevated preceding development of Hodgkin disease; only a small minority of patients are seronegative for EBV. Infection with EBV appears to increase the risk of Hodgkin disease by a factor of two to four. EBV is associated with more than one half of cases of mixed-cellularity Hodgkin disease and approximately one quarter of cases of the nodular sclerosing subtype and is rarely associated with lymphocyte-predominant Hodgkin disease. Immunohistochemical studies have localized EBV to the Reed-Sternberg cells and their variants, the pathognomonic malignant cells of Hodgkin disease.

Failure to control EBV infection may result from host immunologic deficits. The prototype is the *X-linked lymphoproliferative syndrome (Duncan syndrome),* an X chromosome–linked recessive disorder of the immune system associated with severe, persistent, and sometimes fatal EBV infection. Approximately two thirds of these male patients die of disseminated and fulminating lymphoproliferation involving multiple organs at the time of primary EBV infection. Surviving patients acquire hypogammaglobulinemia, B-cell lymphoma, or both. Most patients die by 10 yr.

A number of other congenital and acquired immunodeficiency syndromes are associated with an increased incidence of EBV-associated B-lymphocyte lymphoma, particularly central nervous system lymphoma. The incidence of lymphoproliferative syndromes parallels the degree of immunosuppression. A decline in T-cell function evidently permits EBV to escape from immune surveillance. Congenital immunodeficiencies predisposing to EBV-associated lymphoproliferations include the X-linked lymphoproliferative syndrome, common-variable immunodeficiency, ataxia-telangiectasia, Wiskott-Aldrich syndrome, and Chédiak-Higashi syndrome. Individuals with acquired immunodeficiencies resulting from anticancer chemotherapy, immunosuppression after solid organ or bone marrow transplantation, or HIV infection have a significantly increased risk of EBV-associated lymphoproliferations. The lymphomas

■ **TABLE 215–1 Correlation of Clinical Status and Serologic Responses to EBV Infection**

	Serologic Response					
		EBV-Specific Antibody				
Clinical Status	***Heterophile Antibodies (Qualitative Test)***	**IgM-VCA**	**IgG-VCA**	**EA-D**	**EA-R**	**EBNA**
Negative reaction	–	<1:8*	<1:10*	<1:10*	<1:10*	<1:2.5*
Susceptible	–	–	–	–	–†	–
Acute primary infection: infectious mononucleosis	+	1:32 to 1:256	1:160 to 1:640	1:40 to 1:160	–†	– to 1:2.5
Recent primary infection: infectious mononucleosis	+/–	– to 1:32	1:320 to 1:1,280	1:40 to 1:160	–†	1:5 to 1:10
Remote infection	–	–	1:40 to 1:160	–‡	– to 1:40	1:10 to 1:40
Reactivation: immunosuppressed or immunocompromised	–	–	1:320 to 1:1,280	–‡	1:80 to 1:320	– to 1:160
Burkitt lymphoma	–	–	1:320 to 1:1,280	–‡	1:80 to 1:320	1:10 to 1:80
Nasopharyngeal carcinoma	–	–	1:320 to 1:1,280	1:40 to 1:160	–§	1:20 to 1:160

The data were obtained from numerous studies. Individual responses outside the characteristic range may occur.

**Or the lowest test dilution.*

†In young children and adults with asymptomatic seroconversion, the anti–early antigen response may be mainly to the EA-R component.

‡A minority of individuals will have the anti–early antigen response mainly to the EA-D component.

§A minority of individuals will have the anti–early antigen response mainly to the EA-R component.

EBV = Epstein-Barr virus; – = negative; + = positive; IgM = immunoglobulin M; IgG = immunoglobulin G; VCA = viral capsid antigen; EA-D = diffuse staining component of EA; EA-R = cytoplasmic restricted component of early antigen; EBNA = EBV-determined nuclear antigens.

Reprinted with permission from Sumaya CV, Jenson HB: Epstein-Barr virus. In: *Manual of Clinical Laboratory Immunology, 4th ed. Rose NR, de Macario EC, Fahey JL, Friedman H, Penn GM (eds): Washington, DC, American Society for Microbiology, 1992, p 570.*

may be focal or diffuse, and they are usually histologically polyclonal but may become monoclonal. Their growth is not reversed on cessation of immunosuppression.

EBV has been linked with a multitude of other tumors; the strongest association of EBV is to primary central nervous system lymphoma and carcinoma of the salivary glands. Other tumors include T-lymphocyte lymphoma, lethal midline granuloma (a T-cell lymphoma), angioimmunoblastic lymphadenopathy–like lymphoma, thymomas and thymic carcinomas derived from thymic epithelial cells, supraglottic laryngeal carcinomas, lymphoepithelial tumors of the respiratory tract and gastrointestinal tract, leiomyosarcoma, and gastric adenocarcinoma. The precise contribution of EBV to these various malignancies is not well defined.

CLINICAL MANIFESTATIONS. The incubation period of infectious mononucleosis in adolescents is 30–50 days. In children it may be shorter. The majority of cases of primary EBV infection in infants and young children are clinically silent. In older patients, the onset of illness is usually insidious and vague. Patients may complain of malaise, fatigue, fever, headache, sore throat, nausea, abdominal pain, and myalgia. This prodromal period may last 1–2 wk. The complaints of sore throat and fever gradually increase until patients seek medical care. Splenic enlargement may be rapid enough to cause left upper quadrant abdominal discomfort and tenderness, which may be the presenting complaint.

The physical examination is characterized by generalized lymphadenopathy (90% of cases), splenomegaly (50% of cases), and hepatomegaly (10% of cases). Lymphadenopathy occurs most commonly in the anterior and posterior cervical nodes, and submandibular lymph nodes and less commonly in the axillary and inguinal lymph nodes. Epitrochlear lymphadenopathy is particularly suggestive of infectious mononucleosis. Symptomatic hepatitis or jaundice is uncommon. Splenomegaly to 2–3 cm below the costal margin is typical; massive enlargement is uncommon.

The sore throat is often accompanied by moderate to severe pharyngitis with marked tonsillar enlargement, occasionally with exudates (Fig. 215–1 [color plate section]). Petechiae at the junction of the hard and soft palate are frequently seen. The pharyngitis resembles that caused by streptococcal infection. Other clinical findings may include rashes and edema of the eyelids. Rashes are usually maculopapular and have been reported in 3–15% of patients. Eighty per cent of patients with infectious mononucleosis will experience a rash if treated with ampicillin or amoxicillin; the reason for this phenomenon is unknown.

COMPLICATIONS. Very few patients with infectious mononucleosis experience complications. The most feared complication is splenic rupture, which occurs most frequently during the 2nd week of the disease. A 0.2% rate has been reported in adults; the rate in children is unknown but is probably much lower. Rupture is commonly related to trauma, which often may be mild. Swelling of the tonsils and oropharyngeal lymphoid tissue may be substantial and cause airway impairment manifest by stridor and interference with breathing. Airway impairment may be treated by administration of corticosteroids; respiratory distress with incipient or actual airway occlusion should be managed by maintaining the airway with intubation in an intensive care setting.

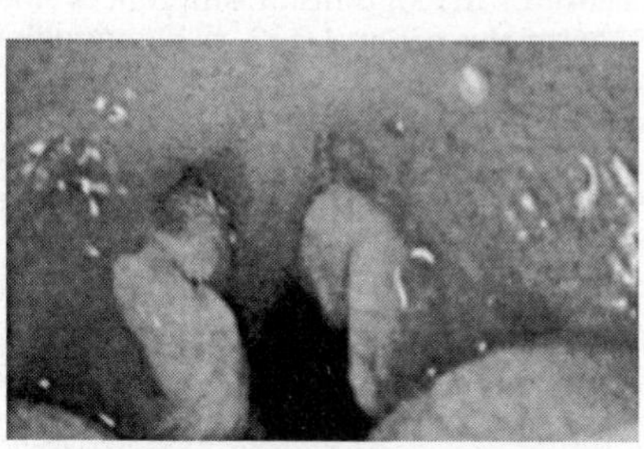

Figure 215–1. Tonsillitis with membrane formation in infectious mononucleosis. See also color section. (Courtesy of Alex J. Steigman, M.D.)

Many uncommon and unusual conditions have been reported to be associated with EBV infectious mononucleosis. Neurologic involvement may be serious with ataxia and seizures. Perceptual distortions of space and size, referred to as the Alice in Wonderland syndrome, may be a presenting symptom. There may be meningitis with nuchal rigidity and mononuclear cells in the cerebrospinal fluid, facial nerve palsy, transverse myelitis, and encephalitis. Guillain-Barré syndrome or Reye syndrome may follow acute illness. Hemolytic anemia, often with a positive Coombs test and with cold agglutinins specific for red cell antigen i, may occur late in the illness. Aplastic anemia is a rare complication that usually presents 1 mo after the onset of illness. The prognosis for eventual recovery is good, although substantial supportive treatment is necessary during the acute stages. Myocarditis or interstitial pneumonia may occur, both resolving in 3–4 wk. Other rare complications include pancreatitis, parotitis, and orchitis.

DIAGNOSIS. The diagnosis of infectious mononucleosis implies primary EBV infection. A presumptive diagnosis may be made by the presence of typical clinical symptoms with atypical lymphocytosis in the peripheral blood. The diagnosis is confirmed by serologic testing.

Differential Diagnosis. Infectious mononucleosis–like illnesses may be caused by primary infection with cytomegalovirus, *T. gondii,* adenovirus, viral hepatitis, HIV, or possibly rubella virus. Cytomegalovirus infection is a particularly common cause in adults. Streptococcal pharyngitis may cause sore throat and cervical lymphadenopathy indistinguishable from that of infectious mononucleosis but is not associated with hepatosplenomegaly. Approximately 5% of cases of EBV-associated infectious mononucleosis have positive throat cultures for group A β-hemolytic streptococci; this represents pharyngeal streptococcal carriage. Failure of a patient with streptococcal pharyngitis to improve within 48–72 hr should evoke suspicion of infectious mononucleosis. The most serious problem in the diagnosis of acute illness arises in the occasional patients with low white cell counts, moderate thrombocytopenia, and even hemolytic anemia. In these patients, bone marrow examination and hematologic consultation are warranted to exclude the possibility of leukemia.

Routine Laboratory Tests. In more than 90% of cases, there is leukocytosis of 10,000–20,000 cells/mm^3, of which at least two thirds are lymphocytes; atypical lymphocytes usually account for 20–40% of the total number. The atypical cells are mature T lymphocytes that have been antigenically activated. Compared with regular lymphocytes microscopically, atypical lymphocytes are larger overall, with larger, eccentrically placed indented and folded nuclei with a lower nuclear-cytoplasm ratio. Although atypical lymphocytosis may be seen with many of the infections usually causing lymphocytosis, the highest degree of atypical lymphocytes is classically seen with EBV infection. Other syndromes associated with atypical lymphocytosis include acquired cytomegalovirus infection (as contrasted to congenital cytomegalovirus infection), toxoplasmosis, viral hepatitis, rubella, roseola, mumps, tuberculosis, typhoid, mycoplasma infection, malaria, as well as some drug reactions. Mild thrombocytopenia to 50,000–200,000 platelets/mm^3 occurs in more than 50% of patients, but only rarely are values low enough to cause purpura. Mild elevation of hepatic transaminases occurs in approximately 50% of uncomplicated cases but is usually asymptomatic without jaundice.

Heterophile Antibody Test. Heterophile antibodies agglutinate cells from species different from those in the source serum. The transient heterophile antibodies seen in infectious mononucleosis, also known as Paul-Bunnell antibodies, are IgM antibodies detected by the Paul-Bunnell–Davidsohn test for sheep red cell agglutination. The heterophile antibodies of infectious mononucleosis agglutinate sheep or, for greater sensitivity, horse red cells but not guinea pig kidney cells. This adsorption property differentiates this response from the heterophile response found in patients with serum sickness, rheumatic diseases, and some normal individuals. Titers greater than 1:28 or 1:40 (depending on the dilution system used) after absorption with guinea pig cells are considered positive.

The sheep red cell agglutination test is likely to be positive for several months after infectious mononucleosis; the horse red cell agglutination test may be positive for as long as 2 yr. The most widely used method is the qualitative, rapid slide test using horse erythrocytes. It detects heterophile antibody in 90% of cases of EBV-associated infectious mononucleosis in older children and adults but in only up to 50% of cases in children younger than 4 yr because they typically develop a lower titer. Approximately 5–10% of cases of infectious mononucleosis are not caused by EBV and are not uniformly associated with a heterophile antibody response. The false-positive rate is less than 10%, usually resulting from erroneous interpretation. If the heterophile test is negative and an EBV infection is suspected, EBV-specific antibody testing is indicated.

Specific EBV Antibodies. EBV-specific antibody testing is useful to confirm acute EBV infection, especially in heterophile-negative cases, or to confirm past infection and determine susceptibility to future infection. Several distinct EBV antigen systems have been characterized for diagnostic purposes (Fig. 215–2). Table 215–1 summarizes serologic responses that are expected in various situations. The EBNA, EA, and VCA antigen systems are most useful for diagnostic purposes. The acute phase of infectious mononucleosis is characterized by rapid IgM and IgG antibody responses to VCA in all cases and an IgG response to EA in most cases. The IgM response to VCA is transient but can be detected for at least 4 wk and occasionally up to 3 mo. The laboratory must take steps to remove rheumatoid factor, which may cause a false-positive IgM VCA result. The IgG response to VCA usually peaks late in the acute phase, declines slightly over the next several weeks to months, and then persists at a relatively stable level for life.

Anti-EA antibodies are usually detectable for several months but may persist or be detected intermittently at low levels for many years. Antibodies to the diffuse-staining component of EA, EA-D, are found transiently in 80% of patients during the acute phase of infectious mononucleosis and reach high titers in patients with nasopharyngeal carcinoma. Antibodies to the cytoplasmic-restricted component of EA, EA-R, emerge transiently in the convalescence from infectious mononucleosis and often attain high titers in patients with EBV-associated Burkitt lymphoma, which in the terminal stage of the disease may be exceeded by antibodies to EA-D. High levels of antibodies to EA-D or EA-R may be found also in immunocompromised patients with persistent EBV infections and active EBV replication. Anti-EBNA antibodies are the last to develop in infectious mononucleosis and gradually appear 3–4 mo after the onset of illness and remain at low levels for life. Absence of anti-EBNA when other antibodies are present implies recent infection, while the presence of anti-EBNA implies infection occurring more than 3–4 mo previously. The wide range of individual antibody responses and the various laboratory methods used can occasionally make interpretation of an antibody profile difficult. The detection of IgM antibody to VCA is the most valuable and specific serologic test for the diagnosis of acute EBV infection and is generally sufficient to confirm the diagnosis.

TREATMENT. There is no specific treatment for infectious mononucleosis. Therapy with high doses of intravenous acyclovir decreases viral replication and oropharyngeal shedding during the period of administration but does not affect the severity of symptoms or the eventual clinical course. Rest and symptomatic therapy are the mainstays of management. Bed rest is necessary only when the patient has debilitating fatigue. As soon as there is definite symptomatic improvement, the patient should be allowed to begin resuming normal activities. Because blunt abdominal trauma may predispose patients to splenic rupture, it is customary and prudent to advise withdrawal from contact sports and strenuous athletic activities during the first 2–3 wk of illness or while splenomegaly is present.

Short courses of corticosteroids (less than 2 wk) may be helpful for complications of infectious mononucleosis, but their use has not been evaluated critically. Some appropriate indications include incipient airway obstruction, thrombocytopenia with hemorrhaging, autoimmune hemolytic anemia, and seizures and meningitis. A recommended dosage is prednisone 1 mg/kg/24 hr (maximum 60 mg/24 hr) or equivalent for 7 days and tapered over another 7 days. There are no controlled data to show efficacy of corticosteroids in any of these conditions. In view of the potential and unknown hazards of immunosuppression for a virus infection with oncogenic complications, corticosteroids should not be used in usual cases of infectious mononucleosis.

PROGNOSIS. The prognosis for complete recovery is excellent if no complications ensue during the acute illness. The major symptoms typically last 2–4 wk followed by gradual recovery. Second attacks of infectious mononucleosis caused by EBV

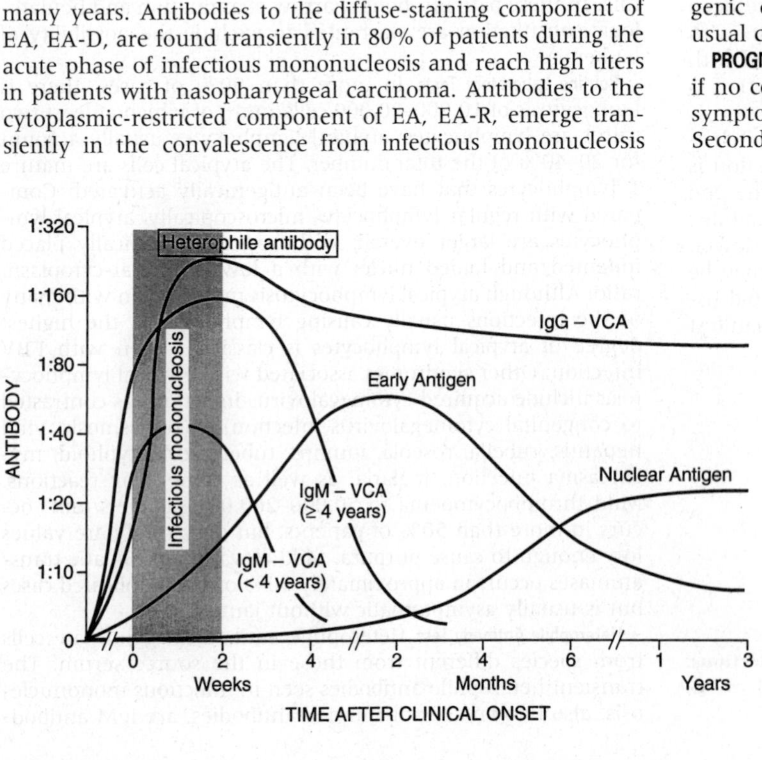

Figure 215–2. Schematic representation of the development of antibodies to various Epstein-Barr virus antigens in patients with infectious mononucleosis. The titers are geometric mean values expressed as reciprocals of the serum dilution. The immunoglobulin M (IgM) response to viral capsid antigen (VCA) is divided because of the significant differences noted according to age of the patient. (IgG = immunoglobulin G) (Reprinted with permission from Sumaya CV, Jenson HB: Epstein-Barr virus. *In* Rose NR, de Macario EC, Fahey JL, Friedman H, Penn GM [eds]: Manual of Clinical Laboratory Immunology, 4th ed. Washington, DC, American Society for Microbiology, 1992, p 570.)

have not been documented. Fatigue, malaise, and some disability that may wax and wane for several weeks to a few months are common complaints even in otherwise unremarkable cases. Occasional persistence of fatigue for a few years after infectious mononucleosis is well recognized. At present, there is no specific evidence linking EBV infection to chronic fatigue syndrome (see Chapter 661).

Alpert G, Fleisher GR: Complications of infection with Epstein-Barr virus during childhood: A study of children admitted to the hospital. Pediatr Infect Dis 3:304, 1984.
Andiman WA: Epstein-Barr virus-associated syndromes: A critical reexamination. Pediatr Infect Dis 3:198, 1984.
Gaffey MJ, Weiss LM: Association of Epstein-Barr virus with human neoplasia. Pathol Annu 27:55, 1992.
Horwitz CA, Henle W, Henle G, et al. Clinical and laboratory evaluation of cytomegalovirus-induced mononucleosis in previously healthy individuals: Report of 82 cases. Medicine 65:124, 1986.
Marshall GS, Gesser RM, Yamanishi K, et al: Chronic fatigue syndrome in children: Clinical features, Epstein-Barr virus and human herpesvirus 6 serology and long term follow-up. Pediatr Infect Dis J 10:287, 1991.
Schlossberg D (ed): Infectious Mononucleosis. New York, Springer-Verlag, 1989.
Straus SE, Tosato G, Armstrong G, et al: Persisting illness and fatigue in adults with evidence of Epstein-Barr virus infection. Ann Intern Med 102:7, 1985.
Sumayer TA, Grierson H, Pirruccello ST, et al: X-linked lymphoproliferative disease. Am J Dis Child 147:1242, 1993.
Sumaya CV, Ench Y: Epstein-Barr virus infectious mononucleosis in children: I. Clinical and general laboratory findings. Pediatrics 75:1003, 1985.
Sumaya CV, Ench Y: Epstein-Barr virus infectious mononucleosis in children: II. Heterophil antibody and viral-specific responses. Pediatrics 75:1011, 1985.

CHAPTER 216
Influenza Viral Infections

Peter Wright

Influenza viral infections cause a broad array of respiratory illnesses that are responsible for significant morbidity and mortality in children.

ETIOLOGY. Influenza viruses are classified as Orthomyxoviridae. They are large, single-stranded RNA viruses with a segmented genome encased in a lipid-containing envelope. The two major surface proteins that determine the serotype of influenza, the hemagglutinin and neuraminidase, project as spikes through the envelope. Influenza viruses are divided into three types: A, B, and C. Influenza types A and B are the primary influenzal pathogens and causes of epidemic disease. Influenza type C is a sporadic cause of predominantly upper respiratory tract disease. Influenza types A and B are further divided into serotypically distinct strains that circulate on a yearly basis through the population.

EPIDEMIOLOGY. Influenza A viruses have a complex epidemiology involving animal hosts that serve as a reservoir for diverse strains with potential for infecting the human population. The segmented nature of the influenza genome allows reassortment to occur between an animal and human virus when coinfection occurs. Thus, potentially any of 13 hemagglutinins and 9 neuraminidases residing in animal reservoirs may be introduced into humans. In addition, avian hosts that are migratory may be responsible for spread of disease. Influenza B has a lesser capacity for major antigenic change and no identified animal reservoir.

When a virus identified by a novel and serologically distinct hemagglutinin or neuraminidase enters the population, there is potential for a pandemic of influenza with excess morbidity and mortality on a global scale in a largely nonimmune population. The most dramatic pandemic in recent history occurred in 1918 when influenza was estimated to have killed more than 20 million people. More common is the almost yearly variation in the antigenic composition of the surface proteins, which confers a selective advantage to a new strain and results in localized epidemics of disease with mortality largely confined to the elderly and to those with underlying cardiopulmonary disease. Each year's strain is novel for infants because they have no pre-existing antibody except for maternally transferred antibody in the very young.

The attack rate and frequency of isolation of influenza is highest in young children. As many as 30–50% of children have serologic evidence of infection in a typical year. Children undergoing primary exposure to an influenza strain have much higher and more prolonged shedding of the virus than adults, making them extremely effective transmitters of infection. Influenza is a disease of the colder months of the year in temperate climates; spread appears to occur by small-particle aerosol. Transmission through a community is rapid, with the highest incidence of illness occurring within 2–3 wk of introduction. It is marked by increased school absenteeism and the yearly peak in visits to the pediatrician. Influenza has been implicated in hospital spread of infection and may complicate the original illness that required hospitalization.

On a country or global basis, one or two predominant strains spread to create the annual epidemic. At present, influenza type A strains with the H1N1 and H3N2 serotypes and type B strains are cocirculating, and either type may be predominant in any one year, making predictions about the serotype and severity of the upcoming influenza season very difficult. Strain variants are identified by their hemagglutinin and neuraminidase serotypes, by the geographic area from which they were originally isolated, by their isolate number, and by year of isolation. Thus, the current influenza vaccine for 1994–1995 is trivalent, having strains identified as A/Shangdong/9/93(H3N2), A/Texas/36/91(H1N1), and B/Panama/46/90.

PATHOLOGY. Influenza causes a lytic infection of the respiratory epithelium with loss of ciliary function, decreased mucus production, and desquamation of the epithelial layer. These changes permit secondary bacterial invasion either directly through the epithelium or, in the case of the middle ear space, through obstruction of the normal drainage through the eustachian tube. Influenza types A and B have been reported to cause myocarditis, and influenza type B can cause myositis. When influenza type B is accompanied by the administration of salicylates, the fatty liver, cerebral edema, and mitochondrial changes that are the hallmarks of Reye syndrome can be seen.

PATHOGENESIS. The incubation period of influenza can be as short as 48–72 hr. The virus attaches to sialic acid residues on cells via the hemagglutinin and, via endocytosis, makes its way into vacuoles, where, with progressive acidification, there is fusion to the endosomal membrane and release of the viral RNA into the cytoplasm. The RNA is transported to the nucleus and transcribed. Newly synthesized RNA is returned to the cytoplasm and translated into proteins, which are transported to the cell membrane. This is followed by budding of virus through the cell membrane. The packaging mechanisms for the segmented genome are not well understood. A proteolytic cleavage of the hemagglutinin occurs at some point in the assembly and release of the virus which is essential for successful reinfection and amplification of virus titer. In humans, this replicative cycle is confined to the respiratory epithelium. With primary infection, virus replication continues for 10–14 days. Implicit in successful replication in the respiratory tract is the assumption that key proteolytic enzymes exist at this site. The successful cleavage of hemagglutinin has been demonstrated by respiratory secretions, but the cellular origin of the enzyme remains undefined.

The exact immune mechanisms involved in termination of

primary infection and protection against reinfection are not well understood. The extremely short incubation period of influenza and its growth on the mucosal surface pose particular problems for invoking a protective immune response. Antigen presentation must be primarily at mucosal sites acting through the bronchial associated lymphoid tract. The major humoral response is directed against the hemagglutinin and high serum antibody levels generated by inactivated vaccine correlate with protection. Mucosally produced immunoglobulin (Ig) A antibodies are presumably directed at the same antigenic sites and are thought to be the most effective and immediate response that can be generated to protect against influenza. Unfortunately, measurable IgA antibodies against influenza persist for a relatively short period, and symptomatic reinfection with influenza can be seen at intervals of 3–4 yr. Although heterotypic immunity can be demonstrated in the mouse through cell-mediated immune mechanisms directed toward common internal proteins, heterotypic immunity has not been shown in humans.

CLINICAL MANIFESTATIONS. Influenza types A and B cause predominantly a respiratory illness. The onset of illness is abrupt and is marked by coryza, conjunctivitis, pharyngitis, and dry cough (Table 216–1). The predominant symptoms may localize anywhere in the respiratory tract, producing an isolated upper respiratory tract illness, croup, bronchiolitis, or pneumonia. More so than any of the other respiratory viruses, influenza is accompanied by systemic signs of high fever, myalgia, malaise, and headache. Many of these symptoms may be mediated through cytokine production by the respiratory tract epithelium instead of reflecting systemic spread of the virus. The typical duration of the febrile illness is 2–4 days. Cough may persist for longer periods of time, and evidence of small airway dysfunction is often found weeks later. Other family members or close contacts often have a similar illness. Influenza is a less distinct illness in younger children and infants, with manifestations that may be localized to any region of the respiratory tract. The children may be highly febrile and toxic in appearance, prompting a full diagnostic workup. In spite of the distinctive features of influenza, the illness is often indistinguishable from that caused by other respiratory viruses such as respiratory syncytial virus, parainfluenza virus, and adenovirus.

LABORATORY FINDINGS. The clinical laboratory abnormalities associated with influenza are nonspecific. A relative leukopenia is frequently seen. Chest radiographs show evidence of atelectasis or infiltrate in about 10% of children.

■ **TABLE 216–1 Relative Frequency of Symptoms and Signs during Classic Influenza in Older Children and Adolescents**

Variable	Occurrence
Symptoms	
Chilly sensation	++++
Cough	+++
Headache	+++
Sore throat	+++
Prostration	++
Nasal stuffiness	++
Diarrhea	++
Dizziness	+
Eye irritation or pain	+
Vomiting	+
Myalgia	+
Signs	
Fever	++++
Pharyngitis	+++
Conjunctivitis (mild)	++
Rhinitis	++
Cervical adenitis	+
Pulmonary rales, wheezes, or rhonchi	+

++++ = 76–100%; +++ = 51–75%; ++ = 26–50%; and + = 1–25%.

DIAGNOSIS AND DIFFERENTIAL DIAGNOSIS. The diagnosis of influenza depends on epidemiologic and clinical considerations. In the context of an epidemic, the clinical diagnosis of influenza in a young child with fever, malaise, and respiratory symptoms can be made with some certainty. The laboratory confirmation of influenza can be made in three ways. If seen early in the illness, virus can be isolated from the nasopharynx by inoculation of the specimen into embryonated eggs or a limited number of cell lines that support the growth of influenza. The presence of influenza in the culture is confirmed by hemadsorption, which depends on the capacity of the hemagglutinin to bind red cells. Rapid diagnostic tests for influenza A are being introduced that use antigen capture in an enzyme-linked immunosorbent assay format. The diagnosis can be confirmed serologically with acute and convalescent sera drawn around the time of illness and tested by hemagglutination inhibition.

COMPLICATIONS. Otitis media and pneumonia are common complications of influenza in young children. Acute otitis media may be seen in up to 25% of cases of culture-documented influenza. Pneumonia accompanying influenza may be a primary viral process. An acute hemorrhagic pneumonia may be seen in the most severe cases, as may have been frequent with the highly virulent strain seen in 1918. The more common cause of pneumonia is probably secondary bacterial infection through the damaged epithelial layer. Unusual clinical manifestations of influenza include acute myositis seen with influenza type B, which follows the acute respiratory illness by 5–7 days and is marked by muscle weakness and pain, particularly in the thigh muscles, and myoglobinuria. Myocarditis also follows influenza, and toxic shock syndrome is associated with influenza type B and staphylococcal colonization. Influenza is particularly severe in children with underlying cardiopulmonary disease including congenital and acquired valvular disease, myocardiopathy, bronchopulmonary dysplasia, asthma, cystic fibrosis, and neuromuscular diseases affecting the accessory muscles of breathing. Virus is shed for longer periods of time in children receiving cancer chemotherapy and children with immunodeficiency.

PREVENTION. An inactivated influenza vaccine becomes available each summer with changes in formulation that reflect the strains anticipated to circulate in the coming year. When the vaccines are released, the American Committee on Immunization Practices publishes guidelines for their use. Current guidelines include the administration of vaccine intramuscularly to children 6 mo of age and older in chronic care facilities; those with chronic disorders of the pulmonary or cardiovascular system, including asthma; those with chronic metabolic diseases (including diabetes mellitus), renal dysfunction, hemoglobinopathies, or immunosuppression (including immunosuppression caused by medications); and children receiving long-term aspirin therapy who may be at risk for Reye syndrome after influenza. In addition, vaccine is recommended for individuals who may transmit influenza to persons at high risk, including health care workers and household members. The split-virus vaccine is recommended for children younger than 12 yr. Two doses of vaccine are recommended for primary immunization of children younger than 8 yr. The dosage is divided in half to a volume of 0.25 mL for children younger than 3 yr. Live, attenuated intranasally administered vaccines are in clinical trials and have been demonstrated to have an efficacy comparable to that of inactivated vaccine. Their ease of administration could serve to increase their use. Amantadine hydrochloride is the only licensed antiviral drug for influenza type A. It has been used prophylactically in high-risk patients and their care providers during influenza epidemics and in immunodeficient persons and those for whom the influenza vaccine is contraindicated.

TREATMENT. Amantadine hydrochloride can be used in the control of influenza type A outbreaks, in institutions, and for therapy in individual cases. If given within the first 48 hr, it decreases the severity and duration of influenzal symptoms. Confusion and inability to concentrate or sleep are seen in a minority of people given amantadine hydrochloride. Drug resistance develops fairly quickly during a course of therapy, but it is not widespread among circulating viruses. Because amantadine hydrochloride has no efficacy against influenza type B, knowledge of the circulating strain is essential to the rational use of the drug.

Adequate fluid intake and rest are important components in the management of influenza. Non-salicylate-containing antipyretics can be used for high fever. The most difficult question is the appropriate timing of consultation with a health care provider. Bacterial superinfections are common, and antibiotic therapy should be administered. Bacterial superinfections should be suspected with recrudescence of fever, prolonged fever, or deterioration in clinical status. With uncomplicated influenza, children should feel at their worst over the 1st 48 hr.

PROGNOSIS. The prognosis for recovery is excellent although full return to normal levels of activity and freedom from cough usually requires weeks rather than days.

Edwards KM, Dupont WD, Westrich MK, et al: A randomized controlled trial of cold-adapted and inactivated vaccines for the prevention of influenza A disease. J Infect Dis 169:68, 1994.

Glezen PW, Couch RB: Interpandemic influenza in the Houston area (1974–76). N. Engl J Med 298:587, 1978.

Hall CB, Dolin R, Gala CL, et al: Children with influenza A infection: Treatment with rimantadine. Pediatrics 80:275, 1987.

Prevention and Control of Influenza: Part I, Vaccines, recommendations of the Advisory Committee on Immunization Practices (ACIP). MMWR 43:RR-9, 1994.

Webster RG, Bean WJ, Gorman OT, et al: Evolution and ecology of influenza A viruses. Microbiol Rev 152, 1992.

Wright PF, Bryant JD, Karzon DT: Comparison of influenza B/Hong Kong virus infections among infants, children and young adults. J Infect Dis 141:430, 1980.

Wright PF, Ross KB, Thompson J, et al: Influenza A infections in young children. N Engl J Med 296:829, 1977.

CHAPTER 217

Parainfluenza Virus

Peter Wright

Viruses in the parainfluenza family are common causes of respiratory illness in infants and young children. They cause a spectrum of upper and lower respiratory tract illnesses, but are particularly associated with laryngotracheitis, bronchitis, and croup.

ETIOLOGY. There are four viruses in the parainfluenza family that cause illness in humans, designated types 1–4. The viruses have a nonsegmented, single-stranded RNA genome with a lipid-containing envelope derived from budding through the cell membrane. The major antigenic moieties are envelope spike proteins that exhibit hemagglutinating (HN protein) and cell fusion (F protein) properties.

EPIDEMIOLOGY. Parainfluenza viruses are spread from the respiratory tract by aerosolized secretions or direct hand contact with secretions. By age 3 yr, most children have experienced infection with types 1, 2, and 3. Type 3 is endemic and can cause disease in the infant younger than 6 mo. Serious illness is seen with parainfluenza type 3 in the immunocompromised child. Types 1 and 2 are more seasonal. They occur in the summer and fall and alternate years in which their serotype is most prevalent. Parainfluenza type 4 is more difficult to grow in tissue culture; thus, its epidemiology is less well defined. However, it does not appear to be a major cause of illness.

PATHOLOGY. Parainfluenza viruses replicate in the respiratory epithelium without evidence of systemic spread. The propensity to cause illness in the upper large airways is presumably related to enhanced replication in the larynx, trachea, and bronchi compared with other viruses. The destruction of cells in the upper airways can lead to secondary bacterial invasion and resultant bacterial tracheitis. Eustachian tube obstruction can lead to secondary bacterial invasion of the middle ear space and acute otitis media.

PATHOGENESIS. Illness caused by parainfluenza occurs shortly after inoculation with the virus. The mechanisms by which viral injury occurs are not known. Some parainfluenza viruses induce cell to cell fusion. During the budding process, cell membrane integrity is lost, and viruses can induce cell death through the process of apoptosis. The severity of illness correlates with the amount of viral shedding. Immune destruction of virally infected cells may also occur but appears to be less important with mucosal than systemic infection. The level of immunoglobulin A antibody is the best predictor of susceptibility to infection. Reinfection is seen particularly with parainfluenza type 3 as mucosal immunity wanes. The inability of children with serious T-cell defects to clear parainfluenza type 3 suggests a cell-mediated component of immunity.

CLINICAL MANIFESTATIONS. Most parainfluenza virus infections are confined to the upper respiratory tract. Selected signs, symptoms, and clinical diagnoses, based on a culture from young children with respiratory illness, are shown in Table 217–1. The relative frequency of parainfluenza type 3 compared with types 1 and 2 is consistent with other epidemiologic studies. This relatively mild-appearing illness is belied by a spectrum of rarer but more serious illnesses that result in hospitalization. The parainfluenza viruses account for 50% of hospitalizations for croup and 15% of cases of bronchiolitis and pneumonia. Parainfluenza type 1 causes more cases of croup, whereas parainfluenza type 3 causes a broad spectrum of lower respiratory tract diseases. Clinical descriptions of croup, bronchitis, bronchiolitis, and pneumonia are presented in Chapters 170, 327, and 332. Parainfluenza virus infections are not associated with high fever. Aside from low-grade fever, systemic complaints are rare. The illness usually lasts 4–5 days;

■ TABLE 217–1 Frequency of Clinical Signs and Symptoms in Children with Parainfluenza Virus Infections

Variable	Type 1 (N = 81)	Type 2 (N = 33)	Type 3 (N = 158)
Signs and Symptoms			
Coryza	60 (74)	24 (73)	129 (82)
Cough	59 (73)	20 (61)	122 (77)
Irritability	36 (44)	9 (27)	81 (51)
Anorexia	28 (35)	11 (33)	49 (31)
Hoarseness	14 (17)	3 (9)	14 (8)
Rales or rhonchi	1 (1)	3 (9)	10 (6)
Wheezing	6 (8)	3 (9)	14 (8)
Temperature ≥38° C	28 (35)	3 (9)	49 (31)
Temperature ≤39° C	8 (10)	1 (3)	10 (6)
Diagnosis			
Upper respiratory tract	71 (88)	30 (91)	136 (86)
Pharyngitis	15 (19)	6 (18)	14 (8)
Acute otitis	26 (32)	9 (27)	72 (46)
Croup or LTB	11 (14)	2 (6)	9 (6)
Bronchiolitis	1 (1)	3 (9)	8 (5)
Pneumonia	0	0	3 (2)
Hospital Admissions	3	0	1

Values in parentheses represent percentages.
LTB = laryngotracheobronchitis.

however, virus may be recovered in low titers for 2–3 wk. Rarely, parainfluenza viruses have been implicated in parotitis.

LABORATORY FINDINGS. There are no distinctive hematologic or chemistry findings. The laboratory diagnosis of parainfluenza virus infection can be accomplished by inoculation of nasal secretions into tissue culture, with presumptive diagnosis based on finding a hemadsorbing agent and final serotypic diagnosis based on hemadsorption inhibition. Direct immunofluorescent staining has been used in some centers to identify infected cells in secretions rapidly.

DIAGNOSIS. The diagnosis of parainfluenza virus infection is based on clinical and epidemiologic criteria in most pediatric settings. The virus should be specifically sought in persistent pneumonias in immunosuppressed children. The radiographic "steeple" sign of progressive narrowing of the subglottic region is characteristic of parainfluenza virus infections.

COMPLICATIONS. In more febrile children and those with more severe respiratory compromise, the possibility of a bacterial tracheitis with purulent material below the epiglottis and vocal cords should be considered. The high frequency of otitis complicating parainfluenza virus means that careful pneumatic otoscopy should be performed in all children with suspected parainfluenza virus infection.

PREVENTION. Work is progressing with both live and subunit parainfluenza type 3 vaccines. The live vaccines include a cold-adapted virus of human origin and a bovine parainfluenza virus, which is attenuated because of host range adaptation. The measure of protection afforded by vaccines will be difficult to assess because symptomatic reinfection is seen and the frequency of serous infection in the general population is low. Nonetheless, it is clear that prevention of acute respiratory illness that results from parainfluenza virus is a worthwhile goal.

TREATMENT. The possibility of rapid respiratory compromise during severe croup should influence the level of care given (see Chapter 332.1) The differentiation between croup and epiglottitis is discussed in Chapter 332. Careful attention to symptomatic care is important as is a description for parents of the parameters of increasing respiratory distress that should lead to reassessment by a health care provider. Humidification and exposure to cold air are both classically associated with a decrease in mucosal edema and liquification of secretions that may relieve obstruction; however, their value has never been proved in a controlled trial. Aerosolized racemic epinephrine may temporarily improve aeration, but one must be convinced that the improvement will be sustained before discharging the child. Recent studies have suggested that aerosolized or systemic steroids were helpful in the management of croup in the emergency room setting and after hospitalization. The indications for antibiotics are limited to well-documented secondary bacterial infections of the middle ears or lower respiratory tract.

Ribavirin has some antiviral activity against parainfluenza virus and should be considered in the immunocompromised child with persistent pneumonia.

PROGNOSIS. The prognosis for full recovery is excellent in the normal child. No long-term pulmonary residua of parainfluenza virus infection have been described.

Denny FW, Murphy TF, Clyde WA Jr, et al: An 11-year study in a pediatric practice. Pediatrics 71:871, 1983.

Hall CB, Geiman JM, Breese BB, et al: Parainfluenza infections in children: Correlation of shedding with clinical manifestations. J Pediatr 91:194, 1993.

Landau LI, Geelhoed GC: Aerosolized steroids for croup. N Engl J Med 33:322, 1994.

Skolnik NS: Treatment of croup: A critical review. Am J Dis Child 143:1045, 1989.

Smith CB, Purcell RH, Bellanti JA, et al: Protective effect of antibody to parainfluenza type 1 virus. N Engl J Med 275:1145, 1966.

CHAPTER 218

Respiratory Syncytial Virus

Kenneth McIntosh

Respiratory syncytial virus (RSV) is the major cause of bronchiolitis (Chapter 338) and pneumonia in infants younger than 1 yr. It is the most important respiratory tract pathogen of early childhood.

ETIOLOGY. RSV is a medium-sized, membrane-bound RNA virus that develops in the cytoplasm of infected cells and matures by budding from the plasma membrane. It belongs to the family *Paramyxoviridae,* along with parainfluenza, mumps, and measles viruses but is classified in a separate genus: the pneumoviruses.

Although different strains of RSV show some antigenic heterogeneity, this variation is primarily seen in only one of the two surface glycoproteins, and the virus behaves in the human host like a single serotype.

RSV grows in a number of types of tissue culture, in which it produces characteristic syncytial cytopathology. Specimens for culture should be delivered rapidly on wet ice to the laboratory because the virus is heat labile and very susceptible to destruction by freezing and thawing.

EPIDEMIOLOGY. The occurrence of annual outbreaks and the high incidence of infection during the first months of life are unique among human viruses. RSV is distributed worldwide and appears in yearly epidemics. In temperate climates these epidemics occur each winter and last 4–5 mo. During the remainder of the year infections are sporadic and uncommon. Epidemics usually peak in January, February, or March, but peaks have been recognized as early as December and as late as June. At these times hospital admissions for bronchiolitis and pneumonia of infants younger than 1 yr increase and decrease in proportion to the number of RSV infections in the community. In the tropics, the epidemic pattern is less clear.

Placentally transmitted antibody probably has some protective effect, particularly when present in high concentration. This may account for the fact that severe infections are uncommon in the first 4–6 wk of life. Nevertheless, serum antibody is not fully protective, and the age at which an infant undergoes first infection depends also on the opportunities for exposure. It is estimated that in an urban setting about half of the susceptible infants undergo primary infection in each epidemic. Thus, infection is almost universal by the 2nd birthday. Reinfection occurs at a rate of 10–20% per epidemic throughout childhood; the frequency is lower in adults. In situations of high exposure such as day-care centers, attack rates are higher: nearly 100% for first infections and 60–80% for second and subsequent infections.

Estimates of the severity of primary infections have emerged from studies of outbreaks in nurseries and institutions. Under these circumstances asymptomatic infection is rare. Most infants experience coryza and pharyngitis, usually with fever and occasionally with otitis. In 10–40% of patients the lower respiratory tract is involved to a varying degree. Bronchitis, bronchopneumonia, and bronchiolitis all occur. Calculations based on hospital admissions in the United States and Britain yield a ratio of 1–3 infants hospitalized with bronchiolitis or pneumonia for every 100 primary infections with the virus.

Reinfection may occur as early as a few weeks after recovery but usually takes place during subsequent annual outbreaks. The severity of illness during reinfection is probably as much influenced by age as by prior experience with this virus; older children are generally less ill. Nevertheless, several instances of severe RSV bronchiolitis occurring twice in succession have been recorded.

Bronchiolitis is the most common clinical diagnosis in infants hospitalized with RSV infections, although the syndrome is often indistinguishable from RSV pneumonia in infants, and, indeed, the two frequently coexist. All RSV diseases of the lower respiratory tract (excluding croup) have their highest incidence in the 2nd–7th mo of life and decrease in frequency thereafter. The syndrome of bronchiolitis becomes uncommon after the 1st birthday; acute infective wheezing attacks after that age are often termed "wheezy bronchitis," "asthmatoid bronchitis," or, simply, asthma attacks. Viral pneumonia is a persistent problem throughout childhood, although RSV becomes less prominent as the etiologic agent after the 1st year. RSV is responsible for 45–75% of cases of bronchiolitis, 15–25% of childhood pneumonias, and 6–8% of cases of croup.

Bronchiolitis and pneumonia resulting from RSV are more common in boys than in girls by a ratio of about 1.5:1. Racial factors make little difference. Lower respiratory tract disease, however, occurs more often and earlier in life in low socioeconomic groups and in crowded living conditions.

The incubation period from exposure to 1st symptoms is about 4 days. The virus is excreted for variable periods, probably depending on severity of illness and immunologic status. Most infants with lower respiratory tract illness shed virus for 5–12 days after hospital admission. Excretion for 3 wk and longer has been documented. Spread of infection occurs when large, infected droplets, either airborne or conveyed on hands, are inoculated in the nose or conjunctiva of a susceptible subject. RSV is probably introduced into most families by school children undergoing reinfection. Typically, in the space of a few days older siblings and one or both parents acquire colds, but the infant becomes more severely ill with fever, otitis, or lower respiratory tract disease.

Hospital cross infection during RSV epidemics is important. Virus is usually spread from child to child on the hands of caregivers. Symptomatic, infected adults have also been implicated in the spread of the infection.

PATHOLOGY AND PATHOGENESIS. Bronchiolitis is characterized by virus-induced necrosis of the bronchiolar epithelium, hypersecretion of mucus, and round cell infiltration and edema of the surrounding submucosa. These changes result in formation of mucous plugs obstructing bronchioles with consequent hyperinflation or collapse of the distal lung tissue. In interstitial pneumonia, infiltration is more generalized, and epithelial necrosis may extend to both the bronchi and the alveoli. Infants are particularly apt to experience small airway obstruction because of the small size of the normal bronchioles.

Several facts suggest immunologic injury as a factor in the pathogenesis of bronchiolitis caused by RSV: (1) infants dying of bronchiolitis have shown both immunoglobulin and virus in the injured bronchiolar tissues; (2) children who received a highly antigenic, inactivated, parenterally administered RSV vaccine experienced, on subsequent exposure to wild-type RSV, more severe and more frequent bronchiolitis than did their age-matched controls; (3) bronchiolitis merges into asthma in older infants, and RSV is a frequently recognized cause of acute asthma attacks in children 1–5 yr old; and (4) immunoglobulin E (IgE) antibody directed toward RSV has been found in the secretions of convalescent infants with bronchiolitis.

It is not clear what role, in addition to the destructive effect of the virus and the attendant host response, is played by superimposed bacterial infection. In most infants with bronchiolitis, with or without interstitial pneumonia, clinical experience suggests that bacteria play an insignificant role.

CLINICAL MANIFESTATIONS. The first signs of infection of the infant with RSV are rhinorrhea and pharyngitis. Cough may appear simultaneously but more often appears after an interval of 1–3 days, at which time there may also be sneezing and a low-grade fever. Soon after the cough has developed, the child begins to wheeze audibly. If the disease is mild, the symptoms may not progress beyond this stage. Auscultation often reveals diffuse rhonchi, fine rales, and wheezes. Rhinorrhea usually persists throughout the illness, with intermittent fever. Roentgenograms of the chest at this stage are frequently normal.

If the illness progresses, cough and wheezing increase, and air hunger and evidence of hyperexpansion of the chest and of intercostal and subcostal retraction occur. The respiratory rate increases, and cyanosis occurs. Signs of severe, life-threatening illness are central cyanosis, tachypnea of more than 70 breaths/min, listlessness, and apneic spells. At this stage the chest may be greatly hyperexpanded and almost silent to auscultation because of poor air exchange.

Chest roentgenograms of infants hospitalized with RSV bronchiolitis are normal in about 10% of cases; air trapping or hyperexpansion of the chest occurs in about 50%. Peribronchial thickening or interstitial pneumonia is seen in 50–80%. Segmental consolidation occurs in 10–25%. Pleural effusion is rarely, if ever, seen.

In some infants the course of the illness may be more like that of pneumonia. In these instances, the prodromal rhinorrhea and cough are followed by dyspnea, poor feeding, and listlessness, with a minimum of wheezing and hyperexpansion. Although the clinical diagnosis is pneumonia, wheezing is often present intermittently and the chest roentgenogram may show air trapping.

Fever is an inconstant sign in RSV infection. Rash and conjunctivitis each occur in a few cases. In young infants, particularly those who were born prematurely, periodic breathing and apneic spells have been distressingly frequent signs, even with relatively mild bronchiolitis. It is likely that a small portion of deaths included in the category of sudden infant death syndrome are due to RSV infection.

RSV infections in profoundly immunocompromised hosts may be severe at any age. The mortality associated with RSV infection in the 1st few weeks after bone marrow or solid organ transplantation may be as high as 50%.

Routine laboratory tests offer little helpful information in most cases of bronchiolitis or pneumonia caused by RSV. The white cell count is normal or elevated, and the differential count may be normal or shifted either to the right or left. Bacterial cultures usually grow normal flora. Hypoxemia is frequent and tends to be more marked than anticipated on the basis of the clinical findings. When it is severe, it is frequently accompanied by hypercapnia and acidosis.

DIAGNOSIS. Bronchiolitis is a clinical diagnosis. The involvement of RSV in any particular child's disease can be suspected with varying degrees of certainty from the season of the year and the presence of a typical outbreak at the time. Other features that may be helpful are the age of the child (aside from RSV, the only respiratory virus that attacks infants frequently during the first few months of life is parainfluenza virus type 3) and the family epidemiology (colds in siblings and parents).

The diagnostic dilemma of greatest import is the question of possible bacterial or chlamydial involvement. When bronchiolitis is mild or when infiltrates are absent by roentgenogram, there is little likelihood of a bacterial component. In infants 1–4 mo of age, interstitial pneumonitis may be caused by *Chlamydia trachomatis* (Chapter 197). In this instance there may be a history of conjunctivitis, and the illness tends to be of subacute onset. Coughing is prominent; wheezing is not. There may also be eosinophilia. Fever is usually absent.

Consolidation without other signs or with pleural effusion is considered of bacterial origin until proved otherwise. Other signs pointing to bacterial pneumonia are elevation of the neutrophil count, depression of the white cell count in the presence of severe disease, ileus or other abdominal signs, high fever, and circulatory collapse. In such instances there is rarely any doubt about the need for antibiotics.

Definitive diagnosis of RSV infection is based on the detection of virus or viral antigens in respiratory secretions. The specimen should be put on ice, taken directly to the laboratory, and processed for antigen detection or inoculated onto susceptible cell monolayers. An aspirate of mucus from the child's posterior nasal cavity is the optimal specimen. Nasopharyngeal or throat swabs are also acceptable. A tracheal aspirate is unnecessary.

PROGNOSIS. The mortality of hospitalized infants with RSV infection of the lower respiratory tract is about 2%. The prognosis is clearly worse in young, premature infants or those with underlying disease of the neuromuscular, pulmonary, cardiovascular, or immunologic system.

Many children with asthma have a history of bronchiolitis in infancy. There is recurrent wheezing in 33–50% of children with typical RSV bronchiolitis in infancy. The likelihood of recurrence is increased in the presence of an allergic diathesis (eczema, hay fever, or a family history of asthma). In bronchiolitis in patients older than 1 yr there is an increasing probability that, though it may be virus induced, this is the first of multiple wheezing attacks that will later be called asthma.

TREATMENT. In uncomplicated cases of bronchiolitis, treatment is symptomatic. Humidified oxygen is usually indicated for hospitalized infants because most are hypoxic. Many infants are slightly to moderately dehydrated; therefore, fluids should be carefully administered in somewhat greater than maintenance amounts. Often intravenous or tube feeding is helpful when sucking is difficult. Most infants seem to breathe better when propped up at an angle of 10–30 degrees.

Bronchodilators should not be routinely used. However, a trial of albuterol aerosols should be made in wheezing children and bronchodilators administered if aerosols are beneficial. Corticosteroids are not indicated except as a last resort in critical cases. Sedatives are rarely necessary.

In most instances antibiotics are not useful, and their indiscriminate use in presumed viral bronchiolitis and pneumonia should be discouraged. Interstitial pneumonia in infants 1–4 mo old may be chlamydial, and erythromycin (40 mg/kg/24 hr) may, therefore, be beneficial. When infants with interstitial pneumonia are older, or when consolidation is found, parenteral antibiotics may be indicated. In the critically ill child antibiotics may also be indicated.

The antiviral drug ribavirin, delivered by small-particle aerosol and breathed, along with the required concentration of oxygen, for 20 of 24 hr per day for 3–5 days, has a modest beneficial effect on the course of RSV pneumonia. Shortened hospital stay and reduced mortality have not been demonstrated, and long-term effects are still unknown. Its use is, therefore, indicated only in very sick infants or in high-risk infants, such as those with underlying cyanotic congenital heart disease, significant bronchopulmonary dysplasia, or severe immunodeficiency. It should be administered early in the course of the infection.

PREVENTION. Within the hospital the most important preventive measures are aimed at blocking nosocomial spread. During RSV season high-risk infants should be separated from infants with respiratory symptoms. Separate gowns and gloves and careful handwashing should be used for the care of all infants with suspected or established RSV infection.

Attempts to develop useful inactivated or attenuated vaccines have been unsuccessful. Indeed, the insufficiency of protection following natural RSV infection diminishes the likelihood that an attenuated vaccine will prevent subsequent disease. Trials of monthly high-titered intravenous Ig have demonstrated some reduction in the severity of RSV infections in high-risk infants. Passive immunoprophylaxis appears to be a promising approach to prevention.

Glezen WP, Paredes A, Allison JE, et al: Risk of respiratory syncytial virus infection for infants from low-income families in relationship to age, sex, ethnic group and maternal antibody level. J Pediatr 98:708, 1981.

Groothuis JR, Simoes EAF, Levin MJ, et al: Prophylactic administration of respiratory syncytial virus immunoglobulin to high-risk infants and young children. N Engl J Med 329:1524, 1993.

Hall CB, Douglas RG Jr, Geiman JM, et al: Nosocomial respiratory syncytial virus infections. N Engl J Med 293:1343, 1975.

Hall CB, McBride JT, Walsh EE, et al: Aerosolized ribavirin treatment of infants with respiratory syncytial virus infection. N Engl J Med 308:1443, 1983.

Henderson FW, Collier AM, Clyde WA Jr, et al: Respiratory-syncytial-virus infections, reinfections and immunity: A prospective, longitudinal study in young children. N Engl J Med 300:530, 1979.

Hertz MI, Englund JA, Snover D, et al: Respiratory syncytial virus-induced acute lung injury in adult patients with bone marrow transplants. Medicine 68:269, 1989.

Holberg CJ, Wright AL, Martinez FD, et al: Risk factors for respiratory syncytial virus–associated lower respiratory illnesses in the first year of life. Am J Epidemiol 133:1135, 1991.

Loda FA, Clyde WA, Glezen WP, et al: Studies on the role of viruses, bacteria and *M. pneumoniae* as causes of lower respiratory tract infections in children. J Pediatr 72:161, 1968.

McIntosh K: Bronchiolitis and asthma: Possible common pathogenetic pathways. J Allergy Clin Immunol 57:595, 1976.

Simpson W, Hacking PM, Court SDM, et al: Radiological findings in respiratory syncytial virus infection in children: II. The correlation of radiological categories with clinical and virological findings. Pediatr Radiol 2:155, 1974.

CHAPTER 219
Adenoviruses

Kenneth McIntosh

Adenoviruses cause 5–8% of acute respiratory disease in infants, plus a wide array of other syndromes including pharyngoconjunctival fever, follicular conjunctivitis, epidemic keratoconjunctivitis, hemorrhagic cystitis, acute diarrhea, intussusception, and encephalomyelitis. Only a third of the 37-plus serotypes have been associated with disease. Although fatalities are rare, they are associated with infections by certain serotypes (particularly type 7) and with infections in severely immunocompromised hosts.

ETIOLOGY. Adenoviruses are DNA viruses of intermediate size, which are classified into subgenera A to G. Types 1–39 are in subgenera A to E, type 40 is subgenus F, and type 41 is subgenus G. The virion has an icosohedral coat made up of several proteins, the most abundant of which is the "hexon," a cross-reacting antigen common to all mammalian adenoviruses. The "penton" confers type specificity, and antibody to it is protective. It is also cytotoxic in tissue culture, and toxic properties have been ascribed to it in vivo as well. Adenoviruses can also be classified by the "fingerprints" their DNA make on gels after being digested with restriction endonucleases, and this classification generally conforms to their antigenic types.

All adenovirus types except types 40 and 41 grow in primary human embryonic kidney cells, and most grow in HEp-2 or HeLa cells, producing a typical destructive cytopathic effect. Types 40 and 41 (and other serotypes as well) grow in 293 cells, a line of human embryonic kidney cells into which certain "early" adenovirus genes have been introduced.

Many adenovirus types, but particularly the common childhood types (1, 2, and 5), are shed for prolonged periods from both the respiratory and gastrointestinal tracts. These types also establish low-level and chronic infection of the tonsils.

EPIDEMIOLOGY. Adenoviral infections are distributed worldwide. They occur year-round but are most prevalent in spring or early summer and again in midwinter in temperate climates. Certain types tend to occur in epidemics, notably types 4 and 7 in epidemics of febrile respiratory disease, types 3, 7, and 21 in severe pneumonia, type 3 in pharyngoconjunctival fever, type 11 in cystitis, and types 8, 19, and 37 in epidemic keratoconjunctivitis. For unexplained reasons, adenovirus types 3 and 7 cause frequent severe epidemics of pneumonia in the children of northern China, with mortality rates of 5–15%.

Over 60% of school-age children have antibodies to the common respiratory types. Almost all adults have serum antibody to types 1–7. Infections with types 1 and 2 tend to occur during the 1st yr or 2 of life, and types 3 and 5 occur a little later. Spread occurs by the respiratory and fecal-oral routes, although it is not clear whether spread is by large- or small-particle aerosol. Hospital outbreaks of respiratory disease and keratoconjunctivitis have been described.

PATHOLOGY AND PATHOGENESIS. Adenoviruses are one of the few "respiratory" viruses that grow well in the epithelium of the small intestine. Although mucosal surfaces are the primary target early in infection, it is likely that viremia is common, accompanying fever. Viremia is, however, of little consequence except in rare instances or in the immunocompromised patient.

Adenoviral pneumonia produces characteristic microscopic changes, with dense lymphocytic infiltrates, destruction of the bronchial and bronchiolar epithelium, focal necrosis of mucous glands, hyaline membrane formation, and several types of nuclear inclusion bodies.

CLINICAL MANIFESTATIONS. Adenoviruses cause a wide array of syndromes:

Acute Respiratory Disease. This is the most common manifestation of adenovirus infection in children and adults. Acute respiratory infections in infants and children are not clinically distinctive and are usually caused by types 1, 2, 3, 5, or 6. They are usually mild but may be complicated or severe. Primary infections in infants are frequently associated with fever and respiratory symptoms and in some series are complicated by otitis in more than half of the patients. Adenovirus respiratory infections are associated with a significant incidence of diarrhea.

Pharyngitis is a characteristic clinical syndrome, and adenoviruses can be identified in 15–20% of children with isolated pharyngitis, mostly in preschoolers and infants. The pharyngitis may be exudative and is often febrile. Most cases are due to type 1, 2, 3, or 5.

Pneumonia is uncommon but 7–9% of hospitalized children with acute pneumonia have adenovirus infection. Any of the "respiratory" types can cause pneumonia, but severe infections are most likely due to type 3, 7, or 21. Such infections have a mortality as high as 10%, and survivors may have residual airway damage, manifested by bronchiectasis, bronchiolitis obliterans, or, rarely, pulmonary fibrosis.

A *pertussis-like syndrome* has been described in association with adenovirus infections. In such instances adenoviruses frequently accompany *Bordetella pertussis* as coinfecting agents, but they may also be causative on their own. In many cases this illness represents activation of latent or low-level chronic respiratory or tonsillar infection by the virus. With improved methods for detecting *B. pertussis,* doubt has increased that adenovirus (or any respiratory virus) can produce the classic pertussis syndrome on its own.

Pharyngoconjunctival fever is a clinically distinct syndrome that occurs particularly in association with type 3 adenoviral infection. Features include a high fever that lasts 4–5 days, pharyngitis with characteristic involvement of pharyngeal lymphoid tissue, conjunctivitis, preauricular and cervical adenopathy, and rhinitis. Nonpurulent conjunctivitis occurs in 75% of patients and is manifested by inflammation of both the bulbar and palpebral conjunctivae of one or both eyes; it often persists after the fever and other symptoms have resolved. Headache, malaise, and weakness are common, and there is considerable lethargy after the acute stage.

Conjunctivitis and Keratoconjunctivitis. Adenovirus is one of the most common causes of follicular conjunctivitis and keratoconjunctivitis. The former is a relatively mild illness. The latter, which may occur in epidemics, is associated with infection by adenovirus types 8, 19, and 37. The disease may cause corneal opacities that last several years.

Gastrointestinal Infections. Adenoviruses can be found in the stools of 5–9% of children with acute diarrhea. About one half of these are the "enteric" types, 40 or 41. It is also clear that enteric infection with any adenovirus serotype is often asymptomatic, so the causative role in these episodes is frequently uncertain.

The pathogenesis of intussusception is thought by many to include enlarged lymph nodes as an initiating factor. Adenoviruses have been recovered from mesenteric lymph nodes at surgery and also from surface cultures in a higher percentage of children with intussusception than from controls. Adenoviruses have also been found in the appendices of children with appendicitis. Whether these findings represent acute etiologic relationships or are manifestations of a protracted, low-level intestinal infection analogous to that described in the tonsils is not clear.

Hemorrhagic Cystitis. This syndrome has a sudden onset of bacteriologically sterile hematuria, dysuria, frequency, and urgency lasting 1–2 wk. Infection with adenovirus types 11 and 21 has been found in some affected children and young adults.

Reye Syndrome and Reye-like Syndromes. Typical Reye syndrome has followed demonstrated adenovirus infection of several serotypes, particularly in very young children. In addition, several cases of a *Reye-like syndrome* have been reported, all of which are caused by infection with adenovirus type 7. The latter disease, which is frequently fatal, is characterized by severe bronchopneumonia, hepatitis, seizures, and disseminated intravascular coagulation. Circulating adenovirus penton antigen has been found in several patients and has been implicated in the pathogenesis.

Infections in Immunocompromised Hosts. Adenoviruses are important pathogens in the immunocompromised host. This includes those with either B- or T-cell deficiencies. In B cell–deficient children, a chronic meningoencephalitis very similar to that caused by enteroviruses has been described. In T cell–deficient patients, regardless of whether this deficiency is congenital, acquired, or iatrogenic, fulminant hepatitis and pneumonia, frequently with a fatal outcome, have been described. There is also a close association between adenovirus infection and both hemorrhagic cystitis and tubulointerstitial nephritis in immunosuppressed children.

DIAGNOSIS AND DIFFERENTIAL DIAGNOSIS. The laboratory diagnosis of adenovirus infection in children may be made by culture (or other method of identifying the presence of the virus), demonstration of a rise in serum antibody level, or some combination of the two. If virus is found in a "privileged" site, such as blood, urine, or cerebrospinal fluid, or in a biopsy of the lung or liver, the implication of infection with disease and organ damage is strong. Likewise, detection of certain adenovirus types in respiratory secretions (type 7 or 21) probably indicates their etiologic involvement. The presence of untyped virus or the common childhood types in respiratory secretions or stool does not, however, indicate clinical adenovirus infection because these viruses may be excreted chronically and asymptomatically. In these instances, discovery of a coincident rise in antibody by either complement fixation or some more type-specific test is helpful in assigning a specific microorganism to disease. Adenovirus infection may also be considered etiologic if a rise in antibody is found between sera drawn in the acute stage and in convalescence from a patient with an appropriate illness. Adenovirus infection often results in a high erythrocyte sedimentation rate and white cell count.

Differential diagnosis is complex and depends on which syndrome is seen.

PREVENTION AND TREATMENT. Vaccines that contain either killed or live virus have been developed to prevent types 4 and 7 infections in military recruits. These vaccines have not, however, been used in children. There are at present no recognized antiviral agents that are effective in treating adenovirus infections. Ribavirin can inhibit viral growth of some strains in vitro, but evidence of its clinical efficacy is lacking.

Brandt CD, Kim HW, Jeffries BC, et al: Infections in 18,000 infants and children in a controlled study of respiratory tract disease: II. Adenovirus pathogenicity in relation to serologic type and illness syndrome. Am J Epidemiol 90:484, 1970.

Brandt CD, Kim HW, Rodriguez WJ, et al: Adenoviruses and pediatric gastroenteritis. J Infect Dis 151:437, 1985.

Edwards KM, Bennett SR, Garner WL, et al: Reye's syndrome associated with adenovirus infections in infants. Am J Dis Child 139:343, 1985.

Kelsey DS: Adenovirus meningoencephalitis. Pediatrics 61:291, 1978.

Ladisch S, Lovejoy FH, Hierholzer JC, et al: Extrapulmonary manifestations of adenovirus type 7 pneumonia simulating Reye syndrome and the possible role of an adenovirus toxin. Pediatrics 95:348, 1979.

Michaels MG, Green M, Wald ER, et al: Adenovirus infection in pediatric liver transplant recipients. J Infect Dis 165:170, 1992.

Nelson KE, Gavitt F, Batt MD, et al: The role of adenoviruses in the pertussis syndrome. J Pediatr 86:335, 1975.

Numazaki Y, Kumasaki T, Yano N, et al: Further study on acute hemorrhagic cystitis due to adenovirus type H. N Engl J Med 289:344, 1973.

Ruuskanen O, Meurman O, Sarkkinen H: Adenoviral diseases in children: A study of 105 hospital cases. Pediatrics 76:79, 1985.

Similä S, Ylikorkala O, Wasz-Hockert O: Type 7 adenovirus pneumonia. J Pediatr 79:605, 1971.

Van R, Wun CC, O'Ryan ML, et al: Outbreaks of human enteric adenovirus types 40 and 41 in Houston day care centers. J Pediatr 120:516, 1992.

CHAPTER 220

Rhinovirus

Kenneth McIntosh

Rhinoviruses, collectively the most common cause of the "common cold" in adults, represent a smaller proportion of infections in young children because of the frequency of other viral respiratory infections. Also rhinoviral infections in young children often do not produce respiratory illness. However, rhinoviruses spread readily, producing illness in nursery and other school groups, and these children provide a major link in their spread within families.

ETIOLOGY. There are 111 serologically distinct rhinoviruses, all members of the *Picornavirus* family of small RNA viruses. They are best identified by inoculating human embryonic kidney or human diploid cell cultures with nasal secretions from infected individuals and waiting to observe a cytopathic effect. Routine serologic testing for acquisition of antibody is not practical because of the multiplicity of types and infrequency of their cross-reactivity.

Several cross-sectional studies indicate that a low percentage of control children or children with diarrhea (1%) yield rhinoviruses at the time of sampling; similarly, only 2.2% of children with respiratory tract illness yield rhinoviruses. In longitudinal studies, however, 75% of pediatric rhinovirus infection is associated with illness, usually rhinitis or the pharyngitis-bronchitis syndrome. Rhinoviruses have also occasionally been associated with serious lower respiratory tract disease, particularly in infants with underlying illnesses. They are frequent precipitants of asthma in children and chronic bronchitis in adults.

EPIDEMIOLOGY. Rhinoviruses are distributed worldwide with no predictable pattern of infection by serotype. Multiple types may be present in a community at one time.

In temperate climates the incidence of rhinoviral infection peaks in September and again in April or May, but some infections occur year-round. The peak incidence in the tropics occurs during the rainy season.

Rhinoviruses are recovered in highest concentration in nasal secretions, and experimental infection is most easily accomplished by nasal or conjunctival instillation. Infection via aerosol is less efficient. Virus persists for several hours in secretions on hands or other surfaces. Transmission probably occurs when infected secretions carried on contaminated fingers are rubbed into the nasal or conjunctival mucosa. More recent evidence also implicates spread through prolonged contact with aerosols produced by talking, coughing, or sneezing.

PATHOGENESIS. The peak nasal inflammatory response occurs when virus growth is at its greatest, 2–4 days after experimental infection. Immune responses include specific nasal immunoglobulin (Ig) A and serum IgG antibody, which may contribute to modifying the illness and limiting viral shedding. Interferon and a nonspecific factor induced by infection with a heterotypic rhinovirus may be a part of the resistance mechanism. Usually the inflammatory response is limited to the nose, throat, and upper bronchial passages, but pneumonia has occurred.

CLINICAL MANIFESTATIONS. The primary clinical response to rhinoviral infection, like that to most respiratory viral infections, is the *common cold* (see Chapter 327.1). There is an incubation period of 2–4 days; then sneezing, nasal obstruction and discharge, and sore throat ensue. Cough and hoarseness occur in 30–40% of cases. Headache and other systemic symptoms are not as common as in influenza. Fever is neither as frequent nor as high as in primary infections with respiratory syncytial virus, parainfluenza virus, influenza virus, or adenovirus. Symptoms are worse in the first 2–3 days of illness and last for a week in a majority of patients; they persist for over 14 days in 35% of young children.

COMPLICATIONS. These are like those of any infection causing edema and inflammation in the nasopharyngeal area. They include otitis media, sinusitis, local spread down the respiratory tract, bacterial superinfection, and, in certain atopic children, acute wheezing. In one study rhinoviruses were the most common virus recovered from the middle ear fluids of infants and children with otitis media.

DIAGNOSIS AND DIFFERENTIAL DIAGNOSIS. Because other viral agents can produce the same manifestations, a clinical diagnosis is only presumptive. Laboratory diagnosis is not practical under ordinary circumstances. If any question exists, bacterial cultures should be taken to exclude streptococcal infection.

TREATMENT AND PREVENTION. There is no specific preventive or ameliorative treatment. Careful hand washing and avoidance of manual nose and eye manipulation is the best approach to reducing spread. For relief of acute symptoms, a mild analgesic and saline or decongestant nose drops may be used for a short time. Interferon administered by nasal spray may be of value in preventing rhinovirus infection.

Arola M, Ziegler T, Ruuskanen O, et al: Rhinovirus in acute otitis media. J Pediatr 113:693, 1988.

Dick EC, Jennings LC, Mink KA, et al: Aerosol transmission of rhinovirus colds. J Infect Dis 156:442, 1987.

Douglas RM, Moore BW, Miles HB, et al: Prophylactic efficacy of intranasal alpha$_2$-interferon against rhinovirus infections in the family setting. N Engl J Med 314:65, 1986.

Ketler A, Hall CE, Fox JP, et al: The Virus Watch Program: A continuing surveillance of viral infections in metropolitan New York families: VIII. Rhinovirus infections: Observations of virus excretion, intrafamilial spread and clinical response. Am J Epidemiol 90:244, 1969.
McMillan JA, Weiner LB, Higgins AM, et al: Rhinovirus infection associated with serious illness among pediatric patients. Pediatr Infect Dis J 12:321, 1993.

CHAPTER 221

Hepatitis A Through E

John D. Snyder and Larry K. Pickering

DEFINITION. Viral hepatitis is a major health problem in developing and developed countries. Recent advances in the field of molecular biology have aided identification and understanding of the pathogenesis of the five viruses that are now known to cause hepatitis as their primary disease manifestation. These hepatotropic viruses are designated hepatitis A, B, C, D, and E (Table 221–1). Many other viruses can cause hepatitis as part of their clinical spectrum including herpes simplex (see Chapter 211), cytomegalovirus (see Chapter 214), Epstein-Barr (see Chapter 215), varicella (see Chapter 213), human immunodeficiency (see Chapter 223), rubella (see Chapter 208), adenovirus (see Chapter 219), enteroviruses (see Chapter 209), and arboviruses (see Chapter 225). Hepatic involvement with these viruses is usually only one component of a multisystem disease.

The five hepatitis viruses are a heterogenous group of viruses that cause similar acute clinical illness. Hepatitis A, C, D, and E are RNA viruses representing four different families, and hepatitis B is a DNA virus (Table 221–2). Hepatitis A and E are not known to cause chronic illness, whereas hepatitis B, C, and D cause important morbidity and mortality through chronic infections. In the United States, hepatitis A virus (HAV) appears to cause most cases of hepatitis in children. Hepatitis B probably accounts for about one third of cases in children, whereas hepatitis C is found in approximately 20%. Hepatitis D occurs in only a small percentage of children who must also have active hepatitis B virus (HBV) infection. Hepatitis E has not been reported in children who have lived and traveled only in the United States.

HEPATITIS A

ETIOLOGY. HAV is a 27-nm diameter, RNA-containing virus that is a member of the *Picornavirus* family. It was isolated originally from stools of infected patients. Laboratory strains of HAV have been propagated in tissue culture. Acute infection is diagnosed by detecting immunoglobulin (Ig)M (IgM) antibodies (anti-HAV) by radioimmunoassay (Fig. 221–1) or, rarely, by identifying viral particles in stool.

■ TABLE 221–1 Hepatitis Nomenclature

Hepatitis	Identified Antigens	Antibodies
A	HAV	Anti-HAV*
B	HBsAg*	Anti-HBsAg*
	HBcAg	Anti-HBcAg*
		IgM anti-HBcAg*
	HBeAg*	Anti-HBeAg*
C	—	Anti-HCV*
D	—	Anti-HDV*
E	—	Anti-HEV

**Assays are commercially available.*
HAV = hepatitis A virus; HBsAg = hepatitis B surface antigen; HBcAg = hepatitis B core antigen; HBeAg = hepatitis B e antigen; IgM = immunoglobulin M; HCV = hepatitis C virus; HDV = hepatitis D virus; HEV = hepatitis E virus.

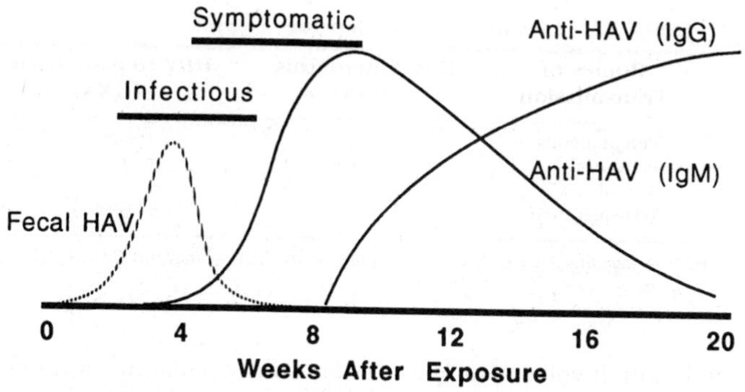

Figure 221–1. Pattern of response to hepatitis A virus (HAV) infection. (IgM = immunoglobulin M; IgG = immunoglobulin G.)

EPIDEMIOLOGY. HAV infections occur throughout the world but are most common in developing countries, where the prevalence rate approaches 100% in children by the age of 5 yr. In the United States, approximately 30% of the adult population have evidence for previous HAV infection; the rates of infection are similar in the 1st, 2nd, and 3rd decades of life. Hepatitis A causes only acute hepatitis. The illness is much more likely to be symptomatic in adults; most infections in children younger than 5 yr are asymptomatic or have mild, nonspecific manifestations. The transmission of HAV is almost always by person-to-person contact. Spread is predominantly by the fecal-oral route; percutaneous transmission is a rare occurrence and maternal-neonatal transmission is not recognized as an epidemiologic entity. HAV infection during pregnancy or at the time of delivery does not appear to result in complications of pregnancy or clinical disease in the newborn. The infectivity of human saliva, urine, and semen is unknown. In the United States, increased risk of infection is found in households, day-care centers, household contacts of children in day-care centers, and homosexual populations. Common-source foodborne and waterborne outbreaks have occurred, including several resulting from contaminated shellfish. Fecal excretion of the virus occurs late in the incubation period, reaches its peak just before the onset of symptoms, and is minimal in the week after the onset of jaundice. The mean incubation period for HAV is about 4 wk.

PATHOLOGY. The acute response of the liver to HAV is similar to that of the other four hepatitis viruses. The entire liver is involved with necrosis, most marked in the centrilobular areas, and increased cellularity, which is predominant in the portal areas. The lobular architecture remains intact, although balloon degeneration and necrosis of parenchymal cells occur initially. Fatty change is rare. A diffuse mononuclear cell inflammatory reaction causes expansion in the portal tracts; bile duct proliferation is common, but bile duct damage is not often found. Diffuse Kupffer cell hyperplasia is present in the sinusoids along with infiltration of polymorphonuclear leukocytes and eosinophils. Neonates respond to hepatic injury by forming giant cells. In fulminant hepatitis, total destruction of the parenchyma occurs, leaving only connective tissue septa. By 3 months after the onset of acute hepatitis resulting from HAV, the liver usually is normal morphologically.

Other organ systems can be affected during HAV infection. Regional lymph nodes and the spleen may be enlarged. The bone marrow may be moderately hypoplastic, and aplastic anemia has been reported. Small-intestine tissue may show changes in villous structure, and ulceration of the gastrointestinal tract can occur, especially in fatal cases. Acute pancreatitis and myocarditis have been reported rarely, and renal, joint,

■ TABLE 221–2 Features of the Hepatitis Viruses

Routes of Transmission	HAV Enterovirus (RNA)	HBV Hepadnavirus (DNA)	HCV Flavivirus (RNA)	HDV Incomplete (RNA)	HEV Calicivirus (RNA)
Percutaneous	+	++++	++++	++++	0
Fecal-oral	++++	0	0	0	++++
Sexual	+	+	+	+	+
Transplacental	0	+++	+	0	?

HAV = hepatitis A virus; HBV = hepatitis B virus; HCV = hepatitis C virus; HDV = hepatitis D virus; HEV = hepatitis E virus; + = minimal; +++ = moderate; ++++ = frequent.

and skin involvement may result from circulating immune complexes.

PATHOGENESIS. Injury in acute hepatitis is caused by several mechanisms. The initial injury in hepatitis A is thought to be cytopathic. Regardless of the mechanism of initial injury to the liver, damage from the five hepatitis viruses is evident in three main ways. The first is a reflection of injury to the hepatocytes, which release alanine aminotransferase (ALT, formerly serum glutamate pyruvate transaminase) and aspartate aminotransferase (AST, formerly serum glutamic-oxaloacetic transaminase) into the bloodstream. The ALT is more specific to the liver than the AST, which also can be elevated after injury to erythrocytes, skeletal muscle, or myocardial cells. The height of elevation does not correlate with the extent of hepatocellular necrosis and has little prognostic value. In some cases, a falling aminotransferase level may predict a poor outcome if the decline occurs in conjunction with a rising bilirubin and prolonged prothrombin time (PT). This combination of findings indicates that massive hepatic injury has occurred, resulting in few functioning hepatocytes. Another enzyme, lactate dehydrogenase is even less specific to liver than AST and usually is not helpful in evaluating liver injury. Viral hepatitis is also associated with cholestatic jaundice, in which both direct and indirect bilirubin levels are elevated. Jaundice results from obstruction of biliary flow and damage to hepatocytes. Elevations of serum alkaline phosphatase, 5′-nucleotidase, γ-glutamyl transpeptidase, and urobilinogen all can reflect injury to the biliary system. Abnormal protein synthesis by hepatocytes is reflected by increased PT. Because of the short half-life of these proteins, the PT is a sensitive indicator of damage to the liver. Serum albumin is another liver-manufactured serum protein, but its longer half-life limits its relevance for monitoring acute liver injury. Cholestasis results in a decreased intestinal bile acid pool and decreased absorption of fat-soluble vitamins. Hepatic injury also may result in changes in carbohydrate, ammonia, and drug metabolism.

CLINICAL MANIFESTATIONS. The onset of HAV infection usually is abrupt and is accompanied by systemic complaints of fever, malaise, nausea, emesis, anorexia, and abdominal discomfort. This prodrome may be mild and often goes unnoticed in infants and preschool-age children. Diarrhea often occurs in children, but constipation is more common in adults. Jaundice may be so subtle in young children that it can be detected only by laboratory tests. When they occur, jaundice and dark urine usually develop after the systemic symptoms. In contrast to HAV infections in children, most HAV infections in adults are symptomatic and can be severe. Symptoms of HAV infection include right upper quadrant pain, dark-colored urine, and jaundice. The duration of symptoms usually is less than 1 mo, and appetite, exercise tolerance, and a feeling of well-being gradually return. Almost all patients with HAV infection will recover completely, but a relapsing course can occur for several months. Fulminant hepatitis leading to death is rare, and chronic infection does not occur.

DIAGNOSIS. The diagnosis of HAV infection should be considered when a history of jaundice exists in family contacts, friends, schoolmates, day-care playmates, or school personnel or if the child or family has traveled to an endemic area. The diagnosis is made by serologic criteria; liver biopsies rarely are performed. Anti-HAV is detected at the onset of symptoms of acute hepatitis A and persists for life (Fig. 221–1). The acute infection is diagnosed by the presence of IgM anti-HAV, which can be detected for 3–12 mo; thereafter, IgG anti-HAV is found. The virus is excreted in stools from 2 wk before to 1 wk after the onset of illness. Rises are almost universally found in ALT, AST, bilirubin, alkaline phosphatase 5′-nucleotidase, and γ-glutamyl transpeptidase and do not help to differentiate the cause. The PT should always be measured in a child with hepatitis to help assess the extent of liver injury; prolongation is a serious sign mandating hospitalization.

DIFFERENTIAL DIAGNOSIS. The possible causes of hepatitis vary somewhat by age. Physiologic jaundice, hemolytic disease, and sepsis in neonates usually are distinguished easily from hepatitis (see Chapters 89 and 96–98). After the immediate newborn period, infection remains an important cause of hyperbilirubinemia, but metabolic and anatomic causes (biliary atresia and choledochal cysts) also must be considered. The introduction of pigmented vegetables into the infant's diet may result in carotenemia, which may be mistaken for jaundice.

In later infancy and childhood, hemolytic-uremic syndrome may be mistaken initially for hepatitis (see Chapter 472). Reye and Reye-like syndromes present in a similar fashion to acute fulminating hepatitis (see Chapter 306). Jaundice also may occur with malaria, leptospirosis, and brucellosis and with severe infection in older children, particularly in those with malignant disorders or with immunodeficiency. Gallstones may obstruct biliary drainage and cause jaundice in adolescents as well as in children with chronic hemolytic processes. Hepatitis may be the initial presentation of Wilson disease, cystic fibrosis, α_1-antitrypsin deficiency, and Jamaican vomiting sickness. The liver may be involved in collagen vascular diseases including systemic lupus erythematosus.

Medications, including acetaminophen overdose, valproic acid, and various hepatotoxins, can be associated with a hepatitis-like picture. Drugs well tolerated in healthy children may cause hepatic dysfunction in children with certain illnesses.

COMPLICATIONS. Children almost always recover from HAV infection. Rarely, fulminant hepatitis (see Chapter 309) can occur, in which a progressive rise in serum bilirubin is accompanied by an initial rise in aminotransferases followed by a fall to normal or low values. Hepatic synthetic function decreases and the PT becomes prolonged, often accompanied by bleeding. The serum albumin falls, causing edema and ascites. The ammonia usually rises and the sensorium becomes altered, progressing from drowsiness to stupor and then deep coma. Progression to end-stage disease and death can occur in less than 1 wk, or can develop more insidiously.

PREVENTION. The recent development of highly immunogenic and safe formalin-killed vaccines marks a major advance in the prevention of hepatitis A. Vaccination of young children in endemic areas is unnecessary because the disease is almost always asymptomatic or mild and confers lifelong immunity. In industrialized countries, vaccination of high-risk children may be of benefit because these children can become carriers of the disease and could infect older siblings and parents who are at greater risk for more severe disease. Vaccination will be of special value to unexposed travelers from developed countries when they travel to hepatitis A–endemic areas.

Enteric precautions should be observed for hospitalized, infected patients who are incontinent of stool or who are in diapers. Careful hand washing is necessary, particularly after changing diapers and before preparing or serving food. Persons infected with HAV are contagious for about 1 wk after onset of jaundice. There is no need to isolate older, continent children, but their stools and fecally contaminated materials should be treated with precautions, and strict hand washing should be practiced.

Standard pooled Ig is effective in modifying clinical manifestations of HAV infection. The prophylactic value is greatest when given early in the incubation period and declines thereafter. Guidelines for hepatitis A prophylaxis are included in Table 221–3. Ig is recommended for all susceptible individuals traveling to developing countries. Unimmunized household contacts should receive a single intramuscular dose of Ig as soon as possible after exposure. This is effective in preventing clinical hepatitis, although infection may still occur. Giving Ig more than 2 wk after exposure is not indicated.

Ig is not recommended routinely for sporadic, nonhousehold exposures (e.g., protection of hospital personnel or schoolmates). Mass administration of Ig to schoolchildren has been used when epidemics have been school centered. When HAV occurs in a child-care center with children not yet toilet trained, Ig should be administered to all children and personnel. It also is advisable to administer Ig to family members of children in diapers.

■ TABLE 221–3 Hepatitis A Prophylaxis

Variable	Dose
Before Exposure (Travelers to Endemic Regions)	
<3-mo trip	Ig: 0.02 mL/kg Vaccine*
≥3-mo trip	Ig: 0.06 mL/kg every 4–6 mo Vaccine*
After Exposure	
Household and intimate contacts	Ig: 0.02 mL/kg within 2 wk
Day care or custodial care	Ig: 0.02 mL/kg within 2 wk
Common-source outbreaks	Ig: 0.02 mL/kg within 2 wk
Casual contact	None

**When available, the vaccine will replace the need for Ig for travelers.*
Ig = immunoglobulin.

HEPATITIS B

ETIOLOGY. HBV is a 42-nm diameter member of the hepadnavirus family, a noncytopathogenic, hepatotropic group of DNA viruses. HBV has a circular, partially double-stranded DNA genome composed of approximately 3,200 nucleotides. Four genes have been identified: the S, C, X, and P genes. The surface of the virus includes two particles designated hepatitis B surface antigen (HBsAg): a 22-nm diameter spherical particle and a 22-nm wide tubular particle with a variable length of up to 200 nm. The inner portion of the virion contains hepatitis B core antigen (HBcAg) and a nonstructural antigen called hepatitis B e antigen (HBeAg), a nonparticulate–soluble antigen derived from HBcAg by proteolytic self-cleavage. Replication of HBV occurs predominantly in the liver but also occurs in lymphocytes, spleen, kidney, and pancreas.

EPIDEMIOLOGY. Worldwide, the areas of highest prevalence of HBV infection are subSaharan Africa, China, parts of the middle East, the Amazon basin, and the Pacific Islands. In the United States, the Eskimo population in Alaska has the highest prevalence rate. An estimated 300,000 new cases of HBV infection occur in the United States each year, with the 20- to 39-yr age group at greatest risk. The number of new cases in children is low but is difficult to estimate because the majority of infections in children are asymptomatic. The risk of chronic infection is related inversely to age; although less than 10% of infections occur in children, these infections account for 20–30% of all chronic cases.

The most important risk factor for acquisition of hepatitis B infection in children is perinatal exposure to an HBsAg-positive mother. The risk of transmission is greatest if the mother also is HBeAg positive; 70–90% of their infants become chronically infected if untreated. During the neonatal period, hepatitis B antigen is present in the blood of 2.5% of infants born to affected mothers, indicating that intrauterine infection occurred. In most cases, antigenemia appears later, suggesting that transmission occurred at the time of delivery; virus contained in amniotic fluid or in maternal feces or blood may be the source. Although most infants born to infected mothers become antigenemic from 2–5 mo of age, some infants of HBsAg-positive mothers are not affected until later ages.

HBsAg has been demonstrated inconsistently in milk of infected mothers. Breast-feeding of unimmunized infants by infected mothers does not appear to confer a greater risk of hepatitis on offspring than does artificial feeding despite the possibility that cracked nipples may result in the ingestion of contaminated maternal blood by the nursing infant.

Other important risk factors for HBV infection in children include intravenous acquisition by drugs or blood products, sexual contact, institutional care, and contact with carriers. Chronic HBV infection, which is defined as being HBsAg positive for 6 or more mo, is associated with chronic liver disease and with primary hepatocellular carcinoma, the most important cause of cancer-related death in the Orient.

HBV is present in high concentrations in blood, serum, and serous exudates and in moderate concentrations in saliva, vaginal fluid, and semen. For these reasons, efficient transmission occurs through blood exposure and sexual contact. The incubation period ranges from 45–160 days, with a mean of about 100 days.

PATHOLOGY. The acute response of the liver to HBV is the same as that for all the hepatitis viruses. Persistence of histologic changes in patients with hepatitis B, C, or D indicates development of chronic liver disease. Chronic hepatitis is discussed in Chapter 307.

PATHOGENESIS. Hepatitis B, unlike the other hepatitis viruses, is a noncytopathic virus that probably causes injury by immune-mediated mechanisms. The first step in the process of acute hepatitis is infection of hepatocytes by HBV, resulting in the appearance of viral antigens on the cell surface. The most important of these viral antigens may be the nucleocapsid antigens, HBcAg and HBeAg, a cleavage product of HBcAg. These antigens, in combination with class I major histocompatibility (MHC) proteins, make the cell a target for cytotoxic T-cell lysis.

The mechanism for development of chronic hepatitis is less well understood. To permit hepatocytes to continue to be infected, the core protein or MHC class I protein may not be recognized, the cytotoxic lymphocytes may not be activated, or some other as yet unknown mechanism may interfere with destruction of hepatocytes. For cell-to-cell infection to continue, some virus-containing hepatocytes must survive.

Immune-mediated mechanisms also are involved in the extrahepatic conditions that can be associated with HBV infections. Circulating immune complexes containing HBsAg can occur in patients who experience associated polyarteritis, glomerulonephritis, polymyalgia rheumatica, mixed cryoglobulinemia, and the Guillain-Barré syndrome.

Mutations of HBV are more common than for the usual DNA viruses, and a series of mutant strains have been recognized. The most important is one that results in failure to express HBeAg and has been associated with development of severe hepatitis and perhaps more severe exacerbations of chronic HBV infection.

CLINICAL MANIFESTATIONS. Many cases of HBV infection are asymptomatic, as evidenced by the high carriage rate of serum markers in persons who have no history of acute hepatitis. The usual acute, symptomatic episode is similar to HAV and hepatitis C virus (HCV) infections but may be more severe and is more likely to include involvement of skin and joints. The first clinical evidence of HBV infection is elevation of ALT, which begins to rise just before the development of lethargy, anorexia, and malaise, about 6–7 wk after exposure. The illness may be preceded in a few children by a serum sickness–like prodrome including arthralgia or skin lesions, including urticarial, purpuric, macular, or maculopapular rashes. Papular acrodermatitis, the Gianotti-Crosti syndrome, also may occur. Other extrahepatic conditions associated with HBV infections include polyarteritis, glomerulonephritis, and aplastic anemia. Jaundice, which is present in about 25% of infected individuals, usually begins about 8 wk after exposure and lasts for about 4 wk. In the usual course of resolving HBV infection, symptoms are present for 6–8 wk. The percentage of people in whom clinical evidence of hepatitis develops is higher for hepatitis B than for hepatitis A, and the rate of fulminant hepatitis also is greater. Chronic hepatitis also occurs, and the chronic active form can result in cirrhosis and hepatocellular carcinoma.

On physical examination, skin and mucous membranes are icteric, especially the sclera and the mucosa under the tongue. The liver usually is enlarged and tender to palpation. When the liver is not palpable below the costal margin, tenderness can be demonstrated by striking the rib cage over the liver gently with a closed fist. Splenomegaly and lymphadenopathy are common.

DIAGNOSIS. The serologic pattern for HBV is more complex than for HAV and differs depending on whether the disease is acute, subclinical, or chronic (Fig. 221–2). Table 221–1 summarizes the several antigens and antibodies that can be used to confirm the diagnosis of acute HBV infection. Routine screening for hepatitis B requires assay of at least two serologic markers. HBsAg is the first serologic marker of infection to appear and is found in almost all infected persons; its rise coincides closely with the onset of symptoms. HBeAg is often present during the acute phase and indicates a highly infectious state. Because HBsAg levels fall before the end of symptoms, IgM antibody to hepatitis B core antigen (IgM anti-HBcAg) also is required because it rises early after infection

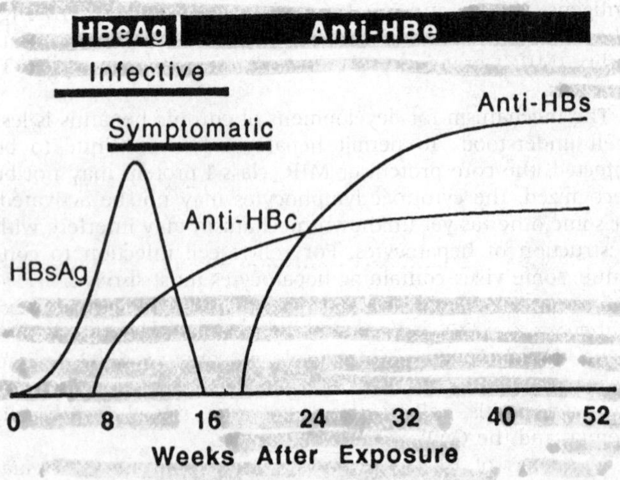

Figure 221–2. Pattern of response to hepatitis B virus infection. (HBeAg = hepatitis B e antigen; HBsAg = hepatitis B surface antigen; HBc = hepatitis B core antigen.)

and persists for many months before being replaced by IgG anti-HBcAg, which persists for years. IgM anti-HBcAg usually is not present in perinatal HBV infections. Anti-HBcAg is the most valuable single serologic marker of acute HBV infection because it is present almost as early as HBsAg and continues to be present later in the course of the disease when HBsAg has disappeared. Only anti-HBsAg is present in persons immunized with hepatitis B vaccine, whereas anti-HBsAg and anti-HBcAg are detected in persons with resolved infection.

DIFFERENTIAL DIAGNOSIS. See discussion of hepatitis A.

COMPLICATIONS. Acute fulminant hepatitis occurs more frequently with HBV than with the other hepatitis viruses, and the risk of fulminant hepatitis is further increased when there is coinfection or superinfection with HDV. Mortality from fulminant hepatitis is greater than 30%. Liver transplantation is the only effective intervention; supportive care aimed at sustaining the patient while providing the time needed for regeneration of hepatic cells is the only other option.

HBV infections also can result in chronic hepatitis, which can lead to cirrhosis and primary hepatocellular carcinoma (see Chapter 457.2). Interferon alpha-2b is available for treatment of chronic hepatitis B in persons 18 years of age or older with compensated liver disease and HBV replication. Membranous glomerulonephritis with deposition of complement and HBeAg in glomerular capillaries is a rare complication of HBV infection.

PREVENTION. Universal immunization of infants with hepatitis B vaccine is now recommended by the American Academy of Pediatrics (AAP) and the U.S. Public Health Service because selective strategies failed to prevent the substantial morbidity and mortality associated with HBV infection. The neonatal period has been targeted because more than 90% of infants who acquire the infection perinatally will become chronic carriers. The risk of acquiring the chronic carrier state diminishes with age; 50% of older children and 10% of adults who become infected will become chronic carriers. Two recombinant DNA vaccines are available in the United States; both have proven to be highly immunogenic in children. The original plasma-derived vaccine is equally immunogenic but is no longer manufactured in the United States.

Infants born to HBsAg-positive women should receive vaccine at birth, 1 mo, and 6 mo of age (Table 221–4). The first dose should be accompanied by administration of 0.5 mL of hepatitis B immunoglobulin (HBIG) as soon after delivery as possible because the effectiveness decreases rapidly with increased time after birth. The AAP recommends that infants born to HBsAg-negative women receive the first dose of vaccine at birth, the second at 1–2 mo of age, and the third between 6 and 18 mo of age.

The methods of prevention of hepatitis B infection depend on the conditions under which the person is exposed to hepatitis B, and the dose is dependent on the age of the person (see Table 221–3). Recommendations for immune prophylaxis of contacts of HBV-infected people are included in Table 221–3.

HEPATITIS C

ETIOLOGY. HCV is now recognized as the cause of almost all of the parenterally acquired cases of what was previously known as non-A, non-B hepatitis. The virus has not been isolated but has been cloned using recombinant DNA technology. Molecular biologic analysis has demonstrated that HCV is a single-strand RNA virus that has been classified as a separate genus within the *Flaviviridae* family. HCV is an enveloped virus, 50–60 nm in size, that is transmitted mainly by blood or blood products, intravenous drug use, and sexual contact. Chronic liver disease is common in infected individuals.

EPIDEMIOLOGY. The most important risk factors for HCV transmission in the United States are the use of intravenous drugs (40%), transfusions (10%), and occupational and sexual expo-

■ **TABLE 221–4 Indications and Dosing Schedule for Hepatitis B Vaccine and Immunoglobulin**

	Vaccine			HBIG	
Group at Risk	***Recombivax HB* (μg)**	***Engerix-B* (μg)**	**Schedule**	***Dose* (mL)**	***Schedule***
Neonates					
Infants of HBsAg-positive women	5.0	10	Birth, 1–6 mo	0.50	Within 12 hr of birth
Infants of HBsAg-negative women	2.5	10	Birth, 1–2 mo, 6–18 mo (AAP)	None	
Contact with Acute HBV					
Intimate					
<11 yr old	2.5	10	Exposure, 1–6 mo	0.06	Exposure
11–19 yr old	5.0	20	Exposure, 1–6 mo	0.06	Exposure
≥20 yr old	10.0	20	Exposure, 1–6 mo	0.06	Exposure
Household	None	None	None	None	
Casual	None	None	None	None	
Contact with Chronic HBV					
Intimate and household					
<11 yr old	2.5	10	Exposure, 1–6 mo	None	
11–19 yr old	5.0	20	Exposure, 1–6 mo	None	
≥20 yr old	10.0	20	Exposure, 1–6 mo	None	
Casual	None	None		None	
Immunosuppressed or Dialysis Patients	40	40	Exposure, 1–6 mo	None	

HBsAg = hepatitis B surface antigen; AAP = American Academy of Pediatrics; HBV = hepatitis B virus; HBIG = hepatitis B immunoglobulin.

sure (10%). The remaining 40% of patients have no known associated risk factors. Perinatal transmission has been described but is uncommon except when the mother is HIV infected or has a high titer of HCV RNA. Although HCV testing has made blood transfusions much safer, testing of blood may result in only a modest decline in HCV cases because transfusions account for only a small percentage of HCV infections. Large population serosurveys in the United States indicate that approximately 1% of the adult population has evidence for previous HCV infection. The incubation period is 7–9 wk (range, 2–24 wk).

PATHOLOGY. The pattern of acute injury is similar to that of the other hepatitis viruses. In chronic cases, lymphoid aggregates or follicles in portal tracts are seen either alone or as part of a general inflammatory infiltration of the tracts.

PATHOGENESIS. HCV appears to cause injury primarily by cytopathic mechanisms, but immune-mediated injury also may occur. The cytopathic component appears to be mild, because the acute form is typically the least severe of all hepatitis virus infections; HCV rarely is fulminant.

CLINICAL MANIFESTATIONS. The clinical pattern of the acute infection is usually similar to that of the other hepatitis viruses. HCV is the most likely hepatitis virus to cause chronic infection; about two thirds of post-transfusion infections and about one third of sporadic, community-acquired cases will become chronic. Typically, a fluctuating pattern of aminotransferase elevations occurs in about 80% of those in whom chronic HCV develops. Although chronic elevations of aminotransferase levels are common, chronic HCV will progress to cirrhosis in only about half of the patients, or about 25% of all those initially infected. Primary hepatocellular carcinoma can develop in patients with cirrhosis, but HCV is less effective than HBV in causing primary hepatocellular carcinoma. The hepatocellular carcinoma associated with HCV probably results from chronic inflammation and necrosis rather than an oncogenic effect of the virus.

DIAGNOSIS. The clinically available serologic assays for HCV are based on development of antibodies to HCV antigens because no detectable antigens have been found in blood. The assays are used mainly for detection of chronic hepatitis C because they remain negative for at least 1–3 mo after the clinical onset of illness. The second-generation assays are the current standard and test for three of the five known antigenic epitopes. They have improved sensitivity over the first-generation tests but still have a 10% false-negative rate. Assays for viral RNA (polymerase chain reaction [PCR], in situ hybridization) are costly, time consuming, and available only in research situations.

DIFFERENTIAL DIAGNOSIS. See discussion of hepatitis A.

COMPLICATIONS. The risk of fulminant hepatitis is low with HCV, but the risk for chronic hepatitis is the highest among the hepatitis viruses. The usual chronic course is mild even when cirrhosis develops; long-term follow-up indicates that the overall mortality of persons with transfusion-acquired HCV is no different from that of noninfected controls. Interferon alpha-2b is available for treatment of chronic hepatitis in persons 18 yr of age or older with compensated liver disease who have a history of blood or blood product exposure or who are HCV antibody positive or both.

PREVENTION. There is no vaccine available, and none may be developed because animal studies suggest that HCV infection does not lead to protective immunity; the same individual can be infected multiple times with the same virus. Ig has not proven to be of benefit. Ig manufactured in the United States does not contain antibodies to HCV because blood and plasma donors are screened for anti-HCV, and exclusion of the HCV positive persons from the donor pool is recommended.

HEPATITIS D

ETIOLOGY. Hepatitis D virus (HDV), the smallest known animal virus, is considered defective because it cannot produce infection without a concurrent HBV infection. The 36-nm diameter virus is incapable of making its own coat protein; its outer coat is composed of excess HBsAg from HBV. The inner core of the virus is single-stranded circular RNA, which expresses the HDV antigen.

EPIDEMIOLOGY. HDV infection cannot occur without HBV as a helper virus. Two patterns of infection are seen. Transmission usually occurs by intrafamilial or intimate contact in areas of high prevalence, which are primarily developing countries. In areas of low prevalence, such as the United States, the percutaneous route is far more common. Hepatitis D infections are uncommon in children in the United States but must be considered when fulminant hepatitis occurs. In the United States, HDV infection is found most frequently in parenteral drug abusers, hemophiliacs, and persons immigrating from southern Italy, parts of eastern Europe, South America, Africa, and the Middle East. The incubation period for HDV superinfection is about 2–8 wk; with coinfection, the incubation period is similar to that of HBV infection.

PATHOLOGY. There are no distinguishing features of liver disease in HDV hepatitis except that the damage is usually more severe.

PATHOPHYSIOLOGY. In contrast to HBV, HDV causes injury directly by cytopathic mechanisms. Many of the most severe cases of hepatitis B appear to be due to combined infection with HBV and HDV. Coinfection with HBV and HDV occurs most frequently in areas of high prevalence. The second mechanism of pathogenesis is superinfection of a person who has chronic HBV, which is more common in developed countries.

CLINICAL MANIFESTATIONS. The symptoms of hepatitis D infection are similar to but usually more severe than those of the other hepatitis viruses. The clinical outcome for HDV infection depends on the mechanism of infection. In coinfection, acute hepatitis, which is much more severe than for HBV alone, is common, but the risk for chronic hepatitis is low. In superinfections, acute illness is rare, whereas chronic hepatitis is common. However, the risk of fulminant hepatitis is highest in superinfection. Hepatitis D should be considered in any child who experiences acute hepatic failure.

DIAGNOSIS. The virus has not been isolated, and no circulating antigen has been identified. The diagnosis is made by detecting IgM antibody to HDV; the antibodies to HDV develop about 2–4 wk after coinfection and about 10 wk after superinfection. PCR assays for viral RNA are available but only as a research tool.

DIFFERENTIAL DIAGNOSIS. See discussion of hepatitis A.

COMPLICATIONS. HDV must be considered in all cases of fulminant hepatitis.

PREVENTION. There is no vaccine for hepatitis D. However, because HDV cannot occur without hepatitis B infection, HBV prevention eliminates HDV. HBIG and hepatitis B vaccines are used for the same indications as hepatitis B (see Table 221–3).

HEPATITIS E

ETIOLOGY. Hepatitis E virus (HEV) has not been isolated but has been cloned using molecular techniques. This RNA virus has a nonenveloped, sphere shape with spikes and is similar to the caliciviruses. Infection is associated with shedding of 27- to 34-nm particles in the stool.

EPIDEMIOLOGY. Hepatitis E is the epidemic form of what was formally called non-A, non-B hepatitis. Infection is transmitted enterically, the highest prevalence has been reported in the Indian subcontinent, the Middle East, and Southeast Asia, especially in areas with poor sanitation. In the United States, the only reported cases have been in persons who have visited or emigrated from endemic areas. The mean incubation period is about 40 days (range, 15–60 days).

PATHOLOGY. The pathologic findings are similar to those of the other hepatitis viruses.

PATHOGENESIS. HEV appears to act as a cytopathic virus.

CLINICAL MANIFESTATIONS. The clinical illness in hepatitis E is similar to that of hepatitis A, the other enterically transmitted virus, but it is often more severe. Both viruses produce only acute disease; chronic illness does not occur. In addition to causing more severe illness than HAV, hepatitis E affects older patients, with a peak incidence between 15 and 34 yr. Another important clinical difference is that HEV has a high fatality rate in pregnant women.

DIAGNOSIS. Recombinant DNA technology has resulted in the development of an antibody to HEV particles, but serologic tests are not yet commercially available. IgM antibody to viral antigen becomes positive after about 1 wk of illness.

DIFFERENTIAL DIAGNOSIS. See discussion of hepatitis A.

COMPLICATIONS. HEV is associated with a high prevalence of death in pregnant women.

PREVENTION. No vaccines are available, and there is no evidence that Ig is effective in preventing hepatitis E infections. However, Ig pooled from patients in endemic areas may prove to be effective.

A-Kader HH, Balistreri WF: Hepatitis C virus: Implications to pediatric practice. Pediatr Infect Dis J 12:853, 1993.

Ballistreri WF: Viral hepatitis. Pediatr Clin North Am 35:637, 1988.

Bancroft WH: Hepatitis A vaccine. N Engl J Med 327:488, 1992.

Carman WF, Thomas HC: Genetic variation in hepatitis B virus. Gastroenterology 102:711, 1992.

Centers for Disease Control and Prevention. Protection against viral hepatitis. MMWR 39:1, 1990.

Choo Q-L, Kuo G, Weiner AJ, et al: Isolation of a cDNA clone derived from a blood-borne non-A, non-B viral hepatitis genome. Science 24:359, 1989.

De Franchisl R, Meucci G, Vecchi M, et al: The natural history of asymptomatic hepatitis B surface antigen carriers. Ann Intern Med 118:191, 1993.

Hall AJ: Hepatitis in travellers: Epidemiology and prevention. Br Med Bull 49:382, 1993.

Hall CB, Halsey NA: Control of hepatitis B: To be or not to be? Pediatrics 90:274, 1992.

Hall CB, Margolis HS: Hepatitis B immunization: Premonitions and perceptions of pediatricians. Pediatrics 91:841, 1993.

Hoofnagle JH, Bisceglie AM: Serologic diagnosis of acute and chronic viral hepatitis. Semin Liv Dis 11:73, 1991.

Innis BL, Snitbhan R, Kunasol P, et al: Protection against hepatitis A by an inactivated vaccine. JAMA 271:1328, 1994.

Krawczynshi K: Hepatitis E. Hepatology 17:932, 1993.

Kuo G, Choo Q-L, Alter HJ, et al: An assay for circulating antibodies to a major etiologic virus of human non-A, non-B hepatitis. Science 23:362, 1989.

Levy RN, Sawitshy A, Florman AL, et al: Fatal aplastic anemia after hepatitis. N Engl J Med 273:1118, 1965.

Polish LB, Gallagher M, Fields HA, et al: Delta hepatitis: Molecular biology and clinical and epidemiological features. Clin Microbiol Rev 6:211, 1993.

Proceedings of a symposium—Hepatitis B today: New guidelines for the pediatrician. Pediatr Infect Dis J 12:427, 1993.

Ramalin G, Swami V, Purcell RH: Waterborne non-A, non-B hepatitis. Lancet 1:571, 1988.

Rizetto M, Durazzo M: Hepatitis delta virus infections: Epidemiological and clinical heterogeneity. J Hepatol 13:S116, 1991.

Seef LB, Buskell-Bales Z, Wright EC, et al: Long-term mortality after transfusion-associated non-A, non-B hepatitis. N Engl J Med 327:1906, 1992.

Sherlock S, Dooley J: Viral hepatitis. *In:* S Sherlock, J Dooley (eds): Diseases of the Liver and Biliary System. London, Blackwell Scientific, 1993, pp 260–292.

Wright R: Viral hepatitis: Comparative epidemiology. Br Med Bull 46:548, 1990.

CHAPTER 222

Rotavirus and Other Agents of Viral Gastroenteritis

Dorsey M. Bass

Diarrhea is probably the leading cause of childhood mortality in the world, accounting for 5–10 million deaths per year. In early childhood, the single most important cause of severe dehydrating diarrhea is rotavirus infection. Rotavirus and other gastroenteritis viruses are not only major causes of pediatric mortality but also lead to significant morbidity as a result of malnutrition. Worldwide, up to 1 million deaths per year are estimated to occur from rotavirus infection alone. In the United States, rotavirus causes millions of episodes of diarrhea per year with 70,000 hospitalizations and more than 100 deaths.

ETIOLOGY. Rotavirus, astrovirus, adenovirus, and caliciviruses, such as the Norwalk agent, are the known, medically important pathogens of human viral gastroenteritis.

Rotaviruses cause disease in virtually all mammals and birds. The virus is a wheel-like, double-shelled icosahedron containing 11 segments of double-stranded RNA. The diameter of the particles by electron microscopy is approximately 80 nm. Rotaviruses are classified by group (A, B, C, D, E), subgroup (I or II), and serotype. Group A, which has no antigenic relationship to the other groups, includes the common human pathogens as well as a variety of animal viruses. Group B rotavirus is reported as a cause of severe disease in infants and adults in China but not elsewhere. Occasional human outbreaks of group C rotavirus are reported. The other groups are limited to animal strains. Rotavirus strains are species specific and do not cause disease in heterologous hosts. Subgrouping of rotaviruses is determined by the antigenic structure of the inner capsid protein, vp6. Serotyping of rotaviruses, as determined by classic cross-neutralization serology, depends on the outer capsid glycoprotein, vp7. This type of serotype is often referred to as the "G" type (for glycoprotein). Recently, many investigators have also reported P types for rotavirus (the "P" refers to the structure of the other rotavirus outer capsid protein, vp4). Although both vp4 and vp7 can elicit neutralizing immunoglobulin (Ig) G antibodies, the role of these antibodies in protective immunity remains unclear.

Astroviruses are the second most important agent of viral gastroenteritis in young children. The recent availability of convenient immunoassays for astrovirus infection has allowed investigators to demonstrate its high incidence in both the developing and developed worlds. Astroviruses are small, approximately 30-nm diameter particles with a characteristic central five- or six-pointed star when viewed by electron microscopy. The virion contains single-stranded RNA of positive sense. The capsid consists of three structural proteins. There are five known human serotypes.

Enteric adenoviruses are the third most common cause of viral gastroenteritis in infants and children. Although many adenovirus serotypes exist and are found in stool, especially during and after typical upper respiratory tract infections, only serotypes 40 and 41 cause gastroenteritis. These strains do not cause respiratory symptoms and are very difficult to grow in tissue culture. They are 80-nm diameter, icosahedral viruses with a relatively complex single-stranded DNA genome.

Norwalk virus is another small 27- to 35-nm virus that is the most common cause of gastroenteritis outbreaks in older children and adults. It has a single structural protein and positive-sense, single-stranded RNA genome. It appears to be closely related to *caliciviruses*. Variant but closely related calicilike viruses have been named for locations of outbreaks: Snow Mountain, Montgomery County, Sapporo, and so on. Other caliciviruses may cause a rotavirus-like illness in young infants. Caliciviruses and astroviruses are sometimes referred to as small round viruses on the basis of appearance on electron microscopy.

Several other viruses that may cause diarrheal disease in animals have been postulated but not yet well established as human gastroenteritis viruses. These include coronaviruses and pestiviruses. Picobirnaviruses, another group of small 30-nm, double-stranded RNA viruses, have been reported to be found in 10% of patients with human immunodeficiency virus–associated diarrhea.

EPIDEMIOLOGY. Rotavirus infection is most common in winter months in temperate climates. Peak incidence spreads from the west to the east in the United States. Unlike other winter viruses such as influenza, this wave of increased incidence is not due to a single prevalent strain or serotype. Typically, several serotypes predominate in a given community for one or two seasons while nearby locations may harbor unrelated strains. Most clinical cases occur in children younger than 2 yr (but older than 3 mo), with serologic evidence of infection developing in virtually all children by age 4 or 5 yr. Subclinical infections are common in newborn nurseries and in adults with intimate contact with infected children. Some rotavirus strains have stably colonized newborn nurseries where for years virtually all newborns have been infected with the colonizing strain without any overt illness. Rotavirus and the other gastroenteritis viruses spread efficiently via a fecal-oral route, and outbreaks are common in children's hospitals and day-care centers. The virus is shed in stool at very high concentration before and for days after the clinical illness. Very few infectious virions are needed to cause disease in a susceptible host.

The epidemiology of astroviruses is not as thoroughly studied as rotavirus, but it is a common cause of mild to moderate watery diarrhea in children and infants and an uncommon pathogen in adults. Hospital outbreaks are common. Enteric adenovirus gastroenteritis occurs year-round, mostly in children younger than 2 yr. Nosocomial outbreaks occur but are less common than in rotavirus and astrovirus. Norwalk virus is best known for causing large explosive outbreaks among older children and adults, particularly in settings such schools, cruise ships, and hospitals. Often a single food, such as shellfish or water used in food preparation, is identified as a source.

PATHOLOGY AND PATHOPHYSIOLOGY. Viruses that cause human diarrhea selectively infect and destroy villus tip cells in the small intestine. Biopsies of the small intestines show variable degrees of villus blunting and round cell infiltrate in the lamina propria. Observed pathologic changes may not correlate with the severity of clinical symptoms and usually resolve before the resolution of diarrhea. The gastric mucosa is not affected despite the commonly used term "gastroenteritis," although delayed gastric emptying has been documented during Norwalk virus infection.

In the small intestine, the upper villus enterocytes are differentiated cells, which have both digestive functions such as hydrolysis of disaccharides and absorptive functions such as the transport of water and electrolytes via glucose and amino acid cotransporters. The crypt enterocytes are undifferentiated cells, which lack the brush border hydrolytic enzymes and are net secretors of water and electrolytes. Selective viral infection of intestinal villus tip cells thus leads to (1) an imbalance of the ratio of intestinal fluid absorption to secretion, and (2) malabsorption of complex carbohydrates, particularly lactose. Most evidence supports the first mechanism as the most important factor in the genesis of viral diarrhea.

In the normal host, extra-intestinal infection is quite rare, although immunocompromised patients may experience hepatic and renal involvement. The increased vulnerability of infants (compared with older children and adults) to severe morbidity and mortality from gastroenteritis viruses may relate to a number of factors including decreased intestinal reserve function, lack of specific immunity, and decreased nonspecific host defense mechanisms such as gastric acid and mucus. Viral enteritis greatly enhances intestinal permeability to luminal macromolecules and has been postulated to increase the risk of food allergies.

CLINICAL MANIFESTATIONS. Rotavirus infection typically begins after an incubation period of fewer than 48 hr with mild to moderate fever and vomiting followed by the onset of frequent watery stools. Vomiting and fever typically abate during the 2nd day of illness, but diarrhea often continues for 5–7 days. The stool is without gross blood or white cells. Dehydration may develop and progress rapidly, particularly in infants. Malnourished children and children with underlying intestinal disease such as short-bowel syndrome are particularly likely to acquire severe rotavirus diarrhea. Rarely, immunodeficient children will experience severe and prolonged illness. Although most newborns infected with rotavirus are asymptomatic, some outbreaks of necrotizing enterocolitis have been associated with the appearance of a new rotavirus strain in the affected nurseries.

The clinical course of astrovirus appears to be quite similar to that of rotavirus with the notable exception that the disease tends to be milder, with less significant dehydration. Adenovirus enteritis tends to cause diarrhea of longer duration, often

10–14 days. The Norwalk virus has a short (12-hr) incubation period. Vomiting and nausea tend to predominate in illness associated with the Norwalk virus, and the duration is brief, usually 1–3 days of symptoms. The clinical and epidemiologic picture of Norwalk virus often closely resembles so-called food poisoning from preformed toxins such as *Staphylococcus aureus* or *Bacillus cereus*.

LABORATORY FINDINGS. Isotonic dehydration with acidosis is the most common finding in children with severe viral enteritis. The stools are free of blood and leukocytes. Although the white cell count may be moderately elevated secondary to stress, the marked left shift seen with invasive bacterial enteritis is absent.

DIAGNOSIS AND DIFFERENTIAL DIAGNOSIS. The differential diagnosis includes other infectious causes such as bacteria and protozoa. Occasionally surgical conditions such as appendicitis, bowel obstruction, and intussusception may initially mimic viral gastroenteritis. In most cases, a satisfactory diagnosis can be made on the basis of the clinical and epidemiologic features. Commercial immunoassays, which offer approximately 90% specificity and sensitivity, are available for group A rotavirus and enteric adenovirus. More obscure cases can be studied by electron microscopy of stools, RNA electrophoresis, nucleic acid hybridization, and polymerase chain reaction assays. The diagnosis of viral gastroenteritis should always be questioned in patients with persistent high fever, blood or white cells in the stool, or persistent severe or bilious vomiting (especially in the absence of diarrhea).

TREATMENT. Avoiding and treating dehydration are the main goals in treatment of viral enteritis (see Chapter 56). A secondary goal is maintainance of the nutritional status of the patient (see Chapter 43).

Rehydration can be accomplished in most patients via the oral route. Modern rehydration solutions containing appropriate quantities of sodium and glucose promote optimum absorption of fluid from the gut. There is no evidence that a particular carbohydrate source (i.e., rice) or addition of amino acids improves the efficacy of these solutions for children with viral enteritis. Other clear liquids such as flat soda, fruit juice, and sports drinks are inappropriate for rehydration of young children with significant stool loss. Rehydration via the oral (or nasogastric if needed) route should be done over 6–8 hr and feedings begun immediately thereafter. Rehydration solution should be continued as a supplement to make up for ongoing excessive stool losses. Initial intravenous fluids are required for the infant in shock or the occasional child with intractable vomiting.

After rehydration has been achieved, resumption of a normal diet for age has been shown to result in a more rapid recovery from viral gastroenteritis. Prolonged (>12 hr) administration of exclusive clear liquids or dilute formula is without clinical benefit and actually prolongs the duration of diarrhea. Breast-feeding should be continued even during rehydration. Selected infants may benefit from lactose-free feedings (such as soy formula or lactose-free cow's milk) for several days, although this is not necessary for most children. The use of hypocaloric diets low in protein and fat such as BRAT (bananas, rice, cereal, applesauce, and toast) have not been shown to be superior to a regular diet.

There is no role for drug treatment of viral gastroenteritis. Controlled studies have shown no benefit from antiemetics or antidiarrheal drugs, and there is a real risk of serious side effects. Obviously, antibiotics are similarly of no benefit. Immunoglobulins have been administered orally to both normal and immunodeficient patients with severe rotavirus gastroenteritis, but this treatment is currently considered experimental therapy.

PREVENTION. Good hygiene reduces the transmission of viral gastroenteritis, but even in the most hygienic societies virtually all children become infected as a result of the efficiency of infection of the gastroenteritis viruses, particularly rotavirus. Strict hand-washing and isolation procedures can help control nosocomial outbreaks. The role of breast-feeding in prevention or amelioration of rotavirus infection is probably small given the variable protection observed in a number of studies.

The most promising prospect for prevention is the development of an effective vaccine. To date, a number of live rotavirus vaccine candidates have been extensively tested. Most have been animal or human-animal hybrid rotaviruses that are attenuated in humans. None have consistently protected infants in a variety of settings, but new candidates are under development. A successful rotavirus vaccine would substantially reduce morbidity and mortality among children throughout the world.

Blacklow NR, Greenberg HB: Viral gastroenteritis. N Engl J Med 325:252, 1991.
Gore SM, Fontaine O, Pierce NP: Impact of rice based ORS on stool output and duration of diarrhea: Meta-analysis of 13 clinical trials. BMJ 304:287, 1992.
Herrmann JE, Taylor DN, Echeverria P, et al: Astroviruses as a cause of gastroenteritis in children. N Engl J Med 24:1757, 1991.
Haffejee IE: Cow's milk-based formula, human milk, and soya feeds in acute infantile diarrhea: A therapeutic trial. J Pediatr Gastroenterol Nutr 10:193, 1990.

CHAPTER 223

Human Immunodeficiency Virus

Wade Parks

Pediatric acquired immunodeficiency syndrome (AIDS) is caused by human immunodeficiency virus (HIV) type 1 (HIV-1). HIV-1 infects $CD4^+$ T lymphocytes predominantly; depletion of $CD4^+$ lymphocytes results in immunodeficiency. Most children with HIV-1 infection are diagnosed between 2 mo and 3 yr of age. HIV-1 transmission usually occurs by contact with infected cells in blood and body fluids. HIV-1 has infected more than 1 million people in the United States during the past 15 yr, including about 20,000 children. HIV-1 infection is a worldwide problem with particularly devastating effects in Africa and Asia.

EPIDEMIOLOGY. The three principal pediatric populations at risk for HIV-1 infection are infants born to infected mothers, patients given HIV-1–contaminated blood products before 1985–1986, and adolescents who acquire infection sexually or by the use of intravenous drugs. HIV-1 infection is the fifth leading cause of death in children younger than 15 yr. Pediatric AIDS is the leading cause of death among children from 2–5 yr old in many cities of the eastern United States. Most HIV-1 infection is associated with exposure of the recipient's $CD4^+$ lymphocytes to HIV-1–positive cells from an infected individual. Cell-free transmission can occur, as evidenced by infection of hemophiliacs by antihemophiliac factor. The usual settings for lymphocyte-lymphocyte interaction are with blood transfusion and sexual intercourse.

Perinatal HIV-1 transmission is the leading cause of pediatric AIDS. In the United States, approximately 7,000 infants are born to HIV-1–infected mothers each year, and approximately 2,000 infants become infected. Mothers who transmit HIV-1 are usually well and have normal numbers of $CD4^+$ T lymphocytes and often do not know that they have HIV-1 infection. Every pregnant woman should be considered potentially HIV-1 positive. Opportunities for early recognition of HIV-1 infection are limited because HIV-1–infected women are often of a low socioeconomic class and may not receive adequate prenatal care. Universal screening of all pregnant women for HIV-1 with appropriate counseling and support is strongly recommended now that the efficacy of zidovudine (AZT) for the prevention of transmission is established. The epidemiology of perinatal AIDS parallels that of other sexually transmitted diseases such as gonorrhea and syphilis. Pediatric AIDS is often the first evidence of heterosexually transmitted HIV-1 infection in populations because clinical disease usually occurs within months in the infant but remains clinically silent for years in infected women. In addition to increasing heterosexual transmission of HIV-1 to women in Africa, the United States, and Europe, pediatric AIDS is becoming a major public health problem in Thailand and India.

HIV-1-Contaminated Blood Products. Pediatric patients requiring blood products from the later 1970s until 1985–1986 were at very high risk of HIV-1 infection. More than 75% of severe hemophiliacs, including approximately 10,000 patients in the United States who were transfused before HIV-1 screening, acquired HIV-1 infection. Patients given multiple transfusions for congenital anemias, leukemias or other diseases had an incidence of HIV-1 infection of approximately 8%. The introduction of HIV-1 antibody screening of donors, donor education, and selected exclusion policies has essentially eliminated the risk of HIV-1 transmission in developed countries. Worldwide, HIV-1 screening of blood is still more a goal than a reality.

Sexual Transmission. Multiple sexual contacts, ulcerative lesions of the vagina, cervix, or penis, and receptive anal intercourse increase the risk of transmission. Adolescents acquire HIV-1 by unprotected sexual intercourse and by intravenous drug abuse. HIV-1 infection acquired during adolescence usually causes AIDS in individuals who are 20–30 yr old. There are 65,000 AIDS patients in this age group, and the number of adolescents with AIDS has doubled during the past 5 yr. Surveys of military recruits, Job Corps participants, and blinded seroprevalence studies indicate that as many as 1 in 20 15–20-yr-olds from the northeastern and southern United States are HIV-1 seropositive. Altering HIV-1 transmission among adolescents poses a great challenge because of their relative lack of knowledge about HIV-1 and their risk-taking behavior.

HIV-1 infection is most often a household infection, usually introduced by one of the parents. Parents and siblings should be counseled, examined, and tested for HIV-1. HIV-1–negative siblings and household contacts of HIV-1–positive family members have very little or no risk of becoming HIV-1 positive by casual exposure. Surrogate measures of HIV-1 infection such as absolute or percent $CD4^+$ lymphocyte counts and immunoglobulin (Ig) levels should be used only in conjunction with specific tests for HIV-1 infection with appropriate informed consent. Adolescent infections and other idiopathic HIV-1 infections require systematic public health investigations.

PATHOGEN AND PATHOGENESIS. HIV-1 is a human retrovirus belonging to the *Lentivirinae* subfamily. Retroviruses contain an inner capsid made up of structural proteins referred to by their size. The major structural protein, p24, is detected in serum of infected patients with high viral loads. The virion capsid contains two copies of a single-stranded RNA and a few molecules of reverse transcriptase. The reverse transcriptase is a viral DNA polymerase that incorporates nucleosides into DNA using viral RNA as a template. The reverse transcriptase is the unique target of nucleoside analogs such as zidovudine and dideoxyinosine (ddI) because, in contrast to cellular DNA polymerase I, it does not discriminate between these chain-terminating analogs and natural nucleosides. The HIV-1 transcriptase is error prone and lacks error-correcting mechanisms. Many mutations arise, creating wide genetic variation in HIV-1 isolates even within individual patients. This genetic variation allows the relatively rapid emergence of drug resistance and probably interferes with elimination of the virus by the immune system. HIV-1 requires active cellular DNA replication to integrate into lymphocyte DNA. Intercurrent infections that stimulate T or B-lymphocytes, such as *Pneumocystis carinii*, malaria, and measles, cause a rapid increase in the viral load. The role of cellular DNA synthesis in HIV replication complicates therapeutic approaches based on immune stimulation or bone marrow replacement.

HIV-1 transcription is followed by translation as a capsid polyprotein, which includes a virus-specific protease, PR. PR is a target for antiviral drug development because it differs from cellular proteases and the viral protease is critical for HIV-1 assembly. Several HIV-1 antiprotease drugs have been developed, but drug resistance remains an obstacle to their clinical efficacy. The *tat, rev,* and *nef* proteins of HIV-1 early gene products are likely to be important virulence factors and are targets for genetic approaches to antiviral therapy. Live, attenuated virus vaccines with *nef* deletions have been proposed for immunoprophylaxis.

The major external viral protein of HIV-1 is a heavily glycosylated gp120 protein associated with the transmembrane glycoprotein gp41E. The gp41E is very immunogenic and is used to detect HIV-1 antibodies in diagnostic assays. The gp120 is a complex molecule that includes the highly variable V3 loop. This region is immunodominant for neutralizing antibodies. The gp120 also carries the binding site for the CD4 molecule of T cells in a constant region of the protein. This region is the ligand that enables the virus to infect $CD4^+$ T lymphocytes.

HIV-1 infection and eventual killing of $CD4^+$ T lymphocytes interferes with T- and B-lymphocyte clonal proliferation and effective immunologic memory responses. HIV-1 Tat protein may induce cell death by apoptosis in T cells. $CD4^+$ lymphocyte function is maintained initially through virus-specific immune responses and replenishment of $CD4^+$ cells from lymphocyte precursor populations. HIV-1 also infects macrophages, but their role in pathogenesis remains unclear.

Experimentally, it is not possible to determine the exact timing of HIV-1 transmission from infected mother to child. Reports of first-trimester transplacental transmission are difficult to validate, and an intact placenta seems to be an effective barrier to HIV-1 transmission. Some transmission may occur later in the third trimester, but exposure during labor and delivery is major factor, explaining the minimal differences in transmission rates between cesarean and vaginal deliveries. Early HIV-1 replication has no apparent clinical consequences. Whether tested by virus isolation or by polymerase chain reaction (PCR) for viral nucleic acid sequences, fewer than 50% of HIV-1–infected infants are positive for the virus at birth. The virus load increases by 2–3 mo, and almost all infants have detectable HIV-1 in peripheral blood.

Two possible outcomes follow as viral replication continues during the first few months of life. Severe clinical disease may result when the decline in $CD4^+$ T lymphocytes is very marked and the infant is exposed to a major pathogen. *P. carinii* is an early lethal infection of HIV-1–positive infants in the United States but is not commonly seen in Europe. Severe bacterial infections are also common in HIV-1–infected infants at this stage, and these infants have protracted and severe viral respiratory infections (e.g., respiratory syncytial virus). Infants who are infected at birth and have serious clinical manifestations before 1 yr of age have a relatively poor prognosis. The second possible outcome is a marked lymphoreticular response in which generalized lymphadenopathy with hepatosplenomegaly develops between 1 and 2 yr. This lymphoreticular response may cause alveolitis, the hallmark of HIV-1–associated lymphoid interstitial pneumonitis (LIP). Generalized lymphoreticular hyperplasia is associated with lower viral loads and a more favorable prognosis. This outcome suggests that there may be a relatively effective immune response that partially controls the *chronic, persistent HIV-1 infection.*

Infected infants and children most commonly have a hypergammaglobulinemia (>1.750 g/L) with high levels of anti-HIV-1 antibody. This response may reflect both a dysregulation of T-cell suppression of B-cell synthesis of antibody and an active $CD4^+$ enhancement of B-lymphocyte humoral responses. Similarly, cell-mediated immune responses have been reported; $CD8^+$ lymphocytes mediate killing of HIV-1–infected lymphocytes. In spite of this evidence of clinical and laboratory immune responses, HIV-1–infected patients eventually succumb to the effects of HIV-1 infection. Long-term survivors are not a biologically distinct population.

HIV-1 is present in breast milk. Where reasonable alternatives are available, HIV-1–positive mothers should not breastfeed their infants because it may increase perinatal transmission. However, in developing countries, recommendations to breast-feed remain in place. Cumulatively, perinatal transmission is approximately 30% (range, 15–40%). Recent reports of high maternal viral load as a significant risk factor for transmission are consistent with reports of an increased risk of transmission in HIV-1–positive mothers with low peripheral blood absolute $CD4^+$ lymphocyte numbers (≤200 $CD4^+/mm^3$). However, the overwhelming majority of perinatal transmission is from mothers with normal $CD4^+$ lymphocyte numbers.

CLINICAL MANIFESTATIONS. Infected infants cannot be identified clinically until severe disease occurs or until chronic problems such as diarrhea, failure to thrive, or oral candidiasis suggest an underlying immunodeficiency.

Clinical manifestations of HIV-1 infection are varied because of the secondary immunodeficiency as well as the multisystem involvement associated with this chronic, persistent virus infection. The Centers for Disease Control (CDC) classification system is given in Table 223–1. Infants have chronic conditions, such as failure to thrive, or acute signs, such as respiratory failure. The initial signs may be hepatosplenomegaly, lymphadenopathy and dyspnea, repeated severe bacterial infections, or loss of developmental milestones. Older children may have proteinuria and hematuria associated with nephrotic syndrome or nephritis or signs of cardiac failure.

Initial clinical signs may be mild and include prolonged diarrhea (≥1 mo), protracted oral candidiasis, lymphadenopathy, hepatomegaly, splenomegaly, or decreased growth velocity. Recurrent otitis media is often a mild clinical presentation. Unexpected severity, a prolonged clinical course, failure to respond to appropriate therapy, or recurrence are indications of an underlying immune disorder that may represent HIV-1 infection. At the next level of severity, patients with HIV-1 infection may present with severe life-threatening bacterial infections, including pneumonia or septicemia with organisms like *Streptococcus pneumoniae* or *Salmonella*. Chronic sinusitis in HIV-1–infected infants may also be the major sign of immune dysfunction. This category of moderately severe presentations includes the AIDS-defining LIP.

LIP is defined as reticulonodular pulmonary infiltrates that persist for 2 mo or more with or without hilar adenopathy and that do not respond to antimicrobials in an HIV-1–infected patient. LIP is a distinctive presentation of HIV-1 infection and is probably the most common clinical presentation in children. Histologically, an LIP is an interstitial infiltrate composed of $CD8^+$ lymphocytes. Children with LIP have persistent cough and exertional dyspnea, which may require chronic oxygen. The prognosis of children with LIP is relatively good compared with that of some other clinical presentations, but most infants still die within a few years.

Acute clinical presentations caused by virulent organisms in $CD4^+$ lymphopenic HIV-1–infected patients are referred to as "AIDS-defining" opportunistic infections. The most common and highly lethal opportunistic infection is *P. carinii* pneumonia (PCP). As a primary infection in HIV-1–infected infants, it has a mortality of greater than 70% and is distinguished from PCP *reactivation* in adults with AIDS. This distinction between primary and reactivation infection also distinguishes *Mycobacterium tuberculosis* infections in children and adults with AIDS. The clinical presentation of PCP in HIV-1–infected infants is severe respiratory distress with cough, tachypnea, dyspnea, and hypoxemia with blood gases indicative of an alveolar capillary block (e.g., an interstitial inflammatory process). Chest roentgenograms reveal bilateral diffuse pneumonitis with flattened diaphragms. Diagnosis is usually confirmed by flexible bronchoscopy and bronchoalveolar lavage with appropriate stains for both the cysts and trophozoites. Lactate dehydrogenase levels are usually elevated as well. The differential diagnosis in infants includes herpesviruses (cytomegalovirus, Epstein-Barr virus, herpes simplex virus), respiratory syncytial virus, and severe wheezing-associated respiratory infection. Treatment of PCP infection must be initiated as early as possible, but the prognosis is poor and is not directly correlated with $CD4^+$ lymphocyte numbers. PCP reactivation is seen increasingly in older children who have a more chronic clinical course of HIV-1 infection. PCP prophylaxis (trimethoprim-sulfamethoxazole three times weekly) is recommended for HIV-1–infected pediatric patients with low $CD4^+$ T-lymphocyte counts (≤25% of absolute count).

A second relatively common AIDS-defining opportunistic infection is esophagitis secondary to *Candida albicans. Candida* eosphagitis manifests as anorexia or dysphasia, complicated by weight loss, and is treated with amphotericin B and ketaconazole. Other important opportunistic infections involve the central nervous system, such as *Toxoplasma gondii. Myobacterium avium complex* infection usually causes gastrointestinal symptomatology, and herpesviruses cause retinal, pulmonary, hepatic, and neurologic complications. Worldwide, *M. tuberculosis* and malaria are the major opportunistic pathogens in AIDS patients. Neoplasms are relatively uncommon in pediatric HIV-1–infected patients.

Associated laboratory findings are anemia (<8 g/dL), neutropenia (<1,000/mm^3), and thrombocytopenia (<100,000/mm^3). These abnormalities usually occur in conjunction with $CD4^+$ lymphopenia and hypergammoglobulinemia but may be the presenting feature of HIV-1 infection. Similarly, tests of liver function are often abnormal although usually within threefold of the upper limits of normal.

The age at the initial clinical presentation and the $CD4^+$ lymphocyte count are major factors in prognosis. AIDS-defining infections presenting before 1 yr in lymphopenic infants have a poor prognosis. Conversely, mild signs or symptoms in a child with stable moderately high levels of $CD4^+$ lymphocytes are indicative of a relatively good prognosis.

DIAGNOSIS. Detection of HIV-1 antibody is both extremely sensitive and very specific; however, maternal transplacental IgG in the infant obscures the usefulness of antibody screening for diagnosis except in older children and adolescents. Maternal IgG has a half-life of 20–28 days, and in most infected infants

■ TABLE 223–1 Classification of HIV-1–Infected Pediatric Patients

$CD4^+$ Lymphocyte Count	Signs and Symptoms			
	None	*Mild*	*Moderate*	*Severe**
Normal (≥25%)	N1	A1	B1	C1
Moderate reduction (15–24%)	N2	A2	B2	C2
Severe reduction (<15%)	N3	A3	B3	C3

Children whose HIV-1 infection status is not confirmed are classified with an E (for perinatal Exposure*) before the appropriate classification code.*

**Category C and lymphoid interstitial pneumonitis in category B are reportable to public health officials as acquired immunodeficiency syndrome.*

HIV-1 = human immunodeficiency virus type 1.

a humoral response to HIV-1 develops by 4–6 mo of age. After 6 mo of age, antibodies can be detected by commercial enzyme-linked immunosorbent assays and quantified by Western blots that measure antibody to specific viral polypeptides. Because some mothers transmit extraordinarily high levels of anti-HIV IgG and because the sensitivity of the HIV-1 antibody test is so high, it may be necessary to wait until 15–18 mo of age to identify an HIV-1–exposed, clinically well infant as uninfected by serologic tests unless quantitative antibody studies are performed. Direct detection of virus proteins or nucleic acids are less sensitive but highly specific diagnostic methods; if available, direct detection is recommended for diagnosis or confirmation. The most sensitive tests are PCR to detect HIV-1 nucleic acid sequences and direct virus isolation from peripheral blood. The p24 protein assay is less sensitive, but it is rapid and readily available. In a situation of known exposure, the negative predictive value of diagnostic tests is critical. The uninfected newborn infant of an HIV-1–positive mother should be closely monitored for several weeks before negative laboratory tests are considered definitive. When clinical findings in the patient are consistent with a diagnosis of pediatric AIDS but there is incomplete information regarding exposure, the diagnosis requires laboratory confirmation using methods with high positive predictive value. Pediatric HIV-1 infection is not a clinical diagnosis.

TREATMENT. At present, the goals of intervention in HIV-1–infected patients focus on decreasing viral burden with chemotherapy and improving the immune response. The psychosocial and emotional needs of an HIV-1 child are often beyond the usual resources of health care providers. Team management of the complex medical and social problems is very important with experienced case management as an ideal. In addition to medical care, ethical and confidentiality issues are important concerns.

Currently, two antiretroviral drugs are licensed for use in HIV-1–infected children. Zidovudine, at a maximum of 180 mg/m^2 is administered every 6 hr and dideoxyinosine, 100 mg/m^2, is given twice daily. These drugs reduce the HIV-1 load significantly and are associated with increased CD4$^+$ lymphocyte counts and clinical improvement. Both drugs cause mild neutropenia, but a macrocytic anemia is associated with zidovudine, and pancreatitis occurs in a small proportion of children treated with ddI. The major problem with the use of these reverse transcriptase inhibitors is the development of viral drug resistance. Even with multiple drugs targeted at a single gene product, the virus is able to replicate, undergo mutations, and become resistant to antiviral agents. Multiple drug chemotherapy directed at least at two different gene products operating in different pathways (e.g., integration vs assembly) is likely to be necessary. The most likely viral targets for this approach are the reverse transcriptase and the viral protease. Other interventions commonly used in the care of HIV-1–infected infants are PCP prophylaxis, immune serum globulin (for replacement in patients with demonstrated deficiencies), and licensed viral vaccines.

PREVENTION. The administration of zidovudine to HIV-1–infected pregnant women reduces the transmission of HIV-1 to infants dramatically. The use of zidovudine (100 mg orally five times/24 hr) in HIV-1–positive women from 14 weeks gestation through labor and delivery and for 6 wk in neonates (180 mg/m^2 orally every 6 hr) reduced transmission for 26% in placebo recipients to 8% in zidovudine recipients, a highly significant difference. The U.S. Public Health Service has issued guidelines for the use of zidovudine in HIV-1–positive pregnant women to prevent perinatal HIV-1 transmission. Women who are HIV-1 positive, pregnant with gestations of 14–34 wk, have CD4$^+$ lymphocyte counts of 200/mm^3 or greater, and are not currently on antiretroviral therapy are advised to use zidovudine. HIV-1–positive women who are identified after 34 wk gestation or who are in labor are also encouraged to use zidovudine. Intravenous zidovudine (1-hr loading dose of 2/mg/kg followed by a continuous infusion of 1 mg/kg/hr until delivery) is recommended during labor. In all situations in which the mother received zidovudine to prevent HIV-1 transmission, the infant should receive zidovudine syrup (2 mg/kg every 6 hr for the first 6 wk of life beginning 8–12 hr after birth). If the mother is HIV-1 positive and did not receive zidovudine, zidovudine should be started in the newborn as soon after birth as possible; there is no evidence to support drug efficacy in preventing HIV-1 infection of the newborn after 24 hr. Mothers and children treated with zidovudine should be observed closely for adverse events and registered with the CDC to assess possible long-term adverse events. To date, only mild, revisible anemia has been noted in infants. To implement this approach fully, all women must receive proper prenatal care, and pregnant women must be tested for HIV-1 positivity.

Sexual Transmission. Prevention of sexual transmission involves avoiding the exchange of bodily fluids. Condoms are an integral part of programs that reduce sexually transmitted diseases. Unprotected sex with older partners or with multiple partners is common among HIV-1–infected adolescents.

FUTURE PROSPECTS. The current major issues in pediatric HIV-1 infection are improved treatment of infected children and the need for more effective chemotherapeutic antiretroviral agents or drug combinations. The second current issue is to implement steps that will prevent perinatal transmission, which requires maternal screening and the use of zidovudine prophylaxis. The prevention of adolescent HIV-1 infection is a longer-term goal. Adolescent HIV-1 infection is the most challenging pediatric HIV-related problem.

Blair JF, Hein KK: Public policy implications of HIV/AIDS in adolescents. Future Children 4:73, 1994.
Caldwell MB, Oxtoby MJ, Simonds RJ, et al: 1994 revised classification system for human immunodeficiency virus infection in children less than 13 years of age. MMWR 43:1, 1994.
Li CJ, Friedman DJ, Wang C, et al: Induction of apoptosis in uninfected lymphocytes by HIV-1 Tat protein. Science 268:429, 1995.
MMWR Recommendations and Reports. Recommendations of the U.S. Public Health Service Task Force on the use of zidovudine to reduce perinatal transmission of human immunodeficiency virus. MMWR 43:1, 1994.
Pizzo PA, Wilfert CM: Pediatric AIDS: The Challenge of HIV Infection in Infants, Children and Adolescents, 2nd ed. Baltimore, Williams & Wilkins, 1994.

CHAPTER 224
Human Papillomavirus

Kenneth H. Fife

Papillomaviruses cause a variety of proliferative cutaneous and mucosal lesions ranging from common skin warts to life-threatening respiratory papillomas as well as benign and malignant genital tract lesions. The inability to propagate these pathogens in culture has prevented the application of traditional virologic methods to their study and has slowed progress in the field. Newer molecular techniques have spawned a recent and dramatic increase in our level of understanding.

ETIOLOGY. The papillomaviruses are small (~55 nm), DNA-containing viruses that are ubiquitous in nature, infecting most mammalian and many nonmammalian animal species. At least 75 different types of human papillomaviruses (HPVs) have been identified by DNA sequence homology. The different HPV types typically cause disease in different anatomic sites; about half of the HPV types have been identified in genital tract specimens.

EPIDEMIOLOGY. There are no accurate data on the prevalence of HPV infection, but most individuals are probably infected with one or more HPV types at some time. Common cutaneous and plantar warts are frequently seen in children; genital warts (condylomata acuminata) are the most prevalent viral sexually transmitted disease and are seen in adolescents and adults. Many HPV infections (such as genital warts) are probably spread by direct contact with an infected individual, whereas other infections (such as plantar warts) may be transmitted by contaminated surfaces. The infection that leads to respiratory papillomas is usually acquired intrapartum by passage through a contaminated birth canal. Adolescent mothers are most likely to give birth to children with respiratory papillomatosis. There is no animal reservoir for HPV, so all transmission is presumably person to person.

PATHOLOGY. HPV-infected epithelium shows a proliferation of the spinous layer, causing an increase in the thickness of the epithelium. Proliferation of the dividing (basal) cells is characteristic of dysplastic epithelium. The koilocyte, a ballooned cell with a perinuclear clearing or halo, is characteristic of HPV infection.

CLINICAL MANIFESTATIONS. The typical HPV-induced lesions of the skin are proliferative, papular, and hyperkeratotic (see Chapter 617). They may be single or multiple and are usually localized to a limited anatomic area. On mucosal epithelium, the lesions are softer and may be cauliflower-like. Flat, macular lesions can also be seen on either cutaneous or mucosal epithelium. Some infected epithelium may be inapparent to visual inspection. Dysplastic changes of the uterine cervix (usually without clinical symptoms) are found with increasing frequency in adolescent females. Respiratory papillomatosis may present with hoarseness, dyspnea, stridor, or cough.

DIAGNOSIS. Application of 3% acetic acid to infected epithelium may show whitening ("acetowhite change"), suggesting hyperkeratosis typical of HPV infection. There are no routine laboratory tests that are useful in establishing the diagnosis. Genital warts can be distinguished from condyloma lata of secondary syphilis by syphilis serology (see Chapter 201.1). Biopsy or cytology specimens can be examined for koilocytes or dysplastic changes; some laboratories can stain for papillomavirus capsid antigen, although this is a very insensitive test. HPV DNA testing is usually applied as a research tool, although it is the most sensitive and specific test.

COMPLICATIONS. Respiratory papillomas can occlude the airway, causing respiratory compromise. These lesions may recur within weeks of removal, requiring frequent surgery. Respiratory papillomas may become malignant, especially if they have been treated with radiation. Some genital HPV types (especially HPV 16 and related types) are associated with cervical dysplasia and cervical cancer, although the latter is rare in pediatric patients.

TREATMENT. Most cutaneous warts will resolve spontaneously and may not require treatment. Treatment usually involves surgical removal or physical or chemical destruction of abnormal tissue using cryotherapy, laser vaporization, trichloroacetic acid, or podophyllotoxin. Interferon has been used in some cases of genital and respiratory papillomas, but its role has not been fully established. With all forms of therapy, the recurrence rate is unacceptably high, up to 50% with some types of lesions.

Brown DR, Fife KH: Human papillomavirus infections of the genital tract. Med Clin North Am 74:1455, 1990.

Kashima HK, Shah K: Recurrent respiratory papillomatosis: Clinical overview and management principles. Obstet Gynecol Clin North Am 14:581, 1987.

Kashima HK, Shah F, Lyles A, et al: A comparison of risk factors in juvenile-onset and adult-onset recurrent respiratory papillomatosis. Laryngoscope 102:9, 1992.

zur Hausen H: Viruses in human cancers. Science 254:1167, 1991.

CHAPTER 225

Arboviruses

Scott Halstead

225.1 Dengue Fever and Dengue-Like Disease

Dengue fever, a benign syndrome caused by several arthropod-borne viruses, is characterized by biphasic fever, myalgia or arthralgia, rash, leukopenia, and lymphadenopathy.

HISTORY. Epidemics were common in temperate areas of the Americas, Europe, Australia, and Asia until early in the 20th century. Dengue fever and dengue-like disease are now endemic in tropical Asia, the South Pacific Islands, Northern Australia, tropical Africa, the Caribbean, and Central and South America. Dengue fever occurs frequently among travelers.

ETIOLOGY. There are at least four distinct antigenic types of dengue virus. In addition, three other arthropod-borne (arbo) viruses cause similar or identical febrile diseases with rash (Table 225–1).

EPIDEMIOLOGY. Dengue viruses are transmitted by mosquitoes of the Stegomyia family. *Aedes aegypti*, a daytime biting mosquito, is the principal vector, and all four virus types have been recovered from it. In most tropical areas *Aedes aegypti* is highly urbanized, breeding in water stored for drinking or bathing or in rain water collected in any container. Dengue viruses have also been recovered from *Aedes albopictus*, and outbreaks in the Pacific area have been attributed to several other *Aedes* species. These species breed in water trapped in vegetation. In Southeast Asia and West Africa, dengue may be maintained in a cycle involving canopy-feeding jungle monkeys and *Aedes* spp, which feed on both monkeys and humans.

Dengue outbreaks in urban areas infested with *Aedes aegypti* may be explosive; up to 70–80% of the population may be involved. Most disease occurs in older children and adults. Because *Aedes aegypti* has a limited range, spread of an epidemic occurs mainly through viremic human beings and follows the main lines of transportation. Sentinel cases may infect household mosquitoes, with a large number of nearly simultaneous secondary infections giving the appearance of a contagious disease. Where dengue is endemic, children and susceptible foreigners may be the only persons to acquire overt disease, adults having become immune.

Dengue-like diseases may occur in epidemics. Epidemiologic features depend upon the vectors and their geographic distribution (see Table 225–1). Chikungunya virus is widespread in the most populous areas of the world. In Asia, *Aedes aegypti* is the principal vector; in Africa other Stegomyia may be important vectors. In Southeast Asia, dengue and chikungunya outbreaks occur concurrently. Outbreaks of o'nyong-nyong and West Nile fever usually involve villages or small towns, in contrast to the urban outbreaks of dengue and chikungunya.

PATHOLOGY. Insufficient pathologic material has been obtained from virologically confirmed cases of dengue fever to permit a comprehensive description. Fatalities are rare with chikungunya and West Nile infections; those recorded have been ascribed to viral encephalitis, hemorrhage, or febrile convulsions.

CLINICAL MANIFESTATIONS. Manifestations vary with age and from patient to patient. In infants and young children the

■ TABLE 225–1 Vectors and Geographic Distribution of Dengue-Like Diseases

Genus	Virus and Disease	Vector	Geographic Distribution
Togavirus	Chikungunya	*Aedes aegypti* *Aedes africanus*	Africa, India, Southeast Asia
Togavirus	O'nyong-nyong	*Anopheles funestus*	East Africa
Flavivirus	West Nile fever	*Culex molestus* *Culex univittatus*	Africa, Middle East, India

disease may be undifferentiated or characterized by a 1- to 5-day fever, pharyngeal inflammation, rhinitis, and mild cough. In outbreaks a majority of infected older children and adults have most of the findings described next.

After an incubation period of 1–7 days, there is a sudden onset of fever, which rapidly rises to 39.4–41.1° C (103–106° F), usually accompanied by frontal or retro-orbital headache. Occasionally, back pain precedes the fever. A *transient*, macular, generalized rash that blanches under pressure may be seen during the first 24–48 hr of fever. The pulse rate may be slow relative to the degree of fever. Myalgia or arthralgia occurs soon after the onset and increases in severity. Involvement of the joints may be particularly severe in patients with chikungunya or o'nyong-nyong infection. From the 2nd–6th days of fever, nausea and vomiting are apt to occur, and generalized lymphadenopathy, cutaneous hyperesthesia or hyperalgesia, taste aberrations, and pronounced anorexia may develop.

One to 2 days after defervescence, a generalized, morbilliform, maculopapular rash appears, which spares the palms and soles. It disappears in 1–5 days; desquamation may occur. Rarely there is edema of the palms and soles. About the time this second rash appears, the body temperature, which has previously fallen to normal, may become slightly elevated and establish the biphasic temperature curve.

Epistaxis, petechiae, and purpuric lesions are uncommon but may occur at any stage. Swallowed blood from epistaxis, vomited or passed by rectum, may be erroneously interpreted as gastrointestinal bleeding. In adults and possibly in children, underlying conditions, together with a dengue-induced hemorrhagic diathesis, may lead to clinically significant bleeding. Convulsions may occur during high fever, especially with chikungunya fever.

Infrequently, after the febrile stage, prolonged asthenia, mental depression, bradycardia, and ventricular extrasystoles may occur in children.

LABORATORY DATA. Pancytopenia may occur on the 3rd–4th days of illness; neutropenia may persist or reappear during the latter stage of the disease and may continue into convalescence. White cell counts as low as 2,000/mm³ have been recorded. Platelets rarely fall below 100,000 cells/mm³. Venous clotting, bleeding and prothrombin times, and plasma fibrinogen values are within normal ranges. The tourniquet test infrequently is positive. Mild acidosis, hemoconcentration, increased transaminase values, and hypoproteinemia may occur during some primary dengue virus infections. Classic dengue hemorrhagic fever–dengue shock syndrome may occur in infants born to dengue-immune mothers (see Chapter 225.2). Sinus bradycardia, ectopic ventricular foci, flattened T waves, and prolongation of the PR interval may be observed electrocardiographically.

DIAGNOSIS AND DIFFERENTIAL DIAGNOSIS. *Clinical diagnosis* derives from a high index of suspicion and a knowledge of the geographic distribution and environmental cycles of causal viruses. Exposure to dengue may occur in hotels and during daytime shopping trips in epidemic or endemic areas.

Differential diagnosis includes a number of viral respiratory and influenza-like diseases and the early stages of malaria, scrub typhus, hepatitis, and leptospirosis. Abortive forms of these latter diseases modified by therapy or vaccine may never evolve beyond a dengue-like stage.

Four arboviral diseases have dengue-like courses but without rash: Colorado tick fever, sandfly fever, Rift Valley fever, and Ross River fever. Colorado tick fever occurs sporadically among campers and hunters in the western United States; sandfly fever in the Mediterranean region, the Middle East, southern Russia, and parts of the Indian subcontinent; and Rift Valley fever in North, East, Central, and South Africa. Ross River fever is endemic in much of eastern Australia with epidemic extension to Fiji. In adults, Ross River fever often produces protracted and crippling arthralgia involving weightbearing joints.

Because clinical findings vary and there are many possible causative agents, the term "dengue-like disease" should be used until a specific diagnosis is established. *Etiologic diagnosis* can be made by serologic study or by isolation of the virus from blood leukocytes or serum. Blood for comparative antibody and viral studies should be obtained during the febrile period, preferably early, and during the convalescent phase, 14–21 days after onset. The acute phase serum or plasma may be frozen, optimally at −65° C or colder. Leukocytes should be refrigerated, not frozen. *Serologic diagnosis* depends on a fourfold or greater increase in antibody titer in paired sera by hemagglutination inhibition, complement fixation, enzyme immunoassay, or neutralization test. Carefully standardized immunoglobulin (Ig) M- and IgG-capture enzyme immunoassays are now widely used to identify acute-phase antibodies from patients with primary or secondary dengue infections in single-serum samples. Usually such samples should be collected not earlier than 5 days nor later than 6 wk after onset. It may not be possible to distinguish the infecting virus by serologic methods alone, particularly when there has been prior infection with another member of the same arbovirus group. Virus can be recovered from acute-phase serum after inoculating tissue culture or living mosquitoes. Viral RNA can be detected in blood or tissues by specific complementary DNA probes or amplified first by the polymerase chain reaction (PCR).

PREVENTION AND CONTROL. Attenuated dengue types 1, 2, 3, and 4 vaccines are under development in Thailand, and a killed vaccine for chikungunya is efficacious but not generally available. Prophylaxis consists of avoiding mosquito bites by use of insecticides, repellents, body covering with clothing, screening of houses, and destruction of *Aedes aegypti* breeding sites. If water storage is mandatory, a tight-fitting lid or a thin layer of oil may prevent egg laying or hatching. A larvicide, such as Abate [O,O′-(thiodi-*p*-phenylene) O,O,O,O′-tetramethyl phosphorothioate], available as a 1% sand-granule formation and effective at a concentration of 1 part/million, may be added safely to drinking water. Ultra-low-volume spray equipment effectively dispenses the adulticide malathion from truck or airplane for rapid intervention during an epidemic. Only personal antimosquito measures are effective against mosquitoes in the field, forest, or jungle.

TREATMENT. Treatment is supportive. Bed rest is advised during the febrile period. Antipyretics or cold sponging should be used to keep body temperature below 40° C (104° F). Analgesics or mild sedation may be required to control pain. Because of its effects on hemostasis, aspirin should not be used. Fluid and electrolyte replacement is required when there are deficits caused by sweating, fasting, thirsting, vomiting, or diarrhea.

PROGNOSIS. Primary infections with dengue fever and dengue-like diseases are usually self-limited and benign. Fluid and electrolyte losses, hyperpyrexia, and febrile convulsions are the most frequent complications in infants and young children. The prognosis may be adversely affected by passively acquired antibody or by prior infection with a closely related virus (see Chapter 225.2).

Halstead SB: Dengue: Hematologic aspects. Semin Hematol 19:116, 1982.
Halstead SB: Selective primary health care: Strategies for control of disease in the developing world. XI. Dengue. Rev Infect Dis 6:251, 1984.
Imported dengue—United States, 1991. MMWR 41:725, 1992.
Tsai CJ, Kuo CH, Chen PC, et al: Upper gastrointestinal bleeding in dengue fever. Am J Gastroenterol 86:33, 1991.

225.2 Dengue Hemorrhagic Fever and Dengue Shock Syndrome

(Philippine, Thai, or Singapore Hemorrhagic Fever; Hemorrhagic Dengue; Acute Infectious Thrombocytopenic Purpura)

Dengue hemorrhagic fever, a severe, often fatal, febrile disease caused by dengue viruses, is characterized by capillary permeability, abnormalities of hemostasis, and, in severe cases, a protein-losing shock syndrome. It is currently thought to have an immunopathologic basis.

ETIOLOGY. At least four distinct types of dengue virus (types 1–4) have been isolated from patients with hemorrhagic fever.

EPIDEMIOLOGY. Dengue hemorrhagic fever occurs where multiple types of dengue virus are simultaneously or sequentially transmitted. It is endemic in tropical Asia, where warm temperatures and the practice of water storage in homes result in large, permanent populations of *Aedes aegypti*. Under these conditions infections with dengue viruses of all types are common, and second infections with heterologous types are frequent. After 1 yr of age, nearly all patients with dengue shock syndrome have a secondary rise of antibody against dengue virus, indicating a previous infection with a closely related virus. A 1981 outbreak in Cuba, in which children and adults were equally exposed, has shown that the acute, vascular permeability syndrome occurs almost exclusively in children 14 yr of age and younger. In adults severe disease is more frequently associated with hemorrhagic phenomena. Dengue hemorrhagic fever can occur during primary dengue infections, most frequently in infants whose mothers are immune to dengue.

Nonimmune foreigners, adults or children, exposed to dengue virus during outbreaks of hemorrhagic fever have classic dengue fever or even milder disease. The differences in clinical manifestations of dengue infections between natives and foreigners in Southeast Asia are related more to immunologic status than to racial susceptibility. However, in the Cuban outbreak, dengue hemorrhagic fever and dengue shock syndrome attack rates were low in black children, possibly explaining the seeming absence of the syndrome in dengue-endemic areas of Africa.

PATHOLOGY. Usually no pathologic lesions are found to account for death. In rare instances, death may be due to gastrointestinal or intracranial hemorrhages. Minimal to moderate hemorrhages are seen in the upper gastrointestinal tract, and petechial hemorrhages are common in the interventricular septum of the heart, on the pericardium, and on the subserosal surfaces of major viscera. Focal hemorrhages are occasionally seen in the lungs, liver, adrenals, and subarachnoid space. The liver is usually enlarged, often with fatty changes. Yellow, watery, and at times blood-tinged effusions are present in serous cavities in about three fourths of patients.

Microscopically, there is perivascular edema in the soft tissues and widespread diapedesis of red cells. There may be maturational arrest of megakaryocytes in bone marrow, and increased numbers of them are seen in capillaries of the lungs, in renal glomeruli, and in sinusoids of the liver and spleen.

Dengue virus is usually absent in tissues at the time of death, with rare isolations reported from liver and lymphatic tissues most often in infants younger than 1 yr who have experienced primary infections.

PATHOGENESIS. The pathogenesis is incompletely understood; epidemiologic studies suggest that it is usually associated with secondary dengue type 2, 3, and 4 infections. There is evidence that non-neutralizing antibodies promote cellular infection and enhance severity of the disease. Dengue viruses demonstrate enhanced growth in cultures of human mononuclear phagocytes prepared from dengue-immune donors or in cultures supplemented with non-neutralizing dengue antibody. Monkeys infected sequentially or receiving small quantities of enhancing antibody have enhanced viremias. Retrospective studies of sera from human mothers whose infants acquired dengue hemorrhagic fever or prospective studies on children acquiring sequential dengue infections have shown that the circulation of infection-enhancing antibodies at the time of infection is the strongest risk factor for development of severe disease. Even low levels of neutralizing antibodies, whether from earlier homotypic infection in mothers or heterotypic infections in children, protect infants or children from dengue hemorrhagic fever. Early in the acute stage of secondary dengue infections, there is rapid activation of the complement system. During shock, blood levels of C1q, C3, C4, C5–C8, and C3 proactivators are depressed, and C3 catabolic rates are elevated. The blood clotting and fibrinolytic systems are activated, and levels of factor XII (Hageman factor) are depressed. No specific mediator of vascular permeability in dengue hemorrhagic fever has been identified. A mild degree of disseminated intravascular coagulation, liver damage, and thrombocytopenia may produce hemorrhage synergistically. Capillary damage allows fluid, electrolytes, protein, and, in some instances, red cells to leak into extravascular spaces. This internal redistribution of fluid, together with deficits caused by fasting, thirsting, and vomiting, results in hemoconcentration, hypovolemia, increased cardiac work, tissue hypoxia, metabolic acidosis, and hyponatremia.

CLINICAL MANIFESTATIONS. The incubation period of dengue hemorrhagic fever is presumed to be that of dengue fever. The course is characteristic in the severely ill child. A relatively mild first phase with abrupt onset of fever, malaise, vomiting, headache, anorexia, and cough is followed after 2–5 days by rapid clinical deterioration and collapse. In this 2nd phase the patient usually has cold, clammy extremities, a warm trunk, flushed face, diaphoresis, restlessness, irritability, and midepigastric pain. Frequently, there are scattered petechiae on the forehead and extremities; spontaneous ecchymoses may appear, and easy bruisability and bleeding at sites of venipuncture are common. A macular or maculopapular rash may appear, and there may be circumoral and peripheral cyanosis. Respirations are rapid and often labored. The pulse is weak, rapid, and thready and the heart sounds faint. The liver may enlarge to 4–6 cm below the costal margin and is usually firm and somewhat tender. Fewer than 10% of patients have gross ecchymosis or gastrointestinal bleeding, usually following a period of uncorrected shock.

After a 24- to 36-hr period of crisis, convalescence is fairly rapid in the children who recover. The temperature may return to normal before or during the stage of shock. Bradycardia and ventricular extrasystoles are common during convalescence. Infrequently, there is residual brain damage caused by prolonged shock or occasionally by intracranial hemorrhage. Dengue 3 virus strains circulating in mainland Southeast Asia since 1983 are associated with a particularly stormy clinical syndrome, characterized by encephalopathy, hypoglycemia, markedly elevated liver enzymes, and, occasionally, jaundice.

In contrast to the fairly characteristic pattern in the severely ill child, secondary dengue infections are relatively mild in the majority of instances, ranging from an inapparent infection through an undifferentiated upper respiratory tract or dengue-like disease to an illness similar to that described previously but without apparent shock.

LABORATORY DATA. The most common hematologic abnormalities during clinical shock are a 20% or greater increase in hematocrit over the recovery value, thrombocytopenia, mild leukocytosis (seldom exceeding 10,000/mm^3), prolonged bleeding time, and moderately decreased prothrombin level (seldom to less than 40% of control). Fibrinogen levels may be subnormal and fibrin split-products elevated.

Other abnormalities include moderate elevations of the serum transaminase levels, consumption of complement, mild metabolic acidosis with hyponatremia, and, at time, hypochloremia, slight elevation of serum urea nitrogen, and hypoalbuminemia. Roentgenograms of the chest reveal pleural effusions in nearly all patients.

DIAGNOSIS AND DIFFERENTIAL DIAGNOSIS. In endemic areas hemorrhagic fever should be suspected in children with a febrile illness who exhibit a positive tourniquet test, hemoconcentration, and thrombocytopenia. These may be accompanied by shock and in some instances by hemorrhagic manifestations. Appearance of pleural effusion with evidence of recent dengue infection is pathognomonic. Because many rickettsial diseases, meningococcemia, and other severe illnesses caused by a variety of agents may produce a similar clinical picture, the etiologic diagnosis should be made only when epidemiologic or serologic evidence suggests the possibility of dengue fever. Hemorrhagic manifestations have been described in other diseases of viral or presumed viral origin, including the clinically distinguishable hemorrhagic fevers described in Chapter 225.3.

In both primary and secondary dengue infections, there is a relatively transient appearance of antidengue IgM antibodies. These disappear in 6–12 wk and can be used to time a dengue infection. In secondary dengue infections, most antibody is of the IgG class. The hemagglutination inhibition (HI) test shows a rapid rise or high fixed (1:640 or greater) titers in paired sera.

Prevention. Preventive measures are described in Chapter 225.2. The possibility exists that dengue vaccination may sensitize a recipient so that ensuing dengue infection may result in hemorrhagic fever. Vaccination with yellow fever 17D strain has no effect on the severity of dengue illness, although seroconversion rates to a dengue 2 vaccine were enhanced in yellow fever-immune persons.

TREATMENT. Management requires immediate evaluation of vital signs and degrees of hemoconcentration, dehydration, and electrolyte imbalance. Close monitoring is essential for at least 48 hr because shock may occur or recur precipitously early in the disease. Patients who are cyanotic or have labored breathing should be given oxygen. Rapid intravenous replacement of fluids and electrolytes can frequently sustain patients until spontaneous recovery occurs. When elevation of the hematocrit persists after replacement of fluids, plasma or plasma colloid preparations are indicated. Care must be taken to avoid overhydration, which may contribute to cardiac failure. Transfusions of fresh blood or of platelets suspended in plasma may be required to control bleeding; they should not be given during hemoconcentration but only after evaluation of hemoglobin or hematocrit values. Salicylates are contraindicated because of their effect on blood clotting.

Paraldehyde or chloral hydrate may be required for children who are markedly agitated. Use of pressor amines, α-adrenergic blocking agents, and aldosterone has not resulted in a significant reduction of mortality compared with that observed with simple supportive therapy. See Chapters 60.5 and 438 for treatment of disseminated intravascular coagulation. Steroids do not shorten the duration of disease or improve prognosis in children receiving careful supportive therapy.

Hypervolemia during the fluid reabsorptive phase may be life threatening and is heralded by a fall in hematocrit with wide pulse pressure. Diuretics and digitalization may be necessary.

PROGNOSIS. Death has occurred in 40–50% of patients with shock, but with adequate intensive care deaths should be less than 2%. Survival is directly related to early and intense management.

Burke DS, Nisalak A, Johnson DE, et al: A prospective study of dengue infections in Bangkok. Am J Trop Med Hyg 38:172, 1988.

Dengue hemorrhagic fever: diagnosis, treatment, prevention and control. Geneva, World Health Organization, 1995.

Halstead SB: Immune enhancement of viral infection. Prog Allergy 31:301, 1982.

Halstead SB: Pathogenesis of dengue: Challenges to molecular biology. Science 239:476, 1988.

Killen H, O'Sullivan MA: Detection of dengue virus by in situ hybridization. J Virol Methods 41:135, 1993.

Kliks S, Nimmannitya S, Nisalak A, et al: Evidence that maternal dengue antibodies are important in development of dengue hemorrhagic fever in infants. Am J Trop Med Hyg 38:411, 1988.

Kliks S, Nisalak A, Brandt WE, et al: Antibody-dependent enhancement of dengue virus growth in human monocytes as a risk factor for dengue hemorrhagic fever. Am J Trop Med Hyg 40:444, 1989.

Tassniyom S, Vasanawathana S, Chirawatkul A, et al: Failure of high-dose methylprednisolone in established dengue shock syndrome—A placebo controlled double-blind study. Pediatrics 92:111, 1993.

Thisyakorn U, Nimmannitya S: Nutritional status of children with dengue hemorrhagic fever. Clin Infect Dis 16:295, 1993.

225.3 Other Viral Hemorrhagic Fevers

Viral hemorrhagic fevers are a loosely defined group of clinical syndromes in which hemorrhagic manifestations are either common or especially notable in severe illness. Both the etiologic agents and clinical features of the syndromes differ, but disseminated intravascular coagulation may be a common pathogenetic feature. A list of the more important viral hemorrhagic fevers is given in Table 225–2.

ETIOLOGY. Six of the viral hemorrhagic fevers are caused by arthropod-borne (arbo) viruses (see Table 225–2). Four are togaviruses of the flavivirus group (KFD, OHF, DHF, and YF), and three are bunyaviruses (Congo, Hantaan, and RVF). Junin (AHF), Machupo (BHF), and Lassa (LF) are arenaviruses, a morphologic and ecologic viral group. Ebola (EHF) and Marburg viruses are enveloped, filamentous RNA viruses, which are sometimes branched, unlike any other known virus, and which are now termed filoviruses.

EPIDEMIOLOGY. With rare exceptions, the viruses causing viral hemorrhagic fevers are initially transmitted through a nonhuman agency. Because a specific ecosystem is required for viral survival, these are diseases of place. Although it is commonly thought that all viral hemorrhagic fevers are arthropod borne, eight may be contracted from environmental contamination caused by animals or animal cells or from infected humans (RVF, AHF, BHF, LF, Marburg disease, EHF, and HFRS). Laboratory and hospital infections have occurred with many of these agents. LF and Argentine and Bolivian hemorrhagic fevers are reportedly milder in children than in adults. Dengue hemorrhagic fever (Chapter 225.2) and yellow fever (Chapter 225.4)

■ TABLE 225–2 Viral Hemorrhage Fevers

Mode of Transmission	Disease	Virus
Tick borne	Congo-Crimean HF*	Congo
	Kyasanur Forest disease	Kyasanur Forest disease
	Omsk HF	Omsk
Mosquito borne†	Dengue HF	Dengue (four types)
	Rift Valley fever	Rift Valley fever
	Yellow fever	Yellow fever
Infected animals or materials to humans	Argentine HF	Junin
	Bolivian HF	Machupo
	Lassa fever*	Lassa
	Marburg disease*	Marburg
	Ebola HF*	Ebola
	Hemorrhagic fever with renal syndrome	Hantaan

*Patients may be contagious, nosocomial infections are common.

†Chikungunya virus is associated at low frequency with petechiae, petechial hemorrhages, and epistaxis. More severe hemorrhagic manifestations have been reported in some studies.

HF = hemorrhagic fever.

are well-established pediatric problems. Features of the more common viral hemorrhagic fevers are summarized next.

Tick-Borne Hemorrhagic Fevers. CONGO-CRIMEAN HEMORRHAGIC FEVER (CHF). Sporadic human infection in Africa provided the original virus isolation. Natural foci are recognized in Bulgaria, western Crimea, and the Rostov-on-Don and Astrakhan regions; a somewhat similar disease occurs in Kazakstan and Uzbekistan. Index cases were followed by nosocomial transmission in Pakistan and Afghanistan in 1976, in the Arabian peninsula in 1983, and in South Africa in 1984. In the Commonwealth of Independent States, the vectors are *Hyaloma marginatum* and *H. anatolicum*, which, along with hares and birds, may serve as viral reservoirs. Disease occurs from June to September, largely among farmers and dairy workers.

KYASANUR FOREST DISEASE (KFD). Human cases occur chiefly in adults in an area of Mysore State, India. The main vectors are two Ixodidae ticks, *Haemaphysalis turturis* and *H. spinigera*. Monkeys and forest rodents may be amplifying hosts. Laboratory infections are common.

OMSK HEMORRHAGIC FEVER (OHF). The disease occurs throughout the south central Russia and in northern Rumania. Vectors may include *Dermacentor pictus* and *D. marginatus*, but direct transmission from moles and muskrats to humans seems well established. Human disease occurs in a spring-summer-autumn pattern, paralleling the activity of vectors. OHF occurs most frequently in persons with outdoor occupational exposure. Laboratory infections are common.

Mosquito-Borne Hemorrhagic Fevers. DENGUE HEMORRHAGIC FEVER AND YELLOW FEVER (DHF AND YF). See Chapters 225.2 and 225.4.

RIFT VALLEY FEVER (RVF). The virus causing RVF is responsible for epizootics involving sheep, cattle, buffalo, certain antelopes, and rodents in North, Central, East, and South Africa. The virus is transmitted to domestic animals by *Culex theileri* and several *Aedes* species. Mosquitoes may serve as reservoirs by transovarial transmission. An epizootic in Egypt in 1977–1978 was accompanied by thousands of human infections, principally among veterinarians, farmers, and farm laborers. Smaller outbreaks occurred in Senegal in 1987 and Madegascar in 1990. Humans are most often infected during the slaughter or skinning of sick or dead animals. Laboratory infection is common.

Hemorrhagic Fever Transmitted Through Environmental Contamination. ARENAVIRAL DISEASE. The prototype arenavirus, lymphocytic choriomeningitis virus, establishes a persistent, tolerated infection in the young of the common house mouse, *Mus musculus*, which excretes virus continuously throughout life, contaminating food and fluids and creating a risk of airborne infection. There is evidence that Machupo and Junin viruses have similar host-parasite relationships with South American rodents as the Lassa virus has with African rodents.

ARGENTINE HEMORRHAGIC FEVER (AHF). Hundreds to thousands of cases occur annually from April through July in the maize-producing area northwest of Buenos Aires that reaches to the eastern margin of the Province of Cordoba. Junin virus has been isolated from the rodents *Mus musculus, Akodon arenicola,* and *Calomys laucha laucha*. It infects migrant laborers who harvest the maize and who inhabit rodent-contaminated shelters.

BOLIVIAN HEMORRHAGIC FEVER (BHF). The recognized endemic area consists of the sparsely populated province of Beni in Amazonian Bolivia. Sporadic cases occur in farm families who raise maize, rice, yucca, and beans. In the town of San Joaquin a disturbance in the domestic rodent ecosystem may have led to an outbreak of household infection caused by *Calomys callosus*, ordinarily a field rodent. Mortality rates are high in young children.

LASSA FEVER (LF). Lassa virus has an unusual potential for human-to-human spread and has resulted in many small epidemics in Nigeria, Sierra Leone, and Liberia. Medical workers in Africa and the United States have also contracted the disease. Patients with acute LF have been transported by international aircraft, necessitating extensive surveillance among passengers and crews. The virus is probably maintained in nature in a species of African peridomestic rodent, *Mastomys natalensis*. Rodent-to-rodent transmission and infection of humans probably operate via mechanisms established for other arenaviruses.

MARBURG DISEASE. Until recently, the world experience has been limited to 26 primary and 5 secondary cases in Germany and Yugoslavia in 1967 and to small outbreaks in Zimbabwe in 1975, in Kenya in 1980 and 1988, and in South Africa in 1983. Transmission occurs by direct contact with tissues of the African green monkey, with infected blood, or with human semen. The reservoir and mode of transmission of the virus in nature are unknown.

EBOLA HEMORRHAGIC FEVER. Ebola virus was isolated in 1976 from a devastating epidemic involving small villages in northern Zaire and southern Sudan; smaller outbreaks have occurred subsequently. Outbreaks initially have been nosocomial. Attack rates have been highest in the birth to 1-yr and 15- to 50-yr age groups. The virus resembles Marburg virus. The vertebrate reservoir and mode of transmission to man are unknown. Reston virus, related to Ebola, has been recovered from Philippine monkeys and has caused subclinical infections in workers in monkey colonies in the United States.

HEMORRHAGIC FEVER WITH RENAL SYNDROME (epidemic hemorrhagic fever; Korean hemorrhagic fever). The endemic area includes Japan, Korea, far eastern Siberia, north and central China, European and Asian Russia, Scandinavia, Czechoslovakia, Rumania, Bulgaria, Yugoslavia, and Greece. Although the incidence and severity of hemorrhagic manifestations and the mortality are lower in Europe than in Northeast Asia, the renal lesion is the same. Disease in Scandinavia, nephropathia epidemica, is caused by a different although antigenically related virus associated with *Clethrionomys glariolus*. Cases occur predominantly in the spring and summer. There appears to be no age factor in susceptibility, but because of occupational hazards, young adult men are most frequently attacked. Rodent plagues or evidences of rodent infestation have accompanied endemic and epidemic occurrences. Hantaan virus has been detected in lung tissue and excreta of *Apodemus agrarius coreae*. Antigenically related agents have been detected in laboratory rats, in urban rat populations around the world, the wild rodent *Microtus pennsylvanicus* in North America (Prospect Hill virus), and, most recently, in the deer mouse, in the southern and southwestern United States (Four Corners virus). *Rodent-to-rodent and rodent-to-human transmission presumably occurs via the respiratory route.*

Clinical, Pathologic, and Laboratory Features. OMSK HEMORRHAGIC FEVER AND KYASANUR FOREST DISEASE. After an incubation period of 3–8 days, both diseases begin with sudden onset of fever and headache. In Omsk hemorrhagic fever there is moderate epistaxis, hematemesis, and a hemorrhagic enanthem but no profuse hemorrhage; bronchopneumonia is common. Kyasanur forest disease is characterized by severe myalgia, prostration, and bronchiolar involvement; it often presents without hemorrhage, but occasionally with severe gastrointestinal bleeding. Severe leukopenia and thrombocytopenia occur in both diseases. In many patients recurrent febrile illness may follow an afebrile period of 7–15 days. This second phase takes the form of a meningoencephalitis.

In Kyasanur forest disease, acute degeneration of renal tubules may correlate with the urinary changes noted. There may be focal liver damage. In both diseases vascular dilatation, increased vascular permeability, gastrointestinal hemorrhages, and subserosal and interstitial petechial hemorrhages occur.

CRIMEAN HEMORRHAGIC FEVER. The incubation period of 3–12 days is followed by a febrile period of 5–12 days and a prolonged convalescence. Illness begins suddenly with fever, severe headache, myalgia, abdominal pain, anorexia, nausea, and vomiting. After a day or more fever may subside until the patient experiences an erythematous facial or truncal flush and injected conjunctivae. A second febrile period of 2–6 days then develops with a hemorrhagic enanthem on the soft palate and a fine petechial rash on the chest and abdomen. Less frequently, there are large areas of purpura and bleeding from gums, nose, intestine, lungs, or uterus. Hematuria and proteinuria are relatively rare. During the hemorrhagic stage there is usually tachycardia with weak heart sounds, and in some cases hypotension occurs. The liver is usually enlarged, but there is no icterus. In protracted cases central nervous system signs may include delirium, somnolence, and progressive clouding of consciousness. In convalescence there may be hearing and memory loss. Mortality ranges from 2–50%. Early in the disease leukopenia with relative lymphocytosis, progressively worsening thrombocytopenia, and gradually increasing anemia occur.

RIFT VALLEY FEVER. Most infections have been in adults, in whom disease is dengue-like. Onset is acute, with fever, headache, prostration, myalgia, anorexia, nausea, vomiting, conjunctivitis, and lymphadenopathy. The fever lasts 3–6 days and is often biphasic. Convalescence is often prolonged. In the 1977–1978 outbreak, many patients died after showing signs that included purpura, epistaxis, hematemesis, and melena. At autopsy there was extensive eosinophilic degeneration of the parenchymal cells of the liver.

ARGENTINE AND BOLIVIAN HEMORRHAGIC FEVER AND LASSA FEVER. The incubation period is commonly 7–14 days; the acute illness lasts for 2–4 wk. Clinical illnesses range from undifferentiated fever to the characteristic severe illness. Lassa fever is most often clinically severe in whites. Onset is usually gradual, with increasing fever, headache, diffuse myalgia, and anorexia. During the 1st wk signs frequently include a sore throat, dysphagia, cough, oropharyngeal ulcers, nausea, vomiting, diarrhea, and pains in chest and abdomen. Pleuritic chest pain may persist into the 2nd–3rd wk of illness. In AHF and BHF and less frequently in LF, a petechial enanthem appears on the soft palate 3–5 days after onset and at about the same time on the trunk. The tourniquet test may be positive.

In 35–50% of all patients these diseases may become severe, with persistent high fever, increasing toxicity, swelling of face or neck, microscopic hematuria, and frank hemorrhages from the stomach, intestines, nose, gums, and uterus. A syndrome of hypovolemic shock is accompanied by pleural effusion and renal failure. Respiratory distress resulting from airway obstruction, pleural effusion, or congestive heart failure may occur. Ten to 20% of patients experience late neurologic involvement characterized by intention tremor of the tongue and associated speech abnormalities. In severe cases there may be intention tremors of the extremities, seizures, and delirium. The cerebrospinal fluid is normal. In LF nerve deafness occurs in early convalescence in 25% of cases. Prolonged convalescence is accompanied by alopecia and in AHF and BHF by signs of autonomic nervous system lability, such as postural hypotension, spontaneous flushing or blanching of the skin, and intermittent diaphoresis.

Laboratory studies reveal marked leukopenia, mild to moderate thrombocytopenia, proteinuria, and, in AHF, moderate abnormalities in blood clotting, decreased fibrinogen, increased fibrinogen–split products, and elevated serum transaminases. Pathologically, there is focal, often extensive eosinophilic necrosis of liver parenchyma, focal interstitial pneumonitis, focal necrosis of the distal and collecting tubules, and partial replacement of splenic follicles by amorphous eosinophilic material. Usually bleeding occurs by diapedesis with little inflammatory reaction. Mortality is 10–40%.

MARBURG DISEASE AND EBOLA HEMORRHAGIC FEVER. After an incubation period of 4–7 days, illness begins abruptly with severe frontal headache, malaise, drowsiness, lumbar myalgia, vomiting, nausea, and diarrhea. Five to 7 days later a papular eruption begins on the trunk and upper arms; becomes generalized, often hemorrhagic, and maculopapular; and exfoliates during convalescence. The exanthem is accompanied by a dark red enanthem on the hard palate, conjunctivitis, and scrotal or labial edema. Gastrointestinal hemorrhage occurs as the severity of illness increases. Late in the illness, the patient may become tearfully depressed with marked hyperalgesia to tactile stimuli. In fatal cases, patients become hypotensive, restless, and confused and lapse into coma. Convalescent patients may experience alopecia and have paresthesias of the back and trunk. There is a marked leukopenia with necrosis of granulocytes. Disseminated intravascular coagulation and thrombocytopenia are universal and correlate with severity of disease; there are moderate abnormalities in clotting proteins and elevated serum transaminases and amylase. The mortality of Marburg disease is 25%; that of EHF, 50–90%.

HEMORRHAGIC FEVER WITH RENAL SYNDROME (HFRS). In most cases HFRS is characterized by fever, petechiae, mild hemorrhagic phenomena, and mild proteinuria, followed by relatively uneventful recovery. In 20% of recognized cases the disease may progress through four rather distinct phases. The *febrile phase* is ushered in with fever, malaise, and facial and truncal flushing, lasts 3–8 days, and ends with thrombocytopenia, petechiae, and proteinuria. The *hypotensive phase* of 1–3 days follows defervescence. Loss of fluid from the intravascular compartment may result in marked hemoconcentration. Proteinuria and ecchymoses increase. The *oliguric phase*, usually 3–5 days in duration, is characterized by a low output of protein-rich urine, increasing nitrogen retention, nausea, vomiting, and dehydration. Confusion, extreme restlessness, and hypertension are common. The *diuretic phase,* which may last for days or weeks, usually initiates clinical improvement. The kidneys show little concentrating ability, and rapid loss of fluid may result in severe dehydration and shock. Potassium and sodium depletion may be severe. Fatal cases manifest abundant protein-rich retroperitoneal edema and marked hemorrhagic necrosis of the renal medulla. Mortality is 5–10%.

DIAGNOSIS. Diagnosis depends upon a high index of suspicion in endemic areas. In nonendemic areas histories of recent travel, recent laboratory exposure, or exposure to an earlier case should evoke suspicion of viral hemorrhagic fever.

In all viral hemorrhagic fevers the viral agent circulates in the blood at least transiently during the early febrile stage. The diagnostic specimens required for togaviruses and bunyaviruses are the same as those described in Chapter 225.1 for dengue fever. The principles for etiologic diagnosis of AHF and BHF are similar; acute-phase blood or throat washings from patients can be inoculated intracerebrally into guinea pigs, infant hamsters, or infant mice. Lassa virus may be isolated from the same specimens by inoculation into tissue cultures. In arenavirus infections, group-reactive complement-fixing antibodies and specific neutralizing antibodies appear in convalescent serum 3–4 wk after onset of illness. For Marburg disease and EHF, acute-phase throat washings, blood, and urine may be inoculated into tissue culture, guinea pigs, or monkeys. The virus is readily visualized by electron microscopy, its filamentous structure differentiating it from all other known agents. Specific complement-fixing and immunofluorescent antibodies appear during convalescence. The virus of HFRS is recovered from acute-phase serum or urine by inoculating susceptible tissue cultures and identifying virus by use of fluorescent antibody, enzyme immunoassay, or neutralization tests. A variety of antibody tests using viral subunits are becoming available. These viruses may also be detected in blood or tissues using DNA probes or first amplifying viral RNA by PCR.

Handling blood and other biologic specimens is hazardous and must be left to specially trained personnel. Blood and autopsy specimens should be placed in tightly sealed metal containers, wrapped in absorbent material inside a sealed plastic bag, and shipped on dry ice to laboratories with biocontainment level 4 facilities. Even routine hematologic and biochemical tests should be done with extreme caution.

Further information and advice about management, control measures, diagnosis, and collection of biohazardous specimens can be obtained from Centers for Disease Control, National Center for Infectious Diseases, Special Pathogens Branch, Atlanta, Georgia 30333 (404–639–1115).

DIFFERENTIAL DIAGNOSIS. Mild cases of hemorrhagic fever may be confused with almost any self-limited systemic bacterial or viral infection. More severe cases may suggest typhoid fever, epidemic, murine, or scrub typhus, leptospirosis, or a rickettsial spotted fever, for which effective chemotherapeutic agents are available. Many of them may be acquired in geographic or ecologic locations similar to those that may provide exposure to a viral hemorrhagic fever.

PREVENTION. A live, attenuated vaccine (Candid-I) for Argentine hemorrhagic fever is highly efficacious. A form of inactivated mouse brain vaccine is said to be effective in preventing Omsk hemorrhagic fever. Inactivated RVF vaccines are widely used to protect domestic animals and laboratory workers. An experimental HFRS inactivated vaccine is under development in Korea, and a live, attenuated vaccine is being developed in China. A vaccinia-vector glycoprotein vaccine provides protection against Lassa fever in monkeys. Prevention of CHF transmission by ticks includes careful examination of the skin after exposure with removal of any vectors found. Tight-fitting clothing that fully covers the extremities is helpful, as is the use of tick repellents. Disease transmitted from a rodent-infected environment can be prevented through methods of rodent control; elimination of refuse and breeding sites is particularly successful in urban or suburban areas. CHF, LF, Marburg disease, and EHF may be transmitted in hospital settings. Patients should be isolated until they are virus free or for 3 wk following illness. Patients' urine, sputum, blood, clothing, and bedding should be disinfected. Disposable syringes and needles should be used. Prompt and strict enforcement of barrier nursing may be lifesaving. The fatality rate among medical workers contracting these diseases is 50%.

TREATMENT. The principle involved in all these diseases, especially HFRS, is the reversal of dehydration, hemoconcentration, renal failure, and protein, electrolyte, or blood losses. The contribution of disseminated intravascular coagulation to the hemorrhagic manifestations is unknown, and the management of hemorrhage should be individualized. Transfusions of fresh blood and platelets are frequently given. Good results have been reported in a few patients after the administration of clotting factor concentrates. The efficacy of steroids, ϵ-aminocaproic acid, pressor amines, or α-adrenergic blocking agents has not been established. Sedatives should be selected with regard to the possibility of kidney or liver damage. The successful management of HFRS may require renal dialysis. Ribavirin administered by parenteral route is effective in reducing mortality in LF and HFRS.

Fisher-Hoch SP, Platt GS, Neild GH, et al: Pathophysiology of shock and hemorrhage in a fulminating viral infection (Ebola). J Infect Dis 152:887, 1985.

Hantavirus infection—southwestern United States: Interim recommendations for risk reduction. MMWR 42:1, 1993.

Huggins JW, Hsiang CM, Cosgriff TM, et al: Prospective, double-blind, concurrent, placebo-controlled trial of intravenous ribavirin therapy of hemorrhagic fever with renal syndrome. J Infect Dis 164:1119, 1991.

Lee HW, Lee MC, Cho LS: Management of Korean hemorrhagic fever. Med Prog Sept:15, 1980.

Management of patients with suspected viral hemorrhagic fever. MMWR 37:Suppl 3, 1988.

McCormick JB, King IJ, Webb PA, et al: Lassa fever: Effective therapy with ribavirin. N Engl J Med 314:20, 1986.

225.4 Yellow Fever

Yellow fever is an acute infection characterized in its most severe form by fever, jaundice, proteinuria, and hemorrhage. The virus is mosquito borne and occurs in epidemic or endemic form in South America and Africa. An effective vaccine is available (Chapter 248). Yellow fever epidemics were described in Caribbean ports as early as the 16th century. The virus was probably introduced during the slave trade. Seasonal epidemics occurred in cities located in temperate areas of Europe and America until 1900; epidemics continue to occur in West, Central, and East Africa.

ETIOLOGY. Yellow fever is the prototype of the *Flavivirus* genus of the family *Flaviviridae*. The enveloped virus particles are 35- to 50-nm in diameter and contain an infectious, single-stranded RNA genome.

EPIDEMIOLOGY. Human and nonhuman primate hosts acquire the infection by the bite of infected mosquitoes. After an incubation period of 3–6 days, virus appears in the blood and may serve as a source of infection for other mosquitos. The virus must replicate in the gut and pass to the salivary gland before the mosquito can transmit the virus. Yellow fever virus is transmitted in an urban cycle—human to *Aedes aegypti* to human—and a jungle cycle—monkey to jungle mosquitoes to monkey. Classic yellow fever epidemics in the United States, South America, the Caribbean, and parts of Europe were of the urban variety. Present-day African epidemics are primarily urban. Most of the approximately 200 cases reported each year in South America are jungle yellow fever. In colonial times, attack rates in white adults were very high, suggesting that the ratio of subclinical infections to overt disease is nearly one in this age group. Yellow fever may be less severe in children, with subclinical infections to clinical case ratios of 2:1 or greater. In areas where outbreaks of urban yellow fever are common, most cases involve children because many adults are immune. Transmission in West Africa is highest during the rainy season, from July to November. The migration of nonimmune laborers into endemic regions is a significant factor in some outbreaks.

In tropical forests, yellow fever virus is maintained in a transmission cycle involving monkeys and tree-hole–breeding mosquitoes (*Haemogogus* spp in the Americas, *Aedes africanus* in Africa). In the Americas, most cases involve men who work in forested areas and are exposed to infected mosquitoes. In Africa, the virus is prevalent in moist savanna and savanna transition areas where other tree-hole–breeding *Aedes* vectors transmit the virus between monkeys and humans and between humans.

CLINICAL MANIFESTATIONS. In Africa, inapparent, abortive, or clinically mild infections are frequent; some studies suggest that children experience a milder disease than adults. Abortive infections, characterized by fever and headache, may be unrecognized except during epidemics.

In its classic form, yellow fever begins with sudden onset of fever, headache, myalgia, lumbosacral pain, anorexia, nausea, and vomiting. Physical findings during the early phase of illness, when virus is present in the blood, include prostration, conjunctival injection, flushing of face and neck, reddening of the tongue at the tip and edges, and relative bradycardia. After 2–3 days, there may be a brief period of remission, followed in 6–24 hr by reappearance of fever with vomiting, epigastric pain, jaundice, dehydration, gastrointestinal and other hemorrhages, albuminuria, hypotension, signs of renal failure, delirium, convulsions, and coma. Death may occur between the 7th and 10th days. The fatality rate in severe cases approaches 50%. Some patients who survive the acute phase of illness later succumb to renal failure or myocardial damage. Laboratory abnormalities include leukopenia; prolonged clotting, prothrombin, and partial thromboplastin times; thrombocytopenia; hyperbilirubinemia; elevated serum transaminases; albuminuria; and azotemia. Hypoglycemia may be present in severe cases. Electrocardiogram abnormalities characterized by bradycardia and ST-T changes are described.

PATHOLOGY AND PATHOPHYSIOLOGY. Pathologic changes are seen in the liver and kidney. They include (1) coagulative necrosis of hepatocytes in the midzone of the liver lobule with sparing of cells around the portal areas and central veins; (2) eosinophilic degeneration of hepatocytes (Councilman bodies); (3) microvacuolar fatty change; and (4) minimal inflammation. The kidneys show acute tubular necrosis. In the heart, myocardial fiber degeneration and fatty infiltration are seen. The brain may show edema and petechial hemorrhages. Direct viral injury to the liver results in impaired ability to carry out its functions of biosynthesis and detoxification. This is the central pathogenic event of yellow fever. Hemorrhage is thought to result from decreased synthesis of vitamin K–dependent clotting factors and, in some cases, disseminated intravascular clotting. Renal dysfunction has been attributed to hemodynamic factors (prerenal failure progressing to acute tubular necrosis). The pathogenesis of shock in patients with yellow fever appears to be similar to that described in dengue shock syndrome and the other viral hemorrhagic fevers (Chapter 225.1–225.3).

DIAGNOSIS AND TREATMENT. Yellow fever should be suspected when fever, headache, vomiting, myalgia, and jaundice appear in residents of endemic areas or in unimmunized visitors who have recently traveled (within 2 wk before onset of symptoms) to those areas. Clinically, yellow fever is quite similar to dengue hemorrhagic fever. In contrast to the gradual onset of acute viral hepatitis resulting from types A, B, C, or E hepatitis viruses, jaundice in yellow fever appears after 3–5 days of high fever and is often accompanied by severe prostration. Mild yellow fever is dengue-like and cannot be distinguished from a wide variety of other infections. Jaundice and fever may occur in any of several other tropical diseases including malaria, viral hepatitis, louse-borne relapsing fever, leptospirosis, typhoid fever, rickettsial infections, certain systemic bacterial infections, sickle cell crisis, RVF, CHF, and other viral hemorrhagic fevers. Outbreaks of yellow fever always include cases with severe gastrointestinal hemorrhage.

Specific diagnosis depends on detection of virus or viral antigen in acute-phase blood samples or antibody assays. The IgM enzyme immunoassay is particularly useful. Sera obtained during the first 10 days after onset of symptoms should be kept in an ultra-low-temperature freezer (−60° C) and shipped on dry ice for virus testing. Convalescent-phase samples for antibody tests are managed by conventional means. In handling acute-phase blood specimens, medical personnel must take care to avoid contaminating themselves or others on the evacuation trail (laboratory personnel and others). Postmortem diagnosis is based on virus isolation from liver or blood, identification of Councilman bodies in liver tissue, or detection of antigen or viral genome in liver tissue.

TREATMENT. It is customary to keep yellow fever patients in a mosquito-free area, using mosquito nets if necessary. Patients are viremic during the febrile phase of the illness. Although there is no specific treatment for yellow fever, medical care is directed at maintaining physiologic status: (1) sponging or acetaminophen to reduce high fever, (2) vigorous fluid replacement to make up for losses resulting from fasting, thirsting, vomiting, or plasma leakage, (3) correcting acid-base imbalance, (4) maintaining nutritional intake to lesson the severity of hypoglycemia, and (5) avoiding drugs that are either metabolized by the liver or toxic to the liver, kidney, or central nervous system. Complications of acute yellow fever include severe hemorrhage, liver failure, and acute renal failure. Bleeding should be managed by transfusion of fresh whole blood or fresh plasma with platelet concentrates if necessary. Renal failure may require peritoneal dialysis or hemodialysis.

PREVENTION AND CONTROL. Yellow fever 17D is a live, attenuated vaccine with a long record of safety and efficacy. It is administered as a single 0.5-ml subcutaneous injection at least 10 days before arrival in a yellow fever endemic area (for international travelers, East, West, and Central Africa). All persons traveling to endemic areas should be considered for vaccination, but length of stay, exact locations to be visited, and environmental or occupational exposure may determine the specific risk and individual need for vaccination. Persons traveling from yellow fever–endemic to yellow fever–receptive countries may be required to obtain a yellow fever vaccine (e.g., from South America or Africa to India). Usually countries that require travelers to obtain a yellow fever immunization will not issue a visa without a valid immunization certificate. Information can be obtained from the Centers for Disease Control, Division of Vector-Borne Diseases, Fort Collins, Colorado (303-221-6400). Vaccination is valid for 10 yr for international travel certification, although immunity lasts at least 40 yr and probably for life.

Yellow fever vaccine should not be administered to persons with symptomatic immunodeficiency diseases or to those taking immunosuppressant drugs. Although the vaccine is not known to harm fetuses, its administration during pregnancy is contraindicated. In very young children, there is a small risk of encephalitis and death after yellow fever 17D vaccination. The 17D vaccine should not be administered to infants younger than 4 mo because nearly all neurologic complications occur in this age group. Residence or travel to areas of known or anticipated yellow fever activity (e.g., forested areas in the Amazon basin), which places an individual at high risk, warrants immunization of infants 4–9 mo of age. Immunization of children 9 mo and older is routinely recommended before entry into endemic areas. Vaccination should be avoided for persons with a history of egg allergy; alternatively, a skin test can be performed to determine whether a serious allergy exists that would preclude vaccination.

Monath TP: Yellow fever—A medically neglected disease. Rev Infect Dis 9:165, 1987.

Monath TP, Naridi A: Should yellow fever vaccine be included in the expanded program of immunization in Africa—A cost-effectiveness analysis for Nigeria. Am J Trop Med Hyg 48:274, 1993.

Tsai TF, Paul R, Lyndberg MC, et al: Congenital yellow fever virus infection after immunization in pregnancy. J Infect Dis 6:1520, 1993.

Yellow fever—The global situation. Bull WHO 70:667, 1992.

225.5 Japanese Encephalitis

Japanese encephalitis (JE) is an acute mosquito-borne viral disease of humans as well as horses, swine, and other domestic animals. It is caused by a flavivirus closely related to Murray Valley encephalitis. Synonyms are Japanese B encephalitis (to distinguish the syndrome from von Economo, or type A, encephalitis) and Japanese summer encephalitis. JE virus produces human infection and disease in a vast area of Asia, from northern Japan and eastern Korea, China, Philippines, Taiwan, Indo-China, and the Indonesian archipelago to the Indian subcontinent.

ETIOLOGY. JE virus is placed in the *Flavivirus* genus of the family *Flaviviridae*. JE virions are spherical particles, approximately 50 nm in diameter. They are single, positive-stranded RNA viruses that possess a lipid-containing envelope.

EPIDEMIOLOGY. *Culex tritaeniorhyncus summarosus*, a nighttime-biting mosquito that feeds preferentially on large domestic animals and birds but only infrequently on humans, is the principal vector of zoonotic and human JE in northern Asia. A more complex ecology prevails in southern Asia. From Taiwan to India, *Culex tritaeniorhyncus* and members of the closely related *Culex vishnui* group are vectors.

As evidenced by its ability to replicate in a wide range of vertebrate and invertebrate species, JE is one of the most protean of animal viruses. In Japan, before 1948, horse encephalitis epizootics tended to coincide with human epidemics. Pigs and other large animals may serve as amplifier hosts. Birds are heavily infected with JE viruses. Even bats, snakes, lizards, and amphibians are infected in nature. Human beings are not preferred hosts for the vector and are not involved until a high density of mosquitoes is reached.

Large summer outbreaks of JE have been confined largely to Japan, Korea, China, Okinawa, and Taiwan. Before the introduction of vaccine, the incidence of JE in Japan, Korea, Taiwan, and China varied from 0.1–10.4 hospitalizations per 100,000 population, and the case fatality rate, from 24–92%. The case fatality rate was highest in children aged 5–9 yr and in persons older than 65 yr. Over the past decade, there has been a pattern of steadily enlarging recurrent seasonal outbreaks in Vietnam, Thailand, Nepal, and India. The ecologic setting in Southeast Asia is similar to that in Japan, except that low-level transmission occurs throughout the year. Seasonal rains are accompanied by increases in mosquito populations and increased transmission. Pigs serve as amplifying host. In humans, prior dengue virus infection provides partial protection from clinical JE (see later discussion). The occurrence of JE in persons returning from the Far East is a by-product of rapid air transportation and emphasizes the importance of a travel history in the diagnosis of central nervous system infections.

PATHOGENESIS AND PATHOLOGY. Relatively little is known about the pathogenesis of JE virus in humans. After subcutaneous or intravenous inoculation by the mosquito, the virus replicates in extraneural tissues for 4–6 days. The site of replication is unknown. During viremia, the virus may traverse the blood-brain barrier possibly via olfactory nerve fibers. For reasons not understood, only rarely does virus replicate in or cause functional damage to the central nervous system. Most cases of JE infection either are silent or are accompanied by mild or undifferentiated systems. The ratios of inapparent to overt JE infections has been variously estimated between 25:1 to 1,000:1. Higher ratios have been estimated in Asians who are indigenous to enzootic areas compared with persons of European or African ancestry who have lived for many generations in areas free of JE. On theoretic grounds, JE should exert a genetic selection toward resistance because overt disease occurs predominantly among the young and is accompanied by high rates of mortality or severe disability. Males have overt infections more frequently than females. Children are more susceptible to encephalitis than adults.

The brain and its coverings show edema, congestion, and focal hemorrhages. Neuronal degeneration and necrosis with associated intense neuronophagia are seen in many parts of the central nervous system, including the cerebral cortex, cerebellum, and spinal cord. There is associated perivascular cuffing and infiltration of adjacent damaged nervous tissue. A striking change is the destruction of Purkinje cells in the cerebellum. Other findings may include interstitial pneumonitis, hemorrhages in the lungs, focal hemorrhage in the kidney, perilobular fatty change, and intracytoplasmic hyaline changes in liver cells.

CLINICAL MANIFESTATIONS. After an incubation period that varies between 4 and 14 days, the typical case progresses through four stages: a prodromal illness (2–3 days), an acute stage (3–4 days), a subacute stage (7–10 days), and convalescence (4–7 wk). Onset may be characterized by abrupt headache, respiratory symptoms, anorexia, nausea, abdominal pain, vomiting, and sensory changes, including psychotic episodes. A low-grade fever or minor respiratory symptoms may be the only clinical expressions of JE. The acute stage may be heralded by a high fever. Grand mal seizures are seen in 10–24% of children. They are usually generalized and major motor in type. Parkinsonian-like nonintention tremor and cogwheel rigidity are seen less frequently. There are signs of upper motor neuron involvement and meningeal irritation. Particularly characteristic are rapidly changing central nervous system signs (e.g., hyper-reflexia followed by hyporeflexia or plantar responses that change). The sensory status of the patient may vary from confusion, disorientation, delirium, or somnolence, progressing to coma. There may be oliguria, diarrhea, and relative bradycardia. During this stage a lumbar puncture reveals an elevated leukocyte count within the cerebrospinal fluid that is initially polymorphonuclear but in a few days becomes predominantly lymphocytic. Albuminuria is common. Fatal cases usually progress rapidly to coma, and the patient dies within 10 days. In the subacute stage, the severity of involvement of the central nervous system lessens, but orthostatic pneumonia, urinary tract infections, or bed sores may be management problems and in some instances are life threatening.

After the acute disease, deficits in neural function may persist. These may include spastic paralysis, wasting, fasciculation, cranial nerve involvement, and extrapyramidal tract abnormalities. The duration of illness and the clinical outcome are extremely varied. Convalescence is prolonged with weakness, lethargy, incoordination, tremors, and neuroses. Weight loss may be severe. The frequency of sequelae has been reported to range from 5–70%. The more common sequelae are mental deterioration, severe emotional instability, personality changes, motor abnormalities, and speech disturbances. Sequelae are most common in patients who were younger than 10 yr at the onset of disease. Infants have more severe sequelae than do older children. The frequency of sequelae is directly related to the severity of disease.

DIAGNOSIS AND TREATMENT. The differential diagnosis of patients with involvement of the central nervous system caused by JE virus includes a large number of viral, bacterial, and fungal diseases, neoplasms, and conditions of unknown cause. In the endemic geographic region, the differential diagnosis includes leptospirosis, enterovirus, and mumps meningitis, herpes encephalitis, rabies, dengue shock syndrome, bacterial meningitis, cysticercosis, Reye syndrome, and toxic encephalitides. In children, systemic disease accompanied by high fever may cause convulsions. Primary or secondary neoplasms may affect the central nervous system and resemble viral encephalitis, although the onset of central nervous system dysfunction usually is not acute, and patients rarely are febrile. Postinfectious or demyelinating encephalitides also may produce a picture similar to JE. The results of examination of cerebrospinal fluid, the season of the year, and occupational or other exposure may assist in narrowing the differential diagnosis. The cerebrospinal fluid usually is clear but may contain 100–1,000 white cells per milliliter. An early polymorphonuclear response quickly becomes predominantly mononuclear. Cerebrospinal fluid protein is moderately elevated.

It is important to obtain paired sera to establish the diagnosis in surviving patients and fresh brain tissue for virus isolation in the event of death (see later discussion). Brain may be obtained at postmortem examination using biopsy needles. Virus isolation from brain biopsy has been accomplished successfully in a living patient. A specific diagnosis can be made by virus isolation, identification of antigen in brain by fluorescent antibody technique, or detection of viral RNA by DNA hybridization. Virus recovery is most likely in persons who die early in the disease. Isolation of virus from blood or cerebrospinal fluid is uncommon. Virus isolation is accomplished by inoculating adult or infant mice or a wide range of vertebrate or invertebrate tissue cultures.

When JE is the only flavivirus infection of humans, a serologic diagnosis can be made by demonstrating rising antibodies using the HI test or the enzyme immunoassay (EIA). Elsewhere, IgM-capture EIA or one of several neutralization tests should be used. In mild disease, IgM antibody is replaced by IgC antibodies within 90 days. IgM antibodies may persist for one half to 1 yr after overt encephalitis.

There is no specific therapy for JE. The skillful application of supportive and symptomatic measures is of prime importance. It is very important to anticipate and be prepared for the complications of convulsions, cerebral edema, hyperpyrexia, inadequate respiratory exchange, disturbed fluid and electrolyte balance, hypostatic pneumonia, aspiration and asphyxia, sudden cardiac and respiratory cessation of central origin, and cardiac decompensation.

Airway Obstruction. Obstruction of the airway should be anticipated when there is impairment of swallowing function, resulting in the pooling of secretions. Intubation or tracheotomy and respiratory support may be indicated. See Chapter 60.1.

Cerebral Edema. Increased intracranial pressure is suggested by irregularity of respiration. Reduction of pressure is of prime importance because adequate circulation may preserve cells that are not irreversibly damaged by virus.

Various measures have theoretic potential for this purpose; trial with any one or all of them may be justified. (1) Hydrocortisone can be given in pharmacologic doses. (2) Improved survival and recovery have been claimed with the use of hypothermia. (3) Substances used in an effort to reduce elevated intracranial pressure include mannitol, glycerol, and urea.

Control of Convulsions. In the acute stage, this can be accomplished by the intravenous use of anticonvulsants such as phenobarbital or, in patients older than 6 mo, diazepam (Valium). Other anticonvulsants may be indicated for several months during convalescence. See Chapter 543.

Intake-Output Management. Distension of the bladder must be anticipated and controlled by the Crede maneuver or by catheterization. Constipation and, in particular, fecal impaction should be prevented by the used of mineral oil and enemas. Water and nutrients must usually be administered intravenously in the early stage. Water intoxication or dehydration must be carefully controlled. Vitamins B and C should be included in daily intake. As soon as possible, feeding should be instituted by nasogastric tube.

Antibiotic Therapy. Antibiotics should be used in therapeutic doses when secondary bacterial infection is diagnosed.

Rehabilitation. Physiotherapy, occupational therapy, and corrective surgery should be used as necessary. Patients or parents should be warned that transient, sometimes quite severe emotional and behavior aberrations are common. Children tend to return to normal more quickly when a permissive rather than a too restrictive attitude is adopted. Parents should be encouraged by the prospect of continued albeit slow improvement. The administration of hyperimmune gamma globulin has not proved effective in human beings who manifest the early clinical signs of tick-borne viral encephalitis.

PREVENTION AND CONTROL. Travelers to endemic country who expect short- or long-term stays in rural areas of the endemic region during the expected period of seasonal transmission should be vaccinated. The present schedule for commercially available vaccines licensed in the United States, Japan, and other countries is three doses of 1.0 mL given subcutaneously. The first two doses are given 1 wk apart and the third dose 3 mo later. Reactions to vaccination include headache, malaise, local pain, swelling, and urticaria. All reactions combined occurred in fewer than 1% of vaccinees. Because vaccine is prepared in mouse brain, intensive surveillance should be maintained for central nervous system disease after JE vaccination. No cases of postvaccinal demyelinating encephalitis have been reported.

Commercial pesticides, widely used by rice farmers in Asia, are effective in reducing populations of *C. tritaeniorhyncus*. Fenthion, fenitrothion, and phenthoate are effectively adulticidal and larvicidal. Insecticides may be applied from portable sprayers or from helicopters or light aircraft.

Personal prophylaxis may be effective in reducing exposure to mosquito bites, especially for short-term residents in endemic areas. This consists of avoiding evening outdoor exposure, using insect repellents, covering the body with clothing, and using of bed nets or house screening.

Innis BL, Nisalak A, Nimmannitya S, et al: An enzyme-linked immunosorbent assay to characterize dengue infections where dengue and Japanese encephalitis co-circulate. Am J Trop Med Hyg 40:418, 1989.

Paul WS, Moore PS, Karabatsos N, et al: Outbreak of Japanese encephalitis on the island of Saipan, 1990. J Infect Dis 167:1053, 1993.

Poland JD, Cropp CB, Craven RB, et al: Evaluation of the potency and safety of inactivated Japanese encephalitis vaccine in U.S. inhabitants. J Infect Dis 161:878, 1990.

White NJ, Krishna S, Looareesuwon S: Encephalitis, not cerebral malaria, is likely cause of coma with negative blood smears. J Infect Dis 166:1195, 1992.

CHAPTER 226
Hantavirus Pulmonary Syndrome

Scott Halstead

In June 1993, a newly recognized hantavirus was identified as the etiologic agent of an outbreak of severe respiratory illness in the southwestern United States. Now called the hantavirus pulmonary syndrome (HPS), sporadic cases have been identified from a wide area in the western and southern United States. HPS is characterized by a febrile prodrome followed by the rapid onset of noncardiogenic pulmonary edema and hypotension of shock. More than half the identified patients have died.

ETIOLOGY. Hantaviruses are a genus in the family Bunyaviridae, which are lipid-enveloped viruses with a negative-stranded RNA genome composed of three unique segments. Most cases of HPS have been associated with a single virus, tentatively named Muerto Canyon, isolated originally from deer mice *(Peromyscus maniculatus)* in New Mexico. Two other new hantaviruses have been identified from genetic sequences detected by reverse transcriptase polymerase chain reactions (PCRs) in lung tissue from HPS patients. Human hantavirus infection has been associated with hemorrhagic fever with renal syndrome (HFRS). Several pathogenic viruses that have been recognized within the genus include Hantaan virus, which causes the most severe form of HFRS seen primarily in mainland Asia; Dobrava virus, which causes the most severe form of HFRS seen primarily in the Balkans; Puumala virus, which causes a milder form of HFRS with a high proportion of subclinical infections and is prevalent in northern Europe; and Seoul virus, which results in moderate HFRS and is transmitted predominantly in Asia by urban rats or worldwide by laboratory rats. Prospect Hill, a virus that is widely disseminated in U.S. meadow voles, is not known to cause human disease.

EPIDEMIOLOGY. Persons acquiring HPS generally have a history of recent outdoor exposure or live in an area with large populations of deer mice. Clusters of cases have occurred in individuals who have cleaned houses that were rodent infested. Deer mice are one of the most common North American mammals. Where *P. maniculatus* is found, it is frequently the dominant member of the rodent community. The ages of the approximately 100 known patients have ranged from 12 to 69 yr. It is not known whether absence of disease in young children is a reflection of innate resistance or lack of exposure. Sixty percent of patients were in the 20- to 39-yr age range and 67% were males.

Hantaviruses do not cause apparent illness in their reservoir hosts, which remain asymptomatically infected for life. Infected rodents shed virus in saliva, urine, and feces for many weeks, but the duration of shedding and the period of maximum infectivity are unknown. The presence of infectious virus in saliva, the sensitivity of these animals to parenteral inoculation with hantaviruses, and field observations of infected rodents indicate that biting is important for rodent-to-rodent transmission. Aerosols from infective saliva or excreta of rodents are implicated in the transmission of hantaviruses to humans. Persons visiting animal care areas housing infected rodents have been infected after 5 min exposure. It is possible that hantaviruses are spread through contaminated food and breaks in skin or mucous membranes; transmission to humans has occurred by rodent bites. Person-to-person transmission is not reported.

PATHOGENESIS. HPS is characterized by sudden and catastrophic pulmonary edema, resulting in anoxia and acute heart failure. The virus is detected in pulmonary capillaries, suggesting that pulmonary edema is the direct consequence of virus-induced capillary damage.

CLINICAL MANIFESTATIONS. The HPS is characterized by a prodrome and a cardiopulmonary phase. The mean duration after the onset of prodromal symptoms to hospitalization is 5.4 days. The mean duration of symptoms to death is 8 days (median, 7 days; range, 2–16 days). The most common prodromal symptoms are fever and myalgia (100%), cough or dyspnea (76%), gastrointestinal symptoms including vomiting, diarrhea, and midabdominal pain (76%), and headache (71%). The cardiopulmonary phase is heralded by progressive cough and shortness of breath. The most common initial physical findings are tachypnea (100%), tachycardia (94%), and hypotension (50%). Rapidly progressive acute pulmonary edema, anoxemia, and shock develop in most severely ill patients. The clinical course of the illness in patients who die is characterized by pulmonary edema accompanied by severe hypotension, frequently terminating in sinus bradycardia, electromechanical dissociation, ventricular tachycardia, or fibrillation. Hypotension may be progressive even with adequate oxygenation.

LABORATORY DATA. Laboratory findings include leukocytosis (median, 26,000 white cells per milliliter), an increased hematocrit, thrombocytopenia (median, 64,000 mL), prolonged prothrombin and partial thromboplastin times, an elevated serum lactate dehydrogenase concentration, decreased serum protein concentrations, and proteinuria.

Biosafety level 2 facilities and practices are recommended for laboratory handling of sera. Biosafety level 3 facilities and practices are recommended for handling tissues from suspect patients because the virus may be aerosolized.

DIAGNOSIS AND DIFFERENTIAL DIAGNOSIS. The diagnosis of HPS should be considered in a previously healthy patient presenting with a febrile prodrome and respiratory distress. The diagnosis of HPS is made by serologic tests that detect hantavirus immunoglobulin M antibodies. Hantavirus antigen can be detected in tissue by immunohistochemistry and amplification of hantaviral nucleotide sequences detected by reverse transcriptase polymerase chain reaction (RT PCR). State Health Department or the Centers of Disease Control laboratories should be consulted (see Treatment).

The differential diagnosis includes adult respiratory distress syndrome, pneumonic plague, psittacosis, severe mycoplasmal pneumonia, influenza, leptospirosis, inhalation anthrax, rickettsial infections, pulmonary tularemia, atypical bacterial and viral pneumoniae, legionellosis, meningococcemia, and other sepsis syndromes.

PREVENTION. Avoiding contact with rodents is the only preventive strategy. Rodent control in and around the home is important. Precautions should be observed in handling sera and human or rodent tissue that might contain hantaviruses.

TREATMENT. Management of patients with hantavirus infection requires maintenance of adequate oxygenation and careful monitoring and support of cardiovascular function. The pathophysiology of HPS resembles that of dengue shock syndrome (see Chapter 225). Pressor or inotropic agents should be administered in combination with careful volume replacement to treat symptomatic hypotension or shock while avoiding volume expansion and overhydration. Intravenous ribavirin given early in the course of hemorrhagic fever with renal syndrome is life saving. Its use in HPS is being studied. For treatment advice, one should contact the Special Pathogens Branch, Division of Viral and Rickettsial Diseases, National Center for Infectious Diseases, 1600 Clifton Road, Atlanta, GA 30033; telephone: (404) 639–1115; fax: (404) 639–1118.

PROGNOSIS. Patient fatality rates are about 50%. Severe abnormalities in hematocrit and lactate dehydrogenase levels, hematocrit and partial thromboplastin time, and white cell count and partial thromboplastin time predict mortality with high specificity and sensitivity.

Butler JC, Peters CJ: Hantaviruses and hantavirus pulmonary syndrome. Clin Infect Dis 19:387, 1994.
Childs JE, Ksiazek TG, Koster FT, et al: Serologic and genetic identification of *Peromyscus maniculatus* as the primary rodent reservoir for a new hantavirus in the Southwestern United States. J Infect Dis 169:1271, 1994.
Duchin JS, Koster FT, Peters CJ, et al: Hantavirus pulmonary syndrome: A clinical description of 17 patients with a newly recognized disease. N Engl J Med 330:949, 1994.
Hantavirus pulmonary syndrome—United States, 1993. MMWR 43:46, 1994.
Hughes JM, Peters CJ, Cohen ML, et al: Hantavirus pulmonary syndrome: An emerging infectious disease. Science 262:850, 1994.
Laboratory management of agents associated with hantavirus pulmonary syndrome: Interim biosafety guidelines. MMWR 43, 1994.

CHAPTER 227
Rabies

Stanley A. Plotkin

Human rabies is a viral infection of the central nervous system usually transmitted by contamination of a wound with saliva from a rabid animal and is virtually 100% fatal once symptoms develop.

ETIOLOGY. Rabies virus belongs to the rhabdovirus group. Rabies and several closely related viruses are classified as lyssaviruses. Rabies-related viruses are found in Europe and Africa and are relatively rare. The viral particles resemble striated bullets. Inside the cylinder is the RNA-containing nucleocapsid. The envelope contains a glycoprotein that elicits neutralizing antibodies and acts as a protective antigen in animal experiments.

EPIZOOTIOLOGY AND EPIDEMIOLOGY. Rabies is a widespread infection of warm-blooded animals. In the United States rabies occurs principally in skunks, raccoons, foxes, and bats. Skunks are the principal vectors in the Midwest, Southwest, and California, with distinct northern and southern strains. Raccoon rabies exists in the form of one strain but two loci: one in the Southeast, and the second throughout the Mid-Atlantic states. Fox rabies is found in Canada, Alaska, and New York, with a separate strain in the Southwest. Bat rabies is found in practically every state. In Central and South America dogs are the usual source of exposure. Vampire bats, which bite cattle, are an important part of the cycle of rabies in Latin America. Europe has had an epizootic of fox rabies. In Asia and Africa the principal problem is the rabid dog. Human rabies is still common in Asia and Africa as a result of canine rabies, although poor reporting precludes precise statements as to incidence. The production of numerous monoclonal antibodies to rabies virus strains has revealed considerable antigenic variation in both the glycoprotein and nucleocapsid antigens of the virus. The result has been the identification of variant strains (called rabies-related viruses) and antigenic differences among true rabies virus that correlate with host species or geographic location. For example, strains isolated from cattle rabies in South America resemble bat strains, confirming the transmission of virus from the vampire bat to the cow.

The existence of rabies-free land areas permits health authorities in certain locations to omit vaccination after most dog bites on the grounds that terrestrial rabies has been unknown there for years. The continent of Australia and many islands, including those of the United Kingdom and Hawaii, are totally free of rabies. Human rabies is a rare disease in the United States and western Europe, where the infected animals are largely sylvatic. Most cases in these areas are imparted from other countries. The bat has been a relatively important vector of human infection in recent American rabies cases.

Rabies is a major public health problem in areas in which dogs are uncontrolled. Thus, the great majority of human cases are seen in India, Southeast Asia, and Africa. The exact annual incidence of human rabies is unknown but is likely between 25,000 and 100,000 cases.

PATHOGENESIS AND PATHOLOGY. The means by which rabies virus travels from the wound to the brain are only partially understood. Because the virus attaches to and penetrates cells rapidly in vitro, it is unlikely that it remains dormant in the wound for long periods of time. Moreover, although the virus has been shown to ascend axons from the periphery to the spinal cord, the speed of spread (3 mm/hr) is far too rapid to explain the long incubation period of the disease.

The virus first multiplies in striated muscle cells, to which it attaches via several receptors, probably including the nicotinic acetylcholine receptor. It may be hypothesized that antibody, interferon, and other host factors then act on the virus as it leaves striated muscle; if these factors are insufficiently protective, virus eventually attaches to the nerve. From then on, rabies may be inevitable. The possibility that the virus must overcome another barrier in passing from the first infected neuron to other neurons is indicated by electron microscopic studies of the brain, which demonstrate viral passage from cell to contiguous cell.

The basic lesion in the brain is neuronal destruction in the brain stem and medulla. The cerebral cortex is usually normal in the absence of prolonged anoxia before death. The hippocampus, thalamus, and basal ganglia often show neuronal destruction and glial infiltrates. The most severe pathology is evident in the pons and the floor of the fourth ventricle. The inspiratory muscle spasms that result in the striking symptom of hydrophobia may be due to destruction of brain stem neurons inhibitory to the neurons of the nucleus ambiguus, which control inspiration. Hydrophobia does not occur in other diseases because only rabies combines brain stem encephalitis with an intact cortex and maintenance of consciousness.

The Negri body, long the pathologic hallmark of rabies, is a cytoplasmic inclusion found in neurons; it consists of clumped viral nucleocapsid. The absence of Negri bodies does not exclude rabies; fluorescent antibody stains of brain sections or smears may be positive in their absence.

Transmission. In animals, as in humans, rabies produces encephalitis as the principal symptom. After establishment of the encephalitis, however, the virus spreads down nerves from the brain. It multiplies in many organs, but those important to transmission are the salivary glands. Not all rabid animals have virus in the saliva, and even when it is present, the quantity is variable. Skunks are particularly likely to have large amounts of virus in saliva. Although dogs may have virus in saliva for many days before symptoms occur, transmission to humans from dogs who appeared normal for 10 days or more after a biting incident has not been reported. The variability of virus in saliva explains the fact that less than half of untreated bites by proven rabid animals will result in rabies.

Scratches by the claws of rabid animals are dangerous because animals lick their claws. Saliva applied to a mucosal surface such as the conjunctiva may be infectious.

Bat excreta contain enough rabies virus to pose a danger of rabies to those who enter infested caves and inhale aerosols created by bats. Aerosols of rabies virus inadvertently produced in laboratories are dangerous to laboratory workers.

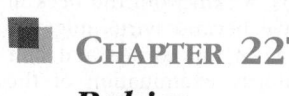

In general, if a biting animal does not die within 10 days, rabies is unlikely, although rarely a rabid terrestrial animal will recover from rabies. Bats, on the contrary, are often infected for long periods without showing symptoms.

Transmission of rabies by corneal transplant from patients with undiagnosed rabies encephalitis to healthy recipients has been recorded with sufficient frequency to warrant exclusion of donors dead from unexplained neurologic disease. Human-to-human transmission is theoretically possible but is poorly documented and rare if it occurs at all.

CLINICAL MANIFESTATIONS. The incubation period of rabies is extremely variable. Exceptionally long incubation periods have been described and a 7-yr incubation period was recently confirmed by strain identification. On the other hand, an incubation period of only 9 days has followed severe exposure. Usually, the incubation period is 20–180 days with the peak at 30–60 days. It tends to be shorter in children and in individuals in whom rabies develops despite vaccination.

There is usually a prodromal phase of rabies, lasting 2–10 days. Common nonspecific symptoms include fever, malaise, headache, anorexia, and vomiting. The patient may be troubled by ill-defined anxiety. Characteristic symptoms at this stage are pain, pruritus, or paresthesia at the site of the wound.

The illness then enters an acute neurologic phase, of either the furious or paralytic variety, which lasts 2–10 days. In the former, *hydrophobia* is a pathognomonic sign. Attempts to swallow liquids, including saliva, result in aspiration into the trachea. Hydrophobia appears to be an exaggerated respiratory tract protective reflex, perhaps mediated by neuronal dysfunction in certain areas of the brain stem. Eventually a psychologic component exacerbates the spasms, and even the sight of water evokes terror. *Aerophobia* may be present and is considered by some also to be pathognomonic of rabies. Aerophobia is elicited by fanning a current of air across the face, which causes violent spasms of the pharyngeal and neck muscles.

The neurologic picture in the typical case may consist of bursts of hyperactivity, disorientation, and bizarre combative behavior, alternating with periods of lucidity. During the lucid periods the patient may be aware of what is happening and may be able to articulate his or her fears. The facial expression is one of grim hopelessness.

Patients may also complain of pharyngeal pain, difficulty in swallowing, and hoarseness. Seizures are common, perhaps on the basis of hypoxia compounded by hyperventilation.

Some rabid patients experience meningismus or even opisthotonos. The cerebrospinal fluid may reflect meningeal irritation, with varying elevations of cells (predominantly lymphocytes) and protein, or may be normal. The peripheral white cell count often shows a polymorphonuclear leukocytosis.

In about 20% of patients, an ascending symmetric paralysis with flaccidity and decreased tendon reflexes dominates the entire acute phase. This course is particularly common after bat bites. In the remainder of patients, paralysis develops toward the end of the acute neurologic phase.

If the patient does not die of cardiorespiratory arrest during the acute stage, he or she slips into coma. With modern intensive care, life may be prolonged, but numerous complications occur during coma. Most significant is myocarditis, manifested by hypotension and arrhythmias. Rabies virus has been recovered from the heart, which shows inflammation at autopsy. Also prominent is pituitary dysfunction expressed as either diabetes insipidus or inappropriate secretion of antidiuretic hormone. Recovery from symptomatic rabies in humans is extremely rare; only four cases have been reported.

DIAGNOSIS AND DIFFERENTIAL DIAGNOSIS. When a patient has a history of having been bitten by an animal, paresthesias at the wound site, and hydrophobia, a clinical diagnosis of rabies is not difficult. Any disease in which there is encephalitis may occasionally cause confusion, such as those caused by arboviruses, enteroviruses, and Herpes simplex. However, if one finds signs of brain stem involvement in a patient whose sensorium is basically clear and who has no signs of a space-occupying lesion, other diagnoses can usually be set aside.

Paralytic rabies may be misdiagnosed as Guillain-Barré syndrome, poliomyelitis, or postrabies vaccine encephalomyelitis. Careful neurologic examination and analysis of the cerebrospinal fluid will often help rule out these diagnoses.

The spasms of tetanus may cause momentary diagnostic confusion, but trismus is not seen in rabies, and hydrophobia is not seen in tetanus. Botulism (wound or ingestion) will cause paralysis, but the absence of sensory changes should exclude rabies.

Perhaps the most confusing differential problem is hysteria in an individual who thinks he or she has rabies. Normal blood gases and the absence of variation in bizarre behavior will suggest pseudorabies.

Laboratory diagnosis is now possible before death. The virus may be demonstrated by fluorescent antibody stain of smears of corneal epithelial cells or sections of skin from the neck at the hairline. These tests are positive because virus migrates down the nerves from the brain; both the cornea and hair follicles are richly innervated. Autopsy examination of the brains of patients with fatal encephalitis should include fluorescent antibody tests for rabies.

Serologic diagnosis is also possible if the patient survives beyond the acute period. Neutralizing antibodies develop eventually in both serum and cerebrospinal fluid and rapidly rise to extremely high levels, for example, more than 100 international units (IU). Vaccination, even with potent vaccine, is unlikely to raise titers above 20 IU.

PROGNOSIS. Although patients can be kept alive for months with intensive care, only a few patients have survived rabies, and the prognosis is bleak.

PREVENTION OF RABIES

PRE-EXPOSURE PROPHYLAXIS. Vaccination of domestic dogs and elimination of strays have resulted in eradication of terrestrial rabies from many areas. If dog control were properly practiced, rabies could be suppressed in much of the world.

Those who are expected to be at risk, such as veterinarians, laboratory workers, and children going to rabies-enzootic areas, can be preimmunized. The cell culture vaccine (see later) will produce virtually 100% response with three doses given at 0, 7, and 28 days. A titer of 0.5 IU has been accepted as protective.

POSTEXPOSURE PROPHYLAXIS. First, a decision must be made about whether rabies prophylaxis is necessary. In many areas of the United States, rabies in mammals has been unknown for years. However, the unprovoked bite of a wild animal should be considered rabid if the animal belongs to a species known to be a rabies host, such as a skunk, fox, raccoon, bat, or coyote. Rodents are very rarely carriers of rabies in the United States. Knowledge of the local epidemiology of rabies is essential to the physician contemplating treatment of a human exposure. Unprovoked bites by bats or other wild animals almost always require immunization; decisions regarding bites from domestic or pet animals should be made after discussion with public health veterinarians.

If a domestic animal such as a dog or cat is the offender, consideration must be given to the question of provocation, to the clinical appearance of the animal if apprehended, and to the rabies vaccination status of the animal. Difficulty in making decisions arises when the biting animal has run away after a seemingly unprovoked attack. Whether the animal was rabid or merely ill-tempered is often impossible to decide. When the animal is under observation, rabies treatment can be withheld until the animal acts abnormally, at which point it should be sacrificed and tested for rabies. However, a wild animal should be killed immediately and its brain examined for rabies antigen by the fluorescent-antibody technique. Table 227–1 may help in making the decision about whether or not to treat.

If rabies prophylaxis is to be given after exposure, prevention depends on three complementary means of reducing the risk. Local treatment (see later) is designed to kill the virus by mechanical and virucidal action. Passive antibody (see later) then provides immediate blockage of attachment of virus to the nerve endings. However, passive antibody ultimately disappears and must be replaced by the active response provided by vaccine. The vaccine must not only produce a primary antibody response but must also overcome the depressive effect of passive antibody on the immune response.

LOCAL TREATMENT. The chief requirement of local treatment is that it be prompt and thorough. Simple mechanical removal by soap and water should be the first step, using copious amounts of solution. Catheters should be inserted for irrigation of puncture wounds. If the mechanical trauma of the local treatment is painful, procaine-type anesthetics may be used to infiltrate the area without adding risk.

The mechanical removal of virus may be followed by application of a virucidal solution such as 1% povidone-iodine or 70% alcohol. In an emergency, any alcoholic liquor of 86 proof or higher may be used. However, most authorities eschew antisepsis and depend on soap and water irrigation.

PASSIVE ANTIBODY. Passive immunization must be given to protect the patient until vaccination produces antibodies. Passive antibody is available in some countries in the form of purified equine immune globulin or human rabies immune globulin. The latter avoids serum sickness reactions to equine protein, which occur in about 1% of recipients of the animal product. The dose for human rabies immune globulin is 20 IU/kg. Up to half of the dose should be infiltrated subcutaneously at the site of bite or scratch; the remainder is injected intramuscularly into the arm or buttocks. The dose for equine immune globulin is 40 IU/kg delivered in the same manner.

Passive immunization should be performed regardless of the interval between rabies exposure and treatment. However, if vaccine was started previously there is no need for passive immunization once 8 days have elapsed. Anaphylaxis is a rare possibility with the equine product, but tests for hypersensitivity should be carried out in the usual manner (consult package insert). Steroids should be avoided if possible in the treatment of reactions because they cause activation of rabies virus in experimental animals.

ACTIVE IMMUNIZATION. Early rabies vaccines were prepared in the central nervous system of animals. Their antigenicity was poor and multiple injections were required. As a result postvaccination encephalitis was a frequent problem. Animal nerve tissue vaccines are still in use in many places in the world, in particular, suckling mouse brain vaccine, which gives fewer neurologic reactions than sheep brain vaccines because it contains less myelin.

However, the major advance in rabies vaccine was the development of cell culture technology, which permitted the production of concentrated vaccines with high antigenic potency and low contamination with cellular proteins. Thus, immunogenicity was improved, allowing reduced numbers of doses, and reactions were reduced. The first widely available cell culture vaccine was produced in human diploid cells (HDCV). This vaccine, and one produced in fetal rhesus diploid cells (RVA), are the only two currently available in the United States. Outside the United States, vaccines produced in Vero (continuous monkey kidney), chick embryo, duck embryo, and other cultured cells are also used.

The schedule recommended for postexposure immunization is five doses given intramuscularly in the deltoid on days 0, 3, 7, 14, and 28. The dose is not reduced for children. Immune responses to the postexposure schedule are regularly seen by the 14th day. However, in situations of exposure to rabies, it is mandatory to provide passive immunization as described previously.

Some individuals are likely to be exposed to rabies because of profession or travel in rabies enzootic areas. For pre-exposure immunization, a three-dose schedule is followed, consisting of intramuscular (1.0 mL) or intradermal (0.1 mL) doses given on days 0, 7, and 28. Care should be taken to give the vaccine in the muscle rather than in the subcutaneous tissue.

Postvaccination antibody titers are not generally needed unless the subject is immunosuppressed or is receiving antimalarial therapy, which may depress the response.

Reaction rates to cell culture vaccines have been low, and neurologic reactions have been rare because no nerve tissue is present in the cell cultures used to grow the virus. Allergic reactions have occurred in less than 0.1% after primary vaccination with HDCV and systemic symptoms such as malaise and fever in only 5–15%. Nevertheless, administration of boosters results in an allergic reaction rate of 6%; accordingly, boosters are no longer routinely recommended, except following rabies exposure, when two doses are given at an interval of 3 days. The RVA vaccine may be useful in those who have reactions to HDCV. Although no controlled study has been done, the efficacy of rabies vaccination is evidently high, judging from the known incidence of disease after untreated bites by infected animals (approximately 15%) and the paucity of vaccine failures. When seen, vaccine failure has usually followed incomplete prophylactic regimens.

TREATMENT OF CLINICAL RABIES. Large doses of interferon and antirabies serum have been advocated, but it is doubtful that

■ **TABLE 227–1 Rabies Postexposure Prophylaxis Guide for the United States**

Animal	Evaluation and Disposition of Animal	Postexposure Prophylaxis Recommendations
Dogs and cats	Healthy and available for 10-day observation	Should not begin prophylaxis unless animal experiences symptoms of rabies*
	Rabid or suspected rabid	Immediate vaccination
	Unknown (escaped)	Consult public health officials
Skunks, raccoons, bats, foxes, and most other carnivores; woodchucks	Regarded as rabid unless geographic area is known to be free of rabies or until animal proven negative by laboratory tests†	Immediate vaccination
Livestock, rodents, ferrets, and lagomorphs (rabbits and hares)	Consider individually	Consult public health officials Bites of squirrels, hamsters, guinea pigs, gerbils, chipmunks, rats, mice, other rodents, rabbits, and hares almost never require antirabies treatment

**During the 10-day holding period, begin treatment with human rabies immune globulin and human diploid cell rabies vaccine or rabies vaccine, adsorbed at first sign of rabies in a dog or cat that has bitten someone. The symptomatic animal should be killed immediately and tested.*

†The animal should be killed and tested as soon as possible. Holding for observation is not recommended. Discontinue vaccine if immunofluorescence test results of the animal are negative.

Modified from Public Health Service Advisory Committee on Immunization Practices: Rabies: Risk, management, prophylaxis, and immunization. MMWR 40:1, 1991.

these substances can affect rabies that has already spread to the brain.

Anderson LJ, Sikes RK, Langkop CW, et al: Prophylactic immunization: Postexposure trial of a human diploid cell strain rabies vaccine. J Infect Dis 142:133, 1980.
Fishbein DB, Robinson LE: Rabies. N Engl J Med 329:1632, 1993.
Houff SA, Burton RC, Wilson RW, et al: Human-to-human transmission of rabies virus by corneal transplant. N Engl J Med 300:603, 1979.
Plotkin SA: Rabies vaccine prepared in human cell cultures: Progress and perspectives. Rev Infect Dis 2:433, 1980.
Plotkin SA, Clark HF: Rabies. *In*: Feigin RD, Cherry JD: Textbook of Pediatric Infectious Diseases, 3rd ed. Philadelphia, WB Saunders, 1992, pp 1657–1666.
Public Health Service Advisory Committee on Immunization Practices: Rabies: Risk, management, prophylaxis, and immunization. MMWR, 40:1, 1991.
Sureau P, Rollin P, Wiktor TJ: Epidemiologic analysis of antigenic variations of street rabies virus: Detection by monoclonal antibodies. Am J Epidemiol 117:605, 1983.
Tsiang H: Pathophysiology of rabies virus infection of the nervous system. Adv Virus Res 42:375, 1993.
Turner GS: A review of the world epidemiology of rabies. Trans R Soc Trop Med Hyg 70:175, 1976.
Warrell DA: The clinical picture of rabies in man. Trans R Soc Trop Med Hyg 70:188, 1976.

CHAPTER 228

*Slow Viral Infections of the Human Nervous System**

David M. Asher

Viruses cause several neurologic diseases that were once considered degenerative. The diseases have symptomatic incubation periods of months to years and durations of overt clinical illness that may also be very long. Although the viruses may be latent in other organs of the body, pathologic changes are found only in the nervous system. Some slow viral infections of the human nervous system are caused by viruses with conventional physical properties—viruses that more often cause acute self-limited illnesses (Table 228–1). Other slow infections are caused by infectious agents of unknown structure, agents that, like viruses, are smaller than bacteria but have an array of physical properties so unlike those of conventional viruses that some authorities have suggested that they not be considered viruses at all.

*All material in this chapter is in the public domain, with the exception of any borrowed figures or tables.

SLOW INFECTIONS WITH CONVENTIONAL VIRUSES

Subacute Sclerosing Panencephalitis

(Dawson Encephalitis)

ETIOLOGY. This chronic encephalitis is caused by a persistent measles virus infection. Dawson was first to describe it clearly and to postulate a viral cause. Subsequently, measles virus was isolated from the brains of patients with subacute sclerosing panencephalitis (SSPE).

EPIDEMIOLOGY. SSPE is a rare disease that occurs worldwide. The disease has been diagnosed in patients aged 6 mo to older than 30 yr, but it affects primarily children and young adolescents. In more than 85% of cases, onset occurs between 5 and 15 yr of age. The average age of onset before 1980 was about 10 yr; between 1980 and 1984 it was almost 14 yr. Acquisition of measles before the age of 18 mo seems to increase the risk of SSPE substantially. The risk among boys is more than twice that among girls, and it is higher among rural children than city children, children with two or more siblings, children of lower socioeconomic status, and mentally retarded children. SSPE was once especially common in the southeastern United States, the Ohio River valley, and some New England states. Recently, cases have been more common in the western United States and in New York City, especially among Hispanic immigrant children. Exposure to birds and other animals has been reported with abnormal frequency in histories of patients with SSPE; the reason is not clear.

Mean annual incidence rates of SSPE in the United States fell markedly from 0.61 cases per 1 million persons younger than 20 yr in 1960 to 0.06 cases per 1 million in 1980. Since 1982 only five or fewer new cases have been registered with the U.S. National SSPE Registry each year from the entire country. The drop roughly parallels the progressive decline in the annual number of measles cases diagnosed since the introduction of live, attenuated measles vaccine in the United States in 1963. The risk of SSPE has been estimated at 8.5 SSPE cases per 1 million cases of measles for a 6-yr period, during which the estimated risk after measles vaccination was only 0.7 cases per 1 million doses of vaccine. The overwhelming advantage of measles vaccination in preventing SSPE is clear.

In a recent case-control study, the lack of vaccination was a highly significant risk factor for SSPE, and in a survey in England and Wales the relative risk of SSPE after measles compared with vaccination was 29 overall; for measles before 1 yr of age it was more than 100. In cases occurring in vaccinated children, it has not been determined whether SSPE resulted from persistent infection with the attenuated measles virus of the vaccine, from undiagnosed wild-type measles infection preceding vaccination, or from vaccine failure and subsequent undiagnosed measles. SSPE continues to occur in ar-

■ TABLE 228–1 Slow Infections of the Nervous System Caused by Conventional Viruses

Disease	Virus	Viral Group
	RNA Viruses	
AIDS encephalopathy	HIV-1	Retrovirus
Kozhevnikov epilepsy (and other chronic forms of tick-borne encephalitis)	Tick-borne encephalitis	Flavivirus
Progressive rubella panencephalitis	Rubella	Rubivirus
Rabies	Rabies	Rhabdovirus
Subacute sclerosing panencephalitis	Measles	Paramyxovirus
Tropical spastic paraparesis and HTLV-I–associated myelopathy	HTLV-I	Retrovirus
	DNA Viruses	
CMV encephalitis	CMV	Herpesvirus
Progressive multifocal leukoencephalitis	JCV	Papovavirus

AIDS = acquired immunodeficiency syndrome; HTLV-I = human T-cell leukemia-lymphoma virus type I; CMV = cytomegalovirus; HIV-1 = human immunodeficiency virus type 1; JCV = J-C virus.

eas of the world in which measles remains unchecked and may be anticipated to increase wherever compliance with vaccination diminishes.

PATHOLOGY. The histopathology of SSPE consists of inflammation, necrosis, and repair. Brain biopsy performed in the early stages of SSPE shows mild inflammation of the meninges and a panencephalitis involving cortical and subcortical gray matter as well as white matter, with cuffs of plasma cells and lymphocytes around blood vessels (Fig. 228–1) and increased numbers of glia throughout. Neuronal loss may not be marked until later in the course of illness, when loss of myelin secondary to neuronal degeneration may be apparent. Intranuclear inclusion bodies surrounded by clear halos (Cowdry type A) may be seen within the nuclei of neurons, astrocytes, and oligodendrocytes. By electron microscopy, the inclusions are seen to contain tubular structures typical of the nucleocapsids of paramyxoviruses. Measles viral antigens can be demonstrated by labeled antibody techniques within the inclusions as well as in cells without inclusions. Lesions may be unevenly distributed throughout the brain, and biopsy is not always diagnostic.

The same findings of inclusion-body panencephalitis are generally present at autopsy; however, late in the disease it may be difficult to find typical areas of inflammation, and the main histopathologic changes are necrosis and gliosis. The disease is believed to begin in the cortical gray matter, progressing then to the subcortical white and gray matter (myoclonus probably results from extrapyramidal involvement) and finally to the lower structures. Although persistent infection of lymphoid tissues with measles virus has been reported, these show no pathologic changes.

PATHOGENESIS. It has been proposed that some mutation may render the measles virus more likely to establish persistent infection, and multiple mutations have been found in isolates from patients with SSPE. However, no consistent genomic abnormalities have been identified in those isolates, and clusters of SSPE cases suggestive of strains of special virulence have been described only rarely. It has also been theorized that patients with SSPE have some subtle predisposing immune deficiency; the markedly increased risk of SSPE after measles in infancy suggests that either immunologic immaturity or persistence of maternal antibodies to measles virus is involved in the later occurrence of the disease.

Complete measles virus particles are not found in the brains of patients with SSPE, and the matrix (M) protein required for the final assembly and budding of virus from the host cells is missing not only from brain tissues of patients but also from cells cultured from their brains; however, the full complement of genetic material needed to code for all proteins, including the M protein, is present and functional. Several studies suggested that M proteins are encoded but that, because of a variety of mutations—mostly U to C shifts—they cannot bind to nucleocapsid, resulting in the accumulation of incomplete measles virus that cannot be cleared either by antibodies or by cell-mediated immunity.

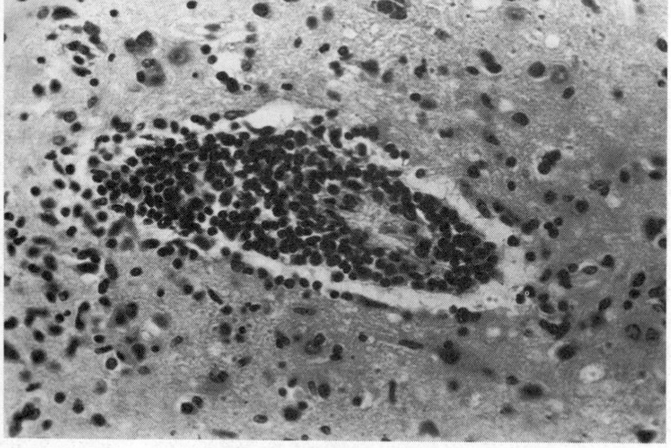

Figure 228–1. A cuff of inflammatory cells surrounds a blood vessel in the cerebral cortex of a child with subacute sclerosing panencephalitis. (Courtesy of Janice Stevens, MD, National Institute of Mental Health, and Peggy Swoveland, MD, University of Maryland School of Medicine.)

CLINICAL MANIFESTATIONS. Children with SSPE generally have a history of typical measles with full recovery several years before the onset of neurologic disease. Measles may have been either mild or severe. Some patients with SSPE have had measles pneumonia, but none has had a history of typical measles encephalitis. The mean interval between measles and onset of SSPE was formerly about 7 yr, but recently it has increased to 12 yr. In vaccinated patients without a history of measles, the mean interval between vaccination and onset of SSPE was 5 yr before 1980 and 7.7 yr between 1980 and 1986.

The clinical picture of SSPE tends to be quite stereotypic; almost 70% of cases have an acute, subacute, or chronic progressive course; fewer than 10% have remissions. The onset is usually insidious, marked by subtle changes in behavior and deterioration of schoolwork, followed by more overtly bizarre behavior and finally by frank dementia.

There is no fever, photophobia, or other findings of acute encephalitis except for occasional complaints of headache. Diffuse neurologic disease becomes progressively more severe. The appearance of massive, repetitive myoclonic jerks, generally symmetric, involving especially the axial musculature and occurring at 5- to 10-s intervals, marks the onset of a second clinical stage of SSPE. The myoclonic jerks appear to be abnormal movements rather than epileptic seizures, but true convulsions can also occur at any stage of the illness. In addition to myoclonic jerks, which tend to disappear as the disease progresses, a variety of other abnormal movements and dystonias have also been observed. Cerebellar ataxia may occur. Retinopathy and optic atrophy may appear, sometimes even before behavioral changes. Dementia progresses to stupor and coma, sometimes with autonomic insufficiency. Patients may be rigid or spastic with decorticate postures, or they may be flaccid.

The speed of progression is highly variable, but in at least 60% of patients the course is inexorable and relatively rapid. The total duration of illness may be as short as a few months, but most patients survive for 1–3 yr after diagnosis, with a mean of about 18 mo. Occasional patients show some spontaneous improvement and live for more than 10 yr. In recent years, the few patients diagnosed with SSPE in the United States tended to have a relatively long survival perhaps because of improvements in chronic care.

LABORATORY DIAGNOSIS. The blood is normal except for elevated titers of antibodies to measles virus; antibodies are of the immunoglobulin (Ig) G and IgM classes and are directed against all the component proteins of measles virus except the M protein. Cell content of the cerebrospinal fluid (CSF) is generally normal, although stained sediments may show plasma cells. Total protein content of the CSF is normal or only slightly elevated; however, the gamma globulin fraction is greatly elevated (usually comprising at least 20% of total protein), resulting in a paretic type of colloidal gold curve. When the CSF is examined by electrophoresis or isoelectric focusing, "oligoclonal" bands of Ig are often observed. IgG and IgM antibodies to measles virus, not normally found in unconcentrated CSF, make up most of the Ig, and these can often be detected in dilutions of 1:8 or more. The complement fixation test has been especially useful for demonstrating antibodies in CSF, but hemagglutination inhibition, immunofluorescence, and other serologic tests, including enzyme-labeled immunosorbent assays (ELISA), are also satisfactory. The normal ratio of titer in serum to titer in CSF is reduced (below 200) for measles antibodies, whereas serum-CSF ratios are normal for other viral antibodies and for albumin, indicating that the increased amounts of measles antibodies in the CSF of patients with SSPE result from synthesis within the nervous system and that the blood-brain barrier is normal.

Early in the course of disease, the electroencephalogram (EEG) may be normal or show only moderate, nonspecific slowing. In the myoclonic stage, most patients with SSPE have "suppression-burst, episodes" in which high-amplitude slow and sharp waves recur at intervals of 3–5 s on a slow background; however, this pattern is not unique to SSPE. Later in the illness, the EEG becomes increasingly disorganized and shows high-amplitude, random dysrhythmic slowing; in terminal disease, the amplitude may fall.

Computed tomograms or magnetic resonance images of patients with SSPE may show variable cortical atrophy and ventricular enlargement, and there may be focal or multifocal low-density lesions in white matter. However, these studies may be normal, especially early in the disease.

Brain biopsy is no longer needed to diagnose SSPE. When performed, it will often show the typical histopathologic findings described earlier. Examination of frozen sections by immunofluorescence technique may demonstrate the presence of measles viral antigens. Persistence of measles virus infection in cultures may be demonstrated by labeled antibody techniques before the complete virus appears. Many specimens fail to yield complete virus. Modifications of the polymerase chain reaction can detect various regions of the measles virus RNA in frozen and even paraffin-embedded brain tissue specimens of patients with SSPE. Nucleic acid hybridization techniques have also been used to demonstrate the measles viral genome.

DIFFERENTIAL DIAGNOSIS. It is most important to rule out potentially treatable illnesses such as bacterial infections and tumors. The diverse cerebral storage diseases and nonstorage poliodystrophies, leukodystrophies, and demyelinating diseases of childhood can also produce progressive dementia with seizures and paralysis resembling SSPE. Early in the course of illness, SSPE must be distinguished from atypical acute viral encephalitides. Other slow viral infections, such as Creutzfeldt-Jakob disease (CJD) and progressive rubella panencephalitis, must be considered in appropriate age groups. The presence of a typical EEG pattern is suggestive of SSPE, as are unusually high levels of measles antibodies in serum. The diagnosis is practically confirmed if measles antibodies are detected in CSF.

COMPLICATIONS. Patients with SSPE have the usual secondary complications associated with incapacitating neurologic diseases, such as pneumonias and decubitus ulcers.

INFECTIVITY AND PRECAUTIONS. The persistent measles infection in SSPE does not result in complete virus particles. Patients with SSPE, therefore, pose no hazard of infection to others, and no special precautions need ordinarily be taken. Blood precautions might be justified under special circumstances.

PREVENTION. Immunization with existing attenuated measles virus vaccines prevents the large majority of cases of SSPE.

PROGNOSIS. As noted earlier, few patients live for more than 3 yr after the diagnosis of SSPE is first made, and those who do survive longer are usually disabled.

THERAPY. Administration of inosiplex may increase the number of patients with prolonged survival and may produce some clinical improvement in the degree of resulting disability (100 mg/kg/24 hr given in divided doses; improvement has been claimed with lower doses as well). Several studies claimed that the progression of SSPE was slowed after intrathecal or intraventricular injections with interferon alpha with or without oral inosiplex. Cimetidine was reported to slow progression in a single study. None of these therapies has been reported to stop the progression of SSPE or to reverse it. Other treatments have been ineffective. The use of anticonvulsants, maintenance of nutritional status, prompt treatment of secondary bacterial infections, physical therapy, and other supportive care may also prolong survival and improve the quality of life for the patient and family. Information on current therapeutic trials can be obtained from the U.S. National SSPE Registry (Dr. Paul R. Dyken, Institute for Research in Childhood Neurodegenerative Diseases, Mobile, Alabama).

Progressive Rubella Panencephalitis

An exceedingly rare chronic encephalitis is associated with persistent rubella virus infection of the brain. Since the disease was first recognized in 1974 20 cases have been reported, all involving males between the ages of 8 and 21 yr at onset; most had typical stigmata of the congenital rubella syndrome including cataracts, deafness, and mental retardation, but two had childhood rubella from which they made a full recovery. No new cases have been described in the United States in recent years presumably resulting from marked reductions in congenital and childhood rubella because of immunization.

CLINICAL MANIFESTATIONS. At onset, progressive rubella panencephalitis resembles SSPE, with insidious changes in behavior and deterioration in school performance. Subsequently, frank dementia and other signs of multifocal brain disease occur, including seizures, cerebellar ataxia, and spastic weakness. Myoclonus and other abnormal movements may occur but are not as common as in SSPE. Retinopathy, similar to that seen in acute rubella, and optic atrophy may occur. The course of illness in progressive rubella panencephalitis is similar to that seen in SSPE, progressing to coma, spasticity, brain stem involvement, and death in 2–5 yr. The peripheral blood is normal in progressive rubella panencephalitis except for elevated titers of antibodies to rubella virus. The CSF shows normal or slightly elevated cell content; CSF protein is slightly elevated, with a marked increase in globulin, which may make up more than 50% of the total protein. Oligoclonal electrophoretic bands of globulin are found in the CSF of progressive rubella panencephalitis patients; the bands resemble those seen in SSPE but consist of antibodies to rubella virus antigens. Antibodies to rubella virus are readily detectable in CSF, often at dilutions of 1:8 or higher. The complement fixation, hemagglutination inhibition, and ELISA techniques should be satisfactory for testing the spinal fluid. Most of the rubella antibodies in the CSF are IgG, although some IgM antibodies have also been detected early in the course of progressive rubella panencephalitis. The serum-CSF ratio of antibody titers to rubella virus is reduced, whereas ratios of titers to measles and other viruses are normal.

The EEG shows a generalized slowing with occasional high-voltage activity, but the suppression-burst pattern of SSPE has not been seen in progressive rubella panencephalitis. Encephalograms (computed tomograms were not available when published cases were studied) show enlargement of all ventricles, especially the fourth, with prominent atrophy of the cerebellum.

PATHOLOGY. Histopathologic changes seen in the brains of patients with progressive rubella panencephalitis are similar to those seen in SSPE, with cuffs of lymphocytes and plasma cells around blood vessels, glial nodules in the cortex, some loss of neurons, an increase in astrocytes throughout the gray matter, and an even greater increase in the white matter. However, in progressive rubella panencephalitis, there are no inclusion bodies, and deposits of material that stains with the periodic acid–Schiff reaction are found around vessels in subcortical white matter.

DIAGNOSIS. Rubella virus has been isolated from brain cell cultures and from separated blood lymphocytes. *Differential diagnosis* of progressive rubella panencephalitis is the same as that for SSPE. The stigmata of congenital rubella syndrome or a history of German measles suggests progressive rubella panencephalitis. Elevated levels of rubella antibodies in serum, the presence of oligoclonal bands of gamma globulins and rubella antibodies in the spinal fluid, and a reduction in the normal serum-CSF ratio for antibodies to rubella virus establish the diagnosis of progressive rubella panencephalitis. Isolation of rubella virus from blood lymphocytes may be attempted. Brain biopsy should not be needed to establish the diagnosis.

Patients with progressive rubella panencephalitis pose no substantial risk of infection to others, although it seems reasonable to avoid exposing rubella-susceptible persons to the blood of patients with the disease. Rubella virus has not been detected in their urine.

OTHER CHRONIC CONVENTIONAL VIRAL INFECTIONS OF THE NERVOUS SYSTEM

CHRONIC TICK-BORNE ENCEPHALITIS (TBE). The virus of TBE, a member of the flavivirus group of small, enveloped RNA viruses, usually causes an acute meningoencephalomyelitis, also called Russian spring-summer encephalitis, that may be of variable severity. As many as 20% of patients recover from acute encephalitis only to experience new signs of progressive neurologic disease months or even years later. Most cases of chronic progressive TBE have been reported from Russia, but two typical patients were described in Japan. Chronic progressive TBE may have the following clinical manifestations: (1) movement or seizure disorders of which epilepsia partialis continua (Kozhevnikov epilepsy) is the most common; (2) paralytic disorders, often with brain stem involvement; and (3) mixed syndromes. The seizure and movement disorders may stabilize or remit, but the progressive paralytic syndrome is usually fatal. The CSF in one patient with chronic TBE contained elevated levels of antibodies to TBE virus. Brain tissue shows panencephalitis without inclusion bodies by light microscopy and no virus-like structures by electron microscopy. Isolation of TBE virus has occasionally been reported from the brain tissue or CSF of patients with chronic post-TBE syndromes, but most attempts to isolate the virus failed.

RASMUSSEN ENCEPHALITIS. Patients with similar types of chronic encephalitis not associated with any known viral infection have been recognized throughout the world. In North America, a syndrome of seizures (especially epilepsia partialis continua), spastic paralysis, and mental retardation associated with chronic encephalitis was described by Rasmussen and colleagues in children, adolescents, and young adults. Patients had no history of preceding acute encephalitis. Computed tomography may show cerebral cortical atrophy or ventricular dilatation, and when brain tissue is resected a panencephalitis without inclusion bodies or virus-like particles is found. A few cases of Rasmussen encephalitis were attributed to infections with Epstein-Barr virus and cytomegalovirus, although those claims were not confirmed. Efforts to isolate viruses from brains of patients with Rasmussen encephalitis have been unsuccessful. One study suggested that an autoimmune process, with circulating antibodies to glutamate receptors, may underlie some cases of Rasmussen encephalitis, and plasma exchanges to reduce the amounts of those antibodies were reported to improve the epilepsy in one patient.

PROGRESSIVE MULTIFOCAL LEUKOENCEPHALOPATHY (PML). This progressive infection of oligodendroglial cells with the JC papovavirus affects immunosuppressed subjects, in whom it is almost invariably fatal. It is even more rare in children than in adults. PML is a well-recognized opportunistic infection frequently complicating acquired immunodeficiency syndrome (AIDS) in adults, but it affects children much less often in spite of the fact that many children have had inapparent infections with the JC virus.

PERSISTENT RETROVIRAL INFECTIONS. The lentivirus human immunodeficiency virus type 1 frequently produces both an acute encephalitis at the time of primary infection and a progressive encephalopathy that is, unfortunately, very common in both adults and children with AIDS (see Chapter 223).

The human T-cell leukemia-lymphoma virus (HTLV-I) has been implicated as the cause of a progressive myelopathy called both tropical spastic paraparesis (TSP) and HTLV-I–associated myopathy (HAM). Although TSP or HAM is much more common among adults, it also occurs in children. HTLV-I may also cause meningoencephalitis and myositis, although these entities have not been observed in children. Recently, an infective dermatitis in children has been attributed to infection with HTLV-I. Infections with HTLV-I are more often completely asymptomatic at least for very long periods of time. The spread of infection with HTLV-I may be reduced by excluding individuals with antibodies to the virus from donating blood and by limiting breast-feeding by infected mothers, when it is practical to do so. HTLV-I is also spread sexually, and campaigns to control HIV may serve to reduce its transmission as well.

SLOW INFECTIONS WITH UNCONVENTIONAL VIRUSES: THE SUBACUTE SPONGIFORM ENCEPHALOPATHIES

The subacute spongiform encephalopathies consist of at least two diseases affecting humans—kuru and CJD and its variant, the Gerstmann-Sträussler-Scheinker (GSS) syndrome—and four affecting animals, the most common and best known of which are scrapie of sheep and bovine spongiform encephalopathy. (It has been proposed that another human neurologic disease—the fatal familial insomnia syndrome—be added to the list; that disease is discussed briefly later under Genetic Counseling.) All spongiform encephalopathies have similarities in clinical manifestations and histopathology, and all are slow infections. The most striking neuropathologic change that occurs in each disease, to a greater or lesser extent, is spongy degeneration of the cerebral cortical gray matter.

Kuru once affected many children and adolescents in a restricted area of Papua New Guinea; its transmission was interrupted 35 yr ago, and it is now found only in older adults. CJD, the most common human spongiform encephalopathy, was formerly thought to occur only in older adults; however, iatrogenically transmitted cases of CJD have been recognized in adolescents and young adults. GSS syndrome, a familial spongiform encephalopathy characterized by striking amyloid plaques and more prominent cerebellar ataxia and a longer mean duration than typical sporadic CJD, may be considered a variant of that disease. GSS has not been diagnosed in children or adolescents.

ETIOLOGY. The spongiform encephalopathies are all slow infections that are transmissible to susceptible animals by inoculation of tissues from affected subjects. Although the infectious agents replicate in some cell cultures, they do not achieve the high titers of infectivity found in brain tissues or cause recognizable cytopathic effects. Most studies of spongiform encephalopathy agents use in vivo assays in which the appearance of typical scrapie or CJD in animals is taken as evidence that the agent is present and intact. Inoculation of the smallest amounts of infectivity of all of these agents in tissues of recipient animals results in the accumulation of large amounts of an agent having the same physical and biologic properties as the original agent.

Until recently, the self-replicating pathogens transmitting the spongiform encephalopathies were generally considered viruses, and they still are by many authorities. However, they display a spectrum of extreme resistance to inactivation by a variety of chemical and physical treatments that is unknown among other viruses. This characteristic stimulated the hypothesis that the spongiform encephalopathy agents might be unique infectious pathogens, probably subviral in size, composed of protein and devoid of nucleic acid. An alternative designation, "prion," has been suggested for such agents. However, the prion hypothesis is not universally accepted. The size and structure of the infectious agent and the presence or absence of a nucleic acid genome have not yet been established. If the spongiform encephalopathy agents ultimately prove to contain nucleic acid genomes, they might still be considered atypical viruses. Until the actual structure of the pathogens is clearly determined, it is less contentious simply to call them agents.

Scrapie-associated fibrils (SAFs) are found in extracts of tissues from a variety of patients and animals with spongiform encephalopathies but not in normal tissues. SAFs resemble but are distinguishable from the amyloid fibrils that accumulate in the brains of patients with Alzheimer disease (AD). A group of antigenically related, low molecular weight proteins, originally designated the "prion protein 27-30" (PrP27-30), are components of SAFs and are consistently found in the amyloid plaques seen in the brains of patients and animals with spongiform encephalopathies. It is not yet clear whether SAF-PrP constitute the complete infectious particle of spongiform encephalopathies or components of those particles or whether they are simply pathologic host proteins not usually separated from the actual infectious entities by currently used techniques. The demonstration that the PrP protein is encoded by a normal host gene favors the last possibility. However, other studies purport to suggest that agent-specific information can be transmitted and replicated in the absence of genetic material independent of the host.

Whatever its relationship to the actual infectious particles, SAF-PrP is extremely important in the pathogenesis of spongiform encephalopathies. It is a glycoprotein that has the physical properties of an amyloid protein. The PrP proteins of several species of animals are very similar in their amino acid sequences and antigenicity but are not identical in structure. The primary structure of PrP is encoded by the host and does not appear to be influenced by the source of the infectious agent provoking its formation. PrP27-30 is derived by cleavage from a larger precursor protein, which differs in properties between normal subjects (in which it is sensitive to digestion with the proteolytic enzyme proteinase K) and those with spongiform encephalopathies (in which it is resistant) but not in primary aminoacid sequence. The function of the PrP precursor in normal cells is unknown. It may play a role in synaptic transmission, but it is not required for life or for relatively normal cerebral function. Expression of PrP does seem to be required for development of scrapie disease in mice and probably for replication of the transmissible agent. The relationship between mutations in the gene coding for PrP and familial spongiform encephalopathies is discussed later under Genetic Counseling.

Attempts to find particles consistent with those of viruses or virus-like agents in brain tissues of humans or animals with spongiform encephalopathies have generally been unsuccessful. Peculiar tubulovesicles have been seen in thin sections and unique tiny particles demonstrated recently in negatively stained extracts of infected brain tissue, but it has not been established that either of those structures is specifically associated with infectivity.

EPIDEMIOLOGY AND MECHANISMS OF TRANSMISSION. The disappearance of kuru among young people suggests that the practice of ritual cannibalism was the most important if not the only mechanism by which the infection spread in Papua New Guinea.

CJD has been recognized worldwide, at rates of 0.25–2 cases per million population per year, with foci of considerably higher incidence among Libyan Jews in Israel, in isolated villages of Slovakia, and in other limited areas. Epidemiologic surveys have investigated several hypothetical mechanisms of spread of CJD, including contamination of meat products with scrapie agent and iatrogenic infection from tissues of patients. The striking resemblance of CJD to scrapie prompted the suggestion that infected sheep tissues might be a source of spongiform encephalopathy in humans. In addition, the outbreak of spongiform encephalopathy among cattle (which were apparently infected by eating scrapie-contaminated bone meal), zoo animals, and domestic cats in Great Britain raised a fear that some strain of the scrapie agent, having crossed a species barrier from sheep to cattle, may have acquired an even broader range of susceptible hosts, posing a potential danger for humans. Although no transmission of spongiform encephalopathy from animals to humans has ever been documented, it seems reasonable to avoid exposing children to meat and meat products likely to be contaminated with spongiform encephalopathy agents.

In contrast, iatrogenic transmission of CJD has been established. Accidental transmission of CJD has occurred by means of contaminated neurosurgical instruments or operating facilities, transplantation of contaminated cornea, contaminated cortical electrodes used during epilepsy surgery, injections of human pituitary growth hormone and human pituitary gonadotropin, and grafts of cadaver dura mater. Pharmaceuticals and grafts derived from or contaminated with human neural tissues, particularly when obtained from unselected donors and from large pools of donors, pose special risks.

Spouses and household contacts of patients are at very low risk of acquiring CJD, although two instances of conjugal CJD have been reported. Medical personnel exposed to brains of patients with CJD may be at some increased risk, and the disease has been recognized in a neurosurgeon, a pathologist, two histopathology technicians, and at least 16 other health care workers.

PATHOLOGY. Typical changes include vacuolation and loss of neurons with hypertrophy and proliferation of glial cells, most pronounced in the cerebral cortex in patients with CJD and in the cerebellum in those with kuru. The lesions are usually most severe in or even confined to gray matter, at least early in the disease. Loss of myelin appears to be secondary to degeneration of neurons. There is usually no inflammation, but there is a marked increase in the number and size of astrocytes. "Amyloid" plaques are found in the brains of all patients with GSS, in at least 70% of patients with kuru, and less commonly in those with CJD. They are most common in the cerebellum but occur elsewhere in the brain as well. The plaques react with antisera prepared against SAF-PrP, and even in the absence of plaques extracellular SAF-PrP has been detected by immunostaining.

PATHOGENESIS. The portal of entry for the kuru agent is thought to be the integument probably through lesions rather than intact skin and mucosa. It is not known whether humans can be infected with spongiform encephalopathies through the intestinal tract. The first site of replication of the agents appears to be the tissues of the reticuloendothelial system. The CJD agent has been detected in human blood, but it is not clear whether "viremia" is responsible for the spread of infection to the nervous system. Limited evidence suggests that in mice the scrapie agent spreads to the central nervous system by ascending peripheral nerves. In human kuru, it seems highly probable that the only portal of exit of the agent from the body, at least in quantities sufficient to infect others, was through tissues exposed during cannibalism. In iatrogenically transmitted CJD, the brains and eyes of patients with CJD have been the sources of contamination. Kidney, liver, lung, lymph node, spleen, and CSF also sometimes contain the agent. At no time during the course of illness have antibodies or cell-mediated immunity to the infectious agents of the spongiform encephalopathies been convincingly demonstrated in either patients or animals.

CLINICAL MANIFESTATIONS. Kuru is a progressive degenerative disease of the cerebellum and brain stem, with less obvious involvement of the cerebral cortex. The first sign of kuru is usually cerebella ataxia followed by progressive incoordination. Coarse shivering tremors are a characteristic manifestation. Variable abnormalities in cranial nerve function appear, with frequent impairment in conjugate gaze and swallowing. Patients die from inanition and pneumonia or from burns from cooking fires, usually less than 1 yr after onset. Although changes in mentation are common, there is no frank dementia or progression to coma as in CJD. There are no signs of acute encephalitis (e.g., no fever, headaches, or convulsions).

CJD occurs throughout the world. Patients initially have either sensory disturbances or confusion and inappropriate behavior, with progression over weeks or months to frank dementia and ultimately coma. Some patients have cerebellar ataxia early in disease, and most experience myoclonic jerking movements. GSS is a familial disease resembling CJD but with more prominent cerebellar ataxia and amyloid plaques; dementia may appear only late in the course. Mean survival of patients with CJD is less than 1 yr from the earliest signs of illness, although about 10% live for more than 2 yr. Patients with GSS tend to survive longer.

LABORATORY FINDINGS. Virtually all patients with CJD have abnormal EEG findings as the disease progresses; the background becomes slow and irregular with diminished amplitude. A variety of paroxysmal discharges may also appear: slow waves, sharp waves, and spike-and-wave complexes; these may sometimes be unilateral or focal as well as bilaterally synchronous. Paroxysmal discharges may be precipitated by loud noise. Many patients have typical periodic suppression-burst complexes of high-voltage slow activity on EEG at some time during the illness. Computed tomography may show cortical atrophy and large ventricles late in the course of CJD. There may be some elevation of CSF protein. Unusual protein spots have been observed in CSF specimens after two-dimensional separation in gels and silver staining; the spots, never identified, are not unique for CJD, but they have not been found in fluids from patients with AD. (Unfortunately, two-dimensional gel separation of CSF proteins remains a research technique.) Abnormal liver function studies in CJD patients sometimes suggest hepatic parenchymal disease.

DIAGNOSIS. Diagnosis of spongiform encephalopathies is most often made on clinical grounds after ruling out other diseases. The presence of abnormal protein spots in CSF may aid in distinguishing between CJD and AD, the most difficult differential diagnosis. Brain biopsy may be diagnostic of CJD, but it should be recommended only if some other potentially treatable disease remains to be excluded. Definitive diagnosis requires microscopic examination of brain tissue obtained at autopsy. The demonstration of SAF or PrP proteins in brain extracts is useful for confirming the histopathologic diagnosis. Transmission of disease to susceptible animals by inoculation of brain suspension is the ultimate diagnostic test for spongiform encephalopathy, although it is usually reserved for cases of special research interest.

PREVENTION, CONTAINMENT, AND DISINFECTION. Universal precautions should be used for handling blood and body fluids. All materials and surfaces known to be contaminated with tissues or CSF from patients suspected of having CJD must be treated with great care. Whenever possible, contaminated instruments should be discarded by careful packaging and transport to sites of incineration. Contaminated tissues and biologic products probably cannot be completely freed of infectivity without destroying their structural integrity and biologic activity; therefore, the medical and family histories of individual tissue donors should be carefully reviewed for dementia. Although no method of sterilization can be relied on to remove all infectivity from contaminated surfaces, exposure to heat, sodium hydroxide, chlorine bleach, concentrated formic acid, and a commercial phenolic disinfectant may markedly reduce infectivity.

TREATMENT. No treatment is effective. Appropriate supportive care should be provided as for other progressive fatal neurologic diseases.

PROGNOSIS. The prognosis of spongiform encephalopathies is uniformly poor. Perhaps 10% of patients survive for a year or even longer, but their quality of life is poor.

GENETIC COUNSELING. Spongiform encephalopathies sometimes run in families, with a pattern of occurrence consistent with an autosomal dominant mode of inheritance. In patients with a family history of CJD, the clinical and histopathologic findings are the same as those seen in sporadic cases. In the United States only about 10% of cases are familial. GSS is always familial. In some affected families, about 50% of siblings and children of a CJD patient eventually acquire the disease; in other families, the "penetrance" of illness is somewhat less.

The gene coding for PrP is closely linked if not identical to that controlling the incubation periods of scrapie in sheep and both scrapie and CJD in mice. The gene encoding the analogous protein in humans, currently designated the PRNP gene, is located on the short arm of chromosome 20. It has an open reading frame of 759 nucleotides (253 codons) in which 10 different point mutations, as well as a variety of inserted sequences encoding extra tandem repeated octapeptides, have been linked to the occurrence of spongiform encephalopathy in families.

Although the interpretation of these findings in regard to the prion hypothesis is in dispute, in affected families with an autosomal dominant pattern of CJD or GSS, subjects who are heterozygous for linked mutations in the PRNP gene clearly have a high probability of acquiring spongiform encephalopathy. The significance of mutations in the PRNP genes of subjects from families that have no history of spongiform encephalopathy is not known. It seems wise to avoid alarming subjects who have miscellaneous mutations in the PRNP gene or their families because the implications are not yet clear.

Another neurologic syndrome, called fatal familial insomnia (FFI), which also occurs with an autosomal dominant pattern of inheritance, was described. Patients with FFI have severe insomnia and progressive autonomic insufficiency, and some have ataxia and myoclonus resembling those in GSS and CJD. Status spongiosus is not a striking finding at autopsy, and cerebral degeneration is largely restricted to thalamic nuclei. The same nucleotide substitution at codon 178 of the PRNP gene associated with CJD in some families has been found in all patients with FFI, linked, however, to a different aminoacid-encoding sequence at codon 129. It has been suggested that FFI be grouped together with the spongiform encephalopathies as a new prion disease. However, thus far, attempts to transmit disease to primates from brain tissues of patients with FFI have been unsuccessful.

OTHER DEGENERATIVE DISEASES OF THE CENTRAL NERVOUS SYSTEM POSSIBLY CAUSED BY UNCONVENTIONAL VIRUSES

It has been claimed that two other human diseases may be caused by infections with agents similar to those causing the spongiform encephalopathies—familial AD of adults and Alper disease of young children. The latter is a convulsive disorder associated with hemiatrophy and status spongiosus of the cerebral gray matter. Attempts to confirm those claims have failed.

Asher DM: Slow viral infections of the central nervous system. *In:* Scheld WM, Whitley RJ, Durack DT (eds): Infections of the Central Nervous System. New York, Raven Press, 1991, pp 145–166.

Asher DM, Gajdusek DC: Virologic studies in chronic encephalitis. *In:* Andermann F (ed) Chronic Encephalitis and Epilepsy: Rasmussen's Syndrome. Boston, Butterworth-Heinemann, 1991, pp 147–158.

Brown P, Cervenakova L, Goldfarb LG, et al: Iatrogenic Creutzfeldt-Jakob disease—An example of the interplay between ancient genes and modern medicine. Neurology 44:291, 1994.

Brown P, Gibbs C Jr, Rodgers-Johnson P, et al: Human spongiform encephalopathy: The NIH series of 300 cases of experimentally transmitted disease. Ann Neurol 35:513, 1994.
Brown P, Kaur P, Sulima MP, et al: Real and imagined clinicopathological limits of prion dementia. Lancet 341:127, 1993.
Dyken PR, Cunningham SC, Ward LC: Changing character of subacute sclerosing panencephalitis in the United States. Pediatr Neurol 5:339, 1989.
Gajdusek DC: Infectious amyloids: Subacute spongiform encephalopathies as transmissible cerebral amyloidoses. *In:* Fields BN, Knipe DM (eds): Virology, Vol 2, 3rd ed. New York, Raven Press, 1995.
Major EO, Amemiya K, Tornatore CS, et al: Pathogenesis and molecular biology of progressive multifocal leukoencephalopathy, the JC virus-induced demyelinating disease of the human brain. Clin Microbiol Rev 5:49, 1992.
Monari L, Chen SG, Brown P, et al: Fatal familial insomnia and familial Creutzfeldt-Jakob disease—Different prion proteins determined by a DNA polymorphism. Proc Natl Acad Sci USA 91:2839, 1994.
Prusiner SB: Genetic and infectious prion diseases. Arch Neurol 50:1129, 1993.
Rasmussen TB: Chronic encephalitis and seizures: Historical introduction. *In:* Andermann F (ed): Chronic Encephalitis and Epilepsy: Rasmussen's Syndrome. Boston, Butterworth-Heinemann, 1991, pp 1–4.
Rogers SW, Andrews PI, Gahring LC, et al: Autoantibodies to glutamate receptor GluR3 in Rasmussen's encephalitis. Science 265:648, 1994.
Rohwer R: The scrapie agent: "A virus by any other name." Curr Top Microbiol Immunol 172:195, 1991.
Wolinsky JS: Subacute sclerosing panencephalitis, progressive rubella panencephalitis, and multifocal leukoencephalopathy. Res Publ Assoc Res Nerv Ment Dis 68:259, 1990.

SECTION 5
Mycotic Infections

CHAPTER 229
Candida

Martin Weisse and Stephen C. Aronoff

MICROBIOLOGY. Candidiasis is caused by several species of the genus *Candida*, which is a part of the larger group of Fungi Imperfecti, or *Deuteromycetes*. *Candida* exists in three morphological forms: oval to round blastospores or yeast cells (3–6 μm in diameter); double-walled chlamydospores (7–17 mm in diameter) usually at the terminal end of a pseudohyphae; and pseudomycelium, which is a mass of pseudohyphae and represents the tissue phase of *Candida*. The most common species implicated in human disease is *C. albicans*, but *C. parapsilosis, C. tropicalis, C. krusei, C. lusitaniae*, and several other species have been reported as pathogens. In addition, *Torulopsis glabrata* has now been subsumed into the genus of *Candida*.

The former genus name was *Monilia*, and the term *moniliasis* is still used occasionally to describe skin or mucous membrane infection caused by *Candida*.

229.1 Neonatal Infection

Thrush, or oral pseudomembranous candidiasis, is a superficial mucous membrane infection that affects approximately 2–5% of normal newborns. Infants acquire *Candida* from their mothers at delivery, and thrush develops 7–10 days later. The use of antibiotics, especially in the 1st year of life, may lead to recurrent or persistent thrush. The plaques of thrush superficially invade the mucosa and may be found on the lips, buccal mucosa, tongue, and palate. Removal of plaques from these surfaces may cause mild punctate areas of bleeding, which helps to confirm the diagnosis. Thrush may cause pain, fussiness, and decreased feeding but may be asymptomatic. Treatment of mild cases may not be necessary. Initial treatment is usually with nystatin suspension; painting the affected areas with gentian violet may be necessary for recalcitrant infections.

Diaper dermatitis is the most common infection caused by *Candida*. Primary infection is generally in the intertriginous areas of the perineum and presents as a confluent, papular erythema with red satellite papules. *Candida* diaper dermatitis is often seen complicating oral antibiotic treatment of otitis media and may also secondarily infect any other noninfectious diaper dermatitis. Many physicians will presumptively treat any diaper rash that has been present for 3 or more days for *Candida*. Treatment is usually with a topical antifungal such as nystatin or clotrimazole (or other); if there is significant inflammation, the addition of hydrocortisone 1% may be useful for the first day or two.

Congenital candidiasis occurs in normal neonates and presents as widespread skin involvement, especially in the intertriginous areas. The rash is maculopapular, with some vesicles and pustules from which *Candida* may be recovered. There is usually little or no mucous membrane involvement, and topical antifungal therapy is usually all that is necessary. Pneumonia only rarely occurs and is a grave prognostic sign. The pathogenesis of congenital candidiasis is presumably an ascending infection from a mother with heavy colonization or vulvar infection with *Candida*.

229.2 Infection in the Normal Host

Oral thrush is usually not a problem for the child older than 12 mo but may occur in the child treated with oral antibiotics. Persistent or recurrent thrush without an obvious predisposing reason, such as recent antibiotic treatment, warrants investigation of an underlying condition such as diabetes mellitus or immunodeficiency. As stated previously treatment is with nystatin or gentian violet.

Paronychia and *onychomycosis* may be due to *Candida*, although this is much less common than periungual infection resulting from *Trichophyton* or *Epidermophyton*. Candidal onychomycoses differ from tinea infections by the propensity to affect the fingernails and not the toenails and the associated paronychia. In addition, once tinea becomes established, it must be treated systemically with griseofulvin, whereas candidal infections often respond to keeping the hands dry and treating with topical antifungal therapy. Systemic therapy with an oral azole antifungal may be necessary, but treatment duration is usually much shorter than that required for tinea onychomycosis.

Vulvovaginitis is a common candidal infection of pubertal and postpubertal females, affecting as many as 75% of females at one time or another (see Chapter 503). Predisposing factors are pregnancy, oral contraceptives, poor hygiene, and oral antibiotics. When prepubertal girls suffer from this condition, a predisposing factor such as diabetes mellitus or prolonged antibiotic treatment is usually present. Clinical manifestations may include pain or itching, dysuria, vulvar or vaginal erythema, an opaque white or cheesy exudate, and thrushlike mucosal plaques. Candidal vulvovaginitis can be effectively treated with either vaginal creams or troches of nystatin, clotrimazole, or miconazole. Oral therapy is usually unnecessary.

Candida has been implicated as a cause of nonspecific complaints such as fatigue, depression, anorexia, intestinal complaints varying from constipation to diarrhea, headaches, and an inability to concentrate, among others. This condition has been called the yeast syndrome, the yeast connection, and *Candida*-related complex. There is no evidence that these symptoms are causally related to *Candida*, and the American Academy of Allergy and Immunology and the Council on Scientific Affairs of the American Medical Association have published statements discouraging the use of antifungal medications in this unproven disease complex.

229.3 Infection in Immunocompromised Patients (See Chapter 173)

HUMAN IMMUNODEFICIENCY VIRUS–INFECTED CHILDREN (see Chapter 223). Oral thrush and diaper dermatitis are the most common candidal infections in children infected with human immunodeficiency virus (HIV), occurring in as many as 50–85% of patients. Infants with symptomatic HIV infection are more than twice as likely to have thrush as infants with indeterminate HIV infection, and the thrush is often much more extensive than in normal children. Besides pseudomembranous candidiasis, three other clinical variants of candidal infection may be observed in these children: atrophic candidiasis, which presents as a fiery erythema of the mucosa or loss of papilla of the tongue; chronic hyperplastic candidiasis, whose symmetrical white plaques cannot be rubbed off; and angular cheilitis, fissuring, and erythema of the angle of the mouth. Topical therapy with nystatin or clotrimazole may be effective for these infections, but gentian violet is often necessary. Symptoms of dysphagia or poor oral intake may indicate that the infection has progressed to the esophagus, necessitating systematic therapy with either ketoconazole or fluconazole.

Candidal dermatitis and onychomycosis are also more common in HIV-infected children. These infections are generally more severe and require more aggressive or prolonged therapy than infections seen in immune-competent children.

PREMATURE INFANTS (see Chapter 98.6). Candida causes significant disseminated disease in 2–5% of premature infants weighing less than 1,500 g. Risk factors associated with candidal sepsis in these patients include prolonged antibiotic therapy, prolonged use of intravascular catheters, intravenous hyperalimentation, and poor nutrition. The presentation of disseminated candidiasis mimics that of any other septic condition, with respiratory distress, apnea, bradycardia, temperature instability, glucose intolerance, or abdominal signs or symptoms. Cutaneous evidence of *Candida* may be seen in as many as half of these patients and manifests as a diffuse erythroderma or vesiculopustules from which the organism can be cultured. Renal involvement is found in more than half of these patients and may manifest as persistent candiduria or ultrasonographically with parenchymal involvement. Ultrasonography or computed tomography may also be helpful in identifying foci in the liver and spleen. Central nervous system involvement occurs in as many as one third of cases, mandating evaluation of the cerebrospinal fluid in all cases of disseminated candidiasis. Because endophthalmitis is seen in 20–50% of cases, retinal examinations should be performed in patients with systemic candidiasis, and patients should be monitored for resolution of retinal lesion. Osteoarthritis is a complication in 20% of cases. Candidal endocarditis is a less common complication but should be considered in patients with central venous catheters that extend into the atrium as well as in those with persistent candidemia. Pneumonia occurs in as many as 70% of patients with disseminated candidemia on the basis of autopsy studies, although some patients will not have radiographic findings of pneumonia at initial evaluation. Cultures from the endotracheal tube may be difficult to interpret because virtually all patients with systemic candiasis will have at least colonization of the endotracheal tube, and respiratory distress may be a manifestation of sepsis in the absence of pneumonia.

ONCOLOGY PATIENTS. Fungal infections, and especially *Candida* infections, are a significant problem in oncology patients who become neutropenic. Although the greatest risk for these patients comes from bacterial pathogens, the risk of candidemia increases dramatically after the 7th day of neutropenia. Blood cultures are notoriously poor at detecting systemic candidemia and are positive in only 5–15% of patients found to have disseminated infection. For this reason, patients who remain febrile after 7 days of antibacterial therapy should be empirically treated with systemic antifungal agents. Patients undergoing bone marrow transplantation are at much higher risk for fungal infections because of the dramatically increased length of time of neutropenia. Prophylactic use of fluconazole has been shown to decrease the incidence of candidemia in bone marrow transplant patients but not in leukemia patients undergoing chemotherapy, in whom an increased infection rate with *C. krusei*, an organism resistant to fluconazole has been noted. The use of granulocyte colony-stimulating factor has made an impact on the duration of neutropenia after chemotherapy and, therefore, on the incidence of candidemia. When *Candida* infection occurs, the lung, spleen, kidney, and liver are involved in more than 50% of cases.

CENTRAL CATHETER INFECTIONS. Central venous catheter infections occur most often in oncology patients but may affect any patient with a central catheter. Neutropenia, the use of broad-spectrum antibiotics, and hyperalimentation are highly associated with candidal central catheter infection. Recovery of *Candida* from the central catheter alone has the same incidence of disseminated infection as when the organism is cultured from both central catheter and peripheral blood. Treating central catheter–related candidemia without removing the central catheter has repeatedly been shown to be extremely difficult and related to increased mortality.

MICROBIOLOGY IN IMMUNOCOMPROMISED PATIENTS. Most cases of candidemia in immunocompromised patients are due to *C. albicans* (70–90%); other more common species include *C. tropicalis* (5–15%), *C. parapsilosis* (3–13%), *C. glabrata* (0–4%), *C. lusitaniae*, *C. krusei*, and *C. guilliermondii* (all <2%). Because *C. albicans* is the most frequently isolated pathogen, a rapid germ tube test should be performed before further tests are done. *C. albicans* is the only species that will form a germ tube when suspended in rabbit or human serum and incubated for 1–2 hr. The other clinically important species can be identified within 48 hr on the basis of results of biochemical tests.

Diagnosis may be presumptive in neutropenic patients with prolonged fever because positive blood cultures are seen only in a minority of patients later found to have disseminated infection. *Candida* grows readily on routine blood culture media, and 90% or more of positive cultures will be identified by

72 hr and 97% or more by 7 days. *Candida* recovered from urine or tracheal secretions may represent colonization but may also represent infection. It is important to remember that when *Candida* infects one organ system it is very likely that other organs are involved as well.

TREATMENT IN IMMUNOCOMPROMISED PATIENTS. Amphotericin B remains the treatment of choice in systemic fungal infections, alone or with the addition of 5-flucytosine, which is especially useful for treating central nervous system infections, parenchymal kidney infections, and osteoarticular infections. Because nephrotoxicity is often seen with amphotericin, some physicians prefer to treat with fluconazole. Fluconazole should not be used in patients with endophthalmitis or in infections caused by *C. krusei* or *C. glabrata* because of the high incidence of fluconazole resistance in these species. Amphotericin is relatively ineffective against *C. lusitaniae* and should not be used in infections caused by this species.

229.4 Chronic Mucocutaneous Candidiasis

Chronic mucocutaneous candidiasis is a heterogeneous group of immune disorders all of which have a primary defect of T-lymphocyte responsiveness to candidal antigen. Endocrinopathies and autoimmune disorders have been associated with this disorder in some patients. Symptoms may begin in the first few months of life or as late as the second decade of life. The disorder is characterized by chronic and severe skin and mucous membrane infections with *Candida*. Systemic candidiasis is rarely a problem; other dermatophytes may cause infection as well. Topical antifungal therapy may be useful early in the course of the disease, but short courses of systemic amphotericin or azole antifungals may be necessary for recalcitrant lesions.

Butler KM, Baker CJ: Candida: An increasingly important pathogen in the nursery. Pediatr Clin North Am 35:543, 1988.
Como KA Dismukes WE: Oral azole drugs as systemic antifingal therapy. N Engl J Med 330:263, 1994.
Crislip MA, Edwards JE: Candidiasis. Infect Dis Clin North Am 3:103, 1989.
Edwards JE, Filler SG: Current strategies for treating invasive candidiasis: Emphasis on infections in nonneutropenic patients. Clin Infect Dis 14(Suppl): S106, 1992.
Eppes SC, Troutman JL, Gutman LT: Outcome of treatment of candidemia in children whose central catheters were removed or retained. Pediatr Infect Dis J 8:99, 1989.
Hughes WT: Systemic candidiasis: A study of 109 fatal cases. Pediatr Infect Dis J 1:11, 1982.
Lecciones JA, Lee JW, Navarro EE, et al: Vascular catheter-associated fungemia in patients with cancer: Analysis of 155 episodes. Clin Infect Dis 14:875, 1992.
Prose NS: Mucocutaneous disease in pediatric human immunodeficiency virus infection. Pediatr Clin North Am 38:977, 1991.

CHAPTER 230
Aspergillosis

Stephen C. Aronoff

Aspergillosis refers to a group of diseases caused by monomorphic, mycelial fungi of the genus *Aspergillus*. Most diseases in children are caused by *A. fumigatus* followed by *A. flavus* and *A. niger*. *A. nidulans* and *A. terreus* have also been implicated in pediatric infections. Aspergilli are distributed worldwide, and spores (conidia) are readily isolated from soil and decaying plants. Outbreaks of invasive disease among immunosuppressed children have occurred after exposure to aerosolized conidia at large construction sites near hospitals and clinics. Infection is usually acquired from inhalation of airborne spores, which colonize the upper and lower respiratory tracts. In the immunosuppressed, infection will widely disseminate hematogenously. Cutaneous infection is also common and may follow wound contamination, intradermal inoculation, or hematogenous dissemination. Ingestion and aspiration may also produce disease. *Aspergillus*-associated diseases may be immunoglobulin (Ig) E mediated (hypersensitivity syndromes), saprophytic (noninvasive), or invasive.

HYPERSENSITIVITY SYNDROMES

Atopic asthma may be precipitated by spores from *Aspergillus* species. Inhalation triggers an IgE-mediated response and bronchospasm. The clinical aspects are nonspecific and include the acute onset of wheezing in the absence of pulmonary infiltrates or fever.

Extrinsic alveolar alveolitis is a hypersensitivity pneumonitis that occurs in nonatopic individuals after repeated exposures to organic dust. *Aspergillus* is one of many organic substances that produces this syndrome ("malt worker's" or "farmer's" lung). The pathogenesis is unknown but is similar to the alveolitis caused by other immunogens and may represent immune-complex disease. The clinical manifestations typically follow exposure by 4–6 hr and include fever, cough, and dyspnea. Physical examination often reveals rhonchi without wheezes. Eosinophilia is absent from blood and sputum, and chest radiograph often shows diffuse interstitial infiltrates. Chronic exposure gradually leads to irreversible pulmonary fibrosis.

Allergic bronchopulmonary aspergillosis (ABA) complicates chronic pulmonary disease in approximately 10% of children with asthma or cystic fibrosis. Chronic mucosal colonization with *A. fumigatus* produces an exaggerated IgG and IgE response, which results in recurrent bronchospasm and proximal, cylindrical bronchiectasis. The diagnosis should be considered in asthmatics and cystic fibrosis patients with recurrent bronchospasm and transient pulmonary infiltrates. Expectoration of mucous spirals containing mycelia is a hallmark of this illness; peripheral eosinophilia is common. The diagnosis of ABA requires fulfillment of the following criteria: (1) reversible paroxysmal bronchiolar obstruction (asthma); (2) immediate cutaneous reactivity to *A. fumigatus* antigens or specific serum IgE to *A. fumigatus* (radioallergosorbent test); (3) elevated total serum IgE; (4) peripheral blood eosinophilia; (5) precipitating serum antibodies against *A. fumigatus*; and (6) proximal bronchiectasis.

Treatment of the hypersensitivity pulmonary syndromes focuses on anti-inflammatory agents, notably glucocorticoid, and bronchodilator therapy. A small study in older adolescents and young adults with ABA demonstrated some potential benefit with the adjunctive use of itraconazole.

SAPROPHYTIC (NONINVASIVE) SYNDROMES

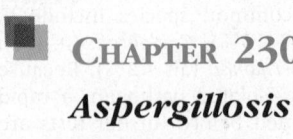

Otomycosis is a chronic condition that predominates in tropical and subtropical regions. Most infections are due to *A. niger* or, less commonly, *A. fumigatus*; coinfection with *Staphylococcus aureus* or *Pseudomonas* species occurs in one third of cases. Otomycosis is rare in infants and children. Most cases are unilateral, and patients present with ear pain, itching of the auditory canal, and a sense of fullness. Otorrhea, decreased hearing, and tinnitus are less common. Examination of the auditory canal typically shows conidial "forests" or mycelial mats. Topical antifungal agents such as nystatin or tolnaftate, dilute acetic acid, and topical steroids are therapeutic; oral itraconazole has been effective, but experience with this agent is limited.

There are three forms of saprophytic *Aspergillus sinonasal disease*. Chronic or indolent sinusitis is confined to one sinus and presents as chronic infection unresponsive to antibacterial therapy. Sinus radiograms are nonspecific, showing mucosal thickening without bony changes. Endoscopic surgery is curative in most cases. Aspergillomas are rare in children. These patients present with long-standing nasal symptoms. Sinus radiographs demonstrate a solitary mass in the ethmoid or maxillary sinus. Bony destruction is variable. Surgical removal of the mass, often endoscopically, is the treatment of choice. Allergic fungal sinusitis involves multiple sinuses and occurs in immunocompetent individuals with histories of multiple sinus surgeries and nasal polyposis. *Aspergillus* species and less often *Curvularia lunata* are etiological. The histology of nasal secretions in these patients reveals thick mucin, eosinophils, and few fungal hyphae. Sinus imaging typically shows multisinus involvement with hypodense areas, occasional calcifications, and occasional bony erosions. The criteria for the diagnosis of allergic fungal sinusitis are immunological and are identical to those of allergic bronchopulmonary aspergillosis; allergic bronchopulmonary aspergillosis may complicate allergic fungal sinusitis. Treatment includes surgical drainage and debridement as well as corticosteroids.

Pulmonary aspergillomas develop in poorly drained bronchi or pre-existing pulmonary cavities that complicate pulmonary tuberculosis, histoplasmosis, blastomycosis, or sarcoidosis; rarely, aspergillomas complicate invasive *Aspergillus* pulmonary disease. Colonization and fungal proliferation without vascular invasion yields an amorphous mycelial mass (mycetoma, fungus ball). Affected children are often asymptomatic, although cough and hemoptysis may be reported. Chest radiographs characteristically demonstrate the air shadow of a pulmonary cavity outlining a rounded mass; these findings may be confirmed by computed tomography of the chest. Management is controversial and may range from watchful waiting of asymptomatic and otherwise healthy children to aggressive surgical resection in patients with profound hemoptysis.

INVASIVE DISEASE

Invasive *Aspergillus* infection is characterized by hyphal infiltration of vascular structures, thrombosis, and focal necrosis. Invasive disease occurs most commonly in the immunocompromised host, particularly in neutropenic children with relapsed leukemia, human immunodeficiency virus, bone marrow transplant recipients, and, less commonly, solid organ recipients. Primary invasive disease may occur at any site in which airborne conidia may colonize and germinate, such as the respiratory tract or skin. In the severely neutropenic child, dissemination follows direct extension from the primary site and hematogenous seeding of distant sites. Sinonasal disease, pulmonary disease, and cutaneous disease are the most common primary infections in children. Otitis is a rare entity. Although systemic amphotericin B remains the recommended treatment for most deep-seated *Aspergillus* infections, outcome appears to hinge on resolution of the underlying neutropenia, remission of the underlying disease, or cessation of immunosuppressive therapy. Itraconazole, a triazole antifungal agent, has appreciable in vitro activity against *Aspergillus* species. In most cases, the experience with this agent for the treatment of children is limited.

Invasive otitis externa associated with *Aspergillus* infection is rare, occurs in the immunosuppressed, and is associated with hearing loss and spread to the petrous portion of the temporal bone and the pinna. Therapeutic options include parenteral antifungal therapy with amphotericin B and surgical debridement; experience with itraconazole is limited.

Invasive or fulminant nasosinusitis is a disease of the immunosuppressed, occurs almost exclusively in patients with profound neutropenia associated with chemotherapy for leukemia or cancer of the head and neck, and is rare in children. Fever, cough, epistaxis, headache, and sinus pain are the most common clinical signs. Examination typically shows nasal crusting with rhinorrhea, sinus tenderness, nasal or oral ulceration, and duskiness or necrosis of the nasal septum or inferior turbinates. Multisinus involvement with opacification or air-fluid levels can be demonstrated radiographically or by computed tomography. Scrapings of the nasal or sinus mucosa demonstrate large numbers of hyphae, and fungal cultures typically yield *A. fumigatus, A. flavus,* or less often *Rhizopus* or *Candida* species. Treatment is not standardized but often includes surgical drainage, intravenous and intranasal amphotericin B, and removal of devascularized, necrotic tissue. Extensive surgical procedures are often hampered by underlying thrombocytopenia and extensive and at times life-threatening hemorrhage. Sporadic successes and failures have been reported in open-label nonrandomized trials with itraconazole; however, comparative data with amphotericin B are not available. Invasive sinusitis carries a poor prognosis for children with relapsed leukemia; better outcomes have been described after resolution of granulocytopenia or remission of the underlying disease.

Invasive pulmonary aspergillosis (IPA) is the most common form of *Aspergillus* infection. The onset of IPA is often insidious in immunocompromised children and may be discovered only at lung biopsy for evaluation of unexplained fever and neutropenia. In both normal hosts and the immunoincompetent, symptomatic IPA presents acutely with fever, cough, dyspnea, and abnormal chest examination; pleuritic chest pain is an infrequent complaint. Chest radiographs often show nodular infiltrates. Coexisting sinusitis is a common finding in neutropenic children with IPA. In children with chronic granulomatous disease, direct extension from the lungs to the chest wall has been reported. The diagnosis is confirmed by the histological demonstration of hyphal invasion of blood vessels and recovery of the mold by culture of the biopsy specimen; recovery of a pure culture of *Aspergillus* species from sputum, bronchial alveolar lavage fluid, or sinuses in the clinical setting of acute pneumonia and sinusitis is highly suggestive. Treatment with high-dose amphotericin B (1 mg/kg/day) for 4–6 weeks or until resolution of neutropenia or remission of the underlying disease is recommended. Itraconazole has been used successfully in a handful of patients in an open, noncomparative fashion.

Cutaneous aspergillosis was the most common form of invasive disease reported in a series of immunocompromised children with invasive aspergillosis. Lesions are typically seen at sites of local trauma such as intravenous sites. Cutaneous disease may result from either direct inoculation of the skin or from hematogenous dissemination. The lesions appear initially as tender erythematous plaques that progress to necrotic eschars or hemorrhagic bullae. In the majority of children with profound neutropenia, cutaneous aspergillosis is sentinel for disseminated disease. The outcome of this form of the disease is poor. Therapy is not standardized but typically includes high-dose, parenteral amphotericin B. Local debridement and topical amphotericin have also been used. Experience with itraconazole is limited.

Fungal endophthalmitis is an important diagnostic finding in immunosuppressed children with disseminated *Aspergillus* infection. Although most patients have no ocular symptoms, pain, photophobia, and diminished visual acuity may occur. Examination of the retina shows focal retinitis, an overlying vitritis, and retinal hemorrhage. Treatment of the underlying immunosuppressive illness, systemic antifungal therapy, vitriectomy, and intraocular amphotericin B are recommended; itraconazole, like amphotericin B, achieves poor intraocular concentrations. Orbital cellulitis rarely complicates invasive sinusitis and follows destruction of the orbital walls and fungal extension into the retro-orbital space. Diplopia, periorbital edema, proptosis, and pain on lateral gaze may occur. Treatment requires a combination of surgical debridement, systemic antifungal therapy, and resolution of the underlying immunosuppressive state. The outcome for this entity is the same as that for fulminant sinusitis. Fungal keratitis and episcleritis are rare problems and follow direct inoculation of spores into the eye. In the absence of significant disseminated disease, topical and intrascleral amphotericin B therapy is recommended.

Cerebral aspergillosis is a rare and almost uniformly fatal complication of disseminated disease. In most cases, infection involves single or multiple foci within the cerebral hemispheres or cerebellum. Patients manifest the acute onset of focal neurological deficits, most often hemiparesis, anterior cranial nerve palsies, or seizures. Progression to herniation is rapid. Meningeal signs are rare and at autopsy arachnoiditis is limited to the area adjacent to the cerebral focus. When performed, cerebrospinal fluid (CSF) studies show a mild mononuclear pleocytosis, elevated CSF protein, and variable degrees of hypoglycorrhachia. Imaging studies demonstrate focal central nervous system (CNS) lesions with variable enhancement (edema). The diagnosis can be established by the acute appearance of CNS symptoms in a patient with proven or suspected invasive aspergillosis or occasionally by CSF or brain biopsy culture. Although cerebral infection is almost universally fatal, treatment with itraconazole was successful in at least one suspected case in a child with chronic granulomatous disease. Alternatively, high-dose amphotericin B combined with flucytosine has also proven effective in a paucity of cases.

Epidural abscess is a rare complication of vertebral osteomyelitis caused by *Aspergillus* species. In two children with epidural abscess, vertebral osteomyelitis and cord compression, surgical decompression and high-dose amphotericin B were curative.

Aspergillosis of the bone is an extremely rare disease and follows direct extension from a surgical or traumatic wound or hematogenous seeding. Involvement of the vertebrae is most common. Osteomyelitis of the rib is rare, occurs in children with chronic granulomatous disease, and represents extension from a pulmonary focus. Surgical drainage is often required. Although comparative studies are not available, initial therapy with amphotericin B plus flucytosine followed by itraconazole is a promising approach.

Endocarditis is a rare form of aspergillosis and can follow contamination at the time of surgery or implantation of a contaminated graft or, uncommonly, may be a manifestation of disseminated aspergillosis. High-dose amphotericin B therapy coupled with surgical removal of infected grafts or prostheses is recommended.

Denning DW, Stevens DA: Antifungal and surgical treatment of invasive aspergillosis: Review of 2121 published cases. Rev Infect Dis 12:1147, 1990.

Neijens HJ, Frenkel J, et al: Invasive *Aspergillus* infection in chronic granulomatous disease: Treatment with itraconazole. J Pediatr 115:1016, 1989.

Walmsley S, Devi S, King S, et al: Invasive *Aspergillus* infections in a pediatric hospital: A ten-year review. Pediatr Infect Dis J 12:673, 1993.

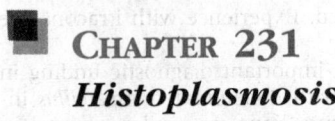

CHAPTER 231
Histoplasmosis

Stephen C. Aronoff

Histoplasma capsulatum is a dimorphic fungi that is found in nature in its mycelial (saprophytic) form and in human tissue as a yeast. The saprophytic form is found in soil throughout the midwestern United States primarily along the Ohio and Mississippi rivers; sporadic cases of human and animal histoplasmosis have been reported from 31 of the 48 contiguous states. In parts of Kentucky and Tennessee, almost 90% of the population older than 20 years have positive skin tests to histoplasmin.

EPIDEMIOLOGY. *H. capsulatum* thrives in soil rich in nitrates such as those areas heavily contaminated with bird droppings or decayed wood. Fungal spores are often carried on the wings of birds. Focal outbreaks of histoplasmosis have been reported after aerosolization of microconidia by construction in areas previously occupied by starling roosts or chicken coops or by chopping decayed wood. Unlike birds, bats are actively infected with histoplasma. Focal outbreaks of histoplasmosis have also been reported after intense exposure to bat guano in caves and along bridges frequented by bats.

PATHOGENESIS AND PATHOLOGY. Inhalation of microconidia is the initial stage of human infection. The conidia reach the alveoli, germinate, and proliferate as yeast. The initial infection is a bronchopneumonia. As the initial pulmonary lesion ages, giant cells form followed by granuloma formation and central necrosis. At the time of spore germination, yeast cells gain access to the reticuloendothelial system via the pulmonary lymphatic system and hilar lymph nodes. Dissemination with splenic involvement typically follows the primary pulmonary infection. In normal hosts, an immune response follows in approximately 2 wk. The initial pulmonary lesion resolves within 2 to 4 mo but may undergo calcification resembling the Ghon complex of tuberculosis, or "buckshot" calcifications involving the lung and spleen may be seen. Unlike tuberculosis, reinfection with *H. capsulatum* occurs and may lead to exaggerated host responses in some cases.

CLINICAL MANIFESTATIONS. There are three forms of human histoplasmosis: acute pulmonary infection, chronic pulmonary histoplasmosis, and progressive disseminated histoplasmosis. *Acute pulmonary histoplasmosis* follows initial or recurrent respiratory exposure to microconidia. The majority of patients are asymptomatic. Symptomatic disease occurs more often in young children; in older individuals symptoms follow exposure to large inocula in closed spaces (e.g., chicken coops or caves) or prolonged exposure (camping on contaminated soil, chopping decayed wood). The prodrome is not specific and usually consists of flulike symptoms: headache, fever, chest pain, and cough. Hepatosplenomegaly occurs more often in infants and young children. Symptomatic infections may be associated with significant respiratory distress and hypoxia, requiring intubation, ventilation, and steroid therapy. Acute pulmonary disease may also present with a prolonged illness (10 days to 3 wk) consisting of weight loss, dyspnea, high fever, asthenia, and fatigue. Ten per cent of patients with acute pulmonary infection present with a sarcoid-like disease that includes arthritis or arthralgia, erythema nodosum, keratoconjunctivitis, or iridocyclitis and pericarditis. Most children with acute pulmonary disease have normal chest radiographs. Individuals with symptomatic disease typically have a patchy bronchopneumonia; hilar adenopathy is variably present. In young children, the pneumonia may coalesce. Focal or buckshot calcifications are convalescent findings of acute pulmonary infection.

Exaggerated host responses to fungal antigens within the lung parenchyma or hilar lymph nodes produce thoracic complications of acute pulmonary histoplasmosis. *Histoplasmomas* are of parenchymal origin and are usually asymptomatic. These fibroma-like lesions are often concentrically calcified and single. Rarely, these lesions may produce broncholithiasis associated with "stone spitting," wheezing, and hemoptysis. In endemic regions, these lesions may mimic parenchymal tumors and are occasionally diagnosed at lung biopsy. *Medistinal granulomas* form when reactive hilar lymph nodes coalesce and mat together. Although these lesions are usually asymptomatic, huge granulomas may compress mediastinal structures, producing symptoms of esophageal, bronchial, or vena cava obstruction. Local extension and necrosis may produce pericarditis or pleural effusions. *Mediastinal fibrosis* is a rare complication of mediastinal granulomas and represents an uncontrolled fibrotic reaction arising from the hilar nodes. Structures within the mediastinum become encased within a fibrotic mass, producing obstructive symptomatology. Superior vena cava syndrome, pulmonary venous obstruction with a mitral stenosis-like syndrome, and pulmonary artery obstruction with congestive heart failure have been described. Dysphagia accompanies esophageal entrapment, and a syndrome of cough, wheeze, hemoptysis, and dyspnea accompanies bronchial obstruction.

Chronic pulmonary histoplasmosis is an opportunistic infection in adult patients with centrilobular emphysema. This entity is rare in children.

Progressive disseminated histoplasmosis is a disease affecting infants and the immunosuppressed. Disseminated disease of infancy occurs almost exclusively in infants younger than 1 yr and follows primary pulmonary infection. Fever is the most common finding and may last for weeks to months before diagnosis. The majority of patients manifest hepatosplenomegaly, anemia, and thrombocytopenia. Pneumonia and pancytopenia are variably present. Although radiographs of the chest are normal in more than half of these children, the yeast can frequently be identified on bone marrow examination.

Children who are immunosuppressed by virtue of disease (e.g., leukemia), drug therapy (e.g., organ transplant recipients), or human immunodeficiency virus (HIV) infection are at increased risk for disseminated histoplasmosis. In non-HIV–infected individuals, disseminated disease presents with unexplained fevers, weight loss, and interstitial pulmonary disease. Extrapulmonary infection is a characteristic of disseminated disease and may include destructive bony lesions, oropharyngeal ulcers, Addison's disease, meningitis, cutaneous infection, and endocarditis. Elevated liver function tests and serum concentrations of angiotensin-converting enzyme may be observed.

Disseminated histoplasmosis in an HIV-infected individual is an infection defining acquired immunodeficiency syndrome. Disseminated disease is often preceded or followed by another opportunistic infection in this patient population. Fever and weight loss occurs in most individuals. In the majority of patients pulmonary disease develops; hepatosplenomegaly, lymphadenopathy, skin rashes, and meningoencephalitis are variably present. A sepsis-like syndrome has been identified in a small number of HIV-infected patients with disseminated histoplasmosis and is characterized by the rapid onset of shock, multiorgan failure, and coagulopathy.

DIAGNOSIS. Recovery of *H. capsulatum* by culture differs with the form of infection. In normal hosts with symptomatic or asymptomatic acute pulmonary histoplasmosis, sputum cultures are rarely obtained and are variably positive; cultures of bronchoalveolar lavage fluid appear to have a slightly higher yield than sputa. Blood cultures are sterile in patients with acute pulmonary histoplasmosis, and cultures from any source are typically sterile in individuals with the sarcoid form of the disease. Yeast forms may be demonstrated histologically in tissue from patients with complicated forms of acute pulmonary disease (mediastinal granuloma, mediastinal fibrosis, and histoplasmoma). Sputum cultures are positive in 60% of adults with chronic pulmonary histoplasmosis. The yeast can be recovered from blood or bone marrow in more than 90% of patients with progressive disseminated histoplasmosis.

The detection of fungal antigen by radioimmunoassay is the best diagnostic study in suspected cases of progressive disseminated histoplasmosis. In HIV infected patients as well as others at risk for disseminated disease, histoplasma-associated antigen can be demonstrated in the urine or blood in more than 90% of cases. False-positive results may occur in individuals with blastomycosis, paracoccidiomycosis, and coccidiomycosis. Sequential measurement of antigen in patients with disseminated disease is useful for monitoring response to therapy. Serum and urine from individuals with acute or chronic pulmonary infections are variably antigen positive.

Seroconversion continues to be useful for the diagnosis of acute pulmonary histoplasmosis, its complications, and chronic pulmonary disease. Serum antibody to yeast and mycelium-associated antigens is classically measured by complement fixation. Although titers greater than 1:8 are found in more than 80% of patients with histoplasmosis, titers of 1:32 and greater are the most significant for recent infection. Complement fixation antibody titers are often not significant early in the infection and do not become positive until 4–6 wk after exposure. Complement fixation titers may be falsely positive in patients with other systemic mycoses and may be falsely negative in the immunocompromised. Antibody detection by immunodiffusion is less sensitive than complement fixation and is used to confirm questionably positive complement fixation titers. Skin testing is useful only for epidemiological studies because cutaneous reactivity is lifelong, and intradermal injection may elicit an immune response in otherwise seronegative individuals.

TREATMENT. Antifungal therapy is not warranted for asymptomatic or mildly symptomatic acute pulmonary histoplasmosis. Mediastinal complications of acute pulmonary infection often require surgical therapy. Sarcoid-like disease with or without pericarditis may be treated with nonsteroidal anti-inflammatory agents.

Amphotericin B continues to be the cornerstone of therapy for progressive disseminated histoplasmosis. In immunocompromised adults and infants with disseminated disease, 35–40 mg/kg total dose is required to minimize relapses. Both ketoconazole and itraconazole have been used successfully to treat progressive disseminated disease in immunocompromised adults. No comparative data with amphotericin B or efficacy data in infected infants are available. Serial measurement of fungal antigen in urine or serum is recommended to ensure adequate treatment.

Relapses in HIV-positive individuals with progressive disseminated histoplasmosis are common. Currently, induction therapy with amphotericin B (10–15 mg/kg total dose; total dose >500 mg in adults) is recommended. Lifelong suppressive therapy may be accomplished with weekly or biweekly amphotericin B (1–1.5 mg/kg/dose) or daily itraconazole (200 mg/day in adults). Ketoconazole is not effective in HIV-infected individuals.

Goodwin RA, Loyd JE, Des Prez, R. Histoplasmosis in normal hosts. Medicine 60:231, 1981.

Leggiadro RJ, Barrett FF, Hughes WT: Disseminated histoplasmosis of infancy. Pediatr Infect Dis J 7:799, 1988.

Wheat J, Hafner R, Wulfsohn M, et al: Prevention of relapse of histoplasmosis with itraconazole in patients with the acquired immunodeficiency syndrome: The NIAID Clinical Trials and Study Group Mycosis Study Group Collaborators. Ann Intern Med 118:610, 1993.

Wheat LJ: Histoplasmosis in Indianapolis. Clin Infect Dis 14(Suppl 1):S91, 1992.

CHAPTER 232
Blastomycosis

Stephen C. Aronoff

ETIOLOGY. *Blastomyces dermatitidis* is a dimorphic yeast that exists in mycelial form in nature and as a yeast in tissue.

EPIDEMIOLOGY. Sporadic infection within endemic regions accounts for the majority of cases of human and canine blastomycosis. The fungus is found throughout the midwestern and southeastern portions of the United States, particularly along the Ohio and Mississippi River valleys, north central Wisconsin, North Carolina, Minnesota, and Illinois. Cases of blastomycosis have been reported rarely outside of North America with the largest concentration in Africa. Although difficult to isolate from soil, *B. dermatitidis* has been recovered from earth enriched with rotted wood, bird droppings, or animal droppings. Soil surrounding bodies of water within the endemic region is particularly rich in fungi. Epidemics are unusual but have been described after excavation of contaminated soil in endemic regions. Individuals who spend large amounts of time in wooded areas within endemic regions, such as hunters or forestry workers, are at highest risk for infection. Blastomycosis in children is decidedly unusual.

The pathogenesis of blastomycosis is similar to that of histoplasmosis. Inhalation of spores results in alveolar inoculation and germination to yeast forms. Although pulmonary macrophages eliminate the majority of spores before infection, those that survive produce pneumonitis and may disseminate hematogenously. The immune response to infection consists of neutrophil and macrophage migration into infected tissue. The resulting "pyogranulomatous" response with associated necrosis and fibrosis is characteristic of blastomycosis.

CLINICAL MANIFESTATIONS. Human blastomycosis presents as a pulmonary or extrapulmonary infection. Three forms of pulmonary infection have been described. *Asymptomatic infection* is rarely identified because of the lack of an inexpensive, reliable screening test. Subclinical infections have been identified serologically during investigations of epidemics. Some of these individuals may exhibit nonspecific symptoms such as weight loss, unexplained fever, and malaise. Chest radiographs often demonstrate an alveolar process that may resemble a parenchymal mass. *Acute pneumonia* is the most common form of human blastomycosis. These patients present with the acute onset of fever, chills, and productive cough; hemoptysis is variably identified. Pleural effusions appear in approximately one quarter to one half of cases, and erythema nodosum may occur during resolution. Alveolar or reticulonodular patterns without hilar adenopathy are often seen on chest radiographs. Diffuse pulmonary disease associated with adult respiratory distress syndrome (ARDS) has been described in a handful of immunocompetent adults with acute pneumonia. *Chronic pneumonia* is characterized by several months of weight loss, cough, night sweats, and fever. The cough becomes productive and may be associated with chest pain; cavitary disease is an uncommon complication of this form of infection.

Extrapulmonary or disseminated disease occurs in immunocompetent individuals and is usually heralded by prior pulmonary symptoms. Laryngeal blastomycosis is relatively common, may follow primary infection of the upper airway, and presents as a laryngeal mass; one episode of laryngeal blastomycosis associated with fungal otitis media and a polyp of the external auditory canal has been reported. Cutaneous disease follows hematogenous or direct inoculation of the subcutaneous tissue and appears as either verrucous or ulcerative lesions. Osteomyelitis occurs in one quarter of extrapulmonary infections and usually involves flat bones such as the skull, vertebrae, and ribs. Central nervous system infection occurs in 10% of extrapulmonary infections and is typified by intracranial abscesses or, rarely, meningitis. Prostatitis and orchitis in males is unusual; endometrial disease is sexually transmitted. Fungal abscesses may form anywhere, including the heart and its surrounding structures, the orbit, and the sinuses.

DIAGNOSIS. Because colonization with *B. dermititidis* does not occur, recovery of the fungus from sputum, bronchoalveolar lavage fluid, pleural fluid, or other sterile sites is diagnostic. Similarly, demonstration of the yeast histologically is diagnostic. Serological diagnosis using complement fixation or immunodiffusion is insensitive and complicated by the high rate of cross-reactivity with anti-*Histoplasma* antibody. An enzyme immunosorbent assay is the most specific serological test and is positive in more than three quarters of cases. Skin testing is unreliable because reactivity wanes over time at an unpredictable rate.

TREATMENT. Uncomplicated acute pneumonia may resolve spontaneously. Itraconazole (200–400 mg/day) or ketoconazole (400–800 mg/day) for 6 mo is curative in the majority of adults with mild to moderate acute lung disease; the former agent appears to be less toxic. The use of azole therapy is limited but promising in chronic pneumonia. Acute pneumonia associated with ARDS and extrapulmonary disease is treated with moderate dosages of amphotericin B (>1.5 g total dose) or induction courses of amphotericin B (500 mg total dose) followed by 5–6 mo of azole therapy. Because of poor cerebrospinal fluid and central nervous system penetration, ketoconazole and itraconazole should be avoided in these situations.

Bradsher RW: Blastomycosis. Clin Infect Dis 14(Suppl 1)S82, 1992.

Dismukes WE, Bradsher RW, Cloud GC, et al: Itraconazole therapy for blastomycosis and histoplasmosis. Am J Med 93:489, 1992.

Istorico LJ, Sanders M, Jacobs RF, et al: Otitis media due to blastomycosis: Report of two cases. Clin Infect Dis 14:355, 1992.

Meyer KC, McManus EJ, Maki DG: Overwhelming pulmonary blastomycosis associated with the adult respiratory distress syndrome. N Engl J Med 329:1231, 1993.

CHAPTER 233
Coccidioidomycosis

(San Joaquin Fever, Valley Fever, Desert Rheumatism, Coccidioidal Granuloma)

Demosthenes Pappagiamis

ETIOLOGY. Coccidioidomycosis is an infection caused by the fungus *Coccidioides immitis* found in the soil of the New World. The minute arthroconidia of its mycelial saprophytic phase airborne in dust are inhaled or, rarely, enter through injured skin. In the infected host they round up into spherules, which develop endospores. Liberation of the latter leads to formation of new spherules, which spread within a host but not to a new host. Viable *C. immitis* does occur in pulmonary cavities, often in the mycelial as well as spherule form, but no cases of person-to-person infection have been discovered. However, the arthroconidia that occur in nature and on the surface of cultures are highly infectious. Although isolation is unnecessary, precautions should be taken with dressings and casts over open lesions to preclude the development of the infective arthroconidia, which occurs in 4–5 days on surface cultures. Within the arid endemic areas of California's San Joaquin Valley, in scattered regions in northern and southern California, in central and southern Arizona, and even in southwestern Texas, many long-time residents have been infected, along with cattle, sheep, dogs, horses, llamas, and wild rodents. Recovery from infection confers permanent immunity except in those with an acquired (natural or iatrogenic) immunodeficiency. Population shifts bring susceptible individuals into endemic areas.

CLINICAL MANIFESTATIONS. Human infection takes three forms: (1) a benign, self-limited, primary infection (60% of infected persons show no clinical manifestations); (2) residual pulmonary lesions; and (3) a rare, disseminating, sometimes fatal disease. The disease tends to be milder in children; however, in those requiring medical attention, dissemination to bones and meninges is fairly common and approaches the incidence of these complications in adults. Laryngeal coccidioidomycosis, although not frequent, has been detected at a proportionately higher rate in children. Maternal-fetal or maternal-neonate infection has been reported.

Primary Coccidioidomycosis. The incubation period varies from 1 to 4 wk, with an average of 10–16 days. Symptoms are influenzal in type; the onset may be insidious or abrupt with malaise, chills, and fever. Chest pain is frequent and may vary from a mere sense of constriction to excruciating pain. Night sweats and anorexia are common. On occasion, there is a persistent dry cough and there may be a painful throat. There also may be headache or backache.

A generalized, fine, macular erythema or urticarial eruption may appear within the 1st day or so. It may be evanescent and present only in the groin. Rarely a vesicular, varicella-like rash has been noted. Most frequently, erythema nodosum occurs with or without erythema multiforme. These lesions develop at the time sensitivity to coccidioidin is maximal, 3–21 days after onset of symptoms. These rashes of acute infection do not contain the organism and may result from hypersensitivity to coccidioidal antigen. Skin lesions may occur, however, in persons otherwise asymptomatic. Other allergic manifestations, arthritis, and phlyctenular conjunctivitis may occur concomitantly.

Chest examination rarely discloses positive findings, even though roentgenography reveals extensive consolidation. Infrequently dullness, a friction rub, or fine rales may be detected. Pleural effusions occur at times and may be massive enough to embarrass respiration; they may develop without preceding respiratory symptoms.

Residual Pulmonary Coccidioidomycosis. Infrequently, a cavity may develop in an area of pulmonary consolidation during the primary infection and then regress. More often, however, after a variably prolonged period a persistent cavity may form. There are often no symptoms, and the diagnosis is made roentgenographically. Occasionally there is mild to moderate hemoptysis, which may recur and be alarming. Rarely, fatal hemorrhage has occurred. Dissemination of the fungus from cavities to other areas is rare. Pulmonary residual "granulomas" sometimes persist. They are not harmful but do pose problems of differentiation from tuberculosis or neoplasms. Infrequently, a chronic progressive fibrocavitary pulmonary disease is seen.

Disseminated or Progressive Coccidioidomycosis (Coccidioidal Granuloma). Certain persons lack ability to localize coccidioidal infection. Dissemination, which is rare and occurs mainly in males, especially in Filipinos, other Asians, and blacks, usually follows the initial illness within 6 mo, often without any interlude. This is analogous to progressive primary tuberculosis. Persons with blood group B may be particularly disposed to dissemination. Certain immunosuppressed states enhance dissemination or bring about relapse of apparently arrested coccidioidomycosis. Dissemination is enhanced if coccidioidal infection is acquired during pregnancy. Skin lesions and cold abscesses, both subcutaneous and osseous, occur. Meningitis is the most serious of the disseminated lesions, being clinically similar to tuberculous meningitis. In whites it is not unusual for meningitis to be the only extrapulmonary lesion. Miliary dissemination and peritonitis may be distinguishable from tuberculosis only by demonstrating the causative agent, though coccidioidal peritonitis may present as a very mild disease. The mortality rate of untreated meningitis is practically 100%, but it is variable with other forms of disseminated coccidioidomycosis.

DIAGNOSIS. Diagnosis of the disseminated infection may be established by biopsy or at autopsy. Sputum is generally so scanty in the primary infection that gastric lavage may be advisable, especially in children. If histological examination demonstrates the characteristic double-contoured spherules with endospores and without budding, the diagnosis is certain. Demonstration of the fungus by culture and its confirmation by a DNA probe, by exoantigen test, or by animal inoculation is also diagnostic. Only especially qualified laboratories should undertake such hazardous procedures.

The sedimentation rate is rapid in patients with both primary and disseminated infections and is helpful in evaluating clinical status. Eosinophilia is common and is proportionately higher with more severe infections. Serum alkaline phosphatase may be elevated in acute coccidioidomycosis even in the absence of obvious systemic dissemination.

Concomitant coccidioidomycosis and other infections (e.g., tuberculosis) can be confounding.

Skin Test. Tests with coccidioidin or spherulin are specific except for occasional cross-reactions with histoplasmosis and blastomycosis. A positive reaction does not distinguish between a recent and an old infection unless it has been preceded within a reasonably short time by a negative test result. However, *a negative skin test does not rule out coccidioidal infection.* Coccidioidin is administered intradermally as 0.1 mL of a 1:1,000, 1:100, or even 1:10 dilution. The reaction generally reaches its peak at 36 hr and should be read at 24 and 48 hr. An area of induration more than 5 mm in diameter is positive. Patients with suspected coccidioidal erythema nodosum are likely to be hypersensitive and should receive the 1:1,000 dilution. Patients with disseminated infections are much less sensitive; even a 1:10 dilution may not elicit a reaction. Dermal sensitivity to coccidioidin is less durable than to tuberculin. There is no danger of disseminating or activating a coccidioidal infection by a strong coccidioidin reaction, although there may be a systemic reaction as well as a local one. Coccidioidin does not evoke antibodies in the human; therefore, the skin test may precede serological tests and will provide information useful in their interpretation. However, negative skin tests should not preclude serological tests. A positive skin test in a healthy individual indicates resistance to reinfection with *C. immitis.*

Blood and Cerebrospinal Fluid Tests. Serum precipitins (immunoglobulin [Ig]M) and complement fixation (IgG) antibodies are detectable in early coccidioidomycosis, and may persist with disseminated coccidioidomycosis. In general, the more severe the infection, the higher the complement fixation titer. Antibodies are generally not demonstrable in asymptomatic acute infections. Rarely, serological tests may be negative in active coccidioidomycosis, for example, in the patient immunosuppressed for renal transplantation or by acquired immunodeficiency syndrome (AIDS). The cerebrospinal fluid findings are similar to those characteristic of tuberculous meningitis (Chapter 199). Fixation of complement by cerebrospinal fluid occurs in 95% of patients with coccidioidal meningitis and is usually diagnostic. Occasionally, epidural coccidioidal lesions may also lead to complement fixation by the cerebrospinal fluid. Complement-fixing antibody may be detected in cisternal and lumbar fluid but may be deceptively absent from the ventricular fluid. Antibodies detectable by complement fixation do not pass the blood-brain barrier (although immunodiffusion may reveal their presence) but are found in cord blood at the same titer as in the mother's blood. Passively transferred antibody disappears from the infant within 6 mo. Coccidioidal precipitin (IgM) has been detected in some neonates of mothers having coccidioidomycosis when there has been no manifestation of disease in the infants.

Roentgenography. During the primary infection roentgenograms of the chest may not reveal pulmonary changes. Hilar adenopathy is frequent, and there may be single or multiple, sharply circumscribed or soft, feathery, small pulmonary densities or larger consolidated areas. Acute respiratory insufficiency may result. Pulmonary cavities, which occur less frequently in children than adults, when present, tend to be thin walled. Pleural effusions are of variable extent. The osseous lesions, usually multiple and with a predilection for cancellous bone, often are widespread and are generally indistinguishable from those of tuberculosis.

PREVENTION. Avoidance of exposure to the arthroconidia although often impractical, is the only means of preventing infection. An available whole killed cell vaccine did not prevent coccidioidomycosis in humans.

TREATMENT. Because most primary coccidioidal infections resolve spontaneously over a variable time period, in the past they have been treated conservatively; activity and symptomatic measures are restricted until the erythrocyte sedimentation rate returns to normal, clinical and roentgenographic improvement are noted, precipitin (IgM) vanishes, and the complement fixation titer of the serum decreases. With the advent of the relatively benign oral azoles, physicians have often initiated therapy with them as soon as coccidioidomycosis is suspected or confirmed. This has been done despite the absence of adequate information that such treatment for primary coccidioidomycosis hastens recovery or decreases the risk of metapulmonary dissemination or development of pulmonary residua (e.g., cavity or solitary nodule).

Pulmonary cavities frequently close spontaneously, but when a cavity persists or is located peripherally, or when there is recurrent bleeding or rupture of the cavity through the pleura, excision should be considered. Coccidioidal cavities with a fluid level, accompanying fever, or hemoptysis should initially be treated with antibacterial antibiotics. Infrequently, bronchopleural fistulas or recurrent cavitation may occur as surgical complications; rarely, dissemination may result. When thoracic surgery is required, perioperative intravenous therapy with amphotericin B may be desirable.

Antifungal chemotherapy is indicated for those at high risk for severe coccidioidomycosis (though there is no assurance that this will prevent dissemination) and those who have recognized metapulmonary dissemination. Currently available chemotherapeutic agents are amphotericin B, as a desoxycholate suspension or in a liposomal or lipid complex form, all parenteral preparations; fluconazole, oral or intravenous; and ketoconazole or itraconazole, both in oral forms. Indications for the use of one or the other of these medications are not clearly defined. However, in the patient with rapidly progressing coccidioidomycosis, amphotericin B should be administered. Amphotericin B, 0.1 to 1.0 mg/kg/24 hr, is given intravenously. Once the full dose is achieved, it can be given every other day or two to three times a week in the face of the frequently reduced renal function owing to its toxicity. Thrombophlebitis is common but can be lessened by the use of indwelling catheters. Anemia resulting from the drug can be effectively treated with transfusion, if necessary, but terminates when treatment is stopped. Agranulocytosis is rare, and hepatic insufficiency develops occasionally, mainly in those with pre-existing liver damage.

Intravenous amphotericin B does not cross the blood-brain barrier in therapeutic amounts, but it may mast the presence of meningitis. Intrathecal (cisternal or lumbar) or intraventricular administration of amphotericin B had been the mainstay of treatment of coccidioidal meningitis. Orally administered fluconazole readily penetrates from the blood into the cerebrospinal fluid, whereas itraconazole does not. Yet fluconazole or itraconazole has proved useful in treating coccidioidal meningitis, although the duration of treatment and of arrest of the meningitis has not yet been defined. Ketoconazole, fluconazole, or itraconazole administered orally (in daily doses of approximately 3–15 mg/kg, 2–7 mg/kg, or 3–6 mg/kg, respectively) has been useful in treating disseminated nonmeningeal coccidioidomycosis that is neither extensive nor progressing rapidly. Although the azoles have increasingly been used to treat children as well as adults with coccidioidomycosis, there is limited information about the effects in younger patients. While ketoconazole can yield hepatic dysfunction and inhibit testosterone synthesis in adults, these effects have not been adequately evaluated in children. Fluconazole is primarily excreted by the kidneys, and itraconazole is metabolized in the liver; these drugs do not significantly affect testosterone or adrenocorticoid synthesis. On the basis of limited experience, coccidioidomycosis in pregnant women should be treated with amphotericin B, which has no apparent adverse effect on the fetus. Until more data are available, azoles should not be given to pregnant patients. The duration of therapy needed with the azoles has not been clearly defined and needs to be determined for individual patients. Relapses have occurred in some patients after favorable clinical responses following therapy for more than a year. The sole indication for parenteral **miconazole** is intrathecal or intraventricular administration for treatment of meningitis.

Chronic pulmonary coccidioidal disease, cavitary or fibrocavitary, has not consistently been improved by the azoles or by amphotericin B. Cavities are often best left alone, but surgical excision may be necessary in some cases.

Other surgical procedures include draining of cold abscesses, removal of infected synovial membranes, and curettage or excision of osseous lesions. Local as well as systemic administration of amphotericin B can be used for coccidioidal osseous and articular disease.

Ampel NM, Wieden MA, Galgiani JN: Coccidioidomycosis: a clinical update. Rev Infect Dis 11:897, 1989.

Bickel KD, Press BH, Hovey LM: Successful treatment of coccidioidomycosis osteomyelitis in an infant. Ann Plast Surg 30:462, 1993.

Boyle JO, Coulthard SW, Mandel RM: Laryngeal involvement in disseminated coccidioidomycosis. Arch Otolaryngol 117:433, 1991.

Galgiani JN: Coccidioidomycosis. West J Med 159:153, 1993.

Harrison HR, Galgiani JN, Reynolds AF Jr, et al: Amphotericin B and imidazole therapy for coccidioidal meningitis in children. Pediatr Infect Dis 2:216, 1983.

Kafka JA, Catanzaro A: Disseminated coccidioidomycosis in children. J Pediatr 98:355, 1981.

Labadie EL, Hamilton RH: Survival improvement in coccidioidal meningitis by high-dose intrathecal amphotericin B. Arch Intern Med 146:2013, 1986.

Pappagianis D: Coccidioidomycosis. *In*: Balows A, et al (eds): Laboratory Diagnosis of Infectious Diseases. New York, Springer-Verlag, 1988.

Pappagianis D, Zimmer BL: Serology of coccidioidomycosis. Clin Microbio Rev 3:247, 1990.

Peterson CM, Schuppert K, Kelly PC, et al: Coccidioidomycosis and pregnancy. Obstet Gynecol Surv 48:149, 1993.

Shafai T: Neonatal coccidioidomycosis in premature twins. Am J Dis Child 132:634, 1978.

Tucker RM, Williams PL, Arathoon EG, et al: Treatment of mycoses with itraconazole. Ann NY Acad Sci 544:451, 1988.

CHAPTER 234
Cryptococcosis

Stephen C. Aronoff

ETIOLOGY AND EPIDEMIOLOGY. Cryptococcosis is an invasive fungal disease caused by a monomorphic, encapsulated yeast. *Cryptococcus neoformans* var *neoformans* is the most common etiological agent worldwide and is the predominant pathogenic species among individuals infected with human immunodeficiency virus (HIV). This species predominates in temperate climates and is found in soil contaminated with avian droppings. *C. neoformans* var *neoformans* is also found on fruits and vegetables and may be carried by cockroaches. *Cryptococcus neoformans* var *gatti* is found mostly in the tropics, under flowering river red gum trees *(Eucalyptus camaldulensis)*. This species causes endemic disease in the tropics in non-HIV–infected individuals. *C. albidus* and *C. laurentii* are rare human pathogens.

Surveillance studies have demonstrated high rates of cryptococcal exposure among pigeon breeders and laboratory personnel who work with cryptococcus. Cryptococcosis is an unusual disease in most individuals, including children. Before the onset of the acquired immunodeficiency syndrome (AIDS) epidemic, cases of cryptococcosis were evenly divided among immunocompetent and immunocompromised individuals. In the United States, cryptococcosis occurs in 5–10% of HIV-infected individuals; higher rates of infection have been reported from less developed countries. Approximately 1% of HIV-infected American children younger than 13 years acquire cryptococcosis, and as many as 6% of HIV-infected adolescents or adults become infected with this fungus. In the vast majority of HIV-infected children, adolescents, and adults who become infected with cryptococcus, this infection is AIDS defining.

PATHOPHYSIOLOGY. Inhalation of fungal spores is the initial event in most cases of cryptococcosis. Local inoculation rarely leads to cutaneous or ophthalmic infection. In most immunocompetent individuals, infection is limited to the lung. In cases in which the immune system fails to contain the infection, dissemination follows with involvement of brain, meninges, skin, eyes, and the skeletal system.

In the lung, cryptococcosis produces granulomas that are often subpleural in location and contain demonstrable yeast forms. In the central nervous system (CNS), cystic cryptococcomas occur in 20% of non-HIV–infected patients with disseminated disease and may be found in the absence of overt meningitis. Granulomas and microabscesses containing yeast occur in cutaneous and bony infection.

CLINICAL MANIFESTATIONS. Although not evident in many instances, *pneumonia* is the most common form of cryptococcosis. Asymptomatic pulmonary infections occur among pigeon breeders, other avian enthusiasts, and laboratory workers. Asymptomatic carriage may occur in patients with underlying chronic lung disease. *Progressive pulmonary disease* is symptomatic and often a prelude to disseminated infection in the immunocompromised. Fever, cough, pleuritic chest pain, and constitutional symptoms occur. Chest radiographs may demonstrate a poorly localized bronchopneumonia, nodular changes, or lobar consolidations; cavities and pleural effusions are rare.

Disseminated infection follows primary pulmonary disease and is seen most often in immunocompromsed individuals, although disseminated infection may occur in otherwise normal children. Although HIV infection is the most common predisposing factor for disseminated cryptococcosis, acute lymphoblastic leukemia, immunosuppression for rheumatic disorders, allogeneic bone marrow transplants, primary immunodeficiencies affecting both T- and B-cell lineages and celiac disease are the major underlying conditions in non-HIV–infected individuals.

Subacute or chronic meningitis is the most common manifestation of disseminated cryptococcal infection. Clinical presentation is variable and prognostic. Good outcomes are associated with the following signs, symptoms, and findings: headache as the initial symptom, normal mental status, absence of predisposing condition, normal cerebrospinal fluid (CSF) opening pressure, normal CSF glucose, CSF white cell count less than 20 cells/mL, negative India ink stain, absence of extraneural infection by culture, and cryptococcal antigen titers in CSF and serum less than 1:32. Overt symptoms of meningitis and HIV infection are predictors of poor outcome. HIV-infected patients typically present with unexplained fevers, headache, and malaise; cryptococcal antigen titers in these individuals often exceed 1:1,024. Computed tomography of the brain will identify cryptococcomas in as many as 30% of patients with disseminated infection and no signs of CNS involvement. The mortality rate for cryptococcal meningitis is between 15 and 30%, with most deaths occurring within several weeks of diagnosis; the fatality rates are higher in HIV-infected individuals and relapse rates exceed 50%. Relapse is unusual in adequately treated, HIV-negative patients. Postinfectious sequelae are common and include hydrocephalus, changes in visual acuity, deafness, cranial nerve palsies, seizures, and ataxia.

Sepsis syndrome is a rare manifestation of cyrptococcosis and occurs almost exclusively in HIV-infected patients. Fever is followed by respiratory distress and multiorgan system disease. This syndrome is often fatal.

Cutaneous disease may accompany disseminated cryptococcosis or local infection. Lesions are often ulcerated, are centrally necrosed, and have raised borders. Early lesions are erythematous, may be single or multiple, and are variably indurated and tender. In HIV-infected patients, cutaneous cryptococcosis may resemble molluscum contagiosum.

Skeletal infection occurs in approximately 5% of individuals with disseminated infection but rarely in HIV-infected patients. The onset of symptoms is insidious and chronic. Bony involvement is typified by soft tissue swelling and tenderness, and arthritis is characterized by effusion, erythema, and pain on motion. Skeletal disease is unifocal in three quarters of cases, and multifocal osteomyelitis or concomitant bone and joint disease occurs from contiguous spread. Vertebral disease is the most common site of infection followed by the tibia, ileum, rib, femur, and humerus.

Chorioretinitis is rare, occurs primarily in adults, and is usually a manifestation of disseminated disease, although direct inoculation of the eye has been described. Eye infection is characterized by the acute loss of visual acuity, eye pain, floaters, and photophobia. On examination, choroiditis with or without retinitis is often noted. Retinovitreal masses and anterior uveitis are seen less commonly. Because eye disease is often a manifestation of disseminated infection, the mortality rate is higher than 20%. Among survivors, only 15% of affected individuals recover full vision.

Lymphonodular disease has been reported in two children, one of whom had an underlying immunodeficiency. This manifestation of cryptococcosis is characterized by disseminated adenopathy including thoracic and abdominal nodes, subcutaneous lesions, liver granulomas, and concomitant pulmonary disease.

DIAGNOSIS. Recovery of the fungus by culture or demonstration of the fungus in histologic section of infected tissue is diagnostically definitive. In disseminated disease, cryptococcal antigen can be readily demonstrated in the serum and CSF. India ink preparations of CSF are useful prognostically but are less sensitive than culture and antigen detection. Skin test antigens are poorly characterized, and the sensitivity and specificity of this test are unknown.

TREATMENT. The normal host with asymptomatic or mild disease limited to the lungs may be closely observed without therapy or treated with oral fluconazole (200–400 mg/day) for 3–6 mo. At present, no comparative data exist and fluconazole is not currently approved by the U.S. Food and Drug Administration for use in children. For normal hosts with progressive pulmonary disease or non-HIV–infected immunosuppressed patients with disease limited to the lungs amphotericin B (15 mg/kg to a maximum of 1.5 g total dose) alone or combined with flucytosine is accepted therapy. Fluconazole is a possible alternative in some of these cases, but the caveats identified earlier apply.

Combination therapy using amphotericin B and flucytosine is recommended for the treatment of CNS and other manifestations of disseminated infection in non-HIV–infected individuals. The total dosage of amphotericin B should exceed 15 mg/kg. Flucytosine (50–150 mg/kg/24 hr) is administered concurrently, and dosage should be adjusted to yield serum concentrations between 50 and 150 μg/mL. Cryptococcal antigen titers should be assayed before therapy is discontinued because serum or CSF values greater than or equal to 1:8 are predictive of relapse. Ventriculoperitoneal shunts may be required for patients with hydrocephalus, and aggressive medical management of increased intracranial pressure may also be required.

Because of the high rate of relapse, disseminated cryptococcosis in HIV-infected patients requires induction and maintenance therapy. Several induction therapies have been described, but data from comparative trials are still forthcoming. Amphotericin B with or without flucytosine in doses similar to those described previously for non-HIV–infected individuals is the best studied regimen for initial therapy. High rates of toxicity from flucytosine may preclude the use of this drug in HIV-infected patients. High-dose fluconazole alone or combined with flucytosine has also been used successfully for initial therapy. Finally, a 2-wk course of amphotericin B (0.7 mg/kg/24 hr) plus flucytosine (100 mg/kg/24 hr) followed by 8 wk of high-dose fluconazole is currently under investigation. Lifelong maintenance therapy with fluconazole is currently recommended and appears to be superior to weekly doses of amphotericin B.

Skeletal infections generally require surgical debridement in addition to systemic antifungal therapy. *Cutaneous infections* are usually treated medically, although surgical biopsy may be required diagnostically. The treatment of *chorioretinitis* also requires systemic antifungal therapy; these regimens should include either fluconazole or flucytosine because both of these agents achieve high drug concentrations in vitreous. In all cases of disseminated disease, duration and selection of antifungal regimens should be guided by HIV status as just noted.

Dismukes WE: Management of cryptococcosis. Clin Infect Dis 17(Suppl 2):S507, 1993.
Leggiadro RJ, Barrett FF, Hughes WT: Extrapulmonary cryptococcosis in immunocompromised infants and children. Pediatr Infect Dis J 11:43, 1992.
Leggiadro RJ, Kline MW, Hughes WT: Extrapulmonary cryptococcosis in children with acquired immunodeficiency syndrome. Pediatr Infect Dis J 10:658, 1991.
Moncino MD, Gutman LT: Severe systemic cryptococcal disease in a child: Review of prognostic indicators predicting treatment failure and an approach to maintenance therapy with oral fluconazole. Pediatr Infect Dis J 9:363, 1990.

CHAPTER 235
Mucormycosis

Stephen C. Aronoff

Mucormycosis *(zygomycosis)* refers to a group of opportunistic mycotic infections characterized by vascular invasion, thrombosis, and necrosis associated with dimorphic fungi of the class Zygomycetes and the order Mucorales. The genuses *Rhizopus, Absidia, Cunninghamella,* and *Mucor* are ubiquitous and found in soil, in decayed plant or animal matter, and on moldy cheese, fruit, or bread. Colonies of Mucorales grow on laboratory media as fluffy white, gray, or brown molds.

EPIDEMIOLOGY. Exposure to fungal spores is common and occasionally causes disease in normal children after insect bites or penetrating injuries with farm equipment. Invasive disease is unusual and occurs almost exclusively in immunocompromised children: diabetics with persistent acidosis, leukemics, steroid recipients, organ transplant recipients, and; those with human immunodeficiency virus infection. Person-to-person spread does not occur.

CLINICAL MANIFESTATIONS. After inhalation of spores from the environment, germination occurs, and local invasion of the nasal mucosa or lung, or both, follows. In severely immunosuppressed individuals, the fungus disseminates hematogenously.

Pulmonary mucormycosis is characterized by fever, tachypnea, and productive cough; pleuritic chest pain and hemoptysis occur variably. Signs of consolidation are found on physical examination. Lobar pneumonia or bilateral infiltrates may be seen on chest radiographs; pleural effusions are not rare. *Rhinocerebral mucormycosis* is rare in children and occurs primarily in individuals with leukemia, diabetes mellitus, or Fanconi anemia. Headache, retro-orbital pain, fever, and nasal discharge are the initial complaints in infected patients. Eye examination demonstrates periorbital edema, proptosis, ptosis, and ophthalmoplegia. The nasal discharge is often dark and bloody; examination of the nasal mucosa reveals black, necrotic areas. Extension beyond the nasal cavity is common. Destructive paranasal sinusitis with intracranial extension can be demonstrated by computed tomographic or magnetic resonance image scanning. Brain abscesses can complicate rhinocerebral infection by direct extension from the nasal cavity and sinuses or disseminated disease. In the former case, frontal or frontotemporal involvement occurs. Occipital or brain stem infection as well as cerebral infection can follow disseminated disease. *Cutaneous mucormycosis* is uncommon and can complicate burns or surgical wounds. Infection presents as an erythematous papule that ulcerates, leaving a black necrotic center.

DIAGNOSIS. Identification of the fungus histologically or recovery of the fungus by culture is required for diagnosis. In lung biopsy specimens and other tissue samples, Mucorales appear as thick-walled, nonseptate, right angle–branched hyphae when stained with silver. Vascular invasion is a hallmark of disease. These fungi may also be identified in secretions by suspending the clinical material in 20% potassium hydrochloride before microscopic examination. The fungi may be grown on standard laboratory media from sputum, bronchioalveolar lavage fluid, skin lesions, or biopsy material.

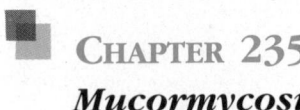

TREATMENT. The optimal therapy for children has not been established. Pulmonary disease has been treated successfully in adults with intermediate doses of amphotericin B (30 mg/kg total dose). Rhinocerebral mucormycosis and brain abscesses caused by Mucorales carry high fatality rates. Correction of the underlying disease, if possible, is a major therapeutic requirement. Extensive surgical debridement and high-dose amphotericin B therapy (1–1.5 mg/kg/24 hr to a total dose of 70 mg/kg) have been associated with successful outcomes. Cutaneous disease requires local debridement and intermediate dosages of amphotericin B (0.5–1 mg/kg/24 hr to a total dose of 30 mg/kg).

Cohen-Abbo A, Bozeman PM, Patrick CC: *Cunninghamella* infections: Review and report of two cases of Cunninghamella in immunocompromised children. Clin Infect Dis 17:173, 1993.
Kline MW: Mucormycosis in children: Review of the literature and report of cases. Pediatr Infect Dis J 4:672, 1985.

CHAPTER 236
Sporotrichosis

Stephen C. Aronoff

Sporotrichosis is an uncommon chronic fungal infection affecting humans and animals and is caused by the dimorphic fungus *Sporothrix schenckii.* The fungus is ubiquitous, although it predominates in the Missouri and Mississippi river valleys and exists in its saprophytic form in living and rotting plant matter. Disseminated infection is unusual, may follow ingestion or inhalation of spores, and occurs in immunocompromised patients. The cutaneous form of sporotrichosis follows intradermal inoculation with spores after fomite (sphagnum moss, barberry, rosebushes, and some grasses) or animal (cats, dogs, rodents, insects, or fish) contact. Sporotrichosis is often an occupational disease among farmers, gardeners, veterinarians, and pet owners. Human-to-human spread has not been reported.

PATHOLOGY. Histologically, sporotrichosis is characterized by noncaseating granulomas and microabscess formation. Oval or cigar-shaped forms are rarely seen in biopsy specimens because of the small number, size, and lack of specific staining techniques.

CLINICAL MANIFESTATIONS. *Cutaneous sporotrichosis* is the most common form of disease in infants and children. *Lymphocutaneous sporotrichosis* accounts for more than 75% of reported cases and occurs after traumatic subcutaneous inoculation. After a variable and often prolonged incubation period (1–12 wk), an isolated, painless erythematous papule develops at the inoculation site, usually an extremity. The initial lesion enlarges and ulcerates. Although the infection may remain limited to the inoculation site (fixed cutaneous sporotrichosis), satellite lesions follow lymphangitic spread and appear as multiple, tender, subcutaneous nodules tracking the lymphatic channels that drain the lesion. These secondary nodules are subcutaneous granulomas that adhere to the overlying skin and subsequently ulcerate. Sporotrichosis does not heal spontaneously, and these ulcerative lesions may persist for years if untreated. Systemic signs and symptoms are uncommon. *Extracutaneous sporotrichosis* is rare in children; pulmonary sporotrichosis, meningitis, osteomyelitis, arthritis, and disseminated disease have been reported in immunocompromised adults.

DIAGNOSIS. Cutaneous and lymphocutaneous sporotrichosis must be differentiated from other causes of nodular lymphangitis: *Mycobacterium marinum, Nocardia brasiliensis, Leishmania brasiliensis,* tularemia, other forms of nocardiosis and atypical mycobacterial infections, other systemic mycoses including coccidioidomycosis, melloidosis, and anthrax. Definitive diagnosis requires isolation of the fungus from the site of infection. In cases of disseminated disease, demonstration of serum antibody against *S. schenkii*–related antigens is diagnostically useful.

TREATMENT. Although comparative trials and extensive experience in children are not available, itraconazole appears to be the treatment of choice for significant infections. Dosages of 100 to 200 mg/24 hr for up to 6 mo may be required for complete resolution. Ketoconazole has also been used successfully for the treatment of cutaneous sporotrichosis; fluconazole appears to be less active in vitro than other azoles.

Kostman JR, DiNubile MJ: Nodular lymphangitis: A distinctive but often unrecognized syndrome. Ann Intern Med 118:883, 1993.
Naqvi SH, Becherer P, Gudipati S: Ketoconazole treatment of a family with zoonotic sporotrichosis. Scand J Infect Dis 25:543, 1993.
Restrepo A, Robledo J, Gomez I, et al: Itraconazole therapy in lymphangitic and cutaneous sporotrichosis. Arch Dermatol 122:413, 1986.
Sharkey-Mathis PK, Kauffman CA, Graybill JR, et al: Treatment of sporotrichosis with itraconazole: NIAID mycoses study. Am J Med 95:279, 1993.

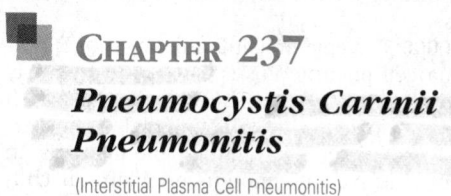

CHAPTER 237
Pneumocystis Carinii Pneumonitis

(Interstitial Plasma Cell Pneumonitis)

Walter T. Hughes

Pneumocystis carinii pneumonia is a life-threatening infection in the lungs of an immunosuppressed host. It is believed to occur in part from activation of latent organisms acquired in early life. Even in the most severe cases, with rare exception, the organisms and the disease remain localized to the lungs.

ETIOLOGY AND EPIDEMIOLOGY. *P. carinii* is a common extracellular parasite found in the lungs of mammals worldwide. The taxonomic placement of this organism has not been established, but it has attributes of fungi and protozoa. The natural habitat and mode of transmission to humans are unknown. Experiments in rats have demonstrated animal-to-animal transmission via the airborne route, but animal-to-human transmission is unlikely because of the host-specific nature of *P. carinii.* Human-to-human transmission has not been demonstrated. Serological surveys show most humans become infected with *P. carinii* before 4 yr of age. In the healthy host, these infections are asymptomatic. Pneumonitis caused by *P. carinii* occurs almost exclusively in severely immunocompromised hosts such as those with malignancies, those with acquired and congenital immunodeficiency disorders, and organ transplant recipients.

Approximately 40% of infants and children and 70% of adults with the acquired immunodeficiency syndrome (AIDS), 12% of children with leukemia, and 10% of patients with organ transplants acquire *P. carinii* pneumonitis, if no prophylaxis is given. Epidemics of interstitial plasma cell pneumonitis resulting from *P. carinii* occured in debilitated infants in Europe during and after World War II. These cases were attributed to malnutrition.

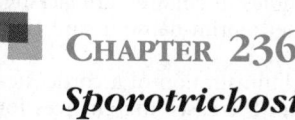

PATHOGENESIS AND PATHOLOGY. Two forms of *P. carinii* are found in the alveolar space: the "cyst" form is 5–8 μm in diameter and may contain up to eight pleomorphic intracystic sporozoites; and the extracystic "trophozoites" are 2 to 5 μ delicate cells derived from excysted sporozoites. *P. carinii* attaches to type I alveolar epithelial cells by adhesive proteins such as fibronectin and mannose-dependent ligand. Alveolar macrophages phagocytize and kill opsonized *P. carinii* organisms, releasing tumor necrosis factor. The histopathology of *P. carinii* pneumonitis is of two types. The first type is infantile interstitial plasma cell pneumonitis, which is seen in epidemic outbreaks in debilitated infants around 3–6 mo of age. Extensive infiltration with thickening of the alveolar septum occurs, and plasma cells are prominent. The second type is a diffuse desquamative alveolar disease found in immunocompromised children and adults. The alveoli contain large numbers of *P. carinii* in a foamy exudate with alveolar macrophages active in the phagocytosis of organisms. The alveolar septum is not infiltrated to the extent of the infantile type, and plasma cells are usually absent.

Cell-mediated immunity has the major role in defense against *P. carinii* pneumonitis as evidenced by its high frequency in severe combined immunodeficiency disorder (attack rates of greater than 40%) and the infrequency of its occurrence in X-linked agammaglobulinemia. Furthermore, studies in patients with AIDS show an increase in the occurrence of *P. carinii* pneumonitis when $CD4^+$ T-lymphocyte counts are below the range of normal. The $CD4^+$ T-lymphocyte count provides a useful indicator for the use of anti–*P. carinii* pneumonitis prophylaxis.

CLINICAL MANIFESTATIONS. The epidemic infantile form of *P. carinii* interstitial plasma cell pneumonitis is seen predominantly in infants between 3 and 6 mo of age. The onset is subtle with tachypnea and no fever, progressing to intercostal, suprasternal, and infrasternal retractions, nasal flaring, and cyanosis. In the sporadic form of *P. carinii* pneumonitis occurring in children and adults with underlying immunodeficiency, the onset is usually abrupt with fever, tachypnea, dyspnea, and cough progressing to nasal flaring and cyanosis. This latter type accounts for the majority of cases, although the severity of clinical expression may vary. Rales are usually absent. Rarely, extrapulmonary sites of *P. carinii* infection may occur (e.g., retina, spleen, bone marrow) but are usually not symptomatic.

The chest radiograph reveals bilateral diffuse alveolar disease with a granular pattern. The earliest densities are perihilar, and progression proceeds peripherally, sparing the apical areas until last.

DIAGNOSIS. A definitive diagnosis requires the demonstration of *P. carinii* in the lung in addition to clinical signs and symptoms of the infection. Methods for obtaining organisms include bronchoalveolar lavage, tracheal aspirates, transbronchial lung biopsy, bronchial brushings, percutaneous transthoracic needle aspiration, and open lung biopsy. Induced sputum samples are useful if *P. carinii* is found, but the absence of the organism does not exclude the infection. The open lung biopsy is the most reliable method, although bronchoalveolar lavage is more practical in most cases. Four stains are in general use: Grocott-Gomori stain and toluidine blue stain the cyst form, polychrome stains such as Giemsa stain the trophozoites and sporozoites, and the fluorescein-labeled monoclonal antibody stains both trophozoites and cysts.

TREATMENT. Without treatment, *P. carinii* is fatal within 3–4 wk of onset in the immunocompromised host. However, survival occurs in 70–90% of cases treated early in the course of the pneumonitis. Trimethoprim (15–20 mg/kg/24 hr) plus sulfamethoxazole (75–100 mg/kg/24 hr) is the treatment of first choice. This fixed-drug combination may be administered intravenously or orally and should be given over a period of about 2 wk for non-AIDS patients and 3 wk for AIDS patients. Unfortunately, adverse reactions frequently occur with trimethoprim-sulfamethoxazole administration, including rash and neutropenia. For patients who cannot tolerate or fail to respond to trimethoprim-sulfamethoxazole, pentamidine isethionate, 4.0 mg/kg/24 hr as a single intravenous dose, may be used. Adverse reactions are frequent and include renal and hepatic dysfunction, hyper- or hypoglycemia, rash, and thrombocytopenia. Atovaquone and trimetrexate glucuronate have been approved by the U.S. Food and Drug Administration for the treatment of adults, but studies in children are lacking. Other effective drugs include trimethoprim-dapsone and clindamycin plus primaquine.

Studies in adults suggest that administration of a corticosteroid along with anti–*P. carinii* drugs increases the chances for survival of moderate and severe cases of *P. carinii* pneumonitis.

PREVENTION. Patients at high risk for *P. carinii* pneumonitis should be placed on chemoprophylaxis. Guidelines have been established by the Centers for Disease Control and Prevention for prophylaxis of HIV-infected infants and children based on age and $CD4^+$ T-lymphocyte counts (see Chapter 223). Patients with severe combined immunodeficiency syndrome, those with organ transplants, and those receiving intensive immunosuppressive therapy for cancer or other diseases are also candidates for prophylaxis. Trimethoprim (5.0 mg/kg/24 hr) plus sulfamethoxazole (25.0 mg/kg/24 hr) is the drug of choice and may be given daily or for 3 days per week. Alternatives for prophylaxis are dapsone or dapsone plus pyrimethamine orally and pentamidine by aerosol. The prophylaxis must be continued as long as the patient is immunocompromised.

Centers for Disease Control. Guidelines for prophylaxis against *P. carinii* pneumonia in children infected with human immunodeficiency virus. MMWR 40:1, 1991.

Conner E, Bagarazzi M, McSherry G, et al: Clinical and laboratory correlates of *Pneumocystis carinii* pneumonia in children infected with HIV. JAMA 265:1693, 1991.

Hughes W. Leoung G, Kramer F, et al: Comparison of atovaquone (566C80) with trimethoprim-sulfamethoxazole to treat *Pneumocystis carinii* pneumonia in patients with AIDS. N Engl J Med 328:1521, 1993.

Hughes WT, Rivera GK, Schell MJ, et al: Successful intermittent chemoprophylaxis for *Pneumocystis carinii* pneumonia. N Engl J Med 316:1627, 1987.

Kovacs A, Frederick T, Church J, et al: CD_4 T-lymphocyte counts and *Pneumocystis carinii* pneumonia in pediatric HIV infection. JAMA 265:1698, 1991.

National Institutes of Health, University of California Expert Panel for Corticosteroids as Adjunctive Therapy for *Pneumocystis carinii*: Consensus statement on the use of corticosteroids as adjunctive therapy for pneumocystis pneumonia in the acquired immunodeficiency syndrome. N Engl J Med 323:1500, 1990.

Sanyal SK, Chebib FS, Gilbert JR, Hughes WT: Sequential changes in vital signs and acid-base and blood-gas profies in *Pneumocystis carinii* pneumonitis in children with cancer: Basis for a scoring system to identify patients who will require ventilatory support. Am J Respir Crit Care Med 149:1092, 1994.

Simmonds RJ, Oxtoby MJ, Caldwell MB, et al: *Pneumocystis carinii* pneumonia among U.S. children with perinatally acquired HIV infection. JAMA 270:470, 1993.

Stavola JJ, Noel GJ: Efficacy and safety of dapsone prophylaxis against *Pneumocystis carinii* pneumonia in human immunodeficiency virus-infected children. Pediatr Infect Dis J 12:644, 1993.

Section 6

Rickettsial Infections

J. Stephen Dumler

Chapter 238

Rickettsiae

CLASSIFICATION. Agents of rickettsial disease were originally grouped together based on the concept that arthropods are an important part of the organisms' life cycle and in part based on the presumed obligate intracellular associations of these agents. Thorough studies of these organisms were greatly hindered because most were difficult or impossible to cultivate; therefore, classification based strictly on this schema is flawed. The advent of molecular taxonomic classification has confirmed a close genetic and phenotypic relationship between some of the genera (*Rickettsia* and *Ehrlichia*) and proved that convergent evolution has yielded characteristics that led to the inclusion of other more diverse genetic and phenotypic genera and species such as *Coxiella* and *Rochalimaea.* In fact, molecular methods of nucleic acid amplification and sequence analysis have shown that a much broader spectrum of rickettsial agents exist that were previously unidentified and that cause significant human disease. In general, three genera are now considered to include important human pathogens in the family Rickettsiaceae: *Rickettsia, Ehrlichia,* and *Coxiella.* Compelling evidence now exists to exclude members of the genera *Bartonella* and *Rochalimaea* from this family; consequently, these bacteria and the diseases that they cause are addressed in separate chapters.

The members of the three genera, which are important human pathogens in the family Rickettsiaceae, are true bacteria that contain DNA and RNA and divide by binary fission. Phylogenetic analysis of the 16S ribosomal DNA sequences indicates that *Rickettsia* and *Ehrlichia* should be classified within the alpha subgroup of purple eubacteria and that *Coxiella burnetii* fits more closely within the gamma subdivision. By ultrastructure, these bacteria have gram negative–type cells walls, and when examined by light microscopy, they appear as small, pleomorphic, gram-negative intracellular bacteria. All of these bacteria have evolved in the context of a eukaryotic intracellular compartment and thus have developed specialized adaptations that permit and enhance survival in their distinctive niches. None have been successfully cultivated on artificial, cell-free medium, and although in vitro cultivation in tissue culture has been accomplished for many of these species (including most of the vasculotropic rickettsiae, *C. burnetii, Ehrlichia chaffeensis,* and *Ehrlichia sennetsu,* the granulocytotropic ehrlichiae and the *Rickettsia typhi*–like ELB rickettsia have never been cultivated in vitro. Members of the genus *Rickettsia* live freely in the cytoplasm of the host cell, whereas those in the genera *Ehrlichia* and *Coxiella* live in membrane-bound vacuoles. Ehrlichiae actively inhibit phagosome-lysosome fusion to grow into a cytoplasmic aggregate of bacteria called a morula, whereas *C. burnetii* tolerates and actively proliferates within the acidified phagolysosome to form aggregates often containing in excess of 100 bacteria.

Rickettsia species contain lipopolysaccharide (LPS) as in other related gram-negative bacteria, and some epitopes in this LPS convey group and genus serologic cross-reactivity. The exception is *R. tsutsugamushi,* which lacks both LPS and peptidoglycan in its cell wall. *C. burnetii* undergo an LPS "phase variation" similar to that described for smooth and rough strains of enterobacteria. Further emphasizing the differences among these genera is the lack of any evidence of LPS or lipo-oligosaccharide components in the genus *Ehrlichia.* Although immunoblot analysis has demonstrated the presence of many species- or genus-specific proteins, no definite function has been ascribed to any of the proteins yet identified. Evidence is now accumulating to suggest that some of the major outer membrane proteins of *Rickettsia* species function as cellular ligands to promote host cell attachment and invasion, and others may serve as structural components. Definite rickettsial virulence factors with proven in vivo significance have yet to be identified.

Rickettsial diseases of humans are separated into groups on the basis of clinical characteristics, etiologic agent, insect vectors, and epidemiology (Table 238–1). Rickettsiae are transmitted among mammalian reservoirs usually by arthropod vectors. Humans are not an essential link in their natural cycle but become chance hosts when they are bitten by an infected vector, scratch or rub infectious arthropod feces into the skin, or inhale or ingest the organism. Rocky Mountain spotted fever (RMSF) is the rickettsial infection most frequently encountered in the United States and accounts for nearly 90% of all rickettsial cases reported each year; sporadic cases of murine typhus, ehrlichiosis, Q fever, rickettsialpox, and epidemic typhus make up the remainder. Boutonneuse fever or other spotted fevers are serologically confirmed in travelers who have been in southern or eastern Africa, the Mediterranean basin, India, or other *Rickettsia*-endemic areas. Epidemic typhus (louse-borne typhus) continues to occur in epidemics wherever human misery, poverty, or pestilence may be identified, as exemplified by recent outbreaks in remote parts of South America. Scrub typhus, caused by *R. tsutsugamushi,* occurs in China, the western Pacific region, the Indian subcontinent, and Australia, where it occasionally poses a risk to travelers who venture into remote rural areas. The presence of indigenous reservoirs and vectors, plus the continuous possibility that new strains of rickettsiae may be introduced from other parts of the world, makes the threat of new outbreaks in the United States a continuing concern. Effective rickettsial vaccines are not available.

PATHOGENESIS. Although grouped together under the name "rickettsial diseases," the pathogenesis of disease caused by the various genera in the family Rickettsiaceae is quite different. Members of the genus *Rickettsia* are vasculotropic and infect endothelial cells, whereas both ehrlichiae and coxiellae reside within phagocytes, which accounts for some of the clinicopathologic differences encountered. The pathogenesis of the vasculotropic rickettsioses is best understood. Once the infectious agent is inoculated through the skin into the dermis via arthropod bite or by contamination of a skin wound with infected arthropod feces, the rickettsiae attach to vascular endothelium via protein ligands. The attached rickettsiae initiate focal host cell membrane injury because of inherent rickettsial phospholipase activity. The membrane damage induces phagocytosis for repair, and the *Rickettsia* is internalized only to gain

■ TABLE 238–1 Rickettsial Diseases of Humans: Summary of Pertinent Features

Group Disease	Causative Agent	Arthropod Vector-Transmission	Hosts	Confirmatory Tests*	Geographic Distribution
Spotted Fever					
Rocky Mountain spotted fever	*Rickettsia rickettsii*	Tick bite	Dogs, rodents	IFA, EIA, DFA, IH, PCR	Western hemisphere
Boutonneuse fever (Mediterranean spotted fever)	*Rickettsia conorii*	Tick bite	Dogs, rodents	IFA, EIA, DFA, IH	Africa, Mediterranean region, India, Middle East
Rickettsialpox	*Rickettsia akari*	Mite bite	Mice	IFA	North America, Russia, Ukraine, Adriatic region, Korea, South Africa
Typhus					
Murine typhus	*Rickettsia typhi*/ELB agent	Rat flea or cat flea feces	Rats, opossums	IFA, EIA, DFA, PCR	Worldwide
Epidemic typhus	*Rickettsia prowazekii*	Louse feces	Humans	IFA, EIA, PCR	Africa, South America, Central America, Mexico, Asia
Brill-Zinnser disease (recrudescent typhus)	*Rickettsia prowazekii*	Reactivation of latent infection	Humans	IFA, EIA	Potentially worldwide; United States, Canada, Eastern Europe
Flying squirrel (sylvatic) typhus	*Rickettsia prowazekii*	Louse or flea of flying squirrel	Flying squirrels	IFA, EIA	Eastern United States
Scrub Typhus					
Scrub typhus	*Rickettsia tsutsugamushi*	Chigger bite	Rodents?	IFA, EIA	Southern Asia, Japan, Indonesia, Australia, Korea, Asiatic Russia, Indian subcontinent, China
Ehrlichiosis					
Human monocytic ehrlichiosis	*Ehrlichia chaffeensis*	Tick bite	Deer, dogs?	IFA, IH, PCR	United States, Europe, Africa
Human granulocytic ehrlichiosis	*Ehrlichia* species closely related to *E. phagocytophila* and *E. equi*	Tick bite	Unknown	IFA, IH, PCR	United States
Sennetsu ehrlichiosis	*Ehrlichia sennetsu*	Unknown	Unknown	IFA	Japan, Malaysia
Others					
Q fever	*Coxiella burnetii*	Ticks?	Cattle, sheep, goats, cats, rabbits	IFA, EIA	Worldwide

**DFA or IH test can be used to detect rickettsiae, ehrlichiae, or coxiellae in tissues samples. PCR may be performed to detect rickettsia, ehrlichia, or coxiella nucleic acids in acute phase blood or tissues using specific oligonucleotide primers. Preferred confirmatory serologic tests include IFA and EIA. Cross-absorption of patient serum with specific rickettsial antigens or defined epitope blocking of species-specific monoclonal antibodies with patient serum may be performed to distinguish among spotted fever and typhus group infections. Cultivation may be attempted by specialized health laboratories.*

IFA = indirect fluorescent antibody assay; EIA = enzyme immunoassay; DFA = direct fluorescent antibody; IH = immunohistology; PCR = polymerase chain reaction.

free access to the cytosol by continued phospholipase-mediated vacuolar membrane lysis. Members of the spotted fever serologic group actively initiate intracellular actin polymerization for directional movement, and rickettsiae may thus easily invade neighboring cells while inducing minimal initial host cell damage. The rickettsiae proliferate and may cause host cell damage by peroxidative membrane alterations or by continued phospholipase activity as in spotted fever group infections or may cause mechanical lysis secondary to the massive numbers of organisms contained within, as in typhus group infections. The presence of the infectious agent initiates the inflammatory cascade including release of cytokines such as tumor necrosis factor-α (TNF-α), (interleukin-1β, and interferon gamma [IFN-γ]) and infiltration of the damaged endothelial cells with lymphocytes, macrophages, and occasionally neutrophils. Local inflammatory and immune responses have been suspected as contributors to vascular injury in the rickettsioses; however, the benefits of effective inflammation and immunity outweigh potential damage mediated by host responses directed toward elimination of local infection. Blockade of TNF-α and IFN-γ action in animal models diminishes survival and increases morbidity of spotted fever group infections probably by abrogating upregulation of nitric oxide synthase and arginine-dependent intracellular killing events. Although infected cells may be sacrificed, the overall effect is beneficial. Similarly, *Rickettsia*-mediated endothelial injury may lead to upregulated expression of procoagulant molecules on the surfaces of endothelial cells to promote platelet adhesion, leukocyte emigration, and coagulation factor consumption, resulting in a clinical syndrome similar to disseminated intravascular coagulation. Vascular changes may occur in any anatomic location and are often detected as a maculopapular or petechial rash or as increased vascular permeability and edema in many organs including lung or brain.

Although patients with ehrlichiosis often present with an illness similar to the vasculotropic rickettsioses, the pathogenesis is clearly different because endothelial cell infection and vasculitis are rare events. The exact pathogenetic mechanisms are poorly understood, but the end result appears to be a diffuse proliferation of mononuclear phagocytes leading to granuloma formation or histiocytic infiltrates and activation of the mononuclear phagocyte system with consumption of platelets and leukocytes. This activation results in moderate to profound leukopenia and thrombocytopenia in the presence of a hypercellular, reactive bone marrow, and fatalities are often associated with severe hemorrhage or secondary infections. Hepatic or other organ-specific injury occurs by an unknown mechanism apparently unrelated to direct infection.

In contrast to these other rickettsial infections, humans acquire *C. burnetii* after inhalation of infectious aerosols. The most frequent presentations of acute Q fever include an influenza-like respiratory illness, a granulomatous illness with hepatitis, and an undifferentiated febrile illness. Pulmonary infection elicits a mild interstitial lymphocytic pneumonitis with a dense macrophage-rich intra-alveolar exudate heavily infected with *C. burnetii.* The infection may elicit granulomas in liver, bone marrow, and other organs, all signs of an acute and usually self-limited infection. As with many other obligate intracellular pathogens, recovery from acute infection may result in nonsterile immunity. One hypothesis suggests that development of debilitating chronic Q fever results after recovery from a mild or inapparent episode of acute Q fever after which the agent is not cleared. The persistence of *C. burnetii* in tissue macrophages at sites of pre-existing vascular damage causes a low-grade smoldering inflammation, which eventually leads to irreversible cardiac valve damage or persistent vascular injury.

DIAGNOSIS. Severe or fatal rickettsial infections are associated with delays in diagnosis and treatment. No single laboratory test completely establishes an early diagnosis. Thus, treatment should not be withheld pending laboratory results for a patient with clinically suspect illness. If a rash is present, a vasculotropic rickettsial infection can be diagnosed as early as day 3 to 4 of illness by immunohistologic demonstration of specific rickettsial antigen in the endothelium in skin biopsies of petechial lesions. The method may be performed by immunofluorescence or by immunoperoxidase and is very specific. Unfortunately, the sensitivity of this method is probably not greater than 70% and can be negatively influenced by prior antimicrobial therapy, biopsy of skin lesions that are less than optimal, or examination of insufficient tissue because the infection may be very focal. Moreover, because approximately 10–15% of patients with RMSF do not have rash or experience atypical rashes, selection of an appropriate biopsy site may be difficult. Evaluation of the coccobacillary morphology of *Rickettsia rickettsii* in its intracellular location should be performed by an experienced individual to avoid a false-positive interpretation of the results. Because cutaneous manifestations of ehrlichiosis and Q fever are infrequent, this method would not be useful for routine diagnosis. Immunocytology has been successful in the identification of ehrlichiae in leukocytes in blood and cerebrospinal fluid, and *C. burnetii* have been demonstrated by immunohistologic methods in tissue samples from occasional patients with Q fever, but the reagents and testing expertise are available only in specialized laboratories.

Molecular diagnostic methods allow a rapid, early diagnosis using polymerase chain reaction (PCR) amplification of rickettsial nucleic acids in acute-phase blood. Unfortunately, evaluations of PCR on blood for *R. rickettsii* nucleic acids demonstrate little additional sensitivity beyond that of immunohistology, probably because the level of rickettsemia is generally very low (<six rickettsia per milliliter of blood). Conversely, PCR on whole blood nucleic acids has proven a useful method for identification of ehrlichiosis, especially given the lack of anatomic localization for biopsy and the propensity of ehrlichiae to infect circulating leukocytes. In monocytic ehrlichiosis, these methods appear to be sensitive (87%) and probably highly specific. In an alternate method, which has been successfully applied for the diagnosis of boutonneuse fever, endothelial cells are isolated from circulating endothelial cells in blood using a monoclonal antibody and are examined for the presence of rickettsiae by immunofluorescence. Unfortunately, these early diagnostic methods are not widely available, and the diagnosis is not excluded by negative results; thus, treatment should not be withheld.

Rickettsiae and coxiellae have been cultivated in tissue culture cells; with the use of centrifugation-assisted shell vial culture and early immunocytologic detection of in vitro infection, a specific diagnosis may be rendered within as few as 48 hr. Some consider rickettsial cultivation hazardous; however, given the widespread application of universal precautions, such methods should be reconsidered for early and specific identification of rickettsial infections. Unfortunately, *E. chaffeensis* has been isolated only two times, each requiring in excess of 30 days for definitive isolation, and, the agent of human granulocytic ehrlichiosis has never been cultivated.

Historically, serology remains the most useful method to confirm infection in a convalescent patient. Paired sera obtained during the acute phase of illness and at least 2–4 wk after the acute illness (convalescent phase) may be tested for antibodies to any of a large number of specific rickettsial or ehrlichial antigens or for *C. burnetii.* A fourfold increase in antibody titer or a single high titer convalescent serum usually provides serologic confirmation in conjunction with a clinically compatible illness. Although members of the genera *Ehrlichia* and *C. burnetii* are antigenically distinct, the genus *Rickettsia* contains several species that demonstrate strong or weak serologic cross-reactions, and using currently available methods a serologic response implicating one species of this genera as the etiologic agent may be difficult to obtain. For the confirmation of infection by *Rickettsia,* the most useful method is the indirect fluorescent antibody (IFA) assay which is highly sensitive and specific. Other sensitive and specific tests include latex agglutination, enzyme-linked immunosorbent assay (ELISA), immunoperoxidase, solid-phase enzyme immunoassay, and indirect hemagglutination. The latex agglutination test is most useful for confirmation in early convalescence because it detects immunoglobulin (Ig)M better than other immunoglobulins. The IFA and enzyme immunoassays can be used to quantitate IgM or IgG. First-generation tests, which include complement fixation and microagglutination methods, use specific rickettsial antigens and generally lack the sensitivity and specificity of later generation tests. So little accurate information may be gained from the insensitive and nonspecific Weil-Felix test, which uses cross-reactive *Proteus* species antigens, that it should be relegated to historical notes only. Protein immunoblot (Western blot) analyses of antirickettsial antibodies have not been proven as a useful adjunct for an etiologic diagnosis down to the species level. However, because all of the vasculotropic rickettsial species of human importance harbor species-specific outer membrane proteins, antibodies present in human serum after infection may effectively block binding of monoclonal antibodies to these species-specific epitopes in a defined epitope-blocking ELISA, which may thus be used to establish an etiologic diagnosis at the genus and species level. Available serologic tests for *Ehrlichia* and *C. burnetii* are largely limited to reference and research laboratories in the United States. Both IFA and ELISA have been used effectively for confirmation of infection.

TREATMENT. Therapy of rickettsial infections has previously been assumed to be monolithic. The dogma of treating with tetracycline, doxycycline, or chloramphenicol regardless of the rickettsial infection must now be questioned. RMSF fever and the other vasculotropic rickettsioses (typhus, rickettsialpox, boutonneuse fever, scrub typhus) are effectively treated with all of these agents, and a cure may be expected if therapy using an adequate dosage is begun on or before the 5th day of disease. However, the use of chloramphenicol is now being questioned because a controlled, retrospective study has shown excess mortality in chloramphenicol-treated patients compared with tetracycline- and doxycycline-treated patients. Moreover, in vitro testing and individual case reports document that ehrlichial susceptibility to chloramphenicol is questionable. This is particularly problematic because the use of tetracycline agents has been discouraged in pediatric patients as a result of the potential for tooth discoloration and other effects on bone. In fact, such abnormalities are cumulative and dose dependent, and a short course of doxycycline or tetracycline provides a small risk for development of these changes. The use of chloramphenicol or tetracycline is best determined for each individual patient's needs.

For some rickettsial infections such as murine typhus or

boutonneuse fever, alternate antimicrobial agents including the fluoroquinolones, ciprofloxacin (200 mg intravenously [IV], or 750 mg orally [PO], every 12 hr), ofloxacin (200 mg PO every 12 hr), and pefloxacin (400 mg IV or PO every 12 hr) are reported to be efficacious or have been successfully used in individual cases. Acute Q fever may be treated similarly; however, chronic Q fever remains quite refractory to most antibiotic therapies and probably requires long-term, multidrug therapy. Other broad-spectrum antibiotics including penicillins, cephalosporins, aminoglycosides, and macrolides are not effective. The use of clarithromycin and azithromycin has not been evaluated. Greater morbidity and excess mortality are associated with the use of sulfonamides; consequently, their use should be discouraged. Most useful antimicrobial agents are rickettsiostatic, and eradication of the rickettsiae depends on development of an adequate immune response. Thus, prophylactic therapy after tick bite or other arthropod bite may only delay the onset of illness and further confound diagnosis.

Specific therapeutic recommendations include doxycycline given in two loading doses (2.2 mg/kg each) at 12-hr intervals PO or IV followed by 2.2 mg/kg/24 hr divided in doses every 12 hr for a maximum dose of 300 mg. Tetracycline is given at 25–50 mg/kg/24 hr in four divided doses for a maximum of 2 g/24 hr). Chloramphenicol is given in a dose of 50–100 mg/kg/24 hr in four divided doses for a maximum of 3 g/24 hr. Therapy should be continued for a minimum of 5 days and until the patient has been afebrile for at least 2–4 days to avoid relapse, especially in those patients treated early. Patients treated with this regimen will usually become afebrile within 48 hr, and thus the entire period of therapy will last less than 10 days. Although no controlled study has been performed to evaluate the use of corticosteroids, patients with central nervous system manifestations resulting from cerebral or meningeal inflammation may benefit from this therapy by a mechanism similar to that reported for other bacterial meningitides. In the most severely affected patients, morbidity usually develops related to vascular permeability; consequently, vigorous supportive therapy with careful hemodynamic monitoring will effectively regulate administration of parenteral fluids and blood or platelet transfusions when required and will avoid life-threatening iatrogenic pulmonary edema. Delayed therapy or diagnosis often results in irreversible rickettsial vascular and end-organ injury.

CHAPTER 239
Spotted Fever Group Rickettsioses

239.1 Rocky Mountain Spotted Fever

EPIDEMIOLOGY. The term *Rocky Mountain spotted fever* is a misnomer because the disease now occurs in almost every state of the continental United States, southwestern Canada, Mexico, Central America, and South America. In the United States, the highest prevalence rates are seen in Oklahoma, North Carolina, Arkansas, Missouri, Tennessee, and Kansas; however, the changing ecology of tick vectors and climate changes may influence the geographic prevalence over different years and decades. Although first recognized as a distinct clinical entity in the Bitterroot region of Montana and in areas of Idaho, only a small percentage of all documented cases are currently reported from the Rocky Mountain region. Habitat associations with disease are predicted by those favored by tick vectors including wooded areas or coastal grassland and salt marshes. Foci of infection have also been well documented in rural and some urban settings such as the South Bronx. Most cases in the United States are documented to occur during seasons with peak tick activity and potential human exposure, especially April through October. The highest incidence of disease occurs in children 5–9 yr of age.

ETIOLOGY AND TRANSMISSION. Ticks are the natural hosts, reservoirs, and vectors of *Rickettsia rickettsii*, the etiologic agent of Rocky Mountain spotted fever. Ticks naturally maintain infection by transovarial transmission (passage of the organism from infected ticks to their progeny) and to a lesser extent by acquisition of rickettsiae when a blood meal is taken from transiently rickettsemic animal hosts such as dogs and rodents. Many species of ticks are capable of sustaining and transmitting the infectious agent to mammalian hosts, including humans, by regurgitation of infected saliva during feeding. The principal hosts of *R. rickettsii* are *Dermacentor variabilis* (the dog tick) in the eastern United States and Canada, *D. andersoni* (the wood tick) in the western United States and Canada, possibly *Amblyomma americanum* (the Lone Star tick) in the south central United States, *Rhipicephalus sanguineus* (the brown dog tick) in Mexico, and *Amblyomma cajennense* in Central and South America.

Dogs may also serve as reservoir hosts for *R. rickettsii* and are important vehicles to bring potentially infected ticks into the environment shared by humans. Serologic studies of patients with Rocky Mountain spotted fever indicate that a high percentage may have contracted the illness from ticks carried by the family dog. Infection is largely transmitted via the bite of an infected tick; however, transmission has occurred by inoculation of tick fluids or feces into open wounds or conjunctivae from the fingers and hands. Fatalities have occurred in laboratory workers exposed to infectious aerosols.

CLINICAL MANIFESTATIONS. The incubation period in children varies from 2–14 days, and the median is 7 days. The illness is initially nonspecific with headache, fever, anorexia, and restlessness. Gastrointestinal symptoms such as nausea, vomiting, diarrhea, or abdominal pain occur frequently (39–63%) early in the disease. Often considered the hallmark of rickettsial infection, skin rash is detected usually after the third day of illness, and the typical clinical triad of headache, fever, and rash is documented in only 3% of all patients at presentation. Approximately 10% of patients have no rash or atypical cutaneous manifestations. The site of tick bite is usually inapparent. Discrete, pale, rose-red blanching macules or maculopapules appear initially and characteristically on the extremities including the ankles, wrists, or lower legs (Fig. 239–1). The rash spreads rapidly to involve the entire body, including soles and palms. After several days, the rash becomes more petechial or hemorrhagic, sometimes palpable purpura (Fig. 239–2). Fever and headache persist and are accompanied by severe myalgia and malaise. Splenomegaly and hepatomegaly are present in approximately 33% of patients. In severe disease, the petechiae may enlarge into ecchymoses, which may become necrotic. Severe vascular obstruction secondary to the rickettsial vasculitis and thrombosis may result in gangrene of digits, ear lobes, the scrotum, the nose, or an entire limb. Central nervous system infection will often yield changes in sensorium, and delirium or coma may supervene. In addition, patients may manifest ataxia, meningismus, or auditory deficits. Other severe manifestations include facial edema, myocarditis, acute renal failure, vascular collapse, and pneumonitis with noncardiogenic pulmonary edema.

In patients with glucose-6-phosphate dehydrogenase defi-

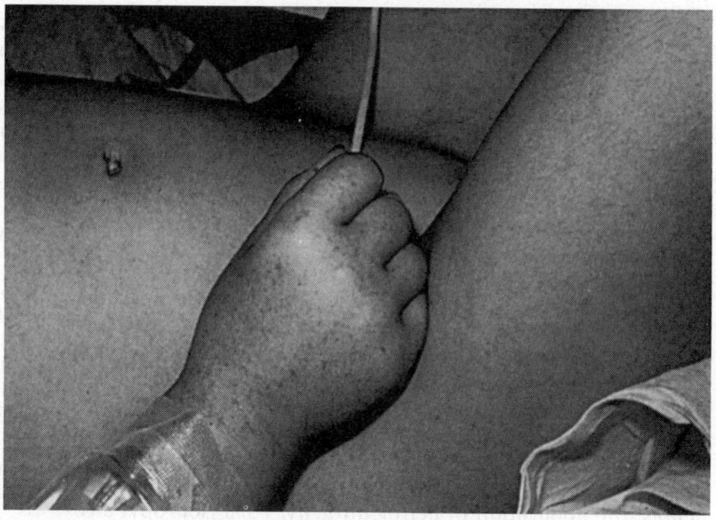

Figure 239–1. Patient with Rocky Mountain spotted fever. Note the predominance of the rash on the extremities. See also color section. (Courtesy of Debra Karp Skopicki, M.D., Baltimore.)

ciency, a rapid and fulminant infection may develop, leading to death in less than 5 days with a clinical course characterized by profound coagulopathy and extensive visceral thrombosis with kidney, liver, or respiratory failure. Clinical features associated with fatal outcome include hepatomegaly, jaundice, stupor, acute renal failure, respiratory distress, and a disseminated intravascular coagulation–like syndrome.

Delays in diagnosis and therapy are significant factors associated with death or severe illness. Before the advent of effective antimicrobial therapy for Rocky Mountain spotted fever, the case fatality rate ranged from 10–40%. More recent statistics have shown a stabilization of this rate fluctuating between 2 and 7%. The fact that fatalities occur despite the availability of effective therapeutic agents indicates the need for vigilant clinical suspicion and a low threshold for early and aggressive therapy in clinically suspect cases. Even with administration of tetracycline or chloramphenicol therapy, delays in therapy may allow sufficient vascular and end-organ damage such that complete recovery may be impossible or that a fatal outcome is inevitable. Early therapy in uncomplicated cases ordinarily leads to a rapid defervescence within 1–3 days and recovery within 7–10 days.

LABORATORY DATA AND DIAGNOSIS. An abnormally low platelet count, normal to slightly low leukocyte count, and low serum sodium concentration are present in about half of patients and may be early suggestive, clues to the diagnosis. Most other clinical laboratory findings are nonspecific and vary depending on the degree of specific organ involvement. Diagnosis may be confirmed in the acute stage by immunohistologic demonstration of *R. rickettsii* in skin biopsy or by the demonstration of *R. rickettsii* nucleic acids in blood by polymerase chain reaction. Because treatment needs to be initiated based on clinical diagnosis alone, the diagnosis is most often confirmed by serology in convalescence. Diagnostic serologies include a fourfold rise in antibody titer (usually indirect fluorescent antibody [IFA] assay), or a single elevated IFA titer of 64 or greater in convalescent serum. A case is considered probable if testing reveals a single titer of 128 or greater by latex agglutination. Weil-Felix testing should not be performed because of the lack of both sensitivity and specificity.

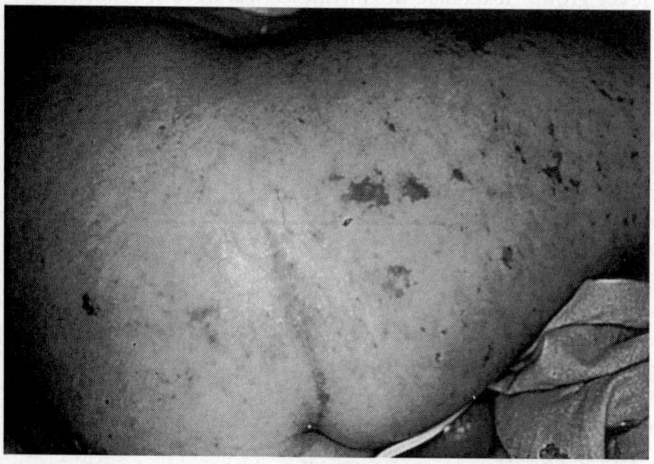

Figure 239–2. Later in the course of Rocky Mountain spotted fever the rash may become hemorrhagic or purpuric. See also color section. (Courtesy of Debra Karp Skopicki, M.D., Baltimore.)

DIFFERENTIAL DIAGNOSIS. The diagnosis of Rocky Mountain spotted fever should be considered in patients presenting during the spring through fall with an acute febrile illness accompanied by headache and myalgia, particularly if they were exposed to known endemic regions, ticks, or forested or tick-infested rural areas or had contact with a dog. A history of tick exposure and the appearance of a rash, especially on the palms or soles, together with laboratory findings of a low serum sodium concentration, normal leukocyte count with a marked left shift, and a relatively low or falling platelet count, are sometimes helpful clues in distinguishing Rocky Mountain spotted fever from some other acute infections. In patients with no rash or in dark-skinned individuals in whom a rash may be difficult to appreciate, the diagnosis may be exceptionally elusive and delayed. On occasion, rickettsial vascular infection predominates in a single organ or system, erroneously suggesting a localized process such as appendicitis or cholecystitis. A thorough evaluation will usually reveal evidence of a systemic process and will avoid unnecessary and potentially detrimental surgical interventions.

Other rickettsial infections are easily confused with Rocky Mountain spotted fever, especially ehrlichiosis and murine typhus. Although murine typhus may be treated similarly, chloramphenicol therapy for ehrlichiosis is controversial, and thus an accurate and thorough clinical evaluation is mandatory in an attempt to differentiate the two entities if this therapy is to be used. Rocky Mountain spotted fever can mimic many diseases. Among the most important to consider in the differential diagnosis are meningococcemia, measles, and enteroviral exanthems. Negative blood cultures may aid in reaching a correct diagnosis; however, *R. rickettsii* may elicit a lymphocytic meningitis, further confounding the diagnosis. Other diseases sometimes included in the differential diagnosis are typhoid fever, secondary syphilis, Lyme borreliosis, leptospirosis, scarlet fever, toxic shock syndrome, rheumatic fever, rubella, Kawasaki disease, idiopathic thrombocytopenic purpura, thrombotic thrombocytopenic purpura, Henoch-Schönlein purpura, hemolytic uremic syndrome, aseptic meningitis, acute gastrointestinal illness, acute abdomen, hepatitis, infectious mononucleosis, and drug reactions.

CONTROL

Because no vaccines are available, prevention of Rocky Mountain spotted fever is best accomplished by elimination of tick infestations of dogs; avoidance of wooded, grassy areas where ticks reside; use of insect repellents; wearing of special protective clothing; and careful inspection of children who have been playing in the woods or fields. Prompt and complete removal of attached ticks will help reduce the risk of transmission because complete exchange of infected tick saliva occurs during the later phases of the blood meal. Contrary to popular beliefs, the application of petroleum jelly, 70% isopropyl alcohol, fingernail polish, or a hot match are not effective in removing ticks from persons or animals. A tick can be safely removed by grasping the mouth parts of the tick at the site of cutaneous contact with a pair of forceps and applying gentle and steady retraction to remove the entire tick and mouth parts. The site of attachment should then be disinfected. Ticks should not be squeezed, crushed, or disrupted because their fluids may be infectious. Disposal may be accomplished by soaking in alcohol or by flushing down the toilet after which one should wash the hands.

239.2 Boutonneuse Fever and Other Spotted Fever Rickettsioses

Also see Chapter 238.

ETIOLOGIC AGENTS AND TRANSMISSION. Among the many members of the spotted fever group of rickettsiae, six or more species aside from *Rickettsia rickettsii* are known to be pathogenic for humans. These agents include the tick-borne typhus agents *R. conorii* (boutonneuse fever), *R. sibericus* (North Asian tick typhus), *R. japonica* (Oriental spotted fever), *R. australis* (Queensland tick typhus), the unnamed Israeli spotted fever rickettsia, and *R. africae* (tick bite fever). *R. akari* (rickettsialpox) is transmitted by the bite of a mite. *R. conorii* is distributed over a large geographic region including India, Pakistan, Russia, Ukraine, Georgia, Israel, Ethiopia, Kenya, South Africa, Morocco, and southern Europe. The disease that it causes is known by various geographically recognized names including boutonneuse fever, Mediterranean spotted fever, Kenya tick typhus, South African tick bite fever, or Indian tick typhus. Similar illnesses occur distributed globally but are caused by distinct yet related species such as *R. sibericus* in Russia, China, Mongolia, and Pakistan, *R. australis* in eastern Australia, *R. japonica* in Japan, and *R. africae* in Africa. In fact, these species are closely related to *R. rickettsii* by analysis of antigens and DNA sequences.

Boutonneuse fever has demonstrated a steadily increasing incidence since 1980 in southern Europe, and in some regions a human seroprevalence rate of 11–26% may be obtained. Transmission occurs after the bite of the brown dog tick, *Rhipicephalus sanguineus*, or other species including *Dermacentor, Haemaphysalis, Amblyomma, Hyalomma*, and *Ixodes*. Peak incidence occurs during July and August in the Mediterranean basin. Many cases of imported infection are documented in travelers to endemic regions, especially in those who go on safaris in high grass and bush land. A strong correlation exists among the incidence of boutonneuse fever, infected ticks, and evidence of infection in both dogs and humans, implicating the household dog as a potential vehicle for transmission.

Rickettsialpox is caused by *R. akari*, which is transmitted by the mouse mite, *Allodermanyssus sanguineus*. Although the mouse host for this mite is widely distributed in cities in the United States, Europe, and Asia, the disease is relatively mild and rarely diagnosed.

CLINICAL MANIFESTATIONS. Patients with boutonneuse fever typically experience fever, headache, myalgias, and a maculopapular rash, which is seen 3–5 days after onset of symptoms. In about 70% of patients, an eschar (tache noire) at the initial site of tick attachment and regional lymphadenopathy will be detected. Although previously considered benign and self-limited, this infection may cause severe disease in up to 6% of affected individuals, characterized by findings similar to those seen in Rocky Mountain spotted fever, including purpuric skin lesions, neurologic signs, respiratory distress, acute renal failure, severe thrombocytopenia, and death in 1.4–5.6%. As in Rocky Mountain spotted fever, a particularly malignant form occurs in patients deficient in glucose-6-phosphate dehydrogenase or in individuals with other underlying debilities such as alcoholic liver disease or diabetes mellitus. The other spotted fever group rickettsioses present similarly, some with an eschar present and some with more aggressive illness. Israeli spotted fever is generally associated with a more severe course, and fatalities in children are well documented. The diagnosis is based on clinical presentation; however, many patients do not recall a tick bite, and many others do not have an eschar or rash at presentation. Thus, the search for the classic clinical triad of fever, rash, and eschar may not often be useful.

Rickettsialpox is generally mild and is best known because of its association with a varicelliform rash. In fact, this rash is probably an aberrant form of a more typical macular or maculopapular rash as seen in other vasculotropic rickettsioses. At presentation, most patients have fever, headache, and chills. In up to 90% of well-documented cases, there may be a papular or ulcerative lesion at the initial site of inoculation, and regional lymphadenopathy may be present. In some patients, the maculopapular rash, which is distributed over the trunk, head, and extremities, may become vesicular. The infection resolves spontaneously even without therapy. Complications and fatalities are rare.

Laboratory diagnosis of these spotted fever group rickettsioses is the same as for Rocky Mountain spotted fever and may be accomplished by immunohistologic demonstration of spotted fever group rickettsiae on skin biopsy, by immunocytologic demonstration of *R. conorii* (and potentially other spotted fever group rickettsiae) in circulating endothelial cells, by in vitro cultivation by centrifugation-assisted shell vial tissue culture, or by the demonstration of serum antibodies to spotted fever group rickettsiae in convalescence. In fact, reagents useful for the diagnosis of Rocky Mountain spotted fever in the United States or boutonneuse fever in Europe, Africa, and Asia may be used effectively for diagnosis of most members of the spotted fever group of rickettsiae. Boutonneuse fever is effectively treated with tetracycline, doxycycline, chloramphenicol, ciprofloxacin, ofloxacin, or pefloxacin.

CHAPTER 240
Typhus Group Rickettsioses

MURINE TYPHUS

Also see Chapter 238.

ETIOLOGY. Murine typhus occurs in a worldwide distribution, especially in warm, coastal ports where it is maintained in a cycle involving rat fleas *(Xenopsylla cheopis)* and rats *(Rattus* species). In the United States, the disease is most prevalent in southern Texas and southern California, although sporadic cases have been reported from most states. The peak incidence occurs during times when rat populations are at the highest during spring, summer, and fall. In the coastal areas of southern Texas, the disease is seen predominantly during March through June and is associated with opossums, cats, and cat fleas *(Ctenocephalides felis)*.

Murine typhus is typically caused by *Rickettsia typhi*, which is transmitted from infected fleas to rats or opossums and back to fleas. Transovarial transmission in fleas is inefficient, and thus transmission depends on distribution by the flea to uninfected mammals, which become transiently rickettsemic and in turn transmit the organism to uninfected fleas. A novel agent within the genus *Rickettsia* has been identified as a cause of murine typhus in southern Texas. The new rickettsia, the ELB agent, is genetically related to both *R. typhi* and *Rickettsia rickettsii*, is capable of highly efficient transovarial transmission in cat fleas and may be found in cat fleas obtained from both areas endemic for murine typhus in the United States. Human acquisition of murine typhus occurs when rickettsiae-infected flea feces contaminate flea-bite wounds.

CLINICAL MANIFESTATIONS. Murine typhus is a moderately severe infection similar to other vasculotropic rickettsioses. The infection in children generally appears to be mild. The incubation period may vary between 1 and 2 wk. The initial presentation is often nonspecific, with fever as the predominant finding. Fewer than half of pediatric patients experience other typically important clues for rickettsiosis including rash (48%), myalgias (29%), vomiting (29%), cough (24%), headache (19%), and diarrhea or abdominal pain (10%). Although neurologic involvement may be a frequent finding in adults with murine typhus, confusion, stupor, coma, seizures, meningismus, and ataxia are seen in less than 5% of infected children. A petechial rash is infrequent, and the usual appearance is that of macules or maculopapules distributed on the trunk and extremities. The rash may involve both soles and palms on rare occasions. Although nonspecific, helpful laboratory findings including mild leukopenia (36%) with moderate left shift, mild to marked thrombocytopenia (50%), hyponatremia (20%), hypoalbuminemia (57%), and elevated serum concentrations of hepatic transaminases such as aspartate aminotransferase (88%) and alanine aminotransferase (83%). Elevations in serum urea nitrogen are usually due to prerenal mechanisms.

Occasionally, patients present with findings suggestive of pharyngitis, bronchitis, hepatitis, gastroenteritis, or sepsis; thus, the differential diagnosis may be extensive. Complications of murine typhus in pediatric patients are infrequent; however, examples of relapse, stupor, facial edema, dehydration, and cerebrospinal fluid pleocytosis have been reported. As for other vasculotropic rickettsioses, delays in diagnosis and therapy are associated with increased morbidity and mortality; thus, diagnosis must be based on clinical suspicion. Confirmation of the diagnosis is usually accomplished in convalescence by indirect fluorescent antibody assay serology; however, polymerase chain reaction amplification of rickettsial nucleic acids in acute phase blood, rickettsial culture by the centrifugation-assisted shell vial assay, and immunohistology on skin biopsy may have some diagnostic utility.

CONTROL. Control of murine typhus has been dependent on elimination of the rat and rat flea reservoir, and this tactic still remains an important component of control. However, with the recognition of cat fleas as potentially significant reservoirs and vectors, the presence of these flea vectors and their mammalian hosts in suburban and urban areas in which close human exposures occur will probably pose increasingly important control problems.

EPIDEMIC TYPHUS, RECRUDESCENT TYPHUS, AND SYLVATIC FLYING SQUIRREL TYPHUS

Also see Chapter 238.

ETIOLOGY AND TRANSMISSION. Humans have long been considered the principal or only reservoir of *Rickettsia prowazekii*, the causative agent of epidemic typhus and its recrudescent form, *Brill-Zinnser disease*. Human body or head lice become infected by feeding on rickettsemic persons. The ingested rickettsiae infect the midgut epithelial cells of the lice and are passed into the feces, which are, in turn, introduced into a susceptible human host through abrasions or perforations in the skin, through the conjunctivae, or rarely through inhalation of dried, infected louse excreta present in clothing, bedding, or furniture. Characteristically, the infection is seen in winter or spring or during times of poor hygienic practices, crowding, war, famine, or civil strife. Sporadic cases of a mild, typhus-like illness have been confirmed to be caused by *R. prowazekii* and are associated with exposure to flying squirrels harboring infected lice or fleas. The *R. prowazekii* isolated from these squirrels appear to be genetically different from isolates obtained during typical outbreaks. In the years 1981–1990, most cases of epidemic typhus have been sporadic, but outbreaks have been identified in Africa (Ethiopia, Nigeria), Mexico, Central America, South America, eastern Europe, Afghanistan, northern India, and China, although reporting of this illness is almost certainly a woeful underestimation.

Epidemic typhus fever may be a mild or severe disease in children. The incubation period is usually fewer than 14 days. The clinical manifestations include fever, severe headache, abdominal tenderness, and rash in most patients, with chills (82%), myalgias (70%), arthralgias (70%), anorexia (48%), nonproductive cough (38%), dizziness (35%), photophobia (33%), nausea (32%), abdominal pain (30%), tinnitus (23%), constipation (23%), meningismus (17%), visual disturbances (15%), vomiting (10%), and diarrhea (7%). The rash is initially pink or erythematous and blanches. In one third of patients, red, nonblanching macules and petechiae appear predominantly on the trunk. Infections identified during the preantibiotic era typically produced a variety of central nervous system findings including delirium (48%), coma (6%), and seizures (1%). Estimates of case fatality rates range between 3.8 and 20% in outbreaks. Brill-Zinnser disease is an unusual form of typhus that becomes recrudescent months to years after primary infection. When rickettsemic, these infected individuals may transmit the agent to lice.

CONTROL. The immediate destruction of vectors with an insecticide is important in the control of an epidemic. Dust containing excreta from infected lice is capable of transmitting typhus, and care must be taken to prevent its inhalation.

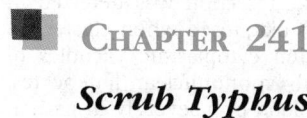

CHAPTER 241

Scrub Typhus

(Tsutsugamushi Fever)

Also see Chapter 238.

ETIOLOGY AND TRANSMISSION. *Rickettsia tsutsugamushi* is the causative agent of scrub typhus. The organism, which is markedly different from the other members of the genus *Rickettsia*, probably represents an excellent example of convergent evolution. Like other vasculotropic rickettsiae, *R. tsutsugamushi* infects endothelium and elicits vasculitis, the predominant clinicopathologic feature of the disease. Scrub typhus occurs mostly in the Far East including areas delimited by a triangle connecting Japan, Pakistan, and northern Australia. Aside from infections in these tropical and subtropical regions, the disease occurs in Korea, the Primorye of far eastern Russia, Tadazhikistan, Nepal, and nontropical China including Tibet. Imported cases in the United States have also been reported. The rickettsia is transmitted via the bite of a trombiculid mite (genus *Leptotrombidium*), which serves as both vector and reservoir. Because transovarial transmission occurs efficiently and transmission of the organism to mites from infected animals is poor, the rodent hosts of these mites are not likely to be involved in natural maintenance of the agent. Although multiple serotypes are known, most share antigenic cross-reactivity with the Karp, Gilliam, or Kato strains.

CLINICAL MANIFESTATION. Scrub typhus may be a mild or severe disease. An incubation period of 6–21 days may pass before the onset of clinical symptoms. At the site of chigger (mite) bite, the rickettsiae proliferate to form a necrotic eschar with an erythematous rim in less than half of cases. The onset of illness is usually manifest by fever, headache, and sometimes myalgia, cough, and gastrointestinal symptoms. Regional or generalized lymphadenopathy is common. A maculopapular rash is also present in less than 50% of patients and involves the trunk and extremities and infrequently the hands or face. Complications include severe meningoencephalitis and interstitial pneumonitis. The case fatality rate in untreated patients may be as high as 7%. The diagnosis is usually confirmed by indirect fluorescent antibody assay or immunoperoxidase serologic tests using various serotypes of *R. tsutsugamushi* as antigen. Therapy includes doxycycline and chloramphenicol, after which prompt (within 24–48 hr) defervescence occurs; however, some reports suggest the emergence of more virulent or potentially antimicrobial resistant strains.

CONTROL. Protective clothing is the most useful mode of prevention of scrub typhus.

CHAPTER 242
Ehrlichiosis

Also see Chapter 238.

EPIDEMIOLOGY AND ETIOLOGY. First recognized as infectious agents of dogs, members of the genus *Ehrlichia* had been largely ignored as important human pathogens until 1987, when the first case of an *Ehrlichia canis*–like infection was detected in humans. This initial infection was diagnosed when clusters of bacteria (morulae) confined within cytoplasmic vacuoles of circulating leukocytes, particularly mononuclear leukocytes, were detected in the peripheral blood of a severely ill patient suffering from suspected Rocky Mountain spotted fever. Serologic tests showed that the agent was antigenically similar to *E. canis*, an ehrlichia of dogs transmitted by a tick that, in the United States, rarely bites humans. In 1990, a new species, *Ehrlichia chaffeensis*, was cultivated and identified as the predominant agent of this infection. Seroepidemiologic investigation has shown that in some geographic areas *E. chaffeensis* infection occurs as frequently as Rocky Mountain spotted fever, and the infection is strongly associated with tick bites. More recently, yet another species of the genus has been implicated as an agent of human disease in the United States. This new human infection was recognized by the observation of ehrlichial morulae present only in circulating neutrophils. Serologic investigation in these cases reveals the lack of *E. chaffeensis* antibodies, and most patients have serologic reactions to *E. equi* or *E. phagocytophila*, previously only known as pathogens of horse and bovine caprine, or ovine granulocytes, respectively. To differentiate between *E. chaffeensis*, which infects predominantly monocytic cells, and infections caused by the neutrophilic ehrlichial pathogen, the names *monocytic ehrlichiosis* and *granulocytic ehrlichiosis* have been applied.

Infections with *E. chaffeensis* have been detected in many of the southern and southern central states in a distribution that parallels that of Rocky Mountain spotted fever. However, infections have also been documented in patients from more northern states, including Washington and Connecticut. Additional suspected cases have been reported with appropriate serologic findings from Portugal in Europe and Mali in Africa. Infections with the granulocytic ehrlichia have only recently been recognized, mostly in northwestern Wisconsin and eastern Minnesota, but additional cases present in Connecticut and Florida suggest that the agent is very widely distributed.

Although the median age of patients infected with monocytic ehrlichiosis is 42 yr, many pediatric patients have been identified. Definite infections of children with the granulocytic ehrlichia have been identified, but the median patient age is 71 yr. As expected, both infections are highly associated with tick bite and tick exposure, and infections are identified predominantly during seasons with tick activity: May through September.

Ehrlichiae are small, pleomorphic, obligate intracellular bacteria that possess gram negative–type cell walls. Genetic analysis of the 16S ribosomal DNA and protein immunoblot investigations indicate that the genus contains at least three separate groups, each denoted by a prototype, *E. canis, E. sennetsu*, and *E. phagocytophila*. These bacteria are pathogens of hematopoietic cells in mammals, and characteristically each species has a specific host cell affinity: *E. chaffeensis* and *E. sennetsu* infect mononuclear phagocytes, and the granulocytic ehrlichia (as well as *E. equi* and *E. phagocytophila*) infects neutrophils. Differences in these host cell affinities may in part explain the clinical findings of rare cells with *E. chaffeensis* in circulating leukocytes, whereas infections with the granulocytic ehrlichia are associated with morulae in up to 40% of circulating neutrophils.

ETIOLOGY AND TRANSMISSION. Investigations of the tick vectors of *E. chaffeensis* show that the predominant species that harbors the organism is *Amblyomma americanum*, the Lone Star tick; however, additional vectors are likely given the presence of *E. chaffeensis* DNA in at least one dog tick (*Dermacentor variabilis*) and the presence of disease outside of the known range of *A. americanum*. The tick vector of granulocytic ehrlichiosis is not known, but *Ixodes* species are the major vector of the related *E. phagocytophila* in Europe. Little is known concerning the transmission of *Ehrlichia* in nature. *E. canis*, a species closely related to *E. chaffeensis*, appears to be maintained solely or predominantly by horizontal tick to mammal to tick transmission because the organism does not invade the female tick ovary and does not appear in larvae from infected females. The implication of these statements suggests that efficient transmission may require persistent infection of mammalian hosts, a situation long recognized in dogs infected with *E. canis*, goats with *E. phagocytophila*, and other hosts of various ehrlichial species. In fact, persistent infection with *E. chaffeensis* has been documented in association with a fatal infection in an adult male patient.

CLINICAL MANIFESTATIONS. Although the average age of patients infected with *E. chaffeensis* is higher than that of patients with Rocky Mountain spotted fever, more than 20 well-defined cases of pediatric infection, including a fatality, have been reported. The incubation period after the last preceding tick bite or tick exposure ranges from 2 days to 3 wk, and tick bite is not documented in nearly one fourth of all patients. The disease usually presents with nonspecific findings including fever and headache in all reported cases. The majority of patients also describe myalgias, anorexia, and nausea or vomiting. Unlike adult patients, nearly two thirds of children with monocytic ehrlichiosis present with a rash. The rash is usually described as macular or maculopapular, although petechial lesions may occur. Photophobia and conjunctivitis may occur, and pharyngitis and cervical lymphadenopathy may be seen in a minority of patients as well. Hepatomegaly and splenomegaly are frequent physical findings; meningitis with a mononuclear cell–predominant pleocytosis is infrequently encountered. Cases with arthritis or arthralgias may suggest Lyme borreliosis or meningococcemia, but this presentation appears to be infrequent. Edema of the face, hands, and feet may contribute to diagnostic uncertainty. Under ordinary circumstances, the illness lasts between 4 and 12 days, and in most published cases hospitalization was required. Well-documented seroconversions in the absence of overt infection have been observed and strongly suggest the occurrence of mild or subclinical infections. Infections of children with granulocytic ehrlichia appear to be infrequent; however, the clinical presentation in adults is very similar to that of adult *E. chaffeensis* infection. Fatal monocytic ehrlichiosis has been demonstrated in only one pediatric patient to date. In this patient a typical course of ehrlichiosis developed that was complicated by a subsequent nosocomial bacterial pneumonia and respiratory failure, a pattern now documented in fatal infections in adults as well. In spite of the Rocky Mountain spotted fever–like presentation of monocytic and granulocytic ehrlichiosis, vasculitis appears to be a rare pathologic finding in these patients. The presence of *Ehrlichia* in organs of the mononuclear phagocyte system and hyperplasia of mononuclear phagocytes in tissues suggest widespread activation of the mononuclear phagocyte system with consequent consumption, destruction, or sequestration of hematopoietic elements as the major pathogenetic event. The exact mechanisms of tissue injury and cellular damage are still unclear.

LABORATORY DATA AND DIAGNOSIS. Characteristically, most children with monocytic ehrlichiosis present with leukopenia (72%), lymphopenia (78%), or thrombocytopenia (80%). Leukocytosis may also occur. In spite of the presence of pancytopenia, examinations usually reveal a cellular or reactive bone marrow. Interestingly, granulomas and granulomatous inflammation are identified in nearly 75% of bone marrows examined from proven cases of *E. chaffeensis* infection. Mild to severe hepatic injury is documented by the frequent (83%) finding of elevated serum aspartate aminotransferase levels. Hyponatremia is present in a minority of cases. Although not yet documented in children, severely affected adults may experience varying degrees of renal failure accompanied by elevations in serum creatinine and urea nitrogen concentrations. A clinical picture similar to that of disseminated intravascular coagulation (DIC) with prolonged activated partial thromboplastin time and prothrombin time, and hypofibrinogenemia has been demonstrated in at least several patients. The first patient and several subsequent pediatric patients with *E. chaffeensis* infection were identified presumptively on the basis of typical *Ehrlichia* morulae in peripheral blood leukocytes (Fig. 242–1). This finding has been too infrequent to be considered a useful diagnostic tool. In contrast, granulocytic ehrlichiosis often presents with a small but significant percentage (1–40%) of circulating neutrophils that contain typical *Ehrlichia* morulae. The distinction between the two infections relies on polymerase chain reaction amplification of species-specific nucleic acids or on the demonstration of specific *E. chaffeensis* or granulocytic ehrlichia (using *E. equi* as a surrogate antigen) serology. In fact, the vast majority of cases of monocytic ehrlichiosis in which the ehrlichiae have been observed in mononuclear cells, especially monocytes, have been infected. In contrast, the morulae in patients infected with granulocytic ehrlichiosis are found almost solely in neutrophils. The current accepted diagnostic criteria for *E. chaffeensis* infection includes a seroconversion with a minimum titer of 64 or a single serum titer (usually convalescent serum) of at least 128 and a clinically compatible illness. Similarly granulocytic ehrlichiosis may be confirmed by a seroconversion or single high titer of *E. equi* or *E. phagocytophila* antibodies. Patients with granulocytic ehrlichiosis will not experience serologic reactions to *E. chaffeensis* or *E. canis*, and thus serodiagnosis of monocytic or granulocytic ehrlichiosis depends on testing with several different ehrlichial antigens. Immunocytologic and immunohistologic methods have been successfully applied in situations in which morulae were suspected in peripheral blood or in cerebrospinal fluid, and polymerase chain reaction amplification may also be used to identify definitively the infectious agent in acute-phase blood from patients with either monocytic or granulocytic ehrlichiosis.

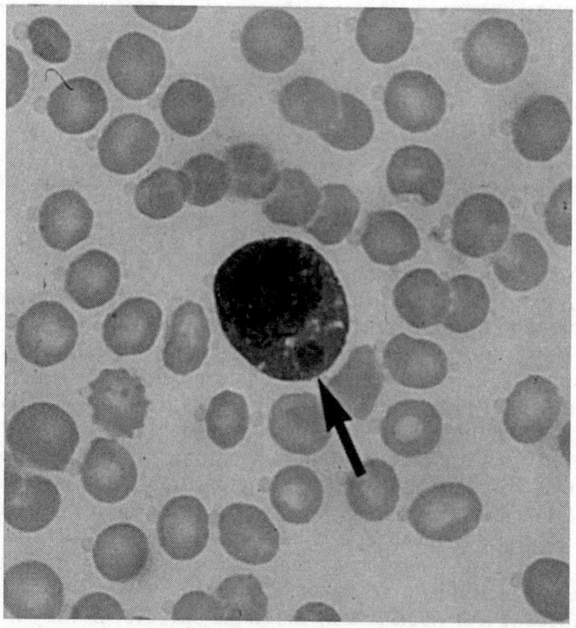

Figure 242–1. ***Ehrlichia* morula in a peripheral blood leukocyte: morula *(arrows)* containing *Ehrlichia chaffeensis* in a monocyte (Wright's stain, original magnification ×1,200). *Ehrlichia chaffeensis* and the human granulocytic ehrlichia have similar morphologies but are serologically and genetically distinct. See also color section.**

DIFFERENTIAL DIAGNOSIS. As for Rocky Mountain spotted fever, a delay in diagnosis or treatment of ehrlichiosis may contribute to increased morbidity or mortality; thus, an early clinical diagnosis is the foundation for therapy. Because of the nonspecific presentation, ehrlichiosis may be mimicked by other arthropod-borne infections such as Rocky Mountain spotted fever, tularemia, babesiosis, Lyme borreliosis, murine typhus, relapsing fever, or Colorado tick fever. When rash and a DIC-like clinical picture predominate, meningococcemia, bacterial sepsis, and toxic shock syndrome may be suspected. Other potential diagnoses considered have included otitis media, streptococcal pharyngitis, infectious mononucleosis, Kawasaki disease, endocarditis, viral syndromes, hepatitis, leptospirosis, Q fever, collagen-vascular diseases, and leukemia.

Chapter 243
Q Fever

Also see Chapter 238.

Q fever is a febrile disease, often without rash, that presents in acute or chronic forms. The acute form is usually associated with an influenza-like illness, interstitial pneumonitis, or granulomatous hepatitis, whereas the chronic form is usually culture-negative endocarditis. The disease is reported worldwide, and unlike infections with other rickettsial organisms, arthropod vectors are rarely implicated in transmission. Immunocompromised patients and patients with underlying cardiac valve or vascular damage or prostheses are at risk for acute and chronic Q fever. The relative risk of disease is correlated with increasing age, such that infected children are infrequently identified.

ETIOLOGY AND TRANSMISSION. Serologic surveys in the United States and elsewhere indicate that many more cases of Q fever occur each year than are recognized. This is not surprising because acute Q fever is nonspecific, specialized laboratory diagnostic tests are required, and it is not currently a notifiable disease in many states. *Coxiella burnetii* may be the cause of between 0.5% and 3% of serologically investigated acute respiratory illnesses or hepatitides in some areas of the United States. Domestic livestock (cattle, sheep, and goats), parturient cats and wild animals such as rabbits, and rarely ticks serve as reservoirs for *C. burnetii* infection. This unusual organism is genetically distinct from members of the genera *Rickettsia* and *Ehrlichia* and is more closely related to *Legionella pneumophila* and the arthropod symbiont *Wolbachia (Francisella) persica. C. burnetii* is highly infectious for humans and animals; even a single organism can cause infection. The usual mode of transmission is via aerosols from dust, straw, cloth contaminated with organisms from birth tissues, by processing of animal products (in abattoirs, hides, wool), or by ingestion of contaminated raw dairy products (fresh cheese or nonpasteurized milk). In Nova Scotia and Maine, exposure to newborn animals (chiefly kittens) has been associated with small outbreaks of Q fever in family settings. In Europe and Australia, exposure to domestic ruminants is the major risk; however, many urban dwellers in France, presumably without significant farm exposure risk, acquire Q fever. Human placental infection is sometimes associated with intrauterine growth retardation or death and may result from primary or reactivation of maternal infection. In fact, because of the quantity of *C. burnetti* released from infected products of conception, obstetric health care workers are at risk for acquiring infection. Immune compromise secondary to cancer therapies, acquired immunodeficiency syndrome, transplantation, hemodialysis, alcoholic liver disease, or chronic granulomatous disease is identified as an underlying factor in more than 20% of patients with acute or chronic Q fever.

CLINICAL MANIFESTATIONS. Acute Q fever develops about 3 wk (range, 14–39 days) after exposure to the causative agent. The severity of illness in children ranges from subclinical infection to a febrile systemic illness with severe frontal headache, arthralgia, and myalgia often accompanied by respiratory symptoms. Most pediatric patients present with fever of unknown origin, and fewer than half of all pediatric patients will have cough or pneumonia. In adults, the pneumonia usually resembles primary atypical or viral pneumonitis or legionnaires disease with a nonproductive cough. Other prominent clinical findings that may lead to diagnostic confusion include fatigue, vomiting, abdominal pain, and meningismus. Hepatomegaly and splenomegaly may be detected in some patients. Laboratory findings may reveal leukopenia with a left shift (>5%) in 50% of patients and thrombocytopenia, which is infrequent. Most children have evidence of mild hepatic injury with increases in serum hepatic aminotransferases that spontaneously normalize after 20 to 30 days. In a review of 170 adult French patients with acute Q fever, 81.8% had fever, and of these patients 62% had elevated serum hepatic transaminase levels, 46% had respiratory involvement, 18% had cutaneous findings, and 11% had neurologic findings that required lumbar puncture for evaluation. Nearly 20% of these patients were afebrile and presented with one or more of hepatic, pulmonic, cutaneous, or neurologic findings. Other series of patients indicate that pulmonary involvement is the most frequent manifestation. Radiographically, the pulmonary consolidations become round and resolve slowly. In children, acute Q fever is a self-limited illness that lasts for 2–3 wk. Severe infections including acute encephalopathy with impairment of consciousness and an abnormal pattern on electroencephalogram and computed tomographic scans of the brain have been reported.

Risk for development of chronic Q fever is strongly correlated with advancing age; thus, children are infrequently diagnosed with chronic Q fever. This is fortunate because chronic Q fever tends to be recalcitrant to therapy and often (23–65%) results in death. Endocarditis, usually present on damaged or prosthetic valves, may occur months to years after acute Q fever or in the absence of any history of Q fever. Chronic Q fever may less frequently present as infections of vascular prostheses and aneurysms, osteomyelitis, undifferentiated fever, pneumonia, and hepatitis or as an isolated purpuric rash. The clinical presentation in children is similar to that of adults. Fever may be absent in up to 15% of cases, and more than 75% of all identified patients have congestive heart failure. Other frequently observed features include marked clubbing of the fingers, hepatomegaly, and splenomegaly. Laboratory findings are usually normal, but leukocytosis, leukopenia, thrombocytopenia, or anemia are seen in a minority of patients. Frequent laboratory abnormalities in chronic Q fever include erythrocyte sedimentation rate greater than 20 mm/hr in 80% of cases, hypergammaglobulinemia in 54% of cases, and hyperfibrinogenemia in 67%. The presence of rheumatoid factors in more than 50%, circulating immune complexes in nearly 90%, and the frequent findings of antiplatelet antibodies, anti–smooth muscle antibodies, antimitochondrial antibodies, circulating anticoagulants, and positive direct Coombs test may suggest an autoimmune process. A variety of other syndromes have been associated with Q fever, including meningoencephalitis, inflammatory pseudotumor of the lung, glomerulonephritis, immune complex vasculitis, hemolytic anemia, and autoimmune disorders.

DIAGNOSIS AND DIFFERENTIAL DIAGNOSIS. Although infrequently diagnosed, Q fever should be considered in children with fever of unknown origin or culture-negative endocarditis who live in rural areas or who are in close contact with domestic livestock, cats, or their products. Isolation and antimicrobial susceptibility testing of *C. burnetii* should be attempted only in specialized biohazard facilities. The diagnosis of Q fever can be confirmed serologically by significant increases in indirect fluorescent antibody titers to phase I and phase II antigens or by a fourfold rise in titer of complement fixation antibody. The inability of the complement fixation test to discriminate between recent and remote infection diminishes its usefulness when acute phase sera are not available. Elevated or rising titers of phase II antibody alone are characteristic of acute Q fever, and the appearance and persistence of elevated titers of phase I and phase II antibody are indicative of chronic Q fever. Elevated titers of phase I immunoglobulin (Ig) A antibody are reported to be diagnostic for Q fever endocarditis; however, one evaluation showed that a phase II IgG titer of 200 or greater is indicative of *C. burnetii* infection and that a phase I IgG titer of less than 800 is inconsistent with chronic Q fever.

The differential diagnosis includes diseases caused by many infectious agents and depends on the clinical presentation. For respiratory disease, *Mycoplasma* pneumonitis, Epstein-Barr virus infection, psittacosis, and legionellosis are included. For granulomatous hepatitis, mycobacterial infections, salmonellosis, visceral leishmaniasis, toxoplasmosis, Hodgkin disease, ehrlichiosis, brucellosis, or autoimmune disorders including sarcoidosis should be considered. Culture-negative endocarditis also suggests infection with *Chlamydia* species, *Brucella* species, or *Rochalimaea* species organisms or nonbacterial endocarditis.

TREATMENT. Most pediatric patients with Q fever experience a self-limited illness that is identified only by retrospective serologic evaluation. However, to prevent potential complications, patients with acute Q fever should be treated within 3 days of onset of symptoms with tetracycline or doxycycline. Later therapy has little effect on the course of the acute infection. Because early laboratory confirmation is not currently available, empiric therapy is warranted in clinically suspected cases. The fluoroquinolones, ofloxacin, and pefloxacin have proven effective, and success with a combination of pefloxacin and rifampin has also been achieved with prolonged (16–21 days) therapy. The efficacy of erythromycin is controversial. Most β-lactams are ineffective; however, individual reports document success with a wide variety of agents including chloramphenicol, trimethoprim-sulfamethoxazole, and ceftriaxone. In anecdotal cases of hepatitis associated with "autoimmune" laboratory findings, prednisone was reported to provide additional clinical benefit.

For chronic Q fever, especially endocarditis, prolonged therapy is mandatory. This usually requires the use of the bacteriostatic drugs tetracycline or doxycycline in combination with bactericidal drugs including rifampin, ofloxacin, or pefloxacin. The use of lysosomotropic alkalinizing agents such as chloroquine may aid in maintaining activity of pH-sensitive antimicrobial agents in the phagolysosomal environment of *C. burnetii*. For patients with heart failure, valve replacement may be warranted and should be accompanied by an effective antibiotic regimen to avoid reinfection of the prosthetic valves. Therapy should be monitored by periodic serologic evaluation; phase I titers less than 200 for IgG and the absence of an IgA titer indicate cure. Even with this evaluation, cure of chronic Q fever in less than 2 yr is unlikely, and thus therapy should be continued for at least 3 yr.

CONTROL. Recognition of the disease in livestock should alert communities to the risk of human infection. Milk from infected herds must be pasteurized at temperatures sufficient to destroy the coxiellae. As environmentally resistant as *C. burnetii* is, it may be inactivated with a solution of 1% Lysol, 1% formaldehyde, or 5% hydrogen peroxide. Special isolation measures are not required because person-to-person transmission is rare, except when exposure to infected products of conception occurs.

Abramson JS, Givner LB: Rocky Mountain spotted fever. Semin Pediatr Infect Dis 5:131, 1994.

Brettman LR, Lewin S, Holzman R, et al: Rickettsialpox: Report of an outbreak and a contemporary review. Medicine 60:363, 1981.

Chen S-M, Dumler JS, Bakken JS, et al: Identification of a granulocytotropic *Ehrlichia* as the etiologic agent of human disease. J Clin Microbiol 32:589, 1994.

Dumler JS. Murine typhus. Semin Pediatr Infect Dis 5:137, 1994.

Dumler JS, Taylor JP, Walker DH: Clinical and laboratory features of murine typhus in south Texas, 1980–1987. JAMA 266:1365, 1991.

Dumler JS, Walker DH: Diagnostic tests for Rocky Mountain spotted fever and other rickettsial diseases. Dermatol Clin 12:25, 1994.

Edwards ME: Ehrlichiosis in children. Semin Pediatr Infect Dis 5:143, 1994.

Everett ED, Evans KA, Henry RB, et al: Human ehrlichiosis in adults after tick exposure: Diagnosis using polymerase chain reaction. Ann Intern Med 120:730, 1994.

Fishbein DB, Dawson JE, Robinson LE: Human ehrlichiosis in the United States, 1985 to 1990. Ann Intern Med 120:736, 1994.

Helmick CG, Bernard KW, D'Angelo LJ: Rocky Mountain spotted fever: Clinical, laboratory, and epidemiological features of 262 cases. J Infect Dis 150:480, 1984.

Marrie TJ (ed): Q Fever, Vol 1: The Disease. Boca Raton, FL, CRC Press, 1990.

Raoult D, Drancourt M: Antimicrobial therapy of rickettsial diseases. Antimicrob Agents Chemother 35:2457, 1991.

Ruiz-Contreras J, Montero RG, Amador JTR, et al: Q fever in children. Am J Dis Child 146:300, 1993.

Schriefer ME, Sacci JB Jr, Dumler JS, et al: Identification of a novel rickettsial infection in a patient diagnosed with murine typhus. J Clin Microbiol 32:949, 1994.

Tissot-DuPont H, Raoult D, Brouqui P, et al: Epidemiologic features and clinical presentation of acute Q fever in hospitalized patients: 323 French cases. Am J Med 93:427, 1992.

Walker DH (ed): Biology of Rickettsial Diseases, Vol 1. Boca Raton, FL, CRC Press, 1988.

Winkler HH: *Rickettsia* species (as organisms). Annu Rev Microbiol 44:131, 1990.

SECTION 7
Parasitic Infections

Adel A. F. Mahmoud

Infectious diseases due to protozoa and helminths are a major cause of morbidity and mortality in infants and children in many parts of the world. The major parasitic infections and their estimated prevalence, mortality, and morbidity are presented in Table XVII–1. The term *parasites* has been used historically and conventionally to refer only to those infectious organisms that belong to the animal kingdom, that is, *protozoa, helminths,* and *arthropods.* Protozoa are unicellular organisms that are able to multiply within their hosts. In contrast, worms or helminths are multicellular and usually do not divide within the human host. These basic biologic differences between protozoa and helminths have important epidemiologic, clinical, and therapeutic implications.

The host-parasite relationship in protozoan and helminthic infections has several unique features. Infection and disease due to these agents must be clearly distinguished. When a parasite invades a host, it may die at once or survive without causing harm to the host (infection). Alternatively, it may survive and produce morbidity (disease) and possibly kill the host. In addition, these organisms have evolved evasive mechanisms against host immune or protective responses. Parasites may cause disease by their physical presence or by competition with the host for specific nutrients. Disease may also result from the host's attempts to destroy the invaders, for example, the host's immunopathologic reaction.

■ **TABLE XVII–1 Estimated Worldwide Prevalence (in Thousands) of the Major Parasitic Infections in Relation to Associated Morbidity and Mortality**

Infection	Prevalence	Morbidity	Mortality
Protozoa			
Amebiasis	500,000	40,000	70
Giardiasis	250,000	500	10
Malaria	2,600,000	150,000	1,500
Trypanosomiasis, African	1,000	10	1
Trypanosomiasis, American	24,000	1,200	60
Toxoplasmosis	800,000	10	0.1
Leishmaniasis	1,000	1,000	1
Helminths			
Ascariasis	700,000	700	10
Hookworms	800,000	1,500	50–60
Filariasis	90,000	1,000	1
Schistosomiasis	300,000	150,000	1,200

Mahmoud AAF: Tropical and Geographical Medicine, 2nd ed. Companion Handbook. New York, McGraw Hill, 1993.
Warren KS, Mahmoud AAF: Tropical and Geographical Medicine. 2nd ed. New York, McGraw-Hill, 1990. ■

CHAPTER 244
Protozoan Diseases

Robert A. Bonomo and Robert A. Salata

Protozoan infections of the intestine cause a wide variety of clinical syndromes, ranging from asymptomatic carrier states to severe disease associated with pathologic lesions in the gastrointestinal tract or other organs (Table 244–1). Infections by the intestinal protozoa are usually acquired orally through fecal contamination of water or food, and they are more endemic in countries with unsanitary water conditions. *Giardia lamblia* and *Cryptosporidium,* however, have recently been recognized as a major cause of epidemics of water-borne diarrhea in North America, and particularly in day-care centers. *Cryptosporidium* infection, and to a lesser extent isosporiasis, have become major causes of diarrhea in patients with the acquired immunodeficiency syndrome (AIDS) (Chapters 223, 244.4, and 286.5). The increased rate of international travel and immigration of children into the United States requires pediatricians to become acquainted with these various syndromes.

244.1 *Amebiasis*

Human infection with *Entamoeba histolytica* is prevalent worldwide; endemic foci are particularly common in the trop-

■ **TABLE 244–1 Important Intestinal Protozoan Infections of Children**

Infection	Etiology	Transmission	Major Clinical Features	Diagnosis
Amebiasis	*Entamoeba histolytica*	Fecal-oral Water-, foodborne	Diarrhea-dysentery Liver abscess	Trophozoites or cysts in stools Serology
Giardiasis	*Giardia lamblia*	Fecal-oral Person-to-person Water-, foodborne	Diarrhea Malabsorption	Cysts in stools Cysts or trophozoites in duodenal aspirate
Cryptosporidiosis	*Cryptosporidium*	Fecal-oral Person-to-person Water-, foodborne Zoonosis	Watery diarrhea Severe diarrhea with malabsorption in AIDS patients	Oocysts in stools (acid-fast staining), small bowel biopsy
Balantidiasis	*Balantidium coli*	Fecal-oral Waterborne Zoonosis	Bloody diarrhea	Trophozoites or cysts in stools
Blastocystis	*Blastocystis hominis*	Fecal-oral Waterborne	Diarrhea Eosinophilia	Organisms in stools
Isosporiasis	*Isospora* sp.	Fecal-oral Zoonosis	Diarrhea in AIDS patients	Oocysts in stools Small bowel biopsy

ics and particularly in areas with low socioeconomic and sanitary standards. *E. histolytica* parasitizes the lumen of the gastrointestinal tract and causes few or no disease sequelae in most infected subjects. In a small proportion of individuals the organisms invade the intestinal mucosa or may disseminate to other organs, especially the liver.

ETIOLOGY. Infection is established by ingestion of parasite cysts. These cysts measure 10–18 μm, contain four nuclei, and are resistant to environmental conditions such as low temperature and the concentrations of chlorine commonly used in water purification; the parasite can be killed by heating to 55° C. Upon ingestion, the cyst, which is resistant to gastric acidity and digestive enzymes, excysts in the small intestine to form eight trophozoites. These are large, actively motile organisms that colonize the lumen of the large intestine and may invade its mucosal lining under conditions that are currently unknown. Trophozoites have an average diameter of 20 μm; their cytoplasm consists of an outer clear zone and an inner densely granular endoplasm containing a spherical nucleus, which has a small central karyosome and fine granular chromatin material. The endoplasm also contains vacuoles, where, in cases of invasive amebiasis, erythrocytes may be seen. Five other species of nonpathogenic *Amoeba* may infect the human gastrointestinal tract: *E. coli, E. hartmanni, E. gingivalis, E. moshkovskii,* and *E. polecki.*

EPIDEMIOLOGY. The prevalence of amebic infections worldwide varies from 5% to 81%, with the highest frequency being in the tropics. Humans are the major reservoir. It is estimated that 12% of the population worldwide is infected with *E. histolytica* (approximately 480 million people). This infection is associated with 50 million cases of symptomatic disease and an annual mortality of 40,000–110,000 deaths/year; amebiasis is the third leading parasitic cause of death on a global scale. Amebic dysentery due to invasion of the intestinal mucosa occurs in approximately 1–17% of infected subjects. Dissemination of the parasites to internal organs such as the liver occurs in an even smaller fraction of infected individuals and is less common in children than in adults.

Although highly endemic in Africa, Latin America, India, and Southeast Asia, amebiasis is not exclusively limited to the tropics. In the United States, amebiasis has been estimated to occur with a prevalence of 1–4% in certain high-risk groups, including chronically institutionalized persons (invasive disease is uncommon in AIDS), mentally retarded children, promiscuous homosexual males, emigrants (especially Mexican Americans) from and travelers to endemic areas, migrant workers, and lower socioeconomic groups in the southern United States. The majority of children infected with *E. histolytica* fall into these risk groups.

The pattern of infection varies in different parts of the world. For example, infection acquired in India, Mexico, or Durban, South Africa, is apparently more virulent than that from other locations. The definition of virulence, geographic strains, and pathogenicity of different amebae, however, remains to be defined.

Food or drink contaminated with *E. histolytica* cysts and direct fecal-oral contact are the most common means of infection. Untreated water and human feces used as fertilizer are important sources of infection. Food handlers carrying amebic cysts may, therefore, play a role in spreading the infection. Direct contact with infected feces also may be responsible for person-to-person transmission.

PATHOGENESIS AND PATHOLOGY. The pathogenicity of *E. histolytica* is believed to be dependent on two mechanisms—cell contact and toxin exposure. Recent work has demonstrated that contact-dependent killing by the trophozoite includes adherence, extracellular cytolysis, and phagocytosis. The galactose-specific lectin receptor is thought to be responsible for mediating attachment to the colonic mucosa. It has been also postulated that amoeba can export pore-forming proteins that form channels in host target-cell membranes. Once *E. histolytica* trophozoites invade the intestinal mucosa, they produce tissue destruction (ulcers) with little local inflammatory response because of the cytolytic capacity of the organism. The organisms multiply and spread laterally underneath the intestinal epithelium to produce the characteristic flask-shaped ulcers. These lesions are commonly seen in the cecum, transverse colon, and sigmoid colon. Amoebae may produce similar lytic lesions if they reach the liver (these are commonly called abscesses although they contain no granulocytes). *E. histolytica* occasionally disseminates to other extraintestinal sites such as the lungs and brain. The contrasts among the extent of tissue destruction by amebae, the absence of a local host inflammatory response, and the demonstration of systemic humoral (antibody) and cell-mediated reactions against the organisms remain a major scientific puzzle.

CLINICAL MANIFESTATIONS. Most infected individuals are asymptomatic, and cysts are found in their feces. Tissue invasion occurs in 2–8% of infected individuals and may be related to the strain of parasites or the nutritional status and intestinal flora of the host. The most common clinical manifestations of amebiasis are due to local invasion of the intestinal epithelium and dissemination to the liver.

Intestinal amebiasis may occur within 2 wk of infection or be delayed for months. The onset is usually gradual with colicky abdominal pains and frequent bowel movements (6–8 movements/24 hr). Diarrhea is frequently associated with tenesmus. Stools are blood-stained and contain a fair amount of mucus with few leukocytes. Generalized constitutional symptoms and signs are characteristically absent, with fever documented in only one third of patients. Acute amebic dysentery occurs in attacks lasting a few days to several weeks; recurrence is very common in untreated individuals. Amebic colitis affects all age groups, but its incidence is strikingly high in children between the ages of 1 and 5 yr. Severe amebic colitis in infants and younger children occurs in tropical and semitropical countries. When young children become infected, they tend to have rapidly progressive illness with frequent extraintestinal involvement and high mortality rates. In contrast to this experience in endemic areas, extraintestinal amebiasis during infancy is rarely seen in the United States.

Occasionally, amebic dysentery is associated with sudden onset of fever, chills, and severe diarrhea, which may result in dehydration and electrolyte disturbances. In a few patients complications such as ameboma, toxic megacolon, extraintestinal extension, or local perforation and peritonitis may occur. The characteristic flask-shaped ulcers with healthy intervening mucosa that occur in most cases may be detected by sigmoidoscopy in 25% of patients.

Hepatic amebiasis is a very serious manifestation of disseminated infection. Although diffuse liver enlargement has been associated with intestinal amebiasis, liver abscess occurs in fewer than 1% of infected individuals and may appear in patients with no clear history of intestinal disease. In children fever is the hallmark of amebic liver abscess. It is frequently associated with abdominal pain, distention, and an enlarged, tender liver. Changes at the base of the right lung, such as elevation of the diaphragm and parenchymal compression, may also occur. Laboratory examination shows a slight leukocytosis, moderate anemia, and nonspecific elevations of liver enzymes. Stool examination for amebae is negative in more than 50% of patients with documented amebic liver abscess. In most cases, computed tomography (CT) imaging, or isotope scans can localize and delineate the size of the abscess cavity. Most patients have a single cavity in the right hepatic lobe, although recent studies employing CT have shown an increased rate of multiple abscesses and left lobe involvement. Amebic liver abscess may be associated with rupture into the peritoneum or thorax, or through the skin when diagnosis and therapy are delayed.

DIAGNOSIS. Patients with invasive amebic colitis test positive for occult blood. Diagnosis is based on detecting the organisms in stool samples, sigmoidoscopically obtained smears, tissue biopsy samples, or, rarely, in aspirates of a liver abscess. Fresh stool samples should be examined within 30 min of passage and screened for motile trophozoites containing erythrocytes. At least three stool samples should be examined by an experienced person. Whenever amebiasis is suspected, an additional stool sample should be preserved in polyvinyl alcohol for further identification and staining of the organisms. Material for microscopic examination may also be obtained by scraping the ulcerated areas of rectal mucosa. Endoscopy and biopsies of suspicious areas should be performed when stool samples are negative and the index of suspicion for amebic colitis remains high. The indirect hemagglutination test may be helpful in the diagnosis of invasive intestinal amebiasis and amebic liver abscess; diagnostic titers of at least 1:128 are reported in 98–100% of cases. Serologic tests may be initially negative in patients presenting with very acute disease.

TREATMENT. Two types of drugs are used to treat infection by *E. histolytica*. The luminal amebicides, such as iodoquinol and diloxanide furoate, are primarily effective in the gut lumen, while metronidazole, chloroquine, and dehydroemetine are effective in the treatment of invasive amebiasis. All individuals with *E. histolytica* trophozoites or cysts in their stools, whether symptomatic or not, should be treated. Diloxanide furoate is the drug of choice for asymptomatic cyst passers. The recommended dose is 10 mg/kg/24 hr orally for 10 days. Toxicity is rare, but the drug should not be used in children under 2 yr of age.

Invasive amebiasis of the intestine, liver, or other organs requires the use of metronidazole, a tissue amebicidal drug; it is administered orally in a daily dose of 50 mg/kg for 10 days. Side effects of this drug include nausea, diarrhea, metallic taste in the mouth, and leukopenia; these are uncommon and disappear on completion of therapy. Metronidazole is also a luminal amebicide but less effective than diloxanide furoate for this purpose. Patients with invasive amebiasis should therefore receive an additional course of the latter drug following metronidazole therapy. If the case is severe or if metronidazole cannot be used, dehydroemetine is the recommended alternative therapeutic agent. It is administered by the subcutaneous or intramuscular route (never intravenously) in a dose of 1 mg/kg/24 hr for 10 days. Patients should be hospitalized when this drug is given because cardiac or renal complications may occur. If tachycardia, T wave depression, arrhythmias, or proteinuria develops, the drug should be stopped. A course of diloxanide furoate is also recommended following completion of dehydroemetine therapy. Chloroquine is also useful in the treatment of amebic hepatic abscess because it is concentrated in the liver. Amebic liver abscesses are treated with specific therapy as outlined earlier; however, aspiration of large lesions or left lobe abscesses may be necessary if rupture is imminent or if the patient shows a poor clinical response 4–6 days after administration of amebicidal drugs. Stool examination should be repeated 2 wk following completion of antiamebic therapy as a test of cure.

Control of amebiasis can be achieved by exercising proper sanitary measures and avoiding fecal-oral contact. Regular examination of food handlers and thorough investigation of diarrhea episodes may identify the source of infection in some communities. There is no prophylactic drug for amebiasis.

Adams EB, MacLeod IN: Invasive amebiasis. I. Amebic dysentery and its complications. Medicine 56:315, 1977.

Adams EB, MacLeod IN: Invasive amebiasis. II. Amebic liver abscess and its complications. Medicine 56:325, 1977.

Aucott JN, Ravdin JI: Amebiasis and "nonpathogenic" intestinal protozoa. Infect Dis Clin North Am 7:467, 1993.

Dykes AC, Ruebush TK, Gorelkin L, et al: Extraintestinal amebiasis in infancy: Report of three patients and epidemiological investigations of their families. Pediatrics 4:799, 1980.

Harrison RH, Crowe PC, Fulginiti VA: Amebic liver abscess in children: Clinical and epidemiologic features. Pediatrics 64:923, 1979.

Jansson A, Gillin F, Kagart U, et al: Coding of hemolysins within the ribosomal RNA repeat on a plasmid in *Entamoeba histolytica*. Science 263:1440, 1994.

Katzenstein D, Rickerson V, Braude A: New concepts of amebic liver abscess derived from hepatic imaging, serodiagnosis, and hepatic enzymes in 67 consecutive cases from San Diego. Medicine 61:325, 1977.

Merritt RJ, Coughlin E, Thomas DW, et al: Spectrum of amebiasis in children. Am J Dis Child 136:785, 1982.

244.2 Primary Amebic Meningoencephalitis

Martin Weisse and Stephen Aronoff

Naegleria, Acanthamoeba, and *Balamuthia* are small, free-living amebas that cause human meningoencephalitis. Amebic meningoencephalitis has two distinct clinical presentations. The more common presentation is that of an acute, usually fatal infection of the central nervous system (CNS) occurring in previously healthy children and young adults; granulomatous amebic meningoencephalitis usually occurs in immunocompromised individuals.

ETIOLOGY AND EPIDEMIOLOGY. The free-living amebas have a worldwide distribution. *Naegleria* has been isolated from a variety of freshwater sources, including ponds and lakes, domestic water supplies, hot springs and spas, thermal discharge of power plants, groundwater, and occasionally from the nasal passages of healthy children. *Naegleria* is an ameboflaggelate that can exist as cysts, trophozoites, and transient flagellate forms. Temperature and environmental nutrient and ion concentrations are the major factors determining at which stage the ameba is found in the environment. Trophozoites are the only stages that are invasive, although cysts are potentially infective because they can convert to the vegetative form very quickly under the right environmental stimuli. There are six species of *Naegleria,* of which only *N. fowleri* has been shown to be pathogenic for humans. *Naegleria* meningoencephalitis was first reported in the United States in 1966, and since that time infection has been reported from every continent. Most of the cases have been contracted during the summer months by previously healthy individuals with a history of swimming in or contact with fresh water before their illness. There are usually only one or two cases reported per year in the United States, with a high of eight cases reported in 1980. Most of the reports have come from the southern and southwestern states, with occasional infections occurring in the Midwest and East.

Acanthamoeba has been isolated from soil, mushrooms and vegetables, brackish and seawater, as well as most of the freshwater sources noted earlier for *Naegleria.* In contrast to *Naegleria, Acanthamoeba* has only a cyst and trophozoite form, of which only the trophozoite form is invasive. Of the 13 species of *Acanthamoeba,* seven are human pathogens. *A. castellanii, A. culbertsoni, A. polyphaga,* and *A. rhysodes* have all been recovered from human infections of both the eye and CNS. *A. astronyxis* and *A. palestinensis* have only been implicated in CNS infection. *A. hatchetti* has only been isolated from the eye. Through 1990, 56 cases of granulomatous amebic encephalitis had been reported worldwide, with 30 in the United States. Nine of these have been in patients with AIDS, and most of the rest have had other immunomodulating conditions such as diabetes mellitus, alcoholism, or radiation therapy. Cases of *Acanthamoeba* keratitis have usually followed incidents of corneal trauma involving flushing with contaminated water, or in contact lens wearers whose lenses have been contaminated with *Acanthamoeba*.

In 1990 an ameba was isolated from the brain of a mandrill baboon that died of meningoencephalitis. Based on immunofluorescent staining, this same organism has been implicated in 35 cases of granulomatous amebic encephalitis that had formerly been without definite diagnosis but attributed to *Acanthamoeba*. This previously undiscovered pathogen has now been named *Balamuthia mandrillaris*.

PATHOGENESIS AND PATHOLOGY. The free-living amebas enter the nasal cavity by inhalation or aspiration of dust or water contaminated with trophozoites or cysts. *Naegleria* gains access to the CNS through the olfactory epithelium and migration up the olfactory nerve to the olfactory bulbs, which are located in the subarachnoid space bathed by the cerebrospinal fluid (CSF). This space is richly vascularized and is the route of spread to other areas of the CNS. Besides evidence of widespread cerebral edema and hyperemia of the meninges, the olfactory bulbs are necrotic, hemorrhagic, and surrounded by a purulent exudate. Microscopically, the gray matter is the most severely affected, with severe involvement in all cases. Fibrinopurulent exudate may be found throughout the cerebral hemispheres, brain stem, cerebellum, and upper portions of the spinal cord. Pockets of trophozoites may be seen in necrotic neural tissue, usually in the perivascular spaces of arteries and arterioles. No cysts are present in the CNS.

The route of invasion and penetration in cases of granulomatous meningoencephalitis, caused by both *Acanthamoeba* and *Balamuthia*, is hematogenous, probably originating from a primary focus in the skin or lungs. Pathologically there is a granulomatous encephalitis, with multinucleated giant cells mainly in the posterior fossa structures, basal ganglia, bases of the cerebral hemispheres, and cerebellum. Both trophozoites and cysts may be found in the CNS lesions, primarily located in the perivascular spaces and invading blood vessel walls. The olfactory bulbs and spinal cord are usually spared.

CLINICAL MANIFESTATIONS. The incubation of *Naegleria* infection may be as short as 2 days or as long as 15 days. Symptoms have an acute onset and are rapidly progressive. There is a sudden onset of severe headache, fever, nausea, and vomiting, signs of meningitis, and then encephalitis. Most cases end in death within 1 wk of onset of symptoms.

Granulomatous amebic meningoencephalitis may occur weeks to months after acquiring the organism. The presenting signs and symptoms are often those of single or multiple space-occupying lesions, and include hemiparesis, personality changes, seizures, and drowsiness. Altered mental status is always a prominent symptom. Headache and fever occur only sporadically, but stiff neck is seen in a majority of cases. Palsies of the cranial nerves may be present.

DIAGNOSIS. The CSF in *Naegleria* infection may mimic that of herpetic encephalitis early in the disease, and later of acute bacterial meningitis, with a neutrophilic pleocytosis, elevated protein, and low glucose. The amebas may be seen on a wet mount of the CSF but are often mistaken for lymphocytes. Strong clinical suspicion early in the course of disease affords the best chance for early treatment and cure. *Naegleria* can be grown on agar enriched with gram-negative bacteria, on which they feed.

In granulomatous meningoencephalitis, examination of the CSF resembles that of aseptic meningitis. The isolation and identification of *Acanthamoeba* from the CNS is the best method of diagnosis. Brain tissue and CSF may be cultured for *Acanthamoeba* using the same agar used for growing *Naegleria*, but *Balamuthia* must be grown on mammalian cell cultures. Immunofluorescence staining of brain tissue can also differentiate between *Acanthamoeba* and *Balamuthia*.

TREATMENT. *Naegleria* infection is nearly always fatal, and early recognition and treatment is crucial to successful therapy. There have only been six treatment survivors, five of whom apparently recovered fully. Amphotericin B in combination with rifampin, sulphadiazine, chloramphenicol, or ketoconazole were the components of the successful regimens.

There is no satisfactory treatment at this time for granulomatous amebic meningoencephalitis. Promising drugs include rifampin and ketoconazole, both of which appear to be effective in vitro and in animal studies of *Acanthamoeba* CNS infection. Acridine derivatives and paramomycin also seem promising in vitro.

Ma P, Visvesvara GS, Martinez AJ, et al: *Naegleria* and *Acanthamoeba* infections: Review. Rev Infect Dis 12:490, 1990.

Visvesvara GS, Schuster FL, Martinez AJ: *Balamuthia mandrillaris*, N.G., n.sp., agent of amebic meningoencephalitis. J Eukaryot Microbiol 40:504, 1993.

Visvesvara GS, Stehr-Green JK: Epidemiology of free-living ameba infections. J Protozool 37:25S, 1990.

Wang A, Kay R, Poon WS, Ng HK: Successful treatment of amoebic meningoencephalitis in a Chinese living in Hong Kong. Clin Neurol Neurosurg 95:249, 1993.

244.3 Babesiosis

Robert A. Bonomo and Robert A. Salata

This malaria-like zoonosis is caused by an intraerythrocytic parasite transmitted by the hard-bodied ticks, members of the genera *Dermacentor, Ixodes,* and *Rhipicephalus.* Over 70 species exist; most are confined to a single specific host. A few, transmitted by multihost ticks, are able to infect humans incidentally. These species (such as *Babesia microti,* a rodent *Babesia* species, and *Babesia divergens,* a cattle species) are responsible for several emerging zoonoses. In addition, babesiosis may be acquired through blood transfusion from an asymptomatically infected host living in an endemic area.

EPIDEMIOLOGY. The primary endemic focus of babesiosis in the United States occurs along the northeast coastal area, centering around Nantucket Island, Martha's Vineyard, Cape Cod, Massachusetts; Long Island and Shelter Island, New York. Epidemiologic surveys in these areas reveal past infection in 2–7% of the population. Cases have also been reported from Georgia and California. The small deer tick, *Ixodes dammini,* serves as the vector for *B. microti,* which is acquired from the white-footed mouse. This is the same deer tick that transmits the agent of Lyme disease *(Borrelia burgdorferi).*

PATHOPHYSIOLOGY. Babesiosis parallels malaria in certain segments of its life cycle. Sporozoites are introduced by tick bites and rapidly invade host red blood cells. Budding forms develop as the protozoan matures and replicates, eventually rupturing the erythrocyte. These daughter forms or mesozoites then infect other red blood cells, and the cycle continues. Conversely, *Babesia* lack an extraerythrocytic stage or sexual forms (gametocytes). Although a ring form may exist in erythrocytes, *Babesia* trophozoites do not contain pigment. Finally, unlike *Plasmodium* species, *Babesia* are present in asynchronous stages in blood.

CLINICAL MANIFESTATIONS. Signs and symptoms follow a variable incubation period of 1–6 wk. A sudden or gradual onset of chills and fever is preceded by malaise, myalgias, and fatigue. Jaundice, dark urine, nausea, and vomiting occur with hemolysis. Mild splenomegaly and/or hepatomegaly occur in a quarter of infected patients. The complications of babesiosis are due to hemolysis, which can lead to renal failure from massive hemoglobinuria and capillary obstruction by parasitized erythrocytes. Laboratory studies show a mild to moderately severe hemolytic anemia, reticulocytosis, nucleated red blood cells on peripheral smear, hyperbilirubinemia, occasional thrombocytopenia, and a near normal white blood cell count; elevation of liver enzymes is found in half of all cases. Infection by *B. divergens* has a more fulminant course than *B. microti*. So far, all known infections with *B. divergens* have occurred in splenectomized hosts living in Europe.

Asymptomatic hosts may demonstrate low levels of parasitemia. In contrast, the most severe forms of babesiosis, including most fatalities, occur in splenectomized hosts. Thus, an intact functioning spleen is apparently necessary to prevent fulminant hemolysis and visceral invasion by Babesia. Complete recovery occurs in several weeks, with or without chemotherapy. One study indicates that babesiosis may be underdiagnosed in children since it follows a less severe course.

DIAGNOSIS. Babesiosis should be suspected in a febrile child with a history of a tick bite who lives in or has traveled to an endemic area or has had a recent blood transfusion. The clinical picture may resemble that of malaria, but peripheral blood smears lack intraerythrocytic pigment, schizonts, gametocytes, or synchronous stages found with malaria. An uncommon finding is the presence of tetrads of mesozoites. Multiple blood smears may be required to demonstrate parasitemia. Microscopic identification of characteristic parasites is facilitated by the use of Giemsa stain. An indirect immunofluorescence serologic test with good reliability is available at the Centers for Disease Control (CDC). In obscure cases, xenodiagnosis may be attempted in hamsters or gerbils. Clinicians should also consider possible co-infection with *Borrelia burgdorferi* because the two organisms share a common vector.

TREATMENT. The recommended therapy for babesiosis is clindamycin (20 mg/kg/24 hr) and quinine (25 mg/kg/24 hr) in combination. The duration of therapy should be 5–10 days. Preliminary animal data suggest that the new macrolide azithromycin may also be effective. For life-threatening situations, exchange blood transfusions may be required. For severe *B. divergens* infections, therapy with pentamidine isoethionate may be tried. Prevention of babesiosis involves avoidance of tick-infested areas, use of protective clothing and insect repellents, and a careful search for and removal of ticks.

Gelfand JA: Babesia. *In:* Mandell GL, Douglas RG Jr, Bennett JE (eds): Principles and Practices of Infectious Diseases, 3rd ed. New York, Churchill Livingstone, 1990, p 2119.

Ruebush TK II: Babesiosis. *In:* Warren KS, Mahmoud AAF (eds): Tropical and Geographical Medicine, 2nd ed. New York, McGraw-Hill, 1990, p 264.

244.4 Cryptosporidiosis and Coccidial Infections

Timothy Flanigan

CRYPTOSPORIDIUM

Cryptosporidium, *Isospora belli*, and *Cyclospora* are all coccidian protozoan parasites that infect the epithelial cells of the digestive tract in many mammalian species and humans, and cause enteritis and diarrhea. Initially, *Cryptosporidium* was thought to be pathogenic almost exclusively in immunocompromised persons, and only a rare cause of disease in immunocompetent individuals. *Cryptosporidium* is now recognized to be a leading protozoal cause of diarrhea in children worldwide and has been reported on all six continents. Among children hospitalized for diarrhea, *Cryptosporidium* is often the third or fourth most frequently detected cause of infectious diarrhea, usually following rotavirus and *Escherichia coli*.

ETIOLOGY. Cryptosporidiosis in humans is initiated by ingestion of the oocysts with subsequent excystation and release of four sporozoites from each oocyst within the gastrointestinal tract. Sporozoites implant immediately in the host epithelial cells and begin a cycle of autoinfection at the luminal surface of the epithelium. The sexual stage of the parasite results in oocysts, which are excreted in the stools, which are immediately infectious to other hosts or can reinfect the same host, even without reingestion. The infectious dose of *Cryptosporidium* may as low as 10 oocysts, which facilitates transmission.

The most common site of *Cryptosporidium* infection in infected individuals is the small intestine, although it is frequently present both in the colon and biliary tract of persons with immunodeficiency. *Cryptosporidium* infects only the epithelial surface of the mucosa and does not invade into the submucosal layer or cause ulcerations. Infection of the epithelial lining of the respiratory tract with associated cough has been reported, although it is uncommon. Chronic involvement of the biliary tract and ampulla of Vater has been associated with cholecystitis, papillary stenosis, and pancreatitis in patients with chronic cryptosporidiosis and AIDS.

EPIDEMIOLOGY. Excluding documented outbreaks, prevalence rates of *Cryptosporidium* infection among children with diarrhea are between 3% and 3.6% in the more industrialized countries of Europe and North America and between 5% and 15% in developing countries. In most studies, children, particularly those less than 2 years of age, appear to have a higher prevalence of infection than adults, with an increase in prevalence in warmer, more humid months. Rates as high as 19% and 36% have been detected in children hospitalized for gastroenteritis in Gaza and Thailand. In a prospective study of Bedoin infants, 45% had acquired *Cryptosporidium* infection by age two. Of great concern, *Cryptosporidium* has been implicated as an etiologic agent of persistent diarrhea in the Third World, with significant morbidity and mortality from malnutrition.

Cryptosporidium infects a number of animals, particularly cows, and can spread from infected animals to humans. Oocysts are infectious when passed in the feces, and person-to-person transmission has been well documented among day-care centers and household contacts. Infected family members are frequently identified during evaluation of day-care center outbreaks; in Michigan, for example, 71% of families with a symptomatic child had additional infected family members.

Cryptosporidium is a common cause of day-care center epidemics of diarrheal illness in the United States. Among six different outbreaks in day-care centers in the United States between 1984 and 1989, children under two had a higher attack rate (usually around 60%) than older children or caregivers. Many cases in child care centers probably remain undetected; in a survey of asymptomatic children in a day-care center (five stools/child were evaluated), a third were found to have *Cryptosporidium* oocysts in stool. Recommendations to prevent outbreaks in child care centers include strict handwashing, use of overclothes or diapers capable of retaining liquid diarrhea, and separation of diapering and food handling areas and responsibilities.

Cryptosporidium has been identified as the etiologic agent of several extensive waterborne outbreaks, usually due to surface infected groundwater sources, often involving farm animals. The oocyst is only 4 μm in diameter, making it difficult to clear through filtration, and it is resistant to routine chlorination. The first documented waterborne outbreak in San Antonio, Texas, had a 34% attack rate and was linked to sewage contamination of a well-water supply that was chlorinated but not filtered. In 1987, an outbreak in Georgia resulted in an estimated 13,000 cases of cryptosporidial enteritis despite the filtered and chlorinated public supply that met established Environmental Protection Agency guidelines. Improved filtering of the water supply ultimately helped terminate the outbreak. An outbreak in Milwaukee, Wisconsin, in 1993 afflicted some 375,000 residents when the spring runoff from grazing lands was not adequately filtered in the public water supply.

CLINICAL MANIFESTATIONS. Typically, acute infection with *Crypt-*

osporidium is characterized by watery diarrhea, crampy epigastric abdominal pain, weight loss, anorexia, and malaise. Diarrhea is the most noteworthy symptom and can range from a few loose bowel movements a day to more than 50 stools with a fluid loss of over 10 L/day. Over 80% of children with cryptosporidiosis will experience vomiting for a duration of 1–15 days. In a majority of patients, diarrhea will be more severe than vomiting, but in one study 40% of patients experienced vomiting for more than 5 days, and in over 15% of patients it lasted more than 10 days. Two patients had persistent vomiting without diarrhea, which required hospitalization for dehydration. Abdominal pain is crampy in nature, which can last from 1 to 10 days. Fever is not uncommon, and it occurs in up to a third of patients. It is usually mild and lasts less than 3 days. Cough in the absence of any lower respiratory tract illness may accompany gastrointestinal symptoms and persist for 1–2 wk.

The subsequent course of clinical illness is determined by the immunocompetence of the infected individual. Immunocompetent persons are susceptible to infection with *Cryptosporidium,* yet the clinical course of enteritis is invariably self-limited and results in complete recovery. On the other hand, individuals with immunodeficiency, such as congenital hypogammaglobulinemia or individuals with severe immunodeficiency related to HIV infection, develop chronic persistent enteritis that ultimately can lead to severe malnutrition, wasting, anorexia, and even death. The relationship between the clinical course of disease and immunodeficiency is illustrated in children who acquire cryptosporidiosis while receiving therapy for hematologous malignancies. The enteritis invariably resolves once the immune system has recovered from the immunosuppressive therapy.

The incubation period may vary from a few days to 2 wk. The duration of illness in immunocompetent hosts ranges from 2 days to a month. Most individuals become asymptomatic within 2 wk, although they may continue to shed oocysts for a longer period.

DIAGNOSIS. Diagnosis is based on identification of the oocysts in stool. Oocysts stain red with varying intensities with a modified acid-fast technique; this technique allows for differentiation of the *Cryptosporidium* oocysts from yeast that are similar in size and shape but are not acid fast. Oocysts can also be detected by a direct immunofluorescent assay that is commercially available and has comparable or slightly better sensitivity than the modified acid-fast stain. Frequently, concentration techniques, such as Sheather sugar flotation, are utilized to detect smaller numbers of oocysts. It is important that laboratory requests specifically mention *Cryptosporidium* when suspected so that appropriate concentration and staining techniques may be performed. The spherical parasite can also be easily identified on biopsy specimens on mucosal surfaces. It is found individually or in clusters on the brush border of mucosal epithelial surfaces, appearing basophilic with hematoxylin and eosin staining. *Cryptosporidium* does not invade below the epithelial layer of the mucosa; therefore, fecal leukocytes are not found within stool specimens.

TREATMENT. Since the diarrheal illness due to cryptosporidiosis is self-limited in immunocompetent patients, no specific antimicrobial therapy is required. Treatment should focus on supportive care only, consisting of rehydration by the oral route or occasionally, if fluid losses are very severe, using intravenous fluid. Oral rehydration solution should be used for children who do not require hospitalization. Patients with severe chronic cryptosporidial enteritis with AIDS or other immunodeficiencies have been treated with a wide variety of chemotherapeutic agents, none of which have been highly effective. Currently two antimicrobial agents, paromomycin and azithromycin, are being evaluated in double-blind, placebo-controlled trials for the treatment of cryptosporidiosis in patients with AIDS.

ISOSPORA

Isospora belli is a coccidian protozoan parasite that causes infection of the gastrointestinal tract in many animals and humans. It appears to be more common in tropical and subtropical climates, such as South America, Africa, and Southeast Asia. It has been implicated as a cause of diarrhea in various institutional outbreaks and in World War II veterans returning from the Pacific. *Isospora* is an infrequent cause of diarrhea in patients with AIDS in the United States but may infect up to 15% of AIDS patients in Haiti.

Infection is acquired through ingestion of the oocysts, after which the parasite invades the intestinal epithelial cell. Oocysts are excreted in stool but are not immediately infectious and must undergo further maturation. Acute illness can begin abruptly with fever, abdominal pain, and watery, nonbloody diarrhea that may last for weeks or months. In patients with AIDS, infections are persistent and resemble the chronic, profuse watery diarrhea of cryptosporidiosis. Eosinophilia, not found with other enteric protozoan infections, may be present. The diagnosis is made by detecting the oocysts on modified acid-fast stain in the stool. The oocyst is significantly larger than *Cryptosporidium* oocysts (25 μm compared with 4 μm). Because oocyst excretion can be intermittent, it may be necessary to examine multiple stools or sample duodenal contents by aspiration or biopsy.

Unlike cryptosporidiosis, isosporiasis responds promptly to treatment with oral trimethoprim-sulfamethoxazole. In patients with AIDS, relapses are common and necessitate maintenance therapy.

CYCLOSPORA

Cyclospora is a newly identified intestinal pathogen of humans that has many of the same features of *Isospora belli* and *Cryptosporidium. Cyclospora* causes a syndrome similar to cryptosporidial enteritis, with watery diarrhea, vomiting, anorexia, malaise, and weight loss. The organism affects both immunocompromised and immunocompetent individuals. Infections appear to be spread through water or food. The primary site of infection is the small intestine; duodenal biopsies show varying degrees of blunting of villi and crypt hyperplasia. The absence of fecal leukocytes and erythrocytes suggests that the infection is noninvasive.

It has only been within the last few years that illness in humans caused by *Cyclospora* infection has been recognized. The majority of isolates from humans have been identified in stool samples obtained from residents of the third world or from travelers returning from developing countries. Infection appears to occur predominantly during the warmer season.

Diagnosis is made by identification of the oocyst in the stool. Oocysts are wrinkled spheres, measure 8–10 μm in diameter, and resemble large *Cryptosporidium.* Formalin-preserved organisms are acid fast, staining with both the Kinyoun and Ziehl-Neelsen methods, but stain best with the modified Carbol Fuchsin acid-fast technique that is used to stain *Cryptosporidium.* Oocysts can also be concentrated by sucrose flotation in Sheather solution. Data with regard to therapy is limited, but it appears that symptoms respond well to trimethoprim-sulfamethoxazole. Many questions remain to be answered about this newly identified pathogen.

SARCOCYSTIS

Human infections due to the coccidian protozoan parasites *Sarcocystis* spp. are rare, asymptomatic, and usually only an incidental finding. Infection occurs worldwide among large mammals and requires two hosts for replication. Sexual reproduction occurs in the intestinal mucosa of the definitive host and results in the shedding of sporocysts in the feces. The intermediate host, on the other hand, ingests feces contaminated with sporocysts, which then invade and infect endothelial cells with subsequent asexual multiplication and the formation of sarcocysts, or cysts, in muscle fiber, usually striated or cardiac. Humans may serve as either a definitive host, with infection of the gut mucosa, or as an intermediate host, with infection of striated muscle. Cysts are usually found incidentally on histologic section of muscle without associated symptoms, but occasionally muscle soreness or swelling may occur. Gastrointestinal infection has not been associated with diarrhea or enteritis.

MacKenzie WR, Huxie NJ, Proctor ME, et al: A massive outbreak in Milwaukee of *Cryptosporidium* infection transmitted through the public water supply. N Engl J Med 331:161, 1994.
Ortega YR, Sterling CR, Gilman RH, et al: Cyclospora—A new protozoan pathogen in humans. N Engl J Med 328:1308, 1993.

244.5 Giardiasis and Other Protozoal Diseases

John Aucott

GIARDIA LAMBLIA

Giardia lamblia is a ubiquitous gastrointestinal protozoa that results in a clinical picture ranging from asymptomatic colonization to acute or chronic diarrheal illness. The infection is more prevalent in children than in adults. *Giardia* is endemic in areas of the world with poor levels of sanitation and is also an important cause of morbidity in the developing world, where it is associated with urban day-care centers, residential institutions for the mentally retarded, and water- and foodborne outbreaks. Giardia is a particularly significant pathogen in people with malnutrition, immunodeficiencies, or cystic fibrosis.

ETIOLOGY. *G. lamblia* infects humans through ingestion of as few as 10 cysts. The mature cyst, measuring approximately 8–10 μm, is thick walled, oval, and contains four nuclei. They are passed in the stools of infected individuals and may remain viable in water for as long as 2 mo. Their viability is not affected by the normal concentrations of chlorine used to purify water for drinking. Upon reaching the upper small intestine, each *Giardia* cyst liberates four trophozoites. Trophozoites colonize the lumen of the duodenum and proximal jejunum, where they attach to the brush border of the intestinal epithelial cells and multiply by binary fusion. The body of the trophozoite is teardrop-shaped and is divided longitudinally by two median rods and contains two oval nuclei anteriorly, a large sucking disk on the ventral surface, and a curved median body posteriorly. Each organism has four pairs of flagella. Different strains of *Giardia* exist, resulting in variation in infectivity, antigenic structure, and isoenzyme patterns. The clinical significance of strains and the apparent capability for antigenic variation remains unknown.

EPIDEMIOLOGY. The prevalence of *Giardia* in several parts of the world varies from 0.5% to 50%, with a prevalence of 19–30% in surveys of day-care centers in the industrialized world. In the developing world *Giardia* is one of the first enteric pathogens to infect infants, with peak prevalence rates of 15–20% in children less that 10 yr old. Humans were thought to be the only reservoir of *G. lamblia,* but it is now believed that the parasite also infects beavers and dogs. *Giardia* is the most common etiologic agent identified by the Centers for Disease Control (CDC) in outbreaks of waterborne disease. Waterborne outbreaks have been linked to the ingestion of surface water treated by faulty or inadequate water purification systems or drinking of untreated mountain stream water by hikers. Attack rates of up to 10% have been reported from epidemics linked to water supplies. Person-to-person, foodborne, and interspecies transmission also occur, resulting in sporadic cases as well as epidemics. Child care centers play an important role in the transmission of urban giardiasis, with secondary attack rates in families as high as 17–30%. The duration of asymptomatic infection is unknown, but some children in child care centers have passed cysts for as long as 6 mo. Giardiasis is an important cause of chronic diarrhea in children with X-linked agammaglobulinemia, suggesting the importance of immunity in controlling giardiasis. The observation that adults living in endemic areas have less symptomatic illness than infants or adult visitors provides evidence of acquired immunity to giardiasis. These is no convincing evidence that patients with acquired immunodeficiency syndrome (AIDS) or selective IgA deficiency have more severe or prolonged disease. Human milk contains cytotoxic free fatty acids and secretary IgA antibodies that may provide protection to nursing infants.

CLINICAL MANIFESTATIONS. The majority of individuals infected with *Giardia* are probably asymptomatic. Symptoms develop 1–3 wk after exposure to the parasite. Giardiasis is more frequently symptomatic in children than in adults. Symptoms occur in 40–80% of infected children after an average incubation period of 8 days. The most common presentation is diarrhea, weight loss, crampy abdominal pain, and failure to thrive or a spruelike illness. The onset of symptoms may be abrupt or gradual; the disease may be self-limited or produce severe protracted diarrhea and malabsorption. Alterations in the digestive function of the brush border are common in those with protracted symptoms. Malabsorption of sugars (such as xylose and disaccharides), fats, and fat-soluble vitamins occurs in more than half of patients who have nonspecific morphologic abnormalities of the small intestinal mucosa, which are similar to those seen in other malabsorptive disorders. Lactose intolerance is common after infection with *Giardia* and may mimic relapse or reinfection. The impact of chronic infection with *Giardia* on children in the developing world is controversial, but some investigators believe *Giardia* infection may affect growth and development in this setting. Trophozoites rarely invade the lamina propria of the intestinal mucosa, and *Giardia* is only rarely reported as a cause of inflammatory diarrhea or fever. Enterotoxin production by *Giardia* has not been demonstrated.

DIAGNOSIS. *G. lamblia* trophozoites or cysts may be found in fecal or duodenal samples obtained from infected children. Fecal leukocytes are not seen in *Giardia* infection. Because cyst excretion is irregular, examination of several fecal samples may be needed. In experienced hands the examination of three formol-ether concentrated samples has a sensitivity of up to 95%. Evaluation by duodenal sampling or biopsy may be necessary for diagnosis. The Entero test is a simple method for detecting *G. lamblia* in duodenal fluid of children that avoids the cost and anesthetic risk of upper intestinal endoscopy. When required, upper intestinal endoscopy is used to obtain specimen by aspiration, brush cytology, and biopsy, all of which have been reported to be highly sensitive. Antigen detection tests are available and are highly sensitive and specific. They are useful in situations where a fecal examination is not necessary to evaluate for other pathogens, for example, when investigating a known outbreak of *Giardia* in a day-care center.

TREATMENT. Most cases of *Giardia* are probably self-limited. When *Giardia* causes symptoms in children or adults, it should be treated because of the potential for chronic or intermittent symptoms. Symptoms or signs of diarrhea, abdominal pain, bloating, or failure to thrive are generally agreed on indications for therapy. Furazolidone (2 mg/kg four times a day for 10 days) is available in pediatric suspension, is well tolerated, and is considered the drug of choice for children. It is only about 80% effective, and therefore patients should be followed carefully for relapse of infection. Metronidazole (5 mg/kg three times a day for 7 days) has been shown to be as effective as furazolidone in the treatment of *Giardia* in children. Metronidazole is available in a liquid suspension and is well tolerated by children. Concerns over mutagenicity of metronidazole in children remain despite lack of evidence of the clinical significance of this concern. Metronidazole is not currently approved by the Food and Drug Administration for the treatment of *Giardia* despite its wide use. Tinidazole has also been evaluated for treatment of infected children; a single oral dose of 50 mg/kg resulted in an 80% cure rate. Quinacrine (2 mg/kg three times a day for 7 days) is highly effective but is less well studied and less well tolerated by young children. Both quinacrine and tinidazole are currently unavailable in the United States. If infection persists or recurs, eradication of the parasite is usually achieved by the use of an agent from an alternative class. Relapse after therapy should be documented by stool examination to distinguish relapse or reinfection from post-*Giardia* lactose intolerance. Rare cases of *Giardia* that were clinically resistant to treatment have been cured with a combination of quinacrine and metronidazole. Patients who fail repeated courses of therapy should be evaluated for possible hypogammaglobulinemia.

There is debate whether asymptomatic persons who harbor *Giardia* should be treated. Arguments for treatment are based on a public health concern for the risk of transmission. Arguments against treatment of asymptomatic individuals include (1) the lack of adverse outcomes in immunocompetent, well-nourished children, (2) the expense and significant side effects associated with treatment, and (3) the lack of any evidence that asymptomatic excretion plays a role of transmission in day-care centers or that treatment decreases the occurrence of *Giardia* during 6–8 mo follow-up periods. Because of these arguments most authorities recommend against treatment of asymptomatic children or adults in settings where rapid reinfection is likely, although this remains controversial. Authorities often advise treatment when reinfection is unlikely, and treatment of high risk individuals such as food handlers is always required.

The recent increase of epidemics of giardiasis requires re-examination of sanitary practices. Adequate filtration of water supplies is the most important factor in preventing waterborne *Giardia*. The concentration of chlorine required for control, particularly in communities that are dependent on surface water but have no sand filtration, needs to be determined. Spread of infection in institutions may be prevented by strict hand washing, treatment of symptomatic carriers, and other infection control practices. Identifying and treating asymptomatic carriers may be considered but is an unproved strategy. No prophylactic medication prevents giardiasis.

BLASTOCYSTIS HOMINIS

Blastocystis hominis is a common protozoan found in 3–18% of all stool specimens submitted to parasitology laboratories. The relationship of *B. hominis* to gastrointestinal symptoms remains controversial. The organism is often found in asymptomatic individuals and often disappears from the stool without specific therapy. *B. hominis* is often found in the presence of other more pathogenic organisms, clouding its etiologic role. *B. hominis* has been reported to be the sole pathogen identified in one series of pediatric patients reporting abdominal pain, diarrhea, weight loss, and vomiting. Illness may be self-limited or may last for months. Immunosuppressed individuals may be more susceptible to symptomatic infection. Physical exam and radiological studies are usually unrevealing. The differential diagnosis includes other parasitic infections, such as *Giardia* and irritable bowel syndrome. Diagnosis is based on the repeated identification of *B. hominis* from stool samples. Some investigators report a correlation of symptoms with greater than five parasites per oil or 400× field. Symptoms may resolve spontaneously without therapy; however, therapy in one study increased the rate of symptomatic resolution from 58% to 90%. When *B. hominis* is repeatedly isolated from persistently symptomatic patients and no other cause of diarrhea can be found, therapy is probably warranted. Metronidazole and diiodohydroxyquin (iodoquinol) have been used with anecdotal success in the therapy of symptomatic infections with *B. hominis*.

DIENTAMOEBA FRAGILIS

Dientamoeba fragilis is a gastrointestinal protozoan whose prevalence may be underestimated because of difficulty in identification and lack of knowledge concerning this parasite. The organism has been found in 4.2% of stools submitted for parasitologic examination in one large study and is more common in individuals under the age of 20. Risk of infection may be increased by poor sanitary conditions, travel, or residence in an institutional setting. *D. fragilis* infection has been found to be associated with *Enterobius vermicularis* infection, suggesting a possible role for transmission through pinworm eggs. Studies have found that up to 90% of children infected with *D. fragilis* are symptomatic. Typical findings include chronic symptoms of abdominal pain, intermittent diarrhea, and anorexia. Infection can also present with acute inflammatory diarrhea containing blood and mucus. An association of *D. fragilis* with fibrosis of the appendiceal wall in patients with appendicitis has also been reported. Peripheral eosinophilia may be present in as many as 50% of cases. The diagnosis is made in 70–85% of cases by examination of three stool samples. The yield may be increased to 90–95% with six samples. Diagnosis with indirect immunofluorescent-antibody assay has been reported as well. Treatment with diiodohydroxyquin 30–40 mg/kg/day for 21 days and tetracycline (in older individuals) is recommended.

GIARDIA LAMBLIA INFECTION

Addiss DG, Mathews HM, Stewart JM, et al: Evaluation of a commercially available enzyme-linked immunosorbent assay for *Giardia lamblia* antigen in stool. J Clin Microbiol 29:1137, 1991.

Bartlett AV, Englender SJ, Jarvis BA, et al: Controlled trial of *Giardia lamblia:* Control strategies in day care centers. Am J Public Health 81:1001, 1991.

Craft JC, Murphy T, Nelson JD: Furazolidone and quinacrine: Comparative study of therapy for giardiasis in children. Am J Dis Child 135:164, 1981.

Farthing MJG, Mata L, Urrutia JJ, et al: Natural history of *Giardia* infection of infants and children in rural Guatemala and its impact on physical growth. Am J Clin Nutr 43:395, 1986.

Hill DR: *Giardiasis.* Issues in diagnosis and management. Infect Dis Clin North Am 7:503, 1993.

Keystone JS, Krajden S, Warren MR: Person-to-person transmission of *Giardia lamblia* in day care nurseries. Can Med Assoc J 119:241, 1978.

Medical Letter: Drugs for parasitic infections. Med Lett Drugs Ther 34:17, 1992.

Nayak N, Ganguly NK, Walia BNS, et al: Specific secretory IgA in the milk of *Giardia lamblia*-infected and uninfected women. J Infect Dis 155:724, 1987.

Paerregaard A, Hjelt K, Krasilnikoff PA: Comparative study of four methods for detecting giardiasis in children. Pediatr Infect Dis J 7:807, 1988.

Pickering LK, Morrow AL: Commentary on treatment of children with asymptomatic and nondiarrheal *Giardia* infection. Pediatr Infect Dis J 10:846, 1991.

Pickering LK, Woodward WE, DuPont JL, et al: Occurrence of *Giardia lamblia* in children in day care centers. J Pediatr 104:522, 1988.

Quiros-Buelna E. Furazolidone and metronidazole for treatment of giardiasis in children. Scand J Gastroenterol 24(Suppl 169):65, 1989.

Upcroft JA, Upcroft P, Boreham PFL: Drug resistance in *Giardia* intestinalis. Int J Parasitol 20:489, 1990.

Webster ADB: Giardiasis and immunodeficiency syndromes. Trans R Soc Trop Med Hyg 74:440, 1980.

BLASTOCYSTIS HOMINIS INFECTION

Markell EK, Udkow MP: *Blastocystis hominis:* Pathogen or fellow traveler? Am J Trop Med Hyg 35:1023, 1986.

Miller RA, Minshew BH: *Blastocystis hominis:* An organism in search of a disease. Rev Infect Dis 10:930, 1988.

O'Gorman MA, Orenstein SR, Proujansky R, et al: Prevalence and characteristics of *Blastocystis hominis* infection in children. Clin Pediatr 32:91, 1993.

Rolston KVI, Winans R, Rodriquez S: *Blastocystis hominis:* Pathogen or not? Rev Infect Dis 11:661, 1989.

***DIENTAMOEBA FRAGILIS* INFECTION**

Chan FTH, Guan MX, Mackenzie AMR: Application of indirect immunofluorescence to detection of *Dientamoeba fragilis* trophozoites in fecal specimens. J Clin Microbiol 31:1710, 1993.

Shein R, Gleg A: Colitis due to *Dientamoeba fragilis*. Am J Gastroenterol 78:634, 1983.

Spencer MJ, Garcia IS, Chapin MR: *Dientamoeba fragilis*, an intestinal pathogen in children? Am J Dis Child 133:390, 1979.

Yang J, Scholten T: *Dientamoeba fragilis*. A review with notes on its epidemiology, pathogenicity, mode of transmission and diagnosis. Am J Trop Med Hyg 26:16, 1977.

244.6 Leishmaniasis

David J. Wyler and Davidson H. Hamer

Infection with different species of *Leishmania* can cause cutaneous lesions, ulcerations of the oronasal mucosa, or visceral dissemination, resulting in fatal complications. Leishmaniasis has a vast geographic distribution, involving millions of people. Diagnosis is typically established by identifying *Leishmania* in infected tissue. Although effective drugs are available for treatment, drug resistance is a problem.

ETIOLOGY. *Leishmania* are protozoal parasites that exist in two morphologically distinct forms (digenetic): the promastigote, which is flagellated and replicates extracellularly within the sandfly vector gut and also in axenic cultures; and the amastigote, which lacks a flagellum and grows within mononuclear phagocytes in the mammalian host. Female vector sandflies (certain *Phlebotomus, Lutzomyia,* and *Psychdopygus* species) become infected by ingesting *Leishmania*-infected macrophages while taking a blood meal. In the sandfly gut, amastigotes exit from the ingested host cells, transform into promastigotes, and replicate. Transmission occurs when promastigotes are subsequently injected into a susceptible host, where they enter mononuclear phagocytes and transform intracellularly into amastigotes. Amastigotes replicate and infect adjacent macrophages. Direct human-to-human transmission rarely occurs when *Leishmania*-infected cells are transferred by blood transfusion, organ transplantation, needle-stick injury, or contact between open skin lesions. In cutaneous leishmaniasis only local replication of amastigotes occurs. In mucocutaneous and visceral disease, dissemination (probably hematogenous) takes places.

PATHOPHYSIOLOGY. *Leishmania* attach to mononuclear phagocytes by a complex process involving parasite- and host-derived macromolecules, including complement components and fibronectin. The parasite is ingested and secondary lysosomes fuse with the parasitophorous vacuole to form a phagolysosome. The pH of this compartment is maintained at about 4.5–5.0. Paradoxically, this typically hostile environment is beneficial to the parasite. *Leishmania* species differ in temperature optima for growth, which may explain why some species disseminate while others are restricted to the cooler parts of the body such as the skin.

Relatively little is known about the basis of skin ulceration in cutaneous leishmaniasis or mucosal and cartilage destruction in mucocutaneous leishmaniasis. The possibility of an autoimmune component in the latter disease has been considered. Several of the complications of visceral leishmaniasis have been traditionally ascribed to the direct effects of infected macrophages in the afflicted organ (including hypersplenism) and to inanition. More recently, the role of overproduction of cytokines (particularly tumor necrosis factor) in the pathogenesis of this disease has captured research attention. New insights can be expected.

Although amastigotes survive and replicate in quiescent mononuclear phagocytes, when these cells are activated they can inhibit parasite replication and may be leishmanicidal. Acquired host defense involves effector $CD4^+$ lymphocytes that impart activation signals to the infected macrophages, either in the form of soluble lymphokines, such as gamma interferon, or by direct cell-to-cell contact. Because some forms of leishmaniasis heal spontaneously while others are chronic and progressive, immunoregulation of the acquired host defense has been extensively investigated. Studies in selected inbred strains of mice infected with *L. major* suggest that a sustained activation of the Th1 helper subset of $CD4^+$ lymphocytes is required for the spontaneous resolution of infection. In contrast, progressive disease is associated with marked stimulation of the Th2 subset and concomitant inhibition of the Th1 subset. As yet, it is not entirely clear that the same immunoregulatory dichotomy occurs in humans, although there is little doubt that anergy to leishmanial antigens accompanies disseminated disease (diffuse cutaneous leishmaniasis and visceral leishmaniasis). Novel approaches to immunization or immunotherapy could result from a better understanding of immunoregulation in leishmaniasis.

CLINICAL MANIFESTATIONS

Visceral Leishmaniasis. This disease, also called kala-azar, is caused by species of *Leishmania* (*L. donovani* complex, *L. chagasi, L. infantum*) that disseminate hematogenously, infecting macrophages in virtually any organ, but particularly in the liver, spleen, bone marrow, and lymph nodes. (It has been recognized recently that *L. tropica,* a traditionally dermatotropic species, can occasionally cause kala-azar.) The infection is zoonotic in most areas. Dogs and other carnivores are the most common reservoirs. In India and East Africa humans are thought to be the reservoir. The disease is found on all continents except Australia, and although epidemiologic features may differ widely, the important clinical features are generally similar in different geographic regions.

Typically, symptoms appear several weeks to 8 mo following the sandfly bite, although incubation periods of up to 10 yr have been reported. Lesions at the inoculation site are rarely observed when the patient first comes to medical attention. The course of the disease can be abrupt (as occurs frequently in young children) or insidious (especially in older children and adults). Oligosymptomatic and asymptomatic forms of the infection have been described in children with positive *Leishmania* serology. Children with subclinical disease may clear the infection spontaneously or may progress to overt disease (especially in the presence of malnutrition or acquired immunodeficiency). Fever is very common. Although it may have periodicity, the pattern is not diagnostically reliable. Vomiting, diarrhea, and a nonproductive cough accompany disease of abrupt onset. Infections with a more protracted course may be characterized by an initial 2–8 wk of fevers and nonspecific systemic complaints, including weakness, anorexia, and vague abdominal problems. Thereafter, the fever may recede and the patient becomes weaker and complains of symptoms related to an enlarged spleen, such as abdominal discomfort and early satiety. The most dramatic finding on physical examination is marked splenomegaly that may reach massive proportions. Hepatomegaly and less frequently lymphadenopathy are associated common features. With time, the hair thins and becomes brittle. The skin becomes dry and scaly and may acquire the gray, ashen appearance from which the Hindi name *kala-azar* ("black sickness") is derived. Petechiae, ecchymoses, and mild edema may appear; jaundice and ascites are rare.

The major complications leading to death, including hemorrhage and bacterial superinfection, result from a decrease in blood elements due to leishmanial infection of the bone marrow and hypersplenism. Anemia, leukopenia, and thrombocytopenia are common. Hypoalbuminemia, a marked polyclonal hypergammaglobulinemia (mostly IgG), circulating immune complexes, and rheumatoid factor are associated laboratory findings. Immune complex glomerulonephritis with proteinuria and microscopic hematuria occurs, although renal disease is uncommon. Secondary amyloidosis and hepatic fibrosis leading to portal hypertension occur rarely. Without treatment, death usually ensues within 2 yr as a result of infectious complications, including pneumonia, tuberculosis, dysentery, and septicemia, or of anemia or hemorrhage.

Post kala-azar dermal leishmaniasis (PKDL) develops in 3–20% of patients after treatment of the visceral infection. The lesions range from depigmented macules on the face and trunk to firm nodules appearing mostly on the nose and around the mouth. They may persist for months or years if untreated. A history of previous kala-azar and isolation of parasites from the lesions help establish this diagnosis.

Kala-azar should be suspected in endemic areas when patients present with enlarging spleens, pancytopenia (especially anemia), and hyperglobulinemia. The infection has occurred in patients with human immunodeficiency virus (HIV) infection residing in temperature regions where transmission occurs (southern Europe) and in travelers to areas with endemic leishmaniasis. The development of kala-azar in these patients (which may be years after exposure) can herald the onset of acquired immunodeficiency syndrome (AIDS).

Kala-azar must be differentiated from malaria, miliary tuberculosis, salmonellosis, acute schistosomiasis, amebic liver abscess, and acute typhus. In the chronic stages it may mimic hepatosplenic schistosomiasis, brucellosis, tropical splenomegaly syndrome, chronic lymphocytic leukemia, lymphoma, malignant histiocytosis, and glycogen storage disease. PKDL may be confused with yaws, syphilis, and leprosy.

Cutaneous Leishmaniasis. This type of infection is traditionally divided into Old World (Mediterranean Basin, Africa, India, China, Soviet Union, and Asia Minor) and New World (primarily Central and South America, excluding Chile and Uruguay). The former is caused by any of a number of species, including *L. tropica* and *L. major;* the latter is caused by the *L. brasiliensis* and *L. mexicana* complexes. In most geographic areas, these parasites are maintained by transmission in nonhuman reservoirs, usually rodents, but human-to-human transmission can also occur.

The characteristic skin lesion begins as an erythematous papule or macule that may ulcerate after several weeks. Unless superinfected with bacteria, the lesions are generally painless, nontender, and not pruritic. In some cases, lymphatic nodules may develop proximal to the lesion. Satellite lesions containing parasites may form adjacent to the primary one. In Old World cutaneous leishmaniasis, spontaneous healing usually occurs over a period of months.

Diffuse cutaneous leishmaniasis (DCL) is a rare form recognized primarily in Ethiopia, Venezuela, and the Dominican Republic. Multiple lesions form on the skin in association with anergy to leishmanial antigens. Defective host defense in these patients is also revealed by a paucity of lymphocytes and a large number of heavily infected macrophages in the lesions. *L. recidiva* is another rare form found in areas of endemic *L. tropica* infection and is manifested by lesions (usually facial) that resemble lupus vulgaris, which may persist for years. In contrast to DCL, the parasites may be difficult to identify in these lesions. The differential diagnosis of cutaneous leishmaniasis includes tuberculosis and atypical mycobacteriosis of the skin, fungal infections, syphilis, yaws, leprosy, basal cell carcinoma, and sarcoidosis.

MUCOCUTANEOUS LEISHMANIASIS (Espundia). This is a complication of cutaneous leishmaniasis acquired in Central and South America. The rate of this complication varies in different geographic areas, from less than 1% to as high as 30% in southern Brazil. *L. braziliensis brasiliensis* is most commonly responsible for this disease. The parasite spreads hematogenously, and the lesions in the oral and nasal mucosa may develop 1 mo to 24 yr (rare cases) after the initial cutaneous lesion. Coryza, nasal stuffiness, or epistaxis are typical presenting complaints. Destructive lesions can involve the lips, tongue, soft palate, nasal septum and bridge, pharynx, larynx, and trachea. Destruction of the nasal septum can lead to perforation or to collapse that gives rise to the so-called tapir nose deformity. Erosion of the nose and lips can cause grotesque facial deformities. Involvement of the larynx, pharynx, or trachea can cause dysphagia and, rarely, asphyxia. Aspiration pneumonia, wound infections, and bacterial meningitis are complications. Mucocutaneous leishmaniasis may resemble syphilis, yaws, histoplasmosis, paracoccidioidomycosis, sarcoidosis, basal cell carcinoma, and midline granuloma.

DIAGNOSIS. When kala-azar is suspected, the diagnosis should be confirmed by biopsy or aspiration of an involved site. Splenic aspiration provides the highest yield (positive in >80% of cases) and is safe but is generally avoided by inexperienced physicians. It should be performed with a small gauge needle and avoided in patients with severe thrombocytopenia (platelets $<40 \times 10^9/L$) or coagulopathy. Bone marrow aspiration is the second most useful procedure (54–86% positive), and liver biopsy may also be helpful (~70% positive). Aspiration of lymph nodes has provided the diagnosis in patients with kala-azar who have lymphadenopathy. By light microscopy, amastigotes appear in Giemsa-stained infected cells as round forms measuring about 2–5 μm in diameter with a characteristic large mitochondrion-associated mass of extrachromosomal DNA (the kinetoplast). Aspirated or homogenized biopsy material should be cultured for up to 4 wk on specialized media. Promastigotes can be observed as motile oblong bodies (20 μm long) in positive cultures.

The *Montenegro skin test* (a test for cutaneous delayed type hypersensitivity response to a killed promastigote preparation called leishmanin) is negative in active kala-azar, only becoming positive after 6–8 wk of successful therapy. Leishmanin is not commercially available but can be obtained from the WHO Leishmaniasis Reference Center, Hadassah Medical Center, Jerusalem, Israel. Serologic tests developed for the diagnosis of kala-azar include complement fixation, fluorescent antibody, indirect hemagglutination, direct agglutination, and ELISA tests. The indirect immunofluorescence antibody test is available from the Centers for Disease Control and Prevention (CDC), Atlanta, Georgia. Serologic tests should not be used to the exclusion of other diagnostic tests, because routine tests are not species specific and may be falsely positive in patients infected with *Trypanosoma cruzi.* On the other hand, leishmanial serologic tests may be falsely negative in AIDS patients with visceral leishmaniasis.

Diagnosis of cutaneous leishmaniasis is best achieved by skin biopsy from the raised edge of a lesion; needle aspirates have also proved useful. Impression smears of biopsy material stained with Giemsa provide the most rapid diagnosis if amastigotes can be identified; identifying parasites on histologic sections may prove more difficult. Some species identifiable on impression smears may fail to grow in culture. The Montenegro test generally becomes positive in 4–6 wk after infection and persists for years; in diffuse cutaneous leishmaniasis it is negative. In leishmaniasis recidiva the reaction is characteristically exuberant. Serology is unreliable in cutaneous leishmaniasis as titers are usually low. In mucocutaneous leishmaniasis organisms may be difficult to identify in tissue. However, the Montenegro test is generally positive, and antibody can be detected by immunofluorescence assay in 90% of such cases.

TREATMENT. The pentavalent antimonial (Sb^v) compounds sodium stibogluconate (Pentostam, Wellcome Foundation, UK; 100 mg Sb/mL; available from CDC) and meglumine antimonate (Glucantime; Rhone Poulenc, France) are the preferred drugs for treating leishmaniasis. Both can be given intravenously or intramuscularly, and they appear to have similar efficacy and toxicities. Effectiveness of treatment depends on the form of leishmaniasis where it was acquired and the immunocompetance of the patient. Failure of pentavalent antimony therapy is common in kala-azar acquired in East Africa, China, and the Mediterranean, and in diffuse cutaneous and mucocutaneous disease in all areas. In addition, drug failures are being increasingly recognized in India and Latin America. Clinical relapse of leishmaniasis following seemingly effective treatment is typical in HIV-infected patients; lifelong suppressive antileishmanial therapy may be necessary.

All forms of visceral, mucocutaneous, and diffuse cutaneous leishmaniasis should be treated. Cutaneous disease acquired in the Old World usually is self-healing and requires treatment only if the lesion progresses, fails to heal in 3–5 mo, is disabling owing to its location, or is cosmetically embarrassing. The safest approach may be to treat all forms of cutaneous leishmaniasis acquired in Central and South America (except uta, a spontaneously healing form of infection found in Peru, and infection acquired in Argentina), because most patients fail to heal spontaneously and some may be at risk for developing mucosal disease. It is not established that treatment of the skin lesion prevents the subsequent development of mucocutaneous leishmaniasis, however. Therefore, patients should be followed even after successful treatment. PKDL and leishmaniasis recidiva are treated in the same way as primary infections.

Precise regimens are difficult to recommend because few careful comparisons have been reported. For most forms of leishmaniasis, 20 mg Sb^v/kg body weight (some suggest to a maximum of 850 mg/24 hr) given once each day intramuscularly or intravenously for 20–40 days should be adequate. Shorter courses have been successful in cutaneous infection acquired in certain regions. For treatment failure or recurrence, one or two repeat courses are often tried and may prove effective. Antimony is rapidly excreted by the kidney (80% in a few hours) with little accumulation in the tissue. Side effects of therapy are dose and duration dependent, and may include arthralgias, fever, rash, elevation of hepatic enzymes, gastrointestinal irritation, pancreatitis, and renal failure. Electrocardiographic changes such as T-wave depression or inversion and prolonged QT interval may herald the onset of arrhythmias but generally are transient and well tolerated with standard regimens.

Alternative antileishmanial therapies are available. Amphotericin B is one of the second-line agents employed in treating all forms of antimony-resistant leishmaniasis. Patients with mucocutaneous or visceral leishmaniasis may require a total dose of 1–3 g; cutaneous disease can often be treated with less. Pentamidine has also been used and is administered intramuscularly, 2–4 mg/kg every other day for 1–25 wk (shorter in American cutaneous leishmaniasis). The addition of gamma-interferon to antimonial therapy shows promise in circumventing treatment failure. Paromomycin has been successful in small series of visceral leishmaniasis cases and merits further study. Although initial studies of allopurinol alone or in combination with pentavalent antimonials were promising, subsequent studies do not support the initial enthusiasm. A variety of other agents (such as liposomal amphotericin B, dapsone, rifampin, trimethoprim-sulfamethoxazole, ketoconazole, and itraconazole) have been employed successfully in isolated cases or in a small series of patients. Their routine use cannot be recommended.

Local therapy of cutaneous leishmaniasis can simplify treatment and reduce the risk of toxicity, goals particularly desirable in children. Topical application of an ointment containing 15% paromomycin and 12% methylbenzathonium chloride has been effective in Old World leishmaniasis and also might be useful in selected cases of New World leishmaniasis in which the risk of subsequent development of mucocutaneous disease is low. Cryosurgery, curettage, intralesional instillation of chemotherapeutic agents, and heat treatment have all had success in the treatment of isolated cases of cutaneous disease.

Adjunctive measures in the treatment of kala-azar include the appropriate management of anemia, infection, and hemorrhage as well as good nutrition. In advanced drug-resistant kala-azar, splenectomy can ameliorate disabling hypersplenism and contribute to clinical cure, especially in small children. Patients with mutilating mucocutaneous disease should be considered for restorative plastic surgery and prostheses only after an extended period of observation following treatment.

In evaluating responses to treatment, assessing both clinical (disappearance of fever, decrease in spleen size, increase in white blood count and hemoglobin) and parasitologic parameters is important. Repeat aspirates or biopsies are useful in assessing a parasitologic "cure," but when the disease progresses despite apparent elimination of parasites, continued treatment is appropriate. Restoration of responsiveness to leishmanin and a fall in antileishmanial antibodies are useful indicators of improvement in the treatment of kala-azar.

PREVENTION. Prevention depends upon a detailed knowledge of the ecology of the reservoirs and vectors of the various forms of leishmaniasis. Treating cases, decreasing human contact with the vector, destroying animal reservoirs, and vector control are important in reducing transmission. Insect repellents and very fine mesh or permethrin-impregnated bed nets can decrease exposure to sandflies. Travelers to endemic areas should be warned of the risk and instructed in methods for preventing acquisition of leishmaniasis. A crude form of vaccination against cutaneous leishmaniasis has been practiced for several generations in the Middle East and Russia; no commercial vaccine is currently available.

Badaro R, Jones TC, Carvalho EM, et al: New perspectives on a subclinical form of visceral leishmaniasis. J Infect Dis 154:1003, 1986.

Badaro R, Falcoff E, Badaro F, et al: Treatment of visceral leishmaniasis with pentavalent antimony and interferon gamma. N Engl J Med 322:16, 1990.

Barral A, Pedral-Sampaio D, Grimaldi G Jr, et al: Leishmaniasis in Bahia, Brazil: Evidence that *Leishmaniasis Amazonensis* produces a wide spectrum of clinical disease. Am J Trop Med Hyg 44:536, 1991.

Berenguer J, Moreno S, Cercenado E, et al: Visceral leishmaniasis in patients infected with human immunodeficiency virus (HIV). Ann Intern Med 111:129, 1989.

Berman JD: Chemotherapy for leishmaniasis: Biochemical mechanisms, clinical efficacy, and future strategies. Rev Infect Dis 10:560, 1988.

Chang KP, Bray RS: Leishmanias. New York, Elsevier, 1985.

El-On J, Halevy S, Grunwald MH, et al: Topical treatment of Old World cutaneous leishmaniasis caused by *Leishmania major:* A double-blind control study. J Am Acad Dermatol 27:227, 1992.

Kager PA, Rees PH, Mangugu FM, et al: Clinical, hematological and parasitological response to treatment of visceral leishmaniasis in Kenya: A study of 64 patients. Trop Geogr Med 36:285, 1984.

Magill AJ, Grogl M, Gasser RA, Jr: Visceral infection caused by *Leishmania tropica* in veterans of Operation Desert Storm. N Engl J Med 328:1383, 1993.

Palma G, Gutierrez Y: Laboratory diagnosis of *Leishmania.* Clin Lab Med 11:909, 1991.

Rees PH, Kager PA, Kyambi JM, et al: Splenectomy in kala azar. Trop Geogr Med 36:285, 1984.

Thakur CP: Epidemiological, clinical and therapeutic features of Bihar kala azar (including post kala azar dermal leishmaniasis). Trans R Soc Trop Med Hyg 78:391, 1984.

244.7 Malaria

David F. Clyde

Malaria results when erythrocytes are invaded by any of four species of protozoan parasites of the genus *Plasmodium.* It is characterized by high fever, which is often intermittent, and by anemia and splenic enlargement. Despite campaigns aimed at eradicating malaria through interruption of the life cycle of the parasite in the mosquito, the disease continues to be the principal health problem of warm climates. Frequently, malaria is imported to the temperate zone countries, where in the summer months, it may be spread by local mosquitoes.

For clinical and diagnostic purposes, malaria may be regarded as two disease entities: the more dangerous one, caused by *Plasmodium falciparum* and formerly termed "subtertian" or "malignant tertian malaria," can produce a variety of acute clinical manifestations and may, if untreated, be fatal within a few days of onset; the other, caused by *P. vivax* or *P. ovale* (benign tertian malaria), or *P. malariae* (quartan malaria), is more typically paroxysmal and almost never fatal. Vivax and ovale infections may recur weeks after apparent cure of a primary attack, in contrast to the other two, which, except in the case of drug-resistant falciparum strains, rarely recrudesce after standard treatment.

ETIOLOGY. Malaria is usually acquired from the bites of previously infected female anopheline mosquitoes. In other instances, malaria has developed following transplacental passage or after the transfusion of infected blood, both of which circumvent the pre-erythrocytic phase of the parasite's development in the liver. The usual evolution of the disease is as follows:

Pre-Erythrocytic Phase. The *sporozoites* injected into the bloodstream by the biting mosquito reach the sinusoids of the liver and enter the cytoplasm of hepatic cells. Growth and nuclear division are rapid, and microscopic cysts *(schizonts)* containing *merozoites* are formed. Most of the cysts of all species rupture at the end of 6–15 days of development, liberating thousands of merozoites to penetrate red blood cells. However, a few *P. vivax* and *P. ovale* forms remain dormant in the liver for weeks or months, paving the way for relapses.

The incubation period (between the infecting mosquito bite and the presence of parasites in the blood) varies with the species; with *P. falciparum* it is 10–13 days; with *P. vivax* and *P. ovale,* 12–16 days; and with *P. malariae,* 27–37 days, depending on the size of the inoculum. Malaria transmitted by the transfusion of infected blood becomes apparent in a shorter time. Clinical manifestations of infection induced by any means may be suppressed for many months by subcurative treatment, particularly in the cases of vivax and quartan malaria.

Erythrocytic Phase. The merozoites that invade red blood cells appear first in stained smears as bluish rings or *(P. malariae)* bands of cytoplasm, with one or occasionally two red dots of nuclear chromatin. The growing parasites are named *trophozoites,* and appearing with them in the red cells are granules of yellow-brown pigment consisting of hematin derived from the hemoglobin consumed by the parasite to meet its protein requirements. The shape of the organism varies during growth until it becomes round and, with the scattered or clumped pigment, almost fills the red blood cell, which, in the case of *P. vivax,* is enlarged and stippled.

The nucleus of the parasite now divides asexually several times; its cytoplasm is arranged around the new nuclei, and the pigment aggregates into large clumps. This segmenter, or mature *schizont (meront),* contains a varying number of merozoites, depending on the species. The erythrocytes containing these merozoites rupture, and naked merozoites, pigment, and erythrocytic debris are freed into the plasma. Those merozoites that escape inactivation by immunoglobulins or phagocytosis enter fresh red blood cells. Thus, an asexual cycle is begun each time a new crop of merozoites invades red cells. This cycle, the duration of which is of considerable clinical importance, lasts 48 hr in falciparum, vivax, and ovale malaria and 72 hr in quartan malaria. The malarial clinical paroxysm takes place only when enough cycles have occurred to produce the amount of parasitic material, pigment, and red cell debris required to induce febrile or other reactions.

Certain of the growing parasites fail to divide, the nucleus remaining intact during the period of maturation. They are differentiated into male or female forms called *gametocytes,* which are of no clinical importance but are capable of infecting mosquitoes feeding on the patient.

Mixed Infections and Broods. In mixed infections one species is usually responsible for the clinical pattern, with falciparum dominating vivax, and vivax dominating quartan; only when sufficient immunity is developed to the dominant strain does the other begin to produce clinical manifestations.

In an infection with a single species, distinct broods may develop. Since the merozoites in the liver are not released simultaneously and the erythrocytic schizonts do not all rupture at the same time, some groups of parasites begin their existence in red blood cells before or after the majority, often maturing in sufficient numbers to produce an independent clinical reaction. In vivax infections single broods will produce a febrile reaction every other day, whereas if two broods develop, there will be daily paroxysms; in falciparum malaria the classic picture of intermittent fever may likewise soon become disrupted.

EPIDEMIOLOGY. Only in regions where the people have gametocytes in their blood can anopheline mosquitoes become infected. Children may be especially important in this respect. Transmission of malaria occurs in most tropical and some temperate zones; although the United States, Canada, Europe, Australia, and Israel are at present free of indigenous malaria, focal outbreaks may occur through infection of local mosquitoes by travelers coming from endemic areas.

Congenital malaria, caused by transfer of the causative agent across the placental barrier, is rare. *Neonatal malaria,* on the other hand, is less uncommon and may result from mingling of infected maternal blood with that of the infant during the birth process.

PATHOLOGY AND PATHOPHYSIOLOGY. The extent of destruction of red blood cells depends upon the duration and severity of the infection. Hemolysis often leads to an increase in the serum bilirubin, and in falciparum malaria it may be sufficiently intense to result in hemoglobinuria *(blackwater fever).* In any malarial infection the degree of anemia is greater than that attributable solely to the destruction of cells by parasites. Autoantigenic changes produced in the red cell by the parasite probably contribute to hemolysis; these changes and increased osmotic fragility occur in all erythrocytes, whether infected or not. Hemolysis may also be induced by quinine or primaquine in persons with hereditary glucose-6-phosphate dehydrogenase deficiency.

The pigment extruded into the circulation upon red blood cell disintegration accumulates in the reticuloendothelial cells of the spleen, the follicles of which become hyperplastic and sometimes necrotic, in the Kupffer cells of the liver, and in the bone marrow, brain, and other organs. Deposition of sufficient pigment and of hemosiderin results in a slate-gray color of the organs.

The malignancy of falciparum malaria is peculiar to that species. The merozoites emerging from the liver are considerably more numerous than those of other species; there are as many in young children as in adults, so that children have a proportionately greater initial wave of infection. Young children are particularly prone to severe, often lethal, parasitemia.

Eight to 18 hr after the parasite has entered the red blood cells, these cells become increasingly sticky and tend to adhere to the endothelial lining of blood sinuses and vessels, especially when the circulation is slow. The sticky cell is thus fixed and unable to return to the general circulation, although the parasite within it matures in the normal manner. As more cells adhere, flow within the vessel is progressively impeded, and occlusion or even rupture may occur.

The site and extent of this interference with vascular function, coupled with a selective localization of parasitized cells in various organs or systems, are responsible for the variety of symptoms from falciparum infections. Thus, pneumonitis, encephalitis, or enteritis may be manifest when the bulk of the infection is in the lungs, brain, or intestinal tract, respectively. In the pregnant woman damage to the placenta may result in the death of the fetus or in premature birth; infants born at full term to infected women have lower birthweights than those of infants born to uninfected mothers living under similar conditions.

The release of merozoites where the circulation is slowed facilitates the invasion of nearby red blood cells, so that falciparum parasitemia may be heavier than that of other species whose rupture of schizonts takes place in the active circulation. Whereas *P. falciparum* invades all erythrocytes irrespective of age, *P. vivax* attacks primarily reticulocytes, and *P. malariae* invades mature red cells, features that tend to limit parasitemia of the latter two forms to less than 20,000 red blood cells/mm^3. Falciparum infections in the nonimmune child may develop densities as high as 500,000 parasites/mm^3.

Successful treatment stops the proliferation of parasites. Specific antibodies are associated with increased levels of immunoglobulin G in the serum of people repeatedly infected with a particular species. Antibody facilitates the phagocytosis of naked merozoites and of parasite-laden erythrocytes, which are ingested by reticuloendothelial cells, by large lymphocytes and neutrophils, and particularly by monocytes. These antibodies do not, however, interfere with the development of the parasite in the liver. Passive immunity, occurring in infants born to mothers who have the disease, limits the severity of attacks of malaria for several weeks after birth. The beneficial effect of this transplacental humoral immunity may be enhanced by persistence of fetal hemoglobin and by a diet limited to milk. Certain hemoglobinopathies are also protective and tend to be genetically selective in endemic malarious regions. *Plasmodium falciparum* may fail to mature in children with the sickle cell trait, and *P. vivax* in those with thalassemia and enzyme deficiencies; *P. falciparum* is unable to attain high densities in children deficient in glucose-6-phosphate dehydrogenase.

CLINICAL MANIFESTATIONS. Children who acquire malaria fall into two groups: those having little or no immunity because of lack of previous contact with the disease, who become seriously ill unless treated; and those having a high degree of tolerance by about 10 yr of age owing to repeated malarial infections in early childhood that they have survived, although there may be impaired growth and development. Tolerance to malaria also appears to be based on inherited factors that modify the severity of the disease; such tolerance is to be found mostly among Africans and persons of African descent. In the partially immune child heavy parasitemia may occur with few symptoms, or an intercurrent infection may initiate renewed activity of a quiescent malarial infection.

In a nonimmune child clinical signs usually appear 8–15 days after infection and may not be distinctive. Behavioral changes such as fretfulness, anorexia, unusual crying, drowsiness, or disturbances of sleep may be observed. Fever may be absent or increase gradually for 1–2 days, or the onset may be sudden with temperature up to 40.6° C (105° F) or higher, with or without prodromal chill. After varying periods of time, the temperature falls to normal or below, and sweating occurs.

The febrile paroxysm may be extremely short or may last for 2–12 hr; its characteristic pattern is usually obscured in children less than 5 yr of age. Complaints include headache, nausea, generalized aching, particularly of the back, and occasionally pain in the abdomen, when the spleen has swollen quickly and is tender. In vivax and quartan infections dominated by a single brood, the fever is the characteristic manifestation, occurring at intervals of 48 hr in the former and 72 hr in the latter. If convulsions occur, they abate when the fever falls. Herpetic lesions of the mouth are not uncommon. The red blood cell count and hemoglobin level may decrease rapidly; leukopenia is variable, but monocytosis is common.

In falciparum infections the fever is less characteristic and may even be continuous; it may be overshadowed by severe manifestations related to the cerebral, pulmonary, intestinal, or urinary systems. Cerebral complications are evidenced by convulsions or coma, the neurologic signs of which in infants and children are those of increased intracranial pressure and symmetric upper motor neuron and brain stem disturbances such as disconjugate gaze and decerebrate and decorticate postures. Except in rare cases when bacterial or viral infections of the central nervous system are superimposed, the cerebrospinal fluid is generally normal. Mortality has been around 20%, and among survivors 18% exhibit such neurologic sequelae as cortical blindness, monoparesis, and speech defects. Children presenting with hypoglycemia, severe convulsions, and prolonged coma are particularly prone to these sequelae. In cases of algid malaria, coma is preceded in the child by shock. Persistent nausea and vomiting, an enlarged and tender liver, and progressive jaundice may evolve into hepatic failure; severe diarrhea may occur; or occasionally the signs of acute appendicitis may be imitated.

The spleen is more commonly enlarged in vivax than in falciparum infections; perisplenitis, infarction, and even rupture may occur, and after repeated attacks the spleen may become very large and hard. *Tropical splenomegaly syndrome* ("hyper-reactive malarial splenomegaly") may constitute an abnormal immune response in malnourished children in developing countries. Enlargement of the spleen, without diminution following antimalarial treatment, is accompanied by lymphocytic infiltration of liver sinusoids and an elevated fluorescent antibody titer for malaria, with or without scanty parasitemia.

Disturbances of renal function are shown by oliguria, and anuria may supervene. The *nephrotic syndrome* is associated with *P. malariae* in children inhabiting endemic malarious areas; the prognosis is poor. *Blackwater fever,* now rarely seen, is associated with *P. falciparum:* hemoglobinuria results from severe and sudden intravascular hemolysis, which may lead to anuria and to death from uremia.

Hypoglycemia may be associated with falciparum malaria. In severe infections, lactic acidosis may develop, presenting with convulsions and impaired consciousness.

DIAGNOSIS. The diagnosis of malaria depends upon the identification of parasites in the blood (Fig. 244–1). In falciparum malaria, only ring forms are likely to be seen initially, crescents (gametocytes) joining them after 10 days; up to 20% of the erythrocytes may be infected. All stages of the other species of

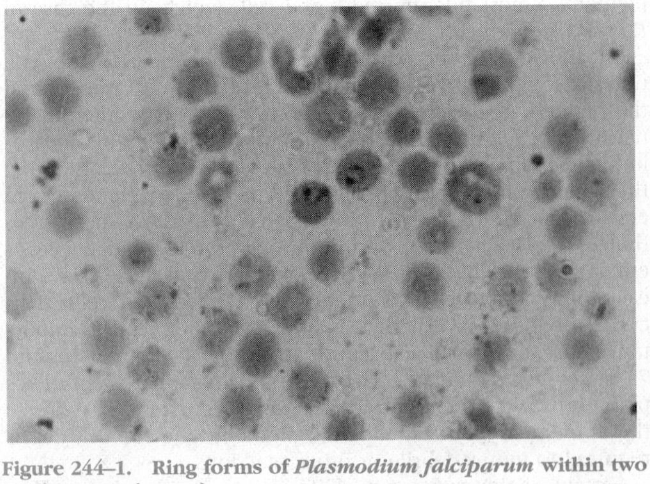

Figure 244–1. Ring forms of *Plasmodium falciparum* within two erythrocytes (*center*).

parasites appear in the blood, but less than 1% of red cells will contain them.

In a blood smear the parasites within the red cells have red chromatin and bluish cytoplasm. In some leukocytes, particularly monocytes, remnants of phagocytized parasites and pigment may be seen. The parasites should first be looked for in thick blood films, since in light infections it may not be possible to find them in the thin film; the latter is best used for species differentiation. Because parasites may not be seen at the height of the fever, examinations should be repeated, preferably at intervals of 12 hr. The most suitable stain is Giemsa diluted 1:25 with distilled water preferably buffered to pH 7.0–7.2. Wright stain may be used, 0.75 g of the powder being repeatedly shaken for 2 days with 65 mL of pure methyl alcohol and 35 mL of pure glycerin.

The presence of species-specific antibodies associated with an elevated level of IgG, persisting for months or years after an acute attack, may be detected serologically, while during an infection the species may be identified by tests involving capture of antigen. A falsely positive Wassermann reaction is found in many cases.

PREVENTION. Natural infection of humans does not occur where breeding of anopheline mosquitoes is prevented, where the adult mosquitoes are kept from contact with people by screens or bed nets, or where they are killed by natural enemies or insecticides before sporozoites have had time to mature. Children visiting endemic malarious areas should be screened from mosquitoes from dusk to dawn, but as this is rarely entirely effective, they should also be given one of the chemoprophylactic drugs *regularly* throughout their stay, commencing 2 wk before the visit and terminating 8 wk after leaving the area. At least during this period, malaria should be suspected if febrile illness or chronic debility affects the child.

Chemoprophylactic drugs in common use are the following: the slightly bitter but extremely safe chlorguanide (proguanil, not available in the United States), taken daily in amounts of 50 mg (in children up to 2 yr), 100 mg (2–6 yr), or 200 mg (older than 6); the tasteless but more toxic pyrimethamine taken weekly in amounts of 6.25 mg (to 2 yr), 12.5 mg (2–6 yr), or 25 mg; and chloroquine taken weekly in amounts of 37.5 mg of the base (to 1 yr), 75 mg (1–2 yr), 112.5 mg (2–6 yr), 150 mg (6–12 yr) or 300 mg. The bitterness of chloroquine diphosphate and sulfate may be disguised if the crushed tablet is mixed with a spoonful of jam or thick syrup. Commercially mixed syrups are available but may not remain stable for long.

Unfortunately, resistance of *P. falciparum* to pyrimethamine and chlorguanide is widely distributed; therefore chloroquine is generally preferred for prophylaxis. When resistance by *P. falciparum* to the latter compound also develops, as in most regions except western Asia and Central America, potentiating combinations of chlorguanide with dapsone (daily) or pyrimethamine with dapsone (weekly) may be indicated; however, their use for periods longer than 6 mo is discouraged because of possible side effects related to antifolate activity. Repetitive use of the combination of pyrimethamine with the long-acting sulfonamides, sulfadoxine and sulfalene, is now considered inadvisable. Children more than 8 yr old may take doxycycline orally 2 mg/kg daily for short periods, but increased photosensitivity to sunlight may occur. Chloroquine should be taken concurrently each week to protect against *P. vivax*. In areas where multidrug resistant *P. falciparum* malaria predominates, the prophylactic use of mefloquine is proposed (pediatric use not yet approved for the United States).

TREATMENT. Therapy falls into four categories: (1) specific chemotherapy for the attack, whether fresh infection, recrudescence, or relapse; (2) supportive treatment and management of complications; (3) specific chemotherapy to prevent late relapse of vivax or ovale infections; (4) specific chemotherapy to destroy or sterilize gametocytes, and thus to protect the community if mosquitoes are present.

1. Clinical cure of all types of malaria and radical cure of falciparum and quartan malaria can be obtained by using the following drug regimens, provided that *P. falciparum* is susceptible: (1) Chloroquine phosphate or hydroxychloroquine sulfate 10 mg base/kg orally, then 5 mg base/kg 6 hr later, then 5 mg base/kg daily for 2 days; or (2) quinine sulfate orally 25 mg/kg/24 hr, in divided doses every 8 hr, for 10–14 days. Children who have inhabited malarious regions and through repeated and prolonged previous infections have acquired some immunity may be cured by using half of the quantities listed. Treatment must be repeated if vomiting occurs within 30 min of ingestion of drugs; persistent vomiting is an indication for parenteral therapy.

Although specific treatment should not usually be undertaken until the diagnosis has been established, many experienced physicians, when confronted with a critically ill or comatose child whose history is suggestive of malaria or exposure thereto, consider it advisable to administer quinine or chloroquine parenterally while awaiting the result of blood film examination.

Parenteral administration of chloroquine or quinine, although hazardous in children bordering on shock, is often essential for those who are vomiting persistently, who are in coma, or who cannot be induced to swallow the drugs even if the bitterness is concealed. Parenteral therapy with anti-malarial drugs should be replaced by oral administration as soon as possible. Quinine dihydrochloride is administered intravenously in a loading dose of 20 mg salt/kg in 10 mg/kg of 5% dextrose over 4 hr, followed by 10 mg salt/kg over 2–4 hr (maximum 1,800 mg/24 hr), until oral therapy can commence. Intramuscular administration has been found equally efficacious. It is desirable to monitor blood glucose levels, as quinine may exacerbate hypoglycemia. When quinine is not available (as in the United States), quinidine gluconate should be administered intravenously, loading dose 10 mg/kg (maximum 600 mg) in normal saline slowly over 1–2 hr, followed by infusion of 0.02 mg/kg/min until oral therapy can commence. It is desirable to monitor for potential side effects by blood pressure and electrocardiogram. If neither quinine nor quinidine is available, chloroquine hydrochloride may be administered intravenously by slow drip in the quantity of 5 mg base/kg in 10 mL/kg of isotonic saline, infused over a 3- to 4-hr period; this dose may be repeated 6 hr later. The volume of saline should be adjusted to the state of hydration of the patient, dehydrated children requiring 20 mL/kg and overhydrated children 5 mL/kg. Administration of chloroquine intramuscularly is not recommended in small children because it has occasionally precipitated convulsions and aggravated shock and resulted in death. It should not be given subcutaneously because of slow absorption by that route.

2. Supportive treatment includes that for hyperpyrexia. Particular attention should be paid to fluid and electrolyte needs (Chapter 56).

Metabolic requirements of the parasite rapidly deplete the reserves of glucose, vitamins, and coenzymes as well as of hemoglobin. Vitamin B_1 may be given, and when the acute phase is passed, ferrous sulfate should be prescribed for a considerable time. Transfusion of packed red cells may be beneficial to children who have had longstanding infections and consequently severe anemia (hemoglobin 5 g/dL or less).

It is essential that children with severe falciparum infections receive fluids intravenously if they are dehydrated or in shock. Rapid expansion of the circulating blood volume is more effective with whole blood than with dextran, plasma, or glucose-saline solution. Renal failure, which may require dialysis, is a rare development. When it is present, no more than one third of the conventional doses of antimalarial drugs should be given until the child is hydrated, out of shock, and urinating; quinine and primaquine are contraindicated in the presence of hemoglobinuria. The judicious use of chloroquine or amodiaquine is indicated for heavy parasitemia.

In the comatose stage of cerebral malaria, in addition to specific parenteral antimalarial treatment, dextran-75 may be useful for the prevention of intravascular sludging. Convulsions may be controlled with paraldehyde or barbiturates.

The nephrotic syndrome associated with quartan malaria is managed by the regimen described in Chapter 481 together with a course of chloroquine.

3. Late relapse of vivax or ovale malaria may occur up to 3 yr after the primary attack and may be prevented by treating the child with primaquine. Because primaquine given at the height of symptoms increases the tendency to vomit and may be immunosuppressive, it should not be given until the 3rd day of the concomitant clinical curative course of chloroquine, amodiaquine, or quinine. Primaquine is given for 14 days in a daily dose of 0.3 mg base/kg; for fear of possible side reactions some authorities prefer not to administer this drug to children less than 3 yr old (or to pregnant women), but to treat the acute attack with chloroquine and then place the patient on a chemoprophylactic regimen for several months.

Children receiving primaquine should be watched for toxic manifestations such as methemoglobinemia, hemolytic anemia, hemoglobinuria in children with G-6-PD deficiency, neutropenia, and renal dysfunction. Hemolytic anemia may be particularly severe in G-6-PD deficient children of eastern Mediterranean or Asian descent, for whom two approaches to anti-relapse treatment are available: primaquine may be given once each wk for 8 wk in a dose of 0.9 mg base/kg; or primaquine may be omitted entirely and chemoprophylaxis given for several months following treatment of the acute attack with chloroquine. Quinacrine (mepacrine) should not be used simultaneously with primaquine. Other synthetic antimalarial drugs are relatively nontoxic in therapeutic doses.

4. Gametocytes, however, do not give rise to symptoms and disappear from the circulation soon after destruction of their asexual precursors by chloroquine, amodiaquine, or quinine. Gametocytes can be destroyed by a single dose of primaquine, 7.5 mg base for children aged 1–3 yr, 15 mg for those aged 4–6 yr, 30 mg for those aged 6–12 yr, and 45 mg for older children; their further development in the mosquito can be inhibited by single doses of chlorguanide or pyrimethamine, provided the parasite is not resistant to these drugs.

Drug resistance is a growing concern. Many strains of *P. falciparum* are now resistant to chlorguanide and to pyrimethamine, but a greater problem is posed by the spread of resistance to chloroquine in this species to most malarious regions. Some strains are also tolerant to quinine. These strains are being introduced into areas that have been free of malaria and may cause focal summer outbreaks. Should the malarial attack not respond to chloroquine by 48–72 hr, quinine or quinidine should be used, 25 mg/kg/24 hr in three doses for 3–7 days. If this has only a temporary effect, the course should be repeated with the addition of (1) on the last day, pyrimethamine and sulfadoxine (combination tablet contains 25 mg and 500 mg, respectively: children aged less than 1 yr receive one tablet, 1–3 yr one tablet, 4–to 8 yr one tablet, 9 yr and older two tablets); or (2), tetracycline 20 mg/kg/24 hr in 4 doses for 7 days (only in children aged 8 yr and older); or (3), clindamycin 20–40 mg/kg/24 hr in three doses for 3 days. These antibiotics have a slow parasiticidal action and should always be accompanied by quinine or quinidine. Also effective against most strains of *P. falciparum* (but not for administration to children weighing less than 15 kg) are mefloquine (25 mg/kg single dose) and halofantrine (8 mg/kg, three doses at 6 hr intervals, repeated in 1 wk). These compounds have not yet been approved for pediatric use in the United States.

Some strains of *P. vivax* in New Guinea and Indonesia have recently been found insensitive to therapeutic doses of chloroquine, necessitating treatment using mefloquine. Licensed for use in many Asian and African countries (but not in the United States) are oral and parenteral compounds related to artemisinine, including artesunate, artemether, and arteether. These are short duration blood schizontocides, acting more rapidly than quinine against *P. falciparum* and requiring several days repetitive use, preferably combined with a dose of mefloquine to deter recrudescence. Of particular pediatric relevance are suppository preparations of artemisinine. There are as yet no proven vaccines available for the prevention or abatement of malaria.

Bondi FS: The incidence and outcome of neurological abnormalities in childhood cerebral malaria: a long-term follow-up of 62 survivors. Trans R Soc Trop Med Hyg 86:17, 1992.
Chongsuphajaisiddhi T: Malaria in paediatric practice. In: Wernsdorfer WH, McGregor I (eds): Malaria. Edinburgh, Churchill Livingstone, 1988, p 889.
Krishna S, Waller DW, ter Kuile F, et al: Lactic acidosis and hypoglycaemia in children with severe malaria: pathophysiological and prognostic significance. Trans R Soc Trop Med Hyg 88:67, 1994.
Miller RD, Greenberg AE, Campbell CC: Treatment of severe malaria in the United States with continuous infusion of quinidine gluconate and exchange transfusion. N Engl J Med 321:65, 1989.
Schapira A, Solomon T, Julien M, et al: Comparison of intramuscular and intravenous quinine for the treatment of severe and complicated malaria in children. Trans R Soc Trop Med Hyg 87:299, 1993.

244.8 Toxoplasmosis

Rima McLeod and Jack S. Remington

Toxoplasma gondii, an obligate intracellular protozoan, is acquired perorally, transplacentally, or, rarely, parenterally in laboratory accidents, by transfusion, or from a transplanted organ. In the immunologically normal child, the acute acquired infection may be asymptomatic, cause lymphadenopathy, or damage almost any organ. Once acquired, the latent encysted organism persists for the lifetime of the host. In the immunocompromised infant or child, either acute acquisition or recrudescence of latent organisms most often causes signs or symptoms related to the central nervous system (CNS). Infection acquired congenitally, if untreated, almost always causes signs or symptoms in the perinatal period or later in life. The most frequent of these signs are due to chorioretinitis and CNS lesions. However, other manifestations, such as intrauterine growth retardation, fever, lymphadenopathy, rash, hearing loss, pneumonitis, hepatitis, and thrombocytopenia, also occur. Congenital toxoplasmosis in babies with human immunodeficiency virus (HIV) infection may be fulminant.

ETIOLOGY. *T. gondii* is a coccidian protozoan. Its tachyzoites are oval or crescent-like, multiply only in living cells, and measure 2–4 × 4–7 μm. Tissue cysts, which are 10–100 μm in diameter, may contain thousands of parasites and remain in tissues, especially the CNS and skeletal and heart muscle, for the life of the host. *Toxoplasma* can multiply in all tissues of mammals and birds, and its disease spectrum is expressed with remarkable similarity in different host species.

Newly infected cats and other Felidae excrete *Toxoplasma* oocysts in their feces. The oocysts are infectious. *Toxoplasma* are acquired by susceptible cats by ingestion of infected meat containing encysted bradyzoites or by ingestion of oocysts excreted by other recently infected cats. The parasites then multiply through schizogonic and gametogonic cycles in the distal ileal epithelium of the cat intestine. Oocysts containing two sporocysts are excreted, and under proper conditions of temperature and moisture, each sporocyst matures into four sporozoites. For about 2 wk the cat excretes 10^5–10^7 oocysts/day, which, in a suitable environment, may retain their viability for a year or more. Oocysts sporulate 1–5 days after excretion and are then infectious. Oocysts are killed by drying, boiling, and exposure to some strong chemicals, but not to bleach. Oocysts have been isolated from soil and sand frequented by cats, and outbreaks associated with contaminated water have been reported. Oocysts and tissue cysts are the sources of animal and human infections (Fig. 244–2).

EPIDEMIOLOGY. *Toxoplasma* infection is ubiquitous in animals and is one of the most common latent infections of humans throughout the world. The incidence varies considerably among people and animals in different geographic areas. Significant antibody titers have been detected in 50–80% of residents of some localities and in fewer than 5% in others. A higher prevalence of infection usually occurs in warmer, more humid climates.

Infection is usually established by the oral route via undercooked or raw meat that contains cysts or by ingestion of oocysts. Freezing meat to −20° C or heating it to 66° C renders the cysts noninfectious. Except for transplacental infection from mother to fetus and, rarely, by organ transplant or transfusion, *Toxoplasma* are not transmitted from person to person.

Transmission to the fetus usually occurs when the infection is acquired by an immunologically normal mother during gestation. Congenital transmission from immunologically normal women infected prior to pregnancy is extremely rare. Immunocompromised women who are chronically infected have transmitted the infection to their fetuses. The incidence of congenital infection in the United States ranges from 1/1,000 to 1/8,000 live births. The incidence of newly acquired infection in a population of pregnant women depends on the risk of becoming infected in that specific geographic area and the proportion of the population that has not been previously infected.

Seronegative transplant recipients who receive an organ (e.g., heart or kidney) from a seropositive recipient have developed life-threatening illness requiring therapy. Seropositive recipients have developed increased serologic titers without associated disease when untreated.

PATHOLOGY. In the acute congenital and acquired forms of toxoplasmosis, histologic changes may occur in almost all tissues. In the congenital form, such changes are especially fre-

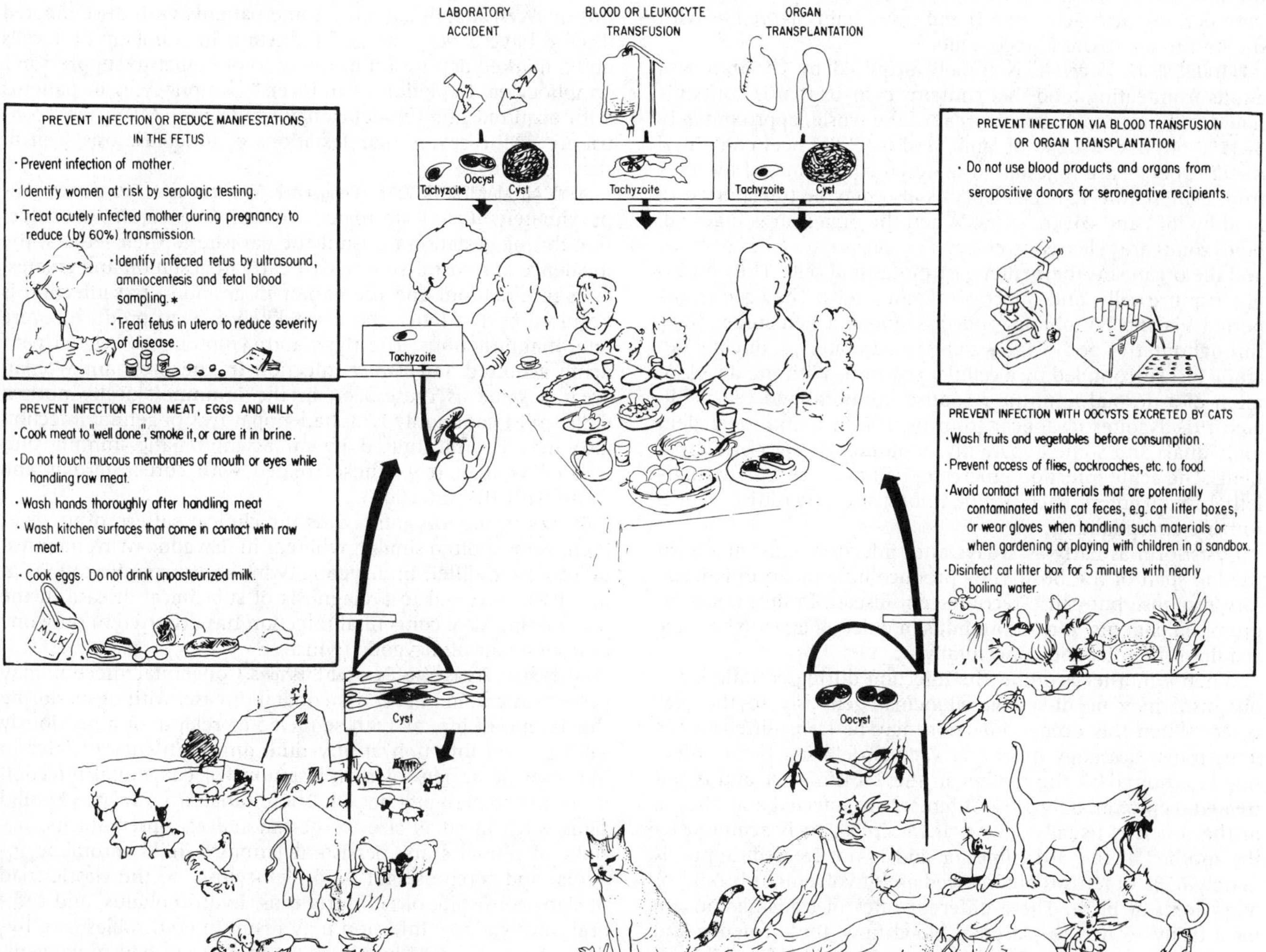

Figure 244–2. Life cycle of *Toxoplasma gondii* and prevention of toxoplasmosis by interruption of transmission to humans. This procedure is no longer recommended unless amniotic fluid PCR testing cannot be performed in a reliable laboratory. (Please see under PCR.)

quent in the CNS, the retina, and the choroid; retinochoroiditis occurs occasionally in acquired toxoplasmosis. During latent infection, *Toxoplasma* in tissues are seen as cysts with little or no associated tissue reaction. In acute infections, intracellular and, in areas of necrosis, extracellular tachyzoites may be noted. Gross or microscopic areas of necrosis may be present in many tissues, especially heart, lungs, skeletal muscle, liver, and spleen. Areas of calcification occur in the brain in patients with congenital toxoplasmosis. In addition, periaqueductal and periventricular vasculitis and necrosis with sloughing of brain tissue may lead to obstruction of the aqueduct of Sylvius or the foramen of Monroe and consequent hydrocephalus. Obstruction of the aqueduct of Sylvius also may occur after the perinatal period.

In acute acquired lymphadenopathic toxoplasmosis, characteristic lymph node changes include reactive follicular hyperplasia with irregular clusters of epithelioid histiocytes that encroach on and blur the margins of germinal centers. Focal distention of sinuses with monocytoid cells also occurs.

Examination of the placenta of infected newborns may reveal chronic inflammation and cysts. Tachyzoites can be seen with Wright or Giemsa stains but are best demonstrated with the immunoperoxidase technique. The tissue cyst stains well with periodic acid-Schiff (PAS) and silver stains as well as with the immunoperoxidase technique.

PATHOGENESIS. *T. gondii* is usually acquired by children and adults from eating food that contains cysts or that is contaminated with oocysts. In many areas of the world, approximately 5–35% of pork, 9–60% of lamb, and 0–9% of beef contain *T. gondii.* Oocysts are ingested in material contaminated by feces from acutely infected cats. Oocysts also may be transported to food by flies and cockroaches. When the organism is ingested, bradyzoites are released from cysts or sporozoites from oocysts, and the organisms then enter gastrointestinal cells. They multiply, rupture cells, and infect contiguous cells. They are transported via the lymphatics and disseminated hematogenously throughout the body. Tachyzoites proliferate, producing necrotic foci surrounded by a cellular reaction. With the development of a normal immune response (humoral and cell-mediated), tachyzoites disappear from tissues. In immunodeficient individuals and some apparently immunologically normal patients, the acute infection progresses and may cause potentially lethal involvement such as pneumonitis, myocarditis, or necrotizing encephalitis.

Cysts form as early as 7 days after infection and remain for the life span of the host. They produce little or no inflammatory response but cause recrudescent disease in immunocompromised patients or chorioretinitis in older children who have acquired the infection congenitally.

When a mother acquires the infection during gestation, the organism may be disseminated hematogenously to the placenta. When this occurs, infection may be transmitted to the fetus transplacentally or during vaginal delivery. If the infection is acquired by the mother in the 1st trimester and is not treated, approximately 17% of fetuses are infected and disease in the infant is usually severe. If the infection is acquired by the mother in the 3rd trimester and is not treated, approximately 65% of fetuses are infected and involvement is mild or inapparent at birth. These different rates of transmission are most likely related to placental blood flow, the virulence and amount of *T. gondii* acquired, and the immunologic ability of the mother to restrict parasitemia.

Almost all congenitally infected individuals have signs or symptoms of infection, such as chorioretinitis, by adolescence if they are not treated in the newborn period. Some more severely involved infants with congenital infection appear to have *Toxoplasma* antigen–specific anergy of their lymphocytes, which may be important in the pathogenesis of their disease. Monoclonal gammopathy of the IgG class has been described in congenitally infected infants, and IgM levels may be elevated in newborns with congenital toxoplasmosis. Glomerulonephritis with deposits of IgM, fibrinogen, and *Toxoplasma* antigen has been reported in congenitally infected individuals. Circulating immune complexes have been detected in sera from an infant with congenital toxoplasmosis and in older individuals with systemic, febrile, and lymphadenopathic forms of toxoplasmosis, but these did not persist after signs and symptoms resolved. Diminished total serum levels of IgA may occur in congenitally infected babies, but no predilection toward associated infections has been noted. The predilection toward predominant involvement of the CNS and eye in this congenital infection has not been fully explained.

There are profound and prolonged alterations in T lymphocyte subpopulations during acute acquired *T. gondii* infection. These have been correlated with disease syndromes but not with disease outcome. Some patients with prolonged fever and malaise have lymphocytosis, increased suppressor T-cell levels, and a decreased helper to suppressor T-cell ratio. These patients may have fewer helper cells even when they are asymptomatic. In some patients with lymphadenopathy, helper cell numbers are diminished for more than 6 mo after onset of infection. Asymptomatic patients also may have abnormal ratios of T-cell subpopulations. Some patients with disseminated disease have a very marked reduction in numbers of T cells and a marked depression in the ratio of helper to suppressor T lymphocytes. Depletion of inducer T lymphocytes in patients with acquired immunodeficiency syndrome (AIDS) may contribute to the severe manifestations of toxoplasmosis seen in these patients.

CLINICAL MANIFESTATIONS. Congenital Toxoplasmosis. TRANSMISSION. Approximately 50% of untreated women who acquire the infection during gestation transmit the parasite to their fetuses; the incidence of transmission is least early in gestation and greatest later in gestation, and the earlier in gestation the infection is acquired by the fetus, the more likely it is to produce severe fetal manifestations. The signs and symptoms associated with acute acquired *Toxoplasma* infection in the pregnant woman are the same as those seen in the immunologically normal child, most commonly lymphadenopathy. Congenital infection also may be transmitted by an asymptomatic immunosuppressed woman (e.g., those treated with corticosteroids and those with HIV infection).

GENETICS. In monozygotic twins the clinical pattern of involvement is most often similar, whereas in dizygotic twins manifestations often differ. In dizygotic twins severe manifestations in one twin have led to a diagnosis of subclinical disease in the other twin. Also, congenital infection has occurred in only one twin of a pair of dizygotic twins.

SPECTRUM AND FREQUENCY OF SIGNS AND SYMPTOMS. Congenital infection may present as a mild or severe neonatal disease, with onset during the 1st mo of life, or with sequelae or relapse of a previously undiagnosed infection at any time during infancy or later in life. A wide variety of manifestations of congenital infection occur in the perinatal period. These range from relatively mild signs, such as small size for gestational age, prematurity, peripheral retinal scars, persistent jaundice, mild thrombocytopenia, and cerebrospinal fluid pleiocytosis, to the classic triad of signs consisting of chorioretinitis, hydrocephalus, and cerebral calcifications. Infection may result in erythroblastosis, hydrops fetalis, and perinatal death. More than half of congenitally infected infants are considered normal in the perinatal period, but almost all such children will have ocular involvement later in life. Neurologic signs in neonates, which include convulsions, sunset sign, and an increase in head circumference disproportionate to other growth parameters, may be associated with substantial cerebral damage. However, such signs also may occur in association with encephalitis without extensive destruction or with relatively mild inflammation adjacent to and obstructing the aqueduct of Sylvius. If such infants are treated promptly, signs and symptoms may resolve, and the child may develop normally.

The spectrum and frequency of manifestations that develop in the perinatal period in infants with congenital *Toxoplasma* infection are presented in Table 244–2. Infection in most of these 210 referred infants was initially suspected because their mothers were identified by a serologic screening program that detected pregnant women with acute acquired *T. gondii* infection. Twenty-one (10%) had severe congenital toxoplasmosis with CNS involvement, eye lesions, and general systemic manifestations. Seventy-one (34%) had mild involvement with normal results on clinical examination other than retinal scars or isolated intracranial calcifications. One hundred and sixteen (55%) had no detectable manifestations. This last figure may reflect the difficulties associated with funduscopic examination of the peripheral retina in infants and young children. These figures represent an underestimation of the relative frequency of severe congenital infection for the following reasons: The most severe cases, including most of those who died, were not referred; therapeutic abortion was often performed when acute acquired infection of the mother was diagnosed early during pregnancy; in utero spiramycin therapy may have diminished the severity of infection; and only 13 infants had CT brain scans and 23% did not have a cerebrospinal fluid examination. Routine newborn examinations are often normal for congenitally infected infants, but more careful evaluations reveal significant abnormalities: Specifically, of 28 infants who were detected by a universal state mandated serologic screening program for *T. gondii* specific IgM, 26 had normal routine newborn examinations and 14 had significant abnormalities with more careful evaluation. These abnormalities included retinal scars (seven infants), active chorioretinitis (three infants), and CNS abnormalities (eight infants).

The clinical spectrum and natural history of untreated congenital toxoplasmosis, which is *clinically apparent* in the 1st yr of life, is presented in Table 244–3. More than 80% of these children had IQs of less than 70, and many had convulsions and severely impaired vision.

■ **TABLE 244–2 Signs and Symptoms in 210 Infants with Proved Congenital Toxoplasma Infection***

Finding	No. Examined	No. Positive (%)
Prematurity	210	
Birthweight <2,500 g		8 (3.8)
Birthweight 2,500–3,000 g		5 (7.1)
Dysmaturity (intrauterine growth retardation)		13 (6.2)
Icterus	201	20 (10)
Hepatosplenomegaly	210	9 (4.2)
Thrombocytopenic purpura	210	3 (1.4)
Abnormal blood count (anemia, eosinophilia)	102	9 (4.4)
Microcephaly	210	11 (5.2)
Hydrocephaly	210	8 (3.8)
Hypotonia	210	12 (5.7)
Convulsions	210	8 (3.8)
Psychomotor retardation	210	11 (5.2)
Intracranial calcifications on x-ray	210	24 (11.4)
Ultrasound	49	5 (10)
Computed tomography of brain	13	11 (84)
Abnormal EEG	191	16 (8.3)
Abnormal CSF	163	56 (34.2)
Microphthalmia	210	6 (2.8)
Strabismus	210	111 (5.2)
Chorioretinitis	210	
Unilateral		34 (16.1)
Bilateral		12 (5.7)

**Data are adapted from Couvreur J, et al: Ann Pediatr (Paris) 31:815, 1984. Table 1. Infants were identified by prospective study of infants born to women who acquired* Toxoplasma *infection during pregnancy.*

■ **TABLE 244–3 Signs and Symptoms Occurring Prior to Diagnosis or During the Course of Untreated Acute Congenital Toxoplasmosis in 152 Infants (A) and in 101 of These Same Children When They Had Been Followed 4 yrs or More (B)***

Signs and Symptoms	Frequency of Occurrence in Patients with "Neurologic" Disease†	"Generalized" Disease‡
A. Infants	***108 Patients (%)***	***44 Patients (%)***
Chorioretinitis	102 (94)§	29 (66)
Abnormal spinal fluid	59 (55)	37 (84)
Anemia	55 (51)	34 (77)
Convulsions	54 (50)	8 (18)
Intracranial calcification	54 (50)	2 (4)
Jaundice	31 (29)	35 (80)
Hydrocephalus	30 (28)	0 (0)
Fever	27 (25)	34 (77)
Splenomegaly	23 (21)	40 (90)
Lymphadenopathy	18 (17)	30 (68)
Hepatomegaly	18 (17)	34 (77)
Vomiting	17 (16)	21 (48)
Microcephalus	14 (13)	0 (0)
Diarrhea	7 (6)	11 (25)
Cataracts	5 (5)	0 (0)
Eosinophilia	6 (4)	8 (18)
Abnormal bleeding	3 (3)	8 (18)
Hypothermia	2 (2)	9 (20)
Glaucoma	2 (2)	0 (0)
Optic atrophy	2 (2)	0 (0)
Microphthalmia	2 (2)	0 (0)
Rash	1 (1)	11 (25)
Pneumonitis	0 (0)	18 (41)
B. Children, 4 yr (or more) old	***70 Patients (%)***	***31 Patients (%)***
Mental retardation	62 (89)	25 (81)
Convulsions	58 (83)	24 (77)
Spasticity and palsies	53 (76)	18 (58)
Severely impaired vision	48 (69)	13 (42)
Hydrocephalus or	31 (44)	2 (6)
microcephalus	12 (17)	3 (10)
Deafness	6 (9)	5 (16)
Normal		

**Adapted from Eichenwald H: A study of congenital toxoplasmosis. In: Siim JC (ed): Human Toxoplasmosis. Copenhagen, Munksgaard, 1960, pp 41–49. Study performed in 1947. The most severely involved institutionalized patients were not included in the later study of 101 children.*

†Patients with otherwise undiagnosed central nervous system disease in the 1st yr of life.

‡Patients with otherwise undiagnosed non-neurologic diseases during the first 2 mo of life.

§Figure outside parentheses = number; figure inside parentheses = percentage.

SKIN. Cutaneous manifestations in infants with congenital toxoplasmosis include petechiae, ecchymoses, or large hemorrhages secondary to thrombocytopenia, and rashes. Rashes may be fine punctate; diffuse maculopapular; lenticular, deep blue-red, sharply defined macular; and diffuse blue papules. Macular rashes involving the entire body, including the palms and soles, exfoliative dermatitis, and cutaneous calcifications have been described. Jaundice due to hepatic involvement with *T. gondii* and/or hemolysis, cyanosis due to interstitial pneumonitis secondary to this congenital infection, and edema secondary to myocarditis or nephrotic syndrome may be present. Jaundice and conjugated hyperbilirubinemia may persist for months.

SYSTEMIC SIGNS. Twenty-five to more than 50% of infants with clinically apparent disease at birth are born prematurely. Low Apgar scores also are common. Intrauterine growth retardation and instability of temperature regulation may occur. Other systemic manifestations include lymphadenopathy; hepatosplenomegaly; signs of myocarditis, pneumonitis, and nephrotic syndrome; vomiting; diarrhea; and feeding problems. Bands of metaphyseal lucency and irregularity of the line of provisional calcification at the epiphyseal plate may occur without periosteal reaction in the ribs, femora, and vertebrae. Congenital toxoplasmosis may be confused with isosensitization causing erythroblastosis fetalis; the Coombs test is usually negative with congenital *T. gondii* infection.

Endocrine Abnormalities. Endocrine abnormalities may occur secondary to hypothalamic or pituitary involvement or end-organ involvement. The following have been reported: myxedema, persistent hypernatremia with vasopressin-sensitive diabetes insipidus without polyuria or polydipsia, sexual precocity, and partial anterior hypopituitarism.

Central Nervous System. Neurologic manifestations of congenital toxoplasmosis vary from massive acute encephalopathy to subtle neurologic syndromes. Toxoplasmosis should be considered as a cause of any undiagnosed neurologic disease in children under 1 yr of age, especially if retinal lesions are present.

Hydrocephalus may be the sole clinical neurologic manifestation of congenital toxoplasmosis and may either be compensated or require correction with shunt placement. Hydrocephalus may present in the perinatal period, progress after the perinatal period, or, less commonly, present later in life. Patterns of seizures are protean and have included focal motor seizures, petit and grand mal seizures, muscular twitching, opisthotonus, and hypsarrhythmia (which may resolve with adrenocorticotropic hormone [ACTH] therapy). Spinal or bulbar involvement may be manifested by paralysis of the extremities, difficulty in swallowing, and respiratory distress. Microcephaly usually reflects severe brain damage, but some children with microcephaly due to congenital toxoplasmosis, who have been treated, appear to function normally in the early years of life. Untreated congenital toxoplasmosis that is symptomatic in the 1st yr of life can cause substantial diminution in cognitive function and developmental delays. Intellectual impairment also occurs in some children with subclinical infection despite treatment with pyrimethamine and sulfonamides for 1 mo. Seizures and focal motor defects may become apparent after the newborn period, even when infection is subclinical at birth.

Cerebrospinal fluid (CSF) abnormalities occur in at least one third of infants with congenital toxoplasmosis. Local production of *T. gondii*-specific antibodies may be demonstrated in CSF fluid of congenitally infected individuals (see later under Diagnosis). CT scan of the brain with contrast enhancement is useful to detect calcifications, determine ventricular size, image active inflammatory lesions, and demonstrate porencephalic cystic structures (Fig. 244–3). Calcifications occur throughout the brain, but there appears to be a special propensity for development of such lesions in the caudate nucleus (i.e., especially basal ganglia area), choroid plexus, and subependyma. Ultrasonography may be useful for following ventricular size in congenitally infected babies. Magnetic resonance imaging (MRI), CT with contrast enhancement, and radionucleotide brain scans may be useful for detecting active inflammatory lesions.

Eyes. Almost all untreated congenitally infected individuals will develop chorioretinal lesions by adulthood, and about 50% will have severe visual impairment. *T. gondii* causes a focal necrotizing retinitis in congenitally infected individuals (Fig. 244–4 [color plate section]). Contractures may occur with retinal detachment. Any part of the retina may be involved, either unilaterally or bilaterally, including the maculae. The optic nerve may be involved, and toxoplasmic lesions that involve projections of the visual pathways in the brain or the visual cortex also may lead to visual impairment. In association with retinal lesions and vitritis, the anterior uvea may be intensely inflamed, leading to erythema of the external eye. Other ocular findings include cells and protein in the anterior chamber, large keratic precipitates, posterior synechiae, nodules on the iris, and neovascular formation on the surface of the iris, sometimes with an associated increase in intraocular pressure and development of glaucoma. The extraocular musculature may also be involved directly, manifest as strabismus, nystagmus, visual impairment, and micro-ophthalmia. The differential diagnosis of lesions resembling ocular toxoplasmosis includes congenital colobomatous defect and other inflammatory lesions due to cytomegalovirus, *Treponema pallidum, Mycobacterium tuberculosis,* or vasculitis. Ocular toxoplasmosis is a recurrent and progressive disease that requires multiple courses of therapy. Couvreur et al have limited data that suggest that occurrence of lesions in the early years of life may be prevented by instituting antimicrobial treatment (with pyrimethamine and sulfonamides in alternate months with spiramycin) during the 1st yr of life.

Ears. Sensorineural hearing loss, both mild and severe, may occur. It is not known whether this is a static or progressive disorder.

Concomitant Infections. Congenital toxoplasmosis in infants with HIV infection usually presents as a severe and fulminant illness with substantial CNS involvement but also may be more indolent in its presentation with focal neurologic deficits or systemic manifestations such as pneumonitis.

Acquired Toxoplasmosis in Immunologically Normal Individuals. Immunologically normal children who acquire the infection postnatally may have no clinically recognizable disease. The most common manifestation is enlargement of one or a few lymph nodes in the cervical region. Cases of *Toxoplasma* lymphadenopathy rarely resemble infectious mononucleosis (due to Epstein-Barr virus, cytomegalovirus, or parvovirus), Hodgkin disease, or other lymphadenopathies. In the pectoral area in older girls and women, the nodes may be confused with breast neoplasms. Mediastinal, mesenteric, and retroperitoneal lymph nodes may be involved. Involvement of intra-abdominal lymph nodes may be associated with fever and mimic appendicitis. Nodes may be tender but do not suppurate. Adenopathy may appear and disappear for as long as 1 yr. When clinical manifestations are apparent, they may include almost any combination of fever, stiff neck, myalgia, arthralgia, maculopapular rash that spares the palms and soles, localized or generalized lymphadenopathy, hepatomegaly, hepatitis, reactive lymphocytosis, meningitis, brain abscess, encephalitis, confusion, malaise, pneumonia, polymyositis, pericarditis, pericardial effusion, and myocarditis. Chorioretinitis, usually unilateral, occurs in approximately 1% of cases. Symptoms may be present for a few days only or may persist many months.

Most patients with malaise and lymphadenopathy recover spontaneously without antimicrobial therapy. Significant organ involvement in immunologically normal individuals is uncommon, but some such individuals have suffered significant morbidity.

Ocular Involvement in the Older Child. In the United States and western Europe, *T. gondii* has been estimated to cause 35% of cases of chorioretinitis. Manifestations include blurred vision, photophobia, epiphora, and, with macular involvement, loss of central vision. Findings due to congenital ocular toxoplasmosis also include strabismus, micro-ophthalmia, microcornea, cataract, anisometropia, and nystagmus. Episodic recurrences are common. See Figure 244–4 and under Congenital Toxoplasmosis.

Toxoplasmosis in the Immunocompromised Patient. Congenital *T. gondii* infection in infants with AIDS is usually a fulminant, rapidly fatal disorder, involving brain and other organs such as the lung and heart. Disseminated *T. gondii* infections also occur in older children who are immunocompromised by AIDS, by malignancies and cytotoxic therapy or corticosteroids, or by immunosuppressive drugs given for organ transplantation. Immunocompromised individuals develop the clinical forms of *Toxoplasma* infection that occur in immunologically normal individuals. Signs and symptoms that are referable to the CNS

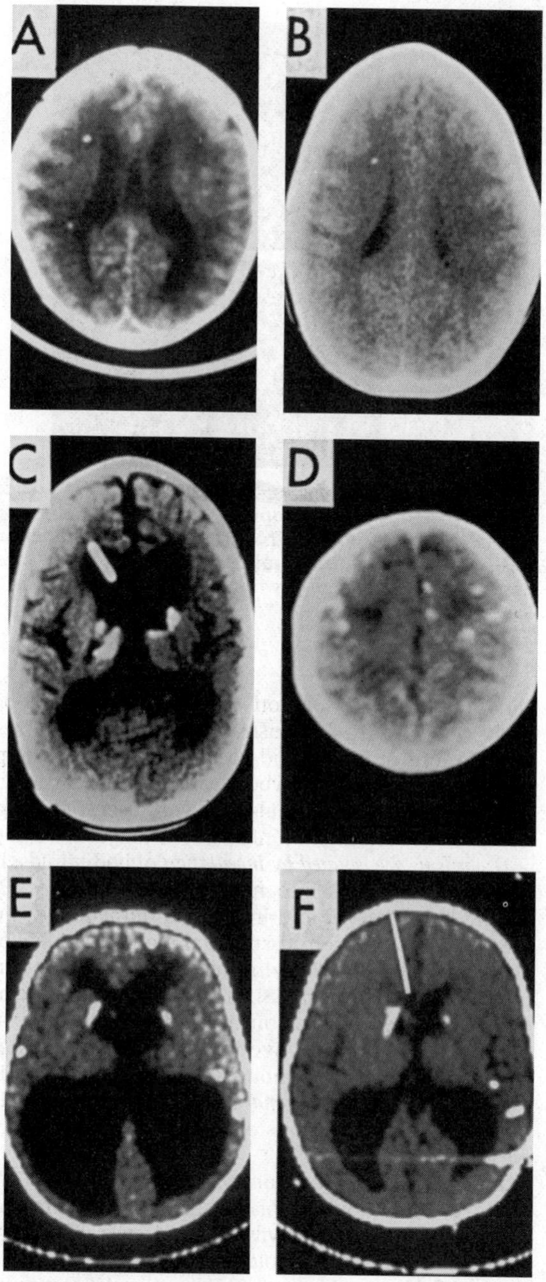

Figure 244–3. Head computed tomography (CT) scans of and historical information in babies with congenital toxoplasmosis. *A*, CT scan at birth that has areas of hypolucency, mildly dilated ventricles, and small calcifications. *B*, CT scan of the same child at 1 yr of age (after antimicrobial therapy for 1 yr). This scan is normal with the exception of two small calcifications. This child's Mental Development Index (MDI) at 1 yr of age was 140 by the Bayley Scales of Infant Development. *C*, CT scan from a 1-yr-old baby who was normal at birth. His meningoencephalitis became symptomatic in the first weeks of life but was not diagnosed correctly and remained untreated during his 1st 3 mo of life. At 3 mo of age, development of hydrocephalus and bilateral macular chorioretinitis led to the diagnosis of congenital toxoplasmosis, and antimicrobial therapy was initiated. This scan shows significant residual atrophy and calcifications. This child has substantial motor dysfunction, developmental delays, and visual impairment. *D*, CT scan obtained during the 1st mo of life of a microcephalic child. Note the numerous calcifications. This child's intelligence quotient (i.e., using the Stanford-Binet Intelligence Scale for children when she was 3 yr old and the Wechsler Preschool and Primary Scale of Intelligence when she was 5 yr old) was 100 and 102, respectively. She received antimicrobial therapy during her 1st yr of life. *E*, CT scan with hydrocephalus owing to aqueductal stenosis (before shunt). *F*, Scan from the same patient as the scan in *E*, after shunt. This child's intelligence quotient (i.e., using the Stanford-Binet Intelligence Scale for children) was approximately 100 when she was 3 and 6 yr old. (Adapted from McAuley J, Boyer K, Patel D, et al: Early and longitudinal evaluations of treated infants and children and untreated historical patients with congenital toxoplasmosis: The Chicago Collaborative Treatment Trial. Clin Infect Dis 18:38, 1994.)

are the most frequent manifestations of severe disease (occurring in 50% of patients), although other organs also may be involved.

Bone marrow transplant recipients present a special problem because active infection in these patients is difficult to diagnose. Specific antibody may not increase in serum or may be absent. In most instances, active infection occurs in a child with prior evidence of latent infection.

Individuals who have antibodies to *T. gondii* and HIV infection are at significant risk of developing toxoplasmic encephalitis, which may be the presenting manifestation of AIDS. In patients with AIDS, toxoplasmic encephalitis is fatal if not treated. Typical findings of CNS toxoplasmosis in patients with AIDS include fever, headache, altered mental status, psychosis, cognitive impairment, seizures, and focal neurologic defects, including hemiparesis, aphasia, ataxia, visual field loss, cranial nerve palsies, and dysmetric or movement disorders. Uncommon findings of CNS or other organ involvement include meningismus, signs referable to involvement of the heart, gastrointestinal tract, testes, panhypopituitarism, and the syndrome of inappropriate antidiuretic hormone. In adult patients with AIDS, toxoplasmic retinal lesions are often large with diffuse necrosis and contain many organisms but little inflammatory cellular infiltrate.

Toxoplasmic encephalitis and congenital toxoplasmosis are a particular problem in such immunocompromised individuals from areas where the incidence of latent infection is high. Specifically, approximately 25–50% of patients with AIDS and *Toxoplasma* antibodies ultimately will develop toxoplasmic encephalitis. The reason only a subpopulation of such latently infected individuals develops toxoplasmic encephalitis is unknown. A diagnosis of presumptive toxoplasmic encephalitis in patients with AIDS should prompt a therapeutic trial of medications effective against *T. gondii* (see Treatment). Clear clinical improvement within 7–14 days and improvement in neuroradiologic studies within 3 wk after therapy is initiated makes the presumptive diagnosis almost certain.

LABORATORY DIAGNOSIS. Diagnosis of acute *Toxoplasma* infection

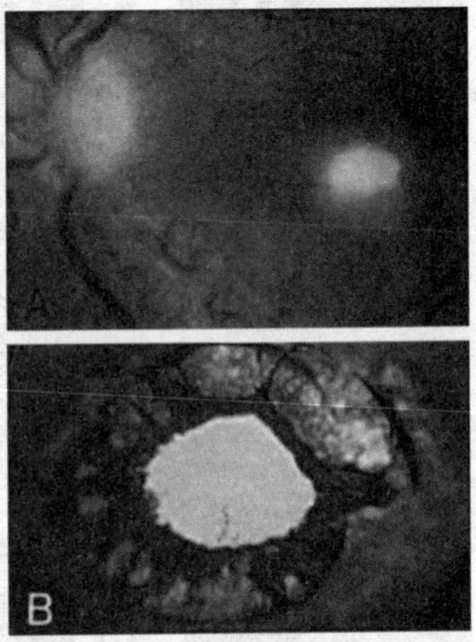

Figure 244–4. Toxoplasmic chorioretinitis. *A*, Active acute lesion by indirect ophthalmoscopy. *B*, Old, quiescent lesion. See also color section. (*B*, adapted from Desmonts G, Remington J: Congenital Toxoplasmosis. *In:* Remington J, Klein J (eds): Infectious Diseases of the Fetus and Newborn Infant, 3rd ed. Philadelphia, WB Saunders, 1991.)

can be made by isolation of *T. gondii* from blood or body fluids and also by demonstration of tachyzoites in sections or preparations of tissues and body fluids, cysts in the placenta or tissues of a fetus or newborn, and characteristic lymph node histology. Serologic tests also are very useful for diagnosis. The CSF is often abnormal in infants with congenital toxoplasmosis.

Organisms are isolated by inoculation of body fluids, leukocytes, or tissue specimens into mice or tissue cultures. Body fluids should be processed and inoculated immediately, but *T. gondii* has been isolated from tissues and blood that have been stored at 4° C overnight. Freezing or treatment of specimens with formalin kills *T. gondii.* Six to 10 days after inoculation, or earlier if mice die, peritoneal fluids should be examined for tachyzoites. If they survive for 6 wk and there is antibody in sera of the inoculated mouse, definitive diagnosis is made by visualization of *Toxoplasma* cysts in mouse brain. If cysts are not seen, subinoculations of mouse tissue into other mice are performed.

T. gondii can also be isolated by *tissue cultures.* Under microscopic examination, the plaques in these preparations are seen to contain necrotic, heavily infected cells with numerous extracellular tachyzoites. Isolation of *T. gondii* from blood or body fluids reflects acute infection. Except in the fetus or neonate it is usually not possible to demonstrate acute infection by isolation of *T. gondii* from tissues such as skeletal muscle, lung, brain, or eye obtained by biopsy or at autopsy.

Diagnosis of acute infection can be made by *demonstration of tachyzoites* in biopsy tissue sections, bone marrow aspirate, or body fluids such as CSF or amniotic fluid. Immunofluorescent antibody and immunoperoxidase staining techniques may be necessary because it is often difficult to see the tachyzoite with ordinary stains. Tissue cysts are diagnostic of infection but do not differentiate between acute and chronic infection; the presence of many cysts suggests recent acute infection. Cysts in the placenta or tissues of the newborn infant establish the diagnosis of congenital infection. Characteristic histologic features are sufficient to establish the diagnosis of toxoplasmic lymphadenitis. Multiple serologic tests may be necessary to confirm the diagnosis of congenital *Toxoplasma* infection or acutely acquired *Toxoplasma* infection. Each laboratory that reports such serologic test results must have established values in their tests that diagnose infection in specific clinical settings, provide interpretation of their results, and assure appropriate quality control before therapy is based on serologic test results. When such serologic test results are used as the basis for therapy, they also should be confirmed in a reference laboratory (e.g., Research Institute, Palo Alto Medical Foundation, CA 415–326–8120).

The *Sabin-Feldman dye test* is sensitive and specific. It measures primarily IgG antibodies. Results should be expressed in International Units (IU/mL) based on international standard reference sera available from the World Health Organization.

The *IgG fluorescent antibody (IgG-IFA) test* measures the same antibodies as the dye test, and the titers tend to be parallel. These antibodies usually appear 1–2 wk after infection, reach high titers (≥1:1,000) after 6–8 wk, and then decline over months to years. Low titers (1:4 to 1:64) usually persist for life. Antibody titer does not correlate with severity of illness. Approximately half of the commercially available IFA kits tested have been found to be improperly standardized and may yield significant numbers of false-positive and false-negative results.

An *agglutination test* (Bio-Merieux, Lyon, France) is available commercially in Europe (e.g., formalin-preserved whole parasites are used to detect IgG). This test is accurate, simple to perform, and inexpensive.

The *IgM fluorescent antibody (IgM-IFA) test* is useful for the diagnosis of acute infection with *T. gondii* in the older child because IgM antibodies appear earlier (often by 5 days after infection) and disappear sooner than IgG antibodies. In most instances, IgM-IFA test antibodies rise rapidly (to levels of 1:50 to >1:1,000) and fall to low titers (1:10 or 1:20) or disappear after weeks or months. However, for some patients they remain positive at low titers for as long as several years. The IgM-IFA test detects *Toxoplasma*-specific IgM in only approximately 25% of congenitally infected infants at birth. IgM antibodies also are often not present in sera of immunodeficient patients with acute toxoplasmosis or in most patients with active toxoplasmosis present only in the eye. Both the IgG-IFA and IgM-IFA tests may show false-positive results owing to rheumatoid factor.

The *double-sandwich enzyme-linked immunosorbent assay (IgM-ELISA)* is more sensitive and specific than the IgM-IFA test for detection of *Toxoplasma* IgM antibodies. In the older child, a level of IgM antibodies against *Toxoplasma* in serum of 1.7 or greater (value of one reference laboratory; each laboratory must establish its own values) indicates that *Toxoplasma* infection has most likely been acquired recently. IgM-ELISA detects approximately 75% of infants with congenital infection. IgM-ELISA avoids both the false-positive results due to rheumatoid factor produced by uninfected infants in utero and false-negative results due to high levels of passively transferred maternal IgG antibody in fetal serum, as occurs in the IgM-IFA test.

The *IgM immunosorbent assay (ISAGA)* combines trapping of a patient's IgM to a solid surface and use of formalin-fixed organisms or antigen-coated latex particles. It is read like an agglutination test and is specific and sensitive. There are no false-positive results due to rheumatoid factor or antinuclear antibodies. IgM antibodies to *Toxoplasma* are detected by the IgM-IFA test for a shorter time than they are by the IgM-ELISA. The IgM ISAGA is more sensitive than the IgM ELISA and may detect specific IgM antibodies before and for longer periods of time than the IgM ELISA. A positive result in *the IgM IFA* is present in sera of about 25% of congenitally infected infants and a positive result in the IgM ELISA is present in sera of about 75% of infants with congenital toxoplasmosis. The *IgA ELISA* is a more sensitive test than the IgM ELISA for detection of congenital infection in the fetus and newborn as well as for detection of acute infection in the fetus and newborn as well as for detection of acute infection in some pregnant women. The IgE ELISA and IgE ISAGA are also useful in establishing the diagnosis of congenital toxoplasmosis or acute acquired *T. gondii* infection. The differential agglutination test (i.e., AC/HS) can be used to differentiate recent and remote infections in adults and older children. In acute infection, there is greater agglutination of acetone-fixed tachyzoites than formalin-fixed tachyzoites. This may be particularly useful in differentiating remote infection in pregnant women, as IgM and IgA antibodies detectable in ELISAs or ISAGAs may remain elevated for prolonged periods (e.g., months to years in adults and older children).

Antibodies measured in *indirect hemagglutination (IHA) tests* are different from those measured in the IFA and dye tests. They may persist for years. However, the IHA test should not be used in infants with suspected congenital infection or in screening for infection acquired during pregnancy because it may be negative for too long a period early during infection.

The level of *Toxoplasma antibody in the aqueous humor* demonstrates local production of antibody during active ocular or CNS toxoplasmosis as follows:

$$C = \frac{\text{antibody titer in body fluid}}{\text{antibody titer in serum}} \times \frac{\text{concentration of gamma globulin in serum}}{\text{concentration of gamma globulin in body fluid}}$$

Significant correlation coefficients [C] are 8 or more (eye), 4 or more (CNS for congenital infection), and over 1 (CNS for patients with AIDS). If the serum dye test titer is 1,000 or more, most often it is not possible to demonstrate significant local antibody production using this formula with either the dye test or the IgM-IFA test titer. IgM antibody may be present in CSF.

Toxoplasma antigen has been detected during acute *Toxoplasma* infection but not in sera of uninfected or chronically infected individuals. Antigen was present in the serum, amniotic fluid, and cerebrospinal fluid in the few infants tested with congenital infections.

Comparative *Western blot* tests of sera from a mother and baby may detect congenital infection. Infection is suspected when the mother's serum and her baby's serum contain antibodies that react with different *Toxoplasma* antigens.

Enzyme-linked immunofiltration assay (ELIFA, using micropore membranes) permits simultaneous study of antibody specificity by immunoprecipitation and characterization of antibody isotypes by immunofiltration with enzyme-labeled antibodies. This method may be capable of detecting 85% of cases of congenital infection in the first few days of life. It is still being evaluated.

Polymerase chain reaction (PCR) is used to amplify the DNA of *T. gondii*, which then can be detected using a DNA probe. Detection of a repetitive *T. gondii* gene, that is, the B1 gene, in amniotic fluid is particularly useful for establishing the diagnosis of congenital *Toxoplasma* infection in the fetus. The sensitivity and specificity of this test using amniotic fluid obtained at ≥18 weeks gestation approached 100% (P Thulliez, personal communication).

Lymphocyte blastogenesis to *Toxoplasma* antigens has been used to diagnose congenital toxoplasmosis if a question persists concerning the diagnosis and other tests are negative.

Laboratory Diagnosis of Congenital Toxoplasmosis. Fetal blood sampling, fetal ultrasound examination (performed every 2 wk during gestation), and analysis of amniotic fluid are used in *prenatal diagnosis* of congenital toxoplasmosis. Abnormalities in the following nonspecific tests suggest that fetal infection is possible: peripheral white blood cell count, number of eosinophils, platelet count, liver function tests (gamma-GTP, LDH), and total IgM. IgM specific for *T. gondii* is usually present only after 24 wk gestation, and *T. gondii* may be isolated from peripheral fetal white blood cells and cells from amniotic fluid. This procedure is no longer recommended unless amniotic fluid PCR testing cannot be performed in a reliable laboratory (see above PCR). *T. gondii* also may be isolated from the placenta.

Serologic tests are also useful in establishing a diagnosis of congenital toxoplasmosis, for example, either persistent or rising titers in the dye test or IFA test or a positive IgM ELISA or ISAGA. The half-life of IgM is 3–5 days, so if there is a placental leak, the level of IgM antibodies in the infant's serum falls significantly within a week. Passively transferred maternal IgG antibodies may require many months to a year to disappear from the infant's serum. The length of time needed for disappearance depends on the magnitude of the original titer. IgG half-life is approximately 30 days. Synthesis of *Toxoplasma* antibody is usually demonstrable by the 3rd mo of life if the infant is untreated. If the infant is treated, synthesis may be delayed until the 9th mo of life, and, infrequently, it may not occur at all. When an infant begins to synthesize antibody, infection may be documented serologically without demonstration of IgM antibodies by computation of the specific "antibody load," that is, the ratio of specific serum antibody titer to the amount of IgG in an infected baby will increase, whereas the ratio will fall as the baby synthesizes IgG if the specific antibody has been passively transferred from the mother.

At birth, when a diagnosis of congenital toxoplasmosis is suspected, the following diagnostic studies should be performed: general, ophthalmologic, and neurologic examinations; head CT scan; attempt to isolate *T. gondii* from the placenta and the infant's white blood cells from umbilical cord blood and buffy coat; measurement of serum *Toxoplasma*-specific IgG, IgM, IgA, and IgE antibodies and the total amount of IgM and IgG in serum; lumbar puncture including analysis of CSF for cells, glucose, protein, *Toxoplasma*-specific IgG and IgM antibodies, and total amount of IgG; evaluation of CSF for *T. gondii* and evaluations of CSF for *T. gondii* by PCR and inoculation into mice. The presence of *Toxoplasma*-specific IgM in CSF that is not contaminated with blood or local antibody production of *Toxoplasma*-specific IgG antibody demonstrated in CSF establishes the diagnosis of congenital *Toxoplasma* infection.

Laboratory Diagnosis of Acute Acquired Toxoplasma Infection in the Immunocompetent Individual. Recent infection is diagnosed by seroconversion from a negative to a positive IgG antibody titer (in the absence of transfer of antibody by transfusion); a serial two-tube rise in *Toxoplasma*-specific IgG titer when sera are obtained 3 wk apart and run in parallel; and the presence of *Toxoplasma*-specific IgM antibody.

Laboratory Diagnosis of Ocular Toxoplasmosis. IgG test titers of 1:4 to 1:64 are usual in older children with active toxoplasmic chorioretinitis. When the retinal lesions are characteristic and serologic tests are positive, the diagnosis is likely.

Laboratory Diagnosis of Toxoplasmosis in the Immunocompromised Individual. IgG antibody titers may be low, and *Toxoplasma*-specific IgM is often absent in immunocompromised individuals with toxoplasmosis. Demonstration of *Toxoplasma* antigens or DNA in serum, blood, and CSF may identity disseminated *Toxoplasma* infection in immunocompromised persons.

Resolution of CNS lesions during a therapeutic trial of pyrimethamine and sulfadiazine has been useful in patients with AIDS. Brain biopsy has been used to establish the diagnosis of toxoplasmic encephalitis when there is no response to this therapeutic trial or to exclude other likely diagnoses in such immunocompromised individuals.

DIFFERENTIAL DIAGNOSIS. Many manifestations of congenital toxoplasmosis occur in other perinatal diseases, especially disease caused by cytomegalovirus. Neither cerebral calcification nor chorioretinitis is pathognomonic. Fewer than 50% of children under 5 yr of age with chorioretinitis satisfy the serologic criteria for congenital toxoplasmosis; the causes of most of the other cases are unknown. The clinical picture in the newborn infant may also be compatible with sepsis, aseptic meningitis, syphilis, or hemolytic disease. In cases of acquired disease, other causes of lymphadenopathic disease must be distinguished from toxoplasmosis.

PREVENTION. Methods of prevention are outlined in Figure 244–2. Counseling women about these methods of avoiding transmission of *T. gondii* during pregnancy can substantially reduce acquisition of infection during gestation. Women who do not have specific antibody to *T. gondii* prior to pregnancy should only eat well-done meat during pregnancy and avoid contact with oocysts excreted by cats. Cats that are kept indoors, maintained on prepared diets, and not fed fresh, uncooked meat should not contact encysted *T. gondii* and shed oocysts. Serologic screening, ultrasound monitoring, and treatment of pregnant women during gestation can also reduce the incidence and perhaps manifestations of congenital toxoplasmosis.

TREATMENT. Therapeutic Agents. Pyrimethamine plus sulfadiazine or trisulfapyrimidines act synergistically against *Toxoplasma*. Combined therapy is indicated to treat many of the forms of toxoplasmosis. However, use of pyrimethamine is contraindicated during the 1st trimester of pregnancy. Spiramycin should be used to prevent transmission of infection to the fetus of acutely infected pregnant women and to treat congenital toxoplasmosis. Pyrimethamine is a folic acid antagonist and therefore produces a dose-related, reversible, and usually gradual depression of the bone marrow, resulting in thrombocytopenia, leukopenia, and anemia. Neutropenia is the most common side effect in treated infants. All patients treated with pyrimethamine should have platelet and peripheral blood cell counts twice weekly. Seizures may occur with overdosage of pyrimethamine. Folinic acid (calcium leukovorin) should always be administered concomitantly with pyrimethamine to prevent suppression of the bone marrow. Potential toxic effects of sulfonamides (e.g., crystalluria, hematuria, and rash) should be monitored. Hypersensitivity reactions occur, especially in patients with AIDS.

Treatment of Congenital Toxoplasmosis. All infected newborns should be treated, whether or not they have clinical manifestations of the infection. In infants with congenital infection, treatment may be effective in interrupting acute disease that damages vital organs. Infants should be treated for 1 yr. For the first 6 mo, oral pyrimethamine (1–2 mg/kg/24 hr for 2 days, then 1 mg/kg/24 hr for 2 mo, then 1 mg/kg/24 hr Monday, Wednesday, and Friday), sulfadiazine or triple sulfonamides (100 mg/kg loading dose, then 100 mg/kg/24 hr in two divided doses), and calcium leukovorin (5–10 mg/24 hr Monday, Wednesday, and Friday) should be administered. In the second 6 mo this regimen is continued or given in alternate months with spiramycin (50 mg/kg twice a day). For infants with moderate to severe involvement the first 6 mo regimen may be continued for a full year or modified to provide pyrimethamine 1 mg/kg/24 hr for the first 6 mo. Pyrimethamine, available only in tablet form, may be crushed and administered in a suspension with juice or food. The effectiveness of these regimens has not been proved, but they are considered reasonable empiric recommendations.* Prednisone (1 mg/kg/24 hr orally in divided doses) has been utilized in addition when active chorioretinitis involves the macula. CSF protein is elevated (≥1,000 mg/dL) at birth, but its efficacy also is not established.

Treatment of Immunologically Normal Older Children with Lymphadenopathy, Severe Symptoms, or Damage to Vital Organs. Patients with lymphadenopathy do not need specific treatment unless they have severe and persistent symptoms or evidence of damage to vital organs. If such signs and symptoms occur, treatment with pyrimethamine, sulfadiazine, and leukovorin should be initiated. Although the optimal duration of therapy is unknown, patients who appear to be immunologically normal but have severe and persistent symptoms or damage to vital organs (e.g., chorioretinitis, myocarditis) need specific therapy until these specific symptoms resolve, followed by therapy for an additional 2 wk. This therapy usually lasts for at least 4–6 wk, and sometimes longer. A loading dose of pyrimethamine for older children is 2 mg/kg/24 hr (maximum 50 mg), given for the first 2 days of treatment. The maintenance dose is 1 mg/kg/24 hr (maximum 25 mg/24 hr). Folinic acid is administered orally at a dosage of 5–20 mg three times/wk (or even daily depending on the white blood cell count). Sulfadiazine or trisulfapyrimidine is administered to children over 1 yr of age with a loading dose of 75 mg/kg/24 hr, and thereafter 50 mg/kg/24 hr.

Treatment of Active Chorioretinitis in Older Children (also see Treatment of Congenital Toxoplasmosis). Such patients should receive pyrimethamine, sulfadiazine, and leukovorin for approximately 1 mo. Within 10 days the borders of retinal lesions should sharpen, and the vitreous haze should disappear in 60–70% of cases. Systemic corticosteroids are administered when lesions involve the macula, optic nerve head, or papillomacular bundle. Photocoagulation has been used to treat active lesions and prevent spread (i.e., most new lesions appear contiguous to old ones). Occasionally vitrectomy and removal of the lens are needed to restore visual acuity.

Treatment of Immunocompromised Patients. Serologic evidence of acute infection in an immunocompromised patient, regardless of whether signs and symptoms of infection are present or tachyzoites are present in tissue, are indications for therapy similar to that described for immunocompetent children with symptoms of organ injury. It is important to establish the diagnosis as rapidly as possible and institute treatment early. In immunocompromised patients other than those with AIDS, therapy should be continued for at least 4–6 wk beyond complete resolution of all signs and symptoms of active disease. Careful follow-up of these patients is imperative because relapse may occur, requiring prompt reinstitution of therapy. Relapse is frequent in patients with AIDS, and suppressive therapy with pyrimethamine and sulfonamides should be continued for life. Therapy usually induces a beneficial response clinically, but it does not eradicate cysts from the CNS and perhaps not from other tissues either.

Treatment of Pregnant Women with *T. gondii* Infection. The immunologically normal pregnant woman who acquired *T. gondii* before conception does not need treatment to prevent congenital infection of her fetus. Treatment of a pregnant woman who acquires infection at any time during pregnancy reduces the chance of congenital infection in her infant by approximately 60%. The medications used are spiramycin and pyrimethamine in combination with sulfadiazine or triple sulfonamides. Because pyrimethamine is potentially teratogenic, spiramycin is administered in the 1st trimester.* The dose of spiramycin is 1 g each 8 hr, given without food; lower doses are less effective.* Toxicity is infrequent. Adverse reactions include paresthesias, rash, nausea, vomiting, and diarrhea. Treatment during the remainder of pregnancy with pyrimethamine and a sulfonamide should be continued at dosages similar to those recommended for therapy of the symptomatic immunocompetent patient. Treatment of the mother of an infected fetus with pyrimethamine and a sulfonamide reduces infection in the placenta and the severity of disease in the newborn.

Chronically infected pregnant women who have been immunocompromised by cytotoxic drugs or corticosteroid therapy have transmitted *T. gondii* to their fetuses. Such women should be treated with spiramycin throughout gestation. The best approach to prevention of congenital toxoplasmosis in the fetus of a pregnant woman with HIV and inactive *T. gondii* infection is unknown. If the pregnancy is not terminated, the

*Information concerning the U.S. National Collaborative Study evaluating these regimens can be obtained by calling 312-791-4152. Spiramycin is available in the United States only through this study or by special permission of the FDA.

*Spiramycin is available in the United States through the FDA (telephone 302–443–7580).

mother should be treated with spiramycin during the first 17 wk of gestation and then with pyrimethamine and sulfadiazine until term. In a study of adult patients with AIDS, a dose of 75 mg pyrimethamine/24 hr and high dosages of intravenously administered clindamycin (1,200 mg/6 hr intravenously) appeared equal in efficacy to sulfonamides and pyrimethamine. Other currently experimental agents include roxithromycin and azithromycin (two new macrolides). These agents have not been used in infants or children.

Azidothymidine (AZT) antagonizes in vitro the toxoplasmacidal effect of pyrimethamine and the synergy of pyrimethamine and sulfadiazine, but the clinical significance of this observation remains to be determined. Therapy with phenobarbital and pyrimethamine may reduce the half-life of pyrimethamine. Sulfadiazine interferes with the metabolism by hepatic microsomal enzymes of other agents such as phenytoin (Dilantin) and warfarin. This prolongs their half-life, and lower dosages of these drugs are therefore likely to achieve therapeutic levels.

Infants with severe systemic and neurologic manifestations of congenital toxoplasmosis, including cerebral calcifications, hydrocephalus, and chorioretinitis, do not have uniformly poor prognoses due solely to their infection, and the usual supportive measures are indicated.

PROGNOSIS. Early institution of specific treatment for congenitally infected infants usually cures the manifestations of toxoplasmosis such as active chorioretinitis, meningitis, encephalitis, hepatitis, splenomegaly, and thrombocytopenia. Hydrocephalus due to aqueductal obstruction may develop or become worse during therapy. Such treatment also may reduce the incidence of some sequelae, such as diminished cognitive or abnormal motor function. Without therapy, chorioretinitis often recurs. Children with extensive involvement at birth may function normally later in life or have mild to severe impairment of vision, hearing, cognitive function, and other neurologic functions. Delays in diagnosis and therapy, perinatal hypoglycemia, hypoxia, hypotension, repeated shunt infections, and severe visual impairment are associated with a poorer prognosis. Prognosis must be guarded but is not necessarily poor for infected babies. Treatment with pyrimethamine and sulfadiazine does not eradicate the encysted parasite. No protective vaccine is available.

Bretagne S, Costa JM, Vidaud M, et al: Detection of *Toxoplasma gondii* by competitive DNA amplification of bronchoalveolar lavage samples. J Infect Dis 168:1585, 1993.

Brooks RG, McCabe RE, Remington JS: Role of serology in the diagnosis of toxoplasic lymphadenopathy. Rev Infect Dis 9:1055, 1987.

Burg JL, Grover CM, Pouletty P, et al: Direct and sensitive detection of a pathogenic protozoan, *Toxoplasma gondii*, by polymerase chain reaction. J Clin Microbiol 27:1787, 1989.

Couvreur J, Desmonts G, Tournier G, et al: Study of homogeneous series of 210 cases of congenital toxoplasmosis in infants aged 0 to 11 months detected prospectively. Ann Pediatr 31:815, 1984.

Daffos F, Forestier F, Capella-Pavlovsky M, et al: Prenatal management of 746 pregnancies at risk for congenital toxoplasmosis. N Engl J Med 318:271, 1988.

Dannemann BR, Vaughan WC, Thulliez P, Remington JS: The differential agglutination test for diagnosis of recently acquired infection with *Toxoplasma gondii*. J Clin Microbiol 28:1928, 1990.

Desmonts G, Couvreur J: Natural history of congenital toxoplasmosis. Ann Pediatr 31:799, 1984.

Desmonts G, Forestier F, Thulliez P, et al: Prenatal diagnosis of congenital toxoplasmosis. Lancet 1:500, 1985.

Donald RGK, Roos DS: Stable molecular transformation of *Toxoplasma gondii*: A selectable dihydrofolate reductase-thymidylate synthase marker based on drug-resistance mutations in malaria. Proc Natl Acad Sci USA 90:11703, 1993.

Grover CM, Thulliez P, Remington JS, et al: Rapid prenatal diagnosis of congenital *Toxoplasma* infection by using polymerase chain reaction and amniotic fluid. J Clin Microbiol 28:2297, 1990.

Guerrina NG, Hsu H, Meissner HC, et al: Neonatal seriologic screening and early treatment for congenital *Toxoplasma gondii* infection. N Engl J Med 330:1858, 1994.

Haentjens M, Sacre L, DeMeuter F: Congenital toxoplasmosis after maternal infection before or slightly after conception. Acta Paediatr Scand 75:343, 1986.

Hohlfeld P, Daffos F, Thulliez P, et al: Fetal toxoplasmosis: Outcome of pregnancy and infant follow-up after in utero treatment. J Pediatr 115:765, 1989.

Israelski DM, Remington JS: Toxoplasmic encephalitis in patients with AIDS. *In:* Sand MA, Volberding PA (eds): The Medical Management of AIDS. Philadelphia, WB Saunders, 1988, pp 193–211.

Koppe JG, Loewer-Sieger DH, De Roever-Bonnet H: Results of 20-year follow-up of congenital toxoplasmosis. Lancet 1:254, 1986.

Luft BJ, Remington JS: Toxoplasmic encephalitis in AIDS. Clin Infect Dis 15:211, 1992.

McAuley J, Boyer K, Patel D, et al: Early and longitudinal evaluations of treated infants and children and untreated historical patients with congenital toxoplasmosis: The Chicago Collaborative Treatment Trial. Clin Inf Dis 18:38, 1994.

McCabe RE, Brooks RG, Dorfman RF, et al: Clinical spectrum in 107 cases of toxoplasmic lymphadenopathy. Rev Infect Dis 9:754, 1987.

McCabe R, Remington JS: Toxoplasmosis: The time has come. N Engl J Med 318:313, 1988.

McGee T, Wolters C, Stein L, et al: Absence of sensorineural hearing loss in treated infants and children with congenital toxoplasmosis. Otolaryngol Head Neck Surg 106:75, 1992.

McLeod R, Hubbel J, Foss R, et al: Serum cerebrospinal and ventricular fluid levels of pyrimethamine in infants treated for congenital toxoplasmosis. Antimicrob Agents Chemother 36:1040, 1992.

McLeod R, Hubbel J, Weller S, et al: Pyrimethamine in the treatment of congenital toxoplasmosis. (In press.)

McLeod R, Mack DG, Boyer K, et al: Phenotypes and functions of lymphocytes in congenital toxoplasmosis. J Lab Clin Immunol 116:623, 1990.

McLeod R, Wisner J, Boyer K: Toxoplasmosis. *In:* Krugman S, Katz S, Wilfert C, Gershon A (eds): Infectious Diseases of Children, 8th ed. St. Louis, MO, LCV Mosby, 1992, pp 518–550.

Mitchell CD, Erlich SS, Mastrucci MT, et al: Congenital toxoplasmosis occurring in infants perinatally infected with human immunodeficiency virus. J Pediatr Infect Dis 9:512, 1990.

Patel DV, Holfels E, Vogel N, et al: Resolution of intracerebral calcifications in children with treated congenital toxoplasmosis. Radiology (In press.)

Remington JS, McLeod R, Desmonts G: Toxolasmosis. *In:* Remington J, Klein J (eds): Infectious Diseases of the Fetus and Newborn Infant. Philadelphia, WB Saunders, 1995, pp 140–268.

Roizen N, Swisher C, Boyer K, et al: Developmental and neurologic outcome in congenital toxoplasmosis. Pediatrics 95:11, 1995.

Saxon SA, Knight W, Reynolds DW, et al: Intellectual deficits in children born with subclinical congenital toxoplasmosis: A preliminary report. J Pediatr 8:2792, 1973.

Swisher CN, Boyer K, McLeod R: Congenital toxoplasmosis. *In:* Bodenstein JB (ed): Seminars in Pediatric Neurology. Philadelphia, WB Saunders. (In press.)

Wilson CB, Remington JS, Stagno S, et al: Development of adverse sequelae in children born with subclinical congenital *Toxoplasma* infection. Pediatrics 66:767, 1980.

Wong SY, Hajdu MP, Ramirez R, et al: The role of specific immunoglobulin E in the diagnosis of acute *Toxoplasma* infection and toxoplasmosis. J Clin Microbiol 31:2952, 1993.

244.9 Trichomoniasis

Robert A. Salata

Trichomonas vaginalis is a sexually transmitted protozoan parasite primarily causing symptomatic vaginitis in women including adolescents. An estimated 3 million American women develop trichomoniasis each year, while the occurrence in males is unknown. The incidence of trichomoniasis is highest among females with multiple sexual partners and in groups with the highest rates of other sexually transmitted infections. Thus, patients found to harbor *T. vaginalis* should be screened for other sexually transmitted pathogens such as *Neisseria gonorrhoeae, Chlamydia trachomatis, Treponema pallidum,* or human immunodeficiency virus (HIV). *Trichomonas vaginalis* is recovered from over two thirds of female partners of infected males and 30–80% of male sexual partners of infected women. Infection appears to be self-limited in men.

Trichomoniasis is occasionally transmitted in some institutional populations, presumably through nonvenereal means. The organism can survive for several hours in moist environments. Trichomoniasis may also be transmitted to neonates during passage through an infected birth canal. It may not be necessary to treat trichomoniasis in the newborn unless symptomatic. Trichomoniasis is rare until menarche, and its presence in a younger child should raise the possibility of sexual abuse.

PATHOGENESIS. Infected vaginal secretions contain 10^1–10^5 protozoa/mL, with many females carrying larger numbers. In fresh preparations, *T. vaginalis* are highly motile and pear-shaped and are most easily recognized by their characteristic twitching motility. The organisms reproduce by binary fission and exist only as vegetative cells, with no cyst forms having been described. *T. vaginalis* activates the alternative pathway of complement and attracts polymorphonuclear neutrophils, which in turn can kill the protozoan. Monocytes and macrophages have been shown to kill trichomonads in vitro, but their role in natural infection is uncertain.

CLINICAL MANIFESTATIONS. The incubation period in females ranges from about 5 to 28 days, and symptoms may begin or exacerbate during menses. About 10–50% of women may asymptomatically harbor the organism. Symptoms most commonly include malodorous vaginal discharge, vulvovaginal irritation, dysuria, and dyspareunia. Abdominal discomfort is an unusual feature and should prompt evaluation for pelvic inflammatory disease. None of these symptoms alone or in combination are sufficient to diagnose trichomoniasis. Spread of trichomoniasis beyond the lower urogenital tract is extremely rare.

Examination of the symptomatic female reveals a copious discharge that pools in the posterior vaginal fornix. The discharge may be yellow and full of bubbles, but mucopurulent cervicitis due to *Chlamydia* may cause a yellow discharge as well. There may be hemorrhages observed, especially with colposcopy. The vaginal discharge in the majority of women has a pH level above 4.5, which is also a feature with bacterial vaginosis.

Most males carrying *T. vaginalis* are asymptomatic; however, this organism can be isolated in 5–15% of men with nongonococcal urethritis, and these patients have symptoms that are indistinguishable from those of nongonococcal urethritis of other causes. Symptomatic males usually have dysuria and scant urethral discharge. Trichomonads occasionally cause epididymitis, prostatic involvement, and superficial penile ulceration.

DIAGNOSIS. The accurate diagnosis of trichomoniasis in both sexes is dependent on the demonstration of the protozoan in genital secretions. In vaginal secretions, trichomonads may be recognized using the wet mount technique, which will identify 60–70% of infected females. Endocervical specimens are unreliable for diagnosis, as the organism is present in only 13% of proven cases. Wet mount examination of material obtained by platinum loop from the anterior urethra will reveal the organism in 50–90% of infected men. Microscopic examination of urine sediment after prostatic massage is of high yield in infected men. A negative wet mount does not exclude the diagnosis of trichomoniasis; the organism may be cultured in a number of liquid and semisolid media if necessary. Serologic testing is plagued by low sensitivity and specificity, and has no current role in the evaluation of the individual patient.

TREATMENT. The drug of choice for therapy of trichomoniasis is a nitroimidazole. In the United States, metronidazole is used, whereas in other countries tinidazole or ornidazole has been used with similar efficacy. Numerous studies have substantiated the efficacy of a single oral 1-g dose of metronidazole in adolescent females; an alternative therapy consists of 250 mg of metronidazole orally three times daily for 7 days. Infected children should receive 15 mg/kg/24hr orally in three divided doses for 7 days. Single oral therapy usually fails to cure 40% of infected males. Metronidazole is contraindicated in the first trimester of pregnancy, while several studies reported the safety of this drug in the last two trimesters. It seems prudent, however, to avoid the drug then as well if this is possible. Symptomatic pregnant women might initially be treated with clotrimazole. The number of putative metronidazole failures appears to be increasing, and in some cases metronidazole-resistant *T. vaginalis* has been documented. In most cases, failure is a consequence of reinfection from an untreated sexual partner or there is noncompliance with multidose therapy.

Lumsden WHR, Robertson DHH, Heyworth R, et al: Treatment failure in *Trichomonas vaginalis* vaginitis. Genitourin Med 64:217, 1988.
Thomason JL, Gelbart SM: Trichomonas vaginalis. Obstet Gyencol 74:536, 1990.

244.10 African Trypanosomiasis

(Sleeping Sickness)

Adel A. F. Mahmoud

The trypanosomiases of tropical Africa are a group of diseases of great social and economic importance. Human infections are caused by two subspecies of *Trypanosoma brucei, T. b. rhodesiense* and *T. b. gambiense,* which are morphologically indistinguishable but differ markedly in their epidemiology and the disease syndromes they cause. Infection with *T. b. rhodesiense* usually results in acute syndromes that run a rapid and, if untreated, fatal course, whereas *T. b. gambiense* infection usually runs a more chronic course, resulting in the typical syndrome of sleeping sickness.

Information on the distribution, prevalence, and mortality rate of African trypanosomiasis is unreliable. Human trypanosomiasis in Africa occurs primarily in the region between latitudes 15 degrees north and 15 degrees south, which corresponds roughly to the area where the annual rainfall (500 mm or more) creates optimal climatic conditions for *Glossina* flies. *T. b. rhodesiense* infection is restricted to the eastern third of the endemic area in tropical Africa, stretching from Ethiopia to the northern boundaries of South Africa; *T. b. gambiense* occurs mainly in the western half of the continent's endemic region.

ETIOLOGY. Human infection is initiated by insect bite; the organisms penetrate intact mucous membranes or skin. The infective metacyclic forms of the trypanosomes are 15 μm long and possess no free flagella. One to 3 wk after a period of local multiplication in the skin, long and slender forms (12–42 μm) can be seen in the peripheral blood; intermediate and stumpy forms also occur. These are flagellated forms with a well-developed undulating membrane. In the early stages of human infection, the organisms multiply rapidly in the blood and lymph nodes. They appear in waves in the peripheral blood, each wave being followed by a crisis. The reappearance of another population of organisms in the blood heralds the formation of a new antigenic variant. Invasion of the central nervous system (CNS) occurs early in *T. b. rhodesiense* infections but late in the Gambian form.

The insect intermediate vectors are species of the tsetse flies of the genus *Glossina.* Inside the flies, the organisms localize in the posterior part of the midgut, where they multiply for about 10 days, then gradually migrate anteriorly where they attach to the walls of the salivary ducts and complete the final stages of development into the infective metacyclic forms. The life cycle within the tsetse fly takes 15–35 days.

Direct transmission to humans has also been reported. It is accomplished either mechanically through contact with the contaminated mouth parts of tsetse flies during feeding or congenitally to infants via the placenta of infected mothers.

EPIDEMIOLOGY. The insect intermediate vector plays a major role in determining the epidemiologic pattern of trypanosomiasis. Several *Glossina* species transmit the infection in different parts of tropical Africa. *Glossina* captured in endemic foci show a low rate of infection, usually under 5%. In the Rhodesian form, which usually runs an acute and often fatal course, chances of transmission to tsetse flies are greatly reduced. However, the ability of *T. b. rhodesiense* to multiply enormously in the bloodstream of humans and to infect other species of mammals helps to maintain its life cycle.

T. b. gambiense infections usually run a chronic protracted course with very low levels of parasitemia. Because of low rates of infection in tsetse flies, the Gambian life cycle necessitates close and repeated contact between humans and insects to permit frequent biting. *T. b. gambiense* is found in a variety of animal reservoirs that may play an important role in the endemicity of the Gambian form of infection.

PATHOLOGY. The initial entry site of the organisms soon develops into a hard, painful, red nodule, a "trypanosomal chancre." Histologically, it contains long, thin trypanosomes multiplying beneath the dermis and is surrounded by a lymphocytic cellular infiltrate. Dissemination into the blood and lymphatic systems follows, with subsequent localization in the CNS. The histopathologic lesions in the brain are those of meningoencephalitis, with increased cellularity of the pia-arachnoid due to lymphocyte infiltration and perivascular cuffing of the blood vessels by the same cell type. In chronic cases the appearance of morular cells (large, strawberry-like cells, supposedly derived from plasma cells) is the most characteristic finding.

CLINICAL MANIFESTATIONS. The clinical presentations vary not only because of the two subspecies of organisms but also because of differences in host response in the indigenous population of endemic areas and in newcomers or visitors. Visitors usually suffer more from the acute symptoms and signs, but in untreated cases death is inevitable for natives and visitors alike. The clinical syndromes of African trypanosomiasis are best described as the trypanosomal chancre, hemolymphatic, and meningoencephalitic stages.

Trypanosomal Chancre. The *site of the tsetse fly bite* may be the first presenting feature. A nodule or chancre develops in 2–3 days; within 1 wk it becomes a painful, hard, red nodule surrounded by an area of erythema and swelling. These nodules are commonly seen on the lower limbs but sometimes also on the head. They subside spontaneously in about 2 wk leaving no permanent scar.

Hemolymphatic Stage. The *most common presenting features* of acute African trypanosomiasis occur at the time of invasion of the bloodstream by the parasites, approximately 2–3 wk after the infection. Irregular episodes of fever, each lasting 1–7 days, are the usual early feature. Attacks may be separated by free intervals of days or even weeks. Headache, sweating, and generalized lymphadenopathy are frequently encountered along with the fever. Enlargement of lymph nodes is one of the most constant signs, particularly in the Gambian form. It most commonly affects the posterior cervical and supraclavicular groups. The lymphadenopathy is painless; the glands are moderately enlarged and are not matted together. Another common feature of trypanosomiasis in whites is the presence of *blotchy, irregular, nonitching, erythematous macules,* which may appear any time following the first febrile episode, usually within 6–8 wk. The majority of macules have a central normal skin area, giving the rash a circinate outline. This skin rash is seen mainly on the trunk and is evanescent, fading in one place only to appear at another site. Examination of the blood during this stage may show anemia, leukopenia with relative monocytosis, and elevated levels of IgM.

Meningoencephalitic Stage. Neurologic symptoms and signs are generally nonspecific. They may precede invasion of the CNS by the organisms and present as irrational and inexplicable anxieties with frequent changes in mood. In untreated *T. b. rhodesiense* infections, invasion of the CNS occurs within 3–6 wk. It is associated with recurrent bouts of headache, fever, weakness, and signs of acute toxemia. Tachycardia from myocarditis and neurologic symptoms such as irritability, insomnia, and personality or mood changes develop. Death occurs in 6–9 mo from secondary infection or cardiac failure.

In the Gambian form cerebral symptoms can be expected to appear within 2 yr after the onset of acute symptoms, although a general increase in drowsiness during the day and insomnia at night reflect the continuous nature of the pathologic processes. Progress is characterized by increasing anemia, leukopenia, and wasting of body musculature. Patients with chronic Gambian trypanosomiasis have an increased susceptibility to secondary infections.

Involvement of the CNS results in a chronic diffuse meningoencephalitis with no localizing symptoms, commonly known as *sleeping sickness.* Drowsiness and an uncontrollable urge to sleep are the major features of this stage of the disease and may become almost continuous in the terminal stages. Associated signs and symptoms also point to involvement of the basal ganglia. Tremor or rigidity with stiff and ataxic gait may occur. Psychotic changes occur in almost one third of untreated patients.

DIAGNOSIS. Definitive diagnosis can be made during the early stages by examination of a fresh, thick blood smear, which will allow visualization of the motile active forms. Dried, Giemsa-stained smears should be examined for the detailed morphology of the organisms. If a thick blood or buffy coat smear is negative, a simple concentration method may help. Ten milliliters of heparinized blood are added to 30 mL of 0.87% ammonium chloride and the mixture is centrifuged at 1,000 g for 15 minutes. The sediment can then be examined fresh or by staining dried smears. Aspiration of an enlarged lymph node can also be used to obtain material for parasitologic examination. In every positive case a sample of cerebrospinal fluid (CSF) should also be examined for the organisms.

TREATMENT. The choice of chemotherapeutic agents depends on the stage of the infection and the causative organisms. The hematogenous forms of both Rhodesian and Gambian trypanosomiasis are susceptible to the action of suramin (Antrypol), which is available as a 10% solution for intravenous administration. A test dose of 10 mg should first be administered intravenously to detect the rare idiosyncratic reactions of shock and collapse. The dose for subsequent injections is 20 mg/kg intravenously, repeated every 5–7 days for a total of five injections. Suramin is nephrotoxic; therefore urine should be examined before each injection. The presence of marked proteinuria, blood, or casts is a contraindication to completion of therapy with suramin. An alternative for treatment of *T. b. gambiense* infection may be eflornithine, administered intravenously 400 mg/kg/24 hr in four divided doses for 14 days followed by 300 mg/kg/24 hr orally for 3–4 wk. Pentamidine, like suramin, is effective only against the hematogenous forms of the trypanosomes; moreover, its activity may be less certain in the Rhodesian form. It is administered intramuscularly as a 10% solution on alternate days for five doses. The dose for each injection is 3–4 mg/kg. Side effects of pentamidine are few; hypotension, faintness, and, occasionally, collapse may occur but can be reversed by administering epinephrine.

If invasion of the central nervous system has occurred, melarsoprol should be used. Melarsoprol contains 18.8% arsenic and is formed from the original arsenical melarsen oxide by the incorporation of dimercaprol (BAL). It is effective against all stages of both Gambian and Rhodesian trypanosomiasis but because of its arsenic content is restricted to use in patients with CNS involvement. It is administered intravenously as a 3.6% solution beginning with 0.4 mg/kg. The drug is given in three courses, each consisting of an injection on each of 3 successive days with a 1-wk interval between courses. According to the tolerance of the patient, the dose should be increased gradually to reach a maximum of 3.6 mg/kg for the 3rd course. Slight reactions such as fever and pains in the chest or abdomen may occur immediately or very soon after an injection of melarsoprol, but they are generally rare. The most important and serious of its toxic effects is encephalopathy and, less commonly, exfoliative dermatitis.

CONTROL. The control of trypanosomiasis in endemic areas of Africa depends on recognition and effective therapy of human infections and on control of the vector. This is complicated by the fact that it involves cattle and humans and by the logistics of applying the available preventive measures.

Pentamidine has been used successfully as a prophylactic drug. A single injection of 3–4 mg/kg will give protection against Gambian trypanosomiasis for at least 6 mo. Its effect against the Rhodesian form, however, is not certain.

Drugs for parasitic infections. Med Lett Drugs Therap 35:111, 1993.
Hajduk SL, Englund PT, Smith DH: African trypanosomiasis. *In:* Warren KS, Mahmoud AAF (eds): Tropical and Geographical Medicine, 2nd ed. New York, McGraw-Hill, 1990, p 268.
Haller L, Adams H, Merouze F, et al: Clinical and pathological aspects of human African trypanosomiasis *(T.b. gambiense)* with particular reference to reactive arsenical encephlopathy. Am J Trop Med Hyg 35:94, 1986.
Greenwood BM, Whittle HC: The pathogenesis of sleeping sickness. Trans R Soc Trop Med Hyg 74:716, 1980.
WHO: Epidemiology and Control of African Trypanosomiasis. Technical Report Series No. 739, Geneva, WHO, 1986.

244.11 American Trypanosomiasis

(Chagas' Disease)

Robert A. Bonomo and Robert A. Salata

Chagas' disease (American trypanosomiasis) is a zoonosis caused by the parasitic, hemoflagellate protozoan *Trypanosoma cruzi.* Endemic to Central America, South America (particularly Brazil, Argentina, Uruguay, Chile, and Venezuela), and Mexico, this illness affects over 20 million people (primarily children and young adults). This insect-transmitted infection is a major health problem largely because it frequently is asymptomatic and essentially untreatable. Primary infection usually occurs in children. Hence, because many families from these areas immigrate to the United States, it is imperative for pediatricians to be well acquainted with this disease and its complications. In addition, cases of transfusion-associated infection are increasingly being reported in the United States.

ETIOLOGY AND PATHOGENESIS. *T. cruzi* has three recognizable morphogenetic phases. Trypomastigotes are the extracellular nondividing forms and amastigotes are the intracellular replicative forms found in mammals. Epimastigotes are found in the midgut of the bloodsucking insects *Triatoma, Rhodnius,* and *Panstrongylus.* Epimastigotes multiply in the midgut and rectum of arthropods and differentiate into metacyclic trypomastigotes. The arthropod vectors for *T. cruzi* are the reduviid insects. These are also variably known as wild bedbugs, assassin bugs, or kissing bugs.

Metacyclic trypomastigotes, the infectious form for humans, are released onto the skin of a human when the insect defecates close to the site of a bite. The trypomastigotes enter the skin or damaged mucous membranes and either enter host cells or are phagocytized by macrophages. Once in the host, they multiply intracellularly as amastigotes and are released into the host's circulation when the cell dies. Amastigotes are approximately 4 μm in diameter and form clusters of oval shapes (pseudocysts) within infected tissues. The bloodstream-borne trypomastigotes circulate until they enter another host cell or are taken up by the bite of another insect. Hence, the life cycle is completed. *T. cruzi* strains have been shown to demonstrate selective parasitism for certain tissues. Most strains are myotropic, invading smooth, skeletal, and heart muscle cells.

Several surface antigens of *T. cruzi* have been identified and have been found to be glycosylated. Sera from infected humans and animals immunoblot with several major surface antigens, suggesting that these antigens may be the dominant components of *T. cruzi.* Biochemical differences between the metabolism of American trypanosomes and mammalian hosts may be exploited for chemotherapy. These trypanosomes are very sensitive to oxidative radicals, and these parasites do not process catalase or glutathione reductase-glutathione peroxidase, which are key enzymes in scavenging free radicals. All trypanosomes also have an unusual NADPH-dependent disulfide reductase. For this reason, drugs that stimulate H_2O_2 generation or prevent its utilization are potential trypanocidal agents.

T. cruzi enter macrophages by a phagocytic mechanism and are initially found in membrane-bound vacuoles. Trypanosomes lyse the phagosome membrane, escape into the cytoplasm, and replicate. Parasite attachment and phagocytosis by macrophages are mediated by protease-sensitive receptors on the surface of the macrophage.

Mechanisms for control of parasitism and resistance are not completely understood. Despite strong acquired immunity, there is no parasitologic cure. Antibodies involved with resistance to *T. cruzi* are related to the chronic phase of infection. These IgG antibodies mediate immunophagocytosis of the parasite by macrophages. Conditions associated with depression of cell-mediated immunity increase the severity of infection with *T. cruzi.* Macrophages probably play a major role in protection against *T. cruzi* infection, especially in the acute phase. Macrophages activated by gamma interferon kill intracellular amastigotes through oxidative mechanisms. Acute Chagas' disease depresses both humoral and cell-mediated immunity. The clinical importance of this depression is uncertain.

EPIDEMIOLOGY. The presence of reservoirs and vectors of *T. cruzi* and the socioeconomic and educational levels of the population are the most important factors in disease transmission. The most common mode of transmission to humans occurs via insect vectors (reduviid bugs). Housing conditions are very important in the transmission chain; the incidence and prevalence of infection depend on the adaptation of the triatomids to human dwellings as well as the vector capacity of the species. The animal reservoirs of reduviid bugs are dogs, cats, rats, opossum, and raccoons. Humans can also be infected transplacentally. *T. cruzi* passes from mother to fetus and can cause congenital Chagas' disease, which is associated with premature birth, abortion, and placentitis. Other modes of transmission are via blood transfusion and through percutaneous injection from laboratory accidents. Breast-feeding is a very uncommon mode of transmission.

CLINICAL MANIFESTATIONS. Chagas' disease occurs in acute and chronic forms. Acute Chagas' disease in children is usually asymptomatic or is associated with a mild febrile illness characterized by fever, malaise, facial edema, and lymphadenopathy. Infants often demonstrate local signs of inflammation at the site of parasite entry (chagomas). Approximately 50% of children come to medical attention with Romaña sign (unilateral, painless eye swelling). The heart, central nervous system (CNS), peripheral nerve ganglia, and reticuloendothelial system are often heavily parasitized. On histologic section, the characteristic pseudocysts are the intracellular aggregates of amastigotes. Hepatosplenomegaly and a cutaneous morbilliform eruption can accompany the acute syndrome. Anemia, lymphocytosis, hepatitis, and thrombocytopenia have been described. Mortality rates are 5–10%, caused by acute myocarditis with resultant heart failure or meningoencephalitis. Children usually undergo spontaneous remission and enter an indeterminant phase with lifelong low-grade parasitemia and development of antibodies to many *T. cruzi* cell surface antigens.

Chronic Chagas' disease is asymptomatic or symptomatic. The most common presentation of chronic *T. cruzi* infection is cardiomyopathy, manifested by congestive heart failure, arrhythmias, and thromboembolic events. Electrocardiographic abnormalities include partial or complete atrioventricular block and right bundle branch block; left bundle bunch block is unusual. Pathologic examination of infected heart muscle reveals muscle atrophy, myonecrosis, myocytolysis, fibrosis, and lymphocytic infiltration. Premature myocardial infarction has been reported and may be secondary to left apical aneurysm embolization or necrotizing arteriolitis of the microvasculature. Autonomic nervous system abnormalities have also been implicated in Chagas' cardiomyopathy. The reduction in acetylcholine and choline acetyltransferase in experimental *T. cruzi* infection lends support to this notion.

Autoimmune abnormalities have been reported in Chagas' cardiomyopathy. Depletion of $CD8^+$ cells accelerates infection. *T. cruzi* infected human peripheral blood mononuclear and endothelial cells synthesize increased levels of interleukins IL-1B, IL-6, and tumor necrosis factor, increasing white blood cell recruitment and smooth muscle cell proliferation, which may be responsible for some of the manifestations of the disease.

The gastrointestinal manifestations of chronic Chagas' disease involve a decrease in Auerbach's and Meissner's plexus. There are also preganglion lesions and a reduction in the number of dorsal motor nuclear cells of the vagus. Sigmoid dilatation, volvulus, and fecalomas are often found. These lesions can be manifested by megacolon. Loss of ganglia in the esophagus results in abnormal dilatation. The esophagus can reach up to 26 times its normal weight and hold up to 2 L of excess fluid; megaesophagus presents with dysphagia, odynophagia, and cough. Esophageal body abnormalities occur independently of lower esophageal dysfunction. Aspiration pneumonia and pulmonary tuberculosis are more common in patients with megaesophagus.

IMMUNOCOMPROMISED HOSTS. *T. cruzi* infections in the immunocompromised host are due to transmission from an asymptomatic donor of blood products or activation of prior infection by immunosuppression. Organ donation to allograft recipients can result in a devastating form of the illness. Cardiac transplantation for Chagas' cardiomyopathy resulted in reactivation, despite prophylaxis with benznidazole and postoperative treatment. Human immunodeficiency virus (HIV) infection also leads to reactivation; cerebral lesions are more common in these patients. In patients in whom the risk of reactivation is real, serologic testing and close monitoring are necessary.

DIAGNOSIS. Microscopic examination of the peripheral blood smear during the acute phase of illness is diagnostic for Chagas' disease. Motile trypanosomes on a fresh preparation of peripheral blood or Giemsa-stained smear will yield the diagnosis. Trypomastigotes are characterized by the presence of one flagellum originating in the kinetoplast, which is an extranuclear, terminally located giant mitochondrion. Serologic testing via complement fixation, indirect immunofluorescence, and ELISA are often used when direct tissue sections or parasitologic techniques do not demonstrate the organism. Mouse inoculation has also been used when repeated peripheral smears are negative. Xenodiagnosis, allowing uninfected reduviid bugs to feed on a patient's blood, and examination of the intestinal contents of reduviid bugs 30 days after the meal detects 100% of cases. PCR-based detection assays employing nuclear and kinetoplast DNA sequences (kDNA) have been developed.

TREATMENT. In treating Chagas' disease, both specific and symptomatic therapy are indicated as well as prevention and treatment of complications. Drug treatment for *T. cruzi* is generally limited to two drugs, benznidazole and nifurtimox. Both have been used to eradicate parasites in the acute stages of infection. Nifurtimox has been used most extensively but whether nifurtimox is effective in the chronic phase of the illness is uncertain. The dose for children is 15–29 mg/kg/24 hr, given in four divided doses for 90–120 days. Benznidazole is as effective as nifurtimox. The recommended dose is 5 mg/kg for 60 days. Allopurinol, a drug that inhibits hypoxanthine oxidase, has also been used. Treatment of heart failure and arrhythmias, as well as the prevention of thromboembolism, requires the use of diuretics, antiarrhythmics, and anticoagulants. Digitalis toxicity occurs frequently in patients with Chagas' cardiomyopathy. Pacemakers may be necessary in cases of severe heart block. A light, balanced diet is recommended for megaesophagus. Megaesophagus is treated by surgery or dilatation of the lower esophageal sphincter. Pneumatic dilatation is the superior mode of therapy. The use of nitrates and nifedipine have been used to reduce lower esophageal sphincter pressure in patients with megaesophagus. Surgical procedures for megaesophagus must be individualized. Treatment of megacolon is surgical and symptomatic.

PREVENTION AND CONTROL. Education of residents in endemic areas, use of bed nets, use of insecticides such as dieldrin or lindane, and the destruction of adobe houses that harbor reduviid bugs are effective methods to control the bug population. Vaccine development has been fruitless and no prophylactic therapy is available. Questionnaire-based screening of potentially infected blood donors from areas endemic for infection reduces the risk of transmission. Potential organ donors should also be screened.

Grant IH, Gold JWM, Wittner M, et al: Transfusion associated acute Chagas' disease acquired in the USA. Ann Intern Med 111:849, 1989.
Kirchhoff LV: Chagas disease: American trypanosomiasis. *In:* Maguire JH, Keystone JS (eds): Infectious Disease Clinics of North America, Vol 7. Philadelphia, WB Saunders, 1993, p 487.
Kirchhoff LV: Trypanosomiasis (Chaga's disease): A tropical disease now in the United States. N Engl J Med 329:639, 1993.
Nickerson P, Orr P, Schroeder ML, et al: Transfusion-associated *Trypanosoma cruzi* in a infection in a non-endemic area. Ann Intern Med 111:851, 1989.
Nogueira N, Coura JR: American trypanosomiasis (Chagas' disease). *In:* Warren K, Mahmoud A (eds): Tropical and Geographical Medicine, 2nd ed. New York, McGraw-Hill, 1989.
Taenias HB, Kirchhoff LV, Simon D, et al: Chagas' disease. Clin Microbiol Rev 5:400, 1992.

CHAPTER 245

Helminthic Diseases

James W. Kazura

NEMATODES

(Roundworms)

Intestinal Nematodes

Infection with intestinal roundworms is the most common type of helminthiasis of humans. Although these infections are more prevalent in tropical and subtropical climates, individuals residing in temperate and cold regions are not spared. Children generally are more heavily infected than adults and are therefore more likely to suffer from the pathologic consequences of these infections. Intestinal nematodes may infect humans either directly by ingestion of mature eggs or indirectly via larval penetration of skin. With the exception of *Strongyloides stercoralis,* the adult stages of these nematodes live in the lumen of the intestinal tract and do not multiply in the human host. Although intestinal nematode infections are not usually associated with peripheral blood eosinophilia, increased eosinophil counts often develop during the phase of infection when parasite larvae migrate through host tissues. The more prevalent intestinal roundworm infections of children will be discussed according to their final location in the gut: small intestine (*Ascaris lumbricoides, Ancylostoma duodenale, Necator americanus,* and *Strongyloides stercoralis*), cecum (*Enterobius vermicularis*), and large intestine (*Trichuris trichiura*).

TREMATODES
(Flukes)

Parasitic trematodes form a group of important human infections that are endemic worldwide but are more prevalent in the less developed parts of the world. Trematodes are characterized by their complex life cycle; sexual reproduction of adult worms in the definitive host is followed by asexual multiplication by the larval stages in the intermediate host. This "alternation of generations" requires that flukes parasitize more than one host (often three) to complete their life cycle.

CESTODES
(Tapeworms)

Human infection with cestodes constitutes a considerable burden of parasitism in many parts of the world. Most commonly adult worms parasitize the gastrointestinal tract, causing little or no clinical morbidity except when they interfere with host nutrition. Major clinical syndromes may occur, however, when humans are infected with the larval stages of some cestodes that disseminate and can cause disease in any internal organ.

245.1 Ascariasis

James W. Kazura

Infection with *Ascaris lumbricoides* is the most prevalent human helminthiasis and produces an estimated 1 billion cases worldwide. Infection is most common in children of preschool or early school age. Ascariasis is ubiquitous; the greatest number of cases occur in countries having warmer climates. Nevertheless, there are approximately 4 million infected individuals, mainly children, in North America.

ETIOLOGY. The infective stage of *A. lumbricoides* is the mature larva-containing egg. It is broadly oval, has a thick shell with an outer mamillated covering, and measures approximately 40 × 60 μm (Fig. 245–1). Eggs are passed in the feces of infected individuals and mature in 5–10 days under favorable environmental conditions to become infective. After ingestion by the human host, larvae are released from the eggs and penetrate the intestinal wall before migrating to the lungs via the venous circulation. They then break through the pulmonary tissues into the alveolar spaces, ascend the bronchial tree and trachea, and are reswallowed. Upon their arrival in the small intestine, the larvae develop into mature adult worms (males measure 15–25 cm × 3 mm and females 25–35 cm × 4 mm). Each female has a lifespan of 1–2 yr and is capable of producing 200,000 eggs/day.

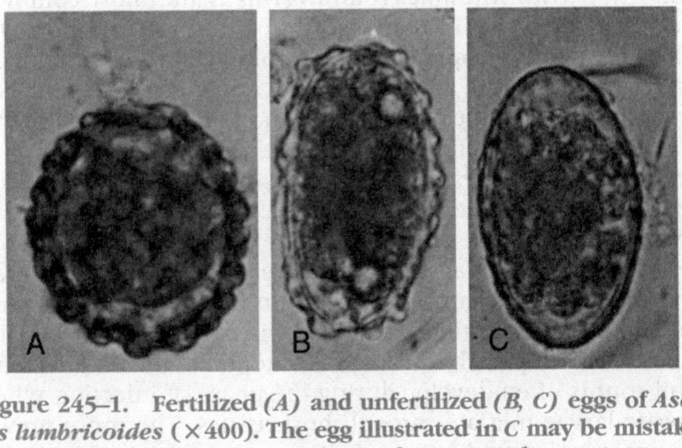

Figure 245–1. Fertilized *(A)* and unfertilized *(B, C)* eggs of *Ascaris lumbricoides* (×400). The egg illustrated in *C* may be mistaken for that of a different nematode or of a trematode.

EPIDEMIOLOGY. Ascariasis, a soil-transmitted infection, depends on dissemination of eggs into environmental conditions that are suitable for their maturation. Promiscuous defecation and use of human manure are the two most important unhygienic practices responsible for the endemicity of ascariasis. The mode of transmission to humans is hand to mouth; the fingers are contaminated by soil contact. Alternatively, food items (particularly those commonly consumed raw) become infected by human fertilizers or by flies. Endemicity of *A. lumbricoides* is aided by the extremely high egg output of worms and their resistance to unfavorable environmental conditions. Eggs have been shown to remain infective in soil for months and may survive cooler weather (5–10° C) for 2 yr. Transmission of ascariasis may occur seasonally or throughout the year.

CLINICAL MANIFESTATIONS. Although disease sequelae occur in only a small proportion of infected individuals, they amount to a significant clinical problem because of the high incidence of ascariasis. Morbidity may be manifested during migration of the larvae through the lungs or be associated with the presence of adult worms in the small intestine. The pathogenesis of pulmonary ascariasis is not known, although a hypersensitivity phenomenon may be involved. Adult worms may cause disease by obstructing the gut or biliary tree and by affecting host nutrition. The nutritional status of children with ascariasis may be affected more by their socioeconomic and nutritional background than by the effects of the *Ascaris* infection.

Pulmonary ascariasis may occur following heavy exposure and is also common in individuals who live in areas with seasonal transmission of infection (seasonal pneumonitis). The most characteristic features are cough, blood-stained sputum, and eosinophilia. This Loeffler-like syndrome may be associated with transient pulmonary infiltrates. In children the differentiation of this syndrome from visceral larva migrans may be difficult, but abdominal symptoms or signs are very rare in pulmonary ascariasis.

The presence of adult worms in the small intestine is associated with vague complaints such as abdominal pain and distention. Intestinal obstruction, although rare, may be due to a mass of worms in heavily infected children; the peak incidence occurs in children 1–6 yr old. The onset is usually sudden, with severe colicky abdominal pain and vomiting, which may be bile stained; these symptoms may progress rapidly and follow a course similar to acute intestinal obstruction of any other etiology. Migration of *Ascaris* worms into the biliary tract has also been reported, particularly occurring in China and the Philippines; the likelihood of this condition increases in heavily infected children. The onset is acute with colicky abdominal pain, nausea, vomiting, and fever. Jaundice is rarely seen.

Steatorrhea and diminished vitamin A absorption have occurred in some *Ascaris*-infected children. A study of Colombian children with moderate infections (30–50 worms) showed that administration of anthelmintic drugs was followed by decreased fat and nitrogen excretion and improved xylose absorption.

DIAGNOSIS. Adult female worms deposit eggs that can be detected by direct fecal smear examination and quantified by the Kato thick smear method. Bisexual infections result in the excretion of mature fertile eggs, whereas infertile eggs are seen in individuals infected with female worms only (Fig. 245–1*B* and *C*). Diagnosis of pulmonary or obstructive ascariasis is based primarily on clinical data and a high index of suspicion.

TREATMENT. Several chemotherapeutic agents are effective against ascariasis; none, however, is useful during the pulmonary phase of the infection. Treatment, particularly of children with heavy infections, should be approached with caution. Piperazine salts (citrate, adipate, or phosphate) are administered orally in a daily dose of 50–75 mg/kg for 2 days. A single dose rather than 2-day regimens is effective in reducing worm loads in infected children. Because piperazine results in neuromuscular paralysis of the parasite and a relatively rapid expulsion of the worms, it is the drug of choice for intestinal or biliary obstruction. Because sporadic hypersensitivity and neurotoxic reactions have been reported with piperazine derivatives, other drugs such as mebendazole (100 mg twice daily for 3 days) should be used for treating uncomplicated intestinal ascariasis. Rarely, surgical treatment may be needed in severe obstructive cases.

CONTROL. Although ascariasis is the most prevalent worm infection worldwide, little attention has been given to its control, partly because of controversy concerning its clinical significance and also because of its unique epidemiologic features. Attempts at reducing worm loads in humans by mass chemotherapy have shown some promise. Because of the high rate of reinfection, chemotherapy has to be repeated at 3- to 6-mo intervals. The feasibility and cost of such an undertaking will have to be evaluated before it can be widely accepted. Sanitary practices directed at treating human feces before it is used as fertilizer and providing hygienic sewage disposal facilities may be the most effective long-term preventive measures against ascariasis.

Louw JH: Abdominal complications of *Ascaris lumbricoides* infestation in children. Br J Surg 53:510, 1966.

Pawlowski ZS: Ascariasis. *In:* Warren KS, Mahmoud AAF (eds): Tropical and Geographical Medicine. New York, McGraw-Hill, 1990, p 369.

Spillman RK: Pulmonary ascariasis in tropical communities. Am J Trop Med Hyg 24:791, 1975.

Stephenson LS, Crompton DWT, Latham MC, et al: Relationship between *Ascaris* infection and growth of malnourished preschool children in Kenya. Am J Clin Nutr 33:1165, 1980.

245.2 Cestodiases

Ronald Blanton

Cestode or tapeworm infections are prevalent on every continent except Antarctica. Unlike many parasites that strictly separate their developmental stages in different host species, some tapeworms can infect humans with the adult worm stage, the invasive intermediate stage, or all stages. Adult tapeworms rarely cause serious morbidity. The intermediate stages, however, are invasive and form cystic structures that result in tissue damage from mass effect or inflammatory reactions. Infection with the adult worm can be easily diagnosed by observing eggs or segments of adult worms in the stool, whereas the invasive stage of the parasite cannot be observed in any easily sampled fluid. Infection with an intermediate stage, therefore, must be diagnosed by serology, imaging, or invasive procedures.

TAENIASIS AND DIPHYLLOBOTHRIASIS

(Giant tapeworms)

ETIOLOGY. The adult beef tapeworm *(Taenia saginata)*, pork tapeworm *(Taenia solium)*, and fish tapeworm *(Diphyllobothrium latum)* are the largest human parasites, ranging in size from 4 to 10 m. Thousands of flattened segments (proglottids) make up the body of adult worms. The most anterior segment of each worm, the scolex, is equipped with suckers and hooklets that serve to anchor the parasite in the intestine. This arrangement is unique for each species. Each of the subsequent segments contains its own reproductive organs and is largely independent of the others. Mature, terminal proglottids are packed with thousands of eggs. The proglottids of taenids (beef and pork tapeworms) generally pass intact in the stool. By contrast, the proglottids of *Diphyllobothrium* often disintegrate in the bowel, and since up to 1 million eggs can be released per day, the eggs are easily observed in stool.

Only the adult forms of the beef and fish tapeworms infect humans. Humans, however, may host both the adult and intermediate forms of the pork tapeworm, and thus *T. solium* is the most serious pathogen in this group. Humans are infected with the adult worms when they consume raw or undercooked pork containing parasitic cysts. Digestion releases the juvenile worms (protoscolices), which then attach to the lumen of the small intestine. *T. solium* is the only giant tapeworm whose scolex is equipped with hooklets in addition to suckers. Humans acquire the intermediate form (cysticercus) when they ingest food or water contaminated with the eggs of *T. solium*. Digestion of the eggshell releases a stage of the parasite that invades the intestinal mucosa and spreads hematogenously to many tissues, but primarily brain and muscle. They develop into small (0.2–0.5 cm), fluid-filled bladders containing a single protoscolex. It is not necessary to consume pork in order to acquire cysticercosis. It only requires ingestion of food or water contaminated with feces containing eggs. Thus the disease may develop in individuals whose religious practices forbid pork consumption. Individuals infected with an adult worm may infect themselves with eggs by the fecal-oral route. Reverse peristalsis in the small intestine has also been implicated as another means of autoinfection.

The life cycle of *D. latum* is distinct from the taenids because it develops in two intermediate hosts. Eggs hatch in fresh water on exposure to light, then newly released parasites are swallowed and develop within small crustaceans (copepods). The parasite passes up the food chain as small fish eat the copepods and are in turn eaten by larger fish. In this way the parasite becomes concentrated in pike, walleye, perch, salmon, and similar fish. Consumption of raw or undercooked fish leads to human infection with adult worms.

EPIDEMIOLOGY. The beef and pork tapeworms are distributed worldwide. Though some person-to-person spread has been documented in the United States, this is uncommon. The risk of infection is much higher in Central America, Africa, India, Indonesia, and China. For both *Taenia* species, human infection is a necessary part of the transmission cycle. The fish tapeworm is much more prevalent in the temperate climates of Europe and Asia, but may be found in cold lakes at high altitude in South America and Africa. In North America, the prevalence is highest in Alaska, Canada, and the northern United States as well as in fish originating there. Part of the Arctic transmission cycle may involve polar bears, seals, walruses, and other fish-loving mammals. Thus, despite attaining adequate levels of hygiene in the human population, infection with the fish tapeworm can continue as a zoonosis.

PATHOGENESIS AND PATHOLOGY. Infection with the adult beef or pork tapeworm alone is an infrequent source of problems. Infection with the cystic, intermediate form (the cysticercus), however, is the most common parasitic cause of central nervous system (CNS) disease. The brain is the organ that is most sensitive to the presence of cysts, but very heavy infections in skeletal or heart muscle can result in myositis. The initial parasite invasion of the brain may cause encephalitis-like symptoms, particularly in children. Otherwise the cysts are frequently silent until they begin to degenerate and a marked inflammatory response precipitates a variety of neurologic complications. Intact cysts may also cause disease when they obstruct cerebrospinal fluid (CSF) flow. The fourth ventricle is the most common site of obstruction.

No signs or symptoms can clearly be attributed to infection

with any adult tapeworm except for *Diphyllobothrium* infection. In some instances (<2%), diphyllobothriasis causes megaloblastic anemia due to vitamin B_{12} and folate absorption by the parasite. The adult efficiently scavenges this vitamin for its own use in the constant production of large numbers of segments and eggs. The parasite also inhibits vitamin B_{12} uptake by inactivating the B_{12}-intrinsic factor complex. Persons who prepare raw fish for home or commercial use or who sample fish prior to cooking are particularly at risk for infection. Other causes of vitamin B_{12} or folate deficiency predispose toward development of symptomatic infection.

CLINICAL MANIFESTATIONS. Apart from nonspecific abdominal symptoms, adult tapeworms cause very little overt morbidity. The protoscolices of the beef tapeworm are motile and will at times produce anal pruritis as they emerge. They are thus more likely to be noticed, causing shock and horror when discovered, but no overt disease.

Cysticerci of *T. solium* are distributed widely in the body. Small cysts can sometimes be palpated under the skin, but they primarily cause disease when located in the brain. Simply stated, any neurologic, cognitive, or personality disorder in an individual from an endemic area may represent neurocysticercosis. Neurocysticercosis can usually be classified based on its clinical presentation and radiologic appearance as parenchymal, intraventricular, meningeal, spinal, or ocular. Parenchymal disease tends to produce focal rather than generalized seizures as well as other focal neurologic deficits. Rarely, there can be cerebral infarction due to obstruction of small terminal arteries or vasculitis. With extensive frontal lobe disease, symptoms of intellectual deterioration with dementia or parkinsonism may not suggest the diagnosis until focal signs appear. There is also a fulminant encephalitis-like presentation, most frequently seen in children and patients with multiple, diffuse parenchymal lesions.

Intraventricular neurocysticercosis is associated with hydrocephalus and acute, subacute, or intermittent signs of increased intracranial pressure without localizing signs. Chronic basilar meningitis is associated with many forms of neurocysticercosis, but some presentations are predominantly meningeal. In addition to signs of meningeal irritation, this form shows increased intracranial pressure due to either edema and inflammation or the presence of a cyst obstructing flow. Racemose cysticercosis is a form of meningeal cysticercosis in which large, lobulated cysts appear in the basal cisterns. Ocular cysticercosis causes decreased visual acuity due to cysticerci floating in the vitreous, retinal detachment, or iridocyclitis. In spinal neurocysticercosis patients present with evidence of cord compression, nerve root pain, transverse myelitis, or meningitis.

Diphyllobothriasis when symptomatic is associated with easy fatigability, fever, edema, glossitis, paresthesias, or signs of dorsal column and corticospinal tract degeneration, that is, loss of vibratory sense, proprioception, and lack of coordination. These neurologic signs may appear in the absence of megaloblastic anemia.

DIAGNOSIS. Parasitologic examination of the stool is useful for diagnosis of fish tapeworm infection but is less sensitive for detecting infection with the adult beef and pork tapeworms. In addition, the eggs of *T. saginata* and *T. solium* (Fig. 245–2) cannot be reliably distinguished. Though often absent from stool, they can be demonstrated by rectal swab or microscopic examination of adhesive tape applied near the rectum, as for diagnosis of pinworm infection. If the parasite is completely expelled, the scolex of each species is diagnostic. With some expertise the proglottids of *T. saginata* can be distinguished from *T. solium*. Fish tapeworm eggs have a distinctive morphology. The eggs are ovoid and have a caplike operculum that opens to release the embryo inside (Fig. 245–3).

Cysticercosis should be suspected in any child with the proper epidemiologic background (residence in an endemic area or with a caretaker from an endemic area) who presents with any neurologic, cognitive, or personality disorder. In particular a seizure, hydrocephalus, unilateral visual impairment, or symptoms of encephalitis are suspicious. Eggs are observed in only 25% of cases of cysticercosis; therefore, imaging studies and, at times, serologic tests are the only way to confirm a clinical suspicion. Plain films may reveal calcifications in muscle or brain consistent with cysticercosis, but these are more often negative in children than adults. Eosinophilia is sometimes observed in the CSF, but this is not a reliable finding. The most useful study is computed tomography (CT) scanning. A solitary parenchymal cyst with or without contrast enhancement and multiple calcifications are the most common findings in children (Fig. 245–4). Intraventricular cysts are found in 11–17% of neurocysticercosis cases. These are difficult to detect because the cyst fluid often has the same density as CSF. Magnetic resonance imaging may (MRI) better detect intraventricular cysts as well as those in the spinal cord by delineating parasite membranes and differences in signal intensity between the fluids. Hydrocephalus on CT scan may indicate intraventricular cysts or may result from meningeal inflammation. Fifty percent of patients have more than one form of disease.

Serologic diagnosis using the ELISA or immunoblot techniques is available in the United States through the Centers for Disease Control (CDC). When possible both serum and CSF should be obtained for testing. CSF has the highest specificity and sensitivity, but the serum is also usually positive. All of the present serologic tests crossreact with other cestode infections and cannot distinguish between intestinal infection with just the adult form and cysticerci in the CNS.

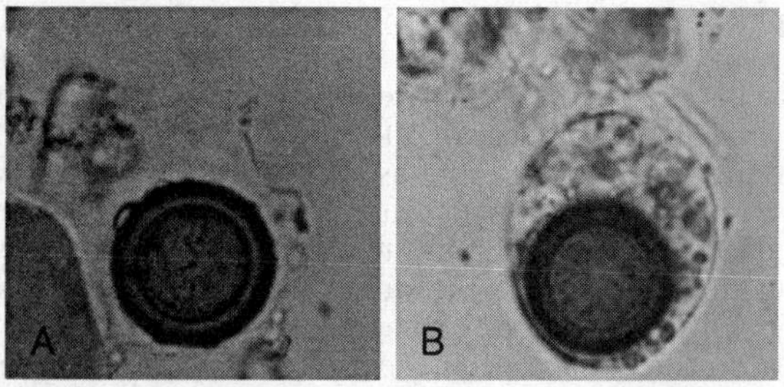

Figure 245–2. Eggs of *Taenia saginata* recovered from fresh feces (×400). The cellular structure in which the egg develops while in the proglottid, more evident in *B* than in *A*, may be retained around the dark prismatic egg membrane that contains the larva. Usually evident in the larva are three pairs of hooklets (*A*), which may occasionally be seen in motion.

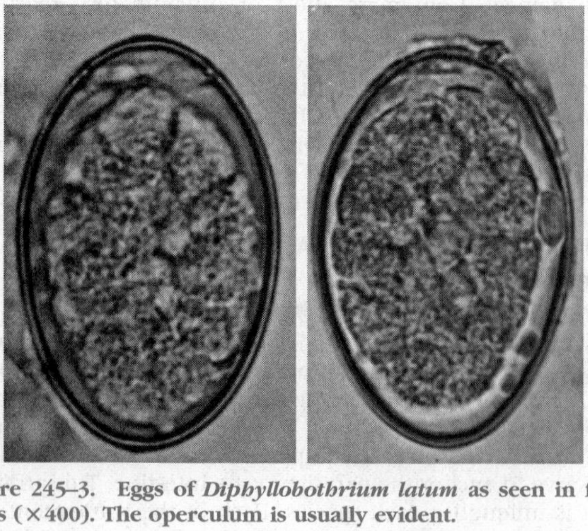

Figure 245–3. Eggs of *Diphyllobothrium latum* as seen in fresh feces (×400). The operculum is usually evident.

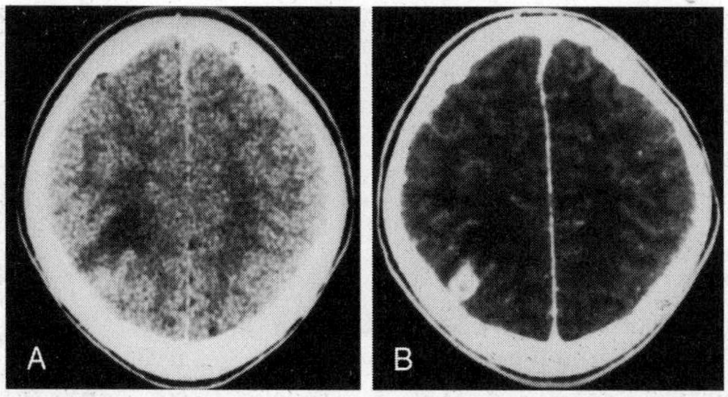

Figure 245–4. CT image of a solitary lesion of neurocysticercosis before (*A*) and after (*B*) contrast enhancement. (Courtesy of Dr. Wendy G. Mitchell and Dr. Marvin D. Nelson, Children's Hospital, Los Angeles.)

DIFFERENTIAL DIAGNOSIS. Clinically the disease presentation can be confused with encephalitis, stroke, meningitis, and many other conditions unless there is clinical suspicion based on travel history or history of contact with another individual who might carry an adult worm. On imaging studies, cysticerci can be mistaken for calcified tuberculomas, toxoplasmosis, or CNS tumor.

PREVENTION. Prolonged freezing or thorough cooking of beef, pork, and fish will kill the parasite. Attention to personal hygiene and avoidance of fresh fruits and vegetables in areas endemic for *T. solium* helps prevent ingestion of eggs. All members of a family of an index case of cysticercosis should be examined for the presence of eggs or signs of disease.

TREATMENT. Infection with adult tapeworms responds to niclosamide or praziquantel. For niclosamide, children weighing 11–34 kg should receive a single dose of two tablets (1 g), and if greater than 34 kg, three tablets. The tablets should be thoroughly chewed after a light meal. Praziquantel is also effective in a single dose of 5–10 mg/kg. Since praziquantel is absorbed and causes the death of cysticerci, it should be administered with great caution in suspected cases of *T. solium* infection.

Two effective anticysticercal drugs are available, albendazole (15 mg/kg/day in three doses for 28 days and taken with a fatty meal to improve absorption) and praziquantel (50 mg/kg/day in three doses for 15 days). The specific treatment of neurocysticercosis, however, depends on the form of the disease. Some issues involving when and how to treat are still not entirely resolved. Children with seizures, no hydrocephalus, and with only calcified, inactive lesions on CT do not require therapy other than antiepileptics. If no anticysticercal drugs will be administered, however, it should also be determined that these patients do not carry adult worms. Active parenchymal lesions may resolve on their own, but a retrospective study of 240 patients indicated that treatment with albendazole or praziquantel was associated with fewer residual seizures on long-term follow-up. Albendazole in several studies appears to produce a somewhat better outcome than praziquantel, and the drug should soon be approved for use in the United States. A worsening of symptoms often follows the use of either drug as the host responds to the dying parasite with increased inflammation. Corticosteroids can ameliorate these effects, but they may decrease praziquantel levels by as much as 50%. In contrast, albendazole levels increase in the presence of corticosteroids. Medical therapy may convert quiescent lesions to active ones or worsen ventricular, ocular, or spinal disease. A ventricular shunt must be placed prior to medical therapy whenever there is evidence of hydrocephalus, or ventricular or spinal disease. Surgery should be limited to placement of shunts, removal of large, solitary cysts for decompression, removal of mobile cysts causing ventricular obstruction, and some cases that fail to respond to medical therapy. Spillage of cyst contents during surgery is not associated with disseminating the parasite as it is with echinococcosis. Ocular cysticercosis is essentially a surgical disease. The outcome is not good in any case and enucleation is frequently required.

Barry M, Kaldjian LC: Neurocysticercosis. Semin Neurol 13:131, 1993.
Del Brutto OH, Sotelo J: Neurocysticercosis: An update. Rev Infect Dis 10:1085, 1988.
Mitchell WG, Crawford TD: Intraparenchymal cerebral cysticercosis in children: diagnosis and treatment. Pediatrics 82:76, 1988.
Richards F, Schantz PM: Laboratory diagnosis of cysticercosis. Clin Lab Med 11:1011, 1991.
Vazquez V, Sotelo J: The course of seizures after treatment for cerebral cysticercosis. N Engl J Med 327:696, 1992.

HYMENOLEPIASIS

(Dwarf Tapeworms)

Infection with *Hymenolepis nana* is very common in developing countries, and, though it rarely causes overt disease, the presence of *H. nana* eggs in stool may serve as a marker for the hygienic conditions a child has experienced. The parasite has its intermediate stages in various hosts, including rodents, ticks, and fleas. Its entire life cycle can be completed, however, in humans. There is thus the potential for hyperinfection with thousands of small adult worms in a single child. Other seemingly benign intestinal worm infections have been shown to retard childhood growth, but the effect of cestode infection on nutritional status and development have not been studied. As with other adult cestodes, *H. nana* can be treated with niclosamide or praziquantel, but the daily dose of niclosamide should be continued for 6 days to eradicate parasites as they develop into adult worms. Praziquantel can be given as a single dose of 25 mg/kg.

245.3 Echinococcosis

Ronald Blanton

ETIOLOGY. Echinococcosis is the most prevalent, serious human cestode infection in the world yet it is a zoonosis. Two species are responsible for two distinct clinical presentations, *Echinococcus granulosus* (cystic hydatid) and the more malignant *E. multilocularis* (alveolar hydatid). Dogs, wolves, dingoes, jackals, coyotes, and foxes are hosts to the small adult worms (2–7 mm), composed of two to six proglottids. These have scolices which are armed with a double row of 35–40 hooks. Eggs from adult worms are passed in stool and contaminate the soil and water, as well as the coat of the dogs themselves. In the case of *E. granulosus*, domestic animals such as sheep, goats, cattle, and camels ingest the eggs while grazing. The intermediate forms penetrate the gut and are carried by the vascular or lymphatic systems to the liver, lungs, and other tissues in the body. Humans are infected with the intermediate stage of the parasite when they ingest food or water contaminated with eggs or from direct contact with infected dogs. The risk for human infection is greatest in the peridomestic dog/sheep cycle. A sylvatic cycle also exists for *E. granulosus* in a wolf/moose cycle in North America but is of less importance for transmission to humans. The transmission cycle of *E. multilocularis* is similar to that of *E. granulosus*, except that this species is mainly sylvatic and uses small rodents as its natural intermediate host. The rodents are consumed by foxes, their natural predators, and sometimes dogs and cats.

EPIDEMIOLOGY. *E. granulosus* thrives in environments as diverse as arctic tundra and the deserts of North Africa. Wherever animals are herded by humans with the help of dogs, there is potential for transmission of this parasite. Cysts have been detected in up to 10% of the population in Northern Kenya and Western China. Among developed countries, the disease is well known in Italy, Greece, and Australia. In the United States there is transmission in Alaska, as well as foci in sheepherding areas of the western states and Isle Royale on Lake Superior, where there is a wolf/moose cycle.

Transmission of *E. multilocularis* occurs primarily in temperate climates of Northern Europe, Siberia, Turkey, and China. There is also an extensive area of transmission in Alaska, Canada, and the central United States as far south as the state of Nebraska. A separate species *(E. vogeli)* causes polycystic disease similar to alveolar hydatidosis in South America.

PATHOGENESIS AND PATHOLOGY. In areas endemic for *E. granulosus* the parasite is often acquired in childhood, but liver cysts require many years to become large enough to detect or cause symptoms. Their growth rate is estimated to be 1 cm/yr. In time, some cysts will reach more than 20 cm in diameter. The right lobe of the liver is the most common site for development of cysts. Cysts can be found in many other sites, however, including bone, brain, and subcutaneous tissues. With cystic hydatidosis from *E. granulosus* infection, the established cyst undergoes internal budding of daughter cysts that remain contained within the larger primary structure. The host surrounds this cyst with a tough, fibrous capsule. The primary cyst also produces a thick lamellar layer that supports a thin germinal layer of cells responsible for budding and production of thousands of juvenile-stage parasites (protoscolices) that remain attached to the wall or are free in the cyst fluid. The fluid in a healthy cyst is clear and watery. After medical treatment it may become thick and bile stained.

Reproduction in *E. multilocularis* resembles a malignancy. The secondary reproductive units bud externally and are not confined within a single, well-defined structure. Further, the cyst tissues are poorly demarcated from those of the host. This makes these cysts unsuitable for surgical removal. The secondary cysts are also capable of distant metastatic spread. The growing cyst mass eventually replaces a significant portion of the liver and compromises adjacent tissues and structures.

CLINICAL MANIFESTATIONS. Many cysts never become symptomatic and regress spontaneously. Those that become symptomatic have relatively nonspecific symptoms early on. Later, there is increased abdominal girth, hepatomegaly, a palpable mass, vomiting, or abdominal pain. The more serious complications, however, are due to compression of adjacent structures, spillage of cyst contents, and location of cysts in sensitive areas such as the reproductive tract, brain, and bone. Jaundice due to cystic hydatid is rare. Though the majority of cysts occur in the liver, the second most common site is the lungs, where cysts produce chest pain, coughing, or hemoptysis. Bone cysts may cause pathologic fractures, and in the genitourinary system they can produce hematuria or infertility.

In alveolar hydatid disease, cyst tissue continues to proliferate and may separate and metastasize distantly. The proliferating mass sufficiently compromises hepatic tissue or the biliary system to cause progressive obstructive jaundice and hepatic failure.

DIAGNOSIS. Because humans are infected only with the intermediate stage of *Echinococcus* species, the parasite cannot be recovered from an easily accessible body fluid. Subcutaneous nodules, hepatomegaly, or a palpable mass may present on physical examination. Ultrasound has proven a very valuable tool in the diagnosis of hydatid disease. Portable machines and generators have made survey of even isolated populations possible. Benign, simple cysts of the liver are relatively common, but the presence of internal membranes suggests hydatid disease. Alveolar disease is less cystic in appearance and resembles a diffuse but solid tumor. The CT scan findings are similar to those of ultrasound (Fig. 245–5) and can at times be useful in distinguishing alveolar from cystic hydatid in areas where both occur.

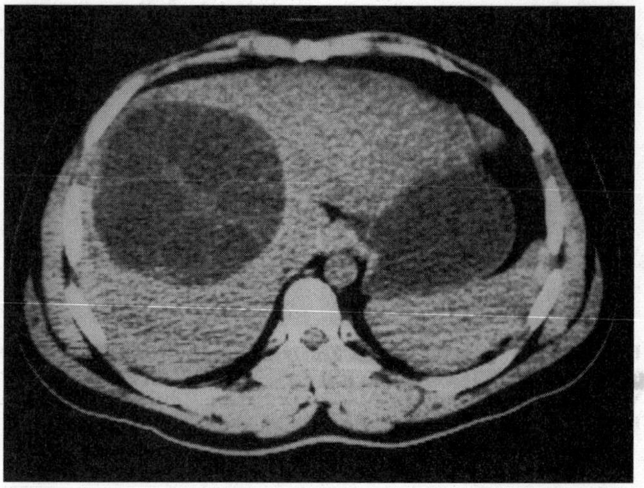

Figure 245–5. CT image of an *E. granulosus* hydatid cyst. The membranes of multiple daughter cysts are visible within the primary cyst structure. (Courtesy of Dr. John R. Haaga, University Hospitals, Cleveland.)

Serologic studies can be useful in confirming a diagnosis of echinococcosis, but the false-negative rate may be as high as 50% in cystic hydatid disease of the lung or where there are only young, intact liver cysts. Most patients with alveolar hydatidosis, however, develop detectable antibody responses. Current tests utilize crude or partially purified antigens that can crossreact in individuals infected with other parasites, such as cysticercosis or schistosomiasis. Antigens based on recombinant DNA technology are being developed and promise greater sensitivity and specificity.

DIFFERENTIAL DIAGNOSIS. Benign hepatic cysts can usually be distinguished from cystic hydatid on ultrasound by the presence of internal structures. The density of hepatic abscesses is distinct from the cystic character of *E. granulosus* infection, but hydatid cysts may be complicated by secondary bacterial infection. Alveolar echinococcosis is often confused with hepatoma and cirrhosis, and also presents features suggestive of pancreatic carcinoma, metastatic liver disease, and cholangitis.

PREVENTION. Important maneuvers to interrupt transmission include avoiding contact with dogs in endemic areas, boiling or filtering water when camping, proper disposal of animal carcasses, and good meat inspection. Strict procedures for disposal of refuse from slaughterhouses must be instituted and followed, so that dogs or wild carnivores do not have access to entrails. Other useful measures are control or treatment of the feral dog population and regular treatment of pets and working dogs in endemic areas with praziquantel.

TREATMENT. Albendazole is the preferred drug for treatment of cystic hydatidosis. The dosage and administration are the same as for cysticercosis, but the course is often repeated for four or more courses with 15-day drug-free intervals. There is no morbid inflammatory response to treatment as there is with cysticercosis, so steroids are not indicated. A positive response is seen in 40–60% of patients. Ultrasound indications of successful therapy are change in shape from spherical to elliptical or flat, progressive increase in echogenicity, and detachment of membranes from the capsule (water lily sign); additional CT criteria are reduction in diameter and augmented density of cyst fluid up to that of other tissues. Though contraindicated in the past, percutaneous drainage of cysts under ultrasound guidance with albendazole therapy has increasingly been used with success for complete resolution of cystic disease. Spillage is surprisingly uncommon. Medical therapy slows the progression of alveolar hydatid, but if feasible, radical surgery for removal of the infected tissue is indicated.

Solitary lesions may be amenable to surgery, particularly after albendazole therapy. Prior to removal, a sample of the cyst fluid is removed for parasitologic examination and the cyst is then injected with a scolicidal agent such as hypertonic saline or cetrimide. Considerable care must be taken to ensure that there is no spillage of cyst contents, because cyst fluid contains viable protoscolices, each capable of producing secondary cysts wherever they lodge. There is also a risk for developing anaphylaxis to spilled cyst fluid as a result of surgery, spontaneous rupture, or trauma. The inner cyst wall is easily peeled from the fibrous layer; the cavity is then topically sterilized and either closed or filled with omentum. Alveolar hydatidosis is frequently incurable by any modality, but radical surgery such as partial hepatectomy or lobectomy may cure early limited disease.

PROGNOSIS. Factors predictive of success with chemotherapy are age of the cyst (>2 yr), low internal complexity of the cyst, and small size. The site of the cyst is not important, except that cysts in bone respond poorly. For alveolar hydatid, unless there is successful radical surgery, the average mortality is 92% by 10 yr after diagnosis.

Filice C, Di Perri G, Strosselli M, et al: Parasitologic findings in percutaneous drainage of human hydatid liver cysts. J Infect Dis 161:1290, 1990.
Gottstein B: *Echinococcus multilocularis* infection: Immunology and immunodiagnosis. Adv Parasitol 31:321, 1992.
Khuroo MS, Dar MY, Yattoo GN, et al: Percutaneous drainage versus albendazole therapy in hepatic hydatidosis: A prospective, randomized study. Gastroenterology 104:1452, 1993.
Teggi A, Lastilla MG, De Rosa F: Therapy of human hydatid disease with mebendazole and albendazole. Antimicrob Agents Chemother 37:1679, 1993.
Todorov T, Mechkov G, Vutova K, et al: Factors influencing the response to chemotherapy in human cystic echinococcosis. Bull WHO 70:347, 1992.

245.4 Dracunculiasis

(Guinea Worm Infection)

James W. Kazura

Dracunculiasis occurs in all areas of the tropics and is especially common in India and West Africa. The parasite, *Dracunculus medinensis,* infects humans when they swallow larva-containing microscopic crustaceans (copepods) living in communal water sites. Adult worms grow to a length of 1 m or more and migrate through the subcutaneous tissues of the lower extremities (or occasionally other sites). An ulcer is produced where they penetrate the skin. The diagnosis is confirmed by identifying larvae contained in washings from the base of the lesion. Administering niridazole (12.5 mg/kg/24 hr for 10 days) or thiabendazole (50 mg/kg/24 hr for 3 days) diminishes the local inflammatory response and permits removal of the helminth. Infection may be prevented by avoiding ingestion of water that humans walk in or use for bathing. Boiling or chlorination kills the organism.

245.5 Enterobiasis

(Pinworm)

James W. Kazura

Enterobius vermicularis infection occurs worldwide and affects individuals of all ages and socioeconomic levels but is especially common in children. Living in congested districts, institutions, or families with pinworm infections predisposes to enterobiasis. The infection is essentially harmless and causes more social than medical problems in affected children and their families.

ETIOLOGY. Humans are infected by ingesting embryonated eggs, which are usually carried on fingernails, clothing, bedding, or house dust. Eggs hatch in the stomach and larvae, and migrate to the cecal region, where they mature into adult worms. *E. vermicularis* are small (1 cm) white worms; the gravid females migrate by night to the perianal region to deposit masses of eggs. Pinworm ova are asymmetric, are flattened on one side, and measure 30 × 60 μm. After a 6-hr maturation period a single-coiled larva can be seen within each ovum. These larvae may remain viable for 20 days.

EPIDEMIOLOGY. Perianal irritation during oviposition by female worms induces scratching. Eggs carried under the fingernails are transmitted directly or disseminated in the environment to infect others. Humans are the only natural hosts of *E. vermicularis.* The prevalence and intensity of infection are low in infants and young children and reach a peak in the 5- to 14-yr-old age group; the prevalence decreases in adulthood because of either reduced exposure or acquisition of immunity.

CLINICAL MANIFESTATIONS. Many local and systemic signs and symptoms have been ascribed to *Enterobius* infection; however, a controlled study of infected children 2–12 yr old failed to document specific syndromes due to *E. vermicularis.* Symptomatic individuals most commonly complain of nocturnal anal pruritus and sleeplessness. The etiology and incidence of perianal and perineal irritation are unknown but may be related to the intensity of infection, to the psychiatric profile of the infected individual and his or her family, or to an allergic reaction to the parasite. Because tissue invasion does not occur in most cases of enterobiasis, eosinophilia is not observed. In a few cases, however, *E. vermicularis* has been recovered from ectopic sites, such as the appendix, female genital tract, and peritoneal cavity.

DIAGNOSIS. Definitive diagnosis is established by either finding the parasite eggs or recovering worms. Eggs can be easily detected on adhesive cellophane tape pressed against the perianal region early in the morning. Repeated examination may be necessary, and in certain situations examination of all family members may be advised. If a worm is seen in the perianal region, it should be preserved in 75% ethyl alcohol until microscopic examination can be performed.

TREATMENT. Drug therapy should be given to all infected and symptomatic individuals. Pyrantel pamoate given at a dose of 11 mg/kg (maximum dose of 1 g) with a repeat dose 2 wk later is recommended. Alternatively, mebendazole given as 100-mg doses on a similar schedule may be used. Repeated treatments every 3–4 mo may be required in situations in which exposure is constant, for example, in children in institutions. While personal cleanliness is a useful general recommendation, there is no proof that it plays a significant role in control of enterobiasis.

Boyer A, Berdknikoff IK: Pinworm infestation in children; the problem and its management. Can Med Assoc J 86:60, 1962.
Drugs for parasitic infection. Med Lett 35:111, 1993.
Weller TH, Sorensen CW: Enterobiasis: Its incidence and symptomatology in a group of 505 children. N Engl J Med 224:131, 1941.

245.6 Eosinophilic Meningitis

Charles H. King

Eosinophilic meningitis is the term commonly given to eosinophilic pleocytosis of the cerebrospinal fluid (CSF) caused by central nervous system (CNS) infection with helminthic parasites. CSF eosinophilic pleocytosis is not unique to parasitic infections; it can be seen in neurosyphilis, multiple sclerosis, viral meningitis, tubercular and fungal meningitis, and in Hodgkin's lymphoma.

ETIOLOGY. Although any tissue-migrating helminth may be the cause of eosinophilic meningitis, the most common cause is inadvertent human infection with the rat lungworm *Angiostrongylus cantonensis*. A second leading cause is transient infection with *Gnathostoma* species, parasites of dogs and cats.

EPIDEMIOLOGY. *Angiostrongylus* is found Southeast Asia, the South Pacific, Japan, and Taiwan. Infection has also been described in Egypt, Ivory Coast, and Cuba. *Gnathostoma* infections are found in Japan, China, India, Bangladesh, and Southeast Asia. Other, less common causes of eosinophilic meningitis include *Trichinella* (Chapter 245.14), *Paragonimus* (Chapter 245.8), and *Toxocara* infection (Chapter 245.13), and *T. solium* in the form of neurocysticercosis (Chapter 245.2). *Angiostrongylus* is acquired by eating raw or undercooked freshwater snails, slugs, prawns, or crabs containing infectious third-stage larvae. Gnathostomiasis is acquired by eating undercooked or raw fish, frog, bird, or snake meat.

CLINICAL MANIFESTATIONS. Patients become ill 1–3 wk after exposure, as the parasites migrate from the gastrointestinal tract to the CNS. There may be fever, peripheral eosinophilia, vomiting, abdominal pain, creeping skin eruptions, or pleurisy. Neurologic symptoms include headache, meningismus, ataxia, cranial nerve palsies, and paresthesias. Radiculitis and/or myelitis may cause paraparesis or incontinence.

DIAGNOSIS AND TREATMENT. The presumptive diagnosis is made by travel and exposure history in the presence of typical clinical and laboratory findings. There is CSF eosinophilic pleocytosis (15–90% of a CSF white cell count over 100/μL). CSF protein is elevated, while the CSF glucose is typically normal. CNS imaging is usually negative with *Angiostrongylus* and *Gnathostoma* infection, although inflammation-associated hydrocephalus may be noted.

Treatment is supportive, as infection is self-limited and anthelmintic drugs do not appear to influence the outcome of infection. Analgesics should be given for headache and radiculitis, and CSF removal or shunting should be performed to relieve hydrocephalus. Corticosteroids have not shown a consistent beneficial effect.

Prognosis is good, with 70% of patients improving sufficiently to leave the hospital in 1–2 wk. The mortality associated with eosinophilic meningitis is less than 1%.

Koo J, Pien F, Kliks MM: *Angiostrongylus (Parastrongylus)* eosinophilic meningitis. Rev Infect Dis 10:1155, 1988.

Salata R, King CH, Mahmoud AAF: Parasitic infection of the central nervous system. *In:* Aminoff MJ (ed): *Neurology and General Medicine.* New York, Churchill Livingstone, 1989, p 643.

Vejjajiva A: Eosinophilic meningitis. *In:* Warren KS, Mahmoud AAF (eds): *Tropical and Geographical Medicine,* 2nd ed. New York, McGraw-Hill, 1990, p 455.

245.7 Filariasis

James W. Kazura

Filariae are threadlike nematodes that may cause significant human morbidity. Disease due to infection with these organisms usually becomes evident years after exposure; it is thus uncommon for children to have clinically significant filariasis.

MALAYAN AND BANCROFTIAN FILARIASIS

Infection with *Brugia malayi, Brugia timori,* or *Wuchereria bancrofti* results in similar clinical syndromes, characterized in the early stages by acute lymphangitis and lymphadenitis, and, later by lymphatic obstruction with hydrocele and elephantiasis (in the case of *W. bancrofti* only). Over 78 million people in developing countries may be infected with these parasites.

ETIOLOGY. Filarial larvae are introduced into humans in secretions of biting mosquitoes. Over months to a year this stage of the helminth develops into adult worms that reside in the lymphatics. Sexually mature adult female worms release large numbers of microfilariae that circulate in the bloodstream. The life cycle of the parasite is completed when mosquitoes ingest these organisms in a blood meal.

EPIDEMIOLOGY. Although as much as 80% of the population of endemic areas may be infected, fewer than 10–20% have clinically significant morbidity. Those who work in areas where there is repeated and chronic exposure to larvae-containing mosquitoes, such as in crowded urban areas with poor sanitation, are most at risk. *W. bancrofti* infection is distributed throughout tropical and subtropical Africa, Asia, and South America, whereas infection with *B. malayi* is restricted to the South Pacific and Southeast Asia. *B. timori* infection occurs in Indonesia. Infection of travelers who spend brief periods of time in endemic areas is rare.

CLINICAL MANIFESTATIONS. The acute stage of infection is characterized by episodes of fever, lymphangitis of an extremity, headaches, and myalgias, which last a few days to several weeks. This syndrome is most frequently observed in young people 10–20 yr old. Chronic manifestations of disease, such as hydrocele and elephantiasis, occur mostly in those over 30 yr old and are a direct result of lymphatic fibrosis and obstruction to lymph flow. The presence of larvae (microfilariae) in the blood is not thought to have any pathologic consequences, except in persons with tropical pulmonary eosinophilia. Children born to microfilaremic mothers may have cellular hyporesponsiveness to microfiliarial antigens.

DIAGNOSIS AND TREATMENT. Demonstrating microfilariae in the blood is the only way to diagnose lymphatic-dwelling filariasis. One milliliter of blood obtained at a time of day when the number of parasites in the circulation is expected to be highest (this varies with the geographic strain of filaria and most commonly occurs around midnight) should be filtered and examined for the organisms.

The use of antifilarial drugs is controversial. There are no controlled studies demonstrating that administration of antifilarial chemotherapy, such as diethylcarbamazine, modified the course of acute lymphangitis. Single doses of diethylcarbamazine (6 mg/kg) may be given to asymptomatic microfilaremic persons to lower the intensity of parasitemia, although the effect of the drug on the acute or chronic pathologic manifestations of the infection has not been established. Repeat doses may be necessary to reduce further the microfilaremia and to kill lymphatic-dwelling adult parasites. Recent studies indicate that a single dose of ivermectin is as effective as diethylcarbamazine in lowering microfilaremia.

INFECTION WITH ANIMAL FILARIAE

Humans may be infected with three types of animal filariae. *Dirofilaria immitis,* the heartworm, is found on all continents and is a common parasite of dogs in many parts of the United States. *D. tenuis, Brugia beaveri,* and other unclassified *Brugia* spp. have also been reported to infect humans. These worms may be introduced into humans by the bite of mosquitoes containing 3rd-stage larvae. The organisms, however, do not undergo normal development in the human host. *D. immitis* are trapped in the lung parenchyma after migrating for several months in the subcutaneous tissues. The pulmonary response consists of granulomas with eosinophils, neutrophils, and tissue necrosis. *D. tenuis* does not leave the subcutaneous tissues, while *B. beaveri* eventually localizes to superficial lymph nodes.

Most human infections with *D. immitis* are discovered incidentally when the chest roentgenogram reveals a solitary pulmonary nodule 1–3 cm in diameter. Definitive diagnosis and cure depend on surgical excision and identification of the nematode within the surrounding granulomatous response. *D. tenuis* and *B. beaveri* infections present as painful, rubbery 1- to 5-cm diameter nodules in the skin of the trunk, extremities, and orbit. Patients often report having been engaged in activities suggestive of exposure to infected mosquitoes, such as working in swampy areas. Diagnosis and management of these infections are similar to those of *D. immitis.*

Kazura JW. Ivermectin and human lymphatic filariasis. Microb Pathog 14:337, 1993.

Steel C, Guinea A, McCarthy JS, et al: Long-term effect of prenatal exposure to maternal microfilaraemia on immune responsiveness to filarial parasite antigens. Lancet 343:890, 1994.

White AT, Newland HS, Taylor HR, et al: Controlled trial and dose finding study of ivermectin for treatment of onchocerciasis. J Infect Dis 156:463, 1987.

245.8 Flukes: Liver, Lung, and Intestine

Charles H. King

CLONORCHIASIS

Infection of bile passages with the Chinese or oriental fluke *Clonorchis sinensis* is endemic in China, other parts of East Asia, and Japan. Humans acquire infection by ingestion of raw or inadequately cooked freshwater fish carrying the encysted metacercariae of the parasite under its scales or skin. These metacercariae excyst in the duodenum and pass through the ampulla of Vater to the common bile duct and bile capillaries, where they mature into hermaphroditic adult worms (3 × 15 mm). *C. sinensis* worms deposit small operculated eggs (14 × 30 μm), which are discharged via the bile duct to the intestine and feces (Fig. 245–6). The eggs mature and hatch outside the body, releasing motile miracidia into local freshwater streams, rivers, or ponds. If these are ingested by specific snails, they will develop into cercariae which are, in turn, released from the snail to encyst under the skin or scales of freshwater fish.

Most *C. sinensis*–infected individuals, particularly those with light infections, are asymptomatic. In heavily infected individuals, localized obstruction of a bile duct results from repeated local trauma and inflammation. In these cases cholangitis and cholangiohepatitis may lead to liver enlargement and jaundice. In Hong Kong, Korea, and other parts of Asia, cholangiocarcinoma is associated with chronic *C. sinensis* infection. Clonorchiasis is diagnosed by examining feces or duodenal aspirates for the parasite eggs. Praziquantel is the drug of choice for treating clonorchiasis (25 mg/kg tid given for 1 day).

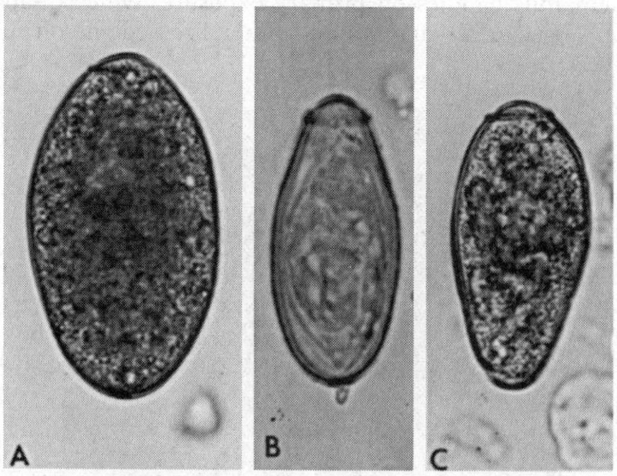

Figure 245–6. Eggs of liver flukes and a lung fluke. ***A, Fasciola hepatica*** **(×400).** ***B, Clonorchis sinensis*** **(×1,000).** ***C, Paragonimus westermani*** **(×400).**

OPISTHORCHIASIS

Infections with species of *Opisthorchis* are clinically similar to those with clonorchiasis. *O. felineus* and *O. viverrini* are liver flukes of cats and dogs that occasionally infect humans through ingestion of metacercariae in freshwater fish. Infection with *O. felineus* is endemic in eastern Europe and Southeast Asia, and *O. viverrini* is found mainly in Thailand. Most individuals are asymptomatic; liver enlargement, relapsing cholangitis, and jaundice may be seen in heavily infected individuals. Diagnosis is based on recovering eggs from stools or duodenal aspirates. Praziquantel, in the same dosage as for clonorchiasis, is the drug of choice.

FASCIOLIASIS

The sheep liver fluke *Fasciola hepatica* infects cattle, other ungulates, and occasionally humans. Infection has been reported in different parts of the world, particularly South America, Europe, Africa, China, and Australia. Although *F. hepatica* is enzootic in North America, reported cases are extremely rare. Humans are infected by ingestion of metacercariae attached to vegetation, especially wild watercress. In the duodenum the parasites excyst; penetrate the intestinal wall, liver capsule, and parenchyma; and wander for a few weeks before entering the bile ducts, where they mature. Adult *F. hepatica* (1 × 2.5 cm) commence oviposition approximately 12 wk after infection; the eggs are large (75 × 140 μm) and operculated, pass to the intestines with bile, and leave the body in the feces (see Fig. 245–6). On reaching fresh water, the eggs mature and hatch into miracidia, which infect specific snail intermediate hosts to multiply into many cercariae. These then emerge from infected snails and encyst on aquatic grasses and plants.

Clinical manifestations usually occur either during the liver migratory phase of the parasites or after their arrival at their final habitat in bile canaliculi. The first phase is characterized by fever, right upper quadrant pain, and hepatosplenomegaly. Peripheral blood eosinophilia is usually marked. As the worms enter bile ducts, most of the acute symptoms subside. On rare occasions, patients may suffer from obstructive jaundice or biliary cirrhosis. *F. hepatica* infection is diagnosed by finding the characteristic eggs in fecal smears or duodenal aspirates. Bithionol (30–50 mg/kg on alternate days for a total of 10–15 doses) is the recommended treatment. In the United States, bithionol is available from the Centers for Disease Control, Atlanta, Georgia.

INTESTINAL FLUKES

Several wild and domestic animal intestinal flukes, such as *Fasciolopsis buski, Nanophyetus salmincola,* and *Heterophyes heterophyes,* may accidentally infect humans. *F. buski* is endemic in the Far East. Humans are infected by ingesting metacercariae encysted on aquatic plants. They hatch and produce large flukes (1 × 5 cm), which inhabit the duodenum and jejunum. Mature worms produce operculated eggs that pass with feces; the organism completes its life cycle through specific snail intermediate hosts. Individuals with *F. buski* infection are usually asymptomatic; heavily infected subjects complain of diarrhea and abdominal pain, and show signs of malabsorption. Diagnosis of fasciolopsiasis and other intestinal flukes is made by fecal examination for eggs. As in other fluke infections, praziquantel is the drug of choice.

LUNG FLUKES
(Paragonimiasis)

Human infection by the lung fluke *Paragonimus westermani* occurs throughout the Far East, in localized areas of West Africa, and in several parts of Central and South America. The highest incidence of pulmonary paragonimiasis occurs in older children and adolescents 11–15 yr of age. Although *P. westermani* is found in many carnivora, human cases are relatively rare and seem to be associated with specific dietary habits, such as eating raw freshwater crayfish or crabs. These crustaceans contain the infective metacercariae in their tissues; they excyst in the duodenum, penetrate the intestinal wall, and migrate to their final habitat in the lungs. Adult worms (5 × 10 mm) encapsulate within the lung parenchyma and deposit brown operculated eggs (60 × 100 μm), which pass into the bronchioles and are coughed up (see Fig. 245–6). Ova can be detected in the sputum of infected individuals or in their feces. If eggs reach fresh water, they hatch and undergo asexual multiplication in specific snails. The cercariae encyst in the muscles and viscera of crayfish and freshwater crabs.

Most individuals infected with *P. westermani* harbor low or moderate worm loads and are asymptomatic. In symptomatic infected children hemoptysis occurs in 98% of cases; other symptoms include cough and production of rust-colored sputum. There are no characteristic physical findings, but laboratory examination usually demonstrates marked eosinophilia. Chest roentgenogram often reveals small patchy infiltrates or radiolucencies in the mid-lung fields; however, the roentgenogram may be normal in one fifth of infected individuals. In rare circumstances lung abscess, pleural effusion, or bronchiectasis may be demonstrable. Extrapulmonary localization of *P. westermani* in the brain, peritoneum, intestines, or pleura may rarely occur. Cerebral paragonimiasis is seen primarily in heavily infected individuals living in highly endemic areas of the Far East; the clinical presentation resembles jacksonian epilepsy or cerebral tumors. Definitive diagnosis of paragonimiasis is made by finding eggs in fecal or sputum smears. The treatment of choice is praziquantel (25 mg/kg) given orally three times in 1 day.

Drugs for parasitic infections. Med Lett 32:23, 1990.
Fischer GW, McGrew GL, Bass JW: Pulmonary paragonimiasis in childhood. JAMA 243:1360, 1980.
Harinasuta T, Bunnag D: Liver, lung, and intestinal trematodiasis. *In:* Warren KS, Mahmoud AAF (eds): Tropical and Geographical Medicine, 2nd ed. New York, McGraw-Hill, 1990, p 473.
Kusner DJ, King CH: Paragonimiasis of the central nervous system. Semin Neurol 13:201, 1993.

245.9 Hookworms

Charles H. King

Three species of hookworm, *Ancylostoma duodenale, Necator americanus,* and *Ancylostoma ceylanicum* infect more than 1 billion people. Infection is endemic in temperate, subtropical, and tropical areas of the world.

ETIOLOGY. Hookworm larvae are found in warm, damp soil and infect the human host by penetrating the skin. Infection may also be acquired by drinking contaminated water or by soil pica. Larvae migrate from the dermis or bowel wall to the venous circulation and are carried to the lungs, where they break into the alveolar spaces, migrate upward, and are then swallowed to reach their final habitat in the upper small intestine. Mature worms develop in 2–4 wk; they are grayish-white and slightly curved and measure 5–13 mm in length. The buccal cavity of *A. duodenale* has pointed, clawed teeth, and that of *N. americanus* has two chitinous plates. These buccal structures help the mature worms attach to the jejunal mucosa and suck blood. In 6–9 wk worms reach sexual maturity and start to deposit eggs, which are excreted in the feces. Mature *A. duodenale* female worms produce about 30,000 eggs/day; daily egg production by *N. americanus* is 9,000. The mean lifespan of adult hookworms is 1–3 yr, although they may occasionally survive up to 9 yr. Hookworm eggs are ovoidal and thin-shelled and measure approximately 36 × 58 μm (Fig. 245–7). When freshly passed, these eggs contain four embryonic segments, which mature into 1st stage larvae that hatch in 1–2 days under favorable environmental conditions. Larvae live in the soil for 1–2 wk, molt twice, and change into infective larvae capable of penetrating human skin.

EPIDEMIOLOGY. Humans are the primary host for the three species of hookworms. Endemicity of infection in any specific geographic location depends on suitability of environmental conditions for hatching of eggs and maturation of larvae, on fecal contamination of soil, and on human contact with contaminated soil. The optimal soil conditions are found in many parts of agrarian tropical countries and also in the southeastern part of the United States.

The morbidity of hookworm infections in endemic areas is sustained primarily by children. In one study half of the children were infected before age 5; 90% were infected by 9 yr of age. Intensity of infection increases up to age 6–7, then stabilizes.

PATHOLOGY AND PATHOGENESIS. Several factors may contribute to the morbidity of hookworm infection; these include worm burden, diet, race, and development of immunity in chronically infected individuals. Anemia, the major pathologic manifestation of infection, is affected primarily by the worm burden and the diet of the host.

Lesions due to hookworm may occur during the migratory phase of infection or may be related to the presence of adult worms in the small intestine. Ground itch or dermatitis results from larval invasion of skin and the subsequent inflammatory response. Mild pulmonary lesions similar to those described in ascariasis may occur during lung migration of larvae; it is questionable whether a Loeffler-like syndrome occurs. The presence of adult worms in the small intestine results in anemia and hypoalbuminemia. The severity of hookworm anemia is related to the intensity of infection and the host's iron balance. Blood loss varies with hookworm species (0.03–0.3 mL of blood lost/worm/day); *A. duodenale* infection causes greater losses than *N. americanus*.

CLINICAL MANIFESTATIONS. Infections are usually asymptomatic; significant clinical disease occurs in only a small percentage of infected individuals. Exposure of skin for the first time to infective larvae may lead to pruritus. Skin reactions vary from erythematous papules on primary exposure, which disappear within 1 wk, to vesiculation and generalized edema on subse-

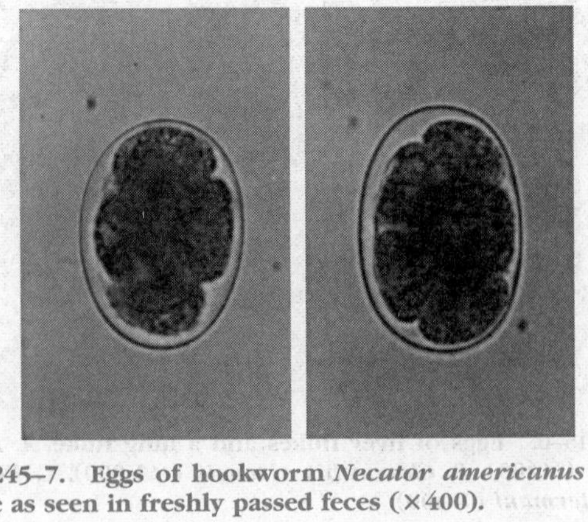

Figure 245–7. Eggs of hookworm *Necator americanus* in early cleavage as seen in freshly passed feces (×400).

quent infections, which may last 1–3 wk. Migration of the larvae through the lungs is associated with few, if any, specific symptoms or signs.

Symptoms of abdominal pain, loss of appetite, indigestion, postprandial fullness, and diarrhea have been attributed to the intestinal phase of hookworm infection. The significant disease sequelae of chronic hookworm infections include anemia, hypoalbuminemia, and edema. Hemoglobin concentrations under 5 g/dL have been associated with heart failure and sudden death. Hypoalbuminemia in excess of that anticipated from whole blood loss may also occur; the attendant decrease in plasma oncotic pressure may lead to edema.

DIAGNOSIS. Direct examination of fecal smears for hookworm eggs provides a qualitative assessment of infection. The Kato thick smear offers a simple technique for quantitation of infection, but because hookworm eggs disappear within 1 hr of preparation, prompt examination of these smears is mandatory. Light hookworm infection may require the use of concentration techniques to detect eggs in the stool. Either zinc sulfate or formalin-ether techniques can be used. Eggs of *A. duodenale* and *N. americanus* are morphologically indistinguishable; the only way to differentiate the species is to allow the eggs to hatch and examine the released larvae.

TREATMENT. Evaluation of intensity of infection and severity of anemia should precede therapy. In children with severe anemia (hemoglobin concentration under 5 g/dL) iron therapy should be given before anthelmintic drugs. Elemental iron is administered orally at a dosage of 2 mg/kg 3 times/day until anemia is corrected. In life-threatening anemia with signs of heart failure, diuretics followed by slow transfusion of packed red cells may be indicated. Mebendazole (100 mg orally twice a day for 3 days or 300 mg as a single dose) or pyrantel pamoate (11 mg/kg up to 1 g as a single dose) will eradicate or significantly reduce the hookworm load.

CONTROL. Eradication or control of hookworm infection depends on sanitation and mass chemotherapy. Seasonal variations in transmission and the hookworm species must also be taken into consideration. Eradication has been achieved in the southeast United States.

Schad GA, Banwell JG: Hookworms in Warren KS. *In:* Mahmoud AAF (eds): Tropical and Geographical Medicine. New York, McGraw-Hill, 1990 p 379.
Ash LR, Orihel TC: Parasites: A Guide to Laboratory Procedures and Identification. Chicago, ASCP Press, 1987.

245.10 Onchocerciasis

James W. Kazura

ONCHOCERCIASIS, LOIASIS, AND TROPICAL PULMONARY EOSINOPHILIA

Infection with *Onchocerca volvulus* (onchocerciasis, river blindness) is a major cause of blindness in West Africa and Central America. The parasite is introduced into humans by blackflies of the genus *Simulium,* which breed in rapidly running water; people who live or work near waterways are thus most likely to be infected. Most individuals are asymptomatic; those with chronic and heavy infections (usually adults over 20 yr old) may suffer from pruritic dermatitis and eye disease (punctate keratitis, corneal pannus formation, chorioretinitis) owing to the presence of microfilariae in subcutaneous and ocular tissues. Firm, nontender subcutaneous nodules containing adult parasites may also be palpable. *O. volvulus* infection is diagnosed by demonstration of parasites in skin snips removed from the buttocks or extremities or by visualization with a slit lamp of microfilariae in the cornea or anterior chamber of the eye. Children with symptomatic skin and/or eye disease should be treated with ivermectin (150 μg/kg as a single dose). Repeat doses 6–12 mo later should be administered if microfilariae in the skin or eye are observed. The drug should not be given to persons with disorders of the central nervous system. The safety of the drug in children less than 5 yr old has not been established.

Loa loa infection occurs in the rain forests of West and Central Africa; the parasite is transmitted to humans by tabanid flies. Adult worms migrate in the subcutaneous tissues and produce painful transient areas of localized edema known as calabar swellings, which tend to appear around the joints of the legs and arms. The parasite occasionally may be directly visualized in the conjunctiva, where it produces an intense inflammatory reaction. Microfilariae are present in highest concentrations in the peripheral circulation between 10 A.M. and 2 P.M.; identification in blood samples is diagnostic. Symptomatic individuals should be given gradually increasing doses of diethylcarbamazine as described for lymphatic filariasis (Chapter 245.8). Therapy should be discontinued and corticosteroids administered if fever, headache, or joint swelling occurs.

Tropical pulmonary eosinophilia (TPE) is a syndrome of filarial etiology in which microfilariae can be found in the lung and lymph nodes. It occurs only in individuals who have lived for at least several months in endemic areas of bancroftian or Malayan filariasis and is most common in Southeast Asia and the South Pacific. Although TPE has been observed in children, 20- to 30-yr-old men are most likely to be affected. Patients present with paroxysmal nonproductive cough, occasional episodes of dyspnea, fever, weight loss, and fatigue. Rales and rhonchi are found on auscultation of the chest; roentgenographic examination may occasionally be normal but usually reveals increased bronchovascular markings, discrete opacities in the middle and basal regions of the lung, or diffuse miliary lesions. Recurrent untreated episodes may result in interstitial fibrosis and chronic respiratory insufficiency. In children hepatosplenomegaly and generalized lymphadenopathy are often seen. Eosinophilia (>2,000/mm^3 blood) with the appropriate history and symptoms suggests the diagnosis. Increased serum IgE levels (>1,000 units/mL) and high titers of antimicrofilarial antibodies in the absence of blood-borne helminths should also be documented. Although microfilariae may be found in sections of lung or lymph node, biopsy is unwarranted in most patients. The clinical response to diethylcarbamazine (5 mg/kg/24 hr for 10 days) is the final criterion for diagnosis because in the majority of patients symptoms improve with this therapy. If they recur, a second course of the drug should be administered. Subjects presenting with chronic symptoms are less likely to show improvement than those who have been ill for a short time.

245.11 Schistosomes

Charles H. King

Five schistosome species infect humans; these are *Schistosoma haematobium, S. mansoni, S. japonicum, S. intercalatum,* and *S. mekongi.* Schistosomiasis infects more than 200 million people, primarily children and young adults. Prevalence is increasing in many areas, as population density increases and new irrigation projects provide broader habitats for vector snails. *S. haematobium* is prevalent in Africa and the Middle East; *S. mansoni* in Africa, the Middle East, the Caribbean, and South America; and *S. japonicum* in China, the Philippines, and Indonesia, with some sporadic foci in parts of Southeast Asia. The other two species are less prevalent. *S. mekongi* is found in the Far East and *S. intercalatum* is found in West and Central Africa.

ETIOLOGY. Humans are infected through contact with water contaminated with cercariae, the free-living infective stage of the parasite. These motile, forked-tail organisms emerge from infected snails and are capable of penetrating intact human skin. In the subcutaneous tissues cercariae change into the next developmental stage (schistosomula) and migrate to the lungs and finally the liver. As they reach sexual maturity, adult worms migrate to specific anatomic sites characteristic of each schistosome species: *S. haematobium* adults are found in the perivesical and periureteral venous plexus, *S. mansoni* in the inferior mesenteric, and *S. japonicum* in the superior mesenteric veins. *S. intercalatum* and *S. mekongi* are found in the mesenteric vessels. Adult schistosome worms (1–2 cm in length) are different from most other flukes in that they exist as separate sexes; the female, however, accompanies the male in a groove formed by the lateral edges of its body. Upon fertilization, female worms begin oviposition in the small venous tributaries. The eggs of the three main schistosome species have characteristic morphologic features: *S. haematobium,* terminal spine; *S. mansoni,* lateral spine; and *S. japonicum,* smaller size with a short curved spine (Fig. 245–8). Eggs reach the lumen of the urinary tract or intestines and are carried to the outside environment, where they hatch if deposited in fresh water. Motile miracidia emerge; they infect specific freshwater snail intermediate hosts and divide asexually. In 4–6 wk the infective cercariae are released in the water.

EPIDEMIOLOGY. Humans are the definitive host for the five clinically important species of schistosomes, although *S. japonicum* may infect some animals such as dogs and cattle. Transmission depends on disposal of excreta, the presence of specific intermediate snail hosts, and the patterns of water contact and social habits of the population. The distribution of infection in endemic areas shows that prevalence increases with age to a maximum in the 10- to 20-yr age group. Furthermore, measuring intensity of infection (by quantitative egg count in urine or feces) demonstrates that the heaviest worm loads are found in the younger age groups. Schistosomiasis, therefore, is most prevalent and severe in children and young adults, who are at maximal risk of suffering from its acute and chronic sequelae.

PATHOLOGY AND PATHOGENESIS. The early manifestations of schistosomiasis are immunologically mediated (dermatitis). Acute schistosomiasis is a febrile illness that represents an immune complex disease associated with early infection and oviposition. However, the major pathology of infection is found in chronic schistosomiasis, where retention of eggs in the host tissues is associated with chronic granulomatous injury. Eggs may be trapped at sites of deposition (urinary bladder, ureters, intestine) or be carried by the bloodstream to other organs, most commonly the liver and less often the lungs and central nervous system. The host response to these eggs involves local as well as systemic manifestations. Granulomas composed of lymphocytes, macrophages, and eosinophils surround the trapped eggs and add significantly to the size of tissue destruction. It has been shown that these granulomas are due to cell-mediated immune responses. Granuloma formation in the bladder wall and at the ureterovesical junction leads to the major disease manifestations of schistosomiasis hematobia: hematuria, dysuria, and obstructive uropathy. Intestinal as well as hepatic granulomas underlie the pathologic sequelae of the other schistosome infections: ulcerations and fibrosis of intestinal wall, hepatosplenomegaly, and portal hypertension due to presinusoidal obstruction of blood flow. Protective immunity against schistosomiasis has been demonstrated in some animal species and may occur in humans.

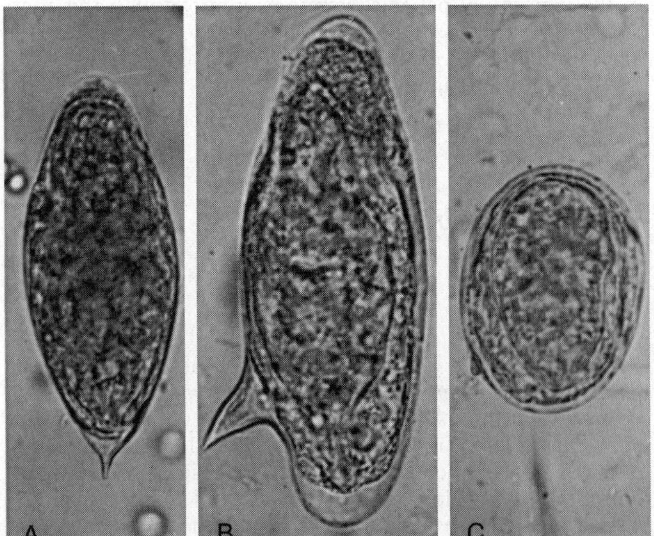

Figure 245–8. Eggs of *Schistosoma haematobium (A), Schistosoma mansoni (B),* and *Schistosoma japonicum (C)* (×320).

CLINICAL MANIFESTATIONS. Most infected individuals suffer no apparent ill health; symptoms occurs mainly in those who are heavily infected. Cercarial penetration of human skin may result in a papular pruritic rash (swimmer's itch). It is more pronounced in previously exposed individuals and involves edema and massive cellular infiltrates in the dermis and epidermis. *Katayama fever* (acute schistosomiasis) may occur, particularly in heavily infected individuals 4–8 wk after exposure; this is a serum sickness-like syndrome manifested by the acute onset of fever, chills, sweating, lymphadenopathy, hepatosplenomegaly, and eosinophilia. Acute schistosomiasis most commonly presents in "northern" visitors to endemic areas who experience primary infection at an older age.

Symptomatic children with chronic schistosomiasis haematobia usually complain of frequency, dysuria, and hematuria. Urine examination shows erythrocytes, parasite eggs, and occasional leukocytes. In endemic areas moderate to severe pathologic lesions have been demonstrated in the urinary tract of more than 50% of infected children. The extent of disease is correlated with the intensity of infection, but significant morbidity can occur even in lightly infected children. The terminal stages of schistosomiasis haematobia are associated with chronic renal failure, secondary infections, and cancer of the bladder.

Children with chronic schistosomiasis *mansoni, japonica, intercalatum,* or *mekongi* may have intestinal symptoms; colicky abdominal pain and bloody diarrhea are the most common. The intestinal phase may, however, pass unnoticed, and the syndrome of hepatosplenomegaly, portal hypertension, ascites, and hematemesis may be the initial presentation. Liver disease is due to granuloma formation and subsequent fibrosis; there is no appreciable liver cell injury, and hepatic function may be preserved for a long time. Schistosome eggs may escape into the lungs causing pulmonary hypertension and cor pulmonale. *S. japonicum* worms may migrate to the brain vasculature and produce localized lesions that cause seizures. Transverse myelitis rarely has been reported in children or young adults with chronic *S. haematobium* or *S. mansoni* infection.

DIAGNOSIS. Schistosome eggs are found in the excreta of infected individuals; quantitative procedures should be used to give an indication of the intensity of infection. Urine should be collected around mid-day (time of maximal egg excretion) and 10 mL filtered through a nucleopore membrane for diagnosis of *S. haematobium* infection. Stool examination by the Kato thick smear procedure is the method of choice for diagnosis and quantification of other schistosome infections.

TREATMENT. Management of children with schistosomiasis should be based on an appreciation of the intensity of infection and the extent of disease. The drug of choice is praziquantel, which is effective against all schistosome species. It is administered orally as a single or divided dose of 40–60 mg/kg.

CONTROL. Transmission in endemic areas may be decreased by reducing the parasite load in the population. The availability of oral, single-dose, effective chemotherapeutic agents may help achieve this goal. Other measures, particularly improved sanitation and focal application of molluscicides, may be useful. Control of schistosomiasis is closely linked to economic and social development.

King CH: Acute and chronic schistosomiasis. Hosp Pract 26:117, 1991.
King CH, Mahmoud AAF: Drugs five years later: Praziquantel. Ann Intern Med 110:290, 1989.
Mahmoud AAF: Schistosomiasis: Clinical Tropical Medicine and Communicable Diseases, Vol 2. London, Bailliere-Tindall, 1987.
Mahmoud AAF, Wahab MFA: Schistosomiasis. *In:* Warren KS, Mahmoud AAF (eds): Tropical and Geographical Medicine, 2nd ed. New York, McGraw-Hill, 1990, p 458.

245.12 Strongyloidiasis

James W. Kazura

Infection with the nematode *Strongyloides stercoralis,* unlike that with other worms, may cause autoinfection with massive parasite invasion of the host and eventual death. This complication is more frequent in malnourished or immunosuppressed children. *S. stercoralis* infection is widely distributed throughout tropical and temperate regions, though it is less common than infection by other intestinal roundworms.

ETIOLOGY. Infected individuals pass larvae in their stools; these parasites may develop into free-living adults in the soil or change into infective filariform larvae. These latter forms penetrate human skin, pass via the bloodstream to the lungs, and follow a pathway similar to hookworm and *Ascaris* larvae until they reach their final habitat in the upper small intestine. Mature worms (2.2 mm in length) burrow into the intestinal mucosa and begin releasing eggs approximately 4 wk after infection. *S. stercoralis* eggs hatch rapidly, and small larvae (225 × 16 μm) are passed in feces. The larvae must undergo morphologic changes in soil to become infective, but these changes may also be accomplished as the parasites are being discharged from the body. Larvae are then capable of infecting the same individual by penetrating the intestinal wall or perianal skin. This unique feature of the *Strongyloides* life cycle allows the parasite to survive for many years inside the same host and occasionally to cause overwhelming infection.

EPIDEMIOLOGY. Humans are the primary hosts of *S. stercoralis.* Transmission of infection and its endemicity depend on suitable soil and climatic conditions and poor sanitary habits. Close contact and poor personal hygiene may be important, because the prevalence of infection is much higher in institutions for the mentally retarded. Host factors such as nutrition and immune status may play a crucial role in the development of the hyperinfection syndrome.

PATHOLOGY AND PATHOGENESIS. The initial penetration of skin by infective larvae usually produces no apparent pathologic lesions. Repeated skin invasion may, however, result in dermatitis; in cases in which autoinfection is established through the skin, a more extensive skin lesion, *larva currens,* may occur. A Loeffler-like syndrome with eosinophilia may be seen during migration of the larvae through the lungs. Eosinophilia may also occur when adult worms burrow into the intestinal mucosa. *Disseminated strongyloidiasis* is a complex pathologic entity due to larval invasion of internal organs accompanied by polymicrobial gram-negative bacteremia.

CLINICAL MANIFESTATIONS. Signs and symptoms of strongyloidiasis occur in only a small percentage of infected individuals or in those with the hyperinfection syndrome. Pulmonary symptoms and skin lesions are usually mild and generally pass un-noticed. Pruritus with a papular erythematous rash may occur. *Larva currens,* a condition due to repeated skin invasion by larvae, is characterized by large erythematous urticarial lesions with rapidly moving edges. These are usually localized to an area within 30 cm of the anus and have a tendency to recur. The typical symptoms, which include abdominal pain, vomiting, and diarrhea, are caused by adult worms in the upper small intestine. These symptoms occur with uncertain frequency and may have an abrupt onset with periodic recurrences. Abdominal pain is often epigastric and may be burning, colicky, or dull in nature. Diarrhea with passage of mucus may alternate with periods of constipation. *Chronic strongyloidiasis* may result in a malabsorption-like syndrome with protein-losing enteropathy and weight loss. Blood eosinophilia is usually associated with and is often the only indication of the intestinal phase of infection.

Disseminated strongyloidiasis occurs in children with predisposing factors such as malnutrition or defects in cell-mediated immunity (lymphomas, Hodgkin disease, and possibly acquired immune deficiency syndrome). The onset is usually sudden, with generalized abdominal pain, distention, fever, and shock due to gram-negative septicemia. Massive invasion of internal organs by the parasite larvae causes extensive tissue destruction. Although leukocytosis may occur in these patients, eosinophilia is often absent.

DIAGNOSIS. Intestinal strongyloidiasis is diagnosed by examining feces or duodenal fluid for the characteristic larvae. Several stool samples should be examined either by direct smear or by a concentration method such as formaldehyde-ether or that of Baermann. Alternatively, duodenal fluid obtained by the pediatric Enterotest or aspiration may provide samples for definitive diagnosis. In children with hyperinfection syndrome, larvae may be found in sputum, gastric aspirates, or, rarely, in small intestinal biopsies. Strongyloidiasis should also be suspected in immunosuppressed patients who suddenly develop signs and symptoms consistent with disseminated infection. A recently described serologic test for *Strongyloides* antibodies may be more sensitive than parasitologic methods for diagnosing intestinal infection, but the utility of this assay in the hyperinfection syndrome has not been determined.

TREATMENT. The most widely used therapeutic agent is thiabendazole. Treatment of infected children should aim at eradication of infection, and therefore subsequent stool examination is essential. Thiabendazole is administered orally in a dose of 25 mg/kg twice daily for 2 days. Courses of up to 2 wk may be needed in those with the hyperinfection syndrome. Ivermectin (200 μg/kg/24 hr) for 1–2 days may be used in children older than 5 yr. The utility of ivermectin for treatment of disseminated infection has not been established.

CONTROL. Sanitary practices designed to prevent soil and person-to-person transmission are the most effective control measures. Because the infection is uncommon, case detection and treatment are also advised. Individuals who will be subjected to immunosuppressive therapy should have a screening examination for *S. stercoralis* and, if infected, be treated with thiabendazole.

Burke JA: Strongyloidiasis in childhood. Am J Dis Child 132:1130, 1978.
Naguira C, Jimenez G, Guerra JG, et al: Ivermectin for human strongyloidiasis and other intestinal nematodes. Am J Trop Med Hyg 40:304, 1989.
Scowden EB, Schaffner W, Stone WJ: Overwhelming strongyloidiasis. Medicine 57:527, 1978.
Smith JD, Goette DK, Odom RB: Larva currens: Cutaneous strongyloidiasis. Arch Dermatol 112:1161, 1976.

245.13 Toxocariasis

James W. Kazura

Tissue-dwelling nematodes infect over 800 million people worldwide. Although morbidity from these helminths primarily afflicts the populations of tropical and developing countries, inhabitants of regions with temperate climates may also be affected. These parasites have a complex life cycle, which in many instances includes an intermediate invertebrate vector. Childhood disease results mainly when children act either as an incidental host in whom the helminth does not undergo its normal development (*Toxocara* sp., *Dirofilaria* sp.) or as the definitive host (filariae, *Dracunculus medinensis*). Infections that are particularly common in childhood (visceral larval migrans) will be discussed first, followed by a discussion of tissue nematodes that cause disease in individuals of all ages (cutaneous larva migrans, *Trichinella spiralis, D. medinensis*) or primarily in adults (human and animal filariae).

VISCERAL LARVA MIGRANS

(Toxocariasis)

Visceral larva migrans is caused by infection with larvae of *Toxocara* sp. It occurs most frequently in children under the age of 10 yr and is characterized by fever, hepatomegaly, pulmonary disease, and eosinophilia.

ETIOLOGY. *Toxocara canis, T. cati,* and *T. leonina* are common parasites of dogs and cats that infect humans when the eggs of the helminth are ingested. Adult worms of *Toxocara* sp. reside in the gastrointestinal tract of dogs and cats, and release large numbers of eggs, which are passed in the feces. Ingestion of eggs by humans is followed by larval penetration of the gastrointestinal tract and migration to the liver, lung, and occasionally other sites (central nervous system, eye, kidney, and heart). *Toxocara* larvae do not develop beyond this stage in the human host.

EPIDEMIOLOGY. Visceral larva migrans is most common in children 1–4 yr of age, particularly those who engage in pica and have close contact with dogs and cats; ocular toxocariasis occurs most frequently in older children. Potential sources of infection are widely distributed in the canine and feline population (an estimated 20% of dogs in the United States excrete *Toxocara* eggs). These animals often defecate in areas where children play (24% of 800 soil samples taken from public parks in Great Britain were found to contain *Toxocara* eggs).

PATHOLOGY. *Toxocara* larvae usually elicit a granulomatous response characterized by large numbers of eosinophils, mononuclear cells, and tissue necrosis. These lesions are found in liver, lung, and other organs through which the helminth migrates. The inflammatory reaction is much less intense in the eye, where lesions consist mainly of mononuclear cells and a few eosinophils.

CLINICAL MANIFESTATIONS. Major symptoms include fever (80%), cough with wheezing (60–80%), and seizures (20–30%). Respiratory distress may be severe enough to warrant hospitalization. Abdominal pain has been noted in occasional patients. Physical findings include hepatomegaly (65–87%), rales and/or rhonchi (40–50%), papular or urticarial skin lesions (20%), and lymph node enlargement (8%). These manifestations subside over a period of several months. Scattered patchy infiltrates are often seen on chest roentgenograms.

Patients with ocular toxocariasis most commonly present with decreased visual acuity (in 75% of cases) and occasionally with strabismus or periorbital edema. In one study unilateral blindness was noted in 6 of 17 patients. Most children do not have concurrent signs and symptoms of visceral disease. Funduscopic examination of the eye usually reveals solitary granulomatous lesions situated in the retina near the optic disc or macula. These may be mistaken for retinoblastomas and have led to inappropriate enucleation. Peripheral retinal lesions with vitreous bands and involvement of the iris have been documented in a few cases.

DIAGNOSIS. The diagnosis is made on the basis of the clinical manifestations and serologic testing. The only reliable and specific test is an enzyme-linked immunosorbent assay (ELISA), which utilizes infective eggs of *T. canis* as antigen. This assay is positive (serum antibody titer ≥1:32) in 78% of cases of visceral larva migrans and in 45% of individuals with a clinical diagnosis of ocular toxocariasis. Eosinophilia (>500/mm^3 blood) occurs in nearly all subjects with the visceral syndrome but is much less common in those with ocular disease. Nonspecific findings include elevations in serum gamma globulins and isohemagglutinins. Although larvae may be found upon examination of tissue sections, biopsy of liver or other organs is generally not indicated because clinical and laboratory data provide enough evidence to make the diagnosis.

TREATMENT. Therapy is not required in the majority of cases, because the signs and symptoms are usually mild and subside over a period of weeks to months. When significant hypoxemia secondary to pulmonary disease occurs, however, the administration of anti-inflammatory drugs (prednisone, 5 mg/kg/24 hr until respiratory function improves) is beneficial. When disease is severe or when larvae lodge in critical locations, such as the eye, the use of drugs exhibiting possible larvicidal activity (diethylcarbamazine, 0.5 mg/kg/24 hr for 3 days, increased gradually to 6 mg/kg/24 hr for 7–10 days) has been advocated. Alternatively, albendazole at doses of 400 mg twice daily for 3–5 days may be used. There is disagreement about the use of anthelmintic drugs in three divided doses, however, since dying larvae theoretically may incite an inflammatory response, which produces more tissue damage than encapsulated, dormant parasites.

CONTROL. Transmission of infection may be prevented by requiring children to wash their hands after playing with pets and instructing them to avoid areas where these animals defecate, particularly children with the habit of pica. Periodic deworming of dogs, especially puppies below the age of 6 mo, also decreases the likelihood of infection.

CUTANEOUS LARVA MIGRANS

(Creeping Eruption)

Cutaneous larva migrans is caused by several larval nematodes not usually parasitic for humans. *Ancylostoma braziliense* (a hookworm of dogs and cats) is the most common of these helminths, but other animal hookworms *(A. caninum, Uncinaria stenocephala,* and *Bunostomum phlebotosum)* and human parasites *(Necator americanus, Ancylostoma duodenale,* and *Strongyloides stercoralis)* may produce the disease. These organisms are widely distributed throughout tropical and subtropical areas of the world. In the United States infections are most prevalent in the South. Parasite eggs are deposited in the feces of animals and hatch to form infective larvae in warm, moist areas, such as near vegetation on beaches or under porches. Humans are infected when the skin comes in contact with these larvae.

CLINICAL MANIFESTATIONS. After penetrating the skin, larvae localize at the epidermal-dermal junction and migrate in this plane, moving at a rate of 1–2 cm/day. The response to the parasite is characterized by raised, erythematous, serpiginous tracks, which occasionally form bullae (Fig. 245–9 [color plate section]). These lesions may be single or multiple, and are usually localized to an extremity, although any area of the body may be affected. As the organism migrates, new areas of involvement may appear every few days. Intense localized pruritus may be associated with the lesions.

DIAGNOSIS AND TREATMENT. Cutaneous larva migrans is diag-

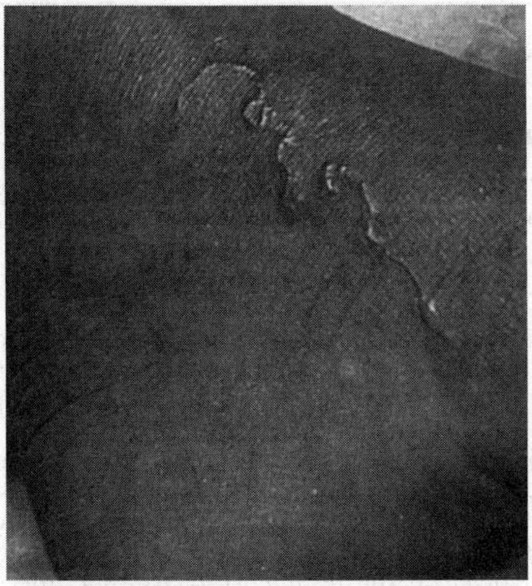

Figure 245–9. Creeping eruption of cutaneous larva migrans. See also color section. (From Korting GW: Hautkrankheiten bei Kindern und Jugendlichen. Stuttgart, Germany, FK Schattauer Verlag, 1969.)

nosed by clinical examination of the skin. Patients are often able to recall the exact time and location of exposure because the larvae produce intense itching at the site of penetration. If left untreated, the larvae die, and the syndrome resolves within a few weeks to several months. Topical application of thiabendazole oral suspension or a 0.5-g tablet triturated with 5 g petroleum jelly may be used if symptoms warrant treatment. Alternatively, oral thiabendazole, 50 mg/kg/24 hr in two doses for 2–5 days may be given. Nausea and vomiting frequently preclude repeated administration of thiabendazole.

Glickman LT: Toxocariasis and related sydromes. *In:* Warren KS, Mahmoud AAf (eds): Tropical and Geographical Medicine. New York, McGraw-Hill, 1990, p 446.

Huntley CC, Costas MC, Lyerly A: Visceral larva migrans syndrome: Clinical characteristics and immunologic studies in 51 patients. Pediatrics 36:623, 1965.

Schantz PM, Glickman LT: Toxocaral visceral larva migrans. N Engl J Med 298:436, 1978.

Zinkham WH: Visceral larva migrans. A review and reassessment indicating two forms of clinical expression: Visceral and ocular. Am J Dis Child 132:627, 1978.

245.14 *Trichinosis*

James W. Kazura

Human infection with *Trichinella spiralis* is fairly common worldwide. Infection is transmitted by ingestion of pork or other meat carrying the parasite. Sporadic epidemics have occurred in North America following ingestion of bear meat. Consumption of horse meat in areas of Europe where this is practiced has also been the source of some outbreaks.

ETIOLOGY. Humans are infected by eating flesh contaminated with viable *T. spiralis* larvae. This stage of the parasite excysts in the stomach and matures to form adult worms within the small intestine. Female *T. spiralis* release large numbers of newborn larvae, which penetrate the gut wall and migrate to striated muscles or occasionally to other sites such as the central nervous system and heart. Larvae that enter muscle cells eventually become encysted and may remain viable for years. The life cycle in nature is maintained by hogs or other animals that ingest garbage containing carcasses of infected rodents.

EPIDEMIOLOGY. *T. spiralis* is found in all areas of the world except Australia and some islands in the South Pacific. Although infection was common in the United States in the past (4% of diaphragms examined post mortem in 1968 contained viable larvae), recent cases have been related to outbreaks resulting from ingestion of undercooked homemade sausage, other pork products, or meat of bears, wild pigs, walruses, and horses. Larvae are destroyed by cooking meat until there is no trace of pink fluid or flesh (this occurs at 55° C) or by storage in a freezer at −15° C for 3 wk. Smoked or salted meat may still contain viable parasites.

PATHOLOGY AND PATHOGENESIS. Adult worms localize in the upper gastrointestinal tract and induce a mucosal inflammatory reaction characterized by a reduced villous-crypt ratio and the presence of eosinophils, neutrophils, and mononuclear cells. This response peaks within the 1st wk of infection, then gradually subsides as adult worms are expelled. In muscle cells migrating larvae elicit a reaction consisting of large numbers of eosinophils and mononuclear cells. These lesions may eventually calcify.

CLINICAL MANIFESTATIONS. The signs and symptoms appear only in heavily infected individuals. Within the 1st wk adult worms in the upper gastrointestinal tract produce gastroenteritis and diarrhea associated with abdominal discomfort. Next, during larval invasion of muscle, periorbital or facial edema (80% of cases), and myalgias occur. Pain is associated with muscle activity; it is most common in the masseters, diaphragm, and intercostals. These signs and symptoms are first noted 10–14 days after infection and last for another 2–3 wk. Heart failure and arrhythmias may occur in patients with exceptionally heavy infestation.

DIAGNOSIS. Periorbital edema, myalgias, fever, and eosinophilia in an individual who gives a history of eating undercooked meat make the diagnosis of trichinosis likely. A history of similar illness in those sharing the food should be sought. Serologic studies such as the bentonite flocculation test (titer of 1:5 or greater) are confirmatory. Biopsy of muscle, usually the deltoid, may reveal larvae upon microscopic examination 3–4 wk after infection. Muscle enzymes such as creatine kinase and lactate dehydrogenase are elevated in 50% of patients.

TREATMENT. There is no clinically established therapy for the syndrome related to larval invasion of muscles. Mebendazole at doses of 200 mg three times per day for 3 days, then 400 mg three times per day for 10 days, may eliminate adult worms from the gut, but evidence for its efficacy against muscle larvae is not well established. Accordingly, the drug is most clearly indicated for treatment of children who are known to have been infected in the preceding 1–3 wk. Corticosteroids may be used in critically ill patients, such as those with myocarditis or central nervous system damage, but evidence of their beneficial effect is equivocal.

245.15 *Trichuriasis*

James W. Kazura

Trichuris trichiura or whipworm causes one of the most common helminthic infections of humans; approximately half a billion cases occur worldwide. Infection is more common in warm climates, but it does exist in North America.

ETIOLOGY. Infection is due to ingesting parasite eggs (Fig. 245–10), which are passed in the stools of infected individuals and mature in 2–4 wk if moisture and temperature conditions of the soil are optimal. Upon ingestion by humans, *Trichuris* eggs hatch, and larvae penetrate the small intestinal villi, where they remain for 3–10 days before slowly moving down the

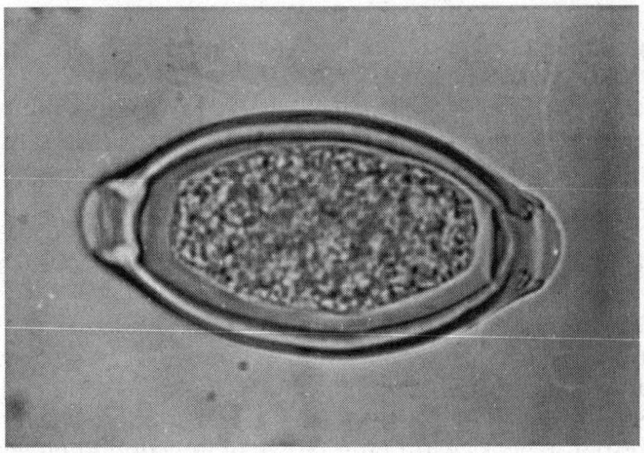

Figure 245–10. Egg of *Trichuris trichiura*, as seen in freshly passed feces (×1,000).

bowel and maturing into adult worms. The final habitats of *T. trichiura* are the cecum and ascending colon. The body is divided into an anterior whiplike portion (hence the term *whipworm*) and a posterior bulky part and measures approximately 40 mm in length. The worms remain in the gut by anchoring the anterior portion of their body to the intestinal mucosa. Egg deposition by maturing females begins 1–3 mo after infection.

EPIDEMIOLOGY. Trichuriasis is most common in poor rural communities lacking sanitary facilities. Humans are the primary hosts; the highest prevalence and intensity of infection occur in children. Transmission of embryonated eggs occurs by contamination of hands, food, or drink. Eggs may also be carried by flies and other insects.

CLINICAL MANIFESTATIONS. Most infected individuals are asymptomatic; however, vague abdominal complaints, colic, and abdominal distention have been associated with infection. Adult *Trichuris* suck approximately 0.005 mL of blood/worm/day. However, only heavy childhood infections produce mild anemia, bloody diarrhea, or, rarely, rectal prolapse. These cases are referred to as massive infantile trichuriasis and are often associated with shigellosis and protozoan infections of the gastrointestinal tract.

DIAGNOSIS AND TREATMENT. Examination of stool smears reveals the characteristic eggs of *T. trichiura*. An oral course of mebendazole (100 mg twice a day for 3 days) produces a cure rate of 70–90% and reduces egg output by 90–99%.

Blumenthal DS: Intestinal nematodes in the United States. N Engl J Med 297:1437, 1977.

Jung RC, Beaver PC: Clinical observations on *Trichocephalus trichiurus* (whipworm) infestation in children. Pediatrics 8:548, 1951.

CHAPTER 246
Antiparasitic Drugs for Children

Robert A. Bonomo and Robert A. Salata

Pediatric parasitic infections constitute a major cause of worldwide morbidity and mortality. It is estimated that humans are infected by over 100 kinds of eukaryotic parasites and that these infections are responsible for over 1 million deaths annually. In the United States and other industrialized countries, parasitic infections in childhood have markedly increased in frequency. The societal and economic impact of this increase is stimulating research into new avenues of treatment. Factors involved in the resurgence of parasitic infections include increasing travel, the frequent use of immunosuppressive drugs, and the greater number of immunocompromised hosts, particularly those with HIV infection. Physicians everywhere may see infections caused by previously unfamiliar parasites.

A discussion of antiparasitic therapy is extremely complex and must take into account the numerous infecting organisms, their complicated life cycles, differences in their metabolism, and the multitude of drugs that are available. An additional problem, particularly in treating infections in pediatric age groups, relates to the paucity of controlled studies demonstrating efficacy and safety of many of the antiparasitic agents. Since clinicians may be unfamiliar with the medications often used in treating parasitic disease, additional information and some medications can be obtained from the Parasitic Disease Drug Service, Division of Host Factors, CDC, Atlanta, GA 30333 (Tel.: 404-639-3670).

Taxonomically, parasites are divided into protozoa and helminths. The protozoa often have complex life cycles but are unicellular. On the other hand, the helminths have highly developed neuromuscular systems, integuments, and digestive tracts. Given these differences, it is not surprising that drugs that are effective against protozoa are not effective against helminths and vice versa. Generally, the susceptibility of parasites to therapeutic agents is associated with taxonomy and metabolism.

The dosage and duration of therapy as well as the major adverse reactions of antiparasitic drugs in treating children are provided in Tables 246–1 (antiprotozoal drugs) and 246–2 (anthelmintic drugs). In every case, the indication for treatment must be weighed against the toxicity of the drug. First-choice and alternative agents have been included. When the first choice drug is clinically ineffective but the alternative therapy is more hazardous, retreatment with the first choice may be the most prudent course.

Drugs for parasitic infections. Med Lett 35:15, 1993.

Van Reken DE, Pearson RD: Antiparasitic agents. *In:* Mandell GL, Douglas RG, Bennett JE (eds): Principles and Practices of Infectious Diseases, 3rd ed. New York, Churchill Livingstone, 1989, pp 398–427.

■ TABLE 246–1 Drugs for Treatment of Protozoan Infections

Infection	Drug	Pediatric Dosage[a]	Adverse Effects
Amebiasis (Entamoeba histolytica)			
Asymptomatic			
Drug of choice:	Diloxanide furoate[b]	20 mg/kg/24 hr in 3 doses for 10 days	Frequent: flatulence Occasional: nausea, vomiting, diarrhea Rare: urticaria, pruritus
Alternatives:	Iodoquinol[c]	30–40 mg/kg/24 hr in 3 doses for 20 days	Occasional: rash, nausea, diarrhea, cramps, anal pruritus Rare: optic atrophy and loss of vision (high doses for months), iodine sensitivity
	Paromomycin	25–30 mg/kg/24 hr in 3 doses for 7 days	Frequent: GI disturbances Rare: 8th nerve dysfunction, azotemia
Intestinal disease			
Drugs of choice:	Metronidazole[d]	30–50 mg/kg/24 hr in 3 doses for 10 days	Frequent: nausea, headache, metallic taste Occasional: vomiting, diarrhea, insomnia, rash, disulfiram-like reaction with alcohol Rare: seizures, encephalopathy, ataxia, leukopenia, peripheral neuropathy
	FOLLOWED BY Diloxanide furoate[b]	20 mg/kg/24 hr in 3 doses for 10 days	See above
Alternatives:	Dehydroemetine[b, e]	1–1.5 mg/kg/24 hr (max. 90 mg/24/hr) IM in 2 doses for up to 5 days	Similar to emetine, but probably less severe
	FOLLOWED BY Diloxanide furoate[b]	20 mg/kg/24 hr in 3 doses for 10 days	See above
	OR Emetine[e]	1 mg/kg/24 hr in 2 doses (max. 60 mg/24 hr) IM for up to 5 days	Frequent: cardiac arrhythmias, precordial pain, muscle weakness, cellulitis at injection site Occasional: diarrhea, vomiting, heart failure, peripheral neuropathy
	FOLLOWED BY Diloxanide furoate[b]	20 mg/kg/24 hr in 3 doses for 10 days	See above
Hepatic abscess			
Drugs of choice:	Metronidazole[d]	35–50 mg/kg/24 hr in 3 doses for 10 days	See above
	FOLLOWED BY Diloxanide furoate[b]	20 mg/kg/24 hr in 3 doses for 10 days	See above
Alternatives:	Dihydroemetine[b, e]	1–1.5 mg/kg/24 hr (max. 90 mg/24 hr) IM in 2 doses for up to 5 days	See above
	FOLLOWED BY Diloxanide furoate[b]	20 mg/kg/24 hr in 3 doses for 10 days	See above
	OR Emetine	1 mg/kg/24 hr in 2 doses (max. 60 mg/24 hr) IM	See above
	Chloroquine phosphate	10 mg base/kg (max. 300 mg base)/24 hr × 2–3 wk	See malaria section
	FOLLOWED BY Diloxanide furoate[b]	20 mg/kg/24 hr in 3 doses for 10 days	See above
Amebic Meningoencephalitis, primarily Naegleria sp.			
Drug of choice:	Amphotericin B[f, g]	1 mg/kg/24 hr, uncertain duration	Frequent: acute reaction (fever, rigors, occasional hypertension and tachypnea), nephrotoxicity, headache, nausea, vomiting, anemia Occasional: renal tubular acidosis, hypomagnesemia Rare: thrombocytopenia and leukopenia
Acanthamoeba spp.	See footnote i		
Babesiosis (Babesis sp.)			
Drugs of choice:	Clindamycin[g]	20–40 mg/kg/24 hr in 3 doses for 7 days	Occasional: anorexia, nausea, vomiting, mild transaminitis, rash, pseudomembranous colitis Rare: fever, eosinophilia, anaphylaxis, Stevens-Johnson syndrome
	PLUS Quinine	25 mg/kg/24 hr in 3 doses for 7 days	Frequent: cinchonism (tinnitus, headache, nausea, abdominal pain, visual disturbances) Occasional: hemolysis anemia, photosensitivity reactions, hypoglycemia, arrhythmias, hypotension, drug fever
Balantidiasis (Balantidium coli)			
Drug of choice:	Tetracycline[g]	>8 years of age: 10 mg/kg qid for 10 days (max. 2 g/24 hr)	Frequent: rash, fever, eosinophilia, GI disturbances, phototoxic reactions, in fetus and young children—staining teeth and retarding bone growth, superinfection with *Candida* Occasional: hepatotoxicity, coagulopathy, increased intracranial pressure in infancy Rare: pseudomembranous colitis
Alternatives:	Iodoquinol[c, g]	30–40 mg/kg/24 hr in 3 doses for 20 days	See above
	OR Metronidazole[d]	35–50 mg/kg/24 hr in 3 doses for 5 days	See above
Blastocystis hominis infection			
Drug of choice:	Iodoquinol[c, g]	30–40 mg/kg/24 hr in 3 doses for 20 days	See above
	OR Metronidazole[d, g]	35–50 mg/kg/24 hr in 3 doses for 10 days	See above
Cryptosporidiosis (Cryptosporidium sp.)	No known effective therapy[h]		

Table continued on following page

■ **TABLE 246–1 Drugs for Treatment of Protozoan Infections** *Continued*

Infection	Drug	Pediatric Dosage[a]	Adverse Effects
***Dientamoeba fragilis* infection**			
Drug of Choice:	Iodoquinol[c] OR	40 mg/kg/24 hr in 3 doses for 20 days	See above
	Tetracycline[g] OR	10 mg/kg qid for 10 days (max. 2 g/24 hr)	See above
	Paromomycin	25–30 mg/kg/24 hr in 3 doses for 7 days	See above
***Entamoeba polecki* infection**			
Drugs of choice:	Metronidazole[d, g] FOLLOWED BY	35–50 mg/kg/24 hr in 3 doses for 10 days	See above
	Diloxamide furoate[b]	20 mg/kg/24 hr in 3 doses for 10 days	See above
Giardiasis (Giardia lamblia)			
Drug of choice:	Furazolidone	1.5 mg/kg qid for 7–10 days	Frequent: nausea, vomiting Occasional: allergic reactions, hypotension, urticaria, fever, hypoglycemia, headache Rare: hemolytic anemia in neonates, polyneuritis, MAO-inhibitor reactions
Alternatives:	Metronidazole[d, g] OR	5 mg/kg tid for 5 days	See above
	Quinacrine HCl	2 mg/kg tid for 5 days (max. 300 mg/24 hr)	Frequent: dizziness, headache, vomiting Occasional: yellow staining of skin, toxic psychosis, insomnia, blood dyscrasias, psoriasis-like rash Rare: Acute hepatic necrosis, convulsions, exfoliative dermatitis, ocular effects
Isosporiasis (Isospora belli)			
Drug of choice:	Trimethoprim-sulfamethoxazole	10 mg/kg/24 hr as TMP in 4 divided oral doses for 3 wk	Frequent: GI disturbances, rash Occasional: cytopenias, hepatotoxicity, renal insufficiency, fever, skin rash (cytopenias and hepatotoxicity occur more frequently in patients with AIDS)
***Leishmaniasis* (*L. braziliensis, L. mexicana,* and mucocutaneous leishmaniasis)**			
Drug of choice:	Stibogluconate sodium[b]	10 mg/kg bid IM or IV (max. 800 mg/24 hr) for 20–28 days	Frequent: myalgias and arthralgias, bradycardia Occasional: diarrhea, rash, pruritus Rare: hepatitis and renal failure, hemolytic anemia, shock, cardiac arrhythmias
Alternative:	Amphotericin B[b]	0.25–1.00 mg/kg/24 hr for up to 8 wk	See above
(*L. donovani*—kala azar, visceral leishmaniasis)			
Drug of choice:	Stibogluconate sodium[b, k] OR	20 mg/kg/24 hr IM or IV (max. 800 mg/24 hr) for 20 days	See above
Alternative:	Pentamidine isoethionate	2–4 mg/kg/24 hr IV or every 2 days IM	Frequent: hypotension, hypoglycemia often followed by diabetes mellitus, vomiting, blood dyscrasias, GI disturbances Occasional: shock, hypocalcemia, liver failure, cardiotoxicity, rash Rare: anaphylaxis, acute pancreatitis
(*L. tropica, L. major*—oriental sore, cutaneous leishmaniasis)			
Drug of choice:	Stibogluconate sodium[c, l]	10 mg/kg/24 hr IM or IV (max. 600 mg/24 hr) for 6–10 days	See above
Alternative:	Topical therapy[l]		
Malaria (Treatment)			
All *Plasmodium* except chloroquine-resistant *P. falciparum*			
ORAL			
Drug of choice:	Chloroquine phosphate[n, o]	10 mg base/kg (max. 600 mg base), then 5 mg base/kg 6 hr later, then 5 mg base/kg/24 hr for 2 days	Occasional: pruritus, vomiting, headache, confusion, rash, corneal opacities, extraocular muscle paralysis, exacerbation of psoriasis, myalgia Rare: irreversible retinal injury (when total dose exceeds 100 g), discoloration of nails and mucous membranes, deafness, neuropathy and myopathy, heart block, blood dyscrasias
PARENTERAL			
Drug of choice:	Quinine dihydrochloride[b] OR	25 mg/kg/24 hr; give one third of daily dose over 2–4 hr, repeat every 8 hr until oral therapy can be started (max. 1,800 mg/24 hr)	See above
	Quinidine gluconate[g, p]	10 mg/kg IV, then 0.02 mg/kg/min IV for 72 hr	Frequent: GI disturbances, cinchonism Occasional: rash, ventricular ectopy, widening of QRS complex and prolonged QT interval, A-V block, headache, delirium, ataxia Rare: cytopenias (especially thrombocytopenia), hypotension, fever, systemic lupus erythematosus See above
Alternative:	Chloroquine HCl[b]	Optimal dosing not determined	See above
Chloroquine-resistant *P. falciparum*			
ORAL			
Drugs of choice:	Quinine sulfate[q, r] PLUS	25 mg/kg/24 hr in 3 doses for 3 days	See above
	Pyrimethamine	<10 kg: 6.25 mg/24 hr for 3 days 10–20 kg: 12.5 mg/24 hr for 3 days 20–40 kg: 25 mg/24 hr for 3 days	Occasional: blood dyscrasias, folic acid deficiency Rare: rash, vomiting, convulsions, shock

■ TABLE 246–1 Drugs for Treatment of Protozoan Infections *Continued*

Infection	Drug	Pediatric Dosage[a]	Adverse Effects
Malaria (Treatment) (Continued)			
	PLUS		
	Sulfadiazine	100–200 mg/kg/24 hr in 4 doses for 5 days (max. 2 g/day)	See trimethoprim-sulfamethoxazole
Alternative:	Quinine sulfate[s]	25 mg/kg/24 hr in 3 doses for 3 days	See above
	PLUS		
	Tetracycline	5 mg/kg qid for 7 days	See above
PARENTERAL			
Drug of choice:	Quinine dihydrochloride[b]	25 mg/kg/24 hr in 3 doses for 3 days	See above
	OR		
	Quinidine gluconate[g, p]	10 mg/kg IV slowly (max. 600 mg), then 0.02 mg/kg/min IV for 72 hr	See above
Prevention of Relapses			
P. vivax and *P. ovale* only			
Drug of choice:	Primaquine phosphate[t]	0.3 mg base/kg/24 hr for 14 days	Frequent: hemolytic anemia in G-6-PD deficiency Occasional: neutropenia, GI disturbances, methemoglobinemia in G-6-PD deficiency Rare: CNS symptoms, hypertension, arrhythmias
Prevention of Malaria[u]			
Chloroquine-sensitive areas			
Drug of choice:	Chloroquine phosphate[n, v]	5 mg/kg base (8.3 mg/kg salt) once per wk, up to maximum adult dose of 300 mg base	See above
Chloroquine-resistant areas			
Drugs of choice:	Mefloquine	<15 kg: not recommended 15–19 kg: ¼ tab (62.5 mg)/wk 20–30 kg: ½ tab (125 mg)/kg 31–45 kg: ¾ tab (187.5 mg)/wk >45 kg: 1 tab (250 mg)/wk	Occasional: GI disturbances, dizziness Rare: problems with fine coordination and spacial discrimination Contraindicated in those with history of seizures, patients using beta blockers or other drugs prolonging cardiac conduction
	OR		
	Chloroquine phosphate[n]	5 mg/kg base (8.3/kg salt) once per wk, up to maximum adult dose of 300 mg base	See above
	PLUS		
	Proguanil[u] (in Africa, south of Sahara)	<2 yr: 50 mg daily 2–6 yr: 100 mg daily 7–10 yr: 150 mg daily 10 yr: 200 mg daily	Occasional: oral ulcerations, vomiting, abdominal pain, diarrhea Rare: hematuria (with large doses)
	Pyrimethamine-sulfadoxine (Fansidar)[x]	2–11 mo: ¼ tablet 1–3 yr: ½ tablet 4–8 yr: 1 tablet 9–14 yr: 2 tablets >14 yr: 3 tablets Take single dose of above for self-treatment of febrile illness when medical care is not immediately available	
	OR		
	Doxycycline[y]	>8 yr of age: 2 mg/kg/24 hr, up to adult dose of 100 mg/24 hr	See above
Pneumocystis carinii pneumonia			
Drugs of choice:	Trimethoprim-sulfamethoxazole	TMP 15–20 mg/kg/24 hr, SMX 75–100 mg/kg/24 hr oral or IV in 4 doses for 14–21 days	See above
Alternatives:	Steroids (prednisone) for severe cases (Po_2>70 mm)		
	Pentamadine isethionate	3–4 mg/kg/24 hr IM or IV for 14–21 days	See above
	Trimethoprim	5 mg/kg q 6 hr × 21 days	See above
	PLUS		
	Dapsone	100 mg qd × 21 days	Frequent: rash, dose-related hemolysis (especially in G-6P-D-deficient patients) Occasional: peripheral neuropathy, nausea, vomiting fever, abdominal pain, insomnia Rare: psychosis, pancreatitis, nephrotic syndrome, male infertility, papillary necrosis, drug-induced SLE
	OR		
	Clindamycin	8–16 mg/kg/24 hr in 3 or 4 divided doses orally or IV for 21 days	Frequent: rash, nausea, vomiting, liver enzyme abnormalities Occasional: *C. difficile*–associated colitis, abdominal pain Rare: polyarthritis, Stevens-Johnson syndrome
	PLUS Pyremethamine	0.3 mg base/kg/24 hr for 21 days	See above
Toxoplasmosis (Toxoplasma gondii)			
Drugs of choice:	Pyrimethamine[z]	2 mg/kg/24 hr for 3 days, then 1 mg/kg/24 hr (max. 25 mg/24 hr) for 4 wk	See above
	PLUS		
	Trisulfapyrimidines	100–200 mg/kg/24 hr for 3–4 wk	See above
Alternative:	Spiramycin	50–100 mg/kg/24 hr for 3–4 wk	Occasional: GI disturbances Rare: allergic reactions
Trichomoniasis (Trichomonas vaginalis)			
Drug of choice:	Metronidazole[d, aa]	15 mg/kg/24 hr orally in 3 doses for 7 days	See above

Table continued on following page

■ TABLE 246–1 Drugs for Treatment of Protozoan Infections *Continued*

Infection	Drug	Pediatric Dosage[a]	Adverse Effects
Trypanosomiasis			
(*T. cruzi*, South American trypanosomiasis, Chagas' disease)			
Drug of choice:	Nifurtimox[b]	1–10 yr: 15–20 mg/kg/24 hr in 4 divided doses for 90 days	Frequent: anorexia, vomiting, weight loss, loss of memory, sleep disorders, tremor, paresthesias, weakness, polyneuritis
		11–16 yr: 12.5–15 mg/kg/24 hr in 4 divided doses for 90 days	Rare: convulsions, fever, pulmonary infiltrate, pleural effusion
Alternative:	Benznidazole[bb]	5–7 mg/kg/24 hr for 30–120 days	Frequent: rash, dose-dependent polyneuropathy, GI disturbances
(*T. gambiense, T. rhodesiense*, African trypanosomiasis, sleeping sickness) hemolymphatic stage			
Drug of choice[bb]:	Suramin[b]	20 mg/kg on days 1, 3, 7, 14, and 21	Frequent: vomiting, pruritus, urticaria, paresthesias, hyperesthesias, photophobia, peripheral neuropathy Occasional: renal insufficiency, blood dyscrasias, shock, optic atrophy
Alternative:	Pentamidine isethionate	4 mg/kg/24 hr IM for 10 days	See above
Late disease with CNS involvement			
Drug of choice:	Melarsoprol[b, dd]	18–25 mg/kg total given over 1 mo; initial dose of 0.36 mg/kg IV, increasing gradually to maximum 3.6 mg/kg at intervals of 1–5 days for total of 9–10 doses	Frequent: myocardial damage, albuminuria, hypertension, Herxheimer reaction, encephalopathy, vomiting, peripheral neuropathy Rare: shock
Alternatives:	Tryparsamide	Unknown	Frequent: nausea, vomiting Occasional: impaired vision, optic atrophy, fever, dermatitis, tinnitus, allergic reactions
	PLUS		
	Suramin[b]	Unknown	See above

[a] *Also see appropriate sections in text.*
[b] *In the United States this drug is available from the CDC Drug Service, Centers for Disease Control, Atlanta, GA 30333; telephone: (404) 639–3670; evenings, weekends, and holidays: (404) 639–2888.*
[c] *Dosage and duration of administration should not be exceeded because of the possibility of optic neuritis; maximum dosage is 2 g/24 hr.*
[d] *Metronidazole is carcinogenic in rodents and mutagenic in bacteria; it should generally not be given in pregnancy (especially in the 1st trimester). Tinidazole, 50 mg/kg (max. 2 g) qd × 3 days is also effective but not available in the United States.*
[e] *Dihydroemetine is probably as effective and less toxic than emetine. Because of cardiac toxicity, patients receiving emetine should have electrocardiographic monitoring during therapy.*
[f] *One patient with a* Naegleria *infection was successfully treated with amphotericin B, miconazole, and rifampin (N Engl J Med 306:346, 1981).*
[g] *Considered an investigational drug for this condition by the U.S. Food and Drug Administration.*
[h] *Octreotide may be effective in controlling diarrhea but not the infection. Paromomycin (25 mg/kg/24 hr) and azithromycin have been sometimes effective in adults, but experience with these two drugs in children is limited.*
[i] *Experimental infections with* Acanthamoeba *sp. have responded to sulfadiazine (Annu Rev Microbiol 25:231, 1971). Amebic keratitis due to* Acanthamoeba *sp. has responded to topical miconazole, 10% propamidine isethionate plus neosporin or oral itraconazole plus topical miconazole (Br J Opthalmol 73:271, 1984; Am J Opthalmol 109:121, 1990). Topical polyhexamethyl biguanidine has been effective (Am J Opthalmol 115:460, 1993). Pentamidine, ketoconazole, flucytosine is effective in vitro against* Acanthamoeba.
[j] *In sulfonamide-sensitive persons, such as many patients with AIDS, pyrimethamine 50–75 mg/day has been effective. In immunocompromised patients it may be necessary to continue therapy indefinitely.*
[k] *In patients with the African form of visceral leishmaniasis, therapy may have to be extended to at least 30 days and may have to be repeated.*
[l] *Ketoconazole 400 mg daily for 4–8 wk has been reported to be effective (Am J Trop Med Hyg 35:491, 1986).*
[m] *Application of heat 39–42° C directly to lesion for 20–32 hr over a period of 10–12 days has been reported to be effective in* L. tropica *minor infections (Am J Trop Med Hyg 33:800, 1984).*
[n] *If chloroquine phosphate is not available, hydroxychloroquine sulfate is as effective; 400 mg of hydroxychloroquine sulfate is equivalent to 500 mg of chloroquine phosphate.*
[o] *In* P. falciparum *malaria, if the patient has not shown a response to conventional doses of chloroquine in 48–72 hr, parasitic resistance to this drug should be considered. Intramuscular injection of chloroquine is painful and can cause abscesses.*
[p] *Optimal dosage for treatment of malaria is currently under investigation. For up-to-date information, telephone the Centers for Disease Control: daytime (404) 488–4046; nights, weekends, holidays (404) 639–2888. Electrocardiographic monitoring is necessary to detect arrhythmias. Some experts consider quinidine more effective than quinine.*
[q] *Quinine alone will usually control an attack of resistant* P. falciparum, *but in a substantial number of infections, particularly with strains from Southeast Asia, it fails to prevent recurrence; the addition of pyrimethamine and sulfadiazine lowers the rate of recurrence.*
[r] *For treatment of* P. falciparum *infections acquired in Thailand, quinine should be given for 7 days instead of 3, combined with 7 days of tetracycline.*
[s] *Quinine plus tetracycline may be the regimen of choice in areas such as Thailand, where resistance to pyrimethamine plus sulfonamides is common.*
[t] *Primaquine phosphate can cause hemolytic anemia, especially in patients whose red cells are deficient in G-6-PD. This deficiency is most common in blacks, Asians, and Mediterranean peoples. Patients should be screened for G-6-PD deficiency before treatment. Primaquine should not be used during pregnancy.*
[u] *At present, no drug regimen guarantees protection against malaria. If fever develops within a year (particularly within the first 2 mo) after travel to malarious areas, travelers should be advised to seek medical attention. Countries with a risk of chloroquine-resistant falciparum malaria continue to increase. Travelers to any of these countries should be advised to avoid mosquito bites by using insect repellants containing diethyltoluamide (DEET) and using mosquito netting when sleeping in exposed areas.*
[v] *For prevention of attack after departure from areas where* P. vivax *and* P. ovale *are endemic, which includes almost all areas where malaria is found (except Haiti), some experts prescribe primaquine phosphate (15 mg base (26.3 mg)/24 hr or, for children, 0.3 mg base/kg/24 hr for 14 days). Others prefer to avoid the toxicity of primaquine and rely on surveillance to detect cases when they occur, particularly when exposure was limited or doubtful. Primaquine can cause hemolytic anemia, especially in patients whose red cells are deficient in G-6-PD. This deficiency is most common in blacks, Asians, and Mediterranean peoples. Patients should be screened for G-6-PD deficiency before treatment. Primaquine should not be used during pregnancy.*
[w] *Proguanil (Paludrine-Ayerst, Canada; ICI) is not available in the United States.*
[x] *Recommmended for travel to Africa south of the Sahara, the Indian subcontinent, South America (except the Amazon basin), Oceania, Hainan Island, and the southern provinces of China. Use of Fansidar, which contains 25 mg of pyrimethamine and 500 mg of sulfadoxine/tablet, is contraindicated in patients with a history of sulfonamide or pyrimethamine intolerance, in pregnancy at term, and in infants less than 2 mo old.*
[y] *Used in Southeast Asia and the Amazon basin. The FDA considers the use of tetracyclines as antimalarials to be investigational. Use of doxycycline is contraindicated in pregnancy and in children less than 8 yr old. Physicians who prescribe doxycycline as malaria chemoprophylaxis should advise patients to limit direct exposure to the sun to minimize the possibility of a photosensitivity reaction. Young children or other travelers who cannot take doxycycline should carry Fansidar.*
[z] *Pyrimethamine is teratogenic in animals. To prevent hematologic toxicity from pyrimethamine, it is advisable to give leucovorin (folinic acid) 10/mg/24 hr by injection or orally. In AIDS patients, therapy should be continued indefinitely. Most authorities would treat congenitally infected newborns for about 1 yr.*
[aa] *Sexual partners should be treated simultaneously. Metronidazole-resistant strains have been reported.*
[bb] *Limited data.*
[cc] *In drug-resistant cases of* T. gambiense *infections, elflornithine (difluoromethylornithine, Merrell Dow) has been used successfully; field trials are now under way (Taelman H, et al: Am J Med 82:607, 1987; Doua F, et al: Am J Trop Med Hyg 37:525, 1987; Pepin J, et al: Lancet 2:1431, 1987). It is highly effective in both CNS and non-CNS infections with* T. gambiense.
[dd] *In frail patients, begin with as little as 18 mg and increase the dose progressively. Pretreatment with suramin has been advocated for debilitated patients.*

■ TABLE 246–2 Drugs for Treatment of Helminthic Infections

Infection	Drug	Pediatric Dosage[a]	Adverse Effects
Angiostrongyliasis			
Angiostrongylus cantanensis			
Drug of choice:	Mebendazole[b, c, d]	100 mg bid for 5 days for children >2 yr	Occasional: diarrhea, abdominal pain Rare: leukopenia, agranulocytosis, hypospermia
Angiostrongylus costaricensis			
Drug of choice:	Thiabendazole[b, c] OR Surgical intervention	25 mg/kg tid for 3 days[e] (max. 3 g/24 hr)	Frequent: nausea, vomiting, vertigo Occasional: leukopenia, crystalluria, rash, hallucinations, olfactory disturbances, erythema multiforme, Stevens-Johnson syndrome Rare: shock, tinnitus, intrahepatic cholestasis, convulsions, angioneurotic edema
Anisakiasis (*Anisakis* sp.)			
Treatment of choice:	Surgical removal		
Ascariasis			
Ascaris lumbricoides (roundworm)			
Drug of choice:	Mebendazole OR	100 mg bid for 3 days for children >2 yr	See above
	Pyrantel pamoate	11 mg/kg once (max. 1 g)	Occasional: GI disturbances, headache, dizziness, rash, fever
Alternative:	Piperazine citrate	75 mg/kg (max. 3.5 g)/24 hr for 2 days	Occasional: dizziness, urticaria, GI disturbances Rare: exacerbation of epilepsy, ataxia, visual disturbances, hypotonia
Capillariasis			
Capillaria philippinensis			
Drug of choice:	Mebendazole[b]	200 mg bid for 20 days	See above
Alternative:	Thiabendazole[b]	25 mg/kg/24 hr for 30 days	See above
Cutaneous Larva Migrans			
Drug of choice:	Thiabendazole	25 mg/kg bid (max. 3 g/24 hr) for 2–5 days and/or topically	See above
Dracunculus medinensis			
(Guinea worm infection)			
Drug of choice:	Metronidazole[b]	25 mg/kg/24 hr (max. 750 mg/24 hr) in 3 doses for 10 days	See Table 246–1
Alternative:	Thiabendazole[b]	25–37.5 mg/kg bid for 3 days	See above
Enterobius vermicularis			
(Pinworm infection)			
Drug of choice:	Pyrantel pamoate	A single dose of 11 mg/kg (max. 1 g) repeated after 2 wk	See above
	OR Mebendazole	A single dose of 100 mg for children >2 yr; repeat after 2 wk	See above
	Albendazole	400 mg once, repeat in 2 wk	Similar to mebendazole
Filariasis			
Wuchereria bancrofti, Brugia malayi, Mansonella, ozzardi, Loa loa			
Drug of choice[g]:	Diethylcarbamazine[h]	Day 1: 1 mg/kg Day 2: 1 mg/kg tid Day 3: 1–2 mg/kg tid Day 4 thru 21: 3 mg/kg tid	Frequent: severe allergic or febrile reaction, GI disturbances Rare: encephalopathy, loss of vision in onchocerciasis
Mansonella perstans			
Drug of choice[i]:	Mebendazole[b]	100 mg bid for 30 days	See above
Topical eosinophilia			
Drug of choice:	Diethylcarbamazine[h]	2 mg/kg tid for 21 days	See above
Onchocerca volvulus			
Drug of choice:	Ivermectin[b, j]	150 μg/kg PO once	Occasional: fever, pruritus, tender lymph nodes Rare: hypotension
Alternatives:	Diethylcarbamazine[h]	0.5 mg/kg tid for 3 days (max. 25 mg/24 hr), then 1.0 mg/kg tid for 3–4 days (max. 50 mg/24 hr), then 1.5 mg/kg tid for 3–4 days (max. 100 mg/24 hr), then 2.0 mg/kg tid for 2–3 wk	See above
	FOLLOWED BY Suramin[k, l]	10–20 mg (test dose) IV, then 20 mg/kg IV at weekly intervals for 5 wk	See Table 246–1
Fluke infection			
Clonorchis sinensis (Chinese liver fluke)			
Drug of choice:	Praziquantel[b]	25 mg/kg tid for 1 day	Frequent: malaise, headache, dizziness Occasional: sedation, abdominal discomfort, fever, sweating, nausea, eosinophilia, fatigue
Fasciola hepatica (sheep liver fluke)			
Drug of choice:	Bithionol	30–50 mg/kg	Frequent: rash, dizziness, headache Occasional: extra heartbeats, lowered blood pressure, liver, bone marrow, kidney toxicity
	Praziquantel[m]	25 mg/kg tid for 2 days	See above

Table continued on following page

■ **TABLE 246–2 Drugs for Treatment of Helminthic Infections** *Continued*

Infection	Drug	Pediatric Dosage[a]	Adverse Effects
Fluke infection (Continued)			
Fasciolopsis buski (intestinal fluke)			
Drug of choice:	Praziquantel[b]	25 mg/kg tid for 1 day	See above
	OR		
	Niclosamide[b]	11–34 kg: a single dose of 2 tablets (1 g) >34 kg: a single dose of 3 tablets (1.5 g)	Occasional: nausea, abdominal pain
Heterophyes heterophyes (intestinal fluke)			
Drug of choice:	Praziquantel[b]	25 mg/kg tid for 1 day	See above
Metagonimus yokogawai (intestinal fluke)			
Drug of choice:	Praziquantel[b]	25 mg/kg tid for 1 day	See above
Opisthorchis viverrini (liver fluke)			
Drug of choice:	Praziquantel[b]	25 mg/kg tid for 1 day	See above
Paragonimus westermani (lung fluke)			
Drug of choice:	Praziquantel[b]	25 mg/kg tid for 2 days	See above
Alternative:	Bithionol[l]	30–50 mg/kg on alternate days for 10–15 doses	Frequent: photosensitivity, vomiting, diarrhea, abdominal pain, urticaria Rare: leukopenia, toxic hepatitis
Gnathostomiasis			
Gnathostoma spinigerum			
Treatment of choice:	Surgical removal		
	OR		
	Mebendazole[b]	Not determined	
	OR		
	Albendazole	400 mg once	See above
Hookworm infection			
Ancylostoma duodenale, Necator americanus			
Drug of choice:	Mebendazole	100 mg bid for 3 days for children >2 yr	See above
	OR		
	Pyrantel pamoate[b]	11 mg/kg (max. 1 g) for 3 days	See above
Schistosomiasis			
S. haematobium			
Drug of choice:	Praziquantel	20 mg/kg bid for 1 day	See above
S. japonicum			
Drug of choice:	Praziquantel	20 mg/kg tid for 1 day	See above
S. mansoni			
Drug of choice:	Praziquantel	20 mg/kg bid 1 day	See above
Alternative:	Oxamniquine	10 mg/kg bid for 1 day[n]	Occasional: headache, fever, dizziness, somnolence, nausea, diarrhea, rash, liver enzyme changes, ECG and EEG changes, orange-red discoloration of urine Rare: convulsions, neuropsychiatric disturbances
S. mekongi			
Drug of choice:	Praziquantel	20 mg/kg tid for 1 day	See above
Strongyloidiasis			
Strongyloides stercoralis			
Drug of choice:	Thiabendazole	25 mg/kg bid (max. 3 g/24 hr) for 2 days[p]	See above
Tapeworm infection			
Adult or intestinal stage (*Diphyllobothrium latum* (fish), *Taenia saginata* (beef),[q] *Taenia solium* (pork), *Dipylidium caninum* (dog)			
Drug of choice:	Niclosamide	11–34 kg: a single dose of 2 tablets (1 g) >34 kg: a single dose of 3 tablets (1.5 g) for 1 day, then 2 tablets for 6 days	See above
		10–20 mg/kg once	See above
Larval or tissue stage	OR		
Hymenolepsis nana (dwarf tapeworm)	Praziquantel	10 mg/kg once	See above
Drug of choice:	Praziquantel	25 mg/kg once	See above
Alternative:	Niclosamide	11–34 kg: a single dose of 2 tablets (1 g) for 1 day, then 1 tablet for 6 days >34 kg: a single dose of 3 tablets (1.5 g) for 1 day, then 2 tablets for 6 days	See above
Echinococcus granulosus			
Treatment of choice:	Surgical resection[r]		
Echinococcus multilocularis			
Treatment of choice:	Surgical resection[s]		
Cysticercus cellulosae (cysticercosis)			
Drugs of choice:[t]	Praziquantel[b]	50 mg/kg/24 hr in 3 doses for 14 days	See above
	Albendazole	15 mg/kg/24 hr in 3 doses × 28 days	See above
Alternative:	Surgery		

■ TABLE 246–2 Drugs for Treatment of Helminthic Infections *Continued*

Infection	Drug	Pediatric Dosage[a]	Adverse Effects
Trichinosis			
Trichinella sourakus			
Drugs of choice:	Steroids for severe symptoms PLUS		
	Thiabendazole[u]	25 mg/kg for 5 days	See above
Trichostrongylus infection			
Drug of choice:	Pyrantel pamoate[b]	11 mg/kg once (max. 1 g)	See above
Alternative:	Thiabendazole[b]	25 mg/kg bid for 2 days	See above
Trichuriasis			
Trichuris trichiuria (whipworm)			
Drug of choice:	Mebendazole	100 mg bid for 3 days for children >2 yr	See above
Visceral Larva Migrans			
Drug of choice:	Diethylcarbamazine[b] OR	2 mg/kg tid for 7–10 days	See above
	Thiabendazole	25 mg/kg bid for 5 days (max. 3 g)	See above
Alternative:	Mebendazole[b]	100 mg bid for 5 days for children >2 yr	See above

[a]*Also see specific sections.*
[b]*Considered an investigational drug for this condition by the U.S. Food and Drug Administration.*
[c]*Effectiveness documented only in animals.*
[d]*Analgesics, corticosteroids, and careful removal of CSF at frequent intervals can relieve symptoms. Albendazole and ivermectin have been used successfully in animals.*
[e]*This dose is likely to be toxic and may have to be decreased.*
[f]*Metronidazole is carcinogenic in rodents and mutagenic in bacteria; it should generally not be given to pregnant women, particularly in the 1st trimester.*
[g]*Several reports indicate that ivermectin may be effective for treatment of* W. bancrofti *(Lancet 1:1030, 1987) and* M. ozzardi *(J Infect Dis 156:662, 1987).*
[h]*Diethylcarbamazine should be administered with special caution in heavy infections with* Loa loa *because it can provoke ocular problems or an encephalopathy. Antihistamines or corticosteroids may be required to decrease allergic reactions owing to disintegration of microfilariae in treatment of all filarial infections, especially those caused by* Onchocerca *and* Loa loa. *Surgical excision of subcutaneous* Onchocerca *nodules is recommended by some authorities before drug therapy is started. Ivermectin may also be effective.*
[i]*Ivermectin may also be effective.*
[j]*Ivermectin in a dose of 200 μg/kg has been reported to be as effective as diethylcarbamazine in decreasing the number of microfilaria and causes fewer adverse ophthalmologic reactions (N Engl J Med 313:133, 1985; J Infect Dis 156:463, 1987). Semiannual to annual prophylaxis appears to be effective in keeping microfilarial counts at low levels.*
[k]*Some Medical Letter consultants use suramin only if ocular microfilariae persist after diethylcarbamazine therapy and nodulectomy.*
[l]*In the United States this drug is available from the CDC Drug Service, Centers for Disease Control, Atlanta, Georgia 30333; telephone (404) 639–3670; evenings, weekends, and holidays: (404) 639–2888.*
[m]*Unlike infections with other flukes,* Fasciola hepatica *infections may not respond to praziquantel. Limited data indicate that albendazole may be effective for this condition.*
[n]*In East Africa the dose should be increased to 30 mg/kg/24 hr, and in Egypt and South Africa to 30 mg/kg/24 hr for 2 days. Neuropsychiatric disturbances and seizures have been reported in some patients (Am J Trop Med Hyg 35:330, 1986).*
[o]*Albendazole or ivermectin has also been effective.*
[p]*In disseminated strongyloidiasis, thiabendazole therapy should be continued for at least 5 days. In immunocompromised patients it may be necessary to continue therapy or use other agents (see footnote o). Albendazole has also been recently shown to be effective.*
[q]*Nicosamide is effective for the treatment of* T. solium, *but, since it causes distintegration of segments and release of viable eggs, its use creates a theoretical risk of causing cysticercosis. It should therefore be followed in 3 or 4 hr by a purge. Quinacrine is preferred by some clinicians because it expels* T. solium *intact.*
[r]*Surgical resection of cysts is the treatment of choice. When surgery is contraindicated, or when cysts rupture spontaneously during surgery, mebendazole (experimental for this purpose in the United States) can be tried (Ann Trop Parasitol 76:165, 1982; Trans R Soc Trop Med Hyg 76:510, 1982). Albendazole has also been reported to be effective (JAMA 253:2053, 1985). Flubendazole has also been used with some success. (Am J Trop Med Hyg 33:627, 1984). Praziquantel and albendazole will kill protoscolices and may be useful in case of a spill during surgery. Recently, percutaneous drainage via ultrasound plus albendazole therapy has been effective in treating hepatic hydatid cysts.*
[s]*Surgical excision is the only reliable means of treatment, although recent reports have been encouraging about the use of albendazole or mebendazole (Am J Trop Med Hyg 37:162, 1987; Bull WHO 64:383, 1986).*
[t]*Corticosteroids should be given for 2–3 days before and during praziquantel therapy. Praziquantel should not be used for ocular or spinal cord cysticercosis. Metrifonate 7.5 mg/kg for 5 days, repeated 6 times at 2-wk intervals, has been reported to be effective for ocular as well as cerebral and subcutaneous disease. Albendazole, 15 mg/kg for 30 days, which can be repeated, has been used successfully (Arch Intern Med 147:738, 1987).*
[u]*The efficacy of thiabendazole for trichinosis is not clearly established; it appears to be effective during the intestinal phase, but its effect on larvae that have migrated is questionable. In the tissue phase, mebendazole 200–400 mg tid for 3 days, then 400–500 mg tid for 10 days, may be effective. Albendazole may also be effective for this indication.*

SECTION 8

Preventive Measures and Infectious Diseases

CHAPTER 247

Immunization Practices

Kenneth J. Bart

Immunization represents one of the most cost-effective means of preventing serious infectious disease. The integration of immunization practices into routine health care services provides pediatricians with control over a substantial proportion of the disease and mortality that plagued the United States and other countries until the second half of the 20th century. The widespread use of vaccines led to the global eradication of smallpox, the elimination of poliomyelitis from the Americas, and the virtual elimination of poliomyelitis from the Western Pacific. In the United States, immunization has almost eliminated congenital rubella syndrome, tetanus, and diphtheria and reduced the incidence of pertussis, rubella, measles, mumps, and *Haemophilus influenzae* type b meningitis dramatically. More than 50 biologic products are licensed in the United States, and 11 antigens are used for routine immunization of infants and children, including diphtheria and tetanus toxoids and pertussis vaccine, trivalent polio, measles, mumps, and rubella vaccines, Hib, and hepatitis B vaccines.

DEFINITIONS AND MECHANISMS. Vaccination means the administration of any vaccine or toxoid. Immunization describes the process of inducing immunity artificially by administering antigenic substances, such as an immunobiologic agent. Administration of an immunobiologic agent cannot be equated automatically with the development of adequate immunity.

Active immunization consists of inducing the body to develop defenses against disease by the administration of vaccines or toxoids that stimulate the immune system to produce antibodies and cellular immune responses that protect against the infectious agent. Passive immunization consists of providing temporary protection through the administration of exogenously produced antibody. Passive immunization occurs through the transplacental transmission of antibodies to the fetus, which provides protection against several diseases for the first 3–6 mo of life, and the injection of immune globulin for specific preventive purposes.

Immunizing agents include vaccines, toxoids, and antibodies containing preparations from human or animal donors (Table 247–1). Most of these agents contain preservatives, stabilizers, antibiotics, adjuvants, and a suspending fluid (Table 247–2).

The principal approaches to active immunization are the use of live, usually attenuated, infectious agents and the use of inactivated or detoxified agents or their extracts or specific products of recombination (hepatitis B). Both approaches have been employed for many diseases (e.g., influenza, poliomyelitis). Live, attenuated vaccines are thought to induce an immunologic response more like that elicited by natural infection than killed vaccines. Inactivated or killed vaccines consist of inactivated whole organisms (e.g., pertussis vaccine), detoxified exotoxins alone (e.g., tetanus toxoid), or endotoxins linked to carrier proteins, soluble capsular material (e.g., pneumococcal polysaccharide) or conjugated capsular material (e.g., Hib conjugate vaccine), or extracts of some component (e.g., hepatitis B) or components of the organism (e.g., subunit influenza).

Because the organisms in live vaccines multiply in the recipient, antigen production increases until it is checked by the onset of the immune response it is intended to induce. In recipients who develop a response, the live, attenuated viruses (e.g., measles, rubella, mumps) are thought to confer lifelong protection with one dose. In contrast, killed vaccines, except for purified polysaccharide antigens, do not induce permanent immunity with one dose. Repeated vaccination and boosters are needed to develop and maintain high levels of antibody (e.g., diphtheria, rabies). Although more antigen is introduced initially in inactivated vaccines, the multiplication of organisms in the host results in a greater antigenic stimulus by live vaccines.

■ TABLE 247–1 Immunizing Agents

Agent	Definition
Vaccine	A suspension of attenuated live or killed microorganisms or antigenic portions of these agents presented to a potential host to induce immunity and prevent disease
Toxoid	A modified bacterial toxin that has been made nontoxic but retains the capacity to stimulate the formation of antitoxin
Immune globulin	An antibody-containing solution derived from human blood obtained by cold ethanol fractionation of large pools of plasma and used primarily for the maintenance of immunity of immunodeficient persons or for passive immunization; available in intramuscular and intravenous preparations
Antitoxin	An antibody derived from the serum of animals from stimulation with specific antigens used to provide passive immunity

■ TABLE 247–2 Constituents of Vaccines

Component	Use and Examples
Preservatives, stabilizers, antibiotics	Constituents can inhibit or prevent bacterial growth or stabilize the antigen. Materials such as mercurials or antibiotics are used. Allergic reactions to any of the additives may occur.
Adjuvants	An aluminum salt is used in some vaccines to enhance the immune response (e.g., toxoids, hepatitis B).
Suspending fluid	Sterile water, saline, or more complex fluids derived from the growing media or biologic system in which the agent is produced (e.g., egg antigens, cell culture ingredients, serum proteins) are used.

DETERMINANTS OF THE IMMUNE RESPONSE. Because the immune response to specific antigens is controlled genetically, individuals cannot be expected to respond equally well to the same vaccine. The extensive polymorphism of the major histocompatibility complex (MHC) in human populations results in the recognition of different epitopes in a complex protein antigen by different individuals. To vaccinate a population effectively, a vaccine must contain epitopes that are processed and bound to the product of at least one MHC allele in every individual.

The nature and magnitude of the response to vaccines or toxoids is determined by the chemical and physical state of the antigen, the mode of administration, the catabolic rate of the antigen, the genetic characteristics of the recipient, host factors (e.g., age, nutrition, gender, pregnancy status, stress, concurrent infections), and the manner in which the antigen is presented. There is a dose-response relationship between antigen concentration and peak response obtained above a threshold.

Vaccines are administered orally, intradermally, subcutaneously, or intramuscularly. The route of administration affects the rapidity and nature of the immune response to a vaccine or toxoid. Parenterally administered vaccines may not induce mucosal secretory IgA. The immunogenicity of some vaccines is reduced when not given by the proper route; for example, administration of hepatitis B vaccine subcutaneously into the fatty tissue of the buttock rather than intramuscularly in the deltoid resulted in substantially lower seroconversion rates.

The schedule of routine immunization by age is based on age-dependent differences in the immune response. The presence of high levels of maternal antibody in the first few months of life or the immaturity of the immune response impairs the initial immune response to some vaccines.

IMMUNE RESPONSE TO VACCINES. The most important protective antibodies include those that inactivate soluble toxic protein products of bacteria (i.e., antitoxins), facilitate phagocytosis and intracellular digestion of bacteria (i.e., opsonins), interact with components of serum complement to damage the bacterial membrane with resultant bacteriolysis (i.e., lysins), prevent proliferation of infectious virus (i.e., neutralizing antibodies), or interact with components of the bacterial surface to prevent adhesion to mucosal surfaces (i.e., anti-adhesions). Many of the structural constituents of microorganisms and exotoxins are antigenic. Most antigens require the interaction of B cells (thymus independent) and T cells (thymus dependent) to generate an immune response (e.g., measles), but some initiate B-cell proliferation and antibody production without the help of T cells (e.g., pneumococcal type III polysaccharide.)

The first step in the induction of a thymus-dependent antibody response is the activation of T helper cells by presentation of an antigen to mononuclear phagocytes or dendritic cells, a step that may be facilitated by the use of an adjuvant. Presentation of an antigen triggers the secretion of a cascade of mediators, called cytokines, which are made by or act on elements of the immune system to stimulate the maturation of naive T helper cells and to communicate between leukocytes, using interleukins (IL) to regulate the immune response.

Depending on the stimulus, T lymphocytes are stimulated to differentiate into one of two subsets: T helper 1 cells (T_H1), which mediate cell-mediated immune responses, or T helper 2 cells (T_H2), which enhance antibody production. T_H1 cells produce IL-2 and interferon-γ, and T_H2 cells produce IL-4, IL-5, and IL-10.

Antibodies formed to vaccine constituents may be of any immunoglobulin class. Antibodies function alone or in conjunction with other components of the immune system (e.g., complement, opsonin) by participating directly in the neutralization of a toxin (e.g., diphtheria); by opsonization of virus (e.g., poliovirus); by initiating or combining with complement and promoting phagocytosis (e.g., pneumococcus, cholera); by reacting with nonsensitized lymphocytes to stimulate phagocytosis; or by sensitizing macrophages to stimulate phagocytosis.

The primary response to a vaccine antigen requires a latent period of several days before humoral and cell-mediated immunity can be detected. Circulating antibodies do not appear for 7–10 days. The immunoglobulin class of the response changes over time. Early-appearing antibodies are usually IgM; later-appearing antibodies are usually IgG. When the antigen is thymus-dependent, IgM and IgG antibodies are secreted initially by B cells, with IgM appearing first. IgM antibodies fix complement, making lysis and phagocytosis possible. The IgM titer falls as the titer of IgG rises during the 2nd wk (or later) after immunogenic stimulation. The switch from IgM synthesis to predominately IgG synthesis in B cells requires T-cell cooperation. IgG antibodies are produced in high concentrations and function in the neutralization, precipitation, and fixation of complement. IgG titers reach a peak within 2–6 wk.

Live pathogens (e.g., polio, rubella) replicate at mucosal surfaces before host invasion and induce secretory IgA at respiratory, gastrointestinal, and other localized sites. IgA antibodies neutralize viruses efficiently, fix complement through the alternative pathway, prevent absorption of organisms (e.g., *Escherichia coli*) to the intestinal wall, and lyse gram-negative bacteria with complement and lysozyme. Most vaccines, except live virus vaccines, do not induce secretory IgA antibodies effectively.

Heightened humoral or cell-mediated responses are elicited by a second exposure to the same antigen. Secondary responses occur rapidly, usually within 4–5 days. The secondary response depends on immunologic memory mediated by T and B cells and is characterized by a marked proliferation of antibody-producing cells or effector T cells. Polysaccharide vaccines, such as that for *Streptococcus pneumoniae*, evoke immune responses that are independent of T cells and are not seen on repeat administration. Linking polysaccharides to proteins converts them to T-cell–dependent antigens that induce immunologic memory and secondary responses to re-vaccination.

The response to vaccines is usually gauged by measuring specific antibody concentrations in the serum. The presence of circulating antibodies correlates with clinical protection for some viral vaccines (e.g., measles, rubella). Antibody titers serve as a dependable indicator of immunity, but seroconversion measures only one parameter of the host response. Although vaccine-induced antibodies (e.g., measles, rubella) decline over time, revaccination or exposure to the organism elicits a secondary response consisting of IgG antibodies with little or no detectable IgM. The anamnestic response suggests that immunity was persistent. The absence of measurable antibody may not mean that the individual is unprotected. In contrast, the presence of antibodies alone is not sufficient to ensure clinical protection after administration of some vaccines and toxoids. A minimal circulating level of antibody is required, such as 0.01 IU/mL of tetanus toxoid.

Independent of antibody production, the stimulation of the immune system by vaccination may elicit unanticipated responses, especially hypersensitivity reactions. Killed measles vaccine induced incomplete humoral immunity and cell-mediated hypersensitivity, resulting in the development of a syndrome of atypical measles in some children after subsequent challenge.

VACCINES FOR ROUTINE USE. The recommended schedule for administration of vaccines in 1994 to infants and children is shown in Table 247–3. Current practice dictates that all children in the United States should receive DTP, polio, measles, mumps, rubella, Hib, hepatitis B, and varicella vaccines unless contraindicated (Table 247–4). Four doses of DTP and three doses of OPV constitute the primary series. A fifth dose of DTP is given at 4–6 yr of age. Adult-formulation tetanus-diphtheria (Td) boosters are recommended every 10 yr thereafter. A fourth dose of OPV is recommended at 4–6 yr of age.

DTP is not given after the 7th birthday. Instead, combined tetanus and diphtheria toxoids (Td) for adult use, containing a smaller amount of diphtheria toxoid, are recommended at 10 yr intervals. DTP and Td should be given intramuscularly, preferably in the anterolateral thigh in young infants and in the thigh or deltoid in older children.

Two types of polio vaccine are licensed in the United States: OPV, a live, attenuated trivalent poliovirus vaccine (Sabin), and IPV, an inactivated (killed) trivalent poliovirus vaccine (Salk). A full course of either vaccine protects the recipient against paralytic poliomyelitis almost without exception. Because rare cases of paralytic poliomyelitis occur in recipients of OPV or in their close contacts, some have advocated returning to IPV for routine immunization of children. However, immunization advisory groups in the United States have continued to recommend OPV for routine immunization of children because of the virtual eradication of poliomyelitis from the United States by OPV and because of the belief that the circulation of wild virus in the community is controlled better by the greater intestinal immunity afforded by OPV.

OPV should not be given to individuals proven or suspected to be immunocompromised, including those with congenital and acquired immunodeficiencies and those whose immune mechanisms are impaired by therapy. OPV should not be given to household contacts of immunocompromised individuals or to subsequent siblings of a child with congenital immunodeficiency until the younger child is shown to be normal.

All newborn infants should be immunized with hepatitis B vaccine. All pregnant women should be screened for hepatitis B carriage, and if the result is positive, their infants should receive hepatitis immune globulin (HBIG) in addition to active immunization.

Delayed Immunization. It is not necessary to restart an interrupted schedule from the beginning or to add an extra dose. Unimmunized infants 2–14 mo of age should be given the same sequence of immunizations and dose intervals recommended for young infants. However, only a single dose of a conjugated Hib vaccine is recommended for those older than 15 mo. When an older unimmunized child is seen in the family, the adequacy of follow-up is doubtful; the simultaneous administration of DTP, OPV, and MMR is reasonable in these circumstances.

Special Vaccines. Annual immunization against influenza is inappropriate for normal children but should be given to children at high risk from infections of the lower respiratory tract. Populations at risk include children with congenital or acquired heart disease (e.g., left to right shunts); disorders that compromise pulmonary function, including cystic fibrosis, severe asthma, neuromuscular and orthopedic conditions that distort or weaken the thoracic cage, and pulmonary dysplasia as a consequence of the neonatal respiratory distress syndrome; chronic azotemic renal disease or the nephrotic syndrome; diabetes mellitus; and chronic, severe anemia, such

■ **TABLE 247–3 Recommended Schedule for Routine Active Vaccination of Infants and Children**

Vaccine	At Birth (Before Hospital Discharge)	1–2 Mo	2 Mo*	4 Mo	6 Mo	6–18 Mo	12–15 Mo	15 Mo	4–6 Yr (Before School Entry)
Diphtheria, tetanus, pertussis (DTP)			DTP†	DTP	DTP		DTaP/DTP‡		DTaP/DTP
Polio, live oral (OPV)			OPV	OPV	OPV§				OPV
Measles, mumps, rubella (MMR)							MMR		MMR#
Haemophilus influenzae type b conjugate									
HbOC/PRP-T†, ¶			Hib	Hib			Hib**		
PRP-OMP¶			Hib	Hib			Hib**		
Hepatitis B††									
Option 1	HepB	HepB‡‡				HepB‡‡			
Option 2		HepB‡‡		Hep‡‡		HepB‡‡			
Varicella									

Adapted from Recommendations from the Advisory Committee on Immunization Practices (ACIP) and those of the Committee on Infectious Diseases (Red Book Committee) of the American Academy of Pediatrics (AAP).

**Can be administered as early as 6 wk of age.*

†*Two DTP and Hib combination vaccines are available (DTP/HbOC [TETRAMUNE] and PRP-T [ActHIB, Omni-HB]) that can be reconstituted with DTP vaccine produced by Connaught).*

‡*This dose of DTP can be administered as early as 12 mo of age provided that the interval since the previous dose of DTP is at least 6 mo. Diptheria and tetanus toxoids and acellular pertussis vaccine (DTaP) is currently recommended only for use as the fourth and/or fifth doses of the DTP series among children 15 mo through 6 yr of age (before the 7th birthday). Some experts prefer to administer these vaccines at 18 mo of age.*

§*The American Academy of Pediatrics (AAP) recommends this dose of vaccine at 6–18 mo of age.*

#*The AAP recommends that two doses of MMR should be administered by 12 yr of age, with the second dose administered preferentially at entry to middle school or junior high school.*

¶*HbOC: Hib TITER (Lederle Praxis); PRP-T: ActHIB, OmniHIB (Pasteur Merieux); PRP-OMP: PedvaxHIB (Merck, Sharp, and Dohme); A DTP/Hib combination vaccine can be used in place of HbOC/PRP-T.*

***After the primary infant Hib conjugate vaccine series is completed, any of the licensed Hib conjugate vaccines may be used as a booster dose at 12–15 mo of age.*

††*For use among infants born to HBsAg-negative mothers. The first dose should be administered during the newborn period, preferably before hospital discharge, but no later than 2 mo of age. Premature infants of HBsAg-negative mothers should receive the first dose of hepatitis B vaccine series at the time of hospital discharge or when the other routine childhood vaccines are initiated. All infants born to HBsAg-positive mothers should receive immunoprophylaxis for hepatitis B as soon as possible after birth.*

‡‡*Hepatitis B vaccine can be administered at the same time as DTP (or DTaP), OPV, Hib, or MMR.*

as thalassemia or sickle cell anemia. Immunodeficient and immunocompromised children may also benefit. The constituents of influenza vaccine change annually because of shifts in prevalent influenza viruses; annual recommendations of the U.S. Public Health Service, published in the *Morbidity and Mortality Weekly Report,* should be consulted for doses and schedules.

The 23-valent pneumococcal vaccine licensed in the United States is not recommended for routine use in children. As with other polysaccharide vaccines, its efficacy is minimal in children younger than 2 yr of age. It is recommended for children older than 2 yr of age who are at risk of severe, life-threatening pneumococcal infection, such as those with sickle cell disease, asplenia syndrome, cerebrospinal fluid leak, and human immunodeficiency virus (HIV) infection or other immunosuppressive disease states. Experience in treating children with sickle cell anemia indicates that the vaccine is useful in children older than 2 yr who have functional or anatomic asplenia. The dose is 0.5 mL intramuscularly or subcutaneously. Reimmunization with pneumococcal vaccine is not indicated, because antibodies persist and reactogenicity is high even as long as 4 yr after the initial dose. The vaccine is probably ineffective in preventing otitis media.

SIMULTANEOUS ADMINISTRATION AND INTERVALS BETWEEN IMMUNIZATIONS. Vaccines can be given safely and effectively at the same time. In general, inactivated vaccines can be administered simultaneously at separate sites, and field observations indicate that simultaneous administration of the most widely used live virus vaccines does not impair antibody responses or increase adverse reactions. Intervals between doses longer than those recommended delay but do not diminish the ultimate protective response. Giving vaccines at shorter than recommended intervals may impair responses. Although recent administration of OPV is not a contraindication to the use of MMR, other live virus vaccines not given together on the same day should be given at least 30 days apart.

Live virus vaccines can interfere with tuberculin test responses. When a tuberculin skin test is indicated, it may be done on the day of immunization or 6 wk later.

USE OF VACCINES IN SPECIAL CIRCUMSTANCES. Pregnancy. Because of theoretical risks to the fetus and the risk of litigation, immunization of pregnant women is usually avoided. Pregnant women can safely receive tetanus and diphtheria toxoids; it is essential to ensure that pregnant women are immune to tetanus, because transfer of maternal antitoxin antibodies is an important means of prevention of neonatal tetanus.

Live virus vaccines should not be given during pregnancy, with the exception of polio and yellow fever vaccines, which are indicated if the risk of exposure is high. Some inactivated virus vaccines, such as those for influenza and hepatitis B, are safe to give to pregnant women.

Breast-feeding. Breast-feeding does not adversely affect the immune response and is not a contraindication for any vaccine. Breast-feeding women may be vaccinated safely. Although live virus vaccines replicate in the mother, most are not excreted in breast milk. Mothers may receive oral polio or yellow fever vaccines without interrupting breast-feeding.

Immunocompromised States. Limited studies of HIV-infected infants and children show no increased risk of adverse events from live or inactivated vaccines. However, immune responses to vaccines such as MMR may not be as vigorous before clinically significant impairment of immune function. IPV should be used when vaccination against polio is indicated because the risk of vaccine-associated poliomyelitis is too great. Care should be taken to ensure that household contacts to be immunized against polio receive IPV and not OPV. It is unnecessary to test for HIV before making immunization decisions for asymptomatic children.

Live, attenuated vaccines are normally contraindicated in other immunocompromised patients, such as those with the congenital immunodeficiency syndromes and patients receiving immunosuppressive therapy. Passive immunization with immunoglobulin preparations and antitoxins are useful in some cases as postexposure prophylaxis or as part of the therapy of established infection.

Passive Immunization. Passive immunization is used to provide temporary immunity in an unimmunized person exposed to an infectious disease when active immunization is unavailable

■ **TABLE 247–4 Vaccination Contraindications and Precautions**

Vaccine	Valid	Invalid
General for all vaccines (DTP/DTaP, OPV, eIPV, MMR, Hib, HBV)	Anaphylactic reaction to a vaccine contraindicates further doses of that vaccine Anaphylatic reaction to a vaccine constituent contraindicates the use of vaccines containing that substance Moderate or severe illnesses with or without a fever	Mild to moderate local reaction (soreness, redness, swelling) after a dose of an injectable antigen Mild acute illness with or without low-grade fever Current antimicrobial therapy Convalescent phase of illnesses Prematurity (use same dosage and indications as for normal, full-term infants) Recent exposure to an infectious disease History of penicillin or other nonspecific allergies or relatives with such allergies
DTP/DTaP	Encephalopathy within 7 days of administration of a previous dose of DTP Fever of ≥40.5° C (105° F) within 48 hr after vaccination with a prior dose of DTP* Collapse or shocklike state (hypotonic-hyporesponsive episode) within 48 hr of receiving a prior dose of DTP* Seizures within 3 days of receiving a prior dose of DTP*† Persistent inconsolable crying lasting ≥3 hr within 48 hr of receiving a prior dose of DTP	Temperature of >40.5° C (105° F) after a previous dose of DTP Family history of convulsions† Family history of an adverse event after DTP administration Family history of sudden infant death syndrome
OPV	Infection with HIV or a household contact with HIV Known immunodeficiency (hematologic and solid tumors; congenital immunodeficiency syndrome; and long term immunosuppressive therapy) Immunodeficient household contact Pregnancy*	Breast-feeding Current antimicrobial therapy Diarrhea
eIPV	Anaphylactic reactions to neomycin or streptomycin Pregnancy*	
MMR‡ and varicella	Anaphylactic reactions to eggs or to neomycin§ Pregnancy Known immunodeficiency (hematologic and solid tumors; congenital immunodeficiency syndrome; and long-term immunosuppressive therapy) Recent (within 3 mo) immunoglobulin administration*	Tuberculosis or positive PPD Simultaneous tuberculosis skin testing# Breast-feeding Pregnancy of mother of recipient Immunodeficient family member or household contact Infection with HIV Nonanaphylactic reactions to eggs or neomycin
Hib	None identified	
HBV		Pregnancy
Influenza	Avoid during 1st trimester of pregnancy on theoretical grounds Anaphylactic reactions to eggs	
Pneumococcus	Has not been evaluated in pregnancy	

Adapted from the recommendations of the Advisory Committee on Immunization Practices (ACIP) and those of the Committee on Infectious Diseases (Red Book Committee) of the American Academy of Pediatrics (AAP) as of October 1992. Sometimes these recommendations vary from those contained in the manufacturers' package inserts. For detailed information, providers should consult the current published recommendations of the ACIP, the AAP, the AAFP, and the manufacturers' package inserts.

**Events or conditions listed as precautions, although not containdications, should be carefully reviewed. The benefits and risks of administering a specific vaccine individual under the circumstances should be considered. If the risks are believed to outweigh the benefits, the immunization should be withheld; if the benefits are believed to outweigh the risks (e.g., during an outbreak or foreign travel), the immunization should be given. Whether and when to administer DTP to children with proven or suspected underlying neurologic disorders should be decided on an individual basis. It is prudent on theoretical grounds to avoid vaccinating pregnant women. However, if immediate protection against poliomyelitis is needed, OPV, not IPV, is recommended.*

†Acetaminophen given before administering DTP and thereafter every 4 hr for 24 hr should be considered for children with a personal or with a family history of convulsions in siblings or parents.

‡There is a theoretical risk that the administration of multiple live virus vaccines (OPV and MMR) within 30 days of one another if not given on the same day will result in a suboptimal immune response. There are no data to substantiate this.

§Persons with a history of anaphylactic reactions after egg ingestion should be vaccinated only with extreme caution. Protocols have been developed for vaccinating persons and should be consulted (J Pediatr 102:196, 1983; J Pediatr 113:504, 1988).

#Measles vaccination may temporarily suppress tuberculin reactivity. If testing cannot be done the day of MMR vaccination, the test should be postponed for 4–6 wk.

DTP = diphtheria and tetanus toxoids and pertussis vaccine; HBV = hepatitis B virus, Hib = Haemophilus influenzae *type b; HIV = human immunodeficiency virus; IPV = injectable polio vaccine; MMR = measles, mumps, rubella vaccine; OPV = oral polio vaccine.*

(e.g., hepatitis A) or has not been given before exposure (e.g., rabies). Passive immunization is used in the treatment of certain disorders associated with toxins (e.g., diphtheria), in certain bites (e.g., snake and spider bites), and as a specific (e.g., Rho[D] immune globulin) or nonspecific (e.g., antilymphocyte globulin) immunosuppressant.

Three types of preparations are used in passive immunization: standard human immune serum globulin (e.g., intravenous or intramuscular gamma globulin), special immune serum globulins with a known antibody content for specific agents (e.g., hepatitis B or varicella-zoster immune globulin), and animal serums and antitoxins.

Postexposure Immunization. For certain infections, active or passive immunization soon after exposure prevents or attenuates the disease (Table 247–5). Measles immune globulin given within 6 days of exposure may prevent or modify infection, and administration of measles vaccine within the first few days after exposure may prevent symptomatic infection. Although clinical manifestations of rubella are minimized by postexposure passive immunization, viremia, fetal infection, and congenital rubella syndrome may not be prevented; the administration of immune globulin is recommended only for women developing rubella during pregnancy who will not consider abortion. Tetanus immune globulin is used in patients with tetanus along with toxoid vaccine for those who have not been immunized. Administration of rabies immune globulin and rabies vaccine in the immediate postexposure period is highly effective. The use of immune globulin within 2 wk of exposure to hepatitis A is likely to prevent clinical illness. HBV immune globulin also prevents disease after exposure.

Persons receiving high doses of immunoglobulin may have impaired responses to some vaccines for as long as 11 mo. High doses of immune globulin may inhibit the efficacy of measles and rubella vaccines; an interval of at least 3 months

■ TABLE 247–5 Recommended Postexposure Immunization with Immunoglobulin Preparations in the United States

Disease	Indicated	Comments
Measles	Yes	Standard human immune globulin is recommended for exposed infants with normal immunocompetence but contraindication to measles vaccine and for immunocompromised patients exposed to measles, regardless of immunization status. Patients should be immunized 3–6 mo after immunoglobulin. Recommended dose of 0.25–0.5 mL/kg IM; maximum, 15 mL
Rubella	No	Efficacy unreliable; therefore, standard human immune globulin is recommended for use only for antibody-negative pregnant women in the 1st trimester with a documented rubella exposure and who will not consider terminating pregnancy. Recommended dose of 0.55 mL/kg IM
Tetanus	Yes	Special human tetanus immune globulin (TIG) has replaced equine tetanus antitoxin because of the risk of serum sickness with equine serum. Recommended dose for postexposure prophylaxis of 250–300 units of TIG Recommended dose for tetanus treatment of 500–3,000 units of TIG
Rabies	Yes	Special human rabies immune globulin (RIG) is preferred over equine rabies antiserum because of the risk of serum sickness, but RIG is not always available. RIG or antiserum is recommended in nonimmunized individuals for all animal bites in which rabies cannot be ruled out and for other exposures to rabid animals. Recommended dose of RIG is 20 IU/kg; recommended dose of antiserum is 40 IU/kg. Rabies vaccine is given as well as on days 0, 3, 7, 14 and 28.
Hepatitis A	Yes	Standard immune serum globulin is given in single dose of 0.02–0.04 mL/kg or up to 0.06 mL/kg every 5 mo for continuous exposure.
Hepatitis B	Yes	Standard immune serum globulin is not reliably effective; special human hepatitis B immune globulin (HBIG) is useful and recommended for neonates born to an infected mother and after mucous membrane or parenteral contact with infected persons or infected blood or serum. Recommended dose for neonates is 0.5 mL IM within 12 hr of birth; recommended dose or percutaneous or mucosal exposure is 0.06–0.12 mL/kg IM.
Non-A, non-B hepatitis	Yes	Standard immune serum globulin may be valuable. Recommended dose is 0.12 mL/kg, up to 10 mL.

Adapted from Recommendations of the Advisory Committee on Immunization Practices (ACIP): Use of vaccines and immmunoglobulins in persons with altered immunocompetence. MMWR 42(RR-4):1, 1993; Rabies prevention—United States, 1991: Recommendations of the Immunization Practices Advisory Committee (ACIP). MMWR 40(RR-1, 1991; Hepatitis B virus: A comprehensive strategy for eliminating transmission in the United States through universal childhood immunization: Recommendations of the Immunization Practices Advisory Committee (ACIP). MMWR 40(RR-13):1, 1991; Rubella prevention: Recommendations of the Immunization Practices Advisory Committee (ACIP). MMWR 39(RR-15):1, 1990.

between administration of immune globulin and vaccine is recommended. Immunoglobulins should not be given for at least 2 wk after MMR. Postpartum vaccination of rubella-susceptible women should not be delayed because of the administration of anti-Rho(D) immune globulin or any other blood product during the last trimester or at delivery. If administration of an immune globulin preparation becomes necessary after vaccination, it should be postponed if possible for at least 14 days to allow vaccine virus replication and development of immunity. Neither OPV nor yellow fever vaccine responses are affected by administration of immune globulin. Immune globulins do not interfere with inactivated vaccines; postexposure passive prophylaxis can be given together with HBV vaccine or tetanus toxoid, resulting in immediate and persistent protection.

Travel. The International Sanitary Regulations allow countries to impose requirements for yellow fever and cholera vaccines as a condition for admission, even though the available killed parenteral cholera vaccine is not an effective public health tool. Travelers should know whether these vaccines are required for entry into the countries on their itinerary to avoid being turned back or immunized at the point of entry. Infants and children should be up to date with all routine immunizations before traveling, especially for polio, measles, and DTP or Td. Pooled human gamma globulin for hepatitis A may be advisable for travelers to some areas. Use of rabies, meningococcal A and C polysaccharide, typhoid, Japanese encephalitis, and plague vaccines should be considered for individuals who expect to go beyond the usual tourist routes or to spend extended time in rural areas in disease-endemic regions.

ADVERSE EVENTS AFTER VACCINATION. Modern vaccines, although safe and effective, are associated with mild to life-threatening adverse effects. Because no vaccine can be expected to be 100% effective, some immunized persons may develop disease after exposure.

Vaccine components, including the protective antigens, animal proteins introduced during vaccine production, and antibiotics or other preservatives or stabilizers, can cause allergic reactions in some recipients. Reactions may be local or systemic, including serious anaphylaxis and urticaria. The most common extraneous allergen is egg protein from vaccines prepared in embryonated eggs, such as measles, mumps, influenza, and yellow fever vaccines. Local or systemic reactions result from too frequent administration of some vaccines, such as tetanus toxoid, Td, DT, or rabies, and are probably caused by antigen-antibody complexes.

The decision to use a vaccine involves assessment of the risk of disease, the benefit of vaccination, and the risk associated with vaccination. These factors may change, requiring continued reassessment of vaccines. Table 247–4 presents a guide to contraindications to immunization and appropriate precautions in the use of specific vaccines.

All adverse events temporally related to vaccination should be reported to the local health department and the vaccine manufacturer. The National Childhood Vaccine Injury Act requires health care providers to report certain suspected adverse events after a mandated vaccine to the Food and Drug Administration's Vaccine Adverse Events Reporting System (Table 247–6). Although a temporal relationship does not establish cause and effect, surveillance is essential to evaluate vaccine safety.

The National Childhood Vaccine Injury Act requires that all mandated vaccinations be recorded by health care providers in the child's permanent medical record, including the date of administration, manufacturer and lot number, and the name of the provider administering the vaccine. Parents also should keep a current immunization record for their children. The act requires that the benefits to the child of vaccination and possible reactions be explained to parents.

The use of mandated vaccines benefits society by reducing morbidity, the cost of care for preventable diseases, and childhood mortality, but these vaccines are associated with severe adverse reactions or sequelae in some children.

The National Childhood Vaccine Injury Compensation Act of 1986 was enacted to ensure fairness to injured persons and protection for federal, state, and local immunization programs, private immunization providers, and vaccine manufacturers. The Act was designed to provide prompt and fair compensation to the families of children who have died or have been injured as a result of routine mandated immunization and to reduce

■ **TABLE 247–6 Reportable Events After Vaccination, as Required by the National Vaccine Injury Act of 1986**

Vaccine or Toxoid	Event	Interval from Vaccination
DTP, DTP/polio combined	Anaphylaxis or anaphylactic shock	24 hr
	Encephalopathy (or encephalitis)*	3 days
	Shock-collapse or hypotonic-hyporesponsive collapse*	3 days
	Residual seizure disorder*	
	Any acute complication or sequela (including death) of above events	No limit
	Events in vaccines described in manufacturer's package insert as contraindications to additional doses of vaccine (e.g., convulsions)†	See package insert
Measles, mumps, and rubella, DT, Td, tetanus toxoid (TT)	Anaplylaxis or anaphylactic shock	24 hr
	Encephalopathy or encephalitis	15 days for measles, mumps and rubella; 3 days for DT, Td, TT
	Residual seizure disorder*	
	Any acute complication or sequela (including death) of above events	No limit
	Events in vaccinees described in manufacturer's package insert as contraindications to additional doses of vaccine†	See package insert
Oral polio vaccine (OPV)	Paralytic polio in a nonimmunodeficient recipient	30 days
	Paralytic polio in an immunodeficient recipient or vaccine-associated community case	6 mo
	Any acute complication or sequela (including death) of the above	No limit
	Events in vaccinees described in manufacturer's package insert as contraindications to additional doses of vaccine	See package insert
Inactivated polio vaccine-enhanced (eIPV)	Anaphylaxis or anaphylactic shock	24 hr
	Any acute complication or sequela (including death) of above events	No limit
	Events in vaccines described in manufacturer's package insert as contraindications to additional doses of vaccine†	See package insert

**Aids to interpretation: Shock-collapse or hypotonic-hyporesponsive collapse may be evidenced by signs or symptoms such as a decrease in or loss of muscle tone, paralysis (partial or complete), hemiplegia, hemiparesis, loss of color or turning pale white or blue, unresponsiveness to environmental stimuli, depression of or loss of consciousness, prolonged sleeping with difficult arousing, or cardiovascular or respiratory arrest. Residual seizure disorder may be considered to have occurred if no other seizure or convulsion unacccompanied by fevers or accompanied by a fever of less than 102° F occurred before the first seizure or convulsion after the administration of the vaccine involved; if in the case of measles, mumps, or rubella-containing vaccines, the first seizure or convulsion occurred within 15 days after vaccination; or in the case of any other vaccine, the first seizure or convulsion occurred within 3 days after vaccination; and if two or more seizures or convulsions unaccompanied by fever or accompanied by a fever of less than 102° F occurred within 1 yr after vaccination. The terms seizure and convulsion include grand mal, petit mal, absence, myoclonia, tonic-clonic, and focal motor seizures and signs. Encephalopathy means any significant acquired abnormality of, injury to, or impairment of function of the brain. Among the frequent manifestations of encephalopathy are focal and diffuse neurologic signs, increased intracranial pressure, or changes in level of consciousness lasting at least 6 hr with or without convulsions. The neurologic signs and symptoms of encephalopathy may be temporary with complete recovery, or they may result in various degrees of permanent impairment. Signs and symptoms such as high-pitched and unusual screaming, persistent inconsolable crying, and bulging fontanels are compatible with an encephalopathy but in and of themselves are not conclusive evidence of encephalopathy. Encephalopathy usually can be documented by slow wave activity on an electroencephalogram.*

†The health care provider must refer to the contraindications section of the manufacturer's package insert for each vaccine.

Adapted from National Childhood Vaccine Injury Act of 1986.

the adverse impact of the tort system on vaccine supply, cost, and innovation and development. The intent is to encourage predictable, speedy, and equitable compensation for persons injured by vaccines.

CONTROL OF VACCINE-PREVENTABLE DISEASES. A continuing task of the pediatrician is to maintain individual immunity and, along with public health workers, herd immunity. The job is not over after the population is fully vaccinated, because it is imperative to immunize subsequent generations as long as the threat of the disease persists. Ongoing surveillance and prompt reporting of disease to local or state health departments are essential to this goal. Most vaccine-preventable diseases are now notifiable, and individual case data are routinely forwarded to the Centers for Disease Control. These data are used to detect outbreaks or other unusual events requiring investigation and to evaluate prevention and control policies, practices, and strategies.

The target population for the common and highly contagious childhood diseases, such as measles, is the whole universe of susceptibles, and the time to immunize is as early in life as feasible. Epidemiologic differences in different settings dictate different strategies of immunization. For example, in the industrialized world, immunization with measles vaccine at 12–15 mo of age is routine because the vaccine protects over 95% of those immunized at this age and the risk of measles morbidity or mortality is low among very young infants. In the developing world, measles fatalities account for a significant proportion of young infant deaths. Immunization in the first few months of life is desirable to close the window of vulnerability between the rapid decline of maternal antibody after 4–5 mo and subsequent vaccine-induced active immunity.

Vaccine failure problems have emerged in measles immunization programs in the developed and the developing world. In the United States, outbreaks of measles have occurred among unvaccinated infants younger than 15 mo, preschoolers from underserved inner-city populations, and among previously vaccinated college students. These outbreaks represent vaccine failure and program failure. Vaccine failures usually represent no primary response to the vaccine, but some are caused by a secondary loss of immunity after immunization, especially after the receipt of unstabilized pre-1980 vaccines or vaccines given with gamma globulin. Program failures represent an inability to reach and immunize the target population, often because no systematic program of immunization exists.

H. influenzae type b is the leading cause of meningitis, epiglottitis, and pneumonia in early childhood. Most severe disease occurs in early childhood, rising sharply after the disappearance of maternally derived antibody. In contrast to measles vaccine, primary failure of Hib vaccine during infancy results from the age-related inability to respond to polysaccharide antigens. To overcome this innate deficit, the protective polysaccharide is coupled with protein to convert it to a T-cell–dependent antigen to which young infants respond.

In some diseases, such as rubella, infection is primarily a threat to the fetus, because young infants and children are not at risk for serious illness. Although it is not clinically necessary to immunize early in life, the goal is to ensure immunity before females enter the reproductive age group. Immunization of all reproductive-age women before pregnancy would be an ideal strategy. Because of the practical difficulties in immunizing all young women, universal childhood immunization is used to reach susceptibles and to interrupt transmission.

DELIVERY OF VACCINES. During the past 20 yr, considerable progress has been made to ensure that every child in the United States is fully immunized by the time of school entry. All 50 states require immunization for school entry, and most have laws addressing attendance at preschool and day-care centers. As a result, up to 98% of all children are immunized against nine vaccine-preventable diseases by the time they enter school, excluding newer vaccines such as HBV and HIB. Despite these successes, only 37–56% of preschoolers in the United States have been completely immunized; the rate is as low as 10% in some communities. The failure to vaccinate preschool children was largely responsible for the resurgence of measles between 1989 and 1991, which included 55,467 cases and over 11,200 admissions to the hospital, with more than 44,100 hospital days and over 130 measles-related deaths. Congenital rubella syndrome also increased from 6 cases in 1988 to 47 in 1991. Outbreaks of pertussis and mumps have increased because of low immunization rates among preschool children.

There are four major barriers to successful infant and childhood immunization within the health care system: low public awareness and lack of public demand for immunization; inadequate access to immunization services; missed opportunities to administer vaccines; and inadequate resources for public health and preventive programs.

The success of immunization makes vaccine-preventable diseases less visible, and parents and health care providers become complacent. Even among the affluent and educated, low levels of immunization may prevail, reflecting a misunderstanding of the continuing threat of diseases with which parents and health care providers have limited experience or an inappropriately greater fear of vaccine adverse reactions than the consequences of vaccine-preventable diseases.

All patients or their parents or guardians should be informed of the benefits and the risks associated with vaccination. The discussion should be carried out in language understood by the recipient or parent or guardian, and ample opportunity for questions and discussion should be given. Vaccine information pamphlets have been developed for measles, mumps, and rubella vaccine or components; diphtheria and tetanus toxoid and pertussis vaccine or components; and oral and inactivated polio vaccines. The National Childhood Vaccine Injury Act requires distribution of these pamphlets. The Public Health Service has developed forms that explain the benefits and risks of vaccination for use with Hib and hepatitis B vaccines. Health care providers can receive copies through local health departments.

Most infants in the United States begin a course of immunization, but a substantial number fail to complete the series on schedule. To ensure that patients receive immunizations on schedule, practitioners should establish recall systems, to ascertain whether needed vaccines have been given. Many areas are developing local and statewide systems in which all children will be enrolled at or shortly after birth. The goals are to allow all providers access to the current immunization status of infants and children and to help remind parents to bring in children for appointments.

STANDARDS FOR PEDIATRIC IMMUNIZATION PRACTICES. Investigation into the resurgence of measles in the United States from 1989 to 1991 indicated that failure to vaccinate preschool children on time was the major cause of the epidemic. These investigations also documented that other significant reasons for the low vaccination rates in children by their 2nd birthday were barriers and obstacles to immunizations that parents faced in getting their children immunized and opportunities missed by health care providers to provide vaccines.

At least three types of missed opportunities exist: when the patient receives some but not all indicated vaccines because the provider is unaware that many vaccines can be administered simultaneously; when inappropriate contraindications are used to deny vaccinations to children in need; and when the patient presents for another reason, such as trauma, and immunization status is not reviewed. To minimize the barriers to immunization and to ensure that all opportunities to vaccinate are taken, in 1992, the National Vaccine Advisory Committee issued 18 standards (Table 247–7), which should be followed by public and private health care providers. These have been endorsed by the U.S. Public Health Service, the American Academy of Pediatrics, and many other professional groups.

Some of the more critical standards include providing vaccines in all health care settings; minimizing prevaccination requirements such as a full physician evaluation when those services are not readily obtainable; screening for contraindications, including a minimum observation of the child, soliciting illness history from the parents, and verbally asking questions about contraindications; use of simultaneous immunization except when, in the judgment of the provider, nonsimultaneous vaccination will not compromise the immunization status of the patient; and regular audits of patient records to determine the vaccination levels of the patients in each provider's practice.

INTERNATIONAL CONSIDERATIONS. Since the establishment of the World Health Organization's Expanded Programme on Immunization (EPI), immunization levels for the six basic children's vaccines have risen from 5% in the early 1980s to approximately 80% worldwide today. Each year, at least 2.7 million deaths from measles, neonatal tetanus, and pertussis and 200,000 cases of paralysis due to polio are prevented. Despite the successes of the EPI, such as the elimination of poliomyelitis from the Americas, many vaccine-preventable diseases remain prevalent in the developing world. Measles, for example, continues to kill an estimated 1.5 million children each year, and cases of diphtheria, whooping cough, polio, and neonatal tetanus still occur at unacceptably high levels. It is estimated that 20–35% of all deaths in children younger than 5 yr of age are associated with vaccine-preventable diseases.

Eight antigens are recommended for routine use in the developing world by the EPI, including BCG, DTP, trivalent polio, and measles vaccines for children and tetanus toxoid for pregnant women. Hib, Japanese B encephalitis, yellow fever, HBV, group A meningococcus, mumps, and rubella are used region-

■ **TABLE 247–7 Standards for Pediatric Immunization Practices**

Standard 1	Immunization services are readily available.
Standard 2	There are no barriers or unnecessary prerequisites to the receipt of vaccines.
Standard 3	Immunization services are available free or for a minimal fee.
Standard 4	Providers use all clinical encounters to screen and, when indicated, immunize children.
Standard 5	Providers educate parents and guardians about immunization in general terms.
Standard 6	Providers question parents or guardians about contraindications and, before immunizing a child, inform them in specific terms about the risks and benefits of the immunizations their child is to receive.
Standard 7	Providers follow only true contraindications.
Standard 8	Providers administer simultaneously all vaccine doses for which a child is eligible at the time of each visit.
Standard 9	Providers use accurate and complete recording procedures.
Standard 10	Providers co-schedule immunization appointments in conjunction with appointments for other child health services.
Standard 11	Providers report adverse events after immunization promptly, accurately, and completely.
Standard 12	Providers operate a tracking system.
Standard 13	Providers adhere to appropriate procedures for vaccine management.
Standard 14	Providers conduct semiannual audits to assess immunization coverage levels and to review immunization records in the patient populations they serve.
Standard 15	Providers maintain up-to-date, easily retrievable medical protocols at all locations where vaccines are administered.
Standard 16	Providers operate with patient-oriented and community-based approaches.
Standard 17	Vaccines are administered by properly trained individuals.
Standard 18	Providers receive ongoing education and training about current immunization recommendations.

ally, depending on the disease epidemiology and resources. Poliomyelitis has been targeted for global eradication by the year 2000.

Because infectious diseases know no geographic or political boundaries, uncontrolled disease anywhere in the world poses a threat to the United States. Vaccines offer the opportunity to control and even eradicate some diseases, and successful eradication means that vaccines are no longer needed. The experience with smallpox shows that the eradication of disease is a remarkably good economic investment. The entire sum that the United States spent for the global smallpox eradication campaign has been recouped, in 1968 dollars, every 2.5 mo since 1971. A similar achievement with polio would save the United States over $300 million each year in vaccine and associated delivery costs, and the goal is feasible.

American Academy of Pediatrics and Peter G, et al (eds): Report of the Committee on Infectious Diseases ("Red Book"), 22d ed. Elk Grove Village, IL, American Academy of Pediatrics 1991.
Centers for Disease Control and Prevention: Recommendations of the Advisory Committee on Immunization Practices (ACIP): General recommendations for routine use. MMWR 43(RR-1):1, 1994.
Standards for pediatric immunization practices. MMWR 41(RR-5):1, 1993.
Health Information for International Travel (published yearly) and *Advisory Memoranda on Travel* (published periodically)

CHAPTER 248
Health Advice for Traveling Children

Robert Bonomo and Robert A. Salata

Each year, more than 40 million American citizens travel, work, or live abroad. Many of these are children. More than 8 million United States citizens travel to developing countries, and over 1 million visit malaria-endemic areas. This major increase in international travel and the resurgence of malaria and other infectious diseases worldwide brings the issues regarding prevention and management of health problems in travelers into the office of every physician caring for children. Many physicians trained in industrialized countries are unfamiliar with the health hazards and rapidly changing information and requirements related to travel. The risks, needs, and requirements for children who are traveling (particularly those younger than 2 yr of age) may sometimes differ from those of adults. The purpose of this section is to provide updated information on pretravel health advice and immunization for traveling children.

GENERAL RECOMMENDATIONS

Parents of traveling children should seek medical consultation well in advance of their departure to obtain a realistic assessment of risks, for immunization and chemoprophylactic measures, and for advice on dealing with disease if it occurs. For traveling with small children, particularly infants, additional concerns relate to inadequate primary immunizations, lack of demonstrated efficacy and safety of many vaccines in infants, excretion of prophylactic drugs in breast milk, and increased morbidity and possible mortality associated with some diseases acquired abroad.

General advice to parents should first include a discussion of *eating and drinking habits*, because most travel-related health problems occur through the ingestion of contaminated food or water. Among the bacterial and protozoan infections children can acquire from contaminated water are *Escherichia coli* infections, shigellosis, salmonellosis, cholera, giardiasis, amebiasis, and cryptosporidiosis. Families must be aware that consumption of chlorinated water may not be entirely free of risk (e.g., giardia, amoeba). Parents should also avoid ice and caution children not to brush their teeth with contaminated water. Boiling water or chemical disinfection with iodine are the most reliable methods to disinfect water. All raw food (e.g., fruits, uncooked vegetables) should be considered contaminated. In particular, children should avoid unpasteurized milk, milk products such as cheese, and uncooked meat or fish. Breastfeeding should be encouraged in infants younger than 6 mo of age if possible.

Consultation should then focus on the common *problems related to travel*, including jet lag, sinus and ear problems, altitude sickness, environmental exposures, the hazards of insects as vectors of many infections (e.g., malaria, yellow fever, dengue, filariasis, trypanosomiasis, onchocerciasis), and the means to avoid these vectors. Exposure to insect bites can be avoided by restricting activities, wearing appropriate attire, and use of insect repellents containing permethrin and *N,N*-diethyl-*m*-touamide (DEET). DEET should be applied carefully to children (<30% concentration) to avoid blistering and encephalopathy. The major cause of serious disability or loss of life are injuries and motor vehicle accidents. The use of safety belts on children should be stressed. When possible, infant seats should be taken along, because many cars in developing countries do not have seat belts. Travelers to remote areas should be warned about venomous animals (snake and scorpion bites can be fatal for infants), rabies (predominantly transmitted by domestic dogs and cats), and exposure to rodents (because of plague). Swimming or diving in contaminated water can result in serious injury and increase the risk of infection. Schistosomiasis, leptospirosis, or primary amoebic meningoencephalitis can result. Most of the illnesses that develop in traveling children are related to behaviors that can be modified with proper advice and supervision by parents.

With acquired immunodeficiency syndrome (AIDS) becoming more prevalent abroad, the hazards of casual sexual encounters for adolescents as well as of needle and blood and blood product exposure should be emphasized. Blood sources in developing countries must be suspect. Although there is global concern about acquiring AIDS by blood transfusion, the systematic screening of blood donations is not yet feasible in developing countries. The universal safety of transfusion services abroad cannot be guaranteed. Children should have their blood typed before departure so that transfusions from family members or travel companions with similar blood types are possible in dire emergencies. Several agencies can provide emergency evacuation to industrialized countries if the situation dictates. The use of biologic products such as clotting factor concentrates or immune globulin should be avoided when manufactured abroad. Insulin-dependent diabetics and hemophiliacs should carry an adequate supply of sterile needles, syringes, and disinfectant swabs. If resuscitation is needed, the use of colloid and crystalloid plasma expanders can be used as a temporizing measure. Human immunodeficiency virus (HIV) is not transmitted through casual contacts, sources of food or water, contact with inanimate objects, mosquitoes, or other insect vectors.

Children with pre-existing medical problems are traveling more extensively and are in greatest need of consultation prior to departure. Conditions on which travel has the greatest impact include chronic cardiopulmonary disease, diabetes, allergies, and gastrointestinal problems, especially diarrhea (malabsorption or inflammatory bowel disease). Special arrangements should be made for patients with bleeding disorders, those on anticoagulation therapy, and those who require hemodialysis.

Children with medical conditions should take with them a brief medical summary. For children requiring care by specialists, an international directory for that specialty can be consulted. A directory of physicians worldwide who speak English and who have met certain qualifications is available from the International Association for Medical Assistance to Travelers (736 Center St., Lewiston, NY 14092; telephone: [716] 754–4883). If medical care is needed urgently when abroad, sources of information include the American embassy or consulate, hotel managers, travel agents catering to foreign tourists, and missionary hospitals. Parents should be counseled, however, to take a sufficient supply of prescription medications for their children and to ensure that bottles are clearly identified. A travel health kit consisting of prescription medications and nonprescription items is also often useful. Travelers also need to ascertain whether their health insurance covers medical care abroad.

IMMUNIZATIONS

General Considerations

Immunization is only one feature of a comprehensive disease prevention program for traveling children (Table 248–1; see Chapter 247). No vaccine is completely safe or effective; benefits and risks must be considered for all immunobiologic agents. One of the most important issues related to vaccinations of traveling children is a modification in the immunization schedule for the unvaccinated or inadequately vaccinated child, especially those less than 2 yr of age. The Centers for Disease Control (CDC) has developed guidelines for immunization for children younger than 2 yr at accelerated intervals to maximize protection. The routine childhood immunizations (i.e., measles, mumps, rubella, hepatitis B, *Haemophilus influenzae* type B conjugate vaccines, diphtheria, tetanus, and pertussis) are most frequently affected and involve alterations in both the minimum age for immunization and the minimum interval between doses (Table 248–2). Issues related to the minimum age at administration also arise for those immunizations that are considered solely because of specific travel-related needs (e.g., cholera, Japanese encephalitis [JE], meningococcal, rabies, typhoid, and yellow fever vaccines and immune globulin).

■ **TABLE 248–1 Immunization for Traveling Children**

Live Attenuated Virus Vaccines*	Inactivated Vaccines	Toxoids	Immunoglobulins
Measles†	Cholera‡	Diphtheria§	Immune globulin
Mumps†	HbCV	Tetanus§	Rabies immune globulin
Rubella†	IPV		
OPV	Hepatitis B		
Yellow fever‡	Japanese encephalitis‖		
	Meningococcal		
	Pertussis§		
	Plague		
	Rabies		
	Typhoid¶		

**Generally contraindicated in immunodeficient children. An exception is measles vaccination which is recommended for both asymptomatic and symptomatic HIV-infected children. Live vaccines should be given simultaneously or at least 30 days apart. Live, attenuated immunizations should not be coadministered with immune globulin (OPV and yellow fever are exceptions); administer these vaccines at least 3 mo after immune globulin use. Immune globulin should be administered no sooner than 2–4 wk after a live virus vaccine is given.*

†Administered together as MMR or separately.

‡May be required for entry into certain countries.

§Administered together as DTP or DT.

‖Only for Asian travelers for >1 mo during high-risk periods.

¶A licensed oral live attenuated typhoid vaccine (Vivotif, Ty21a) can be given to immunocompetent children >6 yr of age.

HbCV = Haemophilus influenzae *type B conjugate vaccine; IPV = injectable polio vaccine (enhanced); OPV = oral polio vaccine.*

■ **TABLE 248–2 Modification of Routine Immunization Schedules for Traveling Children**

Vaccine	Modified Schedule
MMR	Children younger than 6 mo of age should not be vaccinated because of maternal antibodies. Children aged 6–12 mo should receive one dose of measles vaccine before departure and revaccination with MMR at 15 mo of age or at 12 mo if remaining in a high-risk area. If the child is 12–14 mo of age, MMR should be given and revaccination should be considered when the child starts school. Older children who were previously immunized with measles vaccine before 1980 should be revaccinated.
OPV	Children should receive at least three doses at interals of 4–6 wk when time permits. When traveling infants are less than 6 wk old, an initial dose should be given and 3 additional doses at 6, 10, and 14 wk should be administered if remaining in the endemic areas. Children traveling to endemic areas who have received a first or second dose of the primary series should receive their second/third doses 4 wk after their prior dose. Children who have received less than the primary series and who remain in endemic areas should complete the primary series within the endemic area with doses at 4-wk intervals. A booster should be given at 4–6 yr; a supplementary dose–enhanced potency inactivated polio vaccine can be administered as a booster if live vaccines are contraindicated.
HbCV	See Chapters 177 and 247.
DTP	Young infants should receive three doses, the first no sooner than 6 wk and the next two doses at intervals of no less than 4 wk. Children less than 7 yr old who have received fewer than three doses and who will remain in endemic areas should complete their remaining doses at 4-wk intervals. Children older than 1 yr and adolescents should be reimmunized (booster dose) every 10 yr without the pertussis component (dT)

DTP = diphtheria and tetanus toxoids and pertussis vaccine; HbCV = Haemophilus influenzae *type B conjugated vaccine; MMR = measles, mumps, rubella; OPV = oral polio vaccine.*

Pregnant women who travel should avoid live attenuated virus vaccines. If vaccines are to be administered, waiting for the 2nd or 3rd trimester is a reasonable precaution to minimize concern over teratogenicity. Inactivated JE virus vaccine should be given only when the risk of infection outweighs the risk of immunization.

Parents should allow 4–6 wk before departure for optimal administration of vaccines to their children, because some immunizations require multiple doses for full protection and some immunobiologic agents are incompatible with others. In general, inactivated vaccines can be given simultaneously, although both local and systemic adverse reactions may be cumulative. Live attenuated viral vaccines should always be administered together (see Table 248–1); if not administered concurrently, live vaccines should be given at least 30 days apart whenever possible. Inactivated and live vaccines can be given together at any time. The notable exception is yellow fever and cholera vaccines, which should not be given simultaneously or within 3 wk of each other, because the antibody response to both vaccines may be decreased. Because immune globulin can interfere with the replication of live attenuated viruses, live vaccines should not be given within 6 wk and preferably should be delayed until 3 mo after use of immune globulin. Immune globulin preparations do not interfere with the immune response to oral polio or yellow fever vaccines. Immune globulin should be administered no sooner than at least 2 wk and preferably 4 wk after a live virus vaccine is given. Vaccine products produced in eggs may contain an allergenic substance that cause hypersensitivity responses, including anaphylaxis in persons with known egg sensitivity. Screening by history of ability to eat eggs without adverse effect is a reasonable way to identify those at allergic risk from receiving yellow fever, measles, mumps, rubella, or influenza vaccines. Other vaccine components that cause hypersensitivity reactions include other antigens, preservatives (e.g., thimerosal), and antibiotics (e.g., neomycin).

Rapid viral replication after administration of live vaccines occurs in *immunodeficient hosts.* These patients include those with lymphoreticular malignancy, generalized malignancies, or AIDS, or those receiving corticosteroids, cytotoxic agents, or radiation. In general, live virus vaccines and live bacterial vaccines (e.g., BCG oral typhoid) are contraindicated in these individuals. An exception is measles vaccine, which is recommended for both asymptomatic and symptomatic HIV-infected children because of severe, life-threatening measles infection found in children with AIDS. Although children with symptomatic HIV infection should not receive yellow fever vaccine, asymptomatic HIV-infected children may be vaccinated if the risk from yellow fever remains significant. These immunocompromising conditions may also reduce immunologic responses to inactivated vaccines and toxoids; inactivated vaccines and toxoids are not contraindicated in immunodeficient children. Pneumococcal vaccine should be given to any child older than 2 yr of age with HIV infection. *H. influenzae* type B conjugate vaccine can be given as early as 2 mo of age.

Routine Childhood Vaccines and Toxoids

DIPHTHERIA, TETANUS, AND PERTUSSIS. Tetanus is a ubiquitous problem, is a major cause of worldwide neonatal mortality, and is most prevalent in tropical countries. Diphtheria is also endemic in many developing countries. Pertussis is common in the Third World and in some industrialized nations where pertussis immunization is not practiced as widely as in the United States. Guidelines for optimal protection against these three infections in the first year of life are presented in Chapter 247. Protection is attained with three doses of DTP in the first year of life. The immunization schedule for DTP should be modified for young infants and inadequately or unimmunized children according to the guidelines in Table 248–2. For children younger than 7 yr of age with a contraindication to pertussis vaccine, DT should be used. Partially immunized infants for whom further doses of pertussis vaccine are contraindicated should have DT substituted for each of the remaining scheduled DTP doses.

POLIO VACCINE. Eradication of polio will probably occur by the end of the 1990s. Nevertheless, there are areas where polio remains endemic. In most developed nations, the risk of poliomyelitis is usually no different from that seen in the United States, but most developing countries are still endemic for poliomyelitis. Children traveling to such countries are at increased risk for developing poliomyelitis and adequate immunization must be undertaken.

In the United States, a primary series of OPV should be given to individuals less than 18 yr of age (see Chapter 247). Trivalent OPV is the vaccine of choice for all infants and children if there are no contraindications. In cases in which this standard immunization schedule cannot be followed, the age of vaccination can be lowered and the interval between doses can be shortened (see Table 248–2).

Although not considered the vaccine of choice for children, enhanced potency IPV may be indicated for children who are immunocompromised or who are in close contact with immunocompromised individuals. The primary series of enhanced IPV is begun ideally at 8 wk of age with an interval of 8 wk between the 1st two doses and a 12-mo interval between the 2nd and 3rd doses. When necessary, immunization can be started as early as 6 wk of age with a 4-wk interval between the 1st and 2nd doses and between the 2nd and 3rd doses, and a 4th dose administered 6 mo later.

MEASLES, MUMPS, AND RUBELLA VACCINES. Measles is still endemic in many developing countries and in some industrialized nations. Individuals traveling abroad should be immune to measles. Measles vaccine, preferably in combination with mumps and rubella vaccines, should be given to all children at 15 mo of age and older, unless there is a contraindication (see Chapter 247). The age of vaccination should be lowered for children traveling to endemic areas according to the schedule in Table 248–2. Measles in HIV-infected children can be a devastating illness. Consequently, HIV-infected children who travel abroad should be vaccinated.

In the United States, measles vaccine failures have been observed increasingly in children immunized before 1980. These children should be revaccinated, particularly before travel outside the United States.

***HAEMOPHILUS INFLUENZAE* TYPE B CONJUGATE VACCINE.** Severe *H. influenzae* type B infection is most common in children 6 mo to 1 yr of age, but one third of cases of invasive infection are found in children 18 mo of age and older. The risk of developing serious *H. influenzae* infection when traveling outside the United States may be comparable with that found in the United States. See Chapter 247 for the immunization schedule of conjugated *H. influenzae* type B vaccine. Unimmunized children up to 23 mo of age should be vaccinated (see Chapter 247). Children who previously received the polysaccharide vaccine should be revaccinated with *H. influenzae* type B conjugate vaccine.

Special Vaccines for Travel

YELLOW FEVER. Yellow fever is a mosquito-borne viral illness resembling other hemorrhagic fevers but with more prominent liver involvement (see Chapter 225). Yellow fever exists in jungle areas of South America and Africa. In South America, sporadic infection is found in forestry, agricultural, and other occupationally exposed workers. In Africa, the virus is transmitted to young children in the moist savanna zones of West Africa during the rainy season.

Yellow fever vaccine is a live, attenuated vaccine developed in chick embryos and is extremely safe and effective. However, yellow fever vaccine is associated with an increased risk of encephalitis (1%) and other severe reactions in young infants; this vaccine should be delayed until age 9 mo, except when the risk of infection is high. Yellow fever vaccination is required by law by some countries for travelers arriving from endemic areas. Some African countries require evidence of vaccination from all entering travelers. Recommendations can be obtained by contacting state or local health departments or the Division of Vector-Borne Viral Diseases, Centers for Disease Control (CDC), telephone no. (404) 332-4555.

Most countries accept a medical waiver for children who are too young to be vaccinated (<4 mo of age) and for individuals with a contraindication to vaccination, such as immunodeficiency. Children with asymptomatic HIV infection may be vaccinated if exposure to the yellow fever virus cannot be avoided. Vaccine administration should be delayed until 9 mo of age if possible.

The vaccine, made from the attenuated 17D strain, is given as a single 0.5-mL dose. Long-lived, perhaps lifetime immunity develops; however, international travel certificates require proof of immunization within 10 yr. Cholera vaccine given 3 wk before or simultaneously with yellow fever vaccine reduces but does not prevent an antibody response to yellow fever immunization.

CHOLERA VACCINE. Cholera is an acute noninflammatory diarrheal illness caused by *Vibrio cholera* O group 1 acquired through the ingestion of contaminated food or water (see Chapter 185). Severe cases can be characterized by watery diarrhea and vomiting, which can progress to dehydration, shock, acidosis, or death. In children younger than 2 yr of age, cholera is frequently a mild disease. Although there has been continued spread since the 7th worldwide pandemic of cholera of 1961, U.S. travelers rarely contract cholera. The reappearance of cholera in South America and Central America poses additional risks to children traveling to these areas.

Although cholera vaccination (0.2 mL SC or IM ×2 given 1

mo apart if 6 mo–4 yr; 0.3 mL SC or IM ×2 if 5–10 yr; and 0.5 mL SC or IM ×2 if >10 yr) can reduce the rate of illness by 50%, it provides only short-term protection. Vaccine efficacy is low particularly in children younger than 5 yr of age. The World Health Organization (WHO) and the CDC do not recommend cholera vaccination for international travel. Because cholera vaccination is not recommended for children younger than 6 mo of age, a medical waiver should be given before departure. Breast-feeding should be encouraged in cholera-endemic areas. Several new vaccines are being tried. A killed whole-cell oral vaccine given in two doses and a genetically engineered attenuated strain have been studied.

TYPHOID VACCINE. *Salmonella typhi* infection, or typhoid fever, is not uncommon in young children (see Chapter 182). American international travelers are at risk of contracting typhoid, especially in the Indian subcontinent and western South America. Typhoid vaccination is recommended when a person travels to an endemic area and when exposure to contaminated food and water is likely. Vaccination is also recommended for travelers to areas where *Salmonella typhi* is resistant to antimicrobial agents. Pediatricians should be aware that the parenteral vaccine can cause severe systemic reactions and reactions at the site of administration. The heat-phenol-inactivated vaccine (60–80% efficacy), available in the United States, has been widely used for many years and is given as 0.2 mL SC ×2 given 1 mo apart if <10 yr of age; 0.5 mL is used if >10 yr. A newly released parenteral V_1 capsular polysaccharide given as a single dose of 0.5 mL IM for children ≥2 yr appears less toxic. Boosters, 0.1 mL ID of the heat-phenol inactivated vaccine and 0.5 mL IM of the V_1 capsular polysaccharide vaccine are administered at 2 and 3 yr, respectively. In general, typhoid vaccination is not required for international travel. Children 6 mo of age and older who are traveling to a typhoid endemic area should be considered for vaccination with 0.25 mL subcutaneously of the heat-phenol-inactivated vaccine (0.5 mL if older than 10 yr) on two occasions, separated by 4 wk or more. A local reaction to the heat-phenol typhoid vaccination is common and may be associated with fever, headache, and malaise. Hyperpyrexia in reaction to the heat-phenol-inactivated preparation can be severe in young children, and febrile seizures may occur. Acetominophen can be administered as may be done with DTP vaccination.

A licensed oral live-attenuated vaccine (Vivotif, manufactured from the Ty21a strain of *S. typhi*) has undergone field trials among Egyptian and Chilean school children with an estimated efficacy of 67% for at least 4 yr. Because of the lack of efficacy data for children younger than 5 yr of age, Ty21a vaccine is not recommended for children younger than 6 yr. The oral vaccine, given as four enteric-coated capsules qod with boosters recommended every 5 yr, is much less immunogenic in children younger than 4 yr of age, and its efficacy has not been established in children younger than 6 yr of age. It is also not recommended for immunocompromised children; the inactivated vaccine should be used for these children.

MENINGOCOCCAL VACCINE. Meningococcal meningitis is a worldwide disease (see Chapter 178); epidemic disease has been reported in India, Nepal, Saudi Arabia, and sub-Saharan Africa. Cases in American travelers in such areas are infrequent; however, prolonged contact with the local population could increase the risk of infection and makes vaccination a reasonable precaution. Saudi Arabia requires evidence of meningococcal vaccination for travel to parts of that country. Serogroup A is the most common cause of epidemics outside the United States, but serogroup C and, rarely, serogroup B have been associated with epidemics.

Only one vaccine is available in the United States, the quadrivalent A/C/Y/W-135 vaccine. This vaccine is effective against serogroup A in infants younger than 3 mo of age and may be only partially effective in children 3 to 11 mo old. Children younger than 2 yr of age are not protected against serogroup C. A dose of 0.5 mL is given subcutaneously. Children vaccinated before 4 yr of age should be revaccinated after 2 or 3 yr if they remain in an endemic area.

HEPATITIS A. Protection against hepatitis A is recommended for children traveling to developing countries if their travel is done on the usual tourist routes, if they will be eating or drinking water in areas of questionable sanitation, or if they will have contact with local children in settings of poor sanitation. Immunoglobulin is also recommended for children residing in developing countries. Immune globulin is a sterile preparation of IgG antibodies. United States preparations have not been associated with transmission of hepatitis B or HIV infections. Clinical hepatitis may not be symptomatic in young children (<5 yr of age); infected children can, however, transmit infection to older children and adults, in whom it is usually symptomatic. Immunoglobulin should be given at 0.02 mL/kg for a visit of 3 mo or less and 0.06 mL/kg every 5 mo for longer travel. Pretravel anti-hepatitis A IgG antibody screening may be advisable for children who are frequent travelers. Immunoglobulin produced in developing countries may not meet the same standards for purity set in developed countries. Inactivated hepatitis A virus vaccines have been developed and shown to be effective in preventing hepatitis A. Detailed recommendations regarding the use of the hepatitis A vaccine, including in children, are not available before licensure; it is likely that such recommendations will include individuals at risk because of travel.

An alum-absorbed suspension of the formalin-inactivated HM175 strain of hepatitis A virus derived from MRC-5 human diploid fibroblasts recently has been shown to be highly protective. The HM175 vaccine was tested in more than 40,000 children in Thailand and was 95% effective in preventing symptomatic illness. Adverse side effects were limited to pain and tenderness at the site of injection (17.7%), headache (11.7%), and fever (5.7%).

The vaccine should be administered in the deltoid muscle to children 2–18 yr of age who are at risk for acquiring hepatitis A while traveling. Endemic areas include Africa, Asia (except for Japan), Mexico, Central and South America, the Mediterranean Basin, parts of eastern Europe, and the Middle East. In the United States, certain geographic populations, such as the native peoples of Alaska and the Americas, experience cyclic hepatitis A epidemics. Two primary doses (360 ELISA Units/0.5 mL) 1 mo apart and a booster dose between 6 and 12 mo are recommended. Primary immunization should be completed at least 2 wk prior to expected exposure. Recombinant hepatitis B vaccine can be also administered simultaneously. Immunoglobulin can be administered with the inactivated vaccine as well if necessary. It is recommended that immunoglobulin be administered at a separate site and in a separate syringe. The decision to administer IM immunoglobulin or hepatitis A will be dependent on the duration of the trip, vaccine timing, anticipated frequent trips to endemic areas, and cost.

HEPATITIS B VACCINE. Hepatitis B is highly endemic in eastern and southeastern Asia, sub-Saharan Africa, and the Pacific Basin. In certain parts of the world, 8–15% of the population may be chronically infected. Infants and children traveling to such areas may be at risk if they are exposed directly to blood from the local population. Cases in which disease transmission can occur include receipt of blood transfusions not screened for HBsAg, exposure to unsterilized needles, or close contact with local children who have open skin lesions. Adolescents maybe infected through sexual exposure. Exposure to hepatitis B is more likely if the child is living for prolonged periods in the endemic areas. Vaccination for hepatitis B is recommended for all children in the United States and for children staying in an endemic area for 6 mo or longer or who may have the aforementioned exposures or who are not vaccinated. If not already administered as part of regularly scheduled vaccine in early childhood, recombinant hepatitis B vaccine is given in three doses of 0.25 mL each (2nd dose 1 mo after the 1st and the 3rd dose 5 mo after the 2nd dose) for children <10 yr old and 0.5 mL as detailed for children 11–19 yr old. Optimally, vaccination should begin at least 6 mo before departure; some protection occurs by one or two doses.

DELTA HEPATITIS. Because delta hepatitis depends on active hepatitis B replication, hepatitis B vaccine should be protective.

HEPATITIS C. Hepatitis C is a single-stranded RNA virus that has a transmission pattern similar to that of hepatitis B. It remains a major cause of transfusion-associated hepatitis worldwide. However, many cases of hepatitis C occur without an identifiable risk factor. Because no vaccine is available, the traveler should exercise precautions about contact with contaminated body fluids.

RABIES VACCINE. The risk of rabies is currently the highest in countries where rabies in dogs is uncontrolled, including Columbia, Ecuador, El Salvador, Guatemala, India, Mexico, Nepal, Philippines, Thailand, and Vietnam. Rabies is also endemic in most other countries of Africa, Asia, and Central and South America.

Children are at particular risk, because facial bites are more common. Children should be considered for pre-exposure prophylaxis if they will be in endemic areas for more than 1 mo. The major vaccine in the United States is a human diploid cell rabies vaccine (HDCV), which can be administered intradermally or intramuscularly. Pre-exposure prophylaxis is given to individuals at risk as three IM 1-mL doses on days 7 and 28 or 0.1 mL on days 0, 7, and 28. Postexposure prophylaxis is given as five 1-mL doses on days 0, 3, 7, 14, and 28 if unimmunized and in two doses of 1 mL on days 0 and 3, if previously vaccinated. Intramuscular administration is the preferred route for postexposure and pre-exposure immunization in the setting of travel. Rabies immune globulin is also indicated after exposure in unvaccinated children (20 IU/kg), with one half of the dose infiltrated into the wound, when possible, and the other given intramuscularly (see Chapter 227).

JAPANESE ENCEPHALITIS VACCINE. JE is a mosquito-transmitted viral encephalitis with a fatality rate of 20%. The disease occurs primarily in young children and the elderly. It occurs from June to September in temperate zones and throughout the entire year in tropical zones. Worldwide, JE is the leading cause of viral encephalitis and occurs in the People's Republic of China, India, Bangladesh, Nepal, Sri Lanka, Hong Kong, Korea, Japan, Taiwan, Philippines, eastern Russia, and Southeast Asia. In endemic areas, the age-specific incidence is highest in young children. The risk for travelers is associated with the extent of exposure to the mosquito vectors. Since 1981, six cases of JE have been seen among adult expatriate Americans. Fortunately, most cases are asymptomatic, but mortality rates of 50% or significant neurologic sequelae in one third of survivors have been seen in symptomatic cases. A monovalent inactivated vaccine purified from infected suckling mouse brain has been well tolerated and widely used in Asia with an efficacy of greater than 95%. It is administered in a three-dose schedule of 0.5 mL SC on days 0, 7, and 30 for children 1–3 yr and as 1 mL SC in the same schedule for children older than 3 yr. The CDC recommends immunization for travelers with a high risk of exposure to the mosquito vectors and who will stay for several weeks or more in rural endemic areas (especially in areas of rice or pig farming) during transmission season. Those planning prolonged residencies in these areas should also be immunized.

TRAVELERS' DIARRHEA

Travelers' diarrhea, characterized by a 2-fold or greater increase in the frequency of unformed bowel movements, has been observed in as many as 40% of all travelers overseas. Approximately 5 million people per year from industrialized nations who travel abroad develop this illness. A large number of infectious agents (bacteria, viruses, and parasites) have been associated with travelers' diarrhea; enterotoxic *E. coli* is still the most frequent cause. Other bacterial causes include *Shigella, Salmonella, Campylobacter, Vibrio cholerae, Vibrio parahaemolyticus, Aeromonas hydrophilia,* and *Plesiomonas shigelloides.* Protozoan infections such as *Entamoeba histolytica, Giardia lamblia, Cryptosporidium parvum,* and *Isospora* are also found. These parasitic infections are more common in long-term travelers. In some areas, rotavirus has been associated with travelers' diarrhea. The most important risk factor for travelers' diarrhea is the country of destination. High-risk areas (attack rates of 25–50%) are developing countries of Latin America, Africa, the Middle East, and Asia. Intermediate risk occurs in the Mediterranean, China, and Israel, whereas low-risk areas include North America, Northern Europe, Australia, and New Zealand. The disease is usually self-limited and characterized by 3–5 days of nonbloody diarrhea without significant fever.

Careful selection and preparation of food and water can reduce the risk of developing travelers' diarrhea. Breast-feeding is the best alternative for young infants. Great care should be taken in the preparation of formula and selection of pasteurized dairy products for non–breast-fed infants. Carbonated and boiled water is safest. Uncooked vegetables and undercooked meat and fish should be avoided. Fruits should be peeled by parents.

There are few data on the use of antidiarrheal drugs in children. Chemoprophylactic agents have been discouraged in children because potential adverse effects greatly outweight any prophylactic benefit. For example, doxycycline, although effective in prophylaxis, should not be given to children younger than 8 yr of age, because it binds to calcium and is incorporated into growing bones and teeth. Antimicrobial therapy for travelers' diarrhea in infants and young children should be administered in consultation with a physician. This is true particularly if the illness is severe or there is associated high fever or the stools are bloody. If empiric antimicrobial agents are administered by parents in cases of mild illness, trimethoprim (4 mg/kg) and sulfamethoxazole (20 mg/kg) twice each day for 3 days may be effective for infants (2 mo of age or older) and older children. Resistance to trimethoprim-sulfamethoxazole should be considered. Quinolones are contraindicated in children. Furazolidone (5 mg/kg/day in four divided doses) should also be considered, given its efficacy against both bacterial pathogens and *Giardia lamblia.* Antimotility agents like diphenoxylate HCl (Lomotil) should be avoided; mortality and morbidity from infection caused by *Salmonella* and *Shigella* are higher with diphenoxylate HCl therapy.

Dehydration is the greatest threat presented by a diarrheal illness in a small child. Education of parents regarding the symptoms and signs of dehydration is necessary. Parents should carry with them either prepackaged oral rehydration solutions recommended by the WHO or a recipe for a home formula if their children develop an acute, dehydrating diarrheal illness. Pre-existing gastrointestinal disease such as celiac sprue, ulcerative colitis, Crohn disease, and the immunosuppression from HIV can put children at great risk, especially for *Salmonella* infection.

MALARIA CHEMOPROPHYLAXIS

Malaria, a mosquito-borne infection, is the leading parasitic cause of death in children worldwide (see Chapter 244.7). Of the four *Plasmodium* species that infect humans, *P. falciparum* causes the greatest morbidity and mortality. In the United States, a growing number of malaria cases is reported annually for travelers and immigrants. Each year, more than 7 million

United States citizens visit parts of the world where malaria is endemic. Given this major resurgence of malaria, physicians in developed countries are increasingly required to give advice on the prevention, diagnosis, and treatment of malaria.

Malaria transmission occurs primarily between dusk and dawn, and parents should be advised of the importance of *measures to reduce mosquito contact* during these times. Measures to avoid the insect vector, including the use of appropriate clothing, netting, and insect repellents, are extremely important and should be emphasized. Insect repellent should be purchased before departure. The most effective repellents contain DEET. The higher the concentration of DEET, the longer it lasts as a repellent. Toxic encephalopathy, however, has occurred in children exposed to DEET. Frequent application of products containing high concentrations of DEET should be avoided in children.

Prophylactic medication has also been shown to be extremely effective. Unfortunately, only 28% of the 410 American citizens with *P. falciparum* malaria acquired in Africa between 1980 and 1984 were using a recommended drug for prophylaxis. One survey of 4,042 returning American travelers to Africa and Haiti demonstrated that 58% of these individuals did not take recommended prophylactic agents regularly. Travelers are more likely to use prophylactic antimalarial drugs if appropriate recommendations and education are provided to them by physicians before their departure. However, in one survey, only 14% of persons who sought medical advice obtained correct information regarding malaria prevention and prophylaxis.

Resistance of *P. falciparum* to the 1st-line chemoprophylactic agent, chloroquine, is rapidly increasing worldwide. Because of this growing problem of resistance, 2nd-line agents are increasingly used. In the United States, pyrimethamine-sulfadoxine (Fansidar) was given concurrently to travelers visiting areas of chloroquine-resistant *P. falciparum* malaria between 1982 and 1985. During that period, numerous cases of severe cutaneous reactions and seven deaths were reported in individuals taking long-term prophylaxis. As a result, the recommendations for malaria prophylaxis have changed several times during the last few years.

Several factors are important in choosing appropriate chemoprophylactic regimens for malaria. The travel itinerary should be reviewed thoroughly in relation to information regarding areas of risk within a particular country. The risk for acquiring chloroquine-resistant *P. falciparum* should also be determined. Finally, allergic or other known adverse reactions to antimalarial agents should be considered, as well as the availability of medical care during travel.

Chloroquine is still the mainstay of chemoprophylaxis for children traveling to most malaria-endemic areas (Table 248–3). Malaria is fully sensitive to chloroquine only in Haiti, the Dominican Republic, Central America, and the Middle East. *P. vivax, P. ovale,* and *P. malariae* and the other species infecting humans remain chloroquine-sensitive. In areas where *P. falciparum* is developing resistance to chloroquine, sensitive strains coexist. In one study, decreased parasitemia and milder illness were also seen in individuals who took chloroquine but still developed chloroquine-resistant falciparum malaria. Malaria chemoprophylaxis should begin 1–2 wk before departure to ensure adequate serum levels and to screen for adverse effects. Chloroquine should be also continued for 4–6 wk after leaving an endemic area. Chloroquine is manufactured in the United States only in tablet form and tastes quite bitter. Pediatric doses should be carefully calculated per unit body weight because of the risk of severe toxicity. Pharmacists can pulverize tablets and prepare gelatin capsules. Alternatively, mixing pulverized doses in food or drink may facilitate compliance in children. Chloroquine suspension is also widely available overseas. Chloroquine-resistant *P. vivax* organisms have been reported from India and Papua New Guinea.

Parents of children traveling to areas where chloroquine-resistant malaria exists should be warned about the possibility of acquiring resistant malaria, and they should be supplied with **pyrimethamine-sulfadoxine** (Fansidar) for presumptive treatment if a febrile illness develops (see Table 248–3). Fansidar resistance is a problem in sub-Saharan Africa and

■ **TABLE 248–3 Drugs Used in Chemoprophylaxis and Presumptive Treatment of Malaria in Children**

	Drug	Pediatric Dosage
Areas of chloroquine-sensitive *Plasmodium falciparum*	Chloroquine phosphate*	5 mg/kg base (8.3 mg/kg of salt) once per wk, up to maximum adult dose of 300 mg base
Areas of chloroquine-resistant *P. falciparum*	Chloroquine phosphate*	5 mg/kg base (8.3 mg/kg of salt) once per wk, up to maximum adult dose of 300 mg base
	PLUS Proguanil† (East Africa)	<2 yr: 50 mg qd 3–6 yr: 50–75 mg qd 7–10 yr: 100 mg qd >10 yr: 200 mg qd
	PLUS Pyrimethamine-sulfadoxine‡	2–11 mo: ¼ tablet 1–3 yr: ½ tablet 4–8 yr: 1 tablet 9–14 yr: 2 tablets >14 yr: 3 tablets Take single dose of the aforementioned for self-treatment of febrile illness when medical care is not immediately available
	OR Mefloquine§	15–19 kg: ¼ tab/wk (62.5 mg/wk) 20–30 kg: ½ tab/wk (125 mg/wk) 31–45 kg: ¾ tab/wk (187.5 mg/wk) >45 kg: 1 tab/wk (250 mg/wk)
Prevention of relapses	Primaquine phosphate‖	0.3 mg/kg base (0.5 mg/kg of salt) orally, once a day for 14 days, or 0.9 mg/kg base (1.5 mg/kg of salt) orally, once a wk for 8 wk

**If chloroquine phosphate is not available, hydroxychloroquine sulfate is as effective; 400 mg of hydroxychloroquine sulfate is equivalent to 500 mg of chloroquine phosphate.*

†Proguanil (Paludrine-Ayerst, Canada, ICI) is not available in the United States.

‡Recommended for travel to sub-Saharan Africa, the Indian subcontinent, South America (except the Amazon basin), Oceania, Hainan Island, and the southern provinces of China. Pyrimethamine-sulfadoxine (Fansidar) is contraindicated in patients with a history of sulfonamide intolerance, in pregnancy at term, and in infants younger than 2 mo old.

§Mefloquine is not recommended for children less than 15 kg.

‖Primaquine is only recommended to prevent relapse of P. vivax *and* P. ovale *infection. Primaquine phosphate can cause hemolytic anemia, especially in patients with glucose-6-phosphate dehydrogenase (G-6-PD) deficiency. This deficiency is most common in blacks, Asians, and Mediterranean people. Children should be screened for G-6-PD deficiency before treatment.*

Southeast Asia. After giving presumptive treatment with pyrimethamine-sulfadoxine, the parents should seek medical care for the child as soon as possible.

Proguanil, a dihydrofolate reductase inhibitor that is not available in the United States, is recommended by some authorities for prophylaxis against chloroquine-resistant *P. falciparum* in East Africa, especially for children weighing less than 15 kg. Limited data suggest that this drug is not effective in Thailand, the Amazon Basin, Papua New Guinea, and possibly West Africa. Proguanil (see Table 248–3) should be used in combination with weekly chloroquine phosphate.

Mefloquine, a synthetic 4-quinoline related to chloroquine, is highly effective against chloroquine- and pyrimethamine-sulfadoxine–resistant *P. falciparum*. This drug has been approved by the Food and Drug Administration in the United States. In preliminary studies of Peace Corps workers, mefloquine is 67% more effective than chloroquine in malaria endemic areas where chloroquine-resistant *P. falciparum* exists. This drug should not be used in children who weigh less than 15 kg because of insufficient efficacy and tolerance data.

Doxycycline has been recommended for travelers to areas of multidrug-resistant *P. falciparum* (Thailand, Burma, Kampuchea, the Amazon Basin) and for travelers allergic to sulfa drugs. This drug is contraindicated in children less than 8 yr of age. Parents should be discouraged from taking a child on a trip if there will be evening or nighttime exposure in rural areas of countries with chloroquine- (or multidrug-) resistant *P. falciparum* or if the child is allergic to sulfa drugs or is too young to take sulfa drugs.

Primaquine is given to prevent relapses of malaria seen in *P. vivax* or *P. ovale* infection. Prophylaxis is generally indicated for children who have prolonged exposure in malaria-endemic areas (see Table 248–3). Primaquine can cause severe hemolysis in individuals deficient in glucose-6-phosphate dehydrogenase (G-6-PD). Testing for G-6-PD deficiency should be performed in children before administration of primaquine.

Small amounts of antimalarial drugs, including chloroquine and sulfa compounds, are secreted into breast milk of lactating women. The amounts of transferred drug are not considered to be harmful or sufficient to provide adequate prophylaxis against malaria.

Because of changes in the risk of developing malaria, resistance patterns, and recommendations for prophylaxis and treatment, physicians should contact the CDC, Division of Parasitic Diseases, at telephone no. (404) 639–1610 to obtain the most recent information.

Barry M: Medical considerations for international travel with infants and older children. *In*: Gardner P (ed): Infectious Diseases Clinics of North America, Vol 6. Philadelphia, WB Saunders, 1992, p. 389.

DuPont HL and Ericsson CD: Prevention and treatment of traveler's diarrhea. N Engl J Med 328:1821, 1993.

Hill DR: Immunizations. *In*: Gardner P (ed): Infectious Diseases Clinics of North America, Vol 6. Philadelphia, WB Saunders, 1992, p. 291.

Hill DR, Pearson RD: Health advice for international travel. Ann Intern Med 108:839, 1988.

Jong EC and McMullen R: General advice for the international traveler. *In*: Gardner P (ed): Infectious Diseases Clinics of North America, Vol 6. Philadelphia, WB Saunders, 1992, p. 275.

Nahlen BL, Parsonnet J, Preblud SR, et al: International travel and the child younger than two years. II: Recommendations for prevention of travelers' diarrhea and malaria chemoprophylaxis. Pediatr Infect Dis 8:735, 1989.

Preblud SR, Tsai TF, Brink EW, et al: International travel and the child younger than two years. I: Recommendations for immunization. Pediatr Infect Dis 8:416, 1989.

Salata RA, Olds GR: Infectious diseases in travelers and immigrants. *In*: Warren KS, Mahmoud AAF (eds): Tropical and Geographical Medicine, 2nd ed. New York, McGraw-Hill, 1990, pp 228–242.

Schwartz IK: Prevention of malaria. *In*: Gardner P (ed): Infectious Diseases Clinics of North America, Vol 6. Philadelphia, WB Saunders, 1992, p. 313.

The Medical Letter: Advice For Travelers 36:41, 1994.

U.S. Department of Health and Human Services, Public Health Services, Centers for Disease Control: Health Information for International Travel. Health and Human Services Publication, 1993.

Wyler DJ: Malaria chemoprophylaxis for the traveler. N Engl J Med 329:31, 1993.

Wyler DJ: Malaria: Overview and update. Clin Infect Dis 16:449, 1993.

CHAPTER 249
*Infection Control**

Ann M. Arvin

Approximately 5% of all children admitted to pediatric hospitals in the United States acquire an infection in the hospital (nosocomial infection). The consequences can be measured in morbidity, mortality, delayed discharge, and higher hospital costs. The aim of isolation procedures is protection of the patient, other hospitalized children, and the hospital staff. The means of prevention are surprisingly simple. Today, as in the time of Semmelweis, handwashing is the most important measure that can be taken by personnel, who are the passive agents of most nosocomial infections. Physicians, nurses, and other hospital personnel must cooperate to ensure that handwashing is done before and after every patient contact, whether or not the patient is known to be infected. Constant vigilance is required to maintain standards. Adequate separation between patients is also important in reducing nosocomial infection. Recommended isolation systems include universal precautions and category- or disease-specific precautions. Universal precautions (body substance isolation) are of great significance for pediatric and other hospitals. This term means that every patient is assumed to be capable of carrying a bloodborne infection, and all contact with blood or other body fluids containing blood is considered potentially hazardous. Infection with human immunodeficiency virus or hepatitis B virus cannot be predicted from the history or physical examination. Universal precautions should be followed by all health care workers to prevent exposure to blood; to amniotic, pericardial, peritoneal, pleural, synovial, and cerebrospinal fluid; and to semen or vaginal secretions. Gloves are necessary for handling these fluids, and gowns, masks, and goggles are added if circumstances make splashing likely.

Microorganisms are transmitted in a variety of ways. Some are transmitted by direct contact with respiratory or enteric excretions; some by inhalation of small-particle aerosols; some by ingestion of contaminated food or water; some by sexual transmission; some by arthropod bites; and some by inoculation of blood. Category- or disease-specific isolation rules are tailored to fit the type of transmission that is expected and to interpose a block in that transmission. Instructions regarding specific diseases are available from several sources, notably the Report of the Committee on Infectious Diseases (Redbook) of the American Academy of Pediatrics, the Centers for Disease Control, and the American Public Health Association. In addition, each hospital should have an isolation manual, in which recommendations and procedures adapted to local circumstances are given in detail.

Isolation is carried out by means of handwashing, private rooms, gowns, gloves, and masks. Handwashing should be practiced before and after every patient contact, whether or not the patient is known to be infected. Hospital personnel do not need to be infected themselves to infect others; mechanical carriage is enough in the case of agents such as staphylococci and respiratory syncytial virus. Gloves are a useful additional

*Modified from the section in the 14th edition by S. A. Plotkin.

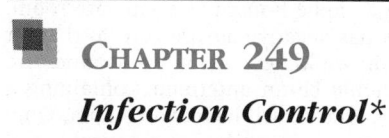

means of reducing nosocomial infection, but they supplement rather than replace handwashing. Gowns are a means of keeping infectious materials off clothing, although in some settings they are used more as reminders that the patient is isolated.

Some patients, usually those with infections transmitted by small-particle aerosols, need to be housed in a separate room. Ideally, an isolation room has negative air pressure so that air is evacuated to the outside while new air enters around and under the door. There should be an anteroom, containing a sink and isolation supplies, which itself has a closed door. Only this type of design can contain infections like varicella and aspergillosis, which are notorious for spreading on air currents.

Many infections transmitted by large-particle aerosols can be contained by bedside isolation using gown and gloves, with masks added only for close contact with secretions or excretions (contact isolation). These methods belong in the category of *enteric and drainage secretion precautions.* Technique is important in maintaining isolation. Individual gowns must be available for each patient and must be removed before leaving the patient's area. Gloves must be put on carefully and removed and discarded without touching other surfaces.

Protective isolation is a form of isolation designed to place a barrier between exogenous microorganisms and an immunosuppressed patient, particularly one who is neutropenic (<500 polymorphonuclear leukocytes/mm^3). Ideally, a patient who needs a protective environment is placed in a laminar air flow room, in which filtered air under positive pressure provides a curtain to keep contamination out. However, patients have endogenous flora that are difficult to control, even when attempts are made to sterilize them with orally administered and topical antibiotics. Moreover, hospital staff who do not practice handwashing may introduce resistant hospital flora.

Education of health care workers about the use and disposal of needles and other sharp instruments is essential to reduce the risk of exposure to bloodborne pathogens. Food and infant formula preparation procedures must be monitored carefully. Attention must be paid to *disinfection* of the physical environment. Although many microorganisms have been shown to persist on inanimate objects for long periods, the role of such persistence in the transmission of human infection is doubtful. Nevertheless, dust should be removed and surfaces cleaned with germicidal solutions. Commercial solutions containing phenol can be used to clean isolation rooms.

Scrupulous cleanliness is needed when aqueous solutions come in contact with the patient or personnel. Water for washing may be contaminated with *Legionella,* sinks and respiratory equipment may be contaminated with gram-negative bacteria, and handwashing solutions are prone to contamination with *Pseudomonas* spp. If infections occur, water-associated sources must be examined.

Every hospital should have an infection control committee and, in addition, an infection control practitioner. The role of the latter is to survey infections on a day-to-day basis, looking for clusters or patterns that indicate epidemic or endemic nosocomial infection. An important aspect of this job is surveillance of surgical infections, which may indicate inadequate sterile technique. The infection control practitioner also attempts to improve isolation practices, institute methods of preventing infection, and educate the staff, including physicians. The role of the infection control committee is to receive reports from the practitioner and to ensure that effective actions are taken. In practice, the chairman of the committee is usually an infection disease specialist or pathologist.

CHAPTER 250

Child Day Care and Communicable Diseases

Larry K. Pickering and Ardythe L. Morrow

An estimated 13 million children 5 yr of age or younger and 60% of school-aged children younger than 13 yr attend some form of child care on a regular basis. Child care facilities can be classified based on the setting and the number, age, and health status of the children enrolled. As defined in the United States, child care facilities consist of child care centers, family child care homes, and special facilities for ill children or children with special needs. Centers are nonresidential settings that provide care and education for preschool-aged children. Center programs may be full day or part day, may expect regular daily attendance, or may be designed for drop-in use. Day care centers are licensed and regulated by the states in which they are located, and each cares for a mean of 68 children. Family child care programs are based in the residence of the care providers and may be large (7–12 children) or small (1–6 children). Day care homes generally are not licensed or registered. Most studies of infectious diseases have been conducted in day care centers.

Epidemiologic studies have established that children in child care are 2–18 times more likely to acquire certain infectious diseases than children not enrolled in child care (Table 250–1). In addition, children in child care are at risk of having more severe illnesses, receiving more antibiotics for longer periods, and acquiring drug-resistant organisms. Transmission of organisms and illness in group care depends on the age and immune status of children involved, season, environmental characteristics of the facilities, and organism characteristics. Rates of infec-

■ TABLE 250–1 Infectious Diseases Studied in the Child Day-Care Setting

Type of Disease or Infection	Examples	Increased Incidence with Child Care
Enteric infection	Diarrhea	Yes
	Hepatitis A	Yes
Respiratory tract infection	Otitis media	Yes
	Sinusitis	Probably
	Pharyngitis	Probably
	Pneumonia	Probably
Invasive bacterial disease	*Haemophilus influenzae* type b	Yes
	Neisseria meningitidis	Probably
	Streptococcus pneumoniae	Not established
Aseptic meningitis	Enteroviruses	Probably
Herpesvirus infections	Cytomegalovirus	Yes
	Varicella-zoster	Yes
	Herpes simplex	Yes
Bloodborne diseases	Hepatitis B	Few case reports
	Human immunodeficiency virus	No cases reported
Vaccine-preventable diseases	Measles, mumps, rubella, diphtheria, pertussis, tetanus	Not established
	Polio	No
	H. influenzae type b	Yes
Skin disease	Impetigo	Probably
	Scabies	Probably
	Pediculosis	Probably
	Ringworm	Probably

tion, duration of illness, and risk of hospitalization tend to decrease among children in day care after they are 3 yr of age.

PATTERNS OF OCCURRENCE. There are several different patterns of occurrence of infectious diseases among children in child care and their contacts. Respiratory tract infections and diarrhea are the most common diseases associated with child care. These infections occur in children, child care staff, and household contacts. Organisms such as enteroviruses (see Chapter 209), which are transmitted by fecal-oral contamination and by respiratory secretions, can infect children and adults. Infections due to hepatitis A virus (HAV) (see Chapter 221) may be inapparent in young children attending child care but may have a major clinical impact on older children and adult contacts, including child care staff and household contacts. Other conditions, such as otitis media (see Chapter 590), varicella (see Chapter 213), and invasive *Haemophilus influenzae* type b disease (see Chapter 77), usually affect children rather than adults. Some infections, such as cytomegalovirus (CMV) (see Chapter 214) and parvovirus B19 (see Chapter 210), may have serious consequences for the fetuses of pregnant women or for certain immunosuppressed hosts. Bloodborne pathogens such as hepatitis B virus (HBV) (see Chapter 221) and human immunodeficiency virus (HIV) (see Chapter 223) can infect all ages but have rarely (HBV) or never (HIV) been reported to be transmitted in the day-care setting.

FREQUENCY OF INFECTIOUS DISEASES IN CHILD CARE. Almost any organism has the propensity to be spread and cause disease in the child care setting, but the organisms listed in Table 250–1 have been studied most extensively. Acute infectious diarrhea is two to three times more common in children in child care than in children cared for in their homes. Outbreaks of diarrhea are common and are caused most frequently by enteric viruses such as rotavirus, enteric adenovirus, astrovirus, or calicivirus or caused by an enteric parasite such as *Giardia lamblia* or cryptosporidium. However, bacterial enteropathogens, such as shigella and *Escherichia coli* O157:H7 also have been associated with outbreaks of diarrhea in some child care settings. HAV infections in children enrolled in child care have resulted in community-wide outbreaks. HAV infections usually are mild or asymptomatic in children and become detected when illness manifests in older children or adults. Enteropathogens and HAV are transmitted in child care facilities by the fecal-oral route and rarely by contaminated food or water. Enteric illness and HAV infections are more common in centers that care for children who are not toilet trained.

Children younger than 2 yr of age attending child care centers have more upper and lower respiratory tract infections than age-matched children not in child care. The organisms responsible for illness are similar to those that circulate in the community and include respiratory syncytial virus, parainfluenza virus, adenovirus, rhinovirus, coronavirus, influenza virus, and parvovirus B19, and less commonly, *Bordetella pertussis* and *Mycobacterium tuberculosis*. The risk of developing otitis media is increased significantly in children attending child care, and the disease is responsible for most of the antibiotic use in children younger than 3 yr of age in child care. Group A streptococcal infection among children in child care is not a common problem, but outbreaks have been reported.

Primary invasive disease due to *H. influenzae* type b has been shown to be more common in children in child care; evidence for increased risk of subsequent or secondary disease due to *H. influenzae* type b in the child care setting is less convincing. There is an indication that the risk of primary disease due to *Neisseria meningitidis* is higher among children in child care than among children cared for at home; the risk for invasive disease due to *Streptococcus pneumoniae* is more common in children in child care. While secondary spread of *S. pneumoniae* and *N. meningitidis* has been reported, the risk to child care children is unknown. An outbreak of aseptic meningitis due to echovirus 30 has been reported among children in a child care center, their parents, and their teachers.

Studies of CMV infection in child care centers have shown that young children shed CMV chronically after acquisition. CMV-infected children often transmit the virus to other children with whom they have contact and to 8–20% of their care providers and mothers per year. Transmission occurs as the result of contact with infected saliva and urine. Varicella frequently is transmitted in child care centers; the role of child care facilities in the spread of herpes simplex, especially during episodes of gingivostomatitis, needs further clarification.

Concern has arisen regarding the potential for transmission of two bloodborne organisms in the child care setting: HBV and HIV. HBV transmission among children in child care has been documented in a few instances, but with implementation of universal immunization of infants with HBV vaccine, concern about this problem will decline. Issues regarding HIV in child care include the potential risk of HIV transmission within the child care setting and risks to the HIV-infected child associated with acquisition of infectious agents. No cases of HIV transmission in out-of-home child care have been reported. Children with HIV infection enrolled in child care facilities should be monitored for exposure to infectious diseases, and their health and immune status should be evaluated frequently.

The most commonly recognized non–vaccine-preventable skin infections or infestations in children in child care are impetigo due to *Staphylococcus aureus* or group A streptococci, pediculosis, scabies, and ringworm. The magnitude of infection or infestation in children in child care is not known.

ANTIBIOTIC USE AND ORGANISM RESISTANCE. The increased frequency of disease in children in child care facilities is associated with increased use of antimicrobial agents. The estimated annual rates of antibiotic use in children in child care range from two to four times higher than in age-matched children cared for at home. The mean duration of antibiotic treatment is four times longer in children in child care. This frequency of antibiotic use combined with the propensity for person-to-person transmission of pathogens in a crowded environment has resulted in an increased prevalence of antibiotic-resistant bacteria such as *Shigella sonnei, S. pneumoniae,* and *E. coli.*

PREVENTION. Written child care center policies designed to prevent or control the spread of infectious agents should be available and reviewed regularly. Standards should be established and implemented for personal hygiene, especially handwashing, maintenance of current immunization records, exclusion policies, targeting frequently contaminated areas for environmental cleaning, and appropriate handling of food.

In the United States, there are ten diseases for which all children should be immunized unless there are contraindications: diphtheria, pertussis, tetanus, *H. influenzae* type b, measles, mumps, rubella, poliomyelitis, HBV, and varicella. High levels of immunization exist among children in licensed child care facilities, probably because there are laws in almost all states of the United States that require age-appropriate immunizations of children attending licensed child care programs. Recommendations for the use of vaccines affect children in the child care setting. Use of *H. influenzae* type b conjugate vaccines has practically eliminated disease due to invasive *H. influenzae* type b organisms. HBV vaccine will impact children in child care centers, and the release of HAV vaccine eventually may decrease this disease among children and adults in the day-care setting. Child care providers should be current for all immunizations routinely recommended for adults. Local health authorities should be notified about cases of communicable disease involving children or child care providers in child care settings.

STANDARDS. Every state has its own standards for licensing and reviewing child care centers and family day-care homes.

In 1992, the American Public Health Association and the American Academy of Pediatrics jointly published the *National Health and Safety Performance Standards: Guidelines for Out-of-Home Child Care Programs* (ISBN 0–87553–205–5). This comprehensive reference book can be used by pediatricians and other health care professionals to guide decisions about infectious disease and other health matters in child care facilities.

Belongia EA, Osterholm MT, Soler JT, et al: Transmission of *Escherichia coli* O157:H7 infection in Minnesota child day-care facilities. JAMA 269:883, 1993.

Berg AT, Shapiro ED, Capobianco LA: Group day care and the risk of serious infectious illness. Am J Epidemiol 133:154, 1991.

Brian MJ, Van R, Townsend I, et al: Evaluation of the molecular epidemiology of an outbreak of multiply resistant *Shigella sonnei* in a day care center using pulsed-field gel electrophoresis and plasmid DNA analysis. J Clin Microbiol 31:2152, 1993.

Cherian T, Steinhoff MC, Harrison LH, et al: A cluster of invasive pneumococcal disease in young children in child care. JAMA 271:695, 1994.

Fornasini M, Reves RR, Murray BE, et al: Trimethoprim-resistant *Escherichia coli* in households of children attending day care centers. J Infect Dis 166:326, 1992.

Frenck Jr, RW, Glezen WP: Respiratory tract infections in children in day care. Semin Pediatr Infect Dis 1:234, 1990.

Helfand RF, Khan AS, Pallansch MA, et al: Echovirus 30 infection and aseptic meningitis in parents of children attending a child care center. J Infect Dis 169:1133, 1994.

Jones DS, Rogers MF: Human immunodeficiency virus infection in children in day care. Semin Pediatr Infect Dis 1:280, 1990.

Mitchell DK, Van R, Morrow AL, et al: Outbreaks of astrovirus gastroenteritis in day care centers. J Pediatr 123:725, 1993.

Osterholm MT, Reves RR, Murphy JR, et al: Infectious diseases and child day care. Pediatr Infect Dis J 11(Suppl):31, 1992.

Osterholm MT: Invasive bacterial diseases and child day care. Semin Pediatr Infect Dis 1:222, 1990.

Pass RF: Day care centers and transmission of cytomegalovirus: New insight into an old problem. Semin Pediatr Infect Dis 1:245, 1990.

Pickering LK, Morrow AL: Contagious diseases of child day care. Infection 19:61, 1991.

Reichler MR, Allphin AA, Breiman RF, et al: The spread of multiply resistant *Streptococcus pneumoniae* at a day care center in Ohio. J Infect Dis 166:1346, 1992.

Reves RR, Morrow AL, Bartlett AV, et al: Child day care increases the risk of clinic visits for acute diarrhea and diarrhea due to rotavirus. Am J Epidemiol 137:97, 1993.

Reves RR, Pickering LK: Impact of child day care on infectious diseases in adults. Infect Dis Clin North Am 6:239, 1992.

Reves RR, Jones JA: Antibiotic use and resistance patterns in day care. Semin Pediatr Infect Dis 1:212, 1990.

Shapiro CN, Hadler SC: Significance of hepatitis in children in day care. Semin Pediatr Infect Dis 1:270, 1990.

Simons RJ, Chanock S: Medical issues related to caring for human immunodeficiency virus-infected children in and out of the home. Pediatr Infect Dis J 12:845, 1993.

Van R, Morrow AL, Reves RR, et al: Environmental contamination in child day care centers. Am J Epidemiol 133:460, 1991.

PART XVIII

The Digestive System

SECTION 1

Clinical Manifestations of Gastrointestinal Disease

Martin Ulshen

CHAPTER 251

Normal Digestive Tract Phenomena

Gastrointestinal function varies with maturity; a symptom that might be abnormal at an older age, such as regurgitation, may be normal in an infant. The fetus can swallow amniotic fluid as early as 12 wk gestation but nutritive sucking in neonates first develops at about 34 wk gestation. The coordinated oral and pharnygeal movements necessary for swallowing solids develop within the 1st mo or two of life in term infants. Prior to this time solids are thrust forward by the tongue, and aspiration is a risk from poor coordination of muscle function. By 1 mo of age, infants appear to show preferences for sweet and salty foods. Infants' interest in solids increases at about 4 mo of age. The current recommendation to begin solids at 6 mo of age is based on nutritional concepts rather than maturation of the swallowing process (Chapter 44). Infants swallow air during feeding and must be stimulated to burp to prevent gaseous distention of the stomach.

A number of normal anatomic variations may be noted in the mouth. A short lingual frenulum ("tongue-tie") may be worrisome to parents but only rarely interferes with eating or speech, generally requiring no treatment. Surface furrowing of the tongue (i.e., a geographic or scrotal tongue) is usually a normal finding. A bifid uvula may be normal or associated with a submucous cleft of the soft palate.

Regurgitation, the result of gastroesophageal reflux, occurs commonly in the first 12–18 mo of life. Effortless emesis may dribble out of the infant's mouth but also may be forceful. In an otherwise healthy infant with regurgitation, volumes of emesis are commonly about 15–30 mL but may occasionally be much larger. In contrast to vomiting, the episode of regurgitation from reflux usually surprises both infant and caretaker. Most often, the infant remains happy, although possibly hungry, after an episode of regurgitation. Episodes may occur from less than one to multiple times per day. If complications develop, gastroesophageal reflux is considered pathologic rather than merely developmental and deserves further evaluation and treatment. These complications include failure to thrive, pulmonary disease (apnea or aspiration pneumonitis), and esophagitis with its sequelae (see Chapters 269 and 270).

Infants and young children may be erratic eaters; this may be a worry to parents. A toddler may eat insatiably after refusing to consume normal amounts of food during previous meals. Infancy and adolescence are periods of rapid growth; high nutrient requirements for growth may be associated with voracious appetites. The reduced appetite of the toddler and preschool child is often a worry to parents who are used to the greater dietary intake during infancy.

The *number, color,* and *consistency of stools* may vary greatly in the same infant and between infants of similar age without apparent explanation. The earliest stools after birth consist of meconium, a dark, viscous, gumlike material. When nursing or formula feedings begin, meconium is replaced by green-brown transition stools, often containing curds, and, after 4–5 days, by yellow-brown milk stools. Stool frequency is extremely variable in normal infants and may vary from 0–7 per day. Breast-fed infants may have frequent, small, loose stools early (transition stools) and then after 2–3 wk may have very infrequent, soft stools. It is possible for a nursing infant to go up to 1–2 wk without any stool and then to have a normal soft bowel movement. The color of stool has little significance except for the presence of blood or absence of bilirubin products. The presence of vegetable matter, such as peas or corn, in the stool of an older infant or toddler ingesting solids is normal and suggests poor chewing and not malabsorption. A pattern of intermittent loose stools, known as "toddler's diarrhea," occurs commonly between 1 and 3 yr of age. Often these children drink frequently (especially juices) and snack throughout the day. Typically the stools occur during the day and not overnight. The volume of fluid intake is often excessive; eliminating between meal liquids and snacks often leads to resolution of the pattern of loose stools.

A *protuberant abdomen* is often noted in infants and toddlers, especially following large feedings. This may result from the combination of weak abdominal musculature, relatively large abdominal organs, and lordotic stance. In the 1st yr of life, it is common to palpate the liver up to 2 cm below the right costal margin. The normal liver is soft in consistency and percusses to normal size for age. A Riedel lobe is a thin projection of the right lobe of the liver that may be palpated low in the right lateral abdomen. A soft spleen tip may also be palpable as a normal finding. In thin, young children, the vertebral column is easily palpable and an overlying structure may be mistaken for a mass. Commonly, pulsation of the aorta can be appreciated. Normal stool can often be palpated in the left lower quadrant in the descending or sigmoid colon.

Blood loss from the gastrointestinal tract is never normal, but swallowed blood may be misinterpreted as gastrointestinal bleeding. Maternal blood may be ingested at the time of birth or later by a nursing infant if there is bleeding near the mother's nipple. Nasal or oropharyngeal bleeding is occasionally mistaken for gastrointestinal bleeding. Red dyes in foods or drinks may give red color to the stool but will not produce a positive test for occult blood.

Jaundice is common in neonates, especially among prematures, and usually results from the inability of an immature liver to conjugate bilirubin, leading to an elevated indirect component (Chapter 88). Persistent elevation of indirect bilirubin levels in nursing infants may be the result of breast milk jaundice, which is usually a benign entity in full-term infants. Elevated direct bilirubin is never normal and suggests liver disease, although in infants it may be the result of extrahepatic infection (e.g., urinary tract infection). The direct bilirubin fraction should account for no more than 15–20% of the total bilirubin. Indirect hyperbilirubinemia, which occurs commonly in normal newborns, tends to give a golden yellow color to the sclerae and skin, whereas direct hyperbilirubinemia produces a greenish-yellow hue.

CHAPTER 252

Major Symptoms and Signs of Digestive Tract Disorders

Disorders of organs outside of the gastrointestinal tract can produce symptoms and signs that mimic digestive tract disorders and should be considered in the differential diagnosis (Table 252–1). Understanding the pathogenesis of symptoms is helpful as specific treatment is not always available and nonspecific management of the symptoms may be necessary.

DISORDERED INGESTION. Disordered ingestion may result from refusal to feed or from swallowing difficulty. Poor weight gain or weight loss suggests a severe process that necessitates further investigation. Dysphagia is difficulty swallowing; occurs at the level of the mouth, oropharynx, or esophagus; and results from a motor disorder (e.g., cerebral palsy or achalasia) or mechanical obstruction (e.g., peptic stricture of the esophagus). The dysphagia in motor disorders may be intermittent and occur with liquids or solids. When solids cause symptoms, they may be washed down with liquids. Ice cold liquids may accentuate symptoms. Liquids will pass without difficulty with a mechanical obstruction but solids that become lodged in the esophagus may require regurgitation. When dysphagia is associated with a delay in passage through the esophagus, the child may be able to point to the level of the chest where the delay occurs; esophageal symptoms may be referred to the suprasternal notch. Therefore, when a child points to the suprasternal notch the impaction may be found anywhere in the esophagus.

Transfer Dysphagia. A complex sequence of neuromuscular events is involved in the transfer of foods to the upper esophagus. Suckling requires the lips to form a tight seal about the nipple while the tongue is displaced posteriorly. As the glottis closes to guard the airway, the soft palate rises to close the nasopharynx, the cricopharyngeal muscles relax, and food passes to the back of the pharynx. Solids similarly require coordinated actions; for large chunks of solid food jaw movement and teeth become factors to consider. Salivary secretions, stimulated by the anticipation and act of ingestion, lubricate foods as they pass through the mouth. It is abnormalities of the muscles involved in the ingestion process, their innervation, strength, or coordination that usually cause transfer dysphagia in infants and children. In such cases, an oropharyngeal problem is almost always part of a more generalized neurologic or muscular problem (botulism, diphtheria, cerebral palsy). Occasionally, painful oral lesions, such as acute viral stomatitis or trauma, will interfere with ingestion. If the nasal air passage is seriously obstructed, the need for air will cause severe distress when suckling. Although severe structural, dental, and salivary abnormalities would be expected to create difficulties, ingestion proceeds relatively well in most affected children if they are hungry.

■ **TABLE 252–1 Some Nondigestive Tract Causes of Gastrointestinal Symptoms in Children**

Anorexia
Systemic disease (e.g., inflammatory, neoplastic)
Iatrogenic—drug therapy, unpalatable therapeutic diets
Depression
Anorexia nervosa
Vomiting
Increased intracranial pressure
Infection (e.g., urinary tract)
Adrenal insufficiency
Pregnancy
Psychogenic
Abdominal migraine
Diarrhea
Infection (e.g., otitis media, urinary)
Uremia
Constipation
Hypothyroidism
Spina bifida
Psychomotor retardation
Dehydration (e.g., diabetes insipidus, renal tubular lesions)
Abdominal pain
Functional recurrent abdominal pain
Pyelonephritis, hydronephrosis, renal colic
Pneumonia
Pelvic inflammatory disease
Porphyria
Angioedema
Abdominal migraine
Familial Mediterranean fever
Sexual or physical abuse
Systemic lupus erythematosus
School phobia
Abdominal distension or mass
Ascites (e.g., nephrotic syndrome, neoplasm, heart failure)
Discrete mass (e.g., Wilms tumor, hydronephrosis, neuroblastoma, mesenteric cyst, hepatoblastoma)
Pregnancy
Jaundice
Hemolytic disease
Gilbert syndrome
Urinary tract infection
Sepsis
Hypothyroidism

Dysphagia. Primary motility disorders causing impaired peristaltic function and dysphagia are rare in children. Motility of the distal esophagus is disordered after repair of tracheoesophageal fistula. Abnormal motility may be seen with collagen-vascular disorders. Achalasia rarely occurs in children. Esophageal web or tracheobronchial remnant may cause dysphagia in infancy. An esophageal stricture secondary to chronic gastroesophageal reflux and esophagitis occasionally presents with dysphagia as the first manifestation. A Schatzki ring is another mechanical cause of recurrent dysphagia presenting after infancy. An esophageal foreign body or a stricture secondary to a caustic ingestion also causes dysphagia.

Regurgitation. Regurgitation is the effortless movement of stomach contents into the esophagus and mouth. It is not associated with distress, and infants with regurgitation are often hungry immediately following an episode. The lower esophageal sphincter (LES) prevents reflux of gastric contents into the esophagus (Chapter 269). Regurgitation is a result of gastroesophageal reflux through an incompetent or, in infants, immature LES. Often this is a developmental process and regurgitation or "spitting" resolves with maturity. Regurgitation should be differentiated from vomiting, which denotes an active reflex process with a different differential diagnosis (Table 252–2).

Anorexia. Hunger and satiety centers are located in the hypothalamus; it seems likely that afferent nerves from the gastrointestinal tract to these brain centers are important determinants of the anorexia that characterizes many diseases of the stomach and intestine. For example, satiety is stimulated by distention of the stomach or upper small bowel, the signal being transmitted by sensory afferents, which are especially dense in the upper gut. Chemoreceptors in the intestine, influenced by the assimilation of nutrients, also affect afferent flow to the appetite centers. Impulses reach the hypothalamus from higher centers, possibly influenced by pain or the emotional disturbance of an intestinal disease. Other regulatory factors include hormones and plasma glucose, which in turn reflect intestinal function.

VOMITING. Vomiting is a highly coordinated, reflex process that may be preceded by increased salivation and begins with involuntary retching. Violent descent of the diaphragm and constriction of the abdominal muscles with relaxation of the gastric cardia actively force gastric contents back up the esophagus. This process is coordinated in the medullary vomiting center, which is influenced directly by afferent innervation and indirectly by the chemoreceptor trigger zone and higher central nervous system (CNS) centers. Many acute or chronic processes can cause vomiting (Table 252–2).

Vomiting caused by obstruction of the gastrointestinal tract is probably mediated by intestinal visceral afferent nerves stimulating the vomiting center. If obstruction occurs below the second part of the duodenum, vomitus is usually bile stained. With repeated vomiting in the absence of obstruction, however, duodenal contents are refluxed into the stomach and the emesis may become bile stained. Congenital and acquired obstructing lesions are noted in Table 252–3. Nonobstructive lesions of the digestive tract can also cause vomiting; most diseases of the upper bowel, pancreas, liver, or biliary tree are capable of provoking emesis. CNS or metabolic derangements may lead to severe, persistent emesis.

DIARRHEA. Diarrhea is best defined as excessive loss of fluid and electrolyte in the stool. A young infant has about 5 g/kg of stool output per day; the volume increases to 200 g/24 hr in an adult. The greatest volume of water is absorbed in the small bowel; the colon concentrates intestinal contents against a high osmotic gradient. The small intestine of an adult may absorb 10–11 L/day of a combination of ingested and secreted fluid, while the colon absorbs about 1/2 L. Disorders that interfere with absorption in the small bowel tend to produce voluminous diarrhea, whereas disorders compromising colonic absorption produce lower volume diarrhea. Dysentery (i.e., small volume, frequent, bloody stools with tenemus and urgency) is the predominant symptom of colitis.

The basis for all diarrhea is disturbed intestinal solute transport; water movement across intestinal membranes is passive and is determined by both active and passive fluxes of solutes, particularly sodium, chloride, and glucose. The pathogenesis of most episodes of diarrhea can be explained by secretory, osmotic, or motility abnormalities or a combination of these (Table 252–4).

Secretory diarrhea is often caused by a secretagogue, such as cholera toxin, binding to a receptor on the surface epithelium of the bowel and thereby stimulating intracellular accumulation of cAMP or cGMP. Some intraluminal fatty acids and bile salts cause the colonic mucosa to secrete through this mechanism. Diarrhea not associated with an exogenous secretagogue may also have a secretory component (e.g., congenital microvillus inclusion disease). Secretory diarrhea tends to be watery and of large volume; the osmolality of the stool can be accounted for by the presence of electrolyte. Secretory diarrhea generally persists even when no feedings are given by mouth.

Osmotic diarrhea occurs after ingestion of a poorly absorbed solute. The solute may be one that is normally not well ab-

■ **TABLE 252–2 Differential Diagnosis of Emesis During Childhood**

Infant	Child	Adolescent
Common		
Gastroenteritis	Gastroenteritis	Gastroenteritis
Gastroesophageal reflux	Systemic infection	Systemic infection
Overfeeding	Toxic ingestion	Toxic ingestion
Anatomic obstruction	Pertussis syndrome	Inflammatory bowel disease
Systemic infection	Medication	Appendicitis
		Migraine
		Pregnancy
		Medication
		Ipecac abuse/bulimia
Rare		
Adrenogenital syndrome	Reye syndrome	Reye syndrome
Inborn error of metabolism	Hepatitis	Hepatitis
Brain tumor (increased intracranial pressure)	Peptic ulcer	Peptic ulcer
Subdural hemorrhage	Pancreatitis	Pancreatitis
Food poisoning	Brain tumor	Brain tumor
Rumination	Increased intracranial pressure	Increased intracranial pressure
Renal tubular acidosis	Middle ear disease	Middle ear disease
	Chemotherapy	Chemotherapy
	Achalasia	Cyclic vomiting
	Cyclic vomiting	Biliary colic
	Esophageal stricture	Renal colic
	Duodenal hematoma	
	Inborn error of metabolism	

■ **TABLE 252–3 Causes of Gastrointestinal Obstruction**

Esophagus	
Congenital:	Esophageal atresia
	Vascular rings
	Schatzki ring
	Tracheobronchial remnant
Acquired:	Esophageal stricture
	Foreign body
	Achalasia
	Chagas disease
	Collagen vascular disease
Stomach	
Congenital:	Antral webs
	Pyloric stenosis
Acquired:	Bezoars/foreign body
	Pyloric stricture (ulcer)
	Chronic granulomatous disease of childhood
	Eosinophilic gastroenteritis
Small Intestine	
Congenital:	Duodenal atresia
	Annular pancreas
	Malrotation/volvulus
	Malrotation/Ladds bands
	Ileal atresia
	Meconium ileus
	Meckel diverticulum with volvulus or intussusception
	Inguinal hernia
Acquired:	Adhesions post surgery
	Crohn disease
	Intussusception
	Distal ileal obstruction syndrome (CF)
Colon	
Congenital:	Meconium plug
	Hirschsprung disease
	Colonic atresia, stenosis
	Imperforate anus
	Rectal stenosis
	Pseudo-obstruction
Acquired:	Ulcerative colitis (toxic megacolon)
	Chagas disease
	Crohn disease

CF = cystic fibrosis.

■ TABLE 252–4 Mechanisms of Diarrhea

Primary Mechanism	Defect	Stool Examination	Examples	Comment
Secretory	Decreased absorption Increased secretion	Watery Normal osmolality Osmolality ≃ [electrolyte]	Cholera, toxigenic *E coli*, carcinoid, VIP,† neuroblastoma	Persists during fasting No stool leukocytes Osmolality ≃ [electrolyte]*
Osmotic	Transport defects; digestive enzyme deficiency; ingestion of unabsorbable solute	Watery, acidic, and reducing substances Osmolality >> [electrolyte]	Lactase deficiency Glucose-galactose malabsorption Lactulose Laxative abuse	Stops with fasting Increased breath hydrogen No stool leukocytes Osmolality >> [electrolyte]*
Increased motility	Decreased transit time	Stimulated by gastrocolic reflex	Irritable bowel syndrome Thyrotoxicosis Postvagotomy Dumping syndrome	
Delayed motility	Bacterial overgrowth		Intestinal pseudo-obstruction	
Combined Mechanisms				
Decreased surface area (osmotic, motility)	Decreased functional capacity	Watery	Short bowel syndrome	May require elemental diet plus parenteral alimentation
Mucosal invasion	Inflammation Decreased colonic reabsorption Increased motility	Blood and increased white blood cells in stool	*Salmonella, Shigella, Amebiasis, Yersinia, Campylobacter*	Dysentery—blood, mucus, and leukocytes

*See text for details.
†VIP = vasoactive intestinal peptide.*

sorbed (e.g., magnesium, phosphate or undigested, unabsorbed sugar, alcohols, or sorbitol) or one that is not well absorbed because of a disorder of the small bowel (e.g., lactose with lactase deficiency or glucose with rotavirus diarrhea). Malabsorbed carbohydrate is typically fermented in the colon and short chain fatty acids (SCFAs) are produced. Although SCFAs can be absorbed in the colon and used as an energy source, the net effect is to increase the osmotic solute load. This form of diarrhea is usually of lesser volume than a secretory diarrhea and stops with fasting. The osmolality of the stool is not solely explained by the electrolyte content, as there is another osmotic component present [the difference between electrolye content (sum of [NA^+], [K^+], and associated anions) and stool osmolality is greater than 50 mOsm] (see Chapter 287). Motility disorders may be associated with rapid or delayed transit, and generally are not associated with large volume diarrhea. Slowed motility may be associated with bacterial overgrowth as a cause of diarrhea. The differential diagnosis of common causes of acute and chronic diarrhea are noted in Table 252–5.

CONSTIPATION. Any definition of constipation is relative, dependent on stool consistency, stool frequency, and difficulty in passing the stool. A normal child may have a soft stool only every 2nd or 3rd day without difficulty; this is not constipation. However, a hard stool passed with difficulty every 3rd day should be treated as constipation. Constipation may arise from defects either in filling or emptying the rectum (Table 252–6).

A nursing infant may have very infrequent stools of normal consistency; this is usually a normal pattern. True constipation in the neonatal period is most likely secondary to Hirschsprung disease, intestinal pseudo-obstruction, or hypothyroidism.

Defective rectal filling occurs when colonic peristalsis is ineffective (e.g., in cases of hypothyroidism or opiate use, and when there is bowel obstruction caused either by a structural

■ TABLE 252–5 Common Causes of Diarrhea*

Infant	Child	Adolescent
Acute		
Gastroenteritis Systemic infection Antibiotic associated	Gastroenteritis Food poisoning Systemic infection Antibiotic associated	Gastroenteritis Food poisoning Antibiotic associated
Chronic		
Postinfectious Seconary disaccharidase deficiency Milk protein intolerance Irritable colon syndrome Cystic fibrosis Celiac disease Short bowel syndrome Factitious	Postinfectious Secondary disaccharidase deficiency Irritable colon syndrome Celiac disease Lactose intolerance Giardiasis	Inflammatory bowel disease Lactose intolerance Giardiasis Laxative abuse (anorexia nervosa)

*Adapted from Behrman RE, Kliegman RM: Nelson Essentials of Pediatrics. Philadelphia, WB Saunders, 1990.

■ TABLE 252–6 Important Causes of Constipation*

Nonorganic (functional); also known as habit or psychogenic constipation
Organic
Intestinal
- Hirschsprung disease
- Anal-rectal stenosis
- Stricture
- Volvulus
- Pseudo-obstruction
- Chagas disease

Drugs
- Narcotic
- Antidepressants
- Psychoactive (thorazine)
- Vincristine

Metabolic
- Dehydration
- Cystic fibrosis (meconium ileus equivalent)
- Hypothyroidism
- Hypokalemia
- Renal tubular acidosis
- Hypercalcemia

Neuromuscular
- Psychomotor retardation
- Absent abdominal muscle
- Myotonic dystrophy
- Spinal cord lesions (tumors, spina bifida, diastematomyelia)
- Amyotonia congenita

Psychiatric
- Anorexia nervosa

*Adapted from Behrman RE, Kliegman RM: Nelson Essentials of Pediatrics. Philadelphia, WB Saunders, 1990.

anomaly or by Hirschsprung disease). The resultant colonic stasis leads to excessive drying of stool and a failure to initiate reflexes from the rectum that normally trigger evacuation. Emptying the rectum by spontaneous evacuation depends on a defecation reflex initiated by pressure receptors in the rectal muscle. Stool retention, therefore, may also result from lesions involving these rectal muscles, the sacral spinal cord afferent and efferent fibers, or the muscles of the abdomen and pelvic floor. Disorders of anal sphincter relaxation may also contribute to fecal retention.

Constipation tends to be self-perpetuating, whatever its cause. Hard, large stools in the rectum become difficult and even painful to evacuate, thus more retention occurs and a vicious circle ensues. Distention of the rectum and colon lessens the sensitivity of the defecation reflex and the effectiveness of peristalsis. Eventually, watery content from the proximal colon may percolate around hard retained stool and pass per rectum unperceived by the child. This involuntary *encopresis* may be mistaken for diarrhea. Constipation does not per se have deleterious systemic organic effects. Urinary tract stasis may accompany severe longstanding cases. Constipation may generate anxiety, having a marked emotional impact on the patient and family.

ABDOMINAL PAIN. Individual children differ greatly in their perception of and tolerance for abdominal pain. This is one reason the evaluation of chronic abdominal pain is frustrating. A child with functional abdominal pain (i.e., no identifiable organic etiology) may be as uncomfortable as one with an organic cause. This distinction is an extremely important part of the medical evaluation, guiding how the work-up is approached and the child is treated. The more specific the pain and the more suggestive of a particular diagnosis, the more likely it will have an organic basis. Normal growth and physical examination (including the rectal exam) are reassuring in a child who is suspected of having functional pain.

A specific cause may be difficult to find, but the nature and location of a pain-provoking lesion can usually be determined from the clinical description. Two types of nerve fibers transmit painful stimuli in the abdomen: In skin and muscle, A fibers mediate sharp localized pain; and C fibers from viscera, peritoneum, and muscle transmit poorly localized, dull pain. These afferent fibers have cell bodies in the dorsal root ganglia, and some axons cross the midline and ascend to the medulla, midbrain, and thalamus. Pain is perceived in the cortex of the postcentral gyrus, which can receive impulses arising from both sides of the body.

Visceral pain tends to be experienced in the dermatome from which the affected organ receives innervation. Painful stimuli originating in the liver, pancreas, biliary tree, stomach, or upper bowel are felt in the epigastrium; pain from the distal small bowel, cecum, appendix, or proximal colon is felt at the umbilicus; and pain from the distal large bowel, urinary tract, or pelvic organs is usually suprapubic. When pain is referred to remote areas supplied by the same neurosegment as the diseased organ, the phenomenon usually means an increased intensity of the provoking stimuli. Parietal pain impulses travel in C fibers of nerves corresponding to dermatomes T6 to L1; such pain tends to be more localized and intense than visceral pain.

In the gut the usual stimulus provoking pain is tension or stretching. Inflammatory lesions may lower the pain threshold, but the mechanisms producing pain of inflammation are not clear. Tissue metabolites released near nerve endings probably account for the pain caused by ischemia. Perception of these painful stimuli can be modulated by input from both cerebral and peripheral sources. Psychologic factors are particularly important. Features of abdominal pain are noted in Tables 252–7 and 252–8.

Gastrointestinal Hemorrhage. Bleeding may occur anywhere along the gastrointestinal tract, and identification of the site may be challenging (Table 252–9). The small intestine, which is most difficult to study, is the least likely site of bleeding. The only exception is the painless bleeding of a Meckel diverticulum, which is not difficult to identify. Erosive damage to the mucosa of the gastrointestinal tract is the most common cause of bleeding, although variceal bleeding secondary to portal hypertension occurs frequently enough to require consideration. Vascular malformations are a rare cause in children; they are difficult to identify.

When bleeding originates in the esophagus, stomach, or duodenum, it may cause *hematemesis.* When exposed to gastric or intestinal juices, blood quickly darkens to resemble coffee grounds; accordingly, the more massive and proximal the bleeding, the more likely it is to be red. Red or maroon blood in stools, *hematochezia,* signifies either a distal bleeding site or massive hemorrhage above the distal ileum. Moderate to mild bleeding from sites above the distal ileum tends to cause blackened stools of tarry consistency, *melena,* and major hemorrhages in the duodenum or above can cause melena.

Children can develop iron deficiency anemia from enteric blood loss even when occult blood is not found in stools on random testing. Gastrointestinal hemorrhage, in itself, rarely causes gastrointestinal symptoms, but brisk duodenal or gastric bleeding may lead to nausea, vomiting, and/or diarrhea. The breakdown products of intraluminal blood may tip the patient into hepatic coma if liver function is already compromised and lead to elevation of serum bilirubin.

ABDOMINAL DISTENTION AND ABDOMINAL MASSES. Enlargement of the abdomen can result from diminished tone of the wall musculature or from increased content—fluid, gas, or solid. Ascites, the accumulation of fluid in the peritoneal cavity, distends the abdomen both in the flanks and anteriorly when it is large in volume. This fluid shifts with movement of the patient and conducts a percussion wave.

Ascitic fluid is usually a transudate with a low-protein concentration resulting from reduced plasma colloid osmotic pressure of hypoalbuminemia, from raised portal venous pressure, or from both. In cases of portal hypertension the fluid leak probably occurs from lymphatics on the liver surface and from visceral peritoneal capillaries, but ascites does not usually develop until the serum albumin level falls. Sodium excretion in the urine decreases greatly as the ascitic fluid accumulates so that additional dietary sodium goes directly to the peritoneal space, taking with it more water. When ascitic fluid contains a high protein concentration, it is usually an exudate caused by an inflammatory or neoplastic lesion.

When fluid distends the gut, either obstruction or imbalance between absorption and secretion should be suspected. Frequently, the factors causing fluid accumulation in the bowel lumen cause gas to accumulate too. The result may be audible gurgling noises. The source of gas is usually swallowed air, but endogenous flora may increase considerably in malabsorptive states and produce excessive gas when substrate reaches the lower intestine. Gas in the peritoneal cavity (pneumoperitoneum), perhaps signaled by a tympanitic percussion note even over solid organs such as the liver, indicates a perforated viscus.

An abdominal organ may enlarge diffusely or be affected by a discrete mass. In the digestive tract such discrete masses may occur in the lumen, in the wall, or in the mesentery. In the constipated child, mobile, nontender fecal masses are often found. The wall of the gut can be affected by anomalies, cysts, or inflammatory disease; gut wall neoplasms are extremely rare in children. The liver may enlarge diffusely in response to many disorders. Discrete liver masses may be islands of regenerating liver tissue in a cirrhotic liver or may be of inflammatory or neoplastic origin.

JAUNDICE (See Chapters 88 and 302).

■ TABLE 252–7 Recurrent Abdominal Pain in Children

Disorder	Characteristics	Key Evaluations
Nonorganic		
Recurrent abdominal pain syndrome (functional abdominal pain)	Nonspecific pain, often periumbilical	Hx and PE; tests as indicated
Irritable bowel syndrome	Intermittent cramps, diarrhea, and constipation	Hx and PE
Nonulcer dyspepsia	Peptic ulcer-like symptoms without abnormalities on evaluation of the upper GI tract	Hx; esophagogastroduodenoscopy
Gastrointestinal Tract		
Chronic constipation	Hx of stool retention, evidence of constipation on exam	Hx and PE; plain x-ray of abdomen
Lactose intolerance	Symptoms may be associated with lactose ingestion; bloating, gas, cramps, and diarrhea	Trial of lactose-free diet; lactose breath hydrogen test
Parasite infection (especially *Giardia*)	Bloating, gas, cramps, and diarrhea	Stool evaluation for o & p; specific immunoassays for *Giardia*
Excess fructose or sorbitol ingestion	Nonspecific abdominal pain, bloating, gas, and diarrhea	Large intake of apples, fruit juice, or candy/chewing gum sweetened with sorbitol
Crohn disease	See Chapter 283	
Peptic ulcer	Burning or gnawing epigastric pain; worse on awakening or before meals; relieved with antacids	Esophagogastroduodenoscopy or upper GI contrast x-rays
Esophagitis	Epigastric pain with substernal burning	Esophagogastroduodenoscopy
Meckel diverticulum	Periumbilical or lower abdominal pain; may have blood in stool	Meckel scan or enteroclysis
Recurrent intussusception	Paroxysmal severe, cramping abdominal pain; blood may be present in stool with episode	Identify intussusception during episode or lead point in intestine between episodes with contrast studies of GI tract
Internal, inguinal, or abdominal wall hernia	Dull abdominal or abdominal wall pain	PE, CT of abdominal wall
Chronic appendicitis or appendiceal mucocele	Recurrent RLQ pain; often incorrectly diagnosed, may be rare cause of abdominal pain	Barium enema, CT
Gallbladder and Pancreas		
Cholelithiasis	RUQ pain, may worsen with meals	Ultrasound of gallbladder
Choledochal cyst	RUQ pain, mass ± elevated bilirubin	Ultrasound or CT RUQ
Recurrent pancreatitis	Persistent boring pain, may radiate to back, vomiting	Serum amylase and lipase ± serum trypsinogen; ultrasound of pancreas
Genitourinary Tract		
Urinary tract infection	Dull suprapubic pain, flank pain	Urinalysis and urine culture; renal scan
Hydronephrosis	Unilateral abdominal or flank pain	Ultrasound of kidneys
Urolithiasis	Progressive, severe pain: flank to inguinal region to testicle	Urinalysis, ultrasound, IVP
Other genitourinary disorders	Suprapubic or lower abdominal pain; GU symptoms	Ultrasound of kidneys and pelvis; gynecologic evaluation
Miscellaneous Causes		
Abdominal migraine	See text; nausea, family Hx migraine	Hx
Abdominal epilepsy	May have seizure prodrome	EEG (may require more than one study, including sleep-deprived EEG)
Gilbert syndrome	Mild abdominal pain (causal or coincidental?); slightly elevated unconjugated bilirubin	Serum bilirubin
Familial Mediterranean fever	Paroxysmal episodes of fever, severe abdominal pain, and tenderness with other evidence of polyserositis	Hx and PE during an episode
Sickle cell crisis	Anemia	Hematologic evaluation
Lead poisoning	Vague abdominal pain ± constipation	Serum lead level
Henoch-Schönlein purpura	Recurrent, severe crampy abdominal pain, occult blood in stool, characteristic rash, arthritis	Hx, PE, urinalysis
Angioneurotic edema	Swelling of face or airway, crampy pain	Hx, PE, upper GI contrast x-rays serum C1 esterase inhibitor
Acute intermittent porphyria	Severe pain precipitated by drugs, fasting, or infections	Spot urine for porphyrins

o & p = ova and parasites; Hx = history; PE = physical exam; RUQ = right upper quadrant; CT = computed tomography; RLQ = right lower quadrant; IVP = intravenous pyelography; EEG = electroencephalogram; abd = abdominal; GI = gastrointestinal; GU = genitourinary.

■ TABLE 252–8 Distinguishing Features of Acute Gastrointestinal Tract Pain in Children

Disease	Onset	Location	Referral	Quality	Comments
Pancreatitis	Acute	Epigastric, left upper quadrant	Back	Constant, sharp, boring	Nausea, emesis, tenderness
Intestinal obstruction	Acute or gradual	Periumbilical—lower abdomen	Back	Alternating cramping (colic) and painless periods	Distention, obstipation, emesis, increased bowel sounds
Appendicitis	Acute	Periumbilical, localized to RL quadrant	Back or pelvis if retrocecal	Sharp, steady	Nausea, emesis, local tenderness, fever
Intussusception	Acute	Periumbilical—lower abdomen	None	Cramping, with painless periods	Hematochezia, knees in pulled-up position
Urolithiasis	Acute, sudden	Back (unilateral)	Groin	Sharp, intermittent, cramping	Hematuria
Urinary tract infection	Acute, sudden	Back	Bladder	Dull to sharp	Fever, costochondral tenderness, dysuria, urinary frequency

■ TABLE 252–9 Differential Diagnosis of Gastrointestinal Bleeding in Childhood

Infant	Child	Adolescent
Common		
Bacterial enteritis	Bacterial enteritis	Bacterial enteritis
Milk protein allergy	Anal fissure	Inflammatory bowel disease
Intussusception	Colonic polyps	Peptic ulcer/gastritis
Swallowed maternal blood	Intussusception	Mallory-Weiss syndrome
Anal fissure	Peptic ulcer/gastritis	Colonic polyps
Lymphonodular hyperplasia	Swallowed epistaxis	
	Mallory-Weiss syndrome	
Rare		
Volvulus	Esophageal varices	Esophageal varices
Necrotizing enterocolitis	Esophagitis	Esophagitis
Meckel diverticulum	Meckel diverticulum	Telangiectasia-angiodysplasia
Stress ulcer, stomach	Lymphonodular hyperplasia	Gay bowel disease
Coagulation disorder	Henoch-Schönlein purpura	Graft-versus-host disease
	Foreign body	
	Hemangioma, arteriovenous malformation	
	Sexual abuse	
	Hemolytic uremic syndrome	
	Inflammatory bowel disease	

Borge A, Nordhagen R, Moe B, et al: Prevalence and persistence of stomach ache and headache among children. Follow-up of a cohort of Norwegian children from 4 to 10 years of age. Acta Paediatr 83:433, 1994.
Cox KC, Ament ME: Upper gastrointestinal bleeding in children and adolescents. Pediatrics 63:408, 1979.
Drossman D: Physical and sexual abuse and gastrointestinal illness: What is the link? Am J Med 97:105, 1994.
Eherer AJ, Fordtran JS: Fecal osmotic gap and pH in experimental diarrhea of various causes. Gastroenterology 103:545, 1992.
Fitzgerald JF: Cholestatic disorders of infancy. Pediatr Clin North Am 35:357, 1988.
Grand RJ, Watkins JB, Torti FM: Development of the human gastrointestinal tract: A review. Gastroenterology 70:790, 1976.
Hall RJC: Normal and abnormal food intake. Gut 16:744, 1975.
Hamilton JR: The pathogenesis of infectious diarrhea. Mod Concepts Gastroenterol 1:335, 1986.
Hyman PE: Gastroesophageal reflux: One reason why baby won't eat. J Pediatr 125:S103, 1994.
Loening-Baucke V: Chronic constipation in children. Gastroenterology 105:1557, 1993.
Rogers B, Arvedson J, Buck G, et al: Characteristics of dysphagia in children with cerebral palsy. Dysphagia 9:69, 1994.
Vandenplas Y: Reflux esophagitis in infants and children: a report from the working group on gastro-oesophageal reflux disease of the European Society of Paediatric Gastroenterology and Nutrition. J Pediatr Gastroenterol Nutr 18:413, 1994.

SECTION 2
The Oral Cavity

David C. Johnsen

The condition of the oral cavity is important to the physical and psychologic health of every child. Timely diagnosis and treatment require close cooperation between physicians and dentists. Many older children have regular dental examinations, but the oral problems of infants that require dental referral are recognized primarily through routine visits to physicians.

All parents of children should receive oral health counseling, particularly on feeding practices, from birth, but certainly before 1 yr of age. Children identified at risk for dental disease (e.g., over 1 yr of age and still sleeping with the nursing bottle) should be referred for dental care. Children should receive a visual oral inspection from a dentist by 18–24 mo of age. Once a rapport with the dentist is established, appointments should be regularly scheduled. Some children with active caries need to be followed every 3 mo. Most children should be seen every 6 mo and some once a year. Oral hygiene instruction should begin at the 1st dental visit. This provides an excellent opportunity to discuss dental disease when parental interest is high, to counsel about avoiding harmful practices, and to initiate measures to prevent dental caries (Chapter 258). ■

CHAPTER 253
Development and Anomalies of the Teeth

INITIATION. The primary teeth form in dental crypts that arise from a band of epithelial cells incorporated into each developing jaw. By the 12th wk of fetal life each of these epithelial bands (the dental laminae) has five areas of rapid growth on each side of the maxilla and the mandible, seen as rounded, budlike enlargements. Organization of adjacent mesenchyme takes place in each area of epithelial growth, and the two elements together are the beginning of a tooth.

The permanent teeth form in two groups. After the formation of the primary crypts, another generation of tooth buds forms lingually from each side for the permanent incisors, cuspids, and premolars, which will erupt into sites previously occupied by primary teeth. This process takes place from about the 5th gestational mo for the central incisors to about 10 mo of age for the second bicuspids. Permanent molars, on the other hand, arise from extension of the dental laminae backward, beyond the site of the second primary molars. Budlike enlargements form for the 1st, 2nd, and 3rd permanent molars at approximately 4 mo of gestation, 1 yr of age, and 4–5 yr of age, respectively.

HISTODIFFERENTIATION-MORPHODIFFERENTIATION. As the epithelial bud proliferates, the deeper surface invaginates, and a mass of mesenchyme becomes partially enclosed. Beginning with the crown, the epithelial cells assume the shape of the tooth they represent and lay down the organic matrix for calcification of dentin. The vascular, nerve, and lymph structures (the dental pulp of the mature tooth) are confined in the mesenchyme of the hollow central portion of the tooth bud.

CALCIFICATION. The deposition of the inorganic mineral crystals of mature enamel and dentin takes place after the organic matrix has been laid down from several sites of calcification that later coalesce. The characteristics of the inorganic portions of a tooth can be altered by (1) disturbances in formation of the matrix, (2) decreased availability of one or more of the minerals involved, or (3) the incorporation of foreign materials. Such disturbances may affect the color, texture, or thickness of the tooth surface.

ERUPTION. At the time of tooth bud formation, each tooth begins a continuous movement outward in relation to the bone. The times of eruption of the human permanent teeth and the times of eruption and shedding of the primary teeth are listed in Table 11–6. The mandibular teeth usually erupt before the respective maxillary teeth, and those of girls generally erupt earlier than those of boys.

253.1 Anomalies Associated with Tooth Development

Both failures and excesses of tooth initiation are observed. *Anodontia,* or absence of teeth, occurs when no tooth buds form. Total anodontia often occurs with ectodermal dysplasia. Partial anodontia results from disturbance of a normal site of initiation (e.g., the area of a palatal cleft) or from genetic failure (frequently familial) to code the formation of specific teeth. Syndromes associated with partial aplasia include Albright osteodystrophy, chondroectodermal dysplasia, cleidocranial dysostosis, Hallermann-Streiff, oto-palato-digital type I, and William. The third molars, maxillary lateral incisors, and mandibular second premolars are the teeth that most commonly fail to form. If the dental lamina produces more than the normal number of buds, *supernumerary teeth* occur, most often in the area of the maxillary central incisors. Because they tend to disrupt the position and eruption of the adjacent normal teeth, their identification as supernumerary teeth by roentgenographic examination is important. Supernumerary teeth occur in Gardner, orofaciodigital, Hallermann-Streiff syndromes, cleidocranial dysplasia, and with cleft lip and palate. *Natal teeth* must be differentiated from supernumerary teeth (see later).

Disturbances during differentiation may result in gross alterations in dental morphology, such as *macrodontia* (large teeth) or *microdontia* (small teeth). The maxillary lateral incisors may assume a slender, tapering shape ("peg-shaped laterals").

Twinning, in which two teeth are joined together, is most often observed in the mandibular incisors of the primary dentition. It may result from gemination, fusion, or concrescence. Gemination is the result of division of one tooth germ to form a bifid or cloven crown on a single root with a common pulp canal; an extra tooth is then present in the dental arch. Fusion is the joining of incompletely developed teeth that, owing to pressure or trauma or crowding, continue to develop as one tooth. Fused teeth are sometimes joined through their entire length; in other cases a single wide crown is supported on two roots. Concrescence is the attachment of the roots of closely approximated adjacent teeth by an excessive deposit of cementum. This type of twinning, unlike the others, is found most often in the maxillary molar region.

Amelogenesis imperfecta, a dominant genetic trait, results in faulty production of the organic matrix. The teeth are covered by only a thin layer of abnormally formed enamel through which the yellow underlying dentin is seen, giving a darkened appearance to the dentition. Usually both primary and permanent teeth are affected. Susceptibility to caries is low, but the enamel is subject to destruction from abrasion. Complete coverage of the crown may be indicated for dentin protection and improved appearance.

Dentinogenesis imperfecta, or hereditary opalescent dentin, is an analogous condition in which the odontoblasts fail to differentiate normally and poorly calcified dentin results. This autosomal dominant disorder may also occur in patients with osteogenesis imperfecta. The junction between the enamel and dentin is altered, the enamel has a tendency to flake away, and the exposed dentin is then susceptible to abrasion. The teeth are opaque and pearly, and the pulp chambers are obliterated by calcification. Both primary and permanent teeth are usually involved. Unless the crowns of these teeth are covered early and completely, the abrasion of chewing often reduces them to the level and contour of the supporting alveolar bone.

Localized disturbances of calcification that correlate with periods of illness or malnutrition are common and analogous to the growth disturbance lines often seen in roentgenograms of long bones. An example is the neonatal line commonly observed on the primary teeth and on the permanent central incisors and tips of cuspids at coronal levels consistent with the stage of calcification at birth. Two general disturbances of the surface of the enamel are also seen. Discoloration of the smooth surface, usually a more opaque white patch, is referred to as *hypocalcification.* A more severe disturbance, *hypoplasia,* may be manifest as pitting or as areas devoid of covering enamel. Hypoplasia is less common in the primary dentition because intrauterine stress is relatively infrequent compared with the frequent occurrence of illness during early infancy when the enamel of the outer third of the permanent incisors, cuspids, and first molars is forming.

In primary dentition, hypoplasias result from disturbances after about 15 wk gestation when the teeth begin to calcify. Enamel hypoplasias have been associated with prematurity. Oxygen deficiency in low birthweight infants has been associated with enamel hypoplasias; the defects follow lines of enamel formation. The association has also been made between enamel hypoplasias in primary teeth and cerebral palsy. One local disturbance associated with enamel hypoplasias is prolonged oral endotracheal intubation. Pressure from the tube interferes with enamel formation in low birthweight infants.

In permanent dentition, hypoplasias have been associated with prolonged illnesses during tooth formation. Systemic conditions, such as kidney failure and cystic fibrosis, have been associated with enamel defects. A local disturbance associated with hypoplasia is trauma to the primary tooth; the force can drive the primary tooth into the developing permanent tooth bud.

Enamel hypoplasia has also been associated with prenatal and postnatal infection, hypothyroidism, head-neck irradiation, local trauma, and dental abscesses. Pitted enamel hypoplasia is a feature of tuberous sclerosis. Dental restoration of such areas is desirable to eliminate the sensitivity of exposed dentin, to prevent caries, and to improve the appearance.

Mottled enamel is found in persons whose early life is spent in areas where the fluoride content of the drinking water is greater than 2.0 parts per million (ppm) and is probably due to ameloblastic dysfunction. It varies from small inconspicuous white patches to severe, brownish discoloration and hypoplasia; the latter changes are usually seen with fluoride concentrations of greater than 5.0 ppm.

Disturbances due to *mineral deficiency* are rare, but irregular dentin and enlarged pulp chambers have been observed with vitamin D–resistant rickets, and hypoplasia has been observed with vitamin D–deficient rickets.

Discolored teeth may result from incorporation of foreign substances into developing enamel. Neonatal *hyperbilirubinemia* may produce blue to black discoloration of the primary teeth, beginning at the neonatal line; the tips of the permanent first molars may also be affected. Porphyria produces a red-brown discoloration. *Tetracyclines* are extensively incorporated into bones and teeth and, if administered during the period of formation of enamel, may result in brown-yellow discoloration and hypoplasia of the enamel. Such teeth fluoresce under ultraviolet light. The period at risk extends from about the 4th mo of gestation to the 10th mo of life for primary teeth, and from about the 4th mo to the 16th yr of life for permanent teeth. Repeated or prolonged therapy with tetracycline has the highest risk. Enamel is completely formed on all but the third molars by about 8 yr of age; accordingly, tetracyclines should not be prescribed for pregnant women or for children under 8 yr of age.

As the teeth penetrate the gums, inflammation and sensitivity sometimes occur *(teething)*. The child may become irritable, and salivation may increase markedly. A blunt, firm object for the infant to bite usually provides some relief; incision of the gums is seldom indicated. There is little evidence that systemic disturbances, such as fever, facial rashes, or mild diarrhea, can result from teething.

Delayed eruption of all teeth may indicate systemic or nutritional disturbances such as hypopituitarism, hypothyroidism, cleidocranial dysostosis, 21-trisomy, progeria, Albright osteodystrophy, incontinentia pigmenti, rickets, and multiple syndromes (Hunter, Dubowitz, Goltz, de Lange, Gardner, Maroteaux-Lamy). Failure of eruption of single or small groups of teeth may arise from local causes such as malpositioning of teeth, supernumerary teeth, cysts, or retained primary teeth. Premature loss of primary predecessors is the most common cause of premature eruption of teeth. If the entire dentition is advanced for age and sex, precocious puberty or hyperthyroidism should be considered.

Natal teeth are observed in approximately 1:2,000 newborn infants; usually there are two in the position of the mandibular central incisors. Natal teeth are present at birth, whereas neonatal teeth erupt in the 1st mo of life. Eruption cysts may precede neonatal teeth. Attachment of natal teeth is generally limited to the gingival margin, with little root formation or bony support; such teeth should not be considered supernumerary until so identified roentgenographically. A natal tooth may be a prematurely erupted primary tooth, in which case early dental eruption may be expected. Natal teeth are associated with cleft palate, Pierre Robin syndrome, Ellis-van Creveld syndrome, Hallermann-Streiff syndrome, pachyonychia congenita, and other anomalies. A family history of natal teeth or premature eruption is present in 15–20% of affected children.

Natal teeth may result in pain and refusal to feed, secondary to looseness and movement, and may produce maternal discomfort due to abrasion or biting of the nipple during nursing. There is danger of detachment with aspiration of the tooth. Because the tongue lies between the alveolar processes during birth, it may become lacerated, and occasionally the tip is amputated (Riga-Fede disease). Decisions regarding extraction of prematurely erupted primary teeth must be made on an individual basis; extraction requires careful dissection of the gingival attachment to prevent tearing of the tissue and excessive hemorrhage.

Exfoliation failure occurs when a primary tooth is not shed prior to the eruption of its permanent successor. The primary tooth may need to be extracted only occasionally if the erupting permanent tooth becomes visible. This occurs most commonly in the mandibular incisor region.

CHAPTER 254

Disorders of the Teeth Associated with Other Conditions

Osteogenesis imperfecta is usually accompanied by hereditary opalescent dentin, also termed *dentinogenesis imperfecta* (Chapter 253.1). Treatment usually involves covering the crowns. In *cleidocranial dysostosis* orofacial variations include frontal bossing, mandibular prognathism, and a broadened base of the nose. Eruption of teeth is usually delayed. The primary teeth are abnormally retained, and the permanent teeth may remain unerupted. Supernumerary teeth are common, especially in the premolar area. Erupted teeth are free of hypoplasia, but variations in size and shape are common. The primary teeth and permanent teeth that do erupt should be restored if they become carious. Patients with this disorder need extensive dental therapy in order to maintain efficient chewing.

In *ectodermal dysplasia* (Chapter 599) the teeth are totally or partially absent. Because alveolar bone does not develop in the absence of teeth, the alveolar processes are usually either totally or partially absent, and the resultant overclosure of the

■ TABLE 254–1 Dental Problems Associated with Selected Medical Conditions

Medical Condition	Common Associated Dental or Oral Condition
• Cleft lip and palate	Missing teeth, extra (supernumerary) teeth, shifting of arch segments, feeding difficulties
• Kidney failure	Mottled enamel (permanent teeth), facial dysmorphology
• Cystic fibrosis	Stained teeth with extensive medication, mottled enamel
• Immunosuppression	Oral candidiasis with potential for systemic candidiasis, cyclosporine induced gingival hyperplasia
• Low birthweight with prolonged oral intubation	Palatal groove, narrow arch
• Heart defects with SBE* susceptibility	Bacteremia from dental procedures or trauma
• Neutrophil chemotactic deficiency	Juvenile periodontitis (loss of supporting bone around teeth)
• Juvenile diabetes (uncontrolled)	Juvenile periodontitis
• Neuromotor dysfunction	Oral trauma from falling; malocclusion (open bite); gingivitis from lack of hygiene
• Prolonged illness (generalized) during tooth formation	Enamel hypoplasia of crown portions forming during illness
• Seizures	Gingival enlargement if phenytoin is used
• Vitamin D–dependent rickets	Enamel hypoplasia

*SBE = subacute bacterial endocarditis.

mandible causes the lips to protrude. Facial development is otherwise not disturbed. Teeth, when present, are small and conical in form. Aplasia of the buccal and labial mucous glands leads to dryness and irritation of the oral mucosa. Persons with ectodermal dysplasia need either partial or full dentures. The vertical height between the jaws is thus restored, improving the position of the lips and facial contours. Masticatory function is restored, and eating habits are therefore improved.

Congenital syphilis affects differentiation of permanent teeth, resulting in screwdriver-shaped incisors, often with central notches in their incisive edges (Hutchinson incisors), and mulberry molars, with lobular occlusal surfaces and narrow, pinched crowns (Chapter 201.1). Dental problems associated with other medical conditions are noted in Table 254–1.

CHAPTER 255
Malocclusion

The oral cavity can be viewed as a masticatory machine. The incisal edges of the anterior teeth are brought into opposition by mandibular closure for the purpose of biting off portions of large food items. The cusps of the opposing posterior teeth interdigitate and slide across each other to reduce foodstuffs to a soft, moist bolus. The cheeks and tongue force the food onto the areas of tooth contact.

The masseter and temporal muscles are the main forces of mandibular closure. Acting in conjunction with the internal pterygoid muscles, they produce high pressures of contact on opposing teeth. If a number of teeth meet simultaneously, the force is distributed over a large area of bone-to-tooth attachment. In malocclusion, when only a few teeth touch, the same force is exerted over a much smaller area. In adulthood, occlusal deformities are a leading cause of loss of teeth. Accordingly, preventive measures in childhood should be directed at establishing proper relationships between upper and lower dental arches for physiologic as well as cosmetic reasons.

Variations in growth patterns are classified into three main types of occlusion (Fig. 255–1). The occlusal relation is determined by observing the positions of the teeth when the jaws are closed and the heads of the mandibular condyles are in the most posterior position within the glenoid fossa. In class I (normal), the cusps of the posterior mandibular teeth interdigitate ahead of and inside the corresponding cusps of the opposing maxillary teeth. This relationship provides a normal facial profile. In class II, the cusps of the posterior mandibular teeth are behind and inside the corresponding cusps of the maxillary teeth. This is the most common occlusal discrepancy; approximately 45% of the population exhibits some degree of this condition. An increased space between upper and lower anterior teeth encourages sucking and tongue-thrust habits. The appearance of a receding chin accompanies the retrognathia. In class III, the cusps of the posterior mandibular teeth interdigitate a tooth or more ahead of their opposing maxillary counterparts. The anterior teeth are directly opposed, or the mandibular incisors protrude beyond the maxillary; a protruding chin accompanies prognathia.

CROSS BITE. Normally the mandibular teeth are in a position just inside the maxillary teeth, so that the outside mandibular cusps or incisal edges meet the central portion of the opposing maxillary teeth. A reversal of this relation is referred to as a "cross bite."

OPEN AND CLOSED BITES. If the posterior mandibular and maxillary teeth make contact with each other but the anterior ones are still apart, the situation is called an "open bite." With the posterior teeth together, if the mandibular anterior teeth occlude inside the maxillary anterior teeth in an overclosed position, the situation is referred to as a "closed bite." Treatment consists of orthodontic correction; a few cases require orthognathic surgery. Optimal timing of treatment varies; earlier treatment generally allows some redirection of the growth pattern. Prognosis with early treatment is good, except in severe cases.

DENTAL CROWDING. Overlap of incisors can result when the jaws are too small for adequate alignment of the teeth. Growth of the jaws is mostly in the posterior aspects of the mandible and maxilla, and there is little growth in the anterior region; inadequate space for the permanent incisor teeth at 7 or 8 yr of age will not resolve with growth of the jaws. Moderate spacing of primary incisors is desirable for adequate alignment of successor teeth; a lack of spacing between primary incisors results in crowded permanent incisors.

THUMB SUCKING. Various and conflicting theories have explained thumb sucking in children, and there are conflicting recommendations for its correction. Prolonged thumb sucking can cause flaring of the maxillary incisor teeth. More than half of children have had a thumb-sucking habit at some time. The prevalence of thumb sucking decreases steadily from the age of 2 yr to approximately 10% by the age of 5.

The likelihood of long-term effect on the developing dentition and face is controversial. The prognosis is good in children with procumbent incisors and acceptable occlusion of the molar and canine teeth; discontinuation of the habit usually results in lessening of the incisor procumbency, with the possibil-

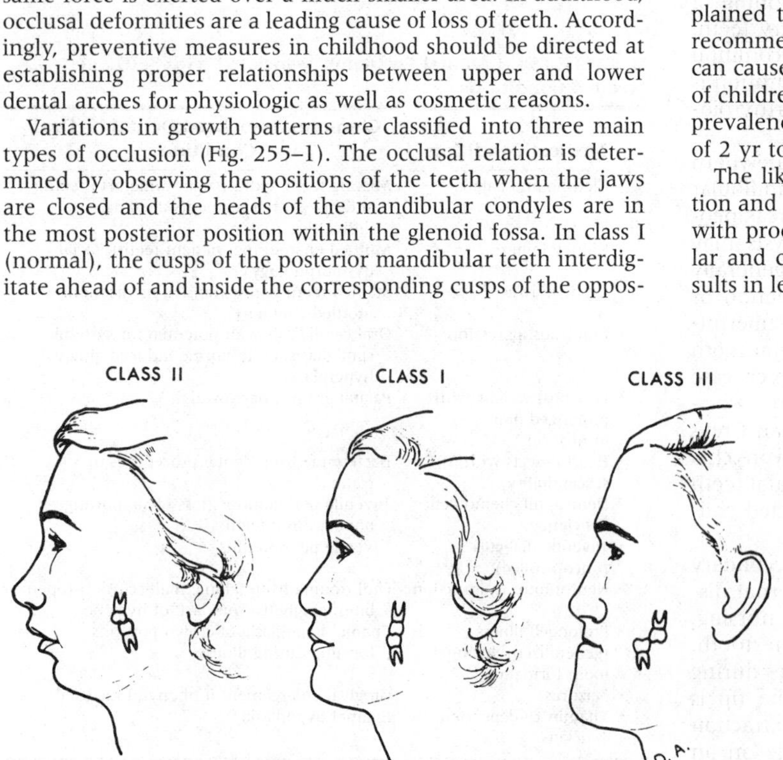

Figure 255–1. Angle classification of occlusion. The typical correspondence between the facial-jaw profile and molar relationship is shown.

ity of an acceptable occlusion. The prognosis is mixed in children with procumbent incisors and a malrelationship of jaws or of posterior teeth; discontinuation of the habit reduces the procumbency of the incisors but will not rectify an already deviant growth pattern. The prognosis worsens with continuation of the habit beyond 6 yr of age. A variety of treatment protocols have been suggested. A common measure is the insertion of an appliance with modest extensions that serves as a reminder when the child attempts to insert the thumb. The greatest likelihood of success occurs in cases in which the child desires to stop.

CHAPTER 256
Cleft Lip and Palate

Clefts of the lip and palate are distinct entities closely related embryologically, functionally, and genetically. Cleft of the lip appears to be due to hypoplasia of the mesenchymal layer, resulting in a failure of the medial nasal and maxillary processes to join. Cleft of the palate appears to represent failure of the palatal shelves to approximate or fuse.

INCIDENCE AND EPIDEMIOLOGY. The incidence of cleft lip with or without cleft palate is about 1:600 births; the incidence of cleft palate alone is about 1:1,000 births. The former is more common in males. Possible etiologies include maternal drug exposure, syndrome-malformation complex, isolated-unknown, or genetic. Genetic factors are of more importance in cleft lip with or without cleft palate than in cleft palate alone. However, both may occur sporadically; the incidence is highest among Asians and lowest among blacks. The incidence of associated congenital malformations and of impairment in development is increased in children with cleft defects, especially in those with cleft palate alone. These findings are partially explained by an increased incidence of conductive hearing impairment in children with cleft palate, due in part to repeated middle ear infections, and by the frequency of cleft defects among children with chromosomal abnormalities. The risks of recurrence of cleft defects within families are discussed in Chapters 66 and 67.

Animal studies suggest that nongenetic influences may be responsible for clefts in a susceptible host at a critical period of organogenesis. Associated malformations are especially frequent in structures derived from the first branchial arch.

CLINICAL MANIFESTATIONS. Cleft lip may vary from a small notch in the vermilion border to a complete separation extending into the floor of the nose. Clefts may be unilateral (more often on the left side) or bilateral, and usually involve the alveolar ridge. Deformed, supernumerary, or absent teeth are associated. The nasal alar cartilage clefts of the lip are frequently associated with deficiency of the columella and elongation of the vomer, producing a protrusion of the anterior aspect of the cleft premaxillary process.

Isolated cleft palate occurs in the midline and may involve only the uvula or may extend into or through the soft and hard palates to the incisive foramen. When associated with cleft lip, the defect may involve the midline of the soft palate and extend into the hard palate on one or both sides, exposing one or both of the nasal cavities as a unilateral or bilateral cleft palate.

TREATMENT. The most immediate problem is feeding; a plastic obturator is fitted soon after birth to aid in control of fluids, to provide a reference plane for suction, and to provide stability for the lateral arch segments. Rapid growth of the dental arches requires the obturator to be refitted every few weeks. Soft artificial nipples with large openings are beneficial to patients with cleft palate. Patients with isolated cleft lip may be breast-fed.

Surgical closure of a cleft lip is usually performed by 2 mo of age, when the infant has shown satisfactory weight gain and is free of any oral, respiratory, or systemic infection. Z-plasty is the most commonly used technique; a staggered suture line minimizes notching of the lip from retraction of scar tissue. The initial repair may be revised at 4–5 yr of age. In many instances, corrective surgery on the nose is delayed until adolescence. Nasal surgery is frequently performed at the time of the lip repair. Cosmetic results depend on the extent of the original deformity, absence of infection, and skill of the surgeon.

Because clefts of the palate vary considerably in size, shape, and degree of deformity, the timing of surgical correction should be individualized. Criteria such as width of the cleft, adequacy of the existing palatal segments, morphology of the surrounding areas (such as width of the oropharynx), and neuromuscular function of the soft palate and pharyngeal walls affect the decision. The goals of surgery are the union of the cleft segments, intelligible and pleasant speech, reduction of nasal regurgitation, and avoidance of injury to the growing maxilla.

In an otherwise healthy child, closure of the palate is usually done prior to 1 yr of age to enhance normal speech development. When surgical correction is delayed beyond the 3rd yr, a contoured speech bulb can be attached to the posterior of a maxillary denture so that contraction of the pharyngeal and velopharyngeal muscles can bring tissues into contact with the bulb to accomplish occlusion of the nasopharynx and help the child to develop intelligible speech. Almost always the cleft crosses the alveolar ridge and interferes with the formation of teeth in the area. The missing elements of the dentition must be replaced by prosthetic devices; alterations of the positions of teeth may also be necessary.

PREOPERATIVE AND POSTOPERATIVE MANAGEMENT. Even the suspicion of infection is a contraindication to operation. If the child is in good nutritional condition and in fluid and electrolyte balance, feeding may be permitted to within 6 hr of the operation (see Chapter 61). During the immediate postoperative period special nursing care is essential. Gentle aspiration of the nasopharynx minimizes the chances of the common complications of atelectasis or pneumonia. The primary considerations in postoperative care are maintenance of a clean suture line and avoidance of strain on the sutures. For these reasons the infant is fed with a medicine dropper, and the arms are restrained with elbow cuffs. A fluid or semifluid diet is maintained for 3 wk, and feeding is done with a dropper or spoon. The patient's hands as well as toys and other foreign bodies must be kept away from the palate.

COMPLICATIONS. Recurrent otitis media and hearing loss are frequent. Excessive dental decay is not unusual. Displacement of the maxillary arches and malpositions of the teeth usually require orthodontic correction.

Speech defects may be present or persist even after good anatomic closure of the palate. Such speech is characterized by the emission of air from the nose and by a hypernasal quality when certain sounds are made. Both before and, at times, after palatal surgery, the speech defect is due to inadequacies in function of the palatal and pharyngeal muscles. The muscles of the soft palate and the lateral and posterior walls of the nasopharynx constitute a valve that separates the nasopharynx from the oropharynx during swallowing and in the production of certain sounds. If the valve does not function adequately, it is difficult to build up enough pressure in the mouth to make such explosive sounds as p, b, d, t, h, y, or the sibilants s, sh, and ch, and such words as "cats," "boats," and "sisters" are not intelligible. After operation or the insertion of a speech appliance, speech therapy may be necessary.

A complete program of habilitation for the child with a cleft lip or palate may require years of special treatment by a team consisting of a pediatrician, plastic surgeon, otolaryngologist, pediatric dentist, prosthodontist, orthodontist, speech therapist, medical social worker, psychologist, child psychiatrist, and public health nurse. Ideally, the child's physician should be responsible for coordination of the use of specialists, and for parental counseling and guidance.

PALATOPHARYNGEAL INCOMPETENCE

The speech disturbance characteristic of the child with a cleft palate can also be produced by other osseous or neuromuscular abnormalities when there is an inability to form an effective seal between oropharynx and nasopharynx during swallowing or phonation. The abnormality may be in the structures of the palate or pharynx or in the muscles attached to these structures. In a child who has previously spoken normally, adenoidectomy may precipitate the speech defect when a submucous cleft palate has not been recognized. In such cases, the adenoid mass may have facilitated a seal when the elevated soft palate made contact with it, this becoming impossible after removal of the adenoids. If there is sufficient reserve neuromuscular function, compensation in palatopharyngeal movement may take place and the speech defect may disappear, although often some symptoms of palatopharyngeal incompetence may persist. In other cases, slow involution of the adenoids may allow for gradual compensation in palatal and pharyngeal muscular function. This may explain why a speech defect does not become apparent in some children who have a submucous cleft palate or similar anomaly predisposing to palatopharyngeal incompetence.

CLINICAL MANIFESTATIONS. The symptoms of palatopharyngeal incompetence are similar to those of a cleft palate, although clinical signs vary. There may be hypernasal speech (especially noted in the articulation of pressure consonants such as p, b, d, t, h, v, f, and s); conspicuous constricting movement of the nares during speech; inability to whistle, gargle, blow out a candle, or inflate a balloon; loss of liquid through the nose when drinking with the head down; and otitis media and hearing loss. Oral inspection may reveal a cleft palate or a relatively short palate with a large oropharynx; absent, grossly asymmetric, or minimal muscular activity of the soft palate and pharynx during phonation or gagging; or a submucous cleft. The latter is suggested by a bifid uvula, by a translucent membrane in the midline of the soft palate (revealing lack of continuity of muscles), by palpable notching in the posterior border of the hard palate instead of a posterior nasal spinous process, or by forward or V-shaped displacement or grooving on the soft palate during phonation or gagging.

Palatopharyngeal incompetence may also be demonstrated roentgenographically. The head should be carefully positioned to obtain a true lateral view; one film is obtained with the patient at rest and another during continuous phonation of the vowel "u" as in "boom." The soft palate contacts the posterior pharyngeal wall in normal function, whereas in palatopharyngeal incompetence such contact is absent.

TREATMENT. In selected cases the palate may be retropositioned or pharyngoplasty performed utilizing a flap of tissue from the posterior pharyngeal wall. Dental speech appliances have also been used successfully.

CHAPTER 257
Syndromes with Oral Manifestations

Many syndromes have distinct or accompanying facial, oral, and dental manifestations (e.g., Apert syndrome, Chapter 542; Crouzon disease, Chapter 542; Down syndrome, Chapter 67).

Pierre Robin sequence consists of micrognathia with glossoptosis (and pseudomacroglossia) and high arched or cleft palate. Posterior displacement of the attachment of the genioglossus muscle to the hypoplastic mandible prevents the normal anchorage of the tongue; in the supine child, under the influence of gravity, the tongue falls back, obstructing the pharynx. A postalveolar cleft of the hard and soft palates is a common but not constant feature, and in some cases the palate is high-arched.

The tongue is usually of normal size, but the floor of the mouth is foreshortened and the buccal cavity is reduced in size. Obstruction of the air passages may occur, particularly on inspiration, and usually requires treatment to prevent suffocation. The infant should be maintained in a prone or partially prone position so that the tongue falls forward to relieve respiratory obstruction. Temporary suturing of the ventral surface of the tongue to the lower lip is usually not necessary; nor is tracheostomy, because sufficient mandibular growth generally takes place within a few mo to relieve the glossoptosis. The feeding of infants with mandibular hypoplasia requires great care and patience but can usually be accomplished without resort to gavage. Often the growth of the mandible will achieve an essentially normal profile within 4–6 yr. Dental anomalies usually require individualized treatment.

In *mandibulofacial dysostosis* (Treacher Collins syndrome or Franceschetti syndrome), the facial appearance is characterized by palpebral fissures sloping downward toward the outer canthi, colobomas of the lower eyelids, sunken cheekbones, blind fistulas opening between the angles of the mouth and the ears, deformed pinnas, atypical hair growth extending toward the cheeks, receding chin, and large mouth. Facial clefts, abnormalities of the ears, and deafness are common. The disorder is autosomal dominant, often with incomplete expression. The mandible is usually hypoplastic; the under-surface is often pronouncedly concave, the ramus may be deficient, and the coronoid and condyloid processes are flat or even aplastic. The palatal vault may be either high or cleft. Infrequently, unilateral or bilateral macrostomia, or failure of embryonic fusion of the maxillary and mandibular processes, may occur. Dental malocclusions are frequent, owing to poor maxillary development and palatal deformity. The teeth may be widely separated, hypoplastic, or displaced or have an open bite. Orthodontic and routine dental treatments are indicated.

Unilateral hypoplasia of the mandible is sometimes part of a syndrome that includes partial paralysis of the facial nerve, macrostomia, blind fistulas between the angles of the mouth and the ears, and deformed ear lobes. Severe facial asymmetry and malocclusion develop because of the absence or hypoplasia of the mandibular condyle on the affected side. Congenital condylar deformity tends to increase with age. Early plastic surgery may be indicated to minimize the deformity.

Facial asymmetries resulting from excessive molding of the cranium or from displacement of the mandible during breech or face presentations are common and are usually self-correcting. Facial asymmetry owing to injury of the growing cartilage or fracture of the condylar head during birth, infancy, or early childhood may be permanent. Traumatic injuries may occur during birth from obstetric forceps placed over the area or may result from blows on the chin during infancy and childhood.

Injuries, acute infections, or arthritis of the growing condylar cartilage may result in partial (fibrous) or complete (bony) *ankylosis of the temporomandibular joint* and failure of that side of the mandible to grow. The normal side, meanwhile, continues to grow and pushes the midline toward the affected side. The midline deviation is exaggerated during mouth opening. Roentgenograms of the affected side reveal an increased preangular notch or displaced condylar head. Bilateral injuries to the growing cartilage result in failure of the mandible and chin to grow downward and forward, causing the entire mandible to be retruded and smaller than normal.

CHAPTER 258
Dental Caries

In otherwise healthy children, tooth decay is a preventable disease.

ETIOLOGY. The development of dental caries is dependent on critical inter-relationships between the tooth surface, dietary carbohydrates, and specific oral bacteria. The decay process is initiated by demineralization of the outer tooth surface, owing to formation of organic acids during bacterial fermentation of dietary carbohydrates. Incipient lesions first appear as opaque white spots; with progressive loss of tooth tissue, cavitation occurs.

An important experimental observation has been that dental caries have microbial specificity; that is, cariogenic potential resides in a group of oral streptococci collectively designated *Streptococcus mutans.* Current knowledge indicates that these organisms initiate most dental caries of enamel surfaces. Once the enamel surface cavitates, other oral bacteria (in particular, the lactobacilli) invade the underlying dentin and cause further destruction of tooth structure through a mixed bacterial infection.

A second important aspect of the etiology of dental caries relates to *frequency* of carbohydrate consumption. Frequency of ingestion is a more important determinant of development of dental caries than is the actual quantity of carbohydrate consumed. For example, cariogenic potential of a nursing bottle of apple juice that is sampled throughout the night or at nap times, or both, is quite different from that of the same volume of apple juice consumed at a single meal. Carbohydrates contained in food products retained orally for a long time may be more cariogenic than those in food products retained for short times (e.g., the sucrose in chewing gum is more cariogenic than the sucrose in cola beverages, as conventionally consumed).

EPIDEMIOLOGY. Recent investigations regarding the prevalence of dental caries in the developed world indicate that its severity has decreased markedly during the last two decades. This decrease is thought to be secondary to advances in prevention, particularly the use of fluorides.

With marked decreases in dental caries it has become apparent that the disease is not evenly distributed among children. Over half of the children in fluoridated areas are free of caries into their teens. Another group of children have dental caries or cavities limited to the grooves and fissures (defects) of the molar teeth. A smaller percentage of children persist with active smooth surface tooth decay.

CLINICAL MANIFESTATIONS. The age-related epidemiology is noted in Figure 258–1. Dental caries usually begins in the pits and fissures of the occlusal (biting) surfaces of the molar teeth. Lesions of short duration cannot be diagnosed by inspection; they are usually detected by probing the affected pit or fissure. In contrast, pit and fissure caries of long duration can usually be detected by inspection and usually present extensive cavitation of the occlusal surface. The second most frequent sites of caries are contact surfaces between the teeth. These areas are difficult to examine, even for the dentist, who usually depends on intraoral radiographs. Caries lesions are least frequently detected in the necks (cervical areas) of the teeth near the gingiva. Cervical decay is uncommon in children with mild to moderate caries but is usually present in cases of *nursing bottle caries* (Fig. 258–2).

There are several significant features of *baby bottle tooth decay* (BBTD). This extensive form of tooth decay occurs from sleeping with the nursing bottle. It is relatively common, occurring in about 15% of medically underserved children in urban and rural areas and in 50% or more in some native American groups. Although an exact prevalence has not been established in suburban populations, BBTD is seen on a regular basis in private pediatric dental offices.

BBTD occurs before 18 mo of age, at a time many children have not visited a dentist, but when many children have visited a pediatrician. This presents the pediatrician with the opportunity to link counseling on nutrition and dental hygiene. Breast-feeding or water bottles at night greatly reduce the occurrence of BBTD. It is the only severe dental disease common in children less than 3 yr of age. Furthermore, children with BBTD are more likely to continue to develop additional cavities on smooth surfaces of teeth. The prevention of this problem can result in the elimination of major dental problems in toddlers and less decay in later childhood. Children more than 1 yr of age who sleep with the bottle should be referred for treatment.

The age at which BBTD occurs is important in dental management. Children under 3 yr of age must often be restrained, sedated, or given general anesthesia. Beyond 3 yr of age children are more cooperative for dental care, and the caries are often less extensive.

COMPLICATIONS. If left untreated, dental caries usually destroys most of the tooth and spreads into contiguous tissues, causing pain and infection. Microbial invasion of the dental pulp (Fig. 258–3) precipitates an inflammatory response (pulpitis) that can elicit significant pain (toothache). Pulpitis can in turn progress to necrosis, with bacterial invasion of the alveolar bone (dental abscess; periapical abscess). This process may be quite painful and is associated with the complications of sepsis and facial space infection (Fig. 258–4). Moreover, periapical infection of a primary tooth may disrupt normal development of the successor permanent tooth.

TREATMENT. Contemporary dental therapeutics can salvage the majority of severely carious teeth. When an extraction is indicated, therapy must also address the problem that teeth surrounding the site of extraction will change their positions in the dental arch. This is particularly important in the primary and mixed dentitions in order to prevent impaction or malposition of permanent successor teeth.

Clinical management of the pain and infection associated with untreated dental caries varies with the extent of involvement and the medical status of the patient. In general, dental infection localized to the dentoalveolar unit can be managed by local measures (e.g., extraction, pulpectomy). Antibiotics are usually not indicated except in those patients with compromised host defenses, impaired wound healing, or risk for endocarditis. In contrast, antibiotics are routinely indicated for dental infections that have spread to structures outside the dentoalveolar unit.

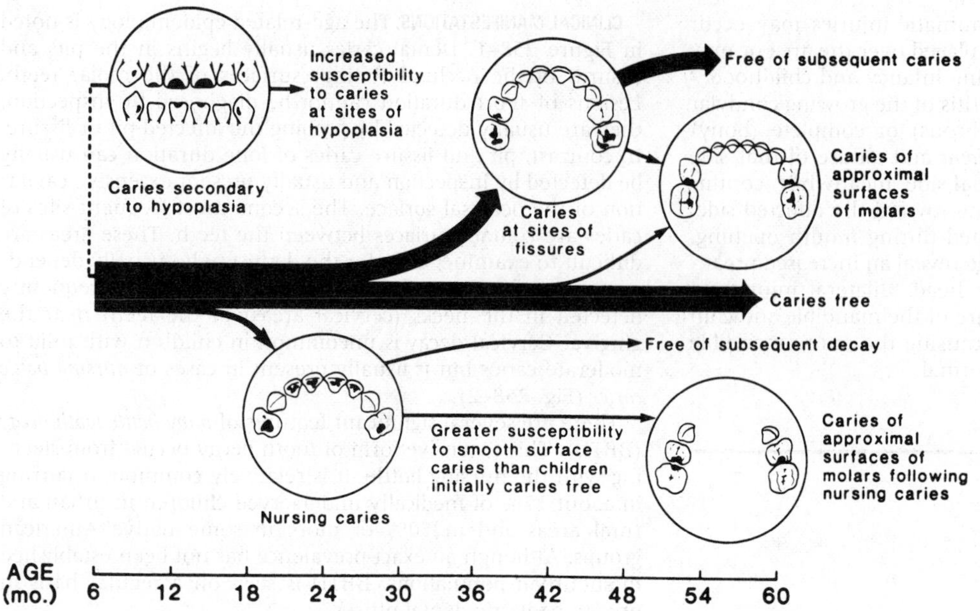

Figure 258–1. Schematic for different kinds of caries and ages when each can start. A significant percentage of children remain caries free. Nursing caries (usually baby bottle tooth decay [BBTD]) begins between 1 and 2 years of age; children with BBTD are at significantly greater risk for future caries than are caries-free children. Pit and fissure caries usually begins after about age 3, with caries of approximating tooth surfaces beginning shortly after. (From Johnsen DC: The role of the pediatrician in identifying and treating dental caries. Pediatr Clin N Am 38:1173, 1991.)

The oral route can usually be used for patients with unremarkable medical histories if the infection does not involve a vital area (e.g., buccal space). If, however, the infection involves a vital area (e.g., submandibular space, which can lead to Ludwig angina; facial triangle, which can lead to cavernous sinus thrombosis; or periorbital space, which can lead to orbital involvement) or oral antibiotics are ineffective, parenteral routes are indicated. Parenteral routes are also indicated for patients with compromised host defenses, with impaired wound healing, or those at risk for endocarditis. Blood cultures should be obtained prior to initiating parenteral antibiotic therapy. Areas of fluctuance should be incised and drained. Exudate should be submitted for culture and Gram stain. Penicillin is the antibiotic of choice, except in patients with a history of allergy to this agent; clindamycin and vancomycin are suitable alternatives for such patients. Finally, the offending tooth must be identified and local treatment should be instituted to ensure resolution of the infection.

Measures for control of pain are adjusted to the need of the patient. Combinations of acetaminophen with codeine given orally are usually adequate.

PREVENTION. Fluoride. The most effective preventive measure against dental caries is fluoridation of communal water supplies to approximately 1.00 ppm. In fluoride-deficient areas similar caries prevention benefits are obtained from dietary fluoride supplements (Table 258–1). The fluoride level of a water supply can usually be obtained by calling the local water board. If the patient uses a private water supply, it may be necessary for the physician or dentist to facilitate a fluoride analysis. The patient's parents should be instructed to use a plastic container for the water specimen (a glass container may impair the accuracy of the fluoride assay). No fluoride prescription should be written for more than a total of 120 mg of fluoride. This provides a daily supply of 1.0 mg of fluoride for 4 mo. Even if a child ingested this entire supply, probably only mild gastric upset would ensue, which can be alleviated by an aluminum hydroxide preparation. Finally, the topical use of fluoride agents applied either professionally or by the patient are beneficial to children at high risk for caries (e.g.,

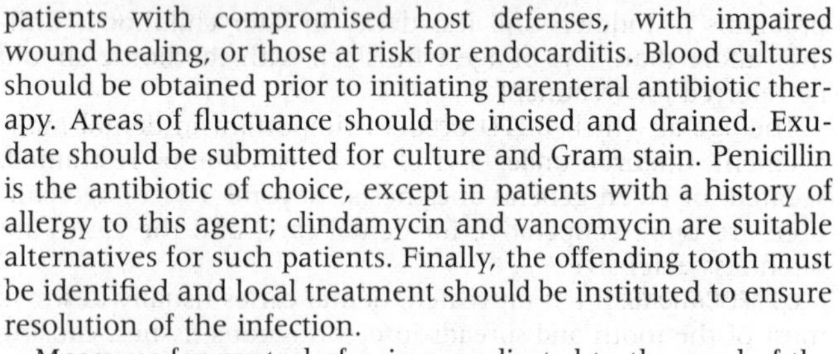

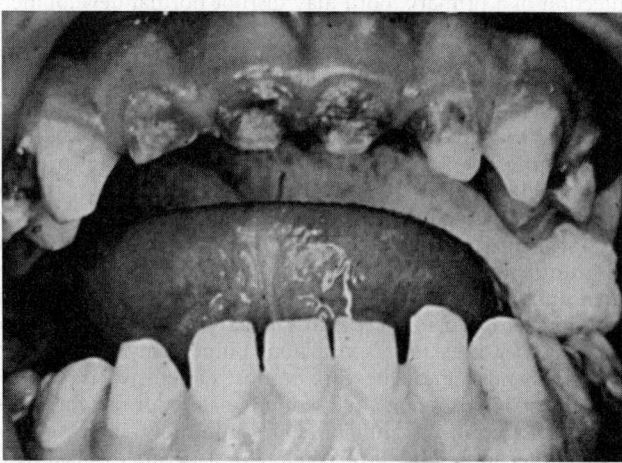

Figure 258–2. Nursing bottle caries.

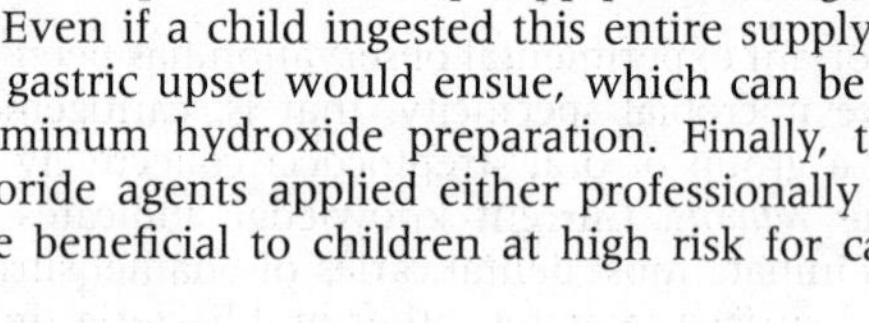

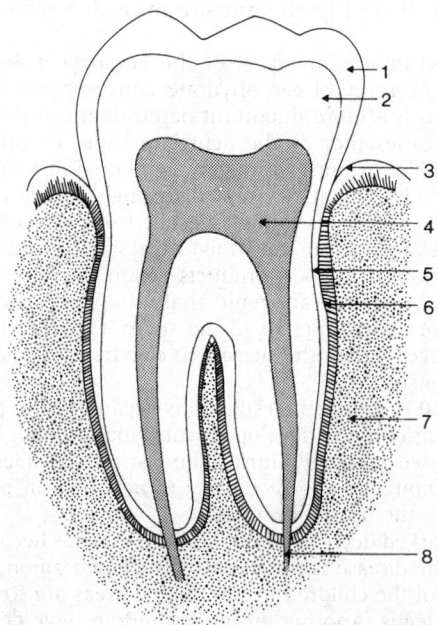

Figure 258–3. Basic dental anatomy: 1 = enamel; 2 = dentin; 3 = gingival margin; 4 = pulp; 5 = cementum; 6 = periodontal ligament; 7 = alveolar bone; 8 = neurovascular bundle.

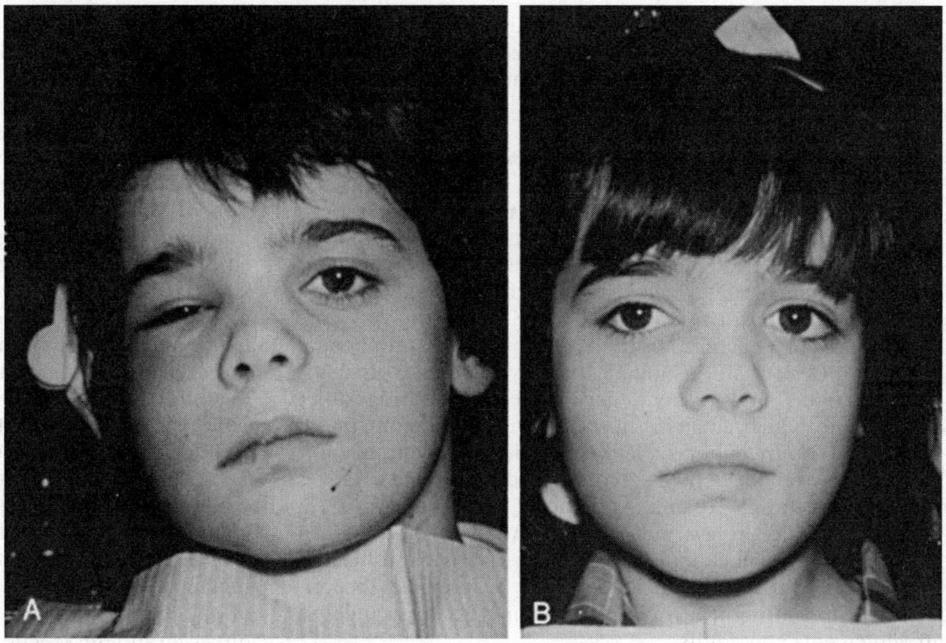

Figure 258–4. *A*, Facial inflammation-infection from the abscess of a maxillary primary molar. *B*, Resolution of the cellulitis in 1 wk with a course of antibiotics and extraction of the tooth.

with xerostomia secondary to tumoricidal doses of head and neck radiation).

Oral Hygiene. Thorough daily brushing and flossing of the teeth helps to prevent dental caries and periodontal disease. Parents should receive professional instruction regarding oral hygiene techniques for children. Studies have shown that most children under 10 yr of age do not have the eye-hand coordination required for adequate oral hygiene; accordingly, parents should assume responsibility for brushing and flossing. The degree of parental involvement should be appropriate to the child's growing ability.

Diet. Decreasing the frequency of carbohydrate ingestion prevents dental caries. Parents and children should be encouraged to avoid between-meal snacks that contain carbohydrates. The use of gum, candy, and soft drinks containing sugar substitutes (mannitol, sorbitol, and aspartame [with precautions]) is an effective approach for the child with a "sweet tooth." In addition, infants should be weaned by 1 yr of age to avoid the problems of nursing bottle caries (see Fig. 258–2). Should this not be possible, bedtime and naptime nursing bottles should contain only water.

Dental Sealants and Plastics. Excellent oral hygiene and optimal fluoride therapy have minimal effect in preventing dental caries in the pits and fissures on the occlusal surfaces of the teeth. The use of sealants has been shown to be effective in the prevention of pit and fissure caries. Sealants are plastic coatings that are professionally applied to the occlusal surfaces of the posterior teeth.

Tooth fissures are the most common sites for dental caries because they are too small to clean mechanically but may support bacterial acid production. Before the dramatic reduction in smooth surface dental caries the use of sealants was not widespread; children who developed smooth surface lesions had dental restorations placed and the sealant removed. With the combination of fluoride and dental sealants today, many children are completely caries free. Sealants are most effective when placed soon after the teeth erupt (usually within 1–2 yr) and when used in children with deep grooves and fissures in the molar teeth, teeth that are currently most susceptible to dental caries. The concept of sealant use is based on the roughening or etching of enamel surfaces with a mild acid and the subsequent attachment of plastics to the tags of enamel that remain. This etching system is also used for a variety of plastic materials that are used to restore fractured teeth, to attach orthodontic brackets, and for intra-tooth restorations.

Identification of High-Risk Patients. Intact salivary gland function is the major host defense against dental caries. Without it, the patient is susceptible to rampant dental caries. Appropriate preventive therapy has been shown to minimize or eliminate development of dental caries in patients with Sjögren syndrome, Mikulicz disease, chronic graft-versus-host disease, and patients receiving long-term therapy with drugs that cause xerostomia. Additional high-risk conditions for caries include gastroesophageal reflux, bulimia, rumination, Prader-Willi syndrome, mental retardation, and dystrophic epidermolysis bullosa. Hereditary fructose intolerance is associated with a reduced incidence of caries, because these patients avoid fructose-containing foods.

■ TABLE 258–1 Supplemental Fluoride Dosage Schedule

	Fluoride in Home Water (ppm)		
Age	**<0.3**	**0.3–0.6**	**>0.6**
Birth–6 mo	0*	0	0
6 mo–3 yr	0.25	0	0
3–6 yr	0.50	0.25	0
6–16 yr	1.0	0.50	0

**Milligrams of fluoride per day.*

CHAPTER 259
Periodontal Diseases

The periodontium includes the gingiva, alveolar bone, and periodontal ligament (see Fig. 258–3). Several distinct diseases of the periodontium occur during childhood and adolescence. These include gingivitis, acute necrotizing ulcerative gingivitis, herpetic gingivostomatitis, cyclosporine- or phenytoin-induced gingival overgrowth, juvenile periodontitis, and acute pericoronitis. Whereas periodontitis has been demonstrated in adults with acquired immunodeficiency syndrome (AIDS), significant periodontal conditions have not been described in children with AIDS.

GINGIVITIS. Cessation of oral hygiene results in the accumulation of a dense bacterial mass (dental plaque) around the cervical areas of the teeth at the gingival margin (gum line). If not removed, this dental plaque will precipitate an inflammatory response of the gingiva, with reddening and swelling of the gingiva, spontaneous gingival hemorrhage, and fetor oris. These clinical signs may vary in severity. Such gingivitis may be localized or generalized; it is reversible when proper oral hygiene measures are instituted. Inability to resolve gingivitis by meticulous oral hygiene necessitates considering other problems in which gingivitis may be a presenting component (e.g., acute nonlymphocytic leukemia, diabetes mellitus, neutropenia, thrombocytopenia, scurvy, and hormonal changes associated with puberty and pregnancy).

Epidemiologic surveys indicate that over half of American school children will experience gingivitis. Gingivitis in healthy prepubertal children is much less likely to progress to periodontitis (resulting in loss of alveolar bone) than is gingivitis in adolescents and adults.

TEETHING. Teething can lead to intermittent localized discomfort in the area of an erupting tooth and subsequent irritability. Low-grade fevers may be associated with teething. Many children go through teething without any apparent problem, whereas others have significant discomfort. There is no proven treatment, although an ice ring for the child to chew on may relieve some discomfort. Similar manifestations can also arise when the first permanent molars erupt at about age 6 yr. These are the largest teeth to penetrate the mucosa and during the mucosal rearrangement to allow eruption of the tooth the gums can become very sore. Parents report that the child has a toothache.

ERUPTION GINGIVITIS. This is an inflammation associated with the eruption of the teeth. Gums can become sore with accompanying bleeding at the gingival margin. Gentle brushing for several days usually resolves the gingivitis. The only associated condition that has long-term consequences is the eruption of a tooth that is well out of alignment in the dental arch. In such cases, formation of normal attached gingiva may not be possible, and either alignment of the tooth orthodontically or gingival grafting can be considered.

ACUTE NECROTIZING ULCERATIVE GINGIVITIS (ANUG; Vincent Infection; Trench Mouth). ANUG is a distinct periodontal disease prone to recurrence, the etiology of which is complex and not fully understood. The dramatic clinical response in its acute phase to penicillin indicates that bacteria are involved. The associated bacteriologic flora is composed of large numbers of oral spirochetes and fusobacteria; it is not clear, however, whether bacteria initiate the disease or are secondary invaders. ANUG develops primarily in young adults and adolescents. It rarely, if ever, develops in healthy children in developed countries. It occurs with surprising frequency, however, among children in southern India and certain African countries. Affected children usually have protein malnutrition. In these children, the lesion may not confine itself to the periodontium but may extend into adjacent tissues causing necrosis of facial structures (cancrum oris, or noma).

Clinical manifestations of ANUG include (1) necrosis and ulceration of erythematous gingiva, in particular, the gingiva between the teeth; (2) an adherent grayish pseudomembrane over the affected gingiva; (3) fetor oris; (4) cervical lymphadenopathy; (5) malaise; and (6) fever. The disease is usually localized, the most common site being the periodontium associated with the mandibular incisor teeth. The condition may be mistaken for acute herpetic gingivostomatitis. ANUG is confined to the periodontium, however, and vesicle formation is not a feature. Dark field microscopy will demonstrate dense spirochete populations in smears of debris obtained from ANUG lesions.

Treatment of ANUG is divided into two phases. The acute phase is managed by antibiotic therapy (penicillin or erythromycin), local debridement, oxygenating agents (direct application of 10% carbamide peroxide in anhydrous glycerol four times a day), and analgesics. Dramatic resolution usually occurs within 48 hr. A 2nd phase of treatment may be necessary if the acute phase of the disease has caused irreversible morphologic damage to the periodontium. Finally, current evidence indicates that this disease represents an endogenous rather than a communicable infection; accordingly, patients need not be managed as contagious.

HERPETIC GINGIVOSTOMATITIS. See Chapter 211.

PHENYTOIN-INDUCED GINGIVAL OVERGROWTH (PIGO, Dilantin Hyperplasia). The use of phenytoin in anticonvulsant therapy is associated with generalized enlargement of the gingiva. The etiology is complex, and not all factors are known. Current evidence indicates that phenytoin (diphenylhydantoin [DPH]) and its metabolites are present in significant quantity in the gingiva of patients treated with DPH. DPH and its metabolites have a direct stimulatory action on gingival fibroblasts in vitro, resulting in accelerated synthesis of collagen. On the other hand, animal models and clinical studies indicate that PIGO does not complicate DPH therapy in most patients who maintain meticulous oral hygiene. This observation suggests that gingivitis plays a role in the pathogenesis of PIGO.

PIGO occurs in 10–30% of patients treated with DPH. Mild *manifestations* involve subtle gingival changes of no consequence to the patient. Severe manifestations may include (1) gross enlargement of the gingiva, sometimes to the point of covering the teeth; (2) edema and erythema of the gingiva; (3) secondary infection, resulting in abscess formation; (4) migration of teeth; and (5) inhibition of exfoliation of primary teeth and subsequent impaction of permanent teeth. Severe PIGO may cause loss of optimal masticatory function and psychologic stress due to the cosmetic effects.

Treatment should be directed toward prevention. Ideally, the drug should be discontinued whenever possible. Patients treated with DPH should receive regular dental follow-up. Meticulous oral hygiene prevents or minimizes PIGO in most cases. The severe form of PIGO is usually treated by gingivectomy; the lesion will recur, however, if excellent oral hygiene cannot be maintained.

JUVENILE PERIODONTITIS (JP). This disease is characterized by rapid alveolar bone loss and is associated with a flora composed of large numbers of *Capnocytophaga, Actinobacillus, Haemophilus,* and *Bacteroides* species. Strains of *Actinobacillus* isolated from human lesions and inoculated into gnotobiotic rodents produced extensive alveolar bone loss in the experimental animals. In addition, the neutrophils of patients with JP have chemotactic and phagocytic defects; JP is associated with certain systemic diseases characterized by defects in neutrophil function (e.g., Down syndrome, diabetes mellitus, Chédiak-Higashi syndrome, Job syndrome, and cyclic neutropenia). Collectively, these data suggest that JP occurs in patients who have impaired host defenses that facilitate colonization by highly periodontopathogenic flora.

JP is exceptionally rare in preschool children who have only primary teeth. In older children it may be localized to the permanent incisors and 6-yr molars or may be generalized; the localized form may be associated with palmar and plantar hyperkeratosis (Papillon-Lefèvre syndrome). The gingiva is usually normal in appearance, but dental radiographs demonstrate alveolar bone loss. Affected teeth demonstrate mobility, which varies with the severity of alveolar bone loss.

The rate of alveolar bone loss in JP is rapid. If left untreated, affected teeth lose their attachment and exfoliate. Treatment approaches vary with the degree of involvement. Patients diagnosed at the onset of the disease are usually managed by local debridement, antibiotic therapy, and meticulous oral hygiene. Patients who have extensive alveolar bone loss at the time of initial diagnosis require extensive periodontal therapy that may include autologous osseous grafting. Prognosis depends on the degree of initial involvement and compliance with therapy.

Prevention of JP is not currently possible, but regular dental evaluations (one to two visits/yr) improve early detection and enhance the likelihood of favorable outcome. Patients with defects of neutrophil function should have such dental surveillance.

ACUTE PERICORONITIS (AP). AP is an acute inflammation of the flap of gingiva that partially covers the crown of an incompletely erupted tooth. Mandibular third molars and less often 2nd molars are common sites of AP. Accumulation of debris and bacteria between the gingival flap and tooth precipitates an inflammatory response. The flap of gingiva may become violently inflamed and edematous. Trismus and severe pain are common. Untreated cases may result in facial cellulitis and peritonsillar abscess, and fatalities have occurred in myelosuppressed patients.

Treatment of AP is in two phases. Treatment of the acute phase includes local debridement and irrigation, hot saline rinses, antibiotic therapy, and relief of the occlusion of the inflamed flap against the opposing jaw. When the acute phase has subsided, therapy is directed at preventing recurrences. This may include extraction of the tooth or resection of the gingival flap. Early recognition of the partial impaction of mandibular 3rd molars and their subsequent extraction will prevent AP.

CHAPTER 260
Dental Trauma

Traumatic oral injuries may be conveniently categorized into three groups: (1) dental injuries, (2) soft tissue injuries (contusions, abrasions, lacerations, punctures, avulsions, burns), and (3) injuries to the body of the jaw bones (mandibular or maxillary fractures or both). This chapter will describe dental injuries.

DENTAL INJURIES

Approximately 10% of all young people between 18 mo and 18 yr of age will sustain significant dental trauma. There appear to be three age periods of predilection: (1) preschool (1–3 yr), usually secondary to falls or child abuse; (2) school aged (7–10 yr), usually from bicycle and playground accidents; and (3) adolescents (16–18 yr), in whom dental trauma is generally secondary to fights, athletic injuries, and automobile accidents. Dental injuries are about twice as common among children with protrusion of teeth as among children with normal occlusion. Children with craniofacial abnormalities or neuromuscular deficits or both are also at increased risk for dental injury. Dental trauma includes injuries to the hard dental tissues and pulp and injuries to the periodontal structure (Fig. 260–1; Table 260–1).

INJURIES TO HARD DENTAL TISSUES AND PULP. Fractures of teeth are uncomplicated or complicated, in accordance with whether the fracture is confined to the hard dental tissues (uncomplicated) or extends through the pulp (complicated). Exposure of the pulp may result in its bacterial contamination, which can lead to infection and pulp necrosis. Pulp exposure complicates therapy and may lower the likelihood of a favorable outcome.

Traumatic blows to the mouth usually strike the maxillary incisor teeth, as they are the most anteriorly located. Fractures of the crowns or roots of these teeth are therefore common.

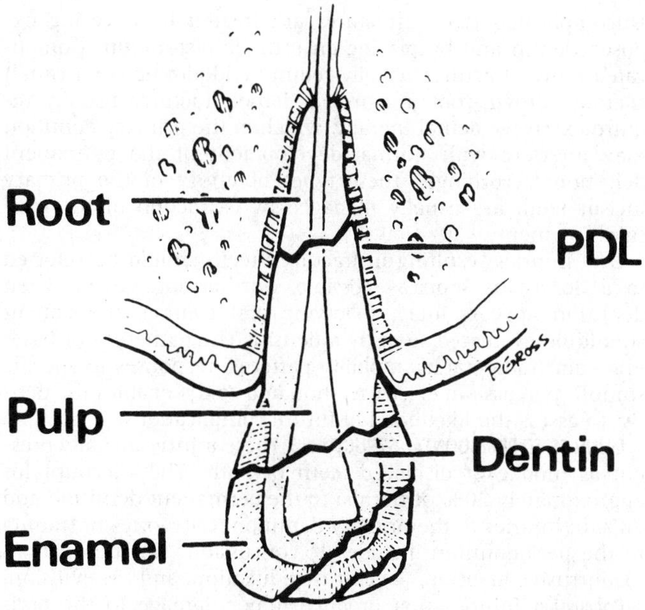

Figure 260–1. Tooth fractures may involve enamel, dentin, or pulp and may occur in the crown or root of a tooth. (From Pinkham JR: Pediatric Dentistry: Infancy Through Adolescence. Philadelphia, WB Saunders, 1988, p 172.)

■ TABLE 260–1 Injuries to Crowns of Teeth

Type of Trauma	Description	Treatment and Referral
Enamel infraction (crazing)	Incomplete fracture of enamel without loss of tooth structure.	Initially may not require therapy but should be assessed periodically by dentist.
Enamel fractures	Fracture of only the outer layer of the tooth (the enamel).	Refer today, tooth may be smoothed or treated to replace fragment.
Enamel and dentin fracture	Fracture of outer enamel and inner dentinal layer of the tooth. The dentin layer is made of tubules that connect to the pulp and may lead to inflammation or necrosis and/or abscess formation. Tooth may be sensitive to cold or air.	Refer today as soon as possible. Area should be treated to preserve the integrity of the underlying pulp.
Enamel, dentin fracture involving the pulp	An exposure of the pulp means it has bacterial contamination, which can lead to necrosis of the pulp and/or abscess. The tooth may have the appearance of bleeding or may display a small red spot.	Refer immediately. The dental therapy of choice depends on the extent of injury, the condition of the pulp, the development of the tooth, time elapsed from injury, and any other injuries to the supporting structures. Therapy is directed toward minimizing contamination in an effort to improve the prognosis.

Injuries to Crowns of Teeth, from Jossell SD, Abrams RG: Managing common dental problems and emergencies. PCNA 38:1325, 1991.

Uncomplicated crown fractures are treated by covering exposed dentin and by placing an esthetic restoration. Complicated crown fractures usually require endodontic (root canal) therapy. Crown-root fractures and root fractures usually require extensive dental therapy, which in the primary dentition may interfere with normal development of the permanent dentition; accordingly, these types of injury of the primary incisor teeth are usually managed by extraction of the fractured segments.

Oral injuries resulting in fractured teeth should be referred to a dentist as soon as possible. Furthermore, even when dentition appears intact following oral trauma, the patient should be evaluated soon by a dentist. The gathering of baseline data (radiographs, mobility patterns, responses to specific stimuli [percussion, electricity, hot, and cold]) enables the dentist to assess the likelihood of future complications.

INJURIES TO PERIODONTAL STRUCTURES. These injuries usually present as mobile or displaced teeth or both. They account for approximately 20% of trauma to the permanent dentition and 70% of injuries to the primary dentition. Categories of trauma to the periodontium include (1) concussion, (2) subluxation, (3) intrusive luxation, (4) extrusive luxation, and (5) evulsion.

Concussion. Injuries that produce minor damage to the periodontal ligament are termed concussions. Teeth sustaining such injuries are without abnormal mobility or displacement but react markedly to percussion. This type of injury usually requires no therapy and resolves without complication. Primary incisors that sustain concussion may change color; this sign usually indicates pulpal degeneration and should be evaluated by a dentist as soon as possible.

Subluxation. This type of injury involves moderate damage to the periodontal ligament. Subluxated teeth exhibit mild to moderate horizontal mobility or vertical mobility or both. Hemorrhage is usually evident around the neck of the tooth at the gingival margin. There is no displacement of the tooth, so that a subluxated tooth retains its normal position in the dental arch. Many subluxated teeth need to be immobilized in order to ensure adequate repair of the periodontal ligament. Immobilization is facilitated by an acrylic splint. Some of these teeth will develop pulp necrosis; this type of injury should be referred to a dentist as soon as possible.

Intrusive Luxation. This type of injury is rare in the permanent dentition but is the most common injury to primary dentition. Intruded primary incisors may give the false appearance of being evulsed (Fig. 260–2). In order to rule out evulsion, an occlusal dental radiograph is indicated (Fig. 260–3). This type of injury should be referred to the dentist as soon as possible.

Extrusive Luxation. This type of injury is characterized by displacement of the tooth from its socket. The tooth is usually displaced to the lingual side, with fracture of the wall of the alveolar socket. These teeth need immediate treatment; the longer the delay, the more likely the tooth will consolidate in its ectopic position. Therapy is directed at reduction (repositioning the tooth) and fixation (acrylic splints). In addition, many such teeth become necrotic and require endodontic therapy. Extrusive luxation in the primary dentition is usually managed by extraction, because complications of reduction and fixation may result in problems with development of permanent teeth.

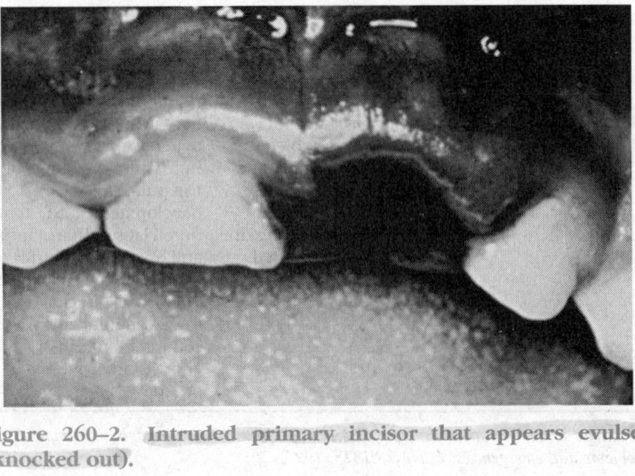

Figure 260–2. Intruded primary incisor that appears evulsed (knocked out).

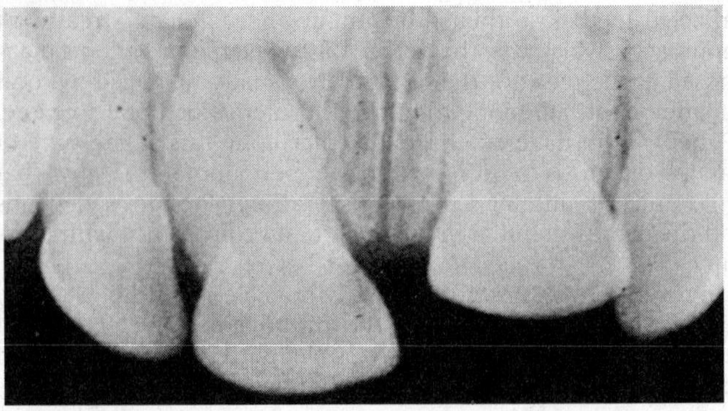

Figure 260–3. Occlusal radiograph documents intrusion of "missing tooth" presented in Figure 260–2.

Evulsion. If evulsed permanent teeth are replanted within 30 min after injury, a greater than 90% success rate may be achieved; whereas if the delay exceeds 2 hr, the failure rate approaches 95%. The likelihood that normal reattachment will follow replantation is related to the viability of the periodontal ligament, and immediate therapy is directed at applying this principle. Parents confronted with this emergency situation can be instructed to

1. *Find the tooth.*
2. *Rinse the tooth.* (Do *not* scrub the tooth. Do *not* touch the root. After plugging the sink drain, hold the tooth by the crown and rinse it under running tap water.)
3. *Insert the tooth into the socket.* (Gently place it back into its normal position. Do not be concerned if the tooth extrudes slightly. If the parent or child is too apprehensive for replantation of the tooth, the tooth should be placed in cow's milk. Milk is the best transport medium to maintain periodontal ligament viability.)
4. *Go directly to the dentist.* (In transit, the child should hold the tooth in place with a finger. The parent should buckle a seatbelt around the child and drive safely. A quick stop may not only result in re-evulsion but may also introduce the complications of ingestion or aspiration.)

After the tooth is replanted, it must be immobilized (acrylic splint) to facilitate reattachment; endodontic therapy is usually required. The initial signs of complications associated with replantation may appear as early as 1 wk post-trauma or as late as several years later. Close dental follow-up is indicated for at least 1 yr.

PREVENTION. To minimize the likelihood of dental injuries:

1. Every child or adolescent who engages in contact sports should wear a mouth protector, which may be constructed by a dentist or purchased at any athletic goods store.
2. Helmets should be worn by children or adolescents with neuromuscular problems or seizures to protect the cranium during falls; they should also have face guards.
3. All children or adolescents with protruding incisors should be evaluated by a pediatric dentist or orthodontist.

Additional Considerations. Children with dental trauma have also sustained head trauma; accordingly, neurologic assessment is warranted. Tetanus prophylaxis should be considered with any injury that disrupts the integrity of the tissues lining the oral cavity. The possibility of child abuse should always be considered.

CHAPTER 261

Common Lesions of the Oral Soft Tissues

OROPHARYNGEAL CANDIDIASIS (OPC, Thrush, Moniliasis). (Chapter 98.6). Oropharyngeal infection with *Candida albicans* is not unusual in neonates who have contact with the organism in the birth canal. Transmission within the newborn nursery may reach epidemic proportions unless appropriate precautions are instituted. The lesions of OPC appear as white plaques covering all or part of the oropharyngeal mucosa. These plaques are removable from the underlying corium, which is characteristically inflamed and hemorrhagic. Discomfort associated with this infection may occasionally interfere with feeding. The diagnosis is confirmed by direct microscopic examination and culture of scrapings from lesions. OPC is usually self-limited in the healthy newborn infant, but treatment with nystatin (1,000,000 units four times a day, applied directly to the lesions) will hasten recovery and reduce the risk of spread to other infants.

OPC is also a major problem during myelosuppressive therapy. Systemic candidiasis (SC), a major cause of morbidity and mortality during myelosuppressive therapy, develops almost exclusively in patients who have had prior oropharyngeal, esophageal, or intestinal candidiasis. This observation implies that prevention of OPC should reduce the incidence of SC. The use of a multiagent regimen for OPC prophylaxis in children receiving bone marrow transplants may be effective in preventing OPC, SC, or candidal esophagitis. The multiagent regimen consists of the following:

1. Debriding all mucous membrane surfaces within the oropharyngeal cavity with one povidone-iodine swabstick four times per day.
2. Subsequently swabbing all mucous membrane surfaces within the oropharyngeal cavity with one large cotton pledget saturated with 500,000 units of nystatin four times per day.

Most of the patients are premedicated with intravenous narcotic analgesics to permit the procedure to be done thoroughly and quickly.

Finally, chronic OPC occurs in children who have certain endocrinopathies, a specific candida immunodeficiency syndrome (associated with cutaneous and nail involvement), acquired immunodeficiency syndrome (AIDS), and nutritional deficiencies or who receive broad spectrum antibiotic therapy that alters the oral flora. In these situations, successful treatment depends also on correction of the underlying problem.

APHTHOUS ULCERS (Canker Sores). The aphthous ulcer is a distinct oral lesion, prone to recurrence. See Chapter 614. The differential diagnosis is noted in Table 261–1.

BOHN NODULES. Bohn nodules are small cystic lesions located along the buccal and lingual aspects of the mandibular and maxillary ridges of the neonate. These lesions arise from remnants of mucous gland tissue. Treatment is not necessary, as the nodules disappear within a few weeks.

DENTAL LAMINA CYSTS. Dental lamina cysts are small cystic lesions located along the crest of the mandibular and maxillary ridges of the neonate. These lesions arise from epithelial remnants of the dental lamina. Treatment is not necessary; they will disappear within a few weeks.

TABLE 261–1 Differential Diagnosis of Oral Ulceration

Condition	Comment
Common	
Aphthous (canker sore)	Painful
Traumatic	Accidents, chronic cheek biter
Hand, foot, mouth disease	Painful, lesions on tongue, anterior oral cavity, hands and feet
Herpangina	Painful, lesions confined to soft palate and oropharynx
Chemical burns	Alkali, acid, aspirin; painful
Uncommon	
Neutrophil defects	Agranulocytosis, leukemia, cyclic neutropenia; painful
Systemic lupus erythematosus	Recurrent, may be painless
Behçet syndrome	Resembles aphthous lesions; associated with genital ulcers, uveitis, etc.
Necrotizing ulcerative gingivostomatitis	Vincent stomatitis; painful
Syphilis	Chancre or gumma; painless
Crohn disease	Aphthous-like; painful
Histoplasmosis	Lingual

MUCOCELE. The mucocele usually appears as a raised bluish vesicle several millimeters in diameter. It occurs most commonly in the lower lip and rarely in the upper lip, palate, buccal mucosa, tongue, or floor of the mouth. It may persist for weeks or months prior to rupture, in which case it usually recurs. This lesion is caused by traumatic laceration of a minor salivary gland duct that permits accumulation of mucus in the soft tissues and subsequent proliferation of granulation tissue to sequester the mucus. Recurrences following surgical excision are largely the result of removing the mucocele without extirpating the minor salivary gland that produced the extravasated mucus.

FORDYCE GRANULES. Almost 80% of adults have multiple, yellow-white granules in clusters or plaquelike areas on the oral mucosa, most commonly on the buccal mucosa or lips. Histologically, normal sebaceous glands are seen in the lamina propria and submucosa. The glands are present at birth, but they hypertrophy and first appear as discrete yellowish papules during the preadolescent period in approximately 50% of children. No treatment is necessary.

CHEILITIS. Dryness of the lips, followed by scaling and cracking and accompanied by a characteristic burning sensation, is common in children. It is usually caused by sensitivity to contact substances (from toys and foods) plus photosensitivity to the sun's rays. It is aggravated by the alternation of wetting with the tongue and drying by the wind, especially in cold weather. Cheilitis also often occurs in association with fever. Frequent application of a bland ointment facilitates healing and is also preventive.

BLACK HAIRY TONGUE (Lingua Nigra). This condition is characterized by an elongation of the filiform papillae into hairlike projections. It is generally concentrated in a triangular area in front of the V-shaped line of circumvallate papillae and is associated with accumulation of debris in that region. The patch may vary from brown to black. The condition is usually chronic but will disappear with regular cleansing of the dorsal tongue. See Chapter 614.

Hairy tongue may also occur during prolonged antibiotic therapy, especially with oral troches. In addition, oral medications that contain bismuth may produce this benign condition.

GEOGRAPHIC TONGUE (Migratory Glossitis). This benign and asymptomatic lesion is characterized by one or more smooth, bright-red patches, often showing a yellow, gray, or white membranous margin upon the dorsum of an otherwise normally roughened tongue. See Chapter 614.

FISSURED TONGUE (Scrotal Tongue). The fissured tongue is a malformation manifested clinically by numerous small furrows or grooves on the dorsal surface. See Chapter 614.

CHAPTER 262

Diseases of the Salivary Glands and Jaws

With the exception of mumps (Chapter 208), disease of the salivary glands is rare in children. Bilateral enlargement of the submaxillary glands may occur in acquired immunodeficiency syndrome (AIDS), cystic fibrosis, malnutrition, and, transiently, during acute asthmatic attacks. Chronic vomiting and aspiration, as in achalasia or bulimia, may be accompanied by enlargement of the parotids. Benign salivary gland hypertrophy has been associated with endocrinopathies; thyroid disease, diabetes, and disorders of the pituitary-adrenal axis are the most frequently encountered.

Newborn infants discharge saliva until swallowing and lip closure are effective. Later, when the irritation of teething is accompanied by increased oral activity, drooling may occur. In some children with neurologic impairment, drooling is never overcome. Increased secretion of saliva occurs as a reflex to anticipated feeding or pain, from irritative lesions in the mouth, in conjunction with nausea, after administration of mercurial compounds, and in encephalitis and chorea.

RECURRENT PAROTITIS. Recurrent idiopathic swelling of the parotid gland may occur in otherwise healthy children. The swelling is usually unilateral, but both glands may be involved simultaneously or alternately; there may be up to 10 or more recurrences. There is little pain. The swelling is limited to the gland and usually lasts 2–3 wk. Subsidence is spontaneous and may be complete or partial. The incidence appears to be higher in the spring.

SUPPURATIVE PAROTITIS. This is usually due to *Staphylococcus aureus* and may be primary or a complication of parotitis due to another cause. It is usually unilateral and may be accompanied by fever. The gland becomes swollen, tender, and painful. Recurrent parotitis may be confused with suppurative parotitis. The latter responds to appropriate antibacterial therapy based on culture of pus obtained from the Stensen duct or by surgical drainage, which is infrequently required.

RANULA. Ranula is a cyst associated with a major salivary gland in the sublingual area. A ranula is a large, soft, mucus-containing swelling in the floor of the mouth. It occurs at any age, including infancy. The cyst should be excised, and the severed duct should be exteriorized.

XEROSTOMIA. Xerostomia (or dry mouth) may be associated with fever, dehydration, ingestion of drugs with anticholinergic activity, chronic graft-versus-host disease, Mikulicz disease, Sjögren syndrome, or tumoricidal doses of radiation when the salivary glands are within the field. Long-term xerostomia renders the patient highly susceptible to dental caries, which can be minimized or eliminated by appropriate preventive measures.

SALIVARY GLAND TUMORS. See Chapter 458.

CAFFEY DISEASE (Infantile Cortical Hyperostosis). See Chapter 644.

OSTEOMYELITIS (Chapter 172). In the newborn infant, facial osteomyelitis tends to occur in the area of the premaxillary suture, but during childhood the mandible is the more common location. The infection is marked by swelling and redness of the oral mucosa or skin, and is associated with pain, fever, and lymphadenopathy. Drainage should be established and the exudate cultured so that an appropriate antibiotic may be administered. Large sequestra may require surgical removal.

RETICULOENDOTHELIOSIS (HISTIOCYTOSIS X) (Chapter 660). Oral lesions may occur in any of the syndromes and may be an early manifestation. Lesions of the jaws may produce pain, swelling, loosening of teeth, and fetid breath. Healing is often delayed after dental extraction.

NEOPLASMS

Benign Tumors. Ossifying fibroma is the most common benign tumor of the jaws. Growth is rapid prior to puberty, after which it may slow or cease. The lesion is painless; a unilateral soft tissue swelling is usually the first sign. Most patients do not require treatment, but if the lesion is extensive, curettage or further surgical correction may be required.

Cysts of the Jaw. These cysts occur with multiple basal cell nevoid syndrome (see Chapter 620).

Malignant Tumors. The malignant primary tumors of the jaws in children include Burkitt lymphoma, osteogenic sarcoma, lymphosarcoma, and, more rarely, fibrosarcoma (see Part XXII).

CHAPTER 263

Diagnostic Roentgenograms in Dental Assessment

The *panoramic roentgenogram* provides a single image of the upper and lower jaws in such a way that all of the teeth and surrounding structures appear on one image. The radiograph includes the mandibular condyle, the inferior border of the mandible, and the maxillary sinuses. The x-ray beam rotates about the patient's head with corresponding movement of the radiographic film during exposure. Panoramic roentgenograms are used to show unerupted teeth, including their angulation and stage of development, cysts of the jaws, fractures, supernumerary (extra) teeth, and missing teeth.

The *cephalometric roentgenogram* positions the child's head in such a way that cranial and facial points and planes can be determined and compared with standards derived from thousands of such roentgenograms. A second major feature is that a child's facial growth can be assessed serially as cephalometric roentgenograms are taken sequentially. A similar protocol for positioning the child is used throughout the world. From the cephalometric roentgenogram the relationships of the upper and lower jaws can be determined as well as the relationships of the jaws to the cranial base, the alignment of the incisor teeth, and the relationship of the teeth to the supporting bone. This information is essential in planning orthodontic care and orthognathic surgical procedures.

Intraoral dental roentgenograms can show one section of the mouth by placing the film within the child's mouth and by directing the beam through the teeth and supporting structures. The individual intraoral roentgenograms can be used to detect dental caries and to show the extent of dental trauma. They also show the position of the supporting bone relative to the teeth as well as the stages of periodontal disease and dental anomalies immediately around the teeth.

Abramson JS, Givner LB: Should tetracycline be contraindicated for therapy of presumed Rocky Mountain spotted fever in children less than 9 years of age? Pediatrics 86:123, 1990.
Berkowitz RJ, Strandjord S, Jones P, et al: Stomatologic complications of bone marrow transplantation in a pediatric population. Pediatr Dent 9:105, 1987.
Bull MJ, Givan DC, Sadove AM, et al: Improved outcome in Pierre Robin sequence: Effect of multidisciplinary evaluation and management. Pediatrics 86:294, 1990.
Flaitz CM: Oral pathologic conditions and soft tissue anomalies. *In:* Pinkham JR (ed): Pediatric Dentistry: Infancy Through Adolescence, 2nd ed. Philadelphia, WB Saunders, 1994, p 29.
Genco RJ, Van Dyke TE, Levine MJ, et al: Molecular factors influencing neutrophil defects in periodontal disease. J Dent Res 65:1379, 1986.
Gihooly JT, Smith JD, Howell LL, et al: Bedside polysomnography as an adjunct in the management of infants with Robin sequence. Plast Reconstr Surg 92:23, 1993.
Greene JC, Louie R, Wycoff SJ: Preventive dentistry. I: Dental caries. JAMA 262:3459, 1989.
Greene JC, Louie R, Wycoff SJ: Preventive dentistry. II: Periodontal diseases, malocclusion, trauma and oral cancer. JAMA 263:421, 1990.
Israele V, Siegel JD: Infectious complications of craniofacial surgery in children. Rev Infect Dis 11:9, 1989.
Johnsen D, Nowjack-Raymer R: Baby bottle tooth decay: Issues, assessment, and an opportunity for the nutritionist. J Am Diet Assoc 89:1112, 1989.
Josell SD, Abrams RG: Pediatric oral health. Pediatr Clin North Am 38: (1049–1350), 1991.
King N, Lee A: Prematurely erupted teeth in newborn infants. J Pediatr 114:807, 1989.
Ross RB: Treatment variables affecting facial growth in complete unilateral cleft lip and palate. Cleft Palate J 24:5, 1987.
Serwint JR, Mungo R, Negrete VF, et al: Child-rearing practices and nursing caries. Pediatrics 92:233, 1993.
Tinanoff N: Dental caries: Etiology, pathogenesis, clinical manifestations, and management. *In:* Wei SHY (ed): Pediatric Dentistry: Total Patient Care. Philadelphia, Lea & Febiger, 1988, p 9.

SECTION 3

The Esophagus

John J. Herbst

CHAPTER 264

Development and Function of the Esophagus

The esophagus develops as a pair of cranial folds in the primitive foregut descends while a single caudal fold ascends to separate the trachea and esophagus, followed by lengthening of the trachea and esophagus. The esophagus transports fluids and solids to the stomach and prevents regurgitation. Its squamous cell lining is suited for this purpose but is susceptible to erosion by refluxed gastric contents.

Swallowing has been observed in utero at 20 wk of gestation, and sucking and swallowing seem to be coordinated by 33–34 wk. The full-term newborn infant has short bursts of sucking followed by swallows. Within a few days (or weeks if premature) the infant is able to swallow and breathe in a coordinated, rhythmic manner during prolonged bursts of sucking.

Swallowing is initiated by a sudden elevation of the posterior portion of the tongue that propels the bolus of food or fluid toward the posterior pharynx. A simultaneous superior and anterior displacement of the larynx and positioning of the epiglottis protects the laryngeal airway, while the nasopharynx is occluded by the soft palate and uvula. The superior esophageal sphincter relaxes, and pharyngeal constrictors help to propel food into the esophagus, where primary peristaltic waves propel food into the stomach. Secondary waves are usually initiated by local distention and serve to empty the esophagus of residual food or of gastric contents. Both of these waves empty the esophagus by propulsive efforts.

In contrast, tertiary waves are nonpropulsive, are abnormal if present in large numbers, and may be associated with chest pain. The distal 1–3 cm of the esophagus has increased tone and serves as the lower esophageal sphincter that prevents reflux but relaxes during deglutition to allow food to enter the stomach.

The *common symptoms and signs* of esophageal disease are cough or choking with swallowing, regurgitation or vomiting, dysphagia, complete inability to swallow, pain on swallowing (odynophagia), and hematemesis. Each can be attributed to one or more defects in the complex coordination of the swallowing sequence.

Diagnostic evaluations include conventional barium swallow roentgenographic studies, which can demonstrate masses impinging on the lumen or demonstrate gastroesophageal reflux. A video esophagram can better demonstrate changing patterns associated with swallowing and esophageal peristalsis. Esophageal manometry permits evaluation of pressure waves in the

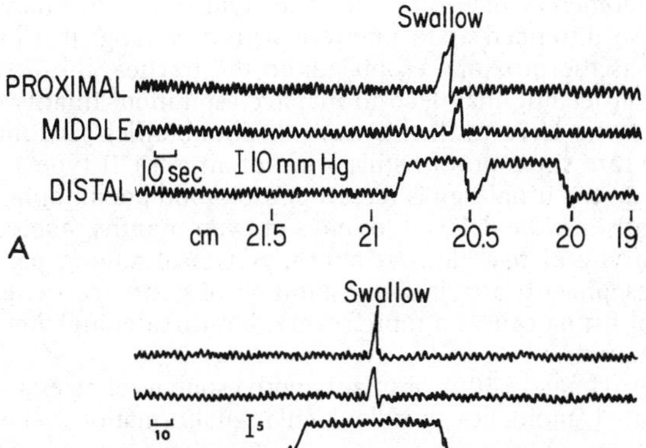

Figure 264–1. *A,* Pressures in the esophagus of a normal infant as recorded with a triple lumen catheter with recording tips 2.5 cm apart. When the distal recording tip was 21.5 cm from the gum line, it was within the lower esophageal sphincter. A swallow initiates a primary peristaltic wave. The pressure wave is detected first in the more proximal catheter and then in the more distal one. A relaxation in the lower esophageal sphincter allows the food to enter the stomach. *B,* Abnormal manometric pattern in a patient demonstrating simultaneous pressure in the two proximal recording tips, characteristic of a tertiary esophageal wave. There is no relaxation of the lower esophageal sphincter. Such a pattern is seen in patients with achalasia.

esophagus, as well as pressure changes in the lower esophageal sphincter, which are decreased in reflux esophagitis and increased in achalasia (Fig. 264–1). Radionuclide scans can evaluate the efficiency of peristalsis in clearing the esophagus and can test for reflux and aspiration. Prolonged monitoring of distal esophageal pH is a very sensitive test for gastric acid reflux. Flexible fiberoptic endoscopy permits biopsy and visualization of the esophagus without general anesthesia; it detects and removes foreign bodies.

CHAPTER 265

Atresia and Tracheoesophageal Fistula

Esophageal atresia occurs in 1 in 3,000–4,500 live births; about one third of affected infants are born prematurely. In more than 85% of cases, a fistula between the trachea and distal esophagus accompanies the atresia (Fig. 265–1*A*). Less commonly, the esophageal atresia or tracheoesophageal fistula may occur alone (Fig. 265–1*B,C*) or in unusual combinations (Fig. 265–1*D,E*). Disorders in the formation and movement of the paired cranial and single caudal folds in the primitive foregut explain the variations in atresia and fistula formation.

CLINICAL MANIFESTATIONS. Atresia of the esophagus should be suspected (1) in cases of maternal polyhydramnios; (2) if a catheter used at birth for resuscitation cannot be inserted into the stomach; (3) if the infant has excessive oral secretions; or (4) if choking, cyanosis, or coughing occurs with an attempt at feeding. Suctioning of excess secretions from the mouth and pharynx frequently results in improvement, but symptoms quickly recur. Unfortunately, the diagnosis is often not made until after the baby has aspirated feedings. When a fistula connects the trachea and distal esophagus, air usually enters the abdomen, which often becomes tympanitic and may become so distended as to interfere with breathing. If a fistula connects the proximal esophagus to the trachea, the first attempt at feeding may lead to massive aspiration. Infants with atresia who have no fistula have scaphoid, airless abdomens. In the rare situation of fistula without atresia ("H type") (Fig. 265–1*C*), the usual sign is recurrent aspiration pneumonia, and diagnosis may be delayed for days or even months. Aspiration of pharyngeal secretions is almost universal among patients with esophageal atresia, but aspiration of gastric contents via a distal fistula causes a more severe, life-threatening chemical pneumonitis.

Approximately 50% of infants with esophageal atresia have associated anomalies. Cardiovascular malformations, skeletal

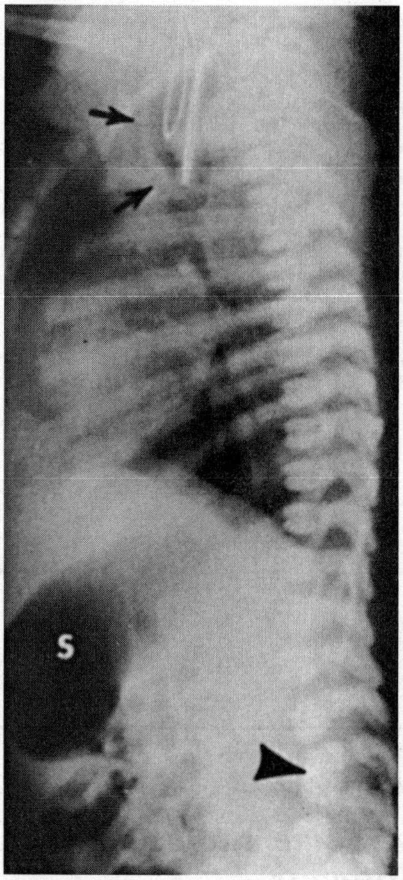

Figure 265–2. Tracheoesophageal fistula. Lateral roentgenogram demonstrating a nasogastric tube coiled *(arrows)* in the proximal segment of an atretic esophagus. The distal fistula is suggested by gaseous dilatation of the stomach (S) and small intestine. The *arrowhead* depicts vertebral fusion, whereas a heart murmur and cardiomegaly suggest the presence of a ventricular septal defect. This patient demonstrated elements of the VATER anomalad. (From Balfe D, Ling D, Siegel M: The esophagus. *In:* Putman CE, Ravin CE (eds): Textbook of Diagnostic Imaging. Philadelphia, WB Saunders, 1988.)

malformations including hemivertebrae and abnormal development of the radius, and renal and urogenital malformations are common; collectively they are known as the VATER syndrome (Chapter 86).

DIAGNOSIS. Diagnosis of esophageal atresia is ideally made in the delivery room, because pulmonary aspiration is a major determinant of prognosis. Inability to pass a catheter into the stomach confirms the suspicion. The catheter usually stops abruptly 10–11 cm from the upper gum line, and roentgenograms show a coiled catheter in the upper esophageal pouch (Fig. 265–2). Occasionally, plain roentgenograms of the chest

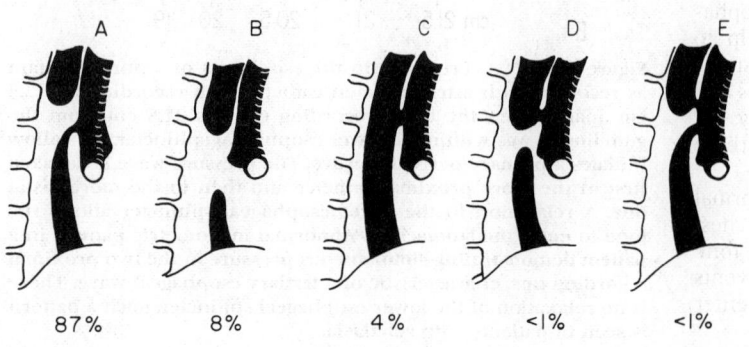

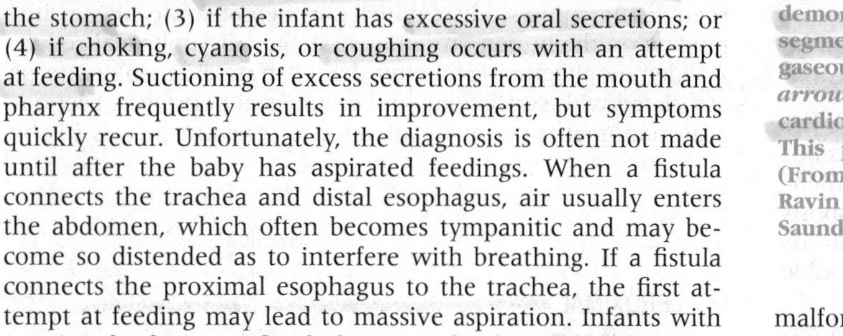

Figure 265–1. Diagrams of the five most commonly encountered forms of esophageal atresia and tracheoesophageal fistula, shown in order of frequency.

show an esophagus dilated with air. The presence of air in the abdomen indicates a fistula between the trachea and the distal esophagus. Contrast medium used for roentgenography should be water soluble; less than 1 mL given under fluoroscopic control is sufficient to outline the blind upper pouch. The contrast medium should then be withdrawn to prevent overflow into the lungs and development of chemical pneumonitis. "H type" fistulas (Fig. 265–1C) may be difficult to demonstrate. A videoesophagram, while filling the esophagus with water-soluble contrast medium, is usually effective. The tracheal orifice of the fistula may be detectable at bronchoscopy. A careful search should be made for associated malformations. Many recommend preoperative cardiac ultrasography to detect cardiac malformations, which are a significant cause of morbidity.

TREATMENT. Esophageal atresia is a surgical emergency. Preoperatively, the patient should be kept prone to decrease any tendency of gastric contents to reach the lungs. The esophageal pouch should be kept empty by constant suction to prevent aspiration of secretions. Careful attention must be given to temperature control, respiratory function, and management of associated anomalies. Occasionally, the patient's condition requires that surgery be performed in stages, the first step usually being ligation of the fistula and insertion of a gastrostomy tube for feeding, and the second being anastomosis of the two ends of the esophagus. Eight to 10 days after a primary anastomosis, oral feedings are usually tolerated. Esophagography at 10 days will help to determine the adequacy of the anastomosis.

Structural malformations of the trachea are common in patients with esophageal atresia and fistula. Tracheomalacia, recurrent aspiration pneumonia, and reactive airway disease are frequently seen. Tracheal development is normal if there is no fistula; esophageal stenosis and severe gastroesophageal reflux are more common in these patients. Failure to thrive, slow feeding, coughing, and choking are common sequelae, especially if primary anastomosis cannot be performed in the immediate neonatal period. Stenosis at the anastomotic site is common and may require dilatations.

CHAPTER 266

Other Disorders of the Esophagus

LARYNGOTRACHEOESOPHAGEAL CLEFT. Rarely, the larynx and upper trachea may fail to separate completely from the esophagus for a variable distance. Symptoms of the resultant laryngotracheoesophageal cleft are similar to those of tracheoesophageal fistula; aphonia should suggest the former. Roentgenographic diagnosis using contrast material is difficult; usually endoscopy is required.

EXTERNAL COMPRESSION. The most common masses impinging on the esophagus are enlarged lymph nodes in the subcarinal area, which may be due to tuberculosis, histoplasmosis, other forms of pulmonary suppuration, or lymphoma. Extrinsic pressure may also be caused by vascular anomalies in the mediastinum (Chapter 386.26).

ESOPHAGEAL DUPLICATION CYSTS. These cysts may cause esophageal compression. Their epithelium may come from any portion of the intestine, and they do not communicate with the esophagus unless there is ulceration from gastric mucosa in the cyst. Two thirds are on the right side of the esophagus. Rarely, duplication cysts may extend through the diaphragm and communicate with the intestine. Diagnosis is usually made by barium esophagography. *Neurenteric cysts* are esophageal duplication cysts that contain glial elements; vertebral anomalies usually accompany these cysts.

CONGENITAL STENOSIS AND WEBS. The embryologic development of these rare lesions is probably similar to atresia. Dysphagia is sometimes delayed until offering of solid foods. Fibromuscular stenosis and filamentous webs respond to dilatation, but must be distinguished from strictures caused by peptic esophagitis (Chapter 270). If there are tracheobronchial remnants in the stenotic area, resection is indicated.

DYSPHAGIA DUE TO NEUROMUSCULAR DISEASE. Many systemic, neurologic, and muscular disorders may give rise to esophageal symptoms. These disorders are listed in Table 266–1 and discussed elsewhere.

CRICOPHARYNGEAL DYSFUNCTION. Spasm of the cricopharyngeal muscle or achalasia of the superior esophageal sphincter may cause intermittent dysphagia, and the increased pressure in the pharynx and upper esophagus may lead to development of a posterior pharyngeal diverticulum. Diagnosis of this idiopathic disorder is made with a videoesophagram or manometric demonstration of a failure of the superior esophageal sphincter to relax during deglutition. Symptoms are relieved by myotomy of the cricopharyngeal muscle, analogous to the procedure used in hypertrophic pyloric stenosis (Chapter 275.1).

CRICOPHARYNGEAL INCOORDINATION OF INFANCY. This incoordination is usually evident soon after birth. Sucking is normal, but affected infants tend to choke and aspirate with deglutition; they generally have small jaws that open poorly. Videoradiography shows repetitive to-and-fro movement of the contrast medium in the posterior pharynx. Careful feedings by spoon or gavage are required until the patient is about 6 mo of age, when symptoms abate. The cause of this disorder is unknown.

BULBAR PALSY (SUPRANUCLEAR OR LOWER MOTOR NEURON). This type of palsy may cause dysphagia. The child has poor sucking with liquids, and chews and swallows solid food with difficulty. With supranuclear bulbar palsy, the jaw jerk is exaggerated and usually signs of generalized spastic cerebral palsy develop. Lower motor neuron disease with flaccid bulbar palsy and facial diplegia constitutes the Möbius syndrome.

PARALYSIS OF THE SUPERIOR LARYNGEAL NERVE. Paralysis has been reported in neonates with dysphagia, diminished esophageal motility, a preference to lie with the head turned to one side, and, in some cases, unilateral facial weakness. The syndrome is thought to be caused when an unusual intrauterine position compresses the nerve between the thyroid cartilage and the hyoid bone. Spontaneous recovery occurs during the 1st yr.

TRANSIENT PHARYNGEAL MUSCLE DYSFUNCTION. This dysfunction is often associated with palatal dysfunction and may be due to delayed normal development or may be associated with cerebral palsy. Choking during feeding and dribbling of formula are the main symptoms. Paralysis of pharyngeal constrictors and a flaccid soft palate are noted in videoradiographic studies.

■ TABLE 266–1 Neuromuscular Disorders That May Cause Dysphagia

Cerebral palsy (more common)
Dermatomyositis
Infections—diphtheria, poliomyelitis, tetanus
Muscular dystrophy (more common)
Myasthenia gravis
Polyneuritis
Familial dysautonomia (Riley-Day) syndrome
Scleroderma
Specific cranial nerve defects (e.g., Möbius syndrome)
Werdnig-Hoffmann disease

Gavage feeding can prevent aspiration (the main complication) and may be required for only a few days or for many weeks. Affected infants often have generalized hypotonia, and other nervous system dysfunctions, especially developmental delays, that often become evident later.

DIFFUSE ESOPHAGEAL SPASM. This spasm may be a cause of chest pain and dysphagia in adolescents. This primary motility disorder has characteristic esophageal contractions noted on manometry simultaneously with midchest, retrosternal pain after swallowing liquids. Tensilon testing may provoke pain. Treatment is usually not needed, except in more severe cases, in which nitrates or calcium channel blocking agents have been successful.

CHAPTER 267

Achalasia

Achalasia is an uncommon motility disorder in which a relative obstruction at the gastroesophageal junction is made worse by a lack of peristaltic waves in the esophagus (see Fig. 264–1*B*). The condition affects primarily adolescents and adults; children under the age of 4 yr constitute fewer than 5% of patients. Ganglion cells are frequently decreased in number and are surrounded by inflammatory cells; a heightened response of the esophageal muscles to methacholine has been interpreted as evidence of degeneration hypersensitivity. Only in Chagas disease has the etiology been well established.

CLINICAL MANIFESTATIONS AND DIAGNOSIS. Symptoms include difficulty in swallowing, regurgitation of food, cough from overflow of fluids into the trachea, and failure to gain weight. Pulmonary infections, including bronchiectasis, may result from persistent aspiration of esophageal contents. Retention of food in the esophagus may cause esophagitis. Achalasia has been reported in siblings, and in association with adrenal insufficiency and alacrima. Air-fluid levels in a dilated esophagus on an upright chest film may suggest the diagnosis. On barium swallow, there is abnormal motility with variable but often massive dilatation of the esophagus, and tapering or breaking at the gastric junction. Frequently, there is no air in the stomach (Fig. 267–1). The diagnosis may be confirmed with esophageal manometry, in which the major findings are incomplete or absent relaxation of the lower esophageal sphincter with swallowing, a lack of primary or secondary propulsive peristaltic waves in the esophagus, and usually an increased lower esophageal sphincter pressure.

TREATMENT. Nifedipine, a calcium channel blocker, will improve esophageal emptying but is recommended only when a brief delay in definitive therapy is indicated. Intrasphincteric injection of botulism toxin also may provide symptomatic relief for as long as 6 mo. Permanent relief of symptoms usually follows surgical division of muscle fibers at the gastroesophageal junction (Heller myotomy). Alternatively, the sphincter may be forcefully dilated with a balloon catheter under fluoroscopic control. Simple bougienage will give only temporary relief and is not recommended. Because the esophageal motility cannot be reversed, any procedure that disrupts the sphincter and relieves obstruction may allow gastroesophageal reflux, esophagitis, and occasional stricture formation.

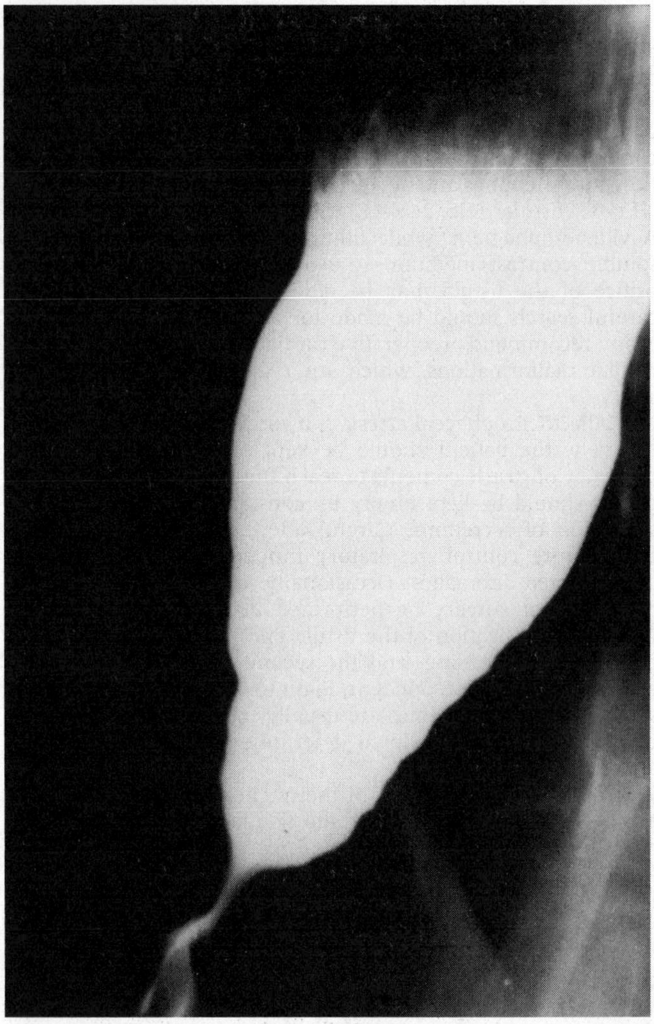

Figure 267–1. Barium esophagogram of a patient with achalasia demonstrating dilated esophagus and narrowing at the lower esophageal sphincter. Note retained secretions layered on top of barium in the esophagus.

CHAPTER 268

Hiatal Hernia

Herniation of the stomach through the esophageal hiatus may occur as a common sliding hernia, in which the gastroesophageal junction slides into the thorax, or be paraesophageal, in which a portion of the stomach (usually the fundus) is insinuated beside the gastroesophageal junction in the hiatus (Fig. 268–1). Sliding hernias are frequently associated with gastroesophageal reflux, especially in retarded children. The relationship to hiatal hernias in adults is unclear. Treatment is not directed at the hernia but at the gastroesophageal reflux.

Paraesophageal hernias may be encountered following fundoplication for gastroesophageal reflux, especially if the edges of a dilated esophageal hiatus have not been approximated. Fullness after eating and upper abdominal pain are the usual symptoms. Infarction of the herniated stomach is rare.

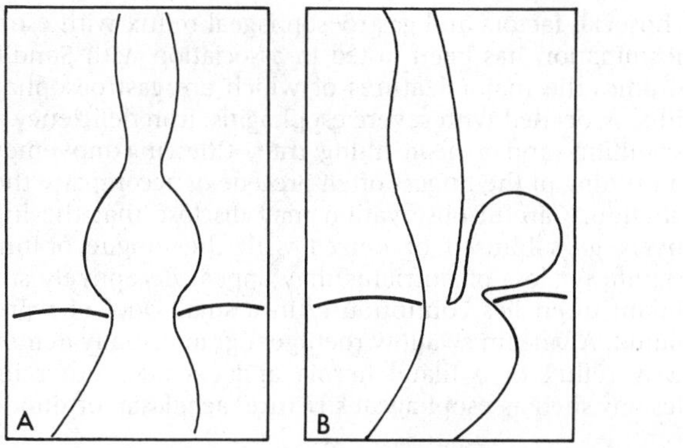

Figure 268–1. Types of esophageal hiatal hernia. *A*, Sliding hiatal hernia, the most common type; *B*, paraesophageal hiatal hernia.

CHAPTER 269

Gastroesophageal Reflux

(Chalasia)

When the lower esophageal sphincter (LES) is not competent, excessive and passive reflux of gastric contents may cause significant symptoms. The term *chalasia* describes free reflux across a dilated sphincter. Although many infants have minor degrees of reflux, about 1:300–1:1,000 have significant reflux and associated complications.

ETIOLOGY. Factors contributing to the competency of the LES include abdominal position of the sphincter, angle of insertion of esophagus into the stomach, and sphincter pressure. Frequent spontaneous drops in sphincter pressure are a major mechanism of reflux, but reflux across a chronically lax sphincter is frequent with esophagitis, while reflux with normal pressure may occur with increased abdominal pressure (coughing, crying, defecating). Reflux is common in normal persons after meals, and the swallowing of saliva to wash away the last traces of acid is an important mechanism for preventing esophagitis. The small reservoir capacity of the infant's esophagus predisposes to vomiting, a much less common problem in adolescents and adults. Patients with abnormal reflux may also demonstrate decreased gastric emptying and reduced acid clearance from the esophagus. Placement of a gastrostomy tube encourages reflux, probably by altering the angle at which the esophagus enters the stomach.

CLINICAL MANIFESTATIONS. The signs and symptoms relate directly to the exposure of the esophageal epithelium to refluxed gastric contents. In 85% of affected infants excessive vomiting occurs during the 1st wk of life; an additional 10% have symptoms by 6 wk. Symptoms abate without treatment in 60% by the age of 2 yr as the child assumes a more upright posture and eats solid foods, but the remainder continue to have symptoms until at least 4 yr of age. Patients with cerebral palsy, Down syndrome, and other causes of developmental delay have an increased incidence of reflux.

Delayed gastric emptying and vomiting occasionally may be forceful because of pylorospasm. Aspiration pneumonia occurs in about one third of patients in infancy, and in those in whom symptoms persist until later childhood chronic cough, wheezing, and recurrent pneumonia are common. There may be rumination (see later). Growth and weight gain are adversely affected in about two thirds of patients.

The major manifestation of esophagitis is hemorrhage; the presence of occult blood in stool is common, hematemesis occurs in some children, but melena is rare. Iron-deficiency anemia is common in patients with severe esophagitis (Chapter 270). Complaints of substernal pain are rare, but dysphagia may cause irritability and anorexia in advanced cases. In untreated patients, esophagitis leads to stricture formation in 5% of cases, and inanition and pneumonia lead to death in another 5%.

Sandifer syndrome, opisthotonus, and other abnormal head posturing are associated with reflux. The head positioning may be a mechanism to protect the airway or reduce acid-reflux–associated pain. Methylxanthines may exacerbate reflux by lowering sphincter tone.

Reflux may rarely cause laryngospasm, apnea, and bradycardia. The relationship between reflux and acute life-threatening events or sudden infant death syndrome (SIDS) remains controversial and may be coincidental (Chapter 657).

DIAGNOSIS. In mild cases, a careful clinical assessment may be sufficient for diagnosis, which is confirmed by assessing the response to therapy. In severe or complex cases, the diagnosis can be confirmed by barium esophagography under fluoroscopic control. The finding of gastric folds above the diaphragm indicates the presence of a hiatal hernia (Fig. 269–1); in children these folds are more readily detected in a collapsed than in a full esophagus. Gastroesophageal reflux is an episodic

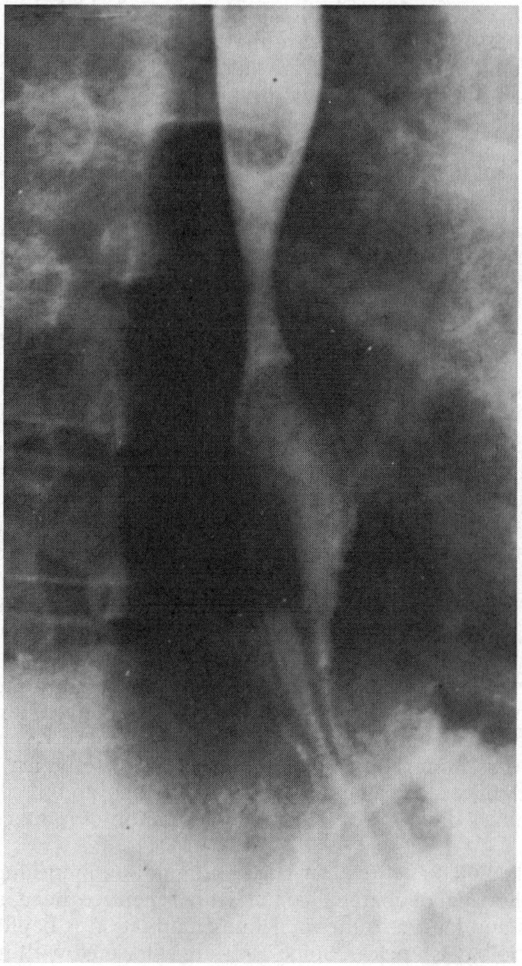

Figure 269–1. Barium esophagogram demonstrating free gastroesophageal reflux. A stricture due to peptic esophagitis is present. Longitudinal gastric folds above the diaphragm indicate the unusual presence of an associated hiatal hernia.

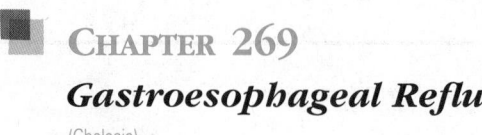

event; accordingly, in many symptomatic patients significant reflux is not demonstrated initially by roentgenography. It is important to use enough barium to approximate the volume of a normal meal. Special maneuvering of the patient is not necessary. Normal children may have a small amount of reflux that is quickly cleared from the esophagus, but recurrent reflux is definitely abnormal. Strictures are easily demonstrated with barium esophagography. Severe esophagitis may be suspected when a ragged mucosal outline is seen on a roentgenogram, but esophagoscopy with biopsy is a superior diagnostic technique for this disorder.

Gastric scintiscans may be used to demonstrate aspiration of gastric contents and can demonstrate reflux, but sensitivity for aspiration and specificity for reflux are not high. Esophagoscopy can evaluate severe reflux and strictures, and esophageal biopsy is a sensitive test for evidence of reflux. Increased thickness of the germinative layer and increased length of dermal papillae are early changes, but intraepithelial neutrophils, eosinophils, ulcer formation, or presence of columnar epithelium (Barrett esophagitis) are seen with more severe disease. The last represents cellular metaplasia and is rarely associated with adenocarcinoma. The frequency and duration of reflux can be documented by continuous monitoring of distal esophageal pH. Although a sensitive test, it is not needed for routine diagnosis, and the costs and complexity of obtaining and scoring the data suggest it is best used to investigate patients with atypical symptoms or to determine if unusual events (coughing, choking, stridor, apnea) are temporally related to reflux episodes.

TREATMENT. A long-term cure may be expected in infants. In older children, symptoms are likely to be chronic, as with adults. Young infants should be kept prone. In older infants and children, raising the head of the bed and keeping the child upright are indicated. Thickening an infant's formula with cereal will decrease crying and the volume of vomitus. Metoclopramide (0.15 mg/kg/dose, qid) will stimulate gastric emptying and esophageal motility and reduce reflux, but drowsiness, restlessness, and extrapyramidal reactions are noted in some children. Domperidone, a similar drug not available in the United States, acts only peripherally. Cisapride (0.2 mg/kg qid) stimulates gastrointestinal motility via serotonin receptors and is as effective as the other prokinetic drugs. If esophagitis is present, antacids, H_2 receptor blockers, or omeprazol are indicated because they will improve symptoms as well as esophageal motility. Omeprazol will most effectively depress acid secretion but is not recommended for prolonged use and is available only as a time-release capsule.

If symptoms do not improve with a prolonged trial of intensive medical therapy, operative therapy may be indicated. Medical therapy may be shortened if recurrent aspiration and apnea do not promptly respond. Stricture formation due to reflux esophagitis will usually require antireflux therapy in addition to bougienage. The Nissen fundoplication or a variation is used in children; percutaneous gastrojejunostomy is a less invasive and potentially beneficial alternative. Reflux is controlled in about 90% of cases. Improvement in respiratory symptoms from reflux depends on the extent to which reflux caused or exacerbated pulmonary problems and if chronic pulmonary disease was initiated by aspiration of refluxed material.

RUMINATION. Repetitive gagging, regurgitation, mouthing, and reswallowing of material, often with repetitive head movements and failure to thrive, defines rumination (Chapter 21). The etiology is unclear. Some cases are associated with mental retardation. Altered interaction with the environment is common, either associated with prolonged lack of stimulation in newborn intensive care units or because of altered relationships with caregivers. There is often an interaction of psychosocial factors and gastroesophageal reflux with esophagitis. Rumination has been noted in association with Sandifer syndrome, the major features of which are gastroesophageal reflux associated with severe esophagitis, iron deficiency anemia, vomiting, and a head-tilting trait. Chewing movements and mouthing of the fingers often precede or accompany the regurgitation. Careful observation may disclose that the infant actively gags himself or herself with the tongue or fingers. A significant loss of nutrients may appear deceptively small; the infant often lies continuously in a small pool of regurgitated liquid. A barium swallow roentgenogram usually demonstrates easy reflux or a hiatal hernia and excludes other intestinal lesions such as esophageal stricture, achalasia, or duodenal ulcer.

Behavioral therapy is routinely used, but medical treatment of reflux is also indicated. In children not responding to intensive medical therapy, an antireflux surgical procedure will routinely stop symptoms.

CHAPTER 270
Esophagitis

Peptic esophagitis due to reflux of gastric acid with pain, blood loss, and occasional stricture formation is the most common form of esophagitis.

Retroesophageal abscess may be caused by perforation of the esophagus (Chapter 271), extension of a retropharyngeal abscess, spinal osteomyelitis, pleuritis, suppuration of mediastinal lymph nodes, pericarditis, or pharyngeal diphtheria. The abscess forms behind and around the esophagus, often displacing it to one side, while compressing the more firmly fixed trachea. Symptoms are dyspnea, brassy cough, dysphagia, pain, swelling and redness in the neck, and occasionally, cervical emphysema. An increased retrotracheal space is visible on plain lateral chest films; barium contrast studies are contraindicated if there is cervical perforation. Local extension, exsanguination following erosion into a great vessel, and asphyxia due to tracheal compression are major complications. Appropriate antibiotics and prompt surgical drainage are important. Cervical drainage along the anterior boarder of the sternocleidomastoid is effective to the level of the fourth dorsal vertebra. Antibiotics alone may be adequate in minor instrumental perforations if initiated immediately and the patient is carefully monitored.

Esophageal candidiasis (moniliasis) is the most common esophageal infection. It is not limited to the immunocompromised patient. *Torulopsis glabrata,* an organism related to *Candida,* may cause esophageal ulcers in patients with AIDS. Oral candidiasis is frequently absent. Barium esophagography in the most severely affected patients may show mucosal irregularities, but esophagoscopy and biopsy are the most sensitive and accurate diagnostic studies. Ketoconazole 3–6 mg/kg/24 hr as a single daily oral dose is usually effective. In immunocompromised patients and in patients with systemic infection, amphotericin and/or flucytosine may be necessary.

Viral esophagitis is usually caused by herpes simplex (HSV), cytomegalovirus (CMV), and occasionally, varicella zoster. Only HSV is common in the normal host. Severe odynophagia and dysphagia are the main symptoms. More than 90% of AIDS patients have evidence of CMV dissemination at autopsy, and 10% of liver and kidney transplant patients develop herpes or CMV esophagitis. Infections are often relatively asymptomatic. Esophagoscopy and biopsy are the best diagnostic tests because superinfection with bacteria and *Candida* is common in the immunocompromised host. Most immunocompetent hosts require only symptomatic therapy with analgesics and antacids. Acyclovir, 750 mg/m²/24 hr, in three intravenous divided doses is effective for herpes simplex and varicella zoster. Ganciclovir, 10 mg/kg/24 hr, given intravenously twice a day, is effective for CMV.

Bacterial esophagitis may occasionally be due to extension of a pharyngeal diphtheria infection or extension from a tubercular lymph node. In immunocompromised hosts other bacteria may invade the esophageal mucosa. These lesions will not respond to other therapy for esophagitis and may serve as a source of sepsis.

CORROSIVE ESOPHAGITIS (See Chapter 666.7). This injury most commonly follows ingestion of household cleaning products. Alkalis (70%), acids (20%), bleaches, detergents, microwave overheated baby bottles, and button mercuric oxide batteries are common agents. Alkalis produce a severe, deep, liquefaction necrosis that affects all layers of the esophagus. Household liquid alkali agents used as drain declogging agents contain 8–10% base, industrial strength usually contains 30–35%, whereas granular agents contain 80% base. Concentrated bases are also used to produce crack-cocaine and may be left on the table in poorly labeled containers. Alkalis have no taste; therefore, a child may ingest a significant amount.

Acidic agents include toilet bowl cleaners, drain decloggers, and rust and stain removers; they contain various acids (sulfuric, hydrochloric, oxalic, acid sulfates) with a range of concentrations (8–65%). Acids taste bitter, thus limiting the total volume of ingestion. Volatile acids (HCl) may produce respiratory symptoms. All acids produce a coagulative necrosis and a thick eschar that usually limits the depth of the esophageal injury to the mucosa and superficial muscularis layers. Both alkalis and acids (more likely) can produce severe gastritis.

The peak age of accidental corrosive ingestion is less than 5 yr of age. Corrosive solutions stored in innocuous-appearing containers (pop bottles) and in open, unlocked areas are risk factors. A history of a child with unobserved access to an open container of such substances, with or without chemical burns of the hands or mouth, should strongly suggest the possibility of caustic ingestion.

Clinical manifestations early on include salivation, refusal to drink, nausea, vomiting, epigastric pain, oral burns or ulcerations, fever, and leukocytosis that may clear in a few days, and rarely, esophageal perforation. Esophageal strictures may develop over a few weeks and cause dysphagia and weight loss.

Emergency *treatment* involves the oral administration of large quantities of fluid (water or milk) to dilute the corrosive agent. Neutralization, induced emesis, and gastric lavage are contraindicated. Edema of the pharynx, larynx, or airway may require urgent endotracheal intubation or tracheostomy. The child should be hospitalized, receive nothing by mouth, and be given intravenous fluids.

Esophagogastroscopy with a flexible fiberoptic endoscope should be performed in all patients within 48 hr to identify those without burns who will not need follow-up and to determine the severity of esophageal burns and gastric antral ulceration. Ampicillin may be given for suspected infection; however, perforation with acute mediastinitis requires broad-spectrum antibiotics and the placement of mediastinal drains. Although prednisone therapy was formerly thought to be effective in reducing the incidence and severity of subsequent stricture formation, a randomized controlled trial did not indicate that prednisone was effective. The risk of stricture formation is related directly to the severity of the injury, as determined by circumferential ulcerations, white plaques, and sloughing of the mucosa. Intraluminal stents may reduce stricture formation in severe esophageal burns.

Early detection and dilatation of developing strictures are an important part of continuing care. Severe strictures that do not respond to dilatation and complete obliteration of the lumen can be treated by colonic interposition. Long-term sequelae, in addition to strictures, include the rare occurrence of esophageal carcinoma.

Prevention is critical because the morbidity may be great. Corrosive compounds should be kept in the original containers and out of the reach of children. Dilute formulations should be used in homes, and industrial strength solutions and solids should be kept at work or locked in a safe, hard-to-reach location.

CHAPTER 271

Esophageal Perforation

Perforation may be spontaneous or due to trauma, endoscopy, dilatation, caustic ingestion, erosion of a tracheostomy or endotracheal tube, or, especially in infants, during a difficult tracheal intubation. Many esophageal perforations are iatrogenic.

Spontaneous perforation may follow sudden increases in esophageal pressure, which occur with violent retching, in automobile accidents, or even with compression in the birth canal. Ninety-five per cent of perforations occur on the left side of the distal esophagus in children but occur more commonly on the right side in neonates. Common symptoms are vomiting followed by severe substernal pain, cyanosis, and shock. Esophagography shows extraluminal water-soluble contrast material.

Violent retching can tear the esophageal mucosa and submucosa, causing hematemesis (Mallory-Weiss syndrome). Esophagoscopy should differentiate this disorder from other more serious forms of upper gastrointestinal bleeding. In children, blood replacement is usually sufficient treatment for this self-limited disease.

CHAPTER 272

Esophageal Varices

Esophageal varices may occur in children as a complication of portal hypertension. The principal signs are recurrent, profuse, bright-red hematemesis, and tarry stools, with signs of intravascular volume depletion. Children with esophageal varices often have another source for acute gastrointestinal hemorrhage. Roentgenographic studies with barium may outline the varices, but esophagoscopy is more precise in diagnosis. Treatment of portal hypertension and acute gastrointestinal bleeding is discussed in Chapter 312.

CHAPTER 273 *Foreign Bodies in the Esophagus* (See Chapter 280)

Children swallow a variety of objects that may lodge in the esophagus, usually below the cricopharyngeal muscle, at the level of the aortic arch or just above the diaphragm. Lodging at any other site should suggest coexistent esophageal disease. Coins are the most commonly ingested object, especially in children less than 5 yr old.

CLINICAL MANIFESTATIONS. The swallowing of a foreign body may provoke an attack of coughing, drooling, and choking. Foreign bodies in the esophagus usually cause pain, dysphagia (especially with solid foods), and occasionally dyspnea, owing to compression of the trachea or larynx. After an initial symptom-free period, edema and inflammation produce symptoms of esophageal obstruction. Pain, fever, and shock develop with perforation.

DIAGNOSIS. Radiopaque foreign bodies are easily diagnosed. Coins and other flat objects are usually seen on edge on lateral films. Symtomatic patients with esophageal foreign bodies should be examined by endoscopy to remove the object and to examine the esophageal mucosa for injury. Asymptomatic patients who swallow radiolucent foreign bodies should be administered a barium swallow. If the object is identified in the stomach, only careful follow-up for passage in the stool is required.

TREATMENT. The usual treatment is removal of the object under direct vision with esophagoscopy. Roentgenography should be repeated just prior to the procedure to make sure the foreign body has not passed into the stomach or been vomited. Sharp objects, such as open safety pins, should be removed emergently, as should disc batteries, since they can cause corrosive injury to the esophagus within 4 hr. Asymptomatic coins may be observed for up to 24 hr after ingestion in expectation that they may pass. An alternative procedure for esophageal coins present for less than 24 hr involves passing a Foley catheter beyond the coin under fluoroscopic control, inflating the balloon, and removing the catheter and coin at the same time.

ESOPHAGEAL ANOMALIES

Berdon WE, Baker DH: Vascular anomalies and the infant lungs: Rings, slings and other things. Semin Roentgenol 7:39, 1972.

Depaepe A, Dolk H, Lechat M, et al: The epidemiology of tracheoesophageal fistula and oesophageal atresia in Europe. Arch Dis Child 68:743, 1993.

Kluth D, Steding G, Seidl W: The embryology of foregut malformations. J Pediatr Surg 22:389, 1987.

Puntis J, Ritson D, Holden C, et al: Growth and feeding problems after repair of esophageal atresia. Arch Dis Child 65:84, 1990.

Reyes H, Meller J, Loeff D: Management of esophageal atresia and tracheoesophageal fistula. Clin Perinatol 16:79, 1989.

HIATAL HERNIA AND GASTROESOPHAGEAL REFLUX

Albanese C, Towbin R, Ulman I, et al: Percutaneous gastrojejunostomy versus Nissen fundoplication for enteral feeding of the neurologically impaired child with gastroesophageal reflux. J Pediatr 123:371, 1993.

Borgstein E, Heij H, Beugelar J, et al: Risks and benefits of antireflux operations in neurologically impaired children. Eur J Pediatr 153:248, 1994.

Byrne WJ: Reflux and related phenomena. J Pediatr Gastroenterol Nutr 8:283, 1989.

Cucchiara S, Gobio-Casali L, Balli F, et al: Cimetidine treatment of reflux esophagitis in children: An Italian multicentric study. J Pediatr Gastroenterol Nutr 8:150, 1989.

Dodds WJ, Dent J, Hogan WJ, et al: Mechanisms of gastroesophageal reflux in patients with reflux esophagitis. N Engl J Med 307:1547, 1982.

Hoeffel JC, Nihoul-Fekete C, Schmitt M: Esophageal adenocarcinoma after gastroesophageal reflux in children. J Pediatr 115:259, 1989.

Orenstein SR: Esophageal disorders in infants and children. Curr Opin Pediatr 5:580, 1993.

Vandenplas Y, Deneyer M, Verlinden M, et al: Gastroesophageal reflux incidence and respiratory dysfunction during sleep in infants: Treatment with cisapride. J Pediatr Gastroenterol Nutr 8:31, 1989.

RUMINATION

Richmond JB, Eddy E, Green M: Rumination: A psychosomatic syndrome of infancy. Pediatrics 22:49, 1958.

Sheagren TG, Mangurten HH, Brea F, et al: Rumination—a new complication of neonatal intensive care. Pediatrics 66:551, 1980.

ACHALASIA

Azizkhan RG, Tapper D, Eraklis A: Achalasia in childhood: A 20-year experience. J Pediatr Surg 15:452, 1980.

Maksimak M, Perlmutter DH, Winter HS: The use of nifedipine for the treatment of achalasia in children. J Pediatr Gastroenterol Nutr 5:883, 1986.

Nakayama DK, Shorter NA, Boyle JT, et al: Pneumatic dilatation and operative treatment of achalasia in children. J Pediatr Surg 22:619, 1987.

Pasricha P, Ravich W, Hendrix T, et al: Intrasphincteric botulism toxin for the treatment of achalasia. N Engl J Med 322:774, 1995.

SWALLOWING AND DYSPHAGIA

Illingworth RS: Sucking and swallowing difficulties in infancy: Diagnostic problems of dysphagia. Arch Dis Child 44:655, 1969.

Milov D, Cynamon H, Andres J: Chest pain and dysphagia in adolescents caused by diffuse esophageal spasm. J Pediatr Gastroenterol Nutr 9:450, 1989.

CORROSIVE ESOPHAGITIS

Anderson KD, Rouse TM, Randolph JG: A controlled trial of corticosteroids in children with corrosive injury of the esophagus. N Engl J Med 323:637, 1990.

Gorman RL, Klein-Schwartz W, Oderda GM, et al: Initial symptoms as predictors of esophageal injury in alkaline corrosive ingestions. Am J Emerg Med 10:189, 1992.

Moore WR: Caustic ingestions: Pathophysiology, diagnosis, and treatment. Clin Pediatr 25:192, 1986.

Wijburg FA, Heymans HSA, Urbanus NAM: Caustic esophageal lesions in childhood: Prevention of stricture formation. J Pediatr Surg 24:171, 1989.

FOREIGN BODIES

Campbell JB, Condon VR: Catheter removal of blunt esophageal foreign bodies in children. Pediatr Radiol 19:361, 1989.

Caravati EM, Bennett DL, McElwee NE: Pediatric coin ingestion: A prospective study on the utility of routine roentgenograms. Am J Dis Child 143:549, 1989.

Litovitz T, Schmitz BF: Ingestion of cylindrical and button batteries: An analysis of 2382 cases. Pediatrics 89:747, 1992.

SECTION 4
Stomach and Intestines

CHAPTER 274
*Normal Development, Structure, and Function**

Martin Ulshen

DEVELOPMENT. The gut matures relatively early in fetal life. In the 4-wk, 3-mm embryo, the primitive foregut and hindgut form a simple tube as the stomach and cecum become distinct. This tube then elongates quickly, protrudes into the umbilical cord, and rotates counterclockwise around the superior mesenteric artery. At 8 wk the caudal end becomes continuous with the rectum, which has evolved from the cloaca, and at 10 wk the bowel rapidly re-enters the abdomen. Later, the colon achieves its mature conformation. Rotations of the midgut and hindgut are independent events. Most structural anomalies of the stomach and intestine are attributable to a delay or aberration in this complex series of events.

The pyloric musculature of the stomach is seen by the 3rd mo of gestation, and parietal and chief cells appear by 14 wk. Intestinal-type cells found in the gastric mucosa gradually disappear during fetal life. Relatively mature villi are seen along the intestine by 12 wk, and by 20 wk the crypts are deep and the enterocytes are columnar with some microvilli. Blood vessels and the nerve supply to the gut are fully developed by 12–13 wk. Intramural ganglia appear first at the proximal end so that if their development is interrupted, the effect will be seen in the distal regions. Peristalsis has been recognized as early as 8 wk, but motility is usually not fully coordinated until near term. Lymphoid tissue has developed by 20 wk.

Some functions develop relatively early in the fetal gut; others mature in postnatal life. In the stomach acid secretion is low in the first 5 hr of life and then increases dramatically by 24 hr after birth; acid and pepsin secretion peak during the first 10 days and decrease from 10–30 days after birth. Intrinsic factor secretion rises slowly during the first 2 wk of life, but at term circulating gastrin levels are inexplicably two- to threefold higher than in adults.

Small intestinal function matures throughout prenatal and postnatal life. Epithelial glucose transport is detectable in the jejunum of the human embryo before 20 wk. In infants, the maximum rate of glucose transport is one quarter that of adults. Disaccharidase activities are measurable in the human fetus at 12 wk; sucrase and maltase achieve maximal activities by the 24th and 32nd wk, respectively; but lactase activity rises later, reaching maximal levels by 36 wk. In many children, particularly of black and Asian races, intestinal lactase activity begins to decline after the first few years of life. Fetal intestine is involved in the daily transport of a large amount of amniotic fluid, and there is significant activity of the Na^+ pump in 10-wk-old human fetal gut. Solute transport is probably adequate but marginal in very young infants. Accordingly, relatively severe functional disturbances in response to small intestinal diseases can be anticipated, whereas older children can be expected to have significant reserve function.

Fat absorption is less efficient in term infants than in older children and even less efficient in premature infants than in those at term. Important determinants of these age-related differences are the relatively slow rates of bile salt synthesis and transport in early life and reduced pancreatic secretion.

The human gut is capable of absorbing antigenically significant quantities of intact protein, particularly during the early weeks of life. Entry of potential protein antigens through the mucosal barrier may play a role in later food- and microbe-induced symptoms.

NORMAL STRUCTURE. The serosal layer of the bowel wall is an extension of the peritoneum that extends distally as far as the rectum. There are two muscle layers: outer longitudinal fibers and inner circular ones; in the colon the longitudinal fibers form bands, or taeniae. The submucosa is a rich matrix for lymph and vascular plexuses, containing lymphoid cells and macrophages and, in the duodenum, Brunner glands. A complex enteric nervous system is an important factor in regulating not only microvascular flow but epithelial function. The mucosa of the small bowel is well designed to absorb nutrients because its absorptive surface has a very large area owing to a multitude of constantly moving villi that extend into the lumen. In children these villi tend to be leaflike rather than finger-shaped projections; thus, the functional surface area of the small intestine probably increases with age. The colonic mucosal surface is flat, with numerous tubular crypts opening into the surface; in the rectum the surface is smooth. The lamina propria, a cellular layer just beneath the epithelium that contains cells capable of phagocytosis and immunoglobulin synthesis, provides a connective tissue core for the epithelium and its vascular supply. Lymphoid tissue is concentrated in Peyer patches, which become more numerous in the distal small bowel. There are several types of epithelial cells in the small intestine: the columnar absorptive cell dominates; goblet cells secrete mucus; endocrine cells secrete certain intestinal hormones; in the crypts there are Paneth cells, whose function is unknown; and over areas of lymphoid aggregation there are "m" cells that have a special capacity to absorb intact, potentially antigenic proteins. The columnar absorptive cell is polarized with a microvillus "brush" border at the luminal surface to which a glycocalyx or "fuzz coat" is tightly adherent. Active cell division of the enterocytes occurs in the crypts, and as cells migrate up the villi, they differentiate. A dramatic shift in gene expression occurs at the crypt-villus junction consistent with differentiation of mature villus enterocytes. The jejunal epithelium is completely renewed in 4–5 days, providing a mechanism for rapid repair after injury; but in the very young infant the process may be slow.

NORMAL FUNCTION. The stomach serves as a reservoir that delivers liquefied, blended, but minimally digested food to the intestine. Initial emulsification of fat and digestion of protein occur here. It also secretes intrinsic factor, essential for the assimilation of vitamin B_{12} in the ileum. The small intestine must process not only ingested nutrients but also a large volume of water and shed epithelial cells. In adults the quantity of water entering the gut lumen is at least seven times the amount ingested.

*Dr. Richard Hamilton authored this chapter in previous editions. His contribution is gratefully appreciated.

Intraluminal digestion depends mainly on the exocrine pancreas. Synthesis and secretion of bicarbonate and digestive enzymes are stimulated by secretin and cholecystokinin, which are released by the upper intestinal mucosa in response to various intraluminal stimuli, among them components of the diet. Digestion is an efficient, fast process, usually completed in the most proximal intestinal segment. Bile salts in the lumen facilitate digestion and are essential for the efficient delivery of products of lipid hydrolysis to the absorptive surface of the epithelium. Emulsification aids digestion, and long-chain monoglycerides and fatty acids usually reach the epithelium in the form of mixed micelles with conjugated bile acids and phospholipid. Sterols such as vitamin D are particularly dependent on these micelles for their absorption; accordingly, diseases such as biliary atresia cause particular difficulties with vitamin D assimilation. Medium-chain triglycerides available in certain specially designed therapeutic diets, on the other hand, do not require micelles, emulsification, or hydrolysis for their absorption.

Carbohydrate, protein, and fat are normally absorbed by the upper half of the small intestine; the distal segments represent a vast reserve of absorptive capacity. Most of the sodium, potassium, chloride, and water is absorbed in the small bowel. Bile salts and vitamin B_{12} are selectively absorbed in the distal ileum and iron in the duodenum and proximal jejunum.

Disaccharides are hydrolyzed by disaccharidases on the outer surface of the microvillus membranes, and resultant monosaccharides are actively transported across the cell, primarily to portal venous drainage. Dipeptides and larger peptides can be hydrolyzed at the brush border surface but may also enter the cell intact before they contact peptidases. The small bowel has active transport pathways for specific groups of amino acids and for oligopeptides, similar to those seen in the renal tubule. Monoglycerides and fatty acids enter the epithelium intact; triglycerides are resynthesized, incorporated with phospholipid and lipoprotein into chylomicrons, and released into lymphatics. Medium-chain triglycerides may be taken up intact and released into the portal stream.

The colon extracts additional water and ions from the luminal contents in order to render the stools partially or completely solid. Stools can then be stored in the rectum until distention triggers a defecation reflex that, when assisted by voluntary relaxation of the external sphincter, permits evacuation.

Berseth CL: Effect of early feeding on maturation of the preterm infant's small intestine. J Pediatr 120:947, 1992.

Grand RJ, Watkins JB, Torti FM: Development of the human gastrointestinal tract; a review. Gastroenterology 79:790, 1976.

Henning SJ: Functional development of the gastrointestinal tract. *In:* Johnson LR (ed): Physiology of the Gastrointestinal Tract. New York, Raven Press, 1987, pp 285–302.

Traber PG: Differentiation of intestinal epithelial cells: lessons from the study of intestine-specific gene expression. J Lab Clin Med 123:467, 1994.

CHAPTER 275

Pyloric Stenosis and Other Congenital Anomalies of the Stomach

Robert Wyllie

The hallmark of gastric obstruction is nonbilious vomiting. Other symptoms include abdominal pain and nausea. Signs of gastric outlet obstruction include abdominal distention and bleeding from secondary inflammation of the gastric or esophageal mucosa.

The most common cause of nonbilious vomiting is infantile hypertrophic pyloric stenosis. Similar symptoms may be associated with a variety of other gastric malformations including pyloric atresia, antral webs, gastric duplications, and gastric volvulus. The differential diagnosis includes gastroesophageal reflux, peptic ulcer disease, salt-wasting adrenogenital syndrome, bezoars, and a variety of other metabolic and motility abnormalities.

275.1 Hypertrophic Pyloric Stenosis

Hypertrophic pyloric stenosis occurs in approximately 3:1,000 live births in the United States; its frequency may be increasing. It is more common in whites of northern European ancestry, less common in blacks, and rare in Asians. Males (especially first born) are affected approximately four times as often as females. The offspring of a mother and to a lesser extent the father who had pyloric stenosis are at higher risk for pyloric stenosis. Pyloric stenosis will develop in approximately 20% of the male and 10% of the female descendants of a mother who had pyloric stenosis. An increased incidence of pyloric stenosis is seen in infants with type B and O blood groups. Pyloric stenosis is associated with other congenital defects including tracheoesophageal fistula.

ETIOLOGY. The cause of pyloric stenosis is unknown, but multiple factors have been implicated. Pyloric stenosis is usually not present at birth and is more concordant in monozygotic than dizygotic twins. Abnormal muscle innervation, breast-feeding, and maternal stress in the third trimester have all been implicated. In addition, elevated serum prostaglandins, reduced levels of pyloric nitric oxide synthase, and infant hypergastrinemia have been found but probably represent secondary phenomena caused by gastric stasis and distention. Exogenous administration of prostaglandin E to maintain patency of the ductus arteriosus has been associated with pyloric stenosis as have eosinophilic gastroenteritis and trisomy 18, Turner, Smith-Lemli-Opitz, and Cornelia de Lange syndromes.

CLINICAL MANIFESTATIONS. Nonbilious vomiting is the initial symptom of pyloric stenosis. The vomiting may or may not be projectile initially but is usually progressive, occurring immediately after a feeding. Emesis may follow each feeding, or it may be intermittent. The vomiting usually starts after 3 wk of age, but symptoms may develop as early as the 1st wk of life and as late as the 5th mo. After vomiting, the infant is hungry and wants to feed again. As vomiting continues, there is a progressive loss of fluid, hydrogen ion, and chloride, leading to a hypochloremic metabolic alkalosis. Serum potassium levels are usually maintained, but there may be a total body potassium deficit. A greater awareness of pyloric stenosis has led to earlier identification of the patient with fewer instances of chronic malnutrition and severe dehydration.

Jaundice associated with a decreased level of glucuronyl transferase is seen in approximately 5% of the infants. The jaundice usually resolves promptly after relief of the obstruction.

The *diagnosis* is established by palpating the pyloric mass. The mass is firm, movable, approximately 2 cm in length, olive shaped, hard, best palpated from the left side, and located above and to the right of the umbilicus in the midepigastrium beneath the liver edge. In the healthy infant, feeding can be an aid to the diagnosis. After feeding there may be a visible gastric peristaltic wave that progresses across the abdomen (Fig. 275–1). After the infant vomits, the abdominal muscula-

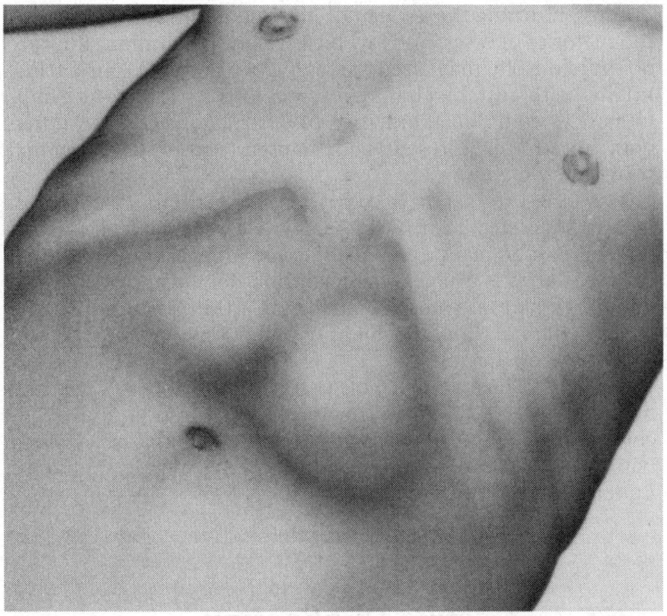

Figure 275–1. Gastric peristaltic wave in an infant with pyloric stenosis.

ture is more relaxed and the "olive" easier to palpate. Sedation may be used to facilitate examination but is usually unnecessary. The diagnosis can be established clinically approximately 60–80% of the time by an experienced examiner.

Imaging procedures are reserved for those infants in whom the diagnosis remains in doubt. Abdominal ultrasonography has replaced barium studies in establishing the diagnosis in difficult cases. Criteria for diagnosis include pyloric muscle thickness greater than 4 mm or an overall pyloric length greater than 14 mm (Fig. 275–2). Ultrasonography has a sensitivity of approximately 90%. When barium studies are performed, they demonstrate an elongated pyloric channel, a bulge of the pyloric muscle into the antrum (shoulder sign), and parallel streaks of barium seen in the narrowed channel, producing a "double tract sign" (Fig. 275–3).

DIFFERENTIAL DIAGNOSIS. The usual case can be diagnosed by the characteristic clinical pattern and the identification of a pyloric mass. Infants who are exceptionally reactive to external stimuli, those fed by inexperienced or anxious caretakers, or those for whom an adequate maternal-infant bonding relationship has not been established may vomit frequently in the early weeks of life. Such infants may come to resemble infants with pyloric stenosis; the vomiting may be persistent and even projectile. Gastric waves are occasionally visible in small, emaciated infants who do not have pyloric stenosis. Chalasia of the esophagus or hiatal hernia usually result in vomiting in the 1st wk of life and can be differentiated from pyloric stenosis by palpation and roentgenographic studies. Adrenal insufficiency may simulate pyloric stenosis, but the absence of a palpable tumor and the metabolic acidosis and elevated serum potassium and urinary sodium concentrations of adrenal insufficiency aid in differentiation. Inborn errors of metabolism may produce recurrent emesis with alkalosis (urea cycle) or acidosis (organic acidemia) and lethargy, coma, or seizures. Vomiting with diarrhea suggests gastroenteritis, but occasionally a patient with pyloric stenosis will have diarrhea. Infrequently, gastroesophageal reflux with or without a hiatal hernia may be confused with pyloric stenosis. Very rarely, a pyloric membrane or pyloric duplication may result in projectile vomiting, visible peristalsis, and, in the case of a duplication, a palpable mass. Duodenal stenosis proximal to the ampulla of Vater results in the clinical features of pyloric stenosis, but there may be no palpable mass.

TREATMENT. The preoperative treatment is directed toward correcting the fluid, acid-base, and electrolyte losses. Intravenous fluid therapy is begun with 0.45–0.9% saline, in 5–10% dextrose, with the addition of potassium chloride in concentrations of 30–50 mEq/L. Fluid therapy should be continued until

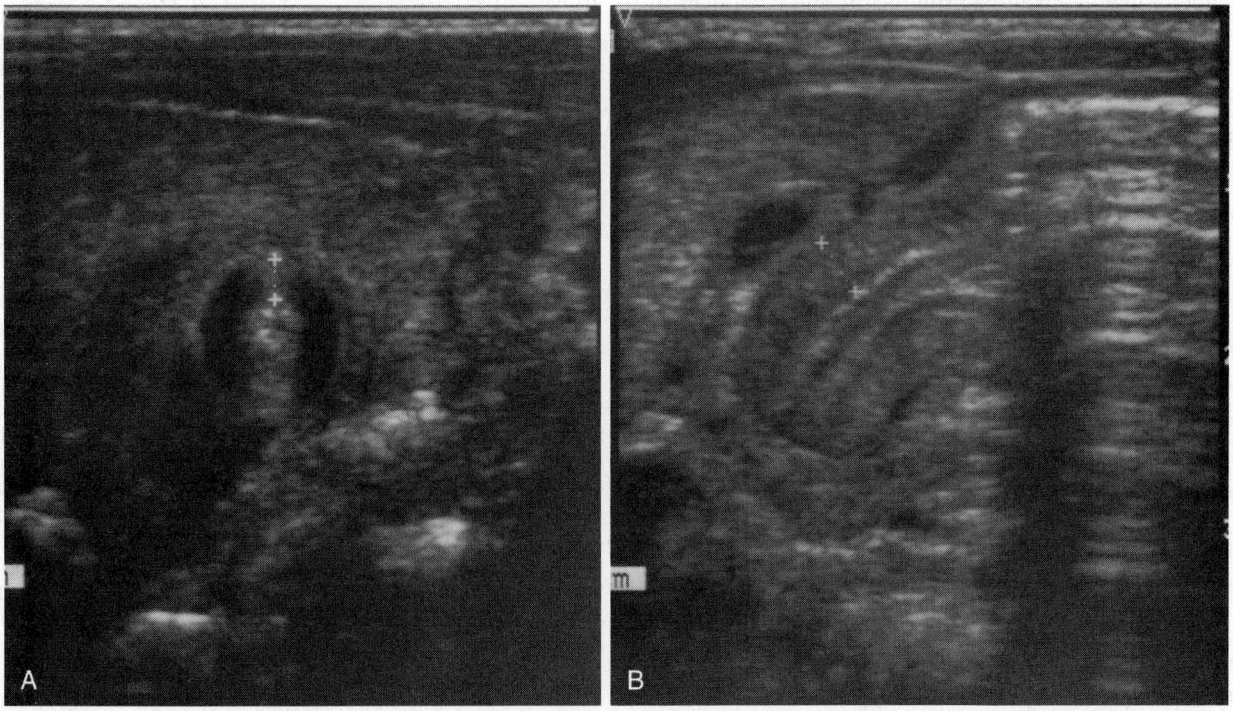

Figure 275–2. *(A)* Transverse sonogram demonstrating a pyloric muscle wall thickness of greater than 4 mm (distance between crosses). *(B)* Horizontal image demonstrating a pyloric channel length greater than 14 mm (wall thickness outlined between crosses) in an infant with pyloric stenosis.

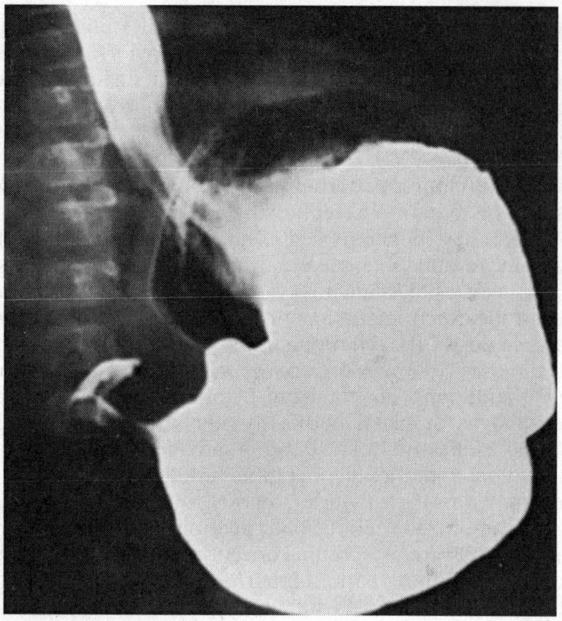

Figure 275–3. Barium in the stomach of an infant with projectile vomiting. The attenuated pyloric canal is typical of congenital hypertrophic pyloric stenosis.

the infant is rehydrated and the serum bicarbonate concentration is less than 30 mEq/dL, which implies that the alkalosis has been corrected. Correction of the alkalosis is essential to prevent postoperative apnea, which may be associated with anesthesia. Most infants can be successfully rehydrated within 24 hr. Vomiting usually stops when the stomach is empty, and only an occasional infant will require nasogastric suction.

The surgical procedure of choice is the Ramstedt pyloromyotomy. The procedure is performed through a short transverse incision or laparoscopically. The underlying pyloric mass is split without cutting the mucosa and the incision closed. Postoperative vomiting may occur in half the infants and is thought to be secondary to edema of the pylorus at the incision site. In most infants, however, feedings can be initiated within 12–24 hr after surgery and advanced to maintenance oral feedings within 36–48 hr of the surgery. Persistent vomiting suggests an incomplete pyloromyotomy, gastritis, hiatal hernia, chalasia, or another cause for the obstruction.

The surgical treatment of pyloric stenosis is curative, with an operative mortality of between 0 and 0.5%. Conservative medical therapy (small frequent feedings, atropine) has been attempted in the past but is associated with slow improvement and a higher mortality. Endoscopic balloon dilation has been successful; these reports need to be confirmed before this practice becomes accepted therapy.

275.2 Congenital Gastric Outlet Obstruction

Gastric outlet obstruction resulting from pyloric atresia and antral webs is uncommon and accounts for less than 1% of all the atresias and diaphragms of the alimentary tract. The cause of the defects is unknown. Pyloric atresia has been associated with epidermolysis bullosa and usually presents in early infancy. The sex distribution is equal.

CLINICAL MANIFESTATIONS. Infants with pyloric atresia present with nonbilious vomiting, feeding difficulties, and abdominal distention during the 1st day of life. Polyhydramnios occurs in the majority of cases, and low birthweight is common. Rupture of the stomach may occur as early as the 1st 12 hr of life. Infants with antral web may present with less dramatic symptoms depending on the degree of obstruction. Older children with antral webs present with nausea, vomiting, abdominal pain, and weight loss.

DIAGNOSIS. The diagnosis of congenital gastric outlet obstruction is suggested by the finding of a large, dilated stomach on abdominal plain roentgenograms. Upper gastrointestinal contrast series is usually diagnostic and demonstrates a pyloric dimple. An antral web may appear as a thin septum near the pyloric channel. In older children, endoscopy has been helpful in identifying antral webs.

TREATMENT. The treatment of gastric outlet obstruction in the neonate starts with the correction of dehydration and hypochloremic alkalosis. Persistent vomiting should be relieved with nasogastric decompression. Operative repair should be undertaken when the patient is stable.

275.3 Gastric Duplication

Gastric duplications are uncommon cystic or tubular structures that usually occur within the wall of the stomach. Most are smaller than 12 cm in diameter and do not usually communicate with the stomach lumen. Associated anomalies occur in up to 35% of the patients. Duplications have been attributed to a failure of recanalization after the solid stage of intestinal development.

The most common *clinical manifestations* are associated with partial or complete gastric outlet obstruction. In 33% of the patients, the cyst may be palpable. Communicating duplications may cause gastric ulceration and be associated with hematemesis or melena.

Gastric duplications are visualized on upper gastrointestinal series as an extrinsic defect usually located along the lesser curve of the stomach. Computed tomography or sonography may be helpful in defining a cystic structure. Surgical excision is the treatment of symptomatic gastric duplications.

275.4 Gastric Volvulus

Gastric volvulus presents with a triad of a sudden onset of severe epigastric pain, intractable retching with emesis, and inability to pass a tube into the stomach. The stomach is tethered longitudinally by the gastrohepatic, gastrosplenic, and gastrocolic ligaments. In the transverse axis, it is tethered by the gastrophrenic ligament and the retroperitoneal attachment of the duodenum. A volvulus occurs when one of these attachments is absent or stretched, allowing the stomach to rotate around itself. In most children, other associated defects are present, including intestinal malrotation, diaphragmatic defects, or asplenia. Volvulus may occur along the longitudinal axis, producing organoaxial volvulus, or along the transverse axis, producing mesenteroaxial volvulus.

CLINICAL MANIFESTATIONS. The clinical presentation of gastric volvulus is nonspecific and suggests high intestinal obstruction. Gastric volvulus in infancy is usually associated with nonbilious vomiting. Acute volvulus may advance rapidly to strangulation and perforation. Chronic gastric volvulus is more common in older children, and the children present with a history of emesis, abdominal pain, and early satiety.

The *diagnosis* is suggested in plain abdominal radiographs by the presence of a dilated stomach. Erect abdominal films demonstrate a double fluid level with a characteristic "beak" near the lower esophageal junction in mesenteroaxial volvulus. In organoaxial volvulus, a single air-fluid level is seen without the characteristic beak. *Treatment* of acute gastric volvulus is emergent surgery once the patient is stabilized. In selected cases of chronic volvulus in older patients, endoscopic correction has been successful.

Kovalivker M, Erez I, Shneider N, et al: The value of ultrasound in the diagnosis of congenital hypertrophic pyloric stenosis. Clin Pediatr 32:281, 1993.
Macdessi J, Oates R: Clinical diagnosis of pyloric stenosis: A declining art. BMJ 306:553, 1993.
Mitchell L, Risch N: The genetics of infantile hypertrophic pyloric stenosis. Am J Dis Child 147:1203, 1993.
Rollins MD, Shields MD, Quinn RJM, et al: Pyloric stenosis: Congenital or acquired? Arch Dis Child 64:138, 1989.
Tack ED, Perlman JM, Bower RJ, et al: Pyloric stenosis in the sick premature infant: Clinical and radiological findings. Am J Dis Child 142:68, 1988.
Touloukian RJ, Higgins E: The spectrum of serum electrolytes in hypertrophic pyloric stenosis. J Pediatr Surg 18:394, 1983.

CHAPTER 276
Intestinal Atresia, Stenosis, and Malrotation

Robert Wyllie

GENERAL CONSIDERATIONS. Intestinal obstruction occurs in approximately 1:1,500 live births. Obstruction may be partial or complete and may arise from intrinsic or extrinsic abnormalities of the gut. Obstruction can be further classified as simple or strangulating. Simple obstruction is associated with the failure of progression of aboral flow of luminal contents. Strangulating obstruction is associated with the impaired blood flow to the intestine in addition to obstruction of the flow of luminal contents. If strangulating obstruction is not promptly relieved, it may lead to bowel infarction and perforation.

Obstruction is typically associated with an accumulation of ingested food, gas, and intestinal secretions proximal to the point of obstruction, leading to distention of the bowel. As the bowel dilates, intestinal absorption decreases and secretion of fluid and electrolytes increases. The shift in fluid and electrolytes results in isotonic intravascular depletion usually associated with hypokalemia. The gut proximal to the obstruction initially demonstrates an increase in contractile activity, which is followed by a marked decrease with hypoactive bowel sounds. The combination of fluid accumulation and hypomotility is associated with nausea and vomiting.

From an anatomic standpoint congenital obstructive lesions of the intestines can be viewed as *intrinsic* (e.g., atresia, stenosis, meconium ileus, and aganglionic megacolon) or *extrinsic* (e.g., malrotation, constricting bands, intra-abdominal hernias, and duplications). An attempt should be made to locate the lesion preoperatively in order to guide the surgical approach.

When the obstruction is *complete,* there should be little difficulty in clinical recognition, but when it is *incomplete,* there may be considerable diagnostic difficulty. Polyhydramnios frequently accompanies high intestinal obstruction, as it does esophageal atresia. When polyhydramnios has been noted, the infant's stomach should be aspirated immediately after birth. Aspiration of 15–20 mL or more of gastric fluid, especially if it is bile stained, is suggestive of a high intestinal obstruction.

Meconium stools may be passed initially if the obstruction is in the upper part of the small intestine or if the obstruction developed late in intrauterine life.

When obstruction is *incomplete* (as, for example, with intestinal stenosis, constricting bands, duplications, and incomplete volvulus), signs (vomiting, abdominal distention, obstipation) may appear shortly after birth or may be delayed an indeterminate time. They may approach in severity those of a completely obstructive lesion, or they may be sufficiently mild and infrequent as to be overlooked until either an acute episode or diagnostic studies disclose the lesion. Incomplete obstruction may present as urgent a need as complete obstruction for surgical intervention.

Atresia refers to complete obstruction of the bowel lumen, and stenosis refers to a partial block of luminal contents. Intestinal atresia is common in the duodenum, jejunum, and ileum and rare in the colon. Intestinal atresia accounts for approximately 33% of all cases of neonatal intestinal obstruction. Atresias affect males and females equally.

Blood flow to the obstructed bowel decreases as the bowel dilates. Blood flow is shifted away from the mucosa with loss of mucosal integrity. Bacteria proliferate in the stagnant bowel with a predominance of coliforms and anaerobes. The rapid proliferation of bacteria coupled with the loss of mucosal integrity allows bacterial translocation across the bowel wall, resulting in endotoxemia, bacteremia, and sepsis.

The *clinical presentation* of intestinal obstruction varies with the cause, level of obstruction, and time between the obstructing event and the patient's evaluation. The classic symptoms of obstruction include nausea and vomiting, abdominal distention, and obstipation. Obstruction high in the intestinal tract involving the duodenum or proximal jejunum results in large-volume, frequent, bilious emesis. Pain is intermittent and is usually relieved by vomiting. The pain is localized to the epigastrium or periumbilical area, and there is little abdominal distention. Obstruction in the distal small bowel leads to moderate or marked abdominal distention with emesis that is progressively feculent. Pain is usually diffuse over the entire abdomen.

No laboratory studies are diagnostic of obstruction or differentiate simple obstruction from obstruction associated with bowel infarction. Obstruction high in the gastrointestinal tract is often associated with hypochloremic metabolic alkalosis. Marked leukocytosis with or without thrombocytopenia, metabolic acidosis, and hematochezia suggests bowel infarction. Serum amylase and lipase determinations should be made to rule out pancreatitis.

Bowel obstruction is almost always suggested on the basis of history and physical examination. Imaging is used to confirm the diagnosis and localize the area of obstruction. Plain supine and erect roentgenographs are the initial studies.

Valuable information on the location of congenital obstructive lesions in the intestine may often be obtained from flat and upright roentgenograms of the abdomen taken without use of contrast media. With completely obstructing lesions there will be distention of the bowel above the obstruction, and there may be a series of fluid levels with superimposed gas in the distended loops in the upright or cross-table lateral position. Pneumoperitoneum may be seen, with free air in the subphrenic regions or over the liver in the left lateral decubitus position. Calcification within the peritoneal cavity usually indicates meconium peritonitis. Rarely, obstruction with intraluminal calcification may be associated with rectourinary fistula, colonic aganglionosis, or intestinal atresia. A characteristic ground-glass appearance in the right lower quadrant with trapped bubbles of air within the obstructing meconium may be seen in patients with meconium ileus. Air is usually demonstrable roentgenographically in the stomach of the normal infant immediately after birth; within 1 hr air may reach the proximal portion of the small intestine and segments of the colon; air may become visible in the distal parts of the colon as early as the 3rd hr or as late as 18 hr. It is difficult to accurately differentiate small from large-bowel obstruction in children younger than 2 yr.

Ultrasonography is helpful in identifying pyloric stenosis and in differentiating it from other causes of proximal obstruction. Contrast studies of the bowel are indicated when plain films or ultrasonograms fail to identify the source of obstruction. Water-soluble contrast studies avoid the risk of barium contamination of the peritoneum when there is a significant chance of perforation not detected by the presence of pneumoperitoneum on plain films. Water-soluble contrast enemas are useful is diagnosing malrotation, meconium ileus, meconium plug, and intussusception. In meconium ileus, meconium plug and intussusception in the enema may be diagnostic and relieve the obstruction. Oral or nasogastric contrast is used to identify obstructing lesions in the proximal bowel (atresia, volvulus, malrotation). Water-soluble agents are used if perforation is suspected.

MANAGEMENT. Infants and children with bowel obstruction suffer from intestinal block and loss of fluid and electrolytes. Those with strangulating vascular obstruction may also manifest intestinal ischemia with sepsis and shock. Initial treatment must be directed at fluid resuscitation and stabilizing the patient. Nasogastric decompression usually provides relief of pain and vomiting. After appropriate cultures, broad-spectrum antibiotics are usually started in neonates with bowel obstruction and those with suspected strangulating infarction. Patients with strangulation must have immediate surgical relief before the bowel infarcts, resulting in gangrene and intestinal perforation. Extensive intestinal necrosis results in short-gut syndrome (Chapter 286.7). Nonoperative conservative management is usually limited to children with suspected adhesions or inflammatory strictures that may resolve with nasogastric decompression or anti-inflammatory medications. If clinical signs of improvement are not evident within 12–24 hr, then operative intervention is usually indicated.

276.1 Duodenal Obstruction

Duodenal atresia is thought to arise from failure to recanalize the lumen after the solid phase of intestinal development during the 4th and 5th wk of gestation. The incidence of duodenal atresia is 1 in 10,000 births and accounts for approximately 25–40% of all intestinal atresias. Half the patients are born prematurely. Duodenal atresia may take several forms, including an intact membrane obstructing the lumen, a short fibrous cord connecting two blind duodenal pouches, or a gap between the nonconnecting ends of the duodenum. An unusual cause of obstruction is a "windsock" web, which is a distensible flap of tissue associated with anomalies of the biliary tract. The membranous form of atresia is most common, with obstruction occurring distal to the ampulla of Vater in the majority of patients. Duodenal obstruction may also be the result of an extrinsic compression such as an annular pancreas or from Ladd bands in patients with malrotation. Down syndrome occurs in 20–30% of the patients with duodenal atresia. Other congenital anomalies that are associated with duodenal atresia include malrotation (20%), esophageal atresia (10–20%), congenital heart disease (10–15%), and anorectal and renal anomalies (5%).

CLINICAL MANIFESTATIONS. The hallmark of duodenal obstruction is bilious vomiting without abdominal distention, which is usually noted on the 1st day of life. Peristaltic waves may be visualized early in the disease process. A history of polyhydramnios is present in half the pregnancies and is caused by a failure of absorption of amniotic fluid in the distal intestine. Jaundice is present in one third of the infants. The diagnosis is suggested by the presence of a "double bubble sign" on plain abdominal radiographs (Fig. 276–1). The appearance is caused by a distended and gas-filled stomach and proximal duodenum. Contrast studies are usually not necessary and may be associated with aspiration if attempted. Contrast studies may occasionally be needed to exclude malrotation and volvulus because intestinal infarction may occur within 6–12 hr if the volvulus is not relieved. Prenatal diagnosis of duodenal atresia is being made with increasing frequency by fetal ultrasonography.

TREATMENT. The initial treatment of infants with duodenal atresia includes naso- or orogastric decompression with intravenous fluid replacement. Echocardiogram and radiology of the chest and spine should be performed to evaluate for associated anomalies. Approximately one third of the infants with duodenal atresia will have associated life-threatening congenital anomalies. Definitive correction of duodenal atresia is usually postponed to evaluate and treat these life-threatening anomalies.

The usual surgical repair for duodenal atresia is duodenoduodenostomy. The dilated proximal bowel may be tapered in an attempt to improve peristalsis. A gastrostomy tube may be placed to drain the stomach and protect the airway. Intravenous nutritional support or a transanastomotic jejunal tube is needed until the infant starts to feed orally. The prognosis is primarily dependent on the presence of associated anomalies.

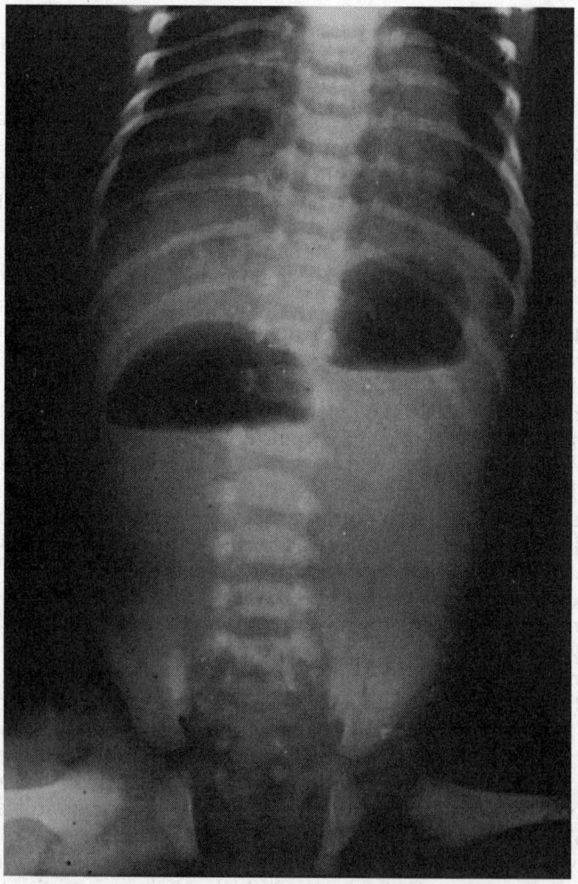

Figure 276–1. Abdominal roentgenogram of a newborn infant held upright. Note the "double bubble" gas shadow above and the absence of gas in the distal bowel in this case of congenital duodenal atresia.

If obstruction is due to Ladd bands with malrotation, an operation is necessary without delay. After division of the abnormal peritoneal folds or bands, the entire large intestine is placed within the left side of the abdomen, after first removing the appendix, with the small bowel on the right—the fetal position of nonrotation. An appendectomy is done to avoid later misdiagnosis of appendicitis. Malrotation may also coexist with an intrinsic duodenal obstruction, such as a membrane or stenosis; this may be identified by passing a nasogastric balloon-tipped catheter into the jejunum below the site of obstruction, inflating the balloon, and slowly withdrawing the catheter. Annular pancreas is best treated by duodenoduodenostomy without dividing the pancreas, leaving as short a defunctioned loop as possible. Duodenal diaphragmatic obstruction is managed by duodenoplasty. The possibility exists that the common bile duct may open on the diaphragm itself.

276.2 Jejunal and Ileal Atresia and Obstruction

Jejunoileal atresias have been attributed to intrauterine vascular obstructive accidents of the bowel. Four different types of jejunal and ileal atresia are encountered (Fig. 276–2). Type I accounts for 20% of the atresias and is an intraluminal diaphragm that obstructs the lumen while continuity is maintained between the proximal and distal bowel. In type II, a small-diameter solid cord connects the proximal and distal bowel, accounting for about 35% of defects. Type III is divided into two subtypes. Type IIIa accounts for approximately 35% of all atresias and occurs when both ends of the bowel end in blind loops accompanied by a small mesenteric defect. Type IIIb is associated with an extensive mesenteric defect and a loss of the normal blood supply to the distal bowel. The distal ileum coils around the ileocolic artery, from which it derives its entire blood supply, producing an "apple peel" appearance. This anomaly is associated with prematurity, an unusually short distal ileum, and a significant foreshortening of the bowel. Type IV is multiple segments of bowel atresia and accounts for approximately 5% of all bowel atresias. Colon atresia has similarities to jejunoileal atresia but is much less common.

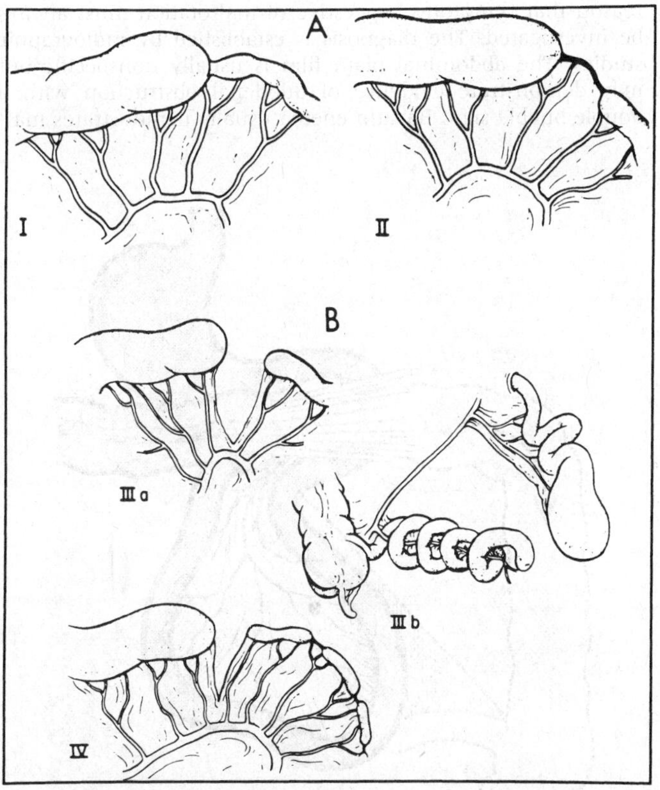

Figure 276–2. *(A, B)* **Classification of intestinal atresia. Type I: Mucosal obstruction caused by an intraluminal membrane with intact bowel wall and mesentery. Type II: Blind ends are separated by a fibrous cord. Type IIIa: Blind ends are separated by a V-shaped mesenteric defect. Type IIIb: "Apple peel" appearance. Type IV: Multiple atresias. (From Grosfeld J: Jejunoileal atresia and stenosis.** ***In:*** **Welch KJ, et al (eds): Pediatric Surgery, 4th ed. Chicago, Year Book Medical Publishers, 1986, p 843.)**

Meconium ileus occurs in newborn infants with cystic fibrosis, but less than 10% of patients with the latter experience meconium ileus. The last 20–30 cm of ileum are collapsed and filled with pellets of pale-colored stool, above which a dilated loop of varying length appears obstructed by meconium with the consistency of thick syrup or glue. Peristalsis fails to propel this very viscid material forward, so that it becomes impacted in the ileum. Volvulus, atresia, or perforation of the bowel may accompany meconium ileus. Perforation in utero produces meconium peritonitis. Intraperitoneal meconium can cause dense adhesions leading postnatally to adhesive intestinal obstruction and may rapidly become calcified.

In 5% of patients with *Hirschsprung disease,* the aganglionic segment involves not only the entire colon but also terminal ileum. This condition causes a dilated small intestine with ganglionated but somewhat hypertrophied walls, a funnel-shaped transitional hypoganglionic zone, and a collapsed distal aganglionic bowel.

CLINICAL MANIFESTATIONS. In contrast to duodenal atresia, extragastrointestinal anomalies are less common in atresias of the remaining intestine. The diagnosis of jejunoileal atresia may be made by prenatal ultrasonograms. Polyhydramnios occurs in 25% of affected patients. Monozygotic twins are at higher risk for atresias than are dizygotic twins or singletons. Premature birth occurs in one third of infants. Most infants become symptomatic during the 1st day of life with abdominal distention and bile-stained emesis or gastric aspirate. Sixty to 75% of the infants will fail to pass meconium. Jaundice has been found in one fifth to one third of the patients. Plain radiographs will demonstrate multiple air-fluid levels or peritoneal calcification associated with meconium peritonitis. Contrast studies of the upper and lower bowel delineate the level of obstruction and differentiate atresia from meconium ileus, meconium plug, and Hirschsprung disease.

In meconium ileus plain films of the abdomen show a typical hazy or ground-glass appearance in the right lower quadrant. Small bubbles of gas trapped in meconium are dispersed within this area. Furthermore, owing to their viscid contents, moderately dilated loops of bowel do not have the air-fluid levels usually seen roentgenographically on the erect projection. If there is meconium peritonitis, patchy calcification may be noted, usually in the flanks. Pneumoperitoneum is most readily seen as free air between the liver and the diaphragm on an upright roentgenogram of the abdomen; if there is a large amount of free air, the entire abdomen may look like a football from distention with air; the ligamentum teres is sometimes clearly visible in the midline.

It is impossible to consistently distinguish small bowel from large bowel by studying plain roentgenograms of the abdomen in newborns and infants. If plain roentgenograms are nonspecific, a barium or Gastrografin study of the colon may be needed to distinguish small- from large-intestine obstructions. A small colon, "microcolon," suggests disuse and the presence of obstruction proximal to the ileocecal valve. Gastrografin enemas should be used with caution in the diagnosis and treatment of meconium ileus because their hyperosmolality may result in dehydration, and undue injection pressure may result in perforation.

TREATMENT. Patients with small-bowel obstruction should be stable and in adequate fluid and electrolyte balance before operation or roentgenographic attempts at disimpaction unless volvulus is suspected. Infections should be treated with appropriate antibiotics. Prophylactic use of antibiotics is indicated and should be given intravenously shortly before surgery.

Ileal or jejunal atresia requires resection of the dilated proximal portion of the bowel followed by end-to-end anastomosis. If a simple mucosal diaphragm is present, jejunoplasty or ileoplasty with partial excision of the web is an acceptable alternative to resection. With meconium ileus an attempt to reduce obstruction with a Gastrografin enema containing polysorbate and a detergent (Tween 80) is usually indicated. The material should be allowed to flow around the pellets of stool in the terminal ileum and into the dilated proximal small bowel containing the obstructing meconium, where it will result in an outpouring of fluid from the bowel wall, dilution of the viscid meconium, and diarrhea. The enema may have to be repeated after 8–12 hr. Resection after reduction is not needed if there have been no ischemic complications.

About 50% of patients with meconium ileus do not adequately respond to Gastrografin enemas and will need a laparotomy. A simple small ileotomy is done within a pursestring suture just large enough to allow the insertion of a No. 10 or No. 12 French catheter. The catheter is used to irrigate and remove the viscid contents of the bowel, using acetylcysteine as a mucolytic agent in concentrations of less than 5%. Once the contents have been aspirated, the pursestring suture is tied and a small drain is placed near the ileostomy, making resections and anastomoses unnecessary.

At laparotomy for pneumoperitoneum, colostomy or ileostomy may be needed at the site of perforation; if the perforation is of the stomach, duodenum, or upper jejunum, primary closure is preferred. Total parenteral nutrition will be required.

276.3 Malrotation

Malrotation is the incomplete rotation of the intestine during fetal development. The gut starts as a straight tube from stomach to rectum. The midbowel (distal duodenum to midtransverse colon) begins to elongate and progressively protrudes into the umbilical cord until it lies totally outside the confines of the abdominal cavity. As the developing bowel rotates in and out of the abdominal cavity, the superior mesenteric artery, which supplies blood to this section of gut, acts as an axis. The duodenum, on re-entering the abdominal cavity, moves to the region of the ligament of Treitz, and the colon that follows is directed to the left upper quadrant. The cecum subsequently rotates counterclockwise within the abdominal cavity and comes to lie in the right lower quadrant. The duodenum becomes fixed to the posterior abdominal wall before the colon is completely rotated. After rotation, the right and left colon and the mesenteric root become fixed to the posterior abdomen. These attachments provide a broad base of support to the mesentery and the superior mesenteric artery, thus preventing twisting of the mesenteric root and kinking of the vascular supply. Abdominal rotation and attachment is completed by 3 mo gestation.

Nonrotation occurs when the bowel fails to rotate after it returns to the abdominal cavity. The first and second portions of the duodenum are in their normal position, but the remainder of the duodenum, jejunum, and ileum occupy the right side of the abdomen while the colon is located on the left. Malrotation and nonrotation are associated with abdominal heterotaxia and the asplenia-polysplenia congenital heart malformation syndrome anomalad (Chapter 387.18).

The most common type of malrotation involves the failure of the cecum to move into the right lower quadrant (Fig. 276–3). The usual location of the cecum is in the subhepatic area. Failure of the cecum to rotate properly is associated with a failure to form the normal broad-based adherence to the posterior abdominal wall. The mesentery including the superior mesenteric artery is tethered by a narrow stalk, which may twist around itself, producing a midgut volvulus. In addition, bands of tissue (Ladd bands) may extend from the cecum to the right upper quadrant, crossing and possibly obstructing the duodenum.

CLINICAL MANIFESTATIONS. The majority of patients present within the 1st yr of life with symptoms of acute or chronic obstruction. Infants often present within the 1st wk of life with bilious emesis and acute bowel obstruction. Older infants present with episodes of recurrent abdominal pain that may mimic colic. Malrotation in older children may present with recurrent episodes of vomiting, abdominal pain, or both. Occasionally, patients present with malabsorption or protein-losing enteropathy associated with bacterial overgrowth. Symptoms are caused by intermittent volvulus or duodenal compression by Ladd bands or other adhesive bands affecting the small and large bowel. Twenty-five to 50% of adolescents with malrotation are asymptomatic. Adolescents who become symptomatic present with acute intestinal obstruction or history of recurrent episodes of abdominal pain with less frequent vomiting and diarrhea.

An acute presentation of small-bowel obstruction is usually the result of volvulus associated with malrotation. This is a life-threatening complication of malrotation, and the main reason that symptoms suggestive of malrotation must always be investigated. The diagnosis is established by radiographic studies. The abdominal plain film is usually nonspecific but may demonstrate evidence of duodenal obstruction with a double bubble sign. Barium enema usually demonstrates mal-

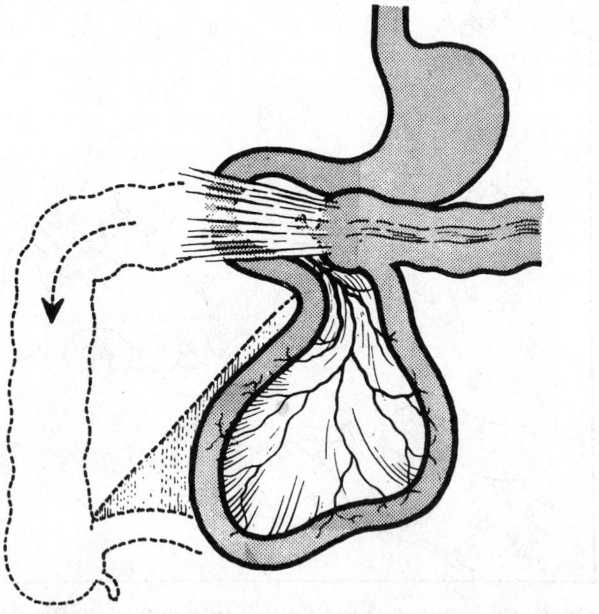

Figure 276–3. The mechanism of intestinal obstruction with incomplete rotation of the midgut (malrotation). The *dotted lines* show the course the cecum should have taken. Failure to rotate has left obstructing bands across the duodenum, and a narrow pedicle for the midgut loop, making it susceptible to volvulus. (From Nixon HH, O'Donnell B: The Essentials of Pediatric Surgery. Philadelphia, JB Lippincott, 1961.)

position of the cecum but may be normal in 10% of patients. Upper gastrointestinal series demonstrates malposition of the ligament of Treitz, confirming the diagnosis of malrotation, and is the initial procedure performed in nonobstructed patients.

The treatment of malrotation is surgical. If a volvulus is present, it is reduced and the duodenum and upper jejunum are freed of any bands and remain in the right abdominal cavity. The colon is freed of adhesions and placed in the right abdomen with the cecum in the left lower quadrant usually accompanied by incidental appendectomy. Extensive intestinal ischemia from volvulus produces the short-gut syndrome (Chapter 286.7). Persistent symptoms after repair of malrotation should suggest a pseudo-obstruction–like motility disorder.

INTESTINAL ATRESIA

Ahlgren L: Apple peel jejunal atresia. J Pediatr Surg 22:451, 1987.
Atwell JD, Klidian AM: Vertebral anomalies and duodenal atresia. J Pediatr Surg 17:237, 1982.
Cragan JD, Martin ML, Waters GD, et al: Increased risk of small intestinal atresia among twins in the United States. Arch Pediatr Adolesc Med 148:733, 1994.
Doolin EJ: Motility abnormality in intestinal atresia. J Pediatr Surg 22:320, 1987.
Duffy LF: Malformation of the gut. Pediatr Rev 13:50, 1992.
Lilien LD, Srinivasan G, Pyati SP, et al: Green vomiting in the first 72 hours in normal infants. Am J Dis Child 140:662, 1986.
Reyes H, Meller J, Loeff D: Neonatal intestinal obstruction. Clin Perinatol 16:85, 1989.
Smith GHH, Glasson M: Intestinal atresia: Factors affecting survival. Aust N Z J Surg 59:151, 1989.

MALROTATION

Coombs RC, Buick RG, Gornall PG, et al: Intestinal malrotation: The role of small intestinal dysmotility in the cause of persistent symptoms. J Pediatr Surg 26:553, 1991.
Devane SP, Coombes R, Smith VV, et al: Persistent gastrointestinal symptoms after correction of malrotation. Arch Dis Child 67:218, 1992.
Ford EG, Senac MO, Srikanth MS, et al: Malrotation of the intestine in children. Ann Surg 215:172, 1992.
Messineo A, MacMillan JH, Palder SB, et al: Clinical factors affecting mortality in children with malrotation of the intestine. J Pediatr Surg 27:1343, 1992.
Rescorla FJ, Shedd FJ, Grosfeld JL, et al: Anomalies of intestinal rotation in childhood: Analysis of 447 cases. Surgery 108:710, 1990.
Schey WL, Donaldson JS, Sty JR: Malrotation of the bowel: Variable patterns with different surgical considerations. J Pediatr Surg 147:40, 1993.
Seashore JH, Touloukian RJ: Midgut volvulus: An ever-present threat. Arch Pediatr Adolesc Med 148:43, 1994.
Weinberger E, Winters WD, Liddell RM, et al: Sonographic diagnosis of intestinal malrotation in infants: Importance of the relative positions of the superior mesenteric vein and artery. AJR 159:825, 1992.

MECONIUM ILEUS

Caniano DA, Beaver BL: Meconium ileus: A fifteen-year experience with forty-two neonates. Surgery 102:699, 1987.
Miller A, Rode H, Cywes S: Management of uncomplicated meconium ileus with T-tube ileostomy. Arch Dis Child 63:390, 1988.
Rescoria FJ, Grosfeld JL, West KJ, et al: Changing patterns of treatment and survival in neonates with meconium ileus. Arch Surg 124:837, 1989.
Venugopal S, Shandling B: Meconium ileus: Laparotomy without resection, anastomosis or enterostomy. J Pediatr Surg 14:715, 1979.
Wagget J, Bishop HC, Koop CE: Experience with Gastrografin enema in the treatment of meconium ileus. J Pediatr Surg 5:649, 1970.

CHAPTER 277
Intestinal Duplications, Meckel Diverticulum, and Other Remnants of the Omphalomesenteric Duct

Robert Wyllie

277.1 Intestinal Duplication

Duplications of the intestinal tract are rare anomalies that consist of well-formed tubular or spherical structures firmly attached to the intestine with a common blood supply. The lining of the duplications resembles that of the gastrointestinal tract. Duplications are located on the mesenteric border and may communicate with the intestinal lumen. Duplications can be classified into three categories: localized duplications, duplications associated with spinal cord defects and vertebral malformations, and duplications of the colon. Occasionally (10–15%) there are multiple duplications.

Localized duplications may occur in any area of the gastrointestinal tract but are most common in the ileum and jejunum. They are usually cystic or tubular structures within the wall of the bowel. The cause is unknown, but their development has been attributed to defects in recanalization of the intestinal lumen after the solid stage of embryologic development. Duplication of the intestine occurring in association with vertebral and spinal cord anomalies (hemivertebra, anterior spina bifida, band connection between lesion and cervical or thoracic spine) is thought to arise from a splitting of the notochord in the developing embryo. Duplication of the colon is usually associated with anomalies of the urinary tract and genitalia. Duplication of the entire colon, rectum, anus, and terminal ileum may occur. The defects are thought to be secondary to caudal twinning with duplication of the hindgut, genital, and lower urinary tracts.

CLINICAL MANIFESTATIONS. Symptoms depend on the size, location, and mucosal lining. Duplications may cause bowel obstruction by compressing the adjacent intestinal lumen, or they may act as the lead point of an intussusception or a site for a volvulus. If they are lined by acid-secreting mucosa, they may cause ulceration, perforation, and hemorrhage of the adjacent bowel. The patient may present with abdominal pain, vomiting, palpable mass, or acute gastrointestinal hemorrhage. Intestinal duplications in the thorax (neuroenteric cysts) may present with respiratory distress. Duplications of the lower bowel may cause constipation or diarrhea or be associated with recurrent prolapse of the rectum.

The *diagnosis* is suspected by the history and physical examination. Radiologic studies such as barium studies, ultrasonography, computed tomography, and magnetic resonance scans are helpful but usually nonspecific, demonstrating cystic structures or mass effects. Radioisotope technetium scanning may localize ectopic gastric mucosa. The *treatment* of duplications is surgical resection and management of associated defects.

277.2 Meckel Diverticulum and Other Remnants of the Omphalomesenteric Duct

A Meckel diverticulum is a remnant of the embryonic yolk sac, which may also be referred to as the omphalomesenteric

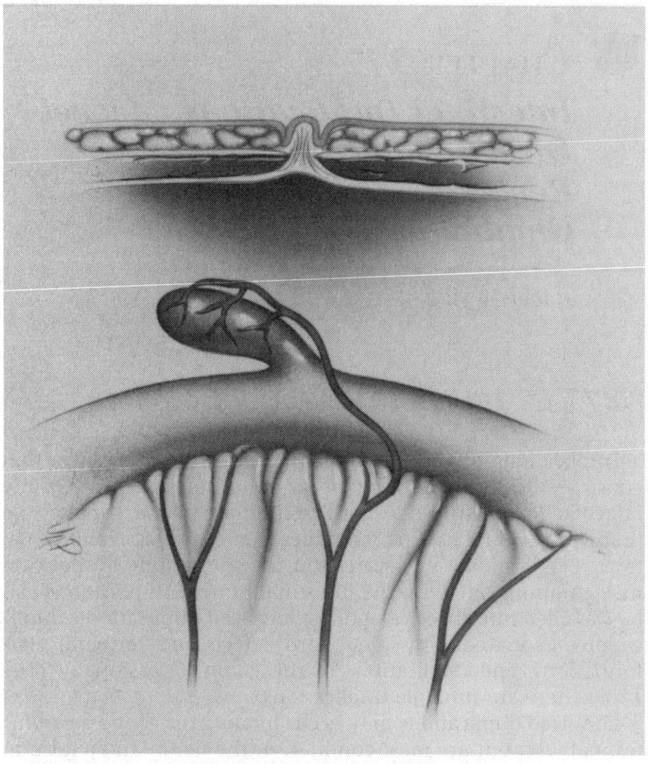

Figure 277–1. Typical Meckel's diverticulum located on the antimesenteric border.

duct or vitelline duct. The omphalomesenteric duct connects the yolk sac to the gut in the developing embryo and provides nutrition until the placenta is established. Between the 5th and 7th wk of gestation, the duct attenuates and separates from the intestine. Just before this involution, the epithelium of the yolk sac develops a lining similar to that of the stomach. Partial or complete failure of involution of the omphalomesenteric duct results in various residual structures. Meckel diverticulum is the most common of these structures and is the most frequent congenital gastrointestinal anomaly, occurring in 2–3% of all infants. A typical Meckel diverticulum is a 3- to 6-cm outpouching of the ileum along the antimesenteric border approximately 50–75 cm from the ileocecal valve (Fig. 277–1). The distance from the ileocecal valve depends on the age of the patient. Other omphalomesenteric duct remnants occur infrequently, including a persistently patent duct, a solid cord, or a cord with a central cyst or a diverticulum associated with a persistent cord between the diverticulum and the umbilicus.

CLINICAL MANIFESTATIONS. Symptoms from a Meckel diverticulum usually arise within the 1st 2 yr of life, but initial symptoms are common during the 1st decade. The majority of symptomatic Meckel diverticula are lined by an ectopic mucosa, including an acid-secreting mucosa, that causes intermittent, painless rectal bleeding by ulceration of the adjacent normal ileal mucosa. Unlike the upper duodenal mucosa, the acid is not neutralized by pancreatic bicarbonate.

The stool is typically described as brick colored or currant jelly colored in appearance. Bleeding may cause significant anemia but is usually self-limited because of contraction of the splanchnic vessels as the patient becomes hypovolemic. Bleeding from a Meckel diverticulum can also be less dramatic with melanotic stools.

Less often, a Meckel diverticulum may be associated with partial or complete bowel obstruction. The most common mechanism of obstruction is when the diverticulum acts as the lead point of an intussusception. This presentation is more common in older male children. Other causes of obstruction may result from intraperitoneal bands connecting residual omphalomesenteric duct remnants to ileum and umbilicus. These bands cause obstruction by internal herniation or volvulus of the small bowel around the band. Occasionally, a Meckel diverticulum may become inflamed (diverticulitis) and present with a picture similar to that of acute appendicitis. Diverticulitis may lead to perforation and peritonitis.

DIAGNOSIS. The diagnosis of omphalomesenteric duct remnants depends on their clinical presentation. If an infant or child presents with significant painless rectal bleeding, the presence of a Meckel diverticulum should be suspected. The confirmation of a Meckel diverticulum can be difficult. Plain abdominal radiographs are of no value, and routine barium studies rarely fill the diverticulum. The most sensitive study is the Meckel radionuclide scan, which is performed after the intravenous infusion of technetium 99m pertechnetate. The mucus-secreting cells of the ectopic gastric mucosa take up pertechnetate, permitting visualization of the Meckel diverticulum (Fig. 277–2). The uptake can be enhanced with a variety of agents including cimetidine, glucagon, and gastrin. The sensitivity of the enhanced scan is approximately 85%, with a specificity of approximately 95%. Other methods of detection include superior mesenteric angiography and technetium-labeled red cells. In patients who present with intestinal obstruction or a picture of appendicitis with omphalomesenteric duct remnants, the diagnosis is rarely made before surgery. The

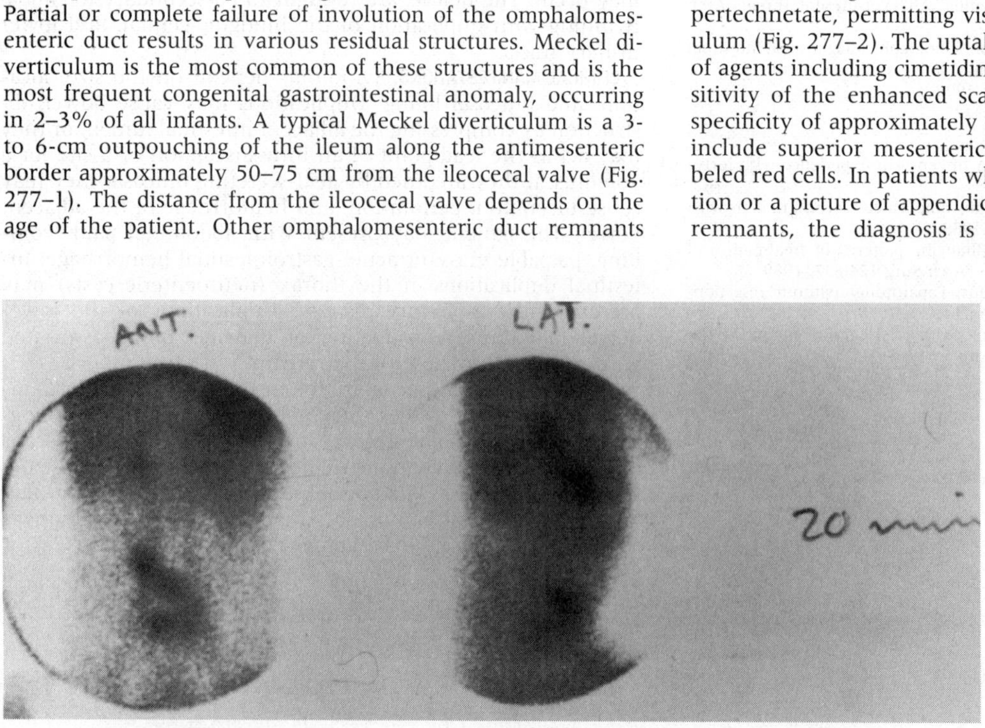

Figure 277–2. Meckel scan demonstrating accumulation of technetium in the stomach (superior right corner) and in the acid-secreting mucosa of a Meckel diverticulum (lower left corner).

treatment of a symptomatic Meckel diverticulum is surgical excision.

Bissler JJ, Klein RL: Alimentary tract duplications in children: Case and literature review. Clin Pediatr 27:152, 1988.
Holcomb GW III, Gheissari A, O'Neill JA Jr, et al: Surgical management of alimentary tract duplications. Ann Surg 209:167, 1989.
St. Vil D, Brandt DL, et al: Meckel's diverticulum in children: A 20-year review. J Pediatr Surg 26:1289, 1991.
Schwartz MZ, Smolens I: Meckel's diverticulum and other omphalomesenteric duct remnants. *In:* Wyllie R, Hyams JS (eds): Pediatric Gastrointestinal Disease: Pathophysiology, Diagnosis and Management. Philadelphia, WB Saunders, 1993, pp 670–676.
Vane DW, West KW, Grosfeld JL: Vitelline duct anomalies: Experience with 217 childhood cases. Arch Surg 122:542, 1987.

CHAPTER 278

Motility Disorders and Hirschsprung Disease

Robert Wyllie

278.1 Chronic Intestinal Pseudo-Obstruction

Chronic intestinal pseudo-obstruction is a group of disorders characterized by signs and symptoms of intestinal obstruction in the absence of an anatomic lesion. Pseudo-obstruction may occur as a primary disease or may be secondary to a large number of conditions that may transiently or permanently alter bowel motility. Pseudo-obstruction represents a wide spectrum of pathologic disorders from abnormal myoelectric activity to abnormalities of the nerves (intestinal neuropathy) or musculature (intestinal myopathy) of the gut. The organs involved may include the entire gastrointestinal tract or may be limited to certain components such as the stomach or colon. The distinctive pathologic abnormalities are considered together because of their clinical similarities.

Most congenital forms of pseudo-obstruction occur sporadically. A few clusters of autosomal dominant or recessive individuals have been reported whose cases are associated with abnormal gut muscle or nerves. Patients with autosomal dominant forms of pseudo-obstruction have variable expressions of the disease. Acquired pseudo-obstruction may follow episodes of acute gastroenteritis presumably resulting in injury to the myenteric plexus.

In congenital pseudo-obstruction, abnormalities of the muscle or nerves can be demonstrated in the majority of cases in which biopsy material is obtained. In muscular disease, the outer longitudinal muscle layer is replaced by fibrous material. In neuronal disease there may be disorganized or hypo- or hyperganglionosis.

CLINICAL MANIFESTATIONS. More than half the children with congenital pseudo-obstruction experience symptoms within the first few months of life. Two thirds of the infants presenting within the first few days of life are born prematurely and about 40% will have malrotation of the intestine. Seventy-five per cent of the children will experience symptoms during the first year of life, and the remainder will present over the next several years. The most common symptoms are abdominal distention and vomiting, which are present in 75% of the infants. Constipation, growth failure, and abdominal pain occur in approximately 60% of patients, and diarrhea occurs in 30–40%. The symptoms wax and wane in the majority of the patients; poor nutrition and intercurrent illness tend to exacerbate symptoms.

The diagnosis of pseudo-obstruction is based on the presence of compatible symptoms in the absence of anatomic obstruction. Plain abdominal radiographs demonstrate air-fluid levels in the small intestine. Neonates with evidence of obstruction at birth will have a microcolon. Contrast studies demonstrate slow passage of barium, and consideration should be given to using water-soluble agents.

Other studies may provide information on the underlying pathophysiology. Esophageal motility is abnormal in about half the patients. Antroduodenal motility and gastric emptying studies are abnormal if the upper gut is involved but do not differentiate pseudo-obstruction from other causes of partial or complete small-bowel obstruction. Colonic motility is abnormal if the colon is involved. Anorectal motility is normal and differentiates pseudo-obstruction from Hirschsprung disease. Intestinal biopsy is not indicated to establish the diagnosis and, if performed, may raise the possibility of future adhesive obstruction with exacerbation of symptoms.

The *differential diagnosis* includes Hirschsprung disease, other causes of mechanical obstruction, psychogenic constipation, neurogenic bladder, and superior mesenteric artery syndrome. Secondary causes of ileus or pseudo-obstruction, such as hypothyroidism, narcotics, scleroderma, Chagas disease, hypokalemia, diabetic neuropathy, amyloidosis, porphyria, angioneurotic edema, and radiation must be excluded.

TREATMENT. Nutritional support is the mainstay of treatment for pseudo-obstruction. Approximately 30–50% require partial or complete parenteral nutrition. Some patients can be managed with intermittent enteral supplementation, whereas others may maintain themselves on selective oral diets. Prokinetic drugs are useful in promoting motility in a small number of children. Cisapride (a 5-hydroxytryptamine receptor antagonist) and erythromycin (a motilin receptor agonist) may enhance gastric emptying and proximal small-bowel motility. Bethanechol, metoclopramide, and domperidone have not been useful.

Symptomatic small-bowel bacterial overgrowth is usually treated with oral antibiotics. Bacterial overgrowth may be associated with steatorrhea and malabsorption. Antibiotics should be used judiciously, however, because they may lead to the emergence of drug-resistant bacteria. Constipation is treated with enemas, suppositories, or bowel softeners. Patients with acid peptic symptoms are treated with acid suppressors (Chapter 282). Surgery, except for gastrostomy or placement of jejunostomy tubes, is generally not helpful. Colectomy in a selective group of children with abnormalities confined to the colon may be curative. Occasional patients with intractable symptoms may need a total bowel resection. In the future, bowel transplantation or electromechanical pacing may benefit selected patients depending on their underlying motility abnormality.

Glassman M, Spivak W, Mininberg D, et al: Chronic idiopathic intestinal pseudo-obstruction: A commonly misdiagnosed disease in infants and children. Pediatrics 83:603, 1989.
Navarro J, Sonsine E, Boige N, et al: Visceral neuropathies responsible for chronic intestinal pseudo-obstruction syndrome in pediatric practice: Analysis of 26 cases. J Pediatr Gastro Nutr 11:179, 1990.
Schuffler MD: Chronic intestinal pseudo-obstruction: Progress and problems. J Pediatr Gastroenterol Nutr 10:157, 1990.
Vargas JH, Sachs P, Ament ME: Chronic intestinal pseudo-obstruction syndrome in pediatrics: Results of a national survey by members of the North American Society of Pediatric Gastroenterology and Nutrition. J Pediatr Gastroenterol Nutr 7:323, 1988.

278.2 Superior Mesenteric Artery Syndrome (Wilkie Syndrome, Cast Syndrome, Arteriomesenteric Duodenal Compression Syndrome)

The existence of the superior mesenteric artery syndrome is debated, with proponents describing an extrinsic compression of the duodenum in children after rapid weight loss and in a supine position. The compression is thought to occur as the mesentery loses its fat and allows the superior mesenteric artery to collapse on the duodenum, compressing it between the superior mesenteric artery anteriorly and the aorta posteriorly. Alternatively, the cause may be that the loss of supporting fat in the second and third portions of the duodenum allows the duodenum to collapse against the spine.

The classic description is of an adolescent who starts vomiting after application of a body cast for orthopedic surgery. Other associated factors include anorexia, prolonged bed rest, weight loss, abdominal surgery, and exaggerated lumbar lordosis. The *diagnosis* is established radiologically with the demonstration of a cutoff of the duodenum just to the right of the midline. The duodenal obstruction may be accompanied by proximal duodenal and gastric dilatation.

Treatment of the acute syndrome involves relief of the obstruction and improved nutrition to alter the anatomic relationships of the duodenum with surrounding structures. Positioning the patient in a lateral or prone position shifts the duodenum away from potential obstructing structures and may allow the resumption of oral intake. Prokinetic agents such as cisapride may be helpful. If repositioning is unsuccessful in relieving symptoms, then a nasojejunal tube may be placed past the point of obstruction and feedings begun. Some patients require total parenteral nutrition to replete lost body fat, and occasional patients may need surgical intervention.

278.3 Congenital Aganglionic Megacolon (Hirschsprung Disease)

Hirschsprung disease or congenital aganglionic megacolon is caused by an abnormal innervation of the bowel, beginning in the internal anal sphincter and extending proximally to involve a variable length of gut. Hirschsprung disease is the most common cause of lower intestinal obstruction in the neonate, with an overall incidence of 1:5,000 live births. Males are affected more often than females (4:1), and there is an increased familial incidence in long segment disease. Hirschsprung disease may be associated with other congenital defects including Down, Laurence-Moon-Bardet-Biedl, and Waardenburg syndromes and cardiovascular abnormalities.

PATHOLOGY. Hirschsprung disease is the result of an absence of ganglion cells in the bowel wall, extending proximally and continuously from the anus for a variable distance. The absence of neural innervation is a consequence of an arrest of neuroblast migration from the proximal to distal bowel. The aganglionic segment is limited to the rectosigmoid in 75% of patients; in 10% the entire colon lacks ganglion cells. Increased nerve endings in the aganglionic bowel result in high concentrations of acetylcholinesterase. Histologically, there is an absence of Meissner and Auerbach plexus and hypertrophied nerve bundles with high concentrations of acetylcholinesterase between the muscular layers and in the submucosa. The disorder has been reproduced in animals by a knockout of the endothelin B receptor.

CLINICAL MANIFESTATIONS. The clinical symptoms of Hirschsprung disease usually begin at birth with the delayed passage of meconium. Ninety-nine per cent of full-term infants pass meconium within 48 hr of birth. Hirschsprung disease should be suspected in any full-term infant (the disease is unusual in preterm infants) with delayed passage of stool. Some infants will pass meconium normally but subsequently present with a history of chronic constipation. Failure to thrive with hypoproteinemia from a protein-losing enteropathy is a less common presentation now that Hirschsprung disease is usually recognized early in the course of the illness. Breast-fed infants may not manifest as severe disease as formula-fed infants.

Failure to pass stool leads to dilatation of the proximal bowel and abdominal distention. As the bowel dilates, intraluminal pressure increases, resulting in decreased blood flow and a deterioration of the mucosal barrier. Stasis allows proliferation of bacteria, which may lead to enterocolitis (*Clostridium difficile, Staphylococcus aureus,* anaerobes, coliforms) with associated sepsis and signs of bowel obstruction. The early recognition of Hirschsprung disease before the onset of enterocolitis is essential in reducing morbidity and mortality.

Hirschsprung disease in older patients must be distinguished from other causes of abdominal distention and chronic constipation (Table 278–1; Fig. 278–1). The history often reveals increasing difficulty with the passage of stools, starting in the 1st few weeks of life. A large fecal mass is palpable in the left lower abdomen, but on rectal examination the rectum is usually empty of feces. The stools, when passed, may consist of small pellets, be ribbon-like, or have a fluid consistency; the large stools and fecal soiling of patients with functional consti-

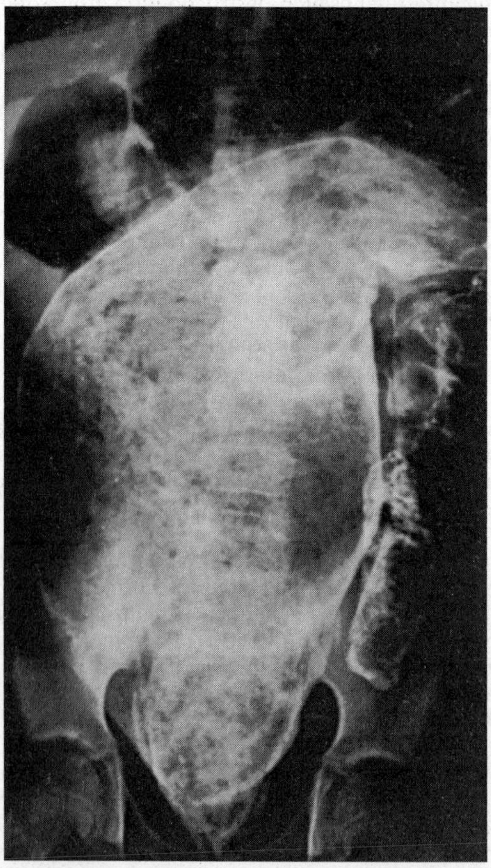

Figure 278–1. Barium enema in a 14-yr-old boy with severe constipation. The enormous dilatation of the rectum and distal colon is typical of acquired functional megacolon.

■ TABLE 278–1 Distinguishing Features of Hirschsprung Disease and Functional Constipation

Variable	Functional (Acquired)	Hirschsprung Disease
History		
Onset constipation	After 2 yr of age	At birth
Encopresis	Common	Very rare
Failure to thrive	Uncommon	Possible
Enterocolitis	None	Possible
Abdominal pain	Common	Common
Examination		
Abdominal distention	Rare	Common
Poor weight gain	Rare	Common
Anal tone	Normal	Normal
Rectal examination	Stool in ampulla	Ampulla empty
Laboratory		
Anorectal manometry	Distention of the rectum causes relaxation of the internal sphincter	No sphincter or paradoxical relaxation or increase in pressure
Rectal biopsy	Normal	No ganglion cells Increased acetylcholinesterase staining
Barium enema	Massive amounts of stool, no transition zone	Transition zone, delayed evacuation (greater than 24 hr)

pation are absent. In infancy Hirschsprung disease must be differentiated from meconium plug syndrome, meconium ileus, and intestinal atresia.

Rectal examination demonstrates normal anal tone and is usually followed by an explosive discharge of foul-smelling feces and gas. Intermittent attacks of intestinal obstruction from retained feces may be associated with pain and fever.

DIAGNOSIS. Rectal manometry and rectal suction biopsy are the easiest and most reliable indicators of Hirschsprung disease. Anorectal manometry measures the pressure of the internal anal sphincter while a balloon is distended in the rectum. In normal individuals rectal distention initiates a reflex drop in internal sphincter pressure. In patients with Hirschsprung disease, the pressure fails to drop, or there is a paradoxical rise in pressure with rectal distention. The accuracy of this diagnostic test is more than 90%, but it is technically difficult in young infants. A normal response in the course of manometric evaluation excludes a diagnosis of Hirschsprung disease; an equivocal or paradoxical response requires a rectal biopsy.

Rectal suction biopsies should be taken no closer than 2 cm to the dentate line to avoid the normal area of hypoganglionosis at the anal verge. The biopsy should contain an adequate sample of submucosa to evaluate for the presence of ganglion cells. The biopsy can be stained for acetylcholinesterase, which may facilitate interpretation. Patients with aganglionosis demonstrate a large number of hypertrophied nerve bundles that stain positively for acetylcholinesterase with an absence of ganglion cells.

The roentgenographic diagnosis of Hirschsprung disease is based on the presence of a transition zone between normal dilated proximal colon and a smaller caliber obstructed distal colon caused by the nonrelaxation of the aganglionic bowel. The transition zone is not usually present before 1 to 2 wk of age and on radiograph is a funnel-shaped area of intestine between the proximal dilated colon and the constricted distal bowel. Radiologic evaluation should be performed without preparation to prevent transient dilatation of the aganglionic segment. Twenty-four-hour delayed films are helpful (Fig. 278–2). If significant barium is still present in the colon, it increases the suspicion of Hirschsprung disease even if a transition zone is not identified. Barium enema examination is useful in determining the extent of aganglionosis before surgery and in evaluating other diseases that present with lower bowel obstruction in the neonate. Full-thickness rectal biopsy may be performed at the time of surgery to confirm the diagnosis and level of involvement.

TREATMENT. Once the diagnosis is established, the definitive treatment is operative intervention. The operative options are to perform a definitive procedure as soon as the diagnosis is established or perform a temporary colostomy and wait until the infant is 6–12 mo old to perform a definitive repair. There are three basic surgical options. The first successful surgical procedure described by Swenson was to excise the aganglionic segment and anastomose the normal proximal bowel to the rectum 1–2 cm above the dentate line. The operation is technically difficult and led to the development of two other procedures. Duhamel described a procedure to create a neorectum, bringing down normally innervated bowel behind the agangli-

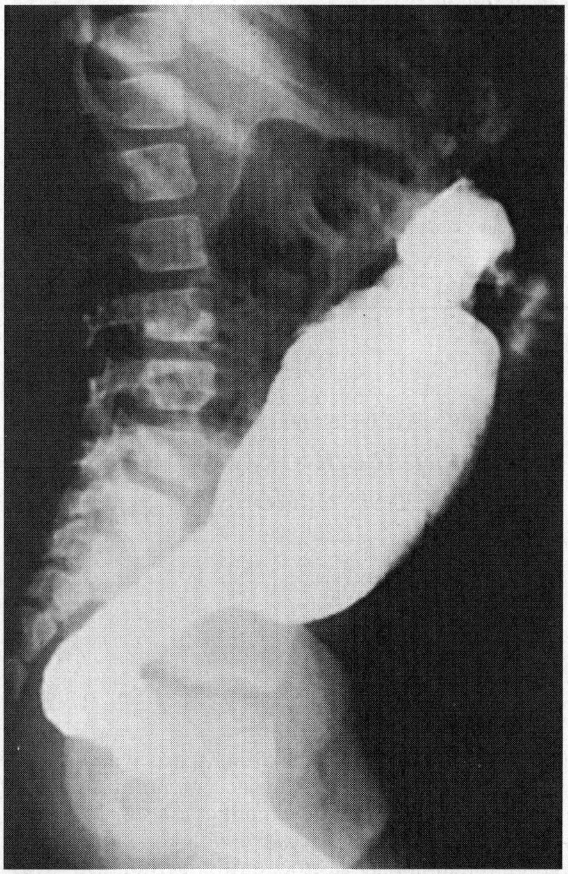

Figure 278–2. Lateral view of a barium enema in a 3-yr-old girl with Hirschsprung disease. The aganglionic distal segment is narrow, with distended normal ganglionic bowel above it.

onic rectum. The neorectum created in this procedure has an anterior aganglionic half with normal sensation and a posterior ganglionic half with normal propulsion. The endorectal pull-through procedure described by Boley involves stripping the mucosa from the aganglionic rectum and bringing normally innervated colon through the residual muscular cuff, thus bypassing the abnormal bowel from within.

In ultrashort segmental Hirschsprung disease, the aganglionic segment is limited to the internal sphincter. The clinical symptoms are similar to those of children with functional constipation. Ganglion cells may be present on rectal suction biopsy, but the rectal motility will be abnormal. Excision of a strip of rectal muscle, including the internal anal sphincter, is diagnostic and therapeutic.

Long-segment Hirschsprung disease involving the entire colon and part of the small bowel represents a difficult problem. Rectal motility studies and rectal suction biopsy will demonstrate findings of Hirschsprung disease, but radiologic studies will be difficult to interpret because no colonic transition zone can be identified. The extent of aganglionosis can be determined accurately by biopsy at the time of laparotomy.

When the entire colon is aganglionic, often together with a length of terminal ileum, ileal-anal anastomosis is the treatment of choice, preserving part of the aganglionic colon to facilitate water absorption, which helps the stools to become firm. The operation of Duhamel is the best for total colonic aganglionosis. The left colon is left in situ as a reservoir, and it is not necessary to anastomose this left colon to the pulled-through small bowel.

The prognosis of surgically treated Hirschsprung disease is generally satisfactory, with the great majority of patients achieving fecal continence. Postoperative problems include recurrent enterocolitis, stricture, prolapse, perianal abscesses, and fecal soiling.

Joseph V, Sim C: Problems and pitfalls in the management of Hirschsprung's disease. J Pediatr Surg 23:398, 1988.

Schofield D, Devine W, Yunis E: Acetylcholinesterase-stained suction rectal biopsies in the diagnosis of Hirschsprung's disease. J Pediatr Gastroenterol Nutr 11:221, 1990.

Srikanth MS, Ford EG, Hirose R, et al: The simple technique of rectal suction biopsy for the diagnosis of Hirschsprung's disease. J Pediatr Surg 28:942, 1993.

Tariq GM, Bereton RJ, Wright VM: Complications of endorectal pull-through for Hirschsprung's disease. J Pediatr Surg 26:1202, 1991.

CHAPTER 279

Ileus, Adhesions, Intussusception, and Closed-Loop Obstructions

Robert Wyllie

279.1 Ileus

Ileus is the failure of intestinal peristalsis without evidence of mechanical obstruction. The lack of normal gut motility interferes with the aboral movement of intestinal contents and in children is most often associated with abdominal surgery or infection (pneumonia, gastroenteritis, peritonitis). Ileus also accompanies metabolic abnormalities, such as uremia, hypokalemia, or acidosis, and occurs with the administration of certain drugs such as vincristine. Ileus may also occur when antimotility drugs such as loperamide are used during episodes of gastroenteritis.

Ileus presents with increasing abdominal distention and initially minimal pain. Pain increases with increasing distention. Bowel sounds are minimal or absent in contrast to early mechanical obstruction when they are hyperactive. Plain abdominal radiographs demonstrate multiple air-fluid levels throughout the abdomen. Serial radiographs usually do not show progressive distention as they do in mechanical obstruction. Contrast radiographs, if done, demonstrate slow movement of the barium through a patent lumen.

Treatment of ileus involves the correction of the underlying abnormality. Nasogastric decompression is used if abdominal distention is associated with pain or to relieve recurrent vomiting. Ileus after abdominal surgical procedures usually results in the return of normal intestinal motility within 24–72 hr. Prokinetic agents such as cisapride or erythromycin may stimulate the return of normal bowel motility and be of assistance to children with prolonged ileus.

279.2 Adhesions

Adhesions are fibrous bands of tissue that are a common cause of postoperative small-bowel obstruction after abdominal surgery. The risk of forming an adhesion that causes obstructive symptoms in childhood has not been well studied but seems to occur in 2–3% of patients after abdominal surgery. The majority of obstructions are associated with single adhesions and can occur anytime after the 2nd postoperative week.

The *diagnosis* is suspected in patients with abdominal pain and a history of intraperitoneal surgery. Nausea and vomiting quickly follow the development of pain. Initially bowel sounds are hyperactive, and the abdomen is flat. The bowel subsequently dilates, producing abdominal distention in most patients, and bowel sounds disappear. Fever and leukocytosis are suggestive of necrotic bowel and peritonitis. Plain roentgenographs demonstrate obstructive features, and contrast studies may be needed to define the cause of obstruction.

Patients with suspected obstruction should have nasogastric decompression, intravenous fluid resuscitation, and broad-spectrum antibiotics in anticipation of surgery. Nonoperative intervention is contraindicated unless the patient is stable with clear evidence of clinical improvement.

279.3 Intussusception

Intussusception occurs when a portion of the alimentary tract is telescoped into a segment just caudad to it. It is the most common cause of intestinal obstruction between 3 mo and 6 yr of age; it is rare in children younger than 3 mo and decreases in frequency after 36 mo. The incidence varies from 1–4/1,000 live births. The male to female ratio is 4:1. A few intussusceptions reduce spontaneously or become autoamputated; if left untreated, most would lead to death.

ETIOLOGY AND EPIDEMIOLOGY. The cause of most intussusceptions is unknown. The seasonal incidence has peaks in spring and autumn. Correlation with adenovirus infections has been noted, and the condition may complicate gastroenteritis. It is postulated that swollen Peyer patches in the ileum may stimulate intestinal peristalsis in an attempt to extrude the mass, thus causing an intussusception. At the peak age of incidence of this condition the infant's alimentary tract is also being introduced to a variety of new materials. In about 5–10% of patients recognizable lead points for the intussusception are found, such as inverted appendiceal stump, Meckel diverticulum, an intestinal polyp, duplication, or lymphosarcoma. Uncommonly, the condition will complicate Henoch-Schönlein purpura, with an intramural hematoma acting as the apex of the intussusception. Rarely, intussusception is postoperative and then always ileoileal. Intussusception occurs in dehydrated patients with cystic fibrosis. Unusual lesions include metastatic tumors, hemangioma, foreign bodies, parasitic infection, and fecolith; they can occur following cancer chemotherapy. Lead points are more common in very young and older patients.

PATHOLOGY. Intussusceptions are most often ileocolic and ileoileocolic, less commonly cecocolic, and rarely exclusively ileal. Very rarely, the appendix forms the apex of an intussusception. The upper portion of bowel, the intussusceptum, invaginates into the lower, the intussuscipiens, dragging its mesentery along with it into the enveloping loop. Constriction of the mesentery obstructs venous return; engorgement of the intussusceptum follows, with edema, and bleeding from the mucosa leads to a bloody stool, sometimes containing mucus. The apex of the intussusception may extend into the transverse, descending, or sigmoid colon—even to and through the anus in neglected cases. This presentation must be distinguished from rectal prolapse. Most intussusceptions do not strangulate the bowel within the first 24 hr but may later eventuate in intestinal gangrene and shock.

CLINICAL MANIFESTATIONS. In typical cases there is sudden onset, in a previously well child, of severe paroxysmal colicky pain that recurs at frequent intervals and is accompanied by straining efforts and loud cries. Initially, the infant may be comfortable and play normally between the paroxysms of pain, but if the intussusception is not reduced, the infant becomes progressively weaker and lethargic. Eventually a shocklike state may develop, with an elevation of body temperature to as high as 41° C (106° F). The pulse becomes weak and thready, the respirations become shallow and grunting, and the pain may be manifested only by moaning sounds. Vomiting occurs in most cases and is usually more frequent early. In the later phase the vomitus becomes bile stained. Stools of normal appearance may be evacuated during the 1st few hr of symptoms. After this time fecal excretions are small or more often do not occur, and little or no flatus is passed. Blood generally is passed in the first 12 hr, but at times not for 1–2 days and infrequently not at all; 60% of infants will pass a stool containing red blood and mucus, the *currant jelly stool.* Some patients have only irritability and alternating or progressive lethargy.

Palpation of the abdomen usually reveals a slightly tender, sausage-shaped mass, sometimes ill defined, which may increase in size and firmness during a paroxysm of pain and is most often in the right upper abdomen, with its long axis cephalocaudal. If it is felt in the epigastrium, the long axis is transverse. About 30% of patients do not have a palpable mass. It is more readily located by bimanual rectal and abdominal palpation between paroxysms of pain. The presence of bloody mucus on the finger as it is withdrawn after rectal examination supports the diagnosis of intussusception. Abdominal distention and tenderness develop as intestinal obstruction becomes more acute. On rare occasions the advancing intestine prolapses through the anus. This prolapse can be distinguished from prolapse of the rectum by the separation between the protruding intestine and the rectal wall, which does not exist in prolapse of the rectum.

Ileoileal intussusception may have a less typical clinical picture, the symptoms and signs being chiefly those of small intestinal obstruction. *Recurrent intussusception* is noted in 5–8% and is more common following hydrostatic than surgical reduction. *Chronic intussusception,* in which the symptoms exist in milder form at recurrent intervals, is more likely to occur with or following acute enteritis and may arise in older children as well as in infants.

DIAGNOSIS. The clinical history and physical findings are usually sufficiently typical for diagnosis. Plain abdominal roentgenograms may show a density in the area of the intussusception. A barium enema will show a filling defect or cupping in the head of barium where its advance is obstructed by the intussusceptum (Fig. 279–1). A central linear column of barium may be visible in the compressed lumen of the intussusceptum, and a thin rim of barium may be seen trapped around the invaginating intestine in the folds of mucosa within the intussuscipiens (coiled-spring sign), especially after evacuation. Retrogression of the intussusceptum under the pressure of the enema and gaseous distention of the small intestine from obstruction are also useful roentgenographic signs. Ileoileal intussusception is usually not demonstrable by barium enema but is suspected because of gaseous distention of the intestine above the lesion. Currently, the use of an "air" enema in the diagnosis and treatment of intussusception is rapidly gaining in popularity in many centers. It is believed to be safer with less risk of perforation, is at least as accurate as a barium enema, and entails less irradiation of the patient.

Real-time sonography may also provide useful diagnostic information: a target or donut configuration of bowel with hypoechoic rims and dense central echogenic core, no movement in the donut, and a rim thickness more than 0.6 cm. An exterior rim thickness more than 1.6 cm is associated with the need for surgical intervention.

DIFFERENTIAL DIAGNOSIS. It may be particularly difficult to diagnose intussusception in a child who already has *gastroenteritis;* a change in the pattern of illness, in the character of pain, or in the nature of vomiting or the onset of rectal bleeding should alert the physician. The bloody stools and abdominal cramps that accompany *enterocolitis* can usually be differentiated from intussusception because the pain is less severe and less regular, there is diarrhea, and the infant is recognizably ill between pains. Bleeding from *Meckel diverticulum* is usually painless. The intestinal hemorrhage of *Henoch-Schönlein purpura* is usually, but not invariably, accompanied by joint symptoms or purpura elsewhere, and the colicky pain may be similar. Because intus-

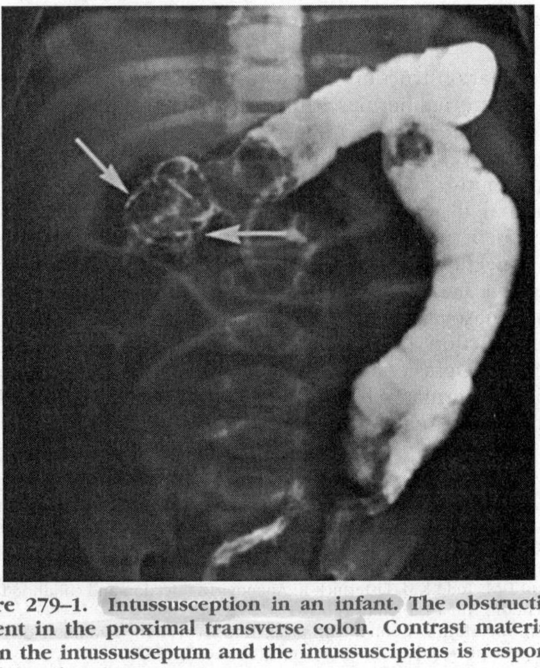

Figure 279–1. Intussusception in an infant. The obstruction is evident in the proximal transverse colon. Contrast material between the intussusceptum and the intussuscipiens is responsible for the coil-spring appearance.

susception may be a complication of this disorder, a barium enema may be required.

TREATMENT. Reduction of the intussusception is an emergency procedure to be carried out immediately after diagnosis and after rapid preparation for operation with fluids and blood for shock and water and electrolytes to replace losses. In more than 75% of cases of short duration, when there are no signs of prostration, shock, intestinal perforation, pneumatosis intestinalis, or peritoneal irritation, it is possible to reduce the intussusception by hydrostatic or pneumatic pressure under fluoroscopic or ultrasonographic guidance and with the consultation and close proximity of a surgeon.

If there is clinical evidence of prolonged intestinal obstruction with peritonitis, hydrostatic reduction of the intussusception should not be attempted because of the risk of perforating the intussuscipiens. In an ileoileal intussusception a barium enema is usually not diagnostic and reduction by the hydrostatic technique may not be possible. Such intussusceptions may develop insidiously as a complication of a laparotomy and require resection. A right-sided transverse paraumbilical or infraumbilical incision gives access to the ascending colon. If manual operative reduction is impossible or the bowel is not viable, resection of the intussusception will be necessary, with end-to-end anastomosis.

PROGNOSIS. Untreated intussusception in infants is almost always fatal; the chances of recovery are directly related to the duration of intussusception before reduction. Most infants recover if the intussusception is reduced within the first 24 hr, but the mortality rate rises rapidly after this time, especially after the 2nd day. Spontaneous reduction during preparation for operation is not uncommon.

The recurrence rate following barium enema reduction of intussusceptions is about 10% and after surgical reduction, about 2–5%; none have recurred after surgical resection. It is unlikely that an intussusception caused by a lesion such as lymphosarcoma, polyp, or Meckel diverticulum will be successfully reduced by barium enema. With adequate surgical management, operative reduction carries a very low mortality rate in early cases.

279.4 *Closed-Loop Obstructions*

Intestinal obstruction may be caused by defects in the mesentery ("internal hernias") through which loops of small bowel may pass and become trapped. Vascular engorgement of the trapped bowel results in intestinal ischemia and gangrene unless promptly relieved. Symptoms include bilious vomiting, abdominal distention, and abdominal pain. Peritoneal signs suggest ischemic bowel. Plain radiographs demonstrate signs of small-bowel obstruction or free air if the bowel has perforated. Supportive management includes intravenous fluids, antibiotics, and nasogastric decompression. Prompt surgical relief of the obstruction is indicated if intestinal gangrene is to be prevented. Occasionally, symptoms can be transient or recurrent if the herniated bowel slides out of the mesenteric defect spontaneously relieving the obstruction.

Akgur FM, Tanyel FC, Buyukpamukcu N, Hicsonmez A: Adhesive bowel obstruction in children: The place and predictors of success for conservative treatment. J Pediatr Surg 26:37, 1991.
Bhisitkul DM, Listernick R, Shkolnik A, et al: Clinical application of ultrasonography in the diagnosis of intussusception. J Pediatr 121:182, 1992.
Bhisitkul DM, Todd KM, Listernick R: Adenovirus infection and childhood intussusception. Am J Dis Child 146:1331, 1992.
Bruce J, Soo Huh Y, Cooney DR, et al: Intussusception: Evolution of current management. J Pediatr Gastroenterol Nutr 6:663, 1987.
Champoux AN, Del Beccaro MA, Nazar-Stewart V: Recurrent intussusception: Risks and features. Arch Pediatr Adolesc Med 148:474, 1994.
den Hollander D, Burge DM: Exclusion criteria and outcome in pressure reduction of intussusception. Arch Dis Child 68:79, 1993.
Ein SH, Stephens CA, Shandling B, et al: Intussusception due to lymphoma. J Pediatr Surg 21:786, 1986.
Lee H-C, Yeh H-J, Leu Y-J: Intussusception: The sonographic diagnosis and its clinical value. J Pediatr Gastroenterol Nutr 8:343, 1989.
Reijnen JAM, Festen C, van Roosmalen RP: Intussusception: Factors related to treatment. Arch Dis Child 65:871, 1990.
Stein M, Alton DJ, Daneman A: Pneumatic reduction of intussusception: 5-year experience. Pediatr Radiol 183:681, 1992.
Stringer MD, Pledger G, Drake DP: Childhood deaths from intussusception in England and Wales, 1984–9. Br Med J 304:737, 1992.

CHAPTER 280

Foreign Bodies and Bezoars

Robert Wyllie

280.1 *Foreign Bodies in the Stomach and Intestine*

Eighty per cent of all foreign body ingestions occur in children, with a peak incidence between the ages of 6 mo and 3 yr. The exact incidence of foreign bodies ingested is unknown; in the United States approximately 1,500 people die annually after ingesting a foreign body.

Coins are the most common foreign body ingested by young children. In older children, teenagers, and adults, fish or chicken bones are the most common objects accidentally ingested. The risk of ingestion increases after alcohol consumption or cold liquids because of a decrease in oral sensory acuity. Repeat ingestion may occur in young children and psychiatrically impaired patients. Of the foreign bodies that come to medical attention, 80–90% will pass through the gastrointestinal tract without difficulty. Ten to 20% will require endoscopic removal or other conservative management, whereas 1% or less will require surgical intervention. Once in the stomach, 95% of all ingested objects pass without difficulty through the remainder of the gastrointestinal tract. Perforation after foreign body ingestion is estimated to be less that 1% of all objects ingested. Perforation tends to occur in areas of physiologic sphincters (pylorus and ileocecal valve), acute angulation (such as the duodenal sweep), congenital gut malformations (webs, diaphragms, or diverticula), or areas of previous bowel surgery.

Patients with nonfood foreign bodies often give a history of ingestion. In young children, there may be a witness. Approximately 90% of foreign bodies are opaque. Radiologic examination is routinely performed to determine the type, number, and location of the suspected objects. Contrast radiographs may be necessary to demonstrate some objects such as plastic parts or toys.

Conservative management is indicated in most foreign bodies that have passed through the esophagus and entered the stomach. Most objects will pass though the intestine in 4–6 days, although some may take as long as 3–4 wk. While waiting for the object to pass, parents are instructed to continue a regular diet and to observe the stools for the appearance of the ingested object. Cathartics should be avoided. Exceptionally long or sharp objects are usually monitored radiologically. Parents or patients should be instructed to report abdominal pain, vomiting, persistent fever, and hematemesis or melena immediately to their physician. Failure of the object to progress over a 3- to 4-wk period seldom implies an impeding perforation but may be associated with a congenital malformation or acquired bowel abnormality.

In older children and adults, oval objects greater than 5 cm in diameter or 2 cm in thickness tend to lodge in the stomach and should be endoscopically retrieved. Thin objects greater than 10 cm in length fail to negotiate the duodenal sweep and should also be removed. In infants and toddlers, objects longer than 3 cm or larger than 20 mm in diameter usually will not pass through the pylorus and should be removed. Open safety pins should also be endoscopically retrieved, but other sharp objects can be managed conservatively.

Children will occasionally place objects in their rectum. Small, blunt objects will usually pass spontaneously, but large or sharp objects will usually need to be retrieved. Adequate sedation is essential to relax the anal sphincter before attempted endoscopic or speculum removal. If the object is proximal to the rectum, observation for 12–24 hr will usually allow the object to descend into the rectum.

Bendig DW, Mackie GG: Management of smooth-blunt foreign bodies in asymptomatic patients. Clin Pediatr 29:642, 1990.
Litovitz T, Shcmitz BF: Ingestion of cylindrical and button batteries: an analysis of 2382 cases. Pediatrics 89:747, 1992.
Webb WA: Management of foreign bodies of the upper gastrointestinal tract. Gastroenterology 94:204, 1988.

280.2 Bezoars

The term *bezoar* refers to an accumulation of exogenous matter in the stomach or intestine. Most bezoars have been found in females with underlying personality problems or in neurologically impaired individuals. The peak age of onset of symptoms is the second decade of life. Bezoars are classified on the basis of their composition. Trichobezoars are composed of the patient's own hair, and phytobezoars are composed of a combination of plant and animal material. Lactobezoars were previously found most often in premature infants and may be attributed to the high casein or calcium content of some premature formulas.

Trichobezoars can become large and form casts of the stomach; they may enter into the proximal duodenum. They present with symptoms of gastric outlet or partial intestinal obstruction including vomiting, anorexia, and weight loss. Patients may complain of abdominal pain, distention, and severe halitosis. Physical examination may demonstrate patchy baldness and a firm mass in the left upper quadrant. Occasionally, patients may have an iron deficiency anemia, hypoproteinemia, or steatorrhea caused by an associated chronic gastritis. Phytobezoars present in a similar manner.

An abdominal plain film may suggest the presence of a bezoar, which can be confirmed on barium or ultrasound examination. Endoscopy provides a definitive diagnosis and a means of therapeutic disruption and removal of the material. If endoscopy is unsuccessful, surgical intervention may be needed. Lactobezoars usually resolve when feedings are withheld for 24–48 hr.

Andrus CH, Ponsky JL: Bezoars: classification, pathophysiology and treatment. Am J Gastroenterol 83:476, 1988.

CHAPTER 281
Anorectal Malformations

Alberto Peña

The term *anorectal malformations* refers to a spectrum of defects. Some are complex, difficult to manage, and associated with important anatomic deficiencies and therefore have a poor functional prognosis. Others are minor and easily treated, having an excellent functional prognosis. The main concerns are future bowel control and urinary and sexual function. Anorectal anomalies occur in about 1:4,000 live births and manifest various grades of anal stenosis—agenesis or rectal agenesis—atresia.

EMBRYOLOGY AND PATHOGENESIS. The origin of the anus and the rectum is an embryologic structure called the cloaca. Lateral ingrowths of this structure form the urorectal septum, separating the rectum dorsally from the urinary tract ventrally. Both systems (rectum and urinary tract) become completely separated by the 7th wk of gestation. At this same time, the urogenital portion of the original cloaca already has an external opening, whereas the anal portion is closed by a membrane that opens by the 8th wk of gestation.

Abnormalities in the development of these processes at varying stages provoke a spectrum of anomalies, most of which affect the lower intestinal tract and the genitourinary structures. Persistence of communication between the genitourinary and rectal portions of the cloaca results in fistulas.

PATHOLOGY AND CLASSIFICATION. Figure 281–1 demonstrates a practical, therapeutic oriented classification of these defects.

Males. **PERINEAL FISTULA.** Perineal (cutaneous) fistula is the simplest defect in both sexes. Patients have a small orifice located in the perineum, anterior to the center of the external sphincter, close to the scrotum in the male or to the vulva in the female. Male patients frequently have in their perineum a "bucket-handle"–type malformation or a "black ribbon"–type structure that represents a subepithelial fistula filled with meconium. These patients usually have a well-formed sacrum, a prominent midline groove, and a prominent anal dimple. The frequency of associated defects affecting other organs is less than 10%. The diagnosis is established by simple perineal inspection. No further investigations are required, and this defect can be repaired without a protective colostomy.

RECTOURETHRAL FISTULA. In cases of rectourethral fistula, the rectum communicates with the lower part of the urethra (bulbar urethra) or the upper part of the urethra (prostatic urethra). The sphincteric mechanism usually is satisfactory; a few patients have poor perineal muscles and a flat-looking perineum. The sacrum may have different degrees of hypodevelopment, particularly in cases of rectourethral prostatic fistula. Most of these patients have a well-formed midline perineal groove and an anal dimple. Those with a rectoprostatic fistula have a poorly developed sacrum and frequently a flat perineum. These patients require a protective colostomy during the newborn period. The complete surgical repair is performed later in life. Rectourethral fistula represents the most frequent anorectal defect seen in male patients.

RECTOVESICAL FISTULA. In patients having rectovesical fistulas, the rectum communicates with the urinary tract at the level of the bladder neck. The sphincteric mechanism is frequently very poorly developed. The sacrum is frequently deformed and often absent. The perineum looks flat. This defect represents 10% of the total number of affected male patients. The prog-

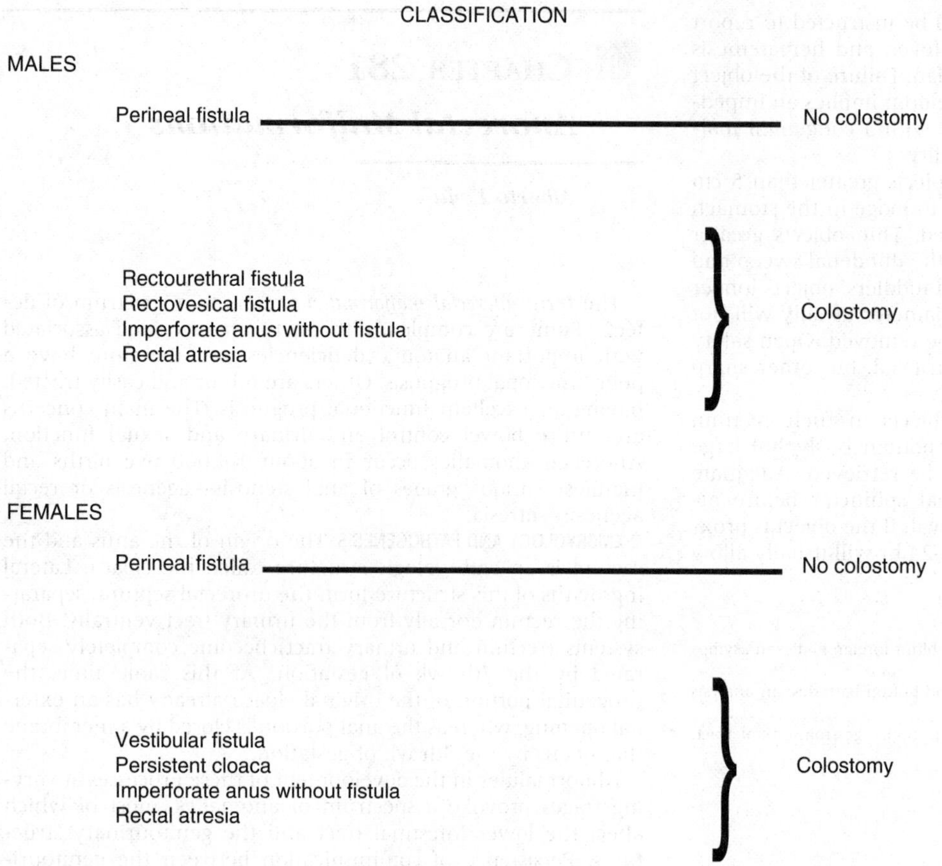

Figure 281–1. Classification of anorectal malformations. (From Kiesewetter WB: *In*: Ravitch MM, et al (eds): Pediatric Surgery, 3rd ed. Chicago, Yearbook, 1979.)

nosis for bowel function is usually poor. A colostomy is mandatory during the newborn period followed by corrective surgical repair later in life.

IMPERFORATE ANUS WITHOUT FISTULA. This defect has the same characteristics in both sexes. The rectum is completely blind and is usually found approximately 2 cm above the perineal skin. The sacrum and the sphincteric mechanism are usually well developed. The functional prognosis is usually good and very similar to those male patients with a rectourethral bulbar fistula. A colostomy is indicated during the newborn period. This defect is frequently associated with Down syndrome.

RECTAL ATRESIA. Rectal atresia is a rare defect occurring in only 1% of anorectal anomalies. It has the same characteristics in both sexes. The unique feature of this defect is that affected patients have a normal anal canal and a normal anus. The defect is frequently discovered while a rectal temperature is being taken. There is an obstruction about 2 cm above the skin level. These patients need a protective colostomy. The functional prognosis is excellent because they have a normal sphincteric mechanism (and normal sensation), which resides in the anal canal.

Females. VESTIBULAR FISTULA. Vestibular fistula is the most frequent defect seen in females. The rectum opens in the vestibule of the female genitalia immediately outside the hymen orifice. Patients are frequently mislabeled as having "rectovaginal fistula." The functional prognosis is excellent. The sacrum is usually normal, and the perineum shows a prominent midline groove and a noticeable anal dimple, all of which indicate that the sphincteric mechanism is intact. A protective colostomy is needed before the corrective surgery, although this colostomy does not need to be performed on an emergency basis because the fistula is frequently competent to decompress the intestinal tract.

PERSISTENT CLOACA. In cases of persistent cloaca, the rectum, vagina, and urinary tract meet and fuse into a single common channel. The perineum shows a single orifice located immediately behind the clitoris. The length of the common channels varies from 1–10 cm; this has important technical and prognostic implications. Patients with short common channels (<3 cm) usually have well-developed sacrums and good sphincters. A common channel longer than 3 cm usually suggests that the patient has a more complex defect and, frequently, has a poor sphincteric mechanism and a poor sacrum. Most patients with cloacas have an abnormally large vagina filled with mucous secretions (hydrocolpos). There are also different degrees of vaginal and uterine septation. A diverting colostomy is indicated at birth; in addition, patients suffering from a cloaca represent a urologic emergency because approximately 90% have associated urologic defects. Before the colostomy, the urologic diagnosis must be established to decompress the urinary tract, if necessary, at the same time the colostomy is created.

The term *rectovaginal fistula* is not used in this classification because true rectovaginal fistulas are extremely unusual defects. This became obvious after the advent of the posterior sagittal surgical approach, which allowed the surgeon to have a direct view of the anatomy.

DIAGNOSIS AND EARLY MANAGEMENT. The most important decision regarding a newborn with an anorectal malformation is whether the patient needs a diverting-decompression colostomy and emergency urinary diversion for an associated obstructed uropathy.

Males. Good clinical evaluation and a urinalysis will provide sufficient information in 80–90% of patients for the surgeon to decide whether a colostomy is needed. If a patient has a perineal or rectourinary fistula, meconium may not be seen at the perineum or in the urine before 16–24 hr after birth. The most distal part of the bowel, in cases of perineal and rectourethral fistulas, is surrounded by voluntary sphincteric muscles; the intraluminal bowel pressure must be high enough to overcome the tone of those muscles before one can see meconium in the urine or in the perineum. At birth the bowel is not distended; therefore, clinical and radiologic evaluations are not reliable during the first 16–24 hr of life. A piece of gauze is placed around the tip of the penis, and the nurse is instructed to check for particles of meconium filtered through this gauze. The presence of meconium in the urine and a flat bottom are considered indications to create a protective colostomy. Clinical findings consistent with the diagnosis of a perineal fistula represent an indication for an anoplasty without a protective colostomy. Sometimes none of the clinical signs already described becomes evident after 24 hr of observation; a radiologic evaluation is then indicated. A cross-table lateral film with the patient in a prone position taken after 16–24 hr of life is valuable for determining the position of the rectal pouch. When this is separated from the skin by more than 1 cm, the patient needs a colostomy. During the first 24 hrs of life, all these patients need an abdominal ultrasound evaluation to identify an obstructive uropathy.

Females. More than 90% of the time, the diagnosis can be established by a meticulous perineal inspection. These patients must be observed during the first 16–24 hr of life. The presence of a single perineal orifice is pathognomonic of a cloaca. A palpable pelvic mass (hydrocolpos) reinforces the suspicions of a cloaca. The diagnosis of a vestibular fistula can be established by a careful separation of the labia to see the vestibule. The rectal orifice is located somewhere between the female genitalia and the center of the sphincter. A perineal fistula is very easy to diagnose; the term *anterior anus,* which is sometimes used for this defect, is inadequate because these are abnormal fistula orifices not surrounded by a normal sphincteric mechanism. Less than 10% of these patients fail to pass meconium through the genitalia or perineum after 24 hr of observation. Those patients may require a cross-table lateral film. They also need an ultrasound study of the abdomen during the first 24 hr of life, because patients with persistent cloaca have the highest incidence of urologic defects.

ASSOCIATED DEFECTS. About 50% of children with anorectal anomalies have a urologic problem. The more serious and complex the anorectal defect, the more frequently it is associated with a urologic anomaly. Male patients with a rectovesical fistula and patients with persistent cloacas have a 90% chance of having a urologic defect. On the other hand, patients with rectoperineal fistula have less than a 10% chance. Urologic evaluation must be established before performing a colostomy. Untreated acidosis and sepsis resulting from an undetected obstructive uropathy may jeopardize the infant.

There is a very good correlation between the degree of sacral development and the final functional prognosis. Patients with absent sacrum will have permanent fecal and urinary incontinence. Different degrees of sacral malformations are associated with important functional sequelae. Spinal abnormalities and different degrees of dysraphism are frequently associated with these defects.

Other associated congenital malformations include esophageal atresia, duodenal atresia, and cardiovascular defects.

TREATMENT. Perineal fistula can be treated by a simple operation called anoplasty without a protective colostomy; the operation can be performed during the newborn period. The fistula orifice is moved back to the center of the external sphincter. Anal dilations are started 2 wk after the operation and gradually increased to reach the size of a normal anus. All other defects are best treated during the newborn period with a protective colostomy. Later in life (1–12 mo), corrective surgical repair is performed.

A posterior sagittal approach uses an electric muscle stimulator to identify objectively the sphincteric mechanism. This approach allows a direct exposure to the internal anatomy, avoiding potential damage to important structures and nerves. A midline incision between both buttocks is used to split all the muscle structures in the midline. The rectum is separated from the genitourinary tract and, in cases of cloaca, the vagina and the urinary tract. The rectum is placed within the limits of the sphincteric mechanism, which is electrically determined. The vagina and urinary tract are also reconstructed in cases of cloacas. Sometimes the rectum is too ectatic to be accommodated within the available space; therefore, the rectum has to be tailored accordingly. In male patients, the malformation can be repaired posterior sagittally 90% of the time. The remaining 10% of patients have a rectovesical fistula; the rectum cannot be reached posterior sagittally; a combined posterior sagittal and abdominal approach is needed. In cases of persistent cloaca, the abdomen must be opened in addition to the posterior sagittal approach in about 30–40% of patients to mobilize a very high rectum or high vagina. Two weeks after corrective surgery, the patients must be subjected to a protocol of anal dilations. These are done twice per day; every week a new size dilator is passed to stretch the anus to normal size.

PROGNOSIS. Patients of both sexes with perineal fistula and rectal atresia should have excellent functional results after the repair of their defects; they should be fully continent. Male patients with rectourethral bulbar fistula and patients of both sexes with imperforate anus without a fistula also have good prognosis. About 80% achieve bowel control between 3 and 4 yr of age. A significant number may occasionally suffer from minimal soiling.

Male patients with rectourethral prostatic fistula have about a 60% chance of having bowel control by the age of 3 yr. Male patients with rectovesical fistula have a poor functional prognosis. Only about 20% have voluntary bowel movements by the age of 3 yr.

A very abnormal sacrum usually means that the patient will suffer from *fecal incontinence.* Very abnormal sacrums are most often associated with rectovesical fistulas or rectoprostatic fistulas. Rarely, one does find a good prognostic type of defect, such as perineal or vestibular fistula, associated with a poor sacrum.

More than 90% of female patients with rectovestibular fistula have voluntary bowel movements by the age of 3 yr. Very few have occasional soiling.

Patients with persistent cloacas with a common channel of less than 3 cm have about an 80% chance of having voluntary bowel movements by the age of 3 yr; most are urine continent. When the common channel is longer than 3 cm, most are fecal incontinent and require intermittent catheterization to empty their bladder. Patients with persistent cloacas with a common channel longer than 3 cm usually have a very abnormal sacrum.

A significant number of patients have fecal incontinence and sometimes *urinary incontinence.* When these patients are old enough to be socially active, a medical program for bowel management and urinary control must be implemented. The use of enemas, suppositories, colonic irrigations, specific diets, and sometimes medications to regulate the motility of the colon will allow them to keep clean for 24 hr, improving their quality of life. Patients with fecal incontinence who have intractable diarrhea are usually refractory to medical management and require a permanent colostomy.

Most patients subjected to an operation to repair an imperforate anus will have different degrees of *constipation.* This symptom is more severe in lower and simpler defects. Patients who had inadequate colostomies (loop colostomies that allow the passing of stool from the proximal into the distal limb of the bowel) may subsequently have constipation. These patients need a diet rich in fiber and, sometimes, laxatives to empty the rectum daily. Ineffective medical treatment may exacerbate the problem; the rectosigmoid continues to enlarge and becomes inefficient in emptying, making the treatment a more difficult task.

Diseth T, Emblem R, Solbraa I, et al: A psychological follow-up of ten adolescents with low anorectal malformation. Acta Paediatr 83:216, 1994.
Narasimharao KL, Prasad GR, Katariya S: Prone cross-table lateral view: an alternative to the invertogram in imperforate anus. AJR 148:127, 1983.
Peña A: Current management of anorectal anomalies. Surg Clin North Am 72:1393, 1992.
Peña A: Posterior sagittal anorectoplasty: results in the management of 322 cases of anorectal malformations. Pediatr Surg Int 3:94, 1988.
Peña A: The posterior sagittal approach: implications in adult colorectal surgery. Dis Colon Rectum 37:1, 1994.
Rich MA, Brock WA, Peña A: Spectrum of genitourinary malformations in patients with imperforate anus. Pediatr Surg Int 3:110, 1988.

CHAPTER 282
Ulcer Disease

John J. Herbst

Ulcer disease is uncommon in children. The true incidence is unknown, but it is higher than estimates from surveys before the endoscopic era of 3.5–14.7/100,000 and much less than the 3% noted in adults older than 45 yr. It is useful to classify ulcers as being primary (peptic) or secondary (caused by factors that affect integrity of the intestinal mucosa). The relationship of conditions such as duodenitis or gastritis to symptoms and ulcer formation is poorly understood.

PATHOLOGY AND PHYSIOLOGY. A number of factors are important in the development of primary ulcer disease, including gastric acidity, blood type O, and high serum levels of pepsinogen I. A family history is noted in 25–50% of children with duodenal ulcers; concordance for duodenal ulcer is 50% for monozygotic twins. Other factors that appear to be important include cigarette smoking, climatic conditions, dietary habits (consumption of alcohol), and emotional strain.

Children with duodenal ulcers have increased acid secretion, but studies do not correlate acid secretion with ulcer size or duration of symptoms. Gastric acidity is often normal or low with gastric ulcers. Tissue resistance, caused in part by cell turnover, mucus production, and bicarbonate secretion, is an important variable regulated and enhanced by local prostaglandin synthesis. Factors that lower resistance to acid-induced injury include anoxia, poor perfusion, bile, and drugs, especially nonsteroidal anti-inflammatory agents that inhibit prostaglandin synthesis.

Helicobacter pylori is an important factor in childhood gastritis and peptic ulcer disease, especially recurrent disease. It is present in gastric mucosa of most patients with chronic peptic ulcer disease. It is more common in lower socioeconomic classes and in individuals from developing countries, and it frequently causes a chronic lymphonodular gastritis. It is unclear whether the organism causes the ulcer or is important in maintaining the ulcer, but eradication of *H. pylori* is associated with healing and long-term cure of recurrent peptic ulcer disease. In general, factors related to acid are more important in duodenal ulcers, whereas tissue resistance is of greater importance in gastric ulcers. Primary peptic ulcers are usually chronic, duodenal, and related to *H. pylori,* whereas secondary ulcers are acute and gastric.

Ulcers may be superficial, erode deeply into the mucosa and submucosa, penetrate a blood vessel and cause hemorrhage, or cause perforation. A very shallow ulcer is considered an abrasion. They are usually 1 cm or less in diameter; a fibrinous coat of leukocytes and red cells covers a zone of fibrinoid necrosis surrounded by an infiltration of acute and chronic inflammatory cells. If inflammation and edema are extensive, acute or chronic gastric obstruction may occur. Most duodenal ulcers occur in the posterior part of the bulb, and most gastric ulcers occur on the lesser curve or antral area. Especially with recurrent peptic ulcers, *H. pylori* bacteria may be seen in adjacent tissue in association with a lymphonodular antral gastritis. Secondary ulcers are often multiple and associated with a diffuse gastritis.

282.1 Primary (Peptic) Ulcers

CLINICAL MANIFESTATIONS. The manifestations of peptic ulcer disease include vomiting, acute and chronic gastrointestinal blood loss, pain, and a strong familial incidence. Only about 15% of adults with symptoms of dyspepsia thought to be compatible with ulcer disease will have ulcers on investigation. The frequency of nonspecific abdominal pain in children and the rarity of ulcer disease suggest a similar situation.

In the 1st mo of life, the two main presentations are gastrointestinal hemorrhage and perforation. Between the neonatal period and 2 yr of age, recurrent vomiting, slow growth, and gastrointestinal hemorrhage are the major symptoms. In preschool-age children, periumbilical postprandial pain is often elicited, whereas vomiting and hemorrhage remain common. After 6 yr of age, the clinical features of ulcer disease are similar to those in adults and commonly include epigastric abdominal pain, acute or chronic gastrointestinal blood loss (hematemesis, hematochezia, or melena) leading to iron deficiency anemia, predominantly male gender, and a strong family history of ulcer disease. The pain is often described as dull or aching in character rather than sharp or burning, as in adults. It may last from minutes to hours, and there are frequent exacerbations and remissions lasting from weeks to months. Nocturnal pain is common. A history of typical ulcer pain with prompt relief after taking antacids is found in less than 33% of patients. Rarely in patients with acute or chronic blood loss, penetration of the ulcer into the abdominal cavity or adjacent organs produces shock, anemia, peritonitis, or pancreatitis.

DIAGNOSIS. An upper gastrointestinal roentgenographic examination is the most useful, regularly available test if symptoms are not acute. It will detect approximately 75% of duodenal ulcers in children on first examination. The duodenal bulb is difficult to examine in infants because of its high posterior position. The ulcer crater should be demonstrated in several films, preferably in a distended bulb. Deformity of the bulb is a good sign of past ulcer disease but does not ensure that current symptoms are due to ulcer disease or that an ulcer is present. Spasm of the bulb with subsequent filling is common and normal; radiographic interpretations such as duodenitis, irritability of the bulb, and pylorospasm should not be interpreted as ulcer disease. Although fewer than 40% of gastric ulcers are demonstrated, primary gastric ulcers are very rare in children.

Gastroduodenoscopy is indicated when roentgenographic findings are questionable or absent in symptomatic patients, when symptoms persist despite radiographic evidence of healing, or with prolonged presence of an ulcer crater. In patients with acute upper gastrointestinal hemorrhage, endoscopy is the procedure of choice if gastric lavage can clear the stomach of obscuring blood and clot. Endoscopy has increased the accuracy of diagnosing ulcers, especially bleeding ulcers, increased the number diagnosed, and made it possible to evaluate the patient for *H. pylori,* and use of various forms of endoscopic cautery (electrocoagulation, heater probe thermal contact) can control bleeding and decrease the chance of a repeat bleed. In patients with active, severe upper gastrointestinal bleeding that precludes endoscopy, angiography can document the site; control of bleeding is possible by embolization (absorbable gelatin [Gelfoam]) of the bleeding vessel or infusing vasoconstrictors into vessels just proximal to the bleeding vessel. Nonetheless, 75–80% of ulcers stop bleeding spontaneously.

The differential diagnosis is extensive but includes esophagitis, giardiasis, pancreatitis, inflammatory bowel disease, cholelithiasis, and recurrent abdominal pain of childhood. Functional, nonspecific pain is common among school-age children but is not associated with weight loss, emesis, blood loss, and preprandial or night pain.

TREATMENT. The goal is to hasten healing of the ulcer, relieve pain, and prevent complications. If present, hemorrhagic shock and anemia must be treated as a first priority. Suppression of gastric acidity is an important factor in treatment. The buffering ability of antacids varies, and recommendations vary widely. Antacids are most effective when given 1 and 3 hr after a meal and at bedtime. The full adult dose of the concentrated liquids is 15 mL per dose. The optimal dose of antacids is controversial and varies with acid secretion; pediatric doses of as much as 1 mL/kg/dose have been recommended. Most antacids are mixtures of magnesium and aluminum salts. The magnesium ion causes diarrhea, whereas the aluminum salts may cause constipation. Aluminum hydroxide binds with dietary phosphates and interferes with their absorption. If large doses of aluminum hydroxide are used over a period of time, complications of phosphate depletion and aluminum toxicity including anorexia, osteomalacia, and osteoporosis may occur. Calcium antacids can cause increased acid secretion after the buffering effect has stopped. Sodium bicarbonate is a very effective acid buffer but is not suitable for chronic use because of the large systemic alkaline and sodium load.

The histamine$_2$ (H_2) receptor blockers offer a convenient alternative, even though they are not officially approved for use in children. Cimetidine (20–40 mg/kg/day in four doses) and ranitidine (4–6 mg/kg/day in two doses) are frequently used liquid preparations. Omeprazol, a potent hydrogen-potassium adenosine triphosphatase pump inhibitor that more completely suppresses acid production, is effective in adults but comes as a single dose in a delayed-release capsule. Neither H_2 blockers nor omeprazol stop the acute hemorrhage but are indicated to prevent recurrences. Anticholinergic drugs inhibit acid secretion only in doses that also cause dry mouth and blurred vision and are not recommended for primary therapy.

Therapy for *H. pylori* is controversial. Approximately half of patients will have long-term cure of ulcers with conventional therapy. It is reasonable that those not responding to therapy and those with recurrent disease be investigated to document the presence of *H. pylori* before therapy. Amoxicillin and metronidazole, usually in combination with bismuth, are added to conventional therapy for 2 wk. Eradication of the organism prevents recurrence of ulcer disease.

Surgery is rarely needed but is indicated in patients with intractable pain or chronic bleeding. Perforation, loss of more than 30% of the blood volume within 48 hr from hemorrhaging that cannot be controlled through embolization or cautery of the bleeding vessel as described earlier, or gastric outlet obstruction that does not improve after 72 hr of nasogastric drainage are indications for immediate surgery. Vagotomy and either pyloroplasty or antrectomy are the procedures most used for chronic ulcer disease in children with acute hemorrhage or perforation; oversewing of the ulcer, often combined with vagotomy or pyloroplasty, is usually recommended.

282.2 Secondary Ulcers

Secondary ulcers occur when normal mucosal protective mechanisms are depressed or disease causes a marked increase in gastric acid or proteolytic enzymes. Secondary ulcers are more than twice as common as primary ulcers in childhood and are much more likely to be gastric. Most secondary ulcers are due to stress, but drugs (nonsteroidal anti-inflammatory agents, including aspirin) are becoming a more common cause.

STRESS ULCERS. In infants, stress ulcers are usually due to sepsis, respiratory or cardiac insufficiency, or dehydration. In older children, they are related to trauma or other life-threatening conditions. Curling ulcers occur in up to 13% of burn patients and are associated with normal gastric secretions. Cushing ulcers follow head trauma or surgery and are associated with gastric hypersecretion. Stress ulcers are often multiple, are associated with hemorrhagic gastritis and erosions, and are often terminal events. Perforation and more often massive hemorrhage are often the initial symptom.

DRUG-RELATED ULCERS. Aspirin and other nonsteroidal anti-inflammatory drugs are an increasing cause of ulcer disease in childhood. Of those patients taking nonsteroidal anti-inflammatory drugs chronically, approximately 25% will experience gastric ulcers and many more will experience erosions.

Alcohol and smoking are known to affect gastroduodenal mucosa adversely and should not be used because of general health concerns. Although there are conflicting studies, a meta-analysis of the literature indicates there is a statistical association between steroid use and ulcer disease in children.

TREATMENT. Treatment of secondary ulcers is similar to that for primary ulcers. Bleeding and less often perforation are common presentations. Maintaining gastric pH above 3.5 in critically ill patients will help prevent ulcer formation. Misoprostol, a prostaglandin analog, may prevent development of gastric ulcers in patients chronically taking nonsteroidal anti-inflammatory drugs; experience in children is limited.

282.3 Zollinger-Ellison Syndrome

This rare syndrome can cause multiple recurrent duodenal and jejunal ulcers and is occasionally associated with diarrhea. Gastric secretion is markedly stimulated by serum gastrin and other hormones secreted by an islet cell tumor or hypertrophy. Hypergastrinemia, albeit lower than Zollinger-Ellison syndrome, may be noted in pyloric stenosis, short-bowel syndrome, hyperparathyroidism, pheochromocytoma, and multiple endocrine neoplasias. Therapy with H_2 drugs or omeprazol can control gastric acid secretion and improve symptoms when these slow-growing tumors cannot be entirely removed.

Caulfield M, Wyllie R, Sivak M, et al: Upper gastrointestinal tract endoscopy in the pediatric patient. J Pediatr 115:339, 1989.
Chiang B-L, Chang M-H, Lin M-I, et al: Chronic duodenal ulcer in children: clinical observation and response to treatment. J Pediatr Gastroenterol Nutr 8:161, 1989.
DeGiacomo C, Fiocca R, Villani L, et al: *Helicobacter pylori* infection and chronic gastritis: clinical, serological, and histologic correlations in children treated with amoxicillin and colloidal bismuth subcitrate. J Pediatr Gastroenterol Nutr 11:310, 1990.
Drumm B, Rhoads JM, Stringer DA, et al: Peptic ulcer disease in children: etiology, clinical findings, and clinical course. Pediatrics 82:410, 1988.
Judd RH: *Helicobacter pylori*, gastritis, and ulcers in pediatrics. Adv Pediatr 39:283, 1992.
Kumar D, Spitz L: Peptic ulceration in children. Surg Gynecol Obstet 159:163, 1984.
Laine L, Peterson W: Bleeding peptic ulcer. N Engl J Med 331:717, 1994.
Meyerovitz MF, Fellows KE: Angiography in gastrointestinal bleeding in children. AJR 143:837, 1984.
Tam PKH, Saing H: The use of H_2-receptor antagonist in the treatment of peptic ulcer disease in children. J Pediatr Gastroenterol Nutr 8:41, 1989.

CHAPTER 283
Inflammatory Bowel Disease

Martin Ulshen

Inflammatory bowel disease (IBD) is a group of idiopathic, chronic disorders that includes Crohn disease and ulcerative colitis. The cause is poorly understood, and the natural course is characterized by unpredictable exacerbations and remissions. The most common time of onset of IBD is during adolescence and young adulthood. A bimodal distribution has been shown with an early onset at 15–25 yr of age and a second smaller peak at 50–80 yr of age. Nonetheless, IBD may begin in the 1st yr of life. IBD is often reported to be more common in urban areas than in rural areas. In developed countries, these disorders are the major causes of chronic intestinal inflammation in children beyond the first few years of life.

There may be genetic and environmental components for the pathogenesis of IBD. The incidence rate among Jews is high but varies geographically. Although incidence rates are low among blacks in Africa, in the United States they are similar to those of whites. The prevalence of Crohn disease in the United States is much lower for Hispanics and Asians than for whites and blacks. The risk of IBD in family members of an affected individual has been reported in the range of 7–22%; a child whose parents both have IBD has a greater than 35% chance of acquiring the disorder. Relatives of an individual with ulcerative colitis have a greater risk of acquiring ulcerative colitis than Crohn disease, whereas relatives of an individual with Crohn disease have a greater risk of acquiring this disorder; the two diseases may occur in the same family. The risk of occurrence of IBD among relatives of individuals with Crohn disease is somewhat greater than for individuals with ulcerative colitis.

Other observations support the importance of genetic factors in the development of IBD. Regarding twins, there is a higher chance that both will be affected if they are monozygotic rather than dizygotic. The concordance rate in twins is higher in Crohn disease than in ulcerative colitis. Genetic disorders that have been associated with IBD include Turner syndrome, Hermansky-Pudlak syndrome, glycogen storage disease type Ib, and a number of immunodeficiency disorders. Environmental factors are important in the cause of IBD and presumably explain discordance among twins and changes in risks among the same race in different geographic regions; the precise factors remain unknown. Individuals migrating to developed countries often appear to acquire the higher rates of IBD associated with these regions.

Mediators of inflammatory states (e.g., cytokines, prostaglandins, and reactive oxygen metabolites) are important in the pathogenesis of IBD. Much of our current therapy is aimed at interfering with this cycle. However, the initiating events that start the inflammatory response remain to be identified.

It is usually possible to distinguish between ulcerative colitis and Crohn disease by a combination of clinical presentation and radiologic, endoscopic, and histopathologic findings (Table 283–1). It is not possible to make a definitive diagnosis in as many as 10% of individuals with chronic colitis; it is best to call this disorder indeterminate colitis. Occasionally, a child will be given a diagnosis of ulcerative colitis on the basis of the clinical findings and even years later it will become apparent that the correct diagnosis is Crohn colitis. In general, the treatments of Crohn disease and ulcerative colitis overlap greatly, but as refinements in treatment are identified, the distinction between these entities becomes more important. The response to treatment may be incomplete.

■ **TABLE 283–1 Comparison of Crohn Disease and Ulcerative Colitis**

Feature	Crohn Disease	Ulcerative Colitis
Rectal bleeding	Sometimes	Common
Abdominal mass	Common	Not present
Rectal disease	Occasional	Nearly universal
Ileal involvement	Common	None (backwash ileitis)
Perianal disease	Common	Unusual
Strictures	Common	Unusual
Fistula	Common	Unusual
Discontinuous (skip) lesions	Common	Unusual
Transmural involvement	Common	Unusual
Crypt abscesses	Less common	Common
Granulomas	Common	Unusual
Risk for colonic cancer	Slightly increased	Greatly increased

Extraintestinal manifestations tend to occur slightly more commonly with Crohn disease than with ulcerative colitis. Growth retardation may be seen in 15–35% of individuals at diagnosis. Of the extraintestinal manifestations that occur with IBD, joint, skin, eye, mouth, and hepatobiliary involvement tend to be associated with colitis whether ulcerative or Crohn colitis. For some of the manifestations, activity correlates with activity of the bowel disease, including peripheral arthritis, erythema nodosum, and anemia. Activity of pyoderma gangrenosum correlates less well with activity of the bowel disease, whereas activities of sclerosing cholangitis, ankylosing spondylitis, and sacroiliitis do not correlate with intestinal disease. Arthritis occurs in three patterns: migratory peripheral arthritis involving primarily large joints, ankylosing spondylitis, and sacroiliitis. The peripheral arthritis of IBD tends to be nondestructive. It may be associated with false-positive antinuclear antibodies. Ankylosing spondylitis begins in the third decade and occurs most commonly in individuals with ulcerative colitis who have human leukocyte antigen B27 phenotype. Symptoms include low back pain and morning stiffness; back, hips, shoulders, and sacroiliac joints are typically affected. Isolated sacroiliitis is usually asymptomatic but is common when a careful search is performed. Among the skin manifestations, erythema nodosum is most common. Individuals with erythema nodosum or pyoderma gangrenosum have a high likelihood of having arthritis as well. Glomerulonephritis and a hypercoagulable state are other rare manifestations that occur in childhood. Cerebral thromboembolic disease has been described in children with IBD. Uveitis occurs in about 5% of children with IBD and is usually asymptomatic and transient; its occurrence does not correlate with activity of bowel disease.

283.1 Chronic Ulcerative Colitis

Ulcerative colitis is an idiopathic chronic inflammatory disorder localized to the colon and sparing the upper gastrointestinal tract. Disease virtually always begins in the rectum and extends proximally for a variable distance. When it is localized to the rectum, the disease is known as ulcerative proctitis, whereas disease involving the entire colon is known as pancolitis. The former disorder is less likely to be associated with systemic manifestations, although it may be less responsive to treatment than more diffuse disease. Ulcerative colitis has been noted to present in infancy, although this is very unusual. One needs to be cautious when evaluating reports of ulcerative colitis in infancy because dietary protein intolerance may be easily misdiagnosed as ulcerative colitis in this age group. Dietary protein intolerance (e.g., cow's milk protein) is a transient disorder, and symptoms are directly associated with the oral intake of the offending antigen.

The incidence of ulcerative colitis has remained constant, in contrast to the increase in Crohn disease, but varies with country of origin. Incidence rates are highest in northern European countries and the United States (~15/100,000) and lowest in Japan and South Africa (~1/100,000). The incidence of ulcerative colitis in Israel varies with the country of origin; those born in Asia or Africa have the lowest risk. The prevalence of ulcerative colitis in northern European countries and the United States varies from 100–200/100,000 population. Men are slightly more likely to acquire ulcerative colitis than women; the reverse is true for Crohn disease. The incidence of ulcerative proctitis is 20–50% of that of ulcerative colitis.

CLINICAL MANIFESTATIONS. Symptoms of mild dysentery (bloody diarrhea with mucus) are the most typical presentation of ulcerative coitis. Symptoms such as tenesmus, urgency, crampy abdominal pain (especially with bowel movements), and nocturnal bowel movements suggest a more severe colitis. The onset may be insidious with gradual progression of symptoms but can be fulminant. Fever, severe anemia, hypoalbuminemia, leukocytosis, and stool frequency of more than six per day all suggest fulminant colitis. Chronicity is an important part of the diagnosis; it is difficult to know whether one is dealing with a subacute, transient colitis or ulcerative colitis when a child has had 3–4 wk of symptoms without an identifiable cause. Symptoms beyond this duration often prove to be secondary to IBD. Occasionally, the presentation of ulcerative colitis may be very mild (e.g., mild rectal bleeding without diarrhea, which is often the result of a localized proctitis). Anorexia, weight loss, and growth failure may be present, although systemic manifestations are more typical of Crohn disease. Extraintestinal manifestations that tend to occur more commonly with ulcerative colitis than with Crohn disease include pyoderma gangrenosum, sclerosing cholangitis, chronic active hepatitis, and ankylosing spondylitis. Any of the extraintestinal disorders described previously for IBD may occur with ulcerative colitis. Iron deficiency may result from chronic blood loss as well as decreased assimilation (either related to decreased intake or decreased absorption). Folate deficiency is unusual but may be accentuated in children treated with sulfasalazine, which interferes with folate absorption. Anemia may be the result of chronic disease without an identifiable deficiency. Secondary amenorrhea is common during periods of active disease in girls past menarche.

The clinical course of ulcerative colitis is marked by exacerbations, often without apparent explanation. Typically, the disease may be quieted with medication but eventually it recurs. Occasionally, the colitis becomes intractable and may then require surgical treatment. It is always important to reconsider the possibility of enteric infection with recurrent symptoms; these infections may mimic a flare-up or actually provoke a recurrence. Nonsteroidal anti-inflammatory drugs may promote exacerbations as well.

It is generally believed that the risk of colon cancer begins to increase after 8–10 yr of disease and may then increase by 0.5–1% per year. The onset of risk is delayed by about 10 yr in individuals with left-sided colitis. Proctitis alone is associated with virtually no increase in risk over the general population. Childhood onset does not appear to increase the risk further. Because colon cancer is usually preceded by changes of mucosal dysplasia, it is recommended to screen patients with ulcerative colitis beyond 10 yr duration with colonoscopy and biopsy every 1–2 yr. The effectiveness of this approach in preventing colon cancer remains to be established. Two concerns about this plan of management have been stated and remain unresolved: (1) the original studies may have overestimated the risk of colon cancer and, therefore, the need for surveillance has been overemphasized and (2) screening for dysplasia may not be adequate for the prevention of colon cancer in ulcerative colitis if some cancers are not preceded by dysplasia. Nevertheless, screening and prophylactic colectomy are the only alternatives.

DIFFERENTIAL DIAGNOSIS. The major differential in establishing the diagnosis of ulcerative colitis is infectious colitis and Crohn colitis. A history of contact with others with gastroenteritis should especially make one consider an infectious cause. Every child with a new diagnosis of ulcerative colitis should have stool cultures for enteric pathogens, stool for ova and parasites, and perhaps serology for ameba (Table 283–2). In the setting of antibiotic use, pseudomembranous colitis secondary to *Clostridium difficile* should be considered. The most difficult distinction is from Crohn disease because the colitis of Crohn disease may initially appear identical to that of ulcerative colitis. The appearance of the colitis or development of small-bowel disease will eventually lead to the correct diagnosis; this may occur years after the initial presentation.

At the onset, the colitis of hemolytic-uremic syndrome (HUS) may be identical to that of early ulcerative colitis. Ultimately, signs of microangiopathic hemolysis (the presence of schistocytes on blood smear), thrombocytopenia, and subsequent renal failure should confirm the diagnosis of HUS. Although Schönlein-Henoch purpura may present with abdominal pain and bloody stools, it is not usually associated with colitis. Behçet syndrome can be distinguished by its typical features. Other considerations, are cathartic colitis, radiation proctitis, human immunodeficiency virus–associated colitis, and ischemic colitis. In infancy, dietary protein intolerance may be confused with ulcerative colitis, although this disorder is a transient problem that resolves on removal of the offending protein from the diet. Hirschsprung disease may produce a colitis usually before or within months after surgical correction, but this complication is unlikely to be confused with ulcerative colitis.

DIAGNOSIS. The diagnosis of ulcerative colitis or ulcerative proctitis requires a typical presentation in the absence of an identifiable specific cause (Tables 283–2 and 283–3) and typical endoscopic and radiologic findings (see Table 283–1). There is no specific test that will confirm the diagnosis; rather one needs to find the right constellation of history and findings in the context of a chronic disorder. One should be hesitant to make a diagnosis of ulcerative colitis in a child who has experienced symptoms for fewer than 3–4 wk. When the diagnosis is made in a child with subacute symptoms, the physician should make a firm diagnosis only when there is evidence of chronicity. Laboratory studies may demonstrate evidence of anemia (either iron deficiency or the anemia of chronic disease) or hypoalbuminemia. Although the sedimentation rate is often elevated, it may be normal even with fulminant colitis. An elevated white count is usually only seen with more severe colitis. A test to distinguish ulcerative colitis from Crohn disease has been described that evaluates the presence of antineutrophil cytoplasmic antibodies in the patient's blood. Although the test is not specific enough to establish a diagnosis, in a study of children with IBD, these antibodies were present in 65% of the children with ulcerative colitis compared with 20% of those with Crohn disease. The test may possibly prove to be a helpful adjunct in reaching a diagnosis. These antibodies persist after colectomy and are also found in healthy relatives of individuals with ulcerative colitis.

Findings of ulcerative colitis can be identified by endoscopic or radiologic examination of the colon, although endoscopy (i.e., sigmoidoscopy or colonoscopy) is more sensitive for mild disease and offers the opportunity for simultaneous biopsy. Certain typical features can be seen on either study, including concentric, diffuse colitis starting in the rectum and extending

■ TABLE 283–2 Infectious Agents Mimicking Inflammatory Bowel Disease

Agent	Manifestations	Diagnosis	Comments
Bacterial			
Campylobacter jejuni	Acute diarrhea, fever, fecal blood, and leukocytes	Culture	Common in adolescents, may relapse
Yersinia enterocolitica	Acute→ chronic diarrhea, right lower quadrant pain, mesenteric adenitis—pseudoappendicitis, fecal blood, and leukocytes Extraintestinal manifestations, mimics Crohn disease	Culture	Common in adolescents as FUO, weight loss, abdominal pain
Clostridium difficile	Postantibiotic onset, watery diarrhea, pseudomembrane on sigmoidoscopy	Culture and cytotoxin	May be nosocomial Toxic megacolon possible
Escherichia coli 0157:H7	Colitis, fecal blood, abdominal pain	Culture and typing	Hemolytic-uremic syndrome
Salmonella	Watery→ bloody diarrhea, food borne, fecal leukocytes, cramps	Culture	Usually acute
Shigella	Watery→ bloody diarrhea, fecal leukocytes, fever, pain, cramps	Culture	Dysentery symptoms
Edwardsiella tarda	Bloody diarrhea, cramps	Culture	Ulceration on endoscopy
Aeromonas hydrophilia	Cramps, diarrhea, fecal blood	Culture	May be chronic Contaminated drinking water
Plesiomonas	Diarrhea, cramps	Culture	Shellfish source
Tuberculosis	Rarely bovine, now *Mycobacterium tuberculosis* Ileocecal area, fistula formation	Culture, PPD, biopsy	May mimic Crohn disease
Parasites			
Entamoeba histolytica	Acute bloody diarrhea and liver abscess, colic	Trophozoite in stool, colonic mucosal flask ulceration, serology	Travel to endemic area
Giardia lamblia	Foul-smelling, watery diarrhea, cramps, flatulence, weight loss; no colonic involvement	"Owl"-like trophozoite and cysts in stool; rarely duodenal intubation	May be chronic
AIDS-Associated Enteropathy			
Cryptosporidium	Chronic diarrhea, weight loss	Stool microscopy	Mucosal findings not like IBD
Isospora belli	As in *Cryptosporidium*		Tropical location
Cytomegalovirus	Colonic ulceration, pain, bloody diarrhea	Culture, biopsy	

FUO = fever of unknown origin; PPD = purified protein derivative; AIDS = acquired immunodeficiency syndrome; IBD = inflammatory bowel disease.

proximally for a variable distance. One should not see skip areas (i.e., areas of normal colon between diseased areas); however, the finding of skip areas must be confirmed histologically before it can be used as evidence against a diagnosis of ulcerative colitis. Endoscopic examination should be done when one suspects this diagnosis. One can use either a flexible sigmoidoscopy to confirm the diagnosis or colonoscopy to evaluate the extent of disease and to rule out evidence of Crohn colitis. A colonoscopy should *not* be performed when fulminant colitis is suspected because of the risk of provoking toxic megacolon or causing a perforation during the procedure. The degree of colitis can be evaluated by the gross appearance of the mucosa. Despite the name of this disorder, one does not generally see discrete ulcers, which would be more suggestive of Crohn colitis. The endoscopic findings of ulcerative colitis result from microulcers, which give the appearance of a diffuse abnormality. The earliest changes are granularity and then loss of the normal vascular pattern. Friability induced on contact with the endoscope may also be seen with a mild colitis. More severe changes include erythema, spontaneous friability, and edema of the mucosa with blunting of mucosal folds. With very severe colitis, pseudopolyps may be seen. Perianal disease, with the exception of mild local irritation or anal fissures associated with diarrhea, should make one think of Crohn disease. The biopsy of involved bowel demonstrates evidence of acute and chronic mucosal inflammation. Typical findings are cryptitis, crypt abscesses, separation of crypts by inflammatory cells, foci of acute inflammatory cells, edema, mucus depletion, and branching of crypts. The last finding is a feature not seen in infectious colitis. Granulomas, fissures, or full-thickness involvement of the bowel wall (usually on surgical rather than endoscopic biopsy) suggests Crohn disease.

Plain radiographs of the abdomen may demonstrate loss of haustral markings in an air-filled colon or marked dilatation with toxic megacolon. Further radiologic studies are often unnecessary if endoscopy has been performed. A double-contrast barium (air) enema is the best of the radiographic studies to identify ulcerative colitis, although it is not as sensitive as endoscopy for mild colitis. Radiologic findings on barium enema demonstrate diffuse, concentric disease with a finely spiculated border representing the microulceration. The earliest changes are fine granularity followed by more coarse granular-

■ TABLE 283–3 Chronic Inflammatory Intestinal Disorders

Infection—see Table 283–2
- Bacterial
- Parasite
- AIDS associated
- Toxin

Immune-Inflammatory
- Congenital immunodeficiency disorders
- Acquired immunodeficiency diseases
- Dietary protein enterocolitis
- Behçet syndrome
- Lymphoid nodular hyperplasia
- Eosinophilic gastroenteritis
- Graft versus host disease

Vascular-Ischemic
- Systemic vasculitis (SLE, dermatomyositis)
- Schönlein-Henoch purpura
- Hemolytic-uremic syndrome

Other
- Prestenotic colitis
- Diversion colitis
- Radiation colitis
- Neonatal necrotizing enterocolitis
- Typhlitis
- Hirschsprung colitis
- Intestinal lymphoma
- Laxative abuse

AIDS = acquired immunodeficiency syndrome; SLE = systemic lupus erythematosus.

ity. With severe disease, "collar button" ulcers with submucosal undermining may be seen. Mucosal folds become thickened and may be completely obliterated to give a smooth-appearing surface, sometimes known as a "lead pipe colon." This appearance is sometimes reversible with treatment. The terminal ileum should appear normal except in children with pancolitis, when the terminal ileum may be dilated with a patulous ileocecal valve (known as "backwash ileitis"). With severe colitis, the colon may become dilated; a diameter of greater than 6 cm, determined radiographically, in an adult suggests toxic megacolon. If it is necessary to examine the colon radiologically in a child with severe colitis (to evaluate the extent of involvement or to try to rule out Crohn disease), it is sometimes helpful to perform an upper gastrointestinal contrast series with small-bowel follow-through and then look at delayed films of the colon. This is much safer than performing a barium enema in the situation of toxic megacolon.

TREATMENT. A medical cure for ulcerative colitis is not available; treatment is aimed at controlling symptoms and reducing the risk of recurrence. The intensity of treatment varies with the severity of the symptoms. In placebo-controlled studies of therapy, about 20–30% of individuals with ulcerative colitis will have spontaneous improvement in symptoms. The first drug to be used with mild colitis is an aminosalicylate, usually sulfasalazine. Sulfasalazine has been used extensively over many years, and its effects are well characterized. It is composed of a sulfur moiety linked to the active ingredient 5-aminosalicylate. This linkage prevents the premature absorption of the medication in the upper gastrointestinal tract, allowing it to reach the colon where the two components are separated by bacterial cleavage. The dose of sulfasalazine is 50–75 mg/kg/day (divided in two to four doses). Generally, the dose is not more than two to three g/day. It is recommended that the dosage gradually increase to full dose over the first week of treatment to avoid gastrointestinal symptoms and to detect sulfa hypersensitivity. Onset of action may be slow (up to several weeks). Sulfasalazine treats colitis; recurrences may be prevented with its use. It is recommended that the medication be continued even when the disorder is in remission. Sulfasalazine is the only drug shown to prevent relapses; it seems likely that this would be true for the newer aminosalicylate preparations.

Hypersensitivity to the sulfa component is the major side effect of sulfasalazine and may occur in up to 10–20% of individuals. This reaction includes varying combinations of skin rash (typically morbilliform), hepatopathy, and fever. Skin manifestations may be as severe as an exfoliative dermatitis (Stevens-Johnson syndrome). Generally these manifestations resolve when the sulfasalazine is discontinued. Other side effects include reversible leukopenia, hemolysis, pancreatitis, headache, nausea and vomiting, and bloody diarrhea. The last manifestation may be difficult to recognize in a child who is being treated for colitis. If a child with ulcerative colitis does not appear to respond to this medication or the colitis seems to worsen, one should consider the possibility that the medication may be contributing to the symptom. A complete blood count should be checked 10–14 days after beginning sulfasalazine to rule out the hematologic side effects. Although desensitization may be successful in individuals with a hypersensitivity reaction, other oral forms of aminosalicylate (olsalazine or delayed release forms of 5-aminosalicylate) are available. The published experience with the newer preparations in children is limited. Perhaps 10–20% of individuals who have an adverse reaction to sulfasalazine will have a similar reaction to another 5-aminosalicylate product; diarrhea is a common side effect. Aminosalicylate may also be given in enema form and is especially useful for proctitis. Hydrocortisone enemas (100 mg) are used to treat proctitis as well. Either form of enema may be administered to older children and is given once a day usually for 2–3 wk. Many children prefer oral medication to enemas.

Children with moderate to severe pancolitis or colitis unresponsive to 5-aminosalicylate therapy should be treated with corticosteroids, most commonly prednisone. The usual starting dose of prednisone is 1–2 mg/kg/24 hr (40 mg should rarely be exceeded). If symptoms are not severe, this medication may be given in a single morning dose to lessen adrenal suppression. With severe colitis, the daily dose may be divided in three or four doses and may be given intravenously. The goal is to taper to an alternate-day dose within 1–3 mo. Persistent symptoms despite steroid treatment or the inability to taper the dose are an indication for the use of other medications or for surgical management. Prolonged use of daily steroids beyond this period is to be avoided because of the many side effects, including growth retardation, adrenal suppression, cataracts, aseptic necrosis of the head of the femur, diabetes mellitus, risk of infection, and cosmetic effects. Colectomy may be necessary in fulminant disease (i.e., greater than six to eight stools in 24 hr, passage of stools during the night, fever, elevated white cell count, anemia, hypoalbuminemia, and tender abdomen) that is unresponsive to medical management for 3–4 wk.

A clear benefit of the use of total parenteral nutrition or continuous enteral elemental diet in the treatment of severe ulcerative colitis has not been noted. Nevertheless, parenteral nutrition is often used so that the patient will be ready for surgery if medical management fails. Other agents that have been used in steroid-unresponsive or steroid-dependent colitis include azathioprine, 6-mercaptopurine (6-MP), metronidazole, and cyclosporine. Azathioprine and 6-MP are the slowest to begin to work. Experience with these medications in the treatment of colitis in children is very limited. With any medical treatment for ulcerative colitis, one should always weigh the risk of the medication or therapy against the fact that colitis may be successfully treated surgically.

Surgical treatment for intractable or fulminant colitis is total colectomy. The optimal approach is to combine colectomy with an endorectal pull-through. In this procedure, the surgeon retains a segment of distal rectum and strips the mucosa from this region. The distal ileum is pulled down and sutured at the internal anus with a J pouch created from ileum immediately above the rectal cuff. This procedure allows the child to maintain continence. Stool frequency is often increased after the procedure but may be improved with loperamide. The major complication of this operation is "pouchitis," which is a chronic inflammatory reaction in the pouch leading to bloody diarrhea, abdominal pain, and occasionally low-grade fever. The cause of this complication is unknown, although it is more frequent when the ileal pouch has been constructed for ulcerative colitis than for other indications (familial polyposis coli).

The concept that ulcerative colitis is primarily a psychogenic disorder is now untenable. However, emotional stresses may contribute to exacerbations. Difficulty adjusting to a chronic disorder is common, and distorted body image should be considered when evaluating the psychological profile of a child with this disorder. Psychosocial support is an important part of therapy of this disorder. This may include adequate discussion of the disease manifestations and management between patient and physician, psychological counseling for the child when necessary, and family support from a social worker or family counselor. Patient support groups have proven very helpful for some families. The largest of these is the Crohn's and Colitis Foundation of America (CCFA), which has local chapters throughout the United States. Children with ulcerative colitis should be encouraged to participate fully in age-appropriate activities, with the exception that activity may be reduced during periods of decreased stamina.

PROGNOSIS. The course of ulcerative colitis is marked by remissions and exacerbations. Most children with this disorder respond initially to medical management. Many children with mild manifestations continue to respond well to medical management and may stay in remission on prophylactic sulfasalazine for long periods of time. However, an occasional child with a mild onset will experience intractable symptoms at a later time. The most serious acute complication is toxic megacolon with the risk of perforation. Beyond the first decade of disease, the risk of development of colon cancer begins to increase rapidly. However, current thinking is that colon cancer may be prevented with surveillance colonoscopies beginning after 8–10 yr of disease.

Braegger C: Immunopathogenesis of chronic inflammatory bowel disease. Acta Paediatr Suppl 395:18, 1994.

Ekbom A, Helmick C, Zack M, et al: Ulcerative colitis and colorectal cancer. N Engl J Med 323:1228, 1990.

Ferry GD, Kirschner BS, Grand RJ, et al: Olsalazine versus sulfasalazine in mild to moderate childhood ulcerative colitis: Results of the Pediatric Gastroenterology Collaborative Research Group Clinical Trial. J Pediatr Gastroenterol Nutr 17:32, 1993.

Kleinman RE, Balistreri WF, Heyman MB, et al: Nutritional support for pediatric patients with inflammatory bowel disease. J Pediatr Gastroenterol Nutr 8:8, 1989.

Korelitz B: Considerations of surveillance, dysplasia and carcinoma of the colon in management of ulcerative colitis and Crohn's disease. Med Clin North Am 74:189, 1990.

Lichtiger S, Present DH, Kornbluth A, et al: Cyclosporine in severe ulcerative colitis refractory to steroid therapy. N Engl J Med 330:1841, 1994.

Markowitz RL, Ment LR, Cryboski JD: Cerebral thromboembolic disease in pediatric and adult inflammatory bowel disease: Case report and review of the literature. J Pediatr Gastroenterol Nutr 8:413, 1989.

Michener W, Wyllie R: Management of children and adolescents with inflammatory bowel disease. Med Clin North Am 74:103, 1990.

North CS, Clouse RE, Spitznagel EL, et al: The relation of ulcerative colitis to psychiatric factors: A review of findings and methods. Am J Psychol 147:947, 1990.

Peppercorn MA: Advances in drug therapy for inflammatory bowel disease. Ann Intern Med 112:50, 1990.

Proujansky R, Fawcett PT, Gibney K M, et al: Examination of anti-neutrophil cytoplasmic antibodies in childhood inflammatory bowel disease. J Pediatr Gastroenterol Nutr 17:193, 1993.

Sartor RB: Cytokines in intestinal inflammation: Pathophysiological and clinical considerations. Gastroenterology 106:533, 1994.

Statter MB, Hirschl RB, Coran AC: Inflammatory bowel disease. Pediatr Clin North Am 40:1213, 1993.

Sugita A, Sachar DB, Bodian C, et al: Colorectal cancer in ulcerative colitis: Influence of anatomical extent and age at onset on colitis-cancer interval. Gut 32:167, 1991.

Treem WR, Hyams JS: Cyclosporine therapy for gastrointestinal disease. J Pediatr Gastroenterol Nutr 18:270, 1994.

283.2 Crohn Disease

(Regional Enteritis, Regional Ileitis, Granulomatous Colitis)

Crohn disease is an idiopathic, chronic inflammatory disorder of the bowel that involves any region of the alimentary tract from the mouth to the anus. Although there are many similarities between ulcerative colitis and Crohn disease, there are also major differences in the clinical course and distribution of the disease in the gastrointestinal tract. The inflammatory process tends to be eccentric and segmental, often with skip areas (i.e., normal regions of bowel between inflamed areas). Whereas inflammation in ulcerative colitis is limited to the mucosa (except in toxic megacolon), gastrointestinal involvement in Crohn disease is transmural. Among children with Crohn disease, the initial presentation most commonly involves ileum and colon (i.e., ileocolitis) but may involve the small bowel alone in about 40% (50% of children have terminal ileitis alone) or colon alone in about 10% (granulomatous colitis). Crohn disease may rarely present in the first years of life. As with ulcerative colitis, Crohn disease tends to have a bimodal age distribution with the first peak beginning in the late teens.

The incidence of Crohn disease has been increasing over the past 10 yr, whereas that of ulcerative colitis has been stable. The proportion of patients with IBD who are being managed for Crohn disease has gradually increased. The reported incidence of Crohn disease is about 3–4/100,000 and prevalence 30–100/100,000. The prevalence of Crohn disease in whites and blacks appears to be 3 to 10 times that of Hispanics and Asians living in the United States.

CLINICAL MANIFESTATIONS. Crohn disease may present in many forms; the manifestations tend to be dictated by the region of bowel involved, the degree of inflammation, and the presence of complications such as stricture or fistula. Children with ileocolitis typically have crampy, abdominal pain and diarrhea, sometimes with blood. Ileitis may present with right lower quadrant abdominal pain alone. Crohn colitis may be associated with bloody diarrhea, tenesmus, and urgency. Systemic signs and symptoms tend to be more common in Crohn disease than in ulcerative colitis. Fever, malaise, and easy fatigability are common. Growth failure with delayed bone maturation and delayed sexual development may precede other symptoms by 1 or 2 yr and are at least twice as likely to occur with Crohn than with ulcerative colitis. Children may present with growth failure as the only manifestation of Crohn disease. Growth retardation is associated with a decrease in lean body mass but preservation of body fat; enteric protein loss and the rate of body protein turnover are increased. Primary or secondary amenorrhea occurs frequently. In contrast to ulcerative colitis, *perianal disease* is common (tags, fistula, abscess). Gastric or duodenal involvement may be associated with recurrent vomiting and epigastric pain. Partial small-bowel obstruction, usually secondary to narrowing of the bowel lumen from inflammation or stricture, may cause symptoms of crampy abdominal pain (especially with meals), borborygmi, and intermittent abdominal distention. Stricture should be suspected if the child notes relief of symptoms in association with a sudden sensation of gurgling of intestinal contents through a localized region of the abdomen. Ureteral obstruction secondary to extension of the inflammatory process is a rare complication of Crohn disease.

Enteroenteric or enterocolonic fistulas (i.e., between segments of bowel) are often asymptomatic but may contribute to malabsorption if they have high output or result in bacterial overgrowth. Enterovesical fistulas (i.e., between bowel and urinary bladder) typically originate from ileum or sigmoid colon and present with signs of urinary infection, pneumaturia, or fecaluria. Enterovaginal fistulas originate from the rectum and cause feculent vaginal drainage. They may be very difficult to manage. Enterocutaneous fistulas (i.e., between bowel and abdominal skin) often are related to surgical anastomoses with leakage. Intra-abdominal abscess may be associated with fever and pain but may have relatively few symptoms. Hepatic or splenic abscess may occur with or without a local fistula. Anorectal abscesses often originate immediately above the anus at the crypts of Morgagni. The patterns of perianal fistulas are complex because of the different tissue planes. Perianal abscess is usually painful, but perianal fistulas tend to produce fewer symptoms than might be anticipated from their appearance. Purulent drainage is commonly associated with perianal fistulas. Psoas abscess secondary to intestinal fistula may present as hip pain, decreased hip extension (psoas sign), and fever.

Extraintestinal manifestations occur more commonly with Crohn disease than with ulcerative colitis; those that are especially associated with Crohn disease include oral aphthous ulcers, peripheral arthritis, erythema nodosum, digital clubbing, episcleritis, renal stones (uric acid, oxalate), and gallstones. Any of the extraintestinal disorders described in the section on IBD may occur with Crohn disease. The peripheral arthritis is nondeforming. In general, the occurrence of extraintestinal manifestations correlates with the presence of colitis.

During periods of active disease, secondary amenorrhea is common in girls past menarche.

Extensive involvement of small bowel, especially in association with surgical resection, may lead to short-bowel syndrome, but this is rare in children. Complications of terminal ileal dysfunction or resection include bile acid malabsorption with secondary diarrhea and vitamin B_{12} malabsorption. Chronic steatorrhea may lead to oxaluria with secondary renal stones. The risk of cholelithiasis is also increased secondary to bile acid depletion.

A disorder with this diversity of manifestations has a major impact on children's lifestyle. Children may repeatedly miss school because of symptoms. The association of pain or diarrhea with eating may limit their interest in participating in many age-appropriate activities. The majority of children with Crohn disease are able to continue with their normal activities, only having to limit activity during periods of increased symptoms.

DIFFERENTIAL DIAGNOSIS. As in patients with ulcerative colitis, the most common diagnoses to be distinguished from Crohn disease are the infectious enteropathies (in the case of Crohn disease: acute terminal ileitis, infectious colitis, enteric parasites, and periappendiceal abscess) (see Tables 283–2 and 283–3). *Yersinia* may cause many of the radiologic and endoscopic findings in the distal small bowel that are seen in Crohn disease. The symptoms of bacterial dysentery are more likely to be mistaken for ulcerative colitis than for Crohn disease. *Giardia* has been noted to produce a Crohnlike presentation including protein-losing enteropathy. Gastrointestinal tuberculosis is extremely rare but can mimic Crohn disease. Foreign body perforation of the bowel (toothpick) may mimic a localized region with Crohn disease. Small-bowel lymphoma may mimic Crohn disease but tends to be associated with nodular filling defects of the bowel without ulceration or narrowing of the lumen. In addition, bowel lymphoma is much less common in children than is Crohn disease. Recurrent functional abdominal pain may mimic the pain of small-bowel Crohn disease. Lymphoid nodular hyperplasia of the terminal ileum (a normal finding) may be mistaken for Crohn ileitis. Right lower quadrant pain or mass with fever may be the result of periappendiceal abscess. This entity may occasionally be associated with diarrhea as well.

Growth failure may be the only manifestation of Crohn disease, and other disorders such as growth hormone deficiency or gluten-sensitive enteropathy need be considered. If arthritis precedes the bowel manifestations, an initial diagnosis of juvenile rheumatoid arthritis may be made. Refractory anemia may be the presenting feature and may be mistaken as a primary hematologic disorder. Leukemia may present with abdominal pain in association with an abnormal blood count and initially may be mistaken for Crohn disease. Chronic granulomatous disease of childhood may cause inflammatory changes in the bowel with granulomas on biopsy. Antral narrowing in this disorder may be mistaken for a stricture secondary to Crohn disease.

DIAGNOSIS. Crohn disease may present with a variety of symptom combinations. At the onset, symptoms may be quite subtle (growth retardation or abdominal pain alone); this explains the fact that, in some cases, the diagnosis is not made until 1 or 2 yr after the start of symptoms. The diagnosis of Crohn disease is dependent on finding typical clinical features of the disorder (history, physical examination, laboratory studies, and endoscopic or radiologic findings), ruling out specific entities that mimic Crohn disease, and demonstrating chronicity. The history may include any combination of abdominal pain (especially right lower quadrant), diarrhea, vomiting, anorexia, weight loss, growth retardation, and extraintestinal manifestations.

Children with Crohn disease often appear chronically ill. They commonly have weight loss and are often malnourished. Linear growth retardation frequently precedes clinical presentation by as much as 1–2 yr; this manifestation may not have been appreciated until the diagnosis is established. Children with Crohn disease often appear pale with decreased energy level and poor appetite; the latter finding sometimes results from an association between meals and abdominal pain or diarrhea. There may be abdominal tenderness, either diffuse or localized to the right lower quadrant. A tender mass or fullness may be palpable in the right lower quadrant. Perianal disease, when present, may be very characteristic. Large anal skin tags (1–3 cm diameter) or perianal fistulas with purulent drainage are suggestive of Crohn disease. Digital clubbing, findings of arthritis, and skin manifestations may be present. A complete blood count commonly demonstrates an anemia, often with a component of iron deficiency. Although the sedimentation rate is often elevated, it may be normal; an elevated platelet count ($>600,000/mm^3$) is seen more commonly. The white cell count may be normal or mildly elevated. The serum albumin may be low and stool α_1-anitrypsin may be elevated consistent with a protein-losing enteropathy.

The choice of colonoscopy or a radiologic study depends on the anticipated location of disease. For small-bowel involvement, an upper gastrointestinal contrast examination with small-bowel follow-through would be the initial area of study. A variety of findings may be apparent on radiologic studies. Plain films of the abdomen may be normal or may demonstrate findings of partial small-bowel obstruction or thumbprinting of the colon wall. Upper gastrointestinal contrast study with small-bowel follow-through may show aphthous ulceration and thickened, nodular folds as well as narrowing of the lumen anywhere in the gastrointestinal tract. Linear ulcers may give a cobblestone appearance to the mucosal surface. Bowel loops are often separated as a result of thickening of bowel wall and mesentery. Terminal ileum is most commonly involved and may be evaluated in this fashion or with reflux into the small bowel during a barium enema study. Diseased regions tend to be eccentric, and normal regions may be found between diseased segments (skip areas).

Other manifestations on radiographic studies that suggest more severe Crohn disease are fistulas between bowel (enteroenteric or enterocolonic), sinus tracts, and strictures. Barium enema may demonstrate mucosal changes in the colon similar to those in the small bowel. The cecum and ascending colon tend to be most commonly involved. Strictures, sinus tracts, and fistulas may also be seen in the colon. Ultrasonogram and computed tomographic (CT) scan are most useful in identifying intra-abdominal abscess. Thickened bowel wall may be seen on CT scan. Magnetic resonance imaging can localize areas of active bowel disease, although this study is probably no better for identifying an abscess. MRI is also useful in evaluating Crohn disease during pregnancy because it does not use ionizing radiation.

Colonoscopy with biopsy can be more helpful than radiologic studies in evaluating colon disease and in establishing a diagnosis when it is uncertain. It is often possible to enter the terminal ileum during colonoscopy; this maneuver may be very helpful in clarifying an equivocal diagnosis of ileal Crohn disease. Findings on colonoscopy may include patchy, nonspecific inflammatory changes (erythema, friability, loss of vascular pattern), aphthous ulcers, linear ulcers, nodularity, and strictures. Findings on biopsy may only be nonspecific inflammatory changes. When the biopsy findings are less striking than the gross appearance of colitis, one should think of the possibility of Crohn disease in which the abnormalities involve deeper layers of tissue. Noncaseating granulomas, similar to those of sarcoidosis, are the most characteristic histologic findings, although they are often not present. Transmural inflammation is also very characteristic but can be identified only in surgical specimens. The presence of colitis or granulomas on blind biopsy of the colon are useful to rule out lymphoma.

TREATMENT. There is no single medical approach to Crohn disease, because of the complexity of the disorder and the variety of its manifestations. The aim of treatment is largely to alleviate symptoms; treatment is dictated by the symptoms present. If disease is largely limited to small bowel, prednisone, 1–2 mg/kg/24 hr, is often the first treatment (maximum dose of 40 mg). If the activity is severe, the steroid dose may be divided during the day or may be given intravenously. Otherwise, a single morning dose will be associated with the least adrenal suppression. The goal is to taper to a single morning alternate-day dose as soon as the disease becomes quiescent. Typically, this occurs by 3–4 wk, although sometimes it may take longer. When an excellent response to the initial prednisone treatment occurs, an immediate change to alternate-day therapy is often well tolerated (changing from prednisone 30 mg everyday to 30 mg every other day). Otherwise, it may be necessary to taper more gradually to alternate-day treatment. This approach is well tolerated without apparent side effects. It is sometimes best to continue to treat a child with poorly controlled disease with 1 mg/kg or less every other day. Adolescents may grow better if they continue with alternate-day treatment rather than repeatedly having the medication dose reduced. Side effects of daily steroid treatment tend to occur more rapidly and be more severe when the serum albumin level is reduced.

Aminosalicylates have been used in the treatment of colon disease and are sometimes more effective than corticosteroids in this region. Sulfasalazine has been used in same dose as for treatment of ulcerative colitis. A delayed release 5-aminosalicylate (Asacol), 50 mg/kg/24 hr; maximum 3 g/24 hr, may be effective in treating small-bowel disease, and prophylactic use of this formulation may reduce the risk of recurrence of symptoms of small-bowel disease (similar to the use of sulfasalazine in ulcerative colitis). Azathioprine, 1–2 mg/kg/24 hr (or its metabolite 6-MP), may be very effective in some individuals who have a poor response to steroids or who are steroid dependent, although some may not respond to these drugs at all. Metronidazole has also been effective in intractable Crohn disease. Both azathioprine and metronidazole may be helpful in the treatment of perianal fistulas. Ciprofloxacin has been used in this situation but should be given only to individuals who have completed bone maturation. Local care of perianal disease with sitz baths should be performed as well. Application of steroid cream may be helpful for mild perianal disease. Cyclosporine has been used for intractable disease but should probably be reserved for limited indications. Diets high in fiber or low in residue or elimination diets have all been tried at one time in the management of Crohn disease, but none has withstood the test of time. Generally, one tries to avoid restricting a child's diet because this often leads to inadequate intake.

The initial onset or a recurrence of Crohn disease may be acute with severe pain, anorexia, fever, abdominal tenderness, and elevated white cell count. In this situation, it is difficult to rule out an infectious process involving the bowel wall (microperforation). In addition to the use of intravenous steroids, broad-spectrum intravenous antibiotic coverage for bowel flora (gram-negative bacteria and anaerobes) should be started initially and discontinued only if it appears that there is not an infectious process. An ultrasonogram or CT study of the abdomen is often necessary to rule out an intra-abdominal abscess. Development of an enteroenteric or colonic fistula may be identified on CT scan, although it is best seen on a conventional small-bowel contrast study.

Careful use of corticosteroids in Crohn disease does not seem to be associated with growth delays; growth retardation appears to be related to the presence of the inflammatory process itself. Nevertheless, the injudicious use of daily steroids may lead to many complications, including growth retardation. Supplying adequate calories in the diet will usually correct growth retardation. High-calorie oral supplements, although effective, are often not tolerated because of early satiety or exacerbation of symptoms (abdominal pain, vomiting, or diarrhea). The use of parenteral nutrients in children with Crohn disease was initially shown to promote growth. The continuous administration of nocturnal nasogastric feedings has been effective with much lower risk of complications. Complex formula may be given at 500 to 1,000 kcal nightly; treatment with 50–80 kcal/kg/night monthly every 4 months has been considered equally effective by some.

Although nutritional therapy traditionally has been considered an adjunct to the management of Crohn disease, it has now been identified as an effective primary treatment. Total parenteral nutrition is effective not only in nutritional repletion but in quieting active disease as well. Controlled trials have compared the use of elemental diet in active Crohn disease with treatment with corticosteroids or total parenteral nutrition. These studies have suggested that the nutritional approach is both as rapid in onset of response and as effective as the other treatments. Elemental diet has also been compared with complex enteral feedings and was superior in inducing remission. Because these diets are relatively unpalatable, they are administered via a nasogastric infusion. With severe, acute disease, they may be given continuously as a 24-hr infusion; the treatment may then be tapered to overnight infusion at home. Repletion should be planned for ideal weight to allow for catch-up growth. Most children are hesitant to use nasogastric infusion, but once it is begun most find it is not difficult. The advantages are that it (1) is relatively free of side effects, (2) avoids the problems associated with corticosteroid therapy, and (3) simultaneously addresses the nutritional rehabilitation. Children may participate in normal daytime activities. A major disadvantage of this approach is similar to that of other therapeutic approaches to Crohn disease: early relapse on discontinuing treatment. In addition, perianal and colon disease has not responded to this treatment plan as well as more proximal disease. Therefore, this approach should be reserved for those with severe nutritional depletion, especially with severe growth failure, and for individuals whose disease is unresponsive to conventional treatment. It is possible that remission induced with nutritional therapy may be maintained with delayed-release 5-aminosalicylate or alternate-day steroid therapy.

Surgical therapy should be reserved for specific indications. Recurrence rate after bowel resection is high (>50% by 5 years), and the risk of requiring additional surgery increases with each operation. Potential complications of surgery include development of fistula or stricture, anastomotic leak, postoperative partial small-bowel obstruction secondary to adhesions, and short-bowel syndrome. Nevertheless, there are situations in which surgery is clearly the treatment of choice. These include localized disease of small bowel or colon that is unresponsive to medical treatment, bowel perforation, stricture with symptomatic partial small-bowel obstruction, and intractable bleeding. Intra-abdominal or liver abscess may sometimes be successfully treated by ultrasonogram or CT-guided catheter drainage and concomitant intravenous antibiotic treatment. Surgical drainage is necessary if this approach is not successful. Perianal abscess often requires drainage unless it opens spontaneously. In general, perianal fistulas should be managed medically. However, a severely symptomatic perianal fistula may require fistulotomy; this procedure should be considered only if the location allows the sphincter to remain undamaged. Growth retardation was once considered an indication for resection; without other indications, this approach has not been shown to be beneficial and medical or nutritional therapy, or both, is preferred.

The approach to surgical resection of bowel for Crohn disease is to remove as small a region as possible. There is no evidence that removing bowel up to margins that are free of disease has a better outcome than removing only the most severely involved areas. The latter approach is preferred because there is less risk for short-bowel syndrome. One approach to symptomatic small-bowel stricture has been to perform a stricturoplasty rather than resection. The surgeon makes a longitudinal incision across the stricture but then closes the incision with sutures in a transverse fashion. This approach is ideal for short strictures without active disease. The rate of reoperation is not higher with this approach than resection, and bowel length is preserved.

Severe perianal disease may be incapacitating and difficult to treat if unresponsive to medical management. Colon diversion may allow the area to be less active, but on reconnection of the colon, disease activity usually recurs. Therefore, surgical treatment of severe perianal disease may require colectomy. Procedures that create a continent ileostomy or endorectal pull-through are generally discouraged in Crohn disease because of the risk of recurrence of the disease in operated bowel. Generally, with colectomy, a conventional ileostomy is performed.

Psychosocial issues for the child with Crohn disease include a sense of being different, concerns about body image, difficulty in not participating fully in age-appropriate activities, and family conflict brought on by the added stress of this disease. Social support is an important component of the management of Crohn disease. There are very active peer support groups for IBD. The largest group is CCFA with local chapters throughout the United States. Parents are often interested in learning about other children with similar problems, but children are often hesitant to participate. Social support and individual psychological counseling are important in the adjustment to a difficult problem at an age that often by itself has difficult adjustment issues. Marital or family problems may predate the onset of Crohn disease or be uncovered by the added family stress of this disease. Patients who are socially "connected" fare better. Ongoing education about the disease is an important aspect of management because children generally fare better if they understand and anticipate.

PROGNOSIS. Crohn disease is a chronic disorder that is associated with high morbidity but low mortality. Symptoms tend to recur despite treatment and often without apparent explanation. One exception is that symptoms of partial small obstruction may occur after a high-residue meal in the presence of a small-bowel stricture. Weight loss and growth failure can usually be improved with treatment and attention to nutritional needs. Up to 15% of individuals with early growth retardation secondary to Crohn disease have a permanent decrease in linear growth. Some of the extraintestinal manifestations may, in themselves, be major causes of morbidity, including sclerosing cholangitis, chronic active hepatitis, pyoderma gangrenosum, and ankylosing spondylitis.

The region of bowel involved may increase with time, although rapid progression typically occurs early and subsequently is slow. Complications of the inflammatory process tend to increase with time and include bowel strictures (small intestine or colon), fistulas (between bowel or enterocutaneous), perianal disease (fistulas, sinus tracts, fissures, and skin tags), and intra-abdominal or retroperitoneal abscess. Nearly all individuals with Crohn disease will eventually require surgery for one of its many complications; the rate of reoperation is high. The time between the onset of symptoms and need for surgery appears to be shorter in children than in adults. Surgery is very unlikely to be curative and should be avoided except for the specific indications noted previously. Repeated small-bowel resection, which may be unavoidable, can lead to malabsorption secondary to short-bowel syndrome. Resection of terminal ileum may result in bile acid malabsorption with diarrhea and vitamin B_{12} malabsorption. Although the risk of colon cancer in individuals with long-standing Crohn colitis may be lower than that associated with ulcerative colitis, it is greater than the risk among the general population.

Despite these complications, most children with Crohn disease lead active, full lives with intermittent flare-up in symptoms.

Ewe K, Press AG, Singe CC, et al: Azathioprine combined with prednisolone or monotherapy with prednisolone in active Crohn's disease. Gastroenterology 105:367, 1993.

Gendre JP, Mary JY, Florent C, et al: Oral mesalamine (Pentasa) as maintenance treatment in Crohn's disease: A multicenter placebo-controlled study. Gastroenterology 104:435, 1993.

Hamilton JR, Bruce GA, Abdourhaman M, et al: Inflammatory bowel disease in children and adolescents. Adv Pediatr 26:311, 1980.

Korelitz B: Considerations of surveillance, dysplasia and carcinoma of the colon in management of ulcerative colitis and Crohn's disease. Med Clin North Am 74:189, 1990.

Markowitz J, Rosa J, Grancher K, et al: Long-term 6-mercaptopurine treatment in adolescents with Crohn's disease. Gastroenterology 99:1347, 1990.

Markowitz RL, Ment LR, Cryboski JD: Cerebral thromboembolic disease in pediatric and adult inflammatory bowel disease: Case report and review of the literature. J Pediatr Gastroenterol Nutr 8:413, 1989.

Mashako MNL, Cezard JP, Navarro J, et al: Crohn's disease lesions in the upper gastrointestinal tract: Correlation between clinical, radiological, endoscopic, and histological features in adolescents and children. J Pediatr Gastroenterol Nutr 8:442, 1989.

Michener W, Wyllie R: Management of children and adolescents with inflammatory bowel disease. Med Clin North Am 74:103, 1990.

Motil KJ, Grand RJ, Davis-Kraft L, et al: Growth failure in children with inflammatory bowel disease: A prospective study. Gastroenterology 105:681, 1993.

Oliva L, Wyllie R, Alexander F, et al: The results of strictureplasty in pediatric patients with multifocal Crohn's disease. J Pediatr Gastroenterol Nutr 18:306, 1994.

Peppercorn MA: Advances in drug therapy for inflammatory bowel disease. Ann Intern Med 112:50, 1990.

Prantera C, Pallone F, Brunetti G, et al: Oral 5-aminosalicylic acid (Asacol) in the maintenance treatment of Crohn's disease. Gastroenterology 103:363, 1992.

Seidman E, LeLeiko N, Ament M, et al: Nutritional issues in pediatric inflammatory bowel disease. J Pediatr Gastroenterol Nutr 12:424, 1991.

Treem WR, Hyams JS: Cyclosporine therapy in gastrointestinal disease. J Pediatr Gastroenterol Nutr 18:270, 1994.

283.3 Behçet Syndrome

Behçet syndrome is a multisystem vasculitis that is very rare in children. Aphthous stomatitis, erythema nodosum, and arthritis are among the most common manifestations. The ulcers are 2–10 mm in diameter and occur anywhere in the mouth or posterior pharynx; intestinal ulceration may mimic Crohn disease. They are covered by white-yellow membranes, have red borders, and are painful. Other signs are genital ulcers, central nervous system involvement, and myositis. Eye findings (iridocyclitis) are less common in children than in adults. Immunosuppressive drugs have been used with mixed success.

Rakover Y, Adar H, Tal I, et al: Behçet disease: Long-term follow-up of three children and review of the literature. Pediatrics 83:986, 1989.

Stringer DA, Cleghorn GJ, Durie PR, et al: Behçet's syndrome involving the gastrointestinal tract: A diagnostic dilemma in childhood. Pediatr Radiol 16:131, 1986.

CHAPTER 284
*Dietary Protein Intolerance (Food Allergy)**

Martin Ulshen

Foods can produce gastrointestinal symptoms in children, but the mechanisms for these manifestations remain partially understood. Dietary components may cause adverse reactions because they are contaminated with microbes or toxins, because they have pharmacologic activity, or because they overload a compromised absorptive or digestive process. The immunologic (allergic) basis of gastrointestinal responses to food is especially problematic. Also see Chapters 145 and 171.

Food allergy is an immunologically mediated response to dietary antigen. Most attention has focused on cow milk protein as the major cause of gastrointestinal food allergy in infants. Several immunologic mechanisms may be involved: immediate anaphylactic hypersensitivity involving immunoglobulin (Ig) E antibodies, antibody-dependent cytotoxic hypersensitivity involving IgM or IgG, immune complex hypersensitivity, and cell-mediated hypersensitivity.

CLINICAL MANIFESTATIONS. Because diagnostic criteria are uncertain, the true incidence is difficult to determine; estimates range from 0.5–1.5%. Food antigen may provoke respiratory, skin, or gastrointestinal symptoms. Gastrointestinal manifestations, with or without involvement of the other two systems, often dominate the clinical picture. Any region of the gastrointestinal tract can be affected.

Mouth. Recurrent shallow, mucosal ulceration and perioral dermatitis have been attributed to allergic responses to food, but usually another cause is found.

Stomach. Intragastric antigen may provoke hemorrhagic and edematous inflammation in the gastric mucosa. Acute vomiting, presumably on the basis of this immediate hypersensitivity, can occur in infants and is usually associated with watery or even bloody diarrhea. In its most fulminant form, this rare syndrome is accompanied by glottic swelling; fatal anaphylactic shock may occur.

Small Intestine. Three syndromes are recognized. *Acute watery diarrhea* may occur as an immediate response to antigen ingestion, with or without vomiting and abdominal cramps. *Chronic diarrhea* and failure to thrive may occur after the ingestion of milk, soy, egg, or fish. A patchy villus lesion in the small intestine is associated with anorexia, chronic diarrhea, and retarded growth. Usually absorptive function is not significantly impaired. *Excessive enteric protein* and *blood loss* may lead to hypoproteinemia and iron deficiency, often without obvious intestinal symptoms. This occurs usually in an older infant at the time of weaning from breast milk, when milk formula feeding is withdrawn, or when ordinary dairy milk feeding is begun. Eosinophilia is common. Manifestations may resolve completely after cow's milk is withdrawn from the diet. A spontaneous "cure" may be evident after reestablishing cow's milk formula or processed milk (evaporated, dried) intake years after the initial manifestations.

Colon. Pancolitis causing bloody diarrhea may occur after cow milk ingestion, usually in young infants. Diarrhea stools contain abundant eosinophils. This syndrome has been seen in exclusively breast-fed infants whose mothers were ingesting cow's milk. The condition should not be confused with eosinophilic gastroenteritis (Chapter 285).

DIAGNOSIS. The diagnosis of dietary protein allergy is clinical. Acute symptoms should subside within 48 hr and chronic symptoms within 1 wk of complete withdrawal of the offending antigen, usually cow's milk. Caution and judgment must be exercised in rechallenging these patients with potential dietary antigens. In a young infant, particularly if an acute response is anticipated, the challenge should be carried out under observation, beginning with a small dose (e.g., 1–5 mL milk) and increasing progressively over a few days provided a response does not occur. For gastrointestinal responses to potential dietary antigen skin tests, circulating antibody titers, complement assays, and coproantibody titers are not of proven diagnostic value. In children with chronic symptoms, some centers use mucosal biopsy to evaluate the response to challenge. It is important to rule out other conditions that may cause similar symptoms, such as enteric infections, lactose intolerance, and other forms of nonspecific inflammatory bowel disease.

The syndromes described for cow's milk intolerance may occur also in response to soy protein. Up to 50% of children intolerant to cow's milk may be intolerant to soy. Because soy is not a commonly used food, most will not be exposed to soy unless they are first found intolerant to cow's milk. The approach to diagnosis is the same as for cow's milk.

TREATMENT. Prolonged breast-feeding reduces the likelihood of later cow's milk intolerance. Treatment consists of removing the offending food from the diet. Breast-feeding mothers may have to go on a cow's milk elimination diet if their infant has manifestations of milk protein allergy. However, in some nursing infants with diet-related colitis, weaning is necessary to stop the symptoms. For the young infant the non-milk-containing dietary formulas consist of various soy feedings and hydrolyzed milk protein feedings. Many children with the enteric protein and blood loss syndrome will benefit by changing from fresh milk to processed (i.e., evaporated, powdered) milk. For rare cases of intolerance to many foods, oral administration of sodium cromoglycate has been reported to suppress intestinal symptoms and permit continued ingestion of the food.

PROGNOSIS. In most cases, food protein intolerance is transitory. About 50% of infants with the conditions described earlier recover within 1 yr and most of the remainder recover within 2 yr.

Esteban MM (ed): Adverse reactions to foods in infancy and childhood [Supplement]. J Pediatr 121:S1–S122, 1992.

Ferguson A: Definitions and diagnosis of food intolerance and food allergy: Consensus and controversy. J Pediatr 121:S7, 1992.

Fontaine SL, Navarro J: Small intestinal biopsy in cow's milk protein allergy in infancy. Arch Dis Child 50:357, 1975.

Hill DJ, Firer MA, Shelton MJ, et al: Manifestations of milk allergy in infancy. J Pediatr 109:270, 1986.

Minford AMB, MacDonald A, Littlewood JM: Food intolerance and food allergy in children: A review of 63 cases. Arch Dis Child 57:742, 1982.

Patrick MK, Gall DG: Protein intolerance and immunocyte and enterocyte interaction. Pediatr Clin North Am 85:17, 1988.

Powell GK: Milk and soy-induced enterocolitis of infancy. J Pediatr 93:558, 1978.

*Dr. Richard Hamilton was the author of this chapter in previous editions. His contribution is gratefully appreciated.

CHAPTER 285
Eosinophilic Gastroenteritis

Martin Ulshen

This entity consists of a group of rare and poorly understood disorders that have in common gastric and small-intestine infiltration with eosinophils and peripheral eosinophilia. The esophagus and large intestine can also be involved. Tissue eosinophilic infiltration can be seen in mucosa, muscularis, or serosa. Mucosal involvement may produce hemorrhage, muscularis involvement may produce strictures and obstruction, and serosal activity produces eosinophilic ascites.

Manifestations of this entity include abdominal pain, vomiting, diarrhea (with or without gross blood), evidence of malabsorption, protein-losing enteropathy (with or without reduced serum albumin and imunnoglobulin levels), delayed growth and poor weight gain, intestinal obstructive symptoms, and eosinophilic ascites. Atopic symptoms, including rhinitis and asthma, are often present, and this condition overlaps clinically the dietary protein hypersensitivity disorders of the small bowel and colon. The mucosal form can be diagnosed by the presence of large numbers of eosinophils in peroral gastric antrum or small-bowel biopsy samples.

The disease usually runs a chronic, debilitating course with sporadic severe exacerbations. A few patients are helped by elimination diets, but most require systemic administration of corticosteroids.

Katz AJ, Golman H, Grand RJ: Gastric mucosal biopsy in eosinophilic (allergic) gastroenteritis. Gastroenterology 73:705, 1977.
Klein NC, Hargrove RL, Sleisinger MN, et al: Eosinophilic gastroenteritis. Medicine 49:299, 1970.
Whitington PF, Whitington GL: Eosinophilic gastroenteropathy in childhood. J Pediatr Gastroenterol Nutr 7:379, 1988.

CHAPTER 286

Malabsorptive Disorders

Martin Ulshen

Malabsorptive disorders or malabsorption syndromes are conditions that cause insufficient assimilation of ingested nutrients either as a result of maldigestion or of malabsorption (Table 286–1). These disorders were previously known as celiac syndromes, but this term is best avoided because of potential confusion with the specific entity celiac disease (gluten-sensitive enteropathy). Disorders that cause generalized defects in assimilation of nutrient tend to present with similar signs and symptoms: abdominal distention; pale, foul-smelling, bulky stools; muscle wasting; poor weight gain or weight loss; and growth retardation (Fig 286–1). Stools may be greasy appearing and may be associated with an oil slick in the toilet; with mild steatorrhea, the stools may appear normal.

Congenital disorders affecting individual intestinal digestive enzymes or transport processes have also been identified. The

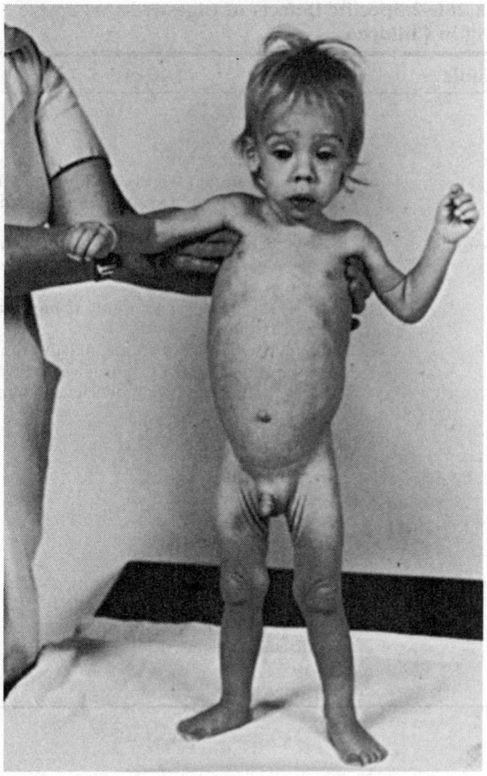

Figure 286–1. An 18-mo-old boy with active celiac disease. Note the loose skin folds, marked proximal muscle wasting, and full abdomen. The child looks ill.

clinical features of these disorders typically differ from those of the generalized malabsorption syndromes, and some present without gastrointestinal symptoms (Table 286–2). The disaccharidase deficiencies are without question the most common of these entities.

286.1 Evaluation of Children with Suspected Intestinal Malabsorption

CLINICAL MANIFESTATIONS. Although many disorders of malabsorption are inherited, it is the child without a family history who presents the greatest diagnostic challenge. Presentation of congenital disorders may include diarrhea and malabsorption from birth (congenital microvillus inclusion disease, glucose-galactose transport defect, congenital chloride diarrhea). Alternatively, the symptoms may not present until the introduction

■ **TABLE 286–1 Generalized Malabsorptive States in Childhood**

Site	More Common	Less Common
Exocrine pancreas	Cystic fibrosis Chronic protein-calorie malnutrition	Shwachman-Diamond syndrome Chronic pancreatitis
Liver, biliary tree	Biliary atresia	Other cholestatic states
Intestine		
Anatomic defects	Massive resection Stagnant loop syndrome	Congenitally short gut
Chronic infection	Giardiasis	Immune deficiency Dietary protein intolerance (milk, soy)
Others	Celiac disease	Tropical sprue Idiopathic diffuse mucosal lesions

■ **TABLE 286–2 Specific Defects of Digestive-Absorptive Function Occurring in Children**

Variable	Disease
Intestinal	
Fat	Abetalipoproteinemia
Protein	Enterokinase deficiency
	Amino acid transport defects (cystinuria, Hartnup disease, methionine malabsorption, blue diaper syndrome)
Carbohydrate	Disaccharidase deficiencies (congenital: sucrase-isomaltase, lactase; developmental: lactase, acquired)
	Glucose—galactose malabsorption (congenital, acquired)
	Glucoamylase deficiency (starch malabsorption)
Vitamin	Vitamin B_{12} malabsorption (juvenile pernicious anemia, transcobalamin II deficiency, Immerslund syndrome)
	Folic acid malabsorption
Ions, trace elements	Chloride-losing diarrhea
	Congenital sodium diarrhea
	Acrodermatitis enteropathica
	Menkes syndrome
	Vitamin D–dependent rickets
	Primary hypomagnesemia
Drug-induced	Sulfasalazine (folic acid malabsorption)
	Cholestyramine (Ca, fat malabsorption)
	Phenytoin (Dilantin) (Ca malabsorption)
Pancreatic	Specific enzyme deficiencies
	Lipase
	Trypsinogen

of a new food (gluten in gluten-sensitive enteropathy, sucrose in congenital sucrase-isomaltase deficiency). A careful history of the time of onset of symptoms and the relationship to diet is helpful. Often, well-intended parents may assume that symptoms are associated with events that may, in fact, be coincidental. If a dietary component is important in the cause of the malabsorption, repetition of symptoms should occur on reintroduction of the substance, and improvement should be reproducibly associated with removal of the offending agent. Frequency, looseness, and quantity of stool can be helpful in formulating a differential diagnosis; however, color, other than the pale stool of fat malabsorption, typically does not provide a clue. Failure to thrive can be caused by many systemic or psychosocial disorders, and one must keep this possibility in mind before making a diagnosis of malabsorption. A common example is the child with chronic, nonspecific diarrhea (toddler's diarrhea) who may inadvisedly receive frequent periods of a clear-liquid diet and lose weight as a result. These children can appear on examination to have a malabsorption syndrome such as gluten-sensitive enteropathy. They typically respond to return to regular diet with improved weight gain.

The usual growth pattern associated with malabsorption and malnutrition demonstrates an initial decrease in weight followed by a deceleration in height velocity (Fig. 286–2). To make this assessment, it is essential to obtain serial weights and heights. Signs of malnutrition may include lethargy, decreased subcutaneous tissue, muscle wasting, edema, and depigmentation of skin and hair. Initially, many infants with fat malabsorption have a voracious appetite. Other offending foods may produce avoidance behaviors if malabsorption produces gaseous distention (carbohydrates); gluten enteropathy frequently produces anorexia. The examination is typically not helpful in making a specific diagnosis, although occasionally features such as digital clubbing (cystic fibrosis, gluten-sensitive enteropathy), severe growth retardation of Shwachman syndrome, or the facial features of the Johannson-Blizzard syndrome can be helpful. A carotenemic infant or toddler would be very unlikely to have fat malabsorption.

LABORATORY MANIFESTATIONS. The most useful screening test for malabsorption is a microscopic examination of stool for fat. This can be performed by mixing a small amount of stool with several drops of water or Sudan red stain. Fat droplets separate and can be easily identified, especially with a Sudan stain. More than six to eight droplets per low-power field is abnormal. Droplets tend to accumulate at the edges of the coverslip. The addition of acetic acid is thought to protonate ionized fatty acids and increase the number of droplets identified with Sudan stain. In disorders with pancreatic insufficiency (cystic fibrosis or Shwachman syndrome), the fat droplets number in the hundreds to thousands. Some malabsorption syndromes, such as gluten-sensitive enteropathy, may not always be associated with fat in the stool. Serum carotene levels have also been used as a screening test for fat malabsorption, but false-negative and false-positive results are common. The child must be receiving carotene in the diet for the test to be valid.

Steatorrhea is most prominent in disorders with pancreatic insufficiency; this finding warrants a sweat chloride test for cystic fibrosis as one of the initial studies. Serum trypsinogen levels have proven to be a good screening test for pancreatic insufficiency. In cystic fibrosis with pancreatic insufficency, the level is greatly elevated early in life but falls so that by 5–7 yr of age most have subnormal values. The levels in children with cystic fibrosis and pancreatic sufficiency are more variable but tend to be normal or elevated. In such children, the trend over time is more helpful than a single value in monitoring pancreatic function. In Shwachman syndrome, the serum trypsinogen level is low.

Other initial studies should include a complete blood count, serum albumin, and serum immunoglobulin levels. A wide range of gastrointestinal disorders can cause hypoproteinemia as a result of decreased ability to assimilate dietary protein, inadequate protein intake, or protein-losing enteropathy (Table 286–3).

A more sensitive test for fat malabsorption is the 72-hr stool collection for fat analysis. A dietary record during this period is used to calculate the fat intake. Many use the diet history as an average 3-day intake and collect stools from the beginning to the end of this period. Fat absorption is calculated by subtracting fat excretion from intake and dividing by fat intake; this fraction is multiplied by 100 to give the percentage of intake that is assimilated, known as the coefficient of fat absorption.

$$\frac{\text{Fat intake} - \text{fat excretion}}{\text{Fat intake}} \times 100.$$

The ability to assimilate dietary fat varies with the maturity of the infant and the kind of fat offered in the diet. A premature infant may absorb only 65–75% of dietary fat, whereas a full-term infant absorbs 90%. Therefore, the finding of fat in the stool on microscopic examination in young infants is not necessarily abnormal. Older children and adults should absorb at least 95% of the fat in a typical diet. Butterfat is absorbed less well than vegetable fat, although human milk fat is absorbed best of all. The decreased ability to assimilate fat by infants reflects a decrease in pancreatic secretion or a decrease in duodenal bile acid levels.

■ **TABLE 286–3 Gastrointestinal Causes of Hypoproteinemia**

Inflammatory bowel disease
Gluten-sensitive enteropathy
Cystic fibrosis
Shwachman syndrome
Disorders with secondary small-bowel mucosal damage (e.g., infectious disorders)
Intestinal lymphangiectasia (primary or secondary)
Hypertrophic gastropathy
Eosinophilic gastroenteropathy (allergic enteropathies)
Trypsinogen or enterokinase deficiency

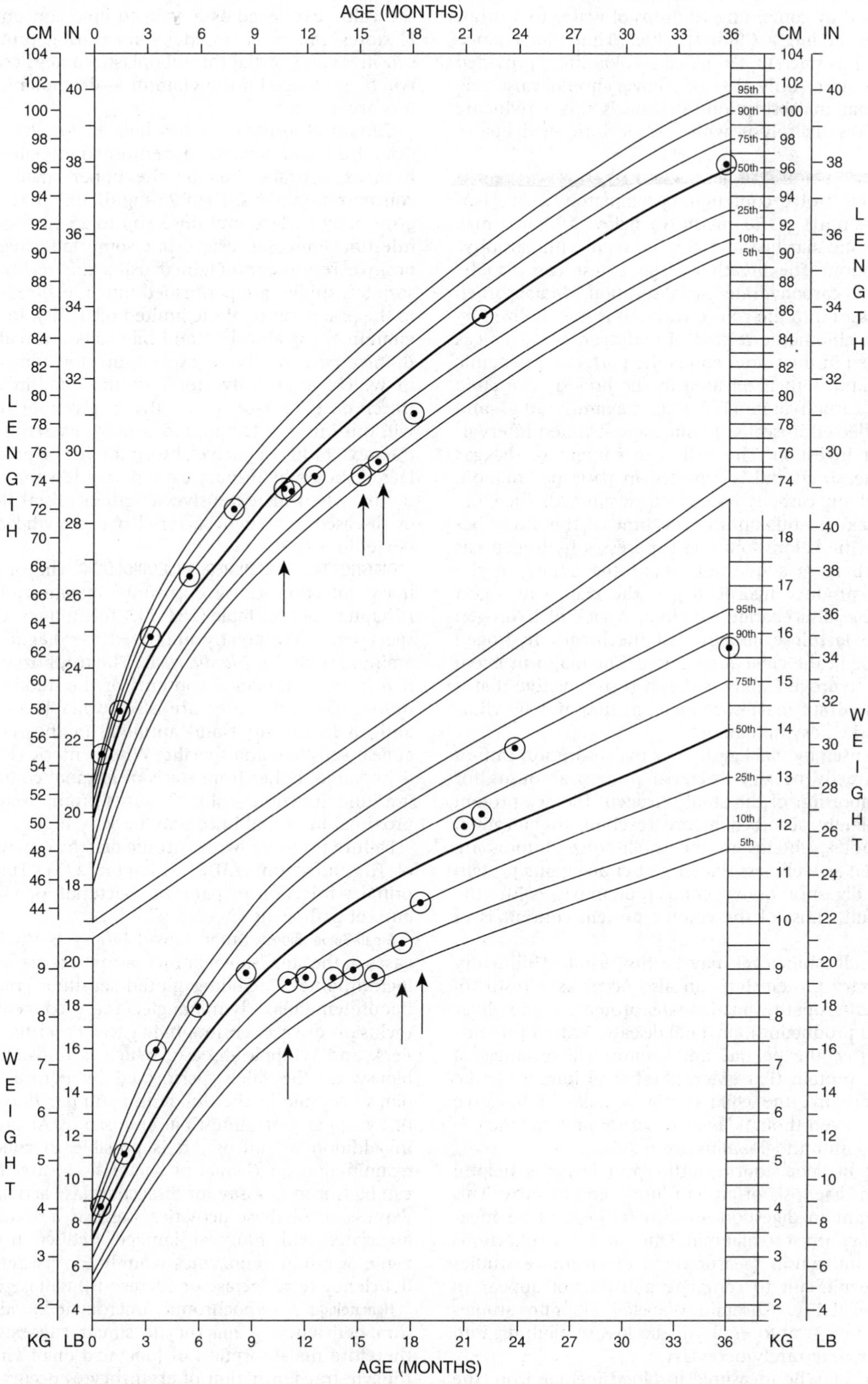

Figure 286–2. Gluten-sensitive enteropathy. Growth curve demonstrates initial normal growth from 0–9 mo, followed by onset of poor appetite with intermittent vomiting and diarrhea after initiation of gluten-containing diet *(single arrow)*. After biopsy-confirmed diagnosis and treatment with gluten-free diet *(double arrow)*, growth improves.

Measurement of carbohydrate in the stool using the Clinitest reagent for reducing substances is simple and can be performed at bedside. This is not a very accurate screening test. The test is easily performed by combining 10 drops of water to 5 drops of stool and then adding a Clinitest tablet. The color change can be quantified as trace to 4+ using a color sheet provided by the manufacturer. Only 2+ or above should raise the possibility of sugar malabsorption. Sucrose is not a reducing sugar and requires hydrolysis with hydrochloric acid before analysis.

Stool pH below 5.6 is also suggestive of carbohydrate malabsorption. Stool electrolye content (approximately 2 × ([sodium] + [potassium]) + 50 mOsm/L) below 290 mOsm/L occurs with osmotic diarrhea and may be seen with carbohydrate malabsorption. The breath hydrogen test can also be used to evaluate carbohydrate malabsorption. Malabsorbed carbohydrate passes into the colon, where it is metabolized by bacteria with stoichiometric release of hydrogen gas. This gas is largely absorbed in the colon, enters the portal and systemic venous return, and is then released in the breath. The child ingests a load of carbohydrate (1–2 g/kg, maximum 50 g), and the breath is collected in sealed plastic bags at timed intervals up to 2 hr after ingestion. The hydrogen content of the gas can be easily measured and is reported in parts per million. Malabsorption of any carbohydrate can be evaluated. The child should not be taking antibiotics at the time of the study because this alters the colon flora and suppresses hydrogen gas production. If there is a question about the ability of the colonic flora to produce hydrogen gas, the child can ingest the nonabsorbable disaccharide lactulose. A lack of hydrogen production with lactulose implies that the breath hydrogen test is not reliable in the child at that time. The major problem with the breath hydrogen study is that it is so sensitive that it identifies carbohydrate malabsorption that may not be clinically important (i.e., asymptomatic).

Protein loss caused by maldigestion or malabsorption cannot be evaluated directly because bacterial protein accounts for such a large proportion of the stool nitrogen. Dietary protein is almost completely absorbed before reaching the terminal ileum. Endogenous proteins in the small-bowel lumen are normally digested as well; less than 1 g of endogenous protein and products of digestion of exogenous protein passes into the colon. As a result, most of the colonic protein content is of bacterial origin.

A low serum albumin level may be the result of difficulty assimilating dietary protein but can also occur as a result of protein-losing enteropathy, inadequate protein intake, liver disease (reduced production), or renal disease. With a protein-losing enteropathy, the peptide and amino acid products of digestion of the protein that enters the bowel lumen can be reabsorbed. Therefore, the child is not actually in negative nitrogen balance even though levels of serum proteins including albumin and immunoglobulins are reduced.

Measurement of spot stool α_1-antitrypsin levels is helpful in establishing a diagnosis of protein-losing enteropathy. This protein is resistant to digestion and, therefore, can be measured in stool in contrast to albumin. One- or 2-day collections of stool for α_1-antitrypsin measurement or clearance studies are much more difficult to complete and do not appear to improve the reliability. Chromium-labeled albumin studies were once the only way to establish the loss of albumin into the stool but now are rarely necessary.

Nutrients that may be measured in blood include iron, the level of which depends on transferrin concentration as well as on absorption; folic acid, the red cell concentration being a more accurate reflection of nutritional status than the serum concentration; calcium and magnesium; vitamin D and its metabolites; vitamin A; and vitamin B_{12}. If the intake of these nutrients is adequate, decreased concentrations will suggest inadequate absorption. It may take years to deplete stores of vitamin B_{12} after absorption is impaired. Vitamin E levels should be measured simultaneous with serum lipid levels and the value expressed as a ratio to lipid concentration. Vitamin K stores can be assessed by measuring prothrombin (more sensitive) and partial thromboplastin times because these times will be prolonged if the vitamin K–dependent coagulation factors are depleted.

Certain absorptive studies help to localize an intestinal lesion. Iron and *D-xylose,* a pentose minimally metabolized in humans, are absorbed by the upper small bowel. A blood concentration of less than 25 mg/dL of xylose 1 hr after a 14.5 g/m² body surface oral dose (up to 25 g) suggests a proximal intestinal mucosal lesion, but some false-negative and false-positive results are obtained using this technique. Xylose absorption studies are performed much less frequently now than in the past because of the limited reliability. In the distal bowel, vitamin B_{12} is absorbed and bile salts are reabsorbed. *Vitamin B_{12} absorption* can be measured directly using the *Schilling test,* in which, after body stores of the vitamin are saturated, a tracer dose of radioactive B_{12} is given by mouth, with or without intrinsic factor, and urinary excretion measured over the next 24 hr. Defective absorption in the presence of intrinsic factor, shown by urinary excretion of less than 5% of the dose, occurs when an extensive length of distal ileum is resected or diseased, or when bacterial overgrowth occurs within the bowel lumen.

DIAGNOSTIC PROCEDURES. MICROBIOLOGIC. The only common primary infection causing chronic malabsorption is giardiasis (Chapter 244.5, Table 281–2). Techniques to fix and stain specimens have greatly improved the diagnostic value of examining stools for *Giardia* cysts. The trophozoite may be identified in fresh duodenal contents or the duodenal mucosa. Immunoassay techniques are also available to identify *Giardia* antigen in the stool and antibody in the serum. These tests appear sensitive and specific. When enteric clearing of bacteria is impaired, either from stasis of luminal contents or impaired immune function, colony counts from bacterial cultures of proximal intestinal juice may be very high.

Failure to thrive, with chronic diarrhea, may be the first sign of HIV infection (AIDS) (Chapter 223). The cause may be primary infection or parasitic, bacterial, or viral opportunistic enterol pathogens.

Small-Bowel Biopsy. Small-bowel biopsy is used to identify diseases of the small-bowel mucosa that are associated with histologic findings, including gluten-sensitive enteropathy, abetalipoproteinemia, lymphangiectasia, congenital microvillus inclusion disease, eosinophilic gastroenteritis, infectious disorders, and Whipple disease, which is unusual in a child. The biopsy can be safely performed by peroral placement of a biopsy capsule in the duodenum (under fluoroscopic control) or by upper gastrointestinal endoscopy. At the time of biopsy, in addition to mucosa, it is possible to collect aspirates for examination for *Giardia* or bacterial culture. Mucosal samples can be frozen to assay for disaccharidase activities later. Diffuse depression of these activities suggests a secondary deficiency associated with mucosal damage. Reduction of a specific enzyme or group of enzymes would be consistent with a specific deficiency (e.g., lactase or sucrase-isomaltase deficiency).

Hematologic. A hypochromic, microcytic blood smear indicates iron deficiency; a macrocytic smear suggests deficiency and therefore malabsorption of folic acid or of vitamin B_{12}. Acanthocyte transformation of erythrocytes occurs in abetalipoproteinemia. A blood smear may also suggest a lymphocyte defect or a neutropenia associated with Shwachman-Diamond syndrome.

Imaging Procedures. Used primarily to identify local lesions in the abdomen, these procedures have limited application to the study of children with malabsorptive disorders. *Plain roentgeno-*

grams and *barium contrast* studies may suggest a site and cause of intestinal stasis. For example, the most common anomaly causing incomplete bowel obstruction is intestinal malrotation, a condition difficult to exclude without a barium enema to locate the cecum. The small intestine should be examined with the use of large quantities of nonflocculating barium and only when a localized lesion, not diffuse disease, is suspected. Although flocculation of normal barium and dilated bowel with thickened mucosal folds have been attributed to diffuse malabsorptive lesions such as celiac disease, these abnormalities are nonspecific and have little diagnostic value. *Ultrasound* can detect alterations in pancreatic mass, biliary tree abnormalities, and stones, even in infants with malabsorption. *Retrograde studies of the pancreatic* and *biliary tree* using contrast injection via endoscopy are reserved for rare cases requiring careful delineation of the biliary tree and pancreatic ducts.

286.2 Chronic Malnutrition

Chronic protein-calorie malnutrition can lead to compromise of pancreatic and small-bowel function. In developed countries, primary malnutrition is rare and chronic digestive disorders account for many cases of malnutrition in children. Environmental deprivation is also an important cause, as are feeding disorders (improper volume or dilution of formula). Protein-calorie malnutrition appears to contribute to the cycle of protracted diarrhea of infancy perhaps through impairment of the functional capacity of the bowel, impairment of immune function, or the development of small-bowel bacterial overgrowth. Worldwide, exocrine pancreatic insufficiency is most often attributable to malnutrition, not to a primary pancreatic disease.

The intestine is remarkably resistant to the effects of protein-calorie malnutrition. Patients with *kwashiorkor* may have a severely flattened small intestinal villus structure, but these abnormalities probably are attributable to coexisting infections and infestations. In *marasmus* villus structure is relatively preserved, although microvillus changes and intracellular electron microscopic abnormalities have been observed. Chronic malnutrition can lead to impaired immune function; perhaps as a consequence, bacterial overgrowth of the upper intestine is seen in malnourished subjects (Chapter 45.1). When oral intake is withheld in experimental animals, intestinal mucosal mass and absorptive function diminish even if nutrient is supplied by the intravenous route. These changes can be reversed by small amounts of oral nutrient. Accordingly, there is a theoretical advantage in delivering nutrients via the gut whenever possible. Recovery from insults to the gastrointestinal tract (viral gastroenteritis) may be prolonged by chronic malnutrition. Certain nutrients, such as glutamine, soluble fiber, short-chain fatty acids, and short-chain triglycerides, may promote small-bowel mucosal growth.

Little is known about the *effect of specific nutritional deficiencies* on the pancreas or intestine; apart from potassium depletion causing ileus and severe dehydration causing constipation, available data suggest a relatively minor clinical effect of a wide range of specific deficiencies. Iron deficiency is associated with enhanced iron uptake at the mucosa and, in a few severe cases, occurrence of mucosal flattening. Deficiencies of vitamin B_{12} and folic acid may cause distortion of enterocyte morphology but no known serious functional abnormalities of the gut. Some hypocalcemic states may be accompanied by steatorrhea and even by ion and water secretion, but this poorly understood relationship is not constant.

Studies from underdeveloped countries suggest that vitamin A supplementation reduces childhood mortality. Improved survival during measles and a reduction in relative risk of contracting diarrheal and respiratory diseases has been identified. The explanation for this finding is uncertain, but children with vitamin A deficiency may have T-cell defects (including a low CD4:CD8 ratio), which can be reversed with vitamin supplementation.

286.3 Liver and Biliary Disorders

Cholestatic liver disease and biliary disorders may lead to fat malabsorption by reducing the duodenal bile acid concentration below the critical micellar concentration. In addition to steatorrhea, patients with these disorders have a propensity to acquire deficiencies of fat-soluble vitamins (vitamins A, D, E, and K). There is no consistent pattern in which these deficiencies occur, except that vitamin A is least likely to be problematic.

Vitamin E deficiency in patients with chronic cholestasis has been associated with a progressive neurologic syndrome, which includes peripheral neuropathy (presenting as loss of deep tendon reflexes and ophthalmoplegia), cerebellar ataxia, and posterior column dysfunction. Early in the course, findings are partially reversible with treatment but late features may not be. It can be difficult to identify vitamin E deficiency because the elevated blood lipid levels of cholestasis can falsely elevate the serum level of vitamin E. Therefore, it is important to measure the ratio of serum vitamin E to total serum lipids if one suspects this deficiency (the normal level for patients younger than 12 yr is greater than 0.6 and for patients 12 yr and older, greater than 0.8). The neurologic disease can be prevented with the use of an oral water-soluble vitamin E preparation (d-α-tocopherol polyethylene glycol-1,000 succinate [TPGS], Liqui-E, Twin Laboratories, Ronkonkoma, NY) at 15–25 IU/kg/24 hr.

Metabolic bone disease can develop secondary to vitamin D deficiency. Simultaneous administration of vitamin D with the water-soluble vitamin E preparation (TPGS) enhances absorption of vitamin D. In young infants, oral vitamin D_3 is given at 1,000 IU/kg/24 hr. After 1 month, if the serum 25-hydroxyvitamin D is low, the same dose of oral vitamin D is mixed with TPGS. It has been recommended that 25-hydroxyvitamin D is then monitored every 3 mo with adjustment of doses as necessary.

Vitamin K deficiency can occur as a result of cholestasis and poor fat absorption. Easy bleeding may be the first sign or a child may be identified before symptoms develop through routine screening of prothrombin (a more sensitive test) and partial thromboplastin times. It is possible for a patient taking the standard oral preparation to acquire a vitamin K–deficient coagulopathy because the currently available oral preparation of vitamin K is not well absorbed. A bile salt–solubilized preparation is under study and may replace the present preparation.

286.4 Intestinal Infections

Malabsorption is a rare consequence of primary intestinal infection in immunocompetent children. Giardiasis is without doubt the most common infectious cause of chronic malabsorption. Symptoms include diarrhea, vomiting, bloating, and gas. Giardiasis should be suspected if a child with persistent acquired malabsorption has family members who have had transient gastroenteritis symptoms at the onset of the child's illness. Children in day care (especially toddlers) are at special risk for *Giardia*, although they may be asymptomatic and pass it on to family members. Cryptosporidiosis can also occur in immunocompetent individuals as can coccidiosis. Infectious causes of malabsorption are especially common in immunocompromised individuals (Chapters 171, 223, 283, and 286.5).

286.5 Immunodeficiency

Gastrointestinal symptoms are a common manifestation of many immune deficiency states, including congenital neutrophil, T and B cell immune deficiencies, conditions of medical immune suppression (cancer and transplantation therapy), and AIDS. The more common congenital disorders associated with bowel disease include severe combined immunodeficiency, agammaglobulinemia, Wiskott-Aldrich syndrome, common variable immunodeficiency disease, and chronic granulomatous disease. Gastrointestinal symptoms of congenital x-linked hypogammaglobulinemia tend to be milder (chronic rotavirus, enterovirus, or giardiasis). Malabsorption occurs in about 10% of individuals with late-onset common variable hypogammaglobulinemia, a primary disorder that presents later in life. Nodular lymphoid hyperplasia may be noted on small bowel radiographs. T-cell abnormalities can also be associated with malabsorption. Selective immunoglobulin (Ig) A deficiency is common, may not always be associated with gastrointestinal symptoms, but may be associated with an increased incidence of gluten-sensitive enteropathy, nodular lymphoid hyperplasia, inflammatory bowel disease, and giardiasis.

Chronic giardiasis and rotavirus infection have been noted to cause malabsorption in children with immune deficiencies. In addition, in children with AIDS, other organisms that can interfere with bowel function include cytomegalovirus, *Mycobacterium avium-intracellularae, Cryptosporidium parvum, Isospora belli,* and *Enterocytozoon bieneusi,* astrovirus, calicivirus, and adenovirus. In addition, HIV itself appears to be a primary bowel pathogen. Disaccharide intolerance is common in HIV-infected children but does not correlate well with enteric infection. Vitamin B_{12} malabsorption has been found to be common in studies of adults with AIDS. Pancreatic insufficiency and steatorrhea have also been described to occur in individuals with AIDS. In addition to the range of infectious causes, in immunosuppressed children diarrhea can be a presentation of toxicity to the drug FK-506 (tacrolimus) or of immunosuppression-induced lymphoproliferative disease.

A congenital deficiency of effective neutrophils predisposes children to at least two different types of gastrointestinal disorders. In patients with neutropenia, a necrotizing enterocolitis may be the cause of fever and right lower quadrant pain and tenderness. This serious problem, which carries a high mortality, is also known as typhlitis; the lesion occurs most often in the lower ileum, cecum, and proximal colon where vascular compromise, mucosal ulceration, and perforation develop. A relationship of this enteropathy to *Clostridium difficile* has been postulated in some cases. In patients with chronic granulomatous disease, phagocytic function is impaired and granulomas may develop throughout the intestine, causing diarrhea and malabsorption. These granulomas, characterized by giant cells and lipid-containing histiocytes, frequently obstruct the gastric antrum.

286.6 Stagnant Loop Syndrome

(Blind Loop Syndrome: Bacterial Overgrowth Syndrome)

These terms describe a condition associated with stasis of small intestinal contents, particularly in the upper regions. Incomplete bowel obstruction, congenital (malrotation with duodenal bands, stenosis, or a diverticulum) or acquired (postoperative intestinal adhesions, long-standing Crohn disease), impairs intestinal motility or causes loss of the normal intestinal mucosal barrier to microorganisms, allowing enteric bacteria to colonize the upper small bowel. These bacteria deconjugate bile salts, which leads to inefficient intraluminal processing of dietary fat and to steatorrhea; they bind vitamin B_{12}, interfering with its absorption; and they may damage the microvillus brush border membrane, diminishing disaccharidase activities.

In addition to symptoms of chronic incomplete bowel obstruction such as distention, pain, and vomiting, the patient may have pale, foul-smelling, bulky stools typical of steatorrhea, a megaloblastic anemia from vitamin B_{12} deficiency, or diarrhea from disaccharidase deficiency. Clinical manifestations often do not suggest chronic intestinal obstruction, but laboratory investigations find the aforementioned functional abnormalities as well as bacterial colonization of the upper intestine and deconjugated bile salts in the upper intestinal juice after a fatty meal. Barium contrast roentgenograms may reveal neither the existence nor the cause of obstruction.

Oral administration of antibiotics may be sufficient to control the problem temporarily. At times, cycling of antibiotics may be effective for a longer period of management. Metronidazole has been used for the treatment of bacterial overgrowth. Other alternatives are nonabsorbable antibiotics for gram-negative bacteria (gentamicin, colistin) and trimethaprim-sulfamethoxazole. In older teenagers, tetracycline or ciprofloxacin might be used. Operative correction of a partial small-bowel obstruction, if present, is the ideal approach.

286.7 Short-Bowel Syndrome

Short-bowel syndrome produces malabsorption and malnutrition after congenital or postnatal loss of at least 50% of the small bowel with or without loss of a portion of the large intestine. Short bowel results in inadequate absorptive surface and compromised bowel function. The condition may not be permanent because the intestine has the capacity for adaptive growth and increase in functional capacity. Adaptation is a gradual process associated with increase in villus height and small-bowel surface rather than lengthening of the bowel.

The small intestine may be congenitally short in conditions in which the bowel is lost in utero, for example, in intestinal malrotation, gastroschisis, and, in some cases, atresia. Most cases involve some surgical resection of the small intestine. Most occur in the neonatal period (necrotizing enterocolitis), although Crohn disease or trauma can account for later onset.

CLINICAL MANIFESTATIONS. The major clinical manifestations are malabsorption and diarrhea. The ability to assimilate nutrients correlates with the length and location as well as the quality of the residual bowel. Carbohydrate malabsorption and steatorrhea are common features resulting in diarrhea and failure to thrive. Large volumes of fluid and electrolyte are normally secreted into the upper gastrointestinal tract and must be reabsorbed. The capacity to reabsorb fluid and electrolyte is usually inadequate in the short-bowel syndrome and results in loss from the gastrointestinal tract with the potential for dehydration, hyponatremia, hypokalemia, and acidosis. The extent of loss is influenced by the presence or absence of the colon in continuity with the small bowel. Trace elements are also poorly absorbed and lost in excess. D-lactic acidosis may occur rarely as a result of fermentation of dietary carbohydrate by luminal bacteria in the small bowel caused by bacterial overgrowth. Patients with this manifestation experience confusion, hyperventilation, and acidosis with an anion gap in the absence of elevated serum lactate as measured by standard techniques (which measure L-lactate). Hypersecretion of acid in the stomach occurs as a result of hypergastrinemia for a transient period after small-bowel resection. However, this condition does not appear to cause problems in infants and children. There is often an associated cholestasis resulting from hyperalimentation and other factors. Cholestasis may contribute to ongoing malabsorption of fat and fat-soluble vitamins.

MANAGEMENT OF SHORT BOWEL. In the late 1960s, about 50% of infants with short bowel survived. Today greater than 90% survive despite the fact that the infants are smaller and have a shorter bowel. The use of total parenteral nutrition has dramatically changed the outcome. These infants cannot maintain adequate nutrition by the enteral route alone and initially must have most of their nutrition given intravenously. Very low amounts of enteral nutrients are given at first as a continuous gastric infusion (1–5 mL/hr depending on the size of the infant). Usually an elemental diet is used at regular strength (20 kcal/oz). This approach is important because there is experimental evidence to suggest that exposure to enteral nutrients contributes to adaptive growth of the small bowel. As tolerated, the quantity can be slowly advanced, perhaps by 1–2 mL/hr each day, as the amount of parenteral nutrition is simultaneously decreased. A level is reached at which diarrhea and malabsorption increase and progression of enteral feedings must be delayed. Bloody diarrhea secondary to a patchy, mild colitis may develop during the progression of enteral feedings. The pathogenesis of this "feeding colitis" is unknown, but it is usually benign. Strictures following neonatal necrotizing enterocolitis may also produce bloody stools (see Chapter 88.2).

When possible, an infant may be given a small amount of formula by mouth to maintain an interest in oral feeding. As children age beyond the first year, it is sometimes possible to add a small amount of solids by mouth (cereal, pureed chicken). For infants with a very short bowel, it may take several years or more until parenteral nutrition can be stopped. An infant with as little as 15 cm of bowel with an ileocecal valve, or 20 cm without, has the potential to survive and eventually be weaned off of parenteral nutrition.

A number of factors appear to influence the length of time until a child is independent of parenteral nutrition. Infants with less than 40 cm of small bowel take twice as long as infants with 40–80 cm of bowel (average of slightly more than 2 yr vs slightly more than 1 yr). The absence of an ileocecal valve doubles the time to complete adaptation, all other factors being equal. The length of residual ileum is inversely correlated with the time until adaptation. Infants with necrotizing enterocolitis and gastroschisis have more difficulty adapting than children with similar bowel resections for other indications.

Bacterial overgrowth is common in infants with a short bowel and may delay progression of enteral feedings (Chapter 286.6). Metronidazole is used empirically, as are nonabsorbable antibiotics that cover gram-negative organisms. Occasionally, a drug that slows gastrointestinal motility, such as loperamide, can be helpful. However, these drugs often do not appear to alter the course. When the small bowel is in continuity with the colon, bile acid malabsorption can cause colonic fluid secretion. In this situation, cholestyramine, 0.25–1 g every 6–8 hr, may be helpful in reducing the watery diarrhea.

LONG-TERM COMPLICATIONS. Long-term complications include those of parenteral nutrition: central catheter infection, thrombosis, hepatotoxicity, and gallstones. For this reason, a continual effort to advance enteral feedings slowly must be considered. Other long-term complications of short bowel include the potential for late vitamin B_{12} deficiency. Stores of vitamin B_{12} acquired in utero are so great that deficiency may not appear until 1 or 10 yr of age. Therefore, it is important to periodically check vitamin B_{12} levels during the first years of life. Gallstones were found in 60% of infants receiving chronic parenteral nutrition who had had terminal ileal resection but in none of the children with an intact ileum. Renal stones can occur as a result of hyperoxaluria secondary to steatorrhea, increased intestinal absorption, and recurrent dehydration.

FUTURE DIRECTIONS IN MANAGEMENT. A number of nutrients have been considered potential stimulants of adaptive growth in experimental animals, but their role in humans remains to be determined. These include glutamine, soluble fiber, short-chain fatty acids, and short-chain triglycerides. Another area of interest, although not yet of clinical use, is the role of peptide growth factors in promoting adaptive growth of the bowel. Bowel-lengthing surgical procedures have been performed with mixed results. Small-bowel transplantation is still in the early stages but has been used in children who appear to be unable to progress off parenteral feedings. Small-bowel and liver transplantation can be performed and is a particular consideration for the child with severe total parenteral nutrition hepatotoxicity.

286.8 *Gluten-Sensitive Enteropathy*

(Celiac Disease)

Gluten-sensitive enteropathy is a disorder in which small-bowel mucosal damage is the result of a permanent sensitivity to dietary gluten. The disorder does not present until gluten products have been introduced into the diet. Typically, the most common period of presentation is between 6 mo and 2 yr of age. Prevalence varies in different regions (it is more frequent in Europe than in the United States), although the incidence appears to be decreasing. In the United States, the incidence is about 1:10,000 live births.

PATHOGENESIS. Three components interact in the pathogenesis: toxicity of certain cereals, genetic predisposition, and environmental factors. The disorder develops only after chronic dietary exposure to the protein gluten, which is found in wheat, rye, oats, and barley. The activity of gluten resides in the gliadin fraction, which contains certain repetitious amino acid sequences (motifs) that lead to sensitization of lamina propria lymphocytes. The evidence that there is a genetic predisposition is that (1) up to 2–5% of first-degree relatives have symptomatic gluten-sensitive enteropathy, (2) as many as 10% of first-degree relatives have asymptomatic damage to small-bowel mucosa consistent with this disorder, and (3) there is an association of the disorder with certain human leukocyte antigen (HLA) types (B8, DR7, DR3, and DQw2). Environmental factors must influence the expression of this genetic predisposition because (1) there is a 30% rate of discordance in monozygotic twins, (2) there is a 70% rate of discordance in HLA-identical siblings, (3) the age of onset among siblings is variable, and (4) the onset of symptoms can be precipitated by gastrointestinal surgery, pregnancy, antibiotic use, or a coincidental diarrheal illness.

The immunologic response to gluten results in villus atrophy, crypt hyperplasia, and damage to the surface epithelium in the small bowel. The injury is greatest in the proximal small bowel and extends distally for a variable distance. The latter observation is undoubtedly the explanation for the variable degree of symptoms and findings of malabsorption among individuals with gluten-sensitive enteropathy. A decrease in absorptive and digestive capacity results from a decrease in small intestinal surface area and a relative increase in immature epithelial cells. Pancreatic secretion is decreased as a result of lowered serum cholecystokinin and secretin levels.

CLINICAL MANIFESTATIONS. The mode of presentation is variable;

the majority present with diarrhea (Table 286–4). Children can have failure to thrive or vomiting as the only manifestation. Perhaps as many as 10% of children referred to endocrinologists for growth retardation without an endocrine or overt gastrointestinal disorder have gluten sensitivity. Anorexia is common and may be the major cause of weight loss or lack of weight gain (Fig 286–2). Infants with gluten-sensitive enteropathy are often, but not always, clingy, irritable, unhappy children who are difficult to comfort. In contrast to infants with cystic fibrosis, they are not interested in food, although this is not always the case. Pallor and abdominal distention are common (see Fig 286–1). Large, bulky stools suggestive of constipation have been described in some children with this condition. Digital clubbing can occur. There is an increased prevalence of gluten-sensitive enteropathy in children with selective IgA deficiency or diabetes mellitus compared with unaffected children. Lymphocytic gastritis occurs in a rare child with gluten-sensitive enteropathy.

EVALUATION. Screening tests for malabsorption are not particularly helpful because they may be normal in a child with gluten-sensitive enteropathy. Anemia and hypoproteinemia may be present. The first serologic tests, including antigliadin antibodies, were not reliable enough. However, the sensitivity and specificity of serum IgA-endomysial antibody testing have approached 100% (except in IgA-deficient patients). Histologic findings on small-bowel biopsy remain the gold standard for diagnosis and biopsy should be performed if one has a high suspicion of gluten-sensitive enteropathy or if serum endomysial antibody is found. The strictest approach to diagnosis is to demonstrate that the biopsy returns to normal within 1–2 yr after starting a gluten-free diet and then to rechallenge with a gluten diet and repeat the biopsy. This approach is now in evolution because it is possible to demonstrate antibody conversion while on a gluten-free diet and only an initial small-bowel biopsy may be necessary.

PATHOLOGY. The diffuse lesion of the upper small intestinal mucosa that characterizes celiac disease is seen in a peroral suction biopsy specimen. Short, flat villi, deepened crypts, and irregular vacuolated surface epithelium with lymphocytes in the epithelial layer are seen by light microscopy. Similar abnormalities occur in other conditions but none is likely to be confused with celiac disease. Infections such as rotavirus enteritis, *Giardia lamblia*, or tropical sprue can cause villus flattening and elongated crypts but not the marked abnormalities of enterocytes. A flat mucosa occurs in kwashiorkor but may represent a response to infestation rather than to undernutrition. Tropical sprue, a poorly understood tropical enteropathy, can cause a lesion that is indistinguishable from that of celiac disease. Some cases of cow's milk protein or soy protein intolerance are associated with lesions similar to those of celiac disease in children. In immune deficiency and eosinophilic gastroenteritis, villi can be partially shortened. Infants with familial enteropathy have short villi, but the crypt dimensions are normal.

TREATMENT. Treatment requires a lifelong, strict gluten-free diet. All wheat, rye, and barley products should be eliminated from the diet; many children tolerate oats. Initially, vitamin and iron supplementation is advisable. When the disorder presents with fulminant diarrhea, initial treatment with oral prednisone can be useful; this approach is rarely necessary. Although the parents of a child with gluten-sensitive enteropathy usually become very knowledgable about diet, initially they need the help of an experienced dietitian. National celiac support groups provide much specific information about the gluten content of foods and medications. Processed foods must be considered carefully because it is common that they contain some gluten. Gluten-free foods are commercially available.

PROGNOSIS. The clinical response to a gluten-free diet of a child with celiac disease is gratifying. Improvement of mood and appetite is followed by lessening of diarrhea. In most cases changes occur within 1 wk of starting therapy, but the response may occasionally be delayed. Older patients and very ill patients tend to respond slowly, but once in remission the celiac child should be treated as a well child. Teenagers often become noncompliant. Unfortunately, this is an age when the disorder tends to be symptomatically quiesent, and a teenager may believe the disorder has resolved. Nevertheless, mucosal damage is present. Subtle manifestations of growth failure or delayed sexual maturation may take place when receiving a gluten-containing diet. Appropriately diagnosed gluten-sensitive enteropathy is a lifelong condition requiring lifelong treatment. The late development of bowel lymphoma in longstanding enteropathy, especially with poor adherence to diet, is possible although controversial. No complications from long-term gluten-free diet treatment are recognized.

■ **TABLE 286–4 Active Childhood Celiac Disease—42 Cases**

Symptoms	No. of Patients
Failure to thrive	36
Diarrhea	30
Irritability	30
Vomiting	24
Anorexia	24
Foul stools	21
Abdominal pain	8
Excessive appetite	6
Rectal prolapse	3
Signs	**No. of Patients**
Height <25th percentile	30
Body weight <25th percentile	37
Wasted muscles	40
Abdominal distention	33
Edema	14
Finger clubbing	11

286.9 Immunoproliferative Small Intestinal Disease

Initially manifesting as intermittent diarrhea in 10- to 30-yr-old males and females in developing countries, this process may progress to a high-grade small intestinal lymphoma.

EPIDEMIOLOGY. Immunoproliferative small intestinal disease is endemic in the Mediterranean basin, Mideast, the Far East, and Africa. Poverty and frequent episodes of gastroenteritis during infancy are antecedent social and medical problems. Sporadic cases occur in Europe and North and South America, predominantly in immigrants from developing countries, although occasionally in native citizens.

PATHOLOGY. Early lesions demonstrate thickened mucosal folds, duodenal or jejunal nodularity, and lymphoplasmacytic infiltrates. The process may be patchy but progresses to diffuse lymphohistiocytic nodules, mesenteric lymph node involvement, the presence of Reed-Sternberg-like cells, and eventually the development of an immunoblastic lymphoma. This process represents an IgA lymphoproliferative disorder progressing to a B-cell lymphoma.

CLINICAL MANIFESTATIONS. Initially, patients have intermittent diarrhea and abdominal pain. Later stages demonstrate persistent chronic diarrhea, malabsorption, weight loss, digital clubbing, and growth failure.

DIAGNOSIS. Endoscopic biopsies of multiple duodenal and jejunal mucosal sites aid in the diagnosis. In addition, a serum marker (α heavy chain paraprotein) of IgA is present in most cases. *Giardia lamblia* may also be present but is not responsible for the lymphoproliferative disorder. Immunosuppressed organ transplant recipients may develop a lymphoproliferative disorder manifesting diarrhea.

TREATMENT. The earliest lesions respond to prolonged (~6 mo) tetracycline therapy. Prelymphomatous stages may be treated with cyclophosphamide with or without prednisone and tetracycline. Lymphomas are treated with a combination of cyclophosphamide, doxorubicin, teniposide, prednisone with or without bleomycin, and vinblastine. Lymphoproliferative disorders in immunosuppressed transplant patients usually improve with reduction of the immunosuppressive drug dose.

PROGNOSIS. Early therapy of antibiotic responsive lesions produces an excellent outcome. Treatment of the later lymphomatous lesions has resulted in a variable but usually poor outcome.

Khojasteh A, Haghighi P: Immunoproliferative small intestinal disease: Portrait of a potentially preventable cancer from the Third World. Am J Med 89:483, 1990.

286.10 Other Malabsorptive Syndromes

INTESTINAL LYMPHANGIECTASIA. This group of disorders is characterized by dilatation of intestinal lymphatic vessels and leakage of lymph into the intestinal lumen and, at times, the peritoneal cavity. Because absorbed fat is normally transferred from the intestine via the lymphatic vessels, children with this disorder have steatorrhea with protein-losing enteropathy and may have lymphocyte depletion. Manifestations may include any combination of hypoalbuminemia, hypogammaglobulinemia, edema, lymphocytopenia, fat malabsorption, and chylous ascites. Intestinal lymphangiectasia can be primary or can result from abdominal or thoracic surgical damage to lymphatic vessels, chronic right-sided heart failure, constrictive pericarditis, retroperitoneal tumor, or malrotation with lymphatic obstruction. Primary intestinal lymphangiectasia is the result of a congenital abnormality of lymphatic drainage from the intestine and may be associated with abnormalities in lymphatic drainage from other regions of the body. Turner and Noonan syndromes have been associated with intestinal lymphangiectasia.

The diagnosis is suggested by the typical findings described previously in association with an elevated fecal α_1-antitrypsin level consistent with protein-losing enteropathy. The characteristic radiologic findings of uniform, symmetric thickening of mucosal folds throughout the small intestine are usually, although not always, present on small-bowel contrast radiographs. The diagnosis is confirmed by the presence of collections of abnormal dilated lacteals with distortion of villi on peroral small-bowel biopsy. The disorder may be seen only in the submucosa, requiring surgical biopsy of the intestine.

MICROVILLUS INCLUSION DISEASE (CONGENITAL MICROVILLUS ATROPHY). Microvillus inclusion disease is a disorder that presents at birth with intractable, watery diarrhea and severe malabsorption. It appears to be the most common cause of persistent diarrhea that begins in the neonatal period. The disorder seems to be inherited in an autosomal recessive pattern. The findings on small-bowel biopsy are the key to the diagnosis and include villus atrophy, crypt hypoplasia, and, on election microscopy, microvillus inclusions in enterocytes. The latter finding is also seen in colonocytes. The somatostatin analog octreotide has been used as treatment and may reduce the volume of stool output in some infants. Epidermal growth factor has been used with equivocal results. Infants with this disorder require total parenteral nutrition for survival and may be candidates for bowel transplantation.

AUTOIMMUNE ENTEROPATHY. Autoimmune enteropathy is a poorly characterized syndrome of chronic diarrhea and malabsorption. If symptoms initially develop after the first 6 mo of life, the disorder is likely to be mistaken for gluten-sensitive enteropathy. Typically, the lack of response to a gluten-free diet leads to further evaluation. Histologic findings in the small bowel include total villus atrophy, crypt hyperplasia, and an increase in chronic inflammatory cells in the lamina propria. Specific serum antienterocyte antibodies may be identified with indirect immunofluorescent staining using normal small-bowel mucosa and the kidney. The colon can also be involved. Extraintestinal autoimmune disorders are usual and include arthritis, membranous glomerulonephritis, thrombocytopenia, and hemolytic anemia. Treatment has included prednisone, azathioprine, cyclophosphamide (Cytoxan), and cyclosporine.

TUFTING ENTEROPATHY. Tufting enteropathy is a disorder that presents in the first weeks of life with persistent watery diarrhea and appears to account for a small fraction of infants with protracted diarrhea of infancy. Onset of symptoms is not immediately after birth as in microvillus inclusion disease. On small-bowel biopsy, the distinctive feature is that 80–90% of the epithelial surface contains focal epithelial "tufts" (teardrop-shaped groups of closely packed enterocytes with apical rounding of the plasma membrane). In other known enteropathies, tufts are seen on 15% or less of the epithelial surface. In this disorder, colonic epithelium shows no abnormality. On electron microscopy of small-bowel epithelium, the major finding is shortening of the microvilli. This does not appear to be an autoimmune enteropathy, and no known enteropathogens have been isolated from the few children described with this entity. The intestinal lesion has not responded to removal of dietary antigens, administration of total parenteral nutrition, or use of immunosuppressive therapy.

TROPICAL SPRUE. This syndrome is characterized by generalized malabsorption associated with a diffuse lesion of the small intestinal mucosa that occurs only in individuals who have lived in or visited certain tropical regions. It occurs in some Caribbean countries but not Jamaica, northern South America, Africa, and parts of Asia. Fever and malaise precede the onset of watery diarrhea. In about 1 wk, acute features subside and chronic malabsorption, intermittent diarrhea, and anorexia lead eventually to severe malnutrition. Signs of malnutrition may include night blindness, glossitis, stomatitis, cheilosis, hyperpigmentation, and edema. Muscle wasting is marked, and the abdomen is often distended. There is evidence of diffuse malabsorption, including steatorrhea and carbohydrate intolerance. Megaloblastic anemia is the result of folate and vitamin B_{12} deficiencies. Biopsy of the small intestinal mucosa shows villus shortening, increased crypt depth, and an increase in chronic inflammatory cells in the lamina propria. Treatment includes nonabsorbable sulfonamides or tetracycline (for 3–4 wks) and folate as well as vitamin B_{12} repletion. The response to treatment is usually excellent.

WOLMAN DISEASE. This rare lethal lipid storage disease leads to lipid accumulation in many organs including the small intestine. In addition to vomiting and hepatosplenomegaly, there may be steatorrhea as the result of lymphatic obstruction (Chapter 72.3).

286.11 Enzyme Deficiencies

ENTEROKINASE DEFICIENCY

Congenital deficiency of this small-intestinal enzyme has been reported in a few children. The disease results in a complete absence of pancreatic proteolytic activity because enterokinase is an essential activator of pancreatic trypsinogens. Affected patients are ill from very early life with severe diarrhea and failure to thrive. Hypoproteinemia is common and may lead to edema. In duodenal fluid tryptic activity is missing while lipase and amylase are normal; in vitro tryptic activity of the fluid can be restored by the addition of enterokinase. Malabsorption of protein is the major defect, although mild steatorrhea has been reported. Pancreatic enzyme replacements restore normal digestive function; much smaller amounts are needed compared to that for pancreatic insufficiency.

DISACCHARIDASE DEFICIENCIES

The disaccharidases are located on the brush border membrane surface of the small bowel. Occasionally, congenital deficiencies occur, but abnormal disaccharidase activities in infants and young children have most often been the result of diffuse acquired lesions of the intestinal epithelium, such as those of infection or celiac disease. In older children and adults, late-onset genetic lactase deficiency is the most common condition with reduced disaccharidase activity.

The response of the patient to significant disaccharidase deficiency (disaccharide intolerance) is similar whatever its cause or the enzymes involved. If disaccharide hydrolysis at the brush border is incomplete, the sugar accumulates in the distal intestinal lumen, where organic acids and hydrogen gas are produced by bacteria. The excess intraluminal sugar and organic acids draw water into the lumen, leading to watery osmotic diarrhea with stools that are frothy, of low pH (pH<5.6), contain excess sugar, and tend to excoriate the buttocks. There may be bloating and borborygmi, but steatorrhea is rare. In some cases, particularly those beyond infancy, gas production causing crampy abdominal pain is the dominant problem, rather than diarrhea.

If the disaccharide involved is a reducing sugar (e.g., lactose), the standard Clinitest examination* will be 2+ or greater in most cases. Disaccharidase activities can be assayed in mucosal biopsy specimens. Breath hydrogen excretion after an oral sugar load is a useful noninvasive technique for detecting disaccharide intolerance (Chapter 286.1).

LACTASE DEFICIENCY. *Congenital* absence of lactase has been reported in very few cases. The usual mechanism for primary lactose intolerance relates to the *developmental* pattern of lactase activity. Because lactase activity rises relatively late in fetal life and begins to fall after the age of 3 yr, intolerance to lactose can be anticipated in very premature infants and in some older children and adults. Approximately 15% of adult whites, 40% of adult Orientals, and 85% of adult blacks in the United States are deficient in intestinal lactase; this is transmitted by autosomal recessive inheritance. Because lactase activity in the mucosa is at best marginal, this enzyme is particularly likely to be depleted *secondary to diffuse mucosal diseases.*

Symptoms occur in response to ingestion of lactose, the sugar in milk. Explosive watery diarrhea is associated with abdominal distention, borborygmi, flatulence, and an excoriated diaper area. A syndrome of recurrent, vague, crampy abdominal pain has also been attributed to lactose intolerance. School- and preschool-age children experience episodic midabdominal pain. Usually, their general health is unaffected, and there is no obvious temporal relationship of pain to milk ingestion or to diarrhea. (Chapter 287.1).

Treatment consists of removal of milk from the diet. In most cases the elimination need not be total; stopping milk ingestion as a beverage is important. A lactase preparation (Lactaid) is available; when added to milk, it allows asymptomatic consumption of modest quantities of milk incubated with the added enzyme. A capsule with lactase activity can also be ingested with meals (Lactaid, Lactrase). Live culture yogurt contains bacteria that produce lactase enzyme and is thus tolerated by lactase-deficient individuals.

SUCRASE-ISOMALTASE DEFICIENCY. The only relatively common congenital deficiency of disaccharidase activities, a combined deficiency of sucrase and isomaltase, is inherited as an autosomal recessive trait and occurs in about 0.8% of North Americans. Symptoms usually begin when a sucrose-containing diet is started. There may be intolerance to starch, but because isomaltase acts only on the branch points of the starch molecule, isomaltase deficiency itself is relatively asymptomatic. The symptoms are bloating, watery diarrhea, and excoriation of the buttocks. Recurrent abdominal pain has not been attributed to sucrose-isomaltose intolerance. Because sucrose is not a reducing sugar, its presence will not be detected in the stool by Clinitest unless the specimen is first hydrolyzed with hydrochloric acid. The morphology of the small intestinal mucosa is normal, but enzyme assays show specific deficiencies of sucrase and isomaltase with normal levels of lactase and maltase. Breath testing usually demonstrates increased hydrogen gas after sucrose ingestion. Affected patients improve quickly after dietary sucrose is reduced to minimal amounts.

286.12 Defects of Absorption or Transport

GLUCOSE-GALACTOSE MALABSORPTION. This rare congenital defect in brush border membrane glucose and galactose-sodium dependent cotransport is inherited as an autosomal recessive trait. It also affects renal tubular epithelium to a mild degree. Severe diffuse mucosal damage, particularly in a young infant, may also impair the glucose-galactose carrier sufficiently to cause intolerance to these sugars. Usually, if mucosal damage is severe enough to impair glucose transport, other absorptive processes are affected.

The symptomatic response to sugar ingestion is similar whether the defect is congenital or secondary. Watery stools follow the ingestion of glucose, breast milk, or conventional formulas because most diet sugars are polysaccharides or disaccharides with glucose or galactose moieties. The patient may be bloated, and, if diarrhea persists, dehydration and acidosis can be severe. The stools are acidic and contain sugar. Patients with the congenital defect tolerate fructose; their small-bowel function and structure are normal in all other aspects.

Treatment consists of rigorous restriction of glucose and galactose and provision of a fructose-containing formula. Later in life limited amounts of glucose or sucrose may be tolerated.

ABETALIPOPROTEINEMIA (Chapter 72.4). This autosomal-recessive condition is associated with severe fat malabsorption from birth. Children fail to thrive during the 1st yr of life and their stools are pale, foul smelling, and bulky. The abdomen is distended, and deep tendon reflexes are absent as a result of a peripheral neuropathy.

Intellectual development tends to be slow. After 10 yr of age, intestinal symptoms are less severe, ataxia develops, and there is a loss of position and vibration senses and the onset of intention tremors. These latter symptoms reflect involvement of the posterior columns, cerebellum, and basal ganglia. In adolescence, an atypical retinitis pigmentosa develops.

Diagnosis rests on finding acanthocytes in the peripheral blood and very low plasma levels of cholesterol (<50 mg/dL). Chylomicrons and very-low–density lipoproteins are not detectable, and the low-density lipoprotein (LDL) fraction is virtually absent from the circulation; there is marked triglyceride accumulation in villus enterocytes in the fasting duodenal mucosa. Usually, there is steatorrhea in younger patients, but

*Ames Company.

other processes of assimilation are intact. Patients lack microsomal triglyceride transfer protein in the small bowel. This protein is required for normal assembly and secretion of chylomicrons. The neuropathy is the result of vitamin E deficiency.

Specific therapy is not available. Large supplements of the fat-soluble vitamins A, D, E, and K should be given. Vitamin E (100 mg/kg/24 hr) and vitamin A (10,000–25,000 IU/day) may arrest the neurologic degeneration. Limiting long-chain fat intake may alleviate intestinal symptoms; medium-chain triglycerides can be used to supplement the fat intake.

HOMOZYGOUS HYPOBETALIPOPROTEINEMIA. This disorder is transmitted as an autosomal dominant trait; the homozygous form is indistinguishable from abetalipoproteinemia. However, the parents of these patients, as heterozygotes, have reduced plasma LDL and apoprotein-β concentrations, unlike the parents of patients with abetalipoproteinemia who have normal levels.

CHYLOMICRON RETENTION DISEASE. In this rare recessive disorder, the processes leading up to the release of chylomicrons from enterocytes appear to be defective. These patients have severe intestinal symptoms with steatorrhea and failure to thrive. Acanthocytosis is rare, and neurologic manifestations are less severe than those observed in abetalipoproteinemia. Plasma cholesterol levels are reduced, but moderately so (<75 mg/dL); fasting triglycerides are normal; but the fat-soluble vitamins, particularly A and E, rapidly deplete. Early aggressive therapy with fat-soluble vitamins is indicated, as for abetalipoproteinemia.

AMINO ACID TRANSPORT DEFECTS. In several of the specific congenital disorders of amino acid transport (Chapter 71) defective intestinal amino acid transport occurs. There appear to be at least three specific small-bowel carriers involved in active transport of amino acids. Amino acid uptake into the intestinal mucosa is defective in *cystinuria,* but these patients have no gastrointestinal symptoms. In *Hartnup disease* malabsorption of tryptophan leads to ataxia, intellectual deterioration, a pellagra-like skin rash, and at times diarrhea. *Methionine malabsorption* is associated with episodes of diarrhea in fair-complexioned, retarded children whose urine has a sweet odor and contains excess α-hydroxybutyric acid. In the *blue diaper syndrome* tryptophan absorption is defective.

VITAMIN B_{12} MALABSORPTION. Several rare congenital defects may affect assimilation of vitamin B_{12}. These conditions are much less common than dietary vitamin B_{12} deficiency or malabsorption secondary to terminal ileal resection or dysfunction. In *juvenile pernicious anemia* intrinsic factor production in the stomach is defective. Vitamin B_{12} malabsorption results, leading to megaloblastic anemia and growth failure. Gastric structure and function are otherwise normal.

Transcobalamin II deficiency is an inherited defect of a protein necessary for intestinal transport of vitamin B_{12}. The result is severe megaloblastic anemia, diarrhea, and vomiting.

Imerslund has described patients in whom ileal absorption of vitamin B_{12} is defective. Ileal structure and function are otherwise normal. Megaloblastic anemia develops toward the end of the 1st yr. Proteinuria is commonly associated.

Treatment of these disorders is to administer vitamin B_{12} by injection: 1,000 μg/wk for transcobalamin II deficiency and 100 μg/mo for the others.

CONGENITAL MALABSORPTION OF FOLIC ACID. A few patients have had folic acid deficiency in infancy as the result of a specific defect in folic acid assimilation. In addition to megaloblastic anemia, they have had cerebral degeneration.

CHLORIDE-LOSING DIARRHEA. This rare specific congenital defect of ileal chloride transport is associated with maternal polyhydramnios. The dominant symptom is severe watery diarrhea beginning at birth, the result of accumulation of chloride ion in the intestinal lumen. Watery diarrhea leads to dehydration and a severe electrolyte disturbance characterized by hypokalemia, hypochloremia, and alkalosis, a most unusual pattern for a child with chronic diarrhea. Other aspects of intestinal absorption are normal. Stools contain chloride in excess of the sum of sodium and potassium. There is no adequate treatment. Potassium supplements and some restriction of chloride intake are advisable.

CONGENITAL SODIUM DIARRHEA. Two patients have been described with profuse watery diarrhea from birth. There was maternal polyhydramnios and neonatal abdominal distention; however, unlike chloride diarrhea, there was acidosis and fecal chloride concentration less than Na^+. Treatment with oral hydration solution was effective in maintaining normal growth. The apparent basis for this rare syndrome is a defect in Na^+/H^+ exchange in the small intestine and colon.

VITAMIN D-DEPENDENT RICKETS. In this autosomal recessive disorder a specific defect in the metabolism of vitamin D causes malabsorption of calcium (Chapter 649). Intestinal function is otherwise normal.

PRIMARY HYPOMAGNESEMIA. This specific intestinal transport defect in magnesium transport causes severe hypomagnesemia and, secondarily, hypocalcemic tetany in infancy. Other aspects of intestinal function are normal. The findings are reversed by large supplements of magnesium, which must be continued indefinitely.

ACRODERMATITIS ENTEROPATHICA. See also Chapter 604. This unusual constellation of clinical findings is due to zinc deficiency secondary to zinc malabsorption. Early in life the patient experiences rashes around mucocutaneous junctions and on the extremities; alopecia, chronic diarrhea, and sometimes steatorrhea may occur. Untreated, the patient fails to thrive. Serum zinc concentration and alkaline phosphatase activity are low. Intestinal mucosal biopsies show Paneth cell inclusions that disappear after treatment. An oral supplement of zinc sulfate, 1–2 mg elemental zinc/kg/24 hr, causes rapid healing of the skin lesions and improvement of diarrhea.

MENKES (KINKY HAIR) SYNDROME. This rare recessively inherited disorder is characterized by growth retardation, abnormal hair, cerebellar degeneration, and early death (Chapter 552.5). Its pathogenesis is unclear, but there is a widespread defect in cellular copper transport that affects the intestine as well as other tissues. Serum copper and ceruloplasmin levels are low, but cellular copper content is increased.

BILE ACID MALABSORPTION. Cases of primary bile acid malabsorption causing diarrhea and steatorrhea from early infancy have occurred. These patients have severe growth retardation and massive steatorrhea based on an apparent congenital defect in ileal bile salt transport.

DRUG-INDUCED ABSORPTIVE DEFECTS. Some drugs have a diffuse impact on the small intestinal epithelium. For example, methotrexate can cause arrest of enterocyte mitoses and result in a mucosal lesion; large doses of neomycin also affect mucosal structure. *Sulfasalazine* interferes with folic acid absorption. *Cholestyramine* binds bile salts and calcium in the intestinal lumen to cause hypocalcemia and steatorrhea. *Phenytoin* interferes with calcium absorption and can cause rickets.

MALABSORPTION SYNDROMES

General Reviews

Ament ME: Malabsorption syndromes in infancy and childhood. J Pediatr 81:685, 1972.
Anderson CM: Malabsorption in children. Clin Gastroenterol 6:355, 1977.
Kleinman RE, Klish W, Lebenthal E, et al: Role of juice carbohydrate malabsorption in chronic nonspecific diarrhea in children. J Pediatr 120:825, 1992.
Riby JE, Fujisawa T, Kretchmer N: Fructose absorption. Am J Clin Nutr 58:748S, 1993.
Wilson FA, Dietschy JM: Differential diagnostic approach to clinical problems of malabsorption. Gastroenterology 61:911, 1971.

Diagnostic Investigations

Ament ME, Berquist WE, Vargus J, et al: Fiberoptic upper endoscopy in infants and children. Pediatr Clin North Am 35:141, 1988.

Barr RG, Perman JA, Schoeller DA, et al: Breath tests in pediatric gastrointestinal disorders: New diagnostic opportunities. Pediatrics 62:393, 1978.

Cobden I, Pothwell J, Axon ATR: Intestinal permeability and screening tests for coeliac disease. Gut 21:512, 1980.

Ghesh SK, Littlewood JM, Goddard D, et al: Stool microscopy in screening for steatorrhea. J Clin Pathol 30:749, 1977.

Hill RE, Cutz E, Cherian G, et al: An evaluation of D-xylose absorption measurements in children suspected of having small intestinal disease. J Pediatr 99:245, 1981.

Hill RE, Hercz A, Corey MD, et al: Fecal clearance of alpha-1-antitrypsin: A reliable measure of protein loss in children. J Pediatr 99:416, 1981.

Katz AJ, Grand RJ: All that flattens is not sprue. Gastroenterology 76:375, 1979.

Khouri M, Huang G, Shiau Y: Sudan stain of fecal fat: New insight into an old test. Gastroenterology 96:421, 1989.

Murphy MS, Eastham EJ, Nelson R, et al: Non-invasive assessment of intraluminal lipolysis using a $^{13}CO_2$ breath test. Arch Dis Child 65:574, 1990.

Riddleshergeг MM: Evaluation of the gastrointestinal tract in the child: CT, MRI, and isotopic studies. Pediatr Clin North Am 35:281, 1988.

Schmerling DH, Farrer JCW, Prader A: Fecal fat and nitrogen in healthy children and in children with malabsorption or maldigestion. Pediatrics 46:690, 1970.

DIGESTIVE TRACT IN CHRONIC MALNUTRITION

Brunser O: Effects of malnutrition on intestinal structure and function in children. Clin Gastroenterol 6:341, 1977.

Durie PR, Forstner GG, Gaskin KJ, et al: Elevated serum immunoreactive pancreatic cationic trypsinogen in acute malnutrition: Evidence of pancreatic damage. J Pediatr 106:233, 1985.

Romer H, Cerbach R, Gomez MA, et al: Moderate and severe protein-energy malnutrition in childhood: Effects on jejunal mucosal morphology and disaccharidase activities. J Pediatr Gastroenterol Nutr 2:459, 1983.

LIVER AND BILIARY DISORDERS

Argao EA, Heubi JE: Fat-soluble vitamin deficiency in infants and children. Curr Opin Pediatr 5:562, 1993.

Hadorn B, Hess J, Troesch V, et al: Role of bile acids in the activation of trypsinogen by enterokinase: Disturbance of trypsinogen activation in patients with intrahepatic biliary atresia. Gastroenterology 66:548, 1974.

Kooh SW, Jones G, Reilly BJ, et al: Pathogenesis of rickets in chronic hepatobiliary disease in children. J Pediatr 94:870, 1979.

SHORT SMALL INTESTINE

Caniano DA, Kanoti GA: Newborns with massive intestinal loss: Difficult choices. N Engl J Med 318:703, 1988.

Goulet OJ, Revillon Y, Jan D, et al: Neonatal short bowel syndrome. J Pediatr 119:18, 1991.

Grant D, Wall W, Mimeault R, et al: Successful small-bowel/liver transplantation. Lancet 335:181, 1990.

Hamilton JR, Reilly BJ, Morecki R: Short small intestine associated with malrotation. A newly described cause of intestinal malabsorption. Gastroenterology 56:124, 1969.

Taylor SF, Sondheimer JM, Sokol RJ, et al: Noninfectious colitis associated with short gut syndrome in infants. J Pediatr 119:24, 1991.

STAGNANT LOOP SYNDROME

Bayes BJ, Hamilton JR: Blind loop syndrome in children. Acta Dis Child 44:76, 1969.

Gracey M: Intestinal microflora and bacterial overgrowth in early life. J Pediatr Gastroenterol Nutr 1:13, 1982.

Soderlund S: Anomalies of midgut rotation and fixation: Clinical aspects based on sixty-two cases in childhood. Acta Pediatr 51:135, 1966.

INFECTIONS CAUSING MALABSORPTION

Ament ME: Diagnosis and treatment of giardiasis. J Pediatr 80:663, 1972.

Liebman WM, Thaler MM, Dehorimier A, et al: Intractable diarrhea of infancy due to intestinal coccidiosis. Gastroenterology 78:579, 1980.

IMMUNODEFICIENCY STATES AND THE INTESTINE

Glover MT, Atherton DJ, Levinsky RJ: Syndrome of erythroderma, failure to thrive and diarrhea in infancy: A manifestation of immunodeficiency. Pediatrics 81:66, 1988.

Kotler DP, Francisco A, Clayton F, et al: Small intestinal injury and parasitic diseases in AIDS. Ann Intern Med 113:444, 1990.

Weikel CS, Gaynes BN, Roche JK: Diarrheal disease in the immunocompromised host. *In*: Guerrant R (ed): Ballière's Clinical Tropical Medicine and Communicable Diseases, Vol 3, p 401. London, Ballière Tindall, 1988.

Yolken RH, Hart W, Oung I, et al: Gastrointestinal dysfunction and disaccharide intolerance in children infected with human immunodeficiency virus. J Pediatr 118:359, 1991.

CELIAC DISEASE

Chan KN, Phillips AD, Mirakian R, et al: Endomysial antibody screening in children. J Pediatr Gastroenterol Nutr 18:316, 1994.

O'Mahony S, Vestey JP, Ferguson A: Similarities in intestinal humoral immunity in dermatitis herpetiformis without enteropathy and in coeliac disease. Lancet 335:1487, 1990.

Report to Working Group of European Society of Paediatric Gastroenterology and Nutrition: Revised criteria for diagnosis of coeliac disease. Arch Dis Child 65:909, 1990.

Rich EJ, Christie DL: Anti-gliadin antibody panel and xylose absorption test in screening for celiac disease. J Pediatr Gastroenterol Nutr 10:174, 1990.

Rossi TM, Albini CH, Kumar V: Incidence of celiac disease identified by the presence of serum endomysial antibodies in children with chronic diarrhea, short stature, or insulin-dependent diabetes mellitus. J Pediatr 123:262, 1993.

Swinson CM, Slavin G, Coles EC, et al: Coeliac disease and malignancy. Lancet 1:111, 1983.

Visakorpi J, Mäki M: Changing clinical features of coeliac disease. Acta Paediatr (Suppl)395:10, 1994.

OTHER SYNDROMES

Klipstein FA, Baker SJ: Regarding the definition of tropical sprue. Gastroenterology 58:717, 1970.

Queloz JM, Capitanio MA, Kirkpatrick JA: Wolman's disease. Radiology 104:357, 1972.

Reifen RM, Cutz E, Griffiths AM, et al: Tufting enteropathy: A newly recognized clinicopathological entity associated with refractory diarrhea in infants. J Pediatr Gastroenterol Nutr 18:379, 1994.

Santiago-Borrero PJ, Maldonado N, Horta E: Tropical sprue in children. J Pediatr 76:470, 1970.

Strober W, Wochner RD, Carbone PP, et al: Intestinal lymphangiectasia: A protein-losing enteropathy with hypogammaglobulinemia, lymphocytopenia and impaired homograft rejection. J Clin Invest 46:1643, 1967.

Vardy PA, Lebenthal E, Shwachman H: Intestinal lymphangiectasis: A reappraisal. Pediatrics 55:842, 1975.

DEFECTS OF ABSORPTION OR TRANSPORT

Levy E, Chouraqui JP, Ray CC: Steatorrhea and disorders of chylomicron synthesis and secretion. Pediatr Clin North Am 35:53, 1988.

Muller DPR, Lloyd JK, Bird AC: Long-term management of abetalipoproteinemia. Arch Dis Child 52:209, 1977.

Rader DJ, Brewer B: Abetalipoporteinemia: New insights into lipoprotein assembly and vitamin E metabolism from a rare genetic disease. JAMA 270:865, 1993.

Scott BB, Miller JP, Losowsky MS: Hypobetalipoproteinemia: A variant of the Bassen-Kornzweig syndrome. Gut 20:163, 1979.

ENTEROKINASE DEFICIENCY

Hadorn B, Tarlow M, Lloyd JD, et al: Intestinal enterokinase deficiency. Lancet 1:812, 1969.

AMINO ACID TRANSPORT DEFECTS

Drummond KN, Michael AF, Ulstrom RA, et al: The blue diaper syndrome: Familial hypercalcemia with nephrocalcinosis and indicanuria. Am J Med 37:928, 1964.

Hooft G, Timmermand J, Snoeck J, et al: Methionine malabsorption syndrome. Ann Pediatr 205:73, 1965.

Milne MD: Hartnup disease. Biochemistry 111:3, 1969.

Morin CL, Thompson MW, Jackson SH, et al: Biochemical and genetic studies in cystinuria: Observations on double heterozygotes of genotype I/II. J Clin Invest 50:1961, 1971.

Whelan DT, Scriver CR: Hyperdibasicaminoaciduria: An inherited disorder of amino acid transport. Pediatr Res 2:525, 1968.

DISACCHARIDASE DEFICIENCIES

Ament ME, Perera DR, Esther L: Sucrase-isomaltase deficiency: A frequently misdiagnosed disease. J Pediatr 83:721, 1973.

Flats G: The genetics of lactose digestion in humans. Adv Hum Genet 16:1, 1987.

Harrison M, Walker-Smith JA: Reinvestigation of lactose intolerant children: Lack of correlation between continuing lactose intolerance and small intestinal morphology, disaccharidase activity and lactose tests. Gut 18:48, 1977.

Lifshitz F: Carbohydrate problems in paediatric gastroenterology. Clin Gastroenterol 6:415, 1977.

Semensa G, Auricchio S: Small intestinal disaccharidases. *In*: Scriver CS, Beaudet AL, Sly WS, et al (eds): The Metabolic Basis of Inherited Disease. New York, McGraw-Hill, 1989, p 2975.

GLUCOSE-GALACTOSE MALABSORPTION

Evans L, Grasset E, Heyman M, et al: Congenital selective malabsorption of glucose and galactose. J Pediatr Gastroenterol Nutr 4:878, 1985.

Fairclough PD, Clark ML, Dawson AM, et al: Absorption of glucose and maltose in congenital glucose-galactose malabsorption. Pediatr Res 12:1112, 1978.

Lindqvist B, Meeuwisse GW, Melin K: Glucose-galactose malabsorption. Lancet 2:666, 1962.

VITAMIN B_{12} MALABSORPTION

Chanarin I: Disorders of vitamin absorption. Clin Gastroenterol 11:73, 1982.

Hall CA: Congenital disorders of vitamin B_{12} transport and their contribution to concepts. Gastroenterology 65:684, 1973.

Hitzig WH, Dohmann V, Pluss HJ, et al: Hereditary transcobalamin II deficiency: Clinical findings in a new family. J Pediatr 85:622, 1974.

Imerslund O: Idiopathic chronic megaloblastic anaemia in children. Acta Paediatr (Suppl) 49:119, 1960.

MacKenzie IL, Donaldson RM, Trier JS, et al: Ileal mucosa in familial selective vitamin B_{12} malabsorption. N Engl J Med 286:1021, 1972.

FOLATE MALABSORPTION

Poncz M, Colman N, Herbert V, et al: Congenital folate malabsorption. J Pediatr 99:828, 1981.

Urbach J, Abrahamov A, Grossowicz N: Congenital isolated folic acid malabsorption. Arch Dis Child 62:78, 1987.

CHLORIDE-LOSING DIARRHEA

Bieberdorf FA, Gorden P, Fordtran JS: Pathogenesis of congenital alkalosis with diarrhea: Implications for the physiology of normal ileal electrolyte absorption and secretion. J Clin Invest 51:1958, 1972.

Holmberg C, Perheentupa J, Launiala K, et al: Congenital chloride diarrhea. Arch Dis Child 52:255, 1977.

CONGENITAL SODIUM DIARRHEA

Booth IW, Murer H, Strange G, et al: Defective jejunal brush border Na^+/H^+ exchange: A cause of congenital secretory diarrhea. Lancet 1:1066, 1985.

Holmberg C, Perheentupa J: Congenital Na^+ diarrhea: A new type of secretory diarrhea. J Pediatr 106:56, 1985.

VITAMIN D-DEPENDENT RICKETS

Hamilton R, Harrison J, Fraser D, et al: The small intestine in vitamin D dependent rickets. Pediatrics 45:364, 1970.

PRIMARY HYPOMAGNESEMIA

Paunier L, Radde IC, Kooh SW, et al: Primary hypomagnesemia with secondary hypocalcemia in an infant. Pediatrics 41:385, 1968.

Stromme JH, Nesbakken R, Normann T, et al: Familial hypomagnesemia. Acta Paediatr Scand 58:433, 1969.

ACRODERMATITIS ENTEROPATHICA

Bohane TD, Cutz E, Hamilton JR, et al: Acrodermatitis enteropathica, zinc and the Paneth cell. Gastroenterology 73:587, 1977.

Moynahan EJ: Acrodermatitis enteropathica: A lethal inherited human zinc-deficiency disorder. Lancet 2:399, 1974.

MENKES SYNDROME

Danks DM: Of mice and men, metals and mutations. J Med Genet 23:99, 1986.

Danks DM, Stevens BJ, Campbell PE, et al: Menkes' kinky-hair syndrome. Lancet 1:110, 1972.

PRIMARY BILE ACID MALABSORPTION

Heubi JE, Balistreri WF, Fondacaro JD, et al: Primary bile acid malabsorption: Defective in vitro ileal active bile acid transport. Gastroenterology 83:804, 1982.

DRUG-INDUCED MALABSORPTION

Franklin JL, Rosenberg HH: Impaired folic acid absorption in inflammatory bowel disease: Effects of salicylazosulfapyridine (Azulfidine). Gastroenterology 64:517, 1973.

Morijiri Y, et al: Factors causing rickets in institutionalized handicapped children on anti-convulsant therapy. Arch Dis Child 56:446, 1981.

Rogers AL, Vloedman DA, Bloom EC, et al: Neomycin-induced steatorrhea. JAMA 197:185, 1966.

Trier JS: Morphologic alterations induced by methotrexate in the mucosa of human proximal intestine. I: Serial observations by light microscopy. Gastroenterology 42:295, 1962.

CHAPTER 287
Chronic Diarrhea

J. Timothy Boyle

Patients with chronic diarrhea present a challenge because of the difficulty in quantifying the symptom, the variability in physical signs, the extensive differential diagnosis, and the myriad diagnostic tests available. Evaluation requires characterization of the diarrhea, establishment of an individualized differential diagnosis, appropriate use of laboratory testing, and in some cases empiric management to arrive at the correct diagnosis.

The classification of diarrhea into acute and chronic types is arbitrary, but usually diarrhea should continue for a minimum of 2 wk before it is considered chronic. This is based on the usual natural history of diarrheal symptoms in both acute bacterial and viral gastroenteritis in the well-nourished, immunocompetent host. Diarrhea is the excessive loss of stool water and electrolytes. In infants, stool volume in excess of 15 g/kg/24 hr is considered diarrhea. By age 3 yr, when stool volume approximates adult output, stool output greater than 200 g/24 hr is considered diarrhea. Because there is variation in stool number, consistency, and volume, chronic diarrhea is usually defined by the parents as a consistent increase in stool frequency, decrease in stool consistency, or increase in stool volume. Frequency and consistency may not be indicators of stool volume. In older children, it is best to collect each day's stools separately so that day-to-day variations are noted. Stool volume is extremely difficult to assess in infants because of the difficulty in separating stool from urine.

CHARACTERIZATION OF DIARRHEA. There are two categories of chronic diarrhea. Diarrhea that stops when feeding (or medication) is discontinued is *osmotic,* whereas diarrhea that persists even if the patient is fasted is *secretory* (see Chapter 252). Disorders causing chronic osmotic diarrhea are common. In contrast, secretory diarrhea is rare and primarily a disorder of infancy. The possibility of secretory diarrhea is suggested when stool frequency is in excess of five times per 24 hr, the diarrhea is characterized as watery and of large volume (saturating more than 75% of the diaper), and the diarrhea occurs throughout the day and night. If secretory diarrhea is a possibility, the patient usually requires hospitalization, complete bowel rest, and intravenous hydration to determine the effects on the stooling pattern; persistence of diarrhea beyond 24–48 hr suggests a secretory cause.

Fresh diarrheal stool has an osmolality of between 280 and 330 mOsm/L regardless of whether the diarrhea is osmotic or secretory. In osmotic diarrhea, the osmolality in diarrheal stool is mainly the unabsorbed or inabsorbable osmotic load. Active transport continues to remove electrolytes, leading to a reduction of electrolyte content of the stool. Active chloride secretion is the basic mechanism leading to secretory diarrhea. Active chloride secretion creates an osmotic gradient in favor of moving fluid passively from the plasma into the intestinal lumen. The osmolality of the diarrheal stool is isosmolar to plasma and can be accounted for by its electrolyte content. If one assumes a constant stool osmolality of 290 mOsm/L in diarrhea stool, the osmotic gap can be calculated by measurement of stool electrolyte concentration. Because sodium (Na^+) and potassium (K^+) are the major stool cations, osmolality is estimated by multiplying the sum of the stool concentrations of Na^+ and K^+ by two. The osmotic gap then equals $290 - 2(Na^+ + K^+)$. In osmotic diarrhea, the stool has a low Na^+ (<50 mEq/L) and an increased osmotic gap (>160 mOsm/L). In secretory diarrhea, the diarrheal stool has a high Na^+ (>90 mEq/L), and the osmotic gap is less than 20 mOsm/L.

287.1 Osmotic Diarrhea

The physician should strive to establish a diagnosis by history, physical examination, laboratory tests, and follow-up. A presumptive diagnosis (overeating, excessive fluid or excessive sorbitol intake, acquired lactose intolerance) is often confirmed by response to management rather than results of diagnostic tests.

Disorders causing chronic osmotic diarrhea can be classified by pathophysiologic mechanism, age of onset, or pattern of presentation.

DIFFERENTIAL DIAGNOSIS OF OSMOTIC DIARRHEA BASED ON PATHOPHYSIOLOGY. Table 287–1 lists the potential mechanisms of osmotic diarrhea and specific disease entities associated with each mechanism. Although most diarrheal disorders affect many intestinal cells, including epithelial cells, neurons, endocrine cells, muscle cells, and inflammatory cells, individual disorders can usually be categorized by one predominant mechanism.

Maldigestion refers to decreased luminal hydrolysis of carbohydrates, lipid, and protein by impaired release; impaired activation or inactivation of pancreatic enzymes; or impaired solubilization of lipids by decrease in luminal bile acids (Chapter 286). The cardinal clinical sign of maldigestion is steatorrhea.

Selective disaccharidase enzyme deficiencies result in impaired hydrolysis of carbohydrate at the enterocyte membrane in the absence of mucosal injury (Chapter 286.11). It can result from congenital absence of a particular enzyme (congenital lactase or sucrase-isomaltase deficiency), loss of activity with age (genetic lactase deficiency), or increase in enterocyte migration rate along the villus-crypt unit (postenteritis lactase deficiency). Because lactase is commonly expressed only in mature enterocytes at the tip of the villus, an increase in enterocyte migration rate (such as can occur in the recovery phase of viral gastroenteritis) may result in the villus tip being populated by less mature enterocytes, which express less lactase activity. Primary lactase and sucrase deficiency present with acid-watery diarrhea. Although there are tests to diagnose isolated lactase and sucrase deficiency, prompt resolution of the diarrhea after restriction of one or the other disaccharide is usually sufficient to make a presumptive diagnosis.

Defect in enterocyte absorption refers to rare, inherited dis-

■ **TABLE 287–1 Differential Diagnosis of Chronic Osmotic Diarrhea on the Basis of Pathophysiology**

Maldigestion	**Noninfectious Colonic Mucosal Inflammation**
Pancreatic insufficiency	Ulcerative colitis
Cystic fibrosis	Crohn disease
Shwachman-Diamond syndrome	Microscopic colitis with crypt distortion
Protein-calorie malnutrition	Lymphocytic colitis
Inactivation of pancreatic enzymes	Collagenous colitis
Zollinger-Ellison syndrome	**Obstruction of Intestinal Lymphatic Vessels**
Impaired activation of pancreatic enzymes	Primary intestinal lymphangiectasia
Enterokinase deficiency	Secondary intestinal lymphangiectasia
Insufficient luminal concentration of bile acids	Cardiovascular anomalies
Cholestatic syndromes	Mesenteric lymphatic obstruction
Bacterial overgrowth	Intestinal inflammatory disease
Resection of ileum	Thoracic duct obstruction
Crohn disease of ileum	**Disorders or Variation of Intestinal Motility**
Selective Disaccharidase Enzyme Deficiencies	Overeating
Acquired lactase deficiency (late onset)	Chronic nonspecific diarrhea (toddler diarrhea)
Postenteritis	Irritable bowel syndrome
Genetic	Dumping syndrome
Sucrase-isomaltase deficiency	Scleroderma
Congenital lactase deficiency	Pseudo-obstruction
Defect in Enterocyte Absorption	**Drug-Induced Diarrhea**
Congenital glucose-galactose malabsorption	Laxatives
Abetalipoproteinemia	Magnesium-containing antacids
Hypobetalipoproteinemia	Cytotoxic agents
Wolman disease	Antibiotics
Acrodermatitis enteropathica	**Endocrine Causes**
Menke disease	Hyperthyroidism
Excessive Sorbitol Ingestion	Zollinger-Ellison syndrome
Enteric Infection	Neuroblastoma, ganglioneuroma, VIPoma
Specific sporadic infection in immunocompetent host	Carcinoid syndrome
Bacterial: *Campylobacter, Salmonella, Yersinia, Plesiomonas, Aeromonas, Clostridium difficile*	Hypoparathyroidism
Parasitic: *Giardia, Cryptosporidium, Blastocystis hominis, Strongyloides stercoralis, Capillaria philippinensis, Entamoeba histolytica, Balantidium coli, Cyclospora* (cyanobacterium-like body)	Addison disease
Small-bowel bacterial overgrowth	Diabetes mellitus
Opportunistic infection in immunocompromised host	**Multiple Causes**
Bacterial: *Mycobacterium avium-intracellulare*	Protein-calorie malnutrition
Parasitic: *Giardia, Cryptosporidium, Isospora belli, Sarcocystis*	
Viral: cytomegalovirus	
Fungal: *Candida*	
Association with immunodeficiency disorders	
Transient hypogammaglobulinemia	
Selective immunoglobulin A deficiency	
Noninfectious Small-Bowel Mucosal Inflammation	
Cow's milk protein allergy	
Soy protein allergy	
Eosinophilic gastroenteritis	
Crohn disease	
Celiac disease	
Immunodeficiency disorders (autoimmune)	
Radiation enteritis	
Graft versus host disease	
Henoch-Schönlein purpura	
Systemic lupus erythematosus	
Tropical sprue	
Whipple disease	

VIP = vasoactive intestinal polypeptide.

orders that affect absorption across the enterocyte membrane or cellular processing of absorbed solutes (Chapter 286.12). Disorders that produce chronic diarrhea are associated with impaired or absent sodium-coupled mucosal uptake of glucose and galactose, impaired lipid processing within the enterocyte, and impaired absorption of specific trace elements.

The polyalcohol sugar *sorbitol* is poorly absorbed by the small intestine and may produce osmotic diarrhea if ingested in large amounts. It occurs naturally in fruits and fruit juices (especially apple, pear, grape) and is also commonly used as a sweetening agent in "sugar-free" and dietetic foods (gum, mints, cough drops, dietetic jams, jellies, and ice cream).

Enteric pathogens cause illness by invasion of the intestinal mucosa, enterotoxin production, cytotoxin production, and mucosal adherence with damage to the microvillus membrane (see Chapter 171). Organisms that invade epithelial cells and the lamina propria provoke a profound local inflammatory response. Enterotoxin causes secretion of electrolytes and water by stimulating cyclic adenosine monophosphate in small intestinal mucosal cells. Cytotoxin triggers inflammation from cell injury as well as elaborating inflammatory mediator substances. Mucosa adherence results in injury to the microvilli and round cell inflammation of the lamina propria. Most bacteria capable of producing chronic enteric infection do so by multiple mechanisms. See discussion of specific infectious agents in Part XVII. In addition to maldigestion described previously, small-bowel bacterial overgrowth also affects the intestinal mucosa (Chapter 286.6). Excessive intraluminal bacteria produce sufficient enzymes and metabolic products to destroy glycoprotein enzymes on the brush border and impair monosaccharide and electrolyte transport. Villus injury results in a patchy, mucosal lesion with segments of subtotal villus atrophy and a marked subepithelial inflammatory response.

The fundamental cause of noninfectious disorders that alter small intestinal mucosal morphology is immunologic. Disorders that affect mucosal morphology may cause both osmotic or secretory diarrhea depending on the degree of villus injury and the length of affected intestine. Altered small intestinal mucosal morphology results in osmotic diarrhea from loss of intestinal absorptive surface as well as functional changes in the absorptive capacity along the villus-crypt unit from increased epithelial turnover. Compensatory attempts at epithelial renewal may result in increased rates of migration up the villus-crypt unit so that immature cells populate the apical villus. Since lactase, fatty acid esterification activity, and lipid-esterifying enzymes are a function of enterocyte maturity, enhanced cell migration may reduce absorptive function independent of absorptive surface area.

Congenital and acquired obstruction of intestinal lymphatic vessels can lead to impaired lymphatic flow from the intestine. The cardinal features of these disorders are hypoalbuminemia, hypogammaglobulinemia, hypolipidemia, and lymphopenia secondary to exudation of protein and lymphocytes into the intestinal lumen. Diarrhea may or may not be an important clinical feature. Primary intestinal lymphangiectasia is rare and may be associated with lymphatic abnormalities elsewhere in the body. Secondary lymphangiectasia may be associated with cardiovascular disease (congestive heart failure, constrictive pericarditis, Budd-Chiari syndrome, Fontan procedure, superior vena cava obstruction), mesenteric lymphatic obstruction (lymphoma, tuberculosis, sarcoidosis, malrotation, radiation therapy), chronic intestinal inflammatory disease, and thoracic duct obstruction (mediastinal tumor).

Disorders or variation of intestinal motility may result in increased transit of food through the intestine overcoming the normal capacity to digest and absorb luminal solutes or slow intestinal transit leading to stasis and bacterial overgrowth. Increased intestinal motor activity may result from abnormal slow-wave pacemaker activity (irritable bowel syndrome), abnormal patterns of spike potential activity (hyperthyroidism, scleroderma, pseudo-obstruction), and excessive bowel distention. The latter may be caused by rapid gastric emptying, overeating, ingestion of large volumes of hypertonic juices, ingestion of commercially prepared nutritional supplements with a high osmolality (>500 mOsm), partial intestinal obstruction, or impaired colonic accommodation. Bowel distention is caused by osmotically active particles holding or pulling water into the intestinal lumen. Disorders that impair transit include small intestinal myopathies or neuropathies that result in diminished intestinal spike-potential excitation or abnormal patterns of spike-potential activity (Chapter 278.1).

Pharmacologic agents may induce diarrhea by multiple mechanisms including (1) presentation of an excessive intraluminal osmotic load (osmotic laxatives such as lactulose, magnesium salts, antacids containing magnesium), (2) a direct toxic effect causing morphologic changes in the mucosa of the small intestine (cytotoxic agents, neomycin), and (3) alteration of intestinal motility (senna, castor oil, quinidine). Drug-induced diarrhea is generally dose related rather than an idiosyncratic reaction. All classes of antibiotics may be associated with diarrhea.

The function of the gastrointestinal tract is influenced in many ways by hormones and by diseases of the endocrine glands. Diarrhea is a common symptom, but its precise mechanism is often unknown. Diseases characterized by excessive secretion of hormones include thyrotoxicosis, Zollinger-Ellison (ZE) syndrome, neuroblastoma, ganglioneuroma, and malignant carcinoid syndrome. Diseases characterized by decreased secretion of hormones include hypoparathyroidism, Addison disease, and rarely diabetes mellitus. Diarrhea associated with hyperthyroidism is primarily caused by hypermotility, which, combined with excessive dietary intake, may also result in steatorrhea. Hypoparathryoidsm and ZE syndrome may also result in steatorrhea.

DIFFERENTIAL DIAGNOSIS OF OSMOTIC DIARRHEA ON THE BASIS OF AGE OF ONSET. Patient age is an especially important factor in the evaluation of chronic osmotic diarrhea (Table 287–2). Although some conditions may become clinically apparent during infancy, their recognition is often delayed beyond 2 yr of age because of mild symptoms. Examples include chronic,

■ TABLE 287–2 Differential Diagnosis of Chronic Osmotic Diarrhea on the Basis of Age of Onset

Infancy	After Infancy	Any Age
Overfeeding	Acquired genetic lactase deficiency	Enteric infection
Milk protein sensitivity	Inflammatory bowel disease	Parasitic
Chronic nonspecific diarrhea	Ulcerative colitis	*Clostridium difficile*
Extraintestinal infection	Crohn disease	*Salmonella, Yersinia*
Otitis media	Irritable bowel syndrome	Bacterial overgrowth
Urinary tract infection	Henoch-Schönlein purpura	Protein-calorie malnutrition
Cystic fibrosis	Collagenous colitis	Excessive sorbitol
Neonatal cholestasis	Scleroderma	Celiac disease
Shwachman-Diamond syndrome	Tropical sprue	Eosinophilic gastroenteritis
Primary lymphangiectasia	Lymphoma	Secondary lymphangiectasia
Sucrase-isomaltase deficiency	Pseudo-obstruction	Lymphocytic colitis
Glucose-galactose malabsorption		Drug-induced enteropathy
Congenital lactase deficiency		Primary immune deficiency
Enterokinase deficiency		Dumping syndrome
Acrodermatitis enteropathica		Hyperthyroidism
Abetalipoproteinemia		Graft versus host disease
Hypobetalipoproteinemia		
Wolman disease		
Menke disease		
Congenital adrenal hyperplasia		

nonspecific diarrhea, cystic fibrosis, and enterokinase deficiency.

DIFFERENTIAL DIAGNOSIS OF OSMOTIC DIARRHEA ON THE BASIS OF THE PATTERN OF PRESENTATION. The pattern of clinical presentation also helps to establish a diagnosis and guide specific diagnostic evaluation and management (Table 287–3).

Chronic Diarrhea After an Acute Enteric Infection. A diagnosis of postinfectious lactose intolerance is reasonable in a previously well infant who experiences persistent diarrhea on resuming a regular lactose-containing diet. The degree of diarrhea does not always correlate with the degree of disaccharidase deficiency. Carbohydrate intolerance is suggested by evidence of an acid pH on touching nitrazine paper directly to the moist, gloved finger after rectal examination. The use of absorbent diapers renders examination of stool water difficult. Clinitest is used to document reducing substances in the stool. The clinical response to the removal of lactose from the diet is an acceptable alternative to stool examination or specific diagnostic tests. Lactose restriction should result in quick resolution of diarrhea within 2–3 days if lactase deficiency is present. One must distinguish lactose intolerance from protein sensitivity; acute gastroenteritis does not trigger milk sensitivity. It is reasonable to switch from cow's milk to soy protein formula if lactose intolerance is suspected because soy formulas contain short-chain starches or sucrose as their source of sugar. Parents must be counseled against the use of dilute formula and excessive supplementation with clear fluids or electrolyte solutions to avoid hyponatremia and postinfectious caloric deprivation, which may prolong diarrhea. Persistent diarrhea despite dietary restriction of lactose suggests a diagnosis other than lactase deficiency. The onset of chronic, nonspecific diarrhea may also be proceeded by an acute diarrheal illness, especially between 3 mo and 1 yr of age.

■ **TABLE 287–3 Patterns of Presentation of Chronic Osmotic Diarrhea**

Chronic Diarrhea After Acute Enteric Infection
Postenteritis lactase deficiency
Starvation stools
Chronic infection: parasitic, *Clostridium difficile, Salmonella, Yersinia*
Chronic, nonspecific diarrhea
Relationship of Diet to Diarrhea
Overeating: chronic, nonspecific diarrhea (toddler diarrhea)
Excessive fluid intake: chronic, nonspecific diarrhea (toddler diarrhea)
Excesive sorbitol intake
Formula or milk intolerance: cow's milk or soy protein sensitivity, congenital or acquired carbohydrate intolerance
Introduction of cereal: celiac disease
Cane sugar intolerance: sucrase-isomaltase deficiency
Risk Factors for Chronic Enteric Infection
Day care
Recent antibiotic therapy
Travel, camping
Protein-calorie malnutrition
Immunodeficiency syndrome
Symptoms of Functional Diarrhea
Normal weight gain and linear growth
Intermittent symptoms
Alternating diarrhea with normal bowel movements or constipation
Feeling of incomplete evacuation
Associated psychosocial stress factors
Family history
History of infantile colic
Symptoms of Maldigestion or Malabsorption
Weight loss
Weight for height ratio less than 5th percentile
Deceleration of weight gain velocity preceding deceleration of linear growth velocity
Associated extraintestinal signs and symptoms
Pulmonary
Hepatobiliary
Recurrent infections
Prior abdominal surgery
Symptoms of Inflammatory Bowel Disease
Evidence of gastrointestinal bleeding
Abdominal pain
Nighttime diarrhea
Tenesmus
Extraintestinal signs and symptoms: fever, arthritis, unexplained rash, oral aphthous ulceration, weight loss

Relationship of Chronic Diarrhea to Diet. Empiric management is often indicated if there is a relationship between diet and the cause of chronic diarrhea. Appropriate dietary change should lead to rapid resolution of the diarrhea. The major cause of chronic diarrhea in early infancy is cow's milk or soy protein sensitivity (Chapter 284). The majority of cases begin within the 1st 3 mo of life and are characterized by gradual onset of watery or blood-tinged mucoid diarrhea. Vomiting, anorexia, and irritability are common associated symptoms.

The usual clinical manifestations of dietary carbohydrate intolerance are watery diarrhea, bloating, flatulence, and crampy abdominal pain (Chapter 286.11). Carbohydrate intolerance is usually secondary to disaccharidase deficiency. Monosaccharide intolerance is rare. Glucose-galactose malabsorption presents as severe osmotic diarrhea in the first week of life, responding only to a modular formula containing fructose. Acquired monosaccharide intolerance in a patient who previously tolerated formulas containing lactose, sucrose, or short-chain starch indicates severe intestinal mucosal injury. Because most commercial formulas do not contain sucrose, diarrhea in patients with sucrase-isomaltase deficiency usually does not begin until introduction of fruits or solid foods into the diet. Rigid exclusion of sucrose from the diet constitutes a valid therapeutic test because diarrheal symptoms resolve within a few days.

Inherited delayed-onset lactase deficiency is a major cause of intolerance of milk products in children older than 4 yr (Chapter 286.11). Another cause of carbohydrate-induced diarrhea, which affects normal individuals without malabsorption, results from excessive ingestion of complex nondigestable carbohydrates that are incompletely absorbed. These substances are particularly found in beans, cabbage, processed bran, and wheat, oat, and rice flour. Diagnosis of carbohydrate intolerance can be confirmed by breath hydrogen testing (Chapter 286.11).

Symptoms of Functional Diarrhea. In infancy, functional diarrhea is termed *chronic, nonspecific diarrhea*; for cases occurring later in childhood, the terms *toddler's diarrhea* and *irritable bowel syndrome* have been used. No anatomic, infectious, inflammatory, or biochemical cause of the clinical syndrome has been described. Diarrhea most commonly begins insidiously with no identifiable precipitating event. Children classically oscillate between normal and watery stools and even between diarrhea and constipation. The condition is associated with other functional motility disorders of early childhood including gastroesophageal reflux and functional constipation and with a history of overeating or excessive fluid intake (>120 mL/kg/24 hr). Stools are rarely expelled during sleep, although it is common for patients to have a watery stool immediately on waking. Parents often describe formed food particles and mucus in the stool. The rates of weight gain and linear growth are normal. Complications of chronic, nonspecific diarrhea are often iatrogenic, resulting from dietary restriction or excessive intake of high-carbohydrate, clear liquids. Excessive manipulation of diet has the potential to result in a secondary or a conditioned feeding disorder.

Irritable bowel syndrome occurs most commonly in adolescents and mimics the disorder seen in adults. An altered bowel pattern is associated with abdominal pain, which is usually relieved by defecation. Loose stools usually follow straining or a sense of urgency and commonly contain mucus. A feeling of incomplete evacuation is characteristic. A positive family history of functional bowel disease is common. Evaluation does not reveal an alternative diagnosis.

Signs and Symptoms Suggesting Maldigestion or Significant Small-Bowel Mucosal Injury. See Chapters 39 and 286 and Table 287–3. The evaluation of malabsorption should proceed with the patient on as normal a diet as possible to avoid masking specific abnormalities. A screening evaluation for the patient with suspected maldigestion or malabsorption without abdominal pain includes a complete blood count, biochemical profile, sweat test, serum for quantitative immunoglobulins, serum for antigliadin antibody, and qualitative stool examination for white cells, neutral and split fat, and guaiac. In addition, enteric infection must be considered. Qualitative evidence of fecal fat by stool examination justifies pancreatic function testing if sweat test and small-bowel morphology are normal (see Chapter 294).

Signs and Symptoms Suggesting Colonic Inflammation. In the absence of enteric infection, any patient with chronic diarrhea associated with abdominal pain should undergo colonoscopy and barium contrast upper gastrointestinal tract series with small-bowel follow-through to rule out Crohn disease and ulcerative colitis (see Chapter 283). Mucosal biopsies should be obtained even in the absence of gross colonoscopic abnormality.

287.2 Secretory Diarrhea

Diagnosis and management of secretory diarrhea are best understood by classifying the various causes by pathophysiologic mechanism (Table 287–4). Primary enteric infection or acquired protein intolerance does not cause chronic secretory diarrhea, although both may act as the stimulus that unmasks a genetic disorder of immune regulation or epithelial cell renewal. There are a few congenital transport defects associated with secretory diarrhea; all have their onset at or soon after birth (see Chapter 286.12). Chronic secretory diarrhea also may occur in patients having enterocolitis complicating Hirschsprung disease or in patients with partial bowel obstruction from stenosis of the small intestine. The exact mechanisms for the protracted diarrhea are unknown. Distended bowel, bacterial stasis, inflammation, and motility abnormalities are contributing factors.

Secretory diarrhea (associated with hypokalemia, flushing spells, and occasionally achlorhydria) may be the predominant clinical manifestation of neural crest tumors in children, including ganglioneuroma, VIPoma, ganglioneuroblastoma, and neuroblastoma (see Chapter 291). Because of elevated plasma levels of vasoactive intestinal polypeptide (VIP) in most reported patients, this polypeptide has been incriminated as the

■ **TABLE 287–4 Differential Diagnosis of Chronic Secretory Diarrhea on the Basis of Pathophysiology**

Congenital Transport Defects
Congenital chloride diarrhea
Congenital sodium diarrhea
Primary bile acid malabsorption
Intestinal Obstruction
Congenital or acquired partial small-bowel obstruction
Hirschsprung disease
Neural Crest Tumors
Enteric Infection
Immunoadherent *Escherichia coli*
Bacterial overgrowth
Idiopathic Villus Atrophy
Congenital microvillus atrophy
Autoimmune enteropathy
Associated with T-cell immunodeficiency
Severe combined immunodeficiency
Common variable immunodeficiency
Acquired immunodeficiency syndrome

secretogogue mediating the diarrhea. Although levels of urinary catecholamines are elevated in most patients, there is no correlation between their level and the development of protracted diarrhea. Gastrinoma, somatostatinoma, glucagonoma, multiple endocrine neoplasias, and carcinoid syndrome, which produce secretory diarrhea in adults, have not been reported to date in children.

Enterotoxin-producing bacteria and viral gastroenteritis are rarely primary causes of secretory diarrhea without antecedent mucosal injury from malnutrition, cow's milk or soy protein allergy, bacterial overgrowth, or primary or secondary immunodeficiency states. Opportunistic pathogens such as cryptosporidium, microsporida, cytomegalovirus, *Isospora belli, Mycobacterium avium-intracellulare* and coccidiosis may evoke a secretory process. Secretory diarrhea has been associated with sporadic colonization of the small bowel by enteropathogenic strains of *Escherichia coli* that are neither enterotoxigenic nor enterovasive but that attach and adhere to the enterocyte brush border (see Chapter 184).

Most causes of chronic secretory diarrhea in the pediatric population are idiopathic and produce both osmotic and secretory diarrhea because of severe mucosal injury. Functional differentiation of the villus-crypt unit explains why secretory diarrhea can develop in cases of severe villus injury (see Chapter 274). Villus cells are primarily absorptive and crypt cells are primarily secretory. Net absorption of solute and water depends on the efficient transport properties of the brush border and basolateral membranes of the enterocytes on the villi and on the ionic permeability of the paracellular pathway (tight junction between epithelial cells and the intracellular space) of the villus to absorb water and chloride actively secreted in the basal state in the crypts. Disorders that destroy enterocytes from the villi can thus result in "leaky membranes" and net secretion. Crypt cell hyperplasia, in an attempt to renew the epithelium in response to injury, may compound the problem by increasing the capacity for active chloride secretion.

Mucosal injury severe enough to cause secretory diarrhea may be caused by genetic defects in epithelial turnover and differentiation or by disorders of immune regulation. In *congenital microvillus atrophy,* there is no evidence of mitotic activity in the crypts. Although the enterocytes retain their columnar shape, electron microscopy reveals shortened and irregular microvilli. The apical cytoplasm of the enterocytes contains electron-dense lysosomal inclusions suggestive of invaginated brush border, raising speculation regarding cell maturation and differentiation. Only immune disorders that include T-cell abnormalities (with or without B-cell abnormality) can result in a degree of mucosal injury severe enough to cause secretory diarrhea. Secretory diarrhea has been described in patients with severe combined immunodeficiency, common variable immunodeficiency, acquired immunodeficiency syndrome, Crohn disease, and autoimmune enteropathy. In autoimmune enteropathy, tests of T- and B-lymphocyte function are characteristically normal. The immunologic marker of this disorder is circulating antienterocyte antibodies. Autoimmune enteropathy resembles Crohn disease in that both small and large bowels are involved; there are similar features of immune activation, and both may respond to immunosuppressive therapy.

DIAGNOSIS. Secretory diarrhea associated with congenital transport defects begins at birth or in the first few days of life, but when it persists, it is referred to as protracted diarrhea (intractable diarrhea of infancy). However, protracted diarrhea also may begin as osmotic diarrhea and evolve to secretory diarrhea. More commonly, this diarrhea begins in the first few weeks of life and is often associated with anorexia and vomiting. Formula change may initially result in transient improvement, but diarrhea recurs. Infants with persistent diarrhea, poor weight gain, or frank weight loss while on a casein hydrolysate formula should be hospitalized. Recurrent use of oral hydration fluids or persistent attempts to find a formula that an infant will tolerate will delay a diagnosis and is a major contributor to malnutrition.

Evaluation of protracted diarrhea requires consideration of infection, anatomic or functional intestinal obstruction, secretory tumor, immune deficiency, and disorder of epithelial turnover and differentiation. Although rarely the primary cause of protracted diarrhea, routine infectious workup is indicated. All patients also should be evaluated for antibodies to human immunodeficiency virus (HIV). Partial intestinal obstruction should be ruled out by a upper gastrointestinal tract series with follow-through examination of the small bowel. Serum VIP levels and urinary vanillylmandelic acid assay are sufficient to screen for possible secretory tumor. Elevated levels should generate a search for a tumor by ultrasonography, computed tomographic scan, and possibly magnetic resonance imaging. Selected laboratory tests should be performed early to evaluate immune function. Delaying increases the risk that secondary factors such as malnutrition, infection, and transfusions will interfere with the interpretation of the results.

Small-bowel and colonic-rectal biopsies are essential to the diagnosis of protracted diarrhea. The biopsy should be performed early in the diagnostic evaluation before the inevitable confounding variables of chronic malnutrition, bacterial overgrowth, or secondary infection ensue. Normal biopsies or mild, nonspecific inflammatory changes that do not significantly alter villus-crypt architecture support aggressive evaluation and management of cellular transport defects, secretory tumors, obstruction, or factitious diarrhea. Duodenal fluid should always be obtained at the time of small-bowel biopsy for aerobic and anaerobic culture. Electron micsoscopy should be performed on all small-bowel biopsies when searching for adherent bacteria, microvillus atrophy, and microvillus inclusions.

FACTITIOUS DIARRHEA. A search for self-induced or factitious diarrhea is appropriate when a reasonable evaluation for chronic diarrhea is nonproductive. Any stools that turn pink on alkalinization or any pink stools that turn colorless with acidification should strongly suggest phenolphthalein (Ex-Lax) ingestion. The presence of other laxative use or abuse can be detected by measuring stool electrolytes, magnesium, sulfate, and chromatographic analysis of anthracene derivatives. Mild superficial colitis has also been described in chronic laxative abuse. A low stool osmolality (less than 280 mOsm/L) implies that water has been added to the stool.

287.3 General Therapeutic Considerations

Only selected management principles are outlined here because treatment principles of specific diseases are discussed elsewhere (Chapters 171 and 286).

Management of chronic diarrhea should be performed in conjunction with providing adequate nutritional support for catch-up or maintenance of normal growth. Protein-calorie malnutrition must be vigorously avoided if possible because it can become a confounding variable slowing or preventing return to normal gut function. Therefore, parents need to be given specific instruction regarding duration of elimination diets. Many parents are so strict in enforcing elimination diets that caloric deprivation ensues. In addition, secondary feeding aversion behavior may become the predominant problem overshadowing the chronic diarrhea.

When fluids are prescribed in the management of diarrhea, attention should be given to the volume of intake as well as to the composition. In infants younger than 2 yr, absorptive capacity can be exceeded by intakes exceeding 200 mL/kg/24 hr. Parents also need to understand that milk protein sensitivity, an inflammatory reaction triggered by the protein in milk, requires strict dietary restriction. In contrast, intolerance to lactose, the sugar in milk, is not an all-or-none phenomenon. There is wide individual variation in symptoms of carbohydrate intolerance independent of enzyme deficiency. Although specific treatment of lactose intolerance is best begun with a strict lactose-free diet, resolution of diarrhea allows for a clearly defined baseline on which to assess an individual's degree of lactose intolerance. In postenteritis lactose intolerance in infancy, standard milk-based formulas should be withheld for a period of 4–6 wk; a commercial lactose-free, milk-based formula or any soy-based formula is substituted. Long-term therapy of lactose intolerance should include the reintroduction of lactose-containing foods, but some lactose-containing foods are better tolerated than others. Unpasturized yogurt, which contains as much or more lactose as whole milk, also contains a microbial β-galactosidase that assists in intraluminal digestion of the sugar. Aged cheeses such as cheddar, swiss, blue, and brie are better tolerated than processed cheeses. High fat–containing foods, which slow gastric emptying and thus delivery of lactose to the small intestine, may be tolerated by some lactose-intolerant patients. Thus, ice cream and whole milk are better tolerated than skim milk. Alternatives for patients who do not tolerate milk include prehydrolyzed milk treated with microbial-derived lactase enzyme or ingestion of this enzyme in tablet form with milk products at mealtime.

Control of chronic, nonspecific diarrhea is best achieved by ingestion of a regular diet and reducing total nonprotein fluid intake to 90 mL/kg/24hr. It may be helpful to give oral loperamide (0.1–0.2 mg/kg/24hr) in two or three divided doses on an as needed basis to patients with chronic nonspecific diarrhea during periods when diarrhea may affect function (e.g., travel). Parents should be specifically told that chronic, nonspecific diarrhea does not affect toilet training.

Appropriate therapy of patients with suspected small-intestine bacterial overgrowth should include consideration of surgical, medical, and nutritional support modalities. Surgery is the appropriate therapeutic choice if there is a surgically correctable cause. Antibiotic therapy is usually initiated with a broad-spectrum antibiotic (e.g., metronidazole, tetracycline, chloramphenicol, ampicillin, and erythromycin in combination with neomycin). Courses of 2 weeks are usually recommended. Improvement in diarrhea should be observed within 1 week provided that dietary restriction of fat and lactose are part of the initial management scheme. Recurrent treatment failure requires intestinal intubation and culture to determine formally microbial sensitivity. Fasting breath hydrogen, glucose breath hydrogen test, or D-xylose test may be used to monitor response to treatment.

The basic principle of the treatment of secretory diarrhea is to maintain nutritional balance. Intravenous nutrition and complete bowel rest should be instituted while diagnostic evaluation proceeds. It is critical to avoid iatrogenic prolongation of malnutrition by blind dietary trials. Refeeding of patients with idiopathic villus atrophy should be postponed until the patient's expected height for weight has returned to the 50th percentile. Refeeding by mouth at that point is essential because of the proven beneficial effects of enteral nutrients on mucosal growth. Pharmacology of idiopathic villus atrophy is generally empiric; the most commonly used agents to decrease fluid transit through the gut are opiates and opiate derivatives. Loperamide is the agent of choice because it has the highest antidiarrheal specificity. Cholestyramine, a strongly basic anion exchange resin that binds bile acids, may protect against direct bile acid–induced injury of the upper small-bowel mucosa and bile acid–induced secretion in the colon. Somatostatin significantly reduces secretory diarrhea caused by neuroendocrine tumors and villus atrophy. Prostaglandin synthetase inhibitors including indomethacin, bismuth subsalicylate, and 5-aminosalicylate have been reported to decrease diarrhea in inflammatory disorders. Anecdotal reports of partial resolution of secretory diarrhea have followed treatment of autoimmune enteropathy with immunosuppressive agents including corticosteroids, azathioprine, and cyclosporine.

Afzalpurkar RG, Schiller LR, Little KH, et al: The self-limited nature of chronic idiopathic diarrhea. N Engl J Med 327:1849, 1992.
Ament ME: Management of chronic diarrhea with parenteral nutrition and enteral infusion techniques. Pediatrics 14:53, 1985.
Anonymous: Chronic diarrhea in children: A nutritional disease. Lancet 1:143, 1987.
Bezerra JA, Duncan B, Udall J: Dietary management of acute diarrhea: Fast or feed. Int Pediatr 5:30, 1990.
Bisset WM, Stapleford P, Long S, et al: Home parenteral nutrition in chronic intestinal failure. Arch Dis Child 67:109, 1992.
Black RE: Persistent diarrhea in children of developing countries. Pediatr Infect Dis J 12:751, 1993.
Cormier-Daire V, Bonnefont J-P, Rustin P, et al: Mitochondrial DNA rearrangements with onset as chronic diarrhea with villous atrophy. J Pediatr 124:63, 1994.
Coulthard M, Searle J, Patrick M, et al: Cyclosporine-responsive enteropathy and protracted diarrhea. J Pediatr Gastroenterol Nutr 10:257, 1990.
Girault D, Goulet O, Le Deist F, et al: Intractable infant diarrhea associated with phenotypic abnormalities and immunodeficiency. J Pediatr 125:36, 1994.
Hill ID, Mann MD, Med M, et al: Use of oral gentamicin, metronidazole, and cholestyramine in the treatment of severe persistent diarrhea in infants. Pediatrics 77:477, 1986.
Househam KC, Bowie DC, Mann MD, et al: Factors influencing the duration of acute diarrheal disease in infancy. J Pediatr Gastroenterol Nutr 10:37, 1990.
Johnston KR, Govel LA, Andritz MH, et al: Gastrointestinal effects of sorbitol as an additive in liquid medications. Am J Med 97:185, 1994.
Lynn RB, Friedman LS: Irritable bowel syndrome. N Engl J Med 329:1940, 1993.
Nathavitharana KA, Green NJ, Raafat F, et al: Siblings with microvillous inclusion disease. Arch Dis Child 71:71, 1994.
Orenstein SR: Enteral versus parenteral therapy for intractable diarrhea of infancy: A prospective, randomized trial. J Pediatr 109:277, 1986.
Phillips AD, Schmitz J: Familial microvillous atrophy: A clinicopathological survey of 23 cases. J Pediatr Gastroenterol Nutr 14:380, 1992.
Roy SK, Haider R, Akbar MS, et al: Persistent diarrhoea: Clinical efficacy and nutrient absorption with a rice based diet. Arch Dis Child 65:294, 1990.
Sanderson IR, Risdon RA, Walker-Smith JA: Intractable ulcerating enterocolitis of infancy. Arch Dis Child 65:295, 1990.
Soave R, Johnson W: Cyclospora: Conquest of an emerging pathogen. Lancet 345:667, 1995.
Thomas AG, Phillips AD, Walker-Smith JA: The value of proximal small intestinal biopsy in the differential diagnosis of chronic diarrhoea. Arch Dis Child 67:741, 1992.
Thompson WG: Irritable bowel syndrome: Pathogenesis and management. Lancet 341:1569, 1993.
Topazian M, Binder HJ: Brief report: Factitious diarrhea detected by measurement of stool osmolality. N Engl J Med 330:1418, 1994.
Treem WR: Chronic nonspecific diarrhea of childhood. Clin Pediatr 31:413, 1992.

Chapter 288

Recurrent Abdominal Pain of Childhood

Martin Ulshen

Recurrent abdominal pain is common in childhood, occurring in at least 10% of preschool- and school-age children. In children younger than 2 yr, the symptom is often associated with an organic cause; however, in older children, only about 10% of cases have an organic cause. Recurrent abdominal pain without an organic cause is often called "functional" abdominal pain. The difficulty for physician, parent, and child is that functional abdominal pain is as uncomfortable and as disruptive to normal activity as organic pain but is often more difficult for the physician to evaluate and manage. The family and the child with functional recurrent abdominal pain may worry about the inability to identify an organic cause. There is a tendency to associate the lack of an obvious organic cause with a more serious prognosis. The physician may become frustrated by the difficulty in identifying an obvious cause of the symptoms and by the pressure from the family to "get to the bottom of the problem." As a result, there is a tendency to perform an excessive evaluation for organic causes when a careful history, social evaluation, and physical examination might suffice. Although it is important to demonstrate to the patient and family that the medical caregivers are considering the symptoms seriously, excessive testing and treatment increase the fear that some life-threatening underlying process must be present. The pattern of the pain and the social setting are often typical when abdominal symptoms are functional, and extensive investigation is not required.

ETIOLOGY. Most often recurrent abdominal pain in childhood is not associated with a specific structural or biochemical (i.e., organic) cause. However, "organic" causes must always be considered in the differential diagnosis because they are amenable to more specific treatments (see Table 252–7). Most children with recurrent abdominal pain syndrome experience pain; a child may occasionally use the symptom as a way to avoid certain activities without actually experiencing pain.

Perception of recurrent abdominal pain is the summation of sensory, emotional, and cognitive input. The dorsal horn of the spinal cord regulates conduction of impulses from peripheral nociceptive receptors to the spinal cord and brain, and the pain experience is further influenced by cognitive and emotional centers. Chronic peripheral pain can produce increased neural activity in higher CNS centers leading to perpetuation of pain. Psychosocial stress can affect pain intensity and quality through these mechanisms. Differences in visceral sensation may lead to differences in perception of pain as well. The child's response to pain can be influenced by stress, personality type, and reinforcement of illness behavior within the family. The same level of discomfort may keep one child home from school, especially if encouraged by caretakers, whereas another child might continue routine activities. There is no evidence of a consistent pattern of psychopathology among children with idiopathic recurrent abdominal pain.

CLINICAL MANIFESTATIONS AND DIAGNOSIS. Typically, the symptoms of nonorganic functional recurrent abdominal pain are nonspecific in character. It is this lack of suggestion of an organic process that is helpful in making a diagnosis of functional abdominal pain. The symptoms do not have any characteristic temporal pattern. Improvement in symptoms during weekends and school vacations suggests functional pain, but the absence of this pattern does not rule out this diagnosis. Two variants of functional abdominal pain are seen more often in adults but may occur in children. *Irritable bowel syndrome* is characterized by abdominal pain associated with intermittent diarrhea and constipation without an organic basis (see Chapter 287). Individuals who have symptoms suggestive of peptic disease and seem to respond to antacid treatment but who have no abnormal findings on upper gastrointestinal tract endoscopy are said to have *nonulcer dyspepsia.* Both constellations of symptoms are seen occasionally in children, especially teenagers.

Identification of a relationship between the pain and either meals or bowel movements may be helpful, especially in considering peptic disease, constipation, and irritable bowel syndrome. Although the occurrence of nocturnal pain has been considered by some an important indicator of organic cause, children with functional pain may awaken during the night with symptoms. Functional abdominal pain tends to be periumbilical in location and is often difficult for the child to characterize. The child can be distracted from the pain. The child may have good periods with remission of symptoms and then recurrence without any apparent reason. In contrast, in many children an association with stressful periods may be obvious.

The child appears well between episodes with a normal physical examination and a history of good growth. The child may appear pale during an episode, but this symptom does not suggest that the cause is more likely to be organic. Frequently, although not always, these children may have certain characteristic psychologic features. They may be described as worriers who tend not to share their concerns with others. Often at school these are children who either are very serious about their work and do very well or, in contrast, have difficulty. Teachers describe these children as their easiest students because they are compliant and are not complainers.

The family may reinforce the symptom by demonstrating excessive concern. This family characteristic may both worry the children and urge physicians to perform more evaluations than might otherwise be considered. The latter approach may further add to the children's and parents' worries. The children's and family's concerns about the possibility of specific organic disorders should always be explored in a nondirect fashion. Often another family member or friend's illness has raised specific concerns.

Children with nonorganic abdominal pain often come from dysfunctional families. In some families, focus on a child's abdominal symptoms may be an unrecognized way of diverting attention from other family stresses, such as marital problems. Sexual abuse as a child is a major cause of recurrent abdominal pain in adults. This possibility should always be considered and not overlooked, especially in a girl whose abdominal symptoms begin in the preteenage or teenage years. Despite these concerns about psychosocial factors, some children with functional abdominal pain appear to be well adjusted and from well-adapted families.

An initial nondirect interview technique often helps to gain a general sense of the likelihood of organicity. The interviewer should elicit a detailed description of the symptom, including character, temporal pattern, severity on a scale ranging from 1–10, associated symptoms, potential initiating events, limitation of activities, and measures that relieve the pain. Functional abdominal pain is typically not associated with other symptoms, although vomiting or headache is sometimes present as a less striking component. The interviewer should be attuned to possible organic causes and should question more specifically about any of these causes if suggested by the initial history.

The onset of recurrent functional abdominal pain may occur at the time of an acute, transient illness, such as gastroenteritis. In this case, the symptoms of the acute illness may serve as a model for ongoing functional symptoms. Family medical history may uncover the possibility of a familial disorder causing abdominal pain but more frequently may uncover models of recurrent abdominal symptoms among close family members. It is common that the relationship of the child's symptoms to those of other family members has not occurred to the parents until identified by the physician. This process also helps the physician to learn how a family copes with medical illness and about their expectations from the physician. Social history is essential because of the association with family stress and dysfunctional families. Although not always necessary, an assessment by a social worker can be a valuable asset. It may be helpful to have an evaluation by a psychologist or psychiatrist as well.

During the physical examination, one must keep in mind possible diagnoses raised by the history. A complete examination (including growth parameters) is important because recurrent abdominal pain may be a manifestation of many different systemic disorders. Weight loss is not consistent with functional pain. Careful assessment of the abdomen for distention, tenderness, organomegaly, or a mass is necessary. A rectal examination should be a routine part of the evaluation for recurrent abdominal pain. Children are unreliable about reporting stool patterns to their parents; the physician may identify a mass of hard stool in the rectum leading to a diagnosis of constipation. Furthermore, a pelvic or abdominal mass may be noted during this examination. Characteristic perianal findings of Crohn disease may be identified at the time of rectal examination. A stool test for occult blood should be done at the time of the rectal examination; otherwise, stool should be collected at home for this evaluation.

Laboratory studies may be unnecessary if the history and physical examination clearly lead to a diagnosis of functional abdominal pain. However, a complete blood count, sedimentation rate, stool test for parasites (including *Giardia*), and urinalysis are reasonable screening studies. If one suspects inflammatory bowel disease, it is important to keep in mind that as many as 50% of children with these disorders may have normal sedimentation rates. The finding of an abnormal sedimentation rate would make one look further for an inflammatory, infectious, or neoplastic disorder. If it appears indicated, an ultrasound examination of the abdomen can give information about kidneys, gallbladder, and pancreas; with lower abdominal pain, a pelvic ultrasonogram may be indicated. An upper gastrointestinal tract x-ray series is indicated if one suspects a disorder of the stomach or small intestine. If peptic disease is suspected, esophagogastroduodenoscopy is the most direct way to establish a diagnosis. However, in the absence of this suspicion, this evaluation is unlikely to identify an abnormality and is usually not necessary.

A wide range of potential organic causes of recurrent abdominal pain (see Table 252–7) must be considered before establishing a diagnosis of functional pain. Among the more common causes are chronic constipation, parasitic infection (*Giardia*), and lactase deficiency. Lactose intolerance is so common that the finding may be coincidental; therefore, one must be cautious in attributing chronic abdominal pain to this condition. Pinworms are not considered to cause abdominal pain. Genitourinary disorders were once found to be common, but this is probably no longer true. Nevertheless, hydronephrosis can occasionally be the cause of unilateral pain without other symptoms.

Crohn disease typically does not present with pain alone. Nevertheless, if the location and characteristics are suggestive, this diagnosis should be considered. When recurrent pancreatitis is the cause, it is often not diagnosed during the first episodes of pain. Serum amylase and lipase should be measured during an episode to rule out pancreatitis. If these are normal but pancreatitis is still suspected, a serum trypsinogen level is more sensitive. An ultrasonogram of the pancreas may show changes suggestive of pancreatitis but may be normal. Peptic ulcer is an unusual cause of chronic abdominal pain and is diagnosed more frequently than it actually occurs; an upper gastrointestinal tract endoscopy should be considered to establish the diagnosis. With any of these disorders, one should expect persistent pain, perhaps accentuated by meals, but not intermittent pain lasting 30 min or less.

Abdominal migraine is a disorder that can cause episodic abdominal pain in children even in the absence of headache. The episodes are very characteristic and almost always include nausea with or without vomiting. Transient fever or diarrhea is less common but can occur with migraine. The episode can last hours but characteristically ends when the child falls asleep and awakens feeling much improved. Episodes may occur several times a week or much less frequently but should not be daily. There is a strong family history of typical migraine headache. There are no specific tests for this disorder; the diagnosis depends on a typical patient and family history. *Abdominal epilepsy* is less common but also can be an unusual cause of recurrent abdominal pain. There may be a repetitious prodrome (the sense of an unusual aroma at the start of an episode). Abnormalities on electroencephalogram (EEG) may be identified but may not be seen on a single study; a sleep-deprived EEG may be required.

An association of chronic *Helicobacter pylori* infection with nonspecific, recurrent abdominal pain in children has been reported. This is of importance not only because of the ability to treat this disorder but because, if there is a causal relationship, a reassessment of the indications for upper gastrointestinal tract endoscopy for recurrent abdominal pain would be required. Nevertheless, it has not yet been shown that this group of children respond to specific treatment of *H. pylori* or that the occurrence of this infection in these children is higher than in a geographically and age-matched control group. The relationship of *H. pylori* with chronic duodenal ulcer is much better established (see Chapter 282).

TREATMENT. If functional bowel disease is diagnosed, the most important component of the treatment is reassurance of the children and family members. Specifically, they need to be reassured that there is no evidence of a serious underlying disorder. Cancer is often an unspoken concern. In this context, a careful history and physical examination help to reassure the parents. Anxiety about the symptom may contribute to focusing on the symptom as well as to reducing the threshold for discomfort. The parents should be instructed to avoid reinforcing the symptom with secondary gain. Furthermore, if pediatric patients have missed school or have been removed from routine activities because of the pain, it is important that they return to regular activities. Medications are generally unhelpful or, at best, offer transient placebo effect. Biofeedback and relaxation techniques have been useful in some children with functional pain.

If lactose intolerance is suspected, a trial of a lactose-free diet for 1 or 2 wk may be both diagnostic and therapeutic. If symptoms improve, the diet should be continued. A fiber supplement often helps the symptoms of irritable bowel. If chronic constipation is identified, it should be treated in the standard fashion (Chapters 21 and 278).

Successful management depends on close follow-up. The family can try new approaches to the child's symptoms without fear that they are being abandoned by the physician if they know that follow-up by telephone or office visit has been arranged. Often it is during the follow-up visits that one truly gets to know the child and understand the symptoms. It is possible that an organic problem may not have been apparent on the initial visit, but with time, the symptom complex becomes more typical.

These approaches often result in reduction or elimination of the abdominal symptoms. However, children with functional abdominal pain are likely to become adults with functional disorders, although the nature of the symptoms may change.

Apley J: The Child with Abdominal Pain. London, Blackwell Scientific, 1975.

Barbero GJ: Recurrent abdominal pain in childhood. Pediatr Rev 4:29, 1982.

Borge A, Nordhagen R, Moe B, et al: Prevalence and persistence of stomachache and headache among children: Follow-up of a cohort of Norwegian children from 4 to 10 years of age. Acta Paediatr 83:433, 1994.

Drossman D: Physical and sexual abuse and gastrointestinal illness: What is the link? Am J Med 97:105, 1994.

Galler JR, Neustein S, Walker WA: Clinical aspects of recurrent abdominal pain in children. Adv Pediatr 27:31, 1980.

Murphy MS: Management of recurrent abdominal pain. Arch Dis Child 69:409, 1993.

Raymer D, Weininger O, Hamilton JR: Psychological problems in children with abdominal pain. Lancet 1:439, 1984.

CHAPTER 289
Acute Appendicitis

Gary E. Hartman

Acute appendicitis is the most common condition requiring emergency abdominal operation in childhood. Diagnosis is difficult in children, a factor contributing to perforation rates of 30–60%. Fifty per cent of children with perforated appendicitis have been seen by a physician before the diagnosis. The risk of perforation is greatest in 1- to 4-yr-old children (70–75%) and lowest in the adolescent age group (30–40%), which has the highest age-specific incidence in childhood. The difficulty in distinguishing appendicitis from other common causes of abdominal pain and the increase in morbidity and mortality accompanying perforation keep appendicitis an important clinical concern of pediatric clinicians.

EPIDEMIOLOGY. Approximately 80,000 children experience appendicitis in the United States annually, a rate of 4 per 1,000 children younger than 14 yr. Appendicitis is rare in third-world countries where diets are high in fiber. However, no causal relationship has been established between dietary fiber and appendicitis. The incidence of appendicitis increases with age, peaking in adolescence and rarely occurring in children younger than 1 yr. A familial predilection to appendicitis has been reported. Males predominate, clustering of cases has occurred, and cases occur more often in the autumn and spring.

ETIOLOGY. Experimentally, ligation (obstruction) of the appendix results in a marked increase of intraluminal pressure, which rapidly exceeds systolic blood pressure. Initial venous congestion progresses to thrombosis, necrosis, and perforation. Clinically, obstruction of the lumen is the prime cause of appendicitis. The obstruction is caused by inspissated fecal material (fecolith). The inspissated material may calcify, leading to a radiographically visible appendicolith (15–20%). Obstruction resulting from mucosal edema may be associated with systemic or enteric viral or bacterial *(Yersinia, Salmonella, Shigella)* infections. Abnormal mucus has been suggested as the cause of the increased incidence of appendicitis in children with cystic fibrosis. Carcinoid tumors, foreign bodies, and *Ascaris* have rarely been implicated as causes of appendicitis.

PATHOLOGY. The pathologic changes in appendicitis progress through three predictable phases. Initially, with luminal obstruction, venous congestion progresses to mucosal ischemia, necrosis, and ulceration. Bacterial invasion with inflammatory infiltrate through all layers of the appendiceal wall characterizes the second phase. Organisms can be cultured from the serosal surface before microscopic perforation. Finally, necrosis of the wall results in perforation and contamination of the peritoneum. The perforation usually occurs at the tip of the appendix, distal to the obstructing fecalith.

Subsequent to perforation, the microbiologic fecal contamination may be confined to the pelvis or the right iliac fossa by the omentum and adjacent loops of small bowel or may spread throughout the peritoneal cavity. Young children have a poorly developed omentum and the local perforation is not usually confinable. Bacterial invasion of the mesenteric veins may result in portal vein sepsis (pylephlebitis) and subsequent liver abscess formation. The inflammatory process associated with perforation may lead to intestinal obstruction or paralytic ileus.

CLINICAL MANIFESTATIONS. The clinical signs and symptoms depend on the pathologic phase of appendicitis at examination. The classic triad consists of pain, vomiting, and fever. In the initial stage of appendiceal obstruction, the pain is periumbilical. Emesis usually follows the onset of pain and is infrequent. Anorexia is more common. Fever is low grade unless perforation with peritonitis has occurred. The sequence of symptoms—pain preceding emesis and fever—is important in distinguishing appendicitis from infectious enteritis, which usually begins with vomiting followed by the crampy pain of hyperperistalsis. Diarrhea, if it occurs, is infrequent and consists of small, mucous stools caused by irritation of the sigmoid colon. Similarly, irritation of the bladder may produce urinary symptoms such as frequency and urgency.

As the inflammation progresses to involve the serosa and overlying peritoneum, the pain migrates to the area of peritoneal irritation, usually the right lower quadrant. If the appendix is retrocecal, the pain will be lateral or posterior and may mimic the symptoms associated with septic arthritis of the hip or psoas abscess. With perforation, the pain becomes generalized unless the contamination is well localized to produce a discrete, usually right lower quadrant, abscess. Palpation of an abdominal or rectal mass indicates abscess formation.

The progression from onset of symptoms to perforation usually occurs over 36–48 hr. If the diagnosis is delayed beyond 36–48 hr, the perforation rate exceeds 65%.

DIAGNOSIS. Physical Examination. History and physical examination should be directed at establishing the findings consistent with appendicitis and excluding alternative diagnoses such as viral gastroenteritis, constipation, urinary tract infection, hemolytic-uremic syndrome, Henoch-Shönlein purpura, mesenteric adenitis, and tubo-ovarian disease.

Pertinent aspects of the history favoring a diagnosis of appendicitis include onset of pain before vomiting or diarrhea, loss of appetite, migration of pain from periumbilical to right lower quadrant, and aggravation of pain during the trip to office or hospital. In excluding alternative diagnoses, it is essential to question the history of constipation, urinary tract symptoms, cough and fever suggesting lower lobe pneumonia, profuse diarrhea, headache, myalgias or other constitutional symptoms of viral syndromes and similar symptoms in other household members. Untreated appendicitis proceeds to perforation within 48–72 hr; therefore, duration of symptoms is very important in the interpretation of physical findings and in the determination of a treatment strategy.

Physical examination should begin with inspection of the child's demeanor as well as the appearance of the abdomen. The child with appendicitis frequently moves tentatively and slowly, hunched forward, and often with a slight limp. The child may protect the right lower quadrant with a hand and be reluctant to climb onto the examining table. Early in appendicitis the abdomen is flat. Discoloration or bruises should suggest abdominal trauma. Abdominal distension indicates a complication such as perforation or obstruction. Auscultation may reveal normal or hyperactive bowel sounds in early appendicitis to be replaced with hypoactive bowel sounds as it progresses to perforation. Severe gastroenteritis usually produces persistently hyperactive bowel sounds.

Palpation of the abdomen should be gentle after the establishment of rapport and is aided by distraction with conversation or the assistance of a parent. The right lower quadrant (McBurney point) should be palpated last after the examiner has had an opportunity to judge the response to examination of quadrants that should not be painful. McBurney point is the junction of the lateral and middle thirds of the line joining the right anterior superior ileac spine and the umbilicus. The most important physical finding in appendicitis is persistent direct tenderness to palpation and rigidity of the overlying rectus muscle. If the child is apprehensive or agitated from prior examination, the abdominal muscles may be diffusely tense, making interpretation of this finding impossible.

Testing for rebound tenderness must be done carefully to be meaningful. Deep abdominal palpation with sudden withdrawal of the examining hand will cause pain or fear in all children and is not recommended. Gentle finger percussion in all four quadrants is a better test of rebound peritoneal irritation in all age groups but particularly in the frightened child. Testing for rebound tenderness and rectal examination should be the final aspects of the abdominal examination. The value of rectal examination in the diagnosis of appendicitis has been questioned. If the history and abdominal examination are convincing for appendicitis, the rectal examination adds little information. However, if the diagnosis is in doubt, particularly in the very young (younger than 4 yr) or in the female adolescent, rectal examination often yields important information.

After the focused abdominal examination, careful examination of the other body regions, including ears, mucous membranes, lungs, and skin, for signs of other diseases should be noted. Careful attention should be made to identify shock from sepsis, dehydration, or both.

LABORATORY FINDINGS. Laboratory evaluation of children with suspected appendicitis usually consists of complete blood count (CBC) and urinalysis. Although many children with appendicitis have a leukocytosis or shift in differential, many others do not. The primary role of laboratory studies is to exclude alternative diagnoses such as urinary tract infection, hemolytic-uremic syndrome, Henoch-Schönlein purpura, and so on. The proximity of the appendix to the ureter may result in inflammatory cells in the urine. Up to 30 white cells per high-power field and 20 red cells have been reported in suppurative appendicitis. The presence of bacteria or pyuria greater than 30 white cells per high-power field suggests true urinary tract infection. Similarly, the presence of significant proteinuria or cast formation argues against appendicitis. Review of the CBC is directed at identification of microangiopathic anemia, thrombocytosis, or thrombocytopenia, all suggesting diagnoses other than appendicitis.

IMAGING STUDIES. The imaging studies that may be helpful in evaluating children with suspected appendicitis include plain radiographs of the abdomen or chest, ultrasonogram, barium enema, and rarely computed tomography (CT). Findings of appendicitis on abdominal films include calcified appendicolith, small-bowel distension or obstruction, and soft tissue mass effect. Severe constipation or lower lobe pneumonia may establish an alternative diagnosis. Graded compression ultrasonography has gained acceptance as a noninvasive study with false-negative and false-positive rates of 8–10% (Fig. 289–1). It is particularly helpful in adolescent girls whose symptoms may be due to pelvic inflammatory disease, ovarian cysts, or torsion. On rare occasions, when clinical examination and ultrasonography are inconclusive, the diagnosis may be aided by barium enema or abdominal CT. Barium enema findings are those of mass effect on the cecum from the inflammatory process and nonfilling or partial filling of the appendiceal lumen. However, many normal children will have nonfilling of the appendix, and this finding must be interpreted with caution. CT of the abdomen may occasionally be helpful in the setting of a complicated perforation with multiple intra-abdominal abscesses. The true value of CT is in the diagnosis, localization, and percutaneous drainage of abscesses occurring in the postoperative period.

DIFFERENTIAL DIAGNOSIS. Accurate diagnosis of children with abdominal pain is facilitated by a thorough and systematic approach. At the conclusion of the history, physical examination, and initial laboratory studies (CBC, urinalysis), patients fall into three groups: those with definite or highly likely appendicitis, those with a definite alternate diagnosis, and those in whom the diagnosis remains uncertain.

Vomiting preceding the pain, large-volume diarrhea, and high fever suggest gastroenteritis caused by viral or bacterial (*Yersinia, Campylobacter*) agents. An abnormal hemogram com-

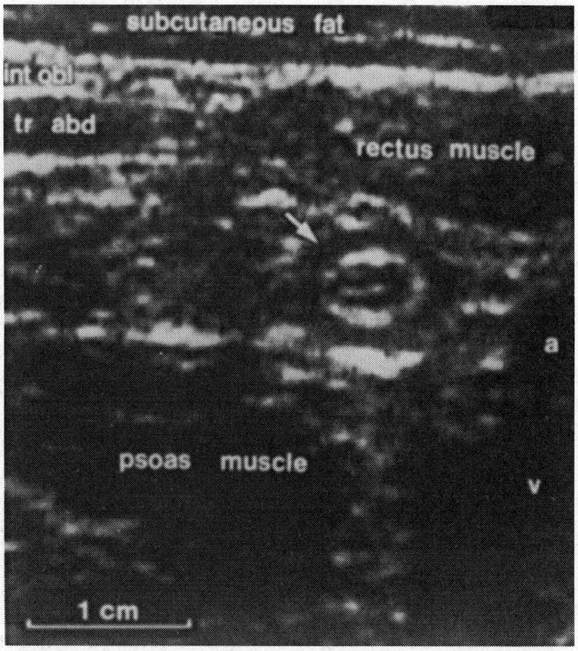

Figure 289–1. A. Graded compression ultrasonogram of acute appendicitis demonstrating edematous enlarged appendix compressed between the abdominal wall and the psoas muscle. (Int obl = internal oblique muscle; tr abd = transverse abdominus muscle; a = right iliac artery; v = right iliac vein.) (From Puylaert JB, Rutgers PH, Laisang RI, et al: A prospective study of ultrasonography in the diagnosis of appendicitis. N Engl J Med 317:666, 1987.)

bined with hemorrhagic skin lesions suggests Henoch-Schönlein purpura or hemolytic-uremic syndrome if renal function and urinalysis are abnormal. Weight loss and prolonged symptoms, especially in a teenager, make inflammatory bowel disease a serious consideration. Torsion of an undescended testis is common, and particular note should be made of testicular location. Follicular cysts of the ovary occur in midcycle and may be painful as a result of rupture, rapid enlargement, or hemorrhage. In pelvic inflammatory disease, the pain is usually suprapubic, bilateral, and of longer duration.

Children with cystic fibrosis have a high incidence of appendicitis but also have a high incidence of intussusception, constipation, and meconium ileus equivalent. Children with malignancies may experience abdominal pain as a result of their chemotherapy, constipation, typhlitis, or appendicitis. If their malignancy is in remission, the signs and symptoms of appendicitis should be the same as those for healthy children. If the malignancy is not controlled, typhlitis is likely if the child is neutropenic. This entity is due to a necrotizing enterocolitis involving the terminal ileum and cecum and usually resolves with recovery of the neutrophil count and conservative management.

Those children with an uncertain diagnosis will require either further diagnostic studies or observation depending on the likelihood of appendicitis and the duration of symptoms. Observation may be done at home or in the hospital. If the diagnosis ultimately is appendicitis, the incidence of perforation is significantly higher (60% vs 30%) if observation is carried out at home.

Once the diagnosis of appendicitis is made or highly suspect, the treatment is surgical appendectomy. Meckel diverticulitis may mimic appendicitis and is usually diagnosed at surgery (Chapter 277.2).

TREATMENT. Children with nonperforated appendicitis require minimal preoperative preparation with intravenous fluids and antibiotics. Although the use of antibiotics in uncomplicated appendicitis is controversial, it has decreased the incidence of postoperative wound infections. Appendectomy should be done within a few hours of establishing the diagnosis and is usually done through a right lower quadrant incision. Laparoscopic appendectomy has been used in children with a complication rate similar to that of open appendectomy. Laparoscopic appendectomy is more expensive but results in a shorter hospital stay, thereby making total cost equivalent. Appendectomy for a nonperforated appendicitis is associated with a low complication rate, rapid recovery, and short (2–3 days) hospitalization.

If the appendix has perforated, especially with generalized peritonitis, significant fluid resuscitation and broad-spectrum antibiotics may be required a few hours before appendectomy. Nasogastric suction should be used if there is significant vomiting or abdominal distension. Antibiotics should cover the commonly encountered organisms (*Bacteroides, Escherichia coli, Klebsiella,* and *Pseudomonas* species). The commonly used intravenous regimens include ampicillin (100 mg/kg/24 hr), gentamicin (5 mg/kg/24 hr), and clindamycin (40 mg/kg/24 hr) or metronidazole (Flagyl) (30 mg/kg/24 hr). Appendectomy is performed with or without drainage of the peritoneal cavity, and the antibiotics are continued for 7–10 days. Occasionally, a localized abscess will be drained by open or percutaneous technique and appendectomy scheduled as a second, elective procedure in 4–6 wk. Contrary to nonperforated appendicitis, the postoperative course is characterized by continued fluid requirement, fever, intra-abdominal abscess formation, sepsis, and prolonged (4–5 days) paralytic ileus.

COMPLICATIONS. Complications occur in 25–30% of children with appendicitis, primarily those with perforation. The most effective method of reducing complications of appendicitis is to reduce the incidence of perforation. Mortality from appendicitis is low (0.5–1%) but does occur. The complications are primarily infectious. Wound infection complicates recovery in 0–2% of children with nonperforated appendicitis and in 10–15% of those with perforated appendicitis. Treatment consists of opening the wound with healing by secondary intention. Further antibiotics are not necessary unless there is associated cellulitis or systemic signs of toxicity. Intra-abdominal abscess is rare in simple appendicitis but occurs in 4–6% of children with perforation. Usually the abscess is solitary and can be drained by CT or an ultrasonogram-guided percutaneous approach. Multiple intra-abdominal abscesses are best treated by open laparotomy with drainage. In the era of current antibiotic therapy, liver abscess from portal vein sepsis is uncommon but may require multiple drainage procedures.

Intestinal obstruction is a common complication and is usually managed with nasogastric suction if it occurs in the early postoperative period. Infertility caused by adhesions or obstruction of the distal fallopian tube is not associated with simple appendicitis but is three to four times more likely after perforation.

Atwood SEA, Hill ADK, Murphy PG, et al: A prospective randomized trial of laparoscopic versus open appendectomy. Surgery 112:497, 1992.

Brender JD, Marcuse EK, Koepsell TD, et al: Childhood appendicitis: factors associated with perforation. Pediatrics 76:301, 1985.

Gilchrist BF, Lobe TE, Schropp KP, et al: Is there a role for laparoscopic appendectomy in pediatric surgery? J Pediatr Surg 27:209, 1992.

Mollitt DL, Mitchum D, Tepas JJ: Pediatric appendicitis: Efficacy of laboratory and radiologic evaluation. South Med J 81:1477, 1988.

Mueller BA, Daling JR, Moore DE, et al: Appendectomy and the risk of tubal infertility. N Engl J Med 315:1506, 1986.

Rothrock SG, Skeoch G, Rush JJ, et al: Clinical features of misdiagnosed appendicitis in children. Ann Emerg Med 20:45, 1991.

Rubin SZ, Martin DJ: Ultrasonography in the management of possible appendicitis in childhood. J Pediatr Surg 25:737, 1990.

Ruff M, Friedland I, Hickey S: *Escherichia coli* septicemia in nonperforated appendicitis. Arch Pediatr Adolisc Med 148:853, 1994.

Tate J, Dawson J, Chung S, et al: Laparoscopic versus open appendectomy: Prospective randomized trial. Lancet 342:633, 1993.

CHAPTER 290
Surgical Conditions of the Anus, Rectum, and Colon

Alberto Peña

In infants and children close inspection of the anal area is as valuable as a digital rectal examination. *Fissures* can be best identified by having a parent hold the infant's hips in acute flexion so that the examiner can separate the patient's buttocks, using both thumbs, gently stretching the anus and everting the lining to expose the fissure. On the other hand, in all cases of constipation, especially when an intrinsic or extrinsic rectal obstruction is possible, a digital examination is indicated, after assessing perianal sensation. Properly done, this should cause little or no discomfort to the patient. A well-lubricated finger is passed over the anus a few times to accustom the patient to the unusual sensation. Then the pulp of the index or fifth finger is pressed against the anus with increasing flexion of the interphalangeal joints and the finger slips easily into the anal canal.

290.1 Anal Fissure

Anal fissure is a small laceration of the mucocutaneous junction of the anus. It is an acquired lesion considered to be secondary to the forceful passage of a hard stool, mainly seen in infancy. Fissures appear to be the consequence and not the cause of constipation.

CLINICAL MANIFESTATIONS. Usually a history of constipation is elicited. At some point the patient has had a painful bowel movement, which may correspond to the actual event of fissure formation after the passing of hard stool. Then, in addition to the primary cause of constipation, the patient becomes a stool holder who tries to voluntarily avoid a bowel movement because of fear of pain. This exacerbates the constipation, and eventually, the passing of a harder and larger stool creates a vicious cycle. Pain on defecation and bright red blood on the surface of the stool may be observed. The diagnosis is established by inspection of the anal area. For this, the infant's hips are held in acute flexion, the patient's buttocks are separated to expand the folds of the perianal skin, and the fissure becomes evident as a minor laceration. Sometimes, peripheral to the laceration, there is a little skin appendage that actually represents epithelialized granulomatous tissue, secondary to the chronic inflammation; this is usually known as a "tag."

TREATMENT. The most important element in the treatment of this condition is for the parents to understand the origin of the laceration and the mechanism of the cycle of constipation. The goal of the treatment is to reverse this cycle, which can be achieved only by guaranteeing that the patient has soft stools to avoid overstretching the anus. The healing process may take several days or even several weeks. One single episode of impaction with passing of a hard piece of stool may exacerbate the problem and recreate the cycle. A stool softener is indicated, but the parents must adjust the dose to the response of the patient. The goal is to avoid both hard stools and diarrhea. Simultaneously, the primary cause of the constipation must be treated when present. There is no scientific basis to support other kinds of treatments, including stretching of the anus, "internal" anal sphincterotomy, or excision of the fissure.

290.2 Perianal Abscess and Fistula

Perineal abscess and fistula can be seen in two different groups of pediatric patients with different cause, pathogenesis, and treatment. These include (1) infants with no predisposing conditions and (2) older children with predisposing conditions. The first group is relatively common and includes infants, usually boys younger than 2 yr. A predisposing illness in this particular age group is rarely seen. This is usually a benign, self-limited condition; the abscess has a communication with one of the crypts of the pectinate line of the anal canal. It is believed that the crypt is the source of contamination, but the exact mechanism is unknown. The abscess eventually drains through an orifice in the perianal area. After this drainage, the inflammation subsides but a fistula remains that communicates with the affected crypt to the perianal external orifice. This can be demonstrated during the surgical treatment. The fistula becomes chronic but usually disappears spontaneously before 2 yr of age. This fistula is located very close to the lumen of the anus, which makes this a very benign condition because the sphincteric mechanism is not affected.

The second group includes patients older than 2 yr with perianal or perirectal abscess and with a predisposing illness, including drug-induced or autoimmune neutropenia, leukemia, acquired immunodeficiency syndrome, diabetes mellitus, Crohn disease, prior rectal surgery (Hirschsprung disease, imperforate anus), or sequelae from the use of immunosuppressant drugs. This is considered a much more serious condition, and the prognosis is intimately related to that of the predisposing disease. The abscess may be deep and may rapidly expand with severe toxic symptoms, particularly when the predisposing illness is associated with immunosuppression. The bacteriology of abscess material reveals a mixed aerobic *(Escherichia coli, Klebsiella pneumoniae, Staphylococcus aureus)* and anaerobic *(Bacteroides species, Clostridium, Veillonella)* flora. Ten to 15% yield pure growth of either *E. coli, S. aureus,* or *Bacteroides fragilis.* Neutropenic patients may also have bacteremia that inconsistently has the same organism as the abscess.

CLINICAL MANIFESTATIONS. The infants with no predisposing conditions have rather mild clinical manifestations, sometimes including low-grade fever, mild rectal pain, and an area of perianal cellulitis. Subsequently, a pustule is formed and the abscess drains through that orifice. This alleviates the symptoms. The inflammation disappears and the pustule heals. However, one or several weeks later, the draining of pus reappears and continues in an intermittent, chronic way. Left alone, this condition usually heals spontaneously before 2 yr of age.

Children with predisposing conditions have a much more serious clinical course. They may or may not have fever depending on their immunologic status. Cellulitis may rapidly expand with warmth, erythema, induration, tenderness, and fluctuation over the ischiorectal fossa, requiring aggressive treatment. Patients may experience severe toxicity and may become septic. In addition, they may show symptoms of the predisposing illness.

TREATMENT. Infants with no predisposing disease usually do not require any treatment because this condition is self-limited. There is no evidence that antibiotics are useful in these patients. Occasionally, when the patient is very uncomfortable, the abscess can be drained under local anesthesia. This alleviates the symptoms of pain and fever but does not eliminate the possibility of a fistula formation. Once a chronic fistula has formed, most recommend a *fistulotomy*, which requires general anesthesia. The anal canal and lower part of the rectum are exposed with an adequate retractor, and a lacrimal probe is passed through the external orifice of the fistula, coming out through one of the crypts. The tissue between the fistula and the lumen of the anal canal is divided with cautery. The wound is left open to spontaneously granulate. This treatment usually runs a 20% chance of recurrence. Conservative management, which consists of observation, is also accepted because in the overwhelming majority of cases the fistula disappears spontaneously before 2 yr of age.

Older children with predisposing diseases may require a more aggressive treatment and treatment of the predisposing condition. Antibiotics must be administered, including a combination that covers enteric gram-negative, *S. aureus*, and fecal anaerobic flora. Wide excision and drainage are mandatory in cases of sepsis and expanding cellulitis.

Fistulas in older patients are seen mainly associated with Crohn disease or in patients with a history of pull-through surgery for the treatment of Hirschsprung disease. Those fistulas are difficult to treat. The treatment is the same as that of the predisposing condition.

290.3 Hemorrhoids

Hemorrhoids in children are uncommon and usually benign. However, when a hemorrhoid is seen, one must suspect portal hypertension. Infants are sometimes brought for consultation after an incidental finding of a hemorrhoid. These follow a very benign course. There are no reports of thrombosis or other complications of hemorrhoids in children; therefore, they should be managed conservatively. Chronic constipation, fecal impaction, or any other kind of irritating local factors must be treated to avoid exacerbation of this condition.

290.4 Rectal Prolapse

Rectal prolapse refers to the exteriorization of the rectal mucosa through the anus. When this extrusion includes all the layers of the rectal wall, it is called *procidentia*. Most cases of rectal tissue protruding through the anus are prolapse and not polyps, intussusception, or other tissue.

Most cases of prolapse are idiopathic. The onset is often between 1–5 yr (mean, 3 yr). Predisposing factors include intestinal parasites (particularly in endemic areas), malnutrition, acute diarrhea, ulcerature colitis, pertussis, Ehlers-Danlos syndrome, meningocele (more frequently associated with procidentia owing to the lack of perineal muscle support), cystic fibrosis, and chronic constipation. Patients treated surgically for imperforate anus may have different degrees of rectomucosal prolapse. This is particularly common in patients with poor sphincteric development.

CLINICAL MANIFESTATIONS. Prolapse of the rectum usually occurs during defecation. Afterward, the prolapse is reduced sometimes spontaneously or manually by the patient or parent. In very severe cases, the prolapsed rectum remains chronically exteriorized, becoming congested and edematous, which makes it more difficult to reduce. Rectal prolapse is usually painless or is associated with a mild discomfort. When the rectum remains prolapsed after defecation, it may be traumatized by underwear and may produce bleeding and wetness. Eventually, the exposed rectum becomes ulcerated. The protruding mass varies from bright red to dark red; it may be as long as 10–12 cm. See Chapter 291 for a distinction from a prolapsed polyp.

TREATMENT. The evaluation should include all the necessary tests to rule out the already stated predisposing conditions. *Reduction of protrusion* is aided by pressure with warm compresses. An easy method of reduction is to cover the finger with a piece of toilet paper, introduce it into the lumen of the mass, and gently push it into the rectum. The finger is then immediately withdrawn. The toilet paper adheres to the mucous membrane, permitting release of the finger; the paper, when softened, is later expelled.

General measures should include careful manual reduction of the prolapse after an episode of defecation, attempts to avoid excessive pushing during bowel movements (with patient's feet off the floor), use of laxatives and stool softeners in cases of constipation, avoidance of inflammatory conditions of the rectum, and treatment of intestinal parasitosis when present. If all this fails to treat idiopathic prolapse, surgical treatment may be indicated. None of the existent operations is considered ideal because each has risks and disadvantages. Therefore, medical treatment should always be tried first. Operations include the placement of a subcutaneous, ringlike band in the perianal area to decrease the diameter of the anus. A significant number of patients become asymptomatic with this treatment; some may experience megacolon owing to a mechanical anal obstruction. Injection of sclerosing substances in the perirectal area has been reported but has the risk of nerve damage and infection. A posterior incision of the rectum, with anchoring of the rectum to the presacral periosteum, represents a useful alternative in severe cases. In cases of procidentia associated with myelomeningocele, the patients may require a laparotomy and an internal fixation of the rectum to the presacral fascia.

290.5 Pilonidal Sinus and Abscess

A dimple located in the midline intergluteal cleft, at the level of the coccyx, is seen relatively frequently in normal infants. There is no evidence that this little pilonidal sinus provokes any problems for the patient. Malignant degeneration of pilonidal sinus cyst has been reported only in patients with chronic infections and abscesses. An open dermal sinus is a benign condition and is usually asymptomatic.

Pilonidal abscesses occur in adolescent patients. Why this condition is not seen in younger patients is unknown. The abscess may require incision and drainage during the acute stage, and subsequently, it requires an en bloc resection to remove all the epithelial tract that caused the problem.

Ashcraft KW, Garred JL, Holder TM, et al: Rectal prolapse: 17 year experience with the posterior repair and suspension. J Pediatr Surg 15:992, 1990.
Grant CS, Al-Salem AH, Anim JT, et al: Childhood fistula-in-ano: a clinicopathological study. Pediatr Surg Int 6:207, 1991.
Longo WE, Touloukian RJ, Seashore JN: Fistula in ano in infants and children: implications and management. Pediatrics 87:737, 1991.
Piazza DJ, Radhakrishnan J: Perianal abscess and fistula-in-ano in children. Dis Colon Rectum 12:1014, 1990.
Pearl RH, Ein SH, Churchill B: Posterior sagittal anorectoplasty for pediatric recurrent rectal prolapse. J Pediatr Surg 24:1100, 1989.
Rakhimov S: Treatment of rectal prolapse in children. Vestn Khir 142:72, 1989.

CHAPTER 291
Tumors of the Digestive Tract

Martin Ulshen

See also Chapter 458.

JUVENILE COLONIC POLYP (RETENTION POLYP, INFLAMMATORY POLYP). This is the most common tumor of the bowel in childhood, present in 3–4% of the population younger than 21 yr. The lesion may appear after 1 yr of age. Most patients become symptomatic between 2 and 10 yr of age, and the lesion is less common beyond 15 yr of age.

Forty per cent or more of these polyps are located proximal to the descending colon. More than half of the children have two or more juvenile polyps. Most juvenile polyps are erythematous, friable, and pedunculated and range in size from a few millimeters to 3 cm. The histology demonstrates hamartomatous proliferation of glandular and stromal elements, marked vascularity, and infiltration with lymphocytes, eosinophils, and polymorphonuclear and plasma cells. These polyps have characteristic mucus-filled cystic glands and are covered by a fragile, single layer of epithelium. The typical juvenile polyp, with no adenomatous change, has no potential for malignancy. However, rare juvenile polyps with an adenomatous component have been reported.

Multiple juvenile colonic polyps occur in families as a dominant trait and are associated with congenital anomalies. These lesions are identical to solitary polyps, but this rare condition may have an increased risk for colonic cancer (see later).

Typical *clinical manifestations* include bright red and painless rectal bleeding during or immediately after a bowel movement. Exsanguinating hemorrhage is rare; bleeding often stops spontaneously. Iron deficiency anemia may be present or, rarely, the initial chief complaint. Lower abdominal pain and cramps are rare and are associated with intussusception or a long pedicle. Prolapse of the polyp appears as a dark, beefy red mass in distinction to the lighter pink mucosal appearance of rectal prolapse. Spontaneous polyp infarction and self-amputation are common, whereas diarrhea and obstruction are uncommon. The *differential diagnosis* includes other forms of intestinal polyposis, Meckel diverticulum, fissure in ano, inflammatory bowel disease, intestinal infections, and coagulation disorders.

The *diagnosis* is often made by rectal examination. Confirmation or identification of more distal polyps is made by sigmoidoscopy. Polyps appear as smooth, pedunculated lesions. Fiberoptic colonoscopy of the entire colon is indicated to identify other polyps. The polyp can be removed during endoscopy. Air-contrast barium enema may also demonstrate distal or multiple polyps. Colonoscopy is preferred because even large polyps may not be seen on otherwise adequate barium studies. Saline enema plus transabdominal ultrasonography may also identify polyps.

Treatment includes the removal of the polyp at colonoscopy by snare cautery or, rarely, by transabdominal polypectomy. Recurrences occasionally are seen.

FAMILIAL POLYPOSIS SYNDROMES. The familial syndromes associated with intestinal polyposis are important because some of them are premalignant states.

Familial Adenomatous Polyposis Coli. This mendelian dominant condition, with reduced penetrance, is premalignant and is characterized by large numbers of adenomatous lesions in the distal large bowel. The incidence is 1:8,000 persons, with usual onset of polyp development late in the 1st decade of life or during adolescence. By definition there are more than 100 (often 1,000) visible adenomas present when the patient is in the 2nd or 3rd decade of life. Congenital hypertrophy of retinal pigment epithelial cells is also present in most patients. The adenomatous polyposis coli (APC) gene is present on the long arm of chromosome 5. On the basis of genetic studies, the APC gene is also responsible for Gardner syndrome. *Turcot syndrome* (primary brain tumor-medulloblastoma and multiple colorectal polyposis) is also associated with germline defects of the APC gene. Some families who do not meet the criteria for adenomatous polyposis coli but who have a high frequency of adenomatous polyps and colonic cancer also have a mutation of the APC gene.

Initially, the polyps are asymptomatic, and many often remain so. When symptomatic, adenomatous polyps cause hematochezia, occasionally cramps, or, rarely, diarrhea. Malignancy arising from pre-existing adenomatous polyps may first appear during adolescence, although they usually appear in young adulthood.

The *diagnosis* should be suspected from the family history. APC gene alterations are detected in 87% of unrelated individuals with familial polyposis coli, suggesting the possibility of presymptomatic testing. The diagnosis is made by direct vision through a colonoscope. The polyps are usually numerous; biopsies demonstrate the adenomatous nature without the inflammatory and cystic finding of juvenile polyps. For a child with a family history of APC, colonoscopy is recommended annually after 10 yr of age.

Management consists of a careful family survey, genetic counseling, and, for confirmed patients with APC, pancolectomy. Current anastomotic methods permit restoration of bowel continuity after resection of all colonic mucosa (ileorectal pull-through). Aspirin, sulindac, and complex resistant starch may slow polyp development; their efficacy is currently unknown.

Peutz-Jeghers Syndrome. This rare dominantly inherited syndrome is characterized by mucosal pigmentation of the lips and gums and hamartomas of the stomach and small bowel. Deeply pigmented discrete freckles are seen at birth or appear during infancy on the lips and buccal mucosa and even around the mouth. Evidence of intestinal lesions may come from bleeding but more commonly may arise from crampy pain associated with obstruction or intussusception.

Family studies and genetic counseling are important. Relatives may be found with either partial or complete manifestations of the syndrome. Intestinal lesions should be excised if they are causing significant symptoms; involvement is usually too extensive to remove all the polyps. Fifty per cent of patients have no family member with the disorder, suggesting a high rate of new mutation. Cancer develops in up to 50% of people having Peutz-Jeghers syndrome, most commonly middle-aged adults. Most of these cancers do not occur in the gastrointestinal tract, and typically the hamartomatous polyps do not contain cancer.

Gardner Syndrome. This dominantly inherited disorder is characterized by multiple intestinal polyps and tumors of the soft tissue and bone, particularly the mandible. Additional features include dental abnormalities, characteristic bilateral pigmented lesions in the ocular fundus, and extracolonic cancers (hepatoblastoma, CNS). Patients with this syndrome have a defect in the APC gene on chromosome 5. Gardner and familial adenomatous polyposis coli syndromes are probably manifestations of the same disease.

The soft tissue lesions and osteomas may appear during childhood, but intestinal polyps usually do not become apparent until early adult life. These polyps may develop anywhere along the digestive tract and are premalignant. Accordingly, aggressive surgical treatment of the intestinal lesions is indicated. Children at risk for Gardner syndrome require the same colon surveillance as in a child having family members with familial polyposis coli. If adenomatous polyps of the colon are identified, colectomy with ileorectal pull-through is currently the recommended approach.

HEMANGIOMA OF THE INTESTINE. These rare benign lesions can cause massive, even fatal hemorrhage. The usual clinical manifestation is painless bleeding beginning in childhood. The blood loss can be subtle and chronic or sudden and massive. Usually, there are no additional intestinal symptoms, but if intussusception occurs, there will be obstructive symptoms. About 50% of patients have cutaneous hemangiomas, and some have a family history of similar lesions. About half of these lesions are in the colon, where they may be seen by colonoscopy. During a period of bleeding selective mesenteric arteriography may be useful in locating a lesion.

LEIOMYOMA. This rare benign tumor occurs most commonly in the stomach and jejunum. It remains asymptomatic for long periods, but if it extends into the lumen, it may cause intussusception.

CARCINOMA. The fact that epithelial tumors of the digestive tract are rare in children argues against an aggressive diagnostic approach to many gastrointestinal symptoms in this age group. Several childhood conditions predispose to development of gastrointestinal adenocarcinoma in adult life; for example, familial polyposis, Gardner syndrome, idiopathic ulcerative colitis, and, to a lesser extent, Crohn disease and disorders associated with chromosomal breaks. The usual site is the colon but gastric lesions are reported. Symptoms are general ill health, abdominal pain, an abdominal mass, and, less frequently, hemorrhage. The tumors tend to be relatively undifferentiated and highly malignant.

LYMPHOSARCOMA OF THE INTESTINE. Of the malignancies of the digestive tract in children, most are lymphosarcomas; some are associated with acquired immunodeficiency syndrome (Chapter 223). The usual site is the lower small intestine. Manifestations are general ill health, abdominal pain, and anemia. Adults with long-standing celiac disease have a relatively high incidence of lymphosarcoma; a beneficial effect of dietary treatment on this relationship has not been proved. Bowel tumors occur with other immunodeficiencies (Wiskott-Aldrich syndrome, transplantation).

CARCINOID TUMORS. These tumors of the enterochromaffin cells of the intestine usually occur in the appendix in children and have very-low-grade malignancy. They cause symptoms similar to those of appendicitis and do not recur after resection, even when the tumor has extended to the muscularis and lymphatics.

Carcinoid tumors outside the appendix commonly metastasize, and the metastatic lesions give rise to the carcinoid syndrome, which is the result of pharmacologically active secretions produced by the tumor. These produce episodic intestinal hypermotility and diarrhea, vasomotor disturbances, and bronchoconstriction. The most important active agent is serotonin, and the diagnosis is usually made by finding high urinary levels of its metabolite, 5-hydroxyindoleacetic acid. These functioning neoplasms are rare in children.

Abrahamson J, Shandling B: Intestinal hemangiomata in childhood and a syndrome for diagnosis: A collective review. J Pediatr Surg 8:487, 1973.
Burn J, Chapman P, Eastham E: Familial adenomatous polyposis. Arch Dis Child 71:103, 1994.
Giardiello FM, Offerhaus JA, Krush AJ: Risk of hepatoblastoma in familial adenomatous polyposis. J Pediatr 119:766, 1991.
Giardiello FM, Welsh SB, Hamilton SR, et al: Increased risk of cancer in the Peutz-Jeghers syndrome. N Engl J Med 316:1511, 1987.
Hamilton S, Liu B, Parsons R, et al: The molecular basis of Turcot's syndrome. N Engl J Med 332:839, 1995.
Leppert M, Burt R, Hughes JP, et al: Genetic analysis of an inherited predisposition to colon cancer in a family with a variable number of adenomatous polyps. N Engl J Med 322:904, 1990.
Nagita A, Amemoto K, Yoden A, et al: Ultrasonographic diagnosis of juvenile colonic polyps. J Pediatr 124:535, 1994.
Postlethwait RW: Gastrointestinal carcinoid tumors—a review. Postgrad Med 40:445, 1966.
Powell SM, Petersen GM, Krush AJ, et al: Molecular diagnosis of familial adenomatous polyposis. N Engl J Med 329:1982, 1993.
Recalde M, Holyoke ED, Elias EG: Carcinoma of the colon, rectum and anal canal in young patients. Surg Gynecol Obstet 139:909, 1974.
Traboulsi EI, Krush AJ, Gardner EJ, et al: Prevalence and importance of pigmented ocular fundus lesions in Gardner's syndrome. N Engl J Med 316:661, 1987.

291.1 Diarrhea from Hormone-Secreting Tumors

Certain hormone-producing tumors cause a marked increase in intestinal secretion leading to severe chronic watery diarrhea (Table 291–1). The secretory diarrhea persists when the patient is placed on nothing by mouth orders. These tumors originate in the APUD cells (*a*mine content, *p*recursor *u*ptake,

■ TABLE 291–1 Diarrhea Caused by Hormone-Secreting Tumors

Name	Site	Hormone	Manifestations	Therapy
APUDomas*				
VIPoma	Pancreas	VIP	Watery diarrhea, achlorhydria, hypokalemia	Somatostatin Resection
Somatostatinoma	Pancreas	Somatostatin	Massive diarrhea†	Resection
Gastrinoma	Pancreas	Gastrin	Peptic ulcer, diarrhea	Cimetidine, omeprazole Tumor resection/gastrectomy
Carcinoid	Intestinal argentaffin cells	Serotonin	Diarrhea,† crampy abdominal pain, flushing, wheezing, cardiac valve damage	Somatostatin Resection
Mastocytoma	Cutaneous, intestine, liver, spleen	Histamine, VIP	Pruritus, flushing, apnea, if VIP is positive, diarrhea	H_1- and H_2-blocking agents, cromolyn, steroids Resection if solitary
Medullary carcinoma	Thyroid	Calcitonin, VIP, prostaglandins	Watery diarrhea	Thyroidectomy
Neurogenic				
Ganglioneuroma, ganglioneuroblastoma	Extra-adrenal sites and adrenals	Catecholamines, VIP	Massive watery diarrhea	Resection
Pheochromocytoma	Chromaffin cells; abdominal > other sites	Catecholamines, VIP	Hypertension, tachycardia, sweating, anxiety, watery diarrhea†	Resection

**APUDoma cells are neural crest cell derivatives of the gastroenteropancreatic endocrine system.*
†Reported only in adults.
APUDoma = amine precursor uptake and decarboxylation of amino acids; VIP = vasoactive intestinal polypeptide.

amino acid *d*ecarboxylation) of the gastroenteropancreatic endocrine system and in adrenal or extra-adrenal neurogenic sites. Neural crest cells are precursors of APUDoma and neurogenic cells.

Diarrhea is massive and results in fluid and electrolyte imbalance and weight loss. *Diagnosis* is based on the presence of secretory watery diarrhea, extraintestinal manifestations, measurement of the suspected hormone or its metabolites in serum or urine, and various imaging techniques. If possible, tumor resection is the treatment of choice. Pharmacologic therapy with hormone antagonists may be palliative (see Table 291–1).

Hamilton JR, Radde IC, Johnson G: Diarrhea associated with adrenal ganglioneuroma: new findings related to the pathogenesis of diarrhea. Am J Med 44:473, 1968.
Kaplan SJ, Holbrook CT, McDaniel HE, et al: Vasoactive intestinal peptide secreting tumors of childhood. Am J Dis Child 134:21, 1980.
Mitchell CH, Sinatra FR, Crast FW, et al: Intractable watery diarrhea, ganglioneuroblastoma and vasoactive intestinal peptide. J Pediatr 89:593, 1976.
Rambaud JC, Modigliani R, et al: Pancreatic cholera: studies on tumor secretions and pathophysiology of diarrhea. Gastroenterology 69:110, 1975.

NODULAR LYMPHOID HYPERPLASIA. Lymphoid follicles in the lamina propria of the gut normally aggregate in Peyer patches. These areas appear as submucosal nodules, which may be visible on barium contrast roentgenograms and mistaken for an abnormality. There are many more Peyer patches in the lower than the upper small bowel. In some patients lymphoid follicles become hyperplastic. The hyperplasia may occur in the colon or extend to the small bowel. Diffuse small-bowel lymphoid hyperplasia may be seen in cases of immunoglobulin deficiency, with and without *Giardia lamblia* infestation. Symptoms are mild. There may be rectal bleeding, diarrhea, and abdominal cramps beginning usually by 3 yr of age.

The major importance of this entity is the similarity of its manifestations to more serious disorders. Lymphoid hyperplasia resolves spontaneously and requires no specific treatment.

Hodgson JR, Hoffman HN, Huizenga KA: Roentgenologic features of lymphoid hyperplasia of the small intestine associated with dysgammaglobulinemia. Radiology 88:883, 1967.
Poley JR, Smith EL: Benign lymphatic hyperplasia of the rectum. South Med J 65:420, 1972.

CHAPTER 292
Inguinal Hernias

Stephen J. Shochat

An inguinal hernia is the most common condition requiring operation in the pediatric age group. The incidence of inguinal hernias in children has not been established but is between 10–20:1,000 live births. The ratio of boys to girls is 4:1. Approximately 50% will present before 1 yr of age; most will be seen in the first 6 mo of life. The most common inguinal hernia in children is an indirect inguinal hernia. Direct hernias are rare and occur in approximately 1% of all inguinal hernias. Femoral hernias are also rare in the pediatric population. Sixty per cent of inguinal hernias are on the right side, 30% are on the left side, and 10% are bilateral. Premature infants have a higher incidence of inguinal hernia, approaching 30%.

EMBRYOLOGY AND PATHOGENESIS. A majority of inguinal hernias in infants and children are indirect resulting from a persistent patency of the processus vaginalis. In the fetus, the gonads begin to develop during the 5th wk of gestation, when the primordial germ cells migrate from the yolk sac to the gonadal ridge. The ligamentous gubernaculum forms and descends on either side of the abdomen at the inferior pole of the gonad and attaches to the internal surface of the labial-scrotal folds. During its course of descent, the gubernaculum passes through the anterior abdominal wall at the site of the future internal inguinal ring and inguinal canal. The processus vaginalis is a diverticular protrusion of the peritoneum that forms just ventral to the gubernaculum and herniates through the abdominal wall with the gubernaculum into the inguinal canal. The testes, which are initially located within the urogenital ridge in the retroperitoneum, descend to the area of the internal ring by approximately 28 wk of gestation. The descent of the testis through the inguinal canal is regulated by androgenic hormones and mechanical factors (increased intra-abdominal pressure). The testes descend into the scrotum by approximately 29 wk of gestation. Each testis descends through the inguinal canal external to the processus vaginalis.

The ovaries also descend into the pelvis from the urogenital ridge but do not exit from the abdominal cavity. The cranial portion of the gubernaculum differentiates into the ovarian ligament, and the inferior aspect of the gubernaculum becomes the round ligament, which passes through the internal ring and into the labia majoris. The processus vaginalis in girls extends into the labia majoris through the inguinal canal, which is also known as the canal of Nuck.

During the last few weeks of gestation or shortly after birth, the layers of the processus vaginalis normally fuse together and obliterate the entrance to the inguinal canal in the vicinity of the internal ring. Failure of obliteration results in a variety of inguinal anomalies, as demonstrated in Figure 292–1. Complete failure of obliteration will lead to a complete inguinal hernia. Obliteration distally with patency proximally will lead to an indirect inguinal hernia. Obliteration proximally with patency distally will lead to an isolated **hydrocele,** also known as a hydrocele of the tunica vaginalis. Obliteration of the processus vaginalis proximally and distally but patency in the midportion of the spermatic cord will lead to a hydrocele of the cord. The term *communicating hydrocele* is confusing and should be discarded because this anomaly is synonymous with a complete inguinal hernia (see Fig. 292–1).

CLINICAL MANIFESTATIONS. An inguinal hernia usually appears as a bulge in the inguinal region and extends toward or into the scrotum. Occasionally, an infant will present with a swelling of the scrotum without a prior bulge in the inguinal region. The parent is usually the first person to notice this bulge, which may be present only during crying or straining. During sleep or when at rest or relaxed, the hernia reduces spontaneously without a noticeable bulge or enlargement of the scrotum. The history of intermittent groin, labial, or scrotal swelling that spontaneously reduces is classic for an indirect inguinal hernia. Occasionally, an inguinal mass will appear suddenly in an infant and will be associated with discomfort. It will be important to distinguish between a hydrocele of the cord and an incarcerated inguinal hernia, but the hydrocele of the cord will not be associated with symptoms of intestinal obstruction such as abdominal distention or vomiting.

Physical examination will reveal an inguinal bulge at the level of the internal or external ring or a scrotal swelling that is reducible or fluctuates in size. The classic method of examining an adult for an inguinal hernia by placing the index finger into the inguinal canal is unnecessary in infants and young children and, in fact, can cause unnecessary discomfort. This is because the internal and external rings are parallel in infants and young children, and a true, well-defined inguinal canal is not present. An inguinal hernia can be identified by

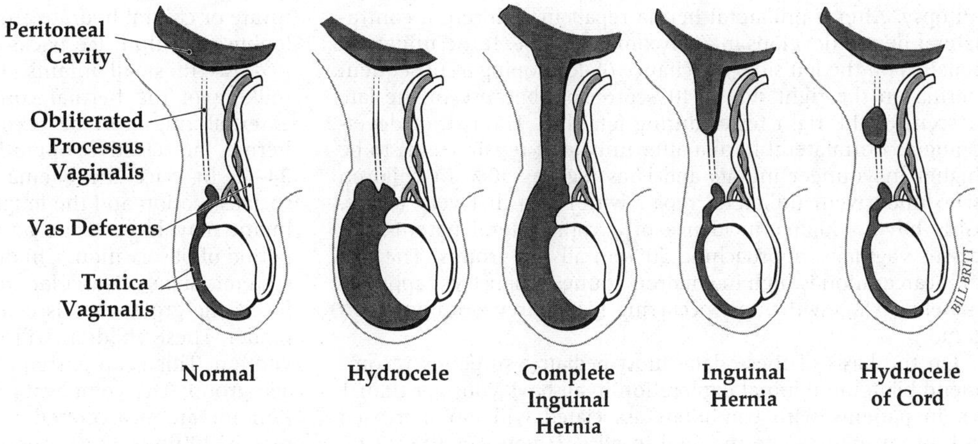

Figure 292–1. Hernias and hydroceles. (Modified from Scherer LR III, Grosfeld JL: Inguinal and umbilical anomalies. Pediatr Clin North Am 40:1122, 1993.)

having the infant lie supine with extended legs and arms over the head. This usually causes the infant to cry, raising the intra-abdominal pressure, which will then demonstrate a bulge over the pubic tubercle (external ring) or a swelling within the scrotum. Older children can be examined standing, which will also increase the intra-abdominal pressure and demonstrate the hernia. Retractile testes are frequent in young infants and children and can resemble an inguinal hernia with a bulge over the external ring. For this reason it is very important to palpate the testes before palpation of the inguinal bulge. This will allow the differentiation between these two entities and avoid an unnecessary operative procedure.

In difficult diagnostic dilemmas, a rectal examination can be extremely helpful in differentiating acute groin abnormalities. The examiner first examines the internal ring on the uninvolved side and then can sweep the index finger or fifth digit toward the internal ring on the involved side. In cases of an indirect inguinal hernia, an intra-abdominal organ can be palpated extending through the internal ring. This technique is quite helpful in distinguishing an incarcerated hernia from an acute hydrocele of the cord or other inguinal abnormalities such as inguinal adenitis.

At times it may be difficult to distinguish a complete inguinal hernia from an isolated hydrocele. These two conditions can usually be differentiated by a careful history. In an infant with a complete inguinal hernia, the scrotal swelling varies during the day, usually being quite large while the child is crying or straining, and disappears or becomes much smaller during relaxation. The isolated hydrocele does not change in size during the day but may gradually disappear over the first year of life. The hydrocele and the complete inguinal hernia both transilluminate and may be difficult to distinguish from each other because occasionally the complete inguinal hernia cannot be reduced manually because of narrowing within a small inguinal canal. In this situation, a classic history is all that is necessary to proceed with operation. In some children with an inguinal hernia, an inguinal bulge or scrotal swelling may not be present at the time of physical examination, and the only finding may be a thickening of the spermatic cord with an associated "silk" sign. The silk sign is elicited by palpating the spermatic cord over the pubic tubercle. The two layers of the peritoneum rubbing together will feel like silk. The silk sign in association with a good history of a hernia can be helpful in diagnosing an inguinal hernia. Occasionally, a full bladder will occlude the internal inguinal ring so that a hernia cannot be demonstrated. Emptying the bladder may be helpful in this situation.

A number of conditions are associated with an increased risk for the development of an indirect inguinal hernia. An increased incidence of inguinal hernias is seen in children with a positive family history of hernias, cystic fibrosis, congenital dislocation of the hip, undescended testes, ambiguous genitalia, hypospadias, epispadias, ascites, and congenital abdominal wall defects. Infants with connective tissue disorders such as Ehlers-Danlos syndrome and mucopolysaccharidosis (Hunter-Hurler syndrome) are at increased risk for inguinal hernia. Female infants with inguinal hernias should be suspected of having testicular feminization because more than 50% of the patients with testicular feminization will have an inguinal hernia. Conversely, the true incidence of testicular feminization in all female infants with hernias is difficult to determine but is approximately 1%. The diagnosis of testicular feminization can be made at the time of operation either by identifying an abnormal gonad within the hernia sac or by performing a rectal examination to palpate a uterus. In the normal female infant, the uterus is easily palpated as a distinct midline structure beneath the symphysis pubis on rectal examination. Chromosome analysis should be reserved for those infants with definite absence of the uterus. All girls with an inguinal hernia should have a rectal examination performed at the time of operation to rule out testicular feminization.

TREATMENT. The treatment of choice for an inguinal hernia is operative repair; an inguinal hernia will not resolve spontaneously. The operation should be carried out electively shortly after diagnosis because of the high risk of later incarceration, especially during the first year of life. Elective inguinal hernia repair can safely be performed in an outpatient setting. Hospitalization should be limited to high-risk patients with cardiac, respiratory, or other medical conditions that would place them at an increased risk after the stress of surgery and anesthesia. Supports and trusses are not indicated and are potentially hazardous. Operation is not indicated for the child with an isolated hydrocele (hydrocele of the tunica vaginalis). There is no indication for operating on a hydrocele except in the infant with a hydrocele of the cord in which there is frequently an associated hernia. An isolated hydrocele often resolves spontaneously within the first year of life; if the hydrocele persists beyond this time, the diagnosis is that of a complete inguinal hernia, which should be treated by an inguinal exploration and herniorrhaphy. Hydroceles should never be aspirated.

There is an ongoing controversy regarding when to proceed with contralateral groin exploration in infants and children with a unilateral indirect inguinal hernia. The incidence of a patent processus vaginalis is approximately 60% at 2 mo of age and 40% at 2 yr of age. A silent patent processus vaginalis is found in approximately 30% of the general population at autopsy. After a unilateral hernia repair in children, a contralateral hernia develops in approximately 30%. If the unilateral repair is on the left side, the chance of developing a subsequent hernia on the right side is 40% probably because of the late descent of the right testes during fetal life. The risk of developing a contralateral hernia after unilateral repair seems to be higher in younger infants and is as high as 50% in children who underwent unilateral repair within the first year of life. Girls have a higher incidence of a contralateral patent processus vaginalis, approaching 50% in all age groups. The risk of incarceration is high in children younger than 1 yr (approximately 30%), with most occurring in children younger than 6 mo.

On the basis of these data, most pediatric surgeons recommend bilateral inguinal exploration in all boys younger than 1 yr, in patients with conditions associated with an increased risk of an inguinal hernia, and in all girls younger than 2 yr. Boys and girls younger than 2 yr presenting with a left inguinal hernia are at higher risk for the development of a contralateral hernia and should have a right-sided exploration. Laparoscopic techniques have been used to visualize the contralateral side, and if this technique is found to be efficacious it may avoid unnecessary contralateral exploration. The decision to perform a bilateral exploration should also depend on the expertise of the surgeon and anesthesiologist and the general condition of the child.

Antibiotic coverage is an important consideration in infants with congenital heart disease and in children with ventriculoperitoneal shunts before operative repair. Ampicillin and gentamicin are the antibiotics of choice for such children, beginning 2 hr before operation and continued in the immediate postoperative period.

Bilateral absence of the vas deferens at the time of herniorrhaphy is an interesting finding in the occasional child with inguinal hernias. Although this condition can be an isolated finding, there is a higher incidence of cystic fibrosis in children with agenesis of the vas deferens. Children with cystic fibrosis also have an increased incidence of inguinal hernias. A sweat chloride should be performed in these infants because an early diagnosis of cystic fibrosis in asymptomatic children may improve the overall prognosis.

COMPLICATIONS. An incarcerated hernia occurs when the contents of the hernia sac cannot be reduced back into the abdominal cavity. The incarcerated organ is usually the intestine, which is associated with signs and symptoms of intestinal obstruction such as vomiting, abdominal distention, constipation, and air-fluid levels on abdominal radiograph. All infants and young children with unexplained intestinal obstruction should be examined for an unrecognized incarcerated hernia. Although the intestines are the most frequent organs involved in an incarcerated hernia, any intra-abdominal organ can become incarcerated, and in young girls the most common organ is the ovary. Once the blood supply to the organ becomes compromised, a strangulated hernia occurs, which is a definite indication for emergency operation.

The incidence of incarceration ranges from 9–20%, with the majority seen within the first yr of life. Approximately half occur within the first yr of life. The incidence of incarceration is higher in girls and in premature infants of both sexes. Incarcerated hernias present with a tender, firm mass in the inguinal canal or the scrotum. The child is fussy, is intolerant of feedings, and cries inconsolably. The skin over the mass may be edematous and slightly discolored but is usually not erythematous or exquisitely tender, as is seen with a strangulated hernia. The hernia should be promptly reduced and can be successfully accomplished in approximately 95% of the cases. It is unusual for a child with an incarcerated inguinal hernia to require an emergency operation. Reduction of an inguinal hernia is aided by sedation with a short-acting barbiturate or chloral hydrate and placing the patient in the Trendelenburg position. Ice packs are not used and have caused fat necrosis in small infants. Once the child is quiet, a gentle milking of the hernial contents toward the internal and/or external rings can be accomplished. After reduction of the hernia, an elective operation should be performed within 24–48 hr once the edema has subsided. Depending on the social situation and the length of time of the incarceration, the infant may have to be admitted to the hospital during this period of observation. Children with strangulated hernias have systemic signs of vascular compromise such as tachycardia and fever; the groin mass is usually erythematous and exquisitely tender. These children will require immediate operative intervention. This is an extremely rare occurrence in the pediatric age group. The complication rate, after an emergency operation for an incarcerated or strangulated hernia, is approximately 20 times that associated with an elected procedure.

In young boys with undescended testes and an associated hernia, incarceration is frequently associated with ischemia and infarction of the testis. For this reason, infants with an undescended testis and associated clinical hernia should have an elective orchiopexy and hernia repair at the time of diagnosis. Young girls can have the ovary and fallopian tube incarcerated within the inguinal canal or the labia majora. If the ovary cannot be reduced, early surgical intervention should be considered because of the possibility of infarction of the ovary.

A unique type of hernia that is extremely rare in infants and young children is a *Richter hernia*. In a Richter hernia, there is an isolated incarceration of the antimesenteric portion of the intestine, and, despite the incarceration and sometimes strangulation, intestinal obstruction is not present. This should be kept in mind in cases in which there is evidence of incarceration or strangulation without intestinal obstruction. The more common situation is that of strangulated omentum, but both conditions should be considered in the infant with a questionable incarcerated hernia and no signs of intestinal obstruction. This problem can be sorted out by performing a rectal examination to determine whether there is evidence of an indirect hernia with contents extending through the internal ring into the inguinal canal.

PREMATURE INFANT. The premature infant has a higher incidence of inguinal hernia and incarceration. Up to 7% of boys born at less than 30 wk gestation have inguinal hernias compared with only 0.6% of male infants born at later than 36 wk gestation. In addition, there is a 20 times greater incidence of hernias in premature infants weighing less than 1,500 g vs larger infants. Because the incidence of incarceration approaches 30% in this patient population, elective hernia repair should be considered before discharge from the neonatal intensive care nursery.

Postoperative apnea is a life-threatening complication of hernia repair in premature infants. The cause of this apnea is unknown but may be due to immaturity of the brain stem ventilatory mechanism. Premature infants with a history of apnea are at extremely high risk for significant respiratory depression after hernia repair. Even in premature infants without prior apnea, there is a significant risk of respiratory arrest and compromise in the postoperative period. The guidelines recommended by pediatric anesthesiologists are that any premature infant younger than 60 wk postconception age should be hospitalized and requires 24-hr postoperative cardiac and respiratory monitoring after herniorrhaphy. Most require general anesthesia, but local anesthetic methods have been attempted with some success; regional anesthesia may also be effective.

PROGNOSIS. The results of inguinal hernia repair in infants and children are excellent. The complication rate after repair of inguinal hernias in children is approximately 2%. The incidence of wound infection approaches 1%, and the recurrence rate is less than 1%. An increased incidence of recurrence is found when there is a history of incarceration or strangulation, in children with connective tissue diseases, and chronic respiratory illness, and when there is increased intra-abdominal pressure, such as infants with a ventriculoperitoneal shunt. Injury to the ileoinguinal nerve or the vas deferens is rare. Testicular compromise is seen in 3–5% of boys who present with an incarcerated hernia.

Gallagher TM: Regional anesthesia for surgical treatment of inguinal hernia repair in preterm babies. Arch Dis Child 69:623, 1993.
Holcomb GW: Laparoscopic evaluation for a contralateral inguinal hernia or a nonpalpable testis. Pediatr Ann 22:678, 1993.
Krieger NR, Shochat SJ, McGowan V, et al: Early hernia repair in the premature infant: long-term follow-up. J Pediatr Surg (in press).
Othersen HB Jr: The pediatric inguinal hernia. Surg Clin North Am 73:853, 1993.
Scherer LR III, Grosfeld JL: Inguinal and umbilical anomalies. Pediatr Clin North Am 40:1121, 1993.
Surana R, Puri P: Is contralateral exploration necessary in infants with unilateral inguinal hernia? J Pediatr Surg 28:1026, 1993.

SECTION 5
Exocrine Pancreas

Steven L. Werlin

Excluding cystic fibrosis, disorders of the exocrine pancreas are uncommon in childhood. Pancreatic disease may be based on traumatic, anatomic (annular pancreas, pancreas divisum), metabolic (Reye syndrome, α_1-antitrypsin deficiency), congenital (Shwachman syndrome, enzyme defects), autoimmune (diabetes mellitus), or inflammatory pathology. A comprehensive discussion of cystic fibrosis is found in Chapter 363. ■

CHAPTER 293
Embryology, Anatomy, and Physiology

The human pancreas develops from evaginations of primitive duodenum beginning at about the 5th wk of gestation. The larger dorsal anlage, which develops into the tail, body, and part of the head of the pancreas, grows directly from the duodenum. The smaller ventral anlage develops as one or two buds from the primitive liver and eventually forms the major portion of the head of the pancreas. At about the 17th wk of gestation, the dorsal and ventral anlage fuse as the buds develop and the gut rotates. The ventral duct forms the proximal portion of the major pancreatic duct of Wirsung, which opens into the ampulla of Vater. The dorsal duct forms the distal portion of the duct of Wirsung and the accessory duct of Santorini, which may empty independently in about 15% of people. Variations in fusion account for the variety of the developmental anomalies of the pancreas.

The pancreas lies transversely in the upper abdomen between the duodenum and the spleen in the retroperitoneum. The head, which rests on the vena cava and renal vein, is adherent to the C loop of the duodenum and surrounds the distal common bile duct. The tail of the pancreas reaches to the left splenic hilum and passes above the left kidney. The lesser sac separates the tail of the pancreas from the stomach.

By the 13th wk of gestation both exocrine and endocrine cells can be identified. Primitive acini containing immature zymogen granules are found by the 16th wk. Mature zymogen granules containing amylase, trypsinogen, chymotrypsinogen, and lipase are present at the 20th wk. Centroacinar and duct cells, which are responsible for water, electrolyte, and bicarbonate secretion, are also found by the 20th wk. The final three-dimensional structure of the pancreas consists of a complex series of branching ducts surrounded by grapelike clusters of epithelial cells. Cells containing glucagon are present at the 8th wk. Islets of Langerhans are first observed at the 12–16th wk.

293.1 Anatomic Abnormalities

An *annular pancreas* results from incomplete rotation of the left (ventral) pancreatic anlage. Patients usually present in infancy with symptoms of complete or partial bowel obstruction. There is frequently a history of maternal polyhydramnios. Some children present with chronic vomiting, pancreatitis, or biliary colic. The treatment of choice is duodenojejunostomy. Division of the pancreatic ring is not attempted because a duodenal diaphragm or duodenal stenosis frequently accompanies annular pancreas. Annular pancreas may be associated with Down syndrome, intestinal atresia, imperforate anus, pancreatitis, and malrotation.

Ectopic pancreatic rests in the stomach or small intestine occur in approximately 3% of the population. Most cases (70%) are found in the upper intestinal tract. Recognized on barium contrast studies by their typical umbilicated appearance, they are rarely of clinical importance. On endoscopy they are typically irregular yellow nodules 2–4 mm in diameter. A pancreatic rest may occasionally be the lead point of an intussusception, produce hemorrhage, or cause bowel obstruction.

Pancreas divisum, which occurs in 5–15% of the population, is the most common pancreatic developmental anomaly. As the result of failure of the dorsal and ventral pancreatic anlagen to fuse, the tail, body, and part of the head of the pancreas drain through the small accessory duct of Santorini rather than the main duct of Wirsung. Most investigators believe that this anomaly may be associated with recurrent pancreatitis when there is a relative obstruction of the outflow of the ventral pancreas. The treatment of choice of recurrent pancreatitis associated with pancreas divisum is endoscopic insertion of an endoprosthesis. If the episodes stop, surgical sphincterotomy is indicated.

Choledochal cysts are dilatations of the biliary tract and usually cause biliary tract symptoms, such as jaundice, pain, and fever. On occasion, the presentation may be that of pancreatitis.

The diagnosis is usually easily made with ultrasonography, computed tomographic scanning, or biliary tract scan. Similarly, a choledochocele, an intraduodenal choledochal cyst, may present with pancreatitis. The diagnosis may be difficult and may sometimes be made only by endoscopic retrograde cholangio-pancreatography.

A number of rare conditions, such as Ivemark and Johanson-Blizzard syndromes, include pancreatic dysgenesis or dysfunction among their features. Many of these syndromes include renal and hepatic dysgenesis along with the pancreatic anomalies. Absence of islet cells and agenesis of the pancreas produce permanent diabetes mellitus, which begins in the neonatal period. Agenesis is also associated with malabsorption.

Hill ID, Lebenthal E: Congenital abnormalities of the exocrine pancreas. *In:* Go ELW, et al (eds): The Exocrine Pancreas: Biology, Pathology, and Diseases. 2nd ed. New York, Raven Press, 1993, pp 1029–1040.

Lans JI, Geenan JE, Johanson JF, Hogan WJ: Endoscopic therapy in patients with pancreas divisum and acute pancreatitis: A prospective, randomized, controlled clinical trial. Gastrointest Endosc 38:430, 1992.

293.2 Physiology

The functional unit of the exocrine pancreas is the acinus. Acinar cells are arranged in a semicircular array around a lumen. Ducts that drain the acini are lined by centroacinar cells and ductular cells. This arrangement allows for the secretions of the various cell types to mix.

The acinar cell synthesizes, stores, and secretes more than 20 enzymes, not all of which have been characterized. These enzymes are stored in zymogen granules, some in inactive forms. The relative concentration of the various enzymes in pancreatic juice is affected and is perhaps controlled by the diet probably by regulating the synthesis of specific messenger RNA. As a general rule, diets high in fat increase the concentration of lipase, a high-protein diet increases pancreatic content of proteases, and a high carbohydrate diet leads to increased content of amylase in the pancreatic juice.

α-*Amylase* splits starch into maltose, isomaltose, maltotriose, and dextrins.

Trypsin and *chymotrypsin,* both endopeptidases, and *carboxypeptidase,* an exopepetidase, are secreted by the pancreas as inactive proenzymes. Trypsinogen is activated in the gut lumen by *enterokinase,* a brush border enzyme. Trypsin can then activate trypsinogen, chymotrypsinogen, and procarboxypeptidase into their respective active forms. Enterokinase is, thus, a key enzyme for exocrine pancreatic function.

Pancreatic *lipase* requires colipase, a coenzyme also found in pancreatic fluid, for activity. Lipase liberates fatty acids from the one and three positions of triglycerides, leaving two—monoglycerides.

The stimuli for *exocrine pancreatic secretion* are neural and hormonal. Acetylcholine mediates the cephalic phase, whereas cholecystokinin (CCK), formerly called pancreozymin, mediates the intestinal phase. CCK is released from the duodenal mucosa by luminal amino acids and fatty acids. Feedback regulation of pancreatic secretion is mediated by pancreatic proteases in the duodenum. Secretion of CCK is inhibited by the digestion of a trypsin-sensitive, CCK-releasing peptide released in the lumen of the small intestine or by a monitor peptide released in pancreatic fluid.

Centroacinar and duct cells secrete water and bicarbonate. Bicarbonate secretion is under feedback control and is regulated by duodenal intraluminal pH. The stimulus for bicarbonate production is *secretin* in concert with CCK. Secretin cells are abundant in the duodenum.

Whereas normal pancreatic function is required for digestion, maldigestion occurs only after considerable reduction in pancreatic function has occurred. For instance, lipase and colipase secretion must be decreased by 90–98% before fat maldigestion occurs.

Although amylase and lipase are present in the pancreas early in gestation, secretion of both amylase and lipase is low in the infant. Adult levels of these enzymes are not reached in the duodenum until late in the 1st yr of life. Thus, digestion of the starch found in many infant formulas depends on the low levels of salivary amylase that reach the duodenum. This explains the diarrhea that may be seen in infants who are fed formulas high in glucose polymers or starch. In contrast, neonatal secretion of trypsinogen and chymotrypsinogen is at about 70% of the level found in the 1-yr-old infant. The low levels of amylase and lipase in duodenal contents of infants may be only partially compensated for by salivary amylase and lingual lipase. This explains the relative starch and fat intolerance of premature infants.

Hadorn HB, Munch G: The exocrine pancreas: Development, physiology and disease. *In:* Anderson CM, Burke V, Gracey M (eds): Pediatric Gastroenterology, 2nd ed. London, Blackwell, 1987.

Lloyd-Still JD, Listernick R, Buentello G: Complex carbohydrate intolerance: Diagnostic pitfalls and approach to management. J Pediatr 112:709, 1988.

Werlin SL: The exocrine pancreas. *In:* Walker WA, Durie PR, Hamilton JE, et al (eds): Pediatric Gastrointestinal Disease, 2nd ed. Philadelphia, Mosby–Year Book, 1995. In press.

CHAPTER 294
Pancreatic Function Tests

Pancreatic function can be measured by direct and indirect methods. Direct stimulation of the pancreas with a test (Lundh) meal of corn oil, skimmed milk powder, and dextrose or with secretin plus cholecystokinin can be performed. A triple-lumen tube is used to isolate the pancreatic secretions in the duodenum. Measurement of bicarbonate concentration and enzyme activity (trypsin, chymotrypsin, lipase, and amylase) is performed on the aspirated secretions. Normal values for children, excluding infants, are well established. Direct stimulation tests are uncomfortable and are not often needed.

A qualitative examination of the stool for *microscopic fat* globules is the most widely practiced screening test for malabsorption. However, analysis of random stool specimens by this method may give both false-positive and false-negative results. A 72-hr collection for *quantitative analysis of fat content* is preferable. The collection is usually performed at home, and the parent is asked to keep a careful dietary record, from which fat intake is calculated. A preweighed, sealable, plastic container is used, which the parent keeps in the freezer. Freezing helps to preserve the specimen but also reduces the odor. Infants are dressed in disposable diapers with the plastic side facing the skin so that the complete sample can be transferred to the container. Normal fat absorption is greater than 93% of intake.

Pancreatic enzyme activities can be measured in stool or duodenal contents. Stool trypsin has been the most commonly measured but is not as reliable as stool chymotrypsin. Neither test is as reliable as fecal fat analysis. Similarly, a random sample of duodenal fluid can be obtained and analyzed for pancreatic enzyme content. The elevated serum levels of trypsinogen found in neonates with cystic fibrosis form the basis of the newborn screening test being adapted in many states. With advancing pancreatic damage serum trypsinogen levels eventually fall below normal.

Bentiromide (*N*-benzoyl-L-tyrosyl-*p*-aminobenzoic acid, Chymex) is a synthetic tripeptide for noninvasive testing of pancreatic enzyme function. After oral ingestion bentiromide is cleaved by chymotrypsin, releasing para-aminobenzoic acid (PABA), which is absorbed and excreted by the kidneys. PABA may be measured in a serum specimen obtained at 90 min.

Pancreatic function can also be measured by *breath tests.* A labeled triglyceride, most commonly ^{14}C-triolein, is ingested and digested by pancreatic lipase in the duodenum liberating $^{14}CO_2$, which is detected in the expired air. Because of the radioactivity and long half-life of ^{14}C, this test is not appropriate for use in children. Research is now ongoing using triolein-labeled with ^{13}C, a stable, nonradioactive isotope. Although this test is safe for pediatric use, detection of $^{13}CO_2$ requires a mass spectrophotometer that is not generally available.

Laufer D, Cleghorn G, Forstner G, et al: The bentiromide test using plasma p-aminobenzoic acid for diagnosing pancreatic insufficiency in young children. Gastroenterology 101:207, 1991.

CHAPTER 295
Disorders of the Exocrine Pancreas

DISORDERS ASSOCIATED WITH PANCREATIC INSUFFICIENCY

Other than cystic fibrosis, conditions that cause pancreatic insufficiency are rare in children. They include Shwachman-Diamond syndrome, isolated enzyme deficiencies, enterokinase deficiency, chronic pancreatitis, and protein-calorie malnutrition (Chapter 286.2).

Cystic Fibrosis

See Chapter 363.

Cystic fibrosis is both the most common lethal genetic disease and the most common cause of malabsorption among white American children. By the end of the 1st year of life, 90% of children with cystic fibrosis have pancreatic insufficiency, leading to malnutrition in many cases. Treatment of the associated pancreatic insufficiency leads to improvement in absorption, better growth, and normalized stools.

Shwachman-Diamond Syndrome

See Chapter 124.

This is an autosomal recessive syndrome (1:20,000 births), consisting of pancreatic insufficiency, neutropenia, which may be intermittent, neutrophil chemotaxis defects, metaphyseal dysostosis, failure to thrive, and short stature. Patients present in infancy with poor growth and greasy, foul-smelling stools that are characteristic of malabsorption. These children can be readily differentiated from those with cystic fibrosis by their normal sweat chloride levels, lack of the cystic fibrosis gene, and characteristic metaphyseal lesions. Despite adequate pancreatic replacement therapy, poor growth frequently continues. Pancreatic insufficiency is often transient, and steatorrhea may spontaneously improve with age (frequently before 4 yr of age). The neutropenia may be cyclic. Recurrent pyogenic infections (otitis media, pneumonia, osteomyelitis, dermatitis, sepsis) are common and are a frequent cause of death. Thrombocytopenia is found in 70% of patients and anemia in 50% of patients. Pathologically, the pancreatic acini are replaced by fat with little fibrosis. Islet cells and ducts are normal. The fatty pancreas has a characteristic hypodense appearance on computed tomographic scan.

Isolated Enzyme Deficiencies

Isolated deficiencies of trypsinogen, lipase, and colipase have been reported, as has enterokinase deficiency. Although enterokinase is a brush border enzyme, deficiency causes pancreatic insufficiency because pancreatic proteases remain inactive. Deficiencies of trypsinogen or enterokinase manifest with failure to thrive, hypoproteinemia, and edema. Isolated amylase deficiency has not been shown to exist as a primary, permanent enzyme deficiency.

SYNDROMES ASSOCIATED WITH PANCREATIC INSUFFICIENCY

Pancreatic agenesis, the *Johanson-Blizzard syndrome* (pancreatic insufficiency, deafness, low birthweight, microcephaly, midline ectodermal scalp defects, psychomotor retardation, hypothyroidism, dwarfism, absent permanent teeth, and aplasia of the alae nasae), Pearson syndrome *(sideroblastic anemia)* with or without splenic atrophy (pancreatic insufficiency), congenital pancreatic hypoplasia, and congenital rubella are rare causes of pancreatic insufficiency. Some children with both syndromic (Alagille) and nonsyndromic paucity of intrahepatic bile ducts may also have pancreatic insufficiency associated with their liver disease. Pancreatic insufficiency has also been reported in duodenal atresia and stenosis and may also be seen in the rare infant with nesidioblastosis who requires 95% pancreatectomy to control hypoglycemia.

Aggett PJ, Cavanagh NPC, Matthew DJ, et al: Shwachman's syndrome: A review of 21 cases. Arch Dis Child 55:331, 1980.
Dupont C, Sellier N, Chochillon C, et al: Pancreatic lipomatosis and duodenal stenosis or atresia in children. J Pediatr 115:603, 1989.
Gaskin KJ, Durie PR, Lee L, et al: Colipase and lipase secretion in childhood-onset pancreatic insufficiency: Delineation of patients with steatorrhea secondary to relative colipase deficiency. Gastroenterology 86:1, 1984.
Hill RE, Durie PR, Gaskin KJ, et al: Steatorrhea and pancreatic insufficiency in Shwachman syndrome. Gastroenterology 83:22, 1982.
Rotig A, Cormier V, Blanche S, et al: Pearson's marrow pancreas syndrome. J Clin Invest 86:1601, 1990.
Schussheim A, Choi SJ: Exocrine pancreatic insufficiency with congenital anomalies. J Pediatr 89:782, 1976.

CHAPTER 296
Treatment of Pancreatic Insufficiency

Treatment of exocrine pancreatic insufficiency by oral replacement would seem rather simple. However, in practice, although creatorrhea can usually be corrected, steatorrhea is difficult to completely correct. This is due to variability of lipase activity in different commercial preparations, inadequate dosage, incorrect timing of doses, lipase inactivation by gastric acid, and the observation that chymotrypsin in the enzyme preparation digests and thus inactivates lipase. At present,

Pancrease, Creon, and Ultrase are the preparations used most widely. These products are enteric-coated preparations that resist gastric acid inactivation.

The dosage of pancreatic replacement for children depends on the amount of food eaten and, thus, can be established only by trial and error. Because these products contain excess protease compared with lipase, the dosage is estimated from the lipase requirement of 1,500 IU/kg/meal. An adequate dose is one that is followed by the return of the stools to normal fat content, size, color, and odor. Enzyme replacement should be given at the beginning of and with the meal. Tablets should be chewed; powder can be mixed with a small quantity of food. Enzyme must also be given with snacks.

When adequate fat absorption cannot be realized, gastric acid neutralization with an antacid or an H_2-receptor blocking agent will prevent gastric acid enzyme inactivation and improve delivery of lipase into the intestine. In selected cases omeprazole, a proton pump inhibitor, is required to normalize digestion. The coating of enteric-coated preparations also protects lipase from acid inactivation.

Untoward effects secondary to pancreatic enzyme replacement therapy include allergic reactions, increased uric acid levels, and kidney stones; colonic strictures have been attributed to high-strength pancreatic enzymes.

Smyth RL, Van Velzen D, Smyth AR, et al: Strictures of the ascending colon in cystic fibrosis and high strength pancreatic enzymes. Lancet 343:85, 1994.

CHAPTER 297
Pancreatitis

After cystic fibrosis, acute pancreatitis is probably the most common pancreatic disorder in children. Mumps, other viral illnesses, drugs, biliary microlithiasis (sludging), and blunt abdominal injuries account for most known etiologies; other causes are uncommon (Table 297–1). Many cases are of unknown etiology or are secondary to a systemic disease process. Child abuse is recognized with increased frequency as a cause of traumatic pancreatitis in young children. Defined causes of pancreatitis include the hemolytic uremic syndrome, Kawasaki syndrome, refeeding after starvation, pancreas divisum, bone marrow transplantation, brain tumor, and head trauma.

PATHOGENESIS. The precise sequence of events leading to pancreatitis is unknown. It is proposed that after an initial insult, such as ductal obstruction, pancreatic proenzymes are activated after co-localization with lysosomal hydrolases within the acinar cell, leading to autodigestion and further activation and release of active proteases. Lecithin is activated by phospholipase A2 into the toxic lysolecithin. Prophospholipase is unstable and can be activated by minute quantities of trypsin. The healthy pancreas is protected by three factors: (1) the process by which pancreatic proteases are synthesized as inactive proenzymes, (2) the process by which digestive enzymes are segregated into secretory granules, and (3) the presence of protease inhibitors.

The histopathologic findings of acute pancreatitis are related to the release of activated proteolytic and lipolytic enzymes. Interstitial edema appears early. Later, as the episode of pancreatitis progresses, localized and confluent necrosis, blood vessel disruption, leading to hemorrhage, and an inflammatory response in the peritoneum may develop.

CLINICAL MANIFESTATIONS. The patient with acute pancreatitis has abdominal pain, persistent vomiting, and fever. The pain is epigastric and steady, often resulting in the child assuming an antalgic position with hips and knees flexed, sitting upright or lying on the side. The child is very uncomfortable and irritable and appears acutely ill. The abdomen may be distended and quite tender. A mass may be palpable. The pain increases in intensity for 24–48 hr, during which time vomiting may increase and the patient may require hospitalization for dehydration and need fluid and electrolyte therapy. The prognosis for the acute uncomplicated case is excellent.

Acute hemorrhage pancreatitis, the most severe form of acute pancreatitis, is rare in children. In this life-threatening condition, the patient is acutely ill with severe nausea, vomiting, and abdominal pain. Shock, high fever, jaundice, ascites, hypocalcemia, and pleural effusions may occur. A bluish discoloration may be seen around the umbilicus (Cullen sign) or in the flanks (Grey Turner sign). The pancreas is necrotic and may be transformed into an inflammatory hemorrhagic mass. The mortality rate, which is approximately 50%, is related to the *systemic inflammatory response syndrome:* shock, renal failure, adult respiratory distress syndrome, disseminated intravascular coagulation, massive gastrointestinal bleeding, and systemic or intra-abdominal infection.

DIAGNOSIS. Acute pancreatitis is usually diagnosed by mea-

■ **TABLE 297–1 Causes of Acute Pancreatitis in Children**

Drugs and Toxins	**Systemic Disease**
Alcohol	α_1-Antitrypsin deficiency
5-Amino salicylate	Bone marrow transplantation
Azathioprine	Brain tumor
L-asparaginase	Carnitine palmitoyltransferase II deficiency
Cimetidine	Crohn disease
Corticosteroids	Cystic fibrosis
DDI	Diabetes mellitus
Erythromycin	Glycogen storage disease type Ia
Estrogen	Head trauma
Furosemide	Hemochromatosis
6-Mercaptopurine	Hemolytic-uremic syndrome
Mesalamine	Schönlein-Henoch purpura
Methyldopa	Homocystinuria
Pentamidine	3-Hydroxy-3 methylglutaryl-coenzyme A lyase deficiency
Scorpion bites	Hyperlipoproteinemia types I and IV
Sulfonamides	Hyperparathyroidism
Sulindac	Isovaleric acidemia
Tetracycline	Kawasaki disease
Thiazides	Malnutrition
Valproic acid	Methylmalonic acidemia
Hereditary Pancreatitis	Periarteritis nodosa
Idiopathic	Peptic ulcer
Infectious	After pancreas transplantation
Coxsackie B virus	Refeeding after malnutrition
Epstein-Barr virus	Systemic lupus erythematosus
Hepatitis A virus	Uremia
Influenza A virus	**Traumatic**
Malaria	Blunt injury
Measles	Child abuse
Mumps	Surgical trauma
Mycoplasma	Total body cast
Rubella	
Reye syndrome: varicella, influenza B	
Obstructive	
Ampullary disease	
Ascariasis	
Biliary microlithiasis (sludging)	
Biliary tract malformations	
Cholelithiasis and choledocholithiasis	
Crohn disease	
Duplication cyst	
ERCP complication	
After liver transplantation	
Pancreas divisum	
Pancreatic ductal abnormalities	
Pancreatic pseudocyst	
Postoperative	
Tumor	

DDI = Dideoxyinosine; ERCP = endoscopic retrograde cholangiopancreatography.

■ TABLE 297–2 Differential Diagnosis of Hyperamylasemia

Pancreatic Pathology
Acute or chronic pancreatitis
Complications of pancreatitis (pseudocyst, ascites, abscess)
Factitious pancreatitis
Salivary Gland Pathology
Parotitis (mumps, *Staphylococcus aureus*, CMV, HIV, EBV)
Sialadenitis (calculus, radiation)
Eating disorders (anorexia nervosa, bulimia)
Intra-Abdominal Pathology
Biliary tract disease (cholelithiasis)
Peptic ulcer perforation
Peritonitis
Intestinal obstruction
Appendicitis
Systemic Diseases
Metabolic acidosis (diabetes mellitus, shock)
Renal insufficiency, transplantation
Burns
Pregnancy
Drugs (morphine)
Head injury
Cardiopulmonary bypass

CMV = cytomegalovirus; HIV = human immunodeficiency virus; EBV = Epstein-Barr virus.

surement of serum amylase and lipase activities. The serum amylase level is typically elevated for up to 4 days. A variety of other conditions may also cause hyperamylasemia without pancreatitis (Table 297–2). The use of the ratio of renal clearances of amylase and creatinine does not improve the sensitivity and specificity of the serum amylase determination. Elevation of the salivary amylase may mislead the clinician into making the diagnosis of pancreatitis in a child with abdominal pain, but the laboratory can separate amylase isoenzymes into pancreatic and salivary fractions. Initially, serum amylase levels are normal in 10–15% of patients. Serum lipase is more specific than amylase for acute inflammatory pancreatic disease and should be determined when pancreatitis is suspected and the amylase level is normal. The serum lipase typically remains elevated 8–14 days longer than serum amylase. Serum lipase may also be elevated in nonpancreatic diseases.

Other laboratory abnormalities that may be present in acute pancreatitis include hemoconcentration, coagulopathy, leukocytosis, hyperglycemia, glucosuria, hypocalcemia, elevated gamma glutamyl transpeptidase, and hyperbilirubinemia.

Roentgenography of the chest and abdomen may demonstrate nonspecific findings. The chest roentgenogram may demonstrate platelike atelectasis, basilar infiltrates, elevation of the hemidiaphragm, left (rarely right)-sided pleural effusions, pericardial effusion, and pulmonary edema. Abdominal roentgenograms may demonstrate a sentinel loop, dilatation of the transverse colon (cutoff sign), ileus, pancreatic calcification (if recurrent), blurring of the left psoas margin, a pseudocyst, diffuse abdominal haziness (ascites), and peripancreatic extraluminal gas bubbles.

Ultrasound and *computed tomographic (CT) scanning* have major roles in the diagnosis and follow-up of children with pancreatitis. Findings may include pancreatic enlargement, a hypoechoic, sonolucent edematous pancreas, pancreatic masses, fluid collections, and abscesses (Fig. 297–1). As many as 20% of children with pancreatitis initially have normal imaging studies. Endoscopic retrograde cholangiopancreatography (ERCP) is essential in the investigation of recurrent pancreatitis, pancreas divisum, sphincter of Oddi dysfunction, and disease associated with gallbladder pathology.

TREATMENT. The aims of medical management are to relieve pain and restore metabolic homeostasis. Meperidine is the drug of choice for pain relief and should be given in adequate doses. Fluid, electrolyte, and mineral balance should be restored and maintained. Nasogastric suction is useful in patients who are vomiting. The patient should be maintained with nothing by mouth. The routine use of antibiotics is of no benefit during the acute phase unless secondary infection is present. The response to treatment is usually complete over 2–4 days. Refeeding may commence when the serum amylase has normalized and clinical symptoms have resolved.

Although surgical therapy of acute pancreatitis is rarely required, the treatment of severe acute pancreatitis may involve total parenteral nutrition and surgical drainage of necrotic material or abscesses. Newer modalities include peritoneal lavage to reduce the risk of secondary infection and the use of trypsin inhibitors. Endoscopic therapy may be of benefit when pancreatitis is caused by anatomic abnormalities, such as strictures or stones.

PROGNOSIS. In adults, poor prognostic factors on admission include blood glucose greater than 200 mg/dL, leukocytosis more than 16,000, serum lactate dehydrogenase more than 700 IU, and SGOT more than 250 IU. High-risk factors within the first 48 hr include a decrease in hematocrit of more than 10%, hypocalcemia less than 8 mg/dL, base deficit more than 4 mEq/L, blood urea nitrogen more than 50 mg/dL, hypoxia (partial pressure of arterial oxygen less than 60 mm Hg), and large 3rd space losses. Prognostic factors have not been

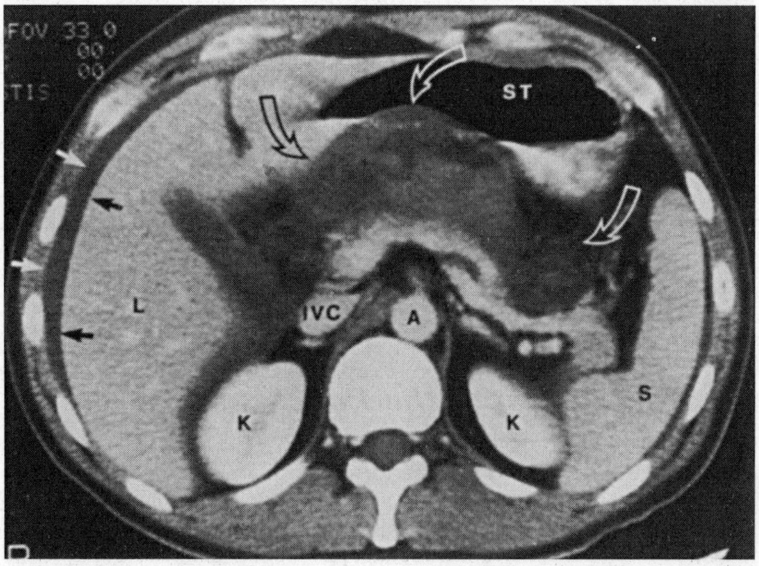

Figure 297–1. Acute pancreatitis. Computed tomography (CT) through the body of the pancreas demonstrates a halo of decreased attenuation around the pancreas that represents a peripancreatic zone of edema and fluid *(curved arrows)*. Note the pancreatic ascites most obvious lateral to the liver *(small arrows)*. If intravenous contrast was administered before the CT scan, the inflamed pancreas would appear more dense (whiter). (L = liver; A = aorta; K = kidney; S = spleen; IVC = inferior vena cava; ST = stomach.) (From Freeny P, Lawson T: The pancreas. *In:* Putman CE, Ravin CE [eds]: Textbook of Diagnostic Imaging. Philadelphia, WB Saunders, 1988.)

developed for children with pancreatitis. These poor prognostic findings are noted in lethal hemorrhagic pancreatitis.

Clavien P-A, Robert J, Meyer P, et al: Acute pancreatitis and normoamylasemia: Not an uncommon combination. Ann Surg 210:614, 1989.
Elistur Y, Hunt J, Chertow B: Hereditary pancreatitis in children in West Virginia. Pediatrics 93:528, 1994.
Ranson JHC, Berman RS: Peritoneal lavage decreases pancreatic sepsis in pancreatitis. Ann Surg 211:708, 1990.
Tein I, Christodoulou J, Donner E, et al: Carnitine palmitoyltransferase II deficiency: A new cause of recurrent pancreatitis. J Pediatr 124:938, 1994.
Weizman Z, Durie PR: Acute pancreatitis in childhood. J Pediatr 113:24, 1988.

297.1 *Chronic Pancreatitis*

Chronic, relapsing pancreatitis in children is frequently hereditary or due to congenital anomalies of the pancreatic or biliary ductal systems. The former disease is transmitted as an autosomal dominant trait with complete penetrance but variable expressivity. Symptoms frequently begin in the 1st decade but are usually mild at the onset. Although spontaneous recovery from each attack occurs in 4–7 days, episodes may become progressively more severe. Hereditary pancreatitis is diagnosed by the presence of the disease in successive generations of a family. An evaluation during symptom-free intervals may be unrewarding until calcifications, pseudocysts, or pancreatic insufficiency develop.

Other conditions associated with chronic relapsing pancreatitis are hyperlipidemia (types I, IV, and V), hyperparathyroidism, ascariasis, and cystic fibrosis. Although it has been thought that most cases of recurrent pancreatitis in childhood are idiopathic, congenital anomalies of the ductal systems, such as pancreas divisum, are probably more common than previously recognized.

A thorough diagnostic *evaluation* of every child with more than one episode of pancreatitis is indicated. Serum lipid, calcium, and phosphorus levels are determined. Stools are evaluated for *Ascaris,* and a sweat test is performed. Plain abdominal films are evaluated for the presence of pancreatic calcifications. Abdominal ultrasound or CT scanning is performed to detect the presence of a pseudocyst. The biliary tract is evaluated for the presence of stones.

ERCP is a technique that can be used to define the anatomy of the gland and is mandatory whenever surgery is considered. This technique should be performed as part of the evaluation of any child with idiopathic, nonresolving, or recurrent pancreatitis and in patients with a pseudocyst before surgery. In these cases, ERCP may detect a previously undiagnosed anatomic defect that may be amenable to endoscopic or surgical therapy. Endoscopic treatments include sphincterotomy, stone extraction, and insertion of pancreatic or biliary endoprostheses. These treatments allow for successful nonsurgical management of conditions previously requiring surgical intervention.

Brown CB, Werlin SL, Geenen JE, et al: The diagnostic and therapeutic role of endoscopic retrograde cholanjeography in children. J Pediatr Gastroenterol Nutr 17:19, 1993.
Rothstein F, Wyllie R, Gauderer M: Hereditary pancreatitis and recurrent abdominal pain of childhood. J Pediatr Surg 20:535, 1985.

CHAPTER 298
Pseudocyst of the Pancreas

Pancreatic pseudocyst formation is an uncommon sequela to acute or chronic pancreatitis. Pseudocysts are sacs delineated by a fibrous wall in the lesser peritoneal sac. They may enlarge or extend in almost any direction, thus producing a wide variety of symptoms (Fig. 298–1).

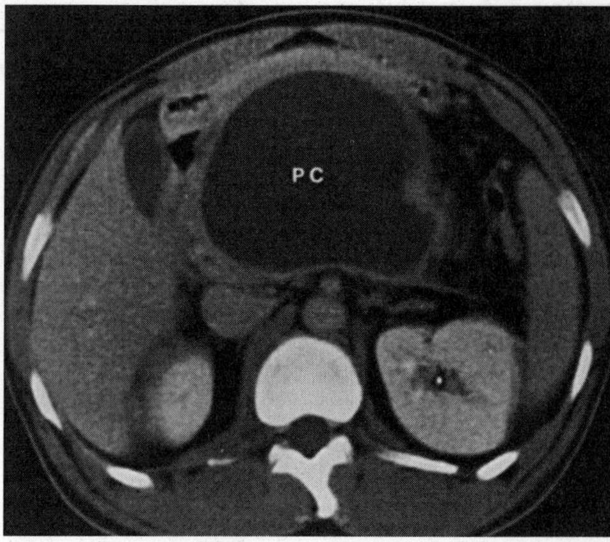

Figure 298–1. Pseudocyst. Follow-up computed tomographic scan 5 mo after the episode of acute pancreatitis demonstrates a large pseudocyst (PC). This large pseudocyst will probably not resolve spontaneously and may need drainage. (From Freeny P, Lawson T: The pancreas. *In:* Putman CE, Ravin CE [eds]: Textbook of Diagnostic Imaging. Philadelphia, WB Saunders, 1988.)

A pancreatic pseudocyst is suggested when an episode of pancreatitis fails to resolve or when a mass develops after an episode of pancreatitis. Clinical features usually include pain, nausea, and vomiting. The most common signs are a palpable mass in 50% of patients and jaundice in 10%. Other findings include ascites and pleural effusions (usually left-sided).

The most useful diagnostic techniques are ultrasonography, computed tomographic scanning, and endoscopic retrograde cholangiopancreatography (ERCP). Because of its ease, availability, and reliability, ultrasonography is the 1st choice. Sequential studies using ultrasonography in adults with pancreatitis have shown that the incidence of pseudocyst formation is greater than previously thought but that most small pseudocysts resolve spontaneously. It is generally recommended that the patient with acute pancreatitis undergo an ultrasonographic evaluation 2–4 wk after resolution of the acute episode for an evaluation of possible pseudocyst formation.

Until recently, the treatment of nonresolving, large pseudocysts has been surgical. However, percutaneous drainage of pseudocysts has now been shown to be safe and effective treatment in most patients. A pseudocyst must be allowed to mature for 4–6 wk before surgical drainage is attempted; however, percutaneous drainage may be attempted earlier. ERCP should precede surgical treatment to help the surgeon plan the approach and define anatomic abnormalities. Endoscopic drainage is an alternative nonsurgical treatment of pancreatic pseudocysts.

Jaffe RB, Arata IA Jr, Matlak ME: Percutaneous drainage of traumatic pancreatic pseudocysts in children. AJR 152:591, 1989.
Millar AJW, Rode H, Studen RJ, et al: Management of pancreatic pseudocysts in children. J Pediatr Surg 23:122, 1988.

CHAPTER 299

Pancreatic Tumors

NEOPLASIA

Pancreatic tumors of childhood include both β and non–β cell tumors. Non-β cell tumors include gastrinomas and VIPomas. Secretion of gastrin by the gastrinoma produces the Zollinger-Ellison syndrome, with intractable peptic ulcer disease or diarrhea (see Table 291–1). The treatment of choice is surgical removal of the tumor. Because most tumors have metastasized by the time of diagnosis, cure is often not possible. The two options that remain are total gastrectomy and treatment with H_2 receptor (cimetidine, ranitidine) or H^+/K^+-ATPase pump (omeprazole) blocking agents that inhibit gastric acid secretion. In appropriate doses, these drugs not only provide symptomatic relief but also avoid the complications of total gastrectomy.

The *watery diarrhea–hypokalemia-acidosis syndrome* is usually produced by the secretion of vasoactive intestinal peptide (VIP) by a non-β cell tumor (VIPoma) (see Table 291–1). VIP levels are frequently, but not always, increased in the serum. Treatment is surgical removal of the tumor. When this is not possible, symptoms may be controlled by the use of octreotide acetate (cyclic somatostatin, Sandostatin), a synthetic analog of somatostatin. Pancreatic tumors secreting a variety of hormones, including glucagon, somatostatin, and pancreatic polypeptide, have also been described.

Pancreatoblastomas, pancreatic adenocarcinomas, cystadenomas, and rhabdomyosarcomas are rarely encountered. The *Frantz tumor* is a papillary cystic tumor that is usually found in girls and young women. Presenting symptoms are usually abdominal pain, mass, or jaundice. The treatment of choice is total surgical removal.

Insulinomas and nesidioblastosis or hyperplasia of the β cells produce symptomatic hypoglycemia. Massive subtotal or total pancreatectomy is the treatment of choice when medical treatment fails (Chapter 77). These children may then develop pancreatic insufficiency or diabetes as a complication of treatment.

SECTION 6

Liver and Biliary System

CHAPTER 300

Development and Function

William F. Balistreri

MORPHOGENESIS. The liver and biliary system originate from a cluster of cells that cap a ventral diverticulum in the primitive foregut. The hepatic anlage (pars hepatis) appears during the 4th wk of gestation as a duodenal diverticulum (Fig. 300–1). Within the ventral mesentery proliferation of cells forms anastomosing hepatic cords, with the network of primitive liver cells, sinusoids, and septal mesenchyme establishing the basic architectural pattern of liver lobule. The solid *cranial* portion of the hepatic diverticulum eventually forms hepatic glandular tissue and the intrahepatic bile ducts; the *caudal* portion (pars cystica) becomes the gallbladder, cystic duct, and common bile duct.

The hepatic lobules are identifiable at the 6th gestational wk. The liver reaches a peak relative size at the 9th wk at about 10% of the fetal weight. The bile canalicular structures that include microvilli and junctional complexes are specialized loci of the liver cell membrane; these appear very early in gestation, and by 6–7 wk large canaliculi bounded by several hepatocytes are seen. The intrahepatic bile ducts are derived through branching of the hepatic duct; formation is complete by the 3rd mo. The cystic duct and the gallbladder are fully recanalized by the 7th–8th wk.

In the hepatic excretory (biliary) system, intercellular bile canaliculi empty into the smallest bile ductules, which unite to form interlobular bile ducts that follow the terminal branches of the portal vein. At the hilum of the liver, the intrahepatic ducts leave the branches of the portal vein and merge to form the *extrahepatic* biliary system. The ducts of the right and left lobes form the common hepatic duct. The common bile duct is formed from the merger of the common hepatic duct and cystic duct; it runs along the right edge of the lesser omentum, terminating as the intramural papilla of Vater. Union of the biliary tract with the pancreatic ducts forms the ampulla of Vater, which, with the sphincter of Oddi, regulates the flow of bile into the intestine, prevents entry of bile into the pancreatic duct, and inhibits reflux of intestinal contents into the ducts.

The transport and metabolic activities of the liver are facilitated by the structural arrangement of liver cell cords (Fig. 300–1*D*), which are formed by rows of hepatocytes, separated by sinusoids that converge toward the tributaries of the hepatic vein (the central vein) located in the center of the lobule. This establishes the pathways and patterns of flow for substances to and from the liver. Plasma proteins and other plasma components are *secreted* by the liver. Absorbed and circulating nutrients arrive through the portal vein or the hepatic artery and pass through the sinusoids and past the hepatocytes to the systemic circulation at the central vein. Biliary components are transported via the series of enlarging channels from the bile canaliculi through the bile ductule to the common bile duct.

Bile secretion has been noted at the 12th gestational wk. The major components of bile vary with stage of development. Near term, cholesterol and phospholipid content is relatively low; and low concentrations of bile acids, the absence of bacterially derived (secondary) bile acids, and the presence of unusual bile acids reflect low rates of bile flow and immature bile acid synthesis.

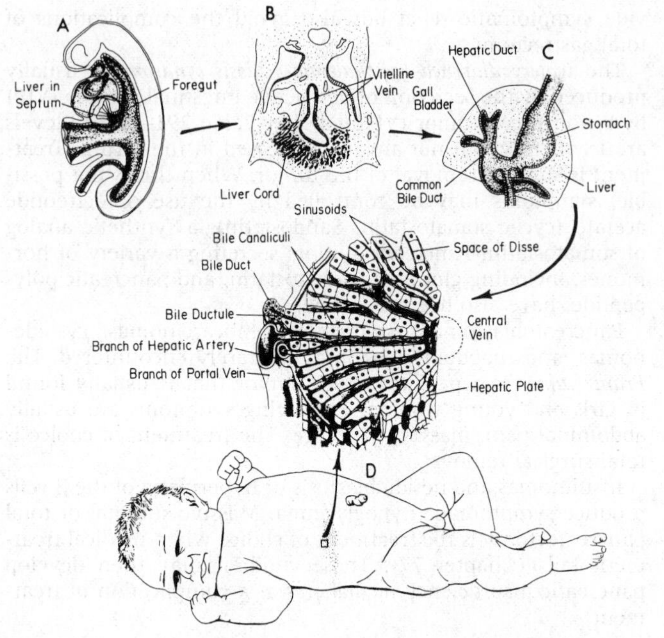

Figure 300–1. Hepatic embryogenesis. ***A,*** **Ventral outgrowth of hepatic diverticulum from foregut endoderm in the 3.5-wk embryo.** ***B,*** **Between the two vitelline veins, the enlarging hepatic diverticulum buds off epithelial (liver) cords that become the liver parenchyma, around which the endothelium of capillaries (sinusoids) align (4-wk embryo).** ***C,*** **Hemisection of embryo at 7.5 wk demonstrating recanalization of the biliary tract.** ***D,*** **Three-dimensional representation of the hepatic lobule as present in the newborn. (From Andres JM, Mathis RK, Walker WA: Liver disease in infants. Parts I and II: Developmental hepatology and mechanisms of liver dysfunction. J Pediatr 90:686 and 964, 1977.)**

Fetal hepatic blood flow is derived from the hepatic artery and from the portal and umbilical veins, which form the portal sinus. The portal venous inflow is directed mainly to the right lobe of the liver; umbilical flow is primarily to the left. The ductus venosus shunts blood from the portal and umbilical veins to the hepatic vein, bypassing the sinusoidal network. The ductus venosus becomes obliterated when oral feedings are initiated. The oxygen saturation is lower in portal than in umbilical venous blood; accordingly, the right hepatic lobe has lower oxygenation and greater hematopoietic activity than the left hepatic lobe. Sinusoidal endothelium is the site of large macrophages, which become the Kupffer (reticulo-endothelial) cell network.

The liver constitutes 5% of body weight at birth but only 2% in the adult. Early in gestation (7th wk), hematopoietic cells outnumber functioning hepatocytes in the hepatic anlage. The hepatocytes are smaller (~20 μm) than at maturity (30–35 μm) and contain less glycogen. Near term, the hepatocytes dominate the organ, and cell size and glycogen content increase. Hematopoiesis is virtually absent by the 2nd postnatal month in full-term infants. As the density of hepatocytes increases with gestational age, the relative volume of the sinusoidal network decreases.

ULTRASTRUCTURE. Our understanding of the ultrastructural anatomy of the hepatocyte (Fig. 300–2) has been made possible through electron microscopy and cell fractionation techniques. Various regions of the hepatocyte *plasma membrane* exhibit specialized functions. For example, bidirectional transport occurs at the sinusoidal surface, where materials reaching the liver via the portal system enter and compounds secreted by the liver leave the hepatocyte. Canalicular membranes of adjacent hepatocytes form bile canaliculi, which are bounded by tight junctions preventing transfer of secreted compounds back into the sinusoid. Abundant *mitochondria* are the sites of oxidation and metabolism of heterogeneous classes of substrates, of fatty acid oxidation, of key processes in gluconeogenesis, and of storage and release of energy. The *nucleus* and *nucleolus* are surrounded by a pair of membranes, the outermost of which adjoins the *endoplasmic reticulum.* The latter is a continuous network of rough- and smooth-surfaced tubules and cisternae, which are the site of various processes, including protein and triglyceride synthesis and drug metabolism. The endoplasmic reticulum is the major part of the *microsomal* fraction obtained by ultracentrifugation of liver homogenate. Low fetal activity of microsomal-bound enzymes accounts for a relative inefficiency of xenobiotic (drug) metabolism. The *Golgi apparatus* is active in protein packaging and possibly in bile secretion. Hepatocyte microbodies *(peroxisomes)* are single-membrane-limited cytoplasmic organelles that contain enzymes such as oxidases and catalase and those that play a role in lipid and bile acid metabolism. The *cytoskeleton,* composed of actin filaments, is distributed throughout the cell and concentrated near the plasma membrane. Microfilaments and microtubules may play a role in receptor-mediated endocytosis, in bile secretion, and in maintaining the architecture and motility of the cell. *Lysosomes* contain numerous hydrolases that play a role in intracellular digestion.

FUNCTIONAL DEVELOPMENT. Several of these metabolic processes are immature in the healthy newborn infant, owing in part to the fetal patterns of activity of various enzymatic processes. Many hepatic functions are carried out for the fetus by the maternal liver, which provides nutrients, serves as a route of elimination of metabolic end products, and is a site of biotransformations. Fetal liver metabolism is devoted primarily to the production of proteins for growth requirements. Toward term, primary functions become production and storage of essential nutrients, excretion of bile, and establishment of processes of elimination. Extrauterine adaptation involves de novo enzyme synthesis. Modulation of these processes depends on substrate and hormonal input via the placenta and on dietary and hormonal input in the postnatal period.

300.1 Metabolic Functions of the Liver

CARBOHYDRATE METABOLISM. The liver stores excess carbohydrate as glycogen, a polymer of glucose readily hydrolyzed to glucose during fasting. Immediately after birth, the infant is dependent on hepatic glycogenolysis; thereafter, the infant is capable of both glycogenolysis and gluconeogenesis. Fetal glycogen synthesis begins at about the 9th wk of gestation, with glycogen stores most rapidly accumulated near term, when the liver contains two to three times the amount of glycogen of adult liver. The majority of this stored glycogen is utilized in the immediate postnatal period. Reaccumulation is initiated at about the 2nd wk of postnatal life, and glycogen stores reach adult levels at approximately the 3rd wk in healthy full-term infants. The fluctuations in serum glucose concentration in preterm infants are due in part to the fact that efficient regulation of the synthesis, storage, and degradation of glycogen develops only near the end of full-term gestation. Dietary carbohydrates such as galactose are converted to glucose, but there is a substantial dependence on gluconeogenesis for glucose in early life, especially if glycogen stores are limited. Gluconeogenic activity is present in the fetal liver but increases rapidly after birth.

PROTEIN METABOLISM. During the rapid fetal growth phase, specific decarboxylases that are rate limiting in the biosynthesis of physiologically important polyamines have higher activities

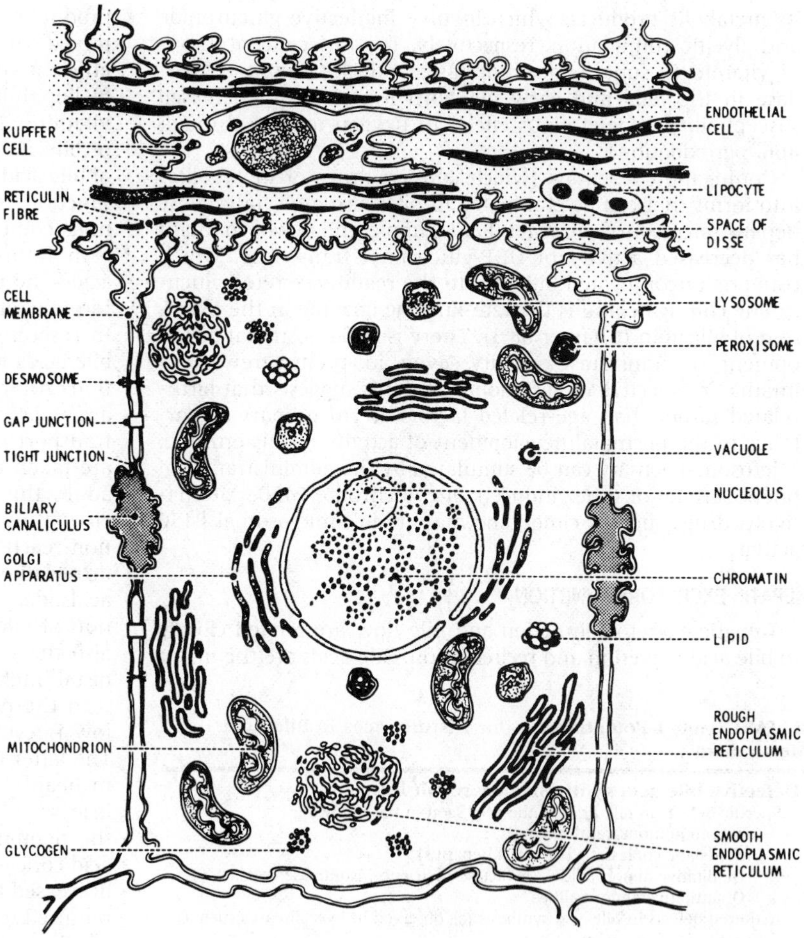

Figure 300–2. Hepatic ultrastructure, conceptualized. Electron microscopic appearance of a normal human liver cell. (From Sherlock S: Hepatic cell structure. *In:* Sherlock S (ed): Diseases of the Liver and Biliary System, Chapter 1. Oxford, Blackwell Scientific, 1981.)

than in the mature liver. The rate of synthesis of albumin and secretory proteins in the developing liver parallels the quantitative changes in endoplasmic reticulum. Synthesis of albumin appears at approximately the 7th–8th wk in the human fetus and increases in inverse proportion to that of α-fetoprotein, which is a dominant fetal protein. By the 3rd–4th mo of gestation, the fetal liver is able to produce fibrinogen, transferrin, and low-density lipoproteins. From this period on, fetal plasma contains each of the major protein classes, at concentrations considerably below those achieved at maturity.

The *postnatal* patterns of development of various proteins are heterogeneous. Lipoproteins of each class rise abruptly in the 1st wk after birth to reach levels that will vary little until puberty. Albumin concentrations are low in the neonate (~2.5 g/dL), reaching adult levels (~3.5 g/dL) after several months. Levels of ceruloplasmin and complement factors increase slowly to adult values during the 1st year. In contrast, transferrin levels at birth are similar to those of the adult, decline for 3–5 mo, and rise thereafter to achieve their final concentrations. Low levels of activity of specific proteins have implications for the nutrition of the infant; for example, a low level of cystathionase activity impairs the trans-sulfuration pathway by which dietary methionine is converted to cystine; accordingly, the latter must be supplied exogenously. Similar dietary requirements may exist for other sulfur-containing amino acids, such as taurine.

LIPID METABOLISM. Fatty acid oxidation provides a major source of energy in early life, complementing glycogenolysis and gluconeogenesis. The newborn infant is relatively intolerant of prolonged fasting, owing in part to a restricted capacity for hepatic ketogenesis. Rapid maturation of the ability of the liver to oxidize fatty acid occurs during the 1st few days of life. Milk provides the major source of calories in early life; this high-fat, low-carbohydrate diet mandates active gluconeogenesis to maintain blood sugar levels. When the glucose supply is limited, ketone body production from endogenous fatty acids may provide energy for hepatic gluconeogenesis and an alternative fuel for brain metabolism. Metabolic processes involving lipid and lipoprotein are predominantly hepatic; liver immaturity or disease affects lipid concentrations and lipoproteins.

BIOTRANSFORMATION. The newborn infant has a decreased capacity to metabolize and detoxify certain drugs, owing to underdevelopment of the hepatic microsomal component that is the site of the specific oxidative, reductive, hydrolytic, and conjugation reactions required for these biotransformations (Chapter 63). The major components of the mono-oxygenase system, such as cytochrome P450, the reduced form of necotinamide-adenine dinucleotide phosphate, and cytochrome C-reductase, are present in low concentrations in fetal microsomal preparations. In the full-term infant, hepatic uridine diphosphate (UDP) glucuronyl transferase and enzymes involved in the oxidation of polycyclic aromatic hydrocarbons have very low activities. Age-related differences in pharmacokinetics vary. For example, the half-life of acetaminophen in a newborn is similar to that of an adult, whereas theophylline has a half-life of approximately 100 hr in the premature infant and 5–6 hr in the adult. These physiologic variables taken together with factors such as binding to plasma proteins and renal clearance are important in determining drug dosage and in the production of toxicity. Dramatic examples of the susceptibility of the newborn infant to drug toxicity are the responses to chloramphenicol (gray syndrome) or to benzoyl alcohol and its metabolic products, which involve ineffective glucuronide and glycine conjugation, respectively. The low concentrations of vitamin E, superoxide dismutase, and glutathione peroxidase in the fetal and early newborn liver lead to increased susceptibility to deleterious effects of oxygen toxicity through lipid peroxidation.

Conjugation reactions (which convert drugs or metabolites into forms that can be eliminated in bile) also are catalyzed by hepatic microsomal enzymes. For example, the newborn infant has decreased activity of UDP-glucuronyl transferase, which converts unconjugated bilirubin to the readily excreted glucuronide conjugate and is the rate-limiting enzyme in the excretion of bilirubin (Chapter 88.3). There is rapid postnatal development of transferase activity, even in prematurely born infants, irrespective of gestational age; this suggests that birth-related rather than age-related factors are of primary importance in the postnatal development of activity of this enzyme. Microsomal activity can be stimulated by the administration of phenobarbital or other inducers of cytochrome P450. Alternatively, drugs such as cimetidine may inhibit microsomal P450 activity.

HEPATIC EXCRETORY FUNCTION

Hepatic excretory function and bile flow are related closely to bile acid excretion and recirculation. Bile acids are the major product of degradation of cholesterol. Their incorporation into mixed micelles with cholesterol and phospholipid creates an efficient vehicle for the solubilization and intestinal absorption of lipophilic compounds, such as dietary fats and fat-soluble vitamins. The secretion of bile acids is the major determinant of bile flow in the mature animal. Accordingly, the maturity of bile acid metabolic processes affects overall hepatic excretory function, including biliary excretion of endogenous and exogenous compounds.

In humans, two bile acids (cholic and chenodeoxycholic acid—the primary bile acids) are synthesized in the liver. Before excretion, they are conjugated with glycine and taurine. In response to a meal, contraction of the gallbladder delivers bile acids to the intestine to assist in fat digestion and absorption. After mediating fat digestion, the bile acids themselves are reabsorbed from the terminal ileum through specific active transport processes. They return to the liver via portal blood, are taken up by liver cells, and are re-excreted in bile. In the adult, this enterohepatic circulation involves 90–95% of the circulating bile acid pool. Bile acids that escape ileal reabsorption reach the colon, where the bacterial flora, through dehydroxylation and deconjugation, produces the secondary bile acids, deoxycholate and lithocholate. In the adult the composition of bile reflects the excretion of not only the primary but also the secondary bile acids, which are reabsorbed from the distal intestinal tract.

In the neonate, there is inefficient ileal reabsorption and a low rate of hepatic clearance of bile acids from portal blood. The latter results in elevated serum concentrations of bile acids in healthy newborns, often to levels that would suggest liver disease in older individuals. The size of the bile acid pool in the neonate is about one half that of the adult, and the bile acid concentration in the proximal intestinal lumen is similarly decreased to levels that are frequently below the concentration required for micelle formation (2 mM); accordingly, absorption of dietary fats and fat-soluble vitamins is reduced but not sufficiently to produce malabsorption. Transient phases of "physiologic cholestasis" and "physiologic steatorrhea" play a role in the nutrition of low-birthweight infants but are of minor importance to healthy full-term newborns.

Beyond the neonatal period, disturbances in bile acid metabolism may be responsible for diverse effects on hepatobiliary and intestinal function (Table 300–1).

■ **TABLE 300–1 Potential Sites for Disturbances in Bile Acid Metabolism**

Defective bile acid synthesis may result from:
- Specific defects in bile acid synthesis as seen in the following:
  - Cerebrotendinous xanthomatosis
  - Intrahepatic cholestasis (neonatal hepatitis)
    - Qualitative abnormalities (reductase deficiency, isomerase deficiency)
    - Quantitative abnormalities
- Acquired defects in bile acid synthesis (as observed in liver diseases such as hepatitis and cirrhosis)

Abnormalities of bile acid delivery to the bowel may be seen in:
- Celiac sprue (sluggish gallbladder contraction)
- Extrahepatic bile duct obstruction caused by the following:
  - Biliary atresia
  - Stricture
  - Stone
  - Malignancy

Interruption of the enterohepatic circulation of bile acids may occur with:
- An external bile fistula
- Ileojejunal exclusion for exogenous obesity or hypercholesterolemia
- Cystic fibrosis
- Contaminated small-bowel syndrome (with bile acid precipitation, increased jejunal absorption, and "short circuiting")
- Entrapment of bile acids in intestinal lumen by:
  - Cholestyramine
  - Trivalent cations (aluminum-containing antacids)
  - Fiber

Bile acid malabsorption
- Primary bile acid malabsorption (absent or inefficient ileal active transport)
  - Intractable diarrhea (infancy)
  - Irritable bowel (adults)
- Secondary bile acid malabsorption
  - Ileal disease or resection
    - Crohn disease
    - Ileal resection
    - Ileal bypass
    - Radiation enteritis
    - Postinfectious enteritis
    - Short-gut syndrome
  - Exogenous bile acid administration (e.g., gallstone dissolution)
  - Cystic fibrosis
- Tertiary bile acid malabsorption
  - Postcholecystectomy
  - Renal failure
  - Drugs

Defective uptake or altered intracellular metabolism
- Parenchymal disease (acute hepatitis, cirrhosis)
  - Regurgitation from cells
  - Portosystemic shunting
- Cholestasis

CHAPTER 301
Manifestations of Liver Disease

William F. Balistreri

PATHOLOGIC MANIFESTATIONS. Alterations in hepatic structure and function can be *acute* or *chronic*, with varying patterns of reaction of the liver to cell injury. The ultimate reaction is cell death, but the hepatocyte has a remarkable capacity for regeneration. Collagen is formed during the healing phase of cellular injury, with excessive growth of fibrous tissue becoming manifest as cirrhosis.

Inflammation or necrosis, or both, of individual hepatocytes can be due to viral infection, drugs or toxins, immunologic disorders, or hypoxia. The evolving process leads to repair, to continuing injury with chronic changes, or in rare cases to massive hepatic damage.

Cholestasis is an alternative or concomitant response to injury. It is defined as the accumulation in serum of substances normally excreted in bile such as bilirubin, cholesterol, bile acids, and trace elements. A liver biopsy demonstrates accumulation of bile and bile pigment in the parenchyma. In extrahepatic obstruction, bile pigment may be visible in the intralobular bile ducts or throughout the parenchyma as bile lakes or infarcts. Cholestasis may also be seen without evidence of bile duct obstruction, when hepatocyte injury or an alteration in hepatic physiology has led to a reduction in the rate of secretion of solute and water. Likely causes may include alterations in the ultrastructure or cytoskeleton of the hepatocyte, alterations in organelles responsible for bile secretion, alterations in enzymatic activity, or alterations in permeability of the bile canalicular apparatus. The end result is clinically indistinguishable from obstructive cholestasis.

Cirrhosis (defined histologically by the presence of bands of fibrous tissue that link central and portal areas and form parenchymal nodules) is a potential end stage of any acute or chronic liver disease. Cirrhosis may be posthepatitic (after acute or chronic hepatitis) or postnecrotic (after toxic injury) or it may follow chronic biliary obstruction (biliary cirrhosis). Cirrhosis may be **macronodular** with nodules of various sizes (up to 5 cm) separated by broad septae, or **micronodular,** with nodules of uniform size (< 1 cm) separated by fine septae. There may also be mixed forms. The progressive scarring of cirrhosis leads to altered hepatic blood flow, with further impairment of liver cell function. In addition, the restriction of blood flow within the liver leads to portal hypertension.

Primary tumors of the liver are discussed in Chapter 457.

The liver may be **secondarily** involved in neoplastic (metastatic) and non-neoplastic (storage diseases and fat infiltration) and infectious processes. The liver may also be affected by chronic passive congestion or acute hypoxia, with hepatocellular damage.

CLINICAL MANIFESTATIONS

Hepatomegaly. Enlargement of the liver can be due to several mechanisms (Table 301–1). Concepts of normal liver size have been based on age-related clinical indices, such as (1) the degree of extension of the liver edge below the costal margin, (2) the span of dullness to percussion, or (3) the length of the vertical axis of the liver, as estimated from imaging techniques. In children, the normal liver edge can be felt up to 2 cm below the right costal margin. In the newborn infant extension of the liver edge more than 3.5 cm below the costal margin in the right midclavicular line suggests hepatic enlargement. Measurement of *liver span* is carried out by percussing the upper margin of dullness and by palpating the lower edge in the right midclavicular line; it may be more reliable than an extension of the liver edge alone, and the two measurements may correlate poorly.

The liver span increases linearly with body weight and age in both sexes. If percussion is used for both the upper and lower borders, the mean liver span is related curvilinearly to age. The span ranges from about 4.5–5 cm at 1 wk of age to approximately 7-8 cm in males and 6–6.5 cm in females by 12 yr of age. The expected span of liver dullness in the midclavicular line in both sexes after 12 yr of age can be calculated as follows: in males, span (cm) $= 0.032 \times$ weight (pounds) $+ 0.18 \times$ height (inches) $- 7.86$; in females, span (cm) $= 0.027 \times$ weight (pounds) $+ 0.22 \times$ height (inches) $- 10.75$. These formulas are not accurate for newborns or younger children. In some persons, the lower edge of the right lobe of the liver extends downward (Riedel lobe) and may be palpable as a broad mass. Downward displacement of the liver by the diaphragm or thoracic organs can create an erroneous impression of hepatomegaly.

Examination of the liver should note the consistency, contour, tenderness, or the presence of any masses or bruits, as well as assessing splenic size.

■ TABLE 301–1 Mechanisms of Hepatomegaly

Increase in the Number or Size of the Cells in the Liver
- Storage
  - Fat: malnutrition, obesity, metabolic liver disease (e.g., diseases of fatty acid oxidation and Reye syndrome–like illnesses), lipid infusion (total parenteral nutrition), cystic fibrosis, diabetes mellitus, medication related
  - Specific lipid storage diseases: Gaucher, Niemann-Pick, Wolman syndromes
  - Glycogen: glycogen storage diseases (multiple enzyme defects); total parenteral nutrition; infant of diabetic mother, Beckwith syndrome
  - Miscellaneous: α_1-antitrypsin deficiency, Wilson disease, hypervitaminosis A, neonatal iron storage (hemochromatosis)

Inflammation
- Hepatocyte enlargement (hepatitis)
  - Viral—acute and chronic
  - Bacterial (sepsis, abscess, cholangitis)
  - Toxic (e.g., drugs)
- Kupffer cell enlargement
- Autoimmune: chronic hepatitis, sarcoidosis, systemic lupus erythematosus, sclerosing cholangitis

Infiltration
- Primary tumors
  - Hepatoblastoma
  - Hepatocellular carcinoma
  - Hemangioma
  - Focal nodular hyperplasia
- Secondary or metastatic tumors
  - Lymphoma
  - Leukemia
  - Histiocytosis
  - Neuroblastoma
  - Wilms tumor

Increased Size of Vascular Space
- Intrahepatic obstruction to hepatic vein outflow
  - Veno-occlusive disease
  - Hepatic vein thrombosis (Budd-Chiari syndrome)
  - Hepatic vein web
- Suprahepatic
  - Congestive heart failure
  - Pericardial disease
  - Tamponade
  - Constrictive pericarditis
  - Hematopoietic: Sickle cell anemia, thalassemia

Increased Size of Biliary Space
- Congenital hepatic fibrosis
- Caroli disease
- Extrahepatic obstruction

Idiopathic (? "Benign")

Ultrasonography can often help in the evaluation of unexplained hepatomegaly; size and consistency can be assessed. Hyperechogenic hepatic parenchyma can be seen with metabolic disease (glycogen storage disease) or fatty liver (owing to malnutrition or hyperalimentation or after corticosteroid therapy).

Ultrasonography can also assess **gallbladder size.** Gallbladder distention may be seen in sick infants who have sepsis. Gallbladder length normally varies from 1.5-5.5 cm (average, 3.0) in infants to 4-8 cm in adolescents; width ranges from 0.5-2.5 cm (mean, 0.8 in neonates) at all ages.

Jaundice. Yellow discoloration of the plasma, skin, and mucous membranes may be the earliest and only sign of hepatic dysfunction; it therefore requires urgent evaluation. Jaundice becomes clinically apparent in children and adults when the serum concentration of bilirubin reaches 2-3 mg/dL. In neonates, higher levels may be found without evident icterus. Icterus may be associated with dark urine or acholic (light-colored) stools.

Bilirubin occurs in plasma in four forms: (1) *unconjugated bilirubin* tightly bound to albumin; (2) *free* or *unbound bilirubin* (the form responsible for kernicterus, because it can cross cell membranes); (3) *conjugated bilirubin* (the only fraction to appear in urine); and (4) δ *fraction* (bilirubin covalently bound to albumin), which appears in serum when hepatic excretion of conjugated bilirubin is impaired in patients with hepatobiliary disease. The δ fraction permits conjugated bilirubin to persist in the circulation and delays resolution of jaundice.

Measurement of serum bilirubin is traditionally via the van den Bergh (diazo) reaction. The terms "direct-reacting" and "indirect-reacting" bilirubin correspond roughly to *conjugated* and *unconjugated* bilirubin, respectively. Routine automated procedures to quantitate *conjugated* bilirubin significantly overestimate the direct reacting fraction at relatively low total bilirubin concentrations. Cholestasis can be excluded by measuring serum bile acids, which will be elevated in the presence of any form of cholestasis.

Jaundice in an infant or older child may reflect accumulation of either unconjugated or conjugated bilirubin. An increase in unconjugated bilirubin may indicate increased production, hemolysis, reduced hepatic removal, or altered metabolism of bilirubin (Table 301–2). Significant accumulations of conjugated bilirubin (>20% of total) reflect decreased excretion by damaged hepatic parenchymal cells or disease of biliary tract, which may be due to sepsis, endocrine or metabolic disease, inflammation of the liver, or obstruction (Table 301–3). In most patients with diseases that tend to produce conjugated hyperbilirubinemia, a portion of the total bilirubin will be present in **unconjugated** form, with near-parallel rises in both fractions.

Pruritus. Intense generalized itching may occur in patients with cholestasis (conjugated hyperbilirubinemia) presumably owing to retained components of bile such as bile acids. Symptomatic relief of pruritus follows administration of bile acid–binding agents such as cholestyramine or choleretic agents such as ursodeoxycholic acid or phenobarbital. Pruritus is unrelated to the degree of hyperbilirubinemia; deeply jaundiced patients may be asymptomatic, and vice versa.

Spider Angiomas. Vascular spiders (telangiectasias), characterized by central pulsating arterioles from which small, wiry venules radiate, may be seen in patients with chronic liver disease. These are presumably reflective of altered estrogen metabolism in the face of hepatic dysfunction.

Palmar Erythema. Blotchy erythema, most noticeable over the thenar and hypothenar eminences and on the tips of the fingers is also noted in patients with chronic liver disease. These may be due to vasodilatation and increased blood flow.

Xanthomata. The marked elevation of serum cholesterol (to levels >500 mg/dL) associated with chronic cholestasis may cause the deposition of lipid in the dermis and subcutaneous tissue. Brown nodules may develop first over the extensor surfaces of the extremities; rarely, xanthelasma of the eyelids develops.

Portal Hypertension. The portal vein drains the splanchnic area (abdominal portion of the gastrointestinal tract, pancreas, and spleen) into the hepatic sinusoids. Pressure is normally slightly higher (~5-10 mm Hg) in the portal vein than in other venous systems in order to overcome the resistance of the sinusoidal system. Portal hypertension is defined as an increase in portal venous pressure to greater than 20 mm Hg (Chapter 312).

Ascites. Ascites may be associated with urinary tract abnormalities, metabolic diseases (such as lysosomal storage diseases), congenital or acquired heart disease, and hydrops fetalis. Intra-abdominal accumulation of fluid is a common manifestation of end-stage liver disease. In patients with significant hepatic disease, sinusoidal blockade caused by cirrhosis increases hydrostatic pressure and transudation of fluid; this may be worsened by hypoalbuminemia (Chapter 312).

Encephalopathy. Metabolic abnormalities may complicate acute or chronic liver disorders, leading to encephalopathy, with neuropsychiatric disturbances that may include neuromuscular dysfunction, altered mentation, altered consciousness, or coma. With chronic liver disease, hepatic encephalopathy may be recurrent and precipitated by intercurrent illness, drugs, bleeding, or electrolyte and acid-base disturbances.

Hepatic encephalopathy is characterized by profound neural inhibition, which may be due to an interaction between γ-aminobutyric acid (GABA, the primary inhibitory neuro-trans-

■ TABLE 301–2 Differential Diagnosis of Unconjugated Hyperbilirubinemia

Increased Production of Unconjugated Bilirubin from Heme

- Hemolytic disease (hereditary or acquired)
  - Isoimmune hemolysis (neonatal; acute or delayed transfusion reaction; autoimmune)
    - Rh incompatibility
    - ABO incompatibility
    - Other blood group incompatibilities
  - Congenital spherocytosis
  - Hereditary elliptocytosis
  - Infantile pyknocytosis
  - Erythrocyte enzyme defects:
    - Glucose-6-phosphate dehydrogenase
    - Pyruvate kinase
    - Hexokinase
  - Hemoglobinopathy
    - Sickle cell anemia
    - Thalassemia
    - Others
  - Sepsis
  - Microangiopathy
    - Hemolytic-uremic syndrome
    - Hemangioma
    - Mechanical trauma (heart valve)
- Ineffective erythropoiesis
- Drugs
  - Vitamin K
  - Maternal oxytocin
  - Phenol disinfectants
- Infection
- Enclosed hematoma
- Polycythemia
  - Diabetic mother
  - Fetal transfusion (recipient)
  - Delayed cord clamping

Decreased Delivery of Unconjugated Bilirubin (in plasma) to Hepatocyte

- Right-sided congestive heart failure
- Portacaval shunt

Decreased Bilirubin Uptake Across Hepatocyte Membrane

- Presumed enzyme deficiency (e.g., Gilbert)
- Competitive inhibition
  - Breast milk jaundice
  - Lucey-Driscoll syndrome
  - Drug-inhibition (radiocontrast material)
- Miscellaneous
  - Hypothyroidism
  - Hypoxia
  - Acidosis

Decreased Storage of Unconjugated Bilirubin in Cytosol (Decreased Y and Z Proteins)

- Competitive inhibition
- Fever

Decreased Biotransformation (Conjugation)

- Neonatal jaundice (physiologic)
- Inhibition (drugs)
- Hereditary (Crigler-Najjar)
  - Type I (complete enzyme deficiency)
  - Type II (partial deficiency)
- Hepatocellular dysfunction

Enterohepatic Recirculation

- Intestinal obstruction
  - Ileal atresia
  - Hirschsprung disease
  - Cystic fibrosis
  - Pyloric stenosis
- Antibiotic administration

Breast Milk Jaundice

■ TABLE 301–3 Differential Diagnosis of Neonatal Cholestasis

Infectious
- Viral hepatitis
  - Hepatitis A, B, C (rare)
  - Cytomegalovirus
  - Rubella virus
  - Herpes simplex 1, 2, 6
  - Varicella virus
  - Coxsackievirus
  - Echovirus
  - Reovirus type 3
  - Parvovirus B19
- Others
  - Toxoplasmosis
  - Syphilis
  - Tuberculosis
  - Listeriosis

Toxic
- Parenteral nutrition related
- Sepsis (e.g., urinary tract) with endotoxemia
- Drug related

Metabolic
- Disorders of **amino acid** metabolism
  - Tyrosinemia
- Disorders of **lipid** metabolism
  - Wolman disease
  - Niemann-Pick disease (type C)
  - Gaucher disease
- Disorders of **carbohydrate** metabolism
  - Galactosemia
  - Fructosemia
  - Glycogenosis IV
- Disorders of **bile acid biosynthesis** (reductase, isomerase)
- Other metabolic defects
  - α_1-Antitrypsin deficiency
  - Cystic fibrosis
  - Idiopathic hypopituitarism
  - Hypothyroidism
  - Zellweger (cerebrohepatorenal) syndrome
  - Neonatal iron storage disease
  - Indian childhood cirrhosis/infantile copper overload
  - Familial erythrophagocytic lymphohistiocytosis
  - Arginase deficiency
  - Mitochondrial DNA depletion

Genetic/Chromosomal
- Trisomy E
- Down syndrome
- Donahue syndrome (leprechaunism)

Intrahepatic Diseases of Unknown Cause
- Intrahepatic cholestasis—persistent
  - "Idiopathic" neonatal hepatitis
  - Alagille syndrome (arteriohepatic dysplasia)
  - Intrahepatic biliary hypoplasia or paucity of intrahepatic bile ducts (nonsyndromic)
  - Byler disease
- Intrahepatic cholestasis—recurrent
  - Familial benign recurrent cholestasis
  - Associated with lymphedema (Aagenaes)
- Congenital hepatic fibrosis/infantile polycystic disease
- Caroli disease (cystic dilatation of intrahepatic ducts)

Extrahepatic Diseases
- Biliary atresia
- Sclerosing cholangitis
- Bile duct stenosis
- Choledochal-pancreaticoductal junction anomaly
- Spontaneous perforation of the bile duct
- Choledochal cyst
- Mass (neoplasia, stone)
- Bile/mucous plug ("inspissated bile")

Miscellaneous
- Histiocytosis X
- Shock and hypoperfusion
- Associated with enteritis
- Associated with intestinal obstruction
- Neonatal lupus erythematosus
- Myeloproliferative disease (21-trisomy)

mitter) and GABA receptors on postsynaptic neurons. With hepatic failure, GABA produced by bacterial flora is not cleared from the blood but crosses the blood-brain barrier and produces inhibition. There may be a simultaneous decrease in excitatory neurotransmission. Other neuroactive or vasoactive compounds, such as glycine or amines, may be synergistic. Alternative theories ascribe a pathogenetic role to ammonia, to synergistic neurotoxins, or to "false neurotransmitters" with plasma amino acid imbalance (Chapter 548).

Endocrine Abnormalities. Endocrine abnormalities are more common in adults with hepatic disease than in children. They reflect alterations in hepatic synthetic, storage, and metabolic functions, including those concerned with hormonal metabolism in the liver. For example, proteins such as those that bind hormones in plasma are synthesized in the liver, and steroid hormones are conjugated in the liver and excreted in the urine; failure of such functions may have clinical consequences. Endocrine abnormalities may also result from malnutrition or specific deficiencies.

Renal Dysfunction. There is a close relationship between hepatic and renal dysfunction. Systemic disease or toxins may affect both organs simultaneously or parenchymal liver disease may produce secondary impairment of renal function, and vice versa. In hepatobiliary disorders, there may be renal alterations in sodium and water economy, impaired renal concentrating ability, and alterations in potassium metabolism. Ascites in patients with cirrhosis may be related to inappropriate retention of sodium by the kidney, with expansion of plasma volume, or to sodium retention mediated by diminished effective plasma volume.

Hepatorenal syndrome is defined as renal failure (azotemia and progressive oliguria) in a patient with cirrhosis (often with refractory ascites) in whom there is no other demonstrable cause of renal failure. This complication represents a complex sequence of compensation and decompensation in end-stage liver disease. The pathophysiology is poorly defined but seems to involve altered renal blood flow and altered hormone metabolism. Intense vasoconstriction of the renal cortical vessels is mediated by hemodynamic, humoral, or neurogenic mechanisms. The urinary sodium concentration is low, and the sediment is normal. In management, a trial of volume expansion is warranted in order to exclude the possibility of prerenal azotemia secondary to volume depletion.

MISCELLANEOUS MANIFESTATIONS OF LIVER DYSFUNCTION. Nonspecific signs of acute and chronic liver disease include (1) anorexia, which is often seen in the patient with anicteric hepatitis and with cirrhosis associated with chronic cholestasis; (2) abdominal pain or distention resulting from ascites, spontaneous peritonitis, or visceromegaly; and (3) bleeding, which may be due to altered synthesis of coagulation factors (biliary obstruction with vitamin K deficiency or excessive hepatic damage) or to portal hypertension. There may be decreased synthesis of specific clotting factors, production of qualitatively abnormal proteins, or alterations in platelet number and function in the presence of hypersplenism. Altered drug metabolism may prolong the biologic half-life of commonly administered medications.

301.1 Evaluation of the Patient with Possible Liver Dysfunction

Adequate evaluation of an infant, child, or adolescent with suspected liver disease involves an appropriate and accurate history, a carefully performed physical examination, and skillful interpretation of signs and symptoms. Further evaluation is aided by judicious selection of diagnostic tests, followed by a liver biopsy or the use of imaging modalities. Most of the so-called liver function tests do not measure specific hepatic functions; a rise in serum aminotransferase (transaminase) activity reflects liver cell injury; an increase in immunoglobulin level reflects an immunologic response to injury; or an elevation in serum bilirubin level may reflect any of several disturbances of bilirubin metabolism outlined in Tables 301–2 and 301–3. Any single biochemical assay provides limited information, which must be placed in the context of the entire clinical and historic picture. The most cost-efficient approach is for the clinician to become familiar with the rationale, implications, and limitations of a selected group of tests, so that specific questions can be answered.

For a patient with suspected liver disease, evaluation addresses the following issues in sequence: (1) Is liver disease present? (2) If so, what is its nature? (3) What is its severity? (4) Is specific treatment available? (5) How can we monitor the response to treatment? and (6) What is the prognosis?

BIOCHEMICAL TESTS. Laboratory tests commonly used to screen for or to confirm the suspicion of liver disease include measurements of serum bilirubin level and of aminotransferase and alkaline phosphatase activities often with determinations of prothrombin time and albumin level. These tests are complementary and provide an estimation of synthetic and excretory functions and may suggest the nature of the disturbance (e.g., inflammation or cholestasis).

Acute liver cell injury (parenchymal disease) in viral hepatitis, drug- or toxin-induced liver disease, shock, hypoxemia, or metabolic disease are best reflected in marked increases in aminotransferase activities. Cholestasis (obstructive disease) involves regurgitation of bile components into serum; accordingly, the serum levels of total and conjugated bilirubin and serum bile acids will be elevated. Elevations in serum alkaline phosphatase and 5′ nucleotidase activities are also sensitive indicators of obstructive processes or of inflammation of the biliary tract.

The severity of the liver disease may be reflected in (1) *clinical signs* (occurrence of encephalopathy, variceal hemorrhage, worsening jaundice, apparent shrinkage of liver mass owing to massive necrosis, or onset of ascites) or in (2) *biochemical alterations* (hypoglycemia, hyper-ammonemia, electrolyte imbalance, continued hyperbilirubinemia, marked hypoalbuminemia, or prolonged prothrombin times unresponsive to parenteral administration of vitamin K).

Measurement of the *conjugated and unconjugated fractions of serum bilirubin* help to distinguish between elevations caused by hemolysis and those caused by hepatic dysfunction. A predominant elevation in the conjugated fraction provides a relatively sensitive index of hepatocellular disease or hepatic excretory dysfunction. Aminotransferase activities are highly sensitive indices of hepatocellular damage. *Alanine aminotransferase* (ALT, serum glutamate pyruvate transaminase) is liver specific, whereas *aspartate aminotransferase* (AST, serum glutamic-oxaloacetic transaminase) is derived from other organs in addition to the liver. In most cases of hepatic disease there are parallel rises in AST and ALT, but sometimes a differential rise or fall can provide useful information. The most marked rises of aminotransferase activities occur with acute hepatocellular injury, such as acute viral hepatitis, hypoxia or hypoperfusion, toxic injury, or Reye syndrome. Following blunt abdominal trauma, elevations in activity of these enzymes may provide an early clue to hepatic injury. In chronic liver disease or in intrahepatic and extrahepatic biliary obstruction, rises in aminotransferase activities may be less marked. In acute hepatitis the rise in ALT may be greater than that of AST, whereas in alcohol-induced liver injury, in fulminant echovirus infection, and in various metabolic diseases, predominant rises in AST have been reported.

Hepatic synthetic function is reflected in *serum protein* levels and in *prothrombin time*. Examination of *serum globulin* concentration and of the relative amounts of the globulin fractions may be helpful. γ-Globulin levels are often high, and increased titers of smooth muscle antibody as well as antimitochondrial antibodies and antinuclear antibodies may be found in patients with autoimmune hepatitis. A resurgence in *α-fetoprotein* levels may suggest hepatoma. Hypoalbuminemia caused by depressed synthesis may complicate severe liver disease and serve as a prognostic factor. Deficiencies of *factor V* and of the *vitamin K–dependent factors (II, VII, IX and X)* may occur in patients with severe liver disease or fulminant hepatic failure. If the prothrombin time is prolonged as a result of intestinal malabsorption of vitamin K (resulting from cholestasis) or decreased nutritional intake of vitamin K, then parenteral administration of vitamin K should correct the coagulopathy leading to normalization within 12 hr. Unresponsiveness to vitamin K would suggest hepatic disease. Persistently low levels of factor VII are evidence of a poor prognosis in fulminant liver disease.

Serum levels of *bile acids* are sensitive indicators of hepatobiliary disease, especially in monitoring patients at high risk for liver injury.

Interpretation of biochemical tests of hepatic structure and function must be made in the context of age-related changes. The activity of *alkaline phosphatase* varies considerably with age, reflecting predominantly the activity of the isoenzyme that originates in bone. Activity of the liver-specific isoenzyme or of *5′ nucleotidase* can be measured; the latter has a similar biliary origin and is not found in bone. An isolated increase in alkaline phosphatase does not indicate hepatic or biliary disease if other liver function test results are normal. *γ-Glutamyl transpeptidase* exhibits high enzyme activity in early life that declines rapidly with age. Cholesterol concentrations increase throughout life. *Cholesterol levels* may be markedly elevated in patients with cholestasis, whether the cause be intrahepatic or extrahepatic. On the other hand, with acute liver disease, such as hepatitis, serum cholesterol levels may be depressed.

Interpretation of *serum ammonia* values must be carried out with caution because of variability in their physiologic determinants and the inherent difficulty in laboratory measurement.

LIVER BIOPSY. The morphologic features of specific hepatic diseases are sufficiently distinctive. Therefore, liver biopsy combined with clinical data can indicate an etiologic diagnosis in most cases. Tissue obtained by percutaneous liver biopsy can be used (1) to provide a precise histologic diagnosis (in patients with neonatal cholestasis, chronic active hepatitis, Reye syndrome, intrahepatic cholestasis (paucity of bile ducts), congenital hepatic fibrosis, or undefined portal hypertension); (2) for enzyme analysis to detect inborn errors of metabolism; and (3) for analysis of stored material (e.g., iron, copper, or specific metabolites). Serial assessments of hepatic status by liver biopsies can monitor responses to therapy or detect complications of treatment with potentially hepatotoxic agents, such as aspirin or nonsteroidal anti-inflammatory agents, antimetabolites, or anticonvulsants.

In infants and children, needle biopsy of the liver is easily accomplished through the percutaneous approach. The amount of tissue obtained, even in small infants, is usually sufficient for histologic interpretation and for biochemical analyses (if the latter are deemed necessary). Percutaneous liver biopsy can be performed safely in infants as young as 1 wk. The patient usually requires only sedation and *local* anesthesia. Contraindications include prolonged prothrombin time, thrombocytopenia, suspicion of a vascular, cystic, or infectious lesion in the path of the needle and severe ascites. If administration of fresh frozen plasma or of platelet transfusions fails to correct a prolonged prothrombin time or thrombocytopenia, open surgical (wedge) biopsy may be considered. The risk of development of a complication such as hemorrhage, hematoma, creation of an arteriovenous fistula, pneumothorax, or bile peritonitis is very small.

HEPATIC IMAGING PROCEDURES. Various techniques help define the size, shape, and architecture of the liver and the anatomy of the intrahepatic and extrahepatic biliary trees. Although imaging may not provide a precise histologic and biochemical diagnosis, specific questions can be answered, such as whether hepatomegaly is related to accumulation of fat or glycogen or is due to a tumor or cyst. These studies may direct further evaluation such as percutaneous biopsy and will make possible prompt referral of patients with biliary obstruction to the surgeon. Choice of imaging procedure should be part of a carefully formulated diagnostic approach, with avoidance of redundant demonstrations by several techniques.

A *plain roentgenographic study* may suggest hepatomegaly, but a carefully performed physical examination gives a more reliable assessment of liver size. The liver may appear less dense than normal in patients with fatty infiltration or more dense with deposition of heavy metals such as iron. A hepatic or biliary tract mass may displace an air-filled loop of bowel. Calcifications may be evident in the liver (parasitic and neoplastic disease), in the vasculature (with portal vein thrombosis), or in the gallbladder or biliary tree (gallstones). Collections of gas may be seen within the liver (abscess), biliary tract, or portal circulation (necrotizing enterocolitis).

Ultrasonography provides information about the size, composition, and blood flow of the liver. Increased echogenicity is observed with fatty infiltration, and mass lesions as small as 1–2 cm may be shown. Ultrasonography has replaced cholangiography in detecting stones in the gallbladder or biliary tree. Even in the neonate ultrasonography can assess gallbladder size, detect dilatation of the biliary tract, and define a choledochal cyst. In infants with biliary atresia, the gallbladder is usually small or absent and the common duct is not visualized. In patients with portal hypertension, ultrasonography can evaluate patency of the portal vein or demonstrate collateral circulation. Relatively small amounts of ascitic fluid can be detected. The use of Doppler ultrasonography has been helpful in determining vascular patency after orthotopic liver transplantation.

Computed tomography (CT) scanning provides information similar to that obtained by ultrasonography but is less suitable for use in patients younger than 2 yr because of the small size of structures, the paucity of intra-abdominal fat for contrast, and the need for heavy sedation or general anesthesia. *Magnetic resonance imaging* (MRI) is a useful alternative. The CT scan or MRI may be more accurate than ultrasonography in detection of focal lesions such as tumors, cysts, and abscesses. When enhanced by contrast medium, CT scanning may reveal a neoplastic mass density only slightly different from that of the normal liver. When a hepatic tumor is suspected, CT scanning is the best method to define anatomic extent, solid or cystic nature, and vascularity. CT scanning can also reveal subtle differences in density of liver parenchyma, the average liver attenuation coefficient being reduced with fatty infiltration. Increases in density may occur with diffuse iron deposition or with glycogen storage. In differentiating obstructive from nonobstructive cholestasis, CT scanning or MRI identifies the precise level of obstruction more frequently than ultrasonography. Either CT scanning or ultrasonography may be used to guide percutaneously placed "fine needles" for biopsies, aspiration of specific lesions, or cholangiography.

Radionuclide scanning relies on selective uptake of a radiopharmaceutical agent. Commonly used agents include (1) technetium 99m–labeled sulfur colloid, which undergoes phagocytosis by Kupffer cells; (2) ^{99m}Tc-iminodiacetic acid agents, which are taken up by hepatocytes and excreted into bile; and (3) gallium 67, which is concentrated in inflammatory and neoplastic cells. The anatomic resolution possible with hepatic scintiscans is generally less than that obtained with CT scanning, MRI, or ultrasonography.

The ^{99m}Tc-sulfur colloid scan may detect focal lesions (e.g., tumors, cysts, or abscesses) greater than 2–3 cm in diameter. This modality may help to evaluate patients with possible cirrhosis in whom hepatic uptake is patchy and in whom there is a shift of colloid uptake from liver to bone marrow.

The ^{99m}Tc-substituted iminodiacetic acid dyes may differentiate intrahepatic cholestasis from extrahepatic obstruction in the neonate. Imaging results are best when scanning is preceded by a 5- to 7-day period of treatment with phenobarbital to stimulate bile flow. Following intravenous injection, the isotope is normally detected in the bowel within 1–2 hr. In the presence of extrahepatic obstruction, excretion of the isotope is delayed; accordingly, serial scans should be made for up to 24 hr following injection. Early in the course of biliary atresia, hepatocyte function is usually good; uptake (clearance) occurs rapidly, but excretion into the intestine is absent. In contrast, uptake is poor in parenchymal liver disease, such as neonatal hepatitis, but excretion into the bile and intestine eventually ensues.

In older infants and children who have undergone liver transplantation, scintigraphy may also help to evaluate the gallbladder, bile ducts, and bile flow. In patients with acute cholecystitis, the gallbladder is not visualized, but the common duct is opacified.

Cholangiography, the direct visualization of the intrahepatic and extrahepatic biliary tree following injection of opaque material, may be required in some patients to evaluate the cause, location, or extent of biliary obstruction. Percutaneous transhepatic cholangiography with a fine needle is the technique of choice in infants and young children. The likelihood of opacifying the biliary tract is excellent in patients in whom CT scanning, MRI, or ultrasonography has shown dilated ducts. Percutaneous transhepatic cholangiography has been used to outline the biliary ductal system.

Endoscopic retrograde cholangiopancreatography is an alternative method of examining the bile ducts in older children. The papilla of Vater is cannulated under direct vision through a fiberoptic endoscope, and contrast material is injected into the biliary and pancreatic ducts to outline the anatomy.

Selective angiography of the celiac, superior mesenteric, or hepatic artery may be used to visualize the hepatic or portal circulation. Both arterial and venous circulatory systems of the liver can be examined. Angiography is frequently required to define the blood supply of tumors before surgery and is useful in the study of patients with known or presumed portal hypertension. The patency of the portal system, the extent of collateral circulation, and the caliber of vessels under consideration for a shunting procedure can be evaluated. MRI can provide similar information.

CHAPTER 302
Cholestasis

William F. Balistreri

302.1 Neonatal Cholestasis

Neonatal cholestasis is defined as prolonged elevation of serum levels of conjugated bilirubin beyond the first 14 days

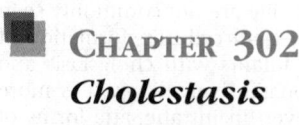

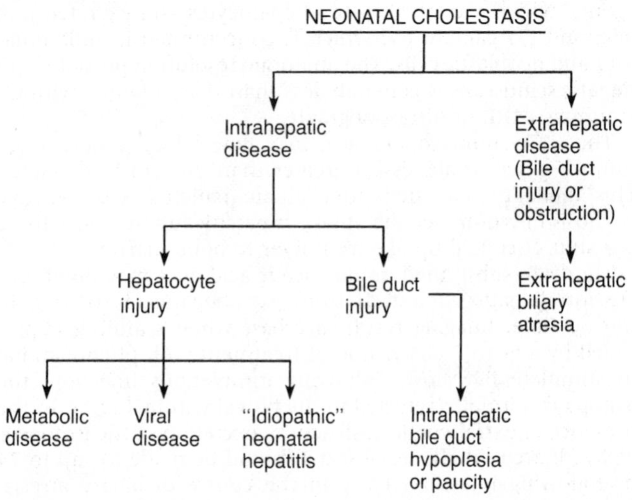

Figure 302–1. Neonatal cholestasis. Conceptual approach to the group of diseases presenting as cholestasis in the neonate. There are areas of overlap—patients with extrahepatic biliary atresia may have some degree of intrahepatic injury. Patients with "idiopathic" neonatal hepatitis may in the future be determined to have a primary metabolic or viral disease.

of life. Cholestasis in the newborn may be due to infectious, genetic, metabolic, or undefined abnormalities giving rise either to mechanical obstruction of bile flow or to functional impairment of hepatic excretory function and bile secretion (Table 301–3). An example of the former is stricture or obstruction of the common bile duct; biliary atresia is the prototypic obstructive abnormality. Functional impairment of bile secretion may result from damage to liver cells or to the biliary secretory apparatus. Neonates with cholestasis may be divided into those with extrahepatic and those with intrahepatic disease (Fig. 302–1). The clinical features of any form of cholestasis are similar. In an affected neonate, the diagnosis of certain entities, such as galactosemia, sepsis, and hypothyroidism, is relatively simple. In most cases, however, the cause of cholestasis is more obscure. Differentiation among *extrahepatic biliary atresia,* idiopathic *neonatal hepatitis,* and *intrahepatic cholestasis* is often particularly difficult.

Mechanisms. The two most likely pathogenetic mechanisms are viral-induced liver injury or metabolic liver disease. There are paradigms for each of these potential mechanisms. For example, metabolic liver disease caused by inborn errors of bile acid metabolism is associated with the accumulation of toxic primitive bile acids and the failure to produce normal choleretic and trophic bile acids. The clinical and histologic manifestations are nonspecific and are similar to those seen in other forms of neonatal hepatobiliary injury. It is also possible that autoimmune mechanisms may be responsible for some of the enigmatic forms of neonatal liver injury. Overall, the mechanisms are not well documented. Some of the histologic manifestations of hepatic injury in early life are not commonly seen in older individuals. For example, giant cell transformation of hepatocytes occurs frequently in infants with cholestasis and may be seen in any form of neonatal liver injury. It is more frequent and more severe, however, in intrahepatic forms of cholestasis (neonatal hepatitis or intrahepatic bile duct paucity). The clinical and histologic findings thought to exist in patients with neonatal hepatitis and in those with extrahepatic biliary atresia have suggested that these diseases are manifestations of a single basic process, with an undefined initiating insult causing inflammation of the liver cells or of the cells within the biliary tract. If bile duct epithelium is the predominant site of disease, cholangitis may result and lead to progressive slcerosis and narrowing of the biliary tree, the ultimate state being complete obliteration *(extrahepatic biliary atresia).* On the other hand, injury to liver cells may present the clinical and histologic picture of *neonatal hepatitis.* This concept does not account for all phenomena, but offers an explanation for well-documented cases of unexpected postnatal evolution of these disease processes; for example, infants initially regarded as having neonatal hepatitis, with a patent biliary system shown on cholangiography, have been later found to have extrahepatic biliary atresia.

Functional abnormalities in the generation of bile flow may also play a role in neonatal cholestasis. Bile flow is directly dependent on effective hepatic bile acid excretion. During the phase of relatively inefficient liver cell transport and metabolism of bile acids in early life, minor degrees of hepatic injury may further decrease bile flow and lead to production of abnormal toxic bile acids. Elective impairment of a single step in the series of events involved in hepatic excretion may produce the full expression of a cholestatic syndrome. A small number of cholestatic syndromes have a familial pattern. For example, Byler disease and benign recurrent cholestasis are presumably related to impaired metabolism or membrane transport of bile acids. Specific defects in bile acid synthesis have been found in infants with intrahepatic cholestasis and in infants with Zellweger syndrome. Severe forms of familial cholestasis have been associated with neonatal hemochromatosis and an aberration in the contractile proteins that comprise the cytoskeleton of the hepatocyte. Sepsis is known to cause cholestasis, presumably mediated by an endotoxin produced by *Escherichia coli.*

Evaluation. (See Table 302–1.) The clinical features of infants with neonatal cholestasis provide very few clues regarding etiology. Affected infants have icterus, dark urine, light or acholic stools, and hepatomegaly, all reflecting decreased bile flow resulting from either liver cell injury or bile duct obstruction. Hepatic synthetic dysfunction may lead to hypoprothrombinemia and a bleeding disorder; administration of vitamin K should be considered in the initial management of cholestatic infants in order to prevent hemorrhage.

Most infants with neonatal cholestasis will come to medical attention in the 1st mo of life. Prompt differentiation of conjugated from unconjugated hyperbilirubinemia is imperative because the finding of cholestasis is more ominous. The initial step in identification of cholestasis is the finding that, of the significantly elevated level of total bilirubin, more than 20% is conjugated bilirubin. The next step is the prompt recognition of any specific or treatable primary causes of cholestasis, such as *sepsis,* an *endocrinopathy* (hypothyroidism or panhypopituitarism), *nutritional hepatotoxicity* caused by a specific metabolic illness (galactosemia), or other *metabolic diseases* (tyrosinemia). Recognition of such entities allows the institution of appropriate therapy and may possibly prevent further injury.

■ TABLE 302–1 Workup for Suspected Neonatal Cholestasis

1. History and physical examination: size and consistency of liver and spleen; presence of other anomalies (cardiac, renal, skin); stool color
2. Blood and urine analysis: fractionated serum bilirubin; serum bile acids; prothrombin time; α_1-antitrypsin phenotype; metabolic screen-urine/serum amino acids, urine reducing substances; thyroxine and thyroid-stimulating hormone; sweat chloride
3. Blood, urine, spinal fluid cultures (bacteria, herpes simplex, CMV, enteroviruses)
4. Serologic studies for evidence of infection (HBsAg, specific viral serology,* and VDRL)
5. Ultrasonography
6. Hepatobiliary scintigraphy
7. Liver biopsy

**Serology for hepatitis A, B, C, E, herpes simplex, CMV, rubella, measles, human herpes virus 6.*

CMV = cytomegalovirus; HBsAg = hepatitis B surface antigen; VDRL = Venereal Disease Research Laboratories.

Hepatobiliary disease may be the initial manifestation of homozygous α-antitrypsin deficiency or of cystic fibrosis. Neonatal liver disease may also be associated with congenital syphilis and specific viral infections, notably enteric cytopathogenic human orphan (ECHO) virus and herpes viruses. The hepatitis viruses (A, B, C) rarely cause neonatal cholestasis.

The final step in the evaluation of the neonate with cholestasis is to differentiate extrahepatic biliary atresia from neonatal hepatitis. Overall, in up to 80% of infants with neonatal cholestasis, extensive evaluation will establish a diagnosis of either biliary atresia or neonatal hepatitis.

NEONATAL HEPATITIS SYNDROME (INTRAHEPATIC CHOLESTASIS). The term *neonatal hepatitis* implies intrahepatic cholestasis (Fig. 302–1), of which we can designate various forms:

1. **Idiopathic neonatal hepatitis,** which can occur in either a sporadic or a familial form, is a disease of unknown cause; most cases are idiopathic. These patients presumably are afflicted with a specific, yet undefined, metabolic or viral disease. In the past, patients with α_1-antitrypsin deficiency were included in this category; however, following characterization of this metabolic disease, it is possible to precisely define this group of patients.
2. **Infectious hepatitis in a neonate** may be shown to be due to a specific virus, such as herpes simplex, enteroviruses, cytomegalovirus, or, rarely, hepatitis B. This accounts for a small percentage of cases of neonatal hepatitis syndrome.
3. Cases of **Intrahepatic bile duct paucity** form a heterogeneous subset of cholestatic diseases that may present as neonatal cholestasis.

INTRAHEPATIC BILE DUCT PAUCITY. Some syndromes characterized morphologically by intrahepatic cholestasis may be clinically manifest either as neonatal hepatitis or as cholestasis in an older child. As the patient matures, clinical and histologic features may suggest a specific syndrome. Many such cases are associated with bile duct "paucity" (often erroneously called intrahepatic biliary atresia), which designates an absence or marked reduction in the number of interlobular bile ducts in the portal triads, with normal-sized branches of portal vein and hepatic arteriole. This unusual histologic feature represents congenital bile duct absence, partial failure of bile duct development, progressive bile duct atrophy, or disappearance of the bile ducts due to segmental destructive processes. Biopsy in early life often reveals an inflammatory process involving the bile ducts; subsequent biopsies then show subsidence of the inflammation with residual reduction in the number and diameter of bile ducts, analogous to the "disappearing bile duct syndrome" noted in adults with immune-mediated disorders.

Recent observations suggest that it is possible to identify distinctive syndromes of isolated intrahepatic bile duct paucity and an intact extrahepatic biliary tree.

Alagille syndrome (arteriohepatic dysplasia) is the most common syndrome incorporating intrahepatic bile duct paucity. Serial assessment of hepatic histology often suggests progressive destruction of bile ducts. Clinical manifestations are expressed in various degrees and may be nonspecific; they include in some patients unusual *facial characteristics* (broad forehead; deep-set, widely spaced eyes; long, straight nose; and underdeveloped mandible). There may also be *ocular* abnormalities (posterior embryotoxon), *cardiovascular* abnormalities (usually peripheral pulmonic stenosis, sometimes tetralogy of Fallot), *vertebral* arch defects and failure of anterior vertebral arch fusion (butterfly vertebrae), and tubulointerstitial *nephropathy.* Other findings such as growth retardation and defective spermatogenesis may reflect nutritional deficiency. The prognosis for prolonged survival is good, but the patients are likely to have pruritus, xanthomata, and neurologic complications of vitamin E deficiency if untreated.

Byler disease is a rare familial form of progressive intrahepatic cholestasis characterized by unique structural abnormalities in the bile canalicular membrane. Affected patients present with failure to thrive, steatorrhea, pruritus, rickets, and low γ-glutamyl transpeptidase levels. Cirrhosis gradually develops.

In **Aagenaes syndrome,** a form of idiopathic familial intrahepatic cholestasis, recurrent cholestasis is associated with lymphedema of the lower extremities.

Zellweger (cerebrohepatorenal) syndrome is a rare autosomal recessive genetic disorder marked by progressive degeneration of the liver and kidneys. The incidence is estimated to be 1:100,000 births; the disease is usually fatal within 6–12 mo. Affected infants have severe, generalized hypotonia and markedly impaired neurologic function with psychomotor retardation. There are an abnormal shape of the head and unusual facies, hepatomegaly, renal cortical cysts, stippled calcifications of the patellae and greater trochanter, and ocular abnormalities. Hepatic cells on ultrastructural examination show an absence of peroxisomes (Chapter 72.2)

Additional cholestatic disorders include neonatal iron storage disease and inborn errors of bile acid metabolism. Defective bile acid metabolism has been postulated to be an initiating or perpetuating factor in neonatal cholestatic disorders; the hypothesis being that inborn errors in bile acid biosynthesis will lead to absence of normal trophic or choleretic primary bile acids and accumulation of primitive (hepatotoxic) metabolities. A new category of metabolic liver disease, **inborn errors of bile acid biosynthesis,** is now a recognizable cause of acute and chronic liver disease; early recognition will allow the institution of targeted bile acid replacement, which will reverse the hepatic injury.

Deficiency of Δ^4-3-oxosteroid-5β reductase, the fourth step in the pathway of cholesterol degradation to the primary bile acids, was first described in a family of four consecutive boys. This disorder is manifest as significant cholestasis and liver failure developing shortly after birth with coagulopathy and metabolic liver injury resembling tyrosinemia. Hepatic histology is characterized by lobular disarray with giant cells, pseudoacinar transformation, and canalicular bile stasis. Mass spectrometry is required to document increased bile acid excretion and the predominance of oxy-hydroxy and oxo-dihydroxy cholenoic acids. Immunoblot analysis of the cytosolic fraction of the liver, using monoclonal antibody against rat Δ^4-3-oxosteroid-4β reductase, will demonstrate an absence of the protein. Treatment with cholic acid and ursodeoxycholic acid is associated with normalization of biochemical, histological, and clinical features.

Deficiency of **3β-hydroxy C_{27}-steroid dehydrogenase isomerase,** the second step in bile acid biosynthesis, causes progressive familial intrahepatic cholestasis. Affected patients usually manifest jaundice with increased aminotransferase levels and hepatomegaly; however γ-glutamyl transpeptidase levels and serum cholylglycine levels are normal. The histology is variable, ranging from giant cell hepatitis to chronic active hepatitis. The diagnosis, suggested by mass spectrometry detection of C^{24} bile acids, which retain the 3β-hydroxy-Δ^5 structure, can be confirmed by determination of 3-HSD activity in cultured fibroblasts using 7α-hydroxy-Δ^5 structure, can be confirmed by determination of 3-HSD activity in cultured fibroblasts using 7α-hydroxyl cholesterol as a substrate. Primary bile acid therapy, administered orally to downregulate cholesterol 7α-hydroxylase activity, limit the production of 3β-hydroxy-Δ^5 bile acids, and facilitate hepatic clearance, has been effective in reversing hepatic injury.

BILIARY ATRESIA

The term *biliary atresia* is imprecise because the anatomy of abnormal extrahepatic bile ducts in affected patients varies markedly. A more appropriate terminology would reflect the pathophysiology, namely *progressive obliterative cholangiopathy.*

There may be distal segmental bile duct obliteration with patent extrahepatic ducts up to the porta hepatis. This is a surgically correctable lesion, but it is uncommon. The most common form of biliary atresia, accounting for approximately 85% of the cases, is obliteration of the entire extrahepatic biliary tree at or above the porta hepatis. This presents a much more difficult problem in surgical management.

INCIDENCE. Biliary atresia has been detected in 1:10,000–15,000 live births, idiopathic neonatal hepatitis in 1:5,000–10,000. Intrahepatic bile duct paucity appears much less commonly, in about 1:50,000–75,000 live births.

DIFFERENTIATION OF IDIOPATHIC NEONATAL HEPATITIS FROM BILIARY ATRESIA. It may be difficult to differentiate clearly infants with biliary atresia, who require surgical correction, from those with intrahepatic disease (neonatal hepatitis) and patent bile ducts. No single biochemical test or imaging procedure is entirely satisfactory. Diagnostic schemata incorporate clinical, historical, biochemical, and radiologic features.

Patients with idiopathic neonatal hepatitis have a familial incidence of approximately 20%, whereas extrahepatic biliary atresia is unlikely to recur within the same family. Some infants with biliary atresia have an increased incidence of other abnormalities, such as the polysplenia syndrome with abdominal heterotaxia, malrotation, levocardia, and intra-abdominal vascular anomalies. Neonatal hepatitis appears to be more common in premature or small for gestational age infants. Persistently acholic stools suggest biliary obstruction (biliary atresia), but patients with severe idiopathic neonatal hepatitis may have a transient severe impairment of bile excretion. On the other hand, consistently pigmented stools rule against biliary atresia. The finding of bile-stained fluid on duodenal intubation also excludes biliary atresia. Palpation of the liver may find an abnormal size or consistency in patients with extrahepatic biliary atresia, which is less common with neonatal hepatitis.

Imaging techniques are generally not helpful, but ultrasonography should be carried out early because it may detect a choledochal cyst or another unsuspected cause of cholestasis associated with dilatation of the biliary tract.

Hepatobiliary scintigraphy using imidodiacetic acid analogs has been used by some clinicians to differentiate biliary atresia from neonatal hepatitis. In biliary atresia, hepatocyte function is intact and uptake of the agent is unimpaired, but excretion into the intestine is absent, whereas in patients with neonatal hepatitis, uptake is sluggish, but excretion into the biliary tract and intestine eventually occurs. Oral administration of phenobarbital (5 mg/kg/day) for 5 days prior to the study enhances biliary excretion of the isotope in patients with neonatal hepatitis.

Liver biopsy provides the most reliable discriminatory evidence. In **biliary atresia,** there are bile ductular proliferation, the presence of bile plugs, and portal or perilobular edema and fibrosis, with the basic hepatic lobular architecture intact. In **neonatal hepatitis,** on the other hand, there is severe, diffuse hepatocellular disease, with distortion of lobular architecture, marked infiltration with inflammatory cells, and focal hepatocellular necrosis; the bile ductules show little alteration. Giant cell transformation is found in infants with either condition and has no diagnostic specificity.

Histologic changes similar to those in idiopathic neonatal hepatitis occur in a variety of diseases, including α_1-antitrypsin deficiency, galactosemia, and, various forms of intrahepatic cholestasis. Although paucity of intrahepatic bile ductules may be detected on liver biopsy even within the first few weeks of life, later biopsies in such patients will reveal a more characteristic pattern.

MANAGEMENT OF PATIENTS WITH SUSPECTED BILIARY ATRESIA. In infants in whom clinical features and liver biopsy suggest biliary obstruction, exploratory laparotomy and direct cholangiography should be done to determine the presence and site of obstruction. For patients in whom a **correctable lesion** is present, direct drainage can be accomplished. When no correctable lesion is found, an examination of frozen sections obtained from the transected porta hepatis can detect the presence of biliary epithelium and determine the size and patency of the residual bile ducts. In some cases, the cholangiogram will indicate that the biliary tree is patent but of diminished caliber, suggesting that the cholestasis is not due to biliary tract obliteration but to bile duct paucity or markedly diminished flow in the presence of intrahepatic disease. In these cases, transection of or further dissection into the porta hepatis should be *avoided.*

For patients in whom **no correctable lesion** is found, the hepatoportoenterostomy procedure of Kasai can be carried out. The rationale for this operation is that minute bile duct remnants, representing residual channels, may be present in the fibrous tissue of the porta hepatis; such channels may be in direct continuity with the intrahepatic ductule system. In such cases, transection of the porta hepatis with anastomosis of bowel mucosa to the proximal surface of the transection may allow bile drainage. If flow is not rapidly established within the first months of life, progressive obliteration and cirrhosis will ensue. If microscopic channels of patency greater than 150 μ in diameter are found, postoperative establishment of bile flow is likely. The Kasai operation is most successful (90%) if performed before 8 wk of life.

Some patients with biliary atresia, even of the "noncorrectable" type, derive long-term benefits from interventions as the Kasai procedure. In most, however, a degree of hepatic dysfunction persists. Patients with biliary atresia usually have persistent inflammation of the intrahepatic biliary tree, which suggests that biliary atresia reflects a dynamic process involving the entire hepatobiliary system. This may account for the ultimate development of complications such as portal hypertension. The short-term benefit of hepatoportoenterostomy is decompression and drainage sufficient to forestall the onset of cirrhosis and sustain growth until a successful liver transplantation can be done (Chapter 313).

MANAGEMENT OF CHRONIC CHOLESTASIS

With any form of neonatal cholestasis, whether the primary disease is idiopathic neonatal hepatitis, intrahepatic bile duct paucity, or biliary atresia, affected patients are at increased risk for chronic complications. These reflect varying degrees of residual hepatic functional capacity and are due directly or indirectly to diminished bile flow:

1. Any substance normally excreted into bile is retained in the liver, with subsequent accumulation in tissue and in serum. Involved substances include bile acids, bilirubin, cholesterol, and trace elements.
2. Decreased delivery of bile acids to the proximal intestine leads to inadequate digestion and absorption of dietary long-chain triglycerides and fat-soluble vitamins.
3. Impairment of hepatic metabolic function may alter hormonal balance and utilization of nutrients.
4. Progressive liver damage may lead to biliary cirrhosis, portal hypertension, and liver failure.

The management of such patients (Table 302–2) is empirical, and the best guide is careful monitoring. At present, no therapy is known to be effective in halting the progression of cholestasis or in preventing further hepatocellular damage and cirrhosis.

A major concern is growth failure, which is related in part to malabsorption and malnutrition resulting from ineffective digestion and absorption of dietary fat. Use of a medium-chain triglyceride-containing formula may improve caloric balance.

With chronic cholestasis and prolonged survival, children

■ **TABLE 302–2 Suggested Medical Management of Persistent Cholestasis**

Clinical Impairment	Management
Malnutrition resulting from malabsorption of dietary long-chain triglyceride	Replace with dietary formula or supplements containing medium-chain triglycerides
Fat-soluble vitamin malabsorption	
Vitamin A deficiency (night blindness, thick skin)	Replace with 10,000–15,000 IU/day as Aquasol A
Vitamin E deficiency (neuromuscular degeneration)	Replace with 50–400 IU/day as oral α-tocopherol or TPGS
Vitamin D deficiency (metabolic bone disease)	Replace with 5,000–8,000 IU/day of D_2 or 3–5 μg/kg/day of 25-hydroxycholecalciferol
Vitamin K deficiency (hypoprothrombinemia)	Replace with 2.5–5.0 mg every other day as water-soluble derivative of menadione
Micronutrient deficiency	Calcium, phosphate, or zinc supplementation
Deficiency of water-soluble vitamins	Supplement with twice the recommended daily allowance
Retention of biliary constituents such as bile acids and cholesterol (itch or xanthomata)	Administer choleretics (Ursodeoxycholic acid, 15–20 mg/kg/day) or bile acid binders (cholestyramine 8–16 g/day)
Progressive liver disease	
Portal hypertension (variceal bleeding, ascites, hypersplenism)	Interim management (control bleeding; salt restriction; spironolactone)
End-stage liver disease (liver failure)	Transplantation

TPGS = D-tocopherol polyethylene glycol-1000 succinate.

with hepatobiliary disease may experience deficiencies of the fat-soluble vitamins (A, D, E, and K). Inadequate absorption of fat and fat-soluble vitamins may be exacerbated by administration of the bile acid binder cholestyramine. Metabolic bone disease is common.

A degenerative neuromuscular syndrome is found with chronic cholestasis caused by malabsorption and therefore deficiency of vitamin E; affected children experience progressive areflexia, cerebellar ataxia, ophthalmoplegia, and decreased vibratory sensation. Specific morphologic lesions have been found in the central nervous system (CNS), peripheral nerves, and muscles. These lesions resemble those found in animals with vitamin E deficiency and are potentially reversible in young children (i.e., those <3–4 yr old). The deficiency may be prevented by the oral administration of large doses (up to 1,000 IU/day) of vitamin E; patients unable to absorb sufficient quantities may require administration of D-tocopherol polyethylene glycol-1000 succinate orally. Serum levels may be monitored as a guide to efficacy; affected children will have low serum vitamin E concentrations, increased hydrogen peroxide hemolysis, and low ratios of serum vitamin E to total serum lipids (<6.0 mg/g for children younger than 12 yr and <0.8 mg/g for older patients).

Serum vitamin A concentrations can usually be maintained at normal levels in patients with chronic cholestasis who received oral supplementation of vitamin A esters. It is essential to monitor the vitamin A status in such patients.

Pruritus is a particularly troublesome complication of chronic cholestasis, often with the appearance of xanthomata. Both features seem to be related to the accumulation of cholesterol and bile acids in serum and in tissues. Elimination of these retained compounds is difficult when bile ducts are obstructed, but if there is any degree of bile duct patency, administration of ursodeoxycholic acid and cholestyramine may increase bile flow or interrupt the enterohepatic circulation of bile acids and thus decrease the xanthomata and ameliorate the pruritus (see Table 302–2). Cholestyramine resin is unpalatable and may have side effects such as constipation, hyperchloremia, and exacerbation of fat-soluble vitamin deficiency. Ursodeoxycholic acid therapy may also lower serum cholesterol levels. The recommended dose is 15 mg/kg/24 hr.

In patients with portal hypertension, variceal hemorrhage and the development of hypersplenism are common. However, episodes of gastrointestinal hemorrhage in patients who have chronic liver disease may be due not to esophageal varices but to gastritis or peptic ulcer disease. Because the management of these various complications differ, differentiation perhaps via endoscopy is necessary before treatment is initiated (Chapter 312).

In patients with **ascites,** initial management consists of dietary salt restriction; sodium intake is limited to 0.5 g (~1–2 mEq/kg/day). It is not necessary to restrict fluid intake in patients with adequate renal output. Diuresis may be maintained by the use of agents, such as furosemide, alone or in combination with spironolactone (3–5 mg/kg/day in four doses). Patients with ascites, but without peripheral edema, are at risk for reduced plasma volume and decreased urine output following diuretic therapy. Tense ascites alters renal blood flow and systemic hemodynamics. Paracentesis and intravenous albumin infusion may improve hemodynamics, renal perfusion, and symptomatology. Follow-up includes dietary counseling and monitoring of serum and urinary electrolyte concentrations (Chapter 315).

In patients with advanced liver disease, hepatic transplantation may have a success rate greater than 85% (Chapter 313). If the operation is technically feasible, it will prolong life and may correct the metabolic error in diseases such as α_1-antitrypsin deficiency, tyrosinemia, or Wilson disease. Success depends on adequate intraoperative, preoperative, and postoperative care and on the cautious use of immunosuppressive agents. Scarcity of donors of small livers severely limits the application of liver transplantation for infants and children. However, the use of *reduced*-size transplants has increased the ability to treat small children successfully.

PROGNOSIS

The prognosis for infants with biliary atresia has been discussed earlier. For patients with idiopathic neonatal hepatitis, the variable prognosis may reflect the heterogeneity of the disease. In **sporadic** cases, 60–70% will recover with no evidence of hepatic structural or functional impairment. Approximately 5–10% will have persistent fibrosis or inflammation, and a smaller percentage will have more severe liver disease, such as cirrhosis. Death of infants usually occurs early in the course of the illness, owing to hemorrhage or sepsis. Of infants with idiopathic neonatal hepatitis of the **familial** variety, only 20–30% will recover; 10–15% will acquire chronic liver disease with cirrhosis. Liver transplantation may be required.

302.2 *Cholestasis in the Older Child*

Acute viral hepatitis accounts for most cases of cholestasis with onset after the neonatal period. Many of the conditions causing neonatal cholestasis may also cause chronic cholestasis in older patients. An adolescent with conjugated hyperbilirubinemia should be evaluated for acute and chronic hepatitis, α_1-antitrypsin deficiency, Wilson disease, liver disease associated with inflammatory bowel disease, and the syndromes of intrahepatic bile duct paucity. Other causes include obstruction caused by cholelithiasis, abdominal tumors or enlarged lymph nodes, or hepatic inflammation resulting from drug ingestion. Management is similar to that proposed for neonatal cholestasis (see Table 302–2).

CHAPTER 303
Metabolic Diseases of the Liver

William F. Balistreri

See also Chapter 70.

Because the liver plays a central role in synthetic, degradative, and regulatory pathways involving carbohydrate, protein, lipid, trace elements, and vitamin metabolism, there are many metabolic abnormalities or specific enzyme deficiencies that affect the liver primarily or secondarily (Table 303–1). Liver disease may arise when absence of an enzyme produces a block in a metabolic pathway, when unmetabolized substrate accumulates proximal to a block, when deficiency develops of an essential substance produced distal to an aberrant chemical reaction, or when synthesis of an abnormal metabolite occurs. The spectrum of pathologic changes includes (1) *hepatocyte injury,* with subsequent failure of other metabolic functions, often eventuating in cirrhosis or liver tumors or both; (2) *storage* of lipid, glycogen, or other products manifest as hepatomegaly, often with complications specific to deranged metabolism (e.g., decreased blood glucose in patients with glycogen storage disease); and (3) absence of structural change despite profound metabolic effects, as with urea cycle defects. The clinical manifestations of metabolic diseases of the liver mimic infections, intoxications, and hematologic and immunologic diseases (Table 303–2). Further clues are provided by family history of a similar illness or by the observation that the onset of symptoms is closely associated with a change in dietary habits (e.g., initiation of ingestion of fructose). In most cases, clinical and laboratory evidence will guide the evaluation. Liver biopsy offers morphologic study and will permit enzyme assays, as well as quantitative and qualitative assays of various other constituents. Such studies require cooperation of experienced laboratories and careful attention to collection and handling of specimens.

■ **TABLE 303–1 Inborn Errors of Metabolism Manifest as Hepatobiliary Dysfunction**

Disorders of Carbohydrate Metabolism
Disorders of **galactose** metabolism
Galactosemia
Disorders of **fructose** metabolism
Hereditary fructose intolerance
Fructose-1,6 DP deficiency
Glycogen storage diseases
Type I
Von Gierke (la)
Type lb
Type III (Cori/Forbes)
Type IV (Andersen)
Type VI (Hers)
Disorders of Amino Acid and Protein Metabolism
Disorders of **tyrosine** metabolism
Transient
Neonatal
Associated with severe liver disease (e.g., cirrhosis)
Nontransient
Hereditary tyrosinemia (type I)
Tyrosinemia, type II
Inherited **urea cycle** enzyme defects
CPS deficiency
OTC deficiency (X-linked dominant)
Citrullinemia
Argininosuccinic aciduria
Argininemia
N-AGS deficiency
Disorders of Lipid Metabolism
Wolman disease
Cholesteryl ester storage disease
Gaucher disease
Niemann-Pick type C
Disorders of Bile Acid Metabolism
Isomerase deficiency
Reductase deficiency
Zellweger syndrome (cerebrohepatorenal)
Disorders of Metal Metabolism
Wilson disease
Hepatic copper overload
Indian childhood cirrhosis
Neonatal iron storage disease (perinatal hemochromatosis)
Disorders of Bilirubin Metabolism
Crigler-Najjar
Type I
Type II—Arias
Dubin-Johnson
Rotor
Miscellaneous
α_1-Antitrypsin deficiency
Cystic fibrosis
Erythropoietic protoporphyria

CPS = Carbamoyl phosphate synthetase; OTC = ornithine transcarbamoylase; N-AGS = N-acetylglutamate synthetase.

■ **TABLE 303–2 Clinical Manifestations that Suggest the Possibility of Metabolic Disease**

Jaundice, hepatomegaly (± splenomegaly), fulminant hepatic failure
Hypoglycemia, organic acidemia, lactic acidemia, hyperammonemia, bleeding (coagulopathy)
Recurrent vomiting, failure to thrive, short stature, dysmorphic features
Developmental delay/psychomotor retardation, hypotonia, progressive neuromuscular deterioration, seizures
Cardiac dysfunction/failure, unusual odors, rickets, cataracts

303.1 Inherited Deficient Conjugation of Bilirubin

(Familial Nonhemolytic Unconjugated Hyperbilirubinemia)

Hepatic glucuronyl transferase activity (Chapter 88.3) is deficient in two genetically and functionally distinct disorders (Crigler-Najjar syndrome) producing congenital nonobstructive, nonhemolytic, unconjugated hyperbilirubinemia. The molecular mechanism of the various Crigler-Najjar syndromes is only partially understood and presumably quite complex. This is due in part to the fact that the activity of multiple glucuronyl transferase isoforms are deficient in various phenotypes of the Crigler-Najjar syndrome. *Low levels of unconjugated hyperbilirubinemia also occur in **Gilbert's syndrome,** a benign disorder, owing to a missense mutation in the transferase gene.*

CRIGLER-NAJJAR SYNDROME (TYPE I GLUCURONYL TRANSFERASE DEFICIENCY). This form is inherited as an autosomal recessive trait. Parents of affected children have partial defects in conjugation as determined by hepatic enzyme assay or by measurement of glucuronide formation, but their serum bilirubin concentrations are normal.

Clinical Manifestations. Severe unconjugated hyperbilirubinemia develops in the homozygous infant during the first 3 days of life, and without treatment serum concentrations of 25–35 mg/dL are reached during the 1st mo. Kernicterus, an almost universal complication of this disorder, is usually first noted in the early neonatal period, but some treated infants have survived childhood without clinical sequelae. Stools are pale yellow. Persistence of unconjugated hyperbilirubinema at levels above 20 mg/dL after the 1st wk of life in the absence of hemolysis should suggest the syndrome.

Diagnosis. The diagnosis of Crigler-Najjar syndrome is based on the early age of onset and the extreme level of bilirubin elevation in the absence of hemolysis. In the bile, bilirubin concentration is less than 10 mg/dL compared with normal concentrations of 50–100 mg/dL, and there is no bilirubin glucuronide. Definitive diagnosis is established by measuring hepatic glucuronyl transferase activity in a liver specimen obtained by a closed biopsy; open biopsy should be avoided because surgery and anesthesia may precipitate kernicterus. Identification of the heterozygous state in the parents is also strongly suggestive of the diagnosis. Differential diagnosis is discussed in Chapter 88.3. Type II disease may be distinguished from type I by the marked decline in serum bilirubin level that occurs in type II disease after 1 wk of treatment with phenobarbital.

Treatment. Serum bilirubin concentration should be kept below 20 mg/dL for at least the first 2–4 wk of life; in low-birthweight infants the levels should be kept lower. This usually requires repeated exchange transfusions and phototherapy. Because the risk of kernicterus persists into adult life, although the serum bilirubin levels required to produce brain injury beyond the neonatal period are considerably higher (usually above 35 mg/dL), phototherapy is generally continued throughout the early years of life. In older infants and children, phototherapy is used mainly during sleep in order not to interfere with normal activities. However, despite the administration of increasing intensities of light for longer periods, the serum bilirubin decrement response to phototherapy decreases with age. Cholestyramine or agar may be used to bind photobilirubin products, thus interfering with the enterohepatic recirculation of bilirubin. Prompt treatment of intercurrent infections, febrile episodes, and other types of illness may help prevent the later development of kernicterus, which may occur at bilirubin levels of 45–55 mg/dL. All type I patients have eventually experienced severe kernicterus by young adulthood, despite vigorous continuous management that maintained neurologic normality during childhood. Orthotopic hepatic transplantation will cure the disease and has been successful in a small number of patients. Other therapeutic modalities have included plasmapheresis, and limitation of bilirubin production. The latter option, inhibiting bilirubin generation, is possible via inhibition of heme oxygenase using metalloporphyrin therapy. Genetically engineered enzymatic replacement therapy remains a potential therapy for the future.

CRIGLER-NAJJAR SYNDROME. GLUCURONYL TRANSFERASE DEFICIENCY TYPE II. This autosomal dominant disease with marked variability of penetrance may present in a manner similar to type I syndrome, or it may be a less severe disorder, occasionally even without neonatal manifestations. Studies have suggested that Crigler-Najjar syndrome type II is caused by homozygous mutation in glucuronyl transferase isoform I activity.

Clinical Manifestations. When this disorder presents in the neonatal period, there is usually unconjugated hyperbilirubinemia during the first 3 days of life; serum bilirubin concentrations may be in a range compatible with physiologic jaundice or may be at pathologic levels. Characteristically, the concentrations remain elevated into and after the 3rd wk of life, persisting in a range of 1.5–22 mg/dL; concentrations in the lower part of this range may create uncertainty as to whether chronic hyperbilirubinemia is present. The onset of kernicterus is unusual. Stool color is normal, and the infants are without clinical signs or symptoms of disease. There is no evidence of hemolysis.

Diagnosis. Bile bilirubin concentration is nearly normal in type II syndrome. Jaundiced infants and young children having type II syndrome respond readily to 5 mg/kg/24 hr of oral phenobarbital with a decrease in serum bilirubin concentration to 2–3 mg/dL within 7–10 days. Those with type I syndrome do not respond.

Treatment. Long-term reduction in serum bilirubin levels can be achieved with chronic administration of phenobarbital at 5 mg/kg/24 hr. The cosmetic and psychosocial benefit should be weighed against the risks of an effective dose of the drug because there is a small long-term risk of kernicterus in the absence of hemolytic disease.

INHERITED CONJUGATED HYPERBILIRUBINEMIA

In inherited conjugated hyperbilirubinemias, which are autosomal recessive disorders characterized by mild jaundice, the transfer of bilirubin and other organic anions from liver to bile is defective. Chronic mild conjugated hyperbilirubinemia is usually detected during adolescence or early adulthood but may occur as early as the 2nd year of life. The results of routine liver function tests are normal. Jaundice may be exacerbated with infection, pregnancy, oral contraceptives, alcohol, or surgery. There is usually no morbidity, and life expectancy is normal; but these disorders may initially present difficult problems in the differential diagnosis of more serious diseases.

DUBIN-JOHNSON SYNDROME. Dubin-Johnson syndrome is considered to be an autosomal recessive inherited defect in hepatocyte secretion of bilirubin glucuronide. The defect in hepatic excretory function is not limited to conjugated bilirubin excretion but also involves multiple organic anions normally excreted from the liver cell into bile. Bile acid excretion is normal and serum bile acid levels are normal. Urinary coproporphyrin excretion is normal in quantity; however, coproporphyrin I constitutes 80% of the total. Coproporphyrin III is normally greater than 75% of the total. Oral and intravenous cholangiography will fail to visualize the biliary tract. The defect is in porphyrin metabolism or excretion with more than 90% of the normal total urinary coproporphyrin excretion occurring as a coproporphyrin I isomer. Roentgenography of the gallbladder is also abnormal. The liver cells contain black pigment similar to melanin.

ROTOR SYNDROME. These patients have an additional deficiency in organic anion uptake. Total urinary coproporphyrin excretion is elevated with a relative increase in the amount of the coproporphyrin I isomer. The gallbladder is normal by roentgenography, and there is no black pigment in liver cells. Sulfabromophthalein excretion is often abnormal.

303.2 Wilson Disease

Wilson disease (hepatolenticular degeneration) is an autosomal recessive disorder characterized by degenerative changes in the brain, liver disease, and Kayser-Fleischer rings in the cornea (Chapter 548). The incidence is 1:500,000–100,000 births. It is fatal if untreated; however, specific, effective treatment is available. Rapid diagnostic investigation of the possibility of Wilson disease in a patient presenting with any form of liver disease, particularly if older than 5 yr, not only will facilitate early institution of management of Wilson disease and related genetic counseling but will also allow appropriate treatment of non-Wilson liver disease once copper toxicosis is ruled out.

PATHOGENESIS. Defective mobilization of copper from lysosomes in the liver cell for excretion into bile is the basis for the multiorgan damage seen in patients with Wilson disease. Relentless accumulation of copper in the liver reaches the point at which the retention capacity is exceeded. Copper then escapes the liver to damage other organs, particularly the brain and kidneys, and accumulates in the cornea, visible as Kaiser-Fleischer rings. The underlying mechanism of liver damage in Wilson disease is presumably oxidant injury to the hepatocyte mitochondria, which is the target organelle in copper-induced toxicity. Lipid peroxidation of the mitochondria resulting from copper overload leads to functional alterations.

The abnormal gene for Wilson disease is on chromosome 13; linkage studies have assigned the Wilson disease locus to chromosome 13 at q14–q21. The gene encodes amino acid structural motifs consistent with a role in copper transport. The cloning of the gene for Wilson disease raises the prospect of precise presymptomatic detection of Wilson disease, timely initiation of therapy, and ultimately gene therapy.

Fetal and neonatal liver normally contains relatively high concentrations of sulfur-rich copper-binding protein (metallothionein) and of copper; serum ceruloplasmin and copper levels are relatively low. The mechanisms responsible for copper homeostasis in older children reach maturity by 2 yr of age. The wilsonian trait may be expressed after this time, but Wilson disease is not clinically manifest before the age of 5 yr.

Altered incorporation of copper into hepatic proteins such as ceruloplasmin is associated with diffuse accumulation of copper in the cytosol of hepatocytes. Later, as liver cells are overloaded, copper is distributed to other tissues, to which it is toxic, primarily as a potent inhibitor of enzymatic processes. Ionic copper inhibits pyruvate oxidase in brain and adenosine triphosphatase in membranes, leading to decreased adenosine triphosphate (ATP)-phosphocreatine and potassium content of tissue. The glycolytic pathway and microsomal membrane ATPases are inhibited.

CLINICAL MANIFESTATIONS. Copper enters the circulation in a non-ceruloplasmin-bound form and accumulates in multiple organs. The symptoms of Wilson disease are due to copper-induced injury in these various organs. Manifestations are variable, with a tendency to familial patterns. The younger the patient, the more likely hepatic involvement will be the predominant manifestation. After the age of 20 yr, neurologic symptoms predominate. Forms of hepatic disease include asymptomatic hepatomegaly (with or without splenomegaly), subacute or chronic hepatitis, or fulminant hepatic failure. Cryptogenic cirrhosis, portal hypertension, ascites, edema, esophageal bleeding, or other effects of hepatic dysfunction (delayed puberty, amenorrhea, or coagulation defect) may be manifestations of Wilson disease.

Neurologic and psychiatric disorders may develop insidiously or precipitously, with intention tremor, dysarthria, dystonia, deterioration in school performance, or behavioral changes. Kayser-Fleischer rings may be absent in young patients with liver disease but are always present in patients with neurologic symptoms. Hemolysis may be an initial manifestation, possibly related to the release of large amounts of copper from damaged hepatocytes; this form of Wilson disease is usually fatal without transplantation. During hemolytic episodes urinary copper excretion and serum copper levels (non-ceruloplasmin bound) are markedly elevated. Manifestations of Fanconi syndrome and progressive renal failure with alterations in tubular transport of amino acids, glucose, and uric acid may be present. Unusual manifestations include arthritis and endocrinopathies, such as hypoparathyroidism.

PATHOLOGY. All grades of hepatic injury occur, with fatty change, ballooned hepatocytes, glycogen granules, minimal inflammation, and enlarged Kupffer cells. The lesion may be indistinguishable from that of chronic active hepatitis. Ultrastructural changes include large, dense mitochondria with altered smooth endoplasmic reticulum.

DIAGNOSIS. The clinical suspicion is confirmed by study of indices of copper metabolism. Wilson disease should be considered in children and teenagers with unexplained acute or chronic liver disease, neurologic symptoms of unknown cause, acute hemolysis, psychiatric illnesses, behavioral changes, Fanconi syndrome, or unexplained bone disease.

The best screening test is to measure the serum ceruloplasmin level. Most patients with Wilson disease will have decreased ceruloplasmin levels. Serum copper may be elevated in early Wilson disease, and urinary copper excretion (usually <40 μg/day) is increased to greater than 100 μg/day and often up to 1,000 μg or more per day. In equivocal cases the response of urinary copper output to chelation may be of diagnostic help; following a 1-g oral dose of D-penicillamine, affected patients will excrete 1,200–2,000 αg/day.

Liver biopsy is of value for examination of the histology and for measurement of the hepatic copper content (normally <10 μg/g dry weight). In Wilson disease hepatic copper content exceeds 250 μg/g dry weight. In healthy heterozygotes, levels may be intermediate.

Family members of patients with proven cases require screening for presymptomatic Wilson disease. Such screening should include determination of the serum ceruloplasmin level and urinary copper excretion. If these results are abnormal or equivocal, liver biopsy should be carried out to determine morphology and hepatic copper content. Genetic testing will be possible in the near future.

TREATMENT. The administration of copper-chelating agents leads to rapid excretion of excess deposited copper in patients with Wilson disease. A major attempt should be made to restrict copper intake to less than 1 mg/day. Foods such as liver, shellfish, nuts, and chocolate should be avoided. If the copper content of the water exceeds 0.1 mg/L, it may be necessary to demineralize the water. Chelation therapy is currently best managed with oral administration of penicillamine (β, β-dimethylcysteine) in a dose of 1 g/day in two doses before meals for adults and 0.5–0.75 g/day for patients younger than 10 yr. In response to D-penicillamine, urinary copper excretion will markedly increase, and there may be slow clinical improvement. Urinary copper levels may become normal with continued administration D-penicillamine, with marked improvement in hepatic and neurologic function and the disappearance of Kayser-Fleischer rings. Toxic effects of penicillamine are uncommon and consist of hypersensitivity reactions (Goodpasture syndrome, systemic lupus erythematosus, polymyositis), interaction with collagen and elastin, deficiency of other elements such as zinc, as well as aplastic anemia and nephrosis. Because penicillamine is an antimetabolite of vitamin B_6, additional amounts of this vitamin are necessary. For those patients who are unable to tolerate penicillamine, triethylene tetramine dihydrochloride (Trien, TETA, Trientine) at a dose of 0.5–2 g/24 hr is an acceptable alternative.

PROGNOSIS. Untreated patients with Wilson disease will die from the hepatic, neurologic, renal, or hematologic complications. The prognosis in patients receiving prompt and continuous D-penicillamine is variable and depends on the time of initiation of and the individual responsiveness to chelation. Liver transplantation should be considered for patients with fulminant liver disease. In asymptomatic siblings of affected patients the expression of the disease can be prevented by early institution of chelation therapy.

303.3 Hepatic Copper Overload Syndrome

Another form of childhood cirrhosis apparently associated with a genetic disturbance in copper metabolism has been described. This syndrome differs from Wilson disease in its earlier onset. Affected children experience progressive lethargy, abdominal distention, and jaundice and die before 6 yr of age. The hepatic histopathology resembles that of Indian childhood cirrhosis.

303.4 Indian Childhood Cirrhosis

Indian childhood cirrhosis is a fatal familial disorder that occurs predominantly in rural India in middle-outcome Hindu families. It has been reported also in the Middle East, in West Africa, and in Central America. It affects children of both sexes, with onset usually at 1–3 yr of age. Hepatomegaly is often the 1st sign; fever, anorexia, and jaundice occur. There is in most cases rapid evolution to cirrhosis and liver failure. Serum immunoglobulin levels and hepatic copper concentrations are markedly elevated. No effective therapy is known.

It has been suggested that excessive dietary copper may play a role in the cause, owing to the use of copper and brass in cooking and for storage of water and milk. The early introduction of copper-contaminated milk into infant diets may explain the epidemiologic features. There may be a predisposing inherited susceptibility.

303.5 Neonatal Hemochromatosis

Neonatal hemochromatosis is a rare form of fulminant liver disease of unknown cause characterized by diffuse increased iron deposition in the liver, pancreas, heart, and endocrine organs without evidence of increased iron intake (ingestion or transfusion). Inheritance is autosomal recessive. Affected infants may be born premature or with intrauterine growth retardation, demonstrate a large placenta, and then manifest a rapidly fatal progressive illness characterized by hepatomegaly, hypoglycemia, hypoprothrombinemia, hypoalbuminemia, and hyperbilirubinemia. Symptoms begin in utero or in the 1st wk of life. The coagulopathy is refractory to therapy with vitamin K. The diagnosis can be confirmed through documentation of extrahepatic siderosis (biopsy of buccal mucosal glands will be laden with iron) or magnetic resonance imaging determination of iron storage in organs such as the pancreas.

The hepatic pathology reveals fibrosis, regenerative nodules, giant cell formation, necrosis, and hepatocellular hemosiderin deposits not unlike those in adult-type hereditary hemochromatosis. Hyperferritinemia is present.

Treatment with chelating agents (deferoxamine) alone is ineffective. Liver transplantation should be an early consideration.

303.6 α-Antitrypsin Deficiency

See also Chapter 354.4.

A small percentage of individuals homozygous for deficiency of the major serum protease inhibitor, α_1-antitrypsin, have neonatal cholestasis and later childhood cirrhosis. α_1-Antitrypsin, a glycoprotein synthesized by the liver, accounts for 80% of the serum α_1-globulin fraction. α_1-Antitrypsin is present in more than 20 different codominant alleles, only a few of which are associated with defective protease inhibitors. The most common allele of the protease inhibitor (Pi) system is M, and the normal phenotype is PiMM. The 2 allele predisposes to clinical deficiency; patients with liver disease are usually PiZZ and have serum α_1-antitrypsin levels less than 2 mg/mL (approximately 10–20% of normal). The incidence of the PiZZ genotype in the white population is estimated at 1:2,000–4,000. Intermediate phenotypes PiMS, PiMZ, and PiSZ are not definitively associated with liver disease. The null genotype has no periodic acid-Schiff (PAS)-positive inclusions and is not associated with liver disease. Of all PiZZ persons, less than 20% will develop neonatal cholestasis. These patients are indistinguishable from other infants with "idiopathic" neonatal hepatitis, of whom they constitute approximately 5–10%.

In affected patients the course of liver disease is highly variable. Jaundice, acholic stools, and hepatomegaly are present during the 1st week of life, but the jaundice usually clears during the 2nd–4th mo. There may follow complete resolution, persistent liver disease, or the development of cirrhosis. Older children may present with manifestations of chronic liver disease or cirrhosis, with evidence of portal hypertension.

The fact that liver disease is not universal suggests a complex pathogenesis. The liver disease may be secondary to retention of the α_1-antitrypsin in the liver.

The diagnosis is best made by determination of a α_1-antitrypsin (Pi) phenotype and confirmed by liver biopsy. PAS-positive disease-resistant intracytoplasmic globules are seen in periportal hepatocytes. Immunofluorescence and immunocytochemical studies have shown this material to be antigenically related to α_1-antitrypsin. It has been suggested that abnormal biosynthesis of the protein or defective glycosylation may interfere with excretion of the product from the rough endoplasmic reticulum into the extracellular space. Electron microscopy shows amorphous deposits (glycoprotein) within dilated rough endoplasmic reticulum.

The pattern of neonatal liver injury may be highly variable. There is hepatocellular damage with giant cell transformation, minimal inflammation, and bile stasis. Varying degrees of portal fibrosis with biliary duct proliferation occur.

Liver transplantation has been curative. There is no other effective therapy for liver disease as yet, but gene therapy may become possible.

CHAPTER 304
Liver Abscess

William F. Balistreri

LIVER ABSCESS. Hepatic abscesses occur in infants in association with sepsis, umbilical vein infection, or vessel cannulation. Beyond infancy, hepatic abscesses occur most commonly in immunosuppressed patients. Of a large series of hepatic abscesses, 40% were found in patients with chronic granulomatous disease, and 20% in otherwise immunosuppressed patients (e.g., leukemia). Pyogenic hepatic abscesses may arise from (1) the portal circulation in patients with pylephlebitis or intra-abdominal sepsis (appendicitis, inflammatory bowel disease); (2) generalized sepsis; (3) cholangitis associated with biliary tract obstruction, such as by gallstones, in inflammatory bowel disease, after a Kasai procedure, and with choledochal cysts; (4) systemic spread from an intra-abdominal infection or contiguous spread (which usually produces large abscesses); and (5) cryptogenic biliary tract infections. Small abscesses (microabscesses) are most commonly secondary to bacteremia, candidemia, or cat-scratch disease. Implicated organisms include predominantly *Staphylococcus aureus, Escherichia coli, Salmonella,* and anaerobic organisms. Symptoms are nonspecific and may suggest systemic infection. There may be fever and pain in the right upper quadrant, and the liver is enlarged and may be tender to percussion. Jaundice is uncommon; serum aminotransferase and alkaline phosphatase activities may be mildly elevated. The erythrocyte sedimentation rate is high, and there is a leukocytosis. The results of blood cultures may be positive. Roentgenographic study of the chest may show elevation of the right hemidiaphragm with decreased mobility. Ultrasound or gallium scans or both may indicate the site of the abscess. In most cases, treatment requires percutaneous ultrasonogram- or CT-guided needle aspiration or surgical drainage. Antibiotic therapy is based on the culture results and Gram stain of the abscess fluid. *Entamoeba histolytica* may also cause hepatic abscesses in symptomatic or asymptomatic patients with amebic infection of the gastrointestinal tract (Chapter 244.1).

CHAPTER 305

Liver Disease Associated with Systemic Disorders

William F. Balistreri

INFLAMMATORY BOWEL DISEASE. Hepatobiliary disease may complicate ulcerative colitis and Crohn disease (see Chapter 283). Both the manifestations and the severity vary. Fatty liver, cholangitis, drug-induced injury, chronic hepatitis, portal fibrosis, cirrhosis, hepatic abscesses, infarction, portal vein thrombosis, sclerosing cholangitis, carcinoma of the biliary tract, and cholelithiasis have all been associated. These complications are more likely to occur in patients with other extraintestinal complications, but there is no correlation with the severity of the inflammatory bowel disease. The cause of abnormalities in liver function in patients with ulcerative colitis or Crohn disease is unknown. Total colectomy has not been beneficial in management of hepatobiliary complications in patients with ulcerative colitis.

Extensive fatty change in the liver has been found, especially in patients with inflammatory bowel disease who are malnourished or chronically incapacitated. Most patients have no symptoms; they have only hepatomegaly as a sign. The chemical abnormalities are mild. The fatty infiltration usually subsides with therapy.

Primary sclerosing cholangitis may be difficult to distinguish from chronic hepatitis in patients with inflammatory bowel disease. The patients may be asymptomatic or have jaundice, pruritus, or abdominal pain. Elevation of alkaline phosphatase or 5′-nucleotidase activities is almost universal. This complication can occur any time in the course of inflammatory bowel disease.

Sclerosing cholangitis (fibrosing inflammation of various segments of the bile ducts) may lead to obliteration of the duct lumen. The clinical and biochemical picture is that of cholestasis, often with intermittent attacks of acute cholangitis (fever, jaundice, right upper quadrant pain, anorexia, weight loss, and pruritus), followed by portal hypertension. This complication is associated with ulcerative colitis and rarely with Crohn disease.

Primary sclerosing cholangitis (*not* associated with inflammatory bowel disease) is uncommon in children. Cholangiography will reveal beading and irregularity of the intrahepatic and extrahepatic bile ducts. Treatment is aimed at improving biliary drainage and attempting to halt the progression of the obliterative process. Symptomatic treatment is required for such complications as pruritus, malnutrition, and infection. There is no definitive treatment; administration of corticosteroids or D-penicillamine has produced inconsistent results. Ursodeoxycholic acid, in a dose of 15 mg/kg/24 hr, may lead to amelioration of pruritus and a decrease in abnormal biochemical values. The course is usually slowly progressive to a fatal outcome if liver transplantation is not carried out.

BACTERIAL SEPSIS. (See Chapters 98 and 168.) This may be complicated by liver disease. The most frequently associated organisms are *Escherichia coli, Klebsiella pneumonia,* and *Pseudomonas aeruginosa.* It is postulated that bacterial endotoxin directly inhibits bile formation by altering the bile canalicular membrane. Clinical manifestations may be subtle and difficult to differentiate from other causes of cholestasis. There is an elevation in the serum bilirubin level, usually predominantly in the conjugated fraction. Serum alkaline phosphatase and aminotransferase activities may be elevated. Liver biopsy shows intrahepatic cholestasis with little or no hepatocyte necrosis. Kupffer cell hyperplasia and an increase in inflammatory cells are also common.

CARDIAC DISEASE. Hepatic congestion and injury may occur as a complication of severe *chronic* or *acute congestive heart failure* (Chapter 399) or *cyanotic heart disease* (Chapter 387). Hepatic dysfunction derives from hypoxemia, systemic venous congestion, and low cardiac output. Hepatic manifestations of left- and right-sided heart failure are similar. With decreased cardiac output, there is decreased hepatic blood flow and centrizonal hypoxia. Hepatic necrosis leads to lactic acidosis, elevated aminotransferase activities, jaundice, prolonged partial thromboplastin time, and possibly hypoglycemia. With right-sided heart failure, increases in right atrial and hepatic venous pressures lead to centrizonal sinusoidal distention that presents a barrier to oxygen diffusion. Hemorrhage, pressure atrophy, and necrosis follow. Jaundice and tender hepatomegaly occur. Ascites may also occur with chronic right-sided congestive heart failure. In patients with shock liver, elevated amino-transferase activities may return rapidly to normal when perfusion and cardiac function improve. A syndrome of fulminant hepatic failure may occur, particularly in patients with aortic coarctation. Hepatic necrosis may be seen in patients with hypoplastic left-sided heart syndrome.

HEMOGLOBINOPATHIES. The patient with *sickle cell anemia* (Chapter 419.1) or *sickle cell thalassemia* (Chapter 419.1) may have hepatic dysfunction owing to acute or chronic viral-associated hepatitis, iron overload, hepatic crises related to severe intrahepatic cholestasis, and ischemic necrosis. In addition, cholelithiasis and a benign form of extreme hyperbilirubinemia have been noted. Hepatic sickle cell crisis or "sickle hepatopathy" may produce intense right upper quadrant pain, fever, leukocytosis, right upper quadrant tenderness, and jaundice. Bilirubin levels may be markedly elevated; alkaline phosphatase activities may be only moderately elevated.

On occasion, children with sickle cell disease experience bilirubin levels exceeding 20 mg/dL; these levels are unaccompanied by severe pain or fever. There is no change in hematocrit or reticulocyte count nor any association with a hemolytic crisis. The clinical course is benign.

CHOLESTASIS ASSOCIATED WITH TOTAL PARENTERAL NUTRITION. The most common metabolic complication of *total parenteral nutrition* (TPN) in premature infants is the development of varying degrees of liver dysfunction. Cholestasis is the most severe form and is potentially fatal. It is the major factor limiting effective long-term use of TPN (Chapter 82).

In *low-birthweight infants,* the incidence of TPN-associated cholestasis is inversely correlated with birthweight. It develops with TPN in almost half of infants with birthweights less than 1,000 g, in 20% of those 1,000–1,500 g, and in 5–10% of those 1,500–2,000 g. The incidence of cholestasis also correlates with the duration of TPN, with onset usually after 2 wk. Respiratory distress, acidosis, hypoxia, necrotizing enterocolitis, short-bowel syndrome, and sepsis seem to enhance the likelihood and severity of cholestasis. Associated illness, the exclusion of enteral intake, and the nature of the underlying disorder that necessitates TPN may also affect the incidence.

The onset is usually insidious, with progressive jaundice and hepatic enlargement or splenomegaly. In low-birthweight infants, the onset of jaundice may overlap the phase of physiologic unconjugated hyperbilirubinemia. Any icteric infant who has received TPN for more than 1 wk should have all bilirubin determinations fractionated. Cholestasis is frequently first detected through routine monitoring of infants receiving TPN. A slow progression of abnormalities is found in biochemical measurements of hepatic function. Serum bile acid concentrations may increase. Rises in serum aminotransferase activities may be a late finding. An elevation in serum alkaline phosphatase activity may be due to rickets, a common complication of TPN in low-birthweight infants.

In addition to cholestasis, biliary complications of intravenous nutrition include cholelithiasis and the development of biliary sludge, associated with thick, inspissated gallbladder contents. These may be asymptomatic.

An effort must be made to differentiate TPN-associated hepatic dysfunction from benign causes of hepatomegaly, such as the deposition of glycogen or fat, which is common with TPN. Serum bilirubin and bile acid levels will remain within the normal range in the latter situation. Consideration of other causes of cholestasis is also appropriate. The group in which TPN-associated cholestasis most frequently occurs (i.e., infants in the neonatal intensive care unit) often receives blood products or drugs. Therefore, hepatic disease related to drug-induced liver disease is a consideration.

The most striking histologic finding in TPN-associated liver disease is canalicular cholestasis, which may begin after less than 2 wk of TPN. Bile duct proliferation may resemble that in biliary atresia. Portal fibrosis is a late finding. Progression of injury to cirrhosis is possible. Milder changes may be reversible with discontinuation of TPN and the initiation of oral feedings.

The pathogenesis of TPN-associated cholestasis is most likely multifactorial. The infant is of low birthweight, is receiving nothing by mouth, may have significant gastrointestinal disease, and often has other systemic complications. The administered nutrient solution has potential toxicity and may induce specific deficiencies. The omission of oral feedings and the absence of intraluminal nutrients blunt the output of the gastrointestinal hormones, which are normal stimulants to bile flow and to development of the hepatobiliary system. Potential hepatotoxins include bacterial endotoxins, specific amino acids or metabolic or degradation products, or copper or manganese; the last two are particularly hepatotoxic.

The goal in management of the infant with TPN-associated cholestasis is to avoid progressive liver injury. It has been shown that with the administration of oral feedings gradual resolution of the liver disease occurs. The initiation of oral feedings of small volume or the infusion of nutrients by continuous nasogastric drip may enhance biliary flow and intestinal motility. This effect may occur even when the enteral intake does not provide the total caloric needs. Improved solutions that meet the specific needs of the neonate may prevent deficiencies and avoid toxicities. In the decision to continue TPN, one must weigh the risk of further hepatic injury against the risk of malnutrition.

In *older children*, TPN-associated cholestasis is less common and less severe than in infants. Hepatic steatosis without cholestasis is often the only abnormality. However, biochemical abnormalities are not uncommon in older patients who are maintained on TPN for prolonged periods, either at home or in the hospital. Patients with chronic intestinal disease, which may be complicated by infection or bacterial overgrowth, are particularly susceptible to hepatic dysfunction. In most such patients, partial enteral alimentation reverses the abnormalities. It may be necessary at any age, when alkaline phosphatase or aminotransferase activities are elevated, to evaluate the underlying liver disease by liver biopsy.

BONE MARROW TRANSPLANTATION. Hepatic dysfunction is common in patients who have undergone *bone marrow transplantation*. Its genesis is multifactorial and may be related to (1) infections (viral, bacterial, or fungal), drugs, parenteral nutrition, chemotherapy, or radiation; (2) veno-occlusive disease (VOD); or (3) graft versus host disease (GVHD); or to any combination of these. Candidates for bone marrow transplantation have often had pre-existing liver disease, such as viral hepatitis, drug-related injury, or malignant infiltration. Percutaneous liver biopsy in such patients may show extensive bile duct injury in GVHD, viral inclusions in cytomegalovirus disease, or the characteristic endothelial lesion in VOD, but the histologic distinction is often unclear. This presents a dilemma because treatment of one suspected complication (e.g., initiation of immunosuppressive therapy for GVHD) may have a deleterious effect if the symptoms are due to another (e.g., fungal or viral infection).

VOD of the liver usually has its onset 1–3 wk after bone marrow transplantation but may appear up to 6 wk afterward. The most characteristic presentation is the onset of rapid weight gain, with ascites, hepatomegaly, right upper quadrant pain, jaundice, and oliguria. Hepatic encephalopathy and fulminant hepatic failure may follow. Less severe forms may be characterized by jaundice and ascites with a slow resolution; a mild form of VOD has histologic changes as the sole manifestation. The diagnosis rests on the exclusion of other diseases, such as congestive cardiomyopathy, constrictive pericarditis, and venous thrombosis (Budd-Chiari syndrome).

Pathologic changes in patients with VOD are best demonstrated using special (trichrome) stains to highlight the central veins. An early lesion is concentric narrowing of the lumina of small central veins, owing to edema in the subendothelial zone. There is a dense, wavy continuous band of collagen in the central veins and centrilobular hemorrhagic necrosis. The lesions may be patchy. The venular changes may progress to complete obliteration. The cause of VOD following bone marrow transplantation is not clear; it may be related to radiation or to antineoplastic drugs, or both. Risk factors for VOD include high-dose conditioning regimens, leukemia, advanced age, and pre-existing liver disease.

Budd-Chiari syndrome involves occlusion of the inferior vena cava or hepatic veins and tributaries; it may be caused by obstruction resulting from a web, mass, or thrombus. The disease has rarely been noted in children; however, a number of associated diseases may increase the risk. These include trauma, coagulopathies, sickle cell anemia, leukemia, polycythemia vera, hepatic abscesses, irradiation, and GVHD. The syndrome is to be regarded as distinct from VOD, which affects the centrilobular and sublobular hepatic veins, sparing the larger veins; it is not associated with thrombosis.

GVHD of the liver may be acute or chronic and is generally concomitant with GVHD in other target organs (Chapter 132.3). Cholestasis and hepatic injury of various degrees occur; there may be hepatic tenderness, dark urine, acholic stools, itching, and anorexia. There are parallel rises in serum bilirubin level and alkaline phosphatase activity; aspartate aminotransaminase elevation is less striking. GVHD is characterized histologically by degeneration and loss of small bile ducts and sparse inflammation, along with cholestasis.

COLLAGEN-VASCULAR DISEASE. Hepatic involvement in patients with *collagen-vascular disease* is uncommon. It has been noted especially in patients with systemic lupus erythematosus. Reactive hepatitis, chronic hepatitis, steatosis, and hepatic infarction have also been described. The association of hepatic injury with drug therapy, such as salicylate use, must be differentiated.

CHAPTER 306
Reye Syndrome and "Reye-like" Diseases

William F. Balistreri

See also Chapter 548.3.

The previously high incidence of this syndrome of acute encephalopathy and fatty degeneration of the liver has decreased markedly. This decline has been attributed to an increased awareness of the highly significant association between this disorder and ingestion of aspirin-containing medications by children with influenza-like illness or varicella. However, investigations of Reye syndrome uncovered a wide variety of previously undefined metabolic diseases whose clinical picture is similar and that need to be considered in the differential diagnosis of acute liver injury mimicking Reye syndrome (Table 306–1).

EPIDEMIOLOGY. Case reports of Reye syndrome were sporadic until 1974, when almost 400 cases were reported in the United States, with a mortality rate of more than 40%. The incidence was increased in direct temporal and geographic relationship to viral epidemics, especially those caused by influenza B and varicella. By 1988 the incidence had declined dramatically; only 20 cases were reported.

Reye syndrome was most commonly seen at approximately 6 yr of age, with most cases in the 4–12-yr age range. There was no gender difference in incidence, but rural and suburban populations appeared to be more frequently affected than urban populations. It is very likely that mild cases were missed and recovered without event. In any case, in the late 1970s Reye syndrome was the most common potentially lethal virus-associated encephalopathy in the United States.

CLINICAL MANIFESTATIONS. Classic Reye syndrome exhibited a sterotypic, biphasic course. It usually occurs in a previously healthy child. A prodromal febrile illness, an upper respiratory tract infection (in 90% of the cases), or chickenpox (in 5–7%) is followed by an interval in which the child has seemingly recovered. The abrupt onset of protracted vomiting then occurs, usually within 5–7 days after the onset of the viral illness. Delirium, combative behavior, and stupor may occur simultaneously or within a few hours after the onset of vomiting.

■ TABLE 306–1 Diseases That Present a Clinical/Pathologic Picture Resembling Reye Syndrome

Metabolic disease
Organic acidurias/defects in hepatic fatty acid oxidation (primary or secondary)
Urea cycle defects (carbamyl phosphate synthetase, ornithine transcarbamylase)
Fructosemia
Defects in fatty acid metabolism
Acyl-CoA dehydrogenase deficiencies
Long chain
Medium chain
Short chain
Systemic carnitine deficiency
Hepatic carnitine palmitoyltransferase deficiency
3-OH, 3-methylglutaryl-CoA lyase deficiency
Central nervous system infections or intoxications (meningitis, encephalitis, toxic encephalopathy)
Hemorrhagic shock with encephalopathy
Drug ingestion (salicylate, valproate)
Toxin (hypoglycin A, valproate)

CoA = coenzyme A.

■ TABLE 306–2 Clinical Staging of Reye Syndrome

Grade	*Symptoms* at Time of Admission
I	Usually quiet, **lethargic** and sleepy, vomiting, laboratory evidence of liver dysfunction
II	Deep lethargy, **confusion,** delirium, combative, hyperventilation, hyperreflexic
III	Obtunded, **light coma** ± seizures, decorticate rigidity, intact pupillary light reaction
IV	Seizures, deepening coma, **decerebrate rigidity,** loss of oculocephalic reflexes, fixed pupils
V	Coma, loss of deep tendon reflexes, respiratory arrest, fixed dilated pupils, **flaccidity/decerebrate** (intermittent); isoelectric electroencephalogram

Neurologic symptoms may rapidly progress to seizures, coma, and death; focal neurologic signs are absent. There is a slight to moderate liver enlargement with abnormalities of hepatic function; the patient remains anicteric. Cerebrospinal fluid is normal except for elevated pressure.

DIAGNOSIS. The clinical features are best reflected in the system of clinical staging that has been proposed (Table 306–2); grades I through III represent mild to moderate illness; grades IV and V represent severe illness. The majority of affected children will have mild illness without progression. The cerebrospinal fluid is normal.

There is explosive release from liver and muscle of such enzymes as aminotransferases, creatine kinase, and lactic dehydrogenase. The activity of the mitochondrial enzyme serum glutamate dehydrogenase is greatly increased. Patients not in coma who have a threefold or higher elevation in serum ammonia level are more likely to progress to coma, as are patients who have hypoprothrombinemia unresponsive to vitamin K. In younger patients, there may be hypoglycemia; however, these patients should be carefully screened for the presence of metabolic disease.

Pathology. The striking and characteristic gross pathologic feature of Reye syndrome is a yellow to white liver, reflective of a high content of triglyceride. Light microscopy shows a uniform foaminess of liver cell cytoplasm with microvesicular fatty accumulation, which may be concealed in routine preparations. Electron microscopic changes include a unique alteration of mitochondrial morphology. At present, biopsy should be carried out to rule out metabolic or toxic liver disease, especially in patients younger than 1–2 yr. Histologic examination of brain tissue reveals a similar pattern of injury. Grossly, there is marked edema.

Pathogenesis. The major site of injury is the mitochondrion. The activities of hepatic intramitochondrial enzymes, including ornithine transcarbamylase (OTC), carbamylphosphate synthetase (CPS), and pyruvate dehydrogenase, are reduced, often to less than half of their normal values. Hyperammonemia may result from acquired decreases in the activities of OTC and CPS.

The reasons for mitochondrial dysfunction are unknown. No toxic factor has as yet been conclusively identified, but studies have suggested an etiologic link among Reye syndrome, use of aspirin, and viral infections. **It is prudent to avoid the use of aspirin as an antipyretic in patients with influenza or varicella.**

TREATMENT. Successful management of Reye syndrome requires (1) precise diagnostic evaluation to exclude disorders resembling Reye syndrome; those disorders, which are more likely to be encountered, include defects in fatty acid oxidation and other metabolic injuries presenting as acute liver failure, (2) control of increased intracranial pressure (ICP) secondary to cerebral edema, which is the major lethal factor.

Early diagnosis may be aided by a high level of clinical suspicion and by assessment of hepatic function in suspected cases. Marked elevation of aminotransferase activities, prolongation of prothrombin time, and elevation of the serum ammonia level above 125–150 μg/dL suggest the diagnosis. It is imperative that cerebral edema be identified and counteracted and that aerobic metabolism be maintained.

Management varies with the severity of the illness. Whereas observation alone may suffice in patients with grade 1 severity, more aggressive therapy will be needed in patients with more severe neurologic deterioration. All patients should initially receive glucose (10–15%) intravenously, because glycogen depletion is common. In patients with cerebral edema, the amount of fluid administered should be restricted to approximately 1500 mL/m^2 day. Hyperthermia should be avoided. Coagulopathy is managed with vitamin K, fresh frozen plasma, and platelet transfusions.

In more severely ill, comatose patients, endotracheal intubation permits adequate oxygenation; hyperventilation induces hypocarbia, which decreases cerebral blood flow by cerebral vasoconstriction. Close monitoring of ICP assists in decisions regarding management. Stimulation of the patient should be minimized because procedures such as suctioning may generate increases in ICP.

An indwelling arterial catheter permits continuous assessment of cerebral perfusion pressure. Osmotherapy (mannitol 0.5–1.0 g/kg every 4–6 hr) should be used to maintain a serum osmolality of 300–320 mOsm/L and to induce cerebral dehydration; the ICP should be held to less than 20 mm Hg and the cerebral perfusion pressure to greater than 50 mm Hg. Pressure (cerebrospinal fluid) monitoring provides an effective guide to therapy with osmotic diuretics and may decrease renal complications resulting from hyperosmolarity. Use of pentobarbital (2.5 mg/kg) to maintain a serum barbiturate level of 20–30 μg/mL may have a protective effect on the central nervous system by decreasing cerebral metabolic demands, decreasing cerebral blood flow, and causing cerebral vasoconstriction. Excessive pentobarbital may reduce cardiac function, lowering blood pressure and, therefore, cerebral perfusion pressure. Pancuronium bromide has been used in the hope of decreasing cerebral blood volume through muscular relaxation and increased peripheral blood pooling.

PROGNOSIS. The duration of disordered cerebral function during the acute stage of illness is the best predictor of eventual outcome. In patients with grade 1 disease, recovery is rapid and complete. In patients with more severe disease there may be subsequent subtle neuropsychologic defects noted (in intelligence, school achievement, visuomotor integration, and concept formation).

DEVELOPMENT OF HEPATIC STRUCTURE AND FUNCTION

Andres JM, Mathis RK, Walker WA: Liver disease in infants: Part I. Developmental hepatology and mechanisms of liver dysfunction. J Pediatr 90:686, 1977.

Andres JM, Mathis RK, Walker WA: Liver disease in infants: Part II. Developmental hepatology and mechanisms of liver dysfunction. J Pediatr 90:964, 1977.

Balistreri WF: Anatomic and biochemical ontogeny of the gastrointestinal tract and liver. *In:* Tsang RC, Nichols BL (eds): Nutrition during Infancy. Philadelphia, Hauley & Belfus, 1987, pp 33–57.

Balistreri WF, Heubi JI, Suchy FJ: Immaturity of the enterohepatic circulation in early life: Factors predisposing to "physiologic" maldigestion and cholestasis. J Pediatr Gastroenterol Nutr 2:346, 1983.

Cox KL, Cheung ATW, Lohse CL, et al: Biliary motility postnatal changes in guinea pigs. Pediatr Res 21:170, 1987.

Fausto N, Mead JE: Regulation of liver growth: Protooncogenes and transforming growth factors. Lab Invest 60:4, 1989.

Gregus Z, Klaassen CD: Hepatic disposition of xenobiotics during prenatal and early postnatal development. *In:* Fox W, Polin RA (eds): Fetal and Neonatal Physiology. Philadelphia, WB Saunders, 1992.

Hutchins GM, Moore GW: Growth and asymmetry of the human liver during the embryonic period. Pediatr Pathol 8:17, 1988.

Jones CT, Rolph TP: Metabolism during fetal life: A functional assessment of metabolic development. Physiol Rev 65:357, 1985.

Kaufman SS: Organogenesis and histologic development of the liver. *In:* Fow W, Polin RA (eds): Fetal and Neonatal Physiology. Philadelphia, WB Saunders, 1992.

Reif S, Lebenthal E: Extracellular matrix modulation of liver ontogeny. J Pediatr Gastroenterol Nutr 12:1, 1991.

Rudolph AM: Hepatic and ductus venosus blood flows during fetal life. Hepatology 3:254, 1983.

Shah RD, Gerber MA: Development of intrahepatic bile ducts in humans: Possible role of laminin. Arch Pathol Lab Med 114:597, 1990.

Suchy FJ, Bucuvalas JC, Novak DA: Determinant of bile formation during development: Ontogeny of hepatic bile acid metabolism and transport. Semin Liver Dis 7:77, 1987.

Townsend SF, Rudolph CD, Rudolph AM: Changes in ovine hepatic circulation and oxygen consumption at birth. Pediatr Res 25:300, 1989.

MANIFESTATIONS OF LIVER DISEASE

A-Kader HH, Ryckman FC, Balistreri WF: Liver transplantation in the pediatric population: Indications and monitoring. Clin Transport 5:161, 1991.

Alvarez F, Bernard O, Brunelle F, et al: Portal obstruction in children. I: Clinical investigation and hemorrhage risk: Portal obstruction in children. J Pediatr 103:696, 1983.

Alvarez F, Bernard O, Brunelle F, et al: Portal obstruction in children. II: Results of surgical portosystemic shunts. J Pediatr 103:703, 1983.

Balistreri WF: The effects of liver disease and nutrition and growth. *In:* Cohen SA (ed): The Underweight Child. Norwalk, CT, Appleton-Century-Crofts, 1986, pp 121–130.

Fonkalsrud EW: Shunt operations for portal hypertension in children. J Pediatr 103:741, 1983.

Oldham KT, Guice KS, Kaufman RA, et al: Blunt hepatic injury and elevated hepatic enzymes: A clinical correlation in children. J Pediatr Surg 19:457, 1984.

Reiff MI, Osborn LM: Clinical estimation of liver size in newborn infants. Pediatrics 71:46, 1983.

Schuval S, Bonagura V: Simultaneous percussion auscultation technique for determination of liver span. Arch Pediatr Adolesc Med 148:873, 1994.

EVALUATION OF THE PATIENT WITH POSSIBLE LIVER DYSFUNCTION

Balistreri WF, Rej R: Liver function. *In:* Burtis C, Ashwood E (eds): Tietz Textbook of Clinical Chemistry, 2nd ed. Philadelphia, WB Saunders, 1993, pp 1449–1512.

Laker MF: Liver function tests. BMJ 301:250, 1990.

Maggiore G, Bernard O, Reily CA, et al: Normal serum β-glutamyl-transpeptidase activity identifies groups of infants with idiopathic cholestasis with poor prognosis. J Pediatr 111:251, 1987.

Newman TB, Easterling J, Goldman ES, et al: Laboratory evaluation of jaundice in newborns. Am J Dis Child 144:364, 1990.

Riddlesberger MM Jr: Diagnostic imaging of the hepatobiliary system in infants and children. J Pediatr Gastroenterol Nutr 3:653, 1984.

Rosenthal P, Henton D, Felber S, et al: Distribution of serum bilirubin conjugates in pediatric hepatobiliary disease. J Pediatr 110:201, 1987.

Sokol RJ: Medical management of infant or child with chronic liver disease. Semin Liver Dis 7:155, 1987.

Spivak W, Sarkar S, Winter D, et al: Diagnostic utility of hepatobiliary scintigraphy with DISIDA in neonatal cholestasis. J Pediatr 110:855, 1987.

SPECIFIC DISEASES OF THE LIVER

Aagenaes O: Hereditary recurrent cholestasis with lymphoedema: Two new families. Acta Paediatr Scand 63:465, 1974.

Alagille D, Estrada A, Hadchovel M, et al: Syndromic paucity of interlobular bile ducts (Alagille syndrome or arteriohepatic dysplasia): Review of 80 cases. J Pediatr 110:195, 1987.

Balistreri WF: Interrelationship between the infantile cholangiopathies and paucity of the intrahepatic bile ducts. *In:* Balstreri WF, Stocker JT (eds): Pediatric Hepatology. Washington, DC, Hemisphere Publishing, 1990, pp 1–18.

Balistreri WF: Neonatal cholestasis. J Pediatr 106:171, 1985.

Balistreri WF, A-Kader HH, Ryckman FC, et al: Biochemical and clinical response to ursodeoxycholic acid administration in pediatric patients with chronic cholestasis. *In:* Paumgartner G, et al: Bile Acids as Therapeutic Agents. Lancaster, UK, Kluwer, 1991, pp. 323–333.

Beath S, Booth I, Kelley D: Nutritional support in liver disease. Arch Dis Child 69:545, 1993.

Danks DM, Campbell PE, Smith AL, et al. Prognosis of babies with neonatal hepatitis. Arch Dis Child 52:368, 1977.

Desmet VJ: Cholangiopathies: Past, present and future. Semin Liver Dis. 7:67, 1987.

Jacquemin E, Dumont M, Bernard O, et al: Evidence for defective primary bile acid secretion in children with progressive familial intrahepatic cholestasis (Byler disease). Eur J Pediatr 153:424, 1994.

Kasai M, Mochizuki I, Ohkohchi N, et al: Surgical limitations for biliary atresia: Indications for liver transplantation. J Pediatr Surg 24:851, 1989.

Lally KP, Kanegaye J, Matsumura M, et al: Perioperative factors affecting the outcome following repair of biliary atresia. Pediatrics 83:723, 1989.

Landing BH: Consideration of the pathogenesis of neonatal hepatitis, biliary atresia, and choledochal cyst: The concept of infantile obstructive cholangiopathy. Prog Pediatr Surg 6:113, 1974.

Laurent J, Gauthier F, Bernard O, et al: Long-term outcome after surgery for biliary atresia: Study of 40 patients surviving for more than 10 years. Gastroenterology 99:1793, 1990.

Mieli-Vergani G, Howard ER, Portmann B, Mowat AP: Late referral for biliary atresia: Missed opportunity for effective surgery. Lancet 1:421, 1989.
Mowat AP, Psacharopoulos HT, Williams R: Extrahepatic biliary atresia versus neonatal hepatitis: Review of 137 prospectively investigated infants. Arch Dis Child 51:763, 1976.
Riely CA: Familial intrahepatic cholestatic syndromes. Semin Liver Dis 7:119, 1987.
Ryckman FC, Noseworthy J: Neonatal cholestatic conditions requiring surgical reconstruction. Semin Liver Dis 7:134, 1987.
Sokol RJ, Heubi JE, Butler-Simon N, et al: Treatment of vitamin E deficiency during chronic childhood cholestasis with oral D-tocopheryl polyethylene glycol-1000 succinate. Gastroenterology 93:975, 1987.
Whitington PF, Balistreri WF: Liver transplantation in pediatrics: Indications, contraindications, and pre-transplant management. J Pediatr 118:169, 1991.
Whitington PF, Whitington GL: Partial external diversion of bile for the treatment of intractable pruritus associated with intrahepatic cholestasis. Gastroenterology 95:130, 1988.

METABOLIC DISEASES OF THE LIVER

Aono S, Yamada Y, Keino H, et al: A new type of defect in the gene for bilirubin uridine 5'-diphosphate-glucuronosyltransferase in a patient with Crigler-Najjar syndrome type I. Pediatr Res 35:629, 1994.
Balistreri WF: Fetal and bile acid synthesis and metabolism: Clinical implications. J Inherit Metab Dis 14:459, 1991.
Balistreri WF: Nontransplant options for the treatment of metabolic liver disease: Saving livers while saving lives. Hepatology 19:782, 1994.
Berglund L, Angelin B, Blomstrand R, et al: Sn-protoporphyrin lowers serum bilirubin levels, decreases biliary bilirubin output, enhances biliary heme excretion and potently inhibits hepatic heme oxygenase activity in normal human subjects. Hepatology 8:625, 1988.
Burchell A: Molecular pathology of glucose-6-phosphatase. FASEB J 4:2978, 1990.
Clayton PT, Leonard JV, Lawson AM, et al: Familial giant cell hepatitis associated with synthesis of 3β, 7α, 12α-trihydroxy-5-cholenoic acids. J Clin Invest 79:1031, 1987.
Crigler JF, Najjar VA: Congenital familial nonhemolytic jaundice with kernicterus. Pediatrics 10:169, 1952.
Crystal RG: α_1-Antitrypsin deficiency, emphysema, and liver disease: Genetic basis and strategies for therapy. J Clin Invest 85:1343, 1990.
Daugherty CC, Setchell KDR, Heubi JE: Resolution of hepatic biopsy alterations in three siblings with bile acid treatment of an inborn error of bile acid metabolism (δ^4-3-oxosteroid 5β-reductase deficiency). Hepatology 18:1096, 1993.
Dubois RS, Rodgerson DO, Hambridge KM: Treatment of Wilson's disease with triethylene tetramine hydrochloride (trientine). J Pediatr Gastroenterol Nutr 10:77, 1990.
Eriksson S: Alpha$_1$-antitrypsin deficiency and the liver. Acta Paediatr 83:444, 1994.
Goldfisher S: Idiopathic neonatal iron storage involving the liver, pancreas, heart and endocrine and exocrine glands. Hepatology 1:58, 1981.
Hoogstraten J, deSha DJ, Knisely AS: Fetal and liver disease may precede extrahepatic siderosis in neonatal hemochromatosis. Gastroenterology 98:1699, 1990.
Joshi V: Indian childhood cirrhosis. Perspect Pediatr Pathol 11:175, 1987.
Kappas A, Drummond GS: Control of heme metabolism with synthetic metalloporphyrins. J Clin Invest 77:335, 1986.
Knisely AS, Magid MS, Dische MR, Cutz E: Neonatal hemochromatosis. Birth Defects 23:75, 1987.
Knisely AS, O'Shea PA, Stocks JF, et al: Oropharyngeal and upper respiratory tract mucosal gland siderosis in neonatal hemochromatosis: An approach to biopsy diagnosis. J Pediatr 113:871, 1988.
Ledley FD: Somatic gene therapy in gastroenterology: Approaches and applications. J Pediatr Gastroenterol Nutr 14:328, 1992.
Lefkowitch JH, Honig CL, King ME, et al: Hepatic copper overload and features of Indian childhood cirrhosis in an American sibship. N Engl J Med 307:271, 1982.
Lindstedt S, Holme E, Lock EA, et al: Treatment of hereditary tyrosinemia type 1 by inhibition of 4-hydroxyphenylpyruvate dioxygenase. Lancet 340:813, 1992.
Makdisi WJ, Wu CH, Wu GY: Methods of gene transfer into hepatocytes: progress toward gene therapy. Prog Liver Dis 10:1, 1992.
McCullough AJ, Fleming CR, Thistle JL, et al: Diagnosis of Wilson's disease presenting as fulminant hepatic failure. Gastroenterology 84:161, 1983.
Perlmutter DH: The cellular basis for liver injury in α_1-antitrypsin inhibitor deficiency. Hepatology 13:172, 1991.
Persico M, Ramano M, Muraca M, et al: Responsiveness to phenobarbital in an adult with Crigler-Najjar disease associated with neurological involvement and skin hyperextensibility. Hepatology 13:213, 1991.
Ritter JK, Yeatman MT, Ferreira P, et al: Identification of a genetic alteration in the code for bilirubin UDP-glucuronosyltransferase in the UGT1 gene complex of a Crigler-Najjar type I patient. J Clin Invest 90:150, 1992.
Sassa S, Fujita H, Kappas A: Succinylacetone and b-aminolevulinic acid dehydratase in hereditary tyrosinemia: Immunochemical study of the enzyme. Pediatrics 86:84, 1990.
Schilsky ML, Scheinberg H, Sternleib I: Prognosis of Wilsonian chronic active hepatitis. Gastroenterology 100:762, 1991.
Setchell KDR, Street JM: Inborn errors of bile acid synthesis. Semin Liver Dis 7:85, 1987.
Setchell KDR, Suchy FJ, Welsh MS, et al: 3-oxosteroid 5β-reductase deficiency described in identical twins with neonatal hepatitis a new inborn error in bile acid synthesis. J Clin Invest 82:2148, 1988.
Sternlieb I: Perspectives on Wilson's disease. Hepatology 12:1234, 1990.
Sveger T: Liver diseases in alpha-1 antitrypsin deficiency detected by screening of 200,000 infants. N Engl J Med 294:1316, 1976.

INFECTIOUS DISORDERS OF THE LIVER

Pineiro-Carrero VM, Andres JM: Morbidity and mortality in children with pyogenic liver abscess. Am J Dis Child 143:1424, 1989.

LIVER DISEASE ASSOCIATED WITH SYSTEMIC DISORDERS

Amedee-Manesme O, Bernard O, Brunelle F, et al: Sclerosing cholangitis with neonatal onset. J Pediatr 111:225, 1987.
Balistreri WF, Bove K: Hepatobiliary consequences of parenteral nutrition. Prog Liver Dis 9:567, 1989.
Buchanan GR, Glader BE: Benign course of extreme hyperbilirubinemia in sickle cell anemia: Analysis of six cases, J Pediatr 91:21, 1977.
Cohen JA, Kaplan MM: Left sided heart failure presenting as hepatitis. Gastroenterology 74:583, 1978.
El-Shabrawi M, Wilkinson ML, Portmann B, et al: Primary sclerosing cholangitis in childhood. Gastroenterology 92:1226, 1987.
Klion FM, Weiner JJ, Schaffner F: Cholestasis in sickle cell anemia. Am J Med 37:829, 1964.
Narkewicz MR, Sokol RJ, Beckwith B, et al: Liver involvement in Alpers disease. J Pediatr 119:260, 1991.
Nemeth A, Ejderhamm J, Glaumann H, et al: Liver damage in juvenile inflammatory bowel disease. Liver 10:239, 1990.
Sisto A, Feldman P, Garel L, et al: Primary sclerosing cholangitis in children: Study of five cases and review of the literature. Pediatrics 80:818, 1987.
Zitelli BJ, et al: Systemic disorders associated with hepatobiliary dysfunction. *In:* Balistreri WF, Stocker JT (eds): Pediatric Hepatology. Washington, DC, Hemisphere Publishing, 1989, pp 203–222.

VENO-OCCLUSIVE DISEASE/GRAFT VERSUS HOST DISEASE

Gentile-Kocher S, Bernard O, Brunnelle F, et al: Budd Chiari syndrome in children: Report of 22 cases. J Pediatr 113:30, 1988.
McDonald GB, Sharma P, Matthews DE, et al: Veno-occlusive disease of the liver after bone marrow transplantation: Diagnosis, incidence, and predisposing factors. Hepatology 4:116, 1984.
Sale GE, Shulman HM: Liver disease after marrow transplantation. *In:* Sale GE, Shulman HM (eds): The Pathology of Bone Marrow Transplantation, Chicago, Year Book Medical Publishers, 1984.
Snover DC, Weisdorf SA, Ramsay NK, et al: Hepatic graft-versus-host disease: A study of the predictive value of the liver biopsy in diagnosis. Hepatology 4:123, 1984.

REYE SYNDROME

Bougneres PF, Rocchiccioli F, Koluraa S, et al: Medium-chain acyl-CoA dehydrogenase deficiency in two siblings with a Reye-like syndrome. J Pediatr 106:918, 1985.
Forsyth BW, Horwitz RI, Acampora D, et al: New epidemiologic evidence confirming that bias does not explain the aspirin/Reye's syndrome association. JAMA 261:2517, 1989.
Greene CL, Blitzer MG, Shapira E: Inborn errors of metabolism and Reye's syndrome: Differential diagnosis. J Pediatr 113:156, 1988.
Hurwitz ES, Barrett MJ, Bergman D, et al: Public health service study of Reye's syndrome and medications: Report of the main study. JAMA 257:1905, 1987.
Lichtenstein PK, Heubi JE, Daugherty CC, et al: Grade I Reye's syndrome: A frequent cause of vomiting and liver dysfunction after varicella and upper-respiratory-tract infection. N Engl J Med 309:133, 1983.
Pollitt RJ: Disorders of mitochondrial B-oxidation: Prenatal and early postnatal diagnosis and the irrelevance to Reye's syndrome and sudden infant death. J Inherit Metab Dis 12:215, 1989.
Reye's syndrome surveillance: United States, 1989. MMWR 40:88, 1991.
Rowe PC, Valle D, Brusilow SW: Inborn errors of metabolism in children referred with Reye's syndrome: A changing pattern. JAMA 260:3167, 1988.
Stanley CA: New genetic defects in mitochondrial fatty acid oxidation and carnitine deficiency. Adv Pediatr 34:59, 1987.
Stanley CA, Hale DE, Coates PM: Medium-chain acylo-CoA dehydrogenase deficiency. *In:* Fatty Acid Oxidation: Clinical, Biochemical and Molecular aspects. New York, Alan R. Liss, 1990, pp 291–302.

CHAPTER 307
Chronic Hepatitis

Frederick J. Suchy

Chronic hepatitis is defined as a continuing hepatic inflammatory process manifested by elevated hepatic transaminase levels, lasting 6 mo or more. The severity is variable; the affected child may have only biochemical evidence of liver dysfunction, may have stigmata of chronic liver disease, or may present in hepatic failure.

Chronic hepatitis can be caused by persistent viral infection, drugs, and autoimmune or unknown factors. Approximately 15–20% of cases are associated with hepatitis B infection (Chapter 221); in this group of patients, unusually severe disease may be caused by superimposed infection with hepatitis D (a defective RNA virus that is dependent on replicating hepatitis B virus). More than 90% of infants infected during the 1st year of life experience chronic hepatitis B infection compared with a rate of 5–10% among older children and adults. Chronic hepatitis may also follow 30–50% of hepatitis C virus infections. Patients receiving blood products or who have had massive transfusions are at increased risk. Hepatitis A virus does not cause chronic hepatitis. Drugs commonly used in children that may cause chronic liver injury include isoniazid, methyldopa, nitrofurantoin, dantrolene, and the sulfonamides.

In most cases, the cause of chronic hepatitis is unknown; in many, an autoimmune mechanism is suggested by the finding of antinuclear and anti-smooth muscle antibodies in serum and by multisystem involvement (including rashes, arthropathy, thyroiditis, and Coombs-positive hemolytic anemia). Histologic features have defined two major subdivisions of chronic hepatitis: *chronic persistent hepatitis* and *chronic active hepatitis.* The pathogenesis of each morphologic form is uncertain, but the criteria defining them predict a benign, self-limited course for chronic persistent hepatitis and a progressive course potentially leading to cirrhosis for chronic active hepatitis. Both forms are to be distinguished from unresolved or prolonged acute viral hepatitis in which clinical and biochemical abnormalities last 2–3 mo; liver biopsy in such cases shows predominantly single cell necrosis in the lobule, with minimal portal and lobular inflammation. In addition, disorders such as Wilson disease and α_1-antitrypsin deficiency must be considered.

307.1 Chronic Persistent Hepatitis

Chronic persistent hepatitis in childhood is a generally benign inflammatory process of the liver. It most commonly follows acute hepatitis caused by hepatitis B or C viruses.

PATHOLOGY. The lobular architecture is always normal. Inflammation is limited to portal triads, and no significant fibrosis or cirrhosis is found.

CLINICAL MANIFESTATIONS. Most pediatric patients with chronic persistent hepatitis are asymptomatic or have nonspecific complaints, such as fatigue or anorexia. Some patients have minimal hepatomegaly or slight right upper quadrant tenderness. Historical features and physical stigmata of drug abuse should be sought in the adolescent.

There are mild to moderate elevations of serum aminotransferase activities and normal or only slightly increased serum bilirubin concentrations (predominantly of the direct-reacting fraction). Serum alkaline phosphatase (hepatic) activity, albumin level, and prothrombin time are normal. Serum globulin and immunoglobulin (Ig) G fraction concentrations are normal or only slightly increased. Tests for anti-smooth muscle and antinuclear antibodies have negative results. As many as one third of patients will be hepatitis B surface antigen (HBsAg) positive, whereas an unknown number are anti-hepatitis C virus positive.

DIAGNOSIS. There is considerable clinical and laboratory overlap between the variants of chronic hepatitis; accordingly, liver biopsy is essential to the diagnosis of chronic persistent hepatitis. Differential diagnosis should include biliary tract disease and the pericholangitis associated with inflammatory bowel disease.

TREATMENT AND PROGNOSIS. The prognosis is good in childhood. In adults chronic persistent hepatitis B and C virus infections are more likely to progress to cirrhosis, liver failure, or hepatocellular carcinoma. Impaired immunity may be responsible for the persistent viral infection. Prednisone therapy is of no benefit. Interferon-α is of some benefit for chronic hepatitis B or C virus. Whether these therapies are indicated for the rare child with progression of chronic persistent hepatitis or if they will reduce the risk for hepatocellular cancer remains to be determined.

307.2 Chronic Active Hepatitis

Chronic active hepatitis is characterized by unresolving inflammation, necrosis, and fibrosis, with the possibility of progression to cirrhosis and liver failure.

ETIOLOGY. Chronic active hepatitis may be caused by chronic infection with hepatitis B or C viruses. Many patients, however, have no evidence of viral infection, drug, or metabolic liver injury as a cause for their liver disease. In many cases, clinical features strongly suggest an autoimmune mechanism.

PATHOLOGY. The histologic features common to untreated cases include (1) inflammatory infiltrates, consisting of lymphocytes and plasma cells, which expand portal areas and often penetrate the lobule; (2) moderate to severe "piece-meal" necrosis of hepatocytes extending outward from the limiting plate; and (3) variable necrosis, fibrosis, and zones of parenchymal collapse spanning neighboring portal triads or between a portal triad and central vein (bridging necrosis). Distortion of hepatic architecture may be severe; cirrhosis may be found in children at the time of diagnosis.

CLINICAL MANIFESTATIONS. The clinical features and course of chronic active hepatitis are extremely variable. Signs and symptoms at the time of presentation include a wide spectrum of disease with a substantial number of asymptomatic patients and some having an acute, even fulminant onset. Some patients acquire chronic active hepatitis following a well-defined episode of hepatitis B infection or post-transfusion hepatitis C infection; and in 25–30% of patients with autoimmune hepatitis, particularly children, the illness may mimic acute viral hepatitis. In most patients, however, the onset is insidious. About half of the patients are younger than 20 yr; most HBsAg-negative patients are female. Patients may be asymptomatic or have fatigue, malaise, behavioral changes, anorexia, and amenorrhea, sometimes for many months before jaundice or stigmata of chronic liver disease are recognized. Extrahepatic manifestations may include arthritis, vasculitis, and nephritis in HBsAg-positive patients, presumably secondary to deposition of hepatitis B antigen-antibody immune complexes.

Thyroiditis, Coombs-positive anemia, arthritis, and rash are common in patients with the autoimmune or "lupoid" variety of chronic active hepatitis. Some patients' initial clinical features may reflect cirrhosis (ascites, bleeding esophageal varices, or hepatic encephalopathy).

There is usually mild to moderate jaundice. Spider telangiectasias and palmar erythema may be present. The liver is often tender and slightly enlarged but may not be felt in patients with cirrhosis. The spleen is commonly enlarged. Edema and ascites may be present in advanced cases. Evidence of involvement of other organ systems may be found. Classic features of autoimmune hepatitis (including cushingoid appearance, acne, hirsutism, and striae) occur in some patients.

LABORATORY MANIFESTATIONS. These reveal moderate elevation (usually less than 1,000 IU/L) of serum aminotransferase activities. Serum bilirubin concentrations (predominantly the direct reacting fraction) are commonly 2–10 mg/dL. Serum alkaline phosphatase activity is normal to slightly increased. Serum γ-globulin levels show marked polyclonal elevations in most patients but may be normal to only slightly increased in HBsAg-positive patients. Hypoalbuminemia is common. The prothrombin time is prolonged, most often as a result of vitamin K deficiency but also as a reflection of impaired hepatocellular function. A normochromic, normocytic anemia, leukopenia, and thrombocytopenia are present and usually become more severe with evolution of portal hypertension and hypersplenism. Serologic (IgG), antigenic, or genomic evidence of hepatitis B, C, or D virus infection may be evident.

Most patients with autoimmune hepatitis have hypergammaglobulinemia. Serum IgG levels usually exceed 16 g/L. Characteristic patterns of serum autoantibodies have been used to define several noninfectious subgroups of chronic active hepatitis. The most common pattern is the formation of non-organ-specific antibodies, such as antiactin (smooth muscle), antinuclear, and antimitochondrial antibodies. Approximately half of these patients are 10–20 yr of age. High titers of a liver-kidney microsomal (LKM) antibody are detected in another form that usually affects children 2–14 yr of age. A subgroup of primarily young women may demonstrate autoantibodies against a soluble liver antigen but not against nuclear or microsomal proteins. Some patients only demonstrate anti-smooth muscle or antinuclear antibodies. Autoantibodies are rare in healthy children so that titers as low as 1:40 may be considered significant for diagnosis. Up to 20% of patients with apparent autoimmune hepatitis may not have autoantibodies at presentation. Antibodies to a cytochrome P450 component of LKM are commonly found in adult patients with chronic hepatitis C infection. Additional less common autoantibodies include rheumatoid factor, anti-parietal cell antibodies, and antithyroid antibodies. A Coombs-positive hemolytic anemia may be present.

DIAGNOSIS. The diagnosis of chronic active hepatitis is established by liver biopsy. The differential diagnosis should include α-antitrypsin deficiency (Chapter 303.6) and Wilson disease (Chapter 303.2). The former disorder must be excluded by performing α_1-antitrypsin phenotyping and the latter by measuring serum ceruloplasmin and 24-hour urinary copper excretion. Other inherited causes of chronic liver disease include tyrosinemia, Niemann-Pick disease type 2, glycogen storage disease type IV, and cystic fibrosis. Chronic active hepatitis may occur in patients with inflammatory bowel disease, but liver dysfunction in such patients is more commonly due to pericholangitis or sclerosing cholangitis. Endoscopic retrograde cholangiography may be required to exclude autoimmune primary sclerosing cholangitis. An ultrasonogram should be done to identify a choledochal cyst or other structural disorders of the biliary system. Dilated or obliterated veins on ultrasonography suggest the possibility of the Budd-Chiari syndrome. The differential diagnosis of chronic liver disease is noted in Table 307–1.

■ **TABLE 307–1 Disorders Producing a Chronic Hepatitis**

Chronic Viral Hepatitis
Hepatitis B
Hepatitis C
Hepatitis D
Autoimmune Hepatitis
Antiactin antibody positive
Anti–liver-kidney microsomal antibody positive
Antisoluble liver antigen antibody positive
Others (includes antibodies to liver-specific lipoproteins or asialoglycoprotein)
Overlap syndrome with sclerosing cholangitis and autoantibodies
Systemic lupus erythematosus
Drug-Induced Hepatitis
Metabolic Disorders Associated with Chronic Liver Disease
Wilson disease
α_1-Antitrypsin deficiency
Tyrosinemia
Niemann-Pick disease type 2
Glycogen storage disease type IV
Cystic fibrosis
Galactosemia

TREATMENT. Controlled studies of the drug treatment of autoimmune forms of chronic active hepatitis have only been conducted in adults, but several retrospective studies in children and adolescents suggest that they benefit from immunosuppressive therapy. It is clear that corticosteroid therapy, with or without low doses of azathioprine, improves the clinical, biochemical, and histologic features in most patients with chronic active hepatitis and prolongs survival in most patients with severe disease. In severe chronic active hepatitis, after exclusion of HBsAg-positive and transfusion-related cases, the course and response to drug therapy appear to be similar whether or not autoimmune features are present.

The goal of treatment is to suppress or eliminate hepatic inflammation with minimal side effects. Prednisone is given at an initial dose of 1–2 mg/kg/day and continued until aminotransferase values return to less than twice the upper limit of normal. The dose should then be lowered in 5-mg decrements over a 4- to 6-wk period, until a maintenance dose of less than 20 mg/day is achieved. In patients who respond poorly, who experience severe side effects, or who cannot be maintained on low-dose steroids, azathioprine (1.5 mg/kg/day, up to 100 mg/day) may be added, with frequent monitoring for bone marrow suppression. Alternate-day corticosteroid therapy should be used with great caution. In adults, this form of treatment produced improvement or even normalization of serum aminotransferase activities, but histologic resolution did not occur.

Histologic progress should be assessed by liver biopsy 6 mo–1 yr after the initiation of treatment because normal results of biochemical tests during therapy do not ensure histologic resolution. Disappearance of symptoms and biochemical abnormalities and either resolution of the necroinflammatory process on biopsy or at least improvement to a pattern of chronic persistent hepatitis justify an attempt at gradual discontinuation of medication. However, there is a high rate of relapse after discontinuation of therapy.

Chronic hepatitis B infection responds poorly to corticosteroid therapy. Recent studies suggest an increased frequency of complications, enhanced viral replication, and a higher death rate in steroid-treated patients. Chronic hepatitis C infection, following blood transfusion, has a fluctuating clinical and biochemical course that may spontaneously improve.

Positive responses to antiviral treatment of chronic hepatitis B and C virus infections have been reported. Doses of intramuscular interferon-α ranging from 5–10 million U/m^2 three times weekly for 16–24 wk have been used successfully in children. Factors predicting a positive response to interferon have included initial serum aminotransferase levels more than twice the upper limits of normal, low levels of hepatitis B DNA in serum, and positivity for hepatitis B e antigen (HBeAg). Patients with long-standing hepatitis B infection and probable integration of viral DNA into the host genome are less likely to benefit from treatment. Unfortunately, many children with perinatal infection often fall into this category. Favorable response to interferon therapy, defined as clearance of HBeAg, hepatitis B-DNA, and DNA polymerase from serum as well as amelioration of the inflammatory liver disease, can be expected in 30–40% of patients. Remission is sustained in only 30–50% of responders, and complete eradication of the infection is unusual. Interferon-α therapy improves liver function in approximately 50% of patients with chronic hepatitis C virus infection. Half of these patients relapse after discontinuation of therapy but usually respond to retreatment. Interferon therapy appears to be well tolerated in children. Fever, myalgias, and malaise are the most common side effects, but patients should be monitored for myelosuppression and the development of autoimmune phenomena (including the development of antinuclear, anti-smooth muscle, and antithyroid antibodies).

PROGNOSIS. Treatment of autoimmune chronic active hepatitis will significantly improve survival in most HBsAg-negative patients. More than 75% of patients can be expected to respond to therapy. In patients meeting the criteria for withdrawal of treatment, 50% can be successfully weaned from medication; in the other 50%, relapse occurs after a variable period of time, but this will usually respond to retreatment. Progression to cirrhosis can occur despite a good response to drug therapy and prolongation of life.

Orthotopic liver transplantation has been successful in patients with end-stage liver disease associated with autoimmune and post transfusion hepatitis C forms of chronic active hepatitis. In contrast, recurrence of severe liver disease is likely following transplantation for chronic hepatitis B infection.

Bach N, Thung SN, Schaffner F: The histological features of chronic hepatitis C and autoimmune chronic hepatitis: A comparative analysis. Hepatology 15:572, 1992.

Bortolotti F, Cadrobbi P, Crivellaro C, et al: Long term outcome of chronic hepatitis type B in patients who acquire hepatitis B infection in childhood. Gastroenterology 99:805, 1990.

Johnson PJ, McFarlane IG, et al: Meeting report: International autoimmune hepatitis group. Hepatology 18:998, 1993.

Lai ME, De Virgilis S, Argiolu F, et al: Evaluation of antibodies to hepatitis C virus in a long term prospective study of posttransfusion hepatitis among thalassemic children: Comparison between first and second-generation assay. J Pediatric Gastroenterol Nutr 16:458, 1993.

Ludwig J: The nomeclature of chronic active hepatitis: An obituary. Gastroenterology 105:274, 1993.

Maggiore G, Veber F, Bernard O, et al: Autoimmune hepatitis associated with anti-actin antibodies in children and adolescents. Pediatric Gastroenterol Nutr 17:376, 1993.

Ruiz-Moreno M, Rua MJ, Castillo I, et al: Treatment of children with hepatitis C with recombinant interferon-α: A pilot study. Hepatology 16:882, 1992.

Ruiz-Moreno M, Rua MJ, Molina J: Prospective, randomized controlled trial of interferon-α in children with chronic hepatitis B. Hepatology 13:1035, 1991.

Sanchez-Urdazpal L, Czaja AJ, van Hoek B, et al: Prognostic features and role of liver transplantation in severe corticosteroid-treated autoimmune chronic active hepatitis. Hepatology 15:215, 1992.

CHAPTER 308

Drug- and Toxin-Induced Liver Injury

Frederick J. Suchy

The liver is the main site of drug metabolism and is particularly susceptible to structural and functional injury following ingestion, parenteral administration, or inhalation of chemical agents, drugs, plant derivatives (home remedies), or environmental toxins. The possibility of drug use or toxin exposure at home or in the parental work place should be explored for every child with liver dysfunction. The clinical spectrum of illness may vary from asymptomatic biochemical abnormalities of liver function to fulminant failure.

Hepatic metabolism of drugs and toxins is mediated by a sequence of enzymatic reactions which, in large part, transform hydrophobic, less excretable molecules into more nontoxic, hydrophilic compounds that can be readily excreted in urine or bile. *Phase 1* of the process involves the enzymatic activation of the substrate to reactive intermediates containing a carboxyl, phenol, epoxide, or hydroxyl group. Mixed-function mono-oxygenase, cytochrome C-reductase, various hydrolases, and the cytochrome P450 system are involved in this process. Nonspecific induction of these enzymatic pathways, which commonly occurs with the administration of certain drugs such as anticonvulsants, may alter the metabolism of other drugs and increase the potential for hepatotoxicity. A single agent may be metabolized by more than one biochemical reaction. The reactive intermediates that are potentially damaging to the cell are enzymatically conjugated in *phase 2* reactions with glucuronic acid, sulfate, or glutathione. Some drugs may be directly metabolized by these conjugating reactions without first undergoing *phase 1* activation. Pathways for biotransformation develop early in life with the possible exception of enzymes for oxidizing polycyclic aromatic hydrocarbons and for forming glucuronide conjugates. Mechanisms for the uptake and excretion of organic ions may also be deficient early in life. Some cases of idiosyncratic hepatotoxicity may occur as a result of aberrations in *phase 1* drug metabolism producing intermediates of unusual hepatotoxic potential combined with developmental, acquired, or relative inefficiency of *phase 2* conjugating reactions. Therefore, children may be more or less susceptible than adults to hepatotoxic reactions; for example, liver injury after the use of the anesthetic halothane is rare in children, and acetaminophen toxicity is unusual in infants compared with adolescents, whereas most cases of fatal hepatotoxicity associated with sodium valproate have been reported in children. In some cases, immaturity of hepatic drug metabolic pathways may prevent degradation of a toxic agent; under other circumstances, the same immaturity might limit the formation of toxic metabolites.

Chemical hepatotoxicity may be (1) *predictable* or (2) *idiosyncratic*. *Predictable* hepatotoxicity implies a high incidence of hepatic injury in exposed individuals, with dose dependency. The agents involved may damage the hepatocyte directly through alteration of membrane lipids (peroxidation) or through denaturation of proteins; such agents include carbon tetrachloride and trichloroethylene. Indirect injury may occur through interference with metabolic pathways essential for cell integrity or through distortion of cellular constituents by covalent binding of a reactive metabolite; examples include the liver injury produced by acetaminophen or by antimetabolites such as methotrexate or 6-mercaptopurine.

Idiosyncratic hepatotoxicity is infrequent and unpredictable. The likelihood of injury is not dose dependent and may occur at any time during exposure to the agent. An idiosyncratic reaction may be immunologically mediated as a result of prior sensitization (hypersensitivity); extrahepatic manifestations of hypersensitivity may include fever, rash, arthralgia, and eosinophilia. Duration of exposure before reaction is generally 1–4 wk, with prompt recurrence of injury on re-exposure.

Studies indicate that arene oxides, generated through oxidative (cytochrome P450) metabolism of aromatic anticonvulsants (phenytoin, phenobarbital, carbamazepine), may initiate the pathogenesis of hypersensitivity reactions. Arene oxides, formed in vivo, may bind to cellular macromolecules, thus perturbing cell function and possibly initiating immunologic mechanisms of liver injury. Idiosyncratic drug reactions in certain patients may reflect aberrant pathways for drug metabolism, with production of toxic intermediates (isoniazid and sodium valproate may cause liver damage through this mechanism). Duration of drug usage prior to liver injury varies (weeks to 1 yr or more), and the response to re-exposure may be delayed.

The *pathologic* spectrum of drug-induced liver disease is extremely wide, is rarely specific, and may mimic other liver diseases. (Table 308–1). Predictable hepatoxins such as acetaminophen produce centrilobular necrosis of hepatocytes. Steatosis is an important feature of tetracycline (microvesicular) and ethanol (macrovesicular) toxicities. A cholestatic hepatitis can be observed with injury caused by erythromycin estolate and chlorpromazine. Cholestasis without inflammation may be a toxic effect of estrogens and anabolic steroids. Oral contraceptives and androgens have also been associated with benign and malignant liver tumors. Some idiosyncratic drug reactions may produce mixed patterns of injury with diffuse cholestasis and cell necrosis. Several antineoplastic drugs and some herbal remedies have produced hepatic veno-occlusive disease. A chronic hepatitis has been associated with the use of methyldopa and nitrofurantoin.

Clinical manifestations may be mild and nonspecific, such as fever and malaise. Fever, rash, and arthralgia may be prominent in cases of hypersensitivity. In the ill, hospitalized patient, the signs and symptoms of hepatic drug toxicity may be difficult to separate from the underlying illness. The differential diagnosis should include acute and chronic viral hepatitis, biliary tract disease, septicemia, ischemic and hypoxic liver injury, malignant infiltration, and inherited metabolic liver disease.

The *laboratory features* of drug- or toxin-related liver disease are extremely variable. Hepatocyte damage may lead to elevations of serum aminotransferase activities and serum bilirubin levels and also to impaired synthetic function as evidenced by decreased serum coagulation factors and albumin. Hyperammonemia may occur with liver failure or with selective inhibition of the urea cycle (sodium valproate). Toxicologic screening of blood and urine specimens may aid in the detection of drug or toxin exposure. Percutaneous liver biopsy may be necessary to distinguish drug injury from complications of an underlying disorder or from intercurrent infection.

Slight elevation of serum aminotransferase activities (generally less than two to three times normal) may occur during therapy with drugs capable of inducing microsomal pathways for drug metabolism. Liver biopsy reveals proliferation of smooth endoplasmic reticulum but no significant liver injury. Liver test abnormalities often resolve with continued drug therapy.

■ TABLE 308–1 Patterns of Hepatic Drug Injury

Disease	Drug
Centrilobular necrosis	Acetaminophen Halothane
Microvesicular steatosis	Valproic acid
Acute hepatitis	Isoniazid
General hypersensitivity	Sulphonamides Diphenylhydantoin
Fibrosis	Methotrexate
Cholestasis	Chlorpromazine Erythromycin Estrogens
Veno-occlusive disease	Irradiation plus Busulfan Cyclophosphamide
Portal and hepatic vein thrombosis	Estrogens Androgens
Biliary sludge	Ceftriaxone
Hepatic adenoma or hepatocellular carcinoma	Oral contraceptives Anabolic steroids

Treatment of drug- or toxin-related liver injury is mainly supportive. Contact with the offending agent should be avoided. Corticosteroids may have a role in immune-mediated disease. Orthotopic liver transplantation may be required for treatment of drug or toxin-induced hepatic failure.

The *prognosis* of drug- or toxin-induced liver injury depends on its type and severity. Injury is usually completely reversible when the hepatotoxic factor is withdrawn. The mortality of submassive hepatic necrosis with fulminant liver failure may, however, exceed 50%. With continued use of certain drugs, such as methotrexate, effects of hepatoxicity may proceed insidiously to cirrhosis. Neoplasia may follow long-term androgen therapy. Rechallenge with a drug suspected of having caused previous liver injury is rarely justified and may result in fatal hepatic necrosis.

Drug-Induced Liver Disease

Kaplowitz N: Drug metabolism and hepatotoxicity. *In:* Kaplowitz N (ed): Liver and Biliary Diseases. Baltimore, MD, Williams & Wilkins, 1992, pp 82–97.

Kaplowitz N, Aw TY, Simon FR, et al: Drug induced hepatotoxicity. Ann Intern Med 104:826, 1986.

Roberts EA: Drug-induced liver disease in children. *In:* Suchy FJ (ed): Liver Disease in Children. St. Louis, CV Mosby 1994, pp 523–549.

Shear NH, Spielberg SP: Anticonvulsant hypersensitivity syndrome: In vitro assessment of risk. J Clin Invest 82:1826, 1988.

Zimmerman HJ (ed): Drug induced liver disease. Semin Liver Dis 1:89, 1981.

CHAPTER 309
Fulminant Hepatic Failure

Frederick J. Suchy

Fulminant hepatic failure is strictly defined as a clinical syndrome resulting from massive necrosis of hepatocytes or from severe functional impairment of hepatocytes in a patient who does not have a pre-existing liver disease. The disorder usually evolves over a period of fewer than 8 wk. Synthetic, excretory, and detoxifying functions of the liver are all severely impaired, with hepatic encephalopathy an essential diagnostic criterion. This narrow definition may be problematic in infants because liver failure in the perinatal period may associated with prenatal liver injury and even cirrhosis. Examples include neonatal iron storage disease, tyrosinemia, and some cases of congenital viral infection. In these disorders, liver disease may be noticed at birth or after several days of apparent well-being. Fulminant Wilson disease also occurs in children who were previously asymptomatic but by definition have pre-existing liver disease. Moreover, in some cases of liver failure, particularly in so-called non-A, non-B hepatitis, the onset of encephalopathy may occur later, from 8–28 wk after the onset of jaundice.

ETIOLOGY. Fulminant hepatic failure is most commonly a complication of viral hepatitis (A, B, D, E, possibly C, and others). An unusually high risk of fulminant hepatic failure occurs in young people who have combined infections with the hepatitis B virus and hepatitis D. Mutations in the precore region of hepatitis B virus (HBV) DNA have been associated with fulminant and severe hepatitis. Hepatitis B is also responsible for some cases of fulminant liver failure in the absence of serological markers of HBV infection but with HBV DNA found in the liver. The hepatitis C and E viruses are uncommon causes of fulminant hepatic failure in the United States. An additional, unidentified virus accounts for the majority of what in the past has been termed fulminant non-A, non-B hepatitis. This form may be the most common cause of fulminant hepatic failure in children. The disease occurs sporadically and usually without the parenteral risk factors of hepatitis B or C. Epstein-Barr virus, herpes simplex virus, adenovirus, enterovirus cytomegalovirus, and varicella zoster infections may produce fulminant hepatitis in children.

A variety of hepatotoxic drugs and chemicals may also cause fulminant hepatic failure. Predictable liver injury may occur after exposure to carbon tetrachloride and *Amanita phalloides* mushroom or after acetaminophen overdose. Idiosyncratic damage may follow the use of drugs such as halothane or sodium valproate. Ischemia and hypoxia resulting from hepatic vascular occlusion, congestive heart failure, cyanotic congenital heart disease, or circulatory shock may produce liver failure. Metabolic disorders associated with hepatic failure include Wilson disease, acute fatty liver of pregnancy, galactosemia, hereditary tryosinemia, hereditary fructose intolerance, neonatal iron storage disease, defects in β-oxidation of fatty acids, and deficiencies of mitochondrial electron transport.

PATHOLOGY. Liver biopsy usually reveals patchy or confluent massive necrosis of hepatocytes. Multilobular or bridging necrosis may be associated with collapse of the reticulin framework of the liver. There may be little or no regeneration of hepatocytes. A zonal pattern of necrosis may be observed with certain insults (e.g., centrilobular damage is associated with acetaminophen hepatotoxicity or with circulatory shock). Evidence of severe hepatocyte dysfunction rather than cell necrosis may occasionally be the predominant histologic finding (e.g., microvesicular fatty infiltrate of hepatocytes is observed in Reye syndrome and in tetracycline toxicity).

PATHOGENESIS. The mechanisms that lead to fulminant hepatic failure are poorly understood. It is unknown why only about 1–2% of patients with viral hepatitis experience liver failure. Massive destruction of hepatocytes may represent both a direct cytotoxic effect of the virus and an immune response to the viral antigens. One third to one half of patients with HBV-induced liver failure become negative for serum hepatitis B surface antigen within a few days of presentation and often have no detectable hepatitis B e antigen or HBV DNA in serum. These findings suggest a hyperimmune response to the virus that underlies the massive liver necrosis. Formation of hepatotoxic metabolites that bind covalently to macromolecular cell constituents is involved in the liver injury produced by drugs such as acetaminophen and isoniazid; fulminant hepatic failure may follow depletion of intracellular substrates involved in detoxification, particularly glutathione. Whatever the initial cause of hepatocyte injury, a variety of factors may contribute to the pathogenesis of liver failure, including impaired hepatocyte regeneration, altered parenchymal perfusion, endotoxemia, and decreased hepatic reticuloendothelial function.

The pathogenesis of hepatic encephalopathy may relate to increased serum levels of ammonia, false neurotransmitters, amines, increased γ-aminobutyric acid receptor activity, or increased circulating levels of endogenous benzodiazepine-like compounds. Decreased hepatic clearance of these substances may produce marked central nervous system (CNS) dysfunction.

CLINICAL MANIFESTATIONS. Fulminant hepatic failure may complicate previously known acute liver disease or be the presenting feature of liver disease. The child with fulminant hepatic failure has usually been previously healthy and most often has no risk factors for liver disease such as hepatitis or blood product exposure. Progressive jaundice, fetor hepaticus, fever, anorexia, vomiting, and abdominal pain are common. A rapid decrease in liver size without clinical improvement is an ominous sign. A hemorrhagic diathesis and ascites may develop. Patients should be closely observed for hepatic encephalopathy, which is initially characterized by minor disturbances of consciousness or motor function. Irritability, poor feeding, and a change in sleep rhythm may be the only findings in infants; asterixis may be demonstrable in older children. The patient is often somnolent or confused or combative on arousal and eventually may become responsive only to painful stimuli. The patient may rapidly progress to deeper stages of coma in which extensor responses and decerebrate and decorticate posturing appear. Respirations are usually increased early, but respiratory failure may occur in stage IV coma (see Table 309–1).

LABORATORY FINDINGS. Serum direct and indirect bilirubin levels and serum aminotransferase activities may be markedly elevated. However, serum aminotransferase activities do not correlate well with the severity of the illness and may actually decrease as the patient deteriorates. The blood ammonia concentration is usually increased. Prothrombin time is always prolonged and often does not improve after parenteral administration of vitamin K. Hypoglycemia can occur, particularly in infants. Hypokalemia, hyponatremia, metabolic acidosis, or respiratory alkalosis may develop.

TREATMENT. Management of fulminant hepatic failure is supportive. No therapy is known to reverse hepatocyte injury or to promote hepatic regeneration.

The infant or child with advanced hepatic coma should be treated in an intensive care unit where continuous monitoring of vital functions is possible. Endotracheal intubation may be required to prevent aspiration, to reduce cerebral edema by hyperventilation, and to facilitate pulmonary toilet. Mechanical ventilation and supplemental oxygen are often necessary in advanced coma. Electrolyte and glucose solutions should be administered intravenously to maintain urine output, to correct or prevent hypoglycemia, and to maintain normal serum potassium concentrations. Hyponatremia is common but is usually dilutional and not a result of sodium depletion. Parenteral supplementation with calcium, phosphorus, and magnesium may be required. Coagulopathy should be treated with parenteral administration of vitamin K and may require fresh frozen plasma; disseminated intravascular coagulation may also occur. Plasmapheresis may permit temporary correction of the bleeding diathesis without resulting in volume overload.

■ **TABLE 309–1 Stages of Hepatic Encephalopathy**

	Stages			
	I	*II*	*III*	*IV*
Symptoms	Periods of lethargy, euphoria; reversal of day–night sleeping; may be alert	Drowsiness, inappropriate behavior, agitation, wide mood swings, disorientation	Stupor but arousable, confused, incoherent speech	Coma IVa responds to noxious stimuli IVb no response
Signs	Trouble drawing figures, performing mental tasks	Asterixis, fetor hepaticus, incontinence	Asterixis, hyperreflexia, extensor reflexes, rigidity	Areflexia, no asterixis, flaccidity
Electroencephalogram	Normal	Generalized slowing, θ waves	Markedly abnormal, triphasic waves	Markedly abnormal bilateral slowing, δ waves, electric-cortical silence

Prophylactic use of antacids or H_2 receptor blockers or both should be considered because of the high risk of gastrointestinal bleeding. Hypovolemia should be avoided and treated with cautious infusions of fluids and blood products. Renal dysfunction may occur from dehydration, from acute tubular necrosis, or from functional renal failure (hepatorenal syndrome). The patient should be monitored closely for infection, including sepsis, pneumonia, peritonitis, and urinary tract infections. At least 50% of patients experience serious infection. Gram-positive organisms *(Staphylococcus aureus, Staphylococcus epidermidis)* are the most common pathogens but gram-negative and fungal infections are also observed. Cerebral edema is an extremely serious complication that responds poorly to measures such as corticosteroid administration and osmotic diuresis. The monitoring of intracranial pressure may be useful in preventing severe cerebral edema, in maintaining cerebral perfusion pressure, and in establishing the suitability of a patient for liver transplantation.

Gastrointestinal hemorrhage, infection, constipation, sedatives, electrolyte imbalance, and hypovolemia may precipitate encephalopathy and should be identified and corrected. Protein intake should be restricted or eliminated. The gut should be purged with several enemas. Lactulose should be given every 2–4 hr orally or by nasogastric tube in doses (10–50 mL) sufficient to cause diarrhea. The dose is then adjusted to produce several acidic, loose bowel movements daily. Lactulose syrup diluted with 1–3 volumes of water may also be given as a retention enema every 6 hr. Lactulose, a nonabsorbable disaccharide, is metabolized to organic acids by colonic bacteria; it probably lowers blood ammonia levels through decreasing microbial ammonia production and through trapping of ammonia in acidic intestinal contents. The oral or rectal administration of a nonabsorbable antibiotic such as neomycin may reduce enteric bacteria responsible for ammonia production. Flumazenil, a benzodiazepine antagonist, may reverse early hepatic encephalopathy.

Controlled trials have shown a worsened outcome of fulminant hepatic failure in patients treated with corticosteroids. A variety of approaches have been used to assist the liver in removing neuroactive toxins such as plasmapheresis or perfusion of the patient's plasma through a column of charcoal or other binding resins. Although the patient may experience an improvement in encephalopathy, there is little evidence that these treatments improve survival. Several liver assist devices containing cultured hepatocytes are also being used experimentally in an effort to allow regeneration of the patient's liver or to temporize until a suitable organ donor becomes available. Orthotopic liver transplantation may be life saving in patients who reach advanced stages of hepatic coma. Reduced-size allografts and living donor transplantation have been important advances in the treatment of infants with hepatic failure.

PROGNOSIS. Children with hepatic failure may fare somewhat better than adults, but overall mortality exceeds 70%. The prognosis may vary considerably with the cause of liver failure and stage of hepatic encephalopathy. With intensive medical support survival rates of 50–60% occur with hepatic failure complicating acetaminophen overdose and with fulminant hepatitis A or B virus infection. In contrast, recovery can be expected in only 10–20% of patients with liver failure caused by non-A, non-B, non-C hepatitis or an acute onset of Wilson disease. In patients who progress to stage IV coma (see Table 309–1) the prognosis is extremely poor. Major complications such as sepsis, severe hemorrhage, or renal failure increase the mortality. Studies indicate that jaundice for more than 7 days before the onset of encephalopathy, a prothrombin time more than 50 s, and a serum bilirubin more than 17.5 mg/dL (300 μmol/L) indicate a poor prognosis irrespective of the initial stage of hepatic coma. Survival of 50–75% is being achieved in patients with the poorest prognosis following orthotopic liver transplantation. Patients who recover from fulminant hepatic failure with only supportive care do not usually experience cirrhosis or chronic liver disease. Aplastic anemia is a common and usually fatal complication of fulminant hepatic failure secondary to sporadic non-A, non-B, non-C hepatitis.

Anonymous: Diuretics or paracentesis for ascites? Lancet ii:725, 1988.
Ascher NL, Lake JR, Emond JC, et al: Liver transplantation for fulminant hepatic failure. Arch Surg 128:677, 1993.
Cade R, Wagemaker H, Vogel S, et al: Hepatorenal syndrome: Studies of the effect of vascular volume and intraperitoneal pressure on renal and hepatic function. Am J Med 82:427, 1987.
Grim G, Katzenschlager R, Schneeweiss B, et al: Improvement of hepatic encephalopathy treated with flumazenil. Lancet ii:1392, 1988.
Lee WM: Acute hepatic failure. N Engl J Med 329:1862, 1993.
Liang TJ, Jeffers L, Reddy RK, et al: Fulminant or subfulminant non-A, non-B viral hepatitis: The role of hepatitis C and E viruses. Gastroenterology 104:556, 1993.
Mullen KD, Szauter KM, Kaminsky-Russ K: "Endogenous" benzodiazepine activity in body fluids of patients with hepatic encephalopathy. Lancet 336:81, 1990.
O'Grady JG, Alexander GJM, Hayllar KN, et al: Early indications of prognosis in fulminant hepatic failure. Gastroenterology 97:439, 1989.
Russell GJ, Fitzgerald JF, Clark JH: Fulminant hepatic failure. J Pediatr 111:313, 1987.
Stanley MM, Ochi S, Lee KK, et al: Peritoneovenous shunting as compared with medical treatment in patients with alcoholic cirrhosis and massive ascites. N Engl J Med 321:1632, 1989.
Terazawa S, Kojima M, Yamanaka T, et al: Hepatitis B virus mutants with precore-region defects in two babies with fulminant hepatitis and their mothers positive for antibody to hepatitis B e antigen. Pediatr Res 29:5, 1991.
Whitington PF: Fulminant hepatic failure in children. *In:* Suchy FJ (ed): Liver Disease in Children. St. Louis, Mosby-Year Book, 1994, pp 180–213.

CHAPTER 310

Cystic Diseases of the Biliary Tract and Liver

Frederick J. Suchy

Cystic lesions of liver parenchyma or of the biliary system may be recognized initially during infancy and childhood. Their classification is not yet satisfactory. Pathologic features may be found in common among several of these disorders, but different patterns of inheritance indicate that their etiology is heterogeneous.

CHOLEDOCHAL CYSTS. These are congenital dilatations of the common bile duct that may cause progressive biliary obstruction and biliary cirrhosis. Cylindrical and spherical cysts of the extrahepatic ducts are the most common types. Segmental or diffuse dilatation can be observed. A diverticulum of the common bile duct or dilatation of the intraduodenal portion of the common duct (choledochocele) is a variant. Cystic dilatation of the intrahepatic bile ducts may be associated with a choledochal cyst.

The pathogenesis of choledochal cysts remains uncertain. Some reports have suggested that junction of the common bile duct and the pancreatic duct before their entry into the sphincter of Oddi may allow reflux of pancreatic enzymes into the common bile duct, causing inflammation, localized weakness, and dilatation of the duct. Other possibilities are that choledochal cysts represent malformations of the common duct or occur as part of the disease spectrum that includes neonatal hepatitis and biliary atresia.

Approximately 75% of cases appear during childhood. The

infant typically presents with cholestatic jaundice; severe liver dysfunction including ascites and coagulopathy can rapidly evolve if biliary obstruction is not relieved. An abdominal mass is rarely palpable. In the older child, the classic triad of abdominal pain, jaundice, and mass occurs in less than 33% of patients. Features of acute cholangitis (fever, right upper quadrant tenderness, jaundice, leukocytosis) may be present. The diagnosis is made by ultrasonography; choledochal cysts have been identified prenatally using this technique.

The treatment of choice is primary excision of the cyst and a Roux-en-Y choledochojejunostomy. Simple drainage into the small bowel is less satisfactory owing to a risk for development of carcinoma in the residual cystic tissue. The postoperative course may be complicated by recurrent cholangitis or stricture at the anastomotic site.

CYSTIC DILATATION OF THE INTRAHEPATIC BILE DUCTS (CAROLI DISEASE). Congenital, saccular dilatation may affect multiple segments of the intrahepatic bile ducts; the dilated ducts are lined by cuboidal epithelium and are in continuity with the main duct system, which is usually normal. Caroli actually described two variants: *Caroli disease,* characterized by ectasias of the intrahepatic bile ducts without other abnormalities and *Caroli syndrome* in which congenital ductal dilatation is associated with features of congenital hepatic fibrosis and the renal lesion of autosomal recessive polycystic renal disease. Caroli syndrome is more common, but both varieties may occur in the same family and are inherited in an autosomal recessive fashion. Choledochal cysts have also been associated with Caroli disease. There is a marked predisposition to ascending cholangitis and calculus formation within the abnormal bile ducts.

Affected patients usually experience symptoms of acute cholangitis as children or young adults. Fever, abdominal pain, mild jaundice, and pruritus occur; and a slightly enlarged, tender liver is palpable. Elevated alkaline phosphatase activity, direct-reacting bilirubin levels, and leukocytosis may be observed during episodes of acute infection. In patients with Caroli syndrome, clinical features may be due to a combination of recurring bouts of cholangitis reflecting the intrahepatic ductal abnormalities and portal hypertensive bleeding resulting from hepatic fibrosis. Ultrasonography shows the dilated intrahepatic ducts, but definitive diagnosis and extent of disease must be determined by percutaneous transhepatic or endoscopic cholangiography.

Cholangitis and sepsis are treated with appropriate antibiotics. Calculi may require surgery. Partial hepatectomy may be curative in rare cases when disease is confined to a single lobe. The prognosis is otherwise guarded, largely owing to difficulties in controlling cholangitis and biliary lithiasis and to a significant risk for developing cholangiocarcinoma.

CONGENITAL HEPATIC FIBROSIS. This is an autosomal recessive disorder characterized pathologically by diffuse periportal and perilobular fibrosis in broad bands that contain distorted bile duct-like structures and that often compress or incorporate central or sublobular veins. The ductlike structures may become dilated to the point of microcyst formation but do not communicate with the biliary tract. Irregularly shaped islands of liver parenchyma contain normal-appearing hepatocytes. Caroli disease and choledochal cysts have been associated (see earlier discussion). About 75% of patients have renal disease, such as renal tubular ectasia, nephronophthisis, or autosomal recessive polycystic renal disease.

The disorder usually has its clinical onset in childhood, with hepatosplenomegaly or with bleeding secondary to portal hypertension. Cholangitis may occur in patients who have associated abnormalities of bile ducts.

Hepatocellular function is well preserved. Serum aminotransferase activities and bilirubin levels are usually normal; serum alkaline phosphatase activity may be slightly elevated. The serum albumin level and prothrombin time are normal. Liver biopsy is usually required for diagnosis.

Treatment of this disorder should focus on control of bleeding from esophageal varices. Infrequent mild bleeding episodes may be managed by endoscopic sclerotherapy or band ligation of the varices. Following more severe hemorrhage, portacaval anastomosis may bring relief of portal hypertension. The prognosis may be greatly improved by a shunting procedure, but survival in some patients may be limited by renal failure.

A **solitary liver cyst** (nonparasitic) rarely occurs in childhood. Abdominal distention and pain may be present, and a poorly defined right upper quadrant mass may be palpable. These benign lesions are best left undisturbed unless they compress adjacent structures or a complication occurs, such as hemorrhage into the cyst.

AUTOSOMAL DOMINANT POLYCYSTIC KIDNEY DISEASE (ADPKD). This disease is associated with multiple cysts of the liver, kidney, and less commonly of other organs. This disorder is autosomal dominant, with a high degree of penetrance. The gene for the disorder has been localized to chromosome 16. The cysts probably arise from defective development of intrahepatic bile ducts, but most do not communicate with the biliary tree. The liver may be of normal size or markedly enlarged. Cysts increase in size from childhood until the 4th or 5th decade of life. Most of the affected children are asymptomatic; the prognosis is determined by the severity of the cystic renal disease. Portal hypertension and obstructive jaundice are rarely produced by large cysts. ADPKD has recently been associated with ductal lesion of Caroli syndrome and with congenital hepatic fibrosis. Autosomal dominant and recessive forms of polycystic kidney disease are not allelic so that unrecognized genetic links between these disorders probably exist.

Subarachnoid hemorrhage may occur from the associated cerebral arterial aneurysms.

AUTOSOMAL RECESSIVE POLYCYSTIC KIDNEY DISEASE (ARPKD) Different forms of ARPKD have been defined according to the age at presentation (perinatal, neonatal, infantile, and juvenile). These subdivisions are recognized on the basis of clinical patterns and probably are not genetically or pathophysiologically distinct. Neonates with the perinatal form die shortly after birth from hypoplastic lungs and pulmonary insufficiency. Renal disease predominates in the neonatal and infantile forms. The kidneys in these patients are markedly enlarged from cysts and function poorly. In surviving patients a progression of the renal and liver disease occurs with increasing amounts of fibrosis. Death from renal failure is common in the first weeks or months of life. Hepatic fibrosis may be progressive but is usually not clinically important in these patients. Portal tracts are enlarged by connective tissue and contain numerous, irregularly dilated bile ducts.

In older children and adults with ARPKD, hepatic disease may be the most significant problem. The typical lesion of congenital hepatic fibrosis and sometimes dilatation of the larger bile ducts (Caroli syndrome) may be present. Hepatic fibrosis and portal vein abnormalities give rise to portal hypertension and gastrointestinal bleeding. Hematemesis or melena may be the presenting feature and can occur as early as the 1st year of life or as late as adolescence. Firm hepatomegaly and splenomegaly are often found. Renal dysfunction as evidenced by impaired ability to concentrate urine and an an elevated blood urea nitrogen may occur in about 20% of these patients. Enlarged kidneys and tubular ectasia rather than large cysts are observed on imaging studies. Long-term survival is possible with successful management of portal hypertension, but outcome can be adversely affected by the additional complications of cholangitis or renal failure.

Variable abnormalities of bile ducts (irregular dilatation, proliferation, cysts) and portal fibrosis may be associated with Meckel syndrome, 17–18 trisomy, tuberous sclerosis, and asphyxiating thoracic dystrophy.

Bancroft JD, Bucuvalas JC, Ryckman FC, et al: Antenatal diagnosis of choledochal cyst. J Pediatr Gastroenterol Nutr 18:142, 1994.

Desmet VJ: Congenital diseases of the intrahepatic bile ducts: Variations on the theme of "ductal plate malformation." Hepatology 16:1069, 1992.
Desmet VJ: What is congenital hepatic fibrosis? Histopathology 20:465, 1992.
Gabow PA: Autosomal dominant polycystic kidney disease. N Engl J Med 329:332, 1993.
Okada A, Nakamura T, Higaki J, et al: Congenital dilatation of the bile duct in 100 instances and its relationship with anomalous junction. Surg Gynecol Obstet 171:291, 1990.

CHAPTER 311

Diseases of the Gallbladder

Frederick J. Suchy

ANOMALIES. The gallbladder is congenitally absent in about 0.1% of the population. Hypoplasia or absence of the gallbladder may be associated with extrahepatic biliary atresia or cystic fibrosis. Duplication of the gallbladder occurs rarely.

ACUTE HYDROPS (Table 311–1). Acute noncalculous, noninflammatory distention of the gallbladder may occur in infants and children. It is defined by the absence of calculi, bacterial infection, or congenital anomalies of the biliary system. The disorder may complicate acute infections, but the cause is often not identified. Hydrops of the gallbladder may also develop in patients receiving long-term parenteral nutrition, presumably as a result of gallbladder stasis during the period of enteral fasting. Hydrops is distinguished from acalculous cholecystitis by the absence of a significant inflammatory process and a generally benign prognosis.

Affected patients usually have right upper quadrant pain with a palpable mass. Fever, vomiting, and jaundice may be present and are usually associated with a systemic illness such as streptococcal infection. Ultrasonography shows a markedly distended, echo-free gallbladder, without dilatation of the biliary tree. Acute hydrops is usually treated conservatively and rarely needs cholecystostomy and drainage. At laparotomy, a large, edematous gallbladder is found that contains white, yellow, or green bile. Obstruction of the cystic duct by mesenteric adenopathy is occasionally observed. Cholecystectomy is required if the gallbladder is gangrenous. Pathologic examination of the gallbladder wall shows edema and mild inflammation. Cultures of bile are usually sterile. Treatment of gallbladder hydrops is usually nonsurgical with a focus on supportive care and managing the intercurrent illness. Spontaneous resolution and return of normal gallbladder usually occur over a period of several weeks.

CHOLECYSTITIS AND CHOLELITHIASIS. *Acute acalculous cholecystitis* is uncommon in children and is usually caused by infection. Reported pathogens include streptococci (groups A and B), gram-negative organisms, particularly *Salmonella,* and *Leptospira interrogans.* Parasitic infestation with ascaris or *Giardia lamblia* may be found. Acalculous cholecystitis may rarely follow abdominal trauma or burn injury or be associated with a systemic vasculitis, such as periarteritis nodosa.

Clinical features include right upper quadrant or epigastric pain, nausea, vomiting, fever, and jaundice. Right upper quadrant guarding and tenderness are present. Ultrasonography discloses an enlarged, thick-walled gallbladder, without calculi. Serum alkaline phosphatase activity and direct-reacting bilirubin levels are elevated. Leukocytosis is usual.

■ **TABLE 311–1 Conditions Associated with Hydrops of the Gallbladder**

Kawasaki disease	Viral hepatitis
Streptococcal pharyngitis	Sepsis
Staphylococcal infection	Henoch-Schönlein purpura
Total parenteral nutrition	Mesenteric adenitis
Prolonged fasting	Necrotizing enterocolitis

■ **TABLE 311–2 Conditions Associated with Cholelithiasis**

Chronic hemolytic disease (sick cell anemia, spherocytosis)
Obesity
Ileal resection or disease
Cystic fibrosis
Chronic liver disease
Prolonged parenteral nutrition
Prematurity with complicated medical or surgical course
Prolonged fasting or rapid weight reduction
Treatment of childhood cancer
Abdominal surgery
Pregnancy

The diagnosis is confirmed at laparotomy. Cholecystectomy and treatment of the systemic infection are required.

Cholelithiasis is relatively rare in otherwise healthy children, occurring more commonly in patients with a variety of predisposing disorders (Table 311–2). Gallstones, composed of a mixture of cholesterol, bile pigment, calcium, and inorganic matrix, are common. In children, more than 70% of gallstones are the pigment type, 15–20% are cholesterol stones, and the remainder are of unknown composition. Stones of pure cholesterol or bile pigment may also occur.

The most important clinical feature is recurrent abdominal pain, which is often colicky and localized to the right upper quadrant. The older child may have intolerance for fatty foods. Acute cholecystitis may be the first manifestation, with fever, pain in the right upper quadrant, and often a palpable mass. Pain may radiate to an area just below the right scapula. A plain roentgenogram of the abdomen may reveal opaque calculi, but radiolucent (cholesterol) stones will not be visualized. Accordingly, ultrasonography is the method of choice for gallstone detection. Cholecystectomy is usually curative; operative cholangiography should be done at the time of surgery to exclude common duct calculi. Dissolution of cholesterol stones with oral chenodeoxycholic acid and extracorporeal lithotripsy are potential alternatives to surgery. Experience in children is limited with these nonoperative therapies. Laparoscopic cholecystectomy is being used successfully in children.

Patients with hemolytic disease (including sickle cell anemia, the thalassemias, and red blood cell enzymopathies) and Wilson disease are at increased risk for black pigment cholelithiasis. Cirrhosis and chronic cholestasis also increase the risk for pigment gallstones. Increasing numbers of sick premature infants are being found to have gallstones; their management is often complicated by such factors as bowel resection, necrotizing enterocolitis, prolonged parenteral nutrition without enteral feeding, cholestasis, frequent blood transfusions, and use of diuretics. Cholelithiasis in premature infants is often asymptomatic and may resolve spontaneously. Brown pigment stones have been found in patients with obstructive jaundice and infected intra- and extrahepatic bile ducts. These stones are usually radiolucent, owing to a lower content of calcium phosphate and carbonate and a higher amount of cholesterol than in black pigment stones.

Cholesterol cholelithiasis in children most frequently affects obese adolescent girls. Cholesterol gallstones are found also in children with disturbances of the enterohepatic circulation of bile acids, including patients with ileal disease and bile acid malabsorption, such as those with ileal resection, ileal Crohn disease, and cystic fibrosis. Pigment stones may also occur in these patients.

Cholesterol gallstone formation seems to result from an excess of cholesterol in relation to the cholesterol-carrying capacity of micelles in bile. Supersaturation of bile with cholesterol leading to crystal and stone formation could result from decreased bile acid or from an increased cholesterol concentration in bile. Other initiating factors that may be important in stone formation include gallbladder stasis, or the presence in bile of abnormal mucoproteins or bile pigments that may serve as a nidus for cholesterol crystallization.

Friesen CA, Roberts CC: Cholelithiasis: Clinical characteristics in children. Clin Pediatr 7:294, 1989.
Heubi JE, Lewis LG: Diseases of the gallbladder in infancy, childhood and adolescence. *In:* Suchy FJ (ed): Liver Disease in Children, 1st ed. St. Louis, Mosby-Year Book, 1994, pp 605–621.
Suchy FJ: Disorders of the biliary tract in infancy and childhood. *In:* Sleisenger MH, Fordtran JS (eds): Gastrointestinal Disease, 5th ed. Philadelphia, WB Saunders, 1993, pp 1747–1964.
Ware RE, Kinney TR, Casey JR, et al: Laparoscopic cholecystectomy in young patients with sickle hemoglobinopathies. J Pediatr 120:58, 1992.

CHAPTER 312
Portal Hypertension and Varices

Frederick J. Suchy

Portal hypertension—defined as an elevation of portal pressure above 10–12 mm Hg—is a major cause of morbidity and mortality in children with liver disease. The normal portal venous pressure is approximately 7 mm Hg. The clinical features of the various forms of portal hypertension may be similar, but the associated complications, management, and prognosis can vary significantly and depend on whether the process is complicated by hepatic insufficiency.

ETIOLOGY. Numerous causes of portal hypertension result from obstruction to portal blood flow anywhere along the course of the portal venous system. The various disorders associated with portal hypertension are outlined in Table 312–1. Portal hypertension may occur as a result of prehepatic, intrahepatic, or posthepatic obstruction to the flow of portal blood.

TABLE 312–1 Causes of Portal Hypertension

Extrahepatic Portal Hypertension
Portal Vein Obstruction
Portal vein thrombosis or cavernous transformation
Splenic vein thrombosis
Increased Portal Flow
Arteriovenous fistula
Intrahepatic Portal Hypertension
Hepatocellular Disease
Acute and chronic viral hepatitis
Cirrhosis
Congenital hepatic fibrosis
Wilson's disease
α_1-Antitrypsin deficiency
Glycogen storage disease type IV
Hepatotoxicity
Methotrexate
Parenteral nutrition
Biliary Tract Disease
Extrahepatic biliary atresia
Cystic fibrosis
Choledochal cyst
Sclerosing cholangitis
Intrahepatic bile duct paucity
Idiopathic Portal Hypertension
Postsinusoidal Obstruction
Budd-Chiari syndrome
Veno-occlusive disease

Extrahepatic portal vein obstruction is an important cause of portal hypertension in childhood. The obstruction may occur at any level of the portal vein. Umbilical infection with or without a history of catheterization of the umbilical vein may be causal in neonates. The infection can spread potentially from the umbilical vein to the left branch of the portal vein and eventually to the main portal venous channel. Intra-abdominal infections including acute appendicitis and primary peritonitis can be causal in older children. Portal vein thrombosis has also been associated with neonatal dehydration and systemic infection. In older children, inflammatory bowel disease can be associated with a hypercoagulable state and portal venous obstruction. Thrombosis of the portal vein has also occurred in association with biliary tract infections and primary sclerosing cholangitis. Portal vein thrombosis has also been associated with hypercoagulable states such as protein C and protein S deficiencies. The portal vein can be replaced by a fibrous remnant or contain an organized thrombus. Obstruction by a web or diaphragm can also occur. In at least half of reported cases there is no defined cause.

Uncommonly, presinusoidal hypertension can be caused by increased flow through the portal system as a result of a congenital or acquired arteriovenous fistula.

There are numerous intrahepatic causes of portal hypertension. Obstruction to flow can occur on the basis of a presinusoidal process including acute and chronic hepatitis, congenital hepatic fibrosis, or schistosomiasis. Portal infiltration with malignant cells or granulomas can also contribute. An idiopathic form of portal hypertension characterized by splenomegaly, hypersplenism, and portal hypertension without occlusion of portal or splenic veins and with no obvious disease in the liver has been described. In some patients, noncirrhotic portal fibrosis has been observed.

Cirrhosis is the predominant cause of portal hypertension and is related to obstruction of blood through the portal vein. There are numerous causes of cirrhosis including recognized disorders such as extrahepatic biliary atresia, metabolic liver disease such as α_1-antitrypsin deficiency, Wilson disease, glycogen storage disease type IV, hereditary fructose intolerance, and cystic fibrosis.

Postsinusoidal causes of portal hypertension are also observed during childhood. The Budd-Chiari syndrome, occurs with obstruction to hepatic veins anywhere between the efferent hepatic veins and the entry of the inferior vena cava into the right atrium. In most cases no specific cause can be found, but the thrombosis can complicate neoplasms, collagen-vascular disease, infection, and trauma. Veno-occlusive disease is the most frequent cause of hepatic vein obstruction in children. In this disorder, occlusion of the centrilobular venules or sublobular hepatic veins occurs. The disorder occurs after total body irradiation with or without cytotoxic drug therapy that is commonly used before bone marrow transplantation. The disease has also occurred after the ingestion of herbal remedies containing the pyrrolizidine alkaloids, which are sometimes taken as medicinal teas.

PATHOPHYSIOLOGY. The primary hemodynamic abnormality in portal hypertension is increased resistance to portal blood flow. This is the case whether the resistance to portal flow has an intrahepatic cause such as cirrhosis or is due to portal vein obstruction. Portosystemic shunting should decompress the portal system and thus significantly lower portal pressures. However, in spite of the development of significant collaterals deviating portal blood into systemic veins, portal hypertension is maintained by an overall increase in portal venous flow and thus maintenance of portal hypertension. A hyperdynamic circulation is achieved by tachycardia, an increase in cardiac output, and a decreased systemic vascular resistance. Splanchnic dilatation also occurs. Overall, the increase in portal flow likely contributes to an increase in variceal transmural pressure. The increase in portal blood flow is related to the contribution of hepatic and collateral flow; the actual portal blood flow reaching the liver is reduced. It is also likely that hepatocellular dysfunction and portosystemic shunting lead to the generation of a variety of humoral factors that cause vasodilatation and an increase in plasma volume.

Many of the portal hypertension complications can be accounted for by the development of a remarkable collateral circulation. Collateral vessels may form prominently in areas in which absorptive epithelium joins stratified epithelium, particularly in the esophagus or anorectal region. The superficial submucosal collaterals, especially those in the esophagus and stomach and to a lesser extent those in the duodenum, colon, or rectum, are prone to rupture and bleeding under increased pressure. In portal hypertension the vascularity of the stomach is also abnormal and demonstrates prominent submucosal arteriovenous communications between the muscularis mucosa and dilated precapillaries and veins. The resulting lesion—a vascular ectasia—has been called *congestive gastropathy* and contributes to a significant risk of bleeding from the stomach.

CLINICAL MANIFESTATIONS. Bleeding from esophageal varices is the most common presentation. In patients with underlying hepatic disease, physical examination may show jaundice and stigmata of cirrhosis such as palmar erythema and vascular telangiectasias. Dilated cutaneous collateral vessels carrying blood from the portal to system circulation may be apparent in the periumbilical region. In the absence of clinical or biochemical features of liver disease and a liver of normal size, portal vein obstruction is most likely. However, well-compensated cirrhosis cannot be completely ruled out under these conditions. An enlarged, hard liver with minimal disturbance of hepatic function suggests the possibility of congenital hepatic fibrosis. Hemorrhage, particularly in children with portal vein obstruction, may be precipitated by minor febrile, intercurrent illness. The mechanism is often unclear; aspirin or other nonsteroidal anti-inflammatory drugs may be a contributing factor by damaging the integrity of a congested gastric mucosa or interfering with platelet function. Coughing during a respiratory illness can also increase intravariceal pressure. The bleeding may become apparent with hematemesis or with melena. Gastrointestinal hemorrhage can also originate from portal hypertensive gastropathy or from gastric, duodenal, peristomal, or rectal varices. Splenomegaly, sometimes with hypersplenism, is the next most common presenting feature in portal vein obstruction and may be discovered first on routine physical examination. Because more than half of patients in many series with portal vein obstruction do not experience bleeding until after 6 yr of age, the diagnosis should be suggested in a child without hepatocellular disease who had a complicated neonatal course and in whom asymptomatic splenomegaly later developed.

Children with portal hypertension, regardless of the underlying cause, may have recurrent bouts of life-threatening hemorrhage. In patients with portal vein obstruction and normal hepatic function, the bleeding usually stops spontaneously. In patients with intrahepatic disease, the combination of portal hypertension and poor liver synthetic ability (coagulopathy) can make bleeding much more difficult to control. Moreover, esophageal hemorrhage and cirrhosis may have injurious effects on the liver, further impairing hepatic function and sometimes precipitating jaundice, ascites, and encephalopathy.

DIAGNOSIS. In patients with established chronic liver disease or in those in whom portal vein obstruction is suspected, an experienced ultrasonographer should be able to demonstrate the patency of the portal vein. In addition, the use of Doppler flow ultrasonography may demonstrate the direction of flow within the portal system. The pattern of flow correlates with the severity of cirrhosis and encephalopathy. Hepatopetal flow is more likely to be associated with variceal bleeding. Ultrasonography is also effective in detecting the presence of esophageal varices. Another important feature of extrahepatic portal vein obstruction is so-called cavernous transformation of the portal vein in which an extensive complex of small collateral vessels have formed to bypass the obstruction. A variety of other imaging techniques also contribute to further definition of the portal vein anatomy but are required less often; computed tomography and magnetic resonance imaging provide similar information to ultrasonography. Selective arteriography of the celiac axis, superior mesenteric artery, and splenic vein may be useful in precise mapping of the extrahepatic vascular anatomy. This is not required to establish a diagnosis but may prove valuable in planning surgical decompression of portal hypertension.

Endoscopy is the most reliable method for detecting esophageal varices and for identifying the source of gastrointestinal bleeding. Although bleeding from esophageal or gastric varices is most common in children with portal hypertension, up to one third of patients, particularly those with cirrhosis, may have bleeding from some other source such as portal hypertensive gastropathy or gastric or duodenal ulcerations. Once a diagnosis of portal hypertension has been established, several endoscopic features of esophageal varices may predict a risk for hemorrhage. There is a strong correlation between variceal size as assessed endoscopically and the probability of hemorrhage. Red spots apparent over varices at the time of endoscopy are a strong predictor of eminent hemorrhage.

TREATMENT. The therapy of portal hypertension can be divided into emergency treatment of potentially life-threatening hemorrhage and prophylaxis directed against prevention of initial or subsequent bleeding. It must be emphasized that many trials of therapy are based on experience with adults with portal hypertension.

The management of the patient with variceal hemorrhage must focus on fluid resuscitation initially in the form of crystalloid infusion followed by the replacement of red cells. Correction of coagulopathy by administration of vitamin K or the infusion of platelets or fresh frozen plasma, or both therapies, may be required. A nasogastric tube should be placed to document the presence of blood within the stomach and to monitor for ongoing bleeding. An H_2 receptor blocker such as ranitidine should be given intravenously to reduce the risk of bleeding from gastric erosions. In most patients, particularly those with extrahepatic portal hypertension and with normal hepatic synthetic function, bleeding usually stops spontaneously. Care should be taken in fluid resuscitation of children after bleeding so as not to produce an excessively high venous pressure and an increased risk for further bleeding.

Pharmacologic therapy to decrease portal pressure may be considered in patients with continued bleeding. Vasopressin, or one of its analogs, has been commonly used and is thought to act by increasing splanchnic vascular tone and thus decreasing portal blood flow. Vasopressin is administered initially with a bolus of 0.33 U/kg over 20 min followed by a continued infusion of the same dose on an hourly basis or a continuous infusion of 0.2 U/1.73 m^2/min. The drug has a half-life of approximately 30 min. Its use may be limited by the side effects of vasoconstriction, which can impair cardiac function and perfusion to the heart, bowel, and kidneys and may also, as a result, exacerbate fluid retention. Nitroglycerin, usually given as a portion of a skin patch, has also been used to decrease portal pressure and, when used in conjunction with vasopressin, may ameliorate some of its untoward effects. The somatostatin analog octreotide is a newer agent in use to decrease splanchnic blood flow with fewer side effects. Although studies in adults are promising, its use and efficacy in children have not been well evaluated.

After an episode of variceal hemorrhage or in patients in whom bleeding cannot be controlled, endoscopic sclerosis of esophageal varices is an important option. In this technique, sclerosants are injected either intravariceally or paravariceally until bleeding has stopped. Although bleeding may be controlled acutely in most cases, further sessions of sclerotherapy are required to achieve temporary obliteration of the varices. Treatments may be associated with further bleeding, bacteremia, esophageal ulceration, and stricture formation. Most centers do not perform endoscopic sclerotherapy of varices prophylactically but use the procedure as a bridge to the time of liver transplantation or until collateral circulation develops in extrahepatic portal vein obstruction. Endoscopic elastic band ligation of varices has recently been introduced as a safer and potentially as effective therapy for obliteration of varices. Experience with the technique in children is limited.

In patients who continue to bleed despite pharmacologic and endoscopic methods to control hemorrhage, a Sengstaken-Blakemore tube may be placed to stop hemorrhage by mechanically compressing esophageal and gastric varices. The device may be the only option to control life-threatening hemorrhage but carries a significant rate of complications and a high rate of bleeding when the device is removed. There is a particularly high risk for pulmonary aspiration, and the tube is not well tolerated in children without significant sedation.

A variety of surgical procedures have been devised to divert portal blood flow and to decrease portal pressure. A portacaval shunt diverts nearly all of the portal blood flow into the subhepatic inferior right vena cava. Although portal pressure is significantly reduced, because of the significant diversion of blood from the liver, there is a marked risk for hepatic encephalopathy in patients with parenchymal liver disease. More selective shunting procedures, such as mesocaval or distal splenorenal shunt, may effectively decompress the portal system while allowing a greater amount of portal blood flow to the liver. The small size of the vessels makes these operations technically challenging in infants and small children, and there is a significant risk of failure as a result of shunt thrombosis. Therefore, orthotopic liver transplantation represents a much better therapy for portal hypertension resulting from intrahepatic disease. A prior portosystemic shunting operation does not preclude a successful liver transplantation but makes the operation technically more difficult. Portosystemic shunting may remain an option in children with extrahepatic portal hypertension, particularly in those patients suffering from potentially life-threatening hemorrhage not effectively controlled by other measures and who reside a great distance from emergency medical care. A transjugular intrahepatic portosystemic shunt, in which a stent is placed between the right hepatic vein and the right or left portal vein, has been used in adults and a few children to control severe variceal bleeding, particularly until liver transplantation can be performed.

Long-term treatment with nonspecific β-blockers such as propranolol has been used extensively in adults with portal hypertension. These agents may act by lowering cardiac output and portal perfusion. There is evidence in adult patients that β-blockers may reduce the incidence of variceal hemorrhage and improve long-term survival. A therapeutic effect is thought to result when the pulse rate is reduced by at least 25%. There is limited published experience with the use of this therapy in children.

PROGNOSIS. Portal hypertension secondary to intrahepatic disease has a poor prognosis. Portal hypertension is usually progressive in these patients and is often associated with deteriorating liver function. Efforts should be directed toward the prompt treatment of acute bleeding and prevention of recurrent hemorrhage with available methods. Ultimately, patients with progressive liver disease and significant esophageal varices will require orthotopic liver transplantation. Liver transplantation might also be considered for patients with portal hypertension secondary to hepatic vein obstruction or resulting from severe veno-occlusive disease.

In patients with portal vein obstruction, episodes of bleeding may become less frequent and severe with age as a collateral circulation develops. Most patients can be managed conservatively with endoscopic sclerotherapy when necessary. Portosystemic shunting procedures may be required in some patients.

Alvarez F, Bernard O, Brunelle F, et al: Portal obstruction in children: I. Clinical investigation and hemorrhage risk. J Pediatr 103:696, 1983.

Alvarez F, Bernard O, Brunelle F, et al: Portal obstruction in children: II. Results of surgical portosystemic shunts. J Pediatr 103:703, 1983.

De Giacomo C, Tomasi G, Burns PN, et al: Ultra sonographic prediction of the presence and severity of esophageal varices in children. J Pediatr Gastroenterol Nutr 9:431, 1989.

Gentil-Kocher S, Bernard O, Brunelle F, et al: Budd-Chiari syndrome in children: Report of 22 cases. J Pediatr 113:30, 1988.

Howard ER, Stringer MD, Mowat AP: Assessment of injection sclerotherapy in the management of 152 children with oesophageal varices. Br J Surg 75:404, 1988.

Maksoud JG, Goncalves EP: Treatment of portal hypertension in children. World J Surg 18:251, 1994.

Sokal E, Van Hoorebeeck N, Van Obbergh L, et al: Upper gastrointestinal tract bleeding in cirrhotic children candidates for liver transplantation. Eur J Pediatr 151:326, 1992.

Webb LJ, Sherlock S: The aetiology, presentation, and natural history of extrahepatic portal hypertension. Q J Med 192:627, 1979.

CHAPTER 313
Liver Transplantation

J. Carlton Gartner, Jr., and Basil J. Zitelli

Orthotopic liver transplantation is standard therapy for end-stage pediatric liver disease. Approximately 350 children undergo the procedure each year in the United States. The most frequent indication for transplantation is cirrhosis from extrahepatic biliary atresia after a failed portoenterostomy (Kasai) procedure. Metabolic liver diseases, of which α_1-antitrypsin deficiency is most frequent, and familial cholestasis are next in frequency (Table 313–1).

Early referral to a transplant center is important so that patients and their families may be treated in a timely fashion. The evaluation procedure includes medical problems (diagnosis, course, complications) as well as psychosocial issues. Scor-

■ TABLE 313–1 Indications for Pediatric Liver Transplantation

Indication	No. Cases
Biliary atresia	145
Metabolic liver disease	42
α_1-Antitrypsin deficiency	27
Tyrosinemia	7
Wilson disease	4
Other	4
Familial cholestasis	19
Fulminant hepatic failure	16
Biliary hypoplasia	13
Hepatitis	12
Cirrhosis, idiopathic	7
Hepatitis, neonatal	5
Sclerosing cholangitis	3
Congenital hepatic fibrosis	2
Carcinoma	2
Miscellaneous	4
Total	270

From Zilell BJ, Gartner JC, Malatack JJ, et al: Liver transplantation in children: A pediatrician's perspective. Pediatr Ann 20:691, 1991.

ing systems that predict death from liver disease are used at different transplant centers, but the most predictive factors are prolonged partial thromboplastin time, ascites, elevated indirect bilirubin levels, and low cholesterol levels. Patients with certain conditions, such as biliary atresia after an unsuccessful Kasai procedure, may undergo transplantation before late complications occur. Early evaluation allows families to live at home and make arrangements to arrive at the center when a donor organ becomes available. Anticipatory guidance to families about the special needs of children with chronic illness may improve the psychosocial outcome after successful surgery.

Pretransplantation management is critical to the success of the procedure and to limiting morbidity from liver disease. Areas of major importance are nutrition, vitamins, immunizations, and general well child care. Patients with liver disease may have malabsorption as well as anorexia. Use of a formula containing medium-chain triglycerides is quite helpful because bile salts are not necessary for their absorption. Caloric requirements may be as high as 150 kcal/kg/24 hr, and nocturnal nasogastric tube drip feedings may be required because of anorexia. Fat-soluble vitamin deficiencies must be prevented. Vitamin E deficiency (ataxia, peripheral neuropathy, gross motor delay) was a major cause of morbidity until the introduction of a new oral vitamin E preparation, which is well absorbed (D-α-tocopherol polyethylene glycol succinate). Vitamin D deficiency is prevented by oral preparations of 25-hydroxyvitamin D_3. Early changes of vitamin A deficiency appear in the conjunctiva and cornea. An oral, water-soluble preparation of vitamin A is available. Vitamin K supplementation and monitoring of prothrombin time are warranted. Parenteral vitamin K is occasionally indicated to ensure that the increased prothrombin time is not related to malabsorption. Serum levels of fat-soluble vitamins E, D, and A should be monitored. Iron status should be evaluated, and zinc deficiency may develop if there is chronic diarrhea. Immunizations, especially those containing live viruses (measles-mumps-rubella, oral polio), should be completed on schedule because immunosuppression after transplantation may prevent administration.

Medical management should also be directed toward control of portal hypertension (varices, gastrointestinal bleeding, ascites). The condition of the patient at the time of transplantation, with the exception of deep coma, may not affect survival but does influence time of recovery and complications.

The success of *transplantation* has been enhanced by better preservation of the organ (up to 18 hr ex vivo), refinements in surgical technique, and advances in immunosuppressive therapy. Most frequently, the biliary tract is connected to a Roux-en-Y loop of jejunum, and direct vascular connections are made. Steroids and either cyclosporine or FK506 are standard therapy to prevent rejection. Compared with cyclosporine, FK506 (tacrolimus) is associated with lower rates of acute rejection and reduced use of corticosteroids but has a higher incidence of drug-related renal impairment, disturbances of glucose metabolism, and neurologic complications. Occasionally, azathioprine is also used. Early complications include recovery from the prolonged surgery with fluid shifts, electrolyte imbalance, renal dysfunction, and hypertension. Although uncommon, vascular complications, such as thrombosis of graft vessels, may be an ominous early problem. After this early phase, infection and organ rejection are the most frequent problems. Bacterial infections are most common, followed by viral (especially cytomegalovirus and adenovirus), fungal, and rarely parasitic *(Pneumocystis carinii)* infections. Hospital stay may be several weeks to several months. One-year survival approximates 85%, but late complications may arise (rejection, cyclosporine- or FK506-induced renal dysfunction, lymphoproliferative disease). The latter is related to Epstein-Barr virus and may resolve if diagnosed early and if immunosuppression can be reduced. Progression to lymphoma may occur.

The prognosis for survivors is very encouraging. Growth improves and stigmata of chronic liver disease resolve. Children and their families resume more normal lives. Close follow-up of medical and psychosocial issues is necessary. Recently, a number of patients have been removed completely from immunosuppressive therapy after prolonged survival. Chimerism between host and graft cells at nonhepatic sites has been demonstrated in many patients, allowing, it is hoped, survival of the graft and freedom from the risk of lymphoproliferative disease.

Burdelski M: Liver transplantation in children. Acta Pediatr Suppl 395:27, 1994.

Codoner-Franch P, Bernard O, Alvarez F: Long term follow-up of growth in height after successful liver transplantation. J Pediatr 124:368, 1994.

Europlan FK 506 Multicenter Liver Study Group. Randomized trial comparing tacrolimus (FK506) and cyclosporine in prevention of liver allograft rejection. Lancet 344:423, 1994.

Malatack JJ, Gartner JC, Urbach AH, et al: Orthotopic liver transplantation, Epstein-Barr virus, cyclosporine, and lymphoproliferative disease: A growing concern. J Pediatr 118:667, 1991.

Starzl TE, Demetris AJ, Murase N, et al: Cell migration, chimerism, and graft acceptance. Lancet 339:1579, 1992.

Whittington PF, Balistreri WF: Liver transplantation in pediatrics: Indications, contraindications, and pretransplant management. J Pediatr 118:667, 1991.

Zitelli BJ, Gartner JC, Malatack JJ, et al: Liver transplantation in children: A pediatrician's perspective. Pediatr Ann 20:691, 1991.

SECTION 7
Peritoneum and Allied Structures

CHAPTER 314
Malformations

Jeffrey S. Hyams

Congenital peritoneal bands may be responsible for intestinal obstruction; numerous other anomalies may occur in the course of the development of the peritoneum but are rarely of clinical importance. Intra-abdominal herniations infrequently occur through ringlike formations produced by anomalous peritoneal bands. Absence of the omentum or its duplication occurs rarely. Omental cysts arise in obstructed lymphatic channels within the omentum. They may be congenital or may result from trauma and are usually asymptomatic. Abdominal pain or partial small-bowel obstruction may result from compression or torsion of the small bowel from traction on the omentum.

CHAPTER 315
Ascites

Jeffrey S. Hyams

Ascites is an accumulation of serous fluid within the peritoneal cavity. Multiple causes of ascites have been described (Table 315–1). In children, hepatic, renal, and cardiac diseases are the most common causes.

The clinical hallmark of ascites is abdominal distention, but this may also be caused by other conditions including gaseous distention, fecal retention, tumor masses, peritoneal hemorrhage, extreme bladder distention, pregnancy, and obesity. Considerable intraperitoneal fluid may accumulate before ascites is detectable by the five classic physical signs: bulging flanks, flank dullness, shifting dullness, fluid wave, and the "puddle sign" (decreased auscultation of high-frequency vibrations in central abdomen when flicking side of abdomen with patient on hands and knees). Umbilical herniation may be associated with tense ascites. Ultrasound examination can detect small amounts of ascites.

The course, prognosis, and treatment of ascites depend entirely on the cause. Patients with any type of ascites are at increased risk for spontaneous bacterial peritonitis.

315.1 Chylous Ascites

Chylous ascites can result from an anomaly, injury, or obstruction of the intra-abdominal portion of the thoracic duct. Although uncommon, it can occur at any age. Causes include congenital malformations, peritoneal bands, generalized lymphangiomatosis, chronic inflammatory processes of the bowel, tumors, enlarged lymph nodes, previous abdominal surgery, and trauma.

In neonates, rapidly progressing abdominal distention is noted along with poor weight gain and loose stools. Peripheral edema is common. Massive chylous ascites may result in scrotal edema, inguinal and umbilical herniation, and respiratory embarrassment.

Diagnosis of chylous ascites depends on the demonstration of milky ascitic fluid obtained via paracentesis after a fat-containing feeding. Fluid analysis will reveal a high protein content, elevated triglycerides, and lymphocytosis. If the patient has had nothing by mouth, the fluid will be serous in appearance. Hypoalbuminemia, hypogammaglobulinemia, and lymphopenia are common.

Treatment includes the provision of a high-protein, low-fat diet supplemented with medium-chain triglycerides that are absorbed directly into the portal circulation. Parenteral alimentation may be necessary if nutrition remains impaired on oral feedings and to decrease lymph flow to facilitate sealing at the point of lymph leakage. Paracentesis should be repeated only if abdominal distention causes respiratory distress. Laparotomy may be indicated to search for the site of the leak if a trial of dietary management has been unsuccessful.

Browse NL, Wilson NM, Russo F, et al: Aetiology and treatment of chylous ascites. Br J Surg 79:1145, 1992.

Griscom NT, Colodny AH, Rosenberg HK, et al: Diagnostic aspects of neonatal ascites: Report of 27 cases. AJR 128:961, 1977.

Unger SW, Chandler JG: Chylous ascites in infants and children. Surgery 93:455, 1983.

TABLE 315–1 Causes of Ascites

Hepatic	**Gastrointestinal**
Cirrhosis	Infarcted bowel
Congenital hepatic fibrosis	Perforation
Portal vein obstruction	**Neoplastic**
Fulminant hepatic failure	Lymphoma
Budd-Chiari syndrome	**Gynecologic**
Lysosomal storage disease	Ovarian tumors
Renal	Ovarian torsion, rupture
Nephrotic syndrome	**Pancreatic**
Obstructive uropathy	Pancreatitis
Perforation of urinary tract	Ruptured pancreatic duct
Peritoneal dialysis	**Miscellaneous**
Cardiac	Systemic lupus erythematosus
Congestive heart failure	Ventriculoperitoneal shunt
Constrictive pericarditis	Eosinophilic ascites
Inferior vena cava web	Chylous ascites
Infectious	Hypothyroidism
Abscess	
Tuberculosis	
Chlamydia	
Schistosomiasis	

CHAPTER 316
Peritonitis

Jeffrey S. Hyams

Inflammation of the peritoneal lining of the abdominal cavity may result from infectious, autoimmune, and chemical processes. Infectious peritonitis is usually defined as primary (spontaneous) or secondary. In primary peritonitis, the source of infection originates outside of the abdomen and seeds the peritoneal cavity via hematogenous or lymphatic spread. Secondary peritonitis arises from the abdominal cavity itself either through extension from or rupture of an intra-abdominal viscus or an abscess within an organ.

Peritonitis in the neonatal period may arise from a transplacental in utero infection; more frequently, it is the result of infection acquired during or shortly after birth. It may be a manifestation of septicemia, a direct extension from an umbilical infection or from perforation of the intestine or necrotizing enterocolitis, or, rarely, the sequel of a ruptured appendix or Meckel diverticulum. Meconium peritonitis is described in Chapter 279.

316.1 Acute Primary Peritonitis

ETIOLOGY AND EPIDEMIOLOGY. Primary peritonitis is a bacterial infection of the peritoneal cavity without a demonstrable intra-abdominal source. Most cases occur in children with ascites resulting from nephrotic syndrome or cirrhosis. Rarely, it may occur in previously healthy children. Most frequently, isolated bacteria include pneumococci, group A streptococci, enterococci, staphylococci, and gram-negative enteric bacteria, especially *Escherichia coli* and *Klebsiella pneumoniae*. The genders are equally affected; most cases occur before 6 yr of age.

CLINICAL MANIFESTATIONS. Onset may be insidious or rapid and is characterized by fever, abdominal pain, vomiting, diarrhea, and a "toxic appearance." Hypotension and tachycardia are common along with shallow, rapid respirations because of discomfort associated with breathing. Abdominal palpation may demonstrate rebound tenderness and rigidity. Bowel sounds are hypoactive or absent. The prior use of corticosteroids may diminish the clinical expression of peritonitis.

DIAGNOSIS AND TREATMENT. Leukocytosis (on complete blood count) with a marked predominance of polymorphonuclear cells is common, although the level of the white cell count may be affected by pre-existing hypersplenism in patients with cirrhosis. Proteinuria is present in subjects with nephrotic syndrome. Roentgenographic examination of the abdomen reveals dilatation of the large and small intestines, with increased separation of loops secondary to bowel wall thickening. Distinguishing primary peritonitis from appendicitis may be impossible in patients without a history of nephrotic syndrome or cirrhosis; accordingly, the diagnosis of primary peritonitis is made only at laparotomy. In a child with known renal or hepatic disease and ascites, the presence of peritoneal signs should prompt a diagnostic paracentesis. Infected fluid usually reveals a white cell count of 250 cells/mm^3 or greater with more than 50% polymorphonuclear cells.

Other peritoneal fluid findings suggestive of primary peritonitis include a pH less than 7.35, arterial-ascitic fluid pH gradient greater than 0.1, and elevated lactate. Gram stain of the ascitic fluid characteristically reveals a single species of gram-positive or, less often, gram-negative bacteria. The presence of mixed bacterial flora on ascitic fluid examination or free air on abdominal roentgenogram in children with presumed primary peritonitis mandates laparotomy to localize a likely intra-abdominal source of the infection. Inoculation of ascitic fluid obtained at paracentesis directly into blood culture bottles will increase the yield of positive cultures. Parenteral antibiotic therapy with cefotaxime and an aminoglycoside should be started promptly with subsequent changes dependent on sensitivity testing (e.g., vancomycin for resistant *Pneumococcus*). Therapy should be continued for 10–14 days.

Culture-negative neutrocytic ascites is a variant of primary peritonitis with a cell count of 500 cells/mm^3, a negative culture, no intra-abdominal source of infection, and no prior treatment with antibiotic. It should be treated in a similar manner as primary peritonitis.

Bhuva M, Ganger D, Jensen D: Spontaneous bacterial peritonitis: An update on evaluation, management and prevention. Am J Med 97:169, 1994.

Gorensek MJ, Lebel MH, Nelson JD: Peritonitis in children with nephrotic syndrome. Pediatrics 81:849, 1988.

Nohr CW, Marshall BG: Primary peritonitis in children. Can J Surg 27:179, 1984.

316.2 Acute Secondary Peritonitis

This is most often due to the entry of enteric bacteria into the peritoneal cavity through a necrotic defect in the wall of the intestines or other viscus as a result of obstruction or infarction or after rupture of an intra-abdominal visceral abscess. Most commonly, it follows perforation of the appendix. Other gastrointestinal causes include incarcerated hernias, rupture of a Meckel diverticulum, midgut volvulus, intussusception, hemolytic-uremic syndrome, peptic ulceration, inflammatory bowel disease, necrotizing cholecystitis, necrotizing enterocolitis, typhlitis, and traumatic perforation. Peritonitis in the neonatal period most often occurs as a complication of necrotizing enterocolitis but may be associated with meconium ileus or spontaneous (or indomethacin-induced) rupture of the stomach or intestines. In postpubertal females, bacteria from the genital tract *(Neisseria gonorrhoeae, Chlamydia trachomatis)* may gain access to the peritoneal cavity via the fallopian tubes, causing secondary peritonitis. The presence of a foreign body, such as a ventriculoperitoneal catheter or peritoneal dialysis catheter, can predispose to peritonitis, with skin microorganisms, such as *Staphylococcus epidermidis, Staphylococcus aureus,* and *Candida albicans,* contaminating the shunt.

CLINICAL MANIFESTATIONS. Similar to primary peritonitis, characteristic symptoms include fever (39.5°C or more), diffuse abdominal pain, nausea, and vomiting. Physical findings of peritoneal inflammation include rebound tenderness, abdominal wall rigidity, a paucity of body motion (lying still), and decreased or absent bowel sounds from a paralytic ileus. Massive exudation of fluid into the peritoneal cavity, along with the systemic release of vasodilatory substances, can lead to the rapid development of shock. A "toxic appearance," irritability, and restlessness are common. Basilar atelectasis as well as intrapulmonary shunting may develop with progression to adult respiratory distress syndrome.

Laboratory studies reveal a peripheral white cell count greater than 12,000 cells/mm^3 with a marked predominance of polymorphonuclear forms. Roentgenograms of the abdomen may reveal free air in the peritoneal cavity, evidence of ileus or obstruction, peritoneal fluid, and obliteration of the psoas shadow.

TREATMENT. Aggressive fluid resuscitation and support of cardiovascular function should begin immediately. Stabilization of the patient before surgical intervention is mandatory. Antibiotic therapy must provide coverage for those organisms that predominate at the site of presumed origin of the infection. For perforation of the lower gastrointestinal tract, a regimen of ampicillin, gentamicin, and clindamycin will adequately address infection by *E. coli, Klebsiella, Bacteroides* species, and enterococci. Alternative therapy could include ticarcillin-clavulanic acid and an aminoglycoside. Surgery should proceed to repair a perforated viscus after the patient is stabilized and antibiotic therapy initiated. Intraoperative peritoneal fluid cultures will indicate whether a change in the antibiotic regimen is warranted.

316.3 Acute Secondary Localized Peritonitis

(Peritoneal Abscess)

ETIOLOGY. Intra-abdominal abscesses may develop within visceral intra-abdominal organs (hepatic, splenic, renal, pancreatic, tubo-ovarian abscesses) or in the interintestinal, periappendiceal, subdiaphragmatic, subhepatic, pelvic, and retroperitoneal spaces. Most commonly, periappendiceal and pelvic abscesses arise from a perforation of the appendix. Transmural inflammation with fistula formation may result in intra-abdominal abscess formation in children with Crohn disease.

CLINICAL MANIFESTATIONS. Prolonged fever, anorexia, vomiting, and lassitude are suggestive of the development of an intra-abdominal abscess. The peripheral white cell count is elevated as is the erythrocyte sedimentation rate. With an appendiceal abscess, there is localized tenderness and a palpable mass in the right lower quadrant.

A pelvic abscess is suggested by abdominal distention, rectal tenesmus with or without the passage of small-volume, mucous stools, and bladder irritability. Rectal examination may reveal a tender mass anteriorly.

Subphrenic gas collection, basal atelectasis, elevated hemidiaphragm, and pleural effusion may be present with a subdiaphragmatic abscess.

Psoas abscess can develop from extension of infection from a retroperitoneal appendicitis, Crohn disease, or a perirenal or intrarenal abscess. Abdominal findings may be minimal, and presentation may include a limp, hip pain, and fever.

Both ultrasound examination as well as computed tomography (CT) scanning can be used to localize intra-abdominal abscesses. Gallium scanning is usually not needed.

TREATMENT. An abscess should be drained and appropriate antibiotic therapy provided. Drainage may be performed under radiologic control (ultrasonogram or CT guidance) and an indwelling drainage catheter left in place. Initial broad-spectrum antibiotic coverage with ampicillin, gentamicin, and clindamycin should be started and can be modified, if necessary, depending on the results of sensitivity testing. The treatment of appendiceal rupture complicated by abscess formation may be problematic because intestinal phlegmon formation can make surgical resection more difficult. Intensive antibiotic therapy for 4–6 wk followed by an interval appendectomy is often the treatment course followed.

Schwartz MZ, Tapper D, Solenberger RI: Management of perforated appendicitis in children: The controversy continues. Ann Surg 197:407, 1983.
Wilson-Storey D, Scobie WG: Appendix masses—A 15 year review. Pediatr Surg Int 4:165, 1989.

CHAPTER 317
Diaphragmatic Hernia

Gary E. Hartman

Herniation of abdominal contents into the thoracic cavity may occur as a result of a congenital or traumatic defect in the diaphragm. Symptomatology and prognosis depend on the location of the defect and associated anomalies. The defect may be at the esophageal hiatus (hiatal hernia), adjacent to the hiatus (paraesophageal), retrosternal (Morgagni), or posterolateral (Bochdalek). Although all of these defects are congenital, the term *congenital diaphragmatic hernia* (CDH) has become synonymous with herniation through the posterolateral foramen of Bochdalek. These lesions usually present with profound respiratory distress in the neonatal period, may be associated with anomalies of other organ systems, and have a significant (40–50%) mortality.

EPIDEMIOLOGY. Reports of the incidence of CDH vary from 1 in 5,000 live births to 1 in 2,000 if stillbirths are included. Defects are more common on the left (70–85%) and are occasionally (5%) bilateral. Malrotation of the intestine and pulmonary hypoplasia occur in virtually all cases and are considered components of the lesion and not associated anomalies. True associated anomalies have been recognized in 20–30% and include central nervous system lesions, esophageal atresia, omphalocele, cardiovascular lesions, and recognized syndromes. In addition to trisomy 21, the lethal syndromes of trisomy 13, trisomy 18, Fryn, Brachmann-de Lange, and Pallister-Killian have been described. Tetrasomy 12p mosaicism (Pallister-Killian syndrome) may have a normal peripheral blood karyotype as a result of infrequent involvement of lymphocytes. This lethal syndrome can be diagnosed by karyotype from amniocentesis or neonatal bone marrow or fibroblasts. Reports of occurrence of CDH in twins, siblings, and offspring are sporadic. An autosomal recessive inheritance mode has been suggested in families with complete agenesis of the diaphragm.

ETIOLOGY. Separation of the developing thoracic and abdominal cavities is accomplished by closure of the posterolateral pleuroperitoneal canals during the 8th wk of gestation. Failure of this canal to close has been the postulated mechanism for the development of congenital posterolateral diaphragmatic hernia. This may be the mechanism in patients with a small diaphragmatic defect. Recent production of unilateral or bilateral diaphragmatic defects in experimental animals by in utero drug exposure suggests an additional mechanism that may explain larger defects. Portions of the diaphragm and the pulmonary parenchyma arise from the developing thoracic mesenchyme, which, if disrupted, may explain the absence of the major portion of a hemidiaphragm and the severe pulmonary hypoplasia that usually accompanies such a large defect.

PATHOLOGY. The pathologic changes in infants with congenital diaphragmatic hernia are not limited to the diaphragm. The diaphragmatic defect may be small and slitlike or include the entire hemidiaphragm. Both lungs are small compared with those of age- and weight-matched controls, with the lung on the side of the defect more severely affected. There is a decrease in number of alveoli and bronchial generations. The pulmonary vasculature is abnormal, with a decrease in volume and marked increase in muscular mass in the arterioles. Although there is some evidence that the pulmonary abnormalities are due to compression by the intrathoracic abdominal viscera, it is not accepted that physical compression is the sole or primary cause. Abnormal development of the mesenchyme is an emerging concept with very different implications.

CLINICAL MANIFESTATIONS. Although many cases are identified by prenatal ultrasonography, the majority of infants with CDH experience severe respiratory distress within the first hours of life. A small group will present beyond the neonatal period. Patients with a delayed presentation may experience vomiting as a result of intestinal obstruction or mild respiratory symptoms. Delayed presentation of right diaphragmatic hernia after a documented episode of group B streptococcal sepsis is a well-described sequence. Occasionally, incarceration of the intestine will proceed to ischemia with sepsis and cardiorespiratory collapse. Unrecognized diaphragmatic hernia has been the cause of sudden death in infants and toddlers.

DIAGNOSIS. Prenatal diagnosis by ultrasonography is common. Careful evaluation for other anomalies should include echocardiography and amniocentesis. Occasionally, a fetus with ultrasonographic diagnosis in utero will have no abnormality on postnatal x-ray film. Parents with the ultrasonographic diagnosis of diaphragmatic hernia must be counseled carefully by a multidisciplinary group with significant experience with this condition if unnecessary terminations and unrealistic expectations are to be avoided.

After birth most infants with diaphragmatic hernia will experience severe respiratory collapse within the first 24 hr. The absence of breath sounds and shift of heart sounds common to CDH and pneumothorax will be accompanied by a scaphoid abdomen in the infants with CDH. Thoracentesis or tube thoracostomy should be withheld if CDH is considered a possibility. Chest x-ray film is usually diagnostic (Fig. 317–1). The lateral view frequently demonstrates the intestine passing through the posterior portion of the diaphragm. Occasionally, congenital cystic lesions of the lung may produce a similar radiographic appearance. Differentiation from diaphragmatic hernia may be accomplished by postnatal ultrasonography or injection of contrast into the stomach or umbilical artery catheter to identify intestine above the diaphragm. In older children, with atypical symptoms, contrast studies of the gastrointestinal tract are usually required. Ultrasonography and fluoroscopy are helpful in distinguishing eventration from true hernia, and computed tomography may be necessary to exclude pneumatoceles or complicated effusions.

TREATMENT. The availability of extracorporeal membrane oxygenation (ECMO), the utility of preoperative stabilization, and advances in in utero therapy have been the major stimuli to *aggressive therapy*. In the past, diaphragmatic hernia was considered a surgical emergency, with urgent operative reduction offering these infants the optimal outcome. Recognition of the role of pulmonary hypertension in addition to hypoplasia and the effects of operative repair on pulmonary function prompted critical re-evaluation of that strategy. It is now clear that the postnatal mass effect of the herniated viscera is a minor factor in the cardiorespiratory compromise compared with the pulmonary hypertension and hypoplasia.

Initial resuscitation should be followed by a period of attempted stabilization with paralysis (pancuronium, 100 μg/kg), modest hyperventilation (partial pressure of carbon dioxide of 25–30 mm Hg) and narcotic sedation (fentanyl, 2–4 μg/kg). Volume resuscitation, dopamine, and bicarbonate (to maintain pH >7.50) may also be helpful. If the infant stabilizes and demonstrates stable pulmonary vascular resistance without significant right to left shunting, repair of the diaphragm is currently performed at 12–24 hr of age. If stabilization is not possible or significant shunting persists, most infants will require ECMO support. Vasoactive drugs (tolazoline, prostaglandins, dopamine) may provide temporary improvement but have been disappointing as definite therapy for the pulmonary hypertension associated with diaphragmatic hernia. Surfactant administration has also been shown to produce a transient improvement in oxygenation in some infants with CDH.

Experience with ECMO in CDH has shown that paralysis and nasogastric suction may produce a dramatic reduction of the volume of herniated viscera. The duration of ECMO for neonates with diaphragmatic hernia is significantly longer than

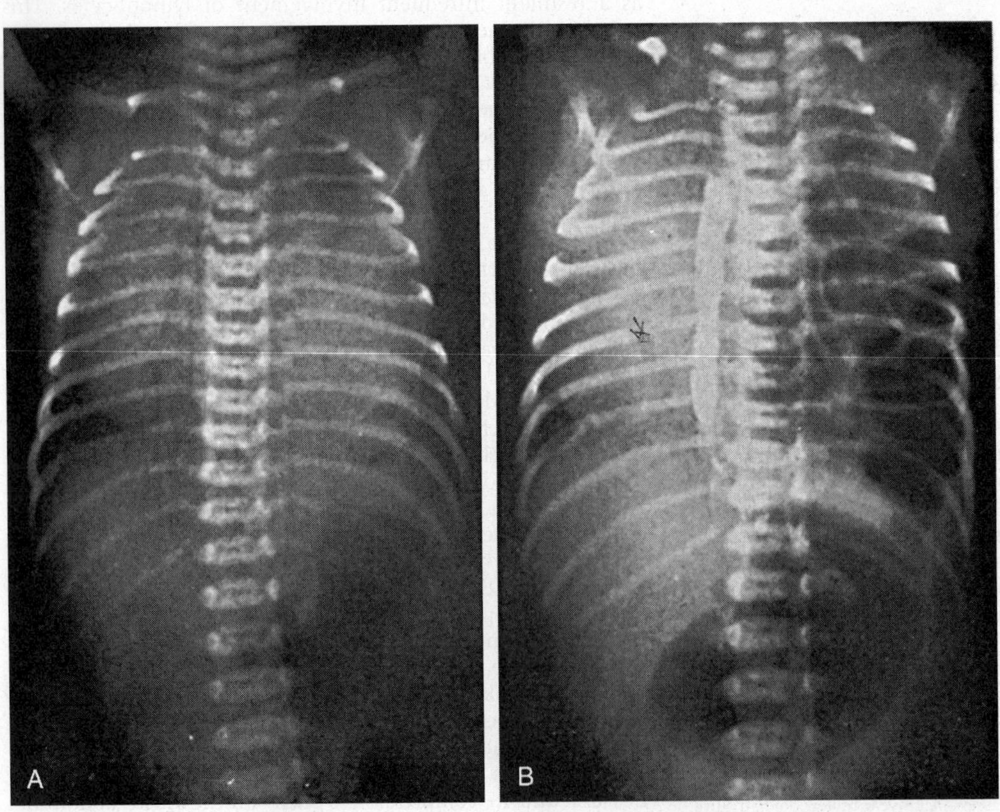

Figure 317–1. Congenital diaphragmatic hernia. *A*, Film exposed shortly after birth: distortion of shadow of the left leaf of the diaphragm with huge, masslike density in left hemithorax displacing the heart to the right. *B*, Film exposed about 20 min after *A*. As the result of swallowed air, coils of air-filled small bowel are now demonstrated in the left hemithorax. The esophagus is outlined by swallowed contrast material. Operative correction was attempted because of extreme dyspnea. Infant died 5.5 hr after birth.

for those with persistent fetal circulation or meconium aspiration and may last up to 3–4 wk. Timing of repair of the diaphragm on ECMO is controversial; some centers prefer early repair to allow a greater duration of postrepair ECMO, whereas many centers defer repair until the infant has demonstrated the ability to tolerate weaning from ECMO. In either case, recurrence of pulmonary hypertension carries a high mortality, and weaning from ECMO support should be cautious. If the patient cannot be weaned from ECMO after repair, options include discontinuing support or experimental therapies such as nitric oxide or single-lung transplantation. High-frequency jet ventilation and oscillatory ventilation have had limited success in newborns with CDH.

The abdominal surgical approach is favored because the accompanying malrotation may be addressed if necessary and the abdominal wall may be left open with skin only closed or a Silastic pouch applied if abdominal pressure is considered excessive. Synthetic patch (polytetrafluoroethylene) is now preferred over autologous muscle transfer or tight primary closure for large defects.

The appreciation of the compressive effects of the herniated viscera and the availability of prenatal diagnosis suggested the utility of in utero measures directed at potentially reversing the pulmonary hypoplasia and, it is hoped, the pulmonary vascular changes. In utero reduction of the herniated viscera has been successfully performed in humans and is currently under prospective study at the Fetal Treatment Center at the University of California in San Francisco. To be considered for in utero reduction, the fetus must be single, diagnosed before 24 wk gestation, and have a normal karyotype and intra-abdominal liver. Reduction is attempted between 24 and 28 wk gestation in appropriate candidates. In experimental animals, occluding the trachea while in utero enhances lung growth by preventing lung fluid egress.

PROGNOSIS. Studies of infants with CDH identified in utero (27–55%) report lower survival than in reports limited to live births (42–66%). From the available studies, it appears that the majority of fetuses with the diagnosis of CDH who do not survive pregnancy die as a result of elective termination. The incidence of spontaneous fetal demise among fetuses diagnosed as having CDH appears to be 7–10%. Of those surviving to delivery, survival appears to range from 42–66% despite current modalities including ECMO. Factors associated with a poor prognosis include associated major anomaly, symptoms before 24 hr of age, distress severe enough to require ECMO, and delivery in a nontertiary center. Initial attempts at intrauterine repair were associated with a low survival (29%), although recent results are reportedly more encouraging.

In the past, survivors of CDH repair were clinically normal, although some abnormalities could be detected by pulmonary function testing. With current treatment modalities, a significant number of survivors are being identified with serious sequelae, primarily pulmonary, neurologic, and growth abnormalities. It is generally accepted that these long-term sequelae are the result of survival of infants with more severe pulmonary compromise than was previously possible. Ten to 20% of CDH survivors are now requiring oxygen therapy at discharge.

Studies have documented abnormalities of pulmonary function in the perioperative period and years after repair. Survivors of CDH repair studied at 6–11 yr of age demonstrated significant decreases in forced expiratory flow at 50% of vital capacity and peak expiratory flow. The lung on the affected side was larger than predicted, suggesting hyperinflation, and had reduced perfusion. These patients had undergone repair before the availability of ECMO. In studies of neonatal pulmonary function, neonates with CDH requiring ECMO demonstrated significantly decreased compliance, dynamic compliance, and tidal volume when compared with those not requiring ECMO. After repair, infants with CDH also had evidence of reactive airway disease. It is now apparent that survivors of CDH have evidence of restrictive lung disease and airway reactivity, which are related to the severity of their initial respiratory failure.

Neurologic abnormalities have been identified in survivors of CDH requiring ECMO. The abnormalities are similar to those seen in neonates treated with ECMO for other diagnoses and include developmental delay, abnormal hearing or vision, seizures, and abnormal CT. The majority of documented neurologic abnormalities are classified as mild or moderate, and the incidence is similar to that of other ECMO survivors.

Growth and nutrition are compromised in CDH survivors who required ECMO. Forty to 50% are at less than the 5th percentile for weight at 2 yr of age. Weight:length ratio was less than the 5th percentile in 40% of survivors at 1 yr and 21% at 2 yr. Nearly all ECMO survivors demonstrated clinical evidence of gastroesophageal reflux, and 20% or more have required fundoplication. Dilation of the esophagus with altered motility that resolves during the first year of life has been correlated with a prenatal history of polyhydramnios.

Other long-term problems occurring in this population include pectus excavatum, scoliosis, fixed pulmonary hypertension, and recurrent herniation. Recurrent hernia formation is common in newborns with large defects requiring synthetic patch repair. Reherniation has been reported in 20–40% of those requiring patch repair and typically occurs within the 1st year.

Survivors of CDH repair, particularly those requiring ECMO support, have a variety of long-term abnormalities that appear to improve with time but require close monitoring and multidisciplinary support.

317.1 Foramen of Morgagni Hernia

The anteromedial diaphragmatic defect through the foramen of Morgagni accounts for 2% or less of diaphragmatic hernias. The transverse colon or small intestine is usually contained in the hernia sac. Symptoms are gastrointestinal and typically occur beyond the neonatal period. Repair is recommended for all patients and can be accomplished by laparotomy.

317.2 Paraesophageal Hernia

Paraesophageal hernia is differentiated from hiatal hernia in that the gastroesophageal junction is in the normal location. The herniation of the stomach alongside or adjacent to the gastroesophageal junction is prone to incarceration with strangulation and perforation. This unusual diaphragmatic hernia should be repaired promptly after identification.

317.3 Eventration

Eventration of the diaphragm consists of a thinned diaphragmatic muscle producing elevation of the entire hemidiaphragm or, more commonly, the anterior aspect of the hemidiaphragm. Most eventrations are asymptomatic and do not require repair. Large or symptomatic eventrations may be repaired by plication by an abdominal or thoracic approach.

Breaux CW, Rouse TM, Cain WS, et al: Improvement in survival of patients with congenital diaphragmatic hernia utilizing a strategy of delayed repair after medical and/or extracorporeal membrane oxygenation stabilization. J Pediatr Surg 26:333, 1991.

Harrison MR, Adzick NS, Estes JM, et al: A prospective study of the outcome for fetuses with diaphragmatic hernia. JAMA 271:382, 1994.

Harrison MR, Adzick NS, Flake AW, et al: Correction of congenital diaphragmatic hernia in utero: VI. Hard-earned lessons. J Pediatr Surg 28:1411, 1993.

Nakayama DK, Motomyama EK, Mutich RL, et al: Pulmonary function in newborns after repair of congenital diaphragmatic hernia. Pediatr Pulmonol 11:49, 1991.

Sweed Y, Puri P: Congenital diaphragmatic hernia: Influence of associated malformations on survival. Arch Dis Child 69:68, 1993.

Van Meurs KP, Robbins ST, Reed VL, et al: Congenital diaphragmatic hernia: Long-term outcome in neonates treated with extracorporeal membrane oxygenation. J Pediatr 122:893, 1993.

Wilcox D, Glick P, Karamanuukian H, et al: Pathophysiology of congenital diaphragmatic hernia: V. Effect of exogenous surfactant therapy on gas exchange and lung mechanics in the lamb congenital diaphragmatic hernia model. J Pediatr 124:289, 1994.

CHAPTER 318
Epigastric Hernia

Gary E. Hartman

Epigastric hernias are defects in the linea alba between the xyphoid and the umbilicus. They are uncommon in childhood, constituting less than 1% of hernias requiring operation. Similar defects below the umbilicus are even more uncommon. These hernias usually contain preperitoneal fat and rarely cause symptoms. They may appear as an intermittent bulge or a midline mass if the fat is incarcerated. Herniation of intestine or other viscera is extremely rare. Repair is indicated for symptomatic hernias or for diagnosis in the case of a mass. Treatment of asymptomatic hernias of the linea alba is less clear. Some believe many will resolve spontaneously and discourage elective repair. Others believe they never resolve and will eventually require repair. Abdominal symptoms other than local pain and tenderness should prompt further diagnostic study rather than repair of the epigastric hernia.

318.1 Incisional Hernia

Hernia formation at the site of a previous laparotomy is uncommon in childhood. Factors associated with an increased risk of incisional hernia include increased intra-abdominal pressure, wound infection, and midline incision. Transverse abdominal incisions are favored because of their increased strength and blood supply, which reduce the likelihood of wound infection and incisional hernia. Although most incisional hernias will require repair, operation should be deferred until the child is in optimal medical condition. Some incisional hernias will resolve, especially those occurring in infants. Some recommend elastic bandaging to discourage enlargement of the hernia and promote spontaneously healing. Newborns with abdominal wall defects represent the largest group of children with incisional hernias. Initial management should be conservative, with repair deferred until about 1 yr of age. Incarceration is very uncommon but is an indication for prompt repair.

Neblett KW, Holcomb TM: Umbilical and other abdominal wall hernias. *In:* Ashcraft, Holder (eds): Pediatric Surgery. Philadelphia, WB Saunders, 1993, pp 557–561.

Robin AP: Epigastric hernia. *In:* Nyhus LM, Condon RE (eds): Hernia. Philadelphia, JB Lippincott, 1989, pp 360–366.

PART XIX

The Respiratory System

SECTION 1

Development and Function

CHAPTER 319

Development of the Respiratory System

Gabriel G. Haddad and J. Julio Pérez Fontán

In air-breathing mammals, the gas-exchanging apparatus is invaginated into alveolar (reptiles, amphibia, mammals) or parabronchial (birds) lungs. Such a design maximizes the contact surface with the atmosphere while limiting excessive water and heat losses through evaporation. For invaginated lungs to be mechanically stable, their gas-exchanging surfaces must be coated with a surface active material, the pulmonary surfactant, which prevents them from sticking to each other (Chapter 87.3). Invaginated lungs also depend on an external mechanism to force air in and out of the gas-exchanging spaces. In mammals and other higher vertebrates, this mechanism resembles a bellows pump operated by muscles. The function of these respiratory muscles is regulated by a network of sensors, which relay mechanical information from the pump itself and chemical information from the blood to a control center in the brain. The pump can, in this manner, generate large and rapid changes in lung ventilation, providing the adaptability demanded by the fast metabolic pace of warm-blooded animals.

The development of the respiratory system encompasses three distinct processes: morphogenesis or formation of all the necessary structures, adaptation to postnatal atmospheric breathing, and dimensional growth. In most mammalian species, the first two processes take place primarily before birth. Growth, in contrast, continues after birth at a pace that is generally dictated by the functional needs of all the other growing organs. The effects of an injury to the respiratory system depend not only on the severity but also on the timing and chronicity of the injury. Insults occurring during morphogenesis, for instance, tend to produce severe and irreversible disruptions of respiratory structure and function, often incompatible with survival. In contrast, injuries that take place during later stages of lung growth are frequently reversible and can be compensated for by the growth process itself.

PRENATAL DEVELOPMENT: MORPHOGENESIS

In the human and other mammals, the morphogenesis of the respiratory system is divided into five periods (Fig. 319–1). The first, or *embryonic period*, begins at approximately 4 wk of gestation, when the primitive airways appear as a ventral outpouching on the endodermal epithelium of the foregut. This outpouching divides almost immediately into two main stem bronchial buds, which burrow rapidly into the mesenchyme separating the foregut from the coelomic cavity. The bronchial buds start to branch, first by monopodal outgrowth (secondary branches grow out of a main branch) and then by asymmetric dichotomy (two secondary branches originate from one main branch).

The peribronchial mesenchyme or *splanchnopleura* plays an essential role in shaping the lungs during the embryonic period. Close contact between this mesenchyme and the epithelium of the bronchial buds is essential for the continued branching of the airways. Although the factors that promote bronchial division are not fully identified, steroid-induced secretion of growth factors by the mesenchymal fibroblasts, specific interactions with acellular components of the mesenchyme, and even direct molecular communications between fibroblasts and endodermal cells across gaps in the basal membrane have been proposed as signaling mechanisms. The interactions between mesenchyme and the bronchial bud endoderm are organ-specific.

The pulmonary vasculature is a mesenchymal derivative. Soon after their appearance, the bronchial buds are surrounded by a vascular plexus, which originates from the aorta and drains into the major somatic veins. This vascular plexus connects with the pulmonary artery and veins to complete the pulmonary circulation at the 7th wk of gestation but retains some aortic connections that form the bronchial arteries. All the supporting structures of the lungs, including the pleura, the septal network of the lungs, and the smooth muscle, cartilage, and connective covers of the airways, originate from the mesenchyme.

Toward the 6th wk of gestation, at the beginning of the

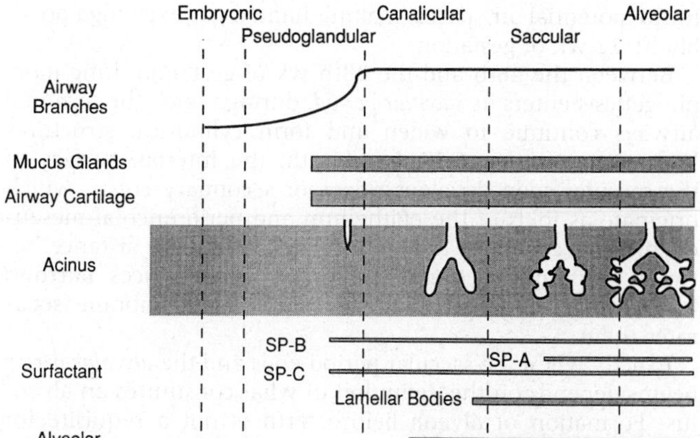

Figure 319–1. Development of various pulmonary structures during the five stages of prenatal lung development (see text).

second or *pseudoglandular period,* the lungs resemble an exocrine gland with a thick stroma crossed by narrow ducts lined by an epithelium of tall cells that almost fill the lumen. The major airways are already present and are in close association with pulmonary arteries and veins. The trachea and the foregut are now separated after the progressive fusion of epithelial ridges growing from the primitive airway. The incomplete fusion of these ridges results in a *tracheoesophageal fistula,* a common congenital malformation. During the pseudoglandular period, the airways continue to branch until the entire conducting airway system is formed, including the primitive bronchioles that eventually give rise to the air-exchanging portions of the lungs. Simultaneously, the pluripotential cells that line the airways differentiate starting from the trachea and main bronchi in a process that also appears to be under some degree of mesenchymal control. They soon form a thinner, pseudostratified epithelium containing ciliated, secretory (Clara), globular, and neuroendocrine (Kulchitsky) cells of neuroectodermal origin. Mucous glands, cartilage, and smooth muscle can be easily distinguished by the 16th wk of gestation.

The diaphragm is formed during this period. Its central tendon originates from the transverse septum, a plate of mesodermal tissue located between the pericardium and the stalk of the yolk sac. Its lateral portions are formed by the pleuroperitoneal folds, which grow from the body wall until they fuse with the esophageal mesentery and the transverse septum. The fusion eliminates the communication between thorax and abdomen and establishes a barrier to the caudal growth of the lungs. Its failure, usually on the left side, causes the *congenital diaphragmatic hernia of Bochdalek.* This defect, which is the most frequent type of diaphragmatic hernia, allows the abdominal organs to enter the primitive pleural cavity and interferes with airway and pulmonary vascular branching. The result is severe hypoplasia of the lung, particularly on the side of the hernia (Chapter 317). Initially membranous, the normal diaphragm is eventually invaded by striated muscle derived from cervical myotomes.

During the third or *canalicular period,* between the 16th and 26–28th wk of gestation, epithelial growth predominates over mesenchymal growth. As a result, the bronchial tree develops a more tubular appearance while its distal regions subdivide further to lay the structural foundations of the pulmonary acinus. The epithelial cells in these regions become more cuboidal and start to express some of the antigen markers that characterize cells as type II pneumocytes. Some cells become flatter and can be identified as potential type I pneumocytes by the presence of a sparse endoplasmic reticulum and abundant cytoplasmic glycogen. The capillaries contained in the distal bronchial mesenchyme form a denser network and grow closer to the potential air spaces, making limited gas exchange possibly by 22 wk of gestation.

Between the 26th and the 28th wk of gestation, lung morphogenesis enters its *saccular period,* during which the terminal airways continue to widen and form cylindrical structures known as saccules. Initially smooth, the internal surface of the saccules soon develops ridges or secondary crests, which originate as folds of the epithelium and peribronchial mesenchyme and contain a double capillary layer. The distance between the capillaries and the potential air spaces narrows further until eventually only a thin basal membrane separates them.

Exactly when the saccular period ends and the *alveolar period* begins depends on the definition of what constitutes an alveolus. Formation of alveoli before birth is not a requisite for survival, as demonstrated by the observation that, in altricial or nonprecocious species, such as the rat or the rabbit, alveoli are not present until several days after birth. In the human fetus, the saccular septation initiated with the appearance of the secondary crests continues at a rapid rate, so that multifaceted structures analogous to the alveoli of the mature lung can be seen at 32 wk of gestation. In more precocious species such as the sheep and the horse, the lungs contain even more alveoli at birth than in humans. There is substantial evidence that the timing and progression of alveolar septation is under endocrine regulation. Thyroid hormones stimulate septation, whereas glucocorticoids impair it in a fashion that, at least in the rat, can be irrevocable (even though they accelerate the thinning of the alveolar capillary membranes). Alveolarization is also influenced by physical stimuli. Both the stretch by the liquid contained in the fetal lung and the periodic distention provided by the action of the respiratory muscles during fetal breathing, for instance, appear to be necessary for the development of the acinus. Their absence when the lungs or chest are compressed (as in the case of a diaphragmatic hernia or oligohydramnios) or when fetal breathing is abolished (by spinal cord lesions, for example) results in *pulmonary hypoplasia* with reduced numbers of alveoli.

ADAPTATION TO AIR-BREATHING

The transition from placental dependence to autonomous gas exchange requires adaptive changes in the lungs. These changes include the production of surfactant in the alveoli, the transformation of the lung from a secretory into a gas-exchanging organ, and the establishment of parallel pulmonary and systemic circulations.

As soon as the newborn takes the first breath of air, an air-liquid interface becomes established inside the lungs. Unless the surface tension generated at this interface is reduced, the walls of the air spaces would tend to stick together, threatening the geometric stability of the lungs. The pulmonary surfactant makes such a reduction possible by forming a hydrophobic lipid monolayer at the very surface of the liquid film that lines the air spaces (Chapter 87.3). Pulmonary surfactant is a heterogeneous mixture of phospholipids and proteins secreted into the saccular or alveolar subphase by the type II pneumocytes. Its presence is first recognized in characteristic secretory organelles known as lamellar bodies as early as the 24th wk of gestation. Surfactant lipids, of which the most abundant is phosphatidylcholine, however, are not detectable in the amniotic fluid until the 30th wk, suggesting that there is a chronological gap between surfactant synthesis and secretion. Labor probably shortens this gap because phospholipids are consistently found in the air spaces of infants born before the 30th wk of gestation. Three apoproteins (SP-A, SP-B, and SP-C) identified in pulmonary surfactant (a fourth lectin-like glycoprotein, SP-D, has been isolated, but its function and regulation are still poorly understood) promote the spreading of the surfactant layer and are therefore essential for the effective reduction of surface tension. Apoproteins also appear to be important for the reuptake and recycling of surfactant products and for the formation of tubular myelin (the structures in which surfactant is stored in the liquid subphase).

Surfactant apoproteins and phospholipids share some, but not all of their regulatory influences. Glucocorticoids, for instance, increase the synthesis of both apoproteins and lipids and, accordingly, their prenatal administration has been used to prevent the respiratory distress syndrome associated with prematurity. Because many actions of the steroids involve direct stimulation of response elements in apoprotein and phospholipid enzyme genes and therefore require messenger RNA production, sufficient time must elapse between steroid administration and birth. Thyroid hormones also enhance the synthesis of phospholipids by a receptor-mediated mechanism, but, unlike the glucocorticoids, they have little or no effect on surfactant apoprotein synthesis. Conversely, β-adrenergic agonists and other agents that raise cellular cyclic AMP content increase apoprotein synthesis and phosphatidylcholine secretion into the air spaces but have no effect on phospholipid synthesis. Insulin, hyperglycemia, ketosis, and androgens may have negative effects on the production of surfactant proteins and phospholipids, thus explaining the high incidence of respiratory distress syndrome in infants of diabetic mothers and the slight maturational delay of the lungs of male compared with female fetuses.

The fetal lung is a secretory organ. Throughout gestation, a Cl^-, K^+, and H^+ enriched fluid is produced in its peripheral air spaces with the help of a Cl^- pump. The presence of this fluid appears to be important for the development of the acinus because chronic drainage of the trachea in experimental animals results in lung hypoplasia. Fluid secretion, however, is incompatible with air-breathing. Accordingly, and in preparation for birth, lung fluid production decreases slowly at the end of gestation. This decrease, which is accelerated by the beginning of labor, denotes a transformation in the ion transfer activities of the pulmonary epithelium from Cl^- (and water) secretion to Na^+ (and water) absorption. In experimental animals, such a transformation can be precipitated by the administration of β-adrenergic agonists at doses that result in serum levels comparable to those found during labor. Stimulation of β-receptors is not the only labor-related signal, because fluid clearance in the fetal lung is delayed by the Na^+ channel blocker amiloride but not by β-blockers. After birth, the still substantial amount of fluid left in the lungs is absorbed over several hours into the circulation either directly through pulmonary vessels or indirectly through an already very effective lymphatic system. The cellular elements responsible for fluid secretion and absorption in the lungs are not fully identified. It is obvious that a mature alveolar epithelium is not essential for fluid secretion, which is already taking place before alveoli or even saccules exist. Alveolar cells, on the other hand, probably play a protagonistic role in fluid absorption. Type II pneumocytes may be involved because they cover a larger portion of the air space surface in the newborn than in the adult, and their metabolic machinery appears to be particularly well adapted to active ion transport.

At birth, the pulmonary circulation changes from a high-resistance to a low-resistance system and, as a consequence, pulmonary blood flow becomes capable of accommodating systemic venous return. The change in resistance is brought about by the combined effects of the mechanical forces applied on the pulmonary vascular walls by the expanding lung tissue and the relaxation of the pulmonary arterial smooth muscle caused by the increased alveolar concentrations of oxygen and probably by endogenous release of vasodilators. The subsequent closure of the foramen ovale and the ductus arteriosus completely separates the pulmonary from the systemic circulation. Arterial oxygen tension then rises sharply and becomes homogeneous throughout the body. Pulmonary vascular resistance continues to decrease gradually during the first few weeks after birth through a process of structural remodeling of the pulmonary vessel musculature.

POSTNATAL DEVELOPMENT

The postnatal development of the lungs can be divided into two phases depending on the relative rates of development of the various components of the lungs. During the first phase, which extends to the first 18 mo after birth, there is an disproportionate increase in the surface and volume of the compartments involved in gas exchange. Capillary volume increases more rapidly than air space volume, and this, in turn, increases more rapidly than solid tissue volume. These changes are accomplished primarily through a process of alveolar septation. This process is particularly active during early infancy and, contrary to previous belief, may reach completion within the first 2 instead of the first 8 yr of life. The configuration of the air spaces becomes progressively more complex, not only because of the development of new septa but also because of the lengthening and folding of the existing alveolar structures. Soon after birth, the double capillary system contained in the alveolar septa of the fetus fuses into one single, denser system. At the same time, new arterial and venous branches develop within the circulatory system of the acinus and muscle starts to appear in the medial layer of the intra-acinar arteries.

During the second phase, all compartments grow more proportionately to each other. Although there is little question that new alveoli can still be formed, the majority of the growth occurs through an increase in the volume of existing alveoli. Alveolar and capillary surfaces expand in parallel with somatic growth. As a result, taller individuals tend to have larger lungs. However, the final size of the lungs and, ultimately, the dimensions of the individual constituents of the acinus are also influenced by factors such as the subject's level of activity and prevailing state of oxygenation (altitude), which allow for a better adaptation of lung structure and function. The same factors are probably operative in the compensatory responses to pulmonary disease and injury.

Bucher U, Reid L: Development of the intrasegmental bronchial tree: the pattern of branching and development of cartilage at various stages of intrauterine life. Thorax 16: 207, 1961.
Gross I: Regulation of fetal lung maturation. Am J Physiol 259:L337, 1990.
Langston C, Kida K, Reed M, et al: Human lung growth in late gestation and in the neonate. Am Rev Respir Dis 129:607, 1984
O'Brodovich H: Epithelial ion transport in the fetal and perinatal lung. Am J Physiol 261:C555, 1991.

CHAPTER 320
Regulation of Respiration

Gabriel G. Haddad

Pediatricians need to be familiar with the general principles of the regulation of respiration because (1) clinical situations involving one or more elements of the respiratory control system are very prevalent, especially in critically ill patients (e.g., apnea, upper airway obstruction, severe asthma, hypoventilation and heart failure, or hypoxemia from various causes); (2) transition from fetal to neonatal life is an extremely complex process during which there are major changes in almost every aspect of respiratory control; and (3) understanding of the neural control of respiration is likely to increase significantly in the next 1–2 decades because of the explosive advances in understanding brain function in general.

THE RESPIRATORY CONTROL SYSTEM IS A NEGATIVE FEEDBACK SYSTEM WITH A CENTRAL CONTROLLER. The overall aim of the respiratory feedback system is to keep blood gas homeostasis in a normal range in the most economical way, from an energy consumption and mechanical standpoint. The term "negative" in this concept refers to the fact that the controller attempts to rectify the deviation from normality. If CO_2 increases, the output of the controller is increased in an attempt to increase ventilation and decrease CO_2. To accomplish this, the feedback system makes use of both an afferent limb and an efferent limb. The afferent limb is made up of tissues (e.g., the airways) that have receptor endings and can send information to the central controller about certain functional parameters, such as the magnitude of stretch of the airways. The carotid bodies that inform the central controller of the status of O_2 represent another important part of the afferent system. Both airway and carotid body sensors have a way to compare signals in order to note differences and feed this information to the central nervous system. The efferent loop is the part of the feedback system that is responsible for the execution of the decision made centrally (i.e., the respiratory muscles and their innervation). There are many muscles of respiration, and the intercostal muscles and the diaphragm are only two of them. Activity and timing of the airway muscles, as is seen later, are very crucial in determining airway resistance and, therefore, the magnitude of ventilation.

THE CENTRAL CONTROLLER INTEGRATES INCOMING AFFERENT INFORMATION AND GENERATES AND MAINTAINS RESPIRATION. These tasks are believed to be in anatomically different locations, but it is not known in precise mechanistic terms how each function takes place. For example, it is not known how the central generation of respiration takes place, where it is located, or how incoming information is integrated. The respiratory controller may be a group of neurons that either form an *emergent network* or are *endogenous* or *conditional bursters*. In the first case, respiratory neurons would not have special properties (e.g., bursting properties) that would make their membrane potential oscillate. Rather, the output of the network that they form would oscillate because of the special *interconnections* and synaptic interactions among these respiratory neurons. In the second case, similar to that of the heart, the respiratory neurons would have special properties that make them *individually* "burst" or oscillate (pacemaker), even if they are disconnected from any other neurons (endogenous burster). A conditional burster is a neuron that oscillates only when exposed to certain chemicals (e.g., neurotransmitters). The properties of the neurons also are very critical in shaping the output of the network itself, irrespective of the properties of the respiratory controller. A number of ideas have emerged regarding the nature and location of the "respiratory center(s)." Two groups of medullary neurons have been considered as potential sites for the initiation of respiration, namely the nucleus tractus solitarius and the nucleus ambiguus (and retroambiguus). At present there is more support for the latter than the former, although the evidence is not strong for either. Another area in the medulla (pre-Bötzinger) may play a major role in the generation of respiration.

It is likely that, independent of the location of the central pattern generator, it is by virtue of the synaptic and cellular/molecular properties of the neurons in these locations that an oscillatory output takes place to drive the phrenic motor pool and the diaphragm. The understanding of the endowment of these cells in terms of properties and their communications becomes exceedingly important to fully appreciate the intricacies of respiratory generation and maintenance.

AFFERENT INFORMATION IS NOT NECESSARY FOR INITIATING RESPIRATION BUT PLAYS AN IMPORTANT ROLE IN MODULATING BREATHING. A multitude of afferent messages converge on the brain stem at any one time. Chemoreceptors and mechanoreceptors in the larynx and upper airways sense stretch, air temperature, and chemical changes over the mucosa and relay this information to the brain stem. Afferent impulses from these areas travel through the superior laryngeal nerve and the tenth cranial nerve (vagus). The superior laryngeal nerve joins and becomes part of the vagal trunk at the nodose ganglion. Changes in O_2 or CO_2 tensions are sensed at the carotid and aortic bodies, and afferent impulses travel through the carotid and aortic sinus nerves. Thermal or metabolic changes are sensed by skin or mucosal receptors or by hypothalamic neurons and are carried through spinal or central tracts to the brain stem for integrative purposes. Furthermore, afferent information to the brain stem need not be only formulated and sensed by the peripheral nervous system. As examples: (1) Sensors of CO_2 lie on the ventral surface of the medulla oblongata and therefore feedback about CO_2 levels comes from the brain stem itself, and (2) emotions and changes in mood that result from central nervous system processing in the limbic system influence respiration through pathways connecting higher brain centers to the brain stem.

The afferent information is not a prerequisite for generating and maintaining respiration. When the brain stem and spinal cord are removed from the body and maintained in vitro, rhythmic phrenic activity can be detected and measured for hours. Other experiments in vivo in which several sensory systems are blocked simultaneously (with local anesthesia to block vagal afferents, 100% O_2 to eliminate carotid discharges, sleep to eliminate wakeful stimuli, and the chronic administration of diuretics to alkalinize the blood) indicate that afferent information is not necessary to stimulate an inherent respiratory rhythm in brain stem respiratory networks. However, both in vitro and in vivo studies also demonstrate that, in the absence of afferent information, the inherent rhythm of the central generator (respiratory frequency) is slow and chemoreceptor afferents play an important part in modulating respiration and rhythmic behavior.

The neonate is more exquisitely sensitive to afferent input than the adult. Laryngeal reflexes are extremely potent in inhibiting respiration in the newborn. Aspiration and stimulation of laryngeal chemoreceptors in premature infants (who lack the ability of a strong cough), especially when these infants are anemic or hypoglycemic or even during normal sleep, can cause life-threatening respiratory events. Similarly, when neonatal animals are deprived of carotid bodies, prolonged and severe apneic episodes are induced, which can prove fatal in a large percentage of these animals.

CENTRAL INTEGRATION AND PROCESSING IN THE BRAIN STEM IS HIERARCHICAL. Respiratory muscles can be recruited to perform different tasks at different times. For example, the diaphragm and some abdominal muscles are activated not only during tidal breathing but also during expulsive maneuvers such as coughing and straining. These actions and others are recruited when an individual attempts to splint the thorax and abdomen. In other conditions, respiratory muscles can be totally inhibited. For example, when delivering a speech, CO_2 responsiveness is decreased substantially because speech muscles are recruited mostly at the expense of other respiratory muscles. Bottle- or breast-feeding in the young is sometimes associated with a reduction in ventilation and a drop in arterial Po_2 because of partial inhibition of respiratory muscles and breathing efforts. Presented with a number of neurophysiologic signals (representing options about various needs), the central controller can enhance or reduce the response to certain stimuli. Therefore, there is a hierarchy that is used by brain stem networks for determining the response of the respiratory system at any one time.

Changes in the state of consciousness modulate the ability of the brain stem to respond to afferent stimuli. For example, trigeminal afferent impulses are less inhibited by cortical influences during quiet sleep than during rapid eye movement (REM) sleep or wakefulness. Thus, the effect of trigeminal stimulation on respiration is more pronounced in quiet sleep. Similarly, age is very important. The response of the brain stem to stimuli varies with maturation and thus with cortical input to brain stem structures.

RESPIRATORY MUSCLES AND CHEST WALL PROPERTIES (e.g., EFFERENT ORGAN) UNDERGO POSTNATAL MATURATION AND CAN FATIGUE. Effective ventilation requires *coordinated interaction* between the respiratory muscles of the chest wall (including the diaphragm and intercostals) and those of the upper airway (including the pharynx and the larynx) under various conditions of altered respiratory drive. In infants, a specific sequential pattern of nerve and muscle activation occurs so that some upper airway muscles contract prior to and during the early part of inspiratory flow: the genioglossus muscle contracts, moving the tongue forward, which prevents pharyngeal obstruction; the vocal cords abduct, reducing inspiratory laryngeal resistance.

Laryngeal muscles also modulate expiratory flow and thus may influence lung volume. Imbalance of pharyngeal and diaphragmatic activities or their responses to chemoreceptor or mechanoreceptor stimulation may contribute to obstructive apnea in infants and children.

Since the *respiratory muscles* are responsible for executing central neural responses and since muscle and chest wall properties change with age in early life, it is likely that neural responses can be influenced by pump properties. Thus, it is important to consider the maturational changes of respiratory muscles and chest wall. One of the important maturational aspects of innervation of respiratory muscles (e.g., in skeletal muscles) is its pattern of innervation. In the adult, one muscle fiber is innervated by one motoneuron. Therefore, if a motoneuron innervates certain muscle fibers (e.g., about 200 muscle fibers in the case of the diaphragm), these fibers do not receive innervation from any other motoneuron. In the newborn, however, each fiber is innervated by two or more motoneurons, and the axons of different motoneurons can synapse on the same muscle fiber—thus the term polyneuronal innervation. Synapse elimination takes place postnatally, and in the case of the diaphragm, the adult type of innervation is reached by several weeks of age depending on the animal species. The time course of polyneuronal innervation of the diaphragm in the human newborn is not known.

The neuromuscular junctional folds, postsynaptic membranes, and acetylcholine receptors and metabolism undergo major postnatal maturational changes. The acetylcholine quantal content per end plate potential is lower in the newborn than in the adult rat diaphragm. The newborn diaphragm is also more susceptible to neuromuscular transmission failure than the adult, especially at higher frequencies of stimulation. Whether this is the result of differences in acetylcholine metabolism between the newborn and the adult or whether this is related to the neuromuscular junction itself is not known.

In addition to an increase in cross-sectional area and muscle mass, *muscle fiber types* in the diaphragm change as a function of gestational and postnatal age. However, there are conflicting reports about the composition of fiber types in young muscle, and it is not known whether human newborn muscles are more oxidative or fatigue resistant than those of the adult. The sarcoplasmic reticulum of the premature diaphragm is, however, underdeveloped compared with that of the adult. This is one major reason for the delay in the release and uptake of Ca^{2+}, which may have functional significance. The poorly developed sarcoplasmic reticulum in the newborn causes increased contraction and relaxation time in neonatal muscle fibers. This increased relaxation time may be an important factor in impeding blood flow, limiting oxidative metabolism, when the muscle is under a load.

The *chest wall* in newborn infants is highly compliant. Because of this and because young infants spend a large proportion of time in REM sleep during which the intercostal muscles are inhibited, there is little splinting of the chest wall for diaphragmatic action. Therefore, with every breath in supine infants (especially in REM sleep), the chest wall is sucked in paradoxically at a time when the abdomen expands. This creates an additional load on the respiratory system and results in a higher work of breathing per minute ventilation in the infant than in the adult. Some believe that this may be an important reason for the newborn's susceptibility to muscle fatigue and respiratory failure.

THE NEWBORN AND YOUNG RESPOND DIFFERENTLY TO STIMULI COMPARED WITH THE MATURE SUBJECT. The young child and neonate respond to various stimuli in a different way from the adult. In response to low O_2, the newborn does not sustain an increase in ventilation, and often ventilation decreases to below baseline levels. CO_2 levels do not increase at a time when ventilation is decreasing, suggesting that ventilation is matching metabolic needs. This neonatal response to low O_2 can be considered as an intermediate response between those of the fetus and the adult; the fetus shuts off all respiratory efforts in response to O_2 deprivation, and the adult hyperventilates as long as the stimulus is present. The mechanism(s) for the lack of sustained increase in ventilation during hypoxia in the newborn is not well understood. In addition to differences in metabolic rate during hypoxemia among neonates and adults, changes in the mechanical properties of the lung and airways, maturation of carotid chemoreceptors, and alterations in the cellular and membrane properties of central neurons have all been proposed as potential individual or combined mechanisms. It is clinically important that neonatal tissues resist O_2 deprivation and do not injure as easily as those of the adult. This is true for the heart and the brain and kidneys, organs known to be sensitive to hypoxia and ischemia in the mature animal or human.

CO_2 response is also reduced in the young. Whether this is a reflection of an inherent difference in their sensitivity or the result of differences in mechanical function is not known.

Although alterations in responsiveness can be secondary to a number of differences between the young and the mature organism, the central neuronal changes with maturation seem especially important. For example, the soma of lumbar and phrenic motoneurons increases with age, and their input resistance (or inverse of membrane conductance) decreases with age. The decrease in input resistance results in major part from the increase in soma size, but other mechanisms, such as a change in the geometry of the dendrites and their outgrowth, a change in the number of ion channels per surface area, and an increase in the number of synapses onto motoneurons, cannot be ruled out. Axonal velocity also increases with age, and action potentials of phrenic and hypoglossal motoneurons decrease in duration. There are also major maturational changes in active cellular properties in some motoneurons or premotor neurons. For example, with increasing postnatal age, neurons in the area of the nucleus tractus solitarius develop cellular properties important for repetitive firing. Changes in neuronal properties could play an important role in the integrative abilities of neuronal cells and, therefore, in their response to stimulation.

CLINICAL IMPLICATIONS

Apnea (See Chapter 87.2). Although there are numerous studies on apnea in the newborn and adult human, there are also a number of controversies. The length of the respiratory pause that has been defined as apnea has varied.

Apnea can be defined statistically as a respiratory pause that exceeds 3 standard deviations of the mean breath time for an infant or a child at any particular age. This definition requires data from a population of infants at that age, lacks physiologic value, and does not differentiate between relatively shorter or longer respiratory pauses. Alternatively, the definition of apnea may be based on the fact that respiratory pauses are associated with cardiovascular or neurophysiologic changes. Such definition relies completely on the functional assessment of pauses and is, therefore, more relevant clinically. Because infants have higher O_2 consumption (per unit weight) than the adult and relatively smaller lung volume and O_2 stores, it is possible that short (e.g., seconds) respiratory pauses that may not be clinically important in the adult can present serious consequences in the very young or premature.

Independent of age group, respiratory pauses are more prevalent during sleep than during the waking state. The frequency and duration of respiratory pauses depend on sleep state in human infants. Respiratory pauses are more frequent and shorter in REM than in quiet sleep and more frequent in younger than in older infants.

Although there is controversy regarding the pathogenesis of respiratory pauses, there is a consensus about certain observations. Normal full-term infants, children, and adult humans exhibit respiratory pauses during sleep. Paradoxically, some believe that the presence of respiratory pauses and breathing irregularity is a "healthy" sign and that the complete absence of such pauses may be indicative of abnormalities. However, prolonged apneas can be life threatening. The pathogenesis of these apneas may relate to the clinical condition of the patient at the time of the apneas, associated cardiovascular (systemic or pulmonary) changes, the chronicity of the clinical condition, the perinatal history, and whether the etiology is central or peripheral. Prolonged apneic spells require therapy and, optimally, treatment should be targeted to the underlying pathophysiology. A septic infant should be treated for the infection and a seizing infant with antiepileptic medication. The child with congenital hypoventilation syndrome (or Ondine curse), in the absence of pharmacologic therapy, should be placed on mechanical ventilation until properly paced with phrenic stimulators (Chapter 377).

Upper Airway Obstruction (Chapter 330). Upper airway obstruction (UAO) during sleep is recognized with increasing frequency in children. In contrast to adults with UAO in whom the etiology of obstruction often remains obscure, many children have anatomic abnormalities. A common cause of UAO in children is tonsillar and adenoidal hypertrophy due to repeated upper respiratory infections. Other associated abnormalities include craniofacial malformations, micrognathia, and muscular hypotonia. The usual site of obstruction in UAO in both infants and adults is the oropharynx, between the posterior pharyngeal wall, the soft palate, and the genioglossus. During sleep (especially REM sleep), upper airway muscles, including those of the oropharynx, lose tone and trigger an episode of UAO.

Snoring with recurrent periods of respiratory pauses commonly occurs during sleep in children. Parents frequently describe periods of increasing chest wall movement without air flow and with cyanosis. In older children the syndrome may include failure to thrive, developmental delay, and poor school performance. Hypertension and daytime hypersomnolence are less common abnormalities in children than in adults. Children with long-standing signs and symptoms of UAO during sleep can present with right ventricular failure and cor pulmonale. The treatment, therefore, varies but should be targeted primarily at the underlying cause of obstruction. Some of these infants will benefit by tonsillectomy and adenoidectomy or, if obese, by a reduction in weight. In some refractory cases, successful treatment has included continuous positive airway pressure applied through the nose.

Haddad GG: Control of breathing in children. *In*: Edelman NH, Santiago T (eds): Contemporary Issues in Pulmonary Disease. New York, Churchill Livingston, 1986, pp 57–80.

Haddad GG: Cellular and membrane properties of brainstem neurons in early life. *In*: Haddad GG, Farber J (eds): Developmental Neurobiology of breathing. Lung Biology in Health and Disease, Vol 53. New York, Marcel Dekker, 1991, pp 591–614.

CHAPTER 321

Respiratory Function and Approach to Respiratory Disease

Gabriel G. Haddad and J. Julio Pérez Fontán

The main function of the respiratory system is to provide adequate gas exchange between the circulating blood and the atmosphere. Respiratory failure is defined in terms of the concentration or partial pressure of oxygen and carbon dioxide in the arterial blood. Nonetheless, respiratory dysfunction frequently occurs with minimal or even the absence of detectable gas exchange aberrations. Most manifestations of respiratory disease in children result from alterations in the mechanical behavior of the chest wall and lungs or from the increase in the work of breathing that these alterations impose.

MECHANICS OF BREATHING

The mechanical function of the respiratory system is analyzed in terms of work and energy. *Work* is a concrete quantity used to characterize the effort needed to move an object. It has the dimensions of force times distance, if the object moves in one dimension, or pressure times volume, if the object moves in three dimensions (as in the case of the lungs and the chest wall). *Energy*, in contrast, is a variable property of objects or systems. It has the same dimensions as work and can be changed into work; however, it is not equivalent to work. The transformation of energy into work is regulated by an *efficiency* factor, which tells how well the system performs.

The definitions of work, energy, and efficiency can be further clarified by applying them to the events that occur during a breath. The process starts with the respiratory muscles using the circulating substrates to obtain energy. A portion of this energy is transformed into mechanical work during muscle contraction; the remainder is used for nonwork activities such as protein synthesis or is simply dissipated as heat. The system is therefore inherently inefficient: It does not transform all the available energy into work. The portion of the energy that is converted into work can be transformed temporarily into kinetic energy, which is associated with movement, or stored, also temporarily, as potential energy.

WORK OF BREATHING. The work performed by the respiratory pump is uniquely defined by how much the volume of the lungs changes when the respiratory muscles generate a given pressure. The volume-pressure relationships of the respiratory system depend on functional properties such as the "suppleness" of the lung and chest wall tissues or the ease with which the airways allow the passage of air. A reasonable approach to characterize these properties is to examine the way in which the associated physicochemical processes handle the energy imparted to the respiratory system during breathing. A substantial portion of the pressure generated by the respiratory muscles is applied to produce reversible rearrangements of the molecular structure of both the alveolar gas-liquid interface and the fibrous network of the lungs. By virtue of their reversibility, the energy used to produce this type of rearrangement during lung inflation is really being stored as potential energy. It therefore remains available for other activities during deflation. In this regard, the respiratory system emulates the elastic behavior of a rubber band, which stores energy when stretched and returns it when it is allowed to recover its original shape.

Another large portion of the effort of the respiratory muscles is directed at producing molecular rearrangements or interactions that are not reversible. The energy spent in such an effort is directly transformed into heat, which is then dissipated into the atmosphere or carried away by the circulating blood. The processes that result in energy dissipation have one thing in common: They only take place in the presence of movement. As a result, the magnitudes of the work and the pressures derived from these processes generally bear a relationship to the rate of gas flow in and out of the lungs. In this regard, the respiratory system exhibits a resistive behavior comparable to that of a household pipe, for which the driving pressure at the water main determines the flow of water. Both the elastic and the resistive components of the work of breathing are usually increased in children with respiratory disease. Establishing a diagnosis and formulating a therapy in these patients is almost always simplified when the clinician distinguishes between conditions that affect primarily the elastic (restrictive respiratory disease) and resistive (obstructive respiratory disease) behaviors of the respiratory system.

ELASTIC PROPERTIES OF THE RESPIRATORY SYSTEM AND RESTRICTIVE DISEASE. The respiratory system exhibits an elastic behavior for two reasons. First, surface tension in the air spaces opposes lung inflation, particularly at low lung volumes when the air spaces are smaller and, in fulfillment of the law of Laplace, the same surface tension causes the inward acting pressure to be greater. By coating the surface of the alveolar film with a monolayer of hydrophobic molecules, surfactant diminishes or neutralizes this pressure in a volume-dependent manner. Conveniently, surfactant is less spread out when the surface area of the alveolar film reaches a minimum, and therefore it is more effective at low than at high lung volumes. Even in the presence of normal amounts of surfactant in the air spaces, surface tension is responsible for approximately 65% of the elastic recoil of the lungs. When surfactant is absent or dysfunctional *(respiratory distress syndrome of the newborn)* (see Chapter 87), elastic recoil becomes markedly increased and atelectasis ensues. The second reason for the elastic behavior of the respiratory system is the presence in the lungs and chest wall of a fibrous network with elastic properties. Disease-related changes in composition *(pulmonary fibrosis)* or architectural arrangement of this network *(lung overdistention)* also increases the elastic recoil of the lungs.

Both surface tension and elastic forces generated by lung fibers depend on the dimensions of the air spaces. Thus it is not surprising that the overall elastic recoil of the lungs is highly dependent on lung volume just like, in the example of the rubber band, tension depends on the extent to which the rubber band is stretched. The relationship between volume and elastic pressure can be obtained easily for the whole respiratory system or independently for the lungs and the chest wall by measuring the corresponding pressure changes while the lungs are passively inflated and deflated in a stepwise manner. All three relationships are sigmoid in shape (Fig. 321–1). Volume increases much less for a given pressure change at low and high volumes than at intermediate volumes, at which normal breathing takes place. In the intermediate volume range, the relationship is steeper and relatively linear, and can therefore be described accurately by a fixed ratio of volume to pressure changes. This ratio defines the concept of *compliance*.

A graphic analysis of the volume-pressure relationships of the lungs and the chest wall clarifies how the mechanical behaviors of these two components interact to shape the volume-pressure relationship of the respiratory system as a whole (Fig. 321–2). Two premises characterize these interactions: First, at any volume the elastic recoil of the respiratory system is equal to the sums of the individual elastic recoils of the lungs and chest wall; and, second, the volume changes experienced by the lungs, the chest wall, and the respiratory system are identical. Based on these premises, it becomes easy to understand, for instance, how pleural pressure (which represents the elastic recoil of the chest wall) may be high in a patient with asthma who has no intrinsic chest wall anomalies but whose lung volume is markedly increased by gas trapping. Because the heart and vessels inside the thorax are exposed to pleural pressure, cardiac output and arterial blood pressure often undergo an exaggerated decrease during inspiration as lung volume increases even further *(pulsus paradoxus)*.

Graphic analysis of the volume-pressure relationships of the lungs and the chest wall also demonstrates some other principles that regulate lung volume. Figure 321–1 shows that each relationship crosses the volume axis at a very different point, regardless of age. The point in question defines the relaxation volume, which is the volume at which no elastic recoil is generated. Under normal conditions, the relaxation volume of

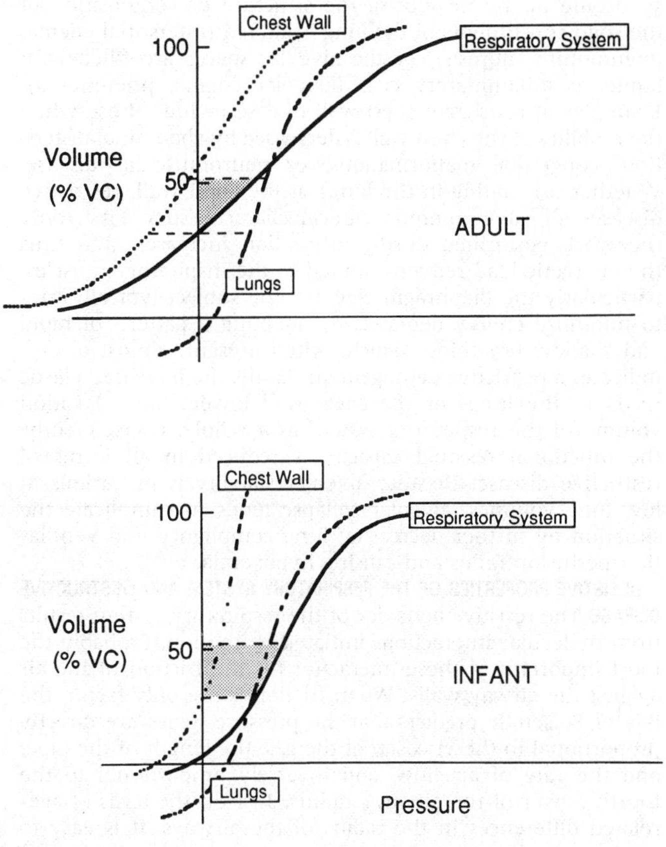

Figure 321–1. Idealized elastic volume-pressure relationships of the lungs, chest wall, and respiratory system in the adult and the infant. Volume is expressed as a proportion of vital capacity (VC). At any volume, the pressure that the respiratory muscles must generate to oppose the elastic recoil of the respiratory system is equivalent to the sum of the recoil pressures of lungs and chest wall individually. The intersection of each relationship with the volume axis corresponds to the relaxation volume of each component (the volume at which the elastic recoil is zero). The volume–elastic pressure relationships of the lungs are similar in the adult and infant. The volume–elastic pressure relationship of the chest wall is steeper in the infant, causing the relaxation volume of the respiratory system to be lower than in the adult. The shaded area represents the elastic work done by the respiratory muscles for a characteristic tidal volume. Note that this work is greater in the infant because the recoil of the chest wall does not contribute to inflate the lungs as it does in the adult. (From Pérez Fontán JJ: Mechanics of breathing. *In*: Gluckman PD, Heymann MA [eds]: Perinatal and Pediatric Pathophysiology: A Clinical Perspective. London, Edward Arnold, 1993.)

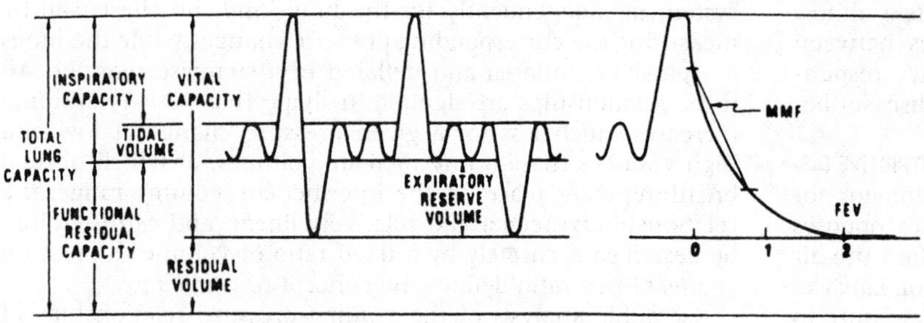

Figure 321–2. *Left,* functional division of total lung capacity. *Right,* flow-time relationship during a forced expiration from vital capacity. FEV represents the volume expired for a given period of time and is often measured at 1 sec. MMF represents the maximal midexpiratory flow rate and is calculated as the average flow for the middle 50% of the forced vital capacity (as shown by the cord in the drawing). (From Doershuk CF, Lough MD. *In:* Lough MD, Doershuk CF, Stern RC [ed]: Pediatric Respiratory Therapy. Chicago, Year Book Medical Publishers, 1974.)

the lungs is considerably smaller than that of the chest wall. This discrepancy has several important mechanical consequences. First, it forces the respiratory system as a whole to adopt a relaxation volume intermediate between that of the lungs and that of the chest wall. After the newborn period, this volume coincides with the *functional residual capacity,* the gas volume of the lungs at the end of a tidal expiration (see Fig. 321–2). In addition, the opposing recoils of the lungs and the chest wall at the relaxation volume of the respiratory system create a negative pleural pressure; this pressure promotes the return of venous blood into the heart and keeps the lung and chest wall attached to each other. If the pleural space were open to the atmosphere and the lungs and the chest wall were allowed to change volume freely without contraction of the respiratory muscles, the lungs would collapse and the chest wall would expand. This happens, with some qualifications, when a *pneumothorax* develops. Finally, for at least a portion of the volume range, the outward-acting recoil of the chest wall helps the expansion of the lungs, thereby reducing energy expenditure during inspiration.

Restrictive disease of the respiratory system occurs whenever the elastic recoil of the lungs or the chest wall is increased at the prevailing lung volumes. Restrictive lung disease occurs when surface tension is abnormally high (respiratory distress syndrome of the newborn), the structure or composition of the solid constituents of the lung is altered (interstitial edema, pneumonitis, fibrosis), or the alveolar spaces are filled with liquid or inflammatory cells (alveolar edema, pneumonia). Examples of restrictive chest wall disease include those when the mobility of the chest wall is decreased by abdominal distention, congenital malformations, or neuromuscular disease. Whether originating in the lungs or the chest wall, restrictive diseases all have common clinical characteristics. First, only the work performed during inspiration increases, and thus the energetic load remains limited to the inspiratory muscles, particularly the diaphragm. Second, the subject typically tries to minimize energy demands by adopting a pattern of rapid and shallow breathing, which, when present, almost always indicates a restrictive derangement. Lastly, the increased elastic recoil of the lungs or the chest wall lowers the relaxation volume of the respiratory system as a whole. Consequently, the functional residual capacity is reduced in all forms of restrictive disease. Because alveolar stability is precarious at low lung volumes, alveolar collapse tends to complicate the situation by further decreasing lung compliance and ventilation/perfusion ratios and causing hypoxemia.

RESISTIVE PROPERTIES OF THE RESPIRATORY SYSTEM AND OBSTRUCTIVE DISEASE. The resistive behavior of the respiratory system results from molecular interactions initiated by motion. Probably the most important of these interactions is the friction of the air against the airway walls. When friction is the only factor, the law of Poiseuille predicts that the pressure losses are directly proportional to the viscosity of the gas, the length of the pipe, and the rate of air flow, and inversely proportional to the fourth power of the airway's radius. Just on the basis of age-related differences in the radius of the airways, it is easy to understand how diseases such as *viral bronchiolitis,* which cause peripheral airway obstruction, increase the work of breathing in newborns and small infants proportionately more than in older children. Molecular interactions within the breathing gas itself, particularly when the flow becomes turbulent in narrow portions of the airways, result in energy dissipation as well. Unlike wall friction, however, the pressure needed to overcome turbulence depends on the density and not on the viscosity of the gas. This is the reason why children with *croup* tend to have less respiratory difficulty when the air that they breathe is replaced with a mixture of oxygen and helium, which has a lower density than air or oxygen. Finally, nonreversible molecular rearrangements within the tissue or the gas-liquid interface play an increasingly more recognized role in the resistive properties of the lungs and the respiratory system as a whole. Their relevance to human disease is not fully understood.

The resistive behavior of the respiratory system can also be analyzed graphically (Fig. 321–3). The volume-pressure relationships of the lungs, chest wall, and respiratory system as a whole form characteristic loops; they show *hysteresis,* which

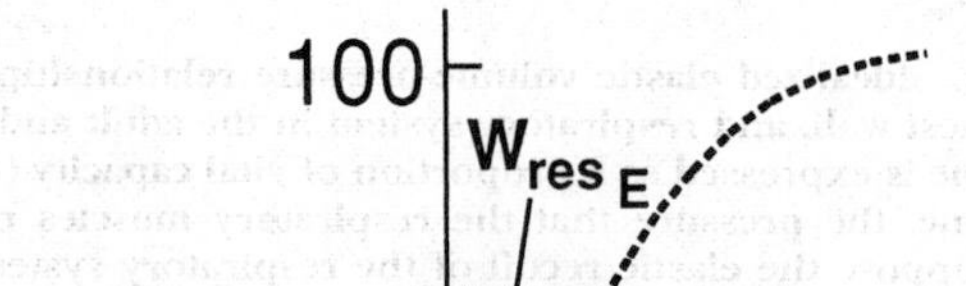

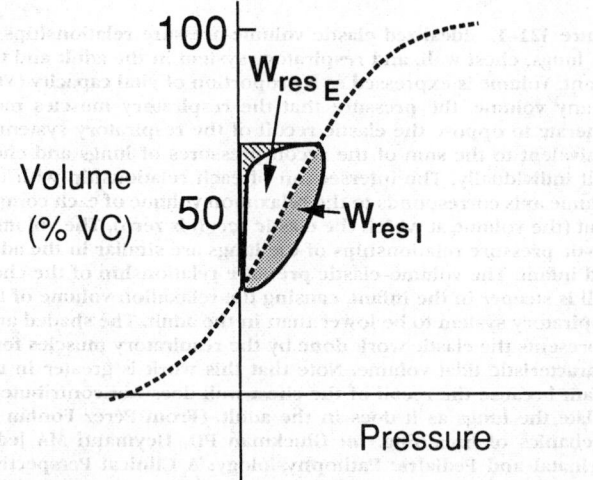

Figure 321–3. Graphic analysis of the resistive behavior of the respiratory system during a tidal breath. In the presence of airway flow, energy dissipation causes the relationship between lung volume (expressed as a proportion of vital capacity [VC]) and the pressure that the respiratory muscles must generate to form a loop (hysteresis). The area enclosed by this loop represents the work done to overcome resistive pressures such as those caused by the friction of the air against the airway walls. Only the inspiratory portion of this work ($Wres_I$), however, is performed by the respiratory muscles. The expiratory portion ($Wres_E$) is done by the energy accumulated in elastic elements of the respiratory system during inspiration. (From Pérez Fontán JJ: Mechanics of breathing. *In:* Gluckman PD, Heymann MA [eds]: Perinatal and Pediatric Pathophysiology: A Clinical Perspective. London, Edward Arnold, 1993.)

means that a relationship has a very different course during inspiration and expiration. Hysteresis always denotes that there is an energy loss from the system. Moreover, the greater the hysteresis, the larger is this energy loss. Accordingly, the width of the loop formed by the pressure-volume relationships of the respiratory system or its components (which has the units of pressure) is often used as a quantitative estimate of resistive behavior. When divided by the rate of gas flow, it yields the *resistance*, a measurement that summarizes various properties that result in the resistive behavior. The graphic analysis of the volume-pressure relationships of the respiratory system also reveals that, even though resistive work is done during inspiration and expiration, only the inspiratory portion of the work represents an energetic burden. Under normal circumstances, expiration does not require the contraction of any muscles; it is passive, which means that all expiratory resistive work is done by the elastic recoil accumulated during inspiration in the lungs and chest wall. However, when expiratory resistance is elevated by disease (asthma, bronchiolitis) or when the subject needs to accelerate the emptying of the lungs to increase ventilation (exercise), then abdominal and other expiratory muscles become engaged. This engagement in a resting child is a good indication of the presence of obstructive respiratory disease.

Proper diagnosis and evaluation of airway obstruction requires additional understanding of the relationships between airway caliber and lung volume. Airway caliber is determined by the coupling of airway wall elasticity and airway transmural pressure. The former depends on the state of health and maturity of the airway tissue (immature airways tend to collapse more easily) and is modulated by the tone of the muscles contained in the airway wall (skeletal muscle for the nose, pharynx, and larynx; smooth muscle for the trachea and bronchi). This tone is in turn regulated by neural efferents, which tend to stiffen the airway walls during inspiration, particularly under conditions in which breathing activity must increase (during exercise, hypoxia, hypercarbia). Airway transmural pressure is the difference between the pressures acting on the inside and the outside of the airway wall. It varies during the respiratory cycle in a fashion that depends on whether the airways are intrathoracic or extrathoracic (Fig. 321–4).

Extrathoracic airways (nose, pharynx, larynx, the extrathoracic portion of the trachea) are exposed to atmospheric pressure on the outside. Because the pressure inside is subatmospheric during inspiration and supra-atmospheric during expiration, the transmural pressure in this portion of the airway tree is always negative (narrowing the airway, or even collapsing it if no muscle tone is present in the airway wall) during inspiration and positive (dilating the airway) during expiration. The outside surface of the intrathoracic airways (trachea, bronchi, alveolar ducts) is exposed either to pleural pressure or to the stresses generated by lung inflation within the lung tissue. These stresses are applied on the airway wall by tissue attachments between the wall and the parenchyma and, when averaged over the airway external surface, they add up to a value very close to the prevailing pleural pressure. Because air only flows in the inspiratory direction if the pressure inside the airways is greater than alveolar pressure and alveolar pressure is always greater than pleural pressure (otherwise, the lungs would have a negative elastic recoil), the transmural pressure of the intrathoracic airways becomes increasingly more positive (dilating the airways) during inspiration. For the alveolar gas to flow in the expiratory direction, the pressure at all points inside the airways must be lower than alveolar pressure. Whether it is higher or lower than pleural pressure, however, depends on the resistive pressure losses upstream from the point in question. If the losses are large, the pressure inside the intrathoracic airways can become lower than pleural pressure. If so, the transmural pressure is

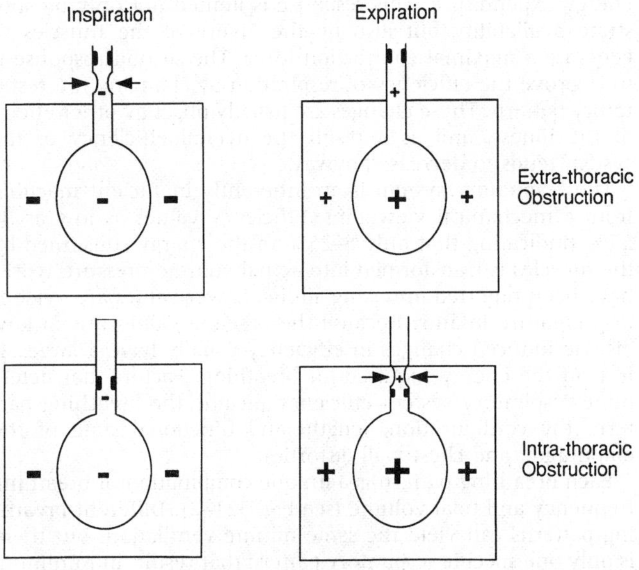

Figure 321–4. Effect of inspiration and expiration on the caliber of the airways during extrathoracic and intrathoracic airway obstruction. Extrathoracic obstruction is exacerbated during inspiration because the pressure inside the airway becomes very negative with respect to the atmospheric pressure outside, causing the airway to collapse *(arrows)*. Intrathoracic obstruction, in contrast, is exacerbated during expiration because the pressure outside the airways (which is similar to pleural pressure) rapidly exceeds the pressure inside, causing the airways downstream from the obstruction point to collapse *(arrows)*. (From Pérez Fontán JJ, Lister G: Respiratory failure. *In:* Toulukian RJ [ed]: Pediatric Trauma, 2nd ed. St. Louis, MO, CV Mosby, 1990.)

negative and the airway tends to collapse, a significant problem if the airway wall is abnormally soft (as in the premature infant or in *bronchomalacia*). The more the subject tries to overcome the resultant increase in expiratory resistance by making use of the expiratory muscles, the more the pleural pressure increases and the more the airway collapses, leading to a situation in which flow cannot increase any more regardless of the effort. The expiratory flow at which such flow limitation occurs is highly reproducible for a given lung volume. Determinations of maximal expiratory flow during respiratory function testing take advantage of this reproducibility to evaluate and follow the function of the intrathoracic airways over time or in response to specific therapies.

Airway obstruction causes an exaggeration of the normal changes in airway caliber (see Fig. 321–4). When the extrathoracic airway is obstructed (croup, foreign body), the pressure inside the airways distal to the narrowing has to become more negative during inspiration to overcome the increased resistance at the point of obstruction. Therefore, the extrathoracic airway collapses downstream from the obstruction, usually causing an audible inspiratory *stridor* as the gas rushes through the obstruction. When the intrathoracic airway is obstructed (asthma, tracheobronchomalacia), the pleural pressure must become more positive during expiration. Because the inside pressure beyond the obstruction decreases, the intrathoracic airways downstream from the obstruction point tend to collapse during expiration, producing an exacerbation of the obstruction, audible expiratory *wheezes*, and flow limitation at low expiratory flows.

RESPONSE TO RESPIRATORY DISEASE: EFFICIENCY OF THE DEVELOPING RESPIRATORY SYSTEM. When the respiratory work load increases in the course of an illness, the respiratory system has two types of responses. The most immediate is to increase the contraction of the respiratory muscles at the cost of increased energy expenditure. This response is limited not only by substrate availability but also by the ability of the muscles to generate a maximal contraction force. The second response is to improve the efficiency of respiration by changing the respiratory pattern. These changes are usually offset by other effects of the illness, and as a result the overall efficiency of the system tends to decrease anyway.

The respiratory system is an inherently inefficient machine from a mechanical viewpoint. Efficiency values as low as 8–25% (indicating that only 8–25% of the energy consumed by the muscles is transformed into actual volume-pressure work) have been reported in resting adults. Lower values are evident in premature infants. Because the baseline values are so low, disease-induced changes in efficiency usually have a large effect on the energy required for breathing. Factors that determine respiratory system efficiency include the breathing pattern; the configuration, length, and functional state of the diaphragm; and chest wall distortion.

Each breathing pattern is a unique combination of breathing frequency and tidal volume (see Fig. 321–2). Different breathing patterns can yield the same minute ventilation, but there is only one specific respiratory pattern that results in minimum energy expenditure at any time. Theoretically, this optimal pattern varies predictably depending on the mechanical characteristics of the respiratory system (Fig. 321–5). Breathing frequency, for instance, increases when elastic recoil becomes greater in the course of a restrictive derangement. In contrast, the frequency decreases when the resistive properties of the respiratory system become exaggerated by airway obstruction. In practice, these theoretical predictions are accurate, and it is therefore possible to categorize respiratory disease as primarily restrictive or obstructive, depending on whether the patient breathes rapidly and shallowly or slowly and more deeply. It is important to remember that breathing pattern is regulated by influences other than energetic considerations. It is common for children with respiratory disease to breathe transiently at frequencies that depart substantially from optimum. Blood gas abnormalities, airway irritation by a poorly positioned endotracheal tube, or crying and agitation can reduce the efficiency of the respiratory system and precipitate respiratory failure.

Like other skeletal muscles, the diaphragm can only develop its maximal force if stretched to an optimal length (Fig. 321–6). This length is attained when the lungs approximate their functional residual capacity (see Fig. 321–2). At this volume, the diaphragm adopts the shape of a dome-capped cylinder. In addition to increasing the volume displaced for a given fiber shortening, this shape allows a direct surface of contact between the diaphragm and the rib cage. Such surface, known as the area of apposition, serves an important function during inspiration. It allows the abdominal contents to push the lower ribs forward and laterally in the inspiratory direction. The shape of the diaphragm in the infant, and particularly in the newborn, may not take advantage of these features (see Fig. 321–6). The lower portion of the rib cage has large anteroposterior and lateral diameters. As a result, the diaphragmatic insertions are spread out, limiting the range of lengths of the diaphragmatic fibers. In addition, radiographic examination of the chest and abdomen suggests that the area of apposition is reduced in early infancy (see Fig. 321–6).

We assume that the chest wall expands uniformly during lung inflation. In reality, not only can different portions of the rib cage and abdomen change volume independently of each other, but they can also do it in opposite directions. Chest wall distortion can occur at all ages and results primarily from the fact that the chest wall does not have a homogeneous composition. Areas with no bony support, like the intercostal spaces, tend to move inward under the effects of negative pleural pressure during inspiration. This movement is exaggerated whenever the pleural pressure becomes more negative than normal in the presence of lung disease, creating visible retractions. The limited ossification of the ribs and sternum makes the chest walls of newborns and infants very compliant (see Fig. 321–1), a feature that facilitates the birth process, but also creates some mechanical liabilities. First, it decreases the relaxation volume of the respiratory system, forcing the newborn to develop strategies to maintain the functional residual capacity within acceptable limits. These strategies, which are generally based on braking expiratory flow, are easily overwhelmed when lung compliance is reduced by disease, when neurologic control is impaired by central nervous system injury or sedation, or when the tone of the chest wall muscles is decreased during REM sleep. Because the functional residual capacity represents the largest oxygen store in the body, its reduction in infants can easily lead to hypoxemia because of the high oxygen consumption rates characteristic of early ages.

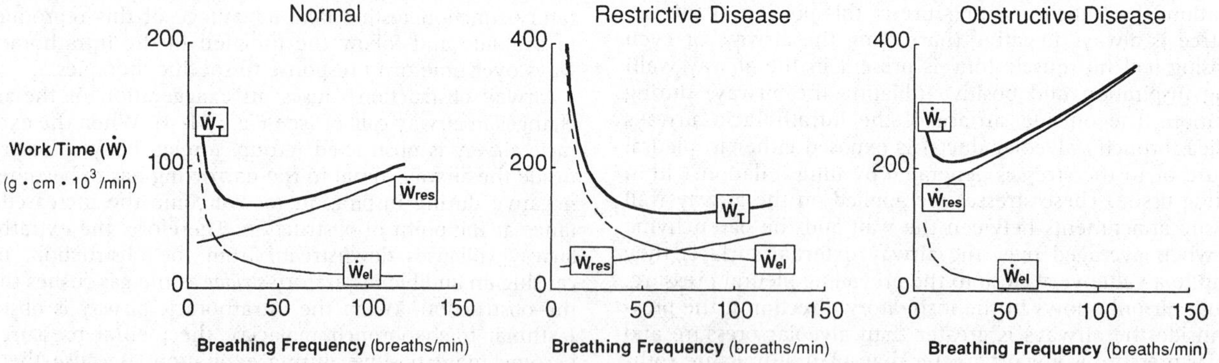

Figure 321–5. Schematic representation of the effects of breathing frequency on the work of breathing per unit of time (Ẇ, breathing power) needed to overcome elastic forces (Ẇel), resistive forces (Ẇres), and their sum ($\dot{W}_T$) in a normal infant and two infants with respiratory disease: one restrictive and the other obstructive. The calculations used to construct the representation are based on typical measurements of respiratory mechanics and on the assumptions that minute alveolar ventilation is constant regardless of the breathing frequency, that breathing pattern is sinusoidal, and that volume- and flow-pressure relationships are linear. Elastic and resistive power decrease and increase, respectively, with frequency. As a result, total power follows a bimodal course, decreasing at low frequencies and increasing at high frequencies. The point at which total power reaches a minimum defines the optimal frequency. This frequency is shifted to lower values in restrictive disease and to higher values in obstructive disease. (From Pérez Fontán JJ: Mechanics of breathing. *In:* Gluckman PD, Heymann MA [eds]: Perinatal and Pediatric Pathophysiology: A Clinical Perspective. London, Edward Arnold, 1993.)

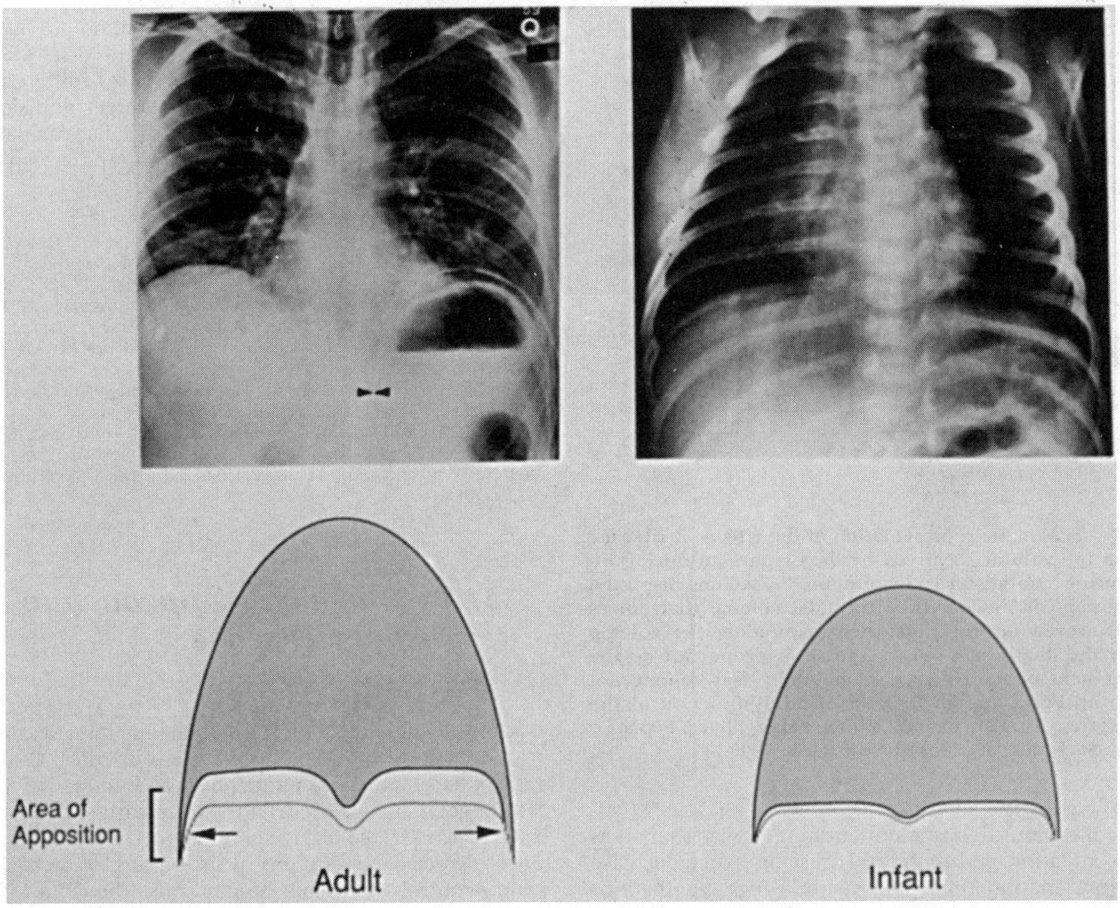

Figure 321–6. Chest radiographs and sketches illustrating the differences in the geometric shapes of the diaphragm of the adult and infant. The diaphragm of the adult *(left)* has the shape of a dome-capped cylinder whose height can be followed in the radiograph of the tip of a catheter inserted in the pleural space *(arrowheads)*. A portion of the diaphragm is apposed to the rib cage, providing a way of transforming the vertical movement of the diaphragm into the anterior and lateral movement of the rib cage in inspiration (see text). The diaphragm of the infant *(right)* is flatter and less capable of displacing large volumes in the vertical direction. In addition, it lacks a substantial area of apposition and thus has limited expanding action on the rib cage.

In addition, a high chest wall compliance promotes increased regional distortion of the rib cage. Because distortion represents a form of work and has a finite energy cost, but does not contribute to lung inflation, it can be considered as a source of inefficiency (Fig. 321–7). The diaphragm may do more work to distort the rib cage than to inflate the lungs in premature infants without lung disease.

GAS EXCHANGE

Gas exchange in the lungs takes place in millions of small units, each constituted by a pulmonary capillary and the neighboring portion of the air space. Because the arterial blood is a weighted mixture of the blood that passes through these units, the arterial concentrations or contents of oxygen and carbon dioxide depend fundamentally on the way in which blood flow and ventilation are matched within the lungs. On one extreme, nonperfused units, which continue to receive ventilation, do not contribute directly to the composition of the arterial blood but waste a portion of the ventilatory effort: They act as dead space. On the other extreme, nonventilated units, which continue to receive blood flow, contaminate the arterial blood with venous blood: They act as a shunt (or promote venous admixture). Between these two extremes, there is usually a wide spectrum of possibilities that define the final composition of the arterial blood. The factors that determine this composition are different for carbon dioxide and oxygen.

The partial pressure of carbon dioxide (P_{CO_2}) in the arterial blood is directly proportional to carbon dioxide production and inversely proportional to alveolar ventilation. The latter can be calculated as the difference of minute ventilation (the amount of gas that enters and leaves the lungs in 1 minute) and dead space ventilation (the portion of the minute ventilation that does not contribute to alveolar gas exchange). Dead space ventilation is usually increased by respiratory disease because of the presence of a large number of gas exchange units with high ventilation/perfusion ratios. If the subject is unable to compensate with a sufficient increase in minute ventilation, the arterial P_{CO_2} rises above its normal values of 33–45 mm Hg.

The partial pressure of oxygen (P_{O_2}) in the arterial blood is influenced by several variables, including the P_{O_2} of the inspired gas, the P_{O_2} of the venous blood, the hemoglobin oxygen capacity, and the respective alveolar gas and capillary blood flows in the lungs. With other factors being constant, increases in gas flow (ventilation) with respect to blood flow (perfusion) augment pulmonary capillary and arterial P_{O_2}. Conversely, decreases in the ventilation/perfusion ratio decrease pulmonary capillary and arterial P_{O_2}. Regional differences in ventilation/perfusion ratios exist in normal lungs. When exaggerated, these differences cause hypoxemia. To un-

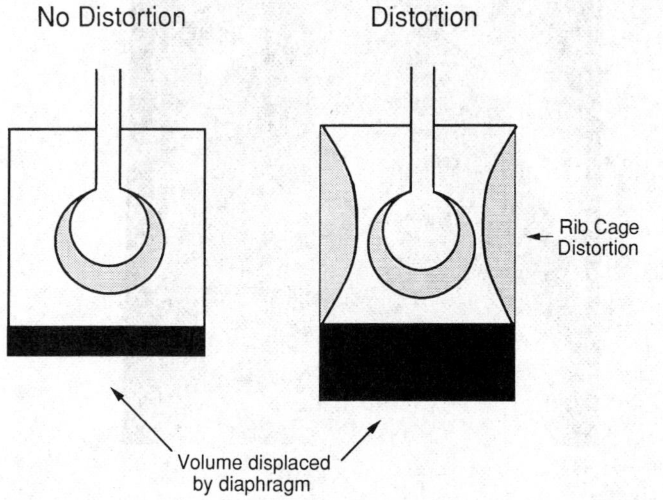

Figure 321–7. Schematic representation of the effects of rib cage distortion on the volume displaced by the diaphragm during inspiration. During a nondistorted inspiration, the volume displaced by the diaphragm is analogous to the tidal volume that enters the lungs. However, during a distorted inspiration, the volume displaced by the diaphragm must increase in proportion to the inward movement of the rib cage to maintain tidal volume unchanged. (From Pérez Fontán JJ: Mechanical dysfunction of the respiratory system. *In:* Fuhrman BP, Zimmerman JJ [eds]: Pediatric Critical Care. St. Louis, MO, Mosby–Year Book, 1992.)

derstand the mechanism, it is important to recognize that areas with a low ventilation/perfusion ratio cause more of a decrease in arterial oxygenation than areas with a high ventilation/perfusion ratio increase it. The reason is that in areas with a low ventilation/perfusion ratio, the hemoglobin-oxygen dissociation curve favors large decreases in the oxygen saturation and content of the capillary blood with small decrements in PO_2. In areas with a high ventilation/perfusion ratio, on the other hand, the oxygen saturation and content in the capillaries changes little, even with large increases in PO_2. As a result, when the oxygen-desaturated blood from areas with a low ventilation/perfusion ratio mixes with oxygenated blood from other areas in the pulmonary veins, the overall oxygen saturation and PO_2 are lower than normal.

Even though the air-blood barrier in the lungs has a lower diffusion conductance for oxygen than for carbon dioxide, the arterial PO_2 is close to the alveolar PO_2 because there is normally enough time for equilibration of oxygen between alveolar gas and capillary blood. However, respiratory disease frequently increases the alveolar-arterial PO_2 difference. This increase is caused by a variable combination of true intrapulmonary shunt in areas where the ventilation/perfusion ratio is zero (alveolar collapse) and ventilation/perfusion mismatch. Diffusion impairment may contribute to hypoxemia in interstitial lung disease in adults, but its contribution is questionable in childhood diseases. The alveolar-arterial PO_2 difference can be calculated at the bedside to quantify the amount of gas exchange impairment by measuring the arterial PO_2 and estimating the alveolar PO_2 (PAO_2) as

$$PAO_2 = PIO_2 - PACO_2/0.8,$$

where PIO_2 represents the partial pressure of inspired oxygen, $PACO_2$ is the arterial partial pressure of carbon dioxide (considered equivalent to the alveolar partial pressure), and 0.8 approximates the normal value of the respiratory quotient (carbon dioxide production/oxygen consumption). The alveolar-arterial PO_2 difference varies with age and is usually less than 5–6 mm Hg in room air for the adolescent and is slightly larger for the younger child and infant. This difference is caused by normal shunt pathways between the pulmonary and systemic circulations. In the term newborn, and particularly in the premature infant, the alveolar-arterial PO_2 difference is even greater. Possible explanations are the larger diffusion distance between the immature saccules and saccular capillaries, heterogeneity of ventilation/perfusion ratios, and airway closure in the supine position.

Bryan AC, Wohl MEB: Respiratory mechanics in children. *In:* Macklem PT, Mead J (eds): The Respiratory System: Mechanics of Breathing. Bethesda, MD, American Physiological Society, 1986, pp 179–191.
Joint Committee of the American Thoracic Society Asembly on Pediatrics and the European Respiratory Society Pediatrics Assembly: Respiratory mechanics in infants: Physiologic evaluation in health and disease. Am Rev Resp Dis 147:474, 1993.
Rysconi F, Castagneto M, Gagliardi L, et al: Reference values for respiratory rate in the first 3 years of life. Pediatrics 94:350, 1994.
Weibel ER: The Pathway for Oxygen: Structure and Function of the Mammalian Respiratory System. Cambridge, MA, Harvard University Press, 1984.
West JB: Ventilation/Blood Flow and Gas Exchange. Oxford, Blackwell Scientific, 1990.

321.1 Diagnostic Approach to Respiratory Disease

Carefully obtained family and personal histories are essential in the diagnosis of respiratory system diseases. Only after the history is obtained can the physical findings be interpreted with a good chance of arriving at the correct diagnosis.

PHYSICAL EXAMINATION. Respiratory dysfunction usually produces detectable alterations in the pattern of breathing. Respiratory control abnormalities may cause the child to breathe at a low rate or periodically. Mechanical abnormalities, on the other hand, produce compensatory changes that are generally directed at maintaining or increasing ventilation. These changes include variable increases in the breathing rate, chest wall retractions, and nasal flaring. Children with restrictive disease breathe at faster rates, and their respiratory excursions are shallow. An expiratory grunt is common, as the child attempts to raise the functional residual capacity by closing the glottis at the end of expiration. Children with obstructive disease take slower, deeper breaths. When the obstruction is extrathoracic (from the nose to the midtrachea), inspiration is more prolonged than expiration, and an inspiratory stridor can usually be heard. When the obstruction is intrathoracic, expiration is more ostensibly prolonged and the patient often has to make use of accessory expiratory muscles. Lung percussion is usually dull in restrictive lung disease and tympanitic in obstructive disease but has limited value in small infants because it cannot discriminate between noises originating from tissues that are close to each other. Auscultation confirms the presence of inspiratory and expiratory prolongation and provides information about the symmetry and quality of air movement. In addition, it often detects abnormal or adventitious sounds such as *stridor* (a predominant inspiratory monophonic noise, usually caused by upper airway obstruction), *rales* or *crackles* (high pitch, interrupted sounds found during inspiration and more rarely during early expiration, which denote opening of previously closed air spaces), or *wheezes* (musical, continuous sounds usually caused by the development of turbulent flow in narrow airway areas).

BLOOD GAS ANALYSIS (See Chapter 324). Cyanosis is influenced by skin perfusion and blood hemoglobin concentration, and is therefore an unreliable sign of hypoxemia. Arterial hypertension, tachycardia, and diaphoresis are late and by no means exclusive signs of hypoventilation. Blood gas exchange is evaluated most accurately by the direct measurement of arterial PO_2, PCO_2, and pH. Although these measurements have no substitute in many conditions, they require arterial puncture and have been replaced to a great extent by noninvasive monitoring. Arterial oxygenation, for instance, can be estimated from skin surface Po_2 determinations, but these are influenced by skin perfusion. Pulse oximetry is used for continuous assessment of arterial oxygen saturation; it has the advantage of providing information about total oxygen content of the arterial blood but is insensitive in the presence of poor perfusion (shock) and to changes in Po_2 at high saturations and inaccurate at low saturations. Arterial Pco_2 can be inferred from end-tidal carbon dioxide concentrations. This method requires some cooperation and is inaccurate in small infants, when the ventilatory rate is high. In addition, it underestimates arterial Pco_2 in the presence of ventilation heterogeneity and is therefore of limited value in patients with asthma, bronchiolitis, and other forms of bronchial obstruction.

The age and clinical condition of the patient need to be taken into account when interpreting blood gas tensions. With the exception of neonates, values of arterial Po_2 lower than 85 mm Hg are usually abnormal for a child breathing room air at sea level. Calculation of the alveolar-arterial oxygen gradient is useful in the analysis of arterial oxygenation, particularly when the patient is not breathing room air or in the presence of hypercarbia. Values of arterial Pco_2 exceeding 45 mm Hg usually indicate hypoventilation or severe ventilation/perfusion mismatch, unless they reflect respiratory compensation for metabolic alkalosis.

RESPIRATORY FUNCTION TESTING (see Chapter 324). The measurement of respiratory function in infants and young children may be difficult by lack of cooperation. Attempts have been made to overcome this limitation by creating standard tests that do not require the patient's active participation (see Chapter 324). Respiratory function tests still provide only a partial insight into the mechanisms of respiratory disease at early ages.

Whether restrictive or obstructive, most forms of respiratory disease cause alterations in lung volume and its subdivision (see Fig. 321–2). Restrictive diseases typically decrease total lung capacity (TLC), which is the total volume of gas contained in the lungs at the end of a maximal inspiration. TLC includes residual volume (the volume of gas contained in the lungs at the end of a forced expiration), which is not accessible to direct determinations. It must therefore be measured indirectly by gas dilution methods or, preferably, by plethysmography. Restrictive disease also decreases vital capacity (VC), which is the total amount of gas that can be inhaled after a forced expiration. VC can be measured by spirometry and is commonly used at the bedside to assess the progression of neuromuscular disorders. Obstructive diseases produce gas trapping and thus increase residual volume and function residual capacity (RC, the volume contained in the lungs at the end of a tidal expiration), particularly when these measurements are considered with respect to TLC.

Measurements of elastic recoil and respiratory compliance require knowledge of the lung volume at which the measurements were made in order to be properly interpreted. Similarly, measurements of airway and total respiratory resistance are technically cumbersome and difficult to interpret because of the large and variable contribution of the upper airway (nose, pharynx, and larynx) and lung and chest wall tissues to these resistances.

Airway obstruction is more frequently evaluated from determinations of gas flow in the course of a forced expiratory maneuver. The peak expiratory flow is reduced in advanced obstructive disease. The wide availability of simple devices that perform this measurement at the bedside makes it useful for assessing children with airway obstruction. Evaluation of peak flows requires a voluntary effort and peak flows may not be altered when the obstruction is moderate or mild. Other gas flow measurements require that the child inhale to TLC and then exhale as far and as fast as possible for several seconds. Cooperation and good muscle strength are therefore necessary for the measurements to be reproducible. The forced expiratory volume in 1 sec (FEV_1) correlates well with the severity of obstructive diseases. The maximal midexpiratory flow rate, the average flow over the middle 50% of the forced vital capacity, is a more reliable indicator of mild airway obstruction. Its sensitivity to changes in residual volume and vital capacity, however, limits its use in children with more severe disease. The construction of flow-volume relationships during the forced vital capacity maneuvers overcomes some of these limitations by expressing the expiratory flows as a function of lung volume.

VENTILATION/PERFUSION STUDIES. The ventilation/perfusion ratio can be examined in children with the help of radionuclide tracers (Chapter 324).

EXERCISE TESTING. Exercise testing is a more direct approach to detect diffusion impairment as well as other forms of respiratory disease. Measurements of heart and respiratory rate, minute ventilation, oxygen consumption, carbon dioxide production, and arterial blood gases during incremental exercise loads often provide invaluable information about the functional nature of the disease. Often a simple assessment of the patient's exercise tolerance in conjunction with other more static forms of respiratory function testing may allow a distinction between respiratory and nonrespiratory disease in children.

SLEEP STUDIES. The sleep state has an important influence on respiratory function, particularly in the newborn and young infant. Polysomnographic studies are often helpful when abnormalities of central respiratory control, muscular disorders, or respiratory complications from gastroesophageal reflux are suspected. These studies, which usually include the simultaneous assessment of ventilatory effort, airway gas flow, gas exchange, and sleep state, are also useful in the diagnosis and management of nocturnal hypoxemia and hypercarbia in children with chronic respiratory disease.

CHAPTER 322

Respiratory Failure

Gabriel G. Haddad and J. Julio Pérez Fontán

Respiratory failure is defined by alterations in the arterial Po_2 and Pco_2. This approach is convenient because blood gas analysis is readily available and easy to interpret. In addition, arterial Po_2 and Pco_2 are tightly regulated by the central nervous system based on the information provided by a complex system of sensors; consequently alterations in their values usually indicate that the mechanisms that execute the regulation are either overwhelmed by the disease or have failed. Defining respiratory failure on the basis of gas exchange alone may have disadvantages. Blood gas tensions alone can be easily misinterpreted. Arterial Po_2 may be normal if the subject is breathing increased inspired oxygen concentrations or decreased without alterations in respiratory function if there is an intracardiac right-to-left shunt. Arterial Pco_2 can also be elevated as a compensatory mechanism in patients with chronic metabolic alkalosis, also in the absence of intrinsic respiratory impairment. Blood gas analysis requires time and should not delay the initiation of lifesaving therapy.

PATHOPHYSIOLOGY. Gas exchange alterations in respiratory failure result from abnormalities either in the mechanical function of the lungs and chest wall or in the respiratory control. Distinguishing between these two possibilities is relatively easy. Mechanical abnormalities typically increase both the ventilatory requirements and the physical effort required to fulfill these requirements. The patient therefore develops tachypnea and rib cage distortion (retractions), makes excessive use of the accessory muscles of respiration (sternocleidomastoid, abdominal muscles), and offers an overall impression of air hunger (dyspnea) resulting from chemoreceptor stimulation and increased respiratory drive. Control abnormalities, on the other hand, are almost always associated with decreased respiratory drive, and therefore produce few or no signs of respiratory difficulty, even in the presence of considerable derangements in gas exchange.

Respiratory failure in children is caused more frequently by abnormalities in the mechanical function of the lungs and the chest wall than by control abnormalities. Both restrictive and obstructive disease increase the work of breathing and therefore raise the energetic demands of the respiratory muscles. If these demands are met, the mechanical abnormality remains compensated. If, on the other hand, the demands exceed the capabilities of the respiratory muscles, respiratory failure develops. In this regard, it is useful to conceive the interplay between work and energy demands as a balance, with the work of breathing on one side and the energy available to the contractile machinery of the respiratory muscles on the other side (Fig. 322–1). The position of the fulcrum depends on the efficiency of the system. Under normal circumstances, energy availability greatly exceeds energy demands and even substantial increases in the work of breathing can be compensated. However, when efficiency is reduced by rib cage distortion, overinflation of the lungs, or respiratory muscle fatigue, insufficient energy is transformed into work and the balance moves in the direction of respiratory failure.

Recognizing the mechanisms that compensate for the increases in the work of breathing is just as important as blood gas analysis for the diagnosis and management of respiratory failure. These mechanisms involve an increased effort on the part of the respiratory muscles. Because the diaphragm, intercostal, and other respiratory muscles are skeletal muscles, their properties are similar to those of the arm and leg muscles used for lifting weights or running. Hence, they can fatigue; the diaphragm can actually fail and stop generating the pressures and ventilation needed to keep up with carbon dioxide production. Although debated, it is possible that neonates have an increased propensity of respiratory muscle fatigue. This probably relates to decreased efficiency caused by mechanical factors such as the high compliance of their chest wall and the small surface of apposition of their diaphragm to the rib cage, rather than to the well-documented maturational changes in the intrinsic properties of the respiratory muscles themselves.

Respiratory muscles can generate enormous pressures and sustain large increases in work for a prolonged period of time; nonetheless, failure of respiratory muscles can occur. Particularly susceptible are the newborn and small infant and children of all ages with malnutrition, decreased perfusion, electrolyte disorders, and hypophosphatemia. Reversing malnutrition, improving blood flow and substrate delivery, and correcting electrolyte abnormalities are therefore important steps to maintain the force-generating ability of the respiratory muscles and to delay respiratory failure. Such considerations are critical in chronic diseases, such as asthma, cystic fibrosis, and bronchopulmonary dysplasia, and in patients being weaned from prolonged ventilatory support.

The muscles of respiration are not just limited to the chest wall and diaphragm. The muscles of the pharynx and larynx, for instance, have a major role in maintaining airway patency during breathing. When these muscles lack appropriate tone, the upper airway collapses during inspiration and sleep apnea/hypoventilation results (see Chapter 330). The diaphragm and the chest wall muscles are, in this case, not in synchrony with the activity of other respiratory muscles and indeed their action is not useful because it is not being translated into ventilation. It is the interaction between these various respiratory muscles that determines the patency of the airways and the amount of flow and ventilation that will be generated.

ETIOLOGY. Frequently, acute respiratory failure occurs in patients who are known to have mild to moderately severe chronic pulmonary disease with normal arterial carbon dioxide

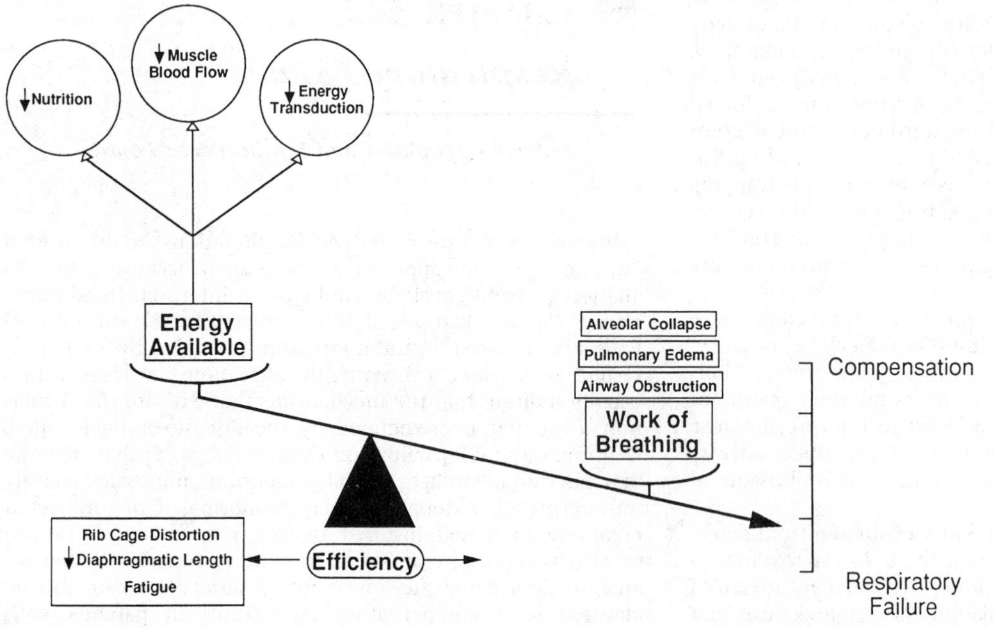

Figure 322–1. Schematic representation of the factors that determine the development of respiratory failure in the presence of abnormalities in the mechanical function of the respiratory system. The balance between the energy available for conversion into work by the respiratory muscles and the work that these muscles must perform depends on the efficiency with which the work is performed. Disease-related abnormalities, such as alveolar collapse, pulmonary edema, and airway obstruction, increase the work of breathing. Similarly, decreased availability of nutrients in malnutrition or when muscle blood flow is limited as well as intrinsic alterations in the transduction of energy by the muscles reduce the energy available. Under these circumstances, decreases in the efficiency of the system caused by rib cage distortion, lung overinflation (which decreases the length of the diaphragmatic fibers), or fatigue can easily displace the fulcrum to the left, precipitating respiratory failure. (From Lister G, Pérez Fontán JJ: Congenital heart disease. *In:* Loughlin GM, Eigen H [eds]: Respiratory Disease in Children: Diagnosis and Management. Baltimore, Williams & Wilkins, 1994.)

tension. During an intercurrent acute illness (e.g., RSV, influenza), such a patient may deteriorate rapidly and develop hypercapnia. Previously well children may also develop acute respiratory failure as a result of pneumonia, epiglottitis or other cause of upper airway obstruction, status asthmaticus, aspiration (including near-drowning), multisystem organ dysfunction with the adult respiratory distress syndrome (see Chapter 60), severe heart failure, or other causes of pulmonary edema (see Chapter 355), and certain poisonings. Patients with cystic fibrosis, bronchopulmonary dysplasia (BPD), or severe scoliosis often develop acute respiratory failure following surgery. Acute central nervous system disease may cause respiratory failure by interfering with the central control of breathing. Severe muscle disease and thoracic abnormalities may result in respiratory failure because of inadequate alveolar ventilation.

CLINICAL MANIFESTATIONS AND DIAGNOSIS. The limited ability of the developing respiratory system to compensate for disease-induced mechanical abnormalities makes the early recognition of respiratory failure essential. Respiratory failure should be anticipated rather than recognized so that alterations in gas exchange can be prevented.

During physical examination, the clinician should avoid interfering with the patient's own mechanisms of compensation. An awake child with upper airway obstruction caused by croup or epiglottitis, for instance, may be more stable in a mother's arms because the increased gas flows generated during crying make breathing mechanically inefficient and can precipitate failure. Similarly, most patients with severe restrictive and obstructive disease tolerate the supine position poorly because the weight of the abdominal organs imposes an additional burden on the diaphragm.

The physical examination is useful in the evaluation of children with respiratory disease (see Chapter 321). In a child suspected of respiratory failure, this evaluation should always start with a quick assessment of the adequacy of ventilation. This assessment includes the presence and vigor of the respiratory movements, breathing rate, extent of the respiratory movements, the presence of cyanosis, and the presence of signs of upper airway obstruction. A child with grossly inadequate respiratory efforts or complete airway obstruction will not survive long unless ventilation of the lungs is restored immediately. In addition, special attention must be paid to the patient's state of conciousness. Hypoxemia and hypercarbia frequently cause lethargy and confusion alternating with agitation. Whether resulting from these or other concurrent mechanisms, central nervous system depression requires immediate attention because it further limits the ability of the respiratory system to deal with mechanical loads and leaves the airway unprotected against obstruction and aspiration of foreign materials.

The patient is usually hyperpneic and cyanotic, and may use the accessory muscles of respiration; most sit up and lean forward to improve leverage for the accessory muscles and to allow easy diaphragmatic movement. Symptoms and signs of the underlying disease are also present. A $Paco_2$ of over 40 mm Hg suggests the possibility of developing acute respiratory failure, and a $Paco_2$ of 50 mm Hg or higher suggests it is imminent. Most patients with acute hypercapnia also have a Pao_2 below 55 mm Hg in room air, suggesting that the oxygen content of the blood may be inadequate to meet the normal needs of the vital organs. Furthermore, at $Paco_2$ levels above 54 mm Hg, diaphragmatic function may be impaired, accelerating the patient's decline.

Acute hypoxemia and hypercapnia result in dilatation of the cerebral blood vessels and increased blood flow, often accompanied by severe headache. The sudden increased work of the accessory muscles of breathing may result in severe lower back pain. Although moderate to severe hypercapnia can cause peripheral vasodilatation, mild to moderate hypoxemia can cause peripheral vasoconstriction, and the patient may complain of cold extremities. Other symptoms of hypoxia include restlessness, dizziness, and impaired thought.

Acute respiratory failure can also result in characteristic multisystem complications. These include gastrointestinal hemorrhage ("stress" ulcer), cardiac arrhythmias (supraventricular arrhythmias), renal failure, and malnutrition.

TREATMENT. The goal of treatment of respiratory failure is the restoration of adequate gas exchange with a minimum of complications. This is achieved by eliminating as quickly as possible the initiating factors. Specific therapy of the initiating and/or underlying disease is essential. Thus respiratory failure caused by cardiogenic pulmonary edema is treated with inotropic medications and diuretics. The child with asthma should be managed with bronchodilators and anti-inflammatory medications. Unfortunately, even in acute illnesses such as these, the response to the treatment is not immediate and frequently the entire function of the respiratory system must be artificially supported.

Hypoxemia is more dangerous than hypercarbia and may be easier to correct. Administration of supplemental oxygen is a safe and wise precaution in all patients at risk for respiratory failure, even if there is no initial evidence of hypoxemia. Oxygen can be administered with face masks, nasal cannulas, hoods, or tents. Face masks are usually not well tolerated by frightened infants and children. Hoods provide more consistent inspired oxygen concentrations than any other device, but they are bulky and limit access to the patient. For this reason, they have limited applicability in the initial treatment in the emergency room.

The indication for ventilatory support in a child with respiratory failure is usually based on the persistence or worsening of gas exchange abnormalities. Mechanical ventilation is necessary in a child with pneumonia who develops severe hypoxemia and hypercarbia because even the most effective antibiotic therapy requires time. On occasion, ventilatory support must be instituted in the absence of alterations in the arterial Pco_2 and Pco_2 when the dysfunction of other systems places gas exchange at jeopardy by severely limiting the compensatory ability of the respiratory system. Cardiovascular shock is a typical example. In this condition, decreased blood flow and substrate delivery to the respiratory muscles may reduce the force that these muscles can develop and can precipitate respiratory failure, even in the absence of substantial mechanical abnormalities of the respiratory system.

Ventilatory support usually (but not always) requires intubation of the trachea with an endotracheal tube or less often a tracheostomy cannula. Regardless of the type of ventilator, the objective of mechanical ventilation is not to normalize arterial blood gas tensions but rather to provide "adequate" gas exchange. The definition of what is "adequate" has changed substantially. At present, there is reasonable consensus among those treating critically ill children that some degree of hypercarbia and hypoxemia is acceptable in order to minimize oxygen- and stretch-induced lung injury. Moderate (permissive) hypercarbia (Pco_2 60–80 mm Hg) has no detectable negative consequences over short periods of time, in part because its effects on the arterial pH are reduced through renal retention of bicarbonate. Moderate hypoxemia (oxygen saturation 85–90%) is similarly well tolerated in otherwise stable patients, particularly if the hemoglobin concentration and the cardiac output are maintained at physiological values and conditions such as fever and agitation, which increase tissue oxygen demands, are avoided. Artificial-mechanical ventilation is usually initiated with conventional volume-driven ventilators; high frequency jet or oscillator ventilators are often used as rescue therapy if conventional ventilators fail to improve oxygenation.

Extracorporeal membrane oxygenation (ECMO) and/or carbon dioxide removal is employed in the treatment of newborns and small infants with life-threatening, refractory respiratory failure that is unresponsive to mechanical ventilation and is expected to resolve in a short period of time (see Chapter 87). ECMO uses an artificial membrane to regulate the oxygen and carbon dioxide content of blood diverted from the patient's central veins. The treated blood is then returned with the help of an artificial pump to the arterial (veno-arterial) or venous (veno-venous) circulation. Because of its risks (from vascular cannulation and anticoagulation) and the fact that its benefits over conventional management in non-neonatal patients have not been unequivocally demonstrated, indications for extracorporeal gas exchange should be contemplated with a great deal of caution. Inhaled nitric oxide may acutely improve oxygenation by reducing increased pulmonary vascular resistance.

Abman SH, Griebel JL, Parker DK, et al: Acute effects of inhaled nitric oxide in children with severe hypoxemic respiratory failure. J Pediatr 124:881, 1994.
Arnold JH, Truog RD, Thompson JE, et al: High-frequency oscillatory ventilation in pediatric respiratory failure. Crit Care Med 21:272, 1993.
Davis SL, Furman DP, Costarino AT: Adult respiratory distress syndrome in children: Associated disease, clinical course, and predictors of death. J Pediatr 123:35, 1993.
DeBruin W, Notterman DA, Magid M, et al: Acute hypoxemic respiratory failure in infants and children: Clinical and pathologic characteristics. Crit Care Med 20:1223, 1992.
Moler FW, Custer JR, Bartlett RH, et al: Extracorporeal life support for severe pediatric respiratory failure: An updated experience 1991–1993. J Pediatr 124:875, 1994.

CHAPTER 323

Defense Mechanisms and Metabolic Functions of the Lung

Gabriel G. Haddad and J. Julio Pérez Fontán

323.1 Defense Mechanisms

The *upper airway* includes the nose, paranasal sinuses, and pharynx; the *lower airway* consists of the remainder of the system from the larynx peripherally. The nose has a relatively large surface area lined with a richly vascular, ciliated epithelium, and by the time the air column reaches the bifurcation of the trachea, up to 75% of the warming and humidification of the inspired air has occurred. During exhalation, heat and moisture are removed from the air stream. Gross filtering of particles larger than 10–15 μm is achieved by the coarse hairs at the nasal orifices, and most inhaled particles larger than 5 μm are impacted on the nasal surface.

Because the larynx is relatively narrow and ringed with cartilage, it is relatively susceptible to obstruction in young children, particularly by inflammation, because the resultant swelling of tissues rapidly encroaches on the lumen and produces inspiratory stridor.

The trachea and bronchi are lined with pseudostratified, ciliated, columnar epithelium and occasional goblet cells. Mucous glands occupy approximately one third the thickness of the airway wall and for the most part lie between the epithelial surface and the cartilage. The trachea is supported by incomplete rings of cartilage with a muscular membrane posteriorly. Irregular plates of cartilage support the bronchi, especially at bifurcations. These diminish and finally disappear in the smallest bronchi. The goblet cells and principally the submucosal glands secrete the mucous layer, which is 2–5 μm in depth and rests on the tips of the cilia. Each ciliated cell has about 275 cilia; movement results from action by microtubules within each cilium. The cilia beat within a periciliary fluid layer at about 1,000 beats/min, moving the mucous blanket toward the pharynx at a rate of approximately 10 mm/min in the trachea. In the respiratory portion of the lung the surface cells gradually become cuboidal and then flat; ciliated cells and goblet cells are usually absent.

The final 25% of the warming and humidifying of the inspired air stream occurs in the trachea and large bronchi. Failure of humidification permits dry air to reach more distal airways. Particles 1–5 μm in size precipitate out on the tracheobronchial mucous blanket so that only particles of 1 μm or less reach the respiratory bronchioles and air spaces, where some may deposit and many will be exhaled.

Respiratory tract secretions are derived primarily from mucous (glycoproteins) and serous cells of the submucosal glands that empty onto the surface epithelium; from goblet cells and Clara cells, the special secreting cells in the surface epithelium of bronchi and bronchioles, respectively; from transudation from the vascular space; and from alveolar fluid, which contributes most of the phospholipid found in tracheobronchial mucus. This mucus is about 95% water.

Beyond infancy, collateral alveolar ventilation can increasingly occur with development of the *pores of Kohn* between alveoli, which provide a means for gas to pass from one lobule to another, perhaps even between segments of lung. Bronchiolar-alveolar communications, known as the *canals of Lambert*, are also found. These anatomic connections may be helpful in preventing or delaying atelectasis.

The defenses of the respiratory system that protect the lung include the filtering of particles, the warming and humidification of inspired air, and the absorption of noxious fumes and gases by the vascular upper airway. The temporary cessation of breathing, reflexly shallow breathing, laryngospasm, or even bronchospasm limits the depth and amount of penetration of foreign matter. Spasm or decreased breathing can provide only brief protection. Aspiration of food, secretions, and foreign bodies are prevented by swallowing and closure of the epiglottis. The respiratory tract distal to the larynx is normally sterile.

CLEARANCE OF PARTICLES. Particles deposited in conducting airways are cleared within hours by the mucociliary mechanism, while clearance of those reaching the alveoli may take several days to months. The latter may be phagocytized by alveolar macrophages and removed from lungs by the mucociliary system or carried into the interstitium for clearance by the lymphocytes into regional nodes or the blood. Some particles penetrate into the interstitium without phagocytosis. Mucociliary clearance may be aided by cough, which provides an effective means by propelling excess mucus up the airways at pressures of up to 300 mm Hg and at flows of up to 5–6 L/sec. Mucus raised by the cough mechanism is usually swallowed by young children but may be expectorated.

DEFENSE AGAINST MICROBIAL AGENTS. Phagocytosis and mucociliary clearance may not be sufficient protection from living agents, such as bacteria and viruses. Additional factors include cellular killing of organisms and immune responses to assist in the phagocytosis-killing process. Alveolar and interstitial macrophages, derived from monocytes, are an essential component of the defense system of the lung. The engulfment and killing of living particles by these macrophages may be enhanced by opsonins or by small lymphocytes. The principal antibody in respiratory secretions is secretory immunoglobulin A (IgA), which is produced by plasma cells in the submucosa of the airways (see Chapter 116). Two molecules of IgA combine with a polypeptide (secretory component) produced by the respiratory epithelium to yield secretory IgA, which is highly resistant to digestion by proteolytic enzymes released after lysis of bacteria and dead cells. IgA can neutralize certain viruses and toxins, and help in the lysis of bacteria. IgA may also prevent antigenic substances from penetrating the epithelial surfaces. Pulmonary secretory IgA reaches adult levels in the first month of life. IgG and IgM are also found in the secretions when lung inflammation occurs.

Lysozyme, lactoferrin, and interferon may also play a defense role in respiratory secretions. In addition, a small fraction of the antibodies of the respiratory surface is made up of immunoglobulin E (IgE), which plays an important role in allergic reactions (Chapter 133).

IMPAIRED DEFENSE MECHANISMS. The phagocytic ability of alveolar macrophages and, in most cases, the mucociliary mechanism can be impaired by ethanol ingestion, cigarette smoke, hypoxemia, starvation, chilling, corticosteroids, nitrogen dioxide, ozone, increased oxygen concentration, narcotics, and some anesthetic gases. The antibacterial killing capacity of the macrophages can be decreased by acidosis, azotemia, and recent acute viral infections, especially rubeola and influenza. Beryllium and asbestos, organic dust from cotton and sugar cane, and gases such as sulfur, nitrogen dioxide, ozone, chlorine, ammonia, and cigarette smoke, are toxic to epithelial cells.

Mucociliary clearance can be reduced by hypothermia, hyperthermia, morphine, codeine, and hypothyroidism. Inhalation of dry gas by mouth breathing during periods of nasal obstruction, after placement of a tracheostomy, or during use of poorly humidified oxygen results in drying of the mucous membrane and slowing of the ciliary beat. Cold air may irritate the tracheobronchial tree.

Damage to the respiratory epithelium may be reversible with rhinitis, sinusitis, bronchitis, bronchiolitis, acute respiratory infections associated with high levels of air pollution, and the epithelial shedding that can occur in asthma, or with some irritants, bronchospasm, edema, congestion, and perhaps mild surface ulceration. However, severe ulceration, bronchiectasis, bronchiolectasis, squamous cell metaplasia, and fibrosis represent serious injury and permanent impairment of the normal clearance mechanism. Other events that can adversely affect the lung include hyperventilation, alveolar hypoxia, pulmonary thromboembolism, pulmonary edema, hypersensitivity reactions, and certain drugs such as salicylates.

Newhouse MT, Bienenstock J: Respiratory tract defense mechanisms. *In*: Baum GL, Wolinsky E (eds): Textbook of Pulmonary Diseases. Boston, Little, Brown, 1989, pp 21–47.
Proctor DF: The upper airways. I: Nasal physiology and defense of the lungs. Am Rev Respir Dis 115:97, 1977.

323.2 Metabolic Functions

The lung contains more than 40 separate cell types. Among these heterogeneous cells, the type I and II pneumocytes, alveolar macrophage, and Clara cell are unique to the lung. The lung can synthesize lipids and proteins, including glycoproteins, secretory antibodies, interferon, proteolytic and fibrinolytic enzymes and activators, collagen, and elastin. Tissue factors such as thromboplastin are found in higher concentration in the lung than in any other organ. Megakaryocytes are concentrated in the lung.

The large alveolar type II pneumocyte synthesizes and releases lung surfactant. Injury to this cell or deficiency in this surfactant pathway results in neonatal respiratory distress syndrome (Chapter 87). A major function of surfactant is to stabilize alveolar air spaces by attenuating surface forces and decreasing their unevenness. Another cell type, the neuroepithelial cell, is present at the airway bifurcation and found in larger proportion in early life. These cells are serotonin rich and have transmitter vesicles that are depleted when exposed to low inhaled O_2 concentration. These cells sense O_2 in the airways through plasma membrane K^+ channels. How they affect respiratory output is not clear at present, although these cells can send afferent information to the central nervous system via the vagus nerve.

Because the lung has the only capillary bed through which the entire blood flow must pass in the normal state, the pulmonary capillary circulation is ideally positioned to control circulating vasoactive hormones. Angiotensin II, up to 50 times more active than its precursor, is converted from angiotensin I during one passage through the pulmonary circulation. Some vasoactive materials, including serotonin, bradykinin, ATP, and prostaglandins E_1, E_2, and F_2, are almost completely removed or inactivated by one passage through the pulmonary circulation, whereas others, such as epinephrine, prostaglandin A_1 and A_2, angiotensin II, and vasopressin, may be minimally affected. Norepinephrine and histamine are taken up to a moderate degree. Failure of inactivation or periodic release of substances such as serotonin, bradykinin, histamine, slow-reacting substance of anaphylaxis (SRS-A), eosinophil chemotactic factor, platelet aggregation factor, endocrine substances, and so forth, may be important in the pathogenesis of some pulmonary disease or as a mediator of secondary effects. These chemicals can contribute to systemic and pulmonary hypertension, systemic hypotension, and pulmonary edema.

Fishman AP: Non-respiratory functions of the lung. Chest 72:84, 1977.
Said SI: The lung in relation to vasoactive hormones. Fed Proc 32:1972, 1973.

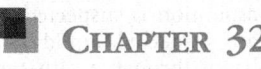

CHAPTER 324
Diagnostic Procedures

Robert E. Wood

RADIOGRAPHIC TECHNIQUES

CHEST ROENTGENOGRAMS. Whenever possible, a posteroanterior and a lateral view (upright and in full inspiration), should be obtained. Portable films, while useful, may give a somewhat distorted image. Expiratory films may easily be misinterpreted, although a comparison of expiratory and inspiratory films may be useful in the evaluation of a child with suspected foreign body (localized failure of the lung to empty reflects bronchial obstruction). If pleural fluid is suspected, decubitus films are indicated. Films taken in a recumbent position are difficult to interpret if there is fluid within the pleural space or a cavity. Oblique views may be advantageous when evaluating the hilum and the area behind the heart, while the apices are best seen in a lordotic view.

COMPUTED TOMOGRAPHY AND MAGNETIC RESONANCE IMAGING. Computed tomography (CT) delineates the internal structure of the thorax in much greater detail than is possible with plain roentgenograms. Technical advances have greatly enhanced the utility of this diagnostic modality (even three-dimensional reconstruction is often feasible), while scan times and radiation exposure have been markedly reduced. CT scans are of particular importance in the evaluation of mediastinal and pleural lesions, solid or cystic parenchymal lesions, and suspected bronchiectasis. Intravenous contrast material can be infused during the scan to enhance vascular structures.

Magnetic resonance imaging (MRI) may be useful for the same disease entities as CT. MRI is an excellent procedure to delineate hilar and vascular anatomy associated with vascular rings or slings.

UPPER AIRWAY FILMS. A lateral view of the neck can yield invaluable information about upper airway obstruction and particularly about the conditions of the retropharyngeal space, supraglottic area, and subglottic space (the latter should also be viewed in a posteroanterior projection). Knowing the phase of respiration during which the film was taken is often essential for accurate interpretation. Patients with suspected obstruction must not be sent unattended to the radiology department.

SINUS, NASAL FILMS. Roentgenographic examination of the sinuses is indicated when sinus disease is suspected. A CT scan will give the most information. Because of the small size and slow development of the frontal and maxillary sinus cavities in children, transillumination is not as successful in documenting sinus disease as are roentgenograms. The need for examining the nasal passages in children is unusual and occurs most often when the neonate presents with obstruction or when tumor or occult foreign body is suspected.

FLUOROSCOPY. Fluoroscopy is especially useful for evaluating stridor and abnormal movement of the diaphragm or mediastinum. Many procedures, such as needle aspiration or biopsy of a peripheral lesion, are also best accomplished with the aid of fluoroscopy. Videotape recording, which does not increase radiation exposure, may allow detailed study, through "replay" capability, during a brief exposure to fluoroscopy.

CONTRAST STUDIES. Barium Swallow. This study, performed with fluoroscopy and spot films, is indicated in the evaluation of patients with recurrent pneumonia, persistent cough of undetermined etiology, stridor, or persistent wheezing. The technique may be modified by using barium of different textures and thickness, ranging from thin liquid to solids, to evaluate swallowing mechanics, especially if aspiration is suspected. If an "H-type" tracheoesophageal fistula is suspected, liquid barium should be injected into the esophagus through a catheter. A contrast esophagram has been used in the evaluation of newborns with suspected esophageal atresia, but this procedure entails a high risk of pulmonary aspiration, and is not usually recommended. Barium swallows are useful in the evaluation of suspected gastroesophageal reflux, but the interpretation may not be straightforward.

Bronchograms. The details of smaller bronchi that cannot be easily evaluated by plain films or even bronchoscopy may be delineated by instilling contrast material directly into the airway. This is indicated in patients with suspected bronchiectasis or airway anomalies who are potential surgical candidates, although for most purposes, CT scanning has supplanted bronchography. Sedation and topical anesthesia, or even general anesthesia, are required; the contrast material is instilled through a catheter (or, preferably, through a flexible bronchoscope) under fluoroscopic control.

Pulmonary Arteriograms. These studies allow detailed evaluation of the pulmonary vasculature and are helpful in assessing pulmonary blood flow and in diagnosing congenital anomalies, such as lobar agenesis, unilateral hyperlucent lung, vascular rings, and arteriovenous malformations and are sometimes useful in evaluating solid or cystic lesions. Real time and Doppler echocardiography are noninvasive methods that often reveal similar information and are performed prior to arteriography.

Aortograms. Thoracic aortograms demonstrate the aortic arch and its major vessels, and the systemic (bronchial) pulmonary circulation. They are useful to evaluate vascular rings and suspected pulmonary sequestration. Although most hemoptysis is from the bronchial arteries, bronchial arteriography is seldom helpful in diagnosing or treating intrapulmonary bleeding in children. Echocardiography with or without CT or MRI is helpful in delineating some of these lesions and should be performed before aortography.

Pneumoperitoneum, Pneumothorax. In selected situations, such as in the evaluation of diaphragmatic eventration, it may be advantageous to inject a small amount of air into the pleural or peritoneal cavity, outlining the limits of the diaphragm or pleural surfaces by air contrast. Rapidly absorbed, the air causes no functional impairment.

Radionuclide Lung Scans. The usual scan uses intravenous injection of material (macroaggregated human serum albumin) that will be trapped in the pulmonary capillary bed. The distribution of radioactivity, proportional to pulmonary capillary blood flow, is useful in evaluating pulmonary embolism and congenital cardiovascular and pulmonary defects. Acute changes in the distribution of pulmonary perfusion may reflect alterations of pulmonary ventilation.

The distribution of pulmonary ventilation may be determined by scanning following the inhalation of a radioactive gas such as ^{133}Xe. After the intravenous injection of ^{133}Xe dissolved in saline, both pulmonary perfusion and ventilation can be evaluated by continuous recording of the rate of appearance and disappearance of the xenon over the lung. Appearance of xenon early after injection is a measure of perfusion, whereas the rate of washout during breathing is a measure of ventilation.

324.1 Endoscopy

LARYNGOSCOPY. Inspection of the glottis is often necessary when evaluating stridor and local upper airway abnormalities. Indirect (mirror) laryngoscopy is useful in older children and adults, but is rarely feasible in infants and small children. Direct laryngoscopy may be performed with a rigid or a flexible instrument; in either case, topical anesthesia and sedation or even general anesthesia are required for an effective and safe examination. Lesions in the subglottic space are difficult to visualize from above the level of the glottis and can easily be missed if the examination is not performed with optimal anesthesia and instrumentation. Flexible (fiberoptic) instruments have some advantage. The larynx can be examined without the anatomic distortion that a rigid laryngoscope sometimes introduces. Airway dynamics can thus be more readily appreciated. Because of the relatively high incidence of synchronous lesions in both upper and lower airways, in most cases it is prudent to examine the lower airway (bronchoscopy), even though the primary indication may be in the upper airway (stridor).

BRONCHOSCOPY. Indications for diagnostic bronchoscopy include recurrent/persistent pneumonia or atelectasis, unexplained and persistent wheezes and infiltrates, the suspected presence of a foreign body, hemoptysis, suspected congenital anomalies, mass lesions, unexplained interstitial disease, pneumonia in the immunocompromised host, or other conditions in which bronchoscopy is the best way to obtain the information necessary for the care of the patient. Indications for therapeutic bronchoscopy include bronchial obstruction by mass lesions, foreign bodies, or mucus plugs, as well as general bronchial toilet and bronchopulmonary lavage. An open tube ("rigid") bronchoscope should be used for extraction of foreign bodies, in patients with massive hemoptysis, or for removal of tissue masses. In most other cases, a flexible bronchoscope offers more utility. Flexible instruments can also be passed through endotracheal or tracheostomy tubes. In most patients, flexible bronchoscopy can be safely and effectively performed with sedation and topical anesthesia.

Complications of bronchoscopy depend on the instrument

used, the procedure performed, and the indication for the procedure. Transient hypoxia, cardiac arrhythmias, laryngospasm, and bronchospasm are the most common complications. Iatrogenic infection, bleeding, and pneumothorax or pneumomediastinum may occur. Following rigid bronchoscopy, subglottic edema is common; this is much less frequent after flexible bronchoscopy, as such instruments are smaller and are less likely to traumatize the subglottic space. Postbronchoscopy croup is treated with oxygen, mist, vasoconstrictor aerosols, and corticosteroids as necessary.

BRONCHOALVEOLAR LAVAGE. Bronchoalveolar lavage (BAL) is a method to obtain a representative specimen of fluid and secretions from the lower respiratory tract, and is useful for the cytologic and microbiologic diagnosis of lung diseases, especially in patients who are unable to expectorate sputum. BAL is performed by gently wedging a flexible bronchoscope into the desired lung segment and sequentially instilling and withdrawing sterile saline in a volume sufficient to ensure that some of the aspirated fluid contains material that originated from the alveolar surface. Nonbronchoscopic BAL can be performed in intubated patients by instilling and withdrawing saline through a catheter passed through the artificial airway and gently wedged (blindly) into a distal airway. Because the methods utilized to perform BAL involve passage through the upper airway, there is a risk of contamination of the specimen by upper airway secretions; careful cytologic examination and quantitative microbiologic cultures are important for correct interpretation of the data. BAL can often obviate the need for more invasive procedures such as open lung biopsy, especially in immunocompromised patients.

THORACOSCOPY. The pleural cavity may be examined through a thoracoscope, which is similar to a rigid bronchoscope. The thoracoscope is inserted through the intercostal space and the lung is partially deflated, thus allowing the operator to view the surface of the lung, the pleural surface of the mediastinum and diaphragm, and the parietal pleura. Multiple thoracoscopic instruments can be inserted, allowing endoscopic lung or pleural biopsy or other operative procedures. Such procedures are much less invasive than an open thoracotomy.

324.2 Thoracentesis

For diagnostic or therapeutic purposes, fluid may be removed from the pleural space by needle puncture. The site of puncture is chosen to maximize the yield of fluid and minimize the risk. The procedure is usually performed while the patient is in a sitting position. First, local anesthetic is injected using a 1.5-inch, No. 22 gauge needle passed just *above* the rib margin to avoid the neurovascular bundle. The pleura may be identified by "touch" or by withdrawing an initial volume of pleural fluid. Then a larger needle is inserted to the same depth through the inferior aspect of the intercostal space. It is often advantageous to pass a plastic catheter through the needle into the pleural space, then withdraw the needle. This allows the operator to move both catheter and patient, thus often collecting more fluid and reducing the possibility of puncture or laceration of the lung. Generally, as much fluid as possible should be withdrawn, and following the procedure an *upright* chest roentgenogram should be obtained.

Complications of thoracentesis include infection, pneumothorax, and bleeding. Thoracentesis on the right may be complicated by puncture or laceration of the capsule of the liver, and on the left, by that of the capsule of the spleen. Specimens obtained should always be cultured, examined microscopically for evidence of bacterial infection, and evaluated for total protein and total differential cell counts. Lactic acid dehydrogenase, glucose, cholesterol, triglyceride (chylous), and amylase determinations may also be useful. If malignancy is suspected, cytologic examination is imperative.

Transudates result from mechanical factors influencing the rate of formation or reabsorption of pleural fluid and generally require no further diagnostic evaluation. *Exudates* result from inflammation or other disease of the pleural surface and underlying lung and require a more complete diagnostic evaluation. In general, transudates have a total protein of less than 3 g/dL or a ratio of pleural protein to serum protein under 0.5, a total leukocyte count of fewer than 2,000 with a predominance of mononuclear cells, and low lactate dehydrogenase levels. Exudates have high protein levels and a predominance of polymorphonuclear cells (although malignant or tuberculous effusions may have a higher percentage of mononuclear cells). Complicated exudates often require continuous chest tube drainage and have a pH less than 7.20. Tuberculous effusions may have low glucose and high cholesterol content.

324.3 Percutaneous Lung Tap

Using a technique very similar to that for thoracentesis, a percutaneous lung tap is the most direct method of obtaining bacteriologic specimens from the pulmonary parenchyma and is the only technique other than open lung biopsy not associated with at least some risk of contamination by oral flora. After local anesthesia, a No. 20 or 22 gauge, 1.5-inch needle attached to a 10-mL syringe containing approximately 1 mL of nonbacteriostatic sterile saline is inserted using aseptic technique through the inferior aspect of an intercostal space in the area of interest. The needle is rapidly advanced into the lung; the saline is injected and reaspirated; and the needle is withdrawn. These actions are performed as quickly as possible. This procedure usually yields a few drops of fluid from the lung, which should be cultured and examined microscopically.

Major indications for a lung tap are roentgenographic infiltrates of undetermined etiology, especially those unresponsive to therapy in immunosuppressed patients who are susceptible to unusual organisms. Complications are the same as for thoracentesis, but the incidence of pneumothorax is higher and somewhat dependent on the nature of the underlying disease process. In patients with poor pulmonary compliance, such as with *Pneumocystis* pneumonia, the rate may approach 30%, with 5% requiring chest tubes. Bronchopulmonary lavage has replaced lung taps for most purposes.

324.4 Lung Biopsy

Lung biopsy may be the only way to establish a diagnosis, especially in protracted, noninfectious disease. In infants and small children an open surgical biopsy is the procedure of choice, and in expert hands it is associated with an extremely low morbidity. As well as ensuring that an adequate specimen can be obtained, the surgeon can inspect the lung surface and choose the site of biopsy. In older patients transbronchial biopsies can be performed using flexible forceps through an endotracheal tube or a bronchoscope, usually with fluoroscopic guidance. This technique is most appropriate when there is diffuse lung disease such as *Pneumocystis* pneumonia. However, because of the small specimens obtained, the diagnosis may be missed more easily than with an open biopsy. Lung biopsy may also be performed with a thoracoscope, depending on the location and nature of the lesion requiring biopsy.

324.5 Transillumination of the Chest Wall

In infants up to at least 6 mo of age, a pneumothorax may often be diagnosed by transillumination of the chest wall using a fiberoptic light probe. Free air in the pleural space often results in an unusually large halo of light in the skin surrounding the probe. This test is unreliable in older patients or in those with subcutaneous emphysema or atelectasis.

324.6 Microbiology

The specific diagnosis of infection in the lower respiratory tract depends on the proper handling of an adequate specimen obtained in an appropriate fashion. Nasopharyngeal or throat cultures are often used but may not correlate with cultures obtained by more direct techniques. Sputum specimens are preferred and are often obtained from patients who do not expectorate by deep throat swab immediately after coughing. Specimens may also be obtained directly from the tracheobronchial tree by nasotracheal aspiration (usually heavily contaminated), by transtracheal aspiration through the cricothyroid membrane (useful in adults and adolescents but hazardous in children), and in infants and children by a sterile catheter inserted into the trachea either during direct laryngoscopy or through an endotracheal tube. A specimen also may be obtained at bronchoscopy. A percutaneous lung tap or an open biopsy is the only way to obtain a specimen that is absolutely free of oral flora.

EXAMINATION OF SECRETIONS. A specimen obtained by direct expectoration is usually assumed to be of tracheobronchial origin, but often, especially in children, it is not from this source. The presence of alveolar macrophages—large, mononuclear cells—is the hallmark of tracheobronchial secretions. Both nasopharyngeal and tracheobronchial secretions may contain ciliated epithelial cells, which are more commonly found in sputum. Nasopharyngeal and oral secretions often contain large numbers of squamous epithelial cells. Sputum may contain both ciliated and squamous epithelial cells.

During sleep, mucociliary transport continually brings tracheobronchial secretions to the pharynx, where they are swallowed. An early morning fasting gastric aspirate often contains material from the tracheobronchial tract that is suitable for culture for acid-fast bacilli.

The absence of polymorphonuclear leukocytes in a Wright-stained smear of sputum or bronchoalveolar lavage (BAL) fluid containing adequate numbers of macrophages is significant evidence against a bacterial infectious process in the lower respiratory tract, assuming the patient has normal neutrophil counts and function. Eosinophils suggest allergic disease. Iron stains may reveal hemosiderin granules within macrophages, suggesting pulmonary hemosiderosis. Specimens should also be examined by Gram stain. Squamous epithelial cells are usually covered with bacteria, which should be ignored. Bacteria within or near macrophages and neutrophils are more significant. Viral pneumonia may be accompanied by intranuclear or cytoplasmic inclusion bodies visible on Wright-stained smears, and fungal forms may be identifiable on Gram or silver stains.

Sweat Testing

See Chapter 363.

324.7 Blood Gas Analysis

(See Chapter 321)

An arterial blood gas analysis is probably the single most useful test of pulmonary function. If multiple samples are to be drawn over a relatively short time, an indwelling arterial line may be placed; constant perfusion with heparinized saline (1 unit/mL, 3–5 mL/hr) may prevent thrombus formation.

Arterial punctures are painful, often resulting in hyperventilation unless local anesthesia is used. The artery should be entered with a No. 21 or 23 gauge straight or scalp vein needle at an angle of approximately 45 degrees. The blood specimen is best collected anaerobically in a heparinized syringe containing only enough heparin solution to displace the air from the syringe. The syringe should be sealed, placed in ice, and carried to the laboratory for immediate analysis.

Arterialized capillary blood may be used if tissue perfusion is good and if great care is taken in collecting and handling the specimen. Under ideal conditions the P_{CO_2} but not the P_{O_2} of arterialized capillary blood correlates with arterial samples. Local vasodilation is produced in the finger, the heel, or the earlobe by warming or by applying nitroglycerin or nicotinic acid cream. When the site has become flushed, blood is collected into a capillary tube from a free-flowing stab wound.

Pulse oximetry, transcutaneous O_2 and CO_2 and end-tidal CO_2 determinations are discussed in Chapter 321.

Venous P_{CO_2} averages 6–8 mm Hg higher than arterial P_{CO_2}, and pH is slightly lower. Venous samples are more useful in managing chronic acid-base disturbances than in managing acute respiratory disease.

324.8 Pulmonary Function Testing

See also Chapter 321.

Ventilation, perfusion, and gas exchange may all be quantified, but in clinical practice measurements of ventilation are the most commonly performed "pulmonary function test."

MEASUREMENT OF VENTILATORY FUNCTION. A *spirometer* is used to measure vital capacity (VC) and its subdivisions and expiratory (or inspiratory) flow rates (see Fig. 321–2). A simple *manometer* can measure the maximal inspiratory and expiratory force a subject generates, normally at least 30 cm H_2O, which is useful in evaluating the neuromuscular component of ventilation. Expected normal values for VC, FRC, TLC, and RV are obtained from prediction equations based on body height.

Flow rates measured by spirometry usually include the volume expired in the 1st sec (FEV_1) and the maximal midexpiratory flow rate (MMEF). More information results from a maximal expiratory flow-volume curve (MEFV), in which expiratory flow rate is plotted against expired lung volume (expressed in terms of either VC or TLC). Flow rates at lung volumes less than about 75% VC are relatively independent of effort. Expiratory flow rates at low lung volumes (less than 50% VC) are influenced much more by small airways than are flow rates at high lung volumes (FEV_1). The flow rate at 25% VC ($\dot{V}_{25}$) is a useful index of small airway function. Low flow rates at high lung volumes associated with normal flow at low lung volumes suggest upper airway obstruction (see Chapters 330, 331, and 332).

Airway resistance (R_{AW}) is measured in a plethysmograph and is expressed as cm H_2O/L/sec. Alternatively, the reciprocal of R_{AW}, *airway conductance* (G_{AW}), may be used. Because airway resistance measurements vary with the lung volume at which they are taken, it is convenient to use specific airway resistance, SR_{AW} ($SR_{AW} = R_{AW} \times$ lung volume), which is nearly constant in subjects older than 6 yr (normally less than 7 sec/cm H_2O).

MEASUREMENT OF GAS EXCHANGE. The *diffusing capacity for carbon monoxide* (DLCO) is related to O_2 diffusion and is measured by rebreathing from a container having a known initial concentration of CO or by using a single breath technique. Decreases in DLCO reflect decreases in effective alveolar capillary surface area or decreases in diffusibility of the gas across the alveolar-capillary membrane. This test is rarely used in pediatrics because primary diffusion abnormalities are unusual in children. *Regional gas exchange* may be conveniently estimated with the perfusion/ventilation xenon scan. Determining *arterial blood gases* will also disclose the effectiveness of alveolar gas exchange.

MEASUREMENT OF PERFUSION (See Chapter 321).

OTHER TESTS OF LUNG FUNCTION (See Chapter 321).

CLINICAL USE OF PULMONARY FUNCTION TESTING. Pulmonary function testing, while rarely resulting in an etiologic diagnosis, is helpful in defining the type of process (e.g., obstruction, restriction) and the degree of functional impairment in following the course and treatment of disease, and in estimating the prognosis. It is also useful in preoperative evaluation and in confirmation of functional impairment in patients having subjective complaints but a normal physical examination. In most patients with obstructive disease, a repeat test after administering a bronchodilator is warranted.

Most tests require some cooperation and understanding by the subject, and interpretation is greatly facilitated if the test conditions and the subject's behavior during the test are known. Accurate testing of children aged 3–6 yr requires great patience by the physician and training of the subject, whereas most children aged 6 yr or older can be tested reliably without excessive difficulty. Infants and young children who cannot or will not cooperate with test procedures can be studied in a limited number of ways, which often require sedation. Flow rates and pressures during tidal breathing, with or without transient interruption of the flow, may be useful to assess some aspects of airway resistance or obstruction, and to measure compliance of the lungs and thorax. Expiratory flow rates may be studied in sedated infants with passive compression of the chest and abdomen with a rapidly inflatable jacket. Gas dilution or plethysmographic methods may also be used in sedated infants to measure FRC and R_{AW}.

Baughman RP (ed): Bronchoalveolar Lavage. St. Louis, MO, Mosby–Year Book, 1992.

Dailey RH, Simon B, Young GP, et al: The Airway: Emergency Management. St. Louis, MO, Mosby–Year Book, 1992.

Holcomb GW III (ed): Pediatric Endoscopic Surgery. Norwalk, CT, Appleton & Lange, 1994.

Hughes WT, Buescher ES: Pediatric Procedures, 2nd ed. Philadelphia, WB Saunders, 1980.

Margolis P, Ferkol T, Marsocci S, et al: Accuracy of the clinical examination in detecting hypoxemia in infants with respiratory illness. J Pediatr 124:552, 1994.

Prakash UBS: Bronchoscopy. New York, Raven Press, 1994.

Putnam CE: Diagnostic Imaging of the Lung. New York, Marcel Dekker, 1990.

Saccomanno G: Diagnostic Pulmonary Cytology. Chicago, American Society of Clinical Pathologists Press, 1986.

SECTION 2

Upper Respiratory Tract

James E. Arnold

In addition to olfaction, the nose provides initial warming and humidification of inspired air. In the anterior nares turbulent air flow and coarse hairs enhance the deposition of large particulate matter; the remaining nasal airways filter out particles as small as 6 μm in diameter. In the turbinate region the air flow becomes laminar and the air stream is narrowed and directed superiorly; thus particle deposition, warming, and humidification are enhanced. Nasal passages contribute as much as 50% of the total resistance of normal breathing. Nasal flaring, a sign of respiratory distress, reduces the resistance to inspiratory flow of air through the nose and may improve ventilation.

The nasal mucosa is more vascular, especially in the turbinate region, than that of the lower airways; however, the surface epithelium is similar, with ciliated cells, goblet cells, submucosal glands, and a covering blanket of mucus. Mucus flows toward the nasopharynx, where the air steam widens, the epithelium becomes squamous, and secretions are wiped away by swallowing; replacement of the mucous layers occurs about every 10 min. In addition to mucous glycoproteins, which provide viscoelastic properties, the nasal secretions contain lysozyme and secretory IgA, both of which have antimicrobial activity.

The *paranasal sinuses* develop in the facial bones as air cells lined with ciliated, mucus-secreting epithelium. Their ostia drain into the middle and superior meatuses and the sphenoethmoid recess of the nose. Development of the sinuses begins at 3–5 mo of gestation but occurs mostly after birth, with the maxillary and ethmoid sinuses being the earliest to form. They are seen on plain roentgenograms by 1–2 yr of age but can be identified on finecut computed tomography (CT) scans in the neonate. The frontal sinuses usually begin their ascent into the frontal bone by the 2nd yr but, along with the sphenoid sinuses, are not readily visible on plain roentgenograms until 5–6 yr of age or later. Growth of the sinuses continues through adolescence; although unusual, asymmetry is most common in the frontal sinuses. Hypoplasia or septa within the maxillary sinuses are seen occasionally. Mucosal thickening greater than 4 mm, air-fluid level, or opacification seen on sinus roentgenograms or computed tomography suggest sinusitis, which can occur alone or in association with other conditions, such as cystic fibrosis (CF), ciliary dyskinesia, or immunodeficiency.

The adenoids on the posterior nasopharyngeal wall and the tonsils at the base of the tongue are directly in line with the mucociliary flow and the air stream, enhancing their protective capabilities. The eustachian tubes, also lined with mucus-secreting, ciliated epithelium, enter the nasopharynx on the lateral walls.

Children and adults breathe through their nose unless nasal obstruction interferes, but most newborns are predominant nasal breathers. ■

CHAPTER 325
Congenital Disorders of the Nose

Congenital structural nasal abnormalities are uncommon compared with acquired malformations. Occasionally, nasal bones are congenitally absent so that the bridge of the nose fails to develop, resulting in nasal hypoplasia. Congenital absence of the nose, complete or partial duplication, or a single centrally placed nostril occasionally occur but usually as a part of malformation syndromes incompatible with life. Rarely, supernumerary teeth may be found in the nose, or teeth may grow into it from the maxilla.

On occasion, nasal bones are sufficiently malformed to produce severe narrowing of the nasal passages. Often such narrowing is associated with a high and narrow hard palate, which is frequently associated with Down syndrome. Children with these defects may have more severe obstruction to airflow during infections of the upper airways and are more susceptible to the development of chronic or recurrent hypoventilation (see Chapter 330). Rarely, the alae nasi may be sufficiently thin and poorly supported to result in inspiratory obstruction.

A wide variety of nasal and midface abnormalities exist that may be part of more extensive craniofacial anomalies. These children are best treated by a team consisting of experienced pediatric, surgical, dental, and rehabilitation specialists.

Choanal atresia, the most common congenital anomaly of the nose, consists of a unilateral or bilateral bony or membranous septum between the nose and the pharynx. Nearly 50% of affected infants have other congenital anomalies (CHARGE syndrome—*C*oloboma, *H*eart disease, *A*tresia choanae, *R*etarded growth and development and/or CNS anomalies, *G*enital anomalies and/or hypogonadism, and *E*ar anomalies and/or deafness). Because newborn infants have a variable ability to breathe through their mouths, the obstruction does not produce the same symptoms in every infant. When only one side is affected, the infant usually does not have severe symptoms at birth and may be asymptomatic for a prolonged period, often until the first respiratory infection, when the diagnosis may be suggested by unilateral nasal discharge or disproportionately severe nasal obstruction.

Infants with bilateral choanal atresia who have difficulty with mouth breathing will make vigorous attempts to inspire, often suck in their lips, and will develop cyanosis. Distressed children then cry (which relieves the cyanosis) and become more calm, only to repeat the cycle after closing their mouths. Those who are able to mouth breathe at once will experience difficulty when sucking and swallowing, becoming cyanotic when they attempt to nurse. Persistent mouth breathing and cyanosis when the mouth is closed (which is relieved when the infant cries) are additional manifestations.

Diagnosis is established by the inability to pass a firm catheter through each nostril 3–4 cm into the nasopharynx. The atresia plate may be seen directly with fiberoptic rhinoscopy. The anatomy is best visualized by using CT scanning.

Treatment consists of promptly providing an oral airway or maintaining the mouth in an open position. Passage of an orogastric tube is often sufficient to prevent the complete opposition of tongue and soft palate and to ensure an open airway. Other techniques use a feeding nipple with large holes at the tip. Once an oral airway is established, the infant can be fed by gavage until breathing and eating without the assisted airway is learned, usually in 2–3 wk. Tracheostomy is rarely indicated. Subsequently, elective operative correction can be done weeks or months later in patients who adapt well to the obstruction. Immediate surgical correction for bilateral choanal atresia is seldom needed. Operative correction of unilateral obstruction may be deferred for several years. Stenosis necessitating reoperation is common.

Congenital defects of the nasal septum, such as *perforation* or *deviation,* are rare. Perforation can be developmental or secondary to infection, such as syphilis or tuberculosis, and to trauma. Septal deviation can be congenital or secondary to birth trauma and may be corrected with immediate realignment using blunt probes, cotton applicators, and topical anesthesia. Formal surgical correction may be required but is usually postponed to avoid disturbance of midface growth. Abnormal formation of the nasal bones is infrequent unless other malformations are also present, such as cleft lip or palate.

Congenital midline nasal masses include *dermoids, gliomas,* and *encephaloceles.* They present intranasally or extranasally and may have intracranial connections. Nasal dermoids often have a dimple on the nasal dorsum, sometimes with hair being present, and predispose to intracranial infections. Gliomas or heterotopic brain tissue are firm, whereas encephaloceles are soft and enlarge with crying or the Valsalva maneuver. Surgical excision is required, and an evaluation to determine intracranial connection is best done with magnetic resonance imaging (MRI).

Poor development of the paranasal sinuses is associated with recurrent or chronic upper airway infection in Down syndrome.

Hughes GB, Sharpino G, Hunt W, et al: Management of the congenital midline mass: A review. Head Neck Surg 2:222, 1980.

Maniglia AJ, Goodwin WJ, Arnold JE, et al: Intracranial abscesses secondary to nasal sinus and orbital infections in adults and children. Arch Otolaryngol Head Neck Surg 115:1424, 1989.

Richardson M, Osguthorpe JD: Surgical management of choanal atresia. Laryngoscope 98:915, 1988.

CHAPTER 326
Acquired Disorders of the Nose

326.1 Foreign Body

Food, crayons, small toys, erasers, paper wads, beads, beans, stones, and other foreign bodies are frequently introduced into the nose by children. Initial symptoms are local obstruction, sneezing, relatively mild discomfort, and, rarely, pain. Irritation results in mucosal swelling, and, because some foreign bodies are hygroscopic and increase in size as water is absorbed, signs of local obstruction and discomfort may increase with time. Infection usually follows and gives rise to a purulent, malodorous, or bloody discharge. Tetanus is a rare complication in nonimmunized children, as is toxic shock syndrome from surgical packings (Chapter 174.3). *Unilateral nasal discharge and obstruction should suggest the presence of a foreign body,* which can often be seen upon examination with a speculum. The patient may also present with a generalized body odor, bromhidrosis. The object is usually situated anteriorly at first, but through unskilled attempts at removal it may be forced deeper into the nose. Removal should be carried out promptly to minimize the danger of aspiration and to prevent local tissue necrosis. It can usually be performed with topical anesthesia, using either forceps or nasal suction. Infection usually clears promptly after the removal of the object, and generally no further therapy is necessary.

326.2 Epistaxis

Nosebleeds are rare in infancy, are common in childhood, and decrease in incidence after puberty. Epistaxis, when it does occur, is often transient and is not very severe; the bleeding often stops spontaneously or with minimal pressure. These isolated episodes of bleeding require no diagnostic evaluation or specific treatment. However, some children develop recurrent epistaxis with mild or moderate bleeding.

ETIOLOGY. Trauma, including picking the nose and foreign bodies, is the most common cause. There is frequently a family history of childhood epistaxis, and susceptibility is increased during respiratory infections and in the winter when dry air irritates the nasal mucosa, resulting in formation of fissures and crusting. Epistaxis is also associated with adenoidal hypertrophy, allergic rhinitis, sinusitis, polyps, and a variety of acute infections. Diseases with paroxysmal and forceful cough, such as cystic fibrosis, may also foster epistaxis. Severe bleeding may be encountered with congenital vascular abnormalities, such as telangiectasias or varicosities, and in children with thrombocytopenia, deficiency of clotting factors, hypertension, renal failure, or venous congestion. Adolescent girls may have epistaxis at the time of menarche.

CLINICAL MANIFESTATIONS. Epistaxis usually occurs without warning, with blood flowing slowly but freely from one nostril or occasionally from both. In children with nasal lesions, bleeding may follow physical exercise. When bleeding occurs at night, the blood may be swallowed and may become apparent only when the child vomits or passes blood in his stools. The source of the bleeding is usually the vascular plexus on the anterior septum (Kiesselbach plexus) or the mucosa of the anterior portions of the turbinates.

TREATMENT. Most nosebleeds stop spontaneously in a few minutes. The nares should be compressed and the child kept as quiet as possible, in an erect position until hemostasis, with the head tilted forward to avoid blood trickling posteriorly into the pharynx. If these measures do not stop the bleeding, local application of a solution of neosynephrine (0.25–1%) with or without topical thrombin may occasionally be useful. If bleeding persists, an anterior nasal pack should be inserted; if bleeding originates in the posterior nares, combined anterior and postchoanal packing is necessary. After bleeding has been controlled, and if a bleeding site is identified, its obliteration by cautery with silver nitrate may prevent further difficulties. As the septal cartilage derives its nutrition from the overlying mucoperichondrium, only one side of the septum should be cauterized at a time to reduce the chance of a septal perforation.

In patients with severe or repeated epistaxis, blood transfusions may be necessary. Otolaryngologic evaluation is indicated for these children and for those with bilateral bleeding or with hemorrhage that does not arise from the Kiesselbach plexus. Profuse epistaxis associated with a nasal mass in a boy near puberty may signal a **juvenile nasopharyngeal angiofibroma.** This unusual tumor has been reported in a 2 yr old and in 30–40 yr olds, but the incidence peaks in adolescent and preadolescent boys. The CT scan with contrast is the best initial evaluation. Arteriography, embolization, and extensive surgery may be needed. Replacement of deficient clotting factors may be required for patients who have an underlying hematologic disorder (see Chapter 432). If a patient lives in a dry environment, a room humidifier may prevent epistaxis.

CHAPTER 327

Infections of the Upper Respiratory Tract

GENERAL CONSIDERATIONS. Upper respiratory tract infections are those primarily affecting the structures of the respiratory tract above the larynx, but most respiratory illnesses affect both the upper and lower portions of the tract simultaneously or sequentially. Pathophysiologic features include inflammatory infiltrates and edema of the mucosa, vascular congestion, increased mucus secretion, and alterations of ciliary structure and function.

Many different microorganisms (chiefly viruses) are capable of causing primary upper respiratory tract disease. The same organism may cause inapparent infection or clinical symptoms of differing severity and extent in accordance with host factors such as age, sex, previous contact with the agent, allergy, and nutritional status. For example, among different members of the same family a single virus may simultaneously produce typical colds in the parents, bronchiolitis in the infant, croup in a somewhat older child, pharyngitis in another, and a subclinical infection in another. Children enrolled in child care are exposed to a wide range of pathogens at an earlier age (see Chapter 35).

ETIOLOGY. Most acute respiratory tract infections are caused by viruses and mycoplasma. An exception is acute epiglottitis. Streptococci and the diphtheria organisms are the major bacterial agents capable of causing primary pharyngeal disease; even in cases of acute tonsillopharyngitis, most illnesses are of nonbacterial origin. Although considerable overlapping exists, some microorganisms are more likely to produce a given respiratory syndrome than others, and certain agents have a greater tendency than others to produce severe disease. Some viruses (e.g., measles) may be associated with varying amounts of upper and lower respiratory tract symptomatology as part of a general clinical picture involving other organ systems.

The **respiratory syncytial virus** (RSV) is the principal single cause of bronchiolitis, accounting for about one third of all cases. It is a common cause of pneumonia, croup, and bronchitis, as well as of undifferentiated febrile disease of the upper respiratory tract (see Chapter 218).

The **parainfluenza viruses** account for most cases of the croup syndrome but may also produce bronchitis, bronchiolitis, and febrile upper respiratory tract disease (see Chapter 217). The **influenza viruses** do not play a large part in the various respiratory syndromes except during epidemics. In infants and children, influenza viruses account for more disease of the upper than the lower respiratory tract.

The **adenoviruses** account for fewer than 10% of respiratory illnesses, many of which are mild or asymptomatic. Pharyngitis and pharyngoconjunctival fever are the most common clinical manifestations in children. However, adenoviruses occasionally cause severe lower respiratory tract infection (see Chapter 219).

The **rhinoviruses** and **coronaviruses** usually produce symptoms limited to the upper tract, most commonly the nose, and account for a significant proportion of the "common cold" syndromes (see Chapter 220).

Coxsackieviruses A and B produce primarily disease of the nasopharynx (see Chapter 209). **Mycoplasma** can produce both upper and lower respiratory tract illness, including bronchiolitis, pneumonia, bronchitis, pharyngotonsillitis, myringitis, and otitis media (see Chapter 196).

Carlo WA, Martin RJ, Bruce EN, et al: Alae nasi activation (nasal flaring) decreases nasal resistance in preterm infants. Pediatrics 72:338, 1983.
Carson JL, Collier AM, Hu SS: Acquired ciliary defects in nasal epithelium of children with acute viral upper respiratory infections. N Engl J Med 312:463, 1985.

327.1 Acute Nasopharyngitis

(Upper Respiratory Tract Infection; URI; the "Common Cold")

Acute nasopharyngitis is the most common infectious condition of children, but its significance depends primarily on the relative frequency with which complications occur. In children this syndrome is more extensive than in adults, often involving the paranasal sinuses and middle ear as well as the nasopharynx.

ETIOLOGY. The illness is caused by more than 200 serologically different viral agents. The principal agents are rhinoviruses (see Chapter 220), which account for more than a third of all colds; coronaviruses are responsible for about 10%. The period of infectivity lasts from a few hours prior to the appearance of symptoms to 1–2 days after the illness has appeared. Group A streptococci are the principal bacterial cause of acute nasopharyngitis. *Corynebacterium diphtheriae, Mycoplasma pneumoniae, Neisseria meningitidis,* and *N. gonorrhoeae* are also primary infectious agents. *Haemophilus influenzae, Streptococcus pneumoniae, Moraxell catarrhalis,* and *Staphylococcus aureus* may infect upper respiratory tract tissues secondarily and are responsible for complications in the sinuses, ears, mastoids, lymph nodes, and lungs. *M. pneumoniae* infections may localize to the nasopharynx and in these cases are difficult to distinguish from viral nasopharyngitis.

EPIDEMIOLOGY. Susceptibility to agents causing acute nasopharyngitis is universal, but for poorly understood reasons it varies in the same person from time to time. Although infections occur throughout the year, in the Northern Hemisphere there are peaks of occurrence in September about the time school opens, in late January, and toward the end of April. Children have an average of five to eight infections a year, and the highest number occurs during the first 2 yr of life. The frequency of acute nasopharyngitis varies directly with the number of exposures, and in nursery schools and day-care centers may be virtually epidemic. Susceptibility may be increased by poor nutrition; purulent complications are increased by malnutrition.

PATHOLOGY. The first changes are edema and vasodilatation in the submucosa. A mononuclear cell infiltrate follows, which, within 1–2 days, becomes polymorphonuclear. Structural and functional changes of cilia result in compromised mucus clearance. In moderate to severe infection, the superficial epithelial cells separate and slough. There is profuse production of mucus, at first thin, later thicker and usually purulent. There may also be anatomic involvement of the upper airways, including occlusion and abnormalities of the sinus cavities.

CLINICAL MANIFESTATIONS. Colds are more severe in young children than in older children and adults. In general, children 3 mo to 3 yr have fever early in the course of infection, occasionally a few hours before localizing signs appear. Younger infants are usually afebrile, and older children may have low-grade fevers. Purulent complications occur with more frequency and severity at younger ages. Persistent sinusitis may occur at any age.

The initial manifestations in infants older than 3 mo of age are the sudden onset of fever, irritability, restlessness, and sneezing. Nasal discharge begins within a few hours, quickly leading to nasal obstruction, which may interfere with nursing; in small infants having a greater dependency on nose breathing, signs of moderate respiratory distress may occur. During the first 2–3 days the eardrums are usually congested, and fluid may be noted behind the drum, whether or not purulent otitis media subsequently occurs. A few infants may vomit, and some have diarrhea. The febrile phase lasts from a few hours to 3 days; fever may recur with purulent complications.

In older children the initial symptoms are dryness and irritation in the nose and not infrequently in the pharynx. These symptoms are followed within a few hours by sneezing, chilly sensations, muscular aches, a thin nasal discharge, and sometimes coughing. Headache, malaise, anorexia, and low-grade fever may be present. Within 1 day the secretions usually become thicker and eventually become purulent. The discharge is irritating, particularly during the purulent phase. Nasal obstruction leads to mouth breathing, and this, through drying of the mucous membranes of the throat, increases the sensation of soreness. In most cases, the acute phase lasts for 2–4 days.

DIFFERENTIAL DIAGNOSIS. The initial manifestations of measles and pertussis—and, to a lesser extent, of poliomyelitis, hepatitis, and mumps—are those of nasopharyngitis. A persistent nasal discharge, particularly if it is bloody, suggests a foreign body or diphtheria and, in infants, choanal atresia or congenital syphilis.

Allergic rhinitis (see Chapter 136) differs from infectious rhinitis in that it is not accompanied by fever: its nasal discharge does not usually become purulent, and it is usually combined with persistent sneezing and itching of the eyes and nose. The nasal mucous membranes in allergic rhinitis are usually pale rather than inflamed, and nasal smears often contain many eosinophils rather than the polymorphonuclear leukocytes associated with infection. In allergic rhinitis, antihistamines may produce rapid and relatively complete disappearance of signs and symptoms; in infectious rhinitis, they produce little consistent benefit and may thicken the secretions making them harder to clear.

Drug abuse, especially with inhaled solvent, cocaine, and marijuana, should also be considered in older children and adolescents.

COMPLICATIONS. These result from the bacterial invasion of the paranasal sinuses and other portions of the respiratory tract. The cervical lymph nodes may also become involved and occasionally suppurate. Mastoiditis, peritonsillar cellulitis, sinusitis, or periorbital cellulitis may occur. The most common complication is otitis media, which is seen in up to 25% of small infants. Although it may occur early in the course of a cold, it usually appears after the acute phase of nasopharyngitis. Thus, otitis media should be suspected if fever recurs. Most viral infections of the upper respiratory tract also involve the lower respiratory tract, and in many cases pulmonary function diminishes even though lower respiratory tract symptoms are inconspicuous or absent. On the other hand, typical laryngotracheobronchitis, bronchiolitis, or pneumonia may develop during the course of acute nasopharyngitis. Viral nasopharyngitis is also a frequent trigger for asthma symptoms in children with reactive airways.

PREVENTION. Effective vaccines are not available. Neither gamma globulin nor vitamin C reduces the frequency or severity of infections, and their use is not recommended.

Because of the ubiquity of the common cold, it is impossible to isolate children from this condition. However, because in the very young infant complications may be relatively serious, some attempt should be made to protect infants from contact with potentially infected persons. Spread of infection is by aerosol (sneezing, coughing) or direct contact with infected material (hands).

TREATMENT. There is no specific therapy. Antibiotics do not affect the course of the illness or reduce the incidence of bacterial complications. Bed rest is generally recommended, but there is no evidence that it shortens the course of the illness or affects the outcome. Acetaminophen or ibuprofen is usually helpful in reducing irritability, aching, and malaise for the first 1–2 days of infection, but excessive use should be avoided. Aspirin given to a child with influenza virus infection increases the risk of developing Reye syndrome and *is not recommended* for children with respiratory tract symptoms.

Most of the distress is owing to nasal obstruction. Attempts should be made to relieve this condition if it interferes with sleep or with fluid or food ingestion. Nasal instillation of medications may be an effective method for relieving nasal obstruction. In infants, instillation of sterile saline may assist with physical removal of excessive mucus. Phenylephrine (0.125–0.25%) is used widely in the United States. More potent, longer acting nose drops, although useful to adults, tend to be irritating and occasionally are hyperexcitative or sedative to infants. Nose drops in oily vehicles should be avoided because they are readily aspirated. The addition of antibiotics, corticosteroids, or antihistamines to nose drops increases their expense and adds nothing to their effectiveness.

Nose drops are best administered 15–20 min before feeding and at bedtime. While the child is supine with the neck extended, 1–2 drops are instilled in each nostril. Because this often produces shrinkage of only the anterior mucous membranes, 1–2 drops can be instilled 5–10 min later. Introducing nasal decongestants by cotton-tipped applicators is not recommended. Older children can use a nasal spray but only under supervision, because such applications tend to be overused. In general, no medication other than saline instilled into the nose should be used for more than 4–5 days; after this time any drug may produce chemical irritation and induce nasal congestion, mimicking acute nasopharyngitis.

Nasal obstruction is difficult to treat in infants. Suction with a soft bulb syringe is occasionally essential to clear the nasal passage sufficiently to permit the young infant to nurse. The best drainage can usually be achieved by placing the infant in the prone position, if this does not further compromise respirations. A highly humidified, heated environment provided by an efficient vaporizer may prevent drying of secretions but has not been demonstrated to have a beneficial effect on cold symptoms of adults.

Orally administered decongestants are also widely used for shrinkage of engorged nasal mucosa and for relief of obstruction. Pseudoephedrine reduces nasal resistance in older children and adults with upper respiratory tract infection; studies in infants and young children have not been reported. Many preparations combine antihistamines and adrenergic agonists. The former have been found effective in some and ineffective in other studies for relief of nasal congestion in children with acute nasopharyngitis. There is no evidence that these drugs prevent otitis media or middle ear effusion.

Most children with acute nasopharyngitis have decreased appetite, but compelling them to eat serves no purpose. Fluids of the child's choice should be offered at frequent intervals. Transient constipation is common but does not require treatment because it disappears rapidly when the child returns to a normal diet.

Doyle WJ, McBride TP, Skoner DP, et al: A double-blind, placebo-controlled trial of the effect of chlorpheniramine on the response of the nasal airway, middle ear, and eustachian tube to provocative rhinovirus challenge. Pediatr Infect Dis J 7:229, 1988.

Fleming DW, Cochi SL, Hightower AW, et al: Childhood upper respiratory tract infections: To what degree is incidence affected by day care attendance? Pediatrics 79:55, 1987.

Forstall GJ, Macklin ML, Yen-Lieberman BR, et al: Effect of inhaling heated vapor on symptoms of the common cold. JAMA 271:1109, 1994.

Gaffey MJ, Kaiser DL, Hayden FG: Ineffectiveness of oral terfenadine in natural colds: Evidence against histamine as a mediator of common cold symptoms. Pediatr Infect Dis J 7:223, 1988.

Gwaltney JM Jr, Phillips CD, Miller RD, et al: Computed tomographic study of the common cold. N Engl J Med 330:25, 1994.

Hutton N, Wilson MH, Mellits ED, et al: Effectiveness of an antihistamine-decongestant combination for young children with the common cold: A randomized, controlled clinical trial. J Pediatr 118:125, 1991.

Monto AS: The common cold. JAMA 271:1122, 1994.

Naclerio RM, Proud D, Kagey-Sobotka A, et al: Is histamine responsible for the symptoms of rhinovirus colds? A look at the inflammatory mediators following infection. Pediatr Infect Dis J 7:218, 1988.

327.2 Acute Pharyngitis

This term refers to all acute infections of the pharynx, including tonsillitis and pharyngotonsillitis. The presence or absence of tonsils does not affect the susceptibility, the frequency, or the course or complications of the illness. Pharyngeal involvement is part of most upper respiratory tract infections and is also found with various acute generalized infections. However, in the strict sense *acute pharyngitis* refers to conditions in which the principal involvement is in the throat. The disease is uncommon under 1 yr of age. The incidence then increases to a peak at 4–7 yr but continues throughout later childhood and adult life. In diphtheria (Chapter 180), herpangina (Chapter 209), adenovirus infection (Chapter 219), and infectious mononucleosis (Chapter 215) pharyngeal involvement may be prominent.

ETIOLOGY. Acute pharyngitis, whether febrile or not, is generally caused by viruses. Group A β-hemolytic streptococcus (Chapter 175) is the only common bacterial causative agent, and, except during epidemics, it accounts for probably fewer than 15% of cases. Mycoplasma and *Arcanobacterium hemolyticum* may also produce pharyngitis. Other bacteria may proliferate during acute viral infections and may therefore be cultured in large numbers from the pharynx of an affected person. Pharyngeal gonococcal infection may occur secondary to fellatio.

CLINICAL MANIFESTATIONS. These differ somewhat, depending on whether streptococci or viruses are the cause. There is, however, much overlapping of signs and symptoms, and it is often impossible to clinically distinguish one form of pharyngitis from another.

Viral pharyngitis is generally considered a disease of relatively gradual onset, which usually has as early signs fever, malaise, and anorexia with moderate throat pain. Sore throat may be present initially but begins more commonly a day or so after the onset of symptoms, reaching its peak by the 2nd to 3rd day. Hoarseness, cough, and rhinitis are also common. Even at its peak, pharyngeal inflammation may be relatively slight, but it is occasionally severe, and small ulcers may form on the soft palate and the posterior pharyngeal wall. Exudates may appear on lymphoid follicles of the palate and tonsils, and may be indistinguishable from those encountered with streptococcal disease. The cervical lymph nodes are often moderately enlarged and firm, and may or may not be tender. Laryngeal involvement is common, but the trachea, bronchi, and lungs are usually not sources of symptoms. White blood cell counts range from 6,000 to above 30,000, an elevated count (16,000–18,000) of predominantly polymorphonuclear cells being common in the early phase of illness. Leukocyte counts have little value in differentiating viral from bacterial disease. The entire illness may last less than 24 hr and does not usually persist for more than 5 days. Significant complications are rare.

Streptococcal pharyngitis in a child over 2 yr often begins with complaints of headache, abdominal pain, and vomiting. These symptoms may be associated with a fever as high as 40° C (104° F); occasionally, a temperature elevation is not noted for 12 hr or so. Hours after the initial complaints, the throat may become sore, and in approximately one third of patients tonsillar enlargement, exudation, and pharyngeal erythema are found. The degree of pharyngeal pain is inconstant and may vary from slight to severe, making swallowing difficult. Two thirds of patients may have only mild erythema, with no enlargement of the tonsils and with no exudate. Anterior cervical lymphadenopathy usually occurs early, and the nodes are often tender. Fever may continue for 1–4 days; in very severe cases the child may remain ill for as long as 2 wk. The physical findings most likely to be associated with streptococcal disease are diffuse redness of the tonsils and tonsillar pillars, with a petechial mottling of the soft palate, whether or not lymphadenitis or follicular exudations are found. These features, although common in streptococcal pharyngitis, are not diagnostic and occur with some frequency in viral pharyngitis.

Conjunctivitis, rhinitis, cough, and hoarseness rarely occur with proven streptococcal pharyngitis, and the presence of two or more of these signs or symptoms suggests the diagnosis of viral infection.

The term **streptococcosis** refers to systemic variations in the presentation of acute streptococcal infections, believed to be related to earlier infection with the β-hemolytic streptococcus. In infants they may take the form of an acute, usually mild episode lasting less than 1 wk and characterized by variable fever (under 39° C [102° F]), mucoserous nasal discharge, and pharyngeal infection. Usually children 6 mo to 3 yr of age are most severely ill. Coryza with postnasal discharge, diffusely reddened pharynx, fever, vomiting, and loss of appetite occurs early. For a few days there is usually fever of 38–39.5° C (100–103° F), which continues irregularly for 4–8 wk, gradually becoming normal. Within a few days of onset, cervical nodes begin to enlarge and become tender; the course of the adenopathy typically parallels that of the fever. Focal complications are common.

DIAGNOSIS AND DIFFERENTIAL DIAGNOSIS. Diagnosis can be made by the rapid detection method for streptococcal antigens or by culture after pharyngeal swabbing. Rapid detection methods may miss 10–15% of culture-proven infections. Therefore, antigen-negative throat swabs from children with compatible clinical features should also be cultured (see Chapter 175).

A syndrome of purulent nasal discharge, pharyngitis, and fever may also be associated with positive pharyngeal cultures for pneumococci or *H. influenzae.* Although this syndrome is probably a complication of viral pharyngitis, some of these patients respond to antibiotics.

When a membranous exudate is present on the tonsils, diphtheria should be considered. The membranous exudate of infectious mononucleosis may resemble that found in the streptococcal infection and the partially immunized child with a diphtheritic infection. Herpangina (Chapter 209) is not usually associated with tonsillar exudates, but rather with many vesiculoulcerative lesions on the anterior pillars, fauces, and soft palate.

Agranulocytosis is often first manifested by symptoms of acute pharyngitis. The tonsils and posterior pharyngeal wall may be covered by a yellow or dirty white exudate. The mucous membranes under this exudate usually become necrotic, and ulceration extends into the mouth and involves the tongue. The lesions are very painful and dysphagia is severe. Enlargement of cervical lymph nodes commonly occurs, as do mucosal hemorrhages.

Children and adolescents who smoke tobacco or marijuana excessively may develop pharyngeal inflammation and sore throat. Allergic rhinitis with a nonpurulent postnasal discharge may also cause a sore throat. Gonococcal pharyngeal infections are usually asymptomatic.

Pharyngoconjunctival fever is discussed in Chapter 219.

COMPLICATIONS. With viral infections the complication rate is low, although purulent bacterial otitis media may occur. In debilitated children both viral and streptococcal infections may lead to large, chronic ulcers in the pharynx. With streptococcal disease, peritonsillar abscess occasionally occurs, as do sinusitis, otitis media, and, rarely, meningitis. Acute glomerulonephritis (Chapter 465.1) and rheumatic fever (Chapter 175.1) may follow streptococcal infections.

Mesenteric adenitis is occasionally associated with pharyngitis of either viral or bacterial origin. This may result in abdominal pain (with or without vomiting) that may closely simulate appendicitis.

TREATMENT. Since even exudative tonsillitis is usually of viral origin, for which there is no specific therapy, the use of antibiotics should be guided by the results of antigen detection tests or cultures, unless there are strong clinical and epidemiologic grounds to suspect a streptococcal infection. Streptococcal pharyngitis is best treated orally with penicillin (125–250 mg of penicillin V three times daily for 10 days). This usually produces prompt clinical response with defervescence within 24 hr and shortens the course of illness by an average of 1.5 days. Erythromycin is a satisfactory alternative if the patient is allergic to penicillin, but erythromycin resistance of group A streptococcal organisms has been documented in the United States.

Most children prefer to remain in bed during the acute phase of the disease. When throat pain is severe, acetaminophen or ibuprofen is often helpful. Gargling with warm saline solution offers some symptomatic relief for throat pain in children old enough to cooperate; in younger children the inhalation of steam occasionally produces similar effects. Because of pain on swallowing, cool bland liquids such as ginger ale are usually more acceptable than solids or hot foods. No attempt should be made to force the child to eat.

The child with a streptococcal infection is noninfectious to others within a few hours after penicillin therapy has begun. Reculturing is not necessary if symptoms abate. A streptococcal carrier is not at risk for rheumatic fever, is unlikely to transmit infection, and does not require treatment unless there is a history of rheumatic fever in the patient or a sibling. The carrier state does make the differentiation of subsequent pharyngitis more difficult. A few children require antibiotic prophylaxis against streptococcal disease, such as those with past history of rheumatic fever (Chapter 175.1).

Breese BB: A simple scorecard for the tentative diagnosis of streptococcal pharyngitis. Am J Dis Child 131:514, 1977.
Kim KS, Kaplan EL: Association of penicillin tolerance with failure to eradicate group A streptococci from patients with pharyngitis. J Pediatr 107:681, 1985.
Schwartz RH, Wientzen RL, Grundfast KM: Sore throat in adolescents. Pediatr Infect Dis 1:443, 1982.

327.3 Acute Uvulitis

Infections of the uvula are infrequent. They are characterized by fever, pain with swallowing, and drooling. Occasionally there are no symptoms or signs referrable to the pharynx. Most cases are due to group A streptococcus or *H. influenzae* type b, often in association with tonsillitis and acute epiglottis, respectively. However, isolated uvulitis has been reported. In general streptococcal uvulitis tends to occur in older children (>5 years), whereas that caused by *H. influenzae* occurs before 5 yr of age. This has become rare owing to the widespread use of conjugate HIB vaccine. In suspected cases blood cultures as well as cultures of the uvula and pharynx are indicated. Young children should be examined carefully for evidence of airway obstruction and treated, initially with an intravenous antibiotic that covers ampicillin-resistant *H. influenzae.* Older children can be treated as indicated for streptococcal pharyngitis.

327.4 Chronic Rhinitis and Nasopharyngitis

The child with persistent or recurring upper respiratory tract infection with or without associated chronic bronchial involvement cannot be placed in any one category; each must be studied to determine, if possible, the most important etiologic or pathophysiologic factors.

Children should recover completely after acute respiratory infections and should appear healthy between episodes. In the chronic cases the child seems to recover from one acute attack only to enter another, or there is more or less persistent rhinitis and cough and a general failure to do well. Such patterns may reflect familial or individual susceptibility or repeated exposure to respiratory infection either within the home or in a day-care school setting.

CHRONIC RHINITIS. Chronic nasal discharge, with or without acute exacerbations, may reflect an underlying disturbance, such as nasal polyps, chronic sinusitis, chronically infected adenoids, cystic fibrosis, dysmotile cilia syndrome, allergy, foreign bodies, deviated septum, various congenital malformations, nasal diphtheria, or syphilis. In addition, the possibility of a chronic debilitating infection or some nutritional, immunologic (Wegener granulomatosis, immunodeficiency), or metabolic (as of the thyroid) deficiency must be considered.

Clinical Manifestations. Symptoms vary, but chronic nasal discharge is common to all cases. In the persistent cases the odor may be foul, and there may be excoriation of the anterior nares and upper lip. Bloody discharge is common in syphilitic and diphtheritic lesions and with foreign bodies but may also occur in other conditions, especially if there is persistent nose picking. Disturbances of taste and smell are frequent. During exacerbations or superimposed infections, fever is common but is otherwise usually absent.

Persistent *allergic rhinitis* is relatively common and may be seasonal (see Chapter 136). The mucous membrane tends to be pale; the soft tissues are swollen and resistant to pressure.

Chronic rhinitis may also result from prolonged or excessive use of topical nasal decongestants (rhinitis medicamentosa).

Atrophic rhinitis is uncommon and is usually associated with some general debilitating condition, or it may be a sequel to long-continued nasal infection. The sense of smell is impaired. There may be little or no discharge but considerable crusting and a sense of dryness in the nose and throat. In some cases there is a profuse, excessively foul nasal discharge **(ozena).**

Treatment. The frequent application to the nares and upper lip of a lanolin, silicone, or petrolatum-base ointment protects against skin excoriation.

In addition, providing humidified air in cold weather may prevent ongoing nasal mucosal damage and foster clearing of the chronic inflammatory state. Otherwise, treatment is directed toward the underlying disturbance. Foci of infection in sinuses, ears, adenoids, or tonsils should be eradicated, and either allergens should be removed from the environment or the patient should be desensitized. Attention should be given to nutritional status, rest, and prevention of exposure to new infections. Although mucosa-shrinking solutions such as phenylephrine and related compounds may provide symptomatic relief, they may also cause further damage. Local antibiotics should be avoided, but systemic administration may be indicated in selected cases.

CHRONIC PHARYNGITIS. Chronic pharyngitis is rare and occurs secondarily to chronic infections of the sinuses, adenoids, or tonsils, although on occasion there is no evidence of infection other than hypertrophied lymphoid tissue on the posterior pharyngeal wall and on the base of the tongue. The latter type of involvement occurs with frequency only in children whose faucial tonsils have been removed; some of these children may also have infected tonsillar tags.

Clinical Manifestations. There are likely to be repeated acute exacerbations; in the intervals there are complaints of throat discomfort such as dryness and raspy irritation. Frequent efforts to clear the throat and the presence of an irritative cough are common. The mucous membrane is usually inflamed, although it is occasionally pale, and the blood vessels are prominent. The pharyngeal wall is frequently covered with a mucopurulent secretion, and the lymphoid tissue is often hypertrophied and has a pebbled appearance.

Treatment. This should be directed toward any disturbance in the sinuses, nose (deformities), adenoids, and tonsils. Attention should also be given to the general nutrition and hygiene of the child.

Wood RA, Doran TF, Schuberth KC: Atopic disease, rhinitis and conjunctivitis, upper respiratory tract infections and insect stings. Curr Opin Pediatr 5:623, 1993.

327.5 Retropharyngeal Abscess

During early childhood the potential space between the posterior pharyngeal wall and the prevertebral fascia contains several small lymph nodes that usually disappear during the 3rd to 4th year of life. The lymphatic channels that communicate with these nodes drain portions of the nasopharynx as well as the posterior nasal passages. With purulent infections of these areas the nodes may become infected; this may, in turn, progress to breakdown of the nodes and to suppuration.

ETIOLOGY. Retropharyngeal abscess may be a complication of bacterial pharyngitis. Less commonly, it occurs after extension of infection from vertebral osteomyelitis or by wound infection following a penetrating injury of the posterior pharynx. Group A hemolytic streptococci, oral anaerobes, and *S. aureus,* in this order, are the most common pathogens.

CLINICAL MANIFESTATIONS. The patient usually has a history of an acute nasopharyngitis or pharyngitis, and the clinical features of the earlier illness may still be present. There is generally an abrupt onset of high fever with difficulty in swallowing, refusal of feeding, severe distress with throat pain, hyperextension of the head, and noisy, often gurgling respirations. Respirations become increasingly labored, and secretions accumulate in the mouth and cause drooling owing to the difficulty in swallowing.

A bulge in the posterior pharyngeal wall is usually apparent. The abscess is sometimes located in an area of the nasopharynx where it may cause nasal obstruction and a bulging forward of the soft palate. A digital examination to determine whether the abscess is fluctuant must be performed with the patient in the Trendelenburg position and with provision for adequate suction in case the abscess ruptures. Retropharyngeal abscesses may not be detectable by simple inspection. However, a lateral roentgenogram of the nasopharynx or neck will reveal the retropharyngeal mass; when an abscess is present, the retropharyngeal soft tissue is more than one half the width of the adjacent vertebral bodies when the patient's neck is extended; air may be seen in the retropharynx, and there is a loss of the normal cervical lordosis.

If left untreated, the abscess may rupture into the pharynx spontaneously, resulting in aspiration of pus. It may also extend laterally and present externally on the side of the neck or dissect along fascial planes into the mediastinum. Death may occur with aspiration, airway obstruction, erosion into major blood vessels, or with mediastinitis.

DIFFERENTIAL DIAGNOSIS. Pressure on the larynx may result in stridor, making retropharyngeal abscess one of the differential diagnostic possibilities in patients with high fever and croup. Many patients have limited neck motion, which may be mistaken for meningismus. Nonfluctuant lymphadenitis may produce a tender bulge in the retropharyngeal space. Tuberculosis of the cervical spine may occasionally produce a lateral retropharyngeal abscess; considerable rigidity of the neck and other signs of spinal involvement are usually present. A computed tomography (CT) scan with contrast may differentiate underlying pathology or identify an early abscess, allowing earlier incision and drainage.

TREATMENT. If the abscess is recognized in the prefluctuant stage, intensive treatment with a semisynthetic penicillin (to cover penicillinase-producing *S. aureus*) may prevent suppuration and abscess formation. Single agent treatment with clindamycin or ampicillin-sulbactam should also be effective. Analgesic drugs may be needed for pain. Because of the risk of airway obstruction, narcotics should be used only with great care. When fluctuance is present, the abscess should be incised and antibiotics should be started; the operation is best performed under general anesthesia.

327.6 Lateral Pharyngeal Abscess

This condition occurs in the space lateral to the pharynx that extends from the hyoid bone to the base of the skull. The carotid vessels and jugular vein may be intimately associated with the abscess.

The patient usually has high fever, trismus, appears acutely ill, and has severe pain and difficulty when swallowing. The bulge in the lateral pharyngeal wall is obvious. Cervical adenitis is usually present, and torticollis toward the side of the abscess due to muscular spasm is common.

Microbiology is identical to that of retropharyngeal abscess. Treatment usually requires lateral neck drainage.

327.7 Peritonsillar Abscess

This abscess occurs in the potential space between the superior constrictor muscle and the tonsil (usually at the superior pole). It is almost always caused by group A β-hemolytic streptococci or oral anaerobes in preadolescent or adolescent patients.

CLINICAL MANIFESTATIONS. The abscess is usually preceded by an attack of acute pharyngotonsillitis. There may be an afebrile interval of several days, or the fever of the primary infection may not subside. The patient has severe throat pain, has trismus because of spasm of the pterygoid muscles, and often refuses to swallow or speak. Occasionally, there is sufficient spasm of the homolateral muscles of the neck to produce torticollis. The fever may be septic and reach 40.5°C (105°F). The affected tonsillar area is markedly swollen and inflamed; the uvula is displaced to the opposite side. In untreated patients the abscess becomes fluctuant within a few days and usually points in the region of the anterior faucial pillar. If the abscess is not incised, spontaneous rupture occurs.

TREATMENT. Antibiotics (usually penicillin) and incision and drainage or aspiration of purulence are required. Outpatient treatment is possible; however, young children usually require general anesthesia and hospitalization. If there is no history of chronic tonsillitis, the chance of recurrence is approximately 10%, and tonsillectomy is not required. If there is a prior history of tonsillitis or a previous abscess, an immediate tonsillectomy should be considered.

327.8 Sinusitis

See also Chapters 136, 137.

Starting in infancy, the maxillary antra and the anterior and posterior ethmoid cells are usually of sufficient size to harbor infection. The frontal sinus is rarely a site of significant infection until the 6th to 10th yr. When there is severe ethmoidal disease in the first few years of life, the development and pneumatization of the frontal sinuses may be curtailed or even completely prevented. The sphenoidal sinus usually does not assume clinical significance until the 3rd to 5th yr of life.

The paranasal sinuses are probably involved in an exudative process in most acute nasal infections, but, as a rule, the sinus involvement does not persist after the nasal infection has subsided unless there has been a pre-existing sinus infection. The incidence of both acute and chronic sinus infections increases in the latter part of childhood. Unrecognized allergic factors, poor sinus drainage such as might occur with septal deviation or adenoid hypertrophy, associated hereditary conditions, immunosuppression, and environmental factors may increase the possibility of sinus infection.

ACUTE PURULENT SINUSITIS

In addition to involvement of the sinuses during acute nasal infections, there may be acute empyema of one or more sinuses. Signs or symptoms often appear 3–5 days after acute rhinitis.

CLINICAL MANIFESTATIONS. Sinusitis should be suspected if a "cold" seems more severe than usual (fever >39°C, periorbital edema, facial pain) or if the "cold" lingers for more than 10 days. A nighttime cough often follows a viral upper respiratory infection, but a daytime cough is more suggestive of sinusitis. Headaches, facial pain, tenderness, and edema are uncommon. An examination after topical decongestants may show pus in the middle meatus that suggests involvement of the maxillary, frontal, or anterior ethmoid sinuses; pus in the superior meatus suggests involvement of the sphenoid or posterior ethmoid cells. Postnasal discharge may result in a sore throat or a persistent cough, especially at night.

In acute *ethmoiditis,* especially in infants and small children, periorbital cellulitis with edema of the soft tissues and redness of the skin is a common manifestation.

Complications are epidural or subdural abscess, meningitis, cavernous sinus thrombosis, optic neuritis, periorbital or orbital cellulitis and abscess, and osteomyelitis.

DIAGNOSIS. Roentgenography is often used but may be misinterpreted. The most common diagnostic findings are air-fluid levels and complete opacification. Mucosa width of 4 mm or greater in children also correlates with the presence of bacteria in sinuses. CT scans are sensitive indicators of sinus disease and may be needed before surgery is planned or if a complication of sinusitis seems likely. In some centers, abbreviated CT studies have replaced the usual sinus series. Sinus roentgenograms (even CT scans) of infants are often misleading. In children it is not necessary initially to puncture a sinus to establish a diagnosis. However, antral puncture is the only reliable method of gathering material for bacterial culture. Indications for sinus aspiration include unresponsiveness to therapy, sinus disease in immunocompromised hosts, or life-threatening complications. Organisms usually recovered in children include *S. pneumoniae, M. catarrhalis,* and nontypable *H. influenzae.* Direct smear of the secretions usually reveals mostly neutrophils but may aid in detecting associated allergy if many eosinophils are present. Nasal swab cultures do not correlate well with cultures of sinus aspirates.

TREATMENT. This consists primarily of effective antimicrobial therapy. Amoxicillin is a reasonable initial choice. In areas in which *H. influenzae* and *M. catarrhalis* producing β-lactamase are common or for treatment failures, trimethoprim-sulfamethoxazole, amoxicillin with potassium clavulanate, erythromycin plus a sulfonamide, and 2nd- and 3rd-generation cephalosporins may be prescribed. Trimethoprim-sulfamethoxazole is ineffective against group A β-hemolytic streptococci. Treatment lasts 14–21 days. Decongestants and antihistamines are not helpful. Sinus drainage and irrigation are reserved for patients who fail usual therapy; who have intraorbital, intracranial, or other complications; or who experience intense pain.

CHRONIC SINUSITIS

Chronic infection of the paranasal sinuses should suggest the possibility of a local or generalized disturbance that facilitates persistence of the infection. A search should be made for nasal deformities, polyps, or infected and hypertrophied adenoids that might cause obstruction, for infected teeth as a source of maxillary sinusitis, for a sinus polyp or mucocele, and for such general disturbances as allergy, cystic fibrosis, and dyskinetic cilia. Chronic or recurrent sinusitis is also common in patients with absence of secretory antibodies (IgA) and in other immunodeficiency states.

CLINICAL MANIFESTATIONS. Symptoms of chronic sinusitis vary considerably but frequently are not prominent. Fever, when present, is low grade. Malaise, easy fatigability, and anorexia may occur. Nasal discharge, which may be bilateral or unilateral, varies from day to day and during the day. Frequently there is sufficient swelling of the middle turbinates to cause substantial nasal obstruction. Postnasal discharge is common and, in the absence of infected adenoids or acute upper respiratory tract infection, is virtually diagnostic. When there is an associated watery nasal discharge or sneezing, the possibility of allergic rhinitis must be considered.

Any of the complications of acute sinusitis may occur with chronic sinusitis. The term *sinobronchitis* is used occasionally to designate the relationship between sinus and lower respiratory tract symptoms; children with this condition may have reactive airways, cystic fibrosis, immunodeficiency, or dyskinetic cilia as the underlying disease. Sinusitis may aggravate asthma. The association of chronic sinusitis with asthma and allergy is more common in patients with extensive disease, often characterized by peripheral eosinophilia.

TREATMENT. In addition to the organisms recovered during acute sinusitis, α-hemolytic streptococci, *S. aureus*, and anaerobes are frequently found on culture of antral aspirates. In general, appropriate antimicrobials should be given for up to 6 wk. Antihistamines and decongestants are often used in addition, especially if there are associated allergic manifestations. Surgery is frequently required.

In cystic fibrosis, panopacification of sinuses is nearly always present but symptomatic disease is unusual. In the absence of symptoms, treatment of sinus disease is not indicated.

Locally obstructive nasal deformities should be corrected, if possible, and infected or hypertrophic adenoid tissue should be removed.

CHAPTER 328
Nasal Polyps

ETIOLOGY. Nasal polyps are benign pedunculated tumors formed from edematous, usually chronically inflamed nasal mucosa. They usually originate from the ethmoid sinus and present in the middle meatus. Occasionally, they appear within the maxillary antrum and can extend to the nasopharynx (antrochoanal polyp). Very large or multiple polyps may completely obstruct the nasal passage.

Cystic fibrosis is probably the most common childhood cause of nasal polyposis; as many as 25% of patients develop polyps. Every child with nasal polyposis should be tested for cystic fibrosis, even in the absence of typical respiratory and digestive symptoms. Nasal polyposis is also associated with chronic sinusitis of other etiologies, chronic allergic rhinitis, and asthma.

CLINICAL MANIFESTATIONS. Obstruction of nasal passages with hyponasal phonation and mouth breathing is prominent. Profuse mucoid or mucopurulent rhinorrhea may also result. An examination of the nasal passages shows glistening, gray, grape-like masses squeezed between the nasal turbinates and the septum. Polyps can be readily distinguished from the well-vascularized turbinate tissue, which is pink or red. Prolonged presence of polyps may widen the bridge of the nose and erode adjacent osseous structures.

TREATMENT. Local or systemic decongestants are not usually effective in shrinking the polyps. Similarly, corticosteroid nose sprays are not usually helpful, although a trial is warranted in recurrent cases. Polyps should be removed surgically if complete obstruction, uncontrolled rhinorrhea, or deformity of the nose appears. If the underlying pathogenic mechanism cannot be eliminated (e.g., cystic fibrosis), the polyps may soon return. More aggressive surgery may reduce the recurrence rate. Antihistamines may be helpful in delaying recurrence owing to allergic causes.

CHAPTER 329
Tonsils and Adenoids

The term *tonsils* is used in its commonly accepted sense of indicating the two faucial tonsils; the term *adenoids* refers to the nasopharyngeal tonsil. The tonsils and adenoids are part of the lymphoid tissues that circle the pharynx and are known collectively as *Waldeyer ring*. This consists of the lymphoid tissue on the base of the tongue (lingual tonsil), the two faucial tonsils, the adenoids, and the lymphoid tissue on the posterior pharyngeal wall. This tissue serves as a defense against infection, but it may become a site of acute or chronic infection.

The principal disturbances of the tonsils and adenoids are infection and hypertrophy. The latter is usually temporary and secondary to infection. The most important issue is if and when they are to be removed. Although both tonsils and adenoids are often removed at the same operation, separate tonsillectomy or adenoidectomy may be indicated, especially in children under 4–5 yr of age. Tonsillar disturbances are uncommon in infancy.

Neoplasms of the tonsils are rare, although 7% of non-Hodgkin lymphomas present in the Waldeyer ring. The nasopharynx is a common site for rhabdomyosarcomas to occur.

Acute infections of the tonsils are considered as acute pharyngitis and are discussed in Chapter 327.2.

CHRONIC TONSILLITIS
(Chronically Hypertrophic and Infected Tonsils)

The management of tonsillitis is of special concern because of its frequency and because tonsils are potentially important to the normal development of the immune system.

CLINICAL MANIFESTATIONS. These vary considerably; the significant features are recurrent or persistent sore throat and obstruction to swallowing or breathing, most often caused by hypertrophied adenoids. There may be a sense of dryness and irritation in the throat, and the breath may be offensive. Constitutional symptoms are not prominent. Rarely, hypertrophied tonsils and adenoids obstructing the upper airway are associated with respiratory distress, chronic hypoxemia, and the development of pulmonary hypertension.

INDICATIONS FOR TONSILLECTOMY. Parents often wrongly attribute frequent respiratory infections, allergic bronchitis, mouth breathing, recurrent purulent or serous otitis, poor appetite, failure to gain weight, or recurrent or chronic fever to chronic tonsillitis. Tonsillectomy and adenoidectomy do not decrease the incidence of these problems during childhood. For children with recurrent throat infections (seven in the past year or five in each of the past 2 years), tonsillectomy decreases the number of throat infections in the subsequent 2 years, compared with no tonsillectomy. However, many children who have not had tonsillectomy also have a decline in the number of throat infections. Until better methods are available to identify those children who will truly benefit from tonsillectomy and adenoidectomy, it seems prudent to avoid surgery in most cases. Factors such as severity of illness and the frequency of missing school need to be considered.

Decision for removal of tonsils should be based on symptoms and signs related directly to hypertrophy, obstruction, and chronic infection in the tonsils and related structures. *Most hypertrophic tonsils actually are normal in size; the misinterpretation results from failure to appreciate that normally tonsils are relatively larger during childhood than in later years.*

Tonsils may virtually meet in the midline in some children who are asymptomatic; tonsils of average size are projected toward the midline when the child is gagged and may be interpreted as being hypertrophic. Alternatively, infection does not always produce hypertrophy, and chronically infected tonsils may be small and embedded behind the faucial pillars. There is no certain way to directly demonstrate whether tonsils are harboring chronic infection. The consistency or size of the tonsils and the presence of cheesy material within the crypts are not reliable guides. Persistent hyperemia of the anterior pillars is a more reliable sign, and enlargement of the cervical lymph nodes is supporting evidence. Persistent enlargement of the node just below and slightly in front of the angle of the jaw is especially significant. Hypertrophy sufficient to obstruct swallowing or breathing is readily detectable; such tonsils practically meet in the midline when the throat is examined without gagging the patient. However, before tonsillectomy is recommended, it should be ascertained that the hypertrophy is chronic and not the result of a recent acute infection. Tonsils can increase in size greatly during an acute infection and recede after its subsidence.

The only absolute indication for a tonsillectomy is to rule out tumor and severe aerodigestive tract obstruction. Tonsillectomy is of no value in the prevention or treatment of acute or chronic sinusitis, chronic otitis media, and middle ear deafness. There is also no evidence to indicate that the removal of tonsils is justified for infections in the lower respiratory tract. No systemic disturbance in itself is an indication for tonsillectomy.

Tonsillectomy in Relation to the Age of the Child. When, on rare occasions, it seems advisable to recommend tonsillectomy for a child 2–3 yr of age, every attempt should be made to postpone the operation. Frequently when the operation is postponed for reasons of age, the apparent need disappears within the next year or so. In the first few years of life the indications for adenoidectomy, although infrequent, are present more often than those for tonsillectomy. Neither procedure should be performed as a prophylaxis against the "common cold" at any age.

Tonsillectomy in Relation to Active Infection. Tonsillectomy should be postponed until 2–3 wk after subsidence of an infection, except in rare cases of acute respiratory obstruction with pulmonary artery hypertension and cor pulmonale.

COMPLICATIONS OF TONSILLECTOMY. The mean duration of postoperative sore throat is 5 days. Referred ear pain and halitosis are common. Minor hemorrhage, postoperative throat infection, or anesthetic complications occur in more than 10% of procedures. Severe hemorrhage or life-threatening complications occur occasionally and are another reason for carefully assessing the indications for surgical intervention. Pulmonary edema also not infrequently occurs after relief of upper airway obstruction with tonsillectomy or adenoidectomy. Therefore, this therapy should be reserved for settings in which postsurgical respiratory failure can be dealt with effectively. Outpatient tonsil and adenoid surgery can be performed safely and may be mandated by insurance carriers; however, surgery for airway obstruction and other conditions requires inpatient surgery and postoperative monitoring, as determined by the pediatrician and surgeon.

ADENOIDAL HYPERTROPHY

(Hypertrophy of Pharyngeal Tonsil; "Adenoids")

Disturbances of the nasopharyngeal lymphoid tissue (adenoids) tend to parallel those of the faucial tonsils. Hypertrophy and infection may occur separately but often occur together; infection is usually primary. The soft adenoid structure, which is normally widespread in the nasopharynx, especially on the posterior wall and the roof, undergoes hypertrophy, and masses of varying size are formed. These masses may almost fill the vault of the nasopharynx, interfere with the passage of air through the nose, obstruct the eustachian tubes, and block the clearance of nasal mucus.

CLINICAL MANIFESTATIONS. Mouth breathing and persistent rhinitis are the most characteristic symptoms. Mouth breathing may be present only during sleep, especially when the child lies supine, when snoring is also likely to occur. With severe adenoid hypertrophy the mouth is kept open during the day as well, and the mucous membranes of the mouth and lips are dry. Chronic nasopharyngitis may be constantly present or recur frequently. The voice is altered with a nasal, muffled quality. The breath is offensive, and taste and smell are impaired. A harassing cough may be present, especially at night, resulting from drainage of pus into the lower pharynx or irritation of the larynx by inspired air that has not been warmed and moistened by passage through the nose. Impaired hearing is common. Chronic otitis media may be associated with infected, hypertrophied adenoids and blockage of the eustachian tube orifices. Chronic mouth breathing predisposes to a narrow, high-arched palate and an elongated mandible. Referrals from orthodontists for evaluation of nasal obstruction and adenoidectomy are frequent.

A small number of young children with marked adenoidal (also tonsillar) enlargement are unable to mouth breathe during sleep. They snort and snore loudly and often display signs of respiratory distress, such as intercostal retractions and nasal flaring. These children are at risk for respiratory insufficiency (hypoxemia, hypercapnia, acidosis) during sleep. Obstructive sleep apnea may result, and some of these children develop pulmonary arterial hypertension and, ultimately, cor pulmonale (see Chapter 330). Lymphoid tissue enlargement of the upper airway with consequent cor pulmonale has been related to cow's milk hypersensitivity in a number of preschool-aged children. Very obese children (e.g., Prader-Willi syndrome) and children with a large or posteriorly placed tongue (e.g., Pierre Robin syndrome) may also develop upper airway obstruction in sleep, mimicking the adenoidal hypertrophy syndrome. Patients with Down syndrome commonly have macroglossia, tonsillar enlargement, and skull base anomalies, which make them susceptible to obstruction.

DIAGNOSIS. During the first few years of life, the size of adenoids can be assessed by digital palpation. Indirect visualization with a pharyngeal mirror is possible in older, cooperative children. Alternatively, the fiberoptic bronchoscope can be used for visualization of the nasopharynx. Lateral pharyngeal roentgenograms are also helpful for detecting nasopharyngeal air column obliteration. The presence of adenoid hypertrophy can be suspected from such symptoms as mouth breathing, snoring, and persistent rhinitis with or without chronic otitis media.

An adenoid tissue abscess is uncommon but may be a cause of protracted fever. Identification and drainage of the abscess have been achieved by digital expression.

TREATMENT. Adenoidectomy may be indicated for symptoms such as persistent mouth breathing, nasal speech, adenoid facies, repeated attacks of otitis media (especially when accompanied by a conductive hearing loss), and persistent or recurring nasopharyngitis when these seem to be related to infected hypertrophied adenoid tissue. Tonsillectomy should not be done routinely for such problems. Chronic serous otitis media may improve after adenoidectomy in some patients. The same precautions for the complete removal and control of bleeding points, such as in tonsillectomy, should be observed.

Boat TF, Polmar SH, Whitman V, et al: Hyperreactivity to cow milk in young children with pulmonary hemosiderosis and cor pulmonale secondary to nasopharyngeal obstruction. J Pediatr 87:23, 1975.
Carson JL, Collier AM, Collier HSS: Acquired ciliary defects in nasal epithelium of children with acute viral upper respiratory infections. N Engl J Med 312:463, 1985.
Coulthard M, Isaacs D: Retropharyngeal abscess. Arch Dis Child 66:1227, 1991.
Crockett DM, McGill TJ, Healy GB, et al: Nasal and paranasal sinus surgery in children with cystic fibrosis. Ann Otol Rhinol Laryngol 96:367, 1987.
Denny FW, Clyde WA: Acute respiratory tract infections: An overview: Pediatrics 17:1026, 1983.
Dingle JH, Badger GF, Jordan WS: Illness in the Home: A Study of 25,000 Illnesses in a Group of Cleveland Families. Cleveland, OH, Press of Western Reserve University, 1964, p 129.
Glasier CM, Ascher DP, Williams KD: Incidental paranasal sinus abnormalities on CT of children: Clinical correlation. AJNR 7:861, 1986.
Johnson F: Bleeding factors and tonsils and adenoid surgery. Arch Otolaryngol 86:584, 1967.
Li K, Kiernon S, Wald ER, et al: Isolated uvulitis due to *Haemophilus influenzae* type b. Pediatrics 74:1054, 1984.
Newman LJ, Platts-Mills TAE, Phillips CD, et al: Chronic sinusitis. JAMA 271:363, 1994.
Paradise JL, Bluestone CD, Backman RZ, et al: Efficacy of tonsillectomy for recurrent throat infection in severely affected children. N Engl J Med 310:674, 1984.
Paradise JL, Bluestone CD, Backman RZ, et al: History of recurrent sore throat as an indication for tonsillectomy. N Engl J Med 298:410, 1978.
Rachelefsky GS: Chronic sinusitis, Am J Dis Child 143:886, 1989.
Simma B, Spehler D, Burger R, et al: Tracheostomy in children. Eur J Pediatr 153:291, 1994.
Spires JR: Treatment of peritonsillar abscess: A prospective study of aspiration vs incision and drainage. Arch Otolaryngol Head Neck Surg 113:984, 1987.
Tinkelman DG, Silk HJ: Clinical and bacteriologic features of chronic sinusitis in children. Am J Dis Child 143:938, 1989.
Wald ER: Acute sinusitis in children. Pediatr Infect Dis 2:61, 1983.

CHAPTER 330
Obstructive Sleep Apnea and Hypoventilation in Children

Carol L. Rosen and Gabriel G. Haddad

Obstructive sleep apnea/hypoventilation (OSA/H) is a common disorder that has become increasingly recognized in children. It is characterized by a combination of prolonged partial upper airway obstruction and intermittent complete obstruction (obstructive apnea) that disrupts normal ventilation and sleep patterns. Habitual snoring, the most common symptom, occurs in 8–10% of all young school children. The incidence of severe OSA/H is estimated to be 1% of these snoring children. However, the exact incidence of clinically significant OSA/H between these two ends of the spectrum is not known. The peak age is 2–5 yr, which coincides with both normal lymphoid hyperplasia and frequent upper respiratory infections. In prepubertal children, the incidence in males and females is similar, which contrasts to the male predominance seen in adults.

PATHOGENESIS. OSA/H occurs when there is a failure to maintain upper airway patency during sleep, which in turn affects blood gas homeostasis. Decreased patency can be complete or incomplete and occurs usually during sleep, although in severe cases obstruction is present in both wakefulness and sleep. Airway patency is normally actively maintained by the dilator muscles of the upper airway, which counterbalance the forces that tend to collapse the upper airway, such as the intraluminal negative pressure generated by the diaphragm and mucosal adhesion forces. Normally, despite the facts that the pharyngeal airway is a collapsible tube and the upper airway muscle tone decreases remarkably during sleep, especially during REM sleep, upper airway patency is maintained and ventilatory output and oxygenation are not impaired. Although sleep plays a permissive role, paO_2 decreases and $paCO_2$ increases only slightly in normal children. However, when certain anatomic factors (adenotosillar hypertrophy, nasal obstruction, obesity, craniofacial anomalies) or neurologic conditions (hypotonia as in trisomy 21, cranial nerve weakness) occur, OSA/H may ensue. This cascade of events is depicted in Figure 330–1; as upper airway muscle activity decreases, the upper airway narrows and upper airway resistance increases in the presence of anatomic or neurologic factors. Episodes of partial or complete airway obstruction result in impaired gas exchange with hypoxemia and hypercapnia. These blood gas abnormalities are potent stimuli for increased ventilatory effort and upper airway muscle activity. Increased effort and airway muscle tone lead to resumption of airway patency. Arousal from sleep may also occur which helps in restoring blood gases. When airflow is restored, oxygen and carbon dioxide levels return to normal. Sleep is re-established, upper airway muscle activity decreases, and the cycle starts again.

The development of OSA/H can have serious cardiorespiratory and neurobehavioral consequences. Chronic hypoxemia

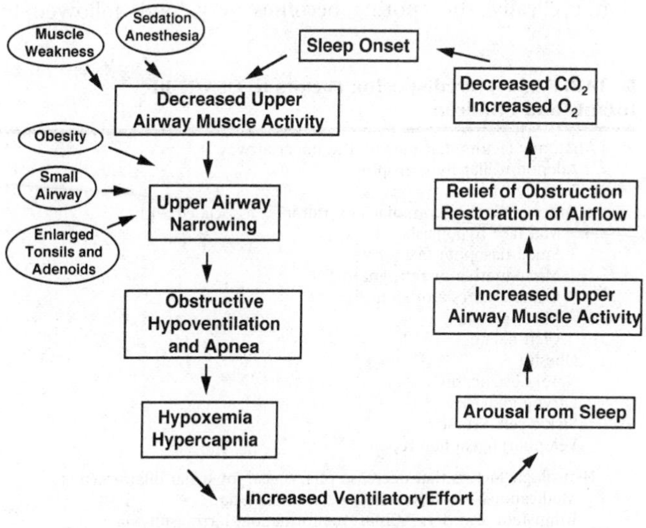

Figure 330–1. Pathophysiology of OSA/H in children.

can lead to polycythemia, growth failure, increased pulmonary artery pressure and pulmonary hypertension, right heart failure, arrhythmias, or even death. Recurrent arousals can lead to sleep fragmentation, loss of normal sleep patterns, and excessive daytime sleepiness. This hypersomnolence can be associated with behavioral problems, impaired school performance, and accidents. Finally, sleep fragmentation itself can suppress arousal responses and further impair the ability to reestablish upper airway patency and restore gas exchange.

Several medical conditions are major risk factors for OSA/H (Table 330–1). In children, the most common anatomic factor that leads to obstruction is adenostonsillar hypertrophy. Other anatomic factors, such as micrognathia, retrognathia, or macroglossia, force the tongue into the oropharyngeal portion of the airway and occlude it. Fat deposition from morbid obesity or congenitally small airway narrow the nasopharynx. Increased resistance from swollen nasal turbinates or choanal stenosis places a greater negative collapsing pressure on the pharyngeal airway. Diminished ventilatory responses to hypoxemia and hypercapnia can attenuate the increase in ventilatory effort and impair an adequate response. Diminished arousal responses can impair the ability to restore upper airway patency (see Fig. 330–1). Finally, sedative medication or general anesthesia can further compromise neural control of the upper airway.

CLINICAL MANIFESTATIONS. The clinical presentation of OSA/H includes a range of symptoms from snoring to severe cardiorespiratory sequelae, but the majority of children with OSA/H do not present with dramatic repetitive obstructive apneas. Instead, obstruction is partial and tonic. Because phasic obstructive apnea is rare, arousals are infrequent and sleep architecture may not be disturbed. For this reason, daytime hypersomnolence, the most common presenting symptom of OSA/H in adults, is rare in children. Because of this more subtle presentation, children often have an unexpected degree of airway obstruction, impairment of gas exchange, and sleep disturbance that is difficult to predict from the clinical history and physical exam alone.

Common clinical manifestations of OSA/H include chronic mouth breathing, snoring, and restlessness during sleep with or without frequent awakening. Children may sleep in unusual positions with the neck hyperextended or with the bottom up in the air to help maintain a patent upper airway. Typically loud snoring is the symptom that most disturbs, and therefore alerts, the parents. Most children with OSA/H breathe normally while awake, but children with the more severe presentation will also have noisy, mildly labored awake breathing that clearly worsens with sleep. Parents will describe that cyclically, the snoring becomes very loud, followed by silence, a snort, an arousal, and resumption of snoring. When snoring is associated with nocturnal breathing difficulties and witnessed respiratory pauses, this triad of symptoms is highly suggestive of OSA/H in children. However, clinical experience suggests that some infants with serious OSA/H have little or no snoring, and their diagnosis depends on the physician's high index of suspicion.

Less common symptoms include daytime hypersomnolence resulting from sleep fragmentation that occurs when obstructive apnea is repeatedly terminated by arousals. Behavioral problems and poor school performance have been described, but the incidence of these problems in OSA/H is unknown. However, it is difficult to recognize excessive sleepiness in young children, who normally have daytime naps and early bed times. Secondary enuresis that disappears after surgical relief of the upper airway obstruction is occasionally seen, but the mechanisms are poorly understood. In contrast to adults, most children with OSA/H are not obese. In fact, some children are underweight or present with failure to thrive. Several factors can contribute to this growth retardation: dysphagia from large tonsils, chronic hypoxemia, higher metabolic expenditure from increased work of breathing, and insufficient growth hormone release in the absence of deep NREM sleep. Children can also present with unexplained right heart failure, but other cardiovascular complications, such as systemic hypertension or life-threatening cardiac arrhythmias, are rarely seen. Finally, in the more severe cases, a relatively minor respiratory illness or infection can trigger an acute episode of respiratory failure.

DIAGNOSIS AND ASSESSMENT. The diagnosis of OSA/H in children is often delayed despite years of symptoms for several reasons: (1) absence of awake symptoms; (2) failure to obtain a sleep history; (3) symptoms of snoring or restless sleep are considered inconsequential; (4) parents may be unaware of the problem because the child's most severe symptoms appear during REM sleep in the last 3rd of the night when parents are asleep; and (5) young children may not generate the loud, disruptive snoring noises of an adult. The diagnosis of OSA/H should be suggested by the clinical presentation. A sleep history should be part of every well child exam, and parental reports of habitual snoring should not be dismissed without further investigation. A sleep and breathing history is also very important for any child with a medical condition that is a risk factor for OSA/H, especially trisomy 21, craniofacial anomalies, or neuromuscular disorders. A home tape recording during sleep may be helpful. However, the history of loud snoring alone is not sufficient to diagnose OSA/H.

The physical examination performed during wakefulness may be entirely normal but should not be used to exclude OSA/H when the clinical history suggests otherwise. Features associated with OSA/H include: unusual facies, mouth breathing, hyponasal speech, macroglossia, cleft palate, or enlarged tonsils. However, snoring, reports of difficulty breathing, and enlarged tonsils are unreliable predictors of the presence or severity of OSA/H in children. Specific craniofacial anomalies may be apparent. A pectus excavatum deformity can develop in longstanding upper airway obstruction. Morbid obesity mechanically loads the chest wall and narrows the upper airway, but OSA/H is not a consistent feature of obesity. The presence of excessive somnolence during the examination requires urgent evaluation. The presence of stridor or hoarse voice can indicate cranial nerve dysfunction and should prompt a meticulous neurologic exam. In particular, cranial nerve dysfunction, weakness, hyper-reflexia, and loss of position and vibratory sense point to brainstem and spinal cord abnormalities. The evaluation would include polysomnography and/or magnetic resonance imaging (MRI) with attention to the brainstem, cervicomedullary junction, and spinal cord.

Laboratory findings such as polycythemia or metabolic alka-

■ TABLE 330–1 Predisposing Factors to OSA/H in Infants and Children

- Anatomic factors that narrow the upper airway
  - Adenotonsillar hypertrophy
  - Trisomy 21
  - Other genetic or craniofacial syndromes associated with
    - Mid face hypoplasia
    - Small nasopharynx
    - Micrognathia or retrognathia
    - Choanal atresia or stenosis
    - Macroglossia
    - Cleft palate
  - Obesity
  - Nasal obstruction
  - Laryngomalacia
  - Sickle cell disease
  - Velopharyngeal flap repair
- Neurologic factors that decrease pharyngeal muscular dilator activity
  - Medications—sedatives or general anesthesia
  - Brainstem disorders—Chiari malformation, birth asphyxia
  - Neuromuscular disease

losis support the diagnosis of OSA/H when present, but in the majority of pediatric patients they are absent. Right ventricular hypertrophy on ECG and dysfunction on echocardiogram are only seen in the severe cases of OSA/H. A lateral soft tissue radiograph of the neck can identify adenoidal tissue but fails to give a three-dimensional, supine view of the airway during sleep. Although computed tomography (CT) or MRI of the nasopharynx displays airway dimensions and fluroscopy or endoscopy shows airway dynamics, these imaging techniques are only "snapshots" of the disorder. When procedures require sedation or anesthesia, extreme caution is required if OSA/H is suspected. Such medications have profound effects on upper airway muscle tone, and sudden respiratory decompensation can occur in these children.

Polysomnography (PSG), an overnight recording of multiple physiologic sensors during sleep is the "gold standard" for the diagnosis of OSA/H. PSG provides a powerful, quantitative, noninvasive assessment of gas exchange impairment, respiratory pattern, thoraco-abdominal movement, and sleep disruption. PSG is especially useful in confirming the diagnosis, in determining the severity of OSA/H, and in documenting the efficacy of treatment. PSG may not be required for diagnostic purposes in all patients. For example, PSG may not be necessary when a child has noisy, awake mouth breathing and tonsils that occlude most of the pharyngeal space; is excessively sleepy; and is observed by skilled personnel to have signs of airway obstruction (apnea and retractions) and hypoxemia. However, in the majority of cases the clinical presentation is not so obvious. Even though PSG may not be required for diagnosis before treatment, it can provide an important clinical baseline to assess the severity and efficacy of treatment, especially in children who are at increased risk for either failure of adenotonsillectomy or operative and postoperative complications. This group includes very young children and children with complex medical problems or craniofacial anomalies.

Several other disorders should be considered in the differential diagnosis of OSA/H or may coexist with this problem. Occasionally, breathing difficulty associated with nocturnal asthma or upper airway obstruction from gastroesophageal reflux may be confused with OSA/H. New onset dysphagia and swallowing difficulties associated with an esophageal foreign body that compresses the airway can masquerade as OSA/H. Stridor due to anatomic airway problems, such as laryngomalacia, vascular ring, intraluminal masses, and vocal cord dysfunction, should be considered. Parasomnia events, such as night terrors or even nocturnal seizures, may be mistaken for arousals associated with OSA/H. Narcolepsy and restless leg syndrome should be considered when PSG fails to document OSA/H in a child with a daytime hypersomnolence.

TREATMENT. Because adenotonsillar hyperplasia is the most common condition associated with pediatric OSA/H, adenotonsillectomy (T&A) provides definitive relief of obstruction in the majority of patients. Children with severe OSA/H who benefit from surgery often demonstrate "catch-up" growth. However, children with underlying problems, such as trisomy 21, craniofacial disorders, extreme obesity, neuromuscular disorders such as cerebral palsy or Chiari malformation, or who present before 2 yr of age are at risk for incomplete resolution of OSA/H after T&A. Even without these risk factors, the parents and health care providers of children who have had T&A should be aware that either persistent or recurring symptoms of OSA/H need reevaluation and possible treatment.

Medical management with nasal continuous airway pressure (CPAP) is an option in children who fail T&A, thus avoiding the need for a tracheostomy. CPAP is safe and well tolerated but requires a motivated family for compliance. PSG is required to select the appropriate pressure level to relieve obstruction. Follow-up PSG should be performed at regular intervals because the long-term stability of CPAP requirements in the growing child is not known. CPAP should not be first line treatment when adenotonsillar hypertrophy is present and absolute contraindications to surgery are absent. CPAP can be useful in the obese child in whom weight loss is desirable but difficult to achieve. Supplemental oxygen may relieve the hypoxemia associated with OSA/H but is clearly insufficient to address the underlying obstruction and hypoventilation.

Pharmacological management has only a limited role in pediatric OSA/H patients. Snoring associated with nasal obstruction can be treated with nasal decongestants and topical steroids, but this management is rarely sufficient to reverse significant OSA/H. Medroxyprogesterone acetate augments ventilatory drive and has been used in the management of the daytime hypoventilation associated with the obesity-hypoventilation syndrome. However, this drug fails to improve nocturnal obstructive symptoms and has adverse effects on growth and pubertal development. Protriptyline is a nonsedating antidepressant with REM suppressant activity that has been tried in adult OSA/H patients. Although it reduces the number of more severe obstructive apnea episodes by decreasing the amount of sleep time spent in REM, it fails to treat the obstructive process and is not recommended.

If serious upper airway obstruction is present in both wakefulness and sleep, tracheostomy is the treatment of choice for vocal cord dysfunction, impaired swallowing, and absent laryngeal protective reflexes. Definitive maxillomandibular reconstructive surgery for children with craniofacial disorders is another therapeutic option but is usually postponed until facial growth is complete. Uvulopalatopharyngoplasty (UPPP), the resection of redundant pharyngeal tissue, has been used to eliminate snoring in adults, but the failure rate is high. Pediatric experience with this surgery has been limited to children with muscular hypotonia and oropharyngeal tissue redundancy, but no controlled studies using objective measures of efficacy have been performed.

Brouillette RT: Assessing cardiopulmonary function during sleep in infants and children. *In*: Beckerman RC et al (eds): Respiratory Control Disorders in Infants and Children. Baltimore, MD, Williams & Wilkins, 1992, pp 125–141.

Dyson M, Beckerman RC, Brouillette RT: Obstructive sleep apnea syndrome. *In*: Beckerman RC et al (eds): Respiratory Control Disorders in Infants and Children. Baltimore, MD, Williams & Wilkins, 1992, pp 212–230.

Guilleminault C, Korobkin R, Winkle R: A review of 50 children with obstructive sleep apnea syndrome. Lung 159:275, 1981.

Marcus C, Omlin K, Basinki D, et al: Normal polysomnographic values for children and adolescents. Am Rev Respir Dis 146:1235, 1992.

Rosen CL, D'Andrea L, Haddad GG: Adult criteria for obstructive sleep apnea do not identify children with serious obstruction. Am Rev Respir Dis 146:1231, 1992.

SECTION 3
Lower Respiratory Tract

CHAPTER 331
Congenital Anomalies

Robert C. Stern

331.1 Laryngeal Anomalies

Complete **atresia of the larynx** is incompatible with life; only rarely can an infant in whom the diagnosis is made at birth be saved by immediate needle tracheostomy and high-pressure transtracheal ventilation. A formal tracheostomy is then performed. Subsequent successful surgical restoration of an adequate upper airway has not been reported. Patients with laryngeal atresia often have other congenital defects that also may be incompatible with life. **Laryngeal webs** are uncommon, occasionally familial, defects resulting from incomplete separation of the fetal mesenchyme between the two sides of the larynx. Most webs occur between the vocal cords. Immediate diagnosis of a complete or nearly complete web is essential to prevent asphyxiation of the newborn. The child may have respiratory distress with severe stridor, and the cry is weak and abnormal in character. The obstruction is often incomplete, with only mild stridor and dyspnea. Direct laryngoscopy is required for prompt diagnosis and treatment. Lysis with a carbon dioxide laser is frequently successful, but surgery is occasionally necessary. Thin supraglottic webs can also be incised, but infants with thicker subglottic or intralaryngeal webs require initial incision, excision, and subsequent dilations, which may be unsuccessful because of reformation of the web. An external approach to divide and excise the web with insertion of silicone or metal is often required. Many surgically treated patients need a tracheostomy for a prolonged period thereafter.

Laryngotracheoesophageal cleft is a rare congenital lesion in which there is a long connection between the airway and the esophagus, sometimes extending to the level of the carina. The lesion is caused by failure of dorsal fusion of the cricoid, which normally is completed by the 8th wk of gestation. Several subtypes have been reported. Type 1 lesions are those above the superior portion of the posterior cricoid plate; type 2 lesions extend to the inferior aspect of the posterior cricoid plate; type 3 includes those that involve the "cervical trachea," and type 4 extend into the thoracic trachea and below. Other anomalies, including unilateral pulmonary hypoplasia, may be present. Symptoms of chronic aspiration, gagging during feeding, and pneumonia suggest H-type tracheoesophageal fistula, but the clinical manifestations are usually more severe and associated with abnormalities in voice. Diagnosis is extremely difficult, but careful roentgenographic studies of swallowing can show aspiration of contrast material into the trachea indicating the need for endoscopic examination of the airway and perhaps the esophagus. The prognosis depends on the severity of the lesion. Some type 1 lesions can be repaired endoscopically. Successful repair of more severe lesions has been reported, but always requires multiple procedures and prolonged tracheostomy.

331.2 Congenital Laryngeal Stridor

(Laryngomalacia and Tracheomalacia)

Stridor persisting or appearing after the first few days of life usually results from disturbances in or adjacent to the larynx. The most common of these, **laryngomalacia** and **tracheomalacia,** are congenital deformities or flabbiness of the epiglottis and supraglottic aperture and weakness of the airway walls, leading to collapse and some airway obstruction with inspiration. Laryngomalacia is the most common congenital laryngeal abnormality. The embryologic origin of the defect is unknown.

CLINICAL MANIFESTATIONS. Noisy, crowing respiratory sounds, usually associated with inspiration, are relatively common during the neonatal period and the first year of life. Stridor, usually present from birth, may not appear until 2 mo in some patients. In symptomatic patients with laryngomalacia, the male to female ratio may be 2.5:1. Symptoms can be intermittent and are worse when the infant lies on his or her back. Some infants merely have noisy breathing, but others have a laryngeal "crow," hoarseness or aphonia, dyspnea, and inspiratory retractions in the supraclavicular, intercostal, and subcostal space. When retractions are severe, thoracic deformity may result. Infants with severe dyspnea may have difficulty nursing, resulting in undernutrition and poor weight gain. Substantial stridor may persist for several months to 1 yr after birth, occasionally becoming slightly worse in the first few months of life and then gradually disappearing with growth and development of the airway.

DIAGNOSIS. Laryngomalacia can usually be diagnosed by direct laryngoscopy. In the first few days of life, differentiating a congenital laryngeal disturbance from neonatal tetany or laryngeal edema secondary to trauma or aspiration at birth may be difficult. The differential diagnosis includes malformations of the laryngeal cartilages or vocal cords, intraluminal webs, generalized severe chondromalacia of the larynx and trachea, tumors of the larynx, mucus retention cysts, branchial cleft cysts, thyroglossal duct remnants, hypoplasia of the mandible, macroglossia, hemangioma, lymphangioma, Pierre Robin syndrome, congenital goiters, and vascular anomalies. Other respiratory tract anomalies may be common in patients with laryngomalacia, especially those who are older than 4 mo at presentation. This prompted the suggestion that full bronchoscopy, rather than laryngoscopy alone, is indicated in these patients.

TREATMENT. Usually no specific therapy is indicated; the condition resolves spontaneously, although there may be difficulty in feeding. In one review, only 4 of 1,415 patients required tracheostomy. Parents should be reassured about the ultimate resolution and counseled to provide slow, careful feedings. A small nipple or dropper or, infrequently, gavage may be required. Most patients seem more comfortable or less noisy lying in a prone position. Severe symptoms may require nasotracheal intubation or, rarely, tracheostomy.

PROGNOSIS. Although laryngomalacia usually resolves clinically by 18 mo of age, some degree of inspiratory obstruction may persist a little longer. Sophisticated pulmonary function testing reveals that minor abnormalities persist, into the teenage years in some patients, but these do not pose any clinically important problems and do not require treatment. However, some patients may develop stridor with respiratory infection, exertion, or crying throughout childhood.

OTHER ANOMALIES. Bifid epiglottis, resulting from cleavage of two thirds or more of the epiglottis, is a rare condition that may not compromise swallowing. It usually does require treatment, however, and is associated with other laryngeal anomalies and with polydactyly. Total absence of the epiglottis is extremely rare. Laryngeal cysts and laryngoceles are occasionally seen; treatment with endoscopic "unroofing" is usually successful.

DuBois JJ, Pokorny WJ, Harberg FJ, et al: Current management of laryngeal and laryngotracheoesophageal clefts. J Ped Surg 25:855, 1990.
Fang SH, Ocejo R, Sin M, et al: Congenital laryngeal atresia. Am J Dis Child 143:625, 1989.
Landing BH: State of the art: Congenital malformations and genetic diseases of the respiratory tract. Am Rev Respir Dis 120:151, 1979.
Macfarlane PI, Olinsky A, Phelan PD: Proximal airway function 8–16 years after laryngomalacia: Follow-up using flow-volume loop studies. J Pediatr 107:216, 1985.
Marcus CL, Crockett DM, Ward SLD: Evaluation of epiglottoplasty as treatment for severe laryngomalacia. J Pediatr 117:706, 1990.
McGill TJI, Healy BG: Congenital and acquired lesions of the infant larynx. Clin Pediatr 17:584, 1978.
Novak RW: Laryngotracheoesophageal cleft and unilateral pulmonary hypoplasia in twins. Pediatrics 67:732, 1981.
Nussbaum E, Maggi JC: Laryngomalacia in children. Chest 98:942, 1990.
Smith RJH, Catlin FI: Congenital anomalies of the larynx. Am J Dis Child 138:35, 1984.

TRACHEOESOPHAGEAL FISTULA

See Chapter 265.

VASCULAR RING

See Chapter 386.26.

331.3 Agenesis or Hypoplasia of the Lung

Bilateral pulmonary agenesis or significant hypoplasia is incompatible with life; hypoplasia is usually associated with anencephaly, diaphragmatic hernias, urinary tract abnormalities, abnormalities of the thumb, deformities of the thoracic spine and rib cage (thoracic dystrophy), renal anomalies (oligohydramnios), right-sided heart malformations, and congenital pleural effusions. Bilateral hypoplasia is found in 10% of all neonatal autopsies (30% of babies younger than 1 wk of age); it plays an important role in the death of many patients with the conditions previously listed. Unilateral agenesis or hypoplasia may have few symptoms and nonspecific findings, resulting in only one third of the cases being diagnosed during life. Left-sided lesions are more common. In unilateral agenesis, the entire pulmonary parenchyma and supporting structures and airways are absent below the level of the carina. A child with unilateral pulmonary hypoplasia usually has a small unexpandable lung. Persistent pulmonary hypertension is often present when pulmonary hypoplasia presents in the newborn period (see Chap. 87.7). Occasional reports of parental consanguinity suggest a genetic basis for at least some of these cases.

There is no specific treatment. Supportive measures including mechanical ventilation and supplemental oxygen may allow sufficient pulmonary parenchymal development to permit survival (25% of the infants in one series). Older patients should be given antibiotics for pulmonary infection and receive annual influenza vaccine. Prognoses for the patients who survive infancy are extremely variable and largely depend on the presence of associated anomalies. The contralateral lung is often larger than normal. The resultant mediastinal shift and associated mortality are greater when the hypoplasia or agenesis involves the right lung. Death may also occur from overwhelming pulmonary infection or from complications of pulmonary hypertension associated with congenital heart disease.

Husain AN, Hessel RG: Neonatal pulmonary hypoplasia: An autopsy study of 25 cases. Pediatr Pathol 13:475, 1993.
Kresch MJ, Markowitz RI, Smith GJW: Respiratory distress and cyanosis in a term newborn infant. J Pediatr 113:937, 1988.
Mardini MK, Nyhan WL: Agenesis of the lung: Report of four patients with unusual anomalies. Chest 87:522, 1985.

LOBAR EMPHYSEMA

See Chapter 354.

331.4 Pulmonary Sequestration

A mass of nonfunctioning embryonic and cystic pulmonary tissue that receives its entire blood supply from the systemic circulation is known as a sequestration. Although most sequestrations do not communicate with functional airways, this is not always the case. Intralobar and extralobar sequestrations probably arise through the same pathoembryologic mechanism as a remnant of a diverticular outgrowth of the esophagus. However, some workers propose that intralobar sequestration is an acquired lesion primarily caused by infection and inflammation, which lead to cystic changes and hypertrophy of a feeding systemic artery. This is consistent with the rarity of this lesion in autopsy series of newborns. Gastric or pancreatic tissue may be found within the sequestration. Cysts may also be present. Other congenital anomalies, including diaphragmatic hernia and esophageal cysts, are not uncommon. Some believe that intralobar sequestration is often a manifestation of cystadenomatoid malformation and have questioned the existence of intralobar sequestration as a separate entity.

Intralobar sequestration is generally found in a lower lobe. Patients usually present with infection. In older patients, hemoptysis is fairly common. A chest roentgenogram during a period when there is no active infection reveals a mass lesion; an air-fluid level may be present. During infection, the margins of the lesion may be blurred. There is no difference in the incidence of this lesion in each lung. Treatment is surgical removal of the lesion, a procedure that usually requires excision of the entire involved lobe. A segmental resection occasionally suffices.

Extralobar sequestration is much more common in males and usually involves the left lung. This lesion is associated strongly with diaphragmatic hernia. Many of these patients are asymptomatic when the mass is discovered by routine chest roentgenogram taken for another reason. Other patients present with respiratory symptoms or heart failure. Surgical resection of the involved area is recommended.

Physical findings in patients with sequestration include an area of dullness to percussion and decreased breath sounds over the lesion. During infection, rales may also be present. A continuous or purely systolic murmur may be heard over the back. If routine chest roentgenograms are consistent with the diagnosis, other procedures are indicated before surgical intervention. Bronchography reveals a mass of intrathoracic tissue without connection to the airways. Ultrasound can help rule out a diaphragmatic hernia. Preoperative aortography is recommended to confirm the diagnosis and to delineate the blood supply of the lesion. However, some workers now believe that Doppler ultrasonography and magnetic resonance imaging are sufficient in most cases. Identifying the blood supply before surgery avoids inadvertently severing this systemic artery, which has accounted for much of the intraoperative mortality in the past.

Case Records of the Massachusetts General Hospital: Case 14–1991. N Engl J Med 324:980, 1991.
Hernanz-Schulman M: Cysts and cystlike lesions of the lung. Radiologic Clin North Am 31:631, 1993.
Nicolette LA, Kosloske AM, Bartow SA, et al: Intralobar pulmonary sequestration: A clinical and pathological spectrum. J Pediatr Surg 28:802, 1993.
Tolkin JB, MacAdam C, Moody S: Extralobar pulmonary sequestration. Am J Dis Child 141:1223, 1987.

331.5 Bronchogenic Cysts

Bronchogenic cysts arise from abnormal budding of the tracheal diverticulum of the foregut and are originally lined with ciliated epithelium. They are most commonly found near a midline structure (e.g., trachea, esophagus, carina), but peripheral lower lobe and perihilar intrapulmonary cysts are not infrequent. Diagnosis may be precipitated by enlargement of the cyst, which causes symptoms by pressure on an adjacent airway. When the diagnosis is delayed until infection occurs, the ciliated epithelium may be lost, and accurate pathologic diagnosis is then impossible. Cysts are rarely demonstrable at birth. Later, some cysts become symptomatic by becoming infected or by enlarging in size and compromising the function of an adjacent airway. Fever, chest pain, and productive cough are the most common presenting symptoms. A chest roentgenogram reveals the cyst, which may contain an air-fluid level. Treatment for symptomatic cysts is surgical excision after appropriate antibiotic management. An asymptomatic cyst discovered incidentally by chest roentgenogram taken for another reason may not require treatment.

Hernanz-Schulman M: Cysts and cystlike lesions of the lung. Radiol Clin North Am 31:631, 1993.

331.6 Bronchobiliary Fistula

This rare anomaly usually presents life-threatening problems during early infancy but diagnosis occasionally has been delayed until adulthood. Females are more commonly affected. The bronchobiliary fistula consists of a fistulous connection between the right middle lobe bronchus and the left hepatic ductal system. All patients have recurrent severe bronchopulmonary infection starting in early infancy. Definitive diagnosis requires endoscopy and bronchography or exploratory surgery. Treatment includes surgical excision of the entire intrathoracic portion of the fistula. If the hepatic portion of the fistula does not communicate with the biliary system or duodenum, the involved segment may also have to be resected. Bronchobiliary communications also occur as acquired lesions resulting from hepatic disease complicated by infection.

Gauderer MWL, Oiticica C, Bishop HC: Congenital bronchobiliary fistula: management of the involved hepatic segment. J Pediatr Surg 28:452, 1993.
Pappas SC, Sasaki A, Minuk GY: Bronchobiliary fistula presenting as cough with yellow sputum. N Engl J Med 307:1027, 1982.
Yamaguchi M, Kanamori K, Fujimura M, et al: Congenital bronchobiliary fistula in adults. South Med J 83:851, 1990.

331.7 Congenital Pulmonary Lymphangiectasis

This disease, characterized by greatly dilated lymphatic ducts throughout the lung, is usually symptomatic with dyspnea and cyanosis in the newborn. Chest roentgenograms reveal punctate and reticular densities. Respiration is compromised because of the space-occupying nature of the lesion and possibly because pulmonary compliance is reduced, increasing the work of breathing. Two forms of the disease—one in which the abnormality is limited to the lung and one in which the pulmonary lymphangiectasis is secondary to pulmonary venous obstruction—are always symptomatic in the neonatal period. Familial occurrence of the first type has been reported. Survival beyond infancy is rare. A third form, in which the pulmonary lymphangiectasis is part of a generalized disease involving other organ systems (e.g., intestine), is associated with milder pulmonary disease and survival to midchildhood and beyond. Definitive diagnosis requires lung biopsy. There is no specific treatment.

Case Records of the Massachusetts General Hospital: Case 31–1989. N Engl J Med 321:309, 1989.
Felman AH, Rhatigan RM, Pierson KK: Pulmonary lymphangiectasis. Am J Roent 116:548, 1972.
Huber A, Schranz D, Blaha I, et al: Congenital pulmonary lymphangiectasia. Pediatr Pulmonol 10:310, 1991.

331.8 Cystic Adenomatoid Malformation

This is the second most common congenital lung lesion; lobar emphysema is the most common. A single lobe of one lung is enlarged and often cystic, compressing the remainder of the ipsilateral lung and frequently causing a mediastinum shift with compression of the contralateral lung. The remaining ipsilateral lung may be hypoplastic as a result of the space-occupying nature of the lesion. There is a slight male preponderance. The lesion probably results from an embryologic insult, usually before the 50th day of gestation, and seems to involve maldevelopment of terminal bronchiolar structures. Histologic examination reveals little normal lung and many glandular elements. Cysts are very common; cartilage is rare. The presence of cartilage may indicate a somewhat later embryologic insult, perhaps extending into the 10th–24th wk.

Cystic adenomatoid malformations can be diagnosed in utero by ultrasound. In one series of 10 such cases, the diagnosis was made at a mean age of 26 wk of gestation (range, 18–36 wk). Polyhydramnios was common (50%). In one case, the malformation resolved spontaneously before birth. Each of the three patients who died after neonatal surgery had hypoplasia of the remaining ipsilateral lung.

The common types of postnatal clinical manifestations include neonatal respiratory distress, recurrent respiratory infection, and pneumothorax. Most patients become symptomatic and die in the newborn period, although a few survive after emergency surgery. Rarely, patients are asymptomatic until midchildhood, when brief episodes of recurrent or persistent pulmonary infection or relatively acute chest pain occur. Breath sounds may be diminished with mediastinal shift away from the lesion on physical examination. Chest roentgenograms reveal a cystic mass with mediastinal shift. Occasionally, an air-fluid level suggests a lung abscess. The lesion may be confused with diaphragmatic hernia in the newborn. Surgical excision of the affected lobe (occasionally a segment) is indicated. After surgery, long-term survival into infancy and even later into childhood has been reported, but these patients may be at increased risk for developing primary pulmonary neoplasms.

Heij HA, Ekkelkamp S, Vos A: Diagnosis of congenital cystic adenomatoid malformation of the lung in newborn infants and children. Thorax 45:122, 1990.
Neilson IR, Russo P, Laberge JM, et al: Congenital adenomatoid malformation of the lung: current management and prognosis. J Pediatr Surg 26:975, 1991.

CHAPTER 332
Acute Inflammatory Upper Airway Obstruction

David M. Orenstein

GENERAL CONSIDERATIONS. Acute inflammation of the upper airway is of greater importance in infants and small children than older children because the airway is smaller, predisposing young children to a relatively greater narrowing than is produced by the same degree of inflammation in an older child. The larynx is composed of four cartilages (i.e., thyroid, cricoid arytenoid, epiglottic) and the soft tissues joining them. The cricoid cartilage encircles the airway just below the vocal cords and defines the narrowest portion of the pediatric upper airway.

Inflammation involving the vocal cords and structures inferior to the cords is called laryngitis, laryngotracheitis, or laryngotracheobronchitis, and inflammation of the structures superior to the cords (i.e., arytenoids, aryepiglottic folds ["false cords"], epiglottis) is called supraglottitis. Croup is a generic term encompassing a heterogeneous group of relatively acute conditions (mostly infectious) characterized by a peculiarly brassy or "croupy" cough, which may or may not be accompanied by inspiratory stridor, hoarseness, and signs of respiratory distress due to various degrees of laryngeal obstruction. Such infection in infants and small children is rarely limited to a single area of the respiratory tract; it usually affects to some degree the larynx, trachea, and bronchi. When there is sufficient involvement of the larynx to produce symptoms, the laryngeal part of the clinical picture is likely to overshadow tracheal or bronchial signs.

332.1 Infectious Upper Airway Obstruction

ETIOLOGY AND EPIDEMIOLOGY. Viral agents account for most acute infectious upper airway obstructions except that associated with diphtheria, bacterial tracheitis, and acute epiglottitis. The parainfluenza viruses account for approximately 75% of cases; adenoviruses, respiratory syncytial, influenza, and measles viruses cause the remaining viral cases. In one study, *Mycoplasma pneumoniae* was recovered from 3.6% of patients who had acute upper airway obstruction. Although *Haemophilus influenzae* type b is the usual cause of acute epiglottitis, *Streptococcus pyogenes, Streptococcus pneumoniae,* and *Staphylococcus aureus* are occasionally implicated. With the near elimination of infections caused by *H. influenzae* type b due to usage of HiB vaccine, the occurrence of epiglottitis has been reduced dramatically. Accordingly, other agents have begun to represent a larger proportion of cases of epiglottitis. Viral epiglottitis is a rare but milder illness. Most patients who have viral croup are between the ages of 3 mo and 5 yr, but disease due to *H. influenzae* and *Corynebacterium diphtheriae* is more common from 3–7 yr of age. The incidence of croup is higher in males, and it occurs most commonly during the cold season of the year. Approximately 15% of patients have a strong family history of croup, and laryngitis tends to recur in the same child.

CLINICAL MANIFESTATIONS. Croup (Laryngotracheobronchitis). Croup, the most common form of acute upper airway obstruction, is caused primarily by viruses. The opportunity for pathologic study is rare; the primary findings appear to be inflammatory edema, destruction of ciliated epithelium, and exudate. Secondary bacterial infection is rare. Most patients have an upper respiratory tract infection for several days before cough becomes apparent. With progressive compromise of the upper airway, a characteristic sequence of symptoms and signs occurs. At first, there is only a mild, brassy cough with intermittent inspiratory stridor. As obstruction increases, stridor becomes continuous and is associated with worsening cough, nasal flaring and suprasternal, infrasternal, and intercostal retractions. As inflammation extends to the bronchi and bronchioles, respiratory difficulty increases, and the expiratory phase of respiration also becomes labored and prolonged. Various degrees of lower respiratory involvement occur. The temperature may be only slightly elevated; it rarely reaches 39–40° C (102–104° F). Symptoms are characteristically worse at night and often recur with decreasing intensity for several days. Older children are usually not seriously ill. Other family members may have mild respiratory illness. The duration of illness ranges from several days to, rarely, several weeks; recurrences are frequent from 3–6 yr of age, decreasing with growth of the airway. Most patients with croup progress only as far as stridor and slight dyspnea before they start to recover. In some, there is worse obstruction. Agitation and crying greatly aggravate the symptoms and signs, and the child prefers to sit up in bed or be held upright.

There may be bilaterally diminished breath sounds, rhonchi, and scattered crackles. With further compromise of the airway, air hunger and restlessness occur and are then superseded by severe hypoxemia, hypercapnia, and weakness, accompanied by decreased air exchange and stridor, tachycardia, and eventual death from hypoventilation. In the hypoxemic child who may be cyanotic, pale, or obtunded, any manipulation of the pharynx, including use of a tongue depressor, may result in sudden cardiorespiratory arrest. This examination therefore should be deferred, and oxygen should be administered until the patient is transferred to a place in the hospital where optimal management of the airway and shock is possible. Occasionally, the pattern of severe laryngotracheobronchitis may be difficult to differentiate from epiglottitis despite the usually more explosive onset and rapid course of the latter; it also requires similar precautions. Roentgenographic examination of the nasopharynx and upper airway may be helpful (Fig. 332–1).

Acute Epiglottitis (Supraglottitis). This dramatic, potentially lethal condition usually occurs in children 2–7 yr old; the peak incidence occurs at about 3.5 yr. It is seen much less commonly since the widespread use of immunization against *H. influenzae* type b. Epiglottitis is characterized by a fulminating course of high fever, sore throat, dyspnea, rapidly progressive respiratory obstruction, and prostration, although respiratory distress is

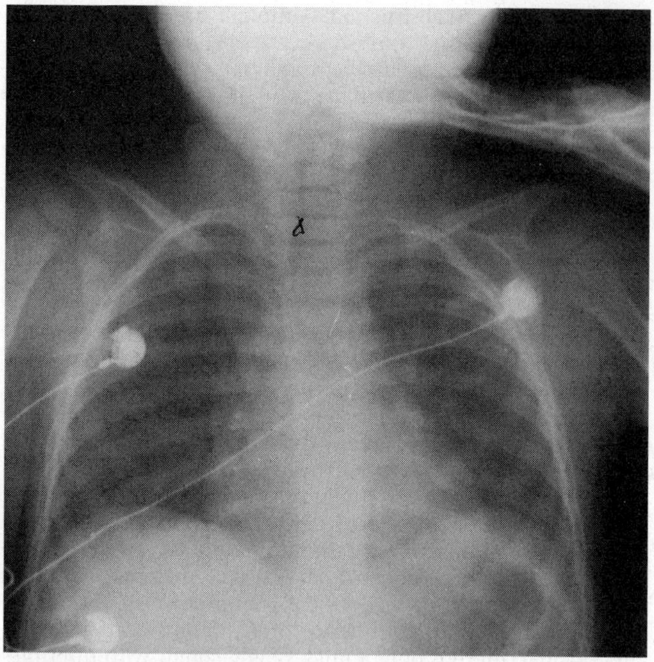

Figure 332–1. Radiograph of an airway of a patient with croup, showing typical subglottic narrowing ("steeple sign").

frequently the first manifestation. Within a matter of hours, it may progress to complete obstruction of the airway and death unless adequate treatment is provided. With adequate treatment, the illness rarely lasts for more than 2–3 days. Often the child, particularly the younger patient, is apparently well at bedtime but awakens later in the evening with high fever, aphonia, drooling, and moderate or severe respiratory distress with stridor. Usually no other family members are ill with acute upper respiratory disease. The older child often complains initially of sore throat and dysphagia. Severe respiratory distress may ensue within minutes or hours of the onset, with inspiratory stridor, hoarseness, brassy cough (less commonly), irritability, and restlessness. Drooling and dysphagia are common. The neck may be hyperextended, although other signs of meningeal irritation are absent. The older child may prefer a sitting position, leaning forward, with the mouth open and the tongue somewhat protruding. Some children may progress rapidly to a shocklike state characterized by pallor, cyanosis, and impaired consciousness.

The physical examination may disclose moderate or severe respiratory distress with inspiratory and sometimes expiratory stridor, flaring of the alae nasi, and inspiratory retractions of the suprasternal notch, supraclavicular and intercostal spaces, and subcostal area. The pharynx may be inflamed, and there may be an abundance of mucus and saliva, which may also result in rhonchi. With progression, stridor and breath sounds may be diminished as the patient tires. A brief period of air hunger with restlessness and agitation may be followed by rapidly increasing cyanosis, coma, and death. Alternatively, the child may have only mild hoarseness and a large, shiny, cherry-red epiglottis brought into view when the posterior portion of the tongue is depressed. Occasionally, an older cooperative child may voluntarily open the mouth wide enough for a direct view of the inflamed epiglottis.

The diagnosis requires visualization of a large, swollen cherry-red epiglottis by direct examination or laryngoscopy. Occasionally, the other supraglottic structures, especially the aryepiglottic folds, may be more involved than the epiglottis itself. Some patients may have reflex laryngospasm and acute complete obstruction, aspiration of secretions, and cardiorespiratory arrest during or immediately after examination of the pharynx with the use of a tongue blade. These examinations should never be undertaken in a child in whom epiglottitis is thought possible without full preparation for immediate endotracheal intubation under controlled conditions. Children with suspected epiglottitis should not be placed in the supine position because of the risk of increased agitation and gravity-induced change in the position of the epiglottis with increased airway obstruction. Arterial blood gas samples should not be obtained before a definitive diagnosis and the establishment of an artificial airway. If the diagnosis is probable on clinical grounds, preparation should be made immediately for examining and controlling the airway, often in the operating room, by physicians skilled in endotracheal intubation, tracheostomy, or both.

Laryngoscopy reveals intense inflammation of the epiglottis and sometimes of the surrounding area as well, including the arytenoids and aryepiglottic folds, vocal cords, and subglottic regions. If epiglottitis is thought to be reasonably possible, although not probable, in a patient with acute upper airway obstruction, the patient should have a lateral roentgenogram of the nasopharynx and upper airway before physical examination of the pharynx (Fig. 332–2). If a roentgenogram shows a normal epiglottis, examination of the epiglottis may be performed while appropriate equipment and personnel are available to control the airway and provide ventilatory support. Patients with suspected epiglottitis should be accompanied by a physician and intubation equipment at all times, including the trip to and from the radiology department.

Establishing an airway by nasotracheal intubation or, less often, by tracheostomy is indicated in patients with epiglottitis, regardless of the degree of apparent respiratory distress, because as many as 6% of children with epiglottitis without an artificial airway die, compared with less than 1% of those with an artificial airway. No clinical features have been recognized that predict fatality. Fulminant pulmonary edema may be associated with acute airway obstruction. The duration of intubation depends on the clinical course of the patient and the duration of epiglottic swelling, as determined by frequent examination using direct laryngoscopy or flexible fiberoptic laryngoscopy. In general, children with acute epiglottitis are intubated for 2–3 days. Because most patients have bacteremia, parenteral antibiotic therapy with cefotaxime, ceftriaxone, or ampicillin with sulbactam (Unasyn) should be instituted

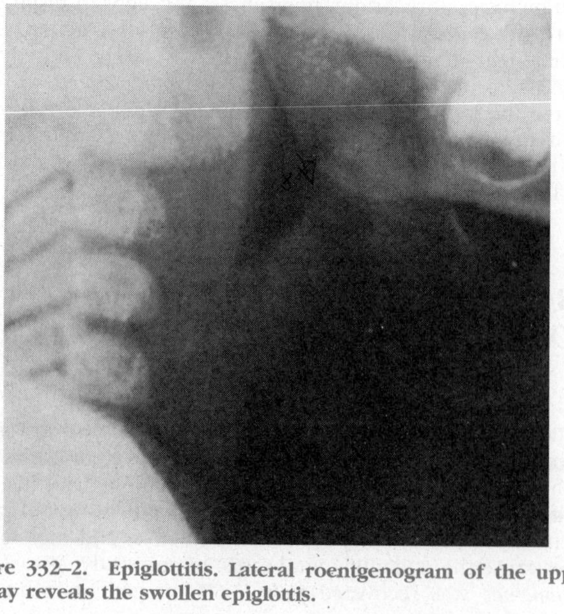

Figure 332–2. Epiglottitis. Lateral roentgenogram of the upper airway reveals the swollen epiglottis.

promptly. Concomitant infection is unusual, but meningitis, pneumonia, cervical adenopathy, or otitis media rarely occur.

Acute Infectious Laryngitis. Laryngitis is a common illness; except for diphtheria, most cases are caused by viruses. The onset is usually characterized by an upper respiratory tract infection during which sore throat, cough, and hoarseness appear. The illness is generally mild; respiratory distress is unusual except in the young infant. Hoarseness and loss of voice may be out of proportion to systemic signs and symptoms. In the rare severe case, the patient may present with severe inspiratory stridor, retractions, dyspnea, and restlessness. As the process progresses, air hunger and fatigue become evident, and the child alternates between periods of agitation and exhaustion. The physical examination is usually not remarkable except for evidence of pharyngeal inflammation and, with respiratory distress, evidence of high respiratory obstruction. Inflammatory edema of the vocal cords and subglottic tissue may be demonstrated laryngoscopically. The principal site of obstruction is usually the subglottic area.

Acute Spasmodic Laryngitis (Spasmodic Croup). Spasmodic croup occurs most often in children 1–3 yr of age and is clinically similar to acute laryngotracheobronchitis, except that findings of infection in the patient and family are frequently absent. The cause is viral in some cases, but allergic and psychologic factors are important in others. Gastroesophageal reflux may play an important role in triggering spasmodic croup, and children with this syndrome deserve careful laryngoscopic examination. The endoscopic documentation of posterior laryngitis (i.e., edema or inflammation of the arytenoid cartilages) suggests reflux. The opportunity for pathologic study is rare; the primary findings appear to be preservation of the epithelium (unlike acute infectious laryngotracheobronchitis) and pale, watery edema. In some cases, there is a familial predisposition to this syndrome.

Occurring most frequently in the evening or night, spasmodic croup begins with a sudden onset that may be preceded by mild to moderate coryza and hoarseness. The child awakens with a characteristic barking, metallic cough, noisy inspiration, and respiratory distress and appears anxious and frightened. Breathing is slow and labored, the pulse is accelerated, and the skin is cool and moist. The patient is usually afebrile. Dyspnea is aggravated by excitement; intermittent episodes of cyanosis are rare. Usually, the severity of the symptoms diminishes within several hours, and the following day, the patient often appears well except for slight hoarseness and cough. Similar, but usually less severe, attacks without extreme respiratory distress may occur for another night or two, eventually concluding in complete recovery. Such episodes often recur several times.

DIFFERENTIAL DIAGNOSIS. These four syndromes must be differentiated from one another and from a variety of other entities that may present upper airway obstruction. *Bacterial tracheitis* is the most important differential diagnostic consideration. *Diphtheritic croup* is rare in North America (see Chapter 180). It is usually preceded by an upper respiratory tract infection for several days. Symptoms usually develop slowly, although respiratory obstruction may occur suddenly; a serous or serosanguineous nasal discharge may occur. Pharyngeal examination reveals the typical gray-white membrane. *Measles croup* almost always coincides with the full manifestations of systemic disease and the course may be fulminant (see Chapter 206).

Sudden onset of respiratory obstruction may be caused by *aspiration of a foreign body* (see Chapter 330). The child is usually 6 mo–2 yr of age. Choking and coughing occur suddenly, usually without prodromal signs of infection, although children with a viral infection can also aspirate a foreign body. A *retropharyngeal* or *peritonsillar abscess* may mimic respiratory obstruction. Roentgenographic examination of the upper airway and chest is essential in evaluating these possibilities and possible causes of *extrinsic compression* of the airway, such as a hematoma from trauma and *intraluminal obstruction* from masses (e.g., cysts, tumors).

Upper airway obstruction is occasionally associated with *angioedema* of the subglottic areas as part of anaphylaxis and generalized allergic reactions, edema following *endotracheal intubation* for general anesthesia or respiratory failure, *hypocalcemic tetany, infectious mononucleosis,* trauma, and tumors or malformations of the larynx. A croupy cough may be an early sign of *asthma.* Psychogenic stridor can also occur. Epiglottitis, with the characteristic manifestations of drooling or dysphagia and stridor can also result from the accidental ingestion of very hot liquid.

COMPLICATIONS. Complications occur in approximately 15% of patients with viral croup. The most common is extension of the infectious process to involve other regions of the respiratory tract, such as the middle ear, the terminal bronchioles, or the pulmonary parenchyma. Bacterial tracheitis may be a complication of viral croup rather than a distinct disease. Interstitial pneumonia may occur, but it is difficult to differentiate on roentgenograms from the patchy areas of atelectasis secondary to obstruction. Bronchopneumonia is unusual unless aspiration of stomach contents has occurred during a period of severe respiratory distress. Although secondary bacterial pneumonia is unusual, suppurative tracheobronchitis is an occasional complication of laryngotracheobronchitis. Pneumonia, cervical lymphadenitis, otitis, or rarely, meningitis or septic arthritis may occur during the course of epiglottitis. Mediastinal emphysema and pneumothorax are the most common complications of tracheotomy.

PROGNOSIS. In general, the length of hospitalization and the mortality rate for cases of acute infectious upper airway obstruction increase as the infection extends to involve a greater portion of the respiratory tract, except in epiglottitis, in which the localized infection itself may prove fatal. Most deaths from croup are caused by a laryngeal obstruction or by the complications of tracheotomy. Untreated epiglottitis has a mortality rate of 6% in some series, but if the diagnosis is made and appropriate treatment is initiated before the patient is moribund, the prognosis is excellent. The outcome of acute laryngotracheobronchitis, laryngitis, and spasmodic croup is also excellent. As a group, children who need to be hospitalized for croup have somewhat increased bronchial reactivity compared with normal children when tested several years later. The differences are small, and their functional importance is unclear.

TREATMENT. Therapy for infectious croup consists primarily of maintaining or providing for adequate respiratory exchange and depends in part on the primary location of the disease and its cause. In the bacterial forms, antibiotic therapy is also important.

Most afebrile children with *acute spasmodic croup* or febrile patients with mild *laryngotracheobronchitis* can usually be safely and effectively managed at home. Treatment of underlying and often unsuspected gastroesophageal reflux may prevent spasmodic croup in children known to be susceptible to it.

The use of steam from a shower or bath in a closed bathroom, steam from a vaporizer, or "cold steam" from a nebulizer (which has a safety and perhaps efficacy advantage) often terminates acute laryngeal spasm and respiratory distress within minutes. The same effect has been observed by many parents as they take their child out into the cold night air on the way to the physician's office. This long-recognized phenomenon may be explained by the upper airway's serving as a heat- and humidity-exchange organ; inspired air that is cooler than body temperature and less than 100% saturated with water vapor results in mucosal cooling, leading to vasoconstriction and lessened edema.

Induction of vomiting by coughing or by syrup of ipecac may

also decrease laryngeal spasm. Although vomiting occasionally appears to break the laryngeal spasm, there is no objective evidence for the effectiveness of ipecac, and respiratory distress may be complicated by vomiting, particularly if the patient aspirates gastric contents.

After the laryngeal spasm has diminished, its return may be prevented by the use of warm or cool humidification near the child's bed for the ensuing 2–3 days.

Children with croup should be hospitalized for any of the following: actual or suspected epiglottitis, progressive stridor, severe stridor at rest, respiratory distress, hypoxemia, restlessness, cyanosis, pallor, depressed sensorium, or high fever in a toxic-appearing child. In all cases, the decision for hospitalization is made because of the need for reliable observation and relatively safe tracheotomy or more often nasotracheal intubation, if either of these becomes necessary.

At home or in the hospital, the patient with croup should be watched carefully for intensification of symptoms of respiratory obstruction. The hospitalized child is usually placed in an atmosphere of cool humidity to lessen irritation and drying of secretions and perhaps to lessen edema. Frequent or continuous monitoring of the respiratory rate is essential, because increasing tachypnea may be the first sign of hypoxemia and approaching total respiratory obstruction. The patient should be disturbed as little as possible. In cases of moderate to severe respiratory distress, parenteral fluids should be given to make up for insensible and respiratory water loss and decrease the risk of vomiting, with its potential for aspiration. Sedatives are usually contraindicated because restlessness is used as one of the principal clinical indices of the severity of obstruction and the need for tracheotomy or nasotracheal intubation. Opiates in particular are contraindicated because they may depress respiration and may dry secretions. Oxygen should be used to alleviate hypoxemia and apprehension, but because the oxygen reduces cyanosis, which is an indication for tracheotomy or nasotracheal intubation, these patients must be observed particularly closely. Expectorants, bronchodilating agents, and antihistamines are not helpful.

Laryngotracheobronchitis and *spasmodic croup* do not respond to antibiotics, and antibiotics are not indicated to prevent suprainfection. Nonurgent tests should be delayed to prevent increased symptoms associated with agitation and anxiety. Racemic epinephrine by aerosol (2.25% solution diluted 1:8 with water in doses of 2–4 mL for 15 min) often results in transient relief of symptoms; close observation and repeated treatments usually are necessary. A child sick enough for hospitalization before administering an aerosol should be hospitalized even if there is a dramatic response to the aerosol, because the obstruction is likely to return after the aerosol's effects have waned. Racemic epinephrine does not cause rebound worsening of obstruction. However, if the aerosol is administered during the worsening phase of the natural history of the child's illness, the obstruction may be worse after the effects have worn off. If the aerosol is administered at what would have been the peak of the obstruction, the child will be better after the aerosol effects have waned. Frequent treatments help all but the sickest children through this illness. Rarely, there is sufficient obstruction to warrant nasotracheal intubation or tracheotomy.

The use of corticosteroids is probably indicated for the hospitalized child with croup. The theoretical basis for corticosteroid treatment in laryngotracheobronchitis is to reduce inflammatory edema and prevent destruction of ciliated epithelium. A metanalysis and another review of 10–13 English language studies suggest some beneficial effect of systemic steroids, particularly if doses of dexamethasone phosphate greater than 0.3 mg/kg are employed. There is no substantial evidence suggesting any adverse effect of corticosteroid treatment. The topical, nonabsorbed, inhaled steroid budesonide (not yet available in the United States) has benefit in treating children with croup. In the very ill child in the intensive care unit, breathing a helium-oxygen mixture, with its lower density and the resultant improved turbulent airflow, may decrease the work of breathing.

Epiglottitis is a **medical emergency.** If diagnosed by inspection of the epiglottis or by roentgenographic examination or if strongly suspected clinically in a severely ill child, it should be treated immediately with an artificial airway placed under controlled conditions, usually in an operating room. All patients should receive oxygen en route to the operating room unless it is contraindicated by the increased agitation caused by the mask. Racemic epinephrine and corticosteroids are ineffective; they do not avert the need for an artificial airway and may dangerously delay definitive treatment. Cultures of blood, epiglottic surface, and in selected cases, cerebrospinal fluid, should be collected at the time of airway stabilization. Ceftriaxone or cefotaxime or a combination of ampicillin and sulbactam should be given parenterally pending culture and susceptibility reports because of the increasing possibility of ampicillin-resistant strains of *H. influenzae* type b. After insertion of the artificial airway, the patient should improve immediately, respiratory distress and cyanosis should disappear, and normal or near-normal blood gases should return. Patients usually fall asleep. The epiglottitis resolves after a few days of antibiotics, and the patient can be weaned from the tracheostomy or nasotracheal tube; antibiotics should be continued for 7–10 days.

Acute laryngeal swelling on an allergic basis responds to epinephrine (1:1,000 dilution in dosage of 0.01 mL/kg to a maximum of 0.3 mL/dose) administered subcutaneously and isoproterenol (1:200 dilution in dosage of 0.01 mL/kg to a maximum of 0.3 mL/dose) administered by aerosol. After recovery, the patient and parents should be instructed in emergency administration of these drugs at home. Corticosteroids are frequently required (1–2 mg/kg/24 hr of prednisone every 6 hr).

Reactive mucosal swelling, severe stridor, and respiratory distress unresponsive to mist therapy may follow *endotracheal intubation* for general anesthesia in children. Intermittent use of racemic epinephrine aerosols or occasional use of corticosteroids may be helpful.

Tracheotomy and Endotracheal Intubation. With the introduction of routine nasotracheal intubation or tracheotomy for epiglottitis, the mortality rate has dropped to almost zero. Both procedures should always be done in an operating room if time permits; prior intubation and general anesthesia greatly facilitate doing a tracheotomy without complications. The choice of procedure should be based on the local expertise and experience with the procedure and the postoperative care involved with each.

Endotracheal intubation or tracheotomy is required for all patients with epiglottitis, but for patients with laryngotracheobronchitis, spasmodic croup, or laryngitis, it is required only for those rare individuals who have increasing signs of respiratory failure secondary to obstruction despite appropriate treatment. Severe forms of laryngotracheobronchitis that require tracheotomy in a high proportion of patients have been reported during severe measles and influenza A virus epidemics. Assessing the need for these procedures requires experience and judgment, because they should not be delayed until cyanosis and extreme restlessness have developed; a pulse rate over 150/min and rising, and an elevated Pco_2, especially in a tiring child, are indications of impending respiratory failure.

The endotracheal tube or tracheostomy must remain in place until edema and spasm have subsided and the patient is able to handle secretions satisfactorily. They should always be removed as soon as possible, usually within a few days. Adequate resolution of epiglottic inflammation that has been accurately confirmed by fiberoptic laryngoscopy, permitting much more rapid extubation, often within 24 hr. There is some evidence that hydrocortisone (50–100 mg/24 hr) or dexamethasone (0.25–0.5 mg/kg/dose every 6 hr prn) and racemic epinephrine may be useful to facilitate extubation or to treat croup associated with extubation.

LARYNGOTRACHEOBRONCHITIS

Denny FW, Murphy TF, Clyde WA Jr, et al: Croup: An 11 year study in a pediatric practice. Pediatrics 71:871, 1984.

Gurwitz D, Corey M, Levison H: Pulmonary function and bronchial reactivity in children after croup. Am Rev Respir Dis 122:95, 1980.

Kairys SW, Olmstead EM, O'Connor GT: Steroid treatment of laryngotracheitis: A meta-analysis of the evidence from randomized trials. Pediatrics 83:683, 1989.

Klassen T, Feldman M, Watters L, et al: Nebulized budesonide for children with mild to moderate croup. N Engl J Med 331:285, 1994.

Singer OP, Wilson WJ: Laryngotracheobronchitis: 2 years' experience with racemic epinephrine. Can Med Assoc J 115:132, 1976.

Skolnik JS: Treatment of croup: A critical review. Am J Dis Child 143:1045, 1989.

Smith MS: Acute psychogenic stridor in an adolescent athlete treated with hypnosis. Pediatrics 72:247, 1983.

Super DM, Cartelli NA, Brooks LJ, et al: A prospective double-blind study to evaluate the effect of dexamethasone in acute laryngotracheitis. J Pediatr 115:323, 1989.

SPASMODIC CROUP

Contencin P, Narcy P. Gastropharyngeal reflux in infants and children: A pharyngeal monitoring study. Arch Otolaryngol Head Neck Surg 118:1028, 1992.

EPIGLOTTITIS

Adams WG, Deaver KA, Cochi SL, et al: Decline in childhood *Haemophilus influenzae* type b (HiB) in the HiB vaccine era. JAMA 269:221, 1993.

Ashcraft CK, Steele RW: Epiglottitis: A pediatric emergency. J Respir Dis 9:48, 1988.

Battaglia JD, Lockhart CH: Management of acute epiglottitis by nasotracheal intubation. Am J Dis Child 120:334, 1975.

Cohen SR, Chai J: Epiglottitis: Twenty-year study with tracheostomy. Ann Otol Rhinol Laryngol 87:1, 1978.

Gorelick MH, Baker MD: Epiglottitis in children, 1979 through 1992. Arch Pediatr Adolesc Med 148:47, 1994.

Kulick RM, Selbst SM, Baker MD, et al: Thermal epiglottitis after swallowing hot beverages. Pediatrics 81:441, 1988.

Molteni RA: Epiglottitis: Incidence of extraepiglottic infection: Report of 72 cases and review of the literature. Pediatrics 58:526, 1976.

Rapkin RH: The diagnosis of epiglottitis: Simplicity and reliability of radiographs of the neck in differential diagnosis of the croup syndrome. J Pediatr 80:96, 1975.

332.2 Bacterial Tracheitis

Bacterial tracheitis, an acute bacterial infection of the upper airway, does not involve the epiglottis but, like epiglottitis and croup, is capable of causing life-threatening airway obstruction. *S. aureus* is the most commonly isolated pathogen. Parainfluenza virus type 1, *Moraxella catarrhalis*, and *H. influenzae* have also been implicated. Most patients are younger than 3 yr of age, although older children have occasionally been affected. There are no clear sex differences in incidence or severity. Bacterial tracheitis usually follows an apparently viral respiratory infection (especially laryngotracheitis). The tracheitis may be a bacterial complication of a viral disease, rather than a primary bacterial illness. This life-threatening entity is probably at least as common as epiglottitis.

CLINICAL MANIFESTATIONS. Typically, the child develops a brassy cough, apparently as part of a viral laryngotracheobronchitis. High fever and "toxicity" with respiratory distress may occur immediately or after a few days of apparent improvement. Usual treatment for croup (e.g., mist, intravenous fluid, aerosolized racemic epinephrine) is ineffective. Intubation or tracheostomy is usually necessary. The major pathology appears to be mucosal swelling at the level of the cricoid cartilage, complicated by copious thick, purulent secretions. Suctioning these secretions, although occasionally affording temporary relief, usually does not sufficiently obviate the need for an artificial airway.

DIAGNOSIS. The diagnosis is based on evidence of bacterial upper airway disease, which includes moderate leukocytosis with many band forms, high fever, and purulent airway secretions, and an absence of the classic findings of epiglottitis.

TREATMENT. Appropriate antimicrobial therapy, which usually includes antistaphylococcal agents, should be instituted in any patient with croup whose course suggests secondary bacterial tracheitis. When bacterial tracheitis is diagnosed by direct laryngoscopy or strongly suspected on clinical grounds, an artificial airway is usually indicated. Supplemental oxygen may be necessary.

COMPLICATIONS. Chest roentgenograms often show patchy infiltrates and may show focal densities. Subglottic narrowing and a rough-ragged tracheal air column can often be demonstrated roentgenographically. If airway management is not optimal, cardiorespiratory arrest can occur. Toxic shock syndrome has been associated with tracheitis (see Chap. 174.3).

PROGNOSIS. The prognosis for most patients is excellent. Most patients become afebrile within 2–3 days of instituting appropriate antimicrobial therapy, but prolonged hospitalization may be necessary. With a decrease in mucosal edema and purulent secretions, extubation can be accomplished safely, and the patient can be observed carefully while antibiotics and oxygen therapy are continued. The mean duration of hospitalization was 12 days in one series.

Denneny JC III, Handler SD: Membranous laryngotracheobronchitis. Pediatrics 70:705, 1982.

Liston SL, Gehrz RC, Siegel LG, et al: Bacterial tracheitis. Am J Dis Child 137:764, 1983.

Nelson WE: Bacterial croup: A historical perspective. J Pediatr 105:52, 1984.

CHAPTER 333

Foreign Bodies in the Larynx, Trachea, and Bronchi

David Orenstein

The air passages of children are common sites for the lodgment of foreign bodies; poor supervision by adults or older siblings is occasionally a contributing factor. The symptoms, physical findings, and complications produced by foreign bodies depend on their nature, location, and the degree of obstruction. For example, a sharp or irritating object lodged in the larynx produces severe local edema and, later, suppurative perichondritis. An obstructing object in a bronchus produces distal atelectasis and later produces bronchiectasis, pulmonary abscess, or empyema.

Most foreign bodies aspirated into the respiratory tract are expelled immediately by reflex cough and never require medical attention. If an object too large to be eliminated by mucociliary clearance is aspirated and is not expelled by coughing, respiratory symptoms inevitably result. A large foreign body that can occlude the upper airway is an immediate threat to life. Smaller objects that lodge in one of the mainstem or lobar bronchi cause more chronic and usually less severe symptoms.

After the initial symptoms, which may have been forgotten, there is often a symptom-free interval that may last from hours to weeks. On occasion, dysphagia may occur from the swelling that results from a foreign body in the region of the larynx. Foreign bodies in the upper esophagus may cause symptoms referable to the air passages by compression or by the overflow of food or secretions into the larynx. Occasionally, an airway foreign body is not diagnosed until it is revealed by pathologic examination of a lobe that has been removed because of chronic bronchiectasis.

LARYNGEAL FOREIGN BODIES

CLINICAL MANIFESTATIONS. A laryngeal foreign body causes a cough that soon becomes croupy, hoarse, and with profound obstruction, aphonia. Hemoptysis, dyspnea with wheezing, and cyanosis may occur. Obstruction resulting from the foreign body alone or its inflammatory reaction may prove fatal if the signs of high respiratory tract obstruction are not promptly recognized and appropriate treatment not given. Hot dogs and bread are two of the most common causes of fatal aspiration. Peanut butter is particularly difficult to remove by cough or instrumentation.

DIAGNOSIS. Roentgenographic and direct laryngoscopic examinations usually reveal or suggest the presence of a foreign body in the larynx (Fig. 333–1). A radioopaque foreign body in the neck is clearly demonstrated on a lateral roentgenogram. When it is lodged anteriorly, it is obviously in the larynx; when it is behind the soft tissue shadows of the larynx, it is in the hypopharynx or the cervical esophagus. The plane in which the foreign body lies is another differential factor in its localization. If it lies in the sagittal plane, it is probably in the larynx. If it is in the coronal plane, it is probably in the esophagus. Even if the foreign body is not radioopaque, high kilovoltage airway films may suggest its presence. Films should always be taken from the lateral and the anteroposterior projections. In some cases, administering a small amount of opaque contrast material orally may be helpful. Direct laryngoscopy with a rigid open-tube endoscope, usually by an otolaryngologist, confirms the diagnosis and provides access for removal of the foreign body. When there is a severe degree of dyspnea, tracheotomy may be advisable before the laryngoscopic examination.

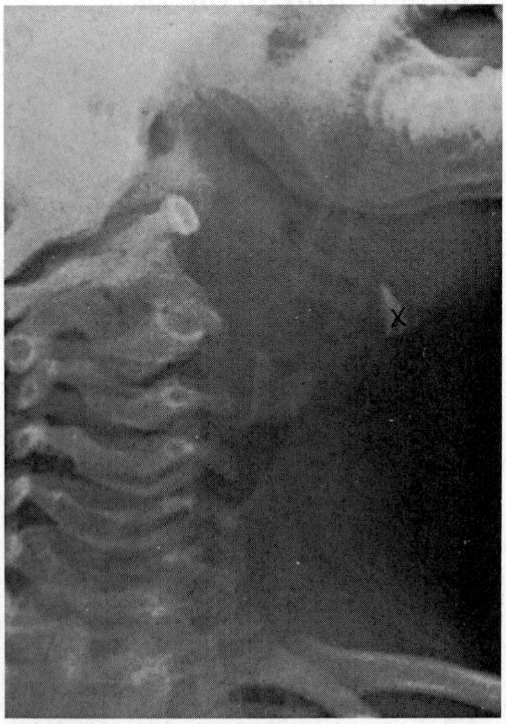

Figure 333–1. Foreign body (fragment of sea shell) in the larynx of a 2-yr-old child treated for "croup" 6 days before the object was suspected. Fortunately, a tracheotomy was not required despite the presence of moderately severe laryngeal edema.

TRACHEAL FOREIGN BODIES

Although a tracheal foreign body may be responsible for cough, hoarseness, dyspnea, and cyanosis, the characteristic signs are wheeze and the audible slap and palpable thud produced by momentary expiratory impaction at the subglottic level. The diagnosis may occasionally be made from the symptoms, physical signs, and roentgenogram of the chest, but in most cases, a definite diagnosis can be made only by bronchoscopy.

BRONCHIAL FOREIGN BODIES

CLINICAL MANIFESTATIONS. The initial symptoms of a bronchial foreign body are usually similar to those of foreign bodies in the larynx or trachea. Cough, wheeze, blood-streaked sputum, and metallic taste with metallic foreign bodies also may be produced by bronchial foreign bodies. The degree of obstruction and the stage in which the patient is seen determine the observed symptoms and pathologic changes. A nonobstructive, nonirritating foreign body may produce few symptoms even after a prolonged time. An obstructive foreign body quickly produces symptoms and signs and pathologic changes. If there is only a slight obstruction (e.g., bypass valve), the passage of air in both directions with only slight interference may produce a wheeze. If the obstruction is greater, one of two pathologic conditions may develop. If the obstruction allows air entry but not exit (i.e., check valve or ball valve obstruction), obstructive overinflation ensues. In the case of complete obstruction, which allows neither air entry nor exit, obstructive atelectasis is produced as the air distal to the obstruction is absorbed. If either condition is allowed to persist, chronic bronchopulmonary disease may develop.

Right and left mainstem bronchial foreign body aspiration occur with roughly equal frequency. There is usually an immediate episode of choking, gagging, and paroxysmal coughing, which may lead to medical consultation. If this acute episode does not occur or is missed or if its importance is underestimated by the parents, a latent period of minutes to months may pass with only occasional cough or slight wheezing; the patient may develop recurrent lobar pneumonia or intractable "asthma," often with bilateral wheezing and many episodes of status asthmaticus. Occasionally, chronic wheezing starts immediately after the aspiration. Rarely, the patient with a foreign body presents with hemoptysis, occasionally months or years after aspiration. History may reveal a forgotten episode of choking while eating or while playing with small objects. Older siblings (3–6 yr of age) may have supplied the aspirated object. The physical examination may reveal a tracheal shift. Breath sounds are decreased on the side of the obstruction, but this sign may not be obvious if there is diffuse wheezing. There may be delayed air entry or exit on the obstructed side, detectable with a two-headed differential stethoscope.

Obstruction of both main bronchi may produce severe dyspnea and even asphyxia. If the foreign body is a vegetable (e.g., peanut), a severe condition known as *vegetal* or *arachidic bronchitis* results, characterized by cough, a septic type of fever, and dyspnea. Chronic suppuration may occur when a bronchial foreign body has been present for a long time.

DIAGNOSIS. Most patients with an airway foreign body have a suggestive history. The possibility of a foreign body must be considered in acute or chronic pulmonary lesions regardless of the history of an aspiration event.

If an object causes complete obstruction in the expiratory phase but allows air to pass in the inspiratory phase, air enters the distal portion of the lung on inspiration but little or none escapes during expiration (i.e., *check or ball valve*). This produces obstructive overinflation (Fig. 333–2). Complete blockage of the bronchus by the object itself or in combination with the inflammatory swelling of the bronchial mucosa results in

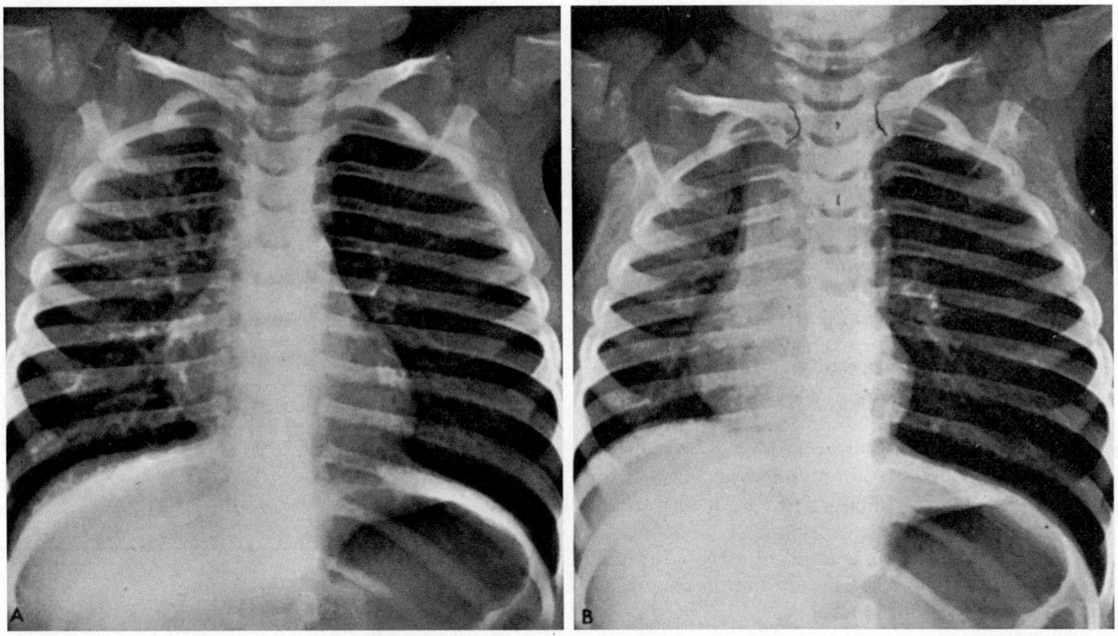

Figure 333–2. Obstructive overinflation due to a peanut fragment in the left mainstem bronchus. *A,* The inspiratory film appears relatively normal except for a slight mediastinal shift to the right. *B,* In expiration, the left lung remains overaerated (i.e., ball-valve mechanism), and the mediastinum moves far to the right.

a *stop valve* obstruction, and the air in the distal portion of the lung is soon absorbed, leaving an area of atelectasis (Fig. 333–3). The physical signs of these results of bronchial obstruction from foreign bodies include limited chest expansion, decreased vocal fremitus, impaired (i.e., atelectasis) or hyperresonant (i.e., overinflation) percussion note, and diminished breath sounds distal to the foreign body. If there is complete obstruction, with a "drowned lung" or with atelectasis, there is absence of vocal fremitus, which may lead to an erroneous diagnosis of empyema. Various degrees of tympany may be demonstrated over areas of obstructive emphysema. Crackles are more likely on the uninvolved side than on the involved one.

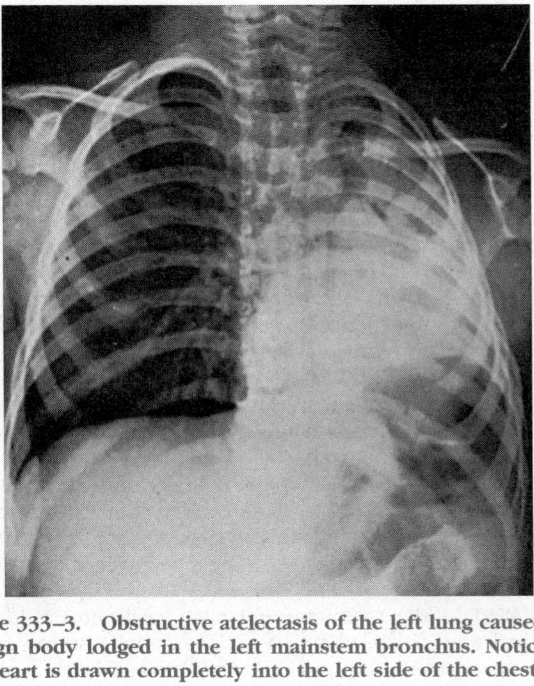

Figure 333–3. Obstructive atelectasis of the left lung caused by a foreign body lodged in the left mainstem bronchus. Notice that the heart is drawn completely into the left side of the chest.

In check valve obstruction, the obstructive overinflation makes it possible to localize a bronchial foreign body by fluoroscopy. The obstructed lung remains expanded during expiration, but the heart and the mediastinum shift to the opposite side as the unobstructed lung empties. The diaphragm is low, flattened, and fixed on the obstructed side; its excursion is free and exaggerated on the unobstructed side. These roentgenographic differences between the lungs are more evident on expiration than on inspiration. With complete obstruction of the bronchus producing obstructive atelectasis, the heart and the mediastinum are drawn toward the obstructed side and remain there during both phases of respiration. The diaphragm on the obstructed side remains high, but that on the unobstructed side moves normally. Films taken at the end of inspiration and of expiration show only a slight difference resulting from the filling and emptying of the unobstructed lung. Even extensive roentgenographic procedures may not completely rule out the presence of a foreign body. The definitive diagnosis of bronchial foreign body is made by direct visualization by bronchoscopy. Flexible fiberoptic bronchoscopy may be employed, particularly if the history and physical examination are equivocal. However, the flexible instrument is generally not useful for foreign body removal, because it does not permit adequate airway control or instrumentation. Therefore, if the history, physical examination, and roentgenograms strongly suggest bronchial foreign body, the diagnostic instrument of choice is the rigid or open-tube bronchoscope.

PROGNOSIS. Foreign bodies lodged in the air passages almost invariably cause serious problems if they are not removed. Fortunately, most can be removed safely by a skilled bronchoscopist. Most patients who are diagnosed and treated quickly recover completely after removal. The incidence of complications, including aspiration pneumonia and airway trauma, and the need for tracheostomy because of subglottic edema, rises significantly if the diagnosis is delayed longer than 24 hr.

PREVENTION. Foreign body aspiration can be prevented. Small objects should be kept out of reach of children who are too young to obey restrictions. Children too young to chew and swallow carefully should not be given small pieces of candy, nuts, or similar food. Similarly, toys containing small or loosely attached parts should not be given to children who are still putting such objects into their mouths. Nuts, which account for more than half of airway foreign bodies, and popcorn are particularly appealing to children, and parents should resist the urge to indulge their young child. Beads, button boxes, and coins should not be given to toddlers as playthings. Safety pins should always be closed and should not be left near a baby or in reach of small children. Balloons are underestimated as potential foreign bodies.

TREATMENT. Endoscopy and removal of the foreign body under direct vision, with a rigid or open-tube bronchoscope should be performed as soon as possible. Rarely, a thoracotomy is necessary to "milk" the object into position for removal by bronchoscopy. Occasionally, especially with long-duration vegetal foreign bodies, lobectomy may be necessary. Biplane fluoroscopy may be helpful when opaque foreign bodies are lodged in peripheral bronchi. Treatment with pulmonary physiotherapy and bronchodilators is not recommended because of the risk of dislodging a distal foreign body, allowing it to move to and obstruct a larger airway, such as a mainstem bronchus, the trachea, or larynx. A delay in instituting endoscopy may increase morbidity by allowing more inflammation to develop around the object.

Treating complications is important to obtaining a good outcome. Secondary infections should be treated with appropriate antibiotics. The outcome of the aspiration of a large foreign body that may be immediately life threatening depends on proper and prompt action taken at the scene of the aspiration.

Emergency treatment of local upper airway obstruction is part of the basic rescuer course in cardiopulmonary resuscitation of the American Heart Association (see Chapter 60). These procedures are used only for children who are aphonic and not breathing. The recommendations for treating infants and young children differ slightly from those for treating teenagers and adults. If the patient can breathe and is able to cough or speak, none of the maneuvers described should be undertaken. For patients who are genuinely choking, the recommendations of the Committee on Accident and Poison Prevention of the American Academy of Pediatrics are as follows. For infants (<1 yr), the repetitive use of four back blows and four chest thrusts is recommended. Abdominal thrusts should not be used. The back blows are delivered while holding the infant with the head lower than the trunk. Four blows are delivered with the heel of the hand between the scapulas. The purpose of this maneuver is to loosen the foreign body. After the back blows, the patient is turned, and four chest thrusts are delivered using the same technique and hand positioning as used for closed cardiac compression (i.e., over the midsternum for infants and slightly lower for older children). This maneuver increases intrathoracic pressure, which may cause expulsion of the foreign body. Blind finger sweeps of the mouth should not be used in infants and young children. Instead, after the administration of the four chest thrusts, the mouth should be opened and a visualized foreign body should be grasped and removed. After each sequence of back blows, chest thrusts, and visual attempt to remove foreign body, rescue breathing should be attempted for the unconscious patient. If unsuccessful, the sequence described above is repeated.

A young child (>1 yr) should be placed on his or her back. The rescuer kneels next to the patient and, using the heel of one hand, performs six to 10 abdominal thrusts by pushing upward and inward from the midabdomen, midway between the umbilicus and the rib cage. If this is unsuccessful, the victim's mouth is opened by using the tongue-jaw lift, and a visualized foreign body is removed. Blind sweeps of the mouth should not be made. Rescue breathing should then be attempted before the entire sequence is repeated. Although there is controversy concerning the precise technique to be used in total upper airway obstruction by a foreign body, pediatricians should provide up-to-date information in these techniques to parents and should urge parents to expect that their baby sitters (including teenagers) are familiar with the symptoms and emergency treatment of foreign body aspiration.

Baker SP, Fisher RS: Childhood asphyxiation by choking or suffocation. JAMA 244:1343, 1980.
Blazer S, Naveh Y, Friedman A: Foreign body in the airway: A review of 200 cases. Am Rev Dis Child 134:68, 1980.
Blumhagen JD, Weisenberg RL, Brooks JG, et al: Endotracheal foreign bodies: Difficulties in diagnosis. Clin Pediatr 19:480, 1980.
Committee on Accident and Poison Prevention: Revised first aid for the choking child. Pediatrics 78:177, 1986.
Esclamado RM, Richardson MA: Laryngotracheal foreign bodies in children. Am J Dis Child 141:259, 1987.
Kloske AM: Respiratory foreign body. *In:* Hilman BH (ed): Pediatric Respiratory Disease: Diagnosis and Treatment. Philadelphia, WB Saunders, 1993, p 513.
Rothman BF, Boeckman CR: Foreign bodies in the larynx and tracheobronchial tree in children. Ann Otol Rhinol Laryngol 89:434, 1980.

CHAPTER 334
Subglottic Stenosis

David M. Orenstein

334.1 Acute Subglottic Stenosis

Acute stenosis may result from an acute infection producing edema of the subglottic region or epiglottis and arytenoids; from inflammation secondary to the inspiration of a vegetal foreign body and especially after instrumentation for the removal of such an object; from edema of an allergic reaction; or from a foreign body lodged in the larynx. Treatment consists of immediate provision of an airway by intubation or tracheotomy, followed by appropriate medical therapy.

334.2 Chronic Subglottic Stenosis

A frequent sequela of high tracheotomy in which damage of the first tracheal ring or cricoid cartilage results in perichondritis and subsequent overgrowth of cartilage or fibrous tissue, chronic stenosis may also result from laryngeal diphtheria, syphilis, tuberculosis, radiation burns, and external trauma. The most common cause is neonatal intubation. Congenital laryngeal stenosis may be transmitted as an autosomal dominant trait in some patients. "Silent" gastroesophageal reflux with aspiration of gastric acid into the subglottic region may be responsible for many cases.

CLINICAL MANIFESTATIONS. The clinical manifestations of chronic laryngeal stenosis may include dyspnea with audible stridor and suprasternal, supraclavicular, and intercostal retractions, or they may be limited to an inability to decannulate a patient's tracheostomy or remove an endotracheal tube. The diagnosis is made by direct laryngoscopy and roentgenographic examination. Scarring and stenosis usually develop in the subglottic region, occasionally with necrosis of cartilage.

TREATMENT. Milder cases may not need treatment. Mild cases of difficulty in decannulating a patient's tracheostomy can be treated by replacing the tracheostomy cannula with a smaller one and closure of this tube, at first partial and then complete, with a cork, which re-educates the patient to mouth breathe and permits the removal of the cannula. If this method is unsuccessful, dilation through a direct laryngoscope may help but should not be done too frequently. For some patients, external surgery with or without the use of an indwelling mold may be necessary. A cricoid-split operation is successful in severe cases. In all cases, patients should be investigated for gastroesophageal reflux, which should be treated aggressively (see Chapter 269). The prognosis for eventual cure is good, but treatment may require months or years.

Landing BH: State of the art: Congenital malformations and genetic diseases of the respiratory tract. Am Rev Respir Dis 120:151, 1979.
Little FB, Kohut RI, Koufman JA, et al: Effect of gastric acid on the pathogenesis of subglottic stenosis. Ann Otol Rhinol Laryngol 94:516, 1985.
McGill TJI, Healy GB: Congenital and acquired lesions of the infant larynx. Clin Pediatr 17:584, 1978.
Proctor DF: The upper airways: 11. The larynx and trachea. Am Rev Respir Dis 115:315, 1977.

CHAPTER 335

Trauma to the Larynx

Robert C. Stern

BIRTH TRAUMA. Laryngeal injury during birth is not infrequent and may result in dislocation of the cricothyroid or cricoarytenoid articulations. Hoarseness and, at times, wheezing or fluttering respiratory sounds are heard. The diagnosis is made by direct laryngoscopic examination. Treatment by direct laryngoscopic manipulations, using a laryngeal dilator, may occasionally be effective, but tracheotomy should be done if there is evidence of hypoxia.

Unilateral or bilateral *recurrent laryngeal nerve paralysis* may also be produced by birth trauma, especially during forceps delivery. Bilateral paralysis is often associated with central nervous system disease (Chiari malformation). Paralysis of one cord may produce only hoarseness and slight stridor without dyspnea. Unilateral paralysis is usually on the left. Bilateral paralysis produces dyspnea with stridor. In unilateral and bilateral vocal cord paralysis, chronic aspiration can lead to recurrent pneumonia. Direct laryngoscopic examination establishes the diagnosis. Tracheotomy is usually necessary for bilateral paralysis. The older child may wear a valvular cannula, or a laryngoplasty with lateral fixation of one vocal cord may be done to improve the airway and permit decannulation if breathing through the larynx has not improved spontaneously.

POSTNATAL TRAUMA. Any trauma, such as that brought about by a fall against a hard object, may produce acute or chronic stenosis of the larynx, as may high tracheotomy and prolonged intubation. Clinically important laryngeal injury is rare in children. Penetrating injuries are usually obvious and require treatment by an otolaryngologic surgeon. Serious nonpenetrating injuries may be deceptive because substantial edema and even a compressing hematoma may give surprisingly few external clues. Laryngeal fracture should be suspected in patients who have hoarseness, hemoptysis, or subcutaneous emphysema after neck trauma. Laryngoscopy and, occasionally, surgical exploration may be indicated in patients who have relatively normal physical findings but whose history is compatible with substantial blunt neck trauma. Most patients with serious laryngeal or upper tracheal injuries require tracheostomy as part of their management; if there are signs of high obstruction, the need may be urgent. The normal voice is frequently not recovered. Similarly, severe thermal injury (after accidental inhalation of steam or smoke) is often best managed with tracheostomy. Ingestion of caustic substances has also been associated with laryngeal lesions.

Acute *overuse of the voice* (e.g., prolonged screaming at a concert or athletic event) may cause transient hoarseness. With cessation of this stress, the voice returns to normal without other treatment. The roles of resting the voice (i.e., whispering or no use of speech at all) or mist in accelerating recovery are not clear. Acute laryngitis is fairly common in older children during mild viral respiratory infections; spontaneous recovery is the rule, and the importance of steam and other therapeutic maneuvers is unknown. Occasionally, a teenager may develop chronic laryngitis from heavy cigarette smoking. The differential diagnosis of persistent hoarse voice includes vocal ("singer's" or "screamer's") nodules, papillomas, and serious tumors such as rhabdomyosarcoma. A laryngeal abscess is a rare cause of persistent hoarseness. These masses are diagnosed by laryngoscopy and may require surgical treatment, which may be followed by voice training. Otolaryngologic consultation is indicated for any child with unexplained continuous hoarseness persisting longer than 1 wk.

Benjamin B: Prolonged intubation injuries of the larynx: Endoscopic diagnosis, classification, and treatment. Ann Otol Rhinol Laryngol 102 (Suppl 160):1, 1990.
Moulin D, Bertrand JM, Buts JP, et al: Upper airway lesions in children after accidental ingestion of caustic substances. J Pediatr 106:408, 1985.

CHAPTER 336

Neoplasms of the Larynx

Robert C. Stern

Papilloma is the most common tumor of the larynx in childhood; it rarely becomes malignant and often disappears after puberty. The pink, warty tumors may grow profusely from any portion of the larynx, although usually from the vocal cords. This disease is caused by the human papillomavirus (see Chapter 224). When maternal vaginal condyloma is present, material containing this virus may be aspirated during delivery, producing disease in a small fraction of exposed infants.

The initial symptom is hoarseness, but dyspnea is likely if the condition is allowed to persist. Asphyxia has occurred. Direct laryngoscopy accomplishes diagnosis (confirmed histologically) and treatment, because the papilloma can be easily removed with forceps. Care should be taken not to damage normal tissue. Cure usually occurs, although rapid recurrence is common at first. Tracheostomy may be required because of recurrences and the threat of aspiration. Cryosurgery and laser surgery have been advocated as alternative or adjuvant therapy. Radical excision and radiation are contraindicated.

Extension of the disease into the lower airways and lungs can occur. The factors that predispose to this complication are unknown. Respiratory papillomatosis is a much more serious disease and carries a high mortality rate. Patients with laryngobronchial papillomatosis who fail to respond to usual treatment may improve after receiving systemic bleomycin. Human leukocyte interferon has been reported to be beneficial for patients with recurrent severe disease. However, in one controlled study, the patients in the treatment group had a better course for 6 mo, but this was not sustained for the next 6 mo. Some success with ribavirin was reported in one 3-yr-old patient. Papilloma may recur many years, even decades, after apparent cure. Malignant degeneration into squamous cell carcinoma has been reported in young children. This complication is more likely after radiation treatment.

Vocal nodules or small tumors may occur in children at the junction of the anterior and middle thirds of the cords. They are usually bilateral and produce slight hoarseness. Spontaneous regression may occur if strenuous use of the voice is avoided. They may be removed under direct laryngoscopic view or treated with laser.

Chaput M, Ninane J, Gosseye S, et al: Juvenile laryngeal papillomatosis and epidermoid carcinoma. J Pediatr 114:269, 1989.
Healy GB, Gelber RD, Trowbridge AL, et al: Treatment of recurrent respiratory papillomatosis with human leukocyte interferon. N Engl J Med 319:401, 1988.
Mehta P, Herold N: Regression of juvenile laryngobronchial papillomatosis with systemic bleomycin therapy. J Pediatr 97:479, 1980.
Morrison GAJ, Kotecha B, Evans NG: Ribavirin treatment for juvenile respiratory papillomatosis. J Laryngol Otol 107:423, 1993.

CHAPTER 337
Bronchitis

Robert C. Stern

337.1 Acute Bronchitis

Although the diagnosis of acute bronchitis is frequently made, this condition may not exist in children as an isolated clinical entity. Bronchitis is associated with several other conditions of the upper and lower respiratory tracts, and the trachea is usually involved. Bronchiolitis (i.e., capillary bronchitis) is an entirely different illness (see Chapter 338).

Asthmatic bronchitis is a form of asthma that is often confused with acute bronchitis. With a variety of upper respiratory tract infections, some children have bronchial spasm and exudation similar to signs in older children with asthma.

Acute tracheobronchitis is commonly associated with an upper respiratory tract infection such as nasopharyngitis but is also associated with influenza, pertussis, measles, typhoid fever (and other salmonelloses), diphtheria, and scarlet fever. An acute, primary, undifferentiated tracheobronchitis also occurs, most commonly in older children and adolescents. It is likely that, except for the bacterial diseases mentioned, acute tracheobronchitis is of viral origin. Pneumococci, staphylococci, *Haemophilus influenzae,* and various hemolytic streptococci may be isolated from the sputum, but their presence does not imply a bacterial cause, and antibiotic therapy does not appreciably alter the course of the illness. Some children appear to be far more susceptible to acute tracheobronchitis than others. The reasons are unknown, but allergy, climate, air pollution, and chronic infections of the upper respiratory tract, particularly sinusitis, may be contributing factors.

The syndrome *bronchiolitis obliterans* may begin with an episode of acute bronchitis, bronchiolitis, or bronchopneumonia and then progress over several weeks to severe chronic pulmonary disease characterized by bronchiolar and bronchial obliteration and bronchiectasis (see Chapter 339).

CLINICAL MANIFESTATIONS. Acute bronchitis is usually preceded by a viral upper respiratory infection. Secondary bacterial infection with *Streptococcus pneumoniae, Moraxella catarrhalis,* or *H. influenzae* may occur. Typically, the child presents a frequent, dry, hacking, unproductive cough of relatively gradual onset, beginning 3–4 days after the appearance of rhinitis. Low substernal discomfort or burning anterior chest pain is often present and may be aggravated by coughing. As the illness progresses, the patient may be bothered by whistling sounds during respiration (probably rhonchi), soreness of the chest, and occasionally by shortness of breath. Coughing paroxysms or gagging on secretions is associated occasionally with vomiting. Within several days, the cough becomes productive, and the sputum changes from clear to purulent. Usually within 5–10 days, the mucus thins, and the cough gradually disappears. The considerable malaise often associated with the illness may continue for 1 wk or more after acute symptoms have subsided.

Physical findings vary with the age of the patient and the stage of the disease. Initially, the child is usually afebrile or has low-grade fever, and there are signs of nasopharyngitis, conjunctival infection, and rhinitis. Later, auscultation reveals roughening of breath sounds, coarse and fine moist rales, and rhonchi which may be high pitched, resembling the wheezing of asthma.

In otherwise healthy children, complications are few, but in undernourished children or those in poor health, otitis, sinusitis, and pneumonia are common.

TREATMENT. There is no specific therapy; most patients recover uneventfully without any treatment. In small infants, pulmonary drainage is facilitated by frequent shifts in position. Older children are more comfortable in high humidity, but there is no evidence that this shortens the duration of illness. Irritating and paroxysmal coughing may cause considerable distress and interfere with sleep. Although suppression of cough may increase the possibility of suppuration, judicious use of cough suppressants (including codeine) may be appropriate for symptomatic relief. Antihistamines, which dry secretions, should not be used, and expectorants are not helpful. Antibiotics do not shorten the duration of the viral illness or decrease the incidence of bacterial complications, although the fact that patients with recurrent episodes may occasionally improve with such treatment suggests that some secondary bacterial infection is present.

Children with repeated attacks of acute bronchitis should be carefully evaluated for the possibility of respiratory tract anomalies, foreign bodies, bronchiectasis, immune deficiency, tuberculosis, allergy, sinusitis, tonsillitis, adenoiditis, and cystic fibrosis.

337.2 Chronic Bronchitis

Although adult chronic bronchitis is defined as 3 mo or more of productive cough each year for 2 or more consecutive yr, there is no such accepted standard for children. Its very existence as a separate entity has been questioned, which emphasizes the importance of searching for an underlying immunologic or mucosal abnormality. A chronic or frequently recurring productive cough usually indicates an underlying pulmonary or systemic disease; affected patients should be evaluated for immune deficiencies, anatomic abnormalities, asthma, environmental disease, upper airway infection with postnasal discharge, cystic fibrosis, ciliary dyskinesis, and bronchiectasis. Cough and wheezing are common, and in one study, all 22 reported patients with chronic bronchitis had evidence of allergic disease. Rarely, bronchial irritation may be secondary to the chronic inhalation of dust or noxious fumes. Tobacco or marijuana smoking is obviously pertinent historical information. Teenagers should be similarly questioned about industrial fumes or automobile exhaust exposure at school or work.

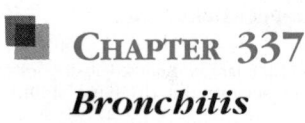

AIR POLLUTION AND CIGARETTE SMOKING. Correlation of a specific pollutant (e.g., NO_2, particulate matter) with a specific childhood respiratory disease or pulmonary symptom is difficult to establish. Any one substance for which such an association is demonstrated may be a marker for one or more other pollutants that are really responsible. However, this does not invalidate the large number of studies indicating that high levels of overall air pollution cause or aggravate lung disease in children. Air pollutants also impair pulmonary function in exercising children and teenagers. Children and parents should be advised of these relationships.

An increased incidence and exacerbations of bronchitis and other forms of acute and chronic lung disease are associated with cigarette smoking. The increased morbidity from respiratory infections in teenagers who smoke is reflected in school and work absences and in functional and pathologic evidence of small airway abnormalities. For example, cigarette smoking is a risk factor for the severity of influenza in young men. Smoking parents, especially those whose children have chronic lung disease, should be advised that they are subjecting their children's lungs to significant amounts of secondhand cigarette smoke in the home; they should be urged to stop smoking.

The Committee on Genetics and Environmental Hazards of the American Academy of Pediatrics has reported that tobacco smoking is one of the most important "sources of environmental contamination and a significant threat to the health of children." It urges physicians to support legislation that would prohibit smoking in public places frequented by children, "particularly in hospitals and other health facilities."

The use of wood-burning stoves also has been associated with a variety of pediatric pulmonary problems. Indoor wood burning results in exposure to particulate matter and polycyclic hydrocarbons. Wheezing and episodic pneumonia have been described in exposed children. In one study, 84% of children exposed to wood-burning stoves (compared with 3% of controls) were reported to have at least one severe respiratory symptom. Systemic problems can also occur if the wood has been treated with toxic materials (e.g., arsenic poisoning has been reported in one family).

Clinical Manifestations. The chief symptom is cough, with or without expectoration. The child usually complains of chest soreness, and characteristically these signs and symptoms are worse at night. Wheezing may also be prominent, and physical findings are similar to those of acute bronchitis. Some patients cough up large, solid, hypereosinophilic mucoid "casts" of the airways, giving rise to the term *plastic bronchitis.* These casts may be related to metaplastic bronchial epithelium, elements of which, together with inflammatory cells and noncellular material, can be found on histologic examination.

Course and Prognosis. The course and the prognosis depend on appropriate management or eradication of any underlying illness. Complications are those of the underlying illness.

Treatment. When an underlying cause for chronic bronchitis is found, this should receive appropriate management. Allergic management may be helpful even when no underlying cause can be discovered. Autogenous vaccines or inhalation of antibiotics is not effective.

Bartecchi CE, MacKenzie TD, Schrier RW: The human cost of tobacco use. N Engl J Med 330:907, 1994.
Braun-Fahrländer C, Ackermann-Liebrich U, Schwartz J, et al: Air pollution and respiratory symptoms in preschool children. Am Rev Respir Dis 145:42, 1992.
Chilmonczyk BA, Salmun LM, Megathlin KN, et al: Association between exposure to environmental tobacco smoke and exacerbations of asthma in children. N Engl J Med 328:1665, 1993.
Christensen W, Hutchins G: Hypereosinophilic mucoid impaction of bronchi in two children under two years of age. Pediatr Pulmonol 1:278, 1985.
Koenig JQ, Covert DS, Hanley QS, et al: Prior exposure to ozone potentiates subsequent response to sulfur dioxide in adolescent asthmatic subjects. Am Rev Respir Dis 141:377, 1990.
Morris K, Morganlander M, Coulehan JL, et al: Wood-burning stoves and lower respiratory tract infection in American Indian children. Am J Dis Child 144:105, 1990.
Perez-Soler A: Cast bronchitis in infants and children. Am J Dis Child 143:1024, 1989.
Samet JM, Marbury MC, Spengler JD: Health effects and sources of indoor air pollution, Parts 1 and 2. Am J Respir Dis 136:1486; 137:221, 1988.
Smith TF, Ireland TA, Zaatari GS, et al: Characteristics of children with endoscopically proved chronic bronchitis. Am J Dis Child 139:1039, 1985.
Taussig LM, Smith SM, Blumenfield R: Chronic bronchitis in childhood: What is it? Pediatrics 67:1, 1981.

CHAPTER 338
Bronchiolitis

David M. Orenstein

Acute bronchiolitis, a common disease of the lower respiratory tract of infants, results from inflammatory obstruction of the small airways. It occurs during the first 2 yr of life, with a peak incidence at approximately 6 mo of age, and in many localities, it is the most frequent cause of hospitalization of infants. The incidence is highest during the winter and early spring. The illness occurs sporadically and epidemically.

ETIOLOGY AND EPIDEMIOLOGY. Acute bronchiolitis is predominantly a viral illness. The respiratory syncytial virus (RSV) is the causative agent in more than 50% of cases (see Chapter 218); parainfluenza 3 virus, mycoplasma, some adenoviruses, and occasionally other viruses produce most of the remaining cases. Adenovirus may be associated with long-term complications, including bronchiolitis obliterans (see Chapter 339) and unilateral hyperlucent lung syndrome (Swyer-James syndrome). There is no firm evidence that bacteria cause bronchiolitis. Occasionally, bacterial bronchopneumonia may be confused clinically with bronchiolitis.

Bronchiolitis occurs most commonly in male infants between 3 and 6 mo of age who have not been breast-fed and who live in crowded conditions. The source of the viral infection is usually a family member with minor respiratory illness. Older children and adults tolerate bronchiolar edema better than infants and do not develop the clinical picture of bronchiolitis even when the smaller airways of their respiratory tract are infected by a virus.

In one report, sophisticated pulmonary function studies were performed for a large population of normal infants. The follow-up analysis revealed that wheezy respiratory illnesses were significantly more common among infants whose initial total respiratory conductance was in the lowest third of those tested. Diminished lung function may play a role in determining which infants with viral infection develop bronchiolitis.

Infants whose mothers smoke cigarettes are more likely to develop bronchiolitis than infants of nonsmoking mothers. Despite the known risks of respiratory infections from child care, infants who stay home with mothers who are heavy smokers are more likely to develop bronchiolitis than infants who attend day care centers.

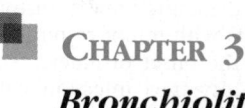

PATHOPHYSIOLOGY. Acute bronchiolitis is characterized by bronchiolar obstruction due to edema and accumulation of mucus and cellular debris and by invasion of the smaller bronchial radicles by virus. Because resistance to airflow in a tube is inversely related to the fourth power of the radius, even minor thickening of the bronchiolar wall in infants may profoundly affect airflow. Resistance in the small air passages is increased during the inspiratory and expiratory phases, but because the radius of an airway is smaller during expiration, the resultant ball valve respiratory obstruction leads to early air trapping and overinflation. Atelectasis may occur when an obstruction becomes complete and trapped air is absorbed.

The pathologic process impairs the normal exchange of gases in the lung. Ventilation perfusion mismatch results in hypoxemia, which occurs early in the course. Carbon dioxide retention (i.e., hypercapnia) does not usually occur except in severely affected patients. The higher the respiratory rate, the lower is the arterial oxygen tension. Hypercapnia usually does not occur until respirations exceed 60/min; it then increases in proportion to the tachypnea.

CLINICAL MANIFESTATIONS. Most affected infants have a history of exposure to older children or adults with minor respiratory diseases within the week preceding the onset of illness. The infant first has a mild upper respiratory tract infection with serous nasal discharge and sneezing. These symptoms usually last several days and may be accompanied by diminished appetite and fever of 38.5–39° C (101–102° F), although the temperature may range from subnormal to markedly elevated. The gradual development of respiratory distress is characterized by paroxysmal wheezy cough, dyspnea, and irritability. Breast- or bottle-feeding may be particularly difficult, because the rapid respiratory rate may not permit time for sucking and swallowing. In mild cases, symptoms disappear in 1–3 days. In the more severely affected patients, symptoms may develop within several hours, and the course is protracted. Other systemic manifestations, such as vomiting and diarrhea, are usually absent.

An examination reveals a tachypneic infant, often in extreme distress. Respirations range from 60–80/min; severe air hunger and cyanosis may occur. The alae nasi flare, and use of the accessory muscles of respiration results in intercostal and subcostal retractions, which are shallow because of the persistent distention of the lungs by the trapped air. The depression of the liver and spleen by the overinflated lungs may result in their being palpable below the costal margin. Widespread fine crackles may be heard at the end of inspiration and in early expiration. The expiratory phase of breathing is prolonged, and wheezes are usually audible. In the most severe cases, breath sounds are barely audible when bronchiolar obstruction is almost complete.

Roentgenographic examination reveals hyperinflation of the lungs and an increased anteroposterior diameter on lateral view. Scattered areas of consolidation are found in about 30% of patients and are caused by atelectasis secondary to obstruction or by inflammation of the alveoli. Early bacterial pneumonia cannot be excluded on radiographic grounds alone.

The white blood cell and differential cell counts are usually within normal limits. Lymphopenia, commonly associated with many viral illnesses, is usually not found. Nasopharyngeal cultures reveal normal bacterial flora. Virus may be demonstrated in nasopharyngeal secretions by antigen detection (e.g., enzyme immunoassay) or by culture.

DIFFERENTIAL DIAGNOSIS. The condition most commonly confused with acute bronchiolitis is asthma. One or more of the following favors the diagnosis of asthma: a family history of asthma, repeated episodes in the same infant, sudden onset without preceding infection, markedly prolonged expiration, eosinophilia, and an immediate favorable response to the administration of a single dose of aerosolized albuterol. Repeated attacks represent an important differential point: fewer than 5% of recurrent attacks of clinical bronchiolitis have viral infections as a cause. Other entities that may be confused with acute bronchiolitis are congestive heart failure, a foreign body in the trachea, pertussis, organophosphate poisoning, cystic fibrosis, and bacterial bronchopneumonias associated with generalized obstructive pulmonary overinflation.

COURSE AND PROGNOSIS. The most critical phase of illness occurs during the first 48–72 hr after the onset of cough and dyspnea. During this period, the infant appears desperately ill, apneic spells occur in the very young infant, and respiratory acidosis is likely to be noticed. After the critical period, improvement occurs rapidly and often dramatically. Recovery is complete in a few days. The case fatality rate is below 1%; death may result from prolonged apneic spells, severe uncompensated respiratory acidosis, or profound dehydration secondary to the loss of water vapor from tachypnea and the inability to drink fluids. Infants with conditions such as congenital heart disease, bronchopulmonary dysplasia, immunodeficiency diseases, or cystic fibrosis have a greater morbidity rate and have a slightly increased mortality rate. The mortality rate is not as great in these "high-risk" infants as it once was. Estimates of mortality among infants with these high-risk conditions who contract RSV bronchiolitis have decreased from 37% in 1982 to 3.5% in 1988. Bacterial complications, such as bronchopneumonia or otitis media, are uncommon. Cardiac failure during bronchiolitis is rare, except in children with underlying heart disease.

A significant proportion of infants with bronchiolitis have hyper-reactive airways during later childhood, but the relation of these two entities, if any, is not understood. The suggestion that a single episode of bronchiolitis may result in very-long-term small airway abnormality requires further investigation. These abnormalities may be partially explained by the finding that infants with low total respiratory conductance are more likely to develop bronchiolitis in response to viral respiratory infection. The infants with bronchiolitis who develop reactive airways are more likely to have a family history of asthma and allergy, a prolonged acute episode of bronchiolitis, and exposure to cigarette smoke.

TREATMENT. Infants with respiratory distress should be hospitalized, but only supportive treatment is indicated. The patient is commonly placed in an atmosphere of cool, humidified oxygen to relieve hypoxemia and reduce insensible water loss from tachypnea; this treatment relieves the dyspnea and cyanosis and allays anxiety and restlessness. Sedatives should be avoided whenever possible because of potential depression of respiration. The infant is usually more comfortable sitting at a 30 to 40 degree angle or with the head and chest slightly elevated so that the neck is somewhat extended. Oral intake must often be supplemented or replaced by parenteral fluids to offset the dehydrating effect of tachypnea. Electrolyte balance and pH should be adjusted by suitable intravenous solutions.

Ribavirin (Virazole), an antiviral agent, has been available for the treatment of RSV infection since 1985. Several controlled trials using high-risk patients showed an improvement in oxygenation and decreased viral shedding. Its use has been recommended for infants with congenital heart disease or bronchopulmonary dysplasia by the Committee on Infectious Diseases of American Academy of Pediatrics (AAP). One study of intubated infants randomized to ribavirin or placebo showed a better outcome for the ribavirin-treated group. Despite these apparently favorable studies and the AAP recommendation, the use of ribavirin remains controversial, even in desperately ill infants. The study of intubated infants, for example, employed water (a known bronchoconstrictor) rather than saline as the placebo, raising important questions about its validity. There has been no convincing evidence of its impact on the duration of hospitalization, requirement for supportive therapies such as oxygen or mechanical ventilation, or mortality. There appears to be generally excellent outcome for even some high-risk infants not treated with ribavirin.

Antibiotics have no therapeutic value unless there is secondary bacterial pneumonia. The low incidence of bacterial complications is not reduced further by antibiotic therapy. Corticosteroids are not beneficial and may be harmful under certain conditions. However, corticosteroids have not been evaluated in patients with severe adenovirus bronchiolitis in whom long-term severe sequelae (e.g., necrotizing lesions) might be more likely. Bronchodilating aerosolized drugs (e.g., albuterol) are frequently used empirically; studies are divided between those that demonstrate benefit and those that demonstrate no benefit or even harm. Epinephrine or other adrenergic agents have a theoretical basis for use, and in two studies, aerosolized epinephrine provided some benefit to infants with bronchiolitis. Chinese herbs have been shown in one study to decrease symptom duration by 2.6 days. Because the obstruction occurs at the bronchiolar level, tracheostomy is not beneficial and involves substantial risks that are not justified in these acutely ill infants. Some patients may progress rapidly to respiratory failure, requiring ventilatory assistance.

Englund J, Piedra P, Ahn Y-M, et al: High-dose, short-duration ribavirin aerosol therapy compared with standard ribavirin therapy in children with suspected respiratory syncytial virus infection. J Pediatr 125:635, 1994.
Gadomski A, Lichenstein R, Horton L, et al: Efficacy of albuterol in the management of bronchiolitis. Pediatrics 93:907, 1994.
Hall CB, McBride JT, Walsh EE, et al: Aerosolized ribavirin treatment of infants with respiratory syncytial viral infection: A randomized double blind study. N Engl J Med 308:1443, 1983.
Kong XT, Fang HT, Jiang GQ, et al: Treatment of acute bronchiolitis with Chinese herbs. Arch Dis Child 68:468, 1993.
Kritjansson S, Lodrup Carlsen KC, Wennergren G, et al: Nebulised racemic adrenalin in the treatment of acute bronchiolitis in infants and toddlers. Arch Dis Child 69:650, 1993.
Martinez FD, Morgan WJ, Wright AL, et al: Diminished lung function as a predisposing factor for wheezing respiratory illness in infants. N Engl J Med 319:112, 1988.
McConnochie KM, Roghmann KJ: Predicting clinically significant lower respiratory tract illness in childhood following mild bronchiolitis. Am J Dis Child 139:625, 1985.
Panitch HB, Callahan CW, Schidlow DV: Bronchiolitis in children. Clin Chest Med 14:715, 1993.
Schuh S, Canny G, Reisman JJ, et al: Nebulized albuterol in acute bronchiolitis. J Pediatr 117:633, 1990.
Wald ER, Dashefsky B: Ribavirin. Red book committee recommendation questioned. Pediatrics 93:672, 1994.
Wheeler JG, Woffard J, Turner RB: Historical cohort evaluation of ribavirin efficacy in respiratory synctial virus infection. Pediatr Infect Dis J 12:209, 1993.

CHAPTER 339
Bronchiolitis Obliterans

David M. Orenstein

In bronchitis obliterans, the bronchioles and smaller airways are injured, and the attempted repair produces large amounts of granulation tissue that causes airway obstruction. Eventually, the airway lumens are obliterated with nodular masses of granulation and fibrosis. The precipitating injury commonly cannot be identified, particularly in children. Some adult cases are related to the inhalation of the oxides of nitrogen or other chemicals. The syndrome has also been associated with connective tissue diseases and some drugs (e.g., penicillamine). Most pediatric cases can be temporally related to pulmonary infection, such as measles, influenza, adenovirus, mycoplasma, and pertussis. Obliterative bronchiolitis is a common and ominous complication of lung transplantation.

CLINICAL MANIFESTATIONS. Initially, cough, respiratory distress, and cyanosis may occur and be followed by a brief period of apparent improvement. Progressive disease is reflected by increasing dyspnea, cough, sputum production, and wheezing. The pattern may resemble bronchitis, bronchiolitis, or pneumonia. The chest roentgenographic findings range from normal to a pattern that suggests miliary tuberculosis. *Swyer-James syndrome* may develop with unilateral hyperlucency and a decrease in pulmonary vascular markings in about 10% of cases. Bronchography shows obstruction of the bronchioles, with little or no contrast material reaching the periphery of the lung. Computerized tomography may reveal the bronchiectasis that occurs in many patients. Pulmonary function test findings are variable, with severe obstruction being most common, but restriction or a combination of obstruction and restriction can be seen. The diagnosis can be confirmed by lung biopsy.

TREATMENT AND PROGNOSIS. There is no specific treatment. The pathology suggests a progressive fibrotic picture that could theoretically be delayed by corticosteroid treatment. Some forms of bronchiolitis obliterans in adults, especially bronchiolitis obliterans organizing pneumonia (BOOP), respond well to corticosteroid treatment. No definitive data about corticosteroid efficacy exist for children. Some patients deteriorate rapidly and die within weeks of the onset of the initial symptoms, but most survive, some with chronic disability.

Epler GR, Colby TV, McLoud TC, et al: Bronchiolitis obliterans organizing pneumonia. N Engl J Med 312:152, 1985.
Hardy KA: Obliterative bronchiolitis. *In:* Hilman BC (ed): Pediatric Respiratory Disease. Diagnosis and Treatment. Philadelphia, WB Saunders, 1993, p 218.
Hardy KA, Schidlow DV, Zaeri N: Obliterative bronchiolitis in children. Chest 93:460, 1988.

339.1 Follicular Bronchitis

Follicular bronchitis is a newly recognized rare problem in children. The etiology is unknown. Most affected children have tachypnea and cough by 6 wk of age. Diffuse crackles are heard on auscultation of the lung fields. Roentgenograms usually reveal a diffuse interstitial pattern, but the picture may be relatively normal. Computed tomography may show subtle interstitial nodules, even in those with normal plain films. The diagnosis is made by lung biopsy. Most children gradually improve, although in some the disorder is life threatening, with a single or recurrent episodes of respiratory failure. Some affected children seem to respond to corticosteroid treatment.

Kinane BT, Mansell AL, Zwerdling RG, et al: Follicular bronchitis in the pediatric population. Chest 104:1183, 1993.

CHAPTER 340
Aspiration Pneumonias and Gastroesophageal Reflux–Related Respiratory Disease

David M. Orenstein

Despite mechanisms for keeping the contents of the gastrointestinal tract out of the respiratory tract (Table 340–1), there are many instances in which dysfunctional swallowing or gastroesophageal reflux can cause or worsen respiratory disease (see Chapter 269). The numerous mechanisms for reflux-associated respiratory disease (Fig. 340–1) include aspiration, with direct mechanical and chemical effects (e.g., obstruction of laryngeal or bronchial lumen, pneumonitis); neurally medi-

■ **TABLE 340–1 Prevention of Respiratory Sequelae due to Reflux**

Structure	Protective Functions	Dysfunctions
Stomach	Antegrade emptying	Delayed gastric emptying
Esophagus and associated structures	Diaphragmatic hiatal tone	Hiatal hernia
Lower esophageal sphincter (LES)	LES tone; differentiates gas from liquid	Hypotensive LES; transient LES relaxations to liquid
Body	Secondary peristalsis	Impaired esophageal clearance
Upper esophageal sphincter (UES)	UES tone; differentiates gas from liquid	Hypotensive UES; transient UES relaxations to liquid
Larynx, pharynx, mouth	Swallow reflex; cord closure; arytenoid-epiglottic approximation	Impaired swallow reflex; impaired cord closure; impaired arytenoid-epiglottic approximation

From Putnam PE, Ricker DH, Orenstein SR: Gastroesophageal reflux. In: *Beckerman RC, Brouillette RT, Hunt CE (eds): Respiratory Control Disorders in Infants and Children. Baltimore, Williams & Wilkins, 1992, p 323.*

ated effects from the airway; and neurally mediated effects from the esophagus.

Respiratory disorders and their therapy can also cause or worsen reflux. The most common mechanism is increasing the gastroesophageal pressure gradient by increasing intragastric pressure, as when the abdominal muscles are tensed with coughing and forced expiratory maneuvers, as in cystic fibrosis, bronchopulmonary dysplasia, or asthma. Much of the increased intra-abdominal pressure is also transmitted to the diaphragm and then to the lower esophageal sphincter, augmenting its antireflux action. Hyperinflation may predispose to reflux by flattening the diaphragm, rendering it less effective in augmenting the lower esophageal sphincter. Intrapleural pressure is more negative than normal with inspiration against an obstructed airway, as occurs in laryngospasm and asthma, favoring movement of gastric contents into the esophagus.

Theophylline and orally administered β-agonist drugs may relax the lower esophageal sphincter and increase gastric acid secretion. Nasogastric tubes used for nutritional supplementation in many children with chronic respiratory disorders predispose the child to gastroesophageal reflux. Mechanical ventilation with tracheal intubation impairs airway protective mechanisms and may predispose the child to aspiration. Mechanically ventilated patients are usually kept supine, a position provocative for reflux. Chest physical therapy and postural drainage increases reflux in children with cystic fibrosis, probably in part because of gravity.

Johannesson N, Andersson K, Joelsson B, Persson C: Relaxation of the lower esophageal sphincter and stimulation of gastric secretion and diuresis by antiasthmatic xanthines. Am Rev Respir Dis 131:26, 1985.

Orenstein DM, Orenstein SR: Gastroesophageal reflux and dysfunctional swallowing. *In:* Loughlin GM, Eigen H (eds): Respiratory Disease in Children. Baltimore, Williams & Wilkins, 1994, p 563.

Schindlbeck N, Heinrich, Clueller-Lissner S: Effects of albuterol (salbutamol) on esophageal motility an gastroesophageal reflux in healthy volunteers. JAMA 260:3156, 1988.

340.1 Aspiration Pneumonia

ASPIRATION OF FOOD AND VOMITUS. Infants with obstructive lesions, such as esophageal atresia or duodenal obstruction; hypotonic, weak, and debilitated infants and children with no obstructive lesions; patients with familial dysautonomia; and patients with impaired consciousness may aspirate, or regurgitate and then aspirate, food and vomitus, causing a chemical pneumonia. Aspiration rarely may be an immediate cause of death by asphyxiation. Hydrochloric acid is an important determinant of lung injury. After aspiration of gastric contents, there frequently is a relatively brief latent period before the onset of signs and symptoms of pneumonia. More than 90% of patients have symptoms within 1 hr, and almost all patients have symptoms within 2 hr. Fever, tachypnea, and cough are common. Apnea and shock may also occur.

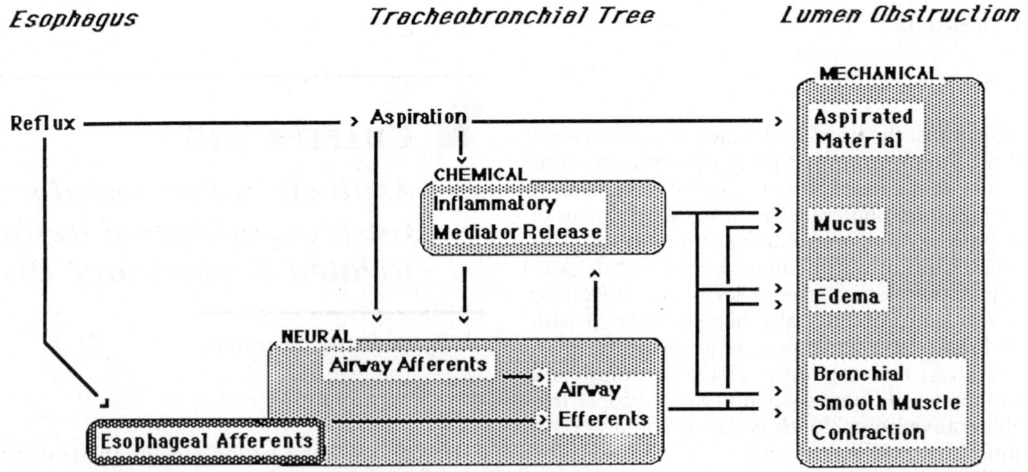

Figure 340–1. Mechanisms of reflux-associated respiratory dysfunction. Reflux may lead to direct pulmonary aspiration of refluxed material, producing mechanical obstruction of the airway lumen. Pulmonary aspiration also leads to the release of chemical mediators of inflammation, which leads to obstruction of the lumen by mucus, mucosal edema, and bronchial smooth muscle contraction. Aspiration stimulates the airway's neural afferents, which influence airway efferents, inducing the release of chemical inflammatory mediators and leading to mucus secretion, edema formation, and bronchial smooth muscle contraction. Reflux can stimulate esophageal afferents, which also influence airway efferents.

Physical examination reveals diffuse crackles, wheezing, and possibly cyanotic features. Chest roentgenograms reveal alveolar and, occasionally, reticular infiltrates that may be localized but often are more extensive and are frequently bilateral. The irritated mucous membrane may also subsequently become the site for bacterial invasion and pneumonia. Aspiration from gastroesophageal reflux occasionally can be demonstrated by barium swallow roentgenography, but radionuclide milk scanning is more sensitive. Bronchoalveolar lavage fluid may be examined for lipid-filled macrophages, lactose, or dyes that had been administered orally to support the diagnosis of reflux-related aspiration, but false-positive and false-negative results limit the usefulness of these methods.

Prophylaxis is essential. Care should be taken to avoid amounts of feedings that overdistend the stomach, especially in infants who are fed by gavage. After being fed, the infant should be placed on the right side. When the infant is supine, the head should be elevated. Critically ill patients may benefit from reduction of gastric acidity with cimetidine or ranitidine.

Treatment by immediate suctioning of the airway and administering oxygen are indicated for aspiration. Endotracheal intubation with suctioning and mechanical ventilation is often required for severe cases. Although the prophylactic use of antibiotics and corticosteroids is advocated by some for patients who have aspirated gastric contents, evidence of their benefit is lacking. Some data suggest that corticosteroid treatment may predispose the patient to pneumonia caused by gram-negative organisms. Previously healthy nonhospitalized patients may become infected with mouth flora (predominantly anaerobes); clindamycin or penicillin is effective therapy. Chronically ill hospitalized patients may be colonized with gram-negative flora (e.g., *Pseudomonas, Escherichia coli, Klebsiella*); additional coverage with an aminoglycoside may be indicated.

Prognosis depends partly on the severity of aspiration and partly on the underlying disease. Most patients demonstrate clearing of infiltrates within 2 wk; the mortality rate for patients with massive aspiration is about 25%.

Brook I, Finegold SM: Bacteriology of aspiration pneumonia in children. Pediatrics 65:1115, 1980.
Colombo J, Hallbert T: Recurrent aspiration in children: Lipid-laden alveolar macrophage quantitation. Pediatr Pulmonol 3:86, 1987.
DeePaso WJ: Aspiration pneumonia. Clin Chest Med 12:269, 1991.
McVeagh P, Howman-Giles R, Kemp A: Pulmonary aspiration studied by radionuclide milk scanning and barium swallow roentgenography. Am J Dis Child 141:917, 1987.
Stagus R, Martin A, Binns S, et al: The significance of fat-filled macrophages in the diagnosis of aspiration associated with gastrooesophageal reflux. Aust Paediatr J 21:275, 1985.
Wolfe JE, Bone RC, Ruth WE: Effects of corticosteroids in the treatment of patients with gastric aspiration. Am J Med 83:719, 1977.

ASPIRATION OF BABY POWDER. Aspiration pneumonia resulting from inhalation of zinc stearate baby powder is rare, because the use of baby powder has decreased and the containers still being used control the outflow of powder. Catastrophic aspirations still occur. Severe respiratory distress almost immediately follows inhalation. Generalized obstructive overinflation with an expiratory type of dyspnea occurs as a result of an inflammatory reaction caused by the zinc stearate powder. After inhalation, the powder is almost immediately drawn into the finer bronchioles because of its extreme lightness; for this reason, suctioning with a bronchoscope is useful to remove the secretions that may subsequently accumulate in the larger air passages. Immediate treatment is oxygen therapy in an atmosphere of high humidity.

The commonly used dusting (i.e., baby) powders today contain magnesium silicate and other silicates; some contain calcium undecylenate. Although not as dangerous as zinc stearate, these powders can also cause serious aspiration pneumonitis. Talc is chemically related to asbestos, and "talcum powder" may contain microscopic asbestos particles, which have the potential to cause malignancy. Systemic corticosteroid treatment appeared to be useful in one patient who had severe dyspnea after aspirating talc.

Cotton WH, Davidson PJ: Aspiration of baby powder. N Engl J Med 313:1662, 1985.
Mofenson HC, Caraccio TR, Okun S, et al: Hazards of baby powder. Pediatrics 78:546, 1986.

PNEUMONITIS FROM OTHER CHEMICALS. Many chemicals, particularly if inhaled in high concentrations, may cause an inflammatory reaction consisting of edema, cellular infiltration, and acute respiratory distress. Prolonged exposure to lower concentrations of these same agents or other chemicals may cause chronic interstitial pneumonitis, characterized by granuloma formation. For example, shellac, polyvinylpyrrolidone (found in hair spray), gum arabic, beryllium, mercury vapors, and chlorine may cause this reaction. Corticosteroids may reduce the inflammatory reaction and prevent fibrosis.

340.2 Hydrocarbon Pneumonia

ETIOLOGY. Hydrocarbons, such as furniture polish, kerosene, charcoal lighter fluid, and gasoline, are occasionally accidentally ingested by young children, causing a secondary pneumonitis. Gasoline may be aspirated by teenagers attempting to siphon gasoline. In general, the lower the viscosity and the higher the volatility of the hydrocarbon compound, the greater is the pulmonary toxicity. In 1990, there were 30,000 hydrocarbon ingestions reported to poison control centers, with four deaths.

PATHOGENESIS. Hydrocarbons are probably aspirated during swallowing, vomiting, or gastric lavage. The low viscosity of hydrocarbons allows them to flow from the hypopharynx into the larynx. Ingestion of large quantities of these bad-tasting liquids is unusual, and gastric lavage is contraindicated unless the hydrocarbon contains poison, such as a potent insecticide e.g., organophosphate. Hydrocarbons may interact with pulmonary surfactant, resulting in alveolar collapse. Alveolar macrophages may also be injured. The pulmonary changes observed in animals after hydrocarbon aspiration are edema, inflammation, and hemorrhage.

CLINICAL MANIFESTATIONS. Coughing and vomiting follow ingestion almost immediately. Within hours, there may be temperature elevation (38–40° C). However, with less extensive aspiration, the onset of pulmonary symptoms and inflammation may be delayed 12–24 hr. The pulmonary findings may include dyspnea, diminished resonance on percussion, suppressed or tubular breath sounds, and crackles. Hypoxemia and cyanosis, caused by inflammation and edema, may be aggravated by the displacement of alveolar gas with vaporized hydrocarbon. Pneumonic involvement is disclosed more frequently by roentgenographic examination than by physical findings. Roentgenograms may occasionally show minimal changes a few hours after ingestion, only to progress rapidly after that time with extensive infiltrates. Despite what may be a stormy clinical course, which averages 2–5 days, recovery occurs in most cases. Systemic symptoms of hydrocarbon ingestion, including somnolence, convulsions, and coma, may occur and sometimes dominate the course (see Chapter 666.4).

COMPLICATIONS. Pneumothorax, subcutaneous emphysema of the chest wall, and pleural effusion, including empyema, have occurred. After the 1st wk, pneumatoceles may develop in areas of extensive consolidation. There may be secondary infection with bacteria or viruses.

TREATMENT. Symptoms and radiologic infiltrates may be delayed, and no patient should be sent home in less than 6 hr, even if there are no symptoms. Patients who are symptomatic when they are first examined, patients who become symptomatic during 6 hr of observation, and all patients who ingested a particularly toxic agent (e.g., furniture polish) should be admitted to the hospital. Patients who are still asymptomatic after 6 hr and who have a normal result on a chest roentgenogram can be observed at home, but parents should be instructed to return the infant or toddler to the hospital if any respiratory symptoms occur. No pulmonary therapy is indicated before symptoms develop.

After ingestion of small to moderate amounts of hydrocarbons, induction of vomiting or gastric lavage is contraindicated because of the risk of aspiration, especially if several hours have elapsed. If a large volume of hydrocarbon is thought to be in the stomach, nasogastric suction performed with great care to avoid aspiration rarely may be necessary to reduce the other dangers of hydrocarbon poisoning, including central nervous system toxicity. The risk of aspiration during gastric lavage or suctioning can be minimized if an endotracheal tube with a balloon cuff can be inserted without inducing vomiting before lavage. For dyspnea, cyanosis, or chemical pneumonitis, supportive measures, including oxygen, physiotherapy, and if necessary, continuous positive airway pressure or other forms of ventilatory assistance, are important components of therapy. A cathartic is usually indicated.

The routine use of antibiotics is not recommended; the occurrence of secondary infection of the affected lung can usually be readily detected by the reappearance of fever on the 3rd–5th day after ingestion and can then be suitably treated with penicillin G and tobramycin. Corticosteroids have no beneficial effect on the course of the illness and may be harmful. Pneumatoceles, when they occur, rarely rupture and do not require treatment. Parents must be reminded to keep cleaning fluids and kerosene in locked cabinets out of reach of children or out of the home.

PROGNOSIS. Although most children survive without complications or sequelae, some progress rapidly to respiratory failure and death.

The prognosis depends on a variety of factors, including the volume of the ingestion or aspiration, the specific agent involved, and the adequacy of medical care. In one series, only 39 of 950 patients developed symptoms; four required assisted ventilation, and two died. Long-term pulmonary function studies several years later are inconclusive, but if lasting damage does occur, the small airways seem to be at greatest risk.

Bergeson PS, Hales SW, Lustgarten MD, et al: Pneumatoceles following hydrocarbon ingestion. Report of three cases and review of the literature. Am J Dis Child 129:49, 1975.

Brown J III, Burke B, Dajani AS: Experimental kerosene pneumonia: Evaluation of some therapeutic regimens. J Pediatr 84:396, 1974.

Guruntz D, Kattan M, Levison H, et al: Pulmonary function abnormalities in asymptotic children after hydrocarbon pneumonitis. Pediatrics 62:789, 1978.

Klein BL, Simon JE: Hydrocarbon poisonings. Pediatr Clin North Am 33:411, 1986.

Litovits T, Bailery K, Schmitz B, et al: 1990 Annual report of the American Association of Poison Control Centers National Data Collection System. Am J Emerg Med 9:461, 1991.

340.3 Lipoid Pneumonia

Lipoid pneumonia is a chronic, interstitial, proliferative inflammation resulting from aspiration of lipoid material; it occurs principally in debilitated infants.

PATHOGENESIS. Factors that may be responsible for aspiration of oil include intranasal instillation of medicated oils, including petroleum jelly; any condition that interferes with swallowing, such as cleft palate, debilitation, or a horizontal position during feeding; and forced feeding, especially the administration of cod liver oil, castor oil, or mineral oil to crying children. In some areas of Saudia Arabia, forced feeding of rendered animal fat (i.e., ghee) to infants is traditional; lipoid pneumonia has followed this practice.

The severity of the pulmonary reaction depends on the kind of oil inhaled. Vegetable oils, such as olive, cottonseed, and sesame oils, are generally the least irritating and produce minimal or no inflammation; however, chaulmoogra, also a vegetable oil, produces extensive damage. Animal oils, because of their high fatty acid content, are the most damaging. Milk aspirated by debilitated infants is one example; cod liver oil also belongs in this category. Liquid petrolatum is chemically inert and is not as irritative as some of the other oils but does act as a foreign body. Excessive use of lip gloss can also cause pneumonitis in teenagers.

The reaction begins as an interstitial proliferative inflammation, and there may be an exudative pneumonia. In the second stage, there is diffuse, chronic, proliferative fibrosis and sometimes superimposed acute infectious bronchopneumonia. In the third stage, there are multiple localized nodules, tumor-like paraffinomas. There are numerous macrophages in the involved areas, with giant cell formation of the foreign body type. The lipoid substance is found in intracellular and extracellular areas. The oil-laden cells may be carried to the hilar lymph nodes.

CLINICAL MANIFESTATIONS. There are no characteristic signs or symptoms; a cough is common, and severe cases may include dyspnea. Unless there is superimposed infection, the physical examination may be normal, although with extensive involvement, there may be some impairment to percussion and a change in voice and breath sounds. Secondary bronchopneumonic infections are common.

The roentgenographic appearance is characteristic (Fig. 340–2). Mild involvement is manifested by an increase in the density and extent of the hilar shadows. With increasing involvement, there is greater density of the perihilar shadows, which widen in all directions. Pulmonary changes may be limited to the right lung, and in the infant who is recumbent most of the time, the changes may be mainly in the right upper lobe.

PROGNOSIS. The prognosis is guarded. It depends on the general condition of the patient, the extent of pulmonary damage, the discontinuation of oil inhalation, and the avoidance of intercurrent infections.

PREVENTION. Intranasal medications in an oily vehicle should not be used. Administration of mineral oil, cod liver oil, and castor oil should be avoided, if possible. Infants who regurgitate or vomit frequently should be placed prone to reduce the likelihood of aspiration.

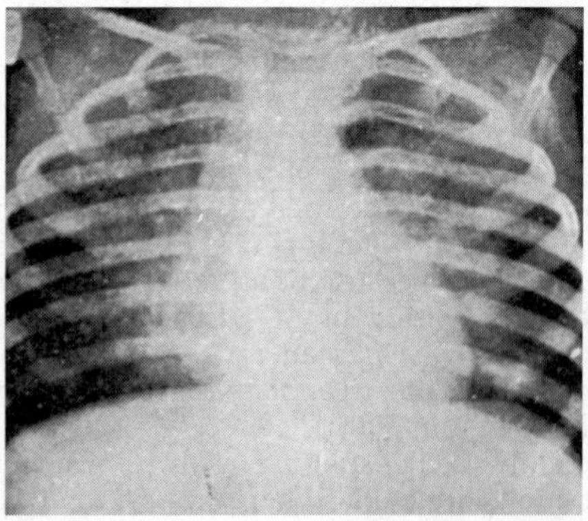

Figure 340–2. Lipoid pneumonia. The roentgenogram shows an increased density radiating from the hilus of each lung in an infant 13 mo of age after intranasal application of liquid petrolatum three times daily for 5 mo.

TREATMENT. There is no specific therapy other than elimination of further exposure.

Annobil SH, Ogunbiyi AO, Benjamin B: Chest radiographic findings in childhood lipoid pneumonia following aspiration of animal fat. Eur J Radiol 16:217, 1993.
Bection DL, Lowe JE, Falleta JM: Lipoid pneumonia in an adolescent girl secondary to use of lip gloss. J Pediatr 105:421, 1984.
Brown AC, Slocum PC, Putthoff SL, et al: Exogenous lipoid pneumonia due to intranasal application of petroleum jelly. Chest 105:968, 1994.
Spickard A III, Hirschmann JV: Exogenous lipoid pneumonia. Arch Intern Med 154:686, 1994.

340.4 Respiratory Disorders Caused or Worsened by Gastroesophageal Reflux or Its Treatment

ASPIRATION PNEUMONIA. Direct aspiration of refluxed materials can cause pneumonia, particularly in children with depressed consciousness (e.g., sleep, general anesthesia, severe mental retardation). Microaspiration may also cause a chemical pneumonitis, asthma-like symptoms, or both.

ASTHMA. Many more children with asthma have abnormal amounts of reflux than healthy control infants. Patients with nocturnal asthma are particularly likely to have reflux. Reflux seems to cause or worsen asthma through vagal pathways originating with acid stimulus of esophageal receptors. Esophageal acidification may not cause bronchospasm directly but may heighten airway responsiveness to other stimuli.

BRONCHOPULMONARY DYSPLASIA. There is some suggestion that reflux may prolong the course of bronchopulmonary dysplasia (BPD) and that treatment of reflux improves pulmonary function in some infants. Physicians should be alert to the possibility of reflux in infants with BPD who are slow to respond to standard treatment or who have prominent nocturnal symptoms.

CYSTIC FIBROSIS. A high proportion of patients with cystic fibrosis may have gastroesophageal reflux. How much of this is related to hyperinflation or to treatment (e.g., postural drainage, bronchodilator drugs) is unclear. There is some suggestion that respiratory disease may improve with treatment of the reflux.

TRACHEOESOPHAGEAL FISTULA. All patients born with tracheoesophageal fistula have esophageal dysmotility, and most have reflux. Some may experience aspiration.

OBSTRUCTIVE APNEA. Obstructive apnea can occur in sleeping or awake infants. In a specific clinical syndrome described in awake infants, shortly after a feeding, the seated or supine infant suddenly stops breathing. These infants are staring, plethoric, often with rigid posturing. Subsequently, they become pale or cyanotic and perhaps hypotonic. Coughing, choking, and gagging are absent.

CENTRAL APNEA AND APPARENT LIFE-THREATENING EVENTS. Many infants with apparent life-threatening events have reflux, and several studies have shown that babies with recurrent respiratory arrest become free of such episodes after treatment for reflux.

STRIDOR. Some infants, particularly those with mild airway compromise from some other cause, such as laryngomalacia, have stridor during episodes of reflux and lessened stridor after antireflux therapy.

Reflux-induced laryngeal inflammation may cause recurrent or spasmodic croup.

HOARSENESS. In adults, inflammation and edema of the larynx, particularly its posterior aspects, is associated with reflux, and their laryngeal symptoms respond to acid suppression therapy. This association probably exists for children.

COUGH. In some adults, cough has been identified as the sole manifestation of reflux and has responded to antireflux therapy. Cough is also associated with reflux in some infants.

HICCUPS. Hiccups have been associated with reflux in adults and children.

RESPIRATORY SIDE EFFECTS OF ANTIREFLUX TREATMENT. Bethanechol, a cholinergic agent that promotes gastric motility and augments lower esophageal pressure, can provoke bronchospasm.

Irwin R, Zawacki J, Curley F, et al: Chronic cough as the sole presenting manifestation of gastroesophageal reflux. Am Rev Respir Dis 140:1294, 1989.
Lew C, Keens T, O'Neal M, et al: Gastroesophageal reflux recovery from bronchopulmonary dysplasia. Clin Res 29:149A, 1981.
Martin M, Grunstein M, Larsen G: The relationship of gastroesophageal reflux to nocturnal wheezing in children with asthma. Ann Allergy 49:318, 1982.
Nielson D, Heldt G, Tooley W: Stridor and gastroesophageal reflux in infants. Pediatrics 85:1034, 1990.
Orenstein DM, Orenstein SR: Gastroesophageal reflux and dysfunctional swallowing. *In:* Loughlin GM, Eigen H (eds): Respiratory Disease in Children. Baltimore, Williams & Wilkins, 1994, p 563.
Putnam P, Orenstein S: Hoarseness in a child with gastroesophageal reflux. Acta Paediatr Scand 81:635, 1992.
Vinocur CD, Marmon L, Schidlow DV, Weintraub WH: Gastroesophageal reflux in the infant with cystic fibrosis. Am J Surg 149:182, 1985.

CHAPTER 341
Silo Filler Disease

Robert C. Stern

The acute or subacute interstitial pneumonia of silo filler disease is caused by inhalation of the oxides of nitrogen, gases most commonly encountered in freshly filled silos, especially corn silos. Nitric and nitrous acids, formed when these gases dissolve, can produce severe burns throughout the respiratory epithelium. A chemical pneumonitis is also involved.

Diagnosis requires a history of entering a silo within 4 wk (usually within 24–100 hr) of its being filled and two or more of the following symptoms at exposure: dyspnea, wheezing, cough, nausea, "choking," or "fatigue." At presentation, which is rarely days or weeks later, one or more of the following should be observed: infiltrates or edema on the chest film; hypoxemia; methemoglobinemia; biopsy or autopsy findings consistent with chemical pneumonitis, including hyperplastic epithelium, widened and edematous interalveolar septa, or alveoli filled with mononuclear cells and fibroblasts. The chest examination reveals rales in about one third of cases. Corticosteroids are usually given, but no controlled data on their efficacy are available. The death rate in patients who present for medical care is 10–20%. This disease is preventable; no one should enter a freshly filled silo for at least 14 days.

Zwemer FL, Pratt DS, May JJ: Silo filler's disease in New York State. Am Rev Respir Dis 146:650, 1992.

CHAPTER 342
Paraquat Lung

Robert C. Stern

Paraquat, a dipyridylium compound used as a weed killer, accumulates selectively in the lung and is highly toxic. The mechanism of toxicity is thought to involve production of a superoxide anion. Death is virtually certain in patients showing radiologic findings; only 11 survivors have been reported. The pulmonary lesion is secondary to systemic absorption through the gastrointestinal tract, skin, or lungs (e.g., smoking contaminated marijuana) and consists of proliferative bronchiolitis, alveolitis, hemorrhage causing intra-alveolar hyaline membranes and fibrosis. Gas exchange is impaired. Some of these patients probably have adult respiratory distress syndrome (see Chapter 60). Paraquat is a corrosive that also causes painful lesions of the mouth and esophagus, renal tubular damage, azotemia, and hematuria. Renal damage may result in prolongation of toxic blood levels, during which time fibroblasts proliferate, filling the terminal air spaces. There is no treatment except for general supportive measures. Oxygen may increase pulmonary toxicity. Lung transplantation was unsuccessful in one patient who died 2 wk later after changes typical of paraquat toxicity had occurred in the transplanted lung. Increased incidence may reflect the large-scale use of paraquat in attempts to kill marijuana plants.

Copland GM, Kolin A, Shulman HS: Fatal pulmonary intra-alveolar fibrosis after paraquat ingestion. N Engl Med 291:290, 1974.
Hudson M, Patel SB, Ewen SWB, et al: Paraquat induced pulmonary fibrosis in three survivors. Thorax 46:201, 1991.

CHAPTER 343

Hypersensitivity to Inhaled Materials

Robert C. Stern

Repeated inhalation of organic dusts may result in chronic pneumonitis that progressively worsens with continued exposure to the antigen. Although the syndrome is most common in adults, it has been reported frequently in children and rarely in infants. Unlike those of asthma, the symptoms of this hypersensitivity syndrome are almost entirely unrelated to bronchospasm (see Chapter 137). Symptoms may result from inhalation of small particles from moldy hay (farmer's lung), maple bark (maple bark stripper's disease), sugar cane fiber (bagassosis), redwood tree bark, pigeon or other bird droppings and feathers (bird fancier's disease), cheese, desiccated pituitary powder, dusty output from air conditioners, and a fungus or mold associated with the specific material to which the patient is exposed.

CLINICAL MANIFESTATIONS. The signs and symptoms are similar in all of these diseases. Within several hours after exposure, cough, dyspnea, chest pain, and sometimes fever occur with few physical findings, although occasional wheezes and moist rales may be audible. Roentgenograms may show minimal emphysema but are usually normal. If no further exposure occurs, the symptoms abate over a period of several days; if contact with the responsible antigen continues, symptoms progress to severe dyspnea and cyanosis associated with diffuse, fine, interstitial or nodular densities and peripheral alveolar infiltrates on chest roentgenogram and occasionally irreversible loss of pulmonary function. The disease should be suspected in children with relatively mild symptoms including cough, fever, and occasional dyspnea, particularly if bronchopneumonia persists despite appropriate treatment with antibiotics.

PATHOLOGY. Histologically, the infiltrate consists of subacute granulomatous inflammation with accumulation of plasma cells, lymphocytes, epithelioid cells, and giant cells of the Langhans type. With continued exposure, inflammatory lesions may be replaced by fibrosis.

DIAGNOSIS. There may be moderate to marked leukocytosis, particularly with acute attacks, elevated serum immunoglobulins (IgG, IgM, and IgA fractions), and a primary restrictive pattern on pulmonary function tests. Arterial blood gas analysis reveals moderate or marked hypoxemia, usually without hypercapnia. Skin testing with the suspected antigen may cause a vigorous delayed hypersensitivity response and is especially useful if an Arthus reaction can be demonstrated histologically by skin biopsy of the test site. Demonstration of a serum precipitin to a given antigen, although characteristic of the disease, is frequently encountered in apparently well persons and is not diagnostic. If the disease is strongly suspected on the basis of clinical findings and environmental history, but serum precipitins are not found by a commercial laboratory, repeat analysis by a specialized laboratory should be considered. Empiric treatment with corticosteroids may be reasonable. Lung biopsy reveals a diffuse fibrotic or granulomatous response. If the antigen is available in purified form, an inhalation challenge may be diagnostic.

TREATMENT. Optimal therapy requires the complete elimination of exposure to the suspected or proven antigen, which includes thoroughly cleaning the home after the source of antigen has been eliminated. The administration of adrenal corticosteroids (e.g., prednisone in initial dosage of 1–1.5 mg/kg/24 hr) usually results in prompt remission of symptoms; continued use for 1–6 mo may prevent the subsequent development of pulmonary fibrosis in cases of chronic exposure. Corticosteroid therapy may be slowly tapered following evidence of recovery of lung function or after several weeks without exposure to a known antigen. If hypersensitivity pneumonitis is strongly suspected but the antigen remains unknown, long-term use of corticosteroid therapy, perhaps on an alternate-day regimen, may be indicated. The patient should be cautioned that re-exposure to the antigen is extremely dangerous even long after apparent complete recovery. Even if treatment is optimal and the exposure is eliminated, some fatalities occur, and a substantial percentage of patients do not completely regain their previous pulmonary status.

Cunningham AS, Fink JN, Schlueter DP: Childhood hypersensitivity pneumonitis due to dove antigen. Pediatrics 58:436, 1976.
Eisenberg JD, Montanero A, Lee RG: Hypersensitivity pneumonitis in an infant. Pediatr Pulmonol 12:186, 1992.
Keith HH, Holsclaw DS, Donsky EH: Pigeon breeder's disease in children: A family study. Chest 79:107, 1981.
O'Connell EJ, Zora JA, Gillespie DN, et al: Childhood hypersensitivity pneumonitis (farmer's lung): Four cases in siblings with long-term follow-up. J Pediatrics 114:995, 1989.
Yee WFH, Castile RG, Cooper A, et al: Diagnosing bird fancier's disease in children. Pediatrics 85:848, 1990.

CHAPTER 344

Pulmonary Aspergillosis

Robert C. Stern

Several species of the genus *Aspergillus* (especially *Aspergillus fumigatus*) are potentially pathogenic. A spectrum of pulmonary manifestations may ensue, depending on the type of exposure and condition of the host (see Chapter 230).

All aspergillus pulmonary disease begins with the inhalation of spores. If neither colonization nor allergy to the organism occurs, there is no disease. If colonization does not occur, but the patient becomes allergic to the organism and has ongoing exposure, an allergic alveolitis may develop. If colonization and infection occur (even without allergy), aspergillus pneumonia develops. Depending on immune status (particularly profound neutropenia), it may progress to invasive disease or necrotizing pneumonia. Hematogenous spread to other organs may occur. However, parenchymal invasion in normal children has been rarely reported. Infection of an extant cavity results in an aspergillus mycetoma.

If colonization with or without infection occurs and the patient develops an allergy to the organism, allergic bronchopulmonary aspergillosis (ABPA) may ensue. ABPA without infection or tissue invasion is the most common aspergillus-related disease in children. Most cases occur in patients with chronic pulmonary disease (e.g., asthma, cystic fibrosis). In some, the immunologic response that leads to ABPA appears to be genetically determined.

CLINICAL MANIFESTATIONS. ABPA should be suspected in an immunosuppressed or chronically ill child who presents relatively acute onset of cough, wheezing, and low-grade fever. The cough may be productive, and occasionally, brown plugs are expectorated that on microscopic examination contain hyphae. Aspergillus can be recovered from this material by culture.

Many patients have multiple precipitin lines on diffusion of serum against aspergillus antigen. The immediate skin test reaction is often strongly positive, and a type III hypersensitivity (Arthus) reaction can usually be demonstrated after skin testing. Chest roentgenograms show transient, occasionally extensive infiltrates. Aspergillus can be strongly suspected in a child with precipitating antibody to aspergillus antigen, a positive result on a skin test, and elevated serum IgE levels. A definite *diagnosis* should be made if there also is substantial eosinophilia or the demonstration of aspergillus-specific IgE or IgG in the patient's serum. Some believe that central bronchiectasis is always present in aspergillosis. However, aspergillus organisms are frequently recovered from cultures of respiratory tract secretions of patients with chronic pulmonary disease who do not have symptoms of ABPA. The recovery of these organisms without typical symptoms and serologic evidence of hypersensitivity is not an indication for treatment.

TREATMENT. The best approach to treatment of ABPA is not clear. Aerosolized amphotericin or direct instillation of amphotericin into the trachea has been recommended, but the correct dosage has not been established. Systemic amphotericin B (0.5–1.0 mg/kg/24 hr, intravenously) or 5-fluorocytosine (50–150 mg/kg/24 hr) may be effective. Although aerosolized corticosteroids have been recommended, only systemic corticosteroid (e.g., prednisone, 0.5 mg/kg/24 hr for 2 wk followed by the same dose on alternate days for 3 mo) is effective and remains the treatment of choice. Itraconazole may be useful when given with systemic corticosteroid. A reasonable goal is the reduction of IgE levels to a range consistent with those seen in asthmatics (without ABPA) who live in the same geographic area. In any case, IgE levels should be obtained immediately after corticosteroid treatment. If, on follow-up, the IgE rises to twice this level or higher, serious consideration should be given to reinstitution of the same regimen described earlier. In patients with underlying asthma, aerosolized bronchodilators, β-agonists, and cromolyn may be helpful.

Aspergillomas may respond to specific antifungal chemotherapy. However, surgical resection with local instillation of amphotericin is considered the treatment of choice. The prognosis, whatever the treatment, depends heavily on the underlying chronic illness. Invasive aspergillosis may be so fulminant that antifungal chemotherapy is not efficacious. Treatment generally consists of amphotericin B combined with 5-fluorocytosine. Treatment should be continued for 2–3 wk.

Bardana EJ, Sobti KL, Cianciulli FD, et al: Aspergillus antibody in patients with cystic fibrosis. Am J Dis Child 129:1164, 1975.
Case Records of the Massachusetts General Hospital: Case 45–1993. N Engl J Med 329:1484, 1993.
Denning DW, Van Wye JE, Lewiston NJ, et al: Adjunctive therapy of allergic bronchopulmonary aspergillosis with itraconazole. Chest 100:813, 1991.
Graves TS, Fink JN, Patterson, R, et al: A familial occurrence of allergic bronchopulmonary aspergillosis. Ann Intern Med 91:378, 1979.
Greenberger PA, Petterson R: Diagnosis and management of allergic bronchopulmonary aspergillosis. Ann Allergy 56:444, 1986.
Yamada H, Kohno S, Koga H, et al: Topical treatment of pulmonary aspergilloma by antifungals. Chest 103:1421, 1993.

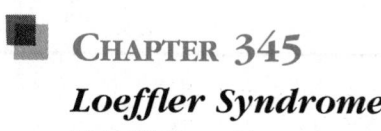

CHAPTER 345
Loeffler Syndrome
(Eosinophilic Pneumonia)

Robert C. Stern

Loeffler syndrome is characterized by widespread transitory pulmonary infiltrations, which roentgenographically vary in size but may resemble those of miliary tuberculosis, and by a blood eosinophilia level that may be as high as 70%. The clinical course is usually not severe and ranges from a few days to several months. There are usually paroxysmal attacks of coughing, dyspnea, pleurisy, and little or no fever. There may be associated hepatomegaly, especially in infants and young children, and biopsy sections of the liver have revealed multiple focal areas of necrosis, granuloma formation, and eosinophilic infiltration. These children have hyperglobulinemia, presumably as the result of hepatic dysfunction and in response to parasitic invasion of tissue. Localized pneumonic consolidation with associated eosinophilia may occur. Autopsy studies have revealed evidence of eosinophilic infiltrations in the lungs and in other organs.

Loeffler syndrome may be an unusual allergic manifestation to a variety of antigens and not a distinct clinical entity. Although certain toxic reactions to drugs (e.g., antibiotics, L-tryptophan, crack cocaine) are included in the Loeffler syndrome, in children, they are usually manifestations of helminthic infections. Perhaps the most common pathogen in this country is the larva of the dog ascarid, *Toxocara canis,* and less often of the cat ascarid, *Toxocara cati* (see Chapter 245.13). Other roundworms may be responsible for the syndrome; these include *Ascaris lumbricoides* (usually responsible for transient pulmonary lesions), *Strongyloides stercoralis,* and hookworms (see Chapter 245). So-called tropical eosinophilia may manifest as Loeffler syndrome and is probably caused by a number of different helminths. Paragonimiasis caused by a lung fluke (see Chapter 245.8) may produce the syndrome and extrapulmonary manifestations. A drug reaction may also result in this syndrome; aspirin, penicillin, sulfonamides, and imipramine are among those implicated.

The hypereosinophilic syndrome, rare in children, is characterized by eosinophilia for more than 6 mo and may be an early manifestation of eosinophilic or acute lymphoblastic leukemia.

One variant of eosinophilic pneumonia is characterized by an acute course of fever and a rapid progression to severe hypoxemia, in addition to the eosinophilia and diffuse pulmonary infiltrates. These young adult patients responded quickly to oral corticosteroids, and none relapsed after the dose was tapered and discontinued.

The differential diagnosis of Loeffler syndrome includes bronchiolitis obliterans, eosinophilic pneumonia with vasculitis (polyarteritis and other collagen diseases); pulmonary eosinophilia with asthma, including allergic bronchopulmonary aspergillosis; tropical pulmonary eosinophilia secondary to infection with filaria; and nonleukemic prolonged pulmonary eosinophilia (i.e., chronic eosinophilic pneumonia). The latter entity is unusual in childhood but has been reported in an infant.

Allen JN, Pacht ER, Gadek JE, et al: Acute eosinophilic pneumonia as a reversible cause of noninfectious respiratory failure. N Engl J Med 321:569, 1989.
O'Sullivan BP, Nimkin K, Gang DL: A fifteen-year-old boy with eosinophilia and pulmonary infiltrates. J Pediatr 123:660, 1993.

CHAPTER 346

Pulmonary Involvement in Collagen Diseases

Robert C. Stern

Rheumatic pneumonia is a rare complication of acute rheumatic fever, rheumatoid arthritis, or other connective tissue diseases, characterized clinically by extensive pulmonary consolidation and rapidly progressive functional deterioration and pathologically by alveolar exudate, inflammatory interstitial infiltrates, and necrotizing arteritis. Physical findings are unexpectedly minimal; often there are no rales. Chest roentgenograms reveal transient areas of infiltrate that resemble pulmonary edema. There is no specific treatment; patients may respond to corticosteroids. If the lesion is diagnosed by lung biopsy, treatment with immunosuppressive agents (e.g., cyclophosphamide [Cytoxan]) may be valuable.

Lovell D, Lindsley C, Langston C: Lymphoid interstitial pneumonia in juvenile rheumatoid arthritis. J Pediatr 105:947, 1984.
Oetgen WJ, Boice JA, Lawless OJ: Mixed connective tissue disease in children and adolescents. Pediatrics 67:333, 1981.
Park S, Nyhan WL: Fatal pulmonary involvement in dermatomyositis. Am J Dis Child 129:723, 1975.
Rajani KB, Aschbacher LV, Kinney TR: Pulmonary hemorrhage and systemic lupus erythematosus. J Pediatr 93:810, 1978.
Serlin SP, Rmisza ME, Gay JH: Rheumatic pneumonia: The need for a new approach. Pediatrics 56:1075, 1975.
Winterbauer RH, De Paso W, Lammert J: Pulmonary disease in rheumatoid arthritis patients. J Respir Dis 10:35, 1989.

CHAPTER 347

Desquamative Interstitial Pneumonitis

Robert C. Stern

The cause of desquamative interstitial pneumonitis is unknown, but it is characterized pathologically by massive proliferation and desquamation of type II alveolar cells and thickening of the alveolar walls. The presence of many macrophages also contributes to filling the alveolar air spaces. The degree of desquamation is far greater than the degree of alveolar wall thickening. Longstanding desquamative interstitial pneumonitis may progress to chronic interstitial fibrosis. Occasionally, there are families with more than one affected child. Most children have a history of preceding upper respiratory infection, although the relationship of the desquamative pneumonitis to these infections of probable viral origin has not been firmly established. Two infants were identified in whom desquamative interstitial pneumonitis and congenital rubella were associated. Circulating immune complexes and alveolar deposition of IgG and complement suggest an immune basis for the disease.

CLINICAL MANIFESTATIONS. Symptoms usually develop slowly. As alveolar function is compromised, tachypnea and dyspnea occur; as the disease progresses, there is a nonproductive cough, anorexia, and weight loss. Cyanosis eventually results; clubbing is not a constant feature, and fever is unusual. Physical findings include tachypnea, nasal flaring, and occasionally fine rales. The use of the accessory muscles of respiration is not as prominent as one would expect in obstructive diseases exhibiting an equal amount of hypoxemia.

LABORATORY MANIFESTATIONS. Chest roentgenograms reveal a diffuse, hazy, ground-glass appearance, particularly at the lung bases, along with poorly defined hilar densities. Viral and bacteriologic cultures and acute and convalescent sera analyses are not helpful diagnostically. Arterial blood samples show hypoxemia; most patients seek medical care before the advent of hypercapnia. Hypoxia at rest is most likely the result of a ventilation-perfusion abnormality, but a diffusion defect eventually occurs, resulting in severe exercise intolerance. Definitive diagnosis requires open lung biopsy.

TREATMENT. Some patients with desquamative interstitial pneumonitis recover without specific treatment. However, the prognosis is guarded when the diagnosis is made before 1 yr of age (8 of 14 died within 4 yr in one report). With worsening pulmonary status or rapid deterioration shown on the chest roentgenogram, an open lung biopsy is important to establish a definitive diagnosis. These patients usually respond to corticosteroid therapy with rapid resolution of symptoms and gradual improvement on roentgenogram. A few corticosteroid-resistant patients are reported, and a variety of other treatments, including immunosuppression, have been proposed; corticosteroid therapy may be less effective in familial cases. Chloroquine phosphate (10 mg/kg/24 hr) has been effective in some corticosteroid-resistant patients, including those with a family history of the disease. Supportive treatment including supplemental oxygen is often necessary. Corticosteroid therapy without a lung biopsy diagnosis is hazardous; chronic viral pneumonitis can present with a similar clinical picture and may be worsened by corticosteroid depression of host defenses. Relapses are reported when therapy is prematurely stopped. A patient treated with lung transplantation developed an unusual alveolar fibrinous exudate, associated with the presence of histiocytes and lymphocytes. These findings suggest an abnormal response to rejection.

Case Records of the Massachusetts General Hospital: Case 49-1993. N Engl J Med 329:1797, 1993.
Farrell PM, Gilbert EF, Zimmerman JJ, et al: Familial lung disease associated with proliferation and desquamation of type II pneumocytes. Am J Dis Child 140:262, 1986.
Stillwell PC, Norris DG, O'Connell EJ, et al.: Desquamative interstitial pneumonitis in children. Chest 77:155, 1980.
Tal A, Maer E, Bar-Ziv J, et al: Fatal desquamative interstitial pneumonitis in three infant siblings. J Pediatr 104:873, 1984.

CHAPTER 348
Hypostatic Pneumonia

Robert C. Stern

Hypostatic pneumonia occurs after prolonged passive pulmonary congestion and may occur postoperatively or in any marasmic state. Lying for a long time in one position favors its development. There is dependent congestion, edema, and pneumonia. The symptoms are not characteristic. There is neither dyspnea nor fever unless these symptoms are secondary to another disorder such as infection or congestive heart failure. The physical signs are principally slight dullness on percussion, feeble respiratory sounds, and the presence of moist rales. Hypostatic congestion is usually a terminal event. There is no specific treatment. Prophylaxis is of the greatest importance; the position of any immobile patient should be changed frequently.

CHAPTER 349
Pulmonary Hemosiderosis

Robert C. Stern

The term "pulmonary hemosiderosis" is used to describe a number of rare conditions characterized by an abnormal accumulation of hemosiderin in the lungs. Hemosiderin deposits follow diffuse alveolar hemorrhage and may occur as a primary disease of the lungs or secondary to cardiac or systemic vascular disease. In children, primary hemosiderosis occurs more frequently than the secondary varieties. There are four types of primary pulmonary hemosiderosis: an idiopathic form, a form associated with cow's milk hypersensitivity (Heiner syndrome), a form occurring in association with myocarditis, and a form associated with progressive glomerulonephritis (Goodpasture syndrome). Three types of secondary pulmonary hemosiderosis are recognized: one occurs with mitral stenosis and chronic left ventricular failure of any cause; one is associated with collagen diseases; and one with hemorrhagic diseases.

IDIOPATHIC PRIMARY PULMONARY HEMOSIDEROSIS. The cause of this illness is unknown. Although the rarely reported familial incidence suggests a possible genetic basis for some cases, other explanations, such as an environmental toxin, are also possible. In one study, insecticides were suspected. Onset usually occurs in childhood, rarely later than early adult life.

Most of the clinical manifestations are related to blood in the alveoli and to the effects of chronic blood loss. Symptoms are those of recurrent or chronic pulmonary disease and include cough, hemoptysis, dyspnea, wheezing, and occasional cyanosis associated with fatigue and pallor. The cough may be productive of bloody sputum, or the infant or child may simply vomit large quantities of blood. During acute attacks, which usually last 2–4 days, the child may be febrile. Digital clubbing is often present.

The usual clinical features of fever, tachycardia, tachypnea, leukocytosis, respiratory distress, and abnormal roentgenographic findings may suggest bacterial pneumonia, and only prolonged follow-up can reveal the correct diagnosis. In some children, the early manifestations of illness are related to chronic iron deficiency anemia, which is often refractory to therapy, and the characteristic pulmonary symptoms do not appear until much later. Paradoxically, the child may have severe pulmonary manifestations without roentgenographic abnormalities, or the roentgenographic picture may be abnormal before pulmonary symptoms have occurred.

The anemia is typically microcytic and hypochromic; serum iron concentrations are low, and there may be elevations in bilirubin, urobilinogen, and reticulocyte count. The stool usually contains occult blood, presumably swallowed. Hemosiderin can usually be demonstrated in macrophages in smears of sputum or material obtained from tracheal or gastric aspirates. Roentgenographic changes range from minimal infiltrates resembling pneumonia to massive pulmonary involvement with secondary atelectasis, emphysema, and hilar lymphadenopathy. The findings may suggest tuberculosis or pulmonary edema, and significant changes may be seen from day to day.

Open lung biopsy may be required to establish the diagnosis by histologic demonstration of intra-alveolar hemorrhage, large numbers of hemosiderin-laden macrophages, alveolar epithelial hyperplasia, interstitial fibrosis, and sclerosis of small vessels. Absence of immunoglobulin or complement deposition on the alveolar basement membrane virtually excludes Goodpasture syndrome, and all biopsy specimens should be subjected to this test. Closed-needle biopsy has been followed by serious complications. Bronchoalveolar lavage may recover cells (e.g., hemosiderin-laden macrophages) compatible with the diagnosis and exclude various infectious diseases mimicking hemosiderosis.

Approximately one half of the patients die within 1–5 yr, usually from acute pulmonary hemorrhage and progressive respiratory failure. A milk-free diet is indicated, pending analysis of serum for precipitins, and also serves as a diagnostic test for cow's milk-related pulmonary hemosiderosis. Corticosteroids (prednisone, 1 mg/kg/24 hr) produce remission in some patients and are of no benefit to others. Maintenance corticosteroid therapy has been used between attacks with variable results. The disease in one patient appeared to respond to combination treatment with azathioprine and corticosteroids.

Acute idiopathic pulmonary hemorrhage has been reported in clusters in Chicago, Cleveland, and other cities. The case definition includes: age less than 1 yr; hemoptysis and/or epistaxis or blood from an endotracheal tube; and no evidence of cardiac or vascular malformation, infection, or trauma. Most affected patients require intensive care and demonstrate anemia, bilateral alveolar infiltrates on chest roentgenograms, and hemosiderin-laden macrophages from bronchoalveolar lavage fluid. No known etiology has been identified. The outcome is usually favorable.

PRIMARY PULMONARY HEMOSIDEROSIS WITH HYPERSENSITIVITY TO COW'S MILK (HEINER SYNDROME). Children affected with this syndrome have the typical picture of idiopathic hemosiderosis, unusually high serum titers of precipitins to multiple constituents of cow's milk, and positive results on intradermal skin tests to various cow's milk proteins. They may also have chronic rhinitis, recurrent otitis media, gastrointestinal symptoms, and growth retardation. The symptoms improve when cow's milk is removed from the diet and return with its reintroduction. Some patients fail to improve at all on a milk-free diet, and others without multiple serum precipitins have improved. Some patients with high titers of milk precipitins and pulmonary hemosiderosis develop cor pulmonale secondary to hypertrophied nasopharyngeal lymphoid tissue. These patients should also have a tonsilloadenoidectomy. In general, patients with hemosiderosis and precipitins to cow's milk have a better prognosis than do those with other forms of the disease, and they may eventually lose their sensitivity to milk. Corticosteroids may be useful, at least during acute bleeding episodes, and cyclophosphamide was effective in a single patient who did not respond to corticosteroids and azathioprine.

PRIMARY PULMONARY HEMOSIDEROSIS WITH MYOCARDITIS. Some patients have various degrees of inflammation of the myocardium associated with pulmonary hemosiderosis, and if significant myocardial disease is present when pulmonary symptoms are first noted, it may be impossible to determine whether the hemosiderosis is a primary or secondary phenomenon. The clinical picture does not differ from that of the idiopathic disease except that the heart may be enlarged and there may be electrocardiographic signs compatible with myocarditis.

PRIMARY PULMONARY HEMOSIDEROSIS WITH GLOMERULONEPHRITIS (GOODPASTURE SYNDROME). This is a disease primarily of young adult males and is rarely observed in children. Initially, the presentation of the disease may be similar to idiopathic pulmonary hemosiderosis with hemoptysis and iron deficiency anemia, but careful study at the time of the initial attack usually reveals proliferative or membranous glomerulonephritis. Biopsies show deposits of IgG along the alveolar basement membranes and the glomerular basement membranes (GBM). Anti-GBM antibody in serum is usually detected by radioimmunoassay. Patients most often have progressive renal disease with hypertension and eventual renal failure and death. The pulmonary disease has improved after bilateral nephrectomy in a few patients but not in others.

SECONDARY PULMONARY HEMOSIDEROSIS. Heart disease producing a chronic increase in pulmonary capillary pressure, such as mitral stenosis, can lead to intrapulmonary hemorrhage and secondary hemosiderosis. Collagen vascular diseases, including periarteritis nodosa and Wegener granulomatosis, may present clinical manifestations of pulmonary hemosiderosis. Occasionally, the vascular changes of polyarteritis are initially limited to the lungs. Other diseases, such as rheumatoid arthritis, may also produce pulmonary hemosiderosis as an effect of generalized diffuse vasculitis. A few patients with anaphylactoid purpura or thrombocytopenic purpura similarly have had hemosiderosis secondary to intrapulmonary hemorrhage with or without hemoptysis.

Beckerman RC, Taussig LM, Pinnas JL: Familial idiopathic hemosiderosis. Am J Dis Child 133:609, 1979.

Boat TF, Polmar SH, Whitman V, et al: Hyperreactivity to cow milk in young children with pulmonary hemosiderosis and cor pulmonale secondary to nasopharyngeal obstruction. J Pediatr 87:23, 1973.

Case Records of the Massachusetts General Hospital: Case 16-1993. N Engl J Med 328:1183, 1993.

CDC: Acute pulmonary hemorrhage among infants—Chicago, April 1992–November 1994. MMWR 44:67, 1995.

Colombo JL, Stolz SM: Treatment of life-threatening primary pulmonary hemosiderosis with cyclophosphamide. Chest 102:959, 1992.

Heiner DC, Sears JW, Kniker WT: Multiple precipitins to cow's milk in chronic respiratory disease. A syndrome including poor growth, gastrointestinal symptoms, evidence of allergy, iron deficiency anemia and pulmonary hemosiderosis. Am J Dis Child 103:634, 1962.

Levy J, Wilmott RW: Pulmonary hemosiderosis. Pediatr Pulmonol 2:384, 1986.

Rossi GA, Balzano E, Battistini E, et al: Long-term prednisone and azathioprine treatment of a patient with idiopathic pulmonary hemosiderosis. Pediatr Pulmonol 13:176, 1992.

CHAPTER 350
Pulmonary Alveolar Proteinosis

Harvey R. Colten and Daphne E. deMello

Pulmonary alveolar proteinosis (PAP) rapidly leads to respiratory failure and is characterized pathologically by the filling of alveolar spaces with a periodic acid–Schiff (PAS)-positive proteinaceous material, rich in lipid. Two clinical childhood forms of PAP are a sporadic type, similar to that described in adults, and a congenital form associated with a genetic deficiency of the lung surfactant apoprotein B (SP-B).

Congenital alveolar proteinosis (CAP) is a fatal respiratory disorder that is immediately apparent in the newborn. Many patients with CAP are homozygous deficient for SP-B, one of the surfactant-associated proteins. Heterozygous SP-B–deficient patients are clinically normal but are identified with molecular diagnostic assays. Although its incidence is not precisely known, CAP may account for almost 1% of all infant deaths within the first 6 mo of life. The frequency of SP-B deficiency among CAP patients is unknown, but the deficiency has been recognized in diverse racial and ethnic groups.

The lungs of infants with congenital SP-B deficiency contain an increased amount and abnormal tissue distribution of the surfactant proteins SP-A and SP-C and lack normal surfactant lipid structures and function. Added to the histopathologic features of alveolar proteinosis are desquamation and hyperplasia of alveolar epithelium, interstitial fibrosis, and impaired alveolarization. SP-A and SP-C accumulate within alveolar spaces, and the amount of SP-C increases within alveolar type II pneumocytes. Ultrastructural findings include decreased lamellar bodies, a lack of tubular myelin, and accumulation of lipid plus SP-A and SP-C between the alveolar epithelium and basement membrane.

SP-B protein is not detected in the lungs of patients with CAP and homozygous SP-B deficiency (Fig. 350–1). Two molecular defects in the SP-B gene have been identified in patients with CAP. The more common defect is a two base pair insertion (121 ins 2) in codon 121 that prevents translation of SP-B protein and generates a restriction fragment length polymorphism (RFLP) that is useful for diagnosis (Fig. 350–2). In a study of affected infants, 6 of 10 carried this mutation. Another SP-B gene defect (deletion of exon 4) has been identified, but its frequency among SP-B deficients is not known.

Typically, the infant with CAP is a full-term newborn who develops rapidly progressive respiratory distress, similar to respiratory distress syndrome of premature infants (see Chapter 87.3). CAP must be differentiated from other pulmonary and cardiac disorders of the newborn, such as persistent fetal circulation, meconium aspiration, infantile respiratory distress syndrome (i.e., hyaline membrane disease), alveolar capillary dysplasia, and congenital heart disease, especially total anomalous

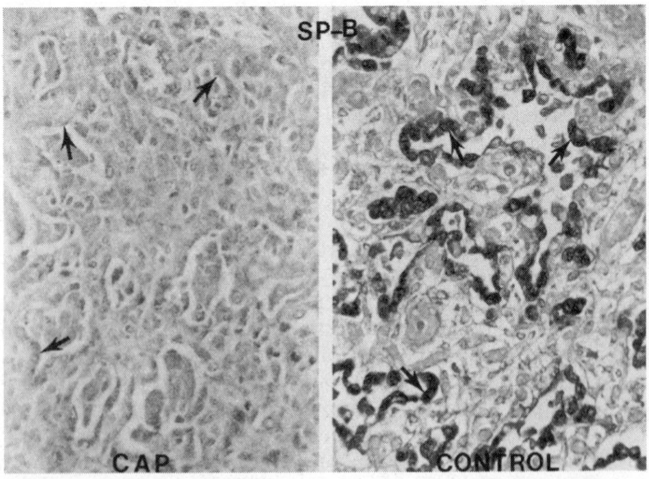

Figure 350–1. Immunostaining of a lung section for surfactant protein B (SP-B). Type II pneumocytes (*arrows*) are negative for SP-B in an infant with congenital alveolar proteinosis (CAP). Intense immunoreactivity for SP-B is present in an age-matched control.

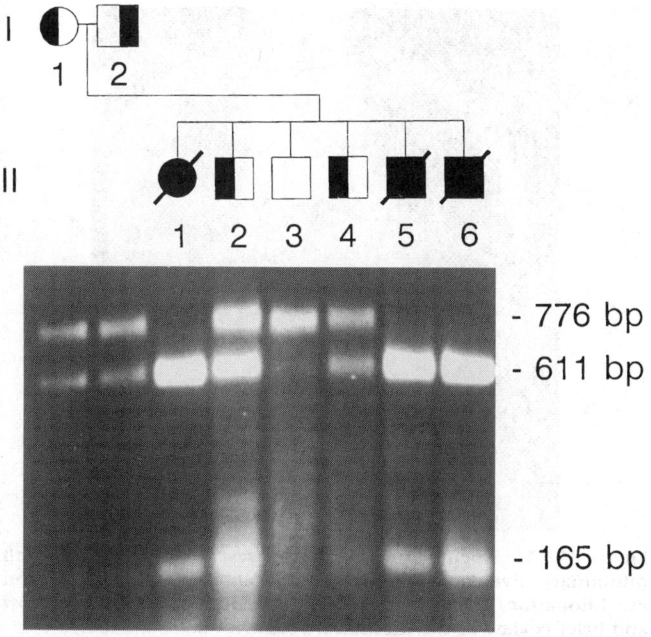

Figure 350–2. **Restriction fragment length polymorphism of a 776–base pair fragment of the SP-B gene in a family with three homozygous deficient patients. From Nogee LM, Garnier G, Dietz HC, et al: A mutation in the surfactant protein B gene as the basis for a fatal neonatal respiratory disease in multiple kindreds. J Clin Invest 93:1860, 1994.**

venous return. Chest roentgenograms characteristically show a fine, diffuse infiltrate radiating from the hilum to the periphery in a "butterfly" distribution. Later, nodular or lobar densities and infiltrates are seen. Positron emission tomography images of SP-B–deficient infants suggest an increase in vascular permeability and protein flux.

DIAGNOSIS. The diagnosis of CAP can be ascertained by lung biopsy. Deficiency of SP-B is established by immunostaining of lung tissue for the surfactant proteins. The common mutation (121 ins 2) in SP-B deficiency can be identified by RFLP analysis of polymerase chain reaction–amplified genomic DNA from the infant's blood, lung tissue, or lavage. The absence of SP-B in lung lavage is also diagnostic. In affected families, an antenatal diagnosis can be established by molecular assays of a chorionic villus biopsy or amniocytes or, late in gestation, by measuring surfactant proteins in amniotic fluid, permitting advance planning of a therapeutic regimen.

TREATMENT. Treatment of CAP with oxygen, supported ventilation or extracorporeal membrane oxygenation (ECMO), is useful but is only a temporizing measure. Replacement therapy with commercially available surfactants containing SP-B is ineffective. The current management of CAP requires ventilatory support, ECMO, or both until a donor lung is available for transplantation. Infants with SP-B deficiency have been successfully treated with lung transplantation. The relative scarcity of available infants' lungs for transplantation, however, suggests that gene therapy is likely to be the treatment of choice in the future. Without transplantation, virtually all patients with CAP die within 6 mo. Without an available lung for transplantation, supportive care is all that can be offered, and the poor prognosis should be explained to the family. Genetic counseling is also important if one of the known mutations of SP-B deficiency has been identified. The risk in future pregnancies of this genetic disorder, which is transmitted as an autosomal recessive trait, must be conveyed, and the availability of antenatal diagnosis and the therapeutic options should be presented.

The *adult form of alveolar proteinosis* is rare in children. It affects males three times as often as females and may be primary (i.e., idiopathic, with no identifiable etiologic factor) or secondary to a variety of inciting agents, including dust, chemicals, and infections in the setting of systemic immunosuppression. The chief differences between the primary and secondary forms of adult PAP are the distribution of the pathologic process, which is diffuse in primary PAP and patchy in secondary PAP, and the amount of alveolar SP-A, which is abundant in primary PAP and scant in secondary PAP. Patients with adult PAP present with dyspnea, fatigue, cough, weight loss, chest pain, or hemoptysis. In the later stages, cyanosis and digital clubbing may be seen. Pulmonary function testing reveals a restrictive pattern, and arterial blood gases show marked hypoxemia with a chronic respiratory alkalosis. The diagnosis is established by lung biopsy, and treatment consists of whole lung bronchoalveolar lavage. Repeated lavage may be necessary, although many patients achieve complete remission after lavage.

DeMello D, Nogee L, Heyman S, et al: Molecular and phenotypic variability in the congenital aveolar proteinosis syndrome associated with inherited surfactant protein B deficiency. J Pediatr 125:43, 1994.
Nogee LM, Garnier G, Dietz HC, et al: A mutation in the surfactant protein B gene as the basis for a fatal neonatal respiratory disease in multiple kindreds. J Clin Invest 93:1860, 1994.
Rosen SH, Castleman B, Liebow AA: Pulmonary alveolar proteinosis. N Engl J Med 258:1123, 1958.
Teja K, Cooper PH, Squires JE, et al: Pulmonary alveolar proteinosis in four siblings. N Engl J Med 305:1390, 1981.

CHAPTER 351

Idiopathic Diffuse Interstitial Fibrosis of the Lung

(Hamman-Rich Syndrome)

Robert C. Stern

Diffuse interstitial pulmonary fibrosis is a rare, chronic, usually fatal disorder of unknown origin, ordinarily observed in adults but occasionally seen in infants and children. Multiple affected individuals in certain families suggest an autosomal dominant genetic basis of inheritance for some of these patients. The disease has been hypothesized to result from an uncontrolled inflammatory process following an otherwise minor insult to the lower respiratory tract. A chronic inflammatory state occurs and leads eventually to progressive fibrosis. Alveolar macrophages, perhaps stimulated by immune complexes, may play a pivotal role by releasing chemotactic factors and stimulants of fibrosis, including fibronectin and alveolar macrophage–derived growth factor.

The clinical pattern is characterized by progressive pulmonary insufficiency resulting from interstitial fibrosis and alveolar-capillary block. The onset is usually insidious, with dyspnea initially occurring only with exercise but later present even at rest. A dry cough is common and may produce blood. The patient is usually afebrile. As the disease progresses, anorexia, weight loss, and fatigability occur, followed by cyanosis, clubbing, cor pulmonale, and right-sided cardiac failure. The lungs are usually clear on auscultation, but occasionally rales are detected. Most children die of respiratory failure after one of the frequent intercurrent pulmonary infections. Serial roentgenograms show progressive, widespread granular or reticular mottling or small nodular densities. Hypoxemia may be present and increases with exercise. There is no increase in airway resistance, and vital capacity, compliance, and diffusion capacity are decreased. Bronchoalveolar lavage fluid contains many inflammatory cells and relatively large numbers of mast cells. ^{67}Ga scans usually have positive results, with the abnormality restricted to the lungs.

The pulmonary pathology is variable. During the early stage of the disease, fibrosis is usually not present, but there is cellular infiltration of the walls of the alveoli, alveolar ducts, and periobronchial tissue by lymphocytes, plasma cells, and occasionally eosinophils. This usually progresses to extensive and diffuse proliferation of fibrous tissue throughout all the lobes of the lung and is associated with organization of intra-alveolar exudate.

Corticosteroids may give some symptomatic relief but do not alter the progression of the disease or improve pulmonary function. Other therapy is also symptomatic. Immunosuppressant drugs have been used with benefit in some adults. A chronic inflammatory state has been demonstrated in the lungs of 50% of first-degree relatives of persons with the autosomal recessive form of the disease. If this finding proves to be predictive of subsequent clinical disease, strategies for preventive treatment might be devised.

Bitterman PB, Rennard SI, Keogh BA, et al: Familial idiopathic pulmonary fibrosis: Evidence of lung inflammation in unaffected family members. N Engl J Med 314:1343, 1986.

Brown CH, Turner-Warwick M: The treatment of cryptogenic fibrosing alveolitis with immunosuppressant drugs. Q J Med 40:289, 1971.

Crystal RG, Bitterman PB, Rennard SI, et al: Interstitial lung disease of unknown cause: Disorders characterized by inflammation of the lower respiratory tract. N Engl J Med 310:154, 1984.

Ivemark BI, Wallgren CG: Diffuse interstitial pulmonary fibrosis (Hamman-Rich syndrome) in an infant. Report of a case with histologic and respiratory studies. Acta Paediatr 51 (Suppl 135):97, 1962.

CHAPTER 352
Pulmonary Alveolar Microlithiasis

Robert C. Stern

This rare disease of unknown etiology often has its onset during childhood, but the clinical manifestations may be delayed until later years. Pulmonary alveolar microlithiasis is characterized by widely disseminated intra-alveolar calculi, which create a characteristic pattern on the roentgenogram (Fig. 352–1). Frequently, the disease is recognized when the roentgenogram is taken for an unrelated illness or when symptoms are still minimal. Definitive diagnosis requires lung biopsy.

The frequent familial incidence (50% of families) and the large percentage (52 [23%] of the 225 reported patients) with Turkish ancestry strongly suggest a genetic basis, at least for some patients. No specific metabolic abnormalities have been identified. Serum calcium and phosphorus are normal. No treatment is available, and patients eventually die during the middle years of adulthood of slowly progressive cardiorespiratory failure, often with superimposed infection. Bronchopulmonary lavage is ineffective. After the patient's diagnosis, other family members should be screened by chest roentgenograms, and parents should be counseled that future children also risk developing the disease. These children require prompt treatment of respiratory infection and should be advised about the dangers of smoking and exposure to industrial fumes. Immunization to measles and pertussis should be completed and yearly influenza vaccine given.

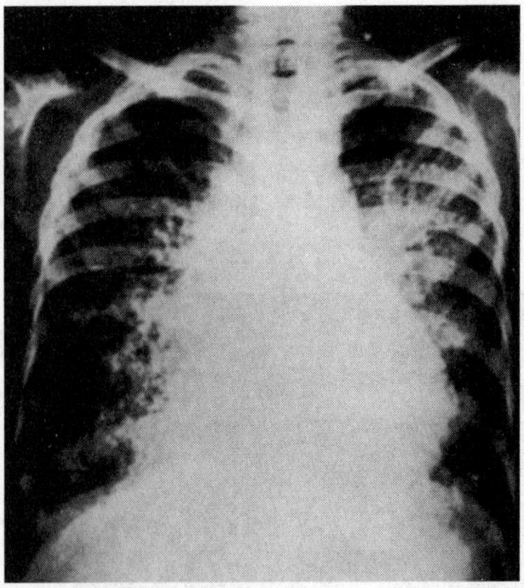

Figure 352–1. Roentgenogram of the chest of a 7-yr-old boy with pulmonary alveolar microlithiasis. (From Clark RB III, Johnson FC: Idiopathic pulmonary alveolar microlithiasis: A case report and brief review of the literature. Pediatrics 28:650, 1961.)

Kino T, Kohara Y, Tsuji S: Pulmonary alveolar microlithiasis: A report in two young sisters. Am Rev Resp Dis 105:105, 1972.

Palombini BC, da Silva Porto N, Wallace CU: Bronchopulmonary lavage in alveolar microlithiasis. Chest 80:242, 1981.

Prakash UBS, Barham SS, Rosenow EC III, et al: Pulmonary alveolar microlithiasis: A review including ultrastructural and pulmonary function studies. Mayo Clin Proc 58:290, 1983.

Ucan ES, Keyf AI, Aydilek R, et al: Pulmonary alveolar microlithiasis: review of Turkish reports. Thorax 48:171, 1993.

CHAPTER 353
Atelectasis

Robert C. Stern

Congenital atelectasis and hyaline membrane disease are discussed in Chapter 87.

ACQUIRED ATELECTASIS

ETIOLOGY. Atelectasis, the imperfect expansion or collapse of air-bearing tissue is not uncommon in infants and children. Collapse results from complete obstruction of the intake of air into the alveolar sacs that usually persists sufficiently long to permit absorption of alveolar air into the blood. In general, the causes may be divided into three groups: external pressure directly on the pulmonary parenchyma or a bronchus or bronchiole; intrabronchial or intrabronchiolar obstruction; and any factor responsible for a continuously decreased amplitude of respiratory excursion or for respiratory paralysis. Bronchoconstriction and increased bronchosecretion due to allergy or other stimuli including embolus and chest wall trauma may also be contributing factors. Exudate formation may be responsible for atelectasis, as in patients with cystic fibrosis.

External Pressure. External factors may operate by direct interference with expansion of lungs (e.g., pleural effusion, pneumothorax, intrathoracic tumors, diaphragmatic hernia) or by external compression of a bronchus completely obstructing ingress of air (e.g., enlarged lymph node, tumors, cardiac enlargement). The right middle lobe is especially likely to become atelectatic because of extrinsic compression from lymph nodes that encircle its bronchus and drain both the middle and upper lobe. Tuberculosis, although it should be considered in any patient with atelectasis, has been replaced by allergic disease or asthma as the most common cause of the right middle lobe atelectasis. In the *right middle lobe syndrome,* intermittent collapse of this lobe occurs in association with exacerbations of asthmatic disease (see Chapter 137).

Intrabronchial or Intrabronchiolar Obstruction. See also Chapter 333. Complete intraluminal obstruction of a bronchus may be produced by a foreign body; by a neoplasm; by granulomatous tissue, as in tuberculosis; or by secretions (including mucous plugs), such as with cystic fibrosis, bronchiectasis, pulmonary abscess, asthma, chronic bronchitis, or acute laryngotracheobronchitis.

Obstruction of one or more bronchioles in a given area may be produced by any of the conditions mentioned, but widespread bronchiolar obstruction is most often produced by bronchiolitis or interstitial pneumonitis and by asthma. Generalized obstructive overinflation is the initial result of such bronchiolar obstructions, but as the pathologic changes progress, some of the bronchioles may become completely obstructed, and there are then interspersed small areas of atelectasis and emphysema. Patchy atelectasis is relatively common in acute bronchiolitis or asthma and is probably always present in advanced chronic diffuse infections, such as the pulmonary infection associated with cystic fibrosis.

Reduced Amplitude of Respiratory Excursion or Respiratory Paralysis. Respiratory compromise may result from interference with the movements of the thoracic cage (e.g., neuromuscular abnormalities as in cerebral palsy, poliomyelitis, spinal muscular atrophy, myasthenia gravis; osseous deformities caused by rickets, scoliosis, kyphosis, scleroderma, overly restrictive casts, and surgical dressings); defective movement of the diaphragm (e.g., paralysis of phrenic nerve, increased abdominal pressure); or restriction of respiratory effort because of postoperative pain.

PATHOLOGY. Atelectatic (airless) areas are firm in consistency and deep red.

CLINICAL MANIFESTATIONS. Symptoms vary with the cause and extent of the atelectasis. A small area is likely to be asymptomatic. When a large area of previously normal lung becomes atelectatic, especially when it does so suddenly, dyspnea accompanied by rapid shallow respirations, tachycardia, and often cyanosis occurs. If the obstruction is removed, the symptoms disappear rapidly. Even atelectasis of an entire lobe may not result in changes in the percussion note because of compensatory expansion of adjacent lung tissue. However, when atelectasis occurs in an area of severe pre-existing disease, the patient may have transient pain but often does not complain of increased dyspnea. No new physical findings may be detected in these patients. However, after partial or complete re-expansion, physical findings of the underlying lung disease, including rales and wheeze, may become evident. Breath sounds are decreased or absent over extensive atelectatic areas.

DIAGNOSIS. The diagnosis can usually be established by roentgenographic examination (Fig. 353–1). Small areas may be indistinguishable from pneumonic consolidations, but those that involve several lobules can usually be identified by the contraction of the area. Bronchoscopic examination reveals a collapsed main bronchus when the obstruction is at the tracheobronchial junction and may also disclose the nature of the obstruction.

PROGNOSIS. If the obstruction disappears spontaneously or is removed, the atelectasis usually disappears unless secondary infection has occurred. The atelectatic area is more susceptible to infection because mucociliary clearance is impaired and cough is ineffective. In persistent cases, bronchiectasis is a frequent complication, and pulmonary abscess is occasionally a complication.

TREATMENT. *Bronchoscopic examination* is immediately indicated if atelectasis is the result of a foreign body or any other bronchial obstruction that may be relieved. It is also indicated when an isolated area of atelectasis persists for several weeks. Usually, it is advisable to suction the orifice of the involved bronchus; occasionally, a **mucous plug** can be removed, with prompt re-expansion. If no anatomic basis for atelectasis is found and no material can be obtained by suctioning, the introduction of a small amount of saline followed by suctioning allows recovery of bronchial secretions for culture and, possibly, for cytologic examination. Frequent *changes in the child's position and deep breathing* may be beneficial. *Oxygen* therapy is indicated when there is dyspnea or substantial hemoglobin desaturation. Morphine and atropine should be avoided if possible.

If the atelectasis is unchanged or only partially helped by bronchoscopy, *postural drainage* and, occasionally, *antibiotics* are indicated. In some situations, such as asthma, *bronchodilator* and *corticosteroid* treatment may accelerate atelectasis clearance. Intermittent positive pressure breathing, incentive inspirometry, and blow bottles have been recommended, but their efficacy remains unproved.

Repeated bronchoscopies may be needed. Postural drainage should be continued at home. *Lobectomy* should not be considered unless chronic infection poses a threat to the remainder of the lung, bronchiectasis is demonstrated radiologically, or systemic symptoms, such as anorexia or fatigue, are persistent. Occasionally, the atelectatic area becomes completely fibrosed; in this case no further treatment is needed.

MASSIVE PULMONARY ATELECTASIS

Massive collapse of one or both lungs is most often a postoperative complication but occasionally results from other causes, such as trauma, asthma, pneumonia, tension pneumothorax, the aspiration of foreign material (either a solid object large enough to obstruct a mainstem bronchus or liquids such as water or blood), following extubation, or paralysis, such as in diphtheria or poliomyelitis. Massive atelectasis is usually produced by a combination of factors: immobilization or decreased use of the diaphragm and the respiratory muscles, obstruction of the bronchial tree, and abolition of the cough reflex.

CLINICAL MANIFESTATIONS. The onset in postoperative cases usually occurs within 24 hr after operation but may not occur for several days, with dyspnea, cyanosis, and tachycardia. The child is extremely anxious and, if old enough, complains of chest pain. Prostration is likely. The temperature may be as high as 39.5–40° C (103–104° F).

The physical signs are characteristic. The chest appears flat on the affected side, where there is also decreased respiratory excursion, dullness to percussion, and feeble or absent breath and voice sounds. Lower lobes are more frequently involved than upper ones. The heart and the mediastinum are displaced toward the affected side. Roentgenograms show the collapsed lung, elevation of the diaphragm, narrowing of the intercostal spaces, and displacement of the mediastinal structures and heart toward the affected side (Fig. 353–2).

PROGNOSIS. Bilateral massive collapse is usually rapidly fatal, although prompt bronchoscopic aspiration and artificial respi-

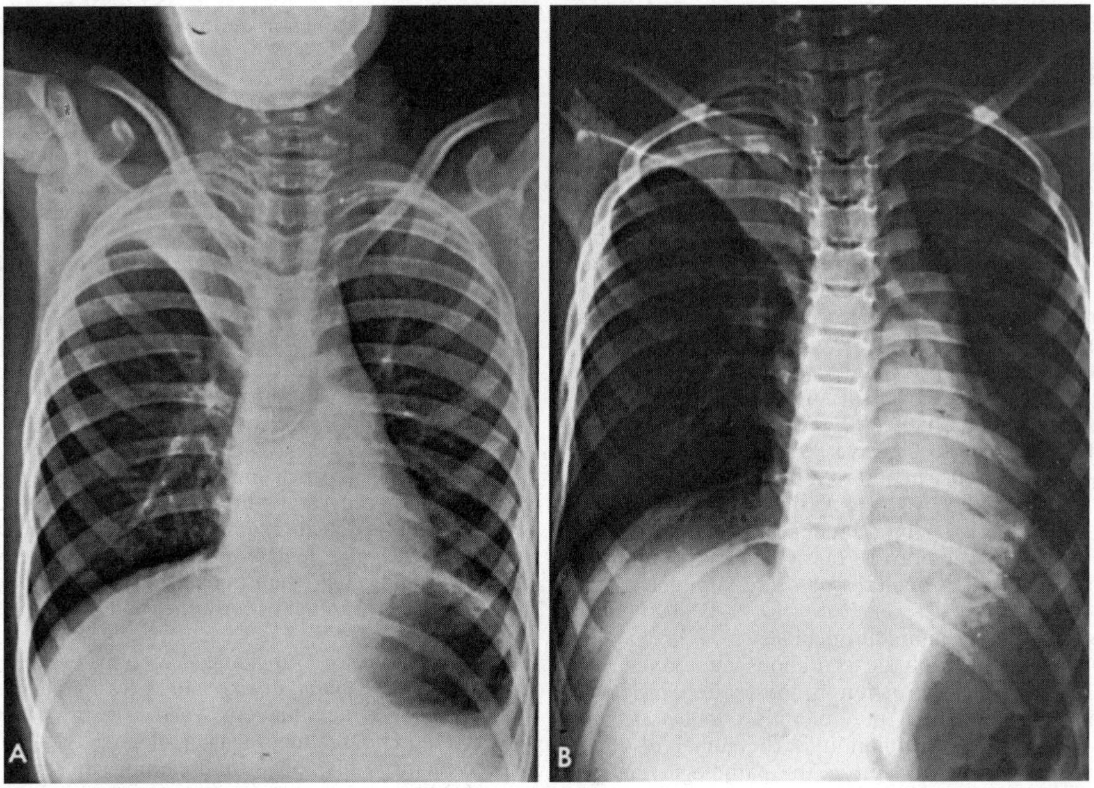

Figure 353–1. Atelectasis that occurred postoperatively and disappeared spontaneously. *A*, The right upper lobe and the left lower lobe are collapsed. *B*, The atelectasis of the left lower lobe is demonstrated on the overpenetrated film.

ration may be lifesaving. In the unilateral cases the prognosis is usually good.

PREVENTION. Prophylaxis is of the greatest importance. The incidence of postoperative atelectasis can be reduced by adequate ventilation during anesthesia. After operation the child's position in bed should be changed frequently, and collections of secretions in the oropharynx should be aspirated; when consciousness returns, the child should be encouraged to breathe deeply. Incentive inspirometers may be useful. Tight thoracic or abdominal binders should be avoided.

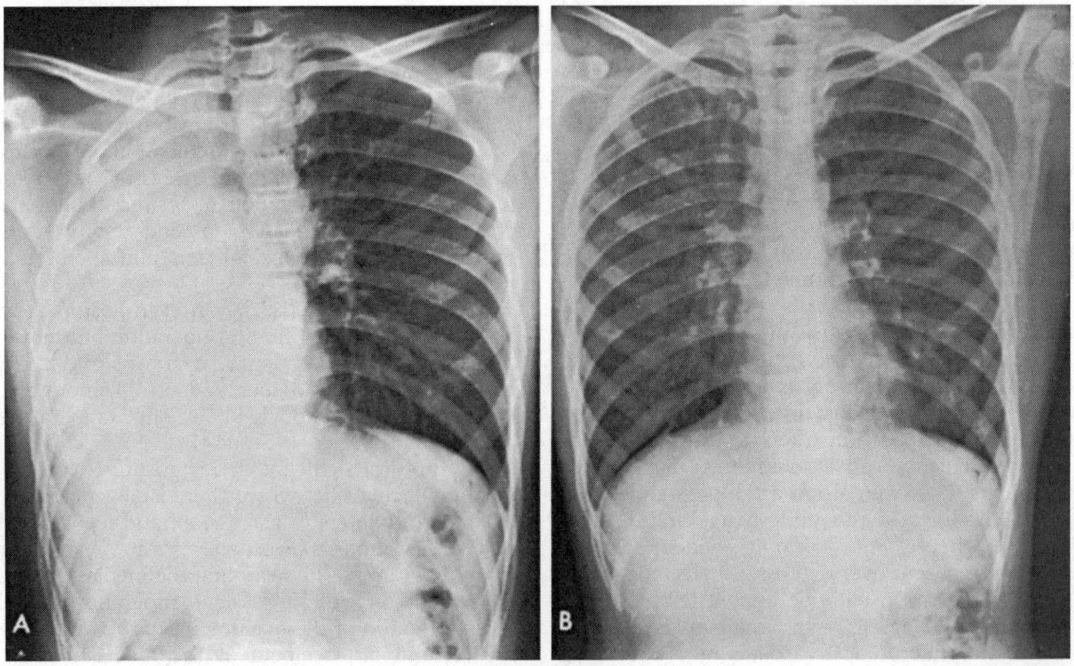

Figure 353–2. *A*, Massive atelectasis of the right lung. The patient is asthmatic. The heart and the other mediastinal structures are shifted to the right during the atelectatic phase. *B*, Comparison study after reaeration following bronchoscopic removal of a mucous plug from the right mainstem bronchus.

TREATMENT. When there is bilateral atelectasis, bronchoscopic aspiration should be performed immediately. When there is only unilateral atelectasis, the child should be placed on the unaffected side; forced coughing or crying while the child is lying on the unaffected side may also be helpful, as is positive pressure ventilation, but when these measures are unsuccessful, bronchoscopic aspiration should be performed.

Relapses are not infrequent, and the child should be kept under constant observation.

Stiller K, Geake T, Taylor J, et al: Acute lobar atelectasis: A comparison of two chest physiotherapy regimens. Chest 98:1336, 1990.

CHAPTER 354

Emphysema and Overinflation

David M. Orenstein

Pulmonary emphysema is distention of airspaces with irreversible disruption of the alveolar septa. It may be generalized or localized, involving part or all of a lung. Overinflation is reversible distention without alveolar rupture.

Compensatory overinflation may be acute or chronic and occurs in normally functioning pulmonary tissue when for any reason a sizable portion of the lung is removed or becomes partially or completely airless, which may occur with pneumonia, atelectasis, empyema, and pneumothorax.

Obstructive overinflation results from partial obstruction of a bronchus or bronchiole, when air leaving the alveoli becomes more difficult than air entry; there is a gradual accumulation of air distal to the obstruction, the so-called bypass, ball valve, or check valve type of obstruction (see Chapter 333).

LOCALIZED OBSTRUCTIVE OVERINFLATION. When a bypass type of obstruction partially occludes the mainstem bronchus, the entire lung becomes overinflated; individual lobes are affected when the obstruction is in a lobar bronchus, and segments or subsegments are affected when their individual bronchi are blocked. Localized obstructions that may be responsible for overinflation include foreign bodies and the inflammatory reaction to them, abnormally thick mucus (e.g., asthma, cystic fibrosis), intrabronchial tuberculosis or tuberculosis of the tracheobronchial lymph nodes, and intrabronchial or mediastinal tumors. When most or all of a lobe is involved, the percussion note is hyper-resonant over the area, and the breath sounds are decreased in intensity. The distended lung may extend across the mediastinum into the opposite hemithorax. Under fluoroscopic scrutiny during expiration, the overinflated area does not decrease in size, and the heart and the mediastinum shift to the opposite side, because the unobstructed lung empties normally.

Unilateral hyperlucent lung may be associated with a variety of cardiac and pulmonary diseases of children, but in some patients, it occurs without easily demonstrable underlying active disease. More than one half the cases follow one or more episodes of pneumonia; a rising titer to adenovirus has been documented in several patients. This condition may follow obliterative bronchiolitis and may include obliterative vasculitis as well, accounting for the greatly diminished perfusion and vascular marking on the affected side.

Patients may present with signs and symptoms of pneumonia, but some are discovered only when a chest roentgenogram is taken for an unrelated reason. A few patients have hemoptysis. Physical findings may include hyper-resonance and decreased breath sounds over the involved area. The chest roentgenogram reveals unilateral hyperlucency and an apparently small lung with the mediastinum shifted toward the more abnormal lung. This condition has been labeled Swyer-James or Macleod syndrome. Some patients show a mediastinal shift away from the lesion with expiration. Bronchiectasis may be demonstrated on a computed tomography scan or by bronchography. In some patients, previous chest roentgenograms have been normal or have shown only an acute pneumonia, suggesting that hyperlucent lung is an acquired lesion. No specific treatment is known; it may become less symptomatic with time.

Congenital lobar emphysema may cause severe respiratory distress in early infancy and may be caused by localized obstruction. Familial occurrence has been reported. Symptoms usually become apparent in the neonatal period but may be delayed for as long as 5–6 mo in 5% of the patients. Some patients remain undiagnosed until school age or beyond. A part, but more often all, of a lobe may be involved; the left upper lobe is most often affected. In many cases, obstruction is not demonstrable, but it is assumed to be produced by a check valve type of mechanism.

Such obstructions have been attributed to defective or overly compliant cartilage in the bronchi, mucosal folds that create a valvelike obstruction, bronchial stenosis, and external compression by aberrant vessels or tumors. A radiolucent lobe and a mediastinal shift are often revealed by roentgenographic examination. If the distention is considerable, the emphysematous lung compresses the unaffected lung below or above it and the opposite lung by extending across the mediastinum (Fig. 354–1). Immediate surgery and excision of the lobe may be lifesaving when cyanosis and severe respiratory distress are present, but some patients respond to medical treatment. Some patients with apparent congenital lobar emphysema have reversible overinflation, without the classic alveolar septal rupture implied in the term "emphysema."

Overinflation of all three lobes of the right lung has been produced by anomalous location of the left pulmonary artery, which impinges on the right mainstem bronchus. Hyperinflation also occurs in patients with the absent pulmonary valve type of tetralogy of Fallot and secondary aneurysmal dilation of the pulmonary artery, which partially compresses the mainstem bronchi. A number of neonates have developed lobar overinflation while being treated for hyaline membrane disease with assisted ventilation, suggesting an acquired cause. Medical management, sometimes with selective intubation of

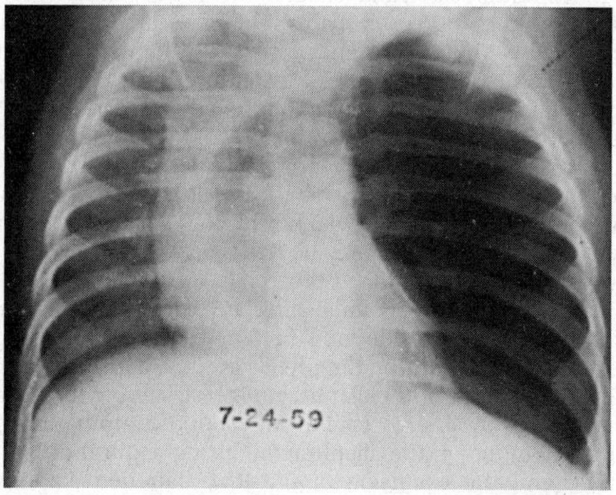

Figure 354–1. Congenital left upper lobe emphysema. Notice the extension of the emphysematous lobe into the left lower lobe and its displacement of the mediastinum toward the right.

the unaffected bronchus or high-frequency ventilation has occasionally been successful and lobectomy has been avoided.

Becroft DM: Bronchiolitis obliterans, bronchiectasis, and other sequelae of adenovirus type 21 infection in young children. J Clin Pathol 24:72, 1971.
Cumming GR, Macpherson RI, Chernick V: Unilateral hyperlucent lung syndrome in children. J Pediatr 78:250, 1971.
Dichnan GL, Short BL, Krauss DR: Selective bronchial intubation in the management of unilateral pulmonary interstitial emphysema. Am J Dis Child 131:365, 1977.
Eigen H, Lemen RJ, Waring WW: Congenital lobar emphysema: long-term evaluation of surgically and conservatively treated children. Am Rev Respir Dis 116:823, 1976.
McBride JT, Wohl MEB, Strieder D, et al: Lung growth and airway function after lobectomy in infancy for congenital lobar emphysema. J Clin Invest 66:962, 1980.
McKenzie SA, Allison DJ, Singh MP, et al: Unilateral hyperlucent lung: The case for investigation. Thorax 35:745, 1980.
Shannon DC, Todres ID, Moylan FMB: Infantile lobar hyperinflation: Expectant treatment. Pediatrics 59:1012, 1977.
Wall MA, Eisenberg JD, Campbell JR: Congenital lobar emphysema in a mother and daughter. Pediatrics 70:131, 1982.

354.1 Generalized Obstructive Overinflation

Acute overinflation of the lung depends on widespread involvement of the bronchioles and is reversible. It occurs more commonly in infants than in children and may be secondary to a number of clinical conditions, including asthma, cystic fibrosis, acute bronchiolitis, interstitial pneumonitis, atypical forms of acute laryngotracheobronchitis, aspiration of zinc stearate powder, chronic passive congestion secondary to a congenital cardiac lesion, and miliary tuberculosis.

Pathology. In chronic overinflation, many of the alveoli are ruptured and communicate with one another, producing distended saccules. Air may also enter the interstitial tissue (i.e., interstitial emphysema), resulting in pneumomediastinum and pneumothorax (see Chapters 366 and 367).

Clinical Manifestations. Generalized obstructive overinflation is characterized by dyspnea, with difficulty in exhaling. The lungs become increasingly overdistended, and the chest remains expanded during expiration. An increased respiratory rate and decreased respiratory excursions result from the overdistention of the alveoli and their inability to be emptied normally through the narrowed bronchioles. Air hunger is responsible for forced respiratory movements. Overaction of the accessory muscles of respiration results in retractions at the suprasternal notch, the supraclavicular spaces, the lower margin of the thorax, and the intercostal spaces. There is scarcely any reduction in size of the overdistended chest during expiration, unlike the flattened chest during inspiration and expiration in cases of laryngeal obstruction. Hoarseness and stridor do not occur with laryngeal obstruction. Cyanosis is common in the severe cases. The percussion note is hyper-resonant, and on auscultation, the inspiratory phase is usually less prominent than the expiratory phase, which is prolonged and roughened. Fine or medium crackles may be heard.

Roentgenographic and fluoroscopic examinations of the chest are a great help in establishing the diagnosis. Both leaves of the diaphragm are low and flattened, the ribs are farther apart than usual, and the lung fields are less dense (Fig. 354–2). The movement of the diaphragm is restricted, which is best demonstrated by fluoroscopic or ultrasound examination. The normal doming of the diaphragm during expiration is decreased, and the excursion of the low, flattened diaphragm in the severe cases is barely discernible. The anteroposterior diameter of the chest is increased, and the sternum may be bowed outward.

354.2 Bullous Emphysema

Bullous emphysematous blebs or cysts (i.e., *pneumatoceles*) result from overdistention and rupture of alveoli during birth or shortly thereafter, or they may be sequelae of pneumonia and other infections. They have been observed in tuberculous lesions while the patient was being treated with specific antibacterial therapy. These emphysematous areas presumably result from rupture of distended alveoli, forming a single or multiloculated cavity. The cysts may become large and may contain some fluid; an air-fluid level may be demonstrated on the roentgenogram. They must be differentiated from pulmonary abscesses. In most cases, the cysts disappear spontaneously within a few months, although they may persist for a year or more. Aspiration or surgery is not indicated except in cases of severe respiratory and cardiac embarrassment.

354.3 Subcutaneous Emphysema

Whenever free air finds its way into the subcutaneous tissue, most commonly as a result of pneumomediastinum or pneumothorax, subcutaneous emphysema occurs. It may be a complication of fracture of the orbit permitting free air to escape from the nasal sinuses. In the neck and thorax, subcutaneous emphysema may follow tracheotomy, deep ulcerations in the pharyngeal region, esophageal wounds, or any perforating lesion of the larynx or trachea. It is occasionally a complication of thoracentesis, asthma, or abdominal surgery. Air rarely may be formed in the subcutaneous tissues by gas-producing bacteria.

If the cause is an air leak from the respiratory system, the problem is usually self-limited and requires no specific treatment. Resolution occurs by resorption of subcutaneous air after elimination of its source. Rarely, dangerous compression of the trachea by air in the surrounding soft tissue requires surgical intervention.

Kress MB, Finklestein AH: Giant bullous emphysema occurring in tuberculosis in childhood. Pediatrics 30:269, 1962.
Nelson WE, Smith LW: Generalized obstructive emphysema in infants. J Pediatr 26:36, 1945.
Victoria MS, Steiner P, Rao M: Persistent pneumatoceles in children. Chest 79:359, 1981.

354.4 α_1-Antitrypsin Deficiency and Emphysema

Homozygous deficiency of α_1-antitrypsin is an important cause of the early onset of severe panacinar emphysema in adults in the 3rd and 4th decades of life and an important cause of liver disease in children, but it rarely causes pulmonary disease in children. α_1-Antitrypsin and other serum antiproteases are thought to be important in the inactivation of proteolytic enzymes released from dead bacteria or leukocytes in the lung. Deficiency leads to accumulation of these enzymes, proteolytic destruction of pulmonary tissue, and development of emphysema. The concentration of proteases (e.g., elastase) in the patients' leukocytes may also be an important factor in determining the severity of clinical pulmonary disease with a given level of α_1-antitrypsin.

The type and concentration of α_1-antitrypsin are inherited

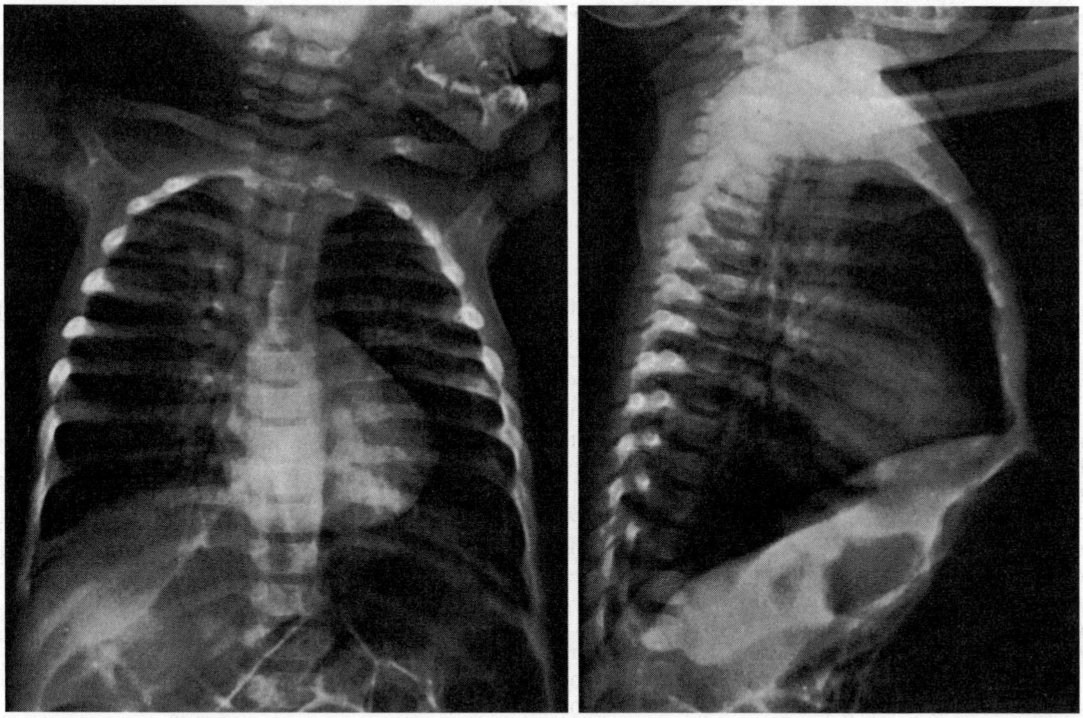

Figure 354–2. Generalized obstructive emphysema (overinflation): dorsal projections of the thorax in inspiratory and expiratory phases of respiration. Notice the relative failure of the lungs to empty in the expiratory phase. The left lung is less obstructed than the right lung (empties to a greater degree in the expiratory phase). This difference between the lungs is not apparent from a study of the diaphragm, which moves very little during respiration; it is evident, however, in the upper portions of the left lung space.

as a series of codominant alleles; the inferred genotype is referred to as the protease inhibitor type (Pi type). Normal persons are classified as Pi type MM. Types null/null and ZZ and, to a lesser extent, other abnormal Pi types, such as SZ, have been associated with early-adult-onset emphysema. Some Pi types are associated with a characteristic form of infantile cirrhosis (see Chapter 303.6), which is considerably more common than childhood onset pulmonary disease.

Most patients who have the Pi-type ZZ defect have little or no detectable pulmonary disease during childhood. A few have very early onset of chronic pulmonary symptoms, including dyspnea, wheezing, and cough, and panacinar emphysema has been documented by lung biopsy. Smoking greatly increases the risk of developing emphysema in most Pi types.

Physical examination may reveal growth failure, an increased anteroposterior diameter of the chest with a hyperresonant percussion note, crackles if there is active infection, and clubbing. Severe emphysema may depress the diaphragm, liver, and spleen, making them more easily palpable. Chest roentgenograms reveal overinflation with depressed diaphragms. Serum has a low trypsin inhibitory capacity, and immunoassay confirms the low level of α_1-antitrypsin.

Danazol, an analog of testosterone, increases hepatic α_1-antitrypsin synthesis, but masculinizing effects make this drug unacceptable for women, and the overall toxicity prevents long-term administration in men. Enzyme replacement appears to be a more promising approach to treatment. α_1-Antitrypsin can be readily purified from pooled human blood, and because it is relatively heat resistant, inactivation of hepatitis and other viruses is easily accomplished. Intravenous administration raises the blood antiprotease level into an acceptable range and results in the appearance of the transfused antiprotease in pulmonary lavage fluid. Severe toxicity has not been reported. The Food and Drug Administration has approved the use of purified blood-derived human enzyme for ZZ and null/null patients. Pure α_1-antitrypsin, produced by recombinant DNA technology, is also available. The aerosolized form appears to be effective, but it is extremely expensive ($20,000–$30,000/yr), and controversy continues over its clinical use. The possibility of more direct therapy with gene insertion has also been suggested.

Nonspecific therapy includes aggressive treatment of pulmonary infection, routine use of pneumococcal and influenza vaccines, bronchodilators, and advice about the risks of smoking.

Treatment is also indicated for other members of the family found to have Pi ZZ phenotypes or null/null even if they are asymptomatic. Persons with the MZ Pi type do not have an increased risk for developing pulmonary disease. The clinical significance of the SZ Pi type is unknown, but nonspecific treatment seems reasonable. All persons with low levels of serum antiprotease should be warned that the eventual development of emphysema is partially related to environmental factors, including exposure to industrial fumes and particularly by cigarette smoking.

Ad hoc Committee on Alpha 1-Antitrypsin Replacement Therapy of the Standards Committee, Canadian Thoracic Society: Current status of alpha-1-antitrypsin replacement therapy: recommendations for the management of patients with severe hereditary deficiency. Can Med Assoc J 146:841, 1992

Bruce RM, Cohen BH, Diamond EL, et al: Collaborative study to assess risk of lung disease in Pi MZ phenotype subjects. Am Rev Respir Dis 130:366, 1984.

Cox DW, Levison H: Emphysema of early onset associated with a complete deficiency of alpha-1-antitrypsin (null homozygotes). Am Rev Respir Dis 137:371, 1988.

Gadek JE, Crystal RG: Experience with replacement therapy in the destructive lung disease associated with severe alpha-1-antitrypsin deficiency. Am Rev Respir Dis 127(Pt 2):545, 1983.

Hubbard RC, Crystal RG: Strategies for aerosol therapy of alpha 1-antitrypsin deficiency by the aerosol route. Lung 168(Suppl):565, 1990.

Setoguchi Y, Jaffe HA, Chu CS, Crystal RG: Intraperitoneal in vivo gene therapy to deliver alpha 1-antitrypsin to the systemic circulation. Am J Respir Cell Mol Biol 10:369, 1994.

Sveger T: Prospective study of children with α_1-antitrypsin deficiency: Eight-year-old follow-up. J Pediatr 104:91, 1984.

CHAPTER 355
Pulmonary Edema

David Orenstein

ETIOLOGY. Pulmonary edema results from the transudation of fluid from the pulmonary capillaries into the alveolar spaces and the bronchioles. It is usually associated with circulatory or neurocirculatory collapse and is often a terminal event in a variety of diseases. Although pulmonary edema may vary in severity, it is an ominous finding even in its mildest stages. It is a common manifestation of left ventricular failure, with the edema resulting from a rise in pulmonary venous pressure, or it may be caused by hypervolemia from a too-rapid or too-large intravenous infusion. It may also be a manifestation of acute or chronic nephritis or, rarely, of upper airway obstruction or pneumonic and other infections with substantial degrees of toxicity. Poisoning by substances such as barbiturates, morphine, epinephrine, and alcohol may be responsible for the development of pulmonary edema, as may the inhalation of toxic gases, such as illuminating gas, ammonia, and nitrogen dioxide, or the ingestion and consequent aspiration of highly volatile hydrocarbons, such as lighter fluid (see Chapter 666.4).

CLINICAL MANIFESTATIONS. The onset is variable but rapid in most cases. The child often complains of difficulty in breathing or a sense of oppression or pain in the chest. Cough is common and often produces a frothy, pink-tinged sputum. There is tachypnea, and the pulse is rapid and weak. The child is usually pale and may be cyanotic. On physical examination, dullness to percussion and moist, bubbly crackles are heard in the lower portions of the chest. There may be wheezing due to peribronchiolar edema early in the course. Chest roentgenograms show a diffuse perihilar infiltrate (butterfly distribution). Engorged lymphatics in intralobular septa, demonstrated as peripheral and horizontal lines (Kerley B), may be evident. Occasionally, one lung is more affected than the other. If the pulmonary edema is superimposed on another pulmonary process (e.g., pneumococcal pneumonia, left-sided heart failure, cystic fibrosis), the clinical and roentgenographic findings of the primary illness may obscure those of the pulmonary edema.

TREATMENT. Treatment is directed at the primary disease causing the pulmonary edema. Administering oxygen relieves some of the dyspnea and chest pain; when possible, it is best accomplished by intermittent positive pressure. Dyspnea can often be relieved by morphine sulfate (0.1 mg/kg). If pulmonary edema is secondary to excessive parenteral administration of fluids or blood or to cardiac failure, administration of diuretics, such as furosemide (1 mg/kg), digitalis, or bronchodilators; rarely, the application of tourniquets or inflated blood pressure cuffs to the extremities; or the withdrawal of blood may be lifesaving.

355.1 High-Altitude Pulmonary Edema

High-altitude pulmonary edema (HAPE) occurs at altitudes above 2,700 m (8,860 ft). Patients with an absent or hypoplastic right pulmonary artery appear particularly vulnerable. The pathogenesis is not fully understood; studies have shown large amounts of high molecular weight proteins, erythrocytes, and leukocytes in bronchoalveolar lavage fluid from mountain climbers with HAPE, suggesting that there is a "large-pore" leak. Total protein concentrations in lung fluid are the same as serum concentrations, also suggesting increased pulmonary capillary permeability. The extreme neutrophil invasion characteristic of other acute pulmonary injuries is not present. Microhemorrhages may also play a role.

The altitude achieved and the rapidity of ascent affect the incidence of HAPE. Cough, shortness of breath, restlessness, vomiting, headache, and chest pain are the most common symptoms and occur within hours of high-altitude exposure. Not all persons are affected, and even affected persons may not develop symptoms with every exposure. Children have an incidence of HAPE two to three times that of adults. Chest roentgenogram reveals bilateral, patchy pulmonary infiltrates.

Oxygen is indicated. Bed rest, diuretics, antibiotics, and corticosteroids have been used, but their efficacy has not been established. Recovery usually occurs within 48 hr, and further residence at a high altitude usually is tolerated without symptoms, but the disease may recur after returning to a high altitude after even a brief visit to lower levels.

Kurland G: Adaptation to high altitude. *In:* Hilman BC (ed): Pediatric Respiratory Disease: Diagnosis and Treatment. Philadelphia, WB Saunders, 1993, p 406.
Rios B, Driscoll DJ, McNamara DG: High-altitude pulmonary edema with absent right pulmonary artery. Pediatrics 75:314, 1985.
Schoene RB, Hackett PH, Henderson WR, et al: High-altitude pulmonary edema: Characteristics of lung lavage fluid. JAMA 256:63, 1986.
Spring CL, Rackow EC, Fein IA, et al: The spectrum of pulmonary edema; differentiation of cardiogenic, intermediate, and no cardiogenic forms of pulmonary edema. Am Rev Respir Dis 124:716, 1981.

CHAPTER 356
Pulmonary Embolism and Infarction

Robert C. Stern

Pulmonary embolism is uncommon in infants and children. Although it often arises from thrombi in the femoral and pelvic veins (often in the postoperative patient), emboli in children and adolescents can also arise from abdominal and head veins. Scoliosis surgery, in particular, may predispose to deep vein thrombosis and pulmonary embolization. Emboli are not uncommon after spinal cord injury, severe burns, prolonged inactivity, or as a complication of intravenous infusions. Pulmonary embolism may be common in sick neonates. The most frequent underlying cause is a medical device, such as an intravenous line, arteriovenous (AV) fistula, or other implanted device; however, emboli also occur in newborns with congenital heart disease and in infants of diabetic mothers. The original source of the embolus may be an infarcted placenta or a thrombus in the umbilical vein, perhaps dislodged by the insertion of a catheter. Asphyxia and subsequent respiratory distress may also predispose to pulmonary embolization in neonates.

In adolescents, recent abortion, drug abuse, hypercoagulation disorders (deficiency of protein C or S, antithrombin III; presence of lupus anticoagulant), or oral contraceptives may be the predisposing problem. As indwelling central venous catheters for home treatment of malignancies and infection become more common, the incidence of associated embolization, including air and clotted blood, may also rise. Urokinase, a thrombolytic drug frequently used to clear these lines, may rarely play a role in embolization if the clots are not totally lysed before the line is flushed.

Intrapulmonary thrombosis may also occur in sickle cell anemia; the subsequent infarction is often difficult to differentiate from pneumonia. Fat emboli are most likely to be derived from fractured bones; they also arise from necrotic tissue in the bone marrow of patients with sickle cell disease. Multiple pulmonary infarcts resulting from small emboli may be associated with severe dehydration in diarrheal disease, cyanotic heart disease, bacterial endocarditis, ventriculoatrial shunts for the treatment of hydrocephalus, and longstanding nutritional deficiencies.

Pulmonary thomboembolism occasionally is responsible for sudden and unexpected death in pediatric patients with a variety of chronic diseases. In one series, a source of the embolus was a central venous catheter. Other patients with chronic heart disease were found to have an intracardiac thrombus at autopsy.

CLINICAL MANIFESTATIONS. Embolism of the pulmonary artery or its larger branches produces a variable clinical picture. The clinical pattern often suggests pneumonia, and the diagnosis may not be made until autopsy. Dyspnea is common, although often transient; pain and collapse are often absent. If present, pain is usually substernal, but it may be pleural and may radiate to the shoulder. Although there are often no physical signs, if the infarct is sufficiently large, there may be impaired resonance and a pleural friction rub. Breath sounds may be distant or absent, and there may be moist rales. Expectorated material, which may be profuse, often contains blood. Large emboli can cause acute right-sided heart failure by raising pulmonary arterial pressure. However, infarction often does not occur, and the classic triad of pleuritic chest pain, hemoptysis, and infiltrate is usually absent in pulmonary embolism. The case fatality rate is high, but recovery may occur even when the area of infarction is relatively large. Secondary infection may result in abscess formation. Emboli carrying bacteria (e.g., right-sided endocarditis) may also be responsible for multiple pulmonary abscesses.

Chest roentgenograms, although useful in ruling out other treatable causes of the patient's symptoms (e.g., pneumothorax), are often normal and rarely diagnostic. In critically ill patients in whom definitive diagnosis is urgent, pulmonary perfusion studies, ventilation scintiphotography, and pulmonary angiogram should be considered; only angiography gives unequivocal evidence of embolism, but its risk must be weighed against the risk of therapy. In addition to the classic physical findings of thrombophlebitis, impedance plethysmography can provide definitive, noninvasive demonstration of lower extremity deep vein thrombosis and assessment of its extent. Radiolabeled fibrinogen, Doppler ultrasound, and contrast venography are also used. In children who are not gravely ill, empiric low-dose heparin therapy when scans are highly probable for pulmonary embolism may be preferable to angiography.

Exchange transfusion should precede arteriography in patients with sickle cell anemia; otherwise, massive, potentially fatal pulmonary thrombosis may occur.

Chronic showers of emboli from ventriculoatrial shunts may cause gradual obliteration of the pulmonary vascular bed and eventually produce pulmonary hypertension. The clinical findings are those of pulmonary hypertension and may include accentuation of the pulmonic component of the 2nd heart sound and the development of pulmonary or tricuspid insufficiency. In severe cases, exercise intolerance and right-sided heart failure occur, indicating that substantial compromise of lung function has already taken place. Serial electrocardiograms that show increasing right ventricular hypertrophy may give an early clue to continuing chronic embolization. Diagnosis may be confirmed by right-sided heart catheterization and determination of pulmonary arterial blood pressure. If chronic embolization is suspected, the shunt should be removed.

The diagnosis of pulmonary embolism is often missed in children, especially if the source of the emboli is not a lower extremity. Pediatricians often wrongly think that embolism is almost exclusively an adult disease. Furthermore, children often have serious underlying diseases whose symptoms and physical findings dominate the patient's course even after embolization has occurred.

TREATMENT. Massive embolization of the larger branches of the pulmonary artery is a medical emergency. The initial treatment objective is cardiovascular support and prevention of circulatory collapse and pulmonary insufficiency by cardiotonic drugs, oxygen, and mechanical ventilation. Surgical removal of pulmonary emboli is unlikely to be successful and should be considered a desperation measure. Thrombolytic therapy may be beneficial. However, if initial treatment, including heparinization, is unsuccessful and the source of the emboli is the lower extremity, a surgical attempt to prevent their access to the inferior vena cava may be worthwhile.

After stabilization and definitive diagnosis, efforts should be made to prevent further embolization. Intravenous heparin (loading dose: 50–75 units/kg; maintenance dose: 25 units/kg/hr) should be given by continuous infusion; the dose should be adjusted to maintain the clotting time at about twice the control value (or the APTT at 1.5 times the control). After 7–10 days of intravenous heparin, 3–6 mo of oral coumarin therapy usually is indicated, unless the source of the emboli has been definitively eliminated. Low molecular weight heparin may be more effective and safer than standard unfractionated heparin. In some patients, it may be prudent to reinstitute coumarin if the situation that led to the original embolus recurs (e.g., surgery, trauma, obesity). The initiation and maintenance of heparin treatment is difficult and potentially dangerous. If the hospital has a rigid algorithm for heparin treatment in adults, pediatricians and house officers may want to consult it when faced with an older child or teenager with probable deep vein thrombosis and pulmonary embolism.

Arnold J, O'Brodovich H, Whyte R, et al: Pulmonary thromboembolic after neonatal asphyxia. J Pediatr 106:806, 1985.
Bernstein D, Coupey S, Schonberg SK: Pulmonary embolism in adolescence. Am J Dis Child 140:667, 1986.
Byard RW, Cutz E: Sudden and unexpected death in infancy and childhood due to pulmonary thromboembolism. Arch Pathol Lab Med 114:142, 1990.
David M, Andrew M: Venous thromboembolic complications in children. J Pediatr 123:337, 1993.
Leizorovicz A, Simonneau G, Decousus H, et al: Comparison of efficacy and safety of low molecular weight heparins and unfractionated heparin in initial treatment of deep venous thrombosis: A meta-analysis. BMJ 309:299, 1994.
Uden A: Thromboembolic complications following scoliosis surgery in Scandinavia. Acta Orthrop Scand 50:175, 1979.

356.1 Hemoptysis

Hemoptysis, the sudden coughing or expectoration of blood or blood-tinged sputum, is a frightening secondary symptom that may result from many possible primary disorders (Table 356–1). The cause can be determined by historical data, physical examination findings, and specific laboratory tests, including a chest roentgenogram and possibly bronchoscopy, depending on the potential primary causes. Hemoptysis must be differentiated from epistaxis (e.g., blood in nares, dripping in the posterior nasopharynx) and hematemesis (e.g., nausea, emesis, abdominal pain and tenderness). Patients with hemoptysis often present with cough, gurgling sounds in the lung, crackles, and signs of the underlying primary disease.

■ **TABLE 356–1 Differential Diagnosis of Hemoptysis**

Primary Disorder	Differential Diagnoses
Infection	Lung abscess
	Pneumonia*
	Tuberculosis
	Bronchiectasis* (cystic fibrosis,* ciliary dyskinesia)
	Necrotizing pneumonia
	Fungus (especially allergic bronchopulmonary aspergillosis or mucormycosis)
	Parasite
	Herpes simplex
Foreign body	Retained object
Congenital defect	Heart defects
	Eisenmenger syndrome
	Abnormal arteriovenous connections
	Arteriovenous malformation
	Telangiectasia (Osler-Weber-Rendu)
	Pulmonary sequestration
	Bronchogenic cyst
Inflammatory autoimmunity	Henoch-Schönlein purpura
	Goodpasture syndrome
	Wegener granulomatosis
	Systemic lupus erythematosus
	Sarcoidosis
Pulmonary hemosiderosis	Idiopathic
	With milk allergy (Heiner syndrome)
Trauma	Contusion*
	Fractured trachea, bronchus
	Gun shot wound
Iatrogenic problem	Postsurgical
	Post-transbronchial lung biopsy*
	Post-diagnostic lung puncture*
Tumors	Benign tumor (e.g., neurogenic, hamartoma, hemangioma, carcinoid)
	Malignant tumor (e.g., adenoma, bronchogenic carcinoma)
	Metastasis (e.g., Wilms tumor, osteosarcoma, sarcoma)
Pulmonary embolus	
Other	Factitious
	Endometriosis
	Coagulopathy*
	Heart failure
	Post surfactant therapy in neonates
	Kernicterus
	Hyperammonemia
	Intracranial hemorrhage
	Epistaxis*

Common cause of hemoptysis.

Treatment includes maintaining a patent airway, providing oxygen, correcting coagulation disorders, bronchoscopy, and arteriographic embolization of the bleeding vessel.

Jones D, Davies R: Massive hemoptysis. Br Med J 300:889, 1990.
Panitch H, Schidlow D: Pathogenesis and management of hemoptysis in children. Int Pediatr 4:241, 1989.

CHAPTER 357

Bronchiectasis

Robert C. Stern

Bronchiectasis refers to permanent dilatation of the subsegmental airways associated with inflammatory destruction of bronchial and peribronchial tissue, accumulation of exudative material in dependent bronchi, and in some cases, distention of dependent bronchi.

ETIOLOGY. Some patients may have *congenital bronchiectasis,* possibly caused by an arrest in bronchial development leading to cyst formation and the destruction of the bronchial wall when the cysts become infected. Alternatively, there may be defective development of the bronchial cartilaginous supports. Tracheobronchomegaly is a rare congenital condition in which the distal trachea and main bronchi are grossly dilated; a similar condition may be associated with recurrent pneumonia.

Most cases of bronchiectasis are acquired after birth, usually resulting from chronic pulmonary infection, but the mechanisms involved are poorly understood. Obstruction of the bronchial tree followed by infection is one likely cause. Measles, pertussis, and pneumonia are rare causes of bronchiectasis. Cystic fibrosis is the most common underlying disease in children with generalized bronchial involvement. Other predisposing factors include aspiration of a foreign body, often a nonopaque one, enlarged bronchopulmonary nodes owing to tuberculosis, recurrent and chronic lung infections, sarcoidosis, neoplasm, lung abscess, localized cysts, emphysema with compression of the other lung, allergy, and asthma. Patients with immunodeficiency syndromes, especially panhypogammaglobulinemia, may have bronchiectasis, usually after repeated attacks of bacterial pneumonia and bronchitis. Recurrent aspiration pneumonitis in familial dysautonomia can lead to bronchiectasis. Primary ciliary dyskinesis (see Chapter 364) results in chronic pulmonary infection which eventually leads to bronchiectasis. Gastroesophageal reflux with chronic aspiration may be a cause of bronchiectasis. Patients with congenital heart disease may develop bronchiectasis secondary to infection related to compression of an airway by an abnormally positioned or very large blood vessel, including those used in shunting procedures.

Reversible bronchiectasis or pseudobronchiectasis occurs commonly after pertussis. Shortly after or during these illnesses, the bronchi may appear cylindrically dilated on bronchography, but if these studies are repeated months later, the changes have disappeared.

PATHOLOGY. The first destructive change is a loss of ciliated epithelium, which is regenerated as cuboidal and squamous epithelium. Concurrently, the elastic tissue within the bronchial walls disappears and thickening occurs because of interstitial edema, fibrosis, and round cell infiltration. In adjacent parenchymal and peribronchial tissue, multiple abscesses may develop, and there is usually characteristic obstructive endarteritis of the small pulmonary vessels. Generally, bronchiectasis follows a segmental distribution, except in cystic fibrosis. The right middle lobe segments, the basal segments of the lower lobes and the lingular segments of the left upper lobe are most frequently affected. The right lower lobe is commonly involved in aspiration of a foreign body, and the right middle lobe is most frequently affected by hilar lymphadenopathy.

CLINICAL MANIFESTATIONS. In symptomatic cases, cough is invariably present and produces copious mucopurulent sputum during acute respiratory infections. The sputum usually is swallowed by young children. Physical activity or change in position, particularly while reclining, often initiates a bout of coughing.

Recurrent infections of the lower respiratory tract are common; they tend to persist and are difficult to control. Anorexia, irritability, and poor weight gain are also common. Fever is much less common. Later in the course, during acute exacerbations, hemoptysis may occur, varying in severity from blood streaked sputum to exsanguinating hemorrhage. Bronchiectasis characteristically follows an intermittently improving and relapsing course.

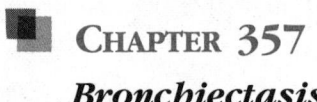

Physical findings are absent or few. Clubbing of the fingers may affect patients with symptoms persisting for more than 1 yr. Moist or musical rales may be heard or elicited by cough; during acute exacerbations physical signs of atelectasis or diffuse pneumonitis are often present. With extensive bronchiectasis, there is persistent dyspnea, and physical development is retarded.

Although there are no pathognomonic findings for bronchiectasis on standard chest radiographs, marked linear streaking ("railroad tracks") with loss of volume ("crowding") is highly suggestive. Bronchography has long been the gold standard for diagnosing bronchiectasis, but it is has been largely replaced by computed tomography (CT). This imaging technique is not quite as sensitive as bronchography but is considerably safer and can be done sequentially to follow the patient's course. A CT scan after inhalation of xenon may prove even more sensitive. Ventilatory and diffusion studies may reveal more widespread or severe pulmonary involvement than suspected otherwise.

Every patient with suspected or proved bronchiectasis should be evaluated for sinusitis, ciliary dyskinesis, immune deficiency diseases, tuberculosis, asthma or other respiratory allergy, and cystic fibrosis. If such a diagnosis cannot be made, these patients should have bronchoscopy to exclude bronchial stenosis, strictures, tumors, and foreign bodies and possibly have bronchography to document the bronchiectasis and determine its extent and severity. A familial deficiency of bronchial cartilage has been proposed as an explanation of some cases of bronchiectasis in childhood and may be suggested by marked dilatation of the 2nd–4th-order bronchi during inspiration and apparent collapse during expiration. Bronchoscopic washings and sputum samples should be cultured for routine pathogens, mycobacteria, and fungi, and a tuberculin skin test should be done.

The *right middle lobe syndrome* consists of subacute or chronic pneumonitis, bronchial obstruction, and atelectasis, and it is generally caused by extrinsic compression of the middle lobe bronchus by hilar nodes, followed by peribronchitis and chronic infection. Bronchiectasis may result. On occasion, this syndrome is related to asthma or congenital anomalies of the bronchi.

Young syndrome is characterized by sinusitis and bronchiectasis, often symptomatic in childhood, and by azoospermia, not detectable until later, when semen analysis can be done. Clubbing is rarely seen. Some patients develop azoospermia after a period of fertility. Urologic procedures to reestablish fertility later have been disappointing. The severity of pulmonary symptoms seems to ameliorate during adolescence or young adult life.

Yellow nail syndrome consists of pleural effusion and lymphedema, associated with discolored nails. Bronchiectasis occurred in 5 of 12 patients in one report.

TREATMENT. Therapy includes elimination of all foci of respiratory infection, effective mucus clearance (e.g., postural drainage), and when indicated, antibiotic therapy. Postural drainage must be carried out intensively as long as secretions are being formed and is one of the most important aspects of management.

Systemic antibiotic therapy should be administered during acute exacerbations in courses of 2–3 wk. Patients with cystic fibrosis may require more prolonged therapy (see Chapter 363). Prolonged treatment for most other patients, increases the risks of acquiring resistant flora and of drug reactions. The appropriate drug is selected on the basis of the antibiotic susceptibility of bacteria isolated from sputum or at bronchoscopy. If no potential pulmonary pathogens are recovered, antibiotics should not be used. Administering antibiotics by aerosol inhalation immediately after appropriate mucus clearance may also be helpful but should not be continued for excessively long periods, because this encourages the establishment of a drug-resistant bacterial flora. *Pseudomonas* can be particularly troublesome. Patients with proven bronchiectasis should be given influenza vaccine every year.

When localized severe disease progresses despite adequate medical management, segmental or lobar resection should be considered, even though the long-term results are often discouraging. Some patients with lobar bronchiectasis, especially those with the right middle lobe syndrome, do very well after lobectomy. Surgery may also be indicated when an intrinsic anatomic obstruction of the bronchus is found or when suppurative lesions result from aspiration of fragmented foreign bodies, especially such vegetal objects as grass fibers or fragments of peanut that elude bronchoscopic removal.

Barker AF, Bardana EJ Jr: Bronchiectasis: Update of an orphan disease. Am Rev Respir Dis 137:969, 1988.
Davis PB, Hubbard VS, McCoy K, et al: Familial bronchiectasis. J Pediatr 102:177, 1983.
Dees SC, Spock A: Right middle lobe syndrome in children. JAMA 197:8, 1966.
Handelsman DJ, Conway AJ, Boylan LM, et al: Young's syndrome: Obstructive azoospermia and chronic sinopulmonary infections. N Engl J Med 310:3, 1984.
Kornreich L, Horev G, Ziv N, Grunebaum M: Bronchiectasis in children: Assessment by CT. Pediatr Radiol 23:120, 1993.
Mitchell RE, Bury RG: Congenital bronchiectasis due to deficiency of bronchial cartilage (Williams-Campbell syndrome): Case report. J Pediatr 87:230, 1975.

CHAPTER 358
Pulmonary Abscess

Robert C. Stern

A lung abscess is a suppurative process resulting in destruction of the pulmonary parenchyma and formation of a cavity containing purulent material. In children they most often result from the *aspiration of infected material* when the local defense mechanisms are overwhelmed by a large number of virulent microorganisms or are compromised by factors such as alcohol, drug abuse, recent surgery (particularly tonsillectomy or adenoidectomy), or systemic disease. Aspirated material containing bacteria that are normal inhabitants of the nasopharynx and oropharynx reaches the most dependent portions of the lung. The posterior segments of the upper lobes and the superior segments of the lower lobes are most frequently involved, and anaerobic bacteria, including bacteroides, *Fusobacterium*, and anaerobic streptococci, are commonly isolated. Occasionally, *pneumonia* caused by aerobic pyogenic microorganisms (*Staphylococcus aureus* and *Klebsiella*) or *bronchial obstruction* due to a tumor or foreign body may be complicated by abscess formation. *Metastatic lung abscess* secondary to bacteremia or to septic emboli from right-sided bacterial endocarditis and septic thrombophlebitis is uncommon in children. Rare causes also include amebic abscess of the lung and infections with *Nocardia*, actinomyces, and mycobacteria.

PATHOLOGY. Lung abscesses occur when pulmonary parenchyma becomes obstructed, infected, and then suppurative and necrotic. Initial inflammatory changes are followed by suppuration and thrombosis of the local blood vessels, which result in necrosis and liquefaction. Granulation tissue forms around the periphery of the abscess and may succeed in walling off the area, but more commonly, the abscess ruptures into a bronchus. Contents of the abscess may then be coughed up or aspirated into other parts of the pulmonary tree, causing additional abscess formation. Sputum is usually fetid. Peripheral abscesses may involve the adjacent pleura, with development of an associated pleural effusion. Abscesses may rupture into the pleural cavity and produce empyema.

CLINICAL MANIFESTATIONS. The onset is generally insidious, with fever, malaise, anorexia, and weight loss. Cough, often associated with hemoptysis and producing copious amounts of foul-smelling or purulent sputum, is characteristic about 10 days after the onset in untreated patients. Lung abscess secondary to staphylococcal and *Klebsiella* pneumonia produces the acute signs and symptoms described for bacterial pneumonia. There may be respiratory distress, spiking fevers, chest pain, and marked leukocytosis. The diagnosis is generally made by roentgenographic examination when a cavity with or without a fluid level surrounded by alveolar infiltration is demonstrated. (Fig. 358–1) Gram stain of the sputum may reveal numerous polymorphonuclear leukocytes and findings consistent with anaerobic microorganisms, such as pleomorphic, slender, gram-negative bacilli (*Bacteroides, Fusobacterium*); gram-negative rods with tapered ends (*Fusobacterium*); large gram-positive bacilli (*Clostridium*); and tiny to small cocci (anaerobic streptococci). Sputum cultures characteristically yield a mixture of anaerobic bacteria. If the abscess is adjacent to the chest wall, particularly if the pathogen is unknown, percutaneous drainage guided by ultrasound or computed tomography can be done as a primary diagnostic procedure. This procedure may also be indicated for patients who are not responding to empiric antibiotic treatment.

TREATMENT. If a predominant aerobic organism is identified, appropriate antibiotic therapy is initiated. However, if lung abscess is secondary to aspiration and the Gram stain is compatible with anaerobic bacteria, treatment with penicillin (100,000 units/kg/24 hr) or clindamycin for an extended period of time (4–6 wk) is the treatment of choice pending the results of anaerobic sputum culture. Alternative treatment in children allergic to penicillin is chloramphenicol or metronidazole. Many consider clindamycin the agent of choice. Appropriate investigation for dental disease should be done in older children and adolescents.

Serial chest roentgenograms show gradual diminution in the size of the abscess cavity over a period of several weeks or months. Most patients are afebrile within 1 wk of institution of appropriate antibiotic therapy. Delayed closure is common. Bronchoscopy is indicated only to identify and remove a foreign body. The routine use of bronchoscopy to facilitate drainage or to obtain culture material is controversial. Chest tube drainage is necessary if empyema occurs. Surgical drainage of a lung abscess is almost never indicated, and resection should be considered only in children with recurrent hemoptysis, a bronchopleural fistula, repeated episodes of infection, or suspicion of malignancy.

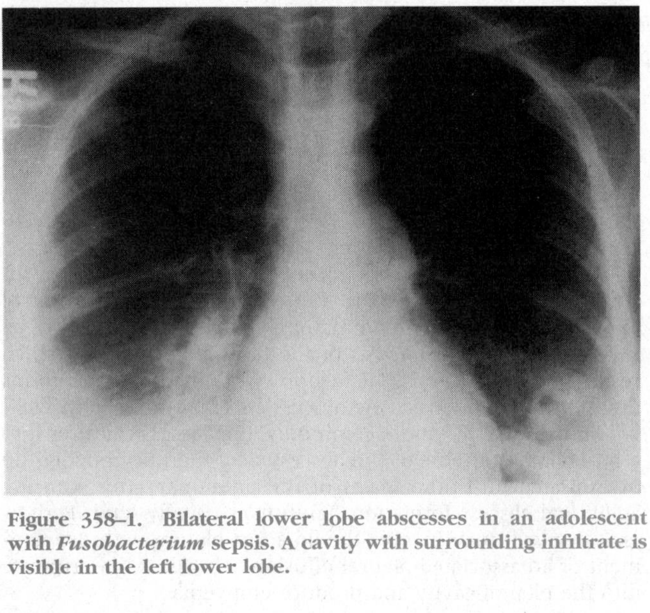

Figure 358–1. Bilateral lower lobe abscesses in an adolescent with *Fusobacterium* sepsis. A cavity with surrounding infiltrate is visible in the left lower lobe.

The overall prognosis for complete recovery from primary lung abscess is excellent. In patients with secondary lung abscess, the prognosis depends heavily on the underlying disease.

Asher MI, Spier S, Beland M, et al: Primary lung abscess in childhood. Am J Dis Child 136:491, 1982.

Brook I, Finegold JM: Bacteriology and therapy of lung abscess in children. J Pediatr 94:10, 1979.

De Boeck K, Van Cauter A, Fivez H, et al: Percutaneous drainage of lung abscess in a malnourished child. Pediatr Infect Dis J 10:163, 1991.

Levine MM, Ashman R, Heald F: Anaerobic (putrid) lung abscess in adolescence. Am J Dis Child 130:77, 1976.

CHAPTER 359

Lung Hernia

Robert C. Stern

Protrusion of the lung beyond its normal thoracic boundaries may be seen in patients with pulmonary diseases such as cystic fibrosis and asthma, which cause frequent cough and generate high intrathoracic pressure, or may result from a congenital weakness of the suprapleural membranes or musculature of the neck. More than one half of congenital lung hernias and almost all acquired hernias are cervical. Congenital cervical hernias usually occur anteriorly through a gap between the scalenus anterior and sternocleidomastoid muscles. Elsewhere, cervical herniation is prevented by the trapezius muscle (posteriorly, at the thoracic inlet) and the three scalene muscles (laterally).

The presenting symptom of a cervical hernia is usually a neck mass noticed while straining or coughing. Some are asymptomatic and detected only when a chest film is taken for another reason. Physical examination is normal except during a Valsalva maneuver, when a soft bulge may be noticed in the neck. In most cases, no treatment is necessary. However, these hernias may cause problems during attempts to place a central venous catheter through the jugular or subclavian veins. Spontaneous resolution can occur.

Paravertebral or parasternal hernias are usually associated with rib anomalies. Intercostal hernias usually occur parasternally, where the external intercostal muscle is absent. Posteriorly, despite the seemingly inadequate internal intercostal muscle, the paraspinal muscles usually prevent herniation. Straining, coughing, or playing a musical instrument may play a role in causing intercostal hernias but, in most cases, there is probably a pre-existing defect in the thoracic wall.

Occasionally surgical treatment for lung hernia is justified for cosmetic reasons. In patients with severe chronic pulmonary disease and chronic cough for whom cough suppression is contraindicated, permanent correction may not be achieved.

Bhalla M, Leitman BS, Forcade C, et al: Lung hernia: Radiographic features. Am J Roentgenol 154:51, 1990.

Bronsther B, Coryllos E, Epstein B, et al: Lung hernias in children. J Pediatr Surg 3:544, 1968.

Jones JG: Cervical hernia of the lung. J Pediatr 76:122, 1970.

CHAPTER 360
Pulmonary Tumors

Robert C. Stern

True carcinoma of the lung is rare in children and adolescents. The youngest patients were 19 yr of age in one series and 20 and 25 yr of age in another series. Heavy and long-duration smoking appears to be the most important risk factor even in these young patients. A variety of primary tumors have been reported, but all are extremely rare. Fewer than 250 cases, including 150 malignancies, have been reported. Bronchial adenoma and carcinoid are the most common primary tumors. Metastatic lesions, such as Wilms tumor, osteogenic sarcoma, and hepatoblastoma are the most common forms of pulmonary malignancy in children (see Part XXII). A high incidence of "inflammatory pseudotumors" clouds the statistics. Patients with symptoms or with roentgenographic or other laboratory findings suggesting pulmonary malignancy should be searched carefully for a tumor at another site before surgical excision is done. Pulmonary tumors may present with fever, hemoptysis, wheezing, cough, pleural effusion, chest pain, dyspnea, or recurrent or persistent pneumonia or atelectasis. Isolated primary lesions and isolated metastatic lesions discovered long after the primary tumor has been removed are best treated by excision. The prognosis varies and depends on the type of tumor involved.

Case records of the Massachusetts General Hospital: Case 50–1989. N Engl J Med 321:1665, 1989.
Case records of the Massachusetts General Hospital: Case 21–1990. N Engl J Med 322:1512, 1990.
Hartman GE, Shochat SJ: Primary pulmonary neoplasms of childhood: A review. Am Thorac Surg 36:108, 1983.
Roviaro GC, Varoli F, Zannini P, et al: Lung cancer in the young. Chest 87:456, 1985.
Wellons HA Jr, Eggleston P, Golden GT, Allen MS: Bronchial adenoma in childhood: Two case reports and review of the literature. Am J Dis Child 130:301, 1976.

360.1 Pulmonary Hemangiomatosis

In this rare and ultimately fatal disease, uncontrolled vascular proliferation causes progressive dyspnea and eventually leads to death from massive hemoptysis or pulmonary hypertension. Its cause is unknown, although infection may play a role. The vascular abnormality involves the smallest (capillary size) vessels in some patients and slightly larger vessels in others. The pathologic angiogenic process may also extend into other intrathoracic tissues (e.g., mediastinum, pericardium, thymus) or the spleen. The patients usually present with hemoptysis or with right-sided heart failure secondary to pulmonary hypertension. Routine chest films are often similar to those seen in interstitial lung disease. The diagnosis is made by pulmonary angiography (which helps to exclude other forms of veno-occlusive disease) and open lung biopsy. The disease can be locally invasive but is not known to metastasize. The primary process appears to be angiogenesis. Most patients die within 1–5 yr from the onset of symptoms.

A substantial and sustained clinical improvement in a 12-yr-old boy treated with recombinant interferon α-2a (initial dose: 1 million units/m^2/24 hr and then raised rapidly to 3 million units/m^2/24 hr) has been reported. Although some hemoptysis was still present, the patient tolerated the treatment well and was still clinically stable 14 mo later. The success of this treatment is additional evidence that the primary lesion is angiogenesis.

Faber CN, Yousem SA, Dauber JH, et al: Pulmonary capillary hemangiomatosis: A report of three cases and a review of the literature. Am Rev Respir Dis 140:808, 1989.
White CW, Sondheimer HM, Crouch EC, et al: Treatment of pulmonary hemangiomatosis with recombinant interferon α-2a. N Engl J Med 320:1197, 1989.

CHAPTER 361
Hiccup

(Singultus)

Robert C. Stern

Hiccup (frequent or rhythmic clonic contraction of the diaphragm) is usually a transient nuisance. Prolonged hiccup, however, can be a diagnostic and therapeutic challenge and can be life threatening. Hiccup can result from a variety of central nervous system diseases (e.g., posterior fossa tumors, brain injury, encephalitis), local irritation along the route of the phrenic nerve or at the diaphragm (e.g., tumor, pleurisy, pneumonia, intrathoracic adenopathy, pericarditis, gastroesophageal reflux, esophagitis), and systemic causes (e.g., alcohol intoxication, uremia). Unusual causes for hiccup include a foreign body or insect in the ear (perhaps by stimulation of the vagus nerve). Hiccups occur frequently in young infants in whom they may be associated with apnea or hyperventilation.

A great many folklore remedies have been used for hiccup. Many of these involve maneuvers that result in aerophagia, breath-holding, pharyngeal stimulation, or that use distraction. For intractable hiccup, a variety of drugs are said to be effective (e.g., haloperidol, metoclopramide, and a variety of anesthetic agents).

Brouillette RT, Thach BT, Abu-Osba YK, et al: Hiccups in infants: Characteristics and effects on ventilation. J Pediatr 96:219, 1980.
Howard RS: Persistent hiccups. BMJ 305:1237, 1992.

CHAPTER 362
Chronic or Recurrent Respiratory Symptoms

Thomas F. Boat and David M. Orenstein

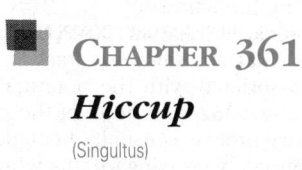

Respiratory tract symptoms such as cough, wheeze, and stridor may occur frequently or persist for long periods in a substantial number of children; others may have persistent and recurring lung infiltrates with or without symptoms. Determining the cause of these chronic findings can be very difficult because symptoms may be caused by a rapid succession of unrelated acute respiratory tract infections or by a single pathophysiologic process, and there is a paucity of easily performed, specific diagnostic tests for many acute and chronic respiratory conditions. Pressure from the affected child's family for a quick remedy because of concern over symptoms related to breathing may complicate diagnostic and therapeutic efforts.

A systematic approach to the diagnosis and treatment of these children consists of assessing whether the symptoms are the manifestation of a minor problem or a life-threatening process; determining the most likely underlying pathogenic mechanism; selecting the simplest effective therapy for the underlying process, which may often be only symptomatic therapy; and carefully evaluating the effect of therapy. Failure of this approach to identify the process responsible or to effect improvement signals the need for more extensive and perhaps invasive diagnostic efforts, including bronchoscopy.

JUDGING THE SERIOUSNESS OF CHRONIC RESPIRATORY COMPLAINTS. Clinical manifestations suggesting that a respiratory tract illness may be life threatening or associated with the potential for chronic disability are listed in Table 362–1. If none of these are detected, the chronic respiratory process is usually benign. Active, well-nourished, and appropriately growing infants who present with intermittent noisy breathing but no other physical or laboratory abnormalities require only symptomatic treatment and parental reassurance. However, benign-appearing but persistent symptoms occasionally may be the harbinger of a serious lower respiratory tract problem, and conversely, a few children (e.g., with infection-related asthma) may have acute recurrent life-threatening episodes but few or no symptoms in the interval. Repeated examinations over an extended period, both when the child appears healthy and when the child is symptomatic, may be helpful in sorting out the severity and chronicity of lung disease.

RECURRENT OR PERSISTENT COUGH. Cough is a reflex response of the lower respiratory tract to stimulation of irritant or cough receptors in the airways' mucosa. The most common cause in children is reactive airways (asthma). Because cough receptors also reside in the pharynx, paranasal sinuses, stomach, and external auditory canal, the source of a persistent cough may need to be sought beyond the lungs. Specific lower respiratory stimuli include excessive secretions, aspirated foreign material, inhaled dust particles or noxious gases, and an inflammatory response to infectious agents or allergic processes. Some of the conditions responsible for chronic cough are listed in Table 362–2.

Characteristics of cough that may aid in distinguishing its origin are presented in Table 362–3. Additional useful information may include a history of atopic conditions (e.g., asthma, eczema, urticaria, allergic rhinitis), a seasonal or environmental variation in frequency or intensity of cough, and a strong family history of atopic conditions, all suggesting an allergic etiology; symptoms of malabsorption or family history indicative of cystic fibrosis; symptoms related to feeding, suggesting aspiration; a choking episode suggesting foreign body aspiration; headache or facial edema associated with sinusitis; and a smoking history in older children and adolescents or the presence of a smoker in the house.

Considerable information pertaining to the cause of chronic cough can be obtained during the physical examination. Posterior pharyngeal drainage combined with a nighttime cough suggests chronic upper airway disease. An overinflated chest suggests chronic airway obstruction, as in asthma or cystic fibrosis. An expiratory wheeze, with or without diminished intensity of breath sounds, strongly suggests asthma or asthmatic bronchitis but may also be consistent with a diagnosis of cystic fibrosis, vascular ring, aspiration of foreign material, or pulmonary hemosiderosis. Careful auscultation during forced expiration may reveal expiratory wheezes that are otherwise undetectable and that are the only indication of underlying reactive airways. Coarse crackles suggest bronchiectasis, including cystic fibrosis, but may also attend an acute or subacute exacerbation of asthma. Clubbing of the digits is seen in most patients with bronchiectasis, but in only a few with other respiratory conditions with chronic cough. Tracheal deviation suggests foreign body aspiration or a mediastinal mass.

■ **TABLE 362–1 Indicators of Serious Chronic Lower Respiratory Tract Disease in Children**

Persistent fever
Ongoing limitation of activity
Failure to grow
Failure to gain weight appropriately
Clubbing of the digits
Persistent tachypnea and labored ventilation
Chronic purulent sputum
Persistent hyperinflation
Substantial and sustained hypoxemia
Refractory roentgenographic infiltrates
Persistent pulmonary function abnormalities
Positive family history

■ **TABLE 362–2 Differential Diagnosis of Recurrent and Persistent Cough in Children**

Recurrent cough
- Increased bronchial reactivity, including allergic asthma
- Drainage from upper airways
- Aspiration syndromes
- Frequently recurring respiratory tract infections
- Idiopathic pulmonary hemosiderosis

Persistent cough
- Postinfection hypersensitivity of cough receptors
- Reactive airways disease (asthma)
- Asthmatic bronchitis
- Chronic sinusitis
- Bronchitis, tracheitis owing to chronic infection, smoking (in older children)
- Bronchiectasis, including cystic fibrosis, primary ciliary dyskinesia, immunodeficiency
- Foreign body aspiration
- Recurrent aspiration owing to pharyngeal incompetence, tracheolaryngoesophageal cleft, tracheoesophageal fistula
- Gastroesophageal reflux, with or without aspiration
- Pertussis syndrome
- Extrinsic compression of the tracheobronchial tract (vascular ring, neoplasm, lymph node, lung cyst)
- Tracheomalacia, bronchomalacia
- Endobronchial or endotracheal tumors
- Endobronchial tuberculosis
- Habit cough
- Hypersensitivity pneumonitis
- Fungal infections
- Inhaled irritants, including tobacco smoke
- Irritation of external auditory canal

■ **TABLE 362–3 Characteristics of a Chronic Cough and Their Etiologic Significance**

Type of Cough	Likely Responsible Condition
Loose (discontinuous), productive	Bronchitis, asthmatic bronchitis, cystic fibrosis, other bronchiectasis
Brassy	Tracheitis, habit cough
With stridor	Laryngeal obstruction, pertussis
Paroxysmal (with or without gagging and vomiting)	Cystic fibrosis, pertussis syndrome, foreign body
Staccato	Chlamydia pneumonitis
Nocturnal	Upper and/or lower respiratory tract allergic reaction, sinusitis
Most severe on awakening in morning	Cystic fibrosis, other bronchiectasis, chronic bronchitis
With vigorous exercise	Exercise-induced asthma, cystic fibrosis, other bronchiectasis
Disappears with sleep	Habit cough, mild hypersecretory states such as in cystic fibrosis and asthma
Tight (wheezy)	Reactive airways

It is essential to allow sufficient examination time to detect a spontaneous cough. If not spontaneous, most children by 4–5 yr of age can cough on request. Asking the child to repeatedly take a maximal breath and forcefully exhale usually induces a cough reflex. Children who cough as often as several times a minute with regularity are likely to have a habit (tic) cough. If the cough is loose, every effort should be made to obtain sputum; most older children can comply. It is sometimes possible to pick up small bits of sputum with a throat swab quickly placed into the lower pharynx while the child coughs with the tongue protruding. Clear mucoid sputum is most often associated with an allergic reaction or asthmatic bronchitis. Cloudy (purulent) sputum suggests a respiratory tract infection but may also reflect increased cellularity (eosinophilia) due to an asthmatic process. Very purulent sputum is characteristic of bronchiectasis. Malodorous expectorations suggest anaerobic infection of the lungs. In cystic fibrosis the sputum, even when purulent, is rarely foul smelling.

Laboratory tests may help to evaluate a chronic cough. Only sputum specimens containing alveolar macrophages should be used for studying lower respiratory tract processes. Sputum eosinophilia suggests asthma, asthmatic bronchitis, or hypersensitivity reactions of lung, but a polymorphonuclear cell response suggests infection; if sputum is unavailable, the presence of eosinophilia in nasal secretions also suggests atopic disease. If most of the cells in sputum are macrophages, postinfectious hypersensitivity of cough receptors should be suspected. Sputum macrophages can be stained for hemosiderin content, diagnostic of pulmonary hemosiderosis, or for lipid content, which in large amounts suggests but is not specific for repeated aspiration. Children whose coughs persist longer than 6 wk should be tested for cystic fibrosis. Sputum culture is helpful but not specific because throat flora may contaminate the sample.

Hematologic assessment may reveal anemia that is the result of pulmonary hemosiderosis or eosinophilia that accompanies asthma and other hypersensitivity reactions of the lung. Infiltrates on chest roentgenogram may suggest cystic fibrosis, bronchiectasis, foreign body, hypersensitivity pneumonitis, or tuberculosis. When asthma equivalent cough is suspected, a trial of bronchodilator therapy may be diagnostic. After the initial evaluation, especially if the cough does not respond to initial therapeutic efforts, more specific diagnostic procedures may be indicated, including an immunologic or allergic evaluation, paranasal sinus imaging, esophagograms, tests for gastroesophageal reflux, special microbiologic studies, evaluation of ciliary morphology and function, and bronchoscopy.

Habit cough ("psychogenic cough tic") needs to be considered in any child with a cough that has lasted for weeks or months, that has been refractory to treatment, that disappears with sleep, and that typically has a harsh, "barking" quality. This cough may be absent if the physician listens outside the examination room, but will reliably appear immediately upon the physician's entering the room and paying attention to the child and the symptom. It typically begins with an upper respiratory infection, but then lingers. The child misses many days of school because the cough disrupts the classroom. This disorder accounts for many unnecessary medical procedures and courses of medication. It is treatable with assurance that lung pathology is absent and that the body has just gotten into the habit of coughing even when it is no longer necessary. This assurance, together with speech therapy techniques that allow the child to reduce musculoskeletal tension in the neck and chest and that increase the child's awareness of the initial sensations that trigger cough, has been very successful, often within minutes. This approach does not depend on deception, unlike a reportedly successful technique that involves wrapping the child's chest with a bedsheet to "strengthen weakened muscles" until the coughing stops. The designation "habit cough" is preferable to "psychogenic cough," because it carries no stigma and since most of these children do not have significant emotional problems. When the cough disappears, it does not re-emerge as another symptom.

RECURRENT OR PERSISTENT WHEEZE. Wheezing is a relatively frequent and particularly troublesome manifestation of obstructive lower respiratory tract disease in children. The site of obstruction may be anywhere from the intrathoracic trachea to the small bronchi or large bronchioles, but the sound is generated by turbulence in larger airways that collapse with forced expiration. Children younger than 2–3 yr of age are especially prone to wheezing, because bronchospasm, mucosal edema, and accumulation of excessive secretions have a relatively greater obstructive effect on their smaller airways. In addition, the very compliant airways in young children collapse more readily with active expiration. Isolated episodes of acute wheezing, such as may occur with bronchiolitis, are not uncommon, but wheezing that recurs or persists for longer than 4 wk suggests other diagnoses (Table 362–4). Most recurrent or persistent wheezing in children is the result of reactive airways disease. Nonspecific environmental factors such as cigarette smoke may be important contributors.

Frequently recurring or persistent wheezing starting at or soon after birth suggests a variety of other diagnoses, including congenital structural abnormalities involving the lower respiratory tract or tracheobronchomalacia. Wheezing that attends cystic fibrosis is most common in the first year of life. Sudden onset of severe wheezing in a previously healthy child should suggest foreign body aspiration.

Repeated examination may be required to verify a history of wheezing in a child with episodic symptoms and should be directed toward assessing air movement, ventilatory adequacy, and evidence of chronic lung disease, such as fixed overinflation of the chest, growth failure, and digital clubbing. Clubbing suggests chronic lung infection and is rarely prominent in uncomplicated asthma. Tracheal deviation from foreign body aspiration should be sought. It is essential to rule out wheezing secondary to congestive heart failure. Allergic rhinitis, urti-

■ TABLE 362–4 Causes of Recurrent or Persistent Wheezing in Children

- Reactive airways disease
  - Atopic asthma
  - Infection associated airway reactivity
  - Exercise-induced asthma
  - Salicylate-induced asthma and nasal polyposis
  - Asthmatic bronchitis
  - Other hypersensitivity reactions:
    - Hypersensitivity pneumonitis
    - Tropical eosinophilia
    - Visceral larva migrans
    - Allergic aspergillosis
- Aspiration
  - Foreign body
  - Food, saliva, gastric contents
  - Laryngotracheoesophageal cleft
  - Tracheoesophageal fistula, H-type
  - Pharyngeal incoordination or neuromuscular weakness
- Cystic fibrosis
- Ciliary dyskinesis
- Cardiac failure
- Bronchiolitis obliterans
- Extrinsic compression of airways
  - Vascular ring
  - Enlarged lymph node
  - Mediastinal tumor
  - Lung cysts
- Tracheobronchomalacia
- Endobronchial masses
- Gastroesophageal reflux
- Pulmonary hemosiderosis
- Sequelae of bronchopulmonary dysplasia
- "Hysterical" airway closure
- Cigarette smoke, other environmental insults

caria, eczema, or evidence of ichthyosis vulgaris suggests asthma or asthmatic bronchitis. The nose should be examined for polyps, which may exist with allergic conditions or cystic fibrosis.

Sputum eosinophilia and elevated serum IgE levels suggest allergic reactions. A response to bronchodilators or related medications is confirmatory of reactive airways. Specific microbiologic studies, special imaging studies of the airways and cardiovascular structures, diagnostic studies for cystic fibrosis, and bronchoscopy should be considered if the response is unsatisfactory.

FREQUENTLY RECURRING OR PERSISTENT STRIDOR. Stridor, a harsh, medium-pitched, inspiratory sound associated with obstruction of the laryngeal area or the extrathoracic trachea, is often accompanied by a croupy cough and hoarse voice. Stridor is most commonly observed in children with croup; foreign bodies and trauma may also cause acute stridor. However, a small number of children develop recurrent stridor or have persistent stridor from the first days or weeks of life (Table 362–5). Most congenital anomalies of large airways that produce stridor become symptomatic soon after birth. Increase of stridor when a child is supine suggests laryngomalacia or tracheomalacia. An accompanying history of hoarseness or aphonia suggests involvement of the vocal cords.

Physical examination for recurrent or persistent stridor is usually unrewarding, although changes of its severity and intensity due to changes of body position should be assessed. Anteroposterior and lateral roentgenograms of the laryngeal and tracheal areas may demonstrate focal narrowing of the air column or extrinsic pressure on the tracheobronchial airways. Occasionally, a specific lesion, such as a laryngocele, can be identified, but in most cases, direct observation is necessary for diagnosis. Undistorted views of the larynx are best obtained with a fiberoptic bronchoscope positioned in the pharynx.

RECURRENT AND PERSISTENT LUNG INFILTRATES. Roentgenographic lung infiltrates due to acute pneumonia usually resolve within 1–3 wk, but a substantial number of children, particularly infants, fail to completely clear infiltrates within a 4-wk period.

■ TABLE 362–5 Causes of Recurrent or Persistent Stridor in Children

Recurrent	Persistent
Allergic (spasmodic) croup	Laryngeal obstruction
Respiratory infections in a child with otherwise asymptomatic anatomic narrowing of the large airways	Laryngomalacia
Laryngomalacia	Papillomas, other tumors
	Cysts and laryngoceles
	Laryngeal webs
	Bilateral abductor paralysis of the cords
	Foreign body
	Tracheobronchial disease
	Tracheomalacia
	Subglottic tracheal webs
	Endotracheal, endobronchial tumors
	Subglottic tracheal stenosis
	Congenital
	Acquired
	Extrinsic masses
	Mediastinal masses
	Vascular ring
	Lobar emphysema
	Bronchogenic cysts
	Thyroid enlargement
	Esophageal foreign body
	Tracheoesophageal fistulas
	Other
	Gastroesophageal reflux
	Macroglossia, Pierre Robin syndrome
	Cri du chat syndrome
	Hysterical stridor

■ TABLE 362–6 Diseases Associated with Recurrent or Persistent Lung Infiltrates Beyond the Neonatal Period

Recurrent or migrating infiltrates	Tracheoesophageal fistula*
Asthma*	Gastroesophageal reflux*
Repeated aspiration*	Foreign body
Hypersensitivity pneumonitis	Lipid aspiration
Pulmonary hemosiderosis*	Immunodeficiency, phagocytic deficiency*
Foreign body	Humoral, cellular, combined immunodeficiency states*
Immunodeficiency, phagocytic deficiency*	Chronic granulomatous disease and related phagocytic defects*
Sickle cell disease	Complement deficiency states*
Cystic fibrosis*	Allergy-hypersensitivity
Persistent infiltrates	Pulmonary hemosiderosis (cow's milk–related, other)*
Congenital infection*	Asthma
Cytomegalovirus	Hypersensitivity pneumonitis (allergic alveolitis)
Rubella	Cystic fibrosis*
Syphilis	Primary ciliary dyskinesia (Kartagener)
Acquired infection	Other bronchiectases
Cytomegalovirus*	Sarcoidosis
Tuberculosis*	Neoplasms (primary, metastatic)
Chlamydia*	Interstitial pneumonitis and fibrosis*
Other viruses*	Usual (Hamman-Rich)
Mycoplasma, ureaplasma*	Desquamative
Pertussis*	Lymphoid (AIDS)
Fungal organisms	Alveolar proteinosis
*Pneumocystis carinii**	Pulmonary lymphangiectasia*
Inadequately treated bacterial infection	α_1-Antitrypsin deficiency
Congenital anomalies	Drug-induced, radiation-induced inflammation and fibrosis
Lung cysts*	Collagen-vascular diseases
Pulmonary sequestration	Eosinophilic pneumonias
Bronchial stenosis	Visceral larva migrans
Vascular ring	Histiocytosis
Congenital heart disease with large left to right shunt	Leukemia
Aspiration	
Pharyngeal incompetence (e.g., cleft palate)*	
Laryngotracheoesophageal cleft*	

**Conditions likely to cause chronic lung infiltrates in infants.*

They may be febrile or afebrile and may present a wide range of respiratory symptoms and signs. Persistent or recurring infiltrates present a diagnostic challenge (Table 362–6).

Symptoms associated with chronic lung infiltrates during the first several weeks of life (but not related to neonatal respiratory distress syndrome) suggest infection acquired in utero or during descent through the birth canal. Early appearance of chronic infiltrates may also be associated with cystic fibrosis or congenital anomalies, which result in aspiration or airway obstruction. A history of recurrent infiltrates, wheezing, and cough may reflect asthma, even in the first year of life.

One uncommon but characteristic syndrome appearing in the first year of life with recurrent lung infiltrates is pulmonary hemosiderosis related to cow's milk hypersensitivity. Children with a history of bronchopulmonary dysplasia frequently have episodes of respiratory distress attended by wheezing and new lung infiltrates. Recurrent pneumonia in a child with frequent otitis media, nasopharyngitis, adenitis, or dermatologic manifestations suggests an immunodeficiency state, complement deficiency, or phagocytic defect. Particular attention must be directed to the possibility that the infiltrates represent lymphocytic interstitial pneumonitis or opportunistic infection associated with human immunodeficiency virus (HIV) infection. A history of paroxysmal coughing in an infant suggests pertussis syndrome or cystic fibrosis. Persistent infiltrates, especially with loss of volume, in a toddler should suggest foreign body aspiration.

Overinflation and infiltrates suggest cystic fibrosis or chronic asthma. A "silent chest" with infiltrates should arouse suspicion of alveolar proteinosis, *Pneumocystis carinii* infection, desquamative interstitial pneumonitis, or tumors. Growth should be carefully assessed to determine whether the lung process has had systemic effects, indicating substantial severity and chronicity as in cystic fibrosis or alveolar proteinosis. Cataracts, retinopathy, or microcephaly suggest in utero infection. Chronic rhinorrhea may be associated with atopic disease, cow's milk intolerance, cystic fibrosis, or congenital syphilis. The absence of tonsils and cervical lymph nodes suggests a combined immunodeficiency state.

Diagnostic studies should be done selectively, based on information obtained from history and physical examination and on a thorough understanding of conditions listed in Table 362–6. Cytologic evaluation of bronchial secretions may be helpful. In patients unresponsive to antibiotics, needle aspiration of the involved area may demonstrate a pathogenic organism. Bronchography, as a rule, is most helpful in identifying surgically approachable focal bronchiectasis and should not be undertaken for routine evaluation of chronic lung infiltrates. Bronchoscopy is indicated for detecting foreign bodies, congenital or acquired anomalies of the tracheobronchial tract, and obstruction by endobronchial or extrinsic masses. Bronchoscopy provides access to secretions that can be studied cytologically and microbiologically. If all appropriate studies have been completed and the condition remains undiagnosed, open lung biopsy may yield a definitive diagnosis.

Optimal medical or surgical treatment of chronic lung infiltrates frequently depends on a specific diagnosis, but chronic conditions may be self-limiting (e.g., severe and prolonged viral infections in infants); in these cases, symptomatic therapy may maintain adequate lung function until spontaneous improvement occurs. Helpful measures include inhalation and physical therapy for excessive secretions, antibiotics for secondary bacterial infections, supplementary oxygen for hypoxemia, and maintenance of adequate nutrition. Because the lung of a young child has remarkable recuperative potential, normal lung function may ultimately be achieved with treatment despite the severity of pulmonary insult occurring during infancy.

Anderson VM, Haesoon L: Lymphocytic interstitial pneumonitis in pediatric AIDS. Pediatr Pathol 8:417, 1988.

Blager F, Gay M, Wood R: Voice therapy techniques adapted to treatment of habit cough: A pilot study. J Communication Disorders 21:393, 1988.

Cloutier MM, Loughlin GM: Chronic cough in children: A manifestation of airway hyperreactivity. Pediatrics 67:6, 1981.

Cohlan S, Stone S: The cough and the bedsheet. Pediatrics 74(1):11, 1984.

Eigen H: The clinical evaluation of chronic cough. Pediatr Clin North Am 29:57, 1982.

Eliasson R, Mossberg B, Camner P, et al: The immotile cilia syndrome. N Engl J Med 297:1, 1977.

Lokshin B, Lindgren S, Weinberger M, et al: Outcome of habit cough in children treated with a brief session of suggestion therapy. Ann Allergy 67:579, 1991.

Morgan WJ, Taussig LM: The child with persistent cough. Pediatr Rev 8:249, 1987.

Orenstein SR, Orenstein DM: Gastroesophageal reflux and respiratory disease in children. J Pediatr 112:847, 1988.

Skoner D, Caliquiri L: The wheezing infant. Pediatr Clin North Am 35:1011, 1988.

Stagno S, Brasfield DM, Brown MB, et al: Infant pneumonitis associated with cytomegalovirus, chlamydia, pneumocystis, and ureaplasma: A prospective study. Pediatrics 68:322, 1981.

CHAPTER 363

Cystic Fibrosis

Thomas F. Boat

Cystic fibrosis (CF) is an inherited multisystem disorder of children and adults, characterized chiefly by chronic obstruction and infection of airways and by maldigestion and its consequences. It is the most common life-threatening recessive genetic trait among whites. A dysfunction of the exocrine glands is the predominant pathogenetic feature and is responsible for a broad, variable, and sometimes confusing array of presenting manifestations and complications.

CF is the major cause of severe chronic lung disease of children and is responsible for most exocrine pancreatic insufficiency during early life. It is also responsible for many cases of nasal polyposis, pansinusitis, rectal prolapse, pancreatitis, cholelithiasis, and insulin-dependent hyperglycemia. CF may present as failure to thrive and occasionally as cirrhosis or other forms of hepatic dysfunction. Therefore, this disorder enters into the differential diagnosis of many pediatric conditions.

GENETICS. CF occurs in approximately 1 of 3,000 white live births and 1 of 17,000 black infants in the United States. The estimated incidence worldwide varies from 1 of 377 live births in parts of Brittany to 1 of 90,000 Asian infants in Hawaii. Generally, the CF gene is most prevalent among Northern and Central Europeans and in individuals who come from these areas.

CF is inherited as an autosomal recessive trait. With the cloning of the CF gene, it is clear that all of the more than 400 gene mutations that contribute to the CF syndrome occur at a single locus on the long arm of chromosome 7. The CF gene codes for a protein of 1480 amino acids, called the CF transmembrane regulator (CFTR). CFTR is expressed largely in epithelial cells of airways, the gastrointestinal tract (including pancreas and biliary system), the sweat glands, and the genitourinary system. CFTR has ion channel and regulatory functions that are perturbed to some extent by the different mutations. The most prevalent mutation of CFTR, occurring in approximately 70% of affected whites, is the deletion of a single phenylalanine residue at amino acid 508 (ΔF508). This mutation is responsible for the high incidence of CF in northern European populations and is considerably less frequent in other populations, such as those in Southern Europe and Israel. Approximately 50% of individuals with CF and Northern European ancestry are homozygous for ΔF508. The remainder of patients have an extensive array of mutation combinations, none of which has a prevalence of more than several per cent, except in circumscribed populations. For example, the W1282X mutation occurs in 60% of the Ashkenazi Jews with CF, and the G542X mutation is more common in Spain. The relationship between genotype and phenotype is discussed in the clinical manifestations section. Using probes for 30 of the most frequent mutations, the genotype of 80–90% of Americans with CF can be ascertained. Other procedures, usually employed only in research laboratories, can be used to increase genotype ascertainment to 95–99%. However, these research methods cannot yet be employed for routine diagnostic studies or screening, and DNA analysis is most useful as a secondary diagnostic tool or for prenatal diagnosis when parental genotypes are known. DNA analysis is also used extensively for carrier detection in CF families and spouses of known carriers. In the latter instance, a small risk remains if the mutation analysis is negative.

The high frequency of the CF gene has been hypothetically ascribed to resistance to the morbidity and mortality associated with cholera through the ages. Cultured CF intestinal epithelial cells homozygous for the ΔF508 mutation are unresponsive to the secretory effects of cholera toxin.

PATHOGENESIS. Four long-standing observations are of fundamental pathophysiologic importance: failure to clear mucous secretions, a paucity of water in mucous secretions, an elevated salt content of sweat and other serous secretions, and chronic infection limited to the respiratory tract. The relationships among these findings were unclear until the early 1980s when it was demonstrated that there is a greater negative potential difference across the respiratory epithelia of CF than of control subjects. Aberrant electrical properties were also demonstrated for CF sweat gland duct epithelium. Subsequent studies demonstrated that the apical membranes of CF epithelial cells are unable to secrete chloride ions in response to cAMP-mediated signals, and that, at least in the respiratory tract, excessive amounts of sodium are absorbed through these membranes (Fig. 363–1). These defects can be traced to dysfunction of an epithelial cell protein, CFTR (Fig. 363–2).

After isolation of the CFTR gene and its characterization, it became clear that cAMP-stimulated chloride conductance was a function of CFTR itself and that this function was absent in epithelial cells with many different mutations of the CFTR gene. CFTR mutations appear to fall into four classes, albeit with some overlap: I, defective CFTR production due to premature transcription termination signals; II, defective CFTR processing and trafficking to the apical membrane (e.g., ΔF508); III, defective regulation of chloride channel function due to mutations in CFTR phosphorylation or ATP-binding sites; and IV, defective chloride conductance due to missense mutations in the membrane-spanning domains of CFTR that line the channel.

The postulated epithelial pathophysiology in airways involves an inability to secrete salt and secondarily secrete water in the face of excessive reabsorption of salt and water. The proposed outcome is insufficient water on the airway surface to hydrate secretions. Desiccated secretions become more viscous and elastic (rubbery) and are harder to clear by mucociliary and other mechanisms. These secretions are retained and obstruct airways, starting with those of the smallest caliber, the bronchioles. Airflow obstruction at the level of small airways is the earliest observable physiologic abnormality of the respiratory system.

Based on evidence for inadequate water secretion by the pancreas, it is likely that similar pathophysiologic events take place in the pancreatic and biliary ducts (and in the vas deferens), leading to desiccation of proteinaceous secretions and

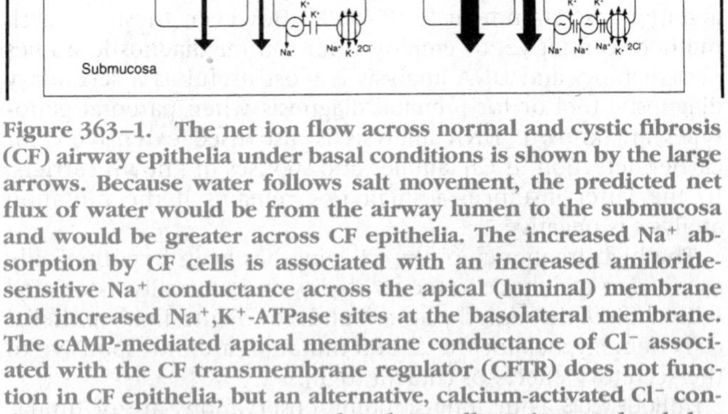

Figure 363–1. The net ion flow across normal and cystic fibrosis (CF) airway epithelia under basal conditions is shown by the large arrows. Because water follows salt movement, the predicted net flux of water would be from the airway lumen to the submucosa and would be greater across CF epithelia. The increased Na^+ absorption by CF cells is associated with an increased amiloride-sensitive Na^+ conductance across the apical (luminal) membrane and increased Na^+,K^+-ATPase sites at the basolateral membrane. The cAMP-mediated apical membrane conductance of Cl^- associated with the CF transmembrane regulator (CFTR) does not function in CF epithelia, but an alternative, calcium-activated Cl^- conductance is present in normal and CF cells. It is postulated that CF cells have a limited ability to secrete Cl^- and absorb Na^+ in excessive amounts, limiting the water available to hydrate secretions and allow them to be cleared from the airways lumen. (From Knowles MR: Contemporary perspectives on the pathogenesis of cystic fibrosis. New Insights into Cystic Fibrosis 1:1, 1993.)

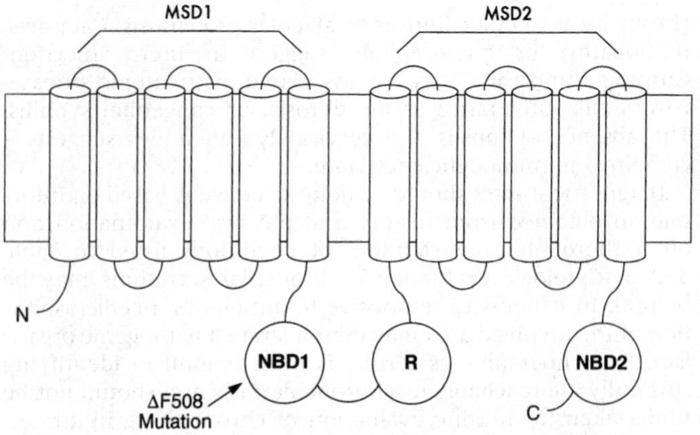

Figure 363–2. The predicted structure of a cystic fibrosis transmembrane regulator (CFTR) shows that the molecule is anchored in the cell membrane by two membrane-spanning domains (MSD1, MSD2). These domains form a channel through which chloride and probably water can pass. Two nucleotide-binding domains (NBD1, NBD2) interact with ATP to provide energy for CFTR functions. The R domain has many sites for phosphorylation by cAMP-dependent kinases. This domain is involved in the regulation of CFTR functions such as chloride conductance. The most common CFTR mutation, ΔF508, is localized to the NBD1 region. This region and the NBD2 site are particularly susceptible to mutation. However, mutations associated with typical manifestations of CF occur in all domains. (From Welsh MJ, Anderson MP, Rich DP, et al: Cystic fibrosis transmembrane conductance regulator. Neuron 8:821, 1992.)

obstruction. Because the function of sweat gland duct cells is to absorb rather than secrete chloride, salt is not retrieved from the isotonic primary sweat as it is transported to the skin surface; chloride and sodium levels consequently are elevated.

Chronic infection in CF is limited to the endobronchial spaces of the airways. The most likely explanation for infection is a sequence of events starting with failure to promptly clear inhaled bacteria and then proceeding to persistent colonization and an inflammatory response in airway walls. These events occur first in small airways, probably because clearance of altered secretions is more difficult from these regions. Chronic bronchiolitis and bronchitis are the initial lung manifestations, but after months to years, structural changes in airway walls produce bronchiolectasis and bronchiectasis.

The agents of airway injury include neutrophil products, such as oxidative radicals and proteases, and immune reaction products. With advanced lung disease, infection may extend to peribronchial lung parenchyma. Several inflammatory products, including proteases, are responsible for the mucus hypersecretion that is characteristic of chronic airways disease.

A finding that is not readily explained is the high prevalence of airways colonization with *Staphylococcus aureus* and *Pseudomonas aeruginosa,* two organisms that rarely infect the lungs of other individuals. There is evidence that the CF airway epithelial cells or surface liquids provide a favorable environment for attachment or induce adherence properties of these organisms. Another puzzle is the propensity for *P. aeruginosa* to undergo mucoid transformation in the CF airways.

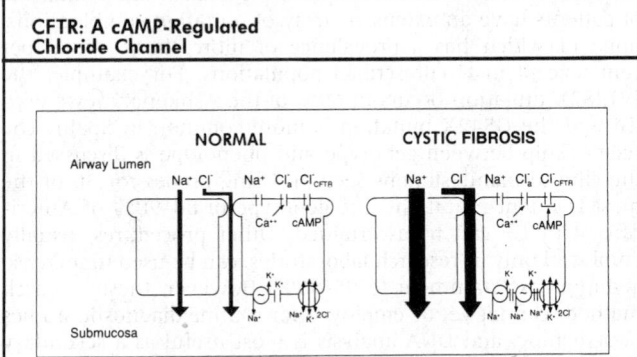

Although functional deficits may occur in cellular immunity, mucosal immune function, and the alternate pathway for complement as lung infection progresses to an advanced stage, the immune system in CF appears to be fundamentally intact. Nutritional deficits, including fatty acid deficiency, have been implicated as predisposing factors for respiratory tract infection. The 10–15% of individuals who retain substantial exocrine pancreatic function have statistically lower sweat chloride values and delayed onset of colonization with *P. aeruginosa.* However, nutritional factors are only in part contributory, because preservation of pancreatic function does not preclude development of typical lung disease.

PATHOLOGY. Striking changes are characteristically observed in the organs that secrete mucus. Eccrine sweat glands and parotid salivary glands, including ducts, are not involved pathologically despite abnormalities in the electrolyte content of their secretory product.

The earliest pathologic lesion in the *lung* is that of bronchiolitis (i.e., mucous plugging and an inflammatory response in the walls of the small airways). With time, mucus accumulation and inflammation extend to the larger airways (bronchitis). Goblet cell hyperplasia and submucosal gland hypertrophy become prominent pathologic expressions of a hypersecretory state, which is most likely a response to chronic airways infection. Organisms appear to be confined to the endobronchial space; invasive bacterial infection is not characteristic. With longstanding disease, evidence of airway destruction such as bronchiolar obliteration, bronchiolectasis, and bronchiectasis becomes prominent. Scanning electron microscopy of the airway surface remains normal, except for scattered areas of squamous cell metaplasia, but freeze-fracture studies have found alterations of tight junctions and apical membrane changes that are probably caused by chronic inflammation. Bronchiectatic cysts and emphysematous bullae or subpleural blebs are frequent with advanced lung disease, the upper lobes being most commonly involved. These enlarged air spaces may rupture and cause pneumothorax. Interstitial disease is not a prominent (common) feature, although areas of fibrosis appear eventually. True emphysema occurs but is not a general pathologic finding. Bronchial arteries are enlarged and tortuous, contributing to a propensity for hemoptysis in bronchiectatic airways. Small pulmonary arteries eventually display medial hypertrophy, which would be expected in secondary pulmonary hypertension.

The *paranasal sinuses* are uniformly filled with secretions, and the lining contains hyperplastic and hypertrophied secretory elements. Polypoid lesions within the sinuses, mucopyocele, and erosion of bone have been reported. The nasal mucosa may contain inflammatory cells, be edematous, and form large or multiple polyps, usually from a base surrounding the ostia of the maxillary and ethmoid sinuses.

The *pancreas* is usually small, occasionally cystic, and often difficult to find at postmortem examination. The extent of involvement varies at birth. In infants, the acini and ducts are often distended and filled with eosinophilic material. In 85–90% of patients, the lesion progresses to complete or almost complete disruption of acini and replacement of exocrine pancreas with fibrous tissue and fat. Infrequently, foci of calcification may be seen on roentgenograms of the abdomen. The islets of Langerhans contain a normal number of β cells, although they may begin to show architectural disruption by fibrous tissue during the 2nd decade of life.

The *intestinal tract* shows only minimal changes. Esophageal and duodenal glands are often distended with mucous secretions. Concretions may form in the appendiceal lumen or cecum. Crypts of the appendix and rectum may be dilated and filled with secretions.

Focal biliary cirrhosis secondary to blockage of intrahepatic bile ducts is uncommon in early life, although it is responsible for occasional cases of prolonged neonatal jaundice. This lesion becomes more prevalent and extensive with age and is found in 25% or more of patients at post mortem. Infrequently, this process proceeds to symptomatic multilobular biliary cirrhosis that has a distinctive pattern of large irregular parenchymal nodules and interspersed bands of fibrous tissue. In addition, approximately 30% of patients have fatty infiltration of the liver, in some cases despite apparently adequate nutrition. At autopsy, hepatic congestion secondary to cor pulmonale is frequently observed. The gallbladder may be hypoplastic and filled with mucoid material and not infrequently contains stones. The epithelial lining often displays extensive mucous metaplasia. Atresia of the cystic duct and stenosis of the distal common bile duct have been observed.

Mucus-secreting *salivary glands* are usually enlarged and display focal plugging and dilation of ducts.

Glands of the uterine cervix are distended with mucus, and copious amounts of mucus collect in the cervical canal. Endocervicitis may be prevalent in teenagers and young women. In more than 95% of males, the body and tail of the epididymis, the vas deferens, and the seminal vesicles are obliterated or atretic.

Generalized amyloidosis has been reported rarely (see Chapter 164).

CLINICAL MANIFESTATIONS. Mutational heterogeneity and environmental factors appear responsible for highly variable involvement of the lung, pancreas, and other organs. A list of presenting manifestations is lengthy (Table 363–1).

Respiratory Tract. Cough is the most constant symptom of pulmonary involvement. At first, the cough may be dry and hacking, but eventually, it becomes loose and productive. In older patients, the cough is most prominent on arising in the morning or after activity. Expectorated mucus is usually purulent. Some patients remain asymptomatic for long periods or seem to have only prolonged acute respiratory infections. Others develop a chronic cough within the first weeks of life or they repeatedly develop pneumonia. Extensive bronchiolitis is attended by wheezing, which is a frequent symptom during the 1st years of life. As lung disease progresses, exercise intolerance, shortness of breath, and failure to gain weight or grow are noted. Exacerbations of lung symptoms eventually require hospitalization for effective treatment. Finally, cor pulmonale, respiratory failure, and death supervene. Colonization with *Pseudomonas (Burkholderia) cepacia* may be associated with particularly rapid pulmonary deterioration and death.

The rate of progression of lung disease is the chief determinant of morbidity and mortality. The course of lung disease, however, is largely independent of genotype. A few mutations (e.g., R117H) may largely spare the lungs. However, early insults to the lungs (e.g., severe viral infections) are more likely to determine the pulmonary outcome.

Early physical findings include increased anteroposterior diameter of the chest, generalized hyper-resonance, scattered or localized coarse crackles, and digital clubbing. Expiratory wheezes may be heard, especially in young children. Cyanosis is a late sign. Common pulmonary complications include atelectasis, hemoptysis, pneumothorax, and cor pulmonale and usually appear beyond the 1st decade of life.

■ **TABLE 363–1 Presenting Manifestations: Indications for Sweat Testing***

Pulmonary	Gastrointestinal
Chronic or productive cough	Meconium ileus, meconium plug syndrome
Recurrent or chronic pneumonia or infiltrates	Steatorrhea, malabsorption
Recurrent bronchiolitis	Rectal prolapse
Atelectasis	Biliary cirrhosis, portal hypertension, bleeding esophageal varices
Hemoptysis	Hypoprothrombinemia beyond newborn period
Infection with *Pseudomonas* (mucoid)	Hypoproteinemia, anasarca
Staphylococcal pneumonia	Deficiency of vitamin A, D, E, or K
Other	Recurrent pancreatitis
Family history of cystic fibrosis	Acrodermatitis enteropathic–like rash
Failure to thrive	
Salty taste when kissed	
Nasal polyps	
Unexplained hypochloremic alkalosis	
Pansinusitis	
Absence of sperm in semen	
Pseudotumor cerebri	

**Individuals with cystic fibrosis may present initially with any of these signs or symptoms.*

Even though roentgenographically the paranasal sinuses are virtually always opacified, acute sinusitis is infrequent. Nasal obstruction and rhinorrhea are common, caused by inflamed, swollen mucous membranes or, in some cases, nasal polyposis. Nasal polyps are most troublesome between 5 and 20 yr of age.

Intestinal Tract. In 10–15% of newborn infants with CF, the ileum is completely obstructed by meconium (meconium ileus). The frequency is greater (~30%) among siblings born subsequent to a child with meconium ileus, but there does not seem to be an association with a particular genotype. Abdominal distention, emesis, and failure to pass meconium appear within the first 24–48 hr of life (see Chapter 88.1). Abdominal roentgenograms (Fig. 363–3) show dilated loops of bowel with air-fluid levels and frequently a collection of granular, "ground glass" material in the lower central abdomen. Rarely, meconium peritonitis results from intrauterine rupture of the bowel wall and can be detected roentgenographically by the presence of peritoneal or scrotal calcifications. Meconium plug syndrome occurs with increased frequency in infants with CF but is less specific than meconium ileus for this condition. Ileal obstruction with fecal material *(distal intestinal obstruction syndrome or meconium ileus equivalent)* occurs in older patients, causing cramping abdominal pain and abdominal distention.

More than 85% of children show evidence of maldigestion due to exocrine pancreatic insufficiency. Symptoms include frequent, bulky, greasy stools and failure to gain weight even when food intake appears to be large. Characteristically, stools contain readily visible droplets of fat. A protuberant abdomen, decreased muscle mass, poor growth, and delayed maturation are typical physical signs. Excessive flatus may be a problem. Several mutations are associated with preservation of some exocrine pancreatic function, most prominently R117H. Individuals homozygous for ΔF508 virtually all have pancreatic insufficiency.

Less common gastrointestinal manifestations include intussusception, fecal impaction of the cecum or appendix with an asymptomatic right lower quadrant mass, and epigastric pain owing to duodenal inflammation. Acid or bile reflux with esophagitis symptoms is common in older children and adults. Subacute appendicitis and periappendiceal abscess have been encountered. Rectal prolapse is relatively frequent. Occasionally, hypoproteinemia with anasarca appears in malnourished infants, especially if children are fed soy-based preparations. Neurologic dysfunction (dementia, peripheral neuropathy) and hemolytic anemia may occur because of vitamin E deficiency. Deficiency of fat-soluble vitamins is occasionally symptomatic. For example, hypoprothrombinemia owing to vitamin K deficiency may result in a bleeding diathesis. Clinical manifestations of other fat-soluble vitamin deficiencies, such as decreased bone density and night blindness, have been noted. Rickets is rare.

Biliary Tract. Biliary cirrhosis becomes symptomatic in only 2–3% of patients. Manifestations may include icterus, ascites, hematemesis from esophageal varices, and evidence of hypersplenism. A neonatal hepatitis-like picture and massive hepatomegaly owing to steatosis have been reported. Biliary colic secondary to cholelithiasis may occur in the 2nd decade of life. Liver disease occurs independent of genotype.

Pancreas. In addition to exocrine pancreatic insufficiency, evidence for hyperglycemia and glycosuria including polyuria and weight loss may appear, especially after 10 yr of age when 8% of individuals develop diabetes. In most cases, ketoacidosis does not occur, but eye, kidney, and other vascular complications have been noted in patients living 10 yr or more after the onset of hyperglycemia. Recurrent acute pancreatitis occurs occasionally in individuals who have residual exocrine pancreatic function.

Genitourinary Tract. Sexual development is often delayed, but only by an average of 2 yr. More than 95% of males are azoospermic because of failure of development of wolffian duct

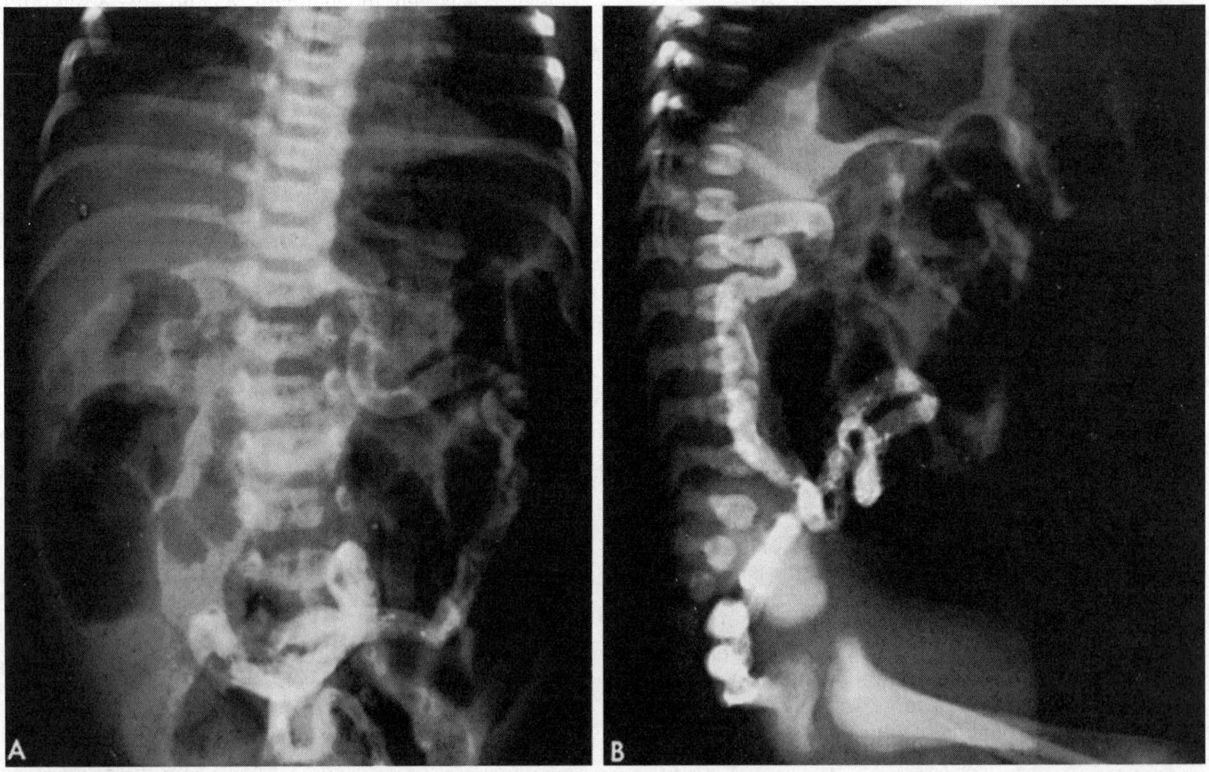

Figure 363–3. *A* and *B*, Contrast enema in a newborn infant with abdominal distention and failure to pass meconium. Notice the small diameter of the sigmoid and ascending colon and dilated, air-filled loops of small intestine. Several air-fluid levels in the small bowel are seen on the upright lateral view.

structures, but sexual function is generally unimpaired. The incidence of inguinal hernia, hydrocele, and undescended testicle is higher than expected. Adolescent females may experience secondary amenorrhea, especially with exacerbations of pulmonary disease. Cervicitis and accumulation of tenacious mucus in the cervical canal have been noted. The female fertility rate is diminished. Pregnancy is generally tolerated well by women with good pulmonary function but may cause a progression of pulmonary disease and even death in those with moderate or advanced lung problems.

Sweat Glands. Excessive loss of salt in the sweat predisposes young children to salt depletion episodes, especially during the time of gastroenteritis and during warm weather. These children present with hypochloremic alkalosis. Frequently, parents notice salt "frosting" of the skin or a salty taste when they kiss the child. A few genotypes (e.g., 3849 + 10 kb C→T) are associated with normal sweat chloride values.

DIAGNOSIS AND ASSESSMENT. The diagnosis of CF has been based for many years on a positive quantitative sweat test ($Cl^- \geq 60$ mEq/L) in conjunction with one or more of the following: typical chronic obstructive pulmonary disease, documented exocrine pancreatic insufficiency, or a positive family history. A diagnosis can also be made for those with typical clinical features and a known CF genotype. DNA analysis, for reasons outlined earlier, cannot alone rule out CF. If sweat chloride values are normal, the documentation of mutations on both chromosomes and a compatible phenotype are sufficient to confirm a diagnosis.

Sweat Testing. The sweat test, using pilocarpine iontophoresis to collect sweat and chemical analysis of its chloride content, remains the standard approach to diagnosis. Indications are enumerated in Table 363–1. The procedure requires care and accuracy. A 3-mA electric current is used to carry pilocarpine into the skin of the forearm and locally stimulate the sweat glands. After washing the arm with distilled water, sweat is collected on filter paper or gauze (or with a capillary tube) that has been placed on the stimulated skin and covered to prevent evaporation. After 30–60 min, the filter paper is removed, weighed, and eluted in distilled water. A chloridometer is recommended for the analysis of chloride in these samples. The amount of sweat collected should be measured and reported. For reliable results, at least 50 mg and preferably 100 mg of sweat should be collected. In infants, it may be necessary to use the upper back to obtain enough sweat. Reliable testing may be difficult in the first few weeks of life because of low sweat rates. Positive results should be confirmed; a negative result should be repeated if suspicion of the diagnosis remains.

More than 60 mEq/L of chloride in sweat is diagnostic of CF when one or more other criteria are present. Values between 40 and 60 mEq/L suggest CF and have been reported in cases with typical involvement. In healthy adults, the sweat chloride values increase slightly, but a value of 60 mEq/L still adequately differentiates CF from other conditions. Chloride concentrations in sweat are somewhat lower in individuals who retain exocrine pancreatic function but remain within the diagnostic range. False-negative test results may be encountered in children with hypoproteinemic edema.

Non-CF conditions associated with elevated concentrations of sweat electrolytes include untreated adrenal insufficiency, ectodermal dysplasia, hereditary nephrogenic diabetes insipidus, glucose-6-phosphatase deficiency, hypothyroidism, hypoparathyroidism, familial cholestasis, pancreatitis, mucopolysaccharidoses, fucosidosis, and malnutrition. Most of these conditions can be easily distinguished from CF by clinical criteria.

Other Diagnostic Tests. The finding of increased potential differences across nasal epithelium, the loss of this difference with topical amiloride application, and documentation of a voltage response to a β-adrenergic agonist have been used to confirm the diagnosis in patients with equivocal or frankly normal sweat chloride values. Failure to sweat when a combination of isoproterenol and atropine is injected into the skin has also been used to characterize CF variants. Both of these tests are considered experimental and are challenging to carry out.

Pancreatic Function. Exocrine pancreatic dysfunction is clinically apparent in many patients. However, documentation is desirable if there are questions about the functional status of the pancreas. Measurement of fat balance with a 3-day stool collection or direct documentation of enzyme secretion after duodenal intubation and pancreozymin-secretin stimulation are reliable measures but are excessively cumbersome or invasive for children and are not used routinely. Quantitation of trypsin and chymotrypsin activity in a fresh stool sample is a useful screening test but is not definitive. Measurement of immunoreactive trypsinogen in serum reliably distinguishes patients with CF, with and without pancreatic insufficiency, after 7 yr of age but not before that time. Other indirect measures of pancreatic enzyme secretion are available but have limited clinical value. Endocrine pancreatic dysfunction may be more prevalent than previously recognized. Some have advocated yearly monitoring of glycosylated hemoglobin levels after 10 yr of age. This approach is more sensitive than spot checks of blood and urine glucose levels.

Radiology. Pulmonary radiologic findings suggest the diagnosis but are not specific. Hyperinflation of lungs occurs early and may be overlooked in the absence of infiltrates or streaky densities. Bronchial thickening and plugging and ring shadows suggesting bronchiectasis usually appear first in the upper lobes. Nodular densities, patchy atelectasis, and confluent infiltrates follow. Hilar lymph nodes may be prominent. With advanced disease, impressive hyperinflation with markedly depressed diaphragms, anterior bowing of the sternum, and a narrow cardiac shadow are noted. Cyst formation, extensive bronchiectasis, dilated pulmonary artery segments, and segmental or lobar atelectasis are often apparent. Computed tomography (CT) of the chest can be used to detect and localize thickening of bronchial airway walls and early bronchiectasis. Typical progression of lung disease is seen in Figure 363–4.

Roentgenograms of paranasal sinuses reveal panopacification and often failure of frontal sinus development.

Pulmonary Function. Pulmonary function studies are not obtained reliably until 5–6 yr of age, by which time most patients show the typical pattern of obstructive pulmonary involvement (see Chapters 321 and 324). Decrease in the midmaximal flow rate is an early functional change, reflecting small airways obstruction. This lesion also affects the distribution of ventilation and increases the alveolar-arterial oxygen difference. The findings of obstructive airway disease and modest responses to a bronchodilator are consistent with the diagnosis of CF at all ages. Residual volume and functional residual capacity are increased early in the course of lung disease. Restrictive changes, characterized by declining total lung capacity and vital capacity, correlate with extensive lung injury and fibrosis and are a late finding. Testing several times a year can be used to evaluate the need for more intensive therapy and the course of the pulmonary involvement. A few patients reach adolescent or adult life with normal routine tests and without evidence of overinflation.

Microbiology. The finding of *S. aureus* or *P. aeruginosa* on culture of the lower airways (e.g., sputum) strongly suggests a diagnosis of CF. In particular, mucoid forms of *Pseudomonas* are virtually diagnostic of CF in children.

Heterozygote Detection and Prenatal Diagnosis. Mutation analysis should be fully informative when testing potential carriers or a fetus, provided that mutations within the family have been previously identified. Testing a spouse of a carrier with a standard panel of probes is approximately 90% sensitive. The rationale for prenatal detection and termination of pregnancy

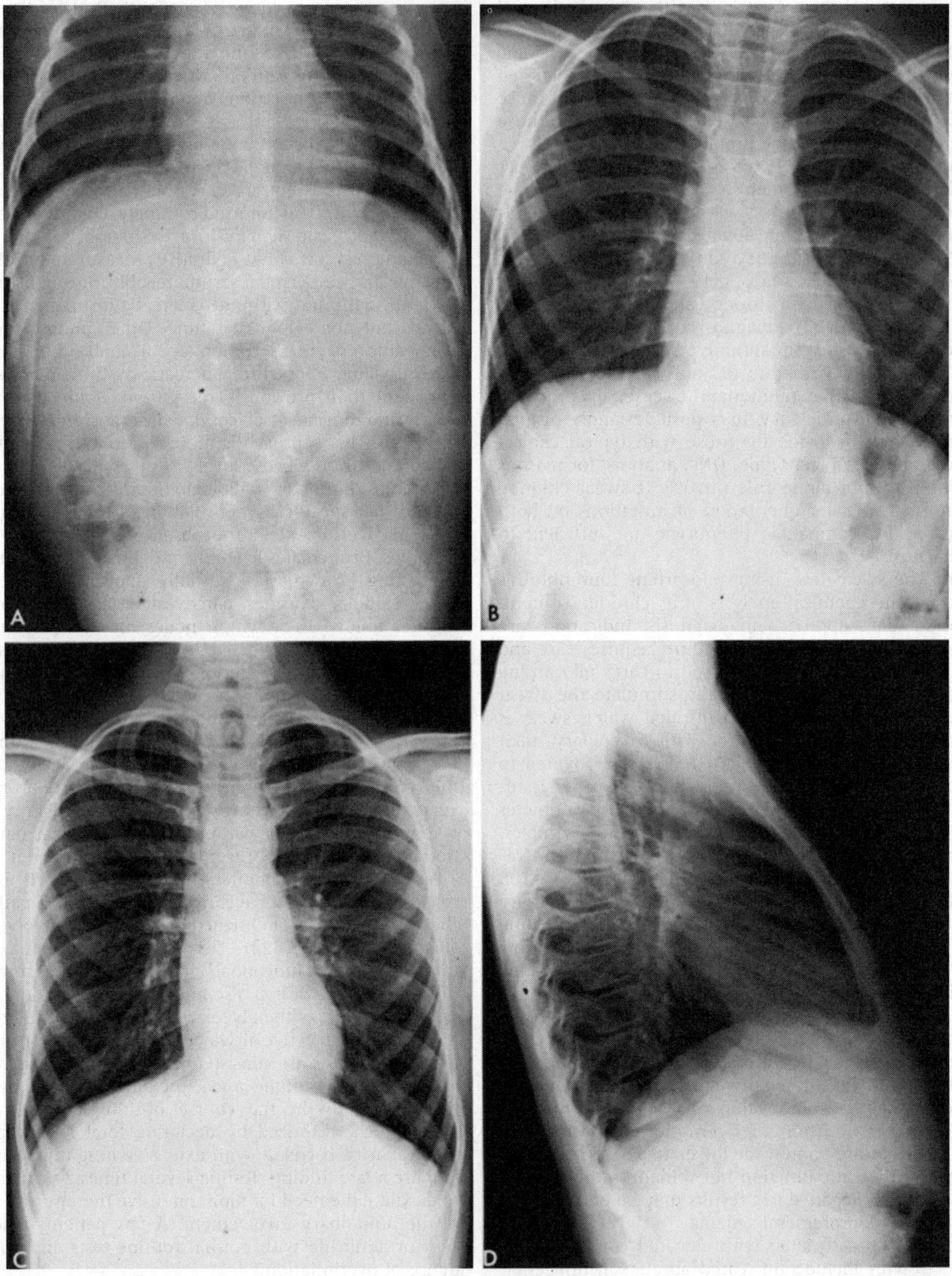

Figure 363–4. Roentgenographic progression of cystic fibrosis lung disease from the diagnosis in an infant to 17 yr of age. *A,* Admitted with cough and wheezing at 2 mo of age. Notice the mild increase in bronchovascular markings, especially in the upper lobe areas. *B,* At age 4 yr, cough was minimal. Bronchovascular markings were mildly increased, and there was some improvement in the upper lobes. The wheeze never recurred. *C* and *D,* At age 13 yr, there was minimal cough and occasional sputum production. The bronchovascular markings were generally further increased, with early bronchiectatic changes in the right upper lobe. The lateral view does not suggest overinflation.

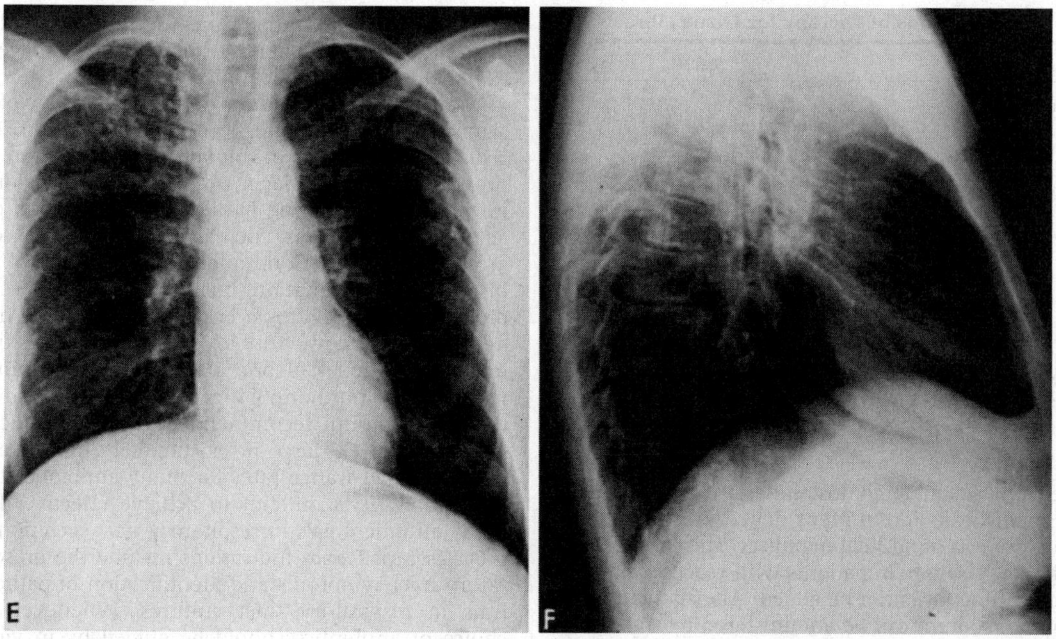

Figure 363–4. *Continued E* and *F,* Age 18 yr. During adolescence, cough and sputum production increased even though outpatient antibiotic therapy was intensified. Small volume hemoptysis, occasional paroxysms of cough, and weight loss as well as increased nodular infiltrates (especially in the right upper lobe, and hyperinflation (as seen on the lateral view) led to the 1st hospitalization since infancy. Height and weight were maintained in the 25th–50th percentile.

is currently a matter of considerable discussion, because expected longevity is approximately 3 decades on average, with promise for even better prognosis in the future.

Newborn Screening. Most newborns with CF can be identified by determination of immunoreactive trypsinogen in blood spots. However, this test is at best only 95% sensitive. Although diagnoses can be made before early nutritional deficiencies and lung disease occur, there is no evidence that early diagnosis improves long-term outcome. The case for routine newborn screening is debatable. A stronger case for screening will emerge when therapies aimed at the fundamental defect are available.

TREATMENT. The treatment plan should be comprehensive and linked to close monitoring and early, aggressive intervention.

General Approach to Care. A period of hospitalization for accurate diagnosis, baseline assessment, initiation of treatment, clearing of the pulmonary involvement, and education of the patient and parents is recommended. The patient is hospitalized for as long as is necessary to reverse pulmonary findings and to achieve steady weight gain. Follow-up outpatient visits are scheduled at least every 3 mo because many aspects of the condition require careful monitoring. An interval history and physical examination should be obtained at each visit. A sputum sample or, if that is not available, a lower pharyngeal swab taken during or after a forced cough is obtained for culture and antibiotic susceptibility studies. Even asymptomatic patients may produce sputum after forced exhalations or pharyngeal stimulation with a swab. Because irreversible loss of pulmonary function from low-grade infection can occur very gradually and without acute symptoms, emphasis is placed on a thorough pulmonary history. Changes in cough frequency or productivity, the appearance of nocturnal cough, the onset of paroxysmal cough with or without vomiting, or hemoptysis all indicate exacerbation of pulmonary infection. New crackles, irritability, decreased activity, decreased appetite, and failure to gain weight may also reflect increased pulmonary infection. All suggest the need for altered or increased antibiotic and physical therapy. Immunoprophylaxis specifically against rubeola, pertussis, and influenza is essential. A nurse, respiratory therapist or physical therapist, social worker, dietitian, and psychologist should participate in the care program. Considerable education and encouragement are required if the patient and parent are to maintain an adequate level of home care.

Because CF patients do not hydrate their secretions adequately, attention in early childhood to oral hydration, especially during warm weather or with acute gastroenteritis, may prevent exacerbation of problems with clearance of mucus from airways. For the same reason, intravenous therapy for dehydration should be initiated early.

The goal of therapy is to maintain a stable condition for prolonged periods. This can be accomplished for most patients by interval evaluation and adjustments of the home treatment program. However, some patients have episodic acute or low-grade chronic lung infection that progresses. For these patients, 2 wk or more of intensive inhalation and physical therapy and intravenous antibiotics is indicated. Intravenous antibiotics may be required infrequently or as often as every 2–3 mo. Significant improvement in pulmonary function and the patient's well-being is usually achieved.

The basic daily care program varies depending on the age of the patient, the degree of pulmonary involvement, other system involvement, and time available for therapy. The major components of this care are pulmonary and nutritional therapy. Because therapy is medication intensive, iatrogenic problems arise frequently. Monitoring for these complications is also an important part of management (Table 363–2).

Pulmonary Therapy. The object is to clear secretions from airways and to control infection. There is a divergence of opinion about specific aspects of therapy. However, the effectiveness of the overall approach, including close supervision, continuity of care, aggressive intervention, and an optimistic outlook, is more important than minor variations in the use of individual measures. When an individual patient is not doing well, every potentially useful aspect of therapy should be considered.

INHALATION THERAPY. Aerosol therapy is used to deliver medications and water to the lower respiratory tract, usually before or after segmental postural drainage. Some agents such as bronchodila-

■ TABLE 363–2 Complications of Therapy for Cystic Fibrosis

Complication	Agent
Renal dysfunction	
Tubular	Aminoglycosides
Interstitial nephritis	Semisynthetic penicillins
Hearing loss	Aminoglycosides
Peripheral neuropathy and/or optic atrophy	Chloramphenicol (prolonged course)
Hypomagnesemia	Aminoglycosides
Hyperuricemia, colonic stricture	Pancreatic extracts (very large doses)
Goiter	Iodine-containing expectorants
Gynecomastia	Spironolactone
Enamel hypoplasia or staining	Tetracyclines (used in first 8 yr of life)

NOTE: Common hypersensitivity reactions to drugs are not included.

tors can be delivered by metered dose inhaler with or without a spacer. The mainstay is intermittent delivery using a small compressor that drives a hand-held nebulizer. The basic aerosol solution is 0.45–0.9% saline. In patients with reactive airways, albuterol or other β-agonists can be added. Alternatively or in addition, cromolyn sodium can be administered by this route. β-Agonists may decrease PaO_2 by increasing ventilation-perfusion mismatch and decrease airway wall tone, resulting in enhanced airway collapse during expiration.

When the airway pathogens are resistant to oral antibiotics or when the infection is difficult to control at home, aerosolized antibiotics may reduce symptoms, especially those referable to tracheitis or bronchitis. Forty to 80 mg of gentamicin, or tobramycin in 1–2 mL of saline has been used two to four times daily in home therapy and also in the hospital in conjunction with intravenous therapy. Some advocate even larger doses of aminoglycosides, up to 600 mg/dose administered with an ultrasonic nebulizer. Carbenicillin (1 g) and ticarcillin (0.5 g) and colistin (20–40 mg) have also been used. Sensitization or resistance to antibiotics may occur, but both are surprisingly infrequent. A preferred but time-consuming regimen is delivery of a bronchodilator, followed by chest physical therapy and then an antibiotic aerosol.

Human recombinant DNase (2.5 mg), given as a single daily aerosol appears to improve pulmonary function, decrease numbers of pulmonary exacerbations, and promote a sense of well-being in patients who have mild to moderate disease and purulent secretions. Improvement has been sustained for 6 mo or more of continuous therapy. Efficacy for patients with severe disease, (e.g., forced vital capacity <40% of predicted) has been difficult to document. Another mucolytic agent, N-acetylcysteine, is toxic to ciliated epithelium, and repeated administration should be avoided.

CHEST PHYSICAL THERAPY (PT). This treatment usually consists of chest percussion combined with postural drainage and derives its rationale from the idea that cough clears mucus from large airways, but that chest vibrations are required to move secretions from small airways where expiratory flow rates are low. Chest PT may be particularly useful for patients with CF because they first accumulate secretions in small airways, even before the onset of symptoms. Improvement of pulmonary function generally cannot be demonstrated immediately after this therapy. However, cessation of chest PT in older children with mild to moderate air flow limitation results in deterioration of lung function within 3 wk and prompt improvement of function when therapy is resumed. Chest PT is recommended one to four times a day, depending on the severity of lung dysfunction. Cough or forced expirations are encouraged after each lung segment is "drained." Mechanical percussors have been designed to assist with therapy and may be useful, especially for adolescents. Voluntary coughing, repeated forced expiratory maneuvers with and without positive expiratory pressure, patterned breathing, use of a handheld Flutter device, and vigorous exercise have all been suggested as additional aids to mucus clearance.

ANTIBIOTIC THERAPY. Antibiotics are the mainstay of therapy designed to control progression of lung infection. The goal is to reduce the intensity of endobronchial infection and to delay progressive lung damage. Differentiation of colonization from infection is a recurring problem, and the usual guidelines for acute chest infections, such as fever, tachypnea, or chest pain, are often absent. Consequently, all aspects of the patient's history and examination, including anorexia, weight loss, and diminished activity, must be used to guide the frequency and duration of therapy. Antibiotic treatment varies from intermittent short courses of one antibiotic to continuous treatment with one or more antibiotics. Dosages are often two to three times the amount recommended for minor infections because patients with CF have proportionately more lean body mass and higher clearance rates for many antibiotics than do other individuals. It is difficult to achieve effective drug levels of many antimicrobials in respiratory tract secretions.

Oral Antibiotic Therapy. Indications include the presence of respiratory tract symptoms and identification of pathogenic organisms in respiratory tract cultures. Whenever possible, the choice of antibiotics should be guided by in vitro sensitivity testing. Common organisms include *S. aureus,* nontypeable *Haemophilus influenzae,* and *P. aeruginosa. P. (Burkholderia) cepacia* is encountered with increasing frequency. The first two can be eradicated from the CF respiratory tract, but *Pseudomonas* is more difficult to treat and rarely is eradicated. The usual course of therapy is 2 wk or more, and maximal doses are recommended. Low-dose, continuous antibiotic therapy is not recommended because organisms tend to develop resistance. Useful oral antibiotics are listed in Table 363–3. Some antimicrobials such as chloramphenicol are effective even when they are not indicated by microbial sensitivity testing. Use of tetracycline should be avoided in children younger than 9 yr of age. The quinolones are the only broadly effective oral antibiotics for *Pseudomonas* infection.

Intravenous Antibiotic Therapy. For the patient who has progressive or unrelenting symptoms and signs despite intensive home measures, intravenous antibiotic therapy is indicated. This therapy is usually initiated in the hospital, but often is completed on an ambulatory basis. Although many patients improve within 7 days, it is usually advisable to extend the period of treatment to at least 14 days. Permanent intravenous access can now be provided for long-term therapy in the hospital or at home.

Intravenous antibiotics commonly used are listed in Table 363–3. In general, treatment of *Pseudomonas* infection requires two drug therapy. A third agent may be required for optimal *S. aureus* coverage. Simultaneous administration of aerosolized antimicrobials can increase endobronchial concentrations. The aminoglycosides have a relatively short half-life in many patients with CF. The initial parenteral dose is noted in Table 363–3, generally given every 8 hr. After blood levels have been determined, the total daily dose should be adjusted. Peak levels of 10 mg/L are desirable, and trough levels should be kept below 2 mg/L to minimize the risk of nephrotoxicity. Changes in therapy should be guided by culture results and by lack of improvement. If patients do not improve, heart failure, reactive airways, and infection with viruses, *Aspergillus fumigatus, Mycobacterium,* or other unusual organisms should be considered. *P. (Burkholderia) cepacia* may be particularly refractory to antimicrobial therapy.

BRONCHODILATOR THERAPY. Reversible airway obstruction occurs in many patients with CF, sometimes in conjunction with frank asthma or acute bronchopulmonary aspergillosis. Reversible obstruction is suggested by improvement of 15% or more in flow rates after inhalation of a bronchodilator. Treatment may

■ TABLE 363–3 Antimicrobial Agents for Cystic Fibrosis Lung Infection

Route	Organisms	Agents	Dosage (mg/kg/24 hr)	Doses/24 hr
Oral				
	Staphylococcus aureus	Cloxacillin	50–100	3–4
		Cefaclor	40–60	3
		Clindamycin	20	3–4
		Erythromycin	50–100	3–4
		Amoxicillin/clavulanate	40	3
	Haemophilus influenzae	Amoxicillin	50–100	3
		Trimethoprim-sulfamethoxazole	20*	2–4
		Chloramphenicol	50–100	3–4
	Pseudomonas aeruginosa	Ciprofloxacin	15–30	3
	Empirical	Tetracycline	50–100	3–4
Intravenous				
	S. aureus	Oxacillin	150–200	4
		Vancomycin	40	4
	P. aeruginosa	Gentamicin or Tobramycin	8–20	1–3
		Amikacin	15–30	2–3
		Netilmicin	6–12	2–3
		Carbenicillin		
		Ticarcillin		
		Piperacillin		
		Mezlocillin		
		Azlocillin	250–450	4–6
		Ticarcillin/clavulanate	250–450	4–6
		Imipenem/cilastatin	45–90	3–4
		Ceftazidime	150	3
		Aztreonam	150	4
Aerosol				
	P. aeruginosa	Gentamicin	40–160†	2–4
		Tobramycin	40–160†	
		Carbenicillin	500–1,000†	

**Quantity of trimethoprim.*
†mg/dose.

include use of β-adrenergic agonists by aerosol. Cromolyn sodium or ipratropium hydrochloride are alternative agents, but their efficacy has not been studied systematically.

Anti-Inflammatory Agents. Corticosteroids are useful for the treatment of allergic bronchopulmonary aspergillosis and other severe reactive airways disease occasionally encountered in patients with CF. Prolonged treatment of standard CF lung disease using an alternate-day regimen initially appeared to improve pulmonary function and diminish hospitalization rates. However, a 4-yr double-blind, multicenter study of this regimen for patients with mild to a moderate lung disease found little efficacy and prohibitive side effects, including growth retardation, cataracts, and abnormalities of glucose tolerance at a dose of 2 mg/kg and growth retardation at 1 mg/kg. Ibuprofen, given chronically (20–30 mg/kg dose, b.i.d.: maximum 1600 mg) over 4 yr duration, is associated with slowing of disease progression of CF.

Endoscopy and Lavage. Treatment of obstructed airways sometimes includes tracheobronchial suctioning or lavage, especially if atelectasis or mucoid impaction is present. Bronchopulmonary lavage may be performed by the instillation of saline or by a mucolytic agent through a fiberoptic bronchoscope. Antibiotics (usually gentamicin or tobramycin) may also be directly instilled at lavage, transiently achieving a much higher endobronchial concentration than can be obtained by using intravenous therapy. There is no evidence for sustained benefit from repeated endoscopic or lavage procedures.

Expectorants. Systemic drugs, such as iodides and guaiphenesin, do not effectively assist with the removal of secretions from the respiratory tract.

Treatment of Pulmonary Complications. A number of pulmonary complications require extra attention or special measures.

Atelectasis. Lobar atelectasis occurs relatively infrequently; it may be asymptomatic and noted only at the time of a routine chest roentgenogram. Aggressive intravenous therapy with antibiotics and increased chest PT directed at the affected lobe may be effective. If there is no improvement in 5–7 days, bronchoscopic examination of the airways may be indicated. If the atelectasis does not resolve, continued intensive home therapy is indicated, since atelectasis may resolve during a period of weeks or months. Persistent atelectasis may be asymptomatic. However, lobectomy should be considered if expansion is not achieved and the patient has progressive difficulty from fever, anorexia, and unrelenting cough. Lobectomy should be performed only after a period of hospitalization for intensive therapy to improve the status of all remaining parts of the lung.

Hemoptysis. Endobronchial bleeding usually reflects airway wall erosion secondary to infection; dilated bronchial arteries are contributory. With increasing numbers of older patients, hemoptysis has become a relatively frequent complication. Blood streaking of sputum is particularly common. Small volume hemoptysis ($<$20 mL) should not trigger panic and is usually viewed as a need for intensified antimicrobial and chest physical therapy. When the hemoptysis is persistent or increases in severity, hospital admission is indicated. Massive hemoptysis, defined as total blood loss of 250 mL or more within a 24-hr period, is rare in the first decade, occurs in less than 1% of adolescents, but requires close monitoring and the capability to rapidly replace blood losses. Chest physical therapy is often discontinued until 12–24 hr after the last brisk bleeding episode and is then reinstituted gradually. Patients should receive vitamin K in the event of an abnormal prothrombin time. During brisk hemoptysis the patient requires a great deal of reassurance that the bleeding will stop. Blood transfusion is not indicated unless there is hypotension or the hematocrit is significantly reduced. Ticarcillin may interfere with platelet function and aggravate hemoptysis. Bronchoscopy has been used in an effort to localize the site of bleeding. However, usually no bleeding site is found. Lobectomy should be avoided, if possible, because functioning lung should be preserved and because it is difficult to be certain of the bleeding site. Bronchial artery embolization can be useful to control persistent, significant hemoptysis.

PNEUMOTHORAX. This is encountered in less than 1% of children and teenagers, but it is more frequently encountered in older patients and may be life threatening. The episode may be asymptomatic but is often attended by chest and shoulder pain, shortness of breath, or hemoptysis. Even mild symptoms should be taken seriously, and a chest roentgenogram should be obtained. If the pneumothorax is smaller than 5–10%, the patient is admitted to the hospital and observed. A pneumothorax greater than 10% or under tension requires rapid, definitive treatment. Because of frequent delayed closure of the air leak and a high rate of recurrence with closed thoracotomy, an open thoracotomy through a small incision with plication of blebs, apical pleural stripping, and basal pleural abrasion is recommended after the first occurrence and within 24 hr of the diagnosis. This procedure is well tolerated even in cases of advanced lung disease. Intravenous antibiotics are begun on admission. The thoracotomy tube is removed as soon as possible, usually on the 2nd or 3rd postoperative day. The patient can then be mobilized, and full postural drainage therapy can be resumed. Recurrences, intraoperative complications, and deaths are rare as a result of this procedure. Closed thoracotomy in conjunction with a sclerosing agent continues to be used by some specialists. Rarely, bilateral simultaneous pneumothorax is encountered; in this case, control of the air leak must be achieved immediately, at least on one side.

ALLERGIC ASPERGILLOSIS. This complication may present with wheezing, increased cough, shortness of breath, or marked hyperinflation on pulmonary function testing (see Chapters 230 and 344). In some patients there are new, focal infiltrates on the chest roentgenogram. The presence of rust-colored sputum, the recovery of aspergillus organisms from the sputum, the demonstration of serum antibodies against *A. fumigatus,* or the presence of eosinophils in a fresh sputum sample support the diagnosis. The serum IgE level may be very high. Treatment is directed at controlling the inflammatory reaction with corticosteroid therapy. This condition is usually self-limited and subsides with several weeks of therapy. For refractory cases, aerosolized amphotericin B or systemic itraconazole may be required.

HYPERTROPHIC OSTEOARTHROPATHY. This complication causes elevation of the periosteum over the distal portions of long bones and bone pain, overlying edema, and joint effusions. Acetaminophen or ibuprofen may provide relief. Control of lung infection usually reduces symptoms. Intermittent arthropathy unrelated to other rheumatologic disorders occurs occasionally in patients, has no recognized pathogenetic basis, and usually responds to nonsteroidal anti-inflammatory agents.

ACUTE RESPIRATORY FAILURE. Acute respiratory failure (see Chapter 322) in patients with mild to moderate lung disease rarely occurs and is usually the result of a severe viral illness such as influenza. Because patients with this complication usually regain their previous status, intensive therapy is indicated. In addition to the aerosol, postural drainage, and intravenous antibiotic treatment, oxygen is required to raise the arterial Po_2 above 50 mm Hg. A rising Pco_2 may require ventilatory assistance. Endotracheal or bronchoscopic suction may be necessary and can be repeated daily. Right-sided heart failure may occur and should be treated vigorously. Recovery is often slow. Intensive intravenous antibiotic therapy and postural drainage should be continued for 1–2 wk after the patient has regained baseline status.

CHRONIC RESPIRATORY FAILURE. Patients usually develop chronic respiratory failure from prolonged slow deterioration of lung function. Although this can occur at any age, it is seen more frequently in adolescent and adult patients. Because a longstanding arterial Po_2 less than 50 mm Hg promotes the development of right-sided heart failure, they usually benefit from low-flow oxygen to raise arterial Po_2 to 55 mm Hg or above. Increasing hypercapnia may prevent the use of optimal FIo_2. These patients do not benefit substantially from continuous ventilator assistance or tracheostomy. Most patients improve somewhat with intensive antibiotic and pulmonary therapy measures and can be discharged from the hospital. Low-flow oxygen therapy at home is needed, especially with sleep. These patients almost always display cor pulmonale and should be maintained on a reduced salt intake and diuretics.

Lung transplantation has become an option for increasing numbers of individuals with CF and end-stage lung disease (see Chapter 402). The majority are now surviving 3 or more years, and lung function as well as quality of life generally improve remarkably. Because of bronchiolitis obliterans and other complications, transplanted lungs cannot be expected to function for the lifetime of a recipient. Individuals with chronic respiratory failure who are on a lung transplant waiting list may be candidates for ventilatory assistance.

RIGHT-SIDED HEART FAILURE. Some patients develop right-sided heart failure as the result of a complication such as an acute viral infection or pneumothorax. Individuals with longstanding, advanced pulmonary disease, especially those with severe hypoxemia (Pao_2 below 50 mm Hg), often develop chronic right-sided heart failure. The mechanisms include hypoxemic pulmonary arterial spasm and loss of pulmonary vasculature with destructive lung disease. Pulmonary artery wall changes contribute to increased vascular resistance with time. Some combination of cyanosis, increased shortness of breath, increased liver size with tender margin, ankle edema, jugular venous distention, an unusual weight gain, increased heart size by chest roentgenogram, or evidence for right-sided heart enlargement by electrocardiogram or echocardiography helps to confirm the diagnosis. Furosemide (1 mg/kg administered intravenously) may result in a good diuresis and confirm the suspicion of fluid retention. Repeated doses may be required at 24- to 48-hr intervals in the initial period to reduce fluid accumulation and accompanying symptoms. Concomitant use of spironolactone may protect against potassium depletion and facilitate long-term diuresis. Hypochloremic alkalosis may complicate respiratory failure and chronic use of loop diuretics. Digitalis is not effective in pure right-sided failure, but it may be useful when there is an associated left-sided dysfunction. The arterial Po_2 should be maintained above 50 mm Hg if at all possible. Loss of respiratory drive may occur during the initial phases of oxygen therapy, and serial arterial blood gases or noninvasive monitoring is required to ensure the continuation of adequate ventilation. Intensive pulmonary therapy including intravenous antibiotics is most important. Initially, the salt intake should be limited to 2 g sodium/24 hr; carbenicillin may be hazardous because of its relatively high sodium content. Fluid overload should be avoided. No clear-cut long-term benefit from pulmonary vasodilators has been demonstrated. In the past, cardiac failure usually meant death within several months. However, the prognosis has been improving, and a number of patients have survived for 5 yr or more after an initial episode of cardiac failure. Lung transplantation is an option for an increasing number of patients with severe cor pulmonale (see Chapter 402).

Nutritional Therapy. Up to 90% of patients have complete loss of exocrine pancreatic function and inadequate digestion of fats and proteins. They require diet adjustment, pancreatic enzyme replacement, and supplementary vitamins.

DIET. Many infants at the time of diagnosis have nutritional deficits. Young infants who present with wheezy breathing and are fed soy protein formulas do not utilize this protein well and may develop hypoproteinemia with anasarca. Infants do well with formulas containing predigested protein and medium-chain triglycerides. A low-fat, high-protein, high-caloric diet was generally recommended in the past for older children. Some children on this diet became deficient in essential fatty acids. With the advent of improved pancreatic enzyme products, normal amounts of fat in the diet are usually tolerated well.

Most individuals have a higher than normal caloric need because of increased work of breathing and perhaps because of increased metabolic activity related to the basic defect. When anorexia of chronic infection supervenes, weight loss occurs. Further encouragement to eat high-caloric foods may be useful, but weight gain generally is not realized unless lung infection is controlled. With advanced lung disease, weight stabilization or gain has been achieved by nocturnal feeding via nasogastric tube or percutaneous enterostomy or by intravenous hyperalimentation. Long-term benefits of these interventions for lung function, quality of life, and psychologic well-being are less clearly substantiated.

PANCREATIC ENZYME REPLACEMENT. Extracts of animal pancreas given with ingested food reduce but do not fully correct stool fat and nitrogen losses. Enzyme dosage and product should be individualized for each patient. The introduction of pH-sensitive enteric-coated enzyme microspheres has been a major advance in patient care. Several strengths, up to 20,000 IU of lipase/capsule are available. Administration of large doses, eg, 5000 IU/kg/meal, has been linked to colonic strictures requiring surgery in a small number of cases. One to three capsules/meal is sufficient for most patients; infants may need only one-half capsule or may prefer pancreatin powder. The microsphere preparations usually are sufficiently effective to permit a liberal diet, which may include homogenized milk. Although patients with CF display bile salt malabsorption, enzyme preparations containing bile salts are infrequently needed. The dose of enzymes required usually increases with age, but some teenagers and young adults may later have a decrease in their requirement.

VITAMIN AND MINERAL SUPPLEMENT. Because pancreatic insufficiency results in malabsorption of fat-soluble vitamins (A, D, E, and K), vitamin supplementation is recommended. Capsules containing adequate amounts of all four vitamins for CF patients are now available. Infants with zinc deficiency and rash have been reported. In addition, attention should be paid to iron status; in one study almost one third of patients with CF had a low serum ferritin concentration.

Treatment of Intestinal Complications

MECONIUM ILEUS (see Chapter 88.1). When meconium ileus is suspected, a nasogastric tube is placed for suction, and the infant is hydrated. In some cases Gastrografin enemas with reflux of contrast material into the ileum have resulted in the passage of a meconium plug and clearing of the obstruction. Use of this hypertonic solution requires careful replacement of water losses into the bowel. Patients who fail this procedure require operative intervention. Individuals who are successfully treated generally have a prognosis similar to that of other patients. Infants with meconium ileus should be treated as having CF until adequate sweat testing can be carried out.

DISTAL INTESTINAL OBSTRUCTION SYNDROME (MECONIUM ILEUS EQUIVALENT) AND OTHER CAUSES OF ABDOMINAL PAIN. Despite appropriate pancreatic enzyme replacement, 2–5% of patients accumulate fecal material in the terminal portion of the ileum and in the cecum, which may result in intermittent or complete obstruction. For intermittent obstruction, pancreatic enzyme replacement should be continued or even increased and laxatives or stool softeners (milk of magnesia, Colace, mineral oil) given. Increased fluid intake is also recommended. Failure to relieve symptoms signals the need for large-volume bowel lavage with a balanced salt solution containing polyethyleneglycol, taken by mouth or by nasogastric tube. When there is complete obstruction, a Gastrografin enema, accompanied by large amounts of intravenous fluids, can be therapeutic. Intussusception, and volvulus must also be considered in the differential diagnosis. Intussusception, usually ileocolic, occurs at any age and often follows a 1- to 2-day history of "constipation." It can often be diagnosed and reduced by a Gastrografin enema. If a nonreducible intussusception or a volvulus is present, laparotomy is required. Repeated episodes of intussusception may be an indication for cecectomy.

Chronic appendicitis with or without periappendiceal abscess may present with recurrent or persistent abdominal pain, raising the question of need for a laparotomy. A lack of acid buffering in the duodenum appears to promote duodenitis and ulcer formation in some children. Bile reflux into the stomach is seen in older patients. Some patients may obtain relief from antacids or H_2 antagonists.

GASTROESOPHAGEAL REFLUX. Because several factors raise intra-abdominal pressure, including cough and obstructed airways, pathologic gastroesophageal reflux is not uncommon and may exacerbate lung disease secondary to reflex wheezing and repeated aspiration. Dietary, positional and medication therapy may help. Cholinergic agonists are contraindicated because they trigger mucus secretion and progressive respiratory difficulty. Fundoplication may improve lung function in selected cases.

RECTAL PROLAPSE. This occurs frequently in infants with CF and less commonly in older children. It is usually related to steatorrhea, malnutrition, and repetitive cough. The prolapsed rectum can usually be replaced manually by continuous gentle pressure with the patient in the knee-chest position. Sedation may be helpful. To prevent an immediate recurrence, the buttocks can be taped closed. Adequate pancreatin replacement, decreased fat and roughage in the diet, and control of pulmonary infection result in improvement. An occasional patient may continue to have rectal prolapse and require surgery.

LIVER DISEASE. Liver function abnormalities associated with biliary cirrhosis can be improved by treatment with ursodeoxycholic acid. Portal hypertension with esophageal varices, hypersplenism, or ascites occurs in 2% or fewer of children with CF (see Chapter 305). The acute management of bleeding esophageal varices includes nasogastric suction and cold saline lavage. Sclerotherapy is recommended after an initial bleed. In the past, significant bleeding has also been treated successfully with portosystemic shunting. Splenorenal anastomosis has been the most effective. Pronounced hypersplenism may require splenectomy. The management of ascites is discussed in Chapter 315.

Obstructive jaundice in newborns with CF requires no specific therapy. Hepatomegaly with steatosis requires careful attention to nutrition and may respond to carnitine repletion. Rarely, biliary cirrhosis proceeds to hepatocellular failure, which should be treated as in other patients with hepatic failure (see Chapters 305 and 309). End-stage liver disease is an indication for liver transplantation in children with CF, especially if pulmonary function is good.

PANCREATITIS. Pancreatitis may be precipitated by fatty meals, alcohol ingestion, or tetracycline therapy. Serum amylase and lipase levels may remain elevated for long periods. Treatment is discussed in Chapter 297.

HYPERGLYCEMIA. Onset occurs most frequently after the 1st decade and is not related to the severity of the disease; ketoacidosis is rarely encountered. Glucose intolerance without urine glucose losses is usually not treated; glycosylated hemoglobin levels should be followed at least annually. With persistent glycosuria and symptoms, insulin treatment should be instituted. Oral antidiabetic agents occasionally are effective. Exocrine pancreatic insufficiency and malabsorption make strict dietary control of hyperglycemia difficult. The development of significant hyperglycemia may adversely affect prognosis.

Other Therapy

NASAL POLYPS (See Chapter 328). These occur in 15–20% of patients with CF, are most prevalent in the 2nd decade of life, and in some are a recurrent problem. Local corticosteroids and nasal decongestants occasionally provide some relief. Allergy

■ TABLE 363–4 Experimental Therapies for Cystic Fibrosis

Class	Agent	Target	Mode of Action
Mucolytics	Gelsolin	Purulent airway secretions	Solubilizes secretions by depolymerizing actin, a PMN product contributing to increased viscosity
Hydrating agents	Amiloride	Airway secretions	Blocks sodium reabsorption by airway epithelial cells
	UTP and its analogs	Airway secretions	Stimulates chloride secretion by airway epithelial cells via a non-CFTR mediated mechanism
Reagents for gene transfer	CFTR-vector constructs	Airway epithelial cells	Expression of normally active CFTR

CFTR = cystic fibrosis transmembrane regulator; PMN = polymorphonuclear lymphocyte; UTP = uridine triphosphate.

skin testing and hyposensitization may be helpful in those with allergic symptoms. When the polyps completely obstruct the nasal airway, rhinorrhea becomes constant, or widening of the nasal bridge is noticed, surgical removal is indicated; polyps may recur promptly after removal but frequently do not grow to the point of obstruction for long periods. Many adults inexplicably stop developing polyps.

SALT DEPLETION. Sweat salt losses can be high, especially in warm arid climates. Children should have free access to salt, and precautions against overdressing infants should be observed. Hypochloremic alkalosis should be suspected in any infant who has had gastroenteritis symptoms, and prompt fluid and electrolyte therapy should be instituted as needed.

MATURATION. Delayed sexual maturation, often associated with short stature, occurs fairly frequently. Although many have severe pulmonary infection or poor nutrition, delayed puberty also occurs in patients with otherwise mild disease and is not well explained. Adolescents with CF should receive specific counseling through their developing years concerning sexual maturation and potential reproductive problems.

SURGERY. Minor surgical procedures, including dental work, should be performed under local anesthesia if possible. Patients with good or excellent pulmonary status can tolerate general anesthesia without any intensive pulmonary measures prior to the surgery. Those with moderate or severe pulmonary infection are usually better off with a 1- to 2-wk course of intensive antibiotic treatment before surgery. If this is impossible, prompt intravenous antibiotic therapy is indicated once it is recognized that major surgery will be required. The total time of anesthesia should be kept to a minimum. After induction, tracheal suctioning is useful and should be repeated at least at the end of the operation. Patients with severe disease require monitoring of their blood gases and may require ventilatory assistance in the immediate postoperative period.

After major surgery, cough should be encouraged and postural drainage treatments should be reinstituted as soon as possible, usually within 24 hr. Adequate analgesia is important if early effective therapy is to be achieved. For those with significant pulmonary involvement, intravenous antibiotics are continued for 7–14 postoperative days. Early ambulation and intermittent deep breathing are important; an incentive spirometer can also be helpful. After open thoracotomy for treatment of pneumothorax or lobectomy, the chest tube is the greatest single obstacle to effective pulmonary therapy and should be removed as soon as possible so that full postural drainage therapy can resume.

New Therapies. Several innovative therapies are under investigation. Some possess the potential for reversing fundamental genetic or pathophysiologic aspects of the disorder and preventing or delaying the onset of airways disease (Table 363–4).

PROGNOSIS. CF remains a life-limiting disorder, although survival has improved dramatically during the last 30–40 yr. Infants with severe lung disease occasionally succumb, but most children survive this difficult period and are relatively healthy into adolescence or adulthood. However, the slow progression of lung disease eventually reaches disabling proportions. National life table data now indicate a median cumulative survival of 30 yr. Male survival is somewhat better than female survival for reasons that are not readily apparent. Survival beyond 20 yr of treatment exceeds 90% if CF is diagnosed and treatment begun before substantial lung damage has occurred.

For the most part, children with CF have good school attendance records and do not need to be restricted in their activities. A high percentage eventually attend and graduate from college. Most find satisfactory employment, and an increasing number marry.

With increasing life span, a new set of psychosocial considerations has emerged, including dependence-independence issues, self-care, peer relationships, sexuality, sterility, substance abuse, educational and vocational planning, financial burdens, and psychologic reactions to anxiety. Many of these issues are best addressed during childhood and early adolescence, prior to the onset of psychosocial dysfunction. With appropriate medical and psychosocial support, children and adolescents with CF generally cope well. Achievement of an independent and productive adulthood is a realistic goal for many.

Collins FS: Cystic fibrosis: molecular biology and therapeutic implications. Science 256:774, 1992.

Colombo C, Apostolo M, Ferrari M, et al: Analysis of risk factors for the development of liver disease associated with cystic fibrosis. J Pediatr 124:393, 1994.

Desmond KJ, Schwenk F, Thomas E, et al: Immediate and long-term effects of chest physiotherapy in patients with cystic fibrosis. J Pediatr 103:538, 1983.

Fitzsimmons SC: The changing epidemiology of cystic fibrosis. J Pediatr 122:1, 1993.

Fuchs JH, Borowitz DS, Christiansen PH, et al: Effect of aerosolized recombinant human DNase on exacerbations of respiratory symptoms and on pulmonary function in patients with cystic fibrosis. N Engl J Med 331:637, 1994.

Haeusler G, Frisch H, Waldhor T, et al: Perspectives of longitudinal growth in cystic fibrosis from birth to adult age. Eur J Pediatr 153:158, 1994.

Knowles MR: Contemporary perspectives on the pathogenesis of cystic fibrosis: From molecular aspects of clinical manifestations. New Insights into Cystic Fibrosis 1:1, 1993.

Knowles M, Gatzy J, Boucher R: Increased bioelectric potential difference across respiratory epithelia in cystic fibrosis. N Engl J Med 305:1489, 1981.

Konstan M, Byrard P, Hoppel C, Davis P: Effect of high-dose ibuprofen in patients with cystic fibrosis. N Engl J Med 332:848, 1995.

Lemna WK, Feldman FL, Kerem B, et al: Mutation analysis for heterozygote detection and the prenatal diagnosis of cystic fibrosis. N Engl J Med 322:291, 1990.

Quinton PM, Bijman J: Higher bioelectric potentials due to decreased chloride absorption in the sweat glands of patients with cystic fibrosis. N Engl J Med 308:1185, 1983.

Ramsey BW, Dorkin HL, Eisenberg JD, et al: Aerosolized tobramycin in patients with cystic fibrosis. N Engl J Med 328:1740, 1993.

Smith RL, van Velsen D, Smyth AR, et al: Strictures of ascending colon in cystic fibrosis and high strength pancreatic enzymes. Lancet 343:85, 1994.

The CF genotype-phenotype consortium: Correlation between genotype and phenotype in patients with cystic fibrosis. N Engl J Med 329:1308, 1993.

Thomassen MJ, Demko AC, Klinger JD, et al: *Pseudomonas cepacia* colonization among patients with cystic fibrosis. Am Rev Respir Dis 131:791, 1985.

Veeze H, Halley D, Bijman J, et al: Determinants of mild clinical symptoms in cystic fibrosis patients. Residual chloride secretion measured in rectal biopsies in relation to genotype. J Clin Invest 93:461, 1994.

Welsh MJ, Anderson MP, Rich DP, et al: Cystic fibrosis transmembrane conductance regulator: A chloride channel with novel regulation. Neuron 8:821, 1992.

Zabner J, Couture LA, Gregory RJ, et al: Adenovirus-mediated gene transfer transiently corrects the chloride transport defect in nasal epithelia of patients with cystic fibrosis. Cell 75:207, 1993.

CHAPTER 364

Primary Ciliary Dyskinesia

Thomas F. Boat

Kartagener described a group of children and adults with situs inversus, chronic sinusitis, and airways disease leading to bronchiectasis. This triad of findings with a familial occurrence (Kartagener syndrome, immotile cilia syndrome) as well as a disorder with similar respiratory tract findings but no situs inversus is the result of absent ciliary and sperm tail motility. The functional abnormality results from changes in the cilia and sperm tails, specifically the absence of arms on the nine peripheral microtubule doublets of the axoneme. These arms are known to contain a cilia-specific ATPase, dynein, required for the differential sliding of microtubules that results in movement of cilia.

Motility may be absent, scattered, or uncoordinated, but all forms of dysmotility result in impaired mucociliary clearance, as demonstrated by inability to clear particles deposited on the respiratory epithelial surface. The most likely pathogenic sequence is airway mucus retention and failure to clear pathogenic organisms, followed by chronic or frequently recurring respiratory tract infections and ultimately, injury to airway walls. Situs inversus occurs in about 50% of individuals with primary cilia dyskinesia (PCD). One hypothesis states that normal rotation of viscera depends on the motion of ciliated gut cells early in development. The absence of ciliary motility allows random rotation.

Other axonenemal abnormalities have been linked to chronic respiratory tract diseases: missing radial spokes that connect central and peripheral microtubules, absence or transposition of microtubules, and random ciliary orientation. Because cilia are highly complex subcellular structures, pathogenic mutations of multiple genes coding for ciliary proteins may occur. However, some of the reported structural abnormalities are observed after injury to ciliated epithelial cells by viral infection or SO_2 exposure. Therefore, definitive evidence that any structural alteration represents a discrete form of PCD awaits the identification of specific gene mutations.

GENETICS. PCD occurs in about 1 of 20,000 whites and has been reported in Japanese patients. It is probably the 3rd most common form of inherited chronic airways disease of white children, following cystic fibrosis (CF) and genetic immunodeficiency states. The inheritance pattern of PCD appears to be autosomal recessive.

CLINICAL MANIFESTATIONS. Individuals with PCD may have respiratory distress during the newborn period but may survive to adulthood without overt chronic sinusitis and airways disease symptoms. A feature that is helpful in differentiating PCD from CF is repeated bouts of acute otitis media or chronic serous otitis. Children diagnosed after several years of life often have been treated with tympanostomy tubes; conductive hearing loss is common. Many children with PCD experience frequent wheezing and may have an initial diagnosis of asthma. The hallmark symptom is a chronic, often loose or productive cough. Sputum can range from mucoid to purulent. The symptoms of acute sinusitis are occasionally encountered. Pneumonia may supervene. Lower respiratory tract symptoms can progress to weight loss, diminished exercise tolerance, and respiratory disability. Respiratory failure in childhood is uncommon, as are lung complications such as pneumothorax and hemoptysis. Lobar atelectasis, occurs frequently. Males are frequently infertile and display absent or poor sperm motility.

DIAGNOSIS. PCD should be suspected in children with chronic or recurring upper and lower respiratory tract symptoms, especially in the presence of substantial middle ear disease. Radiographic or computed tomography (CT) imaging shows involvement of the paranasal sinuses. Chest roentgenograms may demonstrate overinflation, bronchial wall thickening, and peribronchial infiltrates. Bronchiectasis is best detected by CT scanning. The presence of a right-sided heart in a child with chronic respiratory tract symptoms is virtually diagnostic, but this configuration occurs in only 50% of these patients. Pulmonary function testing of older children yields a typical obstructive pattern.

Mucociliary clearance can be assessed in cooperative children by ascertaining the time to taste perception of a saccharin particle placed on the inferior nasal turbinate. Scrapings or brushings of nasal mucosa can be examined directly by light or preferably by phase-contrast microscopy for evidence of motility. In most PCD tissue specimens, little or no ciliary motion is seen. However, because substantial motility has been documented in scrapings of several individuals with absent dynein arms, light microscopic examination of living tissue can only be used as a screening tool. The gold standard is quantitative documentation of abnormal structural elements, such as missing dynein arms or random orientation of cilia in nasal or bronchial biopsies or scrapings. Concordance of ultrastructural abnormalities in cilia and sperm is not complete. To avoid acquired ciliary changes, mucosal specimens should not be obtained until 2 wk after an acute respiratory tract infection. Ultrastructural evaluation should be reserved for highly suspicious cases.

TREATMENT. Therapy is symptomatic. Cough should be encouraged. Chest physiotherapy assists the clearance of mucus. Antibiotics should be prescribed for evidence of infection of sinuses or lower airways. The choice of antibiotics is best dictated by identification and sensitivity testing of pathogenic organisms, often pneumococcus or untypable *Haemophilus influenzae.* Oral antibiotic administration is usually effective. Bronchodilators can be used for symptomatic wheezing or for documentation of reversible airway obstruction. Children should be examined several times each year and followed by periodic chest radiographs and serial pulmonary function testing. Sinus and middle ear symptoms refractory to medical therapy deserve consultation with an otolaryngologist. Surgical intervention may be helpful in selected cases. Prevention of lung infection by measles, pertussis, influenza, and possibly by pneumococcal vaccines is highly desirable. Additional preventive measures include avoidance of cigarette smoke and other airway irritants.

PROGNOSIS. Progression of lung disease appears to be much slower for patients with PCD than for those with CF. With proper treatment, disabling lung disease often can be avoided for long periods. A normal lifespan is possible.

Afzelius BA: A human syndrome caused by immotile cilia. Science 193:317, 1976.

Barlocco EG, Valletta EA, Canciani M, et al: Ultrastructural ciliary defects in children with recurrent infections of the lower respiratory tract. Pediatr Pulmonol 10:11, 1991.

Boat TF, Carson JL: Ciliary dysmorphology and dysfunction—primary or acquired? N Engl J Med 323:1700, 1990.

Carson JL, Collier AM, Hu SS: Acquired ciliary defects in nasal epithelium of children with acute viral upper respiratory infections. N Engl J 312:463, 1985.

Pedersen H, Mygind N: Absence of axonemal arms in nasal mucosal cilia in Kartagener's syndrome. Nature 262:494, 1976.

Rutland J, deIongh RU: Random ciliary orientation: A cause of respiratory tract disease. N Engl J Med 323:1681, 1990.

SECTION 4
Diseases of the Pleura

David M. Orenstein

CHAPTER 365
Pleurisy

The most common cause of pleural effusion in children is bacterial pneumonia (see Chapter 170); heart failure, rheumatologic causes, and metastatic intrathoracic malignancy are the next most common causes. Tuberculous effusion has become much less common with improved screening and antituberculous therapy. A variety of other diseases, including lupus erythematosus, aspiration pneumonitis, uremia, pancreatitis, subdiaphragmatic abscess, and rheumatoid arthritis, account for the remainder of the cases. Males and females are equally affected.

Inflammatory processes in the pleura are usually divided into three types: dry or plastic, serofibrinous or serosanguineous, and purulent pleurisy or empyema.

365.1 Dry or Plastic Pleurisy

Dry or plastic pleurisy may be associated with acute bacterial pulmonary infections or may develop during the course of an acute upper respiratory tract illness. The condition is also associated with tuberculosis and with connective tissue diseases, such as rheumatic fever.

PATHOLOGY. The process is usually limited to the visceral pleura, with small amounts of yellow serous fluid and adhesions between the pleural surfaces. In tuberculosis, the adhesions develop rapidly, and the pleura is often thickened. Occasionally, fibrin deposition and adhesions may be severe enough to produce a fibrothorax that markedly inhibits the excursions of the lung.

CLINICAL MANIFESTATIONS. Signs and symptoms are often overshadowed by the primary disease. The principal symptom is pain, which is exaggerated by deep breathing, coughing, and straining. Occasionally, pleural pain is described as a dull ache, which is less likely to vary with breathing. The pain is often localized over the chest wall and is referred to the shoulder or the back. Pain with breathing is responsible for grunting and guarding of respirations, the child often lying on the affected side in an attempt to decrease respiratory excursions. Early in the illness, a leathery, rough, to-and-fro friction rub may be audible, but this usually disappears rapidly. Occasionally, increased dullness on percussion and suppressed breath sounds are heard if the layer of exudate is thick. Pleurisy may also be asymptomatic and detected only on roentgenograms, showing a diffuse haziness at the pleural surface or a dense, sharply demarcated shadow. The latter finding may be indistinguishable from small amounts of pleural exudate. Chronic pleurisy is occasionally encountered with conditions such as atelectasis, pulmonary abscess, connective tissue diseases, and tuberculosis.

DIFFERENTIAL DIAGNOSIS. Plastic pleurisy must be distinguished from other diseases, such as epidemic pleurodynia or trauma to the rib cage, particularly fracture of a rib, and from lesions of the dorsal root ganglia, tumors of the spinal cord, herpes zoster, gallbladder disease, and trichinosis. Even if evidence of pleural fluid is not found on physical or roentgenographic examination, a pleural tap in suspected cases often results in the recovery of a small amount of exudate, which, when cultured, usually reveals the underlying bacterial cause in cases associated with an acute pneumonia. Patients with pleurisy and pneumonia should always be screened for tuberculosis.

TREATMENT. Therapy should be aimed at the underlying disease. When pneumonia is present, neither immobilization of the chest with adhesive plaster nor therapy with drugs capable of suppressing the cough reflex is indicated. If pneumonia is not present or is under good therapeutic control, strapping of the chest to restrict expansion may afford relief from pain.

365.2 Serofibrinous Pleurisy

Serofibrinous pleurisy is most commonly associated with infections of the lung or with inflammatory conditions of the abdomen or mediastinum. Less commonly, it is found with such connective tissue diseases as lupus erythematosus, periarteritis, or rheumatic fever. On occasion, it is seen with primary or metastatic neoplasms of the lung, pleura, or mediastinum; tumors are commonly associated with a hemorrhagic pleurisy.

CLINICAL MANIFESTATIONS. Because serofibrinous pleurisy is often preceded by the plastic type, the early signs and symptoms may be those of plastic pleurisy. As fluid accumulates, pleuritic pain may disappear, and the patient may become asymptomatic if the effusion remains small, or there may be only the signs and symptoms of the underlying disease. Large fluid collections may produce cough, dyspnea, retractions, tachypnea, orthopnea, or cyanosis. Physical findings depend to some degree on the amount of effusion. Dullness to flatness may be found on percussion. There is a decrease or absence of breath sounds, a diminution in tactile fremitus, a shift of the mediastinum away from the affected side, and occasionally fullness of the intercostal spaces. If the fluid is not loculated, these signs may shift with changes in position. In infants, the physical signs are less definite; instead of decreased or absent breath sounds, bronchial breathing may be heard. If extensive pneumonia is present, crackles and rhonchi may also be audible. Friction rubs are usually detected only during the early or late plastic stage. The process is usually unilateral.

Roentgenographic examination shows a more or less homogeneous density obliterating the normal markings of the underlying lung. Small effusions may cause obliteration only of the costophrenic or cardiophrenic angles or a widening of the interlobar septa. Examinations should be performed with the patient in the supine and upright positions to demonstrate a shift of the effusion with a change in position; the decubitus position may also be helpful. Ultrasound examinations are useful.

DIFFERENTIAL DIAGNOSIS. Thoracentesis should be done when pleural fluid is present or is suspected, unless the effusion is very small and the patient has a classic lobar pneumococcal pneumonia. Examination of fluid is essential to identify acute bacterial infections and may disclose tubercle bacilli. Thoracentesis can differentiate serofibrinous pleurisy, empyema, hydrothorax, hemothorax, and chylothorax. In hydrothorax, the fluid has a specific gravity below 1.015, and evaluation reveals only a few mesothelial cells rather than leukocytes. Chylothorax and hemothorax usually have fluid distinctive in appearance; differentiating serofibrinous from purulent pleurisy is impossible without microscopic examination of the fluid. The fluid of serofibrinous pleurisy is clear or slightly cloudy and contains relatively few leukocytes and, occasionally, some erythrocytes. Cytologic examination may reveal malignant cells. Protein levels greater than 3 g/dL indicate an exudate and are likely to be associated with an infectious process. Similarly, pleural fluid lactic dehydrogenase values higher than 200 IU/L suggest an exudate. Serofibrinous fluid may rapidly become purulent. A pH less than 7.20 suggests an exudate.

COURSE. Unless the fluid becomes purulent, it usually disappears relatively rapidly, particularly with appropriate treatment of bacterial pneumonias. It persists somewhat longer with tuberculosis and connective tissue diseases and may remain or recur for a long time with neoplasms. As the effusion is absorbed, adhesions often develop between the two layers of the pleura, but little or no functional impairment usually results. Pleural thickening may develop and is occasionally mistaken for small quantities of fluid or for persistent pulmonary infiltrates. Pleural thickening may persist for a long time, but the process usually disappears, leaving no residua.

TREATMENT. Therapy is that for the underlying disease, although with large effusions, draining the fluid makes the patient more comfortable. When a diagnostic thoracentesis is done, as much fluid as possible, up to about 1 L, should be removed for therapeutic purposes. Rapid removal of 1 L or more of pleural fluid occasionally has been associated with the ensuing development of re-expansion pulmonary edema. If the underlying disease is adequately treated, further drainage is usually unnecessary, but if sufficient fluid reaccumulates to embarrass the patient's respiration, repeated thoracentesis or chest tube drainage should be performed. In older children with parapneumonic effusion, tube thoracostomy is considered necessary if the pleural fluid pH is below 7.20 or the pleural fluid glucose is below 50 mg/dL. If the fluid is clearly purulent, tube drainage is usually indicated. Systemic acidosis reduces the usefulness of pleural fluid pH measurements. Patients with pleural effusions may need analgesia, particularly after thoracentesis or insertion of a chest tube. Those with acute pneumonia often need supplemental oxygen in addition to specific antibiotic treatment.

Ben-Ami TE, O'Donovan JC, Yousefzadeh DK: Sonography of the chest in children. Radiol Clin North Am 31:517, 1993.
Light RW, Girard WM, Jenkinson SG, et al: Parapneumonic effusions. Am J Med 69:507, 1980.
Wolfe WG, Spock A, Bradford WD: Pleural fluids in infants and children. Am Rev Respir Dis 98:1027, 1968.

365.3 Purulent Pleurisy

(Empyema)

An accumulation of pus in the pleural spaces is most often associated with pneumonia due to staphylococci and less frequently with pneumococci (especially types 1 and 3) and *Haemophilus influenzae*. The relative incidence of *H. influenzae* empyema has decreased since the introduction of HiB vaccination. In pediatric practice, empyema is most frequently encountered in infants and preschool children. The disease may also be produced by rupture of a lung abscess into the pleural space, by contamination introduced from trauma or thoracic surgery, or rarely by mediastinitis or the extension of intra-abdominal abscesses.

PATHOLOGY. Most commonly, purulent pleurisy is an extensive process consisting of a series of loculated areas involving a large portion of one or both pleural cavities. Thickening of the parietal pleura occurs. If the pus is not drained, it may dissect through the pleura into lung parenchyma, producing bronchopleural fistulas and pyopneumothorax, or into the abdominal cavity. Rarely, the pus may dissect through the chest wall (i.e., *empyema necessitatis*). Pockets of loculated pus may eventually develop into thick-walled abscess cavities, or as the exudate organizes, the lung may collapse and become surrounded by a thick, inelastic envelope (i.e., peel).

CLINICAL MANIFESTATIONS. The initial signs and symptoms are primarily those of bacterial pneumonia. Patients treated inadequately or with inappropriate antibiotic agents may have an interval of a few days between the clinical pneumonic phase and the evidence of empyema. Most patients are febrile. In infants, there may be only a moderate exacerbation of respiratory distress. The older child is likely to appear more ill and in greater respiratory difficulty. Physical and roentgenographic findings may be identical to those described for serofibrinous pleurisy, and the two conditions are differentiated only by thoracentesis, which should always be performed when empyema is suspected (see Chapter 365.2). Roentgenographically, finding no shift of fluid with a change of position indicates a loculated empyema. The maximum amount of pus obtainable should be withdrawn by thoracentesis. The appearance of pus produced by different organisms is not distinctive; cultures must always be obtained and gram-stained smears should be examined for the presence of microorganisms. Blood cultures have a high yield (62% in one series), but latex agglutination may also be useful. Leukocytosis and an elevated sedimentation rate may be found.

COMPLICATIONS. With staphylococcal infections, bronchopleural fistulas and pyopneumothorax commonly develop. Other local complications include purulent pericarditis, pulmonary abscesses, peritonitis secondary to rupture through the diaphragm, and osteomyelitis of the ribs. Septic complications such as meningitis, arthritis, and osteomyelitis may also occur. With staphylococcal empyema, septicemia occurs infrequently; it is often encountered in *H. influenzae* and pneumococcal infections.

TREATMENT. Most experts think that, if pus is obtained by thoracentesis, closed drainage should be instituted immediately and controlled by an underwater seal or continuous suction. A catheter with the largest possible internal diameter should be inserted into the site where accumulation of pus is suspected; sometimes several tubes are required to drain loculated areas. Closed drainage is usually continued for about 1 wk, even though small amounts of material continue to drain after this time, probably in response to the presence of the tube in the pleural cavity. Chest tubes that are no longer draining should be removed.

Instilling fibrinolytic agents or proteolytic enzymes into the pleural cavity commonly produces severe systemic reactions in small children and does not promote drainage. Antibiotics should not be instilled into the pleural cavity because they do not improve results obtained with systemic antibiotic therapy alone and are associated with local reactions. Controlling empyema by multiple aspirations of the pleural cavity rather than by closed continuous drainage should not be attempted. If the condition is diagnosed early, thoracentesis and antibiotic treatment alone can bring about complete cure.

Systemic antibiotic therapy is required; the selection of the antibiotic should be based on the in vitro sensitivities of the responsible organism. Infant staphylococcal empyema is best treated by parenteral routes with methicillin or, when applicable, with penicillin G or vancomycin. Pneumococcal infection usually responds to penicillin, ceftriaxone, or cefotaxime but may need vancomycin if penicillin resistance develops; *H. influenzae* responds to cefotaxime, ceftriaxone, ampicillin, or chloramphenicol (see Chapter 177). With staphylococcal infections, resolution of the process is very slow, and systemic antibiotic therapy is required for 3–4 wk. Clinical response in nonstaphylococcal empyema is also slow, even with optimal treatment; little improvement may occur for as long as 2 wk. In patients with inadequately treated empyema, extensive fibrinous changes may take place over the surface of the collapsed lungs, but decortication procedures are rarely indicated. If pneumatoceles form, no attempt should be made to treat them surgically or by aspiration, unless they reach sufficient size to embarrass respiration or become secondarily infected. The long-term clinical prognosis for adequately treated empyema is excellent, and follow-up pulmonary function studies suggest that residual restrictive disease is uncommon.

McLaughlin FJ, Goldmann DA, Rosenbaum DM, et al: Empyema in children: Clinical course and long-term follow-up. Pediatrics 73:587, 1984.
Murphy D, Lockhart CH, Todd JK: Pneumococcal empyema. Am J Dis Child 134:659, 1980.
Redding GJ, Walund L, Walund D, et al: Lung function in children following empyema. Am J Dis Child 144:1337, 1990.
Siegel JD, Gartner JC, Michaels RH: Pneumococcal empyema in childhood. Am J Dis Child 132:1094, 1978.

CHAPTER 366
Pneumothorax

Pneumothorax is the accumulation of extrapulmonary air within the chest. Pneumothorax is uncommon during childhood. It most often results from leakage of air from within the lung. Air leaks can be primary or secondary and can be spontaneous, traumatic, iatrogenic, or catamenial. Pneumothorax in the neonatal period is discussed in Chapter 87.8

A primary spontaneous pneumothorax occurs in someone without trauma or underlying lung disease. Spontaneous pneumothorax with or without exertion (valsalva) occurs occasionally in teenagers and in young adults, most frequently in males who are tall and thin. Families have been described in which many members have had spontaneous pneumothoraces, with the onset ranging from birth to adulthood. Patients with collagen synthesis defects such as Ehlers-Danlos disease and Marfan syndrome are unusually prone to develop pneumothorax.

A pneumothorax arising as a complication of an underlying lung disorder, but without trauma, is a secondary spontaneous pneumothorax. Pneumothorax may occur in pneumonia, usually in connection with empyema; it may also be secondary to pulmonary abscess, gangrene, infarct, rupture of a cyst or an emphysematous bleb (e.g., in asthma), or foreign bodies in the lung. In infant staphylococcal pneumonia, the incidence of pneumothorax is relatively high. It is found in about 5% of hospitalized asthmatic children and usually resolves without treatment. Pneumothorax is a serious complication in cystic fibrosis (CF) (see Chapter 363), occurring in 10–25% of patients older than 10 yr. Pneumothorax also occurs in patients with lymphoma or other malignancies.

External chest or abdominal blunt or penetrating trauma can tear a bronchus or abdominal viscus, with leakage of air into the pleural space.

Iatrogenic pneumothorax can complicate tracheotomy, subclavian line placement, thoracentesis, transbronchial biopsy, or other diagnostic or therapeutic procedures. Pneumothorax may also occur after acupuncture treatment and is classified as iatrogenic or traumatic.

Catamenial pneumothorax, an unusual condition that is by definition associated with menses, results from passage of intra-abdominal air through diaphragmatic defects. When thoracotomy is performed for recurrent pneumothorax of unknown cause in a young woman, an examination of the diaphragm may be appropriate.

Pneumothorax may be associated with a serous effusion (i.e., hydropneumothorax) or a purulent effusion (i.e., pyopneumothorax). Bilateral pneumothorax is rare beyond the neonatal period.

CLINICAL MANIFESTATIONS AND DIAGNOSIS. The onset is usually abrupt, and the severity of symptoms depends on the extent of the lung collapse and on the amount of pre-existing lung disease. Extensive pneumothorax may involve pain, dyspnea, and cyanosis. In infancy, symptoms and physical signs may be difficult to recognize. Moderate pneumothorax may cause little displacement of the intrathoracic organs and few or no symptoms. The severity of pain usually does not directly reflect the extent of the collapse.

Usually, respiratory distress, retractions, and markedly decreased breath sounds over the involved lung are present. The percussion note over the involved area is tympanitic. The larynx, trachea, and heart may be shifted toward the unaffected side. When fluid is present, there is usually a sharply limited area of tympany above a level of flatness to percussion. The presence of amphoric breathing or, when fluid is present in the pleural cavity, of gurgling sounds synchronous with respirations suggests an open fistula connecting with air-containing tissues. Confirmatory evidence is provided when the pneumothorax fills rapidly after it has been aspirated. The diagnosis can usually be established by roentgenographic examination (Fig. 366–1). Scores are often assigned to pneumo-

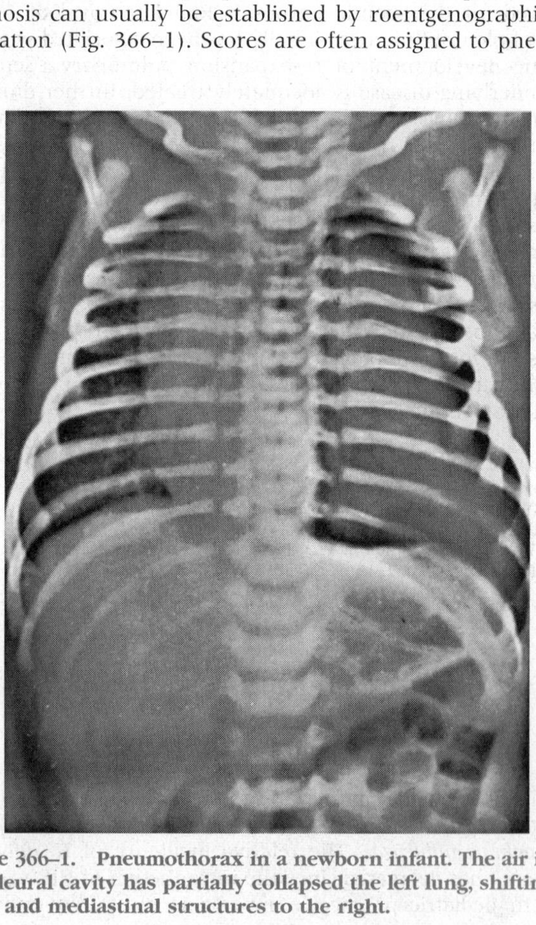

Figure 366–1. Pneumothorax in a newborn infant. The air in the left pleural cavity has partially collapsed the left lung, shifting the heart and mediastinal structures to the right.

thoraces, based on the proportion of a hemithorax filled with extrapulmonary air. A "25% pneumothorax" is one in which the lung occupies only 75% of the hemithorax. Although this provides a rough idea of the extent of leak and collection of extrapulmonary air, it is often misleading. In conditions like CF, in which the lung is relatively noncompliant, much air can accumulate under tension without very much lung collapse. The amount of air outside the lung also varies with time. A roentgenogram taken early shows less lung collapse than one taken later if the leak continues. Expiratory views accentuate the contrast between lung markings and the clear area of the pneumothorax. When considering the possibility of diaphragmatic hernia, a small amount of barium may be necessary to demonstrate that it is not free air but is a portion of the gastrointestinal tract that is in the thoracic cavity.

It is important to determine whether the pneumothorax is under tension (i.e., tension pneumothorax), because this condition limits expansion of the contralateral lung and may compromise venous return. It may be difficult to determine if a pneumothorax is under tension. Evidence of tension includes shift of mediastinal structures away from the side of air leak. A shift may be absent, as in situations in which the other hemithorax resists the shift, such as in the case of bilateral pneumothorax. When the lungs are both stiff, the unaffected lung may not collapse easily, and shift may not occur. On occasion, the diagnosis of tension pneumothorax is made only on the basis of evidence of circulatory compromise or the evidence of an audible "hiss" of rapid exit of air under tension with the insertion of the thoracostomy tube.

DIFFERENTIAL DIAGNOSIS. Pneumothorax must be differentiated from localized or generalized emphysema, from an extensive emphysematous bleb, from large pulmonary cavities or other cystic formations, from diaphragmatic hernia, from compensatory overexpansion with contralateral atelectasis, and from gaseous distention of the stomach; in most cases, a chest roentgenogram differentiates between them.

TREATMENT. Therapy varies with the extent of the collapse and the nature and severity of the underlying disease. A small or even moderate-sized pneumothorax in an otherwise normal child may resolve without specific treatment, usually within about 1 wk. A small (<5%) pneumothorax complicating asthma may also spontaneously resolve. Administering 100% oxygen may hasten resolution by increasing the nitrogen pressure gradient between the pleural air and the blood. Patients with chronic hypoxemia should be monitored closely during the administration of supplemental oxygen. Pleural pain deserves analgesic treatment. Codeine may be justified, but its respiratory depressant effect should be considered. Occasionally, morphine or meperidine is needed. If there is more than 5% collapse or if the pneumothorax is recurrent or under tension, definitive treatment is necessary. Pneumothoraces complicating CF frequently recur, and definitive treatment may be justified with the first episode, even with less than a 5% collapse. Similarly, pneumothorax complicating malignancy and its treatment, if it does not improve rapidly with observation, often necessitates treatment with chemical pleurodesis or open thoracotomy.

Closed thoracotomy (i.e., simple insertion of a chest tube) and drainage of the trapped air through a catheter, the external opening of which is kept in a dependent position under water, is adequate to re-expand the lung in most patients. To prevent recurrences when there have already been pneumothoraces, inducing the formation of strong adhesions between the lung and chest wall by a sclerosing procedure may be indicated. This can be done by the introduction of tetracycline, talc, or silver nitrate into the pleural space (i.e., chemical pleurodesis). Open thoracotomy through a limited incision, with plication of blebs, closure of fistula, stripping of the pleura (usually in the apical lung where the surgeon has direct vision), and basilar pleural abrasion is also an effective treatment for recurring pneumothorax. Stripping and abrading the pleura leaves raw, inflamed surfaces that heal with sealing adhesions. Postoperative pain is comparable to chemical pleurodesis with silver nitrate, but the chest tube can usually be removed within 24–48 hr, compared with the usual 72-hr minimum for closed thoracotomy and pleurodesis. The thoracoscope has permitted a successful surgical approach to blebectomy, pleural stripping, and instillation of sclerosing agents with somewhat less morbidity than the traditional open thoracotomy.

Extensive pleural adhesions help to prevent recurrent pneumothorax, but they also make thoracic surgery, including lung transplantation, difficult. For conditions (e.g., CF) in which lung transplantation may be a future consideration, a stepwise approach to treatment of pneumothorax has been proposed. If the patient is comfortable and the pneumothorax is small, no intervention is warranted. For a larger leak or one that does not resolve, simple thoracostomy tube drainage can be attempted. For continuing leak, or recurrence, the next step could be thoracoscopic blebectomy without pleurabrasion. Only after the failure of these steps should the full aggressive pleural stripping and abrasion be undertaken. At any step during this approach, the patient and family should be given the option of the definitive procedure if they understand it may make lung transplantation difficult or impossible. It should also be kept in mind that the longer a chest tube is in place, the greater the chance of pulmonary deterioration, particularly in a patient with CF, in whom strong coughing, deep breathing, and postural drainage are important. These are all difficult to accomplish with a chest tube in place.

Treatment of the underlying pulmonary disease should begin on admission and should be continued throughout the course of treatment directed at the air leak.

Bernhard WF, Malcolm IA, Berry RW, et al: A study of the pathogenesis and management of spontaneous pneumothorax. Dis Chest 42:403, 1962.

Noyes BE, Orenstein DM: Treatment of pneumothorax in cystic fibrosis in the era of lung transplantation. Chest 101:1187, 1992.

Stern H, Toole AL, Merino M: Catamenial pneumothorax. Chest 78:480, 1980.

Wilson WG, Aylsworth AS: Familial spontaneous pneumothorax. Pediatrics 64:172, 1979.

Yellin A, Benfield IR: Pneumothorax associated with lymphoma. Am Rev Respir Dis 134:590, 1986.

CHAPTER 367

Pneumomediastinum

Pneumomediastinum usually results from alveolar rupture during an acute or chronic pulmonary disease. However, a diverse group of nonrespiratory entities can also cause pneumomediastinum, and in some of these, the lung is not the source of the air. For example, pneumomediastinum has been reported after dental extractions, normal menses, obstetric delivery, diabetes mellitus with ketoacidosis, acupuncture, and acute gastroenteritis. Pneumomediastinum can also result from esophageal perforation or penetrating chest trauma. Occasionally, no underlying cause is found; in an apparently normal child, the pneumomediastinum can present as chest pain associated with subcutaneous air.

After intrapulmonary alveolar rupture, air can dissect through the perivascular sheaths and other soft tissue planes toward the hilum and enter the mediastinum. Pneumomediastinum is rarely a major problem in older children because the mediastinum can be depressurized by escape of air into the neck or abdomen. In the newborn, however, the rate at which air can leave the mediastinum is quite limited, and pneumomediastinum can lead to dangerous cardiovascular compromise or to pneumothorax (see Chapter 366). Acute asthma is the most common cause of pneumomediastinum in older children and teenagers. Simultaneous pneumothorax is unusual in these patients.

The principal clinical manifestations of pneumomediastinum are transient stabbing pains in the chest that may radiate to the neck. Isolated abdominal pain and sore throat also occur. The patient may have dyspnea, but it is difficult to know if this is really a separate symptom or if it is related to the chest pain. Pneumomediastinum is often difficult to detect by physical examination alone. Subcutaneous emphysema, if present, is diagnostic (see Chapter 354.3). Although cardiac dullness to percussion may be decreased, many of these patients' chests are chronically overinflated, and it is unlikely that the clinician can be sure of this finding. A mediastinal "crunch" is occasionally heard but is easily confused with a friction rub. On chest roentgenogram, the cardiac border, highlighted by the mediastinal air, is more distinct than normal, and on the lateral projection, the posterior mediastinal structures are also clearly defined. Subcutaneous air, seen roentgenographically, confirms the pneumomediastinum.

Treatment is directed primarily at the underlying obstructive pulmonary disease. Analgesics are needed occasionally for chest pain. Rarely, subcutaneous emphysema can cause sufficient tracheal compression to justify tracheotomy; the tracheotomy also decompresses the mediastinum.

Church IA, Richards W: Air leak syndromes as complications of respiratory disease in infancy and childhood. Ann Allergy 39:393, 1977.
Sandler CM, Libshitz HI, Marks G: Pneumoperitoneum, pneumomediastinum and pneumopericardium following dental extraction. Radiology 115:539, 1975.
Shahar I, Angelillo VA: Catamenial pneumomediastinum. Chest 90:776, 1986.
Sturtz GS: Spontaneous mediastinal emphysema. Pediatrics 74:431, 1984.

CHAPTER 368
Hydrothorax

In hydrothorax, the fluid is noninflammatory and has a lower specific gravity (1.015) than that of a serofibrinous exudate. It contains less protein and fewer cells and is usually associated with an accumulation of fluid in other parts of the body, such as the peritoneal cavity and the subcutaneous tissues. Hydrothorax is most often associated with cardiac or renal disease, although it may be a manifestation of severe nutritional edema, and it rarely results from venous obstruction by neoplasms, enlarged lymph nodes, or adhesions. Hydrothorax is usually bilateral in cases of renal disease and of nutritional edema; in myocardial disease, it may be bilateral, limited to the right side, or greater on the right than on the left side. The physical signs are those described under serofibrinous pleurisy (see Chapter 365.2), but in hydrothorax, there is more rapid shifting of the level of dullness with changes of position. Treatment is for the primary disorder; aspiration may be necessary when pressure symptoms are notable.

Berger HW, Rammohan G, Neff MS, et al: Uremic pleural effusion. A study in 14 patients on chronic dialysis. Ann Intern Med 82:362, 1975.

CHAPTER 369
Hemothorax

Extensive bleeding into the pleural cavity is rare in children but may result from erosion of a blood vessel in association with inflammatory processes such as tuberculosis and empyema. Hemothorax may complicate a variety of congenital anomalies, including sequestration, patent ductus arteriosus, and pulmonary arteriovenous malformation. It is also an occasional manifestation of intrathoracic neoplasms, blood dyscrasias, and bleeding diatheses, and it may be the result of thoracic trauma, including surgical procedures. Rupture of an aneurysm is unlikely during childhood. Hemothorax also occurs after blunt chest trauma and spontaneously in neonates and in older children. A pleural hemorrhage associated with a pneumothorax is called *hemopneumothorax.*

The diagnosis of a hemothorax can be made only by thoracentesis. In every case, an effort must be made to determine and treat the cause. Surgical intervention may be required to control active bleeding, and transfusion is necessary if blood loss is excessive. Inadequate removal of blood in extensive hemothorax may lead to substantial restrictive disease secondary to deposition and organization of fibrin. A decortication procedure may then be necessary.

Berry RB, Light R: When thoracentesis yields bloody pleural fluid. J Respir Dis 7:18, 1986.
Fleisher GR, Fichman KR, Honig PJ: Hemothorax in a child: an unusual cause of chest pain. Clin Pediatr 17:300, 1978.
Wilimas JA, Presbury G, Orenstein D, et al: Hemothorax and hemomediastinum in patients with hemophilia. Acta Haematol 73:176, 1985.

CHAPTER 370
Chylothorax

Chylothorax results from the escape of chyle from the thoracic duct into the thoracic cavity. The incidence has increased as cardiac surgery is performed on more complex congenital abnormalities; about 50% of these cases are now operative complications resulting from rupture of the thoracic duct. Most of the remainder are associated with chest injury or with primary or metastatic intrathoracic malignancy as a result of the pressure of enlarged lymph nodes or tumor. Less common causes include lymphangiomatosis, restrictive pulmonary diseases, thrombosis of the duct or the subclavian vein, and congenital anomalies of the duct system. Chylothorax can occur in child abuse. In some patients, especially newborns, no specific cause is identified. Chylothorax is rarely bilateral and usually occurs on the left side.

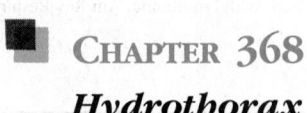

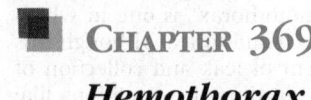

The *clinical manifestations* are those related to the presence of fluid in the thoracic cavity. The diagnosis is established when thoracentesis demonstrates a chylous effusion, a milky fluid containing fat, protein, lymphocytes, and other constituents of chyle. In newborn infants who have not yet been fed, the fluid may be clear. A pseudochylous milky fluid has been reported in cases of serous effusion, in which the fatty material was thought to arise from degenerative changes within the fluid and not from the presence of lymph. This type of fluid may be differentiated from one containing chyle by shaking it with alkalis or ether; the fluid containing chyle tends to become clear. A more definitive test is the quantitation of fluid triglyceride, which is elevated in chylous fluid, and fluid cholesterol, which may be elevated in chronic serous effusions.

Spontaneous recovery has occurred in more than 50% of the reported cases in infants younger than 1 yr of age. Repeated aspirations may be required to relieve the symptoms of pressure. However, chyle reaccumulates quickly, and repeated thoracenteses may cause considerable loss of calories, protein, and lymphocytes. Immunodeficiencies, including hypogammaglobulinemia, and abnormal cell-mediated immune responses have been associated with repeated thoracenteses for chylothorax. Attempts to prevent these problems by intravenous infusion of pleural contents are technically difficult and dangerous and of doubtful benefit. Despite large losses of T lymphocytes, clinical problems of infection are uncommon, but these patients should be protected from potentially dangerous viruses, including cytomegalovirus and live virus vaccines.

Treatment should begin in most cases with a brief period of observation on a low-fat (or medium-chain triglyceride), high-protein diet. For most patients, salt restriction and diuresis are also indicated. The total caloric intake should be above the average requirement, and several times the daily requirements of the various vitamins, especially the fat-soluble vitamins A and D, should be added. If fluid continues to reaccumulate over 1–2 wk, total parenteral nutrition should be instituted and if unsuccessful a more aggressive attempt to locate and ligate the thoracic duct may be indicated. Although even a leaking thoracic duct is difficult to locate, many successful ligations have now been reported for patients with nontraumatic chylothoraces.

Dunkelman H, Sharief N, Berman L, et al: Generalized lymphangiomatosis with chylothorax. Arch Dis Child 64:1058, 1989.
Green HG: Child abuse presenting as chylothorax. Pediatrics 66:620, 1980.
Macfarlane JR, Holman CW: Chylothorax. Am Rev Respir Dis 105:287, 1972.
McWilliams BC, Fan LL, Murphy SA: Transient T-cell depression in post-operative chylothorax. J Pediatr 99:595, 1981.
Van Aerde J, Campbell AN, Smyth JA, et al: Spontaneous chylothorax in newborns. Am J Dis Child 138:961, 1984.

SECTION 5

Neuromuscular and Skeletal Diseases Affecting Pulmonary Function

CHAPTER 371

Pectus Excavatum

David M. Orenstein

Midline narrowing of the thoracic cavity, called pectus excavatum or "funnel chest," is usually an isolated congenital skeletal abnormality but may be a manifestation of a connective tissue disorder, such as Marfan syndrome. The condition may also be acquired. Rarely, it is associated with rickets. It is occasionally associated with upper or lower airway obstruction, and when this is successfully treated or resolves spontaneously, the pectus deformity may lessen or disappear. There have been reports of the coexistence of pectus excavatum and segmental bronchomalacia, particularly in the left mainstem bronchus. Substantial pectus deformity may result in demonstrable restrictive pulmonary disease but usually has little or no functional effect.

Exercise testing has suggested an occasional link between pectus excavatum and exercise limitation. More commonly, exercise intolerance in children with pectus excavatum can be explained by limited habitual activity, related to the parents' fears.

In many patients, the heart is shifted leftward, and in some patients, cardiac function may be adversely affected. Mitral valve prolapse (which may no longer be demonstrable by echocardiography after surgical correction of the pectus) and Wolff-Parkinson-White syndrome appear to be associated abnormalities. The clinical significance of these usually mild cardiac abnormalities is not clear.

Surgical correction of the pectus is not physiologically beneficial for most patients. However, improved exercise capability and normalization of lung perfusion scans and maximal voluntary ventilation have been reported. The functional importance of these findings is not clear. Some patients with very severe deformities may seek repair for cosmetic reasons or psychologic reasons.

Fissure of the sternum is the term used when the halves of the sternum remain separated. *Pigeon breast* (i.e., *pectus carinatum*) is a prominence of the sternum and the cartilaginous parts of the ribs, with lateral depressions of the thorax. A short sternum is a common manifestation of trisomies 18 and 21.

Beiser GD, Epstein SE, Stampfer M, et al: Impairment of cardiac function in patients with pectus excavatum, with improvement after operative correction. N Engl J Med 287:267, 1972.
Castile RG, Staats BA, Westbrook PR: Symptomatic pectus deformities of the chest. Am Rev Respir Dis 126:564, 1982.
Fan L, Murphy S: Pectus excavatum from chronic upper airway obstruction. Am J Dis Child 135:550, 1981.
Godfrey S: Association between pectus excavatum and segmental bronchomalacia. J Pediatr 96:649, 1980.
Park JM, Farmer AF: Wolff-Parkinson-White syndrome in children with pectus excavatum. J Pediatr 112:926, 1988.
Shamberger RC, Welch KJ, Sanders SP: Mitral valve prolapse associated with pectus excavatum. J Pediatr 111:404, 1987.

CHAPTER 372

Asphyxiating Thoracic Dystrophy

(Jeune Syndrome)

David M. Orenstein

See Section 2, Bone and Joints.

Thoracic dystrophy is one manifestation of an autosomal recessive disease that involves a generalized abnormality of skeletal growth. It usually causes life-threatening respiratory difficulties in the newborn period or early infancy. A variety of associated congenital malformations have been reported. Most patients have respiratory distress or infection before 1 yr of age. Older children are occasionally diagnosed when their parents notice an abnormality in the appearance of the chest. A physical examination reveals constriction of the thorax and, usually, short extremities. There is no specific treatment. Surgery to expand the restrictive chest has not been rewarding. However, long-term continuous positive airway pressure was used successfully in one patient. Progressive renal failure occurs frequently among older patients. Respiratory infections should be treated promptly with antibiotics and perhaps with physical therapy. Influenza vaccine should be administered yearly.

Herdman RC, Langer LO: Thoracic asphyxiant dystrophy and renal disease. Am J Dis Child 116:192, 1968.

Oberklaid F, Dantes DM, Mayne V, et al: Asphyxiating thoracic dysplasia: Clinical, radiological, and pathological information on 10 patients. Arch Dis Child 52:758, 1977.

Wiebicke W, Pasterkamp H: Long-term continuous positive airway pressure in a child with asphyxiating thoracic dystrophy. Pediatr Pulmonol 4:54, 1988.

CHAPTER 373

Achondroplasia

David M. Orenstein

Achondroplasia has been associated with several respiratory abnormalities, including recurrent pneumonia, hypoxemia, cor pulmonale, apnea, and sudden unexplained deaths (see Chapter 637). The apneas and sudden deaths may be related to compression of the medulla and upper cervical spinal cord. The chronic and recurrent respiratory problems may be related to constricted middle and upper airways and to relatively small lungs. Children younger than 2 yr of age with achondroplasia are more likely to have reduced thoracic dimensions compared with normal than older children and adults. However, even older patients have smaller vital capacities than their sitting height would predict.

Stokes DC, Pyeritz RE, Wise RA, et al.: Spirometry and chest wall dimensions in achondroplasia. Chest 93:364, 1988.

CHAPTER 374

Kyphoscoliosis

David M. Orenstein

Scoliosis,* including idiopathic adolescent scoliosis, is discussed in Chapter 628. Mild or moderately severe scoliosis does not usually restrict the chest cage enough to affect pulmonary function seriously. Severe scoliosis, however, can dangerously impair function and may be associated with respiratory failure, cor pulmonale, or both. In addition to their restrictive lesion, patients may also have a diffusion abnormality that aggravates hypoxemia. Minor respiratory infections may be life threatening. Pulmonary function worsens with age. Acute respiratory failure, although rare, does occur before 20 yr of age.

Many patients can be managed without mechanical ventilation, and the intermediate-term prognosis is good. Even patients with moderate scoliosis may have unexpectedly severe pulmonary problems immediately after a spinal fusion procedure, because pain and a body cast restrict breathing and interfere with coughing. The magnitude of the postoperative impairment of pulmonary function correlates with the site and magnitude of the surgery and with the preoperative pulmonary abnormality. Patients with severe scoliosis, especially males, may have abnormalities of breathing during sleep, and the resultant periods of hypoxemia may contribute to the eventual development of pulmonary hypertension.

Patients in these categories should be treated as if they had life-threatening pulmonary disease. Influenza vaccine should be given yearly. Careful pulmonary function evaluation is essential before elective surgical procedures, especially before fusion. If pulmonary function is marginal (e.g., vital capacity of less than 40–50% of predicted or less than three times the tidal volume), the patient should receive instruction in and get experience with positive-pressure breathing before surgery. The possibility that the patient may awaken on assisted ventilation with an endotracheal tube should be discussed before surgery. If possible, the patient should actually see the mechanical ventilator and understand how and why it may be used. For patients with marginal pulmonary function, careful postoperative monitoring of blood gases is essential. An occasional patient with extremely severe restrictive disease should have a tracheostomy before surgery. Scoliosis surgery may predispose to deep venous thrombosis and pulmonary embolus.

Leech JA, Ernst P, Rogala EJ, et al: Cardiorespiratory status in relation to mild deformity in adolescent idiopathic scoliosis. J Pediatr 106:143, 1985.

Libby DM, Briscoe WA, Boyce B, et al: Acute respiratory failure in scoliosis or kyphosis: prolonged survival and treatment. Am J Med 73:532, 1982.

Mezon BL, West P, Israels J, et al: Sleep breathing abnormalities in kyphoscoliosis. Am Rev Respir Dis 1222:617, 1980.

Schur MS, Brown JT, Kafer ER, et al: Postoperative pulmonary function in children: comparison of scoliosis with peripheral surgery. Am Rev Respir Dis 130:46, 1984.

CHAPTER 375
Rib Anomalies

David M. Orenstein

The absence or malformation of one to two ribs usually has no substantial effect on pulmonary function and does not require treatment. An absence of multiple ribs is associated with vertebral anomalies and, ultimately, with scoliosis. A portion of lung can herniate through the defect in the chest wall; these hernias are most frequent at the level of the 1st to 5th ribs and are usually anterior (see Chapter 359). The lung may appear as a soft, easily reducible, usually nontender swelling. Minor abnormalities of muscles caused by a loss of their normal attachments are also associated with this lesion. Most rib anomalies are discovered as incidental findings on chest roentgenograms obtained as part of a workup for another illness. When the defect is large and associated with lung hernia, rib splitting and strutting techniques can provide functional and cosmetic improvement.

CHAPTER 376
Neuromuscular Diseases with Hypoventilation

David M. Orenstein

A variety of acute (poliomyelitis, Guillain-Barré syndrome, botulism, spinal cord injury) and chronic (muscular dystrophy, progressive spinal muscular atrophy, myasthenia gravis) neuromuscular diseases can cause respiratory problems (see Chapters 560–567).

CLINICAL MANIFESTATIONS. Alveolar hypoventilation with hypoxemia and respiratory failure is easily recognized, and the need for emergency measures, including mechanical ventilation, is obvious. Arterial blood gas determinations and lung volume measurements confirm its presence and are helpful for proper management. The noninvasive measurement of oxyhemoglobin saturation (pulse oximetry) and end-tidal carbon dioxide can substitute for the painful arterial blood gas test. The vital capacity, which allows assessment of the inspiratory and expiratory muscles, is particularly useful and should be carefully followed. The difference between the vital capacity obtained with the patient lying down and that obtained while sitting offers a rough guide to the strength of the diaphragm. Maximum inspiratory pressure is another easily obtained and valuable measure of the strength of the respiratory muscles.

Chronic, slowly progressive neuromuscular weakness is more likely to cause the insidious onset of respiratory abnormalities that may ultimately become incapacitating or life limiting. With progression of weakness, the patients cannot generate sufficient intrathoracic pressure for effective coughing, or they cannot hold the glottis closed well enough to allow sufficient pressure to build up in the lung. Although tidal volumes may continue to be normal, the progressive decrease in vital capacity also compromises the effectiveness of the cough. Multiple minor episodes of aspiration occur as laryngeal muscles become weaker. With the loss of adequate sigh and a decreased ability of the diaphragm to prevent compromise of the thoracic volume by the abdominal organs, patchy microatelectasis occurs, accompanied by a ventilation perfusion abnormality and hypoxemia. Microatelectasis also appear to be the major cause of decreased lung compliance in these patients. Recurrent or chronic infection then results and further restricts vital capacity. The increased viscosity of infected secretions aggravates the already impaired mucociliary clearance. Progressive loss of pulmonary tissue from the fibrosis associated with chronic infection and the chronic and worsening hypoxemia may lead eventually to pulmonary arterial hypertension and, ultimately, to right-sided heart failure. Weakness of the pharyngeal and laryngeal muscles may result in obstruction when soft tissue, normally retracted during inspiration, partially occludes the upper airway.

TREATMENT. All patients with chronic or progressive muscular weakness require close surveillance for and early treatment of respiratory complications. Prompt antibiotic treatment of upper respiratory infections is indicated. Most patients intermittently require physical therapy, including postural drainage with chest percussion, and parents should be instructed in these techniques. Postural drainage is often effective when used throughout each acute respiratory illness. In some patients, an artificial cough can be accomplished by application of sudden external pressure to the thorax. The usefulness of respiratory muscle training in patients with Duchenne muscular dystrophy has not been demonstrated conclusively. In some patients with advanced neuromuscular disease, however, training of specific muscle groups, such as neck muscles or the pectoralis major, may help with the effectiveness of cough and may permit more sustained periods off mechanical ventilation that could be lifesaving during an electrical failure. Influenza vaccine should be administered annually. However, influenza vaccine should be omitted in the extremely rare instances in which it is suspected of playing a role in the causation of the primary disease (e.g., Guillain-Barré syndrome). Pneumococcal vaccine may be indicated. Theophylline has been shown to increase diaphragm strength and endurance, but its clinical application in patients with dystrophic muscles has not been studied.

A permanent tracheostomy to allow better access to the airway for suctioning can be helpful. Some patients cannot handle secretions and may need a cuffed endotracheal tube or tracheostomy. A small tracheostomy can be plugged when suctioning is not being performed, allowing the patient to breathe and talk around the tube. A standard tracheostomy may alleviate upper airway obstruction and is useful in carefully selected patients. Patients with substantial diaphragmatic weakness may benefit from a mechanical rocking bed to reduce alveolar collapse. Intermittent positive-pressure breathing has also been proposed for this purpose. After pulmonary hypertension and overt right-sided heart failure develop, the prognosis is grave, and treatment with supplemental oxygen and other symptomatic measures allows only temporary improvement.

Ventilator management is indicated for patients whose respiratory failure is likely to be brief (e.g., myasthenia gravis). There is controversy about long-term mechanical ventilation for patients with muscular dystrophy. Such management is routinely employed by many centers and seems well accepted by many patients and families. Those who oppose such treatment point to the fact that these patients have no potential for independent functioning after mechanical ventilation is initiated. Those who support this approach point out that, because the diaphragm is among the last muscles to lose strength, these youngsters had no independent functioning for years before the onset of respiratory failure. However, many such patients and families have had acceptable life quality. The addition of the mechanical ventilator makes little difference to their degree of functioning, but it extends their lives.

Bergofsky EH: State of the art: Respiratory failure in disorders of the thoracic cage. Am Rev Respir Dis 119:643, 1979.
De Troyer A, Deisser P: The effects of intermittent positive pressure breathing on patients with respiratory muscle weakness. Am Rev Respir Dis 124:132, 1981.
De Troyer A, Estenne M, Heilporn A: The mechanism of active expiration in tetraplegic subjects. N Engl J Med 314:740, 1986.
Gilgoff IS, Barras DM, Jones MS, et al: Neck breathing: a form of voluntary respiration for the spine-injured ventilator-dependent quadriplegic child. Pediatrics 82:741, 1988.
Greenberg M, Edmonds J: Chronic respiratory problems in neuromyopathic disorders: the nature and management. Pediatr Clin North Am 21:927, 1974.
Macklem PT: Muscular weakness and respiratory function. N Engl J Med 314:775, 1986.

CHAPTER 377
Central Hypoventilation Syndromes

Gabriel G. Haddad

Patients with any of the central hypoventilation syndromes (CHS) have in common a primary defect in the central nervous system. In addition, patients may have defects in other elements of the respiratory feedback loop (e.g., carotid bodies, peripheral chemosensitivity). There are two forms of the disease: *congenital,* sometimes referred to as Ondine's curse, and *acquired.* In the pediatric age group, unlike in the adult population, most patients have a congenital form. In patients with the congenital form, there are usually no detectable *gross* neurologic abnormalities, including space-occupying lesions, although tumors and arteriovenous (AV) malformations have been described in the brain stem of such patients and other neurologic diagnoses must be considered.

CLINICAL MANIFESTATIONS. Patients with the congenital form present very early in life, often in the first few hours after delivery. Most patients are the products of noneventful pregnancies and are term infants with appropriate weight for gestational age; Apgar scores have been variable. Symptoms of respiratory failure, with slow and irregular respiratory efforts, long respiratory pauses (lasting up to 40 sec), and cyanosis, appear in the first day of life. Cardiac, respiratory, and metabolic diseases are ruled out, drug exposure is absent, and the sepsis workup is negative. One hallmark of this condition is that patients *fail* to respire adequately during *sleep,* not during wakefulness, although patients with the most severe respiratory failure have also been shown to hypoventilate in the waking state as well. In most neonates with this condition, the $Paco_2$ accumulates to very high levels, sometimes up to 80–90 mm Hg, during sleep and drops to normal levels soon after infants awaken. Infants systematically studied using respiratory, neurophysiologic, and cardiac parameters have been shown to have long respiratory pauses, a rather normal tidal volume per breath, and a very low respiratory rate, dropping to as low a level as 8–10/min during sleep, with interspersed respiratory pauses in the first few weeks of life. Respiratory rates are generally normal during wakefulness, and the lowest respiratory rates have been found in non–rapid eye movement (non-REM) or quiet sleep. Because in utero respirations are at their lowest rate during a high-voltage electroencephalogram (non-REM sleep or quiet sleep after birth), it has been speculated that there is an abnormal "persistence of fetal respiration" in this condition.

Because respiratory failure in these infants has a central cause, the hypoxemia that ensues is commensurate with hypoventilation with little or no abnormality in arterial-alveolar (A-a) gradient. However, in some patients, the hypoventilation may be severe enough to produce airway closure, microatelectasis, and an increase in A-a gradient.

In a sizable subset of these infants, abdominal distention, constipation, or complete failure to pass meconium occurs. These patients also have Hirschsprung disease with variable aganglionosis of the colon and small intestine. Whether all patients with congenital CHS have some degree of aganglionosis of the large bowel is unknown.

Patients with CHS, with or without Hirschsprung disease, have a higher heart rate than normal for their age and a heart rate variability that is low with an almost fixed heart rate and little sinus arrhythmia. This raises the question about whether these infants have generalized abnormalities in the autonomic regulation of vital functions. Other anomalies suggesting this possibility, found in these infants on autopsy, include multiple ganglioneuroblastoma of the sympathetic chain and the adrenal medulla.

PATHOGENESIS AND PATHOPHYSIOLOGY. The cause and pathogenesis are unknown. Although there have been reports of familial cases, a specific genetic inheritance mode in CHS is lacking. However, because CHS and Hirschprung disease are rare, the existence of both in the same patients raises the possibility of genetic abnormalities.

Patients with CHS alone or CHS with Hirschsprung disease have no CO_2 sensitivity and no ventilatory response to CO_2 during sleep. During wakefulness, the CO_2 set point is much lower, and they respond to it unless the condition is severe enough to hypoventilate even in the wake state. Patients with CHS and Hirschsprung disease also have been shown to have no sensitivity to O_2 lack or hypoxia. This lack of sensitivity to CO_2 and the respiratory failure do not improve with time, and the oldest children with this syndrome (late teens) still show the same failures. Older children with CHS show an increase in ventilation when they are exercised at various work rates, and the increase in ventilation they exhibit may not be related to anaerobic stimuli (lactate or pH) but rather to neural reflexes (e.g., limb movements) or hormonal cues.

There are at least two main pathways that regulate respiration in animals and humans. One is an automatic or metabolic type of pathway during which the subject's consciousness or sensorium does not play a major role, such as during sleep (except to some degree in REM sleep). The other is more dependent on sensory feedback and on a voluntary type of pathway. In CHS, it would seem that the condition expresses itself best during sleep in which time sensory feedback plays a more minor role. The defect may be in the automatic control system, which resides anatomically mostly in the brain stem. Physiologic evidence indicates that the respiratory failure in these children is mostly based on defects in central mechanisms rather than on peripheral (carotid) mechanisms, although contribution from the interactions between peripheral and central mechanisms may be important in this disease. It is also important that the group of premotor neurons, those that communicate with phrenic or intercostal motoneurons, can be excited enough to drive the respiratory musculature in certain instances (e.g., wakefulness). Although many searches for pharmacologic stimulation have failed, the fact that functional stimulation of the respiratory system is achievable in CHS indicates that pharmacologic or other interventional strategies are potentially important for devising future therapies.

On postmortem examination of some CHS patients, absence of the arcuate nucleus has been seen, but the relation of this anomaly to the disease is not clear. Gliosis in brain stem structures has also been noted, but it is not known whether this is part of a more generalized response of the central nervous system to hypoxia and ischemia that could have resulted from long-term and intermittent respiratory failure or this is part of the basic pathology of CHS.

DIFFERENTIAL DIAGNOSIS. Other neurologic diseases or conditions have to be excluded before this diagnosis is made. Brain stem infarction, tumors, AV malformations, syringomyelia, Leigh necrotizing encephalomyelopathy, olivopontocerebellar degeneration, and Möbius syndrome should be considered.

TREATMENT. Management should include general and nutritional care, ventilatory support, and prevention of cerebral hypoxia, ischemia, and acidosis. Some of these infants can grow and gain developmental and neurologic milestones that are close to normal for age, although neurologic abnormalities persist. It is hard to determine at this stage whether these abnormalities are a result of episodes of hypoxia or part of the spectrum of CHS.

Phrenic nerve pacing has been used in patients after the age of 2 yr. Although there are complications related to pacing, including phrenic nerve fibrosis, infections, and multiple surgeries, a number of these patients have become independent of mechanical ventilators.

Bogousslavsky J, Khurana R, Deruaz JP, et al: Respiratory failure and unilateral caudal brainstem infarction. Ann Neurol 28:668, 1990.

Haddad GG, Mazza NM, Defendini R, et al: Congenital failure of automatic control of ventilation, gastrointestinal motility and heart rate. Medicine (Baltimore) 57:517, 1978.

Mellins RB, Balfour HH, Turino GM, et al: Failure of automatic control of ventilation (Ondine's curse). Medicine (Baltimore) 49:487, 1990.

Mukhopadhyay S, Wilkinson PW: Cerebral arteriovenous malformation, Ondine's curse and Hirschsprung's disease. Dev Med Child Neurol 32:1087, 1990.

Shea SA, Andres LP, Shannon DC, et al: Ventilatory responses to exercise in humans lacking ventilatory chemosensitivity. J Physiol (Lond) 468:623, 1993.

Verloes A, Elmer C, Lacombe D, et al: Ondine-Hirschsprung syndrome (Haddad syndrome). Further delineation in two cases and review of the literature. Eur J Pediatr 152:75, 1993.

Weese-Mayer DE, Silvestri JM, Menzies LJ, et al: Congenital central hypoventilation syndrome: diagnosis, management, and long-term outcome in thirty-two children. J Pediatr 120:381, 1992.

Woos MS, Woo MA, Gozal D, et al: Heart rate variability in congenital central hypoventilation syndrome. Pediatr Res 31:291, 1992.

CHAPTER 378

Obesity

David M. Orenstein

Extreme obesity occasionally causes respiratory embarrassment with somnolence, dyspnea, cyanosis, and, possibly, right-sided heart failure (see Chapter 330). Chest and diaphragmatic excursions are limited, resulting in rapid, shallow breathing; alveolar ventilation is also decreased, resulting in hypoxemia. This syndrome is referred to appropriately as the obesity-hypoventilation syndrome or the Pickwickian syndrome. Ventilation-perfusion abnormalities also contribute to arterial desaturation. Obstructive sleep apnea dominates the clinical picture in many patients. Hypertension and enuresis may be present. Some of these patients appear to have a diminished ventilatory response to hypoxic drive. In those with the *Prader-Willi syndrome,* an abnormal ventilatory response to carbon dioxide has been demonstrated in family members who are otherwise normal, suggesting that the abnormal ventilatory control adds to the respiratory problems caused by the obesity rather than results from them.

Weight loss is the primary goal of treatment (see Chapter 45.2), and, if successful, it alone reduces the pulmonary problems. Some children with hypoventilation and right-sided heart failure secondary to extreme obesity may benefit from treatment with progesterone. This drug stimulates ventilation, perhaps by increasing sensitivity to carbon dioxide. Continuous positive airway pressure administered by nasal prongs may help obese patients with obstructive sleep apnea.

Lopata M, Onal E: Mass loading, sleep apnea, and the pathogenesis of obesity hyperventilation. Am Rev Respir Dis 126:640, 1982.

Orenstein DM, Boat TF, Owens RP, et al: The obesity hypoventilation syndrome in children with the Prader-Willi syndrome: a possible role for familial decreased response to carbon dioxide. J Pediatr 67:765, 1980.

Orenstein DM, Boat TF, Stern RC, et al: Progesterone treatment of the obesity hypoventilation syndrome in a child. J Pediatr 90:477, 1977.

Wilhoit SC, Brown ED, Suratt PM: Treatment of obstructive sleep apnea with continuous nasal airflow delivered through nasal prongs. Chest 85:170, 1984.

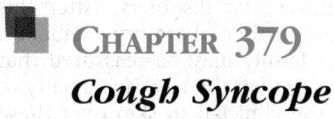

CHAPTER 379

Cough Syncope

David M. Orenstein

Cough syncope has been infrequently reported in children. During a coughing paroxysm in which high intrathoracic pressures are generated, venous obstruction, characterized by redness of the face, is followed by decreased venous return and, ultimately, by decreased cardiac output, which results in transient cerebral hypoxia and syncope. Recovery generally occurs within 10 sec to 2 min. Muscular movements and incontinence occur rarely. Although these events may simulate seizures, the underlying neuronal discharges originate in the reticular formation, unlike involvement of the cerebral cortex in true epilepsy. Asthma is the most common precipitating disease. There is no specific treatment.

Katz RM: Cough syncope in children with asthma. J Pediatr 77:48, 1970.

PART XX

*The Cardiovascular System**

Daniel Bernstein

SECTION 1

Evaluation of the Cardiovascular System

CHAPTER 380

History and Physical Examination

The importance of the history and physical examination cannot be overemphasized in the evaluation of infants and children with suspected cardiovascular disorders. After this assessment, patients may require further laboratory evaluation and eventual treatment or the family may be reassured that no significant problem exists. Although the easy availability of echocardiography may entice the clinician to skip over these preliminary steps, there are several reasons why an initial evaluation by a skilled cardiologist is still preferred: The examination allows the cardiologist to guide the echocardiographic evaluation towards confirming or eliminating specific diagnoses, increasing its accuracy; because most childhood murmurs are innocent, clinical evaluation by a pediatric cardiologist can eliminate unnecessary and expensive laboratory tests; and the cardiologist's knowledge and experience are important in reassuring the patient's family and preventing unnecessary restrictions on healthy physical activity.

HISTORY. A comprehensive cardiac history should start with details of the perinatal period, inquiring as to the presence of cyanosis, respiratory distress, or prematurity. Maternal complications, such as gestational diabetes, medication exposure, or substance abuse, can be associated with cardiac problems. If cardiac symptoms began during infancy, the timing of 1st presentation should be noted, as this can provide a clue as to the specific cardiac condition.

Many of the symptoms of congestive heart failure in infants and children are age specific. In infants, *feeding difficulties* are quite common. The infant having congestive heart failure will often take less volume per feeding and become dyspneic or diaphoretic while sucking. After falling into an exhausted sleep, the baby, inadequately fed, will awaken for the next feeding after a brief period of time. This cycle continues around the clock and must be carefully differentiated from colic or other feeding disorders. Frequent gastroesophageal reflux is also associated with congestive heart failure. Other symptoms and signs include those of *respiratory distress*—rapid breathing, nasal flaring, and chest retractions. In older children, congestive heart failure may initially be manifested by *exercise intolerance,* for example, difficulty in keeping up with peers during sports or the need for a nap after coming home from school, or by poor growth. Eliciting a history of fatigue in an older child requires specific questions about activities, including stair climbing, walking various distances, bicycle riding, and physical education class; information should also be obtained regarding more severe manifestations, such as orthopnea and nocturnal dyspnea.

Cyanosis at rest is often overlooked by parents; it may be considered merely a "deep coloring" or a normal individual variation. In contrast, cyanosis during crying or exercise is more often noted as an abnormal finding by observant parents. However, as many infants and toddlers will turn "blue around the lips" when crying vigorously or during breath-holding spells, this must be carefully differentiated from cyanotic heart disease by inquiring as to the inciting factors, length of episodes, and whether the tongue and mucous membranes also appear cyanotic. Newborns will develop cyanotic extremities when undressed and cold, and this must be carefully differentiated from true cyanosis.

Chest pain is usually not a manifestation of cardiac disease in the pediatric patient, although it is a frequent cause for referral to the pediatric cardiologist, especially in adolescents. Nonetheless, a careful history, physical examination, and, if indicated, laboratory or imaging tests will assist in identifying the etiology of chest pain (Table 380–1).

Cardiac disease may be a manifestation of a known congenital malformation syndrome (Table 380–2) or of a generalized disorder affecting the heart and other organ systems (Table 380–3). *Extracardiac malformations* may be noted in about 25% of infants with congenital heart disease. About 10% of patients have a known chromosomal abnormality, although this percentage will likely increase dramatically as our knowledge of specific gene defects linked to congenital heart disease increases. A careful family history may also reveal early coronary artery disease (familial hypercholesterolemia), generalized muscle disease (muscular dystrophy, dermatomyositis), or relatives with congenital heart disease.

GENERAL PHYSICAL EXAMINATION. This should begin with a general assessment of the patient, with specific attention to the presence of cyanosis, abnormalities of growth, and whether there is evidence of respiratory distress. It is not uncommon for the beginning examiner to place undue emphasis on cardiac murmurs to the exclusion of the rest of the exam. Evaluation of a murmur must always be performed in the context of other physical findings. It is often these associated findings, such as the quality of the pulses or the presence of a ventricu-

*Modified from W. Gersony in 14th edition.

■ TABLE 380–1 Differential Diagnosis of Pediatric Chest Pain

Musculoskeletal (common)
Trauma (accidental, abuse)
Exercise, overuse injury (strain, bursitis)
Costochondritis (Tietze syndrome)
Herpes zoster (cutaneous)
Pleurodynia
Sickle cell anemia vaso-occlusive crisis
Osteomyelitis (rare)
Primary or metastatic tumor (rare)
Pulmonary (common)
Pneumonia
Pleurisy
Asthma
Pneumothorax
Infarction (sickle cell anemia)
Foreign body
Embolism (rare)
Pulmonary hypertension (rare)
Tumor (rare)
Gastrointestinal (rare)
Esophagitis (gastroesophageal reflux)
Esophageal foreign body
Esophageal spasm
Cholecystitis
Subdiaphragmatic abscess
Perihepatitis (Fitz-Hugh–Curtis syndrome)
Peptic ulcer disease
Cardiac (rare)
Pericarditis
Postpericardiotomy syndrome
Endocarditis
Mitral valve prolapse
Aortic stenosis
Arrhythmias
Marfan syndrome (dissecting aortic aneurysm)
Anomalous coronary artery
Kawasaki disease
Cocaine, sympathomimetic ingestion
Angina (familial hypercholesterolemia)
Idiopathic (common)
Anxiety, hyperventilation
Other (common)
Spinal cord or nerve root compression
Breast-related pathology

lar heave, that provide an important clue to a specific cardiac diagnosis.

Accurate measurement of *height and weight,* and plotting on a standard growth chart are important as both cardiac failure and chronic cyanosis often result in failure to thrive. This growth failure is usually manifested predominantly by poor weight gain; if length or head circumference are also affected, additional congenital malformations or metabolic disorders may be present.

Mild *cyanosis* may be too subtle for early detection, and clubbing of the fingers and toes is not usually manifested until late in the 1st yr of life, even in the presence of severe arterial oxygen desaturation. Cyanosis is best observed over the nail beds, lips, tongue, and mucous membranes. Differential cyanosis, manifested by blue lower extremities and pink upper extremities (usually right arm), is seen with right-to-left shunting across a ductus arteriosus in the presence of a coarctation or interrupted aortic arch. Circumoral cyanosis or blueness about the forehead may be the result of prominent venous plexuses in these areas rather than decreased arterial oxygen saturation. The extremities of infants will often turn blue when the infant is unwrapped and cold (acrocyanosis), and this can be distinguished from central cyanosis by examination of the tongue and mucous membranes.

Congestive heart failure in infants and children usually results in some degree of hepatomegaly and occasionally splenomegaly. The sites of presentation of peripheral edema are age dependent. In infants, edema is usually seen around the eyes and over the flanks, especially after first waking in the morning. Older children and teenagers will manifest both periorbital edema and pedal edema. A frequent first complaint for these older patients is that their clothes no longer fit.

The *heart rate* of newborn infants is rapid and subject to wide fluctuations (Table 380–4). The average rate ranges from 120 to 140 beats/min and may increase to 170+ beats/min during crying and activity, or drop to 70–90 beats/min during sleep. As the child grows older, the average pulse rate becomes slower and may be as low as 40/min in athletic adolescents. Persistent tachycardia (over 200/min in neonates, 150/min in infants, or 120/min in older children), bradycardia, or irregular heart beat other than sinus arrhythmia require investigation to exclude pathologic arrhythmias (see Chapter 388).

Careful evaluation of the *character of the pulses* is an important early step in the physical diagnosis of congenital heart disease. A wide pulse pressure with bounding pulses may suggest an aortic runoff lesion, such as patent ductus arteriosus, aortic insufficiency, an arterial-venous communication, or increased cardiac output secondary to anemia, anxiety, or conditions associated with increased catecholamine secretion. Diminished pulses are associated with heart failure, pericardial tamponade, left ventricular outflow obstruction, or cardiomyopathy. The radial and femoral pulses should also be felt simultaneously. Normally the femoral pulse should be appreciated immediately before the radial pulse. In coarctation of the aorta, however, blood flow to the descending aorta may channel through collateral vessels, resulting in the femoral pulse being delayed until after the radial pulse (radial-femoral delay).

The *blood pressure* should be measured in the arms as well as in the legs, the latter on at least one occasion to be certain that coarctation of the aorta is not overlooked. Palpation of decreased femoral and/or dorsalis pedis pulses alone is not reliable to exclude a coarctation. In older children a mercury sphygmomanometer with a cuff that covers approximately two thirds of the upper arm or leg may be utilized for measurement. A cuff that is too small will invariably result in falsely high readings, while a cuff that is somewhat too large will record slightly decreased pressures. Pediatric clinical facilities should be equipped with 3, 5, 7, 12, and 18 cm cuffs to accommodate the large spectrum of pediatric patient sizes. The 1st Korotkoff sounds indicate the systolic pressure. As the cuff pressure is slowly decreased, the sounds usually become muffled before they disappear. The diastolic pressure may be recorded when the sounds become muffled (preferred) or when they disappear; the former is usually higher and the latter lower than the true diastolic pressure. For lower extremity blood pressure determination, the stethoscope is placed over the popliteal artery. Ordinarily, the pressure recorded in the legs with the cuff technique is about 10 mm Hg higher than in the arms.

In infants the blood pressure can be obtained by auscultation, palpation, or the *flush method.* The last technique is most feasible in a restless infant. A cuff of appropriate size is placed around the upper arm or thigh. The distal limb is squeezed and the cuff rapidly inflated so that blanching is noted. The cuff is then gradually deflated. At the point at which the limb flushes red, the blood pressure obtained corresponds to a systolic value slightly below that found by the direct arterial or auscultatory method. Also available are ultrasonic (Doppler) and oscillometric (Dinamap) devices, which, if used properly, provide accurate measurements in infants as well as children.

Blood pressure varies with the age of the child and is closely related to height and weight. Significant increases occur during adolescence, and there are many temporary variations before the more stable levels of adult life are attained. Exercise, excitement, coughing, and straining may raise the systolic pressures of children as much as 40–50 mm Hg above their usual levels. Variability of blood pressure among children of approxi-

■ **TABLE 380–2 Congenital Malformation Syndromes Associated with Congenital Heart Disease**

Syndrome	Features
Chromosomal Disorders	
21-Trisomy (Down syndrome)	Endocardial cushion defect, VSD,* ASD†
22p-Trisomy (cat eye syndrome)	Miscellaneous, total anomalous pulmonary venous return
18-Trisomy	VSD, ASD, PDA,‡ coarctation of aorta, bicuspid aortic or pulmonary valve
13-Trisomy	VSD, ASD, PDA, coarctation of aorta, bicuspid aortic or pulmonary valve
9-Trisomy	Miscellaneous
XXXXY	PDA, ASD
Penta X	PDA, VSD
Triploidy	VSD, ASD, PDA
XO (Turner syndrome)	Bicuspid aortic valve, coarctation of aorta
Fragile X	Mitral valve prolapse, aortic root dilatation
Duplication 3q2	Miscellaneous
Deletion 4p	VSD, PDA, aortic stenosis
Deletion 9p	Miscellaneous
Deletion 5p (cri du chat syndrome)	VSD, PDA, ASD
Deletion 10q	VSD, TOF,§ conotruncal lesions‖
Deletion 13q	VSD
Deletion 18q	VSD
Syndrome Complexes	
CHARGE association (*c*oloboma, *h*eart, *a*tresia choanae, *r*etardation, *g*enital and *e*ar anomalies)	VSD, ASD, PDA, TOF, endocardial cushion defect
DiGeorge sequence, CATCH 22	Aortic arch anomalies, conotruncal anomalies
Alagille syndrome (arteriohepatic dysplasia)	Peripheral pulmonic stenosis
VATER association (*v*ertebral, *a*nal, *t*racheoesophageal, *r*adial, and *r*enal anomalies)	VSD, TOF, ASD, PDA
FAVS (*f*acio-*a*uriculo-*v*ertebral *s*pectrum)	TOF, VSD
CHILD (*c*ongenital *h*emidysplasia with *i*chthyosiform erythroderma, *l*imb *d*efects)	Miscellaneous
Mulibrey nanism (*mu*scle, *li*ver, *br*ain, *ey*e)	Pericardial thickening, constrictive pericarditis
Asplenia syndrome	Complex cyanotic heart lesions with decreased pulmonary blood flow, transposition of great arteries, anomalous pulmonary venous return, dextrocardia, single ventricle, single atrioventricular valve
Polysplenia syndrome	Acyanotic lesions with increased pulmonary blood flow, azygos continuation of inferior vena cava, partial anomalous pulmonary venous return, dextrocardia, single ventricle, common atrioventricular valve
Teratogenic Agents	
Congenital rubella	PDA, peripheral pulmonic stenosis
Fetal hydantoin syndrome	VSD, ASD, coarctation of aorta, PDA
Fetal alcohol syndrome	ASD, VSD
Fetal valproate effects	Coarctation of aorta, hypoplastic left side of the heart, aortic stenosis, pulmonary atresia, VSD
Maternal phenylketonuria	VSD, ASD, PDA, coarctation of aorta
Retinoic acid embryopathy	Conotruncal anomalies
Others	
Apert syndrome	VSD
Autosomal dominant polycystic kidney disease	Mitral valve prolapse
Carpenter	PDA
Conradi	VSD, PDA
Crouzon	PDA, coarctation of aorta
Cutis laxa	Pulmonary hypertension, pulmonic stenosis
de Lange	VSD
Ellis-van Creveld	Single atrium, VSD
Holt-Oram	ASD, VSD; 1st-degree heart block
Infant of diabetic mother	Hypertrophic cardiomyopathy, VSD, conotruncal anomalies
Kartagener	Dextrocardia
Meckel-Gruber	ASD, VSD
Noonan	Pulmonic stenosis, ASD, cardiomyopathy
Pallister-Hall	Endocardial cushion defect
Rubinstein-Taybi	VSD
Scimitar	Hypoplasia of the right lung, anomalous pulmonary venous return to the inferior vena cava
Smith-Lemli-Opitz	VSD, PDA
Thrombocytopenia and absent radius (TAR)	ASD, TOF
Treacher Collins	VSD, ASD, PDA
Williams syndrome	Supravalvular aortic stenosis, peripheral pulmonic stenosis

**VSD = ventricular septal defect.*
†ASD = atrial septal defect.
‡PDA = patent ductus arteriosus.
§TOF = tetralogy of Fallot.
‖Conotruncal = TOF, pulmonary atresia, truncus arteriosus, transposition of the great arteries.

■ TABLE 380–3 Cardiac Manifestations of Systemic Diseases

Systemic Disease	Cardiac Complications
Inflammatory Disorders	
Sepsis	Hypotension, myocardial dysfunction, pericardial effusion, pulmonary hypertension
Juvenile rheumatoid arthritis	Pericarditis, rarely myocarditis
Systemic lupus erythematosus	Pericarditis, Libman-Sacks endocarditis, coronary arteritis, coronary atherosclerosis (with steroids), congenital heart block
Scleroderma	Pulmonary hypertension, myocardial fibrosis, cardiomyopathy
Dermatomyositis	Cardiomyopathy, arrhythmias, heart block
Kawasaki disease	Coronary artery aneurysm and thrombosis, myocardial infarction, myocarditis, valvular insufficiency
Sarcoidosis	Granuloma, fibrosis, amyloidosis, biventricular hypertrophy, arrhythmias
Lyme disease	Arrhythmias, myocarditis
Löffler hypereosinophilic syndrome	Endomyocardial disease
Inborn Errors of Metabolism	
Refsum	Arrhythmia, sudden death
Hunter-Hurler	Valvular insufficiency, heart failure, hypertension
Fabry	Mitral insufficiency, coronary artery disease with myocardial infarction
Glycogen storage disease IIa (Pompe disease)	Short P-R interval, cardiomegaly, heart failure, arrhythmias
Carnitine deficiency	Heart failure, cardiomyopathy
Gaucher	Pericarditis
Homocystinuria	Coronary thrombosis
Alkaptonuria	Atherosclerosis, valvular disease
Morquio-Ullrich	Aortic incompetence
Scheie	Aortic incompetence
Connective Tissue Disorders	
Arterial calcification of infancy	Calcinosis of coronary arteries, aorta
Marfan	Aortic and mitral insufficiency, dissecting aortic aneurysm, mitral valve prolapse
Congenital contractural arachnodactyly	Mitral insufficiency or prolapse
Ehlers-Danlos	Mitral valve prolapse, dilated aortic root
Osteogenesis imperfecta	Aortic incompetence
Pseudoxanthoma elasticum	Peripheral arterial disease
Neuromuscular Disorders	
Friedreich ataxia	Cardiomyopathy
Duchenne dystrophy	Cardiomyopathy, heart failure
Tuberous sclerosis	Cardiac rhabdomyoma
Familial deafness	Occasionally arrhythmia, sudden death
Neurofibromatosis	Pulmonic stenosis, pheochromocytoma, coarctation of aorta
Riley-Day	Episodic hypertension, postural hypotension
Von Hippel-Lindau	Hemangiomas, pheochromocytomas
Endocrine-Metabolic Disorders	
Graves	Tachycardia, arrhythmias, heart failure
Hypothyroidism	Bradycardia, pericardial effusion, cardiomyopathy, low-voltage ECG
Pheochromocytoma	Hypertension, myocardial ischemia, myocardial fibrosis, cardiomyopathy
Carcinoid	Right-sided endocardial fibrosis
Hematologic Disorders	
Sickle cell anemia	High-output heart failure, cardiomyopathy, cor pulmonale
Thalassemia major	High-output heart failure, hemochromatosis
Hemochromatosis (1° or 2°)	Cardiomyopathy
Others	
Cockayne	Atherosclerosis
Familial dwarfism and nevi	Cardiomyopathy
Jervell and Lange-Nielsen	Prolonged Q-T interval, sudden death
Leopard (lentiginosis)	Pulmonic stenosis, prolonged Q-T interval
Progeria	Accelerated atherosclerosis
Rendu-Osler-Weber	Arteriovenous fistula (lung, liver, mucous membrane)
Romano-Ward	Prolonged Q-T interval, sudden death
Weill-Marchesani	Patent ductus arteriosus
Werner	Vascular sclerosis, cardiomyopathy

mately the same age and body build should be expected, and serial measurements should always be obtained in the evaluation of a patient with hypertension (Figs. 380–1 to 380–6).

In cooperative older children, inspection of the jugular venous pulse wave provides information about the *central venous pressure* and right atrial pressure. The neck veins should be inspected with the patient sitting at a 90 degree angle. Under these conditions the external jugular vein should not be visible above the clavicles unless venous pressure is elevated. Increased venous pressure transmitted to the internal jugular vein may appear as venous pulsations without visible distention; such pulsation is not seen in normal children reclining at an angle of 45 degrees. Because the great veins are in direct communication with the right atrium, changes of pressure and volume of this chamber are also transmitted to the veins. The one exception occurs in superior vena caval obstruction, in which venous pulsatility is lost.

CARDIAC EXAMINATION. The heart should be examined in a systematic manner starting with *inspection and palpation.* Much can be learned prior to auscultation that can narrow the list of differential diagnoses. A **precordial bulge** to the left of the

■ **TABLE 380–4 Pulse Rates at Rest**

Age	Lower Limits of Normal		Average		Upper Limits of Normal	
Newborn	70/min		125/min		190/min	
1–11 mo	80		120		160	
2 yr	80		110		130	
4 yr	80		100		120	
6 yr	75		100		115	
8 yr	70		90		110	
10 yr	70		90		110	
	Girls	*Boys*	*Girls*	*Boys*	*Girls*	*Boys*
12 yr	70	65	90	85	110	105
14 yr	65	60	85	80	105	100
16 yr	60	55	80	75	100	95
18 yr	55	50	75	70	95	90

sternum with increased precordial activity suggests cardiac enlargement. A **substernal thrust** indicates the presence of right ventricular enlargement; an **apical heave** is noted with left ventricular hypertrophy. A **hyperdynamic precordium** suggests a volume load such as that found with a large left-to-right shunt. In contrast, a **silent precordium** with a barely detectable apical impulse suggests a pericardial effusion or severe cardiomyopathy.

The relationship of the apical impulse to the midclavicular line, determined with the child in the prone position, is also helpful in the estimation of cardiac size: The apical impulse moves laterally and inferiorly with enlargement of the left

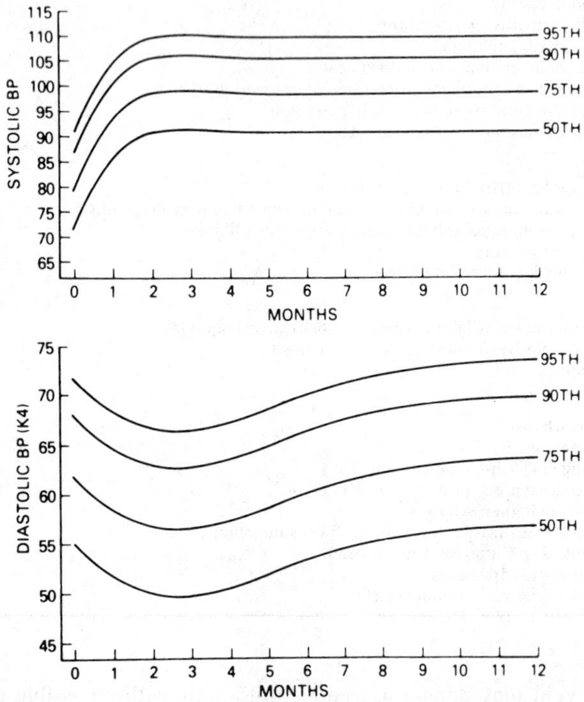

90TH PERCENTILE													
SYSTOLIC BP	87	101	106	106	106	105	105	105	105	105	105	105	105
DIASTOLIC BP	68	65	63	63	63	65	66	67	68	68	69	69	69
HEIGHT CM	51	59	63	66	68	70	72	73	74	76	77	78	80
WEIGHT KG	4	4	5	5	6	7	8	9	9	10	10	11	11

Figure 380–1. Age-specific percentiles of BP measurements in boys—birth to 12 mo of age; Korotkoff phase IV (K4) used for diastolic BP. (From National Heart, Lung, and Blood Institute, Bethesda, MD: Report of the second task force on blood pressure control in children—1987. Reproduced by permission of Pediatrics. Vol 79, p 1. Copyright © 1987.)

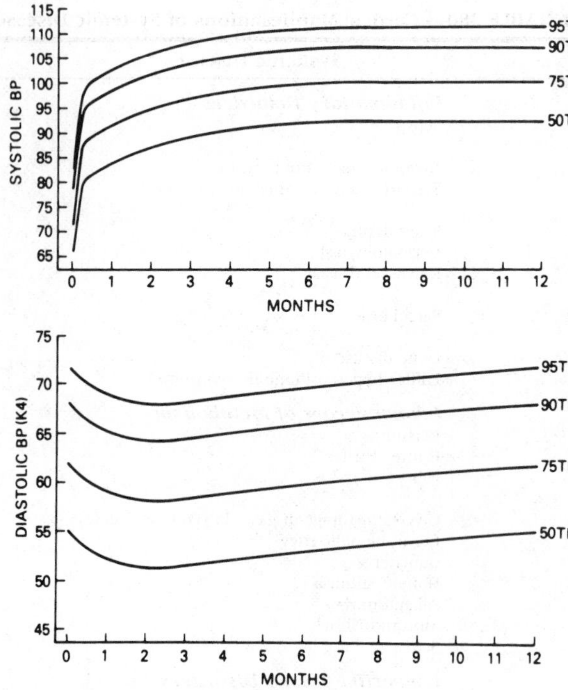

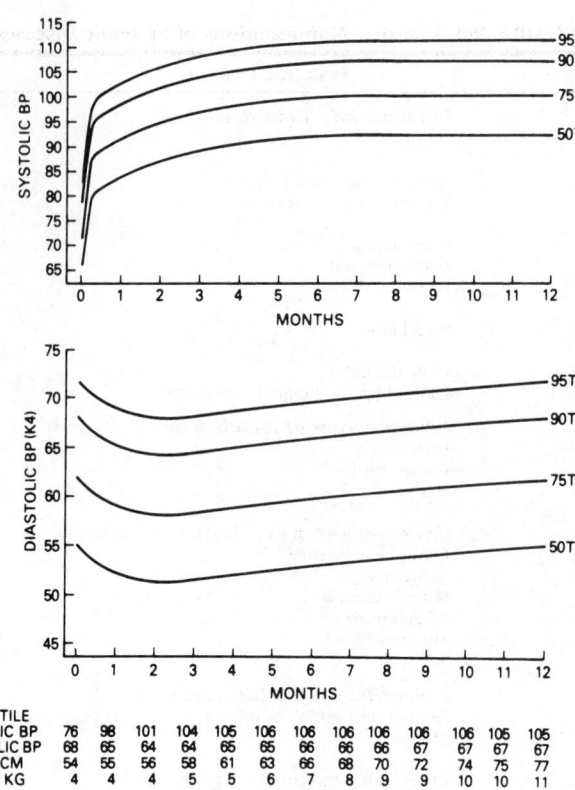

90TH PERCENTILE													
SYSTOLIC BP	76	98	101	104	105	106	106	106	106	106	106	105	105
DIASTOLIC BP	68	65	64	64	65	65	66	66	66	67	67	67	67
HEIGHT CM	54	55	56	58	61	63	66	68	70	72	74	75	77
WEIGHT KG	4	4	4	5	5	6	7	8	9	9	10	10	11

Figure 380–2. Age-specific percentiles of BP measurements in girls—birth to 12 mo of age; Korotkoff phase IV (K4) used for diastolic BP. (From National Heart, Lung, and Blood Institute, Bethesda, MD: Report of the second task force on blood pressure control in children—1987. Reproduced by permission of Pediatrics. Vol 79, p 1. Copyright © 1987.)

ventricle. Right-sided apical impulses signify dextrocardia, tension pneumothorax, or left-sided thoracic space-occupying lesions (e.g., diaphragmatic hernia).

Thrills are the palpable equivalent of murmurs, and correlate with the area of maximum auscultatory intensity of the murmur. It is important to palpate the suprasternal notch and neck for **aortic bruits,** which may indicate the presence of aortic stenosis or, when less prominent, pulmonary stenosis. Right lower sternal border and apical systolic thrills are characteristic of ventricular septal defect and mitral insufficiency, respectively. Diastolic thrills are occasionally palpable in the presence of atrioventricular valvular stenosis. The timing and localization of thrills should be carefully noted.

Auscultation is an art that can be improved upon with practice and determination. The diaphragm of the stethoscope is placed firmly on the chest for high-pitched sounds; a lightly placed bell is optimal for low-pitched sounds. The physician should initially concentrate on the characteristics of the individual heart sounds and their variation with respirations, and later on murmurs. The patient should be supine, lying quietly, and breathing normally. The 1st heart sound is best heard at the apex, whereas the 2nd sound should be evaluated at the upper left and right sternal borders. The 1st heart sound is caused by the closure of the atrioventricular valves (mitral and tricuspid); the 2nd sound is caused by the closure of the semilunar valves (aortic and pulmonary; Fig. 380–7). During inspiration the decrease in intrathoracic pressure results in increased filling of the right side of the heart, increasing right ventricular ejection time and thus delaying pulmonary valve closure; thus the splitting of the 2nd heart sound increases during inspiration and decreases during expiration.

Often the 2nd heart sound appears to be single during expi-

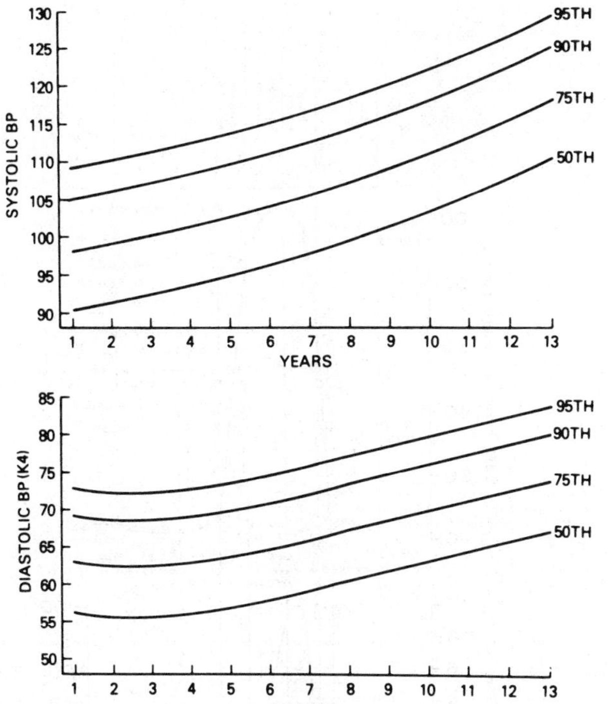

90TH PERCENTILE													
SYSTOLIC BP	105	106	107	108	109	111	112	114	115	117	119	121	124
DIASTOLIC BP	69	68	68	69	69	70	71	73	74	75	76	77	79
HEIGHT CM	80	91	100	108	115	122	129	135	141	147	153	159	165
WEIGHT KG	11	14	16	18	22	25	29	34	39	44	50	55	62

Figure 380–3. Age-specific percentiles for BP measurements in boys—1–13 yr of age; Korotkoff phase IV (K4) used for diastolic BP. (From National Heart, Lung, and Blood Institute, Bethesda, MD: Report of the second task force on blood pressure control in children—1987. Reproduced by permission of Pediatrics. Vol 79, p 1. Copyright © 1987.)

ration. The presence of a normally split 2nd sound is strong evidence against the diagnosis of an atrial septal defect, defects associated with pulmonary artery hypertension, severe pulmonary valve stenosis, aortic and pulmonary atresia, and truncus arteriosus. Wide splitting is noted in atrial septal defect, pulmonary stenosis, Ebstein anomaly, total anomalous pulmonary venous return, tetralogy of Fallot, and right bundle branch block. An accentuated pulmonic component of the 2nd sound with narrow splitting signifies pulmonary hypertension. A single 2nd sound occurs in pulmonary or aortic atresia or severe stenosis, truncus arteriosus, and often in transposition of the great arteries.

A 3rd heart sound is best heard with the bell at the apex in mid-diastole. A 4th sound, occurring in conjunction with atrial contraction, may be heard just prior to the 1st heart sound in late diastole. The 3rd sound may be normal in an adolescent with a relatively slow heart rate, but in a patient with the clinical signs of congestive heart failure and tachycardia, it may be heard as a gallop rhythm and may merge with a 4th heart sound, known as a summation gallop. A **gallop** rhythm is attributed to poor compliance of the ventricle with an exaggeration of the normal 3rd sound associated with ventricular filling.

Ejection clicks, which are heard in early systole, are related to dilatation of, or hypertension in, the aorta or pulmonary artery. They are heard so close to the 1st heart sound that they may be mistaken for a split 1st sound. Aortic ejection clicks are best heard at the left mid to right upper sternal border and are constant in intensity. They occur in conditions in which the aorta is dilated (e.g., aortic stenosis, tetralogy of Fallot, truncus arteriosus). Pulmonary ejection clicks, associated with mild to moderate pulmonary stenosis, are best heard at the left mid to upper sternal border and vary with respirations, often disappearing with inspiration. In contrast, split 1st heart sounds are usually heard best at the lower left sternal border. A midsystolic click heard at the apex, often preceding a late systolic murmur, suggests mitral valve prolapse.

Murmurs should be described as to their intensity, pitch, timing (systolic or diastolic), variation in intensity, time to peak intensity, area of maximal intensity, and radiation to other areas. Auscultation for murmurs should be carried out across the upper precordium, down the left or right sternal border, and out to the apex and left axilla. Auscultation should also always be performed in the right axilla and over the back. **Systolic murmurs** are classified as ejection, pansystolic, or late systolic according to the timing of the murmur in relation to the 1st and 2nd heart sounds. The intensity of systolic murmurs is graded from I to VI: I, barely audible; II, medium intensity; III, loud but no thrill; IV, loud with a thrill; V, very loud but still requires the stethoscope to be on the chest; and VI, so loud that the murmur can be heard with the stethoscope off the chest.

Systolic ejection murmurs start a short time after a well-heard 1st heart sound, increase in intensity, peak, and then decrease in intensity; they usually end before the 2nd sound. However, in patients with severe aortic or pulmonary stenosis, the murmur may extend beyond the 1st component of the 2nd sound, thus obscuring it. Pansystolic or holosystolic murmurs begin almost simultaneously with the 1st heart sound and continue throughout systole, on occasion becoming gradually decrescendo. It is helpful to remember that after the closure of the atrioventricular valves (the 1st heart sound), there is a brief period during which ventricular pressure increases

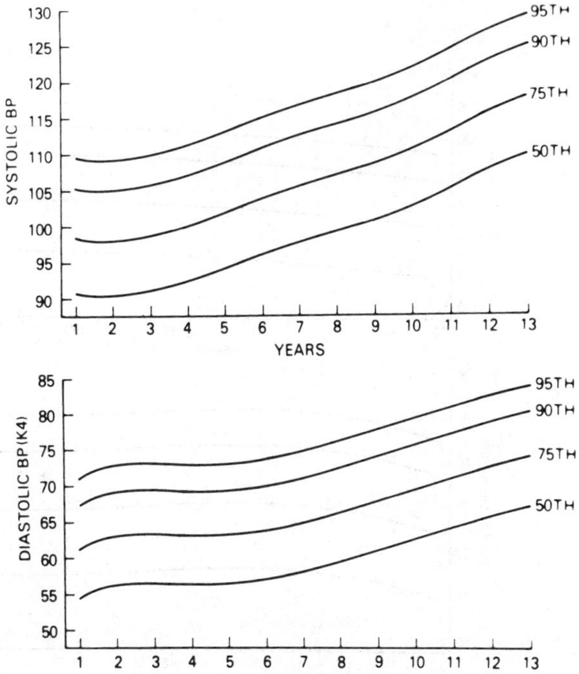

90TH PERCENTILE													
SYSTOLIC BP	105	105	106	107	109	111	112	114	115	117	119	122	124
DIASTOLIC BP	67	69	69	69	69	70	71	72	74	75	77	78	80
HEIGHT CM	77	89	98	107	115	122	129	135	142	148	154	160	165
WEIGHT KG	11	13	15	18	22	25	30	35	40	45	51	58	63

Figure 380–4. Age-specific percentiles of BP measurements in girls—1–13 yr of age; Korotkoff phase IV (K4) used for diastolic BP. (From National Heart, Lung, and Blood Institute, Bethesda, MD: Report of the second task force on blood pressure control in children—1987. Reproduced by permission of Pediatrics. Vol 79, p 1. Copyright © 1987.)

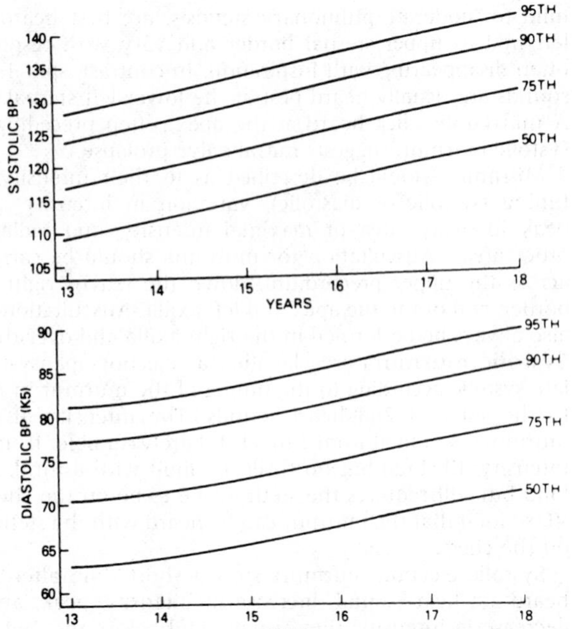

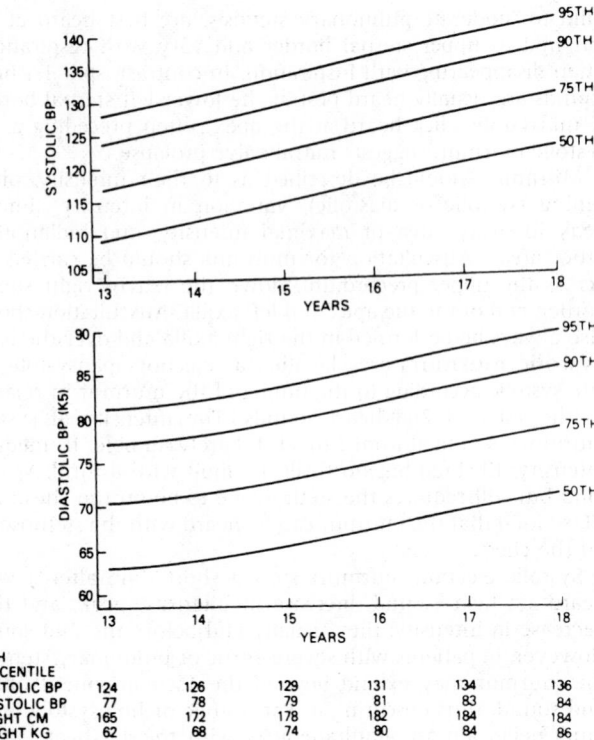

90TH PERCENTILE						
SYSTOLIC BP	124	126	129	131	134	136
DIASTOLIC BP	77	78	79	81	83	84
HEIGHT CM	165	172	178	182	184	184
WEIGHT KG	62	68	74	80	84	86

Figure 380–5. Age-specific percentiles of BP measurements in boys—13–18 yr of age; Korotkoff phase V (K5) used for diastolic BP. (From National Heart, Lung, and Blood Institute, Bethesda, MD: Report of the second task force on blood pressure control in children—1987. Reproduced by permission of Pediatrics. Vol 79, p 1. Copyright © 1987.)

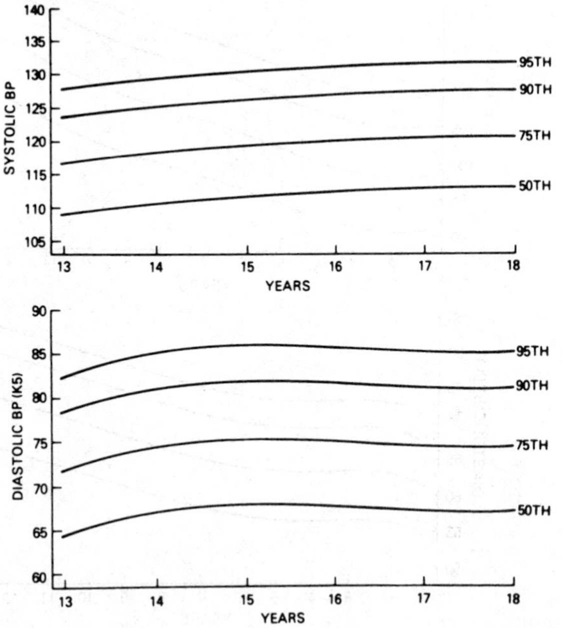

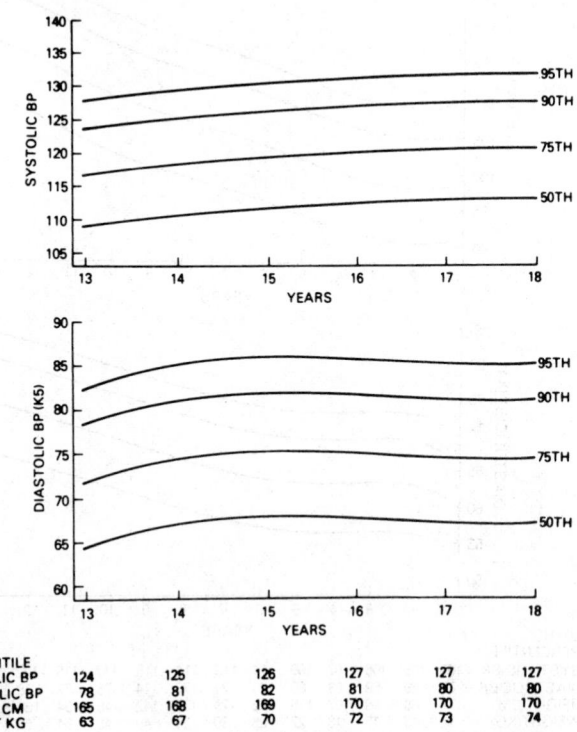

90TH PERCENTILE						
SYSTOLIC BP	124	125	126	127	127	127
DIASTOLIC BP	78	81	82	81	80	80
HEIGHT CM	165	168	169	170	170	170
WEIGHT KG	63	67	70	72	73	74

Figure 380–6. Age-specific percentiles of BP measurements in girls—13–18 yr of age; Korotkoff phase V (K5) used for diastolic BP. (From National Heart, Lung, and Blood Institute, Bethesda, MD: Report of the second task force on blood pressure control in children—1987. Reproduced by permission of Pediatrics. Vol 79, p 1. Copyright © 1987.)

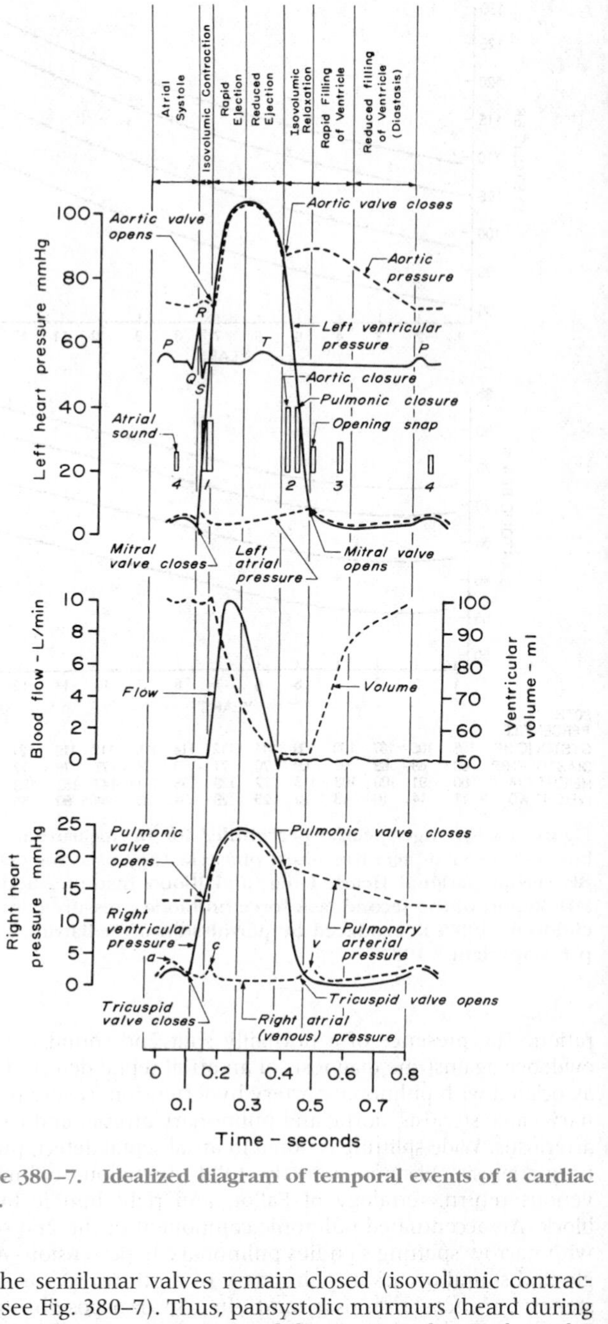

Figure 380–7. Idealized diagram of temporal events of a cardiac cycle.

but the semilunar valves remain closed (isovolumic contraction; see Fig. 380–7). Thus, pansystolic murmurs (heard during both isovolumic contraction and the ejection phases of systole) cannot be caused by flow across the semilunar valves, because these valves are closed during isovolumic contraction. Pansystolic murmurs are thus related to blood exiting the contracting ventricle via either a ventricular septal defect or atrioventricular (mitral or tricuspid) valve insufficiency. Systolic ejection murmurs usually imply increased flow or stenosis across a semilunar (aortic or pulmonary) valve. In infants with rapid heart rates, it is often difficult to distinguish between ejection and pansystolic murmurs. However, if a clear 1st heart sound can be appreciated, the murmur is most likely ejection in nature.

A continuous murmur is a systolic murmur that continues or "spills" into diastole and indicates continuous flow, such as in the presence of a patent ductus arteriosus or other aortopulmonary communication. This should be differentiated from a to-and-fro murmur, which indicates that the systolic component of the murmur ends at or before the 2nd sound and the diastolic murmur begins after semilunar valve closure (e.g., aortic or pulmonary stenosis combined with insufficiency). A late systolic murmur begins well beyond the 1st heart sound and continues until the end of systole. Such murmurs may be heard after a midsystolic click in patients with mitral valve prolapse and insufficiency.

Several types of **diastolic murmurs** (also graded I–VI) can be identified:

1. A high-pitched, blowing, decrescendo diastolic murmur along the left sternal border, beginning with S2. This murmur is associated with aortic insufficiency or, if pulmonary arterial pressure is high, with pulmonary valve insufficiency.
2. Early, short, lower-pitched diastolic murmurs along the left mid and upper sternal border are the more common murmurs heard with pulmonary valvular insufficiency. These murmurs are typically noted after surgical repair of the pulmonary outflow tract in defects such as tetralogy of Fallot or in patients with absent pulmonary valve syndrome.
3. A rumbling mid-diastolic murmur at the left mid and lower sternal border may be due to increased blood flow across the tricuspid valve, such as occurs with atrial septal defect (ASD) or, less often, because of actual stenosis of this valve.
4. A rumbling mid-diastolic murmur at the apex follow the 3rd heart sound is caused by increased transmitral flow in conditions with large left-to-right shunts at the ventricular or great vessel level, or with increased flow because of mitral insufficiency.
5. A longer diastolic rumbling murmur at the apex, accentuated at the end of diastole (presystolic), usually indicates anatomic mitral valve stenosis.

The absence of a precordial murmur does not rule out significant congenital or acquired heart disease. Congenital heart defects, some of which are ductal dependent, may not demonstrate a murmur if the ductus arteriosus closes. These lesions include pulmonary or tricuspid valve atresia and transposition of the great arteries. Murmurs may seem insignificant in patients with severe aortic stenosis, ASD, anomalous pulmonary venous return, atrioventricular septal defects, coarctation of the aorta, or anomalous insertion of a coronary artery. Careful attention to other components of the physical examination (cyanosis, pulses, precordial impulse, heart sounds) will increase the index of suspicion of congenital heart defects in these cases. In contrast, loud murmurs may be present in the absence of structural heart disease, for example, in patients with a large noncardiac arteriovenous malformation, myocarditis, severe anemia, or hypertension.

Many murmurs are not associated with significant hemodynamic abnormalities. These are referred to as functional, normal, insignificant, or innocent (the preferred term) murmurs. During routine random auscultation, over 30% of children may have an *innocent murmur*; this percentage increases when auscultation is carried out under nonbasal circumstances (high cardiac output due to fever, infection, anxiety). The most common innocent murmur is a medium-pitched, vibratory or "musical," relatively short systolic ejection murmur, which is heard best along the left lower and midsternal border, and has no significant radiation to the apex, base, or back. Short systolic ejection murmurs at the base and the continuous sound of a venous hum are other examples of common but insignificant murmurs heard in childhood.

The most common innocent murmur is heard most frequently from 3 to 7 yr of age. The murmur occurs during ejection and is musical, frequently sounding like the vibration of a tuning fork; it is brief in duration, may be attenuated in the sitting or prone position, and is intensified by fever, excitement, or exercise. Innocent pulmonic murmurs are also common in children and adolescents, and originate from normal turbulence during ejection into the pulmonary artery. They are higher pitched, blowing, brief, early systolic murmurs, grade I–II in intensity, and are best detected in the 2nd left parasternal space with the patient in the supine position. The *venous hum* is another example of a common innocent murmur heard during childhood. This is produced by turbulence of blood in the jugular venous system; it has no pathologic significance and may be heard in the neck or anterior portion of the upper chest. It consists of a soft humming sound heard in both systole and diastole, and can be exaggerated or made to disappear by varying the position of the head or can be decreased by lightly compressing the jugular venous system in the neck. These simple maneuvers are sufficient to differentiate a venous hum from the murmurs produced by organic cardiovascular disease, particularly a patent ductus arteriosus.

The lack of significance of an innocent murmur should be discussed with the child's parents. It is important to offer complete reassurance because lingering doubts about the importance of a cardiac murmur may have profound effects on child-rearing practices, most often in the form of overprotectiveness. An underlying fear that a cardiac abnormality is present may negatively affect a child's self-image and subtly influence personality development. The physician should explain that the innocent murmur is simply a "noise" and does not indicate the presence of a significant cardiac defect. When asked, "Will it go away?", the best response is to state that because the murmur has no meaning, it does not matter whether it "goes away" or not. However, with growth, innocent murmurs are less well heard and often disappear completely.

At times, additional studies may be indicated to rule out a congenital heart defect, but "routine" electrocardiogram, chest roentgenogram, and/or echocardiographic examination for well children with innocent murmurs should be avoided.

CHAPTER 381
Laboratory Evaluation

381.1 Radiologic Assessment

The chest roentgenogram may provide information about cardiac size and shape, pulmonary blood flow (vascularity), pulmonary edema, and associated lung and thoracic anomalies that may be associated with congenital syndromes (skeletal dysplasias, extra or deficient numbers of ribs, previous cardiac surgery). Variations are due to differences in body build, the phase of respiration or of the cardiac cycle, abnormalities of the thoracic cage, position of the diaphragm, or pulmonary disease.

The most frequently used measurement of cardiac size is the maximal width of the cardiac shadow in a posteroanterior chest film taken during midinspiration. A vertical line is drawn down the middle of the sternal shadow, and perpendicular lines are drawn from the sternal line to the extreme right and left borders of the heart; the sum of the lengths of these lines is the *maximal cardiac width.* The *maximal chest width* is obtained by drawing a horizontal line between the right and left inner borders of the rib cage at the level of the top of the right diaphragm. When the maximal cardiac width is more than half the maximal chest width (*cardiothoracic ratio* >50%), the heart is usually enlarged. Cardiac size should be evaluated only when the film is taken during inspiration and with the patient in an upright position. Diagnosis of "cardiac enlargement" on expiratory or prone films is a common cause of unnecessary referrals and laboratory studies.

The cardiothoracic ratio is a less useful index of cardiac enlargement in infancy than in older children because the horizontal position of the heart may increase the ratio to more than 50% in the absence of true enlargement. Furthermore, the thymus may overlap not only the base of the heart, but virtually the entire mediastinum, thus obscuring the true cardiac silhouette.

The lateral chest roentgenogram may be helpful in infants, as well as in older children with pectus excavatum or other conditions that result in a narrow anteroposterior chest dimension. In these situations the heart may appear quite small in the lateral view, suggesting that the apparent enlargement in the posteroanterior projection was due to either the thymic image (anterior mediastinum only) or flattening of the cardiac chambers as a result of a structural chest abnormality.

In the posteroanterior view, the left border of the cardiac shadow consists of three convex shadows produced, from above downward, by the aortic knob, the main and left pulmonary arteries, and the left ventricle (Fig. 381–1). In cases of moderate to marked left atrial enlargement, the atrium may project between the pulmonary artery and the left ventricle. The outflow tract of the right ventricle (the pulmonary conus) does not contribute to the shadows formed by the left border of the heart. The aortic knob is not as easily seen in infants and children as in adults. However, the side of the aortic arch (left or right) often can be inferred as being opposite to the side of the midline from which the air-filled trachea is visualized. This is an important observation as a right-sided aortic arch is often present in cyanotic congenital heart disease, particularly in tetralogy of Fallot. Three structures contribute to the right border of the cardiac silhouette; from above downward they are the superior vena cava, the ascending aorta, and the right atrium.

Enlargement of cardiac chambers or major arteries and veins results in prominence of areas where these structures are normally outlined on the chest roentgenogram. These abnormal roentgenographic findings should always be complemented by an electrocardiogram, which is a more sensitive and accurate index of ventricular *hypertrophy.*

It is also important to assess the degree of *pulmonary vascularity* as represented by the intrapulmonary shadows. Angiocardiographic studies have shown that the hilar shadows are mainly vascular. Pulmonary overcirculation is usually associated with left-to-right shunt lesions, whereas pulmonary undercirculation is associated with obstruction of the outflow tract of the right ventricle.

The esophagus is closely related to the great vessels, and visualization with barium helps to delineate these structures in selected situations, such as coarctation of the aorta and vascular ring. However, echocardiographic examination best defines specific intracardiac chamber anatomy and enlargement. Thus, routine esophagograms and fluoroscopy are no longer necessary for the evaluation of most cardiac abnormalities and are now mostly limited to the diagnosis of vascular rings.

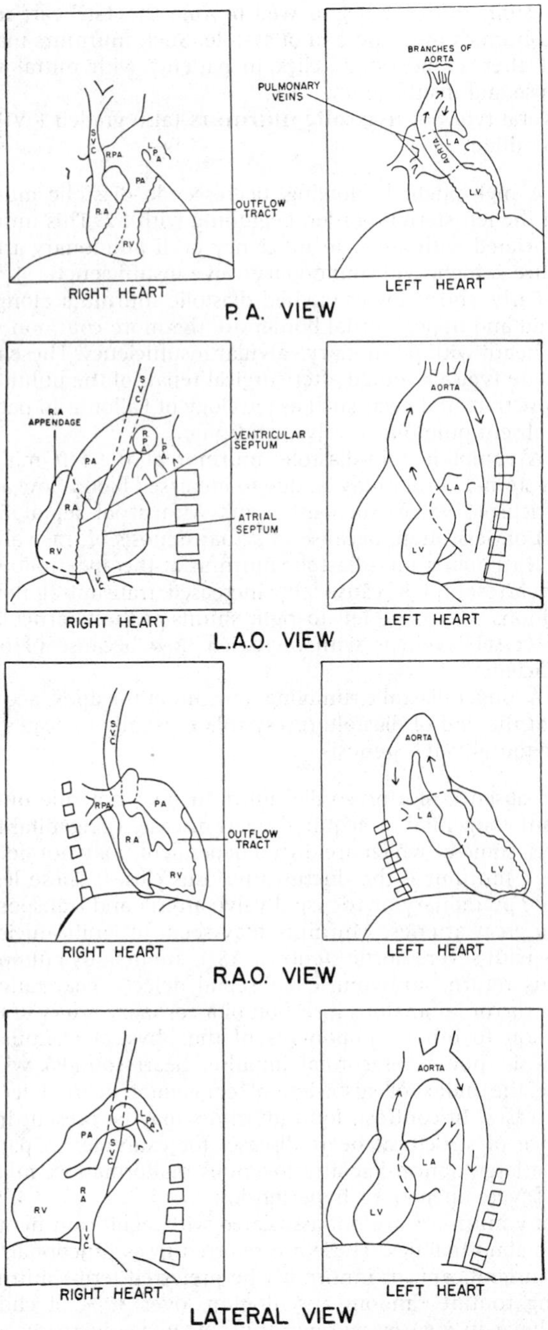

Figure 381–1. Idealized diagrams showing normal position of the cardiac chambers and great blood vessels. P.A. = posteroanterior; L.A.O. = left anterior oblique; R.A.O. = right anterior oblique; SVC = superior vena cava; RA = right atrium; RV = right ventricle; PA = pulmonary artery; RPA = right pulmonary artery; LPA = left pulmonary artery; LA = left atrium; LV = left ventricle; IVC = inferior vena cava. (Adapted and redrawn from Dotter and Steinberg: Radiology 53:513, 1949.)

381.2 Electrocardiogram (ECG)

Changes in cardiac anatomy and hemodynamics soon after birth are reflected in the evolution of the ECG of the neonate. Because vascular resistances in the pulmonary and systemic circulations are nearly equal in the fetus at term, the intrauterine work of the heart results in virtually an equal mass of both the right and left ventricles (see Chapter 382). After birth, systemic vascular resistance rises when the placental circulation is eliminated, and pulmonary vascular resistance falls when the lungs expand. These changes are effected over a period of hours or days, and are eventually reflected in the ECG as the right ventricular wall begins to thin.

The ECG demonstrates these anatomic and hemodynamic features principally by changes in the QRS and T-wave morphology. It is recommended that a 13-lead ECG be carried out in pediatric patients, including either lead V_3R or V_4R. These right precordial leads are extremely important in the evalua-

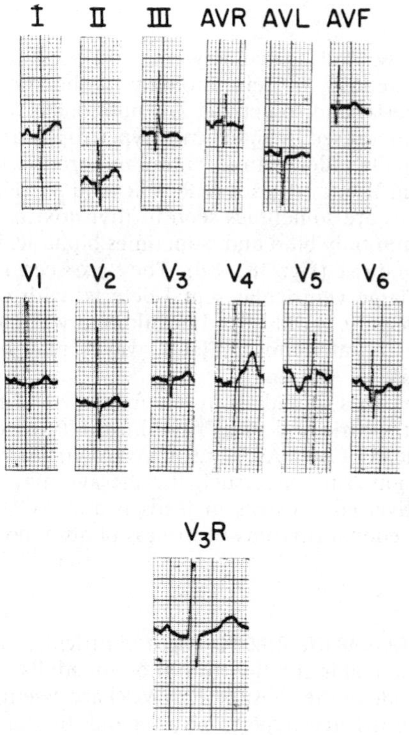

Figure 381–2. Electrocardiogram in a normal neonate less than 24 hr of age. Note the dominant R wave and upright T waves in leads V_3R and V_1. (V_3R paper speed = 50 mm/sec.)

tion of right ventricular hypertrophy in childhood. On occasion, lead V_1 is positioned too far leftward to reflect right ventricular forces accurately and may display the usual R/S pattern of the mid-precordial leads. This problem is particularly present in premature infants in whom the ECG electrode gel may produce contact between all of the precordial leads. At the same time, V_3R or V_4R may reflect a dominant R or S pattern, which is also important diagnostically.

During the 1st days of life, right axis deviation, large R waves, and upright T waves in the right precordial leads (V_3R or V_4R and V_1) are normally seen (Fig. 381–2). When pulmonary resistance decreases and right ventricular pressure reaches its normal level, the right precordial T waves become negative. In the great majority of instances this occurs within the first 48 hr of life. If upright T waves persist in leads V_3R, V_4R, or V_1 beyond 1 wk of life, this represents an abnormal finding, indicating right ventricular hypertrophy or strain, sometimes even in the absence of QRS voltage criteria. The T wave in V_1 should never be positive before 6 yr of age and may remain negative into adolescence. This finding represents one of the most important yet subtle differences between the pediatric and adult ECG.

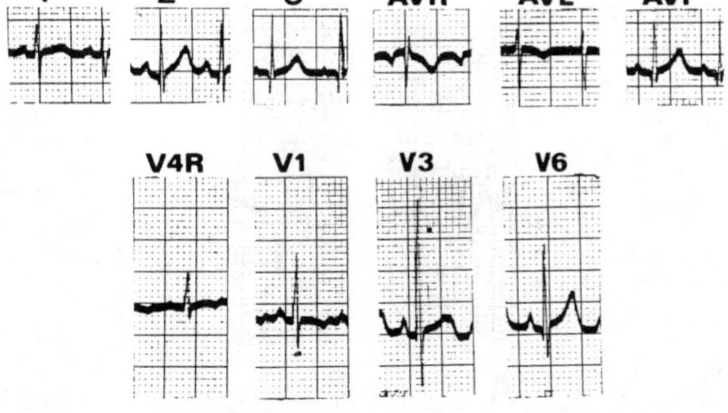

Figure 381–3. Electrocardiogram of a normal infant. Note the tall R and small S waves in V_4R and V_1 and the inverted T wave in these leads. There is also a dominant R wave in V_6.

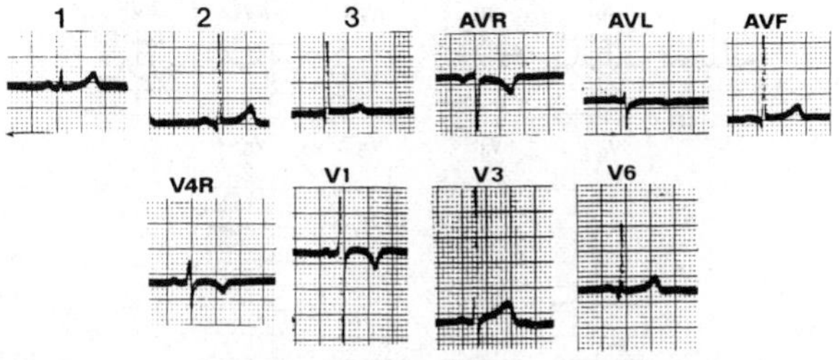

Figure 381–4. Electrocardiogram of a normal child. Note the relatively tall R waves and inversion of the T waves in V_4R and V_1.

In the frontal plane leads of the standard ECG, the mean QRS axis in the newborn normally lies in the range of +110 to +180 degrees. The right-sided chest leads reveal a larger positive (R) than negative (S) wave and may do so for months or years because the right ventricle remains relatively thick throughout infancy. Furthermore, owing to proximity, the voltage recorded by the right precordial leads is influenced to a greater extent by right ventricular depolarization. Left-sided leads (V_5 and V_6) also reflect right-sided dominance in the early neonatal period when the RS ratio in these leads may be less than 1. However, because the left precordial leads are in direct proximity to the left ventricle, a dominant R wave reflecting left ventricular forces quickly becomes evident within the 1st few days of life (Fig. 381–3). Over the years, the QRS axis gradually shifts leftward and right ventricular forces slowly regress. As the left ventricle becomes dominant, the ECG evolves to the characteristic pattern of the older child (Fig. 381–4), and finally the typical adult electrocardiogram emerges (Fig. 381–5).

With the growth of the infant there is a slow regression of right ventricular dominance and an increase in left ventricular forces. Leads V_1, V_3R, and V_4R will display a prominent R wave until 6 mo to 8 yr of age. The majority of children will have an RS ratio greater than 1 in lead V_4R until they are 4 yr of age. The T waves are inverted in V_4R, V_1, V_2, and V_3 during infancy and may remain so into the middle of the 2nd decade of life and beyond. The processes of right ventricular thinning and left ventricular growth are best reflected in the QRS-T pattern over the right precordial leads. Thus, the diagnosis of

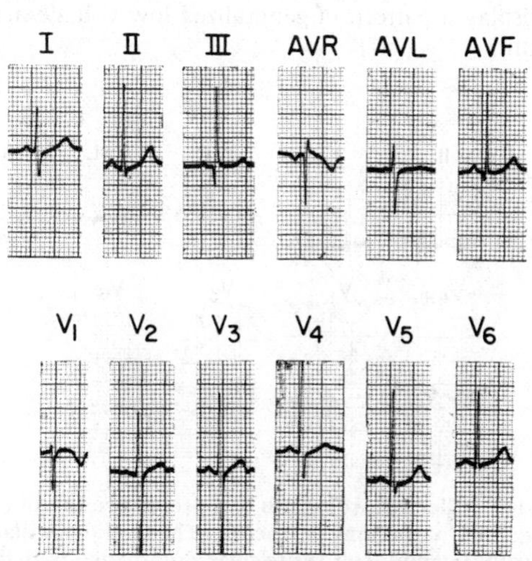

Figure 381–5. Normal adult electrocardiogram. Note the dominant S wave in lead V_1. This pattern in an infant would indicate the presence of left ventricular hypertrophy.

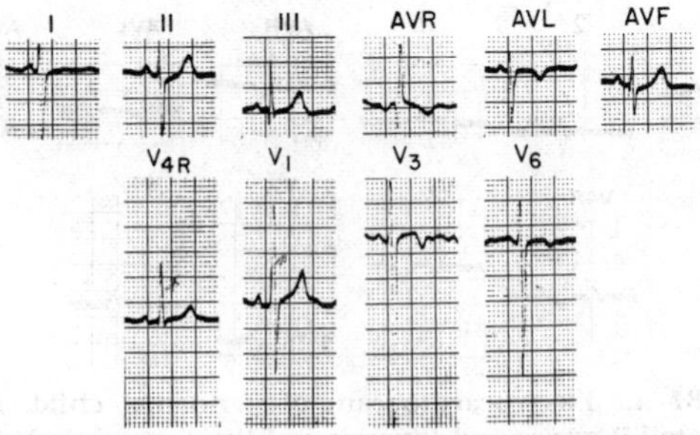

Figure 381–6. Electrocardiogram of an infant with right ventricular hypertrophy (tetralogy of Fallot). Note the tall R waves in the right precordium and deep S waves in V_6. The positive T waves in V_4R and V_1 are also characteristic of right ventricular hypertrophy.

right or left ventricular hypertrophy in the pediatric patient can be made only with an understanding of the normal developmental physiology of these chambers at various ages until adulthood is reached.

Ventricular hypertrophy may result in increased voltage in the R and S waves in the chest leads. However, the height of these deflections is governed by the proximity of the specific electrode to the surface of the heart, and by the sequence of electrical activation through the ventricles, resulting in variable degrees of cancellation of forces, as well as by hypertrophy of the myocardium. Because the chest wall in infants and children as well as in adolescents may be relatively thin, the diagnosis of ventricular hypertrophy should not be based on voltage changes alone in the entire pediatric age range.

The diagnosis of pathologic right ventricular hypertrophy is difficult in the 1st week of life, as physiologic right ventricular hypertrophy is a normal finding. Serial tracings are often necessary to determine whether marked right axis deviation and potentially abnormal right precordial forces or T waves, or both, will persist beyond the neonatal period (Fig. 381–6). In contrast, an adult ECG pattern seen in a neonate suggests left ventricular enlargement (see Fig. 381–5). The exception is the premature infant, who may display a more "mature" ECG than his or her full-term counterpart (Fig. 381–7) as a result of lower pulmonary vascular resistance secondary to underdevelopment of the medial muscular layer of the pulmonary arterioles. Thus, the electrocardiogram may simulate that of the older child, with left ventricular dominance manifested by a more mature R-wave progression across the precordium (qR in V_6, R/S ratio in V_4R, V_3R and V_1 ≤ 1). Some premature infants display a pattern of generalized low voltage across the precordium.

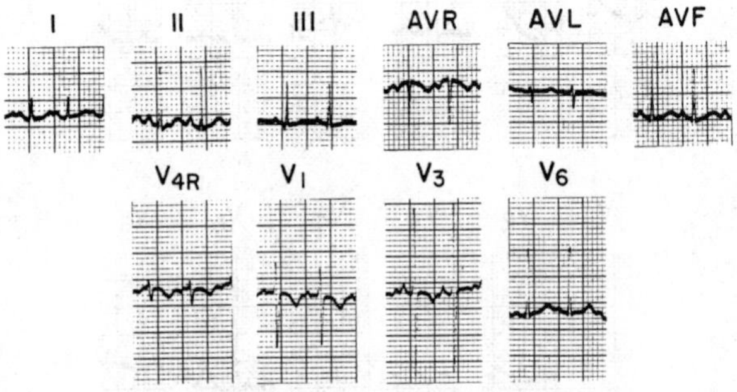

Figure 381–7. Electrocardiogram of a premature infant (weight 2 kg and age 5 wk at the time of tracing). The cardiovascular system was clinically normal. Left ventricular dominance is manifest by R-wave progression across the chest simulating tracings obtained from older children. Compare with the tracing from a normal full-term infant, Figure 381–3.

P WAVE

Tall, narrow, and spiked P waves are seen in congenital pulmonary stenosis, Ebstein anomaly of the tricuspid valve, tricuspid atresia, and sometimes cor pulmonale. These abnormal waves are caused by right atrial hypertrophy and/or dilatation, are usually taller than 2.5 mm, and are most obvious in standard lead II and in leads V_4R, V_3R, and V_1 (Fig. 381–8*A*). Similar waves are sometimes seen in thyrotoxicosis. Widened P waves, commonly bifid and sometimes biphasic, indicate left atrial enlargement (Fig. 381–8*B*). They are seen in some patients with large ventricular septal defects, with communications between the aorta and the pulmonary circulation, and with severe mitral stenosis. Flat P waves may be found in hyperkalemia.

The P wave axis should always be measured. With a normal position of the atria and sinus rhythm, the P wave should be upright in leads I and AVF, and inverted in lead AVR. With atrial inversion (situs inversus), the P wave may be inverted in lead I. Inverted P waves in leads II and AVF are seen in nodal or junctional rhythms regardless of atrial position.

QRS COMPLEX

RIGHT VENTRICULAR HYPERTROPHY. Right ventricular surface leads of infants and children differ from those of adults, and tracings of the right side of the chest (V_4R or V_3R) are essential. Diagnosis of right ventricular hypertrophy depends on the demonstration of the following changes, which may occur singly or in combination (see Fig. 381–6): (1) a qR pattern in the right ventricular surface leads; (2) a positive T wave in leads $V_{3-4}R$ and V_1–V_3 between the ages of 6 days and 6 yr; (3) a monophasic R wave in V_3R, V_4R, or V_1; (4) an rsR′ pattern in the right precordial leads, often with a tall secondary R wave (this pattern is frequently associated with right ventricular volume overload, as typically seen in atrial septal defect); (5) age-corrected increased voltage of the R wave in leads $V_{3-4}R$ and/or of the S wave in leads V_{6-7}; (6) marked right axis deviation (>120 degrees beyond the newborn period); (7) a complete reversal of the normal adult precordial RS pattern; and (8) right atrial enlargement. At least two of these changes should be present to support a diagnosis of right ventricular hypertrophy. In general, if a pattern of right ventricular hypertrophy in the newborn and young infant persists or even becomes more prominent into early childhood, abnormal right ventricular hypertrophy is present. In contrast, the infant who displays the pattern of a "normal" electrocardiogram for an older child may have left ventricular hypertrophy.

Abnormal hemodynamics can be correlated with abnormal electrocardiographic patterns. Obstruction to right ventricular and pulmonary flow (e.g., pulmonary stenosis) is associated with a systolic overload pattern, characterized by tall, pure R waves in the right precordial leads. In older children the T

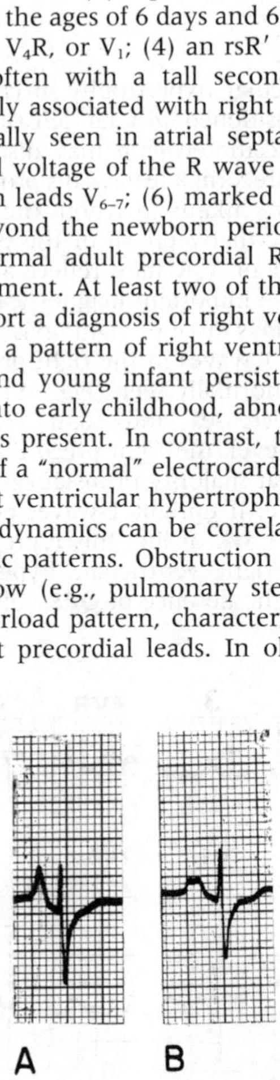

Figure 381–8. Atrial enlargement. *A*, Peaked narrow P waves characteristic of right atrial enlargement. *B*, Wide bifid M-shaped P waves typical of left atrial enlargement.

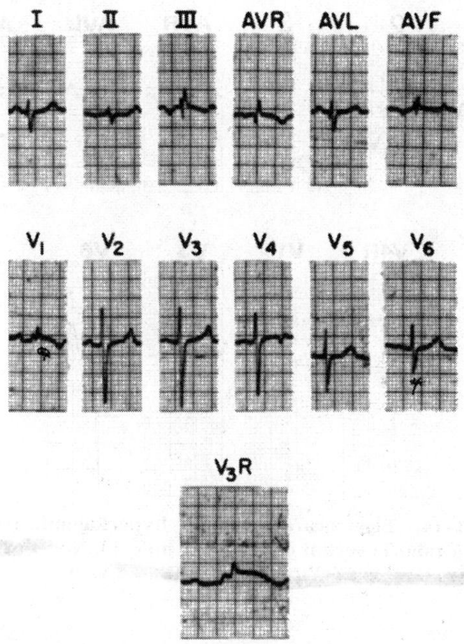

Figure 381–9. **Electrocardiogram showing right ventricular conduction delay characterized by an rsR' pattern in V_1 and a deep S wave in V_6. (V_3R paper speed = 50 mm/sec.)**

waves in these leads are initially upright and later become inverted. In infants and children less than 6 yr of age, T waves in $V_{3-4}R$ and V_1 are abnormally upright. In contrast, diastolic overload of the right ventricle (e.g., with atrial septal defect) is characterized by an rsR′ pattern and right ventricular conduction delay (Fig. 381–9). Patients with mild to moderate pulmonary stenosis may also exhibit an rsR′ in the right precordial leads.

LEFT VENTRICULAR HYPERTROPHY. The following features indicate the presence of left ventricular hypertrophy (Fig. 381–10): (1) depression of the S-T segments and inversion of the T waves in the left precordial leads (V_5, V_6, and V_7), known as a left ventricular strain pattern; these findings suggest the presence of a severe lesion and significant myocardial abnormality; (2)

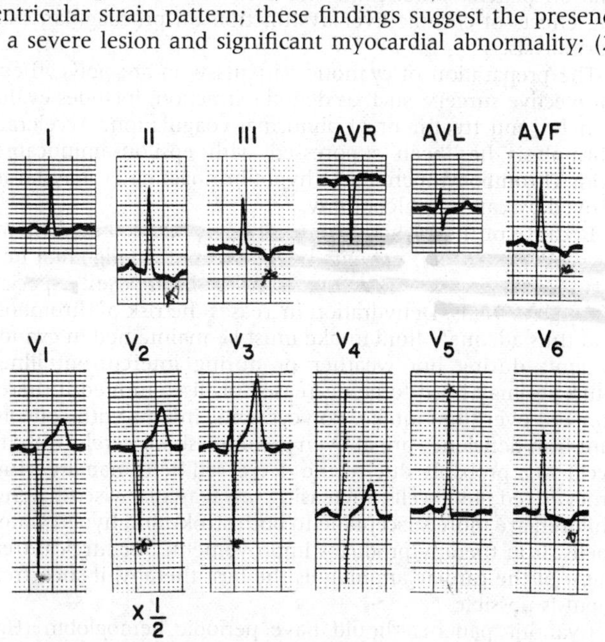

Figure 381–10. **Electrocardiogram showing left ventricular hypertrophy in a 12-yr-old child with aortic stenosis. Note the deep S wave in V_1–V_3 and tall R in V_5. Also, T-wave inversion is present in II, III, AVF, and V_6.**

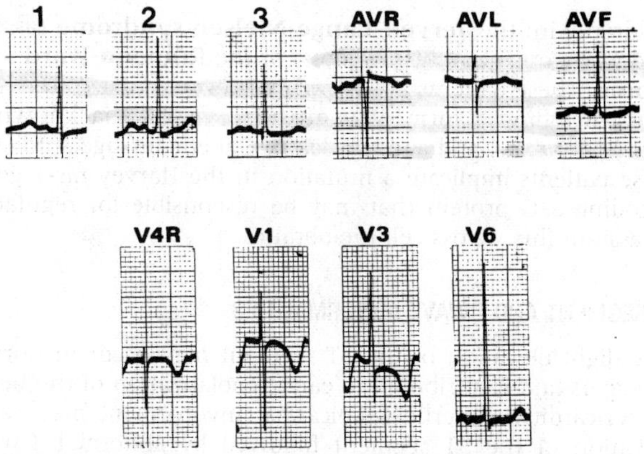

Figure 381–11. **Electrocardiogram in hypocalcemia and hypokalemia (serum calcium 1.8 mEq/L; serum potassium 2.2 mEq/L at the time of tracing). Note the prolongation of electrical systole owing to long S-TU segment. This graph also shows left ventricular hypertrophy.**

increase in magnitude of initial forces to the right (i.e., a deep Q wave in the left precordial leads); (3) increased voltage of the S wave in V_3R and V_1 and/or the R wave in V_{6-7}. It is important to emphasize that evaluation of left ventricular hypertrophy should not be based on voltage criteria alone. The concepts of systolic and diastolic overload, although not always consistent, are also useful in evaluating left ventricular enlargement. Severe systolic overload of the left ventricle is suggested by straightening of the ST segments and inverted T waves over the left precordial leads; diastolic overload may result in tall R waves, a large Q wave, and normal T waves over the left precordium.

BUNDLE BRANCH BLOCK. Complete right bundle branch block may occur as a congenital finding or as an acquired finding after surgery for congenital heart disease, especially when a right ventriculotomy has been performed. Congenital left bundle branch block is rare; this pattern is occasionally seen with cardiomyopathy.

Q-T INTERVAL

The duration of the Q-T interval varies with the cardiac rate; a corrected Q-T interval (Q-T_c) can be calculated by dividing the measured Q-T interval by the square root of the cycle length of the R-R interval. The normal Q-T_c should be less than 0.45. It is often lengthened in children with hypokalemia and hypocalcemia; in the former instance, a U wave may be noted at the end of the T wave (Figs. 381–11 and 381–12). A prolonged Q-T interval (Fig. 381–13) may be also be seen in

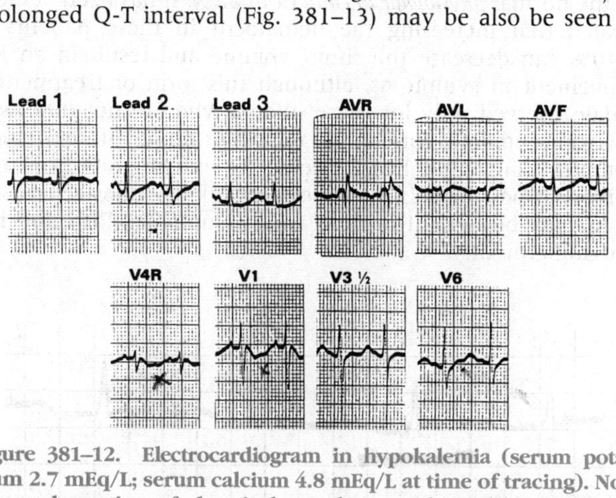

Figure 381–12. **Electrocardiogram in hypokalemia (serum potassium 2.7 mEq/L; serum calcium 4.8 mEq/L at time of tracing). Note the prolongation of electrical systole as evidenced by a widened TU wave; also the depression of the ST segment in V_4R, V_1, and V_6.**

children with the **Jervell-Lange-Nielsen syndrome** (associated with congenital hearing loss) or the **Romano-Ward syndrome.** These patients are at high risk for ventricular arrhythmias, including a form of ventricular arrhythmia known as *torsade de pointes,* and sudden death. Genetic linkage studies in these patients implicate a mutation in the Harvey *ras*-1 gene, encoding a G protein that may be responsible for regulating potassium flux across cell membranes.

ST SEGMENT AND T-WAVE ABNORMALITIES

A slight elevation of the ST segment may occur in normal teenagers and is attributed to early repolarization of the heart. In pericarditis, superficial epicardial involvement may cause elevation of the ST segment followed by abnormal T-wave inversion as healing progresses. Administration of digitalis is associated with sagging of the ST segment and abnormal inversion of the T wave.

Depression of the ST segment may also occur in any condition that produces myocardial damage, for example, anemia, carbon monoxide poisoning, endocardial fibroelastosis, aberrant origin of the left coronary artery from the pulmonary artery, glycogen storage disease of the heart, myocardial tumors, and mucopolysaccharidoses. Aberrant origin of the left coronary artery from the pulmonary artery may lead to changes indistinguishable from those of acute myocardial infarction in adults. Similar changes may occur in patients with other rare abnormalities of the coronary arteries and with cardiomyopathy without anatomic abnormalities of the coronary arteries. These may be misread in young infants because of the unfamiliarity of pediatricians with this "infarct" pattern, and thus a high index of suspicion must be maintained in infants with symptoms compatible with coronary ischemia.

In any form of carditis simple inversion of the T wave may occur. Hypothyroidism may produce flat or inverted T waves in association with generalized low voltage. In hyperkalemia the T waves are commonly of high voltage and are tent-shaped (Fig. 381–14).

381.3 Hematologic Data

Evaluation of hematologic findings as part of the assessment of the cardiovascular system should be carried out with an awareness of the normal variations in infancy (see Chapter 405). In acyanotic infants with large left-to-right shunts, the onset of congestive heart failure often coincides with the nadir of the normal *physiologic anemia* of infancy. It has been demonstrated that increasing the hematocrit in these patients to >40% can decrease the shunt volume and result in an improvement in symptoms, although this form of treatment is today reserved only for those infants who are not otherwise surgical candidates (premature infants or those with extremely complex congenital heart disease for whom only palliative surgery is possible). In these selected infants, booster transfusions may be helpful in decreasing symptomatology and improving growth.

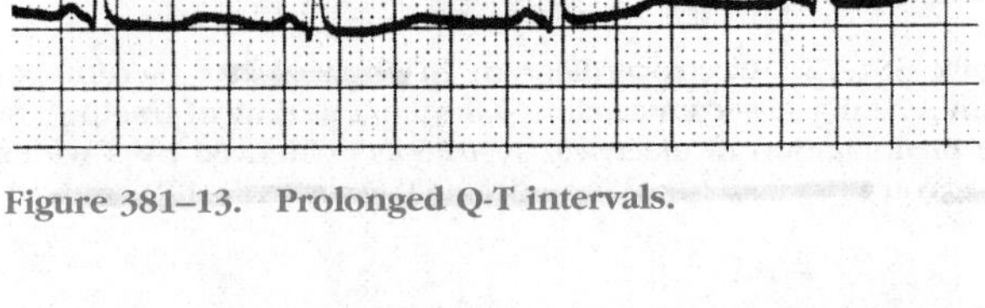

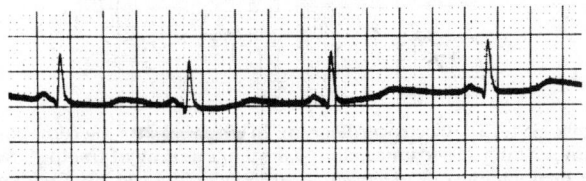

Figure 381–13. Prolonged Q-T intervals.

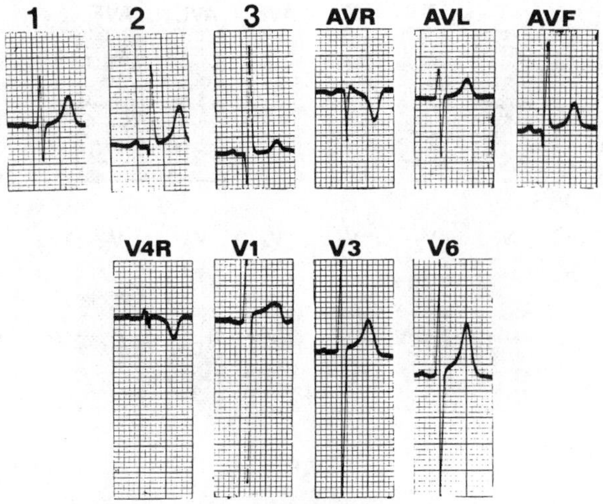

Figure 381–14. Electrocardiogram in hyperkalemia (serum potassium 6.5 mEq/L; serum calcium 5.1 mEq/L). Note the tall, tent-shaped T waves, especially in leads I, II, and V_6.

Although it had been widely believed that the erythrocyte sedimentation rate is low in patients with congestive heart failure, this is not a reliable clinical marker, and patients with heart failure can have normal and even increased sedimentation rates.

Persistent *polycythemia* after the 1st mo of life is frequently noted in patients with right-to-left shunts and cyanosis. Patients with marked polycythemia have a delicate balance between intravascular thrombosis and a bleeding diathesis; this abnormal hemostasis should be recognized and may need to be treated prior to any surgical procedure. The most frequent abnormalities are accelerated fibrinolysis, thrombocytopenia, abnormal clot retraction, hypofibrinogenemia, prolonged prothrombin time, and prolonged partial thromboplastin time. These abnormalities occur singly or in combination, and may be related to the severity of the polycythemia. Abnormal coagulation may be related to the effects of hypoxia and polycythemia on platelet production and consumption combined with the effects of chronic liver dysfunction on procoagulants and fibrinolysis.

The preparation of cyanotic patients who are polycythemic for elective surgery, such as dental extraction, includes evaluation for and treatment of abnormal coagulation. Accelerated fibrinolysis has been suppressed with epsilon-aminocaproic acid. Thrombocytopenia and hypofibrinogenemia may be improved by careful phlebotomy.

Because of the high viscosity of polycythemic blood (hematocrit [Hct] >65%), patients having cyanotic congenital heart disease are at risk to develop vascular thromboses, especially of cerebral veins. Dehydration increases the risk of thrombosis, and thus adequate fluid intake must be maintained in cyanotic patients during hot weather or during intercurrent illness. Diuretics may need to be decreased or discontinued if there is concern over fluid intake. Polycythemic infants with concomitant iron deficiency are at even greater risk for cerebrovascular accidents, probably due to the decreased deformability of microcytic red blood cells, increasing intravascular viscosity. Such children are more susceptible to both stroke and hypercyanotic spells. Iron therapy produces improvement, but surgical treatment of the cardiac anomaly is the best therapy, if such treatment is possible.

Cyanotic patients should have periodic hemoglobin (Hgb) and Hct determinations. Increasing polycythemia, often associated with headache, fatigue, and/or dyspnea, is one indication for palliative or corrective surgical intervention. Among cyanotic patients with inoperable conditions, phlebotomy may be required to treat individuals whose Hct has risen to the 65–70% level, usually when the polycythemia is associated with symptoms, for example, headache. This procedure is not without risk, especially in patients with extreme elevation of pulmonary vascular resistance. Because these patients do not tolerate wide fluctuations in circulating blood volume, the phlebotomy should be performed in the same way as an exchange transfusion; blood is replaced with fresh frozen plasma or albumin. Initially, these patients may require frequent phlebotomies (often weekly) until the Hct is stabilized at the desired level (approximately 60%). Subsequently, phlebotomies may be necessary at intervals of only 3–5 wk. Whether to perform routine phlebotomies for polycythemic patients who are asymptomatic is currently a matter of controversy.

381.4 Echocardiography

Echocardiography is an extremely important technique in the diagnosis of congenital and acquired cardiac disease in infants and children. The echocardiographic examination can also be used to evaluate cardiac contractile function (both systolic and diastolic); gradients across stenotic valves; the direction of flow across a shunt; the patency of coronary arteries; the presence of vegetations due to endocarditis; the presence of pericardial fluid, cardiac tumors, or chamber thrombi; prosthetic valve function; septal hypertrophy; aortic root dimensions; and the effects of cardiotonic or cardiotoxic drugs. Echocardiography may also be used to assist in performance of pericardiocentesis, balloon atrial septostomy (see Chapter 381.7), and endocardial biopsy, and in the placement of flow-directed pulmonary arterial (Swan-Ganz) monitoring catheters. Transesophageal echocardiography can be used to monitor ventricular function in patients during difficult surgical procedures and can provide an immediate assessment of the results of surgical repair of congenital heart lesions. Fetal echocardiography can determine the presence of a congenital heart lesion, often as early as at 17–19 wk of gestation, and can evaluate fetal cardiac arrhythmias. A complete echocardiographic examination usually employs a combination of M-mode, two-dimensional real-time imaging, and pulsed, continuous and color Doppler flow studies.

M-MODE ECHOCARDIOGRAPHY

M mode echocardiography identifies the dimensions and motion of intracardiac structures (opening and closing of valves, movement of free walls and septa), the anatomy of valves, and the presence of endocarditis vegetations larger than 2–3 mm. M mode can define the presence or absence of individual structures and their relationships to one another (Fig. 381–15) and can evaluate cardiac function (Table 381–1).

TWO-DIMENSIONAL ECHOCARDIOGRAPHY

Two-dimensional (2-D) echocardiography provides a realistic real-time image of cardiac structures. With 2-D echocardiogra-

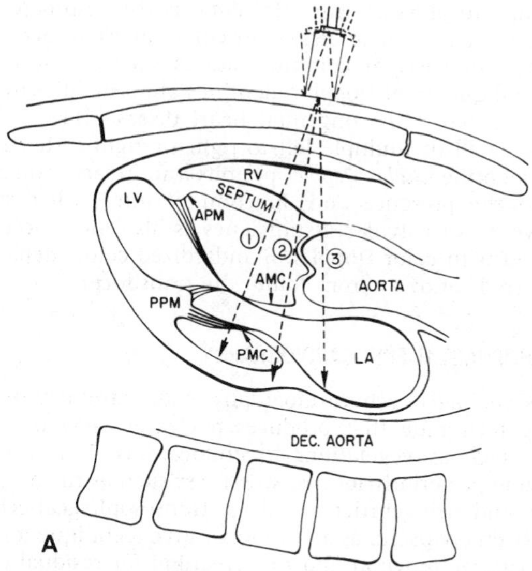

Figure 381–15. **Normal echocardiograms.** ***A*, Diagram of sagittal section of heart showing structures traversed by echo beam in positions (1), (2), and (3). AMC = anterior mitral cusp; APM = anterior papillary muscle; Dec. aorta = descending aorta; LA = left atrium; LV = left ventricle; PMC = posterior mitral cusp; PPM = posterior papillary muscle; RV = right ventricle. *B*, Echocardiogram from transducer position (1); this is the best view to evaluate the interventricular septum (S) and for measurement of the right ventricular dimension (RVED) as well as of the left ventricular dimension (LVED) in end diastole (Dd) and end systole (Ds). CW = chest wall. *C*, Normal septal aortic and mitral aortic relationships obtained when transducer is swept from positions (1) through (3) of A. A = aortic valve; LA = left atrium; LV = left ventricle; MV = mitral valve; RV = right ventricle; S = interventricular septum. Note the continuity of the anterior mitral leaflet with the posterior wall of the aorta and of the ventricular septum with the anterior wall of the aorta.**

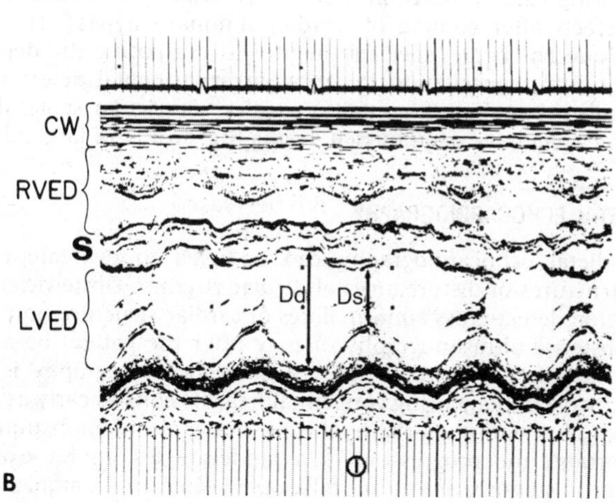

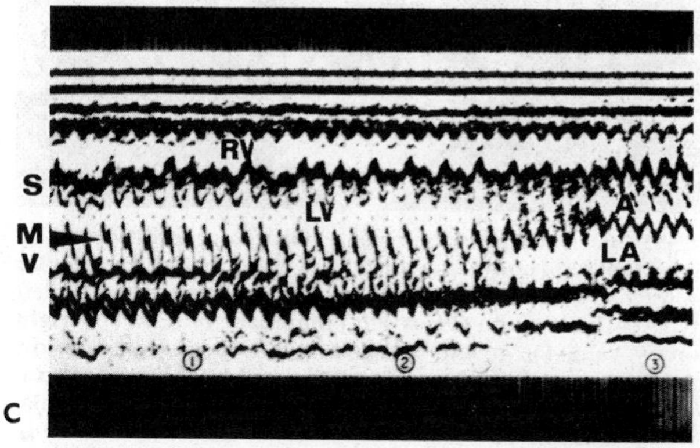

■ **TABLE 381–1 Echographic Measurement of Cardiovascular Performance**

1. Per cent shortening = $\frac{\text{LVED} - \text{LVES}}{\text{LVED}} \times 100$ (see Fig. 381–15)

   LVED = left ventricular end-diastolic dimension; LVES = left ventricular end-systolic dimension. (*Normal*, 28–38%.)

2. Mean VCF = $\frac{\text{LVED} - \text{LVES}}{\text{LVED} \times \text{ET}}$

   VCF = mean velocity of circumferential fiber shortening (expressed as circumference [circ] per second); LVED and LVES as in (1) above; ET = ejection time. (*Normal values:* neonates, 1.51 ± 0.04 [SE] circ/sec; children [5–15 yr], 1.34 ± 0.03 [SE] circ/sec.)

3. Systolic time intervals (a) $\frac{\text{LPEP}}{\text{LVET}}$ (normal range is 0.3–0.39; average, 0.35).

   (LPEP = left ventricular pre-ejection period; LVET = left ventricular ejection time.) (b) $\frac{\text{RPEP}}{\text{RVET}}$ (normal range is 0.16–0.30; average, 0.24). (RPEP = right ventricular pre-ejection period; RVET = right ventricular ejection time.) These ratios are indirect indices of changes in afterload, preload, contractility, and electromechanical delay.

4. Isovolemic contraction (ICT) may be derived from the following regression equation: ICT = 53 − 0.22 × heart rate (SE ± 7.3). ICT is increased in left ventricular myocardial disease and decreased in aortic runoff (e.g., patent ductus arteriosus).

5. Right and left ventricular outflow obstruction may be quantitated by Doppler estimation of the velocity of blood flow (V) across the stenotic segment. The peak systolic ejection gradient (PSEG) = $4V^2$.

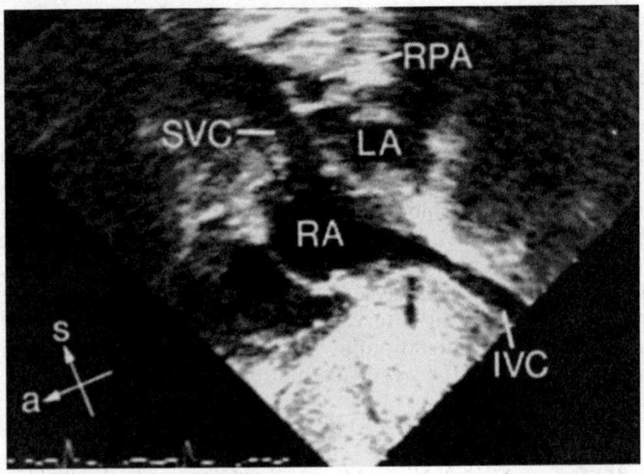

Figure 381–17. Right parasagittal normal echocardiographic plane view showing the junction of the inferior and superior venae cavae with the right atrium. a = anterior; IVC = inferior vena cava; LA = left atrium; RA = right atrium; RPA = right pulmonary artery; s = superior; SVC = superior vena cava. (From Sanders SP: Echocardiography. *In:* Long WA [ed]: Fetal and Neonatal Cardiology. Philadelphia, WB Saunders, 1990.)

phy the contracting heart is imaged in several standard views (subxiphoid, Fig. 381–16; parasagittal, Fig. 381–17; parasternal, Fig. 381–18; suprasternal, Fig. 381–19) that emphasize specific structures (e.g., chambers, valves, septa, great vessels, myocardium). Such images resemble those seen in angiography. Two-dimensional echocardiography is even superior to angiography in several areas, for example, in imaging the atrioventricular valves and their chordal attachments.

DOPPLER ECHOCARDIOGRAPHY

Doppler echocardiography is an ultrasound technique that identifies blood flow rather than morphology. It displays flow in cardiac chambers and vascular channels based on the change in frequency imparted to a sound wave by the movement of erythrocytes. In *pulsed Doppler* and *continuous wave Doppler,* the speed and direction of blood flow in the line of the echo beam change the transducer's reference frequency. This frequency change can be translated into volumetric flow (L/min) data used to estimate systemic or pulmonary blood flow and into pressure (mm Hg) data used to estimate gradients across semilunar or atrioventricular valves, or across septal defects or vascular communications such as shunts. The directional quality of Doppler identifies abnormalities in blood flow associated with congenital heart disease (Fig. 381–20). Because small or multiple left-to-right or right-to-left shunts can be identified, *color Doppler* permits a more accurate assessment of the presence and direction of intracardiac shunts. The severity of valvular insufficiency is also more accurately evaluated with color Doppler. Standardized colors depict flow toward (red) or away from (blue) the transducer.

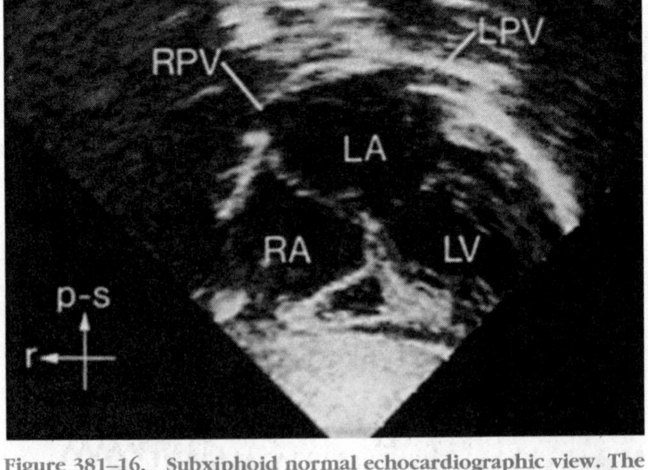

Figure 381–16. Subxiphoid normal echocardiographic view. The anterior angulation shows the mitral valve and the left ventricular inflow tract. Note the pulmonary veins connecting with the left atrium. LA = left atrium; LPV = left pulmonary vein; RPV = right pulmonary vein; LV = left ventricle; p-s = posterior-superior; r = right; RA = right atrium. (From Sanders SP: Echocardiography. *In:* Long WA [ed]: Fetal and Neonatal Cardiology. Philadelphia, WB Saunders, 1990.)

TRANSESOPHAGEAL ECHOCARDIOGRAPHY

Transesophageal echocardiography is an extremely sensitive imaging technique that produces a clearer view of smaller lesions, such as vegetations in endocarditis. It is useful in visualizing posteriorly located structures such as the atria, aortic root, and atrioventricular valves. Transesophageal echo has been extremely useful as an intraoperative technique for monitoring cardiac function and for screening for residual cardiac defects after coming off cardiopulmonary bypass. This technique has been especially helpful in evaluating the degree of residual regurgitation in atrioventricular septal defect repairs and in searching for small muscular ventricular septal defects that may have been missed during the closure of larger defects.

FETAL ECHOCARDIOGRAPHY

Fetal echocardiography can be used to evaluate cardiac structures or disturbances of cardiac rhythm. Obstetricians will often detect gross abnormalities of cardiac structure on routine obstetric ultrasonography or may refer the patient because of unexplained hydrops fetalis. Fetal echocardiography is often capable of diagnosing congenital heart lesions as early as 17–19 wk of gestation. Serial fetal echos have also demonstrated the intrauterine progression of a moderate lesion, for example, aortic stenosis, into a more severe lesion, for example, hypo-

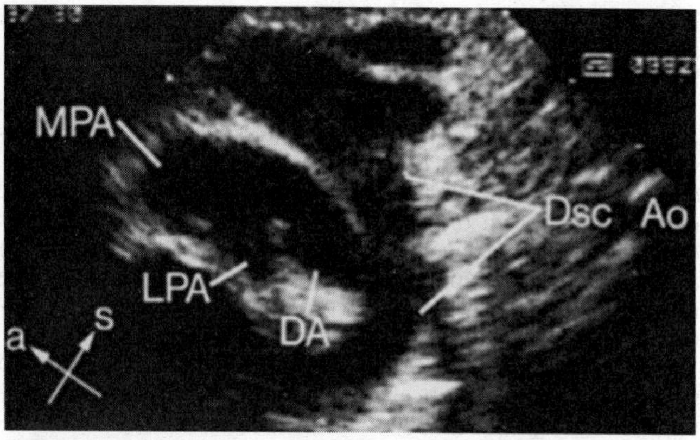

Figure 381–18. Normal high parasternal, parasagittal echocardiographic plane view for imaging the ductus arteriosus. a = anterior; DA = ductus arteriosus; Dsc Ao = descending aorta; LPA = left pulmonary artery; MPA = main pulmonary artery; s = superior. (From Sanders SP: Echocardiography. *In:* Long WA [ed]: Fetal and Neonatal Cardiology. Philadelphia, WB Saunders, 1990.)

plastic left heart. M-mode echocardiography can diagnose rhythm disturbances in the fetus and can determine the success of antiarrhythmic therapy administered to the mother. A screening fetal echocardiogram is recommended for patients with a previous child or a 1st degree relative with congenital heart disease and for patients who are at higher risk of having a child with cardiac disease (e.g., insulin-dependent diabetics, patients with exposure to certain drugs during pregnancy).

OVERVIEW

Used with a careful clinical evaluation and other laboratory methods, echocardiography has in many cases eliminated the need for preoperative cardiac catheterization. It has now become routine in many centers for patients with lesions such as atrial septal defect (ASD) or patent ductus arteriosus (PDA) to be operated on without cardiac catheterization, and this has now extended to many other cardiac lesions. However, in cases in which information from the cardiac examination is not consistent with the echocardiogram, cardiac catheterization is an important tool to confirm the anatomic diagnosis and to evaluate the degree of physiologic derangement (e.g., the size of the left-to-right shunt or the degree of valvular stenosis).

Sophisticated echocardiographic methods of assessing left ventricular systolic and diastolic function, for example, end-systolic wall stress and dobutamine stress echocardiography, have proved useful in the serial assessment of patients at risk for development of ventricular dysfunction. These patients include those receiving anthracycline drugs for cancer chemotherapy, patients at risk for iron overload, and patients being monitored for rejection after heart transplantation.

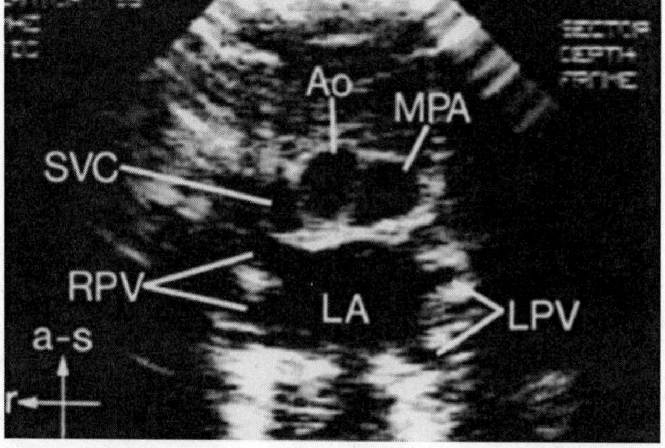

Figure 381–19. Suprasternal notch normal echocardiographic view. Pulmonary veins connecting with the left atrium. Ao = aorta; a-s = anterior-superior; LA = left atrium; LPV = left pulmonary vein; MPA = main pulmonary artery; RPV = right pulmonary vein; r = right; SVC = superior vena cava. (From Sanders SP: Echocardiography. *In:* Long WA [ed]: Fetal and Neonatal Cardiology. Philadelphia, WB Saunders, 1990.)

381.5 Exercise Testing

The normal cardiorespiratory system adapts to the extensive demands of exercise with a severalfold increase in oxygen consumption and cardiac output. Because there is a large reserve capacity for exercise, significant abnormalities of cardiovascular performance may exist without symptoms at rest or during ordinary activities. Generally, patients are evaluated in a resting state, during which significant abnormalities of cardiac function may not be appreciated or, if detected, their implications for quality of life may not be recognized. Permission for children with cardiovascular disease to participate in various forms of physical activity is unfortunately frequently based on subjective criteria. Exercise testing can play an important role in evaluating symptoms, quantitating the severity of cardiac abnormalities, and assisting in the management of these patients, including prescribing a rational physical activity schedule.

Exercise studies are usually performed on a graded treadmill apparatus using timed intervals of increasing grade and speed (e.g., the Bruce protocol). Younger children may be studied on a bicycle ergometer. Many laboratories now have the capacity to measure cardiac output and pulmonary function noninvasively during exercise.

As the child grows, the capacity for work increases with body size and skeletal muscle mass. All indices of cardiopulmo-

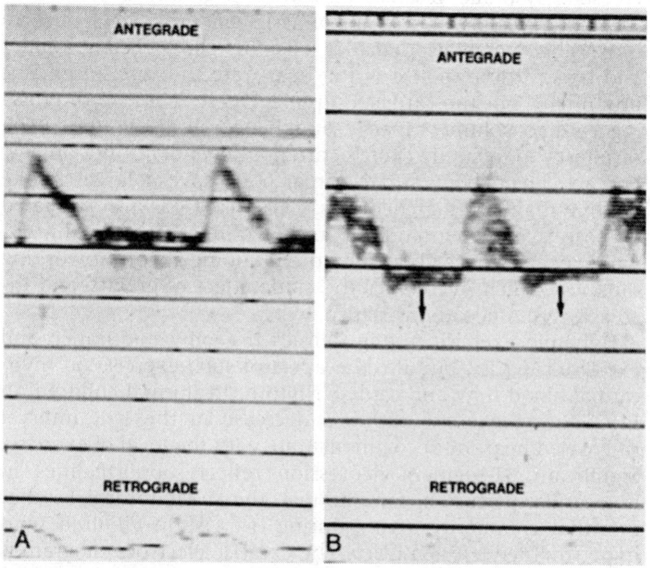

Figure 381–20. Patent ductus arteriosus. *A,* Doppler flow in the proximal descending aorta of normal infant demonstrating the normal antegrade systolic and diastolic flow. *B,* Doppler flow configuration in an infant with patent ductus arteriosus reveals antegrade systolic but retrograde diastolic flow (*arrows*).

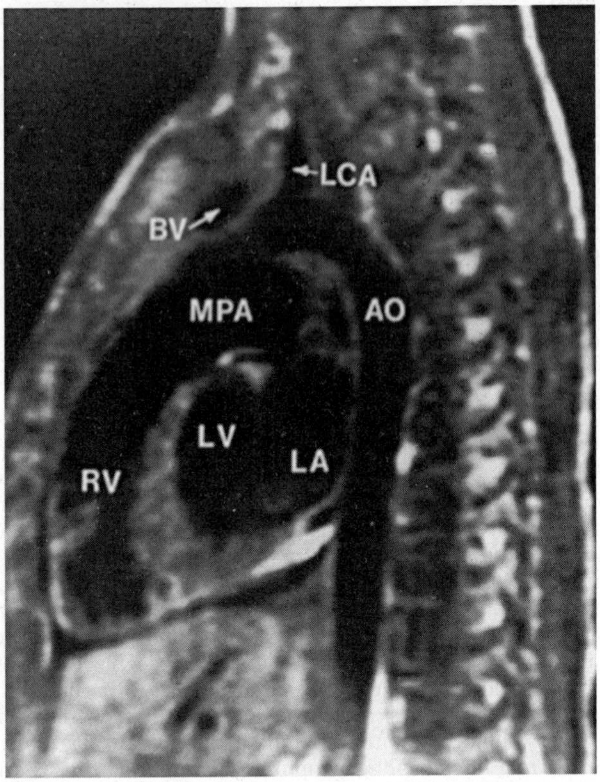

Figure 381–21. Sagittal normal MRI image. AO = aorta; BV = brachiocephalic vein; LA = left atrium; LCA = left coronary artery; LV = left ventricle; MPA = main pulmonary artery; RV = right ventricle. (From Bisset GS III: Cardiac and great vessel anatomy. *In:* El-Khoury GY, Bergman RA, Montgomery WJ: Sectional Anatomy by MRI/CT. New York, Churchill Livingstone, 1990, pp 219–243.)

nary function, however, do not increase in a uniform manner. A major response to exercise is an increase in cardiac output, principally as a result of increased heart rate, but stroke volume, systemic venous return, and pulse pressure are also increased. Systemic vascular resistance is greatly decreased as the blood vessels in working muscle dilate as a response to increasing metabolic demands. As the child becomes older and larger, the response of the heart rate to exercise remains prominent, but the cardiac output increases because of growing cardiac volume capacity and hence stroke volume. The responses to dynamic exercise are not dependent only on age. For any given body surface area, boys have a larger stroke volume than size-matched girls. This increase is also mediated by posture. Augmentation of stroke volume with upright, dynamic exercise is facilitated by the pumping action of working muscles, which overcomes the static effect of gravity and increases systemic venous return.

Dynamic exercise testing defines not only endurance and exercise capacity, but also the effect of such exercise on myocardial blood flow and cardiac rhythm. In normal children an ECG during exercise shows a decrease in the R-R interval (increased heart rate) commensurate with the level of exercise. Significant ST-segment depression reflects abnormalities in myocardial perfusion, for example, the subendocardial ischemia that commonly occurs during exercise in children with hypertrophied left ventricles. The exercise electrocardiogram is considered abnormal if ST-segment depression is ≥2 mm and extends for at least 0.06 sec after the J point (onset of ST segment) in conjunction with a horizontal-, upward-, or downward-sloping ST segment.

Provocation of rhythm disturbances during an exercise study is an important method for evaluating selected patients with known or suspected rhythm disorders. The effect of pharmacologic management can also be tested in this manner.

Conditions in which exercise testing may be helpful include: (1) left ventricular outflow obstruction, such as valvular, subvalvular, and supravalvular aortic stenosis, hypertrophic cardiomyopathy, and coarctation of the aorta; (2) chronic volume overload of the left or right ventricle, such as atrioventricular or semilunar valve incompetence and left-to-right shunts; (3) arrhythmias; (4) hypertension; and (5) patients who have undergone open heart surgical correction of complex congenital heart lesions, for example, the Fontan operation.

A physician should be present during the exercise test to supervise its performance, and adequate emergency equipment must be immediately available (e.g., defibrillator, medications, IV fluids, etc.). Indications for termination of a study are (1) failure or inadequacy of the electrocardiographic monitoring; (2) onset of serious arrhythmias, such as ventricular or supraventricular tachycardia; (3) premature beats (>25% of beats) precipitated or aggravated by exercise; (4) development of heart block; (5) precipitation of pain, headache, dizziness, or syncope; (6) ST-segment depression or elevation of 3 mm or more; (7) inappropriate hypertension (systolic pressure >230 mm Hg or diastolic pressure >120 mm Hg in older children); (8) inappropriate fall of blood pressure; (9) development of cutaneous vascular insufficiency (e.g., pallor); or (10) severe fatigue.

381.6 Magnetic Resonance Imaging (MRI) and Radionuclide Studies

Magnetic resonance imaging is helpful in the diagnosis and management of patients with congenital heart disease. It produces tomographic images of the heart in any projection (Figs. 381–21and 381–22) by portraying the response of tissues in

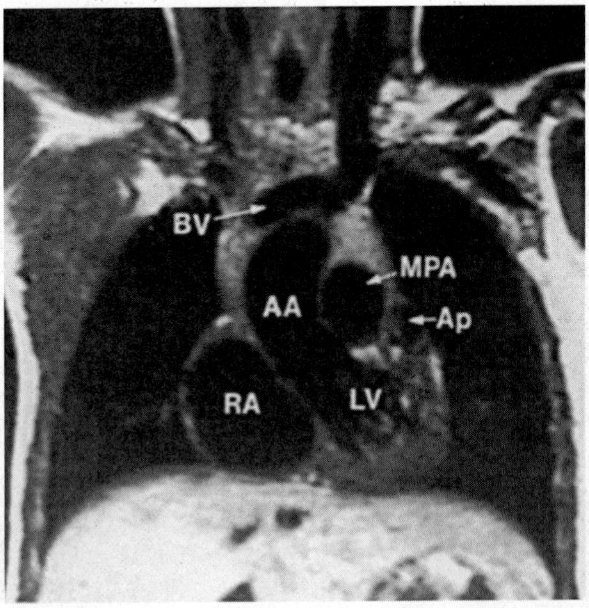

Figure 381–22. Coronal plane, normal MRI image. AA = ascending aorta; Ap = left atrial appendage; BV = brachiocephalic vein; LV = left ventricle; MPA = main pulmonary artery; RA = right atrium. (From Bisset GS III: Cardiac and great vessel anatomy. *In:* El-Khoury GY, Bergman RA, Montgomery WJ: Sectional Anatomy by MRI/CT. New York, Churchill Livingstone, 1990, pp 219–243.)

a homogeneous magnetic field when exposed to bursts of radiofrequency energy. The gray-scale intensity of each individual picture element in an image is related to the concentration, motion, and chemical microenvironment of hydrogen nuclei in that element. Excellent contrast resolution of fat, myocardium, and lung, as well as moving blood from blood vessel walls, is obtained.

This noninvasive method of cardiac imaging provides diagnostic imagery in malformations of the great vessels, including coarctation of the aorta, proximal branch pulmonary artery stenosis, and transposition of the great arteries, as well as simple and complex cardiac malformations, including aortic stenosis, pulmonary stenosis, atrial septal defect, ventricular septal defect, tetralogy of Fallot, single ventricle, and inversion of the ventricles. MRI has been particularly useful in evaluating distal branch pulmonary artery anatomy and anomalies of pulmonary venous return.

New developments in MRI include cine MRI and in vivo magnetic resonance (MR) spectroscopy. Cine MRI allows acquisition of images in several tomographic planes. Within each plane, images are obtained at different phases of the cardiac cycle. Thus, when displayed in a dynamic "cine" format, changes in wall thickening, chamber volume, and valve function can be displayed and analyzed. Blood flow velocity and blood flow volume can be approximated. Phosphorus *MR spectroscopy* provides a means of demonstrating relative concentrations of high-energy metabolites, for example, adenosine triphosphate (ATP), adenosine diphosphate (ADP), inorganic phosphate (P_i), and phosphocreatine, within regions of the working myocardium. Other new MRI techniques under evaluation include a method for estimation of oxygen saturation in the various cardiac chambers, thus allowing the calculation of shunt volumes.

MRI complements information provided by echocardiography and cineangiography. With further development in rapid image acquisition, and spectroscopic techniques, MRI should reduce the need for invasive angiography or tissue biopsy during cardiac catheterization.

Radionuclide angiography may be used to detect and quantify shunts and to analyze the distribution of blood flow to each lung. *Gated blood pool scanning* can be used to calculate hemodynamic measurements, to quantify valvular regurgitation, and to detect regional wall motion abnormalities. *Thallium imaging* can be used to evaluate cardiac muscle perfusion. These methods can be used at the bedside of the seriously ill child and can be employed serially, with minimal discomfort and low radiation exposure. They are particularly useful in quantifying the volume of blood flow distribution between the two lungs in patients with abnormalities of the pulmonary vascular tree or after a shunt (Blalock-Taussig or Glenn) operation.

381.7 Cardiac Catheterization

Cardiac catheterization is an important tool in the diagnosis of congenital heart disease. With this technique the various chambers of the heart, great vessels, and veins are entered and blood samples are obtained for measuring oxygen saturation. Pressures are measured, and contrast is injected to delineate structures. Major indications for cardiac catheterization include: (1) presurgical evaluation of cardiac anatomy and shunt size, (2) evaluation of pulmonary vascular resistance and its reactivity to vasodilators or oxygen, (3) follow-up after surgical repair or palliation of complex congenital heart lesions, (4) myocardial biopsy for diagnosis of cardiomyopathy or screening for cardiac rejection after transplantation, (6) interventional cardiac catheterization, and (7) electrophysiologic study and/or transcatheter ablation (see Chapter 388).

Although the risks are low, cardiac catheterization involves potential complications for the patient and should not be used without an opportunity for benefit. In many instances echocardiography, MRI or radionuclide studies may be used in lieu of multiple cardiac catheterizations in individual patients who require careful monitoring of their hemodynamic status. Within the last 10 yr these noninvasive tests have begun to supplant cardiac catheterization in evaluating many patients prior to surgery. Although the number of preoperative cardiac catheterization procedures has declined with improvements in echocardiography, the number of postoperative procedures has increased with the advent of new palliative surgical procedures to repair extremely complex congenital heart lesions. Finally, interventional cardiac catheterization has replaced surgical repair in many cases (e.g., pulmonary or aortic valve stenosis, re-coarctation of the aorta) and in others is used as an adjunct to complex surgical repairs (branch pulmonary artery stenosis, the fenestrated Fontan operation [see Chapter 387.5]).

Cardiac catheterization should be performed with the patient in as close to a basal state as possible. Children are routinely sedated during these studies, but deep anesthesia is avoided if possible, as depression of cardiovascular function by various anesthetic agents may distort the calculations of hemodynamic measurements, including cardiac output, pulmonary and systemic vascular resistances, and shunt ratios.

If cardiac catheterization is performed on a critically ill infant with congenital heart disease, a surgical team should be alerted in the event that an operation is required immediately afterward. The complication rate of cardiac catheterization and angiography is greatest among critically ill infants; they must be studied in a thermally neutral environment and treated quickly for hypothermia, hypoglycemia, acidemia, or excessive blood loss. Development of soft, flow-directed balloon-tipped catheters has greatly decreased the frequency of complications from catheter manipulation in eras past, such as severe arrhythmias, cardiac perforation, and intramyocardial injection of contrast material.

In most instances catheterization involves both the left and the right sides of the heart. The catheter is passed into the heart under fluoroscopic guidance through a percutaneous entry point in the femoral vein. In infants and in a large number of older children, the left side of the heart can be accessed by passing the catheter across a patent foramen ovale to the left atrium and left ventricle. If the foramen is closed, the left side of the heart can also be catheterized by passing the catheter retrograde via a percutaneous entry into the femoral artery. The catheter can be manipulated through abnormal intracardiac defects (ASDs, ventricular septal defects [VSDs]) or into malpositioned great vessels (e.g., transposition of the great vessels). Complete hemodynamics can be calculated (Table 381–2) through data obtained at catheterization: cardiac output, intracardiac left-to-right and right-to-left shunts, and systemic and pulmonary vascular resistances. The normal circulatory dynamics are depicted in Figure 381–23.

INDICATOR DILUTION AND APPEARANCE TECHNIQUES

If a bolus of an indicator material is injected intravenously or into the right side of the heart, it traverses the pulmonary circulation and enters the left side of the heart and then the arterial circulation. This indicator material may then be detected in the arterial blood. A continuous record of the circulation of indicator in normal subjects shows two peaks (Fig. 381–24). The time between the instant of injection and the detection of the indicator in arterial blood is known as the appearance time and is a measure of the circulation time. The 1st peak of the indicator curve is due to the passage of indicator past the arterial detectors. The 2nd peak is due to recircula-

■ TABLE 381–2 Normal Values and Formulas for Determination of Hemodynamics in Cardiac Catheterization

1. Cardiac index 3.0–5.0 L/min/m²
2. Arteriovenous oxygen difference 4.5 ± 0.7 mL/dL
3. Oxygen consumption 140–160 mL/m²/min
4. Arterial oxygen saturation 94–100%
5. Difference in oxygen content between venae cavae and right atrium <1.9 vol %
6. Difference in oxygen content between right atrium and right ventricle <0.9 vol %
7. Difference in oxygen content between right ventricle and pulmonary artery <0.5 vol %
8. Normal mean left atrial pressure 4–8 mm Hg
9. Pulmonary arteriolar resistance 50–150 dyn sec cm⁻⁵ (1 unit = 80 dynes)
10. Cardiac output mL/min =
$$\frac{O_2 \text{ intake (mL/min)}}{\left\{\begin{array}{l}O_2 \text{ content of arterial blood (vols \%)} \\ \text{minus } O_2 \text{ content of mixed venous blood}\end{array}\right.} \times 100$$
11. Cardiac index = cardiac output (L/min)/m² of body surface area
12. Pulmonary artery flow =
$$\frac{O_2 \text{ intake (mL/min)}}{\left\{\begin{array}{l}O_2 \text{ content of pulmonary venous blood (vols \%)} \\ \text{minus } O_2 \text{ content of pulmonary arterial blood (vols \%)}\end{array}\right.} \times 100$$
If a pulmonary venous sample is not available, it is assumed to be saturated to 95% of capacity
13. Systemic flow =
$$\frac{O_2 \text{ intake (mL/min)}}{\left\{\begin{array}{l}\text{systemic arterial } O_2 \text{ content (vols \%)} \\ \text{minus arterial venous } O_2 \text{ content (vols \%)}\end{array}\right.} \times 100$$
14. Effective pulmonary artery flow =
$$\frac{O_2 \text{ intake (mL/min)}}{\left\{\begin{array}{l}\text{pulmonary venous } O_2 \text{ content (vols \%)} \\ \text{minus mixed venous } O_2 \text{ content (vols \%)}\end{array}\right.} \times 100$$
15. Total left to right shunt = pulmonary artery flow minus effective pulmonary artery flow
16. Total right to left shunt = systemic flow minus effective pulmonary artery flow
17. Pulmonary arteriolar resistance $R = \frac{PA - PC}{PF}$

Where R = pulmonary arteriolar resistance (resistance units)
PA = mean pulmonary artery pressure in mm Hg
PC = mean pulmonary "capillary" pressure in mm Hg
PF = pulmonary flow in L/min/m²

tion through the systemic arterial and venous systems, the pulmonary circulation, and reappearance in the arterial tree. If the concentration of circulating indicator is known, the cardiac output can be computed.

The *thermodilution method* for measuring cardiac output is the most commonly used indicator dilution technique. A known change in heat content of the blood is induced at one point in the circulation (usually the right atrium or inferior vena cava), and the resultant change in temperature is detected at a point downstream (usually the pulmonary artery). The injectate is usually room-temperature saline. This method is used to measure cardiac output in the catheterization laboratory in patients without shunts. When combined with the dye dilution technique, it can also be used to measure the volume of regurgitant flow across diseased mitral or aortic valves. Monitoring the cardiac output by the thermodilution method is also useful in managing critically ill infants and children in an intensive care setting after cardiac surgery or in the presence of shock. In this case a triple-lumen flow directed thermodilution (Swan-Ganz) catheter is used for both cardiac output determinations and for measurement of pulmonary arterial and pulmonary capillary wedge pressures.

ANGIOCARDIOGRAPHY

The great blood vessels and individual cardiac chambers may be visualized by selective angiocardiography, that is, injection of contrast material into specific cardiac chambers or great vessels. This method allows identification of structural abnormalities without interference from the superimposed shadows of normal chambers. Photofluoroscopy with image intensification has made possible simultaneous cardiac catheterization and selective angiocardiography. The preferred method is a combination of photofluoroscopy with closed-circuit television to allow visualization of the cardiac silhouette and the cardiac catheter as it passes through various heart chambers. After the cardiac catheter is introduced into the chamber to be studied, a small amount of contrast medium is rapidly injected and cineangiograms are exposed at 30–60 frames/Chap. Biplane cineangiocardiography allows detailed evaluation of specific cardiac chambers and blood vessels in two planes simultaneous with the injection of a single bolus of contrast material. This technique is now standard in pediatric cardiac catheterization laboratories and allows one to minimize the volume of contrast material used, which is safer for the patient. Various angled views (e.g. left anterior oblique, cranial angulation) are utilized to best display specific anatomic features in individual lesions.

The rapid injection of contrast medium under pressure into the circulation is not without risks, and each injection should be carefully planned. Contrast agents consist of hypertonic solutions, some containing organic iodides, which can cause complications, including nausea, a generalized burning sensation, central nervous system symptoms, and allergic reactions. Intramyocardial injection is generally avoided by careful placement of the catheter prior to injection. Hypertonicity of the

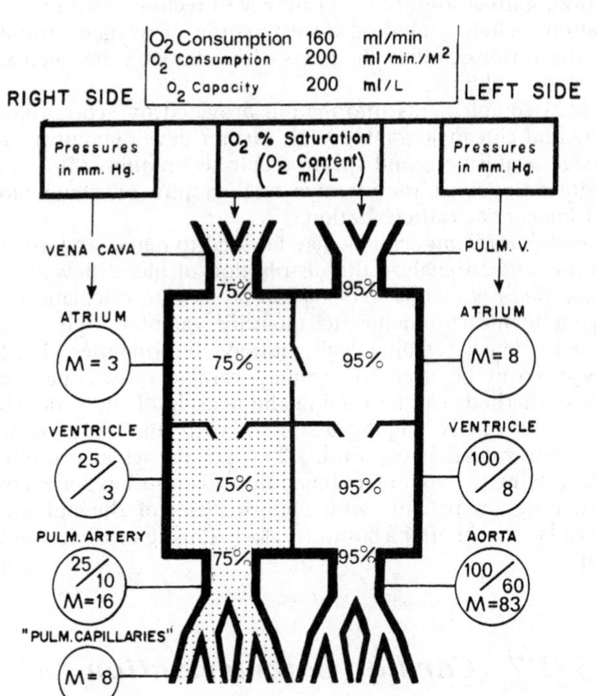

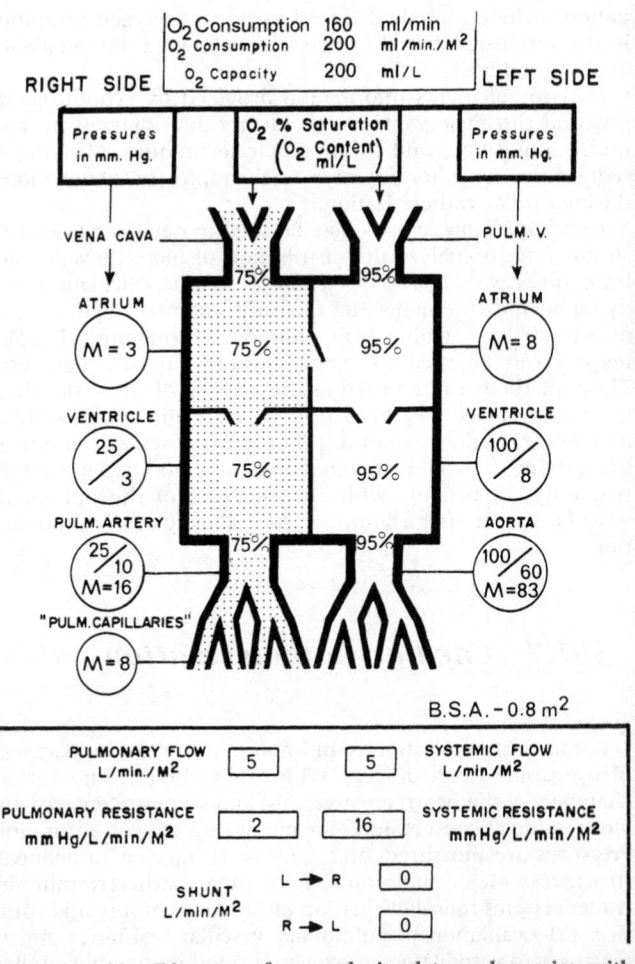

Figure 381–23. Diagram of normal circulatory dynamics with pressures, oxygen contents, and percentage of saturations. (Modified from Nadas AS, Fyler DC: Pediatric Cardiology, 3rd ed. Philadelphia, WB Saunders, 1972.)

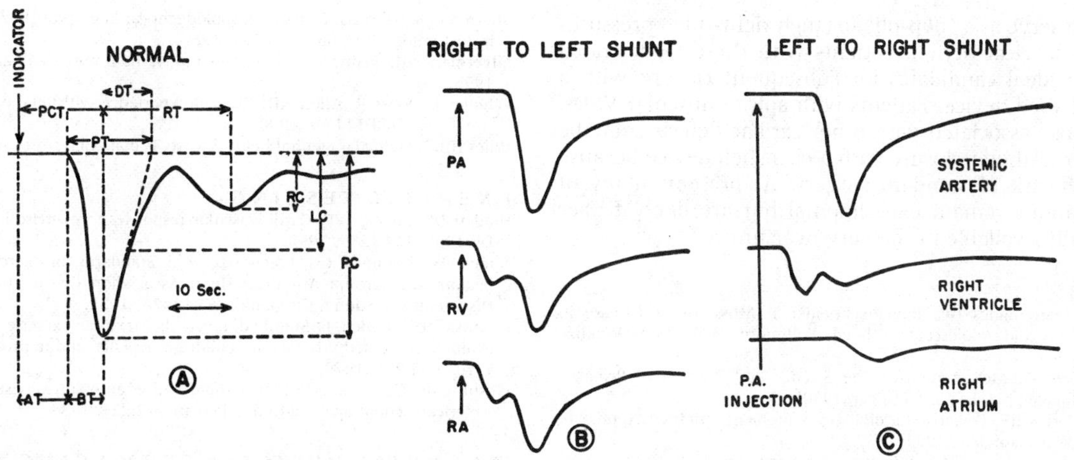

Figure 381–24. Idealized diagrams of indicator dilution curves. *A,* Normal curve showing the time and concentration components. The instant of indicator injection in the right side of the heart is shown by an *arrow* at the top left. The curve is obtained from the indicator detector in a systemic artery. AT = appearance time; BT = build-up time; DT = disappearance time; LC = least concentration; PC = peak concentration; PCT = peak concentration time; PT = passage time; RC = maximal recirculation concentration; RT = recirculation time. Extrapolation of declining slope of concentration is easier if the curve is plotted on a logarithmic scale. Cardiac output may be computed by the formula 601/c(PT), where 1 = amount of indicator, c = mean concentration of indicator, PT = passage time. *B,* Localization of *right to left shunt.* The instant of the injection of the indicator is shown by *arrows.* The example illustrates the shunt at ventricular levels. Site of injection: PA = pulmonary artery; RA = right atrium; RV = right ventricle. Indicator detector in systemic artery in all instances. PA injection (i.e., downstream from the shunt level) shows a normal appearance time. RV and RA injections (i.e., at and upstream from shunt level) show early appearance times. *C,* Localization of *left to right shunt.* Example illustrates shunt at ventricular level. Indicator injected into distal pulmonary artery (PA) in all instances. In the upper tracing the indicator detector is in a systemic artery, and the curve shows a prolonged disappearance time. The middle curve is from the indicator detected in the right ventricle and shows an early appearance time because of ventricular septal defect. The right atrial curve shows a normal appearance time.

contrast medium may result in transient myocardial depression and a drop in blood pressure, and soon afterward tachycardia, an increase in cardiac output, and a shift of interstitial fluid into the circulation. This shift can transiently increase the symptoms of congestive heart failure in critically ill patients.

Idealized diagrams of the normal angiocardiogram are shown in Figure 381–1. The indications for performing cardiac catheterization for individual congenital heart lesions are outlined in the discussion of each individual lesion.

INTERVENTIONAL CATHETERIZATION

Nonsurgical treatment of certain cardiac defects that until now required intraoperative repair has become possible with interventional cardiac catheterization. Interventional techniques include balloon dilatation of stenotic valves and arteries, embolization of abnormal vascular connections, and catheter closure of intracardiac defects. The procedure most often utilized is balloon valvuloplasty. A special catheter with a sausage-shaped balloon at the distal end is passed through an obstructed valve. The balloon is rapidly filled with a mixture of contrast material and saline solution, resulting in tearing of the stenotic valve tissue, usually at the site of inappropriately fused raphe. Valvular pulmonary stenosis can now be treated successfully by balloon angioplasty in most patients and has replaced surgical repair as the initial procedure of choice. The clinical results of this procedure are similar to those obtained by open heart surgery without the need for a sternotomy or prolonged hospitalization. Balloon valvuloplasty for aortic stenosis has also yielded excellent results, although, as with surgery, aortic stenosis often recurs as the child grows and may require multiple procedures. One complication of both valvuloplasty and surgery is the creation of significant valvular insufficiency. This complication has more serious implications when it occurs on the aortic as compared with the pulmonary side of the circulation because regurgitation is less well tolerated at systemic arterial pressures.

There is general agreement that balloon angioplasty represents the procedure of choice for patients with restenosis of a coarctation of the aorta after earlier surgery. However, there is still controversy as to whether angioplasty is the best procedure for native (unoperated) coarctation of the aorta because of reports of later aneurysm formation. The risk of angioplasty and valvuloplasty procedures on the left side of the heart are higher in younger patients, especially infants less than 1 yr of age, because of complications at the site of femoral arterial catheterization. Newer, low-profile catheters have significantly reduced but not eliminated these complications. Other applications of the balloon angioplasty technique include amelioration of mitral stenosis, dilatation of surgical conduits (Mustard or Senning atrial baffles), relief of branch pulmonary arterial narrowing, dilatation of venous obstructions, and the long-utilized balloon atrial septostomy (Rashkind procedure) for transposition of the great arteries (see Chapter 387.9).

Interventional cardiac catheterization techniques using coils and detachable balloons also have been developed for obliteration of arteriovenous shunts and pulmonary collateral vessels, which may be detrimental after surgical repair of pulmonary atresia and VSD. In patients with branch pulmonary arterial stenoses, previously mixed results with balloon angioplasty alone have been supplanted with the use of intravascular stents, which once placed can be dilated to successively greater sizes as the patient grows.

There is also increasing experience with catheter-introduced umbrella devices or buttons to close PDAs and secundum atrial septal defects. Foam plugs and coils may also be introduced to close a PDA. High-risk patients undergoing the Fontan operation (see Chapter 387.5) often have a small fenestration created in the baffle between the right and left sides of the circulation to serve as a "pop-off" for high right-sided pressures in the early surgical period. Patients with these "fenestrated Fontans" are ideal candidates for subsequent closure with a catheter-delivered device. Patients with apical muscular VSDs, especially those associated with other cardiac defects, may be candidates for catheter closure with a clamshell device because of the higher risk of standard surgery. At present, many of these applications remain experimental but are likely to become generally available in the very near future.

GENERAL

Adams FH, Emmanouilides GC, Riemerschneider T: Moss' Heart Disease in Infants, Children and Adolescents, 4th ed. Baltimore, Williams & Wilkins, 1989.
Garson A, Bricker JT, McNamara DG: The Science and Practice of Pediatric Cardiology. Philadelphia, Lea and Febiger, 1990.
Gessner IH, Victorica BE: Pediatric Cardiology: A Problem Oriented Approach. Philadelphia, W.B. Saunders, 1993.
Gillette PC: Congenital heart disease. Pediatr Clin North Am 37:1, 1990.
Hohn AR, Dwyer KM, Dwyer JH: Blood pressure in youth from four ethnic groups: The Pasadena Prevention Project. J Pediatr 125:368, 1994.
Rosner B, Prineas RJ, Loggie MH, et al: Blood pressure nomograms for children and adolescents, by height, sex, and age, in the United States. J Pediatr 123:871, 1993.
Selbst SM: Chest pain in children. Pediatrics 75:1068, 1985.
Shea S, Basch CE, Gutin B, et al: The rate of increase in blood pressure in children 5 years of age is related to changes in aerobic fitness and body mass index. Pediatrics 94:465, 1994.
Zuberbuhler JR: Clinical Diagnosis in Pediatric Cardiology. Edinburgh, Churchill Livingstone, 1981.

CARDIAC SOUNDS AND PHONOCARDIOGRAPHY

McNamara DG: Value and limitations of auscultation in the management of congenital heart disease. Pediatr Clin North Am 37:93, 1990.
Mills P, Craige E: Echophonocardiography. Prog Cardiovasc Dis 20:337, 1989.
Newburger JW, Rosenthal A, Williams RG, et al: Noninvasive tests in the initial evaluation of heart murmurs in children. N Engl J Med 308:61, 1983.

ELECTROCARDIOGRAM AND VECTORCARDIOGRAM

Garson A: The Electrocardiogram in Infants and Children: A Systematic Approach. Philadelphia, Lea & Febiger, 1983.
Garson A, Dick M, Fournier A, et al: The long QT syndrome in children: An international study of 287 patients. Circulation 87:1866, 1993.
Liebman J, Plonsey R, Yoram R: Pediatric and Fundamental Electrocardiography. Boston, Martinis Nijhoff, 1987.
Lipman BF, Massey EF: Clinical Scalar Electrocardiography. Chicago, Year Book Medical Publishers, 1984.
Marriott H: Rhythm Quizlets Self Assessment. Philadelphia, Lea & Febiger, 1987.
Schwartz PJ, Moss AJ, Vincent GM, et al: Diagnostic criteria for the long QT syndrome: An update. Circulation 88:782, 1993.

ECHOCARDIOGRAPHY

Fyfe DA, Kline CH: Fetal echocardiographic diagnosis of congenital heart disease. Pediatr Clin North Am 37:45, 1990.
Hatle L, Angelsen B: Doppler Ultrasound in Cardiology, Physical Principles and Clinical Applications. Philadelphia, Lea & Febiger, 1985.
Klewer SE, Goldberg SJ, Donnerstein RL, et al: Dobutamine stress echocardiography: A sensitive indicator of diminished myocardial function in asymptomatic doxorubicin-treated long-term survivors of childhood cancer. J Am Coll Cardiol 19:394, 1992.
Popp RL: Echocardiography. N Engl J Med 323:101, 1990.
Seward JB, Tajik AJ, Edwards WD, et al: Two-Dimensional Echocardiographic Atlas. I: Congenital Heart Disease. New York, Springer-Verlag, 1987.
Sherman FS, Sahn DJ: Pediatric Doppler echocardiography 1987: Major advances in technology. J Pediatr 110:333, 1987.
Silverman NH: Pediatric Echocardiography. Baltimore, Williams and Wilkins, 1993.
Wheller JJ, Reiss R, Allen HD: Clinical experience with fetal echocardiography. Am J Dis Child 144:49, 1990.
Wiles HB: Imaging congenital heart disease. Pediatr Clin North Am 37:115, 1990.

EXERCISE TESTING

Braden DS, Strong WF: Cardiovascular responses to exercise in children. Am J Dis Child 144:1255, 1990.
James FW, Blomqvist CG, Freed MD, et al: Standards for exercise testing in the pediatric age group: American Heart Association Council on Cardiovascular Disease in the Young. Circulation 66:1377A, 1982.
Rozanski JJ, Dimich I, Steinfeld L, et al: Maximal exercise stress testing in evaluation of arrhythmias in children: Results and reproducibility. Am J Cardiol 42:951, 1979.
Washington RL, et al: Normal aerobic and anaerobic exercise data for North American school-age children. J Pediatr 112:223, 1988.

MAGNETIC RESONANCE IMAGING AND NUCLEAR MEDICINE

Didier D, Higgins CB, Fisher MR, et al: Congenital heart disease: Gated MR imaging in 72 patients. Radiology 158:227, 1986.
Dilworth LR, Aisen AM, Mancini GB: Determination of left ventricular volumes and ejection fraction by nuclear magnetic resonance imaging. Am Heart J 113:24, 1987.
Fletcher BD, Jacobson MD, Nelson AD, et al: Gated magnetic resonance imaging of congenital cardiac malformations. Radiology 150:137, 1984.
Hurwitz RA: Quantitation of aortic and mitral regurgitation in the pediatric population: Evaluation by radionuclide angiography. Am J Cardiol 51:252, 1983.

CARDIAC CATHETERIZATION

Allen HD, Mullins CE. Results of the Valvuloplasty and Angioplasty of Congenital Anomalies Registry. Am J Cardiol 65:772, 1990.
Benson LN, Freedom RM: Interventional cardiac catheterization. Curr Opin Pediatr 1:106, 1989.
Bridges ND, Perry SB, Keane JF, et al: Preoperative transcatheter closure of congenital muscular ventricular septal defects. N Engl J Med 324:1312, 1991.
Freedom RM, Culham JAG, Moes CAF: Angiocardiography of Congenital Heart Disease. New York, Macmillan, 1984.
Gray DT, Fyler DC, Walker AM, et al: Clinical outcomes and costs of transcatheter as compared with surgical closure of patent ductus arteriosus. N Engl J Med 329:1517, 1993.
Kan JS, White RI, Mitchell SE, et al: Treatment of restenosis of coarctation by percutaneous transluminal angioplasty. Circulation 68:1087, 1983.
Lock JE, Keane JF, Fellows KE: The use of catheter intervention procedures for congenital heart disease. J Am Coll Cardiol 7:1420, 1986.
Lock JE, Keane JF, Fellows KE: Diagnostic and Interventional Catheterization in Congenital Heart Disease. Dordrecht, The Netherlands, Martinus Nijhoff, 1987.
Mullins CE, Nihill MR, Vick GW, et al: Double balloon technique for dilatation of valvular or vessel stenosis in congenital and acquired heart disease. J Am Coll Cardiol 10:107, 1987.
O'Laughlin MP, Slack MC, Grifka RG, et al: Implantation and intermediate-term follow-up of stents in congenital heart disease. Circulation 88:605, 1993.
Radtke W, Lick J: Balloon dilation. Pediatr Clin North Am 37:193, 1990.
Rao PS: Balloon valvuloplasty and angioplasty in infants and children. J Pediatr 114:907, 1989.
Rao PS, Thapar MK, Galal O, et al: Follow-up results of balloon angioplasty of native coarctation in neonates and infants. Am Heart J 120:1310, 1990.
Stanger P, Heymann MA, Tarnoff H, et al: Complications of cardiac catheterization of neonates, infants, and children: A three year study. Circulation 50:595, 1974.
Suarez J, Pan M, Sancho M, et al: Percutaneous transluminal balloon dilatation for discrete subaortic stenosis. Am J Cardiol 58:619, 1986.
Waldman JD, Karp RB. How should we treat coarctation of the aorta? Circulation 87:1043, 1993.

SECTION 2

The Transitional Circulation

Daniel Bernstein

CHAPTER 382

The Fetal and Neonatal Circulation

THE FETAL CIRCULATION

Much of the information concerning the fetal circulation has been derived from animal studies, especially those in fetal sheep. Although there may be some species differences, the human fetal circulation and its adjustments after birth are probably qualitatively very similar to those of other large mammals.

In the fetal circulation, the right and left ventricles exist in a parallel circuit as opposed to the series circuit of the newborn or adult (Figure 382–1*A*). In the fetus, gas and metabolite exchange are provided for by the placenta. The lungs do not provide gas exchange, and vessels in the pulmonary circulation are vasoconstricted. There are three cardiovascular structures unique to the fetus that are important for maintaining this parallel circulation: the ductus venosus, foramen ovale, and the ductus arteriosus.

Oxygenated blood returning from the placenta, with a Po_2 of about 30–35 mm Hg, flows to the fetus through the umbilical vein. Approximately 50% of umbilical venous blood enters the hepatic circulation, whereas the rest bypasses the liver and joins the inferior vena cava via the *ductus venosus,* where it partially mixes with poorly oxygenated inferior vena caval blood derived from the fetal lower body. This combined lower body plus umbilical venous blood flow (Po_2 of about 26–28 mm Hg) enters the right atrium and is directed preferentially across the *foramen ovale* to the left atrium (Fig. 382–1*B*). This blood then flows into the left ventricle and is ejected into the ascending aorta. Fetal superior vena caval blood, which is considerably less oxygenated (Po_2 of 12–14 mm Hg), enters

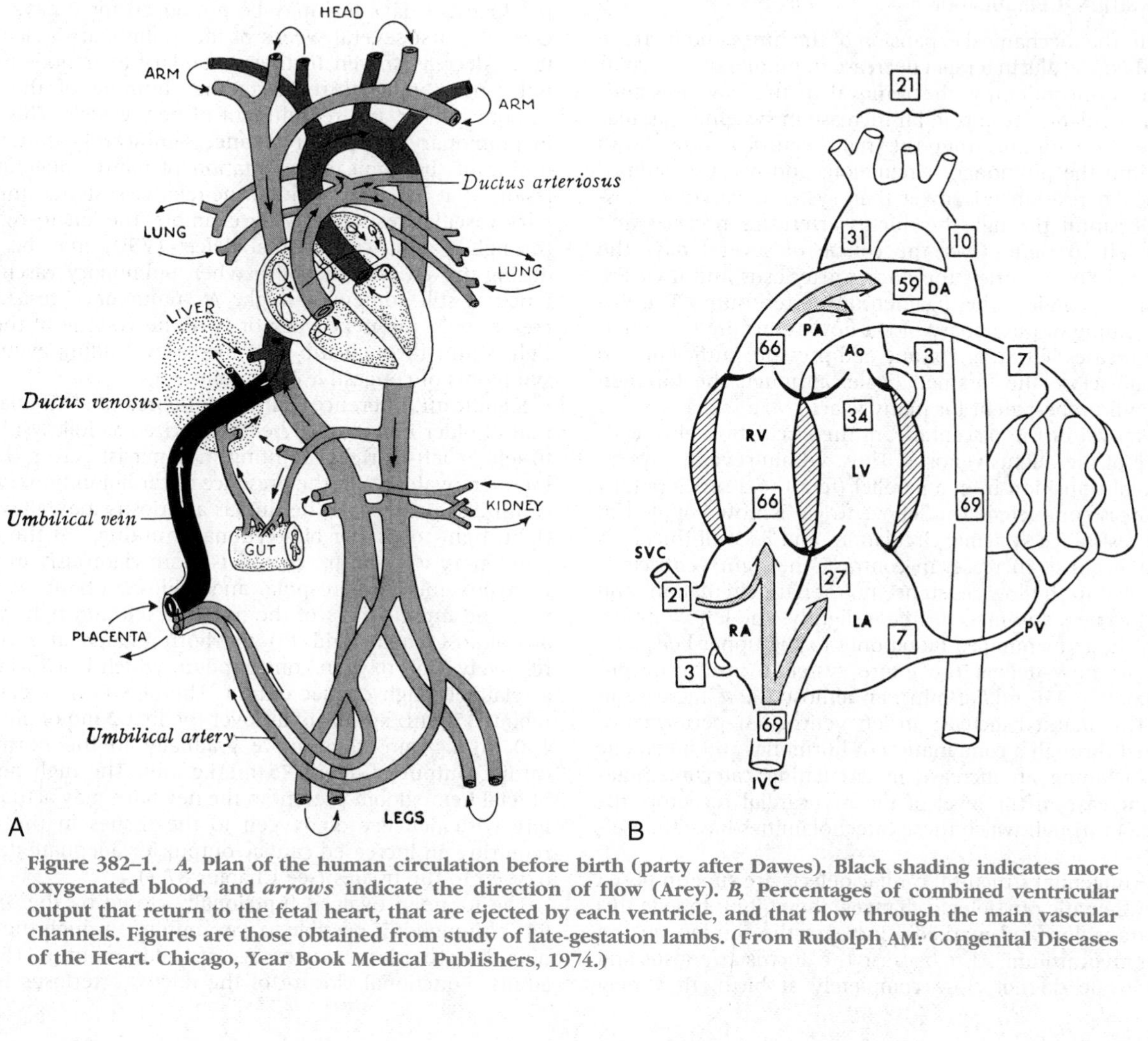

Figure 382–1. *A,* Plan of the human circulation before birth (party after Dawes). Black shading indicates more oxygenated blood, and *arrows* indicate the direction of flow (Arey). *B,* Percentages of combined ventricular output that return to the fetal heart, that are ejected by each ventricle, and that flow through the main vascular channels. Figures are those obtained from study of late-gestation lambs. (From Rudolph AM: Congenital Diseases of the Heart. Chicago, Year Book Medical Publishers, 1974.)

the right atrium and preferentially traverses the tricuspid valve, rather than the foramen ovale, and flows primarily to the right ventricle.

From the right ventricle this blood is ejected into the pulmonary artery. Because the pulmonary arterial circulation is vasoconstricted, only about 10% of right ventricular outflow enters the lungs. The major portion of this blood (which has a Po_2 of about 18–22 mm Hg) bypasses the lungs and flows through the *ductus arteriosus* into the descending aorta to perfuse the lower part of the fetal body as well as to return to the placenta via the two umbilical arteries. Thus, the fetal upper body (including the coronary and cerebral arteries, and those to the upper extremities) is perfused exclusively from the left ventricle with blood having a slightly higher Po_2 than the blood perfusing the lower fetal body, which is derived mostly from the right ventricle. Only a small volume of blood from the ascending aorta (10% of fetal cardiac output) flows across the aortic isthmus to the descending aorta.

The total fetal cardiac output—the combined ventricular output (CVO) of both the left and right ventricles—amounts to about 450 mL/kg/min. Approximately 65% of descending aortic blood flow returns to the placenta; the remaining 35% perfuses the fetal organs and tissues. In the sheep fetus, right ventricular output is approximately two times that of the left ventricle. In the human fetus, with a larger percentage of blood flow going to the brain, right ventricular output is probably closer to 1.3 times left ventricular flow. Thus, during fetal life the right ventricle is not only pumping against systemic blood pressure but is performing a greater volume of work than the left ventricle.

THE TRANSITIONAL CIRCULATION

At birth, the mechanical expansion of the lungs and increase in arterial Po_2 results in a rapid decrease in pulmonary vascular resistance. Concomitantly, the removal of the low resistance placental circulation results in an increase in systemic vascular resistance. The output from the right ventricle now flows entirely into the pulmonary circulation, and because pulmonary vascular resistance is lower than systemic vascular resistance, the shunt through the ductus arteriosus reverses and becomes left to right. Over the course of several days the high arterial Po_2 constricts the ductus arteriosus and it closes, eventually becoming the ligamentum arteriosum. The increased volume of pulmonary blood flow returning to the left atrium increases left atrial volume and pressure sufficiently to functionally close the foramen ovale, although the foramen may remain probe-patent for many years.

The removal of the placenta from the circulation also leads to closure of the ductus venosus. Thus, within several days an almost total transition from a parallel (fetal) to a series (adult) circulation is completed. The left ventricle is now coupled to the high resistance systemic circulation, and its wall thickness and mass begin to increase. In contrast, the right ventricle is now coupled to the low resistance pulmonary circulation, and its wall thickness and mass decrease slightly. The left ventricle, which in the fetus pumped blood only to the upper body and brain, must now deliver the entire systemic cardiac output (approximately 350 mL/kg/min), an almost 200% increase in output. This marked increase in left ventricular performance is achieved through a combination of hormonal and metabolic signals, including an increase in circulating catecholamines and an increase in the level of the myocardial receptors (β-adrenergic) through which these catecholamines have their effect.

When congenital structural cardiac defects are superimposed on these dramatic physiologic changes, they often impede this smooth transition and markedly increase the burden on the newborn myocardium. Also, because the ductus arteriosus and foramen ovale do not close completely at birth, they may remain patent in certain congenital cardiac lesions. Patency of these fetal pathways may provide either a life-saving pathway for blood to bypass a congenital defect (e.g., a patent ductus in pulmonary atresia or coarctation of the aorta or a foramen ovale in transposition of the great vessels) or may present an additional stress to the circulation (patent ductus arteriosus in a premature infant, pathway for right-to-left shunting in infants with pulmonary hypertension). The cardiologist has available pharmacologic means to either maintain these fetal pathways (e.g., prostaglandin E_1) or to hasten their closure (indomethacin).

NEONATAL CIRCULATION

At birth the fetal circulation must immediately adapt to extrauterine life as gas exchange is transferred from the placenta to the lung (see Chapter 87). Some of these changes are virtually instantaneous with the 1st breath, and others are effected over hours or days. After an initial slight fall in systemic blood pressure, there is a progressive rise with increasing age. The heart rate slows as a result of a baroreceptor response to an increase in systemic vascular resistance when the placental circulation is eliminated. The average central aortic pressure in the term neonate is 75/50 mm Hg.

With the onset of ventilation a marked decrease in pulmonary vascular resistance occurs due to both active (Po_2-related) and passive (mechanical-related) vasodilation. In the normal neonate, closure of the ductus arteriosus and the fall of pulmonary vascular resistance result in a fall of pulmonary arterial and right ventricular pressures. The major decline of pulmonary resistance from the high fetal levels to the low "adult" levels in the human infant at sea level usually occurs within the first 2–3 days but may be prolonged for 7 days or more. Over the first several weeks of life, pulmonary vascular resistance decreases even further secondary to remodeling of the pulmonary vasculature, including thinning of the vascular smooth muscle and recruitment of new vessels. This decrease in pulmonary vascular resistance significantly influences the timing of the clinical presentation of many congenital heart lesions that are dependent on the relative systemic and pulmonary vascular resistances. For example, the left-to-right shunt through a ventricular septal defect (VSD) may be minimal during the 1st wk after birth when pulmonary vascular resistance is still somewhat high. As pulmonary resistance decreases over the next week or two, the volume of the left-to-right shunt through the VSD increases, leading eventually to symptoms of congestive heart failure.

Significant differences between the neonatal circulation and that of older infants may be summarized as follows: (1) right-to-left or left-to-right shunting may persist across the patent foramen ovale; (2) in the presence of cardiopulmonary disease, continued patency of the ductus arteriosus may allow left-to-right, right-to-left, or bidirectional shunting; (3) the neonatal pulmonary vasculature constricts more vigorously in response to hypoxemia, hypercapnia, and acidosis; (4) the wall thickness and muscle mass of the neonatal left and right ventricles are almost equal; and (5) newborn infants at rest have a relatively high oxygen consumption, which is associated with a relatively high cardiac output. The newborn cardiac output (about 350 mL/kg/min) falls over the first 2 mo of life to about 150 mL/kg/min, then more gradually to the normal adult cardiac output of about 75 mL/kg/min. The high percentage of fetal hemoglobin present in the newborn may actually interfere with delivery of oxygen to the tissues in the neonate, requiring an increased cardiac output for adequate delivery of oxygen to the tissues (see Chapter 87.1).

The foramen ovale is functionally closed by the 3rd mo of life, although it is possible to pass a probe through the overlapping flaps in a large percentage of children and in 15–25% of adults. Functional closure of the ductus arteriosus is usually complete by 10–15 hr in the normal neonate, although the ductus may remain patent much longer in the presence of congenital heart disease, especially associated with cyanosis. In premature newborn infants an evanescent systolic murmur with late accentuation or a continuous murmur may be audible, and in the context of the respiratory distress syndrome, the presence of a patent ductus arteriosus should be suspected (see Chapter 87.3).

The normal ductus arteriosus differs morphologically from the adjoining aorta and pulmonary artery in that the ductus has a significant amount of circularly arranged smooth muscle in its medial layer. During fetal life, patency of the ductus arteriosus appears to be maintained by the combined relaxant effects of low oxygen tension and endogenously produced prostaglandins, specifically prostaglandin E_2 (PGE_2). In the full-term neonate, oxygen is the most important factor controlling ductal closure. When the Po_2 of the blood passing through the ductus reaches about 50 mm Hg, the ductal wall constricts; the mechanisms by which oxygen activates ductal constriction are not completely understood. The effects of oxygen on the ductal smooth muscle may be direct or mediated by its effects on prostaglandin synthesis. Gestational age also appears to play an important role; the ductus of the premature infant is less responsive to oxygen, even though its musculature is developed.

CHAPTER 383

Persistence of Fetal Circulatory Pathways

(Neonatal Pulmonary Hypertension) (See also Chapter 87.7)

Pulmonary hypertension may persist in the newborn under a variety of different circumstances and as a result of a number of different underlying mechanisms. Pulmonary vasoconstriction and hypertension following perinatal hypoxia can result in right-to-left shunting via a patent foramen ovale or ductus arteriosus. This primary hypertension syndrome is also known as *persistent fetal circulation* (PFC) and may be associated pathologically with increased muscularization of the pulmonary arterial bed. In addition, pulmonary hypertension may be a secondary feature of a variety of primary cardiac and pulmonary diseases.

The numerous disease entities that result in pulmonary hypertension can be classified on the basis of anatomic and physiologic causes in order to formulate a rational approach to diagnosis and management. The term *persistent pulmonary hypertension of the newborn* (PPHN) is applied to all of these causes but is not a specific diagnosis.

Pulmonary venous hypertension may occur in infants having a variety of congenital defects that cause pulmonary venous obstruction in the first few days of life. These include stenosis of the pulmonary veins, total anomalous pulmonary venous return with obstruction, cor triatriatum, congenital mitral stenosis, and supravalvular mitral membrane. Infants with left ventricular failure because of a well-defined cardiac lesion can also have pulmonary arterial hypertension. Severe forms of coarctation of the aorta, aortic valve disease, and cardiomyopathy are included in this group. Infants with transient left ventricular dysfunction secondary to hypoxia can also present with both congestive heart failure and pulmonary arterial hypertension.

Hyperviscosity syndrome occurs in patients with polycythemia, which may be secondary to maternal-fetal or fetal-fetal transfusion or due to perinatal hypoxemia (see Chapter 89.3).

Persistence of the fetal circulation occurs in patients with pulmonary vascular constriction (with or without increased pulmonary vascular smooth muscle) but who have no evidence of parenchymal pulmonary disease or a cardiac lesion. Some infants have both a pulmonary vascular constrictive component and pulmonary parenchymal disease. These infants should be classified according to the primary disease entity, for example, meconium aspiration syndrome with secondary pulmonary vascular constriction and right-to-left shunting (see Chapter 87.7).

An anatomically *hypoplastic pulmonary vascular bed* leads to elevated pulmonary resistance and is another cause of persistent pulmonary hypertension of the newborn. This may occur with congenital pulmonary hypoplasia but is also seen secondary to diaphragmatic hernia or other space-occupying intrathoracic masses, and other diseases. Once hypoxia occurs in these patients, the resulting pulmonary vascular constriction may add to the increased pulmonary resistance and exacerbate the cyanosis.

Infants with *congenital heart lesions* in whom there is nonrestrictive communication between the systemic and pulmonary sides of the circulation have pulmonary hypertension. These patients include those with large ventricular septal defects, and double outlet or single ventricles without associated pulmonic stenosis. Such infants develop medial muscular hypertrophy of small pulmonary vessels and are at risk of developing pulmonary vascular disease (see Chapter 386.28).

Perinatal hypoxemia associated with anatomic and physiologic abnormalities results in persistent pulmonary hypertension of mixed etiologies. For example, infants with diaphragmatic hernia have ipsilateral pulmonary hypoplasia and contralateral pulmonary vasoconstriction, both of which contribute to high pulmonary resistance, hypertension, and right-to-left shunting. Some preterm infants with severe respiratory distress syndrome may also be cyanotic on the basis of pulmonary vasoconstriction, pulmonary hypertension, and right-to-left shunting at the ductus arteriosus and foramen ovale in the first few days of life.

Barst RJ, Gersony WM: The pharmacological treatment of patent ductus arteriosus: A review of the evidence. Drugs 38:250, 1989.

Dawes GS: Fetal and Neonatal Physiology. Chicago, Year Book Medical Publishers, 1968.

Freed MD, Heymann MA, Lewis AB, et al: Prostaglandin E in infants with ductus arteriosus-dependent congenital heart disease. Circulation 64:899, 1981.

Gersony WM: Neonatal pulmonary hypertension: Pathophysiology, classification, and etiology. Clin Perinatol 11:517, 1984.

Gersony WM, Peckham GH, Ellison RC, et al: Effects of indomethacin in premature infants with patent ductus arteriosus: Results of a national collaborative study. J Pediatr 102:895, 1983.

Rudolph AM: Distribution and regulation of blood flow in the fetal and neonatal lamb. Circ Res 57:811, 1985.

Teitel D, Iwamoto HS, Rudolph AM: Effects of birth-related events on central blood flow patterns. Pediatr Res 22:557, 1987.

SECTION 3
Congenital Heart Disease

CHAPTER 384
Epidemiology of Congenital Heart Disease

INCIDENCE. Congenital heart disease occurs in approximately 8 of 1,000 live births. The incidence is higher among stillborns (2%), abortuses (10–25%), and premature infants (about 2% including ventricular septal defect [VSD], but excluding transient patent ductus arteriosus [PDA]). This overall incidence does not include mitral valve prolapse, the PDA of the preterm infant, and bicuspid aortic valves (present in about 0.9% of adult series). Among infants with congenital cardiac defects, there is a wide spectrum of severity: About 2–3 out of 1,000 total newborn infants will be symptomatic with heart disease in the 1st yr of life. The diagnosis is established by 1 wk of age in 40–50% of patients with congenital heart disease and by 1 mo of age in 50–60% of patients. Since palliative or corrective surgery has evolved, the number of children surviving with congenital heart disease has increased dramatically. Table 384–1 summarizes the relative frequency of specific lesions.

Most congenital defects are well tolerated during fetal life because of the parallel nature of the fetal circulation. Even severe cardiac defects, for example, severe hypoplasia of the left ventricle, can usually be well compensated for by the fetal circulation. It is only after the maternal circulation is eliminated, the fetal pathways (ductus arteriosus and foramen ovale) closed or restricted, and the cardiovascular system independently sustained that the full hemodynamic impact of an anatomic abnormality becomes apparent (see Chapter 387.17). One major exception is the case of regurgitant lesions, most commonly of the tricuspid valve. In these lesions, for example, Ebstein anomaly (see Chapter 387.8), the parallel fetal circulation cannot adequately compensate for the volume load imposed on the right heart. In utero heart failure, often with fetal pleural effusions and ascites (hydrops fetalis), may occur.

Although the immediate perinatal period marks the time of the most significant transitions in the circulation, the infant's circulation continues to undergo change after birth, and these later changes may also have a hemodynamic impact on cardiac lesions and their apparent incidence. For example, as pulmonary vascular resistance falls over the 1st several weeks of life, left-to-right shunting through intracardiac defects increases and symptoms become more apparent. The relative significance of various defects can also change dramatically with growth; some ventricular septal defects may become much smaller as the child ages. Alternatively, stenosis of the aortic or pulmonary valve, which may be mild in the newborn period, may become worse if valve orifice growth does not keep pace with patient growth. The physician should be aware of the spectrum of severity for the various congenital heart malformations and their evolution with time, and always be alert for associated congenital malformations, which can adversely affect the patient's prognosis (see Table 380–2).

■ TABLE 384–1 Relative Frequency of Congenital Heart Lesions*

Lesions	% of All Lesions
Ventricular septal defect	25–30
Atrial septal defect (secundum)	6–8
Patent ductus arteriosus	6–8
Coarctation of aorta	5–7
Tetralogy of Fallot	5–7
Pulmonary valve stenosis	5–7
Aortic valve stenosis	4–7
d-Transposition of great arteries	3–5
Hypoplastic left ventricle	1–3
Hypoplastic right ventricle	1–3
Truncus arteriosus	1–2
Total anomalous pulmonary venous return	1–2
Triscuspid atresia	1–2
Single ventricle	1–2
Double-outlet right ventricle	1–2
Others	5–10

Excluding patent ductus arteriosus in preterm neonate, bicuspid aortic valve, peripheral pulmonic stenosis, mitral valve prolapse.

ETIOLOGY. The etiology of most specific congenital heart defects is still unknown. However, recent advances in molecular genetics may soon permit identification of specific chromosomal abnormalities associated with many of these defects. It has long been appreciated that genetic factors played some role in congenital heart disease; for example, certain types of VSDs (supracristal) are more common in children of Asian background. Furthermore, the recurrence risk of congenital heart disease increases from 0.8% to about 2–6% if a 1st degree relative (parent or sibling) is affected. Currently, approximately 3% of patients with congenital heart disease have an identifiable single gene defect, such as Marfan or Noonan syndrome. Five to eight per cent of patients with congenital heart disease have an associated chromosomal abnormality: Heart disease is found in greater than 90% of patients with trisomy 18, 50% of patients with trisomy 21, and 40% of those with XO (Turner syndrome).

Two to four per cent of cases of congenital heart disease are associated with environmental or adverse maternal conditions and teratogenic influences, including maternal diabetes mellitus, phenylketonuria, systemic lupus erythematosus, congenital rubella syndrome, and drugs (lithium, ethanol, thalidomide, anticonvulsant agents) (see Table 380–3). Associated noncardiac malformations noted in identifiable syndromes may be seen in as many as 25% of patients with congenital heart disease (see Table 380–2).

GENETIC COUNSELING. Parents who have a child with congenital heart disease require counseling regarding the probability of a cardiac malformation occurring in subsequent children (see Chapter 69). With the exception of syndromes known to be due to a single gene mutation, most congenital heart disease is the result of a multifactorial inheritance pattern, which results in a low risk of recurrence. There is an approximately 0.8% incidence of congenital heart disease in the normal population, and this incidence increases to 2–6% for a 2nd pregnancy following the birth of a child with congenital heart disease, depending on the type of lesion in the 1st child. When two siblings have congenital heart disease, the risk for a 3rd affected child may reach 20–30%. In general, when a 2nd child is found to have congenital heart disease, it will tend to be of a similar class as the lesion that was discovered in the

1st instance. However, the degree of severity may be quite disparate, and associated defects may be variable. Certain cardiac lesions, for example, left-sided obstructive lesions, may be associated with a much higher rate of recurrence because of the presence of mild and clinically silent defects, for example, a bicuspid aortic valve, in other family members.

Fetal echocardiography has improved the rate of detection of congenital heart lesions in high risk patients (see Chapter 81.5). However, the resolution and accuracy of fetal echocardiography is not perfect. Furthermore, congenital heart lesions may evolve during the course of the pregnancy, for example, moderate aortic stenosis with a normal-sized left ventricle at 18 wk may evolve into aortic atresia with a hypoplastic left ventricle by 34 wk because of decreased flow through the left heart during the later half of gestation.

The question often arises as to whether a woman with congenital heart disease, either unoperated or operated, will be able to carry a fetus to term. The major factor in determining this is the mother's cardiovascular status. In the presence of a mild congenital heart defect, or after successful repair of a more severe lesion, normal childbearing is likely. The increased hemodynamic burden on a patient with poor cardiac function may result in significantly increased risk to the mother as well as to the fetus. The incidence of spontaneous abortion in the presence of severe congenital heart disease is high, especially when the patient is cyanotic. The maternal risk in these situations is also quite high. Therefore, it is important to discuss various methods of birth control with young women with repaired or palliated congenital heart lesions. Antibiotic prophylaxis against endocarditis is also indicated at the time of delivery.

CHAPTER 385
Evaluation of the Infant or Child with Congenital Heart Disease

The initial evaluation of the infant or child with suspected congenital heart disease involves a systematic approach with three major components. First, congenital cardiac defects can be divided into two major groups based on the presence or absence of cyanosis, which can be determined by physical examination, aided by transcutaneous oximetry. Second, these two groups can be further subdivided based on whether the chest radiograph shows evidence of increased, normal, or decreased pulmonary vascular markings. Finally, the electrocardiogram can be used to determine whether right, left, or biventricular hypertrophy exists. The character of the heart sounds and the presence and character of any murmurs further narrows the differential diagnosis. The final diagnosis is then confirmed by echocardiography and/or cardiac catheterization.

ACYANOTIC CONGENITAL HEART LESIONS

Acyanotic congenital heart lesions can be classified according to the predominant physiologic load they place on the heart. Although many congenital heart lesions induce more than one physiologic disturbance, it is helpful to focus on the primary load abnormality for purposes of classification. The most common lesions are those that produce a *volume load,* and the most common of these are the left-to-right shunt lesions. Atrioventricular valve regurgitation and some of the cardiomyopathies are other causes of increased volume load. The second major class of lesions causes an increase in *pressure load,* most commonly secondary to ventricular outflow obstruction (e.g., pulmonic or aortic valve stenosis) or narrowing of one of the great vessels (e.g., coarctation of the aorta). The chest radiograph and electrocardiogram are useful tools for differentiating between these major classes of volume and pressure overload lesions.

LESIONS RESULTING IN INCREASED VOLUME LOAD. The most common lesions in this group are those that cause left-to-right shunts: atrial septal defect (ASD), ventricular septal defect (VSD), atrioventricular septal defects (AVSD, AV canal), and patent ductus arteriosus (PDA). The pathophysiologic common denominator in this group is a communication between the systemic and pulmonary sides of the circulation, resulting in the shunting of fully oxygenated blood back into the lungs. This shunt can be quantitated by calculating the ratio of pulmonary to systemic blood flow, or $Q_p:Q_s$. Thus, a 2:1 shunt usually implies that there is twice the normal pulmonary blood flow.

The direction and magnitude of the shunt across such a communication depends on the size of the defect and the relative pulmonary and systemic pressures and pulmonary and systemic vascular resistances. These factors are dynamic and may change dramatically with age: Intracardiac defects may grow smaller with time; pulmonary vascular resistance, which is high in the immediate newborn period, decreases to normal adult levels by several weeks of life; chronic exposure of the pulmonary circulation to high pressure and blood flow will result in a gradual increase in pulmonary vascular resistance (Eisenmenger physiology, see Chapter 386.28). Thus, in a lesion such as a large VSD, there may be little shunting and few symptoms during the 1st wk of life. When the pulmonary vascular resistance declines over the next several weeks, the volume of the left-to-right shunt increases, and symptoms begin to appear.

The increased volume of blood in the lungs decreases pulmonary compliance and increases the work of breathing. Fluid leaks into the interstitial space and alveoli, causing pulmonary edema. The infant develops the symptoms we refer to as "heart failure," such as tachypnea, chest retractions, nasal flaring, and wheezing. However, the term *heart failure* is a misnomer; total left ventricular output is actually several times greater than normal, although much of this output is ineffective because it returns directly to the lungs. To maintain this high level of left ventricular output, heart rate and stroke volume are increased, mediated by an increase in sympathetic nervous system activity. The increase in circulating catecholamines, combined with the increased work of breathing, result in an elevation in total body oxygen consumption, often beyond the oxygen transport ability of the circulation. This leads to the additional symptoms of sweating, irritability, tachycardia, and failure to thrive. If left untreated, pulmonary vascular resistance eventually begins to rise, and by several years of age the shunt volume will decrease and eventually reverse to right-to-left.

Additional lesions that impose a volume load on the heart include the regurgitant lesions and the cardiomyopathies. Regurgitation of the atrioventricular valves is most commonly encountered in patients with partial or complete atrioventricular septal (AV canal) defects. In this lesion, the combination of a left-to-right shunt with atrioventricular valve regurgitation increases the volume load on the heart and leads to more severe symptomatology. Isolated regurgitation of the tricuspid valve is seen in Ebstein anomaly (see Chapter 387.8). Regurgitation of one of the semilunar valves is usually also associated with stenosis; however, aortic regurgitation may be encountered in patients with a VSD directly under the aortic valve (supracristal VSD).

As opposed to the left-to-right shunts, in which intrinsic

cardiac muscle function is usually either normal or increased, in the cardiomyopathies heart muscle function is decreased. Cardiomyopathies may affect systolic contractility, diastolic relaxation, or both. Decreased cardiac function results in increased atrial and ventricular filling pressures, and pulmonary edema occurs secondary to increased capillary pressure. The major etiologies of cardiomyopathy in infants and children include viral myocarditis, a large range of metabolic disorders, and endocardial fibroelastosis.

LESIONS RESULTING IN INCREASED PRESSURE LOAD. The pathophysiologic common denominator of these lesions is an obstruction to normal blood flow. The most common are obstructions to ventricular outflow: valvar pulmonic stenosis, valvar aortic stenosis, and coarctation of the aorta. Less common are obstruction to ventricular inflow: tricuspid or mitral stenosis and cor triatriatum. Ventricular outflow obstruction can occur at the valve, below the valve (e.g., double-chambered right ventricle, subaortic membrane), or above it (e.g., branch pulmonary stenosis or supravalvar aortic stenosis). Unless the obstruction is severe, cardiac output will be maintained and symptoms of heart failure will be either subtle or absent. This compensation involves an increase in cardiac wall thickness (hypertrophy).

The clinical picture is quite different when obstruction to outflow is severe, usually encountered in the immediate newborn period. The infant may become critically ill within several hours of birth. Severe pulmonic stenosis in the newborn period (critical PS) results in signs of right-sided heart failure (hepatomegaly, peripheral edema) and cyanosis due to right-to-left shunting across the foramen ovale. Severe aortic stenosis in the newborn period (critical AS) presents with signs of left-sided heart failure (pulmonary edema, poor perfusion), right-sided failure (hepatomegaly, peripheral edema), and may progress rapidly to total circulatory collapse.

In older children, coarctation of the aorta usually presents with upper body hypertension and diminished pulses in the lower extremities. In the immediate newborn period, the presentation of coarctation may be delayed due to the presence of a patent ductus arteriosus. In these patients, the aortic end of the ductus may serve as a conduit for blood flow to partially bypass the obstruction. These infants become symptomatic when the ductus finally closes.

CYANOTIC CONGENITAL HEART LESIONS

This group of congenital heart lesions can also be further divided based on pathophysiology: whether pulmonary blood flow is decreased (tetralogy of Fallot, pulmonary atresia with intact septum, tricuspid atresia, total anomalous pulmonary venous return with obstruction) or increased (transposition of the great vessels, single ventricle, truncus arteriosus, total anomalous pulmonary venous return without obstruction). As with the acyanotic lesions, the chest radiograph is a valuable tool for differentiating between these two categories.

CYANOTIC LESIONS WITH DECREASED PULMONARY BLOOD FLOW. These lesions must include both an obstruction to pulmonary blood flow (at the tricuspid valve, right ventricular, or pulmonary valve level) and a pathway by which systemic venous blood can shunt right to left and enter the systemic circulation (via a patent foramen ovale, ASD, or VSD). Common lesions in this group include tricuspid atresia, tetralogy of Fallot, and various forms of single ventricle with pulmonary stenosis. In these lesions, the degree of cyanosis depends on the degree of obstruction to pulmonary blood flow. If the obstruction is mild, cyanosis may be absent at rest. However, these patients may develop hypercyanotic ("tet") spells during conditions of stress. In contrast, if the obstruction is severe, pulmonary blood flow may be dependent on the patency of the ductus arteriosus. When the ductus closes during the 1st few days of life, the neonate presents with profound hypoxemia and shock.

CYANOTIC LESIONS WITH INCREASED PULMONARY BLOOD FLOW. In this group of lesions, there is no obstruction to pulmonary blood flow. Cyanosis is caused by either abnormal ventricular-arterial connections or by total mixing of systemic venous and pulmonary venous blood within the heart. Transposition of the great vessels (TGV) is the most common of the former group of lesions. In TGV, the aorta arises from the right ventricle and the pulmonary artery from the left ventricle. Systemic venous blood returning to the right atrium is pumped directly back to the body, and oxygenated blood returning from the lungs to the left atrium is pumped back into the lungs. The persistence of fetal pathways (foramen ovale and ductus arteriosus) allows for a small degree of mixing in the immediate newborn period; however, when the ductus begins to close, these infants develop extreme cyanosis.

The total mixing lesions include those cardiac defects with a common atria or ventricle, total anomalous pulmonary venous return, and truncus arteriosus. In this group, deoxygenated systemic venous blood and oxygenated pulmonary venous blood mix completely in the heart, resulting in equal oxygen saturations in the pulmonary artery and aorta. If there is no obstruction to pulmonary blood flow, these infants present with a combination of cyanosis and heart failure. In contrast, if pulmonary stenosis is present, these infants present with cyanosis alone, similar to patients with tetralogy of Fallot.

CHAPTER 386
Acyanotic Congenital Heart Disease

The Left-to-Right Shunt Lesions

386.1 Atrial Septal Defect

Atrial septal defects (ASDs) can occur in any portion of the atrial septum (secundum, primum, or sinus venosus). Rarely there may be near absence of the atrial septum, creating a functional single atrium. In contrast, an isolated patent foramen ovale is usually of no hemodynamic significance and is not considered an ASD. However, if right atrial pressure is increased secondary to another cardiac anomaly (e.g., pulmonary stenosis or atresia, tricuspid valve abnormalities, right ventricular dysfunction), venous blood may shunt across the patent foramen ovale into the left atrium with resultant cyanosis. Because of the anatomic structure of a patent foramen ovale, blood normally is not shunted from the left atrium to the right atrium. However, in the presence of a large volume load or a hypertensive left atrium, or both, there may be enough dilatation of the foramen ovale to result in a significant atrial left-to-right shunt. An isolated patent foramen ovale does not require surgical treatment but may be a risk for paradoxical systemic embolization in later life.

386.2 Ostium Secundum Defect

This defect, in the region of the fossa ovalis, is the most common form of ASD and is associated with normal atrioventricular valves. Although late myxomatous changes in the mitral valve have been described, this is only rarely an important clinical consideration. The defects may be single or multiple, and in symptomatic older children openings of 2 cm or more in diameter are not unusual. Large defects may extend inferiorly toward the inferior vena cava and ostium of the coronary sinus, superiorly toward the superior vena cava, or posteriorly. Females outnumber males 3:1. Partial anomalous pulmonary venous return may be an associated lesion.

PATHOPHYSIOLOGY. The degree of left-to-right shunting is dependent on the size of the defect and also on the relative compliances of the right and left ventricles, and relative vascular resistances in the pulmonary and systemic circulations. In large defects, a considerable shunt of oxygenated blood flows from the left to the right atrium. This blood is added to the usual venous return to the right atrium and is pumped by the right ventricle to the lungs. In large defects, pulmonary blood flow is usually 2–4 times systemic blood flow. The paucity of symptoms in infants with ASDs is related to the structure of the right ventricle in early life when its muscular wall is thick and less compliant, thus limiting the left-to-right shunt. As the infant becomes older, the right ventricular wall becomes thinner as a result of its lower pressure-generating requirements, and the left-to-right shunt across the ASD increases. The large blood flow through the right side of the heart results in enlargement of the right atrium and ventricle and dilatation of the pulmonary artery. Despite the large pulmonary blood flow, the pulmonary arterial pressure remains normal because of the absence of a high pressure communication between the pulmonary and systemic circulations. Pulmonary vascular resistance remains low throughout childhood, although it may begin to increase in adulthood. The left ventricle and aorta are normal in size. Cyanosis is only seen occasionally in adults who have the complicating features of pulmonary vascular disease.

CLINICAL MANIFESTATIONS. A child with an ostium secundum defect is most often asymptomatic, and the lesion may be discovered inadvertently during a physical examination. Even an extremely large secundum ASD rarely produces clinically evident heart failure in childhood; in older children varying degrees of exercise intolerance may be noted. Often the degree of limitation may go unnoticed by the family until after surgical repair, when the child's activity level increases markedly. In older infants and children the physical findings are usually characteristic but subtle and require careful examination of the heart and special attention to the heart sounds.

The pulses are normal. A right ventricular systolic lift is usually palpable from the left sternal border to the midclavicular line. There is a loud 1st heart sound and sometimes a pulmonic ejection click. In most patients the 2nd heart sound at the upper left sternal edge is widely split and fixed in its splitting in all phases of respiration. This auscultatory finding is characteristic and is due to the defect producing a constantly increased right ventricular diastolic volume and a prolonged ejection time. The systolic murmur is of the ejection type, medium pitched, without harsh qualities, seldom accompanied by a thrill, and best heard at the left mid and upper sternal border. It is produced by the increased flow across the right ventricular outflow tract into the pulmonary artery. A short, rumbling mid-diastolic murmur produced by the increased volume of blood flow across the tricuspid valve is often audible at the lower left sternal border. This finding, which may be subtle and heard best with the bell of the stethoscope, is an excellent diagnostic sign and usually indicates a shunt ratio of at least 2:1.

DIAGNOSIS. The chest *roentgenogram* shows varying degrees of enlargement of the right ventricle and atrium depending on the size of the shunt; the left ventricle and aorta are of normal size. The pulmonary artery is large, and the pulmonary vascularity is increased. These signs vary and may not be conspicuous in mild cases. Cardiac enlargement is often best appreciated on the lateral view, because the right ventricle protrudes anteriorly as its volume increases. The *electrocardiogram* shows volume overload of the right ventricle with right axis deviation or a normal axis, and a minor right ventricular conduction delay (usually an rsR′ pattern in the right precordial leads).

The *echocardiogram* shows findings characteristic of right ventricular volume overload, including increased right ventricular end-diastolic dimension and an abnormal motion of the ventricular septum. The normal septum moves posteriorly during systole and anteriorly during diastole. With right ventricular overload and normal pulmonary vascular resistance, the septal motion is reversed, that is, anterior movement in systole, or the motion is intermediate so that the septum remains straight. The location and size of the atrial defect are readily appreciated by two-dimensional scanning, and the shunt is confirmed by pulsed and color flow Doppler. Patients with classic features of a secundum ASD, including echocardiographic identification of a well-defined defect, need not be catheterized prior to surgical closure.

If the diagnosis is suspect or the shunt size cannot be determined reliably from noninvasive tests, *cardiac catheterization* will confirm the presence of the defect and allow measurement of the shunt ratio. The oxygen content of blood from the right atrium will be much higher than that from the superior vena cava. This feature is not specifically diagnostic because it may occur with partial anomalous pulmonary venous return to the right atrium, with a ventricular septal defect (VSD) in the presence of tricuspid insufficiency, with atrioventricular septal defects associated with left ventricular-to–right atrial shunts, and with aorta-to–right atrial communications (e.g., ruptured sinus of Valsalva aneurysm). The physical signs produced by the latter three anomalies generally differ greatly from those of ASDs, and their presence can usually be confirmed by selective angiocardiography. Occasionally, mixing of blood is incomplete in the right atrium, and the principal site of shunt appears to be at the ventricular level, even though a VSD is not present.

The catheter can usually be manipulated into the left atrium via the defect. Streaming of inferior vena caval blood across the defect to the left atrium may occur with uncomplicated ASDs. This small right-to-left shunt may be demonstrated by indicator dilution curves but only rarely results in significant arterial desaturation or cyanosis. The pressures in the right side of the heart are usually normal, but small to moderate pressure gradients may be measured across the right ventricular outflow tract. In the absence of associated organic pulmonary stenosis, they are caused by functional stenosis related to excessive blood flow and are usually less than 25 mm Hg. The pulmonary vascular resistance is almost always normal. The shunt is variable depending on the size of the defect, but it may be of considerable volume (as high as 20 $L/min/m^2$). Cineangiography, performed with the catheter through the defect and in the right upper pulmonary vein, will demonstrate the defect. Alternatively, pulmonary angiography will demonstrate the defect on the levophase (return of contrast to the left side of the heart after passing through the lungs).

PROGNOSIS AND COMPLICATIONS. Secundum ASDs are well tolerated during childhood; symptoms usually do not appear until the 3rd decade or later. Pulmonary hypertension, atrial dysrhythmias, tricuspid or mitral insufficiency, and heart failure are late manifestations; these symptoms may first appear during the increased volume load of pregnancy. Infective endocarditis is extremely rare. Postoperative complications, such as late heart failure and atrial fibrillation, are more common in patients operated on after 20 yr of age.

Secundum ASDs are usually isolated, although they may be associated with partial anomalous pulmonary venous return, pulmonary valvular stenosis, VSD, pulmonary arterial branch stenosis, and persistent left superior vena cava, as well as mitral valve prolapse and insufficiency.

TREATMENT. Surgery is advised for all symptomatic patients and also for asymptomatic patients with a shunt ratio of at least 2:1. The timing for elective closure is usually at some time prior to entry into school. Closure is carried out at open heart surgery, and the mortality rate is less than 1%. Repair is preferred during early childhood because the surgical mortality and morbidity are greater in adulthood when late signs are present. Eliminating the increased risks of pregnancy is another important reason to intervene early in females. Mild symptoms with exercise and submaximal physical performance during sports activities are also prevented by early elective repair. Occlusion devices, implanted transvenously at cardiac catheterization, have been used in experimental trials to successfully close secundum ASDs. In patients with small secundum ASDs with minimal left-to-right shunts, the general consensus is that closure is not required. It is unclear at present whether the persistence of a small ASD into adulthood increases the risk for stroke enough to warrant prophylactic closure of all of these defects.

The results after operation in children with large shunts are excellent. Symptoms disappear rapidly, and physical development frequently appears enhanced. The heart size decreases to normal, and the electrocardiogram shows decreased right ventricular forces. Late arrhythmias are less frequent in patients who have had early repair.

386.3 Sinus Venosus Defect

The defect is situated in the upper part of the atrial septum in close relation to the entry of the superior vena cava. Often, one or more pulmonary veins (usually from the right lung) drain anomalously into the superior vena cava. Sometimes the superior vena cava straddles the defect; some systemic venous blood then enters the left atrium. The hemodynamic disturbance, clinical picture, electrocardiogram, and roentgenogram are similar to those of secundum ASD. The diagnosis can usually be made by two-dimensional echocardiography. If cardiac catheterization is carried out to better define the venous drainage, the catheter may enter a right pulmonary vein directly from the superior vena cava. Anatomic correction usually requires the insertion of a patch to close the defect while incorporating the entry of anomalous veins into the left atrium; surgical results are generally excellent.

386.4 Partial Anomalous Pulmonary Venous Return

A varying number of pulmonary veins may enter the systemic venous circulation or the right atrium and produce a left-to-right shunt of oxygenated blood, which may be further augmented if there is an associated ASD. Partial anomalous pulmonary venous return usually involves some or all of the veins from only one lung, more often the right. An associated ASD usually is of the sinus venosus type (see Chapter 386.3). The history, physical signs, electrocardiogram, and roentgenographic findings are indistinguishable from those of an isolated ostium secundum ASD. Occasionally, an anomalous vein draining into the inferior vena cava is visible roentgenographically as a crescentic shadow of vascular density along the right border of the cardiac silhouette (scimitar syndrome); in these cases an ASD is usually not present. The finding of a sinus venosus ASD by echocardiography is often accompanied by the identification or suspicion of associated partial anomalous pulmonary venous return. See Chapter 387.14 for a discussion of total anomalous pulmonary venous return. Echocardiography usually confirms the diagnosis. Magnetic resonance imaging (MRI) is also useful for defining pulmonary venous drainage. At cardiac catheterization, the presence of anomalous pulmonary veins may be demonstrated by selective pulmonary arteriography.

The prognosis is excellent, similar to that for ostium secundum ASDs. When a large left-to-right shunt is present, surgical repair is performed. The associated ASD should be closed in such a way as to direct the pulmonary venous return to the left atrium. A single anomalous pulmonary vein without an atrial communication may be difficult to redirect to the left atrium and, if the shunt size is small, may be left unoperated.

386.5 Atrioventricular Septal Defects

(Ostium Primum and AV Canal or Endocardial Cushion Defects)

These abnormalities are grouped together because they represent a spectrum of a basic embryologic abnormality, a deficiency of the atrioventricular (AV) septum. The *ostium primum defect* is situated in the lower portion of the atrial septum and overlies the mitral and tricuspid valves. In most instances there is also a cleft in the anterior leaflet of the mitral valve. The tricuspid valve is usually functionally normal, although some anatomic abnormality of the septal leaflet is usually present. The ventricular septum is intact.

AV septal defect, also known as AV canal defect or endocardial cushion defect, consists of contiguous atrial and ventricular septal defects with markedly abnormal AV valves. The degree of valve abnormalities varies considerably; in the complete form of AV septal defect there is a single AV valve, common to both ventricles, and consisting of an anterior and a posterior bridging leaflet related to the ventricular septum, with a lateral leaflet in each ventricle. The lesion is common among children with Down syndrome and may occasionally occur with pulmonary stenosis (see Chapters 386.14 and 387.2).

Transitional varieties of these defects also occur. They include ostium primum defects with clefts in the anterior mitral and septal tricuspid valve leaflets, minor ventricular septal deficiencies, and, less commonly, ostium primum defects with normal AV valves. In some patients, the atrial septum is intact, but the inlet ventricular septal defect simulates that found in the full AV septal defect. These defects are also commonly associated with deformities of the AV valves.

PATHOPHYSIOLOGY. The basic abnormality in patients with *ostium primum defects* is the combination of a left-to-right shunt across the atrial defect with mitral (or occasionally tricuspid) insufficiency. The shunt is usually moderate to large. The degree of mitral insufficiency is usually mild to moderate. Pulmonary arterial pressures are usually normal or only mildly increased. The physiology of this lesion is, therefore, very similar to that of an ostium secundum ASD.

In *AV septal defects* the left-to-right shunt is both transatrial and transventricular. Additional shunting may occur directly from the left ventricle to the right atrium because of the absence of the AV septum. Pulmonary hypertension and an early tendency to increase pulmonary vascular resistance are common. AV valvular insufficiency increases the volume load due to regurgitation of blood from the ventricles to both atria. Some right-to-left shunting may also occur at both the atrial and ventricular levels, and lead to mild but significant arterial desaturation. With time, progressive pulmonary vascular disease will increase the right-to-left shunt so that clinical cyanosis develops (Eisenmenger physiology, see Chapter 386.28).

CLINICAL PRESENTATION. Many children with *ostium primum defect* are asymptomatic, and the anomaly is discovered during a general physical examination. In patients with moderate shunts and trivial mitral insufficiency, the physical signs are similar to those of the secundum ASD, but with an additional apical holosystolic murmur due to mitral insufficiency.

A history of exercise intolerance, easy fatigability, and recurrent pneumonias may be obtained, especially in infants with large left-to-right shunts and severe mitral insufficiency. In these patients cardiac enlargement is moderate or marked, and the precordium is hyperdynamic. The auscultatory signs produced by the left-to-right shunt include a normal or accentuated 1st sound; wide, fixed splitting of the 2nd sound; a pulmonary systolic ejection murmur sometimes preceded by a click; and a low-pitched mid-diastolic rumbling murmur at the lower left sternal edge and/or apex due to increased flow through the atrioventricular valves. Mitral insufficiency may be manifested by an apical holosystolic murmur that radiates to the left axilla.

With *complete AV septal defects,* congestive heart failure and intercurrent pulmonary infection usually appear in infancy. During these episodes minimal cyanosis may be evident. The liver is enlarged and the infant shows signs of failure to thrive. Cardiac enlargement is moderate to marked, and a systolic thrill is frequently palpable. A lift may be present at the lower left sternal border. The 1st heart sound is normal or accentuated. The 2nd heart sound is widely split if pulmonary flow is massive. A low-pitched, mid-diastolic rumbling murmur is audible at the lower left sternal edge, and a pulmonary systolic ejection murmur is produced by the large pulmonary flow. The apical holosystolic murmur of mitral insufficiency may also be present.

DIAGNOSIS. Chest *roentgenograms* of children with complete AV septal defects often show marked cardiac enlargement caused by prominence of both ventricles and the right atrium. The pulmonary artery is large, and the pulmonary vascularity is increased.

The *electrocardiograms* of children with complete AV septal defects are distinctive. The principal abnormalities are (1) superior orientation of the mean frontal QRS axis with left axis deviation to the left upper or right upper quadrant, (2) counterclockwise inscription of the superiorly oriented QRS vector loop, (3) signs of biventricular hypertrophy or isolated right ventricular hypertrophy, (4) right ventricular conduction delay (RSR′ in leads V_3R and V_1), (5) normal or tall P waves, and (6) occasional prolongation of the P-R interval (Fig. 386–1).

The *echocardiogram* is characteristic and shows signs of right ventricular enlargement with encroachment of the mitral valve echo on the left ventricular outflow tract; this corresponds to the angiographic "goose-neck" deformity. In normal hearts, the tricuspid valve inserts slightly more towards the apex than the mitral valve. In AV septal defects, both valves insert at the same level due to the absence of the AV septum. In complete AV septal defects, the ventricular septal echo is also deficient and the common AV valve is readily appreciated (Fig. 386–2). Pulsed and color flow Doppler echo will demonstrate left-to-right shunting at atrial, ventricular, or ventricular-to-atrial levels and semiquantitate the degree of AV valve insufficiency. Echocardiography will also aid in assessing for the presence of commonly associated lesions such as patent ductus arteriosus (PDA) or coarctation of the aorta.

Cardiac catheterization and *angiocardiography* may be required to confirm the diagnosis. These studies demonstrate the magnitude of the left-to-right shunt, the severity of pulmonary hypertension, the degree of elevation of pulmonary vascular resistance, and the severity of insufficiency of the common AV valve. By oximetry, the shunt is usually demonstrable at the atrial level; in some patients, increased oxygen saturations are noted only in the right ventricle because of streaming of blood across the primum defect just proximal to the tricuspid valve. The arterial oxygen saturation is normal or mildly reduced unless severe pulmonary vascular disease is present. Children with ostium primum defects usually have normal or only moderate elevation of pulmonary arterial pressure. On the other hand, complete AV septal defects are associated with right ventricular and pulmonary hypertension, and in older patients with increased pulmonary vascular resistance.

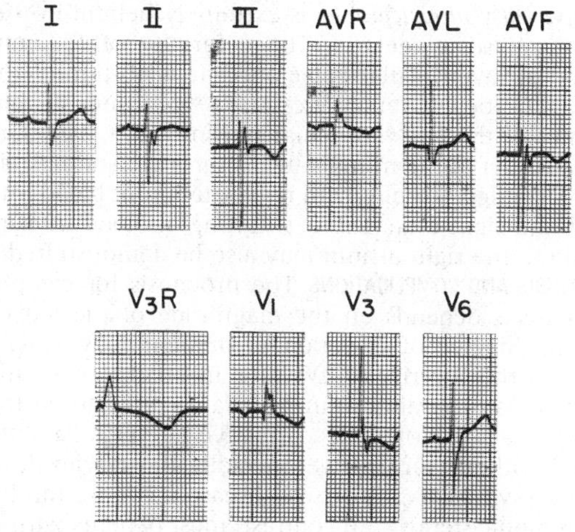

Figure 386–1. Electrocardiogram from a child with an atrioventricular canal. Note the QRS axis of −60 degrees, and the RV conduction delay; RSR′ in V_1 and V_3R. (V_3R paper speed = 50 mm/sec.)

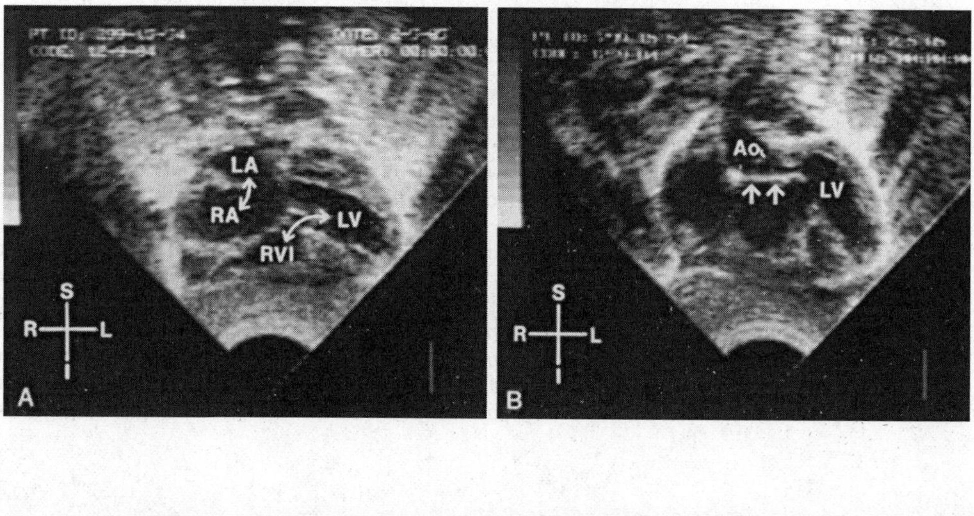

Figure 386–2. Atrioventricular defect. *A,* Four-chamber view demonstrating both an interatrial and interventricular septal defect contributing to the large central communication of this lesion (*arrows*). *B,* Left ventricular long axis projection demonstrating the typical goose-neck deformity created by the anterior leaflet of the mitral valve (*arrows*). RA = right atrium; LA = left atrium; RVI = right ventricular inflow; LV = left ventricle; R = right; L = left; S = superior; I = inferior; Ao = aorta.

Selective left ventriculography is extremely helpful in the diagnosis of AV septal defects. The deformity of the mitral or common atrioventricular valve and the distortion of the outflow tract of the left ventricle causes a "goose-neck"–appearing deformity of the left ventricular outflow tract. The abnormal anterior leaflet of the mitral valve is serrated, and mitral insufficiency is noted, usually with regurgitation of blood into both the left and right atria. Direct shunting of blood from the left ventricle to the right atrium may also be demonstrated.

PROGNOSIS AND COMPLICATIONS. The prognosis for complete AV septal defects depends on the magnitude of the left-to-right shunt, the degree of elevation of pulmonary vascular resistance, and the severity of AV valve insufficiency. Death from congestive cardiac failure during infancy used to be frequent before the advent of early corrective surgery. Patients who survived without surgery were usually those who developed pulmonary vascular obstructive disease, or more rarely those with pulmonic stenosis. In contrast, most patients with ostium primum defects and minimal AV valve involvement are asymptomatic or have only minor, nonprogressive symptoms until they reach the 3rd to 4th decade of life, similar to the course of patients with secundum atrial septal defects.

TREATMENT. Ostium primum defects are approached surgically from an incision in the right atrium. The cleft in the mitral valve is located through the atrial defect and is repaired by direct suture. The defect in the atrial septum is usually closed by insertion of a patch prosthesis. The surgical mortality rate for ostium primum defects is low. Surgical treatment for complete AV septal defects is more difficult, especially in infants with congestive cardiac failure and pulmonary hypertension. However, successful open heart correction of these defects can be accomplished even in infancy. The atrial and ventricular defects are patched closed and the AV valves reconstructed. Complications are uncommon and include surgically induced heart block requiring placement of a permanent pacemaker, excessive narrowing of the left ventricular outflow tract requiring surgical revision, and eventual worsening of mitral regurgitation requiring replacement with a prosthetic valve.

386.6 Ventricular Septal Defect

This is the most common cardiac malformation, accounting for 25% of congenital heart disease. Defects may occur is any portion of the ventricular septum; however, the majority are of the membranous type. These defects are in a posteroinferior position, anterior to the septal leaflet of the tricuspid valve. Defects between the crista supraventricularis and the papillary muscle of the conus may be associated with pulmonary stenosis and the other manifestations of tetralogy of Fallot (see Chapter 387.2). Defects superior to the crista supraventricularis (supracristal) are less common; they are found just beneath the pulmonary valve and may impinge on an aortic sinus, causing aortic insufficiency. Defects in the midportion or apical region of the ventricular septum are muscular in type and may be single or multiple (Swiss-cheese septum).

PATHOPHYSIOLOGY. The physical size of the defect is a major, but not the only, determinant of the size of the left-to-right shunt. The shunt magnitude is also determined by the level of pulmonary vascular resistance compared with systemic vascular resistance. When a small communication is present (usually <0.5 cm^2), the defect is called *restrictive* and right ventricular pressure is normal. The higher pressure in the left ventricle drives the shunt left-to-right; however, the size of the defect limits the magnitude of the shunt. In large *nonrestrictive* defects (usually >1.0 cm^2), right and left ventricular pressures are equalized. In these defects, the direction of shunting and the shunt magnitude are determined by the ratio of pulmonary to systemic vascular resistances.

After birth, in the presence of a large VSD, the pulmonary vascular resistance may remain higher than normal and thus the size of the left-to-right shunt may be limited. As pulmonary vascular resistance falls in the 1st few weeks after birth because of the normal involution of the media of the small pulmonary arteries and arterioles, the size of the left-to-right shunt increases. Eventually, a large left-to-right shunt ensues, and clinical symptoms become apparent. In most cases during early infancy, the pulmonary vascular resistance is only slightly elevated, and the major contribution to pulmonary hypertension is the extremely large pulmonary blood flow. In some patients with a large VSD, pulmonary arteriolar medial thickness remains increased. With continued exposure of the pulmonary vascular bed to high systolic pressure and high flow, pulmonary vascular obstructive disease begins to develop. When the ratio of pulmonary to systemic resistance approaches 1:1, the shunt becomes bidirectional, signs of heart failure abate, and the patient becomes cyanotic (Eisenmenger physiology, see Chapter 386.28). These progressive increases in pulmonary resistance are rarely seen in the present era when prolonged pulmonary hypertension is prevented by early surgical intervention in patients with large VSDs.

The magnitude of intracardiac shunts is usually described by the ratio of pulmonary to systemic blood flow. If the left-to-right shunt is small (pulmonary to systemic flow ratio $<1.75:1$), the cardiac chambers will not be appreciably enlarged and the pulmonary vascular bed will likely be normal. If the shunt is large (flow ratio $>2.5:1$), left atrial and ventricular volume overload occur, as well as right ventricular and pulmonary arterial hypertension. The pulmonary arterial trunk, left atrium, and left ventricle are enlarged because of the large volume of pulmonary blood flow.

CLINICAL MANIFESTATIONS. The clinical presentation of patients with a VSD varies according to the size of the defect and the pulmonary blood flow and pressure. *Small defects with trivial left-to-right shunts and normal pulmonary arterial pressures* are the most common. These patients are asymptomatic, and the cardiac lesion is usually found during a routine physical examination. Characteristically, there is a loud, harsh, or blowing left parasternal holosystolic murmur, heard best over the lower left sternal border and frequently accompanied by a thrill. In a few instances the murmur ends well before the 2nd sound, presumably because of closure of the defect during late systole. The left-to-right shunt may be limited in the neonate because of higher right-sided pressures, and therefore the systolic murmur may not be audible during the 1st few days of life. In premature infants, however, the murmur may be heard early because pulmonary vascular resistance decreases more rapidly. In patients with small VSDs, the chest *roentgenogram* is usually normal, although minimal cardiomegaly and a borderline increase in pulmonary vasculature may be observed. The *electrocardiogram* is usually normal but may suggest left ventricular hypertrophy. The presence of right ventricular hypertrophy is a warning that the defect is not small and that pulmonary hypertension is present or that there is an associated lesion such as pulmonic stenosis.

Large defects with excessive pulmonary blood flow and pulmonary hypertension are responsible for dyspnea, feeding difficulties, poor growth, profuse perspiration, recurrent pulmonary infections, and cardiac failure in early infancy. Cyanosis is usually absent, but duskiness is sometimes noted during infections or crying. Prominence of the left precordium and sternum is common, as are cardiomegaly, a palpable parasternal lift, an apical thrust, and a systolic thrill. The holosystolic murmur may be similar to that of smaller defects, although it is usually less harsh and more blowing in nature due to the absence of a significant pressure gradient across the defect. It is even less likely to be audible in the newborn period. The pulmonic component of the 2nd heart sound may be increased, indicating pulmonary hypertension. The presence of a mid-diastolic, low-pitched rumble at the apex is caused by increased blood flow across the mitral valve and indicates a left-to-right shunt of approximately 2:1 or greater. This murmur is best appreciated with the bell of the stethoscope. In large VSDs, the chest *roentgenogram* shows gross cardiomegaly with prominence of both ventricles, the left atrium, and pulmonary artery. The pulmonary vascular markings are increased and frank pulmonary edema may be present. Pleural effusions may be present. The *electrocardiogram* shows biventricular hypertrophy; P waves may be notched or peaked.

DIAGNOSIS. The *two-dimensional echocardiogram* will show the position and size of the VSD. In very small defects, especially of the muscular septum, the defect itself may be difficult to image and is only visualized by color Doppler examination. A thin membrane (ventricular septal aneurysm) consisting of tricuspid valve tissue can partially cover the defect and limit the amount of the left-to-right shunt. The echo is also useful in estimating the shunt size by examining the degree of volume overload of the left atrium and left ventricle; the extent of their increased dimensions reflects the size of the left-to-right shunt. Pulsed Doppler examination will show if the VSD is pressure restrictive by calculating the pressure gradient across the defect. This will allow estimation of right ventricular pressure and help to determine whether the patient is at risk for the development of early pulmonary vascular disease.

The effects of a VSD on the circulation can also be demonstrated by *cardiac catheterization*. However, this diagnostic procedure is not required in most cases. Catheterization is usually performed when a comprehensive clinical evaluation leaves continued uncertainty regarding the size of the shunt or when laboratory data do not fit well with the clinical findings. Catheterization is also useful for detecting the presence of associated cardiac defects.

When catheterization is performed, oximetry will demonstrate an increase in oxygen content in blood obtained from the right ventricle as compared with that from the right atrium; because some defects eject blood almost directly into the pulmonary artery, this increase is occasionally apparent only when pulmonary arterial blood is sampled (streaming). Small shunts may not result in a detectable increase in oxygen saturation in the right ventricle but may be demonstrated by indicator dilution tests (see Fig. 381–24). Small, restrictive defects are associated with normal right-sided heart pressures and pulmonary vascular resistance. Large, nonrestrictive defects are associated with equal or near-equal pulmonary and systemic systolic pressures. Pulmonary blood flow may be 2–4 times systemic blood flow. In these patients, the pulmonary vascular resistance will be only minimally elevated, because resistance is equal to the pressure divided by the flow. If Eisenmenger syndrome is present, pulmonary artery systolic and diastolic pressures will be elevated, the degree of left-to-right shunting will be minimal, and desaturation of blood in the left ventricle will be encountered. The size, location, and number of ventricular defects are demonstrated by left ventriculography. Contrast medium will pass across the defect(s) to opacify the right ventricle and pulmonary artery.

PROGNOSIS AND COMPLICATIONS. The natural course of a VSD depends to a large degree on the size of the defect. A significant number (30–50%) of small defects will close spontaneously, most frequently during the 1st yr of life. The vast majority of defects that close will do so before age 4 yr. These defects will often have ventricular septal aneurysms limiting the magnitude of the shunt. Most children with small defects remain asymptomatic without evidence of an increase in heart size, pulmonary arterial pressure, or resistance. One of the long-term risks for these patients is that of infective endocarditis. Endocarditis occurs in fewer than 2% of children with VSD, is more common in adolescents, and is rare in children under 2 yr of age. The risk is independent of the VSD size.

It is less common for moderate or large defects to close spontaneously, although even defects large enough to result in heart failure may become smaller and rarely will close completely. More commonly, infants with large defects have repeated episodes of respiratory infection and congestive heart failure despite optimal medical management. Heart failure may be manifested in many of these infants, primarily by failure to thrive. In some growth failure may be the only symptom. Pulmonary hypertension occurs as a result of high pulmonary blood flow. These patients are at risk for developing pulmonary vascular disease with time if the defect is not repaired.

A small number of patients with VSD develop acquired infundibular pulmonary stenosis, which then protects the pulmonary circulation from the short-term effects of pulmonary overcirculation and the long-term effects of pulmonary vascular disease. In these patients the clinical picture changes from that of a VSD with a large left-to-right shunt to a VSD with pulmonary stenosis. The shunt may diminish in size, become balanced, or even become a net right-to-left shunt (see Chapter 387.2). These patients must be distinguished from those who are developing Eisenmenger physiology.

TREATMENT. In patients with small defects, parents should be reassured of the relatively benign nature of the lesion, and the child should be encouraged to live a normal life, with no restrictions of physical activity. Surgical repair is not recommended. As a protection against infective endocarditis, the integrity of primary and permanent teeth should be carefully maintained; antibiotic prophylaxis should be provided for dental visits (including cleanings), tonsillectomy, adenoidectomy, and other oropharyngeal surgical procedures as well as for instrumentation of the genitourinary and lower intestinal tracts (Table 386–1). These patients can be followed by a combination of clinical examinations and occasional noninvasive laboratory tests until the defect has closed spontaneously. The electrocardiogram is an excellent means of screening these patients for possible pulmonary hypertension or pulmonic stenosis indicated by right ventricular hypertrophy.

In infants with a large VSD, medical management has two aims: to control congestive heart failure and to prevent the development of pulmonary vascular disease. These patients may show signs of repeated or chronic pulmonary disease and often fail to thrive. Therapeutic measures are aimed at the control of heart failure symptoms and the maintenance of normal growth (see Chapter 399). If early treatment is successful, the shunt may diminish in size with spontaneous improvement, especially during the 1st yr of life. The clinician must be alert to not confuse clinical improvement due to a decrease in defect size with clinical improvement due to the development of Eisenmenger physiology. Because surgical closure can be carried out at low risk in most infants, medical management should not be pursued in symptomatic infants after an unsuccessful trial. Furthermore, pulmonary vascular disease is prevented when surgery is performed within the 1st yr of life. Thus, large defects associated with pulmonary hypertension should be closed electively at between 6 and 12 mo of age, or earlier if symptoms warrant. Results of primary surgical repair are excellent, and complications resulting in long-term problems (e.g., residual ventricular shunts requiring reoperation or heart block requiring a pacemaker) are extremely rare. Pulmonary arterial banding with repair in later childhood is now reserved only for complicated cases. Surgical risks are higher for defects in the muscular septum, particularly apical defects and multiple (Swiss cheese-type) defects. These patients may require pulmonary arterial banding if symptomatic, with subsequent debanding and repair of multiple VSDs at an older age. Catheter occlusion devices are currently being tested to close apical muscular VSDs.

■ **TABLE 386–1 Recommendations for Prevention of Bacterial Endocarditis***

Dental Procedures and Surgery of Upper Respiratory Tract	
(1) For most patients: Oral amoxicillin	*Adults:* 3 g 1 hr before a procedure and 1.5 g 6 hr after the initial dose *Children:* 50 mg/kg 1 hr before a procedure and 25 mg/kg 6 hr after the initial dose†
(2) Penicillin allergy: Oral erythromycin	*Adults:* 1 g 2 hr before a procedure and 500 mg 6 hr after the initial dose *Children:* 20 mg/kg 2 hr before a procedure and 10 mg/kg 6 hr after the initial dose†
or Oral clindamycin	*Adults:* 300 mg 1 hr before a procedure and 150 mg 6 hr after the initial dose *Children:* 10 mg/kg 1 hr before a procedure and 5 mg/kg 6 hr after the initial dose†
(3) High-risk patients:‡ Parenteral ampicillin plus gentamicin (IV or IM)	*Adults:* Ampicillin 2 g 30 min before a procedure§ Gentamicin 1.5 mg/kg 30 min before a procedure§ *Children:* Ampicillin 50 mg/kg 30 min before a procedure†§ Gentamicin 2 mg/kg 30 min before a procedure§
(4) High-risk penicillin-allergic patients: Vancomycin (IV)	*Adults:* 1g infused slowly in 1 hr, initiated 1 hr before a procedure; no repeat dose needed *Children:* 20 mg/kg infused as adults; no repeat dose needed†
Gastrointestinal and Genitourinary Tract Surgery and Instrumentation	
(1) For most patients: Parenteral ampicillin plus gentamicin (IV or IM)	*Adults:* Ampicillin 2 g 30 min before a procedure§ Gentamicin 1.5 mg/kg 30 min before a procedure§ *Children:* Ampicillin 50 mg/kg 30 min before a procedure†§ Gentamicin 2 mg/kg 30 min before a procedure
(2) Penicillin allergy: Parenteral vancomycin plus gentamicin	*Adults:* Vancomycin 1 g infused slowly over 1 hr before a procedure‖ Gentamicin 1.5 mg/kg 30 min before a procedure‖ *Children:* Vancomycin 20 mg/kg infused slowly over 1 hr before a procedure† Gentamicin 2 mg/kg 30 min before a procedure‖
(3) Oral regiman for low-risk patients: Amoxicillin	*Adults:* 3 g 1 hr before a procedure and 1.5 g 6 hr later *Children:* 50 mg/kg 1 hr before a procedure and 25 mg 6 hr later†

Adapted from JAMA 264:2919, 1990, Copyright 1990, American Medical Association, and from Med Lett Drug Ther 31:112, 1989.

Oral regimens are less expensive, more convenient, and safer than parenteral routes. Amoxicillin is recommended because of excellent bioavailability and good activity against streptococci and enterococci. Parenteral routes are more effective and are recommended by some authorities for high-risk patients.

**Prophylaxis is recommended for patients with previous endocarditis, valvular heart disease, prosthetic heart devices, idiopathic hypertrophic subaortic stenosis, mitral valve prolapse with regurgitation, cardiac transplantation (possibly), and congenital heart disease, except for an isolated secundum atrial septal defect and for patients who have recovered at least 6 mo from surgery for a patent ductus arteriosus or simple atrial septal defect without a patch.*

†Maximal doses for children should not exceed adult doses.

‡High risk includes prosthetic valves, previous endocarditis, continuous penicillin prophylaxis for rheumatic fever, surgically constructed systemic-pulmonary shunts, or conduits.

§Additional parenteral (ampicillin and gentamicin), or more often oral dose (amoxicillin), should be given 6–8 hr after the initial dose in high-risk patients. The dose of gentamicin should not exceed 80 mg.

‖Additional dose may be repeated 8 hr after the initial dose.

After obliteration of the left-to-right shunt the hyperdynamic heart becomes quiet, cardiac size decreases toward normal (Fig. 386–3), thrills and murmurs are abolished, and pulmonary artery hypertension regresses. The patient's clinical status improves markedly. Most infants begin to thrive and cardiac medications are no longer required. Catch-up growth occurs in the majority over the next 1–2 yr. In some instances after successful operation, systolic ejection murmurs of low intensity may persist for months. The long-term prognosis after surgery is excellent.

386.7 Ventricular Septal Defect with Aortic Insufficiency

In this syndrome, the VSD is complicated by prolapse of the aortic valve into the defect and aortic insufficiency. It accounts for approximately 5% of patients with VSD; a considerably larger incidence is reported among Asian children. The septal defect, which may be small or moderate in size, is usually supracristal in location, that is, anterior and directly below the pulmonary valve in the outlet septum, superior to the crista supraventricularis. In occasional cases the VSD is membranous. The right, or less often the noncoronary, aortic cusp prolapses into the defect and may partially or even completely occlude it. This may limit the amount of left-to-right shunting and give the false impression that the defect is not large. Aortic insufficiency is most often not recognized until late in the 1st decade of life or beyond.

Early congestive heart failure secondary to a large left-to-right shunt rarely occurs, but without operation severe aortic insufficiency and left ventricular failure may ensue. The murmur of a supracristal VSD is usually heard at the mid to upper left sternal border as opposed to the lower left sternal border, and sometimes must be distinguished from that of pulmonic stenosis. The physical signs of aortic insufficiency (diastolic murmur and wide pulse pressure), when present, are added to those of the VSD. This clinical presentation needs to be distinguished from PDA or other defects associated with aortic runoff.

The *clinical manifestations* vary widely, from trivial aortic regurgitation and small left-to-right shunt in the asymptomatic child to the symptomatic adolescent with florid aortic incompetence and massive cardiomegaly. Many cardiologists recommend closure of all supracristal ventricular septal defects at the time of diagnosis, even in the asymptomatic child, in an attempt to prevent the development of aortic regurgitation. Patients already having significant aortic incompetence require surgical intervention to prevent irreversible left ventricular dysfunction. Surgical options depend on the degree of damage to the valve and include valvuloplasty for mild involvement,

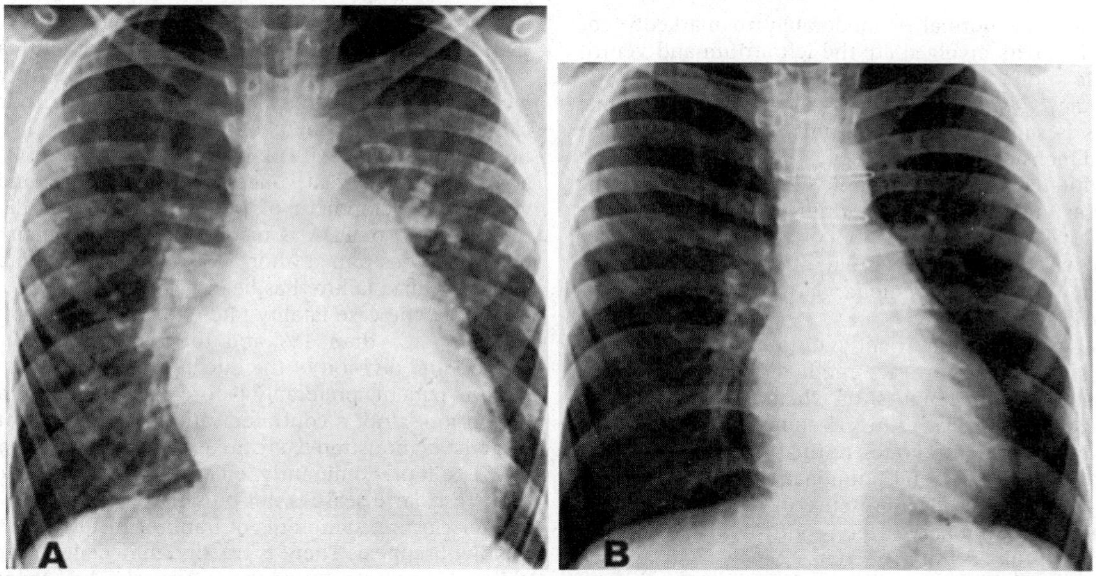

Figure 386–3. *A,* Preoperative roentgenogram in a ventricular septal defect with a large left-to-right shunt and pulmonary hypertension. Significant cardiomegaly, prominence of the pulmonary arterial trunk, and pulmonary overcirculation are evident. *B,* Three years after surgical closure of the defect. There is a marked decrease in the heart size, and the pulmonary vasculature is normal.

and replacement with a prosthesis or homograft, or aortopulmonary translocation (see Chapter 386.16) for severe involvement.

386.8 Patent Ductus Arteriosus (PDA)

During fetal life most of the pulmonary arterial blood is shunted through the ductus arteriosus into the aorta (see Chapter 382). Functional closure of the ductus normally occurs soon after birth, but if the ductus remains patent when pulmonary vascular resistance falls, aortic blood is shunted into the pulmonary artery. The aortic end of the ductus is just distal to the origin of the left subclavian artery, and the ductus enters the pulmonary artery at its bifurcation. Female patients outnumber males 2:1. PDA is one of the most common congenital cardiovascular anomalies associated with maternal rubella infection during early pregnancy. It is a common problem in neonatal intensive care units, where it has several major sequelae in the premature infant (see Chapter 87.3).

When a term infant is found to have PDA, there is deficiency of both the mucoid endothelial layer and the muscular media of the ductus. In the premature infant, however, the patent ductus usually has a normal structural anatomy; in these infants patency is the result of hypoxia and immaturity. Thus a PDA persisting beyond the 1st few weeks of life in a term infant will rarely close spontaneously, whereas in the premature infant, if early pharmacologic or surgical intervention was not required, spontaneous closure would occur in most instances. An obligatory PDA is seen in 10% of patients with other congenital heart lesions. An isolated PDA is also more common in patients born at high altitude.

PATHOPHYSIOLOGY. As a result of the higher aortic pressure, blood flow through the ductus goes from the aorta to the pulmonary artery. The extent of the shunt depends on the size of the ductus and on the ratio of pulmonary to systemic vascular resistances. In extreme cases, 70% of the left ventricular output may be shunted through the ductus to the pulmonary circulation. If the PDA is small, the pressures within the pulmonary artery, the right ventricle, and the right atrium are normal. However, if the PDA is large, pulmonary artery pressures may be elevated to systemic levels during both systole and diastole. These patients are at extremely high risk of developing pulmonary vascular disease if left unoperated. There is a wide pulse pressure due to runoff of blood into the pulmonary artery during diastole.

CLINICAL MANIFESTATIONS. There are usually no symptoms associated with a small patent ductus. A large defect will result in congestive heart failure similar to that encountered in infants with a large VSD. Retardation of physical growth may be a major manifestation in infants with large shunts.

A large PDA will result in striking physical signs attributable to the wide pulse pressure, most prominently bounding arterial pulses. The heart is normal in size when the ductus is small but moderately or grossly enlarged in cases with a large communication. The apical impulse is prominent and, with cardiac enlargement, is heaving. A thrill, maximal in the 2nd left interspace, is often present and may radiate toward the left clavicle, down the left sternal border or toward the apex. It is usually systolic but also may be palpated throughout the cardiac cycle. The classic continuous murmur has been variously described as being like machinery, a humming top, or rolling thunder in quality. It begins soon after onset of the 1st sound, reaches maximal intensity at the end of systole, and wanes in late diastole. It may be localized to the 2nd left intercostal space or radiate down the left sternal border or to the left clavicle. When there is increased pulmonary vascular resistance, the diastolic component of the murmur may be less prominent or absent. In patients with a large left-to-right shunt, a low-pitched mitral mid-diastolic murmur may be audible, owing to the increased volume of blood flow across the mitral valve.

If the left-to-right shunt is small, the *electrocardiogram* is normal; if the ductus is large, left ventricular or biventricular hypertrophy is present. The diagnosis of an isolated, uncomplicated PDA is untenable when right ventricular hypertrophy is noted.

Roentgenographic studies commonly show a prominent pulmonary artery with increased intrapulmonary vascular markings. The cardiac size depends on the degree of left-to-right shunting; it may be normal or moderately to markedly enlarged. The chambers involved are the left atrium and ventricle. The aortic knob is normal or prominent.

The *echocardiographic* view of the cardiac chambers is normal if the ductus is small. With large shunts, left atrial and left ventricular dimensions are increased. The left atrial size is usually quantitated by comparison to the size of the aortic root, known as the LA:Ao ratio. Scanning from the suprasternal notch allows direct visualization of the ductus. Doppler examination will demonstrate systolic and/or diastolic retrograde turbulent flow in the pulmonary artery and aortic retrograde flow in diastole.

The clinical pattern is sufficiently distinctive to allow an accurate diagnosis by noninvasive methods in most patients. In patients with atypical findings, or when associated cardiac lesions are suspected, cardiac catheterization may be indicated. *Cardiac catheterization* demonstrates normal or increased pressures in the right ventricle and pulmonary artery, depending on the size of the ductus. The presence of oxygenated blood shunting into the pulmonary artery confirms a left-to-right shunt. Samples of blood from the venae cavae, right atrium, and right ventricle should have normal oxygen contents. The catheter may pass from the pulmonary artery through the ductus into the descending aorta. Injection of contrast medium into the ascending aorta shows opacification of the pulmonary artery from the aorta and identifies the ductus.

DIAGNOSIS. The diagnosis of uncomplicated PDA is usually not difficult. However, there are other conditions that, in the absence of cyanosis, produce systolic and diastolic murmurs in the pulmonic area and must be differentiated. The characteristics of a venous hum are described in Chapter 380. An aorticopulmonary window defect rarely may be clinically indistinguishable from a patent ductus, although in most cases the murmur is only systolic and is loudest at the right upper sternal border rather than at the left. Similarly, a sinus of Valsalva aneurysm that has ruptured into the right side of the heart or pulmonary artery, coronary arteriovenous fistulas, and an aberrant left coronary artery with massive collaterals from the right coronary display dynamics similar to that of the PDA with a continuous murmur and a wide pulse pressure. Sometimes the murmur is not maximal in the pulmonary area but is heard along the lower left sternal border. Truncus arteriosus with torrential pulmonary flow also has an "aortic runoff" physiology. Pulmonary branch stenosis can be associated with systolic and diastolic murmurs, but the pulse pressure will be normal. A peripheral arteriovenous fistula also results in a wide pulse pressure, but the distinctive murmur of a PDA is not present. VSD with aortic insufficiency and combined rheumatic aortic and mitral insufficiency may be confused with a PDA, but the murmurs should be differentiated by their to-and-fro rather than continuous nature. The combination of a large VSD and a PDA results in findings more like those in isolated VSD. Echocardiography should be able to eliminate these other diagnostic possibilities. If a ductus is suspected clinically but not visualized on echo, a cardiac catheterization is usually indicated.

PROGNOSIS AND COMPLICATIONS. Patients with a small PDA may live a normal span with few or no cardiac symptoms; however, late manifestations may occur. Spontaneous closure of the ductus after infancy is extremely rare. *Congestive cardiac failure* most often occurs in early infancy in the presence of a large ductus but may occur late in life even with a moderate-sized communication. The chronic left ventricular volume load is less well tolerated with aging.

Infective endarteritis may be seen at any age. Pulmonary or systemic emboli may occur. Rare complications include aneurysmal dilatation of the pulmonary artery or the ductus, calcification of the ductus, noninfective thrombosis of the ductus with embolization, and paradoxic emboli. Pulmonary hypertension (Eisenmenger syndrome) usually occurs in patients with a large PDA who do not undergo surgical treatment.

TREATMENT. Irrespective of age, patients with PDA require surgical closure. In patients with a small PDA, the rationale for closure is prevention of endarteritis or other late complications. In patients with a moderate to large PDA, closure is accomplished to treat congestive heart failure, and/or to prevent the development of pulmonary vascular disease. Once the diagnosis of PDA is made, surgical treatment should not be unduly postponed after adequate medical therapy of congestive cardiac failure has been instituted.

Because the case fatality rate with surgical treatment is considerably less than 1% and the risk without it is greater, ligation and division of the ductus are indicated in the asymptomatic patient, preferably before 1 yr of age. Pulmonary hypertension is not a contraindication to operation at any age if it can be demonstrated at cardiac catheterization that the shunt flow is still predominantly left-to-right and that severe pulmonary vascular disease is not present.

After closure, symptoms of frank or incipient cardiac failure rapidly disappear. There is usually immediate improvement in physical development of the infant who had failed to thrive. The pulse and blood pressure return to normal, and the machinery-like murmur disappears. A functional systolic murmur over the pulmonary area may occasionally persist; it may represent turbulence in a persistently dilated pulmonary artery. The roentgenographic signs of cardiac enlargement and pulmonary overcirculation will disappear over several months and the electrocardiogram becomes normal.

Transcatheter closure in the cardiac catheterization laboratory using either a Teflon plug, an occlusional umbrella, or intravascular coils has been successfully used in selected centers and eliminates the risks of surgery. A relatively new approach involves the use of thoracoscopic surgical techniques to ligate the ductus without the need for a large lateral thoracotomy.

PATENT DUCTUS ARTERIOSUS IN LOW-BIRTHWEIGHT INFANTS (see Chapters 82.2 and 87.3)

386.9 Aorticopulmonary Window Defect

This defect consists of a communication between the ascending aorta and main pulmonary artery. The presence of pulmonary and aortic valves and an intact ventricular septum distinguishes this anomaly from truncus arteriosus (see Chapter 387.15). Symptoms similar to those of a large VSD or of PDA appear during early infancy and include recurrent pulmonary infections, congestive heart failure, and, occasionally, minimal cyanosis. The defect is usually large and the cardiac murmur is systolic with a mid-diastolic rumble, reflecting the increased blood flow across the mitral valve. In the rare instance when the communication is somewhat smaller and pulmonary hypertension is absent, the signs can mimic a PDA; a wide pulse pressure, cardiac enlargement, and a right and left upper sternal border continuous murmur may be present. The electrocardiogram shows either left or biventricular hypertrophy. Roentgenographic studies demonstrate cardiac enlargement and prominence of the pulmonary artery and intrapulmonary vasculature. The echocardiogram shows large-volume left-sided heart chambers, and the window defect can often be delineated, especially with color flow Doppler.

Cardiac catheterization reveals a left-to-right shunt at the level of the pulmonary artery, as well as hyperkinetic pulmonary hypertension, because the defect is almost always large. Selective aortography with injection of contrast medium into the ascending aorta demonstrates the lesion, and manipulation of the catheter from the main pulmonary artery directly to the ascending aorta and brachiocephalic vessels is also diagnostic.

The aorticopulmonary window defect is surgically corrected during infancy using cardiopulmonary bypass. If surgery is not carried out in infancy, survivors carry the risk of progressive pulmonary vascular obstructive disease, similar to that of other patients who have large intracardiac or great vessel communications.

386.10 Coronary-Arterial Fistula

A congenital fistula may exist between a coronary artery and an atrium, ventricle (especially the right), or pulmonary artery. Sometimes multiple fistulas exist. Regardless of the recipient chamber, the clinical signs are similar to those of PDA, although the machinery-like murmur may be more diffuse. When a coronary artery empties directly into the right side of the heart, there is often only a small left-to-right shunt at the atrial or ventricular level. The involved coronary artery is often dilated or aneurysmal. The anatomic abnormality is demonstrable by injection of contrast medium into the ascending aorta. Treatment consists of surgical abolition of the fistula.

386.11 Ruptured Sinus of Valsalva Aneurysm

When one of the sinuses of Valsalva of the aorta is weakened by congenital or acquired disease, an aneurysm may form and eventually may rupture, usually into the right atrium or ventricle. This condition is extremely rare in childhood. The onset is usually sudden. The diagnosis is suspected in a patient who develops symptoms of acute congestive heart failure, associated with a new loud to-and-fro murmur. Cardiac catheterization demonstrates the left-to-right shunt at the atrial or ventricular level. Injection of contrast medium into the ascending aorta demonstrates the site of the aneurysm and rupture. Urgent surgical repair is usually required. This condition is often associated with infective endocarditis.

The Obstructive Lesions

386.12 Pulmonary Valve Stenosis with Intact Ventricular Septum

Various forms of right ventricular outflow obstruction with intact ventricular septum exist. The most common is valvular pulmonary stenosis. In this entity the valve cusps are deformed to various degrees, resulting in incomplete opening during systole. The valve may be bicuspid or tricuspid with the leaflets partially fused together and with an eccentric outlet. This fusion may be so severe as to leave only a pinhole central opening. If the valve is not severely thickened, it produces a domelike obstruction to right ventricular outflow during systole. Isolated infundibular stenosis, supravalvular pulmonary stenosis, and branch pulmonary artery stenosis are less commonly encountered. In some instances when pulmonary valve stenosis is the dominant lesion, a small associated VSD is present, and this condition is better classified as pulmonary stenosis with VSD than as tetralogy of Fallot. In addition, pulmonary stenosis and ASD are occasionally seen as associated defects. The clinical and laboratory findings will reflect the dominant lesion, but it is important to rule out these associated anomalies. Pulmonary stenosis as a result of valve dysplasia is the common cardiac abnormality of *Noonan syndrome* (see Chapters 535–538).

PATHOPHYSIOLOGY. The obstruction to outflow from the right ventricle to the pulmonary artery results in increased systolic pressure and wall stress, leading to hypertrophy of the right ventricle. The severity of these abnormalities depends on the size of the restricted valvular opening. In severe cases, right ventricular pressure may be much higher than systemic systolic pressure, whereas in milder obstruction right ventricular pressure is only mildly or moderately elevated. Pulmonary arterial pressure is normal or decreased. *Arterial oxygen saturation will be normal unless there is an intracardiac communication, such as a VSD or ASD.* In severe pulmonic stenosis, markedly decreased right ventricular compliance may lead to right-to-left shunting at the atrial level through a foramen ovale. This is seen most often in the neonate and is referred to as critical pulmonic stenosis.

CLINICAL MANIFESTATIONS. With mild or moderate stenosis there are usually no symptoms. Growth and development are most often normal, and usually older infants and children with pulmonary stenosis appear to be especially well developed and healthy. If the stenosis is severe, there may be signs of right-ventricular failure and exercise intolerance. In the neonate or young infant with critical pulmonic stenosis, signs of right ventricular failure may be more prominent and cyanosis is often present due to shunting at the foramen ovale.

With mild pulmonary stenosis the venous pressure and pulse are normal. The heart is not enlarged; the apical impulse is normal, and the right ventricular impulse is not palpable. A relatively short pulmonary systolic ejection murmur is maximally audible over the pulmonic area and may radiate minimally to the lung fields bilaterally. The murmur is usually preceded by a pulmonic ejection click, which is heard best at the left upper sternal border during expiration. The 2nd heart sound is split with a pulmonary element of normal intensity that may be slightly delayed. The *electrocardiogram* is normal or characteristic of mild right ventricular hypertrophy; there may be inversion of the T waves in the right precordial leads. The only abnormality demonstrable *roentgenographically* is poststenotic dilatation of the pulmonary artery. *Two-dimensional echocardiography* shows right ventricular hypertrophy, a domed valve, and Doppler studies demonstrate a right ventricular–pulmonary artery gradient of 30 mm Hg or less.

In moderate pulmonic stenosis the venous pressure may be slightly elevated, with an intrinsic "a" wave noted in the jugular pulse. A right ventricular lift may be palpable at the lower left sternal border. As the degree of stenosis worsens, the systolic ejection murmur is prolonged later into systole, and becomes louder and harsher (higher frequency). The murmur will radiate to both lung fields. With more severe limitation in valve motion, a pulmonic ejection click will not be appreciated. The 2nd heart sound is split, with a delayed and diminished pulmonary component that may not be audible. The *electrocardiogram* reveals varying degrees of right ventricular hypertrophy, sometimes with a prominent spiked P wave. *Roentgenographically,* the heart can vary from normal size to mildly enlarged because of prominence of the right ventricle; intrapulmonary vascularity may be normal or decreased. The *echocardiogram* will show a thickened pulmonic valve with restricted systolic motion. The Doppler exam will show a ventricular-pulmonary arterial pressure gradient in the 30–60 mm Hg range. Mild tricuspid regurgitation may be present and allows confirmation of the right ventricular systolic pressure.

In severe stenosis, mild to moderate cyanosis may be noted if there is an interatrial communication. If hepatic enlargement and peripheral edema are present, they are an indication of right ventricular failure. Elevation of the venous pressure is common and is caused by a large presystolic jugular "a" wave. The heart is moderately or greatly enlarged, and there is a conspicuous sternal and parasternal right ventricular lift that frequently extends to the midclavicular line. A loud and long systolic ejection murmur, frequently accompanied by a thrill, is maximally audible in the pulmonic area and may radiate widely over the entire precordium, to both lung fields, into the neck, and to the back. The peak of the murmur occurs later in systole as valve opening becomes more restricted (late systolic accentuation). The murmur frequently encompasses the aortic component of the 2nd sound but is not preceded by an ejection click. The pulmonary element of the 2nd sound is usually inaudible.

The *electrocardiogram* shows gross right ventricular hypertrophy, frequently accompanied by a tall, spiked P wave. *Roentgenographic studies* confirm the cardiac enlargement and prominence of the right ventricle and atrium. Prominence of the pulmonary artery segment is due to poststenotic dilatation (Fig. 386–4). The intrapulmonary vascularity is decreased. The *two-dimensional echocardiogram* shows severe deformity of the pulmonary valve and right ventricular hypertrophy. In the late stages of the disease, dysfunction of the right ventricle is seen and the ventricle may become dilated. Doppler studies demonstrate a large gradient across the pulmonary valve. Tricuspid regurgitation may also be prominent. Fortunately, the classic findings of severe pulmonary stenosis in older children are now rarely seen because of early intervention. The signs of critical pulmonic stenosis are usually encountered in the neonatal period.

Cardiac catheterization demonstrates an abrupt pressure gradient across the pulmonary valve. The pulmonary arterial pressure is either normal or low. The severity is graded based on the right ventricular systolic pressure or the pressure gradient. A gradient of 10–30 mm Hg in mild cases, 30–60 mm Hg in moderate cases, and greater than 60 mm Hg, or with right ventricular pressure greater than systemic pressure in severe cases. If the cardiac output is low or a significant right-to-left shunt exists across the atrial septum, the pressure gradient may underestimate the degree of valve stenosis. In severe and in some moderate cases, the right atrial pressure shows a prominent, frequently giant, "a" wave. *Selective right ventriculography* clearly demonstrates the valve obstruction. The flow of contrast medium through the stenotic valve in ventricular systole produces a narrow jet of dye that fills the dilated pulmonary artery. Abnormalities in both structure and motion of the pulmonary valve are visible. In mild to moderate stenosis the doming of the valve in systole is readily seen. Subvalvular hypertrophy that may intensify the obstruction may occasionally be present. The angiogram will also indicate whether the ventricular septum is intact.

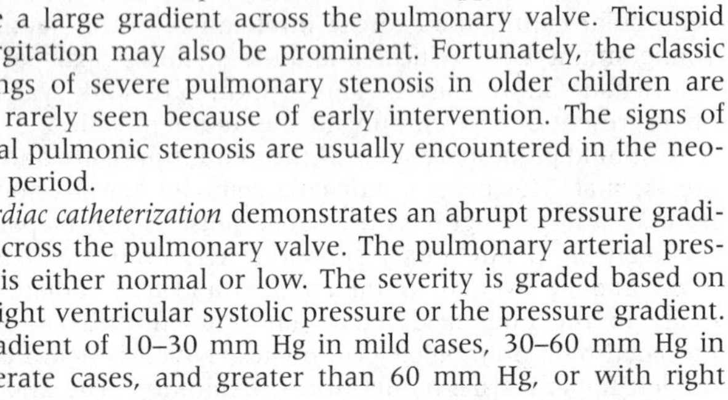

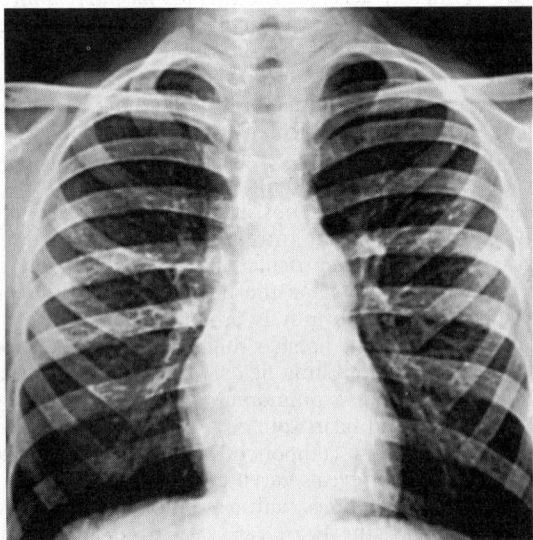

Figure 386–4. Roentgenogram in valvular pulmonary stenosis with a normal aortic root. The heart size is within normal limits, but there is poststenotic dilatation of the pulmonary artery.

PROGNOSIS AND COMPLICATIONS. Congestive cardiac failure, the most common complication, occurs only in severe cases and most often during the 1st mo of life. The development of cyanosis from a right-to-left shunt across a foramen ovale is most often seen in infancy when the stenosis is very severe. Infective endocarditis is a risk but not common in childhood.

Children with mild or moderate stenosis can lead a normal life, but their progress should be evaluated at regular intervals. Patients who have small gradients rarely show progression and do not need intervention, but children having moderate stenosis are more likely to develop a more significant gradient as they grow older. Worsening of obstruction may also be due, in part, to the development of secondary subvalvular muscular and fibrous tissue hypertrophy. In untreated severe stenosis the course may abruptly worsen with the development of right ventricular dysfunction and cardiac failure. Infants with critical pulmonic stenosis require urgent catheter balloon valvuloplasty or surgical valvotomy.

TREATMENT. Patients with moderate or severe isolated pulmonary stenosis require relief of the obstruction. Balloon valvuloplasty is the initial treatment of choice for the vast majority of patients (Fig. 386–5). Patients with severely thickened pulmonic valves, especially common in those with Noonan syndrome, may require surgical intervention instead. In the neonate with critical pulmonic stenosis, emergency treatment with either balloon valvuloplasty or surgical valvotomy is warranted.

Excellent results are obtained in the majority of instances. The gradient across the pulmonary valve is reduced markedly or abolished. In the early period after balloon valvuloplasty a small to moderate residual gradient may remain due to muscular infundibular narrowing; it nearly always resolves with time. A short early decrescendo diastolic murmur at the mid to upper left sternal border due to pulmonary valvular insufficiency may be heard. The degree of insufficiency is usually not clinically significant. There appears to be no difference between valvuloplasty and surgery in patient status at late follow-up, and recurrence is unusual after successful treatment.

386.13 Infundibular Pulmonary Stenosis and Double-Chamber Right Ventricle

Infundibular pulmonary stenosis is caused by muscular or fibrous obstruction in the outflow tract of the right ventricle. The site of obstruction may be close to the pulmonary valve or well below it; an infundibular chamber may be present between the right ventricular cavity and the pulmonary valve. In a significant number of cases, a VSD may have been present initially and later closed spontaneously. When the pulmonary

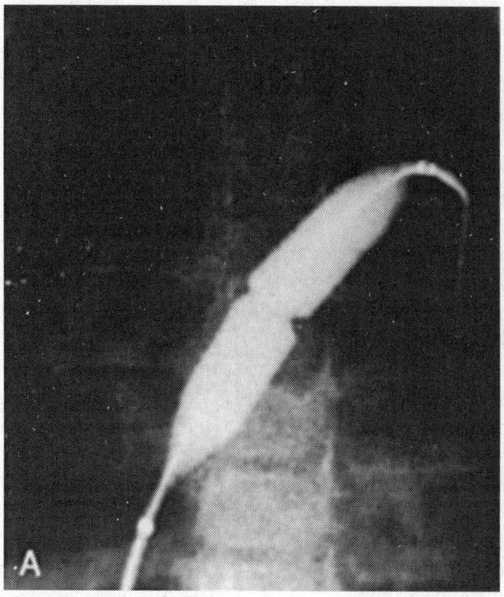

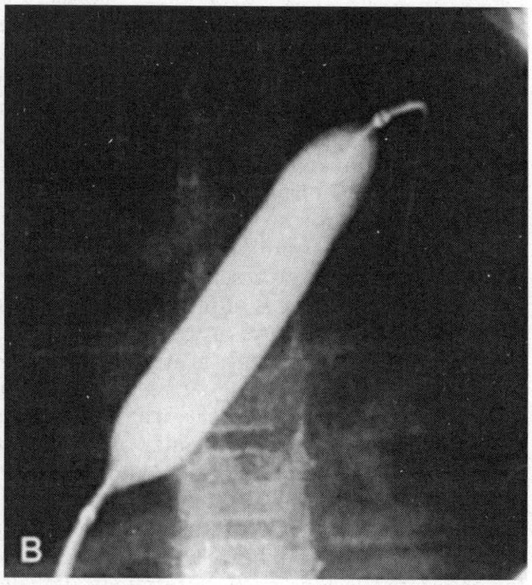

Figure 386–5. Balloon pulmonary valvuloplasty. *A*, Hourglass shape of the balloon at the start of inflation. *B*, Full balloon inflation. The left pulmonary artery is protected from the sharp tip of the catheter with a flexible-tip guidewire. (From Lababidi Z: Neonatal catheter palliations. *In:* Long WA [ed]: Fetal and Neonatal Cardiology. Philadelphia, WB Saunders, 1990, p. 707.)

valve is also stenotic, the combined defect is primarily classified as valvular stenosis with secondary infundibular hypertrophy. The *hemodynamics* and *clinical manifestations* of patients with isolated infundibular pulmonary stenosis are similar, for the most part, to those described under isolated valvular pulmonary stenosis (see Chapter 386.12).

A more common variation of right ventricular outflow obstruction below the pulmonary valve is that of double-chamber right ventricle. In this condition there is a muscular band in the mid right ventricular region, which divides the chamber into two parts and creates obstruction between the inlet and outlet portions. There is often an associated VSD that may close spontaneously. Obstruction is not usually seen early in life but may progress rapidly in a similar manner to the progressive infundibular obstruction observed with tetralogy of Fallot.

The *diagnosis* of isolated right ventricular infundibular stenosis or double-chamber right ventricle can be made by echocardiography and/or cardiac catheterization and angiography. At catheterization, when contrast material is injected into the right ventricle, the site of the stenosis is demonstrated. The ventricular septum must be evaluated to determine whether an associated VSD is present. The prognosis for untreated cases of severe right ventricular outflow obstruction is similar to that for valvular pulmonary stenosis (see Chapter 386.12). Thus, when obstruction is moderate to severe, surgery is indicated. After operation the pressure gradient is abolished or markedly reduced and the long-term outlook is excellent.

386.14 Pulmonary Stenosis in Combination with an Intracardiac Shunt

Valvular or infundibular pulmonary stenosis, or both, may be associated with either an ASD or a VSD. In these patients, the clinical features depend on the degree of pulmonary stenosis, which will determine whether the net shunt is left to right or right to left.

The presence of a large left-to-right shunt at the atrial or ventricular level is evidence that the pulmonary stenosis is mild. These patients will present with symptoms similar to those with an isolated ASD or VSD. However, with increasing age, worsening of the obstruction may limit the shunt, resulting in a gradual improvement in symptoms. Eventually, particularly in patients with pulmonary stenosis and VSD, further increase in the obstruction may lead to right-to-left shunting. When a patient being followed with a VSD develops evidence of decreasing heart failure and increased right ventricular forces on the electrocardiogram, the clinician must differentiate between the development of increasing pulmonary stenosis versus the onset of pulmonary vascular disease (Eisenmenger syndrome).

These anomalies are readily repaired surgically. Defects in the atrial or ventricular septa are closed, and the pulmonary stenosis is relieved by resection of infundibular muscle and/or pulmonary valvotomy as indicated. Patients with a predominant right-to-left shunt will present with symptoms similar to those patients with tetralogy of Fallot (see Chapter 387.2).

386.15 Peripheral Pulmonary Arterial Stenosis

Single or multiple constrictions may occur anywhere along the major branches of the pulmonary arteries and may be mild, extensive, localized, or multiple. Frequently, these defects are associated with other types of congenital heart disease, including valvular pulmonic stenosis, tetralogy of Fallot, PDA, VSD, ASD, and supravalvular aortic stenosis. A familial tendency has been recognized in some patients with peripheral pulmonic stenosis. A high incidence is found in infants with the congenital rubella syndrome. Supravalvular aortic stenosis with pulmonary arterial branch stenosis has also been observed with idiopathic hypercalcemia of infancy (Williams syndrome).

With a mild constriction there is little effect on the pulmonary circulation. With multiple severe constrictions there is an increase in pressure in the right ventricle and in the pulmonary artery proximal to the site of obstruction. When the anomaly is isolated, the *diagnosis* is suspected by the presence of murmurs in widespread locations over the chest, both anteriorly or posteriorly. These murmurs are usually systolic but may be continuous. Most often, the physical signs are dominated by the associated anomaly, such as tetralogy of Fallot. If the stenosis is severe, there is electrocardiographic evidence of right ventricular and right atrial hypertrophy.

In the immediate newborn period, a mild and transient

form of peripheral pulmonic stenosis may be present. Physical findings are usually limited to a soft systolic ejection murmur, which can be heard over either or both lung fields. It is the absence of other physical findings of valvular pulmonic stenosis (right ventricular lift, soft pulmonic second sound, systolic ejection click, murmur loudest at the upper left sternal border) that supports this diagnosis. This murmur will usually disappear by 1–2 mo.

On *roentgenogram*, cardiomegaly and prominence of the main pulmonary artery are present in severe cases. Generally, the pulmonary vasculature is normal; in some cases small intrapulmonary vascular shadows are seen, which may be shown by pulmonary arteriography to be areas of poststenotic dilatation. Pressure gradients across the areas of obstruction are demonstrable by *cardiac catheterization*. These gradients may not be easily identified if right ventricular outflow obstruction coexists, as the pressure in the main pulmonary artery is normal or low in such patients.

Severe obstruction of the main pulmonary artery and its primary branches can be relieved during corrective surgery for associated lesions such as tetralogy of Fallot or valvular pulmonary stenosis. If peripheral pulmonic stenosis is isolated, it may be treated by catheter balloon dilatation. When peripheral obstruction occurs distally in the intrapulmonary vessels, it is usually not amenable to surgical repair. These obstructions are often multiple and are best treated with repeat balloon angioplasty, although there is a high rate of recurrence. The more recent introduction of expandable intravascular stents, placed by catheter in the distal pulmonary arteries, and then dilated with a balloon to the appropriate size, may prevent restenosis.

386.16 Aortic Stenosis

PATHOPHYSIOLOGY. *Congenital aortic stenosis* accounts for about 5% of cardiac malformations recognized in childhood, but an abnormality of the aortic valve (bicuspid) is one of the most common congenital heart lesions identified in adults. Aortic stenosis is more common in males (3:1). In most cases, aortic stenosis is valvular, the leaflets are thickened, and the commissures are fused to varying degrees.

Subvalvular (subaortic) stenosis with a discrete fibrous shelf below the aortic valve is also an important form of left ventricular outflow tract obstruction. This lesion is frequently associated with other forms of congenital heart disease and is notable for rapid progression in severity. It is virtually never diagnosed during early infancy and may develop despite prior documentation of no left ventricular outflow tract gradient. Subvalvular aortic stenosis may become apparent after successful surgery for other congenital heart defects (e.g., coarctation of the aorta, PDA, and VSD), may develop in association with mild lesions that have not been surgically repaired, and may occur as an isolated abnormality.

Supravalvular aortic stenosis, a less common type, may be sporadic, familial, or associated with Williams syndrome, which includes mental retardation, elfin facies (full face, broad forehead, flattened bridge of nose, long upper lip, and rounded cheeks) and idiopathic hypercalcemia of infancy (see Chapter 67). Stenoses of other arteries may also be present.

CLINICAL MANIFESTATIONS. Symptomatology among patients with aortic stenosis depends on the severity of the obstruction. Aortic stenosis that presents in early infancy is termed *critical aortic stenosis* and is associated with severe left ventricular failure. These infants present with signs of low cardiac output. Congestive heart failure, cardiomegaly, and pulmonary edema are severe, and the pulses are weak in all extremities. Urine output may be diminished. Because the cardiac output is decreased, the intensity of the murmur at the right upper sternal border may be minimal. In contrast, most children with less severe forms of aortic stenosis will remain asymptomatic and display a normal growth and development pattern. The murmur is usually discovered during routine physical examination. Rarely, an older child with previously undiagnosed severe obstruction to left ventricular outflow will present with fatigue, angina, dizziness, or syncope. Sudden death has been reported with aortic stenosis but usually occurs in patients with severe left ventricular outflow obstruction in whom surgical relief has been delayed.

The physical findings are dependent on the degree of obstruction to left ventricular outflow. In mild stenosis, the pulses, heart size, and apical impulse are all normal. With increasing degrees of severity, the pulses will become diminished in intensity and the heart may be enlarged with a left ventricular apical thrust. In mild to moderate valvular aortic stenosis, there is usually an early systolic ejection click, best heard at the apex and left sternal edge. Unlike the click associated with pulmonic stenosis, its intensity does not vary with respirations. Clicks are unusual in more severe aortic stenosis or in discrete subaortic stenosis. In severe stenosis the 1st heart sound may be diminished due to decreased compliance of the thickened left ventricle. Normal splitting of the 2nd heart sound is present in mild to moderate obstruction. In patients with severe obstruction, the intensity of aortic valve closure is diminished and, rarely in children, the 2nd sound may be split paradoxically (becoming wider in expiration). A 4th heart sound may be audible when the obstruction is severe.

The intensity, frequency, and duration of the systolic ejection murmur is another indication of severity. Generally, the louder, harsher (higher frequency), and longer the murmur, the greater the degree of obstruction. The typical murmur is audible maximally at the right upper sternal border and radiates to the neck and down the left sternal border. It is usually accompanied by a thrill in the suprasternal notch. In patients with subvalvular aortic stenosis, the murmur may be maximal along the left sternal border or even at the apex. A soft decrescendo diastolic murmur indicative of mild aortic insufficiency is often present when the obstruction is subvalvular or in patients with a bicuspid aortic valve. Occasionally, an apical short mid-diastolic rumbling murmur is audible, even in the presence of a normal mitral valve; however, this should always raise the suspicion of associated mitral stenosis.

DIAGNOSIS. The diagnosis can usually be made on the basis of the physical examination, and the severity of obstruction is confirmed by laboratory tests. If the pressure gradient across the aortic valve is small, the *electrocardiogram* (ECG) is likely to be normal. The ECG may occasionally be normal, even with more severe obstruction, but evidence of left ventricular hypertrophy and strain (e.g., inverted T waves in the left precordial leads) is usually present if severe stenosis is long-standing. *Roentgenograms* frequently show a prominent ascending aorta, but the aortic knob is normal. The heart size is usually normal. Valvular calcification has been noted only in older children. *Echocardiography* will identify both the site and severity of the obstruction. Two-dimensional imaging will show left ventricular hypertrophy, the thickened and domed aortic valve, the number of valve leaflets, and a subaortic membrane, if present. Associated anomalies of the mitral valve or aortic arch will be detected. In the absence of left ventricular failure, the shortening fraction of the left ventricle may be increased because the ventricle is hypercontractile. In infants with critical aortic stenosis, the left ventricular shortening is usually decreased and the endocardium may be bright, indicating the development of endocardial fibroelastosis (see Chapter 395). Doppler studies will show the specific site of obstruction and determine the peak systolic left ventricular outflow tract gradient. When severe aortic obstruction is associated with left ventricular dysfunction, the Doppler-derived aortic valve gradient may not reflect the severity of the obstruction due to the low cardiac output.

Graded exercise testing is useful in evaluating the severity of left ventricular outflow tract obstruction in older children. As the severity of the gradient increases, working capacity decreases, systolic blood pressure fails to rise adequately, diastolic blood pressure may rise, and ST-segment depression can occur. Because patients with severe aortic stenosis may deny symptoms and have normal electrocardiograms and chest roentgenograms, serial echocardiograms and graded exercise tests may be valuable in determining the timing of cardiac catheterization and surgical or balloon catheter valvuloplasty.

Left heart cardiac catheterization demonstrates the magnitude of the pressure gradient from the left ventricle to the aorta. The site of obstruction is best identified by selective left ventriculography. The aortic pressure curve is abnormal if obstruction is severe. In patients with severe obstruction and decreased left ventricular compliance, the left atrial pressure is increased and there may be pulmonary hypertension. Most infants with critical aortic stenosis do not require diagnostic cardiac catheterization. When a critically ill infant with left ventricular outflow tract obstruction undergoes cardiac catheterization, left ventricular function is often markedly decreased. As with the echocardiogram, the gradient measured across the stenotic aortic valve may be less than severe because of low cardiac output. Actual measurement of the cardiac output by thermodilution and calculation of valve area is helpful in these cases.

PROGNOSIS. The prognosis is good in most children with mild to moderate aortic stenosis. In a small number of patients having a severe obstruction, sudden death has occurred. In such instances there is usually evidence of gross left ventricular hypertrophy. Neonates having critical aortic stenosis who die from congestive heart failure frequently have endocardial fibroelastosis of the left ventricle. Infants who present after the 1st wk or two of life respond well to relief of stenosis, and left ventricular function improves. Reoperations on the aortic valve are often required later in childhood or in adult life, and many patients will eventually require valve replacement.

There may be some danger in allowing patients with significant aortic stenosis to participate in active competitive sports, but otherwise they should lead normal lives. The status of each patient should be reviewed annually and intervention advised if progression of signs or symptoms occurs. Lifetime prophylaxis against infective endocarditis is required.

TREATMENT. Balloon valvuloplasty is indicated for children having moderate to severe valvular aortic stenosis to prevent progressive left ventricular dysfunction and the risks of syncope and sudden death. It is generally agreed that valvuloplasty should be advised when the peak systolic gradient between the left ventricle and aorta exceeds 60 mm Hg at rest, assuming a normal cardiac output. A lesser gradient is required for the more rapidly progressive subaortic obstructive lesions. Outside of the neonatal period, surgical treatment is usually reserved for valves that are not amenable to balloon therapy, usually those that are extremely thickened. Whether surgical or catheter treatment has been carried out, aortic insufficiency or calcification with restenosis is likely to occur years or even decades later, eventually requiring reoperation and often aortic valve replacement.

In the neonatal period, balloon valvuloplasty is made more difficult by problems of arterial access. The risk of femoral arterial complications is much higher than in older children, although the development of low-profile balloons has reduced this risk substantially. Currently, both surgical and catheter approaches are being used at different centers for critical aortic stenosis in the newborn period.

Discrete subaortic stenosis can be resected without damage to the aortic valve, the anterior leaflet of the mitral valve, or the conduction system. This type of obstruction is usually not easily amenable to catheter treatment. Relief of supravalvular stenosis is also achieved surgically, and the results are excellent if the area of obstruction is discrete and is not associated with a hypoplastic aorta.

After either catheter or surgical relief of aortic stenosis, recurrence of obstruction or development of aortic insufficiency is common. When recurrence occurs it may not be associated with early symptoms. Signs of recurrent stenosis include electrocardiographic signs of left ventricular hypertrophy, increase in echo Doppler gradient, deterioration of echocardiographic indices of left ventricular function, and recurrence of signs or symptoms during graded exercise. Evidence of significant aortic regurgitation includes symptoms of congestive heart failure, cardiac enlargement on roentgenogram, and left ventricular dilatation on echocardiogram. The choice of reparative procedure depends on the relative degrees of stenosis and regurgitation.

When aortic valve replacement is necessary, the choice of procedure often depends on the age of the patient. Porcine and homograft valves tend to calcify more rapidly in younger children; however, they do not require chronic anticoagulation. In contrast, mechanical prosthetic valves are much longer lasting, yet require anticoagulation, which can be difficult to manage in young children. In adolescent girls who are nearing childbearing age, consideration of the teratogenic effects of warfarin may warrant the use of a homograft valve. None of these options is perfect for the younger child who requires valve replacement, because they will not grow with the patient. An operation being used by many centers is aorto-pulmonary translocation—the Ross procedure. This involves removing the pulmonary valve and using it to replace the abnormal aortic valve. A homograft valve is then placed in the pulmonary position. The possible advantage of this procedure is the potential for growth of the translocated "neo-aortic" valve and the longer longevity of the homograft valve when placed in the lower pressure pulmonary circulation.

386.17 Coarctation of the Aorta

Constrictions of the aorta of varying degrees may occur at any point from the transverse arch to the iliac bifurcation, but 98% occur just below the origin of the left subclavian artery at the origin of the ductus arteriosus (juxtaductal coarctation). The anomaly occurs twice as often in males as in females. Coarctation of the aorta may be a feature of Turner (XO) syndrome (see Chapter 538) and is associated with bicuspid aortic valve in over 70% of patients. Mitral valve abnormalities, for example, a supravalvar mitral ring or parachute mitral valve, and subaortic stenosis are not uncommon associated lesions. When this group of left-sided obstructive lesions occurs together, they are referred to as Shone complex.

PATHOPHYSIOLOGY. Coarctation of the aorta can occur as a discrete juxtaductal obstruction or as a tubular hypoplasia of the transverse aorta starting at one of the head or neck vessels and extending to the ductal area (preductal coarctation). Often, both components are present. It is postulated that coarctation is initiated in fetal life by the presence of a cardiac abnormality that results in decreased blood flow anterograde through the aortic valve (e.g., bicuspid aortic valve, VSD).

After birth, in a discrete juxtaductal coarctation, ascending aortic blood will flow through the narrowed segment to reach the descending aorta, although left ventricular hypertension and hypertrophy will result. In the 1st few days of life, the patent ductus arteriosus may serve to widen the juxtaductal area of the aorta and provide a temporary relief from the obstruction. In these infants net left-to-right ductal shunting occurs and they are acyanotic. In contrast, with more severe juxtaductal coarctation or in the presence of transverse arch hypoplasia, right ventricular blood is ejected through the ductus to supply the descending aorta, as it does during fetal life. Perfusion of the lower body is then dependent on right ventricular output (Fig. 386–6). In this situation the femoral pulses are palpable, and differential blood pressures may not be helpful in making the diagnosis. However, the ductal right-to-left shunting will be manifest as differential cyanosis, with the upper extremities pink and the lower extremities blue.

Such infants may have severe pulmonary hypertension and high pulmonary vascular resistance. Signs of heart failure are prominent. Occasionally, severely hypoplastic segments of the aortic isthmus may become completely atretic, resulting in an **interrupted aortic arch** with the left subclavian artery arising either proximal or distal to the interruption. In the past, coarctation associated with arch hypoplasia was referred to as "infantile type" because it usually presented in early infancy due to its severity. "Adult type" referred to the isolated juxtaductal coarctation, which, if mild, usually did not present until later childhood. These terms have been replaced with the more accurate anatomic terms mentioned earlier describing the location and severity of the defect.

The blood pressure is elevated in the vessels that arise proximal to the coarctation; the blood pressure as well as pulse pressure below the constriction are lower. Hypertension is not due to the mechanical obstruction alone, but also involves renal mechanisms. Unless operated on in infancy, coarctation of the aorta usually results in the development of an extensive collateral circulation, chiefly from the branches of the subclavian, the superior intercostal, and the internal mammary arteries. The thoracic and subscapular branches of the axillary artery may also enlarge as collateral channels. These vessels unite with the intercostal branches of the descending aorta and inferior epigastric branches of the femoral artery to create channels for arterial blood to bypass the area of coarctation. The vessels contributing to the collateral circulation may become markedly enlarged and tortuous by early adulthood.

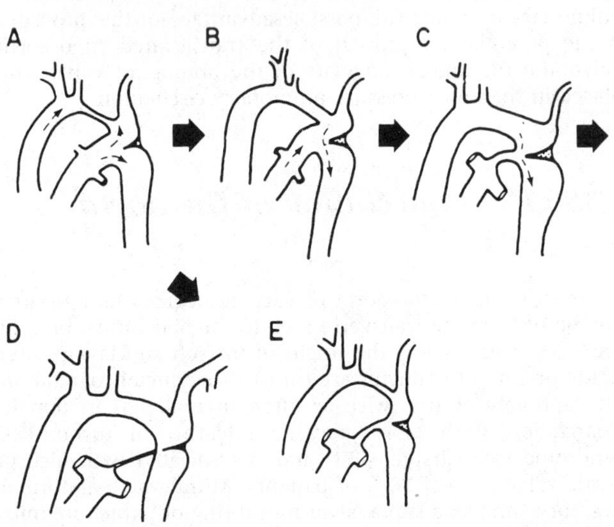

Figure 386–6. Metamorphosis of coarctation. *A,* Fetal prototype. No flow obstruction. *B,* Late gestation. The aortic ventricle increases the output and dilates the hypoplastic segment. Antegrade aortic flow bypasses the shell via a ductal orifice. *C,* Neonate. Ductal constriction initiates the obstruction by removing the bypass and by increasing antegrade arch flow. *D,* Mature juxtaductal stenosis. Bypass completely obliterated; intimal hypoplasia on the edge of the shell aggravates stenosis. Collaterals develop. *E,* Infantile-type fetal prototype persists. An intracardiac left-sided heart obstruction precludes an increase in antegrade aortic flow before or after birth. Both isthmal hypoplasia and contraductal shelf are present. Lower body flow often depends on patency of the ductus. (From Gersony WM: Coarctation of the aorta. *In:* Adams FH, Emmanouilides GC, Riemenschneider T [eds]: Moss Heart Disease in Infants, Children, and Adolescents, 4th ed. Copyright 1989, the Williams & Wilkins Co., Baltimore.)

CLINICAL MANIFESTATIONS. Coarctation of the aorta recognized after infancy rarely is associated with significant symptomatology. An occasional child will complain about weakness and/or pain in the legs after exercise, but in most instances even patients with severe coarctation will be asymptomatic. Older children are frequently brought to the cardiologist's attention when found to be hypertensive on a routine physical examination.

The classic sign of coarctation of the aorta is a disparity in pulsations and blood pressures of the arms and legs. The femoral, popliteal, posterior tibial, and dorsalis pedis pulses are weak (or absent in 40% of patients), in contrast to the bounding pulses of the arms and carotid vessels. The radial and femoral pulses should always be palpated simultaneously for the presence of a radial-femoral delay. Normally, the femoral pulse occurs slightly before the radial pulse. A radial-femoral delay occurs when blood flow to the descending aorta is dependent on collaterals; thus the femoral pulse will be felt after the radial pulse. In normal persons the systolic blood pressure in the legs obtained by the cuff method is 10–20 mm Hg higher than that in the arms. In coarctation of the aorta the blood pressure in the legs is lower than that in the arms; frequently, it is difficult to obtain. This differential in blood pressures is common in patients with coarctation over 1 yr of age, about 90% of whom have systolic hypertension in an upper extremity greater than the 95th percentile for age. It is very important to determine the blood pressure in each arm; a pressure higher in the right arm than the left suggests involvement of the left subclavian artery in the area of coarctation. Occasionally, the right subclavian may arise anomalously from below the area of coarctation, resulting in a left arm pressure higher than the right. With exercise, there is a more prominent rise of systemic blood pressure and the upper-to-lower extremity pressure gradient will increase.

The precordial impulse and heart sounds are usually normal; however, the presence of a systolic ejection click or thrill in the suprasternal notch suggests the presence of a bicuspid aortic valve. A short systolic murmur is often heard along the left sternal border at the 3rd and 4th intercostal spaces. The murmur is well transmitted to the left infrascapular area and occasionally to the neck. Often, the typical murmur of mild aortic stenosis can be heard in the 3rd right intercostal space. Occasionally more significant degrees of obstruction across the aortic valve will be present. The presence of a low-pitched mid-diastolic murmur at the apex suggests the presence of mitral valve stenosis. Among older patients with well-developed collateral blood flow, systolic or continuous murmurs may be heard over the left and right sides of the chest laterally and posteriorly. In these patients, a palpable thrill can occasionally be appreciated in the intercostal spaces on the back.

In contrast, neonates or infants with more severe coarctation, usually including some degree of transverse arch hypoplasia, will usually present with signs of lower body hypoperfusion, acidosis, and severe heart failure. This presentation may be delayed until after closure of the ductus arteriosus. If detected before ductal closure, patients may exhibit differential cyanosis, best demonstrated by simultaneous transcutaneous oximetry of upper and lower extremities. On physical examination, the heart is large, and there is a systolic murmur heard along the left sternal border with a loud 2nd heart sound.

DIAGNOSIS. The findings on *roentgenographic examination* depend on the age of the patient and on the effects of hypertension and collateral circulation. In infants with severe coarctation there is cardiac enlargement and pulmonary congestion. During childhood the findings are not striking until after the 1st decade, when the heart tends to be mildly or moderately enlarged because of left ventricular prominence. The enlarged left subclavian artery commonly produces a prominent shadow in the left superior mediastinum. Notching of the inferior border of the ribs from pressure erosion by enlarged collateral vessels is common by late childhood, except in the upper and lower two to three ribs. In most instances there is an area of poststenotic dilatation of the descending aorta. On a barium esophogram, this may be demonstrated by displacement of the esophagus and by discontinuity of the lateral margin of the aorta below the arch.

The *electrocardiogram* is usually normal in young children but reveals evidence of left ventricular hypertrophy in older patients. Neonates and young infants will display right or biventricular hypertrophy. Most often, the diagnosis can be made by a careful evaluation of the pulses in all major accessible peripheral arteries and by comparative blood pressure determinations in the arms and legs. The segment of coarctation can usually be visualized by two-dimensional *echocardiography;* associated anomalies of the mitral and aortic valve can also be demonstrated, if present. The descending aorta will be hypopulsatile. Color Doppler is useful for demonstrating the specific site of the obstruction. Pulsed and continuous-wave Doppler will determine the pressure gradient directly at the area of coarctation. However, in the presence of a patent ductus arteriosus, the pressure gradient may be underestimated. *Cardiac catheterization* with selective left ventriculography and aortography is useful in selected patients with additional anomalies and as a means of visualizing collateral blood flow. In cases well defined by echocardiography, diagnostic catheterization is usually not required.

PROGNOSIS AND COMPLICATIONS. Abnormalities of the aortic valve are present in most patients. Bicuspid aortic valves are common but usually do not produce clinical signs unless the stenosis is significant. The association of a PDA and coarctation of the aorta is also common. Ventricular and atrial septal defects may be suspected by signs of a left-to-right shunt. Mitral valve abnormalities are also occasionally seen, as is subvalvular aortic stenosis.

Severe neurologic damage or even death rarely may occur from associated cerebrovascular disease. Subarachnoid or intracerebral hemorrhage may result from rupture of congenital aneurysms in the circle of Willis, of other vessels with defective elastic and medial tissue, or of normal vessels; these accidents are secondary to the hypertensive state. Abnormalities of the subclavian arteries may include involvement of the left subclavian artery in the area of coarctation, stenosis of the orifice of the left subclavian artery, and anomalous origin of the right subclavian artery.

Untreated, the great majority of older patients with coarctation of the aorta would succumb between the ages of 20 and 40 yr; some live well into middle life without serious handicap. The common serious complications are related to the hypertensive state, which may result in premature coronary artery disease, congestive heart failure, hypertensive encephalopathy, or intracranial hemorrhage. Heart failure may be worsened by associated anomalies. Infective endocarditis or endarteritis is a significant complication in adults. Aneurysms of the descending aorta or of the enlarged collateral vessels are not unusual. In infants with severe coarctation, congestive heart failure, and hypoperfusion may be life threatening and require immediate medical intervention.

TREATMENT. In neonates with severe coarctation of the aorta, closure of the ductus often results in hypoperfusion, acidosis, and rapid deterioration. These patients should be started on an infusion of prostaglandin E_1 in an attempt to reopen the ductus and re-establish adequate lower extremity blood flow. Once a diagnosis has been confirmed and the patient stabilized hemodynamically, surgical repair should be performed. Older infants who present with congestive heart failure but who are not hypoperfused should be managed with anticongestive measures to improve their clinical status prior to surgical intervention.

Older children with significant coarctation of the aorta should be treated relatively soon after diagnosis. Delay is unwarranted, especially after the 2nd decade, when the operation may be less successful because of decreased left ventricular function and degenerative changes. Nevertheless, if cardiac reserve is sufficient, satisfactory repair is possible well into midadult life. Associated valvular lesions increase the hazards of late surgery.

The procedure of choice for isolated juxtaductal coarctation of the aorta is controversial. In many centers, operation is the procedure of choice, and several surgical techniques are used. The area of coarctation can be excised and a primary reanastomosis performed. Often the transverse aorta can be splayed open and a side-to-end anastamosis performed to increase the effective cross-sectional area of the repair. The subclavian flap procedure, which involves division of the left subclavian artery and its incorporation into the wall of the repaired coarctation, is used by some centers, often in the younger age group. Other centers favor a patch aortoplasty, in which the area of coarctation is enlarged with a roof of prosthetic material. Rarely, if the length of aortic constriction precludes primary anastomosis, a homograft or Dacron graft may be utilized.

After operation there is a striking increase in the amplitude of pulsations in the lower extremities. In the immediate postoperative course, "rebound" hypertension is common and usually requires medical management. This exaggerated hypertension gradually subsides and in most patients antihypertensive medications can be discontinued. Residual murmurs are common and may be due to associated cardiac anomalies, to a residual flow disturbance across the repaired area, or to collateral blood flow. Rare additional operative problems include spinal cord injury due to aortic cross-clamping if there are poorly developed collaterals, chylothorax, diaphragm injury, and laryngeal nerve injury. If a left subclavian flap is employed, the radial pulse and blood pressure in the left arm will be diminished or absent.

In some centers, balloon angioplasty has been used for treatment of "native" or unoperated coarctation. Early reports of results in these patients indicate good relief of the obstruction; however, several have reported the subsequent development of aortic aneurysms. Revised techniques have reduced the incidence of this complication, although the use of angioplasty in native coarctation remains controversial.

Repair of coarctation in the 2nd decade of life or beyond may be associated with a higher incidence of premature cardiovascular disease, even in the absence of residual cardiac abnormalities. There may be early onset of adult hypertension, which has occurred even in patients with adequately resected coarctation.

Although restenosis in older patients who had an adequate coarctectomy is extremely rare, a number of infants with end-to-end anastomoses carried out urgently in the 1st mo of life require revision later in childhood. Long-term follow-up is still incomplete; thus, all patients should be followed carefully for development of recoarctation. Should recoarctation occur, balloon angioplasty is the procedure of choice. In these patients, scar tissue from prior surgery makes reoperation more difficult yet makes balloon angioplasty safer because of the lower incidence of aneurysm formation. Relief of obstruction with this technique is usually excellent.

POSTCOARCTECTOMY SYNDROME. Postoperative mesenteric arteritis may be associated with hypertension and abdominal pain in the immediate postoperative period. The pain varies in severity and may be associated with anorexia, nausea, vomiting, leukocytosis, intestinal hemorrhage, bowel necrosis, and small bowel obstruction. Relief is usually obtained with antihypertensive drugs (nitroprusside, esmolol, captopril) and intestinal decompression; corticosteroids may help to alleviate the symptoms and thus avoid surgical exploration for bowel obstruction.

386.18 Coarctation with Ventricular Septal Defect

Coarctation in the presence of VSD results in both increased preload and afterload on the left ventricle, and patients with this combination of defects will present either at birth or in the 1st mo of life, often with intractable cardiac failure. The magnitude of the left-to-right shunt is dependent on the ratio of pulmonary to systemic vascular resistance. However, in the presence of a coarctation, the resistance to systemic outflow is elevated by the obstruction, markedly increasing the volume of the shunt. The clinical presentation is that of a seriously ill infant with tachypnea, failure to thrive, and typical findings of heart failure. Often there is not a marked difference in blood pressures between the upper and lower extremities because the cardiac output may be low. Although medical management may be helpful initially, early surgical repair is necessary.

In most cases coarctation is the major anomaly causing the severe symptoms, and resection of the coarcted segment will result in marked improvement. Some centers repair the coarctation through a left lateral thoracotomy and at the same time place a pulmonary artery band to decrease the ventricular level shunt. Some centers do not band the pulmonary artery initially, as a number of patients will improve sufficiently so that further surgery is not required during early infancy. However, if heart failure makes it difficult to manage these infants after surgery, open repair of the VSD is then performed. Other centers routinely repair both the VSD and coarctation at the same surgery through a midline sternotomy. When it is determined that a complicated VSD is present (multiple VSDs, apical muscular VSD), pulmonary arterial banding may be performed at the time of coarctation repair to avoid open heart surgery during infancy for these complex ventricular septal abnormalities.

386.19 Coarctation with Other Cardiac Anomalies

Coarctation often occurs in infancy associated with other major cardiovascular anomalies, including hypoplastic left heart, severe mitral or aortic valvular disease, transposition of the great arteries, and variations of double outlet or single ventricle. Severe coarctation may also be associated with endocardial fibroelastosis. The clinical manifestations depend on the effects of the associated malformations as well as the coarctation itself.

Coarctation of the aorta associated with severe mitral and aortic valve disease may have to be treated within the context of the hypoplastic left heart syndrome, even if the left ventricular chamber is not severely hypoplastic. Such patients usually have a long segment of narrow transverse aortic arch with or without an isolated coarctation at the site of the ductus arteriosus. Coarctation of the aorta with transposition of the great arteries or single ventricle may be repaired alone or in combination with other palliative measures.

386.20 Congenital Mitral Stenosis

This relatively rare anomaly can be isolated or associated with other defects, the most common being aortic stenosis and coarctation of the aorta. The mitral valve may be funnel-shaped, with thickened leaflets and chordae tendineae that are shortened and deformed. Other mitral valve anomalies associated with stenosis include parachute mitral valve due to a single papillary muscle and double-orifice mitral valve.

Symptoms usually appear within the first 2 yr. These infants are underdeveloped and usually have obvious dyspnea secondary to congestive heart failure; cyanosis and pallor are common. Some patients, whose symptoms are mainly wheezing, may have been followed with a diagnosis of reactive airway disease. Heart enlargement due to dilatation and hypertrophy of the right ventricle and left atrium is common. Most patients have rumbling diastolic murmurs followed by a loud 1st sound, but the auscultatory findings may be relatively obscure. The 2nd sound is loud and split. An opening snap of the mitral valve may be present. The *electrocardiogram* reveals right ventricular hypertrophy with normal, bifid, or spiked P waves. *Roentgenograms* usually show left atrial and right ventricular enlargement and pulmonary congestion. The *echocardiogram* is characteristic, showing thickened mitral valve leaflets, a diminished E-F slope on the M-mode mitral echogram, and an enlarged left atrium with a normal or small left ventricle. Two-dimensional echo examination shows a significant reduction of the mitral valve orifice in diastole. Doppler studies demonstrate a pressure gradient across the mitral orifice. At *cardiac catheterization* there is an increase in right ventricular, pulmonary arterial, and pulmonary capillary wedge pressures. Associated anomalies, such as aortic stenosis and coarctation, are demonstrated. *Angiocardiography* may show delayed emptying of the left atrium and the small mitral orifice.

The prognosis for untreated patients is poor; the majority of children succumb during the first 2 yr of life. The results of surgical treatment have been mixed; a mitral valve prosthesis is usually required, which will require replacement as the child grows. These patients must be anticoagulated with warfarin and complications of over- and under-anticoagulation are fairly common in infancy.

386.21 Pulmonary Venous Hypertension

A variety of lesions may result in chronic pulmonary venous hypertension, which when extreme may result in pulmonary arterial hypertension and right-sided heart failure. These lesions include congenital mitral stenosis, mitral insufficiency, total anomalous pulmonary venous return with obstruction, left atrial myxomas, cor triatriatum (stenosis of the common pulmonary vein), individual pulmonary venous stenosis, and supravalvular mitral ring or web. In these conditions, early symptoms can be confused with chronic pulmonary disease, as there may be no specific cardiac findings on physical examination. However, subtle signs of pulmonary hypertension may be present. The *electrocardiogram* shows right ventricular hypertrophy with spiked P waves. *Roentgenographic studies* reveal cardiac enlargement and prominence of the pulmonary veins in the hilar region, the right ventricle and atrium, and the main pulmonary artery; the left atrium is normal in size or only slightly enlarged.

The *echocardiogram* may demonstrate a left atrial myxoma, cor triatriatum, or a mitral valve abnormality. *Cardiac catheterization* excludes the presence of a shunt and demonstrates pulmonary hypertension with an elevated pulmonary arterial wedge pressure. The left atrial pressure is normal if the lesion is at the level of the pulmonary veins but is elevated if the lesion is at the level of the mitral valve. Selective pulmonary arteriography usually delineates the anatomic lesion. Cor triatriatum, left atrial myxoma, and supravalvular mitral webs can all be successfully managed surgically.

The differential diagnosis includes pulmonary veno-occlusive disease, an idiopathic process that produces obstructive lesions in the pulmonary veins of children and young adults. The etiology is uncertain. The patient is initially thought to have left-sided heart failure on the basis of congested lungs with apparent pulmonary edema. Dyspnea, fatigue, and pleural effusions are common; cyanosis, digital clubbing, syncope, and hemoptysis are variable findings. The left atrial pressure is normal, but the pulmonary arterial wedge pressure is usually elevated. However, a normal wedge pressure may be encountered because of the formation of collaterals or if the wedge recording is performed in an uninvolved segment. Angiographically, the pulmonary veins return normally to the left atrium, but one or more pulmonary veins are narrowed, either focally or diffusely.

Lung biopsy demonstrates pulmonary venous and, occasionally, arterial involvement. Pulmonary veins and venules demonstrate fibrous narrowing or occlusion, and there may be pulmonary artery thrombi. Therapy is nonspecific and disappointing, and survival ranges from weeks to months in infants and from months to years in adults. Attempts at surgical repair, balloon dilation, and transcatheter stenting have not significantly improved the prognosis of these patients. Combined heart-lung transplantation (see Chapter 402) remains the only moderately successful therapeutic option.

The Regurgitant Lesions

386.22 Pulmonary Valvular Insufficiency and Congenital Absence of the Pulmonary Valve

Pulmonary valvular insufficiency most often accompanies other cardiovascular diseases or may be secondary to severe pulmonary hypertension. Incompetence of the valve is an expected result after surgery for right ventricular outflow tract obstruction, for example, pulmonary valvotomy in patients with valvar pulmonic stenosis and valvotomy with infundibular resection in patients with tetralogy of Fallot. Isolated congenital insufficiency of the pulmonary valve is a rare anomaly. These patient are usually asymptomatic because the insufficiency is usually mild.

The prominent physical sign is a decrescendo diastolic murmur at the upper and mid left sternal border, which has a lower pitch than the murmur of aortic insufficiency due to the lower pressures involved. Roentgenograms of the chest show prominence of the main pulmonary artery and, if the insufficiency is severe, right ventricular enlargement. The electrocardiogram is normal or shows minimal right ventricular hypertrophy. Pulsed and color Doppler studies demonstrate retrograde flow from the pulmonary artery to the right ventricle during diastole. The diagnosis can be made at cardiac catheterization if necessary. There is a low pulmonary arterial diastolic pressure. Selective pulmonary arteriography shows the incompetent valve, but this is difficult to evaluate in mild cases because the catheter crossing the valve usually results in some iatrogenic insufficiency during the injection. Isolated pulmonary valvular incompetence is usually well tolerated and does not require surgical treatment. When pulmonary insufficiency is severe, especially if there is also significant tricuspid insufficiency, replacement with a homograft may become necessary to preserve right ventricular function.

Congenital absence of the pulmonary valve is usually associated with a VSD, often in the context of tetralogy of Fallot (see Chapter 387.2). In many of these neonates, the pulmonary arteries become widely dilated and compress the bronchi, causing recurrent episodes of wheezing, pulmonary collapse, and pneumonitis. The presence and degree of cyanosis is variable. Florid pulmonary valvular incompetence may not be well tolerated, and death may occur from a combination of bronchial compression, hypoxemia, and heart failure. Correction involves plication of the massively dilated pulmonary arteries along with intracardiac correction using a homograft.

386.23 Congenital Mitral Insufficiency

This anomaly may be isolated but is more often associated with other anomalies, including PDA, coarctation of the aorta, VSD, corrected transposition of the great vessels, anomalous origin of the left coronary artery from the pulmonary artery, endocardial fibroelastosis, or Marfan syndrome. Mitral insufficiency is common in patients with atrioventricular septal defects (see Chapter 386.5). Mitral insufficiency can also be seen with severe left ventricular dysfunction, secondary to dilatation of the valve ring.

In isolated mitral insufficiency, the mitral valve annulus is usually dilated, the chordae tendineae are short and may insert anomalously, and the valve leaflets are deformed. When mitral incompetence is clinically significant, the left atrium enlarges as a result of the regurgitant flow and the left ventricle becomes hypertrophied and dilated. Pulmonary venous pressure is increased and ultimately results in pulmonary hypertension and right ventricular hypertrophy and dilatation. Mild lesions produce no symptoms; the only abnormal sign is the holosystolic murmur of mitral incompetence. However, severe regurgitation results in symptoms that can appear at any age. These include poor physical development, frequent respiratory infections, fatigue on exertion, and episodes of pulmonary edema or congestive heart failure. Often these patients will have been followed with a diagnosis of reactive airway disease because of the similarity in pulmonary symptoms.

The typical high-pitched (often referred to as a "cooing dove") apical holosystolic murmur of mitral insufficiency is present, usually associated with an apical low-pitched, mid-diastolic rumbling murmur, indicating increased diastolic flow across the mitral valve. The pulmonary component of the 2nd heart sound is accentuated in the presence of pulmonary hypertension. The *electrocardiogram* usually shows bifid P waves, signs of left ventricular hypertrophy, and sometimes signs of right ventricular hypertrophy. *Roentgenographic examination* shows enlargement of the left atrium, which at times is massive. The left ventricle is prominent, and the pulmonary vascularity is normal or prominent. The *echocardiogram* demonstrates the enlarged left atrium and ventricle. Although motion of the mitral valve is excessive, with a steep E-F slope on M mode, this sign is not diagnostic. Color Doppler will demonstrate the extent of insufficiency, and pulsed Doppler of the pulmonary veins will detect retrograde flow when mitral insufficiency is severe. *Cardiac catheterization* shows an elevated left atrial pressure. Pulmonary artery hypertension of varying severity may be present. Selective left ventriculography reveals the severity of mitral regurgitation.

Mitral valvuloplasty can result in striking improvement in symptoms and heart size, but in some patients installation of a prosthetic mechanical mitral valve may be necessary. Prior to surgery, associated anomalies must be identified. In children beyond 3–4 yr, it may be difficult to exclude rheumatic fever as the cause of mitral insufficiency.

386.24 Mitral Valve Prolapse

This distinctive syndrome results from an abnormal mitral valve mechanism that causes billowing of one or both mitral leaflets, especially the posterior cusp, into the left atrium toward the end of systole. The abnormality is almost always congenital but may not be recognized until adolescence or adulthood. Mitral valve prolapse is more common in girls, may be inherited as an autosomal dominant trait with variable expression, and, thus, may affect siblings. It is common in patients with Marfan syndrome, straight back syndrome, pectus excavatum, and scoliosis. The dominant abnormal signs are auscultatory, although occasional patients may present with chest pain or palpitations. The apical murmur is late systolic and may be preceded by a click, but these signs vary in the same patient so that at times only the click is audible. In the standing or sitting position the click may appear earlier in systole and the murmur may be more prominent in late systole. Arrhythmias, primarily unifocal or multifocal premature ventricular contractions, may occur.

The *electrocardiogram* is usually normal but may show biphasic T waves, especially in leads II, III, AVF, and V_6; the T-wave abnormalities may vary at different times in the same patient. The *chest roentgenogram* is normal. The *echocardiogram* shows a characteristic posterior movement of the posterior mitral leaflet during mid or late systole, or pansystolic prolapse of both anterior and posterior mitral leaflets. These M-mode echocardiographic findings must be interpreted cautiously because the appearance of minimal mitral prolapse may be a normal variant. Two-dimensional real-time echocardiography shows that both the free edge and the body of the mitral leaflets move posteriorly in systole toward the left atrium. The presence and severity of mitral regurgitation can be assessed by Doppler echo.

This lesion is not progressive in childhood, and specific therapy is not indicated. The patient may be at risk to develop infective endocarditis. Antibiotic prophylaxis is recommended during surgery and dental procedures (see Table 386–1).

Adults (more often males than females) with mitral valve prolapse are at increased risk for cardiovascular complications (sudden death, arrhythmia, cerebrovascular accidents, progressive valve dilatation, heart failure, and endocarditis) in the presence of thickened and redundant mitral valve leaflets.

Often, confusion exists concerning the diagnosis of mitral valve prolapse. The high frequency of mild prolapse on the echocardiogram in the absence of clinical findings suggests that in these cases true "mitral valve prolapse syndrome" is not present. These patients and their parents should be reassured of this effect, and no special recommendations should be made regarding management or frequent laboratory studies. Otherwise, 15–20% of the general population would be labeled as having a significant, albeit mild, lesion. Endocarditis prophylaxis is indicated only in substantiated cases, usually those with mitral insufficiency.

386.25 Tricuspid Regurgitation

Isolated tricuspid regurgitation is usually associated with Ebstein anomaly of the tricuspid valve. Ebstein anomaly may present either without cyanosis or with varying degrees of cyanosis depending on the severity of the tricuspid regurgitation and the presence of an atrial level communication (patent foramen ovale or ASD). In general, older children tend to present with the acyanotic form, whereas, if detected in the newborn period, Ebstein anomaly is usually associated with severe cyanosis (see Chapter 387.8).

Tricuspid regurgitation often accompanies right ventricular dysfunction. When the right ventricle dilates due to volume overload and/or intrinsic myocardial disease, the tricuspid annulus also enlarges, resulting in valve insufficiency. This form of regurgitation may improve if the cause of the right ventricular dilatation is corrected, or it may require surgical plication of the valve annulus. Tricuspid regurgitation is also encountered in newborns with perinatal asphyxia. The etiology is thought to be related to an increased susceptibility of the papillary muscles to ischemic damage, leading to transient papillary muscle dysfunction.

Additional Congenital Heart Lesions

386.26 Anomalies of the Aortic Arch

RIGHT AORTIC ARCH. In this abnormality the aorta curves to the right, and, if it descends on the right side of the vertebral column, it is usually associated with other cardiac malformations. It is found in about 20% of cases of tetralogy of Fallot and is also common in truncus arteriosus. A right aortic arch without other cardiac anomalies is not associated with symptoms. It can often be visualized on roentgenograms. The trachea is deviated to the left of the midline rather than to the right, as in the presence of a normal left arch. On a barium esophogram, the esophagus is indented on its right border at the level of the aortic arch.

VASCULAR RINGS. Congenital abnormalities of the aortic arch and its major branches result in the formation of vascular rings around the trachea and esophagus with varying degrees of compression. The following are the more common anomalies: (1) double aortic arch (Figs. 386–7 and 386–8), (2) right aortic arch with left ligamentum arteriosum, (3) anomalous innominate artery arising further to the left on the arch than usual, (4) anomalous left carotid artery arising further to the right than usual and passing anterior to the trachea, and (5) anomalous left pulmonary artery (vascular sling). In the latter anomaly, the abnormal vessel arises from an elongated main pulmonary artery or from the right pulmonary artery. It courses between and compresses the trachea and esophagus. Associated congenital heart disease may be present in 5–50% of patients, depending on the vascular anomaly.

CLINICAL MANIFESTATIONS. If the vascular ring produces compression of the trachea and esophagus, symptoms are frequently present during infancy. Wheezing respirations tend to be chronic and are aggravated by crying, feeding, and flexion of

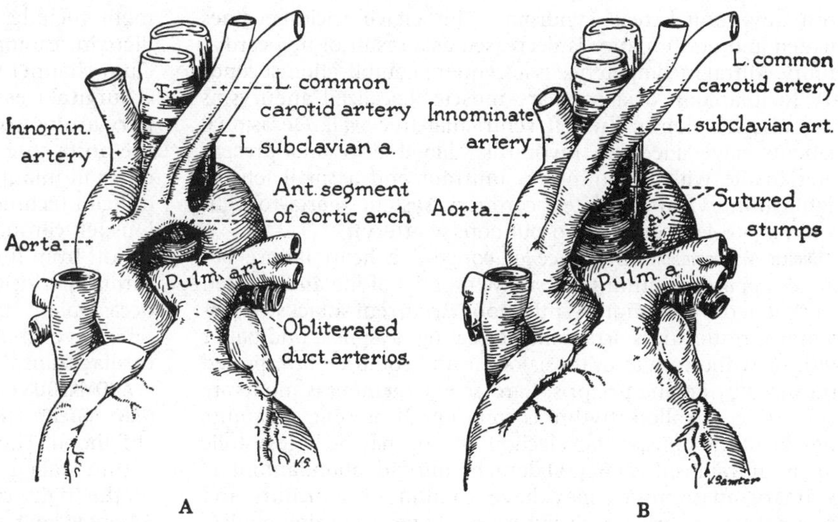

Figure 386–7. Double aortic arch. *A*, Small anterior segment of the double aortic arch (most common type). *B*, Operative procedure for the release of the vascular ring.

the neck. Extension of the neck tends to relieve the noisy respiration. Vomiting is frequent. There may be a brassy cough, and pneumonia is common. Sudden death from aspiration is a threat. Roentgenographic examination of the barium-filled esophagus and aortography identify the anomaly (see Fig. 386–8). An aberrant right subclavian artery is commonly seen but does not cause compression of the trachea. Diagnosis is confirmed by two-dimensional echocardiography, MRI, or angiography during cardiac catheterization. Bronchoscopy may be used to determine the extent of airway narrowing.

TREATMENT. Surgery is advised for symptomatic patients who have roentgenographic evidence of tracheal compression. The anterior vessel is usually divided in patients with double aortic arch (see Fig. 386–7). Compression produced by a right aortic arch and left ligamentum arteriosum is relieved by division of the latter. Anomalous innominate or carotid arteries cannot be divided; the tracheal compression is usually relieved by attaching the adventitia of these vessels to the sternum. An anomalous left pulmonary artery is corrected during cardiopulmonary bypass by division at its origin and reanastomosis to the main pulmonary artery after it has been brought in front of the trachea. In this condition, severe tracheomalacia may be present and may require reconstruction of the trachea as well.

386.27 Anomalous Origin of the Coronary Arteries

ANOMALOUS ORIGIN OF THE LEFT CORONARY ARTERY FROM THE PULMONARY ARTERY. In this anomaly the blood supply to the left ventricular myocardium is severely compromised. Soon after birth, as the pulmonary arterial pressure falls, the perfusion pressure to the left coronary artery becomes inadequate; myocardial infarction and fibrosis may result. In some cases, interarterial collateral anastomoses develop between the right and left coronary arteries. Blood flow in the left coronary artery is then reversed, and it empties into the pulmonary artery, resulting

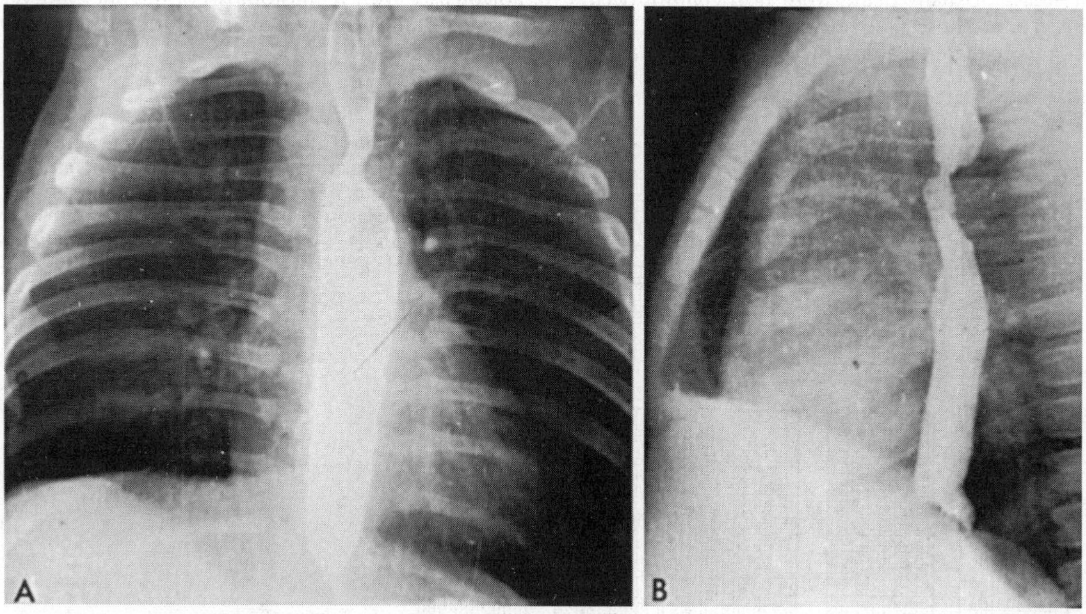

Figure 386–8. Double aortic arch in an infant aged 5 mo. *A*, Anteroposterior view. The barium-filled esophagus is constricted on both sides. *B*, Lateral view. The esophagus is displaced forward. The anterior arch was the smaller and was divided at operation.

in a "myocardial steal" syndrome. The left ventricle becomes dilated and performance is decreased as a result of myocardial injury. Mitral incompetence is a frequent complication secondary to infarction of a papillary muscle. Localized aneurysms may also develop in the left ventricular free wall. Occasional patients have adequate myocardial blood flow and present later in life with a continuous murmur and a small left-to-right shunt via the dilated coronary system (aorta-to-right coronary-to-left coronary-to-pulmonary artery).

Clinical Manifestations. Evidence of congestive heart failure becomes apparent within the 1st few months of life and is often precipitated by respiratory infection. Recurrent attacks of discomfort, restlessness, irritability, sweating, dyspnea, and pallor with or without mild cyanosis occur and could be interpreted as caused by angina pectoris. Cardiac enlargement is moderate to massive. A gallop rhythm is common. If present, murmurs may be of the nonspecific, ejection type or may be holosystolic due to mitral insufficiency. Older patients with abundant intercoronary anastomoses may have continuous murmurs and minimal left ventricular dysfunction. However, during adolescence they may present with angina during exercise. Rare cases with anomalous right coronary artery may present in this manner.

Diagnosis. *Roentgenographic examination* confirms the cardiomegaly, but the contour is not specific unless there is a complicating ventricular aneurysm. The *electrocardiogram* resembles the pattern described in lateral wall myocardial infarction in adults. A QR pattern followed by inverted T waves is seen in leads I and aVL. The left ventricular surface leads (V_5 and V_6) may also show deep Q waves and exhibit elevated ST segments and inverted T waves (Fig. 386–9). In older patients, exercise study is helpful, as ST-T–wave changes or symptoms, or both, occur. *Two-dimensional echocardiography* may suggest the diagnosis, especially with the help of color Doppler, but is not always reliable. *Cardiac catheterization and aortography* are diagnostic; there is immediate opacification of only the right coronary artery. Generally, this vessel is large and tortuous. After filling of the intercoronary anastomoses, the left coronary artery is opacified and contrast can be seen to enter the pulmonary artery. Selective pulmonary arteriography may also opacify the origin of the anomalous left coronary artery. Selective left ventriculography usually demonstrates a dilated left ventricle that empties poorly.

Treatment and Prognosis. Usually death from heart failure occurs within the first 6 mo. Those who survive usually have abundant intercoronary collateral anastomoses. Medical management includes standard therapy for heart failure (diuretics, digoxin, captopril) and for controlling ischemia (nitrates, calcium channel blockers, beta-blocking agents).

Surgical treatment consists of detaching the anomalous coronary artery from the pulmonary artery and anastomosing it to the aorta to establish normal myocardial perfusion. The seriously ill infant with a tiny left coronary artery may present a difficult technical problem. In past years ligation of the anomalous left coronary artery at its origin was carried out to prevent runoff from the coronary circuit and possibly to increase myocardial perfusion by the collateral circulation. This operation occasionally may still be required in some cases. In patients who have already sustained a significant myocardial infarction, cardiac transplantation is the only surgical option.

ANOMALOUS ORIGIN OF THE RIGHT CORONARY ARTERY FROM THE PULMONARY ARTERY. This anomaly rarely manifests in infancy or early childhood. The left coronary artery is enlarged while the right is thin walled and mildly enlarged. In early infancy perfusion of the right coronary artery is from the pulmonary artery, whereas later, perfusion is from collaterals of the left coronary vessels. Angina and sudden death can occur in adolescence or adulthood. When recognized, this anomaly should be repaired by reanastomosis of the right coronary artery to the aorta.

ECTOPIC ORIGIN OF THE CORONARY ARTERY FROM THE AORTA WITH ABERRANT PROXIMAL COURSE. The aberrant artery may be a left, right, or major branch coronary artery. The site of origin may be the wrong sinus of Valsalva or a proximal coronary artery. The ostium may be hypoplastic, slitlike, or of normal caliber. The aberrant vessel may pass anteriorly, posteriorly, or between the aorta and right ventricular outflow tract; it may tunnel in the conal or interventricular septal tissue. Obstruction due to hypoplasia of the ostia, tunneling between the aorta and right ventricular outflow tract or interventricular septum, and acute angulation produce focal myocardial fibrosis or myocardial infarction. Unobstructive vessels produce no symptoms. Patients with this extremely rare abnormality may manifest myocardial infarction, ventricular arrhythmias, sudden death in young adult or adolescent athletes, angina pectoris, and syncope.

Diagnostic evaluation should include an electrocardiogram, stress testing, two-dimensional echocardiography, and cardiac catheterization with selective coronary angiography.

Treatment is indicated for obstructed vessels and includes aortoplasty with reanastomosis of the aberrant vessel or, more often, coronary artery bypass grafting using the internal mammary artery.

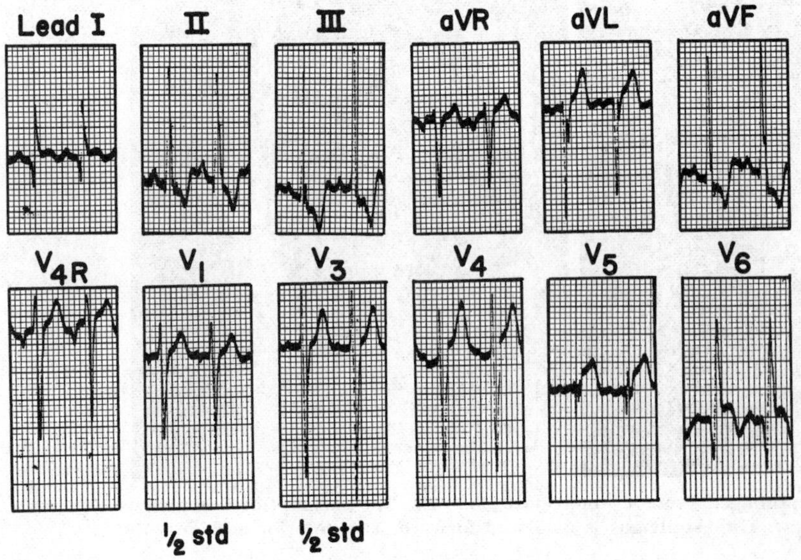

Figure 386–9. Electrocardiogram of a 3-mo-old child with anomalous origin of the left coronary artery from the pulmonary artery. Lateral myocardial infarction is present as evidenced by abnormally large and wide Q waves in leads I, V_5, and V_6, elevated ST segment in V_5 and V_6, and inversion of TV_6.

386.28 Pulmonary Vascular Disease (Eisenmenger Syndrome)

PATHOPHYSIOLOGY. The term *Eisenmenger syndrome* refers to those patients with a VSD whose shunts have become partially or totally right to left as a result of the development of pulmonary vascular disease. This physiologic abnormality also can occur with ASD, AV septal defect, PDA, or with any other communication between the aorta and pulmonary artery. However, pulmonary vascular disease with isolated ASD is rare and does not occur until late in adulthood.

In normal neonates, within a few weeks of life the structure of the pulmonary arterioles changes to that of the adult with a thin wall and a large lumen, and the pulmonary vascular resistance falls to normal adult levels. In Eisenmenger syndrome, the pulmonary vascular resistance either remains high or, after having decreased during early infancy, rises thereafter because of increased shear stress on pulmonary arterioles. This phenomenon is primarily the result of prolonged elevation of pulmonary pressure and results in severe obliterative intimal lesions in these vessels. Factors playing a role in the rapidity of development of pulmonary vascular disease include increased pulmonary arterial pressure, increased pulmonary blood flow, and the presence of hypoxia or hypercarbia. Early in the course of disease in most of these patients, pulmonary hypertension (elevated pressure in the pulmonary arteries) is the result of markedly increased pulmonary blood flow (hyperkinetic pulmonary hypertension). This form of pulmonary hypertension decreases with pulmonary vasodilators and/or oxygen. In contrast, with the development of Eisenmenger syndrome, pulmonary hypertension is the result of pulmonary vascular disease (obstructive pathologic changes in the pulmonary vessels). This form of pulmonary hypertension is usually only minimally or not at all responsive to pulmonary vasodilators or oxygen.

PATHOLOGY AND PATHOPHYSIOLOGY. The pathologic changes of Eisenmenger syndrome occur in the small pulmonary arterioles and muscular arteries (<300 μm) and are graded based on histology (Heath-Edwards classification): Type 1 changes involve medial thickening alone, type 2 changes consist of medial and intimal thickening, and type 3 includes both plus plexiform lesions secondary to hypoplasia of the medial layer of small muscular arteries. Medial hypoplasia predisposes the arteries to aneurysmal dilatation associated with severe pulmonary arterial hypertension. Plexiform lesions indicate severe, irreversible pulmonary vascular obstructive disease. Eisenmenger physiology is defined by an absolute elevation of pulmonary arterial resistance to >12 Wood units (resistance units indexed to body surface area) or by a ratio of pulmonary to systemic vascular resistance ≥ 1.0.

Pulmonary vascular disease occurs more rapidly in patients with trisomy 21 who have left-to-right shunts. It also significantly complicates the natural history of those patients with elevated pulmonary venous pressure due to mitral stenosis or left ventricular dysfunction, any patient with transmission of systemic pressure to the pulmonary circulation via an intraventricular or great vessel level shunt, and those patients chronically exposed to low Po_2 (high altitude). Patients with cyanotic congenital heart lesions associated with unrestricted pulmonary blood flow are at particular risk.

CLINICAL MANIFESTATIONS. Symptoms usually do not occur until the 2nd or 3rd decade of life, although a more fulminant course may occur. Many patients survive for decades with minimal symptoms. Irreversible pulmonary vascular obstruction results in high pulmonary vascular resistance. Intracardiac or extracardiac communications that normally would shunt left to right develop right-to-left shunting as pulmonary vascular resistance exceeds systemic vascular resistance. Cyanosis becomes apparent, and dyspnea, fatigue, and a tendency toward dysrhythmias begin to occur. In the late stages of the disease, heart failure, chest pain, headaches, syncope, and hemoptysis may be seen. Physical examination reveals a right ventricular heave and a narrowly split 2nd heart sound with a loud pulmonic component. A palpable pulmonary artery pulsation may be present at the left upper sternal border. A soft systolic ejection murmur or a holosystolic murmur of tricuspid regurgitation may be audible along the left sternal border. An early decrescendo diastolic murmur of pulmonary insufficiency may also be heard along the left sternal border. The degree of cyanosis depends on the stage of the disease.

DIAGNOSIS. Cyanotic patients will have various degrees of polycythemia depending on the severity and duration of hypoxia. *Roentgenographically,* the heart varies in size from normal to greatly enlarged; the latter occurs usually late in the course of the disease. The main pulmonary artery is usually very prominent (Fig. 386–10). The pulmonary vessels are enlarged in the hilar areas and taper rapidly in caliber in the peripheral branches. The right ventricle and atrium are prominent. The *electrocardiogram* shows marked right ventricular hypertrophy. The P wave may be tall and spiked.

The *echocardiogram* shows a thick-walled right ventricle and will demonstrate the underlying congenital heart lesion. Two-dimensional echo will assist in eliminating from consideration lesions such as obstructed pulmonary veins, supramitral membrane, or mitral stenosis. By M-mode echocardiogram, the right-sided systolic time interval shows a significant increase in the ratio of the pre-ejection period to ejection time because of the increased pulmonary vascular resistance. The pulmonary valve echo will show a characteristic early midsystolic closure, the "W sign." Doppler studies will demonstrate the direction of the shunt and the presence of a typical hypertension wave form in the main pulmonary artery. If present, tricuspid regurgitation can be used in the Doppler examination to estimate the pulmonary arterial pressure. Pulmonary regurgitation can also be semi-quantified.

Cardiac catheterization usually shows a bidirectional shunt at

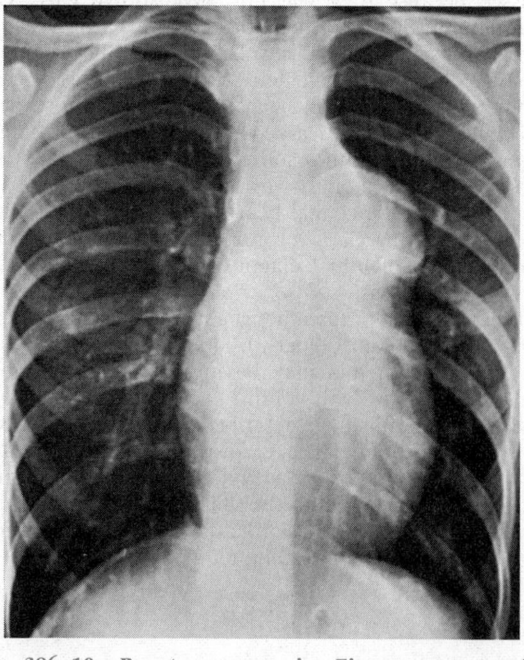

Figure 386–10. Roentgenogram in Eisenmenger syndrome caused by a patent ductus arteriosus. The heart size is normal, the pulmonary artery segment is dilated, and the pulmonary vascularity is normal or slightly increased.

■ TABLE 386–2 Extracardiac Complications of Cyanotic Congenital Heart Disease and Eisenmenger Physiology

Problem	Etiology	Therapy
Polycythemia	Persistent hypoxia	Phlebotomy
Relative anemia	Nutritional deficiency	Iron replacement
CNS abscess	Right-to-left shunting	Antibiotics, drainage
CNS thromboembolic stroke	Right-to-left shunting or polycythemia	Phlebotomy
Low-grade DIC, thrombocytopenia	Polycythemia	None for DIC unless bleeding, then phlebotomy
Hemoptysis	Pulmonary infarct, thrombosis, or rupture of pulmonary artery plexiform lesion	Embolization
Gum disease	Polycythemia, gingivitis, bleeding	Dental hygiene
Gout	Polycythemia, diuretic agent	Allopurinol
Arthritis, clubbing	Hypoxic arthropathy	None
Pregnancy complications: abortion, fetal growth retardation, prematurity, maternal illness	Poor placental perfusion, poor ability to increase cardiac output	Bed rest, pregnancy prevention counseling
Infections	Associated asplenia, DiGeorge syndrome, endocarditis	Antibiotics
	Fatal RSV pneumonia with pulmonary hypertension	Ribavirin
Failure to thrive	Increased oxygen consumption, decreased nutrient intake	Treat heart failure; correct defect early, increased caloric intake
Psychosocial adjustment	Limited activity, cyanotic appearance, chronic disease, multiple hospitalizations	Counseling

CNS = central nervous system; DIC = disseminated intravascular coagulation; RSV = respiratory syncytial virus.

the site of the defect. The systolic pressures are usually equal in the systemic and pulmonary circulations. The pulmonary capillary wedge pressure will be normal unless a left-heart obstructive lesion or left ventricular failure is the etiology for the pulmonary artery hypertension. The arterial oxygen saturation is decreased, reflecting the magnitude of the right-to-left shunt. Response to vasodilator therapy (oxygen, nitroprusside, prostaglandins) may identify patients with hyperdynamic pulmonary hypertension. Selective angiocardiography can locate the site of the shunt, but these studies are usually avoided in these patients because of increased risk and the accuracy of modern echocardiography. Selective pulmonary artery injections may be necessary if pulmonary venous obstruction is suspected because of a high wedge pressure.

TREATMENT. The best management of patients who are at risk of developing late pulmonary vascular disease is prevention by surgical elimination of large intracardiac or great vessel communications during infancy. However, some patients may be missed because they will not have shown early clinical manifestations. Some of these infants never decrease their pulmonary vascular resistance substantially at birth and therefore never develop enough left-to-right shunting to become clinically apparent. This is a particular risk in those patients with congenital heart disease who live at high altitude. It is also a risk in infants with trisomy 21, who are at risk of earlier development of pulmonary vascular disease. Because of the high incidence of congenital heart disease associated with trisomy 21, some physicians recommend routine echocardiography at the time of initial diagnosis, even in the absence of other clinical findings.

Medical treatment of Eisenmenger syndrome is entirely symptomatic (Table 386–2). Older children and adolescents with significant polycythemia may be improved by cautious, repeated phlebotomies with volume replacement. Several small clinical trials in adults have described short-term benefits from chronic calcium channel blocker, prostaglandin, or prostacyclin therapy; however, there is as yet no significant experience with the use of these agents in children. Combined heart-lung or bilateral lung transplantation is the only surgical option for many of these patients (see Chapter 402).

CHAPTER 387
Cyanotic Congenital Heart Disease

387.1 Evaluation of the Critically Ill Neonate with Cyanosis and Respiratory Distress (also see Chapter 83)

The severely ill neonate with a combination of cardiorespiratory distress and cyanosis presents a diagnostic challenge. The clinician must perform a rapid, systematic evaluation to determine whether congenital heart disease is a potential etiology, so that potentially life-saving measures can be instituted. Because of the decreased ventilatory reserve of the neonate, the likelihood of developing acidosis is high, and these patients are at particular risk for progressing rapidly to circulatory collapse. The differential diagnosis of cyanosis in the newborn period includes the following entities.

CARDIAC DISEASE. Congenital heart disease is responsible for cyanosis when obstruction to right ventricular outflow causes intracardiac right-to-left shunting or when complex anatomic defects, unassociated with pulmonary stenosis, cause admixture of pulmonary and systemic venous return in the heart. Cyanosis from pulmonary edema may also develop in patients with heart failure due to left-to-right shunts, although the degree is usually less severe. In addition, cyanosis may be caused by persistence of fetal pathways, for example, right-to-left shunting across the foramen ovale and ductus arteriosus in the presence of pulmonary outflow tract obstruction or persistent pulmonary hypertension of the newborn (see Chapter 87.7).

CENTRAL NERVOUS SYSTEM DISEASE. Irregular shallow breathing, secondary to central nervous system (CNS) depression, results in reduced alveolar ventilation, an abnormally low alveolar oxygen tension, and elevated P_{CO_2}. Intracranial hemorrhage accounts for most cases of this type of cyanosis; drug administration is another cause.

PULMONARY DISEASE. Intrapulmonary diseases, such as hyaline membrane disease, atelectasis, and pneumonitis, cause inflammation, collapse, and fluid accumulation in alveoli, resulting in incompletely oxygenated blood returning via the pulmonary veins to the systemic circulation. These pulmonary diseases may also increase right-sided pressures, worsening the degree of cyanosis due to right-to-left shunting at the ductal or foramen ovale level. Upper airway obstructions may also result in cyanosis owing to reduced pulmonary ventilation.

HEMOGLOBINOPATHIES. Methemoglobinemia (see Chapter 419.7) is a rare cause of cyanosis, resulting in arterial desaturation because of a decrease in the oxygen binding capacity of hemoglobin. Unlike the other causes of cyanosis, in methemoglobinemia the arterial Po_2 is normal.

DIFFERENTIAL DIAGNOSIS. Successful initial evaluation of the cyanotic infant begins with careful observation of the infant's breathing pattern. Weak or irregular respiration is often associated with a weak sucking reflex and a CNS problem. Convulsions and general depression strongly also suggest a CNS etiology. The infant with primary cardiac or pulmonary disease, on the other hand, displays vigorous or labored respirations with tachypnea. The differential diagnosis between pulmonary and cardiac cyanosis may be difficult, especially within the 1st days of life.

The *hyperoxia test* is one method of distinguishing cyanotic congenital heart disease from pulmonary disease. Neonates with congenital heart disease will usually not raise their arterial Pao_2 significantly during administration of 100% oxygen. If the Pao_2 rises above 150 mm Hg during 100% oxygen administration, an intracardiac shunt can usually be excluded, although some patients with cyanotic congenital heart lesions may be able to transiently increase their Pao_2 above 150 mm Hg because of intracardiac streaming patterns. In contrast, patients with pulmonary disease will generally increase their Pao_2 significantly as ventilation-perfusion inequalities, but not intracardiac shunts, are overcome by oxygen administration. Infants with only a CNS disorder will completely normalize their Pao_2 during artificial ventilation.

Although a significant heart murmur usually suggests a cardiac basis for cyanosis, several of the more severe cardiac defects, for example, simple transposition of the great vessels, may not be associated with a murmur. The chest roentgenogram may be helpful in the differentiation of pulmonary from cardiac disease and, in the latter, will indicate whether pulmonary blood flow is increased, normal, or decreased. This distinction is important in the differentiation of the various congenital heart lesions that cause cyanosis in the neonate.

Two-dimensional echocardiography has become the definitive noninvasive test to determine whether congenital heart disease is present. The information obtained by this technique is essential in avoiding unnecessary cardiac catheterization and angiography in the absence of a cardiac defect as well as in making a specific diagnosis when congenital heart disease is present. If echocardiography is not immediately available, the clinician caring for a cyanotic newborn should not hesitate to start a prostaglandin infusion (for a possible ductal dependent lesion) if cyanotic heart disease is suspected on clinical grounds alone. However, because of the risk of hypoventilation associated with prostaglandin use, a practitioner skilled in neonatal endotracheal intubation should always be readily available.

Cyanotic Lesions Associated with Decreased Pulmonary Blood Flow

387.2 Tetralogy of Fallot

Tetralogy of Fallot classically consists of the combination of (1) obstruction to right ventricular outflow (pulmonary stenosis), (2) ventricular septal defect (VSD), (3) dextroposition of the aorta with septal override, and (4) right ventricular hypertrophy. Obstruction to pulmonary arterial blood flow is usually at both the right ventricular infundibulum (subpulmonic area) and pulmonary valve. The main pulmonary artery is often smaller than usual, and there may be various degrees of branch pulmonary artery stenoses as well. Complete obstruction of right ventricular outflow (pulmonary atresia) with VSD is also classified as an extreme form of tetralogy of Fallot.

PATHOPHYSIOLOGY. The pulmonary valve annulus may be of nearly normal size or may be quite small. The valve itself is often bicuspid and, occasionally, is the only site of stenosis. More commonly, there is hypertrophy of the subpulmonic muscle, the crista supraventricularis, which contributes to the infundibular stenosis and results in an infundibular chamber of variable size and contour. When the right ventricular outflow tract is completely obstructed (pulmonary atresia), the anatomy of the branch pulmonary arteries is extremely variable; there may be a main pulmonary artery segment in continuity with the right ventricular outflow, separated by a fibrous but imperforate pulmonary valve, or the entire main pulmonary artery segment may be absent. Occasionally the branch pulmonary arteries may be discontinuous. In these more severe cases, pulmonary blood flow may be supplied by a patent ductus arteriosus (PDA) and by major aortopulmonary collateral arteries (MAPCAs) arising from the aorta.

The VSD is usually nonrestrictive and large, located just below the aortic valve, and related to the posterior and right aortic cusps. Rarely the VSD may be in the inlet portion of the ventricular septum (atrioventricular septal defect variety). The normal fibrous continuity of the mitral and aortic valves is usually maintained. The aortic arch is right sided in about 20% of instances; the aortic root is almost always large and overrides the VSD to a varying degree. When the aorta over-rides more than 50%, and if there is a significant muscular separation between the aortic valve and the mitral annulus (subaortic conus), this defect is usually classified as a form of double-outlet right ventricle; however, the pathophysiology is the same as tetralogy of Fallot.

Systemic venous return to the right atrium and right ventricle is normal. When the right ventricle contracts in the presence of marked pulmonary stenosis, blood is shunted across the VSD into the aorta. Persistent arterial desaturation and cyanosis result. The pulmonary blood flow, when severely restricted by the obstruction to right ventricular outflow, may be supplemented by the bronchial collateral circulation (MAPCAs) and, especially in the immediate newborn period, by a PDA. The peak systolic and diastolic pressures in each ventricle are similar, and at a systemic level a large pressure gradient occurs across the obstructed right ventricular outflow tract, and the pulmonary arterial pressure is usually lower than normal. The degree of right ventricular outflow obstruction determines the timing of onset of symptoms, the severity of cyanosis, and the degree of right ventricular hypertrophy. When obstruction to right ventricular outflow is mild to moderate and there is a balanced shunt across the VSD, the patient may not be visibly cyanotic (acyanotic or "pink" tetralogy of Fallot).

CLINICAL MANIFESTATIONS. Infants with mild degrees of right ventricular outflow obstruction may initially present with congestive heart failure caused by a ventricular level left-to-right shunt. Often cyanosis is not present at birth, but with increasing hypertrophy of the right ventricular infundibulum and growth, cyanosis occurs later in the 1st yr of life. It is most prominent in the mucous membranes of the lips and mouth, and in the fingernails and toenails. In infants with severe degrees of right ventricular obstruction, cyanosis is noted immediately in the neonatal period. In these infants pulmonary blood flow may be dependent on flow through the ductus arteriosus. When the ductus begins to close in the 1st few hours or days of life, severe cyanosis and circulatory collapse may occur. Older children with long-standing cyanosis may have extreme cyanosis, with a dusky blue skin surface, gray sclerae with engorged blood vessels (suggesting mild conjunctivitis), and clubbing of the fingers and toes. The extracardiac manifestations of long-standing cyanotic congenital heart disease are described in Table 386–2.

Dyspnea occurs on exertion. Infants and toddlers will play actively for a short time and then sit or lie down. Older children may be able to walk a block or so before stopping to rest. Characteristically, children assume a squatting position for the relief of dyspnea due to physical effort; the child is usually able to resume physical activity within a few minutes. These findings occur most often in patients with significant cyanosis at rest.

Paroxysmal hypercyanotic attacks (*hypoxic, "blue," or "tet" spells*) are a particular problem during the first 2 yr of life. The infant becomes hyperpneic and restless, cyanosis increases, gasping respirations ensue, and syncope may follow. The spell occurs most frequently in the morning upon first awakening or following episodes of vigorous crying. Temporary disappearance or decrease in intensity of the systolic murmur is usual as flow across the right ventricular outflow tract diminishes. The spells may last from a few minutes to a few hours but are rarely fatal. Short episodes are followed by generalized weakness and sleep. Severe spells may progress to unconsciousness and, occasionally, to convulsions or hemiparesis. The onset is usually spontaneous and unpredictable. Spells are associated with a reduction of an already compromised pulmonary blood flow, which when prolonged results in severe systemic hypoxia and metabolic acidosis. Infants who are only mildly cyanotic at rest are often more prone to develop hypoxic spells because they have not developed the homeostatic mechanisms to tolerate rapid lowering of arterial oxygen saturation, for example, polycythemia.

Depending on the frequency and severity of hypercyanotic attacks, one or more of the following procedures should be instituted in sequence: (1) placement of the infant on the abdomen in the knee-chest position, making certain that there is no constricting clothing; (2) administration of oxygen; and (3) injection of morphine subcutaneously in a dose not in excess of 0.2 mg/kg. Calming the infant, while holding the child in a knee-chest position, may abort progression of an early spell. Premature attempts to obtain blood tests may cause further agitation and be counterproductive.

Since metabolic acidosis develops when the arterial Po_2 is below 40 mm Hg, rapid correction (within several minutes) with intravenous administration of sodium bicarbonate is necessary if the spell is unusually severe and there is lack of response to the foregoing therapy. Recovery from the spell is usually rapid once the pH has returned to normal. Repeated blood pH measurements may be necessary because rapid recurrence of acidosis may occur. β-Adrenergic blockade by intravenous administration of propranolol (0.1 to a maximum of 0.2 mg/kg) has been used successfully in some patients with severe spells, especially spells accompanied by tachycardia. Drugs that increase systemic vascular resistance, such as intravenous methoxamine or phenylephrine, will improve right ventricular outflow, decrease the right-to-left shunt, and thus improve the symptoms, but their use has been limited and should not be allowed to delay needed surgery.

Growth and development may be delayed in patients with severe untreated tetralogy of Fallot. Stature and nutritional status are usually below average for age. Puberty is delayed in unoperated patients.

The pulse is usually normal, as are the venous and arterial pressures. The left anterior hemithorax may bulge anteriorly due to right ventricular hypertrophy. The heart is usually normal in size, and there is a *substernal right ventricular impulse*. In 50% of cases a *systolic thrill* is felt along the left sternal border in the 3rd and 4th parasternal spaces. The *systolic murmur* is frequently loud and harsh; it may be transmitted widely, especially to the lungs, but is most intense at the left sternal border. The murmur may be either ejection or holosystolic and may be preceded by a click. The murmur is caused by turbulence through the right ventricular outflow tract. It tends to become louder, longer, and harsher as the severity of pulmonary stenosis increases from mild to moderate; however, it can actually become less prominent with severe obstruction, especially during a hypercyanotic spell. The 2nd heart sound is either single or the pulmonic component is soft. Infrequently a continuous murmur may be audible.

DIAGNOSIS. *Roentgenographically,* the typical configuration as seen in the anteroposterior view consists of a narrow base, concavity of the left heart border in the area usually occupied by the pulmonary artery, and normal heart size. The hypertrophied right ventricle causes the rounded apical shadow to be uptilted so that it is situated higher above the diaphragm than normal. The cardiac silhouette has been likened to that of a boot or wooden shoe (**coeur en sabot**) (Fig. 387–1). The hilar areas and lung fields are relatively clear, because of diminished pulmonary blood flow and/or the small size of the pulmonary arteries. The aorta is usually large, and in about 20% of instances the aorta arches to the right instead of to the left; this results in an indentation of the leftward-positioned air-filled tracheobronchial shadow in the anteroposterior view or may be confirmed by displacement of the barium-filled esophagus to the left.

The *electrocardiogram* demonstrates right axis deviation and evidence of right ventricular hypertrophy. The latter is found in the right precordial chest leads, where the configuration of the QRS complex is Rs, R, qR, qRs, or rsR′ and the T wave may be positive. The P wave is tall and peaked, or sometimes bifid (see Fig. 381–6).

Two-dimensional echocardiography establishes the diagnosis (Fig. 387–2) and provides information as to the extent of aortic over-ride of the septum, the location and degree of the right ventricular outflow tract obstruction, the size of the proximal branch pulmonary arteries, and the side of the aortic arch. The echo is also useful in determining whether a patent ductus arteriosus is supplying a portion of the pulmonary blood flow. It may obviate the need for catheterization.

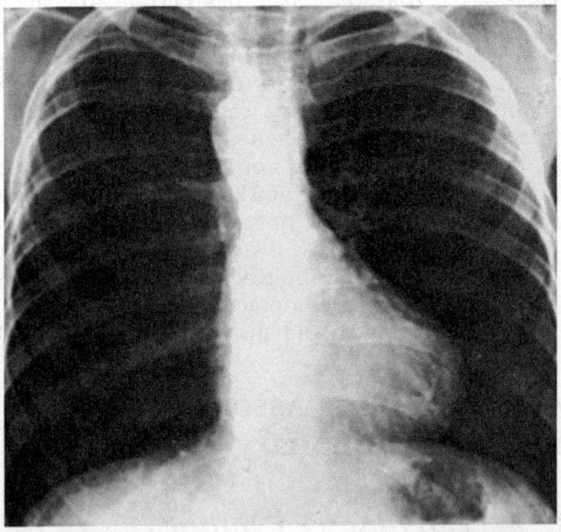

Figure 387–1. Roentgenogram of an 8-yr-old boy with tetralogy of Fallot. Note the normal heart size, some elevation of the cardiac apex, concavity in the region of the main pulmonary artery, right aortic arch, and diminished pulmonary vascularity.

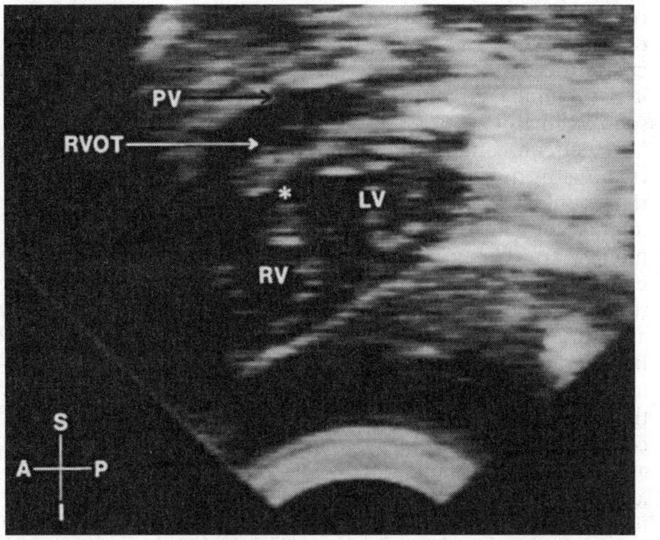

Figure 387–2. Tetralogy of Fallot. This short axis subxiphoid two-dimensional echocardiographic projection demonstrates the anterior/superior displacement of the outflow ventricular septum resulting in stenosis of the subpulmonic right ventricular outflow tract and associated anterior ventricular septal defect. LV = left ventricle; PV = pulmonary valve; RV = right ventricle; RVOT = right ventricular outflow tract; A = anterior; P = posterior; S = superior; I = inferior; asterisk = interventricular septal defect.

Cardiac catheterization demonstrates systolic pressure in the right ventricle equal to systemic pressure, with a marked decrease in pressure as the catheter enters the pulmonary artery or, in some cases, the infundibular chamber beyond the obstruction. The mean pulmonary arterial pressure is commonly 5–10 mm Hg; the right atrial pressure is usually normal. The level of arterial oxygen saturation depends on the magnitude of the right-to-left shunt; in a moderately cyanotic patient at rest it is usually 75–85%. In the absence of a left-to-right shunt, samples of blood from the venae cavae, right atrium, right ventricle, and pulmonary artery will be similar in oxygen content.

Selective right ventriculography best demonstrates the anatomy of tetralogy of Fallot. The contrast medium outlines the heavily trabeculated right ventricle. The infundibular stenosis varies in length, width, contour, and distensibility (Fig. 387–3). The pulmonary valve is usually thickened, and the annulus may be small. Among patients with pulmonary atresia and VSD, the anatomy of the pulmonary vessels may be extremely complex. Complete and accurate information regarding the anatomy of the pulmonary arteries is very important in evaluating these children as surgical candidates.

Left ventriculography demonstrates the size of the left ventricle, the position of the VSD, and the over-riding aorta; it also confirms mitral-aortic continuity, ruling out double-outlet right ventricle. *Aortography* or *coronary arteriography* will outline the course of the coronary arteries. In 5–10% of patients with tetralogy of Fallot, an aberrant major coronary artery crosses over the right ventricular outflow tract; this artery must be not be cut during surgical repair. Delineation of normal coronary arteries by angiography is most important when considering surgery in young infants who may need a patch across the pulmonary valve annulus. Echocardiography can in many cases delineate the coronary artery anatomy.

PROGNOSIS AND COMPLICATIONS. Patients with tetralogy of Fallot prior to correction are susceptible to several serious complications. *Cerebral thromboses,* usually occurring in the cerebral veins or dural sinuses and occasionally in the cerebral arteries, are more common in the presence of extreme polycythemia. They may also be precipitated by dehydration. Thromboses occur most often in patients under the age of 2 yr. These patients may have iron deficiency anemia, frequently with hemoglobin and hematocrit levels in the normal range. Therapy consists of adequate hydration and supportive measures. Phlebotomy and volume replacement with fresh frozen plasma are indicated in the extremely polycythemic patient. Heparin is of little value and is contraindicated in hemorrhagic cerebral infarction. Physical therapy should be instituted as early as possible.

Brain abscess is less common than cerebral vascular events. Patients are usually over the age of 2 yr. The onset of the illness is often insidious with low-grade fever and/or a gradual change in behavior. In some patients there is an acute onset of symptoms, which may develop after a recent history of headache, nausea, and vomiting. Epileptiform seizures may occur; localized neurologic signs depend on the site and size of the abscess, and the presence of increased intracranial pressure. The sedimentation rate and white blood cell count are usually elevated. Computed tomography (CT), magnetic resonance imaging (MRI), or ultrasonography confirms the diagnosis. Massive antibiotic therapy may help to keep the infection localized, but surgical drainage of the abscess is almost always necessary (see Chapter 554).

Bacterial endocarditis occurs in unoperated patients in the right ventricular infundibulum or on the pulmonic, aortic, or, rarely, tricuspid valves. Endocarditis may complicate palliative shunts or, among patients with corrective surgery, any residual pulmonic stenosis or residual VSD. Antibiotic prophylaxis is essential prior to and after dental and certain surgical procedures associated with a high incidence of bacteremia (see Table 386–1).

Congestive heart failure is not a usual feature of patients with tetralogy of Fallot. It may occur, however, in the young infant with "pink" or acyanotic tetralogy of Fallot. As the degree of pulmonary obstruction worsens with age, the symptoms of heart failure resolve and eventually the patient develops cyanosis, often by 6–12 mo of age. These patients are at increased risk for hypercyanotic spells at this time.

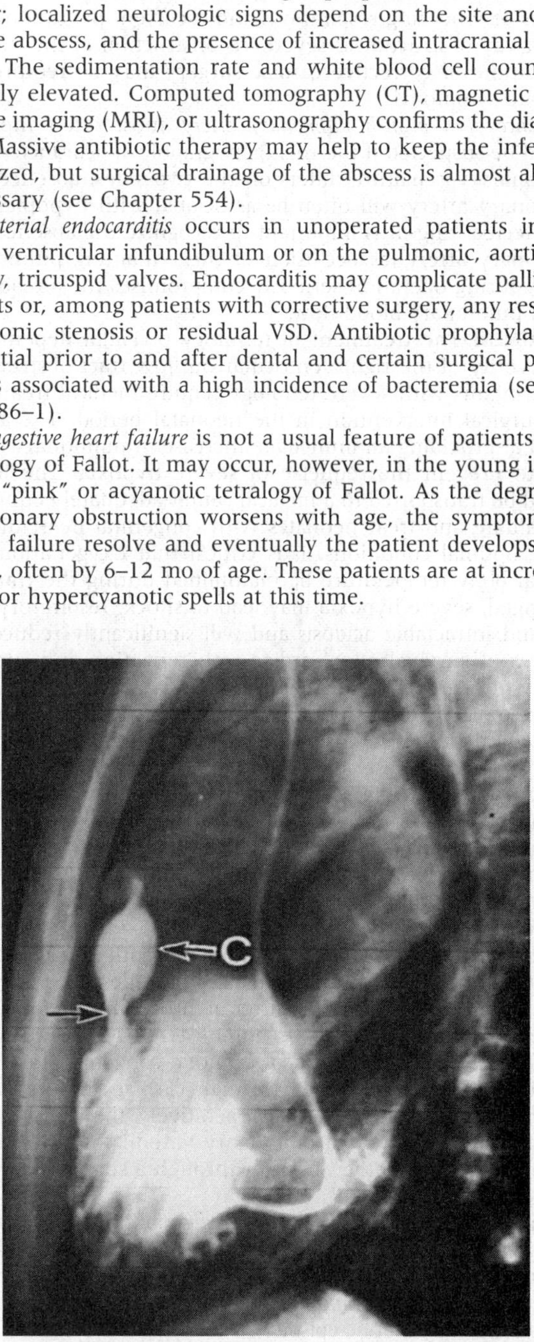

Figure 387–3. Lateral view of a selective right ventriculogram in a patient with tetralogy of Fallot. The *arrow* points to infundibular stenosis that is below the infundibular chamber (C).

ASSOCIATED CARDIOVASCULAR ANOMALIES. An associated PDA may be present and defects in the atrial septum are occasionally seen. A right aortic arch occurs in approximately 20% of cases of tetralogy of Fallot, and other anomalies of the pulmonary arteries and aortic arch may also be seen. Persistence of a left superior vena cava draining into the coronary sinus may be noted. Multiple ventricular septal defects occasionally are present and must be diagnosed prior to corrective surgery. Tetralogy may also occur with atrioventricular septal defects, often associated with Down syndrome.

Congenital absence of the pulmonary valve produces a distinct syndrome, usually marked by signs of upper airway obstruction; cyanosis may be mild, the heart is large and hyperdynamic, and a loud to-and-fro murmur is present. Marked aneurysmal dilatation of the main and branch pulmonary arteries results in compression of the bronchi and produces stridorous or wheezing respirations and recurrent pneumonias. If the airway obstruction is severe, reconstruction of the trachea at the time of corrective cardiac surgery may be required to alleviate symptoms.

Absence of a branch pulmonary artery, most often the left, should be suspected if the roentgenographic appearance of the pulmonary vasculature differs on the two sides; absence of a pulmonary artery will often be associated with hypoplasia of the affected lung. It is important to recognize the absence of a pulmonary artery, as occlusion of the remaining pulmonary artery during operation seriously compromises the already reduced pulmonary blood flow.

TREATMENT. The treatment of tetralogy of Fallot depends on the severity of the right ventricular outflow tract obstruction. Those infants with severe tetralogy require medical treatment and surgical intervention in the neonatal period. Therapy is aimed at providing an immediate increase in pulmonary blood flow to prevent the sequelae of severe hypoxia. The infant should be transported to a medical center adequately equipped to evaluate and treat neonates with congenital heart disease under optimal conditions. It is critical that oxygenation and normal body temperature be maintained during the transfer. Prolonged, severe hypoxia may lead to shock, respiratory failure, and intractable acidosis and will significantly reduce the chances of survival after cardiac catheterization and surgery, even when surgically amenable lesions are present. Cold increases oxygen consumption, which places a further stress on the cyanotic infant, whose oxygen delivery is already limited. Finally, blood glucose levels should be monitored, as infants with cyanotic heart disease are more likely to develop hypoglycemia.

Infants with marked right ventricular outflow tract obstruction may deteriorate rapidly because as the ductus arteriosus begins to close pulmonary blood flow is further compromised. The administration of prostaglandin E_1 (0.05–0.20 μg/kg/min), a potent and specific relaxant of ductal smooth muscle, causes dilatation of the ductus arteriosus and provides adequate pulmonary blood flow until a surgical procedure can be performed. This agent should be administered intravenously as soon as the clinical suspicion of cyanotic congenital heart disease is made and continued through cardiac catheterization and the preoperative period. Postoperatively, the infusion may be continued briefly as a pulmonary vasodilator to augment flow through a palliative shunt or through a surgical valvulotomy.

Infants with less severe right ventricular outflow tract obstruction who are stable and awaiting surgical intervention require careful observation. The prevention or prompt treatment of dehydration is important to avoid hemoconcentration and possible thrombotic episodes. Paroxysmal dyspneic attacks in infancy may be precipitated by a relative iron deficiency; iron therapy may decrease their frequency and also improve exercise tolerance and general well-being. Red blood cell indices should be maintained in the normocytic range. In the past, oral propranolol (1 mg/kg every 6 hr) had been used to decrease the frequency and severity of hypercyanotic spells, but it is preferable to refer the patient for surgical treatment as soon as spells begin.

In general, infants presenting with symptoms and severe cyanosis in the 1st mo of life have marked obstruction of the right ventricular outflow tract or pulmonary atresia. In these infants the most common procedure is a systemic-to-pulmonary artery shunt, performed to augment pulmonary artery blood flow. The rationale of this palliative surgery is to decrease the amount of hypoxia and to improve linear growth as well as to augment the growth of the branch pulmonary arteries. In several centers, corrective open heart surgery in early infancy is being performed in critically ill patients as long as they have normal coronary artery anatomy. The advantages of corrective surgery in early infancy versus a palliative shunt and correction in later infancy are still controversial. For infants who can be maintained until 6–12 mo of age, full correction is a reasonable primary alternative when the pulmonary arteries are of sufficient size and no other complicating great vessel abnormalities are present.

The modified **Blalock-Taussig** shunt is currently the most common aorto-pulmonary shunt procedure and consists of a Gore-Tex conduit anastomosed side to side from the subclavian artery to the homolateral branch of the pulmonary artery. Sometimes the conduit is brought directly from the ascending aorta to the main pulmonary artery and is called a central shunt. The Blalock-Taussig operation can be successfully performed in the newborn period using 4–5 mm diameter shunts and has been utilized successfully in premature infants. The original Blalock-Taussig shunt consisted of a direct anastamosis of the subclavian artery to a branch pulmonary artery. Other shunt procedures include a side-to-side anastomosis of the ascending aorta and right pulmonary artery (Waterson) and anastomosis of the descending aorta and left pulmonary artery (Potts). These procedures are rarely done because of a higher frequency of complicating congestive heart failure and a higher risk for the development of pulmonary hypertension as well as greater technical difficulties in closing these shunts during subsequent corrective surgery.

Usually, the postoperative course of patients with a successful shunt procedure is relatively uneventful. However, postoperative complications following a lateral thoracotomy, such as chylothorax, diaphragmatic paralysis, and Horner syndrome, may occur. *Chylothorax* may require repeated thoracocentesis and, on occasion, reoperation in order to ligate the thoracic duct. *Diaphragmatic paralysis* due to injury to the phrenic nerve may result in a more difficult postoperative course. Prolonged ventilator support and vigorous physical therapy may be required, but diaphragmatic function will usually return in 1–2 mo unless the nerve was completely divided. Surgical plication of the diaphragm may be indicated. *Horner syndrome* is usually temporary and does not require treatment. Postoperative *cardiac failure* may be caused by a large sized shunt; its treatment is described in Chapter 399. Vascular problems, other than a diminished radial pulse and occasional long-term arm length discrepancy, are rarely seen in the upper extremity supplied by the subclavian artery used for the anastomosis.

After a successful shunt procedure, cyanosis diminishes. The development of a continuous murmur over the lung fields after the operation indicates a functioning anastomosis. However, a good shunt murmur may not be heard until several days after surgery. The duration of symptomatic relief is variable. As the child grows, more pulmonary blood flow is needed and the shunt may eventually become inadequate. When increasing cyanosis develops, a corrective operation should be performed if the anatomy is favorable. However, if this is not possible (e.g., because of hypoplastic branch pulmonary arteries) or if the 1st shunt lasts only a brief period in a small infant, a second aorto-pulmonary anastomosis may be required on the opposite side.

Corrective surgical therapy consists of relief of the obstruction of the right ventricular outflow tract by removing obstructive muscle bundles and patch closure of the VSD. If the pulmonary valve is stenotic, a valvotomy is performed. If the pulmonary valve annulus is very small or the valve is extremely thickened, a valvectomy may be performed and a transannular patch placed across the pulmonary valve ring. When there is a previously established systemic to pulmonary shunt, it must be obliterated prior to cardiotomy. The surgical risk of **total correction** is currently under 5%. A right ventriculotomy is performed in most patients, although in some centers a transatrial-transpulmonary approach reduces the long-term risks of a ventriculotomy. The presence of a previous Blalock-Taussig shunt does not increase the operative risk. Increased bleeding in the immediate postoperative period is common in polycythemic patients but should not seriously affect the outcome. The operative risks may be somewhat higher in small infants because these are usually the patients with the more severe forms of right ventricular outflow tract obstruction.

After successful total correction, patients are generally asymptomatic and are able to lead unrestricted lives. Immediate postoperative problems include right ventricular failure, transient heart block, residual VSD with left-to-right shunting, myocardial infarction from interruption of an aberrant coronary artery, and disproportionately increased left atrial pressure due to residual collaterals. Postoperative heart failure (particularly in patients with a transannular outflow patch) requires a positive inotropic agent such as digoxin. The long-term effects of isolated, surgically induced pulmonary valvular insufficiency are unknown, but insufficiency is generally well tolerated. Patients with marked pulmonary valve insufficiency will have moderate to marked cardiac enlargement. Patients having a severe residual gradient across the right ventricular outflow tract may require reoperation, but mild to moderate obstruction is virtually always present and does not require reintervention.

Follow-up of patients 5–20 yr after operation indicates that the marked improvement in symptomatology is generally maintained. However, even asymptomatic patients have working capacities, maximal heart rates, and cardiac outputs that are lower than those of controls. These abnormal findings are more common in patients who had placement of a transannular outflow tract patch and may be less frequent when surgery is undertaken at an early age.

Conduction disturbances are also frequent after operation. The atrioventricular node and the bundle of His and its divisions are in close proximity to the VSD and may be injured during surgery. Permanent complete heart block following surgery is rare. When present, it should be treated by placement of a permanently implanted pacemaker. Bifascicular block occurs in about 10% of patients; the long-term significance is uncertain, but in most instances there are no clinical manifestations. The additional finding of transient complete heart block in the immediate postoperative period, however, appears to be associated with an increased incidence of late-onset complete heart block and sudden death. However, unexpected cardiac arrest rarely occurs many years after surgery in patients without postoperative bifascicular block or transient complete heart block. A number of children will display premature ventricular beats following repair of tetralogy of Fallot. These are of concern in patients with residual hemodynamic abnormalities; 24-hr ECG (Holter) monitoring studies should be performed to be certain that occult short episodes of ventricular tachycardia are not occurring. In addition, exercise studies may be useful in provoking cardiac arrhythmias that are not apparent at rest. In the presence of complex ventricular arrhythmias or severe residual hemodynamic abnormalities, prophylactic antiarrhythmia therapy is warranted. Dilantin, propranolol, or combinations of these agents are most often used.

387.3 Pulmonary Atresia with Ventricular Septal Defect

PATHOPHYSIOLOGY. This condition is an extreme form of tetralogy of Fallot. The pulmonary valve is atretic, rudimentary, or absent, and the pulmonary trunk is atretic or hypoplastic. The entire right ventricular output is ejected into the aorta. Pulmonary blood flow is then dependent on a PDA or on bronchial collateral vessels. The ultimate prognosis of this lesion depends on the degree of development of the branch pulmonary arteries. If these are well developed, surgical repair with an artificial conduit between the right ventricle and pulmonary arteries is feasible. If the pulmonary arteries are moderately hypoplastic, the prognosis is more guarded, and extensive reconstruction may be required. If the pulmonary arteries are severely hypoplastic, heart-lung transplantation may be the only available therapy.

CLINICAL MANIFESTATIONS. Patients with pulmonary atresia and VSD present with similar findings to those with severe tetralogy of Fallot. Cyanosis usually appears within the first few hours or days after birth; the prominent systolic murmur of tetralogy is usually absent; the 1st heart sound is frequently followed by an ejection click caused by the enlarged aortic root; the 2nd sound is moderately loud and single; and continuous murmurs of a PDA or bronchial collateral flow may be heard over the entire precordium, both anteriorly and posteriorly. Most patients are severely cyanotic and require urgent prostaglandin E_1 infusion and palliative surgical intervention; some patients have congestive heart failure caused by increased pulmonary blood flow via bronchial collateral vessels; and some infants have adequate pulmonary blood flow and can be managed like patients with uncomplicated tetralogy of Fallot.

The chest *roentgenogram* will demonstrate a small or enlarged heart, depending on the degree of pulmonary blood flow, a concavity at the position of the pulmonary arterial segment, and often the reticular pattern of bronchial collateral flow. The *electrocardiogram* shows right ventricular hypertrophy. The *echocardiogram* identifies aortic over-ride, a thick right ventricular wall, and atresia of the pulmonary valve. Pulsed and color Doppler echocardiography show absence of forward flow through the pulmonary valve, with pulmonary blood flow being supplied by the ductus arteriosus or by bronchial collaterals. At cardiac catheterization, *right ventriculography* reveals a large aorta, opacified immediately by passage of the contrast medium through the VSD, with no dye entering the lungs through the right ventricular outflow tract. The pathway of pulmonary blood flow from the aorta to the lungs (ductus or collaterals) is also demonstrated.

TREATMENT. The surgical procedure of choice depends on whether there is an adequate main pulmonary artery segment and on the size of the branch pulmonary arteries. In patients with small branch pulmonary arteries, surgical intervention is directed toward increasing pulmonary blood flow in the hope that this will stimulate pulmonary artery growth. Two options are currently considered: an aortopulmonary (Blalock-Taussig or central) shunt; or the establishment of a connection from the right ventricle directly to the pulmonary artery, either by patch "unroofing" of the outflow tract or by implanting a homograft conduit. There is controversy as to whether this type of bypass stimulates the growth of the pulmonary arteries better than a standard shunt operation.

For the patient to be a candidate for full repair, the pulmonary arteries must be of adequate size to accept the full volume of right ventricular output. Complete repair includes closure of the VSD and placement of a homograft (usually aortic, sometimes pulmonic) from the right ventricle to the pulmonary artery. At the time of reparative surgery, any previous shunts are ligated. Because of growth and the development of intimal tissue proliferation, conduit replacement is usually required in later life; sometimes multiple conduit replacements are required. Often, patients have malformations of the primary divisions of the pulmonary arteries in the form of hypoplasia, multiple branch stenoses, absence of a pulmonary artery, and large bronchial collaterals. These vessels are difficult to reconstruct surgically, even after early anastomotic procedures. Some patients with severe tetralogy of Fallot or pulmonary atresia require surgical or catheter obliteration of MAPCAs.

Acquired total atresia of the right ventricular outflow tract may occur after an aorto-pulmonary shunt anastomosis for tetralogy of Fallot. In this case, the systolic murmur due to pulmonary stenosis will become attenuated and then disappear. The completeness of obstruction can be confirmed by right ventriculography at the time of cardiac catheterization. Corrective surgery of the right ventricular outflow tract can be performed in a manner similar to that utilized for congenital pulmonary atresia.

387.4 Pulmonary Atresia with Intact Ventricular Septum

PATHOPHYSIOLOGY. In this anomaly the pulmonary valve leaflets are completely fused to form a membrane and the right ventricular outflow tract is atretic. Because there is no VSD, there is no egress of blood from the right ventricle. Right atrial pressures increase and blood shunts via the foramen ovale into the left atrium, where it mixes with pulmonary venous blood and enters the left ventricle. The combined left and right ventricular output is pumped solely by the left ventricle into the aorta. The only source of pulmonary blood flow occurs via a PDA. The right ventricle is usually hypoplastic, although the degree of hypoplasia varies considerably. Patients who have a very small right ventricular cavity also have a small tricuspid valve annulus, limiting right ventricular inflow. These patients may have sinusoidal channels within the right ventricular wall that communicate directly with the coronary arterial circulation. The high right ventricular pressure results in desaturated blood flowing retrograde via collaterals into the coronary arteries and to the aorta. Patients with intermediate-sized or large ventricular cavities may have tricuspid insufficiency, which serves to decompress the right ventricle.

CLINICAL MANIFESTATIONS. As the ductus arteriosus closes in the first hours or days of life, infants with pulmonary atresia and intact ventricular septum become markedly cyanotic. Untreated, most patients die within the 1st wk of life. Physical examination reveals severe cyanosis and respiratory distress. The 2nd heart sound is single and loud. Often there are no murmurs; sometimes a systolic or continuous murmur can be heard secondary to ductal blood flow.

In the *electrocardiogram*, the frontal QRS axis almost always lies between 0 and +90 degrees. The tall, spiked P waves indicate right atrial enlargement. QRS voltages are consistent with left ventricular dominance or hypertrophy; right ventricular forces are decreased in proportion to the decreased size of the right ventricular cavity. Most patients with small right ventricles have decreased right ventricular forces; however, occasionally, patients with larger right ventricular cavities may show evidence of right ventricular hypertrophy. The chest *roentgenogram* shows decreased pulmonary vascularity, the degree depending on the size of the branch pulmonary arteries and the patency of the ductus or size of bronchial collaterals. The heart may be variable in size. Two-dimensional *echocardiogram* is useful in estimating the right ventricular dimensions and the size of the tricuspid valve annulus, which are of prognostic value. Echocardiography can often demonstrate sinusoidal channels if they are large. *Cardiac catheterization* demonstrates right atrial and right ventricular hypertension. Ventriculography demonstrates the size of the right ventricular cavity, the atretic right ventricular outflow tract, the degree of tricuspid regurgitation, and the intramyocardial sinusoids filling the coronary vessels.

TREATMENT. Infusion of prostaglandin E_1 is usually effective in keeping the ductus arteriosus open prior to intervention, thus reducing hypoxemia and acidemia prior to surgery. Pulmonary valvotomy is carried out to relieve outflow obstruction whenever possible, but in order to preserve adequate pulmonary blood flow an aortopulmonary shunt is usually done during the same procedure. Some groups have reported success by unroofing the right ventricular outflow tract and patch grafting. The aim of surgery is to encourage growth of the right ventricular chamber by allowing some forward flow through the pulmonary valve, while utilizing the shunt to ensure adequate pulmonary blood flow. Later, if the tricuspid valve annulus and right ventricular chamber are of adequate size, a more extensive valvotomy is carried out and the shunt is taken down. If the right ventricular chamber is minuscule, a modified Fontan procedure (see Chapter 387.5) may be used to allow blood to flow to the pulmonary artery directly from the vena cavae, bypassing the hypoplastic ventricle. When retrograde coronary perfusion occurs from the right ventricle via myocardial sinusoids the prognosis may be grave. Arrhythmias, coronary ischemia, and sudden death are not uncommon in these patients. Associated coronary artery abnormalities may be expected. Some of these infants have benefitted from heart transplantation.

387.5 Tricuspid Atresia

PATHOPHYSIOLOGY. In tricuspid atresia there is no outlet from the right atrium to the right ventricle, and the entire systemic venous return enters the left heart by means of the foramen ovale or an associated atrial septal defect (ASD). Left ventricular blood usually flows into the right ventricle via a VSD. Pulmonary blood flow (and thus the degree of cyanosis) depends on the size of the VSD and the presence and severity of pulmonic stenosis. Pulmonary blood flow may be augmented by, or totally dependent on, a PDA. The inflow portion of the right ventricle is always missing in these patients, but the outflow portion is of variable size. If the ventricular septum is intact, the right ventricle is completely hypoplastic and pulmonary atresia is present (see Chapter 387.4). Most patients with tricuspid atresia present in the early months of life with decreased pulmonary blood flow and cyanosis. Less often, a large VSD in the absence of right ventricular outflow obstruction can lead to high pulmonary flow, and these patients present with mild cyanosis and congestive heart failure. One variant of tricuspid atresia is associated with transposition of the great arteries (TGA). In this case, left ventricular blood flow enters directly into the pulmonary artery, whereas systemic blood flow must traverse the VSD and right ventricle to reach the aorta. In these patients pulmonary blood flow is usually increased and congestive heart failure develops early. If the VSD is restrictive, aortic blood flow may be compromised.

CLINICAL MANIFESTATIONS. Cyanosis is usually evident at birth, especially if pulmonary blood flow is limited. There may be an increased left ventricular impulse, in distinction to the majority of other causes of cyanotic heart disease, in which there is usually an increased right ventricular impulse. The majority of patients have holosystolic murmurs audible along the left sternal border; the 2nd heart sound is usually single. The diagnosis is suspected in 85% of patients before 2 mo of age. In older patients, cyanosis, polycythemia, easy fatigability, exertional dyspnea, and occasional hypoxic episodes occur as a result of compromised pulmonary blood flow. Patients with tricuspid atresia are at risk for spontaneous closure of the VSD; as it becomes smaller there is a marked increase in cyanosis.

Roentgenographic studies show either pulmonary undercirculation (usually with normally related great vessels) or overcirculation (usually with transposed great vessels). Left axis deviation and left ventricular hypertrophy are almost invariably present on the *electrocardiogram,* except when there is transposition of the great arteries. The combination of cyanosis and left axis deviation is highly suggestive of tricuspid atresia. In the right precordial leads the normally prominent R wave is replaced by an rS complex. The left precordial leads show a qR complex, followed by a normal, flat, diphasic, or inverted T wave. RV_6 is normal or tall, and SV_1 generally deep. The P waves are usually biphasic, with the initial component tall and spiked in lead II. The *two-dimensional echocardiogram* reveals the presence of a fibromuscular membrane in place of a tricuspid valve, the variably small right ventricle, VSD, and the large left ventricle and aorta. The degree of obstruction at the level of the VSD or right ventricular outflow tract can be determined by direct measurement and by Doppler examination. If blood flow is dependent on a patent ductus, this can be determined by color flow and pulsed Doppler examination.

Cardiac catheterization shows normal or slightly elevated right atrial pressure with a prominent "a" wave. If the right ventricle is entered through the VSD, the pressure may be lower than the left, reflecting the restrictive nature of the ventricular communication in these patients. With right atrial angiography there is immediate opacification of the left atrium from the right atrium followed by left ventricular filling and visualization of the aorta. Absence of direct flow to the right ventricle results in an angiographic filling defect between the right atrium and the left ventricle. The presence or absence of associated transposition of the great vessels is also demonstrated by selective left ventriculography.

TREATMENT. The management of patients with tricuspid atresia depends on the adequacy of pulmonary blood flow. Severely cyanotic neonates should be maintained on an infusion of prostaglandin E_1 until a surgical aorto-pulmonary shunt procedure can be performed to increase pulmonary blood flow. The Blalock-Taussig procedure (or its variations, see Chapter 387.2) is the preferred anastomosis. Some patients with restrictive atrial level communications are benefitted by a Rashkind balloon atrial septostomy (see Chapter 387.10). Infants with increased pulmonary blood flow due to unobstructed pulmonary outflow (usually those patients with aortopulmonary transposition) require pulmonary arterial banding to decrease the symptoms of congestive heart failure and to protect the pulmonary bed from development of pulmonary vascular disease. Infants with just adequate pulmonary blood flow, who are well balanced between cyanosis and pulmonary overcirculation, can be watched closely for the development of increasing cyanosis. This may occur as the VSD begins to get smaller and indicates the need for surgical intervention.

The next stage of palliation for patients with tricuspid atresia involves the creation of an anastomosis between the superior vena cava and the pulmonary arteries (*bidirectional Glenn shunt*). This procedure is most often performed after the patient has shown signs of outgrowing a previous aorto-pulmonary shunt, usually at between 4 and 12 mo of age. The benefit of the Glenn shunt is that it reduces the volume work on the left ventricle and may lessen the chances of the patient developing left ventricular dysfunction later in life. Some centers advocate performing the Glenn anastamosis at an even earlier age (2–4 mo); however, the benefit of this approach has not yet been confirmed in long-term follow-up studies.

The modified Fontan operation is the preferred approach to later surgical management. It is often performed at between 1.5 and 3 yr of age, usually after the patient is ambulatory. In the past, this procedure was performed by anastomosing the right atrium to the pulmonary artery. Today, a modification, known as a *caval-pulmonary isolation procedure,* is performed. This involves anastomosing the inferior vena cava to the pulmonary arteries via a baffle that runs along the lateral wall of the right atrium (Fig. 387–4). The advantage of this approach is that blood flows by a more direct route into the pulmonary arteries, decreasing the possibility of right atrial dilatation and markedly reducing the incidence of postoperative pleural effusions. At the time of surgery, the ASD or foramen ovale is also closed. In this completed repair, desaturated blood flows from both vena cavae directly into the pulmonary arteries. Oxygenated blood returns to the left atrium, enters the left ventricle, and is ejected into the systemic circulation. The volume load is completely removed from the left ventricle and the right-to-left shunt is abolished. The Fontan procedure is contraindicated in very young infants and in patients with elevated pulmonary vascular resistance (>4 Wood units/m^2), in those with pulmonary artery hypoplasia, and in patients with left ventricular dysfunction. It is also important that the patient be in sinus rhythm and not have significant mitral insufficiency.

Postoperative problems after a Fontan procedure include marked elevation of systemic venous pressure, fluid retention, and pleural or pericardial effusions. Pleural effusions used to persist for more than 3 wk in 30–40% of patients. The development of the caval-pulmonary isolation procedure has reduced this risk to approximately 5%. Late complications include residual obstruction, causing superior or inferior vena caval syndrome, vena caval or pulmonary artery thromboembolism, protein-losing enteropathy, and supraventricular arrhythmias (atrial flutter, paroxysmal atrial tachycardia), occasionally associated with sudden death. The late development of left ventricular dysfunction may occur, often in the teen or young adult years.

387.6 Double-Outlet Right Ventricle (DORV) with Pulmonary Stenosis

This anomaly is characterized by both the aorta and pulmonary artery arising from the right ventricle; the only outlet from the left ventricle is via a VSD into the right ventricle. The aortic and mitral valves are separated by a smooth muscular conus, similar to that seen under the normal pulmonary valve. The VSD is inferior to the crista supraventricularis. The aorta may over-ride the VSD by a variable amount, but is at least 50% committed to the right ventricle. This defect may be viewed as part of a continuum with tetralogy of Fallot, depending on the degree of aortic override. The physiology is similar to that in tetralogy of Fallot. The history, physical examination, electrocardiogram, and roentgenograms are as described in Chapter 387.2. The two-dimensional *echocardiogram* demonstrates both great vessels arising from the right ventricle and mitral-aortic valve discontinuity. Doppler examination demonstrates the degree of pulmonic stenosis and the

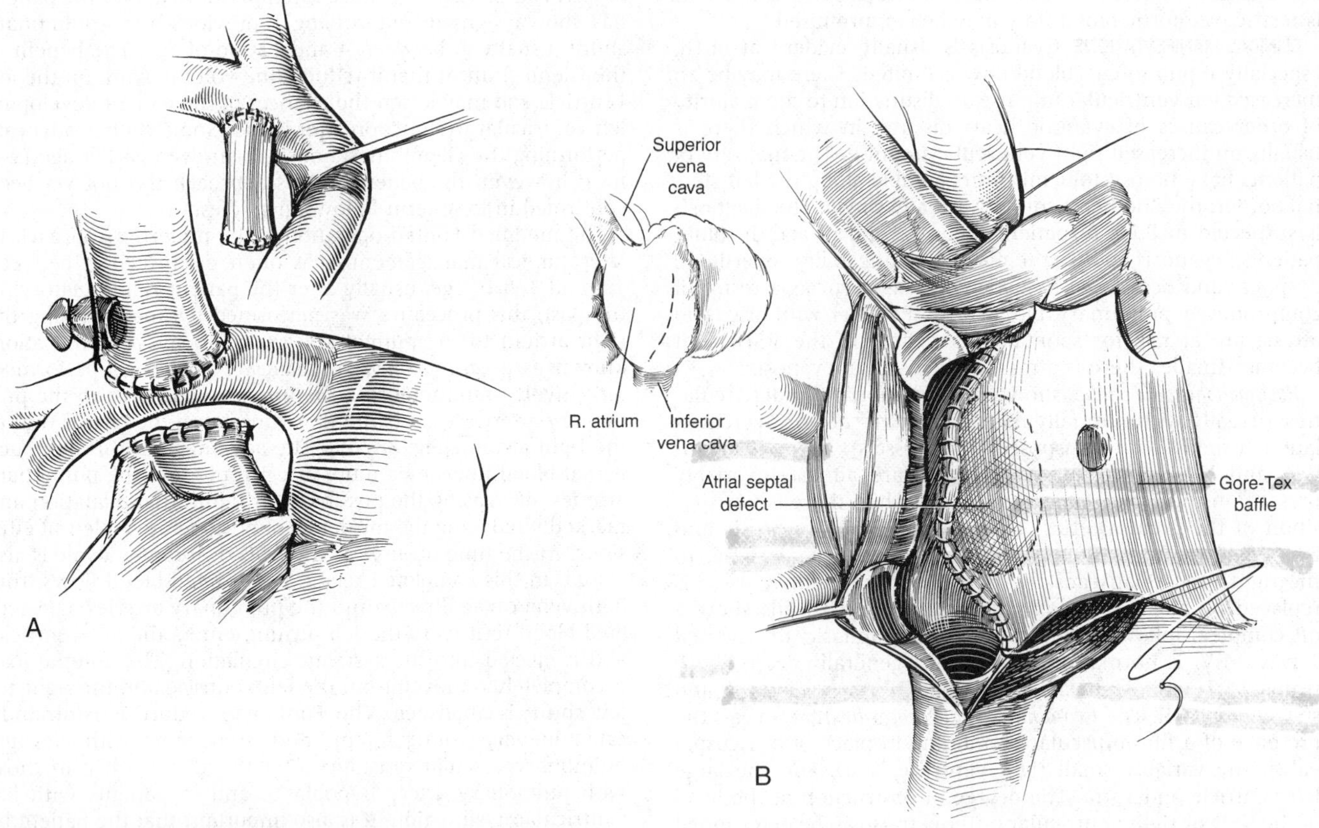

Figure 387–4. ***A,*** **The superior vena cava–to–right pulmonary anastomosis is completed with running absorbable suture.** ***B,*** **Placement of baffle to convey inferior vena caval blood along the lateral wall of the right atrium to the superior vena caval orifice. A 4 mm fenestration is made on the medial aspect of the polytetrafluoroethylene baffle. (From Castaneda AR, Jonas RA, Mayer Jr JE, Hanley FL: Single-ventricle tricuspid atresia.** ***In:*** **Cardiac Surgery of the Neonate and Infant. Philadelphia, WB Saunders, 1994.)**

presence of a ductus arteriosus. At *cardiac catheterization,* angiography shows that the aortic and pulmonary valves lie in the same horizontal body plane and that the anteriorly displaced aorta arises predominantly or exclusively from the right ventricle. Surgical correction consists of creating an intraventricular tunnel so that the left ventricle ejects blood through the VSD, through the tunnel, and into the aorta. The pulmonary obstruction is relieved either with an outflow patch or with a pulmonary or aortic homograft conduit (*Rastelli operation*). In small infants palliation with an aortopulmonary shunt will provide symptomatic improvement and allow for adequate growth (see Chapter 387.2).

387.7 Transposition of the Great Arteries with Ventricular Septal Defect and Pulmonary Stenosis

This combination of anomalies may mimic tetralogy of Fallot in its clinical presentation (see Chapter 387.2). However, because of the transposition, the site of obstruction is in the left as opposed to the right ventricle. The obstruction can be either valvular or subvalvular; the latter type may be dynamic, related to the interventricular septum or atrioventricular valve tissue, or acquired, as in patients with transposition and VSD after pulmonary arterial banding.

Clinical manifestations vary in age of onset from soon after birth to later infancy, depending on the degree of pulmonic stenosis, and include cyanosis, decreased exercise tolerance, and poor physical development. They are similar to those described under tetralogy of Fallot; however, the heart may be more enlarged. The pulmonary vasculature as seen on roentgenogram is dependent on the degree of pulmonary obstruction but is often relatively normal. The electrocardiogram usually shows right axis deviation, right and left ventricular hypertrophy, and sometimes tall, spiked P waves. Echocardiography confirms the diagnosis and is useful in sequential evaluation of the degree and progression of the left ventricular outflow tract obstruction. Cardiac catheterization shows that the pulmonary arterial pressure is low and the oxygen saturation in the pulmonary artery exceeds that of the aorta. Selective right and left ventriculography demonstrates the origin of the aorta from the right ventricle, the origin of the pulmonary artery from the left ventricle, the VSD, and the site and severity of the pulmonary stenosis.

Neonates presenting with cyanosis should be started on an infusion of prostaglandin E_1. The preferred surgical *treatment* in hypoxemic infants is an aorto-pulmonary shunt. When necessary, balloon atrial septostomy is performed to improve atrial-level mixing and to decompress the left atrium (see Chapter 387.10). The patient can then be followed clinically until between 2 and 6 yr of age, when a Rastelli operation is the preferred corrective procedure. The Rastelli procedure achieves physiologic and anatomic correction by (1) patch closure of the VSD, directing left ventricular flow to the aorta; and (2) connection of the right ventricle to the pulmonary artery by ligating the proximal pulmonary artery and placing an extracardiac homograft conduit between the right ventricle and the distal pulmonary artery (Fig. 387–5). The conduit

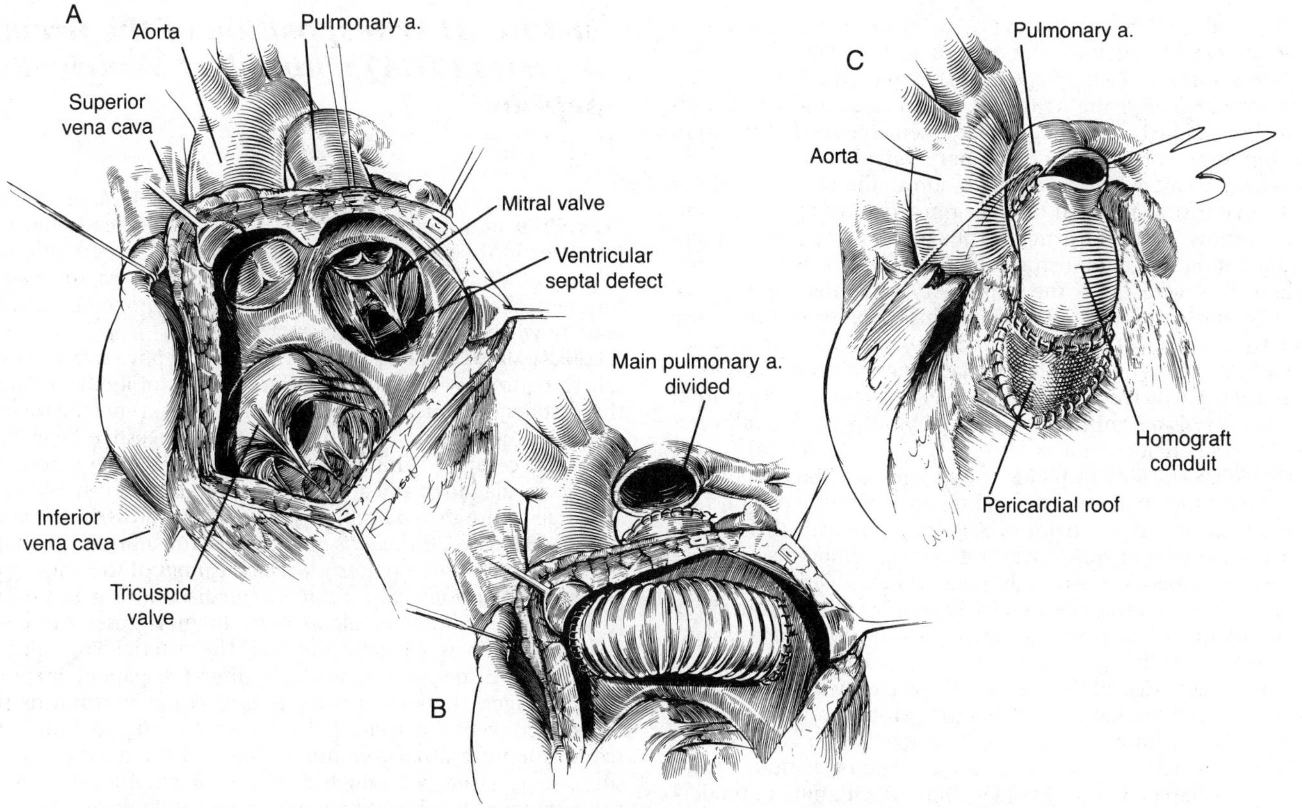

Figure 387–5. *A,* Taussig-Bing type of DORV with subpulmonary stenosis necessitating repair by the Rastelli technique. *B,* Main pulmonary artery is divided and oversewn proximally. The pulmonary valve lies within the baffle pathway. *C,* Completion of the Rastelli repair with a right ventricle–to–pulmonary artery allograft conduit. (From Castaneda AR, Jonas RA, Mayer Jr JE, Hanley FL: Single-ventricle tricuspid atresia. *In:* Cardiac Surgery of the Neonate and Infant. Philadelphia, WB Saunders, 1994.)

may eventually become stenotic or functionally restrictive with growth of the patient and require revision. Surgical correction by the Mustard operation (see Chapter 387.10) with simultaneous closure of the VSD and relief of left ventricular outflow obstruction may be an alternative when the position of the VSD is not suitable for a Rastelli operation. This more complex procedure carries a higher risk. Patients with milder degrees of pulmonary stenosis amenable to simple valvotomy may be able to undergo complete correction with an arterial switch procedure (see Chapter 387.10).

387.8 Ebstein Anomaly of the Tricuspid Valve

PATHOPHYSIOLOGY. This anomaly consists of downward displacement of an abnormal tricuspid valve into the right ventricle. The anterior cusp of the valve retains some attachment to the valve ring, but the other leaflets are adherent to the wall of the right ventricle. The right ventricle is thus divided into two parts by the abnormal tricuspid valve: the first, a thin-walled "atrialized" portion, is continuous with the cavity of the right atrium; the second consists of normal ventricular myocardium. The right atrium is huge, and the tricuspid valve is usually regurgitant, although the degree is extremely variable. The effective output from the right side of the heart is decreased because of the poorly functioning small right ventricle, tricuspid valve regurgitation, and variable degrees of obstruction of the right ventricular outflow tract produced by the large, sail-like, anterior tricuspid valve leaflet. Sometimes right ventricular function is so compromised that it is unable to open the pulmonary valve in systole, producing "functional" pulmonary atresia. The increased volume of right atrial blood shunts through the foramen ovale to the left atrium, producing cyanosis.

CLINICAL MANIFESTATIONS. The severity of symptoms and the degree of cyanosis depends on the degree of displacement of the tricuspid valve and the severity of right ventricular outflow tract obstruction. In many patients, symptoms are mild and the only complaint is fatigue. Cardiac dysrhythmias are frequent, the most common being numerous extrasystoles or attacks of paroxysmal tachycardia, usually supraventricular. A right-to-left shunt through the foramen ovale is responsible for cyanosis and polycythemia. The venous pressure may be normal or increased if there is tricuspid insufficiency. On palpation, the precordium is quiet. A holosystolic murmur is audible over most of the anterior left side of the chest due to tricuspid regurgitation. A gallop rhythm is common, often associated with multiple clicks at the lower left sternal border. A scratchy diastolic murmur may also be heard at the left sternal border. This murmur is superficial and may mimic a pericardial friction rub.

Although some patients may be asymptomatic until well into adult life, newborn infants with Ebstein anomaly often present with severe cyanosis, massive cardiomegaly, and long systolic murmurs. Death may occur as a result of cardiac failure and hypoxemia. In some of these neonates, spontaneous improvement will occur as pulmonary vascular resistance falls normally, improving the ability of the right ventricle to provide pulmonary blood flow. The majority, however, are dependent on a PDA for pulmonary blood flow.

DIAGNOSIS. The *electrocardiogram* usually shows right bundle branch block without increased right precordial voltage, normal or tall and broad P waves, and a normal or prolonged P-R interval. Sometimes the pattern of the Wolff-Parkinson-White syndrome (see Chapter 388) is present. On *roentgenographic examination* the heart size varies from normal to massive, box-shaped cardiomegaly due to enlargement of the right atrium and ventricle. The pulmonary vasculature can be normal or decreased. *Echocardiography* shows the displaced tricuspid valve tissue, a dilated right atrium, and any right ventricular outflow tract obstruction. Pulsed and color Doppler examination will demonstrate the degree of tricuspid regurgitation. In severe cases, the pulmonary valve may appear immobile and pulmonary blood flow may come solely from the ductus arteriosus. *Cardiac catheterization* and *selective angiocardiography* confirm the presence of a large right atrium and abnormal tricuspid valve and any right-to-left shunt at the atrial level. There is a significant risk of arrhythmia during catheterization and angiographic studies.

PROGNOSIS AND COMPLICATIONS. The prognosis in Ebstein anomaly is extremely variable, depending on where the patient falls within the broad spectrum of severity seen with this defect. For the neonate or infant with intractable symptoms and cyanosis, the prognosis is usually poor. Patients with milder degrees of Ebstein anomaly usually survive well into adult life.

TREATMENT. Neonates with severe hypoxia who are prostaglandin dependent have recently been treated by surgical patch closure of the tricuspid valve, atrial septectomy, and placement of an aorto-pulmonary shunt (Starnes procedure). This operation creates a functional tricuspid atresia, which can then be further repaired with first a Glenn and then a Fontan operation (see Chapter 387.5). In older children with mild or moderate disease, control of supraventricular dysrhythmias is of primary importance. In these patients, surgical treatment is seldom necessary until adolescence or young adulthood. Repair or replacement of the abnormal tricuspid valve with closure of the ASD is then carried out.

Cyanotic Lesions Associated with Increased Pulmonary Blood Flow

387.9 D-Transposition of the Great Arteries (TGA)

In this anomaly the systemic veins return normally to the right atrium and the pulmonary veins to the left atrium. The connections between the atria and ventricles are also normal (known as concordant). However, the aorta arises from the right ventricle and the pulmonary artery from the left ventricle. In d-TGA, the aorta is usually anterior and to the right of the pulmonary artery. Desaturated blood returning from the body to the right side of the heart inappropriately goes right out of the aorta and back to the body again, whereas oxygenated pulmonary venous blood returning to the left side of the heart is returned directly to the lungs. Thus, the systemic and pulmonary circulations consist of two parallel circuits. The only means of survival in these newborns are provided by the foramen ovale and the ductus arteriosus, which permit some mixture of oxygenated and deoxygenated blood. About half of patients with TGA will also have a VSD, which provides for much better mixing. The clinical presentation and hemodynamics vary in relation to the presence or absence of associated defects. TGA occurs in 1 of 5,000 live births and is more common in infants of diabetic mothers and in males (3:1). Prior to the modern era of corrective or palliative surgery, the mortality was greater than 90% within the 1st yr of life.

387.10 D-Transposition of the Great Arteries (TGA) with Intact Ventricular Septum

This anomaly is also referred to as simple TGA or isolated TGA. Prior to birth, oxygenation of the fetus is nearly normal, but after birth, once the ductus begins to close, the minimal mixing of the systemic and pulmonary blood via the patent foramen ovale is insufficient and severe hypoxemia ensues, usually within the 1st few days of life.

CLINICAL MANIFESTATIONS. Cyanosis and tachypnea are most often recognized within the 1st hours or days of life. Untreated, the vast majority of these infants would not survive the neonatal period. Hypoxemia is usually severe; congestive heart failure is less common. This condition is a medical emergency, and only early diagnosis and appropriate intervention can avert the sequelae of prolonged severe hypoxemia, acidosis, and death.

DIAGNOSIS. The *electrocardiogram* shows the normal neonatal right-sided dominant pattern. *Roentgenograms* of the chest may show mild cardiomegaly, a narrow mediastinum, and normal to increased pulmonary blood flow. In most cases the chest roentgenogram is virtually normal. The arterial Po_2 value is low and does not rise appreciably after the patient breathes 100% oxygen (hyperoxia test). *Echocardiography* confirms the transposed ventricular-arterial connections. In addition, the size of the intra-atrial communication and the ductus arteriosus can be visualized and the degree of mixing assessed by color Doppler. If echocardiography is not fully diagnostic, cardiac catheterization and angiographic study should be carried out to confirm the diagnosis and to eliminate associated lesions.

Cardiac catheterization shows right ventricular pressure to be systemic, as this ventricle is supporting the systemic circulation. The blood in the left ventricle and pulmonary artery has a higher oxygen saturation than that in the aorta. The degree of arterial desaturation is variable but is most often extremely low. Depending on the age at catheterization, the left ventricular and pulmonary arterial pressures can vary from systemic level to less than 50% of systemic level pressures. *Right ventriculography* demonstrates the anterior and rightward aorta originating from the right ventricle as well as the intact ventricular septum. Anomalous coronary arteries are noted in 10–15%. *Left ventriculography* shows that the pulmonary artery arises exclusively from the left ventricle.

TREATMENT. Immediately upon suspicion of the diagnosis of transposition, an infusion of prostaglandin E_1 (PGE_1) should be initiated to maintain the patency of the ductus arteriosus and to improve oxygenation (dosage, 0.05–0.20 μg/kg/min). Because of the risk of apnea associated with prostaglandin infusion, an individual skilled at neonatal endotracheal intubation should be readily available. Hypothermia intensifies the metabolic acidosis resulting from hypoxemia. Prompt correction of acidosis and hypoglycemia is essential.

Infants who remain severely hypoxic or acidotic despite prostaglandin infusion should be taken immediately to the cardiac catheterization laboratory for performance of a Rashkind balloon atrial septostomy (Fig. 387–6). Some centers perform the Rashkind procedure in the neonatal nursery under echocardiographic guidance. In all patients in whom any significant delay in operation is necessary, a Rashkind atrial septostomy is usually performed. At most centers the arterial switch (Jatene) operation is performed within the first 2 wk of life. If the arterial switch is planned immediately, catheterization and atrial septostomy may be avoided.

A successful Rashkind atrial septostomy should result in a rise in Pao_2 to 35–50 mm Hg and the elimination of the usual preseptostomy pressure gradient across the atrial septum.

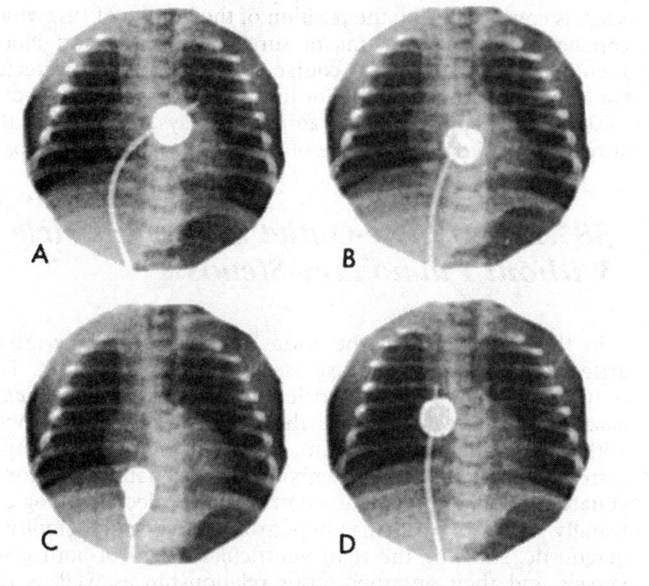

Figure 387–6. Balloon septostomy (Rashkind). Four frames from a continuous cinema that show the creation of an atrial septal defect in a hypoxemic newborn infant with transposition of the great arteries and intact ventricular septum. *A,* Balloon inflated in the left atrium. *B,* The catheter is jerked suddenly so that the balloon ruptures the foramen ovale. *C,* Balloon in the inferior vena cava. *D,* Catheter advanced to the right atrium to deflate the balloon. The time from A to C is less than 1 sec.

Some patients with transposition of the great arteries with associated anomalies may also require balloon atrial septostomy due to poor mixing, even through a VSD. Others may benefit by decompression of the left atrium to alleviate the symptoms of increased pulmonary blood flow and left-sided heart failure.

The **arterial switch (Jatene) procedure** is the surgical treatment of choice for neonates with d-TGA and an intact ventricular septum. The operation is usually performed within the first 2 wk of life. The reason for this urgency is that as pulmonary vascular resistance drops after birth, the pressure in the left ventricle (connected to the pulmonary vascular bed) will also drop. This results in a gradual decrease in left ventricular mass over the 1st few weeks of life. If the arterial switch operation is attempted after the left ventricular pressure has dropped too far, the left ventricle will be unable to generate adequate pressure to support the systemic circulation. The operation involves dividing the aorta and pulmonary artery just above the sinuses and reanastomosing them in their correct anatomic positions. The coronary arteries are then removed from the old aortic root along with a button of aortic wall and reimplanted in the old pulmonary root (the "neoaorta"). By using a button of great vessel tissue, the surgeon avoids having to suture directly on the coronary artery. Rarely, a two-stage arterial switch procedure may be employed in patients over 2–3 wk of age who already have a reduction of left ventricular muscle mass and pressure.

The arterial switch procedure has a survival rate of 90–95% for uncomplicated d-TGV. The arterial switch restores the normal physiologic relationships of systemic and pulmonary arterial blood flow and eliminates the long-term complications of the atrial switch procedure (see later). Although the risk of coronary artery injury and subsequent myocardial damage is present at the time of the arterial switch procedures, complications are rare. Most often ventricular function is excellent, sinus rhythm is maintained, and most patients remain asymptomatic. Intraoperative transesophageal echocardiography has been used at some centers to monitor ventricular function as the patient is being weaned from cardiopulmonary bypass to ensure that coronary perfusion has not been compromised.

Previous operations for d-TGV consisted of some form of atrial switch procedure (Mustard or Senning operation). In older infants these procedures produced excellent early survival (about 85–90%) but significant long-term morbidity. Atrial switch procedures reverse blood flow patterns at the atrial level by the surgical formation of an intra-atrial baffle, allowing systemic venous blood to be directed to the left atrium, left ventricle, and then via the pulmonary artery into the lungs. The baffle also permits oxygenated pulmonary venous blood to cross over to the right atrium, right ventricle, and aorta. The atrial switch procedures involve significant atrial surgery and may result in the late development of atrial conduction disturbances, sick-sinus syndrome with brady-tachyarrhythmias, paroxysmal atrial tachycardia, atrial flutter, sudden death, superior or inferior vena caval syndrome, edema, ascites, and protein-losing enteropathy. Atrial switch operations are now reserved for patients who are not candidates for the arterial switch operation, for example, those with TGV and significant pulmonic stenosis.

387.11 Transposition of the Great Arteries with Ventricular Septal Defect

If the VSD is small, the clinical manifestations, laboratory findings, and treatment are similar to those described earlier. Many of these small defects will eventually close spontaneously.

When the VSD is large and nonrestrictive to ventricular ejection, significant mixing of oxygenated and deoxygenated blood usually occurs and *clinical manifestations* of congestive cardiac failure are seen. The onset of cyanosis may be subtle and frequently delayed, and its intensity is variable. With careful observation, cyanosis can usually be recognized within the 1st mo of life, but some infants may remain undiagnosed for several months. The murmur is holosystolic and generally indistinguishable from that produced by a large VSD in patients with normally related great arteries. In contrast to patients with TGV and intact septum, the heart is usually significantly enlarged.

The cardiomegaly, narrow mediastinal waist, and increased pulmonary vascularity are demonstrated roentgenographically. The electrocardiogram shows prominent P waves and isolated right ventricular hypertrophy or biventricular hypertrophy. Occasionally, dominance of the left ventricle is present. Usually, the QRS axis is to the right, but sometimes it is normal or even to the left. The diagnosis can be confirmed by echocardiography and the extent of pulmonary blood flow can also be assessed by the degree of enlargement of the left atrium and ventricle. The *diagnosis* also may be confirmed by cardiac catheterization and angiocardiography. Right and left ventriculography indicate the presence of arterial transposition and demonstrate the site and size of the ventricular septal defect. Peak systolic pressures are equal in the two ventricles, the aorta, and the pulmonary artery. The left atrial pressure may be much higher than right atrial pressure, indicating a restrictive atrial level communication.

At the time of cardiac catheterization, a Rashkind balloon atrial septostomy may be performed, even in cases in which adequate mixing is occurring at the ventricular level, in order to decompress the left atrium. Surgical treatment is advised soon after diagnosis, usually within the first 2–4 mo of life, as congestive heart failure and failure to thrive are difficult to manage in these patients, and pulmonary vascular disease can develop unusually rapidly. Patients with this combination of defects are usually maintained on digitalis and diuretic therapy to lessen the symptoms of heart failure while awaiting surgical repair.

The patient with TGA and a VSD without pulmonic stenosis can be managed without pulmonary artery banding but with early neonatal atrial septostomy, if needed, and an arterial switch procedure combined with VSD closure. In these patients, the arterial switch operation can be performed after the first 2 wk of life because the VSD results in equal pressure in both ventricles and there is little regression in left ventricular muscle mass, thus permitting adequate left ventricular performance following surgical correction.

Without treatment, the *prognosis* is poor; the majority of patients succumb in the 1st yr of life because of congestive heart failure, hypoxemia, and pulmonary hypertension. In the past, some survived infancy with medical therapy alone but often developed pulmonary vascular disease. The clinical picture and treatment of these patients are similar to those described with Eisenmenger syndrome secondary to an isolated large VSD (see Chapter 386.28).

387.12 L-Transposition of the Great Arteries

(Corrected Transposition)

This malformation consists of discordant atrioventricular relationships (ventricular inversion) and transposition of the great arteries. Desaturated systemic venous blood is returned to a normally positioned right atrium, from which it passes through a bicuspid atrioventricular (mitral) valve into a right-sided ventricle that has the architecture and smooth wall morphology of the normal left ventricle. Because there is also transposition, desaturated blood ejected from this left ventricle enters the transposed pulmonary artery and flows into the lungs. Oxygenated pulmonary venous blood returns to a normally positioned left atrium, passes through a tricuspid atrioventricular valve into a left-sided ventricle, which has the morphology of a normal right ventricle, and is then ejected into the transposed aorta. The pulmonary artery lies in a medial position and the ascending aorta lies to the left (hence, l- or levo-transposition) and lateral, almost in the same horizontal plane. The double inversion of atrioventricular and ventriculoarterial relationships results in desaturated right atrial blood reaching the lungs, and oxygenated pulmonary venous blood appropriately flowing to the aorta. Thus, the circulation is physiologically "corrected." Without other defects, the hemodynamics would be nearly normal. However, in almost every instance associated anomalies coexist; most common are VSD, abnormalities of the left atrioventricular (tricuspid) valve, pulmonary valvular and/or subvalvular stenosis, and atrioventricular conduction disturbances (complete heart block).

CLINICAL MANIFESTATIONS. Symptoms and signs are determined by the associated lesions. If the pulmonary outflow is unobstructed, clinical signs will be similar to those of an isolated VSD. If there is pulmonary stenosis, clinical signs will be similar to tetralogy of Fallot. Posteroanterior chest roentgenograms may suggest the abnormal position of the great arteries; the ascending aorta occupies the upper left border of the cardiac silhouette and has a straight profile. In addition to atrioventricular conduction disturbances, the electrocardiogram may show abnormal P waves; absent QV_6; initial Q waves in leads III, aVR, aVF, and V_1; and upright T waves across the precordium.

Surgical *treatment* of the associated anomalies, most often the VSD, is complicated by the position of the bundle of His, which can be injured at the time of surgery, causing heart block. Identification of the usual course of the bundle in corrected transposition (running superior to the defect) has been accomplished by mapping of the conduction system so that the surgeon can avoid the bundle of His during open heart repair.

387.13 Double-Outlet Right Ventricle Without Pulmonary Stenosis

In this anomaly both the aorta and the pulmonary artery arise from the right ventricle (see also Chapter 387.6). The only outlet from the left ventricle is through a VSD. The *clinical manifestations* closely simulate that of an uncomplicated VSD with a large left-to-right shunt, although there may be mild systemic desaturation due to mixing of oxygenated and deoxygenated blood in the right ventricle. The electrocardiogram usually shows biventricular hypertrophy. Echocardiography is diagnostic, showing the right ventricular origin of both great vessels and their anteroposterior relationship as well as the position of the VSD. Cardiac catheterization and left ventricular angiography demonstrate the proximity of the VSD to the aorta, resulting in most of left ventricular blood being ejected directly into the systemic circulation. The angiogram will also confirm the lack of mitral-aortic fibrous continuity and shows the aortic valve displaced superiorly, at the same level as the pulmonary valve. It is important to differentiate this condition from a simple VSD.

Surgical correction is accomplished by creation of an intracardiac tunnel: blood is then ejected from the left ventricle via the VSD into the aorta. Pulmonary arterial banding may be required in infancy, followed by surgical correction during the preschool years. When there is associated pulmonary stenosis, there is more marked cyanosis and decreased pulmonary blood flow.

In **double-outlet right ventricle with transposition of the great arteries** (also known as the **Taussig-Bing anomaly**) the VSD is above the crista supraventricularis (supracristal or subarterial VSD) and is either directly subpulmonary or related to both pulmonary and aortic valves (doubly committed VSD). These patients develop cardiac failure early in infancy and are at risk for the development of pulmonary vascular disease and cyanosis. Cardiomegaly is usual, and there is a parasternal systolic ejection murmur, sometimes preceded by an ejection click and a loud closure of the pulmonary valve. Left-sided obstructive lesions are frequent, including coarctation of the aorta, interruption of the aortic arch, and a restrictive VSD, which obstructs left ventricular ejection. The electrocardiogram shows right axis deviation and right, left, or biventricular hypertrophy. The roentgenogram documents cardiomegaly, a large left atrium, and prominence of the pulmonary artery and pulmonary vasculature. The anatomic features of the anomaly and associated abnormalities are best demonstrated by a combination of echocardiography and selective right and left ventriculography. Palliation by pulmonary arterial banding in infancy will permit surgical correction at a later age, which may be accomplished by a Rastelli procedure (see Chapter 387.15) or by an arterial switch procedure (see Chapter 387.10).

387.14 Total Anomalous Pulmonary Venous Return (TAPVR)

PATHOPHYSIOLOGY. Abnormal development of the pulmonary veins may result in either partial or complete anomalous drain-

■ TABLE 387–1 Anomalous Pulmonary Venous Return

% and Site of Connection	% with Severe Obstruction
Supracardiac (50)	
Left superior vena cava (40)	40
Right superior vena cava (10)	75
Cardiac (25)	
Coronary sinus (20)	10
Right atrium (5)	5
Infracardiac (20)	95–100
Mixed (5)	

age into the systemic venous circulation. Partial anomalous pulmonary venous return is usually an acyanotic lesion (see Chapter 386.4). However, total anomalous pulmonary venous return produces total mixing of systemic venous and pulmonary venous blood flow within the heart and thus produces cyanosis.

In TAPVR there is no direct pulmonary venous connection into the left atrium, and all of the blood returning to the heart (the systemic and pulmonary venous blood) returns to the right atrium. The abnormal point of entry may be the right atrium directly, the superior or inferior vena cava or one of their major tributaries, or a persistent left superior vena cava that opens into the coronary sinus. The pulmonary veins may also join a common trunk (descending vein) that descends below the diaphragm and enters the venous circulation via the portal vein, ductus venosus, or inferior vena cava. This form of anomalous venous drainage is most commonly associated with obstruction, usually as the ductus venosus closes after birth, although supracardiac anomalous veins may also become obstructed.

In all forms of TAPVR there is mixing of oxygenated and deoxygenated blood before or at the level of the right atrium. Right atrial blood either passes into the right ventricle and pulmonary artery or passes through an ASD or patent foramen ovale into the left atrium. The right atrium and ventricle and the pulmonary artery are usually enlarged, whereas the left atrium and ventricle may be normal in size or small and less compliant. The presentation of total anomalous pulmonary venous return depends on the presence or absence of obstruction of the venous channel(s) (Table 387–1). If the pulmonary venous return is obstructed, severe pulmonary congestion and pulmonary hypertension occur, and rapid deterioration is common unless surgical intervention occurs.

CLINICAL MANIFESTATIONS. Three major clinical patterns of TAPVR are seen. Some infants present in the neonatal period with severe obstruction to pulmonary venous return. This is most prevalent in the infracardiac group (see Table 387–1). Cyanosis is prominent, and there is severe tachypnea. There may be no murmurs present on physical examination. These infants are usually severely ill and may fail to respond to mechanical ventilation. Rapid diagnosis and surgical correction are necessary. Another group of patients also presents with congestive heart failure in early life, but in these infants there is a large left-to-right shunt; obstruction to pulmonary venous return is only mild or moderate. Because pulmonary artery hypertension is present, these infants will be severely ill. Systolic murmurs along the left sternal border are audible, and there may be a gallop rhythm. A continuous murmur is occasionally heard along the upper left sternal border over the pulmonary area. Cyanosis is mild. The third group of patients with TAPVR are those in whom pulmonary venous obstruction is not present at all. In this situation there is total mixing of systemic venous and pulmonary venous blood and a large net left-to-right shunt. Pulmonary hypertension is absent, and these patients are less likely to be severely symptomatic during infancy. Clinical cyanosis is usually mild or absent.

DIAGNOSIS. The *electrocardiogram* demonstrates right ventricular hypertrophy (usually a qR pattern in V_4R and V_1, and the P waves are frequently tall and spiked). *Roentgenograms* are pathognomonic in older children if the pulmonary veins enter the innominate vein and persistent left superior vena cava (Fig. 387–7). There is a large supracardiac shadow, together with the cardiac shadow, forming a *snowman* appearance. The supracardiac shadow is produced by the dilated left superior vena cava, left innominate vein, and right superior vena cava. However, this appearance is not helpful for diagnosis in early infancy because of the presence of the thymus. In most cases of total anomalous pulmonary venous return without obstruction, the heart is enlarged, the pulmonary artery and right ventricle are prominent, and the pulmonary vascularity is increased. In neonates having severe cyanosis due to marked pulmonary venous obstruction (usually infradiaphragmatic),

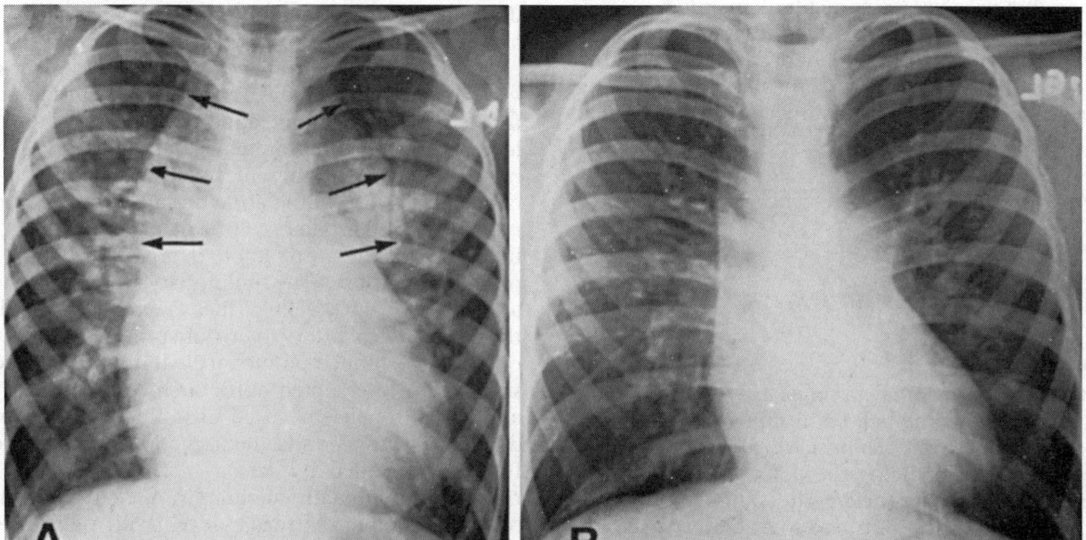

Figure 387–7. Roentgenograms of total anomalous pulmonary venous return to the left superior vena cava. *A*, Preoperative. *Arrows* point to the supracardiac shadow, which produces the snowman or figure 8 configuration. Cardiomegaly and increased pulmonary vascularity are evident. *B*, Postoperative, showing decrease in size of the heart and supracardiac shadow.

the chest roentgenogram demonstrates a perihilar pattern of pulmonary edema and a small heart. This appearance can be confused with primary pulmonary disease. The differential diagnosis includes persistent pulmonary hypertension of the newborn, respiratory distress syndrome, pneumonia (bacterial, meconium aspiration), pulmonary lymphangiectasia, and other heart defects (hypoplastic left heart syndrome).

The *echocardiogram* reflects the right ventricular overload and is usually able to identify the pattern of abnormal pulmonary venous connections. The abnormal venous channel may be seen in either supracardiac or infracardiac locations. The demonstration of a venous channel in the abdomen with Doppler showing flow away from the heart is pathognomonic of TAPVR below the diaphragm. Shunting occurs almost exclusively right to left at atrial level.

Cardiac catheterization shows that the oxygen saturations of blood in both atria, both ventricles, and the aorta are more or less similar. An increase in systemic venous saturation occurs at the site of entry of the abnormal pulmonary venous channel. In older patients the pulmonary arterial and right ventricular pressures may be only moderately elevated, but in infants who present with pulmonary venous obstruction, pulmonary hypertension is usual. *Selective pulmonary arteriography* shows the anatomy of the pulmonary veins and their point of entry into the systemic venous circulation.

TREATMENT. Surgical correction of total anomalous pulmonary venous return during infancy is indicated. Prior to surgery, infants may be stabilized with prostaglandin (PGE_1) to dilate the ductus venosus and the ductus arteriosus; some may require balloon atrial septostomy; however, this is of little or no benefit in the presence of pulmonary venous obstruction. Surgically, the common pulmonary venous trunk is anastomosed directly to the left atrium, the atrial septal defect is closed, and the connection to the systemic venous circuit is interrupted. Results have been generally good, even for critically ill neonates. If the postoperative hemodynamics are normal, the prognosis is excellent. The postoperative period may be complicated by pulmonary vascular hypertensive crises. In some patients, especially those in whom diagnosis may have been delayed, persistent pulmonary hypertension may occur and the long-term prognosis in these patients is poor. Long-term complications include restenosis of the pulmonary venous channel to left atrial communication. This is especially a problem in patients with stenosis of the individual pulmonary veins, in whom the prognosis is particularly guarded.

Without treatment, the prognosis for the great majority of patients with total anomalous pulmonary venous return is poor, and survival beyond infancy is unusual in the presence of pulmonary hypertension. Death is due to congestive heart failure. Patients who survive beyond 2 yr of age are those who do not have obstruction and pulmonary arterial hypertension, and they may remain asymptomatic for many years.

387.15 Truncus Arteriosus

PATHOPHYSIOLOGY. In this anomaly a single arterial trunk (truncus arteriosus) arises from the heart and supplies the systemic, pulmonary, and coronary circulations. A VSD is always present, with the truncus over-riding the defect, receiving blood from both right and left ventricles. The number of truncal semilunar valve cusps varies from two to as many as six. The pulmonary arteries may arise together from the posterior left side of the persistent truncus arteriosus and then divide into left and right pulmonary arteries (type I truncus arteriosus). In types II and III there is no main pulmonary artery and the right and left pulmonary arteries arise from separate orifices in the posterior (type II) or lateral (type III) sides of the truncus arteriosus. Type IV truncus has no identifiable connection between the heart and pulmonary arteries, and pulmonary blood flow derives from major aorto-pulmonary collateral arteries (MAPCAs) arising from the transverse or descending aorta; this form has also been called *pseudotruncus* but is essentially a form of pulmonary atresia with a VSD (see Chapter 387.3).

Both ventricles are at systemic pressure and both eject blood into the truncus. When the pulmonary vascular resistance is relatively high immediately after birth, pulmonary blood flow may be normal; however, as pulmonary resistance drops over the 1st mo of life, blood flow to the lungs is greatly increased and congestive heart failure ensues. Because of the large volume of pulmonary blood flow, clinical cyanosis is usually minimal. If untreated, the pulmonary resistance will eventually increase, pulmonary blood flow decreases, and cyanosis becomes more apparent (Eisenmenger physiology, see Chapter 386.28). The truncal valve is occasionally incompetent, significantly complicating medical and surgical management.

CLINICAL MANIFESTATIONS. The clinical signs of truncus arteriosus vary with age, depending on the level of the pulmonary vascular resistance. In the newborn period, signs of congestive heart failure are usually absent, and a murmur and minimal cyanosis are the presenting signs. In the majority of infants beyond the immediate newborn period, pulmonary blood flow is torrential and the clinical picture is dominated by signs of congestive heart failure: dyspnea, fatigue, recurrent respiratory infections, and poor physical growth. Untreated, these patients usually die during infancy. Cyanosis is minimal. The runoff of blood from the truncus to the pulmonary circulation may result in a wide pulse pressure and bounding pulses. This may be further exaggerated by truncal valve insufficiency. The heart is usually enlarged, and the precordium is hyperdynamic. The 2nd heart sound is loud and single. A systolic ejection murmur, sometimes accompanied by a thrill, is usually audible along the left sternal border. The murmur is frequently preceded by an early systolic ejection click. In the presence of truncal valve insufficiency, a high-pitched early diastolic decrescendo murmur is heard at the upper right and mid-left sternal border. An apical mid-diastolic rumbling murmur, caused by increased flow through the mitral valve, is audible with the bell of the stethoscope. In older children with restricted pulmonary blood flow secondary to the development of pulmonary vascular obstructive disease, progressive cyanosis, polycythemia, and clubbing develop. The manifestation is seen in patients having DiGeorge syndrome (see Chapter 118.1).

DIAGNOSIS. The *electrocardiogram* shows right, left, or combined ventricular hypertrophy. There is also considerable variation in the roentgenographic appearance of the chest. Cardiac enlargement is due to prominence of both ventricles. The truncus may produce a prominent shadow that follows the normal course of the ascending aorta and aortic knob; the aortic arch is to the right in almost 50% of patients. Sometimes a high bulge, left of the aortic knob, is produced by the main or left pulmonary artery. The pulmonary vascularity will increase after the 1st few weeks of life. *Echocardiography* demonstrates the large truncal artery over-riding the VSD and the pattern of origin of the branch pulmonary arteries. Associated anomalies, such as an interrupted aortic arch, can be ruled out. Pulsed and color Doppler are used to evaluate for the presence and degree of truncal valve regurgitation. The diagnosis may be further confirmed by *cardiac catheterization* and by selective right and/or left ventriculography. A left-to-right shunt is demonstrated at the ventricular level, with right-to-left shunting into the truncus. Systolic pressures in both ventricles and the truncus are similar. Angiocardiography reveals the large truncus arteriosus, defines more precisely the origin of the pulmonary arteries, and allows assessment of the competence of this valve.

PROGNOSIS AND COMPLICATIONS. Without surgery, many of these patients succumb during infancy or by the 1st or 2nd yr of life. If pulmonary blood flow is restricted by the development of pulmonary vascular disease, the patient may survive into early adulthood.

TREATMENT. Open heart repair of truncus arteriosus is accomplished in infancy. In the 1st few weeks of life many of these infants can be managed with anticongestive medications; however, as pulmonary vascular resistance falls, heart failure symptoms worsen and surgery is indicated, usually at 4–8 wk of life. Delay of surgery much beyond this period may increase the likelihood of development of pulmonary vascular disease. At surgery, the VSD is closed, the pulmonary arteries are separated from the truncus, and continuity is established between the right ventricle and the pulmonary arteries with a homograft conduit (Rastelli repair). Immediate surgical results are excellent, but after repair in infancy the conduit must be replaced, often several times, as the child grows. In older patients who have already developed pulmonary vascular obstruction, routine surgical treatment is contraindicated and heart-lung transplantation is the only available option.

387.16 Single Ventricle

(Double-Inlet Ventricle, Univentricular Heart)

PATHOPHYSIOLOGY. With a single ventricle, both atria empty through a common valve or via two separate atrioventricular valves into a single ventricular chamber. This chamber may be of left, right, or indeterminate ventricular anatomic characteristics. The aorta and pulmonary artery both arise from this single chamber. Associated cardiac anomalies are frequent and vary considerably. Transposition of the great arteries and presence of a rudimentary outlet chamber below one of the great vessels occur in the vast majority of patients. Pulmonary stenosis or atresia is also common.

CLINICAL MANIFESTATIONS. The clinical picture is variable, depending on the associated intracardiac anomalies and hemodynamics in the individual patient. If the pulmonary outflow is obstructed, the presentation may be similar to that of tetralogy of Fallot: marked cyanosis without heart failure. If the pulmonary outflow is unobstructed, the presentation will be similar to that of transposition with VSD: minimal cyanosis with marked heart failure.

In patients with pulmonary stenosis, cyanosis is present in infancy and increases in intensity during childhood, when clubbing and polycythemia also appear. Dyspnea and fatigue are frequent, cardiomegaly is mild or moderate, a left parasternal lift is palpable, and a systolic thrill is common. The systolic ejection murmur is usually loud; an ejection click may be audible, and the 2nd heart sound is single and loud.

When a single ventricle is associated with an unobstructed pulmonary outflow tract, pulmonary blood flow is torrential. These patients present in early infancy with tachypnea, dyspnea, failure to thrive, and recurrent pulmonary infections. Cyanosis is only mild or moderate. Cardiomegaly is generally marked, and a left parasternal lift is palpable. The systolic ejection murmur is generally not intense, and the 2nd heart sound is loud and closely split. A 3rd heart sound is common and may be followed by a short mid-diastolic rumbling murmur caused by increased flow through the atrioventricular valves. The development of pulmonary vascular disease in patients who have not been operated on may restrict pulmonary blood flow so that cyanosis increases in intensity, heart size decreases, and signs of cardiac failure appear to improve (Eisenmenger physiology, see Chapter 386.28).

DIAGNOSIS. The *electrocardiogram* is nonspecific. P waves are normal, spiked, or bifid. The precordial lead pattern suggests right ventricular hypertrophy, combined ventricular hypertrophy, or sometimes left ventricular dominance. The initial QRS forces are usually to the left and anterior. *Roentgenographic examination* confirms the degree of cardiomegaly. If present, a rudimentary outflow chamber may produce a bulge on the upper left border of the cardiac silhouette in the posteroanterior projection. In the absence of pulmonary stenosis, the pulmonary vasculature is increased. In the presence of pulmonary stenosis, the pulmonary vasculature is diminished. A large main pulmonary artery with rapid attenuation of the size of the peripheral pulmonary arteries occurs in the presence of severe pulmonary vascular disease. Absence or near absence of the ventricular septum is the principal *echocardiographic* sign. The echocardiogram can usually determine whether the single ventricle has features of right, left, or mixed morphology. The presence of a rudimentary outflow chamber under one of the great vessels can be determined, and pulsed Doppler can be used to determine whether there is any obstruction to flow through this communication (bulboventricular foramen).

If *cardiac catheterization* is performed, the arterial oxygen saturation will be decreased in the presence of severe pulmonary stenosis or obstructive pulmonary hypertension but may be near normal when pulmonary blood flow is unimpeded. The pressure in the ventricular chamber is at the systemic level; a gradient may be demonstrated across the entrance to a rudimentary outflow chamber. Pressure measurements and angiography will demonstrate whether pulmonary stenosis is present. Severe pulmonary hypertension may be demonstrated in older patients in the absence of pulmonary stenosis. Selective ventriculography is diagnostic.

PROGNOSIS AND COMPLICATIONS. Unoperated, some patients succumb during infancy from congestive heart failure. Others may survive to adolescence and early adult life but finally succumb to the effects of chronic hypoxemia, or, in the absence of pulmonary stenosis, to the sequelae of pulmonary vascular disease. Patients with moderate pulmonary stenosis have the best prognosis, because pulmonary blood flow, although restricted, is still adequate.

TREATMENT. If pulmonary stenosis is severe, an aorto-pulmonary shunt is indicated. If pulmonary blood flow is unrestricted, pulmonary arterial banding is used to control heart failure and to prevent progressive pulmonary vascular disease. The Glenn shunt followed by a modified Fontan operation (cavo-pulmonary isolation procedure, see Chapter 387.5) is the ultimate treatment of choice for children whose pulmonary resistance is low, either secondary to pulmonary stenosis or after pulmonary artery banding. If subaortic stenosis is present secondary to a restrictive rudimentary outflow chamber, surgical relief can be provided by anastomosing the proximal pulmonary artery to the side of the ascending aorta (Damus-Stansyl-Kaye operation).

387.17 Hypoplastic Left Heart Syndrome

PATHOPHYSIOLOGY. This term is used to describe a closely related group of anomalies that include underdevelopment of the left side of the heart (e.g., atresia of the aortic or mitral orifice) and hypoplasia of the ascending aorta. The left ventricle may be small and nonfunctional, or totally atretic; the right ventricle maintains both pulmonary and systemic circulations. Pulmonary venous blood passes through an atrial defect or dilated foramen ovale from the left to the right side of the heart, where it mixes with systemic venous blood. When the ventricular septum is intact, which is almost always the case, all of the right ventricular blood is ejected into the main pulmonary artery; the descending aorta is supplied via the ductus arteriosus, with flow from the ductus also filling the ascending aorta and coronary arteries in a retrograde fashion. In the presence of a VSD and a patent but small aortic orifice, right ventricular blood is ejected to the small left ventricle and ascending aorta, as well as to the pulmonary artery. The major hemodynamic abnormalities are inadequate maintenance of the systemic circulation and, depending on the size of the atrial level communication, either pulmonary venous hypertension (restrictive foramen ovale) or pulmonary overcirculation (ASD).

CLINICAL MANIFESTATIONS. Although cyanosis may not always be obvious in the first 48 hr of life, a grayish blue color of the skin is soon apparent, a mix of cyanosis and hypoperfusion. Most infants are diagnosed in the 1st few hours or days of life. If the ductus arteriosus partially closes, signs of systemic hypoperfusion and shock predominate. Signs of congestive heart failure will usually appear within the 1st few days or weeks of life and include dyspnea, hepatomegaly, and low cardiac output. All of the peripheral pulses are weak or absent. Cardiac enlargement is usual, with a palpable right ventricular parasternal lift. A nondescript systolic murmur is usually present. Extracardiac anomalies, particularly renal and CNS, may be present.

DIAGNOSIS. On the chest *roentgenogram,* the heart is variable in size in the 1st days of life, but cardiomegaly develops rapidly and is associated with increased pulmonary vascularity. The *electrocardiogram* may show only the normal right ventricular dominance initially, but later P waves become prominent and right ventricular hypertrophy is usual. The *echocardiogram* is diagnostic (Fig. 387–8). There is absence or hypoplasia of the mitral valve and aortic root, a variably small left atrium and posterior (left) ventricle, a large right atrium and anterior (right) ventricle, and an easily identifiable tricuspid valve. The size of the atrial communication, by which pulmonary venous blood leaves the left atrium, can be assessed directly and by pulsed and color flow Doppler. Suprasternal notch views identify the small ascending aorta and transverse aortic arch, and may also demonstrate a discrete coarctation of the aorta in the juxtaductal area. Doppler demonstrates the absence of anterograde flow in the ascending aorta and the presence of retrograde flow via the ductus arteriosus. These findings are so characteristic that the diagnosis of hypoplastic left heart syndrome can usually be made without the need for cardiac catheterization. If a catheterization is necessary, the hypoplastic ascending aorta can be well demonstrated by aortography.

PROGNOSIS AND COMPLICATIONS. Patients most often succumb during the first months of life, usually during the 1st week or two. Occasionally patients may live for months or rarely years. One third of infants with hypoplastic left heart syndrome have evidence of either a major or minor CNS abnormality. Other dysmorphic features may be found in up to 40%. Thus, careful preoperative evaluation (genetic, neurologic, and ophthalmologic) should be performed in those patients being considered for either standard surgical or transplant therapy.

TREATMENT. There is variable success in the surgical therapy of hypoplastic left heart syndrome. Management options include palliation (the Norwood procedure), heart transplantation, and, in some patients, supportive expectant care.

If a *Norwood procedure* is to be performed, preoperative medical management includes correction of acidosis and hypoglycemia, maintenance of the patency of the ductus arteriosus with prostaglandin E_1 to support systemic blood flow, and prevention of hypothermia. A Rashkind balloon atrial septostomy may be indicated if surgery is delayed.

The Norwood procedure is usually performed in three stages. The first stage (Fig. 387–9) includes an atrial septectomy and transection and ligation of the distal main pulmonary artery; the proximal pulmonary artery is then connected to the transversely opened hypoplastic aortic arch, forming a "neo-aorta," and the coarcted segment of the aorta is repaired. A synthetic aorto-pulmonary shunt connects the aorta to the main pulmonary artery at the bifurcation of the left and right pulmonary arteries to provide controlled pulmonary blood flow. The operative risk for the first-stage Norwood procedure is high and varies greatly among centers, although the best reported results demonstrate a better than 75% survival.

The second stage consists of a Glenn anastamosis, connecting the superior vena cava to the pulmonary arteries (see Chapter 387.5). This is followed by a modified Fontan procedure (cavo-

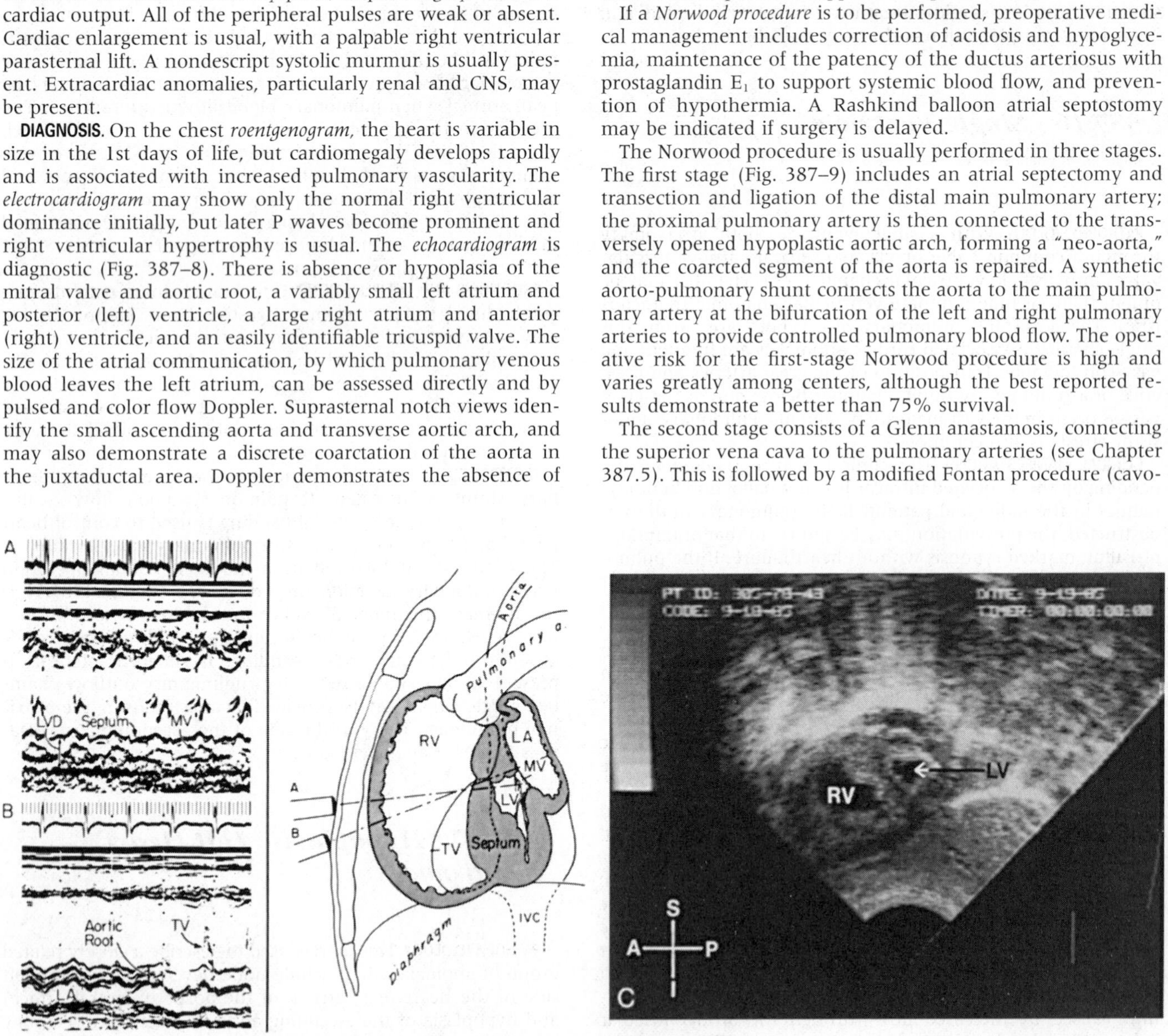

Figure 387–8. Echocardiogram from a neonate with aortic valve atresia. The idealized diagram in the center shows the small left ventricle and aorta. Echogram *A* (from transducer position *A*) shows minute left ventricular dimension (LVD) containing a small mitral valve (MV). Echogram *B* shows a small aortic root and left atrium. *C,* Subxiphoid ventricular short axis two-dimensional echocardiographic projection demonstrates thick-walled, hypoplastic left ventricle in patient with aortic atresia and severe mitral stenosis. LV = left ventricular cavity; RV = right ventricular cavity.

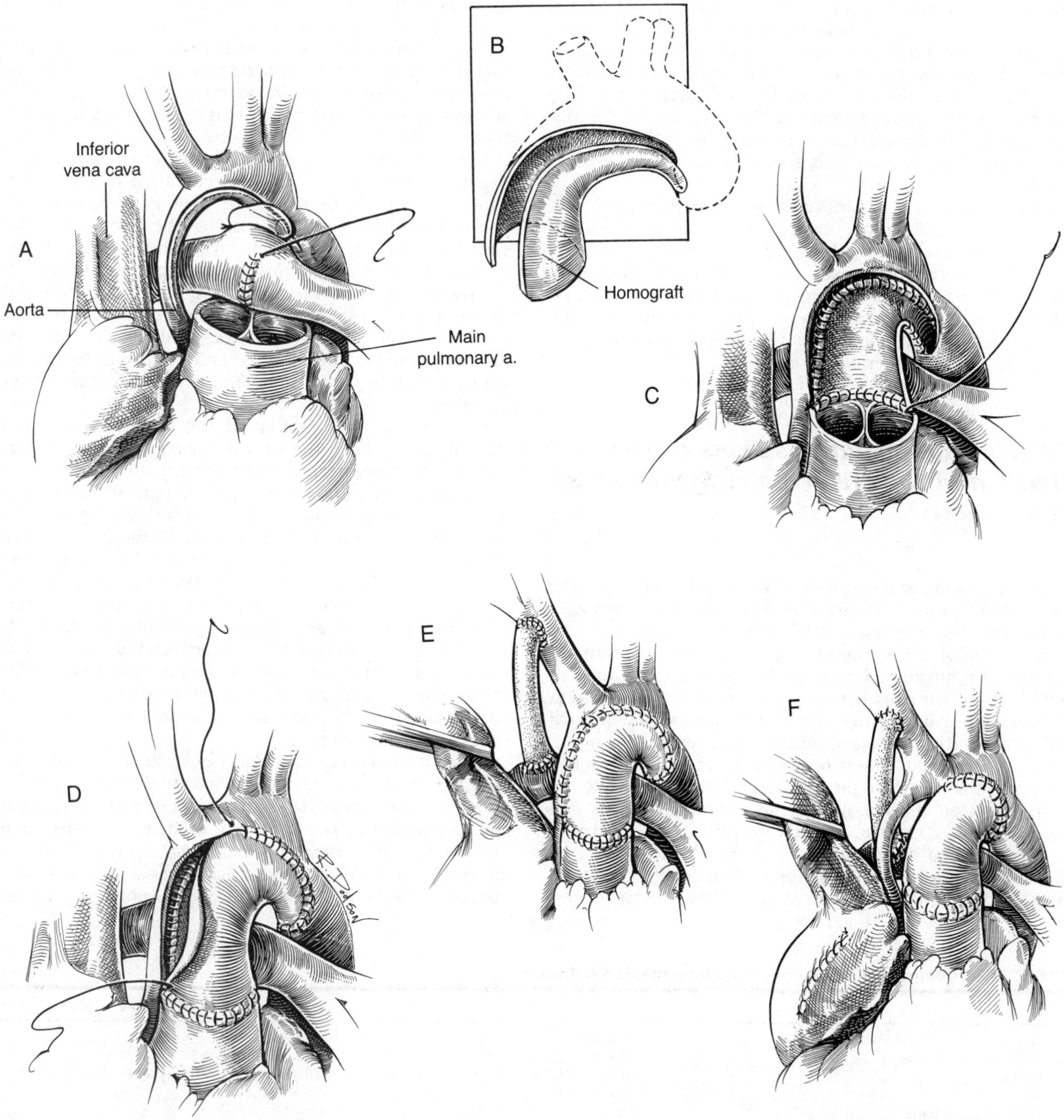

Figure 387–9. Current techniques for first-stage palliation of the hypoplastic left heart syndrome. *A,* Incisions used for the procedure, incorporating a cuff of arterial wall allograft. The distal divided main pulmonary artery may be closed by direct suture or with a patch. *B,* Dimensions of the cuff of the arterial wall allograft. *C,* The arterial wall allograft is used to supplement the anastomosis between the proximal divided main pulmonary artery and the ascending aorta, aortic arch, and proximal descending aorta. *D* and *E,* The procedure is completed by an atrial septectomy and a 3.5 mm modified right Blalock shunt. *F,* When the ascending aorta is particularly small, an alternative procedure involves placement of a complete tube of arterial allograft. The tiny ascending aorta may be left in situ, as indicated, or implanted into the side of the neoaorta. (From Castaneda AR, Jonas RA, Mayer Jr JE, Hanley FL: Single-ventricle tricuspid atresia. *In:* Cardiac Surgery of the Neonate and Infant. Philadelphia, WB Saunders, 1994.)

pulmonary isolation) connecting the inferior vena cava to the pulmonary arteries via an intra-atrial baffle. After the third stage, all systemic venous return enters the pulmonary circulation directly. Pulmonary venous flow enters the left atrium and is directed across the atrial septum to the tricuspid valve and subsequently the right (now the systemic) ventricle. Blood leaves the right ventricle via the "neo-aorta," which supplies the systemic circulation. Coronary blood flow is provided by the old aortic root, now attached to the "neo-aorta." The risk of completing all three stages is considerable, and the long-term results of the Norwood procedure remain to be demonstrated.

An alternate therapy is cardiac transplantation, either in the immediate neonatal period, obviating stage I of the Norwood procedure, or after a successful stage I Norwood procedure is performed as a bridge to transplantation. After transplantation, patients will usually have normal cardiac function and no symptoms of heart failure; however, these patients have the chronic risks of organ rejection and life-long immunosuppressive therapy (see Chapter 401).

387.18 Abnormal Positions of the Heart and the Heterotaxy Syndromes

(Asplenia, Polysplenia)

The classification and diagnosis of abnormal cardiac position is best performed using a segmental approach. This begins with determination of the *visceroatrial situs* by roentgenographic demonstration of the position of the abdominal organs and of the tracheal bifurcation for recognition of the right and left bronchi. The atrial situs is related to the situs of the viscera and lungs. In **situs solitus,** the viscera are in their normal position (stomach and spleen on the left, liver on the right), the three-lobed right lung is on the right, and the two-lobed left lung on the left; the right atrium is on the right, while the left atrium is on the left. When the abdominal organs and lungs are reversed, known as **situs inversus,** the left atrium is to the right and the right atrium to the left. If the visceroatrial situs cannot be readily determined, a condition known as **situs indeterminus** or **heterotaxia** exists. The two major variations are **asplenia syndrome** (right isomerism or bilateral right-sidedness), associated with a centrally located liver, absent spleen, and two morphologic right lungs; and **polysplenia syndrome** (left isomerism or bilateral left-sidedness), associated with multiple small spleens, absence of the intrahepatic portion of the inferior vena cava, and bilateral morphologic left lungs. The heterotaxia syndromes are usually associated with severe congenital heart lesions: ASDs, pulmonary stenosis or atresia, and anomalous systemic venous or pulmonary venous return (Table 387–2).

The next segment is the *localization of the ventricles,* which depends on the direction of development of the embryonic cardiac loop. Initial protrusion of the loop to the right (d-loop) carries the future right ventricle to the right, while the left ventricle remains on the left. With situs solitus, this yields normal atrioventricular connections (right atrium connects to right ventricle, left atrium to left ventricle). Protrusion of the loop to the left (l-loop) carries the future right ventricle to the left and the left ventricle to the right. In this case, in the presence of situs solitus, the right atrium connects with the left ventricle and the left atrium with the right ventricle (*ventricular inversion*).

The final segment is that of the *great vessels.* With each type of cardiac loop, the ventricular-arterial relations may be regarded as either normal (right ventricle to pulmonary artery, left ventricle to aorta) or transposed (right ventricle to aorta, left ventricle to pulmonary artery). A further classification can be made depending on the position of the aorta relative to the pulmonary artery, normally to the right and posterior. In transposition, the aorta is usually anterior, and either to the right of the pulmonary artery (d-transposition) or to the left (l-transposition). These segmental relationships can be determined by echocardiographic and angiographic studies demonstrating both atrioventricular and ventriculoarterial relationships. The clinical manifestations of these syndromes of abnormal cardiac position are dominated by their associated cardiovascular anomalies.

Dextrocardia occurs when the apex of the heart points to the right; levocardia (the normal situation) when the apex points to the left. **Dextrocardia without associated situs inversus** and **levocardia in the presence of situs inversus** are most often complicated by severe malformations that include various combinations of single ventricle, arterial transposition, pulmonary stenosis, ASDs and VSDs, atrioventricular septal de-

■ **TABLE 387–2 Comparison of Cardiosplenic Heterotaxia Syndromes**

	Asplenia	Polysplenia
Spleen	Absent	Multiple
Sidedness (isomerism)	Bilateral right	Bilateral left
Lungs	Bilateral trilobar with eparterial bronchi	Bilateral bilobar with hyparterial bronchi
Sex	Male (65%)	Female ≥ male
Right-sided stomach	Yes	Less common
Symmetric liver	Yes	Yes
Partial intestinal rotation	Yes	Yes
Dextrocardia (%)	30–40	30–40
Pulmonary blood flow	Decreased	Increased
Severe cyanosis	Yes	No
Transposition of great arteries (%)	60–75	15
Total anomalous pulmonary venous return (%)	70–80	Rare
Common atrioventricular valve (%)	80–90	20–40
Single ventricle (%)	40–50	10–15
Absent inferior vena cava with azygos continuation	No	Characteristic
Bilateral superior vena cava	Yes	Yes
Other common defects	PA, PS	Partial anomalous pulmonary venous return, ventricular septal defect, double-outlet right ventricle
Risk of sepsis	Yes	No
Howell-Jolly and Heinz bodies, pitted erythrocytes	Yes	No
Absent gallbladder; biliary atresia	No	Yes
Mortality	High	Moderately high if symptomatic

PA = pulmonary atresia; PS = pulmonary stenosis.

fect, anomalous pulmonary venous return, tricuspid atresia, and pulmonary arterial hypoplasia or atresia. Surveys of older children and adults indicate that dextrocardia with situs inversus and with normally related great arteries (so-called mirror-image dextrocardia) is most often associated with a functionally normal heart, although congenital heart disease of a less severe nature is common.

Anatomic or functional abnormalities of the lung, diaphragm, and thoracic cage may result in displacement of the heart to the right (*dextroposition*), mimicking dextrocardia. However, in this case the cardiac apex is pointed normally to the left. This is less often associated with congenital heart lesions, although hypoplasia of a lung may be accompanied by anomalous pulmonary venous return from that lung.

The electrocardiogram is difficult to interpret in the presence of lesions with discordant atrial, ventricular, and great vessel anatomy. Diagnosis usually requires detailed echocardiographic, hemodynamic, and angiographic studies. There may be mutations in the connexin 43 gap junction gene. Prognosis and treatment of patients with one of the cardiac positional anomalies are determined by the underlying defects. Asplenia increases the risk of serious infections such as endocarditis and requires antibiotic prophylaxis.

Other Congenital Heart Malformations

387.19 Pulmonary Arteriovenous Fistula

Fistulous vascular communications in the lungs may be large and localized, or multiple, scattered, or small. The most common form of this unusual condition is the **Osler-Weber-Rendu syndrome** (hereditary hemorrhagic telangiectasia), which is also manifested by angiomas of the nasal and buccal mucous membranes, gastrointestinal tract, or liver. The usual communication is between the pulmonary artery and pulmonary vein; direct communication between the pulmonary artery and left atrium is extremely rare. Desaturated blood in the pulmonary artery is shunted through the fistula into the pulmonary vein, bypassing the lungs, enters the left heart, and results in systemic arterial desaturation and sometimes clinical cyanosis. The shunt across the fistula is at low pressure and resistance, so that pulmonary arterial pressure is normal; cardiomegaly and heart failure are not present.

The *clinical manifestations* depend on the magnitude of the shunt. Large fistulas are associated with dyspnea, cyanosis, clubbing, a continuous murmur, and polycythemia. Hemoptysis is rare, but when it occurs may be massive. Features of the Osler-Weber-Rendu syndrome occur in about 50% of patients (or other family members) and include recurrent epistaxis and gastrointestinal tract bleeding. Transitory dizziness, diplopia, aphasia, motor weakness, or convulsions may result from cerebral thrombosis, abscess, or paradoxic emboli. Soft systolic or continuous murmurs may be audible over the site of the fistula. The electrocardiogram is normal. Roentgenographic examination of the chest may show opacities produced by large fistulas; multiple small fistulas may be visualized by fluoroscopy (as abnormal pulsations), MRI, or CT scan. Selective pulmonary arteriography demonstrates the site, extent, and distribution of the fistulae.

Treatment by excision of solitary or localized lesions by lobectomy or wedge resection results in complete disappearance of symptoms. However, in most instances fistulas are so widespread that surgery is not possible. If there is a direct communication between the pulmonary artery and left atrium, it can be obliterated by division and suture.

387.20 Ectopia Cordis

In the most common thoracic form of ectopia cordis the sternum is split and the heart protrudes outside the chest. In other forms the heart protrudes through the diaphragm into the abdominal cavity or may be situated in the neck. Associated intracardiac anomalies are common. Death occurs in the 1st days of life in most instances, usually from infection, cardiac failure, or hypoxemia. Surgical therapy for neonates without overwhelmingly severe cardiac anomalies consists of covering the heart with skin without compromising venous return or ventricular ejection. Palliation of associated defects is also often necessary. Occasional patients with the abdominal type have survived to adulthood.

387.21 Diverticulum of the Left Ventricle

In this rare anomaly a diverticulum of the left ventricle protrudes into the epigastrium. The lesion may be isolated or associated with complex cardiovascular anomalies. A pulsating mass is visible and palpable in the epigastrium. Systolic or systolic-diastolic murmurs produced by blood flow in and out of the diverticulum may be audible over the lower sternum and the mass. The *electrocardiogram* shows a pattern of complete or incomplete left bundle branch block. *Roentgenograms* of the chest may or may not show the mass. Associated abnormalities include defects of the sternum, abdominal wall, diaphragm, and pericardium. Surgical treatment of the diverticulum and of associated cardiac defects can be utilized in selected cases. Occasionally a diverticulum may be small and not associated with clinical signs or symptoms. These small diverticuli are diagnosed at the time of echocardiographic examination for other indications.

387.22 Primary Pulmonary Hypertension

PATHOPHYSIOLOGY. This disorder, of unknown origin, is characterized by pulmonary vascular obstructive disease and right-sided heart failure. It may occur at any age, although most pediatric patients present between 10 and 20 yr of age. A genetic component may be present, and there is evidence in some cases of an immunologic disorder. Pulmonary hypertension is associated with precapillary obstruction of the pulmonary vascular bed due to hyperplasia of the muscular and elastic tissues, and to a thickened intima of the small pulmonary arteries and arterioles. Atherosclerotic changes may be found in the larger pulmonary arteries. For the diagnosis of primary pulmonary hypertension, other causes of pulmonary-related heart disease (cor pulmonale) must be absent. This disease is rare in childhood, except in the setting of a chronic indwelling intravascular catheter, where severe pulmonary hypertension may result from myriads of minute microemboli. Primary pulmonary hypertension must also be differentiated from elevated pulmonary pressure resulting from persistent obstruction of the upper airway (e.g., gross enlargement of the tonsils and adenoids), liver disease, or chronic pulmonary parenchymal disease. Female patients outnumber males 1.7:1.

Pulmonary hypertension places an afterload burden on the right ventricle, which results in right ventricular hypertrophy. Dilatation of the pulmonary artery is present, and pulmonary valve insufficiency may occur. In the later stages of the disease, the right ventricle begins to dilate, tricuspid insufficiency develops, and cardiac output is decreased.

CLINICAL MANIFESTATIONS. The predominant symptoms include effort intolerance and fatigability; occasionally, there is precordial chest pain, dizziness, syncope, or headaches. Peripheral cyanosis may be present and is associated with cold extremities; in the late stages of the disease, the patient may have a gray appearance associated with low cardiac output. Arterial oxygen saturation is usually normal. If right-sided heart failure has supervened, the jugular venous pressure is elevated, and hepatomegaly and edema are present. Jugular venous "a" waves are present, and when there is functional tricuspid insufficiency, a conspicuous jugular "cv" wave and systolic hepatic pulsations are manifest. The heart is moderately enlarged, and there is a right ventricular heave. The 1st heart sound is often followed by an ejection click emanating from the dilated pulmonary artery. The 2nd heart sound is closely split, loud, and sometimes booming; it is frequently palpable at the upper left sternal border. A presystolic gallop rhythm may be audible at the lower left sternal border. The systolic murmur is soft and short, and is sometimes followed by a blowing diastolic murmur due to pulmonary insufficiency. In later stages, a holosystolic murmur of tricuspid insufficiency will be appreciated at the lower left sternal border.

Chest roentgenograms reveal a prominent pulmonary artery and right ventricle (Fig. 387–10). The pulmonary vascularity in the hilar areas may be prominent and contrast with the peripheral lung fields, which are clear. The electrocardiogram shows right ventricular hypertrophy with spiked P waves.

DIAGNOSIS. At cardiac catheterization this condition must be differentiated from Eisenmenger syndrome (see Chapter 386.28), which is associated with a communication between the left and right sides of the heart or great arteries, as well as from left-sided obstructive lesions that result in pulmonary venous hypertension (see Chapter 386.21). The presence of pulmonary artery hypertension with a normal pulmonary capillary wedge pressure is diagnostic of primary pulmonary hypertension. The risks of cardiac catheterization may be high in severely ill patients with primary pulmonary hypertension; syncope, bradycardia, or death may occur after pulmonary artery angiography (which should rarely be done in the most severely ill individuals).

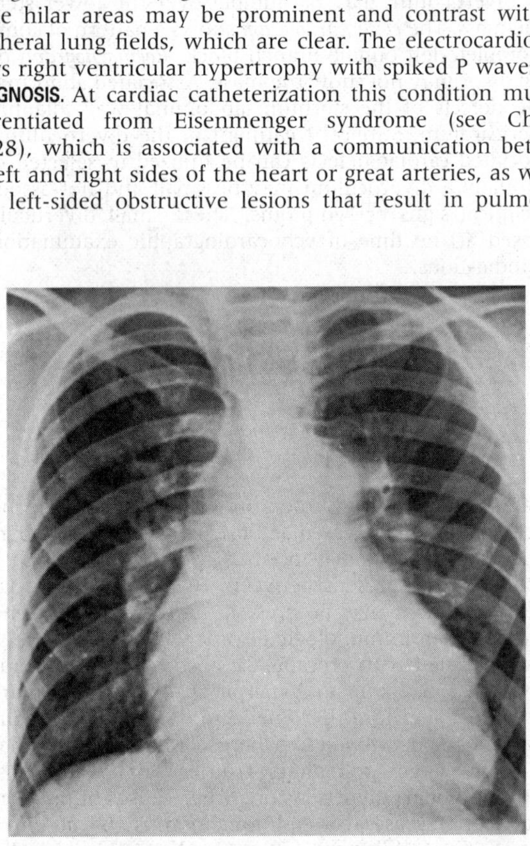

Figure 387–10. Roentgenogram in primary pulmonary hypertension. Note the moderate cardiac enlargement, dilatation of the pulmonary artery, and relative pulmonary undervascularity in the outer two thirds of the lung fields.

PROGNOSIS AND TREATMENT. Primary pulmonary hypertension is progressive, and often there is no specific treatment. Some success has been reported using oral calcium channel blocking agents in children who demonstrate pulmonary vasoreactivity when these agents are administered during catheterization. Continuous intravenous prostacyclin may also provide temporary relief. The only hope for many of these patients is heart-lung or lung transplantation (see Chapters 401 and 402). In patients with severe pulmonary hypertension and low cardiac output, the terminal event is most often sudden and related to a lethal arrhythmia.

387.23 General Principles of Treatment of Congenital Heart Disease

Most patients who have mild congenital heart disease require no treatment. The parents and child should be made aware that a normal life is expected and that no restriction of the child's activities is necessary. Overprotective parents may use the presence of a mild congenital heart lesion or even a functional heart murmur as a means to excessively control their child's activities. Although he or she may not express fears overtly, the child may become quite anxious regarding early death or debilitation, especially when an adult member of the family develops symptomatic heart disease. The family may have an unexpressed fear of sudden death, and the rarity of this manifestation should be emphasized in discussions directed at improving their understanding of the child's congenital heart defect. The difference between congenital heart disease and degenerative coronary disease in adults should be emphasized. General health maintenance, including a well-balanced diet, prevention of anemia, and the usual immunization program, should be encouraged.

Even patients with moderate to severe heart disease need not be markedly restricted in physical activities. Physical education should be modified appropriately to the child's capacity to participate. Rough, competitive sports should be discouraged. Patients having severe heart disease with decreased exercise tolerance usually tend to limit their own activities. Transportation to school may be helpful so that fatigue will not interfere with classroom activities. Dyspnea, headache, and fatigability in cyanotic patients may be a sign of increasing hypoxemia and may require some limitation of activities among those for whom specific medical or surgical treatment is not available. Routine immunizations should be given with the inclusion of influenza vaccine; however, patients who might be considered candidates for heart or heart-lung transplantation should not receive live viral vaccinations.

Bacterial infections should be treated vigorously, but the presence of congenital heart disease is not an appropriate reason to use antibiotics indiscriminately. Prophylaxis against infective endocarditis should be carried out during dental procedures, during instrumentation of the urinary tract, and prior to lower gastrointestinal tract manipulation.

Treatment of iron deficiency anemia is especially important in cyanotic patients who will show improved exercise tolerance and general well-being with adequate hemoglobin levels. On the other hand, these patients should also be carefully observed for excessive polycythemia. Cyanotic patients should avoid situations in which dehydration may occur, which will lead to increased viscosity and will increase the risk of stroke. Diuretics may need to be decreased or temporarily discontinued during episodes of acute gastroenteritis. High altitudes and sudden changes in thermal environment should also be avoided. Phlebotomy with volume replacement should be carried out in symptomatic patients with severe polycythemia (hematocrit >65%); however, the use of routine phlebotomy in the absence of symptoms is controversial. Patients with severe congenital heart disease or a history of rhythm disturbance should be carefully monitored during anesthesia for even routine surgical procedures. Women with nonrepaired severe congenital heart disease should be counseled on the risks associated with childbearing and on the use of contraceptives and tubal ligation. Pregnancy may be extremely dangerous for patients having chronic cyanosis and/or pulmonary artery hypertension. However, women with mild to moderate heart disease and many of those who have had corrective surgery can have normal pregnancies.

The treatment for congestive heart failure is described in Chapter 399, for paroxysmal hypercyanotic attacks in Chapter 387.2, and for cardiac arrhythmias in Chapters 388 and 389. Appropriate surgical procedures for specific cardiac lesions are discussed in the relevant chapters of this section. Cardiac transplantation for children and adolescents is discussed in Chapter 401.

POSTOPERATIVE MANAGEMENT. After successful open heart surgery, the postoperative course depends on numerous factors. The severity of the congenital heart defect, the age and condition (especially nutritional status) of the patient prior to surgery, the events in the operating room, and the quality of the postoperative care will influence the patient's course following surgery. Many patients will have a benign postoperative period without complications, but others may be in a precarious state for hours or days after the operation. Intraoperative factors that influence survival and that should be noted when a patient returns from the operating room include the duration of cardiopulmonary bypass, the duration of aortic cross-clamping (the period of time during which the heart is not being perfused), or the duration of profound hypothermia (usually used in infants: the period of time during which the entire body is not being perfused).

Immediate postoperative care should be provided in an in-

■ **TABLE 387–3 Systems Approach to Postoperative Care Following Surgery for Congenital Heart Disease**

System and Problem	Etiology	Treatment or Prevention
Nervous System		
Coma	Global ischemia	Monitor and treat increased intracranial pressure
	Prolonged anesthetic effect	Reverse anesthesia
	Hypoglycemia	Glucose
Focal lesions	Emboli (air, thrombi)	
Seizures	Metabolic (hyponatremia, hypoglycemia), ischemic, embolic disturbances	Phenytoin, correct metabolic disturbances
Diaphragm paralysis	Phrenic nerve injury	Respiratory care
Vocal cord paralysis	Traction on recurrent laryngeal nerve	Respiratory care
Horner syndrome	Dissection of subclavian artery with sympathetic chain injury	None
Paraplegia	Postcoarctation repair with spinal artery ischemia	Avoid ischemia
Pain	Surgical trauma	Fentanyl, morphine
Anxiety	Stress	Versed, Valium
Respiratory System		
ARDS* postpump syndrome	Unknown; possible release of vasoactive substances by cardiopulmonary bypass	PEEP†, mechanical ventilation, oxygen
Pulmonary edema	Heart failure, left-sided obstructions, fluid overload	Diuresis, PEEP, mechanical ventilation, inotropic agents
Pleural effusions	Hemothorax	Thoracocentesis
	Early serous effusion	Thoracocentesis
	Delayed postpericardiotomy	Anti-inflammatory agents
Chylothorax	Injury to thoracic duct	NPO‡, or medium-chain triglyceride diet
		Rarely surgical ligation of thoracic duct
Atelectasis	Hypoventilation, poor cough	Chest physiotherapy, PEEP
Pneumonia	Aspiration, nosocomial, bacteremia	Identify bacterial/viral (respiratory syncytial virus) etiology; specific antimicrobial therapy
Pulmonary hypertension	Repair of TAPVR, Norwood 1st stage, 21-trisomy; prior preoperative pulmonary hypertension	Hyperventilation, hyperoxia, fentanyl, nitroprusside, prostaglandins
Stridor	Vocal cord edema, paralysis	Steroids, rarely tracheotomy
Cardiovascular System		
Bradycardia, sick sinus, atrioventricular block	Injury to interatrial or interventricular conduction system	Atropine, isoproterenol, pacemaker
Right bundle branch block	Right ventriculotomy	Atrial approach to ventricular septal defect repair of tetralogy of Fallot
Tachyarrhythmias	Supraventricular, junctional tachycardia	Antiarrhythmic agents
	Ventricular tachycardia	Defibrillation, antiarrhythmic agents
Poor cardiac output	Cardiogenic—right ventriculotomy or cardiac stun (prolonged pump and cross-clamp time) or infarction	Inotropic agents, support preload, reduce afterload
	Hypocalcemia	Calcium
	Hypovolemia	Support preload
Pericardial tamponade	Pericardial effusion, acute hemorrhage	Pericardiocentesis
	Serous postpericardiotomy	Anti-inflammatory agents
Hypertension	Stress-pain	Analgesia
	Postcoarctectomy syndrome	Nitroprusside
Mesenteric arteritis	Postcoarctectomy syndrome	NPO, nitroprusside

Table continued on following page

■ TABLE 387–3 Systems Approach to Postoperative Care Following Surgery for Congenital Heart Disease *Continued*

System and Problem	Etiology	Treatment or Prevention
Renal-Metabolic System		
Prerenal oliguria	Hypovolemia Poor cardiac output	Fluid administration Inotropic agents
Renal failure	Hypotension, prolonged pump-cross clamp time, acute tubular necrosis	Improve blood pressure, diuretics
Edema	Fluid resuscitation, capillary leak, poor cardiac output, elevated systemic venous pressure	Diuresis, inotropic agents
Hyponatremia	Dilutional, SIADH§ Diuretics	Fluid restriction Fluid restriction
Hyperglycemia	Hypothermia-inhibition of insulin	None needed
Hypoglycemia	Rebound following hyperglycemia, hepatic failure	Glucose infusion
Hematologic System		
Hemorrhage	Abnormal PT,‖ PTT,** thrombocytopenia Surgical leak	Correct coagulopathy Reoperation, suture
Shunt thrombosis	Poor cardiac output, hypovolemia	Fluids, heparin
Anemia (usually reflecting reduced blood volume)	Hemorrhage, hemolysis	Transfuse packed red blood cells
Graft-versus-host disease	Infusion of viable leukocytes to patients with DiGeorge syndrome	Irradiate blood products
Infectious Diseases		
Wound infection (cutaneous, costochondral, sternotomy, mediastinitis, vascular lines, chest tubes)	Contamination in operating room	Antibiotics
Endocarditis	*Staphylococcus epidermidis, Corynebacterium,* contamination in operating room	Antibiotics
Cystitis, pyelonephritis	Contamination of indwelling urinary catheter	Antibiotics, remove catheter
Hepatitis	Blood borne: Cytomegalovirus, Epstein-Barr virus, hepatitis B and hepatitis C viruses	Screen blood products
Postperfusion syndrome (fever, hepatosplenomegaly, atypical lymphocytes, lymphadenopathy, transient rash)	Cytomegalovirus, Epstein-Barr virus	Screen blood products
Psychosocial Conditions		
Anxiety, separation	Age-related, fears, etc.	Preparedness (videotape, play acting); parent visitation, sedation

**ARDS = adult respiratory distress syndrome.*
†PEEP = positive end-expiratory pressure.
‡NPO = nothing per os (by mouth).
§SIADH = syndrome of inappropriate antidiuretic hormone.
‖ PT = prothrombin time.
***PTT = partial thromboplastin time.*

tensive care unit staffed by a team of physicians, nurses, and technicians experienced with the unique problems encountered after open heart surgery. The preparation for postoperative monitoring begins in the operating room, where the anesthesiologist or surgeon will place an arterial catheter to allow direct arterial pressure measurements and arterial sampling for blood gas determination. A venous catheter is also positioned in the superior vena cava via the jugular vein or inferior vena cava via the femoral vein, and is used for measuring central venous pressure and for infusions of cardioactive medications. Left atrial or pulmonary artery catheters may be inserted directly into these cardiac structures and used for pressure monitoring purposes. Flow-directed thermodilution monitoring (Swan-Ganz) catheters are sometimes used for monitoring pulmonary capillary wedge pressure and cardiac index. Temporary pacing wires are placed on the atrium and ventricle in case temporary heart block occurs. Transcutaneous oximetry provides for continuous monitoring of arterial oxygen saturation.

Functional failure of one organ system may cause profound physiologic and biochemical changes in another (Table 387–3). Respiratory insufficiency, for example, will lead to hypoxia, acidosis, and hypercarbia, which in turn will compromise cardiac, vascular, and renal function. The latter problems will not be able to be managed successfully until adequate ventilation is re-established. Thus, it is essential that the primary source of each postoperative problem be identified and treated.

Respiratory failure is a major postoperative complication encountered after open heart surgery. Cardiopulmonary bypass carried out in the presence of pulmonary congestion results in decreased lung compliance, copious tracheal and bronchial secretions, atelectasis, and increased breathing efforts. Because fatigue and subsequently hypoventilation and acidosis may rapidly ensue, mechanical positive-pressure endotracheal ventilation may be continued following open heart surgery for a minimum of several hours in relatively stable patients, and up to 2–3 days or more in severely ill patients, especially infants. Patients with certain congenital heart lesions may also have airway abnormalities, which could make extubation more difficult.

The electrocardiogram should be monitored continuously during the postoperative period. A change in the heart rate may be the 1st indication of a serious complication, such as hemorrhage, hypothermia, hypoventilation, or congestive heart failure. *Cardiac rhythm disorders* must be diagnosed quickly because a prolonged untreated arrhythmia may add a severe hemodynamic burden to the heart in the critical early postoperative period. Injury to the heart's conduction system during surgery can cause postoperative complete heart block. This complication is usually temporary and is treated with surgically placed pacing wires that can later be removed. Occasionally, complete heart block is permanent. If heart block persists beyond 10–14 days postoperatively, it requires the insertion of a permanent pacemaker. Tachyarrhythmias are a more common problem in postoperative patients. Any of the arrhythmias in Section 4 may occur.

Congestive heart failure with poor cardiac output (see Table 387–3) following cardiac surgery may be secondary to respiratory failure, serious arrhythmias, myocardial injury, blood loss, hypervolemia or hypovolemia, or a significant residual hemodynamic abnormality. Treatment specific to the etiology should be instituted. Catecholamines, digoxin, nitroprusside, and diuretics are the cardioactive agents most often used in patients with myocardial dysfunction in the early postoperative period (see Chapter 399). Amrinone and milrinone, phosphodiesterase inhibitors, can be used in patients with severe cardiogenic shock (Chapter 400). In patients who are unresponsive to standard pharmacologic treatments, various ventricular assist devices are available, depending on the patient's size. If pulmonary function is adequate, an intra-aortic balloon counterpulsation pump, or an external or implantable left ventricular assist device (LVAD), may be utilized. If pulmonary function is inadequate, then extracorporeal membrane oxygenation (ECMO) may be utilized. These extraordinary measures are useful in maintaining the circulation until cardiac function improves, usually within 2–3 days. They have also been used with some success as a bridge to transplantation in patients with severe nonremitting postoperative cardiac failure.

Acidosis secondary to low cardiac output, renal failure, or hypovolemia must be prevented or promptly corrected. An arterial pH below 7.30 may result in a decrease in cardiac output with an increase in lactic acid production and may be the forerunner of a series of arrhythmias or cardiac arrest.

Kidney function may be compromised by congestive heart failure and further impaired by prolonged cardiopulmonary bypass (see Table 387–3). Blood and fluid replacement, cardiac inotropic agents, and sometimes vasodilators will usually reestablish normal urine flow in patients with hypovolemia or cardiac failure. Dopamine is a useful inotropic agent because it also increases renal blood flow directly. Renal failure secondary to tubular injury may require temporary peritoneal dialysis.

Neurologic abnormalities can occur after cardiopulmonary bypass, especially in the neonatal period. Seizures may present when the patient awakens from sedation and usually can be controlled with phenytoin (Dilantin) or phenobarbital. In the absence of other neurologic signs, isolated seizures in the immediate postoperative period usually carry a good prognosis. Thromboembolism and stroke are rare but serious complications of open-heart surgery. Learning disabilities may occur.

The *postpericardiotomy syndrome* may occur toward the end of the 1st postoperative week or sometimes be delayed until weeks or months after operation. This febrile illness is characterized by pericarditis and pleurisy, which in most instances is self-limiting and associated with a benign course. When pericardial fluid accumulates, the potential danger of cardiac tamponade should be recognized (see Chapter 397). Rarely, arrhythmias may also occur. Symptomatic patients usually respond to salicylates or indomethacin and bed rest. Occasionally steroid therapy is required. A prolonged illness or late recurrences are not unusual.

Hemolysis of mechanical origin is rarely seen after repair of certain cardiac defects, for example, atrioventricular septal defects or after the insertion of a mechanical prosthetic valve. It occurs secondary to unusual turbulence of blood at increased pressure. Reoperation may be necessary in rare patients with severe and progressive hemolysis who require frequent blood transfusions, but in most instances the problem slowly regresses.

Infection is another potential postoperative problem. Patients are usually covered with a broad-spectrum antibiotic for the initial postoperative period. Potential sites of infection include pulmonary (usually related to postoperative atelectasis), the subcutaneous tissues at the incision site, the sternum, and the urinary tract (especially after an indwelling catheter has been in place). Sepsis with infective endocarditis is an infrequent complication but can be difficult to manage (see Chapter 390).

PROGNOSIS. Patients who have had palliative procedures for extremely complex heart disease may lead limited but productive lives. These patients require careful follow-up and various restrictions depending on the severity of their disease. The great majority of congenital heart defects can be corrected by open heart surgery or interventional catheterization (balloon angioplasty, device closure); in most patients cardiac dynamics are improved and symptoms disappear. Some patients may develop late complications or require reoperation. Children who have undergone repair of complex cardiac lesions should be followed closely with appropriate laboratory tests. After successful repair of simple lesions with no evidence of residual abnormalities, such as PDA, ASD, or valvular pulmonary stenosis, patients require very few specific follow-up studies and should be encouraged to lead full and active lives. Unfortunately, problems obtaining life and health insurance persist for many patients with operated congenital heart defects, even if totally corrected.

INCIDENCE AND ETIOLOGY

Dennis NR, Warren J: Risks to offspring of patients with some common congenital heart defects. J Med Genet 18:8, 1981.

Driscoll DA, Budarf MC, Emanuel BS: A genetic etiology for DiGeorge syndrome: Consistent deletions and microdeletions of 22q11. Am J Human Genet 50:924, 1992.

Hoffman JIE: Congenital heart disease: Incidence and inheritance. Pediatr Clin North Am 37:25, 1990.

Lin AE, Garver KL: Genetic counseling for congenital heart defects. J Pediatr 113:1105, 1988.

Morris CD, Menashe VD: 25-year mortality after surgical repair of congenital heart defect in childhood: A population-based cohort study. JAMA 266:3447, 1991.

Noonan JA: Syndromes associated with cardiac defects. Cardiovasc Clin 11:97, 1980.

Nora JJ, Nora AH: Maternal transmission of congenital heart disease: New recurrence risk figures and the questions of cytoplasmic inheritance and vulnerability to teratogens. Am J Cardiol 59:459, 1987.

Somerville J: Congenital heart disease in the adolescent. Arch Dis Child 64:771, 1989.

van Mierop LHS, Kutsche LM: Cardiovascular anomalies in DiGeorge syndrome and importance of neural crest as a possible pathogenetic factor. Am J Cardiol 58:133, 1986.

Whittemore R, Hobbins JC, Engle MA: Pregnancy and its outcome in women with and without surgical treatment of congenital heart disease. Am J Cardiol 50:641, 1982.

ATRIAL SEPTAL DEFECT AND ATRIOVENTRICULAR SEPTAL DEFECT

Clapp SK, Perry BL, Farooki ZQ, et al: Surgical and medical results of complete atrioventricular canal: A ten-year review. Am J Cardiol 59:454, 1987.

Marino B, Vairo U, Corno A, et al: Atrioventricular canal in Down syndrome. Am J Dis Child 144:1120, 1990.

Makoney L, Truesdell SC, Krzmarzick TR, et al: Atrial septal defects that present in infancy. Am J Dis Child 140:1115, 1986.

Murphy JG, Gersh BJ, McGoon MD, et al: Long-term outcome after surgical repair of isolated atrial septal defect: Follow-up at 27–32 years. N Engl J Med 323:1645, 1990.

Radzik D, Davignon A, van Doesburg N, et al: Predictive factors for spontaneous closure of atrial septal defects diagnosed in the first 3 months of life. J Am Coll Cardiol 22:851, 1993.

Santon E: Repair of atrioventricular septal defects in infancy. J Thorac Cardiovasc Surg 91:505, 1986.

VENTRICULAR SEPTAL DEFECT

Beerman LB, Park SC, Fischer DR, et al: Ventricular septal defect associated with aneurysm of the membranous septum. J Am Coll Cardiol 5:118, 1985.

Hornberger LK, Sahn DJ, Krabill KA, et al: Elucidation of the natural history of ventricular septal defects by serial Doppler color flow mapping studies. J Am Coll Cardiol 13:1111, 1989.

Leung MP, Beerman LB, Siewers RD, et al: Long term follow-up after aortic valvuloplasty and defect closure in ventricular septal defect with aortic regurgitation. Am J Cardiol 60:890, 1987.

Moller JH, Patton C, Varco RL, et al: Late results (30 to 35 years) after operative closure of isolated ventricular septal defect from 1954 to 1960. Am J Cardiol 68:1491, 1991.

Ramaciotti C, Keren A, Silverman NH: Importance of pseudoaneurysms of the ventricular septum in the natural history of isolated perimembranous ventricular septal defects. Am J Cardiol 57:268, 1986.

Weidman WH, Blount SG Jr, DuShane JW, et al: Clinical course in ventricular septal defect. Circulation 56:156, 1977.

Weidman WH, Gersony WM, Nugent EW, et al: Indirect assessment of severity in ventricular septal defect. Circulation 56(Suppl):24, 1977.

PULMONARY STENOSIS

Benson LN, Freedom RM: Interventional cardiac catheterization. Curr Opin Pediatr 1:106, 1989.

Nugent EW, Freedom RM, Nora JJ, et al: Clinical course in pulmonary stenosis. Circulation 56(Suppl):38, 1977.

AORTIC STENOSIS

Donner R, Black I, Spann JF, Carabello BA: Improved prediction of peak left ventricular pressure by echocardiography in children with aortic stenosis. J Am Coll Cardiol 3:349, 1984.
Doyle EF, Arumugham P, Lara E, et al: Sudden death in young patients with congenital aortic stenosis. Pediatrics 53:481, 1974.
Edmunds LH, Wagner HR, Heyman MA: Aortic valvulotomy in neonates. Circulation 61:421, 1980.
Leichter DA, Sullivan I, Gersony WM: "Acquired" discrete subvalvular aortic stenosis: Natural history and hemodynamics. J Am Coll Cardiol 14:1539, 1989.
McCue CM, Spicuzza TJ, Robertson LW, et al: Familial supravalvular aortic stenosis. J Pediatr 73:889, 1968.
Radtke W, Lock J: Balloon dilation. Pediatr Clin North Am 37:193, 1990.
Sandor GG, Olley PM, Trusler GA, et al: Long-term follow-up of patients after valvotomy for congenital valvular aortic stenosis in children: A clinical and actuarial follow-up. J Thorac Cardiovasc Surg 80:171, 1980.
Zeevi B, Keane JF, Castaneda AR, et al: Neonatal critical valvar aortic stenosis: A comparison of surgical and balloon dilation therapy. Circulation 80:831, 1989.

MITRAL VALVE ANOMALIES

American Academy of Pediatrics: Mitral valve prolapse and athletic competition of children and adolescents. Pediatrics 95:789, 1995.
Bisset GS, Schwartz DC, Meyer RA, et al: Clinical spectrum and long-term follow-up of isolated mitral valve prolapse in 119 children. Circulation 62:423, 1980.
Devereux RB, Kramer-Fox R, Kligfield P: Mitral valve prolapse: Causes, clinical manifestations, and management. Ann Intern Med 111:305, 1989.
Glesby MJ, Pyeritz RE: Association of mitral valve prolapse and systemic abnormalities of connective tissue: A phenotypic continuum. JAMA 262:523, 1989.
Marks AR, Choong CY, Sanfilippo AJ, et al: Identification of high-risk and low-risk subgroups of patients with mitral-valve prolapse. N Engl J Med 320:1031, 1989.

PULMONARY VASCULAR DISEASE

Friedman WF, Heiferman M: Clinical problems of pulmonary vascular disease. Am J Cardiol 56:31, 1982.
Hoffman JIE, Rudolph AM, Heymann MA: Pulmonary vascular disease with congenital heart lesions: Pathologic features and causes. Circulation 64:873, 1981.

TETRALOGY OF FALLOT AND PULMONARY ATRESIA

Dabizzi RP, Caprioli G, Aiazzi L, et al: Distribution and anomalies of coronary arteries in tetralogy of Fallot. Circulation 61:95, 1980.
Garson A, Nihill MR, McNamara DG, et al: Status of the adult and adolescent after repair of tetralogy of Fallot. Circulation 59:1232, 1976.
Kirklin JW, Blackstone EH, Kirklin JK, et al: Surgical results and protocols in the spectrum of tetralogy of Fallot. Ann Surg 198:251, 1983.
McCaughan BC, Danielson GK, Driscoll DJ, et al: Tetralogy of Fallot with absent pulmonary valve: Early and late results of surgical treatment. J Thorac Cardiovasc Surg 89:280, 1985.
Oku H, Shirotani H, Sunakawa A, et al: Postoperative long term results in total correction of tetralogy of Fallot: Hemodynamics and cardiac function. Ann Thorac Surg 41:413, 1986.
Pacifico AO, Saro ME, Bargeron LM Jr, et al.: Transatrial-transpulmonary repair of tetralogy of Fallot. J Thorac Cardiovasc Surg 74:382, 1987.
Pinsky WW, Arciniegas E: Tetralogy of Fallot. Pediatr Clin North Am 37:179, 1990.
Rocchinl AP: Hemodynamic abnormalities in response to supine exercise in patients after operative correction of tetralogy of Fallot after early childhood. Am J Cardiol 48:325, 1981.
Zhao HX, Miller DC, Reitz BA, et al: Surgical repair of tetralogy of Fallot. J Thorac Cardiovasc Surg 89:204, 1985.

TRANSPOSITION OF THE GREAT ARTERIES

Bowyer JJ, Busst CM, Till JA, et al: Exercise ability after Mustard's operation. Arch Dis Child 65:865, 1990.
Deanfield JE: Transposition of the great arteries: To switch or not to switch? Curr Opin Pediatr 1:85, 1989.
Duncan WJ, Freedom RM, Rowe RD, et al: Echocardiographic features before and after the Jatene procedure (anatomical correction) for transposition of the great vessels. Am Heart J 102:227, 1981.
Gillette PC, Kugler JD, Gutgesell HP, et al: Mechanisms of cardiac arrhythmias after the Mustard operation for transposition of the great arteries. Am J Cardiol 45:1225, 1980.
Hayes CJ, Gersony WM: Arrhythmias after the Mustard operation for transposition of the great arteries: A long term study. J Am Coll Cardiol 7:133, 1986.
Kirklin JW, Colvin EV, McConnell ME, et al: Complete transposition of the great arteries: Treatment in the current era. Pediatr Clin North Am 37:171, 1990.
Pacifico AD, Stewart RW, Bargeron LM: Repair of transposition of great arteries with ventricular septal defect by an arterial switch operation. Circulation 68:49, 1983.
Quaegebeur JM, Rohmer J, Ottenkamp J, et al: The arterial switch operation. J Thorac Cardiovasc Surg 92:361, 1986.
Rashkind WJ, Miller WW: Creation of an atrial septal defect without thoracotomy: A palliative approach to complete transposition of the great vessels. JAMA 196:991, 1966.
Rastelli GC, McGoon DC, Wallace RB: Anatomic correction of transposition of the great arteries with ventricular septal defect and subpulmonary stenosis. J Thorac Cardiovasc Surg 58:545, 1969.
Wilcox BR, Ho SY, Macartney FJ, et al: Surgical anatomy of double-outlet right ventricle with situs solitus and atrioventricular concordance. J Thorac Cardiovasc Surg 82:405, 1981.

TRICUSPID ATRESIA

Fontan F, Deville C, Quaegebeur J, et al: Repair of tricuspid atresia in 100 patients. J Thorac Cardiovasc Surg 85:647, 1983.
Girod DA, Fontan F, Deville C, et al: Long-term results after the Fontan operation for tricuspid atresia. Circulation 75:605, 1987.
Mair DD: The Fontan procedure: The first 20 years. Curr Opin Pediatr 1:94, 1989.
Marino B, Marcelletti C: The cavopulmonary anastomosis in congenital heart disease: A consideration of the classic and bidirectional palliations. Curr Opin Pediatr 2:973, 1990.
Sade RM, Fyfe DA: Tricuspid atresia: Current concepts in diagnosis and treatment. Pediatr Clin North Am 37:151, 1990.

EBSTEIN ANOMALY

Mair DD, Seward JB, Driscoll DJ, et al: Surgical repair of Ebstein's anomaly: Selection of patients and early and later operative results. Circulation 72:70, 1985.
Starnes VA, Pitlick PT, Bernstein D, et al: Ebstein's anomaly appearing in the neonate. J Thorac Cardiovasc Surg 101:1082, 1991.
Zuberbuhler JR, Allwork SP, Anderson RH: The spectrum of Ebstein's anomaly of the tricuspid valve. J Thorac Cardiovasc Surg 77:202, 1979.

TOTAL ANOMALOUS PULMONARY VENOUS RETURN

Delisle G, Masahiko A, Calder AL, et al: Total anomalous pulmonary venous connection: Report of 93 autopsied cases with emphasis on diagnostic and surgical considerations. Am Heart J 91:99, 1976.
Duff DG, Nihill MR, McNamara DG: Infradiaphragmatic total anomalous pulmonary venous return. Review of clinical and pathological findings and results of operation in 28 cases. Br Heart J 39:619, 1977.
Gersony WM: Presentation, diagnosis and natural history of total anomalous pulmonary venous drainage. *In:* Godman MJ, Marguis RM (eds): Paediatric Cardiology. Edinburgh, Churchill Livingstone, 1979.
Turley K, Tucker WY, Ullyot DJ, et al: Total anomalous pulmonary venous connection in infancy: Influence of age and type of lesion. Am J Cardiol 45:92, 1980.

HYPOPLASTIC LEFT HEART SYNDROME

Bailey LL, Gundry SR: Hypoplastic left heart syndrome. Pediatr Clin North Am 37:137, 1990.
Chiavarelli M, Gundry SR, Razzouk AJ, et al: Cardiac transplantation for infants with hypoplastic left heart syndrome. JAMA 270:2944, 1993.
Glauser TA, Rorke LB, Weinberg PM: Congenital brain abnormalities associated with the hypoplastic left heart syndrome. Pediatrics 85:984, 1990.
Norwood WI, Lang P, Hansen D: Physiologic repair of aortic atresia-hypoplastic left heart syndrome. N Engl J Med 308:23, 1983.
Starnes VA, Griffin ML, Pitlick PT, et al: Current approach to hypoplastic left heart syndrome: Palliation, transplantation or both? J Thorac Cardiovasc Surg 104:189–195, 1992.

DEXTROCARDIA AND LEVOCARDIA

Britz-Cunningham SH, Shah MM, Zuppan CW, et al: Mutation of the connexin 43 gap-junction gene in patients with heart malformations and defects of laterality. N Engl J Med 332:1323, 1995.
Liberthson RR, Hastreiter AR, Sinha SN, et al: Levocardia with visceral heterotaxy-isolated levocardia: Pathologic anatomy and its clinical implications. Am Heart J 85:40, 1973.
Rose V, Izukawa T, Moes CAF: Syndromes of asplenia and polysplenia: A review of cardiac and non-cardiac malformations in 60 cases with special reference to diagnosis and prognosis. Br Heart J 37:840, 1975.

OTHER LESIONS

Bertrand J-M, Chartrand C, Lamarre A, et al: Vascular ring: Clinical and physiological assessment of pulmonary function following surgical correction. Pediatr Pulmonol 2:378, 1986.
Rich S, Dantzker DR, Ayres SM, et al: Primary pulmonary hypertension: A national prospective study. Ann Intern Med 107:216, 1987.
Rubin LJ, Mendoza J, Hood M, et al: Treatment of primary pulmonary hyperten-

sion with continuous intravenous prostacyclin (epoprostenol). Ann Intern Med 112:485, 1990.

PRINCIPLES OF TREATMENT

Bard H, Fourow JC, Gagnon C, et al: Hypoxemia and increased fetal hemoglobin synthesis. J Pediatr 124:941, 1994.
Chang AC, Hanley FL, Lock JE, et al: Management and outcome of low birthweight neonates with congenital heart disease. J Pediatr 124:461, 1994.
Engle MA, Zabriskie JB, Seuterfit LB, et al: Viral illness and post-pericardiotomy syndrome: A prospective study in children. Circulation 62:1151, 1980.
Ferry PC: Neurologic sequelae of cardiac surgery in children. Am J Dis Child 141:309, 1987.
Gersony WM, Krongrad E: Evaluation and management of patients after surgical repair of congenital heart disease. Progr Cardiovasc Dis 18:39, 1975. Also *In:* Rosenthal EH, Sonnenblick EH, Lesch M (eds): Postoperative Congenital Heart Disease. New York, Grune & Stratton, 1975, p 145.
McCartney FT, Taylor JFN, Graham GR, et al: The fate of survivors of cardiac surgery in infancy. Circulation 62:80, 1980.
Musewe NN: The role of transesophageal echocardiography in pediatrics. Curr Opin Pediatr 2:977, 1990.
Ruttenberg HD: Indications for exercise restrictions in patients with congenital heart disease. Curr Opin Pediatr 4:833, 1992.
Rigby ML: The trend to primary repair of congenital heart defects in the first 3 months of life. Curr Opin Pediatr 1:82, 1989.
Schwarz SM, Gewitz MH, See CC, et al: Enteral nutrition in infants with congenital heart disease and growth failure. Pediatrics 86:368, 1990.
Thomson AH, Beardsmore CS, Firmin R, et al: Airway function in infants with vascular rings: Preoperative and postoperative assessment. Arch Dis Child 65:171, 1990.
Tynan M: Fetal and pediatric cardiac surgery. Curr Opin Pediatr 2:982, 1990.
Wiles HB: Imaging congenital heart disease. Pediatr Clin North Am 37:115, 1990.

SECTION 4

Cardiac Arrhythmias

CHAPTER 388

Disturbances of Rate and Rhythm of the Heart

Pediatric arrhythmias may be transient or permanent, congenital (in a structurally normal or abnormal heart) or acquired (rheumatic fever, myocarditis), caused by a toxin (diphtheria), cocaine or theophylline, proarrhythmic or antiarrhythmic drugs, or be a sequela of surgical correction of congenital heart disease. The major risks of any arrhythmia are those of severe tachycardia or bradycardia leading to decreased cardiac output, or the risk of degeneration into a more severe arrhythmia, for example, ventricular fibrillation. These complications may lead to syncope, which itself can be dangerous under certain circumstances (e.g., swimming, driving), or to sudden death. Thus, when a patient presents with an arrhythmia, one of the major issues in management is to determine whether the particular rhythm disturbance is prone to deteriorate into a life-threatening tachyarrhythmia or bradyarrhythmia. Some rhythm abnormalities, such as single premature atrial and ventricular beats, are common among children without heart disease and in the great majority of instances do not pose a risk to the patient.

An increasing number of pharmacologic agents are available for treating dysrhythmias in adults, but most have not been used extensively in children. Problems with frequency of administration, compliance, side effects, and variable responses still remain, and selection of an appropriate agent involves a great deal of empiricism. However, most rhythm disturbances in children can be reliably controlled with a single agent. The most commonly used agents are listed in Table 388–1. For patients with tachyarrhythmias that are resistant to medical therapy, transcatheter radiofrequency ablation or surgical intervention are available. The specific indications for these procedures, especially in younger children, are currently under investigation. For patients with bradyarrhythmias, implantable pacemakers have become more reliable and significantly smaller, allowing their use even in premature infants. Automatic implantable cardioverter-defibrillators (AICDs) are now available for use in high-risk patients with sudden-onset ventricular tachycardia or fibrillation.

Sinus arrhythmia represents a normally physiologic variation in impulse discharges from the sinus node related to respirations. There is a slowing of heart rate during expiration and an acceleration during inspiration. Occasionally, if the sinus rate becomes slow enough, there will be an escape beat from the atrioventricular junctional region (Fig. 388–1). Irregularities of sinus rhythm are commonly seen in premature infants, especially bradycardia associated with periodic apnea. Sinus arrhythmia is exaggerated during convalescence from febrile illness and by drugs that increase vagal tone, such as digitalis; it is usually abolished by exercise or by atropine. Some children have great variation in heart rate during sinus arrhythmia, which should not be confused with a significant rhythm disorder.

Sinus bradycardia is due to slow discharge of impulses from the sinus node. In general, a sinus rate under 90/min in neonates and under 60/min thereafter is considered to be sinus bradycardia. It is commonly seen in athletes, and in healthy individuals it is without significance. Sinus bradycardia may occur in systemic disease, for example, myxedema, and will

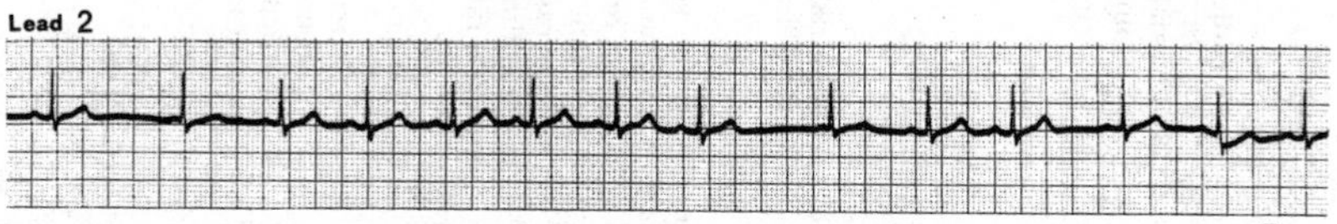

Figure 388–1. Sinus arrhythmia with junctional escape beat. Note the variation in P-P interval with little change in P morphology or P-R interval. When the sinus rate is slow enough, the atrioventricular junction takes over and produces escape beats. This rhythm is normal.

■ TABLE 388–1 Commonly Used Antiarrhythmic Drug Schedules in Pediatric Patients

		Oral Administration		Intravenous Administration*		Comments and Side Effects				
Drug	Indications	*Maintenance Dose*	*Maximal Maintenance Dose*	*Loading Dose*	*Maximal Dose*	*Comments*	*Side Effects*	*Drug Interactions*	*Proarrhythmias*	*Drug Level*
Digoxin	SVT,[1] atrial flutter, atrial fibrillation	0.01–0.02 mg/kg/24 hr q 12 hr	0.5 mg	0.025–0.05 mg/kg/24 hr q 4–8 hr	0.5 mg	Oral loading dose 0.04–0.07 mg/kg/24 hr q 8 hr; see text for age-related differences	APC, VPC, bradycardia, AV block, nausea, vomiting, anorexia; prolongs P-R interval	Quinidine, amiodarone, verapamil, increase digoxin levels Diuretic, amphotericin-induced hypokalemia increases digoxin arrhythmia	Induces APC, VPC, accelerated AV junctional tachycardia	1–2 ng/mL
Quinidine sulfate	SVT,[1] atrial fibrillation, atrial flutter, VPC	20–60 mg/kg/24 hr q 6 hr	2.4 g	—	—	—	Nausea, vomiting, diarrhea, fever, cinchonism, QRS and Q-T prolongation, AV block, asystole, syncope, thrombocytopenia, hemolytic anemia, SLE, blurred vision, convulsions, allergic reactions, exacerbation of periodic paralysis	Enhances digoxin effects	Yes, torsades de pointes	2–7 µg/mL
Quinidine gluconate	Digoxin, verapamil or propranolol must be given first to prevent ventricular tachycardias, as quinidine slows atrial rate	20–60 mg/kg/24 hr q 8–12 hr	2.0 g	10–15 mg/kg as 250 µg/kg/min	20 mg/min to 1.0 g	Oral test dose 2 mg/kg				
Procainamide	SVT,[1] atrial fibrillation, atrial flutter; VPC, ventricular tachycardia[2]	50–100 mg/kg/24 hr q 4–6 hr or q 6 hr†	6.0 g	10–20 mg/kg as 300 µg/kg/min	20 mg/min to 1.0 g	Intravenous maintenance 20–80 µg/kg/min	P-R, QRS, Q-T interval prolongation, anorexia, nausea, vomiting, rash, fever, agranulocytosis, thrombocytopenia, Coombs-positive hemolytic anemia, SLE, hypotension, exacerbation of periodic paralysis	Toxicity increased by amiodarone, cimetidine	Yes, torsades de pointes	4–10 µg/mL
Disopyramide	SVT,[1] atrial fibrillation, atrial flutter, VPC	8–12 mg/kg/24 hr q 6 hr or q 12 hr†	1.2 g	—	—	—	Anticholinergic effects, urinary retention, blurred vision, dry mouth, Q-T and QRS prolongation, hepatic toxicity, negative inotropic effects, agranulocytosis, psychosis, hypoglycemia	—	Yes, torsades de pointes	2–8 µg/mL

Phenytoin	Digoxin-induced arrhythmias with heart block	3–6 mg/kg 24 hr q 12 hr	600 mg	10–15 mg/kg as 250 μg/kg/min	20 mg/min to 1.0 g	—	Rash, gingival hyperplasia, ataxia, lethargy, vertigo, tremor, macrocytic anemia, bradycardia with rapid push	Amiodarone, oral anticoagulants, cimetidine, nifedipine, disopyramide increase toxicity Phenytoin decreases effect of quinidine, mexiletine, furosemide, disopyramide	No	5–20 μg/mL
Lidocaine	VPC, ventricular tachycardia,[2] ventricular fibrillation[3]	—	—	1 mg/kg; repeat q 5 min for 3 times	50–75 mg	Intravenous maintenance 30–50 μg/kg/min	CNS effects, confusion, convulsions, high-degree AV block, asystole, coma, paresthesias, respiratory failure	Propranolol, cimetidine, tocainide increase toxicity	No	1.5–6 μg/mL
Verapamil	SVT[1]	4–10 mg/kg/24 hr q 8 hr	480 mg	0.075–0.15 mg/kg q 20 min for 2 times	5 mg	Contraindicated in ventricular tachycardia, severe CHF, and atrial fibrillation with WPW; use with caution in infants	Bradycardia, asystole, high-degree AV block, P-R prolongation, hypotension, CHF	Use with beta-blocking agent or disopyramide exacerbates or precipitates CHF; increases digoxin levels and toxicity	No, but may increase AV block	—
Propranolol	SVT,[1] VPC	1–4 mg/kg/24 hr q 6 hr	Not established	0.1–0.15 mg/kg	1 mg/min to 10 mg	Long-acting beta blocking agents (nadolol, atenolol) are preferred for long-term therapy (less frequent administration and fewer CNS side effects)	Bradycardia, loss of concentration or memory, bronchospasm, hypoglycemia, hypotension, heart block, CHF	Use with disopyramide or verapamil exacerbates or precipitates CHF	No	—
Adenosine	SVT[1]	—	—	50–300 μg/kg; begin with 50 μg/kg and increase by 50–100 μg/kg/dose if no effect; 6–12 mg in adolescents	Must be given as rapid IV push, repeat at higher dose if no effect	Because of short half-life adverse effects (chest pain, dyspnea, facial flushing) last <1 min; may see transient bradycardia, rarely transient asystole, VPC	May be less effective in patients receiving theophylline. Increased heart block with carbamazepine	—	—	—
Bretylium	Ventricular tachycardia,[2] ventricular fibrillation[3]	—	—	5 mg/kg, then 5–10 mg/kg q 6 hr	30 mg/kg	—	Hypotension, sinus bradycardia, increased sensitivity to catecholamines with transient arrhythmias	Possible hypertension with concurrent sympathomimetic amines	No	—

[1]*Vagotonic maneuvers (placing face in iced saline or ice bag over the face) may be attempted first. If the patient is severely compromised and critically ill, cardioversion is treatment of choice for SVT, atrial flutter, and atrial fibrillation.*
[2]*Cardioversion is treatment of choice for sustained ventricular tachycardia with significant hemodynamic compromise. Some cardiologists try chest thump and/or IV lidocaine. If heart block is present, a temporary ventricular pacemaker may be needed.*
[3]*Defibrillation is treatment of choice.*
**Intravenous administration of antiarrhythmic drugs should always be given slowly with constant monitoring of blood pressure and an electrocardiogram, particularly in patients with compromised cardiac, renal, or hepatic function. The dose must be modified in patients with abnormal renal or hepatic function.*
†*Sustained-release preparations available for clinical use.*
AV = atrioventricular node; SVT = supraventricular tachycardia; SLE = systemic lupus erythematosus–like illness, ANA positive; VPC = ventricular premature contraction; APC = atrial premature contraction; IV = intravenous; WPW = Wolff-Parkinson-White pre-excitation; CHF = congestive heart failure; CNS = central nervous system.

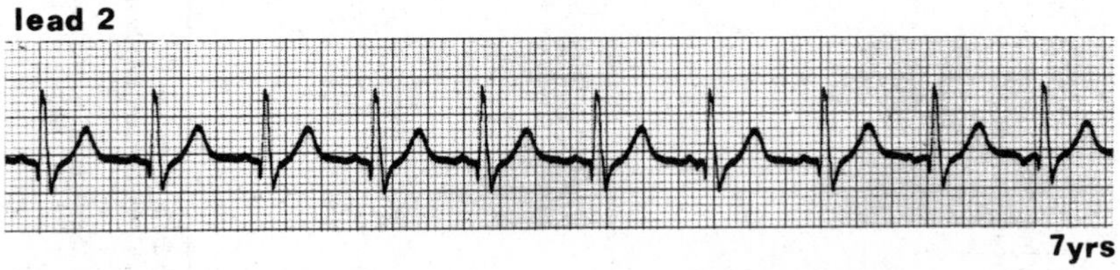

Figure 388–2. Wandering atrial pacemaker. Note the change in P wave configuration in the 7th, 9th, and 10th beats. The 7th P wave may represent a fusion between the sinus P and the ectopic atrial pacemaker seen in the 10th beat.

resolve when the disorder is under control. Sinus bradycardia must be differentiated from sinoatrial and atrioventricular (A-V) block. Children having sinus bradycardia significantly increase their heart rate with exercise to well over 100/min, whereas patients with A-V block are unable to do so. Low-birthweight infants display great variation in sinus rate. Sinus bradycardia is common in these infants and may be associated with junctional escape beats. Premature atrial contractions are also frequent. These rhythm changes, especially bradycardia, appear more commonly during sleep and are not associated with symptoms. No therapy is usually necessary.

Wandering atrial pacemaker (Fig. 388–2) is defined as an intermittent shift in the pacemaker of the heart from the sinus node to another part of the atrium. This is not uncommon in childhood and usually represents a normal variant. It may also be seen in patients with central nervous system disturbances, for example, subarachnoid hemorrhage.

Extrasystoles are produced by the discharge of an ectopic focus that may be situated anywhere in atrial, junctional, or ventricular tissue. Usually, isolated extrasystoles are of no clinical or prognostic significance. Under certain circumstances premature beats may be due to organic heart disease (inflammatory, ischemic, fibrotic, etc.) or to drug toxicity, especially with digitalis.

Premature atrial complexes (PACs) are not uncommon in childhood, even in the absence of cardiac disease. Depending on the degree of prematurity of the beat (coupling interval) and the preceding R-R interval (cycle length), premature atrial complexes may result in either a normal or a prolonged QRS complex. The latter occurs when the premature impulse is conducted to the ventricle while the specialized ventricular conducting system is partially refractory (Fig. 388–3), and these atrial extrasystoles must be distinguished from premature ventricular complexes. Careful scrutiny of the electrocardiogram for a premature P wave preceding the QRS that has a different contour from the other sinus P waves is essential for diagnosis. Atrial premature complexes most often reset the sinus node pacemaker, and therefore the length to the next sinus beat is similar to the normal sinus cycle length (no compensatory pause).

Premature ventricular complexes (PVCs) may arise in any region of the ventricles. They are characterized by premature, widened, bizarre QRS complexes that are not preceded by a P wave (Fig. 388–4). When all premature beats have identical contours, they are classified as unifocal in origin. When PVCs vary in contour, they are designated as multifocal. Ventricular extrasystoles are usually, but not always, followed by a compensatory pause (the interval between the beat preceding the extrasystole and the beat following it is equal to twice the normal sinus cycle length). The presence of fusion beats, that is, complexes that are intermediate in morphology between normal sinus beats and PVCs, is a clue to the ventricular origin of the extrasystole. Extrasystoles produce a smaller stroke and pulse volume than normal and, if very premature, may not be audible with a stethoscope or palpable at the radial pulse. When frequent, extrasystoles may assume a definite rhythm, for example, alternating with normal beats (bigeminy) or occurring after two normal beats (trigeminy). Most patients are unaware of single premature ventricular contractions, although some may be aware of a "skipped beat" or a sudden "turnover" or "tickle" over the precordium. This sensation is due to the increased stroke volume of the normal beat following a compensatory pause. Anxiety, a febrile illness, or ingestion of various drugs or stimulants may cause premature ventricular beats.

It is important to distinguish PVCs that are benign from those that are likely to degenerate into more severe dysrhythmias. The former usually disappear during the tachycardia of exercise. If they persist or become more frequent during exercise, the arrhythmia may have greater significance. The following criteria are indications for further investigation of PVCs that could require suppressive therapy: (1) two or more ventricular premature beats in a row, (2) multifocal origin, (3) increased ventricular ectopic activity with exercise, (4) R on T phenomenon (premature ventricular depolarization occurs on the T wave of the preceding beat), (5) presence of underlying heart disease, and (6) unusual patient awareness of beats associated with marked anxiety. The basis of therapy for benign PVCs is convincing reassurance that the arrhythmia is not the result of structural heart disease; sedatives or suppressive agents may be used in selected cases. Most malignant PVCs are usually secondary to another medical problem, for example, electrolyte imbalance, hypoxia, drug toxicity, cardiac injury, or an intraventricular catheter. Successful treatment includes correction of these underlying abnormalities. An intravenous lidocaine drip is the first line of therapy. The choice of a

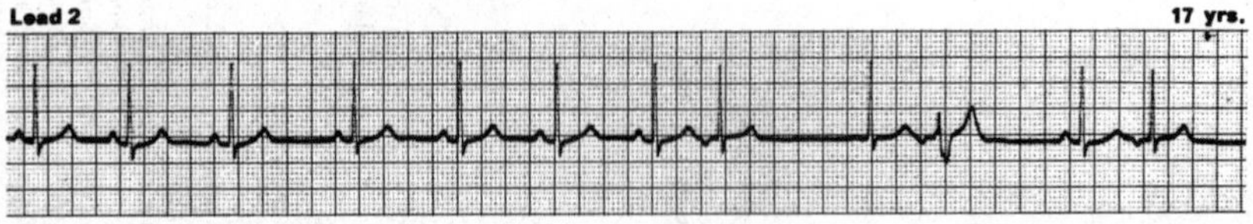

Figure 388–3. Premature atrial contraction (PAC). QRS complexes—the 8th, 10th, and final—in this strip are preceded by a P wave that is inverted, denoting an ectopic origin of atrial depolarization. Note that the 8th and final QRS complexes resemble those of sinus origin, whereas the 10th is aberrantly conducted. This is a function of the preceding cycle length that influences the refractory period of the bundle branches. Note that the pause after the PAC is longer than two P-P intervals, implying that the premature atrial depolarization has invaded and discharged the sinus node, and reset it, so that it fires later.

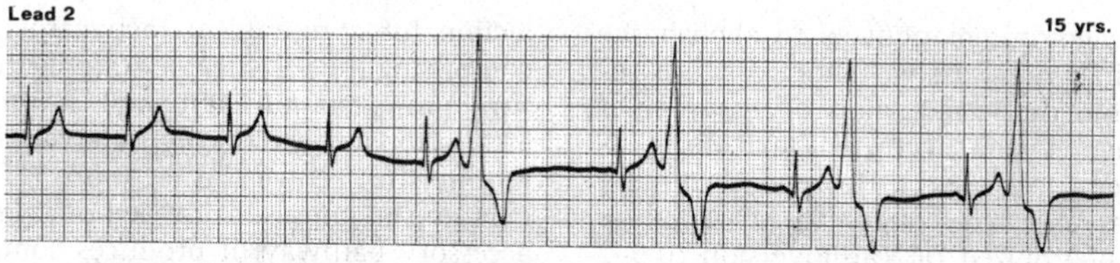

Figure 388–4. Premature ventricular contractions (PVC) induced by hyperventilation. Note that the premature beat is wide and has a completely different morphology from that of the sinus beat. The premature beat is not preceded by a P wave, and the pause following it is fully compensatory (i.e., the P-P interval containing the PVC equals two sinus cycles); this indicates that the sinus mechanism has not been disturbed by the premature beats.

maintenance oral antiarrhythmic agent is determined empirically or at electrophysiologic study.

388.1 Tachyarrhythmias

SUPRAVENTRICULAR TACHYARRHYTHMIAS

(SVT, Paroxysmal Atrial Tachycardia)

Re-entry within the A-V node is the most common mechanism of paroxysmal atrial tachycardia. The tachycardia is initiated by a premature atrial beat that is conducted through a bypass tract within the A-V node. The ventricular response induces an echo beat, which returns to the atrium via a retrograde tract within the A-V node. This echo beat is in turn transmitted back to the ventricle and so on (Fig. 388–5).

CLINICAL MANIFESTATIONS. SVT is characterized by an abrupt onset and cessation; it may be precipitated by an acute infection and usually occurs when the patient is at rest. Attacks may last only a few seconds or may persist for hours. The cardiac rate usually exceeds 180/min and occasionally may be as rapid as 300/min. The only complaint may be awareness of the rapid cardiac rate. Many children tolerate these episodes extremely well, and it is unlikely that short paroxysms are a danger to life. If the rate is exceptionally rapid or if the attack is prolonged, precordial discomfort and congestive heart failure may supervene.

In *young infants,* the diagnosis may be more obscure because of their inability to communicate about their symptoms. Furthermore, the cardiac rate at this age is normally rapid and even in the absence of tachyarrhythmia increases greatly with crying. Infants with SVT often present with congestive heart failure as the tachycardia goes unrecognized for a long time. The cardiac rate during paroxysms is frequently in the range of 200–300/min. If the attack lasts 6–24 hr or more with an extremely fast heart rate, the infant may become acutely ill, with an ashen color, and be restless and irritable. Tachypnea and hepatomegaly are the prominent signs of cardiac failure, and there may be fever and leukocytosis. When tachycardia occurs in the fetus, it can cause severe cardiac failure and is one of the major cardiac etiologies for hydrops fetalis (Fig. 388–6).

SVT in neonates usually presents with a narrow QRS complex (less than 0.08 sec). The P wave is visible on a standard electrocardiogram in only 50–60% of neonates with SVT but is visible with a transesophageal lead in most patients. Differentiation from sinus tachycardia may be difficult; if the rate is greater than 230 beats/min and there is an abnormal P wave axis (the normal P wave is positive in leads I and AVF), SVT is more likely. The heart rate in SVT also tends to be unvarying, whereas in sinus tachycardia the heart rate will vary with changes in vagal and sympathetic tone. Differentiation from ventricular tachycardia is critical, because digoxin can precipitate ventricular fibrillation in patients with ventricular tachycardia. The absence of P waves and presence of wide QRS complexes that are dissimilar to the QRS complex during sinus rhythm are more diagnostic of ventricular tachycardia.

SVT may be noted in the anatomically normal heart or may be associated with a bypass tract in one of the pre-excitation syndromes (Wolff-Parkinson-White or Lown-Ganong-Levine). SVT may occur in the presence of congenital heart disease, more commonly with Ebstein anomaly of the tricuspid valve and corrected transposition of the great vessels. In children, SVT may be precipitated by exposure to sympathomimetic amines contained in over-the-counter decongestants.

TREATMENT. Vagal stimulation by facial submersion in iced saline or an ice bag over the face may abort the attack. Older

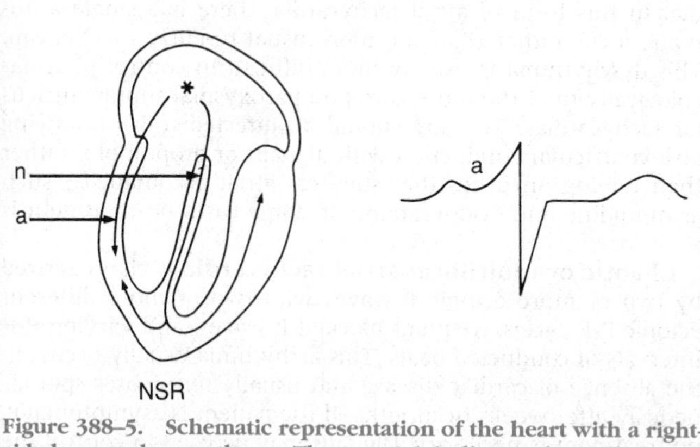

Figure 388–5. Schematic representation of the heart with a right-sided anomolous pathway. The *asterisk* indicates the initiation of the sinus beat. The *arrows* indicate the direction and spread of excitation. The electrocardiographic complex shown represents a fusion beat that combines activation over the normal (n) and accessory (a) pathways. The latter inscribes the δ wave.

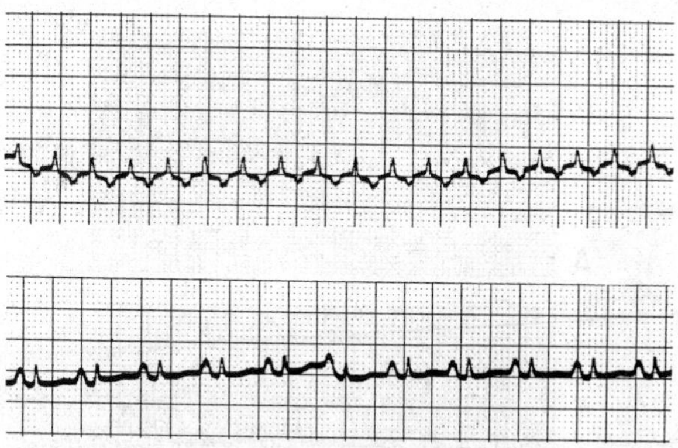

Figure 388–6. The upper tracing shows paroxysmal supraventricular or atrial tachycardia (PAT) with a ventricular rate of 230/min. The lower tracing shows sinus rhythm after D-C cardioversion. Note that during the tachycardia, the T wave is deformed by an inverted, presumably retrograde, P wave. The QRS morphology is unchanged during the tachycardia. Low voltage is due to peripheral edema in a 1-day-old infant who had intrauterine tachycardia and hydrops fetalis.

children may be taught vagotonic maneuvers to abolish the paroxysm, such as straining, the Valsalva maneuver, breath-holding, drinking ice water, or the adoption of a particular posture. When these measures fail, several pharmacologic alternatives are available (see Table 388–1). However, in urgent situations when symptoms of severe congestive heart failure have already occurred, synchronized DC cardioversion (0.5–2 watt-sec/kg) is recommended as the initial management. In stable patients, adenosine, administered by rapid intravenous push, is the treatment of choice, because of its rapid onset of action and minimal effects on cardiac contractility. Other drugs that have been used for initial treatment of SVT include infusions of phenylephrine (Neo-Synephrine) or edrophonium (Tensilon), which increase vagal tone through the baroreflex, and the antiarrhythmics, quinidine, procainamide, and propranolol. Calcium channel blockers such as verapamil (0.1–0.2 mg/kg) have also been used in the initial treatment of SVT in older children. However, verapamil may reduce cardiac output and produce hypotension and cardiac arrest in infants under 1 yr of age; therefore, it is contraindicated in this age group.

Once the patient has been converted to sinus rhythm, a longer acting agent is then selected for maintenance therapy. In infants, digoxin is the mainstay of therapy as it slows conduction within the A-V node and thus interrupts the re-entrant circuit. In older children with evidence of a pre-excitation syndrome, digoxin may increase the rate of anterograde conduction of impulses through the bypass tract. These patients are usually managed long-term with agents such as propranolol, procainamide, or quinidine.

If cardiac failure occurs due to prolonged tachycardia in an infant with a normal heart, cardiac function usually returns to normal after sinus rhythm is reinstituted, although this may take several weeks. Infants presenting with SVT within the first 3–4 mo of life have a lower incidence of recurrence than those presenting at a later age. These patients are usually treated for a minimum of 1 yr after diagnosis, after which the antiarrhythmic agents can be tapered and the patient watched for signs of recurrence.

Between attacks some children may exhibit the electrocardiographic changes of one of the pre-excitation syndromes, most commonly the *Wolff-Parkinson-White (WPW) syndrome*. These include a short P-R interval and slow upstroke of the QRS (delta wave) (Fig. 388–7). Although most often present in a normal heart, this syndrome may also be associated with Ebstein anomaly, corrected transposition (l-TGA, ventricular inversion), and cardiomyopathy. The syndrome causes a predilection for a re-entrant tachycardia. The anatomic substrate comprising the re-entrant circuit is the A-V node and an accessory pre-excitation pathway, a muscular bridge connecting atrium to ventricle on the right or left lateral cardiac border or within the ventricular septum (Fig. 388–5). During sinus rhythm the impulse is carried over both the A-V node and the accessory pathway; it produces some degree of fusion of the two depolarization fronts that results in an abnormal QRS. During tachycardia an impulse is usually carried anterograde through the A-V node, resulting in a normal QRS complex, and in retrograde fashion through the accessory pathway, reaching the atrium and perpetuating the tachycardia. In these cases, only after cessation of the tachycardia are the typical features of Wolff-Parkinson-White syndrome recognized (see Fig. 388–7). However, when rapid anterograde conduction occurs through the pre-excitation pathway during tachycardia and the retrograde re-entry pathway to the atrium is via the A-V node, the tachycardiac complexes are wide and the potential for more serious arrhythmias is greater, especially should atrial fibrillation occur. Patients can usually be successfully treated with a single antiarrhythmic agent, such as propranolol, procainamide, or quinidine.

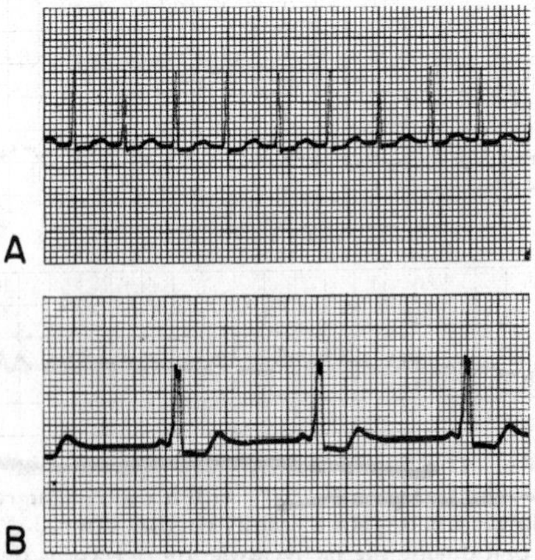

Figure 388–7. *A*, PAT in a child with Wolff-Parkinson-White (WPW) syndrome. Note the normal QRS complexes during the tachycardia. *B*, Later the typical features of WPW are apparent (short P-R interval, δ wave, and wide QRS).

Twenty-four–hour ECG (Holter) recordings are useful in monitoring the course of therapy and in detecting brief runs of tachycardia that may be asymptomatic. A brief assessment of arrhythmia control can be performed at the bedside using *transesophageal pacing*. More detailed *electrophysiologic (EP) studies*, performed in the cardiac catheterization lab, are often indicated in patients with refractory supraventricular tachyarrhythmias. During an EP study, multiple electrode catheters are placed into different locations in the heart. By comparing the timing of premature beats in different leads, the location of an ectopic focus or bypass tract can be identified. The tachyarrhythmia can be induced by pacing and different pharmacologic agents can be tested for their ability to inhibit the arrhythmia. These studies are necessary prerequisites before radiofrequency ablation.

Radiofrequency ablation of an accessory pathway is another treatment option for patients in whom multiple agents are required or if arrhythmia control is poor. The overall initial success rate has been reported to be as high as 83% in a large multicenter study. Surgical excision of bypass tracts can also be successfully carried out in selected patients.

OTHER ATRIAL TACHYARRHYTHMIAS

Ectopic atrial tachycardia is an uncommon tachycardia in childhood. It is characterized by a variable rate (seldom greater than 200), identifiable P waves with an abnormal axis, and chronicity in either a sustained or intermittent tachycardia. In this form of atrial tachycardia, there is a single automatic focus rather than the more usual re-entry mechanism. This dysrhythmia is usually more difficult to control pharmacologically than the more common paroxysmal supraventricular tachycardias. Therapy should be directed toward slowing atrioventricular conduction with digitalis or propranolol rather than relying on drugs that suppress atrial automaticity, such as quinidine and disopyramide. In some cases no treatment is necessary.

Chaotic or multifocal atrial tachycardia is characterized by two or more ectopic P waves with two or more different ectopic P-P cycles, frequent blocked P waves, and varying P-R intervals of conducted beats. This arrhythmia usually occurs in the absence of cardiac disease and usually terminates spontaneously after weeks or months. If the patient is asymptomatic, no treatment is necessary. Digitalis may be used to control the ventricular rate.

Accelerated junctional ectopic tachycardia (JET) is an arrhythmia in which the junctional rate exceeds that of the sinus node so that atrioventricular dissociation results. This arrhythmia is most often recognized in the early postoperative period following cardiac surgery and may be extremely difficult to control. Reduction of the infusion rate of catecholamines and control of fever are important adjuncts to management. JET often disappears spontaneously without specific treatment. Junctional tachycardia may also be a sign of digitalis intoxication, and when this occurs the drug should be discontinued. Recurrent JET in a patient with decreased ventricular function carries a guarded prognosis.

Atrial flutter is a regular or regularly irregular tachycardia due to atrial activity at a rate of 250–400/min. These contractions may be due to a circus rhythm in the atria and may be produced by an irritable focus in the atrial muscle similar to that responsible for paroxysmal atrial tachycardia and atrial extrasystoles. Because the atrioventricular node cannot transmit such rapid impulses, there is virtually always some degree of A-V block, and the ventricles respond to every 2nd–4th atrial beat. Occasionally, the response will be variable and the rhythm will appear irregular.

In older children atrial flutter usually occurs in the setting of congenital heart disease; however, neonates with atrial flutter frequently have normal hearts. Atrial flutter may occur during acute infectious illnesses but is most often seen in patients with large stretched atria, such as those associated with long-standing mitral or tricuspid insufficiency, tricuspid atresia, Ebstein anomaly, or rheumatic mitral stenosis. Atrial flutter also can occur after palliative or corrective intra-atrial surgery. Uncontrolled atrial flutter may precipitate congestive heart failure. Carotid sinus pressure or iced saline submersion usually produces a temporary slowing of the cardiac rate. The diagnosis is confirmed by electrocardiography, which demonstrates the rapid and regular atrial saw-toothed flutter waves. Atrial flutter usually converts immediately to sinus rhythm by DC cardioversion, and this is usually the treatment of choice. Digitalis slows the ventricular response in atrial flutter by prolonging conduction time through the A-V node. Occasionally, the rhythm will then convert to atrial fibrillation. After full digitalization, quinidine or procainamide may be added to convert to sinus rhythm. Neonates with normal hearts, who respond to digoxin, may be treated for 1 yr, after which the medication can often be discontinued.

Atrial fibrillation is produced by a mechanism similar to that causing atrial flutter; the atrial excitation is chaotic and more rapid (300–500/min) and produces an irregularly irregular ventricular response and pulse (Fig. 388–8). This rhythm disorder is most often the result of a chronically stretched atrial myocardium. Atrial fibrillation occurs most frequently in older children with rheumatic mitral valve disease. It also is seen rarely as a complication of intra-atrial surgery, with left atrial enlargement secondary to left atrioventricular valve insufficiency, in conditions producing atrial flutter, and in patients with the Wolff-Parkinson-White syndrome. Thyrotoxicosis, pulmonary emboli, and pericarditis should be suspected in a previously normal older child or adolescent who presents with atrial fibrillation. The best initial treatment is digitalization, which will restore the ventricular rate to normal, although the atrial fibrillation usually persists. Digoxin is not given if Wolff-Parkinson-White syndrome is present. Normal sinus rhythm may then be restored with quinidine sulfate, procainamide, or by DC cardioversion.

VENTRICULAR TACHYARRHYTHMIAS

Ventricular tachycardia (VT) is considerably less common than supraventricular tachycardia in pediatric age patients. VT is defined as at least 3 PVCs at greater than 120 beats/min. It may be paroxysmal or incessant (present most of the day). It may be associated with myocarditis, anomalous origin of a coronary artery, arrhythmogenic right ventricular dysplasia, mitral valve prolapse, primary cardiac tumors, cardiomyopathy, prolonged Q-T interval of either congenital or acquired (proarrhythmic drugs) etiology, Wolff-Parkinson-White syndrome, or drugs (cocaine, amphetamine); develop many years after intraventricular surgery (tetralogy of Fallot, ventricular septal defect [VSD]); or occur without obvious organic heart disease. VT must be distinguished from supraventricular tachycardia with aberrancy or rapid conduction over an accessory pathway (Table 388–2). The presence of capture and fusion beats helps confirm the diagnosis. Although some children tolerate rapid ventricular rates for many hours, this arrhythmia should be promptly treated because hypotension and degeneration into ventricular fibrillation may result. Lidocaine and cardioversion (1–2 watt-sec/kg) are methods of choice for rapid treatment. Bretylium is an alternative drug if the arrhythmia is refractory to lidocaine (see Table 388–1). It is critical to search for and correct any underlying abnormalities, for example, electrolyte imbalance, hypoxia, or drug toxicity if treatment is to be successful. Quinidine, procainamide, and propranolol are useful for chronic therapy. In the neonatal period, ventricular tachycardia may be associated with anomalous left coronary artery or with a myocardial tumor; for the latter, resection is usually curative.

Ventricular fibrillation is a chaotic dysrhythmia that results in death unless an effective ventricular beat is rapidly restored. A thump on the chest sometimes restores sinus rhythm. Usually external cardiac massage with artificial ventilation and DC defibrillation are necessary. Electrophysiologic study is usually indicated for patients who have developed ventricular fibrillation unless a clearly reversible cause is identified. For patients who are refractory to pharmacologic therapy, an automatic implantable cardioverter-defibrillator (AICD) can be inserted.

388.2 Bradyarrhythmias

Sinus arrest and sinoatrial block may cause a sudden pause in the heart beat. The former is presumed to be caused by failure of impulse formation within the sinus node and the latter by a block between the sinus impulse and the sur-

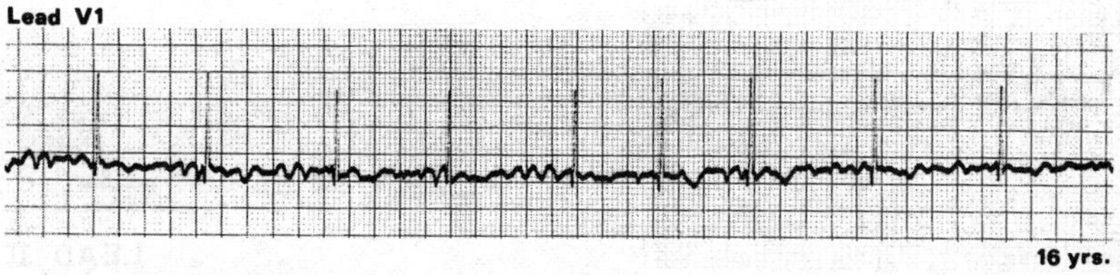

Figure 388–8. Atrial fibrillation, characterized by absence of P waves; presence of fibrillatory waves, which are grossly irregular, rapid undulations; and an irregular ventricular response. Fibrillatory waves may not be visible in all leads and should be carefully sought in every tracing with irregular R-R intervals. (The coexisting qR in V_1 is diagnostic of right ventricular hypertrophy in this patient with Eisenmenger syndrome.)

■ TABLE 388–2 Diagnosis of Tachyarrhythmias

	Electrocardiographic Findings			
	Heart Rate/Min	*P Wave*	*QRS Duration*	*Regularity*
Sinus tachycardia	<225	Always present Normal axis	Normal	Rate varies with respiration
Atrial tachycardia	180–320	Present—50% Superior axis common	Normal or prolonged (RBBB* pattern)	Regular
Atrial fibrillation	120–180	Fibrillatory waves	Normal or prolonged (RBBB pattern)	Irregularly irregular
Atrial flutter	Atrial: 250–400 Ventricular response variable: 100–320	Saw-toothed flutter waves	Normal or prolonged (RBBB pattern)	Regular ventricular response (e.g., 2:1, 3:1, 3:2, etc.)
Ventricular tachycardia	120–240	Absent or atrioventricular dissociation	Usually prolonged	Slightly irregular

RBBB = right bundle branch block.

rounding atrium. These arrhythmias are rare in childhood, except as manifestations of digitalis intoxication or in patients who have had extensive atrial surgery.

Atrioventricular block may be divided into three forms. In 1st-degree block, the P-R interval is prolonged but all of the atrial impulses are conducted to the ventricle. In 2nd-degree block, some impulses are not conducted to the ventricle. In one variant of 2nd-degree block, known as the Wenckebach type (also called Mobitz type I), the P-P interval remains constant and the P-R interval increases progressively until a P wave is not conducted. In the cycle following the dropped beat, the P-R interval is again shorter (Fig. 388–9). In Mobitz type II, occasional atrial beats are not conducted to the ventricle; this conduction defect has more potential to cause syncope and may be progressive. In 3rd-degree block (complete heart block), no impulses from the atria reach the ventricles.

Congenital complete atrioventricular block in children is most often caused by autoimmune injury of the fetal conduction system by maternally derived IgG antibodies (anti-SSA/Ro, anti-SSB/La) in a mother with overt or, more often, asymptomatic systemic lupus erythematosus (SLE). Rarely rheumatoid arthritis, dermatomyositis, or Sjögren syndrome is the primary autoimmune process. Autoimmune disease accounts for 60–70% of all congenital complete heart block and about 80% of cases where there is a structurally normal heart. Complete heart block is also seen in patients with complex congenital heart disease, abnormal embryonic development of the conduction system, myocardial tumors, myocarditis, myocardial abscess due to endocarditis, long QT syndrome, postsurgical repair of congenital heart disease involving the ventricular septum, and Kearns-Sayre syndrome. The incidence of congenital complete heart block is 1 in 20,000–25,000 live births; a high fetal wastage rate may cause an underestimation of its true incidence. In some infants of mothers with SLE, complete heart block is not present at birth but develops within the first 3–6 mo after birth. The arrhythmia is occasionally suspected in the fetus and may produce hydrops fetalis. The dissociation between atrial and ventricular contractions can be diagnosed by fetal echocardiography. At greatest risk for serious illness are infants with associated congenital heart disease who in the 1st wk of life develop congestive heart failure.

In older children with otherwise normal hearts, the condition is commonly asymptomatic, although attacks of syncope may occur. Older infants may develop night terrors, tiredness with frequent naps, and irritability. The peripheral pulse is prominent as a result of the compensatory large ventricular stroke volume and peripheral vasodilatation; the systolic blood pressure is elevated. Jugular venous pulsations occur irregularly and may be large when the atrium contracts against a closed tricuspid valve (cannon wave). Exercise and atropine produce an acceleration of 10–20 beats/min or more. Systolic murmurs are frequent along the left sternal border, and apical mid-diastolic murmurs are not unusual. Heart block in itself results in cardiac enlargement simply on the basis of increased diastolic ventricular filling.

The *diagnosis* is confirmed by electrocardiogram; the P waves and QRS complexes have no constant relation (Fig. 388–10). The QRS duration may be prolonged or may be normal if the heart beat is initiated high in the His bundle.

The *prognosis* for congenital complete heart block is usually favorable; patients who have been observed to the age of 30–40 yr have lived normally active lives. However, some patients have episodes of dizziness with or without syncope **(Stokes-Adams attacks)**; this complication requires the implantation of a permanent cardiac pacemaker. The indications for implanting a pacemaker include the development of symptoms, progressive cardiac enlargement, or prolonged pauses.

Neonates with ventricular rates ≤50 beats/min, evidence of hydrops, or the development of heart failure after birth require *cardiac pacing*. Atropine, isoproterenol, or epinephrine may be used to try to temporarily increase the heart rate while arranging for pacemaker placement. Patients with complete heart block and a wide QRS ventricular response should be paced prior to receiving antiarrhythmic drugs, as these may suppress the escape focus. Transthoracic epicardial pacemaker implants have been traditionally used in infants; however, transvenous placement of pacemaker leads is gaining acceptance for older infants and young children.

Postsurgical complete atrioventricular block can occur after

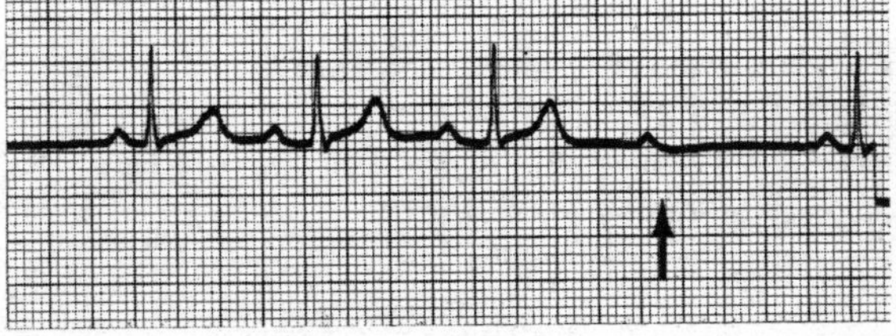

Figure 388–9. Wenckebach phenomenon (Mobitz I). The P-R interval gradually lengthens until the 4th P wave in the cycle is not conducted to the ventricle *(arrow)*. The ensuing P-R interval is once again normal.

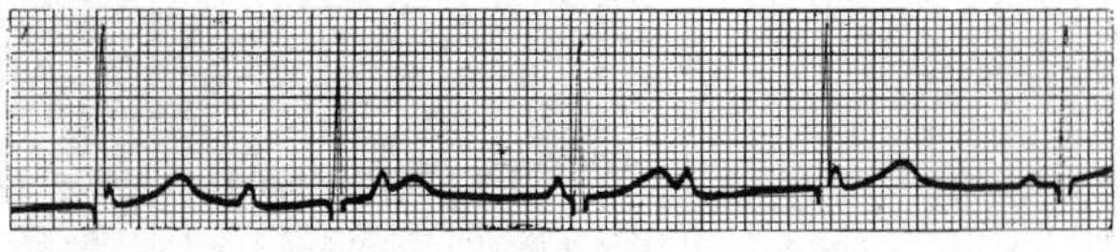

Figure 388–10. Complete atrioventricular block. The ventricular rate is regular at 53/min. The atrial rate varied from 65 to 95/min (probably sinus arrhythmia). The QRS morphology is normal, which is usual in congenital A-V block.

any open heart procedure requiring suturing near the atrioventricular valves or crest of the ventricular septum. Because postoperative heart block may be transient, the patient should be maintained with temporary pacing wires inserted at the time of surgery until at least 10–14 days, after which it is much less likely that sinus rhythm will return.

CHAPTER 389
Sick Sinus Syndrome

The sick sinus syndrome is the result of abnormalities in the sinus node and/or atrial conduction pathways as outlined in Figure 389–1. This syndrome may occur in the absence of congenital heart disease and has been reported in siblings but is most commonly seen after surgical correction of congenital heart defects, especially the Mustard procedure for transposition of the great arteries. The *clinical manifestations* depend on the heart rate. Most patients remain asymptomatic without treatment. Dizziness and syncope can occur during periods of marked sinus slowing with failure of junctional escape (Fig. 389–2). Supraventricular tachycardias may alternate with bradycardias (bradycardia-tachycardia syndrome), causing palpitations, exercise intolerance, or dizziness. *Treatment* must be individualized. In general, aside from digitalis, drug therapy to control tachyarrhythmias (e.g., propranolol, quinidine, procainamide) may suppress sinus and atrioventricular nodal function to the degree that symptomatic bradycardia may be produced. Therefore, insertion of a demand ventricular pacemaker in conjunction with drug therapy is usually necessary for symptomatic patients.

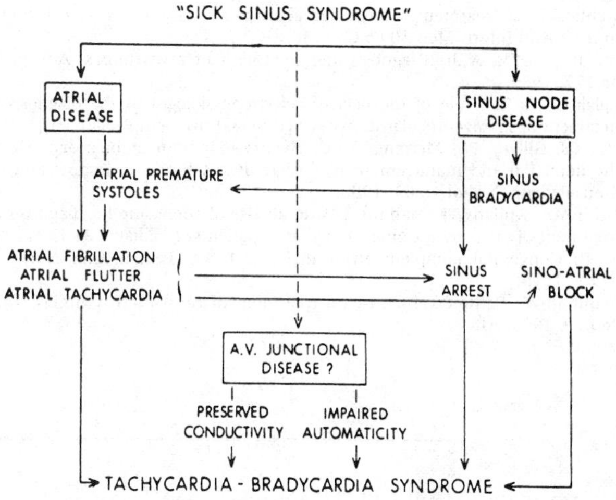

Figure 389–1. Factors resulting in the sick sinus syndrome. (From Kaplan BM, Langendorf R, Lev M, et al: Am J Cardiol 31:497, 1973. Reproduced by permission of Technical Publishing Company.)

Akhtar M, Shenasa M, Jazayeri M, et al: Wide QRS complex tachycardia: Reappraisal of a common clinical problem. Ann Intern Med 109:905, 1988.

Benson DW Jr, Smith WM, Dunnigan A, et al: Mechanisms of regular, wide QRS tachycardia in infants and children. Am J Cardiol 49:1778, 1982.

Brooks R, Burgess JH: Idiopathic ventricular tachycardia: A review. Medicine 67:271, 1988.

Case C, Crawford F, Gillette P: Surgical treatment of dysrhythmias. Pediatr Clin North Am 37:79, 1990.

Deal BJ, Keane JF, Gillette PC, et al: Wolff-Parkinson-White syndrome and supraventricular tachycardia during infancy: Management and follow-up. J Am Coll Cardiol 5:130, 1985.

Dewey RC, Capeless MA, Levy AM: Use of ambulatory electrocardiographic monitoring to identify high-risk patients with congenital complete heart block. N Engl J Med 316:835, 1987.

Dick M: Complete heart block in children. Curr Opin Pediatr 2:957, 1990.

DiMarco JP, Miles W, Akhtar M, et al: Adenosine for paroxysmal supraventricular tachycardia: Dose ranging and comparison with verapamil. Ann Intern Med 113:104, 1990.

Dungan WT, Garson A Jr, Gillette PC: Arrhythmogenic right ventricular dysplasia: A cause of ventricular tachycardia in children with apparently normal hearts. Am Heart J 102:745, 1981.

Dunnigan A, Benson DW Jr, Banditt DG: Atrial flutter in infancy: Diagnosis, clinical features, and treatment. Pediatrics 75:725, 1985.

Fried MD: Advances in the diagnosis and therapy of syncopy and palpitations in children. Curr Opin Pediatr 6:368, 1994.

Garson A, Gillette PC, McNamara DG: Supraventricular tachycardia in children: Clinical features, response to treatment and long-term follow-up in 217 patients. J Pediatr 98:875, 1981.

Garson A Jr, Gillette PC, Titus JL, et al: Surgical treatment of ventricular tachycardia in infants. N Engl J Med 310:1443, 1984.

Garson A Jr, Randall DC, Gillette PC, et al: Prevention of sudden death after repair of tetralogy of Fallot: Treatment of ventricular arrhythmias. J Am Coll Cardiol 6:221, 1985.

Gillette PC, Garson A, Kugler JD: Wolff-Parkinson-White syndrome in children: Electrophysiologic and pharmacologic characteristics. Circulation 60:1487, 1979.

Gow R: Ventricular arrhythmias in infants and children. Curr Opin Pediatr 2:963, 1990.

Griffith MJ, Linker NJ, Garratt CJ, et al: Relative efficacy and safety of intravenous drugs for termination of sustained ventricular tachycardia. Lancet 336:670, 1990.

Hayes CJ, Gersony WM: Arrhythmias after the Mustard operation for transposition of the great arteries: A long-term study. J Am Coll Cardiol 7:133, 1986.

Johnson WH, Dunnigan A, Fehr P, et al: Association of atrial flutter with orthodromic reciprocating fetal tachycardia. Ann J Cardiol 59:374, 1987.

Josephson ME: Antiarrhythmic agents and the danger of proarrhythmic events. Ann Intern Med 111:101, 1989.

Kaminer SJ, Pickoff AS, Dunnigan A, et al: Cardiomyopathy and the use of implanted cardio-defibrillators in children. PACE 13:593, 1990.

Kirk CR, Gibbs JL, Thomas R: Cardiovascular collapse after verapamil in supraventricular tachycardia. Arch Dis Child 62:1265, 1987.

Kugler JD, Danford DA, Deal BJ, et al: Radiofrequency catheter ablation for tachyarrhythmias in children and adolescents. N Engl J Med 330:1481, 1994.

Figure 389–2. Sick sinus syndrome with brady-tachycardia. Note the bursts of supraventricular tachycardia, probably multifocal in origin, followed by long periods of sinus arrest and by sinus bradycardia.

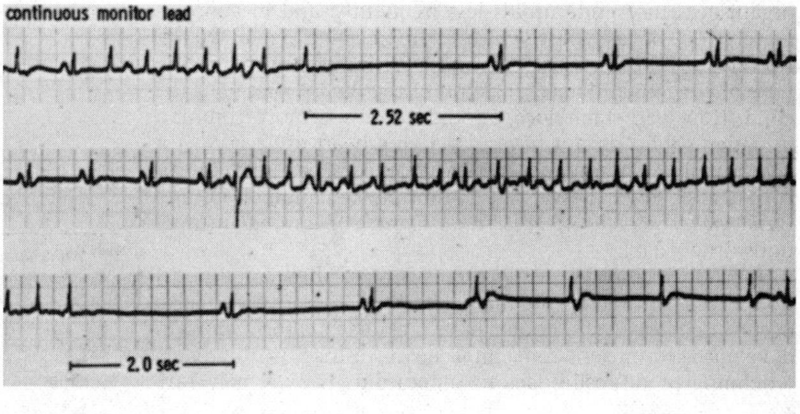

Marchlinski FE: Treatment of sustained ventricular arrhythmias: Which therapy to use? Ann Intern Med 109:522, 1988.
Perry JC, Garson A Jr: Diagnosis and treatment of arrhythmias. Adv Pediatr 36:177, 1989.
Pongiglione G: The role of the pediatric electrophysiologist in the diagnosis and treatment of supraventricular tachydysrhythmias. Curr Opin Pediatr 1:124, 1989.
Porter CJ, Gillette PC, McNamara DG: Twenty-four hour ambulatory ECG's in the detection and management of cardiac dysrhythmias in infants and children. Pediatr Cardiol 1:203, 1980.
Ralston MA, Knilans TK, Hannon DW, et al: Use of adenosine for diagnosis and treatment of tachyarrhythmias in pediatric patients. J Pediatr 124:139, 1994.
Ross B: Congenital complete atrioventricular block. Pediatr Clin North Am 37:69, 1990.
Scheinman M: Catheter and surgical treatment of cardiac arrhythmias. JAMA 263:79, 1990.
Sreeram N, Wren C: Supraventricular tachycardia in infants: Response to initial treatment. Arch Dis Child 65:127, 1990.
Tchou PJ, Kadri N, Anderson J, et al: Automatic implantable cardioverter defibrillators and survival of patients with left ventricular dysfunction and malignant ventricular arrhythmias. Ann Intern Med 109:529, 1988.
Till J, Shinebourne EA, Rigby ML, et al: Efficacy and safety of adenosine in the treatment of supraventricular tachycardia in infants and children. Br Heart J 62:204, 1989.
Van Hare GF, Lesh MD, Scheinman M, et al: Percutaneous radiofrequency catheter ablation for supraventricular tachycardia in children. J Am Coll Cardiol 17:1613, 1991.
Wellens HJJ, Brugada P, Penn OC: The management of preexcitation syndromes. JAMA 257:2325, 1987.
Zipes DP: Guidelines for clinical intracardiac electrophysiologic studies. J Am Coll Cardiol 14:1827, 1989.

SECTION 5
Acquired Heart Disease

CHAPTER 390
Infective Endocarditis

Infective endocarditis includes the entities referred to as acute and subacute bacterial endocarditis (see Chapters 174 and 175) as well as infections of nonbacterial endocarditis such as those caused by viruses, fungi, and other agents. It remains a significant cause of morbidity and mortality among children and adolescents despite the advances in the management and prophylaxis of the disease with antimicrobial agents. The inability to eradicate infective endocarditis by prevention or early treatment stems from several factors: The nature of the infecting organisms has changed over the years; physicians, dentists, and the public are not sufficiently aware of the threat of infective endocarditis and the preventive measures available; diagnosis may be difficult when delayed; and special risk groups have emerged, which include an increasing number of intravenous narcotics users, survivors of cardiac surgery, and patients with lowered resistance to infection who require intravascular catheters.

ETIOLOGY. In the past, *Streptococcus viridans* was the agent most commonly responsible for endocarditis in pediatric patients. However, *Staphylococcus aureus* has become increasingly more common and is now the leading causative agent in some series, accounting for approximately 39% of episodes. Other organisms cause endocarditis less frequently, and in approximately 10% of cases blood cultures are negative (Table 390–1). No relationship exists between the infecting organism and the type of congenital defect, duration of the illness, or age of the child. However, staphylococcal endocarditis is more common in patients who do not have underlying heart disease; *S. viridans* is more common after dental procedures, group D enterococcus after lower bowel or genitourinary manipulation, and *Pseudomonas aeruginosa* or *Serratia marcescens* among intravenous drug users.

EPIDEMIOLOGY. Infective endocarditis is most often a complication of congenital or rheumatic heart disease but can also occur in children who do not have a cardiac malformation. In developed countries, congenital heart disease is the overwhelming predisposing factor. Endocarditis is extremely rare in infancy, and when it occurs in this age group it is usually closely following open heart surgery.

Patients with congenital cardiac lesions that have a high velocity of blood ejected through a hole or stenotic orifice are most susceptible to endocarditis. Vegetations are usually formed at the site of the endocardial or intimal erosion that results from the turbulent flow. Thus, children with ventricular septal defects (VSDs), left-sided valvular disease, and systemic-pulmonary arterial communications (including palliative shunts) are at the highest risk. Therefore, tetralogy of Fallot, VSD, aortic stenosis, patent ductus arteriosus (PDA), transposi-

■ **TABLE 390–1 Bacterial Agents in Pediatric Infective Endocarditis**

Common: Native Valve or Other Cardiac Lesions
Streptococcus viridans group (*S. mutans, S. sanguis, S. mitis*)
Staphylococcus aureus
Group D streptococcus (enterococcus) (*S. bovis, S. faecalis*)
Uncommon: Native Valve or Other Cardiac Lesions
Streptococcus pneumoniae
Haemophilus influenzae
Staphylococcus epidermidis
Coxiella burnetii (Q fever)*
Neisseria gonorrhoeae
*Brucella**
*Chlamydia psittaci**
*Chlamydia trachomatis**
*Chlamydia pneumoniae**
HACEK group†
*Streptobacillus moniliformis**
*Pasteurella multocida**
Campylobacter fetus
Culture negative (10% of cases)
Prosthetic Valve
Staphylococcus epidermidis
Staphylococcus aureus
Streptococcus viridans
Pseudomonas aeruginosa
Serratia marcescens
Diphtheroids
Legionella species*
HACEK group†
Fungi‡

**These fastidious bacteria plus some fungi may produce culture-negative endocarditis. Detection may require special media, incubation for more than 7 days, or serology.*

†HACEK group includes Haemophilus *species* (H. paraphrophilus, H. parainfluenzae, H. aphrophilus), Actinobacillus actinomycetemcomitans, Cardiobacterium hominis, Eikenella corrodens, Kingella *species.*

‡Candida *species,* Aspergillus *species,* Pseudallescheria boydii, Histoplasma capsulatum.

tion of the great arteries, and palliative shunts are the most frequent structural lesions associated with endocarditis. In older patients, congenital bicuspid aortic valves and mitral valve prolapse pose additional risks for endocarditis. Surgical correction of congenital heart disease may reduce but does not eliminate the risk of endocarditis, with the exception of repair of a simple atrial septal defect (ASD) or PDA. Children who have had a valve replacement or valved conduit repair are at particularly high risk.

In approximately 30% of patients with infective endocarditis, a predisposing factor is recognized. A surgical or dental procedure can be implicated in approximately two thirds of these cases in which the potential source of bacteremia is identified. Poor dental hygiene in children with cyanotic heart disease results in a greater risk for endocarditis. The occurrence of endocarditis directly following heart surgery is relatively low, but it is frequently an antecedent event.

CLINICAL MANIFESTATIONS (Table 390–2). The early symptoms and signs are usually mild, especially when *S. viridans* is the infecting organism. Prolonged fever, without other manifestations (except occasionally weight loss), persisting for as long as several months, may often be the only medical history. Alternatively, the onset may be acute and severe, with high, intermittent fever and prostration. Usually, however, the onset and course vary between these two extremes. The symptoms are usually nonspecific and consist of low-grade fever with afternoon elevations, fatigue, myalgia, arthralgia, headache, and at times chills, nausea, and vomiting. New or changing heart murmurs are common, particularly when there is associated congestive heart failure. Splenomegaly is relatively common, and petechiae may occur. Serious neurologic complications, such as emboli, cerebral abscesses, mycotic aneurysms, and hemorrhage, are most often associated with staphylococcal disease. These complications are manifested by meningismus, increased intracranial pressure, altered sensorium, and focal neurologic signs. Myocardial abscesses may also occur with staphylococcal disease and may rupture into the pericardium. Pulmonary and other systemic emboli are infrequent, except with fungal disease. Many of the classic skin manifestations develop late in the course of the disease; hence, they are seldomly seen in the appropriately treated patient. These include *Osler nodes* (tender, pea-sized intradermal nodules in the pads of the fingers and toes), *Janeway lesions* (painless small erythematous or hemorrhagic lesions on the palms and soles), and *splinter hemorrhages* (linear lesions beneath the nails). These lesions probably represent vasculitis produced by circulating antigen-antibody complexes.

The identification of infective endocarditis will most often be based on a high index of suspicion in the evaluation of an infection in a child with an underlying contributory factor.

■ TABLE 390–2 Manifestations of Infective Endocarditis

History
Prior congenital or rheumatic heart disease
Preceding dental, urinary, or intestinal procedure
Intravenous drug use
Central venous catheter
Prosthetic heart valve

Symptoms
Fever
Chills
Chest pain
Arthralgia/myalgia
Dyspnea
Malaise
Night sweats
Weight loss
CNS* manifestations (stroke, seizures, headache)

Signs
Elevated temperature
Tachycardia
Embolic phenomena (Roth spots, petechiae, splinter nailbed hemorrhages, Osler nodes, CNS or ocular lesions)
Janeway lesions
New or changing murmur
Splenomegaly
Arthritis
Heart failure
Arrhythmias
Metastatic infection (arthritis, meningitis, mycotic arterial aneurysm, pericarditis, abscesses, septic pulmonary emboli)
Clubbing

Laboratory
Positive blood culture
Elevated erythrocyte sedimentation rate; may be low with heart or renal failure
Elevated C-reactive protein
Anemia
Leukocytosis
Immune complexes
Hypergammaglobulinemia
Hypocomplementemia
Cryoglobulinemia
Rheumatoid factor
Hematuria
Azotemia, high creatinine (glomerulonephritis)
Echocardiographic evidence of valve vegetations, prosthetic valve dysfunction or leak, or myocardial abscess

*CNS = *central nervous system.*

LABORATORY FINDINGS. The critical information for appropriate treatment of infective endocarditis is obtained from blood cultures. All other laboratory data are secondary in importance (see Table 390–2). Blood cultures should be obtained as promptly as possible and should be drawn even if the child feels well and has no other physical findings. Three to five separate blood collections should be obtained after careful preparation of the phlebotomy site. Contamination presents a special problem, as bacteria found on the skin may themselves cause infective endocarditis. The timing of collections is not important because bacteremia can be expected to be relatively constant. In 90% of cases of endocarditis, the etiologic agent is recovered from the first two blood cultures. The laboratory should be notified that endocarditis is suspected as the blood may need to be cultured on enriched media for a longer than usual time (>7 days) to detect nutritionally deficient and fastidious bacteria or fungi. Antimicrobial pretreatment of the patient reduces the yield of blood cultures to 50–60%. The microbiology laboratory should be notified if the patient has received antibiotics so that more sophisticated methods can be used to recover the offending agent. Other sites that may be cultured include cutaneous lesions, urine, synovial fluid, abscesses, and, in the presence of manifestations of meningitis, the cerebrospinal fluid. Serologic diagnosis is necessary in patients with unusual or fastidious microorganisms (see Table 390–1).

DIAGNOSIS. There should be a high index of suspicion in evaluating infection in a child with an underlying contributing factor. The combination of M-mode, two-dimensional, and transesophageal echocardiography has enhanced the ability to diagnose endocarditis. M mode can detect valvular vegetations larger than 2–3 mm. Two-dimensional echocardiography can identify the size, shape, location, and mobility of the lesion; when combined with Doppler studies, the presence of valve dysfunction (regurgitation, obstruction) can be determined and its effect on left ventricular performance quantified. Echocardiography may also be helpful in predicting embolic complications, as lesions greater than 1 cm and fungating masses are at greatest risk for embolization. The absence of vegetations does not exclude endocarditis, and vegetations are often not visualized in the early phases of the disease or in patients with complex congenital heart lesions.

PROGNOSIS AND COMPLICATIONS. In the preantibiotic era, infective endocarditis was a fatal disease. Despite the use of antibiotic agents, the mortality remains at 20–25%. Serious morbidity occurs in 50–60% of children with documented infective endocarditis; the most common is cardiac failure caused by vegetations involving the aortic or mitral valve. Myocardial abscesses and toxic myocarditis may also lead to congestive heart failure without characteristic changes in auscultatory findings. Systemic emboli, often with central nervous system manifestations, are a major threat. Pulmonary emboli may occur in children with VSD or tetralogy of Fallot, although massive life-threatening pulmonary embolization is rare. Other complications include mycotic aneurysms, rupture of a sinus of Valsalva, obstruction of a valve secondary to large vegetations, acquired VSD, and heart block as a result of involvement of the specialized conduction system.

TREATMENT. Antibiotic therapy should be instituted immediately on diagnosis. When virulent organisms are responsible, small delays may result in progressive endocardial damage and a greater likelihood of severe complications. The choice of antibiotics, method of administration, and length of treatment are outlined in Table 390–3. High serum bactericidal levels must be maintained long enough to eradicate organisms that are growing in relatively inaccessible avascular vegetations. Between 5 and 20 times the minimum in vitro inhibiting concentration must be produced at the site of infection to destroy bacteria growing at the core of these lesions. Several weeks are required for a vegetation to organize completely; thus, therapy must be continued through this period so that recrudescence can be avoided. A total of 4–6 wk of treatment is recommended, with serumcidal levels by tube dilution of at least 1:8 after a dose of antibiotic. Depending on the clinical and laboratory responses, antibiotic therapy may require modification, and in some instances more prolonged treatment is required. With highly sensitive *S. viridans* infections, shortened regimens, including oral penicillin for some portion, have been more recently recommended.

Bed rest should be instituted and should be extended if congestive heart failure occurs. Similarly, digitalis, restriction of salt intake, and diuretic therapy should be utilized when indicated.

Surgical intervention during the course of infective endocarditis is an integral part of management in cases in which severe aortic or mitral valve involvement leads to intractable heart failure. Rarely, a mycotic aneurysm, rupture of an aortic sinus, or dehiscence of an intracardiac patch requires emergency operation. Other surgical indications include failure to sterilize the blood despite adequate antibiotic levels, a myocardial abscess, recurrent emboli, and failure of medical management. Although antibiotic therapy should be administered for as long

■ **TABLE 390–3 Treatment of Infective Endocarditis**

Etiologic Agent	Drug	Dose	Route	Duration of Therapy (Weeks)
Streptococcus viridans, S. bovis (Minimal inhibitory concentration [MIC] ≤0.1 μg/mL)	(1) Penicillin G *or*	200,000–300,000 U/kg/24 hr q 4 hr not to exceed 20 million U/24 hr	IV	4–6
	(2) Penicillin G	As above no. 1	IV	2–4
	plus gentamicin	3–7.5 mg/kg/24 hr q 8 hr not to exceed 80 mg/24 hr	IV	2
S. viridans, S. bovis (MIC ≥0.1 μg/mL)	(3) Penicillin G	As above no. 2	IV	4–6
	plus gentamicin	As above no. 2	IV	2
S. viridans or enterococcus (*S. bovis* or *S. faecalis*) (MIC >0.5 μg/mL)	(4) Penicillin G *or*	As above no. 2	IV	4–6
	ampicillin	300 mg/kg 24 hr q 4–6 hr not to exceed 12 g/24 hr	IV	4–6
	plus gentamicin	As above no. 2	IV	4–6
*S. viridans, S. bovis** (penicillin allergy†)	(5) Vancomycin	40–60 mg/kg/24 hr q 8–12 hr not to exceed 2 g/24 hr	IV	4–6
	plus (6) gentamicin if resistant*	As above no. 2	IV	4–6
Staphylococcus aureus	(7) Nafcillin *or*	200 mg/kg/24 hr q 4–6 hr not to exceed 12 g/24 hr	IV	6–8
	oxacillin	As above no. 2		
	plus optional gentamicin		IV	1–2
S. aureus (methicillin resistant) (penicillin allergy)	(8) Vancomycin	As above no. 5	IV	6–8
	plus optional trimethoprim-sulfamethoxazole	12 mg/kg/24 hr trimethoprim q 8 hr not to exceed 1 g/24 hr	IV, PO	4–8
S. aureus (with prosthetic device, methicillin sensitive)‡	(9) Nafcillin	As above no. 7	IV	6–8
	plus gentamicin	As above no. 2	IV	2
	plus optional rifampin	10–20 mg/kg/24 hr q 12 hr not to exceed 600 mg/24 hr	PO	≥6
S. aureus (with prosthetic device, methicillin resistant)	(10) Vancomycin	As above no. 5	IV	6–8
	plus gentamicin	As above no. 9	IV	2
	plus optional rifampin	As above no. 9	PO	≥6
S. epidermidis	(11) Vancomycin	As above no. 5	IV	6–8
	plus optional rifampin	As above no. 9	PO	6–8
Haemophilus species	(12) Ampicillin	As above no. 4	IV	4–6
	plus optional gentamicin	As above no. 2	IV	2–4
Unknown	(13) Vancomycin	As above no. 5	IV	6–8
Postoperative	plus gentamicin	As above no. 2	IV	2–4
Nonoperative	(14) Nafcillin *or*	As above no. 7	IV	6–8
	vancomycin	As above no. 5	IV	6–8
	plus gentamicin	As above no. 2	IV	2–4
	plus optional ampicillin	As above no. 4	IV	6–8

**Add gentamicin for relatively resistant organisms. Monitor vancomycin peaks 1 hr after infusion (30–45 μg/mL). Adjust dose according to vancomycin levels.*
†Desensitization should be considered for patients who are allergic to penicillin. Cephalosporins are not recommended.
‡May require valve (device) replacement.

as possible prior to surgical intervention, active infection is not a contraindication if the patient is critically ill as a result of severe hemodynamic deterioration from infective endocarditis. Removal of vegetations and, in some instances, valve replacement may be lifesaving, and sustained antibiotic administration will most often prevent reinfection. Replacement of infected prosthetic valves carries a higher risk.

Fungal endocarditis is difficult to manage and most often has a poor prognosis regardless of treatment. It has been encountered after cardiac surgery, especially in severely debilitated or immunosuppressed patients. The drugs of choice are amphotericin B and flucytosine. Surgery to excise infected tissue is occasionally attempted, usually with limited success.

PREVENTION. Antimicrobial prophylaxis prior to and after various procedures, including dental cleaning and other forms of dental manipulation, reduces the incidence of infective endocarditis in susceptible patients. However, proper general dental care and oral hygiene are most important in decreasing the risk of infective endocarditis in susceptible individuals. Vigorous treatment of sepsis and local infections, and careful asepsis during cardiac surgery and catheterization, will also reduce the incidence of infective endocarditis. See Table 386–1 for recommended antibiotic regimens.

Bisno AL, Dismukes WE, Durack DT, et al: Antimicrobial treatment of infective endocarditis due to viridans streptococci, enterococci, and staphylococci. JAMA 261:1471, 1989.

Dinubile MJ: Surgery in active endocarditis. Ann Intern Med 96:650, 1982.

Elward K, Hruby N, Christy C: Pneumococcal endocarditis in infants and children: Report of a case and review of the literature. Pediatr Infect Dis J 9:652, 1990.

Geva T, Frand M: Infective endocarditis in children with congenital heart disease: The changing spectrum, 1965–1985. Eur Heart J 9:1244, 1988.

van Hare GF, Ben-Shachar G, Liebman J, et al: Infective endocarditis in infants and children during the past 10 years: A decade of change. Am Heart J 107:1235, 1984.

Heimberger TS, Duma RJ: Infections of prosthetic heart valves and cardiac pacemakers. Infect Dis Clin North Am 3:221, 1989.

O'Callaghan C, McDougall P: Infective endocarditis in neonates. Arch Dis Child 63:53, 1988.

Saiman L, Prince A, Gersony WM: Pediatric infective endocarditis in the modern era. J Pediatr 122:847, 1993.

Shulman ST, Amren DP, Bisno AL, et al: Prevention of bacterial endocarditis. Am J Dis Child 139:232, 1985.

Stanton BF, Baltimore RS, Clemens JD: Changing spectrum of infective endocarditis in children. Am J Dis Child 138:720, 1984.

Wall TC, Peyton RB, Corey GR: Gonococcal endocarditis: A new look at an old disease. Medicine 68:375, 1989.

Walterspiel JN, Kaplan SL: Incidence and clinical characteristics of "culture-negative" infective endocarditis in a pediatric population. Pediatr Infect Dis 5:328, 1986.

Weinstein MP, Stratton CW, Ackley A, et al: Multicenter collaborative evaluation of a standardized serum bactericidal test as a prognostic indicator of infective endocarditis. Am J Med 78:262, 1985.

CHAPTER 391
Rheumatic Heart Disease

Rheumatic involvement of the valves and endocardium is the most important manifestation of rheumatic fever (see Chapter 175.1). The valvar lesions begin as small verrucae composed of fibrin and blood cells along the borders of one or more of the heart valves. The mitral valve is affected most often, followed in frequency by the aortic valve; right-sided heart manifestations are rare. As the inflammation subsides, the verrucae tend to disappear and leave scar tissue. With a repeated attack of rheumatic fever, new verrucae form near the previous ones, and the mural endocardium and chordae tendineae become involved.

PATTERNS OF VALVULAR DISEASE

Mitral Insufficiency

PATHOPHYSIOLOGY. This is the result of structural changes that usually include some loss of valvular substance and shortening and thickening of the chordae tendineae. During acute rheumatic fever with severe cardiac involvement, congestive heart failure is most often caused by a combination of the mechanical effects of severe mitral insufficiency coupled with inflammatory disease that may involve the pericardium, myocardium, endocardium, and epicardium. Because of the high volume load and inflammatory process, the left ventricle becomes large and inefficient. The left atrium dilates as blood regurgitates into this chamber. Increased left atrial pressure results in pulmonary congestion and symptoms of left-sided heart failure. In most cases mitral insufficiency is in the mild to moderate range. Even in those patients in whom insufficiency is severe at the onset, there is usually spontaneous improvement with time. The resultant chronic lesion is most often mild or moderate in severity, and the patient will be asymptomatic. Over half of patients with mitral insufficiency during an acute attack will no longer have the murmur of mitral involvement 1 yr later. However, in patients with severe chronic mitral insufficiency the pulmonary arterial pressure becomes elevated, and enlargement of the right ventricle and atrium and subsequent right-sided heart failure will occur.

CLINICAL MANIFESTATIONS. The principal physical signs of mitral insufficiency depend on its severity. With mild disease, signs of heart failure will not be present, the precordium will be quiet, and auscultation will reveal a holosystolic murmur at the apex, radiating to the axilla. With severe mitral insufficiency, signs of chronic congestive heart failure, including fatigue, weight gain, weakness, and dyspnea on exertion, may be noted. The heart is enlarged with a heaving apical left ventricular precordial impulse and often an apical systolic thrill. The 1st heart sound is normal; the 2nd heart sound may be accentuated if pulmonary hypertension is present. A 3rd heart sound is usually prominent. There is rarely a midsystolic ejection click, as seen in patients with nonrheumatic mitral valve prolapse. A holosystolic murmur is heard at the apex radiating to the axilla and the sternal edge. In addition, a short mid-diastolic rumbling murmur follows the 3rd heart sound; it is caused by increased blood flow from the volume-loaded left atrium across the mitral valve as a result of the massive insufficiency. The presence of a diastolic murmur associated with mitral insufficiency does not necessarily mean that mechanical mitral stenosis is present. The latter lesion takes many years to develop and is characterized by a diastolic murmur of greater length with presystolic accentuation. In a young child with mitral insufficiency and no history suggestive of acute rheumatic fever, the differential diagnosis between a congenitally abnormal valve and rheumatic mitral involvement on the basis of the physical examination may be difficult.

The electrocardiogram and roentgenograms are normal if the lesion is mild. With more severe insufficiency, the *electrocardiogram* shows prominent bifid P waves, signs of left ventricular hypertrophy, and associated right ventricular hypertrophy if pulmonary hypertension is present. *Roentgenographically,* there is prominence of the left atrium and ventricle. When pulmonary hypertension or congestive heart failure are present, the pulmonary artery segment and right-sided heart chambers are prominent. Congestion of perihilar vessels, a sign of pulmonary venous hypertension, may also be evident. Calcification of the mitral valve is rare in children. *Echocardiography* shows enlargement of the left atrium and ventricle, and Doppler study demonstrates the severity of the mitral regurgitation.

Cardiac catheterization and left ventriculography are considered only if there is rapid progression of the disease and surgical treatment is contemplated, and if diagnostic questions regarding other valves are not totally resolved on the basis of noninvasive assessment. The cardiac output is normal or decreased in severe lesions. The degree of opacification of the left atrium during left ventriculography is used as a qualitative assessment of the severity of mitral insufficiency.

COMPLICATIONS. Severe mitral insufficiency may result in cardiac failure that may be precipitated by progression of the rheumatic process, the onset of atrial fibrillation with rapid ventricular response, or infective endocarditis. After many years, the effects of chronic mitral insufficiency may become manifest clinically without a new rheumatic event. Right-sided heart failure may be accompanied by tricuspid or pulmonary valve insufficiency. Occasional atrial or ventricular extrasystoles are seen. Atrial fibrillation is more common when mitral insufficiency is associated with a large left atrium. Patients with atrial fibrillation usually require anticoagulation for prevention of thromboemboli and stroke.

TREATMENT. In most patients with mitral insufficiency, prophylaxis against recurrences of rheumatic fever is all that is required because the lesions are mild and well tolerated (see Chapter 175.1). The treatment of complicating heart failure, arrhythmias, and infective endocarditis is described elsewhere. Afterload-reducing agents (hydralazine, captopril) may be especially useful. Surgical treatment is indicated in patients who, despite adequate medical therapy, suffer from recurrent episodes of heart failure, dyspnea with moderate activity, and progressive cardiomegaly, often with pulmonary hypertension. Although annuloplasty provides good results in some children and adolescents, valve replacement may be required. Activity should not be restricted in children having mild mitral incompetence. Prophylaxis against bacterial endocarditis is warranted in these patients for dental or other surgical procedures. The routine antibiotics taken by these patients for rheumatic fever prophylaxis are insufficient to prevent endocarditis.

Rheumatic Mitral Stenosis

(Congenital mitral stenosis is described in Chapter 386.20.)

PATHOPHYSIOLOGY. Mitral stenosis of rheumatic origin results from fibrosis of the mitral ring, commissural adhesions, and contracture of the valve leaflets, chordae, and papillary muscles over a significant period of time. It usually takes 10 yr or more for the lesion to become fully established, although the process may occasionally be accelerated. Rheumatic mitral stenosis is seldom encountered prior to adolescence and usually is not recognized until adult life. Mitral stenosis is recognized clinically if the valvular orifice is reduced to 25% or less of the expected normal. Such reductions result in increased pressure and enlargement and hypertrophy of the left atrium. The increased pressure causes pulmonary venous hypertension, increased pulmonary vascular resistance, and pulmonary hypertension. Right ventricular and atrial dilatation and hypertrophy ensue and are followed by right-sided heart failure.

CLINICAL MANIFESTATIONS. Generally, there is a good correlation between symptoms and the severity of obstruction. Patients with mild lesions are asymptomatic. More severe degrees of obstruction are associated with effort intolerance and dyspnea. Critical lesions can result in orthopnea, paroxysmal nocturnal dyspnea, and overt pulmonary edema. These symptoms may be precipitated by uncontrolled tachycardia, atrial fibrillation, or pulmonary infections. Congestive heart failure is usually but not invariably associated with moderate or severe pulmonary hypertension. Right ventricular dilatation may result in functional tricuspid insufficiency, hepatomegaly, ascites, and edema. Hemoptysis due to ruptured bronchial or pleurohilar veins and, occasionally, pulmonary infarction may occur. Blood-streaked sputum appears during episodes of pulmonary edema. With chronic severe mitral stenosis, cyanosis and a malar flush are noted.

The jugular venous pressure is increased in the presence of congestive heart failure, tricuspid valve disease, or severe pulmonary hypertension. The heart size is normal with minimal disease. Moderate cardiomegaly is usual with severe mitral stenosis and sinus rhythm, but cardiac enlargement can be massive, especially when atrial fibrillation and heart failure supervene. The apical impulse is normal, but a parasternal right ventricular lift is palpable when pulmonary pressure is high. The principal auscultatory findings are a loud 1st heart sound, an opening snap of the mitral valve, and a long, low-pitched, rumbling mitral diastolic murmur with presystolic accentuation at the apex. The mitral diastolic murmur may be virtually absent in patients who are in congestive heart failure. A holosystolic murmur owing to tricuspid insufficiency may also be audible. In the presence of pulmonary hypertension, the pulmonic component of the 2nd heart sound is accentuated. An early diastolic murmur may be caused by associated aortic insufficiency or secondary pulmonary valvular insufficiency (Graham Steell murmur).

Electrocardiograms and *roentgenograms* are normal if the lesion is mild; as the severity increases, there are prominent and notched P waves and varying degrees of right ventricular hypertrophy. Atrial fibrillation is a common late manifestation. Moderate or severe lesions are associated with roentgenographic signs of left atrial enlargement, prominence of the pulmonary artery and right-sided heart chambers, and a normal or small aorta and left ventricle; there may be calcifications noted in the region of the mitral valve. Severe obstruction is associated with a redistribution of pulmonary blood flow so that the apices of the lung have a greater perfusion (the reverse of normal). Septal lines at the costophrenic angles may also be present. *Echocardiography* shows distinct narrowing of the mitral orifice during diastole and left atrial enlargement. *Cardiac catheterization* quantitates the diastolic gradient across the mitral valve and the degree of elevation of pulmonary arterial pressure.

TREATMENT. Surgery is indicated when there are clinical signs and hemodynamic evidence of severe obstruction but prior to the severe manifestations outlined earlier. Surgical or balloon catheter mitral valvotomy generally yields good results; valve replacement is avoided unless absolutely necessary. Balloon valvuloplasty is indicated in symptomatic, stenotic, pliable, noncalcified valves of patients without atrial arrhythmias or thrombi.

Aortic Insufficiency

In chronic rheumatic aortic insufficiency, sclerosis of the aortic valve results in distortion and retraction of the cusps. Regurgitation of blood results in a volume overload with dilatation and hypertrophy of the left ventricle. Combined mitral and aortic insufficiency are more common than aortic involvement alone. Left ventricular failure may eventually occur.

CLINICAL MANIFESTATIONS. Symptoms are unusual except in severe aortic insufficiency. The large stroke volume and forceful left ventricular contractions may result in palpitations. Excessive sweating and heat intolerance are related to vasodilatation. Dyspnea on effort can progress to orthopnea and pulmonary edema; angina may occur during heavy exertion. In adolescents with severe insufficiency, nocturnal attacks with sweating, tachycardia, chest pain, and hypertension may occur.

The pulse pressure is wide with bounding peripheral pulses. The systolic blood pressure is elevated, and the diastolic pressure is lowered. In severe aortic insufficiency, the heart is enlarged and there is a left ventricular apical heave. There may be a diastolic thrill. The typical murmur begins immediately with the 2nd heart sound and continues until late in diastole. The murmur is heard over the upper and middle left sternal border with radiation to the apex and to the aortic area. Characteristically, it has a hollow, high-pitched blowing quality. Generally, the murmur is more easily audible in full expiration, with the diaphragm of the stethoscope placed firmly on the chest and the patient leaning forward. Occasionally, it may be louder in the recumbent position. A systolic ejection murmur sometimes preceded by a click is frequent and is produced by the large stroke volume. An apical presystolic murmur (Austin Flint) resembling that of mitral stenosis is sometimes heard and is the result of the large regurgitant aortic flow in diastole that prevents the mitral valve from opening fully.

Roentgenograms show enlargement of the left ventricle and aorta. The *electrocardiogram* may be normal but in advanced cases reveals signs of left ventricular hypertrophy and strain with prominent P waves. The *echocardiogram* shows a large left ventricle and diastolic mitral valve flutter or oscillation caused by regurgitant flow hitting the valve leaflets. The two-dimensional (2-D) echocardiogram shows the abnormal aortic valve, and Doppler studies demonstrate the degree of aortic runoff into the left ventricle. *Cardiac catheterization* is seldom necessary and is undertaken only when surgery is contemplated because of a progressive lesion.

PROGNOSIS AND TREATMENT. Mild and moderate lesions are well tolerated. Many adolescents with severe regurgitation are symptom free and tolerate advanced lesions into the 3rd–4th decades. Unlike mitral insufficiency, aortic insufficiency does not regress. Patients with combined lesions during the episode of acute rheumatic fever may have only aortic involvement 1–2 yr later. Treatment in most cases consists of prophylaxis against the recurrence of acute rheumatic fever and occurrence of infective endocarditis. The patient is encouraged to lead as active and normal a life as possible. Surgical intervention (valve replacement) should be carried out well in advance of the onset of congestive heart failure, pulmonary edema, or angina, when there are signs of decreasing myocardial performance as manifested by increasing left ventricular dimensions on the echocardiogram. When early symptoms are present, when there are ST-T wave changes on the electrocardiogram, or when there is evidence of decreasing left ventricular ejection fraction, then surgery is considered.

Tricuspid Valvular Disease

Primary tricuspid involvement is rare following rheumatic fever. *Tricuspid insufficiency* secondary to right ventricular dilatation resulting from severe left-sided lesions can occur in patients in whom surgery is not carried out. The signs produced by tricuspid insufficiency include prominent pulsations of the jugular veins with a "c-v" wave, systolic pulsations of the liver, and a blowing holosystolic murmur in the 4th and 5th left parasternal spaces that increases in intensity during inspiration. Concomitant signs of mitral or aortic valve disease, with or without atrial fibrillation, are frequent. Signs of tricuspid insufficiency decrease or disappear when heart failure produced by the left-sided lesions is successfully treated. However, tricuspid valvuloplasty may be required in some cases.

Pulmonary Valvular Disease

Pulmonary insufficiency occurs on a functional basis secondary to pulmonary hypertension or dilatation of the pulmonary artery. This is a late finding with severe mitral stenosis. The murmur (Graham Steell murmur) is similar to that of aortic insufficiency, but the peripheral arterial signs (bounding pulses) are absent. The correct diagnosis is confirmed by 2-D echocardiography and Doppler studies.

Anonymous: Acute rheumatic fever at a Navy training center—San Diego, California. MMWR 37:101, 1988.

Barnett LA, Cunningham MW: A new heart-cross-reactive antigen in *Streptococcus pyogenes* is not M protein. J Infect Dis 162:875, 1990.

Dajani AS, Bisno AL, Chung KJ, et al: Prevention of rheumatic fever: A statement for health professionals by the Committee on Rheumatic Fever, Endocarditis and Kawasaki Disease of the Council on Cardiovascular Disease in the Young, the American Heart Association. Pediatr Infect Dis J 8:263, 1989.

Durack DT, Kaplan EL, Bisno AL: Apparent failures of endocarditis prophylaxis. JAMA 205:2218, 1983.

Gersony WM, Hayes CJ: Bacterial endocarditis in patients with pulmonary stenosis, aortic stenosis, or valvular septal defect. Circulation 56(Suppl):84, 1977.

Griffiths SP, Gersony WM: Acute rheumatic fever in New York City (1969 to 1988): A comparative study of two decades. J Pediatr 116:882, 1990.

Markowitz M, Kaplan EL: Reappearance of rheumatic fever. Adv Pediatr 36:39, 1989.

Quinn RW: Comprehensive review of morbidity and mortality trends for rheumatic fever, streptococcal disease, and scarlet fever: The decline of rheumatic fever. Rev Infect Dis 11:928, 1989.

Veasy LG, Wiedmeier SE, Orsmond GS, et al: Resurgence of acute rheumatic fever in the intermountain area of the United States. N Engl J Med 316:421, 1987.

Westlake RM, Graham TP, Edwards KM: An outbreak of acute rheumatic fever in Tennessee. Pediatr Infect Dis J 9:97, 1990.

SECTION 6

Diseases of the Myocardium

The status of the myocardium is a critical factor in the prognosis of cardiac disease. Unlike in adults, where ischemic myocardial damage is often a prominent component of cardiac disease, in children the myocardium is relatively unimpaired in the majority of congenital heart lesions. In some congenital lesions, for example, left-to-right shunts, myocardial function may actually be supranormal. However, in children with unoperated congenital heart disease, long-standing volume or pressure load or chronic hypoxia may lead to eventual myocardial dysfunction. In addition to injury resulting from congenital heart lesions, the myocardium may also be directly affected by infections, mesenchymal diseases, endocrine disorders, metabolic and nutritional diseases, neuromuscular diseases, blood diseases, tumors, hypertension, and primary congenital anomalies (Table 392–1). ■

■ TABLE 392–1 Etiology of Myocardial Disease

Familial-Hereditary	**Connective Tissue—Granulomatous Disease**
Carnitine deficiency syndromes*	Systemic lupus erythematosus
Mitochondrial myopathy syndromes*	Scleroderma
Hypertrophic cardiomyopathy*	Churg-Strauss vasculitis
Duchenne muscular dystrophy*	Rheumatoid arthritis
Other muscular dystrophies (Becker, limb girdle)	Rheumatic fever
Myotonic dystrophy	Sarcoidosis
Kearns-Sayre (progressive external ophthalmoplegia)	Amyloidosis
Friedreich ataxia	Dermatomyositis
Mucopolysaccharidosis	Periarteritis nodosa
Hemochromatosis	**Drugs—Toxins**
Fabry disease	Adriamycin*
Pompe disease	Cyclophosphamide
Primary endocardial fibroelastosis	Chloroquine
Infection	Ipecac (emetine)
Virus: coxsackievirus A and B,* adenovirus,* human immunodeficiency virus (HIV), echovirus, rubella, varicella, influenza, mumps, Epstein-Barr, measles, poliomyelitis	Iron overload (hemosiderosis)
Rickettsiae: psittacosis, *Coxiella*, Rocky Mountain spotted fever	Sulfonamides
Bacteria: diphtheria, *Mycoplasma*, meningococcus, leptospirosis, Lyme disease, typhoid fever, tuberculosis, *Streptococcus*, listeriosis	Mesalezine
Parasites: Chagas disease, toxoplasmosis, Loa loa, *Toxocara canis*, schistosomiasis, cysticercosis, *Echinococcus*, trichinosis	Chloramphenicol
Fungi: histoplasmosis, coccidioidomycosis, actinomycosis	Hypersensitivity reaction
Metabolic, Nutritional, Endocrine	Alcohol
Beriberi (thiamine deficiency)	Irradiation
Keshan disease (selenium deficiency)	**Coronary Arteries**
Kwashiorkor	Kawasaki disease*
Hypothyroidism	Medial necrosis
Hyperthyroidism	Anomalous left coronary artery
Carcinoid	**Other**
Pheochromocytoma	Anemia*
Hypercholesterolemia	Sickle cell anemia (sickling)*
Infant of diabetic mother*	Hypereosinophilic syndrome (Löffler syndrome)
	Endomyocardial fibrosis
	Ischemia-hypoxia
	Peripartum cardiomyopathy
	Idiopathic dilated cardiomyopathy (familial, enteroviral, autoimmune)
	Arrhythmogenic right ventricular dysplasia (familial and nonfamilial)
	Uhl right ventricular anomaly
	Histiocytoid (oncocytic, lipidotic) cardiomyopathy
	Acute eosinophilic necrotizing myocarditis

**Relatively common etiology of myocarditis-cardiomyopathy.*

CHAPTER 392

Noninfectious Conditions Causing Myocardial Damage

(Table 392–1)

MUCOCUTANEOUS LYMPH NODE SYNDROME (KAWASAKI DISEASE). (See Chapter 152.2.) The arteritis associated with Kawasaki disease initially involves small arterioles, but in the 2nd and 3rd wk of illness medium-sized arteries become inflamed and aneurysmal dilatation of the coronary arteries may occur. During the healing phase, alternate areas of coronary dilatation and stenosis may result and can lead to myocardial infarction and death. Myocarditis is a less common manifestation of Kawasaki disease but, when present, manifests as congestive heart failure relatively early in the course.

AUTOIMMUNE DISEASES. *Rheumatic carditis* is described in Chapter 175.1. The cardiovascular manifestations of rheumatoid arthritis, disseminated lupus erythematosus, periarteritis nodosa, dermatomyositis, and scleroderma are described in Part XVI.

ENDOCRINE DISORDERS. Hyperthyroidism (see Chapter 523) produces tachycardia, vasodilatation, a wide pulse pressure, cardiac enlargement, and, occasionally, atrial fibrillation. Hypothyroidism seldom produces gross cardiac involvement in children, but the electrocardiogram is characterized by bradycardia; low voltage of all complexes, especially of the P and T waves; left axis deviation; and prolonged electrical systole. These signs may disappear within 1 mo after initiation of adequate thyroid therapy.

METABOLIC AND NUTRITIONAL DISEASES. Among vitamin deficiency diseases, *beriberi* (Chapter 45.3) causes the most conspicuous cardiac damage. In patients with malnutrition the deficiencies are often multiple, and it may be difficult to separate the cardiac lesion of one nutritional disease from that of another (see Chapters 412 and 413). Other nutritional and metabolic causes of cardiac dysfunction include selenium (see Chapter 43.6) and taurine deficiency and carnitine deficiency (Chapters 43.3 and 72.1).

NEUROMUSCULAR DISEASES. Heart disease is common in *Friedreich's ataxia* (see Chapter 547.1). In some patients effort intolerance, chest pain, and heart failure have been the presenting symptoms, caused by primary myocardial disease that chiefly affects the left ventricle and results in congestive or restrictive cardiomyopathy. Arrhythmias may also occur and consist of atrial tachycardia or fibrillation or extrasystoles. Varying degrees of cardiomegaly, left ventricular prominence, and pulmonary congestion are demonstrable roentgenographically.

In *muscular dystrophy* (see Chapter 560.1) 50% of children have postmortem evidence of myocardial involvement similar to that of the striated muscle. In Duchenne muscular dystrophy cardiac symptoms are usually overshadowed by peripheral muscular and pulmonary complications. The electrocardiogram is, however, frequently abnormal and may reveal tachycardia, abnormalities of the P waves, a short P-R interval, and abnormal Q and T waves. Minimal evidence of right or left ventricular hypertrophy may also be noted. Some patients develop congestive heart failure, although these symptoms must be distinguished from those caused by pulmonary failure. In the less severe forms of muscular dystrophy, for example, Becker dystrophy, cardiac involvement may be more prominent and may be the primary cause of exercise intolerance and respiratory symptoms. Patients with these muscular dystrophies have been shown to have mutations of the dystrophin gene, located on the X chromosome. Other X-linked dilated cardiomyopathies have been described, also associated with deletions of the dystrophin gene, but without associated skeletal muscle involvement. Some limited experience with heart transplantation exists in patients with mild Becker dystrophy.

BLOOD DISEASES. In infants and children, anemia is the most common blood disease associated with cardiac involvement. Although the cardiac output increases when the hemoglobin is below about 7 g/dL, significant cardiac enlargement occurs only with an extreme reduction in hemoglobin, to 3–4 g or less. The heart rate is rapid, the pulse pressure widened, and the venous pressure increased. A systolic flow murmur at the apex or along the left sternal border is usual; diastolic murmurs may occur in the same areas, and a gallop rhythm is also common. Electrocardiographic changes include depressed ST segments and flat T waves. Occasionally, only minimal signs and symptoms are present when extreme states of anemia have developed gradually. In patients with congenital heart lesions, anemia can place an extra stress on the heart's ability to maintain adequate oxygen delivery and can result in considerable worsening of heart failure symptoms. *Treatment* is directed toward the cause of the anemia. If blood transfusions are indicated in the presence of cardiomegaly or heart failure, only small volumes (5 mL/kg) of packed red blood cells should be administered at any one time (see Chapters 412 and 413–430). Sometimes it is more prudent to use exchange transfusion to avoid an acute increase in blood volume.

GLYCOGEN STORAGE DISEASE. Cardiac as well as skeletal muscles are affected in the generalized form of glycogen storage disease known as type II or Pompe disease (see Chapter 73.1). Cardiomegaly is massive; murmurs are insignificant. Pulmonary atelectasis with secondary infection is common and is related to compression by the enlarged heart. The *electrocardiogram* is characteristic and shows prominent P waves, a short P-R interval, massive QRS voltage, signs of isolated left or biventricular hypertrophy, and intraventricular conduction delays. *Roentgenograms* confirm the striking cardiomegaly with prominence of the left ventricle. The echocardiogram shows severe ventricular hypertrophy. The prognosis is poor.

HURLER SYNDROME. In this disorder mucopolysaccharides accumulate in many organs, including the heart and great vessels (see Chapter 74). The most pronounced lesions are found in the valves and coronary arteries, but abnormalities in the pericardium and aorta are not uncommon. The heart may be moderately enlarged, with electrocardiographic signs of left ventricular hypertrophy. Cardiac murmurs may result from insufficiency and stenosis of the mitral and aortic valves. Sometimes the pulmonary and tricuspid valves are also involved. Coronary arterial disease may result in angina and perhaps explain the frequent occurrence of sudden death. The prognosis is poor.

CALCINOSIS OF THE CORONARY ARTERIES. This is a rare disease of infancy. The coronary arteries are tortuous and calcareous, and the ventricles, especially the left, are hypertrophied. Other blood vessels may be similarly involved. The onset of cardiac failure is sudden; death usually occurs in infancy.

DOXORUBICIN (ADRIAMYCIN) CARDIOTOXICITY. This chemotherapeutic agent can cause both acute myocarditis and a chronic cardiomyopathy. The most common manifestation is a severe, chronic, dose-dependent cardiomyopathy, which occurs in about 30% of patients when the total cumulative dose exceeds 550 mg/m^2 but may be seen occasionally, even in patients with doses as low as 200 mg/m^2. Some echocardiographic indices of left ventricular function (wall stress) show abnormalities in as many as 65% of children receiving doses above 220 mg/m^2.

Cardiomyopathy may become manifest months or even years after doxorubicin treatment. Cardiomegaly is due principally to left ventricular and left atrial enlargement. T wave flattening or inversion is nonspecific evidence of cardiac involvement. Early changes in cardiac function, even in the absence of symptoms, may be detected by serial echocardiograms or radionuclide scans, but no method is totally able to predict which patients are at risk. The child's condition may remain clinically stable for many years, even with a decreased fractional shortening. However, once symptoms of congestive heart failure develop, the case fatality rate is as high as 30–50%. Cardiac transplantation has been used with success in these patients (see Chapter 401).

Acute myocarditis is less common and usually occurs during the course of administration of the drug. It is frequently reversible, and the long-term prognosis may be somewhat better. Supportive treatment consists of anticongestive medications such as digoxin, diuretics, and afterload-reducing agents.

IPECAC CARDIAC TOXICITY. This occurs with chronic intentional ipecac abuse secondary to anorexia nervosa or bulimia nervosa. Manifestations are probably caused by the emetine component of ipecac and include chest pain, tachycardia, dyspnea, hypotension, arrhythmias, flattening and inversion of T waves, ST segment abnormalities, prolongation of Q-T and P-R intervals, cardiac failure, and potentially death. Differentiating the cardiac abnormalities owing to ipecac from those of chronic starvation, abnormal diets, and electrolyte abnormalities may be difficult.

CHAPTER 393
Viral Myocarditis

Myocarditis refers to inflammation, necrosis, or myocytolysis that may be caused by many infectious, connective tissue, granulomatous, toxic, or idiopathic processes affecting the myocardium with or without associated systemic manifestations of the disease process or involvement of the endocardium or pericardium (see Table 392–1). Coronary pathology is uniformly absent. The most common manifestation is congestive heart failure, although arrhythmias and sudden death may be the first detectable signs. Viral infections are the most common etiology.

ETIOLOGY AND EPIDEMIOLOGY. The incidence of viral myocarditis in children is unknown, as many mild cases may go undetected. Viral myocarditis is typically a sporadic but occasionally epidemic illness. Its manifestations are to some degree age dependent: In early infancy, viral myocarditis often occurs as an acute, fulminant disease; in toddlers and young children, it occurs as an acute but less fulminant myopericarditis; and in older children and adolescents, it is often asymptomatic and comes to clinical attention primarily as a precursor to idiopathic dilated cardiomyopathy. The most common etiologic agents are coxsackievirus B and adenovirus, although almost every known viral agent has been implicated in myocarditis.

PATHOPHYSIOLOGY. Acute viral myocarditis may produce a fulminant inflammatory process characterized by cellular infiltrates, cell degeneration and necrosis, and subsequent fibrosis. Viral myocarditis may also become a chronic process with persistence of viral RNA or DNA (but not infectious virus particles) in the myocardium. Chronic inflammation is then perpetuated by the host immune response, which includes T lymphocytes activated against viral-host antigenic alterations. Such cytotoxic lymphocytes and natural killer cells, together with persistent and possibly defective viral replication, may impair myocyte function without obvious cytolysis. Alternatively, the persistent viral infection may alter major histocompatibility complex antigen expression, with resultant exposure of neoantigens to the immune system. In addition, some viral proteins may share antigenic epitopes with host cells, resulting in autoimmune damage to the antigenically related myocyte. The net final result of chronic viral-associated inflammation is often dilated cardiomyopathy.

CLINICAL MANIFESTATIONS. The presentation depends on the age and acute or chronic nature of the infection. The *neonate* may present with fever, severe heart failure, respiratory distress, cyanosis, distant heart sounds, weak pulses, tachycardia out of proportion to the fever, mitral insufficiency caused by dilatation of the valve annulus, a gallop rhythm, acidosis, and shock. There may be evidence of viral hepatitis, aseptic meningitis, and an associated rash. In the most fulminant form, death may occur within 1–7 days of the onset of symptoms. The chest roentgenogram demonstrates an enormously enlarged heart and pulmonary edema; the electrocardiogram reveals sinus tachycardia, reduced QRS complex voltage, and ST segment and T wave abnormalities. Arrhythmias may be the first clinical manifestation and in the presence of fever and a large heart strongly suggest acute myocarditis.

The *older patient* with acute myocarditis may also present with acute congestive heart failure; however, more commonly patients will present with the gradual onset of congestive heart failure or the sudden onset of ventricular arrhythmias. In these patients, the acute infectious phase has usually passed and an idiopathic dilated cardiomyopathy is present (see Chapter 396).

DIAGNOSIS. The sedimentation rate and heart enzymes (CPK, LDH) may be elevated in acute or chronic myocarditis. Coxsackievirus IgM is present transiently in 50–60% of patients with acute myocarditis and may persist for 5–10 yr in some patients with dilated cardiomyopathy. Echocardiography will demonstrate poor ventricular function and often a pericardial effusion, mitral valve regurgitation, and the absence of coronary artery or other congenital heart lesions. Myocarditis can be confirmed by endomyocardial biopsy. This is performed during cardiac catheterization and can also detect other causes of cardiomyopathy (carnitine deficiency, storage disease, mitochondrial defects); as many as 50% of clinically suspected cases of myocarditis have another diagnosis. The use of the polymerase chain reaction (PCR) to identify viral RNA or DNA has allowed the viral etiology of many of these formerly "idiopathic" cases to be determined.

DIFFERENTIAL DIAGNOSIS. The predominant diseases mimicking acute myocarditis include carnitine deficiency, hereditary mitochondrial defects, idiopathic dilated cardiomyopathy, pericarditis, endocardial fibroelastosis, and anomalies of the coronary arteries (see Table 392–1).

TREATMENT. The approach to treating acute myocarditis involves supportive measures for severe congestive heart failure (see Chapter 399). Dopamine or epinephrine may be helpful if there is poor cardiac output with systemic hypotension. However, all inotropic agents, including digoxin, should be used with caution as patients with myocarditis may be more susceptible to the arrhythmogenic properties of these agents. Digoxin is often started at half the normal dosage. Pericardiocentesis should be performed if there is evidence of cardiac tamponade. Arrhythmias should be treated as noted in Table 388–1. For infants and children having cardiogenic shock, extracorporeal membrane oxygenation (ECMO) may be indicated. In larger adolescents, implantation of a left ventricular assist device has been performed, usually as a bridge to cardiac transplantation, which is the treatment of choice in patients with refractory heart failure (see Chapter 401). The role of corticosteroids for treatment of acute viral myocarditis is still controversial. In a small series of pediatric patients, treatment with prednisone (2 mg/kg daily, tapered to 0.3 mg/kg daily over 3 mo) was effective in reducing myocardial inflammation and in improving cardiac function. However, relapse may occur when immunosuppression is discontinued. Trials are currently under way evaluating the efficacy of intravenous gamma globulin.

PROGNOSIS. The outcome of the symptomatic neonate with acute viral myocarditis remains poor, with a mortality between 50% and 70%. Patients with lesser symptoms may have a somewhat better prognosis, and complete resolution has been described. The outcome of older patients with chronic dilated cardiomyopathy associated with prior viral infection is also poor without therapy. These patients continue to have inflammation, fibrosis, and deteriorating cardiac function. Although spontaneous resolution may occur in 10–20%, as many as 50% of untreated older patients will die within 2 yr of presentation and 80% within 8 yr without cardiac transplantation.

CHAPTER 394
Nonviral Causes of Myocarditis

BACTERIAL INFECTIONS. In *diphtheria* (see Chapter 180) the toxin of the bacillus may produce peripheral circulatory failure or toxic myocarditis within the first 2 wk of the disease. In addition to therapy for diphtheria, treatment for cardiogenic shock is essential. Diphtheritic toxic myocarditis is characterized by the development of atrioventricular block, bundle branch block, or extrasystoles. Congestive heart failure occurs later and is associated with cardiac enlargement and a gallop rhythm. In addition to the arrhythmia, the electrocardiogram shows ST segment depression and T wave inversion in most leads. The immediate prognosis is grave (about 50% mortality). Treatment includes strict bed rest until all signs of myocarditis have disappeared and management of arrhythmias, including cardiac pacing. Digitalis is reserved for patients with frank congestive heart failure but must be used with care because of the possibility of increased myocardial sensitivity.

In many *systemic bacterial infections,* circulatory involvement is manifested as peripheral circulatory collapse or toxic myocarditis. Toxic myocarditis, as evidenced by tachycardia, a gallop rhythm, and cardiac enlargement, may complicate pneumonia, infective endocarditis, and septicemia. A myocardial depressant factor may produce an acute toxic cardiomyopathy. The prognosis depends on the ability to control the primary infection.

RICKETTSIAL DISEASES. *Rocky Mountain spotted fever* (see Chapter 239.1) may be complicated by hypotension and peripheral vascular collapse. This complication has been attributed to the general vasculitis characteristic of the disease, but acute myocarditis may be a contributing factor.

PARASITIC AND FUNGAL INFECTIONS. Lesions in the myocardium have been described in association with *histoplasmosis, coccidioidomycosis, toxoplasmosis,* and *trichinosis.* In these conditions the cardiac lesion seldom produces clinical signs of myocarditis. *Actinomycosis* may involve the pericardium and myocardium by direct contiguity to a pulmonary abscess. *Hydatid cysts* of the pericardium may be found on routine roentgenograms of the chest and usually produce symptoms only when they rupture. *Schistosomiasis* may produce pulmonary hypertension and cor pulmonale. *Cruz trypanosomiasis* (Chagas disease) may produce either acute or subacute myocarditis and can lead to sudden death.

CHAPTER 395
Endocardial Fibroelastosis

This condition has been called fetal endocarditis, endocardial fibrosis, prenatal fibroelastosis, elastic tissue hyperplasia, and endocardial sclerosis. In *primary* endocardial fibroelastosis (EFE) there is no apparent predisposing valvular lesion or other congenital heart abnormality. In *secondary* EFE severe congenital heart disease of the left-sided obstructive type (e.g., aortic stenosis or atresia, forms of hypoplastic left heart syndrome, or severe coarctation of the aorta) is present. In secondary EFE the ventricular cavity is often contracted, whereas in the primary disease a dilated left ventricular chamber is seen, usually during infancy. However, in young adults a contracted form of primary EFE has been observed. No etiology for primary EFE has been established.

Pathologically, there is a white, opaque fibroelastic thickening of the endocardium, virtually always in the left ventricle, which frequently obscures the trabeculation of the inner surfaces of the cardiac chamber. The lesion may spread to involve the valves. Microscopically, the lesion consists of a fibroelastic thickening of the endocardium and may result in subendocardial degeneration or necrosis of muscle with vacuolation of muscle fibers. The involved valve leaflets are characterized by a myxomatous proliferation with an increase in collagenous elements.

The *clinical manifestations* are variable. Infants, usually younger than 6 mo of age, who apparently had been in good health, develop severe congestive heart failure, often precipitated by a respiratory infection. Affected infants may manifest dyspnea, cough, anorexia, hepatomegaly, edema, failure to thrive, and recurrent pulmonary infections. Chronic congestive heart failure can be controlled for some time by digitalis and diuretics; however, most patients eventually succumb. Infants in whom valvular lesions or associated congenital cardiovascular defects are predominant usually expire in the 1st mo of life. *Roentgenograms* confirm significant cardiac enlargement (Fig. 395–1). The electrocardiogram is abnormal, with changes indicative of left atrial and left ventricular hypertrophy with strain. The echocardiogram shows a bright-appearing endocardial surface and a dilated, poorly functioning left ventricle.

Treatment is directed toward alleviation of congestive heart failure and prevention of intercurrent infections. End-stage EFE, with signs of heart failure despite a maximal medical regimen, is an indication for cardiac transplantation (see Chapter 401).

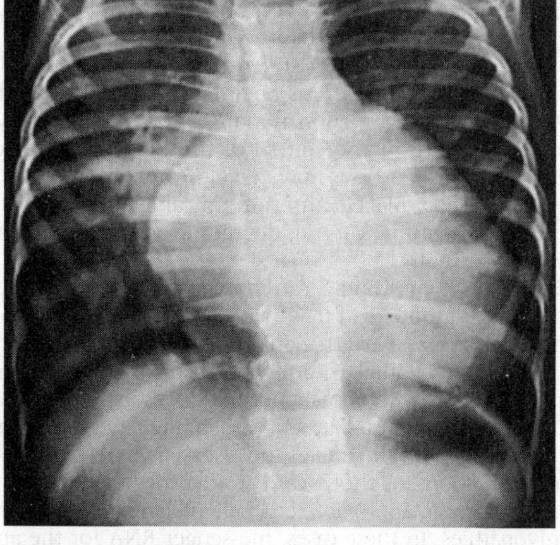

Figure 395–1. Roentgenogram of a 7-mo-old girl with endocardial fibroelastosis. Note the enlargement of the heart, without a distinctive contour and clear lung fields.

CHAPTER 396
The Primary Cardiomyopathies

Heart muscle disease, in the absence of congenital heart disease, hypertension, acquired valve processes, abnormal coronary arteries, infection, or other systemic illnesses, is classified as a primary cardiomyopathy (see Table 392–1). Primary cardiomyopathy may be classified as *hypertrophic* (both obstructive and nonobstructive forms), *dilated* (idiopathic, postinfectious, endocardial fibroelastosis), or *restrictive* (endomyocardial fibrosis, Löffler eosinophilic endomyocardial syndrome, hemochromatosis, Fabry disease, pseudoxanthoma elasticum). They often manifest with an insidious onset of congestive heart failure, chest pain, dyspnea, arrhythmias, or sudden death. Other categories include arrhythmogenic right ventricular dysplasia and oncocytic cardiomyopathy, which predominantly manifest with ventricular arrhythmias or sudden cardiac death. The prevalence of cardiomyopathy in the newborn period is 10 in 100,000 live births, whereas for all children the prevalence is 36.5 per 100,000 for dilated cardiomyopathy and 2.5 per 100,000 for hypertrophic cardiomyopathy.

HYPERTROPHIC CARDIOMYOPATHY

PATHOPHYSIOLOGY. This condition is also known as idiopathic hypertrophic subaortic stenosis or asymmetric septal hypertrophy. Massive ventricular hypertrophy with principal involvement of the ventricular septum characterizes the disease, but all portions of the left ventricle, and sometimes of the right ventricle, are affected. Varying degrees of myocardial fibrosis are also present. The mitral valve is displaced anteriorly by hypertrophy of the papillary muscles, and the left ventricular cavity is distorted by the massive generalized hypertrophy. Microscopically, patchy areas of abnormally thick and short muscle fibers are arranged in circular collections and interspersed among normal as well as hypertrophied muscle fibers. Electron microscopy shows a disarray of myofibrils and myofilaments. An excessive response to calcium or to excessive calcium ion channels may be responsible for myocyte hypertrophy in some patients.

The hypertrophic, fibrosed, stiff muscle has a decreased distensibility so that there is resistance to left ventricular filling, but systolic pumping function remains intact (or even hyperdynamic) until late in the course of the disease. Obstruction to left ventricular outflow may develop owing to apposition of the abnormally placed anterior mitral leaflet against the hypertrophied septum. Varying degrees of mitral valve insufficiency are common.

EPIDEMIOLOGY. Hypertrophic cardiomyopathy has been recognized in all age groups and may occur in many members of the same family, although overt manifestations are present in only about one third of affected individuals discovered through a screening process. In some patients the disease is transmitted in an autosomal dominant pattern with a high degree of penetrance, whereas in other families the disease is genetically heterogeneous. Mutations of the β cardiac myosin heavy-chain gene are responsible for approximately half of familial hypertrophic cardiomyopathies. In these cases, messenger RNA for the abnormal gene may be detected in peripheral blood lymphocytes by the polymerase chain reaction (PCR), resulting in diagnosis before clinical signs become evident. Specific mutations in the myosin gene have now been linked to particular phenotypes: This may eventually allow prediction of which patients are likely to suffer from arrhythmias and sudden death. Other gene alterations associated with hypertrophic cardiomyopathy include those of the mitochondrial respiratory chain enzymes.

In childhood, hypertrophic cardiomyopathy may be somewhat different from the adult disease: There is a greater tendency for right ventricular outflow obstruction to occur. The left ventricular wall may be diffusely thickened, as opposed to only the septal portion, and a pure autosomal dominant inheritance pattern is less often seen.

In *infants of diabetic mothers*, a transient form of hypertrophic cardiomyopathy may be encountered with or without left ventricular outflow tract obstruction. The increased left ventricular mass usually regresses within several months. Premature infants who are receiving *corticosteroids* for chronic lung disease may also develop a transient hypertrophic cardiomyopathy, which resolves rapidly with cessation of steroid therapy.

CLINICAL MANIFESTATIONS. Many children are asymptomatic and are first evaluated only because of a heart murmur. In others the clinical pattern is dominated by weakness, fatigue, dyspnea on effort, palpitations, angina pectoris, dizziness, and syncope. There is risk of sudden death even in asymptomatic children. The pulse is brisk because of the early systolic ejection of blood from the ventricle. There is a prominent left ventricular lift and double apical impulse. The 1st and 2nd heart sounds are usually normal. The rarity of systolic ejection clicks helps to differentiate hypertrophic obstructive cardiomyopathy from valvular aortic stenosis. The systolic murmur is ejection in type and of medium intensity; it is heard maximally at the left sternal edge and apex. The murmur may increase shortly after exercise is discontinued, during the Valsalva maneuver, or during assumption of the erect position.

DIAGNOSIS. The *electrocardiogram* shows left ventricular hypertrophy with or without ST segment depression and T wave inversion. Signs of the Wolff-Parkinson-White syndrome and other intraventricular conduction defects may be present. *Roentgenograms* show mild cardiomegaly with prominence of the left ventricle. The *echocardiogram* shows asymmetric left ventricular hypertrophy, predominantly affecting the interventricular septum; systolic anterior motion of the anterior leaflet of the mitral valve; and premature closure of the aortic valve. Sometimes symmetric left ventricular hypertrophy occurs. Doppler studies will demonstrate the presence of a left ventricular outflow tract gradient, which usually occurs in mid to late systole, when the muscular obstruction to the outflow is maximal.

At *cardiac catheterization*, left ventricular outflow tract obstruction may not be present. When a systolic gradient is present, its severity may be variable, even during a relatively short study. The obstruction may be intensified by administration of isoproterenol, amyl nitrite, or nitroglycerin. Left ventriculography shows encroachment on the left ventricular cavity by the hypertrophied muscle, especially by the interventricular septum. Midsystolic cavity obliteration occurs in the more severe cases. Mitral insufficiency is common. A discrete obstruction with secondary muscular hypertrophy should be ruled out, as surgical management of discrete subaortic stenosis is effective (see Chapter 386.16). The *prognosis* of hypertrophic cardiomyopathy is unpredictable, especially in the asymptomatic patient, who may remain stable for years. Some patients will progress to chronic congestive heart failure, and others are at risk for sudden death caused by arrhythmia.

TREATMENT. There is no standardized therapy. Competitive sports and strenuous physical activity should be discouraged. Digitalis is contraindicated in most patients. Aggressive diuresis or the infusion of isoproterenol or other inotropic agents should also be avoided. β-Adrenergic blocking agents (propranolol) and calcium channel blocking agents (verapamil) have been used with some apparent success in decreasing the degree of outflow obstruction, but obliteration of a left ventricular outflow tract gradient does not necessarily affect the long-term prognosis. Calcium channel blockers should not be used during infancy. A pacemaker has been used in some older patients. Surgical ventricular septal myotomy or resection of the left ventricular outflow tract has been successfully accomplished in some patients, especially in those with disabling angina or syncope and in some with severe obstruction at rest (gradient exceeding 70 mm Hg). Mitral valve replacement may be needed if obstruction cannot be alleviated.

IDIOPATHIC DILATED CARDIOMYOPATHY

PATHOPHYSIOLOGY. This condition is characterized by massive cardiomegaly as a result of the extensive dilatation of the ventricles, most prominently the left. Varying degrees of ventricular hypertrophy are also present. The etiology is unknown and is probably multifactorial; a remote history of viral disease in some patients suggests that the disease may be a sequela of a previous myocarditis. Patients with dilated cardiomyopathy may have carnitine deficiency; thus, urine and serum levels should be obtained. Genetic mitochondrial disease and other metabolic abnormalities affecting the myocardium may also result in dilated cardiomyopathy as a final common pathway. X-linked dilated cardiomyopathy usually presents during adolescence in male patients and has been found to be associated with a mutation in the dystrophin gene. Myocardial biopsy early in the disease process may be useful; however, a specific etiology is rarely found when biopsies are obtained after long-standing disease. The viral etiology of many of these "idiopathic" cases is now being uncovered with PCR. If a family history suggests one of the familial myopathies, DNA studies on both affected and nonaffected family members may be able to determine a specific gene deletion.

CLINICAL MANIFESTATIONS. All age groups may be affected. Usually the onset is insidious, but sometimes symptoms of congestive heart failure occur suddenly. Irritability, anorexia, cough owing to pulmonary congestion, and dyspnea with mild exertion are common. When the disease is fully established, the skin is cool and pale, the arterial pulse volume is decreased, the pulse pressure is reduced, and tachycardia is present. The jugular venous pressure is increased, and hepatomegaly and edema are common. The heart is enlarged, and holosystolic murmurs of mitral and tricuspid insufficiency may be present. A summation gallop rhythm is usually audible.

DIAGNOSIS. The *electrocardiogram* shows a combination of atrial enlargement, varying degrees of left ventricular hypertrophy, and nonspecific T wave abnormalities. The *roentgenogram* confirms the cardiomegaly. Pulmonary congestion and pleural effusions may also be present. The *echocardiogram* shows dilatation of the left atrium and ventricle, and poor contractility. The right ventricle may also be affected. Doppler studies show decreased flow velocity through the aortic valve and mitral regurgitation. In long-standing cases, evidence of pulmonary hypertension may exist.

PROGNOSIS AND MANAGEMENT. The course of the disease is usually progressively downhill, although some patients may remain stable for years. Vigorous treatment for heart failure (see Chapter 399) may result in a temporary remission, but relapses are common, and in time patients tend to become resistant to therapy. At this point, the prognosis for survival beyond a year is poor. Cardiac transplantation has been used very successfully in this group of patients as well as in patients with other forms of cardiomyopathy (see Chapter 401). Serious complications include arrhythmias as well as pulmonary and/or systemic emboli from intracardiac thrombi. Patients with severely depressed myocardial function should receive systemic anticoagulation with warfarin.

RESTRICTIVE CARDIOMYOPATHIES

Poor ventricular compliance is the major abnormality, and inadequate filling of the ventricular cavities occurs during diastole. This results in *clinical manifestations* that closely simulate those of constrictive pericarditis (see Chapter 397). In its full-blown these form, restrictive cardiomyopathy results in dyspnea, edema, ascites, hepatomegaly, increased venous pressure, and pulmonary congestion. The heart is mildly or moderately enlarged, and murmurs are nonspecific. The electrocardiogram shows prominent P waves, often normal QRS voltage, ST segment depression, and T wave inversion. Roentgenographic examination shows mild to moderate cardiomegaly. *Differential diagnosis* from constrictive pericarditis is critical, as the latter can be treated surgically. *Löffler hypereosinophilic syndrome* produces severe multisystem dysfunction (skin, lung, nervous system, liver), and the predominant cause of death is cardiomyopathy. This restrictive cardiomyopathy produces endocardial fibrosis of the mitral and tricuspid valves and of the right and left ventricles. Subsequent formation of endocardial thrombi results in embolization. Löffler syndrome should be distinguished from nonrestrictive, nonfibrotic acute *eosinophilic necrotizing myocarditis*, an acute rapidly fatal illness, and from *hypersensitivity myocarditis* (characterized by fever, rash, tachycardia, eosinophilia, drug allergy, and arrhythmias). Steroids and cytotoxic agents (hydroxyurea) may be beneficial in the hypereosinophilic syndromes. Anticoagulant therapy may reduce the incidence of thromboembolism.

The *prognosis* for restrictive cardiomyopathy is generally poor. Treatment is directed toward relief of edema with diuretics; calcium channel blocking agents may be used to increase diastolic compliance. Cardiac transplantation is the last management option.

CHAPTER 397
Diseases of the Pericardium

Major diseases that involve the pericardium are noted in Table 397–1. In some instances the involvement of the pericardium is only one manifestation of a more generalized illness, and the prominence of the pericardial component will vary depending on the disease entity.

PATHOPHYSIOLOGY. Pericardial inflammation results in an accumulation of fluid in the pericardial space. The fluid varies according to the etiology of the pericarditis and may be serous, fibrinous, purulent, or hemorrhagic. *Cardiac tamponade* occurs when the amount of pericardial fluid reaches a level that compromises cardiac function. In a healthy child there is normally 10–15 mL of fluid in the pericardial space, whereas in an adolescent with pericarditis an excess of 1,000 mL of fluid may accumulate. For every small increment of fluid the pericardial pressure rises slowly, but once a critical level is reached there is a rapid rise in pressure, culminating in severe cardiac compression. Inhibition of ventricular filling during diastole, elevated systemic and pulmonary venous pressures, and, if untreated, eventual compromised cardiac output and shock occur.

CLINICAL MANIFESTATIONS. The first symptom of pericardial disease is often precordial pain. The major complaint is a sharp, stabbing sensation over the precordium and often the left shoulder and back; the pain may be exaggerated by lying supine and relieved by sitting, especially leaning forward. Because there is no sensory innervation of the pericardium, the pain is probably referred pain from diaphragmatic and pleural irritation. Cough, dyspnea, and fever may also occur. The

■ TABLE 397–1 Etiology of Pericardial Disease

Congenital Anomalies
Absence (partial, complete)
Cysts
Mulibrey nanism (*mu*scle, *li*ver, *br*ain, *ey*e) with congenital pericardial thickening and constriction

Infectious
Viral (coxsackievirus B, Epstein-Barr virus)
Bacterial (streptococcus, pneumococcus, staphylococcus, meningococcus, mycoplasma, tularemia)
Immune complex (meningococcus, *H. influenzae*)
Tuberculosis
Fungal (histoplasmosis, actinomycosis)
Parasitic (toxoplasmosis, echinococcus)

Connective Tissue Diseases
Rheumatoid arthritis
Rheumatic fever
Systemic lupus erythematosus
Systemic sclerosis
Sarcoidosis

Metabolic-Endocrine
Uremia
Hypothyroidism
Chylopericardium

Hematology-Oncology
Bleeding diathesis
Malignancy (primary, metastatic)
Radiotherapy induced

Other
Trauma (penetrating or blunt injury)
Postpericardiotomy (cardiac surgery)
Aortic dissection
Idiopathic
Familial Mediterranean fever

presence of symptoms or signs associated with other organs and systems depends on the basic etiology of the pericarditis.

On physical examination, many of the findings relate to the degree of fluid accumulation in the pericardial sac. The presence of a friction rub is helpful but may be a variable sign in acute pericarditis, becoming apparent only after the effusion is reduced. When the effusion is larger, muffled heart sounds may be the only auscultatory finding. Narrow pulses, tachycardia, neck vein distention, and an increased *pulsus paradoxus* suggest significant fluid accumulation.

The pulsus paradoxus is caused by the normal slight decrease in systolic arterial pressure during inspiration. With cardiac tamponade this normal phenomenon is exaggerated, probably because of decreased filling of the left side of the heart with the inspiratory phase of respiration. The degree of the pulsus paradoxus is determined with a mercury manometer. The patient is told to breath normally, without exaggeration. Allowing the manometer to slowly fall, the first Korotkoff sound will initially be heard intermittently (varying with respirations). This first point is noted and the manometer then allowed to fall until the first Korotkoff sound is heard continuously. The difference between these two systolic pressures is the pulsus paradoxus. A pulsus paradoxus of >20 mm Hg in a child with pericarditis is a reliable indicator of the presence of cardiac tamponade; a 10–20 mm Hg change is equivocal. An increased pulsus paradoxus may also be seen in patients with severe dyspnea of any etiology, with pulmonary disease (emphysema or asthma), in obese individuals, or in patients being ventilated with a positive-pressure respirator. In these patients the paradoxic pulse is due to a marked increase in intrathoracic pressure. The etiology of a paradoxic pulse in a child on a ventilator after cardiac surgery may therefore be difficult to assess.

DIAGNOSIS. The specific findings depend on the underlying disease. The effects of pericarditis on the *electrocardiogram* are multiple. Low voltage of the QRS complexes results from a damping effect of the pericardial fluid. Pressure on the myocardium by fluid or exudate produces a current of injury that results in mild elevation of ST segments. Generalized T wave inversion occurs as a consequence of associated myocardial inflammation. The ST segment and T wave changes with pericarditis are more generalized than those seen with myocardial infarction, and the ST segment elevations tend to precede the T wave changes. *Electrical alternans,* demonstrated by a variable QRS complex amplitude, may be present. There may be an interval when the electrocardiogram is in a transitional phase and appears to be normal. This may occur during the acute phase of the illness prior to diagnosis. In some instances clear-cut abnormalities are never identified.

A relatively large pericardial effusion must be present to cause an enlarged cardiac shadow with the usual "water-bottle" configuration on *chest roentgenogram* (Fig. 397–1). In most instances the lung fields are clear. With constrictive pericardial disease the heart is relatively small and calcification may be present.

The *echocardiogram* is a sensitive technique for evaluating the size and progression of pericardial effusions. Normally, the pericardium is closely adherent to the epicardium, and the two layers can only be narrowly separated by the ultrasound beam. In patients with pericardial effusion, a clear, echo-free space is recorded between the epicardium and pericardium. A posterior effusion is recorded behind the left ventricular epicardium and ends at the junction of the left ventricle and left atrium. An anterior effusion will be recorded between the chest wall and the anterior right ventricular wall. The presence of both an anterior and posterior effusion generally indicates that a large collection of fluid is present. Flattening of septal motion and collapse of the right ventricular outflow during diastole are signs of pericardial tamponade.

DIFFERENTIAL DIAGNOSIS. Viral and Acute Benign Pericarditis. These entities are considered synonymous because most episodes of acute benign pericarditis follow or coincide with viral illness. Viruses recognized to cause pericarditis include Coxsackievirus B, influenza, echovirus, and adenovirus. The pathogenesis is unclear but may be related to a hypersensitivity reaction to the viral disease. However, pericardial inflammation is not necessarily the precursor of a generalized inflammatory process. Most cases are mild, and recovery occurs within several weeks. Only symptomatic treatment, usually with nonsteroidal antiinflammatory agents such as indomethacin, is indicated. In rare instances the patient will be severely ill, and cardiac tamponade may ensue. There are also patients in whom a chronic relapsing illness occurs. The differential diagnosis between these patients and those with collagen vascular disease may be difficult. The latter patients respond dramatically to corticosteriods or nonsteroidal anti-inflammatory agents; milder forms may be controlled with aspirin. The clinical course may vary from months to 1–2 yr, during which time patients are dependent on drug therapy for suppression of the pericarditis. Ultimately, these patients will improve and the prognosis is good.

The clinical differential diagnosis between acute pericarditis and myocarditis may be difficult, and usually each includes a component of the other. However, management of these conditions is quite different; anti-inflammatory treatment and urgent response to cardiac tamponade are appropriate in the former, and therapy for congestive heart failure is required in the latter. The echocardiogram can demonstrate the size of the pericardial effusion and also indicate the presence of myocardial dysfunction.

Purulent Pericarditis. This is most often associated with bacterial infections such as pneumonia, epiglottitis, meningitis, or osteomyelitis. There usually are signs and symptoms of the primary infection. Once the purulent process is established, if untreated the course is fulminant, terminated by acute cardiac tampon-

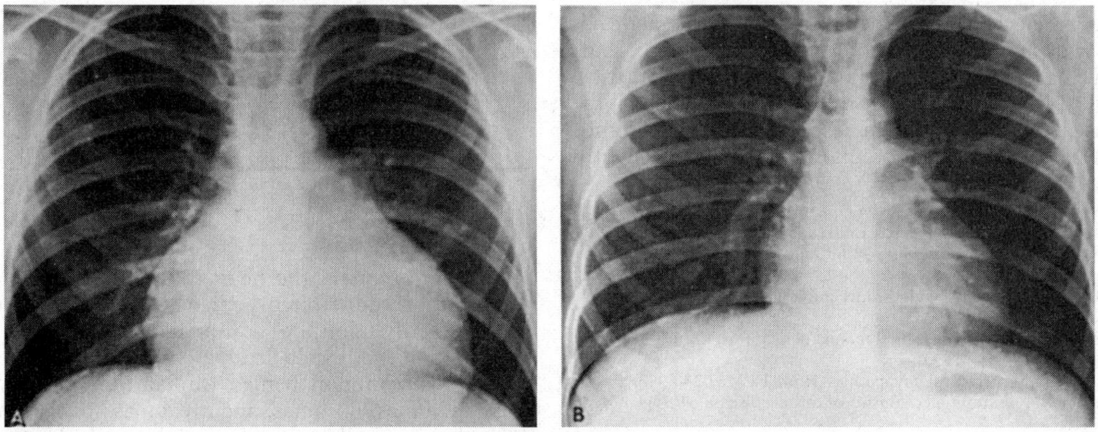

Figure 397–1. Roentgenograms in acute nonspecific pericarditis. *A*, Increase in cardiopericardial shadow caused by pericardial effusion. *B*, One month later after complete recovery.

ade and death. Open pericardial drainage is required, along with appropriate intravenous antibiotics. Although closed pericardial aspiration provides a sample of the exudate for diagnostic purposes and may be lifesaving in the face of severe cardiac compression, without open drainage and removal of adhesions, tamponade will almost invariably recur. Open pericardial drainage has significantly increased survival in patients with this disease. Rarely, with infections that are identified extremely early and with pericardial fluid that is more of a transudate than an exudate, multiple pericardial taps and antibiotic therapy have been successful. The most common organisms implicated in purulent pericarditis are *Staphylococcus aureus, Haemophilus influenzae* type b, and *Neisseria meningitidis.* (For treatment, see Chapters 174, 177, and 178, respectively.) *Tuberculous pericarditis* rarely occurs in children. Extensive treatment with antituberculous chemotherapy is required (see Chapter 199). *Immune complex mediated pericarditis* (sterile) may occur 5–7 days after the initiation of therapy for severe systemic or meningeal infection with meningococcus or *H. influenzae* type b. Therapy includes anti-inflammatory agents and pericardiocentesis, if tamponade develops.

Acute Rheumatic Fever. Pericarditis occurs in acute rheumatic fever as a component of pancarditis (see Chapters 175.1 and 391). It is associated with acute valvulitis. Pericarditis and other manifestations of acute rheumatic pancarditis respond to therapy with steroids. Cardiac tamponade is extremely rare.

Juvenile Rheumatoid Arthritis. Pericarditis is not an uncommon manifestation of juvenile rheumatoid arthritis (see Chapter 148). Rarely, pericarditis may be the only manifestation and precede the onset of arthritis by months or even years. Differentiation of rheumatoid pericarditis from that seen with other collagen vascular disease, particularly lupus erythematosus, may be difficult. Treatment consists of steroids or salicylates, which may be needed on a long-term basis.

Uremia. Uremic pericarditis occurs only in the presence of prolonged severe renal failure and results from chemical irritation of the pericardium secondary to the metabolic abnormalities. It may culminate in cardiac tamponade or cause, recurrent hypotension during hemodialysis. If adequate relief of uremic pericarditis does not occur with hemodialysis, pericardiectomy is recommended.

Neoplastic Disease. Neoplastic pericardial effusion is seen in patients with Hodgkin disease, lymphosarcoma, and leukemia, and results from direct neoplastic invasion of the pericardium. Cardiac tamponade may occur late in the course of the illness. Rarely, pericardial infiltration is the initial manifestation of neoplastic disease. Patients with malignancy may also develop pericarditis as a result of radiation therapy to the mediastinum.

Postpericardiotomy Syndrome (Chapter 387.23). Pericardial effusions are usually seen 1–2 wk following open heart surgery and in some echocardiographic series has been diagnosed in as many as 15% of postoperative patients. The syndrome is a nonspecific hypersensitivity reaction to trauma to the pericardium and the epicardial surface of the heart. High titers of anti-heart antibodies have been reported to correlate with clinical signs of the syndrome. Patients may present with low-grade fever, lethargy, loss of appetite, and precordial or pleural chest pain. In most children, the syndrome is a relatively short illness and responds well to therapy with aspirin or other nonsteroidal anti-inflammatory agents. Corticosteroids are very rarely needed and reserved for the more severe cases. Treatment is maintained for 1–3 mo, but recurrences may be seen as long as 1 yr postoperatively and require reinstitution of therapy.

397.1 Constrictive Pericarditis

In most instances constriction occurs months or years after the initial pericarditis, but occasionally it may be an acute, rapidly progressive process. Constrictive pericarditis most often occurs without an immediate preceding illness or generalized systemic disease.

The *clinical manifestations* occur as a result of impairment of diastolic ventricular filling, compromise of myocardial contractility, and resultant depression of cardiac function. Hepatomegaly and ascites may be out of proportion to the other signs and symptoms, and thus suggest chronic liver disease. However, liver function studies are only mildly abnormal, and careful physical examination reveals other sometimes subtle findings of constriction, including neck vein distention, narrow pulses, quiet precordium, distant heart sounds, a faint pericardial friction rub, and increased pulsus paradoxus. Typical findings become apparent gradually and thus may be easily overlooked. The auscultatory presence of an early pericardial knock and the appearance of calcification of the pericardium on chest roentgenogram are the more obvious manifestations. Protein-losing enteropathy with hypoproteinemia and lymphopenia may be seen in association with severe constriction.

Constrictive pericarditis may be difficult to distinguish from chronic restrictive cardiomyopathy (Chapter 396). Impaired myocardial function occurs with both conditions. However, the myocardial disease of constrictive pericarditis is almost always reversible with pericardiectomy. At times, a definite diagnosis can be made only by exploratory thoracotomy and direct examination of the pericardium.

Radical pericardiectomy with decortication of the pericardium over a wide area of the heart, including the systemic and pulmonary veins, is the only effective treatment for constrictive pericarditis. In most patients surgical intervention elicits a rapid response, characterized by increased cardiac output and prompt diuresis. The long-term prognosis is usually excellent.

Bonow RO, Dilsizian V, Rosing DR, et al: Verapamil-induced improvement in left ventricular diastolic filling and increased exercise tolerance in patients with hypertrophic cardiomyopathy: Short- and long-term effects. Circulation 72:853, 1985.
Gersony WM, Hordof AH: Infective endocarditis and diseases of the pericardium. Pediatr Clin North Am 25:831, 1978.
Hara KS, Ballard DJ, Ilstrup DM, et al: Rheumatoid pericarditis: Clinical features and survival. Medicine 69:81, 1990.
Kelly DP, Strauss AW: Inherited cardiomyopathies. N Engl J Med 330:913, 1994.
Lange LG, Schreiner GF: Immune mechanisms of cardiac disease. N Engl J Med 330:1129, 1994.
Muir P, Nicholson F, Tilzey AJ, et al: Chronic relapsing pericarditis and dilated cardiomyopathy: Serological evidence of persistent enterovirus infection. Lancet 1:804, 1989.
Nishimura RA, Connolly DC, Parkin TW, et al: Constrictive pericarditis: Assessment of current diagnostic procedures. Mayo Clin Proc 60:397, 1985.
Sinzobahamvya N, Ikeogu MO: Purulent pericarditis. Arch Dis Child 62:696, 1987.
Anonymous: Cardiac biopsy in myocarditis. Lancet 336:283, 1990.
Anonymous: Dilated cardiomyopathy and enteroviruses. Lancet 336:971, 1990.
Bowles NE, Richardson PJ, Olsen EGJ, et al: Detection of coxsackie-B-virus-specific RNA sequences in myocardial biopsy samples from patients with myocarditis and dilated cardiomyopathy. Lancet 1:1120, 1986.
Caforio ALP, Stewart JT, McKenna WJ: Idiopathic dilated cardiomyopathy: Rational treatment awaits better understanding of pathogenesis. Br Med J 300:890, 1990.
Chan KY, Iwahara M, Benson LN, et al: Immunosuppressive therapy in the management of acute myocarditis in children: A clinical trial. J Am Coll Card 17:458, 1991.
Chen S-C, Tsai CC, Nouri S: Carditis associated with *Mycoplasma pneumoniae* infection. Am J Dis Child 140:471, 1986.
Chow LC, Dittrich HC, Shabetai R: Endomyocardial biopsy in patients with unexplained congestive heart failure. Ann Intern Med 109:535, 1988.
Dunnigan A, Staley NA, Smith SA, et al: Cardiac and skeletal muscle abnormalities in cardiomyopathy: Comparison of patients with ventricular tachycardia or congestive heart failure. J Am Coll Cardiol 10:608, 1987.
Gilbert EM, Anderson JL, Deitchman D, et al: Long-term β-blocker vasodilator therapy improves cardiac function in idiopathic dilated cardiomyopathy: A double-blind, randomized study of bucindolol versus placebo. Am J Med 88:223, 1990.
Imperato-McGinley J, Gautier T, Ehlers K, et al: Reversibility of catecholamine-induced dilated cardiomyopathy in a child with a pheochromocytoma. N Engl J Med 316:793, 1987.
Katz AM: Cardiomyopathy of overload: A major determinant of prognosis in congestive heart failure. N Engl J Med 322:100, 1990.
Lipshultz SE, Colan SD, Gelber RD, et al: Late cardiac effects of doxorubicin therapy for acute lymphoblastic leukemia in childhood. N Engl J Med 324:808, 1991.
Maron BJ, Tajik AJ, Ruttenberg HD, et al: Hypertrophic cardiomyopathy in infants: Clinical features and natural history. Circulation 65:7, 1982.
McCaffrey FM, Braden DS, Strong WB: Sudden cardiac deaths in young athletes. Am J Dis Child 145:177, 1991.
Muntoni F, Cau M, Ganau A, et al.: Brief report: Deletion of the dystrophin muscle-promoter region associated with X-linked dilated cardiomyopathy. N Engl J Med 329:921, 1993.
Parrillo JE: Heart disease and the eosinophil. N Engl J Med 323:1560, 1990.
Parrillo JE, Cunnion RE, Epstein SE, et al: A prospective, randomized, controlled trial of prednisone for dilated cardiomyopathy. N Engl J Med 321:1061, 1989.
Rosenzweig A, Watkins H, Hwang D-S, et al: Preclinical diagnosis of familial hypertrophic cardiomyopathy by genetic analysis of blood lymphocytes. N Engl J Med 325:1753, 1991.
Scott GB, Hutto C, Makuch RW, et al: Survival in children with perinatally acquired human immunodeficiency virus type 1 infection. N Engl J Med 321:1791, 1989.
Solomon SD, Jarcho JA, McKenna W, et al: Familial hypertrophic cardiomyopathy is a genetically heterogeneous disease. J Clin Invest 86:993, 1990.
Spicer RL, Rocchini AP, Crowley DC, et al: Hemodynamic effects of verapamil in children and adolescents with hypertrophic cardiomyopathy. Circulation 67:413, 1983.
Thiene G, Nava A, Corrado D, et al: Right ventricular cardiomyopathy and sudden death in young people. N Engl J Med 318:129, 1988.
de Vivo DC, Tein I: Primary and secondary disorders of carnitine metabolism. Int Pediatr 5:134, 1990.
Wagner JA, Sax FL, Weisman HF, et al: Calcium-antagonist receptors in the atrial tissue of patients with hypertrophic cardiomyopathy. N Engl J Med 320:755, 1989.
Young LHY, Joag SV, Zheng L-M, et al: Perforin-mediated myocardial damage in acute myocarditis. Lancet 336:1019, 1990.

CHAPTER 398
Tumors of the Heart

Primary tumors of the heart are rare in infancy and childhood and are most often benign. Clinical manifestations depend primarily upon the location of the tumor and, to a lesser extent, upon the histologic type.

The most common benign cardiac tumors in children are rhabdomyomas, fibromas, and myxomas. *Rhabdomyomas* occur as single or usually multiple nodules embedded in chamber walls. They may remain clinically unimportant or even regress but also may cause mechanical obstruction, heart failure, or arrhythmias. They may be familial and are often found in association with **tuberous sclerosis**. Most rhabdomyomas are seen in infants under 1 yr of age. Incessant ventricular tachycardia in an infant younger than 2 yr of age should raise the suspicion of a small endocardial or epicardial rhabdomyoma or *Purkinje cell tumor. Fibromas* are usually solitary nonencapsulated nodules, located in the ventricles; they can be massive. The treatment of rhabdomyomas and fibromas depends on their location and size. Small asymptomatic tumors in the myocardial wall or ventricular septum may be observed for growth or regression. Large tumors that show signs of obstructing blood flow and those producing ventricular arrhythmias should be removed. Large and diffuse tumors may interfere with cardiac performance. Removal of large lesions is often difficult because insufficient normal myocardium may remain. Cardiac transplantation may be the only recourse for patients with extensive tumors.

Myxomas develop in intracavitary locations, most frequently (90%) in the left atrium. Most occur in females (75%). These tumors are solid, smooth, pedunculated masses (1–8 cm) that attach to the interatrial septum, protrude into the atrial chamber, and, by their position relative to the mitral valve, cause intermittent obstruction and a clinical picture consistent with mitral stenosis (syncope, heart failure, atrial fibrillation). A myxoma should be considered in the presence of fainting spells, a positional character (supine vs. erect) to the murmur, or evidence of systemic embolization. Atrial myxomas can also manifest fever, malaise, arthralgias, and systemic emboli mimicking endocarditis, rheumatic fever, or systemic lupus erythematosus. Laboratory features include a high sedimentation rate, hematuria, and echocardiographic evidence of the tumor. Atrial myxomas may be associated with multiple pigmented skin lesions (lentiginosis), myxoid fibroadenomas of the breast, cutaneous myxomas, and adrenal pigmented nodules. Some are associated with various cutaneous and connective tissue lesions and testicular tumors or pituitary adenomas. Treatment consists of surgical excision, which must include all of the base of the tumor to prevent recurrence.

Other benign tumors include *papillomas,* which are attached to valve leaflets and may present in the neonate; *lipomas,* which are situated in ventricular walls; and *mesotheliomas,* which may involve the atrioventricular node and cause abnormalities of electrical conduction, including complete heart block.

Primary malignant cardiac tumors in children are almost exclusively *sarcomas.* These tumors are usually located in the right side of the heart, atrial septum, right atrial wall, or root of the pulmonary artery. They may extend either into the adjacent chamber to cause obstruction to blood flow or into the pericardial cavity to produce effusion or tamponade. The heart also may be involved in the metastatic dissemination of a noncardiac malignancy, such as leukemia or lymphoma, or in Wilms tumor by direct extension of the tumor into the right atrium via the inferior vena cava.

Physical examination will reflect the location and size of the tumor if it interferes with blood flow. Conduction system involvement can be assessed by electrocardiography. Two-dimensional echocardiography is diagnostic and allows excellent visualization of the location and extent of the tumor. Doppler studies evaluate the extent of blood flow obstruction caused by the tumor. Cardiac catheterization may provide further information about the anatomy of the tumor and the hemodynamic effects. When indicated, surgical intervention is directed toward complete removal of the tumor, relief of obstruction, and control of any arrhythmias. Long-term outcome depends upon the type of tumor, completeness of surgical removal, and the postsurgical integrity of the normal cardiac structures and myocardium.

Bini RM, Westaby S, Bargeron LM, et al: Investigation and management of primary cardiac tumors in infants and children. J Am Coll Cardiol 2:351, 1983.
Birnbaum S, McGahan JP, Janos GG, et al: Fetal tachycardia and intramyocardial tumors. J Am Coll Cardiol 6:1358, 1985.
Coltart DJ, Billingham ME, Popp RL, et al: Left atrial myxoma: Diagnosis, treatment and cytological observations. JAMA 234:950, 1975.
Danoff A, Jarmark S, Lorber D, et al: Adrenocortical micronodular dysplasia, cardiac myxomas, lentigines, and spindle cell tumors: Report of a kindred. Arch Intern Med 147:443, 1987.
Felner JM, Knopf WD: Echocardiographic recognition of intracardiac and extracardiac masses. Echocardiography 2:1, 1985.
Garson A Jr, Gillette PC, Titus JL, et al: Surgical treatment of ventricular tachycardia in infants. N Engl J Med 310:1443, 1984.

SECTION 7

Cardiac Therapeutics

CHAPTER 399

Congestive Heart Failure

Heart failure is defined as a state in which the heart cannot deliver an adequate cardiac output to meet the metabolic needs of the body. In early stages of heart failure, various compensatory mechanisms are evoked to maintain normal metabolic function (cardiac reserve). As these mechanisms become ineffective, increasingly severe clinical manifestations result.

PATHOPHYSIOLOGY. The heart can be viewed as a pump with an output proportional to its filling volume and inversely proportional to the resistance against which it pumps. As the ventricular end-diastolic volume increases, the healthy heart will increase cardiac output until a maximum is reached and cardiac output can no longer be augmented (the Frank-Starling principle; Fig. 399–1). The increased stroke volume obtained in this manner is due to the stretching of myocardial fibers, but also results in increased wall tension, which increases myocardial oxygen consumption. Hearts working under various types of stress will function along different Frank-Starling curves. Cardiac muscle with a compromised intrinsic contractility will require a greater degree of dilatation to produce an increased stroke volume and will not achieve the same maximal cardiac output as normal myocardium. If a cardiac chamber is already dilated because of a lesion causing an increased preload (e.g., a left-to-right shunt or valvular insufficiency), there will be little room for further dilatation and augmentation of cardiac output. The presence of lesions that result in increased afterload to the ventricle (aortic or pulmonic stenosis, coarctation of the aorta) will decrease cardiac performance, resulting in a depressed Frank-Starling relationship. The ability of the immature heart to increase cardiac output in response to increased preload is somewhat less than that of the mature heart. Thus, premature infants will be more compromised by a left-to-right ductal level shunt than a full-term infant would.

Systemic oxygen transport (SOT) is calculated as the product of the cardiac output (CO) and the systemic oxygen content (C_aO_2). The cardiac output can be calculated as the product of heart rate and stroke volume (HR × SV). The primary determinants of stroke volume are the *afterload* (pressure work), *preload* (volume work), and *contractility* (intrinsic myocardial function). Abnormalities of heart rate can also compromise cardiac output, including both bradyarrhythmias and tachyarrhythmias, which shorten the diastolic time interval for filling of the ventricles. Alterations in the oxygen carrying capacity of the blood (e.g., anemia or hypoxemia) will also lead to a decrease in SOT and, if compensatory mechanisms are inadequate, can also result in decreased delivery of substrate to the tissues, a form of cardiac failure.

In some cases of heart failure, the CO is normal or increased, yet because of decreased C_aO_2 (secondary to anemia) or increased oxygen demands (secondary to hyperventilation, hyperthyroidism, or hypermetabolism), there is an inadequate amount of oxygen being delivered to meet the body's needs. This condition, *high-output failure,* results in the development of signs and symptoms of congestive heart failure when there is no basic abnormality in myocardial function and the cardiac output is greater than normal. It is also seen with large systemic arteriovenous fistulas. These diseases reduce peripheral vascular resistance and cardiac afterload, and increase myocardial contractility. Heart "failure" results when the demands for cardiac output exceed the ability of the heart to respond. Chronic severe high-output failure may eventually result in a decrease in myocardial performance as the metabolic requirements of the myocardium itself are not met.

One major compensatory mechanism for increasing cardiac output is an increase in sympathetic tone, secondary to increased adrenal secretion of circulating epinephrine and increased neural release of norepinephrine. The initial beneficial effects of sympathetic stimulation include increased heart rate and myocardial contractility, which both serve to increase cardiac output. Because of localized vasoconstriction, blood flow may be redistributed from the cutaneous, visceral, and renal beds to the heart and brain. However, prolonged increases in sympathetic stimulation can have deleterious effects as well, including hypermetabolism, increased afterload, arrhythmogenesis, increased myocardial oxygen requirements, and direct myocardial toxicity. Peripheral vasoconstriction can result in decreased renal, hepatic, and gastrointestinal tract function.

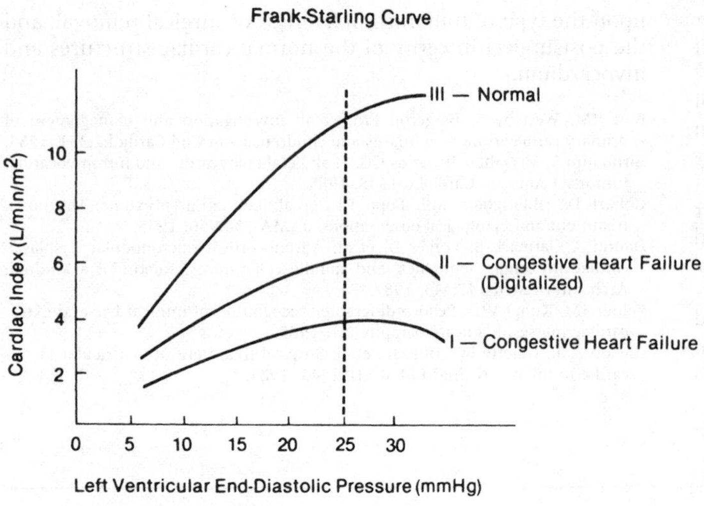

Figure 399–1. As the left ventricular end-diastolic pressure (LVED) increases, cardiac index increases, even in the presence of congestive heart failure, until a critical level of LVED is reached. Adding an inotropic agent (digoxin) shifts the curve from I to II. (From Gersony WM, Steep CN: *In*: Dickerman JD, Lucey JF [eds]: Smith's The Critically Ill Child: Diagnosis and Medical Management, 3rd ed. Philadelphia, WB Saunders, 1984.)

CLINICAL MANIFESTATIONS. These depend on the degree of cardiac reserve under various conditions. A critically ill infant or child who has exhausted his compensatory mechanisms to the point where he can no longer achieve sufficient cardiac output to meet the basal metabolic needs of the body will be symptomatic at rest. Other patients may be comfortable when quiet but are incapable of increasing cardiac output in response to even mild activity without developing significant symptoms. On the other hand, it may take rather vigorous exercise to compromise cardiac function in children who have less severe heart disease. A thorough history is extremely important both in making the diagnosis of heart failure and in evaluating the possible causes. Parents who are observing their infant on a daily basis may not recognize subtle changes that have occurred over the course of days or weeks. Cyanosis may be considered merely "a deep coloring" and not recognized as an abnormal finding. The history of a young infant should also focus on feeding (see Chapter 380). The infant with congestive heart failure often takes less volume per feeding, becomes dyspneic while sucking, and may perspire profusely. Eliciting a history of fatigue in an older child requires specific questions about activity.

In children the signs and symptoms of congestive heart failure are similar to those in adults. These include fatigue, effort intolerance, anorexia, abdominal pain, and cough. Dyspnea is a reflection of pulmonary congestion. Elevation of systemic venous pressure may be gauged by clinical assessment of the jugular venous pressure and liver enlargement. Orthopnea and basilar rales may be present; edema is usually discernible in dependent portions of the body, or anasarca may be present. Cardiomegaly is invariably noted. A gallop rhythm is common; other auscultatory findings are specific to the basic cardiac lesion.

In infants congestive heart failure may be more difficult to identify. Prominent manifestations include tachypnea, feeding difficulties, poor weight gain, excessive perspiration, irritability, weak cry, and noisy, labored respirations with intercostal and subcostal retractions as well as flaring of the alae nasi. The signs of cardiac pulmonary congestion may be indistinguishable from those of bronchiolitis, including wheezing as the most prominent finding. Pneumonitis with or without atelectasis is common, especially of the right middle and lower lobes, due to bronchial compression by the enlarged heart. Hepatomegaly nearly always occurs, and cardiomegaly is invariably present. In spite of pronounced tachycardia, a gallop rhythm can frequently be recognized. The other auscultatory signs are those produced by the underlying cardiac lesion. Clinical assessment of the jugular venous pressure in infants may be difficult because of the shortness of the neck and the difficulty of observing a relaxed state. Edema may be generalized, usually involving the eyelids as well as the sacrum, and less often the legs and feet. The differential diagnosis is age dependent (Table 399–1).

DIAGNOSIS. *Roentgenograms of the chest* show cardiac enlargement. The pulmonary vascularity is variable depending on the etiology of the heart failure. Infants and children having large left-to-right shunts will have exaggeration of the pulmonary arterial vessels to the periphery of the lung fields, whereas patients having cardiomyopathy may have a relatively normal

■ **TABLE 399–1 Etiology of Heart Failure**

Fetal
Severe anemia (hemolysis, fetal-maternal transfusion, parvovirus B19–induced anemia, hypoplastic anemia)
Supraventricular tachycardia
Ventricular tachycardia
Complete heart block

Premature Neonate
Fluid overload
Patent ductus arteriosus
Ventricular septal defect
Cor pulmonale (bronchopulmonary dysplasia)
Hypertension

Full-Term Neonate
Asphyxial cardiomyopathy
Arteriovenous malformation (vein of Galen, hepatic)
Left-sided obstructive lesions (coarctation of aorta, hypoplastic left side of the heart)
Large mixing cardiac defects (single ventricle, truncus arteriosus)
Viral myocarditis

Infant-Toddler
Left-to-right cardiac shunts (ventricular septal defect)
Hemangioma (arteriovenous malformation)
Anomalous left coronary artery
Metabolic cardiomyopathy
Acute hypertension (hemolytic-uremic syndrome)
Supraventricular tachycardia
Kawasaki disease

Child-Adolescent
Rheumatic fever
Acute hypertension (glomerulonephritis)
Viral myocarditis
Thyrotoxicosis
Hemochromatosis-hemosiderosis
Cancer therapy (radiation, Adriamycin)
Sickle cell anemia
Endocarditis
Cor pulmonale (cystic fibrosis)
Cardiomyopathy (hypertrophic, dilated, postviral)

pulmonary vascular bed early in the course of their disease. Fluffy perihilar pulmonary markings suggestive of venous congestion and acute pulmonary edema are usually seen only with more severe degrees of heart failure.

Chamber hypertrophy by *electrocardiography* may be helpful in assessing the etiology of congestive heart failure but does not establish the diagnosis. In cardiomyopathies, left or right ventricular ischemic changes may correlate well with clinical and other noninvasive parameters of ventricular function. Low-voltage QRS morphology with ST-T wave abnormalities may also suggest myocardial inflammatory disease but can also be seen with pericarditis. The electrocardiogram is the best tool for evaluating rhythm disorders as a potential cause of heart failure.

Echocardiographic techniques are very useful in assessing ventricular function. The most commonly used parameter is the fractional shortening, determined as the difference between end-systolic and end-diastolic diameters divided by the end-diastolic diameter. The normal fractional shortening is between 28% and 40%, compared with the normal ejection fraction (which measures volume) of 55–65% measured by angiography. The pre-ejection/ejection period ratio (PEP/EP), measured by M-mode echo, should be less than 40%. A long pre-ejection time with a very short ejection time usually denotes myocardial failure. Doppler studies can be used to calculate cardiac output. *Radionuclide studies* are also useful, because the ejection fraction can be determined by injecting a radioisotope (e.g., ^{99m}Tc) into a vein and measuring end-diastolic volume and systolic volume by counts over the ventricles.

Arterial oxygen levels may be decreased when ventilation/perfusion inequalities occur secondary to pulmonary edema. When heart failure is severe, respiratory and/or metabolic *acidosis* may be present. Infants with congestive heart failure often display *hyponatremia* caused by renal water retention. Total body sodium may be actually increased. Chronic diuretic treatment can decrease serum sodium levels even further.

TREATMENT. The underlying cause of cardiac failure must be removed or alleviated if possible. If the etiology is a congenital cardiac anomaly amenable to surgery, medical treatment is indicated to prepare the patient for operation and in the immediate postoperative period while the heart is recovering from the effects of cardiopulmonary bypass. If the etiology is a cardiomyopathy, medical management will provide a temporary relief from symptoms and allow the patient time to wait for a heart donor if cardiac transplantation is indicated.

General Measures. Strict bed rest is rarely necessary except in extreme cases, but it is important that the child rest often and sleep adequately. Most older patients feel better sleeping in a semi-upright position. For infants with congestive heart failure, an infant chair may be advisable. After patients begin to respond to treatment, restrictions on activities can often be modified within the context of the specific diagnosis and the patient's ability. For patients with severe pulmonary edema, positive-pressure ventilation may be required along with other drug therapy. Beta-adrenergic agonists, such as dopamine, epinephrine, and dobutamine, along with afterload reducing agents (e.g., nitroprusside, captopril), may be required in an intensive care setting.

Diet. Infants having congestive heart failure may fail to thrive because of both increased metabolic requirements and decreased caloric intake. Increasing daily calories is an important aspect of their management. Increasing the number of calories per ounce of infant formula (or supplementing breast feedings) may be beneficial. Many infants will not tolerate an increase beyond 24 calories per ounce because of diarrhea or because these formulas provide too large a solute load for compromised kidneys.

Severely ill infants may lack sufficient strength for effective sucking because of extreme fatigue, rapid respirations, and generalized weakness. In these circumstances, nasogastric feedings may be helpful. In many children with cardiac enlargement, gastroesophageal reflux is a major problem. The use of continuous drip nasogastric feedings at night, administered by pump, may improve caloric intake while decreasing the problems with reflux. Occasionally, medical or surgical intervention to correct reflux is necessary (Nissen fundoplication). Continued malnutrition may be an important factor in the decision to undertake earlier surgical intervention in patients who have an operable congenital heart lesion.

The use of very low sodium formulas in the routine management of infants with congestive heart failure is not recommended, because these preparations are often poorly tolerated. The use of more potent diuretic agents allows more palatable standard formulas to be used for nutrition while controlling salt and water balance by chronic diuretic administration. Most older children can be managed with "no added salt" diets and abstinence from foods containing large amounts of sodium. A strict extremely low sodium diet is rarely required.

Digitalis. Digoxin is the digitalis glycoside used most often in the pediatric patient. The half-life of 36 hr is long enough to allow daily or twice daily administration and short enough to limit toxic effects from overdosage. It is absorbed well by the gastrointestinal tract (60–85%), even in infants. When taken with or after meals the rate of absorption may be somewhat retarded, but the amount of digoxin absorbed is almost always unchanged. Absorption is greater for the elixir than for tablets. An initial effect can be seen as early as 30 min after administration, and the peak effect for oral digoxin is at approximately 2–6 hr. When the drug is administered intravenously, the initial effect is seen in 15–30 min and the peak effect occurs at 1–4 hr. The drug crosses the placenta, and therefore the fetus with heart failure, for example, secondary to arrhythmia, can be treated via administration of digoxin to the mother. Digoxin is eliminated by the kidney and dosing must be adjusted based on the patient's renal function. The rate of excretion is proportional to the glomerular filtration rate. After intravenous administration, 50–70% is excreted unchanged in the urine. The half-life of digoxin may be up to 6 days in patients with renal shutdown, who must utilize slower hepatic excretion pathways.

Rapid digitalization of infants and children in congestive heart failure may be carried out intravenously. The dose depends on the patient's age (Table 399–2). The recommended schedule is to give one half of the total digitalizing dose immediately and the succeeding two one-quarter doses at 12 hr intervals later. The electrocardiogram must be closely monitored and rhythm strips obtained prior to each of the three digitalizing doses. Digoxin should be discontinued if a new rhythm disturbance is noted. A significant prolongation of the PR interval is not in itself an indication to withhold digitalis, but a delay in administering the next dose or a reduction in the dosage should be considered depending on the patient's clinical status. Serum digoxin determination is helpful when digitalis toxicity is suspected, although it may be less reliable in infants. ST segment or T wave changes are commonly noted with digitalis administration and should not affect the digitalization regimen. Baseline serum electrolyte levels should be measured prior to and after digitalization. Hypokalemia and hypercalcemia exacerbate digitalis toxicity. Because hypokalemia is relatively common in patients receiving diuretics, the potassium level should be followed closely in patients receiving a potassium-wasting diuretic, for example, furosemide, in combination with digitalis.

Maintenance digitalis therapy is started approximately 12 hr after full digitalization. The daily dosage is divided in two and given at 12-hr intervals for more consistent blood levels and more flexibility in case of toxicity. The dosage is one quarter of the total digitalizing dose. For patients who are initially

■ **TABLE 399–2 Dosage of Drugs Commonly Used for the Treatment of Congestive Heart Failure**

Drug	Dosage
Digoxin	
Digitalization (PO) (3 divided doses)	Premature 0.02–0.025 mg/kg Neonate (≤1 mo) 0.03–0.04 mg/kg Infant or child 0.04–0.05 mg/kg Adolescent or adult 1.0–1.5 mg in divided doses
Digitalization (IV) (Timing of dosage variable, depending on clinical indications)	75% of PO dose
Maintenance	¼ of digitalizing dose, divided q 12 hr
Furosemide	
IV	1–2 mg/dose, prn
PO	1–4 mg/kg/24 hr, qd, bid, or qid
Bumetanide	
IV	0.01–0.1 mg/kg/dose
PO	0.05–0.1 mg/kg/24 hr q 6–8 hr
Chlorothiazide (PO)	20–50 mg/kg/24 hr, bid, or qid
Spironolactone (PO)	2–3 mg/kg/24 hr, bid, or tid
β Agonists (IV)	
Isoproterenol	0.01–0.5 μg/kg/min
Dopamine	2–20 μg/kg/min
Dobutamine	2–20 μg/kg/min
Amrinone (IV)	0.75 mg/kg bolus over 2–3 min 5–10 μg/kg/min
Afterload-reducing agents	
Nitroprusside (IV)	0.5–8 μg/kg/min
Hydralazine	
IV	0.1–0.5 mg/kg
PO	0.5–7.5 mg/kg/24 hr, tid
Captopril (PO)	0.5–6 mg/kg/24 hr, qid

Note: Pediatric doses based on weight should not exceed adult doses.

digitalized intravenously, maintenance digoxin can be given orally once oral feedings are tolerated. Because absorption from the gastrointestinal tract is less certain, the oral maintenance dose is usually 20–25% higher than when digoxin is used parenterally (see Table 399–2). The normal daily dosage of digoxin for older children (>5 yr of age) calculated by body weight should not exceed the usual adult dose of 0.2–0.5 mg/24 hr.

Patients who are not critically ill may be digitalized initially by the oral route, and in most instances digitalization is completed within 24 hr. When slow digitalization is desirable, for example, in the immediate postoperative period, initiation of a maintenance digoxin schedule without a prior loading dose will achieve full digitalization in 7–10 days. This often can be carried out on an outpatient basis.

If an infant improves significantly on digitalis over a period of a few months and the need for the drug appears to be lessening (e.g., a ventricular septal defect [VSD] that is becoming smaller), the dosage is not increased as the child gains weight. If the clinical status warrants, the drug is eventually discontinued.

Measurement of a *serum digoxin level* is useful under several circumstances: (1) when a standard dose of digoxin is not having beneficial therapeutic effects; (2) when an unknown amount of digoxin has been administered or ingested accidentally; (3) when renal function is impaired or if drug interactions are possible (e.g. quinidine); (4) when there is a question regarding compliance; and (5) when a toxic response is suspected. Blood is usually drawn immediately prior to a dose but at minimum 4 hr after the last dose so that tissue/plasma equilibration has occurred. A normal blood level in an infant is approximately 2–4 ng/mL and in older children 1–2 ng/mL. Exceeding these levels will not generally add significantly to the management of congestive heart failure and only increase the risk of toxicity. In suspected toxicity, elevated serum digoxin levels are not in themselves diagnostic of toxicity but must be interpreted as an adjunct to other clinical and electrocardiographic findings (rhythm and conduction disturbances). Nausea and vomiting are somewhat less frequent in the pediatric patient. Hypokalemia, hypomagnesemia, hypercalcemia, cardiac inflammation due to myocarditis, and prematurity may all potentiate digitalis toxicity. A cardiac arrhythmia that develops in a child who is taking digitalis also may be related to the primary cardiac disease rather than to the drug. However, any form of arrhythmia occurring following the institution of digitalis therapy must be considered to be drug related until proven otherwise. Succeeding doses should be withheld until the question is resolved.

Diuretics. These agents interfere with reabsorption of water and sodium by the kidneys, which results in the reduction of circulating blood volume and thereby reduces pulmonary fluid overload and ventricular filling pressures. They are most often used in conjunction with digitalis therapy in patients with severe congestive heart failure.

Furosemide is the most commonly used diuretic in patients with heart failure. It inhibits the reabsorption of sodium and chloride in the distal tubules and the loop of Henle. Patients requiring acute diuresis should be given intravenous or intramuscular furosemide at an initial dose of 1–2 mg/kg. This usually results in rapid diuresis and prompt improvement in clinical status, particularly if symptoms of pulmonary congestion are present. Chronic furosemide therapy is then prescribed at a dose of 1–4 mg/kg/24 hr given between 1 and 4 times a day. Careful monitoring of electrolytes is necessary with long-term furosemide therapy, because there may be significant loss of potassium. Potassium chloride supplementation is usually required unless the potassium-sparing diuretic spironolactone is given concomitantly. When furosemide is administered every other day, dietary potassium supplementation may be adequate to maintain normal serum potassium levels. Chronic administration of furosemide may cause contraction of the extracellular fluid compartment, resulting in a "contraction alkalosis" (see Chapter 56.8). Under these circumstances, acetazolamide, a carbonic anhydrase inhibitor, may be useful.

Spironolactone is an inhibitor of aldosterone and enhances potassium retention. It is usually given orally in 2–3 divided doses of 2–3 mg/kg/24 hr. Combinations of spironolactone and chlorothiazide are commonly used for convenience and because they eliminate the need for potassium supplementation, which is often poorly tolerated.

Chlorothiazide is used occasionally for diuresis in children with less severe, chronic congestive heart failure. It is less immediate in action and less potent than furosemide, and it affects the reabsorption of electrolytes only in the renal tubules. The usual dose is 20–50 mg/kg/24 hr in divided doses. Potassium supplementation is often required if this agent is used alone.

Afterload-Reducing Agents. This group of drugs reduces ventricular afterload by decreasing peripheral vascular resistance, thereby improving myocardial performance. Some of these agents also decrease systemic venous tone, significantly reducing preload. Afterload reducers are especially useful in children with congestive heart failure secondary to cardiomyopathy and in patients with severe mitral or aortic insufficiency. They may also be effective in patients with congestive heart failure secondary to left-to-right shunts. They are usually not used in the presence of stenotic lesions of the left ventricular outflow tract. Afterload-reducing agents are most often used in conjunction with other anticongestive drugs, such as digoxin and diuretics.

Nitroprusside should be administered only in an intensive care setting and for as short a period of time as possible. Its short intravenous half-life makes it ideal for titrating the dose in critically ill patients. Peripheral arterial vasodilatation and afterload reduction are the major effects, but venodilatation causing a decrease in venous return to the heart may also be beneficial. Blood pressure must be continuously monitored by means of an intra-arterial line, as sudden hypotension can occur with overdosage. Nitroprusside is contraindicated when hypotension pre-exists. As the drug is metabolized, small amounts of circulating cyanide are produced, which are detoxified in the liver to thiocyanate, which is excreted in the urine. However, when high doses of nitroprusside are administered for several days, toxic symptoms related to thiocyanate poisoning may occur, such as fatigue, nausea, disorientation, and muscular spasm. If nitroprusside use is prolonged, blood thiocyanate levels should be monitored; values >10 μg/dL are consistent with clinical symptoms of toxicity.

Hydralazine is a direct arteriolar smooth muscle relaxant and has virtually no effects on preload. It is occasionally administered together with a venodilating agent, such as one of the nitrate derivatives. The usual oral dose of hydralazine is 0.5–7.5 mg/kg/24 hr in three divided doses. Many patients require increasing dosage with time in order to maintain the peripheral dilating effects (tachyphylaxis). Adverse reactions with hydralazine include headache, palpitations, nausea, and vomiting. In addition, systemic lupus erythematosus occasionally occurs after administration of large doses of hydralazine over prolonged periods; these manifestations are reversible when the drug is discontinued.

Captopril is an orally active angiotensin-converting-enzyme (ACE) inhibitor that produces marked arterial dilatation by blocking the production of angiotensin II, resulting in significant afterload reduction. Venodilatation and consequent preload reduction have also been reported. This agent also interferes with aldosterone production and thereby also helps control salt and water retention. The oral dose is 0.5–6 mg/kg/24 hr given in 2–3 divided doses. The adverse reactions to captopril include hypotension and its sequelae (e.g., syncope, weakness, and dizziness). A maculopapular pruritic rash is encountered in 5–8% of patients, but the drug may be continued because the rash often disappears spontaneously with time. Neutropenia and renal toxicity also occur.

β-Adrenergic Agonists. *Isoproterenol,* an intravenous preparation used for treating low cardiac output, has both central and peripheral β-adrenergic effects, and therefore enhances myocardial contractility and also reduces cardiac afterload. The drug is administered in an intensive care setting, where the dose is titrated between 0.01 and 0.5 μg/kg/min. Continuous determinations of arterial blood pressure and heart rate are mandatory, and measuring cardiac output at the bedside with a pulmonary thermodilution catheter may also be helpful in assessing drug efficacy. Because isoproterenol has a marked chronotropic effect, it should not be used in patients who already have significant tachycardia. Children receiving isoproterenol must be carefully monitored for atrial or ventricular premature depolarizations. Often, as isoproterenol or other β-adrenergic agonist treatment is withdrawn, digoxin therapy is added for continued inotropic effect.

Dopamine has fewer chronotropic and arrhythmogenic effects than isoproterenol. In addition, it results in selective renal vasodilatation, particularly useful in patients with the compromised kidney function that is often associated with low cardiac output. At a dose of 2–10 μg/kg/min, dopamine results in increased contractility with little peripheral vasoconstrictive effects. However, if the dose is increased beyond 15 μg/kg/min, its peripheral α-adrenergic effects may result in vasoconstriction. At high doses dopamine may also cause an increase in pulmonary vascular resistance.

Dobutamine, a derivative of dopamine, is also used to treat low cardiac output. It causes direct inotropic effects with a moderate (albeit less than isoproterenol) reduction in peripheral vascular resistance. Dobutamine can be used as an adjunct to dopamine therapy in order to avoid the vasoconstrictive effects of high-dose dopamine. Dobutamine is also less likely to cause cardiac rhythm disturbances. The usual dose is 2–20 μg/kg/min.

Phosphodiesterase Inhibitors. *Amrinone* is useful in treating patients with low cardiac output who are refractory to standard therapy. It works by inhibition of phosphodiesterase, preventing the degradation of intracellular cAMP. Amrinone has both positive inotropic effects on the heart and significant peripheral vasodilatory effects and has generally been used as an adjunct to dopamine or dobutamine therapy in the intensive care unit. It is given at an initial loading dose of 0.75 mg/kg intravenously followed by an intravenous infusion of 5–10 μg/kg/min. A major side effect is hypotension secondary to peripheral vasodilatation. The hypotension can usually be managed by the administration of intravenous fluids to restore adequate intravascular volume. A second side effect is thrombocytopenia; the severity appears to be related to both the rate of infusion and the duration of therapy. It is reversible when the drug is discontinued or the rate of infusion is decreased.

CHAPTER 400
Cardiogenic Shock

(See also Chapter 60.3)

Cardiogenic shock may occur as a complication of (1) severe cardiac dysfunction, often following surgery; (2) septicemia; (3) severe burns; (4) immunologic disease (anaphylaxis); (5) hemorrhage or dehydration; (6) severe debilitation; and (7) acute central nervous system disorders. It is characterized by low cardiac output and hypotension, resulting in inadequate tissue perfusion.

Treatment is aimed at reinstitution of adequate cardiac output and peripheral perfusion to prevent the untoward effects of prolonged ischemia to vital organs as well as management of the underlying cause. Under physiologic conditions, the cardiac output is increased as a result of sympathetic discharge, which increases heart rate. However, in the presence of cardiogenic shock with marked tachycardia, heart rate will not increase further and may reduce cardiac output by decreasing diastolic filling time. Cardiac output must be increased by increasing stroke volume. If the rate of fluid administration is increased, the central venous pressure and ventricular filling pressure (preload) increase and the Frank-Starling mechanism results in an increased stroke volume. Optimal filling pressure is variable and depends on a number of extracardiac factors, including ventilatory support with high positive end-expiratory pressure, peak inspiratory pressure, and intra-abdominal pressure. The increased pressure necessary to fill a relatively noncompliant ventricle should also be considered, particularly after open heart surgery. If incremental fluid administration does not result in improved cardiac output, abnormal myocardial contractility and/or an abnormally high afterload must be implicated as the cause of the low cardiac output.

Myocardial contractility will improve when treatment of the basic cause of shock is instituted, hypoxia is eliminated, and acidosis is corrected. However, dopamine, epinephrine, and dobutamine will improve cardiac contractility, increase heart rate, and ultimately increase cardiac output (see Chapter 399).

The use of cardiac glycosides to treat acute low cardiac

■ **TABLE 400–1 Treatment of Cardiogenic Shock**

Goal—to improve peripheral perfusion by increasing cardiac output
Cardiac output = Heart rate × stroke volume

	Determinants of Stroke Volume		
	Preload	***Contractility***	***Afterload***
Parameters measured	CVP, PCWP	CO, BP	CO, BP
Abnormal physiologic manifestations	Low CVP or PCWP ↓ CO ↓ BP	High CVP or PCWP ↓ CO ↓ BP	High CVP or PCWP ↓ CO → ↑ BP
Treatment to improve cardiac output	Volume expansion Crystalloid, colloids Whole blood	Catecholamines Dopamine, 5–20 μg/kg/min Dobutamine, 2.5–20 μg/kg/min	Vasodilatation Nitroprusside, 0.5–8 μg/kg/min Hydralazine, 0.5 mg/kg

CVP = central venous pressure; PCWP = pulmonary capillary wedge pressure; CO = cardiac output; BP = blood pressure; ↓ = decreased; → = normal; ↑ = increased.

output states should be avoided. Digoxin has a slower effect than do the catecholamines, even with intravenous administration. In addition, adverse effects may result from larger doses and toxicity is less predictable, depending on myocardial and serum potassium and calcium levels. Because it is quite common for patients with cardiovascular shock to have compromised renal perfusion, the administration of digoxin may result in high persistent blood levels because it is excreted in the kidneys. When digoxin is required for these patients, a lower and less frequent dosage should be used and serum digoxin levels must be monitored frequently.

Patients with cardiogenic shock may have a marked increase in systemic vascular resistance, resulting in high afterload and poor peripheral perfusion. If increased systemic vascular resistance is persistent and the administration of positive inotropic agents alone does not improve tissue perfusion, the use of afterload-reducing agents may be appropriate, for example, nitroprusside used in combination with dopamine. In these patients, use of a pulmonary thermodilution catheter to measure cardiac index and to calculate systemic vascular resistance can be indispensable in guiding therapeutic decisions.

Some patients with cardiogenic shock may benefit from intra-aortic balloon counterpulsation, which reduces afterload by mechanical means and also increases diastolic coronary perfusion. Patients with reversible ventricular failure, for example, those in the immediate postoperative state, may also benefit from extracorporeal membrane oxygenation (ECMO).

Sequential evaluation and management of cardiovascular shock is mandatory (see Chapter 60.3). Table 400–1 outlines the treatment of acute cardiac circulatory failure under most circumstances. The treatment of infants and children with low cardiac output following cardiac surgery depends on the nature of the operative procedure and the patient's status after surgery (see Chapter 387.23).

Artman M, Graham T: Guidelines for vasodilator therapy of congestive heart failure in infants and children. Am Heart J 113:121, 1987.
Awan NA, Miller RR, Mason DT: Comparison of effects of nitroprusside and prazosin on left ventricular function and the peripheral circulation in chronic refractory congestive heart failure. Circulation 57:152, 1978.
Benzing G III, Helmsworth JA, Schreiber JT, et al: Nitroprusside after open-heart surgery. Circulation 54:467, 1976.
Dickerman JD, Lucey JF: Smith's The Critically Ill Child, 3rd ed. Philadelphia, WB Saunders, 1985.
Doering W: Quinidine-digoxin interaction: Pharmacokinetics, underlying mechanism and clinical implications. N Engl J Med 301:401, 1979.
Friedman WF, George BL: Medical progress: Treatment of congestive heart failure by altering loading conditions of the heart. J Pediatr 106:697, 1985.
Goodwin JF: Prospects and predictions for the cardiomyopathies. Circulation 50:210, 1974.
Greenwood RD, Nadas AS, Fyler DC: The clinical course of primary myocardial disease in infants and children. Am Heart J 92:549, 1976.
Harris LC, Nghiem QX: Cardiomyopathies in infants and children. Prog Cardiovasc Dis 25:255, 1972.
Harrison DG, Bates JN: The nitrovasodilators: New ideas about old drugs. Circulation 87:1461, 1993.
Hayes CJ, Butler VP Jr, Gersony WM: Serum digoxin studies in infants and children. Pediatrics 52:561, 1973.
Hernandez A, Burton RM, Pagtakhan RD, et al: Pharmacodynamics of ^{3}H-digoxin in infants. Pediatrics 44:418, 1969.
Lang D, von Bernuth G: Serum concentration and serum half-life of digoxin in premature and mature infants. Pediatrics 59:902, 1977.
Lister G, Moreau G, Moss M, et al: Effects of alterations of oxygen transport on the neonate. Semin Perinatol 8:192, 1984.
Loggie JMH, Kleinman LI, VanMaanen EF: Renal function and diuretic therapy in infants and children. J Pediatr 86:485, 657, 825, 1975.
Perkin RM, Levin DL: Shock in the pediatric patient. Part I. Clinical pathophysiology. J Pediatr 101:163, 1982.
Perkin RM, Levin DL: Shock in the pediatric patient. Part II. Therapy. J Pediatr 101:319, 1982.
Zaritsky A, Chernow B: Use of catecholamines in pediatrics. J Pediatr 105:341, 1984.

CHAPTER 401
Pediatric Heart Transplantation

Over 2000 heart transplants have been performed on children worldwide. Survival for children compares favorably with that in adults: 75% at 1 yr and 72% at 5 yr (Fig. 401–1). As new therapeutic regimens are introduced, the long-term outlook for pediatric heart transplant recipients continues to improve. A small but growing number of children are surpassing 10 yr survival.

INDICATIONS. Heart transplantation is performed in infants and children with end-stage cardiomyopathies who have become refractory to medical therapy and for patients with some forms of complex congenital heart disease for whom standard surgical procedures are extremely high risk (e.g., hypoplastic left heart syndrome). The cardiomyopathies account for 66% of heart transplants in the pediatric age group, although the percentage of patients with congenital heart lesions is gradually increasing. As a secondary procedure, heart transplantation is used in children who have previously undergone conventional surgery for congenital heart lesions and who later develop myocardial dysfunction.

RECIPIENT AND DONOR SELECTION. Potential heart transplant recipients must be free of serious noncardiac medical problems, such as neurologic disease, systemic infection, severe hepatic or renal disease, or severe malnutrition. Many children with ventricular dysfunction may develop pulmonary hypertension and even pulmonary vascular disease, which would preclude heart transplantation. For this reason, pulmonary vascular resistance is measured at cardiac catheterization, both at rest and in

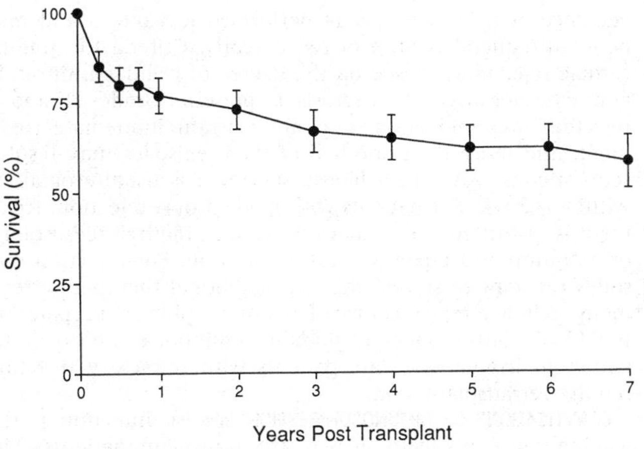

Figure 401–1. Survival after pediatric heart transplantation. Data based on 74 patients transplanted at Stanford University since the introduction of cyclosporine immunosuppression in 1980.

response to vasodilators. Those patients with fixed elevated pulmonary vascular resistance (>5–8 Wood units) may be at too high a risk for heart transplantation and are then considered candidates for heart-lung transplantation (Chapter 402). A comprehensive social service consultation is an important component of the recipient evaluation. Because of the complex post-transplant medical regimen, the family must have a history of medical compliance. Detailed informed consent always should be obtained.

Donor shortage is a serious problem for both adults and children. There is a national registry of transplant recipients in the United States, and allografts are matched by ABO blood group and body weight. HLA matching is not currently feasible for heart transplantation; however, with modern immunosuppression it may offer only minimal advantage. Physicians caring for a patient who may be a potential donor should contact the organ donor coordinator at a transplanting institution, who can best judge the appropriateness of organ donation and has experience in interacting with donor families. Contraindications for organ donation include prolonged cardiac arrest with cardiac dysfunction, systemic illness or infection, and pre-existing severe cardiac disease. A history of resuscitation alone or reparable congenital heart disease is not an automatic exclusion for donation.

The decision of when to place a patient on the transplant waiting list is based on many factors, including: extremely poor ventricular function (left ventricular fractional shortening of <10%, where normal is 28–40%), poor response to medical anticongestive therapy, multiple hospitalizations for heart failure, arrhythmia, progressive deterioration of renal or hepatic function, early stages of pulmonary vascular disease, and poor nutritional status. In patients awaiting transplantation, those with poor left ventricular function (fractional shortening <15%) are placed on oral anticoagulants (usually warfarin) to reduce the risk of mural thrombosis and thromboembolism.

PERIOPERATIVE MANAGEMENT. At surgery, both donor and recipient hearts are excised so as to leave the posterior portions of the atria containing the venae cavae and pulmonary veins. The aorta and pulmonary artery are divided above the level of the semilunar valves. The anterior portion of the donor's atria are then connected to the remaining posterior portion of the recipient's atria, avoiding the need for delicate suturing of the venae cavae or pulmonary veins. Finally, the donor and recipient great vessels are connected via end-to-end anastomoses.

In the immediate postoperative period, immunosuppression is most commonly achieved using a four drug regimen: cyclosporine (10 mg/kg/24 hr), azathioprine (2 mg/kg/24 hr), and prednisone started at 0.6 mg/kg/24 hr and tapered to 0.2 mg/kg/24 hr over the first 6 wk. An antilymphocyte preparation is usually used in the first 1–2 wk, most commonly the monoclonal murine antihuman T lymphocyte antibody (OKT3). Steroids are often increased briefly after discontinuation of OKT3 therapy. In children who do not develop significant graft rejection, steroids can then be further tapered to an alternate-day regimen after the first 6–12 mo, and in many patients steroids can be totally eliminated. In some centers, steroids are not routinely included as part of maintenance immunosuppression but are added later for the treatment of acute rejection episodes. Early experience with newer immunosuppressive agents, such as FK506, suggests that they may be able to significantly reduce the steroid requirement.

In noncomplicated cases, most pediatric heart transplant recipients can be extubated within the first 48 hr post-transplant and are out of bed within 3–4 days. These patients are often discharged as soon as 2 wk post-transplantation. In patients with pre-existing high risk factors, postoperative care is usually considerably prolonged.

DIAGNOSIS AND MANAGEMENT OF ACUTE GRAFT REJECTION. Post-transplant management consists of adjusting medications to maintain a balance between the risk of rejection and the side effects of overimmunosuppression. Next to infection, acute graft rejection is the second leading cause of death in both adult and pediatric heart transplant recipients. The incidence of acute rejection is greatest within the first 3 mo after transplantation and decreases considerably thereafter. Most pediatric patients will experience at least one episode of acute rejection within the 1st yr after transplantation, usually at the time of weaning of one of their immunosuppressive medications.

Clinical manifestations of acute rejection may include fatigue, fluid retention, fever, diaphoresis, abdominal symptoms, and a gallop rhythm. The electrocardiogram may show reduced voltage, atrial or ventricular arrhythmias, or heart block. Roentgenographic examination may show an enlarged heart, effusions, or pulmonary edema. However, cyclosporine has modified the clinical course of rejection, and most rejection episodes now occur without any detectable clinical symptoms. On echocardiogram, indices of systolic left ventricular function usually do not deteriorate until rejection is fairly severe. Newer techniques evaluating wall thickening and left ventricular diastolic function show early promise as predictors of early rejection. However, most transplant centers do not rely on echocardiography alone in rejection surveillance.

Myocardial biopsy is the only reliable method of monitoring patients for rejection. Biopsies are taken from the right ventricular side of the interventricular septum and can be performed relatively safely, even in small infants and children. In older children, myocardial biopsies may be performed as often as every 1–4 wk during the first 3–6 mo post-transplant. The frequency is then reduced to three or four biopsies per year unless the patient has an episode of rejection. In infants, surveillance biopsies are usually performed less often, and may be as infrequent as once or twice yearly. Criteria for grading cardiac rejection is based on the degree of cellular infiltration and whether myocyte necrosis is present. Grades 1 and 2 rejection are mild enough to not warrant immediate treatment, and more than one half of these episodes may resolve spontaneously. A repeat biopsy specimen is usually obtained within 1–2 wk. For patients with grade 3 or 4 rejection, treatment is instituted with either intravenous methylprednisolone or a "bump and taper" of oral prednisone. For rejection episodes resistant to steroid therapy, additional therapeutic regimens include a repeat course of an antilymphocyte preparation (OKT3 or antithymocyte globulin), methotrexate, or total lymphoid irradiation. Rare patients with refractory rejection require retransplantation.

COMPLICATIONS OF IMMUNOSUPPRESSION. Infection. Infection is the leading cause of death in pediatric transplant patients (Fig. 401–2). The incidence of infection is greatest in the first 3 mo post-transplant, during the time when immunosuppressive doses are highest. Viral infections are the most common, especially cytomegalovirus, which accounts for as many as 25% of infectious episodes. Cytomegalovirus infection may occur as a primary infection in patients without prior exposure to the virus or as a reactivation. Severe cytomegalovirus infection can be disseminated, associated with pneumonitis, and may provoke an episode of acute graft rejection or graft coronary disease (see later). Many centers use several weeks of intravenous gancyclovir as prophylaxis in any patient receiving a heart from a donor who is positive for cytomegalovirus.

Most normal childhood viral illnesses are well tolerated and usually do not require special treatment. Otitis media and routine upper respiratory tract infections can be treated in the outpatient setting, although fever or symptoms prolonged beyond the usual course require further investigation. Varicella exposure is treated with varicella immune globulin (VZIG), and if the patient develops clinical varicella infection, treatment with intravenous acyclovir will attenuate the illness.

Bacterial infections are the next most frequent, with the lung being the most common site of infection (35%), followed by the blood, urinary tract, and, less commonly, the sternotomy site. Other sources of post-transplant infection include fungi (14%) and protozoa (6%). The incidence of serious infections is lower in those children who can be managed without steroids.

Growth Retardation. Patients requiring chronic steroid administration usually manifest decreased linear growth. Alternate-day steroid regimens will usually result in improved linear growth. In patients who develop rejection when steroids are weaned, other immunosuppressants (methotrexate, total lymphoid irradiation) have shown promise as steroid-sparing agents.

Hypertension. This is extremely common in patients treated with cyclosporine. It is due to a combination of plasma volume expansion and defective renal sodium excretion. Corticosteroids usually potentiate cyclosporine-induced hypertension.

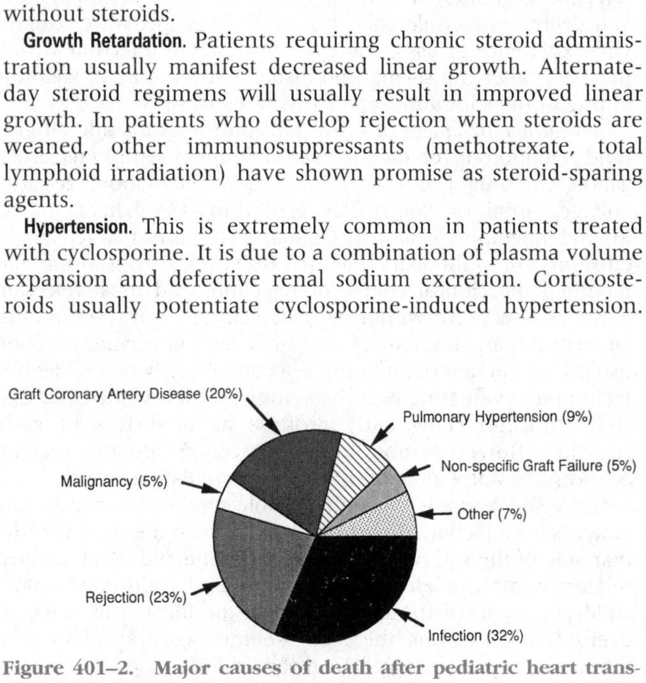

Figure 401–2. Major causes of death after pediatric heart transplantation. Data from Stanford University.

Patients are usually managed with a combination of a diuretic and a vasodilator. Agents that work via calcium channel blockade have the additional advantage of possibly attenuating graft coronary disease (see later). Some of the newer immunosuppressive agents, for example, FK506, are reported to have less renal toxicity.

Renal Function. Chronic administration of cyclosporine can lead to a tubulointerstitial nephropathy in adults, but severe renal dysfunction is rare in children. Most pediatric-age patients gradually increase their serum creatinine during the 1st post-transplant year; however, if renal dysfunction occurs, it usually responds to a decrease in cyclosporine dosage.

Neurologic Complications. Neurologic side effects of cyclosporine include tremor, myalgias, paresthesias, and rarely seizures. These complications can be treated with reduced doses of cyclosporine and occasionally with oral magnesium supplementation. Intracranial infections pose a significant risk, especially because some of the more common signs, such as nuchal rigidity, may be absent in immunosuppressed patients. The most common organisms are *Aspergillus, Cryptococcus neoformans,* and *Listeria monocytogenes.* Aseptic meningitis can be seen days or weeks following OKT3 administration and is usually self-limiting.

Tumors. One of the serious complications limiting long-term survival in pediatric heart transplant patients is the risk of neoplastic disease. The most common is post-transplant lymphoproliferative disease (LPD). LPD is associated with infection by Epstein-Barr virus. It usually responds rapidly to reduction in immunosuppression and acyclovir, and only occasionally requires chemotherapy.

Chronic Rejection. Accelerated graft coronary vascular disease is a manifestation of chronic graft rejection and occurs in 0–30% of children. It is thought to be a form of immunologically mediated vessel injury and is a diffuse process with a high degree of distal vessel involvement. Because the transplanted heart has been denervated, patients do not develop symptoms such as angina pectoris during ischemic episodes, and thus most centers perform coronary angiography annually to screen for abnormalities. Standard coronary artery bypass procedures are usually not helpful because of the diffuse nature of the process, and repeat heart transplantation has been the only effective treatment. The calcium channel blocker diltiazem may be able to either prevent or delay the onset of graft coronary disease in adult transplant patients.

Other Complications. Corticosteroids usually result in Cushingoid facies, steroid acne, and striae. Cyclosporine can cause a subtle change in facial features, hypertrichosis, and gingival hyperplasia. These cosmetic features can be particularly disturbing to adolescents and may be the motivation for noncompliance. Many of these complications are dose related and will improve as immunosuppressive medications are weaned. Osteoporosis and aseptic necrosis are additional reasons for reducing steroid dosage as soon as possible.

Rehabilitation. Despite the potential risks of immunosuppression, the prospect for rehabilitation in pediatric heart transplant recipients is excellent. Between 90% and 100% of pediatric heart transplant recipients have no functional limitations in their daily lives. As many as one quarter of pediatric transplant patients have never been hospitalized for illness after their initial transplant operation.

Pediatric heart transplant recipients can attend day care or school and participate in noncontact competitive sports and other age-appropriate activities. Standardized measurements of ventricular function are close to normal. Because the transplanted heart is denervated, the increase in heart rate and cardiac output during exercise is slower in transplant recipients, and maximal heart rate and cardiac output responses are mildly attenuated. These subtle abnormalities are rarely noticeable by the patient.

Growth of the transplanted heart is excellent, although a mild degree of ventricular and septal hypertrophy is commonly seen even years after transplantation. The sites of the atrial and great vessel anastomoses grow without developing obstruction. However, in neonates transplanted for the hypoplastic left heart syndrome, juxtaductal aortic coarctation may recur.

In children, the psychological adjustment to heart transplantation is usually good, as assessed by standardized psychological testing. There is sometimes a problem with noncompliance once patients reach adolescence, resulting in life-threatening rejection. Early intervention by social service counselors may be able to reduce this risk.

CHAPTER 402

Heart-Lung and Lung Transplantation

Over 200 heart-lung and over 100 lung transplants have been performed in children at almost 30 institutions worldwide. Indications include several forms of complex congenital heart disease associated with pulmonary hypoplasia, Eisenmenger syndrome, primary pulmonary hypertension, and end-stage parenchymal lung disease (bronchopulmonary dysplasia, interstitial fibrosis, and cystic fibrosis). Patients with pulmonary hypertension and some forms of parenchymal lung disease may also be candidates for single or double lung transplantation if right ventricular function is preserved. In some patients with Eisenmenger physiology, lung transplantation can be performed in combination with repair of intracardiac defects. However, patients with cystic fibrosis are not candidates for single lung grafts because of the risk of infection from the diseased contralateral lung. Patients are selected with many of the same criteria as for heart transplant recipients (see Chapter 401).

Post-transplant immunosuppression is achieved with a triple-drug regimen, similar to that for heart transplantation; however, many groups avoid steroids during the early postoperative period to promote better airway healing. Unlike patients with isolated heart transplants, few patients with lung transplants can be weaned off of steroids. Prophylaxis against infection is achieved with trimethoprim/sulfamethoxazole or aerosolized pentamidine. Gancyclovir prophylaxis is used for recipients of a cytomegalovirus (CMV)-positive donor.

Pulmonary rejection is very common in heart-lung transplant recipients, whereas heart rejection is encountered less often than in those patients with isolated heart transplants. Symptoms of lung rejection may include fever and fatigue, although many episodes are minimally symptomatic. Surveillance for rejection is performed by following pulmonary functions (FVC, FEV_1, $FEV_{25\%-75\%}$), systemic arterial oxygen tension, chest roentgenograms, and by serial transbronchial biopsy. Routine biopsies are performed frequently in the first 3 mo, and then quarterly afterwards. Because of technical limitations, biopsies are not performed in infants, who are followed with clinical criteria alone.

Initial results in children demonstrate 55% 1-yr and 40% 5-yr survival rates; however, improved patient selection and postoperative management are continually improving these survival statistics. As in isolated heart transplantation, infection remains the leading cause of early death, accounting for nearly half of all mortality in the 1st yr post-transplant. Other causes of early morbidity and mortality include tracheal complications, pulmonary venous obstruction, donor lung dysfunction (DLD), bleeding, and acute rejection. *Obliterative bronchiolitis* (OB), thought to be a form of chronic rejection, remains a major limitation to long-term survival in a significant number of patients. Between 10% and 50% of long-term survivors of lung transplantation develop OB. Increasing immunosuppression has markedly reduced the incidence of OB in many centers. Additional late complications include the development of airway stenosis, accelerated graft coronary artery disease (although less common than in isolated heart transplantation), and other side effects of chronic immunosuppression (Chapter 401).

Postoperative indices of cardiopulmonary function and exercise capacity show significant improvement. Problems of donor availability are even more severe with lung transplantation. Living-related lung transplantation, in which a lobe from a parent is transplanted into a child, may partially alleviate this problem.

HEART TRANSPLANTATION

Addonizio LJ, Gersony WM, Robbins RC, et al: Elevated pulmonary vascular resistance and cardiac transplantation. Circulation 76(Suppl V):52, 1987.

Bailey LL, Assaad AN, Trimm RF, et al: Orthotopic transplantation during early infancy as therapy for incurable congenital heart disease. Ann Surg 208:279, 1988.

Baum D, Bernstein D, Starnes VA, et al: Pediatric heart transplantation at Stanford: Results of a 15 year experience. Pediatrics 88:203, 1991.

Bernstein D, Starnes VA, Baum D: Pediatric Heart Transplantation. *In*: Barness L (ed): Advances in Pediatrics, Vol 37. Chicago, Year Book, 1990, pp 413–433.

Bernstein D, Baum D, Berry G, et al: Neoplastic disorders after pediatric heart transplantation. Circulation, in press.

Billingham M, Cary N, Hammond M, et al: A working formulation for the standardization of nomenclature in the diagnosis of heart and lung rejection: Heart rejection study group. J Heart Transplant 9:587, 1990.

Fricker FJ, Griffith BP, Hardesty RL, et al: Experience with heart transplantation in children. Pediatrics 79:138, 1987.

Gao SZ, Schroeder JS, Alderman EL, et al: Clinical and laboratory correlates of accelerated coronary artery disease in the cardiac transplant patient. Circulation 76(Suppl 5):56, 1987.

Grattan MT, Moreno-Cabral CE, Starnes VA, et al: Cytomegalovirus infection is associated with cardiac allograft rejection and atherosclerosis. JAMA 261:3561, 1989.

Green M, Wald ER, Fricker FJ, et al: Infections in pediatric orthotopic heart transplant recipients. Pediatr Infect Dis 8:87, 1989.

Hotson JR, Enzmann DR: Neurologic complications of cardiac transplantation. Neurol Clin 6:346, 1988.

Lawrence KS, Fricker FJ: Pediatric heart transplantation: Quality of life. J Heart Transplant 6:329, 1987.

Schroeder JS, Gao SZ, Alderman EL: A preliminary study of diltiazem in the prevention of coronary artery disease in heart transplant recipients. N Engl J Med 3:164, 1993.

Starnes VA, Griffin ML, Pitlick PT, et al: Current approach to hypoplastic left heart syndrome: Palliation, transplantation or both? J Thorac Cardiovasc Surg 104:189, 1992.

Uzark K, Crowley D, Behrendt D, et al: Effects of pediatric heart transplantation on the family. Circulation 76(Suppl IV):145, 1987.

Woo K, Emery J, Peabody J: Cortical hyperostosis: A complication of prolonged prostaglandin infusion in infants awaiting cardiac transplantation. Pediatrics 93:417, 1994.

Wood AJ, Maurer G, Niederberger W, et al: Cyclosporine: Pharamacokinetics, metabolism, and drug interactions. Transplant Proc 15(Suppl 1):2409, 1983.

LUNG TRANSPLANTATION

Health Technology Assessment: Institutional and Patient Criteria for Heart-Lung Transplantation. Washington, DC, U.S. Dept. of Health and Human Services, No. 1, May 1994.

Lawrence EC: Diagnosis and management of lung allograft rejection. Clin Chest Med 11:269, 1990.

Reitz BA, Wallwork JL, Hunt SA, et al: Heart-lung transplantation: Successful therapy for patients with pulmonary vascular disease. N Engl J Med 306:557, 1982.

Starnes VA, Lewiston NJ, Luikart H, et al: Current trends in lung transplantation: Lobar transplantation and expanded use of single lungs. J Thorac Cardiovasc Surg 104:1060, 1992.

Starnes VA, Oyer PE, Bernstein D, et al: Heart, heart-lung, and lung transplantation in the first year of life. Ann Thorac Surg 53:306, 1992.

Spray TL, Mallory GB, Canter CE, et al: Pediatric lung transplantation for pulmonary hypertension and congenital heart disease. Ann Thorac Surg 54:216, 1992.

Theodore J, Starnes VA, Lewiston NJ: Obliterative bronchiolitis. Clin Chest Med 11:309, 1990.

SECTION 8
Diseases of the Peripheral Vascular System

CHAPTER 403
Diseases of the Blood Vessels (Aneurysms and Fistulas)

KAWASAKI DISEASE (see Chapters 152.2 and 392)

Aneurysms of the coronary arteries may complicate Kawasaki disease and are the leading cause of morbidity in this disease.

Other than in Kawasaki disease, aneurysms are not common in children and occur most frequently in the aorta in association with coarctation of the aorta, patent ductus arteriosus, and Marfan syndrome, and in intracranial vessels (see Chapter 553). They may also occur secondary to an infected embolus; infection contiguous to a blood vessel; trauma; congenital abnormalities of vessel structure, especially of the medial wall; and arteritis, for example, polyarteritis nodosa and Takayasu arteritis (see Chapter 152).

ARTERIOVENOUS FISTULAS

These may be limited to small cavernous hemangiomas or may be extensive (see Chapters 461.2 and 600). The most common sites in infants and children are intracranial, hepatic, pulmonary, in the extremities, and in vessels in or near the thoracic wall. These fistulas, though usually congenital, may follow trauma or be a manifestation of hereditary hemorrhagic telangiectasia (Osler-Weber-Rendu syndrome). Femoral arteriovenous fistulas are a rare complication of percutaneous cardiac catheterization.

CLINICAL MANIFESTATIONS. These occur only in association with large arteriovenous communications when arterial blood flows into a low-pressure venous system, increasing local venous pressure and decreasing arterial flow beyond the fistula. Systemic arterial resistance falls because of the runoff of blood through the fistula. Compensatory mechanisms include tachycardia and increased stroke volume so that cardiac output rises. The total blood volume is also increased. In large fistulas, left ventricular dilatation, a widened pulse pressure, and congestive heart failure occur. Injection of contrast material into an artery proximal to the fistula confirms the diagnosis.

Large *intracranial arteriovenous fistulas* most often occur in the newborn infant in association with a vein of Galen malformation. The large intracranial left-to-right shunt results in congestive heart failure secondary to the demand for extremely high cardiac output. Patients with smaller communications may not have cardiovascular manifestations but later develop hydrocephalus (see Chapter 542.11) or seizure disorders. The newborn infant with a large symptomatic intracranial arteriovenous fistula has a grave prognosis; some will survive with medical management but are subject to later complications caused by the intracranial mass. The diagnosis can be made by auscultation of a continuous murmur over the cranium. Older children with more diffuse intracranial arteriovenous malformations may be recognized on the basis of intracranial calcification and a high cardiac output, without frank cardiac failure.

Hepatic arteriovenous fistulas may be localized or generalized in the liver. The fistula may be located between the hepatic artery and ductus venosus or portal vein. Congenital hemorrhagic telangiectasia may also be associated. Large arteriovenous fistulas are associated with an increased cardiac output and heart failure. Hepatomegaly is usual, and systolic or continuous murmurs may be audible over the liver.

Peripheral arteriovenous fistulas usually involve the extremities and are associated with disfigurement, swelling of the extremity, and visible hemangiomas. Some are located in areas that result in upper airway obstruction. Because only a small minority result in large arterial runoff, cardiac failure is not common.

TREATMENT. *Medical management* of congestive heart failure is initially helpful in the neonate with these conditions; with time the size of the shunt may diminish and symptoms spontaneously regress. Hemangiomas of the liver often completely disappear with time. This abnormality is occasionally treated with steroids, epsilon-aminocaproic acid, interferon, local compression, embolization, or local radiation; the beneficial effects of this management are not firmly established, as individual patients display marked variations in clinical course without treatment. *Catheter embolization* is rapidly becoming the treatment of choice for many patients with a symptomatic arteriovenous fistula. Often, multiple procedures are necessary before the flow is significantly reduced. *Surgical removal* of a large fistula may be attempted in the presence of severe cardiac failure and lack of improvement with medical treatment. However, surgical treatment may be contraindicated or unsuccessful when the lesion is extensive and diffuse, or is located in a position where adjoining tissue may be injured during the surgery or related procedures.

CHAPTER 404
Systemic Hypertension

Albert W. Pruitt

Systemic hypertension, a sign of underlying pathophysiology, is recognized more commonly in adults (the prevalence is 10–15% in the adult population) than in children and adolescents. Untreated essential or primary hypertension increases the risk of myocardial infarction, stroke, and renal failure in affected individuals. To increase early detection of hypertension, blood pressure measurement should be a part of the periodic physical examination in children, and careful inquiry of family history of hypertension should be undertaken.

Blood pressure is the product of peripheral vascular resistance and cardiac output. Accurate measurement of blood pressure requires attention to the comfort of the patient and is dependent on the quality of the equipment and the skill of the observer (see Chapter 380). Many patients of all ages have some level of anxiety associated with initial measurements of blood pressure. Depending upon age and desire, the patient may be seated or supine, but subsequent measurements taken for comparison should be obtained with the patient in the same position. Especially in young children, careful attention to cuff size is necessary. The bladder of the pressure cuff should nearly encircle the upper arm, but its ends should not overlap; the cuff should cover at least two thirds of the length of the upper arm. Although systolic pressure is indicated by the appearance of the 1st Korotkoff sound, the true diastolic pressure probably lies between the muffling and the disappearance of sound as the cuff pressure is decreased. Doppler and oscillometric techniques may be used satisfactorily in infants and young children. Because blood pressure often decreases as the patient becomes comfortable with the procedure, repeated measurements are necessary for accuracy.

Because systemic blood pressure gradually increases with age and correlates with weight and height throughout childhood and adolescence, reference standards (see Figs. 380–1 to 380–6) are necessary for interpretation of values obtained during physical examinations. Pressure that is consistently above the 95th percentile for age is abnormal and requires further evaluation. Blood pressure should be obtained in all four extremities to evaluate the presence of coarctation of the aorta (Chapter 386.17). Unless there is need for urgency because of marked elevation of pressure or evidence of a systemic complication, sequential measurements of blood pressure should be obtained over a period of weeks before concluding that the patient has systemic hypertension. Ambulatory blood pressure monitoring may be especially useful in adolescents who in the office setting have borderline hypertension.

ETIOLOGY AND PATHOPHYSIOLOGY. An increase in cardiac output or peripheral resistance results in an increase in blood pressure, although if one of these factors increases while the other decreases, blood pressure may not increase. When the cause of the increase in pressure can be explained by an associated disease, the hypertension is referred to as *secondary*; the term *primary* or *essential hypertension* implies that no known underlying disease is present. However, it is recognized that many factors, such as heredity, salt intake, stress, and obesity, may play a role in the development of essential hypertension.

Essential hypertension is more commonly recognized in adolescents than younger children and appears to have a strong family component. It probably not a single entity, so it is likely that several pathogenic mechanisms are involved. In experimental settings, normotensive children of hypertensive parents may show abnormal physiologic responses that are similar to those of their parents. When subjected to stress or competitive tasks, the offspring of hypertensive adults, as a group, respond with greater increases in heart rate and blood pressure than do children of normotensive parents. Similarly, some children of hypertensive parents may excrete higher levels of urinary catecholamine metabolites or may respond to sodium loading with greater weight gain and increases in blood pressure than those without a family history of hypertension. The abnormal responses in children with affected parents tend to be greater in the black population than in white subjects. As other possible markers for the development of subsequent hypertension, erythrocyte sodium transport, free calcium concentration in platelets and leukocytes, urine kallikrein excretion, and sympathetic nervous system receptors have been investigated.

Categorization of essential hypertension according to the level of plasma renin activity (high, normal, low) has been useful in understanding the pathophysiology and in developing treatment regimens in adults; similar large studies have not been conducted in adolescents with primary hypertension. A large number of adult patients with essential hypertension appear to be especially sensitive to salt intake. The mechanism of salt sensitivity is not clear and may involve the chloride ion rather than sodium. A subgroup of salt-sensitive individuals appear to have impaired ability for urinary excretion of a sodium load. Atrial natriuretic peptides stimulate sodium excretion by the kidneys; their role in the maintenance of normal blood pressure and the development of hypertension is being investigated.

Tracking of blood pressure is likely to occur as children develop, so that over time individuals maintain their relative ranking of blood pressure with respect to their peers. Therefore, children and young adolescents with pressure above the 90th percentile for age often become adults with elevated pressure. Adolescents with essential hypertension may progress from a high cardiac output and normal systemic vascular resistance state to the adult pattern of normal cardiac output with elevated systemic vascular resistance. There are racial differences, however, and black adults with hypertension have greater elevations in peripheral resistance, whereas hypertensive white adults show predominantly an increase in cardiac output.

Secondary hypertension is more common than essential hypertension in infants and children. Both transient and chronic hypertension may accompany diseases, as listed in Tables 404–1 and 404–2. The etiology of hypertension varies with age. For example, elevated pressure in the newborn is most often associated with high umbilical artery catheterization and renal artery obstruction due to thrombus formation. Hypertension during early childhood is also usually secondary, but in later childhood and in adolescents it is more often primary. The level of blood pressure is also helpful in distinguishing secondary from primary hypertension; in general, adolescents

■ TABLE 404–1 Conditions Associated with Transient or Intermittent Hypertension in Children

Renal
- Acute postinfectious glomerulonephritis
- Anaphylactoid (Henoch-Schönlein) purpura with nephritis
- Hemolytic-uremic syndrome
- Acute tubular necrosis
- After renal transplant (immediate and during episodes of rejection)
- After blood transfusion in patients with azotemia
- Hypervolemia
- After surgical procedures on genitourinary tract
- Pyelonephritis
- Renal trauma
- Leukemic infiltration of kidney
- Obstructive uropathy associated with Crohn disease

Drugs and Poisons
- Cocaine
- Oral contraceptives
- Sympathomimetic agents
- Amphetamines
- Phencyclidine
- Corticosteroids and ACTH
- Cyclosporine treatment post-transplantation
- Licorice (glycyrrhizic acid)
- Lead, mercury, cadmium, thallium
- Antihypertensive withdrawal (clonidine, methyldopa, propranolol)
- Vitamin D intoxication

Central and Autonomic Nervous System
- Increased intracranial pressure
- Guillain-Barré syndrome
- Burns
- Familial dysautonomia
- Stevens-Johnson syndrome
- Posterior fossa lesions
- Porphyria
- Poliomyelitis
- Encephalitis

Miscellaneous
- Pre-eclampsia
- Fractures of long bones
- Hypercalcemia
- Postcoarctation repair
- White cell transfusion
- Extracorporeal membrane oxygenation (ECMO)
- Chronic upper airway obstruction

■ TABLE 404–2 Conditions Associated with Chronic Hypertension in Children

Renal
Chronic pyelonephritis
Chronic glomerulonephritis
Hydronephrosis
Congenital dysplastic kidney
Multicystic kidney
Solitary renal cyst
Vesicoureteral reflux nephropathy
Segmental hypoplasia (Ask-Upmark kidney)
Ureteral obstruction
Renal tumors
Renal trauma
Rejection damage following transplantation
Postirradiation damage
Systemic lupus erythematosus (other connective tissue diseases)
Vascular
Coarctation of thoracic or abdominal aorta
Renal artery lesions (stenosis, fibromuscular dysplasia, thrombosis, aneurysm)
Umbilical artery catheterization with thrombus formation
Neurofibromatosis (intrinsic or extrinsic narrowing of vascular lumen)
Renal vein thrombosis
Vasculitis
Arteriovenous shunt
Williams Beuren syndrome
Endocrine
Hyperthyroidism
Hyperparathyroidism
Congenital adrenal hyperplasia (11β-hydroxylase and 17-hydroxylase defect)
Cushing syndrome
Primary aldosteronism
Dexamethasone-suppressible hyperaldosteronism
Pheochromocytoma
Other neural crest tumors (neuroblastoma, ganglioneuroblastoma, ganglioneuroma)
Diabetic nephropathy
Liddle's syndrome
Central Nervous System
Intracranial mass
Hemorrhage
Residual following brain injury
Quadriplegia
Essential Hypertension
Low renin
Normal renin
High renin

with essential hypertension have diastolic pressures at or slightly above the 95th percentile for age.

Approximately 75–80% of children with secondary hypertension have a *renal abnormality.* Urinary tract infection is present in 25–50% of these patients and is often related to an obstructive lesion of the urinary tract. This hypertension may be associated with sodium retention, renin secretion, or a decrease in bradykinin production. A proportion of children with chronic pyelonephritis do not develop hypertension until they become azotemic. Other children, however, demonstrate elevated blood pressure during an episode of acute pyelonephritis; the infection may simply unmask essential hypertension.

Other renal parenchymal lesions associated with hypertension include acute and chronic glomerulonephritis, congenital renal lesions, tumors, and trauma. The reduced glomerular filtration rate of nephritis results in salt and water accumulation, whereas mass lesions (cysts, solid tumors, hematoma) may impair perfusion of portions of the kidney and stimulate renin production by the juxtaglomerular apparatus. There is also evidence that both Wilms tumor and juxtaglomerular cell tumor (hemangiopericytoma) secrete renin or a pressor substance without feedback control.

Renovascular lesions such as coarction of the aorta and renal artery stenosis, result in hypertension through stimulation of the *renin-angiotensin-aldosterone system.* Renin is a proteolytic enzyme secreted by juxtaglomerular cells that converts the α_2-globulin, angiotensinogen, to angiotensin I. Renin secretion is affected to some extent by afferent arteriolar perfusion pressure in the kidney, sodium concentration in plasma and tubular urine, sympathetic nervous system activation, and other factors, such as prostaglandins, potassium intake, and atrial natriuretic peptides. Angiotensin I possesses little physiologic activity and is rapidly converted to angiotensin II by angiotensin-converting enzyme (ACE). This converting enzyme is also responsible for the metabolic degradation of vasodilating kinins. Angiotensin II is a potent vasoconstrictor and also stimulates aldosterone secretion; both effects lead to increased blood pressure.

Endocrinopathies linked with hypertension involve the thyroid, parathyroid, and adrenal glands. Systolic hypertension and tachycardia are common in hyperthyroidism, but diastolic pressure is usually not elevated. Hypercalcemia, whether secondary to hyperparathyroidism or other causes, often results in mild elevation in pressure because of an increase in vascular tone. Adrenocortical disorders (aldosterone secreting tumors, adrenal hyperplasia, Cushing syndrome) may produce hypertension if there is an increased mineralocorticoid effect due to an increased amount of active precursors, aldosterone, or cortisol.

Catecholamine-secreting tumors give rise to hypertension because of the cardiac and vascular effects of epinephrine and norepinephrine. Children with pheochromocytoma usually have sustained rather than intermittent hypertension (see Chapter 533). The tumor may be unilateral or bilateral and may arise in the adrenal medulla or in other chromaffin cells. Approximately 5% of patients with neurofibromatosis will develop pheochromocytoma. Hypertension is much less frequent with other neural crest tumors but may result from catecholamine secretion or interference with renal perfusion.

Excess catecholamines appear to play a role in intermittently elevating blood pressure in patients with Guillain-Barré syndrome, poliomyelitis, burns, and Stevens-Johnson syndrome. Autonomic instability is suggested by episodic increases in urinary excretion of catecholamine metabolites. Sympathetic outflow from the central nervous system is also affected by intracranial lesions.

A number of *drugs of abuse, therapeutic agents,* and *toxins* may increase blood pressure. Inhalation or mucosal application of cocaine may provoke rapid increase in blood pressure and result in seizures or intracranial hemorrhage. Transient hypertension often accompanies phencyclidine use and may become persistent in chronic abusers of amphetamines. Tobacco use may also increase blood pressure. Sympathomimetic agents used as nasal decongestants, appetite suppressants, and stimulants for attention deficit disorder produce peripheral vasoconstriction and varying degrees of cardiac stimulation. Individuals vary in their susceptibility to these effects. Oral contraceptives are a common cause of hypertension in adolescent females. Although as many as 15% of patients who take oral contraceptives may develop hypertension, the incidence may be reduced through the use of low-estrogen preparations. Estrogen likely contributes to the pathogenesis through stimulation of hepatic synthesis of angiotensinogen and subsequent activation of the renin-angiotensin-aldosterone system. In addition, there may be a direct effect by estrogen on salt and water retention. The nephrotoxicity of cyclosporine used as an immunosuppressant is the likely explanation for the hypertension observed in patients after cardiac, bone marrow, and, in some cases, renal and liver transplantation. The coadministration of steroids appears to increase the incidence of hypertension in such patients. Licorice, not licorice flavoring, contains glycyrrhizic acid, which acts on the distal tubule in a manner similar to that of aldosterone. Blood pressure may be elevated in patients with poisoning by a heavy metal; there is also interest in the effect of subtoxic levels of lead on vascular tone.

CLINICAL MANIFESTATIONS. Preadolescents and adolescents with primary hypertension rarely have clinical evidence of disease until the blood pressure elevation is detected, usually at the time of a routine examination or during physical evaluation prior to athletic participation. In addition to having a mild elevation in pressure, many affected individuals are somewhat overweight. Blood pressure is often at the highest level in such patients while they are supine.

The pressure in children with secondary hypertension may be only a few millimeters above the 95th percentile for age or may be markedly elevated. Unless the pressure has been sustained or is rising rapidly, hypertension will usually not produce symptoms. Therefore clinical manifestations of the underlying disease, such as growth failure in children with chronic renal disease, most frequently draw attention to the blood pressure. With substantial elevation, however, headache, dizziness, changes in vision, and seizures may occur. Hypertensive encephalopathy is suggested by the presence of vomiting, temperature elevation, ataxia, stupor, and seizures. Regardless of the cause of the hypertension, cardiac and renal function deteriorate in the face of marked increases in blood pressure.

Young children and infants with unexplained heart failure or seizures should have their blood pressure measured. Such patients often cannot communicate symptoms such as headache, and their behavior may not be considered abnormal until the complications of hypertension are present. Often, in retrospect, after blood pressure has been lowered, parents of hypertensive infants will comment that their child had been increasingly irritable before the hypertension was recognized.

Specific manifestations of the diseases associated with hypertension (see Tables 404–1 and 404–2) are discussed in their respective sections. Routinely measuring and recording blood pressure in infants, children, and adolescents will result in identification of affected patients before symptoms of hypertension develop.

DIAGNOSIS. Essential hypertension is suggested by the patient's age, level of blood pressure, weight, family history, and the paucity of signs and symptoms of underlying disease. It is uncommon to make this diagnosis in children younger than 10 yr of age. Before a patient is diagnosed as hypertensive, several recordings of blood pressure should be obtained. If the pressure is only mildly elevated on the first visit, measurement on two or three occasions over the ensuing weeks may reveal that the initial elevation was related to apprehension; such patients, however, need annual evaluation, as they may subsequently develop sustained hypertension. Excess body weight is associated with essential hypertension; except with disorders of the adrenal cortex, patients with secondary hypertension are rarely obese. Heredity is also a strong determinant of blood pressure; therefore, an adolescent with mild elevation of pressure and a definite family history of essential hypertension rarely needs evaluation for underlying disease. Adolescents suspected of having essential hypertension require regular measurement of blood pressure to determine the course of the evaluation over time. If the pressure continues to rise over several weeks or months of observation, additional diagnostic studies are indicated.

If age, level of blood pressure, or symptomatology suggests that secondary hypertension is likely, the initial focus should be the urinary tract. Measures of growth are important, as is a history of intermittent febrile illnesses, which might suggest recurring infection of the urinary tract. Physical examination should determine the presence of flank masses or abdominal bruits. Lower extremity blood pressure should be compared with that in the arm to rule out coarctation of the aorta. Screening tests should include complete blood count, urinalysis, serum electrolytes, blood urea nitrogen, serum creatinine, and uric acid. Urine culture should be obtained even if the sediment is unremarkable. Chest roentgenography, echocardiography, and electrocardiography are helpful in assessing cardiac response to the elevated pressure.

Renal imaging is discussed in Chapters 491–494. Whereas a renal ultrasound will provide a comparison of kidney size and a view of the anatomy of the collecting system, an intravenous pyelogram is not adequate for detecting differences in renal perfusion. A radionuclide scan is helpful in distinguishing variation in perfusion of the two kidneys. Renal angiography can demonstrate lesions in the main arteries or in the segmental branches; at angiography, venous blood samples should be collected from both renal veins and the inferior vena cava for assay of plasma renin activity. Doppler ultrasound may demonstrate arterial and venous blood flow.

Peripheral plasma renin activity is a useful screening test for both renovascular and renal parenchymal disease. Normal values gradually decrease with age and vary between laboratories. A suppressed value suggests excess mineralocorticoid effect, and an elevated value is associated with renal or renovascular involvement. One approach to the adolescent with hypertension is noted in Figure 404–1. A pregnancy test may be useful in the sexually active female who is noted to be hypertensive.

COURSE AND PROGNOSIS. The natural history of essential hypertension that is first detected during adolescence is under investigation; many such patients will probably continue to have essential hypertension as adults. Collaborative studies in adults with essential hypertension have shown the value of drug therapy in reducing the incidence of congestive heart failure, renal failure, and stroke. A similar reduction in incidence of myocardial infarction has not been proved. That lack of effect is most likely due to antecedent coronary artery disease that is well established before blood pressure is controlled. Drug-induced alteration of serum lipids may exacerbate this problem. Detection and intervention at an earlier age with drugs that do not increase serum lipids should improve outcome.

Prognosis for secondary hypertension is primarily determined by the nature of the underlying disease and its responsiveness to specific therapy. For example, survival in patients with underlying chronic renal diseases is often determined by the patients' response to dialysis and transplant programs. In patients with hyper-reninemic hypertension (e.g., renovascular disease), evaluation of renal vein renin activity may help predict prognosis. A discrepancy in renin secretion between the two kidneys of more than 1.5:1 suggests that the kidney producing the higher level is primarily responsible for the hypertension. Surgical correction of the lesion on the involved side yields a high probability of marked improvement or resolution of the hypertension. The prognosis after surgical repair of coarctation is variable. Although the majority of patients will establish normal systemic blood pressure following surgery, some will have persistently elevated pressure. The long-term outcome is favorable for neonates who develop hypertension as a complication of umbilical artery catheterization. Few of these infants require therapy beyond 12 mo of age, and most show marked improvement in renal perfusion.

PREVENTION. The prevention of high blood pressure may be viewed as a part of the prevention of cardiovascular disease. Several risk factors for cardiovascular disorders have been identified and include obesity, elevated serum cholesterol, high dietary sodium intake, sedentary life style, alcohol abuse, and tobacco use. Beginning in childhood and continuing through adolescence, it is especially important to discourage cigarette smoking because of the pulmonary and cardiovascular consequences. The increase in arterial wall rigidity and increase in blood viscosity that are associated with cigarette smoking may contribute to the adverse effect of tobacco use on blood pressure. Population approaches to prevention of essential hypertension include reduction in sodium intake and increase in physical activity through school-based programs.

TREATMENT. Both nonpharmacologic and pharmacologic approaches to treatment are useful in managing a patient with

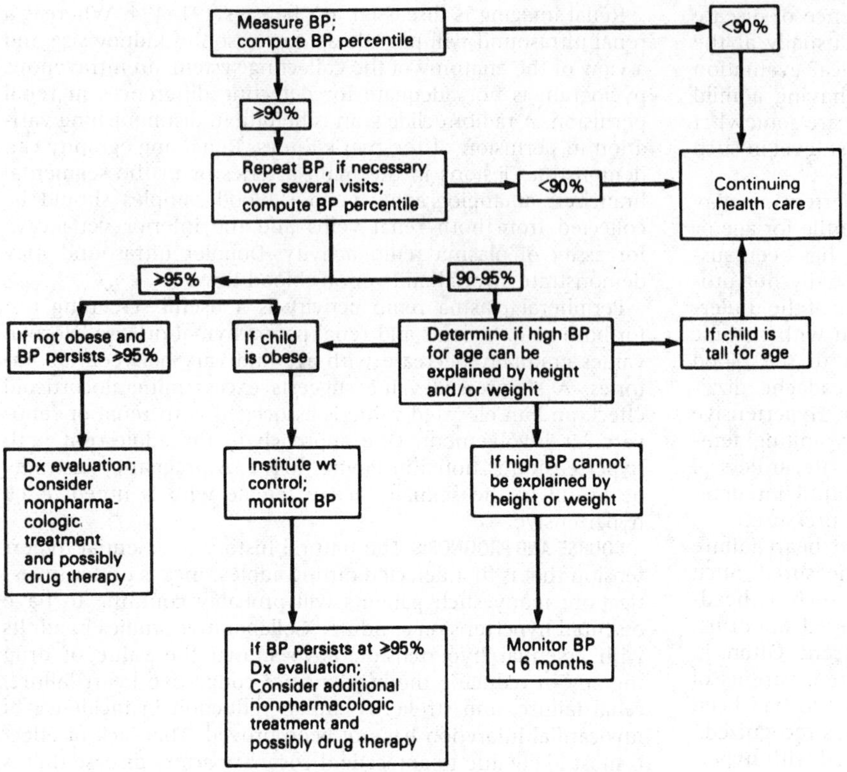

Figure 404–1. Algorithm for identifying children with high BP. Note that whenever BP measurement is stipulated, the average of at least two measurements should be used. (From National Heart, Lung, and Blood Institute, Bethesda, MD: Report of the second task force on blood pressure control in children—1987. Reproduced by permission of Pediatrics. Vol 79, p 1. Copyright © 1987.)

elevated blood pressure. Adolescents with essential hypertension are usually best managed initially with *nonpharmacologic* therapy. Intervention will focus on the factors that were cited as important in prevention. Because many patients with mild elevation of pressure are overweight, weight reduction may result in up to 5–10 mm Hg reduction in systolic pressure and 5 mm Hg reduction in diastolic pressure. A reduction in sodium intake will often lower elevated pressure by about 5 mm Hg. A consistent program of aerobic exercise also has been noted to reduce blood pressure in groups of patients with mild essential hypertension. In view of these benefits and the undesirable effects of many antihypertensive drugs, a well-supervised program of nonpharmacologic therapy should be enthusiastically prescribed for most young patients with essential hypertension. Adolescent patients also should be counseled about the adverse effects of tobacco and alcohol on blood pressure. When the patient will not cooperate with the non-drug approach or the reduction of pressure is not adequate, antihypertensive agents should be prescribed. If, however, the adolescent complies poorly with changes in diet and activity, it is likely that long-term compliance with a drug regimen will be unsatisfactory.

For children with secondary hypertension and for selected patients with essential hypertension, *pharmacologic* therapy will be required. A number of antihypertensive drugs are available for hypertensive emergencies and for chronic therapy (Table 404–3). In lowering blood pressure of a patient during a hypertensive crisis, it is important to select an agent with a rapid and predictable onset of action and to carefully monitor the blood pressure as it is reduced. Because hypertensive encephalopathy is a possible complication of hypertensive emergencies, antihypertensive agents with minimal central nervous system side effects should be chosen so as to avoid confusion between symptoms of disease and adverse effects of drug. Intravenous administration of the antihypertensive is often preferred in order to permit titration of the fall in blood pressure as the drug is administered. Because too rapid reduction in blood pressure may interfere with adequate organ perfusion, a stepwise reduction of pressure should be planned. In general the pressure should be reduced by about one third of the total planned reduction during the 1st 6 hr and the remaining amount over the following 48–72 hr.

In most hypertensive emergencies, the drugs of choice are intravenous labetalol or nitroprusside, or sublingual nifedipine. Labetalol blocks both the α_1-receptor and the β-receptors; with a single dose followed by continuous infusion, controlled reduction in blood pressure can be achieved. Similar control is possible with an infusion of nitroprusside. Nifedipine has rapid onset of action, but its short duration of action must be anticipated. Because nifedipine is available only as a liquid within a capsule, administration to children has presented some difficulty. Although the drug has often been placed in the sublingual space in order to achieve rapid absorption, gastrointestinal absorption is also sufficiently rapid to be effective in a hypertensive crisis. Intravenous hydralazine and diazoxide, when given at intervals, are alternative agents for the management of acute hypertensive episodes, but such an approach may not provide the desired gradual reduction in blood pressure. Most patients with hypertensive crisis have chronic or acute renal disease; management of blood pressure also requires careful attention to fluid balance and requires diuresis. Intravenous furosemide is usually effective, even though glomerular filtration may be impaired.

In selecting a drug regimen for long-term use, an understanding of the underlying pathophysiology is helpful. Drugs with different sites and mechanisms of action are available to specifically alter that pathology. For example, excessive activity of the renin-angiotensin-aldosterone system may be affected by a β-blocking drug (e.g., propranolol) for suppression of renin secretion, an angiotensin-converting enzyme (ACE) inhibitor (e.g., captopril), or, rarely, an aldosterone antagonist (e.g., spironolactone). ACE inhibitors are useful, not only in patients with high renin hypertension that is secondary to renovascular or renal parenchymal disease, but also in patients with high renin essential hypertension. Excess angiotensin production is the likely cause of most hypertension in the

■ TABLE 404–3 Antihypertensive Drugs*

Drug	Mechanism of Action	Dosage Range	Route	Duration	Side Effects
Vasodilators					
Hydralazine	Relax arteriolar smooth muscle	0.4–0.8 mg/kg/dose	IV	2–4 hr	Tachycardia, nausea
		0.5–2 mg/kg and increase to max 200 mg/24 hr	PO	6–8 hr	Drug-induced lupus
Diazoxide	Relax smooth muscle	2–5 mg/kg/dose, max 100 mg	IV	6–24 hr	Tachycardia, hypotension, hyperglycemia
Nitroprusside	Dilatation of arterioles and venules	0.5–8.0 μg/kg/min	IV	With infusion	Thiocyanate production, rarely hypothyroidism
Minoxidil	Arteriolar dilatation	0.2–1.0 mg/kg/24 hr, max 50 mg/24 hr	PO	12–24 hr	Hypertrichosis, fluid retention
Adrenergic Blockade					
Phentolamine	α-Receptor blockade	0.1 mg/kg/dose, max 5 mg	IV	1 hr	Reflex tachycardia
Phenoxybenzamine	α-Receptor blockade	2–5 mg/24 hr	PO	6–12 hr	Tachycardia may progress to arrhythmia
Prazosin	α-Receptor blockade	1-mg initial dose, may increase to 15 mg/24 hr	PO	8–12 hr	First-dose orthostatic hypotension
Propranolol	β-Receptor blockade	0.025–0.1 mg/kg/dose	IV	6–8 hr	Bronchospasm, bradycardia, vivid dreams
	Reduces renin release	0.25–1.0 mg/kg/dose	PO		
Labetalol	α-β Blockade	Titrate 0.2–2 mg/kg/hr (based on adult dose)	IV	With infusion	Orthostasis, dizziness, bronchospasm
		100–400 mg (adult)	PO	12 hr	
Sympatholytic Agents					
α-Methyldopa	Decrease sympathetic tone	10 mg/kg/24 hr and increase	PO	6–8 hr	Sedation, hepatic dysfunction, positive Coombs reaction
Clonidine	2-α Agonist in CNS	3–5 μg/kg/dose	PO	6–8 hr	Sedation, constipation, rebound withdrawal, hypertension
Renin-angiotension					
Captopril	Converting enzyme inhibition of angiotensin II synthesis	0.1–0.3 mg/kg/dose and increase to max 2 mg/kg/dose	PO	8 hr	Proteinuria, neutropenia, rash, dysgeusia
Enalaprilat	Same as captopril	0.005–0.010 mg/kg/dose	IV	8–12 hr	Transient hypotension
Enalapril	Same as captopril	Not determined	PO	12–24 hr	Hypotension
Calcium Channel					
Nifedipine	Calcium channel blocker	0.2–0.5 mg/kg, max 10–20 mg	PO Sub†	Repeat q 30–60 min	Facial flushing, tachycardia
Verapamil	Calcium channel blocker	120–240 mg (adults)	PO	12–24 hr	Limited pediatric experience
Diuretic Agents					
Hydrochlorothiazide	Diuresis	1–2 mg/kg/24 hr	PO	12–24 hr	Hypokalemia, hyperuricemia, hypercalcemia
Furosemide	Diuresis	1 mg/kg/dose	IV	4–6 hr	Hypokalemia, alkalosis
		2 mg/kg/dose	PO	4–6 hr	

**Adapted from Med Lett Drugs Ther 1:25, 1989; 31:31, 1989.*
†Sublingual.

neonate that follows partial occlusion of a renal vessel by thrombus. Captopril is an effective agent in most of these patients, but it must be used with careful attention to renal function. α-Blocking agents (phentolamine, phenoxybenzamine) are beneficial in patients with neural crest tumors and high circulating levels of catecholamines. In such patients, β-blocking drugs are also needed to control cardiac rate, or an agent with dual blocking action (labetalol) may be used. Sympathetic blockade with labetalol is also efficacious in patients who experience marked stimulation of the cardiovascular system from high doses of cocaine.

Young patients with essential hypertension who require drug therapy may be treated initially with a diuretic or a β-blocking agent. Patients with volume-dependent hypertension usually respond adequately to diuretics; those with high-renin, high cardiac output physiology respond best to β-blockers. If the pressure is not lowered adequately, a calcium channel blocker may be added to the diuretic and an ACE inhibitor may replace the β-blocker. Chronic use of diuretics may result in elevation of serum lipids, but long-term investigations of that effect in children are not available. β-Blocking agents have also been associated with changes in serum lipids, and some studies suggest a reduction in exercise tolerance in patients treated with propranolol.

Because of the effect of most diuretics on serum lipids and the tendency of some β-blocking drugs to produce bronchospasm and sleep disturbances, the ACE inhibitors and calcium channel blockers may be considered for initial therapy in the adolescent with significant hypertension. Although captopril has been used more often in the pediatric and adolescent populations, newer ACE inhibitors have a longer duration of action and require less frequent administration of drug. Because enalapril has no sulfhydryl group, side effects such as neutropenia and rash may be less than with captopril.

In patients with longstanding or poorly controlled hypertension, the underlying pathophysiology is often complex. Such patients frequently require trials of combinations of antihypertensive agents in order to gain control of markedly elevated or labile pressure. The basic principle of combination antihypertensive therapy is the coadministration of drugs with different sites or mechanisms of action. Because compliance may become a problem, the drug regimen should be as simple as possible and should take advantage of longer acting agents when available. Drug calendars, parental supervision, and close patient-physician communication also will help to ensure that the medications are taken as prescribed.

Percutaneous balloon angioplasty of lesions that produce renal artery stenosis may cure as many as 50% of patients with fibromuscular dysplasia. Angioplasty is not successful for renal artery stenosis because of atherosclerotic plaques. If angioplasty is unsuccessful for fibromuscular dysplasia, the kidney may be removed and the renal artery repaired and then reimplanted to maintain renal function.

Arroll B, Beaglehole R: Does physical activity lower blood pressure: A critical review of the clinical trials. J Clin Epidemiol 45:439, 1992.

Capolan MS, Cohn RA, Langman CB, et al: Favorable outcome of neonatal aortic thrombosis and renovascular hypertension. J Pediatr 115:291, 1989.
Devereux RB: Does increased blood pressure cause left ventricular hypertrophy or vice versa? Ann Intern Med 112:157, 1990.
Dimsdale JE: Reflections on the impact of antihypertensive medications on mood, sedation, and neuropsychologic functioning. Arch Intern Med 152:35, 1992.
Farine M, Arbus GS: Management of hypertensive emergencies in children. Pediatr Emerg Care 5:51, 1989.
Ganguly A: Glucocorticoid-suppressible hyperaldosteronism: An update. Am J Med 88:321, 1990.
Gillman MW, Ellison RC: Childhood prevention of essential hypertension. Pediatr Clin North Am 40:179, 1993.
Greydanus DE, Rowlett JD: Hypertension in adolescence. Adolesc Health Update 6:1, 1993.
Harshfield GA, Alpert BS, Pullman DA, et al: Ambulatory blood pressure readings in children and adults. Pediatrics 94:180, 1994.
Houtman PN, Dillon MJ: Screening for hypertension in fit children. J Hum Hypertens 5:345, 1991.
Houtman PN, Dillon MJ: Medical management of hypertension in childhood. Child Nephrol Urol 12:154, 1992.
Ingelfinger JR: Pediatric hypertension. Curr Opin Pediatr 6:198, 1994.
Jung FF, Ingelfinger JR: Hypertension in childhood and adolescence. Pediatr Rev 14:169, 1993.
Kotchen JM, Holley J, Kotchen TA: Treatment of high blood pressure in the young. Semin Nephrol 9:296, 1989.
Ramsay LE, Waller PC: Blood pressure response to percutaneous transluminal angioplasty for renovascular hypertension: An overview of published series. Br Med J 300:569, 1990.
Schneeweiss A: Cardiovascular drugs in children. II. Angiotensin-converting enzyme inhibitors in pediatric patients. Pediatr Cardiol 11:199, 1990.
Sinaiko AR: Pharmacologic management of childhood hypertension. Pediatr Clin North Am 40:195, 1993.
Stanley JC: Surgical intervention in pediatric renovascular hypertension. Child Nephrol Urol 12:167, 1992.
Task Force on Blood Pressure Control in Children: Report of the second task force on blood pressure control in children—1987. Pediatrics 79:1, 1987.
Waeber B, Niederberger M, Nussberger J, et al: Ambulatory blood pressure monitoring in children, adolescents and elderly people. J Hypertens 9:572, 1991.
Weir MR: Impact of age, race, and obesity on hypertensive mechanisms and therapy. Am J Med 90:3S, 1991.
Wilson PD, Ferencz C, Dischinger PC, et al: Twenty-four-hour ambulatory blood pressure in normotensive adolescent children of hypertensive and normotensive parents. Am J Epidemiol 127:946, 1988.
Wolfish NM, Delbrouck NF, Shanon A, et al: Prevalence of hypertension in children with primary vesicoureteral reflux. J Pediatr 123:559, 1993.
Zerin JM, Hernandez RJ: Renal imaging in children with persistent hypertension. Pediatr Clin North Am 40:165, 1993.

PART XXI

Diseases of the Blood

SECTION 1

Development of the Hematopoietic System

Robert D. Christensen ▪ *Robin K. Ohls*

It is intuitive that hematopoietic regulation in the human fetus differs markedly from that in the adult. While in the adult, homeostatic maintenance is a prime function of hematopoietic regulation, constant and dramatic changes characterize hematopoiesis in the embryo and fetus. For instance, the incredible rate of somatic growth in the fetus and the resultant need to constantly increase the red cell mass necessitates an extraordinary erythropoietic effort. Also, the relatively low oxygen tensions but high metabolic rates of fetal tissues demand a system of oxygen delivery different from that present in adults. Another marked difference is the sterile intra-amniotic environment, which results in a low demand for neutrophils and obviates the need for maintenance of a large neutrophil reserve in the embryo and early fetus. Improved familiarity with developmental hematopoietic regulation aids in interpretation of postnatal hematologic data; it also results in appreciation of the erythropoietic and granulocytopoietic capacities and limitations of prematurely delivered neonates.

Developmental hematopoiesis can be viewed as occurring in three anatomic stages: mesoblastic, hepatic, and myeloid. Mesoblastic hematopoiesis occurs in extraembryonic structures, principally in the yolk sac, and begins between the 16th and 19th days of gestation. By about 6 wk of gestation the extraembryonic sites of hematopoiesis begin to ablate and hepatic hematopoiesis is initiated. By the 10th–12th wk, mesoblastic hematopoiesis ceases and a small amount of hematopoiesis is evident in the bone marrow. The liver, however, remains the predominant hematopoietic organ until the last trimester of pregnancy.

The anatomic site of hematopoiesis does not simply transfer from yolk sac to liver to marrow. Rather, each organ subsequently houses quite distinct hematopoietic populations. For instance, at 18–20 wk of gestation over 85% of the cells in the fetal liver are erythroid and virtually no neutrophils are present. In contrast, at the same time less than 40% of the cells within the bone marrow are erythroid and up to 15% are neutrophils. Thus not only does the anatomic site of hematopoiesis change during gestation, but the populations of cells generated at those sites are distinct. The mechanisms responsible for the changing anatomic sites of hematopoiesis and for the differences in hemic cells produced in the mesoblastic, hepatic, and myeloid sites have not been determined. Regardless of gestational age or anatomic location, production of all hematopoietic tissues begins with pluripotent stem cells that are capable of both self-renewal and clonal maturation into all blood cell lineages. Progenitor cells differentiate under the influence of hematopoietic growth factors, which include those listed in Table XXI–1.

GRANULOCYTOPOIESIS. Mesenchymal cells with some of the properties of macrophages are present in the first month of gestation. Some aspects of embryonic tissue remodeling take place by the actions of such cells. Whether these early phagocyte-like cells are derived from the same lineage as macrophages and neutrophils (by way of the progenitor termed the *colony forming unit–granulocyte-macrophage*; CFU-GM) is not known. Thus, although some cells with phagocytic properties may be present in the embryo, essentially no neutrophils are observed until midtrimester. In fact, blood obtained from human fetuses in utero during midtrimester contain very low concentrations of neutrophils. In fetuses of 20 wk gestation, Forestier et al reported a mean absolute blood neutrophil concentration of only 190/mm^3, a range of 0–490/mm^3, and a mode concentration of zero. Concordant with the low circulating concentrations of neutrophils, one study reported that no mature neutrophils were present in the liver of normal human fetuses electively aborted at 14–24 wk gestation. Similarly, Keleman observed no neutrophils in the liver or bone marrow of human abortuses until 16–18 wk gestation and thereafter observed significantly lower concentrations of mature neutrophils in the bone marrow of human fetuses (up to 22 wk gestation) than in the marrow of term neonates or adults.

Despite the near absence of neutrophils in the first and second trimester fetus, CFU-GM are abundant in fetal liver, bone marrow, and blood. In rodents, the number of CFU-GM per gram of body weight is far fewer in animals delivered prematurely than in those delivered at term and is lower in term animals than in adults. The quantity of CFU-GM per gram of body weight in the developing human fetus has not been reported. Thus, it is not clear whether, as in experimental animals, preterm human infants have a relatively small supply of granulocytic progenitors. The venous blood of adults contains about 20–300 CFU-GM/mL. In contrast, the blood of term infants contains about 2,000 CFU-GM/mL, and even higher concentrations are noted in the blood of infants delivered prematurely. The high concentrations of CFU-GM in fetal blood do not indicate a large total body quantity of CFU-GM. It is likely that a significant percentage of the fetal CFU-GM are in the circulation, while the liver and marrow contain relatively low concentrations.

When fetal CFU-GM are cultured in vitro in the presence of recombinant granulocyte–colony stimulating factor (G-CSF), they undergo maturation into colonies of neutrophils. CFU-GM of fetal origin often clonally mature into larger colonies, containing more cells, than do CFU-GM obtained from the bone marrow of adults. The physiologic role of G-CSF includes upregulation of neutrophil production, and this appears to be the case for the fetus and neonate as well as for adults. Thus, the low quantities of circulating and storage neutrophils in the midtrimester human fetus may be due in part to low production of G-CSF. Supporting this hypothesis are observations of poor production of G-CSF by cells of human fetal origin. Monocytes isolated from the blood of adults produce G-CSF when stimulated with a variety of inflammatory mediators such as bacterial lipopolysaccharide (LPS) or interleukin-1 (IL-1). In contrast, monocytes isolated from the umbilical cord blood of preterm infants, and from the liver and bone marrow of aborted fetuses up to 24 wk gestation, generate only small quantities (10–100 times less per cell) of G-CSF protein and mRNA after LPS or IL-1 stimulation. Despite the poor capacity to generate G-CSF, it is clear that G-CSF receptors on the surface of neutrophils of newborn infants are equal in number and affinity to those on adult neutrophils.

Thus, no granulocytopoiesis appears to be present in the human embryo, and granulocyte production is a very minor component of hematopoiesis in the fetus even up through the 22nd–24th wk of gestation. This is not due to the absence of neutrophil progenitor cells but rather to a relative lack of the major neutrophil regulatory growth factor, G-CSF. On this basis one might anticipate that newborn infants who are delivered extremely prematurely would be at significant risk for serious bacterial infection. Indeed, of all the risk factors for neonatal infection analyzed by the national collaborative study on neonatal infections, premature birth showed the strongest correlation.

ERYTHROPOIESIS. The synthesis of erythrocytes requires a constant supply of

■ TABLE XXI–1 Characteristics of Hematopoietic Growth Factors

Growth Factors	Molecular Mass (kD)	Chromosomal Location	Principal Target Cell
I. Erythropoietin	30–39	7q11–22	CFU-E, fetal BFU-E
II. Colony Stimulating Factors			
G–CSF	18–22	17q11.2–21	CFU-G, CFU-MIX, mature neutrophil
GM–CSF	18–30	5q23–31	CFU-MIX, CFU-GM, BFU-E, monocyte, mature neutrophil
M-CSF	45–70 Dimer of 2 subunits	5q33.1	CFU-M, macrophage
SCF	36	12	CFU-Mix, BFU-E, CFU-GM, mast cell
III. Interleukins			
IL-1	17	Alpha 2q13 Beta 2q13–21	Hepatocyte, macrophage, lymphocyte
IL-2	15–20	4q26–27	T cell, cytotoxic lymphocyte
IL-3	14–30	5q23–31	CFU-MIX, CFU-Meg, CFU-GM, BFU-E, macrophage
IL-4	16–20	5q23–31	T cell, B cell
IL-5	46 Dimer of 2 subunits	5q23–31	CFU-Eo, B cell
IL-6	19–26	7p21–24	CFU-MIX, CFU-GM, BFU-E, monocyte, B cell, T cell, cytotoxic lymphocyte
IL-7	25	8q12–13	B cell
IL-8	8–10	4	Neutrophil, endothelial cell, T cell
IL-9	16	5q31–32	BFU-E, CFU-MIX
IL-10	18.7	1	Macrophage, lymphocyte
IL-11	23	19q13	CFU-Meg, B cell, keratinocyte
IL-12	70–75 Dimer of 2 subunits	?	T cell, NK cell, macrophage
IL-13	?	5q	LAK cell
IV. Thrombopoietin	35–38	3q27–28	Megakaryocyte progenitor, megakaryocyte

G-CSF, granulocyte–colony-stimulating factor; GM-CSF, granulocyte-macrophage–colony-stimulating factor; M-CSF, macrophage–colony-stimulating factor; SCF, stem cell factor.

amino acids, certain lipids, iron, specific vitamins, and trace nutrients. The rate of erythrocyte production is regulated primarily by the hormone erythropoietin (Epo). Epo is a 30–39 kD glycoprotein that binds to specific receptors on the surface of erythroid precursors and stimulates their differentiation and clonal maturation into mature erythrocytes. In the human fetus, Epo is produced principally by cells of monocyte/macrophage origin residing in the liver. Postnatally Epo is produced almost exclusively by peritubular cells of the kidney. The lack of importance of the renal contribution to Epo production in the fetus is illustrated by the normal serum Epo concentrations and normal hematocrits of anephric fetuses. It is not known what factors regulate the switch of Epo production from the liver to the kidney.

Studies of bone marrow cells in tissue culture have added to our understanding of erythropoietic regulation. When bone marrow cells are placed in semi-solid media culture systems for 5–7 days, the Epo-sensitive precursors, termed *colony forming units–erythroid* (CFU-E) clonally mature into clusters containing 30–100 normoblasts. Erythroid-specific progenitors that are less well differentiated than CFU-E, hence more primitive cells, are termed *burst forming units–erythroid* (BFU-E). Twelve to 14 days after bone marrow cells are placed in semi-solid culture systems, BFU-E will have developed into large clusters of normoblasts, each containing 200 to over 10,000 normoblasts. BFU-E from human fetuses respond in a slightly different fashion than BFU-E isolated from adults. Specifically, BFU-E of fetal origin generally develop into erythroid clones more rapidly and generally develop substantially more normoblasts than do BFU-E of adult origin. Also, BFU-E from adult bone marrow require a combination of Epo plus another factor, such as IL-3 or GM-CSF, in order to clonally mature, while many fetal BFU-E mature in the presence of Epo alone. Cellular differentiation as the red cell attains maturity includes condensation and extrusion of the nucleus and production of hemoglobin. Ninety percent of the dry weight of the mature red cell is hemoglobin.

HEMOGLOBIN. The combustion that is essential to life requires that tissues receive a constant supply of oxygen. The evolutionary development of oxygen-carrying proteins, the hemoglobins, has increased the ability of blood to give fluid transport to this gas. Furthermore, the combination of oxygen with and its dissociation from hemoglobin are accomplished without expenditure of metabolic energy.

Hemoglobin is a complex protein consisting of iron-containing heme groups and the protein moiety, globin. A dynamic interaction between heme and globin gives hemoglobin its unique properties in the reversible transport of oxygen. The hemoglobin molecule is a tetramer made up of two pairs of polypeptide chains, each chain having a heme group attached. The polypeptide chains of various hemoglobins are of chemically different types. For example, the major hemoglobin (Hb) of the normal adult (Hb A) is made up of alpha (α) and beta (β) polypeptide chains, one pair of each. Hb A can therefore be represented as $\alpha_2\beta_2$. α and β chains differ in both the number and sequence of amino acids, and their synthesis is directed by separate genes.

Within the red blood cells of the embryo, fetus, child, and adult, six different hemoglobins may normally be detected: the embryonic hemoglobins, Gower-1, Gower-2, and Portland; the fetal hemoglobin, Hb F; and the adult hemoglobins, Hb A and A_2. The electrophoretic mobilities of hemoglobins vary with their chemical structures. The time of appearance and quantitative relationships among the hemoglobins are determined by complex developmental processes (Fig. XXI–1). Two sets of genes for α polypeptide chains are located on human chromosome 16. β, γ, and δ genes are closely linked on chromosome 11. Two pairs of alleles, located on chromosome 16, provide the genetic information for the structure of the α chain.

EMBRYONIC HEMOGLOBINS. The blood of early human embryos contains two slowly migrating hemoglobins, Gower-1 and Gower-2, and Hb Portland, which has Hb F–like mobility. The zeta (ζ) chains of Hb Portland and Gower-1 are structurally quite similar to α chains. Both Gower hemoglobins contain a unique type of polypeptide chain, the epsilon (ϵ) chain. Hb Gower-1 has the structure $\zeta_2\epsilon_2$ and Gower-2, $\alpha_2\epsilon_2$. Hb Portland has the structure $\zeta_2\gamma_2$. In embryos of 4–8 wk gestation the Gower hemoglobins predominate, but by the 3rd mo they have disappeared.

FETAL HEMOGLOBIN. Hb F contains γ polypeptide chains in place of the β chains of Hb A and can be represented as $\alpha_2\gamma_2$. Its resistance to denaturation by strong alkali is usually used in its quantitation. After the 8th gestational wk Hb F is the predominant hemoglobin; in the 6-mo-old fetus it constitutes 90% of the total hemoglobin. Then a gradual decline occurs, so that at birth Hb F averages 70% of the total. Synthesis of Hb F decreases rapidly postnatally, and by 6–12 mo of age only a trace is present. Less than 2.0% can be detected by alkali denaturation in older children and adults. Hb F is heterogeneous because of two types of γ chains, whose synthesis is directed by two sets of genes. The chains differ at position 136 in the presence of either a glycine (Gγ) or an alanine (Aγ) residue. In the newborn the relative proportion or ratio of Gγ to Aγ chain is 3:1.

ADULT HEMOGLOBINS. Some Hb A ($\alpha_2\beta_2$) can be detected in even the smallest embryos. Accordingly, it is possible as early as 16–20 wk gestation to make a prenatal diagnosis of major β-chain hemoglobinopathies, such as thalassemia major. Prenatal diagnosis is based on techniques that examine the rates of synthe-

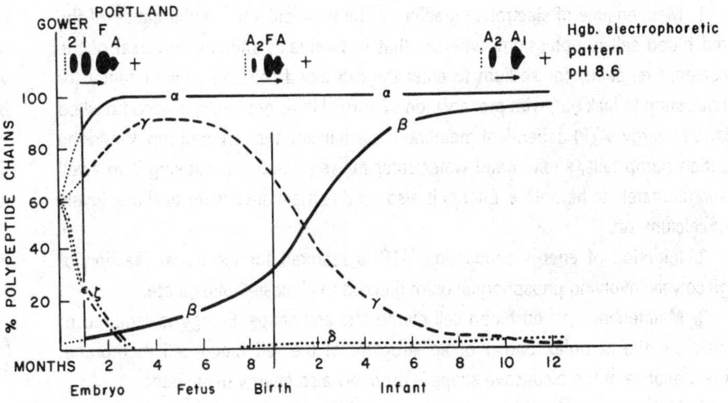

Figure XXI–1. Proportions of the various human hemoglobin polypeptide chains through early life. The hemoglobin electrophoretic pattern typical for each period is also shown. (Modified from Pearson HA: Recent advances in hematology. J Pediatr 69:466, 1966.)

sis of β chains or the structure of newly synthesized β chains. Earlier diagnosis is possible using molecular biology techniques and sampling of chorionic villus tissue or amniotic fluid if DNA structural defects are a cause of the hemoglobinopathies. Similarly, gene deletion disorders such as the α-thalassemias are detectable by the same method.

By the 6th mo of gestation there is about 5–10% of Hb A present. A steady increase follows so that at term Hb A averages 30%. By 6–12 mo of age the normal adult hemoglobin pattern appears. The minor adult hemoglobin component Hb A_2 contains delta (δ) chains and has the structure $\alpha_2\delta_2$. It is seen only when significant amounts of Hb A are also present. At birth less than 1.0% of Hb A_2 is seen, but by 12 mo of age the normal level of 2.0–3.4% is attained. Throughout life the normal ratio of Hb A to A_2 is about 30:1.

NORMAL RELATIONSHIPS AMONG THE HEMOGLOBINS. During fetal life and early childhood the rates of synthesis of γ and β chains and the amounts of Hb A and Hb F are inversely related. This relationship has been attributed to a "switch mechanism" similar to genetic regulatory mechanisms in bacteria, but the genetic, biologic, and developmental processes that direct a switchover from predominantly γ-chain synthesis in utero to predominantly β-chain synthesis after birth are unclear. It is not certain whether the mechanisms involve selective genetic inhibition or facilitation. It has been shown that differential selection and amplified production of red blood cell precursors derived from BFU-E result in considerable Hb F production. This may be the basis for the increased levels of Hb F that occur in many anemias when there is severe erythropoietic stress. Alternative explanations involve more basic genetic regulators in the DNA sequences that flank the hemoglobin gene complexes.

ALTERATIONS OF THE HEMOGLOBINS BY DISEASE. Because hemoglobins containing epsilon chains are normally present only very early in intrauterine life, they are largely of theoretical interest. Small amounts of the Gower hemoglobins have been detectable in a few newborn infants with 13/15-trisomy. Increased levels of Hb Portland have been found in cord blood of stillborn infants with homozygous α-thalassemia.

Levels of fetal hemoglobin may be influenced by various factors. Because the fetal hemoglobin level is elevated during the 1st year of life, a knowledge of its normal decline is important (Fig. XXI–2). In persons heterozygous for β-thalassemia (β-thalassemia trait) the postpartum decrease of Hb F is retarded; about 50% of such persons have elevated levels of Hb F (more than 2.0%) in later life. In homozygous thalassemia (Cooley anemia) and in hereditary persistence of fetal hemoglobin, large amounts of Hb F are characteristically found. In patients with major β-chain hemoglobinopathies (e.g., Hb SS, SC), Hb F is usually increased, particularly during childhood. Finally, moderate elevations of Hb F may be seen in many diseases accompanied by hematologic stress, such as hemolytic anemias, leukemia, and aplastic anemia, because of a minor population of red blood cells that contains increased amounts of Hb F, as can be demonstrated by the acid-elution staining technique of Kleihauer and Betke. Tetramers of γ chains (γ_4 or Hb Barts) or β chains (β_4, Hb H) may be seen in α-thalassemia syndromes.

The normal adult level of Hb A_2 (2.4–3.4%) is seldom altered. Levels of Hb A_2 exceeding 3.4% are found in most persons with the β-thalassemia trait and in those with megaloblastic anemias secondary to vitamin B_{12} and folic acid deficiency. Decreased Hb A_2 levels are found in those with iron deficiency anemia and α-thalassemia.

METABOLISM OF THE RED BLOOD CELL. The nucleated red blood cells in bone marrow participate in various metabolic functions, including active protein synthesis. After extrusion of the nucleus much of this metabolic ability is lost, including the ability to synthesize proteins. Loss of the nucleus makes the red blood cell a better vessel for oxygen transport, but it imposes on the red blood cell a finite life span, because the cell cannot replace or repair its vital enzymatic proteins. The mature red cell contains more than 40 enzymes. Many of these are essential for cellular viability, but genetically determined deficiencies of others, such as catalase, do not interfere with normal survival.

The mature red blood cell is not metabolically inert. It has no mitochondria, however, and ATP generation cannot occur by oxidative phosphorylation in Krebs cycle reactions. Rather, glucose is taken up and lactic acid produced mostly by anaerobic glycolysis (Embden-Meyerhof pathway); about 10% of glucose is metabolized oxidatively through the pentose phosphate pathway. At least five functions for ATP generated by glucose metabolism are essential to normal cell viability:

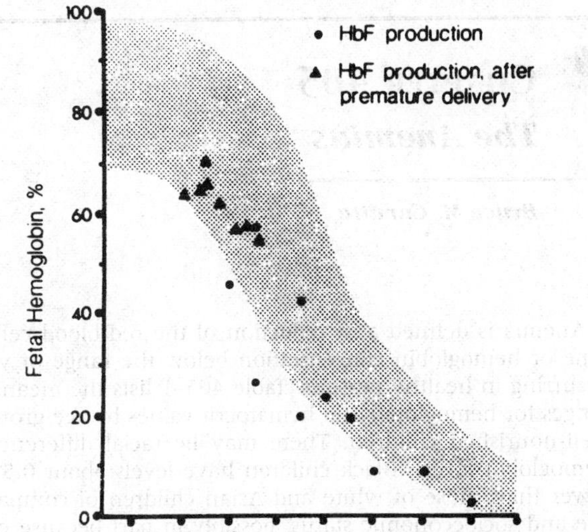

Figure XXI–2. Postnatal changes in percentage of fetal hemoglobin (Hb F) *(shaded area)*. The triangles represent postnatal production by reticulocytes in premature infants, and the dots represent cord and postnatal reticulocyte production in term infants. The percentage Hb F present reflects Hb F production over the previous weeks, whereas the rate of Hb F production is a result of the current proportion of Hb F produced by reticulocytes present, and is thus lower as the Hb F to adult hemoglobin (Hb A) switch progresses. (From Brown MS: Fetal and neonatal erythropoiesis. *In*: Stockman JA, Pochedly C (eds): Developmental and Neonatal Hematology. New York, Raven Press, 1988, p 258.)

1. Maintenance of electrolyte gradients. The principal intracellular cation of the red blood cell is potassium, whereas that in plasma is sodium. Reversal of the constant tendency for sodium to enter the red blood cell and concomitantly for potassium to leak out, with preservation of normal ionic gradients, is accomplished by an energy (ATP)-dependent membrane mechanism, the cation pump. When the cation pump fails, sodium and water enter the red blood cell, causing it to swell and ultimately to hemolyze. Energy is also used to maintain low intracellular levels of calcium ion.

2. Initiation of energy production. ATP is required for the initial reaction of glycolysis involving phosphorylation of glucose to glucose-6-phosphate.

3. Maintenance of red blood cell membrane and shape. Energy is required to maintain the complex phospholipid structure of the red blood cell membrane. Maintenance of the biconcave shape is probably also energy dependent.

4. Maintenance of heme iron in the reduced (ferrous) form. Oxidative potentials within the red blood cell may cause oxidation of the iron of hemoglobin. Hemoglobin containing ferric iron (methemoglobin) is ineffective in oxygen transport. Moreover, if perioxides and other oxidant substances are not inactivated, hemoglobin may be denatured and precipitated. Cells containing such denatured hemoglobin (Heinz bodies) are rapidly removed from the circulation. Protection of the red cell from the effects of oxidation ultimately depends on NADPH and NADH. These compounds are continually regenerated by activities of the glycolytic pathway and pentose shunt. In many genetically determined deficiencies of glycolytic and pentose pathway enzymes, hemolytic states occur because the energy necessary to perform these vital functions cannot be generated.

5. Maintenance of the levels of organic phosphates such as 2,3-diphosphoglycerate (2,3-DPG) and ATP within the red blood cells. These compounds interact with hemoglobin and have profound effects on oxygen affinity.

THROMBOPOIESIS. Like other hemic cells, megakaryocytes are produced following clonal maturation of committed progenitors, termed *colony forming units–megakaryocyte* (CFU-Meg), into megakaryoblasts. This blast cell is similar in appearance to other primitive committed cells, but DNA synthesis is generally more rapid and occurs without cell division, a process referred to as *endomitosis.* Megakaryoblasts grow considerably in size within a few days, with a single nucleus that may have 4–16 times the normal DNA content. The cytoplasm also increases in volume and cellular organelles appear. Long strips of cytoplasm are peeled off the body of the cell and ultimately break up into platelets. Epo, interleukin-6 (IL-6), and interleukin-11 (IL-11) have been shown to induce platelet formation. Thrombopoietin, a 353 amino acid protein with some homology to erythropoietin and interferons (alpha, beta), promotes megakaryocyte progenitor expansion and differentiation. Unlike the blood concentrations of erythrocytes and neutrophils, platelet concentrations remain constant from 18 wk gestation through term, with a range of 150,000–450,000/mm^3.

Aster RH: What makes platelets go? The cloning of thrombopoietin. Transfusion 35:1, 1995.
Athens JW: Granulocytes—Neutrophils. *In*: Lee RG, Bithell TD, Forester J, Athens JW, Leukins JN (eds): Wintrobe's Clinical Hematology, Vol 9. Philadelphia, Lea & Febiger, 1993, pp 239–236.
Bailie KEM, Irvine AD, Bridges JM, et al: Granulocyte and granulocyte-macrophage colony stimulating factors in cord and maternal serum at delivery. Pediatr Res 35:164, 1994.
Cairo MS: Therapeutic implications for dysregulated colony-stimulating factor expression in neonates. Blood 82:2269, 1993.
Carbonell F, Calvo W, Fliedner TM: Cellular composition of human fetal bone marrow. Acta Anat 113:371, 1982.
Forestier F, Daffos F, et al: Hematological values of 163 normal fetuses between 18 and 30 weeks of gestation. Pediatr Res 20:342, 1986.
Holbrook ST, Christensen RD: Hematopoietic growth factors. Adv Pediatr 39:23, 1991.
Keleman E, Janossa M: Macrophages are the first differentiated blood cells formed in human embryonic liver. Exp Hematol 8:996, 1980.
Keleman E, Calvo W, Fliedner TM: Atlas of Human Hemopoietic Development. Berlin, Springer-Verlag, 1979.
Liechty KW, Schibler KR, Ohls RK et al: The failure of newborn mice infected with *Escherichia coli* to accelerate neutrophil production correlates with their failure to increase transcripts for granulocyte colony-stimulating factor and interleukin-6. Biol Neonate 64:31, 1993.
Metcalf D: Hematopoietic regulators: redundance or subtlety? Blood 82:3515, 1993.
Nathan DG: The beneficence of neonatal hematopoiesis [editorial]. N Engl J Med 321:1190, 1989.
Nathan DG: Regulation of hematopoiesis. Pediatr Res 27:423, 1990.
Oski FA: The erythrocyte and its disorders. *In*: Nathan DG, Oski FA (eds): Hematology of Infancy and Childhood, Vol 4. Philadelphia, WB Saunders, 1993, pp 18–43. ■

CHAPTER 405
The Anemias

Bruce M. Camitta

Anemia is defined as a reduction of the red blood cell volume or hemoglobin concentration below the range of values occurring in healthy persons. Table 405–1 lists the means and ranges for hemoglobin and hematocrit values by age groups of well-nourished children. There may be racial differences in hemoglobin levels. Black children have levels about 0.5 g/dL lower than those of white and Asian children of comparable age and socioeconomic status, possibly in part because of the relatively high incidence of α- and β-thalassemia traits in blacks. Alternatively, higher levels of red blood cell 2,3-diphosphoglycerate (2,3-DPG) have been found in black children, which, if not an adaptive mechanism to anemia, would permit better oxygen delivery and a lower hemoglobin.

Although a reduction in the amount of circulating hemoglobin deceases the oxygen-carrying capacity of the blood, few clinical disturbances occur until the hemoglobin level falls below 7–8 g/dL. Below this level pallor becomes evident in the skin and mucous membranes. Physiologic adjustments to anemia include increased cardiac output, increased oxygen extraction (increased arteriovenous oxygen difference), and a shunting of blood flow toward vital organs and tissues. In addition, the concentration of 2,3-DPG increases within the red blood cell. The resultant "shift to the right" of the oxygen dissociation curve, by reducing the affinity of hemoglobin for oxygen, results in more complete transfer of oxygen to the tissues. The same shift may also occur at high altitude. When moderately severe anemia develops slowly, surprisingly few symptoms or objective findings may be evident, but weakness, tachypnea, shortness of breath on exertion, tachycardia, cardiac dilatation, and congestive heart failure ultimately result from increasingly severe anemia, regardless of its cause.

Anemia is not a specific entity but results from many underlying pathologic processes. A useful classification of the anemias of childhood divides them into three large groups by the red cell mean corpuscular volume (MCV): microcytic, macrocytic, or normocytic. The red cell size changes with age and before an anemia can be specifically characterized with respect to red blood cell size, normal developmental changes in the MCV should be understood (see Table 405–1). Table 405–2 classifies the important anemias of childhood by the MCV. Anemias in childhood may also be classified by variations in cell size and shape, as reflected by alterations in the red blood cell distribution width (RDW). The RDW, as determined by the use of electronic cell counting technology, is the coefficient of variation of red blood cell size (standard deviation of the MCV ÷ mean MCV × 100). Knowledge of both the MCV and the RDW can be helpful in the initial classification of anemias of childhood (Table 405–3). In every case of significant anemia it is essential to review the appearance of red blood cells on a peripheral blood smear (Fig. 405–1). Specific morphologic features may point to the underlying diagnosis. In addition,

■ **TABLE 405–1 Hematologic Values During Infancy and Childhood**

	Hemoglobin (g/dL)		Hematocrit (%)		Reticulocytes (%)	MCV (fl)	Leukocytes (WBC/mm³)		Neutrophils (%)		Lymphocytes (%)	Eosinophils (%)	Monocytes (%)
Age	*Mean*	*Range*	*Mean*	*Range*	*Mean*	*Lowest*	*Mean*	*Range*	*Mean*	*Range*	*Mean**	*Mean*	*Mean*
Cord blood	16.8	13.7–20.1	55	45–65	5.0	110	18,000	(9,000–30,000)	61	(40–80)	31	2	6
2 wk	16.5	13.0–20.0	50	42–66	1.0		12,000	(5,000–21,000)	40		63	3	9
3 mo	12.0	9.5–14.5	36	31–41	1.0		12,000	(6,000–18,000)	30		48	2	5
6 mo to 6 yr	12.0	10.5–14.0	37	33–42	1.0	70–74	10,000	(6,000–15,000)	45		48	2	5
7–12 yr	13.0	11.0–16.0	38	34–40	1.0	76–80	8,000	(4,500–13,500)	55		38	2	5
Adult													
Female	14	12.0–16.0	42	37–47	1.6	80	7,500	(5,000–10,000)	55	(35–70)	35	3	7
Male	16	14.0–18.0	47	42–52		80							

**Relatively wide range.*
fl, femtoliters; MCV, mean corpuscular volume; WBC, white blood cells.

■ **TABLE 405–2 Classification of Anemia**

Microcytic
- Iron deficiency
- Thalassemias
- Lead poisoning
- Chronic disease
  - Infection
  - Cancer
  - Inflammation
  - Renal disease
- Vitamin B_6 responsive
- Copper deficiency
- Sideroblastic (some)
- Hemoglobin E

Normocytic
- Decreased production
  - Aplastic anemia
    - Congenital
    - Acquired
  - Pure red cell aplasia
    - Congenital (Diamond-Blackfan)
    - Acquired (transient erythroblastopenia)
  - Bone marrow replacement
    - Leukemia
    - Tumors
    - Storage diseases
    - Osteopetrosis
    - Myelofibrosis
- Blood loss
  - Internal or external
- Sequestration
- Hemolysis: Intrinsic RBC abnormalities
  - Hemoglobinopathies
  - Enzymopathies
  - Membrane disorders
    - Hereditary spherocytosis
    - Acquired: Paroxysmal nocturnal hemoglobinuria
- Hemolysis: Extrinsic RBC abnormalities
  - Immunologic
    - Passive (hemolytic disease of the newborn)
    - Active: Autoimmune
  - Toxins
  - Infections
  - Microangiopathic
    - Disseminated intravascular coagulation (DIC)
    - Hemolytic uremic syndrome
    - Hypertension
    - Cardiac disease

Macrocytic
- Normal newborn (spurious)
- Reticulocytosis (spurious)
- Vitamin B_{12} deficiency
- Folate deficiency
- Oroticaciduria
- Myelodysplasia
- Liver disease
- Hypothyroidism
- Vitamin B_6 deficiency (some)
- Thiamine deficiency

■ **TABLE 405–3 Proposed Classification of Anemic Disorders Based on Red Blood Cell Mean (MCV) and Heterogeneity (RDW)*†‡**

Microcytic Homogeneous (MCV low, RDW normal)†	Microcytic Heterogeneous (MCV low, RDW high)	Normocytic Homogeneous (MCV normal, RDW normal)	Normocytic Heterogeneous (MCV normal, RDW high)	Macrocytic Homogeneous (MCV high, RDW normal)	Macrocytic Heterogeneous (MCV high, RDW high)
Heterozygous thalassemia Chronic disease	Iron deficiency Hb S–β-thalassemia; hemoglobin H; red cell fragmentation	Normal Chronic disease, chronic liver disease; nonanemic hemoglobinopathy (e.g., AS, AC); transfusion; chemotherapy; chronic myelocytic leukemia; hemorrhage; hereditary spherocytosis	Mixed deficiency Early iron deficiency anemia; anemic hemoglobinopathy (e.g., SS, SC); myelofibrosis; sideroblastic	Aplastic anemia Preleukemia	Folate deficiency Vitamin B_{12} deficiency; immune hemolytic anemia; cold agglutinin; high count

**Modified from Bessman JD, Gilmer P, Gardener F: Improved classification of anemias by MCV and RDW. Am J Clin Pathol 80:322, 1983.*
†MCV = mean corpuscular volume.
‡RDW = red blood cell distribution width.
AS = sickle cell trait, AC = hemoglobin C trait, SS = sickle cell anemia, SC = hemoglobin SC disease.

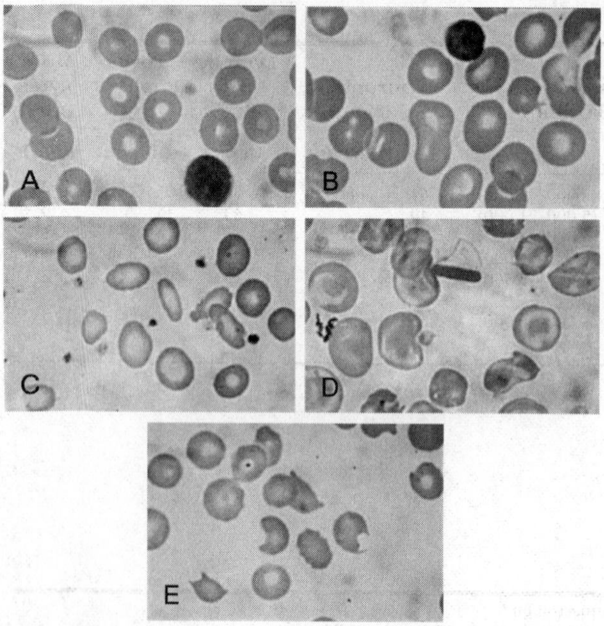

Figure 405–1. Morphologic abnormalities of the red blood cell. *A*, Normal. *B*, Macrocytes (folic acid or vitamin B_{12} deficiency). *C*, Hypochromic microcytes (iron deficiency). *D*, Target cells (Hb CC disease). *E*, Schizocytes (hemolytic-uremic syndrome). (Provided by Dr. E. Schwartz.) See also color section.

the presence of polychromatophilia, which correlates roughly with the degree of reticulocytosis, indicates that the marrow is able to respond to red cell loss or destruction.

Koerper MA, Mentzer WC, Brecher G, Dallman PR: Developmental change in red blood cell volume: Implication in screening infants and children for iron deficiency and thalassemia trait. J Pediatr 89:580, 1976.
Nathan DG, Oski FA: Hematology of Infancy and Childhood, 4th ed. Philadelphia, WB Saunders, 1993.
Oski FA, Naiman JL: Hematologic Problems in the Newborn, 3rd ed. Philadelphia, WB Saunders, 1982.

SECTION 2

Anemias of Inadequate Production*

Elias Schwartz

When oxygen delivery by red cells to tissues is decreased, a variety of mechanisms, including expanded cardiac output, increased production of 2,3-diphosphoglycerate (2,3-DPG) in red cells, and higher levels of erythropoietin, help the body to modify the deficiency. Red cell production by the bone marrow in response to erythropoietin (EPO) may expand severalfold and may compensate for mild to moderate reductions in red cell life span. In a variety of anemias, the bone marrow loses its usual capacity for sustained production and expansion of the red blood cell mass. In these instances, absolute reticulocyte numbers in the peripheral blood are decreased. If the normal reticulocyte percentage of total red cells during most of childhood is about 1.0%, and the expected red cell count is approximately 4.0 $\times 10^6/mm^3$, then the normal absolute reticulocyte number should be about 40,000/mm^3. In the face of anemia, EPO production and the absolute number of reticulocytes should rise. A normal or low absolute number or percentage of reticulocytes in response to anemia indicates relative bone marrow failure or ineffective erythropoiesis (e.g., megaloblastic anemia, thalassemia). Measurement of the serum transferrin receptor (TfR) level or examination of the bone marrow will distinguish between these possibilities, because TfR is elevated with increased red blood cell (RBC) turnover in the marrow in ineffective erythropoiesis and is decreased in marrow RBC hypoproliferation. ■

CHAPTER 406

Congenital Hypoplastic Anemia

(Diamond-Blackfan Syndrome)

This rare condition usually becomes symptomatic in early infancy, frequently with pallor in the neonatal period, but may first be noted later in childhood. About 50% of children are diagnosed by 2 mo of age, and 75% by 6 mo. The most characteristic features are macrocytic anemia, reticulocytopenia, and a deficiency or absence of red blood cell (RBC) precursors in an otherwise normally cellular bone marrow.

ETIOLOGY. Although in 20% of patients a hereditary basis is suggested by instances of familial occurrence, no distinct genetic defect has been identified and dominant and recessive patterns have been noted in different families. Males and females are affected in equal numbers. Erythropoietin (EPO) levels are elevated, even more than expected for the degree of anemia. Although immunologic mechanisms have been suggested as the cause of suppression of red cell precursors, the abnormalities are most likely due to sensitization by transfu-

*Drs. Howard Pearson and James A. Stockman were authors of these sections in previous editions. Their contributions are gratefully acknowledged.

sions. Most evidence indicates that the primary defects are in the erythroid precursor and are not due to immunologic damage to normal stem cells. Cytokines and their receptors on red cells, such as those for EPO stem cell factor (SCF), interleukin-3 (IL-3), and granulocyte-macrophage–colony-stimulating factor (GM-CSF), are possible candidates for genetic defects in this disorder, but investigations thus far have not been positive. High levels of EPO are present in serum and urine. Chromosomes are usually normal. Although addition of SCF to marrow from many of these patients results in improved growth of erythroid colonies (burst-forming units–erythrocyte, BFU-E), no defects have been found in the genes in patients for SCF or its receptor, *c-kit*, nor does prednisone correct the anemias in mice with deficiencies of SCF or *c-kit*. Erythroid progenitors in this disorder have an unusual sensitivity to withdrawal of EPO with resultant increased apoptosis (programmed cell death) accompanied by accelerated DNA fragmentation.

CLINICAL MANIFESTATIONS. Many affected infants appear pale even in the first few days of life, but hematopoiesis must be generally adequate in fetal life. Profound anemia usually becomes evident by 2–6 mo of age, occasionally somewhat later. The liver and spleen are not enlarged initially. About one third of affected children have congenital anomalies, most commonly dysmorphic facies or defects of the upper extremities, including triphalangeal thumbs. The abnormalities are diverse, with no specific pattern emerging in the majority of those affected.

LABORATORY FINDINGS. The RBCs are usually macrocytic with elevated levels of folic acid and vitamin B_{12}. Assay of RBCs reveals a pattern characteristic of a "young" erythrocyte population, including elevated fetal hemoglobin (Hb F) and increased expression of "i" antigen. Adenosine deaminase (ADA) activity is increased in RBCs of patients with this disorder. These findings may help distinguish congenital RBC aplasia from acquired transient erythroblastopenia of childhood (Chapter 408). Thrombocytosis and occasionally neutropenia may also be present initially. Reticulocytes are diminished, even when the anemia is severe. Red blood cell precursors are markedly reduced in the marrow in most patients, while other marrow elements are usually normal. Serum iron levels are elevated. Bone marrow culture shows markedly reduced numbers of colony-forming units–erythrocyte (CFU-E) and BFU-E.

DIFFERENTIAL DIAGNOSIS. Congenital hypoplastic anemia must be differentiated from other anemias with low reticulocyte counts. The anemia of the convalescent phase of hemolytic disease of the newborn may, on occasion, be associated with markedly reduced erythropoiesis. This terminates spontaneously at 5–8 wk of age. Aplastic crises characterized by reticulocytopenia and by decreased numbers of RBC precursors, frequently caused by B19 parvovirus infections, may complicate various types of hemolytic disease, but usually after the first several months of life. Infection with this virus in utero may also cause pure red cell aplasia in infancy, even with hydrops fetalis at birth. The syndrome of transient erythroblastopenia of childhood may be differentiated from Diamond-Blackfan syndrome by its relatively late onset and by biochemical differences in RBCs (Chapter 408).

PROGNOSIS. The outlook is best in those who respond to corticosteroid therapy. About one half of the patients are long-term responders. In the others, survival depends on transfusions. Some children in each group may eventually have spontaneous remissions (about 14%). By late childhood, children who do not respond to corticosteroids may have had 100 or more transfusions, and hemosiderosis may result unless adequate chelation therapy for excess iron is carried out appropriately. The liver and spleen enlarge, and secondary hypersplenism with leukopenia and thrombocytopenia may occur in children who are not chelated adequately or in those with chronic hepatitis acquired from transfusions. The complications of chronic transfusions are similar to those seen in β-thalassemia major, and prevention and treatment of iron overload should be equally aggressive in both groups of transfused patients (see Chapter 419.9).

TREATMENT. Corticosteroid therapy is frequently beneficial if begun early, with three fourths of patients responding initially. The mechanism of its effect is unknown.

Prednisone in three or four divided doses totaling 2 mg/kg/24 hr is used as an initial trial. Red blood cell precursors appear in bone marrow 1–3 wk after therapy is begun, and then normoblastosis and a brisk peripheral reticulocytosis occur. The hemoglobin may reach normal levels in 4–6 wk. The dose of corticosteroid may then be reduced gradually by tapering divided doses and then by eliminating all except a single, lowest effective daily dose. This dose should then be doubled, used on alternate days, and tapered still further while maintaining the hemoglobin level at 10 g/dL or above. In some patients, very small amounts of prednisone, as low as 2.5 mg, may be sufficient to sustain adequate erythropoiesis.

In patients who do not respond to corticosteroid therapy, transfusions at intervals of 4–8 wk are necessary to sustain life. Chelation therapy for iron overload with deferoxamine administered subcutaneously via a battery-powered portable pump should be begun when excess iron accumulation is reflected by serum ferritin levels >1,000 mg/dL, but preferably after 5 yr of age, because the medication may interfere with normal growth. A newer, oral iron chelator, deferiprone (L1), is in clinical trials in Canada and elsewhere, and may offer an easier alternative if it is shown to be effective and to have acceptable toxicity. Other therapies, including androgens, cyclosporin A, cyclophosphamide, antithymocyte globulin (ATG), high-dose intravenous immunoglobulins, erythropoietin, and IL-3 have not had a consistent beneficial effect and may have a high incidence of side effects. High-dose intravenous methylprednisolone has been beneficial in some patients. Splenectomy may decrease the need for transfusion if hypersplenism or isoimmunization has developed. Bone marrow transplantation has a role in children who do not respond to corticosteroids and who have a histocompatible donor, but the risks of death related to transplant and chronic graft-versus-host disease must be weighed against the risks and difficulties of chronic transfusion and iron chelation therapy. The rate of engraftment is high, providing further evidence that immunosuppression is not the primary cause of this disorder.

406.1. Pearson Marrow-Pancreas Syndrome

This form of congenital hypoplastic anemia may be initially confused with Diamond-Blackfan syndrome or transient erythroblastopenia of childhood. The marrow failure usually appears in the neonatal period and is characterized by a macrocytic normochromic anemia, elevated Hb F and red cell adenosine deaminase, vacuolated erythroblasts and myeloblasts in the marrow, and occasional neutropenia and thrombocytopenia. Other features are failure to thrive, insulin-dependent diabetes mellitus, and exocrine dysfunction due to fibrosis of the pancreas, lactic acidosis, renal Fanconi syndrome with vacuolated tubular cells, muscle and neurologic impairment, and, frequently, early death. This multiorgan disorder has been shown to be due to mitochondrial DNA (mtDNA) deletions, with heterogeneity in different tissues and between patients. This heterogeneity accounts for the variable clinical picture, and a change in proportions of mtDNA types in tissues over time may result in spontaneous improvement of red cell hypoproliferation.

CHAPTER 407

Acquired Pure Red Blood Cell Anemias

A number of forms of acquired anemia with reticulocytopenia and reduced red blood cell (RBC) precursors in the marrow have been described. Most of these are rare in childhood, and the causes of most of them are uncertain. In some cases in adults, remission has followed removal of a tumor of the thymus. Association with thymoma has been reported in a child. The presence of a complement-dependent antibody cytotoxic for erythroblasts in some adults, and rarely in children, has suggested the use of high-dose intravenous immunoglobulin (IVIG) or immunosuppressive therapy. The acquired pure RBC anemias may respond to therapy with corticosteroids, and a trial is indicated in any chronic case.

Large doses of chloramphenicol may inhibit erythropoiesis. Reticulocytopenia, erythroid hypoplasia, and vacuolated pronormoblasts in the marrow are reversible effects of this drug. This effect differs from the idiosynchratic and rare development of severe aplastic anemia in recipients of the drug.

Episodes of acute failure of erythropoiesis may follow various viral infections. B19 parvovirus is the best documented viral cause of red cell aplasia (Chapter 210). This small, single-stranded DNA virus is the cause of fifth disease (erythema infectiosum), usually manifested in children by facial erythema and a maculopapular rash on the trunk and, occasionally, by joint pains or arthritis. It may also be associated with systemic necrotizing vasculitis in some children. The virus is particularly infective and cytotoxic for erythroid progenitor cells in the marrow, interacting specifically with the red cell P antigen as a receptor. Characteristic nuclear inclusions in erythroblasts and giant pronormoblasts can be seen with light microscopy of bone marrow. Hemophagocytosis may also be seen in the marrow, perhaps accounting for the occasional granulocytopenia and thrombocytopenia. Because infection with this virus is usually transient, with recovery usually occurring in less than 2 wk, anemia is not present or not noticed in otherwise normal children, in whom the life span of peripheral red cells is 110–120 days. In patients with hemolysis, such as that due to hereditary spherocytosis or sickle cell disease, in whom red cell life span is much shorter, a cessation of erythropoiesis due to parvovirus infection may cause severe anemia, the "aplastic crisis" seen in these diseases. Recovery from moderate to severe anemia is usually spontaneous, heralded by a wave of nucleated red cells and subsequent reticulocytosis in the peripheral blood. Occasionally, a red cell transfusion may be necessary for marked symptoms due to anemia. Rarely, persistence of parvovirus infection may occur in patients unable to mount an adequate antibody response to the virus, as in children with congenital immunodeficiency diseases, those being treated with immunosuppressive agents, and those with acquired immunodeficiency syndrome (AIDS). The resultant pure red cell aplasia may be severe. The viral infection in these chronically infected patients may be treated with high-dose IVIG, which contains neutralizing antibody to the virus. Different clinical manifestations of infection with this virus and destruction of erythroid precursors occur with infections in utero, in which there is increased fetal wastage in the first and second trimesters, and babies may be born with hydrops fetalis and viremia. Congenital infection may also cause congenital pure red cell aplasia due to induction of tolerance. The presence of persistent congenital parvovirus infection needs to be detected by examination of bone marrow DNA because immunologic tolerance to the virus may prevent the usual development of specific antibodies (Chapter 210).

Other viruses causing suppression of erythropoiesis usually affect the production of at least one other hematopoietic cell as well and may also cause increased destruction of peripheral blood cells by immunologic mechanisms. These include hepatitis virus (non-A, non-B, non-C), Epstein-Barr virus, cytomegalovirus, and the human immunodeficiency virus.

CHAPTER 408

Transient Erythroblastopenia of Childhood (TEC)

This syndrome of severe, transient hypoplastic anemia occurs mainly in previously healthy children between 6 mo and 3 yr of age, with most above 12 mo of age at onset; it is more common than congenital hypoplastic anemia. The cause of this acquired decrease in red cell production is not clear, although it frequently follows a viral illness. Parvovirus infections, which may cause hypoplasia in children with hemolytic anemia, does not appear to be commonly associated with TEC. Reticulocytes and bone marrow erythroid precursors are markedly decreased, while white blood cell and platelet numbers are usually normal. Mean corpuscular volume (MCV) is usually normal for age, and fetal hemoglobin (Hb F) levels are normal before the recovery phase. Red cell adenosine deaminase (ADA) levels are normal in this disorder, while they may be elevated in congenital hypoplastic anemia. Differentiation from the latter disease may be difficult, but differences in age of onset and in age-related MCV, Hb F, and ADA may be helpful.

Most children recover within 1–2 mo and recurrence is rare. Red cell transfusions may be necessary for severe anemia (Hb level <3.5 g/dL) in the absence of signs of early recovery. The anemia develops slowly, and marked symptoms usually only develop with severe anemia. Corticosteroid therapy does not appear to be of any value in this disorder.

CHAPTER 409

Anemia of Chronic Disorders and Renal Disease

Anemia complicates a number of chronic systemic diseases associated with infection, inflammation, or tissue breakdown. Examples of such conditions include chronic pyogenic infections, such as bronchiectasis and osteomyelitis; chronic inflammatory processes, such as rheumatoid arthritis, systemic lupus erythematosis, and ulcerative colitis; malignancies; and advanced renal disease. In the latter, an additional major component is decreased production of erythropoietin (EPO) due to damage of the cells producing this cytokine. Despite diverse underlying causes, the erythroid abnormalities are similar. Red blood cell (RBC) life span is moderately decreased, reflecting increased RBC destruction by a hyperactive reticuloendothelial system. The increased hemolysis is less important, however, than a relative failure of bone marrow response, reflecting both hypoactivity of marrow and an EPO production inadequate for the degree of anemia. In addition, there are abnormalities of iron metabolism, including defective iron release from tissues into the plasma. Suppression of the erythroid response in the marrow appears to be primarily due to an increase in tumor necrosis factor (TNF) acting on bone marrow stromal cells to produce interferon (IFN)-β as a primary mediator and an increase in interleukin-1 (IL-1) acting on T cells to produce IFN-γ as a primary mediator. Recombinant human EPO (r-HuEPO) can overcome this effect if the EPO level in a patient is <500 mUnits/mL. TNF and IL-1 decrease EPO production in perfused kidneys and hepatoma cells, corresponding to the two sites of EPO production, accounting for the inadequate EPO response in this type of anemia. The specific stimulant of increased TNF and IL-1 production in these patients has not been identified.

CLINICAL MANIFESTATIONS. Although the important symptoms and signs are those of the underlying disease, the quality of life may be affected by the mild to moderate anemia present (see Chapter 405).

LABORATORY FINDINGS. Hemoglobin concentrations usually range from 6 to 9 g/dL. The anemia is usually normochromic and normocytic; in about one third of patients, modest hypochromia and microcytosis may be seen. Absolute reticulocyte counts are normal or low, and leukocytosis is common. Free erythrocyte protoporphyrin (FEP) levels are frequently elevated and provide a sensitive reflection of derangements of iron metabolism. They return to normal after successful treatment of the primary disease. The serum iron level is low, without the increase in total iron-binding capacity seen in iron deficiency. This pattern of low serum iron and low to normal iron-binding protein is a regular and valuable diagnostic feature. Serum ferritin may be elevated. The bone marrow has normal cellularity; the RBC precursors are low to adequate, marrow hemosiderin may be increased, and granulocytic hyperplasia may be present. A frequent clinical challenge is to identify concomitant iron deficiency in the patient with an inflammatory disease. A trial of iron therapy may be needed to resolve the issue, although there may not be a response, even with iron deficiency, when inflammation due to the primary disease persists. This is a common problem, particularly in disorders such as juvenile rheumatoid arthritis, in which treatment may result in gastrointestinal blood loss and consequent iron deficiency.

TREATMENT AND PROGNOSIS. Because these anemias are secondary to other disease processes, they do not respond to iron or hematinics unless there is concomitant deficiency. Transfusions raise the hemoglobin concentration only temporarily and are rarely indicated. If the underlying systemic disease can be controlled, the anemia is corrected spontaneously. Recombinant human erythropoietin can increase the hemoglobin level and improve activity and the sense of well-being in patients with end-stage renal failure and in those with anemia of chronic inflammation. Treatment with iron is frequently necessary for an optimal EPO effect.

CHAPTER 410
Congenital Dyserythropoietic Anemias

These rare inherited normocytic or macrocytic anemias display multinuclearity and abnormal chromatin patterns in red blood cell precursors. Three major types have been distinguished, with considerable variation within each type and overlap among them. Type I (about 15% of cases) is defined by binuclearity of erythroblasts, thin internuclear chromatin bridges between separate erythroblasts, and megaloblastic morphology. Red cells are macrocytic. Type II (more than 60% of cases) has erythroblastic multinuclearity and a positive acidified serum (Ham) test, but only to 30% of sera. The sugar water test, frequently positive in paroxysmal nocturnal hemoglobinuria, where the Ham test is also positive, is negative in this disorder. Red blood cells in type II (HEMPAS: *h*ereditary *e*rythroblastic *m*ultinuclearity associated with a *p*ositive *a*cidified *s*erum lysis test) are strongly agglutinated by anti-i antibody. The primary defect in some patients with this variant is in a gene for enzymes involved in biosynthesis of asn-linked oligosaccharide chains of glycoproteins, including those in the red cell membrane and in transferrin. Types I and II appear to be inherited as autosomal recessive traits. Type III (about 15% of cases) has pronounced erythroid multinuclearity with DNA content up to 24 times normal in marrow. It appears to be inherited as an autosomal dominant trait in some families and as recessive in others. In each type there are variable degrees of anemia (sometimes first noted in adolescence or adult life), ineffective erythropoiesis, and increased intestinal uptake of iron. Findings of chronic hemolysis, such as intermittent jaundice, gallstones, and splenomegaly, are common. Blood transfusions may occasionally be needed for severe anemia. Splenectomy may help patients with anemia severe enough to require chronic transfusions. Restriction of iron intake and iron chelation therapy should be of value in patients with iron overload.

CHAPTER 411
Physiologic Anemia of Infancy

The normal newborn has higher hemoglobin and hematocrit levels with larger red cells than older children and adults. Within the first week of life a progressive decline in hemoglobin level begins, which persists for approximately 6–8 wk. The result of this decline is generally referred to as *physiologic anemia of infancy.* Several factors are operative. First, there is abrupt cessation of erythropoiesis with onset of respiration at birth, when the arterial oxygen saturation rises toward 95%. Concomitantly, levels of erythropoietin (EPO) are low, perhaps due to the liver being the major site of EPO production in the neonatal period, rather than the kidney, and the relative insensitivity of the liver to EPO release with tissue hypoxia. In addition, EPO has a decreased half-life and an increased volume of distribution in newborns. A shortened survival of the fetal red blood cell (RBC) also contributes to the development of physiologic anemia. Furthermore, the sizable expansion of blood volume that accompanies rapid weight gain during the first 3 mo of life adds to the need for increased red cell production. In addition, red cell function is influenced by the higher levels of serum phosphate in newborns than later on in infancy. Red cell phosphate and 2,3-diphosphoglycerate (2,3-DPG) increase, facilitating release of oxygen from the normal adult hemoglobin (Hb A) that is present and decreasing tissue hypoxia. When the hemoglobin level has fallen to 9–11 g/dL at 2–3 mo of age in full-term infants, erythropoiesis resumes. This "anemia" should be viewed as a physiologic adaptation to extrauterine life.

The premature infant also develops a physiologic anemia. The same factors are operative as in term infants, but they are exaggerated. The decline in hemoglobin level is both more extreme and more rapid. Minimal hemoglobin levels of 7–9 g/dL commonly occur by 3–6 wk of age, and in very small premature infants levels may be even lower (Chapter 89).

In the preterm infant, the inability to produce compensatory amounts of EPO accounts in part for the greater decline in hemoglobin concentrations, but frequent phlebotomies in sick infants for diagnostic and monitoring purposes, particularly in very small infants, are a major cause of anemia and the need for repeated transfusions. When premature infants are transfused with adult blood containing Hb A, the shift of the oxygen dissociation curve as a result of the presence of Hb A facilitates delivery of oxygen to the tissues. Accordingly, the definition of anemia and the need for transfusion in the premature infant must be based not only on hemoglobin level but also on oxygen requirements and the ability of the infant's circulating hemoglobin to release oxygen.

The marginal erythropoietic equilibrium responsible for physiologic anemia can add to anemia accompanying processes with increased hemolysis, such as congenital hemolytic states, which may be associated with severe anemia in the early weeks of life. Late hyporegenerative anemia, with absence of reticulocytes, may occur in infants with rhesus factor (Rh) hemolytic disease, perhaps due to low serum EPO levels. Bone marrow hypoplasia may also occur following intrauterine transfusions, also accompanied by low EPO levels. Therapy with recombinant human EPO (r-HuEPO; 200 IU/kg tiw 200–250 IU/kg three times per week SC), 2–3 mg/kg/24 hr of iron and 0.5–1 mg/24 hr of folate, may accelerate recovery. Some infants with bronchopulmonary dysplasia may develop anemia associated with deficient production of EPO, and a trial of EPO in such patients may be warranted.

Dietary factors may also aggravate physiologic anemia. Deficiency of folic acid superimposed on the physiologic process may result in more severe anemia. Vitamin E deficiency and therapy do not appear to play a role in anemia of prematurity, despite early suggestions to the contrary. A controlled and blinded study of oral vitamin E administration (25 IU dl-α-tocopherol, colloidal aqueous solution) to infants less than 1,500 g showed no difference in hemoglobin levels, reticulocytes, red cell morphology, or platelet counts. Breast milk and modern formulas appear to provide adequate vitamin E. Supplemental iron starting about at approximately 4 mg/kg/24 hr for preterm babies 4–8 wk old and by 4 mo in full-term infants should not cause significant hemolysis due to oxidation.

Unless there has been significant perinatal blood loss, iron deficiency should not be considered as a cause of anemia in the first 3 mo of life. Assuming an infant is born with adequate iron stores, dietary iron deficiency cannot be a cause of anemia until these iron stores have been exhausted. In the absence of blood loss, this does not occur until the birthweight has approximately doubled.

TREATMENT. As a developmental process, physiologic anemia usually requires no therapy other than ensuring that the diet of the infant contains the essential nutrients for normal hematopoiesis, especially folic acid and iron. A premature infant who is feeding well and growing normally rarely needs transfusion unless there has been significant iatrogenic blood loss. Assessment of the overall clinical condition, including growth rate, and monitoring of hematocrit are better guides to transfusion of red cells than are formulas regarding blood loss from phlebotomy. Red cell transfusions consistently do not appear to affect the course of apneic spells and bradycardia, and the beneficial effects noted in some reports are probably due to the effect of volume expansion. The number of donors for an infant should be minimized. The optimal level of hematocrit for premature infants is not settled. In general, raising the hemoglobin to about 30%, particularly if the red cells have a high percentage of Hb A, should suffice for adequate tissue oxygen delivery due to transfused blood. Anemia seen in very low birthweight preterm infants may be related to a relative deficiency of EPO, and clinical trials indicate that infants between 800 and 1,300 g who do not have severe illnesses who are treated with r-HuEPO and iron during the first 6 wk of life, at doses about 250 IU/kg three times per week subcutaneously, require fewer transfusions.

CHAPTER 412
Megaloblastic Anemias

The megaloblastic anemias have in common certain abnormalities of red blood cell (RBC) morphology and maturation. The RBCs at every stage of development are larger than normal and have an open, finely dispersed nuclear chromatin and an asynchrony between maturation of nucleus and cytoplasm, with the delay in nuclear progression being more evident with further cell divisions. Megaloblastic morphology may be seen in a number of conditions; almost all cases in children result from a deficiency of folic acid, of vitamin B_{12}, or of both. Both substances are cofactors required in the synthesis of nucleoproteins, and deficiencies result in defective synthesis of DNA and, to a lesser extent, RNA and protein. Ineffective erythropoiesis results from arrest in development or premature death of cells in the marrow. In the peripheral blood, red cells are large (increased mean corpuscular volume, MCV) and frequently oval, hypersegmented neutrophils appear, and giant platelets may also be found. In the marrow, the late nucleated megaloblastic red cell may appear well hemoglobinized but still retains an immature nucleus, rather than the usual clumped chromatin. Giant metamyelocytes and bands are also present in the marrow. Megaloblastic anemias due to malnutrition are relatively uncommon in the United States.

412.1 Folic Acid Deficiencies

MEGALOBLASTIC ANEMIA OF INFANCY

This disease is caused by a deficient intake or absorption of folic acid (see also Chapters 43 and 45). Folates are abundant in many foods, including green vegetables, fruits, and animal organs (liver, kidney). Folic acid is absorbed throughout the small intestine, after pteroylglutamate reacts with membrane-associated folate-binding proteins. Pteroylpolyglutamates, found in cabbage, lettuce, and other foods, are absorbed less efficiently than pteroylmonoglutamate (folic acid). Pteroylpolyglutamate hydrolase activity in the brush border aids the conversion to the monoglutamate. The specific nature of folate receptors and transport through the intestinal cell is not clear. Surgical removal or disorders of the small intestine may lead to folate deficiency. There is an active enterohepatic circulation. Much of the folate in the plasma is loosely bound to albumin. Pteroylglutamate is not biologically active. It is reduced by dihydrofolate reductase to tetrahydropteroylglutamate (tetrahydrofolate), which is transported into tissue cells and polyglutamated. Dietary deficiency is usually compounded by rapid growth or infection, which may increase folic acid requirements. The normal adult daily requirement is about 100 μg/24 hr, which rises to 350 μg/24 hr in pregnancy. The requirements on a weight basis are higher in the pediatric age range in comparison to adults due to the increased needs of growth. The needs are also increased with accelerated tissue turnover, as in hemolytic anemia. Human and cow's milks provide adequate amounts of folic acid. Goat's milk is clearly deficient; folic acid supplementation must be given when it is the main food. Unless supplemented, powered milk may also be a poor source of folic acid.

CLINICAL MANIFESTATIONS. Mild megaloblastic anemia has been reported in very low birthweight infants, and routine folic acid supplementation is advised. Megaloblastic anemia has its peak incidence at 4–7 mo of age, somewhat earlier than iron deficiency anemia, although the two may be present concomitantly in infants with poor nutrition. Besides having the usual clinical features of anemia, affected infants with folate deficiency are irritable, fail to gain weight adequately, and have chronic diarrhea. Hemorrhages due to thrombocytopenia occur in advanced cases. Folic acid deficiency may accompany kwashiorkor, marasmus, or sprue.

LABORATORY FINDINGS. The anemia is macrocytic (MCV >100 fl). Variations in RBC shape and size are common (see Fig. 405–1*B*). The reticulocyte count is low, and nucleated RBCs demonstrating megaloblastic morphology are often seen in the blood. Neutropenia and thrombocytopenia may be present, particularly in long-standing deficiencies. The neutrophils are large, some with hypersegmented nuclei; more than 5% of neutrophils have five or more nuclear segments. Normal serum folic acid levels are 5–20 ng/mL; deficiency is accompanied by levels less than 3 ng/mL. Levels of RBC folate are a better indicator of chronic deficiency. The normal RBC folate level is 150–600 ng/mL of packed cells. Levels of iron and vitamin B_{12} in serum are usually normal or elevated. Serum activity of lactic acid dehydrogenase (LDH) is markedly elevated. The bone marrow is hypercellular because of erythroid hyperplasia. Megaloblastic changes are prominent, although some normal RBC precursors may also be found. Large, abnormal neutrophilic forms (giant metamyelocytes) with cytoplasmic vacuolization are seen, as well as hypersegmentation of the nuclei of megakaryocytes.

TREATMENT. When the diagnosis is established, or in severely ill children, folic acid may be administered orally or parenterally in a dose of 1–5 mg/24 hr. If the specific diagnosis is in doubt, 50–100 μg/24 hr of folate may be used for a week as a diagnostic test, or 1 μg/24 hr of cyanocobalamin parenterally for suspected vitamin B_{12} deficiency. Because a hematologic response can be expected within 72 hr, transfusions are indicated only when the anemia is severe or the child is very ill. Folic acid therapy should be continued for 3–4 wk. If juvenile pernicious anemia is present or if the anemia recurs after therapy, the prolonged use of folic acid should be avoided, because in pernicious anemia folic acid may produce a partial response to the anemia without decreasing the neurologic abnormalities.

MEGALOBLASTIC ANEMIA OF PREGNANCY

Folate requirements increase markedly during pregnancy, in part to meet fetal needs. Decreases in serum and RBC folate levels occur in as many as 25% of pregnant women at term and may be aggravated by infection. Folate supplementation, 1 mg/24 hr, is often advocated, particularly during the last trimester. Mothers with folate deficiency may have babies with normal folate stores due to selective transfer of folate to the fetus via placental folate receptors.

FOLIC ACID DEFICIENCY IN MALABSORPTION SYNDROMES

Diffuse inflammatory or degenerative disease of the intestine may reduce intestinal pteroylpolyglutamate hydrolase activity as well as markedly impair absorption of folate. Celiac disease, chronic infectious enteritis, and enteroenteric fistulas may lead to folic acid deficiency and megaloblastic anemia. Measurement of serum folate is used to assess small intestinal absorptive functions in malabsorptive disorders. Oral folic acid supplements of 1 mg/24 hr may be indicated in these states (see Chapter 286).

CONGENITAL FOLATE MALABSORPTION

An autosomal recessive defect in the intestinal absorption of folic acid and an associated inability to transfer folate from the plasma to the central nervous system has been associated with megaloblastic anemia, convulsions, mental retardation, and cerebral calcifications. Infants present at 2–3 mo of age with severe megaloblastic anemia. Early and intensive treatment with intramuscular folinic acid (5-formyltetrahydrofolate) is important to correct the hematologic defect and to try to prevent neurologic deterioration.

FOLIC ACID DEFICIENCY ASSOCIATED WITH ANTICONVULSANTS AND OTHER DRUGS

Many patients have low serum levels of folic acid during therapy with certain anticonvulsant drugs (e.g., phenytoin, primidone, phenobarbital), but they usually do not develop anemia. Frank megaloblastic anemia is rare and responds to folic acid therapy, even if administration of the offending drug is continued. Absorption of folic acid is impaired by anticonvulsant drugs, but there is also increased utilization of folate. Megaloblastic anemia has been seen in users of oral contraceptives, but the cause is not clear.

A number of drugs have antifolic acid activity as their primary pharmacologic effect and regularly produce megaloblastic anemia. Methotrexate binds to dihydrofolate reductase and prevents the formation of tetrahydrofolate, the active form. Pyrimethamine, used in the therapy of toxoplasmosis, and trimethoprim, used for treatment of a variety of infections, may induce folic acid deficiency and, occasionally, megaloblastic anemia. Therapy with folinic acid (5-formyl-tetrahydrofolate) is usually beneficial.

CONGENITAL DIHYDROFOLATE REDUCTASE DEFICIENCY

This has been reported in several patients who were unable to form biologically active tetrahydrofolate and who developed severe megaloblastic anemia in early infancy. These patients were successfully treated with large doses of folic acid or folinic acid. Deficiency of methylene tetrahydrofolate reductase has been described in some patients with homocystinuria who had no hematologic abnormalities.

412.2 Vitamin B_{12} (Cobalamin) Deficiency

Vitamin B_{12} is derived from cobalamin in food, mainly animal sources, secondary to production by microorganisms. Humans cannot synthesize vitamin B_{12}. The cobalamins are released in the acidity of the stomach and combine there with R proteins and intrinsic factor (IF), traverse the duodenum, where pancreatic proteases break down the R proteins, and are absorbed in the distal ileum via specific receptors for IF-cobalamin. In addition, some vitamin B_{12} from large doses may diffuse through mucosa in the intestine and mouth. In plasma, vitamin B_{12} is bound to transcobalamin (TC) II, the physiologically important transporter, as well as to TCI and TCIII. TCII-cobalamin enters cells by receptor-mediated endocytosis, and cobalamin is converted to active forms important in the transfer of methyl groups and DNA synthesis.

Vitamin B_{12} deficiency may therefore result from inadequate intake, surgery involving the stomach or terminal ileum, lack of secretion of intrinsic factor by the stomach, consumption or inhibition of the B_{12}-intrinsic factor complex, abnormalities involving the receptor sites in the terminal ileum, or abnormalities of TCII. Although TCI binds 80% of serum cobalamin, a deficiency of this protein results in low serum B_{12} levels but not in megaloblastic anemia (see Chapter 74).

Because vitamin B_{12} is present in many foods, dietary deficiency is rare. It may be seen in cases of extreme dietary restriction (strict vegetarians: "vegans") in which no animal products are consumed. Vitamin B_{12} deficiency is not commonly seen in kwashiorkor or infantile marasmus. Cases occur in breast-fed infants whose mothers have deficient diets or pernicious anemia.

JUVENILE PERNICIOUS ANEMIA

This rare autosomal recessive disorder results from an inability to secrete gastric intrinsic factor or secretion of a functionally abnormal IF. It differs from the typical disease in adults in that the stomach secretes acid normally and is histologically normal.

CLINICAL MANIFESTATIONS. The symptoms of juvenile pernicious anemia become prominent at 9 mo to 11 yr of age. This interval is consistent with exhaustion of the stores of vitamin B_{12} acquired in utero. As the anemia becomes severe, weakness, irritability, anorexia, and listlessness occur. The tongue is smooth, red, and painful. Neurologic manifestations include ataxia, paresthesias, hyporeflexia, Babinski responses, clonus, and coma.

LABORATORY FINDINGS. The anemia is macrocytic, with prominent macro-ovalocytosis of the RBCs (see Fig. 405–1*B*). The neutrophils may be large and hypersegmented. In advanced cases neutropenia and thrombocytopenia, simulating aplastic anemia or leukemia, are seen. Serum vitamin B_{12} levels are <100 pg/mL. Concentrations of serum iron and serum folic acid are normal or elevated. Serum LDH activity is markedly increased. Moderate elevations (2–3 mg/dL) of serum bilirubin levels may be seen. Excessive excretion of methylmalonic acid in the urine (normal amount, 0–3.5 mg/24 hr) is a reliable and sensitive index of vitamin B_{12} deficiency. In contrast to many adult cases with pernicious anemia, serum antibodies directed against parietal cells or intrinsic factor cannot be detected in children with this disorder. Gastric acidity may be reduced initially but returns to normal when vitamin B_{12} therapy is instituted. Intrinsic factor activity is absent in gastric secretion.

Absorption of vitamin B_{12} is usually assessed by the Schilling test. When a normal person ingests a small amount of vitamin B_{12} into which ^{57}Co has been incorporated, the radioactive vitamin combines with the IF in stomach secretions and passes to the terminal ileum, where absorption occurs. Because the absorbed vitamin is bound to TCII and incorporated into tissues, little or none is normally excreted in the urine. If a large dose (1 mg) of nonradioactive vitamin B_{12} is injected parenterally after 2 hr ("flushing dose"), 10–30% of the previously absorbed radioactive vitamin appears in the urine in 24 hr. Children with pernicious anemia usually excrete 2% or less under these conditions. To confirm that absence of IF is the basis of the B_{12} malabsorption, 30 mg of IF is given with a second dose of radioactive vitamin B_{12}. Normal amounts of radioactive vitamin should now be absorbed and flushed out in the urine. On the other hand, when vitamin B_{12} malabsorption results from absence of ileal receptor sites or other intestinal causes, no improvement in absorption is seen with intrinsic factor. Occasionally, gastric disorders may impair absorption of cobalamin incorporated in food but not the pure tracer. A *food Shilling test*, using labeled eggs produced by hens injected with radioactive vitamin B_{12}, may be used to investigate the presence of such disorders. The Schilling test result remains abnormal in pernicious anemia, even when therapy has completely reversed the hematologic and neurologic manifestations of the disease.

TREATMENT. A prompt hematologic response follows parenteral administration of vitamin B_{12} (1 mg), usually with reticulocytosis in 2–4 days, unless there is concurrent inflammatory disease. The physiologic requirement for vitamin B_{12} is 1–5 μg/24 hr, and hematologic responses have been observed with these small doses, indicating that administration of a minidose may be used as a therapeutic test when the diagnosis of vitamin B_{12} deficiency is in doubt. If there is evidence of neurologic involvement, 1 mg should be injected intramuscularly daily for at least 2 wk. Maintenance therapy is necessary throughout the patient's life; monthly intramuscular administration of 1 mg of vitamin B_{12} is sufficient. Oral therapy may succeed because of mucosal diffusion with high doses, but it is not generally advisable due to uncertainty of absorption.

TRANSCOBALAMIN DEFICIENCY

Transcobalamin II is the principal physiologic transport vehicle for vitamin B_{12}. The role of TCII in B12 transport is similar to that of transferrin (Tf) for iron; specific receptors for TCII and Tf exist on cells needing vitamin B_{12} or iron. A congenital deficiency is inherited as an autosomal recessive condition, with failure to absorb and transport vitamin B_{12}. Severe megaloblastic anemia occurs in early infancy. Therapy requires massive parenteral doses of vitamin B_{12}.

VITAMIN B_{12} MALABSORPTION DUE TO INTESTINAL CAUSES

Cases have been reported of familial occurrence of absence or defect of the receptor for IF-B_{12} in the terminal ileum, in some instances associated with proteinuria *(Imerslund syndrome)*. Histology of the stomach is normal, and intrinsic factor and acid are present in gastric secretions. Parenteral treatment with vitamin B_{12} monthly corrects the deficiency.

Surgical resection of the terminal ileum, inflammatory diseases such as regional enteritis, neonatal necrotizing enterocolitis, and tuberculosis may also impair absorption of vitamin B_{12}. When the terminal ileum has been removed, lifelong parenteral administration should be used if the Schilling test indicates that vitamin B_{12} is not absorbed.

An overgrowth of intestinal bacteria within diverticula or duplications of the small intestine may cause vitamin B_{12} deficiency by consumption of or competition for the vitamin or by splitting of its complex with intrinsic factor. In these cases hematologic response may follow appropriate antibiotic therapy. Similar mechanisms may operate when the fish tapeworm *Diphyllobothrium latum* infests the upper small intestine. When megaloblastic anemia occurs in these situations, the serum vitamin B_{12} level is low, the gastric juice contains intrinsic factor, and the abnormal Schilling test result is not corrected by addition of exogenous intrinsic factor.

VITAMIN B_{12} DEFICIENCY IN OLDER CHILDREN

In some cases of vitamin B_{12} malabsorption in adolescence, atrophy of the gastric mucosa, and achlorhydria have been noted. These cases may be related to the syndrome of malabsorption of vitamin B_{12} occurring in combination with cutaneous candidiasis, hypoparathyroidism, and other endocrine deficiencies. The serum contains antibodies against intrinsic factor and parietal cells. An abnormal Schilling test is corrected by addition of exogenous intrinsic factor. Parenteral vitamin B_{12} should be administered regularly to these patients.

412.3 Rare Megaloblastic Anemias

Oroticaciduria is a rare genetically determined defect in pyrimidine biosynthesis associated with severe megaloblastic anemia, neutropenia, failure to thrive, and crystalluria, caused by excretion of orotic acid (Chapter 75). Physical and mental retardation are frequently present. The anemia is refractory to vitamin B_{12} or folic acid but responds promptly to administration of the pyrimidine uridine (100–150 μg/kg/24 hr). The basic defects, which involve many tissues, include deficiencies of orotate phosphoribosyl transferase and orotidine-5-phosphate decarboxylase, enzymes essential for the formation of uridine-5′-phosphate. Inheritance is autosomal recessive. Megaloblastic anemia can also occur in the *Lesch-Nyhan syndrome*, in which regeneration of purine nucleotides is blocked (Chapter 75).

Cases of *thiamine-responsive* and *thiamine-dependent megaloblastic anemia* have been reported. Administration of thiamine, 100 mg/day, produced a brisk reticulocyte response and a sustained increase in hemoglobin level. Sensorineural deafness and diabetes mellitus were associated.

Megaloblastic anemia has also been seen in a group of children with inability to convert cobalamin to its biologically active metabolites, adenosylcobalamin and methylcobalamin, perhaps due to a deficiency in a cobalamin reductase. The disorder is called the *cobalamin C variant* and is characterized by neurologic abnormalities, methylmalonic aciduria, and homocystinuria. Abnormalities are usually noted in the early weeks of life, and include failure to thrive, lethargy, hypotonia, macrocytosis with megaloblastic bone marrow changes and anemia or pancytopenia, and hepatic dysfunction. Serum cobalamin levels are elevated. The megaloblastic changes may reverse and other symptoms may improve with hydroxycobalamin treatment, 1 mg/24 hr IM initially, gradually changed to a dose every month.

CHAPTER 413
Iron Deficiency Anemia

Anemia resulting from lack of sufficient iron for synthesis of hemoglobin is the most common hematologic disease of infancy and childhood. Its frequency is related to certain basic aspects of iron metabolism and nutrition. The body of the newborn infant contains about 0.5 g of iron, whereas the adult content is estimated at 5 g. To make up for this discrepancy, an average of 0.8 mg of iron must be absorbed each day during the first 15 yr of life. In addition to this growth requirement, a small amount is necessary to balance normal losses of iron by shedding of cells. Accordingly, to maintain positive iron balance in childhood, about 1 mg of iron must be absorbed each day.

Iron is absorbed in the proximal small intestine, mediated in part by the duodenal protein mobilferrin. Because absorption of dietary iron is assumed to be about 10%, a diet containing 8–10 mg of iron is necessary for optimal nutrition. Iron is absorbed two to three times more efficiently from human milk than from cow's milk, perhaps due in part to differences in calcium content. Breast-fed infants may, therefore, require less iron from other foods. During the first years of life, because relatively small quantities of iron-rich foods are taken, it is often difficult to attain sufficient iron. For this reason the diet should include such foods as infant cereals or formulas that have been fortified with iron, both of which are very effective in preventing iron deficiency. Formulas with 7–12 mg Fe/L for full-term infants and premature infant formulas with 15 mg/L for infants <1,800 g at birth are effective. Infants breast fed exclusively should receive iron supplementation from 4 mo of age. At best, the infant is in a precarious situation with respect to iron. Should the diet become inadequate or external blood loss occur, anemia ensues rapidly.

Adolescents are also susceptible to iron deficiency because of high requirements due to the growth spurt, dietary deficiencies, and menstrual blood loss. In several affluent countries about 40% of adolescent girls and 15% of boys have serum ferritin levels less than 16%, reflecting low bone marrow iron stores.

ETIOLOGY. Low birthweight and unusual perinatal hemorrhage are associated with decreases in neonatal hemoglobin mass and stores of iron. As the high hemoglobin concentration of the newborn falls during the first 2–3 mo of life, considerable iron is reclaimed and stored (Chapter 89). These reclaimed stores are usually sufficient for blood formation in the first 6–9 mo of life in term infants. In low-birthweight infants or those with perinatal blood loss, stored iron may be depleted earlier, and dietary sources become of paramount importance. Anemia caused solely by inadequate dietary iron is unusual before 4–6 mo but becomes common at 9–24 mo of age. Thereafter, it is relatively infrequent. The usual dietary pattern observed in infants with iron deficiency anemia is the consumption of large amounts of cow's milk and of foods not supplemented with iron.

Blood loss must be considered a possible cause in every case of iron deficiency anemia, particularly in the older child. Chronic iron deficiency anemia from occult bleeding may be caused by a lesion of the gastrointestinal tract, such as a peptic ulcer, Meckel diverticulum, a polyp or hemangioma, or by inflammatory bowel disease. In some geographic areas hookworm infestation is an important cause of iron deficiency. Pulmonary hemosiderosis may be associated with unrecognized bleeding in the lungs and recurrent iron deficiency after treatment with iron. Chronic diarrhea in early childhood may be associated with considerable unrecognized blood loss. Some infants with severe iron deficiency in the United States have chronic intestinal blood loss induced by exposure to a heat-labile protein in whole cow's milk. Loss of blood in the stools each day can be prevented either by reducing the quantity of whole cow's milk to 1 pint/24 hr or less, by using heated or evaporated milk, or by a milk substitute. This gastrointestinal reaction is not related to enzymatic abnormalities in the mucosa, such as lactase deficiency, or to typical "milk allergy."

Characteristically, involved infants develop anemia that is more severe and occurs earlier than would be expected simply from an inadequate intake of iron.

Histologic abnormalities of the mucosa of the gastrointestinal tract, such as blunting of the villi, are present in advanced iron deficiency anemia and may cause leakage of blood and decreased absorption of iron, further compounding the problem.

CLINICAL MANIFESTATIONS. Pallor is the most important clue to iron deficiency. Blue sclerae are also common, although also found in normal infants. In mild to moderate iron deficiency (hemoglobin levels of 6–10 g/dL) compensatory mechanisms, including increased levels of 2,3-diphosphoglycerate (2,3-DPG) and a shift of the oxygen dissociation curve, may be so effective that few symptoms of anemia are noted, although there may be increased irritability. Pagophagia, the desire to ingest unusual substances such as ice or dirt, may be present. In some children, ingestion of lead-containing substances may lead to concomitant plumbism. When the hemoglobin level falls below 5 g/dL, irritability and anorexia are prominent. Tachycardia and cardiac dilatation occur, and systolic murmurs are often present.

The spleen is enlarged to palpation in 10–15% of patients. In long-standing cases, widening of the diploë of the skull similar to that seen in congenital hemolytic anemias may occur. These changes resolve slowly with adequate replacement therapy. The child with iron deficiency anemia may be obese or may be underweight, with other evidence of poor nutrition. The irritability and anorexia characteristic of advanced cases may reflect deficiency in tissue iron, because with iron therapy striking improvement in behavior frequently occurs before significant hematologic improvement.

Iron deficiency may have effects on neurologic and intellectual function. A number of reports suggest that iron deficiency anemia, and even iron deficiency without significant anemia, affect attention span, alertness, and learning of both infants and adolescents, but it is not absolutely clear whether iron deficiency is usually causal or whether it helps to identify infants whose suboptimal behavior has another basis. It is also not clear whether the defects that are observed persist after adequate treatment, because the results of controlled studies are conflicting.

Monoamine oxidase (MAO), an iron-dependent enzyme, plays a crucial role in neurochemical reactions in the central nervous system. Iron deficiency produces decreases in the activities of enzymes such as catalase and cytochromes. Catalase and peroxidase contain iron, but their biologic essentiality is not well established. It is not possible to measure iron in vivo in the enzymatic compartment easily and accurately, yet this is a vital area of iron metabolism.

LABORATORY FINDINGS. In progressive iron deficiency, a sequence of biochemical and hematologic events occurs. First, the tissue iron stores represented by bone marrow hemosiderin disappear. The level of serum ferritin, an iron-storage protein, provides a relatively accurate estimate of body iron stores in the absence of inflammatory disease. Normal ranges are age dependent, and decreased levels accompany iron deficiency. Next, there is a decrease in serum iron (also age dependent), the iron-binding capacity of the serum increases, and the percent saturation falls below normal (also varies with age). When the availability of iron becomes rate limiting for hemoglobin synthesis, a moderate accumulation of heme precursors, free erythrocyte protoporphyrins (FEP), results.

As the deficiency progresses, the red blood cells (RBCs) become smaller than normal and their hemoglobin content decreases. The morphologic characteristics of RBCs are best quantified by the determination of mean corpuscular hemoglobin (MCH) and mean corpuscular volume (MCV). Developmental changes in MCV require the use of age-related standards for diagnosis of microcytosis (see Table 405–1). With increasing deficiency the RBCs become deformed and misshapen and present characteristic microcytosis, hypochromia, poikilocytosis, and increased red cell distribution width (RDW); see Fig. 405–1*C*). The reticulocyte percentage may be normal or moderately elevated, but absolute reticulocyte counts indicate an insufficient response to anemia. Nucleated RBCs may occasionally be seen in the peripheral blood. White blood cell counts are normal. Thrombocytosis, sometimes of a striking degree (600,000–1,000,000/mm^3), may occur or, in a few cases, thrombocytopenia. The mechanisms of these platelet abnormalities are not clear. They appear to be a direct consequence of iron deficiency, perhaps with associated gastrointestinal blood loss or associated folate deficiency, and they return to normal with iron therapy and dietary change. The bone marrow is hypercellular, with erythroid hyperplasia. The normoblasts may have scanty, fragmented cytoplasm with poor hemoglobinization. Leukocytes and megakaryocytes are normal. Hemosiderin cannot be demonstrated in marrow specimens by Prussian blue staining. In about a third of cases occult blood can be detected in the stools.

DIFFERENTIAL DIAGNOSIS (see Table 405–2). Iron deficiency must be differentiated from other hypochromic microcytic anemias. In lead poisoning associated with iron deficiency, the red cells are morphologically similar, but coarse basophilic stippling of the RBCs, an artifact of drying the slide, is frequently prominent. Elevations of blood lead, free erythrocyte protophyrin, and urinary coproporphyrin levels are seen (Chapter 665). The blood changes of β-thalassemia trait resemble those of iron deficiency (Chapter 419.9), and RDW is usually normal or only slightly elevated. α-Thalassemia trait occurs in about 3% of blacks in the United States and in many Southeast Asian peoples. The diagnosis requires direct identification of DNA defects or difficult globin synthesis studies after the newborn period. The diagnosis can be assumed when a case of familial hypochromic microcytic anemia with normal levels of Hb A2 and Hb F, and normal hemoglobin electrophoresis, is refractory to iron therapy. In the newborn period infants with the α-thalassemia trait have 3–10% Barts and the MCV is decreased (Chapter 419.9). Thalassemia major, with its pronounced erythroblastosis and hemolytic component, should present no diagnostic confusion. Hb H disease, a form of α-thalassemia with hypochromia and microcytosis, also has a hemolytic component due to instability of the beta-chain tetramers resulting from a deficiency of alpha globin. The RBC morphology of chronic inflammation and infection, though usually normochromic, may be microcytic, but in these conditions both the serum iron level and iron-binding ability are reduced, and serum ferritin levels are normal or elevated. Elevations of FEP level are not specific to iron deficiency and are observed in patients with lead poisoning, chronic hemolytic anemia, the anemia associated with chronic disorders, and some of the porphyrias.

TREATMENT. The regular response of iron deficiency anemia to adequate amounts of iron is an important diagnostic and therapeutic feature. Oral administration of simple ferrous salts (sulfate, gluconate, fumarate) provides inexpensive and satisfactory therapy. There is no evidence that addition of any trace metal, vitamin, or other hematinic substance significantly increases the response to simple ferrous salts. For routine clinical use the physician should be familiar with an inexpensive preparation of one of the simple ferrous compounds. The therapeutic dose should be calculated in terms of elemental iron; ferrous sulfate is 20% elemental iron by weight. A daily total of 6 mg/kg of elemental iron in three divided doses provides an optimal amount of iron for the stimulated bone marrow to use. Better absorption may result when medicinal iron is given between meals. Intolerance to oral iron is uncommon. A parenteral iron preparation (iron dextran) is an effec-

■ **TABLE 413–1 Responses to Iron Therapy in Iron Deficiency Anemia**

Time After Iron Administration	Response
12–24 hr	Replacement of intracellular iron enzymes; subjective improvement; decreased irritability; increased appetite
36–48 hr	Initial bone marrow response; erythroid hyperplasia
48–72 hr	Reticulocytosis, peaking at 5–7 days
4–30 days	Increase in hemoglobin level
1–3 mo	Repletion of stores

tive form of iron and is usually safe when given in a properly calculated dose, but the response to parenteral iron is no more rapid or complete than that obtained with proper oral administration of iron, unless malabsorption is present.

While adequate iron medication is given the family must be educated about the patient's diet, and the consumption of milk should be limited to a reasonable quantity, preferably 500 mL (1 pint)/24 hr or less. This reduction has a dual effect: The amount of iron-rich foods is increased, and blood loss from intolerance to cow's milk proteins is prevented. When the reeducation of child and parent is not successful, parenteral iron medication may be indicated. Iron deficiency can be prevented in high-risk populations by providing iron-fortified formula or cereals during infancy.

The expected clinical and hematologic responses to iron therapy are described in Table 413–1.

Within 72–96 hr after administration of iron to the anemic child, peripheral reticulocytosis is seen. The height of this response is inversely proportional to the severity of the anemia. Reticulocytosis is followed by a rise in the hemoglobin level, which may increase as much as 0.5 g/dL/24 hr. Iron medication should be continued for 8 wk after blood values are normal. Failures of iron therapy occur when the child does not receive the prescribed medication, when iron is given in a form that is poorly absorbed, or when there is continuing unrecognized blood loss, such as intestinal or pulmonary loss, or with menstrual periods. An incorrect original diagnosis of nutritional iron deficiency may be revealed by therapeutic failure of iron medication.

Because a rapid hematologic response can be confidently predicted in typical iron deficiency, blood transfusion is indicated only when the anemia is very severe or when superimposed infection may interfere with the response. It is not necessary to attempt rapid correction of severe anemia by transfusion; the procedure may be dangerous because of associated hypervolemia and cardiac dilatation. Packed or sedimented red cells should be administered slowly in an amount sufficient to raise the hemoglobin to a safe level at which the response to iron therapy can be awaited. In general, severely anemic children with hemoglobins under 4 g/dL should be given only 2–3 mL/kg of packed cells at any one time (furosemide may also be administered as a diuretic). If there is evidence of frank congestive heart failure, a modified exchange transfusion employing fresh-packed RBCs should be considered, although diuretics followed by slow infusion of packed red cells may suffice.

CHAPTER 414

Other Microcytic Anemias

SIDEROBLASTIC ANEMIAS

The sideroblastic anemias are a heterogeneous group of hypochromic, microcytic anemias whose basic defects may be abnormalities of heme metabolism. Serum iron levels are increased. In the bone marrow ringed sideroblasts are found; these are nucleated red blood cells with a perinuclear collar of coarse hemosiderin granules that represent iron-laden mitochondria.

Pearson syndrome, a combination of refractory sideroblastic anemia with vacuolization of marrow precursor cells and exocrine pancreatic dysfunction, is caused by a variety of deletions in mitochondrial DNA (Chapter 406.1). Acquired sideroblastic anemias occur in adults with various inflammatory and malignant processes, or with alcoholism.

A form of sideroblastic anemia transmitted as an X-linked recessive trait becomes symptomatic by late childhood. Splenomegaly is usually present. Free erythrocyte protoporphyrin (FEP) levels are not elevated. Some cases of sideroblastic anemia are responsive to pyridoxine (vitamin B_6) given in doses of 200–300 mg/24 hr, although other findings of vitamin B_6 deficiency are not observed. In one kindred with *X-linked pyridoxine-responsive sideroblastic anemia,* a thr-to-ser substitution was identified at amino acid residue 388 of erythroid 5-aminolevulinate synthease (ALS), near the pyridoxal phosphate cofactor binding site, affecting heme precursor synthesis. In another kindred, with a son and daughter with *pyridoxine-refractory sideroblastic anemia,* the ALS gene on the X chromosome of the son was normal, and the children each received a different X chromosome, indicating a different autosomal defect.

LEAD POISONING (See Chapter 665)

RARE TYPES OF HYPOCHROMIC MICROCYTIC ANEMIA

Isolated cases are known of hypochromic, microcytic anemia with other abnormalities of iron metabolism; some cases have had defects in iron mobilization or reutilization. *Congenital absence of iron-binding protein* (atransferrinemia) is associated with severe hypochromic anemia despite iron overload and requires lifelong transfusions. Iron is absorbed normally and is deposited in the visceral organs rather than in bone marrow.

Several patients have had refractory hypochromic anemia associated with lymphatic tumors or lymphoid hyperplasia. Correction of the anemia followed removal of the abnormal lymphatic tissue in these patients. (See also Chapter 407.)

GENERAL

Hoffman R, Benz EJ, Shattil SJ, et al: Hematology: Basic Principles and Practices, 2nd ed. New York, Churchill Livingstone, 1995.

Miller DR, Baehner RL: Blood Diseases of Infancy and Childhood, 6th ed. St. Louis, MO, CV Mosby, 1990.

Nathan DG, Oski FA: Hematology of Infancy and Childhood, 4th ed. Philadelphia, WB Saunders, 1993.

Williams WJ, Beutler E, Erslev AJ, Lichtman MA: Hematology, 4th ed. New York, McGraw-Hill, 1990.

PURE RED CELL ANEMIAS

Özsoylu S: High-dose intravenous corticosteroid treatment for patients with Diamond-Blackfan syndrome resistant or refractory to conventional treatment. Am J Pediatr Hematol Oncol 10:217, 1988.

Perdahl EV, Naprstek BL, Wallace WC, et al: Erythroid failure in Diamond-Blackfan anemia is characterized by apoptosis. Blood 83:645, 1994.

Saunders EF, Olivieri N, Freedman MH: Unexpected complications after bone marrow transplantation in transfusion-dependent children. Bone Marrow Transplant 12(Suppl 1):88, 1993.

Superti-Furga A, Schoenle E, Tuchschmid P, et al: Pearson bone marrow-pancreas syndrome with insulin-dependent diabetes, progressive renal tubulopathy, organic aciduria and elevated fetal haemoglobin caused by deletion and duplication of mitochondrial DNA. Eur J Pediatr 152:44, 1993.

Young NS, Alter BP: Aplastic Anemia: Acquired and Inherited. Philadelphia, WB Saunders, 1994.

ANEMIA OF CHRONIC DISEASE

Means RT, Krantz SB: Progress in understanding the pathogenesis of the anemia of chronic disease. Blood 80:1639, 1992.

PHYSIOLOGIC ANEMIA OF INFANCY

Bifano EM, Smith F, Borer J: Relationship between determinants of oxygen delivery and respiratory abnormalities in preterm infants with anemia. J Pediatr 120:292, 1992.

Maier RF, Obladen M, Scigalla P, et al: The effect of epoetin beta (recombinant human erythropoietin) on the need for transfusion in very-low-birth-weight infants. N Engl J Med 330:1173, 1994.

Shannon K: Recombinant erythropoietin in anemia of prematurity: Five years later. Pediatrics 92:614, 1993.

Zipursky A, Brown EJ, Watts J, et al: Oral vitamin E supplementation for the prevention of anemia in premature infants: A controlled trial. Pediatrics 79:61, 1987.

MEGALOBLASTIC ANEMIAS

Beck WS: Diagnosis of megaloblastic anemia. Annu Rev Med 42:311, 1991.

Chanarin I, Deacon R, Lumb M, et al: Cobalamin and folate: Recent developments. J Clin Pathol 45:277, 1992.

Kruhne T, Bubl R, Baumgartner R: Maternal vegan diet causing a serious infantile neurological disorder due to vitamin B_{12} deficiency. Eur J Pediatr 150:205, 1991.

Mitchell GA, Watkins D, Melancon SB, et al: Clinical heterogeneity in cobalamin C variant of combined homocystinuria and methylmalonic aciduria. J Pediatr 108:410, 1986.

Poncz M, Colman N, Herbert V, et al: Therapy of congenital folate malabsorption. J Pediatr 98:76, 1981.

MICROCYTIC ANEMIA

Cox TC, Bottomley SS, Wiley JS, et al: X-linked pyridoxine-responsive sideroblastic anemia due to A THR^{388}-TO-SER substitution in erythroid 5-aminolevulinate synthase. N Engl J Med 330:675, 1994.

Dobbing J: Brain, Behavior, and Iron in the Infant Diet. London, Springer-Verlag, 1990.

Fomon SJ, Ziegler EE, Nelson SE: Erythrocyte incorporation of ingested ^{58}Fe by 56-day-old breast-fed and formula-fed infants. Pediatr Res 33:573, 1993.

Hall RT, Wheeler RE, Benson J, et al: Feeding iron-fortified premature formula during initial hospitalization to infants less than 1800 grams birth weight. Pediatrics 92:409, 1993.

Hallberg L, Hulten L, Lindstedt G, et al: Prevalence of iron deficiency in Swedish adolescents. Pediatr Res 34:680, 1993.

Idjradinata P, Pollitt E: Reversal of developmental delays in iron-deficient anaemic infants treated with iron. Lancet 341:1, 1993.

Oski FA: Iron deficiency in infancy and childhood. N Engl J Med 329:190, 1993.

Walter T, Dallman PR, Pizarro F, et al: Effectiveness of iron-fortified infant cereal in prevention of iron deficiency anemia. Pediatrics 91:976, 1993.

SECTION 3

Hemolytic Anemias

George B. Segel

Hemolysis is defined as the premature destruction of red cells. If the rate of destruction exceeds the capacity of the marrow to produce red cells, anemia results. The normal red cell survival is 110–120 days, and approximately 1% of the red cells (the senescent ones) are removed each day and replaced by the marrow to maintain the red cell count. During hemolysis the red cell survival is shortened, and increased marrow activity results in a heightened reticulocyte percentage and number. Hemolysis should be suspected as a cause of anemia if an elevated reticulocyte count is present in the absence of bleeding or administration of hematinic therapy. The marrow can increase its output two- to threefold acutely with a maximum of six- to eightfold if hemolysis is long-standing. The reticulocyte index quantifies the magnitude of the marrow production in response to hemolysis and is calculated as follows:

$$\frac{\text{observed hematocrit}}{\text{normal hematocrit}} \times \frac{1}{\mu} \times \text{reticulocyte \%},$$

where μ is a maturation factor related to the severity of the anemia. In the absence of hemolysis the reticulocyte index is 1.0, representing normal marrow activity.

As anemia becomes more severe, there is more erythropoietin stimulation of erythropoiesis, and *reticulocytes* are released from the marrow earlier, spending more than one day as reticulocytes in the blood. In terms of quantifying the marrow response, it is inappropriate to count reticulocytes produced yesterday in today's calculation of the reticulocyte index. The maturation factor, μ, provides this correction. The usual marrow response in a chronic hemolytic anemia is reflected by a

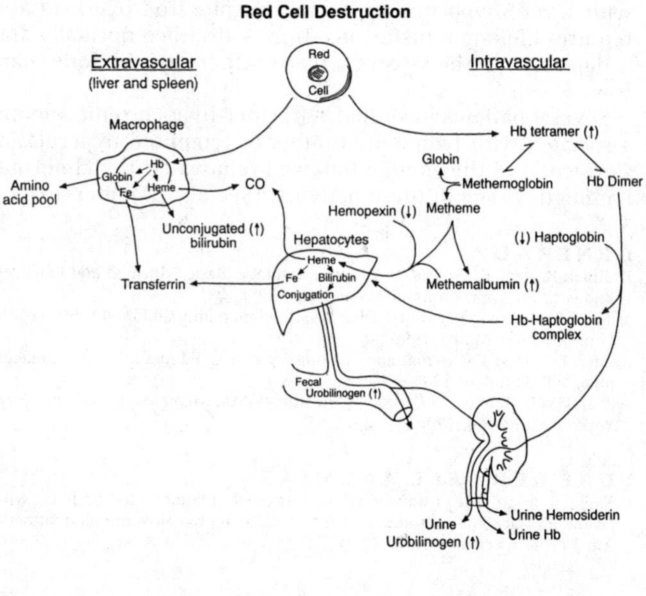

Figure XXI–3. Red cell destruction and the catabolism of hemoglobin (Hb) based on the description by Hillman and Finch. (From Hillman RS, Finch CA: Red Cell Manual. Philadelphia, FA Davis, 1983.)

■ **TABLE XXI–2 Hemolytic Anemias and Their Treatment**

Diagnosis	Defect	Laboratory Tests	Treatment
Cellular Defects			
Membrane Defects			
Hereditary Spherocytosis	Cytoskeletal protein defects Frequently involve vertical interactions of spectrin ankyrin, protein 3	Spherocytes on blood film Negative Coombs Test eliminates immune hemolysis Increased incubated osmotic fragility Abnormal cytoskeletal protein analysis	If Hb > 10 g/dl and retic. < 10%–None If severe anemia, poor growth, aplastic crises and age < 2 years–transfusion If Hb < 10 g/dl and retic. > 10% or massive spleen-splenectomy, preferably > age 6 but earlier if necessary Folic acid 1 mg qd
Hereditary Elliptocytosis	Cytoskeletal protein defects Frequently involve horizontal interactions of spectrin, protein 4.1, glycophorin C	Elliptocytes on blood film Red cells mildly heat sensitive Abnormal cytoskeletal protein analysis	Mild types–no treatment Chronic hemolysis–Transfusion and splenectomy as recommended for spherocytosis (above) Folic acid 1 mg qd
Hereditary Pyropoikilocytosis	Cytoskeletal protein defects Homozygous or double heterozygous abnormality in horizontal interactions of α spectrin	Extreme variation in red cell size and shape on blood film Thermal sensitivity-fragmentation at 45°C for 15 min	Transfusion and splenectomy as recommended for spherocytosis (above) Folic acid 1 mg qd
Hereditary Stomatocytosis	Cytoskeletal protein defects Decreased protein 7.2b (one subset) Abnormal red cell cation and water content	Stomatocytes on blood film	Response to splenectomy variable (see text) Folic acid 1 mg qd
Paroxysmal Nocturnal Hemoglobinuria	Primary acquired marrow disorder Red cells unusually sensitive to complement mediated lysis	Ham test, sucrosis lysis test Marrow aspirate and biopsy to assess cellularity Decreased decay accelerating factor	Folic acid 1 mg qd Mild cytopenias–no treatment Chronic hemolysis and other cytopenias-Prednisone 60 mg qd initially, then taper if possible; chronic 15–40 mg qod Iron for secondary iron deficiency Androgens–Halotestin 10–30 mg qd Marrow transplant for pancytopenia
Enzyme Deficiencies			
Pyruvate Kinase Deficiency	Decreased or abnormal enzyme	PK assay-decreased Vmax or rarely high Km variant	If severe anemia with symptoms, poor growth and age < 2 years-transfusion Splenectomy > age 6 but earlier if necessary Folic acid 1 mg qd
G6PD Deficiency	A type: age labile enzyme Mediterranean type: no enzyme activity in circulating red cells	G6PD assay	Avoid oxidant stress to red cells Transfusion if acute anemia is symptomatic
Hemoglobin Abnormalities (For discussion of hemoglobinopathies see sections on these topics)			
Extracellular Defects			
Autoimmune			
Autoimmune hemolytic anemia "Warm" antibody	Alteration in membrane surface antigen (Rh) or abnormal response of B-lymphocytes, causing autoantibody formation	Spherocytes on blood film Positive direct Coombs test to IgG "warm" antibody directed against red cell Positive indirect Coombs test and antibody detectable in plasma Thermal amplitude 35–40° C Some complement (C3b) may be detected on red cells Tests for underlying disease	If Hb >10 g/dL + retic <10%—none Severe anemia may require transfusion Prednisone 2 mg/kg/24 hr IVIG Danazol Splenectomy Immunosuppressives Folic acid 1 mg/24 hr if chronic
"Cold" antibody	"Cold" or IgM autoantibody directed against I/i antigen system	Agglutination or rouleaux on blood film Positive direct Coombs test to complement (C3b) Tests for underlying disease Serology for infectious mononucleosis; anti-i present Serology for *Mycoplasma pneumoniae;* anti-I present	If Hb >10 g/dL + retic <10%—none Severe anemia may require transfusion Avoid exposure to cold If severe: immunosuppressives and plasmapheresis Prednisone—*less* effective Splenectomy—*not* useful Folic acid 1 mg/24 hr if chronic
Fragmentation Hemolysis			
DIC, TTP, HUS	Direct damage to red cell membrane	Fragments on blood film	Treat underlying condition Transfusion: but transfused cells also will have shortened life span
Extracorporeal membrane oxygenation	Direct damage to red cell membrane	Fragments on blood film	Supportive Transfusion until ECMO discontinued
Prosthetic heart valve	Direct damage to red cell membrane	Fragments on blood film	Folic acid 1 mg/24 hr Iron for secondary iron deficiency
Burns—thermal injury	Direct damage to red cell membrane	Spherocytes on blood film	Supportive Transfusion
Hypersplenism	Effects of sequestration, ↓ pH, lipases and other enzymes, and macrophages on red cells	Thrombocytopenia and neutropenia	Treat underlying condition—cytopenias usually mild Splenectomy if complicating other anemia, e.g., thalassemia major Folic acid 1 mg/24 hr
Plasma Factors			
Liver disease	Alteration in plasma cholesterol and phospholipids	Target cells or spiculated red cells on blood film Abnormal liver function tests	Treat underlying condition Transfusion: but transfused cells also will have shortened life span Folic acid 1 mg/24 hr
Abetalipoproteinemia	Absence of apolipoprotein β Vitamin E deficiency and heightened sensitivity to oxidative damage	Acanthocytes on blood film Absent chylomicrons, VLDL and LDL	Vitamin E (A, K, and D) Folic acid 1 mg/24 hr Dietary restriction of triglycerides
Infections	Toxic effects on red cells	Associated symptoms and signs Cultures	Antibiotics Supportive
Wilson disease	Effect of copper on red cell membrane, usually self-limited	Spherocytes on blood film Copper, ceruloplasmin Penicillamine challenge and urine copper excretion	Penicillamine Supportive Transfusion if acute anemia is symptomatic

ECMO, extracorporeal membrane oxygenation; retic, reticulocyte count; DIC, disseminated intravascular coagulation; TTP, thrombotic thrombocytopenic purpura; HUS, hemolytic uremic syndrome; VLDL, very low density lipoproteins; LDL, low density lipoproteins; IVIG, intravenous immunoglobin.

Modified from Asselin BL, Segel GB: Rakel R (ed): Conn's Current Therapy. Philadelphia, WB Saunders, 1994, pp 338–339.

reticulocyte index of 3–4, with a maximum of 6–8 corresponding to maximal marrow output.

The *erythroid hyperplasia* resulting from chronic hemolytic anemia in children, especially thalassemia, may be so extensive that the medullary spaces may expand at the expense of the cortical bone. These changes may be evident on physical examination or on x-rays of the skull and long bones. A propensity to fracture long bones can occur also.

The *direct assessment of the severity of hemolysis* requires measurement of the red cell survival using red cells tagged with the radioisotope $Na_2{}^{51}CrO_4$. The normal value for the ^{51}Cr half-life is 25–35 days. This value is less than the expected half-life of 50–60 days because of the elution of ^{51}Cr from the labeled red cells at the rate of about 1% per day.

Several other plasma, urinary, or fecal chemical alterations reflect the presence of hemolysis. The *degradation of hemoglobin* results in the biliary excretion of heme pigments and increased fecal urobilinogen (Fig. XXI–3). Elevations of serum unconjugated bilirubin also may accompany hemolysis.

Gallstones composed of calcium bilirubinate may be formed in children as young as 4 yr of age. There are three heme-binding proteins in the plasma that are altered during hemolysis (Fig. XXI–3). Hemoglobin binds to haptoglobin and hemopexin, both of which are reduced. Oxidized heme binds to albumin to form methemalbumin, which is increased. When the capacity of these binding molecules is exceeded, free hemoglobin appears in the plasma and can be seen easily if the red cells are sedimented in a capillary hematocrit tube. If present, free hemoglobin in the plasma is prima-facie evidence of intravascular hemolysis. When the tubular reabsorptive capacity of the kidney for hemoglobin is exceeded, free hemoglobin appears in the urine. Even in the absence of hemoglobinuria, there may be iron loss resulting from reabsorbed hemoglobin and the shedding of renal epithelial cells containing hemosiderin. This may lead to secondary iron deficiency during chronic intravascular hemolysis. When hemoglobin is degraded an alpha-methene bridge is broken in the cyclic tetrapyrrole of the heme moiety with release of carbon monoxide (CO) (Fig. XXI–3). The quantitation of CO in the blood or expired air provides a dynamic measure of the hemolytic rate. The end-tidal CO is being evaluated in several research laboratories but is not used in clinical laboratories to quantify hemolysis.

The hematocrit during hemolysis is dependent on the severity of the hemolysis and on the increased marrow production of red cells. The shortened red cell life span and heightened red cell production result in a marked susceptibility to *"aplastic" or "hypoplastic" crises*, characterized by erythroid marrow failure and reticulocytopenia, accompanied by a rapid fall in hemoglobin and hematocrit. The most common cause of aplastic crises is the parvovirus, which is erythrocytotropic in marrow culture in vitro (see Chapters 210 and 419). Aplastic crises may produce a precipitous and life-threatening fall in the hematocrit, which usually lasts 10–14 days. Such transient erythroid marrow failure has little effect in persons with a normal red cell life span but has a proportionately greater effect as the red cell life span is shortened by hemolysis. A second infection with parvovirus is uncommon, but other infections may compromise the erythroid marrow output, resulting in various degrees of hypoplasia or hypoplastic crises.

The hemolytic anemias may be classified as either (1) cellular, resulting from intrinsic abnormalities of the membrane, enzymes, or hemoglobin; or (2) extracellular, resulting from antibodies, mechanical factors, or plasma factors. Most of the cellular defects are inherited (paroxysmal nocturnal hemoglobinuria is acquired), and most of the extracellular defects are acquired (abetalipoproteinemia with acanthocytosis is inherited). Table XXI–2 shows the most common hemolytic anemias, their underlying defects, the diagnostic laboratory tests, and the current recommendations for treatment. ■

CHAPTER 415

Hereditary Spherocytosis (HS)

George B. Segel

Hereditary spherocytosis is a common cause of hemolysis and hemolytic anemia with a prevalence of approximately 1:5,000 in people of Northern European extraction. It is the most common familial and congenital abnormality of the red cell membrane. Affected individuals may be asymptomatic without anemia and with minimal hemolysis, or may have a severe hemolytic anemia. Hereditary spherocytosis has been described in most ethnic groups but is most common among persons of Northern European origin.

ETIOLOGY. Hereditary spherocytosis usually is transmitted as an autosomal dominant and, less frequently, as an autosomal recessive disorder. There is a high rate of new mutations, and as many as 25% of patients may have no previous family history. The most common molecular defect is an abnormality of spectrin, which is a major component of the cytoskeleton responsible for red cell shape. A recessive defect has been described in α-spectrin; dominant defects in β-spectrin and in protein 3; and dominant and recessive defects in ankyrin. A deficiency in spectrin, protein 3, or ankyrin results in uncoupling in the "vertical" interactions of the lipid bilayer skeleton and the loss of membrane microvesicles (Fig. 415–1). The loss of membrane without a proportional loss of volume causes sphering of the red cells and an associated increase in cation permeability, cation transport, and ATP utilization, and an increase in glycolytic metabolism. The decreased deformability of the spherocytic red cells impairs cell passage from the splenic cords to the splenic sinuses, and the spherocytic red cells are destroyed prematurely in the spleen. Splenectomy markedly improves the red cell life span and cures the anemia.

CLINICAL MANIFESTATIONS. Hereditary spherocytosis may be a cause of hemolytic disease in the newborn and present with anemia and hyperbilirubinemia sufficiently severe to require phototherapy or exchange transfusions. The severity in infants and children is variable. Some patients remain asymptomatic into adulthood, while others may have severe anemia with pallor, jaundice, fatigue, and exercise intolerance. In severe cases there may be expansion of the diploë of the skull and the medullary region of other bones, but to a lesser extent than seen in thalassemia major. After infancy the spleen is usually enlarged, and pigmentary (bilirubin) gallstones may form as early as age 4–5 yr. At least 50% of unsplenectomized patients ultimately form gallstones, although, for the most part, they remain asymptomatic. Because of the high red cell turnover and heightened erythroid marrow activity, children with hereditary spherocytosis are susceptible to aplastic crisis, primarily due to parvovirus, and to hypoplastic crises associated with a variety of other infections. Such erythroid marrow failure may result rapidly in profound anemia (hematocrit $<10\%$), high output heart failure, hypoxia, cardiovascular collapse, and death.

LABORATORY FINDINGS. Evidence for hemolysis includes reticulocytosis and hyperbilirubinemia. The hemoglobin level usually is 6–10 g/dL, but it can be in the normal range. The reticulocyte count often is heightened to 6–20%, with a mean of approximately 10%. The mean corpuscular volume is normal, while the mean corpuscular hemoglobin concentration often is increased (36–38 g/dL red cells). The red cells on the blood film vary in size and include polychromatophilic reticulocytes and spherocytes (Fig. 415–2*A*). The spherocytes are smaller in diameter and on the blood film are hyperchromic as a result of the high hemoglobin concentration. The central pallor is less conspicuous than in normal cells. Spherocytes may be the

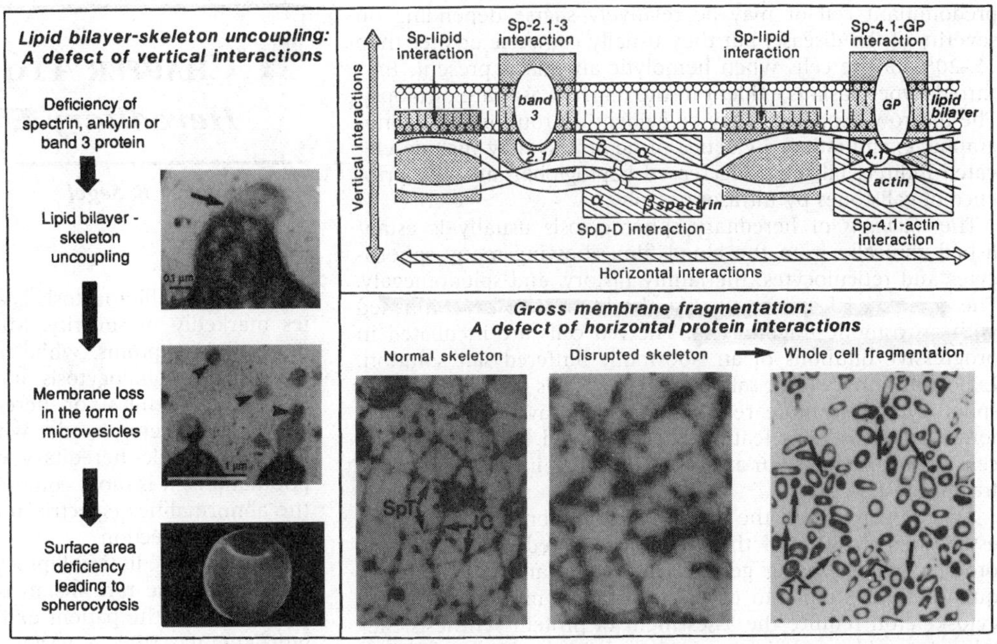

Figure 415–1. Vertical and horizontal interactions of membrane proteins and the pathobiology of the red cell lesion in hereditary spherocytosis (HS) and hereditary elliptocytosis/hereditary pyropoikilocytosis (HE/HPP). *Left*: A defect of vertical or transverse interactions as exemplified by the red cell membrane lesion in HS. Partial deficiencies of spectrin, ankyrin (band 2.1), or band 3 protein lead to uncoupling of the membrane lipid bilayer from the underlying skeleton *(arrow)* followed by a formation of spectrin-free microvesicles of approximately 0.2–0.5 μm in diameter *(arrowheads)*. These vesicles can be visualized by transmission electron microscopy, but they are not seen during examination of blood films. The subsequent loss of cell surface and a decrease in the surface/volume ratio leads to spherocytosis. *Right*: Defect of horizontal or parallel interactions of skeletal proteins as exemplified by the membrane lesion in hemolytic forms of HE associated with a defect of spectrin heterodimer self-association. The molecular lesion involving a weakened self-association of spectrin heterodimers to tetramers represents a horizontal defect of the stress-supporting protein interactions. It leads to a disruption of the membrane skeletal lattice and, consequently, whole cell destabilization followed by red cell fragmentation and poikilocytosis. Such fragments are readily seen on stained blood films. (Modified from Palek J, Jarolim P: Clinical expression and laboratory detection of red blood cell membrane protein mutations. Semin Hematol 30:249, 1993.)

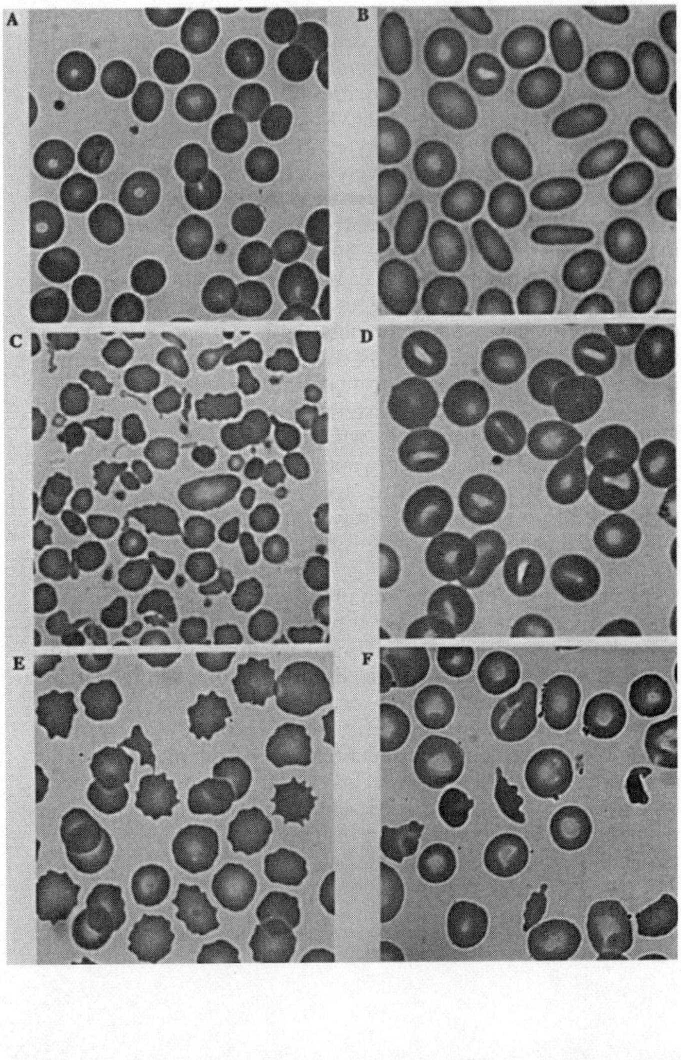

Figure 415–2. Morphology of abnormal red cells. *A*, Hereditary spherocytosis; *B*, hereditary elliptocytosis; *C*, hereditary pyropoikilocytosis; *D*, hereditary stomatocytosis; *E*, acanthocytosis; *F*, fragmentation hemolysis. See also color section.

predominant cell or may be relatively sparse depending on severity of the disease, but they usually comprise greater than 15–20% of the cells when hemolytic anemia is present. Erythroid hyperplasia is evident in the marrow aspirate or biopsy. The marrow expansion may be evident on routine roentgenographic examination. Evidence of hemolysis may include elevated indirect bilirubin, decreased haptoglobin, and the presence of gallstones by ultrasonography.

The *diagnosis* of hereditary spherocytosis usually is established clinically from the blood film, showing many spherocytes and reticulocytes, the family history, and splenomegaly. The presence of spherocytes in the blood can be confirmed with an osmotic fragility test. The red cells are incubated in progressive dilutions of an isoosmotic buffered salt solution. Exposure to hypotonic saline causes red cells to swell, and the spherocytes lyse more readily than biconcave cells in hypotomic solutions. This feature is accentuated by depriving the cells of glucose for 24 hr at 37° C, a so-called incubated osmotic fragility test.

As a research tool, the specific protein abnormality can be established in 80% of these patients by red cell membrane protein analysis using gel electrophoresis and densitometric quantitation. Studies to define the underlying defects in the cytoskeleton require the assessment of protein synthesis, stability, assembly, and binding to the other membrane proteins.

DIFFERENTIAL DIAGNOSIS. The major alternative consideration when large numbers of spherocytes are seen on the blood film is immune hemolysis. Isoimmune hemolytic disease of the newborn, particularly due to ABO incompatibility, mimics hereditary spherocytosis. The detection of antibody on the infant's red cells using a direct Coombs test should establish the diagnosis of immune hemolysis. Other autoimmune hemolytic anemias also are characterized by spherocytes, and there may be evidence of a previously normal hemoglobin, hematocrit, and reticulocyte count. Rare causes of spherocytosis include thermal injury, clostridia septicemia with exotoxemia, and Wilson disease, each of which may present with a transient hemolytic anemia (see Tables 405–2, XXI–2).

TREATMENT. Since the spherocytes in hereditary spherocytosis are destroyed almost exclusively in the spleen, splenectomy eliminates most of the hemolysis associated with this disorder. After splenectomy, the spherocytes may be more numerous, increasing the osmotic fragility, but the anemia, reticulocytosis, and hyperbilirubinemia resolve. Whether all patients with hereditary spherocytosis should undergo splenectomy has become controversial. Some hematologists do not recommend splenectomy for those patients whose hemoglobin values are >10 g/dL and whose reticulocyte counts are <10%. Folic acid, 1 mg/24 hr, should be administered to prevent secondary folic acid deficiency. For patients with more severe anemia and reticulocytosis or those with hypoplastic or aplastic crises, splenectomy is recommended after age 5–6 yr to avoid the heightened risk of postsplenectomy sepsis in younger children. Vaccines for encapsulated organisms such as pneumococcus, meningococcus, and *Haemophilus influenzae* should be administered prior to splenectomy, and prophylactic penicillin (age ≤5 yr: 125 mg/12 hr; age >5 yr through adulthood: 250 mg/12 hr) administered thereafter. Postsplenectomy thrombocytosis is commonly observed but needs no treatment and usually resolves spontaneously. In one report partial splenectomy provided substantial increases in Hb and reductions in the reticulocyte count with potential maintenance of splenic phagocytic and immune function. This technique, if substantiated, would be particularly useful for those children less than 5 yr of age with severe disease and could be employed in older patients with mild disease.

CHAPTER 416
Hereditary Elliptocytosis

George B. Segel

Hereditary elliptocytosis is an uncommon disorder that varies markedly in severity. Mild hereditary elliptocytosis produces no symptoms, while more severe varieties may result in neonatal poikilocytosis and hemolysis, chronic or sporadic hemolytic anemias, or hereditary pyropoikilocytosis (HPP), which is a severe disorder with microspherocytosis and poikilocytosis. While hereditary elliptocytosis is rare in western populations, it is more commonly found in West Africa, where the abnormalities (spectrin mutations) may provide resistance to malarial infection.

ETIOLOGY. Hereditary elliptocytosis is inherited as a dominant disorder. In the rare instances wherein two abnormal alleles are inherited, the patient exhibits a particularly severe hemolytic anemia, HPP. A variety of molecular defects has been described in hereditary elliptocytosis that produce abnormalities of α- and β-spectrin and defective spectrin heterodimer self-association (see Fig. 415–1). Such defects in the horizontal protein interactions result in gross membrane fragmentation, particularly in homozygous HPP. Less commonly, mutations in protein 4.1 and glycophorin C may produce elliptocytosis.

CLINICAL MANIFESTATIONS. Elliptocytosis may be noted as an incidental finding on a routine blood film and not be associated with clinically significant hemolysis (see Fig. 415–2*B*). The diagnosis of hereditary elliptocytosis is established by the findings on the blood film, the autosomal dominant inheritance pattern, and the absence of other causes of elliptocytosis, such as iron, folic acid, or B_{12} deficiencies. Hemolytic elliptocytosis may produce neonatal jaundice, even though characteristic elliptocytosis may not be evident at that time. The blood of the affected newborn may show bizarre poikilocytes and pyknocytes. The usual features of a chronic hemolytic process with elliptocytosis are seen later as anemia, jaundice, splenomegaly, and osseous changes. Cholelithiasis may occur in later childhood, and aplastic crises have been reported. The most severe form is HPP, which is characterized by extreme microcytosis (mean corpuscular volume [MCV] 50–60 fl/cell), with extraordinary variation in the cell size and shape, and primarily microspherocytic rather than elliptocytic cells (see Fig. 415–2*C*). These patients inherit a mutant spectrin from one parent, who has mild or no elliptocytosis, and a partial spectrin deficiency from the other parent, who is hematologically normal.

LABORATORY FINDINGS. The blood film is the most important test to establish hereditary elliptocytosis (see Fig. 415–2*B*). The red cells show various degrees of elongation and may actually be rod shaped. Ovalocytes, in contrast to elliptocytes, are less elongated and may reflect a condition termed *Southeast Asian ovalocytosis* (SAO), which is associated with a mutant protein 3 but does not cause hemolysis. In addition to elliptocytosis, other abnormal red cell shapes may be present depending on the severity of hemolysis. They include microcytes, spherocytes, and other poikilocytes. The reticulocyte count reflects the severity of hemolysis, and erythroid hyperplasia and indirect hyperbilirubinemia may be present. Increased thermal instability is characteristic of HPP, wherein the abnormal spectrin denatures and the cells lyse at 45–46° C instead of the usual 49–50° C. The specific protein abnormality can be established by protein separation and analysis techniques.

TREATMENT. If hereditary elliptocytosis represents a morphologic abnormality on the blood film without hemolysis, no treatment is necessary. Patients with chronic hemolysis should receive folic acid 1 mg/24 hr to prevent secondary folic acid deficiency. Splenectomy decreases the hemolysis and should be considered if the Hb is <10 g/dL and the reticulocyte count is >10%. The red cells on the blood film may be more abnormal after splenectomy even though Hb increases and the reticulocytes decrease (see Chapter 415).

CHAPTER 417
Hereditary Stomatocytosis

George B. Segel

Hereditary stomatocytosis is a rare condition in which the red cells are cup-shaped. On stained blood film they present a mouthlike slit in place of the usual circular area of central pallor (Fig. 415–2*D*). Acquired stomatocytosis may be seen in several conditions, especially liver disease. Hereditary stomatocytosis may be associated with alterations in red cell hydration status or with deficiency in Rh antigens. The hydrocytic or overhydrated variety is associated with abnormalities within the region of protein 7, but the basic pathophysiology has not been defined. There may be hemolytic anemia associated with hereditary stomatocytosis, but splenectomy is not consistently effective as treatment. Symptomatic thrombocytosis may complicate splenectomy if the hemolysis is not decreased. Furthermore, a subgroup of patients has developed the life-threatening tendency to in situ thrombosis postsplenectomy, which may be related to abnormal adherence of the stomatocytic red cells to vascular endothelium as well as to the thrombocytosis.

CHAPTER 418
Other Membrane Defects

George B. Segel

PAROXYSMAL NOCTURNAL HEMOGLOBINURIA (PNH)

ETIOLOGY. Paroxysmal nocturnal hemoglobinuria reflects a clonal abnormality of a marrow stem cell that affects multiple blood cell lines. The disease is not inherited; it is an acquired disorder of hematopoiesis characterized by a defect in proteins of the cell membrane that renders the red cells (and other cells) susceptible to damage by serum complement. The deficient membrane–associated proteins include decay accelerating factor, the C8 binding protein, and other proteins that normally impede complement lysis at various steps. The underlying defect involves the glycolipid anchor that maintains these proteins on the cell surface, and various mutations in the *PIG-A* gene involved in glycolipid biosynthesis have been identified in PNH patients.

CLINICAL MANIFESTATIONS. PNH is a rare disorder, particularly in children, but 26 patients with a mean age of 13 yr (0.8–21.4 yr) were diagnosed at Duke University Medical Center between 1966 and 1991. Approximately 60% of these patients presented with marrow failure, while the remainder had either intermittent or chronic anemia, often with prominent intravascular hemolysis. Nocturnal and morning hemoglobinuria are classic findings in adults if hemolysis is worse during sleep. However, chronic hemolysis is more common in PNH in spite of its name. In addition to chronic hemolysis, thrombocytopenia and leukopenia often are present. Pyogenic infection, thrombosis, and thromboembolic phenomena are serious complications. Abdominal, back, and head pain may be prominent complaints. Hypoplastic or aplastic pancytopenia may precede or follow the onset of PNH, and the clonal disorder rarely progresses to acute myelogenous leukemia. The predicted survival for children is 80% for 5 yr, 60% for 10 yr, and 28% for 20 yr, and the mortality is related primarily to the development of aplastic anemia and/or thrombotic complications.

LABORATORY FINDINGS. The diagnosis of PNH is established by a positive result in the acid serum (Ham) or the sucrose lysis test, which activate the alternate and classical pathways of complement lysis, respectively. Hemosiderinuria is seen frequently and reflects the intravascular hemolysis (see Fig. XXI–4). Markedly reduced levels of red cell acetylcholinesterase activity are also found, and the reduced levels of *decay accelerating factor* are diagnostic.

TREATMENT. Splenectomy is not indicated. Glucocorticoids such as prednisone (2 mg/kg/24 hr) have been used to treat acute hemolytic episodes and should be tapered as soon as the hemolysis abates. Prolonged anticoagulation therapy may be of benefit when thromboses occur. Because there is chronic loss of iron as hemosiderin in the urine, iron therapy may be necessary. Androgens such as halotestin and danazol, and antithymocyte globulin, have been used to treat marrow aplasia. Bone marrow transplantation has been successful in treating some cases.

ACANTHOCYTOSIS

Acanthocytosis is characterized by red cells with irregular circumferential pointed projections (Fig. 415–2*E*). This morphologic finding is seen with alterations in the cholesterol/phospholipid ratio in some patients with liver disease, and in congenital abetalipoproteinemia associated with malabsorption, neuromuscular abnormalities, and retinitis pigmentosa (Chapters 72.4, 286.12). It also is associated with the rare X-linked McLeod syndrome with absence of the Kx (Kell) antigen, late onset myopathy, neurologic abnormalities, splenomegaly, and hemolysis with acanthocytosis.

GENERAL

Nathan DG, Oski FA: Hematology of Infancy and Childhood, 4th ed. Philadelphia, WB Saunders, 1993.

Oski FA, Naiman JL: Hematologic Problems of the Newborn, 3rd ed. Philadelphia, WB Saunders, 1982.

Stockman JA III, Pochedly C: Developmental and Neonatal Hematology. New York, Raven Press, 1988.

HEMOLYTIC ANEMIAS

Asselin BL, Segel GB: Nonimmune Hemolytic Anemia. *In:* Rakel R (ed): Conn's Current Therapy. Philadelphia, WB Saunders, 1994, p 336.

Dacie JV: The Haemolytic Anemias, 3rd ed. New York, Grune & Stratton, 1985.

Hillman RS, Finch CA: Red Cell Manual. Philadelphia, FA Davis, 1974.

HEREDITARY SPHEROCYTOSIS AND OTHER MEMBRANE PROTEINS

Eber SW, Lande WM, Iarocci TA, Mentzer WC, Hohn P, Wiley JS, Schroter W: Hereditary stomatocytosis: consistent association with an integral membrane protein deficiency. Br J Haematol 72:452, 1989.

Eber SW, Armbrust R, Schroter W: Variable clinical severity of hereditary spherocytosis: Relation to erythrocytic spectrum concentration, osmotic fragility, and autohemolysis. J Pediatr 117:409, 1990.

Kelleher JH, Lerban NLC, Mortimer PP: Human serum "parvovirus": A specific cause of aplastic crisis in children with hereditary spherocytosis. J Pediatr 102:722, 1983.

Manno CS, Cohen AR: Splenectomy in mild hereditary spherocytosis: Is it worth the risk? Am J Pediatr Hematol Oncol 11:300, 1989.

Palek J, Jarolim P: Clinical expression and laboratory detection of red blood cell membrane protein mutations. Semin Hematol 30:249, 1993.
Tchernia G, Gauthier F, Mielot F, Dommergues JP, Yvart J, Chasis JA, Mohandas N: Initial assessment of the beneficial effect of partial splenectomy in hereditary spherocytosis. Blood 81:2014, 1993.

PAROXYSMAL NOCTURNAL HEMOGLOBINURIA
Miyata T, Yamada N, Irda Y, et al: Abnormalities in PIG-A transcripts in granulocytes from patients with paroxysmal nocturnal hemoglobinuria. N Engl J Med 330:249, 1994.
Rosse WF: Paroxysmal nocturnal hemoglobinuria and decay-accelerating factor. Annu Rev Med 41:431, 1990.
Ware RE, Hall SE, Rosse WF: Paroxysmal nocturnal hemoglobinuria with onset in childhood and adolescence. N Engl J Med 325:991, 1991.

CHAPTER 419
Hemoglobin Disorders

George R. Honig

The clinical disorders that result from abnormalities of the globin genes comprise a diverse group of hematologic diseases. Normal hemoglobins are tetrameric molecules containing pairs of α or α-like and β or β-like globin-heme subunits. The normal postnatal hemoglobins include hemoglobin (Hb) A ($\alpha_2\beta_2$), Hb F ($\alpha_2\gamma_2$), and Hb A_2 ($\alpha_2\delta_2$). The embryonic hemoglobins, which usually disappear before birth, include Hb Gower-1 ($\zeta_2\epsilon_2$), Hb Gower-2 ($\alpha_2\epsilon_2$), and Hb Portland ($\zeta_2\gamma_2$) (see also Part XXI, Section 1). The genes for the α and ζ chains are encoded on chromosome 16; those for the β group have been localized to chromosome 11. The nucleotide sequences of all these genes have been determined, and many globin-gene abnormalities have been characterized at the molecular level.

The hemoglobin disorders are subdivided into three major groups. The structural abnormalities, including the hemoglobinopathies, result from changes in the amino acid sequences of the globin chains. Most have a single amino acid substitution; in others, however, amino acids may be deleted or inserted, or other, more complex, structural changes may be present. The thalassemias are expressed as quantitative defects, in which the synthesis of one or more of the globin chains is decreased or, in the most severe forms, is totally suppressed. The hereditary persistence of fetal hemoglobin (HPFH) syndromes is characterized by elevated levels of Hb F continuing throughout adult life. Almost all these abnormalities result from the same types of molecular defects: Nucleotides may be substituted, deleted, or inserted into globin-gene DNA.

HEMOGLOBIN STRUCTURAL ABNORMALITIES
(Hemoglobinopathies)

Approximately 600 structural variants of hemoglobin have been identified. Most are rare but a few, including some severely pathologic forms, occur with high frequency in certain populations. Many abnormal hemoglobins are readily identified by electrophoresis, but some are electrophoretically "silent" and require other laboratory studies for identification. Many hemoglobin variants that have abnormal electrophoretic mobility, including benign and pathologic forms, exhibit very similar electrophoresis findings and cannot be specifically identified by this means alone.

419.1 Sickle Cell Hemoglobinopathies

Sickle hemoglobin (Hb S) differs from normal adult hemoglobin by a substitution of glutamic acid at the 6th position of its β chains by valine. In the oxygenated state Hb S functions normally. When this hemoglobin is deoxygenated, an interaction between the β6 valine and complementary regions on the β chains of an adjacent molecule results in the formation of highly ordered molecular polymers; these elongate to form filamentous structures, which aggregate into rigid, crystal-like rods. This process of molecular polymerization is responsible for the spiny, brittle character of sickle erythrocytes under conditions of decreased oxygenation. Certain other abnormal hemoglobins, notably Hb C, Hb D Los Angeles, and Hb O Arab, participate in the molecular polymerization of deoxy-Hb S. Hb A does so to a smaller degree, but fetal hemoglobin (Hb F) does not.

Erythrocytes of heterozygous (sickle cell trait) individuals have been shown to resist invasion by malarial parasites, which appears to have provided protection against the frequently lethal *Plasmodium falciparum* form of the disease. The β^s gene is found in high frequency in those living in regions in which *P. falciparum* malaria has been endemic, including many parts of Africa, the Mediterranean area, and parts of Turkey, the Middle East, and India. In individuals from several geographic areas, the sickle mutation has been shown to exist in genetic linkage with discrete sets of closely associated markers. Some of these Hb S "haplotypes" appear to be predictive of the degree of severity of the sickle cell disease. Those associated with particularly mild disease produce significantly higher levels of fetal hemoglobin. Patients with sickle cell disease who coinherit genes for α-thalassemia may also have disease of modified severity.

Hb S is readily identified by electrophoresis. A confirmatory solubility test excludes other abnormal hemoglobins with similar electrophoretic mobility. Although affected newborns express only small quantities of Hb S, because of the predominance of Hb F at birth, the sickle cell syndromes can nevertheless be identified reliably in the newborn by electrophoretic methods. Neonatal screening programs for the detection of infants with sickle cell disease are widely established in the United States. These disorders can also be determined antenatally using amniocyte or chorionic villus DNA by methods that identify the specific β^s nucleotide substitution.

SICKLE CELL ANEMIA
(Homozygous Hb S)

This disorder is characterized by severe chronic hemolytic disease resulting from premature destruction of the brittle, poorly deformable erythrocytes. Other manifestations of sickle cell anemia are attributable to ischemic changes resulting from vascular occlusion by masses of sickled cells. The clinical course of affected children is typically associated with intermittent episodic events, often referred to as "crises."

CLINICAL MANIFESTATIONS. Affected newborns seldom exhibit clinical features of sickle cell disease; hemolytic anemia gradually develops over the 1st 2–4 mo, parallelling the replacement of much of the fetal hemoglobin by Hb S. Other clinical manifestations are uncommon prior to 5–6 mo of age. Acute sickle dactylitis, presenting as the *hand-foot syndrome,* is frequently the 1st overt evidence that sickle cell disease is present in the infant. Its associated findings include painful, usually symmetric, swelling of the hands and feet. The underlying abnormality is ischemic necrosis of the small bones, believed to be caused by a choking off of the blood supply as a result of the rapidly expanding bone marrow. Roentgenograms are not informative in the acute phase, but later show evidence of extensive bony destruction and repair (Fig. 419–1).

Acute painful vaso-occlusive episodes represent the most frequent and prominent manifestation of sickle cell disease. Most patients experience some pain on a nearly daily basis. Episodes of severe pain that require hospitalization and parenteral analgesic administration average about one per year in children with Hb SS, but this interval varies considerably, with some patients never experiencing severe pain and others requiring hospital admission with such frequency as to become seriously disabled. In young children pain often involves the extremities; in older patients head, chest, abdominal, and back pain occur more commonly. In an individual patient pain tends to recur in a limited number of sites. Intercurrent illnesses accompanied by fever, hypoxia, and acidosis, all of which promote the deoxygenation of Hb S, may precipitate sickle pain episodes, but acute pain also develops frequently without an apparent antecedent event. Sickle-related abdominal pain may mimic that of an acute surgical condition.

More extensive vaso-occlusive events in these patients can produce gross ischemic damage. Acute pain episodes may progress to infarction of bone marrow or bone. Splenic infarcts are common in children between 6 and 60 mo, causing pain and contributing to the process of "autosplenectomy." Pulmonary infarction, often occurring in association with pneumonitis or microscopic fat emboli (from bone marrow infarction) may produce the severe clinical picture of *acute chest syndrome.* Strokes caused by cerebrovascular occlusion are among the most catastrophic acute events and are a frequent cause of hemiplegia. As many as 10% of children with sickle cell anemia, mainly pre-adolescent and older patients, exhibit sequelae of cerebrovascular occlusion. Ischemic damage may also affect the myocardium, liver, and kidneys. Renal function is progressively impaired by diffuse glomerular and tubular fibrosis, and hyposthenuria accompanied by polyuria are characteristic findings in patients over 5 yr of age. Renal papillary necrosis and nephrotic syndrome also develop occasionally. *Priapism* is a relatively frequent complication that results from the pooling of blood in the corpora cavernosa, causing obstruction of the venous outflow.

Young children with Hb SS may have splenic enlargement associated with their hemolytic disease, with progression to the syndrome of hypersplenism accompanied by worsening anemia and sometimes thrombocytopenia. *Acute splenic sequestration* is a distinct and episodic event that occurs in infants and young children with sickle cell anemia. For unknown reasons large amounts of blood become acutely pooled in the spleen, which becomes massively enlarged, and signs of circulatory collapse rapidly develop. Blood transfusions in the acute phase may be lifesaving.

Altered splenic function in young children with sickle cell disease is a significant factor leading to their increased susceptibility to meningitis, sepsis, and other serious infections, mainly caused by pneumococci and *Haemophilus influenzae.* In the absence of specific antibody to the polysaccharide capsular antigens of these organisms, splenic activity is essential for removing these bacteria when they invade the blood. In spite of frequent enlargement of the spleen in young patients with Hb SS, its phagocytic and reticuloendothelial functions have been shown to be markedly reduced. As an additional risk factor, children with sickle cell disease have also been shown to have deficient levels of serum opsonins of the alternate complement pathway, against pneumococci. Children with sickle cell disease also have increased susceptibility to *Salmonella* osteomyelitis (due, in part, to bone necrosis).

In common with patients having other forms of chronic hemolytic anemia, children with Hb SS are at risk of developing a rapid, potentially life-threatening decrease in their hemoglobin level (aplastic episodes) in association with parvovirus infection (see Chapter 210).

An additional group of sickle cell sequelae is attributable primarily to the hemolytic anemia that accompanies this disorder. *Hemolytic crisis* may occur with concomitant G-6-PD deficiency (Chapter 420.3). Cardiomegaly is invariably present in older children, often caused partly by sickle-related cardiomyopathy. Increased iron absorption contributes to parenchymal damage of the liver, pancreas, and heart. Symptomatic gallstone formation is common in adolescent and adult patients, occasionally occurring in children as young as 5 yr of age.

By midchildhood most patients are underweight, and puberty is frequently delayed. Chronic leg ulcers are relatively uncommon in children, usually occurring only in late adolescence.

LABORATORY FINDINGS. Hemoglobin concentrations usually

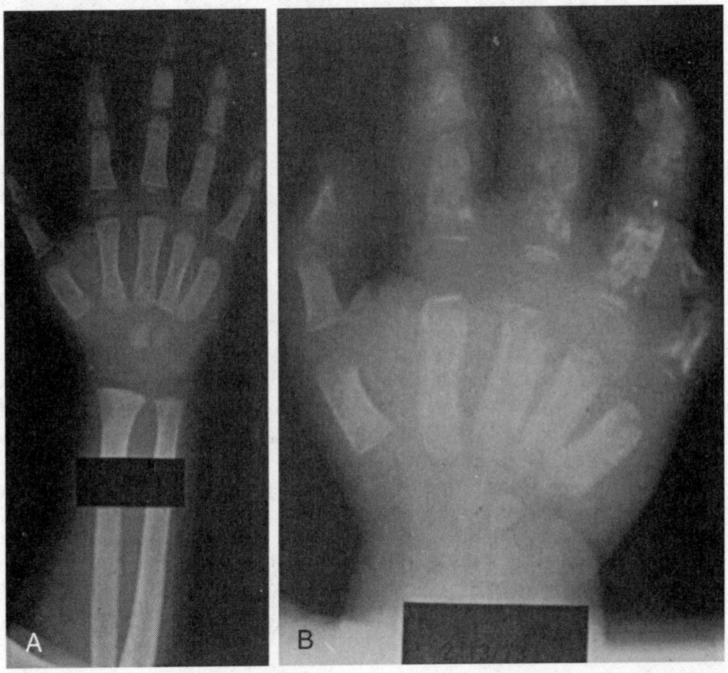

Figure 419–1. Roentgenograms of an infant with sickle cell anemia and acute dactylitis. *A*, The bones appear normal at the onset of the episode. *B*, Destructive changes and periosteal reaction are evident 2 wk later.

range from 5 to 9 g/dL. The peripheral blood smear typically contains target cells, poikilocytes, and irreversibly sickled cells (Fig. 419–2*A*). These findings allow Hb SS and most of the other forms of sickle cell disease to be readily distinguished from sickle cell trait and other clinically benign conditions. Reticulocyte counts usually range from 5% to 15%, and nucleated red cells and Howell-Jolly bodies are often present. The total white blood cell count is elevated to 12,000–20,000/mm³, with a predominance of neutrophils. The platelet count is usually increased; the sedimentation rate is slow. Other changes include abnormal liver function test results, hyperbilirubinemia, and diffuse hypergammaglobulinemia. The bone marrow is markedly hyperplastic and shows erythroid predominance. Roentgenograms show expanded marrow spaces and osteoporosis.

DIAGNOSIS. The diagnosis is established by hemoglobin studies. Electrophoresis at an alkaline pH demonstrates a characteristic mobility, intermediate between those of Hb A and Hb A_2. To distinguish Hb S from other hemoglobins with similar electrophoretic properties, another (confirmatory) test is required, such as electrophoresis at an acidic pH, a sickle cell preparation in which sickling is observed when the cells are deoxygenated or, most commonly, a hemoglobin solubility test. In the Hb S solubility test a measured amount of hemoglobin is added to a concentrated buffer that contains a reducing agent; a turbid precipitate forms when more than about 15% Hb S is present.

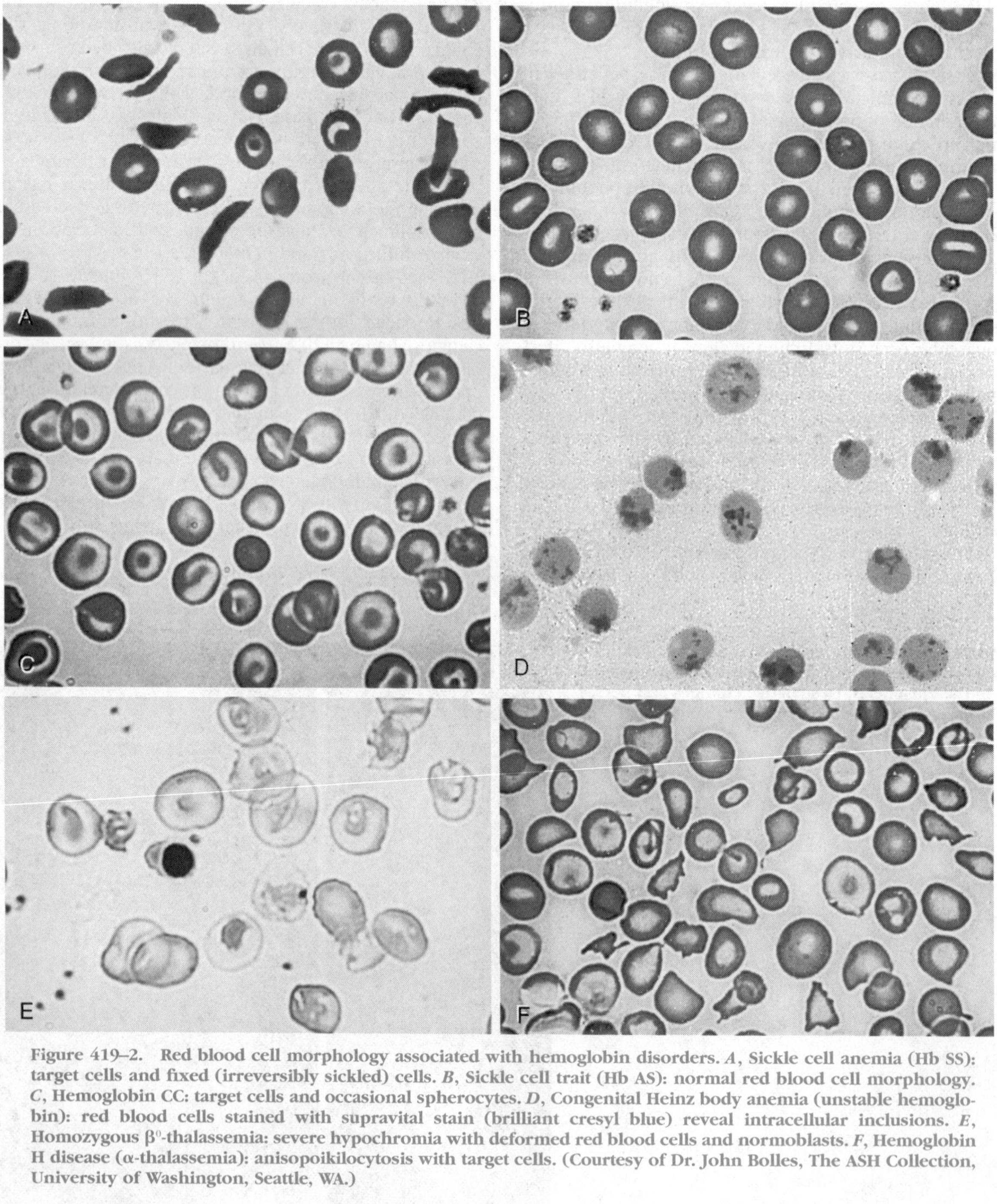

Figure 419–2. Red blood cell morphology associated with hemoglobin disorders. *A*, Sickle cell anemia (Hb SS): target cells and fixed (irreversibly sickled) cells. *B*, Sickle cell trait (Hb AS): normal red blood cell morphology. *C*, Hemoglobin CC: target cells and occasional spherocytes. *D*, Congenital Heinz body anemia (unstable hemoglobin): red blood cells stained with supravital stain (brilliant cresyl blue) reveal intracellular inclusions. *E*, Homozygous β^0-thalassemia: severe hypochromia with deformed red blood cells and normoblasts. *F*, Hemoglobin H disease (α-thalassemia): anisopoikilocytosis with target cells. (Courtesy of Dr. John Bolles, The ASH Collection, University of Washington, Seattle, WA.)

Beyond infancy, red cells from patients with Hb SS contain Hb with between 2% and 20% Hb F and normal quantities of Hb A_2. Hb A is notably absent. The identification of Hb S in each parent provides additional supportive evidence for the diagnosis of sickle cell anemia.

DIFFERENTIAL DIAGNOSIS. The various clinical manifestations of sickle cell disease, including limb pain, heart murmurs, hepatosplenomegaly, and anemia, may suggest a number of other diagnoses, including rheumatic fever or rheumatoid arthritis, osteomyelitis, and leukemia. In patients who have a Hb SS electrophoresis pattern and concomitant microcytosis (MCV <78 fL), possibilities that require consideration include iron deficiency or a combination of Hb S with α- or β^{o}-thalassemia (Table 419–1).

TREATMENT. Measures directed toward the prevention of serious complications of sickle cell disease are among the most important elements of patient management. Maintaining full immunization status of these children is particularly important. Administration of a polyvalent pneumococcal vaccine may be beneficial, but unfortunately the forms of these vaccines currently available appear to be poorly immunogenic in children with Hb SS who are under the age of 5 yr. *Haemophilus influenzae* immunization has been shown to be efficacious in infants with sickle cell disease, and this as well as hepatitis B immunizations are indicated. Prophylactic penicillin G is highly effective in preventing serious pneumococcal infections and should be administered to all young children with sickle cell disease. The penicillin is given orally, twice daily, starting in early infancy and continuing at least to the age of 6 yr. Parents of these children also need to be aware of the need to bring the child promptly to medical attention for acute illness, especially with fever above 39° C. Because of the substantial risk of life-threatening bacterial infections, prompt parenteral antibiotic therapy is generally indicated for infants and young children with an acute onset of high fever. Patients older than 6 mo, excluding those with temperatures above 40° C or who appear seriously ill, generally can be managed effectively on an outpatient basis. In low-risk, well-appearing children, after blood cultures are obtained, intravenous ceftriaxone is given, and the dose is repeated the following day. Parents and caretakers of these children should also be informed about the manifestations of acute splenic sequestration and the need for immediate medical attention for the child with rapid splenic enlargement and pallor.

Painful episodes can frequently be managed with oral acetaminophen, alone or with codeine. More severe episodes may require hospitalization and the parenteral administration of narcotics. Anti-inflammatory agents, ketorolac or, less often, corticosteroids, may decrease or eliminate the need for narcotic analgesics. Epidural analgesia has also been used to manage pain from severe vaso-occusive crisis. Any dehydration and/or acidosis should be rapidly corrected by the intravenous route. Blood transfusions are seldom indicated for painful episodes, and it is doubtful whether transfusion can ameliorate the course of a pain crisis. For patients with disabling chronic pain, for those with ischemic organ damage (acute chest, priapism) or stroke, or in preparation for major surgery, however, transfusions of normal red blood cells can provide symptomatic relief and prevent further ischemic complications. For patients with stroke, cardiomyopathy, and other severe complications, chronic long-term transfusion regimens are a mainstay of therapy. It is important to select the minimum amount of blood necessary to achieve the desired Hb S percentage. These patients also often require iron chelation treatment to prevent the development of hemosiderosis. Packed red blood cell transfusions are specifically indicated for acute splenic sequestration and aplastic episodes. Repeated episodes of splenic sequestration are also an indication for splenectomy.

Bone marrow transplantation from a normal donor can be curative in patients with sickle cell disease, but the risks and morbidity associated with this procedure limit its application to highly selected patients. European experience, from more than 40 young children without chronic organ damage, has shown a high success rate following transplantation. In the United States, fewer patients have been transplanted, most of whom had severe consequences of vaso-occlusive events; all were improved, but some have had neurologic complications post-transplantation.

Chemotherapy regimens that stimulate fetal hemoglobin synthesis have been employed with beneficial effect, on an

■ **TABLE 419–1 Clinically Important Sickle Cell Syndromes***

Sickle Cell Disorder	Hemoglobin Composition (%)	Hb A_2 Level	Erythrocyte Volume (MCV)†	Clinical Severity	Clinical Features
Hb SS	Hb S: 80–95 Hb F: 2–20	Normal	Normal	++ to ++++	See text
Hb S-β^{0}-thalassemia	Hb S: 75–90 Hb F: 5–25	Increased	Decreased	++ to ++++	Generally indistinguishable from SS
Hb S-β^{+}-thalassemia	Hb S: 5–85 Hb A: 10–30 Hb F: 5–10	Increased	Decreased	+ to +++	Generally milder than SS
Hb SS with α-thalassemia trait (−,α/ −,α)	Hb S: 80–90 Hb F: 10–20	Normal	Decreased	++ to ++++	May be milder than SS
Hb SC	Hb S: 45–50 Hb C: 45–50 Hb F: 2–5	Normal	Normal	+ to +++	Generally milder than SS; higher frequency of bone infarcts and proliferative retinal disease
Hb SO Arab	Hb S: 50–55 Hb O: 40–45 Hb F: 2–15	Normal	Normal	++ to ++++	Generally indistinguishable from SS
Hb SD Los Angeles	Hb S: 45–50 Hb D: 30–40 Hb F: 5–20	Normal	Normal	++ to ++++	May be as severe as SS
Hb S/HPFH‡	Hb S: 65–80 Hb F: 15–30	Normal	Normal	0 to +	Usually asymptomatic
Hb AS‡	Hb S: 32–45 Hb A: 52–65	Normal	Normal	0 to +	Asymptomatic

**Adapted from Honig GR, Adams JG III: Human Hemoglobin Genetics. Vienna, Springer-Verlag, 1986.*
†MCV = mean corpuscular volume.
‡These conditions do not ordinarily produce sickle cell disease.

experimental basis, in a number of children with sickle cell disease. These agents, which include hydroxyurea and butyrate, offer considerable promise of more effective means for treating these patients.

OTHER SICKLE CELL SYNDROMES

Sickling disorders of varying degrees of severity result from Hb S existing in combination with other abnormal hemoglobins or thalassemias (see Table 419–1). Several of these syndromes, including Hb SD Los Angeles, Hb SO Arab, and Hb S–β^o-thalassemia, present a clinical picture virtually indistinguishable from that of sickle cell anemia. Most of the others produce less severe manifestations.

Hb SC disease results from the concurrence of genes for Hb S and Hb C. Painful episodes and other vaso-occlusive manifestations are usually less severe in this condition than those associated with Hb SS. Most affected children have persistent splenomegaly, and bone infarcts occur more frequently than in those with Hb SS. Septicemia may also occur. Retinal vascular changes, predominantly in adolescents and adults, may lead to hemorrhage with retinal detachment. The hemoglobin concentration averages 9–10 g/dL, with the blood smear showing target cells and characteristic spindle-shaped red cells.

419.2 Sickle Cell Trait

(Heterozygous Hb S; Hb AS)

Heterozygous expression of the sickle hemoglobin gene is usually associated with a totally benign clinical course. About 8% of American blacks have sickle cell trait, with 35–45% of their hemoglobin consisting of Hb S. This low level of Hb S is insufficient to produce sickling manifestations under usual circumstances, but under conditions of severe hypoxia vaso-occlusive complications may occur. Splenic infarcts and other ischemic sequelae may occur in Hb AS individuals after flying at high altitudes in unpressurized aircraft and from hypoxia associated with general anesthesia. Hyposthenuria is usually present in older children and adults. Occasionally, gross hematuria develops in otherwise well individuals. The hematologic findings in sickle cell trait are indistinguishable from normal (see Fig. 419–2*B*). The diagnosis is established by hemoglobin electrophoresis, with confirmatory sickle testing.

419.3 Other Hemoglobinopathies

HEMOGLOBIN C

Hemoglobin C ($\alpha_2\beta_2{}^6$lysine) occurs in about 2% of American blacks. In the heterozygous state (Hb AC) no anemia or disease is present, but increased numbers of target cells are seen in the peripheral blood. In the homozygous individual (Hb CC disease) a moderately severe hemolytic anemia with hemoglobin levels from 8 to 11 g/dL, a reticulocytosis of 5–10%, and splenomegaly are regularly observed. The peripheral blood contains striking numbers of target cells and occasional spherocytes (see Fig. 419–2*C*).

HEMOGLOBIN E

Hemoglobin E ($\alpha_2\beta_2{}^{26}$lysine) is prevalent in populations from Southeast Asia, particularly Thailand and Cambodia. Homozygous Hb E disease is characterized by hemolytic anemia with prominent target cells, microcytosis, and moderate to severe splenomegaly. The syndrome of Hb E–β^0-thalassemia may be expressed as a severe Cooley anemia–like disorder; electrophoresis shows the presence of only Hb E and Hb F.

419.4 Unstable Hemoglobin Disorders

(Congenital Heinz Body Anemia)

A substantial group of abnormal hemoglobins, most of which are uncommon or rare, are characterized by molecular instability, leading to denaturation and precipitation of hemoglobin within the red cells. In the more severe forms of these disorders, amorphous masses of the denatured hemoglobin, known as Heinz bodies, attach to the red blood cell membrane, damaging the cell and shortening its survival. The Heinz bodies, which are particularly prominent following splenectomy, can be visualized by supravital staining of the red blood cells with brilliant cresyl blue (see Fig. 419–2*D*). These hemolytic anemias are inherited in an autosomal dominant mode, but many of the severe forms apparently occur as new mutations.

Most of the severe types involve the hemoglobin β chains, and hemolysis first becomes apparent at 3–6 mo after birth, when Hb F is replaced by adult hemoglobin. Anemia with increased reticulocytes, jaundice, and splenomegaly are characteristically present, becoming more pronounced with infections or following exposure to oxidant drugs or chemicals. With some of the unstable β-chain abnormalities, hemolysis is accompanied by excretion of darkly pigmented dipyrrolic compounds in the urine. In contrast to the clinical picture of chronic hemolytic disease typically associated with the highly unstable hemoglobins, some of the less severe abnormalities (e.g., Hb Zurich and Hb Hasharon) produce mild and usually inapparent anemia. With fever, infections, or exposure to oxidant conditions, however, these individuals may experience acute hemolytic episodes similar to those associated with G-6-PD deficiency.

Some unstable hemoglobins can be detected by electrophoresis, but many of them comigrate with Hb A. Heating at 50° C or treating the hemolysate with a 17% buffered solution of isopropanol produces a precipitate of the unstable hemoglobin, and screening tests based on these methods are used to detect these abnormalities. Examples include Hb Koln, Hb Hammersmith, and Hb Abraham Lincoln. Splenectomy is sometimes of benefit in these patients, particularly those with severe splenomegaly.

419.5 Abnormal Hemoglobins with Increased Oxygen Affinity

Almost 100 different rare, abnormal hemoglobins have been identified that have increased oxygen affinity, as indicated by a leftward displacement of their oxygen dissociation curves. Because of their increased oxygen affinity, these hemoglobins release oxygen poorly to the tissues, resulting in hypoxia at the tissue level. The hypoxic stimulus increases erythropoietin production, with the development of secondary erythrocytosis. Hemoglobin levels in affected individuals typically range from 16 to 19 g/dL. Some of these variants can be demonstrated by electrophoresis, but many of them have normal electrophoretic properties (e.g., Hb Chesapeake, Hb Malmo, Hb Kempsey).

419.6 Abnormal Hemoglobins Causing Cyanosis

Several rare hemoglobin variants with markedly decreased oxygen affinity have been identified. The oxygen dissociation curves of blood from affected individuals are significantly displaced to the right. Examples of these abnormalities, which produce benign cyanosis, include Hb Kansas and Hb Beth Israel.

An additional group of abnormal hemoglobins that cause cyanosis is the Hb M group. These variants all have amino acid substitutions at positions in the molecule that are close to the heme groups. The structural changes in these hemoglobins have the effect of stabilizing the heme iron atoms in the ferric (Fe^{3+}) state, rendering them incapable of binding oxygen. The Hb M syndromes are characterized by a brown color of the blood, even when fully oxygenated, and by cyanosis. Two of the Hb M variants, Hb M Saskatoon and Hb M Hyde Park, are also unstable and produce chronic hemolytic anemia. The Hb M variants that result from β-chain substitutions, such as Hb M Saskatoon, have an onset of cyanosis beginning at 4–6 mo of age, whereas the α-chain variants, such as Hb M Iwate, produce cyanosis that is apparent at birth. The autosomal dominant mode of inheritance of these abnormalities helps distinguish them from other causes of congenital cyanosis.

Methemoglobinemias resulting from Hb M can be differentiated from other forms of methemoglobinemia by characteristic changes in the spectral absorption patterns of hemoglobin solutions and by the presence of normal levels of methemoglobin reductase (diaphorase) (see Chapter 419.7). Electrophoresis can demonstrate some (but not all) of the Hb M variants. These are clinically benign abnormalities, except for the hemolytic disease that accompanies two of the Hb M group, and no treatment is required.

419.7 Hereditary Methemoglobinemia

The iron of both oxygenated and deoxygenated hemoglobin is normally in the ferrous state, which is essential for its oxygen-transporting function. Oxidation of hemoglobin iron to the ferric state yields methemoglobin, which is nonfunctional and imparts a brown color to the blood; in sufficient concentration it causes cyanosis. The blood of healthy persons contains methemoglobin, but the intraerythrocytic methemoglobin-reducing system maintains its concentration at less than 2% of the total hemoglobin.

HEREDITARY METHEMOGLOBINEMIA WITH DEFICIENCY OF NADH CYTOCHROME b5 REDUCTASE. Four types of enzymopenic hereditary methemoglobinemia have been identified. All have a recessive mode of inheritance. In type I, the most frequent of these rare disorders, a deficiency of cytochrome b5 reductase is limited to erythrocytes, and cyanosis is the only consequence. Type II is a severe, progressive disorder that accounts for approximately 10% of patients with hereditary methemoglobinemia. In this disorder the deficiency of cytochrome b5 reductase is generalized to all tissues. Affected individuals present with methemoglobinemia and severe encephalopathy, appearing before 1 yr of age, and with mental retardation, microcephaly, retarded growth, attacks of bilateral athetoid movements, strabismus, opisthotonos, and generalized hypertonia. In type III disease, the enzyme deficiency is demonstrable in erythrocytes, platelets, lymphocytes, and granulocytes. Clinically, cyanosis is the only manifestation. Type IV disease results from a deficiency of erythrocyte cytochrome b5 and is associated with chronic cyanosis.

Clinically, cyanosis may vary in intensity with season and diet. The time of onset of cyanosis also varies; in some patients it appears at birth, in others as late as adolescence. Although up to 50% of the total circulating hemoglobin may be in the form of nonfunctional methemoglobin, little or no cardiorespiratory distress occurs in these patients, except on exertion.

Daily oral *treatment* with ascorbic acid (200–500 mg in divided doses) gradually reduces the quantity of methemoglobin to about 10% of the total pigment and alleviates the cyanosis as long as therapy is continued. Chronic high doses of ascorbic acid have been associated with hyperoxaluria and renal stone formation. Methylene blue given intravenously (1–2 mg/kg) promptly eliminates both methemoglobin and cyanosis, and this effect can be maintained by the daily oral administration of methylene blue (3–5 mg/kg).

419.8 Syndromes of Hereditary Persistence of Fetal Hemoglobin (HPFH)

These disorders are characterized by the production of elevated levels of Hb F beyond the neonatal period. At least 20 distinct forms of HPFH have been identified, affecting many different ethnic groups. Various molecular abnormalities have been determined as the cause for these conditions; for example, the common African forms result from extensive DNA deletions that encompass the entire β-globin gene. The normal changeover from γ-globin synthesis to β-chain synthesis consequently cannot take place in individuals with these affected chromosomes. In heterozygotes for the common African types, the level of Hb F is 15–30%. These types are characterized by a uniform distribution of Hb F in the red cells (pancellular HPFH) as compared with some of the other forms, in which the Hb F is unevenly distributed (heterocellular HPFH). Rare homozygotes for the African deletion HPFH forms have 100% Hb F in their red blood cells. Except for mild microcytosis they have normal hematologic findings. Individuals who have genes for both sickle hemoglobin and African pancellular HPFH have levels of Hb S in their red blood cells that are similar to those in patients with sickle cell anemia (see Table 419–1). This combination, however, is clinically benign, presumably because the elevated Hb F in all the red blood cells inhibits the sickling process.

419.9 Thalassemia Syndromes

The thalassemias are a heterogeneous group of heritable hypochromic anemias of varying degrees of severity. Underlying genetic defects include total or partial deletions of globin chain genes and nucleotide substitutions, deletions, or insertions. The consequences of these various changes are a decrease or absence of mRNA for one or more of the globin chains or the formation of functionally defective mRNA. The result is a decrease or total suppression of hemoglobin polypeptide chain synthesis. Approximately 100 distinct mutations are known that produce thalassemia phenotypes; many of these mutations are unique to localized geographic regions. In general, the globin chains synthesized in thalassemic red blood cells are structurally normal. In severe forms of α-thalassemia abnormal homotetramer hemoglobins (β_4, or γ_4) are formed, but their component globin polypeptides have a normal structure. Conversely, a number of abnormal hemoglobins also produce thalassemia-like hematologic changes. In characterizing the expression of the various thalassemia genes, superscript designations are used to distinguish those that produce a demonstrable globin chain product, although at decreased levels (e.g., β^+-thalassemia), from those in which the synthesis of the affected globin chain is totally suppressed (e.g., β^0-thalassemia).

Thalassemia genes are remarkably widespread, and these abnormalities are believed to be the most prevalent of all human genetic diseases. Their main distribution includes areas bordering the Mediterranean Sea, much of Africa, the Middle East, the Indian subcontinent, and Southeast Asia. From 3% to 8% of Americans of Italian or Greek ancestry and 0.5% of black Americans carry a gene for β-thalassemia. In some regions of Southeast Asia as many as 40% of the population have one or more thalassemia genes. The geographic areas in which thalassemia is prevalent closely parallel the regions in which *Plasmodium falciparum* malaria was formerly endemic. Resistance to lethal malarial infections by carriers of thalassemia genes apparently represented a strong selective force that favored their survival in these areas of endemic disease.

HOMOZYGOUS β^0-THALASSEMIA

(Cooley Anemia; Thalassemia Major)

CLINICAL MANIFESTATIONS. Homozygous β^0-thalassemia usually becomes symptomatic as a severe, progressive hemolytic anemia during the 2nd 6 mo of life. Regular blood transfusions are necessary in these patients to prevent the profound weakness and cardiac decompensation caused by the anemia. Without transfusion life expectancy is no more than a few years. In untreated cases or in those receiving infrequent transfusions at times of severe anemia, hypertrophy of erythropoietic tissue occurs in medullary and extramedullary locations. The bones become thin and pathologic fractures may occur. Massive expansion of the marrow of the face and skull (Fig. 419–3) produces characteristic facies. Pallor, hemosiderosis, and jaundice combine to produce a greenish-brown complexion. The spleen and liver are enlarged by extramedullary hematopoiesis and hemosiderosis. In older patients the spleen may become so enlarged that it causes mechanical discomfort and secondary hypersplenism. Growth is impaired in older children; puberty is delayed or absent because of secondary endocrine abnormalities. Diabetes mellitus resulting from pancreatic siderosis may also occur. Cardiac complications, including intractable arrhythmias and chronic congestive failure caused by myocardial siderosis, are common terminal events. With modern regimens of comprehensive care for these patients, many of these complications can be prevented and others ameliorated and delayed in their onset.

LABORATORY FINDINGS. The red cell morphologic abnormalities in untransfused patients with homozygous β^0-thalassemia are extreme. In addition to severe hypochromia and microcytosis (see Fig. 419–2*E*), many bizarre, fragmented poikilocytes and target cells are present. Large numbers of nucleated red blood cells circulate, especially after splenectomy. Intraerythrocytic inclusions, which represent precipitated excess α chains, are also seen after splenectomy. The hemoglobin level falls progressively to lower than 5 g/dL unless transfusions are given. The unconjugated serum bilirubin level is elevated. The serum iron level is high, with saturation of the iron-binding capacity. A striking biochemical feature is the presence of very high levels of fetal hemoglobin in the red blood cells (Table 419–2). Dipyrrolic compounds render the urine dark brown, especially after splenectomy.

TREATMENT. Transfusions are given on a regular basis to maintain the hemoglobin level above 10 g/dL. This "hypertransfusion" regimen has striking clinical benefits; it permits normal activity with comfort, prevents progressive marrow expansion and cosmetic problems associated with facial bone changes, and minimizes cardiac dilatation and osteoporosis. Transfusions of 15–20 mL/kg of packed cells are usually necessary every 4–5 wk. Cross-matching should be performed to forestall alloimmunization and prevent transfusion reactions. The use of packed red blood cells that are relatively fresh (less than 1 wk in CPD anticoagulant) is desirable. Even with meticulous care, febrile reactions to transfusions are common. These can be minimized with the use of erythrocytes reconstituted from frozen blood or the use of leukocyte filters, and by the administration of antipyretics before transfusions.

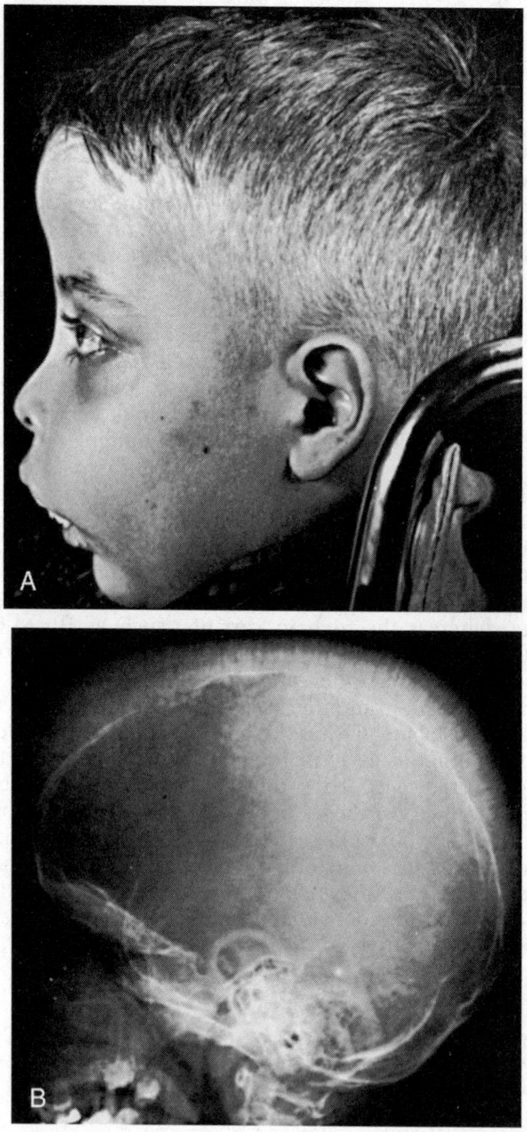

Figure 419–3. *A*, Facial deformities in an inadequately transfused patient with thalassemia major (Cooley anemia). Severe maxillary hyperplasia and malocclusion are present. *B*, Roentgenogram of the skull demonstrates the maxillary overgrowth and shows prominent widening of the diploic spaces, with the "hair-on-end" appearance caused by vertical trabeculae. These changes can be prevented by an appropriate transfusion regimen.

Hemosiderosis is an inevitable consequence of prolonged transfusion therapy because each 500 mL of blood delivers about 200 mg of iron to the tissues that cannot be excreted by physiologic means. Myocardial siderosis is a significant contributing factor in the early death of these patients. Hemosiderosis can be decreased or even prevented with the parenteral ad-

■ TABLE 419–2 Clinical and Hematologic Features of the Principal Forms of Thalassemia*

Type of Thalassemia	Globin-Gene Expression	Hematologic Features	Clinical Expression	Hemoglobin Findings
β-Thalassemias				
β^0 homozygous	β^0/β^0	Severe anemia; nomoblastemia (see Fig. 419–2*E*)	Cooley anemia	Hb F >90% No Hb A Hb A_2 increased
β^+ homozygous	β^+/β^+	Anisocytosis, poikilocytosis; moderately severe anemia	Thalassemia intermedia	Hb A: 20–40% Hb F: 60–80%
β^0 heterozygous	β/β^0	Microcytosis, hypochromia, mild to moderate anemia	May have splenomegaly, jaundice	Increased Hb A_2 and Hb F
β^+ heterozygous	β/β^+	Microcytosis, hypochromia, mild anemia	Normal	Increased Hb A_2 and Hb F
β silent carrier, heterozygous	β/β^+	Normal	Normal	Normal
δβ heterozygous	$\delta\beta/(\delta\beta)^0$	Microcytosis, hypochromia, mild anemia	Usually normal	Hb F: 5–20% Hb A_2: normal or low
γδβ heterozygous	$\gamma\delta\beta/(\gamma\delta\beta)^0$	Newborn: microcytosis hemolytic anemia normoblastemia Adult: similar to heterozygous δβ	Newborn: hemolytic disease with splenomegaly Adult: similar to heterozygous δβ	Normal
α-Thalassemias				
α silent carrier	$-,\alpha/\alpha,\alpha$	Mild microcytosis or normal	Normal	Normal
α trait	$-,\alpha/-,\alpha$ or $-,-/\alpha,\alpha$	Microcytosis, hypochromia, mild anemia	Usually normal	Newborn: Hb Barts (γ_4), 5–10% Child or adult: normal
Hb H disease	$-,\alpha/-,-$	Microcytosis, inclusion bodies by supravital staining; moderately severe anemia (see Fig. 419–2*F*)	Thalassemia intermedia	Newborn: Hb Barts (γ_4), 20–30% Child or adult: Hb H (β_4), 4–20%
α-hydrops fetalis	$-,-/-,-$	Anisocytosis, poikilocytosis; severe anemia	Hydrops fetalis; usually stillborn or neonatal death	Hb Barts (γ_4), 80–90%; no Hb A or Hb F

Adapted from Honig GR, Adams JG III: Human Hemoglobin Genetics. Vienna, Springer-Verlag, 1986.

ministration of the iron-chelating drug, deferoxamine, which forms an iron complex that can be excreted in the urine. A sustained high blood level of deferoxamine is needed for adequate iron excretion. The drug is administered subcutaneously over an 8- to 12-hr period using a small portable pump (during sleep), 5 or 6 nights/wk. Patients who adhere to this regimen can maintain serum ferritin levels of lower than 1,000 ng/mL, which is well below the toxic range. Lethal complications of hepatic and myocardial siderosis can thus be prevented or significantly delayed. An orally effective iron chelating agent, deferiprone, has been shown to have effectiveness similar to that of deferoxamine. Because of concerns about possible toxicity (agranulocytosis, arthritis, arthralgia), this drug is not currently available in the United States.

Hypertransfusion therapy prevents massive splenomegaly resulting from extramedullary erythropoiesis. Splenectomy eventually becomes necessary, however, because of the size of the organ or because of secondary hypersplenism. Splenectomy increases the risk of severe, overwhelming sepsis, and therefore the operation should be performed only for significant indications (see Chapter 442) and should be deferred as long as possible. The most important indication for splenectomy is an increased need for transfusions, indicating an element of hypersplenism. A transfusion requirement exceeding 240 mL/kg of packed red blood cells/yr is usually evidence of hypersplenism and is an indication for considering splenectomy. Immunization of these patients with hepatitis B vaccine, *H. influenzae* type b vaccine, and pneumococcal polysaccharide vaccine is desirable, and prophylactic penicillin therapy is also advocated.

Bone marrow transplantation is curative in these patients and has been performed with increasing success, even in patients who have been transfused extensively. This procedure, however, carries considerable risks of morbidity and mortality and generally can only be used for patients who have nonaffected histocompatible siblings.

OTHER β-THALASSEMIA SYNDROMES

The homozygous expression of milder (β^+) thalassemia genes produces a Cooley anemia–like syndrome of lesser severity ("thalassemia intermedia"; see Table 419–2). Skeletal deformities and hepatosplenomegaly develop in these patients, but their hemoglobin levels are usually maintained at 6–8 g/dL without transfusion. Nevertheless, they may develop severe hemosiderosis, attributable to their greatly increased gastrointestinal iron absorption. For such patients, who do not receive deferoxamine chelation therapy, a low-iron diet is indicated.

Several structurally abnormal hemoglobins produce β-thalassemia–like hematologic changes and, when present in combination with a gene for β-thalassemia, also result in a thalassemia intermedia syndrome. The most prevalent are the Hb Lepore variants, which are composed of α chains and hybrid δβ fusion globin chains. The Lepore hemoglobins are identified by electrophoresis, in which they exhibit Hb S–like mobility.

Most forms of heterozygous β-thalassemia are associated with mild anemia. The hemoglobin concentration typically averages 2–3 g/dL lower than age-related normal values. The red blood cells are hypochromic and microcytic, with poikilocytosis, ovalocytosis, and often basophilic stippling. Target cells may be present but usually are not prominent and are not specific for thalassemia. The mean corpuscular volume (MCV) is low, averaging 65 fL, and the mean corpuscular hemoglobin (MCH) values are also low (<26 pg). A mild decrease in red blood cell survival can be shown, but overt signs of hemolysis are usually absent. The serum iron level is normal or elevated.

Individuals with thalassemia trait are often misdiagnosed as having iron deficiency anemia and may be inappropriately treated with iron for extended periods. More than 90% of persons with β-thalassemia trait have diagnostic elevations of Hb A_2 of 3.4–7%. About 50% of these individuals also have slight elevations of Hb F, about 2–6%. In a small number of otherwise typical cases, normal levels of Hb A_2 with Hb F levels ranging from 5% to 15% are found, representing the δβ type of thalassemia (see Table 419–2). The "silent carrier" form of β-thalassemia produces no demonstrable abnormality in heterozygous individuals (see Table 419–2), but the gene for this condition, when inherited together with a gene for β^0-thalassemia, results in a thalassemia intermedia syndrome.

A rare type of deletion defect, which involves the γ-, δ-, and β-globin genes, produces a clinical picture similar to that of the δβ thalassemia trait in heterozygous individuals. In the newborn period, however, this defect is accompanied by significant hemolytic disease with microcytosis, normoblastemia, and splenomegaly (see Table 419–2). The hemolytic process is self-limited, but supportive transfusions may be required.

α-THALASSEMIA

Microcytic anemias resulting from deficient synthesis of α-globin chains are prevalent in Africa, Mediterranean area countries, and much of Asia. Deletions of α-globin genes account for most of these abnormalities. Four α-globin genes are present in normal individuals, and four distinct forms of α-thalassemia have been identified corresponding to deletions of one, two, three, or all four of these genes (see Table 419–2).

Deletion of a single α-globin gene produces the silent carrier α-thalassemia phenotype. No hematologic abnormality is usually evident, except for mild microcytosis. Approximately 25% of African-Americans have this form of α-thalassemia.

Individuals lacking two α-globin genes exhibit the features of α-thalassemia trait, with mild microcytic anemia. In affected newborns, small quantities of Hb Barts (γ_4) can be identified by hemoglobin electrophoresis. Beyond about 1 mo of age Hb Barts is no longer detectable, and the levels of Hb A_2 and F are characteristically normal. Inclusions of precipitated hemoglobin may be visualized in red blood cell smears, however, following supravital staining.

The deletion of three of the four α-globin genes is associated with a thalassemia intermedia–like syndrome, Hb H disease. Microcytic anemia in this condition is accompanied by abnormal red blood cell morphology (see Fig. 419–2*F*), with prominent intracellular inclusions present in the red blood cells following supravital staining. Hemoglobin H (β_4) is highly unstable; it can be readily identified by electrophoresis, but, unless special measures are taken to prevent its precipitation during sample preparation, it may escape detection.

The most severe form of α-thalassemia, resulting from deletion of all the α-globin genes, is accompanied by a total absence of α-chain synthesis. Because hemoglobins F, A, and A_2 all contain α chains, none of these hemoglobins are produced. Hb Barts (γ_4) accounts for most of the hemoglobin in affected infants, and, because γ_4 has a high oxygen affinity and therefore cannot transport oxygen to the tissues, these infants are severely hypoxic. Their red blood cells also contain small quantities of the normal embryonic Hb Portland ($\zeta_2\gamma_2$), which functions as an oxygen transporter. Most of these infants are stillborn, and most who are born alive die within a few hours. These infants are severely hydropic, with congestive heart failure and massive generalized edema. Those that survive with aggressive neonatal management are also transfusion-dependent.

The types of α-thalassemia genes vary among affected populations, and these differences account for the α-thalassemia syndromes that predominate in specific population groups. In African-Americans α-thalassemia genes are prevalent, with almost all affected individuals having the deletion arrangement (−,α) that produces a single α-locus chromosome. In this population, therefore, α-thalassemia occurs mainly as the silent carrier phenotype (−,α/α,α) or as the α-thalassemia trait (−,α/−,α). Chromosomes with deletions of both of the α loci (−,−) are prevalent in both Mediterranean and Asian populations, and Hb H disease (−,α/−,−) therefore occurs with significant frequency in both groups. The two α-locus deletion defects in Asians are often accompanied by retention of the ζ-globin genes (i.e., ζ,−,−), whereas those from Mediterranean countries usually are not (−,−,−). The latter type of defect, therefore, cannot support the synthesis of Hb Portland ($\zeta_2\gamma_2$), which appears to be essential for the intrauterine survival of fetuses with the hydrops fetalis form of α-thalassemia. Accordingly, the hydrops fetalis form is seen almost exclusively in infants of Asian ancestry. An acquired α-thalassemia syndrome, which may be associated with a large deletion involving the α-globin genes, includes Hb H disease accompanied by mental retardation, microcephaly, and hypogonadism.

A number of abnormal hemoglobins also produce α-thalassemia–like changes. The α-chain variant Hb Constant Spring occurs commonly in Far Eastern populations and is frequently observed in patients with Hb H disease, who have the genotype ($\alpha^A,\alpha^{Co\ Sp}/-,-$). The gene for Hb G Philadelphia, which is the most prevalent α-chain abnormality of African-Americans, usually occurs on a single-locus chromosome ($-,\alpha^G$). Individuals who express this abnormal hemoglobin therefore also exhibit α-thalassemia–like hematologic changes.

419.10 Hemochromatosis

Excessive storage of iron, primarily in the form of hemosiderin in parenchymal cells, can result in impairment of the structure and function of the liver, heart, gonads, skin, and joints. *Idiopathic hemochromatosis,* which has an autosomal recessive mode of inheritance, usually does not become clinically apparent until adult life. More severe forms, however, may present during childhood. The underlying metabolic defect in this disorder is unknown. Symptomatic individuals exhibit massive iron stores with the classical clinical triad of cirrhosis, bronzing of the skin, and diabetes mellitus. Serum ferritin levels are characteristically greatly elevated, with increased transferrin saturation. The gene for this disorder is frequently linked to HLA types A-3, B-7, and B-14, and, in families with an affected individual, this association provides an opportunity for screening sibs prior to the onset of symptomatic iron storage. With treatment by repeated phlebotomy, organ damage can be prevented.

Neonatal hemochromatosis is an acquired syndrome resulting from severe liver disease arising prenatally. A variety of forms of fetal hepatopathy can give rise to this clinical entity, which consists of severe liver dysfunction or liver failure, accompanied by massive iron stores and siderosis. Most of these infants have had a fatal outcome, although some have survived.

Transfusion-induced hemosiderosis, in patients chronically transfused for congenital or acquired anemia, can produce clinical and pathologic features quite similar to those of patients with thalassemia (see Chapter 415.9).

HEMOGLOBIN DISORDERS

Bunn HF, Forget BG: Hemoglobin: Molecular, Genetic, and Clinical Aspects. Philadelphia, WB Saunders, 1986.

Honig GR, Adams JG III: Human Hemoglobin Genetics. Vienna, Springer-Verlag, 1986.

Weatherall DJ, Clegg JB, Higgs DR, et al: The hemoglobinopathies. *In:* Scriver CR, Beaudet AL, Sly WS, Valle D (eds): The Metabolic Basis of Inherited Disease, 6th ed. New York, McGraw-Hill, 1989.

SICKLE CELL DISEASE

Charache S, Lubin B, Reid CD (eds): Management and Therapy of Sickle Cell Disease. Washington, DC, U.S. Dept. of Health and Human Services. NIH pub. no. 92–2117, 1992.

Charache S, Terrin ML, Moore RD, et al: Effect of hydroxyurea on the frequency of painful crises in sickle cell anemia. N Engl J Med 332:1317, 1995.

Collins AF, Fassos FF, Stobie S, et al: Iron-balance and dose-response studies of the oral iron chelator 1,2-dimethyl-3-hydroxypyrid-4-one (L-1) in iron-loaded patients with sickle cell disease. Blood 83:2329, 1994.

Gaston MH, Verter JI, Woods G, et al: Prophylaxis with oral penicillin in children with sickle cell anemia. N Engl J Med 314:1593, 1986.

Griffin TC, McIntire D, Buchanan GR: High-dose intravenous methylprednisolone therapy for pain in children and adolescents with sickle cell disease. N Engl J Med 330:733, 1994.

Honig GR: Sickling syndromes in children. Adv Pediatr 23:271, 1976.

Johnson FL, Mentzer WC, Kalinyak KA, et al: Bone marrow transplantation for sickle cell disease. The United States experience. Am J Pediatr Hematol Oncol 16:22, 1994.

Marcinak JF, Frank AL, Labotka RL, et al: *Haemophilus influenzae* type B vaccine in children with sickle cell disease: Antibody persistence after vaccination at age one and one-half to six years. Pediatr Inf Dis J 10:157, 1991.
Newborn screening for sickle cell disease and other hemoglobinopathies. Pediatrics 83:813, 1989.
Ohene-Frempong K: Stroke in sickle cell disease: Demographic, clinical, and therapeutic considerations. Semin Hematol 28:213, 1991.
Pearson HA, Spencer RP, Cornelius EA: Functional asplenia in sickle cell anemia. N Engl J Med 281:293, 1969.
Platt OS, Brambilla DJ, Rosse WF, et al: Mortality in sickle cell disease. N Engl J Med 330:1639, 1994.
Powars D: Natural history of sickle cell disease—the first ten years. Semin Hematol 12:267, 1975.
Powars D, Hiti A: Sickle cell anemia. β_s gene cluster haplotypes as genetic markers for severe disease expression. Am J Dis Child 147:1197, 1993.
Serjeant GR, Serjeant BE, Thomas PW, et al: Human parvovirus infection in homozygous sickle cell disease. Lancet 341:1237, 1993.
Sickle Cell Disease Guideline Panel: Sickle Cell Disease: Screening, Diagnosis, Management, and Counseling in Newborns and Infants. Clinical Practice Guideline No. 6. Rockville, MD, Agency for Health Care Policy and Research pub. no. 93–0562, 1993.
Vermylen C, Cornu G: Bone marrow transplantation for sickle cell disease. The European experience. Am J Pediatr Hematol Oncol 16:18, 1994.
Wilimas JA, Flynn PM, Harris S, et al: A randomized study of outpatient treatment with ceftriaxone for selected febrile children with sickle cell disease. N Engl J Med 329:472, 1993.
Wong W-Y, Overturf GD, Powars DR: Infection caused by *Streptococcus pneumoniae* in children with sickle cell disease: Epidemiology, immunologic mechanisms, prophylaxis, and vaccination. Clin Infect Dis 14:1124, 1992.

METHEMOGLOBINEMIA

Jaffe ER, Hultquist DE: Cytochrome b_5 reductase deficiency and enzymopenic hereditary methemoglobinemia. *In:* Scriver CR, Beaudet AL, Sly WS, Valle D (eds): The Metabolic Basis of Inherited Disease, 6th ed. New York, McGraw-Hill, 1989.

THALASSEMIA

Lucarelli G, Galimberti M, Polchi P, et al: Marrow transplantation in patients with thalassemia responsive to iron chelation therapy. N Engl J Med 329:840, 1993.
Modell B, Berdoukas V: The Clinical Approach to Thalassaemia. London, Grune & Stratton, 1984.
Nathan D: An orally active iron chelator. N Engl J Med 332:953, 1995.
Olivieri NF, Matsui D, Koren G, et al: Reduction of tissue iron stores and normalization of serum ferritin during treatment with the iron chelator L1 in thalassemia intermedia. Blood 79:2741, 1992.
Piomelli S, Hart D, Graziano J, et al: Current strategies in the management of Cooley's anemia. Ann NY Acad Sci 445:256, 1985.
Sharon BI, Honig GR: Management of congenital hemolytic anemias. *In:* Rossi EC, Simon TL, Moss GS (eds): Principles of Transfusion Medicine. Baltimore, Williams & Wilkins, 1991.
Weatherall DJ: The Thalassemias. *In:* Stamatoyannopoulos G, Nienhuis AW, Majerus PW, Varmus H (eds): The Molecular Basis of Blood Diseases. Philadelphia, WB Saunders, 1994.
Wilkie AOM, Buckle VJ, Harris PC, et al: Clinical features and molecular analysis of the α thalassemia/mental retardation syndromes. I. Cases due to deletions involving chromosome band 16p13.3. Am J Hum Genet 46:1112, 1990.

HEMOCHROMATOSIS

Bothwell TH, Charlton RW, Motulsky AG: Hemochromatosis. *In:* Scriver CR, Beaudet AL, Sly WS, Valle D (eds): The Metabolic Basis of Inherited Disease, 6th ed. New York, McGraw-Hill, 1989.
Knisely AS: Neonatal hemochromatosis. Adv Pediatr 39:383, 1992.
Saddi R, Schapira G: Hemochromatosis, Idiopathic. *In:* Buyse ML (ed): Birth Defects Encyclopedia. Cambridge, MA, Blackwell, 1990.

CHAPTER 420

Enzymatic Defects

George B. Segel

DEFICIENCIES OF ENZYMES OF THE GLYCOLYTIC PATHWAY

A variety of red cell enzymatic defects produce hemolytic anemias, characterized by a lack of spherocytes and few distinguishing features on the blood film. Deficiencies of most of the enzymes in both the anaerobic Embden-Meyerhof pathway and the oxidative pentose phosphate shunt have been described (Fig. 420–1). The most common glycolytic enzyme defect as a cause of hemolytic anemia is pyruvate kinase deficiency, although it is a rare disorder with only 300–400 cases reported.

420.1 Pyruvate Kinase Deficiency

A congenital hemolytic anemia occurs in persons homozygous for an autosomal recessive gene that causes either a marked reduction in red cell pyruvate kinase (PK) or production of an abnormal enzyme with decreased activity. Generation of adenosine triphosphate (ATP) within the red cell is impaired and low levels of ATP, pyruvate, and NAD^+ are seen (see Fig. 420–1). The concentration of 2,3-diphosphoglycerate (2,3-DPG) is increased, which is beneficial in facilitating oxygen release from hemoglobin but detrimental in inhibiting hexokinase as well as enzymes of the pentose shunt. In addition, there is an unexplained decrease in the sum of the adenine (ATP, ADP, and AMP) and pyridine (NAD^+ and NADH) nucleotides, which further impairs glycolysis. As a consequence of decreased ATP, the red cell cannot maintain the potassium and water content; the cells become rigid, and the red cell life span is considerably reduced.

ETIOLOGY. The human PK gene has been mapped to chromosome 1q21, and a variety of mutations involve this structural gene, which codes for a protein with 543 amino acids and forms a functional tetramer. Most affected patients are compound heterozygotes for two different PK gene defects. The many possible combinations likely account for the variability in clinical severity.

CLINICAL MANIFESTATIONS AND LABORATORY FINDINGS. The clinical manifestations vary from a severe neonatal hemolytic anemia to mild, well-compensated hemolysis noted first in adulthood. Severe jaundice and anemia may occur in the neonatal period, and kernicterus has been reported. The hemolysis in older children and adults varies in severity, with hemoglobin values from 8 to 12 g/dL associated with some pallor, jaundice, and splenomegaly. These patients usually do not require transfusion. A severe form of the disease has a relatively high incidence among the Amish of the midwestern United States.

Polychromatophilia and mild macrocytosis reflect the elevated reticulocyte count. Spherocytes are uncommon, but a few spiculated pyknocytes are usually present. Nonincubated osmotic fragility is normal. Autohemolysis is moderately or markedly increased, but addition of glucose does not regularly correct the abnormality as it does in hereditary spherocytosis.

Diagnosis relies on demonstration of a marked reduction of pyruvate kinase (PK) activity or an increase in the Michaelis-Menten dissociation constant (Km) for its substrate, phosphoenolpyruvate, in the red cells. Other red cell enzyme activities are normal or elevated. There are no abnormalities of hemoglobin. The white cells have normal PK activity and must be excluded from hemolysates used to measure PK activity. Heterozygous carriers usually have moderately reduced levels of PK activity.

TREATMENT. Exchange transfusions may be indicated for hyperbilirubinemia in the newborn. Transfusions of packed red cells are necessary for severe anemia or for aplastic crises. If the anemia is consistently severe or if frequent transfusions are required, splenectomy should be performed after 5–6 yr of age. Although not curative, the operation may be followed by higher hemoglobin levels and by strikingly high (30–60%) reticulocyte counts. Deaths resulting from overwhelming

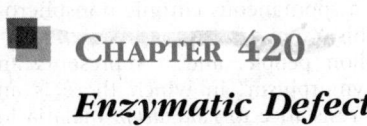

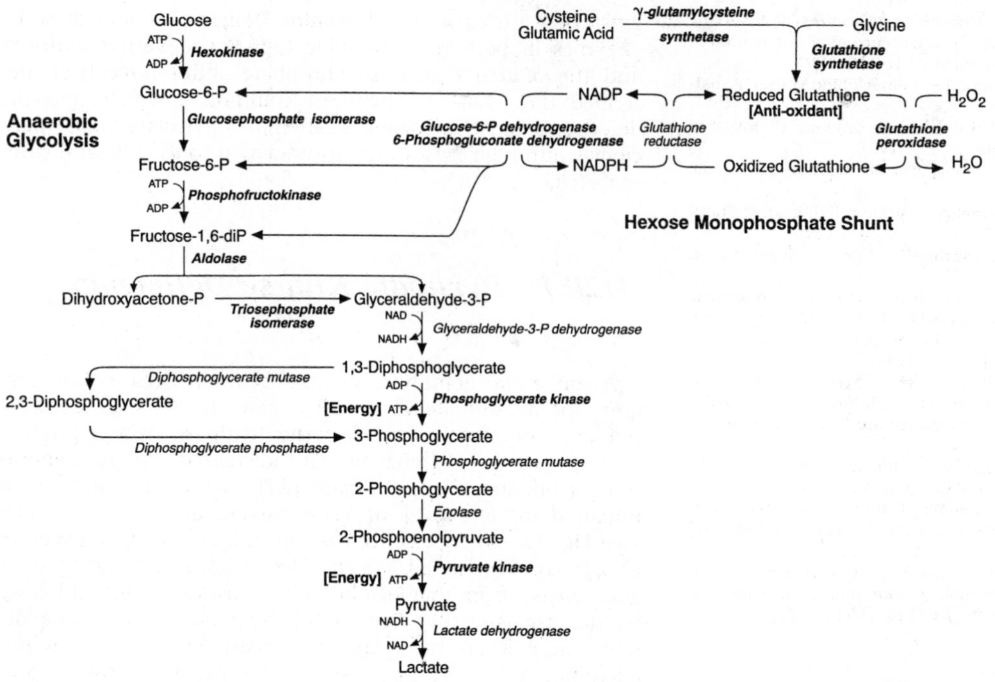

Figure 420–1. Red cell metabolism. Glycolysis and the pentose phosphate pathway. The enzyme deficiencies clearly associated with hemolysis are shown in bold type.

pneumococcal sepsis have followed splenectomy so that immunization with vaccines for encapsulated organisms should be given prior to splenectomy, and prophylactic penicillin should be administered after splenectomy.

420.2 Other Glycolytic Enzyme Deficiencies

Chronic nonspherocytic hemolytic anemias of varying severity have been associated with deficiencies of other enzymes in the glycolytic pathway, including hexokinase, glucose phosphate isomerase, and aldolase, which are inherited as autosomal recessive disorders. *Phosphofructokinase (PFK) deficiency* occurs primarily in Ashkenazi Jews in the United States and results in hemolysis associated with a myopathy classified as glycogen storage disease type VII (see Chapter 73.5). Clinically, a hemolytic anemia is complicated by muscle weakness, exercise intolerance, cramps, and possibly myoglobinuria. Enzyme assays for PFK are low in red cells and muscle.

Triose phosphate isomerase (TPI) deficiency is an autosomal recessive disorder affecting multiple systems. Affected patients have hemolytic anemia, cardiac abnormalities, and lower motor neuron and pyramidal tract impairment without mental retardation. They usually die in early childhood. The TPI gene has been cloned and sequenced and is localized on chromosome 12.

Phosphoglycerate kinase (PGK) is the first ATP-generating step in glycolysis. At least 12 kindreds now have been described with PGK deficiency, which is the only glycolytic enzyme inherited on the X chromosome. The affected males have progressive extrapyramidal disease, seizures, and variable mental retardation in conjunction with hemolytic anemia. The gene for PGK is particularly large, spanning 23 kilobases, and a variety of mutations producing single amino acid substitutions result in PGK deficiency.

DEFICIENCIES OF ENZYMES OF THE PENTOSE PHOSPHATE PATHWAY AND RELATED COMPOUNDS

The most important function of the pentose pathway is to maintain glutathione in its reduced state as protection against oxidation of the red cell (Fig. 420–1). About 10% of the glucose taken up by the red cell passes through this pathway to provide the NADPH necessary for conversion of oxidized glutathione (GSSG) to reduced glutathione (GSH). The maintenance of GSH is essential for the physiologic inactivation of oxidant compounds, such as hydrogen peroxide, that accumulate within the red cell. If glutathione, or any compound or enzyme necessary for maintaining it in the reduced state, is decreased, the SH groups of the red cell membrane are oxidized, and the hemoglobin becomes denatured and may precipitate into red cell inclusions called *Heinz bodies.* Once Heinz bodies have formed, an acute hemolytic process results from damage to the red cell membrane by the precipitated hemoglobin, the oxidant agent, and the action of the spleen. The damaged red cells then are rapidly removed from the circulation.

420.3 Glucose-6-Phosphate Dehydrogenase (G-6-PD) and Related Deficiencies

G-6-PD deficiency is the most important disease of the pentose phosphate pathway and is responsible for two clinical syndromes, an episodic hemolytic anemia induced by infections or certain drugs and a spontaneous chronic nonspherocytic hemolytic anemia. This X-linked enzyme deficiency affects more than 200 million people, and it represents an example of "balanced polymorphism" in which there is an evolutionary advantage of resistance to *Falciparum* malaria in heterozygous females that outweighs the small negative effect of affected hemizygous males.

The deficiency is caused by inheritance of any of a large number of abnormal alleles of the gene responsible for the synthesis of the G-6-PD molecule. The G-6-PD gene has been cloned and sequenced, and the mutations causing episodic versus chronic hemolysis have been identified (Fig. 420–2). Milder disease is associated with mutations near the amino terminus of the G-6-PD molecule, and chronic nonspherocytic

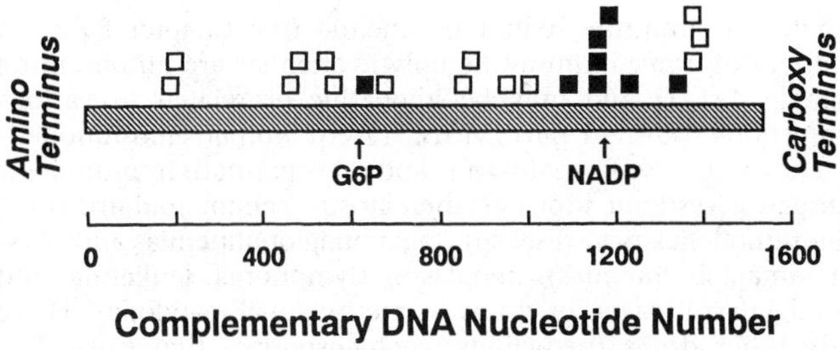

Figure 420–2. Nucleotide substitutions that cause G-6-PD deficiency. Solid squares denote mutations that cause hereditary nonspherocytic hemolytic anemia. Open squares indicate the location of mutations that cause enzyme deficiency but hemolytic anemia only under conditions of stress. The putative binding sites for glucose-6-phosphate (G-6-P) and nicotinamide-adenine dinucleotide phosphate (NADP) are indicated by *arrows*. Note that the mutations that produce nonspherocytic hemolytic anemia are almost all clustered between nucleotides 1089 and 1361, surrounding the NADP-binding domain. The exception is a mutation at nucleotide 637, which is adjacent to the putative G-6-P binding domain at nucleotide 605. (Modified from Beutler E: Glucose-6-phosphate deficiency. N Engl J Med 324:169, 1991.)

hemolytic anemia with mutations clustered near the carboxy terminus. The normal enzyme found in most populations is designated G-6-PD B$^+$. A normal variant designated G-6-PD A$^+$ is common in the African-American population. More than 100 distinct enzyme variants of G-6-PD are associated with a wide spectrum of hemolytic disease.

EPISODIC OR INDUCED HEMOLYTIC ANEMIA

ETIOLOGY. Synthesis of red cell G-6-PD is determined by a gene on the X chromosome. Diseases involving this enzyme occur, therefore, more frequently in males than in females. About 13% of male African-Americans have a mutant enzyme (G-6-PD A$^-$) that results in a deficiency of red cell G-6-PD activity to 5–15% or less of normal. Italians, Greeks, and other Mediterranean, Middle Eastern, African, and Asian ethnic groups also have a high incidence, ranging from 5% to 40%, of a variant designated G-6-PD B$^-$ (G-6-PD Mediterranean). The G-6-PD activity of the homozygous female or the hemizygous male is less than 5% of normal. The heterozygous female has an intermediate enzymatic activity and, as an example of random X chromosome inactivation (Lyon hypothesis), has two populations of red cells; one is normal and the other is deficient in G-6-PD activity. Most heterozygous females do not have clinical hemolysis after exposure to oxidant drugs. Rarely, the majority of the red cells are G-6-PD deficient in a heterozygous female because of random inactivation of the normal X chromosome.

There is considerable variation in the defect among various racial groups. For example, the defect in African-Americans is less severe than in affected whites. In African-Americans, the electrophoretically distinct enzyme variant is unstable in vivo, and its activity is decreased primarily in the older red cells in the circulation. The enzyme activity of red cells containing the variant enzyme (G-6-PD B$^-$) in whites is very low, often less than 1% of normal in the entire red cell population. A third common mutant enzyme with markedly reduced activity (G-6-PD Canton) occurs in about 5% of Chinese. A large number of other rare enzyme variants have been associated with drug-induced hemolysis.

CLINICAL MANIFESTATIONS. In the usual pattern of G-6-PD deficiency, symptoms develop 24–48 hr after the patient has ingested a substance that has oxidant properties. Drugs that have these properties include aspirin, sulfonamides, and antimalarials such as primaquin (Table 420–1). In some patients, ingestion of fava beans, a Mediterranean dietary staple, may also produce an acute and severe hemolytic syndrome called *favism*. This results from oxidative products derived from two glucosidic compounds, vicine and convicine, which are hydrolyzed to divicine and isouramil, ultimately producing H_2O_2 and other reactive oxygen products.

The degree of hemolysis varies with the inciting agent, the amount ingested, and the severity of the enzyme deficiency in the patient. In severe cases hemoglobinuria and jaundice result, and the hemoglobin concentration may fall precipitously and be life threatening. In the A$^-$ variety (African-Americans) some spontaneous recovery may be observed, even if administration of the drug is continued. This is the result of the age-labile enzyme, which is abundant and more stable in younger red cells. The associated reticulocytosis produces a compensated hemolytic process. Infection also may result in hemolysis, and significant hemolysis may occur even when no exposure to drugs can be documented (see Chronic Hemolytic Anemias Associated with Deficiencies of G-6-PD . . .). In A$^-$G-6-PD deficiency spontaneous hemolysis may occur in premature, but not term, infants. In Greek and Chinese newborns with the G-6-PD B$^-$ and Canton varieties, the deficiency of G-6-PD is an important cause of hyperbilirubinemia and potential kernicterus. When a pregnant woman ingests oxidant drugs, they may be transmitted to her G-6-PD–deficient fetus, and hemolytic anemia and jaundice may be apparent at birth.

LABORATORY FINDINGS. The onset of acute hemolysis results in a precipitous fall in hemoglobin and hematocrit. If the episode is severe, the hemoglobin binding proteins such as haptoglobin are saturated, and free hemoglobin may appear in the plasma and subsequently in the urine (see Fig. XXI–3). Unstained or supravital preparations of red cells reveal Heinz bodies (precipitated hemoglobin), which are not visible on the Wright-stained blood film. Because cells containing these inclusions are rapidly removed from the circulation, they are not seen after the first 3–4 days of illness. The blood film reveals a few fragmented cells and polychromatophilic cells (bluish large red cells), representing the reticulocytosis, which often is substantial (5–15%).

DIAGNOSIS. This depends on direct or indirect demonstration of reduced G-6-PD activity in red cells. By direct measurement, enzyme activity in affected persons is 10% of normal or less, and the reduction of enzyme is more extreme in whites and Asians than in African-Americans. Satisfactory screening tests are based on decoloration of methylene blue and on reduction of methemoglobin. Immediately after a hemolytic episode, reticulocytes and young red cells predominate. These young cells have significantly higher enzyme activity than do older cells in the A$^-$ variety. Testing may, therefore, have to be deferred for a few weeks before a diagnostically low level of enzyme can be shown. The diagnosis can be suspected when the G-6-

■ **TABLE 420–1 Agents Precipitating Hemolysis in Glucose-6-Phosphate Dehydrogenase Deficiency**

Medications	***Others***
Antibacterials	Acetophenetidin
Sulfonamides	Vitamin K analogs
Trimethoprim-sulfamethoxazole	Methylene blue
Nalidixic acid	Probenecid
Chloramphenicol	Acetylsalicyclic acid
Nitrofurantoin	Phenazopyridine
Antimalarials	**Chemicals**
Primaquine	Phenylhydrazine
Pamaquine	Benzene
Chloroquine	Naphthalene
Quinacrine	**Illness**
	Diabetic acidosis
	Hepatitis

Reproduced from Asselin BL, Segel GB. In: *Rakel R (ed): Conn's Current Therapy. Philadelphia, WB Saunders, 1994, p 341.*

PD activity is within the low normal range in the presence of a high reticulocyte count. G-6-PD variants also can be detected by electrophoretic analysis.

PREVENTION AND TREATMENT. Prevention of hemolysis constitutes the most important therapeutic measure. When possible, males belonging to ethnic groups in which there is a significant incidence of G-6-PD deficiency (e.g., Greeks, southern Italians, Sephardic Jews, Filipinos, southern Chinese, African-Americans, and Thais) should be tested for the defect before known oxidant drugs are given. The usual doses of aspirin and trimethoprim sulfamethoxazole do not cause clinically relevant hemolysis in the A^- variety. However, aspirin administered for acute rheumatic fever (60–100 mg/kg/day) may produce a severe hemolytic episode. When hemolysis has occurred, supportive therapy may require blood transfusions, although recovery is the rule when the oxidant agent is removed.

CHRONIC HEMOLYTIC ANEMIAS ASSOCIATED WITH DEFICIENCIES OF G-6-PD OR RELATED FACTORS

Chronic nonspherocytic hemolytic anemia has been associated with profound deficiency of G-6-PD caused by enzyme variants, particularly those defective in quantity, activity, or stability. The gene defects leading to chronic hemolysis are located primarily in the region of the NADP binding site near the carboxy terminus of the protein (see Fig. 420–2). These include the Loma Linda, Tomah, Iowa, Beverly Hills, Nashville, Riverside, Santiago de Cuba, and Andalus variants. Occasionally persons with G-6-PD B^- (Mediterranean) enzyme deficiency have chronic hemolysis, and the hemolytic process may worsen following ingestion of oxidant drugs. The location of the gene defect in these patients has not been defined. Splenectomy is of little value in these types of chronic hemolysis.

Other enzyme defects may impair the regeneration of GSH as an oxidant "sump" (see Fig. 420–1). A mild, chronic nonspherocytic anemia has been reported in association with decreased red cell glutathione (GSH) resulting from γ-glutamylcysteine synthetase or glutathione synthetase deficiencies. 6-Phosphogluconate dehydrogenase deficiency has been associated primarily with drug-induced hemolysis, and hemolysis with hyperbilirubinemia has been related to a deficiency of glutathione peroxidase in newborn infants.

CHAPTER 421

Hemolytic Anemias Resulting from Extracellular Factors

George B. Segel

AUTOIMMUNE HEMOLYTIC ANEMIAS

A number of agents and disorders with the ability to damage red cells may lead to their premature destruction (see Table XXI–2). Among the most clearly defined are antibodies associated with immune hemolytic anemias. The hallmark of this group of diseases is a positive direct Coombs test, which detects a coating of immunoglobulin or components of complement on the red cell surface. The most important immune hemolytic disorder in pediatric practice is hemolytic disease of the newborn (erythroblastosis fetalis), caused by transplacental transfer of maternal antibody active against the red cells of the fetus, that is, isoimmune hemolytic anemia (see Chapter 89.2). A variety of other immune hemolytic anemias are autoimmune (Table 421–1) and may be idiopathic or related to various infections (Ebstein-Barr virus, rarely human immunodeficiency virus, cytomegalovirus, and mycoplasma), immunologic diseases (systemic lupus erythematosus, rheumatoid arthritis), immunodeficiency diseases (agammaglobulinemia and dysgammaglobulinemias), neoplasms (lymphoma, leukemia, and Hodgkin's disease), or drugs (α-methyldopa, levodopa). There are other drugs (penicillins, cephalosporins) that cause immune hemolysis that is not autoimmune. The antibodies are "drug dependent" and usually (though not always) have no "specificity" for red cell membrane antigens.

AUTOIMMUNE HEMOLYTIC ANEMIAS ASSOCIATED WITH "WARM" ANTIBODIES

ETIOLOGY. In the autoimmune hemolytic anemias, abnormal antibodies are directed against red cells, but the pathogenetic mechanisms are uncertain. The autoantibody may be produced as an inappropriate immune response to a red cell antigen or to another antigenic epitope similar to a red cell antigen. Alternatively, an infectious agent may in some way alter the red cell membrane so that it becomes "foreign" or antigenic to the host.

In most instances of warm antibody hemolysis, no underlying cause can be found, and it is called primary or idiopathic (Table 421–1). If the autoimmune hemolysis is associated with an underlying disease such as a lymphoproliferative disorder, systemic lupus erythematosus, or immunodeficiency, it is called secondary. In as many as 20% of cases of immune hemolysis, drugs may be implicated.

Drugs that cause hemolysis via the "hapten" mechanism (e.g., penicillin or sometimes cephalosporins) bind tightly to the red cell membrane (Table 421–1). Antibodies to the drug, either newly or previously formed, bind to the drug molecules on red cells, mediating their destruction in the spleen. In other cases, certain drugs, such as quinine and quinidine, do not bind to red cells but rather form part of a "ternary complex," consisting of the drug, a red cell membrane antigen, and an antibody that recognizes both (see Table 421–1). α-Methyldopa may incite true autoantibodies by unknown mechanisms.

CLINICAL MANIFESTATIONS. Autoimmune hemolytic anemias may

■ TABLE 421–1 Diseases Characterized by Immune-Mediated Red Cell Destruction

I. Autoimmune Hemolytic Anemia due to Warm Reactive Autoantibodies
- Primary (idiopathic)
- Secondary
  - Lymphoproliferative disorders
  - Connective tissue disorders (especially systemic lupus erythematosus)
  - Nonlymphoid neoplasms (e.g., ovarian tumors)
  - Chronic inflammatory diseases (e.g., ulcerative colitis)

II. Autoimmune Hemolytic Anemia Due to Cold Reactive Autoantibodies (Cryopathic Hemolytic Syndromes)
- Primary (idiopathic) cold agglutinin disease
- Secondary cold agglutinin disease
  - Lymphoproliferative disorders
  - Infections (*Mycoplasma pneumoniae*, infectious mononucleosis)
- Paroxysmal cold hemoglobinuria
  - Primary (idiopathic)
  - Congenital or tertiary syphilis
  - Viral syndromes (most common)

III. Drug-Induced Immune Hemolytic Anemia
- Hapten/drug adsorption
- Ternary (immune) complex
- True autoantibody induction

Modified from Packman CH: Autoimmune hemolytic anemias. In: *Rakel R (ed): Conn's Current Therapy. Philadelphia, WB Saunders, 1995, p 305.*

occur in either of two general clinical patterns. The first is an acute transient type lasting 3–6 mo that occurs predominantly in children, ages 2–12, and accounts for 70–80% of patients. It is frequently preceded by an infection, usually respiratory. The onset may be acute, with prostration, pallor, jaundice, pyrexia, and hemoglobinuria, or may be more gradual in onset, with primarily fatigue and pallor. The spleen is usually enlarged and is the primary site for destruction of IgG-coated red cells. Underlying systemic disorders are unusual in this group. A consistent response to glucocorticoid therapy, low mortality, and full recovery are characteristic of the acute form. The other clinical pattern involves a prolonged and chronic course, which is more frequent in infants and in children older than 12 yr. Hemolysis may continue for many months or years. Abnormalities involving other blood elements are common, and the response to glucocorticoids is variable and inconsistent. Mortality is about 10%, often attributable to an underlying systemic disease.

LABORATORY FINDINGS. In many cases the anemia is profound, with hemoglobin levels <6 g/dL. Considerable spherocytosis and polychromasia are present. More than 50% of the circulating red cells may be reticulocytes, and nucleated red cells usually are present. In some cases a low reticulocyte count may be present, particularly early in the episode. Leukocytosis is common. The platelet count is usually normal, but occasionally there is concomitant immune thrombocytopenic purpura *(Evans syndrome).* The prognosis of patients with Evans syndrome is poor, as many develop chronic disease, including some with systemic lupus erythematosus.

The direct Coombs test is strongly positive, and free antibody can sometimes be demonstrated in the serum (indirect Coombs test). These antibodies are active between 35° C and 40° C ("warm" antibodies) and most often belong to the IgG class. They do not require complement for activity and usually do not produce agglutination in vitro; they are "incomplete." Antibodies from the serum and those eluted from the red cells react with red cells of many persons, in addition to the patient. They often have been regarded as nonspecific panagglutinins, but careful studies have revealed specificity for red cell antigens of the Rh system in 70% (~50% adults) of patients. Complement, particularly C3b, may be detected on the red cells in conjunction with IgG. Occasionally, the Coombs test is negative because of the limited sensitivity of the Coombs reaction. A minimum of 260–500 molecules of IgG is necessary on the red cell membrane to produce a positive reaction. Special tests are required to detect the antibody in cases of "Coombs negative" autoimmune hemolytic anemia.

TREATMENT. Transfusions usually are only of transient benefit but may be required initially by the severity of the anemia until the effect of other treatment is observed. It may be extremely difficult to find compatible blood; blood in which the red cells give the least positive in vitro reaction by the Coombs technique should be chosen. Sometimes it is necessary to give blood that is "incompatible" as judged by the cross-matching. Failure to transfuse a profoundly anemic infant or child may lead to serious morbidity and even death.

Those patients with mild disease and compensated hemolysis may not require any treatment. If the hemolysis is severe and results in significant anemia or symptoms, treatment with glucocorticoids is initiated. Glucocorticoids decrease the rate of hemolysis by blocking Fc receptors on macrophages, decreasing the production of the autoantibody, and perhaps by enhancing the elution of antibody from the red cells. Prednisone or its equivalent is administered in a dose of 2 mg/kg/24 hr. In some patients with severe hemolysis, doses up to 6 mg/kg/24 hr of prednisone may be required to reduce the rate of hemolysis. Treatment should be continued until the rate of hemolysis decreases, and then the dose is gradually reduced. If relapse occurs, resumption of full dosage may be necessary. The disease tends to remit spontaneously within a few weeks or months. The Coombs test may remain positive, even after hemolysis has subsided. When hemolytic anemia remains severe despite glucocorticoid therapy, or if very large doses are necessary to maintain a reasonable hemoglobin level, intravenous immunoglobulin and danazol may be tried. Splenectomy may be beneficial but is complicated by a heightened risk of infection with encapsulated organisms, particularly if the patient's age is less than 2 yr. Prophylaxis is indicated with appropriate vaccines (pneumoccocal, meningococcal, and *Haemophilus influenzae*) prior to splenectomy and with penicillin after splenectomy. Immunosuppressive agents have been of some benefit in chronic cases refractory to conventional therapy. Various plasmapheresis techniques may be used in refractory cases, but generally are not helpful.

COURSE AND PROGNOSIS. The acute variety of idiopathic autoimmune hemolytic disease in childhood varies in severity but is self-limited, and mortality from untreatable anemia is rare. Approximately 30% of patients develop chronic hemolysis, often associated with an underlying disease, such as systemic lupus erythematosus, lymphoma, or leukemia. The mortality in the chronic patients depends on the primary disorder.

AUTOIMMUNE HEMOLYTIC ANEMIAS ASSOCIATED WITH "COLD" ANTIBODIES

Red cell antibodies that are more active at low temperatures and agglutinate red cells at temperatures below 37° C have been called "cold" antibodies. They are primarily of the IgM class and require complement for activity. The highest temperature associated with red cell agglutination is called the *thermal amplitude.* A higher thermal amplitude results in hemolysis with less severe exposure to a cold environment. High antibody titers are associated with high thermal amplitude.

Cold Agglutinin Disease

Cold antibodies usually have specificity for the oligosaccharide antigens of the I/i system. They may occur in primary or idiopathic cold agglutinin disease, secondary to infections such as *Mycoplasma pneumoniae* and infectious mononucleosis, or secondary to lymphoproliferative disorders. Following mycoplasma pneumonia, the anti-I levels may increase considerably and, occasionally, enormous increases may occur to titers of 1:30,000 or greater. The antibody has specificity for the I antigen and reacts poorly with human cord blood cells, which possess the i antigen but exhibit low levels of I. Occasionally patients with infectious mononucleosis develop cold agglutinin disease, and the antibodies in these patients often have anti-i specificity. Spontaneous red cell agglutination is observed in the cold, and red cell aggregates are seen on the blood film. The mean corpuscular volume (MCV) may be spuriously elevated because of cell agglutination. The severity of the hemolysis is related to the thermal amplitude of the antibody, which itself is partly dependent on the IgM antibody titer.

When very high titers of cold antibodies are present and active near body temperature, severe intravascular hemolysis with hemoglobinemia and hemoglobinuria may occur and be heightened upon exposure of the patient to cold. Each IgM molecule has the potential to active a C1 molecule so that large amounts of complement are found on the red cells in cold agglutinin disease. These sensitized red cells may undergo intravascular complement lysis or be destroyed both in the liver and spleen.

Cold agglutinin disease is less common in children than in adults, and it more frequently results in an acute, self-limited episode of hemolysis. Glucocorticoids are much less effective in cold agglutinin disease and are not particularly useful. Patients should avoid exposure to cold and be treated for any underlying disease. In the infrequent patients with severe hemolytic disease the treatment includes immunosuppression and plasmapheresis. Unfortunately, splenectomy is not useful in cold agglutinin disease.

Paroxysmal Cold Hemoglobinuria

This form of hemolytic anemia is mediated by the Donath-Landsteiner hemolysin, which is an IgG cold-reactive autoantibody with anti-P specificity. This antibody fixes large amounts of complement in the cold, and the red cells lyse as the temperature is increased. Most reported cases are self-limited and are associated with viral infections, and they are now rarely seen associated with congenital or acquired syphilis. This disorder may account for 30% of immune hemolytic episodes among children. Treatment includes transfusions for severe anemia and avoidance of cold ambient temperatures.

CHAPTER 422

Hemolytic Anemias Secondary to Other Extracellular Factors

(See Table XXI–2)

George B. Segel

FRAGMENTATION HEMOLYSIS. Red cell destruction occurs in this group of diseases because of mechanical injury as the cells traverse a damaged vascular bed. This may be microvascular when red cells are sheared by fibrin in the capillaries during intravascular coagulation or when there is renovascular disease in the hemolytic-uremic syndrome or thrombotic thrombocytopenic purpura. Larger vessels may be involved in the Kasabach-Merritt syndrome (giant hemangioma and thrombocytopenia) or when a replacement heart valve is poorly epithelialized. The blood film shows many "schistocytes" or fragmented cells as well as polychromatophilia, reflecting the reticulocytosis (see Fig. 415–2*F*). Secondary iron deficiency may complicate the intravascular hemolysis because of urinary iron loss (see Fig. 405–1*C*, XXI–4). Treatment should be directed toward the underlying condition, and the prognosis depends on the effectiveness of this treatment. The benefit from transfusion is transient because the transfused cells are destroyed as quickly as those produced by the patient.

THERMAL INJURY. Extensive burns may directly damage the red cells and result in hemolysis with spherocytosis.

RENAL DISEASE. The anemia of uremia is multifactorial in origin. Erythropoietin production may be decreased and the marrow suppressed by toxic metabolites. Furthermore, the red cell life span often is shortened owing to retention of metabolites and organic acidemia.

LIVER DISEASE. Change in the ratio of cholesterol to phospholipids in the plasma may result in changes in the composition of the red cell membrane and shortening of the red cell life span. Some patients with liver disease have many target red cells on the blood film, while others have a preponderance of spiculated cells.

TOXINS AND VENOMS. Bacterial sepsis due to *Haemophilus influenzae*, staphylococci, and streptococci may be complicated by accompanying hemolysis. A particularly severe hemolytic anemia has been observed in clostridial infections and results from a hemolytic clostridial toxin. Large numbers of spherocytes may be seen on the blood film in this condition. Spherocytic hemolysis also may be seen after bites with a variety of snakes, including cobras, vipers, and rattlesnakes, which have phospholipases in their venom. Large numbers of bites by insects such as bees, wasps, and yellow jackets also may cause spherocytic hemolysis by a similar mechanism (see Chapter 668).

WILSON'S DISEASE. An acute and self-limited episode of hemolytic anemia may precede by years the onset of hepatic or neurologic symptoms in Wilson's disease. This appears to result from the toxic effects of free copper on the red cell membrane. The blood film often (but not always) shows large numbers of spherocytes, and the Coombs test is negative. Because early diagnosis of Wilson's disease permits prophylactic treatment with penicillamine and prevention of hepatic and neurologic disease, the correct assessment of this rare type of hemolysis is most important.

ENZYMATIC DEFECTS OF RED CELL

Arese P, De Flora A: Pathophysiology of hemolysis in glucose-6-phosphate dehydrogenase deficiency. Semin Hematol 27:1, 1990.

Beutler E: Glucose-6-phosphate dehydrogenase deficiency. N Engl J Med 324:169, 1994.

Tanaka KR, Zerez CR: Red cell enzymopathies of the glycolytic pathway. Semin Hematol 27:165, 1990.

AUTOIMMUNE HEMOLYTIC ANEMIA

Buchanan GR, Boxer LA, Nathan DG: The acute and transient nature of idiopathic immune hemolytic anemia in childhood. J Pediatr 88:780, 1976.

Flores G, Cunningham-Rundles C, Newland AC, Bussel JB: Efficacy of intravenous immunoglobulin in the treatment of autoimmune hemolytic anemia: results in 73 patients. Am J Hematol 44:237, 1993.

Packman CH: Autoimmune hemolytic anemia. *In:* Rakel R (ed): Conn's Current Therapy. Philadelphia, WB Saunders, 1995, pp 305–312.

Packman CH, Leddy JP: Acquired hemolytic anemia due to warm-reacting antibodies. *In:* Beutler E, Lichtman MA, Coller BS, Kipps TJ (eds): Hematology. McGraw-Hill, 1995, New York, pp 677–685.

SECTION 4

Polycythemia

(Erythrocytosis)

Bruce M. Camitta

Polycythemia exists when the red blood cell count, the hemoglobin level, and the total red blood cell volume all exceed the upper limits of normal. In postpubertal children, a hemoglobin >16 g/dL and a total red blood cell mass >35 mL/kg indicate polycythemia. Measurement of the total red blood cell volume by radioisotopic techniques is essential in the differential diagnosis of polycythemia. True polycythemia is characterized by increases of both the red blood cell and total blood volumes. A decrease in plasma volume, such as occurs in acute dehydration and burns, may result in a high hemoglobin. However, these situations are more accurately designated hemoconcentration because the red blood cell mass is not increased and normalization of the plasma volume restores the hemoglobin to normal levels.

PRIMARY POLYCYTHEMIA (Polycythemia Rubra Vera). This myeloproliferative disorder has been reported in only a few children. In vitro cultures of erythroid precursors of affected persons do not require added erythropoietin to stimulate growth. Diagnostic criteria are increased total red blood cell volume, arterial O_2 saturation ≥92%, and splenomegaly. Supportive laboratory abnormalities include: thrombocytosis, leukocytosis, increased leukocyte alkaline phosphatase, and increased vitamin B_{12} or increased unsaturated B_{12} binding capacity. Treatment includes phlebotomy and (if necessary) antiproliferative chemotherapy. The disease may be complicated by bleeding or thrombosis. It may evolve into myelofibrosis or acute leukemia. Prolonged survival is not unusual.

SECONDARY POLYCYTHEMIA. The differential diagnosis of secondary polycythemia is shown in Table XXI–3. Polycythemia may be present in any clinical situation associated with chronic arterial oxygen desaturation. *Hypoxia* of the kidney results in increased production of erythropoietin, which stimulates production of red blood cells. Cardiovascular defects involving right-to-left shunts and pulmonary diseases interfering with proper oxygenation are the most common causes of hypoxic polycythemia. Clinical findings usually include cyanosis, hyperemia of sclerae and mucous membranes, and clubbing of the fingers. As the hematocrit rises above 65%, symptoms of hyperviscosity may require phlebotomy. On the other hand, the increased demand for red cell production may cause iron deficiency. Iron-deficient red cells are more rigid, further increasing the risk of intracranial thrombosis in these patients. Since microcytosis may occur only as a late manifestation of iron deficiency in children with hypoxic polycythemia, routine periodic assessment of iron status, with treatment of iron deficiency, should be performed in these patients. Living at high altitudes also causes hypoxic polycythemia; the hemoglobin level increases about 4% for each rise of 1,000 m in altitude.

More subtle forms of hypoxia may also cause polycythemia. Congenital methemoglobinemia resulting from a deficiency of cytochrome b5 reductase may cause cyanosis and polycythemia (see Chapter 419.7). This condition is transmitted as an autosomal recessive trait. Most affected individuals are asymptomatic. Neurologic abnormalities may be present in patients whose enzyme deficit is not limited to hematopoietic cells. Dominantly transmitted polycythemia is caused by hemoglobins that have increased oxygen affinity. Cyanosis is uncommon in these patients. See Chapter 419.6.

Polycythemia has also been associated with benign and malignant *lesions that secrete erythropoietin.* Exogenous or endogenous excess of *anabolic steroids* also may cause polycythemia. In several families benign polycythemias have been transmitted as dominant or recessive conditions, the bases of which are not known.

When the hematocrit exceeds 65–70% (hemoglobin >23 g/dL) there is a marked increase in blood viscosity. Periodic phlebotomies may prevent or decrease symptomatology. Apheresed blood should be replaced with plasma or saline to prevent hypovolemia in patients accustomed to a chronically elevated total blood volume.

■ **TABLE XXI–3 Differential Diagnosis of Polycythemia**

- **Primary—Polycythemia Vera**
- **Secondary**
  - Neonatal
    - Normal intrauterine environment
    - Twin-twin or maternal-fetal hemorrhage
    - Infants of diabetic mothers
    - Intrauterine growth retardation
    - Neonatal thyroid toxicosis
    - Adrenal hyperplasia
    - Trisomy 21
  - Hypoxia
    - Altitude
    - Cardiac disease
    - Lung disease
    - Central hypoventilation
  - Hemoglobinopathy
    - High O_2 affinity variants
    - Methemoglobin reductase deficiency
    - Chronic carbon monoxide exposure
  - Hormonal
    - Malignant tumors
      - Renal, hepatic, adrenal, cerebellar, other
    - Renal disease
      - Cysts, hydronephrosis
    - Adrenal disease
      - Virilizing hyperplasia, Cushing syndrome
    - Anabolic steroid therapy
  - Familial
- **Spurious—Plasma Volume Decrease**

Erslev AJ: Secondary polycythemia (erythrocytosis). *In:* Williams WJ, Beutler E, Erslev AJ, Lichtman MA (eds): Hematology, 4th ed. New York, McGraw-Hill, 1990, p 705.

Erslev AJ: Hemoglobinopathies producing erythrocytosis. *In:* Williams WJ, Beutler E, Erslev AJ, Lichtman MA (eds): Hematology, 4th ed. New York, McGraw-Hill, 1990, p 717.

Hathaway WE: Neonatal hyperviscosity. Pediatrics 72:567, 1983.

Danish EH, Rasch CA, Harris JW: Polycythemia vera in childhood: Case report and review of the literature. Am J Hematol 9:421, 1980.

SECTION 5

The Pancytopenias

Philip A. Pizzo

Pancytopenia can result from either a failure of production of hematopoietic progenitors, their destruction, or the replacement of the bone marrow by tumor or fibrosis. Although selective cytopenias are important clinical entities (see Chapters 124, 406–410, and 439), pancytopenia refers to a loss of all marrow elements. The clinical consequences include anemia, neutropenia, and thrombocytopenia and, depending on the degree and duration of their impairment, can lead to serious illness and death. Pancytopenia can be constitutional, arising as a consequence of an inherited genetic defect affecting hematopoietic progenitors, or can be acquired, as a consequence of either direct destruction of progenitors, immune-mediated damage to either hematopoietic progenitors or their nurturing microenvironment, or the suppression of or crowding out of progenitors by tumor cells or fibrosis. In this section, the constitutional and acquired pancytopenias will be considered separately. Because the principles of supportive care are generally independent of the etiology of the pancytopenia, they are presented at the conclusion of this section. ■

CHAPTER 423

The Constitutional Pancytopenias

ETIOLOGY. Although Fanconi anemia is the best recognized constititional pancytopenia, a number of other infrequent genetic disorders have also been implicated. These genetic syndromes (Table 423–1) include various modes of inheritance and may be associated with a number of congenital abnormalities, especially of the bones, kidneys, and heart. Because the hematologic manifestations of the congenital pancytopenias may not become manifested until the first years to even decades of life, a genetic predisposition to bone marrow failure should be considered in all cases of aplastic anemia in children (see later). These disorders can be autosomal recessive (e.g., Fanconi anemia, dyskeratosis congenita), X linked, or autosomal dominant (e.g., dyskeratosis congenita). Several of these genetic disorders may present initially with a single cytopenia and subsequently progress to pancytopenia (e.g., Shwachman-Diamond syndrome, amegakaryocytic thrombocytopenia, reticular dysgenesis). In addition, there are a number of inheritable familial marrow dysfunction syndromes that have been associated with pancytopenia (which can also be autosomal recessive, autosomal dominant, or X linked), and aplastic anemia also occurs in association with other genetic disorders (e.g., Down, Dubowitz, and Seckel syndromes). Thus, pancytopenia can be either the primary disease manifestation or can emerge as a rare complication during the course of another illness. Because of the chromosomal fragility or defective repair mechanisms that may be associated, several of these disorders can also be complicated by cancer or other organ dysfunction(s).

EPIDEMIOLOGY. Although the true incidence of these disorders

■ **TABLE 423–1 Inherited Bone Marrow Failure Syndromes**

Feature	Fanconi Anemia	Dyskeratosis Congenita	Shwachman-Diamond Syndrome	Amegakaryocytic Thrombocytopenia
Cases reported	700	150	175	36
Male/female	1.3	4.7	1.8	2.6
Genetics	Autosomal recessive	X linked; autosomal recessive, dominant	Autosomal recessive	X linked, or autosomal recessive
Physical abnormalities (%)	50–75	100	40	40
Hand/arm anomalies (%)	50	15	<2	0
Median age (yr) at diagnosis of initial hematologic disease	8	16	<1	<1 wk
First hematologic manifestation	Pancytopenia	Pancytopenia	Neutropenia	Thrombocytopenia
Bone marrow	Aplastic	Aplastic	Hypocellular or myeloid arrest	Absent or small megakaryocytes
Aplastic anemia (%)	>90	50	20	45
Leukemia (%)	9	0	5	6
Liver disease (%)	4	0	0	0
Cancer	5	7	0	0
Hb F	Increased	Increased	Increased	Increased
Chromosomes	Breaks increased with clastogens	Normal	Normal	Normal
Spontaneous remissions	Very rare	None	Very rare	None
Treatment, responses	Androgens, 50%, transient	Androgens, 50%, transient	Steroids or androgens, 50%, transient	None
Prognosis	Poor	Poor	Fair	Poor
Prenatal diagnosis	Chromosomes	Xq28 RFLP	Neutropenia	Thrombocytopenia
Long-term survival after hematologic disease (%)	<10	<30	40	0
Predicted median survival age (yr)	16	32	35	4

RFLP = restriction fragment length polymorphism.

Modified from Alter BP, Young NS: The bone marrow failure syndromes. In: *Nathan DG, Oski FA (eds): Hematology of Infancy and Children, 4th ed. Philadelphia, WB Saunders, 1993.*

is unknown, the constitutional pancytopenias are rare. The most common disorder is Fanconi anemia, of which approximately 700 cases have been described, in contrast to only about 36 cases for amegakaryocytic thrombocytopenia. Depending on geography, the heterozygote frequency of Fanconi anemia ranges from 1:100 to 1:300. The familial aplastic anemias are much less common.

PATHOLOGY AND PATHOGENESIS. One of the hallmarks of Fanconi anemia is evidence of spontaneous or clastogenic-induced chromosome breaks (100%). Lymphoid, hematopoietic (including progenitors), and fibroblast cells from patients with Fanconi anemia demonstrate a number of cytogenetic abnormalities, including defective DNA repair and an increased susceptibility of hematopoietic cells to oxidant stress. Although the specific molecular defect has not been fully identified, it is likely that it is present in progenitor cells and almost certainly plays a role in the heightened risk of these patients to develop malignancies. Depressed levels of granulocyte-macrophage–colony-stimulating factor (GM-CSF), stem cell factor, and interleukin-6 (IL-6) also have been observed in children with Fanconi syndrome, suggesting that an abnormal cytokine network contributes to the pathogenesis of the bone marrow failure in these patients.

Chromosome breakage has also been observed in approximately 10% of patients with dyskeratosis congenita, and decreased hematopoietic cytokines have been found in some patients with the Shwachman-Diamond syndrome. However, the pathogenesis of these disorders and that of the familial marrow dysfunction syndromes remain undefined.

CLINICAL MANIFESTATIONS. A variety of physical abnormalities accompany most of the congenital pancytopenias, particularly Fanconi anemia and dyskeratosis congenita. Patients having Fanconi anemia are characterized by hyperpigmentation and café-au-lait spots, skeletal abnormalities (especially absent or hypoplastic thumbs), short stature, and a wide array of integumentary and organ abnormalities. *Dyskeratosis congenita* is also very commonly associated with hyperpigmentation as well as nail dystrophy of both the hands and feet, leukoplakia, and a number of ocular abnormalities, including epiphora, blepharitis, and cataracts. The relative frequencies of these abnormalities are compared in Table 423–1. Approximately 14–25% of patients with the cytogenetic abnormalities of Fanconi anemia lack the major physical stigmata of the Fanconi syndrome and have been designated as having the "Estren-Damashek" subtype. A diversity of cutaneous, skeletal, growth, and organ abnormalities can also be found in 30–40% of the other congenital and familial pancytopenias, although they do not follow any uniform pattern.

LABORATORY FINDINGS. Depending on the specific disorder, thrombocytopenia, leukopenia, lymphopenia, or anemia generally precedes the onset of pancytopenia. Further, hematologic abnormalities may precede or follow elucidation of other physical defects. As noted earlier, chromosomal breaks occur in all patients with Fanconi anemia compared with 10% of those with dyskeratosis congenita. Children with Fanconi anemia and dyskeratosis congenita generally have macrocytosis as well as mild poikilocytosis and anisocytosis, and their red blood cells contain higher levels of hemoglobin F than are found in acquired aplasia. The age of onset of hematologic abnormalities ranges from infancy to adolescence. Once peripheral pancytopenia is evident, bone marrow examination generally confirms a hypoplastic or aplastic state comparable to that seen in acquired aplastic anemias.

Additional laboratory examination should include skeletal radiographs as well as examination of the genitourinary tract and, depending on the diagnosis, more detailed examination of the eyes, gastrointestinal tract, heart, teeth, and gonads (in males).

DIAGNOSIS. The presence of characteristic skeletal and cutaneous abnormalities coupled with short stature should suggest the diagnosis of congenital pancytopenia even in the absence of hematologic problems. In contrast, when a child presents with evidence of bone marrow failure, a genetic or familial defect should always be considered and evaluated by cytogenetic examination, including chromosomal breakage. This is particularly important because a number of individuals with congenital pancytopenias may occasionally not have any of the physical abnormalities that are considered characteristic of these syndromes (see Table 423–1).

COMPLICATIONS. The major complications related to the congenital pancytopenias include the consequences of bone marrow failure, a heightened risk for leukemia and other cancers, and organ complications that are specific to the primary defect (e.g., liver problems in Fanconi syndrome, malabsorption in Shwachman-Diamond syndrome). Infection and/or bleeding represent the major hematologic manifestations leading to life-threatening complications (see Chapter 425). Depending on their degree and duration, the hematologic abnormalities may respond to supportive care initially, but when pancytopenia ensues (depending on the syndrome this will occur in 20–90% of patients), more aggressive therapies are required. As more knowledge is gained about the molecular and cellular pathogenesis of these syndromes, it may be possible to delay some of the hematologic complications (see later).

TREATMENT. The traditional backbone of therapy for patients with congenital anemias has been steroids and androgens (especially oxymetholone or nandrolone), alone or in combination. Although 50–75% of patients show some evidence of improvement with androgens, relapse is common and complications (especially hepatic tumors or obstructive liver disease) occur. Improvements in red blood cells generally precede those in white blood cells, and it may take months to achieve a maximum benefit. These therapies have been shown to prolong life by approximately 2 yr and hence can only be considered palliative.

The only "curative" therapy to date has been bone marrow transplantation. However, patients with congenital pancytopenias also have an increased predisposition to malignancy, and the preparative regimens generally used during bone marrow transplantation can adversely impact this susceptibility. Accordingly, lower doses of alkylating agents in the preparative regimens appear to be appropriate. Encouraging results have been reported when GM-CSF was administered subcutaneously to children with Fanconi anemia and pancytopenia. A significant increase in the neutrophil count was observed in 6 of 7 patients who were treated at the Boston Children's Hospital, and this was sustained for more than a year without any evidence of leukemia. Additional follow-up is important, and it is possible that treatment of these patients with multiple cytokines (erythropoietin, IL-3, IL-6) may offer additional benefits. Ultimately, the best hope for these children will emerge from an understanding of the molecular defects that produce the syndromes and, once identified, gene therapy may become a feasible consideration.

PROGNOSIS. Once marrow failure develops, the prognosis is guarded. Although bone marrow transplantation and hematopoietic growth factor reconstitution offer some hope, neither overcome the risks for subsequent cancer or other organ complications.

GENETIC COUNSELING. Once an index case has been identified, genetic counseling is important and must be oriented to the patterns of inheritance and the prospect for prenatal diagnosis. Based on the presence of cytogenetic and chromosomal breakage or, in the case of amegakaryocytic thrombocytopenia, fetal blood platelet counts, a diagnosis can be suspected or confirmed.

CHAPTER 424
The Acquired Pancytopenias

ETIOLOGY AND EPIDEMIOLOGY. A variety of drugs, chemicals, toxins, infectious agents, radiation, or immune disorders can result in pancytopenia, either by the direct destruction of hematopoietic progenitors, by disruption or destruction of the supporting marrow microenvironment and its necessary growth factors, or by the direct or indirect (e.g., virus-related) immune-mediated destruction of marrow elements (Table 424–1). Whenever a child presents with pancytopenia, a careful history of exposure to known risk factors should be obtained. The possibility of a genetic predisposition to bone marrow failure should always be considered, even in the absence of the classic physical findings associated with Fanconi anemia and the other congenital pancytopenias (see Chapter 423). The overall incidence of acquired aplastic anemia is relatively low, with an approximate cumulative annual incidence in both children and adults, in the United States and Europe, of 2–6 cases per million per year.

A number of drugs can result in transient (albeit severe) and predictable bone marrow depression. Most notable, of course, are antineoplastic agents (e.g., anthracyclines, alkylators, antimetabolites) as well as certain antibiotics (e.g., chloramphenicol). Permanent damage can also be done if sufficient doses of these agents are administered and is more likely with certain agents (e.g., benzene). Aplastic anemia or pancytopenia can follow the administration of a great many different kinds of drugs and chemicals (including certain insecticides, antibiotics, anticonvulsants, nonsteroidal anti-inflammatory agents, antihistamines, sedatives, and metals). The relative frequency of aplastic anemias ranges from approximately 1:25,000–40,000 for chloramphenicol to 1:350,000 for cimetidine, and it is even less frequent for other agents. A genetic predisposition may exist that increases the likelihood of pancytopenia following exposure to the drug or chemical.

A number of viruses can either directly or indirectly result in bone marrow failure. The B19 parvovirus is classically associated with pure red cell aplasia, but in patients with sickle cell disease or in other compromised hosts (e.g., with cancer or AIDS), it can result in a transient aplastic crisis (Chapters 210 and 407). Pancytopenia can also be associated with hepatitis virus (both hepatitis B virus [HBV] and hepatitis C virus [HCV]), as well as with dengue virus, presumably consequent to the immune activation that accompanies these virus infections. Herpes viruses, particularly Epstein-Barr virus (EBV) and cytomegalovirus (CMV), can result in bone marrow failure, either in genetically predisposed patients (e.g., those with the X-linked lymphoproliferative syndromes with EBV) or caused by bone marrow graft rejection with CMV. The human immunodeficiency virus (HIV) has also been associated with a number of hematologic abnormalities, including anemia, neutropenia, thrombocytopenia, and pancytopenia.

Although extremely uncommon in children, patients with evidence of bone marrow failure should also be evaluated for paroxysmal nocturnal hemoglobinuria (PNH) and collagen-vascular diseases that may be accompanied by this complication. Pancytopenia without peripheral blasts may be due to bone marrow replacement by leukemic or neuroblastoma malignant cells.

PATHOLOGY AND PATHOGENESIS. The hallmark of aplastic anemia is peripheral pancytopenia coupled with a hypoplastic or aplastic bone marrow. The severity of the disease is related to the degree of myelosuppression. Severe aplastic anemia is defined as a condition in which two or more cell components have become seriously compromised (i.e., an absolute neutrophil count $<500/mm^3$, a platelet count $<20,000/mm^3$, a reticulocyte count $<1\%$ after correction for the hematocrit) in a patient whose bone marrow biopsy is hypocellular. As noted earlier, bone marrow failure can result from a variety of etiologies and mechanisms. For example, it can be a consequence of stem cell failure that is either related to a drug, toxin, or virus or that has resulted from either cell-mediated or antibody-dependent cytotoxicity. Abnormalities of the supporting microenvironment resulting from drugs, toxins, viruses, or immune-mediated mechanisms can also cause bone marrow failure. A loss of critical hematopoietic growth factors can contribute to the marrow failure state.

CLINICAL MANIFESTATIONS, LABORATORY FINDINGS, AND DIFFERENTIAL DIAGNOSIS. Acquired pancytopenia is usually characterized by anemia, leukopenia, and thrombocytopenia with the consequent increased risks of fatigue, cardiac failure, infection, and bleeding. Other treatable disorders, such as cancer, collagen-vascular disorders, PNH, or infections that may respond to specific therapies (e.g., intravenous gamma globulin for parvovirus) should be considered in the differential diagnosis. Careful examination of the peripheral blood smear for red blood cell, leukocyte, and platelet morphology is important. In children, the possibility of a congenital pancytopenia must always be considered and chromosomal breakage should be evaluated (see earlier). The presence of fetal hemoglobin suggests a congenital pancytopenia but is not diagnostic. To rule out PNH, a Ham test should be performed. Bone marrow examination should include both an aspiration and a biopsy, and the marrow should be carefully evaluated for cellularity and morphology. The presence of more than 70% lymphocytes has a poor prognosis.

COMPLICATIONS. The major complications of severe pancytopenia are predominantly related to the risk of life-threatening bleeding due to prolonged thrombocytopenia or to infection secondary to protracted neutropenia. Patients with protracted neutropenia due to bone marrow failure are at risk not only

■ **TABLE 424–1 A Classification of the Aplastic Anemias**

Acquired
- *Secondary*
  - Radiation
  - Drugs and chemicals
    - Predictable: cytotoxic agents, benzene
    - Idiosyncratic: chloramphenicol, anti-inflammatory drugs, antiepileptics, gold
  - Viruses
    - Epstein-Barr virus (infectious mononucleosis)
    - Hepatitis
    - Parvovirus
    - Human immunodeficiency virus (HIV)
  - Immune diseases
    - Eosinophilic fasciitis
    - Hypoimmunoglobulinemia
  - Thymoma
  - Pregnancy
  - Paroxysmal nocturnal hemoglobinuria
  - Preleukemia
- *Idiopathic*

Inherited
- Fanconi anemia
- Dyskeratosis congenita
- Shwachman-Diamond syndrome
- Reticular dysgenesis
- Amegakaryocytic thrombocytopenia
- Familial aplastic anemias
- Preleukemia, myelodysplasia, monosomy 7
- Nonhematologic syndromes (e.g., Down, Dubowitz, and Seckel syndromes)

Modified from Alter BP, Young NS: The bone marrow failure syndromes. In: Nathan DG, Oski FA (eds): Hematology of Infancy and Childhood, 4th ed. Philadelphia, WB Saunders, 1993.

for serious bacterial infections but also for invasive mycoses. The general principles of supportive care that have evolved from the treatment of cancer patients suffering malignancy or chemotherapy-related myelosuppression should be fully extended to the care of patients with acquired pancytopenias (Chapter 425).

TREATMENT. As with the congenital pancytopenias, the treatment of the child with acquired pancytopenia requires comprehensive supportive care coupled with an attempt to treat the underlying marrow failure. The major therapies include the use of antithymocyte globulin (ATG), either alone or with corticosteroids, cyclosporine, bone marrow transplantation, and the use of one or more hematopoietic colony-stimulating factors. For patients with a matched sibling donor, allogeneic bone marrow transplantation offers a 45–70% chance of long-term survival. The risks associated with this approach include the immediate complications of the transplantation, graft-versus-host-disease (which increases with patient age), and the increased risk for subsequent cancers (Chapter 132). Since only a quarter to a third of patients will have a matched donor, the use of bone marrow registries for unrelated donors and unmatched donors has also been successfully pursued. Alternatively, ATG (without transplantation) has had a response rate of 45%, and the survival rate of these patients (60%) is not significantly different from that in patients who have undergone bone marrow transplantation. The use of hematopoietic growth factors, while successful in some patients, has not had a major impact to date, although it remains possible that combinations of cytokines will have a greater effect, at least in patients who do not have significant stem cell depletion. Other therapies that have been used in the past with inconsistent results include androgens, cyclophosphamide, and plasmapheresis.

PROGNOSIS. Although spontaneous recovery rarely occurs, patients with severe pancytopenia have an extremely poor prognosis unless they respond to treatment.

PANCYTOPENIAS CAUSED BY MARROW REPLACEMENT

Processes that either infiltrate or replace the bone marrow can also present as or result in an acquired pancytopenia. This can occur either preceding or during a malignancy (classically either neuroblastoma or leukemia in children) or as a consequence of osteoporosis (marble bone disease), myelofibrosis, or myelodysplasia. Although uncommon, evidence of a hypoplastic anemia can precede, generally by months (and only rarely by a year), the onset of acute leukemia. This is important to appreciate in evaluating and monitoring children who present with what appears to be an acquired aplastic anemia. Similarly, it is important to consider the prospect that the apparent bone marrow failure may be due to a collagen vascular disease (e.g., rheumatoid arthritis) or an underlying myelodysplastic syndrome, making morphologic examination of the peripheral blood and the bone marrow critically important. Chromosomal analysis, which, in the case of certain myelodysplastic syndromes, might reveal clonality, can be particularly helpful. The management and prognosis of these children is dictated by the appropriate diagnosis and management of the true underlying disease.

CHAPTER 425
Infectious and Other Complications of Pancytopenia

RISK FACTORS FOR INFECTION. Although neutropenia (defined as a polymorphonuclear neutrophil count $<500/mm^3$) is the single most important risk factor associated with an increased incidence of infection, other abnormalities contributing to the likelihood of infection include alterations of phagocyte function, perturbations of physical defense barriers, and changes in humoral or cellular immunity. The risk for infection can also be increased through alterations of the endogenous microflora by new and potentially more serious pathogens that have been acquired from the air, food, water, or contacts with other patients or care providers. Recognizing these risks is important in developing rationale approaches to supportive care of these patients.

PREDOMINANT ORGANISMS RESPONSIBLE FOR INFECTION. The pancytopenic patient can be vulnerable to infection from bacteria, fungi, viruses, and parasites. Because virtually any organism may cause infection in the severely pancytopenic host, any isolate should be considered a possible pathogen if associated with a clinical site or setting suggestive of infection. Bacteria are the predominant causes of new fevers when the neutropenic patient first becomes febrile. During the last decade gram-positive bacteria (especially coagulase negative staphylococci, *Staphylococcus aureus*, enterococci, and streptococci) have become more frequent than gram-negative organisms (especially *Pseudomonas aeruginosa*). There can be considerable variation in the predominant bacterial isolates from hospital to hospital, so the physician should be aware of the distribution of pathogens and their antimicrobial sensitivities at the center where the patient is being treated. Fungi (especially *Candida* and *Aspergillus*) represent important secondary pathogens, especially in patients with prolonged neutropenia. Patients with acquired aplastic anemia are similar to cancer patients with prolonged neutropenia in having a heightened risk for these invasive mycoses.

The patterns of risk may also vary according to the treatment the patient is receiving. For example, when cyclosporine and prednisone are administered to the patient with acquired aplastic anemia or those undergoing allogeneic bone marrow transplantation, the patient's susceptibility to virus and fungal infections is heightened (e.g., an increased risk for cytomegalovirus [CMV] approximately 50 days post bone marrow transplantation or for varicella zoster virus [VZV] after the first 100 days of transplantation).

HIGH- AND LOW-RISK PATIENTS. Patients with less than 7–10 days of neutropenia can be considered low risk, whereas those with longer durations are high risk. The former includes primarily patients with transient pancytopenia following infection or drugs. The most common drugs resulting in transient neutropenias include antimicrobial agents (penicillins, cephalosporins, trimethoprim-sulfamethoxazole) and antiviral agents (ganciclovir) and, most notably, the antineoplastic agents (e.g., anthracyclines, antimetabolites, antifols, alkylators). Similarly, virus infections (rubella, influenza, CMV, Epstein-Barr virus [EBV]) can also result in transient periods of neutropenia. Accordingly, it is imperative to assess the causative factors resulting in the neutropenia or pancytopenia in defining the approach to patient management. Patients whose duration of neutropenia exceeds 10 days generally fall into a high-risk category, although this can be modulated by the factors that contributed to the bone marrow failure. These patients have a higher frequency of secondary infectious complications, need more prolonged courses of antimicrobial therapy, and need additions or modifications in the initial therapeutic regimen.

INITIAL MANAGEMENT OF THE NEUTROPENIC PATIENT WHO BECOMES FEBRILE. Initial Therapy. The prompt initiation of empirical broad-spectrum antibiotics as soon as the neutropenic patient becomes febrile (e.g., a single oral temperature >38.5° C or three elevations >38° C during a 24 hr period) is important. Patients should undergo a careful examination, and appropriate pre-antibiotic cultures and a chest radiograph should be obtained. The antibiotics chosen should be directed at the predominant organisms and their sensitivity patterns at the hospital where the patient is being treated. The goal is to provide effective coverage for the major pathogens; not all organisms can or need to be covered by the empirical regimen. Although less frequent, gram-negative bacteria are often more pathogenic, and bactericidal agent(s) whose spectrum encompasses the most common organisms (*Escherichia coli, Klebsiella pneumoniae,* and *Pseudomonas aeruginosa*) should be administered. Gram-positive organisms tend to have somewhat lower morbidity, and anaerobes are usually infrequent as primary isolates, although they can be important in mixed infections in certain sites (e.g., necrotizing gingivitis, perianal cellulitis). No particular empirical antibiotic regimen has proved clearly superior, and the choice of which antibiotics to use depends on the center where the patient is being treated and the preferences and expertise of the physician. Even patients with indwelling catheters can be successfully treated with β-lactam antibiotics, with the caveat that vancomycin be added if a gram-positive organism is isolated that would benefit from its addition.

Criteria for Modifying Initial Therapy. Patients with prolonged neutropenia are at continued risk for the development of second or even multiple infections. Scrupulous and frequent re-assessment of these patients, determining whether new sites of infection have occurred that require additions to or modifications of the primary regimen, is essential to a successful outcome. For patients with fever and neutropenia that persist beyond 1 wk, empirical antifungal therapy is an important addition to the antibiotic regimen and has resulted in a reduction of significant fungal infections. The drug of choice is amphotericin B, initially at doses of 0.5–0.6 mg/kg/24 hr. Most centers begin empirical amphotericin B if the patient is still febrile and neutropenic after 7 days of antibiotic therapy, even if a site of infection was previously identified; some clinicians advocate starting empiric antifungal therapy on day 4 of persistent fever. Breakthrough infections due to *Aspergillus* can occur and require either higher doses of amphotericin (1.5 mg/kg/24 hr) or alternate regimens (e.g., lipid-associated amphotericin, itraconazole). In addition, patients who recover from neutropenia but who remain febrile may have hepatosplenic candidiasis, even though they may have received empirical amphotericin B as part of their management.

MANAGEMENT OF SITES OF INFECTION. Catheter-Associated Infections. Indwelling intravenous access devices are increasingly used in the care of patients with pancytopenia, especially those undergoing transplantation. These devices can be associated with infectious complications, including bacteremias, exit site infections, or tunnel infections. The risk and patterns of infections are comparable regardless of whether the device is externalized (e.g., Hickman- or Groshan-type catheters) or is subcutaneously implanted (e.g., Port-a-Cath, Medi-Port). The infections are predominantly due to gram-positive bacteria (especially coagulase negative staphylococci or *S. aureus*), but gram-negative infections also occur (most notably *P. aeruginosa, Acinetobacter,* or Enterobacteriaceae). Rapidly growing mycobacteria (*Mycobacterium chelonei-fortuitum* complex) also, occasionally, can be associated with exit site infections. Catheter-related *Candida* infections may occur, and, infrequently, *Aspergillus* may also cause an exit site infection. Neutropenic patients who have indwelling catheters should have blood cultures drawn from each lumen and from a peripheral vein. Their initial antibiotic management should be like that for other febrile neutropenic patients.

If an organism is isolated from the catheter, it is frequently possible to treat the patient successfully without removing the device. However, there are several caveats to this approach. First, if there is evidence of a tunnel infection, it is virtually always necessary to remove the catheter. Second, if after starting appropriate antibiotics, the blood cultures remain persistently positive for more than 48 hr, the catheter should be removed. Third, certain organisms nearly always require the removal of the device because treatment failures are otherwise common; these include certain *Bacillus* species and *Candida* spp. It is important to remember that patients with double- or triple-lumen devices should have the antibiotics rotated daily so that each of the ports or lumens is infused. Treatment failures have occurred when this is not routinely done.

Pneumonias. Lower respiratory tract infections can pose difficult management issues when they occur in the febrile neutropenic patient. The general approach depends on whether the patient was recovering or not from neutropenia when the infiltrate was detected and whether it had a localized or diffuse radiographic pattern. When a new localized infiltrate appears in a previously untreated febrile neutropenic patient, appropriate cultures should be obtained and the patient should be begun on broad-spectrum antibiotic therapy. If the infiltrate is progressing after 72 hr of this empirical therapy, a more invasive diagnostic procedure is warranted (e.g., bronchoscopy or even open lung biopsy). Second, if a new infiltrate appears in a neutropenic patient who is already on broad-spectrum antibiotics, and especially if that infiltrate is progressing and the patient is not showing signs of recovery from neutropenia, a fungal process (especially aspergillosis) should be strongly considered. Ideally such patients should undergo a definitive diagnostic procedure (although a positive sputum or bronchoalveolar lavage for *Aspergillus* would essentially establish the diagnosis in this setting) so that future management can be appropriately guided. If this cannot be done, however, the patient should be started empirically on a high dose (1–1.5 mg/kg/24 hr) of amphotericin B.

In contrast, patients who develop a new infiltrate while recovering from neutropenia can be more conservatively managed. It is likely in these patients that the infiltrate represents a "lighting-up" of a previously undetectable occult pneumonitis. If the patient is clinically stable and afebrile, close observation is appropriate. As more cytokines are used in the future, it is probable that such radiographic findings may be more commonly observed.

Interstitial pneumonias are more commonly associated with viral infections or *Pneumocystis carinii* pneumonia. These can be especially problematic in patients who have undergone allogeneic bone marrow transplantation, in whom CMV pneumonia can be associated with serious morbidity and mortality. These appear to be potentially preventable by using CMV seronegative blood products and by prophylaxis with ganciclovir. If CMV pneumonitis does occur in the post-transplant setting, treatment should include ganciclovir plus either intravenous immunoglobin (IVIG) or CMV-specific immunoglobulin.

Gastrointestinal (GI) Infections. Although the GI tract is an important reservoir for many of the organisms that cause infection in the compromised host, it is not commonly a site of infection. However, several GI-associated syndromes require special consideration. *Hepatosplenic candidiasis* is most commonly associated with persistent or recurrent fever in a patient who is recovering from neutropenia. Frequently the patient has a rebound leukocytosis, elevated alkaline phosphatase, and right upper quadrant (RUQ) abdominal discomfort. The diagnosis can be inferred by finding "bull's eye" lesions in the liver or spleen by ultrasound, computed tomography (CT), or magnetic resonance imaging (MRI). The diagnosis is confirmed by biopsy observation of a characteristic granulomatous lesion. Successful treatment often requires prolonged courses of amphotericin B. Lipid-associated formulations of amphotericin B are currently being evaluated as a means to shorten the length of therapy. Fluconazole is best reserved for continuation therapy in patients who have had an "induction" course with amphotericin B, because treatment failures have occurred with fluconazole.

Another GI syndrome in the neutropenic cancer patient is *typhlitis* (or *cecitis*). This is manifested as acute right lower quadrant (RLQ pain), often with rebound tenderness, mimicking acute appendicitis. This is most frequently caused by gram-negative bacterial infection of the cecum and requires intensive medical therapy. In some cases, surgical resection of the necrotic cecum has been life-saving, even though the patient must be considered a poor operative risk because of neutropenia and, frequently, thrombocytopenia. It is important in these patients to consider the possibility that the symptoms might be caused by *Clostridium difficile*, because this can generally be more simply treated with oral vancomycin or metronidazole.

Perianal cellulitis has become less common, but when it occurs it can pose a significant therapeutic challenge. These infections are often mixed, with aerobic gram-negative bacteria, enterococci, and anaerobes comprising the major isolates. Antibiotic therapy should encompass these organisms. The patient should be closely monitored. Surgical drainage should be reserved for those with progressive cellulitis or those who have a drainable collection after recovery from neutropenia.

DURATION OF ANTIMICROBIAL THERAPY. There are no clear guidelines on the appropriate duration of antimicrobial therapy for pancytopenic patients who are likely to remain neutropenic for protracted periods. In general, it is best to limit the duration of antibiotics whenever feasible. For example, if the patient defervesces promptly after the initiation of empirical antibiotics but does not have a defined source of infection, antibiotics should not be extended beyond 3–4 days, with the understanding that careful monitoring is necessary when the antibiotics are discontinued. Patients who have a defined site of infection should be treated until the resolution of the infectious focus, usually 10–14 days. However, patients who remain persistently febrile and neutropenic should continue on antibiotics (and potentially on empirical antifungal therapy), especially during the period when therapy has been administered for the underlying marrow failure (e.g., antithrombocyte globulin [ATG], cyclosporine, transplantation).

NONINFECTIOUS COMPLICATIONS. Blood product support is also integral to the management of the patient with pancytopenia. Balanced against the need to appropriately support the patient is the importance of decreasing antigenic exposure, especially in patients who are candidates for bone marrow transplantation. Children with pancytopenia should be monitored closely and should receive packed red blood cell transfusion when their hemoglobin is <8.0 gm/dL. Platelet transfusion is indicated when the platelet count falls below 10,000–20,000/mm^3 or when there is evidence of bleeding in a child whose platelet count is <50,000/mm^3. It is preferable to use irradiated blood products, especially in children who are receiving immunosuppressive regimens or who are candidates for transplantation.

Alter BP, Young NS: The bone marrow failure syndromes. *In:* Nathan DG, Oski FA (eds): Hematology of Infancy and Childhood, 4th ed. Philadelphia, WB Saunders, 1993, pp 216–316.

DiBartolomeo P, DiGirolama G, Olioso P, et al: Allogeneic bone marrow transplantation for Fanconi anemia. Bone Marrow Transplant 16:53, 1992.

Guinan EC, Lopez KD, Huhn RD, et al: Evaluation of granulocyte-macrophage colony-stimulating factor for treatment of pancytopenia in children with Fanconi anemia. J Pediatr 124:144, 1994.

Pizzo PA: Management of fever in patients with cancer and treatment-induced neutropenia. N Engl J Med 328:1323, 1993.

Socie G, Henry-Anar M, Bacigalupo A, et al: Malignant tumors occurring after treatment of aplastic anemia. N Engl J Med 329:1152, 1993.

Weinberger M, Elattar I, Marshall D, et al: Patterns of infection in patients with aplastic anemia and the emergence of aspergillus as a major cause of death. Medicine 71:24, 1992.

Wevrick R, Clark CA, Buckwald M: Cloning and analysis of the murine Fanconi anemia group cDNA. Hum Mol Genet 2:655, 1993.

SECTION 6

Blood and Blood Component Transfusions

Ronald G. Strauss

Blood transfusions frequently are life-saving, and modern intensive care of premature neonates, children with cancer, and transplant recipients would be impossible without them. However, transfusions are not without risks, and they should be given only when true benefits are likely, that is, to correct a deficiency or defect of a blood component that has caused a clinically significant problem. The principles of transfusion support for children and adolescents are similar to those for adults, but neonates and infants have many special needs. Accordingly, each of these two age groups will be discussed separately within each section. Many of the transfusion guidelines provided are updated versions of those formulated originally by the Pediatric Hemotherapy Committee of the American Association of Blood Banks. ■

CHAPTER 426
Red Blood Cell Transfusions

Red blood cells (RBCs) are the most frequently transfused blood component. They are given to increase the oxygen carrying capacity of the blood and to maintain satisfactory tissue oxygenation. Guidelines for RBC transfusions in *children and adolescents* are similar to those for adults (Table 426–1). However, transfusions may be given more stringently to children because hemoglobin levels are lower in normal children than in adults and, except in defined circumstances, children do not usually have underlying cardiorespiratory diseases. Thus, children should have unimpaired abilities to compensate for RBC loss. In the perioperative period, for example, it is unnecessary for children to maintain hemoglobin levels ≥80 g/L, a level frequently desired for adults. There should be a compelling reason to administer any postoperative RBC transfusion, as most children (without continued bleeding) can quickly restore their RBC mass if given iron therapy. As is true for adults, the most important measures in the treatment of acute hemorrhage, occurring with surgery or injury in children, are first to control the hemorrhage and to restore tissue perfusion, with crystalloid and/or colloid solutions. Then, if the patient's condition remains unstable, RBC transfusions may be indicated. In acutely ill children with severe pulmonary disease requiring assisted ventilation, it is a common practice to maintain the hemoglobin level close to the normal range. Although this recommendation seems logical, its efficacy has not been documented by scientific studies.

With anemias that develop slowly, the decision to transfuse RBCs should not be based solely on blood hemoglobin levels, as children with chronic anemias may be asymptomatic despite very low hemoglobin levels. Patients with iron deficiency anemia, for example, often are treated successfully with oral iron alone, even at hemoglobin levels below 50 g/L. Factors other than hemoglobin concentration that should be considered in the decision to transfuse RBCs include: (1) the patient's symptoms, signs, and functional capacities; (2) the presence or absence of cardiorespiratory and central nervous system disease; (3) the cause and anticipated course of the anemia; and (4) alternative therapies. In anemias that are likely to be permanent, one must also consider the effects of anemia on growth and development, and the potential toxicity of repeated transfusions. RBC transfusions for disorders such as sickle cell anemia and thalassemia are discussed in Chapters 419.1 and 419.9.

For the *neonate,* clearly established indications for RBC transfusions, based on controlled scientific studies, do not exist.

TABLE 426–1 Guidelines for Pediatric RBC Transfusions

Children and Adolescents
Acute loss >15% circulating blood volume
Hemoglobin <80 g/L* in perioperative period
Hemoglobin <130 g/L and severe cardiopulmonary disease
Hemoglobin <80 g/L and symptomatic chronic anemia
Hemoglobin <80 g/L and marrow failure
Infants Within First 4 Mo of Life
Hemoglobin <130 g/L and severe pulmonary disease
Hemoglobin <100 g/L and moderate pulmonary disease
Hemoglobin <130 g/L and severe cardiac disease
Hemoglobin <100 g/L and major surgery
Hemoglobin <80 g/L and symptomatic anemia

**Hematocrit calculated as Hb mg/dL × 3 = 24%.*

Generally, RBCs are given to maintain a blood hemoglobin believed to be most desirable for each neonate's clinical status (Table 426–1). It is widely recognized that this clinical approach is imprecise, but more physiologic indications, such as RBC mass, available oxygen, and measurements of oxygen delivery and tissue extraction, are not usually available in clinical practice. Because definitive data are limited, it is important that pediatricians critically evaluate neonatal RBC transfusions in light of the pathophysiology involved.

During the first weeks of life, all neonates experience a decline in circulating RBC mass caused by both physiologic factors and, in sick premature infants, by phlebotomy blood losses. In healthy term infants, the nadir hemoglobin value rarely falls below 9 g/dL at an age of approximately 10–12 wk. This decline occurs earlier and is more pronounced in premature infants, even in those without complicating illnesses, in whom the mean hemoglobin concentration falls to approximately 8 g/dL in infants of 1.0–1.5 kg birthweight and to 7 g/dL in infants <1.0 kg. A key reason the nadir hemoglobin values of premature infants are lower than those of term infants is the former group's relatively diminished erythropoietin output (EPO) in response to anemia. These issues and the indications for the administration of recombinant EPO are discussed in Chapters 87, 89.1, and 405. Despite the promise of EPO therapy, many low birthweight premature infants need RBC transfusions (Table 426–1). In neonatal patients with severe respiratory disease, defined as those requiring relatively large quantities of oxygen and ventilator support, it is customary to maintain the blood hemoglobin >130 g/L (hematocrit >40%). Proponents believe that transfused RBCs containing adult hemoglobin, with their superior interaction with 2,3-diphosphoglycerate, leading to better oxygen offloading than that of fetal hemoglobin, are likely to provide optimal oxygen delivery throughout the period of diminished pulmonary function. Although this practice is widely recommended, little evidence is available to establish its efficacy or to define its optimal use (i.e., the best hemoglobin level for each degree of pulmonary dysfunction). It seems logical to presume that infants with less severe cardiopulmonary disease require less vigorous support; hence, the lower hemoglobin level suggested for those with only moderate disease. Consistent with the rationale for optimal oxygen delivery in neonates with severe respiratory disease, it seems logical to maintain the hemoglobin >130 g/L (hematocrit >40%) in neonates with severe cardiac disease leading to either cyanosis or congestive heart failure.

Definitive studies are not available to establish the optimal hemoglobin level for neonates facing *major surgery.* However, it seems reasonable to maintain the hemoglobin >100 g/L (hematocrit >30%) because of limited ability of the neonate's heart, lungs, and vasculature to compensate for anemia, the inferior offloading of oxygen due to the diminished interaction between fetal hemoglobin and 2,3-diphosphoglycerate, and the developmental impairment of neonatal renal, hepatic, and neurologic function. This transfusion guideline is simply a recommendation and should be applied with flexibility to individual infants facing different kinds of surgery.

Stable neonates do not require RBC transfusions unless they exhibit clinical problems attributable to anemia. Proponents of RBC transfusions for symptomatic anemia believe that the low RBC mass contributes to tachypnea, dyspnea, apnea, tachycardia, bradycardia, feeding difficulties, and lethargy, and that these problems can be alleviated by transfusing RBCs. However, it is important to remember that anemia is only one of several possible causes for these problems, and RBC transfusions should be given only when clinical problems seem to be manifestations of anemia (i.e., not otherwise explained).

The *RBC product of choice* for children and adolescents is the standard suspension of RBCs isolated from whole blood by centrifugation and stored in an anticoagulant/preservative medium at an hematocrit value of about 60%. The usual dose is 10–15 mL/kg, but transfusion volumes vary greatly depending on clinical circumstances (e.g., continued vs. arrested bleeding, hemolysis, etc.). For neonates, the product of choice is a packed RBC concentrate (hematocrit of 70–90%) infused slowly (2–4 hr) at a dose of about 15 mL/kg body weight. Because of the small quantity of extracellular fluid given at these high hematocrit values and the slow rate of transfusion, the type of anticoagulant/preservative medium selected is believed not to pose risks for the majority of premature infants. Similarly, the traditional use of relatively fresh RBCs (<7 days of storage) is being challenged in hopes that donor exposure can be diminished by using a single unit of RBCs for each infant, regardless of the duration of RBC storage. Neonatologists who object to this practice and insist on transfusing fresh RBCs generally are fearful of the rise in plasma potassium (K^+) that occurs in banked RBCs during extended storage. After 42 days of storage, plasma K^+ levels are ≅50 mEq/L (0.05 mEq/mL), a value that, at first glance, seems alarmingly high. However, the dose of bioavailable K^+ transfused (i.e., that in the extracellular fluid) is quite small. An infant weighing 1.0 kg, given a 15 mL/kg transfusion of packed RBCs (hematocrit 80%), will receive 3 mL of extracellular fluid that contains only 0.15 mEq of K^+, and it will be transfused slowly. However, this rationale may not apply to large-volume transfusions in which greater doses of K^+ may be harmful, especially if infused rapidly.

CHAPTER 427

Platelet Transfusions

Guidelines for platelet (PLT) support of children and adolescents with quantitative and qualitative PLT disorders are similar to those for adults (Table 427–1), in which the risk of life-threatening bleeding following injury or occurring spontaneously can be related to the severity of thrombocytopenia. PLT transfusions should be given to patients with PLT counts <50 × 10^9/L when they are bleeding or are scheduled for an invasive procedure. Studies in thrombocytopenic patients with bone marrow failure indicate that spontaneous bleeding increases markedly when PLT levels fall below 20 × 10^9/L. For this reason, many pediatricians recommend prophylactic PLT transfusions to maintain a PLT count >20 × 10^9/L in children with thrombocytopenia due to bone marrow failure. This threshold has been challenged, and some favor a PLT transfusion trigger of 5–10 × 10^9/L for uncomplicated patients. However, severe thrombocytopenia commonly occurs in association with fever, antimicrobial therapy, active bleeding, need for an invasive procedure, disseminated intravascular coagulation, and other severe clotting abnormalities, situations in which the PLT count at which transfusions are given needs to be raised.

■ TABLE 427–1 Guidelines for Pediatric Platelet Transfusions

Children and Adolescents
PLTs <50 × 10^9/L and bleeding
PLTs <50 × 10^9/L and invasive procedure
PLTs <20 × 10^9/L and marrow failure with additional hemorrhagic risk factors
Qualitative PLT defect and bleeding or invasive procedure
Infants Within First 4 Mo of Life
PLTs <100 × 10^9/L and bleeding
PLTs <50 × 10^9/L and invasive procedure
PLTs <20 × 10^9/L and clinically stable
PLTs <100 × 10^9/L and clinically unstable

PLTs, platelets.

Qualitative PLT disorders may be inherited or acquired (e.g., in advanced hepatic or renal insufficiency or following cardiopulmonary bypass). In such patients, PLT transfusions are justified only if significant bleeding occurs. Prophylactic administration of PLTs is not justified unless an invasive procedure is planned. In these cases, a bleeding time of greater than twice the upper limit of laboratory normal may be taken as diagnostic evidence that PLT dysfunction exists, but this test is poorly predictive of hemorrhagic risk or the need to transfuse PLTs. In these patients, alternative therapies, particularly desmopressin acetate, should be considered to avoid PLT transfusions.

In the *neonate,* hemostasis is quantitatively and qualitatively different than that of older children, and the potential exists for either serious hemorrhage or thrombosis. About 25% of neonates managed in intensive care units will exhibit blood PLT counts <150 × 10^9/L at some time during admission. Although multiple pathogenetic mechanisms are involved in these sick neonates, the predominant one is accelerated PLT destruction. Blood PLT counts <100 × 10^9/L pose significant clinical risks for premature neonates. In one study infants with birthweight <1.5 kg and a blood PLT count <100 × 10^9/L were compared with nonthrombocytopenic infants of similar birthweight. The bleeding time was prolonged at PLT counts <100 × 10^9/L, and PLT dysfunction was suggested by bleeding times that were disproportionately long for the degree of thrombocytopenia present. Hemorrhage was greater in thrombocytopenic infants compared to controls. Of particular importance, the incidence of intracranial hemorrhage in thrombocytopenic infants with birthweight <1.5 kg was 78% versus 48% for nonthrombocytopenic infants of similar size. Moreover, the extent of hemorrhage and neurologic morbidity was greater in the thrombocytopenic group. However, in a randomized trial designed to address this issue, maintaining the blood PLT count at >150 × 10^9/L versus transfusing PLTs only when the PLT count fell below 50 × 10^9/L did not diminish the incidence of intracranial hemorrhage (28% vs. 26%). Few clinical trials have been reported to establish the efficacy of therapeutic PLT transfusions in high-risk, thrombocytopenic neonates. Although basic questions regarding the relative risks of different degrees of thrombocytopenia in various clinical settings are only partially answered, guidelines acceptable to many neonatologists are listed in Table 427–1.

The ideal goal of most PLT transfusions is to raise the PLT count to >50 × 10^9/L, and for neonates to >100 × 10^9/L. This can be achieved consistently by the infusion of 10 mL/kg of standard platelet concentrates, prepared either by centrifugation of fresh units of whole blood or by automated plateletpheresis, for infants and children weighing up to 30 kg. For larger children, the appropriate dose is four to six pooled concentrates from whole blood units or one apheresis unit. PLT concentrates should be transfused as rapidly as the patient's overall condition permits, certainly within 2 hr. Patients requiring multiple PLT transfusions should receive filtered (leukocyte-reduced) blood products, including PLT concentrates, to diminish alloimmunization and PLT refractoriness.

Routinely reducing the volume of platelet concentrates for infants and small children by additional centrifugation steps is both unnecessary and unwise. The calculations to prove it is unnecessary are as follows: (1) All PLT concentrates contain approximately 10 × 10^9 PLTs/10 mL; (2) because the blood volume of an infant or child is about 70 mL/kg, a 1 kg neonate will have 70 mL of circulating blood; (3) in this example, transfusion of 10 mL/kg PLT concentrate will add 10 × 10^9

PLTs to 70 mL of blood, a number calculated to increase the PLT count by 143 × 10^9/L. Acknowledging that post-transfusion PLT recovery is not perfect, this calculated increment is quite consistent with the increment observed clinically. Generally, 10 mL/kg is not an excessive transfusion volume, providing the intake of other intravenous fluids, medications, and nutrients is monitored and adjusted. It is important to minimize transfusion of Group O PLTs to group A or B recipients, as passive anti-A or -B can lead to hemolysis. Although proven methods exist to reduce the volume of platelet concentrates when truly warranted, additional processing should be performed with great care because of probable platelet loss, clumping, and dysfunction caused by the additional handling.

CHAPTER 428

Neutrophil (Granulocyte) Transfusions

Guidelines for granulocyte transfusions (GTX) are listed in Table 428–1. Although GTX are used sparingly by many pediatricians, the ability to collect markedly higher numbers of neutrophils from donors stimulated with recombinant granulocyte colony-stimulating factor has led to renewed interest. GTX should be reconsidered at institutions where neutropenic patients continue to die of progressive bacterial and fungal infections, despite the optimal use of antimicrobial agents and recombinant myeloid growth factors.

The role of GTX added to antibiotics for patients with severe neutropenia (<0.5 × 10^9/L) due to bone marrow failure is similar for both adults and children. Infected neutropenic patients usually respond to antibiotics alone, provided bone marrow function recovers early in infection. Because children with newly diagnosed leukemia respond rapidly to induction chemotherapy, only rarely are they candidates for GTX. In contrast, infected children with sustained bone marrow failure (i.e., malignant neoplasms resistant to treatment, aplastic anemia, and bone marrow transplant recipients) may benefit when GTX are added to antibiotics. The use of GTX for bacterial sepsis that is unresponsive to antibiotics in patients with severe neutropenia (<0.5 × 10^9/L) is supported by most of the seven controlled studies reported to date (see Chapter 168).

Children with qualitative neutrophil defects (neutrophil dysfunction) usually have adequate numbers of blood neutrophils but are susceptible to serious infections because their cells kill pathogenic microorganisms inefficiently. Neutrophil dysfunction syndromes are rare, and no definitive studies have been reported to establish the efficacy of GTX. However, several patients with progressive, life-threatening infections have improved strikingly with the addition of GTX to antimicrobial therapy. These disorders are chronic, and because of the risk of inducing alloimmunization, GTX are recommended only when infections are clearly unresponsive to antimicrobial drugs.

Neonates are unusually susceptible to severe bacterial infections, and several defects of neonatal body defenses have been reported as possible contributing factors (see Chapter 98). Abnormalities of neonatal neutrophils include absolute and relative neutropenia, diminished chemotaxis, abnormal adhesion and aggregation, defective cellular orientation and receptor capping, decreased deformability, inability to alter membrane potential during stimulation, imbalances of oxidative metabolism, and a diminished ability to withstand oxidant stress. These abnormalities are accentuated in sick premature neonates, and it is logical to consider GTX. Neonates exhibiting fulminant sepsis, relative neutropenia (<3.0 × 10^9/L during the first week of life; <1.0 × 10^9/L thereafter), and a severely diminished neutrophil marrow storage pool (<10% of nucleated marrow cells being postmitotic neutrophils) are at particularly great risk of dying if treated only with antibiotics. Therapeutic GTX have been evaluated in several studies, with four of the six reports of controlled studies finding a significant benefit for GTX. Alternative therapies include intravenous immunoglobulin (IVIG) and recombinant myeloid growth factors. Results of studies evaluating IVIG have been mixed. Currently data are insufficient to determine the proper role of recombinant myeloid growth factors in treating these neonates.

Once the decision to provide GTX has been made, an adequate dose of fresh leukapheresis cells must be transfused. Neonates and infants weighing less than 10 kg should receive 1–2 × 10^9/kg neutrophils per GTX. Larger infants and children should receive a total dose of at least 1 × 10^{10} neutrophils per each GTX; the preferred dose for adolescents is 2–3 × 10^{10} per GTX. GTX should be given daily until either the infection resolves or the blood neutrophil count rises to >0.5 × 10^9/L.

■ TABLE 428–1 Guidelines for Pediatric Granulocyte Transfusions

Children and Adolescents
Neutrophils <0.5 × 10^9/L and bacterial infection unresponsive to appropriate antimicrobial therapy
Qualitative neutrophil defect and infection (bacterial or fungal) unresponsive to appropriate antimicrobial therapy
Infants Within First 4 Mo of Life
Neutrophils <3.0 × 10^9/L (1st wk of life) or <1.0 × 10^9/L (thereafter) and fulminant bacterial infection

CHAPTER 429

Transfusions of Fresh Frozen Plasma

Guidelines for fresh frozen plasma (FFP) transfusions in children (Table 429–1) are similar to those for adults. FFP is transfused to replace clinically significant deficiencies of plasma proteins, for which more highly purified concentrates are not available. Transfusion of FFP is efficacious for the treatment of deficiencies of clotting factors II, V, VII, X, and XI. Factor XIII and fibrinogen deficiencies are treated with cryoprecipitate. Requirements for FFP vary with the specific factor being replaced, but a starting dose of 15 mL/kg is usually satisfactory. Transfusion of FFP is no longer recommended for

■ TABLE 429–1 Guidelines for Pediatric FFP Transfusions

Infants, Children, Adolescents
Severe clotting factor deficiency and bleeding
Severe clotting factor deficiency and invasive procedure
Emergency reversal of warfarin effects
Dilutional coagulopathy and bleeding
Anticoagulant protein (AT-III, protein C and S) replacement
Plasma exchange replacement fluid for thrombotic thrombocytopenic purpura

AT-III, Antithrombin III.

treatment of patients with severe hemophilia A or B, because safer factor VIII and IX concentrates are available. Moreover, mild to moderate hemophilia A and certain types of von Willebrand disease can be treated with I-deamino-(8-D-arginine)-vasopressin (DDAVP) (see Chapters 432 and 432.5). An important use of FFP, albeit rare in children, is for the rapid reversal of warfarin effects in patients who are actively bleeding or who require emergency surgery (i.e., in whom functional deficiencies of factors II, VII, IX, and X cannot be rapidly reversed by vitamin K). Results of screening coagulation tests (prothrombin, activated partial thromboplastin, and thrombin times) may be assumed erroneously, to reflect the integrity of the coagulation system, and test abnormalities may be used inappropriately to justify FFP transfusions. Test results should be related to the clinical condition of the patient. Transfusion of FFP in patients with chronic liver disease and prolonged clotting times is not recommended unless bleeding is present or an invasive procedure is planned.

While its major benefit has been in the treatment of bleeding associated with clotting factor deficiencies, FFP also contains several anticoagulant proteins (antithrombin III, protein C, and protein S), whose deficiencies have been associated with thrombosis. In selected situations, FFP may be appropriate as replacement therapy in patients with these disorders. However, when available, purified concentrates are preferred. Other indications for FFP include replacement fluid during plasma exchange in patients with thrombotic thrombocytopenic purpura or other disorders for which FFP is likely to be beneficial (e.g., plasma exchange in a patient with bleeding and a severe coagulopathy). FFP is not indicated for correction of hypovolemia or as immunoglobulin replacement therapy, because safer alternatives exist (e.g., albumin solutions and intravenous immunoglobin [IVIG], respectively).

In *neonates,* FFP transfusions merit special considerations. Clotting times are prolonged due to developmental deficiency of clotting proteins, and FFP should be transfused only after reference to normal values expected for the birthweight and age of the infant in question. The indications for FFP in neonates include: (1) reconstitution of red blood cell (RBC) concentrates to simulate whole blood for use in massive transfusions (e.g., exchange transfusion or cardiovascular surgery), (2) hemorrhage secondary to vitamin K deficiency, (3) disseminated intravascular coagulation with bleeding, and (4) bleeding in congenital coagulation factor deficiency when more specific treatment is either unavailable or inappropriate. The use of prophylactic FFP transfusions to prevent intraventricular hemorrhage in premature infants is not recommended. Although still used occasionally as a suspending agent to adjust the hematocrit values of RBC concentrates prior to use for small-volume RBC transfusions to neonates, FFP offers no apparent medical benefit over the use of sterile solutions for this purpose. This practice should be discouraged. In addition, the use of FFP in partial exchange transfusion for the treatment of neonatal hyperviscosity syndrome is unnecessary, as safer colloid solutions are available.

CHAPTER 430

Risks of Blood Transfusions

Although the risks of allogeneic blood transfusions are extraordinarily low, transfusions must be given judiciously. The risk of transfusion-associated human immunodeficiency virus (HIV) is nearly zero, with estimates ranging from 1:300,000 to 1:1,000,000 donor exposures. The risk of viral hepatitis (non-A, non-B,B,C,D) is about 1:3,000 to 1:5,000 donor exposures. Transfusion-associated cytomegalovirus can be eliminated by transfusing cellular blood products, filtered with leukocyte-depletion filters, or by selecting blood from donors seronegative for antibody to cytomegalovirus. Additional infectious risks include syphilis, parvovirus B19, Epstein-Barr virus, and Chagas' disease. Other transfusion-associated risks of a noninfectious nature that may occur in infants include fluid overload, graft-versus-host disease, electrolyte and acid-base imbalances, iron overload, increased susceptibility to oxidant damage, exposure to plasticizers, hemolysis when T-antigen activation of red blood cells (RBCs) has occurred, immunosuppression, and alloimmunization, although alloimmunization to RBC and leukocyte antigens seems to be very uncommon in infants. Some adverse effects are seen only in massive transfusion settings such as exchange transfusions, where relatively large quantities of blood are needed, and are rare in the small-volume transfusions usually given.

Premature infants are known to have immune dysfunction, but their risk of post-transfusion graft-versus-host disease is not well established. The postnatal age of the infant, the number of immunocompetent lymphocytes in the transfusion product, the degree of human leukocyte antigen (HLA) compatibility between donor and recipient, and other as yet poorly described phenomena may determine which infants are truly at risk and should receive gamma-irradiated cellular products. For all patients, directed donations with blood from first-degree relatives should be irradiated because of the risk of engraftment with HLA haploidentical lymphocytes. Cellular blood products given as intrauterine and exchange transfusions are irradiated, as are transfusions for patients with severe congenital immunodeficiency disorders and recipients of bone marrow transplants. Other groups potentially at risk, but for whom no conclusive data are available, are patients receiving T-cell antibody therapy (antithymocyte globulin or OKT3), recipients of organ allografts, patients infected with HIV, and cancer patients receiving immunosuppressive drug regimens. Current practice utilizes gamma radiation from a cesium, cobalt, or linear acceleration source at doses ranging from 2,500 to 5,000 cGy; a minimum dose of 2,500 cGy is required. All cellular blood components should be irradiated, but frozen "acellular" products such as fresh frozen plasma and cryoprecipitated antihemophilic factor (AHF) do not require it.

Andrew M, Castle V, Saigal S, et al: Clinical impact of neonatal thrombocytopenia. J Pediatr 110:457, 1987.
Andrew M, Vegh P, Caco C, et al: A randomized, controlled trial of platelet transfusions in thrombocytopenic premature infants. J Pediatr 123:285, 1993.
Blanchette VS, Hume HA, Levy GJ, et al: Guidelines for auditing pediatric blood transfusion practices. Am J Dis Child 145:787, 1991.
College of American Pathologists Task Force: Practice parameter for the use of fresh-frozen plasma, cryoprecipitate, and platelets. JAMA 271:777, 1994.
Dodd RY: The risk of transfusion-transmitted infection [editorial]. N Engl J Med 327:419, 1992.
Liu EA, Mannino FL, Lane TA: Prospective, randomized trial of the safety and efficacy of a limited exposure transfusion Program for Premature neonates. J Pediatr 125:92, 1994.
Strauss RG: Current status of granulocyte transfusions to treat neonatal sepsis. J Clin Apheresis 5:25, 1989.
Strauss RG: Perinatal platelet and granulocyte transfusions. *In:* Kennedy MS, Wilson SM, Kelton JG (eds): Perinatal Transfusion Medicine. Arlington, VA, American Association of Blood Banks, 1990, p 123.
Strauss RG: Transfusion therapy in neonates. Am J Dis Child 145:904, 1991.
Strauss RG: Granulocyte transfusions. *In:* Rossi EC, Simon TL, Moss GS (eds): Principles of Transfusion Medicine. Baltimore, MD, Williams and Wilkins, 1991, p 287.
Strauss RG: Therapeutic granulocyte transfusions in 1993. Blood 81:1675, 1993.
Strauss RG: Selection of white cell-reduced blood components for transfusions in early infancy. Transfusion 33:352, 1993.
Strauss RG: Erythropoietin and neonatal anemia [editorial]. N Eng J Med 330:1227, 1994.
Strauss RG, Levy GJ, Sotelo-Avila C, et al: National survey of neonatal transfusion practices: II Blood component therapy. Pediatrics 91:530, 1993.

SECTION 7
Hemorrhagic and Thrombotic Diseases

James J. Corrigan

The blood is in dynamic equilibrium between fluidity and coagulation. This balance must be precisely maintained to ensure that neither excessive bleeding nor thrombosis occurs spontaneously or following trivial trauma. The hemostatic mechanism is complex: It involves local reactions of the blood vessels, the several activities of the platelet, the interaction of specific coagulation factors, inhibitors, and the fibrinolytic proteins that circulate in the blood. The vascular endothelium is the primary barrier against hemorrhage. When small blood vessels are transected, active vasoconstriction and local tissue pressure control minute areas of bleeding, even without mobilization of the coagulation process. The platelet, however, is essential for maintenance of small blood vessels and for the control of hemorrhage from small-vessel injury. More extensive injury and involvement of larger blood vessels require the participation of the coagulation system to provide a firm, stable, fibrin clot. Within this process natural inhibitors in plasma and a competent fibrinolytic system are needed to prevent excessive clot formation and to remove the clot. ■

CHAPTER 431
Hemostasis

SCHEMA OF HEMOSTASIS

The classic schema of hemostasis includes vascular response and platelet plug formation (the primary hemostatic mechanism) and the formation of a stable fibrin clot (the secondary hemostatic mechanism). Coagulation proceeds in three phases: In phase I, thromboplastin is formed by the interaction of certain coagulation factors, phospholipids, and tissue juice (which contains tissue factor); in phase II prothrombin (factor II) is converted to thrombin (factor IIa); and in phase III, soluble fibrinogen is converted by thrombin to fibrin. This simple scheme has been expanded, but retention of the concept as a basic three-phase reaction has merit. Table 431–1 lists the more common coagulation factors and their synonyms. A comprehensive representation of hemostasis is depicted in Fig. 431–1.

Following vascular injury, vasoconstriction occurs and a platelet plug forms. The platelets must first stick to the injured endothelium (adhesion). They require a plasma factor (von Willebrand factor) to be adhesive. After adhesion, the platelets undergo a release reaction in which certain intraplatelet factors(e.g., adenosine diphosphate [ADP], thromboxane A_2) are released into the surrounding area. These materials cause aggregation of platelets and the eventual formation of the platelet plug. In phase I of the coagulation scheme there are two pathways to the formation of thromboplastin (factor Xa, and factor V plus phospholipid complex) called the intrinsic (or plasma) and extrinsic (or tissue) pathways. The intrinsic pathway involves the successive enzymatic conversion of the inactive forms of factors XII, XI, and IX. (Two other plasma proteins are also involved in the activation of factor XII and factor XI—prekallikrein for factor XII and high-molecular-weight kininogen for factor XI.) The activated factor IX (factor IXa) interacts with factor VIII, calcium, and phospholipid to activate factor X. Factor Xa interacts with factor V, calcium, and phospholipid, and becomes the active complex that converts prothrombin (factor II) to thrombin. This active complex has been called prothrombinase (preferred), prothrombin activator, and thromboplastin. The extrinsic pathway involves the conversion of factor VII to factor VIIa by tissue factor (a phospholipid protein complex). In the extrinsic pathway factor VIIa activates factor X directly.

Phase II of coagulation involves the enzymatic cleavage of factor II into smaller molecules, one of which is thrombin (factor IIa). This step requires factor II as substrate for the factor Xa-factor V-phospholipid-calcium complex.

In phase III thrombin splits four small peptides (two fibrinopeptide A and two fibrinopeptide B) from fibrinogen, producing fibrin monomers. These monomers then polymerize spontaneously to form fibrin. Factor XIIIa (formed by the action of thrombin on factor XIII) causes covalent bonding of the fibrin strands, which produces a stable clot.

There are at least three clinically important, naturally occurring coagulation inhibitors: antithrombin III, protein C, and protein S. Antithrombin III inhibits activated coagulation factors that have a serine moiety in their active site, such as thrombin, factor Xa, factor IXa, factor XIa, and factor XIIa. Protein C, when activated (protein Ca), inhibits factor V and factor VIII, using protein S as its cofactor.

■ **TABLE 431–1 The Coagulation Factors**

International Numbers	Synonyms	Comment
I	Fibrinogen	Number rarely used—congenital deficiency known (afibrinogenemia)
II	Prothrombin	Number rarely used—congenital deficiency known
III	Thromboplastin	No specific factor identified
IV	Calcium	Number rarely used
V	Labile factor, proaccelerin	Congenital deficiency known (parahemophilia, Owren disease)
VI	Activated labile factor, accelerin	No longer differentiated from factor V
VII	Stable factor, SPCA, proconvertin	Congenital deficiency known
VIII	Antihemophilic factor (AHF) or globulin (AHG)	Hemophilia A (classic hemophilia)—results from congenital deficiency
IX	Christmas factor, plasma thromboplastin component (PTC)	Hemophilia B—results from congenital deficiency
X	Stuart-Prower factor	Congenital deficiency known
XI	Plasma thromboplastin antecedent, PTA	Congenital deficiency known
XII	Hageman factor	No clinical symptoms associated with congenital deficiency
XIII	Fibrin-stabilizing factor	Congenital deficiency known

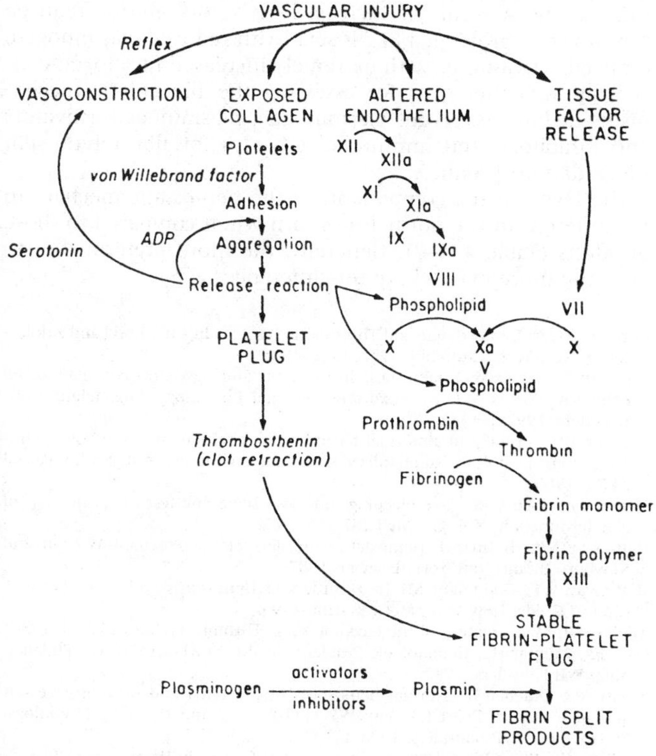

Figure 431–1. Diagrammatic representation of the hemostatic mechanism. (From Nathan DG, Oski FA: Hematology of Infancy and Childhood, 3rd ed. Philadelphia, WB Saunders, 1987, p 1294.)

The fibrinolytic system is composed of plasminogen, activators, and inhibitors. Plasminogen must be converted to plasmin, which is the active proteolytic enzyme, by activators (such as tissue-type plasminogen activator and urinary-type plasminogen activator). This reaction is modulated by plasminogen activator inhibitors (PAIs) and by α_2-antiplasmin (α_2-plasmin inhibitor). Plasmin's function is to lyse fibrin, a process that produces soluble fibrin degradation (split) products.

EVALUATION OF THE PATIENT WITH A SUSPECTED HEMOSTATIC DEFECT

HISTORY AND PHYSICAL EXAMINATION. The focus of the history and physical examination is to determine whether the suspected defect is acquired or congenital (inherited) and which mechanism appears to be affected (primary or secondary hemostatic mechanism). The history should determine the site or sites of bleeding, the severity and duration of the hemorrhage, the age of onset, what was done to control the bleeding, whether the bleeding was spontaneous or induced, the family history, a drug history, the patient's experiences with prior trauma (e.g., surgical procedures, biopsies, venipunctures, dental extraction) and, in females, a detailed menstrual history. The physical examination should determine the characteristics of the bleeding (e.g., petechiae, ecchymoses, hematomas, hemarthroses, mucous membrane bleeding) and identify signs of a primary systemic disease. The characteristic bleeding manifestations in a patient with a defective primary hemostatic mechanism (platelet–blood vessel interaction) are mucous membrane bleeding (e.g., epistaxis, hematuria, menorrhagia, gastrointestinal), petechiae in the skin and mucous membranes, and multiple, small, ecchymotic lesions. The typical bleeding signs in a patient with a defective secondary hemostatic mechanism (coagulation system) are deep bleeding into joints and muscles, large spreading ecchymotic lesions, and hematomas.

LABORATORY TESTS. Patients who are hemorrhaging or who have a history suggestive of a hemostatic disorder should have a platelet count, bleeding time, prothrombin time, and activated partial thromboplastin time (APTT) performed. These screening studies should identify most hemostatic defects, although there are exceptions. More specific tests may be needed to define the defect more precisely.

Certain previously used tests are no longer employed either because they lack sensitivity and specificity or because the current techniques are less cumbersome and the results are easier to interpret. Tests that are now rarely used are the tourniquet test, whole blood clotting time, prothrombin consumption time, and thromboplastin generation test.

Bleeding Time. The bleeding time is the best test for assessing the vascular and platelet phases of hemostasis. It has been standardized by the use of a template that regulates the length and depth of the skin incision. A blood pressure cuff is applied to the arm and inflated to 40 mm Hg for children, 30 mm Hg for term newborns, and 20 mm Hg for preterm babies, and an incision is made using a template and scalpel blade. At 30-sec intervals drops of blood are blotted from the margin of the incision. Normally, blood flow stops within 4–8 min.

Platelet Count. A platelet count is essential in the evaluation, because thrombocytopenia is the most common cause of a defective primary hemostatic mechanism that produces a significant bleeding diathesis in children. There is a linear relationship between the bleeding time and the platelet count, that is, the lower the platelet count, the more prolonged the bleeding time. Using a template, bleeding time in this relationship can be determined as

$$\text{Bleeding time (min)} = 30.5 - \frac{\text{Platelet count (per uL)}}{3{,}850}.$$

If the bleeding time is disproportionate to the platelet count, a qualitative platelet defect should be suspected. Patients with a platelet count above 50×10^9/L rarely have significant bleeding.

Platelet Aggregation and Other Tests. If a platelet function defect is detected, further in vitro studies can be carried out, including platelet aggregation tests using activators (e.g., ADP, collagen, epinephrine, thrombin, and/or ristocetin), clot retraction, prothrombin consumption test (for platelet factor 3), ATP and serotonin release, and others.

The three phases of coagulation can be individually assessed by simple, reliable tests.

Thrombin Time. Phase III can be evaluated by the thrombin time, the time required for plasma to clot after the addition of bovine or human thrombin (factor IIa). The normal thrombin time ranges from 15 to 20 sec in most laboratories. Prolongation of the thrombin time occurs with hypofibrinogenemia, or dysfunctional fibrinogen (dysfibrinogenemia), or by substances that interfere with fibrin polymerization (e.g., heparin, certain fibrinolytic degradation products). If heparin contamination is the cause, the heparin can be inactivated by various neutralizing agents and the test repeated, or the thrombin time can be determined using a snake venom (reptilase) in place of the thrombin. Reptilase is a thrombin-like enzyme that is not affected by heparin. Fibrinogen also can be measured by chemical, immunologic, and heat precipitation methods.

Prothrombin Time. Phase II of coagulation is assessed by the prothrombin time, the time taken for plasma to clot after the addition of exogenous thromboplastin (tissue factor) and calcium. The normal prothrombin time ranges from 11.5 to 14 sec. If phase III is intact, a prolonged prothrombin time indicates a deficiency involving factors II, V, VII, and/or X. Specific assays are available for all these factors. The prothrombin time, however, does not reflect the activity of factors XII, XI, IX, VIII, or XIII.

Activated Partial Thromboplastin Time. Phase I, the most complex part of the coagulation mechanism, is evaluated by the activated

■ TABLE 431–2 Hemostatic Mechanisms of the Newborn*

Component	Newborn Level
Coagulation factors	
Fibrinogen	Lower limit of normal
Factors II, VII, IX, X, XI, XII, high molecular weight kininogen, and prekallikrein	Very low
Factors V and XIII	Normal
Factor VIII and von Willebrand factor	Normal to increased
Inhibitors	
Antithrombin III	Low
Proteins C and S	Low
Fibrinolytic components	
Plasminogen	Low
Plasminogen activators	Low
Plasminogen activator inhibitors	Normal
Plasmin inhibitors	Normal to increased
Platelets	
Quantitative	Normal
Qualitative (function)	Impaired

Compared with those of older children and adults.

partial thromboplastin time (APTT). The APTT is the time required for the clotting of plasma that has been activated by incubation with an inert activator (e.g., kaolin, celite, ground glass, ellagic acid) when calcium and platelets (or a lipid substitute for platelets) are added. The normal APTT ranges from 25 to 40 sec. This test is a simple, inexpensive, and reliable way to assess the adequacy of factors XII (and prekallikrein, high-molecular-weight kininogen), XI, IX, and VIII. The APTT does not assess factor VII or factor XIII activity. If phase III and phase II are intact, a prolonged APTT represents either a deficiency or an inhibitor in the intrinsic pathway.

Mixing Study. The next test to be performed is a mixing study. In this study, normal plasma is added to the patient's plasma and the APTT is carried out on the mixture. If the resulting APTT is normal (i.e., the patient's abnormal APTT is corrected), then a deficiency state is present. If, however, the mixture's APTT remains prolonged, an inhibitor is present. Correction of the abnormal APTT in the mixing study in a patient with a bleeding disorder indicates a deficiency of factor VIII, IX, or XI or, in a patient without a bleeding disorder, indicates a deficiency of factor XII, prekallikrein, or high-molecular-weight kininogen. If the mixing study does not correct (or worsens with incubation) and the patient has a bleeding disorder, an inhibitor against factors VIII, IX, or XI should be suspected. If the patient has no hemorrhagic manifestations, the inhibitor is probably the lupus anticoagulant. Assays for each coagulation factor are available and are needed to identify the specific factor involved and the severity of the defect. Severity is graduated as follows: severe—activity less than 1% of normal (also reported as less than 1 unit/dL or less than 0.01 unit/mL); moderate—activity greater than 1% but less than 5% of normal (or 1–5 units/dL); and mild—activity greater than 5% of normal (or greater than 5 units/dL). Normal levels in most laboratories for these factors are between 50% and 150% (50–150 units/dL).

Other Tests. There are no screening tests for the natural inhibitors of the coagulation mechanism. Specific functional and immunologic assays are available for measuring the plasma levels of antithrombin III, protein C, and protein S.

Screening tests for overall fibrinolysis are insensitive. Such tests include the whole blood clot lysis time and the plasma clot lysis time. The euglobulin clot lysis time (ELT) is used by most laboratories to assess fibrinolysis. In this test a euglobulin fraction of plasma is made (usually by acetic acid precipitation) and the fraction is clotted with calcium or thrombin. The time for clot lysis is determined (usually from 2 to 4 hr). The euglobulin fraction has clotting factors, fibrinogen, plasminogen, and plasminogen activators, but no inhibitors. A short ELT can be a result of increased activators and/or reduced fibrinogen; a prolonged ELT is seen with reduced plasminogen, reduced activator, or with extremely increased fibrinogen concentration. Other tests for assessing the fibrinolytic mechanisms include assays for plasminogen, plasminogen activators and inhibitors, and immunologic assays for fibrinolytic split (degradation) products.

The levels of the components of the hemostatic mechanism are different in the normal newborn when compared to those of adults (Table 431–2). Generally, the more preterm the infant, the more marked are the differences.

Corrigan JJ, Jr: Hemorrhagic and Thrombotic Diseases in Childhood and Adolescence. New York, Churchill Livingstone, 1985.

Corrigan JJ, Jr: Normal hemostasis in the fetus and newborn: coagulation. *In:* Polin RA, Fox WW (eds): Fetal and Neonatal Physiology. Philadelphia, WB Saunders, 1992, p 1368.

Feusner JH: Normal and abnormal bleeding times in neonates and young children utilizing a fully standardized template technique. Am J Clin Pathol 74:73, 1980.

Harker LA, Slichter SJ: The bleeding time as a screening test for evaluation of platelet function. N Engl J Med 287:155, 1972.

Hathaway WE, Bonnar J: Hemostatic Disorders of the Pregnant Woman and Newborn Infant. New York, Elsevier, 1987.

Hathaway WE, Goodnight SH Jr: Disorders of Hemostasis and Thrombosis. A Clinical Guide. New York, McGraw-Hill, 1993.

Mielke CH: Measurement of the bleeding time. Thromb Haemost 52:210, 1984.

Oski FA, Naiman JL: Hematologic Problems in the Newborn, 3rd ed. Philadelphia, WB Saunders, 1982.

Stuart MJ, Graeber JE: Normal hemostasis in the fetus and newborn: vessels and platelets. In: Polin RA, Fox WW (eds): Fetal and Neonatal Physiology. Philadelphia, WB Saunders, 1992, p 1372.

Williams CE, Short PE, George AJ, et al: Critical Factors in Haemostasis. Evaluation and Development. Chichester, England, Ellis Horwood, 1988.

CHAPTER 432
Phase I Disorders: The Hemophilias

The hemophilias are the most common and serious of the congenital coagulation disorders. They are associated with genetically determined deficiencies of factors VIII, IX, or XI.

432.1 Factor VIII Deficiency

(Classic Hemophilia; Hemophilia A; Antihemophilic Factor [AHF] Deficiency)

About 80% of cases of hemophilia are hemophilia A, which is caused by a defective gene carried on the X chromosome. About 75% of patients with hemophilia A have a proportionate reduction in factor VIII activity and factor VIII antigen (protein). They are classified as CRM (cross-reacting material) negative (CRM−) or reduced (CRMred). The remaining 25% of patients have reduced factor VIII activity, but the antigen is present and these patients are classified as CRM^+. Numerous mutations in gene structure have been described. The most common are large deletions and missense mutations. The others include small deletions, insertions, internal gene segment duplications, splice-site mutations, and nonsense point mutations. Except for the missense mutations, most of these appear to prevent the synthesis of factor VIII antigen. In the mis-sense mutations the factor VIII protein is synthesized with variable functional activity of Factor VIII. To date, it is estimated that deletions account for 2.5–10% of mutations causing hemophilia A. The remaining mutations are mostly single nucleotide substitutions.

This deficiency results in a profound depression of the level of factor VIII coagulation activity in the plasma. Factor VIII is complexed with von Willebrand protein (called the factor VIII–von Willebrand complex) in plasma, with the von Willebrand protein acting as a carrier protein. Patients with hemophilia A and women who are carriers for the disorder have reduced factor VIII activity but normal plasma levels of the von Willebrand protein (in contrast to classic von Willebrand disease, in which both levels are reduced). In the normal population the plasma ratio of factor VIII activity to von Willebrand protein is 1:0. Thus, most female carriers have a ratio of less than one, which can be used for carrier detection and genetic counseling. Carrier and fetal detection has become more precise. The methods employed for the genetic analysis of hemophilia A are based on the detection of DNA sequence variations within or near the gene. An affected male and a heterozygotic mother are used to define the defect(s). Fetal samples can be obtained from DNA extracted from chorionic villi (8–11 wk) or from cells aspirated by amniocentesis (midtrimester). A combination of DNA-based methods and assays of factor VIII activity is usually used for carrier detection and prenatal diagnosis. However, it is estimated that 6–20% of women are still misclassified.

In 80% of cases the family history is positive for the disease. Sporadic cases may represent a new mutation. The clinical severity depends on the level of factor VIII activity in the plasma: Severe cases have less than 1% (1 unit/dL) of normal activity; moderate cases have 1–5% (1–5 units/dL); and mild cases have 6–30% (6–30 units/dL). The degree of severity tends to be consistent within a given family.

CLINICAL MANIFESTATIONS. Because factor VIII does not cross the placenta, a bleeding tendency may be evident in the neonatal period. Hematomas after injections and bleeding from circumcision are common, but many affected newborns exhibit no clinical abnormalities. As ambulation begins, excessive bruising occurs. Large intramuscular hematomas result from minor trauma. A relatively minor traumatic laceration, as of the tongue or lip, which bleeds persistently for hours or days, is frequently the event that leads to diagnosis. Of patients with severe disease, 90% have had clear clinical evidence of increased bleeding by 1 yr of age.

The hallmark of hemophilia is hemarthrosis. Hemorrhages into the elbows, knees, and ankles cause pain and swelling and limit movement of the joint; these may be induced by relatively minor trauma but often appear to be spontaneous. Repeated hemorrhages may produce degenerative changes, with osteoporosis, muscle atrophy and, ultimately, a fixed, unusable joint. Spontaneous hematuria is a troublesome but not usually serious complication. Intracranial hemorrhage and bleeding into the neck constitute life-threatening emergencies.

Patients with factor VIII activities greater than 6% (6 units/dL) do not have spontaneous symptoms. These patients, with "mild hemophilia," may experience only prolonged bleeding following tooth extractions or dental work, surgery, or injury.

LABORATORY FINDINGS. The only significant laboratory abnormalities occur in coagulation tests and reflect a serious deficiency of factor VIII. The partial thromboplastin time (PTT) is greatly prolonged. The platelet count, bleeding time, and prothrombin time are normal. Mixing studies using normal plasma show a correction of the PTT. A specific assay for factor VIII activity confirms the diagnosis.

TREATMENT. Prevention of trauma is an important aspect of care for the hemophilic child. During early life the crib and playpen should be padded, and the child should be carefully supervised while learning to walk. As he or she becomes older, physical activities that do not entail a risk of trauma should be encouraged. It is important that a course between overprotection and permissiveness be followed. Aspirin and other drugs that affect platelet function may provoke hemorrhage and must be avoided by hemophilic patients. Because children with severe hemophilia are exposed to blood products throughout life, they should be immunized against hepatitis B virus. The vaccine may be given in the newborn period.

Replacement Therapy. When bleeding episodes occur, replacement therapy is essential to prevent pain, disability, or life-threatening hemorrhage. The aim of therapy is to increase factor VIII activity in the plasma to a level that secures hemostasis. Currently, this can be done only by the intravenous infusion of fresh frozen plasma or of plasma concentrates.

Therapy of the hemophilic patient has been considerably facilitated by the development of factor VIII concentrates; these permit fairly precise estimation of the dosage necessary to attain hemostatic levels. By definition, 1 mL of normal plasma contains 1 unit of factor VIII. Because the plasma volume is about 45 mL/kg, it is necessary to infuse 45 units/kg of factor VIII to increase its level in the hemophilic recipient from 0–100% (0–100 units/dL). A dose of 25–50 units/kg of factor VIII is usually given to raise the recipient's level to 50–100% (50–100 units/dL) of normal. Because the half-life of factor VIII in the plasma is about 8–12 hr, repeated infusions can be given, as necessary, to maintain the desired level of activity.

Several factor VIII concentrates are available (Table 432–1). The most inexpensive of these is cryoprecipitate, which can be prepared in the blood bank from fresh plasma. The yield from 250 mL of fresh plasma is one bag of cryoprecipitate, which usually contains 75–125 units of factor VIII; there may, however, be marked variability in the content of bags. One bag of cryoprecipitate/5 kg of body weight raises the recipient's level to about 50% (50 units/dL) of normal. Because cryoprecipitate is produced from single units of whole blood, the risk of blood-borne diseases such as hepatitis B and AIDS (Chapters 221–223) is lower than with concentrates prepared from large plasma pools. Factor VIII concentrates that are produced by recombinant technology and those that are prepared by monoclonal antibody techniques (Table 432–1) are more expensive than cryoprecipitate but are safer with regard to the transmission of infectious organisms. These concentrates are dispensed as lyophilized powders in bottles of 250–500 units that can be reconstituted just prior to use; they are tremendously useful and convenient. Their potency and relatively low protein content permit rapid restoration of normal hemostatic levels with very small volumes. Commercial factor VIII concentrates also contain anti-A and anti-B isohemagglutinins; when massive amounts are given to persons of blood group A or B, hemolysis may occur.

When the hemophilic child has significant bleeding, replacement therapy should be promptly instituted (Table 432–2). First-aid measures should include application of cold and pressure, but these should not substitute for adequate replacement therapy. For ordinary hemarthroses, it is necessary to raise the factor VIII level to about 50% (50 units/dL) and to maintain it at least above 5% (5 units/dL) for 48–72 hr. A single infusion of 20–30 units/kg of factor VIII concentrate suffices, permitting the "one-shot" therapy of ordinary bleeding episodes. Immobilization is initially indicated, but passive exercise should be started within 48 hr to prevent joint stiffness and fibrosis. The need for aspiration of blood from the joint is controversial. When the skin overlying the joint is tense because therapy has been delayed the aspiration of blood, after adequate factor VIII has been given, may provide relief of pain. Replacement therapy is the most important aspect of the management of hemarthrosis, because equally good results have been obtained by some who routinely practice joint aspiration and by others

■ TABLE 432–1 Factor VIII and Factor IX Concentrates

Factor	Manufacturer	Process
Factor VIII Products		
A. Immuaffinity Purified		
Monoclate P	Armour	Pasteurized
Hemofil M	Baxter-Hyland	Solvent-detergent
Method M	Baxter-Hyland for American Red Cross	Solvent-detergent
B. Intermediate Purity and High Purity		
Koate-HP	Cutter	Solvent-detergent
Humate-P	Behringwerke	Pasteurized
Melate SD	N.Y. Blood Center	Solvent-detergent
Alphanate	Alpha	Solvent-detergent
N.Y. Blood Center	N.Y. Blood Center-Melville Biologics	Solvent-detergent
C. Porcine		
Hyate:C	Porton/Speywood	Polyelectrolyte chromatography
D. Genetically Engineered		
Recombinate AHF	Baxter	Genetically engineered
KoGENate AHF	Cutter	Genetically engineered
Factor IX Products		
E. Factor IX Concentrates		
AlphaNine	Alpha	Heated in N-heptane solution
AlphaNine SD (Enew)	Alpha	TNBP and polysorbate 80
Mononine (Emono)	Armour	Sodium triocyanate, ultrafiltration
F. Factor IX Complex Concentrates		
Konyne 80	Cutter	Dry heat
Proplex T	Baxter-Hylane	Dry heat
Profilnine HT	Alpha	Heated in N-heptane solution
Bebulin VH	Immuno	Vapor heated
G. Activated Complex Concentrates		
Autoplex T	Baxter-Hyland	Dry heat
Feiba VH	Immuno	Vapor heated

who do not. Aggressive replacement therapy with factor VIII and careful orthopedic management of hemarthroses can prevent much severe deformity and crippling, which are now less common than in the past.

When hemorrhage occurs in vital areas such as the brain or neck, or when major surgery is contemplated, intensive therapy using factor VIII concentrates for 2 wk is indicated to maintain the plasma level above 50% (50 units/dL). ϵ-Aminocaproic acid, 50–100 mg/kg every 6 hr, may be indicated in conjunction with replacement therapy for oral mucous membrane hemorrhage and dental extraction. Venipuncture should be performed only from superficial veins; aspiration from femoral or internal jugular veins is hazardous and has led to several deaths. There is compelling evidence that early treatment with factor VIII concentrates reduces disability and deformity as well as the amount and duration of replacement treatment necessary for bleeding episodes. Parents, or the older patient, can be trained to give intravenous infusions or concentrates at home, with substantial decreases in hospitalization, morbidity, and risk of blood-transmitted diseases.

■ TABLE 432–2 Recommendation for Treatment of Hemophilia Patients (in this table, listing includes products proved hepatitis safe)

Classification of Patient	Factor Needed VIII	IX
1. New patient—no inhibitors—HIV neg.	A/D	E/F
2. Old patient—previous exposures to blood products—HIV neg.—no inhibitors	A/B/D/	F/E
3. Old patient—previous exposures to blood products—HIV neg.—with inhibitors	F (G)(C)	G
4. Old patient—HIV positive—with inhibitors	A (B)	F
5. Old patient—HIV positive—with inhibitors	F (G)(C)	G
6. Factor VIII patient inducing immune tolerance	A/D/B	N/A
7. Mild disease/infrequent user of factor	A/D*	N/A

Letters refer to available products listed in Table 432–1. The list in the table is in priority order. For example, A/B/D, means that a product listed under A is usually used in preference to a product listed under B, and this is usually used in preference to a product listed under D.

A letter in parentheses in the list implies a product is usually used under unusual conditions. The preceding letter refers to a product listed under that letter that is usually a standard treatment for that classification of patient.

N/A = not applicable.

**DDAVP fails or is inappropriate.*

Home treatment with periodic assessment and counsel from the physician represents optimal or ideal management for the hemophilic child and family, and this enlightened management may permit the present generation of hemophilic children to enter adult life without major physical or psychologic crippling. On the other hand, some long-term complications may result from modern therapy. Abnormalities of hepatic enzyme activities are found in 50% of patients. Instances of chronic active hepatitis and cirrhosis have been reported. A high proportion of patients now have antibodies against hepatitis B and C viruses, and many older patients have antibodies against the AIDS virus (human immunodeficiency virus, HIV). These findings are the basis for recommending active immunization against HBV. Hypertension and renal disease with hematuria occur in many adult patients; their causes have not been defined.

Desmopressin (DDAVP; Stimate) causes an increase in factor VIII in patients with mild hemophilia A and in some patients with moderate disease. The recommended dose is 0.3 μg/kg body weight, which raises the factor VIII level 25–50% above the baseline. It should only be given once every 1–2 days and only for minor bleeding episodes, such as oral bleeding, dental extractions, and small hematomas. It is ineffective in hemarthrosis, central nervous system bleeding, and for sustaining factor VIII levels after major surgery.

Factor VIII Inhibitors. Ten to 15% of patients with hemophilia become refractory to factor VIII therapy because a circulating inhibitor or antibody develops. The development of inhibitors is not related to the number of plasma transfusions, and replacement therapy should not be withheld in hope of avoiding this. These inhibitors are IgG globulins and are specifically active against factor VIII. The inhibitors may be of low titer and transient, or of extremely higher titer and very persistent. The "Bethesda unit" of inhibition is the amount of inhibitory activity in 1 mL of plasma that reduces the factor VIII level in 1 mL of normal plasma from 1 to 0.5 unit. It is almost impossible to overpower a high-titer inhibitor but, when life-threatening hemorrhage occurs, massive doses of factor VIII concentrates or plasmapheresis with replacement with factor VIII should be given and may be of temporary benefit. Immunosuppressive therapy is of no value.

Another attempt at therapy of the hemophilic child who has developed a factor VIII inhibitor involves the use of factor IX concentrates (Konyne; Autoplex; Feiba), which apparently contain amounts of a factor VIII bypassing principle. These activated coagulants enter the coagulation cascade distal to the level of factor VIII (see Fig. 431–1) and thus bypass the effects of the inhibitor. The activities of various preparations, however, and even of different lots of the same preparation, vary markedly. Thrombosis is a possible complication.

Porcine factor VIII (Hyate: C) is effective in hemophilia A patients with inhibitors. This animal factor VIII provides adequate factor VIII activity in patients with less than 50 Bethesda units of inhibitor. The usual starting dose is 100–150 porcine units/kg. Reported side effects include mild fever, nausea, headache, flushing, and occasional vomiting.

Immune tolerance may potentially be achieved with combined therapy including intravenous immunoglobulin, cyclophosphamide, and factor VIII.

PRENATAL DIAGNOSIS. Each male fetus of a mother who carries hemophilia has a 50% risk of having the disease. Prenatal diagnosis is possible through examination of the blood of the (male) fetus, which can be obtained at fetoscopy at 20–22 wk of gestation. Fetal plasma is assayed for von Willebrand protein and for factor VIIIc; as in the older patient, a markedly higher von Willebrand protein level compared to the factor VIIIc level identifies an affected male. It is now possible to identify a fetus with hemophilia by examining DNA polymorphisms in amniotic fluid fibroblasts. Trophoblastic biopsy in fetuses at risk may permit the diagnosis of hemophilia as early as 10–12 wk of gestation.

432.2 Factor IX Deficiency

(Christmas Disease; Hemophilia B)

Factor IX is produced by the liver and is one of the vitamin K–dependent coagulation factors. About 12–15% of the hemophilias result from a genetically determined deficiency of factor IX.

CLINICAL MANIFESTATIONS. This disease is clinically indistinguishable from factor VIII deficiency (hemophilia A); joint and muscle hemorrhages are characteristic. It is transmitted as an X-linked recessive trait, and the severity is related to the level of coagulant activity of the factor in plasma.

Hemophilia B patients are classified as CRM^+, CRM−, or CRMred; the majority (75%) are CRM−. More than 230 mutations have been described. The CRM− mutations tend to be large gene deletions, frameshift mutations, splice-site mutations, and nonsense mutations. The CRM^+ mutations (having normal or excess factor IX antigen) have had prevention of propeptide cleavage, mutations within the Gla (gamma carboxy glutamic acid) domain, and mutations within the growth factor domain or activation peptide region.

Factor IX is normally reduced in the plasma of newborns and slowly increases into the adult range after several months. Thus, unlike factor VIII, which is at normal or above-normal levels at birth, mild or moderate hemophilia B is difficult to diagnose in the newborn period, but severe hemophilia B (less than 1% factor IX activity) can be diagnosed in the newborn. Although female carriers can be identified by factor IX coagulation assays, detection is more specific by using monoclonal antibody or DNA analysis techniques. As with hemophilia A, the best method is the detection of DNA sequence variations.

LABORATORY FINDINGS. The partial thromboplastin time is usually abnormally prolonged. The bleeding time and prothrombin time are normal. Specific factor IX assay is necessary to distinguish the deficiency from that of hemophilia A and to define the severity of the defect.

TREATMENT. Replacement of factor IX is accomplished by infusions of fresh frozen plasma (FFP) or a factor IX concentrate. Because the half-life of factor IX is longer than factor VIII (about 24 hr), it may be administered less frequently. Also, the dose-response relationship to factor IX is different than that for factor VIII. One unit of factor IX/kg raises the plasma factor IX from 1–1.2% of normal (factor VIII, 1 unit/kg, can raise the plasma factor VIII by 2%). Thus, to achieve 100% (100 units/dL) activity in a patient with severe hemophilia B, an infusion of 100 units of factor IX/kg is needed. Fresh frozen plasma has about 1 unit of factor IX/mL, whereas the concentrates contain considerably more factor IX in less volume. Concentrates that are heat-treated continue to have the risk of transmitting hepatitis B and C viruses. Their use is preferred when levels of factor IX greater than 30% (30 units/dL) are needed. All patients with hemophilia B should receive the hepatitis B vaccine.

Episodes of thrombosis have occurred after use of the concentrates, especially in the postoperative patient with underlying liver disease, presumably because the concentrates contain coagulants.

432.3 Factor XI Deficiency

(Hemophilia C)

Factor XI deficiency is the least common type of hemophilia and is found in 2–3% of all hemophilia patients. Factor XI deficiency is transmitted as an incomplete autosomal recessive disease that affects males and females. Only homozygous patients have a bleeding diathesis. Postoperative and post-trauma hemorrhage is characteristic. Patients may also have epistaxis, hematuria, and menorrhagia. Spontaneous bleeding is rare.

Homozygous patients with factor XI deficiency have a prolonged partial thromboplastin time, and normal bleeding and prothrombin times. The factor XI level is 1–10% (1–10 units/dL), whereas heterozygous patients have factor XI levels of 30–65% (30–65 units/dL).

The half-life of factor XI in vivo is 40–80 hr. Replacement therapy for bleeding episodes is carried out with fresh frozen plasma. Plasma therapy in a dose of 10–15 mL/kg every 24 hr is effective.

432.4 Factor XII Deficiency

(Hageman Factor Deficiency)

Homozygous occurrence of an autosomal gene results in a profound deficiency of factor XII. Despite markedly abnormal test results of the 1st phase of coagulation (PTT and clotting times), affected persons have no clinical abnormalities of bleeding; in fact, some patients have a thrombotic tendency.

■ TABLE 432–3 Genetic and Laboratory Findings in von Willebrand Disease

	Parameter						
Type	**BT**	**VIII-C**	**vW-Ag**	**R-Cof**	**RIPA**	**Multimer Structure**	**Mode of Inheritance**
I (classic)	P†	R	R	R	R	N	AD
II							
A	P	N/R	N/R	R	R	Abn	AD
B	P	N/R	N/R	N/R	I	Abn	AD
III	P	R	R	R	R	Variable	AR

BT, Bleeding time; VIII-C, factor VIII coagulant activity; vW-Ag, von Willebrand antigen (protein); R-Cof, ristocetin cofactor; RIPA, ristocetin-induced platelet aggregation (agglutination); P, prolonged; R, reduced; N, normal; I, increased; N/R, normal or reduced; Abn, abnormal; AD, autosomal dominant; AR, autosomal recessive.

432.5 Von Willebrand Disease

(Vascular Hemophilia)

This disease is not as common as hemophilia A (factor VIII deficiency) but is probably more frequent than hemophilia B (factor IX deficiency). It occurs in both sexes and is inherited as an autosomal dominant trait. A few families with severe disease have been described in which the genetic transmission was autosomal recessive. The disease is caused by underproduction of von Willebrand protein or, in some families, by the synthesis of a dysfunctional protein. The von Willebrand protein contains a platelet-adhesive component (von Willebrand factor) and also the protein functions to carry factor VIII in the plasma.

There are at least three major varieties of von Willebrand disease, based on genetic and laboratory studies (Table 432–3). Types I and II are autosomal dominant and type III is autosomal recessive. Types I (classic von Willebrand disease) and III show reduced factor VIII activity, reduced von Willebrand protein and function, and usually a normal multimer structure of the von Willebrand protein on gel electrophoresis. Type II can have normal or reduced factor VIII activity, normal or reduced von Willebrand protein, reduced von Willebrand factor activity, and a loss of large and intermediate-sized multimers on electrophoresis.

CLINICAL MANIFESTATIONS. These include nosebleeds, bleeding from gums, menorrhagia, prolonged oozing from cuts, and increased bleeding after trauma or surgery. Spontaneous hemarthroses are very rare.

LABORATORY FINDINGS. The bleeding time is prolonged in all von Willebrand syndromes. The platelet count and prothrombin time are normal. The partial thromboplastin time may be normal but usually is mildly to moderately prolonged. Type I patients (classic von Willebrand disease) have reduced plasma levels of von Willebrand protein, von Willebrand factor activity, and factor VIII activity. The platelets in von Willebrand disease have decreased adhesiveness and do not aggregate when the antibiotic ristocetin is added to platelet-rich plasma (because von Willebrand factor is missing), unlike platelets from normal individuals. Rare patients may show increased reactivity to ristocetin (type II B).

TREATMENT. Therapy consists of replacement of the von Willebrand factor using fresh frozen plasma or cryoprecipitate. Cryoprecipitate is the preferred form of therapy for serious bleeding or for preparation for surgery. The recommended dose is two to four bags of cryoprecipitate/10 kg, which can be repeated every 12–24 hr, depending on the bleeding episode to be treated or prevented. Patients with mild to moderate type I von Willebrand disease who have minor bleeding manifestations (e.g., epistaxis), or who are to undergo certain surgical procedures (e.g., dental extraction), may be given DDAVP as for those with hemophilia A.

CHAPTER 433
Phase II Disorders

Factors II (prothrombin), V, VII, and X are involved in the 2nd phase of coagulation and are designated the prothrombin complex. These factors are produced in the liver, and all except factor V require vitamin K for normal synthesis. The vitamin is necessary for the γ-carboxylation of glutamic acid residues, which converts the inactive precursors into their biologically active forms. These precursors are also known as PIVKA (protein induced by vitamin K absence) and preprotein. For example, factor II's precursor is called PIVKA-II, or prefactor II.

Deficiency of a factor in the prothrombin complex is rare and is inherited in an autosomal recessive manner. The production of a functionally abnormal factor II (dysprothrombinemia) is inherited as an autosomal dominant trait. Patients with a deficiency in one or more of these factors have bleeding manifestations similar to those of the hemophilias, except that there is a high prevalence of spontaneous central nervous system bleeding in those with factor VII deficiency.

LABORATORY FINDINGS. The laboratory tests reveal a prolonged prothrombin time in these patients. Patients with factor II, V, and X deficiency also have a prolonged partial thromboplastin time (PTT). In contrast, patients with factor VII deficiency have a normal PTT. Bleeding time, platelet count, and platelet function tests are normal.

TREATMENT. Therapy consists of replacement of the deficient factor or factors with fresh frozen plasma. There is no factor concentrate available for factor V replacement. Severe cases of factor II, VII, or X deficiency may need a prothrombin complex concentrate (Proplex γ, Konyne) for control of hemostasis. These deficiencies are refractory to vitamin K therapy.

CHAPTER 434
Phase III Disorders

CONGENITAL AFIBRINOGENEMIA

This rare hemorrhagic disorder is caused by an autosomal recessive gene. Despite totally incoagulable blood, these patients usually do not have severe spontaneous hemorrhages or hemarthroses, but trauma or surgery may be followed by severe bleeding. Therapy with 100 mg/kg of fibrinogen provides a hemostatic plasma level. Because the plasma half-life of fibrinogen is 3–5 days, frequent infusions are not necessary. Cryoprecipitate contains fibrinogen and is used effectively for therapy. Each cryoprecipitate bag contains between 225 and 250 mg of fibrinogen/bag. Thus, four to five bags provide 1 g of fibrinogen.

CONGENITAL DYSFIBRINOGENEMIAS

A number of abnormal fibrinogens with defective function may be associated with thrombotic and bleeding states. Inheritance is as a dominant trait. The thrombin time is prolonged, but chemical or immunologic methods reveal normal levels of fibrinogen.

FACTOR XIII DEFICIENCY
(Fibrin-Stabilizing Factor Deficiency)

Deficiency of factor XIII has its onset most often in infancy, with bleeding after separation of the umbilical cord stump. Gastrointestinal, intracranial, and intra-articular hemorrhages are the most common clinical manifestations. Routine coagulation studies are normal. Factor XIII deficiency is diagnosed by finding an abnormal solubility of the clot in 5 M urea solution. These patients can be treated with fresh frozen plasma or cryoprecipitate.

Corrigan JJ Jr: The vitamin K-dependent proteins. *In:* Barness LA (ed): Advances in Pediatrics. Chicago, Year Book Medical Publishers, 1981, p 57.

Fricke WA, Lamb MA (guest eds): Clotting factor concentrates in clinical practice. Semin Thromb Hemost 19:1, 1993.

Hilgartner MW, Pochedly C (ed): Hemophilia in the Child and Adult, 3rd ed. New York, Raven Press, 1989.

Hoyer LW: Hemophilia A. N Engl J Med 330:38, 1994.

Kasper CK: Treatment of factor VIII inhibitors. Prog Hemost Thromb 9:57, 1989.

Kogan SC, Doherty M, Gitschier J: An improved method for prenatal diagnosis of genetic diseases by analysis of amplified DNA sequences. Application to hemophilia A. N Engl J Med 317:985, 1987.

Lozier JN, Brunkhous KM: Gene therapy and hemophilias. JAMA 271:47, 1994.

Mammen EF: Congenital coagulation disorders. Semin Thromb Hemost 9:1, 1983.

Mannucci PM: Desmopressin: A nontransfusional form of treatment for congenital and acquired bleeding disorders. Blood 72:1449, 1988.

Stamatoyannopoulos G, Nienhuis AW, Majerus PW, Varmus H: The Molecular Basis of Blood Diseases. Philadelphia, WB Saunders, 1994.

CHAPTER 435
Postneonatal Vitamin K Deficiency

Vitamin K deficiency rarely occurs after the neonatal period, although "late" hemorrhagic disease has been reported in breast-fed children. Intestinal malabsorption of fats and prolonged administration of broad-spectrum antibiotics may result in vitamin K deficiency; cystic fibrosis and biliary atresia may be complicated by disorders of the prothrombin complex. Prophylactic administration of water-soluble vitamin K orally is indicated in these situations (2–3 mg/24 hr for children and 5–10 mg/24 hr for adolescents and adults). In those with advanced liver disease synthesis of the factors of the prothrombin complex may be compromised by hepatocellular damage, so vitamin K therapy is often ineffective in correcting these disorders in these individuals. The anticoagulant properties of dicumarol and related anticoagulants depend on interference with vitamin K and the formation of factors II, VII, and X. Rat poison (superwarfarin) produces a similar deficiency. Vitamin K is a specific antidote.

The laboratory manifestations of vitamin K deficiency are prolonged prothrombin and partial thromboplastin times. The platelet count, bleeding time, and plasma fibrinogen level are normal. If needed, specific assays for factors II, VII, IX, and X or for detecting the noncarboxylated protein precursors of the vitamin K-dependent coagulation factors can be performed.

CHAPTER 436
Liver Disease

Coagulation abnormalities are common in patients with liver disease, estimated to be as high as 85%. Only 15% of patients, however, have significant clinical bleeding states. The severity of the coagulation abnormality appears to be directly proportional to the extent of hepatic cell damage. The most common mechanism causing the defect is decreased synthesis of the coagulation factors. Almost all the coagulation factors are produced only in the liver except, apparently, factor VIII, which can be produced in other organs. Severe liver disease characteristically has normal to increased (not reduced) levels of factor VIII activity in plasma. Rare causes of coagulation defects in hepatic disease are disseminated intravascular coagulation or hyperfibrinolysis.

The treatment of the coagulopathy of liver disease consists of replacement with fresh frozen plasma and cryoprecipitates. Fresh frozen plasma (10–15 mL/kg) can be expected to correct all clotting factor defects except fibrinogen. For fibrinogen correction, cryoprecipitates are recommended (four to five bags/10 kg). Because a reduction in the vitamin K dependent coagulation factors is common in those with acute and chronic liver disease, vitamin K therapy can be given a trial. The vitamin K can be given orally, subcutaneously, or intravenously (not intramuscularly) in a dose of 1 mg/24 hr for infants, 2–3 mg for children, and 5–10 mg for adolescents and adults. An inability to correct the coagulopathy indicates that the coagulopathy may be caused by a reduction in one or more of the non–vitamin K dependent proteins, or because the liver is severely impaired and cannot produce the precursor vitamin K proteins.

CHAPTER 437
Inhibitors

Acquired circulating anticoagulants (inhibitors) are defined as abnormal endogenous components of blood that inhibit the coagulation of normal blood. These anticoagulants are usually specific types of gamma globulin and may represent autoantibodies. The circulating anticoagulant may affect coagulation, either by neutralizing a specific coagulation factor directly or by acting against certain reaction sites in the coagulation pathway. When the anticoagulant acts against a specific coagulation factor (e.g., factor VIII or IX), the patient has a clinical bleeding picture similar to that of the congenital deficiency state. Usually no or minimal bleeding is noted in patients in whom the anticoagulant is directed toward a reaction site.

Circulating anticoagulants are uncommon in otherwise normal children. They are found in patients with systemic lupus erythematosus (SLE) or lymphomas, or in those with penicillin or other drug reactions. Spontaneous inhibitors have been reported in children following incidental viral infections.

LABORATORY FINDINGS. Inhibitors against specific coagulation factors usually affect factor VIII, IX, or XI (a phase I defect). The partial thromboplastin time (PTT) is prolonged and the test does not correct with the addition of normal plasma. The prothrombin time is normal. Specific factor assays determine which factor is involved.

The most common inhibitor against a reaction site is the so-called lupus anticoagulant. Although this inhibitor is found in patients with SLE, it may also occur spontaneously and in other disease states. This anticoagulant does not cause bleeding but paradoxically has been reported to be associated with a thrombotic tendency. It produces a prolonged PTT and it may also result in a prolonged prothrombin time. The addition of normal, platelet-poor plasma does not correct the abnormal tests, but the addition of platelets neutralizes the anticoagulant. On rare occasions there can be an associated hypoprothrombinemia (reduced factor II).

TREATMENT. Management of the patient with an inhibitor against a coagulation factor is the same as for the hemophilia patient who develops an alloantibody against factor VIII or IX. Infusions of a prothrombin complex concentrate (Konyne) or activated prothrombin complex concentrate (Autoplex; Feiba) may be needed to control significant bleeding manifestations. Spontaneous inhibitors, usually following a viral infection, tend to disappear with a few weeks to months. Inhibitors seen with an underlying disease disappear when the primary disease is treated.

CHAPTER 438

Consumption Coagulopathy

(Disseminated Intravascular Coagulation Syndromes)

Consumption coagulopathy refers to a large group of conditions, including disseminated intravascular coagulation (DIC). Consequences of this process include widespread intravascular deposition of fibrin, which may lead to tissue ischemia and necrosis, a generalized hemorrhagic state, and hemolytic anemia.

ETIOLOGY. A number of pathologic processes may incite episodes of DIC, including hypoxia, acidosis, tissue necrosis, shock, and endothelial damage (Fig. 438–1). Accordingly, it is not surprising that a large number of diseases have been reported to be associated with DIC, including incompatible blood transfusions, septic shock (especially gram-negative), rickettsial infections, snakebite, purpura fulminans, giant hemangioma, malignancies, and acute promyelocytic leukemia.

CLINICAL MANIFESTATIONS. Most frequently DIC accompanies a severe systemic disease process. Bleeding frequently first occurs from sites of venipuncture or surgical incision, with associated petechiae and ecchymoses. Tissue thrombosis may involve many organs and can be most spectacular as infarction of large areas of skin and subcutaneous tissue or of kidneys. Anemia caused by hemolysis may develop rapidly.

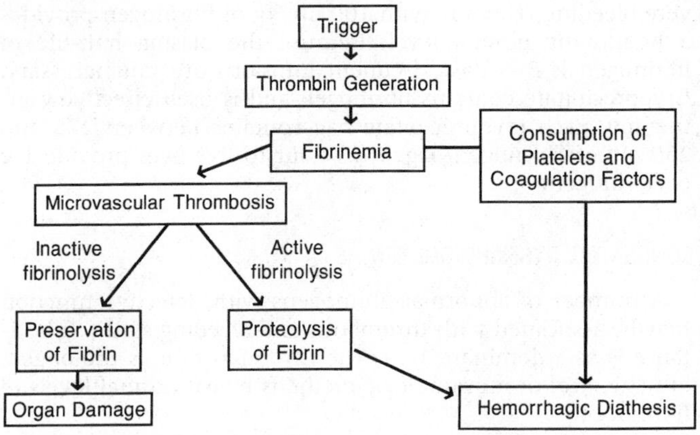

Figure 438–1. Disseminated intravascular coagulation.

LABORATORY FINDINGS. There is no well-defined sequence of events. The consumption coagulation factors (II, V, VIII, and fibrinogen) and platelets may be consumed by the ongoing intravascular clotting process, with prolongation of the prothrombin, partial thromboplastin, and thrombin times. Platelet counts may be profoundly depressed. The blood contains fragmented burr and helmet-shaped red blood cells (schizocytes), changes referred to as microangiopathic. In addition, because the fibrinolytic mechanism is activated, fibrin split products (FSP) appear in the blood. Table 438–1 presents the laboratory findings in children with the three common acquired coagulation defects. The D-dimer assay is equally sensitive and more specific for DIC than the fibrin degradation product (FDP) test. D-dimer is a neo-antigen formed following the thrombin-initiated generation of fibrin from fibrinogen, followed by cross-linking of fibrin by factor VIII and plasmin digestion of the cross-linked fibrin.

TREATMENT. The most important component of therapy is control or reversal of the process that initiated the DIC. Infection, shock, acidosis, and hypoxia must be treated promptly and vigorously. If the underlying problem can be controlled bleeding quickly ceases, and there is improvement of the abnormal laboratory findings. Blood components are used for replacement therapy in patients who have hemorrhage. This may consist of platelet infusions (for thrombocytopenia), cryoprecipitates (for hypofibrinogenemia), and/or fresh frozen plasma (for replacement of other coagulation factors and natural inhibitors).

In some patients the treatment of the primary disease may

■ **TABLE 438–1 Laboratory Findings in Disseminated Intravascular Coagulation, Vitamin K Deficiency, and Liver Disease**

	Disorder		
Test	***DIC***	***Vitamin K Deficiency***	***Liver Disease***
PTT	P	P	P
PT	P	P	P
TT	P	N	P
Platelet count	L	N	N/L
FSPs	+	—	±
Fibrinogen	L	N	L
Factor VIII	L	N	N/I

DIC, Disseminated intravascular coagulation; PTT, partial thromboplastin time; PT, prothrombin time; TT, thrombin time; FSPs, fibrinolytic split products; P, prolonged; N, normal; L, low; N/L, normal or low; +, present; −, absent; ±, present or absent; I, increased.

be inadequate or incomplete, or the replacement therapy may not be effective in controlling the hemorrhage. When this occurs the DIC may be treated with anticoagulants to prevent ongoing consumption of factors. Heparin is the drug of choice and can be administered on an intermittent or continuous intravenous treatment schedule. Using the intermittent intravenous schedule, heparin is given in a dose of 75–100 units/kg every 4 hr. With the continuous schedule, 50–75 units of heparin/kg is given as a bolus followed by a continuous infusion of 15–25 units/kg/hr. The duration and effectiveness of heparin therapy can be judged by serial measurements of the platelet count and plasma fibrinogen concentration.

Heparin has been found to be an effective drug in children with DIC associated with purpura fulminans and promyelocytic leukemia. Lower doses (10–15 units/kg/hr without a loading dose) are used for those with progranulocytic leukemia. Heparin is not indicated and has been reported to be ineffective in septic shock, snake envenomation, heat stroke, massive head injury, and incompatible blood transfusion reaction.

Bernini JC, Buchanan GR, Ashcroft J: Hypoprothrombinemia and severe hemorrhage associated with lupus anticoagulant. J Pediatr 123:937, 1993.
Corrigan JJ Jr: Coagulation inhibitors. Am J Pediatr Hematol Oncol 2:281, 1980.
Corrigan JJ Jr: Disseminated intravascular coagulation: Pathogenesis, diagnosis, and management. *In:* Lusher JM, Barnhart MI (eds): Acquired Bleeding Disorders in Children: Abnormalities of Hemostasis. New York. Masson, 1981, p 27.
Gerson, WT, Dikerman JD, Bovill EG, et al: Severe acquired protein C deficiency in purpura fulminans associated with disseminated intravascular coagulation: treatment with protein C concentrate. Pediatrics 91:418, 1993.
Hathaway WE, Bonnar J: Hemostatic Disorders of the Pregnant Woman and Newborn Infant. New York. Elsevier, 1987.
Owen CA Jr: Coagulation disorders associated with hepatocellular disease. *In:* Lusher JM, Barnhart MI (eds): Acquired Bleeding Disorders in Children: Abnormalities of Hemostasis. New York, Masson, 1981, p 41.
Shapiro SS, Thiagarajan P: Lupus anticoagulants. Prog Hemost Thromb 6:263, 1982.

CHAPTER 439
Platelet and Blood Vessel Disorders

Platelets are non-nucleated, cellular fragments produced by the megakaryocytes of the bone marrow. The large size of the megakaryocyte reflects its polyploidy. As the megakaryocyte reaches maturity, fragmentation of the cytoplasm occurs and large numbers of platelets are liberated. In the circulation they have a life span of 7–10 days. The platelet has a number of intrinsic antigens, which are distinct from those of the red blood cell, and some are shared by the leukocytes.

The platelets are intimately involved in both the vascular and clotting aspects of hemostasis. They are necessary for integrity of the vascular endothelium; when small blood vessels are transected, platelets accumulate at the site of injury, forming a hemostatic plug. Platelet adhesion is initiated by contact with extravascular components such as collagen. Release of thromboxane (a prostaglandin derivative) and endogenous ADP causes firm aggregation. Serotonin and histamine liberated during these processes increase local vasoconstriction. Platelets have a phospholipid with partial thromboplastin activity, which makes an important contribution to coagulation. They also transport other blood coagulation factors through absorption to the platelet surface. Finally, the platelet is necessary for normal clot retraction.

The normal platelet count is 150–400 $\times$ 10^9/L. Lower counts indicate thrombocytopenia, either caused by inadequate production or by excessive destruction or removal of platelets. Inadequate production is almost always a result of marrow dysfunction, with decreases in the number of megakaryocytes. By contrast, in the thrombocytopenias caused by increased destruction, the megakaryocytes are quantitatively normal or increased. The hypomegakaryocytic thrombocytopenias result from aplasia of the marrow or from its infiltration by abnormal or neoplastic tissue. Because of the grave prognosis of such disorders, bone marrow aspiration is indicated in those with significant, unexplained thrombocytopenia. Bone marrow aspirations can usually be performed without serious bleeding, even in patients with severe thrombocytopenia, because thromboplastins in tissue juice usually effect hemostasis.

439.1 Congenital Thrombocytopenias

WISKOTT-ALDRICH SYNDROME

Wiskott-Aldrich syndrome consists of eczema, thrombocytopenic hemorrhage, and increased susceptibility to infection because of an immunologic defect that is transmitted as an X-linked recessive trait (see Chapter 119). The bone marrow contains a normal number of megakaryocytes, but many have bizarre nuclear morphology. Homologous platelets survive normally when transfused into these patients, but autologous platelets have a shortened life span and are small in size. Wiskott-Aldrich syndrome may represent an unusual circumstance in which thrombocytopenia results from abnormal platelet formation or release, despite quantitatively adequate numbers of megakaryocytes. Splenectomy has often been followed by overwhelming sepsis and death, but significant improvement in thrombocytopenia occurs after splenectomy. Prophylactic use of penicillin is essential postsplenectomy. About 5% of patients with Wiskott-Aldrich syndrome develop lymphoreticular malignancies. A few cases have been reported to benefit from the administration of transfer factor or from bone marrow transplantation.

OTHER INHERITED THROMBOCYTOPENIAS

Other types of inherited thrombocytopenias have been described. Some are X linked and some have autosomal transmission. Responses to therapy, including splenectomy, have usually been disappointing. The inordinately high mortality of young males splenectomized for presumed idiopathic thrombocytopenic purpura (ITP) suggests that, even without other stigmata, X-linked thrombocytopenia may represent a variant of Wiskott-Aldrich syndrome. Thus, the young thrombocytopenic male must be carefully studied before a diagnosis of ITP is made. A platelet survival study may be indicated in such patients.

THROMBOPOIETIN DEFICIENCY

A few patients have had chronic thrombocytopenia attributed to deficiency of a megakaryocyte maturation factor contained in normal plasma. Plasma infusions repeatedly produced a sustained rise in the platelet count. In somewhat similar cases, episodic thrombocytopenia and microangiopathic hemolysis were reversed by infusions of plasma.

THROMBOCYTOPENIA WITH CAVERNOUS HEMANGIOMA
(Kasabach-Merritt Syndrome)

Some infants with large, cavernous hemangiomas of the trunk, extremities, or abdominal viscera have severe thrombocytopenia and other evidence of intravascular coagulation (see Chapter 600). Histologic and isotopic studies indicate that platelets are trapped and destroyed within the extensive vascular bed of the tumor. The peripheral blood reveals thrombocytopenia and red blood cell fragments, and the bone marrow contains adequate numbers of megakaryocytes. Spontaneous thrombosis within the tumor may lead to obliteration of the vascular channels and spontaneous recovery; radiation therapy in a single dose of 600–800 rad (6–8 Gy) may accelerate this process, but repeated courses may be necessary. When anatomically feasible, external compression or total excision may be attempted, but surgery can be associated with uncontrollable hemorrhage. Corticosteroids and interferon may hasten involution and warrant trial, especially in the young infant. Splenectomy is contraindicated.

CONGENITAL HYPOPLASTIC THROMBOCYTOPENIA WITH ASSOCIATED MALFORMATIONS

(Thrombocytopenia Absent Radius [TAR] Syndrome)

Severe thrombocytopenia associated with aplasia of radii and thumbs, and with cardiac and renal anomalies, occurs as a familial condition. Severe hemorrhagic manifestations are evident in the first days of life. Hemoglobin levels are normal; leukocytosis and even leukemoid reactions have been found in some patients. Megakaryocytes are absent from the bone marrow.

The anomalies in this disease are similar to those observed in Fanconi pancytopenia, in which the hematologic abnormalities are not usually observed until the 3rd to 4th year of life. In this disorder chromosomes do not reveal the abnormalities found in Fanconi syndrome (see Chapter 423). No infants with congenital hypoplastic thrombocytopenia have been reported to develop full-blown Fanconi syndrome, nor have both conditions been observed in the same family.

439.2 Congenital Platelet Function Defects

Hemorrhagic disease resulting from congenital disorders of platelet function are not common. The inheritance pattern is not known for many of these disorders. The defects can be in adhesion, aggregation, and platelet coagulant activity.

CLINICAL MANIFESTATIONS. The clinical manifestations are similar to those encountered in patients with thrombocytopenia and consist of mucous membrane bleeding (epistaxis, oral cavity bleeding, menorrhagia, gastrointestinal and genitourinary hemorrhage), skin petechiae, and small ecchymoses.

LABORATORY FINDINGS. The laboratory test results are variable and reflect the functional defect, but all functional defects have a prolonged bleeding time, normal prothrombin time, normal PTT, and either a normal or moderately reduced platelet count. The defects can be defined by specific in vitro platelet function tests. Patients with platelet factor 3 deficiency, however, have a normal bleeding time but an abnormal prothrombin consumption test.

TREATMENT. Treatment of the bleeding disorders in these patients is difficult. Platelet transfusions are usually required to control significant hemorrhage.

BERNARD-SOULIER SYNDROME

This autosomal recessive inherited platelet adhesion defect is characterized by moderate thrombocytopenia, large platelets, and decreased ristocetin-induced platelet agglutination (aggregation) that is not corrected by the addition of von Willebrand factor.

GLANZMANN THROMBASTHENIA

This autosomal recessive inherited platelet disorder is characterized by a normal platelet count, absent in vitro aggregation with all agonists, and absent clot retraction.

OTHER DEFECTS

Defects in the normal platelet release reaction have been described, caused by platelet granule deficiency, impaired platelet arachidonic acid metabolism, or an impaired secretion of intraplatelet agonists. Laboratory studies reveal a normal platelet count and abnormal in vitro aggregation. The deficient granule variety can be detected by using electron microscopic techniques.

439.3 Inherited Blood Vessel Defects

Bleeding secondary to defective blood vessels is uncommon in childhood. Disorders such as hereditary hemorrhagic telangiectasia and Ehlers-Danlos syndrome can cause significant mucous membrane and skin bleeding. All laboratory tests for hemostasis are usually normal in these patients.

439.4 Acquired Thrombocytopenias

IDIOPATHIC THROMBOCYTOPENIC PURPURA

Acute idiopathic thrombocytopenic purpura (ITP), the most common of the thrombocytopenic purpuras of childhood, is associated with petechiae, mucocutaneous bleeding, and, occasionally, hemorrhage into tissues. There is a profound deficiency of circulating platelets, despite adequate numbers of megakaryocytes in the marrow.

ETIOLOGY. The disease often appears to be related to sensitization by viral infections; in about 70% of cases there is an antecedent disease such as rubella, rubeola, or viral respiratory infection. The interval between infection and onset of purpura averages 2 wk. As with the adult form, it seems probable that an immune mechanism is the basis for the thrombocytopenia. Platelet antibodies can be detected in some acute cases. Increased amounts of IgG have been found bound to platelets and may represent immune complexes absorbed on the platelet surface. No consistently reliable test currently exists for the serologic diagnosis of ITP.

CLINICAL MANIFESTATIONS. The onset is frequently acute. Bruising and a generalized petechial rash occur 1–4 wk after a viral infection or in some cases without antecedent illness. The bleeding is typically asymmetric and may be most prominent over the legs. Hemorrhages in mucous membranes may be prominent, with hemorrhagic bullae of the gums and lips. Nosebleeds may be severe and difficult to control. The most serious complication is intracranial hemorrhage, which occurs in fewer than 1% of cases. The liver, spleen, and lymph nodes are not enlarged. Except for the signs of bleeding, the patient appears clinically well. The acute phase of the disease associated with spontaneous hemorrhages lasts for only 1–2 wk. Thrombocytopenia may persist, but spontaneous mucocutaneous hemorrhages subside. Sometimes the onset is more insidious, with moderate bruising and few petechiae.

LABORATORY FINDINGS. The platelet count is reduced below 20 $\times$ 10^9/L. The few platelets observed on blood smear are large (megathrombocytes) and reflect increased marrow production. Those tests that depend on platelet function, such as the bleeding time and clot retraction, yield abnormal results. The white count cell count is normal, and anemia is not present unless significant blood loss has occurred.

Bone marrow aspiration, if indicated, reveals normal granulocytic and erythrocytic series and, frequently, modest eosinophilia. Normal or increased numbers of megakaryocytes are seen. Some of these are immature, with deep basophilic cytoplasm; platelet budding may be scanty, but there is no pathognomonic or diagnostic megakaryocyte morphology. The changes seen reflect increased megakaryocytic turnover.

DIFFERENTIAL DIAGNOSIS. ITP must be differentiated from aplastic or infiltrative processes of the bone marrow. Marrow aplasia or replacement is unlikely if the physical examination and blood count are normal, except for thrombocytopenia. Significant enlargement of the spleen suggests primary liver disease with congestive splenomegaly, lipidosis, or reticuloendotheliosis. Thrombocytopenic purpura may be an initial manifestation of systemic lupus erythematosus, AIDS, or lymphoma, but this sequence is unusual in young children. In adolescents the possibility is greater, and serologic studies for systemic lupus erythematosus and AIDS are indicated. Genetically determined thrombocytopenias must be considered in infants (particularly males) found to have low platelet counts.

TREATMENT. ITP has an excellent prognosis, even when no specific therapy is given. Within 3 mo 75% of patients recover completely, most within 8 wk. Severe spontaneous hemorrhages and intracranial bleeding (<1% of patients) are usually confined to the initial phase of the disease. After the initial acute phase, spontaneous manifestations tend to subside. About 90% of affected children have regained normal platelet counts 9–12 mo after onset, and relapses are unusual.

Fresh blood or platelet concentrates have transient benefit because transfused platelets survive only briefly, but they should be administered when life-threatening hemorrhage occurs.

When the disease is mild and hemorrhages of the retina or mucous membranes are not present, no specific therapy may be indicated. The affected child should be protected from falls or trauma. Vitamins K and C have no therapeutic effect.

Gamma Globulin. Infusions of intravenous gamma globulin (Sandoglobulin; Gamimune N) are followed by sustained rises of platelet count. Large doses of intravenous gamma globulin (400 mg/kg for 5 days) induce remission of many cases of acute and, occasionally, chronic ITP. A randomized control trial demonstrated the effectiveness of intravenous immune globulin G (IVIG), 1 g/kg/24 hr for 1 or 2 consecutive days, in reducing the frequency of severe thrombocytopenia (platelet count $\leq$20 $\times$ 10^9/L).

Corticosteroid Therapy. Although corticosteroid therapy has not decreased the number of chronic cases, it is beneficial because it reduces the severity and shortens the duration of the initial phase. In more severe cases, therapy with a corticosteroid, such as prednisone in a dose of 1–2 mg/kg/24 hr in divided doses or its equivalent, is indicated. Some authorities recommend an examination of bone marrow to exclude leukemia prior to initiating prednisone. The necessity for corticosteroid therapy in mild cases has been debated, although the platelet count returns to a hemostatic level more rapidly with such therapy. This therapy is continued until the platelet count is normal or for 3 wk, whichever comes first. At this point steroid therapy should be discontinued, even if the platelet count remains low. Prolonged corticosteroid therapy is not indicated and may depress the bone marrow, in addition to producing cushingoid changes and growth failure. If thrombocytopenia persists for 4–6 mo, a 2nd short course of corticosteroid therapy or intravenous immunoglobulin may be given.

Whether the initial therapy of choice in acute ITP is no therapy, intravenous gamma globulin, or corticosteroids is now being reassessed. Splenectomy should be reserved for chronic patients, defined as thrombocytopenia persistent for more than 1 yr, and for severe cases that do not respond to corticosteroids. Considerable improvement can usually be expected. If the hemorrhagic manifestations are severe, or if intracranial hemorrhage is suspected, larger doses of prednisone (5–10 mg/kg/24 hr) and intravenous gamma globulin can be used. Platelet transfusions may provide temporary control of bleeding, but sustained platelet counts are rarely achieved.

DRUG-INDUCED THROMBOCYTOPENIAS

A number of drugs can cause thrombocytopenia, either as a result of an immune-mediated process (with the drug functioning as a hapten) or of megakaryocyte injury. Drugs commonly used in pediatrics that can cause thrombocytopenia include carbamazepine (Tegretol), phenytoin (Dilantin), sulfonamides, trimethoprim-sulfamethoxazole, and chloramphenicol.

HEMOLYTIC-UREMIC SYNDROME

See also Chapter 474.

This acute disease of infancy and early childhood usually follows an episode of acute gastroenteritis. Shortly thereafter signs and symptoms of hemolytic anemia, thrombocytopenia, and acute renal insufficiency develop.

LABORATORY FINDINGS. The hemolytic anemia is associated with characteristically bizarre red blood cell morphology. Many of the red blood cells are contracted and distorted, with a prominence of spherocytes, burr cells, and helmet-shaped forms (see Fig. 415–2*F*). A depressed platelet count, despite normal numbers of megakaryocytes in the marrow, indicates excessive peripheral destruction. Tests of the coagulation mechanism are usually normal. Protein, red blood cells, and casts are present in the urinary sediment, and grave renal damage is reflected by anuria and azotemia.

TREATMENT. For a discussion of the management of uremia and anuria, see Chapter 474. Transfusions are indicated for severe anemia. Corticosteroid and heparin therapy do not affect survival or prognosis.

THROMBOTIC THROMBOCYTOPENIC PURPURA

This rare and serious disease is similar to the hemolytic-uremic syndrome. Diffuse embolism and thrombosis of the small blood vessels of the brain are evidenced by shifting neurologic signs such as aphasias, blindness, and convulsions. The prognosis is grave. Laboratory findings include thrombocytopenia and a hemolytic anemia associated with distorted and fragmented red blood cell microangiopathy. Plasmapheresis and plasma infusions are effective in 60–70% of cases. Corticosteroids and splenectomy are reserved for refractory cases.

Other Causes

Thrombocytopenia is a common complication of viral and bacterial (especially septicemia) infections, disseminated intravascular coagulation, and, rarely, heparin therapy.

NEONATAL THROMBOCYTOPENIA

Thrombocytopenia of the newborn may indicate primary disease in the infant's hematopoietic system or may be a result of the transfer of abnormal factors from the mother.

Association with Infection

Thrombocytopenia may occur in various fetal and neonatal infections and may be responsible for serious spontaneous bleeding. These include viral infections (especially rubella and cytomegalic inclusion disease), protozoal infections (e.g., toxoplasmosis), syphilis, and bacterial infections, especially those caused by gram-negative bacilli. Hemolysis is usually also present in infants with prominent anemia and jaundice. The liver and spleen are considerably enlarged. The bone marrow changes are variable, but reduced numbers of megakaryocytes may be seen.

Immune Neonatal Thrombocytopenia

About 30% of infants born of mothers with active idiopathic thrombocytopenic purpura have thrombocytopenia resulting from the transplacental transfer of antiplatelet antibodies. Rarely, infants with neonatal disease have been born of mothers with past histories of ITP (but who had splenectomy) who have normal platelet counts and whose disease has been inactive for many years. Petechiae are not present initially but appear in a generalized distribution within a few minutes after birth. Bleeding from the bowel or kidney and intracranial hemorrhage may occur. In mild cases there may be few abnormal findings. Hepatosplenomegaly is not present. The duration of the thrombocytopenia is 2–3 mo.

Therapy is not strikingly successful, but intravenous immunoglobulin, exchange transfusions, or platelet transfusions may be of temporary value in arresting acute bleeding. Corticosteroid therapy has not been proved beneficial. Because of the self-limited nature of the disease, splenectomy is contraindicated. Corticosteroid therapy given to the mother 1 wk prior to delivery or administration of intravenous gamma globulin to the mother late in pregnancy may reduce the severity of the disease in the mother and perhaps in the infant.

When the fetus has platelet antigens that the mother does not have, **alloimmunization** may occur. If maternal antibodies to fetal platelet antigens reach a sufficiently high titer, enough may cross the placenta to produce thrombocytopenia in the fetus. The disease may be familial, and first-born infants are frequently affected. Clinical signs include petechiae and other hemorrhagic manifestations. Antiplatelet antibodies can be demonstrated in about 50% of cases using sensitive tests. The PLA-1 antigen is most frequently involved. Infants born to mothers with antiplatelet alloantibodies are the most severely affected. Exchange transfusion is temporarily effective in stopping bleeding. Intravenous gamma globulin given to the affected newborn may be helpful. If compatible platelets can be obtained (these are most easily procured by preparing washed platelet concentrates from the mother), they offer specific, effective therapy. Infants born of successive pregnancies may be affected. Elective cesarean section has been advocated to spare the infant's head the trauma of delivery. Percutaneous umbilical blood sampling will diagnose fetal thrombocytopenia and permits fetal platelet transfusions with maternal platelets.

When the mother has drug-induced thrombocytopenia, both antibody and drug may cross the placenta and cause neonatal thrombocytopenia. Corticosteroid therapy, and especially exchange transfusions, should be considered when bleeding manifestations are severe.

439.5 Acquired Platelet Function Disorders

Acquired disorders of platelet function are caused by toxic metabolic products (e.g., in uremia), autoantibodies, immune complexes, fibrin split (degradation) products (FSPs), and drugs. These patients have a prolonged bleeding time and abnormalities in platelet aggregation tests.

The most common acquired defect is caused by drugs. Some drugs produce an irreversible reduction of prostaglandin synthesis within the platelet by inhibition of cyclo-oxygenase enzymes. This prevents the release of endogenous ADP and of the prostaglandin derivative thromboxane, which are essential for platelet aggregation. The abnormality can be most easily demonstrated with a platelet aggregometer, by which an ablation of the so-called secondary wave of platelet aggregation can be demonstrated. The most important drug that produces this effect is aspirin. The effect is not dose related. Abnormal platelet aggregation can be demonstrated in adults within 1 hr of ingestion of as little as 300 mg of aspirin. The abnormality persists for 4–6 days, or until the platelets that have been exposed to the drug have been replaced. Usually the effects of these drugs produce no clinical problems, although prolongation of bleeding time is frequently seen. If the patient has an underlying bleeding disorder such as hemophilia or undergoes surgery, however, hemorrhage may occur. Aspirin or other drugs that inhibit platelet aggregation are contraindicated in these circumstances and should be replaced with other agents, such as acetaminophen, when indicated. Aspirin may have transplacental effects on platelet function in the newborn, producing, rarely, neonatal hemorrhage; maternal aspirin consumption should be avoided during the last trimester of pregnancy.

439.6 Acquired Vascular Disorders

The most common cause of a vascular type of nonthrombocytopenic purpura is Schönlein-Henoch syndrome or anaphylactoid purpura (Chapter 152.1). This acute inflammatory process of unknown origin involves the small blood vessels of the skin, joints, gut, and kidney. The striking centrifugal distribution of the rash and involvement of the legs and buttocks are characteristic, particularly when combined with arthritis, nephritis, or gastrointestinal bleeding. The petechiae should be differentiated from those of early meningococcemia or of septicemia caused by other microorganisms. Toxic vasculitis may produce a hemorrhagic rash as a reaction to drugs such as arsenicals and iodides. Similar findings may occur during viral or rickettsial infections.

Treatment of this self-limited condition is supportive. Corticosteroids can be effective in controlling the painful edema, gastrointestinal pain, and arthritis, but not the vasculitic skin rash.

439.7 Thrombocytosis

Platelet counts in excess of $750 \times 10^9/L$ may be designated as thrombocytosis. Markedly elevated counts may accompany hemorrhage, iron deficiency anemia, hemolytic anemias, and primary myeloproliferative disorders. Acute and chronic inflammatory states may be accompanied by elevated platelet counts. Platelet counts exceeding $600 \times 10^9/L$ are regularly observed in those with Kawasaki disease. Persons with asplenia and children with sickle cell anemia often have somewhat elevated platelet counts. After splenectomy for ITP or hemolytic anemia, the platelet count often rises precipitously and may exceed $1,000 \times 10^9/L$ 10–14 days postoperatively. Generally, no specific therapy such as anticoagulation is necessary because thrombosis is extremely rare. The use of aspirin (or dipyridamole), which inhibits platelet function, may be considered if factors predisposing to thrombosis are present.

A case of primary thrombocytosis associated with thrombotic episodes and myocardial infarction has been described.

Ballin A, Andrew M, Ling E, et al: High-dose intravenous gamma globulin therapy for neonatal autoimmune thrombocytopenia. J Pediatr 112:789, 1988.
Blanchette VS, Luke B, Andrew M, et al: A prospective, randomized trial of high dose intravenous immune globulin G therapy, oral prednisone therapy, and no therapy in childhood acute immune thrombocytopenic purpura. J Pediatr 123:989, 1993.
Buchanan GR: Childhood acute idiopathic thrombocytopenic purpura: How many tests and how much treatment required? J Pediatr 106:928, 1985.
Burrows RF, Kelton JG: Fetal thrombocytopenia and its relation to maternal thrombocytopenia. N Engl J Med 329:1463, 1993.
George JN, Nurden AT, Phillips DR: Molecular defects in interactions of platelets with the vessel wall. N Engl J Med 311:1084, 1984.
Halperin DS, Doyle JJ: Is bone marrow examination justified in idiopathic thrombocytopenic purpura? Am J Dis Child 142:508, 1988.
Heath HW, Pearson HA: Thrombocytosis in pediatric outpatients. J Pediatr 114:805, 1989.
Imbach P: A multicenter European trial of intravenous immune globulin in immune thrombocytopenic purpura in childhood. Vox Sang 49:25, 1985.
Weiss HJ: Congenital disorders of platelet function. Semin Hematol 17:228, 1980.
Vain NE, Bedros AA: Treatment of isoimmune thrombocytopenia of the newborn with transfusion of maternal platelets. Pediatrics 63:107, 1979.

CHAPTER 440
Thrombotic Disorders

CLINICAL MANIFESTATIONS AND DIAGNOSIS. The occlusion of a blood vessel with a platelet plug or fibrin clot may occur in vessels of any size. Capillary and small-vessel occlusion are seen in vasculitic diseases and as complications of disseminated intravascular coagulation; in medium-sized vessels, in homocystinuria, cyanotic congenital heart disease, dehydration, and polyarteritis nodosa; and in larger vessels, in aortic thrombosis, superior vena cava thrombosis in the newborn, deep venous thrombosis, sickle cell anemia, and pulmonary embolism. The mechanism leading to the thrombosis is vessel injury in addition to one or all of the following: abnormal platelet adhesiveness-aggregation; an activated coagulation mechanism; an inactive inhibitor system; an inactive fibrinolytic mechanism; and reduced blood flow. Arterial thrombosis appears to depend on vascular injury and platelet activation, whereas venous thrombosis generally occurs in low-flow conditions associated with activation of the coagulation mechanism or with an impaired inhibitor-fibrinolytic system.

The clinical manifestations reflect organ or tissue injury resulting from the absence or a severe reduction in blood perfusion. In general, vascular occlusive events in children have an acute or sudden onset. The diagnosis is made by angiography. Ultrasound and radionuclide scanning techniques can be used for screening purposes. Other laboratory studies are rarely helpful in diagnosing a thromboembolic event except in two settings: when the event is a result of disseminated intravascular coagulation (in which case the patient demonstrates thrombocytopenia, hypofibrinogenemia, reduced factors II, V, and VIII, and positive fibrin split products (FSPs) and, in rare patients, of congenital deficiencies of natural inhibitors.

CONGENITAL AND INHERITED DEFECTS

The formation of a fibrin clot is regulated by a complex inhibitor system that involves antithrombin III, protein C, a cofactor (probably factor V) for activated protein C (APC), and protein S. By regulating clot formation, these plasma inhibitors prevent spontaneous intravascular coagulation, limit the thrombotic response of the body to injury, and control the extension of existing clots. Reduced plasma levels of any one of these inhibitors leads to a propensity to excessive thrombosis. Also, a reduced ability to remove fibrin clots (congenital hypoplasminogenemia and dysplasminogenemia) and the formation of an unusual fibrin clot (congenital dysfibrinogenemia) can lead to thrombotic diseases. The thromboembolic diseases reported in deficient patients predominantly affect the venous system; arterial forms are rare. Deep vein thrombosis of the legs, pulmonary embolism, thromboses of the pelvic veins and mesenteric veins, and sagittal sinus thrombosis are frequent manifestations. The 1st thromboembolic event usually occurs from 10 to 25 yr of age. A severe neonatal form (see later) has been reported.

Antithrombin III Deficiency

Antithrombin III (AT III) is a plasma inhibitor protein that blocks the enzymatic activity of some serine protease coagulation factors. The activity of this inhibitor is increased by heparin (formally called heparin cofactor activity). AT III is therefore necessary for heparin's anticoagulant activity. AT III is synthesized in the liver, is not vitamin K dependent, and can be consumed during the process of extensive intravascular clotting. Patients with AT III deficiency have AT III activity levels between 20 and 60% of normal. Normal newborns have reduced AT III activity.

Congenital AT III deficiency is an autosomal dominant trait that affects both sexes and has been observed in all races. Homozygous patients have not been described. Diagnosis is by detection of reduced AT III activity in plasma. There are at least two types of hereditary AT III deficiency: type I patients (most common) lack both AT III functional activity and protein, and type II patients lack functional activity but have the protein (a dysfunctional protein).

Treatment of thrombotic events in these patients can be difficult. Mildly deficient patients may respond to intravenous heparin but patients with severe deficiency do not. An infusion of plasma (as a source of AT III) plus heparin can be tried for acute therapy. Early initiation of long-term warfarin therapy is recommended for such patients. Danazol, a synthetic weak androgen, may raise AT III levels in selected patients. The efficacy and safety of this drug have not been established in children. Two AT III concentrates are available for clinical use (ATnativ, Kabi Vitrum, Stockholm; Thrombate III, Miles, Cutter Biological, West Haven, CT). An international unit per kilogram of body weight will raise the plasma activity level by 2–2.5% of normal. The drug must be given by the intravenous route.

Protein C Deficiency

Protein C is a plasma inhibitor protein that, once activated, inhibits clot formation and enhances fibrinolysis. It is synthesized in the liver and is vitamin K dependent. Protein C is converted into an active enzyme by a thrombin-thrombomodulin complex on the endothelial cell surface. Activated protein C (protein Ca or APC) inhibits a plasminogen activator inhibitor, which results in enhanced fibrinolysis and, with protein S as a cofactor, inhibits the clotting ability of factors V and VIII by limited proteolysis. APC thus controls the conversion of factor X to Xa and of prothrombin to thrombin. Thromboembolic disease has been reported in patients with levels that are from 38 to 49% of normal, but not all patients with protein C deficiency have thromboembolic disease. Clinical thrombotic events appear in adolescence.

Congenital protein C deficiency is an autosomal dominant trait. Diagnosis is by detection of reduced protein C activity in plasma. There are two types: Type I patients (most common) have both activity and protein reduced, and type II patients have functionally reduced activity but a normal amount of protein. Acquired deficiency may occur in association with infection.

Treatment includes heparin anticoagulation for thrombosis and chronic oral anticoagulation with warfarin to prevent recurrence of thrombosis. Androgenic drugs (e.g., danazol) have been shown to increase the protein C protein level to normal levels within 10–20 days, but the functional activity remains significantly lower than the antigenic level. Thus, its efficacy has not been established.

Purpura Fulminans Neonatalis

Homozygous protein C–deficient infants are characterized by the abrupt, early onset of subcutaneous ecchymoses and necrosis and by the widespread thrombosis of blood vessels. The thrombosis is accompanied by evidence of disseminated intravascular coagulation. These patients have undetectable levels of protein C, and the parents have values consistent with the heterozygous state. Treatment of this rare, severe condition includes fresh frozen plasma and long-term anticoagulation with warfarin. A similar condition has occurred in an infant with homozygous protein S deficiency.

Protein S Deficiency

Protein S, a vitamin K–dependent plasma protein, is synthesized in the liver and by endothelial cells. It functions as a cofactor for the anticoagulant effect of activated protein C. Protein S exists in the protein-bound and free forms in the plasma; the free form is biologically active. Protein S–deficient patients have been identified by immunologic and functional assays. Patients with recurrent thrombosis have protein S free levels of 15–37% of normal. Transient acquired deficiency may occur during infection.

Congenital protein S deficiency is inherited as an autosomal dominant trait. Homozygous deficiency has been described. Thromboembolic disease may or may not occur in the heterozygotes. Treatment consists of heparin anticoagulation for thrombosis and oral anticoagulants for the prevention of further thrombosis.

Resistance to Activated Protein C (APC)

This disorder occurs due to a deficiency of a cofactor to APC that is inherited as an autosomal dominant trait. Factor V is the cofactor and demonstrates both procoagulant and anticoagulant functions. The latter activity is reduced in patients having resistance to APC by a molecular defect in the protein. The prevalence is about 5%, and the frequency in patients with venous thrombosis ranges from 21% to 64%. Anticoagulant therapy should be individualized.

Plasminogen and Fibrinogen Abnormalities

Both qualitative and quantitative plasminogen abnormalities have been observed in rare patients with thromboembolic disorders. Many abnormal fibrinogens (dysfibrinogenemia) have been discovered that form abnormal clots; the dysfibrinogens appear to be inherited as an autosomal dominant trait. Treatment of thromboses in these disorders consists of the administration of heparin and long-term warfarin to prevent subsequent thrombotic events.

ACQUIRED DEFECTS

Acquired thrombotic and embolic events are usually uncommon in children, in general. But there are increasing reports of thromboembolic disease (TED) in newborns and in patients with specific diseases (Table 440–1). Arterial events usually present as stroke (at any age), a cold and pulseless lower extremity, with or without renal involvement (aortic thrombosis in the newborn), and myocardial infarction, although any arterialized organ can be affected. Venous events usually present as deep venous thrombosis with or without phlebitis, pulmonary embolism, and renal vein thrombosis.

The antiphospholipid antibody syndrome (lupus anticoagulant) may be primary (idiopathic) or associated with systemic lupus erythematosus, infections, drug reactions, or other autoimmune diseases. Associated features include livedo reticularis, thrombocytopenia, recurrent fetal loss and thrombosis (arterial, venous, or both). The activated partial thromboplastin time (APTT) may be prolonged but specific assays are needed to detect the antiphospholipid antibody. Treatment includes warfarin with or without aspirin.

Treatment of TED is designed to remove the thrombus or embolus (e.g., by thrombectomy or thrombolytic agents) or to inhibit the formation and propagation of a thrombus with drugs (anticoagulants).

Venous Thrombosis and Thrombophlebitis

Superficial thrombophlebitis is treated by anti-inflammatory drugs (e.g., nonsteroidal agents), heat compresses, rest, and elevation of the affected part. Patients with deep venous thrombosis or thrombophlebitis are treated with anticoagulation and sometimes with thrombolytic agents. Heparin anticoagulation should be used in a full dose for 7–10 days, with warfarin added for an additional 2–3 mo in those patients with proximal (above the knee) venous thrombosis. Patients with calf vein thrombosis should be treated with heparin for 7 days and then with warfarin or subcutaneous heparin for an additional 6 wk. Acute iliofemoral venous thrombosis in adults is treated with thrombolytic agents followed by anticoagulation with heparin and warfarin. Experience with thrombolytic therapy is limited in children, so its usefulness is unknown.

Pulmonary Embolism (See Chapter 356)

The patient with pulmonary embolism (PE) can be treated with heparin or thrombolytic drugs. Thrombolytic therapy produces a more rapid clinical improvement than heparin therapy, but the overall survival and long-term pulmonary function abnormalities appear to be the same in both treatment groups. If maximal medical management is not successful within 1 hr, embolectomy should be strongly considered.

Arterial Thrombosis

Surgical removal of the clot is the treatment of choice in acute arterial thrombosis or embolism. Surgery may not be

■ TABLE 440–1 Acquired Thromboembolic Disease in Newborns, Children, and Adolescents

Newborn: umbilical catheter-related; renal vein thrombosis; aortic thrombosis; vena cava thrombosis
Nephrotic syndrome: venous thrombosis
Cyanotic heart disease: venous thrombosis
Acyanotic heart disease: arterial embolism from prosthetic valves, mitral valve prolapse, mural thrombi; coronary artery thrombosis in Kawasaki disease and polyarteritis nodosa
Vessel injury: arterial and venous thrombosis
DIC syndromes: microvascular thrombosis
Sickle cell anemia: arterial and venous thrombosis
Homocystinuria: arterial and venous thrombosis
Drugs: L-asparaginase
Pregnancy and oral contraceptives: venous thrombosis
Paroxysmal nocturnal hemoglobinuria
Antiphospholipid-antibody syndrome (lupus anticoagulant)

possible, however, because of the location of the clot, size of the artery, or clinical condition of the patient. In such patients, intra-arterial or intravenous thrombolytic drugs have been used, along with successful removal or partial removal of the clot. The therapeutic plan should include prevention of new clot formation by anticoagulation. Platelet-inhibiting drugs may be beneficial in some patients with arterial diseases that predispose to thrombosis, such as aneurysms, cardiomyopathies (mural thrombi), and cardiac prosthesis.

Stroke

Arterial occlusion in the brain occurs when there is a vascular injury or anomaly or, more commonly, embolization from the heart. Venous thrombosis of cerebral vessels can be seen in those with cyanotic heart disease, inflammatory lesions of the brain, or hyperviscosity states. The therapeutic approach is directed toward the cause of the occlusion. Anticoagulation and/or platelet inhibitor drugs may be used. The presence of a hemorrhagic infarct is a contraindication for anticoagulant therapy. It is not known whether thrombolytic therapy is effective or safe in these children.

ANTICOAGULANT AND THROMBOLYTIC THERAPY

Anticoagulants

Heparin

Heparin enhances the rate by which antithrombin III neutralizes the activities of several of the activated clotting proteins, especially thrombin. The average half-life of intravenously administered heparin is about 60 min in adults and can be as short as 30 min in the newborn. Heparin does not cross the placenta. The half-life of heparin is dose dependent, that is, the higher the dose, the longer the circulating half-life. In thrombotic disease the half-life may be shorter than normal in patients with significant TED (such as pulmonary embolism) and longer than normal in patients with cirrhosis and uremia.

Anticoagulation with heparin is contraindicated in the following circumstances: a pre-existing coagulation defect or bleeding abnormality; a recent central nervous system hemorrhage; bleeding from inaccessible sites; malignant hypertension; bacterial endocarditis; recent surgery of the eye, brain, or spinal cord; and current administration of regional or lumbar block anesthesia. Despite these precautions, the frequency of bleeding in patients given heparin anticoagulation is about 5–10%.

Heparin can be given as an intravenous or subcutaneous injection. It is not effective when taken orally and should not be given as an intramuscular injection. Two techniques can be used to administer the drug intravenously, intermittent bolus or continuous infusion. Using the intermittent schedule, the patient is given 75–100 units/kg of heparin intravenously by bolus every 4 hr. Using the continuous infusion schedule, the patient is given a bolus injection of 50–75 units/kg followed by a continuous infusion of 10–25 units/kg/hr. Both schedules provide adequate anticoagulation, but the continuous method has been reported to have the effect of less anticoagulant-related bleeding.

Various coagulation tests are available to measure the action of heparin, including the APTT, the thrombin clotting time (TCT), and the factor Xa inhibition assay. The APTT is the most frequently used test for monitoring heparin therapy. It is sensitive to small amounts of heparin, is rapid and reproducible, and can be performed in most clinical laboratories. Clinical studies suggest that the APTT should be maintained at 1.5–2 times the patient's own preheparin control APTT.

After initiation of heparin therapy, an APTT should be performed periodically to ensure that adequate anticoagulation has occurred and that the patient's requirements for the drug have not changed. In patients receiving the intermittent bolus schedule, the APTT should be determined 1 hr after the initial infusion and should be greatly prolonged at that time. The next APTT should be performed at the 4th hr, that is, just prior to the next dose of heparin; at that time it should be 5–10 sec longer than the normal control time for the laboratory. If the APTT is very prolonged, the dose of the drug should be reduced by 10%, or, if the APTT is within the normal range, the dose of the heparin should be increased 10% and the test repeated 4 hr later. Using the continuous schedule, the APTT can be performed at any time 4 hr after the continuous infusion has begun. The desired result is an APTT 1.5–2 times the patient's pretreatment value. Dose adjustments of 5–10% can be made during this period to achieve adequate anticoagulation.

Heparin can be neutralized immediately by using protamine sulfate. Because of the rapid clearance rate of heparin, however, most patients can be treated by stopping the infusion. As a general rule, 1 mg of protamine sulfate neutralizes between 90 and 110 units of heparin. Because heparin has a rapid in vivo metabolic decay, only half of the total dose of protamine should be administered. A clotting test is performed to determine whether adequate neutralization has occurred; if not, the additional protamine can be given. Protamine itself is an anticoagulant, thus if too much is given the clotting time may be prolonged. Although excess protamine has an anticoagulant effect, it rarely (if ever) is a cause of clinical bleeding.

Warfarin

The coumarin derivatives are oral anticoagulant drugs that act by decreasing the rate of synthesis of the vitamin K–dependent coagulation factors II, VII, IX, and X. In addition, protein C and protein S (the vitamin K–dependent anticoagulants) are also affected. These drugs inhibit vitamin K–dependent carboxylation of the precursor coagulation proteins. Warfarin probably acts by competitively inhibiting vitamin K metabolism. Following the administration of warfarin, the levels of factors II, VII, IX, and X decrease gradually, according to their half-life. Because factor VII has the shortest half-life, its level is the first to decrease, followed by factor IX, X, and finally II. It generally takes about 4–5 days to provide a reduction in all four coagulation factors to a level consistent with anticoagulation.

The prothrombin time (PT) is the clotting test used to assess warfarin anticoagulation. The previously recommended therapeutic range of maintaining the patient's PT at 2.0–2.5 times the normal control should not be used when commercial rabbit brain is used as the clotting reagent. Current recommendations for mechanical prosthetic heart valves and recurrent systemic embolism are 1.5–2.0; for treatment of deep vein thrombosis or pulmonary embolism, 1.3–1.5; and for prevention of systemic embolism in patients with atrial fibrillation, valvular heart disease, or tissue heart valves, 1.3–1.5 times the control plasma.

The most serious side effect of warfarin is hemorrhage. This is often related to changes in the dose or metabolism of the drug. The addition or removal of certain drugs to the patient's therapeutic regimen can have significant effects on oral anticoagulation. For example, warfarin's effect can be enhanced by the administration of antibiotics, salicylates, anabolic steroids, chloral hydrate, laxatives, allopurinol, vitamin E, and methylphenidate HCl; its effect can be diminished by barbiturates, vitamin K, oral contraceptives, phenytoin, and others. Warfarin-induced bleeding is treated by discontinuation of the drug and the administration of vitamin K. Generally the amount of vitamin K given is equal to the amount of the daily warfarin dose. The vitamin can be administered orally, subcutaneously, or intravenously (not intramuscularly). Correction of the coagulopathy begins within 6–8 hr and should be complete in 24–48 hr. If the patient is having a significant bleeding problem, fresh frozen plasma (15 mL/kg) should be given at the same time the vitamin K is administered.

Coumarin anticoagulants are contraindicated in essentially the same circumstances as those for heparin therapy. The oral anticoagulants cross the placenta and should not be given during pregnancy. Although breast milk contains warfarin, the quantity is insignificant and the drug can be used in the lactating mother.

Thrombolytic Therapy

Thrombolytic therapy involves the removal of blood clots by enzymatic digestion. It is accomplished by the in vivo generation of plasmin through the administration of plasminogen activators such as streptokinase, urokinase, and tissue-type plasminogen activator (TPA). Urokinase and TPA act as direct activators, whereas streptokinase acts by binding to plasminogen, and the streptokinase-plasminogen complex becomes the plasminogen activator. For this therapy to be effective, the patient must have a relatively fresh clot (<7–10 days old), the clot must be accessible to the lytic agent, there must be an adequate amount of plasminogen, and the fibrinolytic inhibitors must not interfere with the reaction. Once plasmin has been formed, it lyses fibrin. The plasmin generated by urokinase and streptokinase can produce a systemic hyperfibrinolytic state; when this occurs, the plasmin can degrade other plasma proteins, including fibrinogen, and factors V and VIII, resulting in a hemorrhagic disorder. TPA is fibrin specific—it acts as an activator within or on a fibrin clot. Clinical trials with TPA suggest that a systemic hyperfibrinolytic state is rarely produced.

Thrombolytic therapy has been reported to be beneficial in those with pulmonary embolism, deep venous thrombosis, certain arterial occlusive events, and occluded access shunts. However, there are few published studies on its use in the pediatric age group.

Andrew M, Marzinotto V, Massicotte P, et al: Heparin therapy in pediatric patients: a prospective cohort study. Pediatr Res 35:78, 1994.
Bithel T: Hereditary dysfibrinogenemia. Clin Chem 31:509, 1985.
Comp PC, Nixon RR, Cooper MR, et al: Familial protein S deficiency is associated with recurrent thrombosis. J Clin Invest 74:2082, 1984.
Corrigan JJ Jr: Neonatal thrombosis and the thrombolytic system: Pathophysiology and therapy. Am J Pediatr Hematol Oncol 10:83, 1988.
D'Angelo A, Vallee PD, Crippa L, et al: Autoimmune protein S deficiency in a boy with severe thromboembolic disease. N Engl J Med 328:1753, 1993.
Gerson WT, Dickerman JD, Bovill EG, et al: Severe acquired protein C deficiency in purpura fulminans associated with disseminated intravenous coagulation: Treatment with protein C concentrate. Pediatrics 91:418, 1993.
Hirsh J, Levine MN: The optimal intensity of oral anticoagulant therapy. JAMA 258:2723, 1987.
Horowitz IN, Galvis AG, Gomperts ED: Arterial thrombosis and protein S deficiency. J Pediatr 121:934, 1992.
Lockshin ME: Answers to the antiphospholipid-antibody syndrome? N Engl J Med 332:1025, 1995.
Mahasandana C, Suvatte V, Chuansumrit TA, et al: Homozygous protein S deficiency in an infant with purpura fulminans. J Pediatr 117:750, 1990.
Marciniak E, Farley CH, DeSimone PA: Familial thrombosis due to antithrombin III deficiency. Blood 43:219, 1974.
McDonald MM, Hathaway WE: Anticoagulant therapy by continuous heparinization in newborn and older infants. J Pediatr 101:451, 1982.
Peters C, Casella JF, Marlar RA, et al: Homozygous protein C deficiency: Observations on the nature of the molecular abnormality and the effectiveness of warfarin therapy. Pediatrics 81:272, 1988.
Svensson PJ, Dahlback: Resistance to activated protein C as a basis for venous thrombosis. N Engl J Med 330:517, 1994.

SECTION 8
The Spleen

James French ■ Bruce M. Camitta

ANATOMY. The splenic precursor is recognizable by 5 wk of gestation. At birth, the spleen weighs approximately 11 g. Thereafter, it enlarges until puberty, reaching an average weight of 135 g before diminishing in size during adulthood. The major splenic components are a lymphoid compartment (white pulp) and a filtering system (red pulp). The white pulp consists of periarterial lymphatic sheaths of T cells with embedded germinal centers containing B cells. The red pulp has partially collapsed endothelial passages (cords of Billroth) and splenic sinuses. Fixed cells, mobile activated barrier cells, and macrophages are found in the red pulp. A marginal zone separates the red and white pulp. The splenic capsule contains smooth muscle and contracts in response to epinephrine. Approximately 90% of the blood delivered to the spleen flows rapidly through a closed vascular network. The other 10% flows more slowly through an open system (the splenic cords) where it is filtered before entering the splenic sinuses. The latter flow can increase greatly in specific diseases.

FUNCTION. Unique anatomy and blood flow enables the spleen to perform its immunologic and filtering functions more effectively. The spleen receives 5–6% of the cardiac output but normally contains only 25 mL of blood. It can retain much more when it enlarges. Factor VIII and platelets are stored in the spleen and can be released by stress or an epinephrine injection.

Hematopoiesis is a major splenic function from 3 to 6 mo of fetal life. It can be resumed in the event of myelofibrosis or severe hemolytic anemia. The spleen removes excess membrane from young red blood cells (RBCs), and loss of this function is characterized by target cells, poikilocytosis, and decreased osmotic fragility. It is also the primary site for destruction of old RBCs; this function is assumed by other reticuloendothelial cells after splenectomy. The spleen also removes damaged and abnormal RBCs. Spherocytes and antibody-coated RBCs and platelets are detained in the marginal zone and red pulp where they are then phagocytosed or lysed. In addition, the spleen removes intracytoplasmic inclusions from RBCs without cell lysis. Functional or anatomic hyposplenia is characterized by continued circulation of cells containing these nuclear remnants (Howell-Jolly bodies) and other debris in the RBC. The latter may appear as "pits" on indirect microscopy.

Immunoglobulin, properdin, and tuftsin are produced in the spleen. The spleen has a minor role in antibody responses to intramuscularly or subcutaneously injected antigens but is required for early antibody production after exposure to intravenous antigens. Thus, young (nonimmune) or hyposplenic individuals are at increased risk from sepsis caused by pneumococci and other encapsulated bacteria. The spleen can also use phagocytosis to trap and destroy bacteria or parasitized RBCs. ■

Chapter 441
Splenomegaly

PHYSICAL EXAMINATION. A soft thin spleen may be palpable in 15% of neonates, 10% of normal children, and 5% of adolescents. However, in most individuals, the spleen must be two to three times its normal size before it is palpable. The spleen is best examined in a supine patient by palpating across the abdomen toward the left costal margin from below as the patient inspires deeply. One should remember that an enlarged spleen may descend into the pelvis, thus necessitating a lower abdominal examination starting point when splenomegaly is suspected. Superficial abdominal venous distention may be present when splenomegaly is the result of portal hypertension. Radiologic detection or confirmation of splenic enlargement is done with ultrasound, computed tomography, or a technetium-99m sulfur colloid scan. The latter also assesses splenic function.

DIFFERENTIAL DIAGNOSIS. Specific causes of splenomegaly are listed in Table 441–1. Unique problems are discussed below.

PSEUDOSPLENOMEGALY. Abnormally elongated mesenteric connections may produce a wandering or proptotic spleen. An enlarged left lobe of the liver or a left upper quadrant mass may be mistaken for splenomegaly. Splenic cysts may contribute to splenomegaly or mimic it; these may be congenital (epidermoid) or acquired (pseudocyst) after trauma or infarction. They are usually asymptomatic and are found on radiologic evaluation. Splenosis after splenic rupture or an accessory spleen may also mimic splenomegaly. Most, however, are not palpable. The syndrome of *congenital polysplenism* includes cardiac defects, left-sided organ anomalies, biliary atresia, and pseudosplenomegaly (see Chapter 387.18).

HYPERSPLENISM. Hypersplenism is characterized by increased splenic function (destruction of circulating cells), which results in peripheral blood cytopenias, increased bone marrow activity, and splenomegaly. It is usually secondary to another disease and may be cured by treatment of the underlying condition or, if absolutely necessary, by splenectomy.

CONGESTIVE SPLENOMEGALY (BANTI SYNDROME). Splenomegaly may result from obstruction in the hepatic, portal, or splenic veins. Wilson disease, galactosemia, biliary atresia, and α_1-antitrypsin deficiency result in hepatic inflammation, fibrosis, and vascular obstruction. Congenital abnormalities of the portal or splenic veins may cause vascular obstruction. Septic omphalitis or umbilical venous catheterization in neonates may also result in secondary obliteration of these vessels. Splenic venous flow may be obstructed by masses of sickled erythrocytes. When the spleen is the site of vascular obstruction, splenectomy cures hypersplenism. However, usually the obstruction is in the hepatic or portal systems, and portocaval shunting may be more helpful, because both portal hypertension and thrombocytopenia contribute to variceal bleeding.

■ TABLE 441–1 Common Causes of Splenomegaly

Infection	
Bacterial:	Typhoid fever, endocarditis, septicemia, abscess
Viral:	Epstein-Barr, cytomegalovirus, and others
Protozoal:	Malaria, toxoplasmosis
Hematologic Processes	
Hemolytic anemia:	Congenital, acquired
Extramedullary hematopoiesis:	Thalassemia, osteopetrosis, myelofibrosis
Neoplasms	
Malignant:	Leukemia, lymphoma, metastatic disease
Benign:	Hemangioma, hamartoma
Infiltration and Storage Diseases	
Lipidoses:	Niemann-Pick, Gaucher diseases
Mucopolysaccharidosis infiltration:	Histiocytosis
Congestion	
Cirrhosis or hepatic fibrosis	
Hepatic portal or splenic vein obstruction	
Congestive heart failure	
Cysts	
Congenital (true cysts)	
Acquired (pseudocysts)	
Miscellaneous	
Lupus erythematosus, sarcoid, rheumatoid arthritis	

Chapter 442
Hyposplenism, Splenic Trauma, Splenectomy

Congenital absence of the spleen is associated with complex cyanotic heart defects, dextrocardia, and heterotopic abdominal organs (Ivemark syndrome; see Chapter 387.18). These patients are at increased risk for sepsis. *Functional hyposplenism* may be seen in normal neonates, especially premature infants. Children with sickle cell hemoglobinopathies may develop splenic hypofunction as early as 6 mo of age. Initially, this is due to vascular obstruction that can be reversed with red blood cell (RBC) transfusions. Eventually, the spleen autoinfarcts, resulting in a fibrotic, permanently nonfunctioning spleen. Functional hyposplenism may also be seen in malaria, after irradiation to the left upper quadrant, and when the reticuloendothelial function of the spleen is overwhelmed (as in severe hemolytic anemias or metabolic storage diseases). Regardless of the cause, patients with functional hyposplenism are at increased risk of sepsis from encapsulated organisms.

TRAUMA. Injury to the spleen may occur with left flank or abdominal trauma. Small splenic capsular tears may produce symptoms such as abdominal or referred left shoulder pain as a result of peritoneal irritation by blood. Larger capsular tears result in more severe blood loss with similar pain and signs of hypovolemia. Previously enlarged spleens (as in infectious mononucleosis) are more likely to rupture with minor trauma.

Treatment of a small capsular injury should include careful observation with attention to changes in vital signs or abdominal findings, serial hemoglobin determinations, and the availability of prompt surgical intervention should the patient deteriorate. RBC transfusion requirements should be minimal (less than 25 mL/kg in 48 hr). These patients are usually hospitalized 10–14 days and have their activities restricted for months. A laparotomy with or without splenectomy is indicated for more marked abdominal bleeding, for clinical instability or deterioration, or when other organ damage is suspected. Partial splenectomy and splenic repairs should be substituted for total splenectomy when feasible.

SPLENECTOMY. Because of the risk of postoperative sepsis, splenectomy should be limited to specific indications. These include splenic rupture, anatomic defects, hemolytic anemias, immune cytopenias, metabolic storage diseases, secondary hypersplenism, and (rarely) surgical indications, including exposure of the left upper quadrant. The major risk of splenectomy is infection, including an increased risk of sudden overwhelming infection (sepsis or meningitis). This latter risk is especially high in children younger than 5 yr old at the time of surgery. The risk of sepsis is slightly less in splenectomies done for trauma, RBC membrane defects, and immune cytopenias than when there is pre-existing immune deficiency (Wiskott-Aldrich syndrome) or reticuloendothelial blockage (storage diseases, severe hemolytic anemias).

Encapsulated bacteria such as *Streptococcus pneumoniae* (more than 60% of cases), *Haemophilus influenzae, Neisseria meningitidis,* and *Escherichia coli* are the most common organisms associated with postsplenectomy sepsis. Streptococci and staphylococci are seen less frequently. Because the spleen is responsible for filtering the blood and early antibody responses, sepsis (with or without meningitis) can progress rapidly, leading to death within 12–24 hr of onset. Splenectomized patients are also at increased risk for contracting protozoal infections such as malaria and babesiosis.

Preoperative, intraoperative, and postoperative management may decrease the risk of postsplenectomy infection. Most important is to be certain of the necessity for splenectomy and, if possible, to postpone the operation until the patient is 5 yr of age or older. Vaccination with pneumococcal (and *H. influenzae* and possibly meningococcal) vaccines before splenectomy may be helpful to reduce postsplenectomy sepsis. In trauma cases, splenic repair or partial splenectomy should be considered in an attempt to preserve splenic function. Partial splenectomy or partial splenic embolization may also be sufficient to ameliorate some forms of hemolytic anemia. Surgical splenosis (distributing small pieces of spleen throughout the abdomen) has been suggested as a way to decrease the risk of sepsis in patients whose splenectomy is necessitated by trauma. However, the splenic tissue that regrows frequently has inadequate function. Postsplenectomy, penicillin (or amoxicillin) prophylaxis at a dose of 250 mg twice a day (erythromycin in penicillin-allergic patients) should be given. Penicillin has been shown to reduce the risk of pneumococcal sepsis in patients with hemoglobin SS, but other populations have not been well studied. The appropriate duration for such prophylaxis is unknown. Although the greatest risk is in the immediate postoperative period, reports of deaths occurring many years after splenectomy suggest that the risk (and need for prophylaxis) may be lifelong. Other postoperative measures include patient and family education, wearing a medical information bracelet, and prompt evaluation and treatment of fevers.

Deodhar HA, Marshall RS: Increased risk of sepsis after splenectomy. BMJ 307:1408, 1993.

Eraklis AJ, Filler RM: Splenectomy in childhood: A review of 1413 cases. J Pediatr Surg 7:382, 1972.

Israel DM, Hassal E: Partial splenic embolization in children with hypersplenism. J Pediatr 124:95, 1993.

Pearson HA: The born-again spleen. N Engl J Med 298:1373, 1978.

Pearson HA: Splenectomy, its risks and role. Hosp Pract 94:85, 1984.

Pearson HA, Spencer RP, Cournelius E: Functional asplenia in sickle cell anemia. N Engl J Med 281:923, 1969.

Shapiro ED, Berg AT: The protective efficacy of polyvalent pneumococcal polysaccharide vaccine. N Engl J Med 325:1453, 1991.

Sherman R: Perspective in management of trauma to the spleen. J Trauma 20:1, 1980.

Tchernia G, Gauthier F: Initial assessment of the beneficial effect of partial splenectomy in hereditary spherocytosis. Blood 81:2014, 1993.

SECTION 9

The Lymphatic System

Alice Rock ■ Bruce M. Camitta

The lymphatic system includes circulating lymphocytes, lymphatic vessels, lymph nodes, spleen, tonsils, adenoids, Peyer patches, and thymus. Lymph, an ultrafiltrate of blood, is collected by lymphatic capillaries that are present in all organs except the brain and the heart. These join to form progressively larger vessels that drain regions of the body. During their course, the lymphatic vessels carry lymph to the lymph nodes. In the nodes, lymph is filtered through sinuses where particulate matter and infectious organisms are phagocytized, processed, and presented as antigens to surrounding lymphocytes. This results in stimulation of antibody production, T-cell responses, and cytokine secretion.

Lymph composition can vary with the site it drains. It is usually clear but, after draining the intestines, may be milky (chylous) because of the presence of fats. The protein content is intermediate between an exudate and transudate. The protein level may be increased with inflammation or when draining the liver or intestines. Lymph also contains variable numbers of small lymphocytes. ■

CHAPTER 443

Abnormalities of Lymphatic Vessels

Abnormalities of the lymph vessels may be congenital or acquired. Signs and symptoms may result from increased lymphatic tissue mass or from leakage of lymph. *Lymphangiectasia* is a dilation of the lymphatics. Pulmonary lymphangiectasia causes respiratory distress. Involvement of the intestinal lymphatics causes hypoproteinemia and lymphocytopenia secondary to loss of lymph into the intestines. *Lymphangioma* (cystic hygroma) is a mass of dilated lymphatics. Some of these lesions also have a hemangiomatous component. *Lymphatic dysplasia* may cause multisystem problems. These include lymphedema, chylous ascites, chylothorax, and lymphangiomas of bone, lung, or other locations. *Lymphedema* is caused by obstruction of lymph flow. Congenital lymphedema may be seen in Turner syndrome, Noonan syndrome, and the autosomal a dominantly inherited Milroy disease. Lymphedema praecox causes progressive lower extremity edema, usually in females 10–25 yr old. Lymphedema has also been seen in association with intestinal lymphangiectasia, cerebrovascular malformation, ptosis, yellow dystrophic nails, distichiasis, and cholestasis. Acquired obstruction of the lymphatics can occur due to tumor, postradiation fibrosis, filariasis, and postinflammatory scarring. Injury to the major lymphatic vessels can cause collection of lymph fluid in the abdomen (chylous ascites) and chest (chylothorax). *Lymphangitis* is an inflammation of the lymphatics draining an area of infection. On examination, tender red streaks extend proximally from the infected site. Regional nodes may also be enlarged and tender. *Staphylococcus aureus* and group A streptococci are the most frequent pathogens.

CHAPTER 444
Lymphadenopathy

Most lymph nodes are not palpable in the newborn infant. With varied antigenic exposure, lymphoid tissue increases in volume so that cervical, axillary, and inguinal nodes are often palpable during childhood. They are not considered enlarged until their diameter exceeds 1 cm for cervical or axillary nodes and 1.5 cm for inguinal nodes. Other lymph nodes usually are not palpable or visualized with usual radiologic procedures.

Lymph node enlargement is due to proliferation of normal lymphoid elements or to infiltration by malignant or phagocytic cells. In most patients, a careful history and a complete physical examination suggest the proper diagnosis. The evaluation should include determining whether a swelling is a lymph node and the characteristics of the node. Nonlymphoid masses (cervical rib, thyroglossal cyst, branchial sinus or cyst, cystic hygroma, goiter, sternomastoid muscle tumor, neurofibroma) occur frequently in the neck, less often in other areas. Acutely infected nodes are usually tender. There may also be erythema and warmth of the overlying skin. Fluctuance suggests abscess formation, and tuberculous nodes may be matted. With chronic infection, most of the above signs are not present. Tumor-bearing nodes are usually firm and nontender and may be matted or fixed to the skin or underlying structures.

Generalized adenopathy (enlargement of more than two noncontiguous node regions) is due to systemic disease (Table 444–1) and is often accompanied by abnormal physical findings in other systems. In contrast, localized adenopathy is most frequently due to infection in the involved node and/or its drainage area (Table 444–2). Regional lymphadenitis as a result of agents other than bacteria may be characterized by atypical anatomic areas, a prolonged course, a draining sinus, lack of prior pyogenic infection, and unusual clues in the history (cat scratches, tuberculosis exposure, venereal disease).

■ TABLE 444–1 Common Causes of Generalized Lymphadenopathy

Infections	
	Bacterial, viral, fungal, other
Autoimmune Diseases	
	Rheumatoid arthritis, lupus erythematosus, dermatomyositis
Malignancies	
	Primary: Hodgkin disease, non-Hodgkin lymphoma, histiocytic disorders
	Metastatic: Leukemia, neuroblastoma, rhabdomyosarcoma, other
Lipid Storage Diseases	
	Gaucher disease, Niemann-Pick disease
Drug Reactions	
Other	
	Sarcoidosis, serum sickness

■ TABLE 444–2 Drainage Areas of Regional Nodes

Abdominal and Pelvic:	Lower extremity, abdomen, pelvic organs
Axillary:	Hand, arm, chest wall, upper and lateral abdominal wall, breast
Cervical:	Tongue, external ear, parotid, superficial tissues of the head and neck, larynx, trachea, thyroid
Epitrochlear:	Hand, forearm
Iliac:	Lower abdomen, part of the genitalia, urethra, bladder
Inguinal:	Scrotum and penis in males, vulva and vagina in females; skin of the lower abdomen, perineum, gluteal region, lower anal canal, lower extremity
Mediastinal:	Thoracic viscera
Occipital:	Posterior scalp
Popliteal:	Knee joint, skin of the lateral lower leg and foot
Preauricular:	Eyelid, conjunctivas, cheek, temporal scalp
Submaxillary/submental:	Teeth, gums, tongue, buccal mucosa
Supraclavicular:	Head, neck, arms, superficial thorax, lungs, mediastinum, abdomen. Right supraclavicular adenopathy is usually due to an intrathoracic problem. Left supraclavicular adenopathy is usually due to an intra-abdominal problem

Evaluation and treatment of lymphadenopathy is guided by the probable etiologic factor, as determined from the history and physical examination. Many patients have a viral infection and need no intervention. If a bacterial infection is suspected, antibiotic treatment covering at least streptococci and staphylococci is indicated. Surgical drainage is required if an abscess forms. The size of involved nodes should be documented before treatment. Failure to decrease in size within 10–14 days suggests the need for further evaluation. In a minority of cases, the cause of lymphadenopathy is not initially evident, and further evaluation may include complete blood count with differential; Epstein-Barr virus, cytomegalovirus, *Toxoplasma*, cat-scratch disease, and sexually transmitted disease titers; antistreptolysin O or anti-DNAase serologic tests; tuberculosis skin test; and chest radiograph. Consultation with infectious disease or oncology specialists may be helpful. Biopsy should be considered if there is persistent or unexplained fever, weight loss, night sweats, hard nodes, fixation of the nodes to surrounding tissues, supraclavicular adenopathy, or mediastinal adenopathy. Biopsy may also be indicated if there is an increase in size over baseline in 2 wk, no decrease in size in 4–6 wk, no regression to "normal" in 8–12 wk, or the development of new signs and symptoms.

Bedros AA, Mann JP: Lymphadenopathy in children. Adv Pediatr 28:341, 1981.
Hilliard RI, McKenobey JBJ, Phillips MJ: Congenital abnormalities of the lymphatic system: A new clinical classification. Pediatrics 86:988, 1990.
Knight PJ, Mulne AF, Vassay LE: When is lymph node biopsy indicated in children with enlarged peripheral nodes? Pediatrics 69:391, 1982.

PART XXII

Neoplastic Diseases and Tumors

William M. Crist

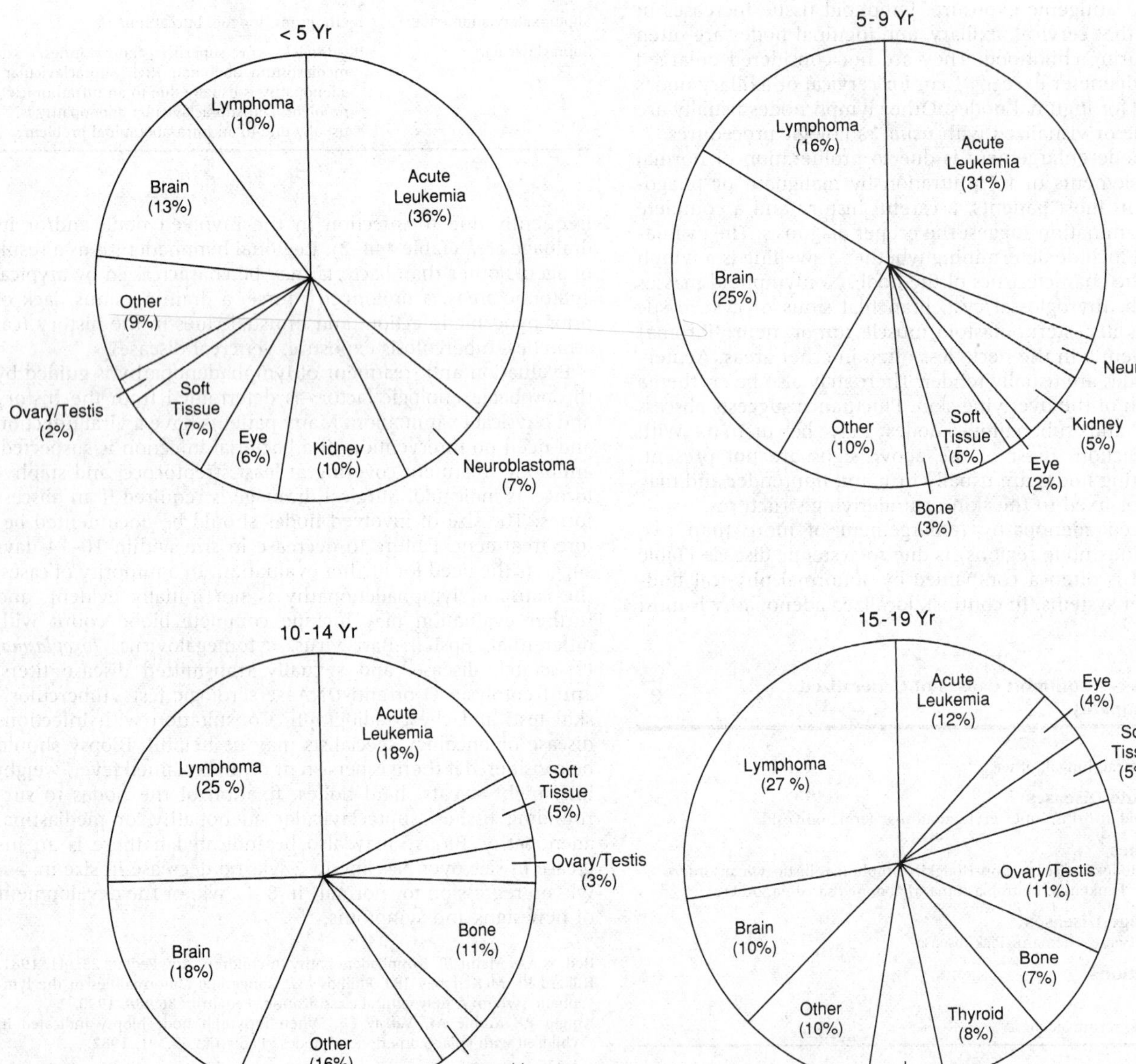

Figure XXII–1. Percentage of primary tumors by site of origin for different age groups. (Adapted from National Cancer Institute Monograph No. 57, SEER Program.)

■ TABLE XXII–1 Incidence and Mortality Rates of Some Common Childhood Cancers: Summary of 15-Yr Trends by Site*

	Average Rate			Average Mortality Rate		
Site	1973–1974	1986–1987	% Change	1973–1974	1986–1987	% Change
Acute lymphoblastic leukemia	2.9	3.3	14.4†	1.4	0.7	−50.7†
Brain and nervous system	2.5	3.2	29.4†	1.0	0.8	−19.2†
Bone	0.7	0.8	12.5†	0.3	0.2	−33.5†
Hodgkin disease	0.8	0.6	−17.5	0.1	0.0	−68.7†
Non-Hodgkin lymphoma	0.8	1.1	31.7	0.4	0.2	−50.2†
Kidney	0.7	0.8	7.5	0.2	0.1	−43.6†
Soft tissue	0.7	0.8	5.2	0.6	0.2	−68.1†
All sites	13.2	14.0	6.1†	5.5	3.6	−35.6†

Rates are per 100,000 whites, ages 0–14 yr, and are age-adjusted to the 1970 standard population in the United States. The mortality rate for every major cancer in children has declined significantly since 1973. The overall cancer mortality rate decreased 36% for children, although the incidence rate increased by 6.1%. As expected with decreasing mortality and increasing incidence rates, the 5-yr relative survival rate has increased from 55.1% in 1974–1976 to 66.8% in 1981–1986.

†*The estimated annual percent change over the 15-yr interval is significantly different from 0 (P<.05).*

(From Ries LAG, Hankey BF, Edwards BK (eds): Cancer Statistics Review 1973–1987. The Surveillance Program Division of Cancer Prevention and Control. NIH publication no. 90-2789. Bethesda, MD, Department of Health and Human Services, 1988.)

Only about 2% of new cases of cancer in the United States occur in children, yet malignancy remains the major cause of death from disease between the ages of 1 and 15 yr because there are approximately 6,500 new cases of cancer annually in this age group. Pediatric cancers differ markedly from adult malignancy in their nature, distribution, and prognosis. Acute lymphoblastic leukemia, central nervous system tumors (see Chapter 555), and sarcomas predominate in children (Table XXII–1); acute and chronic forms of myeloid leukemias, chronic lymphoid leukemia, and carcinomas are more common in adults. The distribution of cases by tumor site varies with age during childhood (Fig. XXII–1).

Because treatment with irradiation, surgery, and chemotherapy can adversely affect growth and development, pediatric oncologists face unique challenges. Given the relative rarity of specific types of childhood cancer and the sophisticated technology and expertise required for diagnosis, treatment, and monitoring of late effects, it is important that all children with cancer be treated with standard clinical protocols in pediatric oncology centers. These centers have the required facilities and expertise and are committed to learning more about the optimal treatment of pediatric malignancy through participation in national clinical trails. Although the results of treatment have improved remarkably over the past quarter century, with substantial decreases in mortality rates, the late effects of therapy and the continuing poor prognosis for specific malignancies demand a concerted and coordinated clinical research effort. ■

Chapter 445
Epidemiology

William M. Crist

The annual incidence rate of malignant tumors in children younger than 15 yr of age was estimated to be 14:100,000 population for the years 1986–1987. Compared with estimates for 1973–1974, the rates in Table XXII–1 show a slight increase in acute lymphoblastic leukemia and a more pronounced rise in central nervous system tumors, with an overall increase of 6.1%. Mortality rates for childhood malignancies during this same period decreased, with significant improvements seen for all tumor types.

In most cases, the precise cause of childhood cancer remains unknown. Specific genetic events associated with tumor development are being identified. Examples include retinoblastoma, which is caused by acquired or inherited mutations in the *Rb* tumor-suppressor gene, and the Li-Fraumeni syndrome, which is characterized by early onset of specific cancers arising from mutations in the p53 tumor-suppressor gene. It is likely that the development of most cancers involves both environmental and genetic factors. However, the cancers of childhood tend to arise in tissues that are not directly exposed to the environment (hematopoietic, nervous, supportive connective tissues), indicating that host factors may be more important.

ENVIRONMENTAL FACTORS (Table 445–1)

IONIZING RADIATION. Increases in the incidence of leukemia followed exposure of children to fallout from the atomic bombs in Hiroshima and Nagasaki (see Chapter 662). The radiation dose and the frequency of leukemia were related in a linear fashion; the type and latency of leukemia were related to age at exposure. Increases in acute lymphoblastic and chronic myeloid leukemias were most dramatic in younger children, whereas acute myeloid leukemia was seen with increased frequency among older children. These leukemias developed relatively quickly, with a peak rate of occurrence 5 yr after exposure. The incidence of breast cancer is also increased among middle-aged women who were younger than 10 yr when exposed. Critical environmental events can cause cancers with long latency periods. The earlier use of radiation therapy for nonmalignant conditions, including "enlarged thymus," large tonsils, or tinea capitis, was associated with an increased risk of cancer, especially thyroid carcinoma. Significant doses of radiation were also given during fluoroscopy before 1955. Leukemia mortality rates for children younger than 5 yr declined substantially during the early 1960s before chemotherapy significantly affected cure rates but after these questionable uses of radiation were curtailed.

Exposure of the fetus to diagnostic x-rays in utero has been associated with a risk ratio of about 1.5 for development of a childhood tumor, but a causal relationship has not been proved. Finally, second malignancies are a risk in patients who have received substantial doses of therapeutic radiation (brain tumors in patients treated with cranial radiation for leukemia).

ULTRAVIOLET RADIATION. Excessive exposure to sunlight with severe sunburning during childhood and adolescence can cause skin cancer later in life. Children who have a genetic predisposition, such as xeroderma pigmentosum or other congenital defects in DNA repair, are at increased risk of having neoplasms develop that are associated with ultraviolet radiation.

DRUGS. Intrauterine exposure to *diethylstilbestrol* (DES) confers an increased risk of clear cell adenocarcinoma of the vagina in the daughters of women given this drug. Also, exposed children of both sexes commonly have malformations of the geni-

■ TABLE 445–1 Environmental Causes of Cancer

Etiology	Cancer
Physical Agents	
Ionizing radiation	Leukemia, thyroid, breast
Ultraviolet irradiation	Melanoma, basal and squamous cell in xeroderma pigmentosum
Chemical Agents	
Cigarette, tobacco	Lung, oropharynx, larynx
Diethylstilbestrol (prenatal)	Vaginal carcinoma in daughter
Asbestos	Mesothelioma
Androgens	Hepatoma
Alkylating agents	Leukemia
Immunosuppressant drugs	Lymphoma
Aflatoxin	Hepatic carcinoma
Vinyl chloride	Hepatic angiosarcoma
Phenytoin	Lymphoma
Prenatal phenytoin	Neuroblastoma
Cyclophosphamide	Bladder cancer, leukemia
Alcohol (fetal alcohol syndrome)	Neuroblastoma
Benzene	Leukemia
Chloramphenicol	Leukemia
Intramuscular iron	Sarcoma at injection site
Microbiologic Agents	
Hepatitis B, C viruses	Hepatic carcinoma
Human immunodeficiency virus	Kaposi sarcoma, lymphoma
Schistosoma haematobium	Bladder carcinoma
Clonorchis sinensis	Biliary tract cancer
Epstein-Barr virus	African Burkitt lymphoma, X-linked immunodeficiency–associated lymphoma, nasopharyngeal carcinoma
Papillomavirus	Cervical cancer
Human T-lymphotropic virus I	T-cell lymphoma
Simian virus 40	Possible ependymoma, choroid plexus tumor

(From Behrman R, Kliegman R (eds): Nelson Essentials of Pediatrics, 2nd ed. Philadelphia, WB Saunders, 1994.)

tal tract (see Chapter 508). DES is currently the only proven human transplacental carcinogen, although two cases of neuroblastoma have been reported in infants with fetal hydantoin syndrome and another has been reported in a child with fetal alcohol syndrome.

Immunosuppressive agents administered after renal or other organ transplantation have been associated with an increased incidence of malignancy (particularly non-Hodgkin lymphoma). The distribution of tumor types in immunosuppressed individuals differs from that in other children, suggesting that immune surveillance may be more effective against some cancers than others.

Treatment of aplastic anemia (especially of the Fanconi type) with *anabolic androgenic steroids* can cause liver tumors, including hepatocellular carcinoma, hepatoma, and hepatic adenoma. The underlying condition may contribute to tumorigenesis because similar tumors have not been reported in athletes who use anabolic steroids to produce muscle hypertrophy. Such athletes may be at risk (see Chapter 105). Cancer chemotherapies, especially alkylating agents and epipodophyllotoxins, can cause second neoplasms, with a cumulative risk as high as 12% at 25 yr post-treatment.

DIET. There is an unexplained association between high fat intake, obesity, and the incidence of cancers of the breast, colon, and uterus in adults. Data to support "preventive" dietary modifications in children are lacking.

VIRUSES

RNA VIRUSES. There is convincing evidence for both vertical and horizontal transmission of lymphatic leukemia and lymphoma associated with type C RNA viruses in animals. Retroviruses also cause leukemia/lymphoma in cats and cows by horizontal transmission. A type of T-cell leukemia seen in adults and, occasionally, in adolescents has been associated with a retrovirus (human T-cell leukemia virus). This form of leukemia is endemic on two islands in southern Japan and also occurs in the Caribbean and sporadically elsewhere, including the United States and Israel. The latency period can be longer than 20 yr. Malignancies such as Kaposi sarcoma and central nervous system lymphoma are noted in patients with acquired immunodeficiency syndrome (AIDS), possibly related to a latent human herpesvirus 8 infection.

DNA VIRUSES. The Epstein-Barr virus (EBV), which causes infectious mononucleosis, is also implicated in Burkitt lymphoma, lymphoepithelioma, and Hodgkin disease. The association is geographic; 90–95% of Burkitt lymphomas in Africa are EBV related versus only 20–30% in the United States. It is thought that chronic stimulation of B lymphocytes by EBV can set the stage for specific chromosomal translocations that contribute to malignant transformation. Chronic malarial infection appears to increase the risk of Burkitt lymphoma by decreasing immune surveillance of genetically altered cells. Hepatitis B virus is associated with adult-onset hepatocellular carcinoma.

PAPOVA VIRUSES. This family of viruses causes warts and papillomas in a variety of tissues. Subtypes of the virus appear to have strong tissue tropisms. Types 6 and 11 are found in lesions of laryngeal papillomatosis and condyloma acuminatum. Although these viral lesions rarely undergo spontaneous malignant transformation, malignant conversion to squamous cell carcinomas is frequent after exposure to a secondary carcinogen, such as cigarette smoke or therapeutic irradiation. Subtypes 16 and 18 appear to be etiologic factors in carcinoma of the uterine cervix.

CHAPTER 446
Molecular Pathogenesis

David N. Shapiro

ONCOGENES. Oncogenes are endogenous human, DNA sequences that arise from normal cellular genes called proto-oncogenes. Proto-oncogenes are normally expressed in many cells, particularly during fetal development, and are thought to play an important role in the regulation of normal cellular growth and development. Like most other genes, proto-oncogenes contain a regulatory region that modulates gene expression and a structural region that encodes a protein product (receptor, growth or transcription factor). Alterations in either region of a proto-oncogene can activate an oncogene, which produces unregulated gene activity and can then contribute directly to tumorigenesis. Structural alterations generally involve a point mutation, small deletion, or gene fusion, resulting from a chromosomal translocation. By contrast, regulatory changes often involve amplification or translocation of a large chromosomal segment that carries a proto-oncogene, resulting in altered expression rather than altered structure.

Oncogene alterations are important as causes of some pediatric malignancies. For example, activating *ras* oncogene point mutations (nucleotide changes) have been found in approximately 33% of embryonal rhabdomyosarcomas. Activated oncogenes are thought to act in a dominant fashion such that a change in a single allele overcomes the effect of the other normal allele.

Regulatory alterations in the expression of proto-oncogenes have also been observed in various pediatric tumors. For example, in Burkitt lymphoma, a characteristic chromosomal translocation, the t(8;14)(q24q32), occurs in which the proto-oncogene C-*myc* is translocated intact from its normal position on chromosome 8 into the vicinity of the immunoglobulin heavy chain locus on chromosome 14. This chromosomal juxtaposition, without structural alteration of the C-*myc* gene, results in deregulated expression of the gene's protein product at an inappropriate time during B-cell differentiation, thereby contributing to tumorigenesis. Increased expression can also occur through gene amplification without chromosomal translocation. For example, amplification of the N-*myc* proto-oncogene in extrachromosomal double-minute chromosomes is seen in a proportion of patients with poor-prognosis neuroblastoma.

Although proto-oncogenes are directly involved in a subset of tumor-specific chromosomal rearrangements and structural alterations (Table 446–1), a more common mechanism of malignant transformation appears to be the creation of chimeric transcription factors. These hybrid transcription factors arise through the fusion of two disparate, nontransforming genes as a result of chromosomal translocation. Presumably, they activate genes not normally expressed in the target tissue, resulting in or contributing directly to malignant transformation. Both the t(11;22) found in Ewing sarcoma and the t(2;13) found in alveolar rhabdomyosarcoma result in the formation of chimeric transcription factors by the fusion of genes located at the translocation breakpoints.

TUMOR-SUPPRESSOR GENES. By contrast with dominantly acting oncogenes, the inappropriate activation of which leads to malignancy, tumor-suppressor genes (also termed antioncogenes or recessive oncogenes) normally downregulate cell growth and require inactivation to allow malignant growth. The concept of tumor-suppressor genes arose from observations of hereditary childhood cancers. In a recessive model of tumorigenesis, Knudson postulated that a susceptibility gene for retinoblastoma is inactivated (deletion or mutation) in the germline of patients with familial retinoblastoma. This germline defect is either inherited from a parent or arises de novo during embryogenesis, with the result that every cell in the individual has one defective allele but is otherwise phenotypically normal. A somatic mutation in the remaining allele would inactivate the putative *Rb* gene and result in tumor formation. By contrast, two independent somatic mutations in the same gene and in the same cell are required in the case of sporadic retinoblastoma.

Several years after Knudson's "two-hit" model was proposed, the *Rb* gene was identified and characterized. It encodes a nuclear phosphoprotein with DNA-binding activity that is critical for cell cycle regulation. The *Rb* gene is expressed in virtually all normal cells, where it functions to regulate cell growth and division negatively, but is absent in cases of retinoblastoma. Since identification of the *Rb* gene, numerous other tumor suppressors have been identified. For example, germline mutations of the p53 tumor-suppressor gene are associated with the Li-Fraumeni syndrome, which is clinically defined by the occurrence of various childhood solid tumors in families that have an excessive occurrence of early-onset breast, bone, brain, and lung cancers. The p53 tumor-suppressor gene product may be a transcription regulatory factor that regulates apoptosis (programmed natural cell death). In the absence of this gene product, apoptosis is absent, cell life is expanded, and tumor cell growth is excessive. The absence of p53 is often associated with aggressive tumors.

OTHER MECHANISMS AND IMPLICATIONS. The associations between underlying genetic disorders and malignancy suggest that mechanisms other than oncogenes or tumor-suppressor genes may be responsible for tumorigenesis. Children with disorders of DNA repair such as xeroderma pigmentosum, ataxia-telangiectasia, Bloom syndrome, and Fanconi anemia are at increased risk for the development of malignancies. Similarly, children with various immunodeficiency states, such as the Wiskott-Aldrich syndrome or congenital X-linked immunodeficiency, have lymphoid malignancies that develop at a substantially higher rate than normal children (Table 446–2).

In evaluating any child with a tumor, look for familial associations, either with malignancy or with any congenital syndrome or abnormality. Syndromes such as neurofibromatosis or hemihypertrophy may not become clinically apparent until the patient is 5–10 yr of age and may not be appreciated when malignancy is diagnosed. In some situations, it may be important to examine the parents and the child or to use newly developed molecular screening procedures to define

■ TABLE 446–1 Molecular Targets of Chromosomal Translocations in Pediatric Malignancies

Disease	Chromosome Abnormality	Molecular Target	Target Gene
Acute Lymphoblastic Leukemia			
B-cell lineage	t(9;22)	*BCR-ABL**	Oncogene
	t(1;19)	*E2A-PBX1**	Transcription factor
	t(8;14), t(2;8), t(8;22)	*IGH, IGK, IGL, myc*	Oncogene
	t(17;19)	*E2A-HLF**	Transcription factor
	t(4;11)	*HRX-AF4**	Transcription factor
	t(11;19)	*HRX-ENL**	Transcription factor
T-cell lineage	t(11;14)	*TTG2-TCRD*	Transcription factor
	t(10;11)	*HOX11-TCRD*	?Transcription factor
	t(1;14)	*TCRD-TAL1*	Oncogene
Lymphoma			
Burkitt	t(8;14), t(2;8), t(8;22)	*IGH, IGK, IGL, myc*	Oncogene
Anaplastic	t(2;5)	*NPM-ALK**	?Oncogene
Chronic Myeloid Leukemia	t(9;22)	*BCR-ABL**	Oncogene
Acute Myeloid Leukemia			
With maturation	t(8;21)	*AML1-ETO**	Transcription factor
Acute promyelocytic	t(15;17)	*PML-RARA**	Transcription factor
With eosinophilia	inv(16)	*CBFβ-MYH11**	Transcription factor
Myelocytic/myelomonocytic	t(11q23;v)	*HRX-various**	Transcription factor
Sarcomas			
Ewing	t(11;22)	*EWS-FLI**	Transcription factor
	t(21;22)	*EWS-ERG**	Transcription factor
Alveolar rhabdomyosarcoma	t(2;13)	*PAX3-FKHR**	Transcription factor

**Gene fusion.*

■ TABLE 446–2 Familial or Genetic Susceptibility to Malignancy

Disorder	Tumor/Cancer	Comment
Chromosomal Syndromes		
Chromosome 11p—(deletion) with sporadic aniridia	Wilms tumor	Associated with genitourinary anomalies, mental retardation
Chromosome 13q—(deletion)	Retinoblastoma	Associated with mental retardation, skeletal malformations: autosomal dominant (bilateral) or sporadic new mutation
Trisomy 21	Lymphocytic or nonlymphocytic leukemia	Risk is 15 times normal
Klinefelter syndrome (47, XXY)	Breast cancer, extragonadal germ cell tumors	
Gonadal dysgenesis XO/XY	Gonadoblastoma	Gonads must be removed; 25% chance of gonadal malignancy
Trisomy 8	Preleukemia	
Noonan syndrome	Schwannoma	
Monosomy 5 or 7	Myelodysplastic syndromes	Recurrent infections may precede neoplasia
DNA Fragility		
Xeroderma pigmentosum	Basal, squamous cell skin cancers	Autosomal recessive; failure to repair solar-damaged DNA
Fanconi anemia	Leukemia	Autosomal recessive; 10% risk for acute myelogenous leukemia; chromosome fragility, positive diepoxybutane test
Bloom syndrome	Leukemia, lymphoma	Autosomal recessive; chromosome fragility; high risk for malignancy
Ataxia-telangiectasia	Lymphoma, leukemia	Autosomal recessive; sensitive to x-radiation, radiomimetic drugs; chromosome fragility
Dysplastic nevus syndrome	Melanoma	Autosomal dominant
Immunodeficiency Syndromes		
Wiskott-Aldrich syndrome	Lymphoma, leukemia	Immunodeficiency; X-linked recessive
X-linked immunodeficiency (Duncan syndrome)	Lymphoma	Epstein-Barr virus is inciting agent
X-linked agammaglobulinemia	Lymphoma, leukemia	Immunodeficiency
Severe combined immunodeficiency	Leukemia, lymphoma	Immunodeficiency; X-linked recessive
Others		
Neurofibromatosis 1	Neurofibroma, optic glioma, acoustic neuroma, astrocytoma, meningioma, pheochromocytoma, sarcoma	Autosomal dominant
Neurofibromatosis 2	Bilateral acoustic neuromas, meningioma	Autosomal dominant
Tuberous sclerosis	Fibroangiomatous nevi, myocardial rhabdomyoma	Autosomal dominant
Hemochromatosis	Hepatoma	Cirrhosis; autosomal dominant/recessive
Retinoblastoma	Sarcoma	Increased risk of secondary malignancy 10–20 yr later
Glycogen storage disease I	Hepatic adenoma	Usually with cirrhosis, autosomal recessive
Familial adenomatous polyposis coli	Adenocarcinoma of colon	Autosomal dominant
Gardner syndrome	Adenocarcinoma of colon; skull and soft tissue tumors	Autosomal dominant
Peutz-Jeghers syndrome	Gastrointestinal carcinoma, ovarian neoplasia	Autosomal dominant
Hemihypertrophy ± Beckwith syndrome	Wilms tumor, hepatoblastoma, adrenal carcinoma	25% develop tumor, most in first 5 yr of life
Tyrosinemia, galactosemia	Hepatic carcinoma	Nodular cirrhosis; autosomal recessive
Multiple endocrine neoplasia syndrome I (Wermer syndrome)	Parathyroid adenoma, pancreatic islet tumor, pituitary adenoma carcinoid	Autosomal dominant; Zollinger-Ellison syndrome
Multiple endocrine neoplasia syndrome II (Sipple syndrome)	Medullary carcinoma of the thyroid, hyperparathyroidism, pheochromocytoma	Autosomal dominant; monitor calcitonin and calcium levels
Multiple endocrine neoplasia III (multiple mucosal neuroma syndrome)	Mucosal neuroma, pheochromocytoma, medullary thyroid carcinoma; Marfan habitus; neuropathy	Autosomal domniant
Rendu-Osler-Weber syndrome	Angioma	Autosomal dominant
von Hippel-Lindau disease	Hemangioblastoma of the cerebellum and retina, pheochromocytoma	Autosomal dominant, mutation of tumor-suppressor gene
Cancer family syndrome	Colonic, uterine carcinoma	Autosomal dominant
Li-Fraumeni syndrome	Bone, soft tissue sarcoma, breast	Mutation of p53 tumor-suppressor gene, autosomal dominant

(From Behrman R, Kliegman R (eds): Nelson Essentials of Pediatrics, 2nd ed. Philadelphia, WB Saunders, 1994.)

abnormalities of potentially important etiologic genes. Awareness of these associations may also protect the parents. One should make sure that the mother of a child with a soft tissue sarcoma knows how to perform breast self-examination. Unfortunately, there are as yet no rules that help prevent the development of cancer in childhood. Trials of pharmacoprevention and nutritional prevention are under way for familial polyposis in an attempt to prevent cancer (see Chapter 291). However, pediatricians can help to avoid cancers in adulthood by encouraging proper nutrition and the avoidance of unhealthy practices such as smoking or exposure to excessive sunlight.

CHAPTER 447

Principles of Diagnosis

William M. Crist and Helen Heslop

Most childhood cancers are curable. The prognosis relates most strongly to tumor type, extent of disease at diagnosis, and the effectiveness of the treatment. Rapid diagnosis ensures that appropriate therapy is given in a timely fashion and optimizes the chances of cure. Because most physicians in general practice rarely encounter children with cancer, they should be alert for an atypical course of a common childhood condition (Table 447–1).

Delays in diagnosis are likely in certain situations. The cardinal symptom of both osteosarcoma and Ewing sarcoma is localized, usually persistent bone-extremity pain. Because these tumors occur during the 2nd decade of life, a time of increased physical activity, the patient often associates the pain with an episode of trauma. Radiologic evaluation can help ensure prompt diagnosis. Tumors of the nasopharynx or middle ear may mimic infection. Prolonged unexplained ear pain, nasal discharge, retropharyngeal swelling, or trismus should be investigated as possible signs of malignancy. Cervical lymph node enlargement is common in children with infection and also with lymphoma. Persistent or progressively enlarging nodes (often painless) suggest lymphoma and indicate the need for biopsy.

The early symptoms of leukemia may be limited to low-grade fever or bone and joint pain. Such pain is intense, awakens the patient, and is often present without objective signs of erythema or swelling. Blood counts, with particular attention to normocytic anemia, neutropenia, or mild thrombocytopenia, may indicate the need for bone marrow examination, even when leukemic blast cells are not seen in the blood smear. Malignancy can also occur in the neonate and should be considered in children with masses or "blueberry muffin" spots on the skin.

When a malignant neoplasm is suspected, the immediate goal is to determine its nature and extent. A tentative diagnosis can often be inferred from the patient's presenting symptoms, age, and tumor location. For example, an abdominal mass is much more likely to be a neuroblastoma or Wilms tumor in a young child than in a child older than 10 yr of age.

A relatively thorough search for metastatic disease usually precedes biopsy of a suspicious lesion. The surgeon can make a more informed choice between an attempt at complete resection and a more limited procedure when the presence or likelihood of disseminated disease is known. The appropriate preoperative studies depend on the tentative diagnosis. Several noninvasive techniques are useful in evaluating for metastatic

■ **TABLE 447–1 Common Manifestations of Childhood Malignancy**

Sign/Symptom	Nonmalignant Condition Mimicked	Significance	Example
Hematologic			
Pallor, anemia	Iron-deficiency anemia, blood loss	Bone marrow infiltration	Leukemia, neuroblastoma
Petechiae, thrombocytopenia	Idiopathic thrombocytopenic purpura	Bone marrow infiltration	Leukemia, neuroblastoma
Fever, pharyngitis, neutropenia	Streptococcal/viral pharyngitis	Bone marrow infiltration	Leukemia, neuroblastoma
Systemic			
Bone pain, limp, arthralgia	Osteomyelitis, rheumatologic disease, trauma	Primary bone tumor, metastasis to bone	Osteosarcoma, Ewing sarcoma, leukemia, neuroblastoma
Fever of unknown origin, weight loss, night sweats	Collagen vascular disease, chronic infection	Lymphoreticular malignancy	Hodgkin disease, non-Hodgkin lymphoma
Painless lymphadenopathy	Epstein-Barr virus, cytomegalovirus	Lymphoreticular malignancy	Leukemia, Hodgkin disease, non-Hodgkin lymphoma, Burkitt lymphoma
Cutaneous lesion	Abscess, trauma	Primary or metastatic disease	Neuroblastoma, leukemia, histiocytosis X, melanoma
Abdominal mass	Organomegaly, hydronephrosis, constipation	Adrenal-renal tumor	Neuroblastoma, Wilms tumor, hepatoblastoma
Hypertension	Renovascular disease, nephritis	Sympathetic nervous system tumor	Neuroblastoma, pheochromocytoma, Wilms tumor
Diarrhea	Inflammatory bowel disease	Vasoactive intestinal polypeptide	Neuroblastoma, ganglioneuroma
Soft tissue mass	Abscess	Local or metastatic tumor	Ewing sarcoma, osteosarcoma, neuroblastoma, rhabdomyosarcoma, eosinophilic granuloma Askin tumor
Vaginal bleeding	Foreign body, coagulopathy	Uterine tumor	Yolk sac tumor, rhabdomyosarcoma
Emesis, visual disturbances, ataxia, headache, papilledema	Migraine	Increased intracranial pressure	Primary brain tumor; metastasis
Chronic ear discharge	Otitis media	Middle or inner ear mass	Rhabdomyosarcoma

Table continued on following page

■ TABLE 447–1 Common Manifestations of Childhood Malignancy *Continued*

Sign/Symptom	Nonmalignant Condition Mimicked	Significance	Example
Ophthalmologic Signs			
Leukocoria	Cataract, glaucoma	White pupil	Retinoblastoma
Periorbital ecchymosis	Trauma	Metastasis	Neuroblastoma
Miosis, ptosis, heterochromia	Third nerve paresis	Horner syndrome: compression of cervical sympathetic nerves	Neuroblastoma
Opsoclonus/ataxia	Drug reaction	Neurotransmitters? Autoimmunity?	Neuroblastoma
Exophthalmos, proptosis	Graves disease	Orbital tumor	Rhabdomyosarcoma
Thoracic Mass			
Anterior mediastinal	Infection (tuberculosis), lymphadenopathy, sarcoidosis	Cough, stridor, pneumonia, tracheal-bronchial compression	Thymoma, teratoma, T-cell lymphoma, thyroid
Posterior mediastinal	Esophageal disease	Vertebral or nerve root compression; dysphagia	Neuroblastoma, neuroenteric cyst

(Modified from Behrman R, Kliegman R (eds): Nelson Essentials of Pediatrics, 2nd ed. Philadelphia, WB Saunders, 1994.)

lesions; bone marrow aspiration, biopsy, or both may be needed. These studies are also used in assessing the disease stage, which is critical in determining the prognosis and treatment plan.

Central to the diagnosis is examination of the histologic type. The initial specimen of tumor tissue should be obtained under conditions that permit full pathologic studies. In some cases, such as suspected lymphomas, fresh tissue may be needed for special studies. These studies take time. It is often impossible to discuss the specific diagnosis with a family immediately after surgery.

The surgeon must search carefully at biopsy, excision, or exploration for evidence of regional dissemination to lymph node groups or to adjacent organs. If total resection is attempted, the pathologist must carefully examine the margins for microscopic residual tumor because subsequent treatment planning depends on this information.

The treatment plan must be carefully explained to parents and, if possible, to the patient. An honest explanation of the facts is the best policy. The child should be told all that he or she can understand and would find useful or wishes to know. Special concerns, such as the possible need to amputate a limb, the loss of hair during chemotherapy, and possible temporary or permanent functional impairment must be anticipated and fully discussed. It may be necessary to repeat explanations several times before distraught family members truly understand what is being said. Throughout treatment, parents, patients, siblings, friends, and medical staff will need help in expressing feelings of anxiety, depression, guilt, and anger.

CHAPTER 448

Principles of Treatment

William M. Crist and Helen Heslop

Treatment of the child with cancer is complex, requiring the expertise of large teams of specialized health care providers (pediatric pathologists, oncologists, radiotherapists, surgeons, radiologists, and a variety of support staff, including nutritionists, social workers, psychologists, and nurses). The best chance for cure exists during the initial course of treatment, and patients should be referred to an appropriate specialized center as soon as possible when the diagnosis of cancer is suspected.

Whenever possible, treatment is given on an outpatient basis. The child should remain at home and in school as much as possible throughout treatment. However, the intensity of many treatment regimens is such that most patients will miss a considerable amount of school in the 1st yr or 2 after diagnosis. Tutoring should be encouraged so the child does not fall behind, and counseling should be provided as appropriate.

Development of selective, highly effective therapy for cancer has been hindered by lack of understanding of the molecular mechanisms underlying malignant transformation and de novo or acquired drug resistance. In spite of discoveries that have clarified these important areas in part, information remains incomplete, and therapy, therefore, continues to be largely empiric. Because of the lack of selectivity of available therapy for malignant vs nonmalignant cells, toxicity remains a troublesome issue.

Local therapy with surgery and/or irradiation is an important component of treatment for most solid tumors, but systemic multiagent chemotherapy is usually necessary because tumor dissemination is generally present, even if undetectable. Similarly, chemotherapy alone is generally insufficient to eradicate gross residual tumors. Hence, most children with malignant tumors require treatment with all three modalities. Unfortunately, most effective treatments have a narrow therapeutic index (ratio of efficacy to toxicity). Therefore, acute and chronic toxicity can be minimized but not avoided entirely.

448.1 Chemotherapy

Drugs for treatment of cancer are selected from several classes of agents, including hormones, antimetabolites, antibiotics, plant alkaloids, and alkylating agents (Table 448–1). All new compounds are studied in animals to assess their efficacy in suppressing tumor growth and their toxicity. The few agents with promise are then studied in phase I clinical trials to assess their toxicity. These studies are usually performed first in adults who have no effective treatment options and who have provided their informed consent. Starting doses are low and are increased to the point of tolerance. Once the maximum tolerated dose is determined, phase II studies, using a fixed dose, are conducted in patients with poor-prognosis disease to assess treatment efficacy in specific tumor types. For

■ TABLE 448–1 Cancer Chemotherapy

Drug*	Action	Metabolism	Excretion	Indication	Toxicity
Antimetabolites					
Methotrexate	Folic acid antagonist; inhibits dihydrofolate reductase	Hepatic	Renal, 50–90% excreted unchanged; biliary	ALL, lymphoma, medulloblastoma, osteosarcoma	Myelosuppression (nadir 7–10 days), mucositis, stomatitis, dermatitis, hepatitis; renal and CNS with high-dose administration; prevent with leucovorin, monitor levels
6-Mercaptopurine (Purinethol)	Purine analog, inhibits purine synthesis	Hepatic; allopurinol inhibits metabolism	Renal	ALL	Myelosuppression, hepatic necrosis, mucositis; allopurinal increases toxicity
Cytarabine (Ara-C)	Pyrimidine analog; inhibits DNA polymerase	Hepatic	Renal	ALL, lymphoma	Myelosuppression, conjunctivitis, mucositis, CNS dysfunction
Alkylating Agents					
Cyclophosphamide (Cytoxan)	Alkylates guanine; inhibits DNA synthesis	Hepatic	Renal	ALL, lymphoma, sarcoma	Myelosuppression, hemorrhagic cystitis, pulmonary fibrosis, inappropriate ADH secretion, bladder cancer, anaphylaxis
Ifosfamide (Ifex)	Similar to cyclophosphamide	Hepatic	Renal	Lymphoma, Wilms tumor, sarcoma, germ cell and testicular tumors	Similar to cyclophosphamide; CNS dysfunction, cardiac toxicity
Antibiotics					
Doxorubicin (Adriamycin) and Daunorubicin (Cerubidine)	Binds to DNA, intercalation	Hepatic	Biliary, renal	ALL, AML, osteosarcoma, Ewing sarcoma, lymphoma, neuroblastoma	Cardiomyopathy, red urine, tissue necrosis on extravasation, myelosuppression, conjunctivitis, radiation dermatitis, arrhythmia
Dactinomycin	Binds to DNA, inhibits transcription	—	Renal, stool; 30% excreted unchanged drug	Wilms tumor, rhabdomyosarcoma, Ewing sarcoma	Tissue necrosis on extravasation, myelosuppression, radiosensitizer, mucosal ulceration
Bleomycin (Blenoxane)	Binds to DNA, cuts DNA	Hepatic	Renal	Hodgkin disease, lymphoma, germ cell tumors	Pneumonitis, stomatitis, Raynaud phenomenon, pulmonary fibrosis, dermatitis
Vinca Alkaloids					
Vincristine (Oncovin)	Inhibits microtubule formation	Hepatic	Biliary	ALL, lymphoma, Wilms tumor, Hodgkin disease, Ewing sarcoma, neuroblastoma, rhabdomyosarcoma	Local cellulitis, peripheral neuropathy, constipation, ileus, jaw pain, inappropriate ADH secretion, seizures, ptosis, minimal myelosuppression
Vinblastine (Velban)	Inhibits microtubule formation	Hepatic	Biliary	Hodgkin disease; Langerhans cell histiocytosis	Local cellulitis, leukopenia
Enzymes					
L-Asparaginase	Depletion of L-asparagine	—	Reticuloendothelial system	ALL	Allergic reaction, pancreatitis, hyperglycemia, platelet dysfunction and coagulopathy, encephalopathy
Pegaspargase	Polyethylene glycol conjugate of L-asparagine	—	As above	As above	Indicated for patients with allergy to L-asparaginase
Hormones					
Prednisone	Unknown; lymphocyte modification?	Hepatic	Renal	ALL; Hodgkin disease, lymphoma	Cushing syndrome, cataracts, diabetes, hypertension, myopathy, osteoporosis, infection, peptic ulceration, psychosis
Miscellaneous					
Carmustine (nitrosourea)	Carbamylation of DNA; inhibits DNA synthesis	Hepatic; phenobarbital increases metabolism, decreases activity	Renal	CNS tumors, lymphoma, Hodgkin disease	Delayed myelosuppression (4–6 wk); pulmonary fibrosis, carcinogenic, stomatitis
Cisplatin (Platinol)	Inhibits DNA synthesis	—	Renal	Gonadal tumors; osteosarcoma, neuroblastoma, CNS tumors, germ cell tumors	Nephrotoxic; aminoglycosides may increase nephrotoxicity, myelosuppression, ototoxicity, tetany, neurotoxicity, hemolytic-uremic syndrome; anaphylaxis
Etoposide (VePesid)	Topoisomerase inhibitor	—	Renal	ALL, lymphoma, germ cell tumor	Myelosuppression, secondary leukemia
Etretinate (Tegison) (vitamin A analog) and tretinoin	Enhances normal differentiation	Liver	Liver	Some leukemias; neuroblastoma	Dry mouth, hair loss, pseudotumor cerebri, premature epiphyseal closure

**Many drugs produce nausea and vomiting during administration, and many cause alopecia with repeated doses.*
ADH = antidiuretic hormone; ALL = acute lymphocytic leukemia; AML = acute myelogenous leukemia; CNS = central nervous system.
(From Behrman R, Kliegman R (eds): Nelson Essentials of Pediatrics, 2nd ed. Philadelphia, WB Saunders, 1994.)

those tumors found to be responsive, phase III trials are designed to incorporate the new agent into regimens with other active drugs, and treatment outcomes are compared with those achieved with standard regimens.

ACUTE COMPLICATIONS AND SUPPORTIVE CARE. Early complications of therapy include metabolic disorders, bone marrow suppression, and immunosuppression. Patients with a large tumor burden may have had substantial breakdown of tumor cells, and renal function can be impaired by tubular precipitates of uric acid crystals (Table 448–2). This problem is seen most often with hematologic malignancies but can occur with large solid tumors (Burkitt lymphoma, germ cell tumor, neuroblastoma). Before initiating therapy, the serum levels of uric acid and creatinine should be measured, adequate hydration should be ensured, and allopurinol (a xanthine oxidase inhibitor) should be given, if necessary, to lower uric acid levels to within the normal range. In the *tumor lysis syndrome,* phosphates and potassium are also released into the circulation in large quantities as cells are lysed by treatment. Symptomatic hyperphosphatemia, hypocalcemia, and hyperkalemia develop in the setting of inadequate renal function.

Tumors that invade and replace bone marrow can cause *pancytopenia;* all chemotherapeutic regimens can produce *myelosuppression.* Anemia can be corrected by transfusions of packed red blood cells and thrombocytopenia, by platelet infusions. Patients receiving immunosuppressive therapy should receive irradiated blood products to prevent graft versus host disease (GVHD). Granulocytopenia (counts less than 500/mm^3) poses the risk of life-threatening infections (Table 448–3). Febrile granulocytopenic patients should be hospitalized and treated with empiric, broad-spectrum intravenous antimicrobial therapy pending the results of appropriate cultures of blood, urine, or any obvious sites of infection (see Chapter 425). Treatment is continued until fever resolves and the granulocyte count rises. If fever persists beyond 1 wk, consideration must be given to a possible fungal infection. Fungal infections caused by Candida and Aspergillus species are common in neutropenic, immunosuppressed patients. Opportunistic organisms such as *Pneumocystis carinii* can produce fatal pneumonia. Prophylactic treatment with trimethoprim/sulfamethoxazole is given when severe immunosuppression is anticipated (see Chapter 173).

Viruses normally of low pathogenicity can produce serious disease in the setting of immunosuppression caused by malignancy or its treatment. Patients should not be given live virus vaccines. Children receiving chemotherapy who are exposed to varicella receive varicella-zoster immunoglobulin and, if clinical disease develops, should be hospitalized and treated with intravenous acyclovir.

Patients undergoing cancer therapy commonly lose 10% or more of their body weight. Patients may reduce their food intake because of treatment-associated nausea and vomiting, and anxious parents should be reassured that the child's poor appetite is not a cause for alarm. *Malnutrition* is a particular risk in patients receiving radiotherapy to the abdomen or head and neck, intensive chemotherapy, or total body irradiation for marrow transplantation. If oral supplementation is inadequate, such patients may require parenteral hyperalimentation. There is no conclusive evidence, however, that hyperalimentation improves the response to therapy.

LATE SEQUELAE (Table 448–4). Late consequences of therapy can cause significant morbidity. Successful surgical resection may require the loss of important functional structures. Irradiation can produce irreversible organ damage, with symptoms and functional limitations depending on the organ involved and the severity of the damage. Many radiation-related problems do not become obvious until the patient is fully grown, for example, when marked asymmetry of irradiated and nonirradiated areas or extremities becomes noticeable. Irradiation of fields that include endocrine organs can cause hypothyroidism or sterility. Cranial irradiation, in sufficient doses, can produce neurologic or intellectual dysfunction and growth retardation from pituitary hormone deficiencies.

Chemotherapy carries the risk of severe organ damage. Of particular concern are leukoencephalopathy after high-dose methotrexate therapy, sterility in male patients treated with alkylating agents, myocardial damage from anthracyclines, pulmonary fibrosis after bleomycin, pancreatitis after asparaginase, and hearing loss associated with cisplatin. These sequelae may be dose related and are usually irreversible. Appropriate baseline testing must be done before these drugs are administered to ensure that there is no pre-existing damage to the organs likely to be affected and to permit monitoring of treatment-induced changes.

Perhaps the most serious late effect is the occurrence of *second cancers* in patients successfully cured of a first malignancy. The risk appears to be cumulative, increasing by about 0.5% per yr to 12% at 25 yr post-treatment. Patients who have been treated for childhood cancer should be examined annually, with particular attention to possible late effects of therapy, including second malignancies.

448.2 Bone Marrow Transplantation

(See also Chapter 132.)

The goal of bone marrow transplantation (BMT) is to replace abnormal cells with normal bone marrow hematopoietic progenitors or to "rescue" the patient after higher than usual doses of marrow-ablative therapy.

In **autologous BMT,** the patient acts as his or her own donor. Marrow is harvested, cryopreserved, and then reinfused after the patient has received intensive chemotherapy. In some cases, peripheral blood stem cells harvested, by leukapheresis after granulocyte or granulocyte-macrophage colony-stimulating factor administration may be used. Autologous BMT may be beneficial in situations in which hematologic toxicity is therapy limiting and dose escalation may improve outcome, for example, acute lymphocytic leukemia, acute myelogenous leukemia, neuroblastoma, Hodgkin disease, non-Hodgkin lymphoma, Ewing sarcoma, and brain tumors. Originally reserved for "salvage therapy" after relapse, autologous BMT is now being evaluated as part of initial consolidation therapy for some malignancies. A problem with this approach is that residual malignant cells in the harvested marrow can contribute to a subsequent relapse, particularly in patients with hematopoietic malignancy or neuroblastoma. Various techniques purge the harvested marrow of residual malignant cells.

In **allogeneic BMT,** marrow is taken from a donor who best "matches" the patient at major histocompatibility complex (MHC) loci. Other than an identical twin (syngeneic transplantation), the best donor is a major MHC-histocompatibility antigen-identical sibling who inherited the same MHC genotype from each parent. Only 20–30% of patients have matched sibling donors, and increasing numbers of transplants are being done using partially matched related donors or matched unrelated donors. The morbidity of these procedures is greater because increased alloreactivity raises the risks of GVHD and marrow rejection. Even with a matched (MHC-identical) sibling donor, there is some degree of alloreactivity because of differences in minor histocompatibility antigens.

In allogeneic transplants, conditioning with chemotherapy and radiation is used not only to eradicate malignancy but also to destroy the recipient's immune system so that engraftment can occur. *Acute regimen-related toxicity* occurs when the pretransplant conditioning regimens cause effects such as mucosi-

■ TABLE 448–2 Oncologic Emergencies

Condition	Manifestations	Etiology	Malignancy	Treatment
Metabolic				
Hyperuricemia	Uric acid nephropathy, gout	Tumor lysis syndrome	Lymphoma, leukemia	Allopurinol; alkalinize urine; hydration and diuresis
Hyperkalemia	Arrhythmias, cardiac arrest	Tumor lysis syndrome	Lymphoma, leukemia	Polystyrene resin (Kayexalate); sodium bicarbonate, glucose and insulin; check for pseudohyperkalemia from leukemic cell lysis in test tube
Hyperphosphatemia	Hypocalcemic tetany; metastatic calcification, photophobia, pruritus	Tumor lysis syndrome	Lymphoma, leukemia	Hydration, forced diuresis; stop alkalinization; oral aluminum hydroxide to bind phosphate
Hyponatremia	Seizure, lethargy; asymptomatic	SIADH; fluid, sodium losses in vomiting, diarrhea, diuresis	Leukemia; CNS tumor	Restrict free water for SIADH; replace sodium if depleted
Hypercalcemia	Anorexia, nausea, polyuria, pancreatitis, gastric ulcers; prolonged PR, shortened QT interval	Bone resorption; ectopic parathormone, vitamin D, or prostaglandins	Hodgkin disease; metastasis to bone	Hydration and furosemide diuresis; corticosteroids; plicamycin; calcitonin; diphosphonates
Hematologic				
Anemia	Pallor, weakness, heart failure	Bone marrow suppression or infiltration; blood loss	Any with chemotherapy	Packed red blood cell transfusion
Thrombocytopenia	Petechiae, hemorrhage	Bone marrow suppression or infiltration	Any with chemotherapy	Platelet transfusion
Disseminated intravascular coagulation	Shock, hemorrhage	Sepsis, hypotension tumor factors	Promyelocytic leukemia; others	Fresh frozen plasma; platelets, correct infection, etc
Neutropenia	Infection	Bone marrow suppression or infiltration	Any with chemotherapy	If febrile, give broad-spectrum antibiotics and G-CSF if appropriate
Hyperleukocytosis (>50,000/mm³)	Hemorrhage, thrombosis; pulmonary infiltrates, hypoxia; tumor lysis syndrome	Leukostasis; vascular occlusion	Leukemia	Leukapheresis; chemotherapy
Graft versus host disease	Dermatitis, diarrhea, hepatitis	Immunosuppression and nonirradiated blood products; bone marrow transplantation	Any with immunosuppression	Corticosteroids; cyclosporine; antithymocyte globulin
Space-Occupying Lesions				
Spinal cord compression	Back pain ± radicular *Cord above T10:* Symmetric weakness, increased DTR; sensory level present; toes up *Conus medullaris* (T10–12): Symmetric weakness, increased knee reflexes, decreased ankle reflexes; saddle sensory loss; toes up or down *Cauda equina* (below L2): Asymmetric weakness, loss of DTR and sensory deficit; toes down	Metastasis to vertebra and extramedullary space	Neuroblastoma; medulloblastoma	MRI or myelography for diagnosis; corticosteroids; radiotherapy; laminectomy; chemotherapy
Increased intracranial pressure	Confusion, coma, emesis, headache, hypertension, bradycardia, seizures, papilledema, hydrocephalus; III and VI nerve palsies	Primary or metastatic brain tumor	Neuroblastoma, astrocytoma; glioma	Computed tomography or MRI for diagnosis; corticosteroids; phenytoin; ventricular-peritoneal shunt; radiotherapy; chemotherapy
Superior vena cava syndrome	Distended neck veins, plethora, edema of head and neck, cyanosis; proptosis; Horner syndrome	Superior mediastinal mass	Lymphoma	Chemotherapy; radiotherapy

SIADH = inappropriate antidiuretic hormone secretion; G-CSF = granulocyte colony-stimulating factor; DTR = deep tendon reflex; MRI = magnetic resonance imaging.
(From Behrman R, Kliegman R (eds): Nelson Essentials of Pediatrics, 2nd ed. Philadelphia, WB Saunders, 1994.)

■ TABLE 448–3 Infectious Complications of Malignancy

Predisposing Factor	Etiology	Site of Infection	Infectious Agents
Neutropenia	Chemotherapy, bone marrow infiltration	Sepsis, shock, pneumonia, soft tissue, proctitis, mucositis	*Staphylococcus aureus, Staphylococcus epidermidis; Escherichia coli, Pseudomonas aeruginosa,* Candida, Aspergillus; anaerobic oral and rectal bacteria
Immunosuppression, lymphopenia, lymphocyte-monocyte dysfunction	Chemotherapy, prednisone	Pneumonia, meningitis, disseminated viral infection	*Pneumocystis carinii, Cryptococcus neoformans,* Mycobacterium; Nocardia, *Listeria monocytogenes,* Candida, Aspergillus, Strongyloides; Toxoplasma, varicella-zoster, cytomegalovirus, herpes simplex
Splenectomy	Staging of Hodgkin disease	Sepsis, shock, meningitis	Pneumococcus, *Haemophilus influenzae*
Indwelling central venous catheter	Nutrition, administration of chemotherapy	Line sepsis, tract or tunnel infection, exit site infection	*S. aureus, S. epidermidis, Candida albicans; P. aeruginosa;* Aspergillus; Corynebacterium JK, *Streptococcus faecalis, Mycobacterium fortuitum, Propionibacterium acnes*

(From Behrman R, Kliegman R (eds): Nelson Essentials of Pediatrics, 2nd ed. Philadelphia, WB Saunders, 1994.)

tis, pneumonitis, veno-occlusive disease, and hemorrhagic cystitis. These complications are more likely in patients who have had extensive prior therapy or who receive highly intensive conditioning.

After transplantation, patients are at risk for a variety of complications. *Marrow rejection* occurs when residual immunocompetent cells survive the conditioning regimen and reject the donor marrow. The likelihood of rejection increases with less intensive conditioning and greater genetic disparity between donor and host. *GVHD* occurs when mature alloreactive T cells in the donor graft recognize host alloantigens. In acute GVHD (1st or 2nd mo post-transplant), the main target organs are the skin, gastrointestinal tract, and liver. Regimens used to prevent GVHD include administration of drugs that interfere with T-cell function (cyclosporine) and removal of mature alloreactive T cells from the infused graft. Even with these measures, acute GVHD occurs in a significant number of patients. Therapy of established GVHD may include steroids or anti–T-cell monoclonal antibodies. Chronic GVHD (3–4 mo post-transplant) involves additional organ systems and often resembles autoimmune diseases such as scleroderma and myasthenia gravis. Severe infection is a risk in patients with immunosuppression related to GVHD and its treatment.

All patients are at risk for life-threatening infection until the recovery of immune function. In the early post-transplant period, neutropenia poses the risk of bacterial or fungal infection. Hematopoietic engraftment generally occurs within 1 mo, but immune recovery is delayed. Hence, the risk of viral and other opportunistic infections persists for several months, particularly in mismatched or unrelated donor transplants. Viral infections often result from reactivation and infection with herpes simplex, varicella zoster, and cytomegalovirus. Antiviral agents (ganciclovir) and immune globulin are often used to prevent infection with cytomegalovirus.

APPLICATIONS OF BMT. In congenital immunodeficiencies, BMT is the only curative option. In hematopoietic malignancies, however, the role of BMT is more difficult to define. Randomized clinical trials are lacking. Most studies that compare the results of chemotherapy with those of BMT are retrospective and cannot control for differences in patient characteristics and supportive care. Hence, treatment decisions are based largely on the patient's history, condition, prognosis, and donor availability.

■ TABLE 448–4 Long-Term Sequelae of Cancer Therapy

Problem	Etiology
Infertility	Alkylating agents; radiation
Second cancers	Genetic predisposition; radiation, alkylating agents
Sepsis	Splenectomy
Hepatotoxicity	Methotrexate, 6-mercaptopurine, radiation
Hepatic veno-occlusive disease	High-dose, intensive chemotherapy (busulfan, cyclophosphamide) ± bone marrow transplant
Amputation	Surgery for osteogenic sarcoma
Scoliosis	Radiation
Pulmonary (pneumonia, fibrosis)	Radiation, bleomycin, busulfan
Myocardiopathy; pericarditis	Doxorubicin, daunomycin; radiation
Leukoencephalopathy	Cranial irradiation ± methotrexate
Cognition/intelligence	Cranial irradiation ± methotrexate
Pituitary dysfunction (isolated growth hormone deficiency, panhypopituitary)	Cranial irradiation
Psychosocial	Stress, anxiety, death of peers; conditioned responses to chemotherapy

(From Behrman R, Kliegman R (eds): Nelson Essentials of Pediatrics, 2nd ed. Philadelphia, WB Saunders, 1994.)

CHAPTER 449

The Leukemias

William M. Crist and Ching-Hon Pui

Leukemias are the most common childhood cancers, accounting for about 33% of pediatric malignancies. Acute lymphoblastic leukemia (ALL) represents about 75% of all cases, with a peak incidence at age 4 yr. Acute myeloid leukemia (AML) accounts for about 20% of leukemias, with an incidence that is stable from birth through age 10 yr, increasing slightly during adolescence. Most of the remaining leukemias are of the chronic myeloid form; chronic lymphocytic leukemia is rarely seen in children. The overall annual incidence of leukemia is 42.1 per million white children and 24.3 per million black children. The difference is due mainly to the lower incidence of ALL among black children. The general clinical features of the leukemias are similar because all involve a severe disruption of bone marrow function. Specific clinical and laboratory features differ, however, and there is marked variability in responses to therapy and in prognosis.

449.1 Acute Lymphoblastic Leukemia

Childhood ALL was the first disseminated cancer shown to be curable with chemotherapy and irradiation. ALL occurs slightly more frequently in boys than in girls. Reports of geographic clusters of childhood leukemia have suggested some shared environmental factor. However, careful review has not supported most of the proposed associations. Lymphoid leukemias occur more often than expected in patients with immunodeficiency (congenital hypogammaglobulinemia, ataxia-telangiectasia) or with constitutional chromosomal defects (trisomy 21).

PATHOLOGY. Cases of ALL are subclassified according to morphologic, immunologic, and genetic features of the leukemic blast cells. Definitive diagnosis is generally based on examination of a bone marrow aspirate. The cytologic appearance of the blast cells is so variable, even within a single specimen, that no completely satisfactory morphologic classification has been devised. The French-American-British (FAB) system distinguishes three morphologic subtypes, L1 to L3. L1 lymphoblasts are predominantly small, with little cytoplasm; L2 cells are larger and pleomorphic with increased cytoplasm, irregular nuclear shape, and prominent nucleoli; and L3 cells have finely stippled and homogeneous nuclear chromatin, prominent nucleoli, and deep blue cytoplasm with prominent vacuolization (Fig. 449–1). Because of the subjective distinction between L1 and L2 blasts and a poor correlation with immunologic and genetic markers, only the L3 subtype is clinically meaningful.

Classification of ALL depends on a combination of cytologic, immunologic, and karyotypic features. With monoclonal antibodies that recognize lineage-associated cell surface and cytoplasmic antigens, the immunophenotype can be determined in most cases. Most are derived from B-progenitor cells; about 15% derive from T-progenitor cells; and 1% are from relatively mature B cells. These immunophenotypes have both prognostic and therapeutic implications. The subtypes of ALL, certain clinical characteristics, and their relative incidence rates are shown in Table 449–1. A few cases cannot be readily classified because they demonstrate antigen expression associated with several different cell lineages (mixed lineage or biphenotypic ALL).

Chromosomal abnormalities can be identified in at least 80–90% of childhood ALLs. The karyotypes of leukemic cells have diagnostic, prognostic, and therapeutic significance. They pinpoint sites for molecular studies to detect genes that may be involved in leukemic transformation. Childhood ALL can also be classified by the number of chromosomes per leukemic cell (ploidy) and by structural chromosomal rearrangements such as translocations.

Another biologic marker with potential usefulness is terminal deoxynucleotidyl transferase (TdT) activity, which is generally demonstrable in B-progenitor–cell and T-cell ALL. Because this enzyme is absent in normal lymphocytes, it can be useful in identifying leukemic cells in difficult diagnostic situations. For example, TdT activity in cells from cerebrospinal fluid may help to distinguish early central nervous system (CNS) relapse from aseptic meningitis.

Most patients with leukemia have disseminated disease at diagnosis, with widespread bone marrow involvement and the presence of leukemic blast cells in circulating blood. Spleen, liver, and lymph nodes are also usually involved. Hence, there is no staging system for ALL.

CLINICAL MANIFESTATIONS. About 66% of children with ALL have had signs and symptoms of their disease for less than 4 wk at the time of diagnosis. The first symptoms are usually nonspecific and include anorexia, irritability, and lethargy. There may be a history of viral respiratory infection or exanthem from which the child has not appeared to recover fully. Progressive bone marrow failure leads to pallor (anemia), bleeding (thrombocytopenia), and fever (neutropenia, malignancy)—the features that usually prompt diagnostic studies.

On initial examination, most patients are pale, and about 50% have petechiae or mucous membrane bleeding. About 25% have fever, which may be ascribed to a specific cause such as upper respiratory infection or otitis media. Lymphadenopathy is occasionally prominent, and splenomegaly (usually extending less than 6 cm below the costal margin) is found in

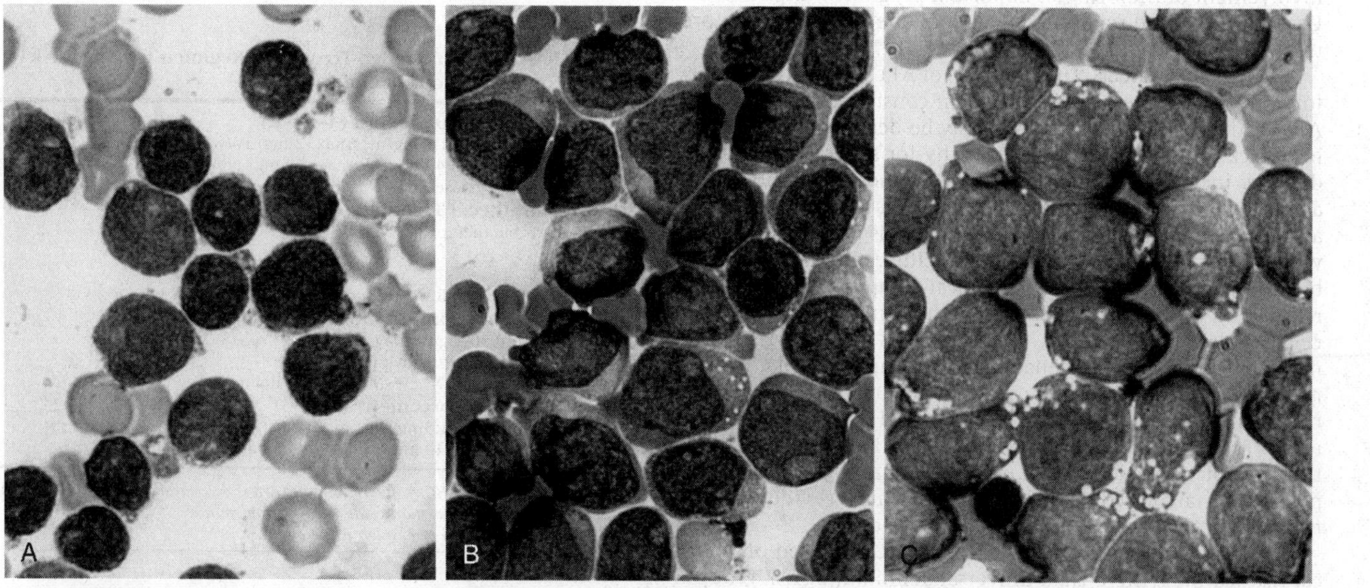

Figure 449–1. Examples of FAB morphologic subtypes of ALL. *A,* L1 blasts are small with scanty cytoplasm; *B,* L2 blasts are larger with more cytoplasm, irregular nuclear membranes, and prominent nucleoli; *C,* L3 blasts have basophilic cytoplasm with vacuolization.

■ **TABLE 449–1 Incidence of the Subtypes of Acute Lymphoblastic Leukemia in a Single Study, with Incidence of Some Clinical Features at the Time of Diagnosis**

Subtype	No. of Patients	%	Age (Median)	Leukocyte Count (× 10^3) (Median)	% Male	% with a Mediastinal Mass	Associated Chromosomal Abnormalities
T(T +)	44	14	7.4 yr	61.2	67.1	38.2	t(11;14)
B (slg +)	2	0.6					t(8;14)
PreB (clg +)	56	18	4.7 yr	12.2	54.8	1.2	t(1;19)
Early preB (T−, slg −, clg−)	209	67	4.4 yr	12.4	56.5	1.0	t(9;22)
Infant early preB	33	NA	< 1 yr	50.0	55	None	t(4;11)

(Adapted from Pullen JD, Boyett JM, Crist WM, et al: Pediatric Oncology Group utilization of immunologic markers in the designation of acute lymphoblastic leukemia subgroups. Influence on treatment response. Ann N Y Acad Sci 428:26, 1983.)

about 66%. Hepatomegaly is less common. About 25% present with significant bone pain and arthralgia caused by leukemic infiltration of the perichondral bone or joint or by leukemic expansion of the marrow cavity. Rarely, signs of increased intracranial pressure, such as headache and vomiting, indicate leukemic meningeal involvement. Children with T-cell ALL are likely to be older and are more often male; 66% have an anterior mediastinal mass, a feature that is strongly associated with this subtype of the disease (Table 449–1).

DIAGNOSIS. On initial examination, most have anemia, although only about 25% have hemoglobin levels below 6 g/dL. Most patients also have thrombocytopenia, but as many as 25% have platelet counts greater than 100,000/mm³. About 50% of patients have white blood cell counts less than 10,000/mm³; about 20% have counts greater than 50,000/mm³. The diagnosis of leukemia is suggested by the presence of blast cells on a peripheral blood smear but is confirmed by examination of bone marrow, which is usually completely replaced by leukemic lymphoblasts. Occasionally, the marrow is initially hypocellular. Cytogenetic studies in these cases may be useful in identifying specific abnormalities associated with preleukemic syndromes. If the marrow cannot be aspirated or the specimen is hypocellular, bone marrow biopsy is required.

A chest radiograph is necessary to determine whether there is a mediastinal mass. Bone radiographs may show altered medullary trabeculae, cortical defects, or subepiphyseal bone resorption. These findings lack clinical or prognostic significance, and a skeletal survey is usually unnecessary. Cerebrospinal fluid should be examined for leukemic cells because early involvement of the CNS has important prognostic implications. Uric acid level and renal function should be determined before treatment is started (see Chapter 448).

DIFFERENTIAL DIAGNOSIS. The diagnosis of ALL is usually straightforward once the possibility has been considered. Inclusion of ALL in the differential diagnosis may be delayed if a child has been sick and febrile with adenopathy for several weeks. The diseases included in the differential diagnosis are those also associated with bone marrow failure, such as aplastic anemia and myelofibrosis. Infectious mononucleosis produces a somewhat similar clinical picture, but careful examination of the blood smear should identify atypical lymphocytes. If doubt remains, a bone marrow aspirate can demonstrate a normal cell population. Infiltration of the marrow by other types of malignant cells can occasionally produce pancytopenia. Pediatric tumors that can infiltrate marrow include neuroblastoma, rhabdomyosarcoma, Ewing sarcoma, and rarely retinoblastoma. These tumor cells are usually found in clumps scattered throughout normal marrow tissue but may occasionally replace the marrow completely. There is usually evidence of a primary tumor in some other site in these cases.

TREATMENT. Contemporary treatment of ALL is based on clinical risk features; there is no universal definition of risk groups. In general, patients with a standard or average risk of relapse are between the ages of 1 and 10 yr, have a white blood cell count under 100,000/mm³, lack evidence of mediastinal mass or of CNS leukemia, and have a B-progenitor–cell immunophenotype. The presence of certain specific chromosomal translocations should be ruled out. The treatment program for standard-risk patients includes administration of induction chemotherapy until the bone marrow no longer shows morphologically identifiable leukemic cells, "prophylactic" treatment of the CNS, and continuation chemotherapy. A sample treatment plan is outlined in Table 449–2.

A combination of prednisone, vincristine (Oncovin), and asparaginase should produce remission in about 98% of children with standard-risk ALL, typically within 4 wk. Fewer than 5% of patients require another 2 wk of induction therapy. Systemic continuation therapy, usually consisting of the antimetabolites methotrexate and 6-mercaptopurine (Purinethol), should be given for 2.5–3 yr.

In the absence of prophylactic treatment, the CNS is the initial site of relapse in more than 50% of patients. Leukemic cells are usually present in the meninges at diagnosis, even if they are not identifiable in the cerebrospinal fluid. These cells survive systemic chemotherapy because of the drug's poor penetration of the blood-brain barrier. Cranial irradiation prevents overt CNS leukemia in most patients but produces late neuropsychologic effects, particularly in younger children. Therefore, standard-risk patients typically receive intrathecal chemotherapy alone to prevent clinical CNS involvement.

Most patients with T-cell ALL relapse within 3–4 yr if treated with a standard-risk regimen. With more intensive multidrug regimens, 50% or more of these patients achieve long-term remission. A goal is to develop targeted therapy that exploits

■ **TABLE 449–2 An Effective Treatment Regimen for Low-Risk Acute Lymphoblastic Leukemia**

Remission Induction (4–6 wk)
- Vincristine 1.5 mg/m² (max. 2 mg) IV/wk
- Prednisone 40 mg/m² (max. 60 mg) po/day
- Asparaginase (*E. coli*) 10,000 U/m²/day biweekly IM

Intrathecal Treatment
- Triple therapy: MTX*, HC*, Ara-C*
- Wkly × 6 during induction and then every 8 wk for 2 yr

Systemic Continuation Treatment
- 6-MP 50 mg/m²/day po
- MTX 20 mg/m²/wk po, IV, IM
- Pulse of MTX ± 6-MP given at higher doses

With Reinforcement
- Vincristine 1.5 mg/m² (max. 2 mg) IV every 4 wks
- Prednisone 40 mg/m²/day po × 7 days every 4 wks

MTX = methotrexate; HC = hydrocortisone; Ara-C = cytarabine; IV = intravenous; po = oral; IM = intramuscular; 6-MP = 6-mercaptopurine.

**The dose of intrathecal medication is age adjusted.*

Age	MTX	HC	Ara-C
≤1 yr	10 mg	10 mg	20 mg
2–8 yr	12.5 mg	12.5 mg	25 mg
≥ 9 yr	15 mg	16 mg	30 mg

the unique characteristics of leukemic T cells. As an example of this approach, monoclonal antibodies to T-cell–associated surface antigens can be conjugated to immunotoxins. The antibody-immunotoxin complex would then attach to T lymphoblasts, undergo endocytosis, and kill the cells.

B-cell cases with L3 morphology and surface immunoglobulin expression once had a poor prognosis. Such patients are best treated with short (3–6 mo) but very intensive regimens developed for advanced B-cell lymphoma. With this approach, cure rates have improved dramatically, from 20% a decade ago to 70% or more.

RELAPSE. The bone marrow is the most common site of relapse, although almost any site can be affected. In most centers, bone marrow is examined at regular intervals to confirm continued remission. If bone marrow relapse is detected, intensive retrieval therapy that includes drugs not used previously may achieve cures in 15–20% of patients, especially those who have had a long first remission (18 mo or more). For patients who experience bone marrow relapse during treatment, intensive chemotherapy followed by bone marrow transplantation from a matched sibling donor offers a better chance of cure. Autologous, mismatched related, or matched unrelated donor transplants are options for those without histocompatible sibling donors (see Chapter 448.2).

The most important extramedullary sites of relapse are the CNS and the testes. The common early manifestations of CNS leukemia are due to increased intracranial pressure and include vomiting, headache, papilledema, and lethargy. Chemical meningitis secondary to intrathecal therapy can produce the same symptoms and must be considered. Convulsions and isolated cranial nerve palsies may occur with CNS leukemia or as side effects of vincristine. Hypothalamic involvement is rare but must be suspected in the presence of excessive weight gain or behavioral disturbances. In most cases, cerebrospinal fluid pressure is elevated, and the fluid shows a pleocytosis due to leukemic cells. If the cell count is normal, leukemic cells may be found in smears of cerebrospinal fluid specimens after centrifugation.

Patients with CNS relapse should be given intrathecal chemotherapy weekly for 4–6 wk until lymphoblasts have disappeared from the cerebrospinal fluid. Doses should be age-adjusted because cerebrospinal fluid volume is not proportional to body surface area (Table 449–2). Cranial irradiation is the only treatment that completely eradicates overt CNS leukemia and should be given after intrathecal therapy. Systemic treatment should also be intensified because these patients are at high risk of subsequent bone marrow relapse. Finally, preventive CNS therapy should be repeated in any patient whose disease has relapsed in the bone marrow or in any extramedullary site.

Testicular relapse generally produces painless swelling of one or both testicles. The patient is often unaware of the abnormality, mandating careful attention to testicular size at diagnosis and during follow-up. The diagnosis is confirmed by biopsy. Treatment should include irradiation of the gonads. Because a testicular relapse usually signals impending bone marrow relapse, systemic therapy should be reinforced for patients who are still undergoing treatment or reinstituted for those who have a relapse after treatment. As noted above, CNS-directed therapy should also be repeated.

PROGNOSIS. Numerous clinical features have emerged as prognostic indicators, only to lose their significance as treatment improves. For example, immunophenotype is important in assigning risk-directed therapy, but its prognostic significance has largely been eliminated by contemporary treatment regimens. Hence, treatment is the single most important prognostic factor. The initial leukocyte count has a consistent inverse linear relationship to the likelihood of cure. Age at diagnosis is also a reliable predictor. Patients older than 10 yr, and those younger than 12 mo who have a chromosomal rearrangement involving the 11q23 region, fare much worse than children in the intermediate age group. Several chromosomal abnormalities influence treatment outcome. Hyperdiploidy with more than 50 chromosomes is associated with a favorable outcome and responds well to antimetabolite-based therapy. Two chromosomal translocations—the t(9;22), or Philadelphia chromosome, and the t(4;11)—confer a poor prognosis. Several investigators advocate bone marrow transplantation during initial remission in patients with these translocations. B-progenitor-cell ALL with the t(1;19) has a less promising prognosis than other cases with this immunophenotype; only 60% of patients will be in remission after 5 yr unless very intensive therapy is used.

449.2 Acute Myeloid Leukemia

Robert A. Krance

AML has an annual incidence of five to six cases per million in children younger than 15 yr. In the United States, this is 350–500 new cases each year. AML constitutes 15–20% of all childhood leukemias but is the predominant neonatal or congenital leukemia. There are no clear racial or gender differences in incidence and, except for a slight increase during adolescence, the distribution of cases by age is consistent throughout childhood.

The incidence of AML exceeds expected rates in certain genetic disorders, including trisomy 21, Fanconi anemia, Diamond-Blackfan anemia, Kostmann syndrome, and Bloom syndrome. Children previously treated for another malignancy are also at increased risk; the incidence of secondary AML approaches 5% after treatment of some malignancies. The incidence of secondary AML peaks within 10 yr of the initial malignancy. Its occurrence is associated with specific therapies (alkylating drugs such as cyclophosphamide, agents that inhibit DNA repair such as etoposide). Radiation therapy given with chemotherapy also increases the risk of secondary leukemia.

CLINICAL MANIFESTATIONS. AML typically presents with signs and symptoms attributable to bone marrow failure. AML must be considered in the evaluation of any patient with pallor, fever, infection, or bleeding. Bone pain is less common than in ALL. Liver and spleen enlargement is common; lymphadenopathy may be present. Unexplained gingival hypertrophy or parotid gland swelling are uncommon but suggestive findings. A localized mass of leukemic cells (chloroma), may develop at any site, but retro-orbital and epidural locations are most likely. Chloroma may precede leukemic cell infiltration of bone marrow. Blood counts are usually abnormal; anemia and thrombocytopenia are often profound. The white blood cell count may be high, low, or normal. Leukemic blasts may be evident on the blood smear.

AML can develop in children who present initially with only anemia, leukopenia, or thrombocytopenia. This presentation, which is more common among adults, is typically termed *myelodysplastic syndrome.* Characteristic features include abnormal morphology of blood and bone marrow cells and the presence of blast cells in the bone marrow. The natural history of myelodysplastic syndrome in children is not well characterized, but most cases evolve into AML. Like secondary AML, myelodysplastic syndrome can develop in children treated for a prior malignancy.

DIAGNOSIS. The presence of at least 30% leukemic blast cells in the bone marrow is necessary for the diagnosis of AML. The morphology and cytochemical analysis (histochemical stain positive for myeloperoxidase, Sudan black, or nonspecific esterase) of the leukemic blasts usually suffice to distinguish AML from ALL. Within the AML category, however, morphology may be variable. For contemporary classification and treatment of AML, leukemic blast cells must be characterized by their expression of cell surface antigens (immunophenotype) and by chromosomal analysis (karyotype). The FAB system divides AML into eight subtypes, M0 to M7 (Table 449–3), which broadly correspond to normal hematopoietic lineages. Among children, the number of patients with the M0, M1, and M2 subtypes approximates the number of M4 and M5 cases; together, these FAB types account for 80% of childhood AMLs. The M3 and M7 subtypes are less common, and M6 is rare. This classification system facilitates study of the clinical course and allows comparisons of various therapies. Specific molecular events underlie some FAB types.

Although hemorrhagic diathesis (disseminated intravascular coagulation at presentation or later) may occur in any of the FAB groups, patients with acute promyelocytic leukemia (M3) are especially at risk. An almost invariant finding in this subtype is translocation of genetic material between chromosomes 15 and 17, producing a fusion gene that includes the gene encoding the α-retinoic acid receptor. Retinoic acid can effectively induce remission in these patients. Translocation between chromosomes 8 and 21, typically present in the M2 subtype, is closely associated with chloroma. Inversion of genetic material in chromosome 16 can be found in M4 AML, in which eosinophilia is a prominent feature.

Myelodysplastic syndrome bears some resemblance to AML, but the bone marrow contains a lower percentage of blast cells and has characteristic dysplastic features, including megaloblastosis. Patients may not be ill at presentation and isolated anemia or leukopenia may bring them to medical attention. Chromosomal changes, including trisomy 8 and complete or partial deletion of chromosome 5 or 7, may be present. Deletion of chromosome 5 or 7 is particularly common in secondary myelodysplastic syndromes and secondary AML.

Juvenile chronic myelogenous leukemia (JCML) is unlike adult-type CML but may have features similar to those of AML and myelodysplastic syndrome. The Philadelphia chromosome is not present in JCML. Nonspecific signs and symptoms include fever, malaise, liver and spleen enlargement, and adenopathy. A chronic desquamative maculopapular skin eruption often predates the diagnosis. Striking elevation of hemoglobin F, which may exceed 50%, and leukocytosis (primarily blood and bone marrow monocytosis) are the predominant findings. JCML is rare in patients older than 5 yr of age and may be more common among children with type 1 neurofibromatosis; familial or hereditary cases have been documented.

TREATMENT. Therapy for AML has improved but remains unsatisfactory. Between 70–80% of patients achieve remission after treatment with chemotherapeutic regimens that include an anthracycline (daunomycin, idarubicin) and cytarabine. Optimal supportive care is critical to afford patients sufficient time to respond to treatment because most nonresponding patients die from infections or chemotherapy-related toxicity. Remission may occur within 2–3 wk after treatment is started but can also take 8–12 wk or longer and may require several courses of chemotherapy. Patients who do not respond to induction therapy are candidates for allogeneic transplantation.

Hemorrhage secondary to pathologic activation of clotting and/or fibrinolytic factors is a particular problem in acute promyelocytic leukemia, but laboratory studies to detect disseminated intravascular coagulation should also be performed for other AML variants. Transfusion of platelets and fresh frozen plasma is mandatory for patients with disseminated intravascular coagulation; the need for heparin or antifibrinolytic therapies is less certain. Retinoic acid as initial treatment for acute promyelocytic leukemia may reduce the risk of hemorrhage but is not curative. Multiagent chemotherapy given as remission induction and consolidation may cure most patients, however.

Once patients achieve remission, the optimal continuation therapy is undefined. Options include autologous or allogeneic bone marrow transplantation or intensive chemotherapy; none of these approaches has demonstrated an absolute survival advantage. Allogeneic bone marrow transplantation during first remission is limited to patients with a suitable sibling donor.

Intrathecal chemotherapy is necessary to prevent CNS relapse. Intrathecal chemotherapy can usually clear leukemic cells from the cerebrospinal fluid in patients who have CNS leukemia at diagnosis (~10% of cases) or who have a CNS relapse, but CNS irradiation may be required to eradicate leukemia permanently.

Because myelodysplastic syndrome is likely to evolve into leukemia, patients are usually treated on AML protocols. If the patient is relatively asymptomatic, therapy may be delayed until symptoms progress. Remission induction is less successful in myelodysplastic syndrome than in AML. Because of this treatment resistance and other considerations, allogeneic marrow transplantation is often the preferred treatment. For similar reasons, allogeneic BMT is recommended for patients with JCML. When a histocompatibility antigen (HLA) genotype-matched donor is not available, a partially matched relative or a matched unrelated donor may be considered.

PROGNOSIS. With aggressive therapy, 40–50% of patients who achieve remission will be long-term survivors (30–40% overall cure rate). Patients who have relapses after receiving chemotherapy or autologous transplantation may be treated with allogeneic transplantation as salvage therapy. Some morphologic and genetic subtypes of AML have a better prognosis.

■ TABLE 449–3 Subtypes of Nonlymphoid Leukemia

Type	FAB Classification
Acute Myeloid Leukemia (AML)	
Myeloblastic, no maturation	M0 and M1
Myeloblastic, some maturation	M2
Hypergranular promyelocytic	M3
Myelomonocytic	M4
Monocytic	M5
Erythroleukemia	M6
Megakaryocytic	M7
Chronic Myelocytic Leukemia (CML)	
Adult form	
Chronic phase	
Blast crisis	
Juvenile form	
Congenital Leukemia	

449.3 Chronic Myelogenous Leukemia

Helen E. Heslop

Chronic myelogenous leukemia (CML) is a clonal malignancy of the hematopoietic stem cell characterized by a specific translocation, the t(9;22)(q34;q1), known as the Philadelphia chromosome. This translocation juxtaposes the *bcr* gene on chromosome 22 with the *abl* gene on chromosome 9, producing a fusion gene that encodes the *bcr-abl* fusion protein. CML is more common in adults and accounts for only 3% of cases of childhood leukemia. In most cases, there are no predisposing features.

CML has a biphasic or triphasic course. During the chronic phase, which lasts for 3–4 yr, white blood cell counts are easily controlled with low-dose chemotherapy. Progression to a myeloid or lymphoid blast crisis that resembles acute leukemia may occur rapidly or may follow an accelerated phase wherein blood counts become difficult to control and additional cytogenetic abnormalities may develop.

PATHOLOGY. CML is characterized by myeloid hyperplasia with increased numbers of differentiating myeloid cells in blood and bone marrow. The pathognomonic Philadelphia chromosome is easily detectable in more than 95% of cases; in most of the remaining patients, Southern blot analysis or polymerase chain reaction techniques reveal the *bcr-abl* rearrangement.

CLINICAL FEATURES. The onset of symptoms is generally insidious, and the diagnosis is often made when a blood count is performed for another reason. Patients may present with splenomegaly (which can be massive) or with symptoms of hypermetabolism, including weight loss, anorexia, and night sweats. Symptoms of leukostasis, such as visual disturbance or priapism, occur rarely.

DIAGNOSIS. Laboratory abnormalities are usually confined initially to elevated white blood cell counts, which may exceed $100,000/mm^3$, with all forms of myeloid cells seen in the blood smear. Platelet counts may also be abnormally high. Other laboratory abnormalities include elevated serum levels of vitamin B_{12} and uric acid and reduced or absent leukocyte alkaline phosphatase activity. The bone marrow is hypercellular, with normal myeloid cells in all stages of differentiation; megakaryocytes may be more numerous. Cytogenetic or molecular studies showing the Philadelphia chromosome confirm the diagnosis.

TREATMENT. In the chronic phase, leukocytosis and symptoms can be controlled by chemotherapy with busulfan (Myleran) or hydroxyurea, but the Philadelphia chromosome is not suppressed. In addition to controlling the leukocytosis, interferon-α also suppresses the Philadelphia chromosome completely, in about 20% of cases, and it appears to lengthen the chronic phase. However, the only curative treatment at present is allogenic bone marrow transplant. The long-term survival rate of pediatric patients who receive an allograft from an HLA-identical sibling in early chronic phase is around 80%. This is the preferred therapy if an appropriate donor is available. When the donor is a partially matched family member or a matched unrelated individual, the transplant-related mortality rate is higher, and the survival rate is around 50–60%. Lymphoid blast crisis can usually be reverted to the chronic phase with standard ALL therapy, whereas myeloid crisis is generally refractory to standard AML chemotherapy; the median survival is only 3–4 mo. If bone marrow transplant is delayed until blast crisis occurs, the survival rate is only 10–20%.

449.4 Congenital Leukemia

Ching-Hon Pui

Congenital leukemia is an extremely rare disease, diagnosed within the first month of life at a rate of 4.7 per million live births. Myeloid leukemia appears to be predominant in this group. Generally, cases present with marked leukocytosis, petechiae, ecchymoses, and extramedullary involvement, with massive hepatosplenomegaly, cutaneous nodules, and CNS leukemia. Neuroblastoma and leukemoid reactions secondary to erythroblastosis fetalis and severe congenital bacterial or viral infection may mimic congenital leukemia, but these can be ruled out by appropriate laboratory studies. More difficult to differentiate is transient myeloproliferative disorder, which occurs primarily in neonates with trisomy 21 or chromosome 21 mosaicism. Most transient myeloproliferative disorders undergo spontaneous remission within a few weeks. Thus, patients should receive only supportive measures initially but require careful follow-up because some will have leukemia months or years later.

Congenital leukemia has a poor prognosis, especially in cases with leukemic cell chromosomal rearrangements affecting the q23 region of chromosome 11. Although the short latency period suggests genetic predisposition, studies suggest that intrauterine exposure to carcinogens is responsible for at least some cases of leukemia in very young children.

CHAPTER 450
Lymphoma

(See Chapters 116 and 444 for related discussion of the immune and lymphatic systems.)

Melissa M. Hudson

Lymphoma is the third most common cancer in children in the United States, with an annual incidence rate of 13.2 per million children. The two broad categories of lymphoma, Hodgkin disease and non-Hodgkin lymphoma (NHL), have different clinical manifestations, treatments, and prognoses.

450.1 Hodgkin Disease

EPIDEMIOLOGY. The age-associated incidence of Hodgkin disease is bimodal. In industrialized countries, the early peak occurs in the middle to late 20s and the 2nd peak after the age of 50 yr. Other epidemiologic features include a higher frequency in males, whites, and patients with underlying immunodeficiency. Familial occurrence has been noted, particularly in same-sex siblings; the reasons for this are unclear. Increasing evidence suggests that Epstein-Barr virus (EBV) may be implicated in pathogenesis, as evidenced by detection of the EBV genomes in some histologic subtypes of Hodgkin disease.

PATHOLOGY. The cardinal histologic feature is the Reed-Sternberg cell (Fig. 450–1). The cell of origin may be an activated antigen-presenting cell such as a lymphoid cell of B- or T-cell origin or even a cell of monocytic lineage. There are four histologic subtypes of Hodgkin disease, each with special clinical and prognostic features. The distribution of subtypes varies with age.

The *nodular sclerosing* variety is the most common form, accounting for 50% of cases in children and 70% in adolescents. Broad bands of collagen divide the involved lymph node into nodular cellular areas. A special cytologic feature is clear spaces surrounding "lacunar cells," variants of the Reed-Sternberg cell. Because of the amount of collagen, the radiographic appearance of these lesions may be slow to normalize, even when the patient responds to therapy.

Hodgkin disease of *mixed cellularity* is the second most common form, affecting 40–50% of patients. It is characterized by an inflammatory background of lymphocytes, plasma cells, eosinophils, histiocytes, and malignant reticular cells; Reed-Sternberg cells are usually abundant. Patients with this subtype

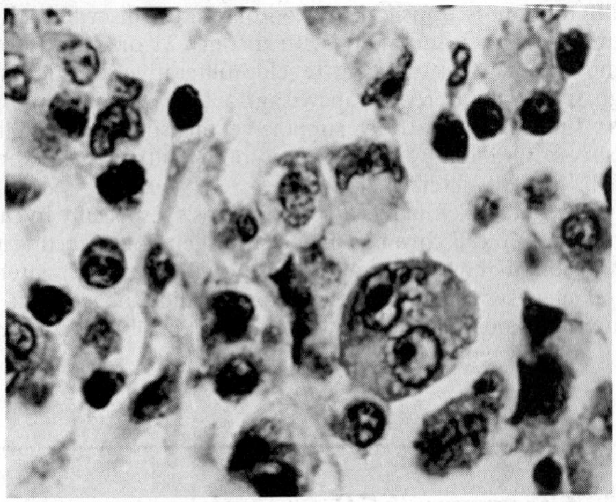

Figure 450–1. Reed-Sternberg cell that contains two nuclei, each with a prominent nucleolus and distinct nuclear membrane. The cytoplasm of this cell is relatively abundant. Other cells present are lymphocytes, plasma cells, and tissue mononuclear cells. Presence of these cells in lymph node tissue is diagnostic of Hodgkin disease.

are more likely to present with advanced disease and extranodal extension.

In the *lymphocyte predominance* variety, most of the cells appear to be mature lymphocytes or a mixture of lymphocytes and benign histiocytes, with only occasional Reed-Sternberg cells. This type affects 10–20% of patients with Hodgkin disease, is more common in males and younger patients, usually presents with clinically localized disease, and has the best prognosis.

The least common and least favorable form is the *lymphocytic depletion* variety, which affects fewer than 10% of patients overall but is a common histologic type in patients infected with the human immunodeficiency virus. Numerous bizarre malignant reticular cells are found, along with Reed-Sternberg cells and relatively few lymphocytes. Patients with this histologic type commonly present with widespread disease involving the bones and bone marrow.

Hodgkin disease usually arises in lymph nodes. Adjacent lymph node areas are the first site of spread, presumably as a result of direct anatomic extension along lymphoid channels. The most common sites of extranodal involvement are lung, bone, bone marrow, and liver.

CLINICAL MANIFESTATIONS. The most common presenting feature is painless enlargement of lymph nodes in cervical, supraclavicular, or occasionally axillary or inguinal areas. The affected nodes are firm, nontender, and usually discrete. Characteristically, there is no evidence of regional inflammation that would explain the lymphadenopathy. Mediastinal lymph node enlargement is common and can produce a cough or other symptoms of airway compression. In younger children, the nodes can be difficult to distinguish from a large, normal thymus, although computed tomography (CT) or magnetic resonance imaging (MRI) of the mediastinum may reveal differences in texture.

About 33% of patients with Hodgkin disease have nonspecific systemic manifestations that include fatigue, pruritus, urticaria, pain that worsens with ingestion of alcohol, lethargy, and anorexia. The specific symptoms of unexplained fever, weight loss of at least 10% in the previous 6 mo, and night sweats are thought to be of prognostic significance and are incorporated in staging assignment by the "B" designation (whereas "A" indicates the absence of any of these symptoms).

Extranodal involvement occurs in 10–15% of patients at diagnosis and is seen most commonly in intrathoracic structures (lung, pleura, pericardium). Lung involvement may be represented radiographically by diffuse fluffy infiltrates that can be difficult to distinguish from disseminated fungal infection. Fever and tachypnea are common with intrathoracic disease, and pulmonary insufficiency may develop.

Rare presentations include intrahepatic biliary obstructive disease. With progression, signs of hepatocellular disease may develop. Extremely advanced bone marrow involvement may result in neutropenia, thrombocytopenia, and anemia. Extradural tumor masses in the spinal canal can cause spinal cord compression. A variety of immune disorders have also been observed, such as autoimmune hemolytic anemia, and thrombocytopenia, and the nephrotic syndrome.

Cellular immunity is impaired by Hodgkin disease and its treatment. Affected patients are at increased risk of infections characteristically seen in immunosuppressed patients (see Table 448–3). Varicella-zoster infections occur in up to 33% of patients and should be treated with intravenous *acyclovir* (Zovirax); fungal infections, such as cryptococcosis, histoplasmosis, and candidiasis, may become disseminated. Humoral immune function may also be transiently depressed after treatment.

DIAGNOSIS. Hodgkin disease should be suspected in patients with persistent unexplained lymphadenopathy. The disease is more common in late childhood and adolescence, when cervical lymphadenopathy resulting from infection is also common. Lymph node biopsy is indicated for persistent lymphadenopathy without evidence of an underlying inflammatory process. Some patients have a history of relatively recent, serologically proved infectious mononucleosis. Hence, enlarged nodes that do not regress after infectious mononucleosis should also be considered for biopsy. Before biopsy is performed, a chest radiograph should be done to explore the possibility of mediastinal involvement and to examine airway patency. Changes in the white blood cell count can include a neutrophilic leukocytosis, lymphopenia, or sometimes eosinophilia and monocytosis. Anemia and thrombocytopenia occur only in patients with disseminated disease. Elevated acute-phase reactants, such as erythrocyte sedimentation rate and serum copper and ferritin levels, may be useful, albeit nonspecific, markers of disease activity.

Once the diagnosis is confirmed, extensive staging procedures are performed to establish the extent of the disease (Table 450–1). Most patients first present with evidence of lymph node enlargement above the diaphragm; therefore, a radiograph and CT scan of the chest should be performed. CT scans may show disease when radiographs appear normal and can also evaluate the extent of pericardial and chest wall involvement.

Abdominal imaging studies (CT or MRI) can indicate the presence of focal lesions in the liver or spleen and node enlargement but cannot define the nature of the underlying process. Liver function tests are unreliable indicators of hepatic disease, and the size of the spleen correlates poorly with

■ **TABLE 450–1 Ann Arbor Staging System for Hodgkin Disease***

Stage I	Involvement of a single lymph node region or of a single extralymphatic organ or site
Stage II	Involvement of two or more lymphoid regions on the same side of the diaphragm; or localized involvement of an extralymphatic organ or site and of one or more lymph node regions on the same side of the diaphragm
Stage III	Involvement of lymph node regions on both sides of the diaphragm, which may be accompanied by localized involvement of an extralymphatic organ or site or by splenic involvement
Stage IV	Diffuse or disseminated involvement of one or more extralymphatic organs or tissues, with or without associated lymph node enlargement

**Stages are further categorized as A or B, based on the absence or presence, respectively, of systemic symptoms of fever and/or weight loss.*

splenic involvement. Lymphangiography is generally accurate in indicating lymph node involvement below the level of the second lumbar vertebra; involved lymph nodes above that level may not take up contrast material because of lymphatic drainage into the thoracic duct. Although lymphangiography can provide useful information about nodal size and architecture, the examination is technically difficult in children, carries some degree of risk, and is available only in selected centers.

Traditionally, a staging laparotomy was performed to determine the presence and extent of abdominal disease. At laparotomy, the spleen is removed, a biopsy is done of the liver, and samples are taken of retroperitoneal and pelvic nodes. For female patients, if radiotherapy to the pelvis is contemplated, the ovaries are moved to a midline position posterior to the uterus to minimize exposure. In about 33% of cases, the clinical disease stage is revised on the basis of such anatomic findings. However, in view of the potential morbidity of the surgery and the long-term risks of splenectomy (see Table 448–3), there is a growing opinion that staging laparotomy is indicated only when the findings will significantly alter therapy.

Bone marrow biopsies should be done in all patients with advanced-stage disease. A bone scan and correlating plain films of abnormal areas define the presence of skeletal metastases and should be considered in patients with bone pain, elevated alkaline phosphatase levels, or extranodal disease identified by other staging modalities.

TREATMENT. Both radiation and chemotherapy are highly effective in the treatment of Hodgkin disease. The goal is to achieve cure while lessening treatment toxicity. For localized (stage I or IIA) disease in patients who have achieved their full growth, radiation to standard fields with doses of 3,500–4,406 cGy may be the treatment of choice. However, as many as 15% of such patients will have recurrences and require combination chemotherapy. Multiagent chemotherapy with nitrogen mustard, vincristine (Oncovin), procarbazine, and prednisone (MOPP), or with doxorubicin (Adriamycin), bleomycin (Blenoxane), vinblastine (Velban), and dacarbazine (ABVD) can produce long-term disease-free periods for patients with advanced disease. The use of alternating noncross-resistant regimens (MOPP/ABVD) in combination with low-dose (2,000–2,500 cGy) radiotherapy has produced cure rates of 70–90% in pediatric patients with advanced-stage disease. This approach is favored by pediatric oncologists for three reasons: (1) potential growth defects and the risk of second solid tumors are reduced by limiting the radiotherapy dose and volume, (2) the risk of infertility and leukemogenesis is decreased by reduced exposure to alkylating agents, and (3) exposure to drugs with potential cardiopulmonary toxicity is limited. Combined-modality regimens with localized radiotherapy and fewer cycles of chemotherapy are being studied to determine whether currently excellent cure rates can be maintained.

PROGNOSIS. With modern treatment, more than 90% of patients with Hodgkin disease achieve an initial complete remission. The likelihood of prolonged remission or cure is related to disease stage at diagnosis. Most patients with stage I/II disease are cured, as are 75–90% of those with stage III disease treated with both chemotherapy and radiation, and 60–85% of those with stage IV disease treated with chemotherapy with or without radiotherapy.

The longer survival of patients has generated concern about late sequelae of treatment (see Table 448–4). Complications of irradiation depend on site, dosage, volume, and age at treatment. Supradiaphragmatic irradiation may lead to restrictive lung capacity, cardiac dysfunction, late-onset breast cancer, or hypothyroidism. Pelvic irradiation can cause sterility despite ovarian and testicular shielding. In the younger child, growth of the vertebral column, clavicles, and breast buds can be affected. Because of concerns regarding growth, standard-dose radiation is rarely given to children. Late pulmonary and cardiac toxicity may also develop after treatment with bleomycin or doxorubicin, respectively. MOPP and other regimens that contain alkylators can cause sterility in male or premature menopause in female patients.

Second malignant tumors are a major concern. The most common second malignant neoplasm in Hodgkin survivors is acute myeloid leukemia (AML). The reported risk of secondary AML ranges from 1.2–13% at 10 yr, with most cases diagnosed 5–10 yr after treatment. The risk of a second malignant solid tumor increases with time after diagnosis, ranging from 13–20% at 15 yr. These tumors usually occur in or at the margins of the radiotherapy field.

A fraction of patients (1–2%) who have undergone splenectomy may have overwhelming sepsis caused by *Streptococcus pneumoniae* or *Haemophilus influenzae*. The risk of this complication has been substantially reduced by routine immunization with pneumococcal and *H. influenzae* B vaccines and by the use of prophylactic antibiotics. Abdominal adhesions may also develop in patients who have had laparotomy, particularly if the abdomen has been irradiated.

450.2 Non-Hodgkin Lymphoma

John T. Sandlund

The NHLs are malignant clonal proliferations of primarily T or B lymphocytes that present with varying degrees of tumor burden. These malignancies should not be confused with polyclonal lymphoproliferative disorders. Both groups of diseases occur with increased frequency in children with inherited immunodeficiency states such as ataxia-telangiectasia, Wiskott-Aldrich syndrome, combined immune deficiencies, and the X-linked lymphoproliferative (XLP) syndrome. The XLP syndrome is characterized by marked sensitivity to EBV-induced diseases, including fatal infectious mononucleosis, which occurs in approximately 57% of cases.

NHL that involves the bone marrow is distinguished from acute lymphoblastic leukemia by the degree of marrow involvement. Patients with greater than 25% marrow replacement are included with acute lymphoblastic leukemia (ALL), and the remaining cases are designated as having NHL with marrow involvement.

PATHOLOGY. The NHLs of childhood, in contrast to those of adults, are usually diffuse, extranodal, high-grade tumors. To eliminate the confusion created by multiple classification schemes, the National Cancer Institute developed a histologic system, which defines three primary subtypes of high-grade NHL: small noncleaved cell (SNCC), lymphoblastic, and large cell.

The SNCC NHLs *(Burkitt and non-Burkitt subtypes)* are B-cell tumors that express surface immunoglobulin and contain one of three characteristic chromosomal translocations—t(8;14), t(2;8), or t(8;22)—each of which involves the c-*myc* oncogene and an immunoglobulin gene (mu heavy chain, kappa light chain, and lambda light chain, respectively). *Lymphoblastic lymphomas* are usually of T-cell origin and may contain a translocation involving a T-cell receptor gene. *Large cell NHLs* occur as T-cell, B-cell or non-B, non-T-cell phenotypes; the t(2;5)(p23;q35) may be present in association with CD30 expression.

CLINICAL MANIFESTATIONS. The presenting signs and symptoms of NHL in children are largely determined by disease site and extent. The most frequent primary sites are the abdomen (31.4%); mediastinum (26%), and the head/neck region, including Waldeyer ring and/or cervical lymph nodes (29%).

Noncervical lymph nodes are the primary sites in 6.5% of cases with skin, thyroid, epidural space, and bone accounting for the remainder (7%).

There is a striking association between histologic subtype and disease site. Lymphoblastic NHL usually occurs in the head and neck region or the anterior mediastinum; SNCC primary tumors arise in the abdomen and/or the head and neck; and large cell NHL may present in any anatomic location. Head and neck primaries are usually painless masses arising from cervical lymph nodes or tonsils. Mediastinal masses may be associated with pleural effusions, respiratory distress, or superior vena cava syndrome (swelling of arms, neck, and face). Abdominal masses usually arise from the ileocecal region and may be associated with abdominal distention, nausea, vomiting, or change in bowel habits, a clinical picture similar to appendicitis or intussusception. Bone marrow involvement may cause anemia or thrombocytopenia and central nervous system disease may result in headache, increased intracranial pressure, or cranial nerve palsies.

DIAGNOSIS. The diagnostic and staging workup of a child with suspected NHL must be expeditious because of the rapid growth rate of these tumors. A tissue diagnosis is necessary before treatment is started. Excisional biopsy or fine-needle aspirate is usually sufficient to evaluate an isolated peripheral node. A mediastinal mass can be evaluated by thoracotomy or mediastinoscopy, parasternal fine-needle aspiration, or thoracentesis (if there is an associated pleural effusion). An open biopsy is usually necessary for abdominal masses, although percutaneous needle biopsy is occasionally feasible.

Once the diagnosis is established, a staging workup must be completed. The most widely used staging system is noted in Table 450–2. The evaluation includes a complete history, physical examination, and numerous laboratory studies (complete blood count and levels of electrolytes, blood urea nitrogen, lactate dehydrogenase [LDH], calcium, phosphorus, and uric acid). Bone marrow and cerebrospinal fluid examinations must be performed. Diagnostic imaging studies include CT of the primary site, chest, abdomen, and pelvis, bone scan, and (in some settings) gallium-67 scan. Staging laparotomy and lymphangiography are not part of the standard evaluation.

TREATMENT. With the development of effective multiagent chemotherapy, most children with NHL are cured. Tumor lysis syndrome is common. A randomized trial comparing two of the first successful treatment regimens (the cyclophosphamide-based COMP regimen and the intensive multiagent LSA_2L_2 regimen) demonstrated that the prognosis for limited-stage disease was excellent with either treatment. However, among patients with advanced-stage disease, those with lymphoblastic NHL had a better outcome when treated with LSA_2L_2; those with SNCC histologic type had a better outcome with COMP.

Current strategies for patients with limited-stage disease focus on reducing morbidity without compromising cure rates. For advanced-stage disease, clinical trials focus on improving treatment outcome with histology-directed therapy that incorporates adequate CNS prophylaxis. The most effective treatments for lymphoblastic disease derive from multiagent regimens designed for the treatment of ALL, delivered over 1–2.5 yr. Cyclophosphamide remains an important component of the highly intensive regimens for SNCC NHL, which are delivered over 2–12 mo. The most effective protocols for large cell NHL usually contain cyclophosphamide, doxorubicin, vincristine, and prednisone (CHOP), given for 12–24 mo. Surgery plays little role in management unless there is a completely resected abdominal mass. Involved field radiation is generally not included in primary therapy.

PROGNOSIS. With modern therapy, the 2-yr event-free survival (EFS) is approximately 90% for children with limited-stage disease and approximately 70% for those with stage III and IV disease. Improvements in the treatment of advanced-stage SNCC NHL have resulted in a 90% 2-yr EFS (70% for those with central nervous system disease). Stage of disease and the log of the serum LDH level at diagnosis have independent prognostic significance.

■ **TABLE 450–2 A Staging System for Non-Hodgkin Lymphoma in Childhood**

Stage I

A single tumor (extranodal) or single anatomic area (nodal), with the exclusion of mediastinum or abdomen.

Stage II

A single tumor (extranodal) with regional node involvement.

Two or more nodal areas on the same side of the diaphragm.

Two single (extranodal) tumors with or without regional node involvement on the same side of the diaphragm.

A primary gastrointestinal tract tumor, usually in the ileocecal area, with or without involvement of associated mesenteric nodes only, which must be grossly (>90%) resected.

Stage III

Two single tumors (extranodal) on opposite sides of the diaphragm.

Two or more nodal areas above and below the diaphragm.

Any primary intrathoracic tumor (mediastinal, pleural, thymic).

Any extensive primary intra-abdominal disease.

Stage IV

Any of the above, with initial involvement of central nervous system and/or bone marrow at time of diagnosis.

(From Murphy SB: Classification, staging, and end results of treatment of childhood non-Hodgkin's lymphomas: Dissimilarities from lymphomas in adults. Semin Oncol 7:332, 1980.)

CHAPTER 451

Neuroblastoma

Victor M. Santana

Neuroblastoma is the most common extracranial solid tumor of childhood, accounting for 8–10% of all childhood cancers, and is the most frequently diagnosed neoplasm in infants. The median age at diagnosis is 2 yr; 90% are diagnosed before the age of 5 yr. The annual incidence is 8.7 per million children, or 500–600 new cases annually in the United States. The incidence is slightly higher in males and in whites. Familial cases occur, and neuroblastoma has also been diagnosed in patients with neurofibromatosis, nesidioblastosis, and Hirschsprung disease.

Microscopic clusters of neuroblasts are normally found in the adrenal gland of fetuses and in about 1 of 200 neonates at autopsy. It is uncertain whether these nodules represent spontaneous regression of congenital neuroblastoma or maturation into asymptomatic benign tumors. The molecular basis for malignant transformation is unknown.

Mass screening programs for infants using measurements of urinary catecholamine metabolites have been conducted in Japan, Canada, and the United States. The value of these studies remains uncertain because most children so detected are asymptomatic and have a good prognosis. The effect of screening, if any, on the disease course in patients with a poor prognosis remains unproven.

PATHOLOGY. Neuroblastomas originate in neural crest cells of the sympathetic nervous system and thus can develop anywhere from the posterior cranial fossa to the coccyx. About 70% of the tumors arise in the abdomen, 50% of these in the adrenal gland. Another 20% arise in the thorax, usually in the posterior mediastinum. The tumor most commonly extends to surrounding tissue by local invasion and to regional lymph nodes via lymphatics. Hematogenous spread to the bone marrow, skeleton, and the liver is frequent. With immunocytologic techniques, tumor cells can be detected in the peripheral blood in more than 50% of children at the time of diagnosis or relapse. Spread to the brain and lungs may occur in rare cases.

Histologically, neuroblastoma consists of small round cells with abundant granules, forming Homer-Wright rosettes, with areas of calcification and necrosis with extensive hemorrhage. Most tumors consist of primitive neuroblastoma cells with little evidence of differentiation. However, with treatment, serial biopsy specimens may contain increasing proportions of mature ganglion cells. The most widely accepted histologic grading system correlates the presence or absence of stroma, the degree of differentiation, the mitotic index, and patient age to clinical outcome. Electron microscopy reveals distinctive features: peripheral dendritic processes, containing longitudinally oriented microtubules, and small, spherical membrane-bound granules with electron-dense cores, representing cytoplasmic neurosecretory granules (catecholamines). These tumors can secrete a variety of neurogenically derived substances, including catecholamines, neuron-specific enolase (NSE), and ferritin. Catecholamine metabolites such as vanillylmandelic acid and homovanillic acid in urine or plasma can serve as indicators of disease. Immunophenotypically, neuroblastomas can be recognized by monoclonal antibodies to cell surface antigens such as glycosphingolipid disganglioside, synaptophysin, NSE, and neurofilament. Cytogenetic abnormalities, present in approximately 80% of cases, include partial deletion of the short arm of chromosome 1, chromosome 17 anomalies, and genomic amplification of the N-*myc* oncogene, an indicator of poor prognosis.

CLINICAL MANIFESTATIONS AND DIAGNOSIS. Neuroblastoma has protean manifestations. Common presentations include a hard, painless mass in the neck; a localized intrathoracic mass found incidentally on a chest radiograph; or a large palpable mass in the flank or abdomen. An abdominal mass may represent an enlarging primary adrenal or retroperitoneal tumor or hepatomegaly secondary to liver involvement. The child often appears chronically ill and may have bone pain from skeletal and bone marrow metastases. About 60–75% of patients have metastatic disease at diagnosis. Metastases to the orbits may cause proptosis and ecchymosis (Fig. 451–1); spread to the dura causes signs of increased intracranial pressure (split sutures may be seen in infants). A primary paraspinal tumor may cause lower limb paresis secondary to epidural extension. Horner syndrome may be present in patients with lesions in the cervical or upper thoracic sympathetic ganglia. A primary tumor in the nasopharynx usually presents with unilateral epistaxis or occlusion of nasal passages. Neonates or infants may present with firm, blue-tinged subcutaneous nodules resembling blueberry muffins.

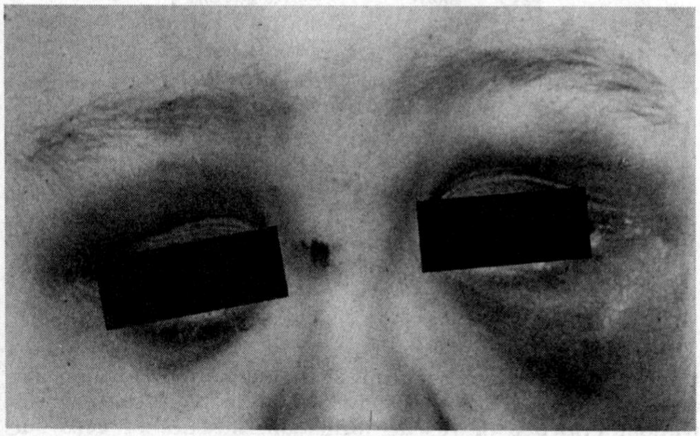

Figure 451–1. Periorbital metastases of neuroblastoma, with proptosis and ecchymoses.

The clinical picture can also reflect tumor-associated metabolic disturbances. An acute cerebellar encephalopathy characterized by cerebellar ataxia, rapid and random eye movements (opsoclonus), and myoclonic jerks occurs in 4% of patients. Severe diarrhea with extreme hypokalemia and achlorhydria may result from production of vasoactive intestinal peptide by tumor cells (see Chapter 291). Elevated levels of catecholamines can cause hypertension.

Physical examination may reveal lymph node enlargement, hepatomegaly, or an abdominal or flank mass. Periorbital ecchymoses (raccoon eyes) and scalp nodules may also be present (Fig. 451–1). A careful neurologic examination is important to ascertain spinal cord involvement. Accurate determination of the extent of disease requires numerous laboratory studies. A complete blood count may reveal anemia or thrombocytopenia from bone marrow infiltration or disseminated intravascular coagulation. Lactate dehydrogenase, serum ferritin, NSE, blood urea nitrogen, or creatinine levels may be elevated, and the coagulation profile (prothrombin and partial thromboplastin times, fibrinogen) may be abnormal. Neuroblastomas are biochemically unique tumors because they possess the enzymes for catecholamine synthesis and catabolism. Homovanillic acid and vanillylmandelic acid are usually excreted in excessive amounts in urine and are the most useful markers of neuroblastoma.

Imaging studies are determined by the suspected site of origin and include a chest radiograph, computed tomography (CT) of the chest and abdomen-pelvis, and bone scintigraphy (Fig. 451–2). CT scans are necessary to document the size and location of any suspected mass, the relationship to adjacent organs (particularly the great vessels), and the feasibility of surgical resection. Magnetic resonance imaging is more accurate in detecting intraspinal extension, vessel encasement or displacement, and bone marrow involvement. Bone scan is also helpful in detecting the primary tumor and in defining the extent of skeletal metastases. Uptake of technetium diphosphonate by the primary tumor can be seen in up to 60% of cases. Imaging using radiolabeled meta-iodobenzylguanidine (MIBG), an analog of catecholamine precursors taken up by catecholamine-producing tumors, can be useful in defining sites of metastasis and in following response.

The diagnosis must be confirmed by tissue biopsy. Bone marrow aspirations and biopsies must be performed before any surgical procedure because they may reveal infiltrating tumor cells (Fig. 451–3). The definitive diagnosis is made by histopathologic studies of tumor tissue or documentation of bone marrow involvement plus increased urine or serum catecholamine levels. Tumor material should be submitted for determination of the DNA content (tumor cell ploidy), the presence of N-*myc* amplification, and cytogenetic analysis.

STAGING. Several staging systems have been used. The Evans and Pediatric Oncology Group (POG) systems and the International Neuroblastoma Staging System are the most widely used. The POG staging system divides tumors into stage A, grossly resected tumor; stage B, localized unresectable tumor; stage C, metastasis to noncontiguous intracavitary lymph nodes; stage D, metastasis beyond lymph nodes; and stage D_s, infants with small adrenal primary with metastatic disease limited to skin, liver, or bone marrow. Neonatal stage D_s has been known to undergo spontaneous remission. The presence of bone involvement at this age is a poor prognostic factor.

TREATMENT. The three main treatment modalities are surgery, chemotherapy, and radiotherapy. For a localized tumor, complete surgical resection, when feasible, is usually curative. Unfortunately, about 70% of patients have relatively advanced disease at diagnosis. Patients with abdominal tumors localized to one side of the midline or crossing the midline without

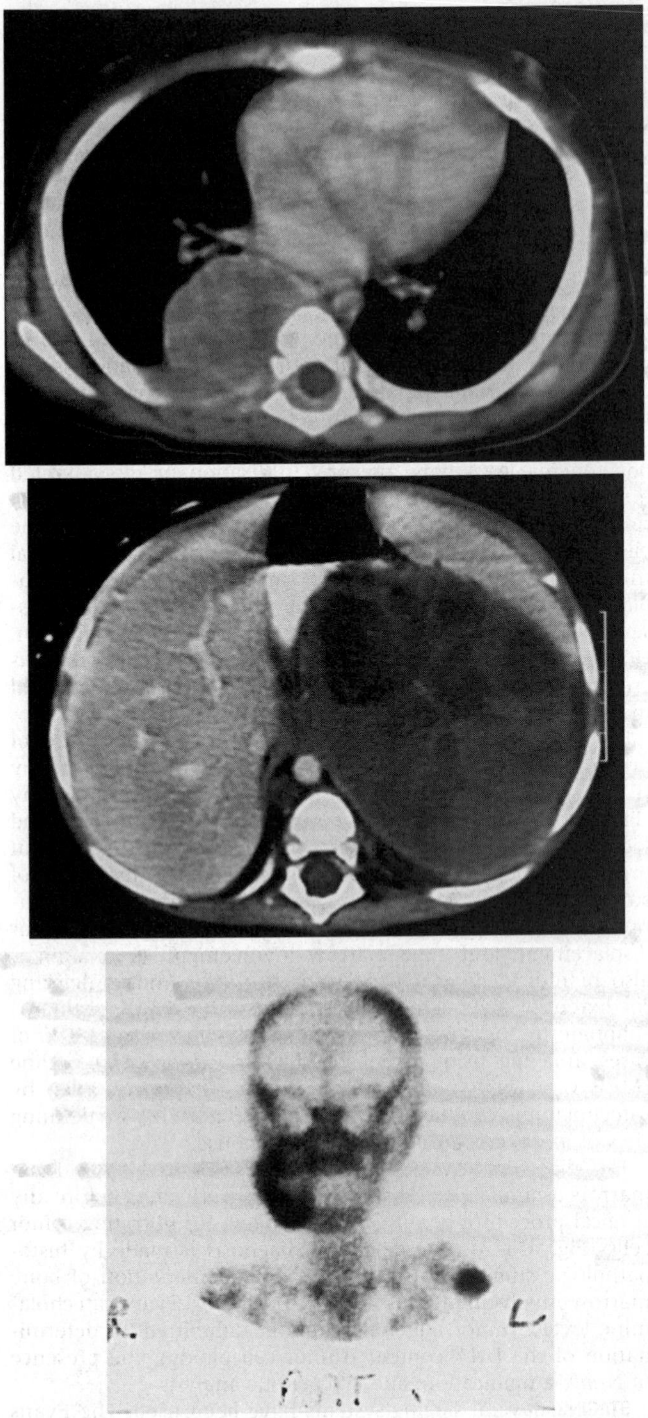

Figure 451–2. ***Top***, **CT scan of a thoracic neuroblastoma with intraspinal extension at diagnosis.** ***Middle***, **CT scan of an adrenal primary with extensive lymph node involvement.** ***Bottom***, **Bone scintigraphy with technetium diphosphonate demonstrating diffuse skeletal involvement.**

encasement of major blood vessels are candidates for primary surgical resection. In children with nonmetastatic neuroblastomas, an important goal of the initial surgical procedure is to determine the status of intracavitary lymph nodes that are not attached to the primary tumor. A liver biopsy should be obtained, particularly in infants. Because chemotherapy can render a large tumor resectable, second-look or delayed surgery is important. Tumors that cause spinal cord compression respond rapidly to chemotherapy, obviating the need for laminectomy.

■ **TABLE 451–1 Four-Year Survival Rates of Infants (<1 yr of age) or Children with Neuroblastoma Treated at St. Jude Children's Research Hospital (1979–1988) According to Extent of Disease (Stage) and Age (> 1 vs < 1 yr)**

	Infants		Children	
Stage*	*4-Yr Survival Rate ± SE (%)*	*No.*	*4-Yr Survival Rate ± SE (%)*	*No.*
A	100	16	100	12
B	100	2	93 ± 7	14
C	88 ± 9	17	36 ± 14	13
D	79 ± 9	33	27 ± 5	94
D_s	73 ± 13	11		

**See neuroblastoma staging section for definitions.*
SE = standard error.
(From Bowman LC, Hancock VM, Santana FA, et al: Impact of Intensified Therapy on Clinical Outcome in Infants and Children with Neuroblastoma: The St. Jude Children's Research Hospital Experience, 1962 to 1988. J Clin Oncol 9:1599, 1991.)

Tumors in the chest may be less aggressive ganglioneuroblastomas amenable to surgery.

The role of surgery in patients with disseminated disease is unclear. Primary resection is not appropriate; delayed or second-look surgery after chemotherapy has been suggested, but the results of this approach are yet to be defined.

Chemotherapy is the mainstay of treatment for unresectable or metastatic disease. Infants (younger than 1 yr of age) with disseminated disease and children with localized unresectable disease have excellent responses to the combination of cyclophosphamide and doxorubicin. For older children with locally advanced and disseminated neuroblastomas, combination chemotherapy (cyclophosphamide, doxorubicin, cisplatin, etoposide, ifosfamide, melphalan, vincristine, and carboplatin in various combinations) produces good initial responses but generally poor overall outcomes. Only 20–25% of children with disseminated disease are alive and disease free at 5 yr postdiagnosis. Experimental approaches include very intensive chemotherapy with or without autologous bone marrow transplantation, the use of radioactive MIBG, and monoclonal antibodies directed against neuroblastoma cell surface proteins. However, relapse remains a major problem.

Most neuroblastomas are radiosensitive; irradiation may be used for local control in addition to systemic chemotherapy in children with regional lymph node disease. Irradiation may also be used for local palliation of metastatic disease.

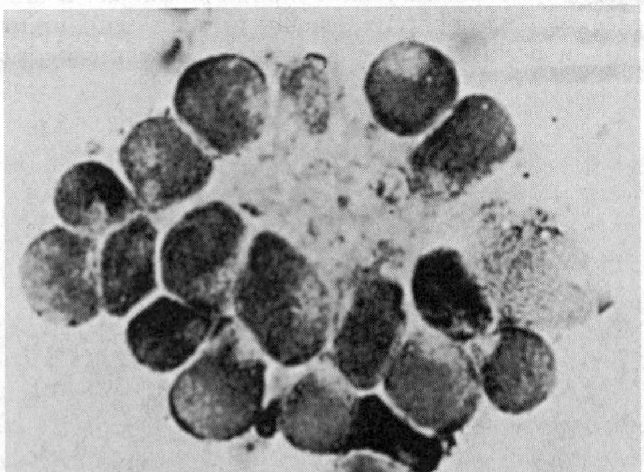

Figure 451–3. Neuroblastoma cells aspirated from the bone marrow. Clumps of cells often contain three or more cells with or without evidence of rosette formation. Rosettes of cells surrounding an inner mass of fibrillary material are characteristic of neuroblastoma.

PROGNOSIS. The identification of specific prognostic factors is important in treatment planning. The most significant predictors of outcome are age and stage (see Table 451–1). Children younger than 1 yr of age fare better than older children with the same disease stage. Survival rates of infants with low-stage disease exceed 90%, and infants with metastatic disease have a long-term survival rate of 50% or greater. Children with low-stage disease have a generally excellent prognosis, regardless of age. The older the patient and the more widespread the disease, the poorer the prognosis is. Despite aggressive conventional treatment or bone marrow transplantation, disease-free survival rates for older children with advanced stage disease rarely exceed 20%.

A variety of biologic and genetic markers such as the tumor cell karyotype, DNA content (ploidy), or N-*myc* copy number have been used to further refine risk-directed therapy. Infants with hyperdiploid tumors (DNA index more than 1) have a survival expectancy of 80% compared with 20% for those with diploid tumors. N-*myc* amplification predicts a poor outcome in all age/stage groups, including patients with localized disease and infants with stage D or D_s disease.

CHAPTER 452
Neoplasms of the Kidney

Patricia D. Shearer and Judith A. Wilimas

452.1 Wilms Tumor

Wilms tumor accounts for most childhood renal neoplasms and occurs with approximately equal frequency in both sexes and in all races, with an annual incidence of 7.8 per million children younger than the age of 15 yr. An important feature of Wilms tumor is its association with congenital anomalies, the most common being genitourinary anomalies (4.4%), hemihypertrophy (2.9%), and sporadic aniridia (1.1%).

Deletions involving one of at least two loci on chromosome 11 have been noted in cells of about 33% of Wilms tumors. Hemizygous constitutional deletions of one of these loci, 11p13, are also associated with two rare syndromes that include Wilms tumor: the *WAGR syndrome* (Wilms tumor, aniridia, genitourinary malformations, and mental retardation) and the *Denys-Drash syndrome* (Wilms tumor, nephropathy, and genital abnormalities). The existence of a second locus, 11p15, may explain the association of Wilms tumor with Beckwith-Wiedemann syndrome, a congenital syndrome characterized by several types of embryonal neoplasms, hemihypertrophy, macroglossia, and visceromegaly (see Chapters 445 and 446). A third locus may be involved in familial Wilms tumor.

PATHOLOGY. Wilms tumor is a solitary growth that occurs in any part of either kidney. In gross appearance, it is sharply demarcated and variably encapsulated. Small areas of hemorrhage are common. The tumors usually distort the renal outline and often compress residual normal kidney into a surrounding thin rim (Fig. 452–1).

The classic microscopic appearance of favorable-histologic Wilms tumor subtype is triphasic, epithelial, blastemal, and stromal elements are present and resemble abortive glomeruli. Anaplasia is found in about 10% of cases, which account for 60% of deaths. This unfavorable histologic subtype, which tends to occur in older, nonwhite patients, features cells three times the normal size, with hyperchromatic nuclei and abnormal mitoses.

Two renal tumors that were previously considered to be unfavorable subtypes of Wilms tumor have been reclassified. *Rhabdoid* tumor, a highly malignant neoplasm composed of cells with fibrillar eosinophilic inclusions, is found most often in very young patients. *Clear cell sarcoma* of the kidney is characterized by a spindle cell pattern with a striking vasocen-

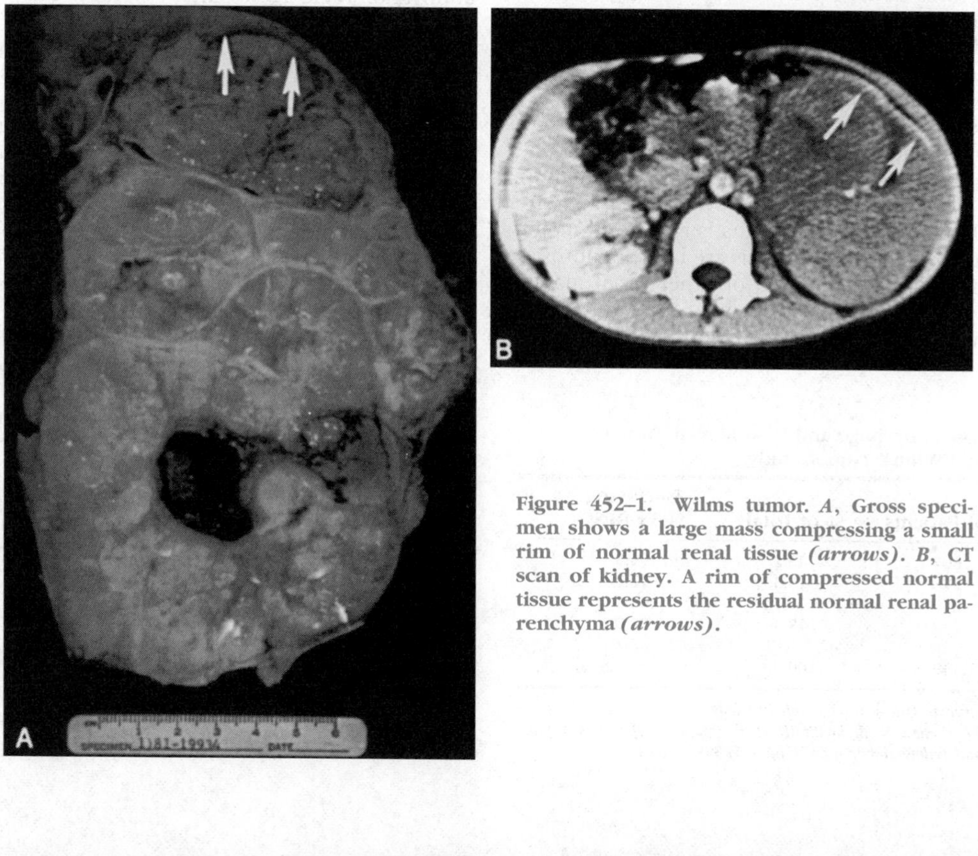

Figure 452–1. Wilms tumor. *A*, Gross specimen shows a large mass compressing a small rim of normal renal tissue *(arrows)*. *B*, CT scan of kidney. A rim of compressed normal tissue represents the residual normal renal parenchyma *(arrows)*.

tric arrangement; it shows a male predominance and a tendency to metastasize to bone.

The staging system most frequently used is that of the National Wilms Tumor Study (NWTS) group. Stage I tumors are limited to the kidney and can be completely excised with the capsular surface intact. The stage II tumor extends beyond the kidney but can be completely excised. In stage III, there is postsurgical residual nonhematogenous extension confined to the abdomen. Stage IV indicates hematogenous metastases, which most frequently involve the lung. Bilateral (usually synchronous) renal involvement is seen in 5–10% of cases (stage V). The relative incidences of stages I to IV and associated survival rates are shown in Table 452–1.

CLINICAL MANIFESTATIONS. The median age at diagnosis of unilateral Wilms tumor is about 3 yr. The most frequent sign is an asymptomatic abdominal or flank mass. The mass is generally smooth and firm and rarely crosses the midline. Masses vary greatly in size at the time of discovery. In one series, the mean diameter was 11 cm. Masses are often discovered by parents or on routine examination. About 50% of affected children have abdominal pain, vomiting, or both. In general, patients with Wilms tumor are slightly older and appear less ill than those with an abdominal mass that is found to be neuroblastoma.

Hypertension, reported in as many as 60% of patients, results from renal ischemia, usually owing to pressure of the tumor on the renal artery. It may be sufficiently severe and prolonged to produce cardiac failure.

DIAGNOSIS. Wilms tumor must be suspected in any young child with an abdominal mass. In 10–25% of cases, microscopic or gross hematuria suggests a renal tumor. Ultrasonography (the initial imaging modality) may indicate that the mass is intrarenal. The major differential diagnostic consideration is neuroblastoma.

Computed tomography (CT) offers several advantages in evaluating a possible Wilms tumor. These include confirmation of intrarenal tumor origin, which usually rules out neuroblastoma; detection of multiple masses; determination of the extent of tumor, including great vessel involvement; and evaluation of the opposite kidney. On CT studies without enhancement, the typical Wilms tumor arises from the kidney as inhomogeneous masses with areas of low density indicating necrosis. Areas of hemorrhage and small focal calcifications are generally less common and less prominent than in neuroblastoma. Tumors enhance slightly after injection of contrast medium. There is often a sharp demarcation between the tumor and normal parenchyma, correlated with a pseudocapsule, and persistent ellipsoid areas of increased attenuation corresponding to the compressed uninvolved renal parenchyma (Fig. 452–1B). Once neuroblastoma is ruled out, major considerations in the differential diagnosis are hydronephrosis, renal cysts, and mesoblastic nephroma or other renal malignancies, such as renal cell carcinoma, sarcoma, and lymphoma.

Pulmonary metastases are evident on chest radiographs in 10–15% of patients at the time of diagnosis. CT scan of the chest is useful, particularly to visualize portions of the lung below the level of the dome of the diaphragm (Fig. 452–2). If hepatic metastases are suspected, CT scan of the abdomen may be helpful. Evaluation of bone and bone marrow should be considered only if the patient has a tumor with unfavorable histologic subtype or has persistent bone pain.

■ TABLE 452–1 Survival by Stage and Histology at Time of Diagnosis in National Wilms' Tumor Study 3

Stage	No. of Patients	% of Total	% Having 4-Yr RFS*
I	607	42.2	96.5
II	278	19.3	92.2
III	275	19.1	86.9
IV	279	19.4	73.0
+ UH			
Total	1,439	100.0	

**RFS = relapse-free survival; UH = unfavorable histology.*

(Data from D'Angio GJ, Breslow N, Beckwith JB, et al: Treatment of Wilms' tumor: Results of the third national Wilms' tumor study. Cancer 64:349, 1989.)

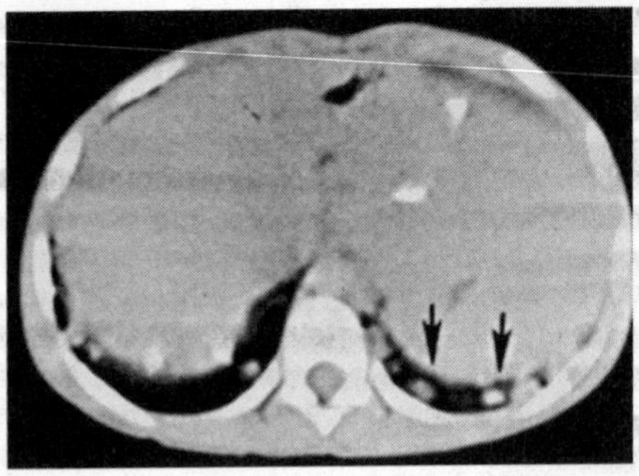

Figure 452–2. Wilms tumor on CT scan of the chest showing metastatic lesions below the dome of the diaphragm *(arrows)*, which would be difficult to visualize on plain radiograph.

Certain rare paraneoplastic syndromes may be associated with Wilms tumor. The tumor may produce erythropoietin, leading to polycythemia; secondary hypercalcemia; and a clinical picture similar to von Willebrand disease.

TREATMENT. The immediate treatment for unilateral tumors is surgical removal of the affected kidney, even if pulmonary metastases are present. At the time of nephrectomy, careful inspection of the other kidney is needed to exclude the possibility of bilateral tumor, and the liver should be evaluated for possible metastasis. The retroperitoneal lymph nodes and renal vein should be examined. Every attempt should be made to remove the tumor without spillage, but because postoperative chemotherapy and radiation can destroy residual tumor, complete resection should not be attempted if the procedure would pose serious risks.

Previously, all patients were treated with postoperative radiation and single-agent chemotherapy. The NWTS group has shown that combination chemotherapy with vincristine (Oncovin) and dactinomycin (Cosmegen) is superior to single-agent therapy in patients with localized disease and that doxorubicin (Adriamycin) is a significant addition to the treatment of patients with advanced disease. For patients with advanced-stage disease, who require radiation in addition to surgery and chemotherapy, the dosage and fields have been modified to reduce the incidence of scoliosis. Pulmonary irradiation and three-drug combination chemotherapy are now recommended for most patients with stage IV disease.

Preoperative therapy is not generally recommended for patients with unilateral disease but is indicated for patients with bilateral tumors to facilitate eventual renal salvage procedures. This approach preserves renal parenchyma and optimizes renal function without compromising survival.

PROGNOSIS. The most significant prognostic variables are histologic subtype and stage (Table 452–1). Recurrence had carried a poor prognosis, although addition of newer agents and salvage regimens may improve outcome for the small group of patients who have a recurrence. The outcome for all patients is optimized by treatment in a pediatric cancer center.

452.2 Other Renal Neoplasms

NEPHROBLASTOMATOSIS. Immature renal elements called nephrogenic rests occur in approximately 33% of unilateral Wilms tumors and in most, if not all, bilateral tumors. These Wilms tumor precursor lesions may be unifocal and deep within the renal parenchyma (intralobar rest) or multifocal (perilobar rest). Subsequent (asynchronous) development of Wilms tumor in the other kidney is more likely in patients with this feature (particularly intralobar rests) at presentation. The finding of nephrogenic rests in one kidney should prompt a careful inspection of the contralateral kidney at the time of surgery and radiographic follow-up with CT scanning.

MESOBLASTIC NEPHROMA. Congenital mesoblastic nephroma is a massive, firm, infiltrative, solitary renal mass, grossly and microscopically resembling a leiomyoma or a low-grade leiomyosarcoma with trapped nephrons. The infiltrative margins are difficult to distinguish histologically from normal or dysplastic renal stroma. Electron microscopy shows the cells to be fibroblasts or myofibroblasts. This tumor accounts for most congenital renal tumors. It occurs more often in males and has been noted to produce renin. The tumor is generally thought to be benign, and resection is adequate therapy. An occasional patient has a very cellular tumor that resembles a clear cell sarcoma. Tumors that recur locally and metastasize would then benefit from chemotherapy and irradiation.

RENAL CELL CARCINOMA. This tumor is rare in the 1st decade of life but occurs occasionally in teenagers. The initial findings are an abdominal mass and hematuria. The microscopic appearance and clinical course are similar to those found in adults with renal cell carcinoma. Complete resection may result in cure, but the prognosis is grim for patients with postoperative residual disease.

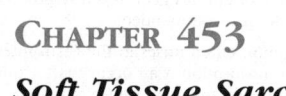

CHAPTER 453
Soft Tissue Sarcomas

William M. Crist

Soft tissue sarcomas have an annual incidence of 8.4 per million white children under the age of 15 yr and about 50% that incidence in black children. Rhabdomyosarcoma accounts for more than 50% of these tumors (Table 453–1). The prognosis is most strongly associated with extent of disease at diagnosis, primary tumor site, and treatment used.

453.1 Rhabdomyosarcoma

EPIDEMIOLOGY. The most common pediatric soft tissue sarcoma, rhabdomyosarcoma accounts for 5–8% of childhood cancers. There are no striking relationships between incidence and demographic features, with the exception of a somewhat higher frequency in males and white children. These tumors can occur at virtually any anatomic site but are most often found in the head and neck (40%), genitourinary tract (20%), extremities (20%), and trunk (10%); retroperitoneal and "other" account for the remainder of primary sites. Both age and tumor histologic type appear related to primary site. For example, extremity lesions are more likely to occur in older children and to have alveolar histologic type.

Rhabdomyosarcoma occurs with increased frequency in patients with neurofibromatosis and has been associated with maternal breast cancer in the Li-Fraumeni syndrome, suggesting a genetic influence.

PATHOLOGY. Rhabdomyosarcoma is thought to arise from the same embryonic mesenchyme as striated skeletal muscle. On the basis of light microscopic appearance, it belongs to the group of "small round cell tumors," which includes Ewing sarcoma, neuroblastoma, primitive neuroectodermal tumor, and non-Hodgkin lymphoma. Definitive diagnosis of a pathologic specimen may require immunohistochemical studies using antibodies to skeletal muscle (desmin, muscle-specific actin) and electron microscopy to distinguish characteristic features.

Determination of the specific histiotype is important in treatment and prognosis. There are four recognized histologic subtypes. The *embryonal* type accounts for about 60% of all cases and has an intermediate prognosis. The *botryoid* type, a variant of the embryonal form in which tumor cells and an edematous stroma project into a body cavity like a bunch of grapes, accounts for 6% of cases and is most often seen in the vagina, uterus, bladder, nasopharynx, and middle ear. *Alveolar* tumors, which account for about 15% of cases, are characterized by the t(2;13) chromosomal translocation. The tumor cells tend to grow in cores that often have cleftlike spaces resembling alveoli. Alveolar tumors occur most often in the trunk and extremities and carry the poorest prognosis. The *pleomorphic* type (adult form) is rare in childhood (1% of cases). About 20% of patients are considered to have *undifferentiated* sarcomas.

CLINICAL MANIFESTATIONS. The most common presenting feature is a mass that may or may not be painful. Symptoms are due to displacement or obstruction of normal structures. Origin in the nasopharynx may be associated with nasal congestion, mouth breathing, epistaxis, and difficulty with swallowing and chewing. Regional extension into the cranium can produce cranial nerve paralysis, blindness, and signs of increased intracranial pressure, with headache and vomiting. When the tumor develops in the face or cheek, there may be swelling, pain, trismus, and, as extension occurs, paralysis of cranial nerves. Tumors in the neck can produce progressive swelling, with neurologic symptoms after regional extension. Orbital primaries are usually diagnosed early in their course because of associated proptosis, periorbital edema, ptosis, change in visual acuity, and local pain. When the tumor arises in the middle ear, the most common early signs are pain, hearing loss, chronic otorrhea, or a mass in the ear canal; extensions of tumor produce cranial nerve paralysis and signs of an intracranial mass of the involved side. An unremitting croupy cough and progressive stridor can accompany rhabdomyosarcoma of the larynx. Because most of these signs and symptoms are also associated with common childhood conditions, the clinician must be alert to the possibility of tumor.

Rhabdomyosarcoma of the trunk or extremities is often first noticed after trauma and may be regarded initially as a hematoma. When the swelling does not resolve or increases, malignancy should be suspected. Involvement of the genitourinary tract can produce hematuria, obstruction of the lower urinary tract, recurrent urinary tract infections, incontinence, or a mass detectable on abdominal or rectal examination. Paratesticular tumors usually present as a painless, rapidly growing mass in the scrotum. Vaginal rhabdomyosarcoma may present as a grapelike mass of tumor tissue bulging through the vaginal orifice (sarcoma botryoides) and can cause urinary tract or large bowel symptoms. Vaginal bleeding or obstruction of the urethra or rectum may occur. Similar findings can be seen with uterine primaries.

Tumors in any location may disseminate early, with presenting symptoms of pain or respiratory distress associated with pulmonary metastases. Extensive bone involvement can produce symptomatic hypercalcemia. In such cases, it may be difficult to identify the primary lesion.

■ TABLE 453–1 Nonrhabdomyosarcoma Soft Tissue Sarcomas

Tissue Type	Tumor	Natural History and Biology
Adipose	Liposarcoma	A very rare tumor. Usually arises in the extremities or retroperitoneum; associated with a nonrandom translocation, t(12;16)(q13;p11). Tends to be locally invasive and rarely metastasizes; wide local excision is the treatment of choice. The role of radiation therapy and chemotherapy in treating gross residual or metastatic disease is not established.
Fibrous	Fibrosarcoma	The most common soft tissue sarcoma in children younger than 1 yr of age. Congenital fibrosarcoma is a low-grade malignancy that commonly arises in the extremities or trunk and rarely metastasizes. Surgical excision is the treatment of choice; dramatic responses to preoperative chemotherapy may occur. In children older than 4 yr, the natural history is similar to that in adults (a 5-yr survival rate of 60%); wide surgical excision and preoperative chemotherapy are commonly used.
	Malignant fibrous histiocytoma	Most commonly arises in the trunk and extremities, deep in the subcutaneous layer. Histologically subdivided into storiform, giant cell, myxoid, and angiomatoid variants. The angiomatoid type tends to affect younger patients and is curable with surgical resection alone. Wide surgical excision is the treatment of choice. Chemotherapy has produced objective tumor regressions.
Vascular	Hemangiopericytoma	Often arises in the lower extremities or retroperitoneum; may present with hypoglycemia and hypophosphatemic rickets. Both benign and malignant histology. Nonrandom translocations t(12;19)(q13;q13) and t(13;22)(q22;q11) have been described. Complete surgical excision is the treatment of choice. Chemotherapy and radiotherapy may produce responses.
	Angiosarcoma	Rare in children; 33% arise in skin, 25% in soft tissue, and 25% in liver, breast or bone. Associated with chronic lymphedema and exposure to vinyl chloride in adults. Survival rate is poor (12% at 5 yr) despite some responses to chemotherapy/radiotherapy.
	Hemangioendothelioma	Can occur in soft tissue, liver, and lung. Localized lesions have a favorable outcome; lesions in lung and liver are often multifocal and have a poor prognosis.
Peripheral nerves	Neurofibrosarcoma	Also known as a malignant peripheral nerve sheath tumor. Develops in up to 16% of patients with NF1; almost 50% occur in patients with NF1. Deletions of chromosome 22q11-q13 or 17q11 and p53 mutations have been reported. Commonly arises in trunk and extremities and is usually locally invasive. Complete surgical excision is necessary for survival; response to chemotherapy is suboptimal.
Synovium	Synovial sarcoma	The most common NRSTS in some series. Often presenting in the 3rd decade, but 33% of patients are younger than 20 yr. Typically arises around the knee or thigh and is characterized by a nonrandom translocation t(X;18)(p11;q11). Wide surgical excision is necessary. Radiotherapy is effective in microscopic residual disease, and ifosfamide-based therapy is active in advanced disease.
Unknown	Alveolar soft part sarcoma	Slow-growing tumor; tends to recur or metastasize to lung and brain years after diagnosis. Often arises in the extremities and head and neck. A myogenic origin has been recently proposed. Resection of primary and metastatic sites, when possible, is recommended.
Smooth muscle	Leiomyosarcoma	The most common pediatric retroperitoneal soft tissue tumor. Often arises in the gastrointestinal tract and may be associated with a t(12;14)(q14;q23) translocation. Can occur with acquired immunodeficiency syndrome and during immunosuppression for renal transplantation. Complete surgical excision is the treatment of choice.

NF = Neurofibromatosis; NRSTS = nonrhabdomyosarcoma soft tissue sarcoma.

DIAGNOSIS. Several months often elapse between the initial symptoms and biopsy. Diagnostic procedures are determined mainly by the area of involvement. With signs and symptoms in the head and neck area, radiographs should be examined for evidence of a tumor mass and for indications of bony erosion. Computed tomographic (CT) scans should be done to identify intracranial extension and may also reveal bony involvement at the base of the skull, which is difficult to visualize radiographically. For abdominal and pelvic tumors, ultrasound examination and CT with oral and intravenous contrast media can help delineate the tumor mass. Cystourethrograms are useful for tumors in the bladder. A radionuclide scan and a full skeletal metastatic survey should be done before definitive surgery. A chest radiograph and CT should be obtained, and bone marrow (aspirate and needle biopsy) should be examined. The results of these studies are used to plan the nature and extent of surgery. The most essential element of the diagnostic workup is examination of tumor tissue.

TREATMENT. Patients with completely resected tumors have the best prognosis. Unfortunately, most rhabdomyosarcomas are not completely resectable. At the initial surgery, tumor margins should be carefully defined, and an appropriate search for regional or metastatic disease (regional lymph nodes, adjacent structures) should be completed, even if the procedure is limited to biopsy. Treatment is based on the primary tumor location and disease stage ("clinical group"). Some patients are given preoperative chemotherapy in an attempt to reduce the extent of surgery and to preserve vital organs, particularly in the genitourinary tract. In group I tumors, complete local excision is followed by chemotherapy to reduce the likelihood of subsequent metastatic disease. For groups II and III (microscopic or gross residual tumor, respectively) surgery is followed by local irradiation and systemic multiagent chemotherapy. Children with metastatic (group IV) rhabdomyosarcoma are treated with systemic chemotherapy and irradiation. Intrathecal chemotherapy is generally given to patients with primary disease in parameningeal sites (nasopharynx, nasal cavity, paranasal sinuses, middle ear, mastoid, pterygopalatine or infratemporal fossae), with intracranial extension.

PROGNOSIS. Among patients with resectable tumor, 80–90% have prolonged disease-free survival. Unresectable tumor localized to certain "favorable" sites (orbit) also has a high likelihood of cure. About 66% of patients with incompletely resected regional tumor also achieve long-term disease-free survival. Patients with disseminated disease have a poor prognosis. Only about 50% achieve remission, and fewer than 50% of these are cured. Older children have a worse prognosis than younger ones.

453.2 Other Soft Tissue Sarcomas

Alberto S. Pappo

The nonrhabdomyosarcoma soft tissue sarcomas (NRSTS) constitute a heterogeneous group of tumors that include 3%

of all childhood malignancies. Because they are relatively rare in children, much of the information regarding their natural history and treatment has been derived from studies of adult patients. In children, the median age at diagnosis is 12 yr, and males predominate (male to female ratio, 2.3:1). The most common histologic types are synovial sarcoma (42%), fibrosarcoma (13%), malignant fibrous histiocytoma (12%), and neurogenic tumors (10%). Table 453–1 describes the clinical features, treatment, and prognosis of the most common NRSTS. These tumors commonly arise in the trunk or lower extremities. Tumor size, stage (clinical group), invasiveness, and histologic grade correlate with survival.

Surgery remains the mainstay of therapy, but a careful search for lung and bone metastases should be undertaken before surgical excision. Lymph node spread is rare, and routine dissection is not recommended. Adjuvant chemotherapy should be considered for high-grade, completely resected tumors, whereas postoperative radiotherapy is used to treat patients with microscopic residual disease. Patients with unresectable or metastatic disease are treated with chemotherapy that includes vincristine (Oncovin), doxorubicin (Adriamycin), ifosfamide (Ifex), cyclophosphamide (Cytoxan), dacarbazine (DTIC-Dome), and dactinomycin (Cosmogen).

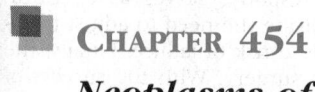

CHAPTER 454
Neoplasms of Bone

William Meyer

Bone tumors are the sixth most common group of pediatric malignancies, with an annual incidence of 5.6 per million population in white children and adolescents and 4.8 per million in blacks. Osteosarcoma (also called osteogenic sarcoma) and the Ewing sarcoma family of tumors account for most primary bone cancers in the pediatric population, with osteosarcoma being slightly more common. Both tumor types occur most often in the 2nd decade of life and show a male predominance. Other associated clinical and demographic features are listed in Table 454–1.

454.1 Osteosarcoma

The development of osteosarcoma has long been associated with periods of rapid bone growth. These tumors are most often diagnosed during adolescence and often occur in the metaphyseal region of rapidly growing bones. Common primary sites are the distal femur, proximal tibia, and proximal humerus. However, osteosarcoma can also arise in flat bones (vertebrae, pelvic bones, mandible) and is sometimes seen in very young children and in adults.

Certain genetic and hereditary conditions are associated with an abnormally high frequency of osteosarcoma. The increased risk among children with bilateral (hereditary) retinoblastoma, originally attributed to prior radiotherapy, has since been associated with loss of the normal *Rb* tumor-suppressor gene. More recent studies also indicate involvement of the p53 gene, inactivation of which favors uncontrolled cell growth. Osteosarcoma is often seen in the Li-Fraumeni syndrome, in which germline mutations of p53 play a central role (see Chapter

■ TABLE 454–1 Comparison of Osteosarcoma and Ewing Sarcoma/Peripheral Neuroepithelioma

Feature	Osteosarcoma	Ewing Sarcoma/Peripheral Neuroepithelioma
Age	Second decade	Second decade
Race	All races	Primarily whites
Sex (M:F)	1.5:1	1.5:1
Cell	Spindle cell–producing osteoid	Undifferentiated small round cell, probably of neural origin
Predisposition	Retinoblastoma, Li-Fraumeni syndrome, Paget disease, radiotherapy	None known
Site	Metaphyses of long bones	Diaphyses of long bones, flat bones
Presentation	Local pain and swelling; often history of injury	Local pain and swelling; fever
Radiographic findings	Sclerotic destruction (less commonly lytic); sunburst pattern	Primarily lytic, multilaminar periosteal reaction ("onion skinning")
Differential diagnosis	Ewing sarcoma, osteomyelitis	Osteomyelitis, eosinophilic granuloma, lymphoma, neuroblastoma, rhabdomyosarcoma
Metastasis	Lung, bones	Lung, bones
Treatment	Chemotherapy Ablative surgery of primary tumor	Chemotherapy Radiotherapy and/or surgery of primary tumor
Outcome	Without metastases: 66% cured; with metastases at diagnosis, ≤20% survival	Without metastases: 60% cured; with metastases at diagnosis, 20–30% survival

446). Other conditions associated with an increased risk of osteosarcoma include Paget disease, enchondromatosis, multiple hereditary exostoses, and osteogenesis imperfecta. Patients who have received local irradiation for Ewing sarcoma are also at risk for subsequent development of osteosarcoma.

PATHOLOGY. Osteosarcoma is a highly malignant spindle cell neoplasm in which the tumor cells produce extracellular osteoid. The tumor arises in the cortical/medullary region of long bones; superficial (periosteal) tumors occur rarely. Tumors typically break through bone cortex and invade surrounding soft tissues (Fig. 454–1). They can also extend into the medullary space, and so-called skip lesions may occur at some distance from the primary tumor mass. Conventional (high-grade) osteosarcomas are classified by *osteoblastic, chondroblastic,* or *fibroblastic* differentiation (or mixture thereof). A rare subtype, *telangiectatic osteosarcoma,* contains blood-filled cystic areas that do not produce calcified osteoid and may be confused radiographically with aneurysmal bone cyst. *Parosteal* osteosarcoma, also a rare variant, is a low-grade, well-differentiated tumor that arises around the peripheral cortex of bone, does not invade the medullary space, and is often curable by surgical resection alone. *Periosteal* osteosarcoma tends to be more pleiomorphic and to behave more aggressively than parosteal osteosarcoma. Finally, in a very small percentage of cases, osteosarcoma may appear synchronously in multiple bones *(multifocal sclerosing osteosarcoma)*; these tumors are almost always osteoblastic and respond poorly to treatment.

CLINICAL MANIFESTATIONS. The most common presenting symptoms are localized pain and swelling. Often, the patient and family ascribe the pain to recent trauma. Physical examination shows local swelling, tenderness, warmth, and limited range of motion when the tumor is adjacent to a joint. Complete blood counts and chemistry profile are usually normal, although serum levels of alkaline phosphatase and/or lactate dehydrogenase are elevated in some patients. Metastases occur most often in lungs and other bones and usually produce few clinical symptoms early in the disease process (Fig. 454–2).

DIAGNOSIS. Persistent, deep, localized pain, particularly when associated with a palpable mass, requires radiologic evaluation.

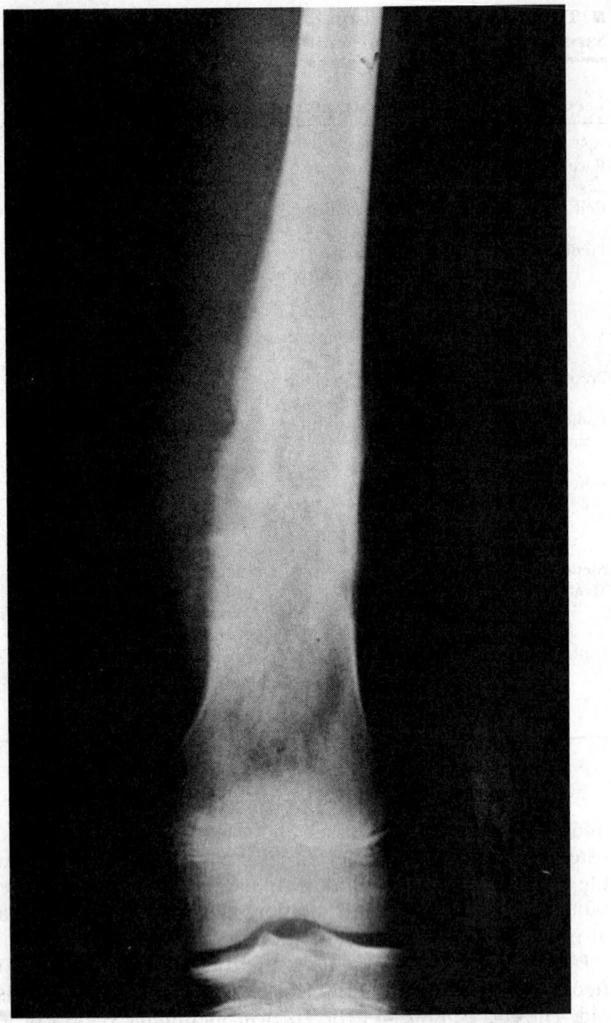

Figure 454–1. Osteosarcoma of the distal portion of the femur. The tumor has broken through the cortex; calcification of the tumor is seen in the surrounding soft tissues.

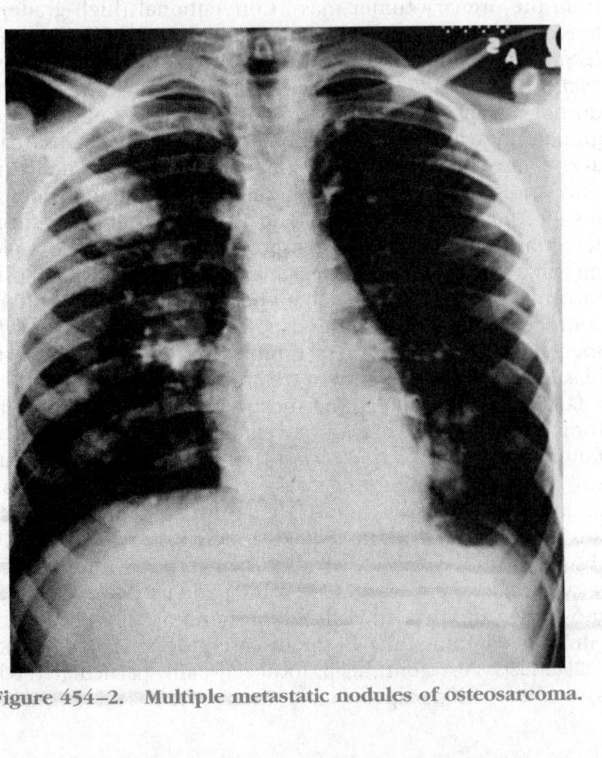

Figure 454–2. Multiple metastatic nodules of osteosarcoma.

A typical lesion is shown in Figure 454–1. Sclerosis of bone and periosteal new bone formation are common. Biopsy is required for diagnosis and should be done by the surgeon who will perform the definitive surgical procedure in a manner that preserves the option of limb-sparing surgery. Many cancer centers complete a thorough staging evaluation before biopsy to avoid distortion of imaging by surgical intervention. Imaging studies include computed tomography (CT) of the lungs to rule out pulmonary metastases, radionuclide bone scan to rule out bony metastases, and magnetic resonance imaging (MRI) of the primary tumor. MRI provides the best assessment of tumor extent within the medullary cavity and in soft tissues.

TREATMENT. Appropriate treatment for osteosarcoma includes chemotherapy and complete surgical resection. Because most osteosarcomas are not radiosensitive, surgery is the mainstay of primary tumor control. Historically, amputation was the preferred method for surgical ablation of tumor. However, amputation alone resulted in 5-yr survival rates of less than 20%, indicating the presence of micrometastases at diagnosis. Intensive treatment with multiagent chemotherapy (doxorubicin, cisplatin, high-dose methotrexate) increased event-free survival rates to more than 60%. Today, cure can be expected in at least 66% of patients without obvious metastases at diagnosis.

The use of aggressive chemotherapy for several weeks before surgical resection provides immediate treatment for occult metastatic disease. The tumor response serves as a critical prognostic indicator that can indicate the need to adjust treatment plans for patients at increased risk of failure. Finally, the approach facilitates limb-sparing surgery. With the success of preoperative chemotherapy, limb salvage is an option for 60–80% of patients at many centers. However, it should be kept in mind that complete resection of tumor remains essential to cure. A variety of surgical techniques are available, with the choice dependent on tumor location, size, and patient age.

Regardless of the surgical procedure used, extensive rehabilitation is crucial. Months of intensive intervention may be needed to attain maximal function. When amputation is necessary, patients should be counseled about phantom sensations before the operation; prosthetic fitting and gait training should occur early in the postoperative period.

PROGNOSIS. The small percentage of patients with parosteal osteosarcomas are usually cured with surgical resection alone, and about 66% of those with high-grade osteosarcomas and no evidence of metastatic disease are cured with effective therapy. A proportion of patients with pulmonary metastases (20–30%) can be treated successfully with salvage therapy if all nodules can be completely resected and aggressive multiagent chemotherapy is given. Patients with fewer tumor nodules have the best prognosis. Children with bony metastatic disease and those with widespread pulmonary disease are not curable with available treatments.

454.2 *Ewing Sarcoma/Peripheral Neuroepithelioma*

William Meyer and Neyssa Marina

Ewing sarcoma, peripheral neuroepithelioma (PN: also known as primitive neuroectodermal tumor [PNET]), and other tumors of similar histologic types constitute a family of highly malignant, small round cell undifferentiated neoplasms that arise most often in bone but can also occur in soft tissues. They are more common in males than females and are rare in black children. Like osteosarcoma, Ewing sarcoma and PN occur most often in the 2nd decade of life.

These tumors may arise in any bone but are found most often in flat bones (pelvis, chest wall, vertebrae) and the diaphyseal region of long bones. The soft tissue tumors occur most often in the trunk, with more than 50% arising in and around the chest. The distinction between a soft tissue and an osseous primary tumor site can be difficult because Ewing sarcomas typically have an extensive soft tissue component. This distinction is not important in terms of treatment. The most frequent sites of metastatic disease are lungs and bones. Less often, the bone marrow is invaded by tumor. At least 25% have clinically apparent metastases at diagnosis.

PATHOLOGY. Special histochemical staining is important in these undifferentiated tumors to rule out rhabdomyosarcoma, neuroblastoma, and lymphoma of bone. Histochemical stains can reveal features consistent with neural differentiation. Positive staining specific for the cell-surface glycoprotein p30/32^{MIC2} (HBA 71) is found in most of these tumors. Other histochemical stains specific for neural differentiation may also give positive results but probably lack prognostic significance. Ewing sarcoma and PN share a specific chromosomal translocation, the t(11;22)(q24;q12), which results in a chimeric *EWS* and *FLi1* gene product. This finding suggests the common origin of these tumors and differentiates them from other histologically similar neoplasms.

CLINICAL MANIFESTATIONS. Most patients present with pain, swelling, and tenderness in the involved site. Fever may be present. Symptoms can be chronic and intermittent, posing the potential for delay in diagnosis. The two conditions most often confused with Ewing sarcoma are eosinophilic granuloma and osteomyelitis. Occasionally, Ewing sarcoma may actually improve transiently with antibiotic therapy. Hence, malignancy must always be considered if bacterial cultures are negative in a case of presumed osteomyelitis.

DIAGNOSIS. The diagnosis of Ewing sarcoma/PN is often suggested by the clinical history and radiologic features. Plain radiographs typically show an aggressive, lytic tumor, often with an associated large soft tissue mass (Fig. 454–3). Confirmation requires surgical biopsy. It is important to obtain sufficient tissue for routine histologic and special histochemical stains. In difficult cases, electron microscopy and chromosomal studies may be required for accurate diagnosis.

Patients must be carefully screened for the presence of metastatic disease at diagnosis. CT scan of lungs is mandatory to rule out pulmonary metastases. Bone scanning should be performed to identify bony metastases. If metastatic disease is suspected, bone marrow examination is required. The extent of the primary lesion is best evaluated with MRI, which is also particularly useful in evaluating the response to therapy.

TREATMENT. Ewing sarcoma and PN are responsive to both radiotherapy and chemotherapy. Therefore, amputation is rarely indicated for local control of primary tumor. However, surgical resection of primary tumor has been associated with improved outcome and should be considered if function can be maintained.

Multiagent chemotherapy is the mainstay of therapy and usually precedes definitive local treatment. There is a benefit to adding ifosfamide (Ifex) and etoposide (VePesid) to standard four-drug chemotherapy with cyclophosphamide (cytoxan), doxorubicin (Adriamycin), vincristine (Oncovin), and dactinomycin (Cosmegen). Increased dose intensity is being studied as a way to improve cure rates. Local radiation therapy to primary and metastatic tumor sites is also imperative for good tumor control. Higher doses of radiotherapy may improve local control rates, but high-dose radiotherapy can also cause failure of bone growth, soft tissue fibrosis, and secondary malignant tumors, particularly osteosarcoma. Bones weakened by tumor involvement and irradiation are at increased risk of pathologic fracture, and heal slowly. Patients should be instructed to avoid vigorous physical activity if the tumor has involved weight-bearing bones. In addition, long-term follow-up is important because tumor recurrence may occur 10 yr or more after diagnosis.

PROGNOSIS. Patients with small extremity tumors and no clinically detectable metastases at diagnosis have a favorable outcome, with cure rates in excess of 70%. Patients with large, centrally located tumors and those with metastatic disease at diagnosis have a poorer prognosis. Although small, single-institution studies report survival rates up to 50% in these two

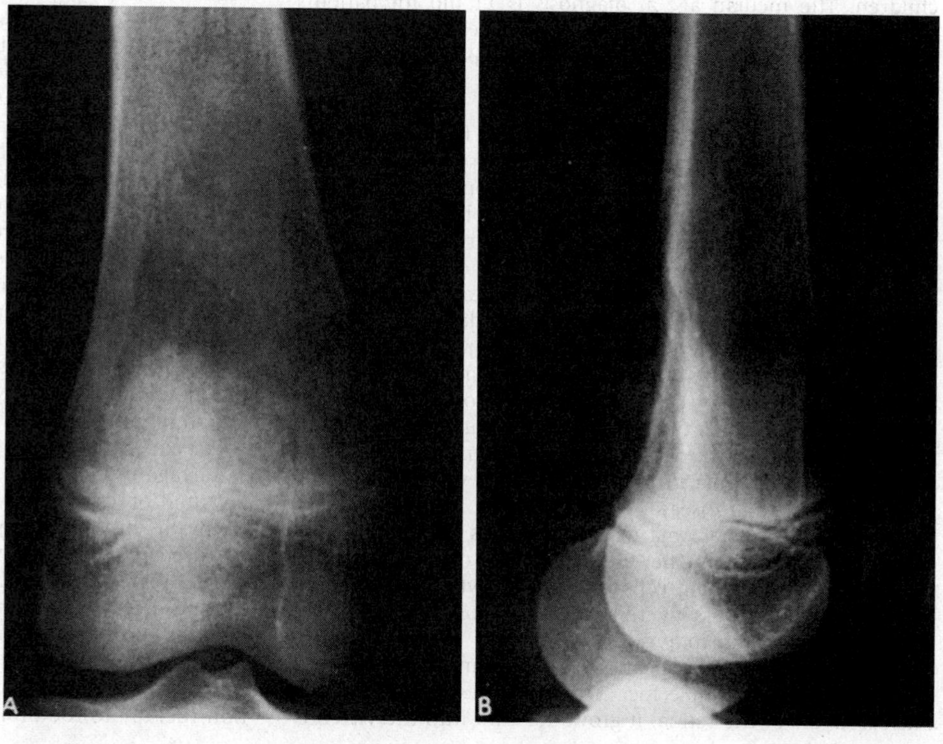

Figure 454–3. Anterior and lateral views of the distal femur of a patient with Ewing sarcoma. The lateral view shows the destruction of cortex, with growth of tumor into the surrounding soft tissues.

higher risk groups, it is unlikely that more than 33% are truly cured with available treatment, given the potential for late relapses.

454.3 Rare Bone Tumors

William M. Meyer

CHONDROSARCOMA. Characterized by the formation of cartilage by malignant spindle cells, chondrosarcoma arises most often in pelvic bones but also occurs in other flat bones of the trunk and in the extremities. Local recurrence is common. The diagnosis can be suspected based on the plain radiographic appearance, but biopsy is necessary to rule out osteosarcoma. The primary treatment, and the only therapy of proven benefit, is complete surgical resection. The tumors arising in the pelvis are often difficult to treat because location precludes complete resection. In such cases, chemotherapy and radiotherapy may produce tumor regression.

FIBROSARCOMA. These rare tumors arise primarily in soft tissue but can also occur in bone. The mainstay of therapy is surgical resection. Some centers use multiagent chemotherapy to prevent distant metastases.

CHAPTER 455

Retinoblastoma

Charles B. Pratt

This tumor occurs in about 1 in 16,000 live births in the United States, with a similar incidence among black and white children. The median age at diagnosis is 11 mo for patients with bilateral tumors and 23 mo for those with unilateral tumors. About 30% of patients with retinoblastoma have bilateral involvement and a dominantly inherited predisposition to the malignancy. Genetic predisposition also occurs in about 20% of patients with unilateral disease. The finding that retinoblastoma occurred in patients with "13q− syndrome" (characterized by growth delay, mental retardation, and facial and other anomalies) helped to localize the retinoblastoma gene to the long arm of chromosome 13 (see Chapter 446).

The *Rb* gene also carries an increased risk of other tumors. For example, in about 1% of the survivors of the hereditary form of retinoblastoma, osteosarcoma will develop by about 10 yr of age. These osteosarcomas may occur at an irradiated site or at a nonirradiated site and are sometimes multifocal. It is estimated that 30% of individuals cured of the hereditary form of retinoblastoma will have a second malignancy within 30 yr. In *trilateral retinoblastoma syndrome,* pineal tumors that are histologically similar to retinoblastoma develop in patients with bilateral ocular disease.

PATHOLOGY. Retinoblastoma usually develops in the posterior portion of the retina. The tumor consists of small, round, closely packed malignant cells with scanty cytoplasm. Rosette formation occurs, possibly reflecting an abortive attempt at formation of rod and cone cells.

Retinoblastoma may appear as a single tumor in the retina but typically has multiple foci. When it arises in the internal nuclear layers of the retina, it grows forward into the vitreous cavity. This endophytic growth is easily seen with the ophthalmoscope. Exophytic tumors (arising in the external nuclear layer and growing into the subretinal space, with detachment of the retina) are hidden, and the diagnosis is more difficult. Tumor fragments may break off from endophytic tumors and float free in the vitreous to "seed" other parts of the retina. Vitreous seeding is associated with large tumors (usually more than 5 disc diameters) and a poor prognosis. Extension of retinoblastoma into the choroid usually occurs with massive tumors and may indicate an increased likelihood of hematogenous metastases. Extension of tumor through the lamina cribrosa and down the optic nerve may lead to central nervous system involvement. Both choroidal and optic nerve invasion increase the risk of metastatic disease.

Because these tumors rarely metastasize before they are detected, the primary concern at diagnosis is generally preservation of useful vision. Accordingly, retinoblastoma is staged by the extent of disease within the eye.

CLINICAL MANIFESTATIONS. Retinoblastoma usually presents with leukocoria, a yellowish white reflex in the pupil caused by tumor behind the lens. Other common findings include diminished or absent vision and strabismus. With more advanced tumor, pupillary irregularity, hyphema, and pain may be present. Proptosis, signs of increased intracranial pressure, or bone pain may occur with very advanced or metastatic disease.

More than 80% of patients with hereditary retinoblastoma have tumors involving both eyes at the time of diagnosis. Multifocal disease involving a single globe is also associated with the hereditary form of retinoblastoma. Asynchronous involvement of both globes rarely appears after 18 mo of age. In the case of familial retinoblastoma, the disease may be discovered on routine funduscopic examination of the offspring or sibling of a patient who has had the disease.

DIAGNOSIS. The finding of leukocoria must be followed by a careful funduscopic examination, which usually requires anesthesia in children. Computed tomographic scan of the orbits should be performed to evaluate the extent of tumor and to assess whether optic nerve or bony structures are involved. Magnetic resonance imaging is of greater value in defining optic nerve invasion. Most intraocular retinoblastomas show evidence of intratumoral calcification. Ultrasonography may aid in the differential diagnosis, which includes other causes of leukocoria such as retinal detachment, persistent hyperplastic primary vitreous, nematode endophthalmitis (ocular larva migrans), bacterial panendophthalmitis, cataract, coloboma of the choroid, and retinopathy of prematurity.

Radionuclide bone scan and examinations of the bone marrow and cerebrospinal fluid for tumor cells are not necessary unless there is physical, radiographic, or histopathologic evidence of extraocular extension. Elevated plasma levels of carcinoembryonic antigen are rarely found at the time of diagnosis; a subsequent rise in levels may indicate recurrence of tumor.

TREATMENT. The standard treatment for unilateral disease is enucleation, although other measures such as cryotherapy and external beam irradiation may be more appropriate for single or multiple small lesions. If the tumors are so small that useful vision might be preserved, irradiation may be preferred. In unilateral disease, however, tumors this small are rare.

For patients with bilateral disease, attempts should be made to salvage useful vision in at least one eye by using radiotherapy and/or cryotherapy. Radiation may be given bilaterally from the outset because the eye that appears to be more involved may have a more dramatic response and be more salvageable. On the other hand, if an eye is so heavily involved that no useful vision remains or if painful glaucoma has developed as a complication, then enucleation is indicated. When enucleation is done, an attempt should be made to resect as much of the optic nerve as possible (10 mm or more). Radiation therapy to the orbit should also be considered if regional extraocular extension of the tumor has been found at the time of enucleation. Radiation therapy requires daily sedation and perhaps daily anesthesia.

Chemotherapy confers no definite benefit in patients whose tumors are localized to the globe. If there is gross or microscopic residual disease in the orbit after enucleation, then chemotherapy with a combination regimen (probably including cyclophosphamide and doxorubicin) should be considered along with radiotherapy. Widespread metastatic disease responds to chemotherapy, although cure is unlikely. Chemotherapy should also be considered for patients whose tumors extensively involve the choroid, sclera, or ciliary body.

PROGNOSIS. The overall survival rate is more than 90%, although survival into the 3rd and 4th decades of life may be decreased considerably by the high incidence of second malignancies. Cures are infrequent for patients with massive orbital disease or extensive optic nerve involvement at diagnosis, who are likely to have intracranial spread and distant metastases. If microscopic examination reveals tumor in the periglobal tissues of the optic nerve, there is a slight chance of long-term survival with irradiation and chemotherapy.

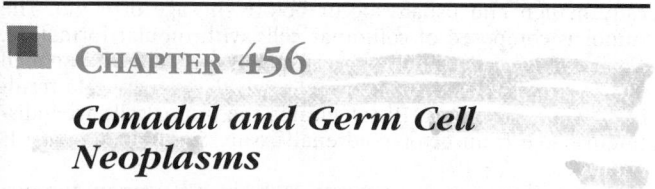

CHAPTER 456

Gonadal and Germ Cell Neoplasms

Neyssa M. Marina

EPIDEMIOLOGY. Malignant gonadal and germ cell tumors are rare in children, accounting for approximately 3% of childhood cancers. This figure underestimates the frequency of germ cell tumors, most of which are benign. For example, sacrococcygeal teratomas are the most common tumor in newborns, with an incidence of 1 in 35,000 live births. The relationship between age and risk varies with tumor types. A female predominance is seen for germ cell tumors in childhood and early adolescence, most likely reflecting the frequency of sacrococcygeal and ovarian tumors in this age group. After age 14 yr, the increased frequency of testicular tumors results in a male predominance. Populations at risk for gonadal or germ cell tumors include males with cryptorchidism and patients with gonadal dysgenesis. There are no other known predisposing features.

PATHOLOGY. Germ cell tumors originate from pluripotent germ cells that give rise to a variety of benign or malignant lesions. Embryonal differentiation of the primordial germ cells results in teratomas or embryonal carcinomas. Extraembryonic differentiation results in choriocarcinoma or yolk sac carcinoma. Hence, the histologic classification of germ cell tumors is based on the differentiation pathway (Fig. 456–1). These tumors are often subclassified by their primary site. Extragonadal tumors, thought to result from aberrant migration of germ cells from the yolk sac into the germinal ridge of the developing fetus, typically are more malignant than gonadal tumors.

Benign lesions, most often cystic teratomas, account for most germ cell tumors. The likelihood of malignancy varies with the primary site and age of the patient. Ovarian germ cell tumors are usually benign in patients younger than 10 yr, about 30% are malignant in adolescents. For sacrococcygeal tumors, the incidence of malignancy increases from 10% at birth to 50–70% at age 2 mo.

Choriocarcinomas are highly malignant tumors that can occur in both gonadal and extragonadal sites. Ovarian choriocarcinoma can develop before puberty, whereas testicular and mediastinal choriocarcinomas are seen only in patients who have reached puberty. Microscopically, the tumor consists of cytotrophoblasts and syncytiotrophoblasts, often with necrosis and hemorrhage. The high serum levels of human chorionic gonadotropin (β-HCG) produced by these tumors provide crucial information at diagnosis and during treatment.

Yolk sac carcinoma is also termed endodermal sinus tumor because it resembles the endodermal sinuses of the rat placenta. Histologically, the presence of Schiller-Duval bodies is diagnostic. Elevated serum levels of α-fetoprotein (AFP) are a consistent biologic marker.

Embryonal carcinoma consists of poorly differentiated cells with an epithelial appearance. It is rare as a pure histologic type in infants and children but occurs fairly frequently admixed with yolk sac carcinoma or teratoma.

Seminomas occur in the testicle and, rarely, in the mediastinum during or after adolescence. Histologically, the tumor is composed of clear cells aggregated in lobules and separated by

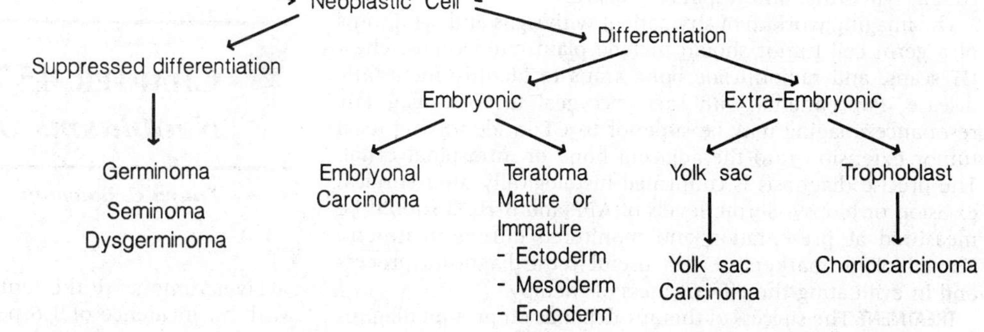

Figure 456–1. Tumors of germ cell origin. (Adapted from Pierce GB, Abeli MR: Embryonal carcinoma of the testis. Pathol Ann 5:27, 1970.)

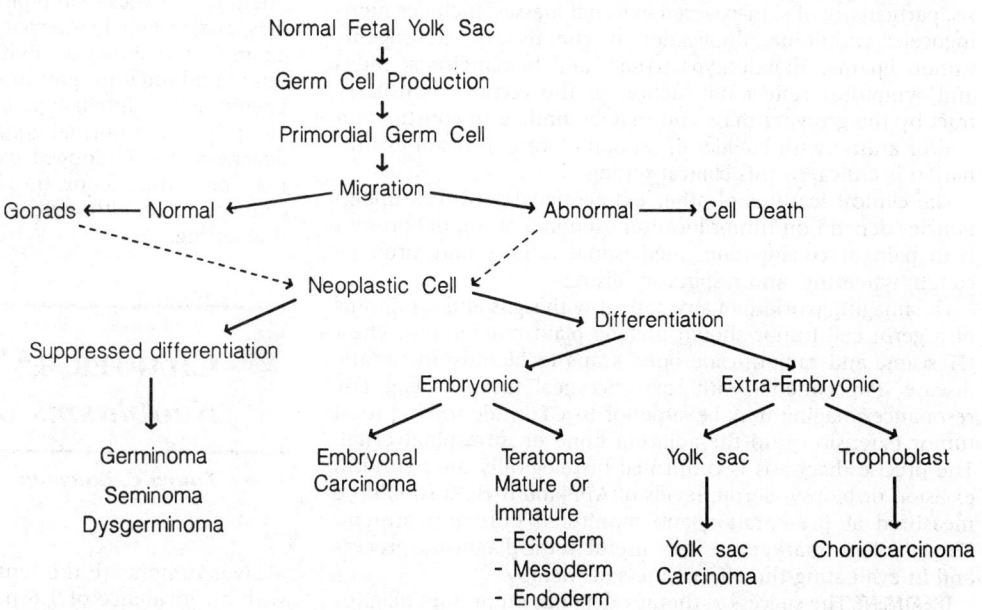

fibrous stroma. There are no associated biologic markers; if the patient has an elevated β-HCG or AFP level, the histologic analysis should be reviewed for the presence of another malignant element. Dysgerminoma, the ovarian counterpart of seminoma, is morphologically and histologically identical to primordial germ cells. Unlike seminomas, these tumors often occur before puberty.

Teratomas are usually benign germ cell tumors that consist of at least two, and sometimes three, germ layers. The degree of malignancy is assessed histologically using a grading system that correlates with the malignant potential and the capacity to metastasize.

CLINICAL MANIFESTATIONS AND DIAGNOSIS. Most germ cell tumors are testicular, ovarian, or sacrococcygeal. Extragonadal tumors also occur, albeit less frequently, in other midline sites (retroperitoneum, mediastinum, head/neck, central nervous system).

Testicular germ cell tumors in infants usually present as a painless mass in the scrotum, with no signs of inflammation. Metastatic disease is rare in this age group. In older boys, swelling of the involved testicle is usually noted over a period of weeks, with pain and tenderness in some cases. Gynecomastia may occur if the tumor secretes β-HCG. Adolescents may present with clinical evidence of metastases to either retroperitoneal lymph nodes or lungs. The chief diagnostic tools are careful physical examination and, because the tumors are usually solid, transillumination. Computed tomography (CT) is used to evaluate the presence of metastatic disease. These studies are followed promptly by surgery (usually, inguinal orchiectomy) and histologic examination.

Patients with *ovarian germ cell tumors* most often present with acute or chronic pain and an enlarged abdomen. In patients who lack symptoms, tumor may first be suggested by an abdominal mass or fullness on routine physical examination. The acute onset of abdominal pain resulting from ovarian torsion can mimic appendicitis or other inflammatory processes. Ultrasound examination to confirm the presence and location of a mass should be followed by CT of the chest, abdomen, and pelvis for staging purposes. Ovarian germ cell tumors can metastasize to the peritoneal cavity by implantation or regional extension but seldom metastasize beyond the abdominal cavity.

Sacrococcygeal germ cell tumors are usually detected at birth or during infancy. Tumors are mainly intrapelvic in only a small percentage of patients; most (90%) have an external component involving the buttocks or sacrum. The differential diagnosis, particularly of skin-covered external masses, includes meningocele, chordoma, duplication of the rectum, neurogenic tumor, lipoma, rhabdomyosarcoma, and hemangioma. Signs and symptoms reflect obstruction of the rectum or urinary tract by the growing mass and may be limited to constipation and/or anuria with bladder distention. A careful rectal examination is critical in this clinical setting.

The clinical features of other extragonadal germ cell malignancies depend on tumor location. Abdominal tumors present with pain or constipation; mediastinal tumors may produce cough, wheezing, and respiratory distress.

The imaging workup of any patient with signs and symptoms of a germ cell tumor should include plain radiographs, chest CT scans, and radionuclide bone scans to identify metastatic disease. For patients with sacrococcygeal tumors, magnetic resonance imaging may be superior to CT in identifying local tumor extension into the adjacent bone or intraspinal canal. The precise diagnosis is confirmed histologically after surgical excision or biopsy. Serum levels of AFP and β-HCG should be measured at presentation and monitored during treatment. These biologic markers are very useful in the diagnostic process and in evaluating the effectiveness of therapy.

TREATMENT. The success of therapy depends on prompt diagnosis and, whenever possible, surgical excision. However, high-risk or unduly disfiguring surgery is avoided because these tumors are very chemosensitive. Traditionally, dysgerminomas and seminomas have been treated with radiotherapy. Chemotherapy offers the option of preserving fertility and is now the preferred therapy. Most patients with malignant germ cell tumors, regardless of stage, should receive combination chemotherapy because of the likelihood of subclinical dissemination at the time of diagnosis. The most commonly used combination (cisplatin, bleomycin, etoposide) produces excellent results with minimal long-term sequelae. Cyclophosphamide (cytoxan) and ifosfamide (Ifex) are also active agents.

PROGNOSIS. Prognosis depends on disease extent at diagnosis and on primary site (gonadal versus extragonadal). With modern therapy, 70–80% of all patients with malignant germ cell tumors will be alive without disease 5 yr after diagnosis. For patients with localized disease and an excellent prognosis, current trials focus on minimizing toxicity. Treatment outcome is less favorable (40–70% 5-yr survival rate) for patients with advanced disease, and clinical studies focus on intensifying therapy. Some patients with recurrent disease can achieve remission or cure with salvage therapy.

OTHER TUMORS OF THE GONADS. Nongerm cell gonadal tumors are uncommon in children. *Sertoli tumors* of the testicle are typically benign and usually occur before the age of 6 mo. The tumor is composed of columnar cells with tubular formation. *Leydig cell tumors* in children are also benign, occurring between the ages of 4–9 yr, with associated sexual precocity as a result of hormone secretion. Histologically, the tumor cells are indistinguishable from ectopic adrenal tissue. Surgical resection is curative.

Benign ovarian cysts represent 50% of all ovarian tumors. Cysts may be found incidentally at laparotomy or on routine physical examination. Occasionally, torsion of the involved ovary can mimic an acute abdomen with abdominal pain, nausea, and vomiting. Other ovarian tumors are rare. The *granulosa-theca cell tumor*, a typically benign lesion, is thought to arise in cells of ovarian stromal origin. It is associated with precocious puberty; endocrine abnormalities resolve after surgery. *Cystadenocarcinoma* of the ovary can be differentiated from other malignant ovarian tumors only by histology. *Hemangiomas* may involve the ovary in rare cases, and ovarian enlargement is the first manifestation of *lymphoma* in a small percentage of cases.

Gonadoblastomas occur only in patients with gonadal dysgenesis. Eighty per cent of affected patients are phenotypic females, usually with evidence of virilization; the remainder are phenotypic males who typically have cryptorchidism, hypospadias, and/or female internal or secondary sex organs. Histologic examination shows a mixture of germ cells and elements resembling immature granulosa or Sertoli cells, with or without Leydig cells or lutein-type cells. The tumor should be removed along with the normal gonad, which may undergo malignant degeneration. Prolonged exogenous hormone administration may be required for the development of secondary sexual characteristics, although secondary uterine cancer is a risk in this setting.

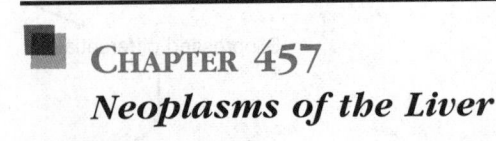

CHAPTER 457
Neoplasms of the Liver

Laura C. Bowman

Liver tumors are the tenth most frequent pediatric tumors, with an incidence of 1.6 per million children. Hepatic malignancy must be distinguished from benign hepatic tumor and non-neoplastic hepatomegaly; metastatic disease must be distinguished from a primary tumor. Almost 50% of primary liver tumors are benign. In children, liver tumors more often represent metastatic disease (neuroblastoma, Wilms tumor) than primary malignancies.

457.1 Hepatoblastoma

Hepatoblastoma is the most common primary malignant liver neoplasm in children. The median age at diagnosis is 1 yr, and most cases occur in children younger than 3 yr. Males are affected more often than females. Hepatoblastoma has been reported in sibling pairs and is also associated with congenital anomalies, including hemihypertrophy, Beckwith-Wiedemann syndrome, diaphragmatic and umbilical hernias, Meckel diverticulum, and renal anomalies. This tumor is composed of immature hepatic epithelial tissue with varying degrees of differentiation. There are four histopathologic subtypes: fetal, embryonal, macrotrabecular, and anaplastic. A mixed subtype contains mesenchymal and squamous elements and may incorporate fibrous tissue, osteoid, cartilage, muscle, and hematopoietic tissue.

CLINICAL AND LABORATORY CHARACTERISTICS. Most children present with an enlarging, asymptomatic abdominal mass. Pain, fever, weight loss, and/or vomiting are present in a minority of cases. Jaundice is rare. An occasional patient presents with isosexual precocious puberty secondary to β-human chorionic gonadotropin hormone secretion. Another rare presentation involves severe osteoporosis with pathologic fractures and vertebral compression fractures. Osteopenia improves with tumor regression or excision.

Sixty-six per cent of patients have elevated serum levels of α-fetoprotein. Significant thrombocytosis, mild anemia, and moderate leukocytosis are also common. Serum alkaline phosphatase, glutamic oxaloacetic transaminase, and glutamic pyruvic transaminase levels are often normal. Radiographs of the abdomen demonstrate hepatic enlargement with intratumor calcification in about 30% of the cases. Computed tomographic scans of the abdomen and chest are essential because 10–20% of patients present with pulmonary or nodal metastatic disease. Most tumors are in the right lobe, although bilobar and multicentric tumors can occur. Angiography to delineate blood supply has largely been replaced by magnetic resonance imaging, which also demonstrates adjacent structures.

TREATMENT AND OUTCOME. Surgical excision of the primary tumor is necessary to achieve a cure but is initially feasible in only 50%. Fortunately, hepatoblastoma is highly chemosensitive, and preoperative chemotherapy allows resection of initially unresectable tumors in 70%. Pulmonary metastases may also respond to chemotherapy; resistant or recurrent pulmonary disease is treated by both surgery and chemotherapy. Successful treatment regimens include cisplatin (Platinol) in combination with either vincristine (Oncovin) and 5-fluorouracil or doxorubicin (Adriamycin). The 3-yr survival rate exceeds 90% in patients with initially resected tumors, is approximately 65% in those with initially unresectable tumors, and is only 10–20% in patients with metastatic disease.

457.2 Hepatocellular Carcinoma

Hepatocellular carcinoma (HCC) occurs most often in older children (12–15 yr), although there is also a peak in incidence before age 4 yr. Approximately 33% have cirrhosis secondary to metabolic abnormalities (galactosemia, tyrosinosis), glycogen storage disease, malnutrition, biliary atresia, or giant cell hepatitis. Pathologically, the tumor is similar to HCC in adults, with tumor cells that are larger than normal hepatocytes and nuclear pleomorphism and prominent nucleoli. The fibrolamellar variant, characterized by a broad fibrous septum and hyaline eosinophilic cytoplasm, is associated with a better prognosis. This variant typically arises in a noncirrhotic liver and is more prevalent in adolescents and young adults.

CLINICAL MANIFESTATIONS AND LABORATORY DATA. Abdominal distention and a right upper quadrant mass are common presenting features. About 50% have abdominal pain; nausea and vomiting are common. Systemic symptoms such as fever, weight loss, and anorexia are more common in HCC than hepatoblastoma. Laboratory findings are similar for the two malignancies, except that thrombocytosis is less common and elevated transaminase levels are more common in HCC. Serum α-fetoprotein is elevated in about 50% but often to a lesser extent than in hepatoblastoma. The imaging workup is the same as that for hepatoblastoma. Intratumor calcification is less common. As in hepatoblastoma, the right lobe is the most common primary site (although HCC is more often multicentric), and lung and lymph nodes are the most common metastatic sites. Hence, differentiation of HCC and hepatoblastoma is often difficult both clinically and pathologically.

TREATMENT AND OUTCOME. Complete surgical excision is the only effective treatment, although complete resection at diagnosis is possible in only 33%; resected tumors recur in approximately 75% of cases. The fibrolamellar variant is more often resectable, which may explain its better prognosis. Responses to chemotherapy with agents such as doxorubicin, etoposide (VePesid), 5-fluorouracil, and cisplatin are seen in 30–40% of cases but are short-lived. The overall prognosis remains very poor.

457.3 Benign Tumors

Cavernous hemangiomas occur most commonly in early childhood and may produce large masses. *Hemangioendothelioma* occurs in the liver as either solitary or multifocal lesions; lesions in other organs, particularly the skin, are common. Large lesions occasionally present with high-output congestive heart failure or thrombocytopenia as a result of platelet sequestration. Other benign liver lesions, in order of frequency, are *mesenchymal hamartoma, focal nodular hyperplasia,* and *liver cell adenoma.* Surgical excision, when feasible, is the usual approach to benign liver lesions. Liver transplantation is a promising therapy for patients with unresectable benign tumors or the rare low-grade malignant tumors that are unlikely to metastasize.

CHAPTER 458
Gastrointestinal Neoplasms

Charles B. Pratt

See also Chapter 291.

458.1 Salivary Gland Tumors

Enlargements of the salivary glands usually result from benign causes such as infection or the formation of mucoceles.

About 66% of tumors that involve the salivary glands are benign hemangiomas, hamartomas, or mixed tumors of salivary glands (pleomorphic adenoma).

Mixed tumors are rare during the 1st decade of life; they occur occasionally during the 2nd decade and are evenly distributed between boys and girls. The gland most often involved is the parotid, and the most frequent presenting manifestation is a mass, usually firm and nontender. Facial nerve paralysis may occur. Treatment is excision of the tumor. The prognosis for disease control is excellent, although recurrence may necessitate a second surgical procedure.

Mucoepidermoid carcinoma, a malignant tumor of the salivary glands, is found primarily during the 2nd decade of life and most frequently involves the parotid gland, usually as a hard, nontender mass. Metastases to regional lymph nodes are unusual and confer a poor prognosis. As with mixed tumors, complete excision produces an excellent prognosis, although local recurrence may necessitate a second surgery. Parotid neoplasms may occur as second malignancies in patients who receive radiation therapy as central nervous system preventive treatment for childhood leukemia.

458.2 Nasopharyngeal Carcinoma

In adults, this tumor is most common in the Far East and North Africa, where it may occur in familial clusters. There is a high degree of association with the Epstein-Barr virus. In the United States, nasopharyngeal carcinoma occurs in or after the 2nd decade of life. Black children in the southern United States appear to have a higher incidence than do white children. Male predominance is observed in adults but not in children. The histologic appearance is that of undifferentiated carcinoma.

The most frequent early finding is cervical adenopathy, which is usually unilateral. Other early symptoms and signs are trismus, epistaxis, sore throat, and difficulty in swallowing. There may be weight loss as a result of dysphagia.

Diagnosis is usually based on biopsy of a cervical node. On careful examination, including computed tomographic (CT) or magnetic resonance imaging scans, it may be possible to locate the primary tumor. Multiple biopsies of the nasopharynx may be required to obtain appropriate tissue. Extension occurs locally to the base of the skull and to the soft tissues surrounding the nasopharynx. Regional lymph node metastases are common, and hematogenous spread to bone and lung may occur.

The primary therapy is irradiation of the involved areas of the nasopharynx, which is curative in more than 50% of cases. A cisplatin (Platinol)/5-fluorouracil/methotrexate chemotherapeutic regimen is also utilized, in schedules similar to those used to treat head and neck carcinomas in adults.

458.3 Carcinoma of the Stomach

This form of gastrointestinal cancer is extremely rare in children. A noticeable mass is the usual symptom; bleeding and gastric obstruction also occur. Malignant lesions affecting the stomach are most often lymphomas or soft tissue sarcomas (leiomyosarcomas). If the lesion is a true carcinoma, resection is the treatment of choice. The responses of adult gastric carcinomas to chemotherapy are generally unsatisfactory.

458.4 Pancreatic Tumors

Pancreatic carcinoma is rarely seen in children and young adults. The usual site of origin is the head of the pancreas, and the initial clinical findings are those of upper abdominal mass, weight loss, pain, and icterus. Obstruction of the common bile duct may lead to obstructive jaundice. Treatment is resection when possible. As in adult patients, the prognosis is poor. These tumors generally do not respond to irradiation. Chemotherapeutic agents (5-fluorouracil, the nitrosoureas, doxorubicin, alkylating agents) may prolong survival or provide palliation in advance disease.

Pancreatoblastoma is an exocrine tumor that behaves in a benign fashion. It is typically located in the head of the pancreas. Because the lesion is encapsulated and does not communicate with pancreatic ducts, it can be removed without interfering with pancreatic function. The symptoms generally are those of an abdominal mass. The prognosis is favorable after resection of these tumors, which must therefore be differentiated from pancreatic carcinoma.

β-Cell endocrine tumors are generally seen in the form of diffuse islet cell malformation or dysplasia (see Chapters 77 and 93.2). Diagnosis is based on the finding of hypoglycemia followed by the demonstration that there are high serum levels of insulin, even at low glucose levels, confirming the autonomous behavior of islet cells. Pancreatectomy is the treatment of choice.

458.5 Colonic Polyps

The juvenile or retention polyp constitutes about 85% of all colorectal polypoid lesions in children. Bright red rectal bleeding (painless) is the most common presenting sign or symptom and occurs in almost all cases. These polyps become symptomatic when children are 3–5 yr of age. Most can be removed through a sigmoidoscope. A new polyp or polyps develops in about 25% of cases. Although these polyps are not premalignant lesions per se, the entity known as *multiple juvenile polyposis* may not be benign. Adenomatous polyps may coexist with these lesions, but true adenomatous polyps of the colon are rare in children, except as part of the familial polyposis or Gardner syndrome (see Chapter 291). Adenomatous polyps are more frequently seen in adult patients and may later be associated with the development of adenocarcinoma of the large bowel.

458.6 Adenocarcinoma of the Colon and Rectum

These cancers represent fewer than 1% of malignant tumors in children, but they can occur during the 1st and 2nd decades of life. Affected patients may present with bloody stools or melena, abdominal pain, anorexia, weight loss, and intestinal obstruction. Signs are often vague, lending to delay in diagnosis. An abdominal mass may be palpable, and hepatomegaly or ascites may be present. The diagnosis can be confirmed by barium enema, direct endoscopic examination, or both. CT scans of the abdomen and pelvis may detect hepatic metastases, retroperitoneal lymphadenopathy, or ovarian metastases. The tumor is rarely confined to the mucosa at the time of diagnosis, usually extending through the serosa with involvement of the regional lymph nodes and peritoneum. Girls can present with or have ovarian metastasis develop after contamination of the peritoneal cavity by tumor spread. Late hematogenous dissemination may occur. Predisposing conditions are familial multiple polyposis, ulcerative colitis, regional enteritis, and the Peutz-Jeghers syndrome. Regular endoscopic examination and prophylactic colectomy may be recommended for these patients. Prognosis is extremely poor for adolescent patients with colorectal carcinoma because of the usual extension of these tumors before diagnosis. Treatment should include 5-fluorouracil/leucovorin/interferon alfa-2a as adjuvant chemotherapy for stage 3 disease and similar agents with therapeutic intent for stage 4 disease. Irradiation is useful in the treatment of rectal carcinomas.

CHAPTER 459
Carcinomas

Charles B. Pratt

CLEAR CELL ADENOCARCINOMA OF THE VAGINA AND CERVIX. This rare tumor has been associated with intrauterine exposure to diethylstilbestrol. Anomalies of the cervix may also occur in affected patients (see Chapter 508).

CARCINOMA OF THE THYROID. Thyroid cancer is discussed in Chapter 524. The incidence is increased in patients who have had head and neck irradiation in childhood. Spontaneous thyroid cancer is more common in girls than boys and is most likely to be papillary in nature and to grow slowly. Medullary carcinoma of the thyroid may occur sporadically or in a familial pattern. In its familial form, it is associated with Marfan-like habitus, mucosal neuromas, and multiple endocrine neoplasias (pheochromocytoma, hyperparathyroidism).

CARCINOMA OF THE ADRENAL GLAND. Adrenocortical carcinoma is rare. It may occur at any age during childhood but is more common during the first few years. Recent reports indicate that this tumor has a relatively high frequency in Brazil. The tumor may be associated with hemangiomas of the skin, hemihypertrophy, urinary tract anomalies, and astrocytomas. Girls predominate among patients with this tumor. The usual presenting symptoms are secondary to the endocrine function of the cancer. Affected children present signs of adrenal hyperfunction (see Chapter 530), which may include Cushing syndrome (see Chapter 530), virilization (see Chapter 529), feminization (see Chapter 532), or a combination of these. Prognosis is dependent on tumor size, extent of tumor, and resectability. The adrenolytic agent mitotane (Lysodren) has demonstrated antitumor activity; other anticancer agents with ill-defined activity against this tumor include cisplatin (Platinol) and etoposide (VePesid).

CARCINOMA OF THE BREAST (see Chapter 112).

CHAPTER 460
Cancer of the Skin

Charles B. Pratt

Cancer of the skin is rare in children but is probably increasing in frequency (see Chapter 620). *Malignant melanoma* may occur during the first 2 decades, with clinical behavior similar to that seen in adults. It usually appears as a rapidly growing, easily traumatized, ulcerated lesion that is darkly pigmented or has changed in color. Melanoma may be found on any part of the body. Certain conditions such as *giant hairy nevi* (bathing trunk nevus) and *dysplastic nevus syndrome* predispose to the development of melanoma. Because malignant melanoma is rare in children, biopsy of a suspicious lesion is indicated initially. If malignancy is found, then wide local resection is indicated and may necessitate skin grafting. Regional lymph nodes should be examined carefully; if they are enlarged, a lymph node dissection should also be performed. For patients with metastatic disease, responses have been seen following chemotherapy with vincristine (Oncovin)/cyclophosphamide (Cytoxan)/dactinomycin (Cosmegen), dacarbazine, cisplatin (Platinol)/etoposide (VePesid), or interferon alfa-2a (Roferon-A).

Xeroderma pigmentosum is an autosomal recessive condition associated with a defective DNA repair mechanism. When the affected person is exposed to sunlight, the ultraviolet radiation produces breaks in DNA, providing an opportunity for mutant malignant growth. The skin is the organ of primary involvement. Multiple skin cancers (basal cell, squamous cell, melanomas) may appear in the exposed areas. Surgical resection of the tumors is necessary, and affected children must be protected as much as possible from sunlight. The *nevoid basal cell carcinoma syndrome* (basal cell nevus syndrome) is discussed in Chapter 620.

CHAPTER 461
Benign Tumors

Alberto S. Pappo

A variety of benign tumors in infants and children present diagnostic challenges. Many of these tumors require treatment. Some, although histologically benign, can be life-threatening.

461.1 Benign Tumors and Tumor-Like Processes of Bone

Like malignant tumors, benign bone lesions can present with pain, local inflammation, and a limp (Table 461–1). High-quality radiographs of the involved area are essential in evaluating the primary bone lesion.

Osteoid osteoma affects children and adolescents 10–25 yr of

■ **TABLE 461–1 Benign Bone Tumors and Cysts**

Disease	Characteristics	Roentgenography	Treatment	Prognosis
Osteochondroma (osteocartilaginous exostosis)	Common; distal metaphysis of femur, proximal humerus, proximal tibia; painless, hard, nontender mass	Bony outgrowth, sessile or pedunculated	Excision, if symptomatic	Excellent; malignant transformation rare
Multiple hereditary exostoses	Osteochondroma of long bones; bone growth disturbances	As above	As above	Recurrences
Osteoid ostoma	Point tenderness; pain relieved by aspirin; femur and tibia; predominantly found in boys	Osteosclerosis surrounds small radiolucent nidus, 1 cm	As above	Excellent
Giant osteoid osteoma (osteoblastoma)	As above, but more destructive	Osteolytic component; size greater than 1 cm	As above	Excellent
Enchondroma	Tubular bones of hands and feet; pathologic fractures, swollen bone; Ollier disease if multiple lesions are present	Radiolucent diaphyseal or metaphyseal lesion; may calcify	Excision or curettage	Excellent; malignant transformation rare
Nonossifying fibroma	Silent; rare pathologic fracture; late childhood adolescence	Incidental roentgenographic finding; thin sclerotic border, radiolucent lesion	None or curettage with fractures	Excellent; heals spontaneously
Eosinophilic granuloma	Age 5–10 yr; skull, jaw, long bones; pathologic fracture; pain	Small, radiolucent without reactive bone; punched-out lytic lesion	Biopsy, excision rare; irradiation	Excellent; may heal spontaneously
Brodie abscess	Insidious local pain; limp; suspected as malignancy	Circumscribed metaphyseal osteomyelitis; lytic lesions with sclerotic rim	Biopsy; antibiotics	Excellent
Unicameral bone cyst (simple bone cyst)	Metaphysis of long bone (femur, humerus); pain, pathologic fracture	Cyst in medullary canal, expands cortex; fluid-filled unilocular or multilocular cavity	Curettage; steroid injection into lesion	Excellent, some heal spontaneously
Aneurysmal bone cyst	As above; contains blood, fibrous tissue	Expands beyond metaphyseal cartilage	Curettage, bone graft	Excellent

(From Behrman R, Kliegman R (eds): Nelson Essentials of Pediatrics, 2nd ed. Philadelphia, WB Saunders, 1994.)

age. There is a male predominance; it usually arises in the femur and tibia. The cardinal clinical feature is pain, which is typically more severe at night and is relieved by aspirin. Signs of inflammation are unusual. The roentgenogram is diagnostic, disclosing a sharply demarcated radiolucent nidus of osteoid tissue surrounded by sclerotic bone. Treatment is surgical; the nidus must be completely removed to prevent recurrence.

Fibrous dysplasia is the most common developmental osseous anomaly. It manifests in late childhood and can be either monostotic or polyostotic. This lesion is frequently seen in association with a pathologic fracture and is a common cause of nonunion. Surgical resection should be postponed until the patient is fully grown because lesions can grow until the adolescent growth spurt is completed. Polyostotic fibrous dysplasia associated with skin hyperpigmentation and endocrine dysfunction is known as Albright syndrome.

Benign fibrous cortical defects occur in 30–40% of children, usually between the ages of 4–8 yr. About 50% are bilateral or multiple, and 90% are located in the distal femur. Nonossifying fibromas are lytic lesions that originate in the metaphyseal regions of long bones. Most are found incidentally on radiographs. The lesions are usually asymptomatic, but chronic bone pain and pathologic fractures may be evident with large lesions. On plain radiographs, they are eccentrically located, are ovoid, and have a loculated portion with a sclerotic medullary border. Treatment is often unnecessary because spontaneous regression can be expected after months or years. Curettage or other interventions may be required for weakened or fractured bones.

Osteochondroma is the most common benign tumor of bone and commonly affects individuals in the 2nd decade of life. It can occur in any bone formed in cartilage but often involves the distal metaphysis of the femur and proximal metaphysis of the tibia. Growth ceases with closure of the neighboring epiphyseal plates, at which time ossification of the cartilaginous cap may occur. A mass may be present, or pain may occur if there is a pathologic fracture. Roentgenographic features are characteristic. Some lesions are pedunculated; others are sessile. In rare cases, reactivation of growth occurs spontaneously, sometimes after a fracture; such lesions should be considered malignant until proved otherwise by occasional biopsy. Lesions that cause pain or disfigurement should be removed. These patients have a small (1%) risk of having chondrosarcomas develop, which are most often associated with lesions in the hip joint area.

Enchondroma is a solitary lesion that involves metacarpals, metatarsals, and phalanges in 35% of the cases. Enchondromas appear as deforming masses or become apparent when they induce pathologic fractures. Radiographs show circumscribed areas of rarefied bone with thinning and often bulging of the cortex and stippled calcification. Lesions in the hands or feet are generally benign; those in the large tubular bones have greater malignant potential and may be difficult to separate histologically from malignant lesions. Treatment consists of curettage for well-contained lesions and autologous bone grafting for extensive lesions in the metacarpals or phalanges. Tumors in long tubular bones and pelvis often require en bloc resection. The presence of multiple enchondromas is known as Ollier disease. These lesions commonly occur in the phalanges and metacarpals but can also be found in the femur, tibia, and iliac crest. A high rate of malignant transformation (up to 50%) has been reported.

Aneurysmal bone cysts can affect any bone. Radiographically, these lesions show a lytic expansile lesion that is well demarcated and lacks a sclerotic ring. Curettage, bone grafting, and cryosurgery are commonly used to remove the cysts.

Simple unicameral bone cysts arise close to the epiphyseal plate and commonly involve the proximal humerus and proximal femur. The cavity is unilocular or multilocular and contains fluid or blood. The origin of the cysts is unknown, although they have been attributed to traumatic hematomas. Symptoms may be absent or scant, and the cysts may be identified because of pathologic fracture. The roentgenographic appearance consists of an area of rarefaction, often pseudoloculated, that does not cross the epiphyseal plate. These cysts may resolve spontaneously. Upper extremity cysts may not need therapy; those of the lower extremity pose a greater risk of fracture and should generally be treated with curettage or excision.

FIBROMATOSES. Fibromatoses account for less than 1% of all pediatric solid tumors, yet they are the most common neoplastic myoblastic-fibroblastic growth in children. Sites of presentation, growth rate, and response to therapy vary markedly, but all fibromatoses tend to infiltrate without destroying neighboring tissue. The juvenile hyalin variant, which affects children 2–5 yr of age, is very rare. It is characterized by the presence of multiple painless cutaneous papules located in the head, back, and extremities. Lesions may continue to appear during adulthood. Surgical excision offers the only definitive treatment. Infantile myofibromatosis commonly affects children during the first 5 yr of life and often arises as a solitary mass located in the soft tissue. These lesions should be removed completely, with negative surgical margins, to prevent local recurrence. For extensive lesions, radiotherapy, tamoxifen (Nolvadex), vincristine (Oncovin), and dactinomycin (Cosmegen) have been used with variable results.

461.2 Hemangioma

Hemangioma is the most common tumor in infants, occurring in 10% of white children and in up to 20% of premature infants weighing less than 1,000 g. Hemangiomas most commonly occur in the skin, are often solitary, predominate in girls, and are rarely fully developed at the time of birth. Nearly 60% are found over the head and neck region. They are characterized by a proliferative growth phase that lasts 6–10 mo and an involutional phase characterized by slow regression of the hemangioma, with nearly 50% of the lesions resolving by age 5 yr and 90% by age 10 yr.

In fewer than 10%, rapidly growing hemangiomas of the head and neck can produce serious or life-threatening complications. Growth of these tumors can produce airway and ear canal obstructions, pressure necrosis of surrounding structures, amblyopia, and feeding difficulties. The tumors can become secondarily infected through the ulceration of overlying skin. If arteriovenous communications of sufficient size develop, congestive cardiac failure can ensue.

Resection of large tumors is frequently difficult because of extensive involvement; complete removal is sometimes impossible. In some cases, prednisone may suppress tumor growth or produce regression. Administration of interferon alfa-2a (Roferon-A) produces significant clinical regressions in most infants with life-threatening hemangiomas. Laser photocoagulation may also offer a treatment alternative in some cases.

Kasabach-Merritt syndrome is a distinct entity characterized by cavernous hemangioma, microangiopathic hemolytic anemia, thrombocytopenia, and consumptive coagulopathy. Treatment is often supportive and should be directed toward improving the coagulopathy using platelets, cryoprecipitate, and fresh frozen plasma and reduction of the size of the hemangioma with steroids. Heparin and antifibrinolytic agents such as aminocaproic acid (Amicar) and tranexamic acid (Amstat) may also be used.

Hemangioendotheliomas of the liver are rare. Initial symptoms include jaundice, vomiting or diarrhea, and abdominal swelling. Radiographs of the abdomen show an enlarged liver and occasionally calcification in the tumor. Radionuclide and computed tomographic scans of liver and spleen show the defect in hepatic tissue; hepatic angiograms show an abnormal vascular pattern. Initial treatment with prednisone and/or radiation has been recommended. Interferon alfa-2a also appears promising. Surgical resection should be considered when the hemangioma is confined to a single lobe, when severe hemorrhage develops, or when congestive heart failure unresponsive to therapy occurs. Hepatic artery catheter embolization has been used in selected patients.

461.3 Lymphatic Malformations

Formerly called lymphangiomas, lymphatic malformations are the second most common benign vascular tumor in children. Lymphatic malformations may be localized or generalized and commonly occur in the cervicofacial region, axilla, and thorax. Like hemangiomas, they appear early in life, with almost all cases evident by the age of 3 yr. They rarely regress spontaneously and may obstruct the aerodigestive tract or expand in size secondary to hemorrhage. The extent of disease should be determined before therapy. Staged surgical resection is recommended because most lesions are diffuse and not easily dissected.

461.4 Thymoma

Thymoma is rare in children and occurs with equal frequency in boys and girls. Frequently associated conditions include myasthenia gravis, red cell aplasia, and hypogammaglobulinemia. With tumor growth, there may be progressive compression of surrounding tissues, leading to the development of cough, dyspnea, dysphagia, and even superior vena cava compression.

Thymomas are slow growing, tend to be locally invasive, and rarely metastasize. The treatment of choice is complete surgical excision. The tumor is radiosensitive, and radiotherapy should be used in cases of invasive disease. Chemotherapy with doxorubicin (Adriamycin), cyclophosphamide (cytoxan), and cisplatin (Platinol) has produced responses in advanced disease.

BONE MARROW TRANSPLANTATION AS THERAPY

Armitage JO: Bone marrow transplantation. N Engl J Med 330:827, 1994.

Bensinger WI: Supportive care in bone marrow transplantation. Curr Opin Oncol 4:614, 1992.

Brenner MK, Heslop HE: Graft-versus-host reactions and bone marrow transplantation. Curr Opin Immunol 3:752, 1992.

Ferrara JLM, Deeg HJ: Mechanisms of disease: Graft versus host disease. N Engl J Med 324:667, 1992.

Johnson FL, Goldman S: Role of autotransplantation in neuroblastoma. Hematol Oncol Clin North Am 7:647, 1993.

Kumar L: Secondary leukemia after autologous bone marrow transplantation. Lancet 345:810, 1995.

Ramsay NKC, Kersey JH: Indications for bone marrow transplantation in acute lymphoblastic leukemia. Blood 75:815, 1990.

Robertson KA: Pediatric bone marrow transplantation. Curr Opin Pediatr 5:103, 1993.

Wingard JR: Advances in the management of infectious complications after bone marrow transplantation. Bone Marrow Transplant 6:371, 1990.

MOLECULAR PATHOGENESIS

Fisher D: Apoptosis in cancer therapy: Crossing the threshold. Cell 78:539, 1994.

Gallie B: Retinoblastoma gene mutations in human cancer. N Engl J Med 330:786, 1994.

Harris C, Hollstein M: Clinical implications of the p53 tumor suppressor gene. N Engl J Med 329:1318, 1993.

Helman LJ, Thiele CJ: New insights into the causes of cancer. Pediatric Clin North Am 38:201, 1991.

Rowley JD, Aster JL, Sklar J: The clinical applications of new DNA diagnostic technology on the management of cancer patients. JAMA 270:2331, 1993.

Skuse G, Ludlow J: Tumour suppressor genes in disease and therapy. Lancet 345:902, 1995.

Solomon E, Borrow J, Goddard AD: Chromosome aberrations and cancer. Science 254:1153, 1991.

Weinberg RA: Tumor suppressor genes. Science 254:1138, 1991.

ACUTE LYMPHOBLASTIC LEUKEMIA

Brisco MJ, Condon J, Hughes E, et al: Outcome prediction in childhood acute lymphoblastic leukaemias by molecular quantification of residual disease at the end of induction. Lancet 343:196, 1994.

Cline MJ: The molecular basis of leukemia. N Engl J Med 330:328, 1994.

Greaves M: A natural history for pediatric acute leukemia. Blood 82:1043, 1993.

Haas OA, Argyriou-Tirita A, Lion T: Parental origin of chromosomes involved in the translocation t(9;22). Nature 359:414, 1992.

Katz JA, Pollok BH, Jacaruso D, et al: Final attained height in patients successfully treated for childhood acute lymphoblastic leukemia. J Pediatr 123:546, 1993.

Pui C-H, Behm FG, Crist WM: Clinical and biologic relevance of immunologic marker studies in childhood acute lymphoblastic leukemia. Blood 82:343, 1993.

Pui C-H, Crist WM: Biology and therapy of acute lymphoblastic leukemia. J Pediatr 124:491, 1994.

Pui C-H, Crist WM, Look AT: Biology and clinical significance of cytogenetic abnormalities in childhood acute lymphoblastic leukemia. Blood 76:1449, 1990.

Pui C-H, Ribeiro RC, Hancock ML, et al: Acute myeloid leukemia in children treated with epipodophyllotoxins for acute lymphoblastic leukemia. N Engl J Med 325:1682, 1991.

Rivera GK, Pinkel D, Simone JV, et al: Treatment of acute lymphoblastic leukemia—30 years' experience at St. Jude Children's Research Hospital. N Engl J Med 329:1289, 1993.

ACUTE MYELOID LEUKEMIA

Creutzig U, Ritter J, Zimmermann M, et al: Does cranial irradiation reduce the risk for bone marrow relapse in acute myelogenous leukemia? Unexpected results of the childhood acute myelogenous leukemia study BFM-87. J Clin Oncol 11:279, 1993.

Hurwitz CA, Schell MJ, Pui C-H, et al: Adverse prognostic features in 251 children treated for acute myeloid leukemia. Med Pediatr Oncol 21:1, 1993.

Van den Berghe H: Morphologic, immunologic and cytogenetic (MIC) working classification of the acute myeloid leukaemias. Br J Haematol 68:487, 1988.

Wells RJ, Woods WG, Lampkin BC, et al: Impact of high-dose cytarabine and asparaginase intensification on childhood acute myeloid leukemia: A report from the Children's Cancer Group. J Clin Oncol 11:538, 1993.

CHRONIC MYELOCYTIC LEUKEMIA

Kantajarian HM, Deisseroth A, Kurzrock R, et al: Chronic myelogenous leukemia: A concise update. Blood 82:691, 1993.

Miller JS, McGlave PB: Therapy for chronic myelogenous leukemia with marrow transplantation. Curr Opin Oncol 5:262, 1993.

Silver RT: Chronic myeloid leukemia. A perspective of the clinical and biological issues of the chronic phase. Hematol Oncol Clin North Am 4:319, 1990.

CONGENITAL LEUKEMIA

Liang D-C, Ma S-W, Lu T-H, et al: Transient myeloproliferative disorder and acute myeloid leukemia: Study of six neonatal cases with long-term follow-up. Leukemia 7:1521, 1993.

Sansone R, Negri D: Cytogenetic features of neonatal leukemias. Cancer Genet Cytogenet 63:56, 1992.

HODGKIN DISEASE

Diehl V, vonKalle C, Fonatsch C, et al: The cell of origin in Hodgkin disease. Semin Oncol 17:660, 1990.

Donaldson SS, Kaplan HS: Complications of treatment of Hodgkin disease in children. Cancer Treat Rep 66:977, 1982.

Gruffermen S, Delzell E: Epidemiology of Hodgkin disease. Epidemiol Rev 6:76, 1984.

Hayes DM, Ternberg JL, Chen PT, et al: Post-splenectomy sepsis and other complications following staging laparotomy for Hodgkin disease in childhood. J Pediatr Surg 21:628, 1986.

Hudson MM, Pratt CB: Risk of delayed second primary neoplasms after treatment of malignant lymphoma. Surg Oncol Clin North Am 2:319, 1993.

Longo DL, Young RC, Wesley M, et al: Twenty years of MOPP chemotherapy for Hodgkin disease. J Clin Oncol 4:1295, 1986.

Santoro A, Bonadonna G, Bonfante V, et al: Alternating drug combinations in the treatment of advanced Hodgkin disease. N Engl J Med 306:770, 1992.

Slivnick DJ, Ellis TM, Nawrocki JF, et al: The impact of Hodgkin disease on the immune system. Semin Oncol 17:673, 1990.

NON-HODGKIN LYMPHOMA

Anderson JR, Wilson JF, Jenkin RDT, et al: Childhood non-Hodgkin lymphoma. The results of a randomized therapeutic trial comparing a 4-drug regimen (COMP) with a 10-drug regimen (LSA_2-L_2). N Engl J Med 308:559, 1983.

Murphy SB: Classification, staging and end results of treatment of childhood non-Hodgkin lymphomas: Dissimilarities from lymphoma in adults. Semin Oncol 7:332, 1980.

Murphy SB, Fairclough D, Hutchison RE, et al: Non-Hodgkin lymphomas of childhood: An analysis of the histology, staging and response to treatment of 338 cases at a single institution. J Clin Oncol 2:186, 1989.

Sandlund JT, Hutchison RE, Crist WM: The non-Hodgkin lymphomas. *In:* Vietti T, Fernbach D (eds): Clinical Pediatric Oncology. St. Louis, CV Mosby, 1991.

Sandlund JT, Pui C-H, Santana VM, et al: Clinical features and treatment outcome for children with CD30-positive large cell non-Hodgkin lymphoma. J Clin Oncol 12:895, 1994.

The Non-Hodgkin Lymphoma Pathologic Classification Project: National Cancer Institute sponsored study of classifications of non-Hodgkin lymphomas. Summary and description of a working formulation for clinical usage. Cancer 49:2112, 1982.

NEUROBLASTOMA

Bowman LC, Hancock ML, Santana VM, et al: Impact of intensified chemotherapy on clinical outcome in infants and children with neuroblastoma: The St. Jude Children's Research Hospital experience, 1962 to 1988. J Clin Oncol 9:1599, 1991.

Brodeur GM, Fong CT: Molecular biology and genetics of human neuroblastoma. Cancer Genet Cytogenet 41:153, 1989.

Brodeur GM, Pritchard J, Berthold F, et al: Revisions of the International Criteria for Neuroblastoma, Diagnosis, Staging, and Response to Treatment. J Clin Oncol 8:1466, 1993.

Johnson FL, Goldman S: Role of autotransplantation in neuroblastoma. Hematol Oncol Clin North Am 7:647, 1993.

Look AT, Hayes FA, Nitschke R, et al: Cellular DNA content as a predictor of response to chemotherapy in infants with unresectable neuroblastoma. N Engl J Med 311:231, 1984.

O'Meara A, Tormey W, Fitzgerald R, et al: Interpretation of random urinary catecholamines and their metabolites in neuroblastoma. Acta Paediatr 83:88, 1994.

Shimada H, Chatten J, Newton WA, et al: Histopathologic prognostic factors in neuroblastic tumors: Definition of subtypes of ganglioneuroblastoma and an age-linked classification of neuroblastoma. J Natl Cancer Inst 73:405, 1984.

WILMS TUMOR

Beckwith JB: Precursor lesions of Wilms tumor: Clinical and biologic implications. Med Pediatr Oncol 21:158, 1993.

Coppes M, Williams ERG: The molecular genetics of Wilms' tumor. Cancer Invest 12:57, 1994.

D'Angio GJ, Breslow N, Beckwith JB, et al: The treatment of Wilms tumor: Results of the third National Wilms' Tumor Study. Cancer 64:349, 1989.

Fishman EK, Hartmen DB, Goldman SM, et al: The CT appearance of Wilms' tumor. J Comput Assist Tomogr 7:659, 1983.

Shearer P, Parham D, Fontanesi J, et al: Bilateral Wilms tumor: Review of outcome, associated abnormalities, and late effects in 36 patients treated at a single institution. Cancer 72:1422, 1993.

SOFT TISSUE SARCOMAS

Fletcher JA: Cytogenetics. *In:* Verweij J, Pinedo HM, Suit HD (eds): Multidisciplinary Treatment of Soft Tissue Sarcomas. Boston, Kluwer Academic Press, 1993, pp. 23–35.

Pizzo PA, Poplack DG. Principles and Practice of Pediatric Oncology. Philadelphia, JB Lippincott, 1993.

Rao BN: Nonrhabdomyosarcoma in children: Prognostic factors influencing survival. Semin Surg Oncol 9:524, 1993.

OSTEOSARCOMA

Frieden RA, Ryniker D, Kenan S, et al: Assessment of patient function after limb-sparing surgery. Arch Phys Med Rehabil 74:38, 1993.

Link MP, Goorin AM, Miser AW, et al: The effect of adjuvant chemotherapy on relapse-free survival in patients with osteosarcoma of the extremity. N Engl J Med 314:1600, 1986.

Marina NM, Pratt CB, Rao BN, et al: Improved prognosis of children with osteosarcoma metastatic to the lung(s) at the time of diagnosis. Cancer 70:2722, 1992.

Meyer WH, Malawer MM: Osteosarcoma. Clinical features and evolving surgical and chemotherapeutic strategies. Pediatr Clin North Am 38:317, 1991.

Meyers PA, Heller G, Healey J, et al: Chemotherapy for nonmetastatic osteogenic sarcoma: The Memorial Sloan-Kettering experience. J Clin Oncol 10:5, 1992.

Meyers PA, Heller G, Healey JH, et al: Osteogenic sarcoma with clinically detectable metastasis at initial presentation. J Clin Oncol 11:449, 1993.

Smith MA, Ungerleider RS, Horowitz ME, et al: Influence of doxorubicin dose intensity on response and outcome for patients with osteogenic sarcoma and Ewing's sarcoma. J Natl Cancer Inst 83:1460, 1991.

EWING SARCOMA

Arai Y, Kun LE, Brooks MT, et al: Ewing's sarcoma: Local tumor control and patterns of failure following limited-volume radiation therapy. Int J Radiat Oncol Biol Phys 21:1501, 1991.

Burgert EO, Jr, Nesbit ME, Garnsey LA, et al: Multimodal therapy for the management of nonpelvic, localized Ewing's sarcoma of bone: Intergroup Study IESS-II. J Clin Oncol 8:1514, 1990.

Cangir A, Vietti TJ, Gehan EA, et al: Ewing's sarcoma metastatic at diagnosis. Results and comparisons of two intergroup Ewing's sarcoma studies. Cancer 66:887, 1990.

Dehner LP: Primitive neuroectodermal tumor and Ewing's sarcoma. Am J Surg Pathol 17:1, 1993.

Fellinger EJ, Garin-Chesa P, Su SL, et al: Biochemical and genetic characterization of the HBA71 Ewing's sarcoma cell surface antigen. Cancer Res 51:336, 1991.

Fellinger EJ, Garin-Chesa P, Triche TJ, et al: Immunohistochemical analysis of Ewing's sarcoma cell surface antigen p30/32MIC2. Am J Pathol 139:317, 1991.

Kretschmar C: Ewing's sarcoma and the "peanut" tumors. N Engl J Med 331:325, 1994.

RETINOBLASTOMA

Grabowski EF, Abramson DH: Intraocular and extraocular retinoblastoma. Hematol Oncol Clin North Am 1:721, 1987.

Howarth C, Meyer D, Hustu HO, et al: Stage-related combined modality treatment of retinoblastoma. Cancer 45:851, 1980.

Knudson AG, Meadows AT, Nichols WW, et al: Chromosomal deletion and retinoblastoma. N Engl J Med 295:1120, 1976.

Pratt CB, Crom DB, Magill et al: Skeletal scintigraphy in patients with bilateral retinoblastoma. Cancer 65:26, 1990.

Pratt CB, Meyer D, Chenaille P, et al: The use of bone marrow aspirations and lumbar punctures at the time of diagnosis of retinoblastoma. J Clin Oncol 7:140, 1989.

Shields CL, Shields JA, Baez K, et al: Optic nerve invasion of retinoblastoma: Metastatic potential and clinical risk factors. Cancer 73:692, 1994.

GONADAL AND GERM CELL NEOPLASMS

Dehner LP: Gonadal and extragonadal germ cell neoplasia of childhood. Hum Pathol 14:493, 1993.

Marina N, Fontanesi J, Kun L, et al: Treatment of childhood germ cell tumors. Cancer 70:2568, 1993.

Norris HJ, Zirkin HJ, Benson WL: Immature (malignant) teratoma of the ovary. Cancer 37:2359, 1976.

GASTROINTESTINAL NEOPLASMS

Drut R, Jones MC: Congenital pancreatoblastoma in Beckwith Wiedermann syndrome. Pediatr Pathol 8:331, 1988.

Fenoglio-Preiser CM, Hutter RVP: Colorectal polyps: Pathologic diagnosis and clinical significance. CA Cancer J Clin 35:322, 1985.

Grosfeld JL, Vane DW, Rescorla FJ, et al: Pancreatic tumors in childhood: Analysis of 13 cases. J Pediatr Surg 25:1057, 1990.

Marin VTW, Salmaso R, Onnis GL: Tumors of salivary glands. Appl Pathol 7:154, 1980.

Naegele RF, Champion J, Murphy S, et al: Nasopharyngeal carcinoma in American children: Epstein-Barr virus-specific antibody titer and prognosis. Int J Cancer 29:209, 1982.

Pao WJ, Hustu HO, Douglass EC, et al: Pediatric nasopharyngeal carcinoma: Long-term follow-up of 29 patients. Int J Radiat Oncol Biol Phys 17:299, 1989.

Powell S, Petersen G, Krush A, et al: Molecular diagnosis of familial adenomatous polyposis. N Engl J Med 329:1982, 1993.

Rao BN, Pratt CB, Fleming ID, et al: Colon carcinoma in children and adolescents: A review of thirty cases. Cancer 55:1322, 1985.

Schimke RN: The multiple endocrine neoplasms syndromes. Cancer Treat Rev 17:249, 1983.

Schwartz MG, Sgaglione NA: Gastric carcinoma in the young. Overviews of the literature. Mt Sinai J Med 51:720, 1984.

NEOPLASMS OF THE LIVER

Douglass EC, Reynolds M, Finegold M, et al: Cisplatin, vincristine, and fluorouracil therapy for hepatoblastoma: A Pediatric Oncology Group Study. J Clin Oncol 11:96, 1993.

Evans AE, Land VJ, Newton WA, et al: Combination chemotherapy (vincristine, Adriamycin, cyclophosphamide, and 5-fluorouracil) in the treatment of children with malignant hepatomas. Cancer 50:821, 1982.

Exelby PR, Filler RM, Grosfeld JL: Liver tumors in children in the particular reference to hepatoblastoma and hepatocellular carcinoma. American Academy of Pediatrics Surgical Survey—1974. J Pediatr Surg 10:329, 1975.

Wineberg AG, Finegold MJ: Primary hepatic tumors of childhood. Hum Pathol 14:512, 1983.

MISCELLANEOUS CARCINOMAS

Greene MH, Clark WH Jr, Tucker MA, et al: High risk of malignant melanoma in melanoma-prone families with dysplastic nevi. Ann Intern Med 102:458, 1985.

Gundlach KK, Keihn M: Multiple basal cell carcinomas and keratocysts: The Gorlin and Goltz syndrome. J Maxillofac Surg 7:299, 1979.

Herbst AL, Robboy SJ, Scully RE, et al: Clear-cell adenocarcinoma of the vagina and cervix in girls: Analysis of 170 registry cases. Am J Obstet Gynecol 119:713, 1974.

Kabayashi M, Satah Y, Irinajin T, et al: Skin tumors in xeroderma pigmentation (1). J Dermatol 9:319, 1982.

Koh HK: Cutaneous melanoma. N Engl J Med 325:171, 1991.

Rao BN, Hayes FA, Pratt CB, et al: Malignant melanoma in children: Its management and prognosis. J Pediatr Surg 25:198, 1990.

Ribeiro RC, Neto RS, Schell MJ, et al: Adrenocortical carcinoma in children: A study of 40 cases. J Clin Oncol 8:66, 1990.

BENIGN TUMORS

Enzinger FM, Weiss SW: Soft Tissue Tumors. St. Louis, CV Mosby, 1988.

Fishman SJ, Mulliken JB: Hemangiomas and vascular malformations of infancy and childhood. Pediatr Clin North America 6:1177, 1993.

Huvos AG: Bone tumors. Diagnosis, Treatment and Prognosis. Philadelphia, WB Saunders, 1991.

Rao BN, Horowitz ME, Parham DM, et al: Challenges in the treatment of childhood fibromatosis. Arch Surg 122:1296, 1987.

PART XXIII

Nephrology

SECTION 1

Structure and Function of the Kidney

Jerry M. Bergstein

CHAPTER 462

Anatomy of the Glomerulus

The kidneys lie in the retroperitoneal space slightly above the level of the umbilicus and range in length and weight, respectively, from approximately 6 cm and 24 g in the full-term newborn to 12 cm or more and 150 g in the adult. The kidney (Fig. 462–1) has an outer layer, the *cortex,* which contains the glomeruli, proximal and distal convoluted tubules, and collecting ducts, and an inner layer, the *medulla,* which contains the straight portions of the tubules, the loops of Henle, the vasa recta, and the terminal collecting ducts (Fig. 462–2).

The blood supply to each kidney usually consists of a main renal artery that arises from the aorta; multiple renal arteries are not uncommon. The main artery divides into segmental branches within the medulla and these into interlobar arteries that pass through the medulla to the junction of the cortex and medulla. At this point, the interlobar arteries branch to form the arcuate arteries, which run parallel to the surface of the kidney. Interlobular arteries originate from the arcuate arteries and give rise to the afferent arterioles of the glomeruli.

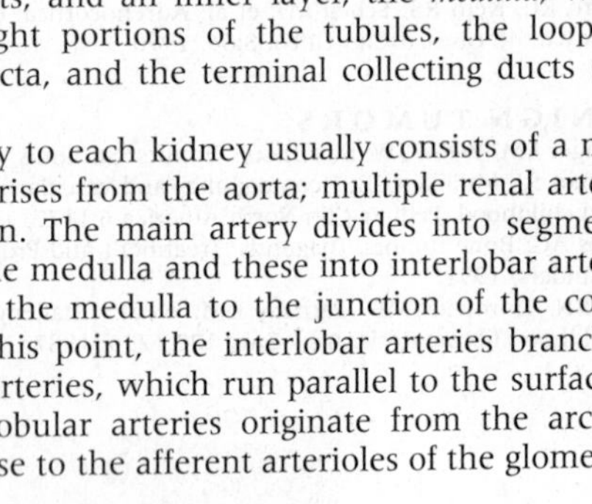

Figure 462–1. Gross morphology of the renal circulation. (From Pitts RF: Physiology of the Kidney and Body Fluids, 3rd ed. Chicago, Year Book Medical Publishers, 1974. Used by permission.)

Specialized muscle cells in the wall of the afferent arteriole, in combination with the lacis cells and that portion of the distal tubule (macula densa) that is adjacent to the glomerulus, form the juxtaglomerular apparatus that controls the secretion of renin. The afferent arteriole divides into the glomerular capillary network, which then merges into the efferent arteriole (Fig. 462–3). The efferent arterioles of glomeruli next to the medulla (juxtamedullary glomeruli) are larger than those in the outer cortex and provide the blood supply (vasa recta) to the tubules and medulla.

Each kidney contains approximately 1 million nephrons (glomeruli and associated tubules). In humans, formation of nephrons is complete at birth, but functional maturation does not occur until later. As no new nephrons can be formed after birth, progressive loss of nephrons may lead to renal insufficiency.

The glomerular network of specialized capillaries serves as the filtering mechanism of the kidney. The glomerular capillaries are lined by endothelial cells (Fig. 462–4) having very thin cytoplasm that contains many holes (fenestrations). The glomerular basement membrane (GBM) forms a continuous layer between the endothelial and mesangial cells on one side and the epithelial cells on the other. The membrane has three layers: (1) a central electron-dense lamina densa; (2) the lamina rara interna, which lies between the lamina densa and the endothelial cells; and (3) the lamina rara externa, which lies between the lamina densa and the epithelial cells. The visceral epithelial cells cover the capillary and project cytoplasmic "foot processes," which attach to the lamina rara externa. Between the foot processes are spaces or filtration slits. The mesangium (mesangial cells and matrix) lies between the glomerular capillaries on the endothelial cell side of the basement membrane and forms the medial part of the capillary wall. The mesangium may serve as a supporting structure for the glomerular capillaries and probably plays a role in the regulation of glomerular blood flow, filtration, and in the removal of macromolecules (such as immune complexes) from the glomerulus, either through intracellular phagocytosis or by transport through intercellular channels to the juxtaglomerular region. The Bowman capsule, which surrounds the glomerulus, is composed of (1) a basement membrane, which is continuous with the basement membranes of the glomerular capillaries and the proximal tubules, and (2) the parietal epithelial cells, which are continuous with the visceral epithelial cells.

462.1 Glomerular Filtration

As the blood passes through the glomerular capillaries, the plasma is filtered through the glomerular capillary walls. The

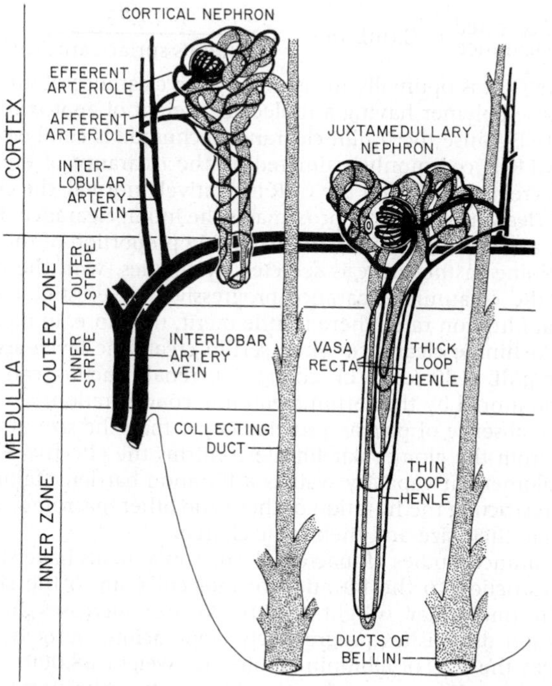

Figure 462–2. Comparison of the blood supplies of cortical and juxtamedullary nephrons. (From Pitts RF: Physiology of the Kidney and Body Fluids, 3rd ed. Chicago, Year Book Medical Publishers, 1974. Used by permission.)

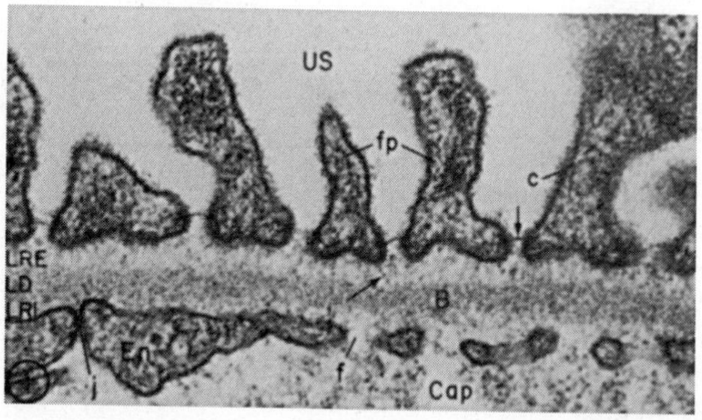

Figure 462–4. Electron micrograph of the normal glomerular capillary (Cap) wall demonstrating the endothelium (En) with its fenestrations (f), the glomerular basement membrane (B) with its central dense layer, the lamina densa (LD) and adjoining lamina rara interna (LRI) and externa (LRE; *long arrow,*) and the epithelial cell foot processes (fp) with their thick cell coat (c). The glomerular filtrate passes through the endothelial fenestrae, crosses the basement membrane, and passes through the filtration slits *(short arrow)* between the epithelial cell foot processes to reach the urinary space (US). (×60,000.) J is the junction between two endothelial cells. (From Farquhar MG, Kanwar YS: Functional organization of the glomerulus: State of the science in 1979. *In:* Cummings NB, Michael AF, Wilson CB [eds]: Immune Mechanisms in Renal Disease. New York, Plenum, 1982. Reprinted by permission.)

ultrafiltrate, which is cell free, contains all the substances in the plasma (electrolytes, glucose, phosphate, urea, creatinine, peptides, low molecular weight proteins) except proteins (like albumin and the globulins) having a molecular weight exceeding 68,000. The filtrate is collected in Bowman space and enters the tubules, where its composition is modified in accordance with body needs until it leaves the kidney as urine.

Glomerular filtration is the net result of opposing forces across the capillary wall. The force for ultrafiltration (glomerular capillary hydrostatic pressure) stems from the systemic arterial pressure, as modified by the tone of the afferent and efferent arterioles. The major force opposing ultrafiltration is the glomerular capillary oncotic pressure, which is created by the gradient between the high concentration of plasma proteins within the capillary and the almost protein-free ultrafiltrate in Bowman space. Filtration may be modified by the rate of glomerular plasma flow, the hydrostatic pressure within Bowman space, and the permeability of the glomerular capillary wall. The permeability, as measured by the ultrafiltration coefficient (K_f), is the product of the water permeability of the membrane and the total glomerular capillary surface area available for filtration.

Although glomerular filtration begins around the 9th week of fetal life, kidney function does not appear necessary for normal intrauterine homeostasis, the placenta serving as the major excretory organ. Following birth, the rate of glomerular filtration increases until growth ceases toward the end of the 2nd decade of life. To facilitate the comparison of the glomerular filtration rates (GFR) of children and adults, the rate is standardized to the surface area (1.73 m^2) of a 70-kg adult. Even after correction for surface area, the GFR of the child does not approximate adult values until the 3rd year of life (Fig. 462–5).

The GFR may be estimated by measurement of the serum creatinine level (Fig. 462–6). Creatinine is derived from muscle metabolism. Its production is relatively constant, and its excretion is primarily through glomerular filtration (although tubular secretion may become important in renal insufficiency). In contrast to the concentration of blood urea nitrogen, the serum creatinine level is minimally influenced by factors (nitrogen balance, state of hydration) other than glomerular function. The serum creatinine is of value in estimating the GFR in the steady state only (e.g., a patient very shortly after the onset of acute renal failure and cessation of urine output may have a normal creatinine level but no effective renal function). The value of the serum creatinine is further compromised by the fact that its level does not rise above normal until the filtration rate falls below 70% of normal.

The precise measurement of the GFR is accomplished by quantitating the "clearance" of a substance that is freely filtered across the capillary wall and that is neither reabsorbed nor secreted by the tubules. The clearance (C_s) of such a substance(s) is that volume of plasma that, when completely

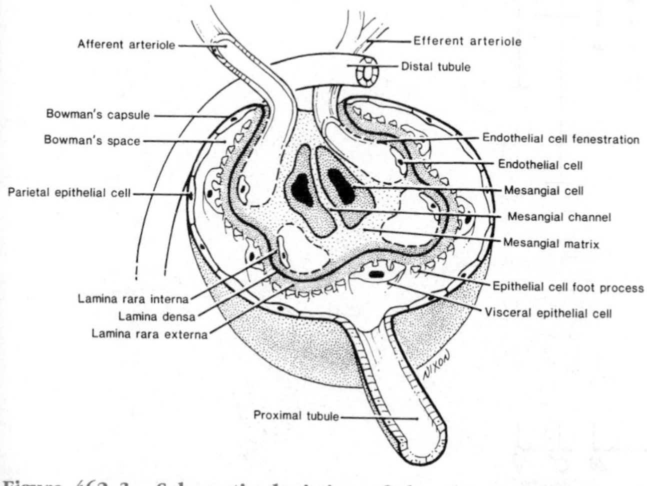

Figure 462–3. Schematic depiction of the glomerulus and surrounding structures.

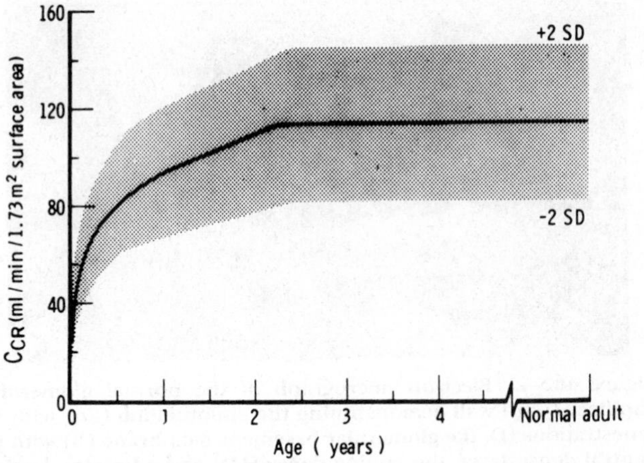

Figure 462–5. Changes in the normal value of the glomerular filtration rate, as measured by the creatinine clearance (C_{CR}), when standardized to mL/min/1.73 m² of body surface area. The *solid line* depicts the mean value, and the shaded area includes two standard deviations. (Reprinted by permission of the publishers from McCrory W: Developmental Nephrology. Cambridge, MA, Harvard University Press. Copyright © 1972 by the President and Fellows of Harvard College.)

"cleared" of the contained substance, would yield a quantity of that substance equal to that excreted in the urine over a specified time. The clearance is represented by the following formula:

$$C_s(\text{mL/min}) = \frac{U_s(\text{mg/mL})V(\text{mL/min})}{P_s(\text{mg/mL})}$$

where C_s equals the clearance of substance s, U_s reflects the urinary concentration of s, V represents the urinary flow rate, and P_s equals the plasma concentration of s. To correct the clearance for body surface area, the formula is

$$\text{Corrected clearance} = C_s(\text{mL/min}) \times \frac{1.73}{\text{Patient's surface area (m}^2)}$$

The GFR is optimally measured by the clearance of inulin, a fructose polymer having a molecular weight of approximately 5,000. Because the inulin clearance technique is cumbersome, the GFR is commonly estimated by the clearance of endogenous creatinine. When the GFR is relatively normal, the creatinine clearance closely approximates the inulin clearance. However, as the GFR declines, an increasing proportion of the total creatinine in the urine is secreted by tubules, with the result that the creatinine clearance progressively overestimates the actual filtration rate. There is little merit, therefore, in measuring creatinine clearance when serum creatinine levels exceed 2.0 mg/dL (180 μmol/L); changes in renal function can then be monitored by the serum creatinine concentration.

The absence of plasma proteins larger than the size of albumin from the glomerular filtrate confirms the effectiveness of the glomerular capillary wall as a filtration barrier. Major factors restricting the filtration of these and other macromolecules include their size and their ionic charge.

Clearance studies of macromolecules in animals have shown no restriction to the filtration of molecules up to the size of inulin (molecular weight 5,000). As size increases further, filtration diminishes progressively, approaching zero for substances the size of albumin (molecular weight 68,000). Morphologic studies suggest that the size-selective filtration barrier resides within the GBM.

The endothelial cell, basement membrane, and epithelial cell of the glomerular capillary wall possess strong negative ionic charges. These anionic charges are a consequence of two negatively charged moieties: proteoglycans (heparan sulfate) and glycoproteins containing sialic acid. Proteins in the blood have a relatively low isoelectric point and carry a net negative charge. Consequently, they are repelled by the negatively charged sites in the glomerular capillary wall, thus restricting filtration.

Arant BS Jr: Postnatal development of renal function during the first year of life. Pediatr Nephrol 1:308, 1987.

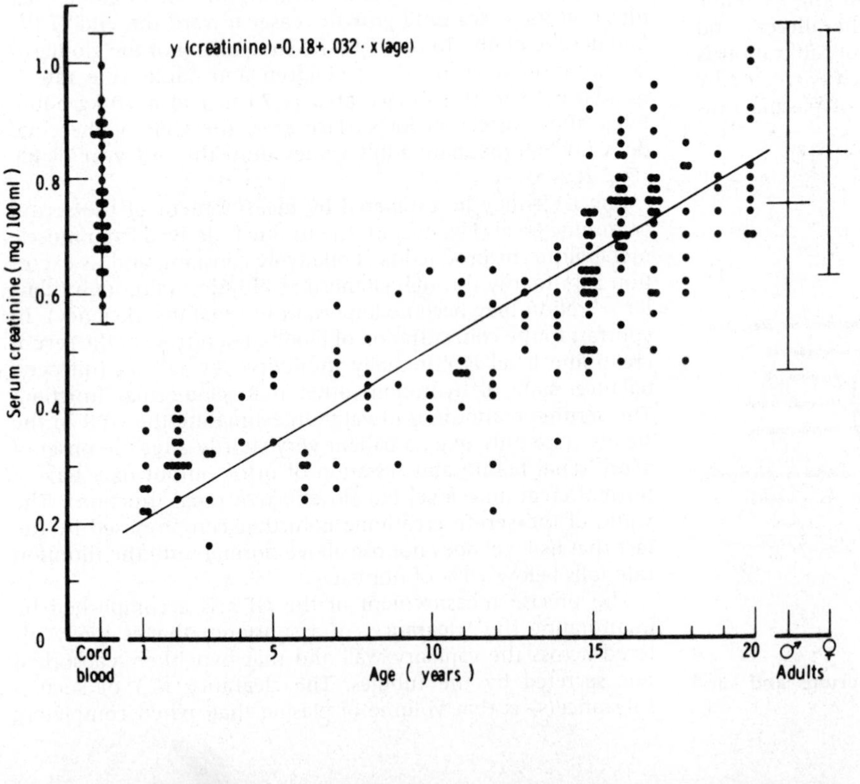

Figure 462–6. The serum creatinine in relation to age. (Reprinted by permission of the publishers from McCrory W: Developmental Nephrology. Cambridge, MA, Harvard University Press. Copyright © 1972 by the President and Fellows of Harvard College.)

Brenner BM, Hostetter TH, Humes HD: Glomerular permselectivity: Barrier function based on discrimination of molecular size and charge. Am J Physiol 234:F455, 1978.
Latta H: An approach to the structure and function of the glomerular mesangium. J Am Soc Nephrol 2:565, 1992.
Perrone RD, Madias NE, Levey AS: Serum creatinine as an index of renal function: new insights into old concepts. Clin Chem 38:1933, 1992.
Renkin EM, Robinson RR: Glomerular filtration. N Engl J Med 290:785, 1974.
Venkatachalam MA, Rennke HG: The structural and molecular basis of glomerular filtration. Circ Res 43:337, 1978.

SECTION 2

Conditions Particularly Associated with Hematuria

Jerry M. Bergstein

Hematuria may be gross (visible to the naked eye) or microscopic (detected only by dipstick or microscopic examination of the urine sediment). Gross hematuria may originate from the kidney, in which case it is generally brown or cola-colored and may contain red blood cell casts, or from the lower urinary tract (bladder and urethra), in which case the urine has a red to pink color and may contain clots. Gross hematuria may be associated with edema, hypertension, and renal insufficiency. This constellation of findings is typical of "the acute nephritic syndrome" and is frequently seen in patients with postinfectious (e.g., poststreptococcal) glomerulonephritis, systemic lupus erythematosus, membranoproliferative glomerulonephritis, anaphylactoid purpura, and rapidly progressive glomerulonephritis. The urine may be colored by pigments other than blood (Table XXIII–1).

In children, microscopic hematuria is most commonly discovered at periodic health examinations, by dipstick or by microscopic examination of the urine sediment. Because the quantitation of blood (actually hemoglobin) on dipsticks is not precise, results should be interpreted as negative (negative or trace readings) or positive (small, medium, and large readings). A positive dipstick test for blood indicates the need for a urinalysis. Microscopic hematuria is defined as more than five red blood cells per high power field in the sediment from 10 mL of centrifuged freshly voided urine.

Asymptomatic microscopic hematuria is found in 0.5–2% of school-aged children, but whether screening for isolated microscopic hematuria can discover occult renal disease is unclear. Because of this uncertainty and its cost, screening urinalysis with microscopic examination of sediment for hematuria or pyuria seems unwarranted in asymptomatic children. On the other hand, a dipstick can detect blood or protein inexpensively, suggesting that this evaluation should be included in health maintenance routines.

■ **TABLE XXIII–1 Urinary Hues**

Dark Yellow	Red food coloring
Concentrated urine	Phenolphthalein
Bile pigments	Urates
	Pyridium
Red	
Blood (red cells or hemoglobin)	**Dark Brown or Black**
Myoglobin	Blood
Porphyrins	Homogentisic acid
Beets	
Blackberries	

■ **TABLE XXIII–2 Causes of Hematuria in Children**

Glomerular Diseases
- Recurrent gross hematuria syndrome
  - IgA nephropathy
  - Idiopathic (benign familial) hematuria
  - Alport syndrome
- Acute poststreptococcal glomerulonephritis
- Membranous glomerulopathy
- Systemic lupus erythematosus
- Membranoproliferative glomerulonephritis
- Nephritis of chronic infection
- Rapidly progressive glomerulonephritis
- Goodpasture disease
- Anaphylactoid purpura
- Hemolytic-uremic syndrome

Infection
- Bacterial
- Tuberculosis
- Viral

Hematologic
- Coagulopathies
- Thrombocytopenia
- Sickle cell disease
- Renal vein thrombosis

Stones and Hypercalciuria

Anatomic Abnormalities
- Congenital anomalies
- Trauma
- Polycystic kidneys
- Vascular abnormalities
- Tumors

Exercise

Drugs

Causes of hematuria are listed in Table XXIII-2. Children with gross hematuria should be hospitalized for evaluation because of the increased likelihood of finding hypertension and renal failure. Children having persistent microscopic hematuria (more than five red blood cells per high power field on three urinalyses at monthly intervals) should undergo further outpatient evaluation. The cost effectiveness of such evaluation remains to be determined. ■

CHAPTER 463
Glomerular Diseases

PATHOGENESIS. Glomerular injury may be the result of immunologic, inherited (presumably biochemical), or coagulation disorders. Immunologic injury is the most common cause and results in *glomerulonephritis,* which is both a generic term for several diseases and a histopathologic term signifying inflammation of the glomerular capillaries. Evidence that glomerulonephritis is caused by immunologic injury includes (1) morphologic and immunopathologic similarities to experimental immune-mediated glomerulonephritis; (2) the demonstration of immune reactants (immunoglobulin and complement components) in glomeruli; and (3) abnormalities in serum complement and the finding of autoantibodies (e.g., anti-glomerular basement membrane [anti-GBM]) in some of these diseases. There appear to be two major mechanisms of immunologic injury: (1) localization of circulating antigen-antibody immune complexes and (2) interaction of antibody with local antigen in situ. In the latter circumstance, the antigen may be a normal component of the glomerulus (e.g., the noncollagenous domain [NC-1] of type IV collagen, which is the putative antigen in human anti-GBM nephritis) or an antigen that has been deposited in the glomerulus.

In immune complex–mediated diseases, antibody is produced against and combines with a circulating antigen that is usually unrelated to the kidney. The immune complexes accumulate in glomeruli and activate the complement system, leading to immune injury. Experimental studies suggest that the complexes may be formed in the circulation and deposited in the kidney. Acute serum sickness in the rabbit is produced by a single intravenous injection of bovine albumin. Within 1 wk after injection, the rabbit produces antibody against bovine albumin, while the antigen remains in the blood in high concentration. As antibody enters the circulation, it forms immune complexes with antigen. While the amount of antigen in the circulation exceeds that of antibody (antigen excess), the complexes formed are small, remain soluble in the circulation, and are deposited in glomeruli. The processes involved in glomerular localization are not well understood but include attributes of the complex (concentration, charge, size), characteristics of the glomerulus (mesangial trapping, negatively charged capillary wall), hydrodynamic forces, and the influence of various mediators (angiotensin II, prostaglandins).

With deposition of immune complexes in glomeruli, rabbits develop an acute proliferative glomerulonephritis. Immunofluorescence microscopy demonstrates granular ("lumpy-bumpy") deposits containing immunoglobulin and complement in the glomerular capillary wall. Electron microscopic studies show these deposits to be on the epithelial side of the GBM and in the mesangium. Over the next few days, as additional antibody enters the circulation, the antigen is ultimately removed from the circulation and the glomerulonephritis subsides. In the rabbit, complement does not participate in the capillary injury, which is largely related to influx of macrophages. In other animal models, complement does play a role in capillary injury.

An example of in situ antigen-antibody interaction is anti-GBM antibody disease, in which antibody reacts with antigen(s) of the GBM. Immunopathologic studies reveal linear deposition of immunoglobulin and complement on the GBM, similar to that seen in Goodpasture disease and certain types of rapidly progressive glomerulonephritis.

The inflammatory reaction that follows immunologic injury results from activation of one or more biochemical mediation systems. Perhaps the most important of these is the complement system, which has two initiating sequences: (1) the classic pathway, which is activated by antigen-antibody immune complexes; and (2) the alternative or properdin pathway, which is activated by polysaccharides and endotoxin. These pathways converge at C3; from that point on, for both, the same sequence leads to lysis of cell membranes (see Fig. 121–1). The major noxious products of complement activation are produced after activation of C3 and include anaphylatoxin (which stimulates contractile proteins within vascular walls and increases vascular permeability) and chemotactic factors (C5a) that direct neutrophils and perhaps macrophages to the site of complement activation, where the cells release substances that damage vascular cells and basement membranes.

The coagulation system may be activated directly, following endothelial cell injury, which bares the thrombogenic subendothelial layer (initiating the coagulation cascade), or indirectly, following complement activation. Fibrin deposits may occur within glomerular capillaries or within Bowman space in crescents. Activation of the coagulation process may activate the kinin system, which also produces chemotactic and anaphylatoxin-like factors.

PATHOLOGY. The glomerulus may be injured by several mechanisms but has only a limited number of histopathologic responses; accordingly, different disease states may produce similar microscopic changes.

Proliferation of glomerular cells occurs in most forms of glomerulonephritis and may be generalized, involving all glomeruli, or focal, involving only some glomeruli while sparing others. Within a single glomerulus, proliferation may be diffuse, involving all parts of the glomerulus, or segmental, involving only some areas but not others. Proliferation commonly involves the endothelial and mesangial cells, and is frequently associated with an increase in the mesangial matrix. Immunofluorescent and electron microscopic studies indicate that mesangial proliferation may result from immune complex deposition within the mesangium. The resultant increase in cell size and number, and in mesangial matrix, may increase glomerular size and narrow the lumina of glomerular capillaries, leading to renal insufficiency.

Crescent formation in Bowman space (capsule) is a result of proliferation of parietal epithelial cells. Crescents develop in several forms of glomerulonephritis (termed *rapidly progressive*) and are thought to be a response to fibrin deposited in Bowman space. New crescents contain fibrin, the proliferating epithelial cells of Bowman space, basement membrane–like material produced by these cells, and macrophages that may play a role in the genesis of glomerular injury. In days to weeks, the crescent is invaded by connective tissue (fibroepithelial crescent); this generally results in glomerular obsolescence. Crescent formation is frequently associated with glomerular cell death (necrosis). The necrotic glomerulus has a characteristic eosinophilic appearance with hematoxylin and eosin stain and usually contains nuclear remnants. Crescent formation is usually associated with generalized proliferation of the mesangial cells and with either immune complex or anti-GBM antibody deposition in the glomerular capillary wall.

In addition to proliferation, certain forms of acute glomerulonephritis show glomerular exudation of blood cells, most commonly neutrophils; eosinophils, basophils, and mononuclear cells may be seen in lesser numbers. The thickened appearance of GBM may result from a true increase in the width of the membrane (as seen in membranous glomerulopathy), from massive deposition of immune complexes that have staining characteristics similar to the membrane (as seen in systemic lupus erythematosus), or from the interposition of mesangial cells and matrix into the subendothelial space between the endothelial cells and the membrane. The latter may give the basement membrane a "split" appearance, as seen in type I membranoproliferative glomerulonephritis and other diseases.

Sclerosis refers to the presence of scar tissue within the glomerulus. Occasionally, pathologists will use this term to refer to an increase in mesangial matrix.

CHAPTER 464
Recurrent Gross Hematuria

In patients having a syndrome of recurrent gross hematuria (RGH), recurrent episodes of generally painless hematuria occur (mild flank pain may be felt). The gross hematuria usually develops 1–2 days after the onset of a presumably viral upper respiratory tract infection. This short latent period between the onset of infection and the appearance of hematuria contrasts with the 7- to 14-day latent period seen in children developing acute poststreptococcal glomerulonephritis. Patients with RGH do not usually have such manifestations of the acute nephritic syndrome as edema, hypertension, or renal insufficiency. Diseases causing RGH may also present with persistent microscopic hematuria without episodes of gross hematuria.

Patients having a first episode of gross hematuria are hospitalized and evaluated for causes of hematuria (Table 464–1). In patients with RGH, routine radiographic and laboratory studies may fail to reveal a cause of hematuria. The gross hematuria resolves over 1–2 wk, but microscopic hematuria usually persists. Later, with another respiratory infection, there is a recurrence of gross hematuria. Renal biopsy is indicated after the second episode to determine the nature of any underlying disease, which will most frequently be IgA nephropathy, idiopathic hematuria, or familial nephritis (Alport syndrome).

■ **TABLE 464–1 Evaluation of the Child with Hematuria**

Step 1: Studies Performed in All Patients
- Complete blood count
- Urine culture
- Serum creatinine level
- 24-hr urine collection for
  - creatinine
  - protein
  - calcium
- Serum C3 level
- Ultrasound or intravenous pyelography

Step 2: Studies Performed in Selected Patients
- DNase B titer or streptozyme test if hematuria is of less than 6 mo duration
- Skin or throat cultures when appropriate
- ANA titer
- Urine erythrocyte morphology
- Coagulation studies/platelet count when suggested by history
- Sickle cell screen in all black patients
- Voiding cystourethrography with infection, or when a lower tract lesion is suspected

Step 3: Invasive Procedures

Renal biopsy indicated for
1. Persistent high-grade microscopic hematuria
2. Microscopic hematuria plus any of the following
   a. diminished renal function
   b. proteinuria exceeding 150 mg/24 hr (0.15 g/24 hr)
   c. hypertension
3. Second episode of gross hematuria

Cystoscopy indicated for
- pink to red hematuria, dysuria, and sterile urine culture

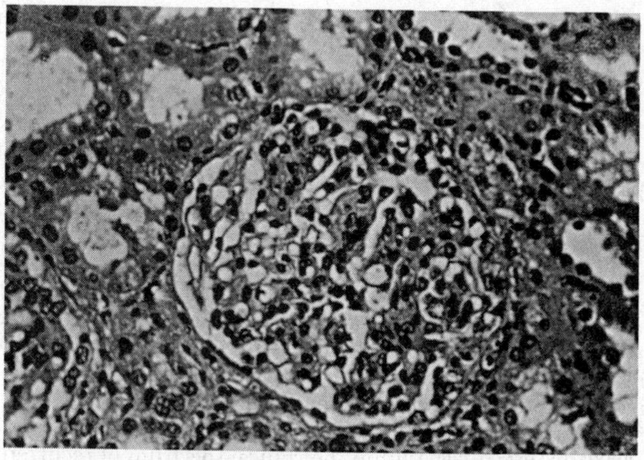

Figure 464–1. Light microscopy of IgA nephropathy demonstrating segmental mesangial proliferation and increased matrix. (×180.)

IgA NEPHROPATHY (BERGER NEPHROPATHY). Patients with this disorder have glomerulonephritis with IgA as the predominant immunoglobulin in mesangial deposits, in the absence of any systemic disease such as systemic lupus erythematosus or anaphylactoid purpura.

Pathology and Pathogenesis. By light microscopy, most kidney biopsies reveal focal and segmental mesangial proliferation and increased matrix (Fig. 464–1). Some show generalized mesangial proliferation, occasionally associated with crescent formation and scarring. IgA is the predominant immunoglobulin deposited in the mesangium (Fig. 464–2), but lesser amounts of IgG, IgM, C3, and properdin are common. Electron microscopic studies confirm these findings.

Most evidence points to an immune complex etiology for IgA nephropathy. If the patient with IgA nephropathy has a kidney transplantation, the nephropathy commonly recurs in the transplanted kidney, indicating the systemic nature of this disorder.

Clinical and Laboratory Manifestations. IgA nephropathy is more common in males than in females (2:1). Patients either present with an episode of gross hematuria or are found to have microscopic hematuria on routine examination. While the gross hematuria lasts, renal function usually remains relatively

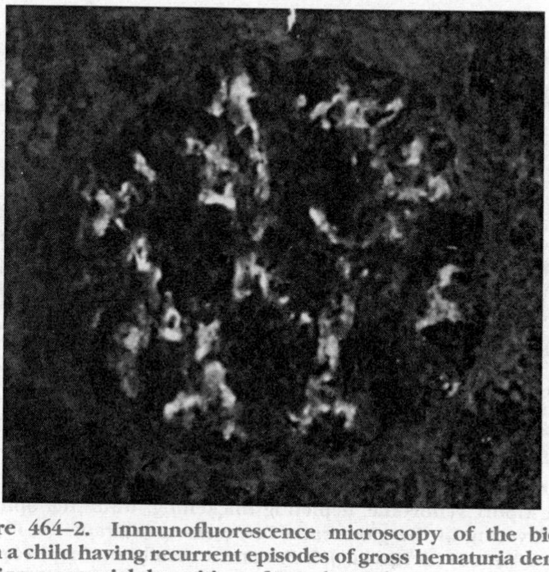

Figure 464–2. Immunofluorescence microscopy of the biopsy from a child having recurrent episodes of gross hematuria demonstrating mesangial deposition of IgA. (×250.)

normal and proteinuria minimal (<1 g/24 hr). Normal serum levels of C3 in IgA nephropathy help to distinguish this disorder from poststreptococcal glomerulonephritis.

Prognosis and Treatment. IgA nephropathy does not lead to significant kidney damage in most patients. Treatment is supportive and activity need not be restricted. Neither the number of episodes of gross hematuria nor the persistence of microscopic hematuria between episodes correlates with the likelihood of progressive disease. Progressive disease develops in 30% of patients, in whom a poor prognosis is associated with hypertension, diminished renal function, or proteinuria exceeding 1 g/24 hr between episodes of gross hematuria, or with histologic evidence of diffuse glomerulonephritis with crescents and scarring. Although controlled studies are lacking, immunosuppressive therapy may be beneficial in certain patients with progressive IgA nephropathy.

IDIOPATHIC HEMATURIA. Within the clinical spectrum of recurrent episodes of gross hematuria, *idiopathic* (benign familial) *hematuria* is defined histologically by normal findings on light and immunofluorescence microscopy. In some patients, electron microscopy demonstrates marked thinning of the glomerular basement membrane (thin basement membrane nephropathy), but the membrane width may be normal in others.

Idiopathic hematuria has an excellent prognosis, but long-term follow-up is required to exclude Alport syndrome. Both disorders may be familial and Alport syndrome may have minimal light microscopic changes, negative immunofluorescence, and thin basement membranes. In patients presumed to have idiopathic hematuria, the development of decreased renal function, proteinuria, or hypertension calls for a second renal biopsy.

ALPORT SYNDROME. This is the most common of several types of hereditary nephritis. There is marked variability in clinical presentation, natural history, histologic abnormalities, and genetic patterns.

Pathology. Kidney biopsies obtained during the first decade of life may show few changes by light microscopy. Later, the glomeruli may develop mesangial proliferation and capillary wall thickening, leading to progressive glomerular sclerosis. Tubular atrophy, interstitial inflammation and fibrosis, and foam cells (nonspecific lipid-laden tubular or interstitial cells) develop if the disease progresses. Immunopathologic studies are usually negative.

In most patients, electron microscopic studies have revealed thickening, thinning, splitting, and layering of the basement membranes of the glomeruli (Fig. 464–3) and tubules, but these lesions are not specific for Alport syndrome and may be absent in certain families that have the typical clinical manifestations of the syndrome.

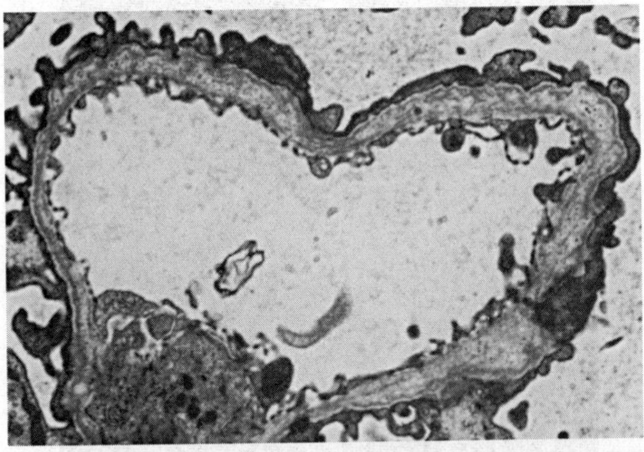

Figure 464–3. Electron micrograph of the biopsy from a child with Alport syndrome, depicting thickening, thinning, splitting, and layering of the glomerular basement membrane. (×16,250.) (From Yum M, Bergstein JM: Basement membrane nephropathy. Hum Pathol 14:996, 1983. Used by permission.)

Clinical Manifestations. Patients with Alport syndrome most commonly present with asymptomatic microscopic hematuria, but recurrent episodes of gross hematuria are not uncommon. In those with microscopic hematuria the development of proteinuria indicates the need for a kidney biopsy, which establishes the diagnosis.

Besides kidney involvement, a minority of patients have sensorineural hearing loss, which may begin in the high frequency range but progresses to involve the speech range and results in deafness. Approximately 10% of patients have eye abnormalities, the most frequent of which are cataracts, anterior lenticonus, and macular lesions.

Genetics. The inheritance of Alport syndrome best fits an X-linked dominant disorder. This explains the more severe clinical course in males than females. However, autosomal dominant transmission also has been described. Up to 20% of patients with Alport syndrome have no family history of renal disease; this suggests a high spontaneous mutation rate for the abnormal gene. In the X-linked form, the disease results from a mutation in the gene that encodes the $\alpha5$ chain of type IV collagen.

Complications. If renal function deteriorates, hypertension, urinary tract infections, and the manifestations of chronic renal failure may appear.

Prevention. Genetic counseling involving the entire family may limit propagation of the genetic abnormality.

Prognosis and Treatment. Males with Alport syndrome commonly develop end-stage renal failure in the 2nd or 3rd decade of life, occasionally in association with hearing loss. There is no specific therapy, but such patients are good candidates for dialysis and kidney transplantation. The development of anti-GBM nephritis in the transplanted kidneys of some patients with Alport syndrome suggests that the GBM of their native kidneys lacks a nephritogenic antigen. Females usually have a normal life span (for this reason, more mothers than fathers transmit the disease to their children) and only subclinical hearing loss.

IDIOPATHIC HYPERCALCIURIA. This disorder may present as RGH, persistent microscopic hematuria, or dysuria in the absence of stone formation. Hypercalciuria (without hypercalcemia) may result from excessive gastrointestinal absorption of normal dietary calcium intake or a defect in renal tubular calcium reabsorption. The precise mechanisms whereby the hypercalciuria causes hematuria or dysuria are unknown. The diagnosis is confirmed by finding a 24-hr urinary calcium excretion exceeding 4 mg/kg. A screening test for hypercalciuria in patients who cannot collect a timed urine specimen may be performed on a random urine specimen by measuring the calcium and creatinine concentrations. In general, a urine calcium to creatinine ratio (mg/mg) exceeding 0.2 suggests hypercalciuria, although normal ratios in infants may be as high as 0.8. Hypercalcemic hypercalciuria due to hyperparathyroidism or vitamin D intoxication must be considered in the differential diagnosis.

Hypercalciuria may lead to *nephrolithiasis.* Oral thiazide diuretics can normalize urinary calcium excretion by stimulating calcium reabsorption in the distal tubule. Such therapy may halt the gross hematuria or dysuria, and prevent nephrolithiasis. However, the precise indications for thiazide treatment remain controversial. In patients with persistent gross hematuria or dysuria, therapy is initiated with chlorothiazide at the dosage of 10–20 mg/kg/24 hr as a single morning dose. The dosage is titrated upwards until the urinary calcium excretion approaches 4 mg/kg/24 hr and the clinical manifestations resolve. After 1 yr of treatment, chlorothiazide is discontinued but may be resumed if gross hematuria, nephrolithiasis, or dysuria recur. During chlorothiazide therapy, the serum potassium should be monitored periodically to avoid hypokalemia. Dietary calcium restriction is not recommended because of the obligate requirement for growth. If low urine citrate levels are noted, supplemental citrate may improve hypercalciuria and its symptoms.

IgA NEPHROPATHY

Andreoli SP, Bergstein JM: Treatment of severe IgA nephropathy in children. Pediatr Nephrol 3:248, 1989.

Berg UB, Widstam-Attorps UC: Follow-up of renal function and urinary protein excretion in childhood IgA nephropathy. Pediatr Nephrol 7:123, 1993.

Ibels L, Györy A: IgA nephropathy: analysis of the natural history, important factor in the progression of renal disease and a review of the literature. Medicine 73:79, 1994.

Levy M, Gonzalez-Burchard G, Broyer M, et al: Berger's disease in children. Medicine 64:157, 1985.

IDIOPATHIC HEMATURIA

Gauthier B, Trachtman H, Frank R, et al: Familial thin basement membrane nephropathy in children with asymptomatic microhematuria. Nephron 51:502, 1989.

Gubler MC, Beaufils H, Noel LH, et al: Significance of thin glomerular basement membranes in hematuric children. Contrib Nephrol 80:147, 1990.

Tiebosch ATMG, Frederik PM, Van Breda Vriesman PJC, et al: Thin-basement–membrane nephropathy in adults with persistent hematuria. N Engl J Med 320:14, 1989.

ALPORT SYNDROME

Bernstein J: The glomerular basement membrane abnormality in Alport's syndrome. Am J Kidney Dis 10:222, 1987.

Feingold J, Bois E: Genetics of Alport's syndrome. Pediatr Nephrol 1:436, 1987.

Grunfeld, J-P: The clinical spectrum of hereditary nephritis. Kidney Int 27:83, 1985.

Kashtan CE, Michael AF: Alport syndrome: from bedside to genome to bedside. Am J Kidney Dis 22:627, 1993.

IDIOPATHIC HYPERCALCIURIA

Alon U, Warady BA, Hellerstein S: Hypercalciuria in the frequency-dysuria syndrome of childhood. J Pediatr 116:103, 1990.

Bonilla-Felix M, Villegas-Medina O, Vehaskari V: Renal acidification in children with idiopathic hypercalciuria. J Pediatr 124:529, 1994.

Garcia CD, Miller LA, Stapleton FB: Natural history of hematuria association with hypercalciuria in children. Am J Dis Child 145:1204, 1991.

Hymes LC, Warshaw BL: Thiazide diuretics for the treatment of children with idiopathic hypercalcemia and hematuria. J Urol 138:1217, 1987.

Sargent JD, Stukel TA, Kresel J, et al: Normal values for random urinary calcium to creatinine ratios in infancy. J Pediatr 123:393, 1993.

CHAPTER 465

Gross or Microscopic Hematuria

465.1 Acute Poststreptococcal Glomerulonephritis

This disease is the classic example of the acute nephritic syndrome: the sudden onset of gross hematuria, edema, hypertension, and renal insufficiency. It was formerly the most common cause of gross hematuria in children, but its frequency has so declined during the last decade that IgA nephropathy now seems to be the most common cause of gross hematuria.

ETIOLOGY AND EPIDEMIOLOGY. Acute poststreptococcal glomerulonephritis follows infection of the throat or skin with certain "nephritogenic" strains of group A beta-hemolytic streptococci. The factors that allow only certain strains of streptococci to be "nephritogenic" remain unclear. During cold weather poststreptococcal glomerulonephritis commonly follows streptococcal pharyngitis, whereas during warm weather the glomerulonephritis generally follows streptococcal skin infections or pyoderma. Epidemics of nephritis have been described in association with both throat (serotype 12) and skin (serotype 49) infections, but the disease is now most commonly sporadic.

PATHOLOGY. As in most forms of acute glomerulonephritis, the kidneys appear symmetrically enlarged. By light microscopy, all glomeruli appear enlarged and relatively bloodless and show diffuse mesangial cell proliferation with an increase in mesangial matrix (Fig. 465–1). Polymorphonuclear leukocytes are common in glomeruli during the early stage of the disease. Crescents and interstitial inflammation may be seen in severe cases. These changes are not specific for poststreptococcal glomerulonephritis.

Immunofluorescence microscopy reveals lumpy-bumpy deposits of immunoglobulin and complement on the GBMs and in the mesangium. By electron microscopy, electron-dense deposits, or "humps," are observed on the epithelial side of the GBM (Fig. 465–2).

PATHOGENESIS. Although morphologic studies and a depression in the serum complement (C3) level strongly suggest that poststreptococcal glomerulonephritis is mediated by immune complexes, the precise mechanisms whereby nephritogenic streptococci induce complex formation remain to be determined. Despite clinical and histologic similarities to acute serum sickness in the rabbit, the finding of circulating immune complexes in poststreptococcal glomerulonephritis is not uniform and complement activation is primarily through the alternative rather than the classic (immune complex–activated) pathway.

CLINICAL MANIFESTATIONS. Poststreptococcal glomerulonephritis is most common in children but rare before the age of 3 yr. The typical patient develops an acute nephritic syndrome 1–2 wk after an antecedent streptococcal infection. The severity of renal involvement may vary from asymptomatic microscopic hematuria with normal renal function to acute renal failure. Depending on the severity of renal involvement, patients may develop varying degrees of edema, hypertension, and oliguria. An encephalopathy or congestive heart failure or both may also develop. The edema is usually the result of salt and water retention, but a nephrotic syndrome may occur. Nonspecific symptoms such as malaise, lethargy, abdominal or flank pain, and fever are common. The acute phase generally resolves within 1 mo following onset, but urinary abnormalities may persist for more than 1 yr.

DIAGNOSIS. Urinalysis demonstrates red blood cells, frequently

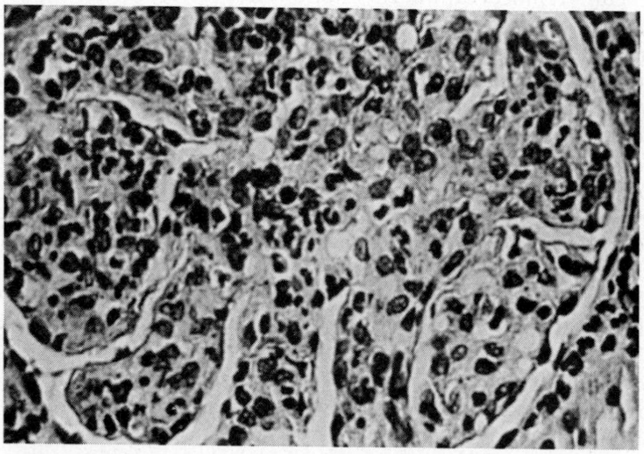

Figure 465–1. Glomerulus from a patient having poststreptococcal glomerulonephritis, appearing enlarged and relatively bloodless and showing mesangial proliferation and exudation of neutrophils. (×400.)

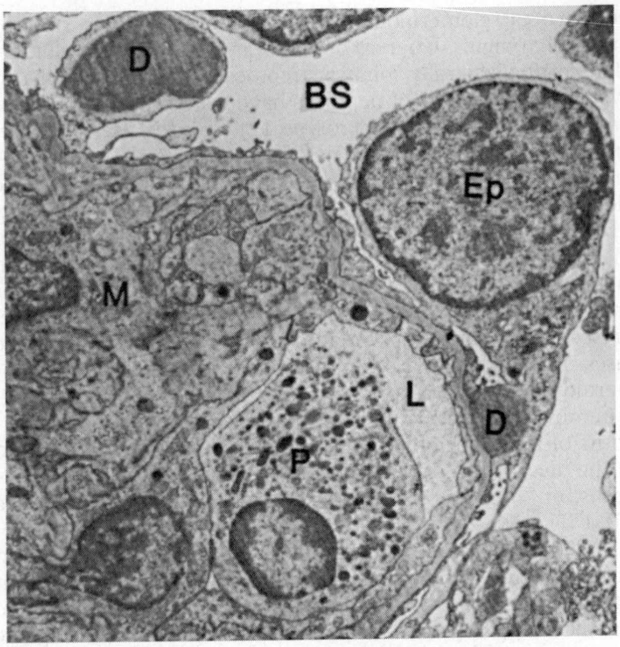

Figure 465–2. Electron micrograph in poststreptococcal glomerulonephritis, demonstrating electron-dense deposits (D) on the epithelial cell (Ep) side of the glomerular basement membrane. A polymorphonuclear leukocyte (P) is present within the lumen (L) of the capillary. BS = Bowman space; M = mesangium.

in association with red blood cell casts and proteinuria; polymorphonuclear leukocytes are not uncommon. A mild normochromic anemia may be present owing to hemodilution and low-grade hemolysis. The serum C3 level is usually reduced.

Confirmation of the diagnosis requires clear evidence of invasive streptococcal infection. Thus, positive throat cultures may support the diagnosis or may simply represent the carrier state. To document streptococcal infection properly, an elevated antibody titer to streptococcal antigen(s) should be confirmed. Although most commonly obtained, determination of the ASO titer may not be helpful because it rarely rises after streptococcal skin infections. The best single antibody titer to measure is that to the DNase B antigen. An alternative is the Streptozyme test (Wampole Laboratories, Stamford, CT), a slide agglutination procedure that detects antibodies to streptolysin O, DNase B, hyaluronidase, streptokinase, and NADase.

In the child with an acute nephritic syndrome, evidence of recent streptococcal infection, and a low C3 level, the clinical diagnosis of poststreptococcal glomerulonephritis is warranted and renal biopsy ordinarily is not indicated. It is important, however, to exclude systemic lupus erythematosus and an acute exacerbation of chronic glomerulonephritis. Considerations for renal biopsy would include the development of acute renal failure or nephrotic syndrome, the absence of evidence for streptococcal infection, the absence of hypocomplementemia, or the persistence of marked hematuria or proteinuria or both, diminished renal function, or a low C3 level for more than 3 mo after onset.

The differential diagnosis of poststreptococcal glomerulonephritis includes many of the causes of hematuria listed in Table XXIII–2. Acute glomerulonephritis may also follow infection with coagulase-positive and -negative staphylococci, *Streptococcus pneumoniae*, gram-negative bacteria, and certain fungal, rickettsial, and viral diseases.

COMPLICATIONS. The complications are those of acute renal failure and include volume overload, circulatory congestion, hypertension, hyperkalemia, hyperphosphatemia, hypocalcemia, acidosis, seizures, and uremia.

PREVENTION. Early systemic antibiotic therapy of streptococcal throat and skin infections will not eliminate the risk of glomerulonephritis. Family members of patients with acute glomerulonephritis should be cultured for group A beta-hemolytic streptococci and treated if culture-positive.

TREATMENT. As there is no specific therapy for acute poststreptococcal glomerulonephritis, the management is that of acute renal failure (Chapter 489.1). Although a 10-day course of systemic antibiotic therapy, generally with penicillin, is recommended to limit the spread of the nephritogenic organisms, there is no evidence that antibiotic therapy affects the natural history of glomerulonephritis. Activity need not be restricted, except during the acute phase of the disease when the complications of acute renal failure may be present, because activity has no detrimental effect on healing.

PROGNOSIS. Complete recovery occurs in more than 95% of children with acute poststreptococcal glomerulonephritis. There is no evidence that progression to chronic glomerulonephritis occurs. Infrequently, however, the acute phase may be very severe and lead to glomerular hyalinization and chronic renal insufficiency. Mortality in the acute stage can be avoided by appropriate management of the acute renal or cardiac failure. Recurrences are extremely rare.

Clark G, White RHR, Glasgow EF, et al: Poststreptococcal glomerulonephritis in children: Clinicopathological correlations and long-term prognosis. Pediatr Nephrol 2:381, 1988.
Heptinstall RH: Pathology of the Kidney, 3rd ed. Boston, Little, Brown, 1983.
Lange K, Seligson G, Cronin W: Evidence for the in situ origin of poststreptococcal glomerulonephritis: Glomerular localization of endostreptosin and the clinical significance of the subsequent antibody response. Clin Nephrol 19:3, 1983.
Vogl W, Renke M, Mayer-Eichberger D, et al: Long-term prognosis for endocapillary glomerulonephritis of poststreptococcal type in children and adults. Nephron 44:58, 1986.

CHAPTER 466
Membranous Glomerulopathy
(Glomerulonephritis)

Membranous glomerulopathy is the most common cause of nephrotic syndrome in adults, but it is uncommon in childhood and a rare cause of hematuria.

PATHOLOGY. By light microscopy, the glomeruli show diffuse thickening of the GBM, without significant proliferative changes (Fig. 466–1). The thickening is presumably due to the production of membrane-like material by the visceral epithelial cells in response to immune complexes deposited on the epithelial side of the membrane. This new material may in certain areas appear as "spikes" on the epithelial side of the basement membrane. Immunofluorescent microscopy demonstrates granular deposits of IgG and C3, which electron microscopy shows to be located on the epithelial side of the membrane.

PATHOGENESIS. Morphologic studies suggest that membranous glomerulopathy is an immune complex–mediated disease, but the mechanism of complex formation and the nature of the antigen within the complexes remain unknown in most patients. Despite close clinical and histologic similarities to the experimental Heymann nephritis, attempts to demonstrate proximal tubular antigen in the deposits have been largely unsuccessful.

CLINICAL MANIFESTATIONS. In children, membranous glomerulopathy is most common in the 2nd decade of life. The disease usually presents as nephrotic syndrome. However, almost all

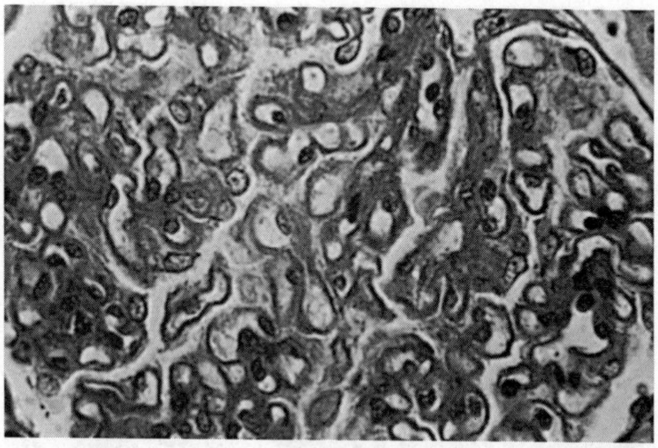

Figure 466–1. Glomerulus from a patient having membranous glomerulopathy, demonstrating diffuse thickening of the glomerular basement membrane in the absence of cellular proliferation. (×400.)

patients have microscopic hematuria and occasional patients suffer gross hematuria. The blood pressure and C3 levels are normal.

DIAGNOSIS. The diagnosis is confirmed by kidney biopsy. The usual indications for biopsy include the presentation of nephrotic syndrome in a child over 8 yr of age or the presence of unexplained hematuria and proteinuria.

Membranous glomerulopathy may occasionally be seen in association with systemic lupus erythematosus, cancer, gold or penicillamine therapy, and syphilis and hepatitis B virus infections. These conditions should be considered in patients having membranous disease, because elimination of the presumed stimulus might lead to resolution of the glomerulopathy. Patients with membranous glomerulopathy are at increased risk of renal vein thrombosis.

TREATMENT. Fortunately, membranous glomerulopathy resolves spontaneously in the majority of children, although some may have persistent proteinuria. The nephrotic state is best controlled with salt restriction and diuretic agents. Studies in adults suggest that immunosuppressive therapy may retard the progressive renal insufficiency observed in some patients.

Austin HA III:.Membranous nephropathy. Ann Intern Med 116:672, 1992.
Latham P, Poucell S, Koresaar A, et al: Idiopathic membranous glomerulopathy in Canadian children: A clinicopathologic study. J Pediatr 101:682, 1982.
Ramirez F, Brouhard BH, Travis LB, et al: Idiopathic membranous nephropathy in children. J Pediatr 101:677, 1982.
Schieppati A, Mosconi L, Perna A, et al: Prognosis of untreated patients with idiopathic membranous nephropathy. N Engl J Med 329:85, 1993.

CHAPTER 467

Systemic Lupus Erythematosus

This systemic disease is characterized by fever, weight loss, rash, hematologic abnormalities, arthritis, and involvement of the heart, lungs, central nervous system, and kidneys. The nonrenal manifestations are discussed in Chapter 150. Kidney disease is one of the most common manifestations of lupus in childhood and may occasionally be the only manifestation.

PATHOGENESIS AND PATHOLOGY. Studies in a mouse (NZB/NZW) strain and in humans suggest that the clinical manifestations of lupus are mediated by immune complexes, which are formed in the circulation and deposited in various organs. Recent studies have revealed aberrations in both B-cell and T-cell function.

Of the several classifications of lupus nephritis, the one offered by the World Health Organization (WHO), which uses light, immunofluorescent, and electron microscopy, is most accepted. In patients with WHO class I nephritis, no histologic abnormalities are detected. In WHO class II (also called mesangial lupus nephritis), some glomeruli have mesangial deposits containing immunoglobulin and complement; light microscopy may be normal (class II-A) or show focal and segmental mesangial hypercellularity and increased matrix (class II-B).

WHO class III (also called focal proliferative lupus nephritis) shows mesangial deposits in almost all glomeruli, and subendothelial deposits (between the endothelial cells and GBM) in some. In addition to focal and segmental mesangial proliferation, occasional glomeruli show capillary wall necrosis and crescent formation.

WHO class IV (also called diffuse proliferative lupus nephritis) is the most common and most severe form of lupus nephritis. All glomeruli contain massive mesangial and subendothelial deposits of immunoglobulin and complement. By light microscopy, all glomeruli show mesangial proliferation. The capillary walls are frequently thickened (owing to subendothelial deposits), creating the "wire-loop" lesion, and commonly show necrosis, crescent formation, and scarring.

WHO class V (also called membranous lupus nephritis) is the least common form of lupus nephritis; it resembles idiopathic membranous glomerulopathy histologically, except for mild to moderate mesangial proliferation.

Transformation of the histologic lesion from one class to another (usually to a more severe class) is common, especially in inadequately treated patients.

CLINICAL MANIFESTATIONS. The large majority of children with systemic lupus are adolescent girls who present with evidence of systemic disease, leading to the ultimate diagnosis. The clinical findings in patients having the milder forms (all class II, some class III) of lupus nephritis include hematuria, normal renal function, and proteinuria of less than 1 g/24 hr. Some patients with class III and all with class IV nephritis have hematuria and proteinuria, with reduced renal function, nephrotic syndrome, or acute renal failure. In some patients with proliferative glomerulonephritis, the finding of normal urinary sediment obscures the renal involvement. Patients with class V nephritis commonly have a nephrotic syndrome.

DIAGNOSIS. The diagnosis of lupus is suggested by the detection of circulating antinuclear antibodies and is confirmed by demonstrating that these antibodies react with native (double-stranded) DNA. In most patients with active disease, C3 and C4 levels are depressed. In view of the lack of clear correlation between the clinical manifestations and the severity of the renal involvement, renal biopsy should be done in all patients with lupus. The findings will guide the selection of immunosuppressive therapy.

TREATMENT. Immunosuppressive therapy in lupus nephritis aims at clinical and serologic remission (normalization of the anti-DNA, C3, and C4 levels). Therapy is initiated in all patients with prednisone, 60 mg/m²/day, divided into three or four doses. In patients having more severe forms of nephritis (some class III, all class IV), azathioprine is added in a once-daily dosage of 2–3 mg/kg. When serologic remission is obtained after 1–2 mo, the dose of prednisone is reduced to 60 mg/m² taken every other day as a single morning dose, being certain that the serologic studies remain normal and renal function stable while the dose is reduced. After a varying period of time, the dose may then be further reduced by 5 mg decrements to 30 mg/m², so long as serologic studies remain normal and renal function stable. The dose of azathioprine may be reduced gradually while serology and renal function are monitored, and may be discontinued after 1 yr. Studies in adults suggest that daily oral or monthly intravenous administration of cyclophosphamide may also be effective in corticosteroid-unresponsive or -toxic patients.

PROGNOSIS. Aggressive immunosuppressive therapy has dramatically improved the prognosis of lupus in childhood, but the disease is controlled, not cured. The risk of relapse, as well as the side effects of chronic immunosuppressive therapy, persists; of special concern are the effects of corticosteroids in teenaged girls. Patients with lupus should be managed in conjunction with specialists in medical centers where both medical and psychologic support can be given to both patients and their families.

Austin HA III, Boumpas DT, Vaughan EM, et al: Predicting renal outcomes in severe lupus nephritis: contributions of clinical and histologic data. Kidney Int 45:544, 1994.

Cameron JS: Lupus nephritis in childhood and adolescence. Pediatr Nephrol 8:230, 1994.

Donadio JV Jr, Glassock RJ: Immunosuppressive drug therapy in lupus nephritis. Am J Kidney Dis 21:239, 1993.

Laitman RS, Glicklich D, Sablay L, et al: Effect of long-term normalization of serum complement levels on the course of lupus nephritis. Am J Med 87:132, 1989.

Levey AS, Lan S-P, Corwin HL, et al: Progression and remission of renal disease in the lupus nephritis collaborative study. Ann Intern Med 116:114, 1992.

McCune WJ, Golbus J, Zeldes W, et al: Clinical and immunologic effects of monthly administration of intravenous cyclophosphamide in severe systemic lupus erythematosus. N Engl J Med 318:1423, 1988.

Schwartz MM, Shu-ping L, Bonsib SM, et al: Clinical outcome of three discrete histologic patterns of injury in severe lupus glomerulonephritis. Am J Kidney Dis 13:273, 1989.

CHAPTER 468
Membranoproliferative (Mesangiocapillary) Glomerulonephritis

The term *chronic glomerulonephritis* implies continuing glomerular injury, such as frequently leads to glomerular destruction and end-stage renal failure. Membranoproliferative glomerulonephritis is the most common cause of chronic glomerulonephritis in older children and young adults.

PATHOLOGY AND PATHOGENESIS. Membranoproliferative glomerulonephritis was initially distinguished from other forms of chronic glomerulonephritis by the finding of hypocomplementemia, in some patients the result of an antibody (called C3 nephritic factor) that activates the alternative complement pathway. Not all patients have hypocomplementemia. Three histologic types are described.

Type I membranoproliferative glomerulonephritis is the most common form; the glomeruli reveal an accentuation of the lobular pattern, due to a generalized increase in mesangial cells and matrix (Fig. 468–1). The glomerular capillary walls appear thickened and, in some areas, duplicated or split, owing to interposition of mesangial cytoplasm and matrix between the endothelial cells and GBM. Crescents may be present; when detected in a high percentage of glomeruli, they indicate a poor prognosis. Immunofluorescent microscopy reveals C3 and lesser amounts of immunoglobulin in the mesangium and along the peripheral capillary walls in a lobular pattern (Fig. 468–2), and electron microscopy confirms the presence of immune complex–like deposits in the mesangial and subendothelial regions.

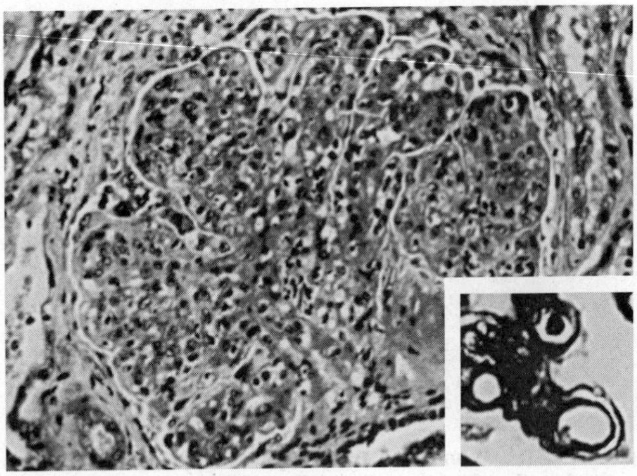

Figure 468–1. Glomerulus from a patient with type I membranoproliferative glomerulonephritis, demonstrating an accentuated lobular pattern, a generalized increase in mesangial cells and matrix, and "splitting" of the glomerular capillary wall *(inset)*. (×250.) (From Kim Y, Michael AF: Idiopathic membranoproliferative glomerulonephritis. Reproduced, with permission, from the Annual Review of Medicine, Vol 31. © 1980 by Annual Reviews, Inc.)

In type II disease, the mesangial changes are less prominent than in type I. The capillary walls demonstrate irregular ribbon-like thickening, owing to dense deposits. Splitting of the membrane is rare, but crescents are common. By electron microscopy, the dense deposits are seen as thickenings of GBM in the region of but distinct from the lamina densa. The deposits are also found in Bowman capsule, mesangium, and tubular basement membranes; their composition is unknown. Immunofluorescent studies show C3, usually with minimal immunoglobulin, along the margin of the dense deposit material.

In type III disease, the light and immunofluorescent microscopic findings resemble those found in type I disease. Electron microscopy reveals contiguous subepithelial and subendothelial deposits, associated with disruption and layering of the lamina densa portion of the basement membrane.

CLINICAL MANIFESTATIONS. Membranoproliferative glomerulonephritis is most common in the second decade of life. The

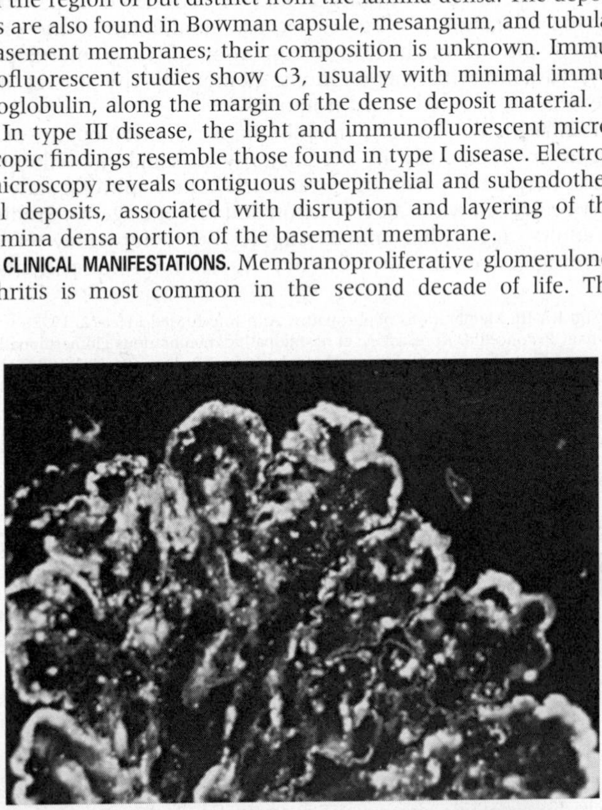

Figure 468–2. Immunofluorescence microscopy in type I membranoproliferative glomerulonephritis, demonstrating granular deposition of C3 along the glomerular basement membranes and in the mesangium. (×610.) (From Kim Y, Michael AF: Idiopathic membranoproliferative glomerulonephritis. Reproduced, with permission, from the Annual Review of Medicine, Vol 31. © 1980 by Annual Reviews, Inc.)

majority of patients present with nephrotic syndrome, and others with gross hematuria or asymptomatic microscopic hematuria and proteinuria. Renal function may be normal to depressed. Hypertension is common. The serum C3 complement level may be decreased.

DIAGNOSIS AND DIFFERENTIAL DIAGNOSIS. The diagnosis of membranoproliferative glomerulonephritis is made by renal biopsy. Indications for biopsy include onset of nephrotic syndrome in a child more than 8 yr of age or persistent microscopic hematuria and proteinuria.

Both membranoproliferative glomerulonephritis and poststreptococcal glomerulonephritis may present gross hematuria, low C3 levels, and elevated antistreptococcal antibody titers (coincidental in patients with membranoproliferative disease); their natural histories will distinguish between the two. Patients with poststreptococcal glomerulonephritis will improve dramatically within 2 mo of onset, whereas in children having membranoproliferative glomerulonephritis, persistent clinical manifestations will lead to kidney biopsy.

PROGNOSIS AND TREATMENT. The outlook for all types of membranoproliferative disease is poor. Complete recovery has been reported, but most patients with type II and many patients with types I and III progress to end-stage renal failure. Types I and II membranoproliferative glomerulonephritis have been found to recur in patients with kidney transplants, suggesting the presence of systemic disorder.

No definitive therapy exists, but stabilization of the clinical course has been reported in some patients receiving long-term alternate-day prednisone therapy.

Bennett WM, Fassett RG, Walker RG, et al: Mesangiocapillary glomerulonephritis type II (dense-deposit disease): Clinical features of progressive disease. Am J Kidney Dis 13:496, 1989.
Ford DM, Briscoe DM, Shanley PF, et al: Childhood membranoproliferative glomerulonephritis type I: limited steroid therapy. Kidney Int 41:1606, 1992.
McEnery PT: Membranoproliferative glomerulonephritis: the Cincinnati experience—cumulative renal survival from 1957 to 1989. J Pediatr 116:S109, 1990.
Tarshish P, Bernstein J, Tobin JN, et al: Treatment of mesangio-capillary glomerulonephritis with alternate-day prednisone—a report of The International Study of Kidney Disease in Children. Pediatr Nephrol 6:123, 1992.

Chapter 469

Glomerulonephritis of Chronic Infection

Occurrence of glomerulonephritis has been recognized during the course of various chronic infections, including subacute bacterial endocarditis (*S. viridans* and other organisms), infected ventriculoatrial shunts for hydrocephalus *(Staphylococcus epidermidis),* syphilis, hepatitis B, hepatitis C, candidiasis, and malaria. In each condition, the infecting organism has low virulence, and the host is chronically seeded with foreign antigen. In the presence of high levels of circulating antigen, the host's antibody response leads to formation of immune complexes, which deposit in the kidneys and initiate the glomerulonephritis.

The histopathologic findings may resemble poststreptococcal, membranous, or membranoproliferative glomerulonephritis. The clinical manifestations are generally those of an acute nephritic or nephrotic syndrome. The C3 level is frequently depressed.

Eradication of the infection before severe glomerular injury occurs usually results in resolution of the glomerulonephritis. Progression to end-stage renal failure has been described.

Arze RS, Rashid H, Morley R, et al: Shunt nephritis: Report of two cases and review of the literature. Clin Nephrol 19:48, 1983.
Chesney RW, O'Regan S, Guyda HJ, et al: Candida endocrinopathy syndrome with membranoproliferative glomerulonephritis: Demonstration of glomerular candida antigen. Clin Nephrol 5:232, 1976.
Hendrickse RG, Adeniyi A: Quartan malarial nephrotic syndrome in children. Kidney Int 16:64, 1979.
Hunte W, Al-Ghraoui F, Cohen RJ: Secondary syphilis and the nephrotic syndrome. J Am Soc Nephrol 3:1351, 1993.
Johnson RJ, Couser WG: Hepatitis B infection and renal disease: clinical, immunopathogenic and therapeutic considerations. Kidney Int 37:663, 1990.
Johnson RJ, Gretch DR, Yamabe H, et al: Membranoproliferative glomerulonephritis associated with hepatitis C virus infection. N Engl J Med 328:465, 1993.
Neugarten J, Baldwin DS: Glomerulonephritis in bacterial endocarditis. Am J Med 77:297, 1984.

Chapter 470

Rapidly Progressive (Crescentic) Glomerulonephritis

The term *rapidly progressive* describes the clinical course of several forms of glomerulonephritis whose unifying abnormality is the presence of crescents in the majority of glomeruli. The natural history in most forms is rapid progression to end-stage renal failure.

CLASSIFICATION. Crescents may be found in several well-defined types of glomerulonephritis, such as poststreptococcal, lupus, membranoproliferative, and the glomerulonephritides of Goodpasture disease, anaphylactoid purpura, and other forms of vasculitis. In these diseases, the typical findings on light, immunofluorescent, and electron microscopic examinations are maintained despite crescent formation, and these histologic findings, in conjunction with appropriate laboratory studies, should reveal the underlying disease. After these recognized forms of glomerulonephritis are excluded, an idiopathic variety of rapidly progressive disease remains.

PATHOLOGY AND PATHOGENESIS. Crescents are found on the inside of Bowman capsule and are composed of the proliferating epithelial cells of the capsule, and of fibrin, basement membrane–like material, and macrophages (Fig. 470–1). The stimu-

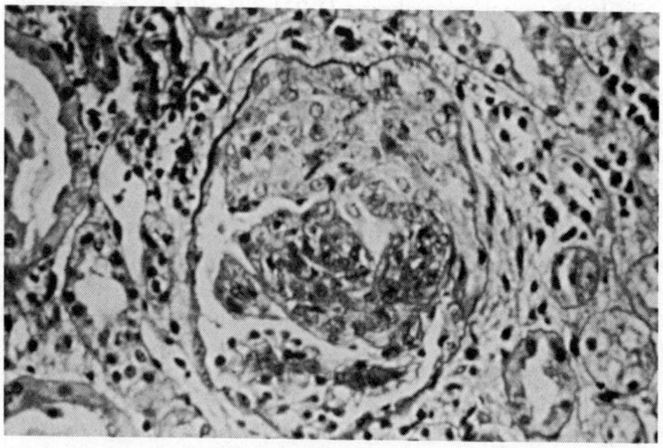

Figure 470–1. Light micrograph of a biopsy specimen from a child with anaphylactoid purpura glomerulonephritis, demonstrating a crescent overlying the glomerulus. (×180.)

lus for crescent formation is presumed to be the deposition of fibrin in Bowman space, probably as a result of necrosis or disruption of the glomerular capillary wall.

In many patients having the idiopathic variety of rapidly progressive disease, no evidence for immunologic mechanisms can be detected; others have antibodies against GBM or deposits of immune complexes on capillary walls. The C3 level is normal.

CLINICAL MANIFESTATIONS. Most patients develop acute renal failure, often after an acute nephritic or nephrotic episode. Progression to end-stage renal failure follows within weeks to months after onset.

DIAGNOSIS AND DIFFERENTIAL DIAGNOSIS. Appropriate serologic studies (ANA, C3, anti-DNase B titers) should be obtained to search for defined types of glomerulonephritis. Rare forms of vasculitis, such as Wegener's granulomatosis and microscopic polyarteritis nodosa, may be suggested by the detection of circulating antineutrophil cytoplasmic antibodies (ANCA). The diagnosis is confirmed by kidney biopsy.

PROGNOSIS AND TREATMENT. Children having rapidly progressive disease associated with poststreptococcal glomerulonephritis may recover spontaneously. We have had success in treating the rapidly progressive nephritis of lupus and of anaphylactoid purpura with prednisone and azathioprine. The prognosis is poor for the remaining types of rapidly progressive glomerulonephritis, although a few patients have been reported to improve with therapy combining pulse methylprednisolone, oral cyclophosphamide, and possibly plasmapheresis.

Jardin HMPF, Leake J, Risdon RA, et al: Crescentric glomerulonephritis in children. Pediatr Nephrol 6:231, 1992.

Kallenberg CGM, Mulder AHL, Tervaert JWC: Antineutrophil cytoplasmic antibodies: a still-growing class of autoantibodies in inflammatory disorders. Am J Med 93:675, 1992.

Roltem M, Fauci AS, Hallahan CW, et al: Wegener granulomatosis in children and adolescents: clinical presentation and outcome. J Pediatr 122:26, 1993.

Srivastava RN, Moudgil A, Bagga A, et al: Crescentric glomerulonephritis in children: a review of 43 cases. Am J Nephrol 12:155, 1992.

CHAPTER 471
Goodpasture Disease

Goodpasture disease (pulmonary hemorrhage and glomerulonephritis associated with antibodies against lung and against globular basement membrane [GBM]) should be distinguished from Goodpasture syndrome (a clinical picture of pulmonary hemorrhage and glomerulonephritis that may be seen with several disorders, including systemic lupus erythematosus, anaphylactoid purpura, polyarteritis nodosa, and Wegener granulomatosis). In some patients, anti-GBM nephritis occurs without pulmonary hemorrhage as one form of rapidly progressive glomerulonephritis.

PATHOLOGY. In most patients, the changes on light microscopy resemble those of rapidly progressive glomerulonephritis; immunofluorescent microscopy shows a continuous linear pattern of IgG along the GBM, typical of anti-GBM antibody (Fig. 471–1).

CLINICAL MANIFESTATIONS. Goodpasture disease is extremely rare in childhood. Hemoptysis is usually the presenting complaint, and pulmonary hemorrhage is a potential cause of death. In days to weeks, hematuria, proteinuria, and progressive renal failure develop. The C3 level is normal.

DIAGNOSIS. The diagnosis is suggested by kidney biopsy. Other diseases that may show linear GBM staining for IgG are excluded when serum is found to contain anti-GBM antibody.

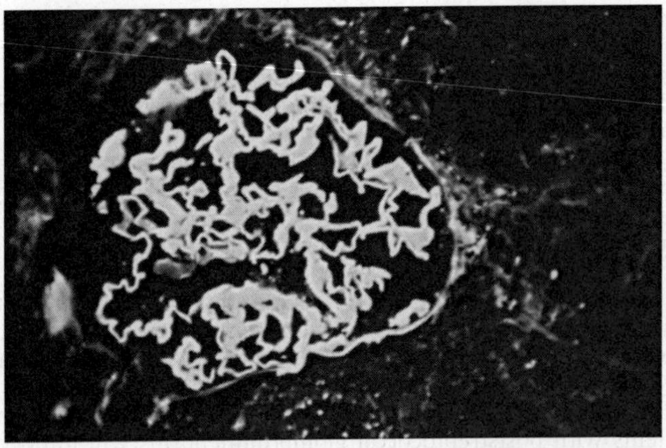

Figure 471–1. Immunofluorescence micrograph demonstrating the continuous linear staining of IgG along the glomerular basement membrane, as found in diseases mediated by antiglomerular basement membrane antibody. (×250.)

PROGNOSIS AND TREATMENT. Patients who survive the pulmonary hemorrhage commonly progress to end-stage renal failure. Rates of survival and recovery of renal function have improved with pulse methylprednisone, oral cyclophosphamide, and plasmapheresis therapy.

Helderman JH: The case of the two disparate diseases: a medical mystery. Am J Nephrol 11:238, 1991.

Herman PG, Balikian JP, Seltzer SE, et al: The pulmonary-renal syndrome. Am J Roentgenol 130:1141, 1978.

Simpson IJ, Doak PB, Williams LC, et al: Plasma exchange in Goodpasture's syndrome. Am J Nephrol 2:301, 1982.

CHAPTER 472
Hemolytic-Uremic Syndrome

The hemolytic-uremic syndrome is the most common cause of acute renal failure in young children, and the incidence is increasing. It was initially believed to be a renal disorder with secondary hematologic manifestations, but recent studies indicate that the syndrome should be regarded as a systemic disease. Hemolytic-uremic syndrome has features common to thrombotic thrombocytopenic purpura, except that the latter tends to occur in young women as a relapsing illness with fever, central nervous system involvement, and cutaneous signs.

ETIOLOGY. The disease most frequently follows an episode of gastroenteritis caused by an enteropathogenic strain of *Escherichia coli* (0157:H7). The reservoir of this organism is the intestinal tract of domestic animals. It is usually transmitted by undercooked meat and unpasteurized milk. Outbreaks have followed ingestion of contaminated apple cider or bathing in a contaminated swimming pool. The organism elaborates a toxin, called verotoxin, which is apparently absorbed from the intestines and initiates endothelial cell injury. It has been associated with other bacterial *(Shigella, Salmonella, Campylobacter, S. pneumoniae), Bartonella,* and viral (coxsackie, ECHO, influenza, varicella, HIV, Epstein-Barr) infections and with endotoxemia. It has been reported also to follow use of oral contraceptives and pyran copolymer, an inducer of interferon. In addition, a hemolytic-uremic type of disorder has been reported to be associated with systemic lupus erythematosus, malignant hypertension, pre-eclampsia, postpartum renal failure, and radiation nephritis. There may be an absence of a plasma factor that stimulates endothelial cell prostacyclin production in familial cases. There are several reports of occurrence in more than one member of a family, but the role of genetic factors in predisposition to the disease is unknown.

PATHOLOGY. The initial changes in the glomeruli include thickening of the capillary walls, narrowing of the capillary lumina, and widening of the mesangium. Electron microscopy shows these changes to be the result of subendothelial and mesangial deposition of a granular, amorphous material of unknown origin. Fibrin thrombi can be found in glomerular capillaries and arterioles and may lead to cortical necrosis.

Severely involved glomeruli progress to partial or total sclerosis; severe vascular involvement may render others obsolescent from ischemia. In these severely involved small arteries and arterioles, concentric intimal proliferation leads to vascular occlusion.

PATHOGENESIS. The primary event in pathogenesis of the syndrome appears to be endothelial cell injury. Capillary and arteriolar endothelial injury in the kidney leads to localized clotting. Evidence for disseminated intravascular coagulation is commonly lacking. The microangiopathic anemia results from mechanical damage to the red blood cells as they pass through the altered vasculature. Thrombocytopenia is due to intrarenal platelet adhesion or damage. Damaged red cells and platelets are removed from circulation by the liver and spleen.

CLINICAL MANIFESTATIONS. The syndrome is most common in children under the age of 4 yr. The onset is usually preceded by gastroenteritis (fever, vomiting, abdominal pain, and diarrhea, which is often bloody) or, less commonly, by an upper respiratory tract infection. This is followed in 5–10 days by the sudden onset of pallor, irritability, weakness, lethargy, and oliguria. Physical examination may reveal dehydration, edema, petechiae, hepatosplenomegaly, and marked irritability.

DIAGNOSIS AND DIFFERENTIAL DIAGNOSIS. The diagnosis of the syndrome is supported by the findings of a microangiopathic hemolytic anemia, thrombocytopenia, and acute renal failure. The hemoglobin is commonly in the range of 5–9 g/dL (50–90 g/L). The blood film reveals helmet cells, burr cells, and fragmented red blood cells (Chapter 439.4). Plasma hemoglobin levels are elevated and plasma haptoglobin levels diminished. The reticulocyte count is moderately elevated; the Coombs test is negative. The white blood cell count may rise to 30,000/mm^3 (30×10^9/L). Thrombocytopenia (20,000–100,000/mm^3; 10^9/L) occurs in more than 90% of patients. Findings on urinalysis are surprisingly mild and usually consist of low-grade microscopic hematuria and proteinuria. Partial thromboplastin time and prothrombin time are usually normal; their prolongation is more commonly due to vitamin K deficiency than to disseminated intravascular coagulation. The severity of the renal involvement, and the complications thereof, vary from mild renal insufficiency to acute renal failure requiring dialysis. Barium contrast roentgenograms (enema) reveal colonic spasm and transient early filling defects. Subsequent intestinal stenosis is a rare sequela.

The sudden onset of acute renal failure in a child should always call this entity to mind. The typical history, clinical picture, and laboratory findings confirm the diagnosis in most patients. Other causes of acute renal failure, especially those that can be associated with a microangiopathic anemia (lupus, malignant hypertension), should be excluded. Except in the rare patient who suffers prolonged renal failure (more than 2 wk) or who fails to develop thrombocytopenia, a renal biopsy is rarely indicated; it should not be performed in the thrombocytopenic patient.

Patients who have bilateral renal vein thrombosis (Chapter 474.3) may be difficult to distinguish from those with the hemolytic-uremic syndrome. Both disorders may be preceded by gastroenteritis, and in both the children may present with dehydration, pallor, and evidence of microangiopathic hemolytic anemia, thrombocytopenia, and acute renal failure. The marked enlargement of kidneys of the child with renal vein thrombosis helps to distinguish the disorders, but angiography may be necessary in obscure cases.

COMPLICATIONS. Complications may include anemia, acidosis, hyperkalemia, fluid overload, congestive heart failure, hypertension, and uremia. In addition, extrarenal involvement may include central nervous system manifestations (irritability, seizures, coma), colitis (melena, perforation), diabetes mellitus, and rhabdomyolysis. The pathogenesis of these complications is unknown; they seem likely to be the result of intravascular thrombosis.

PROGNOSIS AND TREATMENT. With aggressive management of the acute renal failure, more than 90% of patients survive the acute phase, and the majority of these recover normal renal function. It has been difficult to evaluate the results of therapy. Corticosteroids appear to have no value, and experience with platelet inhibitors is so far inconclusive. The treatment has mostly involved anticoagulants, primarily heparin. Analysis of the results fails to demonstrate beneficial effects in most patients, who in any case lack evidence of active hypercoagulation. Fibrinolytic therapy to dissolve intrarenal thrombi would have theoretical benefit, but the risks seem to outweigh the potential gains. Plasmapheresis or the administration of fresh-frozen plasma, or both, has been recommended in hopes of replacing a missing plasma stimulator of prostacyclin production, but results do not as yet permit interpretation.

Careful medical management of the hematologic and renal manifestations, in conjunction with early and frequent peritoneal dialysis, offers the best chance of recovery from the acute phase. Peritoneal dialysis not only controls the manifestations of the uremic state, but also promotes recovery by removing an inhibitor (plasminogen activates inhibitor-1) of fibrinolysis from the circulation, thus allowing endogenous fibrinolytic mechanisms to dissolve vascular thrombi. Long-term observation is necessary to watch for late development of hypertension or chronic kidney disease. Recurrence of the disease is rare.

Bergstein JM, Riley M, Bang NU: Role of plasminogen-activator inhibitor type 1 in the pathogenesis and outcome of the hemolytic uremic syndrome. N Engl J Med 327:755, 1992.

Gianvita A, Perna A, Caringella A, et al: Plasma exchange in children with hemolytic-uremic syndrome at risk of poor outcome. Am J Kidney Dis 22:264, 1993.

Kaplan BS, Trompeter RS, Moake JL (eds): Hemolytic Uremic Syndrome and Thrombotic Thrombocytopenic Purpura. New York, Marcel Dekker, 1992.

Kelles A, Van Dyck M, Proesmans W: Childhood haemolytic uraemic syndrome: long-term outcome and prognostic features. Eur J Pediatr 153:38, 1994.

Martin DL, MacDonald KL, White KE, et al: The epidemiology and chemical aspects of the hemolytic-uremic syndrome in Minnesota. N Engl J Med 323:1161, 1990.

Milford DV, White RHR, Taylor CM: Prognostic significance of proteinuria one year after onset of diarrhea-associated hemolytic-uremic syndrome. J Pediatr 118:191, 1991.

Neild G: Haemolytic uraemic syndrome in practise. Lancet 343:398, 1994.

Siegler RL, Milligan MR, Burningham TH, et al: Long-term outcome and prognostic indicators in the hemolytic-uremic syndrome. J Pediatr 118:195, 1991.

Siegler R, Pavia A, Christofferson R, et al: A 20 year population based study of postdiarrheal hemolytic uremic syndrome in Utah. Pediatrics 94:35, 1994.

CHAPTER 473
Infection as a Cause of Hematuria

Gross or microscopic hematuria may be associated with bacterial, mycobacterial, or viral infections of the urinary tract (Chapter 492). Why the same organism may cause hematuria in one patient with cystitis and not in another is unclear; the occurrence of hematuria may be related to the depth and severity of the inflammatory reaction within the bladder wall.

Urethritis may present gross or microscopic hematuria, usually in conjunction with urgency and urethral discomfort. Urinalysis reveals red blood cells and pyuria. Urine cultures occasionally reveal bacteria, *Ureaplasma,* or *Chlamydia,* but are usually negative. A history of trauma should be sought. The disorder frequently resolves spontaneously. Treatment can be considered with a 10-day course of doxycycline, with a urinary analgesic (phenazopyridine hydrochloride) given for relief of pain. If conservative management fails, cystoscopy may be required to determine the nature of any underlying abnormality.

CHAPTER 474
Hematologic Diseases Causing Hematuria

474.1 Coagulopathies and Thrombocytopenia

Gross or microscopic hematuria may be associated with inherited or acquired disorders of coagulation (e.g., with hemophilias or with disseminated intravascular coagulation or with thrombocytopenia of any cause). In these cases, however, hematuria is almost never the presenting complaint but usually develops after other manifestations (Part XXI, Section 7).

474.2 Sickle Cell Nephropathy

Gross or microscopic hematuria may be seen in children with sickle cell disease or trait. The hematuria presumably results from sickling in the relatively hypoxic, acidic, hypertonic renal medulla, with vascular stasis, diminished blood flow, ischemia, papillary necrosis, and interstitial fibrosis. Additional clinical manifestations of sickle cell nephropathy may include a urinary concentrating defect, renal tubular acidosis and, rarely, a nephrotic syndrome that morphologically resembles focal sclerosis or membranoproliferative glomerulonephritis. The hematuria resolves spontaneously in the majority of patients (Chapter 419.1).

Allon M: Renal abnormalities in sickle cell disease. Arch Intern Med 150:501, 1990.

Bhathena DB, Sondheimer JH: The glomerulopathy of homozygous sickle hemoglobin (SS) disease: morphology and pathogenesis. J Am Soc Nephrol 1:1241, 1991.

Falk RJ, Scheinman J, Phillips G, et al: Prevalence and pathologic features of sickle cell nephropathy and response to inhibition of angiotensin-converting enzyme. N Engl J Med 326:910, 1992.

474.3 Renal Vein Thrombosis

EPIDEMIOLOGY. Renal vein thrombosis seems to occur in two distinct patterns. In newborns and infants, the disease is commonly associated with asphyxia, dehydration, shock, and sepsis; it occurs rarely in infants of diabetic mothers. After infancy, the disease is more commonly associated with the nephrotic syndrome (most frequently with membranous nephropathy), with cyanotic heart disease, and with the use of angiographic contrast agents.

PATHOGENESIS. The disease presumably begins in the intrarenal venous radicles, with both antegrade and retrograde spread. The main renal vein may escape involvement. Thrombus formation is presumably mediated by endothelial cell injury (by hypoxia, endotoxin, or contrast media) in conjunction with a hypercoagulable state (nephrotic syndrome) and diminished vascular blood flow, which may be due to hypovolemia (shock, sepsis, dehydration, or nephrotic syndrome) or to the intravascular sludging of blood that results from polycythemia.

CLINICAL MANIFESTATIONS. The development of renal vein thrombosis in infants is usually heralded by the sudden onset of gross hematuria and unilateral or bilateral flank masses. Older children commonly present with gross or microscopic hematuria and flank pain. The disease is more frequently unilateral than bilateral; bilateral involvement results in acute renal failure.

DIAGNOSIS. The diagnosis is suggested by the development of hematuria and flank masses in a patient with predisposing clinical factors. Most patients will also have a microangiopathic hemolytic anemia and thrombocytopenia. Ultrasonography will show marked enlargement, whereas radionuclide studies reveal little or no renal function in involved kidneys. Doppler flow studies or venacavography of the inferior vena cava may be necessary to confirm the diagnosis in occult cases, but contrast studies should generally be avoided in order to minimize the risk of further vascular damage.

DIFFERENTIAL DIAGNOSIS. The differential diagnosis includes other causes of hematuria (especially the hemolytic-uremic syndrome) or renal enlargement (hydronephrosis, cystic disease, Wilms tumor, abscess, hematoma).

TREATMENT. For unilateral renal vein thrombosis, treatment is supportive and involves correction of fluid and electrolyte abnormalities and treatment of infection. Prophylactic anticoagulation to prevent thrombosis in the remaining kidney is unwarranted, except perhaps in patients with disseminated intravascular coagulation.

Because bilateral renal vein thrombosis frequently leads to chronic renal failure, consideration should be given to use of such measures as thrombectomy or the systemic use of fibrinolytic agents.

PROGNOSIS. In infants, the thrombosed kidney undergoes progressive atrophy, ultimately leaving a small scarred kidney. Nephrectomy should not be performed in the acute phase, and later only if hypertension or chronic infection develops. In older children, the involved kidney may recover function, especially if the thrombosis was associated with nephrotic syndrome or cyanotic heart disease.

Laplante S, Patriquin HB, Robitaille P, et al: Renal vein thrombosis in children: evidence of early flow recovery with Doppler US. Radiology 189:37, 1993.

Mocan H, Beattie TJ, Murphy AV: Renal venous thrombosis in infancy: long-term follow-up. Pediatr Nephrol 5:45, 1991.
Ricci MA, Lloyd DA: Renal venous thrombosis in infants and children. Arch Surg 125:1195, 1990.

CHAPTER 475

Anatomic Abnormalities Associated with Hematuria

CONGENITAL ANOMALIES

Gross or microscopic hematuria may be associated with most types of malformations of the urinary tract. The sudden onset of usually painless gross hematuria after minor trauma to the flank is frequently associated with ureteropelvic junction obstruction or cystic kidneys.

TRAUMA

Blunt or penetrating injury to the abdomen may injure the kidney. Gross or microscopic hematuria, flank pain, and abdominal rigidity may occur; associated injuries may be present. Urethral trauma may result from crushing-type injury, frequently associated with a fractured pelvis, or from direct injury by a foreign object. The injury is suspected when gross blood appears at the external meatus.

Lieu TA, Fleisher GR, Mahboubi S, et al: Hematuria and clinical findings as indications for intravenous pyelography in pediatric blunt renal trauma. Pediatrics 82:216, 1988.
Taylor GA, Eichelberger MR, Potter BM: Hematuria: A marker of abdominal injury in children after blunt trauma. Ann Surg 208:688, 1988.
Yale-Loehr AJ, Kramer SS, Quinlan DM, et al: CT of severe renal trauma in children: Evaluation and course of healing with conservative therapy. AJR 152:109, 1989.

475.1 Autosomal Recessive Polycystic Kidney Disease

Also known as infantile polycystic disease, this rare autosomal recessive disorder may not be detected until after infancy. Besides cysts in the kidneys, cysts may also be found in the liver, with significant liver disease.

PATHOLOGY. Both kidneys are markedly enlarged and grossly show innumerable cysts throughout the cortex and medulla. Microscopic studies show the "cysts" to be dilatations of the collecting ducts. The interstitium and remainder of the tubules may be normal at birth, but development of interstitial fibrosis and tubular atrophy may lead to renal failure.

The majority of patients also have cysts in the liver. In severe cases, the cysts in the liver may be associated with cirrhosis, portal hypertension, and death from ruptured esophageal varices. When the severity of hepatic manifestations exceeds that of renal involvement, the disorder is called *congenital hepatic fibrosis*. Whether infantile polycystic disease and congenital hepatic fibrosis are the opposite ends of the spectrum of a single disorder or distinct autosomal recessive disorders with similar manifestations remains to be determined.

CLINICAL MANIFESTATIONS. The typical patient has bilateral flank masses at birth. The disorder may be associated with oligohydramnios, owing to inadequate formation of urine by the fetus. The oligohydramnios may produce Potter syndrome (flat nose, recessed chin, epicanthal folds, low-set abnormal ears, limb abnormalities), as a result of compression of the fetus, and pulmonary hypoplasia. The pulmonary hypoplasia may produce neonatal respiratory distress, with spontaneous pneumothorax. The association of developmental disorders of the lungs and kidneys is sufficiently frequent to warrant ultrasonic evaluation of the kidneys in all neonates who have spontaneous pneumothorax. Gross or microscopic hematuria and hypertension (which may be severe) are common. Renal function may be normal or diminished, depending on the severity of the renal malformation. Rarely, patients beyond infancy may first present with a nephrogenic diabetes insipidus-like state, renal insufficiency, or hypertension.

DIAGNOSIS. The diagnosis is suggested by the clinical manifestations and is supported by ultrasonography, which shows markedly enlarged and uniformly hyperechogenic kidneys (Fig. 475–1). Because ultrasonic evaluation of the kidneys may fail to define the cysts, intravenous pyelography may be considered. A satisfactory pyelogram will reveal opacification of the dilated collecting ducts. Because these ducts run from cortex to medulla, they will appear as radial streaks similar to the spokes of a wheel. But radiographic studies are rarely able to confirm the diagnosis; therefore, in questionable instances open surgical biopsy of the liver and right kidney may be performed toward the end of the 1st yr of life to confirm the diagnosis and to permit genetic counseling.

The differential diagnosis includes other causes of bilateral renal enlargement, such as multicystic dysplasia, hydronephrosis, Wilms tumor, and renal vein thrombosis.

TREATMENT. The treatment is supportive, including careful management of the hypertension.

PROGNOSIS. Children with severe renal involvement may die in the neonatal period of pulmonary or renal insufficiency. Survivors may live for several years before developing renal insufficiency. During this period, the kidneys shrink in size and the hypertension becomes less severe. When renal failure develops, dialysis and kidney transplantation should be considered. In patients having hepatic fibrosis, cirrhosis may lead to portal hypertension, for which the prognosis is poor.

Cole BR, Conley SB, Stapleton FB: Polycystic kidney disease in the first year of life. J Pediatr 111:693, 1987.

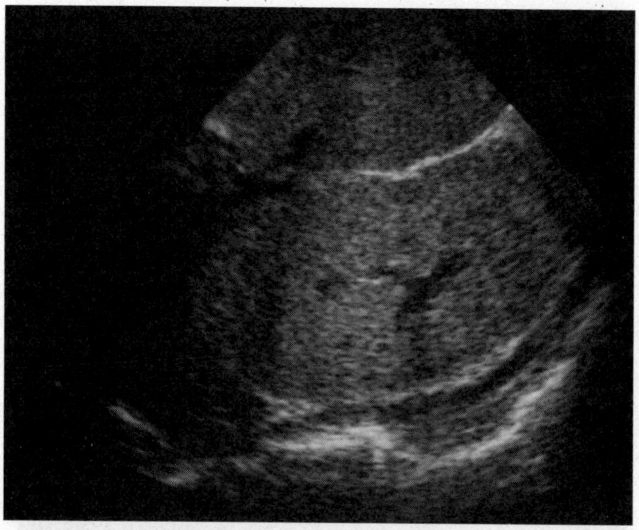

Figure 475–1. Ultrasound examination of a neonate with autosomal recessive polycystic kidney disease demonstrating renal enlargement (9 cm) and increased diffuse echogenicity with complete loss of corticomedullary differentiation due to multiple small cystic interfaces.

Kaariainen H, Koskimes O, Norio R: Dominant and recessive polycystic kidney disease in children: Evaluation of clinical features and laboratory data. Pediatr Nephrol 2:296, 1988.
Kaplan BS, Fay J, Shah V, et al: Autosomal recessive polycystic disease. Pediatr Nephrol 3:43, 1989.
Shaikewitz ST, Chapman A: Autosomal recessive polycystic kidney disease: issues regarding the variability of clinical presentation. J Am Soc Nephrol 3:1858, 1993.

475.2 Autosomal Dominant Polycystic Kidney Disease

Also known as adult polycystic disease, this autosomal dominant disorder is a common cause of end-stage renal failure in adults but is rarely encountered in childhood. In most families the genetic defect seems to involve a locus on the short arm of chromosome 16. In affected adults, both kidneys are enlarged and show cortical and medullary cysts that are primarily dilated tubules. The disease commonly presents in the 4th or 5th decade of life with gross or microscopic hematuria, bilateral flank pain or masses, or both, and hypertension. Associated abnormalities may include hepatic cysts of no clinical significance and aneurysms of the cerebral circulation that may result in intracranial hemorrhage. Children with the disease may present with hematuria or unilateral or bilateral flank masses. Hypertension may develop. The cysts are frequently demonstrable by ultrasonography (Fig. 475–2), intravenous pyelography, or computed tomography (CT) scan. In conjunction with the clinical manifestations and family history, radiographic studies usually confirm the diagnosis. In occult cases, especially those lacking a family history of the disease (the disease has a high spontaneous mutation rate), open renal biopsy may be necessary to confirm the diagnosis. Treatment is supportive. End-stage renal failure frequently develops by the 6th or 7th decade.

Fick GM, Johnson AM, Strain JD, et al: Characteristics of very early onset autosomal dominant polycystic kidney disease. J Am Soc Nephrol 3:1863, 1993.
Gabow P: Autosomal dominant polycystic kidney disease. N Engl J Med 329:332, 1993.
Kaplan BS, Rabin I, Nogrady MG, et al: Autosomal dominant polycystic renal disease in children. J Pediatr 90:782, 1977.

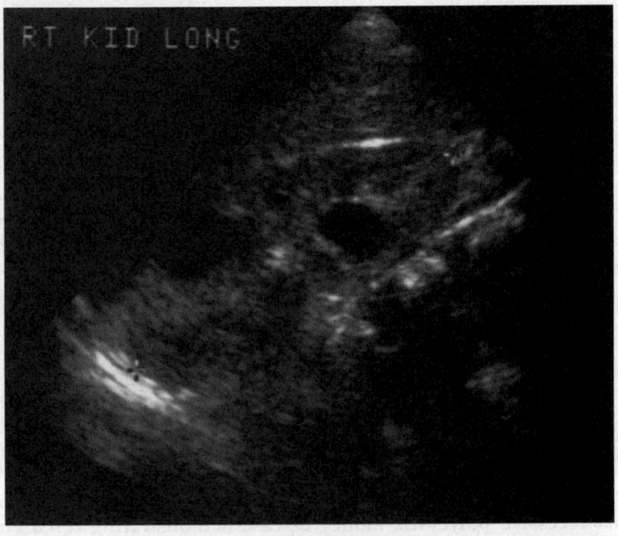

Figure 475–2. Ultrasound examination of an 18-mo-old boy with autosomal dominant polycystic kidney disease demonstrating renal enlargement (10 cm) and two large cysts.

Sedman A, Bell P, Manco-Johnson M, et al: Autosomal dominant polycystic kidney disease in childhood: A longitudinal study. Kidney Int 31:1000, 1987.

475.3 Vascular Abnormalities

Hemangiomas and arteriovenous malformations of the kidneys and lower urinary tract are extremely rare causes of hematuria. They usually present with gross hematuria and the passage of blood clots. Renal colic may develop if the upper tract is involved. The diagnosis is confirmed by angiography.

NEPHROLITHIASIS

(See Chapter 501.)

RENAL TUMORS

(See Chapter 452.)

CHAPTER 476
Miscellaneous Etiologies of Hematuria

476.1 Exercise Hematuria

Gross or microscopic hematuria may follow vigorous exercise. Exercise hematuria is rare in females and can be associated with dysuria. The color of the urine may vary from red to black; myoglobinuria should be excluded. Blood clots may be present in the urine. Findings on urine culture, intravenous pyelography, voiding cystourethrography, and cystoscopy are normal in most patients. This seems to be a benign condition, and the hematuria generally resolves within 48 hr after cessation of exercise. The absence of red blood cell casts or of evidence of renal disease, and the presence of dysuria and blood clots in some patients, suggest that the source of bleeding lies in the lower urinary tract. Rhabdomyolysis with myoglobinuria or march hemoglobinuria should be considered in the differential diagnosis when associated with exercise.

Abarbanel J, Benet AE, Lask D, et al: Sports hematuria. J Urol 143:887, 1990.
Bailey RR, Dann E, Gillies AHB, et al: What the urine contains following athletic competition. N Z Med J 83:309, 1976.
Siegel AJ, Hennekens CH, Solomon HS, et al: Exercise-related hematuria. JAMA 241:391, 1979.

476.2 Drugs

Gross or microscopic hematuria has been associated with the use of various medications. Mechanisms include alterations in the coagulation system (heparin, warfarin, aspirin), tubular damage (penicillins, sulfonamides), and hemorrhagic cystitis (cyclophosphamide).

Northway JD: Hematuria in children. J Pediatr 78:381, 1971.

CHAPTER 477

Evaluation of the Child with Hematuria

A thorough history and physical examination may give clues to the etiology of hematuria. For example, a history of recent upper respiratory, skin, or gastrointestinal infection may suggest acute glomerulonephritis or the hemolytic-uremic syndrome. Frequency, dysuria, and unexplained fevers suggest urinary tract infection. A flank mass may indicate hydronephrosis, cystic disease, renal vein thrombosis, or tumor. Recurrent episodes of gross hematuria suggest IgA nephropathy, idiopathic hematuria, Alport syndrome, or hypercalciuria. Rash and joint pains point toward anaphylactoid purpura or lupus. A history of trauma, of bleeding difficulties, of drug usage, or of kidney disease or high blood pressure in other family members could be useful.

Laboratory evaluation of the child with hematuria is done in steps, beginning with the studies most likely to reveal the etiology (Table 464–1). Depending on the results of the initial group of tests, additional studies may be indicated.

The finding of certain hematologic abnormalities may narrow the differential diagnosis. Anemia may be dilutional (the result of fluid overload in acute renal failure), hemolytic (hemolytic-uremic syndrome, systemic lupus erythematosus), or the result of blood loss (pulmonary hemorrhage in Goodpasture disease, melena in anaphylactoid purpura, hemolytic-uremic syndrome). Confirmation of a hemolytic state (elevated reticulocyte count and plasma hemoglobin level, with a depressed plasma haptoglobin level) indicates additional studies. Observation of the blood film may reveal a microangiopathic process as seen in the hemolytic-uremic syndrome, renal vein thrombosis, vasculitis, and systemic lupus erythematosus. In the latter, the presence of autoantibodies may result in a positive Coombs test, ANA, leukopenia, and multisystem disease. All black children with hematuria should be screened for sickle hemoglobin, even in the absence of anemia. Thrombocytopenia may result from decreased platelet production (malignancies) or increased platelet consumption (lupus, idiopathic thrombocytopenic purpura, hemolytic-uremic syndrome, renal vein thrombosis). Although urinary red blood cell morphology may be normal with lower tract bleeding and dysmorphic from glomerular bleeding, cell morphology does not reliably correlate with the site of hematuria. The best screening test for a bleeding diathesis, however, is a good history; coagulation studies or platelet counts are not routinely obtained unless personal or family history suggests a bleeding tendency.

Urine culture evaluates the possibility of urinary tract infection. Optimally, a timed urine specimen is also collected to measure the creatinine clearance, and protein and calcium excretion. If this is not possible, then determination of the serum creatinine, urine protein by dipstick, and calcium-to-creatinine ratio in a random urine specimen are adequate.

The serum C3 level is determined in all patients, because a low level narrows the differential diagnosis to certain forms of glomerulonephritis: poststreptococcal, lupus, membranoproliferative, and chronic infection. When the hematuria is of less than 6 mo duration, serologic evidence for streptococcal infection should be sought. Throat or skin infections should be cultured for streptococci. An ANA titer should be obtained as a test for lupus.

If the above-mentioned studies do not yield the diagnosis, ultrasound or intravenous pyelography should be carried out to exclude structural abnormalities. Cystography is done only in patients with infection or in patients in whom a lesion of the lower tract is suspected.

The studies in steps 1 and 2, as presented in Table 464–1, will frequently reveal the etiology of the hematuria. In some patients, however, results of all these studies will be normal and no cause for the hematuria will be found. In such patients, despite the lack of a diagnosis, no further studies need be performed. The parents should be reassured that the child does not at that time have evidence of urinary tract disease. Because it remains possible, however, that significant renal disease (e.g., IgA nephropathy, Alport syndrome) may be present, the child with persistent microscopic hematuria should have long-term follow-up, with an annual re-evaluation consisting of history, physical examination, blood pressure determination, urinalysis, creatinine clearance, and determination of protein level in a 24-hr specimen.

Renal biopsy may not yield a definitive diagnosis in children with unexplained low-grade microscopic hematuria and no other laboratory abnormalities. Biopsy is indicated in children with persistent microscopic hematuria associated with decreased renal function, proteinuria, or hypertension; in those children having one or more episodes of unexplained gross hematuria; and in those with persistent high-grade microscopic hematuria.

Cystoscopy is not part of the routine evaluation of hematuria in children. We have found cystoscopy most helpful in patients having bright-red hematuria, dysuria, and sterile urine cultures. In boys, cystoscopy frequently reveals a hemorrhagic lesion in the urethra, probably the result of local trauma. Although neoplasms of the lower urinary tract rarely present as asymptomatic gross hematuria in children, debate persists regarding the need for cystoscopy to exclude the remote possibility of a tumor.

SECTION 3

Conditions Particularly Associated with Proteinuria

Jerry M. Bergstein

Protein may be found in the urine of healthy children. Estimates vary, but a reasonable upper limit of normal protein excretion in healthy children is 150 mg/24 hr (0.15 g/24 hr). Approximately half of this protein derives from the plasma, albumin representing the largest fraction (less than 30 mg/24 hr; 0.03 g/24 hr). The remainder of normal urinary protein is Tamm-Horsfall protein, a mucoprotein of unknown function produced in the distal tubule.

Proteinuria is commonly detected by the dipstick test and is reported as negative, trace, 1+ (closest to 30 mg/dL), 2+ (closest to 100 mg/dL), 3+ (closest to 300 mg/dL), and 4+ (greater than 2,000 mg/dL). Dipsticks detect primarily albuminuria and are less sensitive for (and may miss) other forms of proteinuria (e.g., low molecular weight proteins, Bence Jones protein, gamma globulins). The depth of color of the dipstick reaction increases in a semi-quantitative manner with increasing urinary protein concentrations. Owing to their high sensitivity, dipsticks may detect amounts of protein in the urine that are within normal limits. Because the dipstick reaction cannot accurately measure protein excretion, persistent proteinuria should be quantitated by a more precise method (sulfosalicylic acid) in a timed (preferably 24 hr) urine collection. False-positive test results for proteinuria may be found with both the dipstick test (highly concentrated urine, gross hematuria, contamination with chlorhexidine or benzalkonium, pH over 8.0, phenazopyridine therapy) and the sulfosalicylic acid method (radiographic contrast media, penicillin or cephalosporin therapy, tolbutamide, sulfonamides).

In a semi-quantitative fashion, urinary protein excretion can be estimated by measuring the ratio of urinary protein to creatinine concentrations in a random specimen. Urinary creatinine excretion is constant in patients with relatively normal renal function, as is urinary protein excretion in most disease states. Determination of the ratio is especially helpful in quantitating proteinuria when a timed urine collection is not practicable. Ratios (mg/mg) below 0.5 in children less than 2 yr of age and less than 0.2 in older children suggest normal protein excretion. A ratio greater than 3 suggests nephrotic-range proteinuria.

Abitbol C, Zilleruelo G, Freundlich M, et al: Quantitation of proteinuria with urinary protein/creatinine ratios and random testing with dipsticks in nephrotic syndrome. J Pediatr 116:243, 1990.

CHAPTER 478

Nonpathologic Proteinuria

Proteinuria in excess of 150 mg/24 hr (0.15 g/24 hr) may be divided into two categories (Table 478–1). In the first category, nonpathologic proteinuria, the excessive protein excretion is apparently not the result of a disease state. The level of proteinuria in this category is generally less than 1,000 mg/24 hr (1.00 g/24 hr) and is never associated with edema.

478.1 Postural (Orthostatic) Proteinuria

Children with this disorder excrete normal or slightly increased amounts of protein in the supine position. In the upright position, the amount of protein in the urine may increase 10-fold or more. The proteinuria is usually discovered at routine urinalysis; its etiology is unknown. Hematuria is absent, and the creatinine clearance and C3 complement level are normal. Renal biopsy (not part of the evaluation) is normal or shows mild nonspecific alterations.

In the child having asymptomatic low-grade proteinuria, a study for postural proteinuria should be performed. At bedtime, the child goes to bed without voiding. After 30 min supine, the child voids in this position. This urine is discarded but the time of voiding is recorded as the beginning of the supine collection. The child is then given a large glass of liquid and allowed to sleep. In the morning, the child again voids supine before rising; this ends the supine collection and begins the upright collection, which is terminated at bedtime. The child may have normal daily activities, avoiding the supine position. The protein excretion is measured in the two urine collections, and for each collection the result is calculated as milligrams of protein excreted/minute. A finding of essentially normal protein excretion in the supine collection and increased protein excretion in the upright collection establishes the proteinuria as orthostatic.

Studies in adults suggest that postural proteinuria is a benign process, but similar data are not available for children. Accordingly, long-term follow-up of children is necessary (unless the proteinuria resolves) in order to monitor the patient for evi-

TABLE 478–1 Classification of Proteinuria

Nonpathologic Proteinuria
- Postural (orthostatic)
- Febrile
- Exercise

Pathologic Proteinuria
- Tubular
  - *Hereditary*
  - Cystinosis
  - Wilson disease
  - Lowe syndrome
  - Proximal renal tubular acidosis
  - Galactosemia
  - *Acquired*
  - Antibiotics
  - Interstitial nephritis
  - Acute tubular necrosis
  - Cystic diseases
  - Heavy metal poisoning (mercury, gold, lead, bismuth, cadmium, chromium, copper)
- Glomerular
  - Persistent asymptomatic
  - Nephrotic syndrome
    - Idiopathic nephrotic syndrome
      - Minimal change
      - Mesangial proliferation
      - Focal sclerosis
    - Glomerulonephritis
    - Tumors
    - Drugs
    - Congenital

dence of renal disease (hematuria, hypertension, diminished renal function, or proteinuria exceeding 1 g/24 hr).

Springberg PD, Garrett LE Jr, Thompson AL, et al: Fixed and reproducible orthostatic proteinuria: Results of a 20-year follow-up study. Ann Intern Med 97:516, 1982.

478.2 Febrile Proteinuria

Transient proteinuria may be found in patients having fever in excess of 38.3° C (101° F). The mechanism of proteinuria associated with fever is unknown. The proteinuria does not exceed +2 on the dipstick and may be considered benign if it resolves when the fever abates.

Jensen H, Henriksen K: Proteinuria in non-renal infectious disease. Acta Med Scand 196:75, 1974.
Marks MI, McLaine PN, Drummond KN: Proteinuria in children with febrile illnesses. Arch Dis Child 45:250, 1970.

478.3 Exercise Proteinuria

Proteinuria, like hematuria, may follow vigorous exercise. The level rarely exceeds +2 on the dipstick. The disorder can be considered benign if the proteinuria resolves after 48 hr of rest.

Campanacci L, Faccini L, Englaro E, et al: Exercise-induced proteinuria. Contrib Nephrol 26:31, 1981.
Poortmans JR: Postexercise proteinuria in humans. JAMA 253:236, 1985.

CHAPTER 479
Pathologic Proteinuria

The second category of proteinuria may result from glomerular or tubular disorders.

479.1 Tubular Proteinuria

Healthy individuals filter large amounts of proteins of lower molecular weight than albumin (e.g., lysozyme, light chains of immunoglobulin, β_2-microglobulin, insulin, growth hormone); these are normally reabsorbed in the proximal tubule. Injury to the proximal tubules results in diminished reabsorptive capacity and the loss of these low molecular weight proteins in the urine; such proteinuria rarely exceeds 1 g/24 hr; it is not associated with edema. Tubular proteinuria (see Table 478–1) may be seen in acquired and inherited disorders and may be associated with other defects of proximal tubular function, such as glucosuria, phosphaturia, bicarbonate wasting, and aminoaciduria. Tubular proteinuria rarely presents a diagnostic dilemma because the underlying disease is usually detected before the proteinuria. Asymptomatic patients having persistent proteinuria generally have glomerular rather than tubular proteinuria. In occult cases, glomerular and tubular proteinuria can be distinguished by electrophoresis of the urine. In tubular proteinuria, the low molecular weight proteins migrate primarily in the alpha and beta regions and little or no albumin is detected, whereas in glomerular proteinuria the major protein is albumin.

Alt JM, Von der Heyde D, Assel E, et al: Characteristics of protein excretion in glomerular and tubular disease. Contrib Nephrol 24:115, 1981.
Maack T, Johnson V, Kau ST, et al: Renal filtration, transport, and metabolism of low-molecular-weight proteins: A review. Kidney Int 16:251, 1979.
Waller KV, Ward KM, Mahan JD, et al: Current concepts in proteinuria. Clin Chem 35:755, 1989.

479.2 Glomerular Proteinuria

The most common cause of proteinuria is increased permeability of the glomerular capillary wall. The amount of glomerular proteinuria may range from less than 1 to more than 30 g/24 hr. Glomerular proteinuria may be termed *selective* (loss of plasma proteins of molecular weight up to and including albumin) or *nonselective* (loss of albumin and of larger molecular weight proteins such as IgG). Most forms of glomerulonephritis are accompanied by nonselective proteinuria. Selective proteinuria is seen primarily in minimal-change nephrosis, and in that disease the finding of selective proteinuria increases the likelihood of corticosteroid responsiveness. The determination of urinary protein selectivity is generally of little clinical value, owing to considerable overlap of selectivities among various forms of renal disease.

CHAPTER 480
Persistent Asymptomatic Proteinuria

Persistent asymptomatic proteinuria is defined as proteinuria in an apparently healthy child that occurs without hematuria and persists for 3 mo. The prevalence in school-aged children may be as high as 6%. The amount of proteinuria is usually less than 2 g/24 hr; it is never associated with edema. Causes include postural proteinuria, membranous and membranoproliferative glomerulonephritis, pyelonephritis, hereditary nephritis, developmental anomalies, and "benign" proteinuria.

Evaluation of the child having persistent asymptomatic proteinuria should include urine culture; measurement of creatinine clearance, 24-hr protein excretion, serum albumin, C3 complement levels, and renal ultrasound. In patients with low-grade proteinuria (150–1,000 mg/24 hr [0.15–1.00 g/24 hr]) in whom findings are normal, renal biopsy may not be indicated because evidence for a progressive disease is rarely found. Such patients should have an annual re-evaluation consisting of a physical examination and blood pressure determination, urinalysis, creatinine clearance, and 24-hr protein excretion. Indications for renal biopsy include persistent asymptomatic proteinuria in excess of 1,000 mg/24 hr (1 g/24 hr) or the development of hematuria, hypertension, or diminished renal function.

Dodge WF, West EF, Smith EH, et al: Proteinuria and hematuria in school-age children: Epidemiology and early natural history. J Pediatr 88:327, 1976.
Vehaskari VM, Rapola J: Isolated proteinuria: Analysis of a school-age population. J Pediatr 101:661, 1982.
Yoshikawa N, Kitagawa K, Ohta K, et al: Asymptomatic constant isolated proteinuria in children. J Pediatr 119:375, 1991.

CHAPTER 481
Nephrotic Syndrome
(Nephrosis)

The nephrotic syndrome is characterized by proteinuria, hypoproteinemia, edema, and hyperlipidemia.

ETIOLOGY. Most (90%) children with nephrosis have some form of the idiopathic nephrotic syndrome; minimal-change disease is found in approximately 85%, mesangial proliferation in 5%, and focal sclerosis in 10%. In the remaining 10% of children with nephrosis, the nephrotic syndrome is largely mediated by some form of glomerulonephritis, membranous and membranoproliferative being most common.

PATHOPHYSIOLOGY. The underlying pathogenetic abnormality in nephrosis is proteinuria, which results from an increase in glomerular capillary wall permeability. The mechanism of this increase in permeability is unknown but may be related, at least in part, to loss of negatively charged glycoproteins within the capillary wall. In the nephrotic state, the protein loss generally exceeds 2 g/24 hr and is composed primarily of albumin; the hypoproteinemia is fundamentally a "hypoalbuminemia." In general, edema appears when the serum albumin level falls below 2.5 g/dL (25 g/L).

The mechanism of edema formation in nephrosis is incompletely understood. It seems likely that the edema is initiated by the development of hypoalbuminemia, the result of urinary protein loss. The hypoalbuminemia leads to a decrease in the plasma oncotic pressure, which permits the transudation of fluid from the intravascular compartment to the interstitial space. The reduction in intravascular volume decreases renal perfusion pressure, activating the renin-angiotensin-aldosterone system, which stimulates distal tubular reabsorption of sodium. The reduced intravascular volume also stimulates the release of antidiuretic hormone, which enhances the reabsorption of water in the collecting duct. Because of the decreased plasma oncotic pressure, the reabsorbed sodium and water are lost into the interstitial space, exacerbating the edema. That other factors may also play a role in the formation of the edema is indicated by the observations that some patients with nephrotic syndrome have normal or increased intravascular volume and normal to diminished plasma levels of renin and aldosterone. Hypothetical explanations include an intrarenal defect in sodium and water excretion or the presence of a circulating agent that increases capillary wall permeability throughout the body, as well as in the kidneys.

In the nephrotic state, almost all serum lipid (cholesterol, triglycerides) and lipoprotein levels are elevated. Two factors offer at least partial explanation: (1) the hypoproteinemia stimulates generalized protein synthesis in the liver, including the lipoproteins; and (2) lipid catabolism is diminished, owing to reduced plasma levels of lipoprotein lipase, the major enzyme system that removes lipids from the plasma. Whether lipoprotein lipase is lost in the urine is unclear.

Humphreys MH: Mechanisms and management of nephrotic edema. Kidney Int 45:266, 1994.
Oetliker OH, Mordasini R, Lutschg J, et al: Lipoprotein metabolism in nephrotic syndrome in childhood. Pediatr Res 14:64, 1980.
Tulassay T, Rascher W, Scharer K: Intra- and extrarenal factors of oedema formation in the nephrotic syndrome. Pediatr Nephrol 3:92, 1989.
Wheeler DC, Bernard DB: Lipid abnormalities in the nephrotic syndrome: causes, consequences, and treatment. Am J Kidney Dis 23:331, 1994.

481.1 Idiopathic Nephrotic Syndrome

This syndrome accounts for approximately 90% of nephrosis in childhood. Occasional reports that one of the three histologic types has been transformed into another type suggest that this syndrome may be a single disorder with varying histologic features. It seems more likely, however, that the syndrome represents several diseases having similar clinical manifestations. The resolution of this issue awaits the discovery of the pathogenetic factors. The syndrome has been reported in certain families with a frequency that appears to be increased over that expected, but it does not appear to be inherited.

ETIOLOGY. The cause of the syndrome remains unknown. Early success in controlling nephrosis with "immunosuppressive" drugs suggested that the disease was mediated by immunologic mechanisms, but evidence for classic mechanisms of immunologic injury has been lacking, and it now seems clear that "immunosuppressive" drugs have many effects other than suppression of antibody formation. A few patients have evidence supporting IgE mediation of the disease, but increasing evidence suggests that the syndrome may result from an abnormality in thymus-derived (T-cell) lymphocyte function, perhaps through the production of a factor that increases vascular permeability.

PATHOLOGY. Idiopathic nephrotic syndrome occurs in three morphologic patterns. In minimal-change disease (85%), the glomeruli appear normal or show a minimal increase in mesangial cells and matrix. Findings on immunofluorescent microscopic studies are typically negative. Electron microscopy reveals retraction of the epithelial cell foot processes. More than 95% of children with minimal-change disease respond to corticosteroid therapy.

The mesangial proliferative group (5%) is characterized by a diffuse increase in mesangial cells and matrix. The frequency of mesangial deposits containing IgM and C3 by immunofluorescence is not different from that observed in minimal change disease. Approximately 50–60% of patients with this histologic lesion will respond to corticosteroid therapy.

In biopsies from patients having the focal sclerosis lesion (10%), the majority of glomeruli appear normal or manifest mesangial proliferation. Others, especially those close to the medulla (juxtamedullary), show segmental scarring in one or more lobules (Fig. 481–1). The disease is frequently progressive, ultimately involving all glomeruli, and leads to end-stage renal failure in most patients. Approximately 20% of such patients respond to prednisone or cytotoxic therapy or both. The disease may recur in a transplanted kidney.

CLINICAL MANIFESTATIONS. The idiopathic nephrotic syndrome is more common in boys than in girls (2:1) and most commonly appears between the ages of 2 and 6 yr. It has been reported as early as the last half of the 1st yr of life and is common in adults. The initial episode and subsequent relapses may follow an apparent viral upper respiratory tract infection. The disease usually presents as edema, which is initially noted around the eyes and in the lower extremities, where it is "pitting" in nature. With time, the edema becomes generalized and may be associated with weight gain, the development of ascites and/or pleural effusions, and declining urine output. The

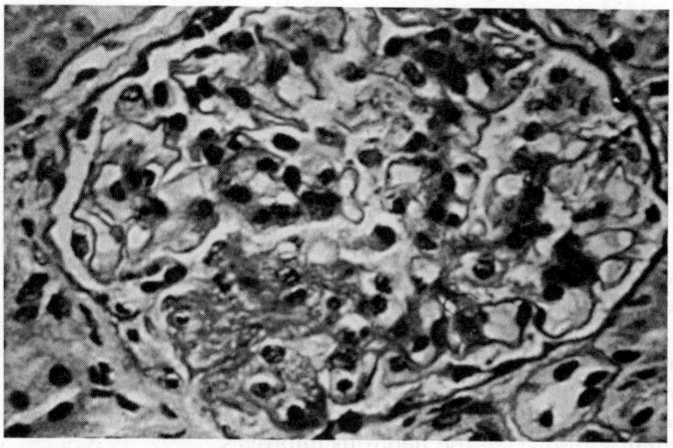

Figure 481–1. Glomerulus from a patient having corticosteroid-resistant nephrotic syndrome, showing mesangial hypercellularity and an area of sclerosis in the lower portion. (×250.)

edema accumulates in dependent sites and appears to shift from the face and back to the abdomen, perineum, and legs as the day progresses. Anorexia, abdominal pain, and diarrhea are common; hypertension is uncommon.

DIAGNOSIS. Urinalysis reveals +3 or +4 proteinuria; microscopic hematuria may be present, but gross hematuria is rare. Renal function may be normal or reduced. The low creatinine clearance is due to diminished renal perfusion resulting from contraction of the intravascular volume and will return to normal when intravascular volume is restored. Protein excretion exceeds 2 g/24 hr. The serum cholesterol and triglyceride levels are elevated, the serum albumin level is generally less than 2 g/dL (20 g/L), and the total serum calcium level is diminished, owing to a reduction in the albumin-bound fraction. The C3 level is normal.

Children with onset of nephrotic syndrome between the ages of 1 and 8 yr are likely to have steroid-responsive minimal-change disease, and corticosteroid therapy should be initiated without renal biopsy. Minimal-change disease remains common in children above the age of 8 yr who present with nephrosis, but membranous and membranoproliferative glomerulonephritis become increasingly common; renal biopsy is recommended in this group to establish a firm diagnosis prior to considering therapy.

COMPLICATIONS. Infection is the major complication of nephrosis; it results from increased susceptibility to bacterial infections during relapse. Proposed explanations include decreased immunoglobulin levels, the edema fluid acting as a culture medium, protein deficiency, decreased bactericidal activity of the leukocytes, "immunosuppressive" therapy, decreased perfusion of the spleen due to hypovolemia, and loss in the urine of a complement factor (properdin factor B) that opsonizes certain bacteria. For reasons that are unclear, **spontaneous peritonitis** is the most frequent type of infection; sepsis, pneumonia, cellulitis, and urinary tract infections may also be seen. *Streptococcus pneumoniae* is the most common organism causing peritonitis; gram-negative bacteria are also encountered. Fever and physical findings may be minimal in the presence of corticosteroid therapy. Accordingly, a high index of suspicion, prompt evaluation (including cultures of blood and peritoneal fluid), and the early initiation of therapy that covers both gram-positive and gram-negative organisms are critical to prevention of life-threatening illness. When in remission, all patients having nephrosis should receive polyvalent pneumococcal vaccine.

Additional complications may include an increased tendency to arterial and venous thrombosis (owing at least in part to elevated plasma levels of certain coagulation factors and inhibitors of fibrinolysis, decreased plasma level of anti-thrombin III, and increased platelet aggregation); deficiencies of coagulation factors IX, XI, and XII; and reduced serum levels of vitamin D.

TREATMENT. The child may be hospitalized with the first episode of nephrosis for diagnostic, educational, and therapeutic purposes. When edema develops, sodium intake is reduced by the initiation of a "no added salt diet." The mother is advised to cook without salt, to hide the salt shaker, and to avoid serving obviously salty foods. Salt restriction is terminated when the edema resolves. Unless the edema is severe, fluid intake is not restricted but need not be encouraged. The child may attend school and participate in physical activities as tolerated. Until corticosteroid-induced diuresis begins, mild to moderate edema can be managed at home with chlorothiazide, 10–40 mg/kg/24 hr, in two divided doses. If hypokalemia develops, an oral potassium chloride supplement or spironolactone (3–5 mg/kg/24 hr divided into four doses) may be added. If the edema becomes severe, resulting in respiratory distress from massive pleural effusions and ascites or in severe scrotal edema, the child should be hospitalized. Sodium restriction should be continued, but further reduction in intake is rarely effective in controlling edema. The swollen scrotum is elevated with pillows to enhance the removal of fluid by gravity. In the past, severe edema was treated with intravenous administration of albumin, followed in some patients by an intravenous dose of furosemide. This type of therapy has now been supplanted by the oral administration of furosemide (1–2 mg/kg every 4 hr) in conjunction with metolazone (0.2–0.4 mg/kg/24 hr in two divided doses); metolazone may act in both the proximal and distal tubules. When using this potent combination, electrolyte levels and renal function must be closely monitored. In some instances of severe edema, intravenous administration of 25% human albumin (1 g/kg/24 hr) may be necessary, but the effect is usually transient and volume overload with hypertension and heart failure must be avoided.

After the diagnosis is confirmed by the appropriate laboratory studies, the pathophysiology and treatment of nephrosis is reviewed with the family to enhance their understanding of the child's disease. Remission is then induced by administration of prednisone, the least expensive corticosteroid, at a dosage of 60 mg/m^2/24 hr (maximum daily dose 60 mg), divided into three or four doses over the day. Divided-dose rather than single-dose therapy is used because some patients who fail to respond to a single daily dose will respond to divided doses. The time needed for response to prednisone averages about 2 wk, the response being defined as the point at which urine becomes free of protein. If the child continues to have proteinuria (2+ or greater) after 1 mo of continuous, daily, divided-dose prednisone, the nephrosis is termed *steroid resistant* and renal biopsy is indicated to determine the precise etiology of the disease.

Five days after the urine becomes free (negative, trace, or 1+ on the dipstick) of protein, the dose of prednisone is changed to 60 mg/m^2 (maximum dose of 60 mg) taken every other day as a single dose with breakfast. This alternate-day regimen is continued for 3–6 mo. The purpose of alternate-day therapy is to maintain the remission using a relatively nontoxic dose of prednisone, thus avoiding frequent relapses of the disease and the cumulative toxicity of frequent courses of daily administration of corticosteroids. After such a period of alternate-day therapy, the prednisone may be discontinued abruptly. Adequate experience indicates that there has been sufficient recovery of pituitary-adrenal axis function that the patient is not at risk for adrenal insufficiency after abrupt withdrawal of the alternate-day prednisone. On the other hand, for up to 1 yr after completing corticosteroid therapy, the child will require corticosteroid supplementation for severe illness or surgery.

Each relapse of the nephrosis is treated in a similar manner.

A relapse is defined as the recurrence of edema and not simply of proteinuria, as many children with this condition will have intermittent proteinuria that resolves spontaneously. A small number of patients who respond to daily, divided-dose therapy will have relapses shortly after switching to or after terminating alternate-day therapy. Such patients are termed *steroid dependent*.

If there are repeated relapses and especially if the child suffers severe corticosteroid toxicity (cushingoid appearance, hypertension, growth failure), then cyclophosphamide therapy should be considered. Cyclophosphamide has been shown to prolong the duration of remission and to prevent relapses in children with frequently relapsing nephrotic syndrome. The potential side effects of the drug (leukopenia, disseminated varicella infection, hemorrhagic cystitis, alopecia, sterility) should be reviewed with the family. The dose of cyclophosphamide is 3 mg/kg/24 hr as a single dose, for a total duration of 12 wk. Alternate-day prednisone therapy is often continued during the course of cyclophosphamide administration. During cyclophosphamide therapy, the white count must be monitored weekly and the drug withheld if the count falls below 5,000/mm^3. Steroid-resistant patients may respond to an extended course (3–6 mo) of cyclophosphamide, pulse methylprednisolone, or cyclosporine.

Renal transplantation is indicated for end-stage renal failure due to steroid-resistant focal and segmental glomerulosclerosis (see Chapter 490). Recurrent nephrotic syndromes develop in 15–55% of patients. Plasma protein absorption onto protein A–based columns may reduce proteinuria in these patients. Protein absorption removes a fraction (<100,000 MW), which enhances renal protein permeability.

PROGNOSIS. Most children with steroid-responsive nephrosis will have repeated relapses until the disease resolves itself spontaneously toward the end of the 2nd decade of life. It is important to indicate to the family that the child will have no residual renal dysfunction, that the disease is generally not hereditary, and that the child (in the absence of cyclophosphamide or chlorambucil therapy) will remain fertile. To minimize the psychologic effects of the nephrosis, we emphasize that when in remission the child is normal and may have unrestricted diet and activity. While the child is in remission it is generally unnecessary to test the urine for protein.

Arbeitsgemeinschaft für Pädiatrische Nephrologie: Cyclophosphamide treatment of steroid dependent nephrotic syndrome: comparison of eight week with 12 week course. Arch Dis Child 62:1102, 1987.
Arbeitsgemeinschaft für Pädiatrische Nephrologie: Short versus standard prednisone therapy for initial treatment of idiopathic nephrotic syndrome in children. Lancet 1:380, 1988.
Berns JS, Gaudio KM, Krassner LS, et al: Steroid-responsive nephrotic syndrome of childhood: A long-term study of clinical course, histopathology, efficacy of cyclophosphamide therapy and effects on growth. Am J Kidney Dis 9:108, 1987.
Dantal J, Bigot E, Boyers W, et al: Effect of plasma protein absorption on protein excretion in kidney-transplant recipients with recurrent nephrotic syndrome. N Engl J Med 330:7, 1994.
Freundlich M, Bourgoignie JJ, Zilleruelo G, et al: Calcium and vitamin D metabolism in children with nephrotic syndrome. J Pediatr 108:383, 1986.
Gorensek MJ, Lebel MH, Nelson JD: Peritonitis in children with nephrotic syndrome. Pediatrics 81:849, 1988.
Habib R, Girardin E, Gagnadoux M-F, et al: Immunopathological findings in idiopathic nephrosis: Clinical significance of glomerular "immune deposits." Pediatr Nephrol 2:402, 1988.
Kaysen G: Nonrenal complications of the nephrotic syndrome. Annu Rev Med 45:201, 1994.
Krensky AM, Ingelfinger JR, Grupe WE: Peritonitis in childhood nephrotic syndrome. Am J Dis Child 136:732, 1982.
Llach F: Hypercoagulability, renal vein thrombosis, and other thrombotic complications of nephrotic syndrome. Kidney Int 28:429, 1985.
Mendoza SA, Tune BM: Treatment of childhood nephrotic syndrome. J Am Soc Nephrol 3:889, 1992.
Ponticelli C, Rizzoni G, Edefonti A, et al: A randomized trial of cyclosporine in steroid-resistant idiopathic nephrotic syndrome. Kidney Int 43:1377, 1993.
Schwartz MM, Korbet SM: Primary focal segmental glomerulosclerosis: pathology, histological variants, and pathogenesis. Am J Kidney Dis 22:874, 1993.
Southwest Pediatric Nephrology Study Group: Focal segmental glomerulosclerosis in children with idiopathic nephrotic syndrome. Kidney Int 27:442, 1985.

481.2 Glomerulonephritis

Nephrotic syndrome may develop during the course of any type of glomerulonephritis but is most common in association with membranous, membranoproliferative, poststreptococcal, lupus, chronic infection (including malaria and schistosomiasis), and anaphylactoid purpura glomerulonephritis. Although the development of a secondary nephrotic syndrome may indicate severe glomerular disease, the nephrotic syndrome frequently resolves if the nephritis improves.

Barsoum RS: Schistosomal glomerulopathies. Kidney Int 44:1, 1993.
Hendrickse RG, Adeniyi A: Quartan malarial nephrotic syndrome in children. Kidney Int 16:64, 1979.
Sitprija V: Nephropathy in falciparum malaria. Kidney Int 34:867, 1988.

481.3 Tumors

See also Chapters 450, 459, and 449.

Nephrotic syndrome has been associated with several extrarenal neoplasms. In patients having solid tumors, such as carcinomas, the glomerular changes resemble membranous glomerulopathy. The renal involvement is presumably mediated by immune complexes composed of tumor antigens and tumor-specific antibodies. In lymphomas (especially Hodgkin disease), minimal-change disease is most commonly found; proliferative lesions have also been described. In patients having the minimal-change lesion, the nephrosis may develop before or after the malignancy is detected, may resolve as the tumor regresses, and may return if the tumor recurs. The mechanism of the nephrosis is unknown; it has been proposed that the tumor produces a lymphokine that increases glomerular capillary wall permeability.

Alpers CE, Cotran RS: Neoplasia and glomerular injury. Kidney Int 30:465, 1986.
Dabbs DJ, Striker L, Mignon F, et al: Glomerular lesions in lymphomas and leukemias. Am J Med 80:63, 1986.

481.4 Drugs

Nephrotic syndrome has developed during therapy with several types of drugs and chemicals. The histologic picture may resemble membranous glomerulopathy (penicillamine, captopril, gold, mercury compounds), minimal-change disease (probenecid, ethosuximide, methimazole, lithium), or proliferative glomerulonephritis (procainamide, chlorpropamide, phenytoin, trimethadione, paramethadione).

481.5 Congenital Nephrotic Syndrome

Nephrotic syndrome is rare during the 1st yr of life. Causes of nephrosis developing during the first 6 mo of life include the congenital nephrotic syndrome, congenital infection (syphilis, toxoplasmosis, cytomegalovirus), and diffuse mesangial sclerosis of unknown etiology (**Drash syndrome**, consisting of nephropathy, Wilms tumor, and genital abnormalities). Nephrosis developing during the last half of the 1st yr is most commonly associated with the idiopathic nephrotic syndrome or drugs. Owing to the diversity of causes of the development of nephrotic syndrome during the 1st year of life, all such patients should have kidney biopsy to determine the precise etiology and severity of the disease.

The congenital nephrotic syndrome (Finnish type) is an autosomal recessive disorder that is most common in populations of Scandinavian descent. The major pathologic feature in some patients is dilatation of the proximal convoluted tubules (microcystic disease), but this is variable, even within the same kindred. The glomeruli show mesangial proliferation and sclerosis. The pathogenesis of the syndrome is unknown; a reduction in the number of heparan sulfate–rich anionic sites has been demonstrated in the glomerular basement membrane. Although proteinuria is present at birth, the nephrotic syndrome becomes apparent within the first 3 mo of life. Additional clinical features include prematurity, an enlarged placenta, respiratory distress, and separation of the cranial sutures. The clinical course is one of persistent edema and recurrent infections. Death due to infection or renal failure is likely by the age of 5 yr. Corticosteroid and immunosuppressive agents are of no value. Treatment is supportive, with the ultimate goal of kidney transplantation. In families at risk, antenatal diagnosis is possible by measuring α-fetoprotein level of the amniotic fluid prior to 20 wk of gestation.

Habib R: Nephrotic syndrome in the first year of life. Pediatr Nephrol 7:347, 1993.

Jadresic L, Leake J, Gordon I, et al: Clinicopathologic review of twelve children with nephropathy. Wilms tumor, and genital abnormalities (Drash syndrome). J Pediatr 117:717, 1990.

Mahan JD, Mauer SM, Sibley RK, et al: Congenital nephrotic syndrome: Evolution of medical management and results of renal transplantation. J Pediatr 105:549, 1984.

Mattoo TK, Al-Sowailem AM, Al-Harbi MS, et al: Nephrotic syndrome in the first year of life and the role of unilateral nephrectomy. Pediatr Nephrol 6:16, 1992.

Rapola J: Congenital nephrotic syndrome. Pediatr Nephrol 1:441, 1987.

Shahin B, Papadopoulou ZL, Jenis EH: Congenital nephrotic syndrome associated with congenital toxoplasmosis. J Pediatr 85:366, 1974.

Sibley RK, Mahan J, Mauer SM, et al: A clinicopathologic study of forty-eight infants with nephrotic syndrome. Kidney Int 27:544, 1985.

Vernier RL, Klein DJ, Sisson SP, et al: Heparan sulfate-rich anionic sites in the human glomerular basement membrane. N Engl J Med 309:1001, 1983.

SECTION 4

Tubular Disorders

CHAPTER 482

Tubular Function

Jerry M. Bergstein

Except for reduced protein levels, the ultrafiltrate of blood that enters the proximal tubule is similar to plasma. Body homeostasis is maintained by tubular reabsorption of salts and water.

SODIUM. After the 1st year of life, the tubules have the reabsorptive capacity to lower the urinary sodium concentration to 1 mEq/L (1 mmol/L). Approximately 65% of filtered sodium is isotonically reabsorbed in the proximal tubule. Glucose and amino acids are also reabsorbed in the proximal tubule in conjunction with sodium transport. An additional 25% of filtered sodium is reabsorbed from the ascending limb of the loop of Henle in association with the active transport of chloride. The remainder of sodium reabsorption is accomplished in the distal tubule and collecting duct, mediated in part by aldosterone. Sodium excretion is closely related to the extracellular fluid volume and may be modified by factors that regulate the extracellular fluid volume.

POTASSIUM. Essentially all of the filtered potassium is reabsorbed, primarily in the proximal tubules. The potassium excreted is derived from distal tubular and collecting duct potassium secretion, as modified by the pH of the extracellular fluid, by aldosterone, and by the urinary flow rate and sodium concentration.

CALCIUM. Approximately 98% of filtered calcium is reabsorbed by the tubules. Proximal tubular reabsorption (65% of the filtered load) is linked to sodium reabsorption. Calcium reabsorption is enhanced by parathyroid hormone, thiazide diuretics, and reduction of the extracellular fluid volume. Calcium excretion is increased by saline infusion and furosemide.

PHOSPHATE. The majority of the filtered phosphate is reabsorbed in the proximal tubule. Reabsorption is inhibited by parathyroid hormone.

MAGNESIUM. About 25% of filtered magnesium is reabsorbed in the proximal tubule; the major site of magnesium reabsorption and the principal moderator of magnesium excretion is the thick ascending limb of Henle.

ACIDIFICATION AND CONCENTRATING MECHANISMS. These are discussed in the sections on renal tubular acidosis and nephrogenic diabetes insipidus (Chapters 483 and 484).

MATURATION OF TUBULAR FUNCTION. At birth and for several months thereafter, tubular functional capabilities are at less than adult levels. Tubular function is adequate for healthy infants, but limitations may contribute to fluid and electrolyte abnormalities in sick infants.

Maximal urinary concentrating capacity in the healthy full-term newborn is 600–700 mOsm/kg (mmol/kg) H_2O. This reduction in concentrating capacity in comparison with older children and adults (who can concentrate to more than 1,000 mOsm/kg [mmol/kg] H_2O) is related to reduced glomerular filtration rate (GFR), to tubular cell immaturity, to reduced nephron length, to reduced medullary solute gradient due to increased medullary blood flow and low urea production, and to diminished tubular responsiveness to antidiuretic hormone. Although the ability of newborn infants to dilute the urine is comparable to that of adults, their capacity to excrete a water load is diminished, owing to the reduced GFR. The capacity of the neonate to excrete sodium, potassium, hydrogen ion, and phosphate is also limited, owing in part to the low GFR and/or immaturity of tubular function.

Hogg RJ, Stapleton FB: Renal tubular function. *In:* Holliday MA, Barratt TM, Vernier RL (eds): Pediatric Nephrology. Baltimore, Williams & Wilkins, 1987, p 59.
McCrory WW: Developmental Nephrology. Cambridge, MA, Harvard University Press, 1972.

CHAPTER 483
Renal Tubular Acidosis

Jerry M. Bergstein

Renal tubular acidosis (RTA) is a clinical state of systemic hyperchloremic acidosis resulting from impaired urinary acidification. Three types exist: distal RTA (type I), proximal RTA (type II), and mineralocorticoid deficiency (type IV). A proposed type III has been found to be a variant of type I.

NORMAL URINARY ACIDIFICATION. After the first few months of life, approximately 85% of the filtered bicarbonate is reabsorbed in the proximal tubules, but in premature infants and neonates such reabsorption of bicarbonate is transiently reduced, and bicarbonate wasting results when the serum bicarbonate level exceeds 20–22 mEq/L (mmol/L). The proximal tubular reabsorption of bicarbonate involves the secretion of hydrogen ion into the tubular lumen in exchange for sodium (Chapter 53). The hydrogen ion combines with filtered bicarbonate to form carbonic acid, which, under the influence of carbonic anhydrase, dissociates into carbon dioxide and water. The carbon dioxide diffuses into the proximal tubular cells, where, under the influence of carbonic anhydrase, it is reconverted to carbonic acid. The carbonic acid dissociates to yield a hydrogen ion that is again secreted to absorb additional bicarbonate, and to yield also a bicarbonate ion that enters the peritubular capillary. The remaining 15% of filtered bicarbonate is reabsorbed in the distal tubule. The normal kidney reabsorbs all filtered bicarbonate, but this does not make the urine acid. Acidification of the urine is mediated by distal tubular secretion of hydrogen ion (which is in part mineralocorticoid-dependent) and of ammonia (which forms ammonium ion in an acidic urine).

PROXIMAL RENAL TUBULAR ACIDOSIS

PATHOGENESIS. Proximal RTA results from reduced proximal tubular reabsorption of bicarbonate, presumably owing to deficient carbonic anhydrase production or hydrogen ion secretion. Rather than reabsorbing the normal 85% of filtered bicarbonate, the proximal tubules in this condition may reabsorb only 60%, thus presenting the distal tubules with 40% rather than the usual 15% of the filtered load. Because the distal tubules can, at a maximum, reabsorb only 15% of the normal filtered load of bicarbonate, up to 25% may be lost in the urine. Proximal RTA is generally more severe than distal RTA, as complete loss of the distal bicarbonate recovery mechanism (which is rare) would waste only 15% of filtered bicarbonate. With urinary bicarbonate loss, the serum bicarbonate level falls until it reaches a level (bicarbonate threshold) at which bicarbonate wasting ceases. At this level (15–18 mEq/L [mmol/L]), the quantity of filtered bicarbonate is reduced to an amount that can be totally reabsorbed by the tubules. Because distal tubular acidification mechanisms remain intact, the urine may then be acidified (pH less than 5.5). Flooding the distal tubule with sodium bicarbonate stimulates sodium reabsorption in exchange for potassium, leading to hypokalemia. Contraction of the extracellular fluid volume (as a result of the loss of sodium bicarbonate) stimulates chloride reabsorption (resulting in hyperchloremia) and aldosterone secretion (enhancing potassium loss).

Proximal RTA (Table 483–1) may occur as an isolated disorder not associated with other diseases or with other abnormalities of proximal tubular function. Isolated proximal RTA may be transient or persistent, sporadic or inherited (usually autosomal dominant). Proximal RTA may also occur as part of a generalized defect in proximal tubular transport (Fanconi syndrome), characterized by glucosuria, phosphaturia, aminoaciduria, carnitinuria, and proximal RTA. A primary form of Fanconi syndrome, also not associated with other disease states, has been reported to show both autosomal dominant and recessive modes of inheritance. Secondary Fanconi syndrome may develop during the course of several inherited or acquired disease states.

Inherited Forms

Cystinosis (Chapters 71.4 and 483.3). This autosomal recessive defect results from the accumulation of cystine within the lysosomes of the bone marrow, liver, spleen, lymph nodes, kidneys, fibroblasts, leukocytes, corneas, and conjunctivae. In the nephropathic variety, initial clinical manifestations may include polyuria and polydipsia (concentrating defect), fever (dehydration), growth retardation, rickets, blond hair and fair skin (diminished pigmentation), and photophobia. Later manifestations may include hypothyroidism, decreased visual acuity, delayed sexual maturation, central nervous system abnormalities, and muscle weakness. Intracellular accumulation of cystine in the kidney leads to progressive renal damage, resulting in end-stage renal failure by the end of the first decade. (See Chapter 483.3 for discussion of therapy.)

Lowe Syndrome. See Chapter 483.4.

Galactosemia (see Chapter 73.5). The renal manifestations of this disorder result from prolonged galactose accumulation in the proximal tubules.

Hereditary Fructose Intolerance (see Chapter 73.3). This autosomal recessive deficiency of fructose 1-phosphate aldolase leads to proximal tubular dysfunction.

Tyrosinemia. Generalized proximal tubular dysfunction is common in hereditary tyrosinemia (see Chapter 71.2).

Wilson Disease. The clinical manifestations of this autosomal recessive disorder include proximal tubular dysfunction; it is discussed in Chapters 303.2 and 547.3.

Medullary Cystic Disease. This disorder is inherited as an autosomal dominant trait, whereas a similar disorder, juvenile nephronophthisis, is inherited as an autosomal recessive trait. Whether these are separate disorders or the same disorder with variable inheritance is uncertain. Children more commonly have the recessive form, whereas the dominant form is more common in adults. The major pathologic finding is cysts in the medulla. As the "cysts" seem to be dilatations of the distal tubules and collecting ducts, some may also be found in the renal cortex. Progressive interstitial inflammation and fibrosis lead to glomerular sclerosis, cortical atrophy, and renal insufficiency. Some children suffer no clinical problems until reaching end-stage renal failure. Others show manifestations of tubular dysfunction such as polyuria and polydipsia (concentrating defect), sodium wasting, and proximal RTA. Red or blond hair is common. Urinalysis may be normal or show minimal abnormalities. Radiographic studies show small, poorly functioning kidneys. The diagnosis is confirmed by biopsy or at nephrectomy if either is warranted in preparation for transplantation.

CAUSES OF ACQUIRED FANCONI SYNDROME. These include tubular toxins such as heavy metals (lead, mercury, cadmium, uranium), outdated tetracycline, proteinuric states (myeloma, nephrotic syndrome), and interstitial nephritis. Excessive parathyroid hormone secretion (primary and secondary hyperpara-

■ **TABLE 483–1 Classification of Renal Tubular Acidosis**

Proximal	Distal	Mineralocorticoid Deficiency*
Isolated	Isolated	Adrenal disorders (↓ A, ↑ R)
Sporadic	Sporadic	Addison disease
Hereditary	Hereditary	Congenital hyperplasia
Fanconi syndrome	Secondary	Primary hypoaldosteronism
Primary	Interstitial nephritis	Hyporeninemic hypoaldosteronism (↓ A, ↓ R)
Secondary	Obstructive	Obstruction
Inherited	Pyelonephritis	Pyelonephritis
Cystinosis	Transplant rejection	Interstitial nephritis
Lowe syndrome	Sickle cell nephropathy	Diabetes mellitus
Galactosemia	Lupus nephritis	Nephrosclerosis
Hereditary fructose intolerance	Ehlers-Danlos syndrome	Pseudohypoaldosteronism (↑ A, ↑ R)
Tyrosinemia	Nephrocalcinosis	
Wilson disease	Hepatic cirrhosis	
Medullary cystic disease	Elliptocytosis	
Acquired	Medullary sponge kidney	
Heavy metals	Toxins	
Outdated tetracycline	Amphotericin B	
Proteinuria	Lithium	
Interstitial nephritis	Toluene	
Hyperparathyroidism		
Vitamin D–deficiency rickets		

**A = aldosterone; R = renin.*

thyroidism, vitamin D–deficient rickets) may also cause proximal RTA, presumably by inhibition of carbonic anhydrase. See also Chapter 483.2.

DISTAL RENAL TUBULAR ACIDOSIS

PATHOGENESIS. The genesis of distal RTA is best explained as a deficiency of hydrogen ion secretion by the distal tubule and collecting duct, although other mechanisms may also be involved. The lack of secreted hydrogen ion reduces the formation of carbonic acid and then carbon dioxide in the tubular lumen. The loss of bicarbonate in the urine may be 5–15% of the filtered load. Owing to the nature of the defect, the pH of the urine cannot be reduced below 5.8 despite severe systemic acidosis. Loss of sodium bicarbonate results in hyperchloremia and hypokalemia. The hypokalemia is usually less severe than that found in proximal RTA because less bicarbonate is wasted. Nephrocalcinosis and nephrolithiasis may be present.

Distal RTA may occur as an isolated condition not associated with any other disorder; as such it may be sporadic or inherited as an autosomal dominant or recessive trait. Secondary distal RTA may develop during the course of several diseases and intoxications involving the distal tubules and collecting ducts (see Table 483–1).

MEDULLARY SPONGE KIDNEY. This noninherited disorder is characterized by cystic dilatation of the terminal portions of the collecting ducts as they enter the renal pyramids. Although renal function and life span are typically normal, the disorder may be complicated by pyelonephritis, hypercalciuria, nephrocalcinosis (Fig. 483–1), nephrolithiasis, impaired concentrating capacity, and distal RTA.

MINERALOCORTICOID DEFICIENCY

PATHOGENESIS. This form of RTA results from inadequate production of or reduced distal tubular responsiveness to aldosterone. The lack of aldosterone effect impairs the establishment across the tubular cell membrane of an electrochemical gradient (with negative electrical potential in the tubular lumen) favorable to hydrogen ion secretion. In the absence of aldosterone-mediated sodium reabsorption, hyperkalemia develops. Hyperkalemia suppresses renal ammonia production, resulting in a reduction of ammonium ion excretion and, thus, net acid excretion. The net effect is a hyperkalemic, hyperchloremic acidosis. The systemic acidosis may render the urine pH acid (less than 5.5).

Mineralocorticoid-deficiency RTA may result from diseases of the adrenal gland (Addison disease, congenital adrenal hyperplasia, primary hypoaldosteronism) in which aldosterone production is deficient. In these disorders, renal function is normal, urinary sodium wasting is common, and the plasma renin level is elevated. Hyporeninemic hypoaldosteronism is a form of RTA that may result from kidney diseases associated with interstitial damage and destruction of the juxtaglomerular apparatus; it may also be observed with volume expansion and prostaglandin inhibition. In these conditions, plasma levels of renin and, as a result, of aldosterone are reduced; renal function may be compromised. Rarely, type IV RTA may be the result of distal tubular unresponsiveness to aldosterone (pseudohypoaldosteronism); plasma renin and aldosterone levels are elevated, renal function is usually normal, and salt wasting is the rule. In adults, this form of RTA may be observed in patients with medullary disease and renal insufficiency.

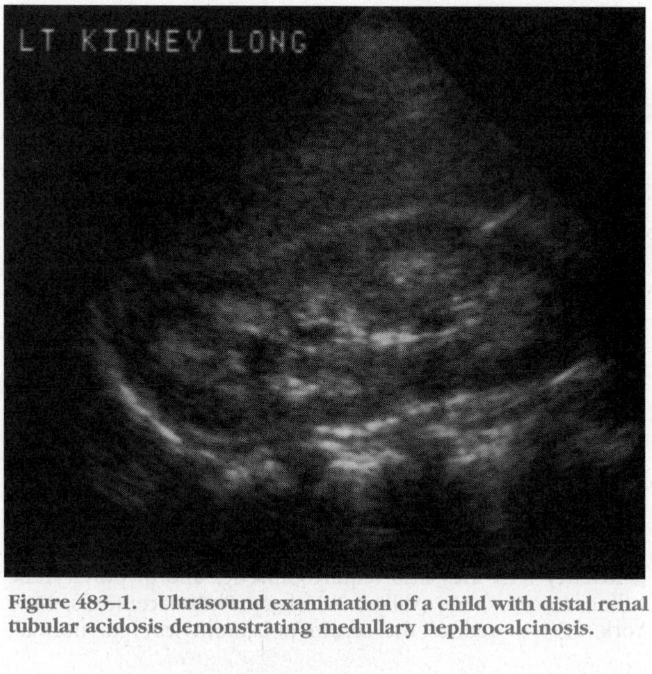

Figure 483–1. Ultrasound examination of a child with distal renal tubular acidosis demonstrating medullary nephrocalcinosis.

CLINICAL MANAGEMENT OF RENAL TUBULAR ACIDOSIS

CLINICAL MANIFESTATIONS. Children having isolated forms of proximal or distal RTA commonly present with growth failure toward the end of the first year of life. Gastrointestinal symptoms are common. Children having secondary forms of proximal or distal RTA may present in a similar fashion or with complaints unique to their fundamental disease. Mineralocorticoid deficiency is usually found as an underlying feature of a primary kidney disease.

Distal RTA is complicated by hypercalciuria, which may lead to nephrocalcinosis, nephrolithiasis, and renal parenchymal destruction. The causes of the hypercalciuria are unknown; potential mechanisms include bone breakdown to release calcium carbonate (the carbonate to be converted to bicarbonate in an attempt to control the acidosis) and diminished levels of urinary citrate (which chelates calcium).

DIAGNOSIS. Before considering the diagnosis of RTA, other causes of systemic acidosis, such as diarrhea, lactic acidosis, diabetes mellitus, and renal failure, should be excluded. The biochemical features of proximal and distal RTA include low serum bicarbonate and potassium levels in association with hyperchloremia. In mineralocorticoid-deficiency RTA, systemic acidosis is associated with hyperkalemia. The anion gap in all forms of RTA is usually normal (see Chapter 53).

Patients suspected of having proximal or distal RTA should be evaluated by comparing the pH (by pH meter) of a first morning urine specimen (collected under mineral oil to prevent the loss of carbon dioxide) with simultaneous measurements of serum electrolytes. In patients who have substantial systemic acidosis (serum bicarbonate less than 16 mEq/L [mmol/L]), a urine pH of less than 5.5 supports the diagnosis of proximal RTA, whereas patients with distal RTA will have a urine pH of 5.8 or greater. The *urinary anion gap* (urine concentrations of sodium plus potassium minus chloride) may be an indirect index of ammonium ion excretion that distinguishes proximal from distal RTA. Normal individuals and patients with proximal RTA have a negative gap during metabolic acidosis due to an increase in ammonium chloride production. Patients with distal RTA have a positive anion gap due to impaired excretion of hydrogen and ammonium ions.

In patients having mild acidosis (serum bicarbonate 17–20 mEq/L [mmol/L]), ammonium chloride loading may be required to distinguish between the two types. In occult cases, measurement of the fractional excretion of bicarbonate after raising the serum bicarbonate to normal by intravenous infusion of bicarbonate should be considered. If proximal RTA is detected, then other defects of proximal tubular function should be sought (glucosuria, phosphaturia, aminoaciduria). When any form of RTA is confirmed, potential underlying causes (see Table 483–1) should be investigated.

TREATMENT. The goals of therapy are correction of the acidosis and maintenance of normal serum bicarbonate and potassium levels. Most patients' conditions can be corrected with oral therapy; in infants having severe acidosis and hypokalemia, intravenous therapy may be required initially. The least expensive and easiest alkalinizing solution for oral use is Shohl solution (Bicitra, Willen Drug Company, Baltimore, MD) containing 1 mEq/mL of "bicarbonate equivalent" as sodium citrate. For patients requiring potassium supplementation, potassium citrate can be added (Polycitra, Willen Drug Company, Baltimore, MD) to form a solution that contains 1 mEq/mL each of sodium and potassium, and 2 mEq/mL of bicarbonate equivalent. Sodium bicarbonate tablets (325 and 650 mg) may be used in older patients. Patients having mineralocorticoid-deficiency RTA may also require diuretics and/or polystyrene sulfonate resin (Kayexalate, Winthrop Pharmaceuticals, New York, NY) to reduce the serum potassium level to normal. Carnitine supplements may be beneficial if serum levels are reduced.

PROGNOSIS. Isolated proximal RTA, although initially more severe than the distal variety, may resolve over the first decade of life. Isolated distal RTA seems to be a lifelong disease; in some instances, renal failure may develop; the prognosis is excellent, however, if the disease is recognized and therapy initiated prior to the development of nephrocalcinosis. A continuing need for alkali therapy and for lifelong monitoring of clinical status is the rule.

Mineralocorticoid-deficiency RTA most frequently results from obstructive uropathy and usually resolves within 12 mo after correction of the obstruction. In other secondary forms of RTA, the ultimate prognosis may depend on the severity of the primary disorder.

Batlle DC, Hizon M, Cohen E, et al: The use of the urinary anion gap in the diagnosis of hyperchloremic metabolic acidosis. N Engl J Med 318:594, 1988.
Burke JR, Inglis JA, Craswell PW, et al: Juvenile nephronophthisis and medullary cystic disease—the same disease (report of a large family with medullary cystic disease associated with gout and epilepsy). Clin Nephrol 18:1, 1982.
Caldas A, Broyer M, Dechaux M, et al: Primary distal tubular acidosis in childhood: clinical study and long-term follow-up of 28 patients. J Pediatr 121:233, 1992.
Chan JCM, Alon U: Tubular disorders of acid-base and phosphate metabolism. Nephron 40:257, 1985.
Charnas LR, Bernardina I, Rader D, et al: Clinical and laboratory findings in the oculocerebrorenal syndrome of Lowe, with special reference to growth and renal function. N Engl J Med 324:1318, 1991.
Kurtzman NA: Acquired distal renal tubular acidosis. Kidney Int 24:807, 1983.
Kurtzman NA: Disorders of distal acidification. Kidney Int 38:720, 1990.
Markello TC, Bernardini IM, Gahl WA: Improved renal function in children with cystinosis treated with cysteamine. N Engl J Med 328:1157, 1993.
O'Neil M, Breslau NA, Pak CYC: Metabolic evaluation of nephrolithiasis in patients with medullary sponge kidney. JAMA 245:1233, 1981.
Rodriguez-Soriano J, Vallo A: Renal tubular acidosis. Pediatr Nephrol 4:268, 1990.
Schneider JA, Katz B, Melles RB: Update on nephropathic cystinosis. Pediatr Nephrol 4:645, 1990.
Steele BT, Lirenman DS, Beattie CW: Nephronophthisis. Am J Med 68:531, 1980.

483.1 Rickets Associated with Renal Tubular Acidosis

Russel W. Chesney

Rickets may be present in primary renal tubular acidosis (RTA), particularly in type II or proximal RTA. Hypophosphatemia and phosphaturia are common in these syndromes, which are characterized by hyperchloremic metabolic acidosis, varying degrees of bicarbonaturia, and frequently hypercalciuria and hyperkaliuria. Bone demineralization without overt rickets usually is detected in type I and distal RTA. In type I there is an inability to form an adequately acid urine at all levels of serum bicarbonate; in type II, there is a lowered renal threshold for bicarbonate and impaired urinary acidification at normal levels of serum bicarbonate (Chapter 53). The metabolic bone disease that occurs in both types may also be characterized by bone pain, growth retardation, osteopenia, and occasionally pathologic fractures. Although acute metabolic acidosis in vitamin D–deficient animals may impair the conversion of 25(OH)D to $1,25(OH)_2D$, resulting in reduced levels of this active metabolite, the circulating levels of $1,25(OH)_2D$ in patients with either type of RTA are normal. If patients with RTA have azotemia and loss of renal mass, serum $1,25(OH)_2D$ levels are often reduced.

Bone demineralization in distal RTA probably relates to dissolution of bone, because the calcium carbonate in bone may serve as a buffer against the metabolic acidosis that is due to the hydrogen ions retained by patients with RTA.

Administration of sufficient bicarbonate to reverse acidosis will stop bone dissolution and the hypercalciuria that is common in distal RTA. Proximal RTA is treated with both bicarbonate and oral phosphate supplements to heal bone disease. Doses of phosphate similar to those used in familial hypophosphatemia should be used (Chapter 648). Vitamin D is needed to offset the secondary hyperparathyroidism that complicates oral phosphate therapy.

483.2 Fanconi Syndrome

(Rickets Associated with Multiple Defects of the Proximal Renal Tubule; de Toni-Debré-Fanconi Syndrome)

Michael E. Norman

Generalized aminoaciduria, renal glycosuria, and phosphaturia resulting in hypophosphatemia characterize Fanconi syndrome. Associated but inconstant renal tubular abnormalities include excessive bicarbonaturia leading to renal tubular acidosis, hyperkaliuria leading to hypokalemia, sodium wasting, uricosuria, proteinuria, and hyposthenuria. Clinical hallmarks are linear growth failure and rickets resistant to doses of vitamin D that are ordinarily adequate for treatment of nutritional deficiency (Chapter 45.3).

ETIOLOGY. Fanconi syndrome occurs with genetically transmitted inborn errors of metabolism (cystinosis, fructose intolerance, galactosemia, glycogenosis, Lowe syndrome, tyrosinemia, and Wilson disease) and with some acquired diseases, including exposure to environmental toxins, for example, heavy metals (Cd, Pb, Hg) or certain drugs (outdated tetracycline, gentamicin, valproic acid, cisplatin, azathioprine). Most commonly, it is idiopathic, and its occurrence in this form may be sporadic or inherited as a mendelian dominant or recessive trait, including X-linked recessive. The following description of the primary idiopathic form is representative of the syndrome in general.

PATHOGENESIS. Studies suggest an abnormality in some final common pathway for normal membrane transport in the proximal renal tubules. There may be deficient energy production, abnormalities in membrane structure, or both, leading to impaired tubular uptake or back-leak of solutes. DNA deletions of respiratory chain genes have been reported, leading to deficient energy production. Also, loss of bicarbonate in the urine leads to proximal RTA (Chapters 483 and 483.1). Renal potassium wasting results from excessive urinary losses of bicarbonate and glucose. Urinary sodium losses are obligatory because of the large excretion of urinary anions. Serum calcium level is normal to low; urinary calcium levels vary. A vasopressin-resistant urinary concentrating defect is often present but is unexplained. A syndrome similar to Fanconi syndrome can be produced in rodents and dogs upon administration of maleic acid, a tubular toxin, and occurs in the Basenji breed of dogs in which excessive urinary losses of amino acids, sugar, and phosphate result from decreased proximal RTA of the glomerular filtrate.

Rickets can result from the combined effects of metabolic acidosis and hypophosphatemia, or from hypophosphatemia alone. Simple calcium deficiency does not appear to play a role in the bone disease. Vitamin D resistance may be due to impaired conversion of vitamin D to its biologically active metabolite, $1,25(OH)_2D_3$, by abnormal proximal tubular cells in the presence of metabolic acidosis (Chapter 483.1).

Microscopic findings are nonspecific. Renal tubules may show dilatation, variation in size and shape, swelling of epithelial cells, and atrophy. Foci of interstitial fibrosis are common. Enlarged mitochondria may be seen on electron microscopy. Typically, glomerular architecture is preserved until late in the disease.

CLINICAL MANIFESTATIONS. Primary Fanconi syndrome typically presents either in the first 6 mo of life or in the 3rd–4th decade. In infancy, vomiting, polydipsia, polyuria, and constipation occur. Episodes of weakness, fever with dehydration, and metabolic acidosis may also occur. Failure to thrive is often pronounced, especially in linear growth. Progressive renal failure is uncommon but has been reported in the Fanconi syndrome.

Roentgenographic signs of rickets or osteopenia may appear despite a history of adequate vitamin D intake and the absence of glomerular insufficiency, indicating a renal tubular cause.

LABORATORY DATA. Usually, a hyperchloremic metabolic acidosis is noted, with normal "anion gap" (Chapter 53), hypokalemia, hypophosphatemia, and hypouricemia. Fractional excretion of phosphate is elevated. Alkaline phosphatase activity is elevated if rickets is present. Glycosuria occurs at normal serum glucose concentrations. There is generalized nonspecific aminoaciduria. Urinary pH is inappropriately elevated, with low levels of urinary ammonia and titratable acid. When the glomerular filtration rate falls late in the course of the disease, there may be a "paradoxic" improvement in the levels of serum electrolytes and an amelioration of aminoaciduria, glycosuria, and phosphaturia.

DIAGNOSIS. There is no definitive diagnostic test for idiopathic Fanconi syndrome. Aminoaciduria, diminished tubular reabsorption of phosphate, and elevated alkaline phosphatase activities accompany other forms of rickets. In a child with stunted growth and rickets refractory to ordinary doses of vitamin D, the presence of renal glycosuria indicates multiple tubular dysfunction. Metabolic acidosis and hypokalemia are corroborative. Fluid deprivation to test urinary concentrating ability is risky in the face of obligatory hyposthenuria, and glucose loading may cause profound symptomatic hypokalemia by shifting potassium into cells.

TREATMENT. The clinical and biochemical expressions vary from one patient to another; accordingly, treatment is not uniform. For patients with secondary Fanconi syndrome, underlying causes should be sought. In those with primary Fanconi syndrome, symptomatic therapy can restore mineral and electrolyte balance, prolong survival, and often permit a normal life. Rickets can be corrected and skeletal deformities prevented, but fully normal growth rates are rarely achieved.

Rickets or osteopenia responds to large doses of vitamin D. The usual starting dose is 5,000 units/24 hr, which should be increased gradually to a maximal dose of 2,000–4,000 units/kg/24 hr. Most patients require at least 25,000 units to heal rickets. Dihydrotachysterol may be substituted for vitamin D at a starting dose of 0.05–0.1 mg/24 hr (1 mg is equivalent to 120,000 units of vitamin D). In recent years, $1,25(OH)_2D_3$ has become the preferred form of vitamin D therapy because of its greater potency and shorter half-life, should hypercalcemia occur. Serum calcium levels must be followed closely (weekly at first, then monthly) to avoid hypercalcemia from vitamin D overdose. Hypophosphatemia can be treated by oral supplementation with 1–3 g of neutral phosphate/24 hr given in 4–5 equally spaced doses through the waking hours. If abdominal pain or diarrhea ensues, therapy should be discontinued temporarily and then reinstituted at a lower dose. Phosphate should not be given without concomitant vitamin D to avoid causing or aggravating hypocalcemia, and causing secondary hyperparathyroidism.

Correcting metabolic acidosis due to excessive bicarbonaturia may require large amounts of alkali. From 2 to 15 mEq/kg/24 hr of alkali may be needed, as sodium bicarbonate solution (1 mEq of base = 1 mL), *Shohl* solution (140 g of citric acid, 90 g of sodium citrate qs to 1 L with water; 1 mEq of base = 1 mL), or *Polycitra* (5 mL = 550 mg of potassium citrate, 500 mg of sodium citrate, 334 mg of citric acid; 2 mEq of base = 1 mL). Doses should be adjusted to raise serum bicarbonate only to near normal levels (18–20 mEq/L). Attempts to normalize serum bicarbonate may exaggerate urinary bicarbonate loss as a result of extracellular fluid volume expansion with excessive sodium loads. Alkali is administered 1–1½ hr after meals in 3–4 divided doses/24 hr, and, if Polycitra is not used, extra potassium should be given at a starting dose of 2–3 mEq/kg/24 hr. Extra salt and water should be provided to counter excessive losses, especially in warm weather.

Chesney RW: Etiology and pathogenesis of the Fanconi syndrome. Miner Electrolyte Metab 4:303, 1980.
Cohn RM, Roth KS: Metabolic Disease: A Guide to Early Recognition. Philadelphia, WB Saunders, 1983, p 258.
Foreman JW, Roth KS: The human renal Fanconi syndrome—then and now. Nephron 51:301, 1989.

483.3 Cystinosis

(Lignac Syndrome; Fanconi Syndrome with Cystinosis)

Michael E. Norman

Cystinosis presents the clinical and laboratory features of Fanconi syndrome with the additional distinctive finding of abnormal accumulation of cystine in various tissues (see also Chapters 70.4 and 483.2).

PATHOGENESIS. The cause is unknown. Increased cellular uptake of cystine results in accumulation in lysosomes, where it cannot be maintained in reduced form. It also appears that there is a failure in lysosomal release of this amino acid. No specific enzyme defect has yet been identified. Tissue levels of cystine do not correlate with the degree of renal tubular dysfunction; accordingly, a simple toxic effect of cystine on tubules is not the cause of Fanconi syndrome in cystinosis.

Cystine is deposited in the reticuloendothelial system, especially in spleen, liver, lymph nodes, and bone marrow, but not in muscle or brain. Deposits occur in renal tubular cells, cornea, and conjunctiva. Cystine also accumulates in peripheral blood leukocytes and fibroblasts. Early renal changes are similar to those of primary Fanconi syndrome; the characteristic "swan neck" lesion consists of atrophy and shortening of the proximal tubule just beneath the glomerulus. Birefringent cystine crystals may be seen in interstitial tissue and rarely in tubular cells; they are sometimes recognizable only on electron microscopy. With advancing renal failure, the kidneys become shrunken and contracted, with glomerular sclerosis and interstitial fibrosis.

CLINICAL MANIFESTATIONS. Cystinosis is inherited as an autosomal recessive trait. There are three clinical patterns in childhood cystinosis. Patients with the *infantile* or *nephropathic form* present with Fanconi syndrome at 3–12 mo of age. A generalized aminoaciduria is found without predominance of cystine. The glomerular filtration rate falls progressively, and chronic renal failure develops within the 1st decade. Severe growth failure and hypothyroidism accompany this state. Distinctive clinical features include blond hair and fair complexion, owing to a defect in melanin synthesis, and photophobia secondary to deposit of cystine crystals on the conjunctivae. The *adolescent* or *intermediate form* is characterized by mild renal involvement, with onset in the 2nd decade and slow progression. Growth failure is not a feature of this form. The *adult type* of cystinosis (benign) causes no renal disease. Cystine crystals may be found in the cornea, bone marrow, and leukocytes.

LABORATORY DATA. Other than the deposition of cystine crystals, laboratory abnormalities are similar to those described for the Fanconi syndrome. Tubular proteinuria characterizes the early phase of nephropathic cystinosis, but glomerular proteinuria supervenes as renal failure ensues.

DIAGNOSIS. In the asymptomatic newborn infant from an affected family the diagnosis of nephropathic cystinosis can be made by measuring the cystine content of leukocytes or fibroblasts, which will be 80–100 times normal. Later, granular and circinate irregularities in the peripheral pigmentation of the retina may be noted. Cystine crystals may be detected in the bone marrow, lymph nodes, conjunctivae, and rectal mucosa. Slit lamp examination shows crystals in the cornea. Prenatal diagnosis can be made by finding an increased concentration of cystine in amniotic fluid cells. Cystinosis must not be confused with cystinuria, which is an inborn error of specific amino acid transport, with neither cystine deposition nor Fanconi syndrome.

TREATMENT. Early on, symptomatic therapy for tubular dysfunction is similar to that for primary Fanconi syndrome. In addition, cysteamine, a sulfhydryl binder, has been shown to lower intracellular cystine in vivo and to slow the rate of progression of renal (glomerular) failure in many children, particularly if it is started prior to the age of 2 yr. It may also attenuate but not reverse some features of the Fanconi syndrome. Cysteamine is bitter tasting and has been replaced by phosphocysteamine, which is more acceptable to children.

For patients with end-stage renal failure, hemodialysis and renal transplantation are recommended. Hemodialysis does not lower tissue cystine levels. Children with cystinosis appear to do as well after kidney transplantation as those with other forms of chronic kidney failure, but long-term survivors may experience progressive photophobia or retinopathy. Cysteamine eye drops may be helpful. Transplantation has increased survival but has been associated with long-term extrarenal manifestations, such as swallowing dysfunction, myopathy, pancreatic endocrine and exocrine insufficiency, and various central nervous system problems (e.g., seizures, cerebral atrophy).

Cohn RM, Roth KS: Metabolic Disease: A Guide to Early Recognition. Philadelphia, WB Saunders, 1983, p 237.
Foreman JW: Cystinosis. Semin Nephrol 9:62, 1989.
Gahl WA: Cystinosis coming of age. Adv Pediatr 33:95, 1986.
Markello TC, Bernadini ME, Gahl WA: Improved renal function in children with cystinosis treated with cysteamine. N Engl J Med 328:1157, 1993.

483.4 Oculocerebrorenal Dystrophy

(Lowe Syndrome)

Michael E. Norman

This rare disorder is transmitted as an X-linked recessive trait. In addition to Fanconi syndrome, organic aciduria, decreased production of urinary ammonia, and occasionally heavy proteinuria occur. Distinctive clinical features include congenital cataracts, glaucoma, and buphthalmos, which lead to severe visual impairment. Severe hypotonia and hyporeflexia appear in the 1st yr. Mental retardation is severe and often progressive. Behavioral abnormalities often supervene. Rickets, marked osteopenia, and pathologic fracture may develop as a result of metabolic acidosis and phosphate depletion.

PATHOGENESIS. The pathogenesis is not known, but recent in vitro studies have suggested an abnormality in collagen metabolism. Pathologic studies have shown splitting of the glomerular basement membranes, with marked variation in their thickness. These changes may not be confined to the kidney.

CLINICAL FEATURES. Early in life the eye abnormalities and mental retardation predominate; the Fanconi syndrome becomes clinically apparent later. If the patient survives childhood, the

Fanconi syndrome may resolve spontaneously, only to be supplanted by chronic renal failure. There is no specific therapy. Treatment is supportive, as in primary Fanconi syndrome, and includes support for the visual, developmental, behavioral, and musculoskeletal complications.

Abbassi V, Lowe CU, Calcagno PL: Oculo-cerebro-renal syndrome: A review. Am J Dis Child 15:145, 1968.
Charnas LR, Gahl WA: The oculocerebral syndrome of Lowe. Adv Pediatr 38:75, 1991.
For advice and support to families with Lowe syndrome, contact the Lowe's Syndrome Association, 607 Robinson Street, West Lafayette, IN 47906.

483.5 Renal Osteodystrophy

Michael E. Norman

The term *renal osteodystrophy* designates the alterations in skeletal growth and remodeling that occur in children with chronic renal disease because of abnormalities in mineral and bone metabolism. These abnormalities include malabsorption of calcium, phosphate retention, hyperfunction of the parathyroid glands; cutaneous, vascular, and visceral calcifications; and impairment in the renal production of biologically active vitamin D. Renal osteodystrophy can occur with tubular dysfunction while glomerular filtration remains intact (Chapters 482, 483, and 483.1) but more commonly follows progressive loss of nephrons, with glomerular insufficiency and uremia.

The condition was formerly called renal (uremic) rickets or renal dwarfism because severe linear growth failure was associated with rickets-like roentgenographic changes. These findings were first thought to be due primarily to a mineralization defect resulting from vitamin D deficiency, but secondary hyperparathyroidism is an equally important contributor to the clinical and roentgenographic findings. Since the advent of pediatric dialysis and kidney transplantation, renal osteodystrophy has emerged as a major complication of chronic renal failure in childhood, along with acidosis, anemia, and caloric deficiency.

PATHOGENESIS. Early in the course of chronic renal insufficiency (glomerular filtration rate 25–50 mL/min/1.73m^2) with a normal dietary intake of phosphorus, there appears to be a phosphate-mediated suppression of renal tubular synthesis of $1,25(OH)_2D_3$, leading to malabsorption of calcium and phosphorus and, through unknown mechanisms, to defective mineralization of osteoid (osteomalacia). Serum calcium is maintained, and serum phosphorus may actually be normal to low as a result of raised parathyroid hormone levels (PTH), leading to increased bone resorption and increased renal phosphate excretion. Proof of this hypothesis comes from studies in which dietary phosphate restriction resulted in raised serum $1,25(OH)_2D_3$ levels and improvement in secondary hyperparathyroidism. At some critical renal threshold, for example, when the glomerular filtration rate falls to approximately 25–30% of normal, the phosphaturic renal response to elevated PTH is lost, and compensatory hyperparathyroidism supervenes in an attempt to restore serum calcium to normal. The consequences are roentgenographic and histologic evidence of exaggerated osteoclast-mediated resorption of bone (osteitis fibrosa). Also, endosteal fibrosis, increased bone turnover, and replacement of regularly textured lamellar bone with disorganized and structurally deficient woven bone are seen. Chronic metabolic acidosis probably contributes to the bony changes by increasing calcium resorption from bone and increasing renal excretion before severe renal failure ensues.

The pathology varies. On biopsy, trabecular bone may show predominant osteomalacia, predominant osteitis fibrosa, or, most commonly, a mixed pattern. Osteitis fibrosa predominates in dialyzed patients. A subgroup of patients has been described in whom fracturing osteomalacia and low bone turnover have resulted from accumulation of aluminum at the mineralization front. These patients have been exposed to either orally administered aluminum phosphate binders or aluminum-containing dialysis solutions. Aluminum blocks bone formation and mineralization, and inhibits PTH release.

Roentgenographic abnormalities at the epiphyseal growth plate may occasionally resemble those of nutritional rickets but are often quite distinct; histologically, they reflect osteitis fibrosa rather than rickets. The growth plate is not actually increased in longitudinal width but appears to be because of the formation of a bar of metaphyseal fibrosis with dysplastic trabeculas. The concomitant defect in mineralization leads to a failure in modeling, with persistence of cartilage, an expanded epiphyseal diameter, and frequent over-riding of the lateral border of the metaphysis.

CLINICAL MANIFESTATIONS. The younger the child at the onset of chronic renal failure and the longer the duration of renal failure,the greater will be the incidence and severity of osteodystrophy. In children with congenital diseases of the kidney, which predominate under the age of 5 yr, the interval between the onset of disease and end-stage renal failure is longer than it is in the glomerulonephritides, which occur later in childhood. However, in children with congenital nephropathies, bone disease is accelerated because it occurs at a time of maximal growth and bone modeling and remodeling.

The earliest sign of renal osteodystrophy is usually growth failure, to which anemia, metabolic acidosis, protein-calorie malnutrition, hormonal disorders, and trace mineral deficiencies associated with chronic renal failure may contribute. Growth failure may occur with no roentgenographic skeletal abnormalities. With advancing (untreated) disease, additional clinical manifestations appear, including muscle weakness, bone pain, bone deformities (pes varus, ulnar deviation of the hands), slipped epiphyses, metaphyseal fractures, metastatic calcification, and pruritus. Genu varum, frontal bossing, and dental abnormalities are particularly evident in young children. Tetany is rare (despite hypocalcemia) because of the combined protective effects of metabolic acidosis and hyperparathyroidism. Osteonecrosis may occur in children with renal disease treated with corticosteroids.

LABORATORY DATA. There may be mild hypocalcemia, but the Ca × P product is usually elevated by increased levels of serum phosphorus. Elevated alkaline phosphatase activity reflects increased bone turnover but is not as reliable a sign in children as in adults.

In roentgenograms of the hands and wrists, subperiosteal erosions of the middle and distal phalanges may be sensitive early indicators of osteitis fibrosa. Erosions may also occur in the distal clavicle and on inner aspects of the distal femur and proximal tibia. Elevated serum levels of PTH generally give the earliest indication of bone disease and may be found when glomerular filtration rates are reduced to as little as 50–75 mL/min/1.73 m^2. The degree of elevation of PTH correlates with roentgenographic and histologic evidence of osteitis fibrosa, but the degree of histologic osteomalacia does not correlate well with chemical abnormalities in serum or with roentgenographic evidence of rickets, osteopenia, or coarsening of trabeculas.

TREATMENT. Renal osteodystrophy can usually be successfully managed by (1) controlling hyperphosphatemia, (2) supplying adequate oral calcium intake, and (3) providing extra vitamin D. Treatment should begin early because growth failure in infancy can greatly influence the attainment of ultimate stature. An unresolved question is whether therapy should be initiated before definite roentgenographic or biochemical abnormalities appear, but recent literature suggests that a raised

PTH level is an indication to begin dietary phosphate restriction.

Hyperphosphatemia should be controlled with oral administration of phosphate binders if dietary restriction is not sufficient. Aluminum-containing binders should be avoided whenever possible because of the risks of aluminum intoxication. However, when there are no satisfactory alternatives, aluminum hydroxide or aluminum carbonate gel can be given at a starting dose of 20–30 mg/kg/24 hr in divided doses with meals and can be subsequently adjusted to keep the serum phosphorus between 4 and 5 mg/dL. The total dose of aluminum should not exceed 50 mg/kg/24 hr. Long-term treatment with high-dose aluminum-containing binders has been reported to cause osteomalacic osteodystrophy and a progressive, irreversible encephalopathy with dementia. Calcium supplementation in the form of calcium carbonate should be added to the diet to provide 1–1.5 g of elemental calcium per day. Calcium carbonate is preferred because it contains the highest percentage of elemental calcium of the available calcium preparations, and it affords some degree of phosphate binding while minimizing calcium absorption, particularly when given with meals. Strict control of acidosis should be achieved by administering sodium bicarbonate. Starting doses are usually 1–2 mEq/kg/24 hr, divided into thirds and given 1 hr after meals (see Chapters 483 and 483.2 for specific agents).

Some form of vitamin D appears necessary for successful treatment of uremic osteodystrophy. The preferred form is $1,25(OH)_2D_3$, although the long-term advantage of this form over dihydrotachysterol (DHT) has not been demonstrated. This therapy is indicated for symptomatic bone disease with hypocalcemia, secondary hypoparathyroidism, and evidence of osteitis fibrosa on roentgenography or bone biopsy. Starting doses are 15–40 ng/kg/24 hr and should be divided and given 8–12 hr apart to reduce the risk of hypercalcemia. Stepwise adjustments in the dose and indefinite biochemical monitoring are indicated, as with DHT treatment (discussed later). The usual maintenance dose of $1,25(OH)_2D_3$ is 0.75–1.50 μg/day. When hypercalcemia ensues, it is usually very short-lived because of the extremely short half-life of $1,25(OH)_2D_3$.

DHT has been favored over vitamin D because it has a better ratio of therapeutic to toxic effects and because its shorter half-life will reduce complications if hypercalcemia occurs. Starting doses are 0.1–0.2 mg/24 hr, and the dosage is increased weekly or biweekly in stepwise fashion to normalize levels of serum calcium and to heal roentgenographic abnormalities. Doses can be lowered once these goals are achieved. Frequent measurements of serum calcium and phosphorus are required, weekly at first, then monthly. The "set-point" of serum calcium at which PTH is released is elevated in chronic renal failure, which may be related to downregulation of vitamin D receptors in the parathyroid gland in chronic renal failure. Thus the therapeutic goal of vitamin D therapy is to raise serum calcium to 10.5–11.0 mg/dL.

Hemodialysis or chronic peritoneal dialysis may either ameliorate or exacerbate bone disease; the effect cannot be predicted. Unrecognized or untreated hypercalcemia may accelerate renal insufficiency or foster metastatic calcification of the tympanic membranes, cornea, conjunctiva, skin, and vascular tree, particularly as the C × P product approaches 75. When hypercalcemia is found, administration of vitamin D must be suspended until the serum calcium level is normal; therapy can then be reinstituted at a lower dose.

Autotransplantation of the parathyroid gland is preferred over parathyroidectomy in carefully selected patients with severe secondary hyperparathyroidism refractory to medical therapy. Indications include severe bone pain, mental aberrations, severe pruritus, fractures, chronic hypercalcemia, and, less commonly, metastatic calcification. In all cases marked elevation of serum PTH levels should be proved prior to surgery.

Foreman JW, Chan JCM: Chronic renal failure in infants and children. J Pediatr 113:793, 1988.
Goodman WG, Coburn JW, Ramirez JA, et al: Renal osteodystrophy in adults and children. *In*: Favus MJ (ed): Primer on the Metabolic Bone Diseases and Disorders of Mineral Metabolism, 2nd ed. New York, Raven Press, 1993, pp 304–323.
Malluche H, Faugere M: Renal osteodystrophy. N Engl J Med 321:317, 1989.
Polinsky MS, Gruskin AB: Aluminum toxicity in children with chronic renal failure. J Pediatr 105:758, 1984.
Mehls O, Salusky IB: Recent advances and controversies in childhood renal osteodystrophy. Pediatr Nephrol 1:212, 1987.

CHAPTER 484
Nephrogenic Diabetes Insipidus

Jerry M. Bergstein

In this disorder the kidney fails to respond to antidiuretic hormone despite elevated blood levels of antidiuretic hormone.

ETIOLOGY. Primary nephrogenic diabetes insipidus is a rare inherited (usually X-linked recessive) disease, characterized by complete tubular unresponsiveness to antidiuretic hormone in males and partial unresponsiveness in females. Partial or complete nephrogenic diabetes insipidus (secondary) may also be associated with disorders that (1) result in loss of the medullary concentrating gradient (acute or chronic renal failure, obstructive and postobstructive uropathy, vesicoureteral reflux, cystic diseases, interstitial nephritis, osmotic diuresis, nephrocalcinosis); or (2) diminish the effect of antidiuretic hormone on the tubules (hypokalemia, hypercalcemia, lithium, amphotericin B, and demeclocycline therapy).

PATHOGENESIS. Concentration of the urine depends on the establishment of a hypertonic renal medulla and the permeability of the distal tubules and collecting ducts to water. The hypertonicity of the medulla is established by a countercurrent mechanism linked to reabsorption of sodium and urea. The permeability of the collecting ducts is regulated by antidiuretic hormone, release of which from the neurohypophysis is triggered primarily by osmosensitive neurons located in the hypothalamus and secondarily by monitors of intravascular volume that reside in the heart, large arteries, kidney, liver, and brain. In the kidney, the hormone acts to increase the permeability of the distal tubules and collecting ducts to water by means of a cyclic adenosine monophosphate–dependent mechanism. This permits water to flow by passive diffusion from the tubule into the hypertonic medullary interstitium of the kidney.

In primary nephrogenic diabetes insipidus, the distal tubule fails to respond normally to antidiuretic hormone, whether endogenous or exogenous. In secondary forms of nephrogenic diabetes insipidus, the hypertonic medullary gradient may be diminished owing to a solute diuresis or inability of tubules to reabsorb sodium chloride and urea. Alternatively, the secondary form may result from induced tubular unresponsiveness to the hormone.

CLINICAL MANIFESTATIONS. Males with primary nephrogenic diabetes insipidus have a dramatic history of polyuria and polydipsia in infancy, often with episodes of hypernatremic dehydration. Females with the primary defect have milder symptoms that may not be detected until later in life. Patients having secondary forms of the disease present with hypernatremia during the course of their primary disorder.

DIAGNOSIS. The diagnosis of primary nephrogenic diabetes insipidus is suspected on clinical history, often with a positive family history in males. Laboratory findings include hypernatremia and dilute urine. If the serum osmolality at initial study exceeds 295 mOsm/kg (mmol/kg) H_2O and concurrent urine osmolality is less than this value, then a dehydration test to establish the diagnosis is unnecessary. The diagnosis is confirmed by administering an intramuscular injection of 0.1–0.2 unit/kg of aqueous vasopressin and measuring the serum and urine osmolality each hour for 4 hr. If the ratio of urine-to-plasma osmolality remains less than 1.0, the patient has nephrogenic diabetes insipidus. If the ratio becomes greater than 1.0, then central diabetes insipidus is suggested, but psychogenic polydipsia must be excluded. Patients with initial serum osmolality levels less than 295 mOsm/kg (mmol/kg) H_2O should be fasted (during the day rather than overnight) until serum osmolality exceeds 295 mOsm/kg (mmol/kg) H_2O; vasopressin is then given as before. The withholding of fluids should be terminated if body weight declines by as much as 3%. In patients suspected of primary nephrogenic diabetes insipidus, appropriate biochemical and radiographic studies should be done to exclude secondary causes.

COMPLICATIONS. As originally described, primary nephrogenic diabetes insipidus was associated with mental retardation. Retardation is more likely the result of repeated episodes of hypertonic dehydration than the consequence of the disease itself. Growth retardation is uniformly present in males with the primary disorder but is usually absent in females. Growth failure was originally thought to result from inadequate caloric intake due to excessive fluid intake, but it now seems that growth failure is intrinsic to the homozygous state. Dilatation of the urinary collecting system may result from excessive urine production. Accordingly, the anatomy of the urinary tract should be examined for evidence of hydronephrosis every few years by renal scan (intravenous pyelography may not visualize the collecting systems when there is rapid flow of large volumes of dilute urine).

TREATMENT. The keys to treatment include the provision of adequate fluid and caloric intake, and reduction of the urinary solute load. These are accomplished by limiting the intake of a low sodium formula (SMA, Wyeth Laboratories, Philadelphia, PA; Similac PM 60/40, Ross Laboratories, Columbus, OH) to only that which is necessary to supply optimal caloric intake for growth. The remainder of the daily fluid requirement (as determined by the maintenance of a normal serum sodium level) is administered as water or fruit juice. The parents should be cautioned that until the child can obtain free access to water, fluids should be offered every 1–2 hr during the day and three times during the night. Once the child becomes old enough to obtain free access to water, the intact thirst mechanism will provide the appropriate stimulus for fluid intake.

In patients with the primary disorder, the urinary volume can be dramatically reduced by diuretic therapy. This paradoxical response results because sodium depletion seems to enhance proximal tubular reabsorption of sodium and water. Less water, therefore, is presented to the defective portion of the tubules. Chlorothiazide (20–40 mg/kg/24 hr in divided doses) in conjunction with moderate salt restriction may significantly reduce the need for fluid intake and the frequency of voiding. The patient should be monitored for the development of hypokalemia. Patients who fail to respond to a low-solute diet and diuretics may be candidates for treatment with inhibitors of prostaglandin synthesis (e.g., indomethacin). This type of therapy is of no value for secondary forms of the disease.

PROGNOSIS. Primary nephrogenic diabetes insipidus is a lifelong disease with a good prognosis if hypernatremic dehydration can be avoided. Genetic counseling should be provided for the family. The prognosis of secondary forms of the disease depends on the nature of the primary disorder. The syndrome may resolve after correction of obstructive lesions.

Gibbons MD, Koontz WW Jr: Obstructive uropathy and nephrogenic diabetes insipidus in infants. J Urol 122:556, 1979.
Jamison RL, Oliver RE: Disorders of urinary concentration. Am J Med 72:308, 1982.
Knoers N, Monnens LAH: Nephrogenic diabetes insipidus: clinical symptoms, pathogenesis, genetics and treatment. Pediatr Nephrol 6:476, 1992.
Libber SL, Harrison H, Spector D: Treatment of nephrogenic diabetes insipidus with prostaglandin synthesis inhibitors. J Pediatr 108:305, 1986.
Rascher W, Rosendahl W, Henrichs IA, et al: Congenital nephrogenic diabetes insipidus—vasopressin and prostaglandins in response to treatment with hydrochlorothiazide and indomethacin. Pediatr Nephrol 1:485, 1987.

CHAPTER 485
Bartter Syndrome

Jerry M. Bergstein

This rare form of renal potassium wasting is characterized by hypokalemia, normal blood pressure, vascular insensitivity to pressor agents, and elevated plasma concentrations of renin and aldosterone. In certain families, the disorder may be inherited as an autosomal recessive trait.

PATHOLOGY. Generalized hyperplasia of the juxtaglomerular apparatus, the site of renin production, is observed in most patients with the syndrome. The renal parenchyma is otherwise normal in most patients; a few have shown nonspecific glomerular disease or interstitial disease or both.

PATHOGENESIS. The etiology is unknown. Currently, the disorder is best explained as a primary defect in chloride reabsorption in the ascending limb of the loop of Henle. The resultant decrease in sodium chloride reabsorption in this portion of the loop will reduce medullary hypertonicity, perhaps explaining the concentrating defect. The defect in chloride reabsorption presents extra sodium chloride to the distal tubule, where sodium is reabsorbed in exchange for potassium; the result is urinary potassium wasting. The induced hypokalemia stimulates the synthesis of prostaglandins (which may account for the vascular insensitivity to pressor agents and the defect in platelet aggregation); these, in turn, activate the renin-angiotensin-aldosterone system by increasing renin release and by stimulating aldosterone synthesis. The latter exacerbates renal potassium wasting.

CLINICAL MANIFESTATIONS. Young children typically present with growth failure, muscle weakness, constipation, polyuria, and dehydration due to urinary salt and water loss. Older children have muscle weakness, or cramps and carpopedal spasms.

DIAGNOSIS. The diagnosis is suggested by the finding of hypokalemia; the serum potassium level is usually less than 2.5 mEq/L (mmol/L). Supportive findings include normal blood pressure; defective platelet aggregation; hypochloremia; metabolic alkalosis; elevated plasma levels of renin, aldosterone, and prostaglandin E_2; and high urinary levels of potassium and chloride. Some patients may also have hypercalciuria, hyperuricemia, hypomagnesemia, and urinary sodium-wasting. The diagnosis is confirmed by the histologic demonstration of hyperplasia of the juxtaglomerular apparatus, but this abnormality is not found in all patients and is most frequently absent in young children.

Bartter syndrome must be differentiated from licorice abuse, laxative or diuretic use, persistent vomiting or diarrhea, pyelonephritis, and diabetes insipidus. Several of these (laxative use, vomiting, diarrhea, diabetes insipidus) are associated with hypovolemia, which results in a low urinary chloride level; whereas Bartter syndrome is associated with an elevated level.

TREATMENT. The goals of therapy are to supply adequate nutrition and to maintain the serum potassium level above 3.5

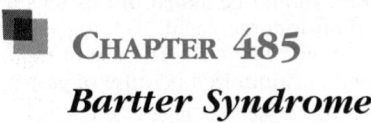

mEq/L (mmol/L). Therapy is initiated with oral potassium chloride supplementation, increasing the dose until the serum potassium level reaches 3.5 mEq/L (mmol/L) or the dosage reaches 250 mEq/24 hr. A reasonably well-tolerated potassium preparation is K-Lyte/Cl (Mead Johnson Company, Evansville IN), flavored effervescent tablets containing 25 or 50 mEq of potassium chloride. Sodium chloride supplementation may also be required in small children. If the serum potassium level remains below 3.5 mEq/L (mmol/L) after reaching a dose of 250 mEq/24 hr of potassium chloride, then triamterene, 5–10 mg/kg/24 hr in divided doses, should be added. If this fails to resolve the hypokalemia, then indomethacin, 3–5 mg/kg/24 hr divided into three doses, should be given. The use of indomethacin is generally avoided or minimized because of gastrointestinal complications.

PROGNOSIS. The long-term prognosis of Bartter syndrome is uncertain. Many patients remain well, but some (especially those with glomerular or interstitial abnormalities) progress to renal insufficiency. Despite severe growth retardation in infancy, normal stature is ultimately obtained. The suggestion that mental retardation occurs in patients who have severe disease in the 1st yr of life remains to be confirmed.

Chan JCM: Bartter's syndrome. Nephron 26:155, 1980.
Dunn MJ: Prostaglandins and Bartter's syndrome. Kidney Int 19:86, 1981.
Gill JR Jr: Bartter's syndrome. Annu Rev Med 31:405, 1980.
Stein J: The pathogenetic spectrum of Bartter's syndrome Kidney Int 28:85, 1985.
Stoff JS, Stemerman M, Steer M, et al: A defect in platelet aggregation in Bartter's syndrome. Am J Med 68:171, 1980.

CHAPTER 486

Interstitial Nephritis

Jerry M. Bergstein

Interstitial nephritis is a histopathologic term signifying inflammation between the glomeruli in the areas surrounding the tubules (the interstitium). Acute and chronic forms are recognized, depending on the nature of the inflammatory infiltrate and the presence or absence of edema and fibrosis. Tubular damage is generally present; glomerular changes may be minimal. Common causes of acute or chronic interstitial nephritis in children are listed in Table 486–1.

ACUTE INTERSTITIAL NEPHRITIS

PATHOLOGY. Whatever the cause of interstitial disease, the interstitial infiltrate is composed of lymphocytes, plasma cells, eosinophils, and occasional neutrophils (Fig. 486–1). The tubules are separated by edema and may show degeneration or frank necrosis. Unless the interstitial nephritis is associated with glomerulonephritis, the glomeruli are normal.

PATHOGENESIS. The genesis of acute interstitial nephritis is poorly understood. When it is due to drug ingestion, failure of the amount of drug administered to correlate with incidence of the syndrome suggests a hypersensitivity reaction. For methicillin, an immunologic mechanism has been suggested in several instances by the finding of anti-tubular basement membrane antibodies. Whether infections cause interstitial inflammation by direct invasion or by other mechanisms remains unclear. In certain forms of glomerulonephritis, tubular basement membrane deposition of immune complexes (lupus, membranoproliferative) or of anti-basement membrane antibodies (Goodpasture, membranous) may initiate the inflammatory reaction. In sarcoidosis and transplant rejection, cell-mediated mechanisms may play a role.

■ **TABLE 486–1 Causes of Interstitial Nephritis**

Acute	Chronic
Drugs	***Drugs***
Penicillin derivatives	Analgesics
Cephalosporins	Lithium
Sulfonamides	***Infections***
Co-trimoxazole	Pyelonephritis
Rifampin	***Disease-Associated***
Phenytoin	Vesicoureteral reflux
Thiazides	Nephrocalcinosis
Furosemide	Prolonged hypokalemia
Allopurinol	Oxalate nephropathy
Cimetidine	Heavy metals
Amphotericin B	Radiation
Nonsteroidal anti-inflammatory drugs	Obstructive uropathy
Infections	Medullary cystic disease
Streptococcal	Sickle cell disease
Pyelonephritis	
Toxoplasmosis	
Diphtheria	
Brucellosis	
Leptospirosis	
Mononucleosis	
Cytomegalovirus	
Disease-Associated	
Sarcoidosis	
Glomerulonephritis	
Transport rejection	
Idiopathic	

CLINICAL MANIFESTATIONS. In hospitalized patients, drugs are the most common cause of acute interstitial nephritis. After a week or so of drug therapy, patients typically present fever and a maculopapular skin rash. Urine output may be normal or diminished. Increased numbers of eosinophils may be detected in the blood or urine or both. Acute renal failure or generalized tubular dysfunction or both may result. Other forms of acute interstitial nephritis present a clinical picture resembling acute glomerulonephritis or acute renal failure, along with manifestations of the initiating disorder. The onset may be preceded by anterior uveitis.

DIAGNOSIS. The diagnosis is confirmed by renal biopsy, although acute interstitial nephritis may not be suspected prior

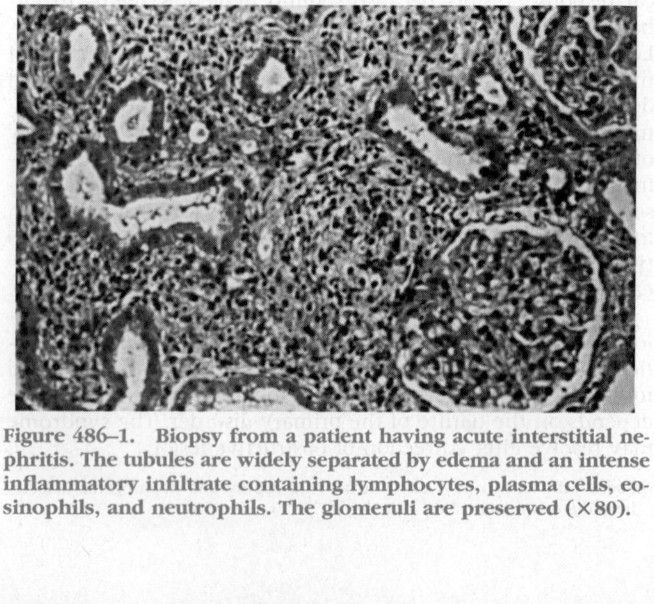

Figure 486–1. Biopsy from a patient having acute interstitial nephritis. The tubules are widely separated by edema and an intense inflammatory infiltrate containing lymphocytes, plasma cells, eosinophils, and neutrophils. The glomeruli are preserved (×80).

to the biopsy. The differential diagnosis includes other causes of acute nephritis or renal failure.

PREVENTION. The development of drug-related interstitial nephritis may be reduced by using alternative therapeutic agents when possible (e.g., the substitution of nafcillin for methicillin).

TREATMENT AND PROGNOSIS. Following appropriate management of the acute renal failure, withdrawal of possible inciting agents, and treatment of precipitating infection, the acute interstitial nephritis may resolve completely, but residual renal dysfunction is not uncommon. In patients suffering severe histologic injury and renal failure, high-dose corticosteroid therapy may bring dramatic improvement.

CHRONIC INTERSTITIAL NEPHRITIS

PATHOLOGY. In chronic interstitial nephritis, the inflammatory infiltrate consists of lymphocytes and plasma cells. The edema of the acute form is replaced by interstitial fibrosis. Tubular dilatation and atrophy are widespread. The glomeruli show partial or total sclerosis, presumably as a result of ischemia.

CLINICAL MANIFESTATIONS. In children, chronic interstitial nephritis usually develops in association with an occult structural abnormality of the kidneys or lower urinary tract (cystic disease, obstruction, reflux). The presenting clinical manifestations may be those of chronic renal failure (nausea, vomiting, pallor, headache, fatigue, hypertension, growth failure) or manifestations of the underlying disorder (urinary tract infection, flank mass).

DIAGNOSIS. The diagnosis is suggested by the presence of chronic renal insufficiency in association with a known cause of the disorder; renal biopsy is not usually indicated.

TREATMENT AND PROGNOSIS. The natural history of chronic interstitial nephritis is progression to end-stage renal failure. Whether elimination of infection or correction of reflux or obstruction will alter this progression is unclear. In adults, avoidance of analgesics (phenacetin) and lithium prior to the development of end-stage renal failure may result in improvement in renal function.

Bunchman TE, Bloom JN: A syndrome of acute interstitial nephritis and anterior uveitis. Pediatr Nephrol 7:520, 1993.
Ellis D, Fried WA, Yunis EJ, et al: Acute interstitial nephritis in children: A report of 13 cases and review of the literature. Pediatrics 67:862, 1981.
Jones CL, Eddy AA: Tubulointerstitial nephritis. Pediatr Nephrol 6:572, 1992.
Neilson EG: Pathogenesis and therapy of interstitial nephritis. Kidney Int 35:1257, 1989.
Sandler DP, Smith JC, Weinberg CR, et al: Analgesic use and chronic renal disease. N Engl J Med 320:1238, 1989.
Toto RB: Acute tubulointerstitial nephritis. Am J Med Sci 299:392, 1990.

SECTION 5

Toxic Nephropathies—Renal Failure

Jerry M. Bergstein

CHAPTER 487

Toxic Nephropathy

Medications, diagnostic agents (iodinated radiographic contrast media), and chemicals may alter the kidneys directly (through reduction of renal blood flow, acute tubular necrosis, intratubular obstruction) or indirectly (through induction of an allergic or hypersensitivity reaction in the vessels or interstitium). Commonly nephrotoxic agents and their clinical manifestations are listed in Table 487–1. Nephrotoxicity is frequently reversible if the noxious agent is removed.

Useful agents should not be withheld because of potential nephrotoxicity, but preventive measures may reduce the risks of nephrotoxicity: (1) in patients with pre-existing renal disease, substitution of ultrasound or isotopic scans for studies using contrast media; (2) substitution of non-nephrotoxic agents for nephrotoxic agents if possible; (3) use of the lowest effective dose of the agent in conjunction with monitoring of

■ TABLE 487–1 Nephrotoxic Compounds*

Nephrotic Syndrome	**Fanconi Syndrome**
Angiotensin converting enzyme inhibitors	Aminoglycosides
Gold salts	Cadmium
Mercurial diuretics	Lead
Mercury compounds	Lysol
Nonsteroidal anti-inflammatory drugs	Mercury
Paramethadione	Nitrobenzene
Penicillamine	Outdated tetracycline
Perchlorate	Salicylate
Probenecid	Uranium
Tolbutamide	**Renal Tubular Acidosis**
Trimethadione	Amphotericin B
Nephrogenic Diabetes Insipidus	Lithium salts
Amphotericin B	Toluene sniffing
Demeclocycline	**Interstitial Nephritis with or without Papillary Necrosis**
Lithium carbonate	Amidopyrine
Methoxyflurane	p-Aminosalicylate
Propoxyphene	Bunamiodyl (papillary necrosis only)

Table continued on following page

■ **TABLE 487–1 Nephrotoxic Compounds*** *Continued*

Interstitial Nephritis with or without Papillary Necrosis (*Continued*)
- Penicillins (especially methicillin)
- Phenacetin
- Phenylbutazone
- Salicylate
- Sulfonamides
- Nonsteroidal anti-inflammatory agents

Renal Vasculitis with or without Glomerular Capillary Involvement
- Hydralazine
- Isoniazid
- Sulfonamides
- Any of the numerous other drugs that may cause a hypersensitivity reaction

Nephrocalcinosis or Nephrolithiasis
- Allopurinol
- Ethylene glycol
- Methoxyflurane
- Vitamin D

Miscellaneous Renal Manifestations, Including Proteinuria, Hematuria, Oliguria, Tubular Necrosis, and Renal Failure
- Acyclovir
- Angiotensin converting enzyme inhibitors
- Arsenic
- Bacitracin
- Cadmium
- Carbon tetrachloride
- Cephaloridine
- Cephalothin
- Cisplatin
- Colistin
- Copper
- Cyclosporine
- Ethylene glycol
- FK 506
- Gentamicin
- Gold salts
- Indomethacin
- Iron
- Kanamycin
- Mercury salts
- Mitomycin C
- Neomycin
- Pentamidine
- Poisonous mushrooms
- Polymyxin B
- Radiocontrast agents
- Streptomycin
- Sulfonamides
- Tetrachlorethylene
- Vancomycin
- Viomycin

**The agents are grouped according to the principal site of injury or manifestations. (Dr. Sean O'Regan assisted in the preparation of this table.)*

the blood level; (4) reduction of the dose in patients with renal insufficiency; (5) avoidance of simultaneous use of several nephrotoxic agents.

Barrett BJ, Carlisle EJ: Metaanalysis of the relative nephrotoxicity of high- and low-osmolality iodinated contrast media. Radiology 188:171, 1993.
Becker BN, Fall P, Hall C, et al: Rapidly progressive acute renal failure due to acyclovir: case report and review of the literature. Am J Kidney Dis 22:611, 1993.
Bennett WM: Lead nephropathy. Kidney Int 28:212, 1985.
Bennett WM, Aronoff GR, Golper TA, et al (eds): Drug Prescribing in Renal Failure, 2nd ed. Philadelphia, American College of Physicians, 1991.
Fer MF, McKinney TD, Richardson RL, et al: Cancer and the kidney: Renal complications of neoplasms. Am J Med 71:704, 1981.
Humes HD: Aminoglycoside nephrotoxicity. Kidney Int 33:900, 1988.
Mendoza SA: Nephrotoxic drugs. Pediatr Nephrol 2:466, 1988.
Murgo AJ: Thrombotic microangiopathy in the cancer patient including those induced by chemotherapeutic agents. Semin Hematol 24:161, 1987.
Porter GA, Bennett WM: Nephrotoxic acute renal failure due to common drugs. Am J Physiol 241:F1, 1981.
Roxe DM: Toxic nephropathy from diagnostic and therapeutic agents. Am J Med 69:759, 1980.
Safirstein R, Winston J, Goldstein M, et al: Cisplatin nephrotoxicity. Am J Kidney Dis 8:356, 1986.
Shah GM, Alvarado P, Kirschenbaum MA, et al: Symptomatic hypocalcemia and hypomagnesemia with renal magnesium wasting associated with pentamidine therapy in a patient with AIDS. Am J Med 89:380, 1990.
Schlondorff D: Renal complications of nonsteroidal anti-inflammatory drugs. Kidney Int 44:643, 1993.
Wedeen RP: Occupational renal disease. Am J Kidney Dis 3:241, 1984.

CHAPTER 488
Cortical Necrosis

Renal cortical (and frequently medullary) necrosis seems to represent a final common result of several types of renal injury. It usually involves both kidneys and may be patchy or involve the entire cortex.

ETIOLOGY. In the newborn, cortical necrosis develops after dehydration, asphyxia, shock, disseminated intravascular coagulation, renal vein thrombosis, or in association with severe congenital heart disease. After the newborn period, cortical necrosis most commonly develops with the hemolytic-uremic syndrome.

PATHOLOGY. Involved portions of the cortex show infarction, with congestion of the glomeruli, thrombosis of the arterioles, and necrosis of the tubules.

PATHOGENESIS. Cortical necrosis seems to develop when endothelial cell injury occurs in conjunction with diminished renal cortical blood flow. Toxins that presumably develop during shock, hemolytic-uremic syndrome, or sepsis (endotoxin) may injure the endothelial cells and initiate intrarenal coagulation, leading to thrombosis and cortical necrosis.

CLINICAL MANIFESTATIONS. Cortical necrosis commonly presents as acute renal failure developing in infants having the above-mentioned predisposing causes. The kidneys are frequently enlarged. Urine output is diminished and may show gross hematuria.

DIAGNOSIS. The diagnosis is supported by the detection on ultrasonography of enlarged, nonobstructed kidneys, which on isotopic renal scan show little or no renal blood flow or function. The differential diagnosis includes other causes of renal failure (Tables 489–1 and 489–2).

TREATMENT AND PROGNOSIS. Therapy is supportive and involves correction of dehydration, asphyxia, and shock and treatment of sepsis. The prognosis depends on the amount of surviving renal cortex.

Chevalier RL, Campbell F, Brenbridge ANAG: Prognostic factors in neonatal acute renal failure. Pediatrics 74:265, 1984.
Guignard JP, Torrado A, Mazouni SM, et al: Renal function in respiratory distress syndrome. J Pediatr 88:845, 1976.
Lerner GR, Kurnetz R, Bernstein J, et al: Renal cortical and renal medullary necrosis in the first 3 months of life. Pediatr Nephrol 6:516, 1992.
Reimold EW, Don TD, Worthen HG: Renal failure during the first year of life. Pediatrics 59:987, 1977.
Rodriguez-Soriano J, Vallo A, Bilbao F, et al: Different functional characteristics of residual nephrons in infantile vs adult diffuse cortical necrosis. Int J Pediatr Nephrol 3:71, 1982.

URINARY TRACT INFECTION IN THE NEWBORN

This subject is reviewed in Chapters 101 and 492.

CHAPTER 489
Renal Failure

489.1 Acute Renal Failure

Acute renal failure develops when renal function is diminished to the point at which body fluid homeostasis can no longer be maintained. Although oliguria (daily urine volume less than 400 mL/m^2) is common, the urine volume may approximate normal (nonoliguric renal failure) in certain types of acute renal failure (aminoglycoside nephrotoxicity). To monitor renal function, it is important to use biochemical studies (BUN, creatinine) as well as measurement of urine volume.

ETIOLOGY. The causes of acute failure are listed in Tables 489–1 and 489–2. In the first category (prerenal), decreased perfusion of the kidney results in decreased renal function; the second category includes diseases of the kidney, while the third is composed primarily of obstructive disorders.

PATHOGENESIS. *Prerenal causes* of acute renal failure produce decreased renal perfusion through decreases in the total or "effective" circulating blood volume. Evidence of kidney damage is absent. Diminished intravascular volume leads to a fall in cardiac output, causing a decline in renal cortical blood flow and glomerular filtration rate (GFR). If, within a certain time, the underlying cause of the hypoperfusion is reversed, then renal function may return to normal. If hypoperfusion persists beyond this critical point, then renal parenchymal damage may develop.

Renal causes of acute renal failure include the rapidly progressive forms of several types of glomerulonephritis (Table 489–2) that are common causes of acute renal failure in older children. Activation of the coagulation system within the kidney, resulting in small vessel thrombosis, may lead to acute renal failure. The hemolytic-uremic syndrome is the most common cause of acute renal failure in toddlers.

The term *acute tubular necrosis* originally described a syndrome of acute renal failure in the absence of arterial or glomerular lesions. The proposed mechanism of the renal failure was necrosis of the tubular cells. Certain agents (heavy metals, chemicals) may indeed cause renal failure by producing tubular cell necrosis, but significant histologic changes are absent in kidneys from patients having other forms of acute tubular necrosis. The precise mechanism of renal failure in these patients is unknown. Proposed mechanisms include alterations in intrarenal hemodynamics, tubular obstruction, and passive backflow of the glomerular filtrate across injured tubular cells into the peritubular capillaries.

Acute interstitial nephritis is an increasingly common cause of acute renal failure and is usually the result of a hypersensitivity reaction to a therapeutic agent. Tumors may produce acute renal failure by infiltration of the kidney or by obstruction of the tubules by uric acid crystals (Chapters 445 and 449).

Developmental abnormalities and hereditary nephritis may be associated with acute renal failure. Inability to conserve sodium and water is common in patients having these disorders, but losses are usually compensated by increased oral intake. If oral intake is compromised (vomiting) and/or extrarenal salt and water loss develops (diarrhea), then these, in conjunction with the obligate urinary salt and water losses, may lead to intravascular volume contraction and renal failure.

Postrenal causes of acute renal failure include obstructions of the urinary tract. With two functioning kidneys, ureteral obstruction must be bilateral to produce renal failure. It is important to recognize that dilatation of the upper collecting system may not occur until several days after acute ureteral obstruction.

■ **TABLE 489–1 Causes of Acute Renal Failure in the Newborn**

Renal dysgenesis	Hemorrhage
Obstructive uropathy	Sepsis
Renovascular accidents	Anoxia
Congenital heart disease	Shock
Dehydration	Renal vein thrombosis

CLINICAL MANIFESTATIONS. The presenting signs and symptoms may be dominated or modified by the precipitating disease. Clinical findings related to the renal failure include pallor (anemia), diminished urine output, edema (salt and water overload), hypertension, vomiting, and lethargy (uremic encephalopathy). Complications of acute renal failure include volume overload with congestive heart failure and pulmonary edema, arrhythmias, gastrointestinal bleeding due to stress ulcers or gastritis, seizures, coma, and behavioral changes.

DIAGNOSIS. A careful history may aid in defining the cause of renal failure. Vomiting, diarrhea, and fever suggest dehydration and prerenal azotemia, but these may also precede development of the hemolytic-uremic syndrome or renal vein thrombosis. Antecedent skin or throat infection suggests poststreptococcal glomerulonephritis. Rash may be found in systemic lupus erythematosus or anaphylactoid purpura. A history of exposure to chemicals and medications should be sought. Flank masses suggest renal vein thrombosis, tumors, cystic disease, or obstruction.

Laboratory abnormalities may include anemia (with the rare exception of blood loss, the anemia is usually dilutional or hemolytic, as seen in lupus, renal vein thrombosis, and the hemolytic-uremic syndrome); leukopenia (lupus); thrombocytopenia (lupus, renal vein thrombosis, hemolytic-uremic syndrome); hyponatremia (dilutional); hyperkalemia; acidosis; elevated serum concentrations of BUN, creatinine, uric acid, and phosphate (diminished renal function); and hypocalcemia (hyperphosphatemia). The serum C3 level may be depressed (poststreptococcal, lupus, or membranoproliferative glomerulonephritis), and antibodies may be detected in the serum to streptococcal (poststreptococcal glomerulonephritis), nuclear (lupus), neutrophil cytoplasmic antigens (ANCA; Wegener granulomatosis, microscopic polyarteritis), or to basement membrane (Goodpasture disease) antigens. Chest roentgenography may reveal cardiomegaly and pulmonary congestion (fluid overload). In all patients presenting in acute renal failure, the possibility of obstruction (which, if detected, is quickly reversed by percutaneous nephrostomy) should be immediately assessed by obtaining a plain roentgenogram study of the abdomen, renal ultrasound, and a radionuclide scan; retrograde pyelography may occasionally be needed to detect occult obstructions. Renal biopsy may ultimately be required to determine the precise cause of renal failure.

TREATMENT. In children with *hypovolemia,* the need for volume replacement may be critical. The initial physical examination of the patient should include a careful assessment of the state of hydration. In some oliguric patients it may be impossible to distinguish whether oliguria is due to hypoperfusion (hypovolemia) or impending acute tubular necrosis. Evaluation of the urine may prove helpful in this regard. In patients with hypovolemia, the urine is concentrated (urine osmolality exceeds 500 mOsm/kg [mmol/L] H_2O), its sodium content is usually less than 20 mEq/L (mmol/L), and the fractional excretion of sodium (urine/plasma sodium concentration divided by the urine/plasma creatinine concentration × 100) is usually less than 1%. By contrast, in patients with tubular necrosis the

■ **TABLE 489–2 Causes of Acute Renal Failure**

Prerenal	Renal	Postrenal
Hypovolemia	Glomerulonephritis	Obstructive uropathy
Hemorrhage	Poststreptococcal	Ureteropelvic junction
Gastrointestinal losses	Lupus erythematosus	Ureterocele
Hypoproteinemia	Membranoproliferative	Urethral valves
Burns	Idiopathic rapidly progressive	Tumor
Renal or adrenal disease with salt wasting	Anaphylactoid purpura	Vesicoureteral reflux
Hypotension	Localized intravascular coagulation	Acquired
Septicemia	Renal vein thrombosis	Stones
Disseminated intravascular coagulation	Cortical necrosis	Blood clot
Hypothermia	Hemolytic-uremic syndrome	
Hemorrhage	Acute tubular necrosis	
Heart failure	Heavy metals	
Hypoxia	Chemicals	
Pneumonia	Drugs	
Aortic clamping	Hemoglobin, myoglobin	
Respiratory distress syndrome	Shock	
	Ischemia	
	Acute interstitial nephritis	
	Infection	
	Drugs	
	Tumors	
	Renal parenchymal infiltration	
	Uric acid nephropathy	
	Developmental abnormalities	
	Cystic disease	
	Hypoplasia-dysplasia	
	Hereditary nephritis	

urine is dilute (osmolality less than 350 mOsm/kg [mmol/L] H_2O), the sodium concentration usually exceeds 40 mEq/L (mmol/L), and the fractional excretion of sodium usually exceeds 1%.

If hypovolemia is detected, intravascular volume should be expanded by the intravenous administration of isotonic saline, 20 mL/kg, over 30 min. In the absence of blood loss or hypoproteinemia, colloid-containing solutions are not required for volume expansion. Following this infusion, the dehydrated patient will generally void within 2 hr. Failure to do so mandates a thorough re-evaluation of the patient. Catheterization of the bladder and determination of the central venous pressure may be helpful. If clinical and laboratory evaluations show that the patient is adequately hydrated, then aggressive diuretic therapy may be considered.

In patients with *impending renal failure* the value of diuretics in preventing development of anuria remains controversial. It seems clear that diuretics have no value in patients with established anuria. In some oliguric patients, furosemide or mannitol or both may increase the rate of urine production. These agents act by altering tubular function, but it should be recognized that the increase in urine flow does not represent an improvement in renal function nor will it affect the natural history of the disease that precipitated the renal failure. On the other hand, enhancement of urine output may be valuable in the management of hyperkalemia and fluid overload.

The pharmacodynamics of furosemide in renal failure are such that the urinary response (which is a function of the dose and blood level obtained) may be delayed for several hours. In the oliguric patient who lacks clinical and laboratory evidence of hypovolemia (and who may have already failed to respond to volume expansion), furosemide may be administered as a single intravenous dose of 2 mg/kg at the rate of 4 mg/per min (to avoid ototoxicity); if no response occurs, a second dose of 10 mg/kg may be given. Bumex may be given (0.1 mg/kg) as an alternative to Lasix. If no increase in urine production is obtained following this dose, then further furosemide therapy is contraindicated. A single intravenous dose of 0.5–1.0 g/kg of mannitol may be given over 30 min in addition to or in place of furosemide. Regardless of the response, no additional mannitol should be given, owing to the risk of toxicity. To increase renal cortical blood flow, dopamine (5 μg/kg/min) may be administered (in the absence of hypertension) in conjunction with diuretic therapy.

Fluid restriction is essential for the patient who fails to obtain adequate urine output following volume expansion or the administration of diuretics. The degree of fluid restriction depends upon the state of hydration. For the patient with oliguria or anuria having a relatively normal intravascular volume, fluid administration should be limited to 400 mL/m^2/24 hr (insensible losses) plus an amount of fluid equal to the urine output for that day. On the other hand, markedly hypervolemic patients may require almost total fluid restriction; omitting the replacement of insensible fluid losses and urine output will aid in diminishing the expanded intravascular volume. Access to the vascular space should be maintained; this is best obtained using an infusion pump at the slowest possible rate. In general, glucose-containing solutions (10–30%) without electrolytes are used as maintenance fluids. The composition of the fluid may be modified in accordance with the state of electrolyte balance. Except in the overhydrated patient, extrarenal (blood, gastrointestinal tract) fluid losses should be replaced, milliliter for milliliter, with appropriate fluids.

In acute renal failure, rapid development of *hyperkalemia* (serum level greater than 6 mEq/L [mmol/L]) may lead to cardiac arrhythmia and death. *The patient should receive no potassium-containing fluid, foods, or medications until adequate renal function is re-established.* The earliest electrocardiographic change seen in patients with developing hyperkalemia is the appearance of tall, peaked T waves. This may be followed by ST-segment depression, prolongation of the P-R and widening of the QRS intervals, ventricular fibrillation, and cardiac arrest.

In children with acute renal failure, procedures to deplete body potassium are initiated when the serum potassium rises to 5.5 mEq/L (mmol/L). To minimize the rate at which the serum potassium rises, all solutions given to the patient should contain high concentrations of glucose. Sodium polystyrene sulfonate resin (Kayexalate), 1 g/kg, should be given orally or by retention enema. This material exchanges sodium for potassium. For best results, the resin should be given orally, suspended in 2 mL/kg of 70% sorbitol. Sorbitol produces an osmotic diarrhea, which will increase fluid and electrolyte losses (the usual patient in renal failure is hypervolemic with increased total body sodium and potassium levels) as well as enhance the movement of the resin through the gastrointestinal tract. Because 70% sorbitol is locally irritating to the rectum, the concentration should be reduced to 20% and the volume increased to 10 mL/kg when it is given by enema. Resin therapy may be repeated every 2 hr, the frequency being limited primarily by the risk of sodium overload.

If the serum potassium rises above 7 mEq/L (mmol/L), emergency measures in addition to Kayexalate must be initiated. The following agents should be given sequentially:

1. Calcium gluconate 10% solution, 0.5 mL/kg intravenously, over 10 min. The heart rate must be closely monitored during the infusion; a fall in rate of 20 beats/min requires stopping the infusion until the pulse returns to the preinfusion rate.
2. Sodium bicarbonate 7.5% solution, 3 mEq/kg intravenously. Possible complications include volume expansion, hypertension, and tetany.
3. Glucose 50% solution, 1 mL/kg, with regular insulin, 1 unit/5 g of glucose, given intravenously over 1 hr. The patient should be monitored closely for hypoglycemia.

Calcium gluconate does not lower the serum potassium but counteracts the potassium-induced increase in myocardial irritability. Bicarbonate lowers serum potassium; the mechanism is not clearly defined. The effect of glucose and insulin is to shift potassium from the extracellular to the intracellular compartment. β-Adrenergic receptor agonists given by aerosol also acutely lower potassium levels. The duration of action of these emergency measures is just a few hours. Persistent hyperkalemia, therefore, especially in patients requiring the emergency measures, should be managed by dialysis.

Moderate *acidosis* is common in renal failure as a result of inadequate excretion of hydrogen ion and ammonia but it rarely requires treatment. Severe acidosis (arterial pH less than 7.15, serum bicarbonate less than 8 mEq/L [mmol/kg]) may increase myocardial irritability and requires treatment. Because of the risks involved in the rapid infusion of alkali, the acidosis should be corrected only partially by the intravenous route, generally giving enough bicarbonate to raise the arterial pH to 7.20 (which approximates a serum bicarbonate level of 12 mEq/L [mmol/L]). The correction formula is

$$\text{mEq NaHCO}_3 \text{ required} = 0.3 \times \text{weight (kg)} \times (12 - \text{serum bicarbonate [mEq/L]})$$

The remainder of the correction, which should be accomplished only after normalization of the serum calcium and phosphorous, may be made by the oral administration of sodium bicarbonate tablets or sodium citrate solution.

In addition to the risks involved in administration of intravenous bicarbonate that have been noted, correction of acidosis with intravenous bicarbonate may precipitate tetany (Chapter 56.9). In patients with renal failure, an inability to excrete phosphorus leads to hyperphosphatemia and a reciprocal hypocalcemia. Acidosis prevents the development of tetany by increasing the ionized fraction of the total calcium. Rapid correction of acidosis will reduce the ionized calcium concentration, resulting in tetany.

Hypocalcemia is treated by lowering the serum phosphorus. Unless tetany develops, calcium is not given intravenously, in order to avoid reaching a calcium × phosphorus product (mg/dL × mg/dL [mmol/L × mmol/L]) of 70 in the serum, the point at which calcium salts are deposited in tissue. To lower the serum phosphorus, a phosphate-binding calcium carbonate antacid is given by mouth, increasing fecal phosphate excretion; common agents include Titralac Liquid (3M Company, St. Paul, MN; starting dose 5–15 mL with meals and before bed) and Os-Cal 500 tablets (Marion Laboratories, Kansas City, MO) or regular strength TUMS (SmithKline Beecham, Pittsburgh, PA); starting dose 1–3 tablets with meals and before bed. The total daily dose should be gradually increased until the serum phosphorus level falls to normal.

Hyponatremia is commonly the result of administration of excessive amounts of hypotonic fluids to the oliguric-anuric patient. Correction may be accomplished by fluid restriction. Patients whose serum sodium levels acutely fall below 120 mEq/L (mmol/L) are at increased risk for developing cerebral edema and central nervous system hemorrhage. In the absence of dehydration, water restriction is essential. When the serum sodium falls below 120 mEq/L (mmol/L), it may be elevated to 125 mEq/L (mmol/L) by the intravenous infusion of hypertonic (3%) sodium chloride, using the following formula:

$$\text{mEq NaCl required} = 0.6 \times \text{weight (kg)} \times (125 - \text{serum sodium [mEq/L]})$$

The risks of administration of hypertonic saline include volume expansion, hypertension, and congestive heart failure; if these occur, they may be treated by dialysis.

Gastrointestinal bleeding may be prevented with calcium carbonate antacids, which also serve to lower the serum phosphorus. Alternatively, intravenous Tagamet (Smith, Kline & French, Philadelphia, PA) may be administered at a dose of 5–10 mg/kg/12 hr.

Hypertension may result from the primary disease process or expansion of the extracellular fluid volume or both. In patients with renal failure and hypertension, salt and water restriction is critical.

In children with severe acute symptomatic hypertension, a useful drug is diazoxide. This potent vasodilator must be given by rapid (less than 10 sec) intravenous injection at a dose of 1–3 mg/kg (maximum dose of 150 mg). A fall in blood pressure is usually seen within 10–20 min; if that following the first injection is insufficient, a second injection may be given 30 min later. More often, nifedipine may be given acutely (0.25–0.5 mg/kg PO). Sodium nitroprusside or labetalol as a continuous intravenous infusion is indicated for hypertensive crises. For less severe hypertension, control of extracellular volume expansion (salt and water restriction, furosemide) and use of beta-blockers (e.g., propranolol; 1–3 mg/kg/12 hr PO) and vasodilators (e.g., apresoline; 0.5–1.5 mg/kg/6 hr IV) are generally effective.

Seizures may be the result of the primary disease process (e.g., systemic lupus erythematosus), hyponatremia (water intoxication), hypocalcemia (tetany), hypertension, or the uremic state itself. If possible, therapy should be directed toward the precipitating cause. Diazepam seems to be the most effective agent in controlling seizures. It should be remembered that its metabolic products are excreted in the urine and may accumulate in patients with renal insufficiency.

Except in the presence of hemolysis (e.g., hemolytic-uremic syndrome, lupus) or bleeding, the *anemia* of acute renal failure is generally mild (hemoglobin 9–10 g/dL [90–100 g/L]), is primarily the result of volume expansion (hemodilution), and does not require transfusion. Blood loss from active bleeding should be replaced appropriately.

In patients with hemolytic anemia or prolonged renal failure, if hemoglobin levels fall below 7 g/dL (70 g/L) blood should be given. In the hypervolemic patient, blood transfusion carries the risk of further volume expansion, which may produce hypertension, congestive heart failure, and pulmonary edema. Slow (4–6 hr) transfusion with fresh (to minimize the amount of potassium administered) packed red blood cells (10 mL/kg) will diminish the risk of hypervolemia. In the presence of severe hypervolemia, anemia should be corrected during dialysis.

The diet of most previously healthy and well-nourished children who suddenly develop acute renal failure should be restricted initially to fats and carbohydrates (gum drops and jelly beans), given the likelihood that the acute renal failure will resolve or respond to therapy within a reasonably brief period of time. Restrictions of sodium, potassium, and water administration have already been mentioned. If renal failure persists beyond 3 days, then an expanded oral diet for renal failure or parenteral hyperalimentation with essential amino acids should be considered.

Indications for *dialysis* in acute renal failure may comprise various combinations of the following factors: acidosis, electrolyte abnormalities (especially hyperkalemia), central nervous system disturbances, hypertension, fluid overload, and congestive heart failure. It appears that the early initiation of dialysis has significantly improved the survival in children with acute renal failure.

Continuous *hemofiltration* is useful in patients with acute renal failure (especially those with unstable cardiopulmonary dynamics, severe coagulopathies, and unavailability of the peritoneal cavity due to surgery or trauma), fluid overload, and severe electrolyte or acid-base disturbances. Hemofiltration is an extracorporeal therapy in which fluid, electrolytes, and small- and medium-sized solutes are continuously removed from the blood over an extended period of time by a process called *convection* or *ultrafiltration* (Fig. 489–1). In convection, water is moved by pressure through a semipermeable membrane, bringing along other molecules (urea). The blood volume is reconstituted by the intravenous infusion of a substitution fluid having a desirable electrolyte composition similar to the blood.

The filter, of which there are several sizes, contains thousands of highly permeable hollow-fiber capillaries that produce a filtrate that is similar to the glomerular filtrate (protein-free, solute concentration similar to the plasma water). The merits of hemofiltration are summarized in Table 489–3.

Hemofiltration is performed by two basic configurations. In *continuous arteriovenous hemofiltration* (CAVH), the blood is pumped through the filter by the patient's heart; the driving force for filtration is the arterial blood pressure. The advantage is that, in the absence of a blood pump, filtration will decrease or stop if the blood pressure falls. Disadvantages include inadequate production of filtrate in patients with marginal cardiac function and the need for long-term arterial catheterization, which may lead to vascular damage. Vascular access is generally obtained by catheterization of the femoral artery and vein, brachial artery and jugular vein, or the umbilical vessels. In *continuous venovenous hemofiltration* (CVVH), blood is moved through the circuit (Fig. 489–1) by a pump. The rate of filtrate formation is dependent on the pressure generated by the pump speed and is independent of the blood pressure. Because filtration will continue despite profound hypotension, the patient's blood pressure must be continuously monitored. Because only venous access is required, double lumen catheters placed into the subclavian or femoral veins may be used.

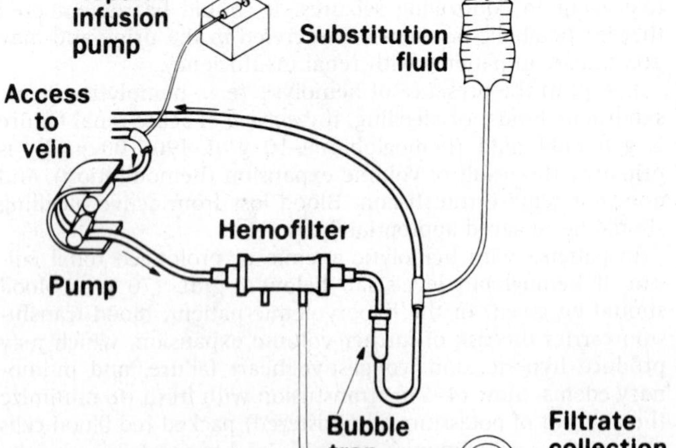

Figure 489–1. Schematic representation of continuous venovenous hemofiltration. (From Amicon, Inc; Diafilter Hemofilters. Beverly, MA, WR Grace, 1990. Used by permission.)

TABLE 489–3 Merits of Continuous Hemofiltration

Advantages	Disadvantages
Hemodynamic stability	Total body heparinization (bleeding)
Avoids rapid osmolar changes and diminished systemic vascular resistance of hemodialysis	Clotting of filter
	Inadequate removal of fluid or solutes in certain patients
Continuous therapy	Infection of access catheter or substitution fluid
Around the clock	
Stabilizes volume and composition of body fluids	Leaking from blood lines
Avoids rapid shifts in electrolyte levels	
Controlled fluid and solute removal	
Slow correction of fluid and electrolyte abnormalities	
Can replace ultrafiltrate with large amounts of hyperalimentation fluid	

In patients undergoing CAVH or CVVH who have inadequate solute removal, dialysate may be circulated through the filter on the ultrafiltrate side of the membrane. This technique is called *hemodiafiltration* and increases solute removal by adding diffusion to convection.

In certain patients with acute renal failure, careful medical management may minimize complications and delay the need for dialysis; other patients will eventually require dialysis for the uremic state itself. The life-threatening complications of uremia are hemorrhage, pericarditis, and central nervous system dysfunction; their precise causes are unknown. The risk of developing these complications correlates more closely with the level of BUN than with that of creatinine.

PROGNOSIS. The prognosis for recovery of renal function depends on the disorder that precipitated the renal failure. In general, recovery of function is likely following renal failure resulting from prerenal causes, the hemolytic-uremic syndrome, acute tubular necrosis, acute interstitial nephritis, or uric acid nephropathy. On the other hand, recovery of renal function is unusual when renal failure results from most types of rapidly progressive glomerulonephritis, bilateral renal vein thrombosis, or bilateral cortical necrosis.

Ellis EN, Pearson D, Robinson L, et al: Pump-assisted hemofiltration in infants with acute renal failure. Pediatr Nephrol 7:434, 1993.
Feld LG, Springate JE, Fildes RD: Acute renal failure. I. Pathophysiology and diagnosis. J Pediatr 109:401, 1986.
Finn WF: Diagnosis and management of acute tubular necrosis. Med Clin North Am 74:873, 1990.
Georgaki-Angelaki HN, Steed DB, Chantler C, et al: Renal function following acute renal failure in childhood: a long term follow-up study. Kidney Int 35:84, 1989.
Hays SR: Ischemic acute renal failure. Am J Med Sci 304:93, 1992.
Myers BD, Moran SM: Hemodynamically mediated acute renal failure. N Engl J Med 314:97, 1986.
Niaudet P, Haj-Ibrahim M, Gagnadoux M-F, et al: Outcome of children with acute renal failure. Kidney Int Suppl 17:148, 1985.
Ronco C: Continuous renal replacement therapies for the treatment of acute renal failure in intensive care patients. Clin Nephrol 40:187, 1993.
Steiner RW: Interpreting the fractional excretion of sodium. Am J Med 77:669, 1984.

489.2 Chronic Renal Failure

ETIOLOGY. The etiology of chronic renal failure in childhood correlates closely with the age of the patient at the time when the renal failure is first detected. Chronic renal failure in children under 5 yr of age is commonly the result of anatomic abnormalities (hypoplasia, dysplasia, obstruction, malformations), whereas after 5 yr of age acquired glomerular diseases (glomerulonephritis, hemolytic-uremic syndrome) or hereditary disorders (Alport syndrome, cystic disease) predominate.

PATHOGENESIS. Regardless of the cause of kidney damage, once a critical level of renal functional deterioration is reached, progression to end-stage renal failure is inevitable. The precise mechanisms resulting in progressive functional deterioration are unclear, but factors that may play important roles include ongoing immunologic injury; hemodynamically mediated hyperfiltration in surviving glomeruli; dietary protein and phosphorus intake; persistent proteinuria; and systemic hypertension.

Ongoing deposition of immune complexes or anti-glomerular basement membrane (GBM) antibodies in the glomerulus may result in persistent glomerular inflammation that leads to eventual scarring.

Hyperfiltration injury may be an important final common pathway of ultimate glomerular destruction, independent of the initiating mechanism of renal injury. Once nephrons are lost for any reason, the remaining nephrons undergo structural and functional hypertrophy mediated, at least in part, by an increase in glomerular blood flow. The increased blood flow in association with dilatation of the afferent arterioles and angiotensin II–induced constriction of the efferent arterioles increase the driving force for glomerular filtration in the surviving nephrons. This beneficial "hyperfiltration" in surviving glomeruli, which serves to preserve renal function, may also damage these glomeruli by mechanisms that are not understood. Potential mechanisms of damage include the direct effect of the elevated hydrostatic pressure on the integrity of the capillary wall, the resultant increase in the passage of proteins across the capillary wall, or both. Ultimately, this leads to changes in the mesangium and epithelial cells with the development of glomerular sclerosis. As sclerosis advances, the remaining nephrons suffer an increasing excretory burden, resulting in a vicious cycle of increasing glomerular blood flow and hyperfiltration. Angiotensin converting enzyme inhibition reduces hyperfiltration by inhibiting angiotensin II production, thereby dilating the efferent arteriole, and may slow the progression of renal failure.

Experimental models of chronic renal insufficiency have shown that a high-protein diet accelerates the development of renal failure, perhaps by means of afferent arteriolar dilatation and hyperperfusion injury. Conversely, a low-protein diet diminishes the rate of functional deterioration. Studies of humans confirm that in normal individuals the GFR correlates directly with protein intake and suggest that restriction of dietary protein may reduce the rate of functional deterioration in chronic renal insufficiency.

Some controversial studies in animal models suggest that dietary phosphorus restriction preserves renal function in chronic renal insufficiency. Whether this beneficial effect is due to the prevention of calcium-phosphate salt deposition in the blood vessels and tissues or to suppression of secretion of parathyroid hormone, a potential nephrotoxin, is unclear.

Persistent proteinuria or systemic hypertension from any cause may directly damage the glomerular capillary wall, leading to glomerular sclerosis and initiation of hyperfiltration injury.

As renal function begins to deteriorate, compensatory mechanisms develop in the remaining nephrons to maintain a normal internal environment. When the GFR falls below 20% of normal, however, a complex constellation of clinical, biochemical, and metabolic abnormalities develop that together constitute the uremic state. The pathophysiologic manifestations of the uremic state are listed in Table 489–4.

■ **TABLE 489–4 Pathophysiology of Chronic Renal Failure**

Manifestation	Mechanisms
Accumulation of nitrogenous waste products (azotemia)	Decline in glomerular filtration rate
Acidosis	Urinary bicarbonate wasting Decreased ammonia excretion Decreased acid excretion
Sodium wasting	Solute diuresis Tubular damage Functional tubular adaption for sodium excretion
Sodium retention	Nephrotic syndrome Congestive heart failure Anuria Excessive salt intake
Urinary concentrating defect	Nephron loss Solute diuresis Increased medullary blood flow
Hyperkalemia	Decline in glomerular filtration rate Acidosis Excessive potassium intake Hypoaldosteronism
Renal osteodystrophy	Decreased intestinal calcium absorption Impaired production of 1,25-dihydroxy-vitamin D by the kidneys Hypocalcemia and hyperphosphatemia Secondary hyperparathyroidism
Growth retardation	Protein-calorie deficiency Renal osteodystrophy Acidosis Anemia Unknown factors
Anemia	Decreased erythropoietin production Low grade hemolysis Bleeding Decreased erythrocyte survival Inadequate iron intake Inadequate folic acid intake Inhibitors of erythropoiesis
Bleeding tendency	Thrombocytopenia Defective platelet function
Infection	Defective granulocyte function Impaired cellular immune functions
Neurologic (fatigue, poor concentration, headache, drowsiness, loss of memory, slurred speech, muscle weakness and cramps, seizures, coma, peripheral neuropathy, asterixis)	Uremic factor(s) Aluminum toxicity
Gastrointestinal ulceration	Gastric acid hypersecretion
Hypertension	Sodium and water overload Excessive renin production
Hypertriglyceridemia	Diminished plasma lipoprotein lipase activity
Pericarditis and cardiomyopathy	Unknown
Glucose intolerance	Tissue insulin resistance

CLINICAL MANIFESTATIONS. In patients developing chronic renal failure from glomerular or hereditary diseases, the renal disease is usually detected because of clinical manifestations apparent prior to the onset of renal insufficiency. The development of renal failure may be insidious, however, in patients having anatomic abnormalities, and their presenting complaints may be nonspecific (headache, fatigue, lethargy, anorexia, vomiting, polydipsia, polyuria, growth failure). Physical examination occasionally may be surprisingly unrewarding, but most patients with chronic renal failure appear pale and weak, and have high blood pressure. Patients having anatomic abnormalities, in whom the renal failure has developed slowly over several years, may also have growth retardation and rickets.

TREATMENT. The management of the child having chronic renal failure requires close monitoring of the patient's clinical (physical examination and blood pressure) and laboratory status. Blood studies to be followed routinely include the hemoglobin (anemia), electrolytes (hyponatremia, hyperkalemia, acidosis),

BUN and creatinine (nitrogen accumulation and level of renal function), calcium and phosphorus levels, and alkaline phosphatase activity (hypocalcemia, hyperphosphatemia, osteodystrophy). Periodic examination of intact parathyroid hormone levels and roentgenographic studies of bone may be of value in detecting early evidence of osteodystrophy. Chest roentgenography and echocardiography may be helpful in assessing cardiac function. Nutritional status may be monitored by periodic evaluation of the serum albumin, zinc, transferrin, folic acid, and iron levels. Optimally, the patient should be managed in conjunction with a medical center capable of supplying medical, nursing, social service, and nutritional support as the patient progresses to end-stage renal failure.

Diet in Chronic Renal Failure. In children with renal insufficiency, the growth rate diminishes when the GFR falls below 50% of normal. The precise cause of growth failure is unknown; a major factor is inadequate caloric intake (less than 70% of recommended dietary allowance). The optimal caloric intake in renal insufficiency is unknown, but an attempt should be made to equal or exceed (in patients with growth failure) the recommended daily caloric allowance for age. Caloric intake can be enhanced by adding to the diet unrestricted amounts of carbohydrate (sugar, jam, honey, glucose polymers: Polycose, Ross Laboratories, Columbus, OH) and fat (medium-chain triglycerides oil: MCT Oil, Mead Johnson and Company, Evansville, IN) as tolerated by the patient. If oral caloric intake is inadequate, intermittent or overnight nasogastric or gastrostomy tube feedings can be initiated. Recombinant human growth hormone therapy combined with optimal dialysis improves linear growth.

When BUN exceeds approximately 80 mg/dL (30 mmol/L of urea), patients may develop nausea, vomiting, and anorexia. These symptoms result from the accumulation of nitrogenous waste products and can be relieved by restricting dietary protein intake. Because children in renal failure continue to require adequate protein intake for growth, protein is provided at the level of 1.5 g/kg/24 hr and should consist of proteins of high biologic value that are metabolized primarily to usable amino acids rather than to nitrogenous wastes. The proteins of highest such biologic value are those of eggs and milk, followed by meat, fish, and fowl. Because cow's milk contains a high concentration of phosphate, moderate restriction or the use of a formula containing a reduced amount of phosphate (Similac PM 60/40, Ross Laboratories, Columbus, OH), sometimes in conjunction with an oral phosphate binder (see subsequent section on renal osteodystrophy), may be indicated.

Owing to inadequate intake or dialysis losses, children with renal insufficiency may become deficient in water-soluble vitamins. These should be routinely supplied, using preparations such as Nephrocaps (Fleming, Fenton, MO). Zinc and iron supplements should be added only after deficiencies are confirmed. Supplementation with fat-soluble vitamins A, E, and K is not required.

Water and Electrolyte Management in Chronic Renal Failure. Until the development of end-stage renal failure requires the initiation of dialysis, water restriction is rarely necessary in children with renal insufficiency, because water needs are regulated by the thirst center in the brain.

Most children with renal insufficiency will maintain normal sodium balance with the sodium intake derived from an appropriate diet. Some patients whose renal insufficiency is a consequence of anatomic abnormalities may waste sodium in the urine and require dietary salt supplementation. On the other hand, patients with high blood pressure, edema, or congestive heart failure may require sodium restriction, sometimes in conjunction with aggressive furosemide therapy (1–4 mg/kg/24 hr).

In most children with renal insufficiency, potassium balance will be maintained until renal function deteriorates to the level at which dialysis is initiated. Hyperkalemia may develop in patients having only moderate renal insufficiency, however, as a result of excessive dietary potassium intake, the development of severe acidosis, or aldosterone deficiency (destruction of the juxtaglomerular apparatus). Hyperkalemia may be controlled by reducing dietary potassium intake and adding oral alkalinizing agents and/or Kayexalate (Winthrop Pharmaceuticals, New York, NY), an oral resin that (in 1 g/kg/dose) binds to and removes potassium from the intestine.

Acidosis in Chronic Renal Failure. Acidosis develops in almost all children with renal insufficiency and need not be treated unless the serum bicarbonate falls below 20 mEq/L (mmol/L). Either Bicitra (1 mL equals 1 mEq of base) or sodium bicarbonate tablets (325 and 650 mg; 325 mg equals 4 mEq of base) may be used to raise the serum bicarbonate above 20 mEq/L (mmol/L).

Renal Osteodystrophy. (See Chapter 483.5.) Renal osteodystrophy commonly develops in association with hyperphosphatemia, hypocalcemia, and elevation of parathyroid hormone levels and serum alkaline phosphatase activity. In general, serum phosphorus levels rise when the GFR falls below 30% of normal. Hyperphosphatemia may be controlled with a low phosphate formula (Similac PM 60/40) and by enhancing fecal excretion by using oral calcium carbonate, an antacid that coincidentally also binds phosphate in the intestinal tract. The usual dosage range is 1–4 tsp (Titralac, 3M Company, St. Paul, MN) or tablets (Os-Cal 500 Tablets, Marion Laboratories, Kansas City, MO; regular strength TUMS, SmithKline Beecham, Pittsburgh, PA) with each meal and before bed. Because aluminum may be absorbed from the gastrointestinal tract, especially in small children, and lead to aluminum poisoning (dementia, osteomalacia), aluminum antacids should be used rarely, if ever, with periodic monitoring of the serum aluminum level.

Hypocalcemia may result from hyperphosphatemia, inadequate dietary intake, and decreased intestinal calcium absorption caused by a deficiency in the active form (1,25-dihydroxycholecalciferol) of vitamin D. If the serum calcium remains low after correction of the serum phosphorus, then oral calcium supplements (Neo-Calglucon Syrup, Dorsey Pharmaceuticals, East Hanover, NJ; Os-Cal Tablets, Marion Laboratories, Kansas City, MO; regular strength TUMS, SmithKline Beecham, Pittsburgh, PA) at a dose of 500–2,000 mg/24 hr can be administered.

Vitamin D is converted to its active form (1,25-dihydroxycholecalciferol) by 1-hydroxylation in the kidney. With severe kidney destruction, insufficient conversion results in vitamin D deficiency. Vitamin D therapy is indicated (1) in patients having persistent hypocalcemia despite reduction of the serum phosphorus below 6 mg/dL (1.90 mmol/L) and the addition of oral calcium supplements; and (2) in patients with osteodystrophy, as indicated by elevated serum alkaline phosphatase and parathyroid hormone levels and roentgenographic evidence of rickets. Therapy may be initiated with one capsule (0.25 μg) per day of the active form of dihydroxy vitamin D (Rocaltrol, Roche Laboratories, Nutley, NJ) or 0.05–0.20 mg/24 hr of dihydrotachysterol solution (DHT Oral Solution, Roxane Laboratories, Columbus, OH), which is metabolized to its active form in the liver. The dose of vitamin D is progressively increased until the serum calcium level and alkaline phosphatase activity are normal, the intact parathyroid hormone is less than twice normal, and roentgenographic healing of the rickets is seen. The dose of vitamin D should then be reduced to the initial level.

Despite adequate nutritional intake and correction of osteodystrophy, electrolyte abnormalities, acidosis, and anemia, many children with chronic renal failure have marked growth retardation. Growth in these patients may be accelerated with recombinant human growth hormone therapy.

Anemia in Chronic Renal Failure. Anemia is common in chronic renal

■ **TABLE 489–5 Merits of Recombinant Human Erythropoietin Therapy**

Benefits	Potential Complications
Avoid blood transfusions	Iron deficiency
Reduced sensitization to histocompatibility antigens	Most require iron therapy
Reduced exposure to infectious diseases	Hypertension
Improved appetite	Seizures
Enhanced physical fitness	Decreased dialyzer clearance
Increased activity during day	Hyperkalemia
Improved sleep	Clotting of vascular access
Improved well-being	

failure and is primarily the result of inadequate erythropoietin production by the failing kidneys, but inadequate dietary intake of iron and folic acid should not be overlooked. In most patients, the hemoglobin level will stabilize in the range of 6–9 g/dL (60–90 g/L); transfusion therapy is not indicated, as this would further suppress erythropoietin production. If the hemoglobin falls below 6 g/dL (60 g/L), 10 mL/kg of packed red blood cells should be administered cautiously (the small volume reduces the risk of circulatory overload). The problem of anemia has been alleviated with the introduction of recombinant human erythropoietin therapy. Erythropoietin can be administered subcutaneously to predialysis and peritoneal dialysis patients, and intravenously to patients on hemodialysis. The goal is to maintain hemoglobin concentration within the range of 10–11 g/dL. The merits of erythropoietin therapy are summarized in Table 489–5.

Hypertension in Chronic Renal Failure. Hypertensive emergencies should be treated with oral nifedipine (0.25–0.5 mg/kg) or intravenous administration of diazoxide (Hyperstat, Schering Corporation, Kenilworth, NJ). The dose of diazoxide is 1–3 mg/kg, up to a maximum of 150 mg; it is given within 10 sec by manual injection. When severe hypertension is associated with circulatory overload, 2–4 mg/kg of furosemide may also be administered at the rate of 4 mg/min. Sodium nitroprusside should be used with great caution in renal insufficiency, owing to the possible accumulation of toxic thiocyanate.

The treatment of sustained hypertension may include a combination of salt restriction (2–3 g/24 hr), furosemide (1–4 mg/kg/24 hr), propranolol (Inderal, Ayerst Laboratories, New York, NY; 1–4 mg/kg/24 hr), hydralazine (Apresoline, CIBA Pharmaceutical Company, Summit, NJ; 1–5 mg/kg), and nifedipine (Pfizer Labs, New York, NY; 0.2–1.0 mg/kg/24 hr). Minoxidil and captopril should be used only in patients whose blood pressure is inadequately controlled with the above-mentioned measures and should be administered with the guidance of a pediatric nephrologist. Captopril may produce hyperkalemia.

Drug Dosage in Chronic Renal Failure. As many drugs are excreted by the kidneys, their administration to patients with renal insufficiency must be altered to maximize effectiveness and minimize the risk of toxicity (Chapter 63).

489.3 End-Stage Renal Failure

The incidence of end-stage renal disease in children is 20 per million population. In the treatment of end-stage renal failure in children, the ultimate goal is a successful kidney transplant (Chapter 490).

Dialysis is generally initiated when the patient's creatinine level approaches 10 mg/dL (900 μmol/L), depending on the patient's clinical status, the results of other laboratory studies, and the availability of a kidney donor. If histocompatibility or other studies reveal that no family donor is available, the patient is placed on a waiting list for a cadaver kidney in the hope that one will become available before dialysis is required. Children are usually hospitalized for initiation of dialysis. If, in preparation for transplantation, bilateral nephrectomies are required (for severe hypertension, vesicoureteral reflux, or chronic pyelonephritis), these may be done at this time.

Continuous ambulatory peritoneal dialysis (CAPD) is the standard technique for the majority of children requiring chronic dialysis. However, some require hemodialysis and the use of long-term indwelling subclavian vein catheters and arteriovenous fistulas created at the wrist.

In CAPD, dialysis across the peritoneal membrane removes excess body water through an osmotic gradient created by the glucose concentration in the dialysate; wastes are removed by diffusion from the peritoneal capillaries into the dialysate. CAPD is not as efficient as hemodialysis, but the fact that it is continuous around the clock (as contrasted with 12–18 hr/wk for hemodialysis) permits the maintenance of satisfactory levels of BUN and creatinine.

Access to the peritoneal cavity is achieved by inserting a soft Tenckhoff catheter through a midline infraumbilical incision; the catheter is brought out through the skin by means of a subcutaneous tunnel and connected to an extension tube that has a spike for insertion into the dialysis bag.

The parents (and patient, if more than 10–12 yr old) are then taught the techniques of spiking the bags of dialysate, allowing the dialysate to run in and dwell in the peritoneal cavity for the prescribed period of time, draining the dialysate back into the dialysate bag, and replacing the used bag of dialysate with a fresh one. Such "exchanges" are performed 3–5 times per day between arising and bedtime. Because the advantages of CAPD seem to far outweigh the risks (Table 489–6), CAPD is the optimal form of chronic dialysis for most children. Modifications of the procedure include mechanical devices for spiking the bags (with or without ultraviolet sterilization during the connection) and Y-shaped dual bag systems. The latter permits drainage of spent dialysate into an empty bag followed by instillation of fresh dialysate from the second bag, after which the patient "disconnects" from the bag system by covering the end of the catheter tubing with a cap containing a povidone iodine–impregnated sponge. These modifications have decreased the frequency of peritonitis and have improved patient acceptance of the technique.

An alternative to CAPD is *continuous cyclic peritoneal dialysis* (CCPD). This procedure reverses the schedule of CAPD by providing the exchanges at night rather than during the day. The exchanges are performed automatically during sleep by a simple cycler machine. This permits an uninterrupted day of activities, a reduction in the number of connections and disconnections (which should decrease the risk of peritonitis), and a reduction in the time required by the patient and parent to perform dialysis, reducing the risk of fatigue and burnout.

The success rate for kidney transplants in children over the

■ **TABLE 489–6 Value of Continuous Ambulatory Peritoneal Dialysis (CAPD)**

Advantages	Disadvantages
Rapid training	Catheter malfunction
Technical simplicity (no machines)	Infection
Greater mobility	Poor appetite
Minimal dietary restriction	Poor body image
Feel better than hemodialysis patients	Parental "burnout" (emotional exhaustion)
Steady state chemistries	Elevated serum lipids
Can live far from medical center	
Cheaper than hemodialysis	
Improved growth rate	
Fewer blood transfusions	

age of 5 yr approximates that for adults, and successful grafts have been performed in children as small as 5 kg. Ongoing research into better and less toxic means to prevent graft rejection should improve these statistics. Psychologic aspects of care of these children are discussed in Chapters 40.1 and 41.

Baldwin DS, Neugarten J: Treatment of hypertension in renal disease. Am J Kidney Dis 5:A57, 1985.
Balteau PR, Peluso FP, Coles GA, et al: Design and testing of the Baxter integrated disconnect systems (IDS). Perit Dial Int 11:131, 1991.
Bennett WM, Aronoff GR, Golper TA, et al (eds): Drug Prescribing in Acute Renal Failure, 2nd ed. Philadelphia, American College of Physicians, 1991.
Brocklebank J, Wolfe S: Dietary treatment of renal insufficiency. Arch Dis Child 69:704, 1993.
Chan JC, McEnery P, Chinchilli V, et al: A prospective, double blind study of growth failure in children with chronic renal insufficiency and the effectiveness of treatment with calcitriol versus dihydrotachysterol. J Pediatr 124:520, 1994.
Chesney RW, Avioli LV: Childhood renal osteodystrophy. *In*: Edelmann CM Jr (ed): Pediatric Kidney Disease, Vol I, 2nd ed. Boston, Little, Brown, 1992, p 647.
Eberst ME, Berkowitz LR: Hemostasis in renal disease: pathophysiology and management. Am J Med 96:168, 1994.
Fine LG: Preventing the progression of human renal disease: Have rational therapeutic principles emerged? Kidney Int 33:116, 1988.
Fine RN, Kohaut EC, Brown D, et al: Growth after recombinant human growth hormone treatment in children with chronic renal failure: report of a multicenter randomized double-blind placebo-controlled study. J Pediatr 124:374, 1994.
Frasier CL, Arieff AI: Nervous system complications in uremia. Ann Intern Med 109:143, 1988.
Geary DF, Haka-Ikse K: Neurodevelopmental progress of young children with chronic renal disease. Pediatrics 84:68, 1989.
Hanna JD, Chan JCM, Gill JR Jr: Hypertension and the kidney. J Pediatr 118:327, 1991.
Hellerstein S, Holliday MA, Grupe WE, et al: Nutritional management of children with chronic renal failure. Pediatr Nephrol 1:195, 1987.
Klahr S, Schreiner G, Ichikawa I: The progression of renal disease. N Engl J Med 318:1657, 1988.
Morrison G, Murray TG: Electrolyte, acid-base, and fluid homeostasis in chronic renal failure. Med Clin North Am 65:429, 1981.
Nissenson AR: Recombinant human erythropoietin and renal anemia: molecular biology, clinical efficacy, and nervous systems effects. Ann Intern Med 114:402, 1991.
Polinsky MS, Kaiser BA, Stover JB, et al: Neurologic development of children with severe chronic renal failure from infancy. Pediatr Nephrol 1:157, 1987.
Port FK, Held PJ, Nolph KD, et al: Risk of peritonitis and technique failure by CAPD connection technique: a national study. Kidney Int 42:967, 1992.
Querfeld U: Disturbances of lipid metabolism in children with chronic renal failure. Pediatr Nephrol 7:749, 1993.
Ritz E, Matthias S, Seidel A, et al: Disturbed calcium metabolism in renal failure—pathogenesis and therapeutic strategies. Kidney Int 42 (Suppl 38):S37, 1992.
Suki WN: Pericarditis. Kidney Int 33:S10, 1988.
Vanholder R, Ringoir S: Infectious morbidity and defects of phagocytic function in end-stage renal disease: a review. J Am Soc Nephrol 3:1541, 1993.

CHAPTER 490
Renal Transplantation

Rodrigo E. Urizar

Chronic dialysis therapy for end-stage renal disease (ESRD) is frequently associated with failure to thrive, social maladaptation, lack of sexual maturation, and chronic encephalopathy (in the very young) and explains the reluctance to dialyze children extensively unless more acceptable alternatives are unavailable. Optimal treatment for children with ESRD is early renal transplantation (RT) from a living related donor (LRD-RT). Although less successful than LRD-RT, cadaveric (CAD) grafts are also used in children.

EPIDEMIOLOGY. The United States Renal Data System (USRDS) documents 20 new ESRD cases per million children each year, peaking at about 11–15 yr of age. Below 1 yr of age the incidence is 0.2 patient/million/year. An estimated 43–45% (up to 58% in 1991) of 2,000 pediatric renal transplants performed in this country used kidneys donated by parents (37%) and, to a lesser extent, by siblings or other relatives (6%). Preemptive renal transplant (RT) (carried out without previous dialysis) constitutes 22% of LRD engraftings. Indications for RT are noted in Table 490–1.

■ TABLE 490–1 Criteria for Performing Living Related Donor or Cadaveric Renal Transplantation in Pediatric Patients

Renal failure, chronic or end-stage renal disease of any etiology
Age, weight dependent to accommodate adult kidney
Good nutritional condition
Absence of
Active infection
Severe mental retardation
Obstructed urinary tract (ileal loops, colonic diversions and bladder augmentation procedures are helpful in many instances)
Gastrointestinal, liver, pancreas, or cardiovascular disease
Serious psychosocial or behavioral problems, and noncompliance with medication and dietary regimen
Sensitization in recipient
Massive obesity

From Mauer SM, Nevins TE, Ascher N: Renal transplantation in children. In: Edelman CM Jr (ed): Pediatric Kidney Disease. Boston, Little Brown, 1992, pp 941–981.

A well-functioning graft (LRD or CAD) may fully rehabilitate the patient. Nonetheless, the expectant graft recipient and/or relatives must understand that renal transplantation is not a permanent cure for ESRD. Furthermore, a poorly functioning transplanted kidney (uncontrollable progressive rejection) is associated with serious morbidity, mortality, and prospective return to, or initiation of, chronic dialysis. The transiency of renal grafts has committed transplant programs to multiple engraftments per patient, a goal seriously hampered by the limited availability of CAD kidneys. The latter may reflect reticence of the lay and professional community (general public, nurses, physicians) toward organ donation.

Causes of ESRD vary with the patient's age and include congenital renal diseases (53%), glomerulonephritides (20%), focal segmental glomerular sclerosis (12%), metabolic diseases (10%), and miscellaneous (5%) (Tables 490–2 and 490–3). Although the glomerulopathies constitute a significant proportion of this population (particularly in 13–17 yr olds), congenital and obstructive processes predominate in the very young (<5 yr).

TREATMENT. Children weighing <15–20 kg have a transperitoneal graft via a midline incision; in those weighing >20 kg, the kidney is placed retroperitoneally in the right iliac fossa. Renal vessels are anastomosed to the external iliac artery and vein, the ureter is reimplanted in the bladder (ureteroneocystostomy), and the lower pole is kept free of interposing intestine. The extraperitoneal kidney facilitates access for future percutaneous biopsies. The donor and recipient clinical laboratory evaluations prior to transplantation are summarized in Table 490–4. Very young age of the recipient may be an obstacle to renal transplantation. Some institutions accept patients 5–6 mo old weighing 5–6 kg to be engrafted with adult

■ TABLE 490–2 Most Frequent Hereditary-Metabolic Diseases of Childhood That Lead to End-Stage Renal Disease

Nephronophthisis—medullary cystic disease
Congenital nephrotic syndrome
Alport syndrome
Nephropathic and juvenile cystinosis
Primary oxalosis with oxaluria
Polycystic kidney disease (both infantile and adult varieties)
Nail-patella syndrome

■ **TABLE 490–3 Individual Glomerulopathies of Childhood That May Progress to Chronic/End-Stage Renal Disease**

Entity	Clinical Manifestation
Idiopathic rapidly progressive GN (crescentic GN, mediated by immune complexes)	Acute progressive renal failure
IgA nephropathies (Berger disease, anaphylactoid or Henoch-Schönlein purpura)	Chronic active GN, nephrotic syndrome, occasionally RPGN
Membranoproliferative glomerulonephritis (idiopathic; types I, II, and III)	Acute and chronic nephritic syndrome, occasionally RPGN
Focal segmental glomerulosclerosis	Nephrotic syndrome, progressive renal failure, acute/chronic active progressive GN, occasionally RPGN
Systemic lupus GN (WHO types 3 & 4)	
Microangiopathic syndromes (hemolytic, uremic, and thrombotic thrombocytopenic purpura syndromes)	Acute, chronic, and occasionally RPGN
Vasculitis (polyarteritis nodosa and Wegener)	Same
Anti-basement membrane antibody diseases (Goodpasture syndrome and idiopathic RPGN)	Acute, progressive renal failure, and RPGN with or without pulmonary renal syndrome

GN, Glomerulonephritis; RPGN, rapidly progressive glomerulonephritis.

kidneys. Small patients transplanted with small kidneys from infant donors do not do as well as expected. Kidney grafts from LRD have significantly better survival than CAD-RT. Approximately 90% of kidneys from LRD function adequately by 1 yr and 80% by the 3rd yr; the figures for CAD-RT are 72% and 65%, respectively. Generally CAD-RT in children is less favorable than in adults. In transplanted patients who are <1 yr of age, the 2 yr graft survival is less than that of older children. Overall, by 39 mo post-transplantation 80% of LRD and 58% of CAD-RT were functional. Approximately 50% of graft failure has been due to rejection (RR). In 26% RR was acute, whereas in 7% recurrence of the original renal disease induced the transplant failure. Although almost any glomerulopathy may redevelop in the graft, focal segmental glomerulosclerosis is observed most frequently (Table 490–5). Thrombosis-related kidney failure occurs in 15% of cases. In patients with LRD-RT, thrombotic episodes developed in very young recipients, presumably due to hemodynamic and/or technical problems. Conversely, graft thrombosis in CAD-RT is unaffected by the recipient age but is proportional to the donor age. In older children, renal failure is frequently due to acute tubular necrosis.

■ **TABLE 490–4 Clinical and Laboratory Evaluation of Prospective Living Related Kidney Donor and Recipient**

Recipient
- Complete history and physical examination—updated immunizations, including pneumococcal and hepatitis B
- Transplant orientation session: patient (if old enough), parents, prospective donors, transplant surgeon or representative, nephrologist or representative, social worker
- Laboratory data
  - Blood group (ABO)
  - Tissue typing (HLA-A, -B, -C, -D/DR), MLC
  - Hepatitis, cytomegalovirus, varicella, Ebstein-Barr virus panel
  - CBC, complement (C3, C4), ANA, quantitative Ig
  - Serum creatinine, electrolytes, cholesterol, liver function tests, coagulation profile, blood sugar
  - Urinalysis, urine and throat cultures
  - Chest x-ray (two-position), bone age films (if not previously available)
  - Neurologic consult and EEG and CT scan of brain (for infants)
  - Dental evaluation
  - Cultures: exit site of all catheters and peritoneal fluid in CAPD patients
  - Complete urologic evaluation for those with obstructive or congenital urinary tract problems
  - 24-hr protein excretion

Donor
- Complete history and physical examination
- Chest x-rays
- Electrocardiogram
- Renal ultrasound (IVP if necessary)
- Laboratory
  - CBC, ESR, ABO blood groups, HLA and MLC testing
  - Coagulation profile
  - Serum creatinine and electrolytes, liver function tests, blood sugar
  - Urinalysis, urine culture, 24-hr urine protein and creatinine excretion
  - Hepatitis, cytomegalovirus, herpes, Ebstein-Barr virus antibody titers
  - Renal angiogram

EEG, electroencephalogram; CT, computed tomography; CAPD, continuous ambulatory peritoneal dialysis; IVP, intravenous pyelogram.

From Mauer SM, Nevins TE, Ascher N: Renal transplantation in children. In: *Edelman CM Jr (ed): Pediatric Kidney Disease. Boston, Little Brown, 1992, pp 941–981.*

HISTOCOMPATIBILITY. The major histocompatibility complex (MHC) genes, present on the short arm of chromosome 6, encode the human leucocyte antigens (HLA) (Fig. 490–1). These are composed of class I proteins (tissue transplantation antigens) and cell mediated immunotoxicity; class II proteins that control induction of immune response; and class III pro-

■ **TABLE 490–5 Renal Diseases That May Recur in the Transplanted Pediatric Patient***

Condition	Results	Graft Damage
FSGS with nephrotic syndrome	Massive proteinuria with nephrosis (20%–30%)	About 50% loss within 1 yr
MPGN	Mostly main dense deposit disease in glomeruli	Possibly 50% loss
Goodpasture syndrome and other RPGN	Rare in children but produce nephritic/nephrotic syndrome	High losses; exact number unknown because of rarity in children
Wegener granulomatosis		
IgA nephropathies	Development of IgA	Graft is seldom lost
HSP and IgA GN	Glomerular deposits	
HUS/TTP	More severe microangiopathy in graft; do not use cyclcosporine A	Occurs frequently but exact number unknown
Hyperoxalosis/oxaluria	Heavy deposits of Ca oxalate; kidney tissue destruction	High losses
Cystinosis	Cystine deposits in macrophages but not in kidney tissue	Good survival
De novo glomerulonephritis	Membranoproliferative	Associated with graft loss
	Type I pattern—chronic rejection	
Membranous glomerulopathy	Associated with chronic rejection reaction	Graft loss
Alport syndrome	Lack of goodpasture; antigen may induce production of antiglomerular basement membrane antibodies by graft	Graft may be lost (lungs are spared)

FSGS, Focal segmental glomerular sclerosis; MPGN, membranoproliferative (or mesangiocapillary) glomerulonephritis; RPGN, crescentic, necrotizing rapidly progressive glomerulonephritis; HUS/TTP, hemolytic uremic thrombotic thrombocytopenic purpura syndromes (microangiopathies).

HSP, Henoch-Schönlein purpura.

From Mauer SM, Nevins TE, Ascher N: Renal transplantation in children. In: *Edelman CM Jr (ed): Pediatric Kidney Disease. Boston, Little Brown, 1992, pp 941–981.*

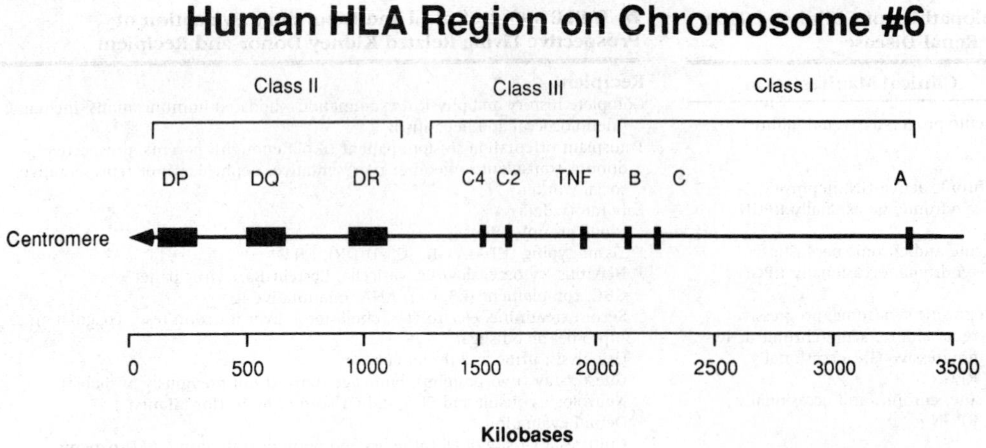

Figure 490–1. Organization of HLA region of chromosome 6. The loci for HLA-A, -B, and -C are found in the class I region. The loci encoding HLA-DR, -DQ, and -DP are found in the class II region, centromeric to class I. In between class I and II are the so-called class III genes, which encode some of the complement proteins as well as some cytokines. (From Grimm PC, Laufer J, Ettenger RB: The immunobiology of renal transplantation. *In:* Edelman CM Jr [ed]: Pediatric Kidney Disease. Boston, Little Brown, 1992, pp 941–981.)

teins, which include tumor necrosis factor (TNF) and complement components (C2 and C4). Each chromosome 6 contains all three classes of proteins: HLA-A, -B, and -C for class I; HLA-DP, -DQ, and -DR for class II; and C2, C4, and TNF for class III. Multiple alleles (polymorphism) exist for each protein: 23(A), 47(B), 8(C), 19(D), 16(DR), 3(DQ), and 6(DP). The A, B, and DR proteins are regarded as the most important in clinical transplantation. The HLA genes concentrated within a defined area of chromosome 6 are inherited as a packet or haplotype. Each individual inherits a haplotype of HLA genes from each parent concurrently, and both contribute to the offspring's HLA profile. The parent donor and child recipient share 50% of the haplotypes; typically a child will have one representative antigen from class I, II, and III loci of each parent, while among siblings all, some, or no haplotypes may be shared (2 haplotype, 1 haplotype, or 0 haplotype match). By definition, in the absence of recombination a child is a 1 haplotype match to each parent and transmission (inheritance) of haplotypes occurs in a codominant Mendelian fashion (Fig. 490–2). In the genetically related donor/recipient pair the probability of a good HLA match increases, while graft loss decreases.

Cellular expression of class I and II antigens, restricted to B and T lymphocytic cells and macrophages, multiplies with inflammation and by the action of lymphokines (interleukins 2, 4, and 5) secreted by T cells. CD4 (T-helper) and CD8 (T-suppressor) cell surface markers have high affinity for MHC (HLA) I (histocompatibility) antigens. When attached to cells displaying class I antigen, they transmit signals to synthesize cytokines or to lyse cells. In the acute and chronic rejection reaction, both cellular and humoral mechanisms damage the graft, whereas antibodies, preformed or induced by T-helper cells, mediate accelerated (hyperacute) forms of the rejection reaction (Fig. 490–3). In the cellular variety the graft is infiltrated by lymphocytes—T-helper and suppressor cells, B lymphocytes, macrophages, plasma cells, and monocytes—resulting in hemorrhage, edema, accumulation of polymorphonuclear leukocytes, activated platelets, and clotting.

Clinically, RR manifests swelling and tenderness of the graft, fever, oliguria, hypertension, and progressive elevation of serum creatinine. Renal ultrasound may reveal an enlarged graft with echogenic cortex, while a renal scan demonstrates decreased blood flow. Graft biopsy will show signs of rejection with relatively intact glomeruli, mild ultrastructural changes, and negative glomerular immunofluorescence. Differentiation between RR, acute tubular necrosis, cyclosporine-A toxicity, and de novo occurrence of the original renal disease in the graft requires a kidney biopsy. *Hyperacute* or *accelerated rejections* are seldom observed because pretransplant crossmatching

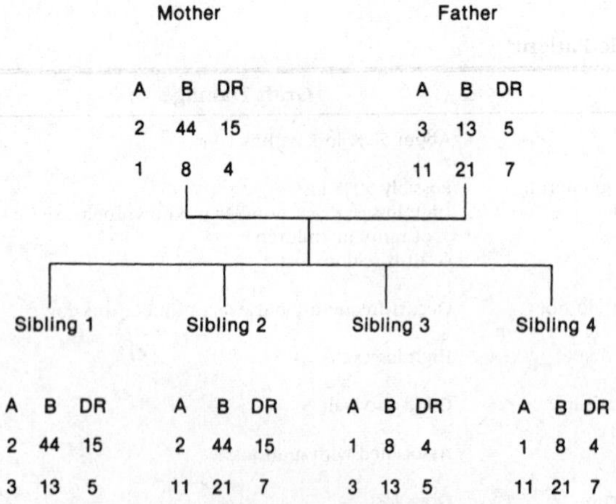

Figure 490–2. Inheritance of haplotypes and HLA profile in four theoretical siblings. Sibling 1 is a 1 haplotype match to siblings 2 and 3, and a 0 haplotype match to sibling 4. (From Terasaki PI, Park MS, Danovitch GM: Histocompatibility testing, crossmatching and allocation of cadaveric kidney transplants. *In:* Danovitch GM [ed]: Handbook of Kidney Transplantation. Boston, Little Brown, 1992, pp 43–66.)

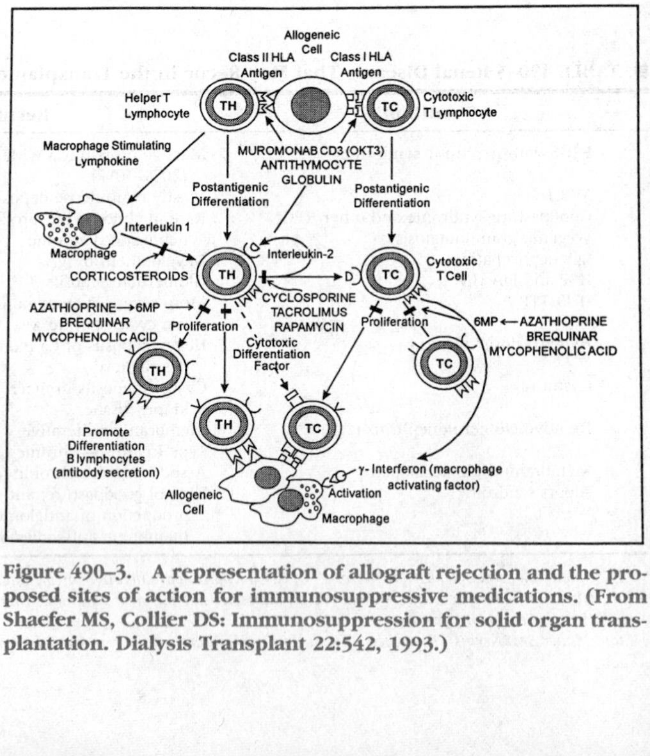

Figure 490–3. A representation of allograft rejection and the proposed sites of action for immunosuppressive medications. (From Shaefer MS, Collier DS: Immunosuppression for solid organ transplantation. Dialysis Transplant 22:542, 1993.)

■ TABLE 490–6 Immunosuppressive Agents

Drug	Dose	Mechanisms	Side Effect(s)
Azathioprine (Imuran)	1–3 mg/kg/day	Specific for T lymphocytes; decreases IgG & IgM antibodies; blocks primary & secondary immune response, both cell and humoral	Bone marrow suppression; hepatotoxicity; pancreatitis
Prednisone and methyl prednisolone	5–10 mg/kg/day 10–1,000 mg IV dose	Antilymphocyte action; decrease IL1; decrease inflammation; decrease fungicidal action; decrease new cell formation; decrease monocyte migration	Psychological disturbances; NaCl retention; volume expansion weight gain (increased appetite); arterial hypertension; myopathy; infections; growth retardation
Cyclosporine (Sandimmune)	10 mg/kg/dose 4–6 mg/kg/day (maintenance)	Fungal undecapeptide inhibits helper T cell, lesser effect on T-suppressors; decreases IL-2	Nephrotoxicity, hepatotoxicity, hypertension, CNS toxicity (tremor, confusion, seizures, coma), IV reaction due to carrier, gingival hyperplasia, hypertrichosis
Tacrolimus (FK506)	0.05–0.1 mg/kg/day continuous IV infusion 0.15–0.3 mg/kg/day BID, PO	As per cyclosporine; used as primary agent or rescue therapy if cyclosporine fails	As per cyclosporine; possible steroid sparing and fewer side effects compared with cyclosporine
Antithymocyte Ig (ATGAM) and Antilymphoblast (MALG)	10–30 mg/kg/day 10–30 mg/kg/day	Horse IgG polyclonal antibody to T lymphocytes Horse IgG antibody to T lymphocytes; same as above	Common to both: chills and fever (15–20%), erythema, pruritus, thrombocytopenia, anaphylactoid reaction, leukopenia Opportunistic infections (delayed side effect common to these drugs)
OKT3 (Orthochlone, Muromonab)	2.5–5.0 mg/day	IgG2a binds to CD3 of T cells; removed by RES	Fever (78%), tachycardia (68%), chills (60%), headaches (40%), hypertension, nausea, vomiting, diarrhea, hypotension, and wheezing

RES, Reticuloendothelial system.
From Shaefer MS, Collier DS: Immunosuppression for solid organ transplantation. Dialysis Transplant 22:542, 1993.

(MLC) detects the presence of pre-existing anti-HLA antibodies. In this condition the kidney becomes dark and soft as it is revascularized. Anti-HLA antibodies bind to endothelium, while renal intravascular coagulation destroys glomeruli and peritubular capillaries. Chronic rejection damages mainly arteries and arterioles, which become thickened with obstructed lumens, while glomeruli undergo ischemic wrinkling of the basement membrane. Mononuclear cells infiltrate the interstitium, and arteriolar walls may display immunoglobulin deposits.

Histocompatibility testing is considered of paramount importance in prolonging the survival of LRD and CAD RT. Having HLA-A, -B, -C, and -D/DR identical with an MLC nonstimulatory sibling donor produces the best graft survival results. The second best is the sibling or parent donor who has one haplotype match.

PRINCIPLES OF IMMUNOSUPPRESSION AND THERAPY OF REJECTION REACTION. Immune system stimulation by foreign protein (renal graft) results in the activation of cell-mediated and humoral-mediated immune inflammation with cell destruction, or RR (Fig. 490–3). (See also Chapter 132.2.) To subdue or control this process, which otherwise results in acute graft loss, the use of immunosuppressive medications is mandatory. The current drugs, doses, mechanism(s) of action, and side effects are listed in Table 490–6 and Figure 490–3. Sequential immunosuppression with azathioprine, cyclosporine, and low dose corticosteroids is the most frequently used protocol. Fifty per cent of pediatric patients with LRD and 65% of those receiving CAD kidneys develop RR. One or more acute episodes occur in all transplants; 62% of first episodes are successfully treated, whereas only 30% can be reversed when four or more crises have occurred. Chronic rejection is relentless and unresponsive to therapy. In addition, concurrent rejection with complications, particularly infection, places patients at higher risk of graft loss or death. If complications occur due to immunosuppression, one should treat the complication and abandon the graft. The use of antithymocyte globulin (ATGAM), prophylactically or in the immediate postoperative period, improves the short-term graft outcome in 50% of pediatric patients. Importantly, 6 mo after LRD or CAD transplant, these children have lower mean serum creatinine levels, the interval from transplant to first RR is lengthened, and the 1 yr graft survival is improved.

GROWTH AND RENAL TRANSPLANTATION. Stunted linear growth and, less often, overt malnutrition are complications of chronic renal failure and of the ESRD-dialysis patient (Chapter 489). Although supportive care improves stamina and a sense of well-being develops, only a successful transplant adequately corrects these abnormalities. Most children awaiting transplantation show retarded growth of −2.8 standard deviations (SD) when 5 yr of age or less, while in those with more than one RT stunting reaches −3.2 SD. Transplant-related accelerated growth, lasting 6–12 mo, is observed in younger children; in adolescents, a growth spurt has not been documented. Weight gain, on the other hand, yields mean values similar to normal adolescents for 2–3 yr. Daily corticosteroid treatment retards growth, even at relatively small doses. Every-other-day prednisone use is unpopular in many transplant centers, allegedly because it may precipitate graft rejection. Nevertheless, the validity and success of the every-other-day corticosteroid regimen has been amply demonstrated in children. Daily steroids may be used for 6 mo in decreasing doses, then switched to every other day and tapered to 0.5–0.2 mg/kg given as a single dose every other day.

Judicious use of recombinant human growth hormone before and after transplantation (Nuprin, now approved by the FDA for use in children) improves linear growth significantly, although there are contradictory data indicating that graft function may decrease.

■ TABLE 490–7 Post-Transplantation Complications in Pediatric Patients

Acute tubular necrosis
Rejection reaction
Technical: vascular, urologic
Recurrence of original renal disease
Drug toxicity (immunosuppressives, antibiotics)
Infection (particularly viral, systemic); wound or urinary tract infection
Bleeding
Pancreatitis
Lymphocele
Urinoma
Bowel obstruction

From Mauer SM, Nevins TE, Ascher N: Renal transplantation in children. In: Edelman CM Jr (ed): Pediatric Kidney Disease. Boston, Little Brown, 1992, pp 941–981.

■ TABLE 490–8 Types of Cytomegalovirus Infection in the Pediatric Renal Transplant Recipient

Type of Infection	Type of Patient	Symptomatic	Prevention
Primary	Seronegative with seropositive kidney, transfusion of leucocytes, blood products transfusion	60%	Avoidance of CMV infection or use active immunization (live attenuated vaccine: Towne strain; not very effective)
Reactivation	Seropositive prior to transplantation	<20%	High titer human hyperimmune anti-CMV globulin (Cytogam)
Superinfection	Seropositive patient transplanted with CMV + kidney	40%	Human IgG concentrates (CMV nonspecific Gamma-gard or Polygam)

CMV, Cytomegalovirus.
From Snydman DR: Prevention of cytomegalovirus-associated diseases with immunoglobulin. Transplant Proc 23:131, 1991.

COMPLICATIONS. Other complications that develop after transplantation are summarized in Table 490–7. Of these, infection is the most common cause of death during the first year after transplantation. Cytomegalovirus (CMV) infection is common. CMV antibody titers must be routinely screened in the donor and recipient. CMV infection may be primary, transmitted by the transplant itself or by blood transfusions, or reactivated by immunosuppression in a seropositive patient (Table 490–8). The latter disease becomes apparent 1–3 mo after transplantation. About 90% may be self-limited and asymptomatic, and 5–10% lead to death; direct tissue damage by CMV may also result in graft loss. In addition, CMV disease usually triggers a rejection reaction. This poses a serious therapeutic dilemma: Although immunosuppression may reactivate the disease, it is indispensable for graft retention. Low dose immunosuppressive agents with the use of antiviral drugs (gancyclovir and anti-CMV immunoglobulin intravenously) control the infection, while kidney biopsy helps monitor the rejection. Immunosuppression must be discontinued in systemic (lung, brain, liver) CMV infection. If rejection is unresponsive, the kidney should be abandoned. Concomitant infection with other viruses (varicella zoster, Epstein-Barr, herpes simplex, hepatitis) requires thorough investigation and treatment. *Pneumocystis carinii* has all but disappeared due to prophylactic use of trimethoprim-sulfamethoxazole, which also prevents bacterial urinary tract infections.

The mortality of transplanted children is 4–4.5%; in 40–45% of these mortality is due to infection. The 2 yr patient survivals for LRD and CAD-RT are 95% and 92%, respectively. Renal diseases that recur in the transplanted kidney are listed in Table 490–5. Pediatric renal transplant patients may develop tumors, mainly lymphomas, sarcomas, and carcinomas, with significant death rates years after the transplant.

Almond PS, Matas A, Gillingham K, et al: Risk factors for chronic rejection in renal allograft recipients. Transplantation 55:752, 1993.
Bartosh SM, Aronson AJ, Swanson-Prewitt EE, et al: OKT3 induction in pediatric renal transplantation. Pediatr Nephrol 7:45, 1993.
Briscoe DM, Kim MS, Lillehei C, et al: Outcome of renal transplantation in children less than 2 years of age. Kidney Int 42:657, 1992.
Cochat P, Castelo F, Glastre C, et al: Outcome of cadaver kidney transplantation in small children. Acta Paediatr 83:78, 1994.
Cole BR: The psychosocial implications of preemptive transplantation. Pediatr Nephrol 5:158, 1991.
Ettenger RB, Rosenthal JT, Marik J, et al: Cadaver renal transplantation in children. Results with long-term cyclosporine immunosuppression. Transplantation 4:329, 1990.
Ettenger RB, Rosenthal JT, Marik JL, et al: Improved cadaveric renal transplant outcome in children. Pediatr Nephrol 5:137, 1991.
Ferraresso M, Kahan BD: New immunosuppressive agents for pediatric transplantation. Pediat Nephrol 7:567, 1993.
Fine RN, Yadin O, Nelson PA, et al: Recombinant growth hormone treatment of children following renal transplantation. Pediatr Nephrol 5:147, 1991.
First MR: Long-term complications after transplantation. Am J Kidney Dis 22:477, 1993.
Gagnadoux MF, Niaudet P, Broyer M: Non-immunologic risk factors in pediatric renal transplantation. Pediatr Nephrol 7:89, 1993.
Gruber SA, Chavers B, Skjel KL, et al: De novo cancer after pediatric kidney transplantation. Transpl Proc 23:1373, 1991.
Harmon WE: Opportunistic infections in children following renal transplantation. Pediatr Nephrol 5:118, 1991.
Harmon WE, Stablein D, Alexander SR, et al: Graft thrombosis in pediatric renal transplant recipients. Transplantation 51:406, 1991.
Harmon WE, Alexander SR, Tejani A, et al: The effect of donor age on graft survival in pediatric cadaver renal transplant recipients. A report of the North American Pediatric Renal Transplant Cooperative Study. Transplantation 54:232, 1992.
Iragorri S, Pillay D, Scrine M, et al: Prospective cytomegalovirus surveillance in pediatric renal transplant patients. Pediatr Nephrol 7:55, 1993.
Lewis R, Podbielski J, Sprayberry S, et al: Stability of renal allograft glomerular filtration rate associated with long-term use of cyclosporine-A. Transplantation 55:1014, 1993.
McEnery PT, Stablein DM, Arbus G, et al: Renal transplantation in children. A report of the North American Pediatric Renal Transplant Cooperative Study. N Engl J Med 326:1727, 1992.
McEnery PT, Alexander SR, Sullivan K, et al: Renal transplantation in children and adolescents: the 1992 annual report of the North American Pediatric Renal Transplant Cooperative Study. Pediatr Nephrol 7:711, 1993.
Morel P, Almond PS, Matas AJ, et al: Long-term quality of life after kidney transplantation in childhood. Transplantation 52:47, 1991.
Norman DJ, Leone MR: The role of OKT3 in clinical transplantation. Pediatr Nephrol 5:130, 1991.
Suthanthiran M, Strom T: Renal transplantation. N Engl J Med 331:365, 1994.
Yadim O, Grimm P, Ettenger RB: Renal transplantation in children. Pediatr Ann 20:657, 1991.

Part XXIV

Urologic Disorders in Infants and Children

Ricardo Gonzalez

Chapter 491

Congenital Anomalies and Dysgenesis of the Kidneys

Almost all premature and full-term infants void within the first 24 hr after birth. If an infant has not voided by the end of the 1st day of life, a search should be initiated for underlying anatomic abnormalities.

The urine of the healthy neonate may have a pH of 5–7 and an osmolality of 60–600 mOsm/kg (mmol/kg) H_2O. It usually has many epithelial cells and may contain an occasional red blood cell. White blood cells should be absent, and the culture should be sterile. Trace amounts of glucose and protein may be found on dipstick testing.

RENAL AGENESIS (APLASIA). *Bilateral agenesis* is not compatible with extrauterine life. The stillborn fetus has the stigmata of severe prenatal renal failure and oligohydramnios; the facies is characteristic (Fig. 491–1). The eyes are widely separated and have epicanthic folds, the ears are low set, the nose is broad and flat, the chin is receding, and there are limb anomalies. The hypoplastic lungs preclude survival. The syndrome of bilateral renal agenesis occurs in 1/3,000 births and accounts for one fifth of newborns with the Potter phenotype. Other common causes of severe prenatal renal failure associated with the Potter phenotype include cystic renal dysplasia and obstructive uropathy. Less common causes are infantile polycystic kidney disease (autosomal recessive), renal hypoplasia, and medullary dysplasia. Agenesis should be distinguished from aplasia, an extreme form of dysplasia in which a nubbin of nonfunctioning tissue is seen capping a normal or abnormal ureter. Clinically this distinction may be difficult. Hereditary renal adysplasia should be differentiated from bilateral renal agenesis because of its genetic implications; this condition has an autosomal dominant inheritance pattern with a penetrance of 50–90% and variable expression. Associated anorectal, cardiovascular, and skeletal abnormalities are seen in both hereditary renal adysplasia and bilateral renal agenesis.

Bilateral renal agenesis should be suspected prenatally when maternal ultrasound demonstrates oligohydramnios, nonvisualization of the bladder, and absent kidneys in the second trimester. Death occurs in the first months of life from uremia or pulmonary insufficiency.

Unilateral renal agenesis is often discovered during the course of an evaluation for other congenital anomalies or for urinary tract symptoms. It should be suspected in newborns with a single umbilical artery. The ureter and the ipsilateral bladder hemitrigone are usually absent. The contralateral kidney undergoes compensatory hypertrophy after birth. Associated anomalies involve the genitourinary system in 40% of cases, the skeletal system in 30%, cardiovascular and gastrointestinal systems in 15% of cases each, and the central nervous and respiratory systems in 10% of cases each. Unilateral aplasia is seen in about 1/1,000 live births; males are affected more than females, and the left kidney is usually absent. Notable among the genitourinary malformations are vaginal atresia or agenesis *(Mayer-Rokitansky syndrome)*, agenesis of the vas deferens, and seminal vesicle cysts. Individuals with solitary kidneys may be at risk for hypertension and proteinuria, and should be followed appropriately.

ANOMALIES IN SHAPE AND POSITION. The normal process of ascent and rotation of the kidney may be incomplete, resulting in

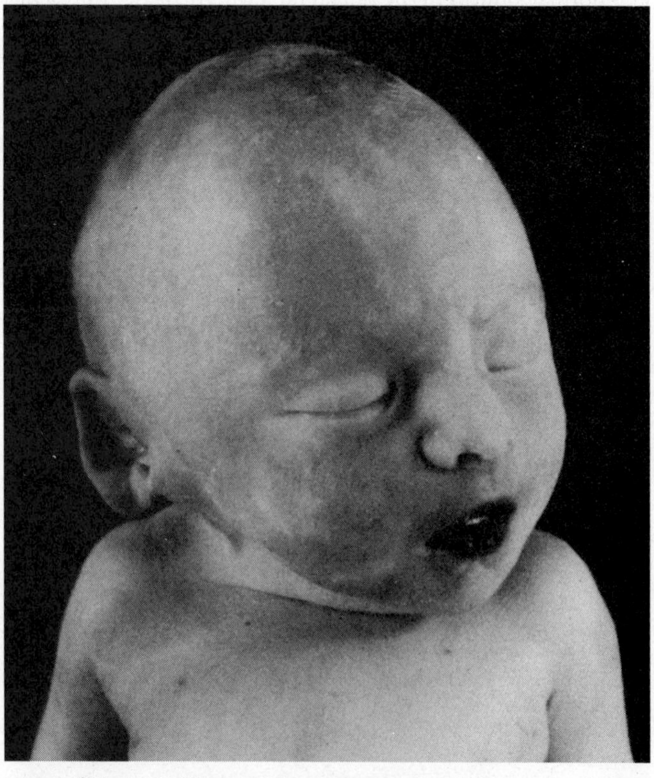

Figure 491–1. Stillborn with renal agenesis exhibiting the characteristic Potter facies. (Courtesy of Barbara Burke, M.D., Department of Laboratory Medicine and Pathology, University of Minnesota Hospital, Minnesota.)

renal ectopia (usually in the pelvis) or nonrotation. The lower poles of the kidneys may fuse in the midline, resulting in a horseshoe kidney (Fig. 491–2). The fusion may be asymmetric, or one kidney may cross the midline, resulting in crossed ectopia with or without fusion.

Horseshoe kidneys occur in 1:500 births but are seen in 7% of patients with Turner syndrome. Horseshoe kidney is one of the many renal anomalies that occur in one third of these patients. Wilms tumors are 2–8 times more frequent in children with horseshoe kidneys than in the general population.

HYPOPLASIA. This term signifies small kidneys having a reduction in the number of nephrons. Hypoplasia is not inherited; it may be unilateral or bilateral. When unilateral, the hypoplasia may involve the entire kidney or portions thereof. In the latter case (segmental hypoplasia or Ask-Upmark kidney), transverse scars may run from the cortex to medulla. Unilateral hypoplasia of either type is one of the more common causes of hypertension in the first decade of life.

Bilateral hypoplasia usually presents with the manifestations of chronic renal failure and is a leading cause of end-stage renal failure during the first decade of life. A history of polyuria and polydipsia is common. Urinalysis may be normal. A rare form of bilateral hypoplasia is called *oligomeganephronia,* in which the number of nephrons is markedly reduced but those present are markedly hypertrophied.

DYSPLASIA. This term indicates altered structural differentiation of the fetal kidney such that it contains cysts, abnormal ducts, undifferentiated mesenchyme, or nonrenal elements (such as cartilage).

Dysplasia may result from *intrauterine obstruction* of the urinary tract (e.g., prune-belly syndrome, ureterocele, urethral valves, ureteropelvic junction). Such dysplasia is usually bilateral and frequently leads to end-stage renal failure.

Another form of the disorder is *multicystic dysplasia.* This may be unilateral or bilateral and is commonly associated with developmental anomalies of the lower tracts or the contralateral normal kidney. In the unilateral form, the patient presents with a nonfunctioning flank mass that appears histologically to be a mass of cysts containing little or no identifiable renal tissue. The mass is usually removed if hypertension or infection develops. Prenatal detection of asymptomatic multicystic dysplasia is common. Bilateral multicystic dysplasia is associated with chronic renal failure; severe cases may show Potter syndrome.

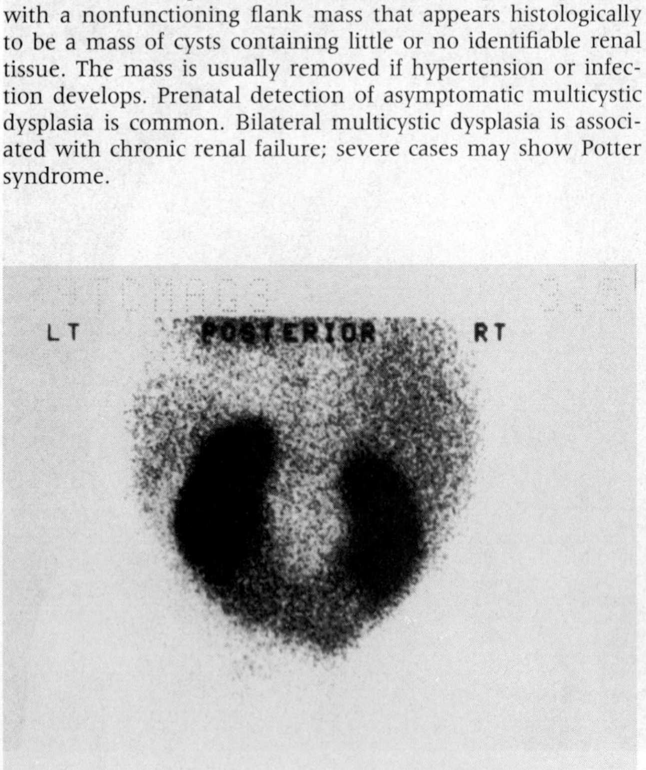

Figure 491–2. Isotopic renogram showing the characteristic configuration of a horseshoe kidney with an isthmus of functioning parenchyma.

Arant BS Jr, Sotelo-Avila C, Bernstein J: Segmental "hypoplasia" of the kidney (Ask-Upmark). J Pediatr 95:931, 1979.
Ashkenazi S, Merlob P, Stark H, et al: Renal anomalies in neonates with spontaneous pneumothorax—incidence and evaluation. Int J Pediatr Nephrol 4:25, 1983.
Carter JE, Lirenman DS: Bilateral renal hypoplasia with oligomeganephronia. Am J Dis Child 120:537, 1970.
Clark DA: Times of first void and first stool in 500 newborns. Pediatrics 60:457, 1977.
McPherson E, Carey J, Kramer A, et al: Dominantly inherited renal adysplasia. Am J Med Genet 26:863, 1987.
Moore ES, Galvez MB: Delayed micturition in the newborn. J Pediatr 80:867, 1972.
Pitts WR, Muecke EC: Horseshoe kidneys: A 40 year experience. J Urol 113:743, 1975.
Ritchey M: Anomalies of the Kidneys *In:* Kelalis PK, King LR, Belman AB (eds): Clinical Pediatric Urology. Philadelphia, WB Saunders, 1992, pp 500–529.
Roodhooft AM, Birnholz JC, Holmes CB: Familial nature of congenital absence and severe dysgenesis of both kidneys. N Engl J Med 310:1341, 1984.
Tarry WF, Duckett JW, Stephens FD: The Mayer-Rokitansky syndrome: Pathogenesis, classification and management. J Urol 136:648, 1986.
Thomas IT, Smith DW: Oligohydramnios, cause of the nonrenal features of Potter's syndrome, including pulmonary hypoplasia. J Pediatr 84:811, 1974.
Vinocur L, Slovis TL, Perlmutter AD, et al: Follow-up studies of multicystic dysplastic kidneys. Radiology 167:311, 1988.
Wilson RD, Baird PA: Renal agenesis in British Columbia. Am J Med Genet 21:153, 1985.

CHAPTER 492

Urinary Tract Infections

PREVALENCE AND ETIOLOGY. The prevalence of urinary infections varies markedly with sex and age. Symptomatic urinary tract infections occur in about 1.4/1,000 newborn infants (see Chapter 101). Urinary tract infections are more common in uncircumcised male infants. Thereafter, infections are much more common in females. Symptomatic and asymptomatic urinary tract infections occur in 1.2–1.9% of school-aged females and are most common in the 7- to 11-yr-old age group (2.5%). Infections are quite rare in males of similar age. Sexually active females are at increased risk for cystitis; both male and female sexually active adolescents may have urethritis.

Urinary tract infections are caused mainly by colonic bacteria. In females 75–90% of all infections are caused by *Escherichia coli,* followed by *Klebsiella* and *Proteus*. Some series report that in males over 1 yr of age, *Proteus* is as common as *E. coli;* others report a preponderance of gram-positive organisms in males. *Staphylococcus saprophyticus* is a proven pathogen in both sexes. Viral infections may also occur.

PATHOGENESIS AND PATHOLOGY. In the neonatal period, bacteria reach the urinary tract via the bloodstream or urethra, whereas later in life they ascend the urinary tract from below. Individual differences in susceptibility to urinary tract infections may be explained by such host factors as production of urethral and cervical antibodies (IgA), and other factors that influence bacterial adherence to the epithelium of the introitus and the urethra. Some of these factors, such as the P blood group phenotype, are genetically determined. Immunosuppression, diabetes, urinary tract obstruction, and chronic granulomatous disease are other factors that increase susceptibility to infections. Once the organisms gain entrance to the bladder, the severity of the infection may reflect the virulence of the bacteria and such anatomic factors as vesicoureteral reflux, obstruction, urinary stasis, and the presence of calculi. With urinary stasis, bacteria have increased opportunity to multiply, because urine is an excellent culture medium. In addition, vesical over-

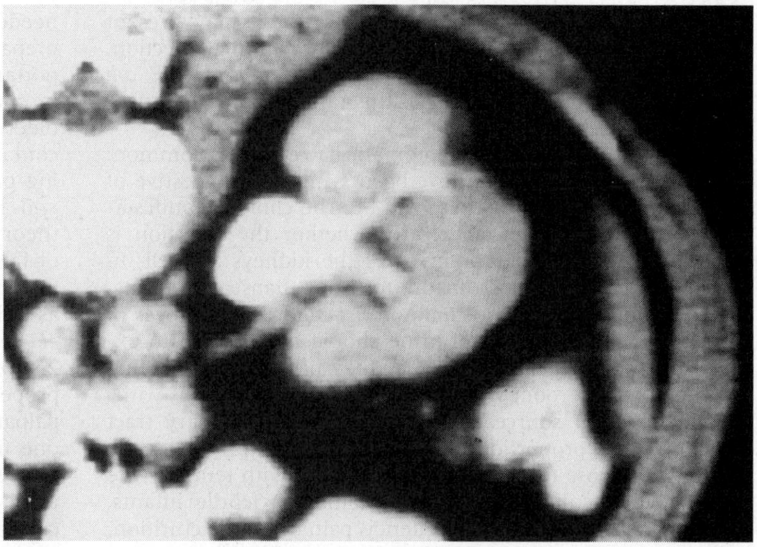

Figure 492–1. CT scan showing an area of parenchymal thinning corresponding to an underlying calyx, characteristic of pyelonephritic scarring or reflux nephropathy.

distention decreases the blood flow to the bladder wall and may decrease the bladder's natural resistance to infection.

Acute bacterial cystitis is characterized by mucosal congestion and edema, occasionally with petechiae and hemorrhage. The inflammatory reaction causes hyperactivity of the detrusor muscle and a decrease in the functional capacity of the bladder. These changes may precipitate vesicoureteral reflux, particularly when the vesicoureteral junction is already abnormally developed. Chronic or frequently recurrent infections may cause changes of *cystitis cystica* in the bladder wall, with characteristic endoscopic and histologic appearances.

Bacteria can reach the kidney from the bladder by way of established vesicoureteral reflux or through transient reflux precipitated by the inflammation of the bladder wall. Patients with the P1 blood group can develop ascending recurrent pyelonephritis in the absence of vesicoureteral reflux, because *E. coli* binds specifically to the P1 antigens on the epithelial cell surface. *Acute pyelonephritis* leads to enlargement of the kidney due to edema and acute inflammatory infiltrates in the medulla and pelvis. If untreated, these changes may lead to the formation of renal microabscesses, which may become confluent. Acute pyelonephritis is always more severe when obstruction is present. These changes may result in the development of renal scars, with the histologic findings commonly known as chronic pyelonephritis; however, prompt treatment of the infection can result in complete healing.

Histologically, *chronic pyelonephritis* is often difficult to distinguish from other causes of end-stage renal scarring, such as medullary cystic disease, ischemia, irradiation, analgesic abuse, and others. The scars can be focal or diffuse. The characteristic finding in chronic pyelonephritis is a cortical scar with an underlying calyceal deformity (Fig. 492–1). Microscopically, the lesions are patchy with glomerular fibrosis, interstitial chronic inflammation, and fibrosis and atrophy of the tubules. Local conditions of the renal medulla, such as high osmolality, which interferes with phagocytic activity of leukocytes, make this region of the kidney more susceptible to infections than the cortex.

Such renal scars are found also in children with vesicoureteral reflux who have no history of urinary tract infection; for this reason some prefer the term *reflux nephropathy* to *chronic pyelonephritis*. In any case, 90% of children with lesions of chronic pyelonephritis have or have had vesicoureteral reflux. Reflux nephropathy or chronic pyelonephritis is the most common cause of arterial hypertension in children; some of the vascular and glomerular changes may be secondary to hypertension rather than to the inflammatory process. In experimental animals, reflux nephropathy occurs only in areas of the kidney where the renal papillae allow reflux of urine from the calyx to the collecting tubules (intrarenal reflux) (Fig. 492–2), which is facilitated by the anatomic configuration of the flat papillae present in the compound calyces; conical papillae usually present in simple calyces help to prevent the occurrence of intrarenal reflux. Autoimmune responses to Tamm-Horsfall protein may also play a role in the development and progression of the pyelonephritic scar.

In addition to the inflammatory changes just described, infection by urea-splitting organisms such as *Proteus* can lead to stone formation. The ammonia derived from urea produces a strongly alkaline urine in which calcium phosphate and triple calcium, magnesium, and ammonium phosphate can precipitate. The calculi act as foreign bodies and help perpetuate the infection. With ureteral obstruction, renal infection can rapidly lead to septicemia, pyonephrosis, and the formation of renal and perirenal abscesses.

Xanthogranulomatous pyelonephritis is a distinct histologic type of renal infection characterized by granulomatous inflamma-

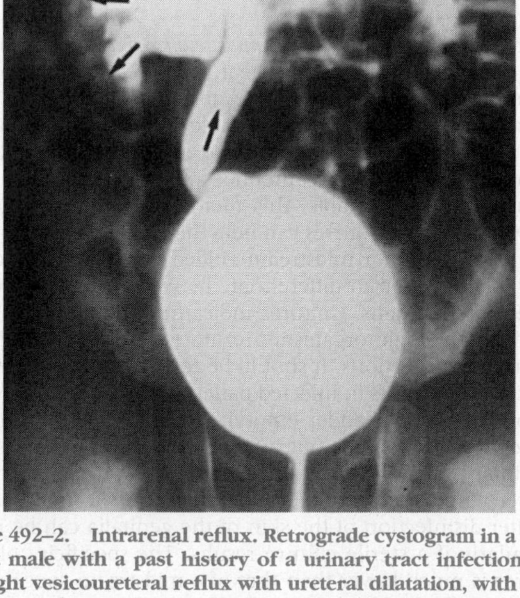

Figure 492–2. Intrarenal reflux. Retrograde cystogram in a young infant male with a past history of a urinary tract infection. Note the right vesicoureteral reflux with ureteral dilatation, with opacification of the renal parenchyma representing intrarenal reflux.

tion with giant cells and foamy histiocytes. It may present clinically as a renal mass or an acute or chronic infection. Renal calculi, obstruction, and infection with *Proteus* or *E. coli* contribute to the development of this rare lesion, which usually requires nephrectomy.

CLINICAL MANIFESTATIONS. Asymptomatic bacteriuria is common; in most cases, either there have been symptoms suggestive of urinary tract infection or there will be. The clinical manifestations often fail to indicate clearly whether the infection is confined to the bladder or involves the kidneys as well. In infancy, fever, weight loss, failure to thrive, nausea, vomiting, diarrhea, and jaundice are common. In children with fever of unknown origin, cultures of urine should be obtained to exclude urinary tract infection. In a study of infants presenting to an emergency room with a temperature >38.3°C but without an apparent source of fever, 7.5% had a urinary tract infection. This proportion was higher for white and female patients, and rose to 17% for white females with temperature >39°C. Urine culture should be obtained in febrile infants. Later in childhood, urinary frequency, pain during micturition, urinary incontinence associated with urgency, bedwetting in a previously dry child, abdominal pain, and foul-smelling urine are common symptoms. Chronic or frequently recurrent cystitis is often responsible for daytime incontinence and other manifestations of bladder instability, which may persist even after the urine has become sterile.

Hematuria is occasionally observed as a sign of hemorrhagic cystitis caused by *E. coli*. In acute pyelonephritis, fever, chills, and flank or abdominal pain and tenderness are common. The kidney may be enlarged. Children with chronic pyelonephritis are often asymptomatic. Arterial hypertension is commonly associated with renal scars. Reflux nephropathy, commonly attributed to the combination of vesicoureteral reflux and infection, is responsible for up to 15% of cases of end-stage renal failure in children in the United States. Sepsis is common in infants and older children with infection and urinary tract obstruction. Hyperammonemia with central nervous system manifestations is a rare complication of urinary tract infections due to *Proteus* and is associated with urinary stasis or obstruction.

LABORATORY DATA. The diagnosis of urinary tract infections depends on the culture of bacteria from the urine. The finding of any bacteria in urine obtained from the bladder or renal pelvis is indicative of infection. An accurate diagnosis may be difficult to establish, owing to the frequent contamination of voided specimens or to prior treatment of the patient with antibiotics.

In toilet-trained children, a *midstream urine culture* obtained after cleansing the urethral meatus with a povidone-iodine solution and rinsing with sterile water or saline is usually satisfactory. In females, the labia should be spread manually to avoid contamination of the urine or contact with the skin. In uncircumcised males, the prepuce must be retracted; if the prepuce is not retractable, this method of urine collection is not reliable. Skillful nurses can help the child's parent to obtain these specimens. For midstream voided specimens, the colony count is often used to differentiate between infected and contaminated specimens. Cultures indicating more than 10^5 colonies/mL of a single organism are more than 90% specific for urinary tract infections. It should be recognized, however, that lower colony counts in infected patients may be due to overhydration, to recent bladder emptying, or to antibiotic therapy; such counts do not rule out infection.

In infants and both circumcised male and female young children, the application of an adhesive, sealed, *sterile collection bag* after disinfection of the skin of the genitalia can be useful, particularly if a sterile culture results. The specificity of these cultures is much lower than that of a midstream specimen.

When greater assurance as to the possibility of infection is needed, a *catheterized specimen* must be obtained. Proper skin preparation and good technique of catheterization are important. The use of a No. 5 French polyethylene feeding tube in infants or of a No. 8 French tube with proper lubrication in older children minimizes the chance of urethral trauma and contamination. Catheterization shortly after spontaneous voiding produces a measure of the residual urine in the bladder and helps assess problems related to bladder emptying. In theory, the normal flora of the distal urethra may be a source of false-positive culture results, but in practice the finding of any colonies grown from bladder urine should be considered as indicative of infection.

The use of a *suprapubic puncture* of the full bladder with a 25- or 22-gauge needle yields reliable results. With the child properly hydrated (when the bladder can be percussed or palpated), the skin is disinfected and a puncture performed one finger-breadth above the pubis in the midline. A syringe is used to aspirate as the needle is inserted; 1 or 2 mL of urine is sufficient for culture. The urine specimen for bacterial culture should be kept refrigerated until the culture is plated to avoid bacterial overgrowth. False-negative findings on urine culture may result from unrecognized antibiotic treatment, dilution from overhydration, or contamination of the specimen with the antiseptic solution.

A urinalysis should be obtained from the same specimen as that cultured. Pyuria (leukocytes in the urine) suggests infection, but infection can occur in the absence of pyuria; accordingly, this finding is more confirmatory than diagnostic. Conversely, pyuria can be present without urinary tract infections. Microscopic hematuria is common in acute cystitis. Casts in the urinary sediment suggest renal involvement. *Proteus* infections consistently produce an alkaline pH.

With acute renal infection, leukocytosis, neutrophilia, and elevated erythrosedimentation rate and C-reactive protein are common. Unfortunately, in children such tests to differentiate upper from lower urinary tract infections as the detection of antibody coated bacteria, response to single-dose antibiotic therapy, and other immunologic and biochemical tests are unreliable. Inability to concentrate the urine is a common but unreliable finding in acute and chronic pyelonephritis. In 30% of infants with renal infections, the serum creatinine level is transiently elevated. Because sepsis is common in renal infections, particularly in infants and with obstruction, blood cultures should be obtained during febrile infections.

IMAGING STUDIES. During acute febrile infection, renal ultrasound should be obtained to rule out hydronephrosis and renal or perirenal abscesses; other indications for this study are when the response to antibiotic therapy is not prompt, when the child is severely ill and toxic, and when the serum creatinine level is elevated. Renal ultrasound is also very sensitive for detecting pyonephrosis, a condition that may require prompt drainage of the collecting system by percutaneous nephrostomy.

When the diagnosis of acute pyelonephritis is uncertain, renal scanning with technetium labled 2,3-dimercaptosuccinic acid (DMSA) or glucoheptanate is useful. The presence of a parenchymal filling defect on the renal scan supports the diagnosis of pyelonephritis but cannot differentiate an acute from a chronic process. The routine use of DMSA scans during the acute episode in children with clinical manifestations of pyelonephritis and positive urine cultures is unnecessary. Computed tomography (CT) is the definitive diagnostic test for acute pyelonephritis. However, a CT scan is seldom necessary to establish such diagnosis.

Approximately 3 wk after treatment of the acute infection, all children should have voiding cystourethrography to assess reflux. Some physicians would restrict such studies to all males and to females under 5 yr of age who have an initial infection; older females would be studied at the time of a second infection. We prefer the former approach, because reflux will be found in 25% of all children under the age of 10 yr who have had symptomatic or asymptomatic bacteriuria; it is more frequently observed in children under 3 yr of age. If it is available, radioisotopic voiding cystourethrography can be used in females; this technique is sensitive and exposes the ovaries to 50- to 100-fold less radiation than would conventional voiding cystourethrography with intermittent fluoroscopic control. In males, radiographic definition of the urethra is important; accordingly, radiographic voiding cystourethrography with fluoroscopic control is recommended for the initial work-up. Renal ultrasound may also be carried out as part of the initial work-up in order to exclude obstruction and to determine kidney size.

If vesicoureteral reflux is present, intravenous pyelography with nephrotomography may be obtained to evaluate kidney size and to detect possible calyceal blunting, ureteral dilatation, and renal scarring. A better alternative to intravenous urography for detection of renal scars is radioisotopic renal scanning with DMSA or glucoheptanate. These diagnostic tests are more sensitive than urography and avoid the possible adverse reactions associated with an intravenously administered contrast medium. Renal scanning is particularly useful in infants and young children, in whom abdominal gas makes the interpretation of urography difficult (Fig. 492–3). Further evaluation of children with infections and reflux or obstructive uropathy will be discussed in other sections.

The frequently performed cystoscopies and measurements of urethral caliber advocated for girls in the past contribute nothing to the therapeutic decisions to be made in children with normal findings on radiographic study or with primary reflux. Narrowing of the female urethra was once postulated to be a contributing factor in the development of urinary tract infections, but the urethras of girls with recurrent urinary tract infections are not narrower than those of girls without infections.

DIFFERENTIAL DIAGNOSIS. Inflammations of the external genitalia, vulvitis, and vaginitis caused by yeast, pinworms, and other agents may be accompanied by symptoms mimicking cystitis. Viral and chemical cystitis must be distinguished from bacterial cystitis on the basis of history and results of urine culture. Radiographically, the hypoplastic or dysplastic kidney, or a small kidney secondary to a vascular accident, may appear similar to a kidney with chronic pyelonephritis. With the latter, however, vesicoureteral reflux is usually present.

Acute hemorrhagic cystitis is frequently caused by *E. coli;* it has been attributed also to adenovirus types 11 and 21. Adenovirus cystitis is more frequent in males; it is self-limiting, with hematuria lasting approximately 4 days. *Eosinophilic cystitis* is a rare form of cystitis of obscure origin that occasionally has been found in children. The usual symptoms are those of cystitis with hematuria, ureteral dilatation, and filling defects in the bladder caused by masses that consist histologically of inflammatory infiltrates with eosinophils.

TREATMENT. Acute cystitis should be treated promptly to prevent its possible progression to pyelonephritis. If the symptoms are severe, a specimen of bladder urine is obtained for culture and treatment is started immediately. If the symptoms are mild or the diagnosis doubtful, treatment can be delayed until the results of culture are known, and the culture can be repeated if the results are uncertain. For example, if midstream culture grew between 10^4 and 10^5 colonies of a gram-negative organism, a second culture may be obtained by catheterization or suprapubic aspiration before treatment is initiated. If treatment is initiated before the results of a culture and sensitivities are available, a 7- to 10-day course of therapy with trimethoprim-sulfamethoxazole (see later) will be effective against most strains of *E. coli.* Nitrofurantoin (5–7 mg/kg/24 hr in 3–4 divided doses) is also very effective and has the advantage of being active against *Klebsiella-Enterobacter* organisms. Amoxicillin (50 mg/kg/24 hr) is also effective as initial treatment but has no clear advantages over the sulfonamides or nitrofurantoin.

In acute febrile infections suggestive of pyelonephritis, the use of broad-spectrum antibiotics capable of reaching significant tissue levels is preferable. If the child is acutely ill, parenteral treatment with cefotaxime (100 mg/kg/24 hr) or ampicillin (100 mg/kg/24 hr) with an aminoglycoside such as gentamicin (3 mg/kg/24 hr in 3 divided doses) is preferable. The potential ototoxicity and nephrotoxicity of aminoglycosides should be considered, and serum creatinine levels must be obtained prior to initiating treatment as well as daily thereafter as long as treatment continues. Treatment with aminoglycosides is particularly effective against *Pseudomonas,* and alkalinization of urine with sodium bicarbonate increases their effectiveness in the urinary tract. The combination of sulfamethoxazole and trimethoprim (Cotrim, Bactrim, Septra), either orally or intravenously, is effective against a variety of gram-negative organisms other than *Pseudomonas* and is considered by some authorities to be the treatment of choice for oral therapy. The oral dosage is 20 mg/kg/24 hr for sulfamethoxazole and 4 mg/kg/24 hr for trimethoprim, given in 2 divided doses. Ciprofloxacin is an alternative agent for resistant microorganisms in patients older than 18 yr.

A urine culture should be obtained a week after the termination of treatment of any urinary tract infection to assure that the urine remains sterile. Given the tendency of urinary tract infections to recur even in the absence of predisposing anatomic factors, follow-up urine cultures should be obtained at 3-mo intervals for 1–2 yr, even when the child is asymptomatic. If recurrences are frequent, prophylaxis against reinfection, using either the sulfamethoxazole-trimethoprim combi-

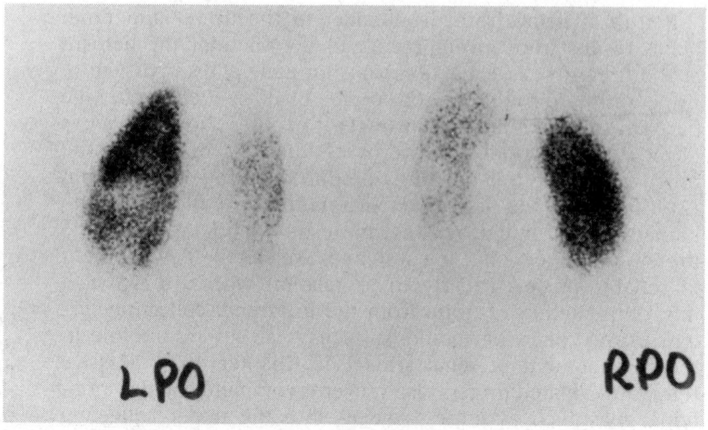

Figure 492–3. DMSA renal scan showing bilateral photopenic areas indicative of renal scarring.

nation or nitrofurantoin at one third the normal therapeutic dose once a day, is often effective. It is important, however, to obtain periodic urine cultures if the child is receiving prolonged prophylactic treatment, in order to rule out asymptomatic infections caused by resistant organisms. Antibacterial prophylaxis is also indicated for as long as vesicoureteral reflux persists (see Chapter 493), or when recurrent cystitis causes such symptoms as incontinence, frequency, and urgency of urination, which are perpetuated by frequent reinfections. Other indications for long-term prophylaxis (neurogenic bladder, urinary tract stasis and obstruction, reflux, and calculi) are discussed in a later chapter. Because the probability of finding vesicoureteral reflux is 25% and the probability of a recurrent infection is 50%, it is logical to continue antibacterial prophylaxis with low dose sulfamethoxazole-trimethoprim combinations or nitrofurantoin until completion of the radiologic evaluation. The prolonged use of any chemotherapeutic agent should be monitored for evidence of toxicity (anemia, leukopenia, and so on). Broad-spectrum antibiotics are usually ineffective for prophylaxis, because the colonic bacteria likely to be responsible for reinfections quickly become resistant to these agents.

The long-term prognosis for urinary tract infections is usually excellent, provided prompt and adequate treatment is instituted when the diagnosis is established. The prompt treatment of acute bacterial pyelonephritis in animals has prevented the development of renal scars. Notwithstanding this usually favorable long-term outcome, children with recurrent urinary tract infections often present difficult and frustrating problems in treatment and prophylaxis. The main consequences of chronic renal damage caused by pyelonephritis are arterial hypertension and renal insufficiency; when they are found they should be treated appropriately. Some children with urinary tract infections void infrequently and many also have severe constipation. Counseling of parents to try to establish more normal patterns of voiding and defecation may be helpful in controlling recurrences.

Children with renal or perirenal abscesses or with infections in obstructed urinary tracts require surgical or percutaneous drainage in addition to antibiotic therapy and other supportive measures.

CHAPTER 493
Vesicoureteral Reflux

Reflux of urine from the bladder to the ureter and renal pelvis results from incompetence of the valvular mechanism at the ureterovesical junction that normally allows passage of urine only from the ureter to the bladder. Reflux can be harmful to the kidneys because (1) it exposes the renal pelvis (which has a normal pressure of less than 10 mm Hg) to the much higher vesical pressures produced during voiding, and (2) it facilitates the passage of bacteria from the bladder to the kidneys. Accordingly, reflux can result in dilatation of the ureter and upper collecting system as well as the development of renal scars, particularly in association with urinary tract infections. Reflux of urine from the intrarenal collecting system to the collecting tubules also plays an important role in the development of renal scars (see Chapter 492). Massive reflux into dilated ureters also prevents complete bladder emptying, inasmuch as urine "voided" into the upper collecting

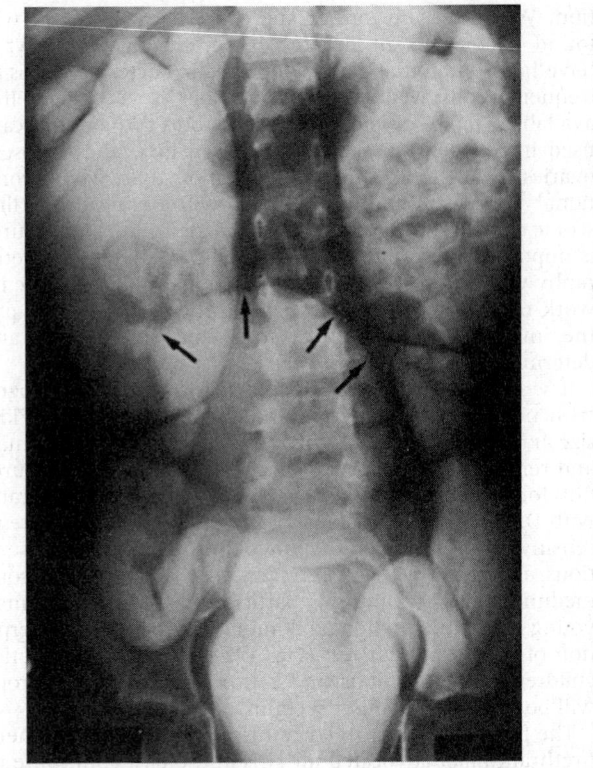

Figure 493–1. Excretory urogram in a male with megaureter-megacystic syndrome. Note the massive ureteral dilatation due to high-grade vesicoureteral reflux. The bladder is very distended, reaching the level of the third lumbar vertebra. There was no urethral obstruction or neurogenic dysfunction.

system rapidly returns to the bladder, with development of progressive bladder dilatation, as in the megaureter-megacystic syndrome (Fig. 493–1). Reflux nephropathy accounts for 15–20% of all end-stage renal failure in children and young adults, and is an important cause of hypertension in children.

CLASSIFICATION. Primary vesicoureteral reflux results from a congenital anomaly of the ureterovesical junction in which the intramural ureteral tunnel is short, the ureteral orifice is placed in a lateral and cephalad direction, and the trigone is underdeveloped. This shortening of the intramural tunnel decreases the efficiency of the valvular mechanism. The degree of vesicoureteral reflux varies with the degree of malformation of the orifice (Fig. 493–2). Conditions such as cystitis and bladder instability may precipitate or perpetuate reflux with a marginally competent ureterovesical junction that would

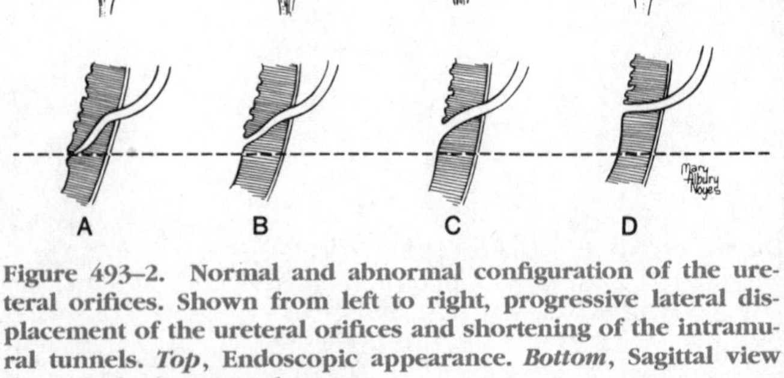

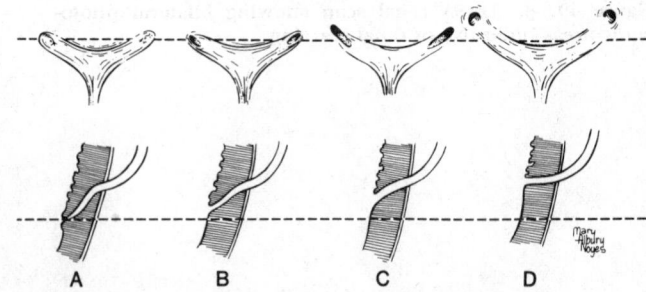

Figure 493–2. Normal and abnormal configuration of the ureteral orifices. Shown from left to right, progressive lateral displacement of the ureteral orifices and shortening of the intramural tunnels. *Top*, Endoscopic appearance. *Bottom*, Sagittal view through the intramural ureter.

■ TABLE 493–1 Classification of Vesicoureteral Reflux

Type	Cause
1. Primary	Congenital incompetence of the valvular mechanism of the vesicoureteral junction
2. Primary associated with other malformations of the ureterovesical junction	Ureteral duplication Ureterocele with duplication Ureteral ectopia Paraureteral diverticula
3. Secondary to increased intravesical pressure	Neurogenic bladder Non-neurogenic bladder dysfunction Bladder outlet obstruction
4. Secondary to inflammatory processes	Severe bacterial cystitis Foreign bodies Vesical calculi Clinical cystitis
5. Secondary to surgical procedures involving the ureterovesical junction	

otherwise not reflux. A wide spectrum of anomalies may be associated (Table 493–1).

With duplication of the ureters and ureterocele, the ureterocele obstructs the upper collecting system, and there is often reflux to the ureter of the lower collecting system and occasionally to the contralateral side. In duplicated systems, reflux is more common in the lower ureter, which enters the bladder higher and more laterally and has a less competent valve. Reflux is always present when the ureter enters a diverticulum (Figs. 493–3 and 493–4).

In cases of congenital neurogenic bladder, such as myelomeningocele and sacral agenesis, reflux is present in one third of the cases at birth and develops eventually in more than half of affected children. Reflux is seen in more than half of cases of posterior urethral valves. Both clinically and experimentally, reflux with increased intravesical pressures (as in bladder outlet obstruction and vesical dysfunction) has severe consequences for the kidney, even in the absence of infection. Reflux is classified into five grades according to its severity and the degree of ureteral dilatation and calyceal deformity (Fig. 493–5). This grading of reflux has prognostic and therapeutic significance.

NATURAL HISTORY. In children with reflux, the incidence of renal scarring or reflux nephropathy increases with the grade

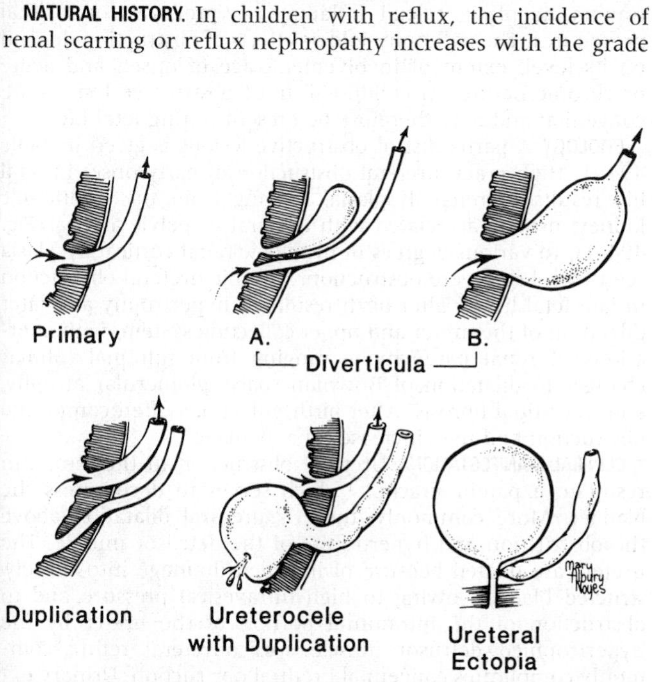

Figure 493–3. Various anatomic defects of the ureterovesical junction associated with vesicoureteral reflux.

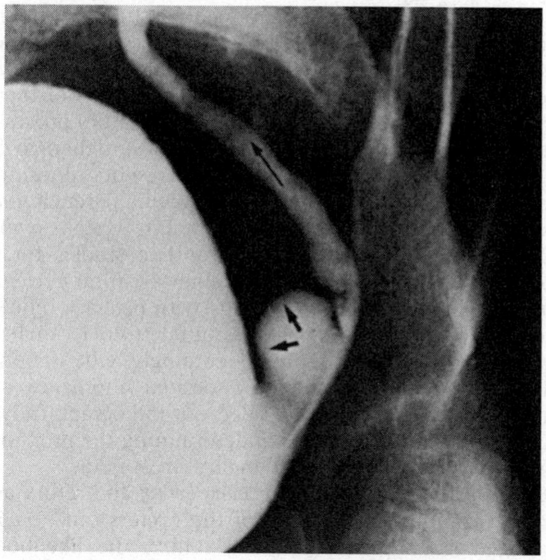

Figure 493–4. Reflux and bladder diverticulum. The voiding cystourethrogram demonstrates left vesicoureteral reflux and a paraureteral diverticulum.

of reflux. Intrarenal reflux seems to increase the risk of scarring. In grades I and II reflux in patients who have no ureteral dilatation, the anatomy of the vesicoureteral region tends to be nearly normal, and in about 80% of cases reflux will cease spontaneously with maturation of the child. With greater degrees of ureteral dilatation and of abnormality of the vesicoureteral junction, the chances of spontaneous disappearance decrease to about 15% in grades III and IV. Reflux may be familial and evaluation of siblings younger than 5 yr is recommended.

CLINICAL MANIFESTATIONS. In the majority of children, reflux is discovered during an evaluation for urinary tract infection. In other children, voiding cystourethrography is part of an evaluation of voiding dysfunction, renal insufficiency, hypertension, or other suspected pathology of the urinary tract. It has become increasingly common to diagnose reflux in asymptomatic siblings of children with reflux.

DIFFERENTIAL DIAGNOSIS. The distinction between primary and secondary reflux is usually easy to make on the basis of history and radiographs. In the case of the child who has reflux, infection, and voiding dysfunction, it may be difficult to determine whether the voiding dysfunction is secondary to infection or the cause of reflux that predisposes to infection. If symptoms do not resolve with antibacterial prophylaxis, treat-

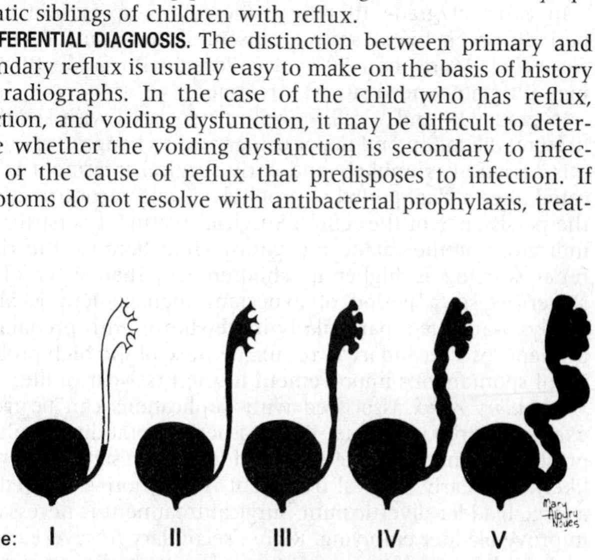

Figure 493–5. Grading of a vesicoureteral reflux. Grade I: reflux into a nondilated distal ureter. Grade II: reflux into the upper collecting system without dilatation. Grade III: reflux into dilated ureter and/or blunting of calyceal fornices. Grade IV: reflux into a grossly dilated ureter. Grade V: massive reflux, with ureteral dilatation and tortuosity and effacement of the calyceal details.

ment with anticholinergics or urodynamic studies of the lower urinary tract (see Chapter 497) may be necessary in such cases.

EVALUATION. Once reflux is diagnosed, graded, and determined to be primary, secondary to other malformations of the vesicoureteral junction, or secondary to inflammatory processes or increased intravesical pressure, it is important then to know the renal size and whether scars are present; ultrasound is indicated to evaluate renal size, and isotopic parenchymal renal scanning is helpful to rule out scars. Intravenous pyelography and tomography are also appropriate studies for these purposes. Blood pressure and baseline creatinine clearance should also be measured. In patients with primary reflux, the degree of abnormality of the intramural tunnel can be predicted from the grade of reflux. Accordingly, when anomalies of the urethra or bladder and associated anomalies of the vesicoureteral junction can be ruled out radiographically, cystoscopy is of little or no value in determining the prognosis or choosing between surgical and medical treatment.

TREATMENT. The treatment of *primary reflux* and reflux associated with complete duplication of the ureters can be considered together. In grades I and II reflux, the likelihood of spontaneous resolution is great, and a long period of expectant treatment is warranted, during which the child must be protected from infection by administration of low doses of an antibacterial medication such as sulfamethoxazole-trimethoprim combination or nitrofurantoin (see Chapter 492). At the beginning of treatment, urine cultures are obtained at monthly intervals; when the efficacy of prophylaxis has been established, cultures can be obtained at 3-mo intervals.

Since asymptomatic bacteriuria and reflux can be harmful, it is important to culture the urine even in the absence of symptoms. Using a radionuclide, voiding cystourethrography is obtained at yearly intervals. A yearly or every-other-year renal ultrasound study is useful to evaluate renal growth. When a radiographic study indicates spontaneous cessation of the reflux, another study made in 3–6 mo should confirm this before antibacterial therapy is discontinued, because reflux is occasionally intermittent. Grade II reflux seldom needs surgical correction, but if antibacterial prophylaxis fails to keep the urine consistently sterile, surgery is indicated. A DMSA renal scan at the end of the treatment period helps select children with residual scars who need long-term follow-up of their blood pressure.

In cases of grade III reflux, the follow-up is similar, but periodic parenchymal scans are useful if new scar formation is suspected. More than 50% of children with grade III reflux may ultimately need surgical treatment.

In grades IV and V reflux (reflux associated with significant ureteral dilatation and upper urinary tract changes), spontaneous cessation is unlikely and early surgical treatment is indicated after a brief period of prophylaxis and reconfirmation of the persistence of the reflux. Surgical treatment is particularly indicated for the infant and young child because the risk of renal scarring is higher in children less than 5 yr of age. Nevertheless, a period of expectant management is almost always warranted, particularly in newborns with prenatal hydronephrosis secondary to reflux, because of the high probability of spontaneous improvement in the first year of life.

Secondary reflux associated with duplications can be treated exactly as primary reflux. When a periureteral diverticulum is present, spontaneous cessation of reflux is significantly less likely, and early surgical treatment is therefore indicated. For a large bladder diverticulum, surgical treatment is necessary to improve bladder emptying. Reflux secondary to severe cystitis, such as that which may accompany foreign bodies or chemical irritation, will usually cease once the primary cause of the cystitis is removed. Iatrogenic reflux usually requires surgical treatment. The treatment of reflux in cases of ureteroceles, posterior urethral valves, and neurogenic bladder is discussed in a later section.

The results of surgical correction of reflux using the Cohen operation are excellent, with greater than 97% success. However, when the ureters are very dilated and other techniques, such as long tunnel reimplantation with psoas hitch of the bladder or reduction ureteroplasty, are necessary, the success rate is lower and obstructive complications more common.

Complications of antireflux surgery include persistence of reflux and obstruction of the distal ureter. Careful follow-up of patients after surgery is therefore required. When only unilateral reflux has been demonstrated, bilateral correction of reflux is usually unnecessary. Reflux may appear transiently on the opposite side after surgery, but it usually ceases spontaneously.

Endoscopic injection of polytetrafluoroethylene (Polytef) under the ureteral orifice has been effective in the short term to control reflux in some children. The safety of Polytef paste injection in the bladder wall remains questionable. Subureteric injection of other substances such as collagen or silicone particles has been used experimentally. The early success rate with a single injection is about 65–70%. The advantages of these techniques include absence of incision and the ability to perform the injection on an outpatient basis. Nevertheless, for now and until a substance for subureteric injection is proven safe and effective, the Cohen reimplantation remains the standard for treatment.

CHAPTER 494
Obstructions of the Urinary Tract

Obstructive lesions of the urinary tract occur at any level from the urethral meatus to the calyceal infundibula. In children, obstruction can be congenital (anatomic) or caused by trauma, neoplasia, calculi, inflammatory processes, or surgical procedures. The pathophysiologic effects of obstruction depend on its level, extent of involvement, age of onset, and acute or chronic nature. In childhood, most obstructive lesions are congenital and may therefore be present during fetal life.

ETIOLOGY. A partial list of obstructive lesions is given in Table 494–1. High-grade ureteral obstruction of early onset in fetal life results in renal dysplasia, ranging from the multicystic kidney, usually associated with ureteral or pelvic atresia (Fig. 494–1), to various degrees of histologic renal cortical dysplasia seen with less severe obstruction. Chronic ureteral obstruction in late fetal life or after birth results in hypertrophy and later dilatation of the ureter and upper collecting system, with alterations of renal parenchyma ranging from minimal tubular changes to dilatation of Bowman space, glomerular atrophy, and interstitial fibrosis. After birth, infections often complicate obstruction and may increase renal damage.

CLINICAL MANIFESTATIONS. Urethral obstruction in the fetus can result in a patent urachus, which serves to decompress the bladder. More commonly, there is urethral dilatation above the obstruction and hypertrophy of the detrusor muscle. The ureters are dilated because of impeded drainage into the obstructed bladder, owing to high intravesical pressure and to obstruction of the intramural portion of the ureter by the hypertrophied detrusor muscle. Vesicoureteral reflux commonly complicates congenital urethral obstruction. Urinary extravasation sometimes occurs in children with congenital obstruction when urine under pressure leaks out of the intrarenal

■ **TABLE 494–1 Types and Causes of Urinary Tract Obstruction**

Location	Cause
Infundibula	Congenital
	Calculi
	Inflammatory (tuberculosis)
	Traumatic
	Postsurgical
	Neoplastic
Renal pelvis	Congenital (infundibulopelvic stenosis)
	Inflammatory (tuberculosis)
	Calculi
	Neoplasia (Wilms tumor, neuroblastoma)
Ureteropelvic junction	Congenital stenosis
	Calculi
	Neoplasia
	Inflammatory
	Postsurgical
	Traumatic
Ureter	Congenital obstructive megaureter
	Ureteral ectopia
	Ureterocele
	Retrocaval ureter
	Ureteral fibroepithelial polyps
	Ureteral valves
	Calculi
	Postsurgical
	Extrinsic compression
	Neoplasia (neuroblastoma, lymphoma, and other retroperitoneal or pelvic tumors)
	Inflammatory (Crohn disease, chronic granulomatous disease)
	Hematoma, urinoma
	Lymphocele
	Retroperitoneal fibrosis
Bladder outlet and urethra	Neurogenic bladder dysfunction (functional obstruction)
	Posterior urethral valves
	Anterior urethral valves
	Diverticula
	Urethral strictures (congenital, traumatic, or iatrogenic)
	Urethral atresia
	Ectopic ureterocele
	Meatal stenosis (males)
	Calculi
	Foreign bodies
	Phimosis
	Extrinsic compression by tumors
	Urogenital sinus anomalies

collecting system, usually through ruptured calyceal fornices, into the subcapsular or perirenal spaces (urinomas) or into the peritoneal cavity (urinary ascites). Bilateral ureteral obstruction or urethral obstruction may cause oligohydramnios and pulmonary hypoplasia. The newborn may exhibit the facies and stigmata of severe prenatal renal failure (see Chapter 491). The immediate prognosis for newborns with severe obstructive uropathy is often more closely related to the degree of pulmonary insufficiency than to the degree of renal damage.

In high-grade urethral obstruction or bilateral ureteral obstruction, there is renal failure. The urinary output may be low, normal, or increased because of tubular dysfunction with decreased concentrating ability. Renal function usually recovers completely following relief of a brief acute obstruction. The potential for recovery of renal function in chronic (including all congenital) cases depends on the degree of dysplasia or irreversible renal damage. In renal failure with obstructive uropathy, both the concentrating ability and the ability of the tubules to excrete hydrogen ions are decreased. Accordingly, infants with renal failure secondary to obstruction may, after relief of obstruction, continue to have polyuria, dilute urine, and chronic acidosis with normal serum creatinine levels.

Hypertrophy and dilatation in the bladder and collecting systems persist long after correction of the obstruction and are often irreversible. Following relief of obstruction in the uremic child, postobstructive diuresis may ensue. This is usually transient and due to the combination of tubular dysfunction and an osmotic diuresis caused by high blood levels of urea.

DIAGNOSIS. Urinary tract obstructions are often silent, and advanced lesions (particularly unilateral ones) can be found in children without symptoms. In the newborn, a palpable abdominal mass is most commonly a hydronephrotic kidney. With infravesical obstructive lesions, the bladder as well as the kidneys may be palpably enlarged. A patent urachus should suggest urethral obstruction. Ascites in the newborn may be caused by intraperitoneal urinary extravasation (see earlier). Prune-belly syndrome (abdominal muscle deficiency and undescended testes) is often accompanied by massive dilatation of the bladder and ureters, and occasionally by infravesical obstruction.

Urinary tract obstruction may be diagnosed prenatally by ultrasonography. In such cases, further ultrasound and, if indicated, a more complete evaluation should be undertaken in the neonatal period. Oligohydramnios and various degrees of pulmonary hypoplasia accompany the more severe cases of urethral or bilateral ureteral obstruction.

Infection and sepsis may be the first indications of an obstructive lesion of the urinary tract. The combination of infection and obstruction poses a serious threat to infants and children, and usually requires parenteral administration of antibiotics and drainage of the obstructed kidney. For this reason, renal ultrasound should be performed for all children during the acute stage of febrile urinary tract infections. Obstructive renal insufficiency can manifest itself by failure to thrive, vomiting, diarrhea, or other nonspecific signs and symptoms. In older children, infravesical obstruction can be associated with overflow urinary incontinence or a poor urinary stream. Acute ureteral obstruction causes flank or abdominal pain, and there may be nausea and vomiting. Chronic ureteral obstruction can be silent or cause vague abdominal or typical flank pain with increased fluid intake. Abdominal ultrasound should be the initial imaging study in all children with abdominal pain. If attention is focused initially on the gastrointestinal tract, the diagnosis of ureteral obstruction is often delayed unnecessarily.

Imaging Studies. The common characteristic of obstruction is the

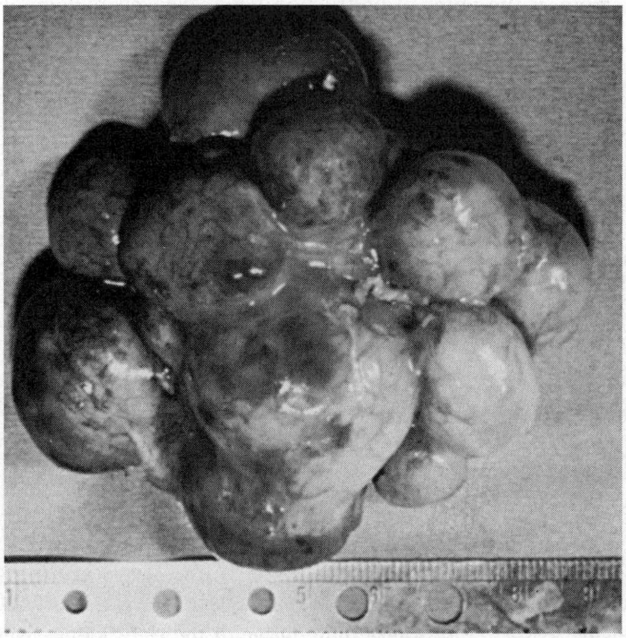

Figure 494–1. Surgical specimen of a multicystic dysplastic kidney associated with ureteral atresia.

presence of a dilated urinary tract. Dilatation is frequently an ultrasonographic finding (Fig. 494–2). However, dilatation is not always indicative of obstruction but may persist after surgical correction or spontaneous resolution of an obstructive lesion. Dilatation may result from vesicoureteral reflux, or it may be a manifestation of abnormal development of the urinary tract, even when there is no obstruction. Renal ultrasound is, nonetheless, useful in the assessment of the presumably obstructed urinary tract, not only as a screening method but also to evaluate renal size and parenchymal thickness, to determine whether ureteral dilatation is present, and to evaluate the bladder. In acute or intermittent obstruction, the dilatation of the collecting system may be minimal and ultrasound may be misleading.

Radioisotopic renography using technetium labeled diethylenetriaminepentaacetic acid (DTPA) gives a gross estimate of differential renal function. In a normal renogram, the isotope is excreted spontaneously, but when dilatation is present it tends to remain in the renal pelvis. If furosemide is administered, the unobstructed system promptly excretes the isotope, whereas the obstructed urinary tract will excrete it slowly or not at all (Fig. 494–3). Because there are many cases of both false-negative interpretations and, more importantly, false-positive interpretations of this test, it should be interpreted cautiously. In the newborn and in cases of compromised renal function, even nonobstructed and nondilated kidneys may fail to respond to furosemide. Isotopic renography with iodine-labeled Hippuran is probably more accurate, but when obstruction is present it exposes the kidneys to unreasonably high doses of radiation and it has been abandoned. MAG3 (^{99}Tc mercaptoacetylglycine) is safe, offers some of the advantages of Hippuran, and provides excellent images in infants.

In older children, the intravenous urogram is still quite useful. The preliminary radiography of the abdomen should be inspected for calculi, spinal abnormalities, or an abnormal intestinal gas pattern. In infravesical obstruction, the bladder wall is irregular or trabeculated because of detrusor hypertrophy. A postvoiding film may show residual bladder urine. In ureteral obstruction, there is dilatation of the collecting system above the obstruction and blunting of the calyces. Concentration of the radiopaque medium on the obstructed side is decreased, and there may be delayed appearance of the dye in the collecting system with progressive increase in dye concentration at the point of obstruction when delayed radiographs are obtained. In high-grade obstruction, the dye may remain in the collecting system after 24 hr.

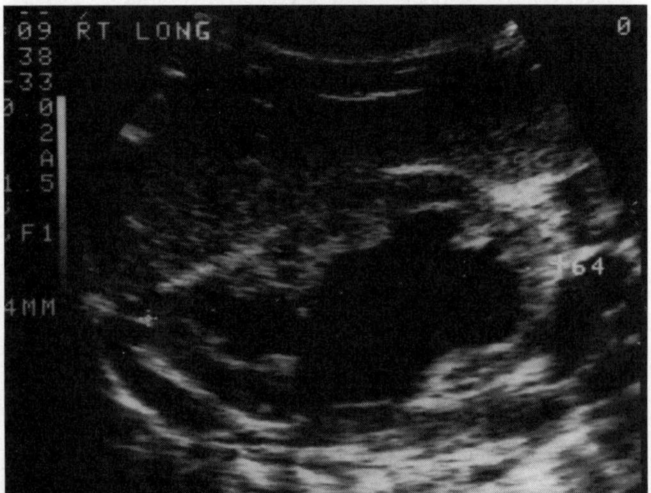

Figure 494–2. Ultrasonographic image of the right kidney with marked pelvic and calyceal dilatation in an infant with ureteropelvic junction obstruction.

Urinary extravasation can be detected in the early or delayed films of a urographic study. When intermittent obstruction is suspected, intravenous urography during an acute episode of pain is often the most valuable diagnostic study.

Pressure Flow Studies. Another way to establish the diagnosis of obstruction of the upper collecting systems in equivocal cases is by performing pressure flow studies, as described by Whitaker. With a No. 22–gauge needle, percutaneous access to the renal pelvis is gained; the collecting system is then perfused with radiopaque dye at a measured flow rate, usually 10 mL/min. The pressures in the renal pelvis and the bladder are monitored during this infusion, and pressure differences exceeding 20 cm of water indicate obstruction. This test usually requires general anesthesia for immobilization. Antegrade pyelography is obtained at the same time, which provides excellent delineation of the anatomy of the collecting system.

Voiding Cystourethrography. In all cases of ureteral dilatation, voiding cystourethrography should be obtained to rule out vesicoureteral reflux as a possible cause of the dilatation. The voiding cystourethrogram is also necessary to rule out urethral obstruction, particularly in cases of posterior urethral valves. In infravesical obstruction in infants, the bladder may be palpable because of chronic distention and incomplete emptying. In older children, the urinary flow rate can be measured in a simple noninvasive way with a urinary flow meter, and decreased flow in the presence of normal bladder contraction is diagnostic of infravesical obstruction. When the urethra cannot be catheterized to obtain a voiding cystourethrogram, one must suspect a urethral stricture or an obstructive urethral lesion other than valves. Retrograde urethrography with dye injected into the urethral meatus will help delineate the anatomy of the urethral obstruction.

SPECIFIC TYPES OF URINARY TRACT OBSTRUCTION

HYDROCALYCOSIS. This term refers to a localized dilatation of the calyx caused by obstruction of its infundibulum. Such obstruction can be developmental in origin or secondary to inflammatory processes (particularly tuberculosis, now rarely seen). In congenital obstructions due to stenosis or extrinsic vascular compressions, the presenting symptom is usually pain, which can be relieved by surgical correction of the obstruction. The diagnosis of infundibular obstruction is usually established by intravenous urography.

OBSTRUCTION OF THE URETEROPELVIC JUNCTION. This is the most common obstructive lesion in childhood and is caused most often by congenital stenosis of the ureteropelvic junction. Ureteral kinks, fibrous bands, and apparently aberrant vessels are usually secondary phenomena caused by dilatation of the pelvis above the obstruction. Ureteropelvic junction obstruction most commonly presents as: (1) maternal ultrasonography revealing fetal hydronephrosis; (2) a palpable renal mass in a newborn; (3) abdominal, flank, or back pain; (4) a febrile urinary tract infection; or (5) hematuria after minimal trauma. Twenty per cent of obstructions are bilateral.

The *diagnosis* of this condition is particularly difficult to establish in the asymptomatic infant in whom dilatation of the renal pelvis is found incidentally in a prenatal ultrasonogram. The recognition of unilateral hydronephrosis in the fetus with a normal contralateral kidney and normal volume of amniotic fluid is not an indication for prenatal intervention or early induction of labor. After birth, the sonographic study is repeated to confirm the prenatal finding. If no dilatation is found after birth, the newborn may have had transient fetal hydronephrosis. However, renal ultrasonograms should be repeated at 3 or 6 mo of age, because the dilatation may be minimal after birth but may become more evident later in life. It is best to perform the first postnatal ultrasound study after the 3rd day

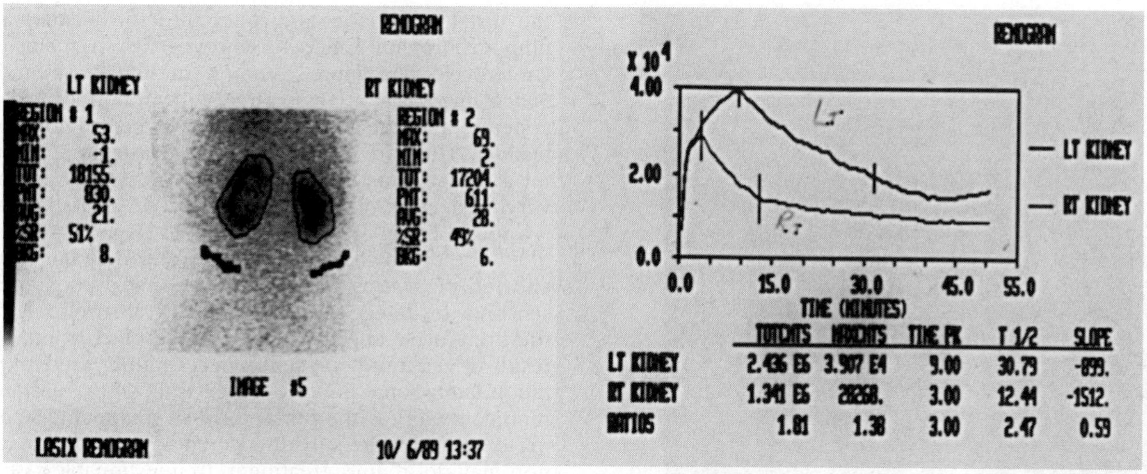

Figure 494–3. DTPA diuresis renogram in a child with left flank pain. The renal function is symmetric. The excretory curve on the right is normal. The kidney excretes the isotope before the injection of furosemide at the 10-min mark. The left kidney retains the isotope and excretes it slowly (T 1/2 30 min) after an injection of furosemide.

of life because oliguria in the newborn may mask the dilatation. If the kidney is hydronephrotic, a period of observation is usually advisable provided that the serum creatinine level and the other kidney are normal. In many infants, mild to moderate hydronephrosis improves with time and may not require treatment, particularly if the calyces are not dilated. However, the natural history of prenatally diagnosed hydronephrosis is incompletely understood and long-term follow-up may be indicated. If the degree of hydronephrosis is marked or if the renal parenchyma is thin, an isotopic renogram will give a gross estimation of the differential renal function. If the function is normal, the infant should be followed with serial ultrasonograms. If there is no improvement, a diuresis renogram after 6–12 mo may help to decide between continued observation or surgical repair. Early surgical repair is indicated in infants in whom the function of the involved kidney is decreased, in those with bilateral involvement or solitary kidneys, and when there is diminished overall renal function. Early repair should also be done when there is a palpable mass.

In older children who present with symptoms, diagnosis is established by intravenous urography (Fig. 494–4). When the kidneys function poorly and are not visualized on the delayed postinjection radiographs, renal ultrasonography will show hydronephrosis. Renography in these cases is useful to determine individual renal function, which is helpful to decide whether to repair or remove the involved kidney. Also, renography provides a baseline to compare postoperative studies. Retrograde pyelography or percutaneous antegrade pyelography on the operating table will establish the point of obstruction. In the *differential diagnosis*, the following entities should be considered: (1) megacalycosis, a congenital nonobstructive dilatation of the calyces without pelvic or ureteric dilatation; (2) vesicoureteral reflux with marked dilatation and kinking of the ureter (voiding cystourethrography should be done on all patients with suspected ureteropelvic junction obstruction); and (3) midureteral or distal ureteral obstructions when the ureter is not well visualized on the urogram.

In the neonate with a renal mass, ureteropelvic junction obstruction must be distinguished from multicystic renal dysplasia, solid renal tumors, and renal vein thrombosis. The clinical picture and imaging studies will help establish an accurate diagnosis. A multicystic dysplastic kidney may mimic a ureteropelvic junction obstruction on ultrasound but invariably shows no function on the radioisotopic renogram. Treatment consists of surgical excision of the obstructed ureteropelvic junction with reanastomosis of the ureter and renal pelvis. The success rate of pyeloplasties is high, but postoperative ultrasound and intravenous urography often show persistent dilatation of the calyces. Diuresis renography is useful for the longitudinal follow-up of these patients.

MIDURETERAL OBSTRUCTION. Congenital ureteral stenosis or ureteral valves can sometimes occur in the midureter. A retrocaval ureter can be partially obstructed; such *circumcaval ureters* are invariably on the right side and represent anomalous development of the vena cava, with persistence of the ventral infrarenal subcardinal veins. Excretory urography shows the right ureter to be medially deviated at the level of the 3rd lumbar vertebra (Fig. 494–5). Surgical treatment is needed only when obstruction is present. Retroperitoneal tumors, fibrosis caused by surgical procedures, inflammatory processes (as in chronic granulomatous disease), and radiation therapy can cause acquired midureteral obstruction.

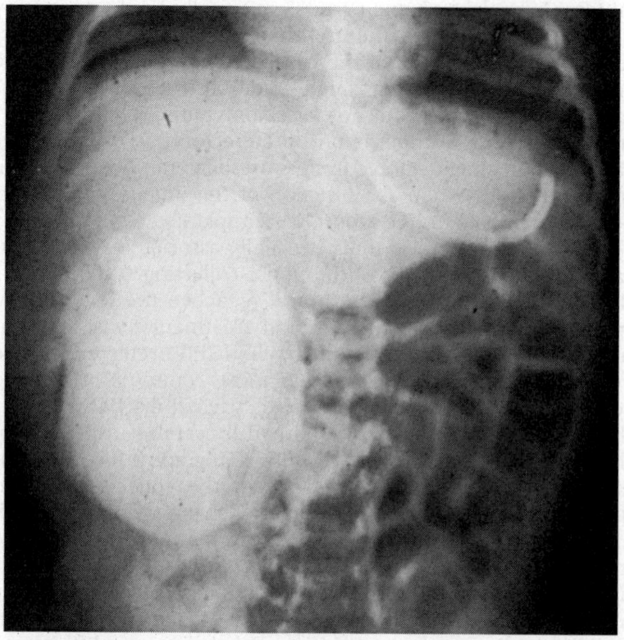

Figure 494–4. Ureteropelvic junction obstruction. Excretory urogram in a newborn, showing dilatation of the right renal pelvis and blunting of the calyces characteristic of a ureteropelvic junction obstruction.

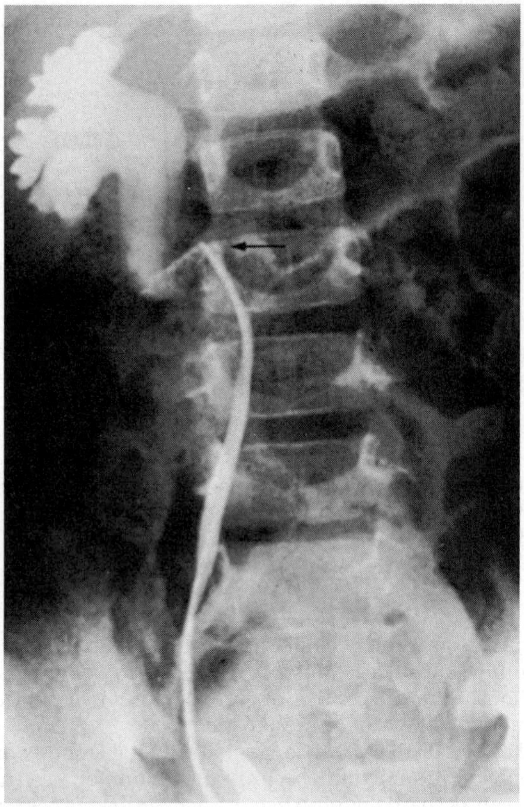

Figure 494–5. Circumcaval ureter. Retrograde pyelogram showing medial deviation of a dilated upper ureter to the level of the 3rd lumbar vertebra, characteristic of a circumcaval ureter.

URETERAL ECTOPIA. An ectopic ureteral orifice can be located anywhere along the path of migration of the mesonephric duct. The ectopic ureter may drain a single collecting system, but more commonly it belongs to the upper moiety of a duplicated collecting system. The ureteral orifice of the upper collecting system is always caudal to that of the lower collecting system. In males, ectopic ureters are usually single; they may enter the bladder neck, the urethra above the external sphincter, the seminal vesicle, or the vas deferens; ectopic ureters are commonly associated with high-grade obstruction and symptoms of urinary tract infection or epididymitis. When the contralateral side is normal, nephroureterectomy is usually indicated. When single ectopic ureters are bilateral, or in the rare unilateral cases when the function of the involved kidney is good, the ectopic ureter should be reimplanted.

In females, ureteral ectopia is usually associated with duplication. When the ureter of the upper collecting system enters the bladder neck or the urethra at or above the level of the sphincter, there is obstruction, and treatment consists of an upper pole nephroureterectomy. When the ureter enters the vestibule, vagina, or uterus, the most common presenting complaint is urinary incontinence or vaginal discharge. In either case, the diagnosis is established by careful inspection of the urogram, renal and bladder ultrasonography (Fig. 494–6), and endoscopy. Although obstructed, the collecting system drained by a duplicated ectopic ureter may be very small and difficult to detect even after careful inspection of the intravenous urogram. A high degree of suspicion is always necessary to establish this diagnosis. In bilateral simple ectopic ureters in the female, there is usually bladder hypoplasia in addition to ureteral obstruction; such cases are difficult to manage and may require bladder reconstruction, urinary diversion, or renal transplantation.

URETEROCELE. Ureterocele is a congenital cystic dilatation of the distal ureter that protrudes into the bladder and has a pinpoint ureteral orifice. Its embryogenesis remains uncertain. Ureteroceles are more common in females than in males. *Simple ureteroceles* are associated with nonduplicated collecting systems, and the orifice is in the expected location in the bladder. They are usually discovered during an investigation for a urinary tract infection. Intravenous pyelography reveals varying degrees of ureteral and calyceal dilatation, and there is a round filling defect in the bladder (Fig. 494–7). In delayed films, the cystic dilatation of the ureter may be clearly visible and full of contrast material. Vesical ultrasonography is very sensitive to detect the ureterocele. Transurethral incision of the ureterocele effectively relieves the obstruction, but it may result in vesicoureteral reflux necessitating ureteral reimplantation later. Some prefer open excision of the ureterocele and reimplantation as the initial form of treatment. Small, simple ureteroceles incidentally discovered without upper tract dilatation may not require treatment. In questionable cases, diuresis renography and pressure flow studies (see earlier) are useful.

More commonly, ureteroceles are associated with ureteral duplication. The ureter involved with the ureterocele drains the upper renal moiety, which frequently functions poorly or is dysplastic because of congenital obstruction. The more cephalad ureter drains the lower renal moiety and frequently refluxes. These *ectopic ureteroceles* may extend submucosally into the posterior urethra. Affected children also present with urinary tract infections. Rarely, large ectopic ureteroceles may cause bladder outlet obstruction and retention of urine; in females, the ureterocele may prolapse from the urethral meatus. Reflux to the ipsilateral lower segment ureter is common. Contralateral reflux is usually present when the bladder neck is obstructed. Both simple and ectopic ureteroceles can be bilateral. Intravenous pyelography usually shows a large filling defect in the bladder corresponding to the ureterocele and characteristic findings of duplication of the collecting systems (poor or absent function of the upper collecting system and caudal displacement of the lower collecting system) (Fig. 494–8). More commonly, these lesions are detected and evaluated with renal and vesical ultrasonography, and isotopic studies to evaluate the function of the various renal segments.

Treatment of ectopic ureteroceles is the excision of the upper

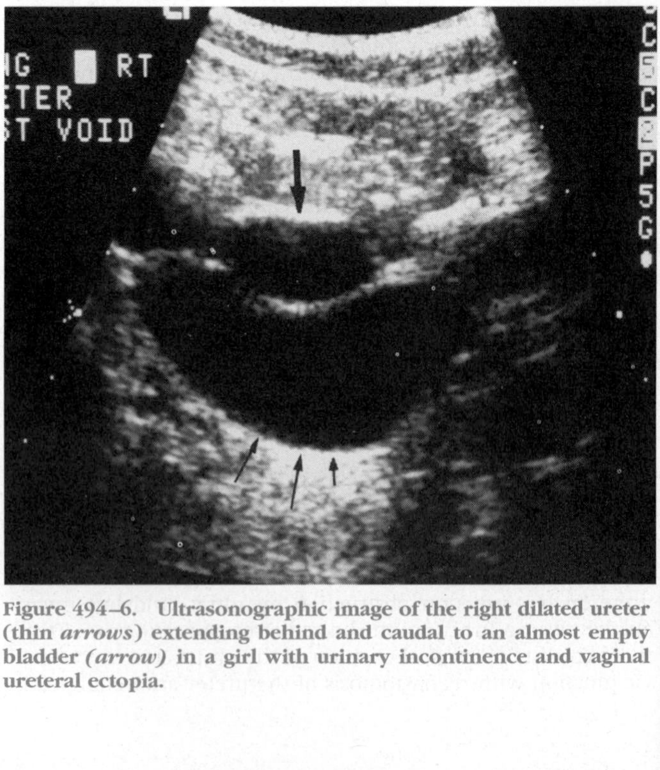

Figure 494–6. Ultrasonographic image of the right dilated ureter (thin *arrows*) extending behind and caudal to an almost empty bladder *(arrow)* in a girl with urinary incontinence and vaginal ureteral ectopia.

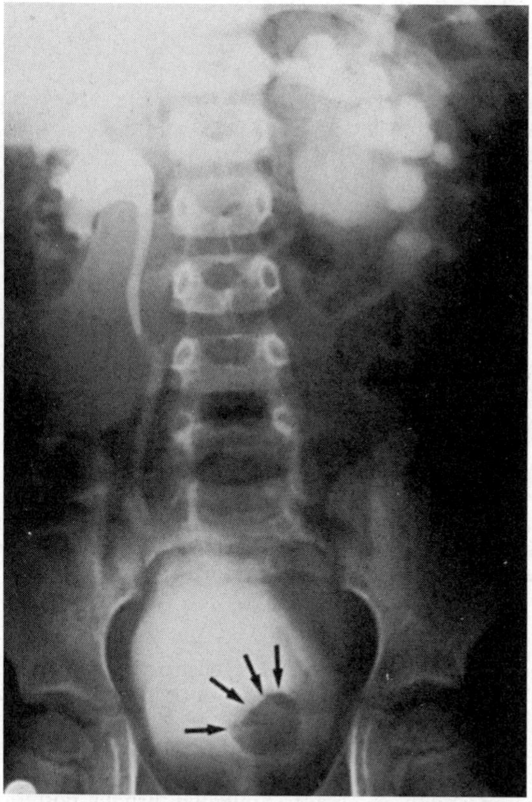

Figure 494–7. Simple intravesical ureterocele. Excretory urogram showing left hydronephrosis and a round filling defect on the left side of the bladder corresponding to a simple ureterocele causing left ureteral obstruction.

collecting system, involving partial nephrectomy and ureterectomy. When the ectopic ureterocele is small and there is low grade or no reflux in the ipsilateral duplicated ureter, the decompressed ureterocele need not be excised and usually will cause no further problems. Large ureteroceles, however, or those with high-grade reflux to the ipsilateral lower ureter, are best treated by excision of the ureterocele and reimplantation of the remaining ureter, plus partial upper moiety nephroureterectomy. This can usually be accomplished in a single operation. In the treatment of an acutely ill, septic infant with an obstructing ureterocele, drainage of the involved collecting system may be necessary, either transureterally or by percutaneous nephrostomy of the upper collecting system.

MEGAURETER. This term refers generally to the dilated ureter. A classification of megaureters is given in Table 494–2. In this section, primary obstructed and nonrefluxing nonobstructed megaureters will be discussed. Megaureters are usually discovered through ultrasonography of the kidneys and the bladder, or intravenous urography done for urinary tract infections, hematuria, or abdominal pain. A careful history, physical examination, and voiding cystourethrography will help to rule out causes of secondary megaureters and refluxing megaureters as well as the prune-belly syndrome. Primary obstructed megaureters and nonobstructed megaureters probably represent opposite extremes of a spectrum of the same anomaly.

Radiographically, the distal ureter is more dilated in its distal segment and tapers abruptly at or above the junction of the bladder (Fig. 494–9). The lesion may be unilateral or bilateral. Dilatation of the upper collecting system and calyceal blunting are suggestive of obstruction. In most cases, however, diuresis renography, pressure flow studies, and careful follow-up are needed to differentiate obstructed from nonobstructed megaureters. Obstructed megaureters require surgical treatment, with tapering and reimplantation of the ureter. The results of surgical reconstruction are usually good, but the prognosis depends on pre-existing renal function and whether complications develop.

PRUNE-BELLY SYNDROME. This syndrome, also called *abdominal muscle deficiency syndrome* or *Eagle-Barrett syndrome,* occurs in approximately 1/40,000 births. The characteristic association of deficient abdominal muscles, undescended testes, and urinary tract abnormalities probably results from severe urethral obstruction in fetal life (Fig. 494–10). Oligohydramnios and pulmonary hypoplasia are frequent complications in the perinatal period. Many affected infants are stillborn. Urinary tract abnormalities include massive dilatation of the ureters and upper tracts, and a very large bladder, with a patent urachus or a urachal diverticulum. There may be vesicoureteral reflux. The prostatic urethra is usually dilated and the prostate is hypoplastic. The anterior urethra may be dilated, resulting in a megalourethra. Rarely, there is urethral stenosis or atresia. The kidneys usually show various degrees of dysplasia, and the testes are usually intra-abdominal. There is often malrotation of the bowel with a universal mesentery. Cardiac abnormalities occur in 10% of cases, and more than 50% have abnormalities of the musculoskeletal system, including limb abnormalities and scoliosis. Only about 3% of patients with prune-belly syndrome are females. In females, anomalies of the urethra, uterus, and vagina are usually present.

One fourth of the patients have demonstrable urethral obstruction at the time of birth. When no obstruction is present, the goal of treatment is the prevention of urinary tract infection. When obstruction of the ureters or urethra can be demonstrated or is suspected, temporary drainage procedures, such as pyelostomies or vesicostomies, may help to preserve renal

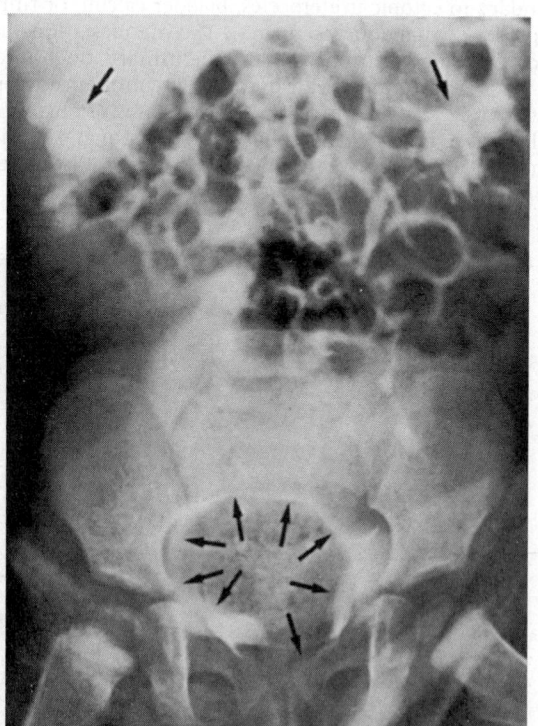

Figure 494–8. Bilateral ectopic ureteroceles. Excretory urogram of a 1-yr-old girl with a history of febrile urinary tract infections. The large filling defect in the bladder represents bilateral ectopic ureteroceles. The visualized portion of the upper urinary tracts reveals only the lower moiety of the duplicated kidneys, with a characteristic drooping lily configuration. The upper moieties drained by the ureters involved in the ureteroceles function poorly and are not opacified. Most cases of ectopic ureteroceles are unilateral.

■ TABLE 494–2 International Classification of Megaureters

	Primary	Secondary
Obstructed	Intrinsic ureteral obstruction	Associated with urethral obstruction or extrinsic lesions
Refluxing	Reflux is only abnormality	Associated with bladder outlet obstruction or neurogenic bladder
Nonrefluxing, nonobstructed	Idiopathic ureteral dilatation	Associated with polyuria (diabetes insipidus) or infection

From King LR: Ureter and ureterovesical junction. In: *Kelalis PP, King LR, Belman AB (eds):* Clinical Pediatric Urology. *Philadelphia, WB Saunders, 1985, p 486.*

function until the child is old enough for reconstructive surgery. Some children with prune-belly syndrome have been found to have classic or atypical posterior urethral valves. Urinary tract infections are frequent and should be treated promptly. Antibacterial prophylaxis is often necessary. Correction of the undescended testis by orchidopexy in these children can be quite difficult and is best accomplished in the 1st yr of life. Reconstruction of the abdominal wall offers cosmetic and functional benefits.

The prognosis ultimately depends on the degree of pulmonary and renal dysplasia. One third of children with prune-belly syndrome are stillborn or die in the first few months of life of pulmonary complications. Of the long-term survivors, one half develop chronic renal failure from dysplasia or complications of infection or reflux, and eventually require renal transplantation. The results of renal transplantation in these patients are favorable.

BLADDER NECK OBSTRUCTION. Bladder neck obstruction is usually secondary to ectopic ureteroceles, bladder calculi, or tumors of the prostate (rhabdomyosarcoma). The manifestations include difficulty voiding, urinary retention, urinary tract infection, and bladder distention with overflow incontinence. Apparent bladder neck obstruction is common in cases of posterior urethral valves, but it seldom has any functional significance. Primary bladder neck obstruction is exceptional in males and, according to current thinking, probably never occurs in females. Functional bladder neck obstruction can also result from nonrelaxation of the bladder neck in neurogenic bladder dysfunction.

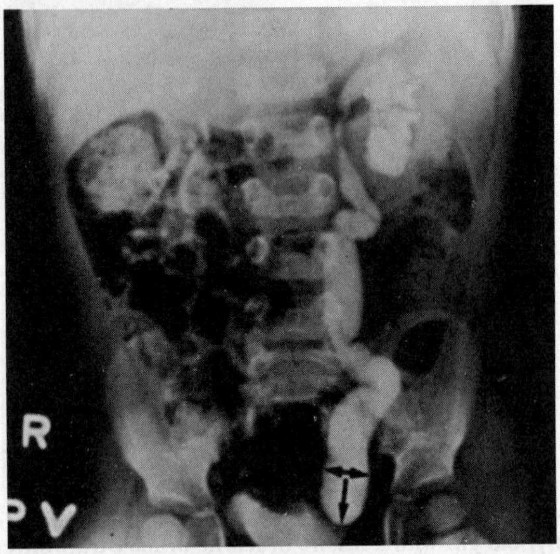

Figure 494–9. Obstructed megaureter. Excretory urogram in a girl with a history of a febrile urinary tract infection. The right side is normal. The left side reveals hydroureteronephrosis with predominant dilatation of the distal ureter. Note the characteristic appearance of the distal ureter. There was no vesicoureteral reflux. The diagnosis of obstruction was confirmed by pressure-flow studies.

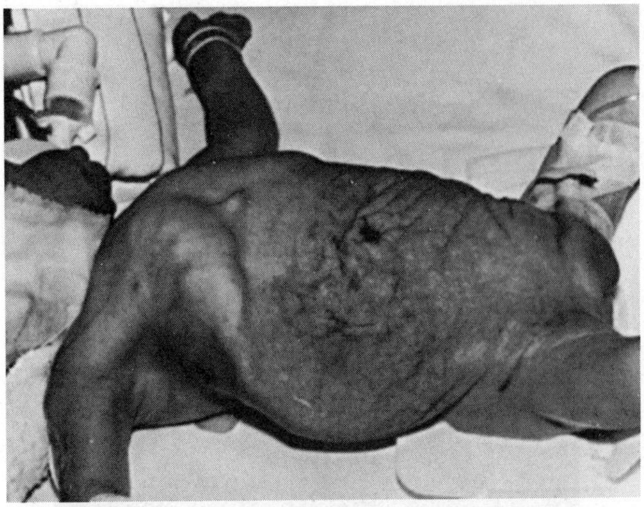

Figure 494–10. Eagle-Barrett syndrome. Photograph of a 1,600-g newborn with the prune-belly syndrome. Note the lack of tonicity of the abdominal wall and the wrinkled appearance of the skin.

POSTERIOR URETHRAL VALVES. The most common types of urethral valves are located in the posterior urethra. They are membranes with an eccentric opening, usually posterior, that arise from the verumontanum in males and extend distally and attach to the anterolateral walls of the urethra. Valves are congenitally abnormal structures of unclear embryologic origin and cause varying degrees of obstruction. The prostatic urethra dilates and the detrusor muscle and bladder neck hypertrophy. There may be vesicoureteral reflux or distal ureteral obstruction resulting from a chronically distended bladder or bladder muscle hypertrophy. The renal changes range from mild hydronephrosis to severe dysplasia; their severity probably depends on the severity of the obstruction and the time of its onset in fetal life. As in other cases of obstruction or renal dysplasia, there may be oligohydramnios and pulmonary hypoplasia.

With increasing frequency, posterior urethral valves are being discovered prenatally when maternal ultrasonography reveals bilateral hydronephrosis, a dilated bladder, and, if the obstruction is severe, oligohydramnios. Prenatal bladder decompression by percutaneous vesicoamniotic shunt or open fetal surgery has been reported. However, experimental and clinical evidence of the possible benefits of fetal intervention is lacking, and these procedures should be considered experimental. Prenatally diagnosed posterior urethral valves carry a worse prognosis than those detected after birth. In the male neonate, posterior urethral valves are suspected when there is a palpably distended bladder and the urinary stream is weak. If the obstruction is severe and goes unrecognized during the neonatal period, infants will present later in life with failure to thrive due to uremia or sepsis caused by infection in the obstructed urinary tract. With lesser degrees of obstruction, children present later in life with difficulty in maintaining urinary continence during the daytime or with urinary tract infections. The diagnosis is established by voiding cystourethrography (Fig. 494–11).

Vesicoureteral reflux is present in two thirds of cases and may be unilateral or bilateral. The prognosis for renal function is worse when reflux is present. Once the diagnosis is established, renal function and the anatomy of the upper urinary tract should be carefully evaluated. In the healthy neonate, a small polyethylene feeding tube (No. 5 French or No. 8

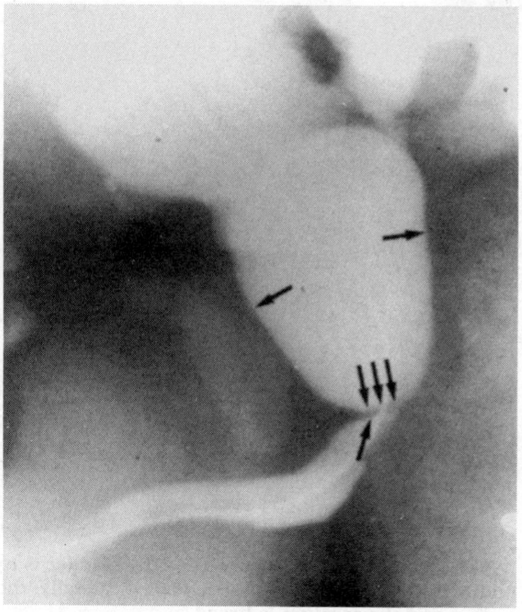

Figure 494–11. Posterior urethral valves. Voiding cystourethrogram in an infant with posterior urethral valves. Note the dilatation of the prostatic urethra and the transverse linear filling defect corresponding to the valves.

French) is inserted in the bladder and left indwelling for several days. If the serum creatinine level remains normal or returns to normal, treatment is by primary ablation of the valves through a transurethral approach or by temporary vesicostomy. If the urethral caliber is insufficient for transurethral ablation, temporary vesicostomy is preferred, to be followed by closure of the vesicostomy and transurethral ablation of the valves at a later date when the growth of the child permits use of urethral instrumentation.

If the serum creatinine level remains high or increases despite bladder drainage by a small catheter, secondary ureteral obstruction, irreversible renal damage, or renal dysplasia should be suspected. In such cases, upper tract drainage by cutaneous pyelostomy or high ureterostomy is necessary. If renal function does not improve, the child should have reconstructive surgery at a relatively early age to prevent infections and restore bladder function before the need for renal transplantation arises. If renal function improves between the ages of 6 mo and 1 yr, the ureters are re-evaluated by pressure flow studies. Distal obstruction caused by hypertrophy of the detrusor muscle may reverse spontaneously; if it persists, however, the child should have ablation of the valves, closure of the pyelostomies, and correction of the distal ureteral obstruction.

Infants presenting later in life with uremia without infection should be evaluated and treated following identical guidelines. In the septic and uremic infant, lifesaving measures must include prompt correction of the electrolyte imbalance and control of the infection by appropriate antibiotics. Drainage of the upper tracts by percutaneous nephrostomy and hemodialysis are frequently required. After the patient's condition becomes stable, step-by-step evaluation and treatment can be undertaken. Prolonged use of intubated nephrostomy drainage is inconvenient for the parents, introduces infection, and is generally detrimental to renal function.

Most children presenting with incontinence can be treated by primary valve ablation. When vesicoureteral reflux is present, expectant treatment and suppressive doses of antibacterial drugs are advisable; however, if reflux persists more than 1 yr after ablation of the valves and if the function of the involved kidney warrants it, surgical correction should be undertaken.

There is some degree of urinary incontinence in up to 50% of children after treatment of posterior urethral valves. Assuming there has been no surgical damage to the sphincter, the dilatation of the prostatic urethra, poor bladder compliance, and polyuria from renal damage are all important factors that contribute to incontinence. Urinary incontinence usually improves with age, particularly after puberty.

The prognosis in the newborn is related to the degree of pulmonary hypoplasia and potential for recovery of renal function. Severely affected infants are often stillborn. Of those who survive the neonatal period, approximately one third will retain some degree of renal insufficiency and many will eventually require renal transplantation. Renal transplantation in children with posterior urethral valves has a lower success rate than transplantation in children with normal bladders, presumably because of the adverse influence of altered bladder function on graft function and survival. Meticulous attention to bladder compliance, emptying, and infection may improve results in the future.

URETHRAL STRICTURES. Urethral strictures *in males* are rarely congenital. They usually result from urethral trauma, either iatrogenic (catheterization, endoscopic procedures, or previous urethral reconstruction) or accidental (straddling injuries or pelvic fractures). Because these lesions may develop gradually, the decrease in force of the urinary stream is seldom noticed by the child or his or her parents. More commonly, the obstruction causes symptoms of bladder instability, hematuria, or dysuria. Catheterization of the bladder is usually impossible. The diagnosis is made by a voiding film obtained during intravenous urography; retrograde urethrography and endoscopy are confirmatory. Endoscopic treatment of short strictures by dilatation or internal urethrotomy is usually successful. Longer strictures surrounded by periurethral fibrosis often require urethroplasty. Repeated endoscopic procedures should generally be avoided, as they may cause additional urethral damage. Noninvasive measurement of the urinary flow rate and pattern is useful for diagnosis and follow-up.

In females, true urethral strictures are exceptional, because the female urethra is protected from trauma, particularly in childhood. In the past it was thought that the urethral ring commonly caused obstruction of the female urethra and urinary tract infection and that affected girls benefited from urethral dilatation. The diagnosis was suspected when a "spinning top" deformity of the urethra was found in the voiding cystourethrogram and was confirmed by urethral calibration. Treatment for this condition invariably included antibiotic therapy, and adequately controlled studies were not done. Moreover, other studies have found no correlation between the radiologic appearance of the urethra in the voiding cystourethrogram and the urethral caliber, and no significant difference in urethral caliber between females with recurrent cystitis and normal age-matched controls. This area remains somewhat controversial, but endoscopy and urethral dilatation are seldom justified solely by the radiologic appearance of the urethra or by a history of recurrent urinary tract infections. Likewise, there is no justification for performing urethral dilatation in girls with diurnal or nocturnal enuresis because there is no evidence that urethral obstruction plays a role in the pathogenesis of these symptoms. The evaluation and treatment of these conditions are discussed in Chapter 497.

ANTERIOR URETHRAL VALVES AND URETHRAL DIVERTICULA IN THE MALE. *Anterior urethral valves* are usually associated with congenital urethral diverticulum. They are considerably rarer than valves of the posterior urethra, but they may cause similar symptoms and have identical effects on the urinary tract. The diagnosis is established on voiding cystourethrography. *Urethral diverticula* are discovered on voiding cystourethrography, often during evaluation for hematuria or urinary tract infections. Many diverticula are believed to arise from dilatations of Cowper glands and ducts. Small diverticula require no treatment; larger ones are usually managed endoscopically.

Fusiform dilatation of the urethra or megalourethra may result from underdevelopment of the corpus spongiosum and support structures of the urethra. This is commonly associated with the prune-belly syndrome.

MALE URETHRAL MEATAL STENOSIS. Congenital stenosis of the urethral meatus in the male is rare. It has in the past probably been overdiagnosed, and unrelated conditions, such as nocturnal enuresis, have been blamed on presumed meatal stenosis. True urethral meatal stenosis (a meatus less than No. 8 French in boys under 4 yr old, or less than No. 10 French in prepubertal boys over the age of 10) usually results from inflammation associated with ammoniacal dermatitis of the glans following neonatal circumcision. Children with hypospadias rarely may have stenosis of the urethral meatus. The treatment of symptomatic urethral meatal stenosis is by a meatoplasty with careful follow-up to avoid reapproximation of the edges of the enlarged meatus. A more common abnormality is the development of a thin ventral membrane that partially covers the meatus and produces dorsal deflection of the urinary stream. Even though the actual meatus is often of normal caliber, these children may require meatoplasty to allow them to aim their urinary stream as desired.

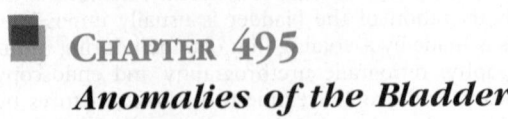

CHAPTER 495
Anomalies of the Bladder

BLADDER EXSTROPHY

Exstrophy of the urinary bladder occurs about once in every 40,000 births. It is more common in boys than in girls. The severity ranges from a small cutaneous fistula in the abdominal wall or simple epispadias to complete exstrophy of the cloaca involving exposure of the entire hindgut and the bladder.

CLINICAL MANIFESTATIONS. These anomalies result when the mesoderm fails to invade the cephalad extension of the cloacal membrane; the extent of this failure determines the degree of the anomaly. In classic bladder exstrophy (Fig. 495–1), the bladder protrudes from the abdominal wall and its mucosa is exposed. The umbilicus is displaced downward, the pubic rami are widely separated in the midline, and the recti muscles are separated. In males there is complete epispadias with a wide and shallow scrotum. Undescended testes and inguinal hernias are common. Females also have epispadias, with duplication of the clitoris and wide separation of the labia. The anus is displaced anteriorly in both sexes, and there may be rectal prolapse. The consequences of untreated bladder exstrophy are total urinary incontinence and an increased incidence of bladder cancer, usually adenocarcinoma. The genital deformities produce sexual disability in both sexes, but particularly in the male. The wide separation of the pubic rami causes a characteristic broad-based gait but no significant disability.

TREATMENT. Management of bladder exstrophy should start at birth. The bladder should be covered with a Silastic shield or another appropriate plastic dressing that will prevent desiccation of the bladder mucosa but allow urinary drainage. Application of gauze or Vaseline-gauze to the bladder mucosa should be avoided. The infant should then be transferred promptly to a center equipped for the treatment of such anomalies.

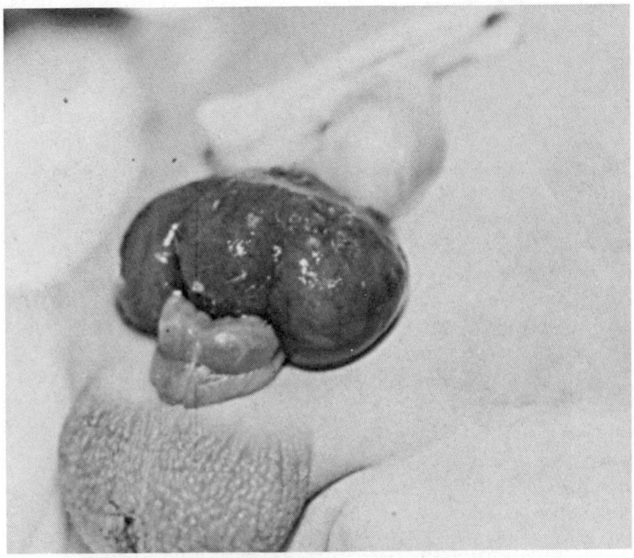

Figure 495–1. Classic bladder exstrophy. The bladder is exposed in the midline; the umbilical cord is displaced caudally; the penis is epispadiac; and the scrotum is broad.

Closure of the exstrophied bladder is the preferred treatment, ideally performed during the first 48 hr of life before permanent changes in the bladder wall are established. At this time the flexibility of the pelvic joints allows precise reconstruction of the bladder and prostatic urethra in the male, with approximation of the pubic rami and reconstruction of the abdominal wall without the iliac osteostomies that are often required in the older child. This treatment can be applied to almost all infants with classic bladder exstrophy. Treatment should be deferred in certain exceptional circumstances when surgery would be excessively risky or complex, such as when the bladder is extremely small or there are upper tract changes, or when there are complex genital anomalies such as complete duplication of the penis.

The purpose of the initial operation is the precise closure of the bladder and prostatic urethra in the male, elongation of the urethral plate and penis, and closure of the abdominal wall. Postoperatively, the infant's upper urinary tract is watched closely for the possible development of hydronephrosis and infection. The majority of such infants have vesicoureteral reflux and should receive antibiotics. When the child is between 1 and 2 yr old, the resulting epispadias is repaired to create an anterior urethra and correct the malformation of the penis. Treatment of the incontinence by bladder neck reconstruction is reserved for children who remain incontinent of urine after they have gained rectal control.

PROGNOSIS. This plan of treatment has yielded less than 15% deterioration of the upper urinary tract and over 70% continence in some centers. This continence rate reflects not only the successful reconstruction but also the quality and size of the bladder. It appears that children who have reconstructive surgery as newborns have a greater chance for obtaining a normally functioning bladder. Children whose sphincters cannot be successfully reconstructed should have artificial sphincters implanted. If the cause of incontinence is a small bladder capacity, an augmentation cystoplasty using a segment of the large bowel will help obtain continence. The exceptional children whose anomaly cannot be reconstructed can have a urinary diversion with a continent abdominal stoma. Ureterosigmoidostomy has been popular in the past and is still employed in some centers; it is attractive because it avoids the need for external urinary diversion. This operation, however, carries a significant risk of chronic pyelonephritis, of upper urinary tract damage, of electrolyte imbalance resulting from absorption of hydrogen ions and chloride in the intestine, and of colonic carcinoma after a long latency period.

Other Exstrophy Anomalies

The more complex cases of *cloacal exstrophy* may have severe abnormalities of the colon and the rectum, and often have a short bowel syndrome. Mortality in infancy is high for such patients, but some can undergo genital reconstruction and others can be helped with permanent urinary diversions and colostomies. Because genital reconstruction in males with cloacal exstrophy is extremely difficult, most authors recommend assigning female gender to such infants.

Epispadias is in the spectrum of exstrophy anomalies. Distal epispadias should be repaired by reconstructing the urethra and the penis. The more severe cases of epispadias also have separation of the pubic rami and urinary incontinence. Such children require surgical reconstructions analogous to those of the 2nd and 3rd stages of management of patients with classic bladder exstrophy.

BLADDER DIVERTICULA

Bladder diverticula usually occur at the ureterovesical junction and are associated with vesicoureteral reflux (see Fig. 483–3). Congenital diverticula in other locations also occur. Bladder diverticula are also commonly associated with distal urethral obstruction or neurogenic bladder dysfunction. Small diverticula require no treatment other than that of the primary disease, whereas large diverticula may contribute to inefficient voiding, residual urine, urinary stasis, and urinary tract infections and should be excised.

URACHAL ANOMALIES

Urachal abnormalities are more common in males than in females. A patent urachus can occur as an isolated anomaly, in which case it should be corrected surgically, or it may be associated with prune-belly syndrome. Other anomalies related to the urachus are cysts and bladder diverticula and umbilical sinus; these should be excised.

CHAPTER 496

Neurogenic Bladder

Neurogenic bladder dysfunction in children is often congenital and may result from myelomeningocele, lipomeningocele, sacral agenesis, or other spinal abnormalities. Acquired diseases and traumatic lesions of the spinal cord are less frequent. Cerebral palsy, central nervous system tumors and their treatment, and pelvic operations such as repair of imperforate anus or excision of a sacrococcygeal teratoma can result in abnormal innervation of the bladder and the sphincters. The two most important consequences of neurogenic bladder dysfunction are upper tract deterioration and urinary incontinence.

Renal damage is the result of lack of coordination between the contraction of the detrusor muscle and the relaxation of the sphincter, normally a function located in the brain stem. This dys-synergia results in functional obstruction of the bladder outlet, leading to high intravesical pressures, bladder muscle hypertrophy and trabeculation, vesicoureteral reflux, and rapid deterioration of the upper tracts. Infection often compounds the problem. For example, vesicoureteral reflux is present in 30% of neonates with myelomeningocele and develops later in life in another 20%. Reflux secondary to neurogenic bladder has much more severe consequences than primary reflux. However, not all children with myelomeningocele (or any other neurologic anomaly) have similar patterns of lower tract dysfunction, so that its occurrence cannot be predicted accurately from the neurologic examination or radiographic appearance of the spine. Accordingly, accurate urodynamic studies (by cystometrography and sphincter electromyography) and radiologic evaluation of the urinary tract are required in every case. If the bladder is atonic or the sphincters are denervated, bladder pressure tends to be low, and vesicoureteral reflux is unlikely to develop, even when bladder emptying is incomplete.

Urinary incontinence in the child with neurogenic bladder can result from total or partial denervation of the sphincter, from bladder hyper-reflexia or poor bladder compliance, from chronic urinary retention, or from a combination of factors. The treatment of children with neurogenic bladder aims at protecting the upper urinary tracts and eventually providing continence. Supravesical diversion, once commonly performed to achieve these goals, yielded unsatisfactory long-term results and is now seldom employed. The neonate with low intravesical pressures and no vesicoureteral reflux can be treated expectantly with follow-up renal ultrasound to detect possible development of hydronephrosis and radioisotopic cystography for the early detection of reflux. Occasionally, limited intravenous pyelography is needed as well. Recurrent urinary tract infections may require prolonged antibiotic prophylaxis (see Chapter 492). Urodynamic studies should be repeated at 6 mo of age to detect possible neurologic changes following repair of the myelomeningocele. The neurologic lesion in myelomeningocele can vary with time owing to tethering of the spinal cord or to development of secondary central changes.

When reflux is present or there are elevated intravesical pressures (indicative of high risk for developing reflux), treatment with antibacterial prophylaxis, intermittent catheterization, and often anticholinergic drugs (oxybutynin 0.2 mg/kg/24 hr in two divided doses) will cure the reflux in up to 40% of patients without ureteral dilation (grades I and II). Children with more severe reflux require corrective surgery followed by intermittent catheterization and anticholinergic drugs. When intermittent catheterization is impossible, as may be the case in male neonates and small infants, when there are urethral abnormalities that preclude catheterization, or when anticholinergics are not well tolerated, a temporary cutaneous vesicostomy provides effective, temporary bladder decompression. Failure of these methods to relieve intravesical pressures is an indication for augmentation enterocystoplasty and intermittent catheterization. Attempts to denervate the bladder to control bladder hypertonicity have yielded unsatisfactory long-term results.

The treatment of incontinence should be tailored to the individual case. If the sphincter tone is sufficient and the bladder has adequate compliance, intermittent catheterization every 4 hr is usually successful in keeping the child dry. Anticholinergic drugs are sometimes needed to relax the bladder and enhance continence. Most children 7–8 yr old who have adequate manual dexterity can learn the technique of intermittent self-catheterization. Bacteriuria is seen in up to 50% of children using intermittent self-catheterization, but it seldom causes symptoms. In the absence of reflux, there seems to be little cause for concern. Antibacterial prophylaxis can often be effective in keeping the urine sterile while intermittent catheterization is used.

When the bladder capacity and compliance are adequate but the urethral resistance is low, implantation of an artificial sphincter is usually successful. This sphincter consists of an inflatable cuff that is placed around the bladder neck, a pressure-regulating balloon implanted in the extraperitoneal space, and a pumping mechanism that is implanted in the scrotum of males and in the labia of females. Sometimes bladder augmentation by enterocystoplasty alone or in combination with other means to increase outlet resistance is necessary, along with intermittent catheterization. With the treatment as outlined earlier and lifelong follow-up, urinary diversion can be avoided in most cases, children can reach a satisfactory degree of continence, and the chances of upper tract deterioration are low (Fig. 496–1).

The more frequent application of *enterocystoplasty* for increasing bladder capacity—not only in children with neurogenic bladder but also in some patients with bladder exstrophy, posterior urethral valves, and other congenital and acquired bladder disorders that result in a small functional bladder capacity—requires that pediatricians be informed about some of the implications of these operations. The bowel segments used to enlarge the bladder are isolated from the right or left side of the colon and the ileum. Most children with augmented bladders require intermittent catheterization for emptying. The urine is usually colonized with gram-negative bacteria, and

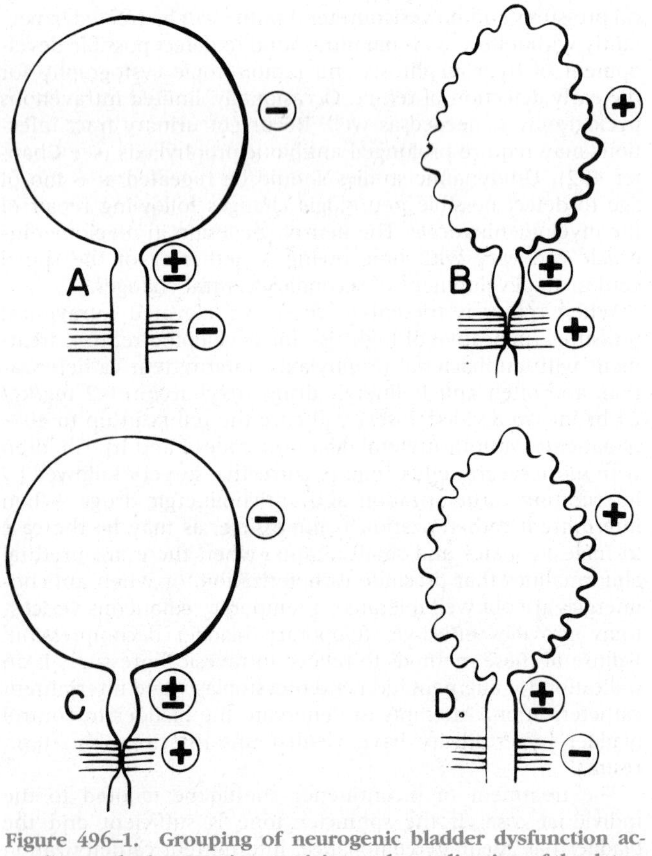

Figure 496–1. Grouping of neurogenic bladder dysfunction according to the innervation, tonicity, and coordination of the detrusor and sphincters described by Guzman. This grouping is based on data from imaging studies, cystometrography, and electromyography of the sphincters. Patients in group B are at risk of developing reflux and hydronephrosis. For guidance in the treatment of incontinence, group *A* benefits from procedures that increase outlet resistance, group *B* from anticholinergics or bladder augmentation surgery, and group *C* from intermittent catheterization, and group *D* requires both increased outlet resistance and pharmacologic or surgical bladder enlargement. Most patients require intermittent catheterization to empty. (Modified from Gonzalez R: Urinary incontinence. *In*: Kelalis PK, King LR, Belman AB (eds): Clinical Pediatric Urology. Philadelphia, WB Saunders, 1992, p 387.)

attempts to sterilize the urine for prolonged periods of time usually fail. Therefore, only symptomatic urinary tract infections should be treated in these patients. Even when there is no reflux, the upper tracts may be colonized as well. However, there is no evidence that chronic bacteriuria in these patients is associated with renal damage. Nevertheless, long-term follow-up is necessary.

The enteric mucosal surface in contact with the urine absorbs ammonium, chloride, and hydrogen ions and loses potassium. Hyperchloremic metabolic acidosis can result and may require medical treatment. Chronic acidosis may compromise skeletal growth. This complication is more common in patients with compromised renal function. To overcome this limitation of enterocystoplasty in patients with chronic renal insufficiency, a gastric segment can be used instead of a segment of the small or large intestine. The stomach secretes chloride and hydrogen ions; thus, pre-existing metabolic acidosis will remain stable or improve. However, the possibility of intractable metabolic alkalosis and peptic ulceration of the augmentation has diminished the enthusiasm for this procedure.

Perforation of the augmented bladder and peritonitis are serious complications that have occurred in up to 10% of patients in some series. Prompt diagnosis and treatment are lifesaving. Although the precise pathogenesis of these perforations remains unclear, meticulous adherence to the prescribed program of intermittent catheterization to avoid bladder overdistention is important.

The potential for malignancy secondary to enterocystoplasty is unknown but, based on past experience with ureterosigmoidostomy and some reported cases, it is prudent to advise yearly endoscopic examinations or urine cytology beginning in the 7th–10th postoperative years.

CHAPTER 497
Voiding Dysfunction

NOCTURNAL ENURESIS (see Chapter 21.3)

Enuresis is the occurrence of involuntary voiding at an age when volitional control of micturition is expected. *Nocturnal enuresis* without overt daytime voiding symptoms affects up to 20% of children at the age of 5 yr; it ceases spontaneously in approximately 15% of the involved children every year thereafter. Its frequency among adults is probably less than 1%. The cause of nocturnal enuresis is not precisely known but appears to involve delayed maturation of the cortical mechanisms that allow voluntary control of the micturition reflex. Children with the disorder produce more urine at night than during the daytime, a reversal of the normal pattern that may be due to an alteration of the circadian rhythm of antidiuretic hormone (ADH) secretion. The reason why enuretic children fail to awaken when the bladder is full is unknown. The disorder can be primary (when the child never has a period of night-time continence) or secondary (developing in a formerly "dry" child following some emotionally disruptive event). Nocturnal enuresis is three times more common in males than in females, and there is often a family history of bedwetting.

The child with nocturnal enuresis should be examined carefully for neurologic and spinal abnormalities. A careful history should be obtained, especially with respect to fluid intake and urinary output. Children with diabetes insipidus, diabetes mellitus, and chronic renal disease may have high obligatory urinary output and a compensatory polydipsia. A complete examination should include palpation of the abdomen and rectal examination after voiding, to assess the possibility of a chronically distended bladder. If possible, the child should be watched during micturition to observe the force and quality of the urinary stream; measurement of the urinary flow rate helps rule out obstructive lesions. Bacteriuria has increased frequency in enuretic girls and, if found, should be investigated and treated (see Chapter 492), though this will not always lead to resolution of bedwetting. Urinalysis should be obtained after an overnight fast and evaluated for specific gravity or osmolality, or both, in order to exclude polyuria as a cause of frequency and incontinence, and to ascertain that the concentrating ability is normal. The absence of glycosuria should be confirmed. Urine culture should be done routinely. If there are no daytime symptoms and if the physical examination, urinalysis, and culture are normal, then further evaluation for urinary tract pathology is not warranted, even in older children.

The best approach to treatment is to assure parents that the problem is self-limited and to eliminate punitive measures that may adversely affect the psychologic development of the child (see Chapter 21.3). Nasal administration at bedtime of desmopressin (DDAVP, 20–40 μg), a synthetic analog of ADH, stops bedwetting in 60–75% of children during its administration but does not cure the condition permanently. DDAVP is more effective when there is a family history of enuresis. The role of imipramine and conditioning alarm devices is very limited.

UNSTABLE BLADDER

Voiding dysfunction not related to neurologic abnormalities or dysfunction is common in children. The child with an unstable bladder usually exhibits urinary frequency, urgency, and episodes of diurnal urinary incontinence with or without bladder pain. Such symptoms are seen also in about 15% of children with nocturnal enuresis, but sometimes the daytime symptoms predominate and certainly always have greater psychosocial consequences, particularly in school-age children. In females, a history of recurrent urinary tract infection is common, but incontinence may persist long after infections are brought under control. It is not clear in these cases if the voiding dysfunction is a sequel of the infections or if the voiding dysfunction disposes to recurrent infections. In other female cases and usually in male cases, there is no antecedent history of infection and the cause of uninhibited bladder is obscure. Many authors attribute it to a delayed maturation of the neurologic mechanisms that modulate the spinal micturition reflex. Bladder outlet obstructions result in detrusor hyper-reflexia and can also lead to uninhibited bladder contractions.

In the evaluation of affected children, a careful history helps rule out the possibility of previous urinary tract infections. Constipation is sometimes associated. Its treatment may lead to improvement of the urinary symptoms. The physical examination is directed at detecting neurologic abnormalities and residual urine after voiding. Urinalysis and urine culture rule out infection and causes of polyuria. Examination of the urinary flow rate by visual inspection of the urinary stream or, ideally, with a uroflowmeter helps rule out gross urethral obstruction. Abdominal ultrasound excludes hydronephrosis and gross bladder abnormalities, and confirms the completeness of bladder emptying. In males, voiding cystourethrography is usually necessary to rule out bladder or urethral abnormalities. If the evaluation rules out significant urinary tract pathology, a therapeutic trial with oxybutynin or other anticholinergic drugs is warranted and often effective. The treatment is usually prolonged and should be interrupted periodically to determine its continued need. If there is a history of cystitis but no other abnormalities such as vesicoureteral reflux that require additional evaluation and treatment, prophylactic antibacterial agents help prevent recurrence of infection, which can exacerbate bladder instability. Children not responding to this simple treatment should be evaluated endoscopically and urodynamically to rule out other possible forms of bladder or sphincter dysfunction.

NON-NEUROGENIC NEUROGENIC BLADDER

This is a more serious but less common disorder involving failure of the external sphincter to relax during voiding, in children without neurologic abnormalities. Children with this syndrome, also called non-neurogenic detrusor/sphincter dyssynergia, exhibit daytime and night-time wetting. There is usually a history of urinary tract infections and constipation, with or without encopresis. Evaluation of affected children usually reveals vesicoureteral reflux, a trabeculated bladder, and decreased urinary flow rate with an intermittent pattern. The pathogenesis of this syndrome appears to involve problems during toilet training, because the syndrome is not seen in children before the age when voluntary micturition occurs. The urodynamic evaluation should be complemented with magnetic resonance imaging of the spine to rule out a neurologic cause for the bladder dysfunction. The treatment is usually difficult and requires appropriate treatment of the reflux with antibacterial prophylaxis. Behavioral modification and encouragement of relaxation during voiding are sometimes useful. Biofeedback has been used successfully in older children to teach relaxation of the external sphincter. Some investigators have recommended intermittent catheterization and anticholinergic drugs to decrease intravesical pressures; others have administered diazepam to facilitate relaxation of the external sphincter. The prognosis for this condition is poor, and many patients develop chronic renal failure. Therefore, aggressive treatment of the bladder dysfunction is often justified and may include antireflux surgery, intermittent catheterization, and bladder augmentation. These children require long-term treatment and careful follow-up.

INFREQUENT VOIDING

Infrequent voiding is a common disorder of micturition, usually associated with urinary tract infections. Affected children, usually girls, void only twice a day rather than the normal three to five times. With bladder overdistention and prolonged retention of urine, growth of bacteria leads to recurrent urinary tract infections. Some such children are constipated. There is sometimes a family history of infrequent voiding. Some of these children also have occasional episodes of incontinence due to overflow or urgency. The etiology of this disorder appears to be behavioral. When the children have urinary tract infections, the treatment is by antibacterial prophylaxis, and encouragement of frequent voiding and of complete emptying of the bladder by double voiding until a normal pattern of micturition is re-established.

OTHER CAUSES OF INCONTINENCE IN FEMALES

Table 497–1 lists other causes of urinary incontinence. *Ureteral ectopia,* usually associated with a duplicated collecting system in girls, can produce urinary incontinence characterized by constant dribbling of urine during day and night, in addition to a normal voiding pattern. Sometimes the urine production from the renal segment drained by the ectopic ureter is small and urinary drainage is confused with watery vaginal discharge. Children with a history of vaginal discharge or inconti-

■ TABLE 497–1 Urinary Incontinence in Childhood

With Complete Bladder Emptying	
Ectopic ureter and fistulas	Neurogenic
Sphincter failure (with total or partial incontinence)	Traumatic Iatrogenic
Urgency Incontinence	
Detrusor hyperactivity is caused by inflammation, neurogenic dysfunction, or detrusor instability secondary to functional or mechanical obstruction	Cystitis Unstable bladder Neurogenic bladder Hyper-reflexia Bladder outlet obstruction Noncompliant bladder, neurogenic or non-neurogenic Detrusor sphincter dys-synergia, neurogenic or non-neurogenic
With Incomplete Bladder Emptying	
Overflow incontinence (incomplete bladder emptying may be due to decompensated obstruction or paralysis of the detrusor muscle)	Bladder outlet obstruction (e.g., posterior urethral valves) Neurogenic detrusor areflexia Detrusor sphincter dys-synergia, neurogenic or non-neurogenic Behavioral
Other	
Combination of above	Multiple factors

nence and an abnormal voiding pattern require careful study. The ectopic orifice is usually difficult to find. On intravenous urography, one may suspect duplication of the collecting system (Fig. 497–1), but the upper collecting system drained by the ectopic ureter usually has poor or very delayed function. Ultrasound and computed tomography (CT) scan of the kidneys help rule out subtle duplication that may not be discovered on intravenous urography. Examination under anesthesia for an ectopic ureteral orifice in the vestibule or the vagina is often necessary (Fig. 497–2). The treatment in these cases is by partial nephroureterectomy, removing the involved segment of the duplicated kidney and the ureter down to the pelvic brim. A short, incompetent urethra may be associated with certain urogenital sinus malformations. The diagnosis of these malformations requires a high index of suspicion and a careful physical examination of all incontinent girls. In these cases, urethral and vaginal reconstruction can often restore continence.

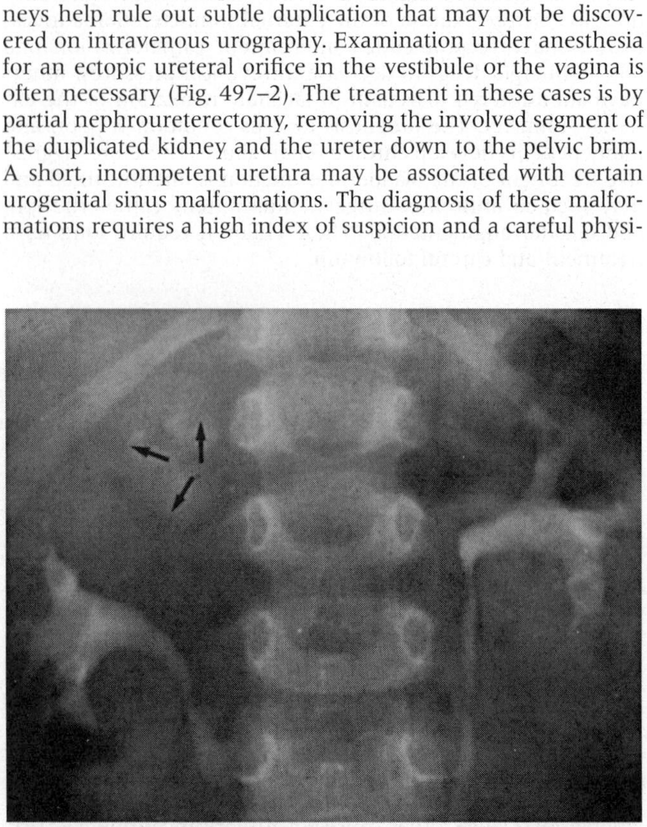

Figure 497–1. Duplication of the right collecting system with ectopic ureter. Excretory urogram in a female presenting with a normal voiding pattern and constant urinary dribbling. The left kidney is normal and the right side, well visualized, is the lower collecting system of a duplicated kidney. On the upper pole opposite the 1st and 2nd vertebral bodies, note the accumulation of contrast material corresponding with a poorly functioning upper pole drained by a ureter opening in the vestibule.

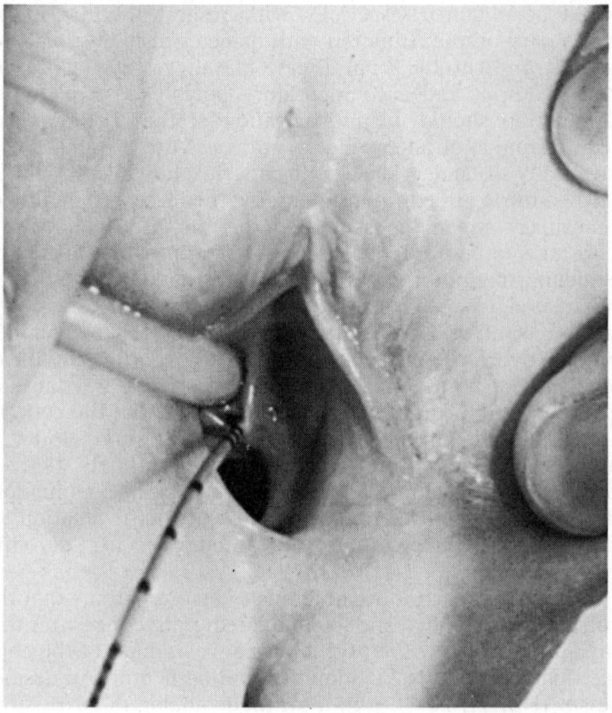

Figure 497–2. Ectopic ureter. The photograph shows an ectopic ureter entering the vestibule next to the urethral meatus. The thin ureteral catheter with transverse marks has been introduced into this ectopic ureter. This girl had a normal voiding pattern and constant urinary dribbling.

CHAPTER 498
Anomalies of the Penis and Urethra

HYPOSPADIAS. Hypospadias occurs in approximately 1 of 500 newborns. In the mildest cases, the urethral meatus opens on the ventral aspect of the glans, there are various degrees of malformation of the glans, and the prepuce is defective ventrally with the appearance of a dorsal hood (Fig. 498–1). With increasing degrees of severity, the penis is curved ventrally (chordee) and the penile urethra is progressively shorter, but the distance between the meatus and the glans may not increase significantly until the chordee is corrected. It is misleading, therefore, to classify hypospadias solely on the basis of the location of the meatus. In some cases, the meatus is at the penoscrotal junction; in extreme cases, the urethra opens in the perineum, the scrotum is bifid and sometimes extends to the dorsal base of the penis (scrotal transposition), and the chordee is extreme (Fig. 498–2). In such cases, there is usually a urethral diverticulum opening at the level of the verumontanum, representing a vestige of mullerian structures. In variant cases, ventral curvature of the penis occurs without a hypospadiac urethral meatus. In these cases, the prepuce is usually hooded and the corpus spongiosum may be underdevel-

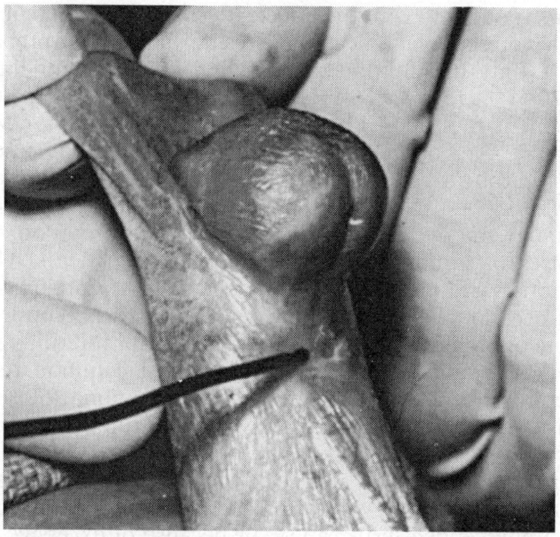

Figure 498–1. Distal hypospadias. Note the urethral meatus in the subcoronal position and the incomplete or hooded prepuce. There was no ventral curvature of the penis in this case.

oped. The megameatus variant has a fully developed prepuce and can be overlooked at the time of the newborn circumcision. Recognition of this variant and avoidance of the circumcision facilitates future reconstruction.

Testes are undescended in 10% of boys with hypospadias. Inguinal hernias are also common. In the newborn period, the differential diagnosis of severe penoscrotal and perineal hypospadias with undescended testes should include other forms of ambiguous genitalia, particularly masculinization of females (congenital adrenal hyperplasia) and gonadal dysgenesis. A karyotype should be obtained in all patients with hypospadias and cryptorchidism (see Chapter 529). The incidence of other anomalies of the genitourinary tract in boys with hypospadias is low, and with the probable exception of the more severe cases of perineal hypospadias, radiographic studies of the urinary tract are not justified.

The *treatment* of hypospadias starts in the newborn period. Routine circumcisions should be avoided, as the foreskin is often essential for repair later in life. Mild cases of hypospadias are usually repaired for cosmetic reasons alone, but with increasing severity repair becomes essential in order to allow the child to void standing, to allow future normal sexual function, and to avoid psychologic consequences of having malformed external genitalia. The ideal age for repair is before the age of 18 mo. Most of these anomalies can now be repaired in a single operation with minimal hospitalization; accordingly, emotional trauma is less likely or severe now than with the older techniques. Repair of hypospadias is a technically demanding operation and should be performed by surgeons with extensive experience.

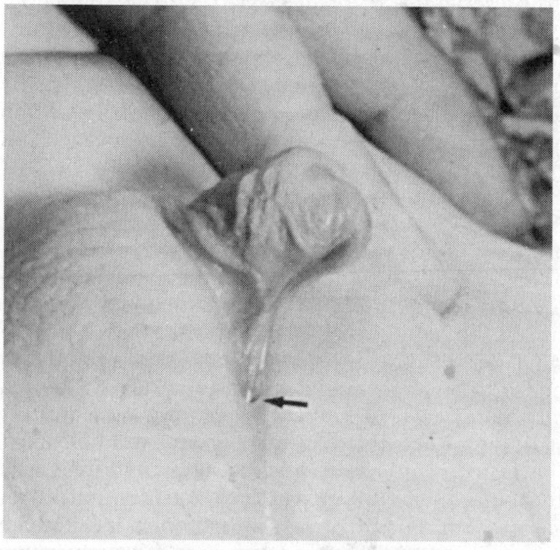

Figure 498–2. Severe perineoscrotal hypospadias. Note the ventral curvature and the underdeveloped ventral surface of the penis, the hooded prepuce, and the urethral meatus in the midline of the bifid scrotum. This child had palpable gonads and a normal chromosome pattern.

AGENESIS AND MICROPENIS. *Agenesis* of the penis is rare and usually associated with anorectal and renal anomalies. If the child is likely to survive the associated anomalies, rearing as a female is recommended, with later genital reconstruction.

The length of the normal newborn penis is 3.5 ± 0.7 cm. *Micropenis* results from primary or secondary testicular failure during fetal life after morphogenesis is complete. Secondary congenital testicular failure is seen in anencephaly, pituitary agenesis, and Kallmann, Noonan, Prader-Willi, and other syndromes. Other cases may be due to the presence of rudimentary testes, dwarfism, or maternal hormone administrations. Treatment options include a trial of hormonal stimulation, or rearing as female, with later genital reconstruction. Adjustment to the male gender role and sexual satisfaction is possible in some of these patients.

PHIMOSIS AND PARAPHIMOSIS. In 90% of uncircumcised males the prepuce becomes retractable by the age of 3 yr. Inability to retract the prepuce before this age is therefore not pathologic and not an indication for circumcision. *Phimosis* is the inability to retract the prepuce at an age when it should normally be retractable. Phimosis can be congenital or a sequel of inflammation. True phimosis usually requires surgical enlargement of the phimotic ring or circumcision. Accumulation of smegma under the infantile prepuce is not pathologic and does not require surgical treatment.

Paraphimosis occurs when a phimotic prepuce is retracted behind the coronal sulcus and this retraction cannot be reduced. This causes venous stasis distal to the corona, with edema leading to severe pain and inability to reduce the foreskin. If discovered early, the condition can be treated by reduction of the foreskin with appropriate lubrication, while the child is under heavy sedation or a short-acting general anesthetic. In some cases, circumcision is required.

CIRCUMCISION. In the United States, circumcision is usually

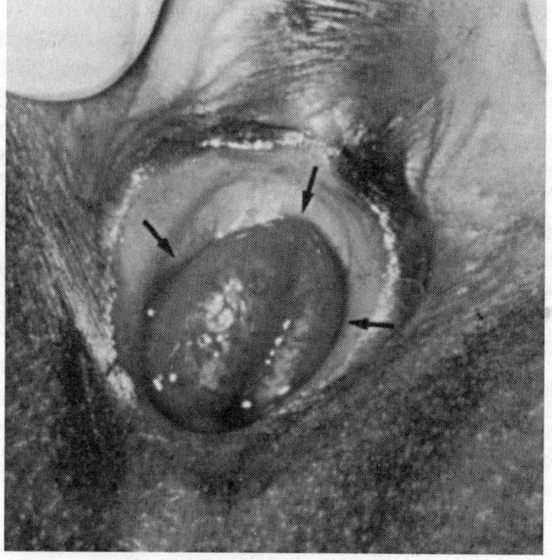

Figure 498–3. Urethral prolapse in a 4-yr-old black girl who had blood spotting on her underwear.

performed for cultural reasons, or because it prevents phimosis, paraphimosis, balanoposthitis, and urinary tract infections. Routine neonatal circumcision carries a very small but real risk of potentially serious complications, including sepsis, amputation of the distal part of the glans, removal of an excessive amount of foreskin, and the occurrence of urethrocutaneous fistulas. Intense debate continues about the cost effectiveness and public health benefits of routine neonatal circumcision (i.e., decrease in the risk of urinary tract infections in male infants with normal urinary tracts from 0.041 to 0.002, prevention of penile cancer, and avoidance of medically indicated circumcision later in life). Proponents of neonatal circumcision also argue that when circumcision is done later in life it is more costly and carries a greater morbidity; however, less than one quarter of circumcisions performed in older children are medically indicated and many children circumcised at birth require revisions for complications or unsatisfactory results.

URETHRAL PROLAPSE. Urethral prolapse is encountered predominantly in black females who exhibit vulvar bleeding (Fig. 498–3). Surgical excision and reapproximation of the mucosal edges is curative.

CHAPTER 499

Disorders and Anomalies of the Scrotal Contents

UNDESCENDED TESTES

UNDESCENDED AND ECTOPIC TESTES. Failure to find one or both testes in the scrotum may indicate any of a variety of congenital or acquired conditions, including true undescended testes, ectopic or maldescended testes, retractile testes, and absent testes.

True undescended testes and *maldescended* or *ectopic* testes can be differentiated from each other only by surgical exploration, and both conditions usually are referred to as cryptorchidism or hidden testes. The true undescended testis is found along the normal path of descent, and the processus vaginalis is usually patent. The ectopic testis has completed its descent through the inguinal canal but ends up in a subcutaneous location other than the scrotum, the most common being a point lateral to the external inguinal ring, below the subcutaneous fascia. Cryptorchidism is present in 0.7% of children after 1 yr of age and in adults. The incidence is high in full-term newborns (3.4%) and increases with prematurity (to 17% in infants with birthweights between 2,000 and 2,500 g and to 100% in those under 900 g). This reflects the fact that testicular descent from the inguinal canal into the scrotum takes place in the 7th mo of gestation. Spontaneous testicular descent does not occur after the age of 1 yr.

The consequences of cryptorchidism include infertility in adulthood, tumor development in the undescended testes, associated hernias, torsion of the cryptorchid testis, and the possible psychologic effects of an empty scrotum. Cryptorchidism is bilateral in up to 30% of cases. Infertility is the rule in adults with untreated bilateral cryptorchidism, and of those treated in childhood less than one third will be fertile. With unilateral undescended testis, the rate of infertility is probably similar to that in the general population.

The undescended testis is often histologically normal at birth, but *failure of development and atrophy* are detectable by the end of the 1st yr of life, and by the end of the 2nd yr the number of germ cells in the affected testis is severely reduced. Surgical correction at an early age results in a greater probability of fertility in adulthood. The patient with cryptorchidism has a 20–44% increase in risk of developing a *malignant testicular tumor* in the 3rd or 4th decade of life. Patients with untreated intra-abdominal cryptorchidism or those who underwent surgical correction during or after puberty are at greatest risk. Although surgical correction of the cryptorchidism may not change the overall risk of malignant transformation, very few cases of tumors have been reported in patients whose operations were performed before 8 yr of age. Carcinoma in situ is occasionally discovered when the testis is biopsied at the time of orchiopexy or during evaluation for infertility later in life; its significance is unclear. The most common tumor developing in undescended testes is the seminoma (60%); in contrast, seminomas represent only 30% of tumors occurring in normally descended testes.

Indirect inguinal hernias always accompany true undescended testes and are common with ectopic testes. *Torsion and infarction* of the undescended testis can occur because of excessive mobility of such testes. The treatment of the unilateral cryptorchid testis is best undertaken early in the 2nd yr of life. Most testes located extra-abdominally can be brought down to the scrotum and the associated hernia corrected with an operation (*orchiopexy*). This can often be performed without hospitalization. When the testis is not palpable, preoperative laparoscopy is used to determine its location. In the majority of cases, orchiopexy of the intra-abdominal testis located immediately inside the internal inguinal ring offers little difficulty, but orchiectomy should be considered in the more difficult cases or when the testis appears to be severely atrophied. Two-stage orchidopexy is sometimes needed in high abdominal testes. Testicular prostheses are available for older children and adolescents when the absence of the gonad in the scrotum may have an undesirable psychologic effect but, the advisability of using silicone implants has been questioned.

Treatment of bilateral undescended testes is identical to the treatment of unilateral undescended testis when the testes are palpable. When testes are not palpable, however, differential diagnosis must be made from absent testes by measuring serum testosterone levels before and after stimulation with human chorionic gonadotropin (hCG). If the testosterone level rises, an abdominal exploration and orchiopexy should be undertaken. A negative response does not rule out the possible existence of intra-abdominal testicular tissue. An attempt is made to preserve these gonads for hormonal production after puberty; the likelihood of preserving fertility is very low.

Hormonal treatment with hCG or luteinizing hormone-releasing hormone (LH-RH) has not replaced surgical treatment of cryptorchidism. Most agree that hormonal stimulation, which induces an early pseudopuberty, succeeds only in bringing down retractile testes (see later). Some believe that preoperative treatment with hCG facilitates surgery. Recent reports on the advantages of hormonal treatment with LH-RH followed by HCG for nonresponders, and early surgery for the 60% of testes that fail to descend, need to be weighed against potential detrimental effects on pubertal penile growth of early exposure of the penile receptors to testosterone.

RETRACTILE TESTES. These testes retract into the inguinal canal in response to an exaggerated cremasteric reflex. The cremasteric reflex is weak or absent at birth. Consequently, when testes that were palpable at birth become nonpalpable later, retractile testes should be suspected. Retractile testes can be brought down by careful palpation when the child is relaxed in a warm room, and scrotal examination is facilitated if the child is in a squatting position. Often more than one examination is required to establish the diagnosis. The retractile testis usually adopts a permanent scrotal position during puberty and has none of the complications commonly associated with the true undescended or ectopic testis.

ABSENT TESTES. Approximately 20% of nonpalpable testes are absent. Congenital absence of the testis is possible, but it is quite rare and may be associated with some degree of feminization of the internal organs on the ipsilateral side. More commonly, the fetal testis disappears some time after the differentiation of the internal and external genitalia has occurred. This vanishing of the testis is usually attributed to a vascular accident that has taken place prenatally or after birth but was not recognized clinically. At exploration, the spermatic vessels and the vas deferens end blindly, usually somewhere in the inguinal region or in the scrotum. Because this condition is analogous to testicular torsion, some authors advocate fixation of the contralateral testis to prevent torsion from occurring in the remaining gonad. In these cases, placement of a testicular prosthesis can be considered as well.

TORSION OF THE TESTIS OR APPENDICES

Testicular torsion requires prompt diagnosis and treatment if the gonad is to survive. Testicular torsion accounts for approximately 40% of all cases of acute scrotal pain and swelling and for the majority of such cases in patients less than 6 yr old. It is caused by an abnormal fixation of the testis to the scrotal envelope. Under normal conditions, the testis is partially covered on its anterior portion by the tunica vaginalis, a serosal membrane derived from the processus vaginalis of the peritoneum. When the tunica vaginalis covers not only the testis but also the epididymis and the distal part of the spermatic cord, the testis is allowed to rotate freely within this serosal space and torsion can occur (bell clapper deformity). This abnormality of the tunica vaginalis is often bilateral.

Testicular torsion produces acute pain and swelling of the scrotum. On examination, the scrotum is swollen, very tender, and often difficult to examine. The cremasteric reflex is absent. The condition can be differentiated from an incarcerated hernia because swelling in the inguinal area is often absent. The differential diagnosis includes torsion of one of the testicular or epididymal appendices (embryologic vestiges), which usually causes less swelling and pain; occasionally a blue dot is observed above the testis and there is localized tenderness in this area. Often, however, differentiation can be made only at the time of surgical exploration. Torsion of the appendices is more common between the ages of 7 and 12 yr.

In children over 13 yr old, the differential diagnosis should include *epididymitis.* In epididymitis, the urinalysis is often abnormal, and there may be an antecedent history of sexual activity or urinary tract infection. Epididymitis is the most common cause of acute scrotal pain and swelling in patients over 18 yr of age. Nevertheless, in the prepubertal or adolescent boy with acute painful and swollen testes, testicular torsion should be considered present until proven otherwise. The accuracy of ultrasonography, color Doppler ultrasound, and isotopic scans in differentiating testicular torsion from other conditions is uncertain, and these diagnostic measures often delay unnecessarily a surgical procedure that can salvage the gonad.

The optimal treatment is prompt surgical exploration. If the testis is explored within 6 hr of torsion, up to 90% of the gonads will survive after detorsion and fixation to the scrotum. Survival decreases rapidly with a delay of more than 6 hr, and such cases usually require orchiectomy. It is probably unwise not to remove a necrotic testis if torsion is confirmed. The contralateral testis should be fixed to the scrotum to prevent future torsion. If torsion of the appendices or epididymis is found, surgical removal of the necrotic appendix will result in cure.

In cases of *neonatal torsion* the mechanism for torsion appears to be different, in that abnormal fixation of the testis to the scrotum is not necessarily present. These torsions are usually extravaginal, as the entire testis and tunica vaginalis rotate within the lax subcutaneous tissue of the scrotum. This type of torsion can occur in utero or be present at birth. Salvage of testes with neonatal torsion is extremely rare. Many authors recommend exploration to remove the necrotic testis and to fix the contralateral side, because there have been some reports of later torsion involving the remaining testis.

VARICOCELE

Dilatation of the pampiniform venous plexus results from valvular incompetence of the spermatic vein. Varicoceles occur predominantly on the left side, are bilateral in 10% of cases, and rarely involve the right side only. Rarely seen before the age of 10 yr, varicoceles are present in 15% of adult males. In some cases, varicoceles cause male subfertility with decreased sperm concentration or motility. Varicoceles are also associated with decrease in size of and characteristic testicular histologic changes in the involved testis.

A large varicocele can be painful, particularly during strenuous physical activity. In the standing position, venous varicosities can be palpated along the spermatic cord. This venous distention increases with the Valsalva maneuver and collapses with recumbency. A fixed varicocele is suggestive of a retroperitoneal tumor. Surgical treatment by ligation of the internal spermatic vein is sometimes required in adolescents to relieve pain or, when there is disparity in testicular size, to allow normal development of the testis. The effect of early surgical correction of varicoceles on future fertility is unknown. Improved testicular growth has been reported after surgery for varicocele in adolescents.

HYDROCELE

Hydrocele is an accumulation of fluid in the tunica vaginalis. When the amount of fluid varies with time, there is communication with the peritoneal cavity. Small hydroceles can disappear by the age of 1 yr, but larger ones often persist and require surgical treatment. Communicating hydroceles should be treated as indirect inguinal hernias.

EPIDIDYMITIS

Acute inflammation of the epididymis presents acute scrotal pain and swelling; it is rare before puberty and should raise the question of a congenital abnormality of the wolffian duct, such as an ectopic ureter entering the vas. After puberty, epididymitis becomes progressively more common and is the principal cause of acute painful scrotal swelling in young adults. Urinalysis usually reveals pyuria. Epididymitis can be bacterial (gonococcus, chlamydia), but often the organism remains undetermined. Treatment is by bed rest and antibiotics. Differentiation from torsion can be very difficult, and in children surgical exploration is usually required.

CHAPTER 500
Trauma to the Genitourinary Tract

Accidental injuries to the genitourinary tract in children are usually the result of blunt trauma from falls, athletic activities, or motor vehicle accidents. In childhood, genitourinary trauma is exceeded in frequency only by trauma to the skeleton and the central nervous system. In more than half of the cases there are also major injuries to the brain, spinal cord, skeleton, lungs, or other intraperitoneal organs. In cases of isolated renal injury, particularly following minor trauma, a pre-existent anomaly such as a horseshoe kidney, renal ectopia, hydronephrosis, or tumor should be suspected. Hematuria, bleeding through the urethral meatus, a flank mass, fractured lower ribs or lumbar transverse processes, or a perineal or scrotal hematoma suggests a major injury to the genitourinary tract in a child with trauma. In lesions involving the renal pedicle, hematuria is often absent.

Evaluation of the patient starts as soon as an adequate airway has been established and the patient is hemodynamically stable. The bladder should be catheterized in all cases except when there is bleeding from the urethral meatus, an indication of potential urethral injury. Straddling injuries are usually associated with trauma to the bulbous urethra. Rupture of the membranous urethra occurs in 3% of cases of pelvic fractures. Passing the catheter in the presence of a urethral injury may increase the extent of the damage and convert a partial tear to a total disruption. Instead, a retrograde urethrogram should be performed by injecting a radiopaque medium into the urethral meatus. Oblique radiographs will demonstrate the extent of the injury and whether urethral continuity is preserved or has been disrupted. Treatment is by suprapubic cystostomy drainage until the hematoma is reabsorbed, followed by urethroplasty when necessary to correct a resulting stricture. Erectile impotence, urethral stricture, and urinary incontinence are the major complications of rupture of the membranous urethra.

When the bladder can be catheterized, cystography is performed by infusing radiopaque medium through the catheter by gravity. If possible, flat and oblique views are obtained; a roentgenogram is also obtained after the bladder is drained. Bladder ruptures can be intraperitoneal or extraperitoneal. All intraperitoneal ruptures require surgical repair. Minor extraperitoneal near-ruptures might be treated by catheter drainage but generally require surgical treatment as well.

Intravenous urography or preferably computed tomography (CT) scanning is next done to evaluate the kidneys. Complete absence of function of the one kidney without contralateral compensatory hypertrophy (indicative of congenital absence) should be regarded as an indication of major injury to the renal pedicle. Renal angiography may be useful immediately before surgical exploration.

Renal injuries are usually classified as minor and major. *Minor renal injuries* include contusion of the renal parenchyma and shallow cortical lacerations not involving the collecting system. The majority of renal injuries fall into this category and can be treated nonoperatively with bed rest and supportive measures. *Major renal injuries* include deep lacerations involving the collecting system, the shattered kidney, and renal pedicle injuries. After the bladder is evaluated by cystography, intravenous pyelography or CT scanning is obtained. The observation of prompt function of both kidneys without extravasation usually excludes major renal injury. When findings on intravenous urography are not diagnostic, however, CT scanning is the ideal method for evaluating these lesions and has largely replaced angiography. CT scanning better defines the extent of injury and also allows evaluation of other intra-abdominal organs.

Major renal injuries may require surgical treatment either during the course of an exploration for other intra-abdominal injuries or as management of the renal injury per se to control bleeding or significant urinary extravasation. Besides loss of renal parenchyma, the main long-term complication of renal injury is arterial hypertension. Children who sustain renal injuries should have periodic measurement of the blood pressure for approximately 1 yr following injury. All penetrating injuries of the kidneys should be surgically explored.

Ureteral injuries are usually iatrogenic. Injuries of the ureter by blunt or penetrating trauma require immediate surgical attention.

Testicular injuries are relatively uncommon in children because of the small size of the testes and their great mobility. Such injuries usually result from athletic activities. Prompt surgical treatment of testicular injuries increases the testicular salvage rate.

CHAPTER 501
Urinary Lithiasis

Urinary lithiasis in children is very common in some parts of the world but rare in the United States. The wide geographic variations in the incidence of lithiasis in childhood appear related to climatic, dietary, and socioeconomic factors. These factors also influence the location of the calculi; primary bladder stones are common in developing countries, whereas upper tract stones predominate in the United States (except in children with pre-existing bladder diseases, such as neurologic dysfunction, obstruction, or previous surgical procedures).

Children with urolithiasis almost always have either gross or microscopic hematuria. In order of frequency, abdominal pain, flank or back pain, and symptoms of urinary tract infection follow. When the diagnosis of urolithiasis is suspected, a plain roentgenogram of the abdomen will detect radiopaque stones, mainly those containing calcium. Cystine stones and infectious stones (composed of struvite) may be faintly radiopaque. Radiolucent stones (uric acid, 2,8-dihydroxyadenine, and xanthine calculi) can be detected by abdominal ultrasonography or as filling defects found in the upper collecting system or bladder on intravenous urography or on computed tomography (CT) scanning of the abdomen. When lithiasis is diagnosed, a complete functional and radiographic evaluation of the urinary tract is made to rule out stasis, obstruction, or infection as predisposing factors. One fourth of children with urinary calculi have vesicoureteral reflux. The best insight into the etiology of lithiasis in a particular patient is the complete chemical and crystallographic analysis of the stone (as obtained by spontaneous passage, or surgical or endoscopic extraction).

A metabolic evaluation for the most common predisposing factors should be undertaken as well, keeping in mind that structural, infectious, and metabolic factors often coexist. Nephrolithiasis may occur in infants treated with furosamide. The basic laboratory studies required are listed in Table 501–1.

The causes of urolithiasis are multiple, and a complete listing is given in Table 501–2. Some of the more frequently encountered types of calculi are discussed here.

CALCIUM STONES. The most common urinary calculi in children in the United States are made of calcium oxalate. Cases in which no metabolic explanation for the stone formation is found are referred to as *idiopathic urolithiasis.* Hypercalciuria often leads to the formation of calcium oxalate stones and may be associated with hypercalcemia (due to hyperparathyroidism, sarcoidosis, immobilization, hypervitaminosis D, or idiopathic causes, and so on) but more often is an isolated phenomenon. Normocalcemic hypercalciuria may result from administration of furosemide (which often leads to stone formation in neonates), or from uncontrolled distal renal tubular

■ TABLE 501–1 Laboratory Tests Suggested to Evaluate Urolithiasis

Serum
Calcium
Phosphorus
Uric acid
Electrolytes and acid-base balance
Creatinine
Alkaline phosphatase
Urine
Urinalysis
Urine culture
Urinary pH
Calcium/creatinine ratio
Spot test for cystinuria
24-hr collection for
creatinine clearance
calcium
phosphorus
oxalate
uric acid
dibasic amino acids (if cystine spot test is positive)

acidosis, total parenteral alimentation, or alkalosis. In most cases, however, hypercalciuria leading to stone disease is idiopathic and may result from a renal tubular calcium "leak," which causes usually mild, secondary compensatory hyperparathyroidism and intestinal hyperabsorption of calcium. Another type of isolated hypercalciuria is related to *primary intestinal hyperabsorption* of calcium, which increases the filtered load of calcium and causes parathyroid inhibition.

■ TABLE 501–2 Classification of Urolithiasis

Renal Tubular Syndromes
Renal tubular acidosis
Distal defect, type I
Carbonic anhydrase inhibitors
Cystinuria
Glycinuria
Enzyme Disorders
Primary hyperoxaluria
Type I, glycolic aciduria
Type II, L-glyceric aciduria
Xanthinuria
Metabolic (enzymatic) hyperuricosuria
2,8-Dihydroxyadeninuria
Hypercalcemic States
Primary hyperparathyroidism
Sarcoidosis
Hypervitaminosis D
Milk-alkali syndrome
Neoplasms
Cushing syndrome
Hyperthyroidism
Idiopathic infantile hypercalcemia
Immobilization
Uric Acid Lithiasis and Related Disorders
Hereditary metabolic hyperuricosuria
Hereditary renal hypouricemia
2,8-Dihydroxyadeninuria
Myeloproliferative disorders
Low urine output states
Nephrolithiasis and Intestinal Disease
Acquired hyperoxaluria
Uric acid lithiasis
Idiopathic Renal Lithiasis
Infected Urolithiasis and Urinary Stasis
Endemic Calculi
Nephrocalcinosis

Modified from Malek RS: Urolithiasis. In: *Kelalis PP, King LR, Belman AB (eds): Clinical Pediatric Urology. Philadelphia, WB Saunders, 1985.*

The precise cause of these disorders remains unclear. Children with hypercalciuria sometimes have recurrent episodes of gross hematuria and flank pain years before the 1st stone is detected; accordingly, the work-up of children with recurrent gross hematuria should include the measurement of urinary calcium. Upper limits of normal are 4 mg/kg/24 hr. A urinary calcium/creatinine ratio in a first morning voided specimen greater than 0.25 is abnormal. A detailed metabolic workup to differentiate the various types of hypercalciuria has been described by Pak. Despite careful evaluation, there remains a group of children who are stone formers, in whom neither metabolic nor anatomic abnormalities can be detected. Calculi of calcium oxalate can also occur in children in whom small bowel disease and malabsorption lead to excessive reabsorption of oxalate in the colon (intestinal hyperoxaluria). Renal stone formation and nephrocalcinosis in primary hyperoxaluria (type 1 or 2) usually begins before the age of 4–5 yr and often runs a progressive course leading to renal failure.

CYSTINURIA. This inborn error of transport of the dibasic amino acids (cystine, ornithine, arginine, and lysine) results in excessive urinary excretion of these products. The only known complication of this familial disease is the formation of calculi, owing to the low solubility of cystine. The sulfur content of cystine gives these stones their faint radiopaque appearance.

STRUVITE STONES. Urinary tract infections caused by urea-splitting organisms (e.g., *Proteus* and occasionally *Klebsiella, Escherichia coli, Pseudomonas,* and others) result in urinary alkalinization and excessive production of ammonia, which can lead to the precipitation of magnesium ammonium phosphate (struvite) and calcium phosphate. The stones act as foreign bodies, causing obstruction and perpetuating infection. Patients with struvite stones may also have metabolic abnormalities that predispose to stone formation. These stones are often associated with reflux and neurogenic bladder dysfunction.

URIC ACID STONES. Calculi containing uric acid represent less than 5% of all cases of lithiasis in children in this country but are more common in less developed areas of the world. Hyperuricosuria with or without hyperuricemia is the common underlying factor in most cases. The stones are radiolucent. The diagnosis should be suspected when there is a persistently acid urine and urate crystalluria. Hyperuricosuria may result from various inborn errors of purine metabolism that lead to overproduction of uric acid, the end product of purine metabolism in humans. Children with the Lesch-Nyhan syndrome and patients with glucose-6-phosphatase deficiency (G-6-PD) form urate calculi as well. In children with short bowel syndrome, and particularly in those with ileostomies, chronic dehydration and acidosis are sometimes complicated by uric acid lithiasis. One of the most common causes of uric acid lithiasis is the rapid turnover of purine with some tumors and myeloproliferative diseases. The risk of uric acid lithiasis is especially great when treatment of these diseases causes rapid breakdown of nucleoproteins. Uric acid calculi or "slush" can fill the entire upper collecting system and cause renal failure and even anuria. In addition, urates also are present within calcium-containing stones. In these cases more than one predisposing factor for stone formation may exist. A related disorder only recently recognized is *2,8-dihydroxyadenine lithiasis,* which results from a deficiency in adenine phosphoribosyltransferase. The stones are radiolucent and can be differentiated from uric acid calculi by mass spectrometry but not by routine chemical analysis. In contrast to uric acid, which is very soluble in alkaline urine, the solubility of 2,8-dihydroxyadenine changes little within physiologic pH ranges.

TREATMENT. The treatment of urinary lithiasis is approached from two perspectives. One aspect is the treatment of the underlying metabolic disorder, infections, or predisposing anatomic factors; the other is the treatment of complications associated with the stone itself, principally obstruction and infection. The simplest and most effective measure to prevent recurrence in all forms of lithiasis is to maintain an adequate state of hydration and diuresis 24 hr a day, in order to keep the urine dilute and to diminish the likelihood of precipitation of stone ingredients.

Alterations of the urine pH can also prevent recurrence of calculi. Cystine is much more soluble when the urinary pH is over 7.5, and alkalinization of urine with sodium bicarbonate or sodium citrate is effective. Recurrence of uric acid lithiasis may likewise be prevented by keeping the urinary pH above 7.5; indeed, hydration, urinary alkalinization, and measures directed at reducing uric acid excretion can cause dissolution of uric acid calculi. Acidification impairs the growth of struvite stones, but this cannot be achieved in practice so long as the stone or an infection by urea-splitting organisms is present.

Whenever possible, and if simple measures fail, specific therapy for any underlying metabolic disorder should be used. Thiazides appear to be effective in controlling primary renal hypercalciuria, but their effectiveness in the treatment of calcium oxalate stones caused by primary hypercalciuria remains debatable. Treatment of renal tubular acidosis controls recurrence of stone disease or nephrocalcinosis. Allopurinol is an inhibitor of xanthinoxidase and is effective in reducing the production both of uric acid and of 2,8-dihydroxyadenine, and can help control recurrence of both types of stones. Rarely, excessive urinary excretion of xanthine with stone formation has been reported during treatment with allopurinol. D-Penicillamine is a chelating agent that binds to cysteine or hemicystine, increasing the solubility of the product. Although poorly tolerated by many patients, it has been reported to be effective in dissolving cystine stones and in preventing recurrences when hydration and urinary alkalinization fail. *N*-acetylcysteine appears to have low toxicity and may be effective in controlling cystinuria, but long-term experience with it is lacking. Other specific therapies for lithiasis include the use of cellulose phosphate to bind calcium in the intestine in cases of primary absorptive hypercalciuria. Poor compliance with treatment and poor tolerance of the medication are significant drawbacks to its use. Pyridoxine has been used in some cases of hyperoxaluria. Salts of phosphate, citrate, magnesium, and other compounds directed at increasing the solubility of calcium oxalate and other stone ingredients in the urine are used in some centers, with varying success. Citrate is especially useful in the presence of hypocitraturia.

Surgical treatment of stone disease has been widespread in the past. Stones must be removed when they cause obstruction of the collecting system, pain, or bleeding, or if they are a factor in perpetuating infections. All struvite stones should be removed, because these carry a significant risk of renal parenchymal destruction and of renal or perirenal abscess formation. Newer modalities of stone removal, both endoscopically and by percutaneous access to the kidney, have been applied on a limited scale in children. Extracorporeal shock wave lithotripsy (ESWL) has been successfully applied to both renal and ureteral stones in children with a success rate of more than 75%.

URINARY TRACT INFECTIONS

Benador D, Benador N, Slosman DO, et al: Cortical scintigraphy in the evaluation of renal parenchymal changes in children with pyelonephritis. J Pediatr 124:17, 1994.

Burbige KA, Retik AB, Colodny AH, et al: Urinary tract infection in boys. J Urol 132:54, 1984.

Chessare JB: Circumcision: is the risk of urinary infection really the pivotal issue? Clin Pediatr (Phila) 31:100, 1992.

Gillenwater YJ, Harrison RB, Kunin CM: Natural history of bacteriuria in school girls: A long term case control study. N Engl J Med 301:396, 1979.

Hoberman A, Chao HP, Keller DM, et al: Prevalence of urinary tract infections in febrile infants. J Pediatr 123:17, 1993.

Newcastle Asymptomatic Bacteriuria Research Group: Asymptomatic bacteriuria in school children in Newcastle upon Tyne. Arch Dis Child 50:90, 1975.

Rushton HG: Genitourinary infections. Non-specific infections. *In:* Kelalis PK, King LR, Belman AB (eds). Clinical Pediatric Urology. Philadelphia, WB Saunders, 1992, p 286.

Sheldon CA, Gonzalez R: Differentiation of upper and lower urinary tract infections. How and when? Med Clin North Am 68:321, 1984.

Sinha B, Gonzalez R: Hyperammonemia in boys with obstructive ureterocele and Proteus infection. J Urol 131:1, 1984.

VESICOURETERAL REFLUX

Edwards D, Normand ICS, Prescod N, et al: Disappearance of vesicoureteric reflux during longterm prophylaxis of urinary tract infection in children. Br Med J 2:285, 1977.

Hjälmas K, Löhr G, Tamminen-Möbius T, et al: Surgical results in the international reflux study (Europe). J Urol 148:1657, 1992.

Jenkins GR, Noe N: Familial vesicoureteral reflux: A prospective study. J Urol 128:774, 1982.

Koff SA, Murtagh DS: Uninhibited bladder in children: Effect of treatment on recurrent urinary tract infection and on vesicoureteral reflux resolution. J Urol 130:1138, 1983.

Nasrallah PF, Nava S, Crawford J: Clinical application of nuclear cystography. J Urol 128:550, 1982.

Noe HN: The long term results of prospective sibling reflux screening. J Urol 148:1739, 1992.

Puri P, O'Donnell R: Endoscopic correction of grades IV and V primary vesicoureteral reflux: 6 to 30 months follow-up in 42 ureters. J Pediatr Surg 2:1087, 1987.

Rance CP, Arbus GS, Balfe JW, et al: Persistent systemic hypertension in infants and children. Pediatr Clin North Am 21:801, 1974.

Ransley PG: Intrarenal reflux: Anatomical, dynamic and radiological studies. Urol Res 5:61, 1977.

Tamminen-Möbius T, Brunier E, Ebel KD, et al: Cessation of vesicoureteral reflux for 5 years in infants and children allocated to medical treatment. J Urol 148:1662, 1992.

OBSTRUCTION

Churchill BM, Krueger RP, Fleischer MH, et al: Complications of posterior urethral valve surgery and their prevention. Urol Clin North Am 10:519, 1983.

Gonzalez R, Chiou RK: The diagnosis of upper urinary tract obstruction in children: Comparison of diuresis renography and pressure flow studies. J Urol 133:1, 1985.

Gonzalez R, Lapointe S, Sheldon CA, et al: Undiversion in children with chronic renal failure. J Pediatr Surg 19:632, 1984.

Hendren WH: Posterior urethral valves in boys: A broad clinical spectrum. J Urol 106:298, 1971.

Homsy YL, Williot P, Danais S: Transitional neonatal hydronephrosis: Fact or fantasy? J Urol 136:339, 1986.

Immergut M, Notman GE: The urethral course of female children with recurrent urinary tract infection. J Urol 99:189, 1965.

Kaplan GW, Sammons TA, King LR: Blind comparison of dilatation urethrotomy and medication alone in the treatment of infection in girls. J Urol 109:917, 1973.

Keating MA, Escala J, Snyder HM, et al: Changing concepts in management of primary obstructive megaureter. J Urol 142:636, 1989.

Kletscher B, deBadiola FIP, Gonźalez R: Outcome of prenatally diagnosed hydronephrosis. J Pediatr Surg 26:455, 1991.

Lockhart JL, Singer AM, Glenn JF: Congenital megaureter. J Urol 122:310, 1979.

Manivel JC, Pettmato G, Reinberg Y, et al: Prune belly syndrome: Clinicopathological study of 28 cases. Pediatr Pathol 9:691, 1989.

Nguyen DH, Aliabadi H, Ercole CJ, et al: Nonintubated Anderson-Hines repair of ureteropelvic junction obstruction in 60 patients. J Urol 142:704, 1989.

Perez-Aytes A, Graham JM, Hersh JH, et al: Urethral obstruction sequence and lower limb deficiency: Evidence for the vascular disruption hypothesis. J Pediatr 123:398, 1993.

Reinberg Y, Castaño I, González R: Prognosis for patients prenatally diagnosed posterior urethral valves. J Urol 148:125, 1992.

Reinberg Y, Chelimsky G, González R: Urethral atresia and the prune belly syndrome. Report of 6 cases. Br J Urol 72:122, 1993.

Reinberg Y, González R: Acute and chronic urinary tract obstruction: Pathophysiology, diagnosis and treatment. *In:* Mandal AK, Jennette JC (eds): Diagnosis and Management of Renal Disease and Hypertension, 2nd ed. In press.

Reinberg Y, Gonzalez R, Fryd D, et al: The outcome of renal transplantation in children with posterior urethral valves. J Urol 140:1491, 1988.

Reinberg Y, Manivel JC, Pettinato G, et al: Development of renal failure in children with the prune belly syndrome. J Urol 145:1017, 1991.

Sullivan M, Halpern L, Hodges CV: Extravesical ureteral ectopia. Urology 11:577, 1978.

Weiss RM: Obstructive uropathy. Pathophysiology and diagnosis. *In:* Kelalis PK, King LR, Belman AB (eds): Clinical Pediatric Urology. Philadelphia, WB Saunders, 1992, p 664.

Whitaker RH: Percutaneous upper urinary tract dynamics in equivocal obstruction. Urol Radiol 2:187, 1981.

Woodhouse CRJ, Kellett JS, Williams DI: Minimal surgical interference in prune belly syndrome. Br J Urol 51:475, 1979.

OTHER DISEASES AND ANOMALIES OF THE BLADDER

Exstrophy

Arap S, Giron DM, Menezes de Goes G: Initial results of the complete reconstruction of bladder exstrophy. Urol Clin North Am 7:477, 1980.

Jeffs RD: Exstrophy and cloacal exstrophy. Urol Clin North Am 5:127, 1978.

Sheldon CA, McKinley R, Hartig P, et al: Carcinoma at the site of the ureterosigmoidostomy. J Dis Colon Rectum 26:55, 1983.

Bladder Diverticula

Johnston JH: Vesical diverticula without urinary obstruction in childhood. J Urol 84:535, 1960.

Urachal Anomalies

Bauer SB, Retik AB: Urachal and related umbilical disorders. Urol Clin North Am 5:195, 1978.

Neurogenic Bladder

Bauer SB: Urodynamic evaluation and neuromuscular dysfunction. *In:* Kelalis PK, King LR, Belman AB (eds): Clinical Pediatric Urology. Philadelphia, WB Saunders, 1985.

Fernandes E, Reinberg Y, Vernier R, et al: Neurogenic bladder in children. Review of pathophysiology and current treatment. J Pediatr 124:1, 1994.

Gonzalez R: Bladder augmentation with sigmoid or descending colon. *In:* Webster GD, Kirby R, King LR, Goldwasser B (eds): Reconstructive Urology. Boston, Blackwell Scientific, 1992, p 443.

Gonzalez R: Urinary incontinence. *In:* Kelalis PK, King LR, Belman BA (eds): Clinical Pediatric Urology. Philadelphia, WB Saunders, 1992, p 384.

Gonzalez R, Nguyen D, Koleliat N, et al: The artificial sphincter AS800 in congenital urinary incontinence. J Urol 142:512, 1989.

Kaplan WE, Firlit CF: Management of reflux in myelodysplastic child. J Urol 129:1195, 1983.

Kass EJ, Koff SA, Diokno AC: Fate of vesicoureteral reflux in children with neuropathic bladders managed by intermittent catheterization. J Urol 125:63, 1981.

Lapides J, Diokno AC, Lowe BS: Follow-up on unsterile intermittent self catheterization. J Urol 111:184, 1974.

Sidi AA, Dykstra DD, Gonzalez R: The value of urodynamic testing in the management of neonates with myelodysplasia: A prospective study. J Urol 135:90, 1986.

Sidi AA, Peng W, Gonzalez R: Vesicoureteral reflux in children with myelodysplasia: Natural history and results of treatment. J Urol 136:329, 1986.

Reconstruction

Peters CA: Bladder reconstruction in children. Curr Opinion Pediatr 6:183, 1994.

Enuresis and Voiding Dysfunction

Allen TD: The non-neurogenic neurogenic bladder. J Urol 117:232, 1977.

Fernandes E, Vernier R, Gonźalez R: The unstable bladder in children. J Pediatr 118:831, 1991.

Mikkelsen EJ, Rappaport JL: Enuresis: Psychopathology, sleep stage and drug response. Urol Clin North Am 7:361, 1980.

Pedersen PS, Hejl M, Kjoller SS: Desamino-D-arginine vasopressin in childhood. Nocturnal enuresis. J Urol 133:65, 1985.

Rushton HG: Enuresis. *In:* Kelalis PK, King LR, Belman AB (eds): Clinical Pediatric Urology. Philadelphia, WB Saunders, 1992, p 365.

OTHER DISEASES AND ANOMALIES OF THE PENIS AND URETHRA

Hypospadias

American Academy of Pediatrics: Report of the task force on circumcision. Pediatrics 84:388, 1989.

Bauer SB, Retik AB, Colodny AH: Genetic aspects of hypospadias. Urol Clin North Am 8:559, 1981.

deBadiola FIP, Anderson K, Gonźalez R: Hypospadias repair in an outpatient setting without proximal diversion. Experience with 113 urethroplasties. J Pediatr Surg 26:461, 1991.

Johnston JH: Abnormalities of the penis. *In:* Williams DI, Johnston JH (eds): Paediatric Urology. London, Butterworth Scientific, 1982, p 435.

Reilly JM, Woodhouse CRJ: Small penis and the male sexual role. J Urol 142:569, 1989.

Rozenman J, Hertz M, Boichis H: Radiological findings of the urinary tract in hypospadias: A report of 770 cases. Clin Radiol 30:471, 1979.

Section on Urology, American Academy of Pediatrics: The timing of elective surgery on the genitalia of male children with particular reference to undescended testes and hypospadias. Pediatrics 56:479, 1975.

Winberg J, Bollgren I, Gotheforrs L, et al: The prepuce: a mistake of nature? Lancet 1(86380):589, 1989.

Wiswell T: Circumcision: An update. Curr Probl Pediatr 22:424, 1992.

DISEASES AND ANOMALIES OF THE SCROTAL CONTENTS

Bartsch G, Frank ST, Marberger H: Testicular torsion: Late results with special regard to fertility and endocrine function. J Urol 124:375, 1980.

Berkowitz GS, Lapinski RH, Dolgun SE, et al: Prevalence and natural history of Cryptorchidism. Pediatrics 92:44, 1993.

Cendron M, Keating MH, Huff DS, et al: Cryptorchidism, orchiopexy and infertility: A critical long-term retrospective analysis. J Urol 142:559, 1989.

Frick J: LHRH and cryptorchidism. Eur J Pediatr 152:528, 1993.

Gonzalez R: Outpatient orchidopexy in children. *In:* Kaye KW (ed): Outpatient Urologic Surgery. Philadelphia, Lea & Febiger, 1985, p 204.

Heinz HA, Voggenthaler J, Weissbach L: Histologic findings in testes with varicocele during childhood and their therapeutic consequences. Eur J Pediatr 133:139, 1980.

Husman DA, CAin MP: Micropenis: Eventual phallic size is dependent upon the timing of androgen administration. J Urol 152:734, 1994.

Lala R, Matarazzo P, Chiabotto P, et al: Combined therapy with LHRH and HCG in cryptorchid infants. Eur J Pediatr 152:531, 1993.

Martin DC: Malignancy on the cryptorchid testes. Urol Clin North Am 9:371, 1982.

Papadotos C, Moutsouris C: Bilateral testicular torsion in the newborn. J Pediatr Surg 71:249, 1967.

Study Group John Radcliffe Hospital: Cryptorchidism: a prospective study of 7500 consecutive male births 1984–8. Arch Dis Child 67:892, 1992.

TRAUMA

Brower P, Paul J, Brosman SA: Urinary tract abnormalities presenting as a result of shunt abdominal trauma. J Trauma 18:719, 1978.

Burrington JD: Childhood trauma. *In:* Holder TM, Ashcroft KLW (eds): Pediatric Surgery. Philadelphia, WB Saunders, 1980, p 149.

Cass AS: Blunt renal trauma in children. J Trauma 23:123, 1983.

Pinhas ML, Gonzales ET: Genitourinary trauma in children. Urol Clin North Am 12:53, 1985.

URINARY LITHIASIS

Abrams SA, Yergey AL, Schanler RJ, et al: Hypercalciuria in premature infants receiving high mineral content diets. J Pediatr Gastroenterol Nutr 18:20, 1994.

Alon US, Scagliotti D, Garola RE: Nephrocalcinosis and nephrolithiasis in infants with congestive heart failure treated with furosemide. J Pediatr 125:149, 1994.

Gearhart JP, Herzberg GZ, Jeffs RD: Childhood urolithiasis: Experiences and advances. Pediatrics 87:445, 1991.

Hoppe B, Hesse A, Neuhaus T, et al: Urinary saturation and nephrocalcinosis in preterm infants: Effect of parenteral nutrition. Arch Dis Child 69:299, 1993.

Hulbert JC, Reddy PK, Gonzalez R, et al: Percutaneous nephrostolithotomy: An alternative approach to the management of pediatric calculous disease. Pediatrics 76:610, 1985.

Meyers DA, Mobley TB, Jenkins JM, et al: Pediatric low energy lithotripsy with lithostar. J Urol 153:453, 1995.

Nijman RJM, Ackaer TK, Scholtneijer RJ, et al: Long-term results of extracorporeal shock wave lithotripsy in children. J Urol 142:609, 1989.

Noe HN, Stapleton FB, Roxy S III: Potential surgical implications of hematuria in children. J Urol 132:737, 1984.

Pak CYC: The spectrum and pathogenesis of hypercalciuria. Urol Clin North Am 8:245, 1981.

Sinno K, Boyce WH, Resnick MI: Childhood urolithiasis. J Urol 121:662, 1979.

Stapleton FB, Rog S, Noe HN, et al: Hypercalciuria in children with hematuria. N Engl J Med 310:1345, 1984.

PART XXV

Gynecologic Problems of Childhood

Joseph S. Sanfilippo

CHAPTER 502

History and Physical Examination

NEONATE. The initial gynecologic assessment of the newborn should begin with the breast examination. Not uncommonly, as a result of maternal endogenous estrogen production, breast tissue is increased in the neonate; nipple discharge may be noted. See Chapter 505. The abdomen is gently palpated for evidence of organomegaly and the external genitalia assessed for any ambiguity. The labia should be grasped gently and separated, allowing inspection of the introitus-hymenal area. Upon completion of the inspection segment of the exam, a rectal examination is performed. A midline structure, indicative of the uterus, is usually palpable, and the adnexa should not be apparent at this time. Abducting the hips with the labia gently retracted frequently facilitates inspection of the introital area. A normal protuberant hymen with associated thin white mucoid discharge from the vagina is often perceptible. In the first few weeks of life, a small amount of vaginal bleeding may occur, reflecting the fall in circulating levels of maternal estrogens.

PREPUBERTAL CHILD. The pediatric or adolescent patient undergoing her first gynecologic examination should be managed with particular care, as the initial encounter may well set the tone for all future gynecologic examinations. If the examination is painful or uncomfortable, or if there is a significant lack of rapport between the patient and the examiner, the child may suffer lasting psychologic consequences. A gentle, caring attitude by the health care provider will go far in enabling the patient to relax at the time and during all future gynecologic examinations.

The history is obtained primarily from the parent(s), who should be integrally involved in the physical examination of a child in this age group. In addition, the patient should have a sense of control over the examination involved, and should experience no discomfort. Ideally, the goals are accomplished by providing an adequate explanation prior to the examination. Much information can be obtained by inspection of the vulvovaginal area. Ideally, the patient is placed in a frog-legged position. If this is not satisfactory, then a knee-chest position with a Valsalva's maneuver allows adequate assessment of the introital (lower-third) vaginal area. Magnification often can be accomplished with use of a colposcope or hand-held magnifying glass; appropriate documentation is also important. Visualizing the vestibule permits assessment of any discharge. Use of an aseptic technique in which an intravenous tubing (butterfly) is passed into a soft #12 bladder catheter, all of which is then attached to a 1 mL tuberculin syringe, allows aspiration of any fluid in the vagina as well as successful lavage. Wet mounts can be obtained and evaluated as indicated as well as cultures for further evaluation of vulvovaginitis. Other instrumentation used for the genital examination include an otoscope and/or Cameron-Myers vaginoscope. Gentle traction on the labia upward and outward further exposes the vaginal introitus and permits assessment. Calcium alginate (Calgi) swabs are also useful, especially for obtaining cultures from the vagina. A number of variations of the normal-appearing hymen occur and care must be taken to determine if there is an imperforate, microperforate, or septated hymen. If an inadequate examination is accomplished in an office-clinic setting, then consideration for sedation or examination under anesthesia is appropriate.

ADOLESCENT. Obtaining a history in this age group may take place initially in the presence of the patient's parent(s). However, the adolescent should be made aware of the concept of confidentiality and be given the opportunity to provide her own history without the parent(s) being present (see Part XIII). This can be accomplished in the examination room prior to the actual physical examination. Concern for the presence of vaginal discharge, the potential for sexually transmitted disease, pregnancy, or menstrual aberration, etc. should be explored. The health care professional must win the confidence of the adolescent, provide a relaxed atmosphere for the examination, and communicate to the teenager one's availability for consultation. Indications for the first pelvic exam in adolescents are addressed in Table 502–1.

The teenager, in a manner similar to that for the pediatric patient, should be involved in the examination. The examination is best performed in the absence of parent(s), but a chaperon should be present, which may serve to neutralize any adverse psychosocial aspects of the situation. Communication should occur between the physician and the patient through-

TABLE 502–1 Suggested Indications for Pelvic Examination in the Adolescent

Age 18
Sexually active
Past or current
Menstrual irregularities
Severe dysmenorrhea
Unexplained abdominal pain
Unexplained dysuria
Abnormal vaginal discharge

Modified from: The adolescent obstetric-gynecologic patient. ACOG Techn Bull 145:3, 1990.

out the examination. The examination should be performed in the dorsal lithotomy position with an effort made to maintain eye contact. Appropriate-sized specula should be available, including the small Pedersen (8 cm in depth). The 4–5 cm pediatric specula is best avoided in that it results in inadequate visualization; however, the pediatric-sized Huffman speculum is appropriate.

Inspection of the vulva is followed by palpation of Bartholin's urethral Skene's glands. The clitoris, which is normally 2–4 mm wide, is then assessed. A clitoris >10 mm in width, especially in the presence of other signs of virilization, is abnormal. The hymenal configuration should also be evaluated. The patient should be told immediately prior to insertion of the speculum that she will experience a pressure sensation. Before touching the introitus, it is useful to touch the inner thigh with the speculum. Trauma to the urethra is to be avoided, and displacement of the fourchette posteriorly further facilitates proper speculum placement. Discussion with the adolescent regarding techniques to relax the perineal musculature is often helpful.

Once the speculum portion of the exam is complete, a bimanual examination is undertaken. In the virginal female, a single digit exam with appropriately lubricated, gloved finger allows proper palpation of the vaginal walls and cervix and bimanual assessment of the uterus and the adnexa. The cul-de-sac is assessed and a rectovaginal examination performed to complete the bimanual exam.

Cavanaugh R: Obtaining a personal and confidential history from adolescents. An opportunity for prevention. J Adolesc Health Care 2:118, 1986.

Greydanus DE: Contraception. *In*: Sanfilippo JS, Lavery JP (eds): Pediatric Adolescent Obstetrics and Gynecology. New York, Springer-Verlag, 1985, p 234.

Phillips S, Bohannon W, Heald F: Teenager's choices regarding the presence of family members during the examination of genitalia. J Adolesc Health Care 7:245, 1986.

Pokorny SF: Pediatric vulvovaginitis. *In*: Kaufman R, Friedrich E, Gardner H (eds): Benign Diseases of the Vulva and Vagina. Chicago, Year Book Medical, 1989, p 55.

Pokorny SF, Stormer J: Atraumatic removal of secretions from the prepubertal vagina. Am J Obstet Gynecol 156:5, 1987.

Sanders JM Jr, Durant RH, Chastain DO: Pediatricians use of chaperons when performing gynecologic examinations on adolescent females. J Adolesc Health Care 10:110, 1989.

Talbot CW: The gynecologic examination of the pediatric patient. Pediatr Ann 15:501, 1986.

CHAPTER 503
Vulvovaginitis

This is the most common childhood or adolescent gynecologic problem. Vulvovaginal irritation results from the lack of labial fat pads and pubic hair for protection of the external genitalia. The labia minora tend to open when the child squats; this, in turn, causes exposure of the more sensitive tissues within the hymenal ring. In addition, the close proximity of the anal orifice to the vagina allows transfer of fecal bacteria to the vulvovaginal area. Masturbation may also be a contributing factor.

The squamous epithelium of the vaginal mucosa is sensitive to steroid hormones. In the relatively low estrogenic environment, the thin atrophic epithelium becomes susceptible to bacterial invasion. Thus, recurrent vulvovaginitis usually ceases once a female child reaches puberty and the pH of the vagina becomes more acidic. In part, this is due to increased production of acetic and lactic acids, a phenomenon accompanied by an increase in superficial cell proliferation and glycogen as well as by enhancement of normal bacterial flora (Table 503–1).

PATHOLOGIC VAGINAL DISCHARGE. In the pediatric patient, vaginal discharge is a common presenting complaint. It is often the primary symptom of vulvitis, vaginitis, or vulvovaginitis. Pruritus, frequent urination, dysuria, or enuresis may be associated signs and symptoms. Vulvitis is manifested primarily by dysuria and pruritus, associated with erythema of the vulva. Vulvitis commonly has a more protracted course than vaginitis; the latter is characterized by discharge without associated dysuria, pruritus, or erythema. Vulvovaginitis involves a combination of these manifestations. The color, odor, and duration of the discharge should be noted. Although there are a number of causes of vulvovaginitis in the pediatric patient, the more common ones include poor perineal hygiene, *Candida* infection, and a foreign body.

NONSPECIFIC VULVOVAGINITIS. Patients with poor perineal hygiene often develop a condition known as nonspecific vulvovaginitis. Overall, nonspecific vulvovaginities account for 70% of all pediatric vulvovaginitis cases. The discharge is characteristically brown or green, has a fetid odor, and is associated with a vaginal pH of 4.7–6.5. In 68% of reported cases, this type of vaginitis is associated with coliform bacteria secondary to fecal contamination. The next most common bacterial organisms associated with nonspecific vulvovaginitis are β-hemolytic *Streptococcus* and coagulase-positive *Staphylococcus*. These organisms are often transmitted manually from the nasopharynx. Clothing, chemicals, cosmetics, and soap products or detergents used for bathing or laundry may also cause irritation that leads to nonspecific vulvovaginitis. Tight-fitting clothing, such as jeans, leotards, and tights, as well as rubber pants or plastic-coated paper diapers, have also been implicated.

Nonspecific vulvovaginitis occasionally can result in chronic infection, which may cause significant psychologic consequences for child and parent alike. The physician should stress the importance of avoiding "vaginal fixation," while encouraging proper perineal hygiene.

Successful *treatment* of nonspecific vulvovaginitis should include instruction in perineal hygiene, switching from tight-fitting underwear, the use of sitz baths with mild soap, and air drying the vulva. The patient should be instructed in appropriate bowel and bladder habits, emphasizing the necessity of wiping fecal material away from the vulvovaginal area. Recurrent vulvovaginitis should be treated with systemic antibiotics such as amoxicillin or cephalosporins. Topical estrogen cream or polysporin ointment is often helpful.

SPECIFIC VULVOVAGINITIS (see Table 503–1). *Gardnerella vaginalis* is the most common organism cultured in the pediatric or adolescent patient with vulvovaginitis, followed by *Candida*. Other identified organisms include enterococci and anaerobic bacteria such as *Peptococcus*, *Peptostreptococcus*, *Veillonella parvula*, *Eubacterium*, *Propionibacterium*, and *Bacteroides* species. Protozoa, helminths, and viruses should also be considered as etiologic agents. Treatment will depend on the offending organism (see Table 503–1).

LABIAL ADHESIONS. In this disorder, the labia minora have a central line of adherence from an area immediately inferior to the clitoris to the fourchette (Fig. 503–1). Labial adhesions are commonly seen in patients under 6 yr of age, and the condition is often asymptomatic. The lesions usually are associated with local inflammation in association with the hypoestrogenic state of the preadolescent. Pooling of urine in the vagina and recurrent vulvovaginitis appear to provide a continuous nidus for recurrent urinary tract infections. Recurrent urinary tract symptoms occur in 20–40% of patients and should be treated. Once the vaginal pH becomes more acidic, as occurs with adolescence, the recurrent labial adhesions almost always disappear.

■ TABLE 503–1 Specific Vulvovaginitis

Organism	Presentation	Diagnosis	Treatment
Enterobiasis (pinworms)	Perineal pruritus (nocturnal) GI symptoms; variable vulvovaginal contamination from feces	Adult worms in stool or eggs on perianal skin	Mebendazole; repeat in 3 weeks if necessary
Giardiasis	Asymptomatic fecal contaminant, vaginal discharge, diarrhea, malabsorption syndrome	Protozoal flagellate (cyst or trophozoites) in feces	Metronidazole or quinacrine
Molluscum contagiosum	Vulvar lesions, nodules with umbilicated area; white core of curdlike material	Isolation of pox virus	Dermal curettage of papule
Phthirus pubis (pediculosis pubis)	Pruritus, excoriation, sky blue macules; inner thigh or lower abdomen	Nits on hair shafts, lice-skin or clothing	Lindane lotion (Kwell)
Sarcoptes scabei (scabies)	Nocturnal pruritus, pruritic vesicles, pustules in runs	Mites; ova black, dots of feces (microscopic)	1% lindane
Shigella species (shigellosis)	Fever malaise, fecal contamination, diarrhea; blood and mucus, cramps, pus in stool	Stools; WBC and RBC, positive for *Shigella*	Trimethoprim and sulfamethoxazole; chloramphenicol, ampicillin, or tetracycline
Staphylococcus and *streptococcus*	Vaginal discharge to vulvovaginal area; spread from primary lesion	Positive culture for appropriate organism	Penicillin or cephalosporin

Sanfilippo J: Adolescent girls with vaginal discharge. Pediatr Ann 15:509, 1986.

Topical estrogen cream applied each evening is the *treatment* of choice and is effective in over 90% of reported cases; as an alternative, polysporin or bacitracin ointment may be applied each evening for 1 wk. Elimination of the agglutination may require 2–8 wk of therapy. Cleansing followed by application of a bland ointment such as petrolatum should continue for 1–2 mo after the adhesions separate. Mechanical separation of the adhesions is advisable only if the adhesions appear to separate easily and if it does not cause significant trauma. Once the adhesions are separated, the patient should be reexamined for any predisposing cause, such as the presence of a vaginal septum.

CANDIDIASIS. *Candida* infection is often associated with a diaper rash. *Candida vulvovaginitis*, while rare in children, must be considered, especially for individuals with chronic mucocutaneous candidiasis. The presence of candida-infected tissue may be indicative of significant immunosuppression. Underlying factors such as diabetes mellitus should be considered. *Treatment* with an imidazole cream (e.g., clotrimazole) is frequently effective, except in cases of chronic mucocutaneous candidiasis.

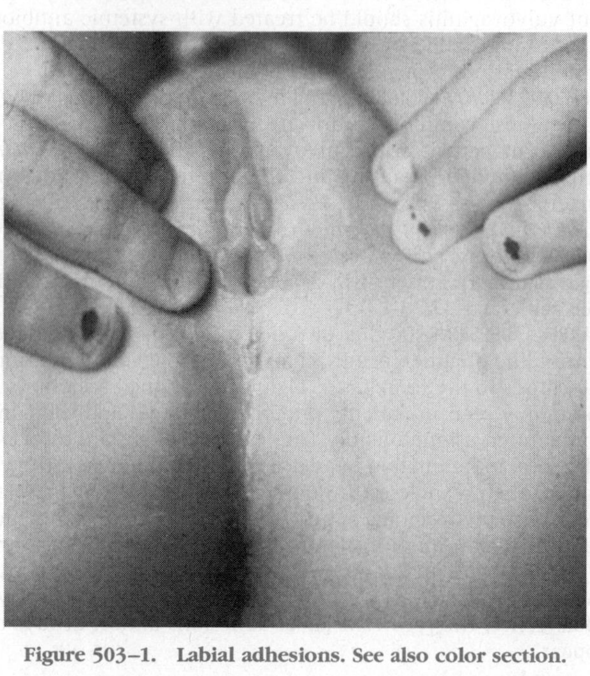

Figure 503–1. Labial adhesions. See also color section.

DIAPER DERMATITIS. This entity is a common problem occurring in the first several weeks of life (see Chapters 597 and 605).

MOLLUSCUM CONTAGIOSUM. This common infection of the skin is associated with the pox virus group (Part XVII, Section 4). Molluscum contagiosum presents as an umbilicated, dome-shaped papule. The central umbilication usually is associated with a pulpy core. Vulvar lesions appear to result from autoinoculation or from close contact (sexual or nonsexual) with an infected individual. The incubation period is 2–7 wk. Diagnosis is confirmed by light microscopic visualization of viral inclusions (molluscum bodies) in the central core. *Treatment* requires elimination of the lesions, usually by application of silver nitrate after gentle curettage; other methods of therapy include cryosurgery or electrocautery.

INTERTRIGO. Intertrigo can occur in the genitocrural areas in association with friction, obesity, and moisture in the area. Miliaria and secondary infection can also occur in association with intertrigo. The affected areas are red and macerated. Careful hygiene, combined with bland emollients, and perhaps a mild corticosteroid, appear to be an effective *treatment*.

IMPETIGO. This entity is commonly identified during the first several weeks of life. It is usually caused by *Staphylococcus aureus*, usually phage group II, especially type 71, which may be acquired from the mother, other relatives, or staff. Impetigo tends to affect the vulva and periumbilical areas, causing lesions or blisters that later become crusted. Extensive spread and complications may ensue if *treatment* with antibiotics is not promptly instituted (Chapter 174).

PITYRIASIS VERSICOLOR. This condition is caused by *Pityrosporon orbiculare* and is manifested by scaly macules on the trunk in postpubertal patients, but lesions have been reported on the face and genital area. The diagnosis is established by visualization on wet prep of hyphae and spores with 10% potassium hydroxide. *Treatment* requires application of topical imidazoles (e.g., clotrimazole).

HERPES SIMPLEX VIRUS (see also Chapter 211). Herpes simplex virus (HSV) types 1 and 2 involve the vulvar area. The types are not exclusively site specific, but type 2 is commonly responsible for genital lesions and type 1, in general, for facial-oral lesions. The infection is characterized by papules, which become vesicles, with the virus affecting the dorsal root ganglia. Differential diagnoses include any eroded or blistering lesions as well as herpes zoster. A definitive diagnosis is established by culturing the virus or visualizing it via electron microscopy. *Treatment* with topical acyclovir reduces viral shedding and accelerates healing.

HUMAN PAPILLOMA VIRUS (HPV). HPV is associated with a number of serotypes, including 6, 11, 16, and 18, which usually are noted in the anogenital region. Types 16 and 18 are particularly associated with malignant and premalignant lesions of the vulva (see Chapter 224). Differential diagnoses include molluscum contagiosum, condyloma accuminatum, and vulvar intraepithelial neoplasia. There must be strong consideration of the possibility of child sexual abuse when these lesions are identified. *Treatment* is usually symptomatic and remains a challenge for clinicians.

LICHEN SCLEROSUS. This is a chronic atrophic skin disease characterized by small, pink to ivory, flat-topped papules that are several millimeters in diameter. The papules appear to coalesce into plaques that become wrinkled and atrophic. The anogenital lesions frequently resemble an hourglass or a "figure 8" (Fig. 503–2). Vesicles and bullae may spread over the vulva with associated hemorrhage. A biopsy is often required for accurate diagnosis.

The onset of lichen sclerosus in most children usually occurs before 7 yr of age. The youngest reported patient was an infant only several weeks old. The onset of menarche often results in spontaneous improvement of the lesions, but the process usually continues. Patients are often intermittently symptomatic, and there is no relationship between menarche and symptomatic improvement or resolution of the disease. Atrophy of the labia minora and clitoral phimosis, as well as contracture of the introitus, may occur.

The cause of lichen sclerosus is unknown, but it is believed to be related to an autoimmune disorder. Positive immunofluorescence for fibrin, serum complement (C′3), or immunoglobulin M (IgM) in involved areas has been demonstrated in 75% of patients.

Treatment is symptomatic; emollients and topical corticosteroids usually provide relief. Topical estrogens and androgens also have been used, but these agents may produce a vaginal discharge as well as other secondary problems, such as breast development and clitoral enlargement. Secondary infection should be treated with antibiotics. Some affected individuals demonstrate what is known as the Koebner phenomenon, the precipitation of lesions secondary to trauma. For relief, these individuals should avoid tight-fitting clothing and genital trauma. Newer treatment modalities include laser vaporization to the level of the first surgical plane.

LICHEN PLANUS. Vulvar lichen planus is often associated with oral mucosal and subcutaneous lesions. The vulvar lesions, characterized by angular violaceous, flat-topped papules, may simulate leukoplakia. In addition, the oral lesions consist of minute white papules that form a lacy pattern and usually are located on the buccal mucosa. The lesions are intensely pruritic and may become excoriated and macerated; erosions and ulcerations may even occur in severe cases. Diagnosis requires biopsy. Exacerbation or recurrence of the lesions is common.

Treatment consists of topical intralesional corticosteroids and antihistamines to control the pruritus. Squamous cell carcinoma may occur with long-standing, hypertrophic, vulvar lichen planus; therefore, long-term follow-up and the histologic examination of any changed or otherwise suspicious area is advisable.

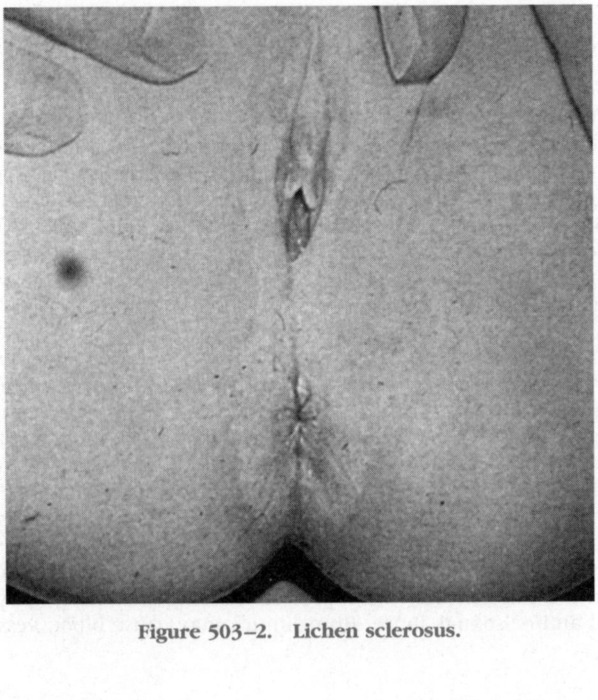

Figure 503–2. Lichen sclerosus.

LICHEN SIMPLEX CHRONICUS (NEURODERMATITIS). This is a chronic, lichenified plaque that causes pruritus. Scratching and inflammation may result, causing a vicious cycle. The condition is rare in children. *Treatment* with antihistamines and topical or intralesional corticosteroids is recommended.

SEBORRHEIC DERMATITIS (see Chapter 605). This presents as erythematous, oily, circumscribed patches that can be found on the face, scalp, and chest as well as on intertriginous areas of the body. There may also be fissures and associated secondary infection around the vulva; secondary bacterial or candidal infection is quite common, causing pain, pruritus, dysuria, and vaginal bleeding. Acute episodes are best treated with sitz baths or topical aluminum acetate solution (Burow solution). Exacerbating factors, such as tight clothing or rubber pants, should be eliminated. Systemic antibiotics with appropriate topical antifungal medication should be administered for secondary infection.

ATOPIC DERMATITIS (see Chapter 138). This affects 3% of all children. The patient presents with hay fever or asthma or both, and generally there is a family history. The vulvar lesion is characterized as a chronic condition accompanied by intense pruritus, erythema, papules, and vesicles, with oozing and crusting of the involved areas. There may be associated circumscribed, lichenified scaly patches on the vulvar area. Pruritus often causes scratching, which results in excoriation of the lesions. Secondary bacterial or candidal infection is common.

Antihistamines are necessary for control of pruritus. Sitz baths with mild soap and lubricants are helpful. Topical corticosteroids such as 1% hydrocortisone are also effective. Secondary bacterial or candidal infections require specific treatment.

CONTACT DERMATITIS (see Chapter 605). In either allergic or irritant contact dermatitis, the vulva may be affected by edematous, erythematous, oozing lesions that are sometimes accompanied by vesicles or pustules. Chronic contact dermatitis is often associated with thickened and lichenified lesions. The clue for correct diagnosis of this condition is the limitation of the dermatitis to the area of contact with the etiologic agent. There may also be a secondary candidal or bacterial infection. Some common etiologic agents are soaps, powders, bubble baths, feminine hygiene sprays, topical medications, toilet paper, rubber, and certain types of clothing. *Treatment* should include avoidance of the offending agents and sitz baths, or compresses with topical aluminum acetate solution (Burrow solution) during acute episodes. Mild topical corticosteroids such as 0.5–1% hydrocortisone cream applied several times daily may further aid healing and alleviate vulvar irritation. Recurrence can be prevented by removal of the offending etiologic agent.

VULVAR PSORIASIS (see Chapter 607). This is frequently associated with lesions of other parts of the body and is characterized by violaceous papules or plaques with a thick adherent silvery scale (Fig. 503–3). The intertriginous areas may show "inverse" psoriasis, a variation that does not occur on the extremities. Vulvar lesions usually are poorly demarcated and may present

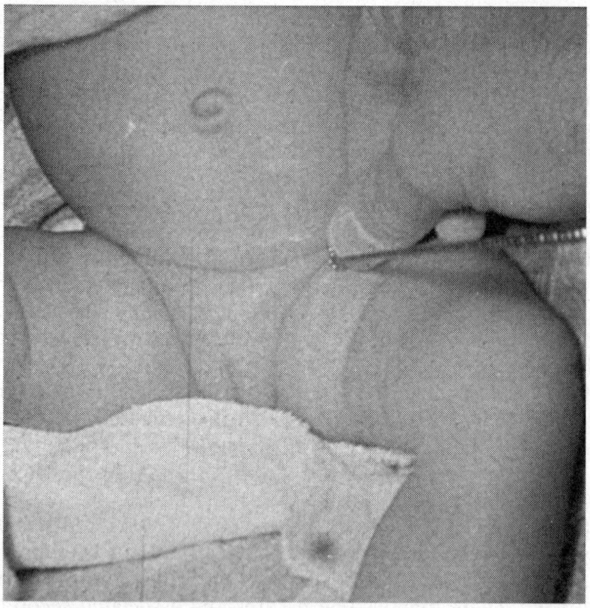

Figure 503–3. Vulvar psoriasis. See also color section.

as scaly patches, most commonly on the mons pubis. The vulvar lesions are often resistant to therapy; therefore, a multifaceted approach is essential. A corticosteroid cream (e.g., 1% hydrocortisone) should be used in conjunction with control of secondary infection and pruritus.

ENTEROBIASIS (see Chapter 245.5). Pinworms *(Enterobius vermicularis)* are helminths that may carry colonic bacteria to the perineum, causing recurrent vulvovaginitis. The female pinworm emerges from the anus to deposit eggs. Vulvovaginitis develops in about 20% of girls infected with *E. vermicularis.* The "scotch tape" test should be used to search for the organism if there is any suspicion or if there is undiagnosed recurrent vulvovaginitis. Victims typically have pruritus and nocturnal episodes of scratching. Treatment consists of pyrantel pamoate (see Table 503–1).

SHIGELLOSIS (see Chapter 183). *Shigella flexneri* and *S. sonnei* cause various gastrointestinal symptoms in association with vaginitis. Forty-seven per cent of patients present with a bloody vaginal discharge and 2% with diarrhea. Systemic antibiotics are the treatment of choice. Bowel colonization with *Shigella* can result in subclinical gastrointestinal symptoms in 10% of household members.

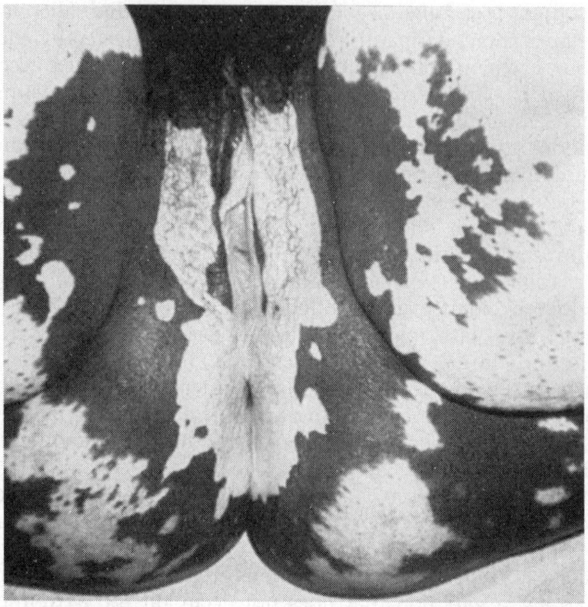

Figure 503–4. Vitiligo. See also color section.

VITILIGO. This presents as sharply demarcated, pink to ivory patches that tend to spread and coalesce (Fig. 503–4). The skin on the patch is smooth with no palpable changes. It may be differentiated from lichen sclerosus because the hyperpigmented patches are asymptomatic. No treatment is necessary unless cosmetic problems result.

Charles V, Charles SX: A case of vulvo-vaginal diphtheria in a girl of seven years. Indian Pediatr 15:257, 1978.

Clark JA, Muller SA: Lichen sclerosus et atrophicus in children: A report of 24 cases. Arch Dermatol 95:476, 1967.

Davis AJ, Goldstein DP: Treatment of pediatric lichen sclerosus with the CO_2 laser. Adolesc Pediatr Gynecol 2:103, 1989.

Gerstner G, Grunberger W, Boschitsch E, et al: Vaginal organisms in prepubertal children with and without vulvovaginitis. Arch Gynecol 231:247, 1982.

Leung AK, Robson WL, Tay-Uyboco J: The incidence of labial fusion in children. J Paediatr Child Health 29:235, 1993.

Murphy T, Nelson J: Shigella vaginitis: Report of 38 patients and review of the literature. Pediatrics 63:511, 1979.

Paradise J, Willis E: Probability of vaginal body in girls with genital complaints. Am J Dis Child 139:472, 1985.

Redmond CA, Cowell CA, Krafchik BR: Genital lichen sclerosus in prepubertal girls. Adolesc Pediatr Gynecol 1:177, 1988.

Williams T, Callen J, Owen L: Vulvar disorders in the prepubertal female. Pediatr Ann 15:588, 1986.

Young SJ, Wells DL, Ogden EJ: Lichen sclerosus, genital trauma and child sexual abuse. Aust Fam Phys IC 22:729, 1993.

CHAPTER 504
Bleeding

A number of entities responsible for isolated vaginal bleeding include exposure to exogenous sex steroids; foreign body; hemorrhagic cystitis; hypothyroidism; precocious puberty; the presence of an ovarian cyst; trauma, which may or may not be associated with sexual abuse; urethral prolapse; and vulvovaginitis, as well as neoplasms, for example, rhabdomyosarcoma, clear cell sarcoma, endodermal sinus tumors, and mesonephric carcinoma (see Chapter 111 for discussion of menstrual problems).

FOREIGN BODY. A foreign body may be responsible for vaginal bleeding in the pediatric patient. The presence of a foul-smelling discharge with associated vaginal bleeding suggests the possibility of a foreign body. A plain roentgenogram or ultrasound of the pelvis is often helpful. Wadded toilet paper is the most common foreign body identified in the vagina. A vaginal foreign body was found in 18% of preadolescent girls with vaginal bleeding with or without discharge and in 50% of those with bleeding and no discharge.

URETHRAL PROLAPSE. Vulvar bleeding can be associated with urethral prolapse, which is characterized by the urethral mucosa protruding through the meatus and forming a hemorrhagic, often sensitive vulvar mass that bleeds easily. The "mass" is separate from the vagina. There may be difficulty with urination, depending on the size of the mass and whether or not it precludes the urethral meatus. The entity responds to topical application of estrogens.

GENITAL TRAUMA. Although most injuries to this area are accidental, concern must be expressed for the possibility of physical and/or sexual abuse. Blunt injury may cause blood vessels beneath the perineal skin to rupture. Blood accumulating under the skin forms a hematoma, which may present as a round, tense, tender mass. Contusion to the vulva usually does not require treatment. A small vulvar hematoma often can be controlled by pressure with an ice pack, complemented by a prescription for analgesics.

Penetrating injuries to the vaginal area warrant further careful evaluation, and once again the possibility of sexual abuse must be seriously considered. A detailed examination may be necessary, especially in the presence of active bleeding. The potential for bowel and/or bladder trauma must also be considered.

GENITAL TUMORS. Benign and malignant tumors of the vulva must be considered when vaginal bleeding occurs in the pediatric patient. A broad spectrum of entities, ranging from capillary hemangiomas through malignancies such as rhabdomyosarcoma, requires appropriate tissue diagnosis and treatment. The most common tumors include endodermal carcinoma, which occurs most often in young children; mesonephric carcinoma, which arises in a remnant of a mesonephric duct and occurs more often in girls age 3 or older; and clear cell adenocarcinoma, which is often associated with a history of antenatal exposure to diethylstilbestrol (see Chapters 456 and 507).

American College of Obstetricians and Gynecologists: Dysfunctional Uterine Bleeding. ACOG Techn Bull 134, Washington, DC, 1985.
Gidwani GP: Vaginal bleeding in adolescence. J Reprod Med 29:419, 1984.
Grant DB: Vaginal bleeding in childhood. Pediatr Adolesc Gynecol 1:173, 1983.
Kerns DL, Terman DL, Larson CS: The role of physicians in reporting and evaluating child sexual abuse cases. Future Children 4:119, 1994.
Muram D, Sanfilippo JS, Hertweck SP: Vaginal bleeding in childhood and menstrual disorders in adolescence. *In*: Sanfilippo JS (ed): Pediatric and Adolescent Gynecology. Philadelphia, WB Saunders, 1994, pp 222–231.

CHAPTER 505
Breast Disorders

The mammary glands are derived from the epidermal layer. Beginning at approximately 6 wk of gestation, epidermal cells migrate to the mesenchyme and form the mammary ridges. Breast buds, lactiferous ducts, and fully developed mammary glands eventually form. Breast development normally occurs in girls between the ages of 8 1/2 and 13 yr. The rate of breast growth varies, and development is often asymmetric. Complete development may not occur until a woman is in her early 20s.

BREAST SELF-EXAMINATION. Early diagnosis is central to improvement in health care for breast abnormalities, including carcinoma. Instruction in breast self-examination should be given during the initial gynecologic evaluation of the adolescent with reinforcement during follow-up visits (Table 505–1).

TABLE 505–1 How to Do Breast Self-Examination*

1. Lie down. Flatten your right breast by placing a pillow under your right shoulder. If your breasts are large, use your right hand to hold your right breast while you do the exam with your left hand.
2. Use the sensitive pads of the middle three fingers on your left hand. Feel for lumps using a rubbing motion.
3. Press firmly enough to feel different breast tissues.
4. Completely feel all of the breast and chest area to cover breast tissue that extends toward the shoulder. Allow enough time for a complete exam. Women with small breasts will need at least 2 minutes to examine each breast. Larger breasts will take longer.
5. Use the same pattern to feel every part of the breast tissue. Choose the method easiest for you. The three patterns preferred by women and their doctors are the circular, clock or oval pattern, the vertical strip, and the wedge.
6. After you have completely examined your right breast, then examine your left breast using the same method. Compare what you have felt in one breast with the other.
7. You may also want to examine your breasts while bathing, when your skin is wet and lumps may be easier to feel.
8. You can check your breasts in a mirror looking for any change in size or contour, dimpling of the skin, or spontaneous nipple discharge.

**Published with permission of The American Cancer Society, Kentucky Division.*

CONGENITAL ANOMALIES. Complete absence of a breast, *amastia,* is rare; more frequently it is unilateral and often associated with other abnormalities, such as **Poland syndrome** (aplasia of the pectoralis muscles, rib deformities, webbed fingers, and radial nerve aplasia). Amastia can be iatrogenic, as a result of the inadvertent excision of a breast bud. *Athelia* is defined as absence of one or both nipples. This condition is also rare and may not be associated with absent breast tissue. Both abnormalities require surgical correction.

Supernumerary breasts (polymastia) and *supernumerary nipples* (polythelia) are relatively common (Fig. 505–1); they occur along the "milk lines" and are usually asymptomatic. There is an association between polythelia and anomalies of the urinary and cardiovascular systems. In general, surgical excision of accessory breasts or nipples is not necessary. However, if the aberrant breasts or nipples become symptomatic, excision may be indicated.

Hypoplasia of the breasts varies in degree from a nearly total absence of breast tissue to well-formed breasts that are considered by the patient to be too small. There are three general causes for poor or absent breast development: (1) The onset of breast development may be delayed, and the breast will develop slowly but will be normal in all other respects; (2)

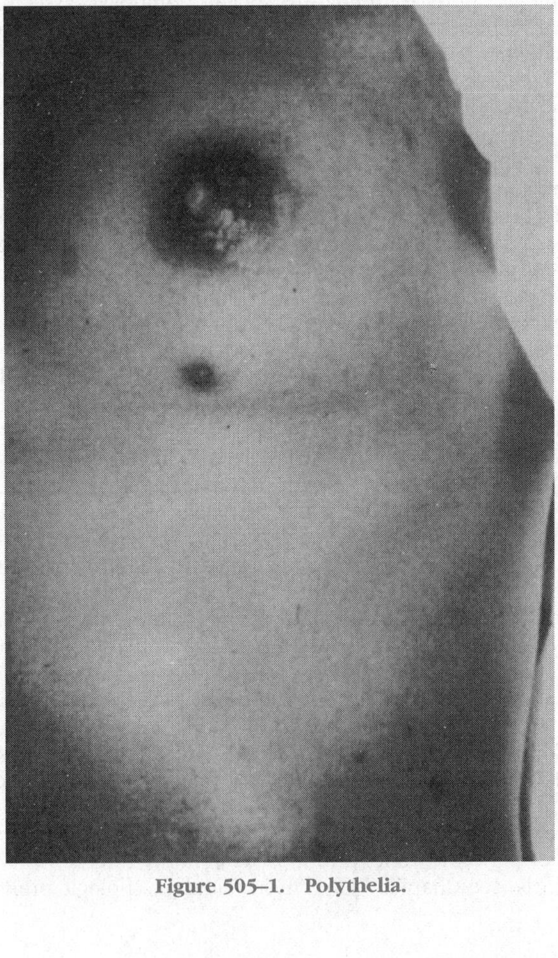

Figure 505–1. Polythelia.

there may be a family history of late breast development; (3) ovarian function may have failed or been suppressed (see Chapter 538). Treatment depends on the underlying cause.

Breast atrophy is seen occasionally in adolescents and is almost uniformly secondary to dietary changes such as occurs with anorexia nervosa. Correction of the underlying problem results in re-establishment of breast tissue.

NEONATAL BREAST ABNORMALITIES. Bilateral breast hypertrophy may occur as a result of elevated circulating endogenous steroid hormones in late gestation. It may be associated with discharge from the nipples known as "witches' milk." Repeated manipulation of the breast can exacerbate the condition. On occasion, the hypertrophy is associated with mastitis caused by a staphylococcal infection; antibiotics should be administered.

MASTODYNIA. Painful breast engorgement (mastodynia) usually is associated with ovulatory cycles; this is uncommon in the adolescent until approximately 18 mo following menarche, the time that may be necessary to establish ovulatory cycles. There is frequently a cyclical pattern to the breast discomfort. Analgesics such as nonsteroidal anti-inflammatory drugs (NSAIDs), including naproxen sodium and ibuprofen, as well as the use of a good support bra, are often helpful in alleviating discomfort.

BREAST MASSES. A retrospective review of breast disease in adolescent females revealed that about 54% have fibroadenomas and 13% have virginal hypertrophy. Fibrocystic or proliferative breast disease occurs in about 24%. Primary rhabdomyosarcoma, metastatic rhabdomyosarcoma, metastatic neuroblastoma, and non-Hodgkin's lymphoma occur in 2–3% of all breast masses in this age group. Other diagnoses include polythelia, accessory breast tissue, mastitis, hemangioma, fat necrosis, and intramammary lymph nodes.

A thorough history and complete physical examination are mandatory for any pediatric or adolescent patient who has a breast mass. The clinical problem should be reviewed with a radiologist prior to rendering specific radiologic assessment. Needle aspiration and biopsy are often essential for evaluation of palpable breast abnormalities. Large breast tumors also occur in adolescents. Although malignancy is often suspected because of rapid growth of the mass and skin ulceration, breast tumors can have varied presentations. Giant fibroadenomas in adolescence may be treated by simple enucleation.

Malignant Tumors. Although rare, breast *cancer* does occur in the adolescent. Early menarche in association with anovulatory cycles is a risk factor. The estrogen-to-androgen ratio appears to be critical, with androgens having a protective effect.

Cystosarcoma phylloides, an uncommon breast tumor in adults, may occur in adolescents. It is characterized by asymmetric breast enlargement in association with a firm, mobile, circumscribed mass. Often the tumor increases rapidly in size and can become quite large. Fixation of the tumor to the skin or chest wall is rare. The majority of these tumors are benign, but malignant cystosarcoma phylloides with metastases has been reported. Excision is the preferred initial therapy in the adolescent patient, regardless of the histologic classification of the lesion. Malignant cystosarcoma is more likely to recur than is a benign lesion. Fatal metastatic cystosarcoma phylloides in an adolescent has been reported.

Breast tumors also may be the first manifestation of relapse (extramedullary) in *acute lymphoblastic leukemia.* Reports in the literature include a case of *radiation-induced sarcoma* of the breast in a female adolescent and a case of *liposarcoma* in a 17-yr-old black female who previously had a total mastectomy.

MACROMASTIA (VIRGINAL HYPERTROPHY). The etiology of massive breast enlargement during puberty and early adolescence is unknown but probably represents an end-organ increased sensitivity to circulating estrogens. It is bilateral, often occurs over a brief period of time, and most commonly affects 13–17-yr-old girls (see Chapter 112). Physical and psychologic problems may occur in the adolescent with macromastia. Posture problems and discomfort often result. Reduction mammoplasty is the treatment of choice but should be delayed until late adolescence to allow for complete breast development. Surgical intervention often necessitates relocation of the nipple, which may result in decreased sensation and altered lactation. In addition, strong emotional support should be provided.

MASTITIS AND ABSCESS. Mastitis and breast abscess may require antibiotic therapy as well as incision and drainage. Coverage should include *Staphylococcus* species.

TRAUMA AND INFLAMMATION. Breast trauma in adolescent females is more common because of the increased number of young women participating in contact sports. The trauma usually takes the form of contusion or hematoma, and often resolves without incident. Occasionally, fat necrosis occurs and results in either late cystic changes in the breast or fibrosis with retraction of skin or the nipple over the injured area. These late changes may mimic those associated with malignancy; biopsy may be the only means of differentiating between the two.

MAMMARY DYSPLASIA. This common lesion is characterized by changes associated with the menstrual cycle. Hormonal imbalance associated with exaggerated responses in the breast tissue, especially in the upper and outer quadrants during the premenstrual phase of the cycle, may account for the problem. The extent of treatment depends on the degree of symptomatology. Danazol (Danocrine), a synthetic androgen, can be beneficial in the adolescent patient; daily dosage ranges from 100 to 800 mg, depending on weight. In addition, methylxanthines and caffeine (e.g., coffee, tea, carbonated drinks) should be eliminated from the diet.

NIPPLE DISCHARGE. This must be carefully evaluated and a distinction made between the presence of galactorrhea ("spontaneous flow of milk") and bloody discharge. Evaluation of galactorrhea in children is the same as for adults. Serum prolactin levels are obtained to rule out the presence of a pituitary prolactinoma (see Chapter 504). If there is suspicion of a pituitary tumor or adenoma based on markedly elevated serum prolactin levels, with or without headaches and bitemporal hemianopsia, appropriate radiologic (computed tomography [CT], magnetic resonance imaging [MRI]) assessment is necessary. Another cause of galactorrhea is hypothyroidism in association with elevated levels of thyroid releasing hormone, which also stimulates prolactin release. Treatment of galactorrhea consists primarily of dopamine agonists such as bromocriptine (Parlodel). Surgical intervention, usually in the form of transsphenoidal hypophysectomy, is rarely required. Galactorrhea secondary to chest wall surgery in an adolescent has also been reported. The galactorrhea occurred for 2 mo and was associated with transient amenorrhea.

Bloody nipple discharge can be indicative of *duct ectasia.* Cytologic assessment and surgical consultation are indicated. Nipple discharge in association with *Montgomery tubercles* also has been reported. These secretions can be episodic and vary in color from clear to brown, but they are usually not milky. This discharge evolves over a period of 3–5 wk and may be associated with breast lumps. This is a benign, self-limited problem. *Intraductal breast papillomas* have been reported in adolescents.

Apter D, Vinko R: Early menarche, a risk factor for breast cancer, indicates early onset of ovulatory cycles. J Clin Endocrinol Metab 57:82, 1983.

Briggs R, Walters M, Rosenthal D: Cystosarcoma phylloides in adolescent female patients. Am J Surg 146:712, 1983.

Cromer B, Frankel M, Kader L: Compliance with breast self-examination and instruction in healthy adolescents. J Adolesc Health Care 10:105, 1989.

Diehl G, Kaplan D: Breast masses in adolescent females. J Adolesc Health Care 6:353, 1985.

Ellegaard J, Bendix-Hanson K, Boesen A, et al: Breast tumor as a first manifestation of extramedullary relapse in acute lymphoblastic leukemia. Scand J Haemotol 33:288, 1984.

Heyman R, Rauh J: Areolar gland discharge in adolescent females appears to be benign. J Adolesc Health Care 4:285, 1983.
Letson G, Moore D: Galactorrhea secondary to chest wall surgery in an adolescent. J Adolesc Health Care 5:277, 1984.
Ngala Kenda J: Fatal metastatic cystosarcoma phylloides in a young woman: Report of a case. Arch Surg 118:871, 1983.
Raganoonan C, Fairbairn J, Williams S, et al: Giant breast tumors of adolescence. Aust NZ J Surg 57:243, 1987.
Simmons P, Wold L: Surgically treated breast disease in adolescent females: A retrospective review of 185 cases. Adolesc Pediatr Gynecol 2:95, 1989.
Watkind F, Giacomantonio M, Salisbury S: Nipple discharge and breast lump related to Montgomery's tubercles in adolescent females. J Pediatr Surg 23:718, 1988.

CHAPTER 506
Hirsutism and Polycystic Ovarian Syndrome

EXCESSIVE ANDROGEN PRODUCTION PRIOR TO PUBERTY. Hirsutism (excessive hair growth) must be distinguished from virilization. The latter involves increased body hair, acne, deepening of the voice, change in body habitus due to increased muscle mass, and clitoromegaly (see Chapter 517). Premature pubarche is defined as the appearance of genital hair or axillary hair, or both, before 8 yr of age. (Chapter 505) Adrenarche, the output of increased androgen from the adrenal gland, usually occurs between 12 and 18 yr of age and is discussed in Chapter 516.

HIRSUTISM IN THE ADOLESCENT. Table 506–1 lists the causes of hirsutism. *Androgen-producing* tumors of adrenal or gonadal origin should be considered when an adolescent presents with excessive hair growth. However, hirsutism is most often *idiopathic* with normal total circulating androgen levels. Sex hormone-binding globulin (SHBG) levels may be decreased in hirsute patients, which allows a higher fraction of bioactive androgens despite normal serum androgen levels. SHBG levels are affected by a number of factors. Androgens, specifically testosterone, cause a decrease in SHBG levels; estrogens and dexamethasone tend to increase SHBG. Futhermore, a decline in SHBG occurs with increasing age, especially from prepuberty to adolescence. Body weight has an inverse correlation with SHBG levels independent of androgen levels.

■ **TABLE 506–1 Causes of Hirsutism**

Peripheral
- Idiopathic
- Partial androgen insensitivity (5-α-reductase deficiency)
- HAIR-AN syndrome (hirsutism, androgenization, insulin resistance, and acanthosis nigricans)
- Hyperprolactinemia

Gonadal
- Polycystic ovary syndrome (PCO, chronic anovulation)
- Ovarian neoplasm (Sertoli-Leydig cell, granulosa cell, thecoma, gynandroblastoma, lipoid cell, luteoma, hypernephroma, Brenner's tumor)
- Gonadal dysgenesis (Turner's mosaic with XY, or H-Y antigen positive)

Adrenal
- Cushing syndrome
- Adrenal hyper-responsiveness
- Congenital adrenal hyperplasia (classic, cryptic, adult onset)
  - 21-hydroxylase deficiency
  - 11-hydroxylase deficiency
  - 3-β-ol-dehydrogenase deficiency
  - 17-ol-dehydrogenase deficiency
- Adrenal neoplasm (adenoma, cortical carcinoma)

Exogenous

Minoxidil	Oral contraceptives
Dilantin	Danazol
Cyclosporin	Androgenic steroids
Anabolic steroids	Psoralens
Diamox	Diazide
Penicillamine	Phenothiazines

Congenital Anomalies
- Trisomy 18 (Edward syndrome)
- Cornelia de Lange syndrome
- Hurler syndrome
- Juvenile hypothyroidism

From Bailey-Pridham DD, Sanfilippo JS: Hirsutism in the adolescent female. Pediatr Clin North Am 36:581, 1989.

HAIR-AN syndrome is the acronym for the association of hirsutism, androgen excess, insulin resistance, and acanthosis nigricans. The pathogenesis of this syndrome is unknown. However, there is a defect in membrane insulin receptors. Elevated androgen levels contribute to the development of acanthosis.

Hyperprolactinemia, a central nervous system disorder, is an occasional cause of hyperandrogenemia (see Chapter 517). Approximately 40% of patients with hyperprolactinemia exhibit androgenic abnormalities. Laboratory findings may include elevated free testosterone due to decreased SHBG levels and increased adrenal production of 17-hydroxyprogesterone and androstenedione following ACTH stimulation.

Polycystic ovary syndrome (PCO, chronic anovulation, Stein-Leventhal syndrome) is the most commonly diagnosed ovarian cause of hirsutism (see Chapter 538). The underlying biochemical cause of PCO is unknown, and controversy exists over whether the basic defect is central (hypothalamic or pituitary regulation of gonadotropins) or ovarian (defect in a peptide hormone, perhaps inhibin, with resultant abnormal feedback to the pituitary gland). The usual hormonal pattern of PCO begins with altered luteinizing hormone release (a luteinizing hormone-to-follicle stimulating hormone ratio of 2:1 or 3:1, shortened pulse frequency, and slightly increased pulse amplitude of luteinizing hormone). Adolescents with hyperandrogenism display an exaggerated luteinizing hormone pulsatility similar to that found in adults with PCO syndrome.

Hirsutism in adolescents can also be due to a heterozygous form of *21-hydroxylase deficiency* (see Chapter 529). This has been called adult-onset congenital adrenal hyperplasia (AO-CAH). Various other forms of *congenital adrenal hyperplasia* and *congenital anomalies* are also associated with hirsutism. Clinically, it may be difficult to distinguish between PCO and AO-CAH.

Ovarian hyperthecosis, which can be familial, may be a variant of PCO. Hyperthecosis is defined as isolated islands of luteinized cells within the ovary contributing to increased androgen production. Ovarian androgen production and peripheral effects are similar to those associated with PCO.

Medications, radiation, and chronic irritation (e.g., the placement of a cast) can also initiate localized, nonendocrinologic hair growth.

Treatment of the Hirsute Patient. Treatment alternatives for idiopathic hirsutism and PCO are outlined in Table 506–2. Hirsutism secondary to hyperprolactinemia is best treated with bromocriptine. In patients with multicystic (polycystic) ovaries and primary hypothyroidism, the polycystic ovaries resolve rapidly with adequate doses of thyroid replacement therapy. If an exogenous cause such as a medication is producing hirsutism, it should be eliminated.

Even when the increased tissue androgen effect is reversed by appropriate treatment, hair follicles converted to terminal hair may still produce that type of hair. Electrolysis may then provide an improved cosmetic appearance, with the assurance that if the underlying abnormality is controlled there should be no new growth of hair.

Cushing syndrome or disease, androgen-producing tumors, and congenital adrenal hyperplasia are discussed in Chapters 529 and 530.

■ **TABLE 506–2 Treatment of Hirsutism: Idiopathic and Polycystic Ovary Syndrome**

Medication	Dose†	Comments
Oral contraceptives (estrogen dominant)	35 μg	Decrease in plasma testosterone, androstenedione, and DHEA-S
Spironolactone	100 mg bid	Decreased androgen production and androgen receptor competition
Medroxyprogesterone acetate-depo (Depo-Provera)	150–250 mg q 2–4 wk	Decreased testosterone production and 17-ketosteroid levels
Cyproterone acetate	Diane, 2 mg Androcur, 100 mg	Decreased plasma testosterone, androstenedione, SHBG, induces "insulinemia"
Dexamethasone	0.25–0.5 mg	Dose adequate if plasma-free testosterone <15 pg/mL
Cimetidine	200–300 mg tid–qid	Decreased serum testosterone, increased serum estradiol
GnRH agonist (Nafarelin)	1,000 μg	Decreased testosterone and androstenedione

From Bailey-Pridham DD, Sanfilippo JS: Hirsutism in the adolescent female. Pediatr Clin North Am 36:581, 1989; with permission.
†Dosages given are for a 70-kg female. Daily dosages are indicated unless otherwise specified.

Apter D, Siegberg R, Laatikainen T: Pulsatile secretion of luteinizing hormone in adolescents with hyperandrogenism. Adolesc Pediatr Gynecol 1:104, 1988.
Belgorosky A, Rivarola M: Progressive increase in non-sex hormone binding globulin-bound testosterone and estradiol from infancy to late prepuberty in girls. J Clin Endocrinol Metab 67:234, 1988.
Boor JT, Herwig J, Schrezenneir J, et al: Familial insulin resistant diabetes associated with acanthosis nigricans, polycystic ovaries, hypogonadism, pigmentary retinopathy, labrinthine deafness, and mental retardation. Am J Med Genet 45:649, 1993.
Judd H, Scully R, Herbst A, et al: Familial hyperthecosis: Comparison of endocrinologic and histologic findings with polycystic ovarian disease. Am J Obstet Gynecol 117:976, 1973.
Kamilaris T, DeBold C, Manolus K, et al: Testosterone secreting adrenal adenoma in a peripubertal patient. JAMA 258:2558, 1987.
Lindsay A, Voorhess M, MacGillivray M: Multicystic ovaries in primary hypothyroidism. Obstet Gynecol 61:433, 1983.
Parker L, Sack J, Fisher D, et al: The adrenarche: Prolactin, gonadotropins, adrenal androgens and cortisol. J Clin Endocrinol Metab 60:409, 1985.
Rosen G, Kaplan B, Lobo R: Menstrual function and hirsutism in patients with gonadal dysgenesis. Obstet Gynecol 71:677, 1988.
Speroff L, Glass RH, Kase NG: Hirsutism. *In*: Speroff L, Glass RH, Kase NG (eds): Clinical Gynecologic Endocrinology and Infertility, 4th ed. Baltimore, Williams & Wilkins, 1989, p 233.
Zumogg B, Freeman R, Coupa S, et al: A chronobiologic abnormality of luteinizing hormone secretion in teenage girls with the polycystic ovary syndrome. N Engl J Med 309:1206, 1983.

CHAPTER 507
Neoplasms

The most common gynecologic neoplasm found in children is of ovarian origin and usually presents as an abdominal mass. The vagina or vulva, or both, may also be the site of benign or malignant lesions in children (see Chapter 504); cervical dyspasia may occur in adolescents. Breast masses are discussed in Chapter 505.

OVARIES. Ovarian tumors are the most frequent type of pelvic neoplasm noted in patients less than 18 yr of age; paraovarian tumors are next in frequency, followed by uterine neoplasms. Most often, the clinical presentation is that of abdominal pain, a mass, or both. In the adolescent, the most common ovarian neoplasm is the *teratoma*. It is usually benign, but malignant teratomas may occur. Calcification on abdominal roentgenogram is often a hallmark of a benign teratoma. During surgery the opposite ovary should be evaluated. If there is any question about the possibility of a neoplasm, biopsy is obtained. Ovarian *adenomas* are the second most common benign ovarian tumor.

With respect to *germ cell tumors*, the most common is the dysgerminoma, followed in incidence by malignant teratomas, endodermal sinus tumors, embryonal carcinomas, mixed cell neoplasms, and gonadoblastomas. Germ cell neoplasms (e.g., immature teratomas, endodermal sinus tumors) are a more aggressive malignancy than dysgerminomas and occur in a significantly higher proportion of younger females (under 10 yr of age). In this age group, 10-yr survival rates determined by life table analyses were 73% for epithelial carcinomas, 44% for sex cord stromal tumors, 73% for dysgerminomas, 33% for malignant teratomas, 39% for endodermal sinus tumors, 25% for embryonal carcinomas, 30% for other germ cell neoplasms, and 100% for gonadoblastomas. Dysgerminomas usually are associated with XY gonadal dysgenesis. Y-DNA probes are becoming increasingly important in their diagnosis. Tumor markers such as α-fetoprotein, carcinoembryonic antigen, and the antigen CA-125 are also used to assess ovarian malignancy.

Surgical excision followed by postoperative chemotherapy and radiotherapy is often necessary. Staging at the beginning of therapy is of the utmost importance. In many cases, a second-look procedure can assist further in the treatment of these neoplasms.

Sex cord stromal tumors comprise 5% of ovarian neoplasms, of which the *granulosa cell tumor* is the most common. Isosexual precocity and occasionally virilization may be observed in the juvenile variety. The characteristic histologic features include nodular architecture, follicle formation, microcysts, cell necrosis, and increased mitotic activity.

Ovarian Follicular Cysts. Such entities occur from birth to puberty and usually disappear spontaneously. By ultrasound the cyst usually presents as a nonechogenic area, frequently larger than 20 mm at its greatest diameter; diffuse swelling of the ovarian parenchyma and follicular enlargement of the cortical zone are also noted.

Ovarian Torsion. Torsion of an adnexum is a complication that must always be considered, and prompt surgical intervention is necessary. Torsion often presents with intermittent sharp abdominal pain that, in many cases, radiates down the ipsilateral extremity. Bilateral ovarian torsion may occur in infancy and should be considered in the differential diagnosis of abdominal pain in the pediatric female patient. When unilateral torsion is diagnosed, oophoropexy (plication) of the contralateral adnexa is recommended.

Autoamputation of the Ovary. This entity presents as a small, calcified free-floating mass associated with an absent adnexa. The child may be asymptomatic, and ultrasound is often helpful in establishing the diagnosis. It has been hypothesized that antenatal or subclinical ovarian torsion leads to necrosis, calcification, and separation of the adnexa from its blood supply.

CERVIX. *Cervical intraepithelial neoplasia* (CIN), diagnosed in sexually active teenagers and young adults, is associated with abnormal cytology in 2–3% of patients. The prevalence of dysplasia and carcinoma in situ is 18.8/1,000 for those 15–19 yr of age. Biopsy-proven cases of all grades of CIN in the teenage population have a prevalence of 13.3/1,000. Sexually transmitted diseases are well correlated with CIN. In a case-controlled study, human papilloma virus infection and altered vaginal flora were consistent findings in patients with CIN.

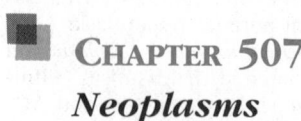

Abnormal Papanicolaou (Pap) smears in adolescents also correlate with significant CIN; abnormal Pap smears should be evaluated and a tissue diagnosis obtained. Colposcopic examination is essential when CIN is diagnosed in the adolescent. Other perhaps somewhat more common pathologic abnormalities of the cervix include cervical polyps and mixed mesodermal tumor. The latter may represent a mixed, heterologous, or homologous sarcoma of the uterine cervix.

UTERUS (Benign and Malignant Tumors of the Uterine Corpus). *Adenocarcinoma* of the corpus is rare in children and adolescents. Vaginal bleeding that is not associated with sexual precocity in the pediatric patient is a frequent sign at presentation. The treatment of malignant tumors consists of hysterectomy, ideally with removal of the ovaries, followed by adjunctive radiotherapy or chemotherapy, or both, depending on the operative findings. Mixed *mesodermal tumors* of the uterus also have been noted. *Leiomyomata* are described in this age group and should be included in the differential diagnosis of an adolescent presenting with a pelvic mass. *Leiomyosarcoma* has also been noted in an adolescent; the presentation is variable, but usually abnormal vaginal bleeding is present.

VAGINA. One of the more common vaginal wall abnormalities is the *Gartner duct (mesonephric) cyst.* Usually it is an incidental finding and requires no specific therapy. In the sexually active patient, excision may be necessary if there is associated dyspareunia. *Paramesonephric (müllerian) duct cysts* often become symptomatic at menarche when the cavity fills with menstrual blood. Women who were exposed to diethylstilbestrol (DES) in utero have a high incidence of *adenosis* of the vagina and cervix (see Chapter 504). These patients have a host of potential reproductive abnormalities, including infertility, habitual abortion, and tubal and uterine cavity abnormalities. *Clear cell adenocarcinoma* of the vagina and cervix is a rare sequela of DES exposure in utero.

Sarcoma botryoides, a vaginal carcinoma that occurs primarily in the pediatric patient, is best treated by surgical excision. Chemotherapy is usually administered postoperatively. Any questionable vulvar lesion should be submitted for histologic examination. *Liposarcoma* of the vulva has been reported in a 15-yr-old girl. *Malignant melanoma* of the vulva has also been described in a 14-yr-old patient.

Ablin A, Issacs H Jr. Germ cell tumors. *In:* Pizzo PA, Poplack DG (eds): Pediatric Oncology. Philadelphia, JB Lippincott, 1989, pp 713–731.
Barber HR: Ovarian cancers in childhood. Int J Radiat Oncol Biol Phys 8:1427, 1982.
Berenson A, Pokorny S, Dutton R: The autoamputated ovary: A rare cause of abdominal calcification. Adolesc Pediatr Gynecol 2:99, 1989.
Biscotti C, Hart W: Juvenile granulosa cell tumors of the ovary. Arch Pathol Lab Med 113:40, 1989.
Brooks J, Livolsi V: Liposarcoma presenting on the vulva. Am J Obstet Gynecol 156:73, 1987.
Copeland LJ, Gershenson DM, Saul PB, et al: Sarcoma botryoides of the female genital tract. Obstet Gynecol 66:262, 1985.
Freedman R, Kopf A, Jones W: Malignant melanoma in association with lichen sclerosus on the vulva of a 14-year-old. Am J Dermatopathol 6:253, 1984.
Graif M, Itzchak Y: Sonographic evaluation of ovarian torsion in childhood and adolescence. AJR 150:647, 1988.
Gribbon M, Ein SH, Mancer K: Pediatric malignant ovarian tumors: A three-year review. J Pediatr Surg 27:480, 1992.
Guijon F, Paraskevas M, Brunham R: The association of sexually transmitted diseases with cervical intraepithelial neoplasia: A case-controlled study. Am J Obstet Gynecol 151:185, 1985.
Hicks ML, Piver S: Conservative surgery plus adjuvant therapy for vulvovaginal rhabdomyosarcoma, diethylstilbesterol, clear cell adenocarcinoma of the vagina and unilateral germ cell tumors of the ovary. Obstet Gynecol Clin North Am 19:219, 1992.
Liapi C, Evain-Biron D: Diagnosis of ovarian follicular cyst from birth to puberty: A report of 20 cases. Acta Paediatr Scand 76:91, 1987.
Rosenfeld WD, Kleinhaus S, Kutcher R, et al: Leiomyoma in a 15-year-old girl. Adolesc Pediatr Gynecol 1:109, 1988.
Roye CF: Abnormal cervical cytology in adolescents: A literature review. J Adolesc Health 13:643, 1992.
Sadeghi S, Hsieh E, Gonn S: Prevalence of cervical intraepithelial neoplasia in sexually active teenagers and young adults: Results of data analysis of mass Papanicolaou screening of 796,337 women in the United States in 1981. Am J Obstet Gynecol 148:726, 1984.
Sagot P, Lopes P, Mensier A, et al: Carbon dioxide laser treatment of cervical dysplasia in teenagers. Eur J Obstet Gynecol Reprod Biol 46:143, 1992.
Starceski P, Lee P, Siever W: Bilateral ovarian pathology and torsion in infancy: Assessment of pubertal and gonadal function. Adolesc Pediatr Gynecol 1:199, 1988.
Young RH, Kozakewich WP, Scully RE: Metastatic ovarian tumors in children: A report of 14 cases and review of the literature. Int J Gynecol Pathol 12:8, 1993.

CHAPTER 508
Developmental Anomalies

EMBRYOLOGY. The *uterus* is formed by fusion of the cordal elements of the müllerian ducts, a process that occurs at 8 wk of gestation. The fusion begins from the cordal end (Müller tubercle) and is completed at the upper level of the fundus. A median septum is present until the end of the 1st trimester of gestation.

The *vagina* is formed from the terminal portion of the uterovaginal canal (müllerian origin), which is met by the posterior aspect of the urogenital sinus (terminal portion of Müller tubercle). Further thickening occurs in the portion of the posterior wall of the urogenital sinus that is in contact with Müller tubercle. The tissue is of combined urogenital and müllerian duct origin and is known as the vaginal epithelial plate. Bilateral evaginations of the vaginal epithelial plate encircle the caudal aspect and form the uterine canal. Canalization of the vaginal plate occurs and proceeds in a caudal direction to form the vagina. The process elongates the vaginal structure, leaving the cranial two thirds of müllerian origin and the caudal one third of urogenital origin.

Common müllerian duct anomalies are defined in Tables 508–1 and 508–2.

CONGENITAL ABSENCE OF THE VAGINA (MAYER-ROKITANSKY-KUSTER-HAUSER SYNDROME). This anomaly is often discovered in adolescents who present with primary amenorrhea. Absence of the vagina has significant anatomic, physiologic, and psychologic implications for the patient and family. Vaginal agenesis is characterized by primary amenorrhea with absence of the vagina and presence of a normal vulva, a duplication anomaly of the uterus, attenuated fallopian tubes, normal ovaries, normal female karyotype, normal female phenotype, and associated anomalies (most frequently renal and skeletal).

INCOMPLETE VERTICAL FUSION OF THE VAGINA. Transverse and longitudinal vaginal septa represent failure of completion of canalization of the vagina. Not uncommonly, the patient presents with amenorrhea and with cyclical pain, which is a result of cryptomenorrhea. Müllerian agenesis must be differentiated from androgen insensitivity (testicular feminization). A serum testosterone level will usually distinguish whether the levels are in the male range, as occurs in androgen insensitivity

■ **TABLE 508–1 Common Müllerian Anomalies**

Hydrocolpos	Accumulation of mucus or nonsanguineous fluid in the vagina
Hemihematometra	Atretic segment of vagina with menstrual fluid accumulation
Hydrosalpinx	Accumulation of serous fluid in the fallopian tube, often an end result of pyosalpinx
Didelphic uterus	Two cervices each associated with one uterine horn
Bicornuate uterus	One cervix associated with two uterine horns
Unicornuate uterus	Result of failure of one müllerian duct to descend

■ TABLE 508–2 Heritable Disorders Associated with Müllerian Anomalies*

Mode of Inheritance	Disorder	Associated Müllerian Defect
Autosomal dominant	Camptobrachydactyly	Longitudinal vaginal septa
	Hand-foot-genital	Incomplete müllerian fusion
Autosomal recessive	Kaufman-McCusick	Transverse vaginal septa
	Johanson-Blizzard	Longitudinal vaginal septa
	Renal-genital-middle ear anomalies	Vaginal atresia
	Fraser syndrome	Incomplete müllerian fusion
	Uterine hernia syndrome	Persistent müllerian duct derivatives
Polygenic/multifactorial	Mayer-Rokitansky-Kuster-Hauser syndrome	Müllerian aplasia
X linked	Uterine hernia syndrome	Persistent müllerian duct derivatives

*From Shulman L, Elias S: Developmental abnormalities of the female reproductive tract: Pathogenesis and nosology. Adolesc Pediatr Gynecol 1:232, 1988.

syndrome. Müllerian agenesis is associated with renal anomalies in 34% and skeletal anomalies in 12% of patients. Unilateral renal agenesis (15%) is the most common abnormality followed by skeletal anomalies, the most frequent of which are vertebral abnormalities. Klippel-Feil syndrome has been reported in association with müllerian agenesis. Müllerian agenesis, with a reported incidence of 1/5,000 to 1/20,000, is more common than androgen insensitivity and second in frequency to gonadal dysgenesis as a cause of primary amenorrhea. There is usually a normal female karyotype of 46 XX but autosomal translocation of chromosomes 12q and 14q occurs. Affected siblings have been reported, as well as families with variable expression of defects in müllerian, renal, and skeletal systems.

An intravenous pyelogram (IVP) is indicated to determine the presence and extent of associated renal anomalies. Skeletal anomalies should also be ruled out. Karyotype determination will help in ruling out other diagnoses, such as androgen insensitivity (46XY). A pelvic ultrasound is helpful in defining the anomaly, and computed tomography (CT) scanning and magnetic resonance imaging (MRI) provide increased refinement in detail. Laparoscopy is usually reserved for evaluation of a pelvic mass and associated abnormalities.

Vaginoplasty is best deferred until the patient has matured and should be supported by counseling for both patient and family. The MacIndoe procedure, the usual treatment of choice, involves the use of a skin graft, usually from the buttocks, to create a vagina after appropriate dissection of the vulvovaginal area. Other procedures have included the use of human amniotic membrane as an allograft and the use of fasciocutaneous flaps for vaginal reconstruction. The artificial vaginal epithelium changes cytologically to an almost normal-appearing vaginal mucosa. Various dilatation procedures result in an increased vaginal size, which ultimately permits intercourse. Squamous cell carcinoma of the reconstructed vagina has been reported and appears to be related to the type of tissue transplanted. Radiotherapy is usually the primary method of treatment for this particular squamous cell carcinoma.

TRANSVERSE VAGINAL SEPTA. The incidence of transverse vaginal septa is approximately 1/80,000 females. The patient presents with amenorrhea, which may be associated with cyclical pelvic pain, and often a pelvic mass as well as *cryptomenorrhea.* The problem is usually asymptomatic until puberty, although it may present in pediatric patients as *hydrometrocolpos.* It may be associated with other congenital anomalies, although this occurs less often than with müllerian agenesis. The most common site of the septum is between the middle and upper thirds of the vagina. These patients have a functional uterus, although their fertility is often compromised; 47% of affected females in one retrospective series had spontaneous abortions. The prognosis is worse for higher obstructions. There is also an increased incidence of endometriosis secondary to retrograde menstruation.

Evaluation of transverse vaginal septa includes careful pelvic examination and often pelvic imaging to delineate the anatomic abnormalities. Treatment is surgical resection of the obstruction from below. Anastomosis of the upper and lower segments should be attempted, if at all possible, to prevent stenosis. A skin graft may be necessary. Often a lucite form is placed in the vagina to maintain patency.

DISORDERS OF LATERAL FUSION. These include a number of anatomic variations of nonobstructive longitudinal septum as well as the obstructed hemivagina. The latter may be associated with a didelphic uterus and often with a pelvic mass, which represents retrograde menstruation associated with the occluded hemivagina. The patient presents with menses that are often cyclical, representing an unobstructed outflow tract from one of the uterine horns.

The incidence of uterine anomalies ranges from 1/100 to 1/1,000. Anomalous development of the uterine cavity may have a host of clinical presentations. The patient may present with primary amenorrhea or with irregular or even regular menses. There may be an asymptomatic pelvic mass or dysmenorrhea. In the adult, pregnancy wastage and infertility may cause the first suspicion of uterine anomaly. Evaluation should include a pelvic ultrasound, IVP, and skeletal inspection for anomalies. Karyotyping and diagnostic laparoscopy may be necessary, depending on the presentation and laboratory assessment. A hysterosalpingogram may be helpful in further delineating the uterine anomaly.

Treatment depends on the specific anomaly and must be individualized accordingly. Traditionally, surgical repair of uterine malformations have included Strassman metroplasty, Jones "wedge" metroplasty, and Tompkins metroplasty. The obstructions to the outflow tract must also be relieved; this may necessitate creation of a vaginal window or excision of a hemivagina. Careful determination of retrograde menstruation in a uterine horn must also be considered and appropriate surgical correction provided.

CONGENITAL ATRESIA OF THE UTERINE CERVIX. The patient often presents at puberty with cryptomenorrhea, amenorrhea, and pelvic pain. This problem is extremely rare and is associated with significant renal anomalies in 5–10% of patients. On examination, there is complete absence of a cervix but the presence of a palpable uterus. Pelvic imaging is helpful in defining the abnormality. Treatment may include laparotomy to create a uterovaginal fistula. If this is impossible, a hysterectomy may be necessary. Other anomalies include mesonephric cysts, which are remnants of the wolffian duct. Incomplete reduplication of internal genitalia and unilateral renal aplasia also have been reported. Each of these patients had a didelphic uterus, in which one uterus emptied into a normally developed vagina and the other into a blind pouch (hemihematometra) or into an atretic vagina (hemihematocolpos). In addition, gastrointestinal (42.9%), respiratory (47.6%), central nervous system (28.6%), cardiovascular (38.1%), and musculoskeletal abnormalities (33.3%) also may be associated.

COMPLETE VULVAR DUPLICATION. This rare congenital anomaly presents in infancy and consists of two vulvas, vaginas, and bladders, a didelphic uterus, a single rectum and anus, and two renal systems.

LABIAL HYPERTROPHY. Elongation of the labia minora can be present at birth. Usually this is of no consequence. Surgical revision may be necessary if the problem is symptomatic.

CLITORAL ABNORMALITIES. Agenesis of the clitoris is rare. Clitoral duplication has been reported and is often associated with pelvic organ abnormalities, including agenesis of other genital structures as well as associated bladder exstrophy.

CLITORAL HYPERTROPHY IN ASSOCIATION WITH AMBIGUOUS GENITALIA. See Chapter 529.

HYMENAL ABNORMALITIES. An imperforate hymen can be present in the pediatric patient and is often associated with mucocolpos; it can also be associated with hydrometrocolpos. Other hymenal abnormalities include cribriform or stenotic hymen.

Bergh P, Breen J, Gregori C: Congenital absence of the vagina—the Mayer-Rokitansky-Kuster-Hauser syndrome. Adolesc Pediatr Gynecol 2:73, 1989.
Freedman M: Uterine anomalies. Semin Reprod Endocrinol 4:39, 1986.
Hopkins M, Marley G: Squamous cell carcinoma of the neovagina. Obstet Gynecol 69:525, 1987.
Horejsi JA: Incomplete reduplication of internal genitalia and unilateral renal aplasia syndrome. Adolesc Pediatr Gynecol 1:42, 1988.
Joshi N, Sotrel G: Diagnostic laparoscopy in apparent uterine agenesis. J Adolesc Health Care 9:403, 1988.
Kucheria K, Taneja N, Kinra G: Autosomal translocation of chromosomes 12q and 14q in müllerian duct failure. Indian J Med Res 87:290, 1988.
Lewis V, Money J: Gender-identity/role. Par A:XY (androgen insensitivity) syndrome and XX (Rokitansky) syndrome, vaginal atresia compared. *In*: Dennerstein L, Burroughs G (eds): Handbook of Psychosomatic Obstetrics and Gynecology. New York, Elsevier Biomedical Press, 1983, p 61.
Morton K, Davies D, Dewhurst J: The use of the fasciocutaneous flap in vaginal reconstruction. Br J Obstet Gynaecol 93:970, 1986.
Rock J, Azziz R: Genital anomalies in childhood. Clin Obstet Gynecol 30:682, 1987.
Shulman LP, Elias S: Developmental abnormalities of the female reproductive tract: Pathogenesis and nosology. Adolesc Pediatr Gynecol 1:230, 1987.
Sorenson S: Estimated prevalence of müllerian anomalies. Acta Obstet Gynecol Scand 67:441, 1988.

CHAPTER 509

Athletic Problems

The most common gynecologic endocrinologic problem in the female athlete is menstrual aberration, usually manifested as amenorrhea or oligomenorrhea. It has been reported that female adolescents who participate in strenuous training have significant alterations in circulating hormone levels and reproductive function. Specific problems include delayed puberty, delayed menarche, and oligoovulation with resultant oligomenorrhea. A significant inverse relationship between plasma estradiol and miles run per week has been reported. Adolescent female runners who train extensively have associated low serum estradiol levels and are predisposed to bone demineralization.

Endogenous opiates (EOP) within the hypothalamus may also play a role in that EOP inhibit gonadotropin-releasing hormone neurons and thus affect LH secretion and reproductive function. Serum cortisol levels also are affected; there is an increase in both eumenorrheic and amenorrheic runners compared with sedentary controls. Overall, athletes appear to have an increase in corticotropin secretion. Body composition and weight loss appear to be integrally involved in the menstrual defect. Amenorrheic runners tend to have less body fat than eumenorrheic runners. Menarche has been reported to be delayed approximately 3 yr in ballet dancers (in comparison with nonathletic adolescents) preparing for a professional career. Delayed puberty in association with endurance training does not appear to be related to significant alteration in follicle-stimulating hormone (FSH) and luteinizing hormone (LH) levels. They are generally in the low to normal range and are essentially the same as in normal prepubertal children (an individual who is 13–16 yr of age). It is important to assess nutritional status and other potential causes before delayed puberty is ruled out.

Baer JT, Taper LJ, Gwazdauskas FG, et al: Diet, hormonal, and metabolic factors affecting bone mineral density in adolescent amenorrheic and eumenorrheic female runners. J Sports Med Phys Fitness 32:51, 1992.
Ding JH, Sheckter CB, Drinkwater BL, et al. High serum cortisol levels in exercise-associated amenorrhea. Ann Intern Med 108:530, 1988.
Warren MD, Brooks-Gunn J, Hamilton LH, et al. Scoliosis and fractures in young ballet dancers. Relation to delayed menarche and secondary amenorrhea. N Engl J Med 314:1348, 1986.

CHAPTER 510

Children with Special Gynecologic Needs

Gynecologic care for the mentally handicapped pediatric or adolescent patient is a challenging task. When the mentally handicapped adolescent presents to the clinician with the problem of "perineal hygiene," an adequate gynecologic examination is required. Outpatient sedation with oral ketamine (Ketalar) and midazolam (Versed) markedly decreases the need for examination under anesthesia. Once an adequate examination, including a Pap smear, is obtained, the various alternative treatments should be discussed.

A number of medical approaches have been proposed to suppress the menses, for example, depomedroxyprogesterone acetate, usually prescribed at a dose of 125 mg/60 kg, injected intramuscularly every 6–12 wk. Other alternatives are the use of oral contraceptives, which will not produce amenorrhea but will result in marked decrease in the quantity of menstrual flow, resulting in a more manageable condition. Before the clinician considers a surgical approach such as hysterectomy, there should be a thorough discussion with parents or custodians after a trial of medical treatment that has not been successful. An ethics advisory committee should be consulted to aid in decisions to sterilize mentally handicapped patients (see also Chapter 3).

Braham D: House of Lords upholds decision to sterilise 17-year-old mentally handicapped girl. Lancet 1:1099, 1987.
Elkins T, Hoyle D, Darnton T, et al: The use of a societally based ethics class advisory committee to aid in decisions to sterilize mentally handicapped patients. Adolesc Pediatr Gynecol 1:190, 1988.
Elkins T, McNeeley S, Rosen D, et al: A clinical observation of a program to accomplish pelvic exams in difficult-to-manage patients with mental retardation. Adolesc Pediatr Gynecol 1:195, 1988.

CHAPTER 511

Gynecologic Imaging

A transabdominal approach with use of a distended bladder to serve as a window allows appropriate identification of the uterus and the ovaries; bladder distention displaces gas-filled

■ **TABLE 511–1 Ovary**

Birth
15 mm long, 3 mm wide, 2.5 mm thick
Ovarian volume 0.7 cm²*
Postpuberty
22.5–5.0 mm in length
1.5–3 cm in width; 0.6–1.5 cm in thickness
Ovarian volume 1.8–5.7 cm²

**Ovarian volume can be determined by using the formula: length × height × width × 0.523.*

Sanfilippo JS, Lavery JP: The spectrum of ultrasound: antenatal to adolescent years. Semin Reprod Endocrinol 6:47, 1988.

bowel loops out of the pelvis with resultant enhanced imaging. A 7.5 or 5 MHz transducer is usually used, the latter being especially helpful with larger children and teenagers. With respect to ovarian assessment, volume is determined by the following formula: length × height × width × 0.523. Normal values are included in Table 511–1. The uterus in the neonate ranges in size between 2.3 and 4.6 cm in length with a maximum anteroposterior diameter of 0.8–2.2 cm (Table 511–2).

■ **TABLE 511–2 Uterus**

Neonate
Length 2.3–4.6 cm
AP diameter 0.8–2.2 cm
Infant to 7 yr of age
Length 2.5–3.3 cm
AP diameter 0.4–1.0 cm

Sanfilippo JS, Lavery JP: The spectrum of ultrasound: antenatal to adolescent years. Semin Reprod Endocrinol 6:47, 1988.

Pelvic masses can be identified either in utero or in the neonate, as well as in the pediatric or adolescent patient. Ovarian cysts and hydrocolpos or hydrometrocolpos appear to be the most common abnormalities noted in neonates. The former is defined as dilatation of the vagina, which usually is associated with the accumulation of serous fluid or urine if there is a urogenital sinus. The latter implies dilatation of both the uterus and the vagina. This may also be associated with vaginal or cervical atresia, stenosis, or an imperforate hymen.

Ultrasonography is a key screening tool, enabling establishment of the appropriate diagnosis of patients presenting with ambiguous genitalia, ovarian or uterine masses, primary amenorrhea, and abdominal and/or pelvic pain. Magnetic resonance imaging as well as computed tomography appear efficacious when further assessment is deemed necessary. Most large ovarian cysts (simple cystic) in children may be safely followed with serial pelvic ultrasonography. Most cysts tend to decrease in size or completely resolve. A solid mass requires a tissue diagnosis.

Siegel MJ, Surratt JT: Pediatric gynecologic imaging. Obstet Gynecol Clin North Am 19:103, 1992.

Warner BW, Kuhn JC, Barr LL: Conservative management of large ovarian cysts in children: the value of serial pelvic ultrasonography. Surgery 112:749, 1992.

PART XXVI

The Endocrine System

SECTION 1

Disorders of the Hypothalamus and Pituitary Gland

Angelo M. DiGeorge ▪ *John S. Parks*

The anterior pituitary gland originates from the Rathke pouch as an invagination of the oral endoderm. It then detaches from the oral epithelium and becomes an individual structure of rapidly proliferating cells. Persistent remnants of the original connection between the Rathke pouch and the oral cavity can develop into craniopharyngiomas, which are the most common type of tumor in this area. Five cell types in the anterior pituitary produce six peptide hormones. Somatotropes produce growth hormone (GH), lactotropes produce prolactin, and thyrotropes make thyrotropin or thyroid-stimulating hormone (TSH). A single transcriptional activation protein, Pit-1, contributes to the embryologic development and differentiated function of these three cell types. Developing under the influence of unidentified differentiation factors, gonadotropes make lutropin or luteinizing hormone (LH) and follitropin or follicle-stimulating hormone (FSH), and corticotropes produce corticotropin (ACTH) and other peptides from the pro-opiomelanocorticotropic (POMC) precursor protein.

ANTERIOR LOBE HORMONES. The protein hormones produced by the anterior pituitary act on other endocrine glands and on certain body cells to affect almost every organ. Anterior pituitary cells are themselves controlled by neuropeptide-releasing and release-inhibiting hormones that are produced by hypothalamic neurons, secreted into the capillaries of the median eminence, and carried by portal veins to the anterior pituitary. Many conditions formerly classified as pituitary in origin are caused by hypothalamic defects. The identification and availability of hypothalamic hormones permits more precise delineation of these conditions.

Human GH is a protein with 191 amino acids. Its gene *(GH1)* is the first in a cluster of five closely related genes on the long arm of chromosome 17 (q22–24). The four other genes have greater than 90% sequence identity with the *GH1* gene. They consist of the *CS1* and *CS2* genes, which encode the same human chorionic somatomammotropin (hCS) protein; a placental growth hormone gene *(GH2)*; and a partly disabled pseudogene *(CSP)*. Syncytiotrophoblastic cells of the fetal placenta produce large quantities of hCS, and placental GH replaces pituitary GH in the maternal circulation after 20 wk of gestation. When the fetal genome lacks the *CS1, CS2, GH2,* and *CSP* genes, hCS and placental GH are absent, but fetal growth and postpartum lactation are normal.

The *GH1* gene is expressed in pituitary somatotropes under the control of two hypothalamic hormones. Growth hormone–releasing hormone (GHRH) stimulates, and somatostatin inhibits, GH release. Alternating secretion of GHRH and somatostatin accounts for the rhythmic secretion of GH. Peaks of GH occur when peaks of GHRH coincide with troughs of somatostatin. When plasma levels of GH are measured by standard radioimmunoassay (RIA), its secretion appears to be pulsatile, but when measured by an ultrasensitive immunoradiometric assay (IRMA), which can measure GH in a previously undetectable range, it is observed to be secreted in a rhythmic fashion with a dominant 2-hr periodicity. The highest levels of GH are achieved during sleep when measured by RIA or IRMA.

The three molecular species of GHRH contain 37, 40, or 44 amino acids. A fully active 29–amino acid synthetic GHRH is available for diagnostic use. Somatostatin exists in 14– and 28–amino acid forms. Somatostatin production is not limited to the hypothalamus. It also acts through autocrine and paracrine mechanisms in the islets of Langerhans and in the gastrointestinal tract. Somatostatin inhibits secretion of insulin, glucagon, secretin, gastrin, vasoactive intestinal peptide (VIP), GH, and thyrotropin. In the pancreatic islets, it is localized to the D cells. Somatostatin-secreting pancreatic tumors (i.e., somatostatinomas) have been reported in adults. A potent, long-acting somatostatin analog, octreotide, which inhibits GH preferentially over insulin, is available to treat patients with GH-secreting tumors. It is also useful in managing patients with gastrinomas, insulinomas, glucagonomas, VIPomas, and carcinoids (see Chapters 77 and 291). ^{123}I-labeled octreotide appears to be useful in localizing somatostatin receptor–positive tumors and their metastases.

GH acts through binding to receptor molecules on the surface of target cells. The GH receptor is a single-chain molecule of 620 amino acids. It has an extracellular domain, a single membrane-spanning domain, and a cytoplasmic domain. Proteolytically cleaved fragments of the extracellular domain circulate in plasma and act as a GH-binding protein. In common with other members of the cytokine receptor family, the cytoplasmic domain of the GH receptor lacks intrinsic kinase activity; instead, GH binding induces receptor dimerization and activation of a receptor-associated Janus kinase (Jak2). Phosphorylation of the kinase and other protein substrates initiates a series of events that leads to alterations in nuclear gene transcription.

The mitogenic actions of GH are mediated through increases in the synthesis of insulin-like growth factor-I (IGF-I), formerly named somatomedin C, a single-chain peptide with 70 amino acids coded for by a gene on the long arm of chromosome 12. IGF-I has considerable homology to insulin. Circulating IGF-I is synthesized primarily in the liver and formed locally in mesodermal and ectodermal cells, particularly in the growth plate of children, where its effect is exerted by paracrine or autocrine mechanisms. Circulating levels of IGF-I are related to blood levels of GH to a large extent, except in the fetus and during the neonatal period. IGF-I circulates bound to several different binding proteins; the major one is a 150-dalton complex (IGF-BP3), which is decreased in GH-deficient children but is in the normal range in children who are short for other reasons. Human recombinant IGF-I is being used experimentally to determine its therapeutic potential. IGF-II is a single-chain protein with 67 amino acids that is coded for by a gene on the short arm of chromosome 11. It has homology to IGF-I, but much less is known about its physiologic roles, although it appears to be an important mitogen in bone cells, where it occurs in a concentration many times higher than that of IGF-I.

Several disorders of growth are caused by abnormalities of the genes that code for the GHRH receptor, Pit-1, GH1, and the GH receptor. No growth disorders have been localized to the genes that code for GHRH, IGF-I, IGF-I receptor, or IGF-II.

Prolactin is composed of 199 amino acids, and its gene is located on chromosome 6. The identity of the prolactin-releasing factor (PRF) is unknown, but evidence suggests that it is localized almost exclusively in the intermediate lobe of the pituitary rather than in the hypothalamus. The major prolactin-inhibiting factor (PIF) is dopamine, and medications that disrupt hypothalamic dopaminergic pathways result in increased serum levels of prolactin. Serum levels of prolactin are increased after administration of thyrotropin-releasing hormone (TRH), in states of primary hypothyroidism, and after disruption of the pituitary stalk, as may occur in children with craniopharyngioma.

The main established role for prolactin is the initiation and maintenance of lactation. Concentrations in amniotic fluid are 10–100 times the levels in maternal or fetal serum. The major source of amniotic prolactin appears to be the decidua. Mean serum levels in children and in fasting adults of both sexes are about 5–20 μg/L, but levels in the fetus and in neonates during the 1st wk of life are usually higher than 200 μg/L.

TSH consists of two glycoprotein chains linked by hydrogen bonding. The α chain is identical to that found in FSH, LH, and chorionic gonadotropin (hCG). The β chain is unique in each of these hormones and confers specificity. The gene for the α chain has been mapped on chromosome 6, that for the β chain of TSH on chromosome 1, and those for the β chains for LH and hCG on chromosome 19. TSH increases iodine uptake, iodide clearance from the plasma, iodotyrosine and iodothyronine formation, thyroglobulin proteolysis, and release of thyroxine (T_4) and triiodothyronine (T_3) from the thyroid. Most of the effects of TSH are mediated by cyclic adenosine monophosphate. Deficiency of TSH results in inactivity and atrophy of the thyroid, and excess results in hypertrophy and hyperplasia.

TRH was the first hypothalamic hormone to be isolated, characterized, and synthesized; it is a tripeptide ([pyro] Glu-His-Pro-NH_2). T_4 and T_3 inhibit TSH secretion by blocking the action of TRH on the pituitary cell. TRH also stimulates the release of prolactin in both sexes. Synthetic TRH is useful for testing pituitary reserves of TSH and prolactin.

ACTH is derived by proteolytic cleavage from a large precursor glycoprotein product of the pituitary gland called POMC. Cleavage of POMC yields ACTH, a single, unbranched glycoprotein chain of 39 amino acids, and β-lipotropin (β-LPH), a 91–amino acid glycoprotein. Further cleavage of ACTH and β-LPH in the pituitary yields yet other hormonal products. The α-melanocyte-stimulating hormone is identical to the first 13 amino acids of ACTH but has no corticotropin activity; cleavage of β-LPH results in neurotropic peptides with morphinomimetic activity (fragment 61–91 is β-endorphin), and β-melanocyte-stimulating hormone consists of a 17–amino acid fragment of β-LPH.

ACTH acts primarily on the adrenal cortex. It produces changes in structure, chemical composition, enzymatic activity, and release of corticosteroid hormones. ACTH release has a diurnal rhythm. The level is lowest between 10 P.M. and 2 A.M., with peak levels reached about 8 A.M.. Levels of β-LPH and of β-endorphin are elevated in patients with increased levels of ACTH. It appears that ACTH rather than FSH is the principal pigmentary hormone in humans.

POMC peptides are also produced in nonpituitary tissues. In the testis, some peptides act as autocrine regulators of androgen-secreting Leydig cells, and others may potentiate or oppose the action of FSH on Sertoli cells.

Secretion of ACTH, β-endorphin, and other POMC-related peptides is regulated by corticotropin-releasing hormone (CRH). CRH is a 41–amino acid peptide found predominantly in the median eminence but also in other areas of the brain and in tissues outside the brain, particularly the placenta. During pregnancy, levels of CRH rise several hundred-fold, increase further during labor and delivery, and then fall to nonpregnant levels within 24 hr. Its source is probably the placenta, which contains the peptide and its mRNA. Synthetic ovine (oCRH) and human CRH (hCRH) have been used clinically. The oCRH is the clinical agent of choice, because responses to it are greater and longer lasting than with hCRH. It is particularly useful in differentiating the different forms of Cushing syndrome.

Gonadotropic hormones include two glycoproteins: LH and FSH. Each has an α subunit and a β subunit. The α subunits of these two hormones and of TSH are identical; specificity of hormone action resides in the β subunit, which is different for each of the three. Receptors for FSH on the ovarian granulosa cells and on testicular Sertoli cells mediate FSH stimulation of follicular development in the ovary and of gametogenesis in the testis. On binding to specific receptors on ovarian theca cells and testicular Leydig cells, LH promotes luteinization of the ovary and Leydig cell function of the testis. The receptors for LH and FSH belong to a class of receptors with seven membrane-spanning protein domains. Receptor occupancy activates adenylyl cyclase through mediation of G proteins.

Hypothalamic control of gonadotropic hormones has long been known, and separate releasing hormones for FSH and LH were once anticipated. Luteinizing hormone–releasing hormone (LHRH), a decapeptide, has been isolated, synthesized, and widely used in clinical studies. Because it leads to the release of LH and FSH from the same gonadotropic cells, it appears that there is only one gonadotropin-releasing hormone.

Secretion of LH is inhibited by androgens and estrogens, and secretion of FSH is suppressed by gonadal production of inhibin, a 31-kD glycoprotein produced by the Sertoli cells. Inhibin consists of α and β subunits joined by disulfide bonds. The β-β dimer (activin) also occurs, but its biologic effect is to stimulate FSH secretion. The biology of these newer hormones is being delineated. In addition to its endocrine effect, activin has paracrine effects in the testis. It facilitates LH-induced testosterone production, indicating a direct effect of Sertoli cells on Leydig cells analogous to the interaction of these cells through the paracrine effects of POMC.

POSTERIOR LOBE HORMONES. The posterior lobe of the pituitary is part of a functional unit, the neurohypophysis, that consists of the neurons of the supraoptic and paraventricular nuclei of the hypothalamus; neuronal axons, which form the pituitary stalk; and neuronal terminals in the median eminence or in the posterior lobe.

The neurohypophysis is the source of arginine vasopressin (AVP, the antidiuretic hormone) and of oxytocin. Both are octapeptides, differing in only two amino acids. These hormones are produced by neurosecretion in the hypothalamic nuclei. Vasopressin derives its name from early observations of its pressor and antidiuretic activities; however, the latter is its physiologically important function. At levels 50–1,000 times those found in blood, it affects blood pressure, intestinal contractility, hepatic glycogenolysis, platelet aggregation, and release of factor VIII. AVP and oxytocin are secreted by separate cells of the supraoptic and paraventricular nuclei. Secreted concurrently in equimolar amounts with these hormones are vasopressin neurophysin (neurophysin II) and oxytocin neurophysin (neurophysin I). Each hormone binds to its respective neurophysin and is transported to the nerve terminals in the posterior pituitary, where it is secreted in the free form. RIAs of the neurophysins provide a direct index of AVP and oxytocin levels in plasma. The concentration of AVP in umbilical cord plasma appears to be a sensitive indicator of fetal stress.

AVP has a short half-life and responds quickly to changes in hydration. The stimuli for AVP release are increased plasma osmolality, perceived by osmoreceptors in the hypothalamus, and decreased blood volume, perceived by baroreceptors in the carotid sinus of the aortic arch. AVP changes the permeability of the renal tubular cell membrane through cAMP. A synthetic analog, desmopressin, combines high potency, selectivity for antidiuretic hormone receptors, and resistance to degradation by proteases. Small amounts administered intranasally are effective therapy for patients with diabetes insipidus. ■

CHAPTER 512
Hypopituitarism

Angelo M. DiGeorge and John S. Parks

This chapter discusses the hypopituitary states associated with a deficiency of growth hormone (GH), with or without a deficiency of other pituitary hormones (Table 512–1). Isolated deficiencies of thyrotropin, corticotropin (ACTH), and gonadotropin are also addressed. Affected children have in common a phenotype of growth impairment that is specifically corrected by replacement of GH.

■ TABLE 512–1 Etiologic Classification of Hypopituitarism

- Developmental defects
  - Anencephaly
  - Holoprosencephaly (i.e., cyclopia, cebocephaly, orbital hypotelorism)
  - Midfacial anomalies (e.g., hypertelorism)
  - Septo-optic dysplasia (de Morsier syndrome)
  - Cleft lip and palate
  - Solitary maxillary central incisor
  - Hall-Pallister syndrome (i.e., hypothalamic hamartoblastoma, imperforate anus, polydactyly)
  - Rieger syndrome
- Genetic defects of GH or GHRH
  - Isolated GH deficiency
    - Autosomal recessive type I
      - Type IA with deletions of the *GH1* gene
      - Type IB with mutations in *GH1* or other genes
    - Autosomal dominant type II with mutations in *GH1* or other genes
    - X-linked type III with or without hypogammaglobulinemia
  - Multiple pituitary deficiencies
    - Autosomal recessive type I
      - GH, TSH, ACTH, LH, and FSH deficiency
      - GH, TSH, and PRL deficiencies with mutations in the Pit-1 gene *(PIT1)*
    - Autosomal dominant type II
      - GH, TSH, and PRL deficiencies with mutations in the Pit-1 gene *(PIT1)*
    - X-linked type III
      - GH, TSH, ACTH, LH, and FSH deficiency
- Destructive lesions
  - Trauma
    - Perinatal trauma (e.g., trauma, anoxia, hemorrhagic infarction)
    - Basal skull fractures
    - Child abuse
  - Infiltrative lesions
    - Tumors
    - Histiocytosis X
    - Craniopharyngioma
    - Hypothalamic tumors
    - Germinoma
    - Optic glioma
    - Pituitary adenomas
    - Sarcoidosis
    - Hemochromatosis
    - Tuberculosis
    - Toxoplasmosis
  - Irradiation (e.g., central nervous system, eyes, middle ears)
  - Surgery
    - Removal of pharyngeal pituitary
    - Surgery for craniopharyngioma and other tumors
  - Vascular lesions
    - Infarctions (e.g., hemoglobinopathy)
    - Aneurysm
  - Autoimmune hypophysitis
- Unresponsiveness to growth hormone
  - Insulin-like growth factor deficiency
  - Laron syndrome with mutations in the GH-receptor gene
- Other functional deficiency
  - Hypothyroidism
  - Psychosocial deprivation

ACTH = corticotropin; FSH = follicle-stimulating hormone; GH = growth hormone; GHRH = growth hormone–releasing hormone; LH = luteinizing hormone; PRL = prolactin; TSH = thyroid-stimulating hormone.

ETIOLOGY. Congenital Defects. Pituitary hypoplasia can occur as an isolated phenomenon or in association with more extensive developmental abnormalities, such as anencephaly, holoprosencephaly (i.e., cyclopia, cebocephaly, orbital hypotelorism), and septo-optic dysplasia (de Morsier syndrome). In Hall-Pallister syndrome, absence of the pituitary gland is associated with hypothalamic hamartoblastoma, postaxial polydactyly, nail dysplasia, bifid epiglottis, imperforate anus, and anomalies of the heart, lungs, and kidneys. In the neonate, symptoms of hypopituitarism with postaxial polydactyly and bifid epiglottis suggest this diagnosis. Hypoplasia of the pituitary with anencephaly has long been known, but recent observations reveal a large residuum of normal pituitary function and suggest that hypoplasia may be secondary to the hypothalamic defect. With hypothalamic-releasing hormones, it is possible to determine whether defects in pituitary function reside in the pituitary or hypothalamus. Deficiency of GH occurs in 4% of all patients with cleft lip or cleft palate and in 32% of those who also have short stature. Midfacial anomalies or the finding of a solitary maxillary central incisor indicate a high likelihood of GH deficiency.

Bilateral or unilateral optic nerve hypoplasia is often associated with hypopituitarism. When it is also associated with absence of the septum pellucidum, the condition is known as septo-optic dysplasia. The fundus exhibits hypoplastic discs with typical double rims and sparse retinal vessels. Endocrine abnormalities are extremely variable. Hormonal deficiency most often involves GH alone, but multiple pituitary deficiencies, including diabetes insipidus, may occur. The defect resides primarily in the hypothalamus. Delay in linear growth may begin as early as 3 mo of age or may not be observed before 3–4 yr of age. Affected newborns often have apnea, hypotonia and seizures, prolonged jaundice, hypoglycemia without hyperinsulinism, and (in males) microphallus. The condition is usually sporadic but has been reported in first cousins. The cause is unknown, but young maternal age and nulliparity are strongly associated factors.

Aplasia of the pituitary without abnormalities of the brain or skull is rare, but affected infants are being increasingly recognized because hypoglycemia occurs early and, in males, there is microphallus. Some infants have shown evidence of the neonatal hepatitis syndrome, but the relationship with hypopituitarism is obscure. The condition has been reported in siblings of both sexes, and consanguinity has been observed in two families; autosomal recessive inheritance is suggested. Studies of some children have placed the defect in the hypothalamus. This may be a heterogeneous group of disorders.

In empty-sella syndrome, a deficient sellar diaphragm leads to herniation of the suprasellar subarachnoid space into the sella turcica, with remodeling of the sella and flattening of the pituitary gland. It may develop after surgery or radiation therapy, or it may be idiopathic. Of 17 pediatric cases, significant hypopituitarism was found in 5. Empty-sella syndrome with an enlarged sella and hypopituitarism has been observed in siblings.

Other syndromes in which short stature is a prominent feature may be associated with deficiency of GH. For example, some patients with Turner, Fanconi, Russell-Silver, Rieger, Williams, or the CHARGE syndrome have hypopituitarism.

Destructive Lesions. Any lesion that damages the hypothalamus, pituitary stalk, or anterior pituitary may cause pituitary hormone deficiency. Because such lesions are not selective, multiple hormonal deficiencies are usually observed. The most common lesion is the craniopharyngioma. Central nervous system germinoma, eosinophilic granuloma, tuberculosis, sarcoidosis, toxoplasmosis, and aneurysms may also cause hypothalamic-hypophyseal destruction. These lesions are frequently associated with roentgenographic changes in the skull. Besides diabetes insipidus, a deficiency of GH and other pituitary hormones may occur in children with histiocytosis, especially if treated with cranial irradiation. Enlargement of the sella or deformation or destruction of the clinoid processes usually indicates a tumor. Intrasellar or suprasellar calcifications usually indicate a craniopharyngioma. Trauma, including child abuse, traction at delivery, anoxia, and hemorrhagic infarction, may also damage the pituitary, its stalk, or the hypothalamus.

Improved survival of children who receive radiotherapy for malignancies of the central nervous system or other cranial structures has resulted in a substantial group of patients with GH deficiency. Children with acute lymphocytic leukemia who have received prophylactic cranial irradiation also belong in this group. Growth typically slows during radiation therapy or chemotherapy, improves for a year or two, and then declines with the development of hypopituitarism. Spinal irradiation contributes to disproportionately poor growth of the trunk. The dose of irradiation and the fractionation schedule used are important determinants of the incidence of hypopituitarism. GH deficiency is almost universal 5 yr after therapy with a total dose of 35–45 Gy. Subtler defects are seen with doses around 20 Gy. Deficiency of GH is the most common defect, but deficiencies of thyroid-stimulating hormone (TSH) and ACTH may also occur. Unlike in other forms of hypopituitarism, puberty is not delayed. A pubertal growth spurt at a normal to early age may lessen clinical suspicion of GH deficiency.

Idiopathic Hypopituitarism. Most patients with hypopituitarism have no demonstrable lesion of the pituitary or hypothalamus. In most, the functional defect is hypothalamic rather than pituitary. The deficiency may be of GH only or of multiple hormones. The condition is most often sporadic. Association with breech birth, forceps delivery, and intrapartum and maternal bleeding suggests that birth trauma and anoxia may be pathogenic factors in some instances.

Genetic Forms of Hypopituitarism. Well-recognized genetic forms of hypopituitarism account for at least 5% of cases. As in idiopathic hypopituitarism, the defect may be limited to GH, or it can involve deficiencies of several other anterior pituitary hormones. Roman numerals are used to denote the mode of inheritance. In the McKusick classification of isolated GH deficiency (IGHD), type I is autosomal recessive, type II is autosomal dominant, and type III is X linked. Similarly, autosomal recessive multiple pituitary hormone deficiency is type I, and the X-linked form is type III.

Among families with autosomal recessive IGHD, some have complete deletions of the *GH1* gene and are considered to have IGHD type IA. Early reports of this disorder stressed the tendency of these children to form antibodies to human GH during treatment and to experience a lessening of growth response. With more widespread application of Southern blotting and polymerase chain reaction techniques for detecting *GH1* gene deletions and with the availability of less antigenic biosynthetic GH preparations, it appears that a minority develop such antibodies. There are several different sizes of deletions, reflecting nonhomologous crossing over at different sites in the *GH* and *CS* gene cluster. The smallest and most common deletions are 6.7 kb long. Other deletion sizes are 7.0, 7.6, and greater than 45 kb. All cases show extreme postnatal growth failure and fail to release GH after stimulation with growth hormone–releasing hormone (GHRH) or more conventional stimuli to GH release.

Autosomal recessive IGHD type IB is heterogeneous with respect to severity and the sites of mutations. Some children have 1- or 2-bp deletions in the *GH1* gene that introduce a frameshift, followed by an early translational stop signal. Homozygosity for this type of *GH1* allele or compound heterozygosity for a small and a large *GH1* deletion results in total absence of GH and a clinical picture equally as severe as that of IGHD type IA. Other families have mutations within the fourth and last intron of the *GH1* gene. These mutations compromise the efficiency of normal pre-mRNA splicing at the usual exon 3 to exon 4 splice boundary. In some IGHD IB families, tracking the restriction fragment length polymorphisms shows that transmission of the disease is not linked to transmission of *GH1* alleles. Attempts to link IGHD IB to defects in the *GHRH* gene have been uniformly unsuccessful. The little mouse model of IGHD IB is caused by a mutation in the gene for the GHRH receptor. It seems likely that some human forms of IGHD result from mutations in the same gene.

Some cases of autosomal dominant IGHD III are caused by mutations in the *GH1* gene. They involve single-base substitutions in intron 3 that result in omission of exon 3 from the spliced mRNA. The predicted protein has a molecular weight of 17,000, lacks amino acids 32 to 71, and lacks one of the cysteine residues involved in formation of intramolecular disulfide bonds. It has been speculated that this mutant protein forms intermolecular bonds with the product of the normal *GH1* allele and interferes with secretion of GH from secretory granules.

The gene responsible for X-linked IGHD III has not been identified. In several families, GH deficiency has been transmitted along with immunoglobulin deficiency. The disorder in these families may involve deletion of several contiguous genes.

Most cases of autosomal recessive and X-linked multiple pituitary hormone deficiency involve underproduction of GH, TSH, ACTH, luteinizing hormone, and follicle-stimulating hormone. Prolactin (PRL) values tend to be normal or high. Other hormones are often released in response to administration of releasing factors. These observations suggest a hypothalamic rather than a pituitary defect, and no candidate genes have been implicated. A subset of familial cases lack GH, TSH, and PRL but have normal secretion of ACTH and gonadotropins. Affected children in several families have been shown to have defects in the gene for the Pit-1 pituitary transcriptional activation protein. Gene deletions and nonsense and missense mutations have been described. Most eliminate binding of Pit-1 to target sequences in the GH, PRL, and β-TSH promoters. At least one mutant protein retains binding activity although it lacks the ability to activate transcription. It may retain some role in pituitary development, because children with this mutation have normal anterior pituitary size on magnetic resonance imaging (MRI). Another mutation, substituting tryptophan for arginine at position 271, exerts a dominant negative effect in vivo and in vitro. It provides an example of multiple pituitary hormone deficiency type II.

Growth Hormone–Receptor Defects. Children with Laron syndrome have all the clinical findings of those with hypopituitarism, but they have elevated levels of circulating GH. Levels of insulin-like growth factor-I (IGF-I) are very low and fail to respond to exogenous hGH. Absence of GH-binding activity confirms the diagnosis and points to an abnormality of the GH receptor. A variety of gene defects have been discovered in different families, ranging from the deletion of several exons of the gene, through nonsense mutations, to missense mutations, and to mutations that alter splicing of pre-mRNA. More than 40 affected individuals in two large Ecuadorian kindreds are homozygous for a base substitution that creates a new splice site and results in a protein that lacks 12 of the amino acids normally found in the extracellular domain. A second kindred living in the Bahamas expresses a different mutation that also introduces a new splice site and results in a nonfunctional protein. Most of the mutations responsible for Laron syndrome produce a loss of GH-binding activity in the membrane receptor and the circulating GH-binding protein representing the extracellular domain of the receptor. The mutant protein in at least one family retains normal affinity for GH binding but lacks the ability to form dimers of GH receptor around a single bound GH molecule. Most parents of children with Laron syndrome are within the normal range for adult stature. With the availability of techniques for screening the GH-receptor gene sequence, it will be interesting to see whether some mutations act in a dominant fashion to cause milder forms of short stature.

CLINICAL MANIFESTATIONS. Patients Without Demonstrable Lesions of the Pituitary. The child with hypopituitarism is usually of normal size and weight at birth. Retrospective studies of children with multiple pituitary hormone deficiencies and those with genetic defects of the *GH1* or *GHR* gene indicate that birth length averages 1 SD below the mean. Children with severe defects in GH production or action fall more than 4 SD below the mean by 1 yr of age. Others with less severe deficiencies may have regular but slow growth in height, with the increments always below the normal percentiles, or periods of lack of growth may alternate with short spurts of growth. Delayed closure of the epiphyses permits growth beyond the age when normal persons cease to grow. Without treatment, adult heights are 4–12 SD below the mean.

Infants with congenital defects of the pituitary or hypothalamus usually present neonatal emergencies such as apnea, cyanosis, or severe hypoglycemia. Microphallus in the male provides an additional diagnostic clue. Deficiency of GH may be accompanied by hypoadrenalism and hypothyroidism, and clinical manifestations of hypopituitarism evolve more rapidly than in the usual hypopituitary child. Prolonged neonatal jaundice is common. It involves elevation of conjugated and unconjugated bilirubin and may be mistaken for neonatal hepatitis.

The head is round, and the face is short and broad. The frontal bone is prominent, and the bridge of the nose is depressed and saddle shaped. The nose is small, and the nasolabial folds are well developed. The eyes are somewhat bulging. The mandible and the chin are underdeveloped and infantile, and the teeth, which erupt late, are frequently crowded. The neck is short and the larynx small. The voice is high pitched and remains high after puberty. The extremities are well proportioned, with small hands and feet. The genitalia are usually underdeveloped for the child's age, and sexual maturation may be delayed or absent. Facial, axillary, and pubic hair usually is lacking, and the scalp hair is fine. Symptomatic hypoglycemia, usually after fasting, occurs in 10–15% of children with panhypopituitarism and those with an IGHD. Intelligence is usually normal. Affected children may become shy and retiring.

Patients with Demonstrable Lesions of the Pituitary. The child is normal initially, and manifestations similar to those seen in idiopathic pituitary growth failure gradually appear and progress. When complete or almost complete destruction of the pituitary gland occurs, signs of pituitary insufficiency are present. Atrophy of the adrenal cortex, thyroid, and gonads results in loss of weight, asthenia, sensitivity to cold, mental torpor, and absence of sweating. Sexual maturation fails to take place or regresses if already present; there may be atrophy of the gonads and genital tract with amenorrhea and loss of pubic and axillary hair. There is a tendency to hypoglycemia and coma. Growth ceases. Diabetes insipidus may be present early but tends to improve spontaneously as the anterior pituitary is progressively destroyed.

If the lesion is an expanding tumor, symptoms such as headache, vomiting, visual disturbances, pathologic sleep, decreased school performance, seizures, polyuria, and growth failure may occur. Growth failure frequently antedates the neurologic signs and symptoms, especially with craniopharyngiomas, but symptoms of hormonal deficit account for only 10% of presenting complaints. In other patients, the neurologic manifestations may precede the endocrinologic, or evidence of pituitary insufficiency may first appear after surgical intervention. In children with craniopharyngiomas, visual field defects, optic atrophy, papilledema, and cranial nerve palsy are common.

LABORATORY DATA. The diagnosis of classic GH deficiency is suspected in cases of profound postnatal growth failure, with heights more than 3 SD below the mean for age and gender. Acquired GH deficiency can occur at any age. There is dramatic slowing of growth, but when the disorder is of short duration, height may still be within the normal range. A strong clinical suspicion is important in establishing the diagnosis, because laboratory measures of GH sufficiency lack specificity. Observation of low serum levels of IGF-I and the GH-dependent IGF-BP3 can be helpful. Values that are in the upper part of the normal range for age effectively exclude GH deficiency. Values for normally growing and hypopituitary children overlap, particularly during infancy and early childhood.

Definitive diagnosis rests on demonstration of absent or low levels of GH in response to stimulation. A variety of provocative tests have been devised that rapidly increase the level of GH in normal children. These include a 20-min period of strenuous exercise or administration of L-dopa, insulin, arginine, clonidine, or glucagon. Peak levels of GH below 7 μg/L are compatible with GH deficiency. The frequency of false-negative responses in normally growing children with any single test is considered to be approximately 20%. If this were true, about 4% of normal children would fail both tests. One study suggests that a majority of normal prepubertal children fail to achieve GH values above 7 μg/L with two pharmacologic tests. The researchers suggest that 3 days of estrogen priming should be used before GH testing to achieve greater diagnostic specificity.

During the 3 decades when hGH was obtained by extraction from human pituitary glands culled at autopsy, its supply was sharply limited, and only patients with classic GH deficiency were treated. With the advent of an unlimited supply of recombinant GH, there has been a marked interest in redefining the criteria for GH deficiency to include children with lesser degrees of deficiency. It has become popular to evaluate the spontaneous secretion of GH by measuring its level every 20 min during a 24- or 12-hr (8 P.M.–8 A.M.) period. Some short children with normal levels of GH when studied by provocative tests show very little spontaneous GH secretion. Such children are considered to have GH neurosecretory dysfunction. With the collection of more normative data, it is clear that frequent GH sampling also lacks diagnostic specificity. There is a wide range of spontaneous GH secretion in normally growing prepubertal children and considerable overlap with the values observed in children with classic GH deficiency. Although the clinical and laboratory criteria for GH deficiency in patients with severe (classic) hypopituitarism are well established, the diagnostic criteria are unsettled for short children with lesser degrees of GH deficiency.

In addition to establishing the diagnosis of GH deficiency, it is necessary to examine other pituitary functions. Levels of TSH, thyroxine (T_4), ACTH, cortisol, dehydroepiandrosterone sulfate, gonadotropins, and gonadal steroids may provide evidence of other pituitary hormonal deficiencies. The defect can be localized to the hypothalamus if there is a normal response to the administration of hypothalamic-releasing hormones for GH, TSH, ACTH, or gonadotropins. When there is a deficiency of TSH, serum levels of T_4 and TSH are low. A normal rise in TSH and PRL after stimulation with thyrotropin-releasing hormone places the defect in the hypothalamus, and absence of such a response localizes the defect to the pituitary. An elevated level of plasma PRL taken at random in the patient with hypopituitarism is also strong evidence that the defect is in the hypothalamus rather than in the pituitary. Some children with craniopharyngioma have elevated PRL levels before surgery, but after surgery, PRL deficiency occurs because of pituitary damage. Antidiuretic hormone deficiency may be established by appropriate studies.

ROENTGENOGRAPHIC EXAMINATION. Roentgenograms of the skull are most helpful when there is a destructive or space-occupying lesion causing hypopituitarism. In patients with nausea, vomiting, loss of vision, headache, or increase in circumference of the head, evidence of increased intracranial pressure may be found. Enlargement of the sella, especially ballooning with erosion and calcifications within or above the sella, may be detected. MRI is indicated in all patients with hypopituitarism. In addition to providing detail about space-occupying lesions, it can define the size of the anterior and posterior pituitary lobes and the pituitary stalk. It is superior to computed tomography in differentiating a full from an empty sella turcica. The posterior pituitary is readily recognized as a bright spot. In many cases of idiopathic multiple pituitary hormone deficiency with prenatal or perinatal onset, the posterior pituitary bright spot it ectopic. It appears at the base of the hypothalamus rather than in the pituitary fossa. This diagnostic technique can provide timely confirmation of suspected hypopituitarism in a newborn with hypoglycemia and micropenis.

Skeletal maturation is markedly delayed in patients with longstanding GH deficiency. The bone age tends to be approximately 75% of chronological age. It may be even more delayed for patients with TSH and GH deficiency. The fontanels may remain open beyond the 2nd yr, and intersutural wormian bones may be found. Long bones are slender and osteopenic. Newer methods of assessing body composition, such as dual photon x-ray absorptiometry, show deficient bone mineralization, deficiencies in lean body mass, and a corresponding increase in adiposity.

DIFFERENTIAL DIAGNOSIS. The causes of growth disorders are legion; systemic conditions such as inflammatory bowel disease, occult renal disease, and Turner syndrome must always be considered. Many theoretical defects of molecular structure resulting in bioinactive GH are possible, but none has been documented at the genetic level. A few otherwise normal children are short (i.e., >3 SD below the mean for age) and grow 5 cm/yr or less but have normal levels of GH in response to provocative tests and normal spontaneous episodic secretion. Most of these children show increased rates of growth when treated with GH in doses comparable to those used to treat children with hypopituitarism. Plasma levels of IGF-I in these patients may be normal or low. Several groups of treated children have achieved final or near final adult heights. On average, they did not exceed the heights predicted from heights and bone ages at the start of treatment. There are no methods that can reliably predict which of these children will become taller as adults and which will have compromised adult height as a result of GH treatment. Such treatment of short children without proven hypopituitarism is undergoing experimental trials.

Constitutional growth delay is one of the variants of normal growth commonly encountered by the pediatrician. Length and weight measurements of affected children are normal at birth, and growth is normal for the first 4–12 mo of life. Growth then decelerates to near or below the 3rd percentile for height and weight. By 2–3 yr of age, growth resumes at a normal rate of 5 cm/yr or more. Studies of GH secretion and other studies are within normal limits. Bone age is closer to height age than to chronological age. Detailed questioning often reveals other family members (frequently one or both parents) with histories of short stature in childhood, delayed puberty, and eventual normal stature. The prognosis for these children to achieve normal adult height is good. Boys with unusual degrees of delayed puberty may benefit from a short course of testosterone therapy to hasten puberty after 14 yr of age. The cause of this variant of normal growth is thought to be persistence of the relatively hypogonadotropic state of childhood (see Chapter 535). Constitutional growth delay can be differentiated from genetic short stature by the level of skeletal maturation, which is consistent with chronological age in the latter condition. Genetic short stature is usually found in other family members. Results of studies of hormones related to growth, however, are normal.

Primary hypothyroidism is usually easily diagnosed on clinical grounds. Responses to GH provocative tests may be subnormal, and enlargement of the sella may be present. Low T_4 and elevated TSH levels clearly establish the diagnosis. Pituitary hyperplasia recedes during treatment with thyroid hormone. Because thyroid hormone is a necessary prerequisite for normal GH synthesis, its levels must always be assessed before GH studies.

Emotional deprivation is an important cause of retardation of growth and mimics hypopituitarism. The condition is known as psychosocial dwarfism, deprivation dwarfism, or reversible hyposomatotropism. The mechanisms by which sensory and emotional deprivation interfere with growth are not fully understood. Functional hypopituitarism is indicated by low levels of IGF-I, by inadequate responses of GH to provocative stimuli, and perhaps by delayed puberty. Appropriate history and careful observations reveal disturbed mother-child or family relations and provide clues to the diagnosis. Proof may be difficult to establish, because the adults responsible often hide from professionals the true situation in the family, and the children rarely divulge their plight. Emotionally deprived children frequently have perverted or voracious appetites, enuresis, encopresis, insomnia, crying spasms, and sudden tantrums. They may be excessively passive or aggressive and are borderline or dull-normal in intelligence. When child-rearing practices are altered or when the child is removed from the domicile of abuse, the rate of growth improves significantly. During this period of catch-up growth, separation of the cranial sutures and other evidence of pseudotumor cerebri may occur; these should not be mistaken for signs of a mass lesion.

The Silver-Russell syndrome is characterized by short stature, frontal bossing, small triangular facies, sparse subcutaneous tissue, shortened and incurved 5th fingers, and in many cases, asymmetry (i.e., hemihypertrophy). Affected children have low birthweights for gestational age. Studies have revealed some degree of GH secretory deficiency in very short children with intrauterine growth retardation, whether or not they have Silver-Russell syndrome. Short-term treatment with GH often results in increased rates of growth, but its long-term benefits are unknown.

TREATMENT. In patients with demonstrable organic lesions, treatment should be directed to the underlying disease process. Evaluation of pituitary function is indicated after surgery or irradiation.

Treatment of children with classic GH deficiency should begin as early as possible. Younger children respond better than older ones, and long-term expectations are better. The recommended dose of hGH is 0.18–0.3 mg/kg/wk. It is administered subcutaneously in six or seven divided doses. Therapy should be continuous until there is no further response, a point usually concomitant with closure of the epiphyses. If the effect of therapy wanes, compliance should be evaluated before the dose is increased. Some patients treated with GH have subsequently developed leukemia. The risk of leukemia in treated patients may be double that in the general population, but this is still under investigation. Other reported side effects include pseudotumor cerebri, slipped capital femoral epiphysis, and worsening of scoliosis. There is an increase in total body water during the first 1–2 wk of treatment. Fasting and postprandial insulin levels are characteristically low before treatment, and they normalize during GH replacement. Development of diabetes mellitus is rare. Older GH-deficient patients treated with cadaver pituitary extracts are at risk for Creutzfeldt-Jakob disease for at least 10–15 yr after therapy. Recombinant GH has eliminated this risk.

Maximal response to GH occurs in the 1st yr of treatment.

With each successive year of treatment, the response tends to decrease. Some patients receiving GH develop reversible hypothyroidism because of enhanced conversion of T_4 to T_3 and decreased levels of TSH. Periodic evaluation of thyroid function is indicated for all patients treated with GH. GHRH is just as effective as GH in the treatment of children with hypopituitarism with a deficiency of GHRH, but multiple daily subcutaneous injections are required. When a depot form becomes available, it may provide a practical form of treatment for this group of children. Recombinant IGF-I may prove useful in the treatment of children with Laron syndrome and possibly those with *GH1* gene deletions and high titers of antibodies.

The doses of GH used to treat children with classic GH deficiency usually enhance growth of many non–GH-deficient children as well. Intensive investigation is in progress to determine the full spectrum of short children who may benefit from treatment with GH. Children with intrauterine growth retardation, chronic renal failure, Noonan syndrome, Turner syndrome, and others experience increases in growth velocity when treated with GH. Girls with Turner syndrome treated with GH appear to have a final height several centimeters greater than that of untreated girls. For children with all other causes of short stature, it is unknown whether GH treatment increases their final height, and treatment of such patients should be confined to prospective clinical trials until further data establish the validity of this expensive, long-term form of therapy.

Replacement should also be directed at other hormonal deficiencies. In TSH-deficient subjects, thyroid hormone is given in full replacement doses. In ACTH-deficient patients, the optimum dose of hydrocortisone should not exceed 10 mg/m²/24 hr. Increases are made during illness or in anticipation of surgical procedures. Therapy can often be deferred until growth has been completed if the deficiency is partial. In patients with a deficiency of gonadotropins, gonadal steroids are given when the bone age reaches the age when puberty usually takes place. For infants with microphallus, one or two 3-mo courses of monthly intramuscular injections of 25 mg of testosterone enanthate may bring the penis to normal size without an inordinate effect on osseous maturation.

Allen DB, Fost NC: Growth hormone therapy for short stature: Panacea or Pandora's box. J Pediatr 117:16, 1990.

Amselem S, Duquesnoy P, Goossens M: Molecular basis of Laron dwarfism. Trends Endocrinol Metab 2:35, 1991.

Berg MA, Guevara-Aguirre J, Rosenbloom AL, et al: Mutation creating a new splice site in the growth hormone receptor genes of 37 Ecuadorian patients with Laron syndrome. Hum Mutation 1:24, 1992.

Brown RS, Vijayalakshmi B, Hayes E: An apparent cluster of congenital hypopituitarism in central Massachusetts: Magnetic resonance imaging and hormonal studies. J Clin Endocrinol Metab 72:11, 1991.

Cacciari E, Tassoni P, Parisi G, et al: Pitfalls in diagnosing impaired growth hormone (GH) secretion: Retesting after replacement therapy of 63 patients defined as GH deficient. J Clin Endocrinol Metab 74:1284, 1992.

Cara JF, Kreiter ML, Rosenfield RL: Height prognosis of children with true precocious puberty and growth hormone deficiency: Effect of combination therapy with gonadotropin releasing hormone agonist and growth hormone. J Pediatr 120:709, 1992.

Clayton PE, Shalet SM: Dose dependency of time of onset of radiation-induced growth hormone deficiency. J Pediatr 118:226, 1991.

Cogan JC, Phillips JA III, Sakati N, et al: Heterogeneous growth hormone (GH) gene mutations in familial GH deficiency. J Clin Endocrinol Metab 76:1224, 1993.

Costin G, Murphree AL: Hypothalamic-pituitary function in children with optic nerve hypoplasia. Am J Dis Child 139:249, 1985.

Dean HJ, Bishop A, Winter JSD: Growth hormone deficiency in patients with histiocytosis. J Pediatr 109:615, 1986.

Donaldson DL, Hallowell JG, Pan E, et al: Growth hormone secretory profiles: Variation on consecutive nights. J Pediatr 115:51, 1989.

Duquesnoy P, Sobrier ML, Duriez B, et al: A single amino acid substitution in the exoplasmic domain of the human growth hormone (GH) receptor confers familial GH resistance (Laron syndrome) with positive GH-binding activity by abolishing receptor homodimerization. EMBO J 13:1386, 1994.

Frasier SD: Human pituitary growth hormone (hGH) therapy in growth hormone deficiency. Endocrinol Rev 4:155, 1983.

Gertner JM, Genel M, Gianfredi SP, et al: Prospective clinical trial of human growth hormone in short children without growth hormone deficiency. J Pediatr 104:172, 1984.

Guevara-Aguirre J, Rosenbloom AL, Fielder PJ, et al: Growth hormone receptor deficiency in Ecuador: Clinical and biochemical phenotype in two populations. J Clin Endocrinol Metab 76:417, 1993.

Hall JG, Pallister PD, Carren SK, et al: Congenital hypothalamic hamartoblastoma, hypopituitarism, imperforate anus, and postaxial polydactyly—a new syndrome? Part 1: Clinical, causal and pathogenetic considerations. Am J Med Genet 7:47, 1980.

Hasegawa Y, Hasegawa T, Aso T, et al: Clinical utility of insulin-like growth factor binding protein-3 in the evaluation and treatment of short children with suspected growth hormone deficiency. Eur J Endocrinol 131:27, 1994.

Herman SP, Baggenstoss AM, Clothier MD: Liver dysfunction and histiologic abnormalities in neonatal hypopituitarism. J Pediatr 87:892, 1975.

Kappy M, Blizzard RM, Migeon CJ: Wilkins: The Diagnosis and Treatment of Endocrine Disorders in Childhood and Adolescence, 4th ed. Springfield, Charles C Thomas, 1994.

Kamijo T, Phillips JA III, Ogawa M, et al: Screening for growth hormone gene deletions in patients with isolated growth hormone deficiency. J Pediatr 118:245, 1991.

Kuroiwa T, Okabe Y, Hasuo K, et al: MR imaging of pituitary dwarfism. Am J Neuroradiol 12:161, 1991.

LaFranchi S: Human growth hormone. Who is a candidate for treatment? Postgrad Med 91:367, 1992.

Laron Z, Lilos P, Klinger B: Growth curves for Laron syndrome. Arch Dis Child 68:768, 1993.

Lesage C, Walker J, Landier F, et al: Near normalization of adolescent height with growth hormone therapy in very short children without growth hormone deficiency. J Pediatr 119:29, 1991.

Littley MD, Shalet SM, Beardwell CG, et al: Radiation-induced hypopituitarism is dose-dependent. Clin Endocrinol 31:363, 1989.

Lovinger RD, Kaplan SL, Grumbach MM: Congenital hypopituitarism associated with neonatal hypoglycemia and microphallus: Four cases secondary to hypothalamic hormone deficiencies. J Pediatr 87:1171, 1975.

Low LC: The therapeutic use of growth-hormone–releasing hormone. J Pediatr Endocrinol 6:15, 1993.

Margalith D, Tze WJ, Jan JE: Congenital optic nerve hypoplasia with hypothalamic-pituitary dysplasia. Am J Dis Child 139:361, 1985.

Marin GM, Domene HM, Barnes KM, et al: The effects of estrogen priming and puberty on the growth hormone response to standardized treadmill exercise and arginine-insulin in normal girls and boys. J Clin Endocrinol Metab 79:537, 1994.

Miller WL, Kaplan SL, Grumbach MM: Child abuse as a cause of post-traumatic hypopituitarism. N Engl J Med 302:724, 1980.

Moell C, Marky I, Hovi L, et al: Cerebral irradiation causes blunted pubertal growth in girls treated for acute leukemia. Med Pediatr Oncol 22:375, 1994.

Money J: The syndrome of abuse dwarfism (psychosocial) or reversible hyposomatotropism. Am J Dis Child 131:508, 1977.

Neely EK, Rosenfeld RG: Use and abuse of human growth hormone. Annu Rev Med 45:407, 1994.

Parks JS, Abdul-Latif H, Kinoshita E, et al: Genetics of growth hormone gene expression. Horm Res 40:54, 1993.

Pfäffle RW, DiMattia GE, Parks JS, et al: Mutation of the POU-specific domain of Pit-1 and hypopituitarism without pituitary hypoplasia. Science 257:1118, 1992.

Radovick S, Nations M, Du Y, et al: A mutation in the POU-homeodomain of Pit-1 responsible for combined pituitary hormone deficiency. Science 257:1115, 1992.

Rapaport EB, Ulstrom RA, Gorlin RJ, et al: Solitary maxillary central incisor and short stature. J Pediatr 91:924, 1977.

Rose SR, Ross JL, Uriarte M, et al: The advantage of measuring stimulated as compared with spontaneous growth hormone levels in the diagnosis of growth hormone deficiency. N Engl J Med 319:201, 1988.

Rosenfeld RG, Rosenbloom AL, Guevara-Aguirre J: Growth hormone (GH) insensitivity due to primary GH receptor deficiency. Endocr Rev 15:369, 1994.

Stanhope R, Albanese A, Hindmarsh P, Brook CG: The effects of growth hormone therapy on spontaneous sexual development. Horm Res 38(Suppl 1):9, 1992.

Tatsumi K, Miyai K, Notomi T, et al: Cretinism with combined hormone deficiency caused by a mutation in the Pit-1 gene. Nature Genet 1:56, 1992.

Walker JM, Bond SA, Voss LD, et al: Treatment of short normal children with growth hormone—a cautionary tale? Lancet 336:1331, 1990.

White MC, Chahal P, Banks L, et al: Familial hypopituitarism associated with an enlarged pituitary fossa and an empty sella. Clin Endocrinol 24:63, 1986.

Wilkinson IA, Duck SC, Gager WE, et al: Empty-sella syndrome. Occurrence in childhood. Am J Dis Child 136:245, 1982.

Wilson DM, Dotson RJ, Neely EK, et al: Effects of estrogen on growth hormone following clonidine stimulation. Am J Dis Child 147:63, 1993.

Zadik Z, Landau H, Limoni Y, et al: Predictors of growth response to growth hormone in otherwise normal short children. J Pediatr 121:44, 1992.

CHAPTER 513
Diabetes Insipidus
(Arginine Vasopressin Deficiency)

Angelo M. DiGeorge

Diabetes insipidus (DI), characterized by polyuria and polydipsia, results from lack of the antidiuretic hormone, arginine vasopressin (AVP). Destruction of the supraoptic and paraventricular nuclei or division of the supraoptic-hypophyseal tract above the median eminence results in permanent DI. Transection of the tract below the median eminence or removal of just the posterior lobe may result in transitory polyuria, but in this case, AVP released into the median eminence prevents occurrence of DI. AVP acts directly on the distal tubules and collecting ducts of the kidney by binding to V_2 receptors, which are G protein coupled before triggering cAMP. The V_2 receptor is also responsible for vasodilator effects of the hormone, for increasing factor VIII activity, and for increasing the concentration of von Willebrand factor in plasma. AVP deficiency may be total or partial, with varying degrees of polydipsia and polyuria.

ETIOLOGY. Any lesion that damages the neurohypophyseal unit may result in DI. Tumors of the suprasellar and chiasmatic regions, particularly craniopharyngiomas (Fig. 513–1), optic gliomas, and germinomas, are common causes; the symptoms of increased intracranial pressure may accompany those of DI or may follow years later. Approximately 25% of patients with Langerhans cell histiocytosis develop DI as a consequence of histiocytic infiltration of the hypothalamus and pituitary. DI is seldom present when histiocytosis is diagnosed but almost always occurs within 4–5 yr. It occurs most often in children with multisystem disease and in those with proptosis. About half of these patients have cytoplasmic antibodies to AVP-producing cells, suggesting an autoimmune response to histiocytic cell invasion of the hypothalamus. Encephalitis, sarcoidosis, tuberculosis, actinomycosis, and leukemia are occasional causes. Injuries to the head, especially basal skull fractures, may produce DI immediately or after a delay of several months. Operative procedures near the pituitary or hypothalamus may result in transitory or permanent DI.

In a few cases, DI is hereditary. An autosomal dominant form is characterized by variable onset, from birth to several years of age, and variable severity within a family and in individuals over time. Symptoms decrease in the 3rd–5th decades. Levels of AVP may be absent (<0.5 pg/mL) or variably decreased. The gene is on chromosome 20, and the preprotein it encodes contains AVP and neurophysin II (NP II), the hormone's carrier protein. This single polypeptide chain is cleaved within secretory granules and then reassembled into an AVP–NP II complex before secretion. Mutations causing autosomal dominant DI have been localized to the NP II moiety. Although the mutation involves only one allele, the mutant AVP–NP II complex disrupts the functioning of the normal allele, resulting in autosomal dominant inheritance. The mutated gene product is thought to be the cause of selective death of the magnocellular neurons in patients with longstanding familial DI.

Wolfram syndrome, also known by the acronym DIDMOD, consists of *d*iabetes *i*nsipidus, *d*iabetes *m*ellitus, *o*ptic atrophy, and *d*eafness. It has an autosomal recessive inheritance pattern, and the gene is located on chromosome 4p. Pathologic studies suggest a degenerative process involving β cells, supraoptic and paraventricular nuclei, the optic nerve, and cranial nerve VIII.

Absence of islet cell antibodies and of the usual HLA haplotypes associated with classic insulin-dependent diabetes mellitus differentiates the cause of this condition from that of the usual type 1 autoimmune diabetes mellitus.

DI occasionally accompanies *septo-optic dysplasia.*

DI has been reported in the newborn infant following asphyxia, intraventricular hemorrhage, intravascular coagulopathy, *Listeria monocytogenes* sepsis, and group B β-hemolytic streptococcal meningitis.

In many instances, the cause of DI cannot be found initially, but disease in only about 20% of affected patients eventually

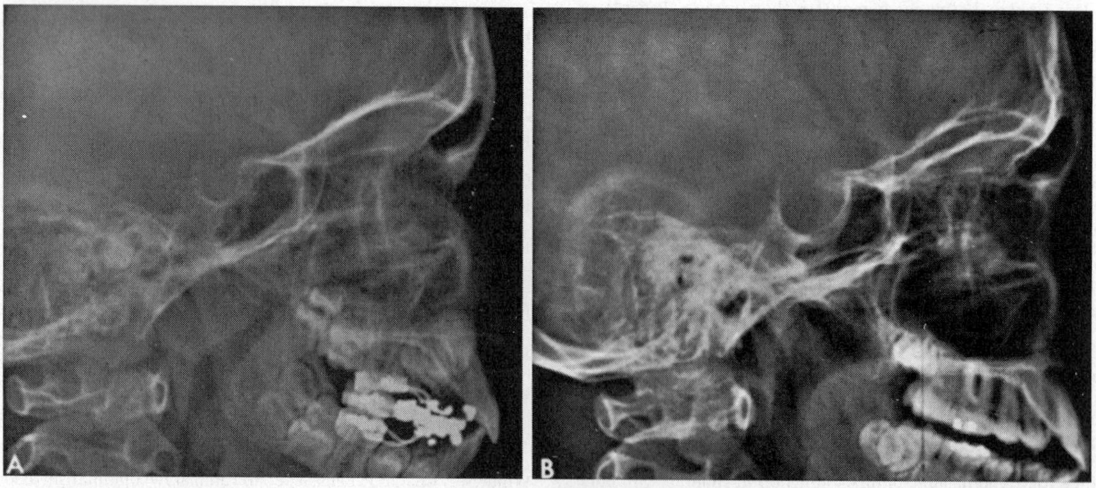

Figure 513–1. *A,* Roentgenograph of the skull of a 9-yr-old boy with polydipsia, polyuria, nocturia, and enuresis. Urine specific gravity was 1.010 after water deprivation. Growth was normal, and the sella turcica was considered roentgenographically to be at the upper limit of normal but was probably enlarged. Over the ensuing 6 mo, the symptoms of diabetes insipidus abated. *B,* The patient returned at 14 yr of age because of growth failure and delay in sexual maturation. Studies revealed a deficiency of growth hormone, gonadotropins, corticotropin, and thyrotropin. Note the enlargement and the thinning of the sella turcica but also the absence of intrasellar or suprasellar calcification. The neurologic and ophthalmologic examinations were normal. There was exacerbation of diabetes insipidus with the administration of hydrocortisone and thyroxine. At surgery, a large craniopharyngioma was found.

is classified as idiopathic. In more than one half of all patients with intracranial tumors, clinical or neuroradiologic signs (or both) are not manifested until 1 yr after DI has been diagnosed, and in 25%, the delay is as long as 4 yr. Periodic reevaluation is required for at least 4 yr before the entity can be called idiopathic. About one third of patients with idiopathic DI have antibodies to AVP-producing cells, suggesting an autoimmune basis for the condition. This idea is further supported by the frequent occurrence in this subgroup of patients of other autoimmune endocrine disorders, especially autoimmune thyroid disease. These autoimmune disorders are particularly evident in adults. DI is increasingly recognized as a terminal event in brain-dead individuals.

CLINICAL MANIFESTATIONS. Polydipsia and polyuria are the outstanding symptoms of DI. In families with the hereditary disorder, the polyuria is often noticed in early infancy. The infant cries excessively and is not satisfied with additional milk but is quieted with water. Hyperthermia, rapid loss of weight, and collapse are common in infancy. Vomiting, constipation, and growth failure may be observed. Dehydration in early infancy may result in brain damage and mental impairment. In children with AVP deficiency, there is wide variation in the manifestations. Severity tends to increase with age, and some affected children are asymptomatic until adolescence. Many affected families accept polydipsia and polyuria as a family habit and do not seek medical attention or may even prefer the symptoms to therapy.

In a child who has acquired bladder control, enuresis may be the first symptom. The excessive thirst is disturbing and interferes with play, learning, and sleep. Children with DI do not perspire; their skin is dry and pale. Anorexia is common; there is a preference for carbohydrates.

Other signs and symptoms depend on the primary lesion; for example, patients with tumors in the region of the hypothalamus may have disturbance of growth, progressive cachexia or obesity, hyperpyrexia, sleep disturbance, sexual precocity, or emotional disorders. Lesions initially causing DI may eventually destroy the anterior pituitary; in such instances, the DI tends to become milder or disappear completely.

LABORATORY DATA. The daily volume of urine may be 4–10 L or more. The urine is pale or colorless; the specific gravity varies from 1.001 to 1.005, with a corresponding osmolality of 50–200 mOsm/kg water. During periods of severe dehydration, the specific gravity may rise to 1.010 and the osmolality to 300. Other renal function studies are normal. Serum osmolality is normal with adequate hydration. During water deprivation tests, patients must be closely observed to prevent surreptitious intake of water and to avoid severe and rapid development of dehydration. In patients with severe deficiency, a 3-hr period of dehydration leads to elevation of plasma osmolality while urine osmolality characteristically remains below plasma levels. Administration of desmopressin or AVP quickly raises urine osmolality. When polyuria is mild and the deficiency is incomplete, urine osmolality may exceed that of plasma, and the response to AVP is attenuated.

Radioimmunoassay for vasopressin is available; plasma levels consistently below 0.5 pg/mL indicate severe neurogenic DI. AVP levels that are subnormal for the concomitant hyperosmolality indicate partial neurogenic DI. The assay is particularly useful in differentiating partial DI from primary polydipsia.

Roentgenograms of the skull may reveal evidence of an intracranial tumor such as calcifications, enlargement of the sella turcica, erosion of the clinoid processes, or increased width of the suture lines. Magnetic resonance imaging (MRI) is indicated for all patients suspected of having DI. T1-weighted MRI images can differentiate the posterior pituitary from the anterior pituitary by the hyperintense signal, also referred to as a bright signal or bright spot. The bright spot is present on scans of most normal patients, but it usually is absent for patients with hypothalamic-neurohypophyseal tract lesions. For patients with autosomal dominant DI, the bright spot is usually present, presumably caused by accumulation of mutant AVP–NP II complex. Thickening of the pituitary stalk may be seen by MRI in patients with DI and Langerhans cell histiocytosis (LCH) or lymphocytic infiltration; in some patients this MRI abnormality may be detected even before other clinical evidence of LCH.

DIFFERENTIAL DIAGNOSIS. Polydipsia, polyuria, and impaired concentration are common in patients with hypercalcemia or potassium deficiency. In the male infant, nephrogenic DI must be differentiated from inherited or acquired AVP deficiency; failure of response to exogenous AVP or desmopressin is a critical differential (see Chapter 484).

Defects in urinary concentrations also occur in a variety of chronic renal disorders. Familial nephronophthisis, in particular, can mimic DI. Elevated plasma levels of urea and creatinine, anemia, and isotonic rather than hypotonic urine are characteristics of primary renal disease.

Compulsive water drinking (i.e., *psychogenic polydipsia*) is rare but may easily be confused with DI. Affected persons are usually able to produce a concentrated urine when fluids are withheld. Occasionally, however, diagnosis is difficult, because prolonged polydipsia lowers the maximal urinary concentrations achievable after dehydration or even after infusion of hypertonic saline solution. As a rule, a urine osmolality greater after dehydration than after administration of AVP alone indicates the ability to secrete vasopressin. If administration of AVP produces a urinary osmolality that is substantially higher than that with dehydration alone, AVP secretion is deficient. This rule seems to apply no matter how low or how high the urinary concentration may be.

Adipsia or *hypodipsia*, as an isolated defect of the thirst center, is extremely rare. Because the osmoreceptors for thirst and AVP occupy contiguous areas of the anterior hypothalamus, hypodipsic hypernatremia is usually associated with defects in antidiuretic function. This most often occurs in patients with hypothalamic tumors, especially germinomas, gliomas, histiocytosis, congenital malformations, and microcephaly. Adipsia seriously complicates the management of problems of water balance.

PROGNOSIS. When DI is diagnosed, the underlying process must be determined. DI itself rarely threatens life, but it may signify a serious underlying condition. It may be only transitory after trauma or surgical intervention in the region of the hypothalamus or pituitary. In some patients with Langerhans cell reticuloendothelioses, spontaneous remission occurs, but in others, DI may be the only residuum long after remission of the primary condition. Amelioration of clinical DI may herald development of anterior pituitary insufficiency. The prognosis of patients with brain tumors depends on the site of the lesion and the type of neoplastic cell.

TREATMENT. The causative factor deserves first consideration in the treatment. Patients with uncomplicated DI may live untreated for years with only the inconvenience of polyuria and polydipsia so long as they have an intact thirst mechanism and are allowed free access to water.

The drug of choice is desmopressin (1-desamino-8-D-arginine vasopressin; DDAVP), a highly effective analog of AVP. This analog is more resistant to degradation by peptidases than native AVP. The antidiuretic activity of DDAVP is 2,000–3,000 times greater than its pressor activity, and 1 μg produces an antidiuresis that lasts 8–10 hr, compared with only 2–3 hr for native AVP. DDAVP is given by a nasal tube delivery system that delivers precise amounts to the nasal mucosa. The usual dose ranges from 5–15 μg, given as a single dose or divided into two doses. Children younger than 2 yr of age require smaller doses (0.15–0.5 μg/kg/24 hr). The dose must be individualized, and it is important that the dosage schedule be adjusted to allow patients to revert to mild polyuria before the next dose is given. For patients requiring over 10 μg/dose, a nasal spray preparation is also available. A parenteral preparation of DDAVP (0.03–0.15 μg/kg) is available and is useful postoperatively, particularly after transsphenoidal surgery, when nasal packing precludes nasal insufflation.

Great care must be taken in patients with DI who are comatose, undergoing surgery, or receiving intravenous fluids for any reason. Regardless of the form of therapy, any effective dose should be repeated only after its effect has worn off and polyuria recurs. Postoperative DI is often transient; daily reassessment of the need for antidiuretic hormone is necessary after it has been initiated.

DDAVP also has an effect on V_2-like extrarenal receptors, resulting in release of factor VIII and von Willebrand factor. Selected patients with mild or moderate hemophilia A or von Willebrand disease can be successfully treated with doses of DDAVP 15 times higher than the dose used for antidiuresis. Desmopressin is being increasingly used in the management of children with enuresis. Some of these children have been said to have nocturnal deficiency of vasopressin secretion, but this is not established. The dose required is slightly higher (20–40 μg) than that used to treat neurogenic DI. It is given as a nasal spray before bedtime.

513.1 Nephrogenic Diabetes Insipidus

(Vasopressin Receptor Defects)

See Chapter 484.

Assadi FK, John EG: Hypouricemia in neonates with syndrome of inappropriate secretion of antidiuretic hormone. Pediatr Res 19:424, 1985.

Czernichow P, Pomerade R, Basmaciogullari A, et al: Diabetes insipidus in children. III. Anterior pituitary dysfunction in idiopathic types. J Pediatr 106:41, 1985.

Dunger DB, Broadbent V, Yeoman E, et al: The frequency and natural history of diabetes insipidus in children with Langerhans-cell histiocytosis. N Engl J Med 321:1157, 1989.

Ganong CA, Kappy MS: Cerebral salt wasting in children. The need for recognition and treatment. Am J Dis Child 147:167, 1993.

Hammond DN, Moll GW, Robertson GL, et al: Hypodipsic hypernatremia with normal osmoregulation of vasopressin. N Engl J Med 315:433, 1986.

Hendricks SA, Lippe B, Kaplan SA, et al: Differential diagnosis of diabetes insipidus: Use of DDAVP to terminate the seven-hour water deprivation test. J Pediatr 98:244, 1981.

Imura A, Nakao K, Shimatsu A, et al: Lymphocytic infunduloneurofibrositis as a cause of central diabetes insipidus. N Engl J Med 329:683, 1993.

Kohn B, Norman ME, Feldman H, et al: Hysterical polydipsia (compulsive water drinking). Am J Dis Child 130:210, 1976.

Laine J, Holmberg C, Anttila M, et al: Types of fluid disorder in children with bacterial meningitis. Acta Paediatr Scand 80:1031, 1991.

Maghrue M, Villa A, Arico M, et al: Correlation between magnetic resonance imaging of posterior pituitary and neurohypophyseal function in children with diabetes insipidus. J Clin Endocrinol Metab 74:795, 1992.

Miller WL: Molecular genetics of familial central diabetes insipidus. J Clin Endocrinol Metab 77:592, 1993.

Repaske DR, Browning JE: A de novo mutation in the coding sequence for neurophysin-II (Pro24→Leu) is associated with onset and transmission of autosomal dominant neurohypophyseal diabetes insipidus. J Clin Endocrinol Metab 79:421, 1994.

Richardson DW, Robinson AG: Desmopressin. Ann Intern Med 103:228, 1985.

Scherbaum WA, Wass JAH, Besser GM, et al: Autoimmune cranial diabetes insipidus: Its association with other endocrine diseases and with histiocytosis X. Clin Endocrinol 25:411, 1986.

Schmitt S, Wichmann W, Martin E, et al: Pituitary stalk thickening with diabetes insipidus preceding typical manifestations of Langerhans cell histiocytosis in children. Eur J Pediatr 152:399, 1993.

Sklar C, Fertig A, David R: Chronic syndrome of inappropriate secretion of antidiuretic hormone in childhood. Am J Dis Child 139:733, 1985.

Toth EL, Bowen PA, Crockford PM: Hereditary central diabetes insipidus: Plasma levels of antidiuretic hormone in a family with a possible osomoreceptor defect. Can Med Assoc J 131:1237, 1984.

Yuasa H, Ito M, Nagasaki H, et al: Glu-47, which forms a salt bridge between neurophysin-II and arginine vasopressin, is deleted in patients with familial central diabetes insipidus. J Clin Endocrinol Metab 77:600, 1993.

Zerbe RL, Robertson GL: A comparison of plasma vasopressin with a standard direct test in the differential diagnosis of polyuria. N Engl J Med 305:1539, 1981.

CHAPTER 514

Inappropriate Secretion of Antidiuretic Hormone

(Hypersecretion of Vasopressin)

Angelo M. DiGeorge

The syndrome of inappropriate secretion of antidiuretic hormone (SIADH) is now recognized as one of the most common aberrations of arginine vasopressin (AVP) secretion. In this condition, plasma levels of AVP are inappropriately high for the concurrent osmolality of the blood and are not suppressed by further dilution of body fluids.

ETIOLOGY. The syndrome is recognized in an increasing number of clinical conditions, particularly those involving the central nervous system, including meningitis, encephalitis, brain tumor and abscesses, subarachnoid hemorrhage, Guillain-Barré syndrome, head trauma, and after transsphenoidal surgery for pituitary tumors. Pneumonia, tuberculosis, acute intermittent porphyria, cystic fibrosis, infant botulism, perinatal asphyxia, use of positive-pressure respirators, and certain drugs such as vincristine and vinblastine also produce the syndrome. The mechanism of the disturbed regulation of AVP in these conditions is not fully understood, but in many instances, there is direct involvement of the hypothalamus. The syndrome has been observed in patients with Ewing sarcoma; with malignant tumors of the pancreas, duodenum, or thymus; and particularly with oat cell carcinoma of the lung. In these instances, the tumor presumably synthesizes and secretes AVP, with the syndrome disappearing when the tumor is removed. In rare cases, no cause for the syndrome has been found.

The syndrome has occurred during chlorpropamide therapy for diabetes mellitus, presumably because this drug potentiates AVP. Patients with diabetes insipidus treated with various antidiuretic preparations readily develop the syndrome during periods of excessive ingestion of fluids or during intravenous fluid therapy.

CLINICAL MANIFESTATIONS. The syndrome is probably most often latent and asymptomatic and forms the basis for the observation that serum sodium levels may be unexpectedly low in conditions such as pneumonia, tuberculosis, and meningitis. Careful attention to fluid replacement in patients with conditions known to be associated with the syndrome may prevent the development of symptoms.

The clinical manifestations are attributable to hypotonicity of body fluids and are those of water intoxication. If the serum sodium level is not below 120 mEq/L, there may be no symptoms. Early, the loss of appetite is followed by nausea and sometimes by vomiting. Irritability and personality changes, including hostility and confusion, may occur. When the serum sodium level falls below 110 mEq/L, neurologic abnormalities or stupor is common, and convulsive seizures may occur. Skin turgor and blood pressure are normal, and there is no evidence of dehydration.

LABORATORY DATA. Serum sodium and chloride concentrations are low, but the serum bicarbonate level usually remains normal. Despite low serum sodium, there is continued renal excretion of sodium. The serum is hypo-osmolar, but the urine is less than maximally dilute, and its osmolality is greater than appropriate for the tonicity of the serum. Hypouricemia is common, probably because of increased urate clearance secondary to volume expansion. Concurrence of hypouricemia with hyponatremia is a clue to the diagnosis of SIADH and is especially helpful in the neonate. Renal and adrenal functions are normal.

TREATMENT. Successful treatment of the underlying disorder (e.g., meningitis, pneumonia) is followed by spontaneous remission. Immediate management of the hyponatremia consists simply of *restriction of fluids*. Sodium should be made available to replace the sodium loss; hypertonic saline solution is usually of little benefit, because even large sodium loads are excreted in the urine. In cases of severe water intoxication, with convulsions or coma, administration of hypertonic saline solution increases osmolality and controls the central nervous system manifestations. In such emergencies, administration of furosemide with 300 mL/m^2 of 1.5% sodium chloride causes a rise in sodium levels and diuresis. Demeclocycline interferes with the action of AVP on the renal tubule. Experience in adults with SIADH indicates that this agent may be useful, but its role in the treatment of children is not established. An 8-yr-old child with chronic SIADH has been successfully treated with single daily doses of furosemide.

514.1 Cerebral Salt Wasting

Children with acute or chronic central nervous system damage may develop a distinctive syndrome of salt wasting. The disorder has been associated with head trauma, central nervous system surgery, tumor, or meningitis. These children, unlike those with SIADH, have hypovolemia, excessive urine flow rate while receiving maintenance fluids, a large net loss of sodium, and a decreased plasma concentration of ADH. Levels of natriuretic hormone (ANH) are increased, but plasma renin and aldosterone levels are decreased; this suggests the syndrome is caused by inappropriate secretion of ANH. Therapy consists of volume-for-volume replacement of the urine loss with a 0.9% or 3% solution of sodium chloride. The condition usually remits but may recur and, in some instances, persists.

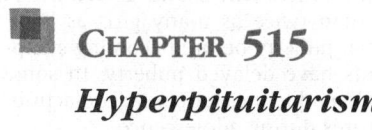

CHAPTER 515
Hyperpituitarism

Angelo M. DiGeorge

Hypersecretion of pituitary hormones is an expected finding in conditions in which deficiency of a target organ gives decreased hormonal feedback, as in primary hypogonadism or hypoadrenalism. In primary hypothyroidism, pituitary hyperfunction and hyperplasia can enlarge and erode the sella and, on rare occasions, increase intracranial pressure. Such changes should not be confused with primary pituitary tumors; they disappear when the underlying thyroid condition is treated. Pituitary hyperplasia also occurs in response to stimulation by ectopic production of releasing hormones such as that seen occasionally in patients with Cushing syndrome, secondary to corticotropin-releasing hormone excess, or in children with acromegaly secondary to growth hormone–releasing hormone (GHRH) produced by a variety of systemic tumors.

Primary hypersecretion of pituitary hormones by a suspected or proved adenoma is rare in childhood. The most commonly encountered pituitary tumors are those that secrete corticotropin, prolactin, or growth hormone (GH). With rare exceptions, pituitary adenomas that secrete gonadotropins or thyrotropin occur in adults. Hypothalamic hamartomas that secrete gonadotropin-releasing hormone are known to cause precocious puberty. It is suspected that some pituitary tumors may result from stimulation with hypothalamic-releasing hormones and in other instances, as in McCune-Albright syndrome, the tumor is caused by constitutive activating mutation of the $G_s\alpha$ gene. Any pituitary tumor may also cause various hormonal deficiencies by compressing pituitary tissue.

PITUITARY GIGANTISM AND ACROMEGALY

In young persons with open epiphyses, overproduction of GH results in gigantism; in persons with closed epiphyses, the result is acromegaly. Often, some acromegalic features are seen with gigantism, even in children and adolescents; after closure of the epiphyses, the acromegalic features become more prominent.

ETIOLOGY. Pituitary gigantism is rare. The cause is most often a pituitary adenoma, but gigantism has been observed in a 2.5-yr-old boy with a hypothalamic tumor that presumably secreted GHRH. Other tumors, particularly in the pancreas, have produced acromegaly by secretion of large amounts of GHRH with resultant hyperplasia of the somatotrophs; GHRH was first isolated from two such pancreatic tumors. The GH-secreting adenomas associated with McCune-Albright syndrome are caused by an activating mutation of the $G_s\alpha$ gene (see Chapter 517).

CLINICAL MANIFESTATIONS. The usual manifestations consist of rapid linear growth, coarse facial features, and enlarging hands and feet. In young children, rapid growth of the head may precede linear growth. Some patients have behavioral and visual problems. In most of the recorded cases, the abnormal growth became evident at puberty, but the condition has been established as early as the newborn period in one child and at 21 mo of age in another. Giants may grow to a height of 8 ft or more. Acromegaly consists chiefly of enlargement of the distal parts of the body, but manifestations of abnormal growth involve all portions. The circumference of the skull increases, the nose becomes broad, and the tongue is often enlarged, with coarsening of the facial features. The mandible grows excessively, and the teeth become separated. The fingers and toes grow chiefly in thickness. There may be dorsal kyphosis. Fatigue and lassitude are early symptoms. Delayed sexual maturation or hypogonadism may occur. Signs of increased intracranial pressure appear later; visual loss may be demonstrable only on careful examination of visual fields.

LABORATORY DATA. GH levels are elevated and may occasionally reach 400 ng/mL. The episodic pattern of secretion and the nocturnal surge may be preserved in some patients. There is usually no suppression of GH levels by the hyperglycemia of a glucose tolerance test. There may be no response, normal responses, or paradoxical responses to various other stimuli. For example, L-dopa may paradoxically decrease GH levels. Administration of thyrotropin-releasing hormone results in increased GH levels in some acromegalics, and in a 5-yr-old giant, it resulted in a threefold increase in levels of GH. Insulin-like growth factor-I (IGF-I) levels are consistently elevated in acromegaly, in one study ranging from 2.6–21.7 U/mL; normal levels are 0.3–1.4 U/mL. Most patients also have marked hyperprolactinemia as a result of plurihormonal adenomas that secrete GH and prolactin.

Adenomas may compromise other anterior pituitary function through growth or cystic degeneration. Secretion of gonadotropins, thyrotropin, or corticotropin may be impaired.

Roentgenograms of the skull may reveal enlargement of the sella turcica and of the paranasal sinuses; computed tomography scans or magnetic resonance imaging (MRI) delineates the tumor. Tufting of the phalanges and increased heel pad thickness are common. Osseous maturation is normal.

DIFFERENTIAL DIAGNOSIS. In the differential diagnosis, hereditary tall stature must be considered; in this condition, there is usually abnormal height in one or both parents or in close relatives. Such tall persons are well proportioned and free of signs of increased intracranial pressure. Excessive growth during preadolescence in obese children is a temporary state; although such children may become tall, they do not attain the height of giants. Children with precocious puberty are often unusually tall but do not develop into giants, because their epiphyses close early and growth ceases prematurely. Patients with tall stature associated with hypogonadism or Marfan syndrome are easily differentiated clinically and have normal levels of GH. Gigantism and increased GH levels may occur in some patients with lipodystrophy, but absence of subcutaneous fat is a characteristic finding; there is increasing evidence of disordered hypothalamic function in this condition. Sotos syndrome, which is more common than pituitary gigantism, can usually be differentiated on clinical grounds.

TREATMENT. Modalities include surgery, irradiation, and medical therapy; there are advantages and disadvantages of each. Octreotide, a long-acting analog of somatostatin, is 45 times more active than the native peptide in suppressing GH secretion. Experience in adults with acromegaly indicates that octreotide persistently suppresses GH and IGF-I concentrations and reduces tumor size in a significant number of patients. This agent may be helpful in some patients as primary therapy or when surgery has not been successful.

SOTOS SYNDROME
(Cerebral Gigantism)

Although it is characterized by rapid growth, there is no evidence that Sotos syndrome is an endocrine disorder. A hypothalamic defect has been suggested as a cause, but none has been demonstrated functionally or at necropsy. Birthweight and length are above the 90th percentile in most affected infants, and macrocrania may be noted. Growth is rapid, and by 1 yr of age, affected infants are over the 97th percentile in height. Accelerated growth continues for the first 4–5 yr and then returns to a normal rate. Puberty usually occurs at the normal time but may occur slightly early. The hands and feet are large, with thickened subcutaneous tissue. The head is large and dolichocephalic, the jaw is prominent, there is hypertelorism, and the eyes have an antimongoloid slant. Clumsiness and awkward gait are characteristic, and affected children have great difficulty in sports, in learning to ride a bicycle, and in other tasks requiring coordination. Some degree of mental retardation affects most patients; in some children, perceptual deficiencies may predominate (Fig. 515–1).

Roentgenograms reveal a large skull, a high orbital roof, a sella of normal size but slightly posterior inclination, and an increased interorbital distance. Osseous maturation is compatible with the patient's height. GH levels and results of other endocrine studies are usually normal; there are no distinctive laboratory markers for the syndrome. Abnormal electroencephalograms are common; other studies frequently reveal a dilated ventricular system.

The cause of the disorder is unknown, nor is it clear whether all patients with this syndrome have the same defect. Most cases are sporadic. Familial cases are usually consistent with autosomal dominant inheritance, occasionally with autosomal recessive inheritance. Affected patients may be at increased risk for neoplasia; hepatic carcinoma and Wilms, ovarian, and parotid tumors have been reported.

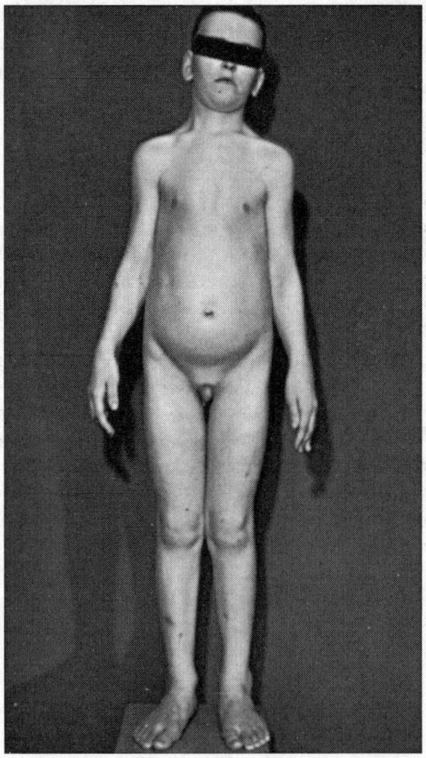

Figure 515–1. Cerebral gigantism in an 8-yr-old boy. The height age was 12 yr; the bone age was 12 yr; IQ was 60; the electroencephalogram had abnormal findings. Notice the prominence of the forehead and the jaw and the large hands and feet. Sexual development was consistent with chronological age. Hormone study results were normal. The adult height was 208 cm (6 ft 10 in); his sexual development was normal. He wears size 18 shoes.

PROLACTINOMA

Prolactin-secreting pituitary adenomas are the most common tumors of the pituitary in adolescents. With the advent of MRI, more of these tumors, particularly microadenomas (<1 cm), are being detected. The most common presenting manifestations are headache, amenorrhea, and galactorrhea. The disorder affects more than twice as many girls as boys; most have undergone normal puberty before becoming symptomatic. Only a few patients have delayed puberty. In some kindreds with type I multiple endocrine neoplasia, prolactinomas are the presenting features during adolescence.

Prolactin levels may be moderately (40–50 ng/mL) or markedly (10,000–15,000 ng/mL) elevated. Most prolactinomas in children have been large (macroadenomas), have caused the sella to enlarge, and in some cases, have caused visual field defects. Approximately one third of patients with macroadenomas develop hypopituitarism, particularly GH deficiency.

Prolactinomas should not be confused with the hyperprolactinemia and pituitary hyperplasia that may occur in patients with primary hypothyroidism, which is readily treated with thyroid hormone (see Chapter 520). Moderate elevations (<200 ng/mL) of prolactin are also associated with a variety of medications, with pituitary stalk dysfunction such as may occur with craniopharyngioma, and with other benign conditions. Treatment for most children has been surgical resection by transfrontal or transsphenoidal approach. However, the management of prolactinoma is becoming increasingly conservative. Some patients can be effectively managed by treatment with bromocriptine, the standard drug for treating hyperprolactinemia. About 80% of adult patients respond with shrinkage of the tumor and marked decreases in serum prolactin levels.

Bale AE, Drum A, Perry DM, et al: Familial Sotos syndrome (cerebral gigantism): Craniofacial and psychological characteristics. Am J Med Genet 20:613, 1985.
Cutler L, Jackson JA, Uz-zafar S, et al: Hypersecretion of growth hormone and prolactin in McCune-Albright syndrome. J Clin Endocrinol Metab 68:1148, 1989.
Daughaday WH: Pituitary gigantism. Endocrinol Metab Clin North Am 21:633, 1992.
Dodge PR, Holmes SJ, Sotos JF: Cerebral gigantism. Dev Med Child Neurol 25:248, 1983.
Ezzat S, Snyder PJ, Young WF, et al: Octreotide treatment of acromegaly. A randomized multicenter study. Ann Intern Med 117:711, 1992.
Guyda H, Robert F, Colle E, et al: Histologic, ultrastructural and hormonal characterization of a pituitary tumor secreting both HGH and prolactin. J Clin Endocrinol Metab 36:531, 1973.
Kane LA, Leinung MC, Scheithaver BW, et al: Pituitary adenomas in childhood and adolescence. J Clin Endocrinol Metab 79:1135, 1994.
Lightner ES, Winter JSD: Treatment of juvenile acromegaly with bromocriptine. J Pediatr 98:494, 1981.
Liuzzi A, Dellabonzana D, Oppizzi G, et al: Low doses of dopamine agonists in the long-term treatment of macroprolactinomas. N Engl J Med 313:636, 1985.
Lu PW, Silink M, Johnston I, et al: Pituitary gigantism. Arch Dis Child 67:1039, 1992.
Moran A, Asa SL, Kovacs K, et al: Gigantism due to pituitary mammosomatotroph hyperplasia. N Engl J Med 323:322, 1990.
Patton ML, Woolf PD: Hyperprolactinemia and delayed puberty: A report of three cases and their response to therapy. Pediatrics 71:572, 1983.
Polymeropoulas MH, Swift RG, Swith M: Linkage of the gene for Wolfram syndrome to markers of the short arm of chromosome 4. Nature Genet 8:95, 1994.
Rajasoorya C, Holdaway IM, Wrightson P, et al: Determinants of clinical outcome and survival in acromegaly. Clin Endocrinol 41:95, 1994.
Rutter SC, Cole TR: Psychological characteristics of Sotos syndrome. Dev Med Child Neurol 33:898, 1991.
Sack J, Friedman E, Tadmor R, et al: Growth and puberty arrest due to prolactinoma. Acta Paediatr Scand 73:863, 1984.
Sadeghi-Nejad A, Wolfsdorf JI, Biller BJ, et al: Hyperprolactinemia causing primary amenorrhea. J Pediatr 99:802, 1981.
Serri O: Progress in management of hyperprolactinoma. N Engl J Med 331:942, 1994.
Tyson D, Reggiardo D, Sklar C: Prolactin-secreting macroadenomas in adolescents. Response to bromocriptine therapy. Am J Dis Child 147:1057, 1993.
Whitaker MD, Scheithaver BW, Hayles AB, et al: The hypothalamus and pituitary in cerebral gigantism. A clinico-pathologic and immunocytochemical study. Am J Dis Child 139:679, 1985.
Zimmerman D, Young WF Jr, Ebersold MJ, et al: Congenital gigantism due to growth hormone–releasing hormone excess and pituitary hyperplasia with adenomatous transformation. J Clin Endocrinol Metab 76:216, 1993.

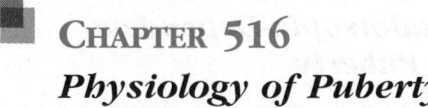

CHAPTER 516
Physiology of Puberty

Angelo M. DiGeorge and Luigi Garibaldi

Between early childhood and approximately 8–9 yr of age (i.e., *prepubertal* stage), the hypothalamic-pituitary-gonadal axis is dormant, as reflected by undetectable serum concentrations of luteinizing hormone (LH) and sex hormones (i.e., estradiol in girls, testosterone in boys). In this phase, the activity of the hypothalamus and pituitary is thought to be suppressed by neuronal restraint pathways and by the negative feedback provided in young children by the minute amounts of circulating gonadal steroids. Evidence of hypothalamic-pituitary-gonadal interaction during the prepubertal period resides in the fact that serum follicle-stimulating hormone (FSH) concentrations are detectable in most children and may be increased (with serum LH concentrations) in children with Turner syndrome or anorchia.

One to 3 yr before the onset of puberty becomes clinically evident, low serum levels of LH during sleep become demonstrable (i.e., *peripubertal* period). This sleep-entrained LH secretion occurs in a pulsatile fashion and probably reflects endogenous episodic discharge of hypothalamic gonadotropin-releasing hormone (GnRH). Nocturnal pulses of LH continue to increase in amplitude and, to a lesser extent, in frequency as clinical puberty approaches. This pulsatile secretion of gonadotropins is responsible for enlargement and maturation of the gonads and the secretion of sex hormones. The appearance of the secondary sex characteristics in *early puberty* is the visible culmination of the sustained, active interaction occurring among hypothalamus, pituitary, and gonads in the peripubertal period. By *midpuberty*, LH pulses become evident even during the daytime and occur at about 90–120-min intervals.

A second critical event occurs in middle or late adolescence in girls, in whom cyclicity and ovulation occur. A positive-feedback mechanism develops whereby rising levels of estrogen in midcycle cause a distinct increase of LH.

The factors that normally activate or restrain the hypothalamic neurons responsible for GnRH secretion (i.e., neurosecretory unit known as *the GnRH pulse generator*) are unknown. It is clear that GnRH is the major, if not the only, hormone responsible for the onset and progression of puberty, because pubertal development can be reproduced in sexually immature or gonadotropin-deficient animals and humans by pulsed administration of GnRH.

The interpretation of the hormonal changes of puberty is complex because of several factors. First, pituitary gonadotropins are heterogeneous and circulate in multiple isoforms, with different half-lives, immunoreactivities, and bioactivities. More-bioactive isoforms of LH may be preponderant during puberty. Second, LH immunoreactivity is variable in different immunoassays, and the results of LH measurements vary widely among laboratories. Third, the pulsatile secretion of gonadotropins and the synergism of FSH and LH in promoting gonadal maturation make interpretation of single serum gonadotropin concentrations difficult. Measurement of gonadotropins in serially obtained (every 10–20 min for 12–24 hr) serum samples or timed urine collections is more meaningful. Fourth, important sex differences exist in the maturation of the hypothalamus and pituitary gland, and serum LH concentrations rise earlier in the course of the pubertal process in boys than in girls.

The age of onset of puberty varies and is more closely correlated with osseous maturation than with chronological age (see Chapter 15). In girls, the breast bud is usually the first sign of puberty (10–11 yr), followed by the appearance of pubic hair 6–12 mo later. The interval to menarche is usually 2–2.5 yr but may be as long as 6 yr. In the United States, at least one sign of puberty is present in approximately 95% of girls by 12 yr of age and in 99% of girls by 13 yr of age. Peak height velocity occurs early (at breast stage II–III, typically between 11 and 12 yr of age) in girls and always precedes menarche. The mean age of menarche is about 12.75 yr. There are, however, wide variations in the sequence of changes involving growth spurt, breast bud, pubic hair, and maturation of the internal and external genitalia.

In boys, growth of the testes (>3 mL in volume or 2.5 cm in longest diameter) and thinning of the scrotum are the first signs of puberty. These are followed by pigmentation of the scrotum and growth of the penis (see Chapter 15). Pubic hair then appears. Appearance of axillary hair usually occurs in midpuberty. In boys, unlike girls, acceleration of growth begins after puberty is well under way and is maximal at genital stage IV–V (typically between 13 and 14 yr of age). In boys, the growth spurt occurs approximately 2 yr later than in girls, and growth may continue beyond 18 yr of age.

Genetic and environmental factors affect the onset of puberty. The drop in menarcheal age in the past century probably reflects better nutrition and improved general health. American black girls are significantly more advanced in development of secondary sex characteristics than white girls. Ballet dancers, gymnasts, runners, and other girl athletes in whom leanness and strenuous physical activity have coexisted from early childhood frequently exhibit a marked delay in puberty or menarche; the same individuals frequently have oligomenorrhea or amenorrhea as adults. This observation supports the thesis that the energy balance is closely related to the activity of the GnRH pulse generator and the mechanisms initiating and sustaining puberty.

Adrenal cortical androgens also play a role in pubertal maturation. Serum levels of dehydroepiandrosterone (DHEA) and its sulfate (DHEAS) begin to rise at approximately 6–8 yr of age, before any increase in LH or sex hormones and before the earliest physical changes of puberty are apparent; this process has been called adrenarche. DHEAS is the most abundant adrenal C-19 steroid in the blood, and its serum concentration remains fairly stable over 24 hr; a single measurement of this hormone is commonly used as a marker of adrenal androgen secretion. Although adrenarche typically antedates the onset of gonadal activity (i.e., gonadarche) by a few years, the two processes do not seem to be causally related, because adrenarche and gonadarche are dissociated in conditions such as central precocious puberty and adrenocortical failure.

CHAPTER 517

Disorders of Pubertal Development

Angelo M. DiGeorge and Luigi Garibaldi

Precocious puberty is difficult to define because of the marked variation in the age at which puberty begins in normal children, particularly if they belong to different ethnic groups. Nevertheless, onset of secondary sexual characteristics before 8 yr of age in girls and 9 yr in boys is generally considered precocious.

Precocious pubertal development may be classified as gonadotropin dependent, also called *true* or *central* precocious puberty, or gonadotropin independent, also called *peripheral* precocious puberty or precocious *pseudopuberty* (Table 517–1). True precocious puberty is always isosexual and involves hypothalamic-pituitary-gonadal activation; the precocity involves secondary sexual characteristics and a gonadotropin-mediated increase in the size and activity of the gonads. In precocious pseudopuberty, some of the secondary sex characteristics appear, but there is no activation of the normal hypothalamic-pituitary-gonadal interplay. In this latter group, the sex characteristics may be isosexual or heterosexual (see Chapters 529, 536, and 539).

Precocious pseudopuberty may induce maturation of the hypothalamic-pituitary-gonadal axis and trigger the onset of true sexual precocity. This mixed type of precocious puberty occurs commonly in conditions such as congenital adrenal hyperplasia and McCune-Albright syndrome, when the bone age reaches the pubertal range (10.5–12.5 yr).

■ TABLE 517–1 Conditions Causing Precocious Puberty

- Gonadotropin-dependent puberty (true precocious puberty)
  - Idiopathic (constitutional, functional)
  - Organic brain lesions
    - Hypothalamic hamartoma
    - Brain tumors, hydrocephalus, severe head trauma
  - Hypothyroidism, prolonged and untreated
- Combined gonadotropin-dependent and gonadotropin-independent puberty
  - Treated congenital adrenal hyperplasia
  - McCune-Albright syndrome, late
  - Familial male precocious puberty, late
- Gonadotropin-independent puberty (precocious pseudopuberty)
  - Females
    - Isosexual (feminizing) conditions
      - McCune-Albright syndrome
      - Autonomous ovarian cysts
      - Ovarian tumors
        - Granulosa-theca cell tumor associated with Ollier disease
        - Teratoma, chorionepithelioma
        - Sex-cord tumor with annular tubules (SCTAT) associated with Peutz-Jeghers syndrome
      - Feminizing adrenocortical tumor
      - Exogenous estrogens
    - Heterosexual (masculinizing) conditions
      - Congenital adrenal hyperplasia
      - Adrenal tumors
      - Ovarian tumors
      - Glucocorticoid receptor defect
      - Exogenous androgens
  - Males
    - Isosexual (masculinizing) conditions
      - Congenital adrenal hyperplasia
      - Adrenocortical tumor
      - Leydig cell tumor
      - Familial male precocious puberty
      - Isolated
      - Associated with pseudohypoparathyroidism
      - hCG-secreting tumors
        - Central nervous system
        - Hepatoblastoma
        - Mediastinal tumor associated with Klinefelter syndrome
      - Teratoma
      - Glucocorticoid receptor defect
      - Exogenous androgen
    - Heterosexual (feminizing) conditions
      - Feminizing adrenocortical tumor
      - Sex-cord tumor with annular tubules (SCTAT) associated with Peutz-Jeghers syndrome
      - Exogenous estrogens
- Incomplete (partial) precocious puberty
  - Premature thelarche
  - Premature adrenarche
  - Premature menarche

517.1 Gonadotropin-Dependent Precocious Puberty

In the past, no causative factor could be found to account for precocious puberty in about 80–90% of girls and 50% of boys. Computed tomography (CT) scans and magnetic resonance images (MRI) have lowered the percentages of children with idiopathic sexual precocity. The condition occurs at least 10-fold more frequently in girls than in boys and is usually sporadic, although some cases are familial.

CLINICAL MANIFESTATIONS. Sexual development may begin at any age and generally follows the sequence observed in normal puberty. In girls, the first sign is development of the breast; pubic hair may appear simultaneously but more often appears later. Maturation of the external genitalia, the appearance of axillary hair, and the onset of menstruation follow. The early menstrual cycles may be more irregular than they are with normal puberty. The initial cycles are usually anovulatory, but pregnancy has been reported as early as 5.5 yr of age (Fig. 517–1).

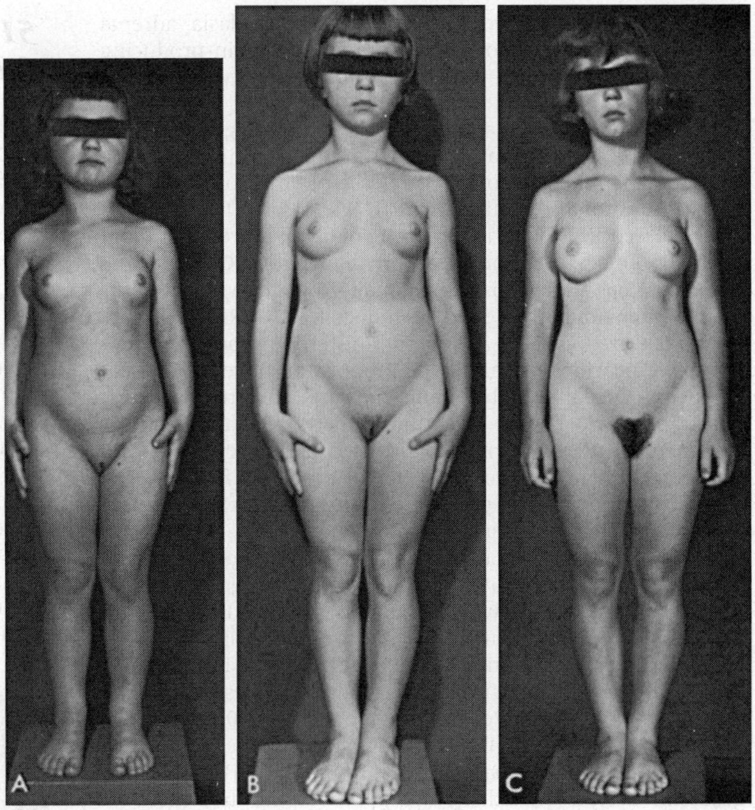

Figure 517–1. Idiopathic precocious puberty. Patient *(A)* at 3 11/12, *(B)* at 5 8/12, and *(C)* at 8 1/2 yr of age. Breast development and vaginal bleeding began at 2 1/2 yr of age. Osseous age was 7 1/2 yr at 3 11/12 and 14 yr at 8 yr of age. Repeated estrogen assays varied between normal prepubertal and adult female levels. Urinary gonadotropins were not demonstrable until the child was 5 yr of age. Intelligence and dental age were normal for chronological age. Growth was completed at 10 yr; ultimate height was 142 cm (56 in).

In boys, enlargement of the testes is followed by enlargement of the penis, appearance of pubic hair, and acne. Erections are common, and nocturnal emissions may occur. The voice deepens, and linear growth is accelerated. Testicular biopsies have shown stimulation of all elements of the testes, and spermatogenesis has been observed as early as 5–6 yr of age.

In affected girls and boys, height, weight, and osseous maturation are advanced. The increased rate of ossification results in early closure of the epiphyses, and the ultimate stature is less than it would have been otherwise. Without treatment, approximately one third of girls and an even larger percentage of boys achieve a height below the 5th percentile as adults. Mental development is usually compatible with chronological age. Emotional behavior and mood swings are not uncommon, but serious psychologic problems are rare.

Although the clinical course is variable, three main patterns of pubertal progression can be identified, at least in girls. Most girls (particularly those younger than 6 yr of age at the onset) have *rapidly progressive* sexual precocity, characterized by rapid physical and osseous maturation, leading to a loss of height potential. Many girls (generally older than 6 yr of age at the onset) have a *slowly progressive variant,* characterized by parallel advancement of osseous maturation and linear growth, with preserved height potential. A small percentage of girls have spontaneously regressive or *unsustained* central precocious puberty. This variability in the natural course of sexual precocity underscores the need for longitudinal observation at the onset of sexual development, before treatment is considered.

LABORATORY DATA. Sensitive immunoradiometric, immunofluorimetric, and chemiluminescent assays for luteinizing hormone (LH) are replacing the traditional LH radioimmunoassays and offer greater diagnostic sensitivity using random blood samples. With these new assays, serum LH concentrations are undetectable in prepubertal children, but they become detectable in 50–70% of girls and possibly a higher percentage of boys with central sexual precocity. Measurement of LH in serial blood samples obtained during sleep has greater diagnostic power than measurement using a single random sample, and the serial samples typically reveal well-defined pulsatile secretion of LH. Intravenous administration of gonadotropin-releasing hormone *(GnRH stimulation test)* is a helpful diagnostic tool, particularly for boys, in whom a brisk LH response with predominance of LH over follicle-stimulating hormone (FSH) occurs in the early phase of precocious puberty. In girls with sexual precocity, the nocturnal LH secretion and the LH response to GnRH may be quite low in the early phase of sexual development, and the LH:FSH ratio may remain low until midpuberty.

As in normal puberty, serum estradiol concentrations are low or undetectable in the early phase of sexual precocity in girls. In boys, serum testosterone levels are detectable or clearly elevated by the time the parents seek medical attention, particularly if an early morning blood sample is obtained. Sex hormone concentrations usually are appropriate for the stage of puberty in both sexes. Osseous maturation is variably advanced, often above 2–3 SD. Pelvic ultrasonography in girls reveals progressive enlargement of the ovaries, followed by enlargement of the uterus, to pubertal size. A CT or MR scan may demonstrate physiologic enlargement of the pituitary gland, as seen in normal puberty.

DIFFERENTIAL DIAGNOSIS. Organic central nervous system (CNS) causes of central sexual precocity should be ruled out by CT or MR scans, particularly in girls younger than 6 yr of age and all boys. However, in children presenting without neurologic signs or symptoms, the CNS lesions causing precocious puberty are rarely malignant and seldom require neurosurgical intervention.

Gonadotropin-independent causes of isosexual precocious puberty must be considered in the differential diagnosis (see Table 517–1). For girls, these include tumors of the ovaries, autonomously functioning ovarian cysts, feminizing adrenal tumors, McCune-Albright syndrome, and exogenous sources of estrogens. For boys, congenital adrenal hyperplasia, adrenal tumors, Leydig cell tumors, chorionic gonadotropin-producing hepatoma, and familial male precocious puberty should be considered.

TREATMENT. The observation that the pituitary gonadotropic cells require pulsatile, rather than continuous, stimulation by GnRH to maintain the ongoing release of gonadotropins provides the rationale for using GnRH agonists for treatment of central precocious puberty. By virtue of being more potent and having a longer duration of action than native GnRH, these GnRH analogs "desensitize" the gonadotropic cells of the pituitary to the stimulatory effect of endogenous GnRH. A variety of analogs are available and, if administered properly, are extremely efficacious in halting the progression of central sexual precocity. Virtually all boys and the large subgroup of girls with rapidly progressive precocious puberty are candidates for treatment. However, girls with slowly progressive puberty do not seem to benefit in terms of height prognosis from GnRH-agonist therapy. Rare patients require treatment for psychologic or social reasons alone.

In the past, treatment required daily subcutaneous or multiple intranasal administrations of the GnRH analog. The advent of depot preparations, which maintain fairly constant serum levels of long-acting GnRH analogs for weeks, has markedly simplified therapy and increased its effectiveness. The preparation approved for this use in the United States, leuprolide acetate (Lupron Depot Ped), is given in a dose of 0.25–0.3 mg/kg (minimum, 7.5 mg) intramuscularly once every 4 wk. Other long-acting preparations (D-Trp6-GnRH [Decapeptyl]; goserelin acetate [Zoladex]) are approved for treatment of precocious puberty in other countries. Fewer than 5% of patients have local side effects from therapy, of which recurrent sterile fluid collection at the sites of injections is the most serious. Most of these patients have no side effects when treatment is changed to daily subcutaneous injections of an aqueous analog (e.g., histrelin acetate [Supprelin], 10 μg/kg/24 hr).

EFFECTS OF TREATMENT. Treatment results in decrease of the growth rate, generally to age-appropriate values, and an even greater decrease of the rate of osseous maturation. Some children, particularly those with greatly advanced (pubertal) bone age, may show marked deceleration of their growth rate and a complete arrest in the rate of osseous maturation. Treatment results in enhancement of the predicted height, although the actual adult height of patients followed to epiphyseal closure is approximately 1 SD below their midparental height. In girls, breast development may regress in those with Tanner stage II–III development. Most commonly, the size of the breasts remains unchanged in girls with stage III–V development or may even increase slightly because of progressive adipose tissue deposition. The amount of glandular tissue decreases. Pubic hair does not progress during treatment. Pelvic sonography demonstrates a decrease of the ovarian and uterine size. In boys, there is decrease of testicular size, variable regression of pubic hair, and decrease in the frequency of erections. Except for a decrease in bone density (of uncertain clinical significance), no serious adverse effects of GnRH analogs have been reported in children treated for sexual precocity.

If treatment is effective, the serum sex hormone concentrations decrease to prepubertal levels (testosterone, <20 ng/dL in boys; estradiol, <10 pg/mL in girls), and the serum LH concentration, as measured by sensitive immunometric assays, decreases to less than 1 IU/L. Moreover, the incremental FSH and LH response to GnRH stimulation decreases below 1–2 IU/L. Serum LH and sex hormone levels remain suppressed for as long as therapy is continued, but puberty resumes promptly when therapy is discontinued. In girls, menarche and ovulatory cycles appear within a few years.

517.2 Precocious Puberty Resulting from Organic Brain Lesions

ETIOLOGY. A wide variety of lesions of the CNS have been associated with gonadotropin-dependent sexual precocity. Postencephalitic scars, tuberculous meningoencephalitis, hydrocephalus, tuberous sclerosis, and severe head trauma have each been etiologic factors. Optic gliomas, astrocytomas, ependymomas, and neurofibromas may cause sexual precocity. How these lesions activate hypothalamic mechanisms that initiate puberty is unknown, but they usually involve the hypothalamus by scarring, invasion, or pressure. Irradiation of the brain (e.g., children with leukemia) hastens the onset of puberty, particularly in girls.

With the advent of CT and MR scans, *hypothalamic hamartoma* has been recognized as one of the most common brain lesions causing true precocious puberty (Fig. 517–2). This congenital malformation consists of ectopically located neural tissue containing GnRH-secretory neurons and functions as an accessory GnRH pulse generator. On MRI, it appears as a small pedunculated mass attached to the tuber cinereum or the floor of the third ventricle or, less often, as a sessile mass (Fig.

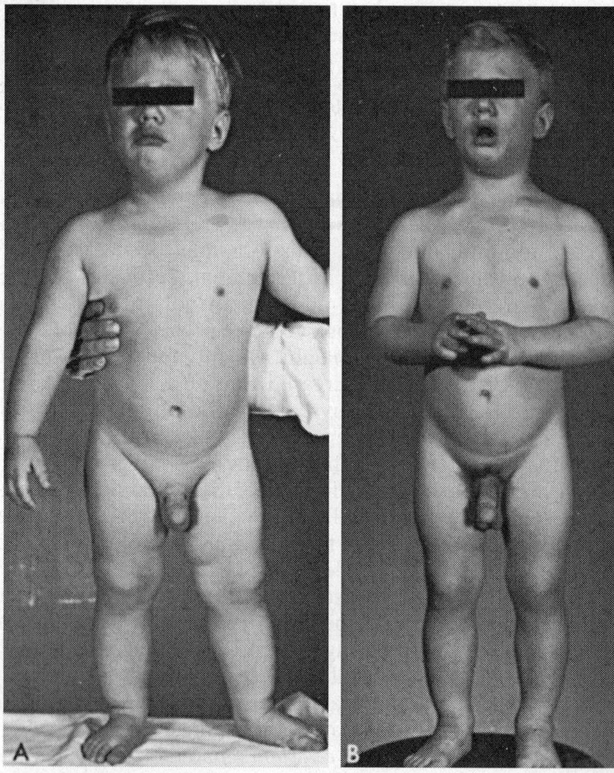

Figure 517–2. Precocious puberty with central nervous system lesion. Photographs at *(A)* 1.5 and *(B)* 2.5 yr of age. Accelerated growth, muscular development, osseous maturation, and testicular development were consistent with the degree of secondary sexual maturation. Urinary gonadotropins were repeatedly negative; 17-ketosteroids were usually 2–3 mg/24 hr. In early infancy, the patient began having frequent spells of rapid, purposeless motion; later in life, he had episodes of uncontrollable laughing with ocular movements. At 7 yr, he exhibited emotional lability, aggressive behavior, and destructive tendencies. Although a hypothalamic hamartoma had been suspected, it was not established until computed tomographic scanning became available, when the patient was 23 yr of age. Epiphyses fused at 9 yr of age; final height was 142 cm (56 in). At 24 yr of age, he developed an embryonal cell carcinoma of the retroperitoneum.

517–3), which remains static in size over the years. This lesion is infrequently associated with gelastic or psychomotor seizures.

About half of the tumors in the pineal region are germinomas or astrocytomas; the remainder consist of a wide variety of histologically distinct tumor types. These tumors cause precocious puberty by interrupting poorly characterized pubertal restraint pathways or, in boys only, by secreting human chorionic gonadotropin (hCG), which stimulates the Leydig cells of the testes. Intracranial hCG-secreting germinomas usually do not produce precocious puberty in girls, presumably because complete ovarian function cannot occur without FSH priming.

CLINICAL MANIFESTATIONS. Some of these tumors (e.g., hypothalamic hamartomas) or malformations remain static in size or grow slowly, producing no signs other than precocious puberty. For lesions causing neurologic symptoms, the neuroendocrine manifestations may be present for 1–2 yr before the tumor can be detected radiologically. Hypothalamic signs or symptoms such as diabetes insipidus, adipsia, hyperthermia, unnatural crying or laughing (gelastic seizures), obesity, and cachexia should suggest the possibility of an intracranial lesion.

The sexual precocity is always isosexual, and the endocrine patterns are generally those found in children without demonstrable organic lesions. In conditions other than hypothalamic hamartoma, growth hormone deficiency may occur and may be masked by the growth-promoting effect of the increased sex hormone levels. Previous series suggested that more than one third of boys but less than 10% of girls with true precocious puberty have an intracranial tumor; accordingly, the diagnosis of idiopathic precocious puberty can be made with less confidence in boys than in girls. Rapidly progressive sexual precocity in very young children suggests the likelihood of a hypothalamic hamartoma.

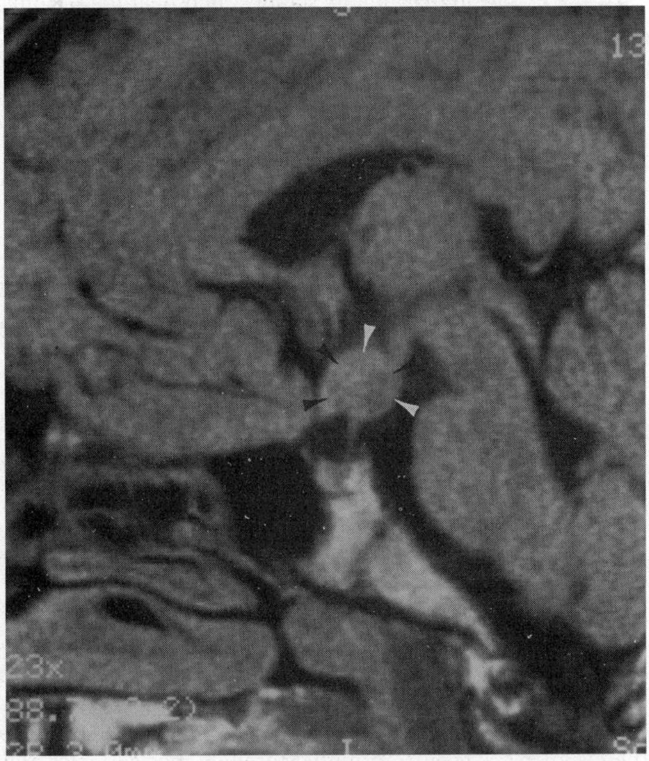

Figure 517–3. Magnetic resonance image of a central nervous system lesion in a child with central precocious puberty. A 6-yr-old girl was referred for stage IV breast development and growth acceleration. Serum luteinizing hormone and estradiol concentrations were in the adult range. The midsagittal T1-weighted image shows an isointense hypothalamic mass *(arrowheads)*, typical of a hamartoma. (From Sharafuddin M, et al: Am J Roentgenol 162:1167, 1994.)

TREATMENT. Neurosurgical intervention is not indicated for hypothalamic hamartomas, except for the rare patients with intractable seizures. For other neurologic lesions, therapy depends on the nature and location of the pathologic process. Regardless of the cause, therapy with GnRH analogs is as effective in children with organic brain lesions causing central precocious puberty as it is in children with idiopathic sexual precocity, and the analogs are the therapy of choice to halt premature sexual development. Combined growth hormone therapy should be considered for patients with associated growth hormone deficiency.

517.3 Syndrome of Precocious Puberty and Hypothyroidism

In children with untreated hypothyroidism, the onset of puberty is usually delayed until epiphyseal maturation has reached 12–13 yr of age. Precocious puberty in a child with untreated hypothyroidism and a prepubertal bone age presents a strikingly unphysiologic association. The phenomenon is not uncommon. Among 54 carefully studied children with primary hypothyroidism, half had varying degrees of isosexual development before attaining a pubertal bone age.

Affected patients have usually had severe hypothyroidism of long duration, with the usual manifestations, including retardation of growth and of osseous maturation. The causes of the hypothyroidism include lymphocytic thyroiditis, thyroidectomy, and overtreatment with antithyroid drugs.

Sexual development in girls consists primarily of breast enlargement and menstrual bleeding; the latter may occur even in girls with minimal breast enlargement. Pelvic sonography may reveal large, multicystic ovaries. Boys have testicular enlargement associated with modest or no penile enlargement and no pubic hair development. Enlargement of the sella, which is typical of longstanding primary hypothyroidism, may be demonstrated by skull film or MRI. Plasma levels of thyroid-stimulating hormone (TSH) are markedly elevated, often over 1,000 μU/mL. Plasma levels of prolactin and FSH LH are mildly elevated while LH levels are low, resulting in a high FSH:LH ratio. As a consequence, unlike in true precocious puberty, testicular enlargement occurs without substantial Leydig cell stimulation and testosterone secretion in affected boys. In affected girls, ovarian estrogen production occurs without a concomitant increase in androgens. The precocious puberty associated with hypothyroidism is an incomplete form of gonadotropin-dependent puberty. The pathogenesis of this type of sexual precocity is unclear, and hypotheses have included "specificity spillover" by the greatly elevated TSH levels (TSH and gonadotropins share identical α-chains) and impaired degradation of FSH and LH. Whatever the mechanism, treatment of the hypothyroidism results in rapid return to normal of the biochemical and clinical manifestations. Macroorchidism (testicular volume >30 mL) may persist in adult life despite adequate L-thyroxine therapy.

517.4 Gonadotropin-Secreting Tumors

HEPATIC TUMORS. About 30 patients with isosexual precocious puberty associated with hepatoblastoma have been recorded.

All have been males, with the age of onset varying from 4 mo–8 yr (average, 2 yr). An enlarged liver or mass in the upper quadrant should suggest the diagnosis. The tumor cells produce hCG, which stimulates the LH receptors in the Leydig cells of the testes. The testicular histology reveals interstitial cell hyperplasia and absence of spermatogenesis. Plasma levels of hCG and α-fetoprotein are usually markedly elevated; they serve as useful markers for following the effects of therapy. Plasma levels of testosterone are elevated, and the FSH and LH levels, as measured by specific, immunometric assays, are low; in the past, LH levels were falsely elevated because of cross-reaction with hCG on radioimmunoassay.

Treatment for these tumors is the same as that for other carcinomas of the liver; survival is usually less than 1 yr from the time of diagnosis. One patient has survived disease free for over 7 yr.

OTHER TUMORS. Chorionic gonadotropin–secreting choriocarcinomas, teratocarcinomas, or teratomas (also called ectopic pinealomas or atypical teratomas) may also cause precocious puberty. These tumors may be located in the CNS, mediastinum, or gonads. They are much more common (10–20-fold) in boys with precocious puberty than in girls. About a dozen boys with mediastinal tumors and precocious puberty had small testes, leading to the diagnosis of Klinefelter syndrome. Why extragonadal tumors (particularly mediastinal) occur more frequently than gonadal tumors in patients with Klinefelter syndrome is unknown. Affected patients often have marked elevations of hCG and α-fetoprotein.

PRECOCIOUS PSEUDOPUBERTY. The adrenal causes of pseudopuberty are discussed in Chapter 532, and the gonadal causes are discussed in Chapters 536 and 539.

517.5 McCune-Albright Syndrome

(Precocious Puberty with Polyostotic Fibrous Dysplasia and Abnormal Pigmentation)

This is a syndrome of endocrine dysfunction associated with patchy cutaneous pigmentation and fibrous dysplasia of the skeletal system. In the first 4 decades after Albright's description of this entity, sexual precocity in girls was the major recognized endocrinopathy. During the past decade, associated pituitary, thyroid, and adrenal aberrations have been increasingly recognized. For many years, the disorder was presumed to originate in the hypothalamus, but clinical and molecular advances have clearly established it as a prototypical model of autonomous hyperfunction of multiple glands. The disorder is caused by a missense mutation in the gene encoding the α-subunit of G_S, the G protein that stimulates cAMP formation. This results in activation of receptors (e.g., corticotropin [ACTH], TSH, FSH, LH receptors) that operate with a cAMP-dependent mechanism. Because the mutation is somatic, rather than genomic, it is expressed differently in different glands or tissues; hence, the variability of clinical expression in different patients.

Precocious puberty has been described predominantly in girls (Fig. 517–4). The average age at onset in affected girls is about 3 yr, but vaginal bleeding has occurred as early as 4 mo of age and secondary sex characteristics have occurred as early as 6 mo. Young girls have suppressed levels of LH and FSH, and there is no response to GnRH stimulation. Estradiol levels vary from normal to markedly elevated (>900 pg/mL), are often cyclic, and may correlate with the size of the cysts. In boys, precocious puberty is less common but has been reported in several instances. Unlike ovarian enlargement in girls, testicular enlargement in boys is fairly symmetric. It is followed by the appearance of phallic enlargement and pubic hair, as in normal puberty. Testicular histology has demonstrated large seminiferous tubules and no or minimal Leydig cell hyperplasia; these findings may simply reflect the fact that biopsy specimens were obtained at an early stage of pubertal development. In girls and boys, when the bone age reaches the usual pubertal age range, gonadotropin secretion begins, and the response to GnRH becomes pubertal. True (gonadotropin-dependent) precocious puberty overrides the antecedent (gonadotropin-independent) precocious pseudopuberty. In girls, menses become more regular, but often not completely, and fertility has been documented.

The hyperthyroidism that occurs in this condition differs from that characteristic of Graves disease. There is an equal distribution among males and females, and the goiters tend to be multinodular. Clinical hyperthyroidism is uncommon in children, but goiters, mildly elevated T_3 levels, suppressed TSH levels, and abnormalities on ultrasound have been reported.

In patients with associated Cushing syndrome, bilateral nodular adrenocortical hyperplasia has occurred in early infancy, antedating the sexual precocity. ACTH levels are low, and adrenal function is not suppressed by large doses of dexamethasone.

At least 17 patients with McCune-Albright syndrome are known who have increased secretion of growth hormone. This increase is manifested clinically by gigantism or acromegaly or by increased rates of growth even in the absence of precocious puberty. Girls and boys are equally affected. Levels of growth hormone are elevated and increase during sleep; they are augmented by TRH and poorly inhibited by oral glucose. Serum levels of prolactin are increased in most patients, but fewer than half of the patients have a demonstrable pituitary tumor.

Of the extraglandular manifestations, phosphaturia, leading to rickets or osteomalacia, is probably the most common. Cardiovascular and hepatic involvement are rare but may be life threatening (e.g., severe neonatal cholestasis).

All patients must be thoroughly investigated. Functioning ovarian cysts often disappear spontaneously; aspiration or surgical excision of cysts is rarely indicated. For girls with persistent estradiol secretion, testolactone, an aromatase inhibitor that interferes with the final step of estrogen biosynthesis, decreases, but does not normalize, estrogen production. Associated therapy with long-acting agonists of GnRH is indicated only for patients whose puberty has shifted from a gonadotropin-independent to a predominantly gonadotropin-dependent mechanism. Cushing syndrome requires adrenalectomy. Octreotide, a long-acting somatostatin inhibitor, has been used to treat the hypersomatotropism. The prognosis is favorable for longevity, but deformities, repeated fractures, pain, and occasional cranial nerve compression may result from the bony lesions.

517.6 Familial Male Gonadotropin-Independent Precocious Puberty

Male-limited autosomal dominant sexual precocity is gonadotropin independent. In the dozen or so described pedigrees, the disorder has been transmitted through affected males and unaffected female carriers of the gene. Signs of puberty appear by 2–3 yr of age. The testes are only slightly enlarged. Testicular biopsies show Leydig cell maturation and, in some instances, marked hyperplasia. Maturation of seminiferous tubules may be present. Testosterone levels are markedly elevated to the same range seen in boys with true precocious puberty; however, baseline levels of LH are prepubertal, pulsatile secretion of LH is absent, and LH does not respond to

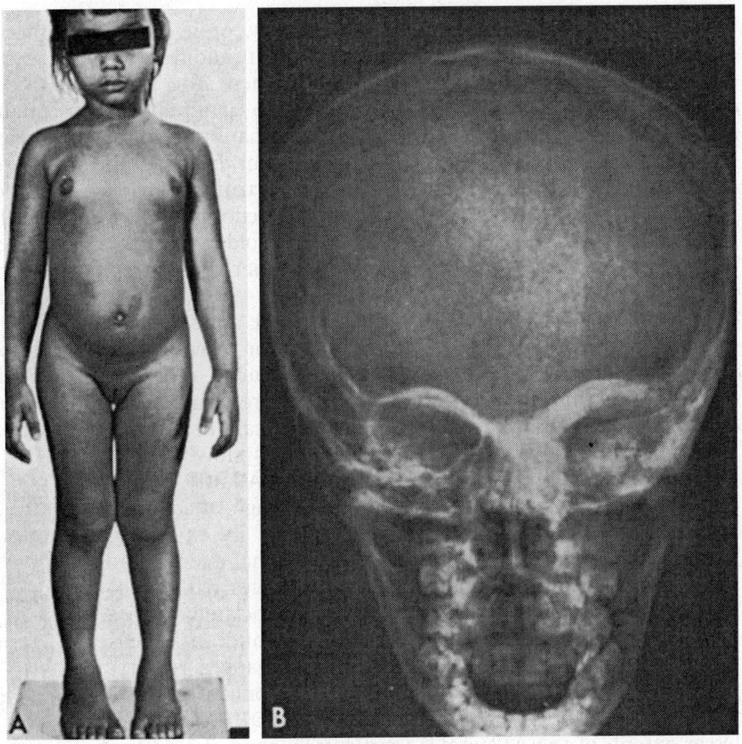

Figure 517–4. Precocious puberty associated with polyostotic fibrous dysplasia (McCune-Albright syndrome) in a girl 4.5 yr of age; at this time, her height age and osseous age were normal. Menarche occurred at 4 yr of age. *A*, Notice the bilateral breast development, the hyperpigmented spots on the abdomen, and the prominence of the left side of the face. *B*, Roentgenograms revealed fibrous dysplasia in the distal end of the left ulna and thickening of the bones about the left orbit and the maxillary portion of the frontal bones shown here.

stimulation with GNRH. The cause for activation of Leydig cells independent of gonadotropin stimulation is a missense mutation of the LH receptor leading to constitutive activation of cAMP production.

Osseous maturation may be markedly advanced; when it reaches the pubertal age range, normal gonadotropin secretion intervenes because maturation of the hypothalamus is enhanced by exposure to abnormal levels of sex hormones. Precocious puberty then becomes gonadotropin dependent. This sequence of events is similar to that occurring in children with McCune-Albright syndrome or in those with congenital adrenal hyperplasia, in whom sexual precocity is initially gonadotropin independent but becomes gonadotropin dependent when maturation of the hypothalamus initiates normal gonadotropin secretion.

Gonadotropin-independent precocious puberty has been diagnosed in two unrelated boys with type IA pseudohypoparathyroidism who had a single mutation of the $G_{s\alpha}$ protein. This mutation is inactivating at normal body temperature and causes pseudohypoparathyroidism, but in the cooler temperature of the testes, it is constitutionally activating, resulting in adenyl cyclase stimulation and production of testosterone. Although this mutation differs from the constitutive LH receptor (mutation), which usually causes familial male gonadotropin-independent precocious puberty, the end result is the same.

TREATMENT. Young boys have been successfully treated with ketoconazole (600 mg/24 hr in 8-hr divided doses), an antifungal drug that inhibits C-17,20-lyase and testosterone synthesis. Other investigators have used a combination of spironolactone (to block androgen action) and testolactone (a competitive inhibitor of aromatase), because estrogens derived from androgens stimulate bone maturation. Unfortunately, these medications are unable to revert the serum testosterone to the normal (prepubertal) concentrations or completely block the testosterone effects. They slow down, but do not halt, the progression of puberty and do not improve the height prognosis. Boys whose GnRH pulse generator has matured become resistant to treatment and require combined therapy with GnRH agonists.

517.7 Incomplete (Partial) Precocious Development

Isolated manifestations of precocity without development of other signs of puberty are not unusual; development of the breasts in girls and growth of sexual hair in both sexes are the two most common forms.

PREMATURE THELARCHE. This term applies to a transient condition of isolated breast development that most often appears in the first 2 yr of life; in some girls breast development is present at birth and persists. Breast development may be unilateral or asymmetric and often fluctuates in degree. Growth and osseous maturation are normal or slightly advanced. The genitalia show no evidence of estrogenic stimulation. The condition is usually sporadic and is rarely familial. Breast development may regress after 2 yr, often persists for 3–5 yr, and is rarely progressive. Menarche occurs at the expected age, and reproduction is normal. Plasma levels of LH and estradiol are below the limits of the assays, but basal levels of FSH and their responses to GnRH stimulation are greater than those seen in normal controls. In contrast, children with true precocious puberty secrete predominantly LH. Ultrasound examination of the ovaries reveals normal size, but a few small (<9 mm) cysts are not uncommon.

In some girls of the same age group, breast development may be associated with definite evidence of systemic estrogen effects, such as growth acceleration or bone age advancement. Pelvic sonography may reveal enlarged ovaries or uterus. This condition has been referred to as *exaggerated* or *atypical thelarche*. It differs from central sexual precocity because it is spontaneously regressive. GnRH stimulation elicits a robust FSH response and a minimal LH response. The pathogeneses of typical and exaggerated forms of thelarche are unclear, although a delay in the transition from the activated (neonatal-infantile) to the inactive (prepubertal) pituitary-ovarian axis may underlie both conditions.

Premature thelarche is a benign condition but may be the

first sign of true or pseudoprecocious puberty, or it may be caused by exogenous exposure to estrogens. In addition to a detailed history, a bone age should be obtained. The serum concentrations of FSH, LH, and estradiol are generally low and not diagnostic. Pelvic ultrasound examination is rarely indicated. Continued observation is important because the condition cannot be readily distinguished from true precocious puberty. Regression and recurrence suggest functioning follicular cysts. Occurrence of thelarche in children older than 3 yr of age most often is caused by a condition other than benign precocious thelarche.

PREMATURE ADRENARCHE. This term applies to the appearance of sexual hair before the age of 8 yr in girls or 9 yr in boys without other evidence of maturation. It is much more frequent in girls than in boys and may occur more frequently in American black girls than in others. Hair appears first on the labia majora; in young children it progresses slowly to the pubic region and finally appears in the axilla. Adult-type axillary odor is common. Affected children are slightly advanced in height and osseous maturation.

Premature adrenarche is an early maturational event of adrenal androgen production. This event coincides with precocious maturation of the zona reticularis, an associated decrease in 3β-hydroxysteroid-dehydrogenase activity, and an increase in C-17,20-lyase activity. These enzymatic changes result in increased basal and ACTH-stimulated serum concentrations of the Δ^5-steroids (17-hydroxypregnenolone and DHEA) and, to a lesser extent, of the Δ^4-steroids (particularly androstenedione) compared with age-matched controls. The levels of these steroids and those of DHEAS are usually comparable to those of children in the early stages of normal puberty.

Premature adrenarche is a benign condition that requires no therapy. However, a few affected patients have one or more features of systemic androgen effect, such as marked growth acceleration, clitoral (girls) or phallic (boys) enlargement, cystic acne, or advanced bone age (>2–3 SD above the mean for age). In these patients with *atypical premature adrenarche*, an ACTH stimulation test with measurement of serum 17-hydroxyprogesterone is indicated to rule out nonclassic congenital adrenal hyperplasia due to 21-hydroxylase deficiency. Epidemiologic and molecular-genetic studies have shown that other enzyme defects (i.e., 3β-hydroxysteroid-dehydrogenase or 11β-hydroxylase deficiencies) are extremely rare in girls with premature pubarche.

Although premature adrenarche is a benign condition, preliminary observations suggest that girls with premature adrenarche are at high risk for hyperandrogenism and polycystic ovarian syndrome as adults.

PREMATURE MENARCHE. Isolated menses without other evidence of sexual development occurs less frequently than premature thelarche or premature adrenarche. The majority of affected girls have only 1–3 episodes of bleeding; puberty occurs at the usual time and menstrual cycles are normal. Plasma levels of gonadotropins are normal, but estradiol levels may be elevated, probably owing to bursts of ovarian activity. Occasional patients are found to have ovarian follicular cysts on ultrasound. Vaginal causes of bleeding such as vulvovaginitis, foreign body, urethral prolapse, and sarcoma botryoides must be ruled out by careful physical examination.

517.8 Medicational Precocity

A variety of medicaments can induce the appearance of secondary sexual characteristics that may be confused with precocious puberty. A careful history focused on exploring the possibility of accidental exposure to or ingestion of sex hormones is important. Precocious pseudopuberty has occurred in both boys and girls from the accidental ingestion of estrogens (including contraceptive pills) and from the administration of anabolic steroids. Estrogens in cosmetics, hair creams, and breast augmentation creams have caused breast development in girls and gynecomastia in boys; estrogens are readily absorbed through the skin. Contamination of vitamin tablets by sex hormones has been reported to cause precocious pseudopuberty. A recent "epidemic" of premature thelarche and precocious pseudopuberty in Puerto Rico has been attributed to contamination of meats, particularly chicken, with estrogens used in animal husbandry but has not been proved. Exogenous estrogens may produce an intense, dark brown color in the areola of the breasts that is not usually seen in endogenous types of precocity. The precocious changes disappear after cessation of exposure to the hormones.

Apter D, Butzow TL, Laughlin GA, et al: Gonadotropin-releasing hormone pulse generator activity during pubertal transition in girls: Pulsatile and diurnal patterns of circulating gonadotropins. J Clin Endocrinol Metab 76:940, 1993.
Barnes ND, Hayles AB, Ryan RJ: Sexual maturation in juvenile hypothyroidism. Mayo Clin Proc 48:849, 1973.
Boepple PA, Frisch LS, Wierman ME, et al: The natural history of autonomous gonadal function, adrenarche, and central puberty in gonadotropin-independent precocious puberty. J Clin Endocrinol Metab 75:1550, 1992.
Breyer P, Haider A, Pescovitz OH: Gonadotropin-releasing hormone agonists in the treatment of girls with central precocious puberty. Clin Obstet Gynecol 36:764, 1993.
Bruder JM, Samuels MH, Bremner WJ, et al: Hypothyroidism-induced macroorchidism: Use of a gonadotropin-releasing hormone agonist to understand its mechanism and augment adult stature. J Clin Endocrinol Metab 80:11, 1995.
Burstein S: Growth disorders after cranial radiation in childhood. J Clin Endocrinol Metab 78:1280, 1994.
Comite F, Pescovitz OH, Rieth KG, et al: Luteinizing hormone-releasing hormone analog treatment of boys with hypothalamic hamartoma and true precocious puberty. J Clin Endocrinol Metab 59:888, 1984.
Conn PM, Crowley WR Jr: Gonadotropin-releasing hormone and its analogues. N Engl J Med 324:93, 1991.
Demir A, Dunkel L, Stenman U, Voutilainen R: Age-related course of urinary gonadotropins in children. J Clin Endocrinol Metab 80:1457, 1995.
DiGeorge AM: Albright syndrome: Is it coming of age? J Pediatr 87:1018, 1975.
Dunkel L, Alfthan H, Stenman U, et al: Developmental changes in 24-hour profiles of luteinizing hormone and follicle-stimulating hormone from prepuberty to midstages of puberty in boys. J Clin Endocrinol Metab 74:890, 1992.
Feuillan PP, Jones J, Cutler GB Jr: Long-term testolactone therapy for precocious puberty in girls with the McCune-Albright syndrome. J Clin Endocrinol Metab 77:647, 1993.
Fontoura M, Brauner R, Prevot C, et al: Precocious puberty in girls: Early diagnosis of a slowly progressing variant. Arch Dis Child 64:1170, 1989.
Garibaldi LR, Aceto T Jr, Weber C: The pattern of gonadotropin and estradiol secretion in exaggerated thelarche. Acta Endocrinol (Copenh) 128:345, 1993.
Garibaldi LR, Picco P, Magier S, et al: Serum luteinizing hormone concentrations, as measured by a sensitive immunoradiometric assay, in children with normal, precocious or delayed pubertal development. J Clin Endocrinol Metab 72:888, 1991.
Grave GD, Cutler GB (eds): Sexual Precocity. New York, Raven Press, 1993.
Harlan WR, Grillo GP, Cornoni-Huntley J, Leaverton PE: Secondary sex characteristics of boys 12–17 years of age. J Pediatr 95:293, 1979.
Harlan WR, Harlan EA, Grillo GP: Secondary sex characteristics of girls 12 to 17 years of age: The US Health Examination Survey. J Pediatr 96:1074, 1980.
Hertz R: Accidental ingestion of estrogens by children. Pediatrics 21:203, 1958.
Holland FJ: Gonadotropin-independent precocious puberty. Endocrinol Metab Clin North Am 20:191, 1991.
Ibanez L, Potau N, Virdis R, et al: Postpubertal outcome in girls diagnosed of premature pubarche during childhood: Increased frequency of functional ovarian hyperandrogenism. J Clin Endocrinol Metab 76:1599, 1993.
Iiri T, Herzmark P, Nakamoto JM, et al: Rapid GDP release from $G_{s\alpha}$ in patients with gain and loss of endocrine function. Nature 371:164, 1994.
Ilicke A, Prager Lewin R, Kauli R, et al: Premature thelarche—Natural history and sex hormone secretion in 68 girls. Acta Paediatr Scand 73:756, 1984.
Jay N, Mansfield MJ, Blizzard RM, et al: Ovulation and menstrual function of adolescent girls with central precocious puberty after therapy with gonadotropin-releasing hormone agonists. J Clin Endocrinol Metab 75:890, 1992.
Kaplan SL, Grumbach MM: Pathophysiology and treatment of sexual precocity. J Clin Endocrinol Metab 71:785, 1990.
Kletter GB, Kelch RP: Disorders of puberty in boys. Endocrinol Metab Clin North Am 22:455, 1993.
Kulin HE: The assessment of gonadotropins during childhood and adolescence: An ongoing struggle. Endocrinologist 4:279, 1994.
Laue L, Jones J, Barnes KM, et al: Treatment of familial male precocious puberty with spironolactone, testolactone, and deslorelin. J Clin Endocrinol Metab 76:151, 1993.

Mahachoklertwattana P, Kaplan SL, Grumbach MM: The luteinizing hormone–releasing hormone–secreting hypothalamic hamartoma is a congenital malformation: Natural history. J Clin Endocrinol Metab 77:118, 1993.
Morris AH, Reiter EO, Geffner ME, et al: Absence of nonclassical congenital adrenal hyperplasia in patients with precocious adrenarche. J Clin Endocrinol Metab 69:709, 1989.
Nakagaware A, Ikeda K, Tsuneyoshi M, et al: Hepatoblastoma producing alpha-fetoprotein and human chorionic gonadotropin. Cancer 56:1636, 1985.
Oerter KE, Manasco P, Barnes KM, et al: Adult height in precocious puberty after long-term treatment with deslorelin. J Clin Endocrinol Metab 73:1235, 1991.
Pescovitz OH, Comite F, Hench K, et al: The NIH experience with precocious puberty: Diagnostic subgroups and response to short-term luteinizing hormone releasing hormone analogue therapy. J Pediatr 108:47, 1986.
Pescovitz OH, Hench KD, Barnes KM, et al: Premature thelarche and central precocious puberty: The relationship between clinical presentation and the gonadotropin response to luteinizing hormone-releasing hormone. J Clin Endocrinol Metab 67:474, 1988.
Premawardhana LD, Vora JP, Mills R, et al: Acromegaly and its treatment in the McCune-Albright syndrome. Clin Endocrinol 36:605, 1992.
Rieter EO, Fuldauer VG, Root AW: Secretion of the adrenal androgen dehydroepiandrosterone sulfate, during normal infancy, childhood and adolescence in sick infants, and in children with endocrinologic abnormalities. J Pediatr 90:766, 1977.
Romshe CA, Sotos JF: Intracranial human chorionic gonadotropin-secreting tumor with precocious puberty. J Pediatr 86:250, 1975.
Rosenfield RL: Selection of children with precocious puberty for treatment with gonadotropin releasing hormone analogs. J Pediatr 124:989, 1994.
Schimke RN, Madigan CM, Silver BJ, et al: Choriocarcinoma, thyrotoxicosis, and the Klinefelter syndrome. Cancer Genet Cytogenet 9:1, 1983.
Schwindinger WF, Levine MA: McCune-Albright syndrome. Trends Endocrinol Metab 4:238, 1993.
Sharafuddin MJ, Luisiri A, Garibaldi LR, et al: MR imaging diagnosis of central precocious puberty: Importance of changes in the shape and size of the pituitary gland. Am J Roentgenol 162:1167, 1994.
Shaul PW, Towbin RB, Chernausek SD: Precocious puberty following severe head trauma. Am J Dis Child 139:467, 1985.
Shenker A, Laue L, Kosugi S, et al: A constitutively activating mutation of the luteinizing hormone receptor in familial male precocious puberty. Nature 365:652, 1993.
Shenker A, Weinstein LS, Moran A, et al: Severe endocrine and nonendocrine manifestations of the McCune-Albright syndrome associated with activating mutations of stimulatory G protein Gs. J Pediatr 123:509, 1993.
Stanhope R, Abdulwahid NA, Adams J, et al: Studies of gonadotropin pulsatility and pelvic ultrasound examination distinguish between isolated premature thelarche and central precocious puberty. Eur J Pediatr 145:190, 1986.
Van Winter JT, Noller KL, Zimmerman D, et al: Natural history of premature thelarche in Olmsted County, Minnesota, 1940 to 1984. J Pediatr 116:278, 1990.
Weinstein LS, Shenker A, Gejman PV, et al: Activating mutations of the stimulatory G protein in the McCune-Albright syndrome. N Engl J Med 325:1688, 1991.

SECTION 2

Disorders of the Thyroid Gland

Angelo M. DiGeorge ■ Stephen LaFranchi

THYROID PHYSIOLOGY. The main function of the thyroid gland is to synthesize thyroxine (T_4) and 3,5,3′-triiodothyronine (T_3). The only known physiologic role of iodine is in the synthesis of these hormones; the recommended dietary allowance of iodine is 40–50 μg/24 hr for infants, 70–120 μg/24 hr for children, and 150 μg/24 hr for adolescents and adults. The daily intake in North America varies from 240 to more than 700 μg. Whatever the chemical form ingested, iodine eventually reaches the thyroid gland as iodide. Thyroid tissue has an avidity for iodine and is able to trap (with a gradient of 100:1), transport, and concentrate it in the follicular lumen for synthesis of thyroid hormone.

Before trapped iodide can react with tyrosine, it must be oxidized; this reaction is catalyzed by thyroidal peroxidase. The thyroid cells also elaborate a specific thyroprotein, a globulin with approximately 120 tyrosine units. Iodination of tyrosine forms monoiodotyrosine and diiodotyrosine; two molecules of diiodotyrosine then couple to form one molecule of T_4, or one molecule of diiodotyrosine and one of monoiodotyrosine to form T_3. Once formed, hormones are stored as thyroglobulin in the lumen of the follicle (colloid) until ready to be delivered to the body cells. Thyroglobulin is a large globular glycoprotein with a molecular weight of about 660,000 and under normal conditions is detectable in the blood of most individuals at nanogram levels. T_4 and T_3 are liberated from thyroglobulin by activation of proteases and peptidases.

The metabolic potency of T_3 is 3–4 times that of T_4. In adults, the thyroid produces approximately 100 μg of T_4 and 20 μg of T_3 daily. Only 20% of circulating T_3 is secreted by the thyroid; the remainder is produced by deiodination of T_4 in the liver, kidney, and other peripheral tissues by type I 5′-deiodinase. In the pituitary and brain, approximately 80% of required T_3 is produced in situ from T_4 by a different enzyme, type II 5′-deiodinase. In the fetal rat, although plasma levels of T_3 are very low, cerebral concentrations increase to almost adult levels. T_3 carries out most of the physiologic actions of the thyroid hormones. T_4 is more abundant, but it binds weakly to nuclear receptors, and most of its physiologic effects occur by conversion to T_3. The level of T_3 in blood is 1/50 that of T_4.

The thyroid hormones increase oxygen consumption, stimulate protein synthesis, influence growth and differentiation, and affect carbohydrate, lipid, and vitamin metabolism. The free hormones enter cells, where T_4 may be converted to T_3 by deiodination. Intracellular T_3 then enters the nucleus, where it binds to thyroid hormone receptors. Thyroid hormone receptors are members of the steroid hormone receptor superfamily that includes glucocorticoids, estrogen, progesterone, vitamin D, and retinoids. Four different isoforms of the thyroid hormone receptor (α 1 and 2, β 1 and 2) are expressed in different tissues; the protein product of the formerly designated *c-erb A* proto-oncogene (now called *THRA2*) has been identified as the α2 thyroid hormone receptor in the brain and hypothalamus. Thyroid hormone receptors consist of a ligand-binding domain (binds T_3), hinge region, and DNA-binding domain (zinc finger). Binding of T_3 activates the thyroid hormone receptor response element, resulting in production of an encoded mRNA and protein synthesis and of secretion specific for the target cell. In this manner, a single hormone, T_4, acting through tissue-specific thyroid hormone receptor isoforms and gene-specific thyroid response elements, can produce multiple effects in various tissues.

About 70% of the circulating T_4 is firmly bound to *thyroxine-binding globulin* (TBG). Less important carriers are thyroxine-binding prealbumin, now named *transthyretin* (TTR), and albumin. Only 0.03% of T_4 in serum is not bound and comprises free thyroxine (FT_4). Approximately 50% of circulating T_3 is bound to TBG, and 50% is bound to albumin; 0.30% of T_3 is unbound or free T_3. Because the concentration of TBG is altered in many clinical circumstances, its status must be considered when interpreting T_4 or T_3 levels.

The thyroid is regulated by thyroid-stimulating hormone (TSH), a glycoprotein produced and secreted by the anterior pituitary. This hormone activates adenylate cyclase in the thyroid gland to effect release of thyroid hormones. TSH is composed of two noncovalently bound subunits (chains): α and β (hTSH-β). The α subunit is common to luteinizing hormone, follicle-stimulating hormone, and chorionic gonadotropin; the specificity of each hormone is conferred by the β subunit. TSH synthesis and release are stimulated by TSH-releasing hormone (TRH), which is synthesized in the hypothalamus and secreted into the pituitary. TRH is found in other parts of the brain besides the hypothalamus and in many other organs; aside from its endocrine function, it seems to serve as a neurotransmitter. TRH, a simple tripeptide, was the first neuropeptide to be identified, synthesized, and used in clinical medicine. In states of decreased production of thyroid hormone, TSH and

TRH are increased. An excess of TRH or of TSH results in hypertrophy and hyperplasia of thyroid cells, increased trapping of iodine, and increased synthesis of thyroid hormones. Exogenous thyroid hormone or increased thyroid hormone synthesis inhibits TSH and TRH production. Except in the neonate, levels of TRH in serum are very low.

Further control of the level of circulating thyroid hormones occurs in the periphery. In many nonthyroidal illnesses extrathyroidal production of T_3 decreases; factors that inhibit thyroxine-5′-deiodinase include fasting, chronic malnutrition, acute illness, and certain drugs. Levels of T_3 may be significantly decreased while levels of T_4 and TSH remain normal. Presumably, the decreased levels of T_3 result in decreased rates of oxygen production, of substrate use, and of other catabolic processes.

Burrow GH, Fisher DA, Larsen PR: Maternal and fetal thyroid function. N Engl J Med 331:1072, 1994.

CHAPTER 518
Thyroid Hormone Studies

Angelo M. DiGeorge and Stephen LaFranchi

SERUM THYROID HORMONES. Methods are available to measure all of the thyroid hormones in sera: thyroxine (T_4), free T_4, triiodothyronine (T_3), free T_3, and the diiodothyronines. A metabolically inert T_3 (3,5′,3′-triiodothyronine), called reverse T_3, is also present in sera. Age must be considered in interpreting results, particularly in the neonate.

Thyroglobulin (Tg) is a glycoprotein dimer that is secreted through the apical surface of the thyrocyte into the colloid. Small amounts escape into the circulation and are measurable in serum. Levels increase with thyroid-stimulating hormone (TSH, also called thyrotropin) stimulation and decrease with TSH suppression. Levels are increased in the neonate, in patients with Graves disease, and in those with endemic goiter. The most marked elevations of Tg occur in patients with differentiated carcinoma of the thyroid. Athyreotic infants may have markedly reduced levels of Tg in serum.

TSH levels in serum are an extremely sensitive indicator of primary hypothyroidism. Radioimmunoassay methods for the measurement of serum levels of TSH have been replaced by immunometric assay methods, which are capable of quantitating the lower limits of normal as well as elevated levels. A 3rd generation of assays (chemiluminescent assays) that can measure complete suppression of TSH is now standard. These sensitive TSH assays obviate the need for thyrotropin-releasing hormone (TRH) stimulation in the diagnosis of most patients with thyroid disorders.

After the neonatal period, normal levels of TSH are below 6 μU/mL. TSH secretion can be stimulated by intravenous administration (7 μg/kg) of TRH. In normal subjects, TRH administration increases baseline levels of TSH within 30 min. In hyperthyroidism, there is no rise in serum levels of TSH in response to TRH because the elevated levels of thyroid hormones block the effect of TRH on the pituitary. In patients with even very mild degrees of thyroid failure, administration of TRH results in an exaggerated TSH response. Patients with pituitary or hypothalamic failure have low basal levels of TSH, although it may not be below the lower range of normal; a normal response to TRH localizes the defect in the hypothalamus.

FETAL AND NEWBORN THYROID. The fetal hypothalamic-pituitary-thyroid system develops independently of maternal influence. By 10–12 wk of gestation, the fetal thyroid is able to concentrate iodine and to synthesize iodothyronines. By the same time, the fetal pituitary contains TSH. Fetal serum T_4 increases progressively from midgestation to approximately 11.5 μg/dL at term. Fetal levels of T_3 are low before 20 wk and then gradually rise to about 60 ng/dL at term. Reverse T_3 levels, however, are very high in the fetus (250 ng/dL at 30 wk) and fall to 150 ng/dL at term. Serum levels of TSH gradually rise to 10 μU/mL at term. Approximately one third of maternal T_4 crosses the placenta to the fetus. Maternal T_4 may play a role in fetal development, especially that of the brain, before the synthesis of fetal thyroid hormones begins. The fetus of a hypothyroid mother may be at risk for neurologic damage, and a hypothyroid fetus may be partially protected by maternal T_4 until delivery.

At birth, there is an acute release of TSH; peak serum concentrations reach 70 μU/mL in 30 min in full-term infants. A rapid decline occurs in the ensuing 24 hr and a more gradual decline within the next 2 days to below 10 μU/mL. The acute increase in TSH produces a dramatic rise in levels of T_4 to approximately 16 μg/dL and of T_3 to approximately 300 ng/dL in about 4 hr. This T_3 seems largely derived from increased peripheral conversion of T_4 to T_3. T_4 levels gradually fall during the first 2 wk of life to 12 μg/dL. T_3 levels then decline during the 1st wk of life to levels under 200 ng/mL. Reverse T_3 levels are maintained for 2 wk (200 ng/dL) and fall by 4 wk to around 50 ng/dL. Small amounts of T_4 cross the placenta but are not sufficient to interfere with a diagnosis of congenital hypothyroidism in the neonate.

SERUM THYROXINE-BINDING GLOBULIN. The thyroid hormones are transported in plasma bound to thyroxine-binding globulin (TBG), a glycoprotein synthesized in the liver. Estimation of TBG levels is occasionally necessary because TBG is increased or decreased in a variety of clinical situations, with effects on the level of thyroxine. TBG binds about 70% of T_4 and 50% of T_3. TBG levels increase in pregnancy and in the newborn period, and with administration of estrogens (oral contraceptives), perphenazine, and heroin and decrease with androgens, anabolic steroids, glucocorticoids, and L-asparaginase. These effects are the results of modulation of hepatic synthesis of TBG. Phenytoin (diphenylhydantoin) is another cause of drug-induced abnormality of thyroid function tests. Phenytoin, an inducer of hepatic enzymes, stimulates hepatic degradation of T_4 and accelerates transport of T_4 into tissues. Phenobarbital has a similar effect. Some drugs, particularly phenytoin, also inhibit binding of T_4 and T_3 to TBG. Decreased or increased levels of TBG also occur as genetic traits (see later). TBG levels may be markedly decreased owing to loss in the urine, as in infants with congenital nephrotic syndrome.

The most commonly used measures of TBG or TBG-binding capacity are variations of the resin triiodothyronine uptake test (RT_3U), a test that allows interpretation of T_4 results, which vary depending on TBG levels; it should never be used as an autonomous test of thyroid function. The product of the serum T_4 concentration and T_3 uptake (thyroxine-resin T_3 index or T_4-RT_3U index) correlates closely with free T_4 concentration in serum. This index increases in hyperthyroidism, decreases in hypothyroidism, and is normal in euthyroid patients with mild abnormalities in the concentration of TBG. Normal values for the index vary among laboratories because T_4 levels and T_3 uptakes are often determined by a variety of kit methods and calculations and expressions of the index vary among laboratories. A radioimmunoassay method for TBG is available.

IN VIVO RADIONUCLIDE STUDIES. Markedly improved direct tests of thyroid function have made radioiodine uptake studies less useful. The iodine-trapping or concentrating mechanism of the thyroid can be evaluated by the radioactive isotope ^{123}I (half-life of 13 hr). The technology allows doses of radioiodine (0.1–0.5 μCi) that are only a fraction of those formerly used. Technetium (^{99m}Tc) is a particularly useful radioisotope for children, because in contrast to iodine, it is trapped but not organified by the thyroid and has a half-life of only 6 hr. Thyroid scanning may be indicated to detect ectopic thyroid tissue, to evaluate thyroid nodules, or to assess the presence of thyroid tissue in questions of thyroid agenesis. These studies should be performed with ^{99m}Tc as pertechnetate because it has the advantages of lower radiation exposure and high-quality scintigrams. Use of ^{131}I in children should be limited to those known to have thyroid cancer.

CHAPTER 519
Defects of Thyroxine-Binding Globulin

Angelo M. DiGeorge and Stephen LaFranchi

Abnormalities in levels of thyroxine-binding globulin (TBG) are not associated with clinical disease and do not require treatment. They are usually uncovered by a chance finding of abnormally low or high levels of thyroxine (T_4) and may be sources of confusion in the diagnosis of hypo- or hyperthyroidism.

TBG deficiency occurs as an X-linked dominant disorder. Congenital TBG deficiency is most often discovered through screening programs for neonatal hypothyroidism that use levels of T_4 as the primary screen. Affected patients have low levels of T_4 and elevated resin triiodothyronine uptake (RT_3U), but levels of free T_4 and thyroid-stimulating hormone (TSH) are normal. The diagnosis is confirmed by the finding of absent or low levels of TBG by radioimmunoassay. The disorder is more readily recognized in males because it is caused by a gene on the short arm of the X chromosome. TBG deficiency occurs in 1 in 2,400 newborn males, of whom 36% have TBG levels below 1 mg/L. Milder forms of TBG deficiency occur in approximately 1 of 42,000 heterozygous females. Complete TBG deficiency (<5 μg/L) occurs much less frequently. Three of eight families with complete TBG deficiency have been found to have a codon mutation (leucine to proline); other patients with reduced affinity of TBG for T_4 have had other point mutations that affect the tertiary structure of the protein.

Elevated TBG is also a harmless X-linked dominant anomaly, occurring in about 1 of 2,500 persons. It has been recognized primarily in adults, but neonatal screening programs are uncovering the condition in the neonate. The level of T_4 is elevated, T_3 is variably elevated, TSH and free T_4 are normal, and RT_3U is decreased. The elevated levels of TBG and normal levels of free T_4 confirm the diagnosis. In neonates, levels of T_4 as high as 95 μg/dL have been found, which decrease to 20–30 μg/dL after 2–3 wk. Such high levels of T_4 are thought to be related in part to the normally elevated levels of TBG in neonates during the 1st mo of life, presumably as an effect of maternal estrogens. Affected patients are euthyroid. Family studies may be indicated to alert other affected individuals. Acquired elevations of TBG occur with pregnancy, estrogen treatment, and hepatitis.

Familial dysalbuminemic hyperthyroxinemia is an autosomal dominant disorder that may be confused with hyperthyroidism. Markedly increased binding of T_4 to an abnormal albumin variant leads to increased serum concentrations of T_4. However, the levels of free T_4, free T_3, and TSH are normal. Levels of T_3 are normal or only slightly elevated. Affected patients are euthyroid.

CHAPTER 520
Hypothyroidism

Angelo M. DiGeorge and Stephen LaFranchi

Hypothyroidism results from deficient production of thyroid hormone or a defect in its receptor (Table 520–1). The disorder may be manifest from birth. When symptoms appear after a period of apparently normal thyroid function, the disorder may be truly "acquired" or may only appear so as a result of one of a variety of congenital defects in which the manifestation of the deficiency is delayed. The term cretinism is often used synonymously with congenital hypothyroidism but should be avoided.

CONGENITAL HYPOTHYROIDISM

Congenital causes of hypothyroidism may be sporadic or familial, goitrous or nongoitrous. In many cases, the deficiency

■ TABLE 520–1 Etiologic Classification of Hypothyroidism

Pit-1 (homeobox protein) mutations
- Deficiency of thyrotropin, growth hormone, and prolactin

Thyrotropin-releasing hormone (TRH) deficiency
- Isolated?
- Multiple hypothalamic deficiencies (e.g., craniopharyngioma)

Thyrotropin (TSH) deficiency
- Mutations in β chain
- Multiple pituitary deficiencies

Thyrotropin unresponsiveness
- $G_s\alpha$ mutation (e.g., type IA pseudohypoparathyroidism)
- Mutation in TSH receptor
  - Mouse (autosomal recessive)
  - Man?

Defect of fetal thyroid development
- Aplasia, ectopia (dysgenesis)

Defect in thyroid hormone synthesis (e.g., goitrous hypothyroidism)
- Iodide transport defect
- Thyroid peroxidase defect
- Thyroglobulin synthesis defect
- Deiodination defect

Iodine deficiency (endemic goiter)
- Neurologic type
- Myxedematous type

Maternal antibodies
- Thyrotropin receptor–blocking antibody (TRBAb)

Maternal medications
- Radioiodine, iodides
- Propylthiouracil, methimazole
- Amiodarone

Autoimmune (acquired hypothyroidism)
- Hashimoto thyroiditis
- Polyglandular autoimmune syndrome, types I, II, and III

Iatrogenic
- Propylthiouracil, methimazole, iodides, lithium, amiodarone
- Irradiation
  - Radioiodine
  - X-rays (neck or whole body)
- Thyroidectomy

Systemic disease
- Cystinosis
- Histiocytic infiltration

Resistance to thyroid hormone (only occasional clinical manifestations of hypothyroidism)

of thyroid hormone is severe, and symptoms develop in the early weeks of life. In others, lesser degrees of deficiency occur, and manifestations may be delayed for months or years.

ETIOLOGY. Thyroid Dysgenesis. Since the establishment of nationwide programs for neonatal screening for congenital hypothyroidism, many millions of neonates have been screened. The prevalence of congenital hypothyroidism has been found to be 1 in 4,000 infants worldwide, lower in black Americans (1 of 20,000) and higher in Hispanics and Native Americans (1 of 2,000). Developmental defects (thyroid dysgenesis) account for 90% of infants in whom hypothyroidism is detected; in about one third, even sensitive radionuclide scans can find no remnants of thyroid tissue *(aplasia)*. In the other two thirds of infants, rudiments of thyroid tissue are found in an ectopic location, anywhere from the base of the tongue *(lingual thyroid)* to the normal position in the neck. Most infants with congenital hypothyroidism are asymptomatic at birth even if there is complete agenesis of the thyroid gland. This situation is attributed to the transplacental passage of moderate amounts of maternal thyroxine (T_4), which provides fetal levels that are 25–50% of normal at birth. These low serum levels of T_4 and concomitantly elevated levels of thyroid-stimulating hormone (TSH) make it possible to screen and detect most hypothyroid neonates.

Little is known about the factors that interfere with the normal migration and development of the thyroid gland. Thyroid dysgenesis occurs sporadically, but familial cases have occasionally been reported. Twice as many females as males are affected. The frequent finding of thyroid dysgenesis confined to only one of a pair of monozygotic twins suggests the operation of a deleterious factor during intrauterine life. For years, it had been proposed that maternal antithyroid antibodies might be that factor, especially because antibodies in patients with autoimmune thyroid disease belong predominantly to the IgG class and can cross the placenta. Although thyroid antimicrosomal antibodies have been detected in some mother-infant pairs, there is little evidence of their pathogenicity. The demonstration of thyroid growth-blocking and cytotoxic antibodies in some infants with thyroid dysgenesis and in their mothers suggests a more likely pathogenetic mechanism. Maternal TSH-binding antibodies as a cause of transient congenital hypothyroidism and of neonatal Graves disease are well established.

Ectopic thyroid tissue (lingual, sublingual, subhyoid) may provide adequate amounts of thyroid hormone for many years or may fail in early childhood. Affected children come to clinical attention because of a growing mass at the base of the tongue or in the midline of the neck, usually at the level of the hyoid. Occasionally, ectopia is associated with thyroglossal duct cysts. It may occur in siblings. Surgical removal of ectopic thyroid tissue from a euthyroid individual usually results in hypothyroidism, because most such patients have no other thyroid tissue. Newborn screening programs may detect these patients and obviate delayed diagnosis.

Thyrotropin Receptor–Blocking Antibody (TRBAb). TRBAb was formerly called thyroid-binding inhibitor immunoglobulin (TBII). An unusual cause of transitory congenital hypothyroidism is the transplacental passage of maternal antibodies that inhibit binding of TSH to its receptor in the neonate. The frequency is approximately 1 of 50,000–100,000 infants. It should be suspected whenever there is a history of maternal autoimmune thyroid disease, including Hashimoto thyroiditis, Graves disease, hypothyroidism on replacement therapy, or recurrent congenital hypothyroidism of a transient nature in subsequent siblings. In these situations, maternal levels of TRBAb should be measured during pregnancy. Affected infants and their mothers often also have thyrotropin receptor–stimulating antibodies (TRSAb) and antiperoxidase (formerly antimicrosomal) antibodies. Technetium pertechnetate and ^{125}I scans may fail to detect any thyroid tissue, mimicking thyroid agenesis, but after the condition remits, a normal thyroid gland is demonstrable after discontinuation of replacement treatment. The half-life of the antibody is 7.5 days, and remission of the hypothyroidism occurs in about 3 mo. Correct diagnosis of this cause of congenital hypothyroidism prevents protracted unnecessary treatment, alerts the clinician to possible recurrences in future pregnancies, and allows the offering of a favorable prognosis to the parents.

Defective Synthesis of Thyroxine. A variety of defects in the biosynthesis of thyroid hormone may result in congenital hypothyroidism; when the defect is incomplete, compensation occurs, and onset of hypothyroidism may be delayed for years. A goiter is almost always present, and the defect is detected in 1 in 30,000–50,000 live births in neonatal screening programs. These defects are genetically determined and are transmitted in an autosomal recessive manner.

DEFECT OF IODIDE TRANSPORT. This rare defect has been reported in nine related infants of the Hutterite sect, and about half the cases are from Japan. Consanguinity has occurred in about one third of the families. In the past, clinical hypothyroidism with or without a goiter often developed in the first few months of life, but in recent years, the condition has been detected in neonatal screening programs. In Japan, however, untreated patients develop goiter and hypothyroidism after 10 yr of age, perhaps because of the very high iodine content (often 19 mg/24 hr) of the Japanese diet.

The energy-dependent mechanisms for concentrating iodide are defective in the thyroid and in the salivary glands. In contrast to other defects of thyroid hormone synthesis, uptake of radioiodine and pertechnetate is low; a saliva:serum ratio of ^{123}I may be required to establish the diagnosis. This condition responds to treatment with large doses of potassium iodide, but treatment with thyroxine is preferable.

THYROID PEROXIDASE DEFECTS OF ORGANIFICATION AND COUPLING. This is the most common of the thyroxine synthetic defects. After iodide is trapped by the thyroid, it is rapidly oxidized to reactive iodine, which is then incorporated into tyrosine units. This process requires generation of H_2O_2, thyroid peroxidase, and hematin (an enzyme cofactor); defects can involve each of these components, and there is considerable clinical and biochemical heterogeneity. In the Dutch neonatal screening program 23 infants have been found with a complete organification defect (1 of 60,000), but its prevalence in other areas is unknown. A characteristic finding in all patients with this defect is a marked decrease in thyroid radioactivity when perchlorate or thiocyanate is administered 2 hr after administration of a test dose of radioiodine. In these patients, perchlorate discharges 40–90% of radioiodine compared with less than 10% in normal individuals. Several mutations in the *TPO* gene have been reported in children with congenital hypothyroidism. Patients with **Pendred syndrome**, a disorder comprising sensorineural deafness and goiter, also have a positive perchlorate discharge, but the precise biochemical defect in these people is unknown.

DEFECTS OF THYROGLOBULIN SYNTHESIS. This heterogeneous group of disorders, characterized by goiter, elevated TSH, low T_4 levels, and absent or low levels of thyroglobulin (Tg), has been reported in 89 patients. Studies in animal models with congenital goiter have disclosed point mutations of the gene for Tg in Afrikander cattle and in Dutch goitrous goats. Analogous molecular defects have been described in a few patients.

DEFECTS IN DEIODINATION. Monoiodotyrosine and diiodotyrosine released from thyroglobulin are normally deiodinated within the thyroid or in peripheral tissues by a deiodinase. The liberated iodine is reused in the synthesis of Tg. Patients with a deficiency of this enzyme develop severe iodine loss from the constant urinary excretion of nondeiodinated tyrosines, leading to hormonal deficiency and goiter. The deiodination defect may be limited to thyroid tissue only or to peripheral tissue only, or it may be universal.

Radioiodine. Hypothyroidism has been reported as a result of inadvertent administration of radioiodine during pregnancy for treatment of cancer of the thyroid or of hyperthyroidism. Although only a few affected infants have been reported, a 1976 mail survey of endocrinologists uncovered 237 women who had inadvertently received therapeutic doses of ^{131}I during the 1st trimester of pregnancy. The fetal thyroid is capable of trapping iodide by 70–75 days. Whenever radioiodine is administered to a woman of child-bearing age, a pregnancy test must be performed before a therapeutic dose of ^{131}I is given, regardless of the menstrual history or putative history of contraception. Administration of radioactive iodine to lactating women is also contraindicated because it is readily excreted in milk.

Thyrotropin Deficiency. Deficiency of TSH and hypothyroidism may occur in any of the conditions associated with developmental defects of the pituitary or hypothalamus (see Chapter 512). More often in these conditions, the deficiency of TSH is secondary to a deficiency of thyrotropin-releasing hormone (TRH). TSH-deficient hypothyroidism is found in 1 of 30,000–50,000 infants, but only 30–40% of these are detected by neonatal thyroid screening. The majority of affected infants have multiple pituitary deficiencies and present with hypoglycemia, persistent jaundice, and micropenis in association with septo-optic dysplasia, midline cleft lip, midface hypoplasia, and other midline facial anomalies.

Pit-1 mutations are a recessive cause of hypothyroidism secondary to TSH deficiency. Affected children also have deficiency of growth hormone and prolactin. Pit-1, a tissue transcription factor, is essential to differentiation, maintenance, and proliferation of somatotrophs, lactotrophs, and thyrotrophs. Examination of prolactin and TSH responses to TRH stimulation can detect these patients. Failure of the prolactin response to TRH should prompt examination of the Pit-1 gene.

A mutation in the TSH-receptor (TSHR) gene has been reported in three siblings with elevated levels of TSH and normal levels of T_4; two of them had been detected during neonatal screening. Despite persistent resistance to TSH through childhood, they remained euthyroid without treatment. Patients in three other reports of presumed TSHR mutations had severe hypothyroidism which required treatment. The disorder is inherited in an autosomal recessive fashion.

Isolated deficiency of TSH is a rare autosomal recessive disorder that has been reported in five sibships. DNA studies in two Japanese children and in three children in two related Greek families have revealed different point mutations in the TSH β-subunit gene.

Thyrotropin Hormone Unresponsiveness. Mild congenital hypothyroidism has been detected in newborn infants who subsequently proved to have type Ia pseudohypoparathyroidism. The molecular cause of resistance to TSH in these patients is the generalized impairment of cAMP activation caused by genetic deficiency of the α subunit of the guanine nucleotide regulatory protein, $G_{s\alpha}$ (see Chapter 526).

Only five instances of isolated TSH unresponsiveness have been detected. Serum levels of T_4 were low, those of TSH by radioimmunoassay and bioassay were elevated, and there was no response to exogenous TSH administration.

Thyroid Hormone Unresponsiveness. An increasing number of patients are being found who have resistance to the actions of endogenous and exogenous T_4 and T_3. Most patients have a goiter, and levels of T_4, T_3, free T_4, and free T_3 are elevated. These findings have often led to the erroneous diagnosis of Graves disease, although most affected patients are clinically euthyroid. The unresponsiveness may vary among tissues. There may be subtle clinical features of hypothyroidism, including mild mental retardation, growth retardation, and delayed skeletal maturation. One neurologic manifestation is an increased association of attention-deficit hyperactivity disorder (ADHD); the converse is not true, however, because individuals with ADHD do not have an increased risk of thyroid hormone resistance. It is presumed that these patients have incomplete resistance to thyroid hormone. TSH levels are diagnostic in that they are not suppressed as in Graves disease but instead are moderately elevated or normal but inappropriate for the levels of T_4 and T_3 when measured by a sensitive TSH assay. A TSH response to TRH occurs in these patients, unlike the situation in Graves disease. The failure of TSH suppression indicates that the resistance is generalized and affects the pituitary gland as well as peripheral tissues. The disorder is most often inherited in an autosomal dominant fashion. More than 40 distinct point mutations in the hormone-binding domain of the β-thyroid receptor have been identified. Different phenotypes do not correlate with genotypes. The same mutation has been observed in individuals with generalized or pituitary resistance, even in different individuals of the same family. Individuals heterozygous for a complete deletion of one *hTR*β allele are normal; a child homozygous for the receptor mutation showed unusually severe resistance. These cases support the dominant negative effect of mutant receptors, in which the mutant receptor protein inhibits normal receptor action in heterozygotes. Elevated levels of T_4 on neonatal thyroid screening should suggest the possibility of this diagnosis. No treatment is usually required unless growth and skeletal retardation are present.

Two infants of consanguineous matings are known to have an autosomal recessive form of thyroid resistance. These infants had manifestations of hypothyroidism early in life, and DNA studies revealed a major deletion of the β-thyroid receptor in one individual. The resistance appears to be more severe in this form of the entity.

On rare occasions, resistance to thyroid hormone may selectively affect the pituitary gland. Because the peripheral tissues are not resistant to thyroid hormones, the patient presents with a goiter and manifestations of hyperthyroidism. The laboratory findings are the same as those seen with generalized thyroid hormone resistance. This condition must be differentiated from a pituitary TSH-secreting tumor. At least one young child has been successfully treated with D-thyroxine therapy.

Other Causes of Hypothyroidism. Congenital hypothyroidism may result from fetal exposure to excessive iodides or antithyroid drugs. This condition is transitory and must not be mistaken for the other forms of hypothyroidism described. In the neonate, topical iodine-containing antiseptics used in nurseries and by surgeons can also cause transient congenital hypothyroidism, especially in low-birthweight infants, and can lead to abnormal results on neonatal screening tests. In older children, the usual sources of iodides are proprietary preparations used to treat asthma. In a few instances, the cause of hypothyroidism was amiodarone, an antiarrhythmic drug with a high iodine content. In most of these instances a goiter is present (see Chapter 522).

CLINICAL MANIFESTATIONS. The clinician is becoming increasingly dependent on neonatal screening tests for diagnosis of congenital hypothyroidism. Laboratory errors occur, however, and awareness of early symptoms and signs must be maintained. Congenital hypothyroidism is twice as common in girls as in boys. Before neonatal screening programs, congenital hypothyroidism was rarely recognized in the newborn since the signs and symptoms are usually not sufficiently developed. It can be suspected and the diagnosis established during the early weeks of life if the initial but less characteristic manifestations are recognized. Birthweight and length are normal, but head size may be slightly increased because of myxedema of the brain. Prolongation of physiologic icterus, caused by delayed maturation of glucuronide conjugation, may be the earliest sign. Feeding difficulties, especially sluggishness, lack of interest, somnolence, and choking spells during nursing, are often present during the 1st mo of life. Respiratory difficulties, due in part to the large tongue, include apneic episodes, noisy respirations, and nasal obstruction. Typical respiratory distress syndrome may also occur. Affected infants cry little, sleep much, have poor appetites, and are generally sluggish. There may be constipation that does not usually respond to treatment. The abdomen is large, and an umbilical hernia is usually present. The temperature is subnormal, often below 35° C (95° F), and the skin, particularly of the extremities, may be cold and mottled. Edema of the genitals and extremities may be present. The pulse is slow; heart murmurs, cardiomegaly, and asymptomatic pericardial effusion are common. Anemia is often present and is refractory to treatment with hematinics. Since symptoms appear gradually, the diagnosis is often delayed.

These manifestations progress; retardation of physical and mental development becomes greater during the following months, and by 3–6 mo of age, the clinical picture is fully developed (Fig. 520–1). When there is only a partial deficiency of thyroid hormone, the symptoms may be milder, the syndrome incomplete, and the onset delayed. Although breast milk contains significant amounts of thyroid hormones, particularly T_3, it is inadequate to protect the breast-fed infant with congenital hypothyroidism, and it has no effect on neonatal thyroid screening tests.

The child's growth is stunted, the extremities are short, and the head size is normal or even increased. The anterior and posterior fontanels are widely open; observation of this sign at birth may serve as an initial clue to the early recognition of congenital hypothyroidism. Only 3% of normal newborn infants have a posterior fontanel larger than 0.5 cm. The eyes appear far apart, and the bridge of the broad nose is depressed. The palpebral fissures are narrow and the eyelids swollen. The mouth is kept open, and the thick and broad tongue protrudes from it. Dentition is delayed. The neck is short and thick, and there may be deposits of fat above the clavicles and between the neck and shoulders. The hands are broad and the fingers short. The skin is dry and scaly, and there is little perspiration. Myxedema is manifest, particularly in the skin of the eyelids, of the back of the hands, and of the external genitalia. Carotenemia may cause a yellow discoloration of the skin, but the scleras remain white. The scalp is thickened, and the hair is coarse, brittle, and scanty. The hairline reaches far down on the forehead, which usually appears wrinkled, especially when the infant cries.

Development is usually retarded. Hypothyroid infants appear lethargic and are late in learning to sit and stand. The voice is hoarse, and they do not learn to talk. The degree of physical and mental retardation increases with age. Sexual maturation may be delayed or may not take place at all.

The muscles are usually hypotonic, but in rare instances generalized muscular hypertrophy occurs *(Kocher-Debré-Sémélaigne syndrome)*. Affected children may have an athletic appearance due to pseudohypertrophy, particularly in the calf muscles. Its pathogenesis is unknown; nonspecific histochemical and ultrastructural changes seen on muscle biopsy return to normal with treatment. Boys are more prone to develop the syndrome, which has been observed in siblings born to a consanguineous mating. Affected patients have hypothyroidism of longer duration and severity.

LABORATORY DATA. Most newborn screening programs in North America measure levels of T_4, supplemented by measurement of TSH when T_4 is low. This approach identifies infants with primary hypothyroidism, those with low thyroxine-binding globulin (TBG) and some with hypothalamic or pituitary hypothyroidism, and infants with hyperthyroxinemia. European and Japanese neonatal screening programs are based on a primary measurement of TSH; this approach misses infants with hyperthyroxinemia, low TBG, and hypothalamic or pituitary hypothyroidism but may detect infants with compensated hypothyroidism (normal T_4, elevated TSH). With any of these assays, special care should be given to the normal range of values for age of the patient, particularly in the first weeks of life. Regardless of the approach used for screening, some infants escape detection because of technical or human errors; clinicians must maintain their vigilance for clinical manifestations of hypothyroidism.

Serum levels of T_4 are low; serum levels of T_3 may be normal and are not helpful in the diagnosis. If the defect is primarily in the thyroid, levels of TSH are elevated, often to above 100 μU/mL. Serum levels of prolactin are elevated, correlating with those of TSH. Serum levels of Tg are usually low in infants with thyroid dysgenesis or defects of Tg synthesis or secretion. Undetectable levels of Tg usually indicate thyroid aplasia.

Special attention should be paid to monoamniotic twins, because in at least four cases neonatal screening failed to detect

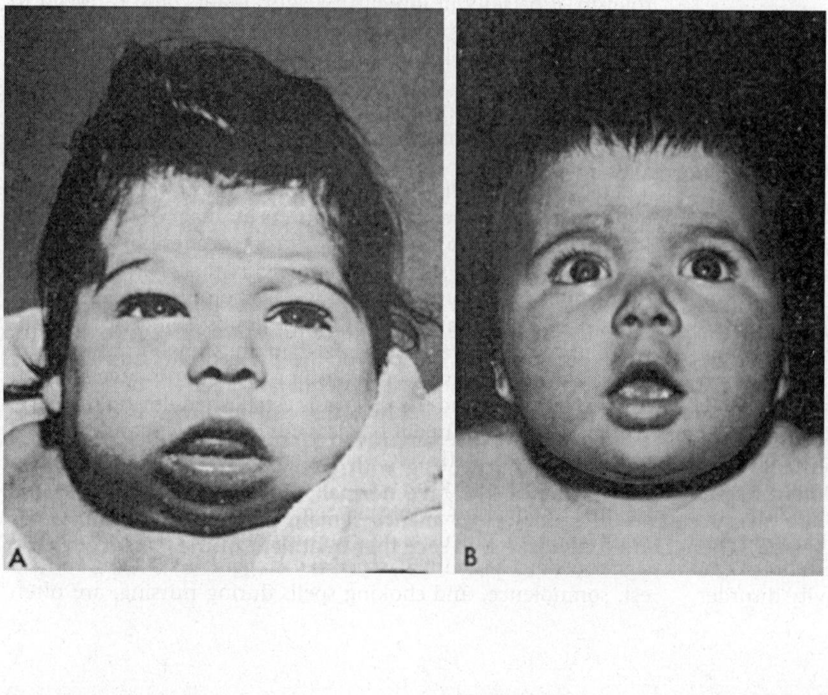

Figure 520–1. Congenital hypothyroidism in an infant 6 mo of age. The infant fed poorly in the neonatal period and was constipated. She had a persistent nasal discharge and a large tongue; she was very lethargic; and she had no social smile and no head control. *A*, Notice the puffy face, dull expression, and hirsute forehead. Tests revealed a negligible uptake of radioiodine. Osseous development was that of a newborn. *B*, Four mo after treatment, notice the decreased puffiness of the face, the decreased hirsutism of the forehead, and the alert appearance.

the discordant twin with hypothyroidism, and the diagnosis was not made until the infants were 4–5 mo of age. Apparently, transfusion of euthyroid blood from the unaffected twin normalized the serum level of T_4 and TSH in the affected twin at the initial screening.

Retardation of osseous development can be shown roentgenographically at birth in about 60% of congenitally hypothyroid infants and indicates some deprivation of thyroid hormone during intrauterine life. For example, the distal femoral epiphysis, normally present at birth, is often absent (Fig. 520–2*A*). In untreated patients, the discrepancy between chronological age and osseous development increases. The epiphyses often have multiple foci of ossification (epiphyseal dysgenesis, Fig. 520–2*B*); deformity ("breaking") of the 12th thoracic or 1st or 2nd lumbar vertebra is common. Roentgenograms of the skull show large fontanels and wide sutures; intersutural (wormian) bones are common. The sella turcica is often enlarged and round; in rare instances there may be erosion and thinning. Delays in formation and eruption of teeth may occur. Cardiac enlargement or pericardial effusion may be present.

Scintigraphy can help to pinpoint the underlying cause in infants with congenital hypothyroidism, but treatment should not be unduly delayed for this study. ^{125}I-sodium iodide is superior to ^{99m}Tc-sodium pertechnetate for this purpose. Neither thyroid ultrasound examination nor serum levels of Tg are reliable alternatives to radionuclide scanning. Demonstration of ectopic thyroid tissue is diagnostic of thyroid dysgenesis and establishes the need for lifelong treatment with T_4. Failure to demonstrate any thyroid tissue suggests thyroid aplasia but also occurs in neonates with TRBAb and in infants with the iodide-trapping defect. A normally situated thyroid gland with a normal or avid uptake of radionuclide indicates a defect in thyroid hormone biosynthesis. Patients with goitrous hypothyroidism may require extensive evaluation, including radioiodine studies, perchlorate discharge tests, kinetic studies, chromatography, and studies of thyroid tissue, if the biochemical nature of the defect is to be determined.

The electrocardiogram may show low-voltage P and T waves with diminished amplitude of QRS complexes and suggest poor left ventricular function and pericardial effusion. The electroencephalogram frequently shows low voltage. In children older than 2 yr of age, the serum cholesterol level is usually elevated.

PROGNOSIS. With the advent of neonatal screening programs for detection of congenital hypothyroidism, the prognosis for affected infants has improved dramatically. Early diagnosis and adequate treatment from the first weeks of life result in normal linear growth and intelligence comparable with that of unaffected siblings. Some screening programs report that the most severely affected infants, as judged by the lowest T_4 levels and retarded skeletal maturation, have slightly reduced IQs and other neuropsychologic sequelae. Without treatment, affected infants become mentally deficient dwarfs. Thyroid hormone is critical for normal cerebral development in the early postnatal months; biochemical diagnosis must be made soon after birth, and effective treatment must be initiated promptly to prevent irreversible brain damage. Delay in diagnosis, inadequate treatment, and poor compliance result in variable degrees of brain damage. When onset of hypothyroidism occurs after 2 yr of age, the outlook for normal development is much better even if diagnosis and treatment have been delayed, indicating how much more important thyroid hormone is to the rapidly growing brain of the infant.

TREATMENT. Sodium-L-thyroxine given orally is the treatment of choice. Because 80% of circulating T_3 is formed by monodeiodination of T_4, serum levels of T_4 and T_3 in treated infants return to normal. This is also true in the brain, where 80% of required T_3 is produced locally from T_4. In neonates, the dose is 10–15 μg/kg (37.5 *or* 50 μg/24 hr). Levels of T_4 and TSH should be monitored and maintained in the normal range. Children with hypothyroidism require about 4 μg/kg/24 hr, and adults require only 2 μg/kg/24 hr.

Later, confirmation of the diagnosis may be necessary for some infants to rule out the possibility of transient hypothyroidism. This is unnecessary in infants with proven thyroid ectopia or in those who manifest elevated levels of TSH after 6–12 mo of therapy owing to poor compliance or an inadequate dose of T_4. Discontinuation of therapy at about 3 yr of age for 3–4 wk results in a marked increase in TSH levels in children with permanent hypothyroidism.

The only untoward effects of sodium-L-thyroxine are related to its dose. An occasional older child (8–13 yr) with acquired hypothyroidism may develop pseudotumor cerebri within the first 4 mo of treatment. In older children, after catch-up growth is complete, the growth rate provides an excellent index of the adequacy of therapy. Parents should be fore-

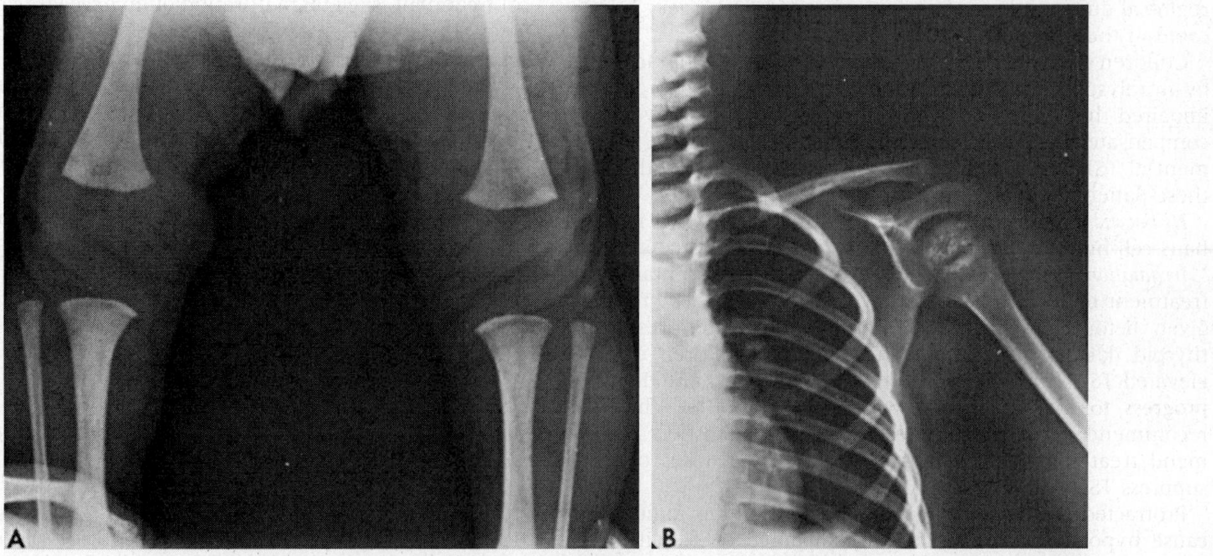

Figure 520–2. Congenital hypothyroidism. *A*, Absence of distal femoral epiphysis in a 3-mo-old infant who was born at term. This is evidence for the onset of the hypothyroid state during fetal life. *B*, Epiphyseal dysgenesis in the head of the humerus in a 9-yr-old girl who had been inadequately treated with thyroid hormone.

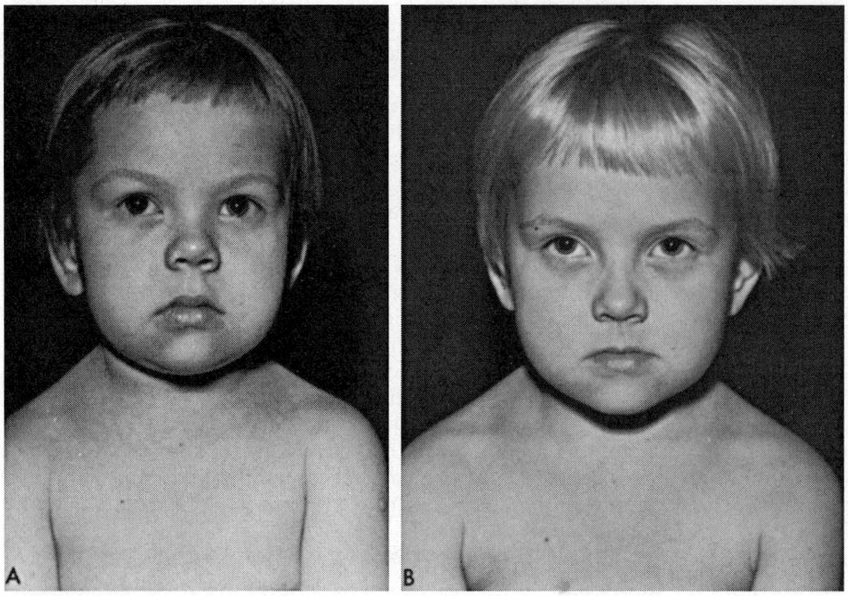

Figure 520–3. *A*, Acquired hypothyroidism in a girl 6 yr of age. She was treated with a wide variety of hematinics for refractory anemia for 3 yr. She had almost complete cessation of growth, constipation, and sluggishness for 3 yr. The height age was 3 yr; the bone age was 4 yr. She had a sallow complexion and immature facies with a poorly developed nasal bridge. Serum cholesterol, 501 mg/dL; radioiodine uptake, 7% at 24 hr; PBI, 2.8 μg/dL. *B*, After therapy for 18 mo, notice the nasal development, the increased luster and decreased pigmentation of hair, and the maturation of face. The height age was 5.5 yr; the bone age was 7 yr. There was a decided improvement in her general condition. Menarche occurred at 14 yr. The ultimate height was 155 cm (61 in). She graduated from high school. The disorder was well controlled with sodium-L-thyroxine daily.

warned about changes in behavior and activity expected with therapy, and special attention must be given to any developmental or neurologic deficits.

ACQUIRED HYPOTHYROIDISM

ETIOLOGY. The most common cause of acquired hypothyroidism is lymphocytic thyroiditis (see Chapter 521). Although typically seen in adolescence, it occurs as early as in the first 2 yr of life. Some patients with congenital thyroid dysgenesis or with incomplete genetic defects in thyroid hormone synthesis may not develop clinical manifestations until childhood and appear to have acquired hypothyroidism; most patients with these conditions are now detected in newborn screening programs. Subtotal thyroidectomy for thyrotoxicosis or cancer may result in hypothyroidism, as may removal of ectopic thyroid tissue. For example, *lingual thyroid, subhyoid median thyroid,* or thyroid tissue in a *thyroglossal duct cyst* usually constitutes the only source of thyroid hormone, and excision results in hypothyroidism. Because subhyoid glands usually mimic thyroglossal duct cysts, a radionuclide scan before surgery is indicated in these patients.

Children with *nephropathic cystinosis,* a disorder characterized by intralysosomal storage of cystine in body tissues, develop impaired thyroid function. Hypothyroidism may be overt, but compensated forms are more common, and periodic assessment of TSH levels is indicated. By 13 yr of age, two thirds of these patients require thyroxine replacement.

Histiocytic infiltration of the thyroid in children with Langerhans cell histiocytoses may result in hypothyroidism.

Irradiation to the area of the thyroid that is incidental to the treatment of Hodgkin disease or other malignancies or that is given before bone marrow transplantation often results in thyroid damage. About one third of such children develop elevated TSH levels within a year after therapy, and 15–20% progress to hypothyroidism within 5–7 yr. Some clinicians recommend periodic TSH measurements, but others recommend treatment of all exposed patients with doses of T_4 to suppress TSH (see Chapter 524).

Protracted ingestion of medications containing iodides can cause hypothyroidism, usually accompanied by a goiter (see Chapter 522). Amiodarone, a drug used for cardiac arrhythmias, consisting of 37% by weight of iodine, causes hypothyroidism in about 20% of treated children. It affects thyroid function directly by its high iodine content as well as by inhibition of 5′-deiodinase, which converts T_4 to T_3. Children treated with this drug should have serial measurements of T_4, T_3, and TSH.

CLINICAL MANIFESTATIONS. Deceleration of growth is usually the first clinical manifestation, but this sign often goes unrecognized (Fig. 520–3). Myxedematous changes of the skin, constipation, cold intolerance, decreased energy, and increased need for sleep develop insidiously. Surprisingly, school work and grades usually do not suffer, even in severely hypothyroid children. Osseous maturation is delayed, often strikingly, which is an indication of the duration of the hypothyroidism.

Some children present with headaches, visual problems, precocious puberty, or galactorrhea. These children usually have hyperplastic enlargement of the pituitary gland, often with suprasellar extension, after longstanding hypothyroidism; this condition may be mistaken for a pituitary tumor (see Chapter 512).

All of these changes return to normal with adequate replacement of T_4, but in children with longstanding hypothyroidism, catch-up growth may be incomplete. During the first 18 mo of treatment, skeletal maturation often exceeds expected linear growth, resulting in a loss of about 7 cm of predicted adult height. The cause for this is unknown.

Diagnostic studies and treatment are the same as those described for congenital hypothyroidism. Measurement of antithyroglobulin and antiperoxidase (formerly antimicrosomal) antibodies may pinpoint autoimmune thyroiditis as the cause. During the 1st yr of treatment, deterioration of school work, poor sleeping habits, restlessness, short attention span, and behavioral problems may ensue, but these are transient; forewarning families about these manifestations enhances appropriate management.

Adams A, Matthews C, Collingwood TH, et al: Genetic analysis of 29 kindreds with generalized and pituitary resistance to thyroid hormone. J Clin Invest 94:506, 1994.

American Academy of Pediatrics: Newborn screening for congenital hypothyroidism: Recommended guidelines. Pediatrics 91:1203, 1993.

Bogner U, Gruters A, Sigle B, et al: Cytotoxic antibodies in congenital hypothyroidism. J Clin Endocrinol Metab 68:671, 1989.

Brent GA: The molecular basis of thyroid hormone action. 331:847, 1994.

Brown RS, Bellisario RL, Mitchell E, et al: Detection of thyrotropin binding inhibitory activity in neonatal blood spots. J Clin Endocrinol Metab 77:1005, 1993.

Burrow GN, Dussault JH (eds): Neonatal Thyroid Screening. New York, Raven Press, 1980.

Codaocioni JL, Cargyon P, Miche-Bechet M, et al: Congenital hypothyroidism

associated with thyrotropin unresponsiveness and thyroid cell membrane alterations. J Clin Endocrinol Metab 50:932, 1980.
Cosman BC, Schullmger JN, Bell JJ, et al: Hypothyroidism caused by topical povidone-iodine in a newborn with omphalocele. J Pediatr Surg 23:356, 1988.
Costigan DC, Holland FJ, Daneman D, et al: Amiodarone therapy effects on childhood thyroid function. Pediatrics 77:703, 1986.
Cutler AT, Benezra-Obeiter R, Brink SJ: Thyroid function in young children with Down syndrome. Am J Dis Child 140:479, 1986.
Dacou-Voutetakis C, Felquate DM, Drakopoulou M, et al: Familial hypothyroidism by a nonsense mutation in the thyroid-stimulating hormone β-subunit gene. Am J Hum Genet 46:988, 1990.
Fisher DA: Management of congenital hypothyroidism. J Clin Endocrinol Metab 72:523, 1991.
Germak JA, Foley TP Jr: Longitudinal assessment of L-thyroxine therapy for congenital hypothyroidism. J Pediatr 117:211, 1990.
Glorieux J, Dussault J, Van Vliet G: Intellectual development at age 12 years of children with congenital hypothyroidism diagnosed by newborn screening. J Pediatr 121:581, 1992.
Grant DB, Fuggle P, Tokar S, Smith I: Psychomotor development in infants with congenital hypothyroidism diagnosed by newborn screening. Acta Med Aust 19:54, 1992.
Gushurst CA, Muehler JA, Green JA, et al: Breast milk iodide: Reassessment in the 1980's. Pediatrics 73:354, 1984.
Hanna CE, Krainz PL, Skeels MR, et al: Detection of congenital hypopituitary hypothyroidism: Ten-year experience in The Northwest Regional Screening Program. J Pediatr 109:959, 1986.
Hauser P, Zametkin AJ, Martinez P, et al: Attention deficit-hyperactivity disorder in people with generalized resistance to thyroid hormone. N Engl J Med 328:997, 1993.
Hopwood NJ, Sauder SE, Shapiro B, et al: Familial partial peripheral and pituitary resistance to thyroid hormone: A frequently missed diagnosis. Pediatrics 78:1114, 1986.
Kleinhaus N, Faber J, Kahana L, et al: Euthyroid hyperthyroxinemia due to a generalized 5′-deiodinase defect. J Clin Endocrinol Metab 66:684, 1988.
LaFranchi SH, Hanna CE, Krainz PL, et al: Screening for congenital hypothyroidism with specimen collection at two time periods: Results of the Northwest Regional Screening Program. Pediatrics 76:734, 1985.
Levine MA, Jap TS, Hung W: Infantile hypothyroidism in two sibs: An unusual presentation of pseudohypoparathyroidism type Ia. J Pediatr 107:919, 1985.
Mandel SH, Hanna CE, Boston BA, et al: Thyroxine binding globulin deficiency detected by newborn screening. J Pediatr 122:227, 1993.
Muir A, Daneman D, Daneman A, et al: Thyroid scanning, ultrasound, and serum thyroglobulin in determining the origin of congenital hypothyroidism. Am J Dis Child 142:214, 1988.
New England Congenital Hypothyroidism Collaborative: Correlation of cognitive test scores and adequacy of treatment in adolescents with congenital hypothyroidism. J Pediatr 124:383, 1994.
Parks JS, Kinoshita EI, Pfaffle RW: Pit-1 and hypopituitarism. Trends Endocrinol Metab 4:81, 1993.
Porterfield SP, Hendrich CE: The role of thyroid hormones in prenatal and neonatal neurological development—current perspectives. Endocr Rev 14:94, 1993.
Refetoff S, Weiss RE, Usala SJ: The syndromes of resistance to thyroid hormones. Endocr Rev 14:348, 1993.
Rivkees SA, Bode HH, Crawford JD: Long-term growth in juvenile acquired hypothyroidism: The failure to achieve normal adult stature. N Engl J Med 318:519, 1988.
Rovet JF, Ehrlich RM, Sorbara DL: Neurodevelopment in infants and preschool children with congenital hypothyroidism: Etiological and treatment factors affecting outcome. J Pediatr Psychol 17:187, 1992.
Smith DW, Klein AM, Henderson JR, et al: Congenital hypothyroidism—signs and symptoms in the newborn period. J Pediatr 87:958, 1975.
Sunthurnepaurkul T, Gottschalk M, Hayashi Y, Refetoff S: Brief report: Resistance to thyrotropin caused by mutations in the thyrotropin-receptor gene. N Engl J Med 332:155, 1995.
Thorpe-Beeston JG, Nicolaides KH, Fetton CV, et al: Maturation of the secretion of thyroid hormone and thyroid-stimulating hormone in the fetus. N Engl J Med 324:532, 1991.
Toft AD: Drug therapy: Thyroxine therapy. N Engl J Med 331:174, 1994.
van der Gaag RD, Drexhage HA, Dussault JH: Role of maternal immunoglobulin blocking TSH-induced thyroid growth in sporadic forms of congenital hypothyroidism. Lancet 1:246, 1985.
VanDop C, Conte FA, Koch TK, et al: Pseudotumor cerebri associated with initiation of levothyroxine therapy for juvenile hypothyroidism. N Engl J Med 308:1076, 1983.
Vulsma T, Gons MH, deVijlder JJM: Maternal-fetal transfer of thyroxine in congenital hypothyroidism due to a total organification defect or thyroid agenesis. N Engl J Med 321:13, 1989.

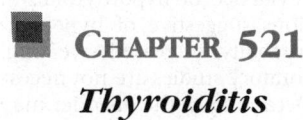

CHAPTER 521
Thyroiditis

Angelo M. DiGeorge and Stephen LaFranchi

LYMPHOCYTIC THYROIDITIS
(Hashimoto Thyroiditis; Autoimmune Thyroiditis)

Lymphocytic thyroiditis is the most common cause of thyroid disease in children and adolescents and accounts for many of the enlarged thyroids formerly designated "adolescent" or "simple" goiter. It is also the most common cause of acquired hypothyroidism, with or without goiter. Its incidence may be as high as 1% among school children.

ETIOLOGY. This is a typical organ-specific autoimmune disease. The condition is characterized histologically by lymphocytic infiltration of the thyroid. Early in the course of the disease, there may be only hyperplasia; this is followed by infiltration of lymphocytes and plasma cells between the follicles and by atrophy of the follicles. Lymphoid follicle formation with germinal centers is almost always present; the degree of atrophy and of fibrosis of the follicles varies from mild to moderate.

Intrathyroidal lymphocyte subsets differ from those in blood. About 60% of infiltrating lymphoid cells are T cells, and about 30% express B-cell markers; the T-cell population is represented by helper ($CD4^+$) and cytotoxic ($CD8^+$) cells. Participation of cellular events in the pathogenesis is clear. Certain HLA haplotypes (HLA-DR4, HLA-DR5) are associated with an increased risk of goiter and thyroiditis, and others (HLA-DR3) are associated with the atrophic variant of thyroiditis. Much remains to be discovered about the disturbance in immunoregulation and how it interacts with genetic predisposition and environmental factors in the pathogenesis of autoimmune thyroid disease.

A variety of different thyroid antigen autoantibodies are also involved in the process. Thyroid antiperoxidase antibodies (TPOAb), formerly called antimicrosomol antibodies, are demonstrable in the sera of 90% of children with lymphocytic thyroiditis and in many patients with Graves disease. For many years TPOAb has been considered nonpathogenic, but evidence now shows that TPOAb inhibit enzyme activity and stimulate natural killer cell cytotoxicity. With the molecular cloning of the *TPO* gene, a new generation of ultrasensitive tests for the measurement of these antibodies is under development.

Antithyroglobulin antibodies occur in a smaller percentage of affected children but are much more common in adults. Thyrotropin receptor–blocking antibodies (TRBAb) are frequently present, especially in patients with hypothyroidism, and it is now believed they are related to the development of hypothyroidism and thyroid atrophy in patients with autoimmune thyroiditis.

CLINICAL MANIFESTATIONS. The disorder is 4–7 times more frequent in girls than in boys. It may occur during the first 3 yr of life but becomes sharply more common after 6 yr of age and reaches a peak incidence during adolescence. The most common clinical manifestations are growth retardation and goiter. The goiter may appear insidiously and may be small or large. In most patients, the thyroid is diffusely enlarged, firm, and nontender. In about one third of the patients, the gland is lobular and may seem to be nodular. Most of the affected children are clinically euthyroid and asymptomatic; some may have symptoms of pressure in the neck. Some children have clinical signs of hypothyroidism, but others who appear clinically euthyroid have laboratory evidence of hypothyroidism. A few children have manifestations suggestive of hyperthyroidism, such as nervousness, irritability, increased sweating, or hyperactivity, but results of laboratory studies are not necessarily those of hyperthyroidism. Occasionally, the disorder may coexist with Graves disease. Ophthalmopathy may occur in lymphocytic thyroiditis in the absence of Graves disease.

The clinical course is variable. The goiter may become smaller or may disappear spontaneously, or it may persist unchanged for years while the patient remains euthyroid. A significant percentage of patients who are euthyroid initially exhibit hypothyroidism gradually within months or years; thyroiditis is the cause of most cases of nongoitrous (atrophic) hypothyroidism.

Familial clusters of lymphocytic thyroiditis are common; the incidence in siblings or parents of affected children may be as high as 25%. Autoantibodies to thyroglobulin (Tg) and human thyroid peroxidase (hTPO) in these families appear to be inherited in an autosomal dominant fashion, with reduced penetrance in males. The concurrence within families of patients with lymphocytic thyroiditis, "idiopathic" hypothyroidism, and Graves disease provides cogent evidence for a basic relationship among these three conditions. The disorder has been associated with many of the other autoimmune disorders more often than would be expected by chance alone. Autoimmune thyroiditis occurs in 10% of patients with type I polyglandular autoimmune syndrome, which consists of hypoparathyroidism, Addison disease, and mucocutaneous candidiasis. The association of Addison disease with insulin-dependent diabetes mellitus or autoimmune thyroid disease or both is known as *Schmidt syndrome* or *type II polyglandular autoimmune disease*. Autoimmune thyroid disease also tends to be associated with pernicious anemia, vitiligo, or alopecia. TPOAb are found in approximately 20% of white and 4% of black children with diabetes mellitus. Autoimmune thyroid disease has an increased incidence in children with congenital rubella. Lymphocytic thyroiditis is also associated with certain chromosomal aberrations, particularly Turner syndrome and Down syndrome. The pathogenetic mechanisms for these associations are not known.

LABORATORY DATA. The definitive diagnosis can be established by biopsy of the thyroid, but this procedure is rarely indicated for clinical purposes alone. Thyroid function tests are often normal, although the level of thyroid-stimulating hormone (TSH) may be slightly or even moderately elevated in some euthyroid individuals. With progressive thyroid failure, a decrease in the levels of thyroxine (T_4) is followed by a decrease in levels of triiodothyronine (T_3) and progressive increases in levels of TSH. The fact that many patients with lymphocytic thyroiditis do not have elevated levels of TSH indicates that the goiter may be caused by the lymphocytic infiltrations or by thyroid growth–stimulating immunoglobulins. In 50% of patients, thyroid scans reveal irregular and patchy distribution of the radioisotope, and in about 60% or more, the administration of perchlorate results in a greater than 10% discharge of iodide from the thyroid gland. Thyroid ultrasonography shows scattered hypoechogenicity in most patients. Most patients with lymphocytic thyroiditis have serum antibody titers to thyroid peroxidase, but the antithyroglobulin test for thyroid antibodies is positive in fewer than 50%. When both tests are used, approximately 95% of patients with thyroid autoimmunity are detected. In general, levels in children and adolescents are lower than those in adults with lymphocytic thyroiditis, and repeated measurements are indicated in questionable instances because titers may increase later in the course of the disease.

Antithyroid antibodies may be found also in almost one half the siblings of affected patients and in a significant percentage of the mothers of children with Down syndrome or Turner syndrome without demonstrable thyroid disease. They are also found in 20% of children with diabetes mellitus and in 23% of children with the congenital rubella syndrome.

TREATMENT. If there is evidence of hypothyroidism, replacement treatment with sodium-L-thyroxine (50–150 μg daily) is indicated. The goiter usually shows some decrease in size but may persist for years. Antibody levels fluctuate in both treated and untreated patients and persist for years. Because the disease may be self-limited in some instances, the need for continued therapy requires periodic re-evaluation. Untreated patients should also be periodically checked. Prominent nodules that persist despite suppressive therapy should be examined histologically because thyroid cancer has occurred in patients with lymphocytic thyroiditis.

OTHER CAUSES OF THYROIDITIS

Specific conditions such as tuberculosis, sarcoidosis, mumps, and cat-scratch disease are rare causes of thyroiditis.

Acute suppurative thyroiditis is uncommon; it is usually preceded by a respiratory infection. The left lower lobe is affected predominantly. Abscess formation may occur. Anaerobic organisms, with or without aerobes, are the most common organisms; *Eikenella corrodens* has been reported. Recurrent episodes or the detection of a mixed bacterial flora suggests that the infection arises from a thyroglossal duct remnant or, more often, from a piriform sinus fistula. Exquisite tenderness of the gland, swelling, erythema, dysphagia, and limitation of head motion are characteristic findings. Systemic manifestations are often absent, and leukocytosis is present. Scintigrams of the thyroid often reveal decreased uptake in the affected areas, and ultrasonography may show a complex echogenic mass. Thyroid function is usually normal, but thyrotoxicosis due to escape of thyroid hormone has been encountered in a child with suppurative thyroiditis resulting from *Aspergillus*. When suppuration occurs, incision and drainage and administration of antibiotics are indicated. After the infection subsides, a barium esophagram is indicated to search for a fistula tract; if one is found, exteriorization is indicated.

Subacute nonsuppurative thyroiditis (deQuervain disease) is rare in children. It is thought to have a viral cause and remits spontaneously. The disorder becomes manifest by a vague tenderness over the thyroid and low-grade fever or by severe pain in the region of the thyroid and systemic manifestations with chills and high fever. Inflammation results in leakage of preformed thyroid hormone from the gland into the circulation. Serum levels of T_4 and T_3 are elevated, and mild symptoms of hyperthyroidism may be present, but radioiodine uptake is depressed. The erythrocyte sedimentation rate is increased. The course is variable, usually passing through a euthyroid to a hypothyroid phase; remission usually occurs in several months. Occasionally, this condition is superimposed on lymphocytic thyroiditis.

Boyages SC, Halpern JP, Maberly GF, et al: Possible role for thyroid autoimmunity. Lancet 2:529, 1989.

Chiovato L, Vitti P, Santini F, et al: Incidence of antibodies blocking thyrotropin effect in vitro in patients with euthyroid or hypothyroid autoimmune thyroiditis. J Clin Endocrinol Metab 71:40, 1990.

Foley TP Jr, Abbassi V, Copeland KC, et al: Brief report: Hypothyroidism caused by chronic autoimmune thyroiditis in very young infants. N Engl J Med 330:466, 1993.

Gutekunst R, Hafermann W, Mansky T, Scriba PC: Ultrasonography related to clinical and laboratory findings in lymphocytic thyroiditis. Acta Endocrinol (Copenh) 121:129, 1989.

Lautenschlager I, Maenpaa J, Nyberg M, et al: Thyroid infiltrating cells in juvenile autoimmune thyroiditis: A follow-up of 1 year. Clin Immunol Immunopathol 49:143, 1988.

Loeb PB, Drash AL, Kenny FM: Prevalence of low titer and "negative" antithyroglobulin antibodies in biopsy-proven juvenile Hashimoto's thyroiditis. J Pediatr 82:17, 1973.

Mangklabruks A, Cox N, DeGroot LJ: Genetic factors in autoimmune thyroid disease analyzed by restriction fragment length polymorphisms of candidate genes. J Clin Endocrinol Metab 73:236, 1991.

Phillips D, McLachlan S, Stephenson A, et al: Autosomal dominant transmission of autoantibodies to thyroglobulin and thyroid peroxidase. J Clin Endocrinol Metab 70:742, 1990.
Rallison ML, Dobyns BM, Keating FR, et al: Occurrence and natural history of chronic lymphocytic thyroiditis in childhood. J Pediatr 86:675, 1975.
Rallison ML, Dobyns BM, Meikle AW, et al: Natural history of thyroid abnormalities: Prevalence, incidence, and regression of thyroid diseases in adolescents and young adults. Am J Med 91:363, 1991.
Riley WJ, Maclaren NK, Lezotte DC, et al: Thyroid autoimmunity in insulin-dependent diabetes mellitus. The case for routine screening. J Pediatr 98:350, 1981.
Yokoyama N, Taurog A, Klee GG: Thyroid peroxidase and thyroid microsomal antibodies. J Clin Endocrinol Metab 68:766, 1989.

CHAPTER 522 *Goiter*

Angelo M. DiGeorge and Stephen LaFranchi

A goiter is an enlargement of the thyroid gland. Persons with enlarged thyroids may have normal function of the gland *(euthyroidism)*, thyroid deficiency *(hypothyroidism)*, or overproduction of the hormones *(hyperthyroidism)*. Goiter may be congenital or acquired, endemic or sporadic.

The goiter often results from increased pituitary secretion of thyrotropic hormone in response to decreased circulating levels of thyroid hormones. Thyroid enlargement may also result from infiltrative processes that may be inflammatory or neoplastic. Goiter in patients with thyrotoxicosis is caused by thyrotropin receptor–stimulating antibodies (TRSAb).

522.1 Congenital Goiter

Congenital goiter is usually sporadic and may result from the administration of antithyroid drugs or iodides during pregnancy for the treatment of thyrotoxicosis. Goitrogenic drugs and iodides cross the placenta and at high doses may interfere with synthesis of thyroid hormone, resulting in goiter and hypothyroidism in the fetus. The concomitant administration of thyroid hormone with the goitrogen does not prevent this effect, because insufficient amounts of thyroxine (T_4) cross the placenta. Iodides are included in many proprietary preparations used to treat asthma; these preparations must be avoided during pregnancy, because they have often been a cause of unexpected congenital goiter. Amiodarone, an antiarrhythmic drug with a 37% iodine content, has also caused congenital goiter with hypothyroidism. Even when the infant is clinically euthyroid, there may be retardation of osseous maturation, low levels of T_4, and elevated levels of thyroid-stimulating hormone (TSH). Because these effects can occur when the mother takes only 100–200 mg of propylthiouracil/24 hr, all such infants should undergo thyroid studies at birth. Administration of thyroid hormone to affected infants may be indicated to treat clinical hypothyroidism, to hasten the disappearance of the goiter, and to prevent brain damage. Because the condition is rarely permanent, thyroid hormone may be safely discontinued after several months.

Enlargement of the thyroid at birth may occasionally be sufficient to cause respiratory distress that interferes with nursing and may even cause death. The head may be maintained in extreme hyperextension. When respiratory obstruction is severe, partial thyroidectomy rather than tracheostomy is indicated (Fig. 522–1).

Goiter is almost always present in the congenitally hyperthyroid infant. These goiters are usually not large; the infant manifests clinical symptoms of hyperthyroidism, and the mother often has a history of Graves disease (see Chapter 523.1).

When no causative factor is identifiable, a defect in synthesis of thyroid hormone should be suspected. One of 30,000–50,000 live births is found in neonatal screening programs to have such a defect. Study of this group of infants is complex. If the infant is hypothyroid, it is advisable to treat immediately with thyroid hormone and to postpone more detailed studies for later in life. Because these defects are transmitted by recessive genes, a precise diagnosis is important for genetic counseling. Monitoring subsequent pregnancies with ultrasound can be useful in detecting fetal goiters (see Chapter 520).

Iodine deficiency as a cause of congenital goiters has become rare but persists in isolated endemic areas. More important is the recent recognition that severe iodine deficiency early in pregnancy may cause neurologic damage during fetal development even in the absence of goiter. The iodine deficiency may result in maternal and fetal hypothyroidism, preventing the partially protective transfer of maternal thyroid hormones.

When the "goiter" is lobulated, asymmetric, firm, or large to an unusual degree, a teratoma within or in the vicinity of the thyroid must be considered in the differential diagnosis (see Chapter 456).

522.2 Endemic Goiter and Cretinism

The association between dietary deficiency of iodine and the prevalence of goiter or cretinism has been recognized for over half a century. A moderate deficiency of iodine can be overcome by increased efficiency in the synthesis of thyroid hormone. Iodine liberated in the tissues is returned rapidly to the gland, which resynthesizes the hormone at a higher rate than normal. This increased activity is achieved by compensatory hypertrophy and hyperplasia, which satisfy the demands of the tissues for thyroid hormone. In geographic areas where deficiency of iodine is severe, decompensation and hypothyroidism may result. It is estimated that 800 million people in developing countries live in areas of iodine deficiency.

Sea water is rich in iodine, and the iodine content of fish and shellfish is also high. Endemic goiter is rare therefore in populations living along the sea. Iodine is deficient in the water and native foods in the Pacific West and the Great Lakes areas of the United States. Deficiency of dietary iodine is even greater in certain Alpine valleys, the Himalayas, the Andes, the Congo, and the highlands of Papua New Guinea. In areas such as the United States, where iodine is provided in foods from other areas and in iodized salt, endemic goiter has disappeared. Iodized salt in the United States contains potassium iodide (100 μg/g) and provides excellent prophylaxis. Further iodine intake in the United States is contributed by iodates used in baking, iodine-containing coloring agents, and iodine-containing disinfectants used in the dairy industry. The recommended daily allowance of iodine for infants is 40–50 μg/24 hr; this amount is exceeded 4-fold in breast-fed infants and 10-fold in infants fed cow's milk in the United States.

CLINICAL MANIFESTATIONS. If the deficiency of iodine is mild, thyroid enlargement does not become noticeable except when there is increased demand for the hormone during periods of rapid growth, as in adolescence and during pregnancy. In regions of moderate iodine deficiency, goiter observed in

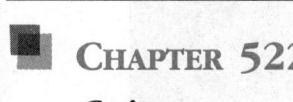

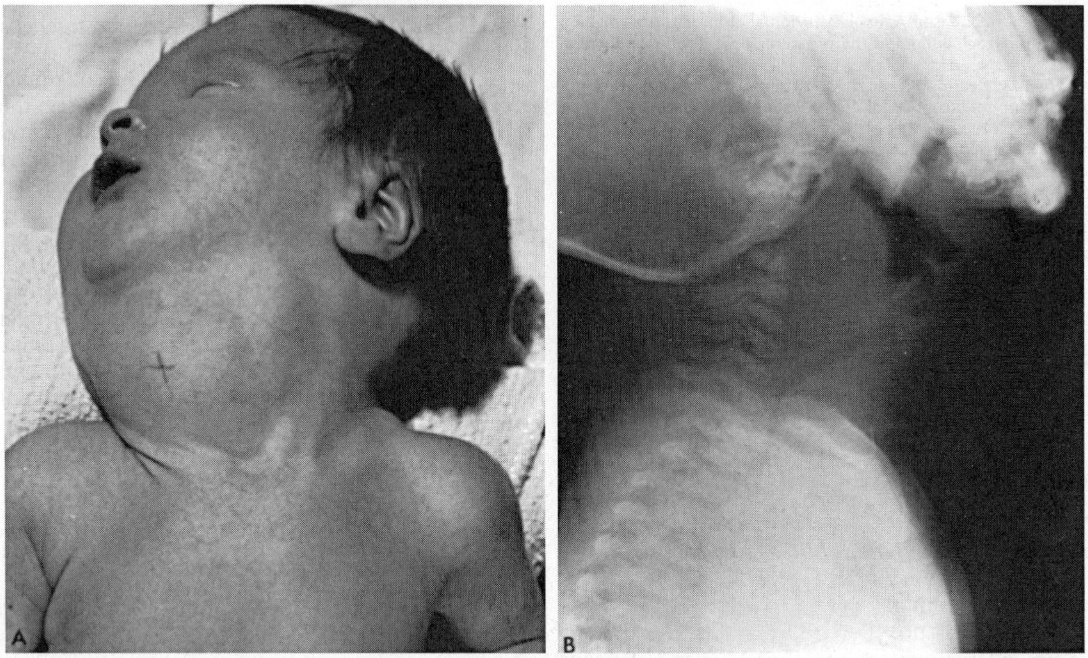

Figure 522–1. Congenital goiter in infancy. *A*, Large congenital goiter in an infant born to a mother with thyrotoxicosis who had been treated with iodides and methimazole during pregnancy. *B*, A 6-wk-old infant with increasing respiratory distress and cervical mass since birth. The operation revealed a large goiter that almost completely encircled the trachea. Notice the anterior deviation and posterior compression of the trachea. Partial thyroidectomy completely relieved the symptoms. It is apparent why a tracheostomy is not adequate treatment for these infants. The cause for the goiter was not found.

school children may disappear with maturity and reappear during pregnancy or lactation. Iodine-deficient goiters are more common in girls than in boys. Where iodine deficiency is severe, as in the hyperendemic highlands of Papua New Guinea, nearly half the population has large goiters, and endemic cretinism is common.

Serum T_4 levels are often low in people with endemic goiter, although clinical hypothyroidism is rare. This is true in New Guinea, the Congo, the Himalayas, and South America. Despite low serum levels of thyroid hormone, serum TSH concentrations are often only moderately increased. In such patients circulating levels of triiodothyronine (T_3) are elevated. Moreover, T_3 levels are also elevated in those patients with normal T_4 levels, indicating a preferential secretion of T_3 by the thyroid in this disease.

Endemic cretinism, the most serious consequence of iodine deficiency, has been recognized for centuries; it occurs only in geographic association with endemic goiter. The term endemic cretinism includes two different but overlapping syndromes, a neurologic type and a myxedematous type. The frequency of the two types varies among different populations; in Papua New Guinea, the neurologic type occurs almost exclusively, but in Zaire, the myxedematous type predominates. Both types are found in all endemic areas, and some individuals have intermediate or mixed features.

The neurologic syndrome is characterized by mental retardation, deaf-mutism, disturbances in standing and gait, and pyramidal signs such as clonus of the foot, Babinski sign, and patellar hyperreflexia. Affected individuals are goitrous but euthyroid, have normal pubertal development and adult stature, and have little or no impaired thyroid function. Individuals with the myxedematous syndrome also are mentally retarded and deaf and have neurologic symptoms, delayed sexual development and growth, myxedema, and absence of goiter; serum T_4 levels are low, and TSH levels are markedly elevated. Delayed skeletal maturation may extend into the 3rd decade or later. Ultrasound examination shows thyroid atrophy.

The pathogenesis of the neurologic syndrome has been attributed to iodine deficiency and hypothyroxinemia during pregnancy leading to fetal and postnatal hypothyroidism. Although some investigators have attributed brain damage to a direct effect of elemental iodine deficiency in the fetus, others believe the neurologic symptoms are caused by fetal and maternal hypothyroxinemia. There is evidence that the human fetal brain has receptors for thyroid hormone before development of the fetal thyroid, and there is also evidence of some transplacental passage of maternal thyroid hormone into the fetus, which normally might ameliorate the effects of fetal hypothyroidism on the developing nervous system. The pathogenesis of the myxedematous syndrome leading to thyroid atrophy is more bewildering. Searches for additional environmental factors that may provoke continuing postnatal hypothyroidism have led to incrimination of selenium deficiency, goitrogenic foods, thiocyanates, and *Yersinia.* Studies from Western China suggest that thyroid autoimmunity may play a role. Myxedematous cretins with thyroid atrophy, but not euthyroid cretins, were found to have thyroid growth–blocking immunoglobulins (TGBI) of the kind found in infants with sporadic congenital hypothyroidism. Others are skeptical about any role of TGBI in goitrogenesis and in endemic goiter.

In many developing countries, administration of a single intramuscular injection of iodinated poppy seed oil to women prevents iodine deficiency during future pregnancies for about 5 yr. This form of therapy given to children under 4 yr of age with myxedematous cretinism results in a euthyroid state in 5 mo. However, older children respond poorly and adults not at all to iodized oil injections, indicating an inability of the thyroid gland to synthesize hormone; these patients require treatment with T_4. In the Xinjiang province of China, where the usual methods of iodine supplementation had failed, iodination of irrigation water has increased iodine in soil, animals, and human beings.

522.3 Sporadic Goiter

The term sporadic goiter encompasses goiters developing from a variety of causes; patients are usually euthyroid but may be hypothyroid. The most common cause of sporadic goiter is lymphocytic thyroiditis (see Chapter 523). Intrinsic biochemical defects in the synthesis of thyroid hormone are almost always associated with goiter. The occurrence of the disorder in siblings, onset in early life, and possible association with hypothyroidism (goitrous hypothyroidism) are important clues to the diagnosis.

IODIDE GOITER. A small percentage of patients treated with iodide preparations for prolonged periods develop goiters. Iodides are commonly included for their expectorant effect in cough medicines and in proprietary mixtures for asthma. Goiters resulting from iodine administration are firm and diffusely enlarged, and in some instances hypothyroidism may develop. In normal subjects acute administration of large doses of iodine inhibits the organification of iodine and the synthesis of thyroid hormone (Wolff-Chaikoff effect). This effect is short-lived and does not lead to hypothyroidism. When iodide administration continues, an autoregulatory mechanism in normal persons limits iodine trapping and permits the level of iodide in the thyroid to fall and organification to proceed normally. In patients with iodide-induced goiter, this escape does not occur because of an underlying abnormality of biosynthesis of thyroid hormone. Persons most susceptible to the development of iodide goiter are those with lymphocytic thyroiditis or with a subclinical inborn error in thyroid hormone synthesis and those who have had partial thyroidectomy.

Lithium carbonate also causes goiters; it is currently widely used as a psychotropic drug. Lithium competes with iodide; the mechanism producing the goiter or hypothyroidism is similar to that described earlier for iodide goiter. Lithium and iodide also act synergistically to produce goiter; their combined use should be avoided.

Amiodarone, a drug used to treat cardiac arrhythmias, can cause thyroid dysfunction with goiter because it is rich in iodine. It is also a potent inhibitor of 5′-deiodinase, preventing conversion of T_4 to T_3. It can cause hypothyroidism, particularly in patients with underlying autoimmune disease; in other patients, it may cause hyperthyroidism.

SIMPLE GOITER (COLLOID GOITER). A few children with euthyroid nontoxic goiters have simple goiters, a condition of unknown etiology not associated with hypothyroidism or hyperthyroidism and not caused by inflammation or neoplasia. The condition predominates in girls and has a peak incidence before and during the pubertal years. Histologic examination of the thyroid either is normal or reveals variable follicular size, dense colloid, and flattened epithelium. The goiter may be small or large. It is firm in consistency in half the patients and is occasionally asymmetric or nodular. Levels of TSH are normal or low; scintiscans are normal; thyroid antibodies are absent. Differentiation from lymphocytic thyroiditis may not be possible without a biopsy, but biopsy is ordinarily not indicated. Therapy with thyroid hormone may help to avoid progression to a large multinodular goiter, although it is difficult to separate any treatment effects from the natural history, which is for the goiter to decrease in size. Untreated patients should be re-evaluated periodically. This condition must be differentiated from lymphocytic thyroiditis (see Chapter 523).

MULTINODULAR GOITER. Rarely, a firm goiter with a lobulated surface and single or multiple palpable nodules is encountered. Areas of cystic change, hemorrhage, and fibrosis may be present. The incidence of this condition has decreased markedly with the use of iodine-enriched salt. A mild goitrogenic stimulus, acting over a long time, is thought to be the cause. Ultrasound examination may reveal multiple echo-free and echogenic lesions that are nonfunctioning on scintiscans. Thyroid studies are usually normal, but TSH may be elevated and thyroid antibodies may be present. The condition occurs in children with McCune-Albright syndrome and has been described in three children (including two siblings) with digital anomalies and cystic renal disease. If the nodules are not suppressed by replacement therapy with T_4, surgery is indicated, because malignancy cannot readily be ruled out.

522.4 Intratracheal Goiter

One of the many ectopic locations of thyroid tissue is within the trachea. The intraluminal thyroid lies beneath the tracheal mucosa and is frequently continuous with the normally situated extratracheal thyroid. The thyroid tissue is susceptible to goitrous enlargement, which involves the normally situated and the ectopic thyroid. When there is obstruction of the airway associated with a goiter, it must be ascertained whether the obstruction is extratracheal or endotracheal. If obstructive manifestations are mild, administration of sodium-L-thyroxine usually causes the goiter to decrease in size. When symptoms are severe, surgical removal of the endotracheal goiter is indicated.

GOITER

Daneman D, Davy T, Mancer K, et al: Association of multinodular goiter, cystic renal disease, and digital anomalies. J Pediatr 107:270, 1985.

Davidson KM, Richards DS, Schatz DA, et al: Successful in utero treatment of fetal goiter and hypothyroidism. N Engl J Med 324:543, 1991.

DeLuca G, Chaussain JL, Job JC: Hyperfunctioning thyroid nodules in children and adolescents. Acta Paediatr Scand 75:118, 1986.

Feuillan PP, Shawker T, Rose SR, et al: Thyroid abnormalities in the McCune-Albright syndrome. Ultrasonography and hormonal studies. J Clin Endocrinol Metab 71:1596, 1990.

Hay ID: Thyroiditis: A clinical update. Mayo Clin Proc 60:836, 1985.

Hayashi Y, Tamai H, Fukata S, et al: A long-term clinical, immunological, and histological follow-up study of patients with goitrous chronic lymphocytic thyroiditis. J Clin Endocrinol Metab 61:1172, 1985.

Matsuura N, Konishi J, Yuri K, et al: Comparison of atrophic and goitrous autoimmune thyroiditis in children: Clinical, laboratory and TSH-receptor antibody studies. Eur J Pediatr 149:529, 1990.

Pharoah POD, Buttfield IH, Hetzel BS: Neurological damage to the foetus resulting from severe iodine deficiency during pregnancy. Lancet 1:308, 1971.

Queen JS, Clegg HW, Council JC, et al: Acute suppurative thyroiditis caused by *Eikenella corrodens*. J Pediatr Surg 23:359, 1988.

Randolph J, Grunt JA, Vawter GF: The medical and surgical aspects of intratracheal goiter. N Engl J Med 268:457, 1963.

Rich EJ, Mendelman PM: Acute suppurative thyroiditis in pediatric patients. Pediatr Infect Dis J 6:936, 1987.

GOITROUS CRETINISM

Abramowicz MJ, Targovnik HM, Cochaux P, et al: Identification of a mutation in the coding sequence of the human thyroid peroxidase gene causing congenital goiter. J Clin Invest 90:1200, 1992.

Benmiloud M, Chaouki ML, Gutekunst R, et al: Oral iodized oil for correcting iodine deficiency: Optimal dosing and outcome indicator selection. J Clin Endocrinol Metab 79:20, 1994.

Bikker H, den Hartog MT, Baas F, et al: A 20-base pair duplication in the human thyroid peroxidase gene results in a total iodide organification defect and congenital hypothyroidism. J Clin Endocrinol Metab 79:248, 1994.

Boyages SC, Halpern JP, Maberly GF, et al: A comparative study of neurological and myxedematous endemic cretinism in Western China. J Clin Endocrinol Metab 67:1262, 1988.

Boyages SC, Halpern JP, Maberly GF, et al: Endemic cretinism: Possible role for thyroid autoimmunity. Lancet 2:529, 1989.

Boyages SC, Halpern JP, Maberly GF, et al: Supplementary iodine fails to reverse hypothyroidism in adolescents and adults with endemic cretinism. J Clin Endocrinol Metab 70:336, 1990.

Couch RM, Dean HJ, Winter JSD: Congenital hypothyroidism caused by defective iodide transport. J Pediatr 106:950, 1985.
Gattereau A, Bernard B, Bellabarba D, et al: Congenital goiter in four euthyroid siblings with glandular and circulating iodoproteins and defective iodothyronine synthesis. J Clin Endocrinol Metab 37:118, 1973.
Illum P, Kiaer HW, Hvidberg-Hansen J, et al: Fifteen cases of Pendred's syndrome. Congenital deafness and sporadic goiter. Arch Otolaryngol 96:297, 1972.
Medeiros-Neto G, Targovnik HM, Vassart G: Defective thyroglobulin synthesis and secretion causing goiter and hypothyroidism. Endocr Rev 14:165, 1993.
Weetman AP: Editorial: Is endemic goiter an autoimmune disease? J Clin Endocrinol Metab 78:1017, 1994.

CHAPTER 523
Hyperthyroidism

Angelo M. DiGeorge and Stephen LaFranchi

Hyperthyroidism results from excessive secretion of thyroid hormone and, with few exceptions, is due to diffuse toxic goiter (Graves disease) during childhood. Two large pedigrees have been reported of nonautoimmune autosomal dominant hyperthyroidism. These patients have thyroid hyperplasia with goiters and suppressed levels of thyroid-stimulating hormone (TSH). Both families have germline mutations of the TSH receptor resulting in constitutively activating (i.e., gain of function) mutations. Different activating mutations have been identified in some cases of thyroid adenomas. Other rare causes of hyperthyroidism that have been observed in children include toxic uninodular goiter (Plummer disease), hyperfunctioning thyroid carcinoma, thyrotoxicosis factitia, subacute thyroiditis, and acute suppurative thyroiditis. Hyperthyroidism occurs in some patients with McCune-Albright syndrome, which is associated with autonomous thyroid adenomas. Suppression of plasma TSH indicates that the hyperthyroidism is not pituitary in origin. Hyperthyroidism due to excess thyrotropin secretion is rare and, in most cases, is caused by pituitary unresponsiveness to thyroid hormone. TSH-secreting pituitary tumors have been reported only in adults. In infants born to mothers with Graves disease, hyperthyroidism may occur as a transitory phenomenon or as classic Graves disease during the neonatal period. Choriocarcinoma, hydatidiform mole, and struma ovarii have caused hyperthyroidism in adults but have not been recognized as causes in children.

523.1 Graves Disease

ETIOLOGY. Enlargement of the thymus, splenomegaly, lymphadenopathy, infiltration of the thyroid gland and of retro-orbital tissues with lymphocytes and plasma cells, and peripheral lymphocytosis are well-established findings in Graves disease. In the thyroid gland, T helper cells ($CD4^+$) tend to predominate in dense lymphoid aggregates; in areas of lower cell density, cytotoxic T cells ($CD8^+$) predominate. The percentage of activated B lymphocytes infiltrating the thyroid is higher than in peripheral blood. A postulated failure of T suppressor cells allows expression of T helper cells, sensitized to the TSH antigen, which interact with β cells. These cells differentiate into plasma cells, which produce thyrotropin receptor–stimulating antibody (TRSAb). TRSAb binds to the receptor for TSH and stimulates cAMP, analogous to TSH itself. In addition to TRSAb, thyrotropin receptor–blocking antibody (TRBAb) may also be produced, and the clinical course of the disease usually correlates with the ratio between the two antibodies.

The ophthalmopathy occurring in Graves disease is caused by antibodies against antigens shared by the thyroid and eye muscle. The antibodies that bind to the extraocular muscles and orbital fibroblasts stimulate the synthesis of glycosaminoglycans by orbital fibroblasts and produce cytotoxic effects on muscle cells.

In whites, Graves disease is associated with HLA-B8 and HLA-DR3; the latter carries a 7-fold relative risk for Graves disease. Therefore, it is not surprising that Graves disease is also associated with other HLA-D3–related disorders such as Addison disease, insulin-dependent diabetes mellitus, myasthenia gravis, and celiac disease. Systemic lupus erythematosus, rheumatoid arthritis, vitilago, idiopathic thrombocytopenic purpura, and pernicious anemia have been described in children with Graves disease. In family clusters, the most frequent association with Graves disease is lymphocytic thyroiditis, autoimmune hypothyroidism, and neonatal hyperthyroidism.

CLINICAL MANIFESTATIONS. About 5% of all patients with hyperthyroidism are under 15 yr of age; the peak incidence occurs during adolescence. Graves disease has begun between 6 wk and 2 yr of age in children born to mothers without a history of hyperthyroidism. The incidence is about five times higher in girls than in boys.

The clinical course in children is highly variable but usually is not so fulminant as in many adults. Symptoms develop gradually; the usual interval between onset and diagnosis is 6–12 mo. The earliest signs in children may be emotional disturbances accompanied by motor hyperactivity. The children become irritable, excitable, and cry easily owing to emotional lability. Their school work suffers as a result of a short attention span. Tremor of the fingers can be noticed if the arm is extended. There may be a voracious appetite combined with loss of or no increase in weight. The size of the thyroid is variable. It may be so little enlarged that it escapes detection initially, but with careful examination, a goiter is found in almost all patients. Exophthalmos is noticeable in most patients but is usually mild. Lagging of the upper eyelid as the eye looks downward, impairment of convergence, and retraction of the upper eyelid and infrequent blinking may be present. The skin is smooth and flushed, with excessive sweating. Muscular weakness is uncommon but may be severe enough to result in falling spells. Tachycardia, palpitations, dyspnea, and cardiac enlargement and insufficiency cause discomfort but rarely endanger the patient's life. Atrial fibrillation is a rare complication. Mitral regurgitation, probably resulting from papillary muscle dysfunction, is the cause of the apical systolic murmur present in some patients. The systolic blood pressure and the pulse pressure are increased. Many of the findings in Graves disease result from hyperactivity of the sympathetic nervous system.

Thyroid "crisis" or "storm" is a form of hyperthyroidism manifested by an acute onset, hyperthermia, and severe tachycardia and restlessness. There may be rapid progression to delirium, coma, and death. "Apathetic" or "masked" hyperthyroidism is another variety of hyperthyroidism characterized by extreme listlessness, apathy, and cachexia. A combination of both forms may also occur. These symptom complexes are rare in children.

LABORATORY DATA. Serum levels of thyroxine (T_4), triiodothyronine (T_3), free T_4, and free T_3 are elevated. In some patients, levels of T_3 may be more elevated than those of T_4. Levels of TSH measured by a sensitive assay are suppressed below normal levels. Thyroid peroxidase antibodies are often present. Most patients with newly diagnosed Graves disease have measurable TSH receptor–stimulating antibodies, and their disappearance predicts remission of the disease. Assays of TSH-receptor antibodies are rarely necessary for diagnosis or management of Graves disease. Radioiodine is rapidly and diffusely concentrated in the thyroid, but this study is rarely necessary. Very young children with Graves disease often have advanced skeletal maturation and craniostenosis.

DIFFERENTIAL DIAGNOSIS. Diagnosis is rarely difficult once it has been considered. Elevated levels of T_4 and free T_4 in association with suppressed levels of TSH are usually diagnostic. The presence of TRSAb establishes the cause as Graves disease.

Most other causes of hyperthyroxinemia are rare but may result in erroneous diagnosis. Patients with elevated thyroxine-binding globulin (TBG) levels or familial dysalbuminemic hyperthyroxinemia have normal levels of free T_4 and TSH. If a thyroid nodule is palpable, or if T_3 is preferentially elevated, a functional thyroid nodule must be considered; radionuclide study is diagnostic. If precocious puberty, polyostotic fibrous dysplasia, or café-au-lait pigmentation is present, the autonomous thyroid disorder of McCune-Albright syndrome is likely. Patients with generalized thyroid hormone unresponsiveness have elevated or normal levels of free T_4, but levels of TSH are inappropriately elevated. Patients with pituitary unresponsiveness to thyroid hormone also have clinical hyperthyroidism, but their levels of TSH are elevated or normal, and they must be differentiated from patients with TSH-secreting pituitary tumors, who have elevated serum levels of the TSH α chain.

When hyperthyroxinemia is caused by exogenous thyroid hormone, levels of free T_4 and TSH are the same as those seen in Graves disease, but the level of thyroglobulin is very low, although in patients with Graves disease, it is elevated.

TREATMENT. Most pediatric endocrinologists recommend medical therapy rather than subtotal thyroidectomy or radioiodine. The two thionamide drugs in widest use are propylthiouracil (PTU) and methimazole (Tapazole). Both compounds inhibit incorporation of trapped inorganic iodide into organic compounds, and they may also suppress levels of TRSAb by directly affecting intrathyroidal autoimmunity. But there are important differences between the two drugs. Methimazole is at least 10 times more potent than PTU on a weight basis and has a much longer serum half-life (6–8 hr vs 0.5 hr); PTU must be administered three times daily, but methimazole can be given once daily. Unlike methimazole, PTU is heavily protein bound and has a lesser ability to cross the placenta and to pass into breast milk; theoretically, PTU is the preferred drug during pregnancy and for nursing mothers. PTU, more than methimazole, inhibits extrathyroidal conversion of T_4 to T_3; this may be advantageous in the treatment of neonatal thyrotoxicosis.

Toxic reactions occur with both drugs; most are mild, but some are life threatening. They are unpredictable and can occur after therapy of any duration. There is increasing evidence that these reactions may be fewer in patients treated with methimazole. Transient leukopenia ($<4,000/mm^3$) is common; it is asymptomatic and not a harbinger of agranulocytosis, and it usually is not a reason to discontinue treatment. Transient urticarial rashes are common. These can be managed by a short period off therapy and restarting the alternate antithyroid drug. The most severe reactions are hypersensitive in nature and include agranulocytosis, hepatitis, hepatic failure, a lupus-like syndrome, glomerulonephritis, and a vasculitis involving the skin and other organs. Although rare, these reactions have been reported with both drugs, and it is probably best to treat unusually hypersensitive patients with radioiodine or thyroidectomy. Cases of congenital skin defects (aplasia cutis) have been seen in infants exposed in fetal life to methimazole, but this association does not appear to be a strong one.

The initial dose of PTU is 5–10 mg/kg/24 hr given three times daily, and that of methimazole is 0.5–1.0 mg/kg/24 hr given once or twice daily. Smaller initial doses should be used in early childhood. Careful surveillance is required after treatment is initiated. Raising serum levels of TSH above normal indicates overtreatment and leads to increased size of the goiter. Clinical response becomes apparent in 2–3 wk, and adequate control is evident in 1–3 mo. The dose is decreased to the minimal level required to maintain a euthyroid state.

Drug therapy may be necessary for 6 yr or longer because there appears to be a remission rate of about 25% every 2 yr. If a relapse occurs, it will usually appear within 3 mo and almost always within 6 mo after therapy has been discontinued. Therapy may be resumed in case of a relapse. Patients over 13 yr of age, boys, and those with small goiters and modestly elevated T_3 levels appear to have earlier remissions.

A β-adrenergic blocking agent such as propranolol (0.5–2.0 mg/kg/24 hr, given three times daily) is a useful supplement in management of severely toxic patients. Thyroid hormones potentiate the actions of catecholamines, which include tachycardia, tremor, excessive sweating, lid lag, and stare. These symptoms abate with use of propranolol, which does not, however, alter thyroid function or exophthalmos.

Operation or radioiodine treatment is indicated when adequate cooperation for medical management is not possible or when adequate trial of medical management has failed to result in permanent remission. Subtotal thyroidectomy, a rather safe procedure, is performed only after the patient has been brought to a euthyroid state. This may be accomplished with PTU or methimazole over 2–3 mo. After a euthyroid state has been attained, 5 drops of a saturated solution of potassium iodide/24 hr are added to the regimen for 2 wk before operation to decrease the vascularity of the gland. Complications of surgical treatment are rare and include hypoparathyroidism (transient or permanent) and paralysis of the vocal cords. The incidence of residual or recurrent hyperthyroidism or of hypothyroidism depends on the extent of the surgery. Some recommend near-total thyroidectomy. The incidence of recurrence will be low, but that of hypothyroidism may exceed 50%.

Radioiodine has proved to be an effective, relatively safe first or alternate therapy for Graves disease in children. Pretreatment with antithyroid drugs is unnecessary; if a patient is on them, they should be stopped 5 days before radioiodine administration. Most children become euthyroid after one dose (88% in one study), but a few may require a second or third treatment dose. Because the full effects of treatment may not be complete for 2–3 mo, adjunctive therapy with a β-adrenergic antagonist is recommended. Although there have been concerns about radiation oncogenesis and genetic damage, follow-up of treated children for as long as 40 yr has not shown this. The risk of benign adenoma may be increased (0.6–1.9% in one study). The major consequence of radioiodine is hypothyroidism, which occurs in 10–20% of patients after the first year and in about 3% per year thereafter.

The ophthalmopathy remits gradually and usually independently of the hyperthyroidism. Severe ophthalmopathy may require treatment with prednisone.

523.2 Congenital Hyperthyroidism

Onset of neonatal hyperthyroidism usually begins prenatally and is present at birth, although it may not be noticed until a few days after birth; occasionally, onset may be delayed for several weeks or more. The mothers of these infants have active Graves disease, Graves disease in remission, or rarely, hypothyroidism and a history of lymphocytic thyroiditis. The condition is caused by transplacental passage of TRSAb, but the clinical onset, severity, and course may be modified by the concurrent presence of TRBAb and by the transplacental passage of antithyroid drugs taken by the mother. Very high levels of TRSAb usually result in classic neonatal hyperthyroidism, but if the infant has been exposed to the antithyroid drugs, onset of symptoms is delayed 3–4 days to allow degradation of the maternally derived antithyroid drug. If TRBAb is also present, onset of hyperthyroid symptoms may be delayed for several weeks.

Neonatal hyperthyroidism occurs in only about 2% of infants born to mothers with a history of Graves disease. The finding of very high levels of TRSAb in these mothers usually predicts the occurrence of an affected infant. Fetal tachycardia and goiter may allow prenatal diagnosis. Unlike Graves disease at all other ages, neonatal hyperthyroidism affects males as often as females. The disorder usually remits spontaneously within 6–12 wk but may persist longer, depending on the levels of TRSAb. Mild asymptomatic hyperthyroxinemia also occurs. Occasionally, classic neonatal Graves disease does not remit but persists for several years or longer. These patients have impressive family histories of Graves disease. In these infants TRSAb transfer from the mother apparently blends with the infantile onset of autonomous Graves disease.

Many of the infants are premature and appear intrauterine growth retarded. Most have goiters. The infant is extremely restless, irritable, and hyperactive and appears anxious and unusually alert. Microcephaly and ventricular enlargement may be present. The eyes are widely opened and appear exophthalmic. There may be extreme tachycardia and tachypnea, and the temperature is elevated. In severely affected infants, there is a progression of symptoms; weight loss occurs despite a ravenous appetite, hepatosplenomegaly increases, and jaundice may become manifest. Cardiac decompensation is common, and severe hypertension may occur. The infant may die if therapy is not instituted promptly. The serum level of T_4 is markedly elevated and TSH is suppressed. Advanced bone age, frontal bossing with triangular facies, and cranial synostosis are common, especially in those infants with persistent clinical manifestations of hyperthyroidism. Prognosis for intellectual development is guarded for infants with cranial synostosis.

Treatment consists of oral administration of Lugol solution (1 drop every 8 hr) and PTU (5–10 mg/kg/24 hr given every 8 hr). If the thyrotoxic state is severe, parenteral fluid therapy, propranolol (2 mg/kg/24 hr, orally in three divided doses), and corticosteroids may be indicated. When propranolol is used during pregnancy to treat thyrotoxicosis, it crosses the placenta and may cause respiratory depression in the newborn infant. If heart failure occurs, digitalization is indicated. After a euthyroid state is reached, only PTU treatment is necessary. The dose should be gradually tapered to keep the infant euthyroid. Most remit by 3–4 mo of age.

Occasionally, neonatal hyperthyroidism does not remit but persists into childhood. These patients may have an impressive family history of hyperthyroidism, but TSH-stimulating antibodies are absent. Advanced osseous maturation, microcephaly, and mental retardation occur when treatment is delayed. It has been recently established that a child with this disorder has a *mutation of the TSH-receptor (TSHR) gene.* A gene-line mutation in the TSHR gene resulted in constitutive activation of the receptor. Persistent and adequate treatment is necessary to prevent irreversible consequences.

Bahn RS, Heufelder AE: Pathogenesis of Graves' ophthalmopathy. N Engl J Med 329:1468, 1993.
Cheron RG, Kaplan MM, Larsen PR, et al: Neonatal thyroid function after propylthiouracil therapy for maternal Graves' disease. N Engl J Med 304:525, 1981.
Cooper DS: Which anti-thyroid drug? Am J Med 80:1165, 1986.
Daneman D, Howard NJ: Neonatal thyrotoxicosis: Intellectual impairment and craniosynostosis in later years. J Pediatr 97:257, 1980.
Darby CP: Three episodes of spontaneous thyroid storm occurring in a nine year-old child. Pediatrics 30:927, 1962.
Duprez L, Parma J, Van Sande J, et al: Germline mutations in the thyrotropin receptor gene cause non-autoimmune autosomal dominant hyperthyroidism. Nature Gene 7:396, 1994.
Foley TP, White C, New A: Juvenile Graves disease: Usefulness and limitations of thyrotropin receptor antibody determinations. J Pediatr 110:378, 1987.
Hamburger JI: Management of hyperthyroidism in children and adolescents. J Clin Endocrinol Metab 60:1019, 1985.
Hashizume K, Ichikawa K, Sakurai A, et al: Administration of thyroxine in treated Graves' disease. Effects on the level of antibodies to thyroid-stimulating hormone receptors and on the risk of recurrence of hyperthyroidism. N Engl J Med 324:947, 1991.
Kopp P, van Sande J, Parma J, et al: Brief report: Congenital hyperthyroidism caused by a mutation in the thyrotropin-receptor gene. N Engl J Med 332:150, 1995.
Levy WJ, Schumacher P, Gupta M: Treatment of childhood Graves' disease: A review with emphasis on radioiodine treatment. Cleve Clin J Med 55:373, 1988.
Lightner ES, Allen HD, Laughlin G: Neonatal hyperthyroidism and heart failure. Am J Dis Child 131:68, 1977.
Lippe BM, Landow EM, Kaplan SA: Hyperthyroidism in children treated with long-term medical therapy: Twenty-five percent remission rate every two years. J Clin Endocrinol Metab 64:1241, 1987.
McKenzie JM, Zakarija M: The clinical use of thyrotropin receptor antibody measurements. J Clin Endocrinol Metab 68:1093, 1989.
Mihailovic V, Feller MS, Kourides IA, et al: Hyperthyroidism due to excess thyrotropin secretion: Follow-up studies. J Clin Endocrinol Metab 50:1135, 1980.
Milham S Jr: Scalp defects in infants of mothers treated for hyperthyroidism with methimazole or carbimazole during pregnancy. Teratology 32:321, 1985.
Perelman AH, Clemons RD: The fetus in maternal hyperthyroidism. Thyroid 2:225, 1992.
Riggs W Jr, Wilroy RS Jr, Etteldorf JN: Neonatal hyperthyroidism with accelerated skeletal maturation, craniosynostosis, and brachydactyly. Radiology 105:621, 1972.
Roti E, Gardini E, Minelli R, et al: Methimazole and serum thyroid hormone concentrations in hyperthyroid patients: Effects of single and multiple daily doses. Ann Intern Med 111:181, 1989.
Stenszky V, Kozma L, Balazs C, et al: The genetics of Graves disease: HLA and disease susceptibility. J Clin Endocrinol Metab 61:835, 1985.
Totterman TH, Karlsson FA, Bengstsson M, et al: Induction of circulating activated suppressor-like T cells by methimazole therapy for Graves disease. N Engl J Med 316:15, 1987.
Viscardi RM, Shea M, Sriwantanakul K, et al: Hyperthyroxinemia in newborns due to excess thyroxine-binding globulin. N Engl J Med 309:897, 1983.
Volpe R, Ehrlich R, Steiner G, et al: Graves' disease in pregnancy years after hypothyroidism with recurrent passive-transfer neonatal Graves' disease in offspring. Therapeutic considerations. Am J Med 77:572, 1984.
Zakarija M, McKenzie JM: Pregnancy-associated changes in the thyroid-stimulating antibody of Graves' disease and the relationship to neonatal hyperthyroidism. J Clin Endocrinol Metab 57:1036, 1983.

CHAPTER 524

Carcinoma of the Thyroid

Angelo M. DiGeorge and Stephen LaFranchi

Carcinoma of the thyroid is rare in children; only 37 new cases among 1 million people are found annually, and about 7% of these occur in children under 18 yr of age. Unlike other malignancies in childhood, thyroid cancer usually has a very indolent course, even after pulmonary metastases have developed.

The thyroid gland of children is unusually sensitive to exposure to external irradiation. There probably is no threshold dose; even 7 Gy increases the incidence of cancer. In the past, about 80% of children with cancer of the thyroid had received irradiation of the neck and adjacent areas during infancy for such benign conditions as "enlarged" thymus, hypertrophied tonsils and adenoids, hemangiomas, nevi, eczema, tinea capitis, and "cervical adenitis." With the disuse of irradiation for benign conditions, this cause of thyroid cancer has vanished. However, the long-term survival of children who have received therapeutic irradiation to areas of the neck for neoplastic disease has now made this cause of thyroid cancer and nodules increasingly prevalent; increased dose, younger age at time of treatment, and female sex are factors that increase the risk of developing thyroid cancer. Long-term risk data for cancer are sparse, but 15–50% of children who have received irradiation and chemotherapy for Hodgkin disease, leukemia, and other malignancies of the head and neck develop elevated levels of thyroid-stimulating hormone (TSH) within the 1st yr of therapy, and 5–20% progress to hypothyroidism during the next 5–7 yr. Most large groups of treated patients have a 10–30% incidence of benign thyroid nodules and an increased incidence of thyroid cancer. Thyroid cancer begins to appear within 3–5 yr after irradiation treatment and reaches a peak in 15–25 yr. It is unknown whether there is a period after which no more tumors develop.

Histologically, the carcinomas are papillary (80%), follicular (17%), medullary (2%), or mixed differentiated tumors. These are usually slow-growing tumors and may remain dormant for years. The type of tumor and the natural course of disease in irradiated and nonirradiated patients are the same, except that multicentricity is more frequent in irradiation-induced cancer. In about 4% of patients with papillary cancer, another family relative is affected. Undifferentiated (anaplastic) thyroid neoplasms are rare in children and usually have a rapidly fatal course.

Girls are affected twice as often as boys. The average age at diagnosis is 9 yr, but the onset may be as early as the 1st yr of life. A painless nodule in the thyroid or in the neck is the usual first evidence of disease. Cervical lymph node involvement is often present at the time of initial diagnosis. Any unexplained cervical lymph node enlargement requires examination of the thyroid, which occasionally has a primary tumor too small to be felt; the diagnosis is based on biopsy results of the lymph node. The lungs are the most common site of metastases beyond the neck. There may be no clinical manifestations referable to them; roentgenographically, they appear as diffuse miliary or nodular infiltrations, principally in the basal portions. They may be mistaken for tuberculosis, histoplasmosis, or sarcoidosis. Other sites of metastases include the mediastinum, long bones, skull, and axilla. Almost all children are euthyroid, but rarely, the carcinoma may be functional and produce symptoms of hyperthyroidism.

A thyroid scan should be performed whenever a thyroid nodule is found. ^{123}I or ^{99m}Tc-pertechnetate is the preferred scanning agent. Most malignant lesions show decreased concentrations of radioisotope ("cold"), but many cold lesions are benign. Serum levels of thyroglobulin (Tg) are often elevated and return to normal after surgical removal of differentiated tumors; this test also permits early detection of metastases. Tg levels do not correlate with any histologic characteristics or with malignancy or benignity of thyroid tumors. Other tests of thyroid function are normal, but Hashimoto thyroiditis has been associated with thyroid cancer.

Because differentiated thyroid carcinoma is a chronic disease with a long survival, optimal therapy is still evolving. There is increasing evidence that small (<2 cm) papillary carcinoma, the least aggressive type, is effectively treated by subtotal thyroidectomy and suppressive doses of thyroid hormone. Papillary carcinomas tend to be multicentric, and several studies show that one half of these children have regional lymph node involvement at presentation. For larger papillary carcinomas, follicular carcinoma, or regional lymph node involvement, near-total thyroidectomy with excision of regional lymph nodes appears to be the treatment of choice. There is no role for radical neck dissection. Thyroidectomy is usually followed by an ^{131}I ablative dose (30–100 mCi).

Many patients with cervical or pulmonary metastases have survived for many years. Pure follicular and mixed papillary and follicular cancers are more aggressive; affected patients may require total thyroidectomy and neck dissection. For any form of therapy, survival or recurrence does not appear to be different for patients with or without involvement of the cervical nodes. Even patients with cervical or pulmonary metastases have survived for many years.

More than 95% of patients are alive 25 yr after initial treatment if the tumor was intrathyroid, less than 2 cm in diameter, and classified as grade 1. Greater tumor size, distant spread, and greater atypia are associated with increased cumulative mortality.

After surgery, all patients should be treated with sodium-L-thyroxine in doses sufficient to suppress TSH. Periodic determinations of Tg levels should also be performed, because Tg is an excellent marker for tumor recurrence in patients taking thyroxine (T_4). If the patient has undergone a total thyroidectomy or ^{131}I ablation, the serum Tg level should be less than 5 ng/mL on T_4 suppressive therapy.

524.1 Solitary Thyroid Nodule

Solitary nodules of the thyroid are uncommon in children. In the past, it was estimated that as many as half were carcinomas, but later studies indicate that there is an approximately 15% incidence of malignancy, perhaps because of decreasing exposure of children to irradiation. Children exposed to irradiation have a high incidence of benign adenoma and carcinoma of the thyroid.

Benign disorders that may present as solitary thyroid nodules include benign adenomas (e.g., follicular, embryonal, Hürthle cell), colloid (adenomatous) nodule, lymphocytic thyroiditis, thyroglossal duct cyst, ectopically located normal thyroid tissue, a single median thyroid, agenesis of one of the lateral thyroid lobes with hypertrophy of the contralateral lobe, thyroid cysts, and abscess. A suddenly appearing or rapidly enlarging thyroid mass may indicate hemorrhage into a benign adenoma. In most cases, the child is euthyroid, and thyroid function studies are normal. A ^{99m}Tc scan is usually indicated. Ultrasound is particularly useful in detecting cystic lesions. When lymphocytic thyroiditis is the cause of the nodule, T_4 may be low, TSH may be elevated, and thyroid antibodies are usually present. The scan may reveal a moth-eaten appearance. Rarely, lymphocytic thyroiditis may be associated with carcinoma of the thyroid.

Some nodules are "cold" on ^{99m}Tc scan, as is the case with carcinoma, but other lesions, such as developmental defects of the thyroid, demonstrate normal uptake. In questionable cases, suppressive therapy with 0.1–0.2 mg daily of sodium-L-thyroxine may be used. Cold nodules that continue to grow over 4–6 mo or that do not reduce in size by 50% in 1 yr should be surgically explored. Fine-needle aspiration to determine the nodule's histology is being used more for children. The rate of false-negative cytologic results ranges from 1–6%, and the false-positive rate is 50%. Surgery without delay is indicated when the nodule is hard or has grown rapidly, when there is evidence of tracheal or vocal cord involvement, or when there is enlargement of adjacent lymph nodes. All persons with a history of head or neck irradiation should have careful examinations of the thyroid at least every 2 yr, indefinitely.

Rarely, thyroid nodules may be functional, producing hyperthyroidism (Plummer disease). The uptake of radionuclide is concentrated in the nodule ("hot" or "warm" nodule), and thyroid function studies indicate that the nodule is functioning autonomously. Such nodules are usually benign, but a few instances of carcinoma in such cases have been reported. T_4

levels are usually normal, but triiodothyronine (T_3) levels are elevated (T_3 toxicosis), and TSH levels are suppressed. Treatment consists of surgical removal of the nodule.

A suppressible functioning nodule in a euthyroid child has been reported only once.

524.2 Medullary Carcinoma

This carcinoma of the thyroid arises from the parafollicular cells (C cells) of the thyroid and accounts for about 2% of thyroid malignancies. The tumor is pleomorphic, with sheets of spindle or small cells with eosinophilic granular cytoplasm. Amyloid is invariably deposited in the stroma, and calcification is common. The most common symptom is goiter or a palpable thyroid nodule. Roentgenograms may reveal dense, conglomerate, homogeneous calcification in the thyroid. Metastases to the regional lymph nodes and to the liver are common, and these also may calcify. Death may result, but long survivals are not uncommon.

The tumors occur sporadically, as a familial autosomal dominant disorder, and as components of two distinct autosomal dominant syndromes. The susceptibility for all these disorders has been mapped to chromosome 10q11.2. When the tumor occurs sporadically, it is usually unicentric, but in the familial form, it is usually multicentric, and it begins as hyperplasia of parafollicular cells. The tumors are often too small to be found by palpation, scintigraphy, or ultrasound examination in at-risk patients in these families. Diagnosis of medullary carcinoma should lead to a careful search for associated tumors, particularly pheochromocytoma. No clinically recognizable manifestations result from the elevated serum levels of calcitonin or from the calcitonin gene–related peptide and the carboxy-terminal flanking peptide (katacalcin) that are associated.

MULTIPLE ENDOCRINE NEOPLASIA (MEN), TYPE IIA. When hyperplasia or carcinoma of C cells is associated with adrenal medullary hyperplasia or pheochromocytoma and parathyroid hyperplasia, it is known as MEN IIA. The inheritance pattern for MEN IIA is autosomal dominant, with a high degree of penetrance and variable expressivity; the gene (*RET* proto-oncogene) was assigned by linkage studies to chromosome 10q11.2, where the *RET* proto-oncogene had also been mapped. At least 19 different specific missense mutations of exons 10 or 11 of the extracellular domain of the *RET* gene have been described for MEN IIA and for cases of medullary carcinoma. In the past, it was necessary to perform repetitive, burdensome biochemical tests of limited value for at-risk individuals in these families, but DNA analysis permits unambiguous identification of carriers of the *RET* proto-oncogene gene. C-cell hyperplasia or tumors usually appear earlier than pheochromocytoma. Pheochromocytomas are frequently bilateral and may be multiple. Adrenal medullary hyperplasia is known to precede pheochromocytoma, but the detectable latent period is short. Hypercalcemia is a late manifestation and indicates hyperparathyroidism. The parathyroids may reveal chief-cell hyperplasia or only hypercellularity.

MULTIPLE ENDOCRINE NEOPLASIA (MEN), TYPE IIB. The distinguishing feature of MEN IIB, also called the *mucosal neuroma syndrome*, is the occurrence of multiple neuromas and a characteristic phenotype associated with medullary carcinoma and pheochromocytoma. This condition is also autosomal dominant, and 93% of families have a missense mutation of the *RET* proto-oncogene. However, the mutation is in exon 16, the tyrosine catalytic domain of *RET*; all patients have had the same point mutation.

The neuromas most often occur on the tongue, buccal mucosa, lips, and conjunctivae. Peripheral neurofibromas and café-au-lait patches may be present, and intestinal ganglioneuromatosis is common. Diffuse proliferation of nerves and ganglion cells is found in mucosal, submucosal, myenteric, and subserosal plexuses involving the small and large bowel as well as the esophagus. The patients may be tall, with arachnodactyly and a Marfan-like appearance. Scoliosis, pectus excavatum, pes cavus, and muscular hypotonia are common. The eyelids may be thickened and everted, the lips patulous and blubbery, the jaw prognathic. Feeding difficulties, poor sucking, diarrhea, constipation, and failure to thrive may begin in infancy or early childhood, many years before the appearance of neuromas or endocrine symptoms.

TREATMENT. Total thyroidectomy is indicated for all children who are shown by DNA studies to carry the gene. Recognition of familial forms of this tumor is critical to the early diagnosis in patients at risk. Evidence suggests that thyroidectomy must be done very early, because medullary carcinoma has been seen in a 6-mo-old child with MEN IIB and in a 3-yr-old child with MEN IIA. Monitoring the levels of calcitonin is useful in detecting metastatic lesions and in following the course of the disease after operation for patients who have developed medullary carcinomas before prophylactic thyroidectomy. Periodic screening for development of pheochromocytoma is indicated.

Ashcroft NW, Van Herle AJ: The comparative value of serum thyroglobulin measurements and iodine ^{131}I total body scans in the follow-up of patients treated with differentiated thyroid cancer. Am J Med 71:806, 1981.

Carney JA, Go VLW, Sizemore GW, et al: Alimentary tract ganglioneuromatosis. A major component of the syndrome of multiple endocrine neoplasia, type 2b. N Engl J Med 295:1287, 1976.

Crile Y Jr, Antunex AR, Esselstyn CB, et al: The advantages of subtotal thyroidectomy and suppression of TSH in the primary treatment of papillary carcinoma of the thyroid. Cancer 55:2691, 1985.

DeGroot LJ: Diagnostic approach and management of patients exposed to irradiation of the thyroid. J Clin Endocrinol Metab 69:925, 1989.

Dobyns BM, Sheline GE, Workman JB, et al: Malignant and benign neoplasms of the thyroid in patients treated for hyperthyroidism: A report of the cooperative thyrotoxicosis therapy follow-up study. J Clin Endocrinol Metab 38:976, 1974.

Eng C, Smith DP, Mulligan LH, et al: Point mutation within the tyrosine kinase domain of the *RET* proto-oncogene in multiple endocrine neoplasia type 2B and related sporadic tumors. Hum Mol Genet 3:237, 1994.

Fleming ID, Black TL, Thompson EI, et al: Thyroid dysfunction and neoplasia in children receiving neck irradiation for cancer. Cancer 55:1190, 1985.

Gagel RF: The impact of gene mapping techniques on the management of multiple endocrine neoplasia type 2. Trends Endocrinol Metab 2:19, 1991.

Gagel RF, Robinson MF, Donovan DT, et al: Medullary thyroid carcinoma: Recent progress. J Clin Endocrinol Metab 76:809, 1993.

Griffiths AM, Mack DR, Byard RW, et al: Multiple endocrine neoplasia IIb: An unusual cause of chronic constipation. J Pediatr 116:285, 1990.

Hempelmann LH, Hall WJ, Phillips M, et al: Neoplasms in persons treated with x-rays in infancy: Fourth survey in 20 years. J Natl Cancer Inst 55:519, 1975.

Hofstra RMW, Landsvater RM, Ceccherini I, et al: A mutation in the *RET* proto-oncogene associated with multiple endocrine neoplasia type 2B and sporadic medullary thyroid carcinoma. Nature 367:375, 1994.

Hung W, Anderson KD, Chandra RS, et al: Solitary thyroid nodules in 71 children and adolescents. J Pediatr Surg 27:1407, 1992.

Keiser HR, Beaven MA, Doppham J, et al: Sipple's syndrome: Medullary thyroid carcinoma, pheochromocytoma and parathyroid disease. Ann Intern Med 78:561, 1973.

Kirk JM, Mort C, Grand DB, et al: The usefulness of serum thyroglobulin in the follow-up of differentiated thyroid carcinoma in children. Med Pediatr Oncol 20:201, 1992.

Kirkland RT, Kirkland JL, Rosenberg HS, et al: Solitary thyroid nodules in 30 children and report of a child with a thyroid abscess. Pediatrics 51:85, 1973.

Lips CJM, Landsvater RM, Höppener JWM, et al: Clinical screening as compared with DNA analysis in families with multiple endocrine neoplasia type 2A. N Engl J Med 331:828, 1994.

Mazzaferri EL: Management of a solitary thyroid nodule. N Engl J Med 328:553, 1993.

Razack MS, Sako K, Shimaoka K, et al: Radiation-associated thyroid carcinoma. J Surg Oncol 14:287, 1980.

Rojeski MT, Gharib H: Nodular thyroid disease. Evaluation and management. N Engl J Med 313:428, 1985.

Samaan NA, Schultz PN, Ordunez NG, et al: A comparison of thyroid carcinoma in those who have and have not had head and neck irradiation in childhood. J Clin Endocrinol Metab 64:219, 1987.

Sazmaan NA, Maheshwari YK, Nader S, et al: Impact of therapy for differentiated carcinoma of the thyroid: An analysis of 706 cases. J Clin Endocrinol Metab 56:1131, 1983.
Scott MD, Crawford JD: Solitary thyroid nodules in childhood: Is the incidence of thyroid carcinoma declining? Pediatrics 58:521, 1976.
Stjernholm MR, Freudenborrg JC, Mooney HS, et al: Medullary carcinoma of the thyroid before age 2 years. J Clin Endocrinol Metab 51:252, 1980.
Sussman L, Librik L, Clayton GW: Hyperthyroidism attributable to a hyperfunctioning thyroid carcinoma. J Pediatr 72:208, 1968.
Vane D, King DR, Boles ET Jr: Secondary thyroid neoplasm in pediatric cancer patients: Increased risk with improved survival. J Pediatr Surg 19:855, 1984.
Zimmerman D, Hay ID, Gough IR, et al: Papillary thyroid carcinoma in children and adults: Long-term follow-up of 1039 patients conservatively treated at one institution during three decades. Surgery 104:1157, 1988.

SECTION 3

Disorders of the Parathyroid Glands

Angelo M. DiGeorge ■ *Stephen LaFranchi*

Parathyroid hormone (PTH) and vitamin D are the principal regulators of calcium homeostasis. Calcitonin and PTH-related peptide (PTHrP) appear to be important primarily in the fetus.

PARATHYROID HORMONE. PTH is an 84-amino acid chain (9,500 dalton), but its biologic activity resides in the first 34 residues. In the parathyroid gland, a pre-pro-PTH (115-amino acid chain) and a proparathyroid hormone (90 amino acids) are synthesized. Pre-pro-PTH is converted to pro-PTH and pro-PTH to PTH. PTH (1–84) is the major secretory product of the gland, but it is rapidly cleaved in the liver and kidney into smaller COOH-terminal, midregion, and NH_2-terminal fragments.

The occurrence of these fragments has complicated the reliable measurement of PTH in serum and has led to the development of a variety of assays. The 1–34 amino-terminal (N-terminal) fragments possess biologic activity but are present in very low amounts in the circulation; assay of these fragments is most useful for detecting acute secretory changes. The carboxy-terminal (C-terminal) and midregion fragments, although biologically inert, are cleared more slowly from the circulation and represent 80% of plasma immunoreactive PTH; values of the C-terminal fragment are 50–500 times the level of the active hormone. The C-terminal assays are effective in detecting patients with hyperparathyroidism, but because C-terminal fragments are removed from the circulation by glomerular filtration, these assays are less useful for evaluating the secondary hyperparathyroidism characteristic of renal disease. Only certain sensitive radioimmunoassays for PTH can differentiate the subnormal concentrations that occur in hypoparathyroidism from normal levels. A sensitive 15-min immunochemiluminometric assay, developed for intraoperative use, can provide the surgeon with useful information.

When serum levels of calcium fall, secretion of PTH increases. PTH stimulates activity of 1α-hydroxylase in the kidney, enhancing production of 1,25-dihydroxycholecalciferol ($1,25[OH]_2D_3$). The increased level of $1,25[OH]_2D_3$ induces synthesis of a calcium-binding protein *(calbindin-D)* in the intestinal mucosa with resultant absorption of calcium. PTH also mobilizes calcium by directly enhancing bone resorption, an effect that requires $1,25[OH]_2D_3$. The effects of PTH on bone and kidney are mediated through binding to specific receptors on the membranes of target cells and through activation of a transduction pathway involving a G protein coupled to the adenylate cyclase system.

PTH-RELATED PEPTIDE. PTHrP is homologous to PTH only in the first 13 amino acids of its amino terminus, 8 of which are identical to PTH. Its gene is on the short arm of chromosome 12, and that of PTH is on the short arm of chromosome 11.

PTHrP, like PTH, activates PTH receptors in kidney and bone cells and increases urinary cAMP and renal production of $1,25[OH]_2D_3$. It is produced in almost every type of cell of the body, including every tissue of the embryo at some stage of development. PTHrP is critical for normal fetal development, and deletion of the gene in mice results in neonatal death and skeletal defects. It appears to have a paracrine or autocrine role, because serum levels are quite low except in a few clinical situations. Cord blood contains levels of PTHrP that are three-fold higher than in serum from adults; it is produced by the fetal parathyroids and appears to be the main agent stimulating maternal-fetal calcium transfer. PTHrP appears to be essential for normal skeletal maturation of the fetus, which requires 30 g of calcium. During pregnancy, maternal absorption of calcium increases from about 150 mg daily to 400 mg during the second trimester.

As in cord blood, PTHrP levels are increased during lactation and in patients with benign breast hypertrophy. Breast milk and pastureized bovine milk have levels of PTHrP that are 10,000 times higher than those of normal plasma. Most instances of the hormonal hypercalcemia syndrome of malignancy are caused by elevated concentrations of PTHrP.

VITAMIN D. See Chapters 43.7 and 483.1

CALCITONIN (CT). CT is a 32-amino acid polypeptide. Its gene is on chromosome 11p and is tightly linked to that of PTH. The CT gene encodes three peptides: CT, a 21-amino acid carboxy-terminal flanking peptide (katacalcin), and a CT gene-related peptide. Katacalcin and CT are cosecreted in equimolar amounts by the parafollicular cells (C cells) of the thyroid gland. CT appears to be of little consequence in children and adults, because very high levels in patients with medullary carcinoma of the thyroid (a tumor arising from the C cells) does not cause hypercalcemia. In the fetus, however, circulating levels are high and appear to augment bone metabolism and skeletal growth; these high levels are probably stimulated by the normally high fetal calcium levels. Unlike the high levels in cord blood and circulating concentrations in young children, levels in older children and adults are quite low. Infants and children with congenital hypothyroidism (and presumed deficiency of C cells) have lower levels of CT than normal children.

Its action appears to be independent of PTH and of vitamin D. Its main biologic effect appears to be the inhibition of bone resorption by decreasing the number and activity of bone-resorbing osteoclasts. This action of CT is the rationale behind its use in treatment of Paget disease. CT is synthesized in other organs, such as the gastrointestinal tract, pancreas, brain, and pituitary. In these organs, CT is thought to behave as a neurotransmitter to impose a local inhibitory effect on cell function. ■

CHAPTER 525
Hypoparathyroidism

Angelo M. DiGeorge

ETIOLOGY (Table 525–1). The normal level of parathyroid hormone (PTH) in cord blood is low; it doubles by the 6th day to reach a level nearly that of normal infants and children. Hypocalcemia is common from 12–72 hr of life, especially in premature infants, in infants with asphyxia at birth, and in infants of diabetic mothers *(early neonatal hypocalcemia)* (see Chapter 50). After the 2nd–3rd day and during the 1st wk of life, the type of feeding is also a determinant of the level of serum calcium *(late neonatal hypocalcemia)*. The role played by the parathyroids in these hypocalcemic infants remains to be clarified, although functional immaturity of the parathyroids has often been invoked as a pathogenetic factor. In a group of infants with *transient idiopathic hypocalcemia* (1–8 wk of age) serum levels of PTH were significantly lower than in normal infants. It is possible that the functional immaturity is a manifestation of a delay in development of the enzymes that convert glandular PTH to secreted PTH; other mechanisms are possible.

Hyperparathyroidism during pregnancy may result in transient hypocalcemia of the newborn infant. It appears that their hypocalcemia results from suppression of the fetal parathyroids by exposure to elevated levels of calcium in maternal serum. Tetany usually develops within 3 wk but may be delayed 1 mo or more if the infant is breast-fed. Hypocalcemia may persist for weeks or months. When the cause of hypocalcemia in young infants is unknown, their mothers should have measurements of calcium, phosphorus, and parathyroid hormone. Most affected mothers are asymptomatic, and the cause of their hyperparathyroidism is usually a parathyroid adenoma.

Aplasia or hypoplasia of the parathyroid glands is often associated with the DiGeorge syndrome and less often with the velocardiofacial (Shprintzen) syndrome. These two syndromes appear to be one and the same condition. Although the most common associations are conotruncal heart defects, thymic hypoplasia, abnormal facies, and cleft palate, the phenotype is variable, and the spectrum continues to widen. Most patients have a deletion within chromosome 22q11. Hypocalcemia usually occurs in the neonatal period and is often transient, but it may recur later or it may not have its onset until later in life. The syndrome and hypocalcemia also occur in some patients with the CHARGE and VATER syndromes, in infants of diabetic mothers, and in infants born to mothers treated with retinoic acid for acne early in pregnancy.

Administration of ^{131}I during pregnancy has resulted in hypoparathyroidism and in hypothyroidism.

Familial Congenital Hypoparathyroidism. Familial clusters of hypoparathyroidism with various patterns of transmission have been described. In two large North American pedigrees, this disorder appears to be transmitted by an X-linked recessive gene. In these families, the onset of afebrile seizures characteristically occurs in infants from 2 wk–6 mo of age. The absence of parathyroid tissue after detailed examination of a boy with this condition suggests it is a defect in embryogenesis.

An autosomal recessive syndrome of hypoparathyroidism with dysmorphic features has been described in Middle Eastern children. Parental consanguinity occurred for almost all of several dozen affected patients. Profound hypocalcemia occurs early in life, and dysmorphic features include microcephaly, deep-set eyes, beaked nose, micrognathia, and large floppy ears. Intrauterine and postnatal growth retardation are severe, and mental retardation is common. The cause is unknown. The autosomal recessive form of hypoparathyroidism that occurs with type I polyglandular autoimmune disease is described subsequently. In a few patients with autosomal recessive inheritance of isolated hypoparathyroidism, mutations of the PTH gene have been found.

Most often, hypoparathyroidism occurs as an autosomal dominant disorder. The gene has been localized to chromosome 3q13, the location of the CA^{2+}-sensing receptor. Inactivating mutations of this receptor result in familial hypocalciuric hypercalcemia and neonatal hyperparathyroidism. In patients with hypoparathyroidism, the mutation in the CA^{2+}-sensing receptor is an activating one, forcing the receptor to an "on" state and depression of PTH secretion. The hypocalcemia is usually mild and does not require treatment beyond childhood.

Another distinct form of autosomal dominant hypoparathyroidism is associated with sensorineural deafness and renal dysplasia.

Surgical Hypoparathyroidism. Removal or damage of the parathyroid glands may complicate thyroidectomy. Hypoparathyroidism has developed although the parathyroid glands have been identified and left undisturbed at the time of operation. This presumably is the result of interference with the blood supply or of postoperative edema and fibrosis. Symptoms of tetany may occur abruptly postoperatively and be temporary or permanent. In some instances, symptoms may develop insidiously and go undetected until months after thyroidectomy. Occasionally, the first evidence of surgical hypoparathyroidism may be the development of cataracts. The status of parathyroid function should be carefully monitored in all patients subjected to thyroidectomy.

Deposition in the parathyroid glands of iron pigment (e.g.,

■ **TABLE 525–1 Etiologic Classification of Hypocalcemia**

Parathyroid hormone (PTH) deficiency
Aplasia or hypoplasia of parathyroids
With 22q11 deletion
DiGeorge syndrome
Velocardiofacial syndrome
Conotruncal-face syndrome
With maternal diabetes mellitus or retinoic acid treatment
With VATER, CHARGE syndromes
With X-linked isolated hypoparathyroidism
PTH gene mutations
Autosomal recessive
PTH receptor defects (pseudohypoparathyroidism)
Type IA (inactivating mutation of $G_{s\alpha}$)
With gonadotropin-independent precocious puberty
Type IB (normal Gs_{α})
Type II (normal cAMP response)
CA^{2+}-sensing receptor defects
Activating mutation (autosomal dominant)
Autoimmune parathyroiditis
Isolated
With Addison disease or mucocutaneous candidiasis (type 1 autoimmune polyendocrinopathy)
Infiltrative lesions
Hemosiderosis (treatment of thassemia)
Copper deposition (Wilson disease)
Unknown cause of hypoparathyroidism
With dysmorphic features in Middle Eastern children
Autosomal recessive
With sensineural deafness and renal dysplasia
Autosomal dominant
Kenny-Caffey syndrome
Vitamin D deficiency (see Chapter 45.3)
Magnesium deficiency
Primary hypomagnesemia
Renal tubular defect
Aminoglycoside therapy
Inorganic phosphate excess
Laxatives

thalassemia) or of copper (e.g., Wilson disease) may produce hypoparathyroidism.

Idiopathic Hypoparathyroidism. The term idiopathic should be reserved for the small residuum of children with hypoparathyroidism for when no etiologic mechanism can be defined. Most children in whom onset of hypoparathyroidism occurs after the first few years of life have an autoimmune condition. Some have incomplete forms of DiGeorge syndrome or the autosomal dominant type of familial hypoparathyroidism.

Autoimmune Hypoparathyroidism. An autoimmune mechanism for hypoparathyroidism is strongly suggested by the finding of parathyroid antibodies and by the frequent association with other autoimmune disorders or organ-specific antibodies. Autoimmune hypoparathyroidism is often associated with Addison disease and chronic mucocutaneous candidiasis. The association of at least two of these three conditions has been tentatively classified as *polyglandular autoimmune disease, type I.* One third of patients with this syndrome have all three components; two thirds have only two of three conditions. The candidiasis almost always precedes the other disorders (70% of cases occur in children younger than 5 yr of age); the hypoparathyroidism (90% after 3 yr of age) usually occurs before Addison disease (90% after 6 yr of age). A variety of other disorders occur at various times; these include alopecia areata or totalis, malabsorption disorder, pernicious anemia, gonadal failure, chronic active hepatitis, vitiligo, and insulin-dependent diabetes. Some of these associations may not appear until adult life. Autoimmune thyroid disease is a rare concomitant.

Affected siblings may have the same or different constellations of disorders (e.g., hypoparathyroidism and Addison disease). The disorder is thought to have an autosomal recessive mode of inheritance, and it occurs more frequently among Finns and Iranian Jews. Patients with Addison disease, whether isolated or part of polyendocrinopathy syndrome type I or type II, have demonstrated adrenal specific 21-hydroxylase autoantibody reactivity.

CLINICAL MANIFESTATIONS. There is a spectrum of parathyroid deficiencies with clinical manifestations, varying from no symptoms to those of complete and longstanding deficiency. Mild deficiency may be revealed only by appropriate laboratory studies. Muscular pain and cramps are early manifestations; they progress to numbness, stiffness, and tingling of the hands and feet. There may be only a positive Chvostek or Trousseau sign or laryngeal and carpopedal spasms. Convulsions with loss of consciousness may occur at intervals of days, weeks, or months. These may begin with abdominal pain, followed by tonic rigidity, retraction of the head, and cyanosis. Hypoparathyroidism is frequently mistaken for epilepsy. Headache, vomiting, increased intracranial pressure, and papilledema may be associated with convulsions and may suggest a brain tumor.

The teeth erupt late and irregularly. Enamel formation is irregular, and the teeth may be unusually soft. The skin may be dry and scaly, and the nails of the fingers and toes may have horizontal lines. Manifestations of a wide variety of other disorders that are not direct consequences of PTH deficiency may also be seen. Mucocutaneous candidiasis, when present, antedates the development of hypoparathyroidism; the candidal infection most often involves the nails, the oral mucosa, the angles of the mouth, and less often, the skin.

Cataracts in patients with longstanding untreated disease are a direct consequence of hypoparathyroidism; other autoimmune ocular disorders such as keratoconjunctivitis may also occur. Manifestations of Addison disease, lymphocytic thyroiditis, pernicious anemia, alopecia areata or totalis, hepatitis, and primary gonadal insufficiency may also be associated with those of hypoparathyroidism.

Permanent physical and mental deterioration occur if initiation of treatment is long delayed.

LABORATORY DATA. The serum calcium level is low (5–7 mg/dL) and the phosphorus elevated (7–12 mg/dL). Blood levels of ionized calcium (approximately 45% of the total) more nearly reflect physiologic adequacy. The serum level of alkaline phosphatase is normal or low, and the level of $1,25[OH]_2D_3$ is usually low, but high levels have been found in some children with severe hypocalcemia. The level of magnesium is normal but should always be checked in hypocalcemic patients. By immunometric assay serum levels of PTH are low. Administration of the synthetic 1–34 fragment of human PTH (teriparatide acetate) results in increased urinary levels of cAMP and phosphate. This response differentiates hypoparathyroidism from pseudohypoparathyroidism. With the advent of very sensitive PTH assays, this test may no longer be necessary. Roentgenograms of the bones occasionally reveal an increased density limited to the metaphyses, suggestive of heavy metal poisoning, or an increased density of the lamina dura. Roentgenograms or computed tomography of the skull may reveal calcifications in the basal ganglia. There is a prolongation of the QT interval on the electrocardiogram, which disappears when the hypocalcemia is corrected. The electroencephalogram usually reveals widespread slow activity; the tracing returns to normal after the serum calcium has been within the normal range for a few weeks unless irreversible brain damage has occurred or unless the parathyroid insufficiency is associated with epilepsy. When hypoparathyroidism occurs concurrently with Addison disease, the serum level of calcium may be normal, but hypocalcemia appears after effective treatment of the adrenal insufficiency.

TREATMENT. Emergency treatment for neonatal tetany consists of intravenous injections of 5–10 mL of a 10% solution of calcium gluconate at the rate of 0.5–1 mL/min. Additionally, 1,25-dihydroxycholecalciferol (calcitrol) should be given. The initial dose is 0.25 μg/24 hr; the maintenance dose ranges from 0.01–0.10 μg/kg/24 hr, to a maximum of 1–2 μg/24 hr. Calcitrol has a short half-life and should be given in two equal divided doses; it has the advantages of rapid onset of effect (1–4 days) and rapid reversal of hypercalcemia after discontinuation in the event of overdosage (i.e., calcium begins to fall in 3–4 days).

After normocalcemia has been achieved, one may wish to continue therapy with vitamin D_2 because it is considerably less costly than calcitriol. The usual doses are 0.1–0.5 mg/24 hr in infants and young children. One milligram of vitamin D_2 has a biologic activity of 40,000 IU. Older children require 1.25–2.50 mg (50,000–100,000 IU) once daily. Vitamin D_2 has a slow onset of effect, and reversal of hypercalcemia after discontinuation of treatment is markedly delayed; its main advantage is its low cost.

An adequate intake of calcium should be ensured. Supplemental calcium can be given in the form of calcium gluconate or calcium glubionate (Neo-Calglucon) to provide 800 mg of elemental calcium daily, but it is rarely essential. Foods with a high phosphorus content such as milk, eggs, and cheese should be reduced in the diet.

Clinical evaluation of the patient and frequent determinations of the serum calcium levels are indicated in the early stages of treatment to determine the requirement for calcitriol or vitamin D_2. If hypercalcemia occurs, therapy should be discontinued and resumed at a lower dose after the serum calcium level has returned to normal. In longstanding cases, repair of cerebral and dental changes is not likely. Pigmentation, lowering of the blood pressure, or weight loss may indicate adrenal insufficiency, which requires specific treatment.

DIFFERENTIAL DIAGNOSIS. *Magnesium deficiency* must be considered in patients with unexplained hypocalcemia. Concentrations of magnesium in serum below 1.5 mg/dL (1.2 mEq/L) are usually abnormal. *Familial hypomagnesemia* with secondary hypocalcemia has been reported in 37 patients, most of whom developed tetany and seizures from 2–6 wk of age. Administration of calcium is ineffective, but administration of magnesium promptly corrects both calcium and magnesium levels. Oral supplements of magnesium are necessary to maintain levels of magnesium in the normal range. The profoundly low levels of magnesium result from a specific defect in intestinal absorption. The disorder appears to be caused by an autosomal recessive gene.

Hypomagnesemia also occurs in malabsorption syndromes and has occurred in granulomatous colitis and cystic fibrosis. Therapy with aminoglycosides causes hypomagnesemia by increasing urinary losses. Patients with autoimmune hypoparathyroidism may have concurrent steatorrhea and low magnesium levels.

It is not clear how low levels of magnesium lead to hypocalcemia. Evidence suggests that hypomagnesemia impairs release of PTH and induces resistance to the effects of the hormone, but other mechanisms also may be operative.

Poisoning with inorganic phosphate leads to hypocalcemia and tetany. Infants administered large doses of inorganic phosphates, either as laxatives or as sodium phosphate enemas, have had sudden onset of tetany, with serum calcium levels below 5 mg/dL and markedly elevated levels of phosphate. Symptoms are quickly relieved by intravenous administration of calcium. The mechanism of the hypocalcemia is not clear.

Hypocalcemia may occur early in the course of treatment of *acute lymphoblastic leukemia*. It is usually associated with hyperphosphatemia (resulting from destruction of lymphoblasts), which is probably the primary cause of hypocalcemia.

Episodic symptomatic hypocalcemia occurs in the *Kenny-Caffey syndrome*, which is characterized by medullary stenosis of the long bones, short stature, delayed closure of the fontanel, delayed bone age, and eye abnormalities. Idiopathic hypoparathyroidism and abnormal PTH levels have been found. Autosomal dominant and autosomal recessive modes of inheritance have been reported.

CHAPTER 526

Pseudohypoparathyroidism

(Albright Hereditary Osteodystrophy)

Angelo M. DiGeorge

In this syndrome, in contrast to the situation in idiopathic hypoparathyroidism, the parathyroid glands are normal or hyperplastic histologically, and they can synthesize and secrete parathyroid hormone (PTH). Serum levels of immunoreactive PTH are elevated when the patient is hypocalcemic. Neither endogenous nor administered PTH raises the serum levels of calcium or lowers the levels of phosphorus. The genetic defects in the hormone receptor–adenylate cyclase system are classified into various types depending on the phenotypic and biochemical findings.

TYPE IA. This type accounts for 50% of patients with pseudohypoparathyroidism (PHP). Affected patients have a genetic defect of the α subunit of the stimulatory guanine nucleotide–binding protein ($G_{s\alpha}$). This coupling factor is required for PTH bound to cell-surface receptors to activate cAMP. Heterogeneous mutations of the $G_{s\alpha}$ gene have been documented. Deficiency of the G unit is a generalized cellular defect and accounts for the association of other endocrine disorders with type IA PHP. The defect is inherited as an autosomal dominant trait, and the paucity of father-to-son transmissions is thought to be due to decreased fertility in males.

Tetany is often the presenting sign. Affected children have a short, stocky build and a round face. Brachydactyly with dimpling of the dorsum of the hand is usually present. The 2nd metacarpal is the least often involved. As a result, the index finger may occasionally be longer than the middle finger. Likewise, the 2nd metatarsal is only rarely affected. There may be other skeletal abnormalities such as short and wide phalanges, bowing, exostoses, and thickening of the calvaria. These patients frequently have calcium deposits and metaplastic bone formation subcutaneously. Moderate degrees of mental retardation, calcification of the basal ganglia, and lenticular cataracts are common in patients who are diagnosed late.

Some members of affected kindreds may have the usual anatomic stigmata of PHP, but serum levels of calcium and phosphorus are normal despite reduced $G_{s\alpha}$ activity and mutations in its gene. This variant of PHP type Ia is called *pseudopseudohypoparathyroidism*. Transition from the normocalcemic to the hypocalcemic form has been observed. These phenotypically similar but metabolically dissimilar patients also have mutations of $G_{s\alpha}$ protein. It is not known what other factors cause clinically overt hypocalcemia.

In addition to resistance to PTH, resistance to the metabolic effects of TSH, gonadotropins, and glucagon may be detected in patients with type IA PHP. Clinical hypothyroidism is uncommon, but basal levels of TSH are elevated, and TRH-stimulated TSH responses are exaggerated. Moderately decreased levels of thyroxine and increased levels of TSH have been detected in newborn thyroid screening programs, leading to the detection of type IA PHP in infancy. In adults, gonadal dysfunction is common, as manifested by sexual immaturity, amenorrhea, oligomenorrhea, and infertility. Each of these abnormalities can be related to deficient synthesis of cAMP secondary to a deficiency of $G_{s\alpha}$, but it is not clear why resistance to other G-protein–dependent hormones (e.g., corticotropin, vasopressin) is much less affected.

Serum levels of calcium are low, and those of phosphorus and alkaline phosphatase are elevated. Levels of both immunoreactive and bioactive PTH are elevated. Definitive diagnosis rests on the demonstration of a markedly attenuated response in urinary phosphate and cAMP after intravenous infusion of the synthetic 1–34 fragment of human PTH (teriparatide acetate).

Type IA with Precocious Puberty. Two boys with type IA PHP were reported to have gonadotropin-independent precocious puberty (see Chapter 517.6). They have a single mutation of $G_{s\alpha}$ rendering the G protein temperature sensitive. At normal body temperature (37° C), the $G_{s\alpha}$ is degraded, resulting in PHP, but in the cooler temperature of the testes (33° C), the $G_{s\alpha}$ results in constitutive activation of the luteinizing hormone receptor and precocious puberty.

TYPE IB. Affected patients have normal levels of G-protein activity and a normal phenotypic appearance. These patients have resistance to PTH but not to other hormones. Serum levels of calcium, phosphorus, and immunoreactive PTH are the same as those in patients with type IA PHP; however, bioactive PTH is not increased. The pathophysiology of the disorder in this group of patients is uncertain. Proposed explanations include production of a defective, biologically inactive hormone, presence of inhibitory PTH peptides, and a defect in the PTH receptor or in the catalytic subunit of adenyl cyclase. It is likely that the cause of the abnormality in this group is heterogeneous.

TYPE II. This type of pseudohypoparathyroidism has been detected in only a few patients and differs from type I in that the urinary excretion of cAMP is elevated both in the basal state and after stimulation with PTH, but phosphaturia does not increase. It appears that cAMP is normally activated, but the cell is unable to respond to the signal.

CHAPTER 527
Hyperparathyroidism

Angelo M. DiGeorge

Excessive production of parathyroid hormone (PTA) may result from a primary defect of the parathyroid glands such as an adenoma or hyperplasia *(primary hyperparathyroidism).*

More often, the increased production of PTH is compensatory, usually aimed at correcting hypocalcemic states of diverse origins *(secondary hyperparathyroidism).* In vitamin D–deficient rickets and in the malabsorption syndromes, intestinal absorption of calcium is deficient, but hypocalcemia and tetany may be averted by increased activity of the parathyroid glands. In pseudohypoparathyroidism, PTH levels are elevated because of mutation in the $G_{s\alpha}$ protein interferes with PTH response. Early in chronic renal disease, hyperphosphatemia results in a reciprocal fall in the calcium concentration with a consequent increase in PTH, but in advanced stages of renal failure, production of $1,25[OH]_2D_3$ is also decreased, leading to increased hypocalcemia and further stimulation of PTH. In some instances, if stimulation of the parathyroids has been sufficiently intense and protracted, the glands may continue to secrete increased levels of PTH for months or years after renal transplantation, with resulting hypercalcemia.

ETIOLOGY. *Primary hyperparathyroidism* is rare in children. When its onset occurs in the neonatal period, it is always caused by generalized hyperplasia of the parathyroid glands, but onset during childhood is usually the result of a single benign adenoma.

Neonatal primary hyperparathyroidism has been reported in fewer than 50 infants. Symptoms develop shortly after birth and consist of anorexia, irritability, lethargy, constipation, and failure to thrive. Roentgenograms reveal subperiosteal bone resorption, osteoporosis, and pathologic fractures. Symptoms may be mild, resolving without treatment, or may have a rapidly fatal course if diagnosis and treatment are delayed. Histologically, the parathyroid glands consist of diffuse hyperplasia. Affected siblings have been observed in three kindreds, and parental consanguinity has been reported in four kindreds.

Many affected infants have been in kindreds with the clinical and biochemical features of *familial hypocalciuric hypercalcemia* (FHH). These infants are homozygous for the mutation in the Ca^{2+}-sensing receptor gene; individuals with one copy of this mutation exhibit autosomally dominant familial hypocalciuric hypercalcemia.

Childhood hyperparathyroidism usually becomes manifest after 10 yr of age and is most frequently caused by a single adenoma. There have been many kindreds in which three or more members have hyperparathyroidism. In such cases of autosomal dominant hyperparathyroidism, most of the affected family members are adults, but children have been involved in about a third of the pedigrees. Some affected patients in these families are asymptomatic and are detected only by careful study. In some kindreds, hyperparathyroidism also occurs as part of the constellation known as the multiple endocrine neoplasia (MEN) syndromes.

MEN type I is an autosomal dominant disorder characterized by hyperplasia or neoplasia of the pancreatic islets (which secrete gastrin, insulin, pancreatic polypeptide, or occasionally glucagon), the anterior pituitary (which usually secretes prolactin), and the parathyroids. In most kindreds, hyperparathyroidism is usually the presenting manifestation, with a prevalence approaching 100% by 50 yr of age but occurring only rarely in children younger than 18 yr of age. In the past, after an affected family was identified, it was necessary to perform repeated metabolic screening for many years to detect other affected family members. With appropriate DNA probes, it is possible to detect carriers of the gene with 99% accuracy as early as birth, avoiding unnecessary biochemical screening programs.

The gene for MEN type I has been localized to 11q13. The gene appears to function as a tumor-suppressor gene and follows the two-hit hypothesis of tumor development. The 1st mutation (germinal) is inherited and is recessive to the dominant allele; this does not result in tumor formation. A 2nd mutation (somatic) is required to eliminate the normal allele, which leads to tumor formation.

MEN type II is also associated with hyperparathyroidism (see Chapter 524).

Transient neonatal hyperparathyroidism has occurred in a few infants born to mothers with hypoparathyroidism (idiopathic or surgical) or with pseudohypoparathyroidism. In each case, the maternal disorder had been undiagnosed or inadequately treated during pregnancy. The cause of the condition is chronic intrauterine exposure to hypocalcemia with resultant hyperplasia of the fetal parathyroid glands. In the newborn, manifestations involve the bones primarily, and healing occurs between 4 and 7 mo.

CLINICAL MANIFESTATIONS. At all ages, the clinical manifestations of hypercalcemia of any cause include muscular weakness, anorexia, nausea, vomiting, constipation, polydipsia, polyuria, loss of weight, and fever. Calcium may be deposited in the renal parenchyma (nephrocalcinosis), with progressively diminished renal function. Renal calculi are common and may produce renal colic and hematuria. Osseous changes may produce pain in the back or extremities, disturbances of gait, genu valgum, fractures, and tumors. Height may decrease from compression of vertebras; the patient may become bedridden. Completely asymptomatic patients are being detected with the use of automated serum calcium determinations.

Abdominal pain is occasionally prominent and may be associated with acute pancreatitis. Parathyroid crisis may occur, manifested by serum calcium levels greater than 15 mg/dL and progressive oliguria, azotemia, stupor, and coma. In infants, failure to thrive, poor feeding, and hypotonia are common. Mental retardation, convulsions, and blindness may occur as sequelae.

LABORATORY DATA. The serum calcium level is elevated; 39 of 45 children with adenomas had levels over 12 mg/dL. The hypercalcemia is more severe in infants with parathyroid hyperplasia; concentrations ranging from 15–20 mg/dL are common, and values as high as 30 mg/dL have been reported. Ionized (Ca^{2+}) calcium levels are often elevated, even when total serum calcium is borderline or only slightly elevated. The serum phosphorus level is reduced to about 3 mg/dL or less, and the level of serum magnesium is low. The urine may have a low and fixed specific gravity, and serum levels of nonprotein nitrogen and uric acid may be elevated. In patients with adenomas who have skeletal involvement, serum phosphatase is elevated, but in infants with hyperplasia the levels of alkaline phosphatase may be normal even when there is extensive involvement of bone.

Serum levels of PTH measured by carboxy-terminal antisera are elevated, especially in relation to the level of calcium. Results may vary markedly from one laboratory to another, depending on the antibody used. Calcitonin levels are normal.

Acute hypercalcemia can stimulate calcitonin release, but with prolonged hypercalcemia, hypercalcitoninemia does not occur.

The most consistent and characteristic roentgenographic findings are resorption of subperiosteal bone, best seen along the margins of the phalanges of the hands. In the skull, there may be gross trabeculation or a granular appearance resulting from focal rarefaction; the lamina dura may be absent. In more advanced disease, there may be generalized rarefaction, cysts, tumors, fractures, and deformities. About 10% of patients have roentgenographic signs of rickets. Roentgenograms of the abdomen may reveal renal calculi or nephrocalcinosis.

DIFFERENTIAL DIAGNOSIS. *Hypercalcemia* of any origin results in a similar clinical pattern; other causes must be differentiated from hyperparathyroidism (Table 527–1). A low serum phosphorus level with hypercalcemia is characteristic of primary hyperparathyroidism; elevated levels of PTH are also diagnostic. With hypercalcemia of any cause except hyperparathyroidism and familial hypocalciuric hypercalcemia, PTH levels are suppressed. Pharmacologic doses of corticosteroids lower the serum calcium level to normal in patients with hypercalcemia from other causes but generally do not affect the calcium level in patients with hyperparathyroidism.

TREATMENT. Surgical exploration is indicated in all instances. All glands should be carefully inspected; if an adenoma is discovered, it should be removed; very few instances of carcinoma are known in children. Most neonates with severe hypercalcemia require total parathyroidectomy; less severe hypercalcemia may remit spontaneously in others. A portion of a parathyroid gland may be autografted into the forearm; four infants treated in this fashion were able to maintain normocalcemia without supplementary treatment, but no long-term outcome has yet been reported. The patient should be carefully observed postoperatively for the development of hypocalcemia and tetany; intravenous administration of calcium gluconate may be required for a few days. The serum calcium level then gradually returns to normal, and under ordinary circumstances, a diet high in calcium and phosphorus needs to be maintained for only several months after operation.

■ TABLE 527–1 Etiologic Classification of Hypercalcemia

- Parathyroid hormone (PTH) excess
  - Primary hyperparathyroidism
    - Adenoma
      - Sporadic
      - Autosomal dominant
    - Hyperplasia or adenoma
      - MEN type I—autosomal dominant; mutation in phospholipase Cβ3 gene
      - MEN type IIA—autosomal dominant; mutation in *RET* proto-oncogene
    - Parathyroid hyperplasia of infancy
      - Homozygous mutation of CA^{2+}-sensing receptor
      - Secondary to maternal hypoparathyroidism
    - Ectopic PTH production
      - Nonendocrine malignancies
- Parathyroid hormone–related peptide (PTHrP) excess
  - Nonendocrine malignancies
  - Benign hypertrophy of breasts
- CA^{2+}-sensing receptor inactivating mutation
  - Heterozygous—familial hypocalciuric hypercalcemia (FHH)
  - Homozygous—neonatal hyperparathyroidism
- Vitamin D excess
  - Iatrogenic
  - Ectopic production
    - Sarcoidosis, tuberculosis, granulomatous lesions, subcutaneous fat necrosis
- Vitamin D sensitivity (?)
  - Idiopathic hypercalcemia of infancy
  - Williams syndrome
- Other
  - Hypophosphatasia
  - Prolonged immobilization
  - Jansen-type metaphyseal chondrodysplasia: mutant PTH-PTHrP receptor
  - Thyrotoxicosis
  - Hypervitaminosis A

Arteriography and selective venous sampling with radioimmunoassay of PTH for preoperative localization and for differentiation of a single adenoma from hyperplasia have been replaced by imaging methods. Computed tomography, real-time ultrasound, and subtraction scintigraphy using ^{99m}Tc pertechnetate and ^{201}Tl have each proved effective in 50–90% of adults. These procedures are rarely required by the expert parathyroid surgeon but may be advisable before re-exploration in cases of persistent or recurrent hyperparathyroidism.

PROGNOSIS. The prognosis is good if the disease is recognized early and there is appropriate surgical treatment. When extensive osseous lesions are present, deformities may be permanent; with renal disease the prognosis is less hopeful. A search for other affected family members is indicated.

Other Causes of Hypercalcemia

FAMILIAL HYPOCALCIURIC HYPERCALCEMIA (FAMILIAL BENIGN HYPERCALCEMIA). Patients with this disorder are usually asymptomatic, and the hypercalcemia comes to light by chance during routine investigation for other conditions. The parathyroid glands are normal, PTH levels are inappropriately normal, and subtotal parathyroidectomy does not correct the hypercalcemia. Serum levels of magnesium are high normal or mildly elevated. The rate of calcium to creatinine clearance is usually decreased despite hypercalcemia. The disorder is inherited in an autosomal dominant manner and is caused by a mutant gene on chromosome 3q2. Penetrance is near 100%, and affected individuals can be diagnosed early in childhood by serum and urinary calcium concentrations. Detection of other affected family members is important to avoid inappropriate parathyroid surgery. The basic defect in this condition results from inactivating mutations in the CA^{2+}-sensing receptor gene. This G-protein–coupled receptor senses the level of free CA^{2+} in the blood and triggers the pathway to increase intracellular CA^{2+}. It appears that this receptor functions in the parathyroid and kidney to regulate calcium homeostasis; inactivating mutations lead to resistance to extracellular Ca^{2+} with mild to moderate hypercalcemia in heterozygotes.

GRANULOMATOUS DISEASES. Hypercalcemia occurs in 30–50% of children with sarcoidosis and less often in patients with other granulomatous diseases such as tuberculosis. Levels of PTH are suppressed, and levels of $1,25[OH]_2D_3$ are elevated. The source of ectopic $1,25[OH]_2D_3$ is the activated macrophage, through stimulation by interferon α from T lymphocytes, which are present in abundance in granulomatous lesions. Unlike renal tubular cells, the 1α-hydroxylase in macrohages is unresponsive to homeostatic regulation. Oral administration of prednisone (2 mg/kg/24 hr) lowers serum levels of $1,25[OH]_2D_3$ to normal and corrects the hypercalcemia.

HYPERCALCEMIA OF MALIGNANCY. Hypercalcemia frequently occurs in adults with a wide variety of solid tumors but is identified much less often in children. It has been reported in infants with malignant rhabdoid tumors of the kidney or congenital mesoblastic nephroma and in children with neuroblastoma, medulloblastoma, leukemia, Burkitt lymphoma, and rhabdomyosarcoma. Serum levels of PTH are rarely elevated. In most patients, the hypercalcemia associated with malignancy is caused by elevated levels of PTHrP. Rarely, tumors produce $1,25[OH]_2D_3$ or PTH ectopically.

MISCELLANEOUS CAUSES OF HYPERCALCEMIA. Hypercalcemia may occur in infants with *subcutaneous fat necrosis.* Levels of PTH are normal. In one infant, the level of $1,25[OH]_2D$ was elevated, and biopsy of the skin lesion revealed granulomatous infiltration, suggesting that the mechanism of the hypercalcemia was akin to that seen in patients with other granulomatous disease. In another infant, although $1,25[OH]_2D$ was normal, PTH was suppressed, suggesting the hypercalcemia was not PTH related. Treatment with prednisone is effective.

Hypophosphatasia, especially the severe infantile form, is usually associated with mild to moderate hypercalcemia. Serum levels of phosphorus are normal, and those of alkaline phosphatase are subnormal. The bones exhibit rachitic-like lesions on roentgenograms. Urinary levels of phosphoethanolamine, inorganic pyrophosphate, and pyridoxal 5′-phosphate are elevated; each is a natural substrate to a tissue-nonspecific (liver, bone, kidney) alkaline phosphatase enzyme. Missense mutations of the gene result in an inactive enzyme in this autosomal recessive disorder.

Idiopathic hypercalcemia of infancy is manifested by failure to thrive and hypercalcemia during the 1st yr of life followed by spontaneous remission. Serum levels of phosphorus and PTH are normal. The hypercalcemia results from increased absorption of calcium. Vitamin D may be involved in the pathogenesis. Both normal and elevated levels of $1,25[OH]_2D$ have been reported. An excessive rise in the level of $1,25[OH]_2D$ in response to PTH administration years after the hypercalcemic phase suggests that vitamin D has a role in the pathogenesis. A blunted calcitonin response to intravenous calcium has also been reported.

Williams syndrome is frequently associated with infantile hypercalcemia. The phenotype consists of feeding difficulties, slow growth, an elfin facies, renovascular disorders, and a gregarious personality. The IQ scores of 50 to 70 is curiously accompanied by enhanced quantity and quality of vocabulary, auditory memory, and social use of language. A submicroscopic deletion at chromosome 7q11.23, which includes deletion of one elastin allele, occurs in 90% of patients and seems to account for the vascular problems. The hypercalcemia and central nervous system symptoms may be caused by deletion of adjacent genes. Hypercalcemia has been successfully controlled with either prednisone or calcitonin.

Hypervitaminosis D resulting in hypercalcemia from drinking milk incorrectly fortified with vitamin D has been reported. Serum levels of 25[OH]D is a better indicator of hypervitaminosis D than $1,25[OH]_2D$ because of its longer half-life.

Prolonged immobilization may lead to hypercalcemia and occasionally to decreased renal function, hypertension, and encephalopathy.

Jansen-type metaphyseal chondrodysplasia is associated with asymptomatic hypercalcemia and hypophosphatemia; a constitutively active mutant PTH-PTHrP receptor appears to be the cause.

Ahonen P, Myllarniemi S, Sipla I, Perheentupa J: Clinical variation of autoimmune polyendocrinopathy-candidiasis-ectodermal dystrophy (APECED) in a series of 68 patients. N Engl J Med 322:1829, 1990.
Berliner BC, Shenker IR, Weinstock MS: Hypercalcemia associated with hypertension due to prolonged immobilization. (An unusual complication of extensive burns.) Pediatrics 49:92, 1972.
Bilaus RW, Murty G, Parkinson DB, et al: Brief report: Autosomal dominant familial hypoparathyroidism, sensorineural deafness, and renal dysplasia. N Engl J Med 327:1069, 1992.
Body JJ, Chanoine JP, Dumon JC, Delange F: Circulating calcitonin levels in healthy children and subjects with hypothyroidism from birth to adolescence. J Clin Endocrinol Metab 77:565, 1993.
Bronsky D, Kiamko RT, Moncado R, et al: Intrauterine hyperparathyroidism secondary to maternal hypoparathyroidism. Pediatrics 42:606, 1968.
Burtis WJ, Brady TG, Orloff JJ, et al: Immunochemical characterization of circulating parathyroid hormone-related protein in patients with hormonal hypercalcemia of cancer. N Engl J Med 322:1106, 1990.
Clapman DS: Why testicles are cool. Nature 371:109, 1994.
Chesney RW: Requirements and upper limits of vitamin D intake in the term neonate, infant, and older child. J Pediatr 116:159, 1990.
Cook JS, Stone MS, Hansen JR: Hypercalcemia in association with subcutaneous fat necrosis of the newborn: Studies of calcium-regulating hormones. Pediatr 90:93, 1992.
Cooper L, Wertheimer J, Levey R, et al: Severe primary hyperparathyroidism in a neonate with two hypercalcemic parents: Management with parathyroidectomy and heterotopic autotransplantation. Pediatrics 78:263, 1986.
Culler FL, Jones KL, Deltos LJ: Impaired calcitonin secretion in patients with Williams syndrome. J Pediatr 107:720, 1985.
Davis RF, Eichner JM, Bleyer WA, et al: Hypocalcemia, hyperphosphatemia, and dehydration following a single hypertonic phosphate enema. J Pediatr 90:484, 1977.
DePapp AS, Stewart AF: Parathyroid hormone related protein. A peptide of diverse physiologic functions. Trends Endocrinol Metab 4:181, 1993.
DiGeorge AM: Congenital absence of the thymus and its immunologic consequences, concurrence with congenital hypoparathyroidism. *In*: Bergsma D, Good RA (eds): Birth Defects. Original Article Series, No. 1, Vol. IV. New York, The National Foundation, 1968.
Driscoll DA, Budarf ML, Emanuel BS: A genetic etiology for DiGeorge syndrome: Consistent deletions and microdeletions of 22q11. Am J Hum Genet 50:924, 1992.
Ewart AK, Morris CA, Atkinson D, et al: Hemizygosity at the elastin locus in a developmental disorder, Williams syndrome. Nature Genet 5:11, 1993.
Finegold DN, Armitage MM, Galiani M, et al: Preliminary localization of a gene for autosomal dominant hypoparathyroidism to chromosome 3q13. Pediatr Res 36:414, 1994.
Fitch N: Albright's hereditary osteodystrophy: A review. Am J Med Genet 11:11, 1982.
Franceschini P, Testa A, Bogetti G, et al: Kenny-Caffey syndrome in two sibs born to consanguineous parents: Evidence for an autosomal recessive variant. Am J Med Gen 42:112, 1992.
Goodyear PR, Frank A, Kaplan BS: Observations on the evolution and treatment of idiopathic infantile hypercalcemia. J Pediatr 105:771, 1984.
Green CG, Doershuk CF, Stern RC: Symptomatic hypomagensemia in cystic fibrosis. J Pediatr 107:425, 1985.
Hanukoglu A, Chalew S, Kowarski AA: Late-onset hypocalcemia, rickets and hypoparathyroidism in an infant of a mother with hyperparathyroidism. J Pediatr 112:751, 1988.
Iiri T, Herzmark P, Nakimoto JM, et al: Rapid GDP release from $G_{s\alpha}$ in patients with gain and loss of endocrine function. Nature 371:164, 1994.
Jacabus CH, Holick MF, Shao G, et al: Hypervitaminosis D associated with drinking milk. N Engl J Med 326:1173, 1992.
Key LL, Thorne M, Pitzer B, et al: Management of neonatal hyperparathyroidism with parathyroidectomy and autotransplantation. J Pediatr 116:923, 1990.
Khosla S, Johansen KL, Ory SJ, et al: Parathyroid hormone-related peptide in lactation and in umbilical cord blood. Mayo Clin Proc 65:1408, 1990.
Kao PC, van Heerden JA, Taylor RL: Intraoperative monitoring of parathyroid procedures by a 15-minute parathyroid hormone immunochemiluminometric assay. Mayo Clin Proc 69:532, 1994.
Larsson C, Shepard J, Nakamura Y, et al: Predictive testing for multiple endocrine neoplasia type I using DNA polymorphism. J Clin Invest 89:1344, 1992.
Law WM Jr, Bollman S, Kumar R, et al: Vitamin D metabolism in familial benign hypercalcemia (hypocalciuric hypercalcemia) differs from that in primary hyperparathyroidism. J Clin Endocrinol Metab 58:744, 1984.
Levine MA, Downs RW Jr, Moses AM, et al: Resistance to multiple hormones in patients with pseudohypoparathyroidism. Association with deficient activity of guanine nucleotide regulatory protein. Am J Med 74:545, 1983.
Levitt M, Gessert C, Finberg L: Inorganic phosphate (laxative) poisoning resulting in tetany in an infant. J Pediatr 82:479, 1973.
Lund B, Soresen OH, Lund B, et al: Vitamin D metabolism in hypoparathyroidism. J Clin Endocrinol Metab 51:606, 1980.
Mallette LE: Synthetic human parathyroid hormone 1–34 fragment for diagnostic testing. Ann Intern Med 109:800, 1988.
Markowitz ME, Rosen JF, Smith C, et al: 1,25-Dihydroxyvitamin D_3-treated hypoparathyroidism: 35 patient years in 10 children. J Clin Endocrinol Metab 55:727, 1982.
Martin TJ, Suva LJ: Parathyroid hormone-related protein in hypercalcaemia of malignancy. Clin Endocrinol 31:631, 1989.
Marx SJ: Familial multiple endocrine neoplasia type 1. Mutation of a tumor suppressor gene. Trends Endocrinol Metab 76:82, 1989.
McKay C, Furman WL: Hypercalcemia complicating childhood malignancies. Cancer 72:256, 1993.
Miller RR, Menke JA, Mentser MI: Hypercalcemia associated with phosphate depletion in the neonate. J Pediatr 105:814, 1984.
Miric A, Vechio JD, Levine MA: Heterogeneous mutations in the gene encoding the α-subunit of the stimulatory G protein of adenylyl cyclase in Albright hereditary osteodystrophy. J Clin Endocrinol Metab 76:1560, 1993.
Morris CA, Demsey SA, Leonard CD, et al: Natural history of Williams syndrome: Physical characteristics. J Pediatr 113:318, 1988.
Patten JL, Johns DR, Valle D, et al: Mutation in the gene encoding the stimulating G protein of adenylate cyclase in Albright's hereditary osteodystrophy. N Engl J Med 322:1412, 1990.
Pollak MR, Brown EM, WuChou YH, et al: Mutations in the human Ca^{2+}-sensing receptor gene cause familial hypocalciuric hypercalcemia and neonatal severe hyperthyroidism. Cell 75:1297, 1993.
Pollak MR, WuChou YH, Marx SJ, et al: Familial hypocalciuric hypercalcemia and neonatal severe hyperparathyroidism. Effects of mutant gene dosage on phenotype. J Clin Invest 93:1108, 1994.
Pronicka E, Gruszczynska B: Familial hypomagnesemia with secondary hypocalcemia—autosomal or X-linked inheritance? J Inherit Metab Dis 14:397–399, 1991.
Radeke HH, Auf'mkolk B, Juppner H, et al: Multiple pre- and postreceptor defects in pseudohypoparathyroidism (a multicenter study with twenty-four patients). J Clin Endocrinol Metab 62:393, 1986.
Rapaport D, Rubin ZM, Huminer D, et al: Primary hyperparathyroidism in children. J Pediatr Surg 21:395, 1986.
Reichel H, Koeffler HP, Norman AW: The role of the vitamin D endocrine system in health and disease. N Engl J Med 320:980, 1989.

Richardson RJ, Kirk JMW: Short stature, mental retardation and hypoparathyroidism: a new syndrome. Arch Dis Child 65:1113, 1990.
Ross AJ III, Cooper A, Attie MF, et al: Primary hyperparathyroidism in infancy. J Pediatr Surg 21:493, 1986.
Sanjad SA, Sakati NA, Abu-Osba YK, et al: A new syndrome of congenital hypoparathyroidism, severe growth failure and dysmorphic features. Arch Dis Child 66:193, 1992.
Schipani E, Kruse K, Juppner H: A constitutively activated mutant PTH-PTHrP receptor in Jansen-type metaphyseal chondrodysplasia. Science 268:98, 1995.
Song YH, Connor EL, Muir A, et al: Autoantibody epitope mapping of the 21-hydroxylase antigen in autoimmune Addison's disease. J Clin Endocrinol Metab 78:1108, 1994.
Stewart AF, Broadus A: Parathyroid hormone-related proteins: Coming of age in the 1990's. J Clin Endocrinol Metab 71:1410, 1990.
Taylor AB, Stern PH, Bell NH: Abnormal regulation of circulating 25-hydroxyvitamin D in the Williams syndrome. N Engl J Med 306:972, 1982.
Whyte MP, Weldon VV: Idiopathic hypoparathyroidism presenting with seizures during infancy: X-linked recessive inheritance in a large Missouri kindred. J Pediatr 99:608, 1981.
Whyte MP: Hypophosphatasia and the role of alkaline phosphatase in skeletal mineralization. Rev 15:439, 1994.
Wilson DI, Burn J, Scambler P, Goodship J: DiGeorge syndrome: Part of CATCH 22. J Med Genet 30:852, 1993.
Winter WE, Silverstein JH, MacLaren NK, et al: Autosomal dominant hypoparathyroidism with variable, age-dependent severity. J Pediatr 103:387, 1983.
Young TO, Satzstein EC, Boman DA: Parathyroid carcinoma in a child: Unusual presentation with seizures. J Pediatr Surg 19:194, 1984.

SECTION 4

Disorders of the Adrenal Glands

Angelo M. DiGeorge ■ Lenore S. Levine

The adrenal gland is composed of two endocrine systems, the medullary and the cortical systems. Mesodermal cells contribute to the development of the adrenal cortex, the gonads, and the liver; these three tissues are active in steroid metabolism in the fetus. Adrenals and gonads have in common certain enzymes involved in steroid synthesis, and an inborn defect in one tissue may also involve the other.

At about the 7th wk of gestation, the primordium of the adrenal cortex is invaded by sympathetic neural elements. About 1 wk later, these cells begin to differentiate into the chromaffin cells capable of synthesizing and storing catecholamines; the methyl transferase, which converts norepinephrine to epinephrine, develops later.

In a fetus of 2 mo, the adrenals are larger than the kidneys, but from the 4th mo, the kidneys grow rapidly, becoming about twice as large as the adrenals by the end of the 6th mo. In the full-term infant, the adrenal gland is one third the size of the kidney, and the combined weight of both glands is 7–9 g.

The adrenal cortex in the fetus and the newborn infant has two histologically distinct components: an outer portion, called the true cortex, and a more central portion, called the "fetal cortex." At birth, the fetal cortex makes up about 80% of the gland. Within a few days, it begins to involute, undergoing a 50% reduction by 2 wk of age and disappearing completely by about 6 mo of age. The major steroids produced by the fetal cortex are dehydroepiandrosterone (DHEA) and its sulfurylated derivative (DHEAS).

The true cortex consists of three zones. In the zona glomerulosa, situated beneath the capsule, there is an alveolar arrangement of the cells; in the broader zona fasciculata, the columns of cells are radially arranged; in the zona reticularis, the cells form a network next to the medulla.

FETOPLACENTAL UNIT. Until near the end of gestation, the fetal adrenal does not possess the 3β-hydroxysteroid dehydrogenase necessary to form progesterone; it uses placental pregnenolone to synthesize cortisol, aldosterone, and particularly DHEAS. The placenta uses the fetal DHEAS to produce estrone and estriol. Estriol is the major estrogen found in maternal urine in pregnancy, especially in the late stages. In instances of fetal adrenal hypoplasia, maternal urinary estriol levels are markedly reduced.

ADRENAL CORTEX. The adrenal cortex secretes various steroid compounds essential to life. Studies indicate that the zona fasciculata and zona glomerulosa behave as two separate glands: corticotropin (ACTH) primarily stimulates the zona fasciculata to secrete cortisol and androgens; the zona glomerulosa is involved primarily in synthesis of aldosterone. The primary stimuli of the zona glomerulosa are the renin-angiotensin system and potassium.

Glucocorticoids have a 21-carbon structure and are produced by the zona fasciculata; they are also referred to as 17-hydroxycorticosteroids or simply as corticosteroids. The principal one is cortisol, also known as compound F or hydrocortisone. Cortisol can be interconverted to cortisone by the enzyme 11β-hydroxysteroid dehydrogenase (11β-OHSD) in peripheral tissues; surprisingly, a deficiency of this enzyme results in heritable forms of apparent mineralocorticoid excess (see Chapter 531).

Glucocorticoids affect the metabolism of most tissues. They attach to specific intracellular receptor proteins, which then bind to the cell nucleus to influence RNA and protein synthesis. Steroid hormone receptors may be found in the cystolic and nuclear fractions of a tissue homogenate. The receptors for glucocorticoids (type II) and mineralocorticoids (type I) are very similar. The type I receptor binds mineralocorticoids and glucocorticoids. It appears that the mineralocorticoid-responsive tissues (e.g., kidney), by converting cortisol to cortisone, exclude the glucocorticoid from the type I receptor. Specificity depends on prereceptor enzyme activity. In many tissues, glucocorticoids have a catabolic effect, resulting in increased degradation of protein; primarily affected are muscles, skin, and connective, adipose, and lymphoid tissues. Glucocorticoids are anabolic in the liver, where they stimulate a number of enzymes, increase protein and glycogen content, and enhance its capacity for gluconeogenesis. Patients with cortisol excess (e.g., Cushing syndrome) have increased glucose production, and those with deficiency of cortisol (Addison disease) have decreased gluconeogenesis, with hypoglycemia. The effects of insulin and androgens are antagonistic to those of glucocorticoids. Glucocorticoids have effects on the immune and nervous systems.

The 17-hydroxycorticosteroids are excreted in urine; cortisol itself is also excreted in urine in amounts less than 1% of the adrenal production. Levels of cortisol and of its precursors and metabolites can be measured by radioimmunoassay and by high-performance liquid chromatography (HPLC) in biologic fluids and tumor tissues. Levels of cortisol in plasma vary with the time of day; after the first few years of life, a circadian rhythm follows that of ACTH.

Glucocorticoid synthesis is regulated primarily by ACTH, with cortisol exerting negative feedback on ACTH secretion. One of the major regulators of ACTH is corticotropin-releasing hormone (CRH).

Many synthetic analogs of cortisone and hydrocortisone are available. Derivatives with an additional double bond in ring A are known as prednisone and prednisolone. They are four times as potent in anti-inflammatory and carbohydrate activity as the natural steroids but have less effect on salt and water retention. Halogenated derivatives have different effects; 9α-fluorohydrocortisone has approximately 15 times more anti-inflammatory activity than hydrocortisone but is more than 125 times as active in salt and water retention. Betamethasone and dexamethasone are approximately 25 times as potent as cortisol and have little effect on the retention of water and electrolytes. These analogs are usually used in pharmacologic doses for their anti-inflammatory or immunosuppressive properties.

Aldosterone, a potent mineralocorticoid, is the 18-aldehyde of corticosterone and is produced primarily in the zona glomerulosa. Its secretion is regulated by activation of the renin-angiotensin system. Renin produced by the juxtaglomerular apparatus of the kidney reacts with renin substrate, an α_2-globulin produced by the liver, to yield the inactive decapeptide, angiotensin. A converting enzyme rapidly changes angiotensin I to the biologically active octapeptide, angiotensin II. Angiotensin II is a pressor agent 50 times more potent than norepinephrine. One of its main functions is to act directly on the adrenal cortex to stimulate the secretion of aldosterone.

In a person with good health and a normal dietary intake, ACTH plays a minor role in the regulation of aldosterone secretion, but under some conditions, as in an anephric man, it may have a more significant effect. Potassium may be equally important in the regulation of aldosterone secretion as the renin-angiotensin system. In studies of aldosterone secretion, dietary potassium and sodium must be rigidly controlled. Aldosterone and renin activity in plasma can be measured by radioimmunoassay.

Sodium deprivation is a potent stimulus to secretion of aldosterone. Changes in intake of sodium result in small changes in blood volume, arterial pressure, and renal blood flow. These changes are sensitively monitored by the juxtaglomerular cells on the renal afferent arterioles, which form the receptor site or volume receptor. Activation of the juxtaglomerular apparatus results in increased output of renin, followed by increased secretion of aldosterone.

The principal action of aldosterone is the maintenance of electrolyte equilibrium, which in turn contributes to the stabilization of blood volume and blood pressure. Aldosterone controls sodium reabsorption (and hence water reabsorption) in the distal tubule of the kidney.

Androgens are produced by the zona fasciculata and zona reticularis. They are capable of increasing retention of nitrogen, potassium, phosphorus, and sulfate. They promote growth and have androgenic effects, which are most conspicuous when adrenal hyperplasia or adrenal tumors induce precocious growth and development of male secondary sex characteristics. The adrenal androgens seem to be partly responsible for the development of axillary and pubic hair in the female.

DHEAS is the most abundant adrenal androgen in the circulation. It is derived from adrenal secretion or from peripheral sulfation of DHEA secreted by the adrenal. DHEAS levels are low during childhood but begin to rise before the other hormonal changes of puberty take place in a process called adrenarche. The zona reticularis is probably the major source of these adrenarcheal changes. Aside from a relationship of these hormones to the growth of sexual hair, their function remains unknown; they do not appear to be an initiator of puberty. Levels are low in patients with Addison disease and in those with adrenal insufficiency secondary to ACTH deficiency. However, administration of ACTH does not acutely increase DHEAS levels, indicating that it is not the corticotropic hormone that initiates adrenarche. For many years, a separate adrenal cortical androgen–stimulating hormone (CASH) has been proposed but has not yet been identified. Marked elevations of DHEAS occur in patients with virilizing adrenal cortical tumors, lesser elevations occur in patients with congenital adrenal hyperplasia, and modest elevations occur in children with isolated precocious adrenarche.

ADRENAL MEDULLA. The principal hormones of the adrenal medulla are the physiologically active catecholamines: dopamine, norepinephrine, and epinephrine. The sequence of their biosynthetic reactions is shown in Figure 533–1. Catecholamine synthesis occurs also in the brain, in sympathetic nerve endings, and in chromaffin tissue outside the adrenal medulla. Metabolites of catecholamines are excreted in the urine. The principal ones are 3-methoxy-4-hydroxy-mandelic acid (VMA), metanephrine, and normetanephrine. Measurement of metanephrines and catecholamines is used to detect functioning tumors of the adrenal medulla.

The proportions of epinephrine and norepinephrine in the adrenal vary with age. In early fetal stages there is practically no epinephrine, and even at birth norepinephrine is predominant. In adults norepinephrine makes up only 10–30% of the pressor amines in the medulla. Both epinephrine and norepinephrine raise the mean arterial blood pressure, norepinephrine without changing the cardiac output. By increasing peripheral vascular resistance, norepinephrine increases systolic and diastolic blood pressures with only a slight reduction in the pulse rate. Epinephrine increases the pulse rate and, by decreasing the peripheral vascular resistance, decreases the diastolic pressure. The hyperglycemic and calorigenic effects of norepinephrine are much less pronounced than those of epinephrine. ■

CHAPTER 528
Adrenocortical Insufficiency

Deficient production of cortisol or aldosterone may result from a wide variety of congenital or acquired lesions of the hypothalamus, pituitary, or adrenal cortex (Table 528–1). Depending on the pathologic lesions, symptoms may be severe or mild, appear abruptly or insidiously, begin in infancy or later, and be permanent or temporary.

ETIOLOGY. Corticotropin Deficiency. Congenital hypoplasia or aplasia of the pituitary is almost always associated with secondary hypoplasia of the adrenals as well as with other hormonal deficiencies. These congenital defects are usually associated with abnormalities of the skull and brain such as anencephaly and holoprosencephaly. Such infants have a considerable residuum of pituitary function, and the hypoplasia of the pituitary is probably secondary to a hypothalamic deficiency of corticotropin-releasing hormone (CRH). The adrenals are characteristically small with normal architecture, a well-defined permanent zone, and a reduced fetal zone. The disorder is usually sporadic, although a few cases of autosomal recessive inheritance have occurred. Isolated deficiency of corticotropin (ACTH) has been reported, including in several sets of siblings. Idiopathic hypopituitarism and destructive lesions in the area of the pituitary, such as craniopharyngioma, are the most common causes of corticotropin deficiency; the defect is in the hypothalamus in many patients. Isolated deficiency of CRH has been documented in an Arabic kindred as an autosomal recessive trait. In rare instances, autoimmune hypophysitis has been the cause of corticotropin deficiency.

Adrenal Hypoplasia Congenita (AHC). Onset of hypoadrenalism usually begins in the neonatal period but may be delayed to 10 yr of age; marked intrafamilial variability of onset has been reported in several instances. Increasing pigmentation, salt-losing symptoms, and low levels of all adrenal steroids are the presenting manifestations. Histologic examination of the hypoplastic adrenal cortex reveals disorganization and cytomegaly, findings not present in the adrenals from corticotropin-deficient patients. The disorder affects primarily boys and has been shown to be caused by a mutation of the DAX-1 gene, a new member of the nuclear hormone receptor family, located on Xp21. It has been known for 20 years that boys with AHC do not undergo puberty owing to hypogonadotropic hypogonadism (HHG), but the reason for this association has been unclear. It is now clear that both AHC and HHG are caused by the same mutated DAX-1 gene. Cryptorchidism, often noted in these boys, is probably an early manifestation of HHG.

AHC also occurs as part of a contiguous deletion syndrome together with Duchenne muscular dystrophy and/or glycerol kinase deficiency.

Familial Glucocorticoid Deficiency. This form of chronic adrenal insufficiency is characterized by isolated deficiency of glucocorticoids, elevated levels of ACTH, and normal aldosterone production. The salt-losing manifestations of most other forms of adrenal insufficiency do not occur; instead, patients present primarily with hypoglycemia, seizures, and pigmentation during the 1st decade of life. The disorder affects both sexes equally and is inherited in an autosomal recessive manner.

■ TABLE 528–1 Etiologic Classification of Adrenocortical Hypofunction

- Corticotropin-releasing hormone deficiency
  - Isolated deficiency
  - Multiple deficiencies
    - Congenital defects (e.g., anencephaly, septo-optic dysplasia)
    - Destructive lesions (e.g., tumor)
    - Idiopathic (e.g., idiopathic hypopituitarism)
- Corticotropin deficiency
  - Isolated
  - Autosomal recessive
  - Multiple deficiencies
    - Pituitary hypoplasia or aplasia
    - Destructive lesions (e.g., craniopharyngioma)
    - Autoimmune hypophysitis
- Primary adrenal hypoplasia or aplasia
  - X-linked
    - With Duchenne muscular dystrophy and glycerol kinase deficiency (Xp21 deletion)
    - With hypogonadotropic hypogonadism (DAX-1 mutation)
- Familial glucocorticoid deficiency
  - Corticotropin-receptor mutations
  - With alacrima, achalasia, and neurologic disorders (triple A syndrome)
- Defects of steroid biosynthesis
  - Lipoid adrenal hyperplasia ($P450_{SCC}$ deficiency)
  - Mutation of steroidogenic acute regulatory protein (StAR)
  - 3β-Hydroxysteroid dehydrogenase deficiency
    - Classic
      - Salt loser
      - Non–salt loser
    - Mild or non-classic
    - Mild
  - 21-Hydroxylase ($P450_{C21}$) deficiency
    - Classic
      - Salt loser
      - Non–salt loser
  - Isolated aldosterone ($P450_{C18}$) deficiency
- Pseudohypoaldosteronism—aldosterone unresponsiveness
- Adrenoleukodystrophy (peroxisomal membrane protein defect)
  - Isolated adrenal involvement
  - With neurologic involvement
- Acid lipase deficiency
  - Wolman disease, fatal neonatal form
- Destructive lesions of adrenal cortex
  - Granulomatous lesions (e.g., tuberculosis)
- Autoimmune adrenalitis (idiopathic Addison disease)
  - Isolated
    - Associated with hypoparathyroidism and/or mucocutaneous candidiasis (type I autoimmune polyglandular syndrome)
    - Associated with autoimmune thyroid disease and insulin-dependent diabetes (type II autoimmune polyglandular syndrome)
- Neonatal hemorrhage
- Acute infection (Waterhouse-Friderichsen syndrome)
- Iatrogenic
  - Abrupt cessation of exogenous corticosteroids or corticotropin
  - Removal of functioning adrenal tumor
  - Adrenalectomy for Cushing disease
  - Drugs
    - Aminoglutethimide
    - Mitotane (o,p′-DDD)
    - Metyrapone
    - Ketoconazole
- Fetal adrenal suppression—maternal hypercortisolism
  - Endogenous
  - Therapeutic

Histologically, there is marked adrenocortical atrophy with relative sparing of the zona glomerulosa. Recently, a number of mutations in the gene for the ACTH receptor have been described in some of these patients.

Another syndrome of ACTH resistance occurs in association with achalasia of the cardia and alacrima (triple A or Allgrove syndrome). These patients also have autonomic dysfunction, mental retardation, and other neurologic disorders that in some instances are progressive. This syndrome is also inherited in an autosomal recessive fashion, but thus far no mutations of the ACTH receptor have been detected. Several mutations in the gene for the ACTH receptor have been described in some of these patients.

Inborn Defects of Steroidogenesis. The most common causes of adrenocortical insufficiency in infancy are the salt-losing forms of congenital adrenal hyperplasia (Chapter 529). More than one half the infants with the 21-hydroxylase defect, all infants with lipoid adrenal hyperplasia, and most infants with a deficiency of 3β-hydroxysteroid dehydrogenase manifest salt-losing symptoms in the newborn period. In these defects, there is a deficiency in the synthesis of both cortisol and aldosterone, and elevated levels of steroids that are precursors to the enzymatic defect.

Isolated Deficiency of Aldosterone. This is a rare autosomal recessive disorder in which conversion of corticosterone (B) to aldosterone is impaired. There are two forms of the disorder, corticosterone methyloxidase I (CMO I) deficiency, in which conversion of B to 18-hydroxycorticosterone (18OHB) is defective, and corticosterone methyloxidase II (CMO II) deficiency, in which there is impaired conversion of 18OHB to aldosterone. The disorders can be differentiated biochemically. In CMO I deficiency, the ratio of B to 18OHB is increased, and 18OHB is usually decreased. In CMO II deficiency, there is overproduction of 18OHB and a markedly increased 18OHB to aldosterone ratio. CMO I and CMO II deficiencies result from mutations in the aldosterone synthase gene *(CYP11B2)*. Aldosterone synthase (P450c18) mediates the three final steps in the synthesis of aldosterone. A number of mutations in the *CYP11B2* gene have been described.

Infants with aldosterone synthase deficiency may have severe electrolyte abnormalities with hyponatnemia, hyperkalemia, and acidosis; with hyper-reninemia, and hypoaldosteronism in the newborn period, or they may present later with failure to thrive and poor growth. Adults often are asymptomatic.

Treatment consists of administration of enough salt or 9α-fluorocortisol (0.05–0.3 mg daily) or both to return plasma renin to normal. With increasing age, the salt-losing manifestations improve, and it appears that therapy may be discontinued; however, levels of plasma renin rise and growth decelerates, indicating chronic salt depletion. The biosynthetic defect persists and can be demonstrated in adults. This autosomal recessive defect is especially frequent in Iranian Jews. Carrier detection and prenatal diagnosis are possible.

Pseudohypoaldosteronism. This salt-losing syndrome also presents in the neonate; however, levels of aldosterone in plasma and urine are markedly elevated. Levels of plasma renin activity are elevated, indicating hyperactivity of the renin-angiotensin system. The defect is target-organ unresponsiveness to aldosterone. Administration of mineralocorticoids is ineffective; the condition is treated by supplementary dietary salt, which may be discontinued as the condition improves, usually by 2 yr of age. The syndrome appears to be heterogeneous. In some patients salt loss involves only the renal tubules, whereas in others the salivary and sweat glands may be involved, and occasionally the colonic mucosal cells may be affected. In the more than 70 reported patients, autosomal dominant and autosomal recessive forms have been identified. In the few patients studied, the gene for the aldosterone receptor was normal.

Addison Disease. Destruction of the adrenal cortex during childhood is one of the more common causes of adrenal insufficiency. Tuberculosis, a common cause of adrenal destruction in the past, has virtually vanished as a cause. The most common cause is autoimmune destruction of the glands. The glands may be so small that they are not visible at autopsy, and only remnants of tissue are found in microscopic sections. Usually, the medulla is not destroyed, and there is marked lymphocytic infiltration in the area of the former cortex. In advanced disease, all adrenal cortical function is lost, but early in the clinical course, isolated cortisol deficiency may antedate aldosterone deficiency and salt-losing manifestations. Most patients have antiadrenal cytoplasmic antibodies in their plasma. About 75% of affected patients have immunoglobulins that block the growth and steroidogenic effects of ACTH. Autoantibodies to 21-hydroxylase have been found in most patients with Addison disease. How the various antibodies act in concert with cell-mediated processes to cause disease is unknown.

Addison disease often occurs as a component of two syndromes, each consisting of a constellation of autoimmune disorders. *Type I autoimmune polyendocrinopathy* is also known as *autoimmune polyendocrinopathy-candidiasis-ectodermal dystrophy* (APECED). Chronic mucocutaneous candidiasis is most often the first manifestation, followed by hypoparathyroidism and then by Addison disease. Other closely associated autoimmune disorders include gonadal failure, alopecia, vitiligo, keratopathy, enamel hypoplasia, nail dystrophy, intestinal malabsorption, and chronic active hepatitis. Hypothyroidism and type I diabetes mellitus occur in fewer than 10% of affected patients. The disorder is inherited as an autosomal recessive disorder and the gene has been assigned to chromosome 21q22.3. Some components of the syndrome continue to develop as late as the 5th decade. The presence of antiadrenal antibodies and steroidal-cell antibodies in these patients usually indicates a high likelihood of developing Addison disease or, in females, ovarian failure.

Type II autoimmune polyendocrinopathy consists of Addison disease associated with autoimmune thyroid disease or insulin-dependent diabetes. HLA-D3 and HLA-D4 predominate in these patients.

Adrenoleukodystrophy. In this disorder, adrenocortical deficiency is associated with demyelination in the central nervous system (see Chapters 72 and 552.3). High levels of very-long-chain fatty acids (VLCFA) are found in tissues and body fluids resulting from impairment of their degradation in the peroxisomes. Neonatal adrenoleukodystrophy (ALD) is an autosomal recessive disorder. Infants present with neurologic deterioration and have or develop evidence of adrenocortical dysfunction. Most patients have severe mental retardation and die before 5 yr of age.

The more frequent form of ALD is an X-linked disorder with various presentations. The most common clinical picture is of a degenerative neurologic disorder appearing in childhood or adolescence and progressing to severe dementia and deterioration of vision, hearing, speech, and gait, with death occurring within a few years. A milder form of X-linked ALD is adrenomyeloneuropathy that begins in later adolescence or early adulthood. Many patients have evidence of adrenal insufficiency at the time of neurologic presentation, but Addison disease may precede the neurologic symptoms by many years. X-linked ALD may present as isolated Addison disease. The therapeutic approaches of uncertain efficacy include diets restricted in VLCFAs and bone marrow transplantation. A putative gene for ALD has been identified, and mutations and deletions of this gene have been described. Definitive proof of the association of the putative gene with the disorder remains to be established.

Hemorrhage Into Adrenal Glands. This may occur in the neonatal period as a consequence of difficult labor or of asphyxia. The hemorrhage may be sufficiently extensive to result in death from exsanguination or from hypoadrenalism. Often, the hemorrhage is asymptomatic initially and is identified by later calcification of the adrenal. On rare occasions, gradual impairment in function resulting from progressive fibrosis or cystic changes may culminate in adrenocortical insufficiency in infancy or childhood. Another cause of hemorrhage into the adrenal glands is the *Waterhouse-Friderichsen syndrome,* the characteristic state of shock resulting from meningococcemia (see Chapter 178).

Abrupt Cessation of Administration of Corticotropin or a Corticosteroid. This condition may result in adrenal insufficiency, manifesting glucocorticoid but not mineralocorticoid deficiency. Symptoms are most likely to occur if these substances have been given in large doses for a long time to patients who are subsequently subjected to stressful situations such as severe infections or surgical procedures.

Drugs. Ketoconazole, an antifungal drug, can cause adrenal insufficiency by inhibiting adrenal enzymes. Rifampicin and anticonvulsive drugs such as phenytoin and phenobarbital reduce the effectiveness and bioavailability of corticosteroid replacement therapy by inducing steroid-metabolizing enzymes in the liver.

CLINICAL MANIFESTATIONS. The age at onset of symptoms and the clinical manifestations depend on the specific etiologic factor involved. In patients with adrenal hypoplasia, defects in steroidogenesis, or pseudohypoaldosteronism, symptoms and signs begin shortly after birth and are those characteristic of salt loss. Failure to thrive, vomiting, lethargy, anorexia, and dehydration occur; circulatory collapse may be fatal.

In older children with Addison disease, the onset is usually more gradual and is characterized by muscular weakness, lassitude, anorexia, loss of weight, general wasting, and low blood pressure. Abdominal pain may simulate an acute abdominal process, and there may be an intense craving for salt. If the condition is not recognized and treated, *adrenal crisis* may supervene. The patient suddenly becomes cyanotic, the skin cold, and the pulse weak and rapid. The blood pressure falls, and respirations are rapid and labored. In the absence of immediate and intensive therapy, the course is rapidly fatal. In patients with inadequately treated chronic adrenal insufficiency, crises may be precipitated by infection, trauma, excessive fatigue, or drugs such as morphine, barbiturates, laxatives, thyroid hormone, or insulin.

Increased pigmentation of the skin should always alert the clinician to the possibility of adrenocortical insufficiency. This manifestation occurs in those conditions in which there are a deficiency of cortisol and excessive secretion of corticotropin, as in primary adrenal hypoplasia, familial glucocorticoid deficiency, adrenoleukodystrophy, and Addison disease. Pigmentation may be first apparent on the face and hands and is most intense around the genitalia, umbilicus, axillae, nipples, and joints. Scars and freckles may be especially pigmented. Areas of depigmentation (vitiligo) may be interspersed with dark areas. The exposed areas of the skin are the most intensely affected, and failure of a suntan to disappear may be the first clue to the condition. In the buccal mucosa the pigmentation is usually bluish brown.

The presenting manifestations may be those of hypoglycemia, particularly in the neonate with congenital adrenal hypoplasia. Patients with adrenocortical insufficiency are deficient in gluconeogenic substrates; the hypoglycemia may therefore be associated with ketosis and confused with ketotic hypoglycemia (see Chapter 77).

In young children with familial glucocorticoid deficiency, salt-losing manifestations do not occur, and the symptoms consist primarily of increased pigmentation and hypoglycemia. Symptoms may begin shortly after birth and almost always appear by 5 yr of age. Many affected children have received other treatment for seizures before the hypoglycemic cause was recognized.

In patients with a deficiency of corticotropin, pigmentation does not occur. Hypoglycemia is the usual presenting manifestation. Hyperkalemia does not occur because of preserved aldosterone secretion, but hyponatremia may occur.

In conditions known to have a genetic basis, it is important to evaluate fully the adrenocortical function of siblings.

LABORATORY DATA. When salt-losing manifestations are present, the levels of sodium and chloride in the serum are usually low and that of potassium elevated, with increased plasma renin activity. Urinary excretion of sodium and chloride is increased, urinary potassium is decreased, and acidosis exists. The nonprotein nitrogen level in plasma is elevated if dehydration is present. Hypoglycemia may be striking or may become manifest only after prolonged fasting. The blood eosinophils may be increased in number. When hemorrhage, adrenal cysts, or tuberculosis has been a causative factor, roentgenograms of the abdomen may reveal calcifications in the area of the adrenals. Ultrasound and computed tomography may also be helpful. A small and narrow roentgenographic shadow of the heart reflects hypovolemia. Electrocardiographic changes reflect potassium levels.

The most definitive test is measurement of the plasma or serum levels of cortisol before and after administration of ACTH; resting levels are low, and no increase occurs after administration of corticotropin. Occasionally, normal resting levels that do not increase after administration of ACTH indicate an absence of adrenocortical reserve. A low initial level followed by a significant response to ACTH may indicate adrenal insufficiency secondary to endogenous insufficiency of ACTH. Levels of ACTH are elevated in disorders of primary cortisol deficiency and are low when the adrenal insufficiency is secondary to a hypothalamic or pituitary disorder. Testing with CRH may be helpful in localizing the defect.

Measurement of plasma or serum levels of cortisol precursors is necessary in infants in whom congenital adrenal hyperplasia is suspected. Aldosterone secretion may be low in patients with salt-losing congenital adrenal hyperplasia, adrenal hypoplasia, or Addison disease. Measurement of aldosterone is necessary in infants suspected of having isolated defects of aldosterone synthesis (in whom it is low) and in those suspected of having pseudohypoaldosteronism (in whom it is usually elevated). In patients with familial glucocorticoid deficiency aldosterone levels are normal and rise appropriately with salt deprivation.

TREATMENT. Treatment for acute adrenal insufficiency or for adrenal crisis must be immediate and vigorous. If the cause of adrenal insufficiency has not been established, a blood sample should be obtained before therapy for determination of levels of cortisol, 17-hydroxyprogesterone, and adrenal androgens. Intravenous administration of 5% glucose in 0.9% saline solution should be given to correct the hypoglycemia and the sodium loss. Concomitantly, a water-soluble form of hydrocortisone, such as hydrocortisone hemisuccinate, should be given intravenously. High levels are achieved instantaneously, and large doses can be used safely. As much as 25 mg for infants and 75 mg for older children should be given intravenously at 6-hr intervals for the first 24 hr. These doses may be reduced during the next 24 hr if progress is satisfactory. Adequate fluid and sodium repletion is achieved by the intravenous saline administration, aided by the mineralocorticoid effect of high doses of hydrocortisone. After the first 48 hr, if oral intake is satisfactory, intravenous fluids may be discontinued and the corticosteroid given orally as cortisol in doses of 5–20 mg at 8-hr intervals. Further reduction can then be accomplished until maintenance levels and a stable clinical situation are achieved. Florinef (9α-flurocortisol), a mineralocorticoid, can be added orally at 0.05–0.3 mg daily.

After the acute manifestations are under control, most patients require chronic replacement therapy for their aldosterone and cortisol deficiencies. The cortisol may be given orally in daily doses of 5–10 mg/24 hr in two or three divided doses for infants and 10–20 mg/24 hr in two or three divided doses for children and adolescents. Florinef is continued orally in doses of 0.05–0.3 mg daily. Measurements of plasma renin activity are useful in monitoring adequacy of mineralocorticoid replacement. During situations of stress, such as periods of infection or operative procedures, the dose of hydrocortisone should be increased.

Overdosage with fluorohydrocortisone results in hypertension and may lead to cardiac enlargement and edema because of excessive retention of sodium chloride and water; excessive loss of potassium may produce weakness or paralysis.

Patients with primary corticotropin deficiency or with familial glucocorticoid deficiency do not require a salt-retaining hormone because their ability to secrete aldosterone is intact. Patients with primary defects in aldosterone synthesis do not require cortisol; a salt-retaining hormone may be required, but in milder forms, the addition of salt to the diet is adequate to maintain homeostasis. In patients with pseudohypoaldosteronism, administration of salt-retaining hormones does not correct the urinary sodium loss; therapy must consist of supplementation with sodium chloride. In newborn infants with adrenal hemorrhage, vitamins K and C and transfusions with whole blood may be indicated.

Patients with apparent Addison disease must be differentiated from those with familial glucocorticoid deficiency and adrenoleukodystrophy (see Chapter 72); absence of salt-losing manifestations and presence of alacrima suggest the former, and elevated levels of very long chain fatty acids are diagnostic for the latter. The presence of antiadrenal antibodies suggests an autoimmune pathogenesis; these patients must be closely observed for the development of other associated autoimmune disorders. Infants with congenital adrenal hypoplasia should undergo chromosomal analysis to search for a deletion of the Xp21 region; elevated levels of creatine phosphokinase indicate an association with Duchenne muscular dystrophy, and elevated levels of triglycerides suggest glycerol kinase deficiency. DNA probe analysis for the gene defect, glycerol kinase enzyme assay, and negative dystrophin staining of muscle tissue permit confirmation of the components of this complex.

Aaltonen J, Bjorses P, Sandkuijl L, et al: An autosomal locus causing autoimmune disease: Autoimmune polyglandular disease type I assigned to chromosome 21. Nature Genet 8:83, 1994.

Ahonen P, Myllarniemi S, Spila I, et al: Clinical variation of autoimmune polyendocrinopathy-candidiasis-ectodermal dystrophy (APECED) in a series of 68 patients. N Engl J Med 322:1824, 1990.

Armanini D, Kuhnle U, Strasser T, et al: Aldosterone-receptor deficiency in pseudohypoaldosteronism. N Engl J Med 313:1178, 1985.

Aubourg P, Chaussain J-L: Adrenoleukodystrophy presenting as Addison's disease in children and adults. Trends Endocrinol Metab 2:49, 1991.

Carey DE: Isolated ACTH deficiency in childhood: Lack of response to corticotropin-releasing hormone alone and in combination with arginine vasopressin. J Pediatr 107:925, 1985.

Carney JA, Hruska LS, Beauchamp GD, et al: Dominant inheritance of the complex of myxomas, spotty pigmentation, and endocrine overactivity. Mayo Clin Proc 61:165, 1986.

Clark AJL, Weber A: Molecular insights into inherited ACTH resistance syndromes. Trends Endocrinol Metab 5:209, 1994.

Corvol P, Funder J: The enigma of pseudohypoaldosteronism. J Clin Endocrinol Metab 79:25, 1994.

Grant DB, Dunger DB, Smith I, Hyland K: Familial glucocorticoid deficiency with achalasia of the cardia associated with mixed neuropathy, long-tract degeneration and mild dementia. Eur J Pediatr 151:85, 1992.

Guiochon-Mantel A, Milgrom E: Cytoplasmic-nuclear trafficking of steroid hormone receptors. Trends Endocrinol Metab 4:322, 1993.

Hay ID: Pubertal failure in congenital adrenocortical hypoplasia. Lancet 2:1035, 1977.

Kirkland RT, Kirkland JL, Johnson CM, et al: Congenital lipoid adrenal hyperplasia in an eight-year-old phenotypic female. J Clin Endocrinol Metab 36:488, 1973.

Kletter GB, Gorski JL, Kelch RP: Congenital adrenal hypoplasia and isolated gonadotropin deficiency. Trends Endocrinol Metab 2:123, 1991.

Kruse K, Sippell WG, Schnakenburg KV: Hypogonadism in congenital adrenal hypoplasia: Evidence for a hypothalamic origin. J Clin Endocrinol Metab 58:12, 1984.

Kuhnle U, Nielsen MD, Tietze U, et al: Pseudohypoaldosteronism in eight families: Different forms of inheritance are evidence for various genetic defects. J Clin Endocrinol Metab 70:638, 1990.

Lee PDK, Patterson BD, Hintz RL, et al: Biochemical diagnosis and management

of corticosterone methyloxidase type II deficiency. J Clin Endocrinol Metab 62:225, 1986.
Linder BL, Esteban NV, Yergey AL, et al: Cortisol production rate in childhood and adolesence. J Pediatr 117:892, 1990.
McCabe ERB, Towbin J, Chamberlain J, et al: Complementary DNA probes for the muscular dystrophy locus demonstrate a previously undetectable deletion in a patient with dystrophic myopathy, glycerol kinase deficiency, and congenital adrenal hyperplasia. J Clin Invest 83:95, 1989.
Moser HW, Moser AE, Singh J, et al: Adrenoleukodystrophy: Survey of 303 cases: Biochemistry, diagnosis, and therapy. Ann Neurol 16:628, 1984.
Mosser J, Lutz Y, Stoeckel ME, et al: The gene responsible for adrenoleukodystrophy encodes a peroxisomal membrane protein. Hum Mol Genet 3:265, 1994.
Muscatelli F, Strom TM, Walker AP, et al: Mutations in the DAX-1 gene give rise to both X-linked adrenal hypoplasia congenita and hypogonadotropic hypogonadism. Nature 372:672, 1994.
Song Y-H, Connor EL, Muir A, et al: Autoantibody epitope mapping of the 21-hydroxylase antigen in autoimmune Addison's disease. J Clin Endocrinol Metab 78:1108, 1994.
White PC: Disorders of aldosterone biosynthesis and action. N Engl J Med 331:250, 1994.
Yao-Hua S, Connor EL, Muir A, et al: Autoantibody epitope mapping of the 21-hydroxylase antigen in autoimmune Addison's disease. J Clin Endocrinol Metab 78:1108, 1994.
Zlotogora J, Shapiro S: Polyglandular autoimmune syndrome type I among Iranian Jews. J Med Genet 29:824, 1992.

CHAPTER 529
Adrenogenital Syndrome

ADRENOCORTICAL HYPERFUNCTION

Four syndromes are attributable to hyperadrenocorticism: the *adrenogenital syndrome, Cushing syndrome, hyperaldosteronism,* and *feminization* (Table 529–1). The adrenogenital syndrome is produced by congenital adrenal hyperplasia and by virilizing adrenocortical tumors.

529.1 Congenital Adrenal Hyperplasia

PATHOGENESIS. When the adrenogenital syndrome is associated with congenital adrenal hyperplasia, it is caused by a family of autosomal recessive disorders of adrenal steroidogenesis leading to a deficiency of cortisol (Fig. 529–1). The deficiency of cortisol results in increased secretion of corticotropin, which leads in turn to adrenocortical hyperplasia and overproduction of intermediary metabolites. Severe and mild forms of these disorders, caused by variations in the severity of the genetic mutations, have been reported.

Deficiency of 21-hydroxylase accounts for 95% of affected patients. This P450 enzyme ($P_{450}c21$) hydroxylates progesterone and 17-hydroxyprogesterone (17-OHP) to yield 11-deoxycorticosterone and 11-deoxycortisol (see Fig. 529–1). There are two steroid 21-hydroxylase genes (*CYP21A* and *CYP21B*), which alternate in tandem with two genes for the fourth component of complement (C4A and C4B) on the short arm of chromosome 6 between the HLA-B and HLA-DR loci. The *CYP21B* gene is the active gene; the *CYP21A* gene is 98% homologous to the *CYP21B* gene but is a pseudogene. The majority of mutations causing 21-hydroxylase deficiency are recombinations (deletions or gene conversions) between the active *CYP21B* gene and the adjacent *CYP21A* pseudogene. The classic disorder occurs in salt-wasting and simple virilizing forms. A milder nonclassic form also occurs, with a high frequency reported among Ashkenazi Jews.

Newborn screening programs, using capillary heel blood on filter paper disks, have been developed to detect 21-hydroxylase deficiency. Data on more than 2 million neonates screened indicate that the disorder occurs in 1 of 20,000 members of the population in Japan, 1 of 10,000–16,000 in Europe and North America, and 1 of 300 in Yupik Eskimos of Alaska. About 75% of affected infants have the salt-losing, virilizing form and 25% have the simple virilizing form of the disorder. The nonclassic form is not detected by newborn screening.

Deficiency of 11β-hydroxylase accounts for 5–8% of cases of adrenal hyperplasia. This $P_{450}c11$ enzyme mediates the 11β-hydroxylation of 11-deoxycortisol to cortisol. This deficit occurs relatively frequently in Israeli Jews of North African origin; in this ethnic group, a point mutation (Arg448 to His) has been found in the *CYP11B1* gene encoded on chromosome 8q22. Other mutations have also been identified. This disorder presents in a classic, severe form and a nonclassic, milder form.

Hypertension is a distinctive clinical feature of the disorder but is absent in the first few years of life. Virilization occurs as in 21-hydroxylase deficiency. The plasma characteristically contains large amounts of both 11-deoxycortisol and DOC. The elevated levels of DOC are thought to cause the hypertension and prevent symptoms of salt losing. Prenatal diagnosis is possible by measuring levels of 11-deoxycortisol in maternal urine during pregnancy or in amniotic fluid, and by DNA probes.

Deficiency of 3β-hydroxysteroid dehydrogenase (*3β-HSD*) occurs in fewer than 5% of patients with adrenal hyperplasia. This enzyme is required for conversion of Δ^5 steroids (pregnenolone, 17-hydroxypregnenolone, dehydroepiandrosterone [DHEA]) to Δ^4 steroids (progesterone, 17-hydroxyprogester-

■ TABLE 529–1 Etiologic Classification of Adrenocortical Hyperfunction

Excess androgen (adrenal hyperplasia)
Congenital adrenal hyperplasia
21-Hydroxylase ($P450_{c21}$) deficiency
11β-Hydroxylase ($p450_{c11}$) deficiency
3β-Hydroxysteroid dehydrogenase defect (females)
Tumor
Carcinoma
Adenoma—isolated testosterone secretion
Excess cortisol (Cushing syndrome)
Bilateral adrenal hyperplasia
Hypersecretion of corticotropin (Cushing disease)
Ectopic secretion of corticotropin
Exogenous corticotropin
Tumor
Carcinoma
Adenoma
Adrenocortical nodular dysplasia
Pigmented nodular adrenocortisol disease (Carney complex)
Excess mineralocorticoid (hypertensive hypokalemic syndrome)
Primary hyperaldosteronism
Aldosterone-secreting adenoma
Bilateral micronodular adrenocortical hyperplasia
Glucocorticoid-suppressible aldosteronism
Tumor
Adenoma
Carcinoma
Desoxycorticosterone excess
Adrenal hyperplasia
11β-Hydroxylase ($P450_{c11}$)
17α-Hydroxylase ($P450_{c17}$)
Tumor (carcinoma)
Apparent mineralocorticoid excess
11β-Hydroxysteroid dehydrogenase deficiency
Excess estrogen (adrenal feminization syndrome)
Carcinoma
Adenoma
Mixed hypercorticism—tumor

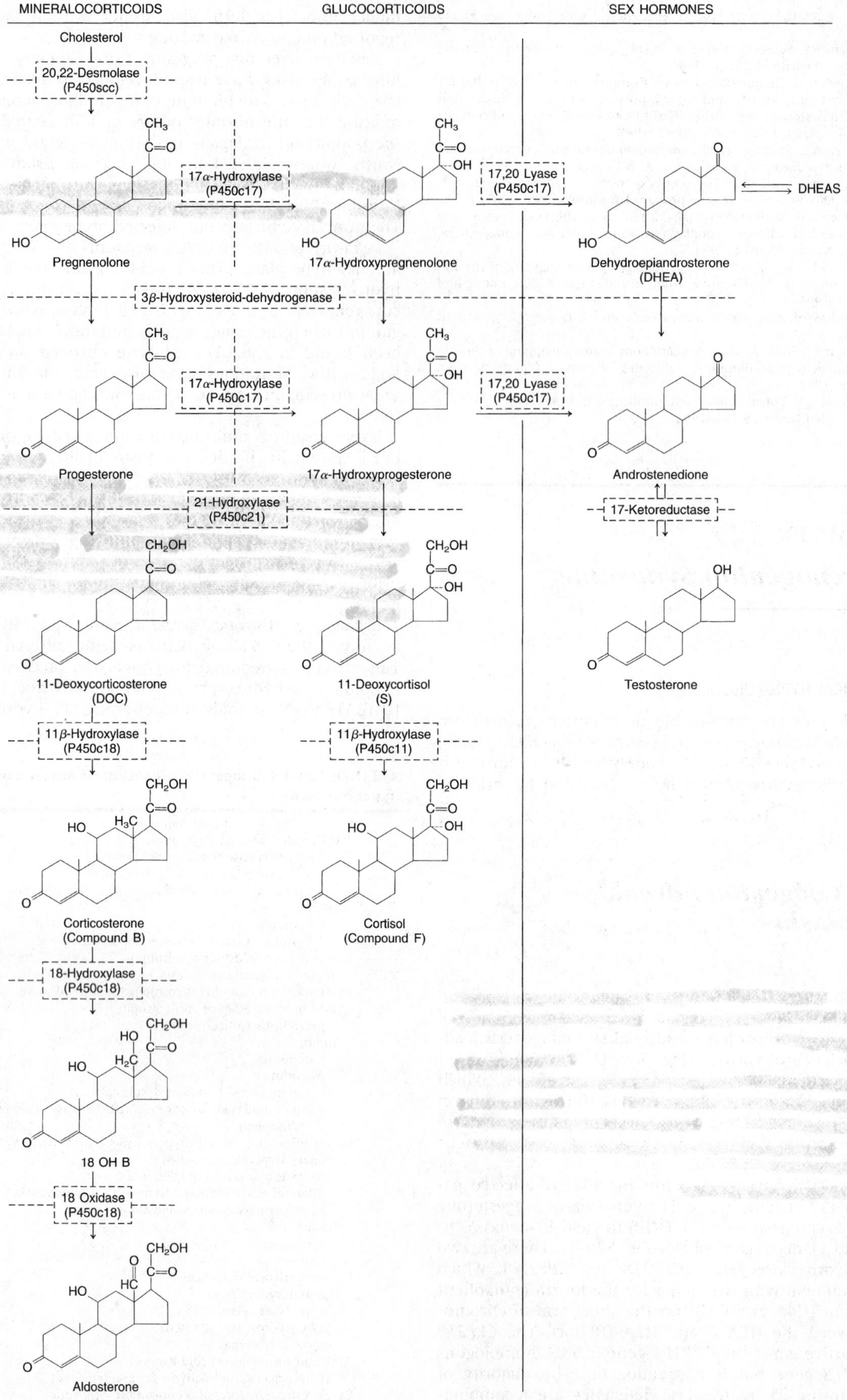

Figure 529–1. The synthesis of cortisol and aldosterone is shown to the left of the vertical line. To the right of the solid vertical line are the predominant adrenal androgens that lead to conversion to testosterone. Note that a single polypeptide, P_{450}c17, catalyzes both 17α-hydroxylase and 17,20-lyase activities. Likewise, polypeptide P_{450}c18 mediates the last three steps in aldosterone synthesis.

one, and androstenedione). Deficiency of [illegible] sults in decreased synthesis of cortisol, aldo[illegible]ns (see Fig. 529–1). The 3β-HSD enzyme ex[illegible] cortex and gonad is encoded by the ty[illegible] located on chromosome 1. A number of mu[illegible] II gene have been described in patients wit[illegible] ciency. Severe and milder forms of the disorder [illegible] classic form of the disease, there is often a salt-w[illegible] in the newborn, boys are incompletely virilized and [illegible] pospadias, and girls are mildly virilized. In the non[illegible] milder form, salt wasting and ambiguity of the genitalia d[illegible] occur, and affected individuals may present with precocio[illegible] pubarche or with hirsutism, menstrual disorders, and infertility. Polycystic ovaries may be found on examination. The hallmark of this disorder is the marked elevation of the Δ^5 steroids preceding the block. Patients may also have elevated levels of 17-hydroxyprogesterone because of the extra-adrenal 3β-HSD activity that occurs in peripheral tissues and may be mistaken for patients with 21-hydroxylase deficiency.

Lipoid adrenal hyperplasia has been reported in more than 32 patients, 18 of whom were Japanese. Failure of cleavage of the side chain of cholesterol results in marked accumulation of cholesterol and lipids in the adrenal cortex, and in failure of synthesis of any adrenal steroids. A single protein termed $P_{450}SCC$ is responsible for all three steps in the conversion of cholesterol to pregnenolone (formerly 20,22-desmolase); the gene is encoded on chromosome 15. The same enzymatic defect is present in the testes, preventing synthesis of testicular hormones. As a consequence, genetic males are phenotypically female and females exhibit no genital abnormality. Salt-losing manifestations are usual, and most infants have died in early infancy. Because adrenal steroid levels are not elevated in this form of adrenal hyperplasia, affected infants are apt to be confused with those with adrenal hypoplasia. In three patients studied, no mutation of the P_{450} gene has been found. Instead, all had a mutation of the gene for steroidogenic acute regulatory protein (StAR), a mitochondrial protein that activates steroidogenesis.

17α-Hydroxylase deficiency has been described in more than 125 patients. A single polypeptide, $P_{450}17$, catalyzes two distinct reactions: 17α-hydroxylation of pregnenolone and progesterone, and the 17,20-lyase reaction mediating conversion of 17α-hydroxypregnenolone and 17α-hydroxyprogesterone to DHEA and Δ^4-androstenedione, respectively, the C-19 steroid precursors of testosterone and estrogen (see Fig. 529–1). The enzyme is encoded on chromosome 10, and the gene is [illegible]xpressed in both the adrenal cortex and the gonads. The [illegible]ciency results in overproduction of DOC, leading to hyper[illegible]n, hypokalemia, and suppression of renin and aldoste[illegible] addition, there is an inability to synthesize normal [illegible] of sex hormones. Affected males are incompletely [illegible]d present as phenotypic females or with sexual [illegible]ale pseudohermaphroditism). Affected females [illegible] with failure of sexual development at the ex[illegible]uberty. Patients have been described with [illegible] combined 17α-hydroxylase–17,20-lyase de[illegible] deficiencies of only one of these activities. [illegible] cloned. At least 15 different genetic lesions [illegible]d. This defect must be considered in the differ[illegible] male pseudohermaphroditism or of testicula[illegible]-Hydroxylase deficiency in females must b[illegible] the differential diagnosis of primary hypogona[illegible]hapter 538).

CLINICAL MANIFESTA[illegible]. Most patients with congenital adrenal hyperplasia have the defect in 21-hydroxylation and exhibit the classic form of the disease. In newborn screening programs, about 75% of infants in whom this condition is detected are salt losers, whereas without screening only about 50% of clinically diagnosed infants are salt losers, presumably because of undiagnosed neonatal deaths.

Patients without Salt Losing. In the *male* the main clinical manifestations are those of premature isosexual development. The infant usually appears normal at birth, but signs of sexual and somatic precocity may appear within the first 6 mo of life or develop more gradually, becoming evident at 4–5 yr of age or later. Enlargement of the penis, scrotum, and prostate, appearance of pubic hair, and development of acne and a deep voice are noted. Muscles are well developed, and bone age is advanced for chronologic age. Although affected patients are tall in early childhood, premature closure of the epiphyses causes growth to stop relatively early, and adult stature is stunted (Fig. 529–2).

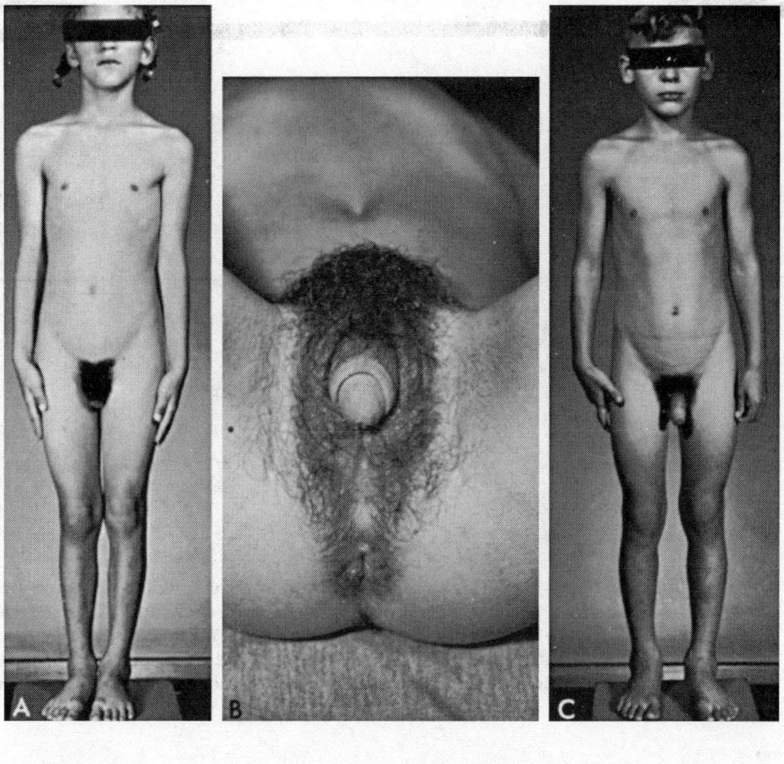

Figure 529–2. *A*, A 6-yr-old girl with congenital virilizing adrenal hyperplasia. The height age was 8.5 yr; the bone age was 13 yr; and urinary 17-ketosteroids were 50 mg/24 hr. *B*, Notice the clitoral enlargement and labial fusion. *C*, Five-yr-old brother of girl in *A* was not considered to be abnormal by the parents. The height age was 8 yr; the bone age was 12.5 yr; and the urinary 17-ketosteroids were 36 mg/24 hr.

The testes are prepubertal in size so that they appear relatively small in contrast to the enlarged penis. Occasionally, ectopic adrenocortical cells in the testes of patients with adrenal hyperplasia become hyperplastic just as the adrenal glands do, producing enlargement of the testes (see Chapter 536). Mental development is usually normal, but the abnormal physical development may result in behavioral problems.

In the *female* congenital adrenal hyperplasia results in female pseudohermaphroditism (Fig. 529–3). Because the disorder of steroidogenesis begins early in fetal life, there is almost always evidence of some degree of masculinization at birth. It is manifested by enlargement of the clitoris and varying degrees of labial fusion. The vagina has a common opening with the urethra (urogenital sinus). The clitoris may be so enlarged that it resembles a penis, and, because the urethra opens below this organ, a mistaken diagnosis of hypospadias and cryptorchidism is sometimes made. Females with a male phenotype have been reported; there is complete labial fusion, a phallic urethra, and an external meatus at the tip of the penis. The severity of the virilization is in general greater in infants who are salt losers than in those who are not. The internal genital organs are those of a normal female.

After birth, the masculinization progresses. Pubic and axillary hair develop prematurely, acne appears, and the voice assumes a masculine quality. Affected girls are tall for their age, and ossification is advanced; they show good muscular development and, in general, have the body build of a boy (see Fig. 529–2). Although the internal genitalia are female, breast development and menstruation do not occur unless the excessive production of androgens is suppressed by adequate treatment.

Several virilized female pseudohermaphrodites whose condition was not diagnosed until adult life have been erroneously reared as males. These patients have behaved in every way as males, including having sexual intercourse; some have had satisfactory (albeit infertile) marriages.

With the *11-hydroxylase defect,* salt-losing manifestations do not occur. Most patients are hypertensive, but several have been normotensive or have had intermittent hypertension only. The disorder has been diagnosed only rarely in early life, but hypertension was not present. Several prepubertal children with this defect presented with gynecomastia. Virilization occurs in all patients and is as severe as with the 21-hydroxylase defect.

Patients with Salt Losing. In patients with the salt-losing variant, symptoms begin shortly after birth with failure to regain birthweight, progressive weight loss, and dehydration. Vomiting is prominent, with anorexia. Disturbances in cardiac rate and rhythm may occur, with cyanosis and dyspnea. Without treatment, collapse and death may occur within a few weeks.

In females, virilization of the external genitalia in an infant with the these manifestations directs attention to the correct diagnosis. In the male, the genitalia appear normal, and clinical manifestations are likely to be confused with those of pyloric stenosis, intestinal obstruction, heart disease, cow's milk intolerance, or other causes of failure to thrive.

Familial homogeneity of defect is usually observed for the salt-losing and non–salt-losing forms. Under conditions of stress or sodium deprivation, salt losing may be provoked in compensated patients.

Patients with the 3β-*hydroxysteroid dehydrogenase* defect are usually salt losers but are less virilized. In females, virilization is usually mild, with slight to moderate clitoral enlargement. It may be mild enough to escape detection. In the male, varying degrees of hypospadias may occur, with or without bifid scrotum or cryptorchidism. Patients with *lipoid adrenal hyperplasia* are salt losers, and their phenotype is female with normal genitalia.

Nonclassic 21-Hydroxylase Deficiency. In this attenuated form, affected females have normal genitalia at birth. Males and females may present with precocious pubarche, early development of pubic and axillary hair. Hirsutism, acne, menstrual disorders, and infertility may develop later in life. Some females and males are completely asymptomatic. About 75% of patients are HLA-B14,DR1. The genetic defect is allelic with classic 21-hydroxylase; a mutation in codon 281 appears to be a marker for the disorder. It is estimated that 1% of North American whites have this disorder, with the highest frequency occurring in Ashkenazi Jews.

LABORATORY DATA. Salt losers may have low serum concentrations of sodium and chloride and elevated levels of potassium and nonprotein nitrogen. Plasma levels of renin are elevated. In classic 21-hydroxylase deficiency, serum levels of 17-hydroxyprogesterone (17-OHP) are markedly elevated and are especially helpful in diagnosis, but they are normally high during the first 2–3 days of life and may range as high as levels found in affected patients; by the 3rd day, however, levels in normal infants fall, and those in affected infants rise to clearly diagnostic levels. Sick, unaffected infants and prematures may have elevated levels of 17-OHP. Blood levels of cortisol are

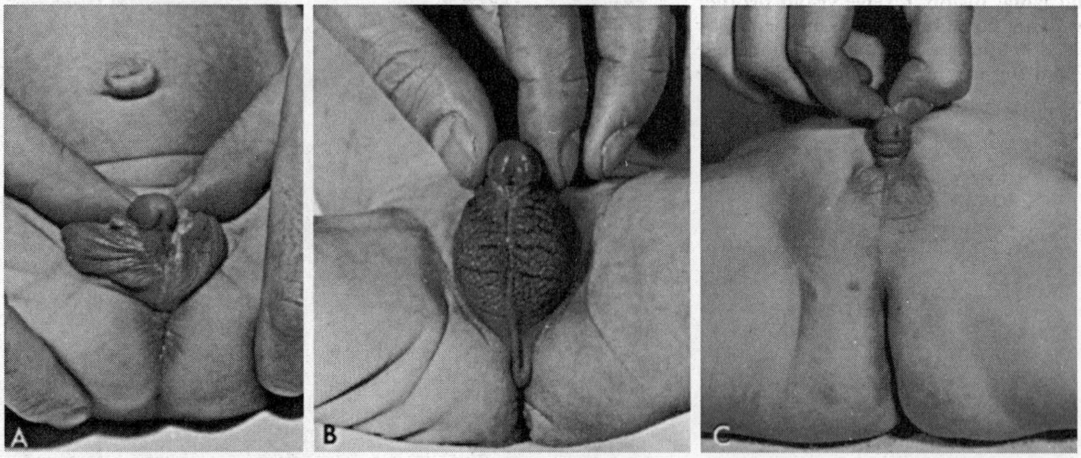

Figure 529–3. Three female pseudohemaphrodites with untreated congenital adrenal hyperplasia. All were erroneously assigned male sex at birth, and each had normal female sex-chromosome complement. Infants *A* and *B* were salt losers and were diagnosed in early infancy. Infant *C* was referred at 1 yr of age because of bilateral cryptorchidism. Notice the completely penile urethra; such complete degrees of masculinization in females with adrenal hyperplasia are rare; most of these infants are salt losers.

usually low in patients with the salt-losing type but are often normal in those with the simple virilizing type. A large part of the virilization is caused by increased levels of testosterone; the excess 17-OHP is partially diverted to androstenedione, which is converted to testosterone in the periphery (see Fig. 529–1). Levels of urinary 17-ketosteroids and pregnanetriol are elevated; 24-hr urine collections are often unnecessary, however, because radioimmunoassay permits measurement in serum or plasma of the levels of the steroids involved in all forms of congenital adrenal hyperplasia.

In the late-onset variant of congenital adrenal hyperplasia, basal circulating levels of 17-OHP are not as high as in the classic form and may even be normal. There is, however, a diagnostic rise in the level 60 min following an intravenous bolus of 0.25 mg of ACTH (1–24).

In patients with the 11-hydroxylase defect, plasma levels of DOC and 11-deoxycortisol (compound S) are elevated.

The 3β-hydroxysteroid dehydrogenase defect is characterized by markedly elevated Δ^5 steroids such as 17-hydroxypregnenolone. 17-OHP levels are also elevated, however, and the condition may be confused with the 21-hydroxylase defect. It is necessary to determine the ratios of Δ^5 to Δ^4 steroids in plasma or urine for definitive diagnosis.

Affected females have an XX karyotype; males have a normal XY chromosome constitution. Injection of contrast medium into the urogenital sinus of female pseudohermaphrodites usually demonstrates a vagina and uterus. Ultrasonography is also helpful.

DIAGNOSIS. Congenital adrenal hyperplasia in an infant or child should always alert one to the diagnosis in later siblings. The salt-losing form of the disorder must be suspected in any infant who fails to thrive and especially in female infants with ambiguous external genitalia. When virilization occurs postnatally in males or females, a virilizing adrenocortical tumor must be considered in the differential diagnosis.

An adrenal tumor may be palpable or suggested on pyelography by displacement of the adjacent kidney. Ultrasound or CT scans may be necessary if hormonal studies have ruled out congenital adrenal hyperplasia. Urinary 17-ketosteroid excretion and plasma levels of dehydroepiandrosterone sulfate (DHEAS) are elevated with congenital hyperplasia and with cortical tumors, but very high values favor the diagnosis of neoplasm. Administration of hydrocortisone quickly reduces these and other elevated steroid levels to normal in patients with congenital adrenal hyperplasia but does not do so in those with a virilizing tumor. Corticosteroids, by inhibiting secretion of corticotropin, reduce the excessive stimulation of the adrenals in patients with hyperplasia, whereas adrenocortical tumors are not subject to pituitary regulation.

In males with adrenal hyperplasia, the testes are small for the degree of virilization, whereas in those with true precocious puberty or with Leydig cell tumors, the testes are enlarged for age.

Females with this condition must be differentiated from those with other causes of ambiguous external genitalia. Only in this condition are adrenal cortical steroid levels elevated. Males with the 3β-HSD defect may be confused with female pseudohermaphrodites because they lack normal virilization of the external genitalia. These male patients are 46XY and also have elevated adrenal cortical steroids.

Detection of the heterozygous carrier of 21-hydroxylase deficiency is possible by measuring the ratio of 17-OHP to 11-deoxycortisol or cortisol 60 min after an intravenous bolus injection of 0.25 mg of ACTH (1–24). In families in which there is an affected individual with 21-hydroxylase deficiency, HLA genotyping provides a reliable basis for counseling. Molecular DNA techniques are now also available.

Prenatal Diagnosis and Treatment. Prenatal diagnosis of 21-hydroxylase is possible in the 1st trimester by performing biopsy of the chorionic villi followed by HLA typing or DNA analysis. In the 2nd trimester, the diagnosis can be established by measuring 17-OHP in amniotic fluid as well as by HLA typing and DNA analysis of amniotic fluid cells. Prenatal treatment of more than 50 affected female infants has been reported. In approximately one fourth, genitalia were normal; in one half, there was mild virilization with clitoromegaly or partial labial fusion; and in one fourth, therapy was unsuccessful and the infants had marked genital virilization. Possible reasons for unsuccessful treatment are late onset of treatment, inadequate dosage, and variations in maternal and placental metabolism of the administered steroid. Recommendations for pregnancies at risk consist of administration of dexamethasone, a steroid that readily crosses the placenta, by the 5th wk of pregnancy in an amount of 1.5 mg/24 hr in two or three divided doses. First-trimester chorionic villus biopsy is then done to determine the sex and genotype of the fetus; therapy is continued only if the fetus is an affected female. It is unknown whether or to what degree such a regimen will be effective or whether there are long-term risks to the treatment.

TREATMENT. Administration of glucocorticoids inhibits excessive production of androgens and stems virilization. A variety of glucocorticoids and dosage schedules have been used for this purpose. We recommend hydrocortisone (10–20 mg/m²/24 hr) administered orally in two or three divided doses. Infants usually require 2.5–5 mg two to three times daily and children 5–10 mg two to three times daily. Doses are individualized by monitoring growth and hormonal levels. Patients with disturbances of electrolyte regulation (salt-losers) and elevated plasma renin activity require a mineralocorticoid and sodium supplementation in addition to the glucocorticoid. Maintenance therapy with 9 α fluorocortisol (0.05–0.3 mg daily) and sodium chloride, 1–3 g, is usually sufficient to normalize plasma renin activity. Non–salt-losing patients may also manifest elevated plasma renin activity and require a mineralocorticoid.

The optimal way to monitor these patients varies with personal preference. Measurements of urinary levels of 17-ketosteroids and pregnanetriol are no longer necessary. Plasma levels of 17-OHP, androstenedione, testosterone, and renin, measured preferably at 9:00 A.M., usually provide adequate indices of control. Monitoring of growth and osseous maturation is equally important.

The administration of hydrocortisone must be continued indefinitely in *all* patients. Increased doses are indicated during periods of stress such as infection or surgery or during periods of decreased salt intake for salt-losing and non–salt-losing patients, including those with the 11-hydroxylase defect because they all have defective adrenal reserve.

The enlarged clitoris of female infants usually requires surgical correction; a good age for this elective surgery is 6–12 mo. Recession of the clitoris is preferred rather than its removal; the clitoris is freed and repositioned beneath the pubis with preservation of the glans, corporal components, and all neural and vascular elements. Parents should be reassured that complete sexual gratification, including orgasm, can be achieved. The menarche occurs at the appropriate age in most girls in whom good control has been achieved. It is not exceptional for adolescents past the age of 16 not to have begun menstruating; such delay is probably related to suboptimal control.

Non–salt-losing children, particularly males, are frequently not diagnosed until 3–7 yr of age, at which time osseous maturation may be 5 yr or more in advance of chronologic age. Institution of treatment slows growth and osseous maturation to more nearly normal rates in some children; in others, especially if the bone age is 12 yr or more, spontaneous gonadotropin-dependent puberty may occur, therapy with hydrocortisone having suppressed production of adrenal androgens and permitted release of pituitary gonadotropins if the appropriate level of hypothalamic maturation is present. This form of superimposed true precocious puberty may now be effectively treated with a luteinizing hormone–releasing hormone analog.

Males who have had inadequate corticosteroid therapy may develop unilateral or bilateral testicular tumors, which may or may not regress with increased dosage. The tumors are thought to arise from adrenal rest cells present in the testes. Prolonged inadequate adrenal suppression may also result in adenomatous changes in the adrenal gland.

529.2 Virilizing Adrenocortical Tumors

Tumors of the adrenal cortex may result in masculinization in girls and precocious pseudopuberty in boys. Hypertension is common, and manifestations of Cushing syndrome may accompany virilization because these tumors frequently secrete excessive cortisol and, less often, mineralocorticoids in addition to androgens.

In males, the symptoms are usually the same as those occurring with non–salt-losing congenital adrenal hyperplasia. It is virtually impossible to differentiate the two conditions on clinical grounds. *In females,* virilizing tumors of the adrenal cause masculinization of a previously normal female, but congenital hyperplasia is almost always associated with genital abnormalities at birth. However, virilization in congenital adrenal hyperplasia may have its onset during childhood, and an adrenal adenoma is known to have caused intrauterine clitoral enlargement and mild labial fusion. Instances of an adrenal cortical carcinoma arising in the newborn period are known.

Tumors of the adrenal (with or without Cushing syndrome) may be associated with hemihypertrophy, usually during the first few years of life. These tumors are also associated with Beckwith-Wiedemann syndrome and other congenital defects, particularly genitourinary tract and central nervous system abnormalities and hamartomatous defects.

Urinary 17-ketosteroids and serum levels of DHEA, DHEAS, and androstenedione are usually elevated, often markedly. Serum levels of testosterone are also usually increased as a result of peripheral conversion of androstenedione, but infants who have had predominantly testosterone-secreting adenomas are known. Many adrenocortical tumors have 11β-hydroxylase deficiency and secrete increased amounts of deoxycorticosterone; these patients are hypertensive, and the tumor is usually malignant. Ultrasound and magnetic resonance studies are indicated and can detect masses as small as 1.3 cm. Carcinomas are three times more common than adenomas. Differentiation between benign and malignant tumors by histologic criteria is often not possible.

The treatment is surgical; a transperitoneal approach is usually recommended. Some of these neoplasms are highly malignant and metastasize widely, but cure with regression of the masculinizing features may follow removal of less malignant encapsulated tumors.

A neoplasm of one adrenal may produce atrophy of the other, because excessive production of cortical hormones by the tumor suppresses ACTH stimulation of the normal gland. Consequently, adrenal insufficiency may follow surgical removal of the tumor. This situation can be avoided by giving 10–25 mg of hydrocortisone every 6 hr, starting on the day of operation and continuing for 3–4 days postoperatively. It may also be necessary to give corticotropin concurrently with cortisol to reactivate the atrophied gland. Adequate quantities of water, sodium chloride, and glucose must also be provided. Rarely, the tumors are bilateral, and in at least five instances the contralateral adrenal was absent; in such instances replacement therapy must be continued indefinitely.

Patients with tumors that are easily resected and weigh less than 150 g have a good prognosis. If the tumor is large or incompletely removed, the prognosis is guarded. Radiotherapy is not generally helpful. Adrenal androgen levels should be measured at monthly intervals to detect recurrences early. Adjuvant therapy with mitotane (o,p′-DDD), an isomer of DDD, is indicated for inoperable tumors and for recurrences. This agent can induce regression of abnormal steroid production in most patients and tumor regression in only 10–20% of patients; only a few long-term survivals are known. In at least eight patients a second primary tumor developed; the central nervous system was the most frequent site.

ADRENAL CORTICAL HYPERFUNCTION

Bitton RN, Cobbs R, Schneider BS: Development of Nelson syndrome in a patient with recurrent Cushing disease: Analysis of secretory behavior of the pituitary tumor. Am J Med 84:319, 1988.

Boston BA, Mandel S, LaFranchi S, Bliziotes M: Activating mutation in the stimulatory guanine nucleotide-binding protein in an infant with Cushing's syndrome and nodular adrenal hyperplasia. J Clin Endocrinol Metab 79:890, 1994.

Bryer-Ash M, Wilson DM, Tune BM, et al: Hypertension caused by an aldosterone-secreting adenoma. Occurrence in a 7-year-old child. Am J Dis Child 138:673, 1984.

Burr IM, Sullivan J, Graham T, et al: A testosterone-secreting tumour of the adrenal producing virilization in a female infant. Lancet 2:643, 1973.

Cara JF, Moshang T Jr, Bongiovanni AM, et al: Elevated 17-hydroxyprogesterone and testosterone in a newborn with 3-beta-hydroxysteroid dehydrogenase deficiency. N Engl J Med 313:618, 1985.

Clark RV, Albertson BD, Munabi A, et al: Steroidogenic enzyme activities, morphology, and receptor studies of a testicular adrenal rest in a patient with congenital adrenal hyperplasia. J Clin Endocrinol Metab 70:1408, 1990.

Comite F, Schiebinger RJ, Alertson BD, et al: Isosexual precocious pseudopuberty secondary to a feminizing adrenal tumor. J Clin Endocrinol Metab 58:435, 1984.

Cutler GB Jr, Lave L: Congenital adrenal hyperplasia due to 21-hydroxylase deficiency. N Engl J Med 323:1806, 1990.

Duck SC: Acceptable linear growth in congenital adrenal hyperplasia. J Pediatr 97:93, 1980.

Eldar-Geva T, Hurwitz A, Velsei P, et al: Secondary biosynthetic defects in women with late-onset congenital adrenal hyperplasia. N Engl J Med 323:855, 1990.

Fallo F, Kuhnle U, Boscaro M, Sonino N: Abnormality of aldosterone and cortisol late pathways in glucocorticoid-remediable aldosteronism. J Clin Endocrinol Metab 79:772, 1994.

Fardella CE, Hum DW, Homoki J, Miller WL: Point mutation of Arg 440 to His in cytochrome P450c17 causes severe 17α-hydroxylase deficiency. J Clin Endocrinol Metab 79:160, 1994.

Funder JW: Mineralocorticoids, glucocorticoids, receptors and response elements. Science 259:1132, 1993.

Fraumeni JF Jr, Miller RW: Adrenocortical neoplasms with hemihypertrophy, brain tumors, and other disorders. J Pediatr 70:129, 1967.

Gomez MT, Malazowski S, Winterer J, et al: Urinary free cortisol values in children and adolescents. J Pediatr 118:256, 1991.

Gomez-Sanchez CE, Gill JR Jr, Ganguly A, et al: Glucocoid-suppressible aldosteronism: A disorder of the adrenal transitional zona. J Clin Endocrinol Metab 67:444, 1988.

Harshfield GA, Alpert BS, Pullam DA: Renin-angiotensin aldosterone system in healthy subjects ten to eighteen years. J Pediatr 122:563, 1993.

Holler W, Scholz S, Knon D, et al: Genetic differences between the salt-wasting simple virilizing and nonclassical types of congenital adrenal hyperplasia. J Clin Endocrinol Metab 60:757, 1985.

Howard CP, Takahashi H, Hayles AB: Feminizing adrenal adenoma in a boy. Case report and literature review. Mayo Clin Proc 52:354, 1977.

Karl M, Lamberts SWJ, Detera-Wadleigh SD, et al: Familial glucocorticoid resistance caused by a splice site deletion in the human glucocorticoid receptor. J Clin Endocrinol Metab 76:683, 1993.

Lee PDK, Winter RJ, Green OC: Virilizing adrenocortical tumors in childhood: Eight cases and a review of the literature. Pediatrics 76:437, 1985.

Levine LS, Pang S: Prenatal diagnosis and treatment of congenital adrenal hyperplasia. J Pediatr Endocrinol 7:193, 1994.

Lifton RP, Dluhy RG: The molecular basis of a hereditary form of hypertension, glucocorticoid-remediable aldosteronism. Trends Endocrinol Metab 4:57, 1993.

Lin D, Sugawara T, Straun JF, et al: Role of steroidogenic acute regulatory protein in adrenal and gonadal steroidogenesis. Science 267:1828, 1995.

Luton LP, Cerdas S, Billaud L, et al: Clinical features of adrenocortical carcinoma, prognostic factors, and the effect of mitotane therapy. N Engl J Med 322:1195, 1990.

Mason JI: The 3β-hydroxysteroid dehydrogenase gene family of enzymes. Trends Endocrinol Metab 6:199, 1993.

Malchoff CD, Javier EC, Malchoff DM, et al: Primary cortisol resistance presenting as isosexual precocity. J Clin Endocrinol Metab 70:503, 1990.

Miller WL: Gene conversions, deletions, and polymorphisms in congenital adrenal hyperplasia. Am J Hum Genet 42:4, 1988.

Miller WL: Molecular biology of steroid hormone synthesis. Endocr Rev 9:295, 1988.

Miller WL: Genetics, diagnosis, and management of 21-hydroxylase deficiency. J Clin Endocrinol Metab 78:241, 1994.

New MI, Lorenzen F, Lerner AJ, et al: Genotyping steroid 21-hydroxylase deficiency: Hormonal reference data. J Clin Endocrinol Metab 57:320, 1983.
Pang S, Levine LS, Stoner E, et al: Nonsalt-losing congenital adrenal hyperplasia due to 3β-hydroxysteroid dehydrogenase deficiency with normal glomerulosa function. J Clin Endocrinol Metab 56:808, 1983.
Pescovitz OH, Comite F, Cassorla F, et al: True precocious puberty complicating congenital adrenal hyperplasia: Treatment with a luteinizing hormone-releasing hormone analog. J Clin Endocrinol Metab 58:857, 1984.
Rescoria FJ, Vane DW, Fitzgerald JF, et al: Vasoactive intestinal polypeptide-secreting ganglioneuromatosis affecting the entire colon and rectum. J Pediatr Surg 23:635, 1988.
Ribeiro RC, Neto RS, Schell MJ, et al: Adrenocortical carcinoma in children: A study of 40 cases. J Clin Oncol 8:67, 1990.
Sanchez R, Rheaume E, LaFlamme N, et al: Detection and functional characterization of the novel missense mutation Y254D in type II 3β-hydroxylase dehydrogenase (3β254D) gene in a female patient with nonsalt-losing 3βHSD deficiency. J Clin Endocr Metab 78:561, 1994.
Speiser PW, Agdere L, Ueshiba H, et al: Aldosterone synthesis in salt-wasting congenital adrenal hyperplasia with complete absence of adrenal 21-hydroxylase. N Engl J Med 324:145, 1991.
Speiser PW, New MI, White PC: Molecular genetic analysis of nonclassic steroid 11-hydroxylase deficiency associated with HLA-B14,DR1. N Engl J Med 319:19, 1988.
Stewart PM, Edwards CRW: Specificity of the mineralocorticoid receptor. Crucial role of 11β-hydroxysteroid dehydrogenase. Trends Endocrinol Metab 1:225, 1990.
Strachan T: Molecular pathology of congenital adrenal hyperplasia. Clin Endocrinol 32:373, 1990.
Sultan C, Descomps B, Garandeau P, et al: Pubertal gynecomastia due to an estrogen-producing adrenal adenoma. J Pediatr 95:744, 1979.
Styne DM, Isaac R, Miller WL, et al: Endocrine, histological and biochemical studies of adrenocorticotropin-producing islet cell carcinoma of the pancreas in childhood with characterization of propiomelanocortin. J Clin Endocrinol Metab 57:723, 1983.
Urabe K, Kimura A, Harada F, et al: Gene conversions in steroid 21-hydroxylase genes. Am J Hum Genet 46:1178, 1990.
White PC, Tusie-Luna Mt, New MI, Speiser PW: Mutations in steroid 21-hydroxylase (CPY21). Hum Mutations 3:373, 1994.
White PC, Pascoe L: Disorders of steroid 11β-hydroxylase isozymes. Trends Endocrinol Metab 3:229, 1992.
Yanase T, Simpson ER, Waterman MR: 17α-hydroxylase/17.20-lyase deficiency: From clinical investigation to molecular definition. J Clin Endocrinol Metab 12:91, 1991.
Wolffraat NM, Drexhage HA, Wiersinga WM, et al: Immunoglobulins of patients with Cushing's syndrome due to pigmented adrenocortical micronodular dysplasia stimulate in vitro steroidogenesis. J Clin Endocrin Metab 66:301, 1988.

CHAPTER 530
Cushing Syndrome

Cushing syndrome, a characteristic pattern of obesity with associated hypertension, is the result of maintenance of abnormally high blood levels of cortisol by hyperfunction of the adrenal cortex. The syndrome may be corticotropin (ACTH) dependent or ACTH independent.

ETIOLOGY. In infants, Cushing syndrome is most often caused by a *functioning adrenocortical tumor,* usually a malignant carcinoma but occasionally a benign adenoma. More than 50% of cortical tumors occur in children 3 yr of age or younger, and 85% occur in children 7 yr or younger. Patients with cortical tumors often exhibit a mixed form of hypercortisolism because of overproduction of other steroids such as androgens, estrogens, and aldosterone.

Primary pigmented nodular adrenocortical disease is a distinctive form of ACTH-independent Cushing syndrome in infants and children. The adrenal glands are small and have characteristic multiple, small (<4 mm in diameter), pigmented (black) nodules containing large cells with cytoplasm and lipofuscin; between the nodules, there is cortical atrophy. Evidence suggests that the condition is caused by circulating immunoglobulins directed toward the ACTH receptor, with ensuing stimulation of adrenal steroidogenesis. This adrenal disorder occurs as a component of the **Carney complex**, an autosomal dominant disorder consisting of centrofacial lentigines, cardiac and cutaneous myxomas, sexual precocity in boys with testicular tumors, functioning pituitary tumors, and pigmented melanotic schwannomas.

ACTH-independent Cushing syndrome with nodular hyperplasia and adenoma formation occurs in cases of McCune-Albright syndrome, with symptoms beginning in infancy or childhood. In a report of an infant with nonpigmented adrenocortical hyperplasia with nodular elements and asymptomatic fibrous dysplasia of the left femur and humerus, an activating mutation in the stimulatory G protein that controls the production of cAMP was detected. Activating mutations have been found in several patients with McCune-Albright syndrome.

In children older than 7 yr of age, *bilateral adrenal hyperplasia,* an ACTH-dependent form of Cushing syndrome, is usually found. This entity is caused by a basophilic adenoma of the pituitary in about 20% of affected children. Covert pituitary adenomas (microadenomas) occur in most patients with Cushing disease, and resection of these tumors results in correction of the hypercorticism. In some children, the pituitary tumors become overt after adrenalectomy *(Nelson syndrome)*; these consist principally of chromophobe cells and produce increased levels of β-lipotropin, β-endorphin, and ACTH. There are only two reports of ACTH-secreting tumors in infants with Cushing syndrome.

Bilateral hyperplasia of the adrenals may also result from *ectopic production of ACTH.* Cushing syndrome has been associated with an islet cell carcinoma of the pancreas in four children, with neuroblastoma or ganglioneuroblastoma in several children, with a hemangiopericytoma arising from the cerebral tentorium in a 7-yr-old boy, with Wilms tumors in two children, and with thymic carcinoid in a 10-yr-old girl.

Prolonged exogenous administration of ACTH or hydrocortisone or its analogs results in a clinical pattern identical to the spontaneous disorder and is frequently referred to as *cushingoid syndrome.*

CLINICAL MANIFESTATIONS. Symptoms may begin in the neonatal period and have been recognized in at least 35 infants younger than 1 yr of age. Early in life, girls outnumber boys 3:1, and adrenocortical tumors (e.g., carcinoma, adenoma, nodular hyperplasia) are the usual causative lesions. The disorder appears to be more severe and the clinical findings more flagrant in infants than when the onset occurs in older children. The face is rounded, with prominent cheeks and a flushed appearance (moon facies). The chin is doubled, there is a buffalo hump, and generalized obesity is common. Signs of abnormal masculinization due to the androgen production of tumors occur frequently; accordingly, there may be hypertrichosis on the face and trunk, pubic hair, acne, deepening of the voice, and enlargement of the clitoris in girls. Growth is impaired, with length falling below the 3rd percentile, except when significant virilization produces normal or even accelerated growth. Hypertension is common and may lead to heart failure. An increased susceptibility to infection may lead to fatal sepsis. Infants with Cushing syndrome, despite a robust appearance, are usually fragile. Occasionally, the condition is associated with hemihypertrophy or other congenital defects.

In older children, bilateral hyperplasia of the adrenals is the most common lesion, and the sex incidence is equal. In addition to obesity, short stature is a common presenting feature. Gradual onset of obesity and deceleration or cessation of growth may be the only early manifestations. Purplish striae on the hips, abdomen, and thighs are common. Pubertal development may be delayed, or amenorrhea may occur in girls past menarche. Weakness, headache, deterioration in school work, and emotional lability may be prominent. Hypertension is usual. Renal stones have occurred in older children and in infants.

LABORATORY DATA. Polycythemia, lymphopenia, and eosinopenia are common. The glucose tolerance test result may be diabetic despite elevated levels of insulin. Levels of serum electrolytes are usually normal, but potassium may be decreased.

Cortisol levels in blood are normally elevated at 8:00 A.M. and decrease to less than 50% by 8:00 P.M. except in children younger than 3 yr of age, in whom a diurnal rhythm is not always established. In patients with Cushing syndrome, this diurnal rhythm is lost, and cortisol levels at 8:00 P.M. are usually elevated. Urinary excretion of free cortisol is almost always increased; normal values are 20–90 μg/24 hr. Urinary excretion of 17-hydroxycorticosteroids is usually increased (>5 mg/m^2/24 hr). In questionable cases, a single-dose dexamethasone suppression test may be helpful; a dose of 0.3 mg/m^2 given at 11:00 P.M. will result in a plasma cortisol level of less than 5 μg/dL at 8:00 A.M. the next morning in normal children.

After the diagnosis of Cushing syndrome has been established, it is necessary to determine whether it is ACTH dependent or independent. ACTH concentrations alone usually are not helpful in the differential diagnosis because of the large range of normal basal levels. The ovine corticotropin-releasing hormone (oCRH) stimulation test is still experimental but seems promising. After an intravenous bolus of oCRH (1 μg/kg), patients with ACTH-dependent Cushing syndrome have an exaggerated ACTH and cortisol response, but those with adrenal tumors show no increase in ACTH and cortisol. Another test consists of administration of dexamethasone, 30 and 120 μg/kg/24 hr, divided into four doses and given for 2 consecutive days each. In children with ACTH-dependent Cushing syndrome, the larger dose suppresses urinary free cortisol or 17-hydroxycorticosteroids to less than 50% of baseline, and serum levels of cortisol decrease to less than 7 μg/dL. Occasional parodoxic results have been reported.

Osseous maturation is usually moderately retarded but may be normal; in virilized children, the bone age is likely to be advanced. Osteoporosis is common and is most evident in roentgenograms of the spine. Pathologic fractures may be detected. Levels of growth hormone, secreted spontaneously and stimulated, are suppressed but return to normal when the hypercortisolism is corrected. Diminution of muscle mass and increased deposition of adipose tissue may be noticed in roentgenograms of the extremities. The thymic shadow is absent because excessive cortisol produces involution. Computed tomography (CT) scanning detects virtually all adrenal tumors larger than 1.5 cm in diameter. Adrenal scintigraphy with radiocholesterol is rarely indicated except for patients with pigmented micronodular adrenal hyperplasia, for whom it may be more accurate than a CT scan. Magnetic resonance imaging is the screening method of choice to detect ACTH-secreting pituitary adenomas; the addition of gadolinium contrast increases the sensitivity of detection. Bilateral inferior petrosal blood sampling to measure concentrations of ACTH before and after CRH administration may be required when a pituitary adenoma is not visualized.

DIFFERENTIAL DIAGNOSIS. Cushing syndrome is frequently suspected in children with obesity, particularly when striae and hypertension are present. The differential diagnosis is complicated by the fact that elevated urinary concentrations of corticosteroids are frequently secondary to obesity itself. Children with simple obesity are usually tall, but those with Cushing syndrome are short or have a decelerating growth rate. The excretion of urinary corticosteroids is rapidly suppressed by oral administration of low doses of dexamethasone in persons with uncomplicated obesity. Elevated levels of cortisol and ACTH without clinical evidence of Cushing syndrome occur in patients with generalized glucocorticoid resistance. Affected patients may be asymptomatic or exhibit hypertension, hypokalemia, and precocious pseudopuberty; these manifestations are caused by increased mineralocorticoid and adrenal androgens in response to elevated ACTH levels. Several mutations of the glucocorticoid receptor have been reported.

TREATMENT. If the lesion is a benign cortical adenoma, unilateral adrenalectomy is indicated. Such adenomas are occasionally bilateral; then the treatment of choice is subtotal adrenalectomy. In either instance, an excellent therapeutic result is achieved by removing the tumor. Adrenocortical carcinomas frequently metastasize, especially to the liver and lungs, and the prognosis may be unfavorable despite removal of the primary lesion. Rarely, the tumors are bilateral and require total adrenalectomy. It is often impossible to differentiate benign from malignant tumors by histologic appearance alone.

Management of Cushing disease is still unsettled. Total adrenalectomy has fallen into disfavor because about 30% of patients develop an expanding pituitary tumor postoperatively. Intense melanosis, markedly elevated serum levels of ACTH (often >1,000 pg/mL), and enlargement of the sella turcica occur *(Nelson syndrome)*. To circumvent this problem, current treatment is directed at the pituitary. External irradiation of the pituitary is advocated by some, but remission is slow and sequelae include hypopituitarism and behavioral changes. The most frequently recommended approach is transsphenoidal pituitary microsurgery. In the hands of an experienced neurosurgeon, selective adenoma resection has produced low morbidity and a good remission rate.

Cyproheptadine, a centrally acting serotonin antagonist that blocks ACTH release, has been used to treat Cushing disease in adults; remissions are usually not sustained after discontinuation of therapy. A child with Cushing disease treated with this agent has had a 3-yr remission after cessation of therapy; further therapeutic trials are needed.

Management of patients undergoing adrenalectomy requires adequate preoperative and postoperative replacement therapy with a corticosteroid. Tumors that produce corticosteroids usually lead to atrophy of the normal adrenal tissue, and replacement with cortisol and ACTH may be required. Postoperative complications have included sepsis, pancreatitis, thrombosis, poor wound healing, and sudden collapse, particularly in infants with Cushing syndrome. Substantial catch-up growth occurs, but adult height is often compromised.

CHAPTER 531
Excess Mineralocorticoid Secretion

The principal mineralocorticoid secreted by the adrenal is aldosterone. Increased secretion may result from a primary defect of the adrenal (primary hyperaldosteronism) or from factors that activate the renin-angiotensin system (secondary hyperaldosteronism). Patients with primary hyperaldosteronism usually have hypertension or hypokalemia; those with secondary hyperaldosteronism do not.

Desoxycorticosterone is a precursor of aldosterone, with only about one thirtieth the sodium-retaining potency of aldosterone (see Fig. 529–1). Overproduction of desoxycorticosterone occurs with two distinct defects of adrenal steroidogenesis. The first defect involves 11-hydroxylation, which also leads [illegible] androgen excess and presents clinically as the hypertensive [illegible] of congenital adrenal hyperplasia (see Chapter 529). The [illegible] defect involves 17-hydroxylation, producing hypogo- [illegible] female and male pseudohermaphroditism in the [illegible] synthesis of androgens and estrogens as well [illegible] aired.

[illegible] steronism encompasses disorders char- [illegible] dosterone secretion independent of the [illegible] These disorders, rare in children, are cha[illegible] hypokalemia, and suppression of the [illegible]

Aldosterone-se[illegible] teral and have been reported in childre[illegible] age; they mainly affect girls.

Bilateral micronodular adre[illegible]*asia* tends to occur in older children. There is increa[illegible]ence that the adrenal is being stimulated by a circulating [illegible]coprotein that appears to originate in the pituitary.

Primary aldosteronism due to unilateral adrenal hyperplasia has been reported infrequently in children.

Glucocorticoid-suppressible aldosteronism, also known as glucocorticoid-remediable aldosteronism, is an ACTH-dependent autosomal dominant form of hyperaldosteronism. The hyperaldosteronism is rapidly suppressed by glucocorticoid administration, with normalization of the biochemical abnormalities and, in young patients, of the hypertension. In this disorder there is marked overproduction of 18-hydroxycortisol and 18-oxocortisol, hybrid steroids having the characteristics of zona glomerulosa and zona fasciculata steroids. The regulation of aldosterone secretion by ACTH and the oversecretion of the hybrid steroids have been explained by recent studies that demonstrated that the disorder is caused by crossover events between the *CYP11B1* gene (which encodes $P_{450}c11$) and the *CYP11B2* gene (which encodes aldosterone synthase or $P_{450}c18$). A "hybrid" gene is produced, having the regulatory sequence of *CYP11B1* and the coding sequences of the aldosterone synthase gene. This results in the ectopic expression of aldosterone synthase in the adrenal fasciculata. At-risk family members should be investigated for this easily treated cause of hypertension. The biochemical abnormality can be demonstrated in normotensive individuals.

CLINICAL MANIFESTATIONS. Some affected children have no symptoms, the diagnosis being established after incidental discovery of moderate hypertension. Others have severe hypertension (up to 240/150 mm Hg), with headache, dizziness, and visual disturbances. Chronic hypokalemia may lead to "clear cell nephrosis," polyuria, nocturia, enuresis, and polydipsia. Muscle weakness and discomfort, tetany, intermittent paralysis, fatigue, and growth failure affect these patients.

LABORATORY STUDIES. Hypertension, hypokalemia, and suppressed plasma renin activity are the hallmarks of hyperaldosteronism. The serum pH, carbon dioxide content, and sodium concentrations may be elevated and the serum chloride and magnesium levels decreased. Serum levels of calcium are normal, even in children who manifest tetany. The urine is neutral or alkaline. Plasma and urine levels of aldosterone are increased, and plasma levels of renin are persistently low. In patients with glucocorticoid-suppressible aldosteronism, urinary and plasma levels of 18-oxocortisol and 18-hydroxycortisol are markedly increased.

DIFFERENTIAL DIAGNOSIS. After establishing the diagnosis of primary aldosteronism, it is necessary to determine the cause. All children should have a therapeutic trial with dexamethasone before invasive studies are done. Daily administration of 0.25 mg every 6 hr results in marked suppression of aldosterone and disappearance of hypertension in those patients with the glucocorticoid-suppressible variant of hyperaldosteronism. If there is no response to dexamethasone, computed tomography (CT) may help to detect an adrenal adenoma, but the tumors are often quite small. If CT scans are normal, adrenal vein catheterization is indicated. High concentrations of aldosterone are found in only one adrenal vein when an adenoma is present and in both when bilateral hyperplasia is the cause. Cortisol levels should be obtained simultaneously to compare adrenal vein aldosterone and cortisol ratios. If adrenal vein catheterization is not successful, exploratory laparotomy may be required to establish the diagnosis.

Hyperaldosteronism occurs in many other conditions in which it is a normal homeostatic response. In such *secondary hyperaldosteronism*, plasma renin activity is high or rises with a low-salt diet, whereas in primary hyperaldosteronism the renin-angiotensin system is suppressed. Increased aldosterone secretion occurs in edematous disorders with reduced effective volume, such as nephrotic syndrome, congestive cardiac failure, and cirrhosis of the liver. Increased secretion of aldosterone also occurs in conditions in which compromise of renal perfusion results in increased secretion of renin, such as in stenosis of the renal artery. Wilms tumor and juxtaglomerular cell tumors may also secrete renin and cause secondary hyperaldosteronism.

In *pseudohypoaldosteronism* the increased levels of aldosterone are due to a deficiency or abnormality of aldosterone receptors, with ensuing activation of the renin-angiotensin system (see Chapter 528).

Barrter syndrome is also characterized by hypokalemic alkalosis, hypochloremia, and hyperaldosteronism, but the blood pressure is normal, and secretion of renin is increased. Growth failure is the usual presenting complaint. The primary defect appears to be deficient reabsorption in the ascending limb of the loop of Henle. Renal biopsy reveals hyperplasia of the juxtaglomerular apparatus. Urinary excretion of prostaglandins has been demonstrated, and it has been suggested that this mediates the hyper-reninemia (see Chapter 485).

11β-Hydroxysteroid dehydrogenase (11β-OHSD) deficiency has been reported in 18 children. Onset occurs in early childhood with failure to thrive, polyuria and polydipsia secondary to the effects of hypokalemia, and severe hypertension. Strokes have occurred in young children. The disorder has been reported in siblings and appears to have a genetic basis. Although clinically the disorder mimics that seen in patients with elevated aldosterone levels, renin and aldosterone levels are low *(low-renin hypertension)*. For several decades, the condition was thought to be caused by production of an undetected mineralocorticoid and was named the *syndrome of apparent mineralocorticoid excess*. However, the disorder is caused by a deficiency of the enzyme that converts cortisol to cortisone. Plasma levels of cortisol are normal, but those of cortisone are low, and the ratio of the urinary tetrahydro products of cortisol to cortisone is characteristically elevated.

How this glucocorticoid defect can cause such profound mineralocorticoid effects has been elucidated. Type I mineralocorticoid receptors (kidney, parotid glands, colon) have equal affinity for aldosterone and cortisol. Under normal conditions, 11β-OHSD acts as a paracrine protector for the mineralocorticoid receptor in the proximal tubules of the kidney; by converting cortisol to cortisone at this site, it can no longer bind to the receptor. In the absence of this enzyme and with failure of conversion of cortisol to cortisone, cortisol binds to the mineralocorticoid receptor and elicits effects similar to those of aldosterone. Another name suggested for this condition is *pseudohyperaldosteronism*. The gene for 11β-OHSD has been cloned. However no mutations in the gene have been detected to date in the patients with this disorder who have been studied. The well-known hypertensive effect of glycorrhetinic acid, a constituent of licorice, is now known to be caused by its inhibition of renal 11β-OHSD.

TREATMENT. Glucocorticoid-suppressible hyperaldosteronism is managed by daily administration of dexamethasone or prednisone. Bilateral adrenal hyperplasia that does not respond to this therapy requires bilateral adrenalectomy; the results are excellent, but adrenal replacement therapy is required. Removal of an aldosterone-secreting adenoma results in cure.

Treatment of secondary hyperaldosteronism is directed to the specific causative disorder.

CHAPTER 532
Feminizing Adrenal Tumors

Adrenocortical tumors have been reported in approximately a dozen boys with excessive production of estrogens and heterosexual precocious puberty. Gynecomastia was the initial manifestation, appearing from 6 mo–7 yr of age. Growth and development were otherwise normal, or concomitant virilization was sometimes evidenced by acne, deep voice, phallic enlargement, and advanced osseous maturation. The testes were not enlarged. Hypertension is common in affected adults but has not been observed in children. The levels of estrogens and often of androgens in plasma and urine are markedly elevated. Tumors may be carcinomas or benign adenomas and may be calcified on roentgenograms. Gynecomastia regresses after removal of the tumor, and hormone values return to normal.

Estrogen-secreting adrenocortical tumors have been reported in at least 12 girls ranging in age from 6 mo–10 yr. The majority of the tumors were adenomas, some of which also elaborated androgens (with virilization) or mineralocorticoids (with hypertension). In addition to elevated plasma and urinary levels of estrogens, there were usually elevated levels of 17-ketosteroids in urine and of Δ^5 adrenal steroids (i.e., dehydroepiandrosterone and its sulfate) in plasma. Plasma gonadotropin levels are suppressed, and GnRH stimulation does not elicit a response. Computed tomography usually localizes the tumor.

CHAPTER 533
Pheochromocytoma

The pheochromocytoma, a catecholamine-secreting tumor, arises from the chromaffin cells. The most common site of origin is the adrenal medulla; tumors may develop, however, anywhere along the abdominal sympathetic chain and are likely to be located near the aorta at the level of the inferior mesenteric artery or at its bifurcation. They also appear in the periadrenal area, the urinary bladder or ureteral walls, the thoracic cavity, and the cervical region. Fewer than 5% of reported instances have occurred in children. Tumors vary from about 1–10 cm in diameter; they are found more often on the right side than on the left. In 20% of affected children, the adrenal tumors are bilateral, and in 30%, tumors are found in both the adrenal and extra-adrenal areas or only in an extra-adrenal area.

Pheochromocytoma is frequently inherited as an autosomal dominant trait. In affected families, the ages of patients at the time of diagnosis have varied from the 1st to 5th decades of life; more than half the patients have had multiple tumors.

Pheochromocytoma is frequently associated with other syndromes or tumors. Approximately 5% of patients with pheochromocytoma have neurofibromatosis. Sporadic and familial instances of pheochromocytoma have been observed in patients with von Hippel–Lindau disease. Early molecular diagnosis of this condition is important, because families predisposed to develop pheochromocytomas have specific missense mutations.

Pheochromocytoma is a component of type IIA and type IIB multiple endocrine neoplasia syndrome; medullary carcinoma of the thyroid usually appears at an earlier age than pheochromocytoma (see Chapter 524). These syndromes are inherited in an autosomal dominant fashion; the condition is caused by a mutation of the *RET* proto-oncogene on chromosome 10q11.2.

CLINICAL MANIFESTATIONS. The clinical features result from excessive secretion of epinephrine and norepinephrine; the clinical picture varies with quantitative variations in their secretion. All patients have hypertension at some time. The hypertension is usually sustained, but it may often be *paroxysmal.* Paroxysms should particularly suggest pheochromocytoma as a diagnostic possibility. When there are paroxysms of hypertension, the attacks are usually infrequent at first but become more frequent and eventually give way to a continuous hypertensive state. Between attacks of hypertension, the patient may be free of symptoms. During attacks, the patient complains of headache and palpitations, and pallor, vomiting, and sweating also occur. Convulsions and other manifestations of hypertensive encephalopathy may occur. In severe cases, precordial pains radiate into the arms, and pulmonary edema and cardiac and hepatic enlargement may develop. The child has a good appetite but because of hypermetabolism does not gain weight, and severe cachexia may develop. Polyuria and polydipsia can be sufficiently severe to suggest diabetes insipidus. Growth failure may be striking. The blood pressure may range from 180–260 systolic and 120–210 diastolic, and the heart may be enlarged. Ophthalmoscopic examination may reveal papilledema, hemorrhages, exudate, and arterial constriction.

LABORATORY DATA. The urine contains protein, a few casts, and occasionally glucose. Gross hematuria suggests that the tumor is in the bladder wall. Polycythemia is occasionally observed. The diagnosis is established by demonstration of elevated plasma or urinary levels of catecholamines and their metabolites.

Pheochromocytomas produce norepinephrine and epinephrine; norepinephrine in plasma is derived, however, from the adrenal gland and adrenergic nerve endings, but epinephrine is derived primarily from the adrenal. In contrast to adults, the predominant catecholamine in children is norepinephrine, and total urinary catecholamine excretion usually exceeds 300 μg/24 hr. The concentrations of catecholamines in urine are directly related to those in the tumor. Urinary excretion of vanillylmandelic acid (VMA, 3-methoxy-4-hydroxymandelic acid), the major metabolite of epinephrine and norepinephrine, and of metanephrine (see Fig. 533–1) are also increased. Catecholamine levels can be measured by radioimmunoassay and high-performance liquid chromatography methods. Excretion of catecholamine metabolites may be similar in children with neuroblastoma and with pheochromocytoma, but levels are usually higher in those with pheochromocytoma. Daily urinary excretion of these compounds by unaffected children increases with age; and vanilla-containing foods and fruits can produce falsely elevated levels of VMA. Certain drugs interfere with fluorometric determinations of catecholamines.

Most tumors in the area of the adrenal are readily localized by echography or by computed tomography or magnetic resonance scans; their frequent bilateral occurrence must not be

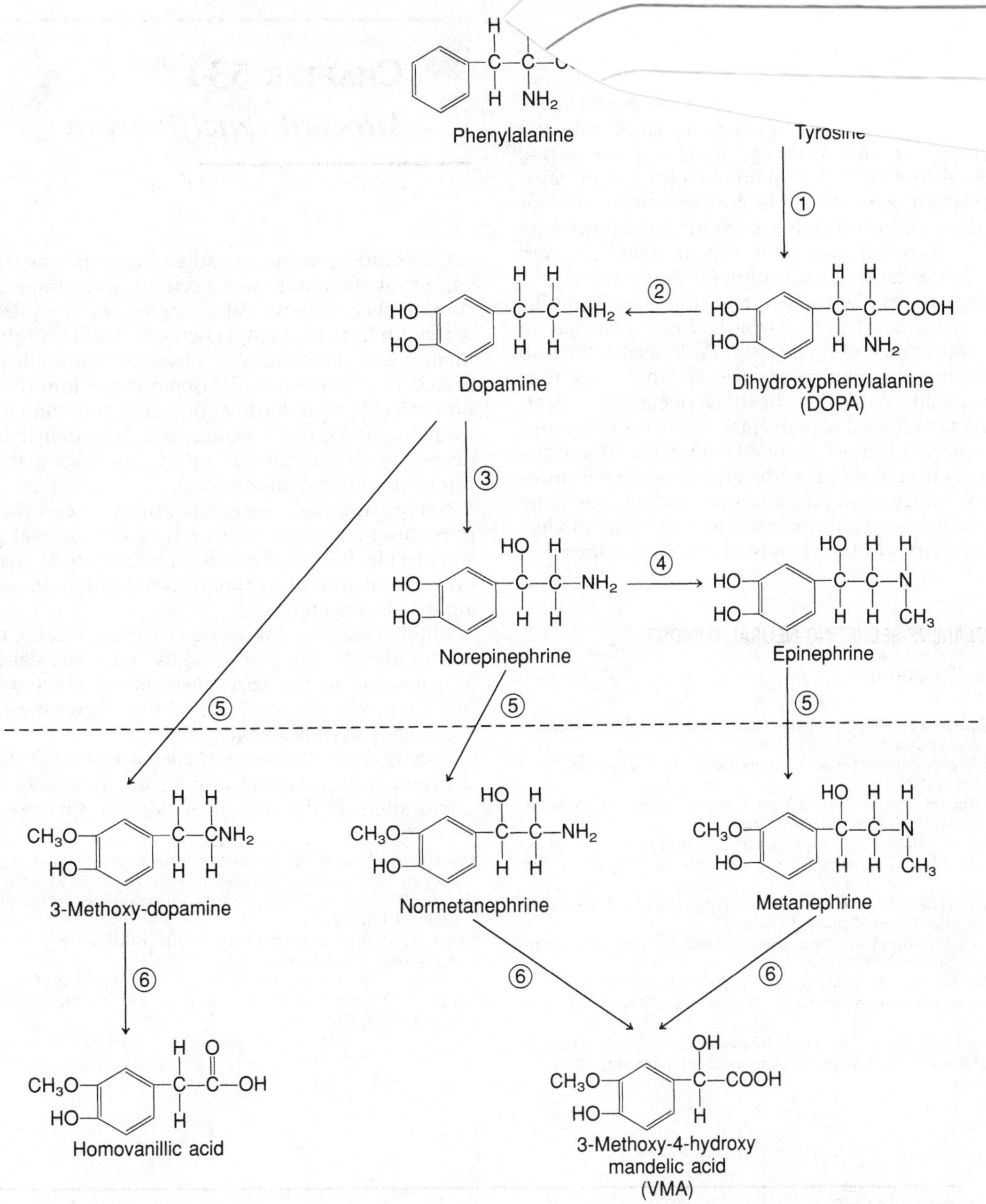

Figure 533–1. Biosynthesis (above dashed line) and metabolism (below dashed line) of the catecholamines: norepinephrine and epinephrine. Enzymes: 1. Tyrosine hydroxylase; 2. Dopa decarboxylase; 3. Dopamine β-oxidase; 4. Phenylethanolamine-*N*-methyl transferase; 5. Catechol-*O*-methyltransferase; 6. Monocrine oxidase.

forgotten. Extra-adrenal tumors, anywhere from the neck to the bladder, may be difficult to detect. ^{131}I-metaiodobenzylguanidine is taken up by chromaffin tissue anywhere in the body and is useful for localizing small tumors. Venous catheterization with sampling of blood at different levels for catecholamine determinations is now only rarely necessary for localizing the tumor.

DIFFERENTIAL DIAGNOSIS. The various causes of hypertension in children, such as renal or renovascular disease, coarctation of the aorta, acrodynia, thallium intoxication, hyperthyroidism, Cushing syndrome, 11β-hydroxylase, 17-hydroxylase, and 11β-hydroxysteroid dehydrogenase deficiency, primary aldosteronism, adrenal cortical tumors, and essential hypertension must be considered. A nonfunctioning kidney may result from compression of a ureter or of a renal artery by a pheochromocytoma. Paroxysmal hypertension may be associated with familial dysautonomia. Urinary excretion of VMA is low in familial dysautonomia because of a defect in release rather than in synthesis of catecholamines. Cerebral disorders, diabetes insipidus, diabetes mellitus, and hyperthyroidism must also be considered in the differential diagnosis. Hypertension in patients with neurofibromatosis may be caused by renal vascular involvement and by concurrent pheochromocytoma.

Neuroblastoma, ganglioneuroblastoma, and ganglioneuroma frequently produce catecholamines. Secreting neurogentic tumors commonly produce hypertension, excessive sweating, flushing, pallor, rash, polyuria, and polydipsia. Diarrhea may be associated with these tumors, particularly with ganglioneuroma, and at times may be sufficiently persistent to suggest the celiac syndrome.

TREATMENT. Removal of these tumors results in cure, but the operation is not without danger. Careful preoperative, intraoperative, and postoperative management is essential. Preoperative α- and β-adrenergic blockade is required. Because these tumors are often multiple in children, a thorough transabdominal exploration of all the usual sites offers the best chance of finding all of them. Appropriate choice of anesthesia and expansion of blood volume with appropriate fluids during surgery are critical to avoid a precipitious drop in blood pressure during operation or within 48 hr postoperatively. Manipulation and excision of these tumors result in marked increases in catecholamine secretion that cause rises in blood pressure and heart rate. Surveillance must continue postoperatively.

Although these tumors often appear malignant histologically, only rarely has malignancy been established unequivocally in a child by the appearance of metastases. Prolonged follow-up is indicated because functioning tumors at other sites may become manifest many years after the initial operation. Examination of relatives of affected patients may reveal other persons harboring unsuspected tumors. In one family with 10 affected individuals, the highest blood pressures and urinary concentrations of catecholamines were found in the children, but some of the affected adults were normotensive and had only moderately elevated urinary concentrations of catecholamines and VMA.

OTHER CATECHOLAMINE-SECRETING NEURAL TUMORS

See Chapters 291 and 451.

Bravo EL: Evolving concepts in the pathophysiology, diagnosis and treatment of pheochromocytoma. Endocr Rev 15:356, 1994.

Kaye TB, Crapo L: The Cushing syndrome: An update on diagnostic tests. Am J Intern Med 112:424, 1990.

Levy SR, Cerdas S, Billard L, et al: Cushing's syndrome in infancy secondary to pituitary adenoma. Am J Dis Child 136:605, 1982.

McArthur RG, Bahn RC, Hayles AB: Primary adrenocortical nodular dysplasia as a cause of Cushing's syndrome in infants and children. Mayo Clin Proc 57:58, 1982.

Magiakou MA, Mastorakos G, Oldfield EH, et al: Cushing's syndrome in children and adolescents. N Engl J Med 331:629, 1994.

Mampalam TH, Tyrell JB, Wilson CB: Transphenoidal microsurgery for Cushing disease. Ann Intern Med 109:487, 1988.

Muguruza MTG, Chrosus GP: Periodic Cushing syndrome in a short boy: Usefulness of the ovine corticotropin-releasing hormone test. J Pediatr 115:270, 1990.

Styne DM, Grumbach MM, Kaplan SL, et al: Treatment of Cushing's disease in childhood and adolescents by transphenoidal microadenomectomy. N Engl J Med 310:889, 1984.

CHAPTER 534
Adrenal Calcification

Calcification within the adrenal glands may occur in a wide variety of situations, some serious and others of no obvious consequence. Adrenal calcifications are often detected as incidental findings in roentgenographic studies of the abdomen in infants and children. The physician may elicit a history of anoxia or trauma at birth. Hemorrhage into the adrenal at or immediately after birth is probably the common factor that leads to subsequent calcification. Although it is advisable to assess the adrenocortical reserve of such patients, there is rarely any functional disorder.

Neuroblastomas, ganglioneuromas, cortical carcinomas, pheochromocytomas, and cysts of the adrenal gland may be responsible for calcifications, particularly if hemorrhage has occurred within the tumor. Calcification in such lesions is almost always unilateral.

In the past, tuberculosis was a common cause of calcification within the adrenals and of Addison disease. Calcifications may also develop in the adrenal glands of children who recover from the Waterhouse-Friderichsen syndrome; such patients are usually asymptomatic.

Infants with *Wolman syndrome,* a rare lipid disorder due to deficiency of lysosomal acid lipase, have extensive bilateral calcifications of the adrenal glands (see Chapter 72.3).

Crocker AC, Vawter GF, Neuhauser EBO, et al: Wolman's disease: Three new patients with recently described lipidosis. Pediatrics 35:627, 1965.

Hill EE, Williams JA: Massive adrenal haemorrhage in the newborn. Arch Dis Child 34:178, 1959.

Jarvis JL, Seaman WB: Idiopathic adrenal calcification in infants and children. Am J Roentgenol 82:510, 1959.

Stevenson J, MacGregor AM, Connelly P: Calcification of the adrenal glands in young children: A report of three cases with a review of the literature. Arch Dis Child 36:316, 1961.

SECTION 5
Disorders of the Gonads

Angelo M. DiGeorge

FUNCTION OF THE TESTES. In the 1st trimester of pregnancy, levels of placental chorionic gonadotropin peak (8–12 wk) and stimulate the fetal Leydig cells to secrete testosterone, the main hormonal product of the testis. This period (8–12 wk) is critical for normal virilization of the XY fetus. Defects in this process of fetal masculinization lead to different forms of male pseudohermaphroditism (see Chapter 540). After masculinization occurs, fetal levels of testosterone decrease but are maintained at low levels in the latter half of pregnancy by luteinizing hormone (LH) secreted by the fetal pituitary; this is required for continued penile growth.

Shortly after birth, a transient increase of gonadotropins, especially LH, occurs, leading to a sharp increase in serum levels of testosterone, which peak at about 1–3 mo of age (80–400 ng/dL). Thereafter, levels of gonadotropins subside, and by 6 mo of age, levels of testosterone decrease to the low prepubertal levels (10–20 ng/mL) that persist until the beginning of puberty. The significance of this "mini-puberty" in the neonate is unknown. Neonates with testicular torsion and atrophy have very low levels of testosterone and markedly elevated levels of follicle-stimulating hormone (FSH) and LH. Development of nocturnal pulsatile secretion of LH marks the advent of puberty (see Chapter 516).

Within specific target cells, about 6–8% of testosterone is converted by 5α-reductase to dehydrotestosterone, another potent androgen (see Fig. 540–1), and about 0.3% is acted on by aromatase to produce estradiol (Fig. 537–1). Approximately half of circulating testosterone is bound to *sex hormone–binding globulin* (SHBG) and half to albumin; only 2% circulates in the free form. Plasma levels of SHBG are low at birth, rise rapidly during the first 10 days of life, and then remain stable until the onset of puberty. Thyroid hormone may play a role in this physiologic increase because neonates with athyreosis have very low levels of SHBG.

Müllerian-inhibiting substance (MIS), also called antimüllerian hormone (AMH), is a glycoprotein hormone secreted by the Sertoli cells of the fetal testes. It causes involution of the embryologic precursors of the cervix, uterus, and fallopian tubes (müllerian ducts) during sexual differentiation. MIS persists after birth; levels remain measurable in serum until puberty, when there is a sharp decline. Several extramüllerian functions have been described.

Inhibin is another glycoprotein hormone secreted by the Sertoli cells of the testes. This hormone consists of α and β subunits and appears to have an important regulatory role in the secretion of FSH. In the 1st yr of life, levels are elevated; then they decrease and rise again during puberty, correlating with those of FSH. The precise role of this hormone has yet to be elucidated.

The functional integrity of the pituitary-testicular axis in the neonate can be assessed by the measurement of FSH, LH, and testosterone levels. In the near future, measurements of MIS and inhibin levels may also become clinically useful. After the neonatal period, the ability of the quiescent prepubertal testes to secrete testosterone can be assessed by administering chorionic gonadotropin (hCG), which stimulates the Leydig cells in a manner analogous to LH. Many different dosage schedules have been devised; a common regimen is intramuscular administration of 3,000 Units/m^2 once daily for 3–5 days.

Clinical patterns of pubertal changes vary widely (see Chapters 15 and 516). In 95% of boys enlargement of the genitalia begins between 9½ and 13½ yr, reaching maturity from 13 to 17 yr. In a small minority of normal boys, puberty begins after 15 yr of age. In 50% of boys, pubic hair is present by 11 yr of age, and by 13–17½ yr, it is equivalent in amount to that of normal adult males. In some boys, pubertal development is completed in less than 2 yr, but in others, it may take longer than 4½ yr. The adolescent growth spurt occurs later in boys than in girls at corresponding levels of sexual maturation; for example, the peak velocity of change in height is not attained in boys until the genitalia are well developed, but in girls the growth rate is usually at its maximum when the nipple and areola have developed but before there is any other significant breast development.

The median age of sperm production *(spermarche)* is 14 yr. This event occurs in midpuberty as judged by pubic hair, testes size, evidence of growth spurt, and testosterone levels. Night-time levels of FSH are in the adult male range at the time of spermarch; the first conscious ejaculation occurs at about the same time.

FUNCTION OF THE OVARIES. The most important estrogens produced by the ovary are estradiol-17β (E_2) and estrone (E_1); estriol is a metabolic product of these two, and all three estrogens may be found in the urine of mature females. Estrogens also arise from androgens in the adrenal gland and in the testis; the pathway for this conversion is shown in Figure 537–1. This conversion explains why in certain types of male pseudohermaphroditism feminization occurs at puberty; in 17-ketosteroid reductase deficiency, for example, the enzymatic block results in markedly increased secretion of androstenedione, which is converted in the peripheral tissues to estradiol and estrone; these estrogens, in addition to those directly secreted by the testis, result in gynecomastia. The ovary also synthesizes progesterone, a progestational steroid; adrenal cortex and testis synthesize progesterone as a precursor for other adrenal and testicular hormones.

Plasma levels of estradiol increase slowly but steadily with advancing sexual maturation and correlate well with clinical evaluation of pubertal development, skeletal age, and rising levels of FSH. Levels of LH do not rise until secondary sexual characteristics are well developed. Estrogens, like androgens, inhibit secretion of both LH and FSH (negative feedback). In females, estrogens also provoke the surge of LH secretion that occurs in the midmenstrual cycle. The capacity for this positive feedback is another maturational milestone of puberty. The average age at menarche in American girls is 12½–13 yr, but the range of "normal" is wide, and 1–2% of "normal" girls have not menstruated by 16 yr of age. Menarche generally correlates closely with skeletal age (see Chapters 516 and 517). Maturation and closure of the epiphysis is at least partially estrogen dependent, as demonstrated by a 28-yr-old, normally masculinized male with incomplete closure of the epiphyses who proved to have complete estrogen insensitivity because of an estrogen receptor defect.

DIAGNOSTIC AIDS. Rapid advances in understanding the hypothalamic-pituitary-gonadal interactions involved with puberty and in the clinical diagnosis of aberrations of pubertal development have been made possible by markedly improved assays for pituitary and gonadal hormones that can be measured in small amounts of blood. With GnRH it is also possible to differentiate between primary pituitary and hypothalamic defects in hypogonadotropic patients.

THERAPEUTIC AIDS. Naturally occurring estrogens administered orally are rapidly destroyed by gastrointestinal and liver enzymes; accordingly, they are usually given as conjugates or esters. The most widely used oral preparations are equine conjugated estrogens (e.g., Premarin) and ethinyl estradiol. Androgens are generally injected as long-acting esters (enanthate, cyclopentylpropionate, or phenylacetate) because of their potency and steady response. Oral preparations, such as methyltestosterone or fluoxymesterone, do not produce as potent an androgenic response. ■

CHAPTER 535 Hypofunction of the Testes

Testicular hypofunction may be primary in the testis (primary hypogonadism) or secondary to deficiency of pituitary gonadotropic hormones (secondary hypogonadism). Patients with primary hypogonadism have elevated levels of gonadotropin (hypergonadotropic); those with secondary hypogonadism have low or absent levels (hypogonadotropic).

535.1 Hypergonadotropic Hypogonadism in the Male

(Primary Hypogonadism)

Defects of androgen production involving the fetal testis and resulting in male pseudohermaphroditism are discussed in Chapter 540.

ETIOLOGY. *Congenital anorchia* occurs in 0.6% of boys with nonpalpable testes (1 of 20,000 males). These boys have normal external genitalia, indicating that a noxious factor damaged the fetal testes of the genetic male fetus sometime after sexual differentiation had taken place (14th wk of fetal life). The condition has been reported in monozygotic twins. Low levels of testosterone (<10 ng/dL) and markedly elevated levels of luteinizing hormone (LH) and follicle-stimulating hormone (FSH) are found in the early postnatal months; thereafter, levels of gonadotropins tend to decrease even in agonadal children, rising to castrate levels as the pubertal years approach. Stimulation with chorionic gonadotropin (hCG) fails to evoke an increase in the levels of testosterone.

A syndrome of *rudimentary testes* has been described in which the testes are exceedingly small; this appears to be inherited as an autosomal or X-linked recessive trait. The cause is unknown. *Atrophy* of the testes may follow damage to the vascular supply as a result of unskillful manipulation of the testes during surgical procedures for correction of cryptorchidism or as a result of bilateral torsion of the testes. *Acute orchitis* in pubertal or adult males with mumps may also damage the testes; usually, only the reproductive function of the testes is impaired. The routine immunization of all prepubertal males with mumps vaccine should prevent this complication.

Testicular damage is a frequent sequela of *chemotherapy* and of *radiotherapy* for cancer. The frequency and extent of damage depend on the agent used, total dosage, duration of therapy, and post-therapy interval of observation. Another important variable is age at therapy; germ cells are less vulnerable in prepubertal than in intrapubertal and postpubertal boys, although nitrosourea administered before the age of 16 yr almost always causes permanent damage to the germinal epithelium with a high likelihood of infertility. Because of these variables, reports of the frequency and degree of testicular damage are often conflicting. Testicular function should be carefully evaluated in adolescents who have prolonged survival after multimodal treatment for cancer in childhood. Replacement therapy with testosterone or counseling concerning fertility may be indicated.

The term hypogonadism has been widely used to describe aspects of children with a variety of syndromes of multiple malformations. The term often refers simply to cryptorchidism, a small phallus, or a scrotal anomaly. In many of these syndromes little is known about the function of the testes; hyper- or hypogonadotropic hypogonadism has been proved in some instances.

Various degrees of hypogonadism also occur in a significant percentage of patients with chromosomal aberrations such as Klinefelter syndrome or XX males.

CLINICAL MANIFESTATIONS. Primary hypogonadism may be suspected at birth if the testes and penis are abnormally small. The condition often is not noticed until puberty is expected and secondary sex characteristics fail to develop. Facial, pubic, and axillary hair is scant or absent; there is neither acne nor regression of scalp hair, and the voice remains high pitched. The penis and scrotum remain infantile and may be almost obscured by pubic fat; the testes are small or absent. Fat accumulates in the region of the hips and buttocks and sometimes in the breasts and on the abdomen. The epiphyses close late in life; therefore, extremities are long. The span is several inches longer than the height, and the distance from the symphysis pubis to the soles of the feet is much greater than from the symphysis to the vertex. This clinical state is also known as *eunuchism*, and the proportions of the body are described as eunuchoid. Many individuals with milder degrees of hypogonadism may be detected only by appropriate studies of the pituitary-gonadal axis.

DIAGNOSIS. Levels of serum FSH and, to a lesser extent, of LH are elevated above age-specific normal values. These elevated levels indicate that even in the prepubertal child there is an active hypothalamic-gonadal-feedback relationship. After the age of 11 yr, FSH and LH levels rise significantly, reaching the postmenopausal range. Plasma testosterone levels are ordinarily low in normal prepubertal children, rising during puberty to attain adult levels. During puberty, these levels correlate better with testicular size and stage of sexual maturity than with age. In patients with primary hypogonadism, testosterone levels remain low at all ages, and there is an attenuated rise or no rise following administration of hCG, although in normal males at any stage of development, hCG produces a significant rise in plasma testosterone.

NOONAN SYNDROME

The term Noonan syndrome has been applied to phenotypic males and females who have certain anomalies that occur also in females with Turner syndrome. These boys and girls have normal karyotypes. The disorder is usually sporadic, but affected siblings of the same and of different genders have been reported. Total or partial expression is present in 20% of relatives. Reports of male-to-male transmission suggest an autosomal dominant gene with variable expressivity. The gene has been mapped to chromosome 12q.

The most common abnormalities are short stature, webbing of the neck, pectus carinatum or pectus excavatum, cubitum valgum, congenital heart disease, and a characteristic facies. Hypertelorism, epicanthus, an antimongoloid palpebral slant, ptosis, micrognathia, and ear abnormalities are common. Other abnormalities such as clinodactyly, hernias, and vertebral anomalies occur less frequently. Moderate mental retardation occurs in 25% of patients. The cardiac defect is most often pulmonary valvular stenosis or atrial septal defect. Features of both Noonan syndrome and type 1 neurofibromatosis have been reported in about a dozen families, but linkage has been excluded. Males frequently have cryptorchidism and small testes; they may be hypogonadal or normal. Puberty is delayed 2 yr on average; adult height is achieved by the end of the 2nd decade and usually reaches the lowest limit of the normal population.

KLINEFELTER SYNDROME

ETIOLOGY. Approximately 1 of 1,000 newborn males has a 47,XXY chromosome complement. The incidence approximates 1% among the mentally retarded, clustering among patients with IQs above 50 and among children admitted to psychiatric hospitals or referred to psychiatric clinics. The chromosomal aberration most often results from meiotic nondisjunction of an X chromosome during parental gametogenesis; the extra X chromosome is maternal in origin in 54% and paternal in origin in 46% of patients. Increased maternal age predisposes to meiotic nondisjunction and to this syndrome, but in most instances, maternal age is not advanced.

The 47,XXY complement is the most common chromosomal pattern in persons with Klinefelter syndrome; some have mosaic patterns: 46,XY/47,XXY; 46,XY/48,XXYY; 45,X/46,XY/46,XXY; or 46,XX/47,XXY. Rarely, occurrence of more than two X chromosomes may result in Klinefelter variants: 48,XXXY; 49,XXXYY; 49,XXXXY; 50,XXXXYY; 47,XXY/48,XXXY; 47,XXY/49,XXXXY; or 48,XXYY karyotype. Even with as many as four X chromosomes, the Y chromosome determines a male phenotype. In most patients with four or five X chromosomes, all the additional chromosomes come from the same parent and are not associated with increased parental age.

CLINICAL MANIFESTATIONS. The diagnosis is rarely made before puberty because of the paucity or subtleness of clinical manifestations in childhood. Because behavioral or psychiatric disorders may often be apparent long before defects in sexual development, the condition should be considered in all boys with mental retardation and in children with psychosocial, learning, or school adjustment problems. Affected children may be anxious, immature, excessively shy, or aggressive; they may engage in antisocial acts. Fire-setting behavior has been observed in some of these children. Problems often first become apparent after the child begins school. The patients tend to be tall, slim, and underweight and to have relatively long legs, but body habitus can vary markedly. The testes tend to be small for age, but this sign may become substantially apparent only after puberty, when normal testicular growth fails to occur. The phallus tends to be smaller than average, and cryptorchidism or hypospadias may occur in a few patients.

Pubertal development may be delayed. Some degree of androgen deficiency is usually detected, although some patients may undergo almost normal masculinization. About 80% of adults have gynecomastia; they have sparser facial hair, most shaving less than daily. Azoospermia and infertility are usual, although rare instances of fertility are known. Height tends to be increased. There is also an increased incidence of pulmonary disease, varicose veins, and cancer of the breast. Mediastinal germ cell tumors have been reported in approximately 40 patients with Klinefelter syndrome; some of these tumors produce HCG and cause precocious puberty in young boys. These may also be associated with leukemia and other hematologic neoplasia.

In a prospective study, a group of children with 47,XXY karyotypes identified at birth exhibited relatively mild deviations from normal during the first 5 yr of life. None had major physical, intellectual, or emotional disabilities; some were inactive, with poorly organized motor function and mild delay in language acquisition.

In adults with XY/XXY *mosaicism*, the features of Klinefelter syndrome are decreased in severity and frequency. Little is known of children with mosaicism, but they have a better prognosis for virilization, fertility, and psychosocial adjustment. The XXYY *male* phenotype is not distinctively different from that of the XXY patient, except that XXYY adults tend to be taller than the average XXY patient.

Klinefelter Variants. When the number of X chromosomes exceeds two, the clinical manifestations, including mental retardation and impairment of virilization, are more severe. The 49,XXXXY variant has been reported in more than 100 patients and is sufficiently distinctive to be detected in childhood. The disorder arises from sequential nondisjunction in meiosis. Affected patients are severely retarded, and many have large malformed ears, a short neck, and a typical facies with wide-set eyes that have a mild mongoloid slant; epicanthus, strabismus, a wide, flat upturned nose, and a large open mouth may also be present. The testes are small and may be undescended, the scrotum is hypoplastic, and the penis is very small. Defects suggestive of Down syndrome (e.g., short in-curved terminal 5th phalanges, single palmar creases, and hypotonia) and other skeletal abnormalities (including defects in the carrying angle of the elbows and restricted supination) are common. The most frequent radiographic abnormalities are radioulnar synostosis or dislocation, elongated radius, pseudoepiphyses, scoliosis or kyphosis, coxa valga, and retarded osseous age. Most patients with such extensive changes have a 49,XXXXY chromosome karyotype; several mosaic patterns have also been observed: 48,XXXY/49,XXXXY (Fig. 535–1); 48,XXXY/49,XXXXY/50,XXXXXY; and 48,XXXY/49,XXXXY/50,XXXXYY.

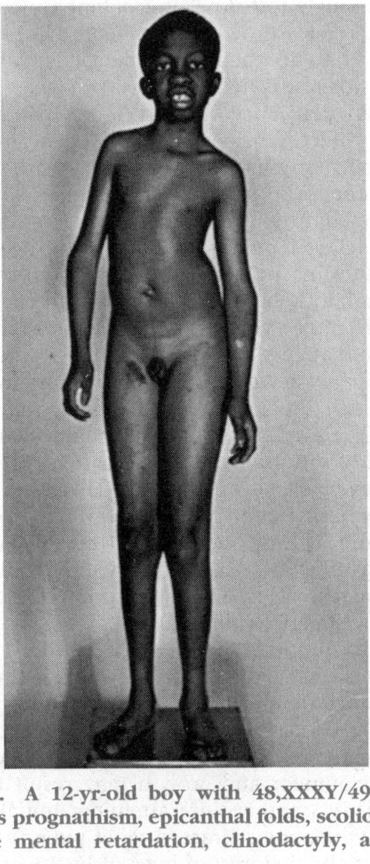

Figure 535–1. A 12-yr-old boy with 48,XXXY/49XXXXY mosaicism who has prognathism, epicanthal folds, scoliosis, very small testes, severe mental retardation, clinodactyly, and radioulnar synostoses.

LABORATORY DATA. The chromosomes should be examined in all patients suspected of Klinefelter syndrome, particularly those attending child guidance, psychiatric, and mental retardation clinics. Before 10 yr of age, boys with 47,XXY Klinefelter syndrome have normal basal plasma levels of FSH and LH. Responses to gonadotropin-stimulating hormone and to hCG are also normal. The testes show normal growth early in puberty, but by midpuberty testicular growth stops, gonadotropins become elevated, and testosterone levels are slightly low. Elevated levels of estradiol resulting in a high estradiol to testosterone ratio account for the development of gynecomastia during puberty.

Testicular biopsy before puberty may reveal only a deficiency or absence of germinal cells. After puberty, the seminiferous tubular membranes are hyalinized, and there is adenomatous clumping of Leydig cells. Azoospermia is characteristic, and infertility is the rule.

TREATMENT. Replacement therapy with a long-acting testosterone preparation should begin at 11–12 yr of age. The enanthate ester may be used in a starting dose of 50 mg injected intramuscularly every 3 wk, with 50-mg increments every 6–9 mo until a maintenance dose for adults (200–250 mg every 3–4 wk) is achieved. For older boys, larger initial doses and increments can achieve more rapid virilization.

XX MALES

More than 150 males with 46,XX chromosome constitution have been identified; the disorder is thought to occur in 1 of 20,000 newborn males. Affected individuals have a male phenotype, small testes, a small phallus, and no evidence of ovarian or müllerian duct tissue; they appear, therefore, to be distinct from the XX true hermaphrodite (see Chapter 540). This disorder resembles Klinefelter syndrome, but stature is greater in the latter. The histologic features of the testes are essentially the same in the two conditions. Patients with the condition usually come to medical attention in adult life because of hypogonadism, gynecomastia, or infertility. Hypergonadotropic hypogonadism occurs secondary to testicular failure.

For 2 decades, it has been theorized that male-determining genes have been translocated from the Y chromosome to the X chromosome. It is now established that in 80% of XX males with normal male external genitalia, one of the X chromosomes carries the testis-determining factor (TDF). This gene has been designated SRY (sex-determining region of the Y). The exchange from the Y to the X chromosome occurs during paternal meiosis, when the short arms of the Y and X chromosomes pair. XX males inherit one maternal X chromosome and one paternal X chromosome containing the translocated male-determining gene. Such exchanges occur because of the proximity of TDF to the pseudoautosomal region where recombination between X and Y chromosomes normally occurs in meiosis. Most XX males who are identified before puberty have hypospadias or micropenis; this group of patients usually lacks Y-specific sequences, suggesting other mechanisms for virilization (see Chapter 540).

45,X MALES

Of the few male patients recognized with a 45,X karyotype, Yp sequences have been translocated to an autosomal chromosome. In one instance, the terminal short arm of the Y chromosome was translocated on to an X chromosome.

XYY MALES

The 47,XYY male does not have hypogonadism; this condition is discussed here for easy comparison with the XXY and the XX male syndromes.

Approximately 1 of 1,000 newborn males has an XYY chromosome pattern. When this disorder was first discovered in adults, studies of XYY individuals in mental or penal institutions created a stereotype of affected individuals as having deviant behavior marked by physical aggressiveness and violence. It now appears that the rate at which XYY males are found in mental or penal settings may be as high as 20 times the rate at which they are born. Adults with this karyotype may be relatively impulsive, antisocial, and likely to break the law, but they are not especially aggressive. Unselected 47,XXY boys detected in screening programs tend to exhibit attention deficits, impulsive behavior, inadequate poor interactions, and poor self-image. Patients with 48,XXYY and 48,XYYY karyotypes also tend to have similar deviant behavior.

The XYY adult has few phenotypic manifestations. He tends to be tall and to have severe nodulocystic acne. In affected persons, genital abnormalities have been observed, but cryptic mosaicism, such as X/XYY, is a possibility in these instances. Prolonged PR intervals on electrocardiography and radioulnar synostosis appear to occur more often than in the general population. No clear-cut endocrine abnormalities have been found. This condition poses a serious dilemma for counseling of parents of infants or children discovered to have this sex chromosome complement. The risks for some developmental disability may not be trivial, but neither do they appear to be as dire as earlier thought.

535.2 Hypogonadotropic Hypogonadism in the Male

(Secondary Hypogonadism)

In hypogonadotropic hypogonadism, there is deficiency of FSH or LH. The primary defect may lie in the anterior pituitary or in the hypothalamus as a deficiency of gonadotropin-releasing hormone. The testes are normal but remain in the prepubertal state because stimulation by gonadotropins is lacking.

ETIOLOGY. Hypopituitarism. Most causes of hypopituitarism may be associated with deficiency of gonadotropins and hypogonadotropic hypogonadism (see Chapter 512). In patients with organic lesions in or near the pituitary (e.g., craniopharyngioma), the gonadotropin deficiency is pituitary in origin. In many patients with "idiopathic" or "familial" hypopituitarism, the defect resides in the hypothalamus and is caused by a deficiency of gonadotropin-releasing hormone (GnRH). Microphallus (<2.5 cm) in the newborn male with growth hormone deficiency suggests the likelihood of gonadotropin deficiency, and diagnostic confirmation is feasible; after 6 mo of age, gonadotropin deficiency cannot be established with certainty until the teenage years.

Isolated Deficiency of Gonadotropin. Usually, this disorder involves the hypothalamus rather than the pituitary. It affects about 1 of 10,000 males and 1 of 50,000 females and encompasses a heterogeneous group of entities. GnRH deficiency may be complete or partial; it may occur sporadically or in families. Kallmann syndrome, one of the most frequent genetic forms of hypogonadotropic hypogonadism, is characterized by its association with anosmia or hyposmia. The X-linked disorder is caused by a mutation of the KAL gene at Xp22.3. The association reflects the failure of olfactory axons and GnRH-expressing neurons to migrate from their common origin in the olfactory placode to the brain. The KAL gene is also expressed in various parts of the brain. It appears that the KAL product functions in the guidance of neuronal migration.

Some kindreds contain anosmic individuals with or without hypogonadism, others contain hypogonadal individuals who are anosmic. Cleft palate, hypotelorism, median facial clefts, neural hearing loss, unilateral renal aplasia, neurologic deficits, and other findings occur in some affected patients. When Kallmann syndrome is caused by terminal or interstitial deletions of the Xp 22.3 region, it may be associated with other contiguous gene syndromes, such as chondrodysplasia punctata, X-linked ichthyosis, or ocular albinism. Autosomal recessive and autosomal dominant forms of Kallmann syndrome have been reported.

Mutations of Gonadotropins. One family with a point mutation of the β subunit of LH and another family with a point mutation of the β subunit of FSH have been reported as causes for isolated hypogonadotropic hypogonadism.

Melatonin-Related Hypogonadism. A 21-yr-old man with delayed puberty, hypogonadotropic hypogonadism, markedly elevated plasma concentration of melatonin, and an enlarged pineal gland has been reported; these findings gradually reverted to normal over several years. This patient tends to support the putative role of the pineal and melatonin in pubertal development.

Other Disorders. Hypogonadotropic hypogonadism is associated with the X-linked form of *congenital adrenal hypoplasia* (Chapter 528) and has been observed in two young men with *polyglandular autoimmune syndrome*. A variety of other syndromes such as Bardet-Biedl, Prader-Willi, multiple lentigines, and several syndromes of ataxia have been reported in association with hypogonadism. Many of these have not been evaluated by current techniques, and the sites of the defects are unknown.

DIAGNOSIS. Levels of gonadotropins and gonadal steroids remain in the prepubertal range, and nocturnal pulsatile secretion of LH does not occur. The gonadotropin response to the standard GnRH stimulation test is markedly blunted. All of these findings are also consistent with those observed in normal adolescents with the variant known as *constitutional delayed puberty*; a variety of tests proposed in the past to separate these two conditions have proved inadequate. Preliminary data suggest that a single test dose of a potent GnRH agonist will evoke a greater release of LH in patients with constitutional growth delay than in those with deficiency of LH; further evaluation of this test is necessary.

Gonadotropin deficiency is likely if the patient has other evidence of pituitary deficiency, such as a deficiency of growth hormone, particularly if it is associated with corticotropin (ACTH) deficiency. The presence of anosmia usually indicates permanent gonadotropin deficiency, but occasional instances of markedly delayed puberty (18–20 yr of age) have been observed in anosmic individuals. Although anosmia may be present in the family or in the patient from early childhood, its existence is rarely volunteered, and direct questioning is necessary in all patients with delayed puberty. Magnetic resonance imaging may detect anomalous olfactory lobes and sulci in some patients. Prolactinomas are increasingly recognized as a cause of delayed puberty and should be ruled out by determination of serum levels of prolactin.

Probes are available to establish the diagnosis in heterozygotes and newborn infants with the X-linked form of Kallmann syndrome. During the first 3–4 mo of life, unaffected infants demonstrate the usual physiologic rise in gonadotropins and gonadal steroids, and the response to GnRH exceeds that seen in prepubertal children.

TREATMENT. Constitutional delayed puberty must be ruled out before a diagnosis of isolated deficiency of GnRH can be established. Testicular volume of less than 4 mL by 14 yr of age occurs in about 3% of boys, but true hypogonadotropic hypogonadism is a rare condition. Even relatively moderate delays in sexual development and growth may result in significant psychologic distress and require attention. Initially, an explanation of the variations characteristic of puberty and reassurance suffice for the majority of boys. If by 15 yr of age there is no clinical evidence of puberty beginning and the testosterone level is less than 50 ng/dL, a brief course of testosterone is indicated. Testosterone enanthate, 100–200 mg intramuscularly once monthly for 4 mo, usually initiates puberty and differentiates constitutional delay in puberty from isolated gonadotropin deficiency. Only rarely is a second course indicated if puberty is not sustained.

Patients with established deficiency of gonadotropins can be treated with the same program of repository testosterone as that used for those with primary testicular deficiency (see Chapter 535.1). With this therapy, the testes will remain small. Treatment with hCG, given subcutaneously or intramuscularly in doses of 500–1,000 IU, three times weekly, stimulates growth of the testes and spermatogenesis. If after 6–12 mo of therapy sufficient growth of the testes has not occurred, human menopausal gonadotropin may be added in doses of 37.5–150 IU, three times weekly. It may require up to 2 yr of treatment to achieve adequate spermatogenesis in adults.

A more physiologic but cumbersome form of treatment consists of episodic administration (subcutaneously or intravenously) of GnRH. Long-term therapy has been used with a programmable peristaltic infusion pump. Most patients require about 2 yr of treatment to maximize testicular growth and to achieve spermatogenesis.

Baker ML, Hutson JM: Serum levels of Mullerian inhibiting substance in boys throughout puberty and in the first two years of life. J Clin Endocrinol Metab 76:245, 1993.
Barkam AL, Kelch RP, Marshall JC: Isolated gonadotrope failure in the polyglandular autoimmune failure. N Engl J Med 312:1535, 1985.
Borghgraef M, Fryns JP, Smeets E, et al: The 49,XXXXY syndrome. Clinical and psychological follow-up data. Clin Genet 33:429, 1988.
Burger HG, Yamada Y, Bangah ML, et al: Serum gonadotropin, sex steroid, and immunoreactive inhibin levels in the first two years of life. J Clin Endocrinol Metab 72:682, 1991.
Clayton PE, Shalet SM, Price DA, et al: Testicular damage after chemotherapy for childhood brain tumors. J Pediatr 112:922, 1988.
Crowne EC, Shalet SM: Management of constitutional delay in growth and puberty. Trends Endocrinol Metab 1:239, 1990.
Dunkel L, Perheentupa J, Virtanen M, et al: Gonadotropin-releasing hormone test and human chorionic gonadotropin test in the diagnosis of gonadotropin deficiency in prepubertal boys. J Pediatr 107:388, 1985.
Ehrmann DA, Rosenfield RL, Cuttler L, et al: A new test of combined pituitarytesticular function using the gonadotropin-releasing hormone agonist Nafarelin in the differentiation of gonadotropin deficiency from delayed puberty: Pilot studies. J Clin Endocrinol Metab 69:963, 1989.
Fechner PY, Marcantonio SM, Jaswaney V, et al: The role of sex-determining region Y gene in the etiology of 46,XX maleness. J Clin Endocrin Metab 76:690, 1993.
Finkel DM, Phillips JL, Snyder PJ: Stimulation of spermatogenesis by gonadotropins in men with hypogonadotropic hypogonadism. N Engl J Med 313:651, 1985.
Grammatico P, Bottoni N, DeSanctis S, et al: A male patient with 48,XXYY syndrome: Importance of distinction from Klinefelter's syndrome. Clin Genet 38:74, 1990.
Hasle H, Jacobsen BB, Asschenfeldt P, Anderson K: Mediastinal germ cell tumour associated with Klinefelter syndrome. A report of care and review of the literature. Eur J Pediatr 151:735, 1992.
Kaplowitz PB: Diagnostic value of testosterone therapy in boys with delayed puberty. Am J Dis Child 143:116, 1989.
Kassai R, Hamada I, Furuta H, et al: Penta X syndrome? A case report with review of the literature. Am J Med Genet 40:51, 1991.
Kulin HE, Frontera A, Demers LM, et al: The onset of sperm production in pubertal boys. Relationship to gonadotropin excretion. Am J Dis Child 143:190, 1989.
Lamelino CA, Reiss AL: 49,XXXXY syndrome: Behavioral and developmental profiles. J Med Genet 28:609, 1991.
Lee MM, Donahue PK: Müllerian inhibiting substance: A gonadal hormone with multiple functions. Endocr Rev 14:152, 1993.
MacDonald M, Hassold T, Harvey J, et al: The origin of 47,XXY and 47,XXX aneupolidy: Heterogeneous mechanisms and role of aberrant recombination. Hum Mol Gen 8:1365, 1994.
Matus-Ridley M, Nicosia SV, Meadows AT: Gonadal effects of cancer therapy in boys. Cancer 55:2353, 1985.
Money J, Franzke A, Borgaonkar DS: XYY syndrome, stigmatization, social class, and aggression. South Med J 68:1536, 1975.
Najjar SS, Takla RJ, Nassar VH: The syndrome of rudimentary testes: Occurrence in five siblings. J Pediatr 84:119, 1974.
Numabe H, Nagafuchi S, Nakahuri Y, et al: DNA analysis of XX and XX-hypospadiac males. Hum Genet 90:211, 1992.
Oerter KE, Kamp GA, Munson PJ, et al: Multiple hormone deficiencies in children with hemachromatosis. J Clin Endocrin Metab 76:357, 1993.
Petit C: Molecular basis of the X-chromosome-linked Kallmann's syndrome. Trends Endocrinol Metab 4:8, 1993.
Pike MG, Hammerton M, Edge J, et al: A family with X-linked ichthyosis and hypogonadism. Eur J Pediatr 148:442, 1989.
Randke MB, Heidemann P, Knupter C, et al: Noonan syndrome: Growth and clinical manifestations in 144 cases. Eur J Pediatr 148:220, 1988.
Prager D, Braunstein GD: X-chromosome-linked Kallmann's syndrome: Pathology at the molecular level. J Clin Endocrinol Metab 76:824, 1993.
Rose SR, Cassorla F, Sherins RJ: Normal neonatal surge of gonadotropins and sex steroids in infants of men with isolated hypogonadotropic hypogonadism. Clin Endocrinol 29:577, 1988.
Rosenfeld RL: Diagnosis and management of delayed puberty. J Clin Endocrinol Metab 70:559, 1990.
Salbenblatt JA, Bender BG, Puck MH, et al: Pituitary-gonadal function in Klinefelter syndrome before and during puberty. Pediatr Res 19:82, 1985.
Seyler LE, Arulananthan K, O'Connor CF: Hypergonadotropic-hypogonadism in the Prader-Labhart-Willi syndrome. J Pediatr 94:435, 1979.
Shalet SM, Hann IM, Lendon M, et al: Testicular function after combination chemotherapy in childhood for acute lymphoblastic leukaemia. Arch Dis Child 56:275, 1981.
Spratt DI, Carr DB, Merriam GR, et al: The spectrum of abnormal patterns of gonadotropin-releasing hormone secretion in men with idiopathic hypogonadotropic hypogonadism: Clinical and laboratory correlations. J Clin Endocrinol Metab 64:283, 1987.
Stanhope R, Brook CGD, Pringle PJ, et al: Induction of puberty by pulsatile gonadotropin-releasing hormone. Lancet 2:552, 1987.
VanDop C, Burstein S, Conte FA, et al: Isolated gonadotropin deficiency in boys: Clinical characteristics and growth. J Pediatr 111:684, 1987.
Weiss J, Axelrod L, Whitcomb RW, et al: Hypogonadism caused by a single amino acid substitution in the β subunit of luteinizing hormone. N Engl J Med 326:179, 1992.

CHAPTER 536

Pseudoprecocity Resulting from Tumors of the Testes

Leydig cell tumors of the testis are rare causes of precocious pseudopuberty. Leydig cells are sparse before puberty; tumors derived from them are more common in the adult. About 50 cases have been reported in children, including one member in each of two pairs of identical twins. These tumors are usually unilateral and benign. Reinke crystalloids are a characteristic microscopic feature but occur in fewer than 50% of Leydig cell tumors.

The clinical manifestations are those of puberty in the male; onset occurs usually from 5–9 yr of age. Gynecomastia has occurred in five patients. The tumor of the testis can usually be readily felt; the contralateral unaffected testis is normal in size for the age of the patient.

Plasma levels of testosterone are markedly elevated. Follicle-stimulating hormone and luteinizing hormone levels are suppressed, and there is no response to gonadotropin-releasing hormone. Ultrasound may aid in the detection of small nonpalpable tumors. Treatment consists of surgical removal of the affected testis. Progression of virilization ceases, and partial reversal of the signs of precocity may occur.

Testicular adrenal rests may develop into tumors that mimic Leydig cell tumors; in the absence of Reinke crystals these two tumors cannot be differentiated histologically. Adrenal rest tumors are usually bilateral and occur in patients with congenital adrenal hyperplasia, usually salt-losing patients, during adolescence or young adult life. The stimulus for the growth of the adrenal rests is inadequate corticosteroid suppressive therapy, and treatment with adequate doses almost always results in their regression. Definite evidence of the origin of these tumors has been achieved by demonstrating their 21-

hydroxylase activity. The misdiagnosis of these tumors in patients with congenital adrenal hyperplasia has led to unnecessary orchidectomy. Successful pregnancy after treatment of adrenal rest tumors by conservative steroid replacement therapy has been reported.

Fragile X syndrome is the most frequent cause of hereditary mental retardation; a cardinal characteristic of the condition is testicular enlargement (macroorchidism), reaching 40–50 mL after puberty. Although the condition has been recognized in a child as young as 5 mo of age, affected boys younger than 6 yr of age rarely have testicular enlargement; by 8–10 yr of age, most have testicular volumes over 3 mL. The testes are enlarged bilaterally, not nodular, and histologically normal. Results of hormonal studies are normal. The gene involved in this condition is located in chromosome Xp17.3, a region that cytogenetically displays a fragile site. Direct DNA analysis permits definitive diagnosis (see Chapter 67).

Sex cord tumors with annular tubules of the testes are increasingly recognized as a cause of breast development in young boys. These tumors usually are associated with Peutz-Jeghers syndrome; they occur bilaterally, are multifocal, and are detectible by ultrasonography. Excessive production of aromatase ($P\text{-}450_{arom}$) has been established as the cause for feminization of these boys.

In boys with *unilateral cryptorchidism*, the contralateral testis is about 25% larger than normal for age.

Carmi R, Meryash DL, Wood J, et al: Fragile-X syndrome ascertained by the presence of macro-orchidism in a 5 month-old infant. Pediatrics 74:883, 1984.

Clark RV, Albertson BD, Monabi A, et al: Steroidogenic enzyme activities, morphology and receptor studies of a testicular rest in a patient with congenital adrenal hyperplasia. J Clin Endocrinol Metab 70:1408, 1990.

Coen P, Kulin H, Ballantine T, et al: An aromatase-producing sex-cord tumor resulting in prepubertal gynecomastia. N Engl J Med 324:317, 1991.

Combes-Moukousky ME, Kottler ML, Valensi P, et al: Gonadal and adrenal catheterization during adrenal suppression and gonadal stimulation in a patient with bilateral testicular tumors and congenital adrenal hyperplasia. J Clin Endocrinol Metab 79:1390, 1994.

Nisula BC, Loriaux DL, Sherins RJ, et al: Benign bilateral testicular enlargement. J Clin Endocrinol Metab 38:440, 1974.

Rosenberg T, Gilboa Y, Golik A, et al: Pseudoprecocious puberty in a young boy due to interstitial cell adenomas of the testis. Helv Paediatr Acta 39:79, 1984.

CHAPTER 537

Gynecomastia

Gynecomastia, or the occurrence of mammary tissue in the male, is a common condition. It is almost always a sign of estrogen-androgen imbalance, but its cause is often obscure. It occurs in most newborn males as a result of stimulation by maternal hormones. The effect disappears in a few weeks.

During midpuberty approximately two thirds of boys develop various degrees of subareolar hyperplasia of the breasts. *Physiologic pubertal gynecomastia* may involve only one breast, and it is not unusual for both breasts to enlarge at disproportionate rates or at different times. Tenderness of the breast is common but transitory. Spontaneous regression may occur within a few mo; it rarely persists longer than 2 yr. Mean concentrations of follicle-stimulating hormone, luteinizing hormone, prolactin, testosterone, estrone, and estradiol are the same as in boys without gynecomastia. When, however, levels are correlated with stage of puberty, a decreased ratio of testosterone to estradiol is found in boys with gynecomastia. Treatment usually consists of reassurance of the boy and his family of the physiologic and transient nature of the phenomenon. Surgical removal of the breast is rarely indicated; when enlargement is striking and persistent and causes serious emotional disturbance to the patient, removal may be justified.

Occasionally, breast development may mimic female breast development (to Tanner stages 3–5) and fails to regress. *Familial gynecomastia* has occurred in several kindreds as an X-linked or autosomal dominant sex-limited trait. Levels of gonadotropins, testosterone, prolactin, and steroid-binding globulins are normal. Increased peripheral conversion of C_{19}-steroids to estrogens (increased aromatization) has been found in familial and sporadic cases of gynecomastia and may explain some instances of this condition (Fig. 537–1).

In young children with gynecomastia, an exogenous source of estrogens must be sought. Accidental or therapeutic exposure to small amounts of estrogens by inhalation, percutaneous absorption, or ingestion may cause gynecomastia. Increased pigmentation of the nipple and areola should suggest this cause. Gynecomastia may also be caused by exogenously administered androgens.

Several other pathologic conditions may cause gynecomastia. It has been observed in children with the 11β-hydroxylase–deficient form of congenital virilizing adrenal hyperplasia. It may be associated with Leydig cell tumors of the testis or with feminizing tumors of the adrenal. More than a dozen boys with the *Peutz-Jeghers syndrome* and gynecomastia had *sex-cord tumors with annular tubules* of the testes. The testis may not be enlarged; the tumor is usually multifocal and bilateral. Excessive aromatase production accounts for the gynecomastia. Gynecomastia occurs in patients with Klinefelter syndrome and with other types of testicular failure (hypergonadotropic states). It is a common finding in boys with certain types of male pseudohermaphroditism, particularly Reifenstein syndrome, the testicular feminization syndrome, and in patients with the 17-ketosteroid reductase defect. When gynecomastia is associated with galactorrhea, a prolactinoma should be considered. In adults gynecomastia occurs with liver cirrhosis, with digitalis therapy for congestive heart failure, with bronchogenic carcinoma, with administration of various nonsteroidal therapeutic agents, and with heavy marijuana smoking. Ketoconazole, an antifungal drug, causes gynecomastia by directly inhibiting testosterone synthesis. In a pubertal boy with fibrolamellar carcinoma of the liver, the associated gynecomastia and elevated estrogen level were attributed to increased aromatization of circulating androgens by the tumor.

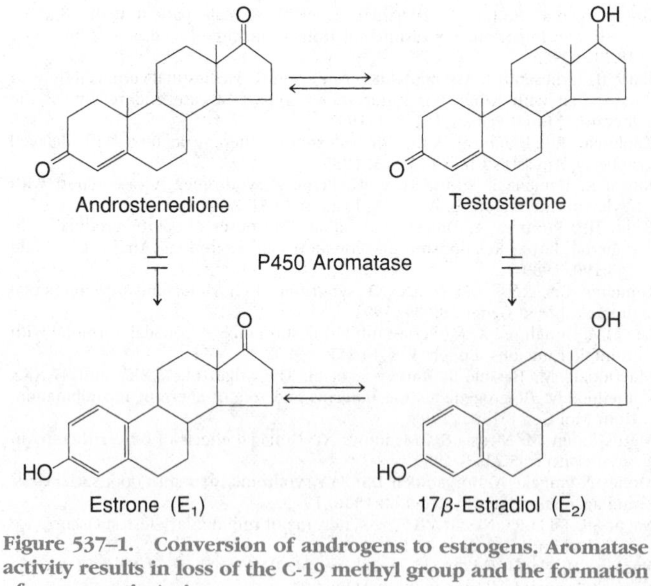

Figure 537–1. Conversion of androgens to estrogens. Aromatase activity results in loss of the C-19 methyl group and the formation of an aromatic A ring.

August GP, Chandra R, Hung W: Prepubertal male gynecomastia. J Pediatr 80:259, 1972.
Berkovitz GD, Guerami A, Brown TR, et al: Familial gynecomastia with increased extraglandular aromatization of plasma $carbon_{19}$-steroids. J Clin Invest 75:1763, 1985.
Bulard J, Mowszowicz I, Schaison G: Increased aromatase in pubic skin fibroblasts from patients with isolated gynecomastia. J Clin Endocrinol Metab 64:618, 1987.
Hochberg Z, Even L, Zadik Z: Mineralocorticoid in the mechanism of gynecomastia in adrenal hyperplasia caused by 11β-hydroxylase deficiency. J Pediatr 118:258, 1991.
Lee PA: The relationship of concentrations of serum hormones to pubertal gynecomastia. J Pediatr 86:212, 1975.
Maclaren NK, Migeon CJ, Raiti S: Gynecomastia with congenital virilizing adrenal hyperplasia (11β-hydroxylase deficiency). J Pediatr 86:579, 1975.
Nydick M, Bustos J, Dale JH Jr, et al: Gynecomastia in adolescent boys. JAMA 178:449, 1961.

CHAPTER 538
Hypofunction of the Ovaries

Hypofunction of the ovaries may be caused by congenital failure of development, postnatal destruction (primary or hypergonadotropic hypogonadism), or lack of stimulation by the pituitary (secondary or hypogonadotropic hypogonadism). Many chronic diseases may result in the latter type.

538.1 Hypergonadotropic Hypogonadism in the Female

(Primary Hypogonadism)

Diagnosis of hypergonadotropic hypogonadism before puberty is difficult. Except in the case of Turner syndrome, most affected patients have no prepubertal clinical manifestations.

TURNER SYNDROME

In 1938, Turner described a syndrome consisting of sexual infantilism, webbed neck, and cubitum valgum in adult females. The chromosomal nature of the condition was discovered in 1959.

PATHOGENESIS. The initial finding of 45,X in patients with Turner syndrome occurs in only about 50% of affected patients. About 15% of patients are mosaics for 45,X and a normal cell line (45,X/46,XX). Other mosaics with isochromosomes, 45,X/46,X,i(Xq); with rings, 45,X/46,X,r(X); or fragments, 45,X/46fra occur less often. The single X is of maternal origin in 75% of 45,X patients. The mechanism of chromosome loss is unknown, and the risk for the syndrome does not increase with maternal age. It is likely that the genes involved in the Turner phenotype are X-linked genes that escape inactivation. There appears to be a locus for stature on distal Xp, close to the pseudoautosomal region. Xp and Xq appear to contain genes for normal ovarian function.

Turner syndrome occurs in about 1 of 1,500–2,500 live-born females. The frequency of the 45,X karyotype at conception is about 3.0%, but 99% of these are spontaneously aborted, accounting for 5–10% of all abortuses. Mosaicism (45,X/46,XX) occurs in a proportion higher than that seen with any other aneuploid state, but the mosaic Turner constitution is rare among the abortuses; these findings indicate preferential survival for mosaic forms.

The normal fetal ovary contains about 7 million oocytes, but these begin to disappear rapidly at about 5 mo of gestation. At birth, there are only 3 million; by menarche, there are 400,000; and at menopause, 10,000 remain. In the absence of one X chromosome, this process is accelerated, and nearly all oocytes are gone by 2 yr of age. In aborted 45,X fetuses, the number of primordial germ cells in the gonadal ridge appears to be normal, suggesting that the normal process is accelerated in patients with Turner syndrome. Eventually, the ovaries are described as "streaks" and consist only of connective tissue, but a few germ cells may persist.

CLINICAL MANIFESTATIONS. In the past, the diagnosis was generally first suspected in childhood or at puberty when sexual maturation failed to occur. Many patients with Turner syndrome are recognizable at birth because of a characteristic edema of the dorsa of the hands and feet and loose skinfolds at the nape of the neck. Significantly low birthweight and decreased length are common. Clinical manifestations in childhood include webbing of the neck, a low posterior hairline, small mandible, prominent ears, epicanthic folds, high arched palate, a broad chest presenting the illusion of widely spaced nipples, cubitum valgum, and hyperconvex fingernails.

Short stature, the cardinal finding in all girls with Turner syndrome, may be present with minimal other clinical manifestations. During the first 3 yr of life, the rate of growth is normal, albeit in the lower percentiles; thereafter, it begins to decelerate and results in significant short stature. Sexual maturation fails to occur at the expected age. The mean adult height is 143 cm (132–155 cm) (Fig. 538–1). Pigmented nevi become more prominent with increasing age.

Associated covert defects are common. Complete cardiologic evaluation, including echocardiography, reveals isolated non-

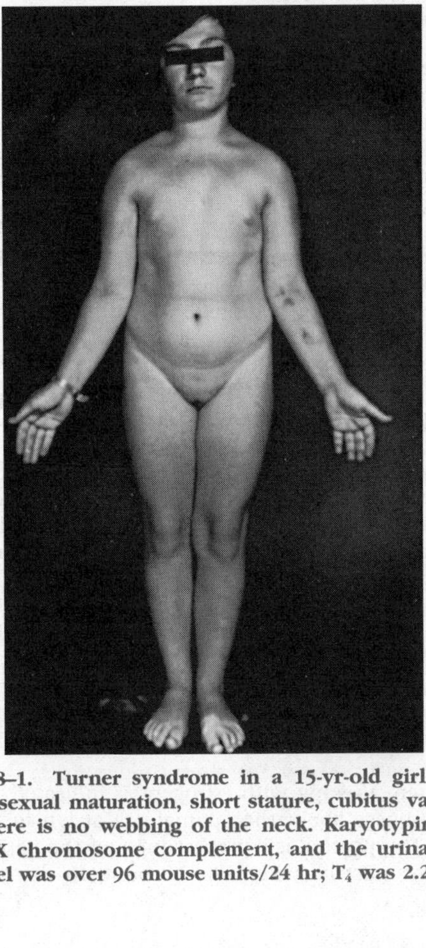

Figure 538–1. Turner syndrome in a 15-yr-old girl exhibiting failure of sexual maturation, short stature, cubitus valgus, and a goiter. There is no webbing of the neck. Karyotyping revealed 45,X/46,XX chromosome complement, and the urinary gonadotropin level was over 96 mouse units/24 hr; T_4 was 2.2 μg/dL.

stenotic bicuspid aortic valves in about one third of patients. Less frequent but more serious defects include aortic stenosis, aortic coarctation, and anomalous pulmonary venous drainage. Approximately one third of patients have renal malformations on ultrasound examination. The more serious defects include pelvic kidney, horseshoe kidney, double collecting system, complete absence of one kidney, and ureteropelvic junction obstruction.

When the ovaries are examined by ultrasound, small but nonstreak ovaries are found in half the patients in the first 4 yr of life; between 4 and 10 yr of age, the ovaries appear as streaks in 90% of patients. Sexual maturation usually fails to occur, but 10–20% of girls have spontaneous breast development, and an occasional girl may even have some menstrual periods. More than 50 pregnancies have been reported for spontaneously menstruating patients with Turner syndrome.

Recurrent bilateral otitis media occurs in about 75% of patients. Sensorineural hearing deficits are common, and the frequency increases with age. Increased problems with gross and fine motor-sensory integration, failure to walk before 15 mo of age, and early language dysfunction often raise questions about developmental delay, but intelligence is normal. However, mental retardation does occur in patients with 45,X/46,X,r(X), because the ring chromosome is unable to undergo inactivation and leads to two functional X chromosomes. In adults, deficits in perceptual spatial skills are more common than they are in the general population.

The presence of a goiter should suggest lymphocytic thyroiditis. Abdominal pain, tenesmus, or bloody diarrhea may represent inflammatory bowel disease; and recurrent gastrointestinal bleeding may indicate gastrointestinal telangiectasia.

In patients with 45,X/46,XX mosaicism, the abnormalities are attenuated and fewer; short stature is as frequent as it is in the 45,X patient and may be the only manifestation of the condition other than ovarian failure (see Fig. 538–1).

LABORATORY DATA. Chromosomal analysis must be considered in all short girls. Patients with a marker chromosome in some or all cells should be tested for DNA sequences at or near the centromere of the Y chromosome. As many as 50% of all 45,X patients may carry Y sequences, but the significance of this finding is unknown. Only patients with a marker chromosome bearing Y sequences require removal of the gonads, because they have a 30% risk of developing gonadoblastomas.

Ultrasound of the heart, kidneys, and ovaries is indicated after the diagnosis is established. The most common skeletal abnormalities are shortening of the 4th metatarsal and metacarpal bones, epiphyseal dysgenesis in the joints of the knees and elbows, Madelung deformity, scoliosis, and in older patients, inadequate osseous mineralization.

Plasma levels of gonadotropins, particularly follicle-stimulating hormone (FSH), are markedly elevated above those of age-matched controls during infancy; at about 2–3 yr of age, a progressive decrease in levels occurs until they reach a nadir at 6–8 yr of age, and by 10–11 yr, they rise to adult castrate levels.

Thyroid antiperoxidase antibodies should be checked periodically, and if positive, levels of thyroxine and thyroid-stimulating hormone should be obtained. Extensive studies have failed to establish that growth hormone deficiency plays a primary role in the pathogenesis of the growth disorder. Mild carbohydrate intolerance in young girls tends to improve with puberty.

TREATMENT. Data indicate that treatment with recombinant human growth hormone (GH) alone or in combination with an anabolic steroid increases height velocity. Many girls may achieve heights of 150 cm or more with early initiation of treatment.

Replacement therapy with estrogens is indicated, but there is little consensus about the optimal age at which to initiate treatment. The psychologic preparedness of the patient to accept therapy must be taken into account. In the past, there was a tendency to delay replacement therapy with estrogens to achieve maximal height. The improved growth achieved by girls treated with GH permits initiation of estrogen replacement at 12–13 yr. Premarin, 0.3–0.625 mg given daily for 3–6 mo, is usually effective in inducing puberty. The estrogen then is cycled (taken on days 1–23), and Provera, a progestin, is added (taken on days 10–23) in a dose of 5–10 mg daily. In the remainder of the calendar month, during which no treatment is given, withdrawal bleeding usually occurs. Other estrogen preparations and regimens of treatment are also in current use.

Prenatal chromosome analysis for advanced maternal age has revealed a frequency of 45,X/46,XX that is 10 times higher than when diagnosed postnatally. Most of these patients have no clinical manifestations of Turner syndrome, and levels of gonadotropins are normal. Awareness of this mild phenotype is important in counseling patients.

Psychosocial support for these girls is an integral component of treatment. The Turner Syndrome Society, which has local chapters in the United States, and similar groups in Canada and other countries provide a valuable support system for these patients and their families in addition to that given by the physician.

Successful pregnancies have been carried to term using ovum donation and in vitro fertilization.

XX GONADAL DYSGENESIS

Some phenotypically and genetically normal females have gonadal lesions identical to those in 45,X patients but without somatic features of Turner syndrome; their condition is termed "pure" gonadal dysgenesis or *pure ovarian dysgenesis*. Here we discuss only those with the XX chromosome constitution. XY gonadal dysgenesis, also termed *Swyer syndrome*, is discussed later in the section on male pseudohermaphroditism. These two conditions are quite distinct entities; in no instance have XX and XY gonadal dysgenesis been reported in the same family.

The disorder is rarely recognized in children because the external genitalia are normal, no other abnormalities are visible, and growth is normal. At pubertal age, sexual maturation fails to take place. Plasma gonadotropin levels are elevated. Delay of epiphyseal fusion results in a eunuchoid habitus. Pelvic ultrasound reveals streak ovaries.

Affected siblings, parental consanguinity, and failure to uncover mosaicism all point to female-limited autosomal recessive inheritance. The disorder appears to be especially frequent in Finland (1 of 8,300 live-born girls). In 24 patients, XX gonadal dysgenesis has been associated with sensorineural deafness *(Perrault syndrome)*. There may be distinct genetic forms of this disorder. Tumors of the gonads have not been reported in these patients. Treatment consists of replacement therapy with estrogens.

45,X/46,XY GONADAL DYSGENESIS

This condition, *mixed gonadal dysgenesis*, has extreme variability, which may extend from a Turner-like syndrome to a male phenotype with a penile urethra; it is possible to delineate three major clinical phenotypes. Short stature is a major finding in all affected patients.

Some patients have no evidence of masculinization; they have a female phenotype and often have the somatic signs of Turner syndrome. The condition is discovered prepubertally when chromosomal studies are made in short girls, or later, when chromosomal studies are made because of failure of sexual maturation. Fallopian tubes and the uterus are present. The gonads consist of intra-abdominal undifferentiated streaks; chromosome study of the streak often reveals an XY cell line.

The streak gonad differs somewhat from that in girls with Turner syndrome; in addition to wavy connective tissue, there are often tubular or cordlike structures, occasional clumps of granulosa cells, and frequently mesonephric or hilar cells.

Some patients have mild virilization manifested only by prepubertal clitorimegaly. Normal müllerian structures are present, but at puberty virilization occurs. These patients usually have an intra-abdominal testis, a contralateral streak gonad, and bilateral fallopian tubes.

Many patients present with frank ambiguity of the genitalia; this is the most frequent phenotype encountered in infants. A testis and vas deferens are found on one side in the labioscrotal fold, and a streak gonad on the contralateral side. Despite the presence of a testis, fallopian tubes are often present bilaterally. An infantile or rudimentary uterus is almost always present.

Other genotypes and phenotypes have been described. About 25% of the more than 200 reported patients have a dicentric Y chromosome (45,X/46,X,dic Y). In some patients, the Y chromosome may be represented by only a fragment (45,X/45,X +fra); application of Y-specific probes can establish the origin of the fragment. It is not clear why the same genotype (45,X/46,XY) can result in such diverse phenotypes.

Patients with a female phenotype present no problem in gender of rearing. Patients who are only slightly virilized are usually assigned a female gender of rearing before a diagnosis is established. Patients with ambiguity of the genitalia are readily confused with various types of male pseudohermaphrodites. In most instances, these patients are best reared as females; the short stature, the ease of genital reconstruction, and the predisposition of the gonad to develop malignancy favor this choice. In some patients followed to adulthood, the putative normal testis proved to be dysgenetic with eventual loss of Leydig and Sertoli cell function.

Gonadal tumors, usually gonadoblastomas, occur in about 25% of these patients, particularly in those with the more female phenotypes. A gonadoblastoma locus has been localized to a region near the centrome of the Y chromosome. These germ cell tumors are preceded by the changes of carcinoma in situ. Accordingly, both gonads should be removed in all patients reared as girls, and the undifferentiated gonad should be removed in the few patients reared as males.

In the past, all patients came to clinical attention because of their abnormal phenotypes. However, 45,X/46,XY mosaicism is found in about 7% of fetuses with true chromosome mosaicism encountered prenatally. Of 76 infants with 45,X/46,XY mosaicism diagnosed prenatally, 72 had a normal male phenotype, 1 had a female phenotype, and only 3 males had hypospadias. Of 12 males whose gonads were examined, only 3 were abnormal. These data must be taken into account when counseling a family in which a 45,X/46,XY infant is discovered prenatally.

XXX, XXXX, AND XXXXX FEMALES

XXX FEMALES. The 47,XXX chromosomal constitution is the most frequent X chromosomal abnormality in females, occurring in almost 1 of 1,000 live-born females. In 68%, this condition is caused by maternal meiotic nondisjunction but most of 45,X and half of the 47,XXY constitutions are caused by paternal sex chromosome errors. The phenotype is that of a normal female; affected infants and children are not recognized.

Sexual development and menarche are normal. Most pregnancies have resulted in normal infants. However, prospective studies of infants diagnosed at birth and followed to young adult life have provided new information about these patients. By 2 yr of age, delays in speech and language become evident, and lack of coordination, poor academic performance, and immature behavior are seen. These girls tend to be tall and gangly, manifest behavior disorders, and are placed in special education classes. There is marked variability within the syndrome, and a small proportion of affected girls are well coordinated, socially outgoing, and academically superior.

XXXX AND XXXXX FEMALES. About 36 females with four X and 23 with five X chromosomes have been described. All have been mentally retarded except for one of the 48,XXXX girls. Commonly associated defects are epicanthal folds, hypertelorism, clinodactyly, simian crease, radioulnar synostosis, and congenital heart disease. Sexual maturation is often incomplete and may not occur at all. Nevertheless, one woman with the tetra-X syndrome gave birth to three normal children, but one of two children of another woman had trisomy 21.

NOONAN SYNDROME

Girls with Noonan syndrome show certain anomalies that also occur in girls with 45,X Turner syndrome, but they have normal 46,XX chromosomes. The most common abnormalities are the same as those described for males with Noonan syndrome (see Chapter 535.1). The phenotype differs from Turner syndrome in several respects. Mental retardation is often present; the cardiac defect is most often pulmonary valvular stenosis or an atrial septal defect rather than an aortic defect; and normal sexual maturation usually occurs but is delayed 2 yr on average; premature ovarian failure occurred in one teenage girl.

OTHER OVARIAN DEFECTS

An increasing number of other young women with no chromosomal abnormality are being found to have streak gonads that may contain only occasional germ cells, if any. Gonadotropins are increased. *Cytotoxic drugs* and exposure of the ovaries to radiation for the treatment of malignancy are increasingly frequent causes of ovarian failure. A study of young women with Hodgkin disease found that combination chemotherapy and pelvic irradiation may be more deleterious than either therapy alone. Teenagers are more likely than older women to retain or recover ovarian function after irradiation or combined chemotherapy; normal pregnancies have occurred after such treatment. Current treatment regimens may result in some ovarian damage in most girls treated for cancer. The LD_{50} for the human oocyte has been estimated to be about 4 Gy.

Autoimmune ovarian failure occurs in 60% of patients older than 13 yr of age with *type I autoimmune polyendocrinopathy* (Addison disease, hypoparathyroidism, candidiasis). Affected girls may not develop sexually, or secondary amenorrhea may occur in young women. The ovaries may have lymphocytic infiltration or appear simply as streaks. Most affected patients have circulating steroid cell antibodies and autoantibodies to 21-hydroxylase.

The condition also occurs in young women as an isolated event or in association with other autoimmune disorders, leading to secondary amenorrhea *(premature menopause)*. About 70% of sera from affected adult patients contains antibodies against the ovaries and oocytes. Some adults treated with immunosuppressive doses of glucocorticoids resume menses and become pregnant; in one case, fertility returned spontaneously 7 yr after onset of autoimmune ovarian failure.

Galactosemia, particularly the classic form of the disease, almost always results in ovarian damage, beginning during intrauterine life. Levels of FSH and luteinizing hormone (LH) are elevated early in life. Ovarian damage had been thought to be caused by fetal accumulation of galactose-1-phosphate, but more recent evidence suggests that deficient UDP-galactose may be the basis for the defect (see Chapter 72).

Ataxia-telangiectasia may be associated with ovarian hypoplasia and elevated gonadotropins; the cause is unknown. Gonadoblastomas and dysgerminomas have occurred in a few girls.

538.2 Hypogonadotropic Hypogonadism in the Female

(Secondary Hypogonadism)

Hypofunction of the ovaries can result from failure to secrete normal levels of gonadotropins. The defect may lie in the anterior pituitary, but as in the male, there is increasing evidence of a hypothalamic defect in most such hypogonadal females.

ETIOLOGY. Hypopituitarism. Destructive lesions in or near the pituitary almost always result in impaired secretion of gonadotropins and other pituitary hormones. In patients with idiopathic hypopituitarism, the defect is usually found in the hypothalamus. In these patients, administration of gonadotropin-releasing hormone (GnRH) results in increased plasma levels of FSH and LH, establishing the integrity of the pituitary gland.

Isolated Deficiency of Gonadotropins. This heterogeneous group of disorders is sorted out with the help of the GnRH test. In most patients, the pituitary is normal, the defect residing in the hypothalamus.

Several sporadic instances of anosmia with hypogonadotropic hypogonadism have been reported. Anosmic hypogonadal females have also been reported in kindreds with Kallmann syndrome, but hypogonadism more frequently affects the males in these families. Mutations of the β subunit of FSH or LH have been reported in single families.

Some autosomal recessive disorders such as the Laurence-Moon-Biedl, multiple lentigines, and Carpenter syndromes appear in some instances to include gonadotropic hormone deficiency. Girls with severe thalassemia may have gonadotropin deficiency due to pituitary damage caused by chronic iron overload secondary to multiple transfusions.

DIAGNOSIS. The diagnosis is not difficult in patients with other deficiencies of pituitary tropic hormones, but it is difficult to differentiate isolated hypogonadotropic hypogonadism from physiologic delay of puberty. Repeated measurements of FSH and LH, particularly during sleep, may reveal the rising levels that herald the onset of puberty.

POLYCYSTIC OVARIES

(Stein-Leventhal Syndrome)

The classic polycystic ovaries syndrome (PCOS) is characterized by obesity, hirsutism, and secondary amenorrhea, with bilaterally enlarged polycystic ovaries, but these manifestations may not all be present. Onset usually occurs at puberty or shortly thereafter; menstrual irregularities and hirsutism are the most frequent complaints. In the reproductive years, the condition is the most common cause of anovulatory infertility. The enlarged ovaries can often be felt on combined rectal and abdominal palpation and are always demonstrable by ultrasound (see Chapter 506).

The cause of the disorder in most patients is unsettled despite intensive investigation. PCOS is a heterogeneous condition that may be associated with several distinct entities, such as 21-hydroxylase deficiency, deficiency of 3β-hydroxysteroid dehydrogenase, and deficiency of ovarian 17-ketoreductase, the enzyme that converts androstenedione to testosterone and estrone to estradiol. However, in most patients with PCOS the elevated plasma level of free testosterone or androstenedione is not suppressed by dexamethasone, ruling out an adrenal cause of the disorder. About 75% of patients have an increased ratio of LH to FSH levels, an increased amplitude and frequency of plasma LH levels, and an exaggerated response to GnRH. Premenarcheal girls may have an early morning rise in LH rather than the characteristic nocturnal one. These perturbances of LH secretion are believed to bring about hyperplasia of theca cells, arrested follicular development, and impaired estradiol production. These effects lead to hyperandrogenemia and irregular cycles or amenorrhea. In patients with congenital virilizing syndromes, the hypothalamic-pituitary axis appears to be programmed for hypersecretion of LH at puberty, leading to hyperandrogenism even when adrenal androgens are adequately suppressed.

Insulin-resistant hyperinsulinemia and *acanthosis nigricans* are associated with PCOS, especially in obese patients. The insulin resistance appears to differ from that which occurs in obesity and in non–insulin-dependent diabetes mellitus; its mechanism remains to be defined.

In the differential diagnosis, adrenal disorders must be ruled out. Basal levels of adrenal steroids may be normal; an ACTH (1–24) stimulation test is necessary to reveal these defects. A deficiency of 17-ketoreductase is suggested when there are affected brothers or when the estrone-estradiol and androstenedione-testosterone ratios are increased. Women treated with valproate for epilepsy before 20 yr of age often have PCOS and elevated testosterone serum levels, but their levels of LH are normal.

The optimal method of treatment is still evolving but usually consists of ovarian suppression by the contraceptive pill. Further suppression can be achieved with tesolactone, a compound with antiandrogen and weak progestin properties. Attention to the obesity is important because its correction often leads to correction of the insulin resistance.

Ahonen P, Myllärniemi S, Sipila I, et al: Clinical variation of autoimmune polyendocrinopathy-candidiasis-ectodermal dystrophy (APECED) in a series of 68 patients. N Engl J Med 322:1829, 1990.

Aittomaki K: The genetics of XX gonadal dysgenesis. Am J Hum Genet 54:844, 1994.

Allanson JE, Hall JG, VanAllen MI: Noonan phenotype associated with neurofibromatosis. Am J Med Genet 21:457, 1985.

Barnes R, Rosenfield RL: The polycystic ovary syndrome: Pathogenesis and treatment. Ann Intern Med 110:386, 1989.

Barnes RB, Rosenfield RL, Ehrmann DA, et al: Ovarian hyperandrogynism as a result of congenital virilizing disorders: Evidence for perinatal masculinization of neuroendocrine function in women. J Clin Endocrinol Metab 79:1328, 1994.

Chang HJ, Clark RD, Bachman H: The phenotype of 45,X/46,XY mosaicism: An analysis of 92 prenatally diagnosed cases. Am J Hum Genet 46:156, 1990.

Franks S: Polycystic ovary syndrome. Trends Endocrinol Metab 1:60, 1990.

Fryns JP, Kleczkowska A, Petit P, et al: X-chromosome polysomy in the female: Personal experience and review of the literature. Clin Genet 23:341, 1983.

Horning SJ, Hoppe RT, Kaplan HS, et al: Female reproductive potential after treatment for Hodgkin's disease. N Engl J Med 304:1377, 1981.

Kocova M, Siegel SF, Wenger SL, et al: Detection of Y chromosome sequences in Turner's syndrome by Southern blot analysis of amplified DNA. Lancet 342:140, 1993.

Krauss CM, Turksoy N, Atkins L, et al: Familial premature ovarian failure due to an interstitial deletion of the long arm of the X chromosome. N Engl J Med 317:125, 1987.

Lack EE, Perez-Atayde AR, Murthy AS, et al: Granulosa theca cell tumors in premenarchal girls: A clinical and pathologic study of ten cases. Cancer 48:1846, 1981.

Linssen WHJP, Bent MJV, Brunner HG, Poels PJE: Deafness, sensory neuropathy, and ovarian dysgenesis: A new syndrome or a broader spectrum of Perrault syndrome. Am J Med Genet 51:81, 1994.

Magenis RE, Tochen ML, Holalan KP, et al: Turner syndrome resulting from partial deletion of Y chromosome short arm: Localization of male determinants. J Pediatr 105:916, 1984.

Massarano AA, Adams JA, Preece MA, et al: Ovarian ultrasound appearances in Turner syndrome. J Pediatr 114:568, 1989.

Matthews CH, Borgato S, Beck-Peccoz P, et al: Primary amenorrhea and infertility due to a mutation in the β-subunit of follicle-stimulating hormone. Nature Genet 5:83, 1993.

May KM, Jacobs PA, Lee M, et al: The parental origin of the extra X chromosome in 47,XXX females. Am J Hum Genet 46:754, 1990.

Migeon BR, Luo S, Jani M, Jeppesen P: The severe phenotype of females with tiny ring X chromosomes are associated with mobility of these chromosomes to undergo X inactivation. Am J Med Genet 55:497, 1994.

Muller J, Shakkeback NE, Ritzen M, et al: Carcinoma in situ of the testis in children with 45,X/46,XY gonadal dysgenesis. J Pediatr 106:431, 1985.

Nicosia SV, Matus-Ridley M, Meadows AT: Gonadal effects of cancer therapy in girls. Cancer 55:2364, 1985.

O'Meara NM, Blackman JD, Ehrmann DA, et al: Defects in β-cell function in functional ovarian hyperandrogenism. J Clin Endocrinol Metab 76:1241, 1993.

Rosenfeld RG, Grumbach MM (ed): Turner Syndrome. New York, Marcel Dekker, 1989.
Saenger P: The current status of diagnosis and therapeutic intervention in Turner syndrome. J Clin Endocrinol Metab 77:297, 1993.
Solh HM, Azoury RS, Najjar SS: Peutz-Jeghers syndrome associated with precocious puberty. J Pediatr 103:593, 1983.
Stokns-Brantsma WH, von Weissenbruch MM, Schoemaker WH, et al: Sexual precocity induced by ovarian follicular cysts. Is autoimmunity involved? Clin Endocrinol 32:603, 1990.
Tanaka Y, Sasaki Y, Nishihira H, et al: Ovarian juvenile granulosa cell tumor associated with Maffucci's Syndrome. Am J Clin Pathol 97:523, 1992.
Yeh J, Rebar RW, Liu JH, et al: Pituitary function in isolated gonadotropin deficiency. Clin Endocrinol 31:375, 1989.
Young RH, Dickersin GR, Scully RE: Juvenile granulosa cell tumor of the ovary. A clinicopathologic analysis of 125 cases. Am J Surg Pathol 8:575, 1984.
Zaloudek C, Norris JH: Granulosa cell tumors of the ovary in children: A clinical and pathological study of 32 cases. Am J Surg Pathol 6:513, 1982.
Zinn AR, Page DC, Fisher EMC: Turner syndrome: The case of the missing X chromosome. Trends Genet 9:90, 1993.

CHAPTER 539
Pseudoprecocity Due to Lesions of the Ovary

Functioning lesions of the ovary consist of benign cysts or malignant tumors. The majority synthesize estrogens; a few synthesize androgens (see Chapter 456).

ESTROGENIC LESIONS OF THE OVARY

These lesions cause isosexual precocious sexual development but account for only a small percentage of all cases of precocity.

Juvenile Granulosa-Cell Tumor

In childhood, the most common neoplasm of the ovary with estrogenic manifestations is the granulosa-cell tumor, although it comprises only 9% of all ovarian tumors. These tumors have distinctive histologic features that differ from those encountered in older women (adult granulosa-cell tumor). Follicles are often irregular, Call-Exner bodies are rare, and luteinization is frequent. The tumor may be solid, cystic, or both. In about a dozen instances, this tumor has been associated with multiple enchondromas *(Ollier disease)* and, in three of these cases, with multiple subcutaneous hemangiomas *(Maffucci syndrome)*.

CLINICAL MANIFESTATIONS. The tumor has been observed in a newborn infant, and in 36 known instances sexual precocity occurred at 2 yr of age or younger; about half of these tumors have occurred before 10 yr of age. They are almost always unilateral. The breasts become enlarged, rounded, and firm and the nipples prominent. The external genitalia resemble those of a normal girl at puberty, and the uterus is enlarged. A white vaginal discharge is followed by irregular or cyclic menstruation. Ovulation, however, does not occur. The presenting manifestation may be abdominal pain or swelling. Pubic hair is usually absent unless there is mild virilization.

A mass is readily palpable in the lower portion of the abdomen in most patients by the time sexual precocity is evident. The tumor may be small, however, and escape detection even on careful rectal and abdominal examination; such tumors are usually detectable by ultrasound.

Plasma estradiol levels are markedly elevated; a 9-yr-old girl with a granulosa-cell tumor had a level of 413 pg/dL, although levels in fully mature women or in children with idiopathic precocious puberty are under 100 pg/dL. Plasma levels of gonadotropins are suppressed and do not respond to gonadotropin-releasing hormone (GnRH) stimulation. Levels of müllerian-inhibiting substance, inhibin, and α-fetoprotein may be elevated. Osseous development is moderately advanced.

The tumor should be removed as soon as the diagnosis is established. Prognosis is excellent because fewer than 5% of these tumors in children are malignant. Vaginal bleeding immediately after removal of the tumor is common. Signs of precocious puberty abate and may disappear within a few months after the operation. The secretion of estrogens returns to normal.

Sex-cord tumor with annular tubules is a distinctive tumor, thought to arise from granulosa cells, that occurs primarily in patients with Peutz-Jeghers syndrome. These tumors are multifocal, bilateral, and benign. The presence of calcifications aids ultrasonographic detection. Increased aromatase production by these tumors results in gonadotropin-independent precocious puberty.

Chorionephithelioma has been reported in only about 20 girls. This very malignant tumor is thought to arise from a preexisting teratoma. The usually unilateral tumor produces large amounts of chorionic gonadotropin (hCG), which stimulates the contralateral ovary to secrete estrogens and progesterone. Elevated levels of hCG are diagnostic.

Follicular Cyst

Small ovarian cysts (<0.7 cm in diameter) are common in prepubertal children. At puberty and in girls with true isosexual precocious puberty, larger cysts (1–6 cm) are often seen; these are secondary to stimulation by gonadotropins. However, similar larger cysts occur occasionally in young girls with precocious puberty in the absence of LH and FSH. Because surgical removal or spontaneous involution of these cysts results in regression of pubertal changes, there is little doubt that they are its cause. The mechanism of production of these autonomously functioning cysts is unknown. Such cysts may form only once, or they may disappear and recur, resulting in waxing and waning of the signs of precocious puberty. They may be unilateral or bilateral. The sexual precocity that occurs in young girls with McCune-Albright syndrome is usually associated with autonomous follicular cysts caused by a somatic-activating mutation of the G protein occurring early in development (see Chapter 517). Gonadotropins are suppressed, and estradiol levels are often markedly elevated, but they may fluctuate widely and even return to normal. GnRH stimulation fails to evoke an increase in gonadotropins. Because gonadotropins are suppressed in these patients, the mechanism of ovarian stimulation is unknown. Ultrasound is the method of choice for the detection and monitoring of such cysts. A short period of observation to ascertain a lack of spontaneous resolution is advisable before cyst aspiration or cystectomy is considered. Cystic neoplasms must be considered in the differential diagnosis.

ANDROGENIC LESIONS OF THE OVARY

Virilizing ovarian tumors are rare at all ages but particularly so in prepubertal girls. The *arrhenoblastoma* has been reported as early as 14 days of age, but fewer than 2 dozen cases have been reported in girls younger than 16 yr of age.

The *gonadoblastoma* occurs exclusively in dysgenetic gonads, particularly in phenotypic females who have a Y chromosome in their genotype (46,XY; 45,X/46,XY; 45,X/46,X fra). The tumor may be bilateral. Virilization occurs with some but not all tumors. The clinical features are the same as those seen in patients with virilizing adrenal tumors and include accelerated growth, acne, clitoral enlargement, and growth of sexual hair.

A palpable, abdominal mass is found only in about 50% of patients. Plasma levels of testosterone and androstenedione are elevated, and those of gonadotropins are suppressed. Ultrasound and computed tomography scans usually localize the lesion. The dysgenetic gonad of phenotypic females with a Y chromosome should be removed prophylactically. When a unilateral tumor is removed, the contralateral dysgenetic gonad should also be removed.

Virilizing manifestations occur occasionally in girls with *juvenile granulosa-cell tumors.*

Dewhurst J, Pryse-Davies J, Helm W, et al: Diagnosis and management of granulosa/theca cell tumors of childhood. Pediatr Adolesc Gynecol 3:131, 1985.

CHAPTER 540

Hermaphroditism

(Intersexuality)

Hermaphroditism implies a discrepancy between the morphology of the gonads and that of the external genitalia. Many chromosomal aberrations resulting in ambiguity of the external genitalia have been discussed earlier in this section. In this chapter, conditions of aberrant sexual differentiation that are imposed on the XX or XY genotype (female and male pseudohermaphrodites) are discussed (Table 540–1). An increasing number of such conditions are understood through advances in the molecular biology of normal sexual differentiation. The category known as true hermaphroditism, with few exceptions, is still a poorly understood heterogeneous group of disorders.

■ **TABLE 540–1 Etiologic Classification of Hermaphroditism**

- Female pseudohermaphroditism
  - Androgen exposure
    - Fetal source
      - 21-Hydroxylase (P-450$_{c21}$) deficiency
      - 11β-Hydroxylase (P-450$_{c11}$) deficiency
      - 3β-Hydroxysteroid dehydrogenase II (3β-HSD II) deficiency
      - Aromatase (P-450$_{arom}$) deficiency
    - Maternal source
      - Virilizing ovarian tumor
      - Virilizing adrenal tumor
      - Androgenic drugs
  - Undetermined origin
    - Associated with genitourinary and gastrointestinal tract defects
- Male pseudohermaphroditism
  - Defects in testicular differentiation
    - Denys-Drash syndrome (mutation in WT1 gene)
    - WAGR syndrome (*W*ilms tumor, *a*niridia, *g*enitourinary malformation, *r*etardation)
      - Deletion of 11p13
    - Camptomelic syndrome (autosomal gene at 17q24.3–q25.1)
    - Mutation in SOX 3 (SRY-related HMO-box genes)
    - XY pure gonadal dysgenesis (Swyer syndrome)
      - Mutation in *SRY* gene (15%)
      - Unknown cause (85%)
    - XY gonadal agenesis
  - Deficiency of testicular hormones
    - Leydig cell aplasia
    - Mutation in LH receptor
    - Lipoid adrenal hyperplasia (P-450$_{scc}$) deficiency
    - Mutation in STAR (steroidogenic acute regulatory protein)
    - 3-β-Hydroxysteroid dehydrogenase II (3β-HSDII) deficiency
    - 17-Hydroxylase/17,20-lyase (P-450$_{c17}$) deficiency
    - Persistent müllerian duct syndrome
      - Gene mutations—müllerian inhibiting substance (MIS)
      - Receptor defects for MIS(?)
  - Defect in androgen action
    - 5α-Reductase II mutations
    - Androgen receptor defects
      - Testicular feminization syndrome
      - Incomplete testicular feminization
      - Reinfenstein syndrome
  - Other
    - Smith-Lemli-Opitz syndrome
      - Defect in conversion of 7-dehydrocholesterol to cholesterol
- True hermaphroditism
  - XX
  - XY
  - XX/XY chimeras

EMBRYONIC SEXUAL DIFFERENTIATION. In normal differentiation, the final form of all sexual structures is consistent with normal sex chromosomes (either XX or XY). A 46,XX complement of chromosomes is necessary for the development of normal ovaries. Both the long and the short arms of X chromosomes bear genes for normal ovarian development. An autosomal gene also appears to play a role in normal ovarian organogenesis and in normal testicular development. A deletion affecting the short arm of the X chromosome produces the typical somatic anomalies of Turner syndrome.

Development of the male phenotype is more complex. Maleness requires a Y chromosome, but only the short arm of the Y chromosome is critical for sex determination; a testis-determining factor (TDF) at this site has been proposed, the gene for which has been cloned and designated *SRY.* During male meiosis, the Y chromosome must segregate from the X chromosome so that both X and Y chromosomes do not occur in the same spermatozoa. The major portion of the Y chromosome is composed of Y-specific sequences that do not pair with the X chromosome. However, a minor portion of the Y chromosome shares sequences with the X chromosome, and pairing does occur in this region. Because the genes and sequences in this area recombine between the sex chromosomes, they behave like autosomal genes; the term *pseudoautosomal* is used to describe the genetic behavior of these genes. The gene for TDF has now been localized adjacent to this pairing and exchange (pseudoautosomal) region of the Y chromosome. When recombination events extend beyond the pseudoautosomal region, X- and Y-specific DNA may be transferred between the chromosomes. Such aberrant recombinations result in X chromosomes carrying TDF, resulting in XX males, or Y chromosomes that have lost TDF, resulting in XY females.

TDF in some unknown way induces the indifferent genital ridge to develop into a testis. The first hormone produced by the fetal testis (6–7 wk) is an inhibiting substance (MIS), a high molecular weight glycoprotein produced by the Sertoli cells. MIS causes the müllerian ducts to regress; in its absence, they persist. By about 8 fetal wk, the Leydig cells of the testis begin to produce testosterone. During this critical period of male differentiation, testosterone secretion is stimulated by placental chorionic gonadotropin (hCG), which peaks at 8–12 wk. In the latter half of pregnancy, lower levels of testosterone are maintained by luteinizing hormone (LH) secreted by the fetal pituitary. Testosterone initiates virilization of the wolffian duct into the epididymis, vas deferens, and seminal vesicle. Development of the external genitalia also requires dihydrotestosterone (DHT), an active metabolite of testosterone. DHT is necessary to fuse the genital folds to form the penis and scrotum. A functional androgen receptor, controlled by an X-linked gene, is required for testosterone and DHT to effect these masculinizing changes.

In the XX fetus, the bipotential gonad does not develop into an ovary until about the 12th wk. This occurs only in the absence of testosterone and MIS. The female phenotype develops independently of the fetal gonads, but maleness is imposed on a basically female potential by the hormones of the fetal testes. Moreover, estrogen is unnecessary for normal prenatal sexual differentiation, as demonstrated by 46,XX patients with aromatase deficiency and by mice without estradiol receptors.

540.1 Female Pseudohermaphroditism

In the female pseudohermaphrodite, the genotype is XX and the gonads are ovaries, but the external genitalia are virilized. Because there is no MIS, the uterus, tubes, and ovaries develop. The mechanisms involved in normal female differentiation are considerably less complex than those required for male differentiation, and the varieties and causes of female pseudohermaphroditism are fewer. Most instances result from exposure of the female fetus to excessive androgens during intrauterine life; and the changes consist principally of virilization of the external genitalia (clitoral hypertrophy and labioscrotal fusion).

CONGENITAL ADRENAL HYPERPLASIA. This is the most common cause of the condition. Females with the 21-hydroxylase and 11-hydroxylase defects are the most highly virilized, although minimal virilization also occurs with the type II 3β-hydroxysteroid dehydrogenase defect. Salt losers tend to have greater degrees of virilization than non–salt-losing patients. Masculinization may be so intense that a complete penile urethra results, and the condition may mimic a male with cryptorchidism (Chapter 529).

AROMATASE DEFICIENCY. Two 46,XX patients with aromatase deficiency have been identified. At birth, both had enlargement of the clitoris and posterior labial fusion. In one instance, maternal serum and urinary levels of estrogen were very low, and serum levels of androgens were high. Cord serum levels of estrogen were also extremely low, but those of androgen were elevated. The second patient also had virilization of unknown etiology since birth, but the aromatase deficiency was not diagnosed until 14 yr of age, when she had further virilization and failed to go into puberty. At that time, she had elevated levels of gonadotropins and androgens but low estrogens, and ultrasonography revealed large ovarian cysts bilaterally. These two patients demonstrate the important role of aromatase in the conversion of androgens to estrogens. In genotypic females, aromatase deficiency during fetal life leads to female pseudohermaphroditism and results in hypergonadotropic hypogonadism at puberty because of ovarian failure to synthesize estrogen (see Section 4 and Fig. 537–1).

MASCULINIZING MATERNAL TUMORS. Rarely, the female fetus has been virilized during fetal life by a maternal androgen-producing tumor. In a few cases, the lesion was a benign adrenal adenoma, but all others were ovarian tumors, particularly androblastomas, luteomas, and Krukenberg tumors. Maternal virilization may be manifested by enlargement of the clitoris, acne, deepening of the voice, decreased lactation, hirsutism, and elevated levels of androgens. In the infant there is enlargement of the clitoris of varying degrees, often with labial fusion. Mothers of children with unexplained female pseudohermaphroditism should undergo measurements of their own levels of plasma testosterone, dehydroepiandrosterone sulfate, and androstenedione.

ADMINISTRATION OF ANDROGENIC DRUGS TO WOMEN DURING PREGNANCY. Testosterone and 17-methyltestosterone have been reported to cause female pseudohermaphroditism in some instances. The greatest number of cases, however, have resulted from the use of certain progestational compounds for the treatment of threatened abortion. In recent years, most of these progestins have been replaced by nonvirilizing ones.

Infants with female pseudohermaphroditism and caudal anomalies have been reported for whom no masculinizing agent could be identified. In such instances, the disorder is usually associated with other congenital defects, particularly of the urinary and gastrointestinal tracts. Y-specific DNA sequences, including *SRY*, are absent.

540.2 Male Pseudohermaphroditism

In the male pseudohermaphrodite, the genotype is XY, but the external genitalia are incompletely virilized, ambiguous, or completely female. When gonads can be found, they are invariably testes; their development may range from rudimentary to normal. Because the process of normal virilization in the fetus is so complex, it is not surprising that there are many varieties of male hermaphroditism.

DEFECTS IN TESTICULAR DIFFERENTIATION

The first step in male differentiation is conversion of the indifferent gonad to a testis. If in the XY fetus there is a deletion of the *short arm of the Y chromosome* or deletion of the male-determining genes, male differentiation does not occur. The phenotype is female; müllerian ducts are well developed, but gonads consist of undifferentiated streaks. By contrast, even extreme deletions of the *long arm of the Y chromosome* (Yq−) have been found in normally developed males, most of whom are azoospermic and have short stature, indicating that the long arm of the Y chromosome normally has genes that prevent these manifestations. In other syndromes in which the testes fail to differentiate, Y chromosomes are morphologically normal.

DENYS-DRASH SYNDROME. The constellation of nephropathy with ambiguous genitalia or Wilms tumor are the major characteristics of this syndrome. Of the 150 reported cases, most have been 46,XY. Müllerian ducts are often present, indicating a global deficiency of fetal testicular function. Patients with 46,XX karyotype have normal external genitalia. The onset of proteinuria in infancy progresses to nephrotic syndrome and to end-stage renal failure by 3 yr of age, with focal or diffuse mesangial sclerosis being the most consistent histopathologic finding. Wilms tumor usually develops in children younger than 2 yr of age and is frequently bilateral. Gonadoblastomas have been reported in six children.

A constitutional point mutation of the Wilms tumor gene *(WT1)*, located at chromosome 11p13, has been found in 34 patients. *WT1* functions as a tumor-suppressor gene and transcriptional factor and is expressed in the genital ridge and fetal gonads.

WAGR SYNDROME. This acronymic syndrome consists of *W*ilms tumor, *a*niridia, *g*enitourinary malformations, and *r*etardation. Only 46,XY males have genital abnormalities, ranging from cryptorchidism to severe deficiency of virilization. Gonadoblastomas have developed in the dysgenetic gonads. Wilms tumor usually occurs by 2 yr of age. These patients have a deletion of one copy of chromosome 11p13, which may be visible on karyotype analysis. The deleted region encompasses the aniridia gene *(PAX6)* and Wilms tumor suppressor gene *(WT1)*, which is critical for testicular development.

CAMPTOMELIC SYNDROME. This form of short-limbed dysplasia is characterized by anterior bowing of the femora and tibia and by malformations of other organs. It is usually lethal in early infancy. About 60% of reported 46,XY patients exhibit sex reversal with completely female phenotype; the external and internal genitalia are female. Some 46,XY patients have ambiguous genitalia. The gonads appear to be ovaries but histologically contain elements of ovaries and testes.

The recently described gene responsible for the condition is

SOX 3 (*SRY*-related HMG-box genes) and is on 17q24.1-q25.1. This gene is structurally related to the testis-determining factor SRY and is involved in both chondrogenesis and control of testis development. Mutation of a single allele in patients studied thus far strongly support the disorder as autosomal dominant.

XY PURE GONADAL DYSGENESIS (SWYER SYNDROME). The designation "pure" distinguishes this condition from forms of gonadal dysgenesis that are of chromosomal origin and associated with somatic anomalies. Affected patients have normal stature and a female phenotype, including vagina, uterus, and fallopian tubes, but at pubertal age, breast development and menarche fail to occur. None of the defects associated with 45,X patients are present. Patients present at puberty with hypergonadotropic primary amenorrhea. Familial cases suggest an X-linked or a sex-limited dominant autosomal transmission. About 15% of patients examined have had mutations of the testis-determining factor gene *(SRY)*, most of which have been confined to the DNA-binding domain. The cause of the condition for most patients is unknown. The gonads consist of almost totally undifferentiated streaks despite the presence of a cytogenetically normal Y chromosome. The primitive gonad cannot accomplish any testicular function, including suppression of müllerian ducts. There may be hilar cells in the gonad capable of producing some androgens; accordingly, some virilization, such as clitoral enlargement, may occur at the age of puberty. The streak gonads may undergo neoplastic changes, such as gonadoblastomas and dysgerminomas, and should be removed shortly after ascertainment, regardless of age.

Pure gonadal dysgenesis also occurs in XX individuals (see Chapter 538).

XY GONADAL AGENESIS SYNDROME (EMBRYONIC TESTICULAR REGRESSION SYNDROME). In this rare syndrome, the external genitalia are slightly ambiguous but more nearly female. Hypoplasia of the labia, some degree of labioscrotal fusion, a small clitoris-like phallus, and a perineal urethral opening are present. No uterus, no gonadal tissue, and usually no vagina can be found. At the age of puberty, no sexual development occurs, and gonadotropin levels are elevated. Most patients have been reared as females. In several patients with XY gonadal agenesis in whom no gonads could be found on exploration, significant rises in testosterone followed stimulation with hCG, indicating Leydig cell function somewhere. Siblings with the disorder are known.

In this condition, it is presumed that testicular tissue was active long enough during fetal life for MIS to inhibit development of müllerian ducts but not long enough for testosterone production to result in virilization. In one patient, no deletion of the Y chromosome was found using Y specific DNA probes. Testicular degeneration seems to occur between the 8th and 12th fetal wk. Regression of the testis before the 8th fetal wk results in Swyer syndrome, between the 14th and 20th wk of gestation the rudimentary testis syndrome, and after the 20th wk of anorchia.

In *bilateral anorchia,* testes are absent, but the male phenotype is complete; it is presumed that tissue with fetal testicular function was active during the critical period of genital differentiation but that sometime later it was damaged. Bilateral anorchia in identical twins and unilateral anorchia in identical twins and in siblings suggest a genetic predisposition. Coexistence of anorchia and the gonadal agenesis syndrome in a sibship is evidence for a relationship between the disorders.

DEFECTS IN TESTICULAR HORMONES

Five genetic defects have been delineated in the enzymatic synthesis of testosterone by fetal testis, and a defect in Leydig cell differentiation has been described. These defects produce male pseudohermaphroditism through inadequate masculinization of the XY fetus (Fig. 540–1). Because levels of testosterone are normally low before puberty, a hCG stimulation test must be used in children to assess the ability of the testes to synthesize testosterone.

LEYDIG CELL APLASIA. Eighteen patients with aplasia or hypoplasia of the Leydig cells have been described. The phenotype is usually female, but there may be mild virilization. Testes, epididymis, and vas are present; the uterus and fallopian tubes are absent. There are no secondary sexual changes at puberty; pubic hair may be normal. Plasma levels of testosterone are low and do not respond to hCG; LH levels are elevated. The Leydig cells of the testes are absent or markedly deficient. The defect may involve lack of receptors for LH. In children, hCG stimulation is necessary to differentiate the condition from testicular feminization. Male-limited autosomal recessive inheritance appears to be the mode of inheritance. A homozygous missense mutation of the LH receptor gene has been found in two patients.

20,22-DESMOLASE DEFICIENCY. This enzyme, now designated P-450_{scc}, is required to cleave the cholesterol side chain early in the biosynthesis of all steroid hormones (see Chapter 529). In its absence, the adrenal is unable to synthesize any steroid. There is marked accumulation of lipids in the adrenal (lipoid adrenal hyperplasia). Affected males have a female phenotype but male genital ducts. Salt-losing manifestations and early adrenal crisis are the presenting manifestations in both genetic males and females. Partial defects with partially virilized males and delayed onset of salt loss have been described. Surprisingly, no mutation has been found in the coding sequence for P-450_{scc}, but a mutation has been found in the gene that codes for steroidogenic (StAR). This protein facilitates cholesterol transport into mitochondria.

3β-HYDROXYSTEROID DEHYDROGENASE DEFICIENCY. Males with this form of congenital adrenal hyperplasia (see Chapter 529) have various degrees of hypospadias, with or without bifid scrotum and cryptorchidism. Affected infants usually develop salt-losing manifestations shortly after birth. Incomplete defects have been reported. These patients have point mutations of the gene for type II 3β-hydroxysteroid enzyme, resulting in impairment of steroidogenesis in the adrenal and gonads. Normal pubertal changes in some boys could be explained by the normally present type I 3β-hydroxysteroid dehydrogenase present in many peripheral tissues.

DEFICIENCY OF 17-HYDROXYLASE/17,20 LYASE. A single enzyme (P-450_{c17}) has both 17-hydroxylase and 17,20 lyase activities in adrenal and gonadal tissues (Chapter 529). Over 125 cases and 15 different genetic lesions have been reported. Genetic males usually present with a complete female phenotype or, less often, with various degrees of virilization from labioscrotal fusion to perineal hypospadias and cryptorchidism. Pubertal development fails to occur in both genetic sexes.

In the classic disorder, there is decreased synthesis of cortisol by the adrenal and of sex steroids by the adrenal and gonads (Fig. 540–1 and see Fig. 529–1). Levels of deoxycorticosterone and corticosterone are markedly increased and lead to the hypertension and hypokalemia characteristic of this form of male pseudohermaphroditism. Although levels of cortisol are low, the elevated corticotropin (ACTH) and corticosterone levels maintain a eucorticoid state, and the renin-aldosterone axis is suppressed. Virilization does not occur at puberty; levels of testosterone are low and those of gonadotropins are increased. Because fetal production of MIS is normal, no müllerian duct remnants are present. In phenotypic XY females, gonadectomy and replacement therapy with hydrocortisone and sex steroids are indicated.

The gene is on chromosome 10, and the defect follows autosomal recessive inheritance. Affected XX females are usually not detected until young adult life, when they fail to experience normal pubertal changes and are found to have hypertension and hypokalemia.

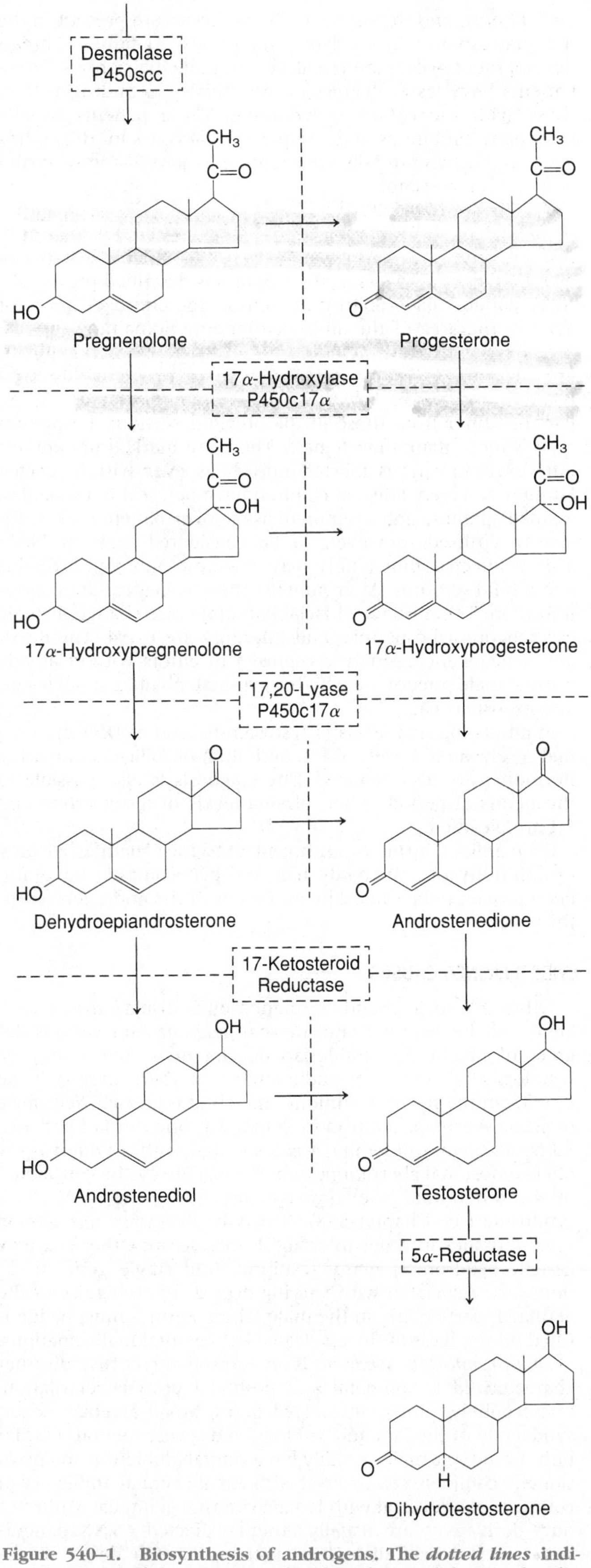

Figure 540–1. Biosynthesis of androgens. The *dotted lines* indicate enzymatic defects associated with male pseudohermaphroditism. The *vertical dotted line* indicates a defect in 3β-hydroxysteroid dehydrogenase. A single polypeptide, P450c17, catalyzes both 17α hydroxylase and 17,20-lyase activities.

DEFICIENCY OF 17-KETOSTEROID REDUCTASE. This enzyme, also called 17β-hydroxysteroid dehydrogenase (I7β-HSD), is the last in the testosterone biosynthetic pathway; it is necessary to convert androstenedione to testosterone. Enzymatic defects in fetal testicular tissue give rise to males with complete or near-complete female phenotype in 46,XY males. Müllerian ducts are absent, and a shallow vagina is present. The diagnosis is based on the ratio of testosterone to androstenedione; in prepubertal children, prior stimulation with hCG is necessary.

The defect is inherited in an autosomal recessive fashion. It is especially common in a highly inbred Arab population in the Gaza strip. The gene for the disorder is at 9q22, and mutations have been delineated. Most patients are diagnosed at puberty because of the failure to menstruate and virilization. Testosterone levels at puberty may approach normal, presumably as a result of peripheral conversion of androstenedione into testosterone; at this time, some patients spontaneously adopt a male gender role.

A late-onset form of 17-ketosteroid reductase deficiency presents as gynecomastia in young adult males.

PERSISTENT MÜLLERIAN DUCT SYNDROME. In this disorder, there is persistence of müllerian duct derivatives in otherwise completely virilized males. More than 150 cases, including siblings and one pair of identical twins, have been reported. The gene has been mapped to chromosome 19. Cryptorchidism is present in 80% of affected males, and during surgery for this or for inguinal hernia, the condition is uncovered when a fallopian tube and uterus are found. The degree of müllerian development is variable and may be asymmetric. Testicular function is normal. About 50% of patients have mutations of the gene coding for MIS and nondetectable MIS. Patients with normal levels of MIS probably have receptor defects. Treatment consists of removal of as many of the müllerian structures as possible without causing damage to the testis, epididymis, or vas deferens. Some affected males develop testicular tumors after puberty.

DEFECTS IN ANDROGEN ACTION

In the following group of disorders, fetal synthesis of testosterone is normal, and defective virilization results from inherited abnormalities in androgen action.

5α-REDUCTASE DEFICIENCY. Decreased production of dihydrotestosterone (DHT) in utero results in severe ambiguity of the external genitalia of the affected male fetus. Biosynthesis and peripheral action of testosterone are normal.

Affected boys have a small phallus, bifid scrotum, urogenital sinus with perineal hypospadias, and a blind vaginal pouch. Testes are in the inguinal canals or labioscrotal folds and are normal histologically. There are no müllerian structures; the vas deferens, epididymis, and seminal vesicles are present. Most affected patients have been identified as females. At puberty, masculinization occurs normally; the phallus enlarges, the testes descend and grow normally, and spermatogenesis occurs. There is no gynecomastia. Beard growth is scanty, acne is absent, the prostate is small, and recession of the temporal hairline fails to occur. The testosterone:DHT ratio is elevated in early infancy and postpubertally or may be demonstrable by hCG stimulation in prepubertal children.

These findings are consistent with studies in animals that show virilization of the wolffian duct to be caused by the action of testosterone itself, although masculinization of the urogenital sinus and external genitalia depends on the action of DHT during the critical period of fetal masculinization. Growth of facial hair and of the prostate also appears to be DHT dependent. The disorder is inherited as an autosomal recessive but is limited to males; normal homozygous females with normal fertility indicate that in females DHT has no role in sexual differentiation or in ovarian function later in life. Mutations of the gene coding for 5α-reductase 2 cause the condition. In 23 interrelated families in the Dominican Republic, although many of the 38 affected males had been reared as females, most assumed a male gender role coincident with masculinization at puberty. It appears that exposures to testosterone in utero, neonatally, and at puberty contribute to the formation of male gender identity. Patients with this condition should be reared as boys whenever practical. Treatment of male infants with DHT resulted in phallic enlargement.

TESTICULAR FEMINIZATION SYNDROME. In this extreme form of failure of virilization, genetic males appear female at birth and are invariably reared accordingly. The external genitalia are female; the vagina ends blindly in a pouch, and the uterus is absent. In about one third of patients, unilateral or bilateral fallopian tube remnants are found. The testes are usually intra-abdominal but may descend into the inguinal canal; they consist largely of seminiferous tubules. At puberty, there is normal development of breasts, and the habitus is female, but menstruation does not occur, and sexual hair is absent. Adult heights of these women are commensurate with those of normal males despite profound congenital deficiency of androgenic effects. Psychosexual orientation of such persons is entirely female.

The testes of affected adult patients produce normal male levels of testosterone and DHT. Failure of normal male differentiation during fetal life reflects defective response to androgens at that time, but the absence of müllerian ducts indicates normal fetal testicular production of MIS. The absence of androgenic effects is caused by a striking resistance to the action of endogenous or exogenous testosterone at the cellular level. In many patients, receptor binding for androgen is undetectable (receptor negative). In other clinically identical patients, receptor binding is qualitatively abnormal or normal (receptor positive).

The disorder follows X-linked recessive inheritance, and the gene encoding the androgen receptor has been localized to Xq11-12. Female heterozygotes are normal, but about 20% have delayed menarche. Most patients with testicular feminization have absent or near-absent androgen binding, and the gene has a point mutation in the DNA-binding or hormone-binding domain of the receptor sequence.

Prepubertal children with this disorder are often detected when inguinal masses prove to be a testis or when a testis is unexpectedly found during herniorrhaphy in a phenotypic female. About 1–2% of girls with an inguinal hernia prove to have this disorder. In infants, elevated gonadotropin levels should suggest the diagnosis. In adults, amenorrhea is the usual presenting symptom. Affected patients should always be reared as females. In prepubertal children, the condition must be differentiated from other types of XY male pseudohermaphroditism in which there is complete feminization. These include XY gonadal dysgenesis (Swyer syndrome), true agonadism, Leydig cell aplasia, and 17-ketosteroid reductase deficiency; all of these conditions, unlike testicular feminization, are characterized by low levels of testosterone as neonates and during adult life and by failure to respond to hCG during the prepubertal years.

The testes should be removed as soon as they are discovered. In one third of patients, malignant tumors, usually seminomas, develop by 50 yr of age. Several 14-yr-old girls have developed seminomas. Replacement therapy with estrogens is indicated at the age of puberty.

Affected girls who have not had their testes removed by the age of puberty develop normal breasts. In these individuals, production of estradiol results from aromatase activity. The absence of androgenic activity also contributes to the feminization of these women.

INCOMPLETE TESTICULAR FEMINIZATION. In this disorder, patients exhibit some degree of masculinization and at birth may have enlargement of the phallus and labioscrotal fusion. The vagina ends blindly, and the uterus is absent. Testes are present in the inguinal canal or in the labioscrotal folds. At puberty, breast development occurs, and axillary and pubic hair grows. These patients have lesser degrees of insensitivity to androgen than those with the complete syndrome. These patients usually have point mutations in the sequence that codes for the androgen receptor, and the disorder represents part of the spectrum of androgen resistance.

REIFENSTEIN SYNDROME. This syndrome and other syndromes of defective virilization are caused by decreased end-organ responsiveness to androgens and are best described as *partial androgen insensitivity.* As in the conditions described previously, these patients have point mutations of the androgen receptor gene in the area of the androgen-binding domain. Treatment with large doses of depot testosterone may increase phallic growth and virilization, particularly in patients with partial receptor resistance. Inheritance is X-linked recessive. These patients differ from those in the previous section; the phenotype is more male than female. There are marked phenotypic differences in various affected individuals, even within affected families. Severely affected children have perineal hypospadias, a small phallus, and cryptorchidism. Most patients are sufficiently virilized, however, to be considered male at birth. Mildly affected individuals may manifest only microphallus and a bifid scrotum. After puberty, there is inadequate masculinization. There is lack of facial hair and voice change. Female escutcheon, azoospermia, and infertility are usual. The disorder is being increasingly recognized in adults with relatively normal male phenotype who have a small phallus, small testes, and azoospermia.

In adults, plasma levels of testosterone and of DHT are normal or elevated. Levels of LH, and often of follicle-stimulating hormone, are also elevated. The diagnosis is also possible in the neonatal period, when plasma levels of testosterone and LH are elevated.

Even milder forms of androgen resistance manifested only by infertility or scant body hair and gynecomastia have also been proven to be caused by mutations of the androgen receptor gene.

UNDETERMINED CAUSES

Other XY male pseudohermaphrodites display much variability of the external and internal genitalia and various degrees of phallic and müllerian development. Testes may be histologically normal or rudimentary, or there may only be one. Even the newer techniques may find no recognized cause of pseudohermaphroditism in as many as one third of patients. Some ambiguity of genitalia is associated with a wide variety of chromosomal aberrations, which must always be considered in the differential, the most common being the 45,X/46,XY syndrome (see Chapter 538). It may be necessary to examine several tissues in order to establish mosaicism. Other complex genetic syndromes, many resulting from single gene mutations, are associated with varying degrees of ambiguity of the genitalia, particularly in the male. These entities must be identified on the basis of the associated extragenital malformations.

Smith-Lemli-Opitz syndrome is an autosomal recessive disorder characterized by prenatal and postnatal growth retardation, microcephaly, ptosis, anteverted nares, broad alveolar ridges, syndactyly of the 2nd and 3rd toes, and severe mental retardation. Genotypic males usually have genital ambiguity and occasionally complete sex reversal with female genital ambiguity or complete sex reversal with female external genitalia. Müllerian duct derivatives are usually absent. Affected 46,XX patients have normal genitalia. These patients have a defect in the terminal step of cholesterol synthesis. A low serum cholesterol level and marked elevation of its precursor, 7-dehydrocholesterol, is diagnostic. The degree of genital defect and severity of the phenotype appears to be related to the enzymatic defect.

The pathogenesis is enigmatic. Dietary methods of treatment are under investigation.

540.3 True Hermaphroditism

In true hermaphroditism, both ovarian and testicular tissues are present, either in the same or in opposite gonads. Affected patients have ambiguous genitalia, varying from normal female with only slight enlargement of the clitoris to almost-male external genitalia.

About 70% of all patients have a 46,XX karyotype; 45% of affected African blacks are 46,XX. Fewer than 10% of true hermaphrodites are 46,XY; in one of these, a mutated *SRY* gene was found. About 20% have 46,XX/46,XY mosaicism. Half of these are derived from more than one zygote and are chimeras (chi 46,XX/46,XY). The presence of paternal and both maternal alleles for some blood groups are demonstrated.

Examination of 46,XX true hermaphrodites with Y-specific probes have detected fewer than 10% with a portion of the Y chromosome including the *SRY* gene. True hermaphroditism is usually sporadic, but a small number of siblings have been reported. The cause of most cases of true hermaphroditism is unknown.

The most frequently encountered gonad in true hermaphrodites is an ovotestis, which may be bilateral; if unilateral, the contralateral gonad is usually an ovary but may be a testis. The ovarian tissue is normal, but the testicular tissue is dysgenetic. The presence and function of testicular tissue can be determined by measuring basal and hCG-stimulated testosterone levels. Patients who are highly virilized, have good testicular function, and have no uterus may be reared as males. If a uterus exists, virilization is mild, and testicular function minimal, assignment of female sex is indicated. Selective removal of gonadal tissue inconsistent with sex of rearing is indicated.

Pregnancies with living offspring have been reported in 46,XX true hermaphrodites reared as females, but male true hermaphrodites are almost always infertile. About 5% of patients develop gonadoblastomas, dysgerminomas, or seminomas; the youngest patient was 14 mo old.

DIAGNOSIS AND MANAGEMENT

In the neonate, ambiguity of the genitalia requires emergency medical attention to decide on the sex of rearing as early in life as possible. While awaiting the results of chromosomal analysis, pelvic ultrasound examination is indicated to determine the presence of a uterus and ovaries. Presence of a uterus and absence of palpable gonads usually suggests a virilized XX female. Search for the source of virilization should be undertaken; this includes studies of adrenal hormones to rule out varieties of congenital adrenal hyperplasia, and occasionally, studies of androgens and estrogens may be necessary to rule out aromatase deficiency. Female pseudohermaphrodites should be reared as females even when highly virilized.

The absence of a uterus, with or without palpable gonads, almost always indicates male pseudohermaphroditism and an XY karyotype. Measurements of levels of gonadotropins, testosterone, and DHT are necessary to determine whether testicular production of androgen is normal. Male pseudohermaphrodites who are totally feminized must be reared as females. However, certain significantly feminized infants, such as those with 5α-reductase deficiency, should be reared as males, because these children virilize normally at puberty. An infant with a comparable degree of feminization resulting from an androgen-receptor defect is best reared as a female. It is more feasible to reconstruct the external genitalia to create a functional female, particularly when a vagina is present, than to create a functional male phallus. Infants with 45,X/46,XY whose phenotype varies from almost completely male to completely female are usually reared as females because they are generally short in stature and have a uterus, and they will require gonadectomy.

When receptor disorders are suspected in the XY male with a small phallus (micropenis), a course of 3 monthly intramuscular injections of testosterone enanthate (25–50 mg) may assist in the differential diagnosis as well as in treatment.

The management of the potential psychologic upheaval that these disorders can generate in the patient or the family is of paramount importance and requires physicians with sensitivity, training, and experience in this field. After the appropriate sex of rearing has been established, parents should be left with no ambiguity in their minds as to the gender of the child.

In some mammals, the female exposed to androgens prenatally or in early postnatal life exhibits aberrant sexual behavior in adult life. Girls who have undergone fetal masculinization from congenital adrenal hyperplasia or from maternal progestin therapy have no such problems in sexual identity, although during childhood, they may appear to prefer male playmates and activities over female playmates and feminine play with dolls in mothering roles.

Affara NA, Chalmers IJ, Ferguson-Smith MA: Analysis of the SRY gene in 22 sex-reversed XY females identifies four new point mutations in the conserved DNA binding domain. Hum Mol Genet 2:785, 1993.

Braun A, Kammerer S, Cleve H, et al: True hermaphroditism in a 46,XY individual, caused by a postzygotic somatic point mutation in the male gonadal sex-determining locus (SRY): Molecular genetics and histological findings in a sporadic case. Am J Hum Genet 52:578, 1993.

Castro-Magana M, Angulo M, Uy J: Male hypogonadism with gynecomastia caused by late-onset deficiency of testicular 17-ketosteroid reductase. N Engl J Med 328:1297, 1993.

Conte FA, Grumbach MM, Ito Y, et al: A syndrome of female pseudohermaphroditism, hypergonadotropic hypogonadism, and multicystic ovaries associated with missense mutations in the gene encoding aromatase ($P450_{arom}$). J Clin Endocrinol Metab 78:1287, 1994.

Coppes MJ, Hober DN, Grundy PE: Genetic events in the development of Wilms' tumor. N Engl J Med 331:586, 1994.

Coppes MJ, Huff V, Pelletier J: Denys-Drash syndrome: Relating a clinical disorder to genetic alterations in the tumor suppressor gene WT1. J Pediatr 123:673, 1993.

Fardella CE, Hum DW, Homoki J, Miller WL: Point mutation of Arg 440 to His in cytochrome P450c17 causes severe 17α-hydroxylase deficiency. J Clin Endocrinol Metab 79:160, 1994.

Griffin JE: Androgen resistance—the clinical and molecular spectrum. N Engl J Med 326:611, 1992.

Hadjiathanasiou CG, Brauner R, Lortat-Jacob S, et al: True hermaphroditism: Genetic variants and clinical management. J Pediatr 125:738, 1994.

Harada N, Ogawa H, Shozu M, Yamada K: Genetic studies to characterize the origin of the mutation in placental aromatase deficiency. Am J Hum Genet 51:666, 1992.

Hawkins JR: The SRY gene. Trends Endocrinol Metab 10:328, 1993.

Imbeaud S, Carre-Eusebe D, et al: Molecular genetics of the persistent Mullerian duct syndrome: A study of 19 families. Hum Mol Genet 3:125, 1994.

Josso N, Boussin L, Knebelmann B, et al: Anti-müllerian hormone and intersex states. Trends Endocrinol Metab 2:227, 1991.

Klocker H, Kaspar F, Eberle J, et al: Point mutation in the DNA binding domain of the androgen receptor in two families with Reifenstein syndrome. Am J Hum Genet 50:1318, 1992.

Kremer H, Karaaij R, Toledo SPA, et al: Male pseudohermaphroditism due to a homozygous missense mutation of the luteinizing hormone receptor gene. Genetics 9:160, 1995.

Krob G, Braun A, Kuhnle U: True hermaphroditism: Geographical distribution, clinical findings, chromosomes and gonadal histology. Eur J Pediatr 153:2, 1994.

Lin D, Sugawara T, Strauss JF, III, et al: Role of steroidogenic acute regulation protein in adrenal and gonadal steroidogenesis. Science 267:1828, 1995.

Lubahn DB, Moyer JS, Golding TS, et al: Alterations of reproductive females but not prenatal sexual development after insertional disruption of the mouse estrogen receptor gene. Proc Natl Acad Sci USA 90:11162, 1993.

McElreavey K, Rappaport R, Vilain E, et al: A minority of 46,XX true hermaphrodites are positive for the Y DNA sequence including SRY. Hum Genet 90:121, 1992.

Martinez-Mora J, Saez JM, Toran N, et al: Male pseudohermaphroditism due to Leydig cell agenesis and absence of testicular LH receptors. Clin Endocrinol 34:485, 1991.

McPhaul MJ, Marcelli M, Zoppi S, et al: The spectrum of mutations in the androgen receptor gene that causes androgen resistance. J Clin Endocrinol Metab 76:17, 1993.

Mueller RF: The Denys-Drash syndrome. J Med Genet 31:471, 1994.

O'Leary TJ, Ooi TC, Miller JD, et al: Virilization of two siblings by maternal androgen-secreting adrenal adenoma. J Pediatr 109:841, 1986.

Poulat F, Scullier S, Goze C, et al: Description and functional implications of a novel mutation in the sex-determining gene SRY. Hum Mutation 3:200, 1994.

Rheume E, Simard J, Morel Y, et al: Congenital adrenal hyperplasia due to point mutations in the type II 3β-hydroxysteroid dehydrogenase gene. Nature Genet 1:239, 1992.

Sakai Y, Yanase T, Okabe Y, et al: No mutation in cytochrome P450 side chain cleavage in a patient with congenital lipoid adrenal hyperplasia. J Clin Endocrin Metab 79:1198, 1994.

Seaver LH, Grimes J, Erickson RP: Female pseudohermaphroditism with multiple caudal anomalies: Absence of Y-specific DNA sequences as pathogenetic factors. Am J Med Genet 51:16, 1994.

Smith EP, Boyd J, Frank GR, et al: Estrogen resistance caused by a mutation in the estrogen-receptor gene in a man. N Engl J Med 331:1056, 1994.

Tammerup N, Schempp W, Meinecke P, et al: Assignment of an autosomal sex reversal locus (SRA1) and camptomelic dysplasia (CMPD1) to 17q24.3-q25.1. Nature Genet 4:170, 1993.

Tint GS, Irons M, Elias ER, et al: Defective cholesterol biosynthesis associated with Smith-Lemli-Opitz syndrome. N Engl J Med 330:107, 1994.

Tsukada T, Inoue M, Tachibana S, et al: An androgen receptor mutation causing androgen resistance in undervirilized male syndrome. J Clin Endocrinol Metab 79:1202, 1994.

Wagner T, Wirth J, Meyer J, et al: Autosomal sex reversal and camptomelic dysplasia are caused by mutations in and around the SRY-related gene SOX9. Cell 79:1111, 1994.

Wilson JD, Griffin JE, Russell DW: Steroid 5α-reductase 2 deficiency. Endocr Rev 14:577, 1993.

SECTION 6

Diabetes Mellitus

Mark A. Sperling

Diabetes mellitus is a syndrome of disturbed energy homeostasis caused by a deficiency of insulin or of its action and resulting in abnormal metabolism of carbohydrate, protein, and fat. It is the most common endocrine-metabolic disorder of childhood and adolescence with important consequences for physical and emotional development. Individuals affected by insulin-dependent diabetes confront serious burdens that include an absolute daily requirement for exogenous insulin, the need to monitor their own metabolic control, and the need to pay constant attention to dietary intake. Morbidity and mortality stem from metabolic derangements and from long-term complications that affect small and large vessels and result in retinopathy, nephropathy, neuropathy, ischemic heart disease, and arterial obstruction with gangrene of the extremities. The acute clinical manifestations can be fully understood in the context of current knowledge about the secretion and action of insulin; genetic and other etiologic considerations point to autoimmune mechanisms as factors in the genesis of type I diabetes, and there is an emerging consensus that the long-term complications are related to metabolic disturbances. These considerations form the basis of therapeutic approaches to this disease.

CLASSIFICATION

Diabetes mellitus is not a single entity but rather a heterogeneous group of disorders in which there are distinct genetic patterns as well as other etiologic and pathophysiologic mechanisms that lead to impairment of glucose tolerance. The National Diabetes Data Group has proposed a classification of diabetes and other categories of glucose intolerance based on contemporary knowledge. This classification has been endorsed and accepted by various diabetes associations throughout the world as well as by pediatric investigators (Table XXVI–1). Three major forms of diabetes and several forms of carbohydrate intolerance have been identified.

TYPE I DIABETES (Juvenile-Onset Diabetes). This condition is characterized by severe insulinopenia and dependence on exogenous insulin to prevent ketosis and to preserve life; it is therefore also termed *insulin-dependent diabetes mellitus* (IDDM). The natural history of this disease indicates that there are preketotic, non–insulin-dependent phases both before and after the initial diagnosis. Although the onset occurs predominantly in childhood, it may come at any age. Hence, such terms as juvenile diabetes, ketosis-prone diabetes, and brittle diabetes should be abandoned in favor of *type I diabetes* or IDDM. Type I diabetes is clearly distinct by virtue of its association with certain histocompatibility antigens (HLA); the presence of circulating antibodies to cytoplasmic and cell-surface components of islet cells; antibodies to insulin in the absence of prior exposure to exogenous injection of insulin; antibodies to glutamic acid decarboxylase (GAD), the enzyme that converts glutamic acid to gamma aminobutyric acid (GABA), found abundantly in the innervation of pancreatic islet; lymphocytic infiltration of islets early in the disease; and other autoimmune diseases. With few exceptions, diabetes in children is insulin dependent and falls into the type I category.

TYPE II DIABETES. Persons in this subclass (formerly known as adult-onset diabetes, maturity-onset diabetes [MOD], or stable diabetes) are not insulin dependent and only infrequently develop ketosis; some may, however, need insulin for correction of symptomatic hyperglycemia, and ketosis may develop in some during severe infections or other stress. This is generally termed *non–insulin-dependent diabetes mellitus* (NIDDM).

Serum concentration of insulin may be normal or moderately depressed; it is generally less when compared to that in controls matched for weight, age, and stage of puberty. In the majority of instances, the onset of non–insulin-dependent diabetes mellitus occurs after age 40, but it may occur at any age. It is rare in childhood and adolescence, when it may become manifest as abnormal glucose tolerance, usually in obese individuals. There appears to be adequate secretion of insulin, but there is also resistance to it, and in some individuals it may represent slowly evolving type I diabetes mellitus. As an initial approach, weight reduction is indicated in children who are obese. Abnormal carbohydrate tolerance may also occur in children who have a strong family history of type II diabetes in a pattern suggestive of dominant inheritance; this pattern of diabetes has been termed *MODY* (maturity-onset diabetes of the young), and it may require treatment with insulin. Most important, in this type of diabetes there is no association with human leukocyte antigens (HLAs), autoimmunity, and/or islet cell antibodies. Although MODY may be heterogenous, a specific genetic disorder involving mutations in the gene encoding pancreatic β cell and liver glucokinase is the cause of hyperglycemia in many affected families. The mutant glucokinase may lead to hyperglycemia by raising the threshold of circulating glucose concentration that induces insulin secretion. A defect in the gene regulating glucose transport into the pancreatic β cell, GLUT-2 transporter, may be responsible for other forms of non–insulin-dependent diabetes mellitus. The molecular genetic basis of NIDDM now includes defects in glucokinase, GLUT-2 glucose transporter, glycogen

■ **TABLE XXVI–1 Summary of Classification of Diabetes Mellitus in Children and Adolescents***

Classification	Criteria
Diabetes mellitus	
1. Insulin-dependent (IDDM, type I)	Typical manifestations: glucosuria, ketonuria, random plasma glucose (PG) >200 mg/dL
2. Non–insulin-dependent (NIDDM, type II)	FPG >140 mg/dL and 2-hr value >200 mg/dL during OGTT on more than one occasion and in absence of precipitating factors
3. Other types	Type I or II criteria in association with certain genetic syndromes (including cystic fibrosis), other disorders, and drugs (see text)
Impaired glucose tolerance (IGT)	FPG <140 mg/dL with 2-hr value >140 mg/dL during OGTT
Gestational diabetes (GDM)	Two or more of following abnormalities during OGTT: FPG >105 mg/dL; 1 hr, >190 mg/dL; 2-hr, >165 mg/dL; 3 hr, >145 mg/dL
Statistical risk classes	
1. Previous abnormality of glucose tolerance	Normal OGTT following a previous abnormal one, spontaneous hyperglycemia or gestational diabetes
2. Potential abnormality of glucose tolerance	Genetic propensity (e.g., identical nondiabetic twin of a diabetic sibling); islet cell antibodies

**Proposed by National Diabetes Data Group (Diabetes 28:1039, 1979) and endorsed by various diabetes associations worldwide.*
PG = plasma glucose; FPG = fasting plasma glucose; OGTT = oral glucose tolerance test.

synthase, insulin receptors, Rad (Ras associated with diabetes), and possibly apolipoprotein C-III.

SECONDARY DIABETES. This subclass contains a variety of types of diabetes, for some of which the etiologic relationship is known. Examples include diabetes secondary to exocrine pancreatic diseases, such as cystic fibrosis; endocrine diseases other than pancreatic diseases (e.g., Cushing syndrome); and ingestion of certain drugs or poisons (e.g., the rodenticide Vacor). Certain genetic syndromes, including those with abnormalities of the insulin receptor, also are included in this category. There are no associations with HLAs, autoimmunity, or islet cell antibodies among the entities in this subdivision.

For all types of diabetes, many believe that the criterion of a fasting blood glucose level in excess of 140 mg/dL is too stringent because normal children do not exceed a fasting blood glucose level of 120 mg/dL.

TYPE I DIABETES MELLITUS

(Insulin-Dependent Diabetes Mellitus [IDDM]; Juvenile-Onset Diabetes)

EPIDEMIOLOGY. Surveys in the United States indicate that the prevalence of diabetes among school-age children is about 1.9 in 1,000. The frequency, however, is highly correlated with increasing age; available data indicate a range of 1 in 1,430 children at 5 yr of age to 1 in 360 children at 16 yr. Data on prevalence and incidence in relation to racial or ethnic backgrounds indicate a range of nearly 30 new cases annually in 100,000 population in Finland to 0.8 in 100,000 in Japan (Fig. XXVI–1). Among American blacks the occurrence of insulin-dependent diabetes has been reported to be only 20–30% of that seen in American whites, although it may be as high as two thirds. These observations have implications for genetic counseling (see later). The annual incidence in the United States is about 12–15 new cases per 100,000 of the childhood population (see Fig. XXVI–1). Males and females are almost equally affected; there is no apparent correlation with socioeconomic status. Peaks of presentation occur in two age groups: at 5–7 yr of age and at the time of puberty. The first peak corresponds to the time of increased exposure to infectious agents coincident with the beginning of school; the latter to the pubertal growth spurt induced by gonadal steroids and increased pubertal growth hormone secretion, which antagonize insulin action, and to the emotional stresses accompanying puberty. These possible cause-and-effect relationships remain to be proved. The prevalence and incidence of insulin-dependent diabetes in childhood in the United States and elsewhere may reflect the distribution of susceptibility genes encoded on the DQ β chain of the HLA system.

Seasonal and long-term cyclic variations occur in the incidence of insulin-dependent diabetes mellitus. Newly recognized cases appear with greater frequency in the autumn and winter months in the Northern and Southern Hemispheres. Seasonal variations are most apparent in the adolescent years. Attempts to link a pattern of long-term cyclicity with the incidence of mumps or other viral infections when allowance was made for a 4-yr time lag have not been successful. There is, however, a definite increased incidence of diabetes in children with congenital rubella. These associations with viral infections suggest a potential role for viruses as direct or indirect triggering mechanisms in the etiology of diabetes.

ETIOLOGY AND PATHOGENESIS. The basic cause of the initial clinical findings in this predominant form of diabetes in childhood is the sharply diminished secretion of insulin. Although basal insulin concentrations in plasma may be normal in newly diagnosed patients, insulin production in response to a variety of potent secretagogues is blunted and usually disappears over a period of months to years, rarely exceeding 5 yr. In certain individuals considered at high risk for the development of type I diabetes, such as the nonaffected identical twin of a diabetic, a progressive decline in insulin-secreting capacity has been noted for months to years before the clinical appearance of symptomatic diabetes, which usually becomes manifest when the insulin-secreting reserve is 20% or less of normal (Fig. XXVI–2).

The mechanisms that lead to failure of pancreatic β-cell function increasingly point to the likelihood of autoimmune destruction of pancreatic islets in predisposed individuals. Type I diabetes has long been known to have an increased prevalence among persons with such disorders as Addison disease,

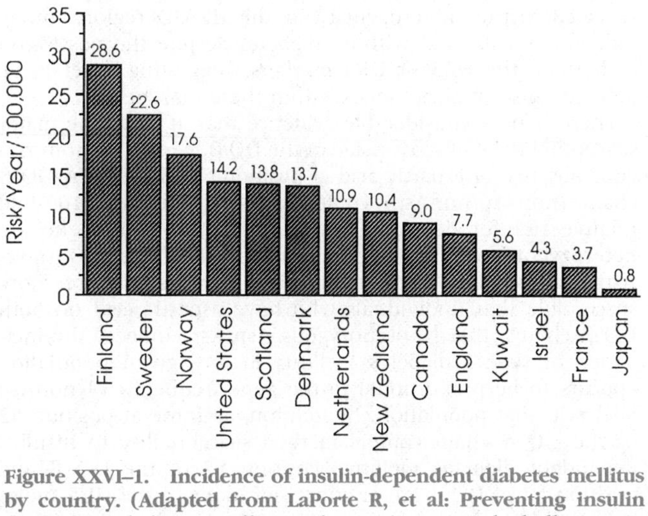

Figure XXVI–1. Incidence of insulin-dependent diabetes mellitus by country. (Adapted from LaPorte R, et al: Preventing insulin dependent diabetes mellitus: The environmental challenge. Br Med J 295:479, 1987.)

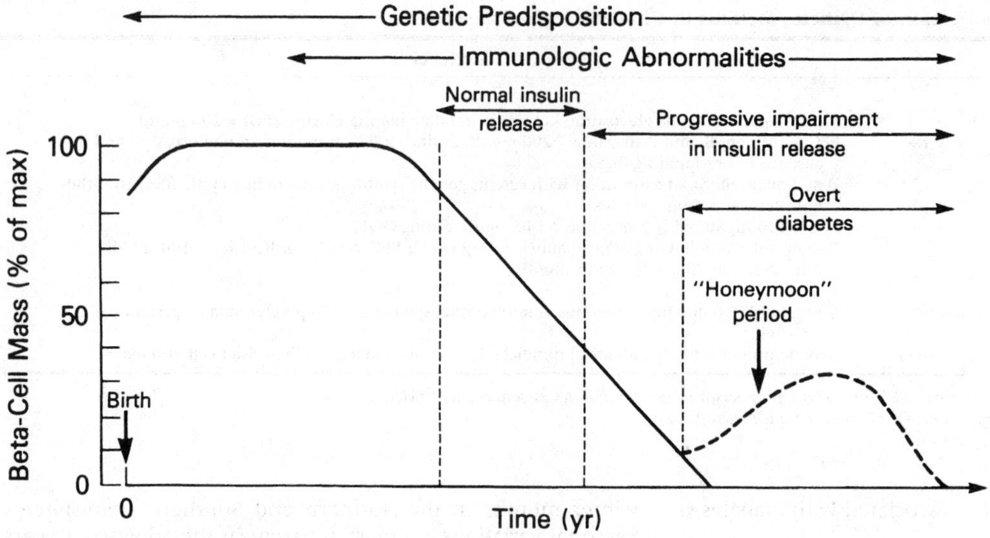

Timing of trigger in relation to immunologic abnormalities is unknown. Note that overt diabetes is not apparent until insulin secretory reserves are <10–20% of normal.

Figure XXVI–2. Proposed scheme of natural history of β-cell defect. (Adapted from Sperling MA [ed]: Physician's Guide to Insulin-Dependent [Type 1] Diabetes Mellitus: Diagnosis and Treatment. Copyright (1988) by the American Diabetes Association. Reprinted with permission.)

Hashimoto thyroiditis, and pernicious anemia, in which autoimmune mechanisms are known to be pathogenic. These conditions, as well as insulin-dependent type I diabetes mellitus, also are known to be associated with an increased frequency of certain HLAs, in particular HLA-B8, -DR3, -BW15, and -DR4. Located on chromosome 6, the HLA system is the major histocompatibility complex, consisting of a cluster of genes that code transplantation antigens and play a central role in immune responses.

Increased susceptibility to a number of diseases has been related to one or more of the identified HLA antigens. Inheritance of HLA-D3 or -D4 antigens appears to confer a two- to threefold increased risk for developing type I diabetes. When both D3 and D4 are inherited, the relative risk for developing diabetes is increased by sevenfold to 10-fold. A rare genetic type of properdin factor B (BfF1) that is closely linked to the HLA system on chromosome 6 is found in more than 20% of type I diabetics but in less than 2% of healthy subjects; thus there is a relative risk factor of 15 for those who inherit this genetic marker. Certain blood groups have also been associated with an increased risk of diabetes. Application of newer molecular genetic techniques through analysis of DNA polymorphisms after digestion by specific restriction endonucleases has revealed further heterogeneity in the HLA-D region among individuals with and without diabetes despite the possession in both of the DR3 or DR4 markers, suggesting a yet to be defined "susceptibility" locus within these markers.

There is now considerable evidence that at least one major susceptibility locus may reside in the DQ β_1 gene. The homozygous absence of aspartic acid at position 57 of the HLA-DQ β chain (nonAsp/nonAsp) confers an approximately 100-fold relative risk for developing type I diabetes. Those who are heterozygous with a single aspartic acid at position 57 (nonAsp/Asp) are less likely to develop diabetes but are more susceptible than individuals who have aspartic acid on both DQ β chains, that is, homozygous Asp/Asp. Indeed, the incidence of type I diabetes mellitus in any given population appears to be proportional to the gene frequency of nonAsp alleles in that population. In addition, arginine at position 52 of the DQ α chain confers marked susceptibility to insulin-dependent diabetes mellitus. Position 57 of the DQ β and position 52 of DQ α are at critical locations of the HLA molecule that permit or prevent antigen presentation to T-cell receptors and activate the autoimmune cascade.

These observations provide a rational framework for the long-recognized association of type I diabetes with genetic factors on the bases of the increased incidence in some families, of the concordance rates in monozygotic twins, and of ethnic and racial differences in prevalence. For example, type I diabetes among American blacks is associated with the same HLA genes as it is in American whites. From multiple family pedigrees and HLA typing data, it has been determined that if a sibling shares both HLA-D haplotypes with an index case, the risk for that individual is 12–20%; for a sibling sharing one haplotype, the risk for developing IDDM is 5–7%; and with no haplotypes in common, the risk is only 1–2%. HLA typing is not recommended for routine practice because of its expense. When coupled with measurement of spontaneous antibodies to insulin, islet cell antibodies including GAD, and assessment of insulin secretory reserve, it may be possible to predict and hence delay or prevent the clinical appearance of IDDM. In general, for purposes of genetic counseling, it can be safely assumed that in whites, the overall recurrence risks to siblings are approximately 6% if the proband is under 10 yr of age and 3% if he or she is older at the time of diagnosis. The risk to offspring is 2–5%, with the higher risk in the offspring of a diabetic father. In American blacks, these risks are only one-half to two-thirds those in whites.

Factors other than pure inheritance must also be involved in evoking clinical diabetes. For example, HLA-D3 or -D4 is found in approximately 50% of the general population and (nonAsp/nonAsp) in approximately 20% of white nondiabetics in the United States, yet the risk for IDDM in these subjects is only one-tenth that in an HLA-identical sibling of an index case with IDDM possessing these markers. Even siblings sharing only one haplotype have a sixfold to 10-fold greater risk of developing IDDM compared with the normal population. In addition, about 10% of patients with IDDM do not possess either HLA-D3 or -D4, although almost all white diabetics lack at least one aspartic acid at position 57 of the DQ β chain. Most compelling is the fact that the concordance rate among identical twins of whom one has insulin-dependent diabetes is only 30–50%, suggesting the participation of environmental triggering factors or other genetic factors such as the postnatal selection of certain autoreactive T-cell clones that bear receptors recognizing "self." This postnatal process occurs within the thymus and implies that identical twins are not identical with respect to the T-cell receptor repertoire they possess.

Triggering factors might include viral infections. In animals, a number of viruses can cause a diabetic syndrome, the appearance and severity of which depend on the genetic strain and immune competence of the species of animal tested. In humans, epidemics of mumps, rubella, and coxsackievirus infections have been associated with subsequent increases in the incidence of type I diabetes; the acute onset of diabetes mellitus, presumably induced by coxsackievirus B4, has been described. The viruses may act by directly destroying β cells, by persisting in pancreatic β cells as slow viral infections, or by triggering a widespread immune response to several endocrine tissues. The virus may induce initial β-cell damage that results in the presentation of previously masked or altered antigenic determinants. It is also possible that the virus shares some antigenic determinants with those present on or in β cells, including GAD, so that antibodies formed in response to the virus may interact with these shared determinants of β cells, resulting in their destruction, an example of molecular mimicry. Molecular mimicry is also invoked as a possible mechanism in bovine serum albumin (BSA)–mediated islet antibodies because many patients with new-onset diabetes have IgG antibodies to BSA, specifically a 17 amino acid peptide that also occurs on islet membranes. Implicit in these findings is the possibility that early exposure to cow milk may be a factor in triggering diabetes, thus explaining the reported lower incidence of diabetes among breast-fed infants. Antecedent stress and exposure to certain chemical toxins have been implicated in the development of IDDM. Histologic examination of pancreas from patients with IDDM who die from incidental causes has revealed lymphocytic infiltration around the islets of Langerhans. Later, the islets become progressively hyalinized and scarred, a process suggesting an ongoing inflammatory response, possibly autoimmune in nature.

Considerable evidence now supports an autoimmune basis for the development of type I diabetes. Some 80–90% of newly diagnosed patients with IDDM have islet cell antibodies (ICA) directed at cell surface or cytoplasmic determinants in their islet cells; the prevalence of these antibodies decreases with the duration of established disease. In contrast, after pancreatic transplantation, ICA may reappear in patients whose sera had become negative for ICA prior to transplantation. Taken together, these findings suggest that ICA disappear as the antigens in the form of pancreatic islets are destroyed and reappear when fresh antigen (transplanted islets) is presented. Studies in identical twins and in family pedigrees demonstrate that the existence of ICA may precede by months to years the appearance of symptomatic IDDM. In vitro, ICA may impair insulin secretion in response to secretagogues and can be shown to be cytotoxic to islet cells, especially in the presence of complement or T cells from patients with type I diabetes. As many as 80% of patients may have antibodies to GAD and 30–40% may have spontaneous anti-insulin antibodies at initial diagnosis. There is also some evidence of abnormal T-cell function with an alteration in the ratio of suppressor to killer T cells at the onset of the disease. These findings suggest that type I diabetes, like other autoimmune diseases such as Hashimoto thyroiditis, is a disease of "autoaggression," in which autoantibodies, in cooperation with complement, T cells, or other factors, induce destruction of the insulin-producing islet cells. Thus, inheritance of certain genes intimately associated with the HLA system on chromosome 6 appears to confer a predisposition toward autoimmune disease, including diabetes, when triggered by an appropriate stimulus such as a virus. Although it is understood that some insulin-dependent diabetic patients have none of the frequently associated HLAs, the evidence in favor of an immune basis of islet cell destruction is sufficiently compelling to have fostered several studies of different immunosuppressive agents in the treatment of newly diagnosed diabetics. These immunosuppressive agents must be considered experimental and should not be viewed as established or recommended therapy. Figure XXVI–2 summarizes current concepts of the etiology of type I diabetes as an autoimmune disease, the tendency toward which is inherited through the HLA system and in which autoimmune destruction of β cells is triggered by an as yet unidentified agent. The slope of decline in insulin varies, and the point at which clinical features appear corresponds to approximately an 80% destruction of the insulin secretory reserve. This process may take months to years, usually in adolescent and older patients, and weeks in the very young patient. Higher titers of spontaneous autoinsulin antibodies and islet cell antibodies are characteristic of the more active islet cell destruction typically seen in the younger patient and may prove useful in predicting evolving diabetes. Though no presently available marker or test can accurately predict the development of type I diabetes mellitus, there is increased evidence that type I diabetes may be predictable. It has been proposed that the presence of high titers of islet cell, GAD, and insulin autoantibodies combined with a markedly diminished first phase response to insulin, corresponding to the 5th percentile or less for age, can be used to reliably predict the onset of IDDM. Though there is disagreement on this point, the data are sufficiently persuasive to have fostered national trials in Europe and the United States to predict and possibly prevent the clinical onset of IDDM through immune intervention strategies. These strategies must be viewed as experimental and not in the domain of clinical practice.

PATHOPHYSIOLOGY. The progressive destruction of β cells leads to a progressive deficiency of insulin, a major anabolic hormone. Its normal secretion in response to feeding is exquisitely modulated by the interplay of neural, hormonal, and substrate-related mechanisms to permit controlled disposition of ingested foodstuff as energy for immediate or future use; mobilization of energy during the fasted state depends on low plasma levels of insulin. Thus, in normal metabolism there are regular swings between the postprandial, high-insulin anabolic state and the fasted, low-insulin catabolic state that affect three major tissues: liver, muscle, and adipose tissue (Table XXVI–2). Type I diabetes mellitus, as it evolves, becomes a permanent low-insulin catabolic state in which feeding does not reverse but rather exaggerates these catabolic processes. It is important to emphasize that liver is more sensitive than muscle or fat to a given concentration of insulin; that is, endogenous glucose production from the liver through glycogenolysis and gluconeogenesis can be restrained at insulin concentrations that do not fully augment glucose utilization by peripheral tissues.

■ TABLE XXVI–2 Influence of Feeding (High Insulin) or of Fasting (Low Insulin) on Some Metabolic Processes in Liver, Muscle, and Adipose Tissue*

	High Plasma Insulin (Postprandial State)	Low Plasma Insulin (Fasted State)
Liver:	Glucose uptake	Glucose production
	Glycogen synthesis	Glycogenolysis
	Absence of gluconeogenesis	Gluconeogenesis
	Lipogenesis	Absence of lipogenesis
	Absence of ketogenesis	Ketogenesis
Muscle:	Glucose uptake	Absence of glucose uptake
	Glucose oxidation	Fatty acid and ketone oxidation
	Glycogen synthesis	Glycogenolysis
	Protein synthesis	Proteolysis and amino acid release
Adipose tissue:	Glucose uptake	Absence of glucose uptake
	Lipid synthesis	Lipolysis and fatty acid release
	Triglyceride uptake	Absence of triglyceride uptake

**Insulin is considered to be the major factor governing these metabolic processes. Diabetes mellitus may be viewed as a permanent low-insulin state that, untreated, results in exaggerated fasting.*

Consequently, with progressive failure of insulin secretion, the initial manifestation is postprandial hyperglycemia; fasting hyperglycemia indicates excessive endogenous glucose production and is a late manifestation reflecting severe insulin deficiency.

Although insulin deficiency is the primary defect, several secondary changes that involve the stress hormones (epinephrine, cortisol, growth hormone, and glucagon) accelerate and exaggerate the rate and magnitude of metabolic decompensation. Increased plasma concentrations of these counter-regulatory hormones magnify metabolic derangements by further impairing insulin secretion (epinephrine), by antagonizing its action (epinephrine, cortisol, and growth hormone), and by promoting glycogenolysis, gluconeogenesis, lipolysis, and ketogenesis (glucagon, epinephrine, growth hormone, and cortisol) while decreasing glucose utilization and glucose clearance (epinephrine, growth hormone, and cortisol). With progressive insulin deficiency, excessive glucose production and impairment of its utilization result in hyperglycemia with glucosuria when the renal threshold of approximately 180 mg/dL is exceeded. The resultant osmotic diuresis produces polyuria, urinary losses of electrolytes, dehydration, and compensatory polydipsia. These evolving manifestations, especially dehydration, represent physiologic stress, resulting in hypersecretion of epinephrine, glucagon, cortisol, and growth hormone that amplifies and perpetuates the metabolic derangements and accelerates metabolic decompensation. The acute stress of trauma or infection may likewise accelerate metabolic decompensation to ketoacidosis in evolving or established diabetes. Hyperosmolality, commonly encountered as a result of progressive hyperglycemia, contributes to the symptomatology, especially to cerebral obtundation in diabetic ketoacidosis. Serum osmolality (in mOsm/kg) can be estimated by the following formula:

$$[\text{Serum Na}^+ \text{ (mEq/L)} + \text{K}^+ \text{ (mEq/L)}] \times 2 + \frac{\text{glucose (mg/dL)}}{18} + \frac{\text{BUN (mg/dL)}}{3}$$

Consideration of serum osmolality has important implications in the therapy of diabetic ketoacidosis.

The combination of insulin deficiency and elevated plasma values of the counter-regulatory hormones is also responsible for accelerated lipolysis and impaired lipid synthesis, with resulting increased plasma concentrations of total lipids, cholesterol, triglycerides, and free fatty acids. The hormonal interplay of insulin deficiency and glucagon excess shunts the free fatty acids into ketone body formation; the rate of formation of these ketone bodies, principally β-hydroxybutyrate and acetoacetate, exceeds the capacity for their peripheral utilization and renal excretion. Accumulation of these ketoacids results in metabolic acidosis and in compensatory rapid deep breathing in an attempt to excrete excess CO_2 *(Kussmaul respirations).* Acetone, formed by nonenzymatic conversion of acetoacetate, is responsible for the characteristic fruity odor of the breath. Ketones are excreted in the urine in association with cations and thus further increase losses of water and electrolytes (Table XXVI–3). With progressive dehydration, acidosis, hyperosmolality, and diminished cerebral oxygen utilization, consciousness becomes impaired, and the patient ultimately becomes comatose. Thus, insulin deficiency produces a profound catabolic state—an exaggerated state of starvation—in which all of the initial clinical features can be explained on the basis of known alterations in intermediary metabolism mediated by insulin deficiency in combination with counter-regulatory hormone excess. Because the counter-regulatory hormonal changes are secondary, the severity and duration of the symptoms reflect the extent of the primary insulinopenia.

CLINICAL MANIFESTATIONS. The classic presentation of diabetes in children is a history of polyuria, polydipsia, polyphagia, and weight loss. The duration of these symptoms varies but is often less than 1 mo. A clue to the existence of polyuria may be the onset of enuresis in a previously toilet-trained child. An insidious onset characterized by lethargy, weakness, and weight loss is also quite common. The loss of weight in spite of an increased dietary intake is readily explicable by the following illustration: The average healthy 10-yr-old child has a daily caloric intake of 2,000 or more calories, of which approximately 50% are derived from carbohydrate. With the development of diabetes, daily losses of water and glucose may be as much as 5 L and 250 g, respectively. This represents 1,000 calories lost in the urine, or 50% of average daily caloric intake. Therefore, despite the child's compensatory increased intake of food and water, the calories cannot be utilized, excessive caloric losses continue, and increasing catabolism and weight loss ensue.

■ TABLE XXVI–3 Fluid and Electrolyte Maintenance Requirements and Estimated Losses in Diabetic Ketoacidosis

	Approximate Daily Maintenance Requirements*	Approximate Accumulated Losses†
Water	1500 mL/m²	100 mL/kg (range 60–100 mL/kg)
Sodium	45 mEq/m²	6 mEq/kg (range 5–13 mEq/kg)
Potassium	35 mEq/m²	5 mEq/kg (range 4–6 mEq/kg)
Chloride	30 mEq/m²	4 mEq/kg (range 3–9 mEq/kg)
Phosphate	10 mEq/m²	3 mEq/kg (range 2–5 mEq/kg)

**Maintenance is expressed in surface area to permit uniformity because fluid requirements change as weight increases. See also Chapter 55.*

†Losses are expressed per unit of body weight because the losses remain relatively constant in relation to total body weight.

Pyogenic skin infections and monilial vaginitis in teenage girls are occasionally present at the time of diagnosis of diabetes. They are rarely the sole clinical manifestations of diabetes in children, and a careful history will invariably reveal the coexistence of polyuria and polydipsia.

Ketoacidosis is responsible for the initial presentation of many (approximately 25%) diabetic children. The early manifestations may be relatively mild and consist of vomiting, polyuria, and dehydration. In more prolonged and severe cases, Kussmaul respirations are present, and there is an odor of acetone on the breath. Abdominal pain or rigidity may be present and may mimic appendicitis or pancreatitis. Cerebral obtundation and ultimately coma ensue. Laboratory findings include glucosuria, ketonuria, hyperglycemia, ketonemia, and metabolic acidosis. Leukocytosis is common, and nonspecific serum amylase may be elevated; serum lipase is usually not elevated. In those with abdominal pain, it should not be assumed that these findings are evidence of a surgical emergency before a period of appropriate fluid, electrolyte, and insulin therapy has been tried to correct dehydration and acidosis; the abdominal manifestations frequently disappear after several hours of such treatment.

DIAGNOSIS. Children in whom the diagnosis of diabetes mellitus must be considered may, for practical purposes, be divided into three general categories: (1) those who have a history suggestive of diabetes, especially polyuria with polydipsia and failure to gain weight or a loss of weight in spite of a voracious appetite; (2) those who have a transient or persistent glucosuria; and (3) those who have clinical manifestations of metabolic acidosis with or without stupor or coma. In all instances the diagnosis of diabetes mellitus is dependent on the demonstration of hyperglycemia in association with glucosuria with or without ketonuria. When classic symptoms of polyuria and polydipsia are associated with hyperglycemia and glucosuria, the glucose tolerance test is not needed to support the diagnosis.

Renal glucosuria may be an isolated congenital disorder or a manifestation of the Fanconi syndrome and other renal tubular disorders due to severe heavy metal intoxication, ingestion of certain drugs (e.g., outdated tetracycline), or inborn errors of metabolism (cystinosis). When vomiting, diarrhea, or inadequate intake of food is a complicating factor in any of these conditions, starvation ketosis may ensue, simulating diabetic ketoacidosis. The absence of hyperglycemia eliminates the possibility of diabetes. It is also important to recognize that not all urinary sugar is glucose, and infrequently galactosemia, pentosuria, and the fructosurias will require consideration as diagnostic possibilities.

The discovery of glucosuria with or without a mild degree of hyperglycemia during a hospital admission for trauma or infection, or even during the associated emotional upheaval, may, but usually does not, herald the existence of diabetes; in most of these instances the glucosuria remits during recovery. Because this circumstance may indicate a limited capacity for insulin secretion, which is unmasked by elevated plasma concentrations of stress hormones, these patients should be rechecked at a later date for the possibility of hyperglycemia or clinical features of diabetes mellitus. In these circumstances, a glucose tolerance test may be useful to establish a diagnosis; glucose tolerance testing should be performed several weeks after recovery from the acute illness using a glucose loading dose adjusted for weight. Evidence indicates that the test is most likely to be abnormal in patients with HLA-DR3 and -DR4, and those in whom islet cell antibodies or insulin autoantibodies are detected.

Screening procedures, such as postprandial determinations of blood glucose or oral glucose tolerance tests, have yielded low detection rates in children, even among those considered at risk, such as siblings of diabetic children. Accordingly, such screening procedures are not recommended in children.

Diabetic ketoacidosis must be differentiated from acidosis and/or coma due to other causes; these causes include hypoglycemia, uremia, gastroenteritis with metabolic acidosis, lactic acidosis, salicylate intoxication, encephalitis, and other intracranial lesions. Diabetic ketoacidosis exists when there is hyperglycemia (glucose greater than 300 mg/dL), ketonemia (ketones strongly positive at greater than 1:2 dilution of serum), acidosis (pH less than 7.30 and bicarbonate less than 15 mEq/L), glucosuria, and ketonuria in addition to the clinical features described. Precipitating factors, even for the initial presentation, include stress such as trauma, infection, vomiting, and psychologic disturbances. Recurrent episodes of ketoacidosis in established diabetics often represent deliberate errors in recommended insulin dosage or unusual stress responses that indicate psychologic disturbances and, at times, pleas to be removed from a home environment perceived to be stressful or intolerable. Diabetic ketoacidosis also should be distinguished from nonketotic hyperosmolar coma.

Nonketotic hyperosmolar coma is a syndrome characterized by severe hyperglycemia (blood glucose greater than 600 mg/dL); absence of or only very slight ketosis; nonketotic acidosis; severe dehydration; depressed sensorium or frank coma; and various neurologic signs that may include grand mal seizures, hyperthermia, hemiparesis, and positive Babinski signs. Respirations are usually shallow, but coexistent metabolic (lactic) acidosis may be manifested by Kussmaul breathing. Serum osmolarity is commonly 350 mOsm/kg or higher. This condition usually occurs in middle-aged or elderly individuals who have "mild" diabetes; among them mortality rates have been as high as 40–70%, possibly in part because of delays in recognition and in institution of appropriate therapy. In children this condition is infrequent; among reported cases there has been a high incidence of pre-existing neurologic damage. Profound hyperglycemia may develop over a period of days, and initially the obligatory osmotic polyuria and dehydration may be partially compensated by increasing fluid intake. With progression of disease, thirst becomes impaired, possibly because of alteration of the hypothalamic thirst center by hyperosmolarity and possibly in some instances because of a pre-existing defect in the hypothalamic osmoregulating mechanism.

The low production of ketones is attributed mainly to the hyperosmolarity, which in vitro blunts the lipolytic effect of epinephrine and the antilipolytic effect of insulin; blunting of lipolysis by the therapeutic use of β-adrenergic blockers may contribute to the syndrome. Depression of consciousness is closely correlated with the degree of hyperosmolarity in this condition as well as in diabetic ketoacidosis; hemoconcentration may also predispose to cerebral arterial and venous thromboses.

Treatment of nonketotic hyperosmolar coma is directed at repletion of the vascular volume deficit and correction of the hyperosmolar state (also see later under management of ketoacidosis). One half isotonic saline (0.45% NaCl) is administered at a rate estimated to replace 50% of the volume deficit in the first 12 hr, and the remainder is administered during the ensuing 24 hr. When the blood glucose concentration approaches 300 mg/dL, the hydrating fluid should be changed to 5% dextrose in 0.2 normal (N) saline. Approximately 20 mEq/L of potassium chloride should be added to each of these fluids to prevent hypokalemia. Serum potassium and plasma glucose concentrations should be monitored at 2-hr intervals for the first 12 hr and at 4-hr intervals for the next 24 hr to permit appropriate adjustments of administered potassium and insulin.

Insulin can be given by continuous intravenous infusion beginning with the second hour of fluid therapy. Because blood glucose may decrease dramatically with fluid therapy alone, the intravenous loading dose should be 0.05 U/kg of regular (fast-acting) insulin followed by 0.05 U/kg/hr of the same insulin, rather than 0.1 U/kg/hr as advocated for patients with diabetic ketoacidosis. During the recovery period, therapy with insulin and diet and monitoring of the patient should be the same as described for patients recovering from diabetic ketoacidosis (see Table XXVI–3 and related text).

TREATMENT. The management of insulin-dependent diabetes mellitus may be divided into three phases depending on the initial presentation: that of ketoacidosis; the postacidotic or transition period for establishment of metabolic control; and the continuing phase of guidance of the diabetic child and his or her family. Each of these phases has separate goals, although in practice they merge into a continuum. For purposes of management, the transition period corresponds to patients presenting with polyuria, polydipsia, and weight loss but without biochemical decompensation to ketoacidosis.

Ketoacidosis. The immediate aims of therapy are expansion of intravascular volume; correction of deficits in fluids, electrolytes, and acid-base status; and initiation of insulin therapy to correct intermediary metabolism. Treatment should be instituted as soon as the clinical diagnosis is confirmed by the presence of hyperglycemia and ketonemia. Determinations of blood pH and electrolytes should also be obtained; an electrocardiogram (ECG) is useful to provide a rapid reference for the existence of hyperkalemia. If sepsis is suspected as a possible precipitating factor, a blood culture should be obtained and the urine examined for the presence of bacteria and leukocytes. A flow sheet to record chronologically the rate and composition of fluid input, urine output, amount of insulin administered, and the acid-base and electrolyte values of the blood is most useful. Catheterization of the bladder is not routinely recommended in children; bag collection or condom drainage permits an assessment of urinary output, but catheterization may be indicated in comatose patients.

Fluid and Electrolyte Therapy (Table XXVI–4). The expansion of reduced intravascular volume and correction of depleted fluid and electrolyte stores are most important in the treatment of

■ **TABLE XXVI–4 Fluid and Electrolyte Therapy for Diabetic Ketoacidosis**

Recommendations for replacement of fluid losses and for maintenance of a 30-kg (surface area 1.0 m^2) child with assumed 10% dehydration. Duration of treatment: 36 hours.

REPLACEMENT FLUIDS	Approximate Accumulated Losses with 10% Dehydration	Approximate Requirements for Maintenance (36 hr)	Approximate Totals for Replacement and Maintenance (36 hr)
Water (mL)	3,000	2,250	5,500
Sodium (mEq)	180	65	250
Potassium (mEq)	150	50	200
Chloride (mEq)	120	45	165
Phosphate (mEq)	90	15	100

REPLACEMENT SCHEDULE (continuous intravenous infusion)

Approximate Duration	Fluid (Composition)	Sodium (mEq)	Potassium (mEq)	Chloride (mEq)	Phosphate (mEq)
Hour 1	500 mL of 0.9% NaCl (isotonic saline)	75	—	75	—
Hour 2	500 mL of 0.45% NaCl (0.5 isotonic saline) plus 20 mEq of KCl	35	20	55	—
Hour 3–12 (200 mL/hr for 10 hr)	2,000 ml of 0.45% NaCl with 30 mEq/L of potassium phosphate	150	60	150	40
Subtotal initial 12 hr	3,000 mL	260	80	280	40
Next 24 hr 100 mL /hr	5% glucose in 0.2% NaCl with 40 mEq/L of potassium phosphate	75	100	75	60
Total over 36 hours	5,400 mL	335	180	355	100

Note: All replacement values should be halved if dehydration is estimated to be 5%. Maintenance requirements remain the same.

ADDITIONAL GUIDELINES

A diabetic flow sheet *with laboratory data appropriately recorded must be maintained in the patient's chart.*

Insulin therapy by continuous low-dose intravenous method: *Priming dose—bolus injection of 0.1 U/kg of regular insulin IV followed immediately by continuous IV infusion of 0.1 U/kg/hr of regular insulin beginning with 2nd hr.*

Directions for making insulin infusion: *Add 50 U of regular insulin to 500 mL of isotonic saline. Flush 50 mL through the tubing to saturate insulin-binding sites. For 30-kg patient, infuse at rate of 30 mL/hr. When the blood glucose concentration approaches 300 mg/dL, continue the insulin infusion at a reduced rate, or add glucose to the infusate until acidosis is resolved, then start insulin therapy by subcutaneous injections of 0.2–0.4 U/kg of insulin at intervals of 6 hr.*

Bicarbonate therapy: *For pH >7.20, no therapy necessary. For pH 7.10–7.20, 40 mEq/m^2 of bicarbonate over 2 hr; then re-evaluate. For pH <7.10, 80 mEq/m^2 of bicarbonate over 2 hr; then re-evaluate. New diabetics, <2 yr of age, with diabetic ketoacidosis and 10% dehydration, or any diabetic with pH <7.00, should be managed in an intensive care unit or equivalent setting.*

diabetic ketoacidosis (DKA). It must be stressed, however, that exogenous insulin is essential to arrest further metabolic decompensation and to restore intermediary metabolism.

Dehydration is commonly on the order of 10%; initial fluid therapy can be based on this estimate, with subsequent adjustments related to clinical and laboratory data. The initial hydrating fluid should be isotonic saline (0.9%). Because of the hyperglycemia, hyperosmolarity is universal in DKA; thus, even 0.9% saline is hypotonic relative to the patient's serum osmolality. A gradual decline in osmolality is desirable because too rapid a decline has been implicated in the development of cerebral edema, one of the major complications of diabetic therapy in children. For the same reason, the rate of fluid replacement is adjusted to provide only 50–60% of the calculated deficit within the initial 12 hr; the remaining 40–50% is administered during the next 24 hr. Also, administration of glucose (5% solution in 0.2 N saline) is initiated when the blood glucose concentration approaches 300 mg/dL in order to limit the decline of serum osmolality and reduce the risk of developing cerebral edema (see later and Table XXVI–4).

Administration of potassium (K^+) should be started early. Total body potassium may be considerably depleted during acidosis, even when the serum potassium concentration is normal or elevated. Whereas potassium moves from intracellular to extracellular sites during acidosis, the reverse occurs during correction of acidosis, particularly when exogenous insulin and glucose are available in the circulation. This shift of potassium back to the intracellular compartment may result in life-threatening hypokalemia. Hence, after the initial fluid replacement of approximately 20 mL/kg of isotonic saline (0.9%) has been provided, potassium should be added to subsequent infusates if urinary output is adequate; serum potassium concentration should then be monitored periodically. An ECG provides a rapid assessment of serum potassium concentration; T waves are peaked in hyperkalemia and are low and associated with U waves in hypokalemia (see Chapter 48). Because the total potassium deficit cannot be replaced within the initial 24 hr of treatment, potassium supplementation should be continued as long as fluids are administered intravenously (see Table XXVI–4).

It is almost inevitable that the patient will receive an excess of chloride, which may aggravate acidosis. The extent of acidosis, however, can be reduced by substitution of phosphate, which is also significantly depleted in DKA. Moreover, phosphate in conjunction with glycolysis is essential for the formation of 2,3-diphosphoglycerate (2,3-DPG), which governs the oxygen dissociation curve. During deficiency of 2,3-DPG, the oxygen dissociation curve is shifted to the left, that is, more oxygen is retained by hemoglobin and less is available to the tissues, a situation that predisposes to lactic acidosis. Acidosis per se tends to shift the oxygen dissociation curve toward the right (Bohr effect) and thus partially "compensates" for 2,3-DPG deficiency. As acidosis resulting from the accumulation of ketones is corrected by the provision of insulin, with or without administration of bicarbonate, the effects of 2,3-DPG deficiency may no longer be "compensated," and the release of oxygen to tissues may again be impaired. Exogenous phosphate, by contributing to the formation of 2,3-DPG, permits the oxygen dissociation curve to shift to the right and thus facilitates release of oxygen to tissues and aids in the correction of acidosis. Furthermore, resistance to insulin action is associated with hypophosphatemia. Hence, we recommend the administration of potassium phosphate as outlined in Table XXVI–4. Because excessive use of phosphate may result in hypocalcemia, serum calcium should be measured periodically. Symptomatic hypocalcemia should be corrected with calcium gluconate and potassium chloride, which should be temporarily substituted for potassium phosphate.

ALKALI THERAPY. With provision of fluids, electrolytes, glucose, and insulin, metabolic acidosis is usually corrected through the interruption of ketogenesis, the metabolism of ketones to bicarbonate, and the generation of bicarbonate by the distal renal tubule. Concerns about the therapeutic administration of bicarbonate center on four issues: (1) alkalosis, by shifting the oxygen dissociation curve to the left, may diminish the release of oxygen to tissues and hence predispose to lactic acidosis; (2) alkalosis accelerates the entry of potassium into cells and hence may produce hypokalemia; (3) provision of bicarbonate according to the calculated base deficit overcorrects and may result in alkalosis; and, perhaps most important, (4) bicarbonate may lead to a worsening of cerebral acidosis while the plasma pH is being restored to normal because HCO_3^- combines with H^+ and dissociates to CO_2 and H_2O. Whereas bicarbonate passes the blood-brain barrier slowly, CO_2 diffuses freely, thereby exacerbating cerebral acidosis and possibly cerebral depression. On the other hand, severe acidosis, with a blood pH of 7.1 or less, diminishes respiratory minute volume, may produce hypotension by means of peripheral vasodilation, impairs myocardial function, and may be a factor in insulin resistance. For these reasons, administration of bicarbonate is recommended only when the pH is 7.2 or below (see Table XXVI–4). At pH 7.1–7.2, 40 mEq of HCO_3^-/m^2, and below pH 7.1, 80 mEq of HCO_3^-/m^2, should be infused over a period of 2 hr; acid-base status should then be reevaluated prior to continuing further alkali therapy. Bicarbonate should not be given by bolus infusion because it may precipitate cardiac arrhythmias.

The major life-threatening complication in children treated for DKA is *cerebral edema*. Clinically, cerebral edema develops several hours after the institution of therapy, when clinical and biochemical indices may suggest improvement. The manifestations are those of raised intracranial pressure and include headache, alteration and deterioration in alertness and conscious state, "delirious outbursts," bradycardia, vomiting, diminished responsiveness to painful stimuli, and diminished reflexes. There may be a change in pupillary responsiveness with unequal pupils or fixed dilated pupils. Polyuria, secondary to development of diabetes insipidus, may be erroneously attributed to osmotic diuresis secondary to hyperglycemia, although diabetes mellitus and diabetes insipidus coexist. Prompt recognition of the condition as it evolves, and prompt therapy with mannitol and hyperventilation, can be lifesaving. Increasingly, evidence points to the conclusion that subclinical cerebral edema occurs in the majority of patients treated with fluids and insulin for DKA, and that in only a minority does it become clinically manifest as a medical emergency.

The evidence that a majority of patients treated for DKA develop subclinical cerebral edema includes increasing cerebrospinal fluid pressure documented by continuous intrathecal monitoring during therapy of DKA in adults and evidence from sequential computed tomography of the head that ventricular size is narrower, compatible with brain swelling, during therapy than several days after recovery from DKA. Excessive use of fluids, excessive use of bicarbonate, compensatory responses to intracellular acidosis through the NA^+/H^+ exchanger, and large doses of insulin during treatment have all been implicated. The reason that a majority have subclinical brain swelling, whereas only a minority (1–2%) manifest clinically apparent cerebral edema, may be related to the intracranial pressure-volume curve, which shows a steep exponential rise in intracranial pressure beyond a critical volume of cerebral volume.

For these reasons, it is prudent to anticipate clinical cerebral edema in all children treated for DKA by limiting the rate of fluid administration to 4.0 $L/m^2/24$ hr or less, avoiding the excessive use of bicarbonate as outlined earlier, and being alert to the clinical manifestations of raised intracranial pressure. Once raised intracranial pressure has become clinically manifest, reduction of the rate of fluid administration, use of mannitol at 10–20 g/m^2 intravenously, repeated at 2- to 4-hr intervals, and hyperventilation are warranted. Preliminary retrospective evidence suggests that these measures, instituted promptly, are lifesaving and may avoid neurologic sequelae.

INSULIN THERAPY. The continuous low-dose intravenous infusion method, in which a priming dose of 0.1 U/kg of regular insulin is followed by a constant infusion of 0.1 U/kg/hr, is outlined in Table XXVI–4. This method is effective, simple, and physiologically sound, and has gained wide acceptance as the preferred method of administering insulin during DKA. It provides a constant steady concentration of insulin in plasma that approximates the peak attained in normal individuals during an oral glucose tolerance test. Presumably, the same steady concentration is attained at the cellular level and permits a steady metabolic response without the fluctuations that must occur with intermittent injections of insulin. Concern that the insulin may adhere to glass and tubing has proved to be unfounded, and effective delivery of insulin can be provided without the use of albumin or gelatin added to the infusate. Moreover, insulin infusion can be provided by gravity drip without the use of a special pump, although such a pump is helpful. A separate infusion set for insulin connected to the infusion line used for fluid and electrolyte therapy is recommended so that adjustments in the dosage of each can be made independently. After the amount of insulin for the initial 6–8 hr has been calculated, this quantity is added to a 250- or 500-mL bottle of 0.9% saline (see Table XXVI–4 for specific instructions).

When the blood glucose concentration approaches 300 mg/dL, the ongoing potassium requirement is added to 5% glucose in 0.2 N saline, and the rate of insulin infusion may sometimes be reduced from 0.1 to 0.05 U/kg/hr providing that the acidosis is being corrected. The rate of insulin infusion should, however, be periodically adjusted according to the patient's recovery from acidosis and the blood glucose response of each individual.

In treating DKA, it is commonly observed that the blood glucose concentration corrects more quickly than the pH or plasma bicarbonate. Insulin must be provided by infusion or subcutaneous injection as long as acidosis persists even if the glucose concentration is approaching 300 mg/dL. It may be necessary to add glucose to the infusate while continuing insulin infusion at a rate of 0.05–0.1 U/kg/hr until the acidosis is corrected. If acidosis persists despite these measures, a cause such as gram-negative sepsis should be considered.

When the acidosis has been corrected, the continuous infusion may be discontinued and insulin given immediately by subcutaneous injection at a dose of 0.2–0.4 U/kg every 6–8 hr while maintaining the glucose infusion until the child can fully tolerate food. Subcutaneous injections of regular insulin at doses of 0.2–0.4 U/kg every 6–8 hr before meals should be continued for a full 24-hr day after the child is eating. The blood glucose level should be monitored before and 2 hr after each meal, and the insulin dose adjusted to maintain the blood glucose concentration in the range of 80–180 mg/dL. The total dose of regular insulin used in this representative day serves as a guide for subsequent insulin treatment with a combination of intermediate- and short-acting insulin as described later.

Insulin treatment during DKA can also be administered by repeated intramuscular or subcutaneous bolus injections; a portion of the dose is also usually injected intravenously. One such regimen based on body weight is outlined in Table XXVI–5; if plasma ketones are only moderately elevated, the recommended doses may be half of those listed. Administrations of insulin as the fast-acting form are repeated every 2–4

■ TABLE XXVI–5 Intermittent Insulin Regimen for Diabetic Ketoacidosis

Blood Glucose	Total Insulin Dose	Intravenous Dose	Intramuscular or Subcutaneous Dose	Frequency
>600 mg/dL	1 U/kg	0.5 U/kg	0.5 U/kg	Every 2–4 hr
300–600 mg/dL	0.5 U/kg	0.25 U/kg	0.25 U/kg	Every 2–4 hr

When blood glucose approaches 300 mg/dL, the intravenous infusion for fluid and electrolyte replacement should contain 5% glucose (see Table XXVI–4 for rate of administration). Continue subcutaneous injections of insulin at 0.2–0.4 U/kg every 6 hr and monitor blood glucose concentration at the same time. If blood glucose concentration rises, increase the next insulin dose by 50%; if glucose concentration falls, decrease the next insulin dose by 50%. Continue this insulin regimen for 24 hr after oral intake of fluid and food is established. See text for subsequent management.

hr, and blood glucose values and acid-base status are monitored as they are during the continuous intravenous insulin approach. When the blood glucose concentration has fallen to approximately 300 mg/dL, subsequent insulin therapy at a dose of 0.2–0.4 U/kg may be given subcutaneously every 6–8 hr while maintaining an infusion of 5% glucose in 0.2 N saline with potassium added (see Table XXVI–4) until the acidosis is resolved and the child can tolerate solid foods. Sips of clear liquid, broth, or carbonated beverages may be given during this interval. Subcutaneous injections of regular insulin at doses of 0.2–0.4 U/kg every 6–8 hr before meals are continued for a full 24-hr day after the child is eating, when the switch to combined intermediate- and short-acting insulins is made as described. Intermediate-acting insulin can usually be begun within 36 hr after commencing therapy for ketoacidosis.

Ketonemia and **ketonuria** may persist despite clinical improvement. The nitroprusside reaction that is routinely used to measure "ketones" reacts with acetoacetate and weakly with acetone but not with β-hydroxybutyrate. The usual ratio of β-hydroxybutyrate to acetoacetate is approximately 3:1, but it is commonly as high as 8:1 or more in patients with DKA. With correction of acidosis, β-hydroxybutyrate dissociates to acetoacetate, which is identified by the nitroprusside reaction. Hence, persistence of ketonuria for a day or more may not reliably reflect the clinical improvement and should not be interpreted as a poor therapeutic response.

Postacidotic Phase or Transition Period for Establishment of Metabolic Control. Diabetic ketoacidosis is usually corrected within 36–48 hr by the foregoing therapeutic regimen. At this time food and fluids are usually tolerated orally, and insulin can be given by subcutaneous injection. The child who presents with classic symptoms and documented hyperglycemia in the absence of clinical dehydration and ketoacidosis can be considered as requiring treatment at this transition stage. For such children, subcutaneous injections of fast-acting insulin are begun at doses of 0.1–0.25 U/kg every 6–8 hr before meals with simultaneous monitoring of the blood glucose concentration and adjustment of the insulin dose for 1–2 days. The initial dose of insulin is lower because these children generally have a lower blood glucose concentration and are more sensitive to insulin than are those presenting with DKA. One to 2 days of fast-acting insulin therapy are needed to estimate the total daily insulin requirement as a guide to the subsequent use of combined intermediate- and short-acting forms.

The aims of therapy during the transitional period are to treat any recognized precipitating cause of DKA such as infection, to stabilize the patient's metabolic control by adjusting the insulin dosage, to institute an appropriate nutritional pattern for the child, and to educate the parents and patient in the principles of diabetic management. These principles include techniques of insulin injection, monitoring of blood and urine glucose levels, monitoring of a urinary ketone spill, understanding the nutritional requirements, recognition of hypoglycemia (insulin shock) and its management, and ability to make adjustments in insulin dosage during minor illnesses and for regularly planned exercise. This education is best carried out by coordinating the participation of the physician, dietitian, and nurse educator, who have special training in diabetes. For newly diagnosed patients, this phase commonly lasts 5–10 days; less time may be required for the stabilization and reeducation of previously diagnosed patients. Ongoing education and adjustment of insulin dosage are continued after discharge from the hospital through patient visits and inquiries by telephone; during this phase, gradual reductions in insulin dosage are frequently required, and the patient should be so advised (see later section on residual β-cell function). The details and rationale for insulin and dietary therapy as well as other aspects of long-term management are provided in the following section on insulin regimens.

The immediate goals in the management of children with type I diabetes are to provide adequate nutrition and exogenous insulin in a manner that prevents polydipsia and polyuria, including nocturia, avoids ketoacidosis and severe hypoglycemia, and permits normal growth and development with an active life pattern. These goals are achievable by most patients and their parents if they come to understand the principles of the pathophysiology and management of this disease. Ongoing supervision by the physician is essential and should be provided in a manner that avoids undue anxiety and psychologic dependence on the part of the child or parents, or a sense of guilt on the part of the parents.

Evidence is now compelling that the long-term complications of diabetes are related to the degree of metabolic control that is achieved. Therefore, one should aim for a metabolism that is as nearly normal as possible. Achievement of a completely normal metabolism, however, is not possible with the standard pattern of treatment that consists of one to two daily injections of insulin and attention to nutritional intake and exercise. In highly motivated individuals and their care providers, however, near-normal metabolism can now be achieved in one of two ways: (1) Monitoring of blood glucose values at home with the appropriate adjustment of insulin dosage 2–3 times a day and paying close attention to nutritional intake can be effective; (2) continuous subcutaneous insulin infusion by means of a pump worn externally that can be programmed to provide a basal rate of delivery with meal-related increments is also an effective means for patients. For the majority of pediatric patients, however, these newer approaches are not available or applicable, and routine management rests on three pillars: the provision of insulin and guidance with respect to its dosage, attention to nutritional intake, and exercise.

Insulin Regimens. The diurnal pattern of insulin concentration in the plasma of normal persons is characterized by a basal level on which are superimposed secretory episodes that coincide with intake of food. Each rise in plasma insulin concentration during feeding is synchronous with and proportional to the rise in blood glucose. Plasma insulin concentrations, however, do not reflect total insulin secretion. Because insulin is secreted into the portal circulation, its first target organ is the liver, the key organ governing the initial disposal of a glucose load (see Table XXVI–2). The liver extracts approximately 50% of the insulin presented to it from the portal circulation.

Currently available forms of insulin and their durations of action are listed in Tables XXVI–6 and XXVI–7. They are classified as short-, intermediate-, and long-acting types; each is available in a concentration of 100 U/mL (U-100); higher concentrations

■ **TABLE XXVI–6 Common Types of Available Insulin**

Product	Form	Strength
Rapid Acting		
Humulin R (regular)*	Human	U-100
Regular Iletin I*	Mixed beef & pork	U-100
Regular Iletin II*	Pork	U-100, U-500
Regular Purified†	Pork	U-100
Regular Standard†	Pork	U-100
Novolin regular (recombinant DNA)†	Human	U-100
Velosulin regular (semisynthetic)†	Human	U-100
Intermediate Acting		
Humulin L (Lente)*	Human	U-100
Lente Iletin I*	Mixed beef & pork	U-100
Lente Iletin II*	Pork	U-100
Humulin N (NPH)*	Human	U-100
NPH Iletin I*	Mixed beef & pork	U-100
NPH Iletin II*	Pork	U-100
Lente Standard†	Beef	U-100
Lente Purified†	Pork	U-100
Novolin Lente (recombinant DNA)†	Human	U-100
NPH (Isophane) Standard†	Beef	U-100
NPH (Isophane) Purified†	Pork	U-100
Novolin NPH (recombinant DNA)†	Human	U-100
Long Acting		
Humulin U (Ultralente)*	Human	U-100
Ultralente†	Beef	U-100
Premixed		
Humulin 70/30*	Human	U-100
Humulin 50/50*	Human	U-100
Novolin 70/30 (recombinant DNA)†	Human	U-100

Onset ½–1 hr, peak effect 2–4 hr, duration 6–8 hr.
Onset 1 –2 hr, peak effect 4–12 hr, duration 24 hr.
Onset 4 –8 hr, peak effect 14–20 hr, duration 24–36 hr.
Onset and duration can vary from person to person.
**Lilly.*
†Novo Nordisk.

are available for the unusual patient who has high resistance to insulin. Appropriate dilutions can be prepared for younger patients requiring low doses. Refinements in manufacture are now responsible for forms of insulin that have distinctly less contamination than formerly by such other pancreatic hormones as proinsulin, glucagon, pancreatic polypeptide, and somatostatin. Antibodies to these and other contaminants have been demonstrated in the sera of insulin-treated diabetics. It is unclear whether the new and more highly purified insulins facilitate metabolic control, but they probably do result in fewer local and systemic allergic reactions, including lipoatrophy and lipohypertrophy. The currently available insulins are extracted from beef and pork pancreas and are marketed separately or as a mixture of the two forms of insulin. Human insulin, synthesized in bacteria via recombinant DNA technology (synthetic) or by chemical modification of pork insulin (semisynthetic), is also routinely available for therapy. Human insulin may be less allergenic and less likely to induce antibody formation, but the limited data available do not indicate any significant advantages over highly purified pork insulin. Human insulin, synthetically produced by recombinant DNA techniques or semisynthetically by chemical modification of porcine insulin, is likely to become the exclusively available insulin.

Because exogenous insulins are injected subcutaneously rather than directly into the portal vein, their rate of absorption may be variable, and because the dose injected is determined empirically, it lacks the precision of endogenously secreted insulin. Therefore, a single injection of intermediate-acting insulin cannot duplicate the pattern of normal insulin secretion, and periods of excessive plasma insulin that may produce hypoglycemia and/or periods of inadequate insulin that permit hyperglycemia are virtually inevitable. Even with injections of regular fast-acting insulin prior to each meal, normalization of blood glucose values is not entirely achieved, although the degree of control is clearly improved. Hence, the regimen of insulin administration selected for the diabetic child must represent a compromise designed to achieve as nearly normal an intermediary metabolism as possible that will permit normal growth and development and avoid frequent hypoglycemic reactions and the consequence of unrestrained hyperglycemia.

At the onset of diabetes, or after recovery from ketoacidosis, the total daily dose of insulin is about 0.5–1.0 U/kg. The actual total daily requirement of insulin is estimated from the representative 24-hr period when regular insulin only was administered before each meal during the transition phase after resolution of ketoacidosis or during the initial management of less severely affected patients as outlined earlier. Long-acting insulins are not often used in children. In most instances, one of the intermediate insulins is employed, but, because of its delayed action, a fast-acting (regular) insulin is usually combined with it. With the single-daily dose combined regimen, approximately two thirds of the total dose is an intermediate-acting insulin (e.g., NPH, lente), and the remainder is regular insulin; the injection is given 30 min before breakfast. The two insulins should always be drawn into the syringe in the same sequence (regular first) so that the residual insulin in the "dead space" is always the same type; thus, greater stability of the patient can be assured once a therapeutic dose is established. Disposable syringes with fine needles, minimal dead space, and easy-to-read calibration for use with U-100 insulin are available. For small children, syringes calibrated to a maximum of 50 U are also available; in some European countries diluted insulins are marketed.

In order to avoid hypoglycemia, the single-daily dose regimen combining intermediate- and short-acting insulin is initially calculated on the basis of two thirds of the total daily

■ **TABLE XXVI–7 Insulins by Relative Comparative Action Curves**

Insulin	Onset (hr)	Peak (hr)	Usually Effective Duration (hr)	Usual Maximal Duration (hr)
Animal				
Regular	0.5–2.0	3–4	4–6	6–8
NPH	4–6	8–14	16–20	20–24
Lente	4–6	8–14	16–20	20–24
Ultralente	8–14	Minimal	24–36	24–36
Human				
Regular	0.5–1.0	2–3	3–6	4–6
NPH	2–4	4–10	10–16	14–18
Lente	3–4	4–12	12–18	16–20
Ultralente	6–10	?	18–20	20–30

dose, or approximately 0.5 U/kg. Step increases or decreases of 10–15% can then be made daily during the initial phase in the hospital until the desired degree of control is achieved. The initial phase of recovery of metabolic equilibrium is characterized by a period of replenishment of body stores of glycogen, protein, and fat that were depleted during the evolution of diabetes. Hence, insulin requirements for the first few days may on occasion be found to be even greater than 1 U/kg/24 hr. Adjustments in the dose of insulin are made in relation to the pattern of blood glucose values monitored before each meal and/or of the excretion of glucose. If the predominant hyperglycemia or glucosuria occurs in late morning, then the quick-acting form of insulin is increased by 10–15%. If the predominant hyperglycemia or glucosuria occurs in late afternoon or evening, then the intermediate-acting insulin is increased by 10–15%. Should hypoglycemic reactions occur between midmorning and noon, the quick-acting form of insulin is reduced by 10–15%, and if hypoglycemia occurs in late afternoon or evening, the intermediate-acting insulin is decreased by 10–15%. In anticipation of increased exercise at home, the daily dose of insulin should be decreased by 10% at the time of discharge from the initial hospitalization.

Although many children can be managed with a single daily injection of insulin, *two daily injections* are now routinely recommended (Fig. XXVI–3). When there is persistent nocturia associated with excessive fasting hyperglycemia and morning glucosuria in response to a single daily injection of insulin, consideration should be given to dividing the total daily dose into two injections. In this plan two thirds of the daily total dose is given before breakfast and one third before the evening meal; each injection consists of intermediate- and short-acting insulins in proportions of 2–3:1. For example, assuming a total daily dose of 1 U/kg for a 30-kg child, 14 U of NPH or lente combined with 6 U of regular insulin would be given before breakfast, and 6 U of NPH or lente with 4 U of regular insulin would be given before the evening meal. As with the single-daily dose regimen, stepwise increases or decreases, each consisting of 10–15%, should be made to minimize hypoglycemic reactions and undue hyperglycemia (see earlier paragraph for guidelines).

Two daily injections of insulin are especially applicable for infants and children under 5 yr of age, in whom intake of food and extent of activity are not always predictable, and for adolescents, especially during the pubertal growth spurt. Two

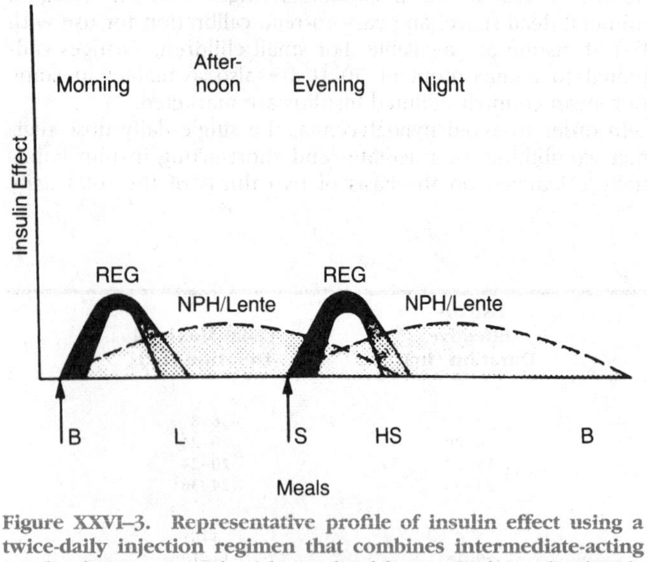

Figure XXVI–3. Representative profile of insulin effect using a twice-daily injection regimen that combines intermediate-acting insulin (NPH or Lente) with regular (short-acting) insulin (REG). (From Sperling MA: Outpatient management of diabetes mellitus. Pediatr Clin North Am 34:919, 1987.)

daily injections tend to result in smoother metabolic control with fewer hypoglycemic reactions and less uncontrolled hyperglycemia. This approach is more effective also when the evening meal is the major one (see later section under Nutritional Management). With an explanation of the rationale, adherence to this twice-daily regimen by patients and parents is usually good, and twice-daily insulin is now considered standard therapy. When compliance is not good, which occurs particularly in adolescents, one injection is preferable to none, because there is evidence that two daily injections may not always result in better metabolic control than one daily injection. The physician should in all instances attempt to determine the regimen that will be in the best interests of the patient. For children who insist on only one daily injection of insulin, the daily dose is adjusted according to carefully kept records of blood or urinary glucose values until the best possible degree of metabolic control is achieved. In this way, confidence in the patient-family-physician relationship is maintained, and a sense of guilt in the patient or family is avoided. In special circumstances, such as highly motivated older adolescents, or with particularly committed, capable parents, three or more daily injections of insulin based on frequent blood glucose monitoring can be administered. This kind of intensive therapy improves glycemic control toward normal and diminishes the risk of microvascular complications, but is often associated with more severe and frequent hypoglycemic reactions.

The *technique of injection of insulin* should be taught to the parents and to the patient when he or she is ready for it. Injections are given subcutaneously, rotating sites on arms, thighs, buttocks, and abdomen in a regular sequence. An appropriate rotation helps to ensure adequate absorption of insulin, prevent fibrosis, and minimize lipodystrophic changes. With this rotation and the availability of the purer, single-peak insulins, lipoatrophy and lipohypertrophy are quite unusual. Younger children may find injections in the abdominal wall difficult or painful. Depending on their physical and psychologic maturity, children over the age of 10–12 yr should be encouraged to administer their own insulin and to monitor their own responses to it. The assumption of responsibility for self-monitoring will be a gradual process in which the parents and child all participate. Once the child has assumed total responsibility, the parents must resist a tendency toward overprotection. Guidelines for adjusting the dose of insulin based on blood or urinary glucose profiles have been outlined earlier, and those for adjusting the dose of insulin with exercise, illness, and "brittle" diabetes are provided in greater detail in the following section. It should be stressed, however, that the adolescent growth spurt is regularly associated with an increase in insulin requirements, which usually become lower when puberty is completed.

Hypersensitivity to insulin is uncommon in children. Local skin reactions are characterized by erythema or urticaria, with burning, itching, and tenderness within hours or sooner after an injection. These reactions usually resolve spontaneously over a period of days but may require a change from mixed beef-pork to pure pork or human insulin, or from NPH to lente insulin because of allergy to protamine in the former; antihistamines may be used if necessary. Generalized reactions with severe urticaria or angioedema are extremely rare and may also resolve spontaneously, but a change in the type of insulin is usually indicated, for example, from a mixed beef-pork preparation to a pure pork or human preparation. Desensitization may also be necessary, as may a course of systemic corticosteroid therapy for 1–2 wk. Rarely, insulin resistance develops in response to a local tissue enzyme that destroys injected insulin. Some of these patients have benefited from the addition of a protease enzyme inhibitor to the insulin solution; others have required chronic intravenous infusion and are best managed in a hospital with a specialized diabetes unit.

After several months of insulin therapy, nearly all patients will have acquired *antibodies to insulin*. In the majority, these do not interfere with the metabolic response. They may, however, promote instability by creating a reservoir of insulin that may be released at unpredictable times. Rarely, children with antibodies develop true resistance to insulin and require more than 2 U of insulin/kg/24 hr. A change to a preparation of pure pork, pure beef, or human insulin usually resolves this problem; in some instances a period of corticosteroid therapy or a course of desensitization may be necessary. Antibodies causing allergy are usually of the IgE class; IgA and IgM antibodies may be responsible for resistance to insulin.

Nutritional Management. Because the word *diet* may connote restriction and denial and constitute a source of anxiety and/or rebellion on the part of parent or patient, its use should be avoided. Instructional discussion can be provided under such terms as *nutritional requirements* and *meal plans*. Actually, there are no special nutritional requirements for the diabetic child other than those for optimal growth and development. However, because the capacity to secrete insulin in response to the intake of food is negligible in the diabetic child, and because the dose of insulin is predicated on caloric intake, regularity of the eating pattern for the determined insulin regimen becomes paramount. In outlining nutritional requirements for the child on the basis of age, sex, weight, and activity, food preferences, including any based on cultural and ethnic background, should be considered. Although general guidelines are usually applicable, individualization for each child should be programmed.

Total recommended *caloric intake* is based on size or surface area and can be obtained from standard tables. The caloric mixture should consist of approximately 55% carbohydrate, 30% fat, and 15% protein. In general, we recommend that approximately 70% of the carbohydrate content be derived from complex carbohydrates such as starch and that intake of sucrose and highly refined sugars be avoided. Complex carbohydrates require prolonged digestion and absorption so that plasma glucose rises slowly, whereas glucose in refined sugars, including those in carbonated beverages, is rapidly absorbed and may cause wide swings in the metabolic pattern; carbonated beverages should therefore be of the sugar-free variety. In the United States the ban on saccharin as an artificial sweetener has been removed pending further evidence of its toxic or teratogenic effect. Although in children there is concern about the potential cumulative effect, available data do not support an association of moderate amounts with bladder cancer. Other non-nutritive sweeteners such as aspartame are used in a variety of products. Sorbitol and xylitol should not be used as artificial sweeteners; they are products of the polyol pathway and are implicated in some of the complications of diabetes.

Diets with a *high fiber content* are useful in improving control of blood glucose in diabetic subjects. Inclusion of about 20–35 g/24 hr of fiber from foods such as vegetables, especially legumes, whole-meal bread, bran cereals, and fruits in the diet of adult diabetics has led to significant reductions in the concentration not only of blood glucose but also of total and LDL cholesterol. In addition, small amounts of sucrose consumed with fiber-rich foods such as whole-meal bread may have no more glycemic effect than their low-fiber, sugar-free equivalents. The concept of biologic equivalence or a "glycemic index" of foods is currently under investigation. When completed, these studies may provide a listing of foods with more predictable and desirable effects on blood glucose and serum lipid patterns for patients with diabetes.

The *intake of fat* is adjusted so that the polyunsaturated/saturated (P/S) ratio is increased to about 1.2:1.0, in contrast to the estimated American average of 0.3:1.0. Dietary fats derived from animal sources are therefore reduced and are replaced by polyunsaturated fats from vegetable sources. Substituting margarine for butter, vegetable oil for animal oils in cooking, and lean cuts of meat, poultry, and fish for fatty meats such as bacon is advisable. The intake of cholesterol is also reduced by these measures and by limiting the number of egg yolks consumed. There is ample evidence that these simple measures reduce serum LDL cholesterol, a predisposing factor to atherosclerotic disease. Less than 10% of calories should be derived from saturated fats, up to 10% from polyunsaturated fats, and the remaining fat-derived calories from monounsaturated fats.

The total daily caloric intake may be divided to provide 20% at breakfast, 20% at lunch, and 30% at dinner, leaving 10% for each of the midmorning, midafternoon, and evening snacks, if they are desired. In older children, the midmorning snack may be omitted and its caloric equivalent added to the lunch. Special brochures and pamphlets describing the exchanges and sample meal plans for children are usually available from regional diabetes associations; their use should be encouraged as part of the educational process. Meal plans are often based on groups of food exchanges; within each of the exchange lists of foods that are principal sources of carbohydrates, proteins, and fats, respectively, there is a wide variety of foods that can be substituted or exchanged. For practical purposes there are few restrictions, so that each child can select a diet based on personal taste or preferences with the help of the physician and/or dietitian. Emphasis should be placed on regularity of food intake and on constancy of carbohydrate intake. Occasional excesses for birthdays and other parties are permissible and are tolerated in order not to foster rebellion and stealth in obtaining desired food. Similarly, cakes, doughnuts, and even candies are permissible on special occasions as long as the food exchange value and carbohydrate content are adjusted in the meal plan. Adjustments in meal planning must be made for anticipated vigorous exercise (see later section, Exercise). Above all, adjustments must constantly be made to meet the needs as well as the desires of each child. Although a consistent eating pattern with appropriate supplements for exercise, for the pubertal growth spurt, and for pregnancy in a diabetic adolescent are important for metabolic control, there is an increased frequency of eating disorders among young women with diabetes. Thus, expectations and educational advice regarding diet must be dealt with in a sensitive, careful manner, especially in adolescents.

Monitoring. Success in the daily management of the diabetic child can be measured to a considerable extent by the competence acquired by the family, and subsequently by the child, in *assuming responsibility* for daily "diabetic care." Their initial and ongoing instruction in conjunction with their supervised experience can lead to a sense of confidence in making intermittent adjustments in insulin dosage for dietary deviations, unusual physical activity, and even for some minor intercurrent illnesses as well as for otherwise unexplained repeated hypoglycemic reactions and excessive glucosuria. Within limits, such acceptance of responsibility should make them independent of the physician for their ordinary care. Independence is good provided that the physician maintains ongoing interested supervision and shared responsibility with the family and with the child.

Self-monitoring is essential to such a plan and necessitates a regimen that includes measurements of blood or urinary glucose and, at times, of ketones, and the keeping of a standardized record of these results and of the corresponding data of dietary deviations, unusual physical activity, hypoglycemic reactions, intercurrent illness, the daily dose of insulin, and other items of possible relevance. Many of these records may be patently unreliable for a number of reasons. There may be self-delusion, reliance on memory with charting just prior to the visit to the physician, attempts to please the physician and avoid rebuke, as well as reluctance to perform some aspects of the blood or urinary tests. In spite of these problems, asking patients to keep records is justified. Initially, following dismissal from the hospital, the parent or patient is apt to be particularly attentive to a prescribed regimen. It is after some months of satisfactory experience that parents or patients tend to become less attentive to detail. When the physician apparently accepts the contrived report, the parent or child may come to find more and more reasons for noncompliance. When the physician mistrusts the report, he may think it justifiable to make evaluations of his own selection (see later). Should his data be counter to those in the parent's or child's report, he can then attempt to clarify the situation with them in such a manner as not to undermine their mutual confidence. Such situations test the physician's skill in the management of patients with persistent but not confining illness.

The *daily tests for glucosuria* are appropriately scheduled to be performed just prior to each of the three major meals and at the time of the evening snack. This timing is designed to secure an estimate of the effect of the prescribed insulin 3–4 hr after each meal. The preciseness of this estimate is increased if the child voids approximately 30 min before the test voiding; the initial specimen is discarded. When reliable measurements consistently indicate 2% or more glucose in the urine for a given portion of the day, the appropriate dose of the short- or intermediate-acting insulin should be increased by 10–15%. Conversely, when urine is consistently free of glucose for any portion of the day, the insulin dose may need to be reduced by 10–15% if hypoglycemic reactions ensue or if the blood glucose concentration, as determined by the glucose oxidase strip, is 60 mg/dL or less. In the absence of symptomatic hypoglycemia or of documented low blood glucose concentrations, absence of glucosuria does not warrant a reduction in insulin dosage; such patients are manifesting desirable metabolic control. Consistent patterns of excessive glucosuria at fixed times in the morning or afternoon are indications for appropriate increases in the morning or evening doses and at times for a change to another type of insulin. When more precise adjustments are deemed necessary, the physician may request a fractional 24-hr collection of urine. The urine should be collected in three fractions: 8.00 A.M. to 2.00 P.M.; 2.00 P.M. to 8.00 P.M.; and 8.00 P.M. to 8.00 A.M. Assessment of volume and semiquantitative or quantitative glucose values in each sample permits a rational basis for adjusting the respective doses of the rapid- and intermediate-acting insulins.

Short-term (daily) blood glucose monitoring has been markedly enhanced by the availability of strips impregnated with glucose oxidase that permit blood glucose measurement from a drop of blood. The blood glucose concentration can be approximated directly by comparison to a color scale or accurately by a portable calibrated reflectance meter. A small spring-loaded device that automates capillary blood-letting in a relatively painless fashion is also commercially available. Parents and patients should be taught to use these devices and to measure blood glucose 3–4 times daily: before breakfast, lunch, and supper, and before retiring at night. Initially, in the hospital the blood glucose measurement should also be performed at 3.00–4.00 A.M. to exclude inappropriate nocturnal hypoglycemia and to avoid the Somogyi phenomenon (see later). Ideally, the blood glucose concentration should range from approximately 80 mg/dL in the fasting state to 140 mg/dL after meals. In practice, however, a range of 60–240 mg/dL is acceptable. Blood glucose measurements that are consistently at or outside these limits, in the absence of an identifiable cause such as exercise or dietary indiscretion, are an indication for a change in the insulin dose. For example, if the fasting blood glucose is high, the evening dose of intermediate-acting insulin is increased by 10–15%; if the noon glucose level exceeds set limits, the morning regular insulin is increased by 10–15%; if the presupper glucose is high, the morning intermediate-acting insulin is increased by 10–15%; and if the prebedtime glucose measurement is high, the evening dose of regular insulin is increased by 10–15%. Similarly, reductions in insulin type and dose should be made if the corresponding blood glucose measurements are consistently below desirable limits.

Daily blood glucose measurements should be continued after discharge from the hospital as long as they are acceptable to the patient. Practical considerations require a reduction in the frequency of blood glucose monitoring at home; few children tolerate capillary blood-letting 4 times daily for prolonged periods. Consequently, after the initial stabilization period of several weeks, when the routine of insulin administration and meal plan has been established, some suggest that home blood glucose monitoring be performed only 2 days per week, varying the days each week to allow a representative profile in time. Monitoring of urine glucose spill is performed on those days when blood glucose measurements are omitted. However, blood glucose measurement should be performed if there are symptoms suggestive of hypoglycemia or if urine glucose spill persists at 2% or greater. In highly motivated adolescents and young adults who become sufficiently knowledgeable about managing their diabetes, self-monitoring of blood glucose levels before and 2 hr after meals, in conjunction with multiple daily injections of insulin, adjusted as necessary, can maintain near-normal glycemia for prolonged periods.

A reliable index of long-term glycemic control is provided by measurement of *glycosylated hemoglobin*. Glycohemoglobin (HbA_{1c}) represents the fraction of hemoglobin to which glucose has been nonenzymatically attached in the bloodstream. The formation of HbA_{1c} is a slow reaction that is dependent on the prevailing concentration of blood glucose; it continues irreversibly throughout the red blood cell's lifespan of approximately 120 days. The higher the blood glucose concentration and the longer the red blood cell's exposure to it, the higher the fraction of HbA_{1c}, which is expressed as a percentage of total hemoglobin. Because a blood sample at any given time contains a mixture of red blood cells of varying ages, exposed for varying times to varying blood glucose concentrations, an HbA_{1c} measurement reflects the average blood glucose concentration during the preceding 2–3 mo. When measured by standardized methods to remove labile forms, the fraction of HbA_{1c} is not influenced by an isolated episode of hyperglycemia. Consequently, as an index of long-term glycemic control, a measurement of HbA_{1c} is superior to measurements of glycosuria or a single blood glucose determination. It is recommended that glycohemoglobin measurements be obtained 3–4 times per year in order to obtain a profile of long-term glycemic control. The more consistently lower the glycohemoglobin level, and hence the better the metabolic control, the more likely it is that microvascular complications such as retinopathy and nephropathy will be less severe, delayed in appearance, or avoided. Depending on the method used for determination, glycohemoglobin values may be spuriously elevated in thalassemia (or other conditions with elevated HbF) and spuriously lower in sickle cell disease. Although values of HbA_{1c} may vary according to the method used for measurement, in normal individuals the HbA_{1c} fraction is usually less than 7%; in diabetics, values of 6–9% represent very good metabolic control, values of 9–12% fair control, and values above 12% poor control.

Exercise. Exercise is an integral component of growth and development. No form of exercise, including competitive sports of any kind, should be forbidden to the diabetic child, who should not be made to feel different or restricted. Examples of athletes with diabetes who have excelled in national or international sports are not rare. A major complication of exercise in diabetic patients is the presence of a hypoglycemic reaction during or within hours after exercise. If hypoglycemia does not occur with exercise, adjustments in diet or insulin are not necessary, and glucoregulation is likely to be improved through the increased utilization of glucose by muscles. The major contributing factor to hypoglycemia with exercise is an increased rate of absorption of insulin from its injection site. Higher insulin levels dampen hepatic glucose production so that it is inadequate to meet the increased glucose utilization of exercising muscle. Regular exercise also improves glucoregulation by increasing insulin receptors. In patients who are in poor metabolic control, vigorous exercise may precipitate ketoacidosis because of the exercise-induced increase in the counter-regulatory hormones.

In anticipation of vigorous exercise, one additional carbohydrate exchange may be taken prior to the exercise, and glucose in the form of orange juice, carbonated beverage, or candy should be available during and after exercise. With experience and trial and error, each child and parent, guided by the physician, should develop an appropriate regimen for regularly planned exercise that is frequently associated with hypoglycemia; in such instances, the total dose of insulin may be reduced by about 10–15% on the day of the scheduled exercise. Prolonged exercise such as long-distance running may require reduction of as much as 50% or more of the usual insulin dose.

Levels of Treatment. The intensity of treatment required for patients with diabetes mellitus must reflect mutually desirable goals negotiated between the physician and the patient and family. These goals may change depending on the age of the patient, his physical and emotional maturity, understanding, commitment, financial resources available to the family, and their health beliefs as well as those of the physician. Goals that are not mutually acceptable are doomed to failure. Minimal levels of treatment are preferable to recurrent hospitalization for diabetic ketoacidosis; intensive therapy carries a significant risk for recurrent hypoglycemia, although it may reduce the risk of microvascular complications. The biochemical and clinical characteristics of minimal, average, and intensive treatment are summarized in Table XXVI–8.

Residual β-Cell Function (Honeymoon Period). After the initial stabilization period some 75% of newly diagnosed diabetic children require progressive reductions in the daily dose of insulin from approximately 1 U/kg to 0.5 U/kg or less. Recurrent hypoglycemia is the manifestation that prompts a reduction in the insulin dose. A minority of children can even maintain normoglycemia for a time without any administered insulin; this complete remission occurs in less than 5% of diabetics, but even in these patients glucose tolerance tests demonstrate abnormal carbohydrate metabolism. The duration of this "honeymoon" phase is variable; it commonly lasts several weeks or months but may last as long as 1–2 yr. Recent investigations clearly demonstrate that residual insulin secretion, measured as C-peptide, is present during this remission period and to some extent in virtually all diabetic children in the initial year of their disease; in approximately 20% there is some C-peptide response even after 5 yr. Stable, well-controlled subjects have higher C-peptide secretion than nonstable subjects, and the required dose of insulin is inversely correlated to the basal or stimulated C-peptide response.

It is not completely clear why this residual insulin secretion is inadequate to prevent the evolution of diabetes, including ketoacidosis, but the reasons presumably relate to stress-provoked secretion of catecholamines that inhibit still further the insulin secretory capacity of the pancreatic β cells. In any event, the clinical remission phase is limited; with isolated exceptions, insulin-dependent diabetes inevitably recurs. Although opinion varies, insulin treatment should be maintained unless a daily dose of 0.1 U/kg still causes hypoglycemia, in which case insulin treatment should be discontinued and the patient periodically tested for the re-emergence of glycosuria. The physician may decide to discontinue insulin treatment completely if it appears to be in the patient's best interests during this period. The patient and family, however, should not be led to believe that the disease is "cured" and should continue to examine the child's urine for glucose.

Hypoglycemic Reactions (Insulin Shock). Virtually all diabetic children experience a hypoglycemic reaction at some time during the course of their disease. Hypoglycemia occurs suddenly or over a span of minutes, in contrast to diabetic ketoacidosis, which develops over hours or days. The symptoms and signs are those due to an outpouring of catecholamines, which include pallor, sweating, apprehension, trembling, and tachycardia, and those due to cerebral glucopenia, which include hunger, drowsiness, mental confusion, seizures, and coma. Mood and personality changes plus some abnormal physical patterns may be characteristic for an individual and provide an early clue to the more pronounced reaction. There is some evidence that these symptoms may occur with a sudden drop in blood glucose to levels that do not meet the criteria for hypoglycemia (<60 mg/dL) in healthy subjects. For the same degree of hypoglycemia, children secrete more catecholamines than adults; children secrete catecholamines at levels of glucose higher than in adults and not traditionally considered as hypoglycemia, for example, 60–70 mg/dL. As blood glucose falls toward these glucose concentrations, subtle impairment in cognitive abilities may occur. However, these subtle effects of mild hypoglycemia do not impair long-term intellectual development.

The occurrence of hypoglycemia in a diabetic child indicates too much insulin relative to food intake and energy expenditure. Common causes include the evolution of the honeymoon phase (see earlier) after the initial diagnosis, deliberate or accidental errors in insulin dosage, inadequate caloric intake, and strenuous and sustained physical activity in the absence of increased caloric intake.

The most important factors in the management of hypoglycemia are an understanding by the patient and family of the symptoms and signs of the reaction, especially of the patient's individual pattern, and avoidance of known precipitating factors. For management of the acute episode a carbohydrate-containing snack or drink such as orange juice or a sugar-containing carbonated beverage or candy (equivalent to 5–10 g of glucose) should be taken. Patients, parents, and teachers should also be instructed in the administration of glucagon; 0.5 mg given intramuscularly is particularly useful when the patient is losing consciousness or is vomiting. If exercise has been the precipitating factor, the patient should be instructed to take additional calories prior to exercise as a preventive measure. If hypoglycemic episodes persist subsequently under similar circumstances, a reduction in the morning and evening dose of insulin by 10–15% for that day is indicated. The avoidance of severe hypoglycemic episodes should be a major

■ **TABLE XXVI–8 Levels of Treatment: Biochemical and Clinical Characteristics**

Minimal
HbA_{1c} 11.0–13.0% and GHb 13.0–15.0%
Many SMBG values of ≥300 mg/dL
Almost constantly positive urine glucose tests
Intermittent spontaneous ketonuria
Average
HbA_{1c} 8.0–9.0% and GHb 10.0–11.0%
Premeal SMBG 160–200 mg/dL
Intermittent positive urine glucose
Rare ketonuria
Intensive
HbA_{1c} 6.0–7.0% and GHb 7.0–9.0%
Premeal SMBG 70 –120 mg/dL; postmeal SMBG <180 mg/dL
Essentially no positive urine glucose or ketones

SMBG = self-monitored blood glucose; HbA_{1c} = glycohemoglobin; GHb = glycosylated hemoglobin.

objective of treatment; they have been implicated in epileptic seizures, and there is an increased frequency of abnormal electroencephalographic changes in diabetics.

The Somogyi Phenomenon, the Dawn Phenomenon, and Brittle Diabetes. Hypoglycemic episodes, which may be mild and manifest as late nocturnal or early morning sweating, night terrors, and headaches alternating rapidly (within 4–5 hr) with ketosis, hyperglycemia, ketonuria, and excessive glucosuria, should suggest the possibility of the **Somogyi phenomenon**. This syndrome has been suitably described as "hypoglycemia begetting hyperglycemia" and is believed to be due to an outpouring of counter-regulatory hormones in response to insulin-induced hypoglycemia. The coexistence of this brittle form of diabetes with daily doses of more than 2 U/kg of insulin suggests the presence of this phenomenon and the need to reduce the dose of insulin. The term *brittle diabetes* implies that control of blood glucose fluctuates widely and rapidly despite frequent adjustments of the dose of insulin.

The Somogyi phenomenon should be distinguished from the **dawn phenomenon**, in which elevations of blood glucose concentration occur between 5.00 and 9.00 A.M. without preceding hypoglycemia. The dawn phenomenon is a normal event and occurs even in patients treated by continuous subcutaneous infusion of insulin unless the rate of insulin infusion is increased in the early morning hours. The dawn phenomenon reflects the waning effects of biologically available insulin, probably as a consequence of increased clearance of insulin and nocturnal surges of growth hormone that antagonize insulin's metabolic effects; the normal early morning rise in cortisol is not responsible for this phenomenon. Together, the Somogyi and dawn phenomena are the most common causes of instability or "brittleness" in diabetic children. To distinguish between the dawn and Somogyi phenomena, blood glucose concentrations should be measured at 3.00 A.M., 4.00 A.M., and 7.00 A.M. If blood glucose concentrations are over 80 mg/dL in the first two samples and markedly higher in the last, then the dawn phenomenon is likely; an increase in the evening dose of intermediate insulin of 10–15% may be helpful. It may also be helpful to delay the evening dose of intermediate-acting insulin by 2–3 hr so that its delayed peak effect coincides with the anticipated timing of the dawn phenomenon, and excessive increases of blood glucose are avoided or blunted. On the other hand, if the 3.00 A.M. or 4.00 A.M. blood glucose measurement is 60 mg/dL or less and rebound hyperglycemia is evident at 7.00 A.M., the Somogyi phenomenon is likely; a reduction of the evening intermediate-acting insulin of 10–15%, or a delay in its injection until approximately 9.00 P.M., is indicated (Fig. XXVI–4).

In other patients with brittle diabetes better control is often achieved by instituting a change from one to two daily injections of insulin or by a change from beef-pork mixtures to pure pork or human insulin, which may circumvent problems with antibodies that bind insulin. Attention should also be directed to psychologic problems that may be the basis for deliberate errors in insulin or nutritional intake.

Psychologic Aspects. Diabetes in a child affects the lifestyle and interpersonal relationships of the entire family. Feelings of anxiety and guilt are common in parents. Similar feelings, coupled with denial and rejection, are equally common in children, particularly during the rebellious teenage years. No specific personality disorder or psychopathology is characteristic of diabetes; similar feelings are observed in families with other chronic disorders.

In children with diabetes these feelings find expression in nonadherence to instructions regarding nutritional and insulin therapy and in noncompliance with self-monitoring. Deliberate overdosage with insulin, resulting in hypoglycemia, or omission of insulin, often in association with excesses in nutritional intake, resulting in ketoacidosis, may be pleas for psychologic help or manipulative attempts to escape an environment perceived as undesirable or intolerable; occasionally they may be manifestations of suicidal intent. Frequent admissions to the hospital for ketoacidosis or hypoglycemia should arouse a suspicion of underlying emotional conflict. Overprotection on the part of parents is common and often is not in the best interests of the patient. Feelings of being different or of being alone are common and may be justified in view of the restrictive schedules imposed by testing of urine and blood, administration of insulin, and nutritional limitations. Furthermore, publicity about the likelihood of developing complications and the decreased lifespan of patients with type I diabetes fosters anxiety. Unfortunately, misinformation abounds about the risks of development of diabetes in siblings or in offspring and of pregnancy in young diabetic women. Even appropriate information often causes further anxiety.

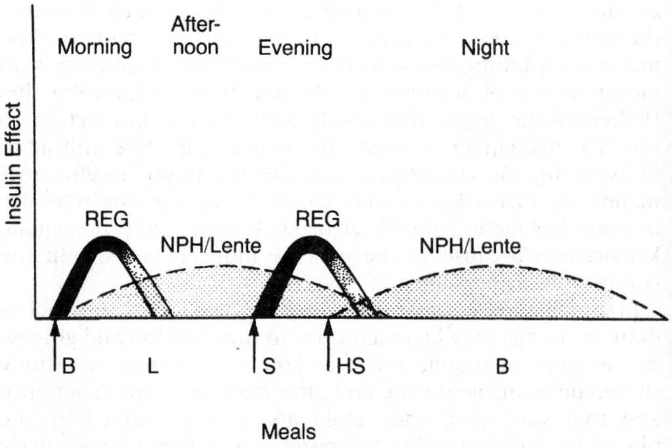

Figure XXVI–4. Three-dose insulin regimen intended to reduce the likelihood of the Somogyi or the dawn phenomenon. The morning dose comprises a combined short- and intermediate-acting insulin of about one half to two thirds of the total daily dose. The short-acting dose before supper covers the anticipated glycemic elevation with dinner. The intermediate-acting insulin is delayed until bedtime so that the peak effect is delayed. (From Schade DS, Santiago JV, Skyler JS, et al: Intensive Insulin Therapy. Princeton, NJ, Excerpta Medica, 1983.)

Many, but not all, of these problems can be averted through continued empathic counseling based on correct information and attempts to build attitudes of normality in the patient and a feeling of being a productive member of society. Recognizing the potential impact of these problems, peer discussion groups have been organized in many locales; feelings of isolation and frustration tend to be lessened by the sharing of common problems. Summer camps for diabetic children afford an excellent opportunity for learning and sharing under expert supervision. Education about the pathophysiology of diabetes, insulin dose, technique of administration, nutrition, exercise, and hypoglycemic reactions can be reinforced by medical and paramedical personnel. The presence of numerous peers with similar problems offers new insights to the diabetic child.

The physician managing a child or adolescent with diabetes should be aware of his pivotal role as counselor and advisor and should anticipate the common emotional problems of his patient. When emotional problems are clearly responsible for poor compliance with the medical regimen, referral for psychologic help may be indicated. Such help is often available in pediatric centers, where psychologists form part of the management team for diabetic children.

Management During Infections. Systemic and local infections are no more common in diabetic children than in nondiabetic ones. During intercurrent illnesses, either infectious or traumatic, diabetic children nearly always require additional insulin, especially during prolonged serious episodes that necessitate inactivity. In the latter situations, when glucosuria is excessive, a good working rule is to add 10–20% of the total daily dose as regular (short-acting) insulin prior to each meal. Subsequent increases or decreases should then be based on careful monitoring of urinary and blood glucose values.

Patients who are vomiting should, nevertheless, take some insulin; approximately 50% of the daily dose is a general rule, followed by careful monitoring of urinary or blood glucose and subsequent adjustments of the dose of insulin as indicated. If vomiting continues and the patient cannot tolerate clear liquids, admission to the hospital and consideration of intravenous therapy with glucose, electrolytes, and insulin are warranted.

Management During Surgery. The objectives of management are prevention of hypoglycemia during anesthesia, of severe loss of fluids, and of diabetic acidosis. The regimens described later are generally applicable, but vigilance and individual adjustments for each patient are necessary to achieve these goals.

When surgery is elective, the patient should be admitted to the hospital 24 hr prior to surgery; during this time the usual nutritional requirements and insulin dose are provided. Supplemental regular insulin may be given to achieve better control of blood glucose when the need is demonstrated. On the morning of surgery an infusion of 5% glucose in 0.45% saline solution plus 20 mEq/L of potassium chloride is begun; initially 1 U of regular insulin is added to the infusate for each 4 g of administered glucose. The rate of infusion should provide maintenance fluid requirements plus estimated losses during surgery. The blood glucose concentration should be monitored at periodic intervals before, during, and after surgery; concentrations of approximately 120–150 mg/dL should be the goal; this can be achieved by varying the rate of infusion of the glucose and electrolyte mixture or the amount of insulin added. This regimen may be discontinued when the patient is awake and capable of taking food and fluid orally. Prior to reinstitution of the patient's usual diet, regular insulin may be administered at a dose of 0.25 U/kg at 6-hr intervals; appropriate adjustments in the dose are based on blood or urinary concentrations of glucose.

An equally effective plan that is particularly useful for surgery of short duration is as follows: On the morning of surgery half of the usual morning dose of insulin is administered subcutaneously, and intravenous infusion of the electrolyte and glucose solution described in the preceding paragraph but minus the insulin is initiated. After surgery, regular insulin in a dose of 0.25 U/kg is administered subcutaneously; subsequent doses at 6-hr intervals are adjusted on the basis of blood glucose concentrations until the patient is ready for his or her usual dietary pattern.

For emergency surgery an intravenous infusion is initiated that provides 5–10% glucose in 0.45% saline solution, 20 mEq of potassium chloride, and 1 U of regular insulin for each 2–4 g of glucose. Blood glucose concentration should be maintained at approximately 120–150 mg/dL. When possible, rehydration and metabolic balance should precede the surgery. After surgery the regimen described earlier can be instituted.

For minor surgery under local anesthesia the usual insulin and dietary regimens can be maintained. If extensive vomiting occurs, the losses can usually be compensated with glucose solution administered intravenously.

NEUROVASCULAR AND OTHER COMPLICATIONS: RELATION TO GLYCEMIC CONTROL. The increasingly prolonged survival of the diabetic child is associated with an increasing prevalence of complications that affect the microcirculation of the eye (retinopathy), the kidney (nephropathy), the nerves (neuropathy), the large vessels (atherosclerosis), and the lens (cataracts). Retinopathy is present in 45–60% of insulin-dependent diabetics after 20 yr of known disease and in 20% after 10 yr; lens opacities are present in at least 5% of those under 19 yr of age. Diabetic nephropathy is also common; it is present in about 40% of patients after 25 yr of insulin-dependent diabetes whose onset occurred in childhood; this complication may account for about 50% of deaths in long-term insulin-dependent diabetics.

Studies implicate possible biochemical pathways that may be responsible for these complications. For example, the process of glycosylation of erythrocytic hemoglobin, which is directly proportional to the blood glucose concentration, also involves other serum and tissue proteins; it has been implicated in basement membrane thickening in the glomeruli. There is evidence that activation of the polyol pathway and disturbances in myoinositol metabolism are related, respectively, to cataracts and to neuropathy. In humans, typical lesions of diabetic nephropathy develop in normal kidneys within several years after they have been transplanted to diabetics with chronic renal failure. By contrast, the early histologic changes of diabetic nephropathy regress when kidneys of a diabetic are transplanted to a nondiabetic recipient with chronic renal failure. Therefore, it appears that the diabetic environment and not the genetic background predisposes to these renal changes. Genetic factors clearly play a role, however, because only 30–40% of patients affected by type I diabetes mellitus eventually develop end-stage renal disease, and only 50% develop proliferative retinopathy.

There is a relationship between the degree of metabolic control and the appearance, progression, and severity of retinopathy, nephropathy, and neuropathy. In the United States, the National Institutes of Health conducted a multicenter randomized trial to compare the effects of intensive treatment versus standard therapy on microvascular complications. Those in the customary treatment group received no more than twice-daily insulin, tested blood glucose once daily, followed standard nutrition and exercise regimens, and maintained a glycohemoglobin level significantly higher than those in the intensively treated group who used multiple (3–4) daily injections of insulin or continuous subcutaneous insulin infusion via programmable pumps coupled with frequent self-monitoring of blood glucose to maintain blood glucose concentrations as near normal as possible. Intensive therapy reduced the risk of developing clinically significant retinopathy, including severe nonproliferative and proliferative retinopathy, by 35–75%. Intensive therapy similarly reduced the development and progression of diabetic nephropathy and the development of neuropathy. However, intensive therapy was associated with a 2- to 3-fold increase in episodes of severe hypoglycemia as well as excessive weight gain. The relationship between development or progression of a microvascular complication was linearly related to the level of glycosylated hemoglobin, suggesting that there is no set point of metabolic control above which complications develop exponentially or below which complications may be avoided. Similar results have been reported from European trials. Moreover, the importance of metabolic control for limiting the development of diabetic nephropathy extends to adolescents and to those who ultimately may require a renal transplant. In such patients, there is a causal relationship between the development of nephropathy in the kidney transplanted to a diabetic recipient and the degree of hyperglycemia. In those whose renal function begins to deteriorate as a result of diabetic nephropathy, the use of angiotensin converting enzyme (ACE) inhibitors protects against deterioration in renal function. These ACE inhibitors are significantly more protective than blood pressure control alone.

Because of this relationship between the development of complications and metabolic control, physicians should encourage their patients to achieve the best possible metabolic control compatible with their psychologic, social, physical, and emotional well-being. Although the preadolescent may be naturally protected against the development of microvascular complications, the principles of metabolic control and their potential impact on future complications must be imparted from the outset.

Other complications described in diabetic children include dwarfism associated with a glycogen-laden enlarged liver **(Mauriac syndrome)**, osteopenia, and a syndrome of limited joint mobility associated with tight, waxy skin, growth impairment, and maturational delay. The Mauriac syndrome is clearly related to underinsulinization; it is now rare because of the availability of the longer-acting insulins. The syndrome of limited joint mobility is frequently associated with the early development of diabetic microvascular complications, such as retinopathy and nephropathy, which may appear before 18 yr of age. None of these complications has been demonstrated in a nondiabetic identical twin, even after 20 yr of recognized diabetes in his or her insulin-dependent twin. As indicated, genetic predisposition to the development of diabetic vascular complications does, however, play a role.

Another rare syndrome associated with diabetes mellitus is the **Wolfram syndrome**, also known as the **DIDMOAD syndrome** because of its major cardinal manifestations of diabetes insipidus, diabetes mellitus, optic atrophy, and deafness. The disease is familial with an autosomal recessive pattern of inheritance. Deletions of mitochondrial DNA have been described in this disorder, suggesting a respiratory chain defect causally related to insulin-requiring diabetes mellitus. Nuclear genetic defects or mitochondrial genetic defects may independently lead to this disease. Magnetic resonance imaging of the brain reveals widespread atrophic changes in patients who manifest the ataxia, nystagmus, seizures, and mental retardation occasionally found in this syndrome.

PROGNOSIS. Type I diabetes mellitus is not a benign disease. In one study of the long-term outcome of 45 children under 12 yr of age at the time of diagnosis, there were several deaths within 10–25 yr of diagnosis: three were directly attributable to diabetes, and two were due to suicide; three patients attempted suicide unsuccessfully. Visual, renal, neuropathic, and other complications were relatively frequent. Furthermore, although diabetic children eventually attain a height within the normal adult range, puberty may be delayed, and the final height may be less than the genetic potential. From studies in identical twins it is apparent that, despite apparently satisfactory control, the diabetic twin manifests delayed puberty and a substantial reduction in height, with a mean difference of 5 cm, when onset of disease occurs before puberty. These observations indicate that in the past, conventional criteria for judging control were inadequate and that adequate control of insulin-dependent diabetes was almost never achieved by routine methods.

The introduction of portable devices that can be programmed to provide continuous subcutaneous infusion of insulin with meal-related pulses is one approach to the resolution of these long-term problems. In selected individuals, nearly normal patterns of blood glucose and other indices of metabolic control including HbA_{1c} have been maintained for several years. This approach, however, should be reserved for highly motivated persons who are committed to rigorous self-monitoring of blood glucose and are alert to the potential complications, such as mechanical failure of the infusion device, causing hyperglycemia or hypoglycemia, and infections at the site of needle implantation.

IMPAIRED GLUCOSE TOLERANCE AND TYPE II NON–INSULIN-DEPENDENT DIABETES

In the classification of diabetes mellitus and other clinical impairments of glucose tolerance proposed by the National Diabetes Data Group (see Table XXVI–1) the term *impaired glucose tolerance* is used to characterize individuals who have a plasma glucose concentration in excess of 140 mg/dL 2 hr after initiation of the standard oral glucose tolerance test but do not have symptoms of diabetes or fasting hyperglycemia. The indication for an oral glucose tolerance test may be the discovery of isolated or intermittent glucosuria or the occurrence of hyperglycemia during a stressful illness or during corticosteroid therapy. Individuals considered at risk for abnormal glucose metabolism may also need to be tested; these include obese children, those who have symptoms suggestive of reactive postprandial hypoglycemia, and close relatives of known diabetics. An oral glucose tolerance test is not indicated in a child who has characteristic diabetic symptoms and a random blood glucose value in excess of 200 mg/dL.

The term *impaired glucose tolerance* is suggested as a replacement for such terms as asymptomatic diabetes, chemical diabetes, subclinical diabetes, borderline diabetes, or latent diabetes in order to avoid the stigma associated with the term diabetes mellitus, which may influence the choice of vocation, eligibility for health or life insurance, and self-image. Furthermore, although impaired glucose tolerance represents a biochemical intermediate between normal glucose metabolism and that of diabetes, experience has shown that few children with impaired glucose tolerance go on to develop diabetes; estimates range 0–10%. There is disagreement about whether the degree of glucose intolerance is useful as a prognostic index of the likelihood of progression, but there is evidence that among the few who do progress, the insulin response during glucose tolerance testing is severely impaired; islet cell or insulin autoantibodies as well as the HLA-DR3 or -DR4 haplotype are commonly found in those who go on to diabetes. In the majority of children with impaired glucose tolerance, particularly the obese, insulin responses during oral glucose tolerance tests are higher than the mean for age-adjusted but not weight-adjusted controls; these individuals have some resistance to the effects of insulin rather than a total inability to secrete it.

In normal children the glucose response during an oral glucose tolerance test is similar at all ages. In contrast, plasma insulin responses during the test increase progressively within the age span of about 3–15 yr and are significantly higher during puberty, so that interpretation of these responses requires comparison with age- and puberty-adjusted criteria.

The performance of the glucose tolerance test should be standardized according to currently accepted criteria. These include at least 3 days of a well-balanced diet containing approximately 50% of calories from carbohydrates; fasting from midnight until the time of the test in the morning; and a dose of glucose for the test of 1.75 g/kg but not more than 75 g. Plasma samples are obtained prior to ingestion of the glucose and at 1, 2, and 3 hr thereafter. The arbitrarily designated response to the test that identifies "impaired glucose tolerance" is a fasting plasma glucose value of less than 140 mg/dL and a value at 2 hr of more than 140 mg/dL. Determination of serum insulin responses during the glucose tolerance test is not a prerequisite for reaching a diagnosis; the magnitude of the response, however, may have prognostic value.

In children with impaired glucose tolerance but without fasting hyperglycemia, repeated oral glucose tolerance tests are not recommended. Investigations in such children indicate that the degree of impaired glucose tolerance tends to remain stable or may actually improve over a period of years, except in patients with markedly subnormal insulin responses. Consequently, apart from reduction in weight for the obese child, no therapy is indicated. In particular, the use of oral hypoglycemic agents should be restricted to investigational studies. If fasting hyperglycemia or characteristic symptoms of diabetes develop, the affected children will have the characteristics of non–insulin-dependent diabetes (type II), previously known as adult-onset diabetes (see Table XXVI–1 and the brief description in text under Classification). Such children may require insulin for control of hyperglycemia, although they generally do not develop ketosis in the absence of exogenous insulin therapy and hence, by definition, are not insulin dependent.

DISEASES ASSOCIATED WITH DIABETES

CYSTIC FIBROSIS (see Chapter 363). Because of improvements in the medical care of children with cystic fibrosis, many survive to the late teen and early adult years. In addition to the primary insufficiency of pancreatic exocrine function, there is an increasing incidence of pancreatic endocrine dysfunction manifested as glucose intolerance that progresses occasionally to overt diabetes mellitus. When hyperglycemia develops, the accompanying metabolic derangements are usually mild, and, if insulin therapy becomes necessary, relatively low doses usually suffice for adequate management. Ketoacidosis is uncommon but may occur with progressive deterioration of islet cell function. Treatment with insulin is the same as that outlined for type I diabetes, but dietary management may be limited by the constraints of the primary disturbance.

AUTOIMMUNE DISEASES. *Chronic lymphocytic thyroiditis* (Hashimoto thyroiditis) is frequently associated with type I diabetes in children. As many as 1 in 5 insulin-dependent diabetics may have thyroid antibodies in their serum; the prevalence is 2–20 times greater than that observed in control populations. Only a small proportion of these diabetics, however, develop clinical hypothyroidism; the interval between diagnosis of diabetes and development of thyroid disease averages about 5 yr. Periodic palpation of the thyroid gland is indicated in all diabetic children; if the gland feels firm or enlarged, serum measurements of thyroid antibodies and thyroid-stimulating hormone (TSH) should be obtained. A TSH level of greater than 10 μU/mL indicates existing or incipient thyroid dysfunction that warrants replacement with thyroid hormone. Deceleration in the rate of growth may also be due to thyroid failure and is in itself a reason for securing serum measurements of thyroxine and TSH concentrations.

When diabetes and thyroid disease coexist, the possibility of *adrenal insufficiency* should also be considered. It may be heralded by decreasing insulin requirements, increasing pigmentation of the skin and buccal mucosa, salt craving, weakness, asthenia, postural hypotension, or even frank addisonian crisis as evidence of primary adrenal failure. This syndrome is most unusual in the 1st decade of life, but it may become apparent in the 2nd decade or later.

Circulating *antibodies to gastric parietal cells* and to intrinsic factor are 2–3 times more common in patients with type I diabetes than in control subjects. There are good correlations of antibodies to gastric parietal cells with **atrophic gastritis** and of antibodies to intrinsic factor with **malabsorption of vitamin B_{12}**. Although the possibility of **megaloblastic anemia** should be considered in children with type I diabetes, its occurrence is rare.

A variant of the *multiple endocrine deficiency syndrome* (see Part XXVI: Section 3) is characterized by type I diabetes, idiopathic intestinal mucosal atrophy with associated inflammation and severe malabsorption, IgA deficiency, and circulating antibodies to multiple endocrine organs, including the thyroid, adrenal, pancreas, parathyroid, and gonads. In addition, nondiabetic family members have an increased frequency of vitiligo, Graves disease, and multiple sclerosis; low complement levels; and a high frequency of antibodies to endocrine tissues.

Type I diabetes may itself be an autoimmune disease.

ACANTHOSIS NIGRICANS WITH INSULIN RESISTANCE TYPE A. This syndrome is characterized by acanthosis nigricans, especially of the axillae and neck, variable degrees of glucose intolerance, including symptomatic diabetes, hirsutism, accelerated growth suggestive of gigantism, and marked endogenous hyperinsulinemia with severe resistance to exogenous insulin. The syndrome occurs predominantly in black females, who commonly present during adolescence for evaluation of menstrual irregularities; many are obese and have laboratory findings suggestive of the polycystic ovary syndrome. The carbohydrate intolerance, hyperinsulinemia, and resistance to exogenous insulin result from a congenitally reduced number of insulin receptors, alteration of their molecular structure, or inability to transduce the insulin signal owing to defects in the receptor's tyrosine kinase activity. Weight reduction may ameliorate the carbohydrate intolerance, but exogenous insulin is usually not helpful.

GENETIC SYNDROMES ASSOCIATED WITH DIABETES MELLITUS

A number of rare genetic syndromes associated with insulin-dependent diabetes mellitus or with carbohydrate intolerance have been described. These syndromes represent a broad spectrum of diseases ranging from premature cellular aging, as in the **Werner** and **Cockayne syndromes** (see Chapter 606), to excessive obesity associated with hyperinsulinism, resistance to insulin action, and carbohydrate intolerance, as in the **Prader-Willi syndrome** (see Chapter 535). Some of these syndromes are characterized by primary disturbances in the insulin receptor or in antibodies to the insulin receptor without any impairment in insulin secretion. Although rare, these syndromes provide unique models with which to study the multiple causes of disturbed carbohydrate metabolism from defective insulin secretion or from defective insulin action at the cell receptor or postreceptor step.

TRANSIENT DIABETES MELLITUS OF THE NEWBORN

Onset of persistent insulin-dependent diabetes before the age of 6 mo is very unusual. The syndrome of transient diabetes mellitus in the newborn infant has its onset in the first weeks of life and persists only several weeks to months before resolving spontaneously. It occurs most often in infants who are small for gestational age and is characterized by hyperglycemia and pronounced glycosuria, resulting in severe dehydration and at times metabolic acidosis but with only minimal or no ketonemia or ketonuria. Insulin responses to glucose or tolbutamide are low to absent; basal plasma insulin concentrations, however, are normal. After spontaneous recovery, the insulin responses to these same stimuli are brisk and normal, implying a functional delay in β-cell maturation with spontaneous resolution. Occurrence of the syndrome in consecutive siblings has been reported. Permanent diabetes does not usually develop, although there are reports of patients with classic type I diabetes who formerly had transient diabetes of the newborn. It remains to be determined whether this association of transient diabetes in the newborn followed much later in life by classical IDDM is a chance occurrence or causally related. This syndrome should be distinguished from severe hyperglycemia that may occur in hypertonic dehydration (see Chapter 56); this occurs usually in infants past the newborn period, who respond promptly to rehydration and have a minimal requirement for insulin.

Administration of insulin is mandatory during the active phase of this syndrome. Intermediate-acting insulin, 1–2 U/kg/24 hr given in two divided doses, usually results in dramatic improvement and accelerated growth and gain in weight. Attempts at gradually reducing the dose of insulin may be made as soon as recurrent hypoglycemia becomes manifest or after 2 mo of age. The parents should be assured of the transient nature of the disease and the excellent prognosis. Rarely, **pancreatic agenesis** may be associated with early but permanent diabetes mellitus as well as malabsorption.

HYPOGLYCEMIA AND DIABETES

The most common type of hypoglycemia in childhood is that occurring in insulin-treated diabetes mellitus. A typical patient may experience several hundred episodes of severe hypoglycemia in the course of lifelong insulin therapy. Almost 30% of patients with insulin-dependent diabetes mellitus have experienced hypoglycemic coma at some stage; about 10% of patients experience severe hypoglycemia once annually, and 3–5% experience repeated severe bouts of hypoglycemia. Although the pathophysiology of diabetes mellitus in childhood, its treatment, and its complications were dealt with earlier in this chapter, several important aspects relating to hypoglycemia in diabetes mellitus warrant emphasis.

Hypoglycemia in insulin-dependent diabetes mellitus represents an imbalance between the effects of insulin and those of the counter-regulatory hormones. In many instances, this imbalance can be predicted. For example, in the honeymoon phase recovery of residual endogenous insulin secretion occurs after initial diagnosis, so that the use of additional exogenous insulin frequently results in hypoglycemia. Reducing the dose of exogenous insulin diminishes the episodes of hypoglycemia. This situation represents an example of absolute insulin excess. Absolute insulin excess also occurs with deliberate or inadvertent errors in insulin dosage, or when patients are not taking food to cover the effect of the injected insulin. Again, such omissions of food may be inadvertent, but they may be deliberate during attempts to lose weight or a manifestation of anorexia nervosa. Hypoglycemia may also occur during or after exercise when increased insulin absorption from the injected site results from increased cardiac output and, hence, increased tissue perfusion. As a result of increased insulin absorption from its injection site, serum insulin levels rise during exercise, whereas they normally fall during exercise in a nondiabetic individual. The increase in insulin concentration accentuates the increased glucose consumption by exercising muscle, while simultaneously inhibiting glucose production via the liver. This inhibition of glucose production occurs despite an increase in the counter-regulatory hormones that occurs with exercise. Normally, the production of counter-regulatory hormones in exercise is exquisitely finely tuned to the needs of the exercising muscle such that the production of glucose and its consumption are equal, resulting in virtually unchanged glucose concentrations during mild to moderate exercise lasting minutes to hours.

Deficiency of counter-regulatory hormones also may occur in diabetes. Most patients with insulin-dependent diabetes mellitus lose their ability to secrete glucagon in response to hypoglycemia after 5 yr or more of diabetes and then rely almost solely on epinephrine secretion. The mechanism for the impairment of glucagon secretion is not clear. Epinephrine deficiency also may develop if the patients develop autonomic neuropathy as part of the diabetes complications or if patients are simultaneously using β-blockers. Intensive insulin therapy also may blunt the capacity for epinephrine responsiveness and is associated with frequent hypoglycemic episodes. Patients with an impaired epinephrine response are at risk for "hypoglycemic unawareness." These patients may not experience anxiety, tachycardia, or other manifestations of epinephrine secretion, and the first sign of hypoglycemia may be cerebral dysfunction, including confusion, that may lead to further errors of inappropriate medication or impair the ability to take measures to counter hypoglycemia so that unconsciousness and coma may follow.

For the same hypoglycemic stimulus, children secrete two to five times as much epinephrine as do adults. This may lead to more intense symptoms of hypoglycemia in such children. Exaggerated epinephrine responses in children relative to adults can also be demonstrated during oral glucose tolerance testing, when the normal nadir of glucose, 3–4 hr after glucose ingestion, results in significantly higher epinephrine secretion in children. In both adults and children, glycemic thresholds for the activation of glucose counter-regulatory systems are higher than the thresholds for symptoms. Nevertheless, the glycemic threshold for epinephrine release in children is higher than in adults, and modest decrements in plasma glucose concentration may cause early impairment in cognitive function before the activation of counter-regulatory mechanisms in the absence of typical hypoglycemic symptoms. Thus, clinicians managing children with diabetes need to be alert to the possibility that symptoms consistent with hypoglycemia can occur at blood glucose concentrations not previously considered in the hypoglycemia range and that the definition of hypoglycemia as 40 mg/dL or less for normal children and adults is not applicable to those with diabetes mellitus. Strict control of diabetes appears to induce delayed release of epinephrine so that glucose counter-regulation becomes impaired.

There is debate about whether treatment with human insulin, rather than the formerly used beef and pork preparations, results in less awareness of acute hypoglycemic symptoms in insulin-dependent diabetes. However, well-controlled studies demonstrate that the symptomatic and hormonal responses to acute hypoglycemia produced by either pork or human insulin are indistinguishable, even after carefully selecting patients who had complained of hypoglycemia unawareness with human insulin.

Physicians caring for patients with insulin-dependent diabetes should be aware of a syndrome of *cerebral glucopenia with hypoglycemic encephalopathy.* In these patients, prolonged severe hypoglycemia that is not recognized or treated may result in seizures and coma that lasts for hours despite correction of blood glucose concentrations. Such patients are often combative and use profane language. Several hours of glucose therapy may be necessary for recovery.

PANCREAS AND ISLET TRANSPLANTATION

In an attempt to cure insulin-dependent diabetes, transplantation of a segment of the pancreas or of isolated islets has been increasingly performed in humans. These procedures are both technically demanding and associated with the risks and complications of rejection and its treatment by immunosuppression. Hence, segmental pancreas transplantation is generally performed in association with transplantation of a kidney for a patient with end-stage renal disease due to diabetic nephropathy in whom the immunosuppressive regimen is indicated for the renal transplant. Several thousand such transplants have been performed worldwide during the past 25 yr. With experience and newer immunosuppressive agents, functional survival of the pancreatic graft may be achieved for up to several years, during which time patients may be in metabolic control with no or minimal exogenous insulin and reversal of some of the microvascular complications. However, because children and adolescents with diabetes mellitus are not likely to have end-stage renal disease from their diabetes, pancreas transplantation as a primary treatment in children cannot be recommended or its risks justified.

Some of the newer antirejection drugs, notably cyclosporin and FK-506, are themselves toxic to the islet of Langerhans, impairing insulin secretion and even causing diabetes. Attempts to transplant isolated islets have been equally challenging because of techniques to harvest sufficient islets and the issue of rejection. Research continues to improve techniques for the yield, viability, and reduction of immunogenicity of the islet of Langerhans for transplantation. Transplantation of islets coated or microencapsulated with a film of protective chemicals that permit diffusion of insulin and nutrients, but prevent T-cell contact and hence avoid rejection, are being investigated.

EPIDEMIOLOGY, ETIOLOGY, PATHOLOGY, CLASSIFICATION, AND PREVENTION

Alberti KGMM: Preventing insulin dependent diabetes mellitus. Br Med J 307:1435, 1993.
Atkinson MA, Bowman MA, Kao KJ, et al: Lack of immune responsiveness to bovine serum albumin in insulin-dependent diabetes. N Engl J Med 329:1853, 1993.
Bach JF: Insulin-dependent diabetes mellitus as an autoimmune disease. Endocr Rev 15:516, 1994.
Chase HP, Garg SK, Butler-Simon N, et al: Prediction of the course of pre-type I diabetes. J Pediatr 118:838, 1991.
Dotta F, Eisenbarth GS: Type I diabetes mellitus: A predictable autoimmune disease with interindividual variation in the rate of β-cell destruction. Clin Immunol Immunopathol 50:LS85, 1989.
Froguel P, Zouali H, Vionnet N, et al: Familial hyperglycemia due to mutations in glucokinase. N Engl J Med 328:697, 1993.
Green A, Gale EAM, Patterson CC: Incidence of childhood-onset insulin-dependent diabetes mellitus: The Eurodiab Ace study. Lancet 339:905, 1992.
Groop LC, Kankuri J, Schalin-Janti C, et al: Association between polymorphism of the glycogen synthase gene and non-insulin dependent diabetes mellitus. N Engl J Med 328:10, 1993.
Harrison LC, Honeyman MC, DeAizpurua HJ, et al: Inverse relation between humoral and cellular immunity to glutamic acid decarboxylase in subjects at risk of insulin-dependent diabetes. Lancet 341:1365, 1993.
Karam JH, Lewitt PE, Young CW, et al: Insulinopenic diabetes after rodenticide (Vacor) ingestion: A unique model of acquired diabetes in man. Diabetes 29:971, 1980.
Keller RJ, Eisenbarth GS, Jackson RA: Insulin prophylaxis in individuals at high risk of type I diabetes. Lancet 341:927, 1993.
LaPorte RE, Dorman JS, Orchard TJ, et al: Preventing insulin dependent diabetes mellitus: The environmental challenge. Br Med J 295:479, 1987.
Lowdell M, Bottazzo GF: Autoimmunity and insulin-dependent diabetes. Lancet 341:1378, 1993.
Maclaren N, Atkinson M: Is insulin-dependent diabetes mellitus environmentally induced? N Engl J Med 327:348, 1992.
Maclaren NK: How, when and why to predict IDDM. Diabetes 37:1591, 1988.
National Diabetes Data Group: Classification and diagnosis of diabetes mellitus and other categories of glucose intolerance. Diabetes 28:1039, 1979.
Reynet C, Kahn CR: Rad: A member of the Ras family overexpressed in muscle of type II diabetic humans. Science 262:1441, 1993.
Riley WJ, Winter WE, Maclaren NK: Identification of insulin-dependent diabetes mellitus before the onset of clinical symptoms. J Pediatr 112:314, 1988.
Rosenbloom AL, Kohrman A, Sperling M: Classification and diagnosis of diabetes mellitus in children and adolescents. J Pediatr 98:320, 1981.
Skyler JS, Marks JB: Immune intervention in type I diabetes mellitus. Diabetes Rev 1:15, 1993.
Sperling MA (ed): Physician's Guide to Insulin-Dependent (Type I) Diabetes Mellitus: Diagnosis and Treatment. Alexandria, VA, American Diabetes Association, 1988.
Tuomi T, Groop LC, Zimmet PZ, et al: Antibodies to glutamic acid decarboxylase reveal latent autoimmune diabetes mellitus in adults with a non-insulin-dependent onset of disease. Diabetes 42:359, 1993.
Weir GC: A defective beta-cell glucose sensor as a cause of diabetes. N Engl J Med 328:729, 1993.

GENETICS

Faas S, Trucco M: The genes influencing the susceptibility to IDDM in humans. J Endocrinol Invest 17:477, 1994.
Leahy JL, Boyd AE II: Diabetes genes in non-insulin dependent diabetes mellitus. N Engl J Med 328:56, 1993.
Reardon W, Ross RJM, Sweeney MG: Diabetes mellitus associated with a pathogenic point mutation in mitochondrial DNA. Lancet 340:1376, 1992.
Tas S, Abdella NA: Blood pressure, coronary artery disease, and glycemic control in type 2 diabetes mellitus: Relation to apolipoprotein-CIII gene polymorphism. Lancet 343:1194, 1994.
Trucco M: To be or not to be ASP 57: That is the question. Diabetes Care 15:5, 1992.
Trucco M, Dorman JS: Immunogenetics of insulin-dependent diabetes mellitus in humans. Crit Rev Immunol 9:201, 1989.
Warram JH, Krolewski AS, Gottlieb MS, et al: Differences in risk of insulin-dependent diabetes in offspring of diabetic mothers and diabetic fathers. N Engl J Med 311:149, 1984.
Wassmuth R, Lernmark A: The genetics of susceptibility to diabetes. Clin Immunol Immunopathol 53:358, 1989.

DIABETIC KETOACIDOSIS

Adrogue HJ, Wilson H, Boyd AE III, et al: Plasma acid-base patterns in diabetic ketoacidosis. N Engl J Med 307:1603, 1982.
Arieff AI: Pathogenesis of lactic acidosis. Diabetes Metab Rev 5:637, 1989.
Duck SC, Wyatt DT: Factors associated with brain herniation in the treatment of diabetic ketoacidosis. J Pediatr 113:10, 1988.
Durr JA, Hoffman WH, Sklar AH, et al: Correlates of brain edema in uncontrolled IDDM. Diabetes 41:627, 1992.
Foster DW, McGarry JD: The metabolic derangements and treatment of diabetic ketoacidosis. N Engl J Med 309:159, 1983.
Harris GD, Fiordalisi I, Finberg L: Safe management of diabetic ketoacidemia. J Pediatr 113:65, 1988.
Harris GD, Fiordalsi I, Harris WL, et al: Minimizing the risk of brain herniation during treatment of diabetic ketoacidemia: A retrospective and prospective study. J Pediatr 117:22, 1990.
Kecskes SA: Diabetic ketoacidosis. Pediatr Clin North Am 40:355, 1993.
Krane EJ, Rockoff MA, Wallman JK, et al: Subclinical brain swelling in children during treatment of diabetic ketoacidosis. N Engl J Med 312:1147, 1985.
Matz R: Cerebral edema in diabetic ketoacidosis. Lancet 2:689, 1987.
Riley LJ, Cooper M, Narins RG: Alkali therapy of diabetic ketoacidosis: Biochemical, physiologic, and clinical perspectives. Diabetes Metab Rev 5:627, 1989.
Rosenbloom AL: Intracerebral crisis during treatment of diabetic ketoacidosis. Diabetes Care 13:22, 1990.
Sperling MA: Diabetic ketoacidosis. Pediatr Clin North Am 31:591, 1984.
Van der Meulen JA, Klip A, Grinstein S: Possible mechanism for cerebral edema in diabetic ketoacidosis. Lancet 2:306, 1987.
Winter RJ, Harris CJ, Phillips LS, et al: Diabetic ketoacidosis: Induction of hypocalcemia and hypomagnesemia by phosphate therapy. Am J Med 67:897, 1979.

MANAGEMENT OF TYPE I DIABETES IN CHILDREN

Arky RA: Nutritional therapy for the child and adolescent with type I diabetes mellitus. Pediatr Clin North Am 31:711, 1984.
Becker DJ, Sperling MA: Sucrose in the diet of children with insulin-dependent diabetes mellitus. J Pediatr 119:586, 1991.
Bolli GB, Gerich JE: The "dawn phenomenon"—a common occurrence in both non-insulin and insulin-dependent diabetes mellitus. N Engl J Med 310:746, 1984.
Bolli GB, Gottesman IS, Campbell PJ, et al: Glucose counterregulation and waning of insulin in the Somogyi phenomenon (posthypoglycemic hyperglycemia). N Engl J Med 311:1214, 1984.
Cerreto MC, Travis LB: Implications of psychological and family factors in the treatment of diabetes. Pediatr Clin North Am 31:689, 1984.
Fels Tinker L, Heins JM, Holler HJ: Commentary and translation: 1994 nutrition recommendations for diabetes. J Am Diet Assoc 94:507, 1994.
Dietary fibre: Importance of function as well as amount. Lancet 340:1133, 1992.
Goldstein DE: Understanding GHb assays: A guided tour for clinicians. Clin Diabetes 4:7, 1986.
Ingersoll GM, Orr DP, Herrold AJ, et al: Cognitive maturity and self-management among adolescents with insulin-dependent diabetes mellitus. Clin Lab Observ 108:620, 1986.
Kovacs M, Feinberg TL, Paulauskas S, et al: Initial coping responses and psychosocial characteristics of children with insulin-dependent diabetes mellitus. J Pediatr 106:827, 1985.
Menon RK, Sperling MA: Childhood diabetes. Med Clin North Am 72:1565, 1988.
Nutrition recommendations and principles for people with diabetes mellitus. Diabetes Care 17:519, 1994.
Sperling MA: Insulin biosynthesis and C-peptide. Am J Dis Child 134:1119, 1980.
Sperling MA: Diabetes in adolescence. Adolescent Medicine: State of the Art Reviews 5:87, 1994.
Stein R, Golberg N, Kalman F, et al: Exercise and the patient with type I diabetes mellitus. Pediatr Clin North Am 31:665, 1984.
Tamborlane WV, Press CM: Insulin infusion pump treatment of type I diabetes. Pediatr Clin North Am 31:721, 1984.
The perfect enemy: Eating and IDDM. Lancet 1:1564, 1990.
Zinman B: The physiologic replacement of insulin. N Engl J Med 321:363, 1989.

LONG-TERM OUTCOME OF CHILDHOOD DIABETES: RELATION OF CONTROL TO DEVELOPMENT OF COMPLICATIONS

Abouna GM, Kremer GD, Daddah SK, et al: Reversal of diabetic nephropathy in human cadaveric kidneys after transplantation into non-diabetic recipients. Lancet 2:1274, 1983.
Browning and diabetic complications. Lancet 1:1192, 1986.
Diabetes Control and Complications Trial: The effect of long-term intensified insulin treatment on the development of microvascular complications of diabetes mellitus. N Engl J Med 329:304, 1993.
Kirschenbaum DM: Glycosylation of proteins: Its implications in diabetic control and complications. Pediatr Clin North Am 31:611, 1984.
Leslie ND, Sperling MA: Relation of metabolic control to complications in diabetes mellitus. J Pediatr 108:491, 1986.
Makita Z, Radoff S, Rayfield EJ, et al: Advanced-glycosylation end products in patients with diabetic nephropathy. N Engl J Med 325:936, 1991.
Nathan DM: Long-term complications of diabetes mellitus. N Engl J Med 328:1676, 1993.
Reichard P, Nilsson BY, Rosenqvist U: The effect of long-term intensified insulin treatment on the development of microvascular complications of diabetes mellitus. N Engl J Med 329:304, 1993.
Roe TF, Costin G, Kaufman FR, et al: Blood glucose control and albuminuria in type I diabetes mellitus. J Pediatr 119:178, 1991.
Rosenbloom AL: Skeletal and joint manifestations of childhood diabetes. Pediatr Clin North Am 31:569, 1984.
Sandman DD, Shore AC, Tooke JE: Relation of skin capillary pressure in patients

with insulin-dependent diabetes mellitus to complications and metabolic control. N Engl J Med 327:760, 1992.

Steffes MW, Sutherland DER, Goetz FC, et al: Study of kidney and muscle biopsy specimens from identical twins discordant for type I diabetes mellitus. N Engl J Med 312:1282, 1985.

Wang PH: Tight glucose control and diabetic complications. Lancet 342:129, 1993.

Wang PH, Lau J, Chalmers TC: Meta-analysis of effects of intensive blood-glucose control on late complications of type I diabetes. Lancet 341:1306, 1993.

White NW, Waltman SR, Krupin T, et al: Reversal of neuropathic and gastrointestinal complications related to diabetes mellitus in adolescents with improved metabolic control. J Pediatr 99:41, 1981.

Winegrad AI: Does a common mechanism induce the diverse complications of diabetes? Diabetes 36:396, 1987.

DISEASES AND SYNDROMES ASSOCIATED WITH DIABETES

Austin A, Kalhan SC, Orenstein D, et al: Roles of insulin resistance and β-cell dysfunction in the pathogenesis of glucose intolerance in cystic fibrosis. J Clin Endocrinol Metab 79:80, 1994.

Bu X, Rotter JI: Wolfram syndrome: A mitochondrial-mediated disorder? Lancet 342:598, 1993.

Didmoad (Wolfram) syndrome. Lancet 1:1075, 1986.

Flier JS, Kahn CR, Roth J: Receptors, antireceptor antibodies and mechanisms of insulin resistance. N Engl J Med 300:413, 1979.

Kinsley BT, Firth RG: The Wolfram syndrome: A primary neurodegenerative disorder with lethal potential. Ir Med J 85:34, 1992.

Lippe BM, Sperling MA, Dooley RR: Pancreatic alpha and beta cell functions in cystic fibrosis. J Pediatr 90:751, 1977.

Low L, Chernausek SD, Sperling MA: Acromegaloid patients with type-A insulin resistance: Parallel defects in insulin and insulin-like growth factor-I receptors and biological responses in cultured fibroblasts. J Clin Endocrinol Metab 69:329, 1989.

Morrison EY, McKenzie K: The mauriac syndrome. West Indian Med J 38:180, 1989.

National Diabetes Data Group: Classification and diagnosis of diabetes mellitus and other categories of glucose intolerance. Diabetes 28:1039, 1979.

Rando TA, Horton JC, Layzer RB: Wolfram syndrome: Evidence of a diffuse neurodegenerative disease by magnetic resonance imaging. Neurology 42:1220, 1992.

Rotig A, Cormier V, Chatelain P, et al: Deletion of mitochondrial DNA in a case of early-onset diabetes mellitus, optic atrophy, and deafness. J Clin Invest 91:1095, 1993.

Sullivan MM, Denning CR: Diabetic microangiopathy in patients with cystic fibrosis. Pediatrics 84:642, 1989.

Winter WE, Maclaren NK, Riley WJ, et al: Congenital pancreatic hypoplasia: A syndrome of exocrine and endocrine pancreatic insufficiency. J Pediatr 109:465, 1986.

Winter WE, Maclaren NK, Riley WJ, et al: Maturity-onset diabetes of youth in black Americans. N Engl J Med 316:285, 1987.

TRANSIENT DIABETES OF THE NEWBORN

Blethen SL, White NH, Santiago JV, et al: Plasma somatomedins, endogenous insulin secretion, and growth in transient neonatal diabetes mellitus. J Clin Endocrinol Metab 52:144, 1981.

Geffner ME, Clare-Salzler M, Kaufman DL, et al: Permanent diabetes developing after transient neonatal diabetes. Lancet 341:1095, 1993.

Pagliara AS, Karl IE, Kipnis DB: Transient neonatal diabetes: Delayed maturation of the pancreatic beta cell. J Pediatr 82:97, 1973.

Schiff D, Colle E, Stern L: Metabolic and growth patterns in transient neonatal diabetes. N Engl J Med 287:119, 1972.

Shield JPH, Baum JD: Is transient neonatal diabetes a risk factor for diabetes in later life? Lancet 341:693, 1993.

HYPOGLYCEMIA AND DIABETES

Amiel SA, Simonson DC, Sherwin RS: Exaggerated epinephrine responses to hypoglycemia in normal and insulin-dependent diabetic children. J Pediatr 110:832, 1987.

Amiel SA, Tamborlane WV, Simonson DC, et al: Defective glucose counterregulation after strict glycemic control of insulin-dependent diabetes mellitus. N Engl J Med 316:1376, 1987.

Bergada I, Suissa S, Dufresne J, et al: Severe hypoglycemia in IDDM children. Diabetes Care 12:239, 1989.

Casparie AF, Elving LS: Severe hypoglycemia in diabetic patients: Frequency, causes, prevention. Diabetes Care 8:141, 1985.

Cryer PE, Binder C, Bolli GB, et al: Hypoglycemia in IDDM. Diabetes 38:1193, 1989.

DCCT Research Group, Bethesda, MD: Epidemiology of severe hypoglycemia in the diabetes control and complications trial. Am J Med 90:450, 1991.

DeFeo P, Gallai V, Mazzota G, et al: Modest decrements in plasma glucose concentration cause early impairment in cognitive function and later activation of glucose counterregulation in the absence of hypoglycemic symptoms in normal man. J Clin Invest 82:436, 1988.

Editorial: Awareness of hypoglycemia in diabetes. Lancet 2:371, 1987.

Gale EAM: Hypoglycemia and human insulin. Lancet 2:1264, 1989.

Gerich JE: Lilly Lecture, 1988. Glucose counterregulation and its impact on diabetes mellitus. Diabetes 37:1608, 1988.

Heller SR, MacDonald IA, Herbert M, et al: Influence of sympathetic nervous system on hypoglycemic warning symptoms. Lancet 2:359, 1987.

Schwartz NS, Clutter WE, Shah SD, et al: Glycemic thresholds for activation of glucose counterregulatory systems are higher than the threshold for symptoms. J Clin Invest 79:777, 1987.

PANCREAS AND ISLET TRANSPLANTATION

Brouhard BH, Rogers DG: Pancreatic and islet replacement therapy for insulin-dependent diabetes mellitus. Clin Pediatr 32:258, 1993.

Robertson RP, Kendall D, Teuscher A, et al: Long-term metabolic control with pancreatic transplantation. Transplant Proc 26:386, 1994.

Sutherland DE: Present status of pancreas transplantation alone in nonuremic diabetic patients. Transplant Proc 26:379, 1994.

Sutherland DE, Gores PF, Farney AC, et al: Evolution of kidney, pancreas, and islet transplantation for patients with diabetes at the University of Minnesota. Am J Surg 166:456, 1993.

Sutherland D, Gruessner A, Moudry-Munns K: International pancreas transplant registry report. Transplant Proc 26:407, 1994.

PART XXVII

The Nervous System

Robert H. A. Haslam

CHAPTER 541
Neurologic Evaluation

The neurologic evaluation seeks to assess the integrity of the central nervous system (CNS) by means of a thorough history and physical examination and thus to determine the location (and causes) of abnormal function. This section highlights those features of the history and neurologic examination that are peculiar to the infant and provides the framework for the history and neurologic examination in the premature, infant, and child.

HISTORY

The history is the most important component of the evaluation of a child with a neurologic problem. The history should carefully document in chronologic order the onset of symptoms and a thorough description of their frequency, duration, and associated characteristics. Most children beyond the age of 3–4 yr are capable of contributing to their history, particularly concerning facts relating to the present illness. It is essential to obtain a comprehensive review of the function and interaction of all organ systems, because abnormalities of the CNS may initially present with clinical manifestations (e.g., vomiting, pain, constipation, or urinary tract disorders) implicating other systems. A detailed history might suggest that the child's vomiting is due to increased intracranial pressure, that the pain behind the eye may be caused by migraine headaches or multiple sclerosis, and that the constipation and urinary dribbling may be due to a spinal cord tumor.

It is important to start with a concise description of the chief complaint within its developmental context. For example, parents may be concerned that their child cannot talk. The seriousness of this problem depends on many factors, including the age of the patient, the normal range of language development for age, the parent/child interaction, function of the auditory system, and the intellectual level of the child. A comprehensive understanding of developmental milestones is essential in order to ascertain the relative importance of the parents' observations (see Chapters 10–16). There is no particular order to the neurologic history; each physician should utilize the method that is personally most comfortable and familiar, but the history should be comprehensive.

Following the chief complaint and history of present illness, a review of the pregnancy, labor, and delivery is indicated, particularly if a congenital disorder is suspected (see Chapters 80–86). Was the mother exposed to a viral illness during the pregnancy and what is the mother's rubella immune status? The history should also include information about the quantity of cigarette and alcohol consumption and drug use (legal and illicit) that are known to have an adverse effect on fetal development. Decreased or absent fetal activity may be associated with the congenital myopathies and other neuromuscular disorders. Seizures in utero occasionally occur and suggest placental insufficiency or rare inborn errors of metabolism, such as pyridoxine dependency. Seizure activity in utero is difficult to evaluate, particularly in the primigravida. The fact that seizures occurred during pregnancy is often made retrospectively after the mother has had an opportunity to observe her infant's seizures. The mother's postpartum health may provide a clue as to the cause of her infant's neurologic problem; for example, maternal fever, drug dependence, cervical or vaginal vesicles (e.g., herpes simplex), hemorrhage, petechiae, or the presence of an abnormal placenta.

The history of the birthweight, length, and head circumference are particularly important. It may be necessary to obtain the infant's hospital records to determine the head circumference, particularly if congenital microcephaly is a consideration, and the Apgar score, for suspected asphyxia. There are, however, several indicators of neurologic dysfunction during the newborn period that can reliably be obtained from the history. The fact that a full-term infant was unable to breathe spontaneously and required ventilatory assistance may suggest a CNS abnormality. A poor, uncoordinated suck or a full-term infant that requires an inordinate amount of time to feed suggests a neurologic disorder requiring careful evaluation. If such an infant requires gavage feeding, there is almost certainly a significant problem. All of the aforementioned abnormalities may be common to the premature infant, particularly the very low birthweight infant, and do not necessarily signify a poor neurologic outcome. Additional important information in the newborn period includes the presence of jaundice, its degree, and management. The physician should also attempt to assess the activity, sleep patterns, the nature of the cry, and the general well-being of the newborn infant from the history.

The most important component of a neurologic history is the child's developmental assessment (see Chapters 10–16). A careful evaluation of a child's developmental milestones usually determines the presence of a global delay in language, gross and fine motor or social skills, or a delay in a particular subset of development. An abnormality in development from birth suggests an intrauterine or perinatal cause. A slowing of the rate of acquisition of skills later in infancy or childhood may imply an acquired abnormality of the nervous system. A loss of skills (regression) over time strongly suggests an underlying degenerative disease of the CNS. The ability of parents to precisely recall the timing of their children's developmental milestones is extremely variable. Some are very reliable and others are uncertain, particularly if the patient in question has a significant neurodevelopmental problem. Table 541–1 provides some guidelines with regard to the upper range of normal skills that are usually recalled by the parents and that,

■ **TABLE 541–1 Screening Scheme for Developmental Delay: Upper Range**

Age (Months)	Gross Motor	Fine Motor	Social Skills	Language
3	Supports weight on forearms	Opens hands spontaneously	Smiles appropriately	Coos, laughs
6	Sits momentarily	Transfers objects	Shows likes and dislikes	Babbles
9	Pulls to stand	Pincer grasp	Plays patty-cake, peek-a-boo	Imitates sounds
12	Walks with one hand held	Releases an object on command	Comes when called	1–2 meaningful words
18	Walks upstairs with assistance	Feeds from a spoon	Mimics actions of others	At least six words
24	Runs	Builds a tower of six blocks	Plays with others	2–3 word sentences

if not present, should alert the physician. It is often helpful to request photographs taken at an earlier age or to review the family's baby book, because milestones for a child may have been dutifully recorded. Parents (particularly mothers) are usually aware when their children have a developmental problem, and the physician should show appropriate concern.

The family history is extremely important in the neurologic evaluation of the child. Parents are sometimes unwilling to discuss, or may be unaware of family members with, debilitating neurologic disorders, particularly if they are institutionalized. However, most parents are extremely cooperative in securing medical information concerning family members, particularly if it may have relevance for their child. The history should document the ages and well-being of all close relatives and the presence of neurologic disease, including epilepsy, migraine, cerebrovascular accidents, and heredofamilial disorders. The sex and age at death of miscarriages or live-born siblings, including the results of postmortem examinations, should be obtained because this information may have a direct bearing on the patient's condition. It should also be determined whether the parents are related, because the incidence of metabolic and degenerative disorders affecting the CNS is increased significantly in children of consanguineous marriages.

Finally, an attempt should be made to learn about the patient as a person. The child's performance in school, both academically and socially, may shed light on the diagnosis, particularly if there has been an abrupt change. A description of the child's personality before and after the onset of symptoms may provide a clue with regard to the cause of the disorder. Discussions with the day-care worker, or kindergarten or school teacher may provide useful information that is not available from the parent.

NEUROLOGIC EXAMINATION

The neurologic examination of a child begins at the outset of the interview. Observation during interaction with the parents, while playing, or during the time when little attention is directed to the child can provide useful information (Chapters 7 and 17). It may be obvious that the child has characteristic facies, an unusual posture, or an abnormality of motor function manifested by a gait disturbance or hemiparesis. Furthermore, much can be learned from observing the child's behavior during the interview. The normally inquisitive child or toddler may play independently but soon wishes to become involved with the interview process. The child with an attention disorder may display inappropriate behaviors in the examining room, whereas the neurologically abnormal child may appear lethargic or disinterested or may show a complete lack of awareness of the environment. The degree of interaction between the parent and the child should be noted. As the neurologic examination of a newborn or premature infant requires a somewhat modified approach from that of the older child, the differences in the examination will be highlighted for both age groups (see also Chapters 7 and 79.2).

The examination should be conducted in a setting that is nonthreatening and enjoyable for the child. The more it seems like a game, the greater will be the degree of cooperation. The child may be most comfortable on a parent's lap or interacting on the floor of the examination room. It is unwise to force the child to sit on the examining table or to demand that all clothes be removed at the beginning of the procedure. Cooperation is essential for a comprehensive neurologic examination; as a child's confidence increases, so too does the level of participation. Several methods may be used to assess *mental status, cognitive function,* and the level of *alertness,* depending on the age of the child. Simple puzzles may be useful. A child's ability to tell a story or to draw a picture is often a powerful method for assessing cognitive function or for determining the developmental level. The manner in which a child plays with toys or explores the function of a new object or game is an excellent indicator of intellectual curiosity. The level of alertness of a newborn infant depends on many factors, including the time of the last feeding, the room temperature, and the gestational age. Prematures less than 28 wk of gestation do not consistently demonstrate periods of alertness, whereas gentle physical stimulation applied to a slightly older infant arouses the child from sleep and results in a brief period of alertness. Sleep and waking patterns are well developed at term.

The examiner must take advantage of the opportunities provided by the patient; if the circumstances permit, evaluation of muscle power and tone or cerebellar function might precede the cranial nerve examination. However, if a hearing assessment is considered to be important for the historical information, attention should be directed initially to that portion of the examination so that full cooperation can be achieved before the interest and curiosity of the child is lost.

THE HEAD. The *size* and *shape* of the head should be documented carefully. The tower-head, or oxycephalic, skull suggests premature closure of sutures and is associated with various forms of inherited craniosynostosis (see Chapter 542.12). A broad forehead may indicate hydrocephalus and a small head microcephaly. The observation of a square or a "box-shaped" skull should suggest chronic subdural hematomas because the longstanding presence of fluid in the subdural space causes enlargement of the middle fossa. Inspection of the scalp should include observation of the venous pattern, because increased intracranial pressure and thrombosis of the superior sagittal sinus can produce marked venous distention.

The infant has two *fontanels* at birth; a diamond-shaped open anterior fontanel that is situated in the midline at the junction of the coronal and sagittal sutures, and a posterior fontanel placed between the intersection of the occipital and parietal bones that may be closed at birth or, at the most, admit the tip of a finger. The posterior fontanel is usually closed and nonpalpable beyond the first 6–8 wk of life; its persistence suggests underlying hydrocephalus or the possibility of congenital hypothyroidism. The anterior fontanel varies greatly in size, but the usual measurement approximates 2 × 2 cm. The average time of closure is 18 mo, but the fontanel may normally close as early as 9–12 mo. A very small or absent anterior fontanel at birth may indicate premature fusion of the sutures of microcephaly, whereas a very large fontanel could signify a variety of problems (see Table 79–1). *The fontanel is normally slightly depressed and pulsatile and is best evaluated when the infant is held upright and is asleep or feeding.* A bulging fontanel is a reliable indicator of increased intracranial pressure, but vigorous crying can cause a protuberant fontanel in a normal infant.

Palpation of the newborn's skull characteristically shows over-riding of the cranial sutures for the first several days of life due to the pressures exerted on the skull during its descent through the pelvis. Marked over-riding of the sutures beyond a few days is cause for alarm and suggests the possibility of an underlying abnormality of the brain. Palpation may uncover cranial defects or *craniotabes,* a peculiar softening of the parietal bone so that gentle pressure produces a sensation similar to indenting a ping-pong ball. Craniotabes is often associated with prematurity.

Auscultation of the skull is an important adjunct to the neurologic examination. *Cranial bruits* are most prominent over the anterior fontanel, temporal region, or the orbits and are best heard by the diaphragm of the stethoscope. Soft symmetric bruits may be discovered in normal children less than 4 yr of age or in association with a febrile illness. Arteriovenous malformations of the middle cerebral artery or vein of Galen may produce a loud bruit. Murmurs arising from the heart or great vessels frequently are transmitted to the cranium. The child with severe anemia is often found to have a skull bruit that disappears when the anemia is corrected. Increased intracranial pressure resulting from hydrocephalus, tumor, subdural effusions, or purulent meningitis frequently produces significant intracranial bruits. *The demonstration of a loud or localized bruit is usually significant and warrants further investigation.*

Transillumination of the cranium is an important diagnostic screening procedure that should be performed on any child 2 yr of age and under who is suspected of having a neurologic disorder. The child should be examined in a dark room with a bright flashlight (with a molded rubber adapter) or with a commercially available transilluminator with a high-intensity light source. The degree of transillumination varies with the patient's age, the area of the skull, and the thickness of the cortical mantle. The newborn or premature infant has a very thin skull, particularly in the frontal region, resulting in greater transillumination. Generally, asymmetric, localized, or diffuse transillumination suggests an underlying pathologic process. Increased transillumination is typically observed in hydranencephaly or marked hydrocephalus with a thin cortical mantle. Porencephalic or arachnoid cysts as well as the Dandy-Walker syndrome are frequently demonstrated by this technique. The result of transillumination is often positive in children with subdural effusions complicating meningitis, and the procedure offers a quick, reliable, and noninvasive method of following their size and dissolution. In contrast, acute subdural hematomas may reveal a decreased area of transillumination due to the viscidity of fresh blood. Transillumination is not routinely used at the bedside since the advent of computed tomography (CT).

The correct *measurement of the head circumference* is important. It should be performed on every patient, at every visit, and should be recorded on a suitable head growth chart. A nondistensible plastic measuring tape should be utilized. The tape is placed over the midforehead and is extended circumferentially to include the most prominent portion of the occiput so that the greatest volume of the cranium is measured. The head circumferences of the parents and siblings should also be recorded if the patient is found to have an abnormally sized skull. Errors in the accurate measurement of a newborn skull are frequent and result from scalp edema, over-riding of the sutures, intravenous fluid infiltration, and the presence of a cephalohematoma. The average rate of head growth in a healthy premature infant is 0.5 cm in the first 2 wk, 0.75 cm during the 3rd wk, and 1.0 cm in the 4th wk and thereafter until the 40th wk of development. The head circumference of the term infant at birth measures 34–35 cm, 44 cm by 6 mo, and 47 cm by 1 yr of age (see Chapters 10 and 11).

CRANIAL NERVES. Olfactory Nerve (1). Anosmia, loss of smell, is most commonly found in association with an upper respiratory tract infection in children and, therefore, is a transient abnormality. A fracture of the base of the skull and cribriform plate as well as a frontal lobe tumor also may produce anosmia. Occasionally, a child who recovers from purulent meningitis or who develops hydrocephalus will have a diminished sense of smell. Rarely, anosmia is congenital. Although not a routine component of the examination, smell can be tested reliably as early as the 32nd wk of gestation. Care should be taken to use appropriate stimuli, such as coffee, peppermint, and peanut butter, that are familiar to the child; strongly aromatic substances should be avoided.

Optic Nerve (2). Examination of the optic disk and retina is an important component of the neurologic examination. In order to visualize a good portion of the retina, dilation of the pupil is necessary. One drop of a combination of 1% cyclopentolate hydrochloride, 2.5% phenylephrine hydrochloride, and 1% tropicamide repeated every 15 min on three occasions effectively produces mydriasis. Mydriatics should not be used if a patient's pupil reaction is necessary to follow the level of consciousness or if a cataract is present. Examination of the retina in an infant is enhanced by providing a nipple or soother and by placing the head on one side. The physician gently strokes the patient to maintain arousal, while examining the closest eye. The older child should be placed in the parent's lap and should be distracted by bright objects or toys that are presented during the ophthalmologic examination. The optic nerve is a salmon-pink color in the child but is a gray-white color in the newborn, particularly in a blond infant. This normal finding may cause confusion and may lead to the improper diagnosis of optic atrophy.

Papilledema rarely occurs in infancy because the skull sutures are capable of separating to accommodate the expanding brain. Papilledema in the older child may be recognized by the following changes in the optic nerve and surrounding retina (Fig. 541–1):

1. The optic nerve becomes hyperemic.
2. The small capillaries that normally cross the optic nerve are no longer visualized as they become constricted.
3. The larger veins become dilated, and the accompanying arterioles become constricted.
4. The border of the optic nerve becomes indistinct from the surrounding retina, particularly along the temporal edge.
5. Subhyaloid, flame-shaped hemorrhages appear in the retina surrounding the optic nerve.
6. In some cases, a macular star develops due to retinal edema in the region of the macula. Visual acuity and color vision remain intact in acute papilledema as contrasted with optic neuritis, but the blind spot is increased in both.

Retinal hemorrhages occur in 30–40% of all full-term newborn infants. The hemorrhages are more common after vaginal delivery compared with infants delivered by cesarean section and are not associated with birth injury or with neurologic complications. They disappear spontaneously by 1–2 wk of age.

Vision (see also Part XXIX). The normal 28-wk-old premature infant blinks when a bright light is directed to the eyes, and by 32 wk the infant maintains eye closure until the light source is removed. At 37 wk, the normal premature turns the head and the eyes to a soft light, and by term, visual fixation and the ability to follow a brilliant target are present. During a period of alertness, optokinetic nystagmus can be demonstrated in the newborn. The visual acuity in the term infant approximates 20/150 and reaches the adult level of 20/20 by about 6 mo of age. Children who are too young to read the standard letters on the Snellen Eye Chart may learn the "E game" by pointing a finger in the direction that the "E" is oriented. Children as young as 2½ or 3 yr of age with normal

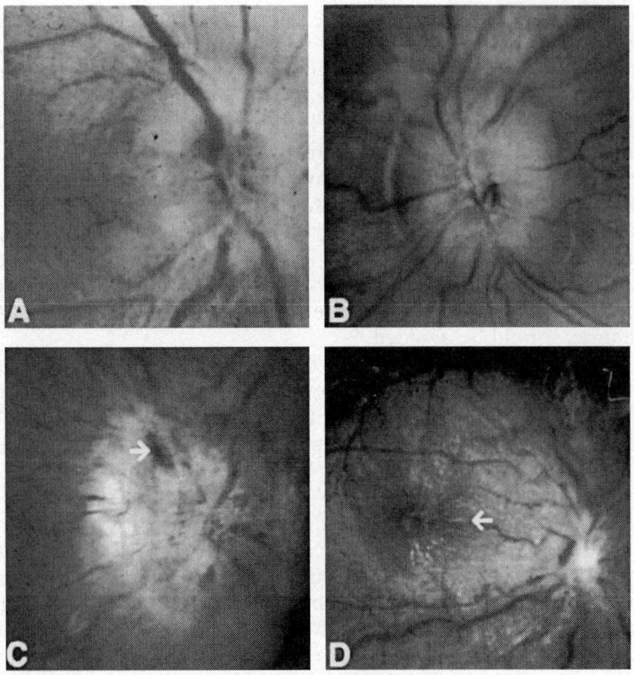

Figure 541–1. *A*, Mild papilledema. Blurred disc margins and venous congestion. *B*, Moderate papilledema. Disc edematous and raised. Vessels buried within substance of nerve tissue. *C*, Severe papilledema. Hemorrhages are evident within disc *(arrow)*, and there are microinfarcts (soft exudates) in the nerve fiber layer. *D*, Macular star *(arrow)* with edema residues distributed within the Henle layer of the macula. See also color section.

vision will identify the objects on the Allen Chart at a distance of 15 or 20 ft. Peripheral vision may be tested in an infant by bringing an object from behind the patient into the peripheral field of vision that normally produces a visual recognition response. The examiner should be assured that the object rather than a sound produces the visual response.

The *pupil* is difficult to examine in the premature due to the poorly pigmented iris and the resistance to lid opening. The pupil reacts to light by the 29th–32nd wk of gestation. The equality of the pupils, their size, and reaction to light may be affected by drugs, a space-occupying brain lesion, metabolic disorders, and abnormalities of the midbrain and optic nerves. *Horner syndrome* is characterized by miosis, ptosis, enophthalmos, and ipsilateral anhidrosis of the face. It may be congenital or may result from a lesion involving the sympathetic nervous system in the brain stem, cervical spinal cord, or the sympathetic plexus in juxtaposition to the carotid artery. Localization of the lesion within the sympathetic nervous system is aided by the pupillary response to a series of topical drugs, incuding cocaine, epinephrine, hydroxyamphetamine, and phenylephrine.

Oculomotor (3), Trochlear (4), and Abducens Nerves (6). The eye is moved by the extraocular muscles that are innervated by the oculomotor, trochlear, and abducens nerves. The oculomotor nerve innervates the superior, inferior, and medial rectus as well as the inferior oblique and the levator palpebra superioris muscles. Complete paralysis of the oculomotor nerve causes ptosis, dilation of the pupil, displacement of the eye outward and downward, and impairment of adduction and elevation. The trochlear nerve supplies the superior oblique muscle, and isolated paralysis causes the eye to deviate upward and outward, often with an associated head tilt. The abducens nerve innervates the lateral rectus muscle so that its paralysis causes medial deviation of the eye and the inability to abduct beyond the midline. In the older child, the *red glass test* is used to assess extraocular palsies. A red glass is placed over one eye, and the patient is requested to follow a white light in all fields of direction. The child sees only one red/white light in the direction of normal muscle function but notes a separation of the red and white images that is greatest in the plane of action of the affected muscle. *Internuclear ophthalmoplegia* results from a lesion in the brain stem and consists of paralysis of medial rectus function of the adducting eye and nystagmus confined to the abducting eye. *Internal ophthalmoplegia* refers to a dilated pupil that is unreactive to light and accomodation but has normal extraocular function, and *external ophthalmoplegia* is associated with ptosis and paralysis of all eye muscles with preservation of the pupillary response. *Nystagmus* is an involuntary rapid movement of the eye that may be horizontal, vertical, rotatory, pendular, or mixed. Jerk nystagmus is used to describe a fast and slow phase. Horizontal nystagmus occurs with an abnormality of the peripheral labyrinth or with a lesion of the vestibular system in the brain stem or cerebellum and as a consequence of drugs, particularly phenytoin. Vertical nystagmus is indicative of brain stem dysfunction.

Complete ocular movement may be demonstrated as early as 25 wk of gestation utilizing the *doll's eye maneuver.* This technique is used to examine horizontal and vertical eye movements in the infant, or the uncooperative or comatose patient. If the head is suddenly turned to the right, the eyes look to the left in a symmetric fashion. Horizontal eye movements in the opposite direction may then be evaluated if the head is turned to the left. Vertical movements may be assessed in a similar fashion by rapid flexion and extension of the head. The normal infant and child will follow a toy or interesting object in all directions. The examiner observes the completeness and flow of the eye movements and determines the presence or absence and the direction of nystagmus, diplopia, opsoclonus, ocular bobbing, or other abnormal eye positions. Premature infants tend to have slightly disconjugate eyes at rest with one eye horizontally displaced from the other by 1 or 2 mm. Skew deviation of the eyes (vertical displacement) is always abnormal and requires investigation. Strabismus is discussed in Chapter 574.

Trigeminal Nerve (5). The sensory distribution of the face is divided into three areas: the ophthalmic area, the maxillary area, and the mandibular area. Each region may be tested by light touch and by pinprick, and may be compared with the opposite side. The corneal response is elicited by touching the cornea with a small pledget of cotton and by observing the eye closure response. Trigeminal nerve function in the premature is best documented by facial grimacing from a pinprick (away from the eye) or by stimulating the nostril with a cotton tip. Motor function may be tested by examination of the masseters, pterygoid, and temporalis muscles during mastication as well as by evaluation of the jaw jerk.

Facial Nerve (7). Decreased voluntary movement of the lower face with flattening of the nasolabial angle on the ipsilateral side indicates an upper motor neuron or supranuclear corticospinal lesion. A lower motor neuron lesion tends to equally involve upper and lower facial muscles. Facial nerve paralysis may be congenital or secondary to trauma, infection, intracranial tumor, hypertension, toxins, or myasthenia gravis. Taste for the anterior two-thirds of the tongue may be tested in the cooperative child by placing a solution of saline or glucose on one side of the extended tongue. The normal child can identify the substance with little difficulty.

Auditory Nerve (8). Screening for hearing loss is an important component of the neurologic examination, because a hearing deficit is not readily recognized by parents (see Chapter 587). A normal newborn will pause briefly during sucking when a bell is presented, but after several stimuli the pauses will cease as habituation occurs. The neurologically abnormal infant will not habituate. The normal hearing infant will turn its head toward a bell, rattle, or crumpled paper and by 3 mo of age will look in the direction of the sound source. The normally intelligent, hard-of-hearing toddler is visually alert and responds appropriately to physical stimuli. Temper tantrums and abnormal speech are common symptoms in a hard-of-hearing child. Audiometry or brain stem–evoked potential testing is mandatory for any child suspected of a hearing loss (see Chapter 587). The risk factors that indicate a need for testing during the first few months of life include a family history of deafness, prematurity, severe asphyxia, use of ototoxic drugs in the newborn period, hyperbilirubinemia, congenital anomalies of the head or neck, bacterial meningitis, and congenital infections due to rubella, toxoplasmosis, herpes, and cytomegalovirus.

Vestibular function may be evaluated by the *caloric test.* Approximately 5 mL of ice water is delivered by syringe into the external auditory canal with the patient's head elevated 30 degrees from the horizontal position. In the obtunded or comatose patient with an intact brain stem, there is prompt deviation of the eyes to the side of the stimulus. A much smaller quantity of ice water (0.5 mL) is used in the alert, awake subject. In the normal subject, introduction of ice water produces nystagmus with the quick component in the opposite direction to the stimulated labyrinth. No response implies severe dysfunction of the brain stem and medial longitudinal fasciculus. If the otoscopic examination reveals a ruptured tympanic membrane, the test should not be performed in that ear.

Glossopharyngeal Nerve (9). This nerve supplies innervation to the stylopharyngeus muscle. An isolated lesion of the ninth cranial nerve is rare. The nerve is tested by observing the gag response to tactile stimulation of the posterior pharyngeal wall. Taste for the posterior one third of the tongue is provided by the sensory portion of the glossopharyngeal nerve.

Vagus Nerve (10). A unilateral injury of the vagus nerve produces weakness and asymmetry of the ipsilateral soft palate and a hoarse voice due to paralysis of a vocal cord. Bilateral lesions may produce respiratory distress as a result of vocal cord paralysis as well as nasal regurgitation of fluids, pooling of secretions, and an immobile, low-lying soft palate. Isolated lesions of the vagus nerve may occur postoperatively following a thoracotomy due to separation of the recurrent laryngeal nerve, and these lesions are not uncommon during the neonatal period in children with the type II Chiari malformation. If a lesion involving the vagus nerve is suspected, visualization of the vocal cords is necessary.

Accessory Nerve (11). Paralysis and atrophy of the sternomastoid and trapezius muscles result from lesions of the accessory nerve. The sternomastoid muscle has two origins, sternal and clavicular, and is tested by forceful rotation of the head and neck against the examiner's hand. Motor neuron disease, myotonic dystrophy, and myasthenia gravis are the most common conditions producing weakness and atrophy of these muscles.

Hypoglossal Nerve (12). The hypoglossal nerve innervates the tongue. Examination of the tongue includes an assessment of its motility, size, and shape and the presence of atrophy or fasciculations. Malfunction of the hypoglossal nucleus or nerve produces wasting, weakness, and fasciculations of the tongue. If the injury is bilateral, tongue protrusion is not possible and dysphagia may be present. Werdnig-Hoffmann disease (infantile spinal muscular atrophy) and congenital anomalies in the region of the foramen magnum are the principle causes of hypoglossal nerve involvement.

MOTOR EXAMINATION. The motor examination includes an assessment of the integrity of the musculoskeletal system and the search for abnormal movements that may indicate an abnormality of the peripheral nervous system or the CNS. The components of the motor examination include testing of strength (power), muscle bulk, tone, posture, locomotion and motility, deep tendon reflexes, and the presence of primitive reflexes, when applicable.

Strength. The testing of muscle strength is relatively straightforward in the cooperative child. It may begin by requesting that the child squeeze the examiner's fingers, flex and extend the wrist and elbow, and adduct and abduct the shoulder against resistance. Shoulder girdle muscle strength may be evaluated in the newborn or infant by supporting the child by the axillae. The patient with weakness will be unable to support body weight and will "slip through" the examiner's hands. Distal power can be tested in the infant by evaluating the palmar grasp; the child with weakness will not adequately grasp or will show abnormalities in the manipulation of objects. A normal 3- to 4-yr-old child will cooperate in the testing of the extension or flexion of the muscles of the foot, knee, and hip. Examination of the pelvic girdle and proximal lower extremity muscles is also performed by observing the child climb steps or stand up from a prone position. Weakness in these muscles causes the child to use the hands to "climb up" the legs in order to assume an upright position, a maneuver called *Gowers' sign* (Fig. 541–2). The infant with diminished power in the lower extremities tends to have decreased spontaneous activity in the legs and refuses to support body weight when suspended by the axillae. It is important not only to assess individual muscle groups but also to carefully compare muscle power between the upper and lower extremities as well as the opposite extremities. Muscle power in a cooperative child is graded by a scale of 0–5 as follows: 0 = no movement, 1 = minimal contraction, 2 = movement only in the horizontal plane (with gravity), 3 = movement against gravity, 4 = movement against gravity and resistance, and 5 = normal strength. Examination of muscle power should include the muscles of respiration. Observation of the action of the intercostal muscles, diaphragmatic movement, and the use of accessory muscles of respiration should be documented. Finally, the evaluation of power should include an assessment of muscle bulk and nutrition. Weakness may be associated with muscle atrophy and fasciculations. Because most infants have an excess of body fat, muscle fasciculations and atrophy are most commonly demonstrated in the denervated tongue in this age group.

Tone. Muscle tone is tested by assessing the degree of resistance when an individual joint is moved passively. Tone undergoes considerable change and assumes different forms depending on age. The premature or newborn infant is relatively hypotonic compared with the child. Tone in this age group is tested by a variety of maneuvers (see Chapter 82 and Fig. 82–3). When the upper extremity of the normal term infant is pulled gently across the chest, the elbow normally does not quite reach the mid-sternum *(scarf sign).* The elbow of the hypotonic infant extends beyond the midline with ease. Measurement of the popliteal angle is a useful method to document tone in the legs of the newborn. The examiner flexes the child's lower extremity on the abdomen and extends the knee. The normal term infant allows extension of the knee to approximately 80 degrees. Abnormalities of tone consist of spasticity, rigidity, and hypotonia.

Spasticity is characterized by an initial resistance to passive movement, followed by a sudden release called the *clasp-knife* phenomenon. Spasticity is most apparent in the upper extremity flexors and lower extremity extensor muscles. It is associated with brisk tendon reflexes and an extensor plantar reflex, clonus, diminished active movements, and disuse atrophy. *Clonus* may be demonstrated in the lower extremity by sudden dorsiflexion of the foot with the knee partially flexed. Whereas sustained clonus is always abnormal, 5–10 beats in the newborn is a normal finding unless the clonus is asymmetric. Spasticity results from a lesion that involves upper motor neuron tracts and may be unilateral or bilateral. *Rigidity,* the result

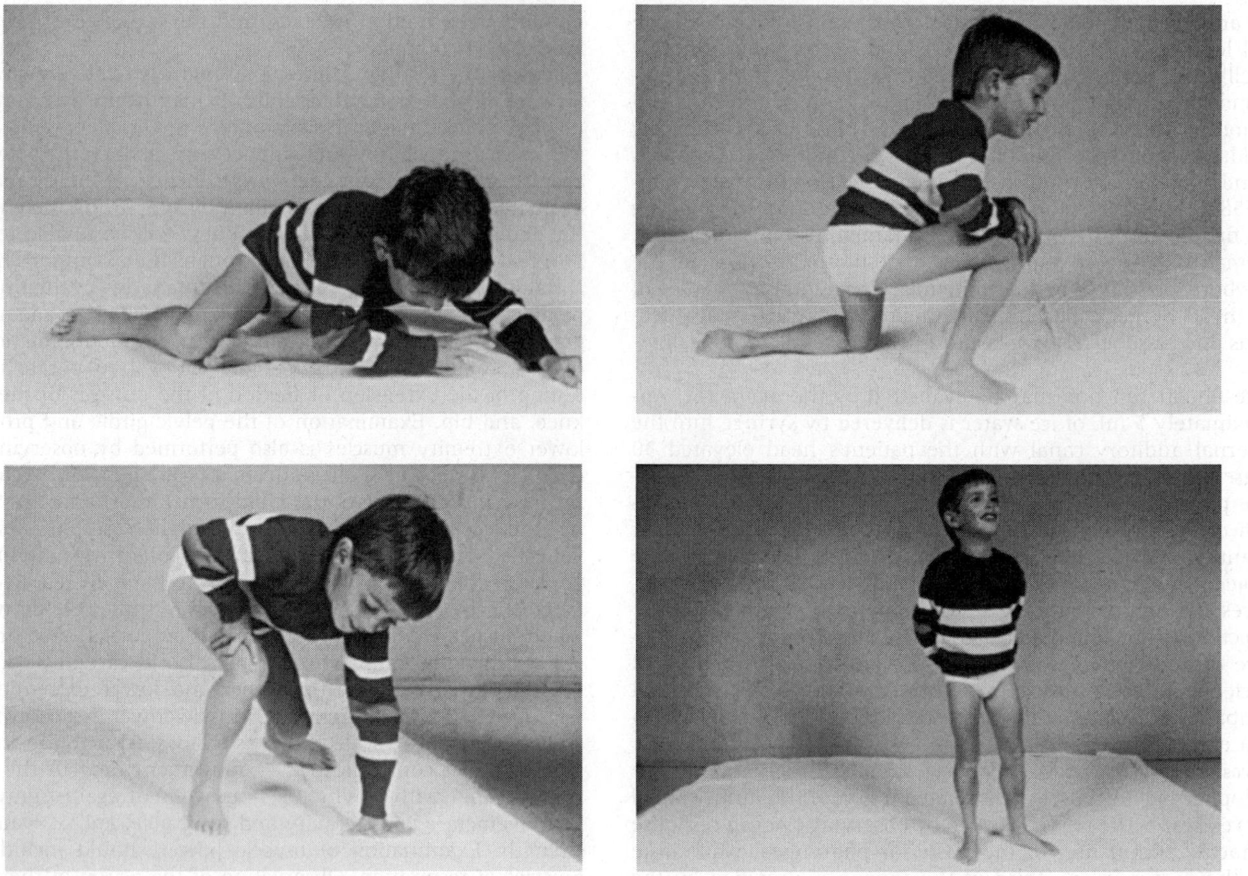

Figure 541–2. Gowers' sign. A boy with hip girdle weakness due to Duchenne muscular dystrophy.

of a basal ganglia lesion, is characterized by a constant resistance to passive movement of both extensor and flexor muscles. As the extremity is undergoing passive movement, a typical *cogwheel* sensation may be evident. The rigidity persists with repetitive passive extension and flexion of a joint and does not "give way" or release, such as with spasticity. The child with spastic lower extremities will drag the legs while crawling (commando style) or will walk on tiptoes. The patient with marked spasticity or rigidity will develop a posture of *opisthotonus,* in which the head and the heels are bent backward and the body bowed forward (Fig. 541–3). *Decerebrate* rigidity is characterized by marked extension of the extremities

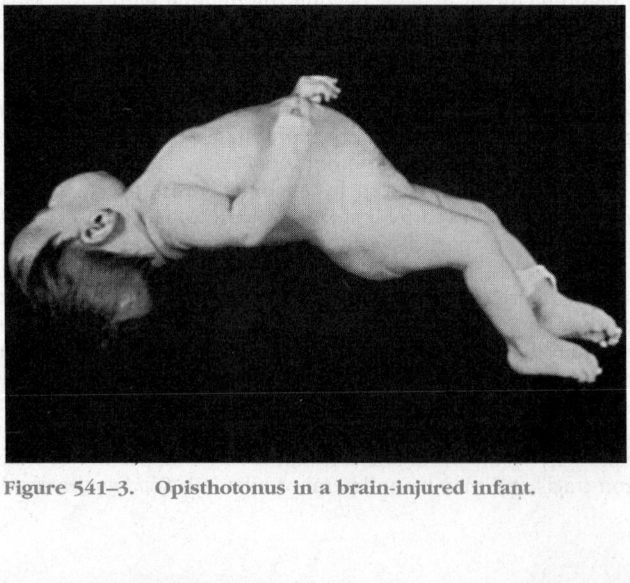

Figure 541–3. Opisthotonus in a brain-injured infant.

resulting from dysfunction or injury to the brain stem at the level of the superior colliculi. *Hypotonia* refers to abnormally diminished tone and is the most common abnormality of tone in the neurologically compromised premature or full-term neonate. The demonstration of hypotonia may reflect pathology of the cerebral hemispheres, cerebellum, spinal cord, anterior horn cell, peripheral nerve, myoneural junction, or muscle. An unusual position or posture by an infant is a reflection of abnormal tone. The hypotonic infant is *floppy* and may have difficulty in maintaining head support or a straight back while sitting. Such infants may assume a *frog-leg* posture in the supine position. The premature infant of 28 wk of gestation tends to extend all extremities at rest, but by 32 wk there is evidence of flexion, particularly in the lower extremities. The normal full-term infant's posture is characterized by flexion of all extremities.

Motility and Locomotion. The premature of less than 32 wk of gestation displays random, slow writhing movements interspersed with rapid, myoclonia-like activity of the extremities. Beyond 32 wk, the motor activity is primarily flexor. Observation of crawling, cruising, walking, or running may uncover movement disorders, most of which are most likely to be apparent during motion and to disappear with rest or sleep. *Ataxia* refers to incoordination of movement or a disturbance of balance. It may be primarily truncal or may be limited to the extremities. Truncal ataxia is characterized by unsteadiness during sitting or standing, and results primarily from involvement of the cerebellar vermis. Abnormalities of the cerebellar hemispheres characteristically cause intention tremor unaffected by visual attention. Ataxia may be demonstrated by the finger-to-nose and heel-to-shin tests, heel-to-toe or tandem walking, and, in the infant, by observation of reaching for or playing with toys. Additional abnormalities associated with cerebellar lesions include dysmetria (errors in measuring distances), rebound (inability to inhibit a muscular action, such as when the examiner suddenly releases the flexed arm and the patient inadvertently strikes the face), and disdiadochokinesia (diminished performance of rapid alternating movements). Hypotonia, dysarthria, nystagmus, and decreased deep tendon reflexes are common features of cerebellar abnormalities. Sensory ataxia is found with diseases of the spinal cord and peripheral nerves. In these disorders, the *Romberg sign* (patient is unsteady with eyes closed but not open) is positive, and there are often related sensory findings including abnormalities in joint position and vibration sense.

Chorea is characterized by involuntary movements of the major joints, trunk, and the face that are rapid and jerky. The child is incapable of extending the arms without producing abnormal movements. There is a tendency to pronate the arms when held above the head. The hand grip contracts and relaxes *(milkmaid sign)*, the speech is explosive and inarticulate, the deep tendon reflexes of the knee are "hung up," and the patient may have difficulty in maintaining protrusion of the tongue. *Athetosis* is a slow, writhing movement that is often associated with abnormalities of muscle tone. It is most prominent in the distal extremities and is enhanced by voluntary activity or emotional upset. Speech and swallowing may be affected. Chorea and athetosis are the result of basal ganglia lesions and are difficult to separate clinically. They may both be prominent in the same patient. *Dystonia* is an involuntary, slow, twisting movement that primarily involves the proximal muscles of the extremities, trunk, and neck.

Deep Tendon Reflexes and the Plantar Response. The deep tendon reflexes are readily elicited in most infants and children. In the premature and term infant, the biceps, knee, and ankle jerks are the most reliable deep tendon reflexes. The ankle reflex is difficult to obtain by percussing the Achilles tendon in this age group. Gentle dorsiflexion of the foot and tapping the plantar surface with the reflex hammer will usually elicit a response. The knee jerk in the infant may produce a crossed adductor response (tapping the patellar tendon in one leg causes contraction in the opposite extremity), which, if present, does not become abnormal until 6–7 mo of age. The deep tendon reflexes are absent or decreased in primary disorders of the muscle (myopathy), nerve (neuropathy), and myoneural junction, and in abnormalities of the cerebellum. They are characteristically increased in upper motor neuron lesions. Asymmetry of deep tendon reflexes suggests a lateralizing lesion. The plantar response is obtained by stimulation of the external portion of the sole of the foot, beginning at the heel and extending to the base of the toes. Firm pressure from the examiner's thumb is a useful method for eliciting the response. The *Babinski reflex* is characterized by extension of the great toe and by fanning of the remaining toes. Too vigorous stimulation may produce withdrawal, which may be misinterpreted as a Babinski response. Most newborn infants show an initial flexion of the great toe upon plantar stimulation. As with adults, asymmetry of the plantar response between extremities is a useful lateralizing sign in infants and children.

Primitive Reflexes. Primitive reflexes appear and disappear in sequence during specific periods of development. Their absence or persistence beyond a given time frame signifies dysfunction of the CNS. Some primitive reflexes, such as the snout or *rooting reflex*, reappear during old age or with specific degenerative diseases involving the cerebral cortex. Although many primitive reflexes have been described, the Moro, grasp, tonic neck, and parachute reflexes are the most important. The *Moro reflex* is obtained by placing the infant in a semi-upright position. The head is momentarily allowed to fall backward with immediate resupport by the examiner's hand. The child will symmetrically abduct and extend the arms, flex the thumbs, followed by flexion and adduction of the upper extremities. An asymmetric response may signify a fractured clavicle, brachial plexus injury, or a hemiparesis. Absence of the Moro reflex in the term newborn is ominous, suggesting significant dysfunction of the CNS. The *grasp* response is elicited by placing a finger or object in the open palm of each hand. The normal infant will grasp the object and with attempted removal, the grip is reinforced. The *tonic neck* reflex is produced by manually turning the head to one side while supine. Extension of the arm occurs on that side of the body corresponding to the direction of the face, while flexion develops in the contralateral extremities. An obligatory tonic neck response, by which the infant remains "locked" in the fencer's position, is always abnormal and implies a disorder of the CNS. The *parachute reflex* is demonstrated by suspending the child by the trunk and by suddenly producing forward flexion as if the child were to fall. The child spontaneously extends the upper extremities as a protective mechanism. The parachute reflex appears before the onset of walking.

SENSORY EXAMINATION. The sensory examination is difficult to interpret in the infant or uncooperative child. Furthermore, the understanding child soon tires of the examination because it requires considerable attention to repetitious and uninteresting tasks. The more this part of the neurologic examination can be made to simulate a game, the greater will be the likelihood that the child will cooperate. Fortunately, disorders involving the sensory system are less common in the pediatric population than among adults, so that this component of the neurologic assessment is less important for infants and children than for the adolescent and adult. While the infant is distracted by a parent or an interesting toy, the examiner touches the patient with a piece of cotton or a sterile pin. The normal child indicates an awareness of the stimulus by pausing during play, withdrawing the extremity, crying, or looking at and touching the stimulated area. Unfortunately, the child quickly loses patience and soon begins to disregard the examiner. It is critical, therefore, that the area in question is tested efficiently and, if necessary, re-examined at an appropriate time.

The identification of a sensory level in association with a *spinal cord lesion* can be very difficult in the infant. Observation may suggest a difference in color, temperature, or perspiration, with the skin cooler and dry below the spinal cord level. Touching the skin lightly above the level evokes a response that is usually in the form of a squirming movement or physical withdrawal. The superficial abdominal reflexes may be absent. A child with a spinal cord lesion may have evidence of rectal sphincter incontinence that is manifested by a patulous anus, by the absence of contraction of the sphincter when the skin in the anal region is stimulated with a sharp object (anal wink), and by a lack of contraction of the anal sphincter during the rectal examination. In males, the presence of the cremasteric reflex is also valuable. Children 4–5 yr of age are capable of detailed sensory testing, including joint position, vibration, temperature, stereognosis, two-point discrimination, double simultaneous extinction, light touch, and pain. The success of the sensory examination depends on the ingenuity and the patience of the examiner.

GAIT AND STATION. Observation of a child's gait is an important aspect of the neurologic examination. The *spastic gait* is characterized by stiffness and by a "tin soldier"-like steppage appearance. The spastic child may walk on tip toes because of tightness or contractures of the Achilles tendons. *Hemiparesis* is associated with a decreased arm swing on the affected side and a lateral circular motion of the leg *(circumduction gait)*. Extrapyramidal movements, such as dystonia or chorea, may become apparent while the child is walking or running. Cerebellar ataxia produces a broad-based unsteady gait and, if severe, the child requires support to prevent falling. Heel-to-toe or tandem walking is performed poorly in patients with abnormalities of the cerebellum. A *waddling gait* results from weakness of the proximal hip girdle. These children often develop a compensatory lordosis and have difficulty in climbing stairs. Weakness or hypotonia of the lower extremities may result in genu recurvatum and flat feet, which causes a clumsy, tentative gait. *Scoliosis* may cause an abnormal gait and can result from disorders of muscle and spinal cord.

GENERAL EXAMINATION

The physical examination of other organ systems is an essential component of the neurologic examination. For example, cutaneous lesions suggest a neurocutaneous syndrome (see Chapter 546), hepatosplenomegaly suggests inborn errors of metabolism, storage diseases, HIV, or malignancy, while various dysmorphic features suggest various syndromes (see Chapter 86). Heart murmurs raise the possibility of rheumatic fever (chorea), tuberous sclerosis (cardiac rhabdomyoma), cerebral abscess or thrombosis (cyanotic heart disease), or cerebral vascular occlusion (endocarditis).

SOFT NEUROLOGIC SIGNS. These signs should be interpreted cautiously because they are present in normal children during various stages of neurodevelopment. A soft neurologic sign may be defined as a particular form of deviant performance on a motor or sensory test in the neurologic examination that is abnormal for a particular age. Testing for the presence of soft neurologic signs involves the observation of a series of timed motor tasks and a comparison of the quality and the precision of the patient's movement with normal controls of similar age and sex. The tests include repetitive and successive finger movements, hand pats, arm pronation-supination movements, foot taps, hopping, and tandem walking. There is considerable variation in the expression of these signs, depending on age, sex, and maturation of the nervous system. For example, minimal choreoathetoid movements in the fingers of the extended arms are normal at 4 yr of age but disappear by 7 or 8 yr of age. The neurodevelopment of girls is more accelerated than that of boys for many motor tasks, including hopping, skipping, and fine balance maneuvers. Although intellectually normal children may demonstrate a soft neurologic sign, the finding of two or more persistent soft signs correlates significantly with neurologic dysfunction, including attention deficit disorder, learning disorders, and cerebral palsy. Because specific soft signs lack association with a particular disability and can occur in the normal child, it is unwise to label a child who manifests several soft neurologic signs. It is more appropriate to monitor such a patient closely and to ensure that a developmental disability has been excluded.

SPECIAL DIAGNOSTIC PROCEDURES

LUMBAR PUNCTURE AND CEREBROSPINAL FLUID EXAMINATION. An examination of the cerebrospinal fluid (CSF) is essential in confirming the diagnosis of meningitis, encephalitis, and subarachnoid hemorrhage and is often helpful in the evaluation of demyelinating, degenerative, and collagen vascular diseases and the presence of tumor cells within the subarachnoid space. Preparation of the patient is important in order to successfully complete the procedure. The skin is thoroughly prepared with a cleansing agent, and the patient is placed in the lateral recumbent position. The physician should be gowned and gloved; the patient should be draped. The neck and legs of the patient are flexed by an assistant to enlarge the intervertebral spaces. The ideal interspace for lumbar puncture (LP) is L3–L4 or L4–L5, which is determined by drawing an imaginary horizontal line from one anterior superior spine of the ilium to the other. The skin and underlying tissue are anesthetized with a local anesthetic. A No. 18- to 22-gauge, 1- to 2-inch, sharp, beveled spinal needle with a properly fitting stylet is introduced into the midsagittal plane directed slightly in the cephalad direction. The stylet is removed frequently as the needle is slowly advanced to determine whether CSF is present. A "pop" is felt as the needle penetrates the dura and enters the subarachnoid space. A manometer and a three-way stopcock may be attached to obtain an opening pressure. The opening pressure in the recumbent and relaxed, less flexed position should be less than 160 mm of water; the range in the flexed lateral decubitus position is 100–280 mm of water. The most common cause of an elevated opening pressure is a crying, uncooperative, and struggling patient. The pressure is recorded most reliably with the child positioned comfortably with the head and the legs extended. Sick neonates may be placed in the upright position for a spinal tap, because decreased ventilation and perfusion abnormalities leading to respiratory arrest are more common in the recumbent position in this age group.

The *contraindications* for performing an LP include: (1) raised intracranial pressure owing to a suspected mass lesion of the brain or spinal cord, which may develop transtentorial herniation or herniation of the cerebellar tonsils following the procedure. Inspection of the eyegrounds for the presence of papilledema is mandatory before proceeding with an LP; (2) symptoms and signs of pending cerebral herniation in a child with probable meningitis. These include decerebrate or decorticate posture, a generalized tonic seizure, abnormalities of pupil size and reaction, with absence of the oculocephalic response and fixed oculomotor deviation of the eyes. Pending herniation is also associated with respiratory abnormalities, including hyperventilation, Cheyne-Stokes, ataxic breathing, apnea, and respiratory arrest. These children must be treated immediately with appropriate IV antibiotics and transported to a critical care unit for stabilization and imaging studies before an LP is contemplated. LP is the primary diagnostic procedure in children with suspected bacterial meningitis in the absence of overwhelming sepsis or shock, or symptoms and signs of brain herniation. As the clinical status of children with untreated bacterial meningitis may rapidly deteriorate, deferral of the LP and appropriate antibiotic therapy while awaiting the results of a CT could be the determining factor between recovery or severe complications and death; (3) *on rare occasions*, an LP is temporarily withheld from a critically ill, moribund patient because the procedure may produce cardiorespiratory arrest. In this situation, blood cultures are drawn; antibiotics and supportive care are administered; and when the patient is stabilized, an LP may be accomplished safely under more controlled circumstances; (4) a skin infection at the site of the LP. If examination of the CSF is urgent in such a patient, a ventricular or cisterna magna tap performed by a skilled physician is indicated; and (5) thrombocytopenia, with a platelet count less than 20×10^9/L may cause uncontrolled bleeding in the subarachnoid or subdural space.

Normal CSF is the color of water. Cloudy CSF results from an elevated white blood cell (WBC) or red blood cell (RBC) count. The normal CSF contains up to five lymphocytes, and the newborn may have as many as 15 per mm^3. Polymorphonuclear (PMN) cells are always abnormal in the child, but 1–2 per mm^3 may be present in the normal neonate. The presence of PMN cells raises suspicion of a pathologic process. An elevated PMN count suggests bacterial meningitis or the early phase of an aseptic meningitis (Chapter 169). CSF lymphocytosis indicates aseptic, tuberculous, or fungal meningitis; demyelinating diseases; brain or spinal cord tumor; immunologic disorders including collagen vascular diseases; and chemical irritation (e.g., postmyelogram, intrathecal methotrexate).

A Gram stain of the CSF is essential in the investigation of suspected bacterial meningitis; an acid-fast stain or India ink preparation is used if tuberculous or fungal meningitis is a possibility. The fluid is placed on appropriate culture media based on the clinical findings and on the CSF analysis.

There are no RBCs in normal CSF. The presence of RBCs

indicates a traumatic tap or a subarachnoid hemorrhage. Bloody CSF should be centrifuged immediately. The supernatant of a bloody tap will be clear, but it will be xanthochromic in the presence of a subarachnoid hemorrhage. Progressive clearing of bloody CSF is noted during the collection of the fluid in the case of a traumatic tap. The presence of crenated RBCs does not differentiate a traumatic tap from a subarachnoid hemorrhage. In addition to a subarachnoid hemorrhage, xanthochromia may result from hyperbilirubinemia, carotenemia, and a markedly elevated CSF protein.

The normal *CSF protein* ranges from 10–40 mg/dL in the child and as high as 120 mg/dL in the neonate. The CSF protein falls to the normal childhood range by 3 mo of age. The CSF protein may be elevated in multiple processes, including infectious, immunologic, vascular, and degenerative diseases as well as tumors of the brain and spinal cord. The CSF protein is increased following a bloody tap by approximately 1 mg/dL for every 1,000 RBC/mm^3. Elevation of CSF immunoglobulin G (IgG), which normally represents approximately 10% of the total protein, is observed in subacute sclerosing panencephalitis, postinfectious encephalomyelitis, and in some cases of multiple sclerosis.

The *CSF glucose* content is about 60% of the blood glucose in the healthy child. In order to prevent a spuriously elevated blood/CSF glucose ratio in a case of suspected meningitis, it is advisable to collect the blood glucose prior to the LP when the child is relatively calm. Hypoglycorrhachia is found in association with diffuse meningeal disease, particularly bacterial and tuberculous meningitis. In addition, widespread neoplastic involvement of the meninges, subarachnoid hemorrhage, fungal meningitis, and, on occasion, aseptic meningitis can produce a low CSF glucose.

The CSF may also be examined for specific *antigens* (e.g., latex agglutination for suspected meningitis) and the investigation of a series of metabolic diseases (e.g., lactate, amino acids, endolase determination).

SUBDURAL TAP. This procedure may be indicated to establish the diagnosis of a subdural effusion or hematoma. A blunt, short-beveled No. 20 gauge needle and stylet are used for the procedure. The subdural space is approached at the lateral border of the anterior fontanel or along the upper margin of the coronal suture at least 2–3 cm from the midline to prevent injury to the underlying sagittal sinus. Following adequate cleansing and preparation of the skull, including shaving of the hair from the operative site, the patient is placed in the supine position and is firmly held by an attendant. The needle and stylet are slowly advanced through the skin and underlying tissue with a z-like movement until the dura is entered with a sudden "popping" sensation. Considerable care is taken to prevent advancement of the needle into the cerebral cortex, which in the infant is approximately 1.5 cm from the skin surface. The attachment of a hemostat approximately 5–7 mm from the beveled end of the needle should provide an adequate safeguard. The subdural fluid, which may squirt out under pressure, is collected and is sent for protein analysis, cell count, and culture. The color of the fluid may be xanthochromic, bright red, or an oily brown (depending on the age of the subdural collections). Bilateral subdural taps may be indicated, because subdural collections are bilateral in most cases. The amount of fluid removed with each tap should be limited to a total of 15–20 mL from each side in order to prevent rebleeding from a sudden shift of the intracranial contents. At the termination of the procedure, a sterile dressing is applied, and the child is placed in a sitting position that tends to prevent leakage of fluid from the puncture site. (See Chapter 169 for a discussion of subdural fluid associated with meningitis.)

VENTRICULAR TAP. A ventricular tap is used for the removal of CSF in the management of life-threatening increased intracranial pressure associated with hydrocephalus, when conservative measures have failed. The procedure should not be undertaken by a pediatrician except when the patient's life is in jeopardy and a neurosurgeon is not available. For the infant, the procedure is similar to a subdural tap. A No. 20 gauge ventricular needle with a stylet is placed in the lateral border of the anterior fontanel and is directed toward the inner canthus of the ipsilateral eye. The needle is advanced slowly, and the stylet is removed frequently to determine the presence of CSF. The ventricle is usually encountered about 4 cm from the skin surface.

NEURORADIOLOGIC PROCEDURES. The *skull roentgenogram* is a useful diagnostic procedure but unfortunately is frequently overlooked in the era of computed tomography (CT) scanning and magnetic resonance imaging (MRI). It may demonstrate fractures, intracranial calcification, craniosynostosis, congenital anomalies, or bony defects and evidence of increased intracranial pressure. Acute increased intracranial pressure is characterized by separation of the sutures, whereas erosion of the posterior clinoid processes, enlargement of the sella turcica, and an increase in convolutional markings indicate longstanding intracranial hypertension. *CT scanning* has revolutionized the neuroradiologic examination of children, obviating pneumoencephalography, and has greatly reduced the requirement for cerebral angiography. CT scanning is a noninvasive procedure that utilizes conventional x-ray techniques. Sedation is usually required for infants and young children, because a lack of head movement is essential during the study. Pentobarbital, 4 mg/kg IM 30 min before the CT scan, with a supplementary dose of 2 mg/kg IM 1–1½ hr later if necessary, is usually effective. Chloral hydrate, 50–75 mg/kg PO 45 min before the procedure, is an alternate method of sedation. CT scanning is useful in demonstrating congenital malformations of the brain, including hydrocephalus and porencephalic cysts, subdural collections, cerebral atrophy, intracranial calcification, intracerebral hematoma, brain tumors and areas of cerebral edema, infarction, and demyelination. The intravenous injection of radiographic contrast medium enhances areas of increased vascular permeability due to abnormalities of the blood-brain barrier and highlights abnormal collections of blood vessels in an arteriovenous malformation. *MRI* is a noninvasive procedure and is especially well suited for the study of neoplasms, cerebral edema, degenerative diseases, and congenital anomalies, particularly of the posterior fossa and spinal cord. MRI is capable of detecting small plaques in patients with multiple sclerosis and areas of localized gliosis in children with uncontrolled seizures. Intracerebral calcifications are not detected by MRI. The contrast agent, gadolinium-DTPA, is useful during MRI, especially to highlight lesions associated with a disrupted blood-brain barrier. *Radionuclide brain scan* utilizes a radioactive material such as ^{99}Tc, which concentrates in regions where the blood-brain barrier has been disrupted. It is useful in the investigation of herpes encephalitis and cerebral abscess. *Positron emission tomography* (PET) provides unique information on brain metabolism and perfusion by measuring blood flow, oxygen uptake, and glucose consumption. PET is an expensive technique that has been utilized primarily in adults, but its use for the study of epilepsy and metabolic and neurobehavioral disorders in the pediatric population holds considerable promise. *Single photon emission computerized tomography* (SPECT), using technetium Tc 99m hexamethyl propylenamine oxime (Tc 99m-HMPAO) is a sensitive and inexpensive technique to study regional cerebral blood flow. SPECT is particularly useful in the investigation of cerebral vascular disease in children (systemic lupus erythematosus), herpes encephalitis, localization of focal epileptiform discharges, and recurrent brain tumors. *Cerebral angiography* is reserved for the study of vascular disorders. The procedure requires a general anesthetic in most children. Cerebral angiography, utilizing subtraction techniques, is particularly useful for the delineation of arteriovenous malformations, aneurysms, arterial occlusions, and venous thrombosis. In most cases, a four-vessel study (internal carotids and vertebral arteries) is accomplished. *MRA* (angiography) may reduce the need for contrast invasive angiography. *Cranial ultrasound*, for the detection of intracranial hemorrhage, hydrocephalus, and intracranial tumors, is limited to the infant with a patent fontanel. The procedure is utilized intraoperatively in older children for the placement of shunts, for the location of small tumors, and for the direction of needle biopsies. *Myelography* was used in the past for the demonstration of congenital anomalies, tumors, and vascular malformations of the spinal cord. MRI is superior in most cases to contrast myelography and is not associated with arachnoiditis, which occasionally complicates the injection of contrast material into the subarachnoid space.

ELECTROENCEPHALOGRAPHY. The *electroencephalogram* (EEG) provides a continuous recording of electrical activity between reference electrodes placed on the scalp. Although the genesis of the electrical activity is not certain, it likely originates from postsynaptic potentials in the dendrites of cortical neurons. Even with amplification of the electrical activity, not all potentials are recorded due to the buffering effect of the scalp, muscles, bone, vessels, and subarachnoid fluid. The EEG waves are classified according to their frequency as delta (1–3/sec), theta (4–7/sec), alpha (8–12/sec), and beta (13–20/sec). These waves are altered by many factors, including age, state of alertness, eye closure, drugs, and disease states. The maturational changes between the neonate and childhood are evident in Figure 541–4. High-voltage slow and sharp waves (K complexes) and sleep spindles (regular 12–14/sec waves) confined to the central regions occur during sleep in the normal EEG. Abnormalities of waveform include spikes and slow waves. Spikes are characteristically paroxysmal, sharp, and of high voltage followed by a slow wave. Spikes and slow waves are associated with epilepsy, but some normal patients may have this EEG finding. Focal spikes are often associated with irritative lesions, including cysts, slow-growing tumors, and glial scar tissue. Epileptiform activity may be enhanced by activation procedures, including hyperventilation, photic stimulation, and sleep deprivation. Slow waves may be focal, in which case a circumscribed lesion such as a hematoma, tumor, infarction, or a localized infectious process may be considered; generalized slow waves suggest a metabolic, inflammatory, or more widespread process.

EEG/polygraphic/video monitoring provides precise characterization of seizure types, which allows for specific medical or surgical management. In addition, the physician is more accurately able to differentiate epileptic seizures from paroxysmal events that mimic epilepsy, including pseudoseizures. EEG/polygraphic/video monitoring provides for the quantification of seizure discharges and for the study of the efficacy of various therapeutic regimens. Finally, polygraphic/EEG with video monitoring simultaneously records physiologic and EEG changes, which is particularly useful in the neonate in whom the characterization of seizures is difficult.

EVOKED POTENTIALS. An evoked potential is an electrical response that follows stimulation of the CNS by a specific stimulus of the visual, auditory, or sensory system. The clinical application of evoked potentials in infants and children has increased dramatically during the last decade. Stimulation of the visual system by a flash or patterned stimulus, such as a black-and-white checkerboard, produces *visual evoked potentials* (VEPs), which are recorded over the occiput and averaged in a computer. Abnormal VEPs result from lesions involving the visual system from the retina to the visual cortex. Neurodegenerative diseases, such as Tay-Sachs, Krabbe, Pelizaeus-Merzbacher disease, and neuronal ceroid lipofuscinoses, show characteristic VEP abnormalities. Lesions of the optic nerve and

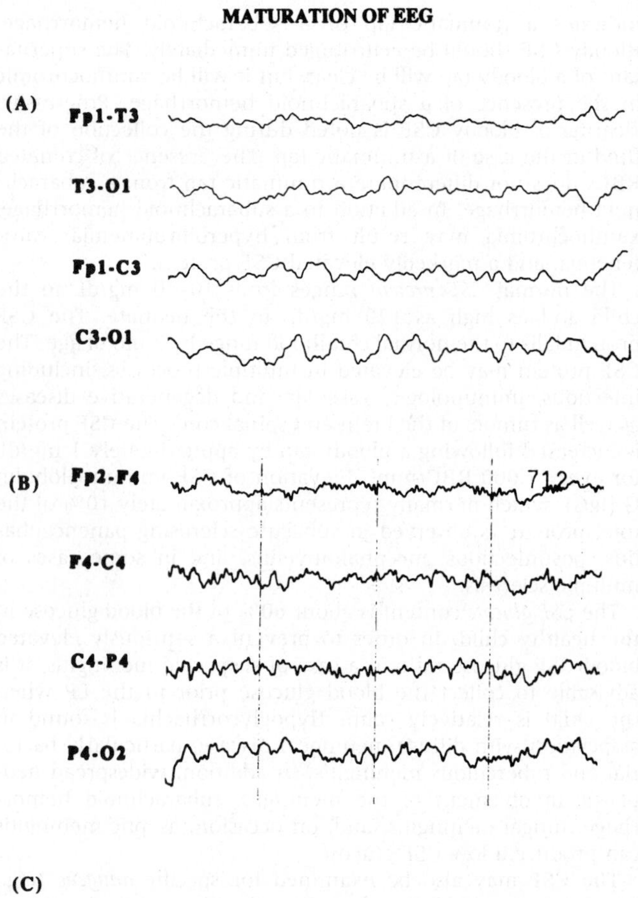

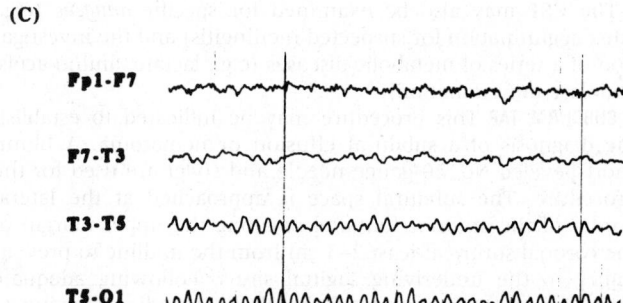

Figure 541–4. *A*, Normal waking record in a term infant. The background rhythm consists of low-amplitude 3- to 4-Hz activity. *B*, An 8-mo-old infant with occipital θ (5 Hz) and superimposed frontal β waves. *C*, Normal 9 yr old. Note the regular α rhythm in the occipital region.

chiasm also produce abnormalities in the VEP response. The VEP, using patterned stimuli, is useful particularly in the assessment of visual function in the at-risk neonate. Flash VEPs are also very useful in predicting outcome in term infants after asphyxia. *Brain stem auditory evoked potentials* (BAEPs) may be used to objectively measure hearing acuity, particularly in the neonate or uncooperative child when routine hearing assessment techniques have failed. The BAEP is abnormal in many neurodegenerative diseases in children and is an important tool in the evaluation of patients with suspected tumors of the cerebellopontine angle. BAEPs are helpful in the assessment of brain stem function in the comatose patient, because the waveforms are unaffected by drugs or by the level of consciousness. They are not accurate in predicting neurologic recovery and outcome. *Somatosensory evoked potentials* (SSEPs) are obtained by stimulating a peripheral nerve (peroneal, median) and by recording the electrical response over the cervical region and contralateral parietal somatosensory cortex. The SSEP determines the functional integrity of the dorsal column–medial-lemniscal system and is useful in monitoring spinal cord function during operative procedures, such as scoliosis, the repair of coarctation of the aorta, and myelomeningocele. SSEPs are abnormal in many neurodegenerative disorders in children and are the most accurate evoked potential in the assessment of neurologic outcome following a severe CNS insult.

Backman DS, Hodges FJ, Freeman JM: Computerized axial tomography in neurologic disorders of children. Pediatrics 59:352, 1977.

Ellis R: Lumbar cerebrospinal fluid opening pressure measured in a flexed lateral decubitus position in children. Pediatrics 93:622, 1994.

Gooding CA, Brasch RC, Lallemand DP, et al: Nuclear magnetic resonance imaging of the brain in children. J Pediatr 104:509, 1984.

Haslam RHA: Role of computed tomography in the early management of bacterial meningitis. J Pediatr 119:157, 1991.

Mizrahi EM: Electroencephalographic/polygraphic/video monitoring in childhood epilepsy. J Pediatr 105:1, 1984.

Packer RJ, Zimmerman RA, Sutton LN, et al: Magnetic resonance imaging of spinal cord disease of childhood. Pediatrics 78:251, 1986.

Portnoy JM, Olson LC: Normal cerebrospinal fluid values in children: Another look. Pediatrics 75:484, 1985.

Taylor MJ: Evoked potentials in paediatrics. *In*: Halliday AM (ed): Evoked Potentials in Clinical Testing, 2nd ed. Edinburgh, Churchill Livingstone, 1993, p 489.

CHAPTER 542

Congenital Anomalies of the Central Nervous System

542.1 Neural Tube Defects

(Dysraphism)

Neural tube defects account for most congenital anomalies of the CNS and result from the failure of the neural tube to close spontaneously between the 3rd and 4th wk of in utero development. Although the precise cause of neural tube defects remains unknown, there is evidence that many factors, including radiation, drugs, malnutrition, chemicals, and genetic determinants, may adversely affect the normal development of the CNS from the time of conception. In some cases, an abnormal maternal nutritional state or exposure to radiation prior to conception may increase the likelihood of a CNS congenital malformation. The major neural tube defects include spina bifida occulta, meningocele, myelomeningocele, encephalocele, anencephaly, dermal sinus, tethered cord, syringomyelia, diastematomyelia, and lipoma involving the conus medullaris.

The human nervous system originates from the primitive ectoderm that also develops into the epidermis. The ectoderm, endoderm, and mesoderm form the three primary germ layers that are developed by the 3rd wk. The endoderm, particularly the notochordal plate and the intraembryonic mesoderm, induces the overlying ectoderm to develop the neural plate during the 3rd wk of development (Fig. 542–1*A*). Failure of normal induction is responsible for most of the neural tube defects. Rapid growth of cells within the neural plate causes further invagination of the neural groove and the differentiation of a conglomerate of cells, the neural crest, which migrate laterally on the surface of the neural tube (see Fig. 542–1*B*). The notochordal plate becomes the centrally placed notochord, which acts as a foundation around which the vertebral column ultimately develops. With the formation of the vertebral column, the notochord undergoes involution and becomes the

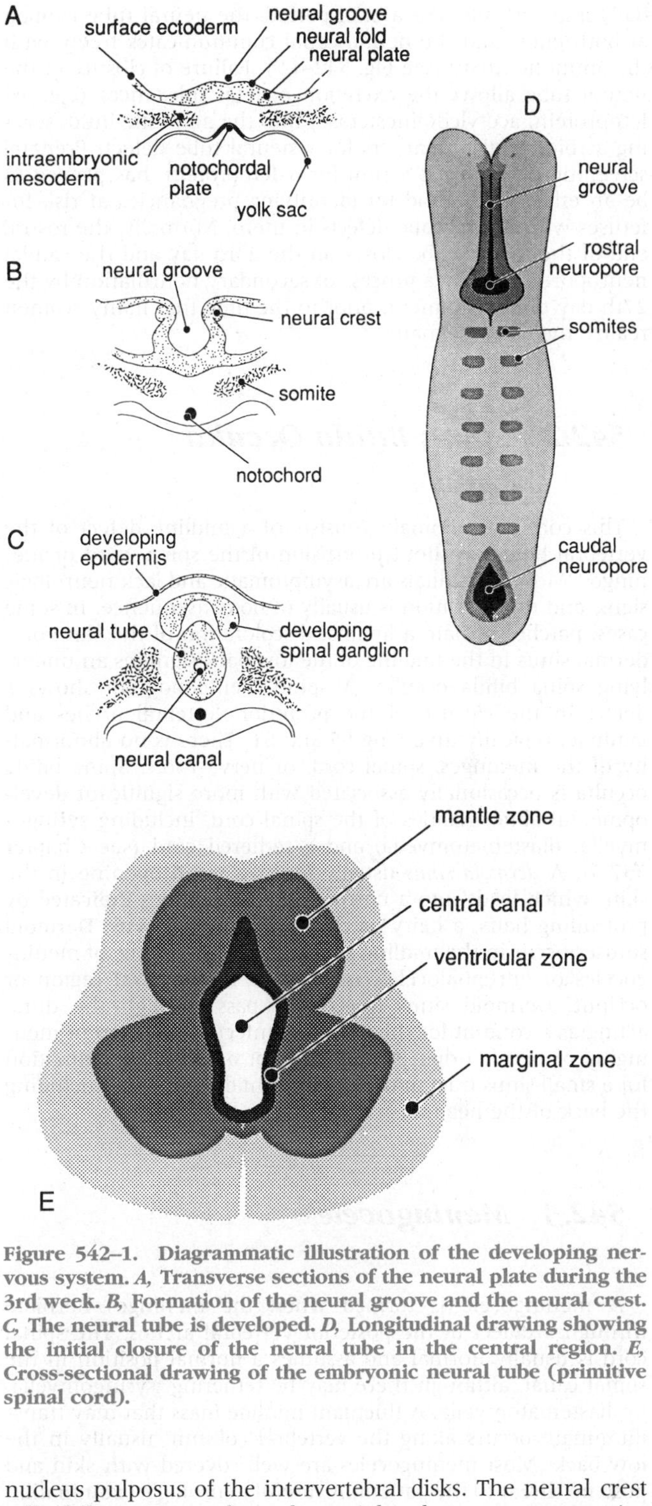

Figure 542–1. Diagrammatic illustration of the developing nervous system. *A*, Transverse sections of the neural plate during the 3rd week. *B*, Formation of the neural groove and the neural crest. *C*, The neural tube is developed. *D*, Longitudinal drawing showing the initial closure of the neural tube in the central region. *E*, Cross-sectional drawing of the embryonic neural tube (primitive spinal cord).

nucleus pulposus of the intervertebral disks. The neural crest cells differentiate to form the peripheral nervous system, including the spinal and autonomic ganglia as well as the ganglia of cranial nerves V, VII, VIII, IX, and X. In addition, the neural crest forms the leptomeninges, as well as Schwann cells, which are responsible for myelinization of the peripheral nervous system. The dura is believed to arise from the paraxial mesoderm.

During the 3rd wk of embryonic development, invagination of the neural groove is completed and the neural tube is formed by separation from the overlying surface ectoderm (see Fig. 542–1*C*). The initial closure of the neural tube is accomplished in the area corresponding to the future junction of the spinal cord and medulla, and moves rapidly both caudally and rostrally. For a brief period, the neural tube is open at both ends, and the neural canal communicates freely with the amniotic cavity (see Fig. 542–1*D*). Failure of closure of the neural tube allows the excretion of fetal substances (e.g., α-fetoprotein, acetylcholinesterase) into the amniotic fluid, serving as biochemical markers for a neural tube defect. Prenatal screening of maternal serum for α-fetoprotein, has proved to be an effective method for identifying pregnancies at risk for fetuses with neural tube defects in utero. Normally, the rostral end of the neural tube closes on the 23rd day and the caudal neuropore closes by a process of secondary neurulation by the 27th day of development, prior to the time that many women realize they are pregnant.

542.2 Spina Bifida Occulta

This common anomaly consists of a midline defect of the vertebral bodies without protrusion of the spinal cord or meninges. Most individuals are asymptomatic and lack neurologic signs, and the condition is usually of no consequence. In some cases, patches of hair, a lipoma, discoloration of the skin, or a dermal sinus in the midline of the low back signifies an underlying spina bifida occulta. A spine roentgenogram shows a defect in the closure of the posterior vertebral arches and laminae, typically involving L5 and S1. There is no abnormality of the meninges, spinal cord, or nerve roots. Spina bifida occulta is occasionally associated with more significant developmental abnormalities of the spinal cord, including syringomyelia, diastematomyelia, and a tethered cord (see Chapter 557.3). A *dermoid sinus* usually forms a small opening in the skin, which leads into a narrow duct, sometimes indicated by protruding hairs, a hairy patch, or a vascular nevus. Dermoid sinuses occur in the midline at the site of occurrence of meningoceles or encephaloceles, that is, the lumbosacral region or occiput. Dermoid sinus tracts may pass through the dura, acting as a conduit for the spread of infection. Recurrent meningitis of occult origin should prompt a careful examination for a small sinus tract in the posterior midline region, including the back of the head.

542.3 Meningocele

A meningocele is formed when the meninges herniate through a defect in the posterior vertebral arches. The spinal cord is usually normal and assumes a normal position in the spinal canal, although there may be tethering, syringomyelia, or diastematomyelia. A fluctuant midline mass that may transilluminate occurs along the vertebral column, usually in the low back. Most meningoceles are well covered with skin and pose no threat to the patient. A careful neurologic examination is mandatory. Asymptomatic children with a normal neurologic examination and full-thickness skin covering the meningocele may have surgery delayed. Prior to surgical correction of the defect, the patient must be thoroughly examined with the use of plain roentgenograms, ultrasound, and computed tomography (CT) scanning with metrizamide or magnetic resonance imaging (MRI) to determine the extent of neural tissue involvement, if any, and associated anomalies, including diastematomyelia, tethered spinal cord, and lipoma. Those patients with leaking cerebrospinal fluid (CSF) or a thin skin covering should undergo immediate surgical treatment to prevent meningitis. A CT scan of the head is recommended for children with a meningocele because of the association with hydrocephalus in some cases. An anterior meningocele projects into the pelvis through a defect in the sacrum. Symptoms of constipation and bladder dysfunction develop owing to the increasing size of the lesion. Female patients may have associated anomalies of the genital tract, including a rectovaginal fistula and vaginal septa. Plain roentgenograms demonstrate a defect in the sacrum and CT scanning or MRI outlines the extent of the meningocele.

542.4 Myelomeningocele

Myelomeningocele represents the most severe form of dysraphism involving the vertebral column and occurs with an incidence of approximately 1/1,000 live births.

ETIOLOGY. The cause of myelomeningocele is unknown, but as with all neural tube closure defects, a genetic predisposition exists; the risk of recurrence after one affected child rises to 3–4% and increases to approximately 10% with two previous abnormal pregnancies. Nutritional and environmental factors undoubtedly play a role in the etiology of myelomeningocele. Studies have provided strong evidence that maternal periconceptional use of folic acid supplementation greatly reduces the incidence of neural tube defects in pregnancies at risk. To be effective, folic acid supplementation should be initiated prior to conception and continued until at least 12 wk of gestation when neurulation is complete. The U.S. Public Health Service has recommended that all women of childbearing age capable of becoming pregnant take 0.4 mg of folic acid daily and that women who have previously had a pregnancy resulting in a neural tube defect be treated with 4 mg of folic acid daily, beginning 1 mo prior to the time the pregnancy is planned. As with any high-risk pregnancy, these patients require careful supervision, counseling, and follow-up. Certain drugs are also known to increase the risk of myelomeningocele. Valproic acid, an effective anticonvulsant, causes neural tube defects in approximately 1–2% of pregnancies if the drug is administered during pregnancy. The normal process of neurulation involves cellular and molecular mechanisms. The developmental regulation of specific genes and their products during the closing of the neural tube has suggested an important role for cytoskeletal microfilaments (actin, fodrin) and proteoglycans (basement membrane hyaluronate). Recent studies have used a number of models for dysraphism, which include rodent mutations and chromosomal aberrations, teratogens (retinoic acid), and interaction between predisposing genetic factors and environmental causative agents. With the notable exception of valproic acid, there are a few teratogens that produce dysraphism in both rodent models and humans.

CLINICAL MANIFESTATIONS. The condition produces dysfunction of many organs and structures, including the skeleton, skin, and genitourinary tract, in addition to the peripheral nervous system and the CNS. A myelomeningocele may be located anywhere along the neuraxis, but the lumbosacral region accounts for at least 75% of the cases. The extent and degree of the neurologic deficit depend on the location of the myelomeningocele. A lesion in the low sacral region causes bowel and bladder incontinence associated with anesthesia in the perineal area but with no impairment of motor function. The newborn with a defect in the mid-lumbar region typically has a saclike cystic structure covered by a thin layer of partially epithelialized tissue (Fig. 542–2). Remnants of neural tissue are visible beneath the membrane, which may occasionally rupture and leak CSF. An examination of the infant shows a flaccid paralysis of the lower extremities, an absence of deep tendon reflexes, a lack of response to touch and pain, and a high incidence of postural abnormalities of the lower extremi-

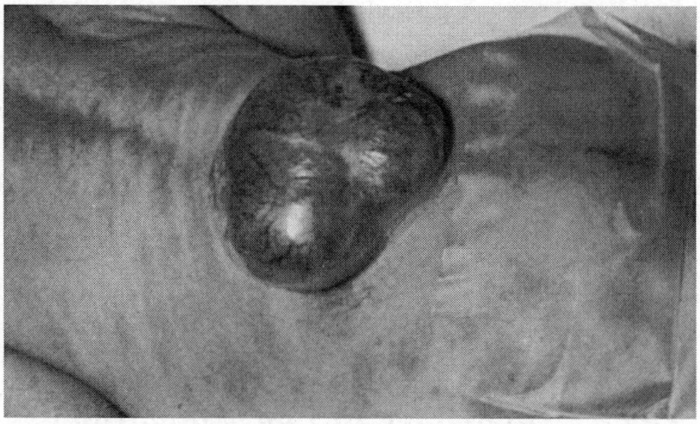

Figure 542–2. A lumbar myelomeningocele is covered by a thin layer of skin.

ties (including club feet and subluxation of the hips). Constant urinary dribbling and a relaxed anal sphincter may be evident. Thus, a myelomeningocele in the mid-lumbar region tends to produce lower motor neuron signs due to abnormalities and disruption of the conus medullaris. Infants with myelomeningocele typically have an increasing neurologic deficit as the myelomeningocele goes higher into the thoracic region. However, patients with a myelomeningocele in the upper thoracic or the cervical region usually have a very minimal neurologic deficit and in most cases do not have hydrocephalus.

Hydrocephalus in association with a type II Chiari defect develops in at least 80% of patients with myelomeningocele. Generally, the lower the deformity in the neuraxis (e.g., sacrum), the less likely will be the risk of hydrocephalus. Ventricular enlargement may be indolent and slow growing or it may be rapid, causing a bulging anterior fontanel, dilated scalp veins, "setting-sun" appearance of the eyes, irritability, and vomiting associated with an increased head circumference. Not infrequently, infants with hydrocephalus and the Chiari II malformation develop symptoms of hindbrain dysfunction, including difficulty feeding, choking, stridor, apnea, vocal cord paralysis, pooling of secretions, and spasticity of the upper extremities, which, if untreated, can lead to death. This *Chiari crisis* is due to downward herniation of the medulla and cerebellar tonsils through the foramen magnum.

TREATMENT. The management and supervision of a child and family with a myelomeningocele require a *multidisciplinary team approach*, including surgeons, physicians, and therapists, with one individual (often a pediatrician) acting as the advocate and coordinator of the treatment program. The news that a newborn child has a devastating condition such as myelomeningocele causes considerable grief and anger in the parents. They need time to learn about the handicap and the associated complications and to reflect on the various procedures and treatment plans. The parents must be given the facts by a knowledgeable individual in an unhurried and nonthreatening setting. If possible, discussions with other parents of children with neural tube defects are helpful in resolving important questions and issues.

In the past, it was advocated that the myelomeningocele should be repaired as soon as possible after birth to preserve neurologic function and to prevent further deterioration. Recent studies indicate similar long-term results with a delay in *surgery* for several days (with the exception of a CSF leak), which allows the parents to begin to adjust to the shock and to prepare for the multiple procedures and inevitable problems that lie ahead. Some centers have attempted to develop criteria for determining which infants will be treated aggressively and which will receive only supportive care. The most-quoted exclusion criteria, developed in the United Kingdom, consist of the following: marked paralysis of the legs; thoracolumbar or thoracolumbosacral lesions; kyphosis or scoliosis; associated birth injury; other congenital defects of the heart, brain, or gastrointestinal tract; and a grossly enlarged head. More recent information suggests that such selective criteria have little prognostic value, and as a result most pediatric centers aggressively treat the majority of infants with myelomeningocele. After the repair of the myelomeningocele, most infants require a shunting procedure for hydrocephalus. If symptoms or signs of hindbrain dysfunction appear, early surgical decompression of the medulla and cervical cord is indicated. Club feet may require casting, and dislocated hips may require operative procedures.

Careful evaluation and reassessment of the *genitourinary system* are some of the most important components of the management. Teaching the parents, and ultimately the patient, to regularly catheterize a neurogenic bladder maintains a low residual volume that prevents urinary tract infections and reflux leading to pyelonephritis and hydronephrosis. Periodic urine cultures and assessment of renal function, including serum electrolytes and creatinine as well as renal scans, intravenous pyelograms, and ultrasounds, are obtained according to the progress of the patient and the results of the physical examination. This approach to urinary tract management has greatly reduced the need for surgical diversionary procedures and has significantly decreased the morbidity and mortality associated with progressive renal disease in these patients. Some children can become continent with the surgical implantation of an artificial urinary sphincter at a later age. Although *incontinence of fecal matter* is common and is socially unacceptable during the school years, it does not pose the same risks as urinary incontinence. Many children can be "bowel-trained" with a regimen of timed enemas or suppositories that allows evacuation at a predetermined time once or twice a day. Also see Chapter 21.

Functional *ambulation* is the wish of each child and parent and may be possible depending on the level of the lesion and on the intact function of the iliopsoas muscles. Almost every child with a sacral or lumbosacral lesion obtains functional ambulation; approximately one half of the children with higher defects will ambulate with the use of braces and canes.

PROGNOSIS. For the child born with a myelomeningocele who is treated aggressively, the mortality rate is approximately 10–15%, and most deaths occur before 4 yr of age. At least 70% of survivors have normal intelligence, but learning problems and seizure disorders are more common than in the general population. Previous episodes of meningitis or ventriculitis adversely affect the ultimate intelligence quotient. Because myelomeningocele is a chronic handicapping condition, periodic multidisciplinary follow-up is required for life.

542.5 Encephalocele

There are two major forms of dysraphism affecting the skull, resulting in protrusion of tissue through a bony midline defect, called *cranium bifidum*. A *cranial meningocele* consists of a CSF-filled meningeal sac only, and a *cranial encephalocele* contains the sac plus cerebral cortex, cerebellum, or portions of the brain stem. Microscopic examination of the neural tissue within an encephalocele is often abnormal. The cranial defect occurs most commonly in the occipital region at or below the inion, but in certain parts of the world frontal or nasofrontal encephaloceles are more prominent. These abnormalities are one tenth as common as neural tube closure defects involving the spine. The etiology is presumed to be similar to that for anencephaly and myelomeningocele, because examples of each have been reported in the same family.

Infants with a cranial encephalocele are at increased risk for developing hydrocephalus due to aqueduct stenosis, a Chiari malformation, or the Dandy-Walker syndrome. Examination may show a small sac with a pedunculated stalk or a large cyst-like structure that may exceed the size of the cranium. The lesion may be completely covered with skin, but areas of denuded skin can occur and require urgent surgical management. Transillumination of the sac may indicate the presence of neural tissue. A plain roentgenogram of the skull and cervical spine is indicated to define the anatomy of the vertebra. An ultrasound is most helpful in determining the contents of the sac, obviating the need for a CT scan in most cases. Children with a cranial meningocele generally have a good prognosis, whereas patients with an encephalocele are at risk for visual problems, microcephaly, mental retardation, and seizures. Generally, children with neural tissue within the sac and associated hydrocephalus have the poorest prognosis. *Meckel-Gruber syndrome* is a rare autosomal recessive condition that is characterized by an occipital encephalocele, cleft lip or palate, microcephaly, microphthalmia, abnormal genitalia, polycystic kidneys, and polydactyly. Encephaloceles may be diagnosed in utero by the determination of α-fetoprotein levels and ultrasound measurement of the biparietal diameter.

542.6 Anencephaly

The anencephalic infant presents a distinctive appearance with a large defect of the calvarium, meninges, and scalp associated with a rudimentary brain, which results from a failure of closure of the rostral neuropore. The primitive brain consists of portions of connective tissue, vessels, and neuroglia. The cerebral hemispheres and cerebellum are usually absent, and only a residue of the brain stem can be identified. The pituitary gland is hypoplastic, and the spinal cord pyramidal tracts are missing due to the absence of the cerebral cortex. Additional anomalies include folding of the ears, cleft palate, and congenital heart defects in 10–20% of cases. Most anencephalic infants die within several days of birth. The incidence of anencephaly approximates 1/1,000 live births, and the greatest frequency is in Ireland and Wales. The recurrence risk is approximately 4% and increases to 10% if a couple has had two previously affected pregnancies. Many factors have been implicated as the cause of anencephaly (in addition to a genetic basis), including low socioeconomic status, nutritional and vitamin deficiencies, and a large number of environmental and toxic factors. It is very likely that several noxious stimuli interact on a genetically susceptible host to produce anencephaly. Fortunately, the frequency of anencephaly has been decreasing during the last two decades. Approximately 50% of anencephalic pregnancies are associated with polyhydramnios. Couples who have had an anencephalic infant should have successive pregnancies monitored, including amniocentesis, determination of α-fetoprotein levels, and an ultrasound examination between the 14th and 16th week of gestation.

Charney EB, Weller SC, Sutton LN, et al: Management of the newborn with myelomeningocele: Time for a decision-making process. Pediatrics 75:58, 1985.
Copp AJ, Brook FA, Estibeiro JP, et al: The embryonic development of mammalian neural tube defects. Prog Neurobiol 35:363, 1990.
Fernandes ET, Reinberg Y, Vernier R, et al: Neurogenic bladder dysfunction in children: Review of pathophysiology and current management. J Pediatr 124:1, 1994.
Haddow JE, Palomaki GE, Knight GJ, et al: Reducing the need for amniocentesis in women 35 years of age or older with serum markers for screening. N Engl J Med 330:1114, 1994.
Hannigan KF: Teaching intermittent self-catheterization to young children with myelodysplasia. Dev Med Child Neurol 21:365, 1979.
Lemire RJ, Beckwith JB, Warkany J: Anencephaly. New York, Raven Press, 1978.
Lorber J, Salfiedl S: Results of selective treatment of spina bifida cystica. Arch Dis Child 56:822, 1981.
McLone DG: Results of treatment of children born with a myelomeningocele. Clin Neurosurg 30:407, 1983.
McLone DG, Czyzewski D, Raimondi AJ, et al: Central nervous system infections as a limiting factor in the intelligence of children with myelomeningocele. Pediatrics 70:338, 1982.
MRC Vitamin Study Research Group: Prevention of neural tube defects: results of the Medical Research Council Vitamin Study. Lancet 338:131, 1991.
Norman D, Brant-Zawadski M, Yeates A, et al: Magnetic resonance imaging of the spinal cord and canal: Potentials and limitations. AJNR 5:9, 1985.
Opitz JM, Howe JJ: The Meckel syndrome. Birth Defects 5:167, 1969.
Robert E, Guibaud P: Maternal valproic acid and congenital neural tube defects. Lancet 2:937, 1982.

542.7 Disorders of Cell Migration

Disorders of cell migration may result in minor abnormalities with little or no clinical consequence (e.g., small heterotopia of neurons) or devastating abnormalities of the CNS (e.g., mental retardation, lissencephaly, schizencephaly). One of the most important mechanisms in the control of neuronal migration is the radial glial fiber system that guides neurons to their proper site. The severity and the extent of the disorder are related to numerous factors, including the timing of a particular insult and a host of environmental and genetic factors. Although abnormalities of lamination of the six layers of the cerebral cortex account for some important neurologic conditions related to cell migration, a brief description of the formation of the spinal cord will highlight the potential for errors in migration.

The embryonic neural tube consists of three zones: ventricular, mantle, and marginal (see Fig. 542–1*E*). The ependymal layer consists of a pluripotential, pseudostratified, columnar neuroepithelium. Specific neuroepithelial cells differentiate into primitive neurons or neuroblasts that form the mantle layer. The marginal zone is formed from cells in the outer layer of the neuroepithelium, which ultimately becomes the white matter. Glioblasts, which act as the primitive supportive cells of the CNS, also arise from the neuroepithelial cells in the ependymal zone. They migrate to the mantle and marginal zones and become future astrocytes and oligodendrocytes. It is likely that microglia originate from mesenchymal cells at a later stage of fetal development when blood vessels begin to penetrate the developing nervous system. A brief description of selected examples of disordered cell migration follows.

LISSENCEPHALY

Lissencephaly or agyria refers to a rare disorder that is characterized by the absence of cerebral convolutions and a poorly formed sylvian fissure, giving the appearance of a 3–4 mo fetal brain. The condition is probably the result of faulty neuroblast migration during early embryonic life and is usually associated with enlarged lateral ventricles and heterotopias in the white matter. There is a four-layered cortex, rather than the usual six, with a thin rim of periventricular white matter and numerous gray heterotopia visible by microscopic examination. Clinically, these infants present with failure to thrive, microcephaly, marked developmental delay, and a severe seizure disorder. Ocular abnormalities are common, including hypoplasia of the optic nerve and microphthalmia. Lissencephaly can occur as an isolated finding or in association with the *Miller-Dieker syndrome* (MDS). These children have characteristic facies, including a prominent forehead, bitemporal hollowing, anteverted nostrils, prominent upper lip, and micrognathia. About 90% of children with MDS have visible or submicroscopic chromosomal deletions of 17p13.3. The CT scan typically shows a smooth brain with an absence of sulci (Fig. 542–3).

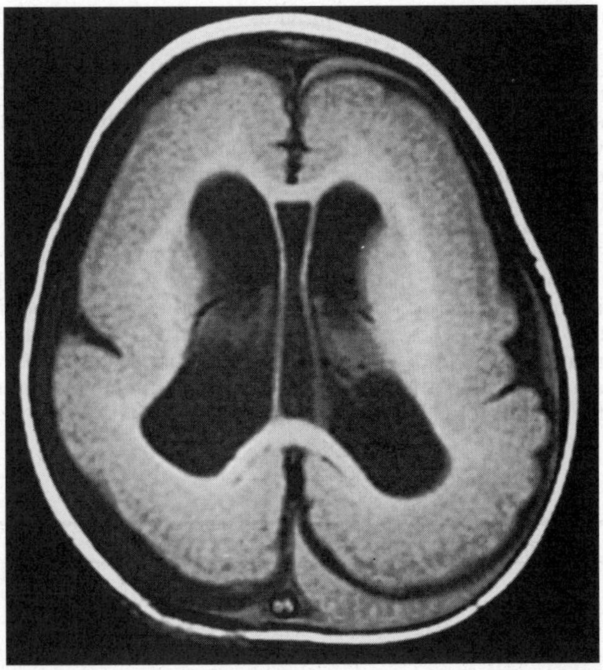

Figure 542–3. MRI of an infant with lissencephaly. Note the absence of cerebral sulci and the maldeveloped sylvian fissures associated with enlarged ventricles.

SCHIZENCEPHALY

Schizencephaly refers to the presence of unilateral or bilateral clefts within the cerebral hemispheres due to an abnormality of morphogenesis. The cleft may be fused or unfused and, if unilateral and large, may be confused with a porencephalic cyst. Not infrequently, the borders of the cleft are surrounded by abnormal brain, particularly microgyria. The CT scan is diagnostic and clearly demonstrates the size and extent of the cleft. Many patients are severely mentally retarded, with seizures that are difficult to control, and microcephalic, with spastic quadriparesis when the clefts are bilateral.

PORENCEPHALY

Porencephaly refers to the presence of cysts or cavities within the brain that result from development defects or acquired lesions, including infarction of tissue. *True porencephalic* cysts are most frequently located in the region of the sylvian fissure and typically communicate with the subarachnoid space, the ventricular system, or both. They represent developmental abnormalities of cell migration and are often associated with other malformations of the brain, including microcephaly, abnormal patterns of adjacent gyri, and encephalocele. These infants tend to have multiple problems, including mental retardation, spastic quadriparesis, optic atrophy, and seizures. *Pseudoporencephalic cysts* characteristically develop during the perinatal or postnatal period and result from abnormalities of arterial or venous circulation. These cysts tend to be unilateral; they do not communicate with a fluid-filled cavity; and they are not associated with abnormalities of cell migration or CNS malformations. Infants with pseudoporencephalic cysts present with hemiparesis and focal seizures during the 1st year of life.

542.8 Agenesis of the Corpus Callosum

Agenesis of the corpus callosum consists of a heterogeneous group of disorders that vary in expression from severe intellectual and neurologic abnormalities to the asymptomatic and normally intelligent individual. The corpus callosum develops from the commissural plate that lies in proximity to the anterior neuropore. An insult to the commissural plate during early embryogenesis causes agenesis of the corpus callosum. When agenesis of the corpus callosum is an isolated phenomenon, the patient may be normal, whereas individuals with neurologic symptoms, including mental retardation, microcephaly, hemiparesis, diplegia, and seizures, have associated brain anomalies due to cell migration defects, such as heterotopias, microgyria, and pachygyria (broad, wide gyri) in addition to the absence of the corpus callosum. The anatomic features are best depicted on a CT scan or by MRI and show widely separated frontal horns with an abnormally highly positioned third ventricle between the lateral ventricles. The MRI precisely outlines the extent of the corpus callosum defect. An absence of the corpus callosum may be inherited as an X-linked recessive trait or as an autosomal dominant trait. The condition may be associated with specific chromosomal disorders, particularly 8-trisomy and 18-trisomy. The *Aicardi syndrome* represents a complex disorder that affects many systems and is typically associated with agenesis of the corpus callosum. These patients are almost all female, suggesting a genetic abnormality of the X chromosome (it may be lethal in males during fetal life). Seizures become evident during the first few months and are typically resistant to anticonvulsants. The EEG shows independent activity recorded from both hemispheres as a result of the absent corpus callosum. All patients are severely mentally retarded and may have abnormal vertebrae that may be fused or only partially developed (e.g., hemivertebra). Abnormalities of the retina, including circumscribed pits or lacunae and coloboma of the optic disk, are the most characteristic findings of the Aicardi syndrome.

542.9 Agenesis of the Cranial Nerves

Absence of the cranial nerves or the corresponding central nuclei has been described in several conditions and includes the optic nerve, congenital ptosis, the Marcus Gunn phenomenon (sucking jaw movements causing simultaneous eyelid blinking; this congenital synkinesis results from abnormal innervation of the trigeminal and oculomotor nerves), the trigeminal and auditory nerves, and cranial nerves IX, X, XI, and XII. *Möbius syndrome* is characterized by bilateral facial weakness, which is often associated with abducens nerve paralysis. Hypoplasia or agenesis of brain stem nuclei as well as absent or decreased numbers of muscle fibers have been reported. These infants present in the newborn period with facial weakness, causing feeding difficulties due to a poor suck. The immobile, dull facies may give the incorrect impression of mental retardation; the prognosis for normal development is excellent in most cases.

542.10 Microcephaly

Microcephaly is defined as a head circumference that measures more than three standard deviations below the mean for age and sex. This condition is relatively common, particularly among the mentally retarded population. Although there are many causes of microcephaly, abnormalities in neuronal migration during fetal development, including heterotopias of neuronal cells and cytoarchitectural derangements, are found in many brains. Microcephaly may be subdivided into two main groups: primary (genetic) microcephaly and secondary (nongenetic) microcephaly. A precise diagnosis is important for genetic counseling and for prediction for future pregnancies.

ETIOLOGY. Primary microcephaly refers to a group of conditions that usually have no other malformations and follow a mendelian pattern of inheritance or are associated with a specific genetic syndrome. These infants are usually identified at birth because of a small head circumference. The more common types include familial and autosomal dominant microcephaly and a series of chromosomal syndromes that are summarized in Table 542–1. Secondary microcephaly results from a large number of noxious agents that may affect the fetus in utero or the infant during periods of rapid brain growth, particularly the first 2 yr of life.

CLINICAL MANIFESTATIONS. A thorough family history should be taken, seeking additional cases of microcephaly or disorders affecting the nervous system. It is important to obtain the patient's head circumference at birth. A very small head circumference implies a process that began early in embryonic or fetal development. An insult to the brain that occurs later in life, particularly beyond the age of 2 yr, is less likely to produce severe microcephaly. Serial head circumference measurements are more meaningful than a single determination, particularly when the abnormality is minimal. In addition, the head circumference of each parent and sibling should be recorded.

The laboratory investigation of the microcephalic child is determined by the history and physical examination. If the cause of the microcephaly is unknown, the mother's serum phenylalanine level should be determined. High phenylalanine serum levels in an asymptomatic mother can produce marked brain damage in the otherwise normal nonphenylketonuric infant. A karyotype is obtained if a chromosomal syndrome is

■ TABLE 542–1 Causes of Microcephaly

Causes	Characteristic Findings
Primary (Genetic)	
1. Familial (autosomal recessive)	• Incidence 1/40,000 births • Typical appearance with slanted forehead, prominent nose and ears; severely mentally retarded and prominent seizures; surface convolutional markings of the brain poorly differentiated and disorganized cytoarchitecture
2. Autosomal dominant	• Nondistinctive facies, upslanting palpebral fissures, mild forehead slanting, and prominent ears • Normal linear growth, seizures readily controlled, and mild or borderline mental retardation
3. Syndromes	
Down (21-trisomy)	• Incidence 1/800 • Abnormal rounding of occipital and frontal lobes and a small cerebellum; narrow superior temporal gyrus, propensity for Alzheimer neurofibrillary alterations, and ultrastructure abnormalities of cerebral cortex
Edward (18-trisomy)	• Incidence 1/6,500 • Low birthweight, microstomia, micrognathia, low-set malformed ears, prominent occiput, rocker-bottom feet, flexion deformities of fingers, congenital heart disease, increased gyri, heterotopias of neurons
Cri-du-chat (5 p-)	• Incidence 1/50,000 • Round facies, prominent epicanthic folds, low-set ears, hypertelorism, and characteristic cry • No specific neuropathology
Cornelia de Lange	• Prenatal and postnatal growth delay, synophrys, thin down-turning upper lip • Proximally placed thumb
Rubinstein-Taybi	• Beaked nose, downward slanting of palpebral fissures, epicanthic folds, short stature with broad thumbs and toes
Smith-Lemli-Opitz	• Ptosis, scaphocephaly, inner-epicanthic folds, anteverted nostrils • Low birthweight, marked feeding problems
Secondary (Nongenetic)	
1. Radiation	• Microcephaly and mental retardation most severe if exposure prior to 15th wk of gestation
2. Congenital infections	
Cytomegalovirus	• Small for dates, petechial rash, hepatosplenomegaly, chorioretinitis, deafness, mental retardation, and seizures • CNS calcification and microgyria
Rubella	• Growth retardation, purpura, thrombocytopenia, hepatosplenomegaly, congenital heart disease, chorioretinitis, cataracts, and deafness • Perivascular necrotic areas, polymicrogyria, heterotopias, subependymal cavitations
Toxoplasmosis	• Purpura, hepatosplenomegaly, jaundice, convulsions, hydrocephalus, chorioretinitis, and cerebral calcification
3. Drugs	
Fetal alcohol	• Growth retardation, ptosis, absent philtrum and hypoplastic upper lip, congenital heart disease, feeding problems, neuroglial heterotopia, and disorganization of neurons
Fetal hydantoin	• Growth delay, hypoplasia of distal phalanges, inner-epicanthic folds, broad nasal ridge, and anteverted nostrils
4. Meningitis/encephalitis	• Cerebral infarcts, cystic cavitation, diffuse loss of neurons
5. Malnutrition	• Controversial cause of microcephaly
6. Metabolic	• Maternal diabetes mellitus and maternal hyperphenylalaninemia
7. Hyperthermia	• Significant fever during 1st 4–6 wk has been reported to cause microcephaly, seizures, and facial anomalies • Pathologic studies show neuronal heterotopias • Further studies showed no abnormalities with maternal fever
8. Hypoxic-ischemic encephalopathy	• Initially diffuse cerebral edema; late stages characterized by cerebral atrophy

suspected or if the child has abnormal facies, short stature, and additional congenital anomalies. CT scanning or MRI may be useful in identifying structural abnormalities of the brain or intracerebral calcification. Additional studies include a fasting plasma and urine amino acid analysis; serum ammonium; *to*xoplasmosis, *r*ubella, *c*ytomegalovirus, and *h*erpes simplex (TORCH) titers of the mother and child; and a urine sample for the culture of cytomegalovirus.

TREATMENT. Once the cause of the microcephaly has been established, the physician must provide accurate and supportive genetic and family counseling. Because many children with microcephaly will also be mentally retarded, the physician must assist with placement in an appropriate program that will provide the maximum development of the child (Chapter 40).

Barth PG: Disorders of neuronal migration. Can J Neurol Sci 14:1, 1987.
Dobyns WB, Reiner O, Carrozzo R, et al: A human brain malformation associated with deletion of L1S1 gene located at chromosome 17p13. JAMA 270:2838, 1993.
Dobyns WB, Stratton RF, Greenberg F: Syndromes with lissencephaly. 1: Miller-Dieker and Norman-Roberts syndromes and isolated lissencephaly. Am J Med Genet 18:509, 1984.
Harwood-Nash DC: Congenital craniocerebral abnormalities and computed tomography. Semin Roentgenol 12:39, 1977.
Haslam RHA: Microcephaly. *In:* Vinken PJ, Bruyn G, Klawans HL (eds): Handbook of Clinical Neurology. Amsterdam, Elsevier Science Publishers, 1987, pp 267–284.
Ledbetter SA, Kuwano A, Dobyns WB, et al: Microdeletions of chromosome: A cause of isolated lissencephaly. Am J Hum Genet 50:182, 1992.
Miller GM, Stears JC, Guggenheim MA, et al: Schizencephaly: A clinical and CT study. Neurology 34:997, 1984.
Molina JA, Mateos F, Merino M, et al: Aicardi syndrome in two sisters. J Pediatr 115:282, 1989.
Naeff RW: Clinical features of porencephaly. Arch Neurol Psychiatry 80:133, 1958.
Nerdich JA, Nussbaum RL, Packer TCJ, et al: Heterogeneity of clinical severity and molecular lesions in Aicardi syndrome. J Pediatr 116:911, 1990.
Parrish ML, Roessmann U, Levinsohn MW: Agenesis of the corpus callosum: A study of the frequency of associated malformations. Ann Neurol 6:349, 1979.
Sudarshan A, Goldie WD: The spectrum of congenital facial diplegia (Moebius syndrome). Pediatr Neurol 1:180, 1985.

542.11 Hydrocephalus

Hydrocephalus is not a specific disease; rather, it represents a diverse group of conditions, which result from impaired circulation and absorption of CSF or, in the rare circumstance, from increased production by a choroid plexus papilloma.

PHYSIOLOGY. The CSF is formed primarily in the ventricular system by the choroid plexus, which is situated in the lateral, third, and fourth ventricles. Although the majority of CSF is produced in the lateral ventricles, approximately 25% originates from extrachoroidal sources, including the capillary endothelium within the brain parenchyma. There is active neurogenic control of CSF formation as the choroid plexus is innervated by adrenergic and cholinergic nerves. Stimulation of the adrenergic system diminishes CSF production, whereas excitation of the cholinergic nerves may double the normal CSF production rate. In the normal child, approximately 20 mL of CSF is produced per hour. The total volume of CSF approximates 50 mL in an infant and 150 mL in an adult. Most of the CSF is extraventricular. CSF is formed by the choroid plexus in several stages; through a series of intricate steps a plasma ultrafiltrate is ultimately processed into a secretion, the CSF.

CSF flow results from the pressure gradient that exists between the ventricular system and venous channels. The intraventricular pressure may be as high as 180 mm of water in the normal state, whereas the pressure in the superior sagittal sinus is in the range of 90 mm of water. Normally, CSF flows from the lateral ventricles through the foramina of Monro into the third ventricle. It then traverses the narrow aqueduct of Sylvius, which is approximately 3 mm in length and 2 mm in diameter in the child, to enter the fourth ventricle. The CSF exits the fourth ventricle through the paired lateral foramina of Luschka and the midline foramen of Magendie into the cisterns at the base of the brain. Hydrocephalus resulting from obstruction within the ventricular system is called *obstructive* or *noncommunicating hydrocephalus*. The CSF circulates from the basal cisterns posteriorly over the cerebellum and cerebral cortex, and anteriorly through the cistern system and over the convexities of the cerebral hemispheres. CSF is absorbed primarily by the arachnoid villi through tight junctions of their endothelium by the pressure forces that were noted earlier. CSF is absorbed to a much lesser extent by the lymphatic channels directed to the paranasal sinuses, along nerve root sleeves, and by the choroid plexus itself. Hydrocephalus resulting from obliteration of the subarachnoid cisterns or malfunction of the arachnoid villi is called *nonobstructive* or *communicating hydrocephalus*.

PATHOPHYSIOLOGY AND ETIOLOGY. Obstructive or noncommunicating hydrocephalus develops most commonly in children because of an abnormality of the aqueduct or a lesion in the fourth ventricle. *Aqueductal stenosis* results from an abnormally narrow aqueduct of Sylvius that is often associated with branching or forking. In a small percentage of cases, aqueductal stenosis is inherited as a sex-linked recessive trait. These patients occasionally have minor neural tube closure defects, including spina bifida occulta. Rarely, aqueductal stenosis is associated with neurofibromatosis. *Aqueductal gliosis* may also give rise to hydrocephalus. As a result of neonatal meningitis or a subarachnoid hemorrhage in a premature infant, the ependymal lining of the aqueduct is interrupted and a brisk glial response results in complete obstruction. Intrauterine viral infections may also produce aqueductal stenosis followed by hydrocephalus, and mumps meningoencephalitis has been reported as a cause in a child. A vein of Galen malformation can expand to a large size and, because of its midline position, obstruct the flow of CSF. Lesions or malformations of the posterior fossa are prominent causes of hydrocephalus, including posterior fossa brain tumors, the Chiari malformation, and the Dandy-Walker syndrome.

Nonobstructive or communicating hydrocephalus most commonly follows a subarachnoid hemorrhage, which is usually the result of intraventricular hemorrhage in the premature infant. Blood in the subarachnoid spaces may cause obliteration of the cisterns or arachnoid villi, and obstruction of CSF flow. Pneumococcal and tuberculous meningitis have a propensity to produce a thick, tenacious exudate that obstructs the basal cisterns, and intrauterine infections may also destroy the CSF pathways. Finally, leukemic infiltrates may seed the subarachnoid space and produce communicating hydrocephalus.

CLINICAL MANIFESTATIONS. The clinical presentation of hydrocephalus is variable and depends on many factors, including the age of onset, the nature of the lesion causing obstruction, and the duration and rate of rise of the intracranial pressure. In the infant, an accelerated rate of enlargement of the head is the most prominent sign. In addition, the anterior fontanel is wide open and bulging, and the scalp veins are dilated. The forehead is broad and the eyes may deviate downward because of the impingement of the dilated suprapineal recess on the tectum, producing the "setting-sun" eye sign. Long-tract signs including brisk tendon reflexes, spasticity, clonus (particularly in the lower extremities), and Babinski sign are common due to stretching and disruption of the corticospinal fibers originating from the leg region of the motor cortex. In the older child, the cranial sutures are partially closed so that the signs of hydrocephalus may be more subtle. Irritability, lethargy, poor appetite, and vomiting are common to both age groups, and headache is a prominent symptom in the older age patient. A gradual change in personality and a deterioration in academic productivity suggests a slowly progressive form of hydrocephalus. Serial measurements of the head circumference indicate an increased velocity of growth. Percussion of the skull may produce a "cracked-pot" or *Macewen sign*, indicating separation of the sutures. A foreshortened occiput suggests the Chiari malformation, and a prominent occiput suggests the Dandy-Walker malformation. Papilledema, abducens nerve palsy, and pyramidal tract signs, which are most evident in the lower extremities, are apparent in most cases.

The *Chiari malformation* consists of two major subgroups. Type I typically produces symptoms during adolescence or adult life and is usually not associated with hydrocephalus. These patients complain of recurrent headache, neck pain, urinary frequency, and progressive lower extremity spasticity. The deformity consists of displacement of the cerebellar tonsils into the cervical canal. Although the pathogenesis is unknown, the prevailing theory suggests that obstruction of the caudal portion of the fourth ventricle during fetal development is responsible. The type II Chiari malformation is characterized by progressive hydrocephalus and a myelomeningocele. This lesion represents an anomaly of the hindbrain, probably due to a failure of pontine flexure during embryogenesis, and results in elongation of the fourth ventricle and kinking of the brain stem, with displacement of the inferior vermis, pons, and medulla into the cervical canal. Approximately 10% of type II malformations produce symptoms during infancy consisting of stridor, weak cry, and apnea, which may be relieved by shunting or by posterior fossa decompression. A more indolent form consists of abnormalities of gait, spasticity, and increasing incoordination during childhood. Plain skull radiographs show a small posterior fossa and a widened cervical canal. CT scanning with contrast and MRI display the cerebellar tonsils protruding downward into the cervical canal and the hindbrain abnormalities. The anomaly is treated by surgical decompression.

The *Dandy-Walker malformation* consists of a cystic expansion of the fourth ventricle in the posterior fossa, which results from a developmental failure of the roof of the 4th ventricle during embryogenesis (Fig. 542–4). Approximately 90% of patients have hydrocephalus, and a significant number of children have associated anomalies, including agenesis of the posterior cerebellar vermis and corpus callosum. Infants present

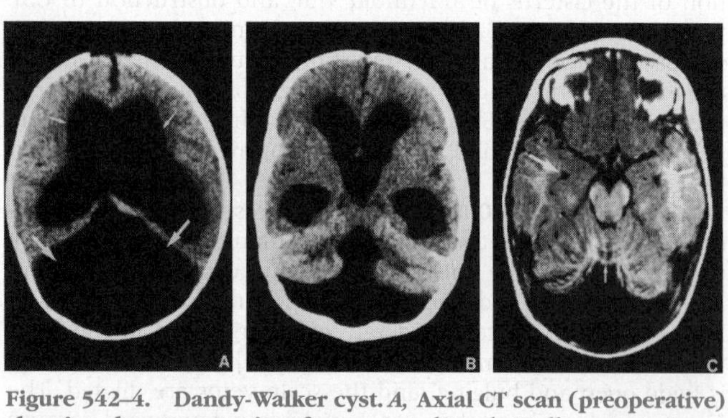

Figure 542–4. Dandy-Walker cyst. *A*, Axial CT scan (preoperative) showing large posterior fossa cyst (Dandy-Walker cyst; *large arrows*) and dilated lateral ventricles *(small arrows)*, a complication secondary to CSF pathway obstruction at the 4th ventricular outlet. *B*, Same patient, with a lower axial CT scan showing splaying of the cerebellar hemispheres by the dilated 4th ventricle (Dandy-Walker cyst). The dilated ventricles proximal to the 4th ventricle again show CSF obstruction due to the Dandy-Walker cyst. *C*, MRI of the same patient showing decreased size of the Dandy-Walker cyst and temporal horns *(arrows)* following shunting. The incomplete vermis *(small arrow)* now becomes recognizable.

with a rapid increase in head size and a prominent occiput. Transillumination of the skull may be positive. Most children have evidence of long-tract signs, cerebellar ataxia, and delayed motor and cognitive milestones, probably owing to the associated structural anomalies. The Dandy-Walker malformation is managed by shunting the cystic cavity (and on occasion the ventricles as well) in the presence of hydrocephalus.

DIAGNOSIS AND DIFFERENTIAL DIAGNOSIS. The investigation of a child with hydrocephalus begins with the history. Familial cases suggest X-linked hydrocephalus secondary to aqueductal stenosis. A past history of prematurity with intracranial hemorrhage, meningitis, or mumps encephalitis is important to ascertain. Multiple café-au-lait spots and other clinical features of neurofibromatosis point to aqueductal stenosis as the cause of hydrocephalus. Examination includes careful inspection, palpation, and auscultation of the skull and spine. The occipitofrontal head circumference is recorded and compared with previous measurements. The size and configuration of the anterior fontanel are noted, and the back is inspected for abnormal midline skin lesions, including tufts of hair, lipoma, or angioma that might suggest spinal dysraphism. The presence of a prominent forehead or abnormalities in the shape of the occiput may suggest the pathogenesis of the hydrocephalus. A cranial bruit is audible in association with many cases of vein of Galen arteriovenous malformation. Transillumination of the skull is positive with massive dilatation of the ventricular system or in the Dandy-Walker syndrome. Inspection of the eyegrounds is mandatory because the finding of chorioretinitis suggests an intrauterine infection such as toxoplasmosis as a cause of the hydrocephalus. Papilledema is observed in older children but is rarely present in infants because the cranial sutures separate as a result of the increased pressure. Plain skull films typically show separation of the sutures, erosion of the posterior clinoids in the older child, and an increase in convolutional markings ("beaten-silver appearance") with longstanding increased intracranial pressure. The CT scan and/or MRI along with ultrasound in the infant are the most important studies to identify the specific cause of hydrocephalus.

The head may appear enlarged secondary to a thickened cranium resulting from chronic anemia, rickets, osteogenesis imperfecta, and epiphyseal dysplasia. Chronic subdural collections can produce bilateral parietal bone prominence. Various metabolic and degenerative disorders of the CNS produce megalencephaly due to abnormal storage of substances within the brain parenchyma. These disorders include lysosomal diseases (e.g., Tay-Sachs, gangliosidosis, and the mucopolysaccharidoses), the aminoacidurias (e.g., maple syrup urine disease [MSUD]), and the leukodystrophies (e.g., metachromatic, Alexander disease, and Canavan disease). In addition, cerebral gigantism and neurofibromatosis are characterized by increased brain mass. Familial megalencephaly is inherited as an autosomal dominant and is characterized by delayed motor milestones and hypotonia but normal or near-normal intelligence. Measurement of the parent's head circumference is necessary to establish the diagnosis. *Hydranencephaly* may be confused with hydrocephalus. The cerebral hemispheres are absent or represented by membranous sacs with remnants of frontal, temporal, or occipital cortex dispersed over the membrane. The midbrain and brain stem are relatively intact (Fig. 542–5). The cause of hydranencephaly is unknown, but bilateral occlusion of the internal carotid arteries during early fetal development would explain most of the pathologic abnormalities. The infant may have a normal or enlarged head circumference at birth that grows at an excessive rate postnatally. Transillumination shows an absence of the cerebral hemispheres. The child is irritable, feeds poorly, develops seizures and spastic quadriparesis, and has little or no cognitive development. A ventriculoperitoneal shunt prevents massive enlargement of the cranium.

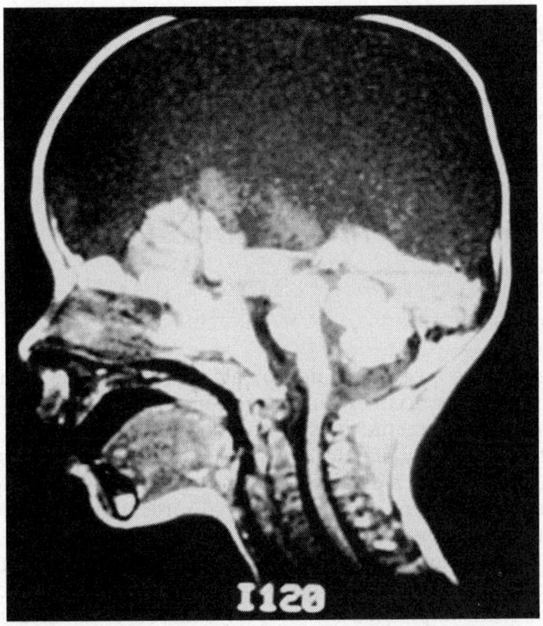

Figure 542–5. Hydranencephaly. MRI showing the brain stem and spinal cord with remnants of the cerebellum and the cerebral cortex. The remainder of the cranium is filled with CSF.

TREATMENT. Therapy for hydrocephalus depends on the cause. Medical management, including the use of acetazolamide and furosemide, may provide temporary relief by reducing the rate of CSF production, but long-term results have been disappointing. Most cases of hydrocephalus require extracranial shunts, particularly a ventriculoperitoneal shunt (occasionally a ventriculostomy will suffice). The major complication of shunts is bacterial infection, usually due to *Staphylococcus epidermidis* (Chapter 174). With meticulous preparation, the shunt infection rate can be reduced to 0–2%. The results of intrauterine surgical management of fetal hydrocephalus have been poor, possibly because of the high rate of associated cerebral malformations in addition to the hydrocephalus.

PROGNOSIS. This depends on the cause of the dilated ventricles and not on the size of the cortical mantle at the time of operative intervention. Hydrocephalic children are at increased risk for a variety of developmental disabilities. The mean intelligence quotient is reduced compared with the general population, particularly for performance tasks as contrasted to verbal abilities. Most children have abnormalities in memory function. Visual problems are common, including strabismus, visuospatial abnormalities, visual field defects, and optic atrophy with decreased acuity secondary to increased intracranial pressure. The visual-evoked potential latencies are delayed and take some time to recover following correction of the hydrocephalus. Although most hydrocephalic children are pleasant and mild mannered, some children show aggressive and delinquent behavior. It is imperative that the hydrocephalic child receive long-term follow-up in a multidisciplinary setting.

Cochrane DD, Myles ST, Nimrod C, et al: Intrauterine hydrocephalus and ventriculomegaly: Associated abnormalities and fetal outcome. Can J Neurol Sci 12:51, 1985.
Cull C, Wyke MA: Memory function of children with spina bifida and shunted hydrocephalus. Dev Med Child Neurol 26:177, 1984.
De Myer W: Megalencephaly in children. Neurology 22:634, 1972.
Dennis M, Fitz CR, Netley CT, et al: The intelligence of hydrocephalic children. Arch Neurol 38:607, 1981.
Fernell E, Hagberg G, Hagberg B: Infantile hydrocephalus epidemiology: an indicator of enhanced survival. Arch Dis Child 70:123, 1994.
Fitzsimmons JS: Laryngeal stridor and respiratory obstruction in association with myelomeningocele. Dev Med Child Neurol 15:533, 1973.
Greene M, Benaceraf B, Crawford J: Hydranencephaly: Ultrasound appearance in utero evolution. Radiology 156:779, 1985.
Hirsch JF, Pierre-Kahn A, Renier D, et al: The Dandy-Walker malformation. J Neurosurg 61:515, 1984.
Hoffman HJ, Hendrick EB, Humphreys RP: Manifestations and management of Arnold-Chiari malformations in patients with myelomeningocele. Childs Brain 1:255, 1975.
Jackson JC, Blumhagen JD: Congenital hydrocephalus due to prenatal intracranial hemorrhage. Pediatrics 72:344, 1983.
Johnson RT, Johnson KP, Edmonds CJ: Virus-induced hydrocephalus: Development of aqueductal stenosis in hamsters after mumps infection. Science 157:1066, 1967.

542.12 *Craniosynostosis*

Craniosynostosis is defined as premature closure of the cranial sutures and is classified as primary or secondary. *Primary craniosynostosis* refers to the closure of one or more sutures due to abnormalities of skull development, whereas *secondary craniosynostosis* results from failure of brain growth and expansion and will not be discussed further. The incidence of primary craniosynostosis approximates 1 per 2,000 births. The cause is unknown in the majority of children; however, genetic syndromes account for 10–20% of cases.

DEVELOPMENT AND ETIOLOGY. A review of skull development is helpful in understanding the genesis of craniosynostosis. During early development, the brain is enveloped by a film of mesenchyme. By the 2nd mo, osseous tissue is evident in that portion of the mesenchyme corresponding to the cranium, and cartilaginous tissue is formed at the base of the skull. The bones of the cranium are well developed by the 5th mo of gestation (frontal, parietal, temporal, and occipital) and are separated by sutures and fontanels. The brain grows rapidly during the first several years of life and is normally not impeded because of equivalent growth along the suture lines. The etiology of craniosynostosis is unknown, but the prevailing hypothesis suggests that abnormal development of the base of the skull creates exaggerated forces on the dura that act to disrupt normal cranial suture development. Dysfunctional osteoblasts or osteoclasts are not responsible for craniosynostosis.

CLINICAL MANIFESTATIONS AND TREATMENT. Most cases of craniosynostosis are evident at birth and are characterized by a skull deformity that is the direct result of premature suture fusion. Palpation of the suture reveals a prominent bony ridge, and fusion of the suture may be confirmed by plain skull roentgenograms or bone scan in ambiguous cases.

Premature closure of the sagittal suture produces a long and narrow skull or *scaphocephaly,* the most common form of craniosynostosis. Scaphocephaly is associated with a prominent occiput and a broad forehead and a small or absent anterior fontanel. The condition is sporadic and more common in males, and often causes difficulties during labor because of cephalopelvic disproportion. Scaphocephaly does not produce increased intracranial pressure or hydrocephalus, and the neurological examination of affected patients is normal.

Frontal plagiocephaly is the next most common form of craniosynostosis and is characterized by unilateral flattening of the forehead, elevation of the ipsilateral orbit and eyebrow, and a prominent ear on the corresponding side. The condition is more common in females and is the result of premature fusion of a coronal and sphenofrontal suture. Surgical intervention produces a cosmetically pleasing result.

Occipital plagiocephaly is most often the result of positioning during infancy and is more common in an immobile or handicapped child, but fusion or sclerosis of the lambdoid suture can cause unilateral occipital flattening and bulging of the ipsilateral frontal bone. *Trigonocephaly* is a rare form of craniosynostosis due to premature fusion of the metopic suture.

These children have a keel-shaped forehead and hypotelorism, and are at risk for associated developmental abnormalities of the forebrain. *Turricephaly* refers to a conical-shaped head due to premature fusion of the coronal and often sphenofrontal and frontoethmoidal sutures. The *kleeblattschädel deformity* is a peculiarly shaped skull that resembles a cloverleaf. These children have very prominent temporal bones, and the remainder of the cranium is constricted. Hydrocephalus is a common complication.

Premature fusion of only one suture rarely causes a neurologic deficit. In this situation, the sole indication for surgery is to enhance the cosmetic appearance of the child, and the prognosis depends on the suture involved and on the degree of disfigurement. Neurologic complications, including hydrocephalus and increased intracranial pressure, are more likely to occur when two or more sutures are prematurely fused, in which case operative intervention is essential.

The most prevalent genetic disorders associated with craniosynostosis include Crouzon, Apert, Carpenter, Chotzen, and Pfeiffer syndromes. *Crouzon syndrome* is characterized by premature craniosynostosis and is inherited as an autosomal dominant trait. The shape of the head depends on the timing and order of suture fusion but most often produces a compressed back-to-front diameter or brachycephalic skull due to bilateral closure of the coronal sutures. The orbits are underdeveloped, and ocular proptosis is prominent. Hypoplasia of the maxilla and orbital hypertelorism are typical facial features.

Apert syndrome has many features in common with Crouzon syndrome. However, Apert syndrome is usually a sporadic condition, although autosomal dominant inheritance may occur. It is associated with premature fusion of multiple sutures, including the coronal, sagittal, squamosal, and lambdoid sutures. The facies tend to be asymmetric, and the eyes are less proptotic compared with Crouzon syndrome. Apert syndrome is characterized by syndactyly of the 2nd, 3rd, and 4th fingers, which may be joined to the thumb and the 5th finger. Similar abnormalities often occur in the feet. All patients have progressive calcification and fusion of the bones of the hands, feet, and cervical spine.

Carpenter syndrome is inherited as an autosomal recessive condition, and the multiple fusion of sutures tends to produce the kleeblattschädel skull deformity. Soft-tissue syndactyly of the hands and feet is always present, and mental retardation is common. Additional, but less common, abnormalities include congenital heart disease, corneal opacities, coxa valga, and genu valgum.

Chotzen syndrome is characterized by asymmetric craniosynostosis and plagiocephaly. The condition is the most prevalent of the genetic syndromes and is inherited as an autosomal dominant trait. It is associated with facial asymmetry, ptosis of the eyelids, shortened fingers, and soft-tissue syndactyly of the 2nd and 3rd fingers.

Pfeiffer syndrome is most often associated with turricephaly. The eyes are prominent and widely spaced, and the thumbs and great toes are short and broad. Partial soft-tissue syndactyly may be evident. Most cases appear to be sporadic, but autosomal dominant inheritance has been reported.

Each of the genetic syndromes is at risk for additional anomalies, including hydrocephalus, increased intracranial pressure, papilledema, optic atrophy due to abnormalities of the optic foramina, respiratory problems secondary to a deviated nasal septum or choanal atresia, and disorders of speech and deafness. Craniectomy is mandatory for the management of increased intracranial pressure, and a multidisciplinary craniofacial team is essential for the long-term follow-up of affected children.

Cohen MM: Craniosynostosis update. Am J Med Genet 4(Suppl):99, 1987.
David DJ, Poswillo D, Simpson D: The Craniosynostoses: Causes, Natural History and Management. Berlin, Springer Verlag, 1982.
Shillito J, Matson BD: Craniosynostosis: A review of 519 surgical patients. Pediatrics 41:829, 1968.

CHAPTER 543
Seizures in Childhood

Seizures are a common neurologic disorder in the pediatric age group and occur with a frequency of 4–6 cases/1,000 children. They are the most common cause for referral to a pediatric neurology practice. The presence of a seizure disorder does not constitute a diagnosis but is a symptom of an underlying central nervous system (CNS) disorder that requires a thorough investigation and management plan. In most children, an etiology for the seizure cannot be determined, and a diagnosis of idiopathic epilepsy is made. Although the outcome for most uncomplicated seizures in children is good, a small number have persistent seizures refractory to drugs, and these pose a diagnostic and management challenge. The terms *seizure* and *convulsion* may be incorrectly used interchangeably with *epilepsy.* A *seizure* (convulsion) is defined as a paroxysmal involuntary disturbance of brain function that may manifest as an impairment or loss of consciousness, abnormal motor activity, behavioral abnormalities, sensory disturbances, or autonomic dysfunction. Some seizures are characterized by abnormal movements without loss or impairment of consciousness. *Epilepsy* is defined as recurrent seizures unrelated to fever or to an acute cerebral insult.

EVALUATION. The *history* should attempt to define factors that may have promoted the convulsion and to provide a detailed description of the seizure and the child's postictal state. Children who have a propensity to develop epilepsy may experience the first convulsion in association with a viral illness or a low-grade fever. Seizures that occur during the early morning hours or with drowsiness, particularly during the initial phase of sleep, are common in childhood epilepsy. In retrospect, irritability, mood swings, headache, and subtle personality changes may precede a seizure by several days. Some parents can accurately predict the timing of the next seizure based on changes in the child's disposition.

Most parents vividly recall their child's initial convulsion and can describe it in detail. The first step in an evaluation is to determine whether the seizure has a focal onset or is generalized. *Focal seizures* may be characterized by motor or sensory symptoms and include forceful turning of the head and eyes to one side, unilateral clonic movements beginning in the face or extremities, or a sensory disturbance such as paresthesias or pain localized to a specific area. Focal seizures in the adult usually indicate a localized lesion, but the investigation of focal seizures during childhood is frequently negative. Motor seizures may be focal or generalized and tonic-clonic, tonic, clonic, myoclonic, or atonic. *Tonic seizures* are characterized by increased tone or rigidity, and atonic seizures are characterized by flaccidity or by lack of movement during a convulsion. *Clonic seizures* consist of rhythmic muscle contraction and relaxation, and myoclonus is most accurately described as shocklike contractions of a muscle. The duration of the seizure and state of consciousness (retained or impaired) should be documented. The history should determine whether an aura preceded the convulsion and the behavior of the child immediately preceding the seizure. The most common aura experienced by children consists of epigastric discomfort or pain and a feeling of fear. The posture of the patient, presence and distribution of cyanosis, vocalizations, loss of sphincter control (particularly of the urinary bladder), and postictal state (including sleep and headache) should be noted.

Some parents can precisely act out or recreate a seizure. The physical portrayal by the parent or caregiver is often surprisingly similar to the actual convulsion and is much more accurate than the verbal description. Aside from the description of the seizure pattern, the frequency, time of day, precipitating factors, and alteration in the type of convulsive disorder are important. Although generalized tonic-clonic seizures are readily documented, the frequency of absence seizures is often underestimated by the parent. A prolonged personality change or intellectual deterioration may suggest a degenerative disease of the CNS, whereas constitutional symptoms, including vomiting and failure to thrive, might indicate a primary metabolic disorder or a structural lesion. It is essential to obtain details of prior anticonvulsant medication and the child's response to the regimen, and to determine whether drugs that may potentiate seizures, including chlorpromazine or methylphenidate, were prescribed.

The *examination* of a child with a seizure disorder should be geared toward the search for an organic cause. The blood pressure is recorded, and the child's head circumference, length, and weight are plotted on a growth chart and compared with previous measurements. The finding of unusual facial features or associated physical findings such as hepatosplenomegaly point to an underlying metabolic or storage disease as the cause of the neurologic disorder. A search for vitiliginous lesions of tuberous sclerosis utilizing an ultraviolet light source, examination for adenoma sebaceum, shagreen patch, multiple café-au-lait spots, or a nevus flammeus, and the presence of retinal phakoma would indicate a neurocutaneous disorder as the cause of the seizure. Localizing neurologic signs such as a subtle hemiparesis with hyper-reflexia, an equivocal Babinski, and a downward-drifting extended arm with eyes closed might suggest a contralateral hemispheric structural lesion, such as a slow-growing temporal lobe glioma, as the cause of the seizure disorder. A unilateral growth arrest of the thumbnail, hand, or extremity in a child with a focal seizure disorder suggests a chronic condition such as a porencephalic cyst, arteriovenous malformation, or cortical atrophy in the opposite hemisphere. The eyegrounds must be examined for the presence of papilledema, retinal hemorrhages, chorioretinitis, coloboma, and macular changes as well as retinal phakoma. Hyperventilation for a 3- or 4-min period produces an immediate seizure in virtually all children with absence epilepsy.

CLASSIFICATION OF SEIZURES

It is important to classify the type of seizure for several reasons. First, the seizure type may provide a clue to the cause of the seizure disorder. In addition, precise delineation of the seizure may allow a firm basis for making a prognosis. The child with generalized tonic-clonic epilepsy is usually readily controlled with anticonvulsants, whereas the patient with partial seizures may fare less well. The infant with benign myoclonic epilepsy has a more favorable outlook than a patient with infantile spasms. Similarly, the school-aged child who has benign partial epilepsy with centrotemporal spikes (rolandic epilepsy) has an excellent prognosis and is unlikely to require a prolonged course of anticonvulsants. The clinical classification of seizures may be difficult because the manifestations of different seizure types may be similar. For example, the clinical features of a child with absence seizures may be almost identical to those of another patient with complex partial epilepsy. The electroencephalogram (EEG) is a useful adjunct to the classification of epilepsy because of the variability of seizure expressivity in this age group. A classification useful in delineating childhood epilepsy is shown in Table 543–1.

■ **TABLE 543–1 International Classification of Epileptic Seizures**

Partial Seizures
Simple partial (consciousness retained)
Motor
Sensory
Autonomic
Psychic
Complex partial (consciousness impaired)
Simple partial, followed by impaired consciousness
Consciousness impaired at onset
Partial seizures with secondary generalization
Generalized Seizures
Absences
Typical
Atypical
Generalized tonic-clonic
Tonic
Clonic
Myoclonic
Atonic
Infantile spasms
Unclassified Seizures

543.1 Partial Seizures

Partial seizures account for a large proportion of childhood seizures, up to 40% in some series. Partial seizures may be classified as *simple* or *complex;* consciousness is maintained with simple seizures and is impaired in patients with complex seizures.

SIMPLE PARTIAL SEIZURES (SPS). Motor activity is the most common symptom of SPS. The movements are characterized by asynchronous clonic or tonic movements, and they tend to involve the face, neck, and extremities. *Versive seizures* consisting of head turning and conjugate eye movements are particularly common in SPS. Automatisms do not occur with SPS, but some patients complain of aura (e.g., chest discomfort and headache), which may be the only manifestation of a seizure. Unfortunately, children have difficulty in describing aura and often refer to it as "feeling funny" or "something crawling inside me." The average seizure persists for 10–22 sec. SPS may be confused with tics; however, *tics* are characterized by shoulder shrugging, eye blinking, and facial grimacing and primarily involve the face and shoulders (Chapter 22). Tics can be briefly suppressed, but partial seizures cannot be controlled. The EEG may show spikes or sharp waves unilaterally or bilaterally, or a multifocal spike pattern in patients with SPS.

RASMUSSEN ENCEPHALITIS. This subacute inflammatory encephalitis, is one cause of *epilepsia partialis continua.* A preceding, nonspecific febrile illness may precede the onset of focal seizures, which may be very frequent or continuous. The onset is usually before age 10 yr. Sequelae include hemiplegia, hemianopsia, and aphasia. The EEG reveals diffuse paroxysmal activity with a slow background. The disease is progressive and potentially lethal, but more often becomes self limited with significant focal neurologic deficits. The disease may be due to autoantibodies that bend to and stimulate the glutamate receptor.

COMPLEX PARTIAL SEIZURES (CPS). A CPS may begin with a simple partial seizure with or without an aura, followed by impaired consciousness, or, conversely, the onset of the CPS may coincide with an altered state of consciousness. An *aura* consisting of vague, unpleasant feelings, epigastric discomfort, or fear is present in approximately one third of children with SPS and CPS. As partial seizures are difficult to document in the infant and child, the frequency of their association with CPS may be underestimated. Impaired consciousness in the infant and child is difficult to appreciate. There may be a brief blank stare or a sudden cessation or pause in activity that is frequently overlooked by the parent. Furthermore, the child is unable to communicate or to describe the periods of impaired consciousness in most cases. Finally, the periods of altered consciousness may be brief and infrequent, and only an experienced observer or an EEG may be able to identify the abnormal event.

Automatisms are a common feature of CPS in infants and children, occurring in approximately 50–75% of cases; the older the child, the greater will be the frequency of automatisms. Automatisms develop following the loss of consciousness and may persist into the postictal phase, but they are not recalled by the child. The automatic behavior observed in infants is characterized by alimentary automatisms, including lip smacking, chewing, swallowing, and excessive salivation. These movements can represent normal infant behavior and are difficult to distinguish from the automatisms of CPS. Prolonged and repetitive alimentary automatisms associated with a blank stare or with a lack of responsiveness almost always indicate CPS in an infant. Automatic behavior in older children consists of semipurposeful, incoordinated, and unplanned gestural automatisms, including picking and pulling at clothing or the bed sheets, rubbing or caressing objects, and walking or running in a nondirective, repetitive, and often fearful fashion.

Spreading of the epileptiform discharge during CPS can result in secondary generalization with a tonic-clonic convulsion. During the spread of the ictal discharge throughout the hemisphere, contralateral versive turning of the head, dystonic posturing, and tonic or clonic movements of the extremities and face including eye blinking may be noted. The average duration of a CPS is 1–2 min, which is considerably longer than an SPS or an absence seizure.

CPS are associated with interictal *EEG* anterior temporal lobe sharp waves or focal spikes, and multifocal spikes are a frequent finding. Approximately 20% of infants and children with CPS have a normal routine interictal EEG. In these patients, a sleep-deprived EEG study, zygomatic leads during EEG, prolonged EEG recording, or study of the hospitalized patient weaned from anticonvulsants are techniques that can be utilized to increase the identification of spikes and sharp waves (Fig. 543–1*A*). In addition, some children with CPS have interictal sharp waves or spikes originating from the frontal, parietal, or occipital lobes. Radiographic studies including computed tomography (CT) scanning and especially magnetic resonance imaging (MRI) are most likely to identify an abnormality in the temporal lobe in a child with CPS. These lesions include mesial temporal sclerosis, hamartoma, postencephalitic gliosis, subarachnoid cysts, infarction, arteriovenous malformations, and a slow-growing glioma.

BENIGN PARTIAL EPILEPSY WITH CENTROTEMPORAL SPIKES (BPEC). BPEC is a common type of partial epilepsy in childhood and has an excellent prognosis. The clinical features, EEG findings, and lack of a neuropathologic lesion are characteristic and readily separate BPEC from CPS. BPEC occurs between the ages of 2 and 14, and has a peak age of onset of 9–10 yr. The disorder occurs in normal children with an unremarkable past history and a normal neurologic examination. There is often a positive family history of epilepsy. The seizures are usually partial, and motor signs and somatosensory symptoms are often confined to the face. Oropharyngeal symptoms include tonic contractions and paresthesias of the tongue, unilateral numbness of the cheek (particularly along the gum), guttural noises, dysphagia, and excessive salivation. Frequently, unilateral tonic-clonic contractures of the lower face accompany the oropharyngeal symptoms, as do clonic movements or paresthesias of the ipsilateral extremities. Consciousness may be intact or impaired, and the partial seizure may proceed to secondary generalization. Approximately 20% of children experience only one seizure, the majority have infrequent seizures, and about one quarter have repeated clusters of seizures. BPEC occurs during sleep in 75% of patients, whereas CPS tends to be observed during the waking hours. The EEG pattern is diagnostic for BPEC and is characterized by a repetitive spike focus localized in the centrotemporal or rolandic area with a normal background activity (see Fig. 543–1*A*). Anticonvulsants are necessary for patients who have frequent seizures but should not be prescribed automatically after the initial convulsion. Carbamazepine is the preferred drug, which is continued for at least 2 yr or until 14–16 yr of age, when spontaneous remission of BPEC usually occurs.

543.2 Generalized Seizures

ABSENCE SEIZURES. Simple (typical) absence (petit mal) seizures are characterized by a sudden cessation of motor activity or speech with a blank facial expression and flickering of the eyelids. These seizures, which are uncommon prior to the age of 5 yr, are more prevalent in girls; they are never associated with an aura; they rarely persist longer than 30 sec; and they are not associated with a postictal state. These features tend to differentiate absence seizures from complex partial seizures. The patient does not lose body tone, but the head may fall forward slightly. Immediately after the seizure, the patient resumes preseizure activity with no indication of postictal impairment. Automatic behavior frequently accompanies simple absence seizures. Hyperventilation for 3–4 min routinely produces an absence seizure. The EEG shows a typical 3/sec spike and generalized wave discharge (see Fig. 543–1*B*). Complex (atypical) absence seizures have associated motor components consisting of myoclonic movements of the face, fingers, or extremities and, on occasion, loss of body tone. These seizures produce atypical EEG spike and wave discharges at 2–2.5/sec.

GENERALIZED TONIC-CLONIC SEIZURES. These seizures are extremely common and may follow a partial seizure with a focal onset (secondary generalization) or occur de novo. They may be associated with an aura suggesting a focal origin of the epileptiform discharge. It is important to inquire about the presence of an aura, because its presence and site of origin may indicate the area of pathology. The patient suddenly loses consciousness and in some cases emits a shrill, piercing cry. The eyes roll back, the entire body musculature undergoes tonic contractions, and the child rapidly becomes cyanotic in association with apnea. The clonic phase of the seizure is heralded by rhythmic clonic contractions alternating with relaxation of all muscle groups. The clonic phase slows toward the end of the seizure, which usually persists for a few minutes, and the patient often sighs as the seizure comes to an abrupt stop. During the seizure, the child may bite the tongue but rarely vomits. Loss of sphincter control, particularly the bladder, is common during a generalized tonic-clonic seizure.

Tight clothing and jewelry around the neck should be loosened, the patient should be placed on one side, and the neck and jaw should be gently hyperextended to enhance breathing. The mouth should not be opened forcibly by an object or by a finger because the patient's teeth may be dislodged and aspirated or significant injury to the oropharyngeal cavity may result. Postictally, the child will initially be semicomatose and typically remain in a deep sleep from 30 min to 2 hr. If the patient is examined during the seizure or immediately postictally, he or she may demonstrate truncal ataxia, hyperactive deep tendon reflexes, clonus, and a Babinski reflex. The postictal phase is often associated with vomiting and an intense bifrontal headache. *Idiopathic seizure* is a term applied when the cause of a generalized seizure cannot be ascertained. Many factors are known to precipitate generalized tonic-clonic sei-

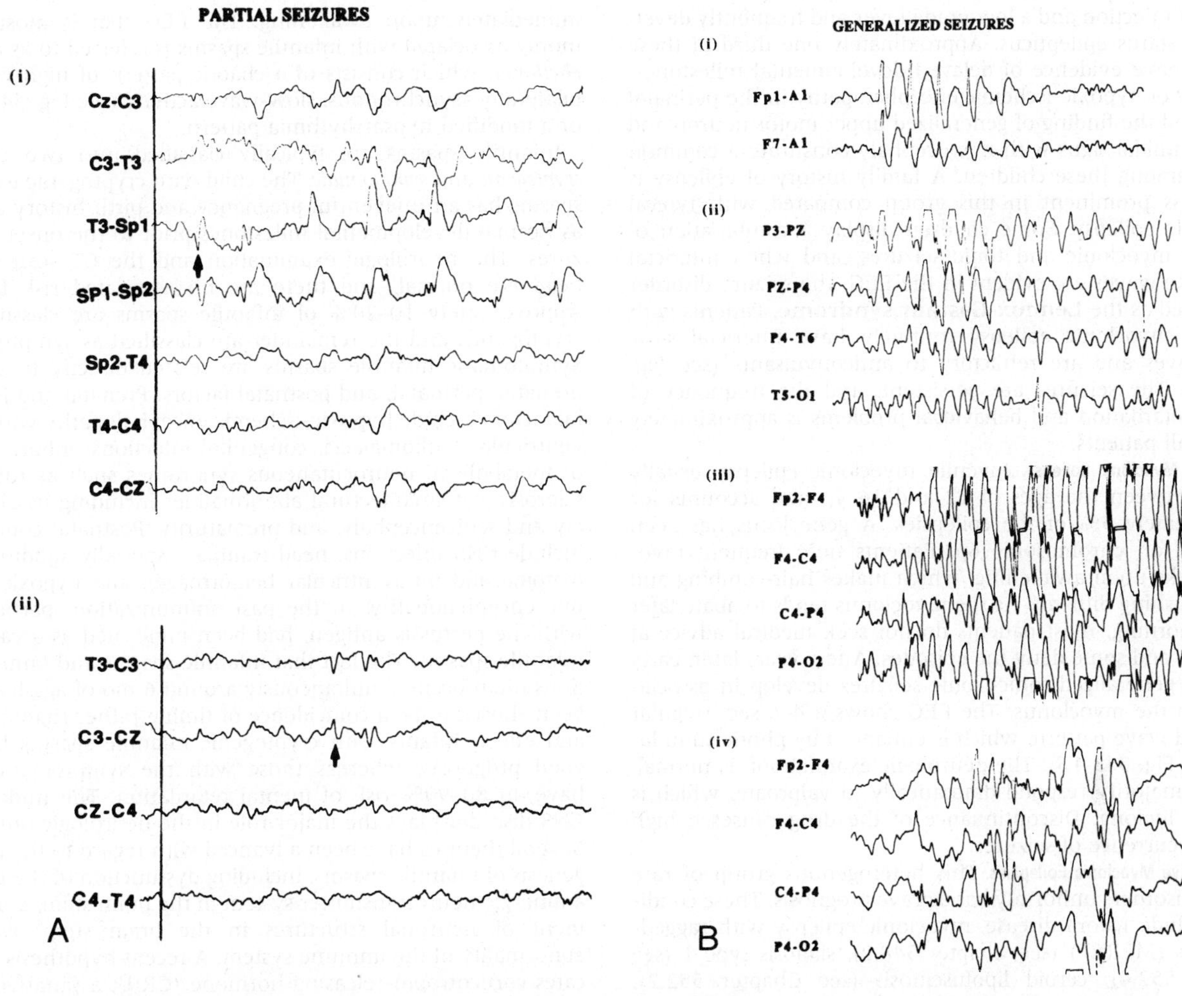

Figure 543–1. *A,* An EEG of partial seizures: (i) spike discharges from the left temporal lobe *(arrow)* in a patient with CPS, (ii) left parietal central spikes *(arrow)* characteristic of BPEC. *B,* Representative EEGs of generalized seizures: (i) 3/sec spike and wave discharge of absence seizures with normal background activity, (ii) complex myoclonic epilepsy (Lennox-Gastaut syndrome) with interictal slow spike waves, (iii) juvenile myoclonic epilepsy showing 6/sec spike and waves enhanced by photic stimulation, and (iv) hypsarrhythmia with an irregular high-voltage spike and wave activity.

zures in children, including low-grade fever associated with infections, excessive fatigue or emotional stress, and various drugs including psychotropic medications, theophylline, and methylphenidate.

MYOCLONIC EPILEPSIES OF CHILDHOOD. This disorder is characterized by repetitive seizures consisting of brief, often symmetric muscular contractions with loss of body tone and falling or slumping forward, which has a tendency to cause injuries to the face and the mouth. Myoclonic epilepsies include a heterogeneous group of conditions with multiple causes and variable outcomes. However, at least five distinct subgroupings can be identified that represent the broad spectrum of myoclonic epilepsies in the pediatric population.

Benign Myoclonus of Infancy. Benign myoclonus begins during infancy and consists of clusters of myoclonic movements confined to the neck, trunk, and extremities. The myoclonic activity may be confused with infantile spasms; however, the EEG is normal in patients with benign myoclonus. The prognosis is good, with normal development and the cessation of myoclonus by 2 yr of age. An anticonvulsant is not indicated. A familial autosomal dominant form is thought to be linked to a locus on chromosome 20.

Typical Myoclonic Epilepsy of Early Childhood. Children who develop typical myoclonic epilepsy are near normal prior to the onset of seizures with an unremarkable pregnancy, labor, and delivery and intact developmental milestones. The mean age of onset is approximately 2½ yr, but the range spreads from 6 mo to 4 yr. The frequency of myoclonic seizures varies; they may occur several times daily or children may be seizure free for weeks. A few patients have febrile convulsions or generalized tonic-clonic afebrile seizures that precede the onset of myoclonic epilepsy. Approximately one half of the patients occasionally have tonic-clonic seizures in addition to the myoclonic epilepsy. The EEG shows fast spike wave complexes of ≥2.5 Hz and a normal background rhythm in most cases. At least one third of the children have a positive family history of epilepsy, which suggests a genetic etiology in some cases. The long-term outcome is relatively favorable. Mental retardation develops in the minority, and more than 50% are seizure free several years later. However, learning and language problems and emotional and behavioral disorders occur in a significant number of these children and require prolonged follow-up by a multidisciplinary team.

Complex Myoclonic Epilepsies. These consist of a heterogeneous group of disorders with a uniformly poor prognosis. Typically, focal or generalized tonic-clonic seizures beginning during the 1st year of life antedate the onset of myoclonic epilepsy. The generalized seizure is often associated with an upper respiratory tract infection and a low-grade fever and frequently develops into status epilepticus. Approximately one third of these patients have evidence of delayed developmental milestones. A history of hypoxic-ischemic encephalopathy in the perinatal period and the finding of generalized upper motor neuron and extrapyramidal signs with microcephaly constitute a common pattern among these children. A family history of epilepsy is much less prominent in this group compared with typical myoclonic epilepsy. Some children display a combination of frequent myoclonic and tonic seizures, and when interictal slow spike waves are evident in the EEG, the seizure disorder is classified as the **Lennox-Gastaut syndrome.** Patients with complex myoclonic epilepsy routinely have interictal slow spike waves and are refractory to anticonvulsants (see Fig. 543–1*B*). The seizures are persistent, and the frequency of mental retardation and behavioral problems is approximately 75% of all patients.

Juvenile Myoclonic Epilepsy. Juvenile myoclonic epilepsy usually begins between the ages of 12 and 16 yr, and accounts for approximately 5% of the epilepsies. A gene locus has been identified on chromosome 6p. Patients note frequent myoclonic jerks upon awakening, which makes hair-combing and tooth-brushing difficult. As the myoclonus tends to abate later in the morning, most patients do not seek medical advice at this stage and some deny the episodes. A few years later, early morning generalized tonic-clonic seizures develop in association with the myoclonus. The EEG shows a 4–6/sec irregular spike and wave pattern, which is enhanced by photic stimulation (see Fig. 543-1*B*). The neurologic examination is normal, and the majority respond dramatically to valproate, which is required lifelong. Discontinuance of the drug causes a high rate of recurrence of seizures.

Progressive Myoclonic Epilepsies. This heterogenous group of rare genetic disorders uniformly has a grave prognosis. These conditions include Lafora disease, myoclonic epilepsy with ragged-red fibers (MERRF) (see Chapter 548.2), sialiosis type 1 (see Chapter 552.4), ceroid lipofuscinosis (see Chapter 552.2), juvenile neuropathic Gaucher disease, and juvenile neuroxonal dystrophy. *Lafora disease* presents in children between 10 and 18 yr with generalized tonic-clonic seizures. Ultimately, myoclonic jerks appear, which become more apparent and constant with progression of the disease. Mental deterioration is a characteristic feature and becomes evident within 1 yr of the onset of seizures. Neurologic abnormalities, particularly cerebellar and extrapyramidal signs, are prominent findings. The EEG shows polyspike-wave discharges, particularly in the occipital region, with progressive slowing and a disorganized background. The myoclonic jerks are difficult to control, but a combination of valproic acid and a benzodiazepine (e.g., clonazepam) is effective in controlling the generalized seizures. Lafora disease is an autosomal recessive disorder, and the diagnosis may be established by examination of a skin biopsy for characteristic periodic acid-Schiff positive inclusions, which are most prominent in the eccrine sweat-gland duct cells.

INFANTILE SPASMS. Infantile spasms usually begin between the ages of 4 and 8 mo and are characterized by brief symmetric contractions of the neck, trunk, and extremities. There are at least three types of infantile spasms: flexor, extensor, and mixed. *Flexor spasms* occur in clusters or volleys and consist of sudden flexion of the neck, arms, and legs onto the trunk, whereas *extensor spasms* produce extension of the trunk and extremities, and are the least common form of infantile spasm. *Mixed infantile spasms,* consisting of flexion in some volleys and extension in others, is the most common type of infantile spasm. Clusters or volleys of seizures may persist for minutes with brief intervals between each spasm. A cry may precede or follow an infantile spasm, accounting for the confusion with colic in a few cases. The spasms occur during sleep or arousal but have a tendency to develop while the patient is drowsy or immediately upon awakening. The EEG that is most commonly associated with infantile spasms is referred to as *hypsarrhythmia,* which consists of a chaotic pattern of high-voltage, bilaterally asynchronous, slow-wave activity (see Fig. 543–1*B*), or a modified hypsarrhythmia pattern.

Infantile spasms are typically classified into two groups: *cryptogenic* and *symptomatic.* The child with cryptogenic infantile spasms has an uneventful pregnancy and birth history as well as normal developmental milestones prior to the onset of seizures. The neurologic examination and the CT scan of the head are normal, and there are no associated risk factors. Approximately 10–20% of infantile spasms are classified as cryptogenic, and the remainder are classified as symptomatic. Symptomatic infantile spasms are related directly to several prenatal, perinatal, and postnatal factors. Prenatal and perinatal factors include hypoxic-ischemic encephalopathy with periventricular leukomalacia, congenital infections, inborn errors of metabolism, neurocutaneous syndromes such as tuberous sclerosis, cytoarchitectural abnormalities including lissencephaly and schizencephaly, and prematurity. Postnatal conditions include CNS infections, head trauma (especially subdural hematoma and intraventricular hemorrhage), and hypoxic-ischemic encephalopathy. In the past, immunization, particularly with the pertussis antigen, had been implicated as a cause of infantile spasms. The fact that infantile spasms and immunizations often occur simultaneously around 6 mo of age has now been shown to be a coincidence of timing rather than a cause and effect. Infants with cryptogenic infantile spasms have a good prognosis, whereas those with the symptomatic type have an 80–90% risk of mental retardation. The underlying CNS disorder plays the major role in the neurologic outcome. Several theories have been advanced with regard to the pathogenesis of infantile spasms, including dysfunction of the monoaminergic neurotransmitter system in the brain stem, derangement of neuronal structures in the brain stem, and an abnormality of the immune system. A recent hypothesis implicates corticotropin-releasing hormone (CRH), a putative neurotransmitter, metabolized in the inferior olive. CRH acts on the pituitary to enhance the release of ACTH; ACTH and glucocorticoids suppress the metabolism and secretion of CRH by a feedback mechanism. It is proposed that specific stresses or injury to the infant during a critical period of neurodevelopment causes CRH overproduction, resulting in neuronal hyperexcitability and seizures. The number of CRH receptors reaches a maximum in the infant brain followed by a spontaneous reduction with age, perhaps accounting for the eventual resolution of infantile spasms, even without therapy. Exogenous ACTH and glucocorticoids suppress CRH synthesis, which may explain their effectiveness in treating infantile spasms. The therapy of infantile spasms follows in the treatment section.

LANDAU-KLEFFNER SYNDROME (LKS). This is a rare condition of unknown etiology, more common in boys, with a mean onset of 5.5 yr. It is characterized by loss of language skills in a previously normal child. At least 70% have an associated seizure disorder. Language regression may be sudden or the speech loss protracted. The aphasia may be primarily receptive or expressive, and auditory agnosia may be so severe that the child is oblivious to everyday sounds. Hearing is normal, but behavioral problems, including irritability and poor attention span, are particularly common. Formal testing often shows normal performance and visual-spatial skills in spite of poor language. The seizures are of several types, including focal or generalized tonic-clonic, atypical absence, partial complex, and occasionally myoclonic. High-amplitude spike and wave discharges predominate and tend to be bitemporal, but can be multifocal or generalized. In the evolutionary stages of the condition, the EEG may be normal. The spike discharges are always more apparent during non-REM sleep, so that a child suspected of LKS should have an EEG during sleep, particularly if the awake record is normal. CT and MRI studies are typically normal, and PET scans have demonstrated either unilateral or bilateral hypometabolism or hypermetabolism. Microscopic examination of surgical specimens has shown minimal gliosis but no evidence of encephalitis.

Valproic acid is the anticonvulsant of choice; however, some children require a combination of valproic acid and clobazam to control the seizures. If the seizures and aphasia persist, a trial of steroids should be considered. One recommended schedule consists of oral prednisone, 2 mg/kg/24 hr for 1 mo, tapered to 1 mg/kg/24 hr for an additional month. With clinical improvement, the prednisone is reduced further to 0.5 mg/kg/24 hr for up to 6–12 mo. It is imperative to initiate speech therapy and maintain treatment for several years, as improvement in language function occurs over a prolonged period. Some centers advocate an operative procedure, subpial transection, when medical management fails, but this procedure requires further study. Methylphenidate should be considered for the patient with severe hyperactivity and inattention. Seizures may be potentiated by methylphenidate; however, anticonvulsants are usually protective. Some children experience a reoccurrence of aphasia and seizures following apparent recovery. Most children with LKS will have a significant abnormality of speech function during adulthood. The onset of LKS at an early age (<2 yr) uniformly tends to be associated with a poor prognosis for recovery of speech.

543.3 Febrile Seizures

Febrile convulsions rarely develop into epilepsy, and they spontaneously remit without specific therapy. They are the most common seizure disorder during childhood, with a uniformly excellent prognosis. However, a febrile convulsion may signify a serious underlying acute infectious disease such as sepsis or bacterial meningitis so that each child must be carefully examined and appropriately investigated for the cause of the associated fever (Chapter 169). Febrile seizures are age dependent and are rare prior to 9 mo and after 5 yr of age. The peak age of onset is approximately 14–18 mo of age, and the incidence approaches 3–4% of young children. There is a strong family history of febrile convulsions in siblings and parents, suggesting a genetic predisposition. Animal studies suggest that arginine vasopressin may be an important mediator in the pathogenesis of hyperthermia-induced seizures.

CLINICAL MANIFESTATIONS. The convulsion is associated with a rapidly rising temperature and usually develops when the core temperature reaches 39°C or greater. The seizure is typically generalized, tonic-clonic of a few seconds to 10-min duration, followed by a brief postictal period of drowsiness. Febrile seizures persisting longer than 15 min suggest an organic cause such as an infectious or toxic process and require a thorough investigation. As the seizure is no longer present by the time that the child reaches the hospital, the physician's most important responsibility is to determine the cause of the fever and to rule out meningitis. *If any doubt exists with regard to the possibility of meningitis, a lumbar puncture with examination of the cerebrospinal fluid (CSF) is indicated.* Viral infections of the upper respiratory tract, roseola, and acute otitis media are most frequently the causes of febrile convulsions.

An EEG is not warranted following a simple febrile seizure because the recording will prove nonepileptiform or normal and that finding will not alter the management. An EEG is indicated for atypical febrile seizures or for the child at risk for developing epilepsy. Atypical febrile seizures include a seizure persisting for more than 15 min, repeated convulsions for several hours or days, and a focal seizure. Approximately 50% of children have recurrent febrile seizures, and a small minority have multiple recurrent seizures. The risk factors for the development of epilepsy as a complication of febrile seizures include a positive family history of epilepsy, initial febrile seizure prior to 9 mo of age, a prolonged or atypical febrile seizure, delayed developmental milestones, and an abnormal neurologic examination. The incidence of epilepsy is approximately 9% when several risk factors are present compared with an incidence of 1% in children who have febrile convulsions and no risk factors.

TREATMENT. The routine management of the normal infant who has simple febrile convulsions includes a careful search for the cause of the fever, active measures to control the fever including the use of antipyretics, and reassurance of the parents. Short-term anticonvulsant prophylaxis is not indicated. Prolonged anticonvulsant prophylaxis for the prevention of recurrent febrile convulsions is controversial and no longer recommended. Antiepileptics such as phenytoin and carbamazepine have no effect on febrile seizures. Phenobarbital has been ineffective in preventing recurrent febrile seizures and may decrease cognitive function in treated children compared with untreated children. Sodium valproate is effective in the management of febrile seizures, but the potential risks of the drug do not justify its use in a disorder with an excellent prognosis irrespective of treatment. Oral diazepam is recommended as an effective and safe method of reducing the risk of reoccurrence of febrile seizures. At the onset of each febrile illness, diazepam, 0.3 mg/kg q8h po (1 mg/kg/24 hr), is administered for the duration of the illness (usually 2–3 days). The side effects are usually minor, but symptoms of lethargy, irritability, and ataxia may be reduced by adjusting the dose.

MECHANISMS OF SEIZURES

Although the precise mechanisms of seizures are unknown, there appear to be several physiologic factors responsible for the development of a seizure. To initiate a seizure, there must be a group of neurons that are capable of generating a significant burst discharge and a GABAergic inhibitory system. Seizure discharge transmission is ultimately dependent upon excitatory glutamateric synapses. Recent evidence suggests that excitatory amino acid neurotransmitters (glutamate, aspartate) may play a role in producing neuronal excitation by acting on specific cell receptors. It is known that seizures may arise from areas of neuronal death and that these regions of the brain may promote the development of novel hyperexcitable synapses that can cause seizures. For example, lesions in the temporal lobe (including slow-growing gliomas, hamartomas, gliosis, and arteriovenous malformations) cause seizures, and when the abnormal tissue is removed surgically, the seizures are likely to cease. Further, convulsions may be produced in the experimental animal by the phenomenon of *kindling.* In this model, repeated subconvulsive stimulation of the brain (e.g., amygdala) leads ultimately to a generalized convulsion. Kindling may be responsible for the development of epilepsy in humans following an injury to the brain. In humans, it has been proposed that recurrent seizure activity from an abnormal temporal lobe may produce seizures in the contralateral normal temporal lobe by transmission of the stimulus via the corpus callosum.

Seizures are more common in the infant and in the immature experimental animal. Certain seizures in the pediatric population are age specific (e.g., infantile spasms), which suggests that the underdeveloped brain is more susceptible to specific seizures than the older child or adult. Genetic factors account for at least 20% of all cases of epilepsy. Utilizing linkage analyses, the chromosomal location of several familial epilepsies has been identified, including benign neonatal convulsions (20q), juvenile myoclonic epilepsy (6p), and progressive myoclonic epilepsy (21q 22.3). It is very likely that in the near future the molecular basis of additional epilepsies, such as benign rolandic epilepsy and absence seizures, will be identified. It is also known that the substantia nigra plays an integral role in the development of generalized seizures. Electrographic seizure activity spreads within the substantia nigra, causing an increase in uptake of 2-deoxyglucose in adult animals, but there is little or no metabolic activity within the substantia nigra when immature animals have a convulsion. It has been proposed that the functional immaturity of the substantia nigra may play a role in the increased seizure susceptibility of the immature brain. Additionally, the gamma aminobutyric acid (GABA)-sensitive substantia nigra pars reticulata (SNR) neurons play a role in preventing seizures. It is likely that substantia nigra outflow tracts modulate and regulate seizure dissemination but are not responsible for the onset of seizures. Additional research will likely focus on the causes of neuronal hyperexcitability, additional inhibitory mechanisms, the search for nonsynaptic mechanisms of seizure propagation, and GABA receptor abnormalities.

DIAGNOSIS OF SEIZURES

The investigation of a seizure depends on many factors, including the age of the patient, the type and frequency of the seizure, and the presence or absence of neurologic findings and constitutional symptoms. The minimum work-up for the first afebrile seizure in an otherwise healthy child includes a fasting glucose, calcium, magnesium, serum electrolytes, and a routine *EEG*. The demonstration of paroxysmal discharges on the EEG during a clinical seizure is diagnostic of epilepsy, but seizures rarely occur in the EEG laboratory. A normal EEG does not exclude the diagnosis of epilepsy, because the interictal recording is normal in approximately 40% of patients. Activation procedures, including hyperventilation, eye closure, photic stimulation, and, when indicated, sleep deprivation and special electrode placement (e.g., zygomatic leads), substantially increase the positive yield. Seizure discharges are more likely to be recorded in the infant and child than in the adolescent or adult.

Prolonged EEG monitoring with simultaneous closed-circuit video recording is reserved for the complicated patient with protracted and unresponsive seizures. It provides an invaluable method for the recording of ictal seizure events that are rarely obtained during routine EEG studies. This technique is extremely helpful in the classification of seizures because it can accurately determine the location and frequency of seizure discharges while recording alterations in the level of consciousness and the presence of clinical signs. Patients with pseudoseizures can be readily distinguished from those with true epilepsy, and the seizure type (e.g., complex partial vs. generalized) can be more precisely identified, which is critical in the investigation of a child who may be a candidate for epilepsy surgery.

The role of *CT scanning* or *MRI* in the investigation of seizures is controversial. The yield in the routine use of these procedures in the patient with a first afebrile seizure and a normal neurologic examination is negligible. In studies of children with chronic seizure disorders, the results are similar. Although approximately 30% of these children show a structural abnormality (e.g., focal cortical atrophy or dilated ventricles), only a small minority benefit from active intervention as a result of CT scanning. Thus, CT scanning or MRI should be reserved for patients in whom an intracranial lesion is suspected on the basis of the history or an abnormal neurologic examination. Prolonged partial seizures, intractability to anticonvulsant therapy, a focal neurologic deficit, and evidence of increased intracranial pressure are indications for neuroimaging studies.

Examination of the CSF is indicated if the seizure is potentially related to an infectious process, subarachnoid hemorrhage, or a demyelinating disorder. Specific metabolic tests are outlined in the sections on neonatal seizures and status epilepticus.

543.4 Treatment of Epilepsy

The first step in the management of epilepsy is to ensure that the patient has a seizure disorder and not a condition that mimics epilepsy (see later). It is sometimes difficult to be certain about the etiology of a paroxysmal event in a normal child. A negative result on a neurologic examination and EEG usually supports the approach of watchful waiting rather than the administration of an anticonvulsant. The true cause of the paroxysmal disorder eventually becomes apparent. Although there is not uniform agreement, most would concur that antiepileptics should be withheld from a previously healthy child with the first afebrile convulsion if there is a negative family history, a normal examination and EEG, and a cooperative and compliant family. Approximately 70% of these children will not experience another convulsion. A recurrent seizure, particularly if it occurs in close proximity to the first seizure, is an indication to begin an anticonvulsant. Table 543–2 suggests an approach to a child with a suspected seizure disorder.

The second step involves the choice of an anticonvulsant. The drug of choice depends on the classification of the seizure, determined by the history and EEG findings. The goal for every patient should be the use of only one drug with the fewest possible side effects for the control of seizures. The drug is increased slowly until seizure control is accomplished or until undesirable side effects develop. The child's serum anticonvulsant level should be monitored during this stage, and the dosage should be altered accordingly. Table 543–3 summarizes the common antiepileptic drugs used in childhood epilepsy and highlights the recommended daily dosage, therapeutic serum levels, and common side effects. A suggested loading dose is indicated for drugs that are useful for the treatment of status epilepticus. The physician should be familiar with the pharmacokinetics of the anticonvulsant and its toxic actions, and should monitor the child on a regular basis to gauge the seizure control while watching for unwanted side effects.

Anticonvulsants that are introduced during childhood may be required during adolescence and the childbearing years. Unfortunately, some anticonvulsants, including phenytoin, valproic acid, carbamazepine, and primidone, are associated with the occurrence of specific birth defects, including facial and limb anomalies and spinal dysraphism. A debate continues with regard to whether the teratogenic effect is secondary to the mother's epilepsy or the anticonvulsant medication. Meanwhile, the pediatrician should counsel the family about the possible relationship and should avoid prescribing an anticonvulsant to a pregnant patient unless it is absolutely necessary.

If complete seizure control is accomplished by an anticonvulsant, a minimum of two seizure-free years is an adequate and safe period of treatment in a patient with no risk factors. Prominent risk factors include age greater than 12 yr at onset, neurologic dysfunction (motor handicap or mental retardation), a history of prior neonatal seizures, and more than 21 seizures before the onset of anticonvulsant therapy. In the child with complete seizure control for a minimum of 2 yr and low risk factors, the chance of recurrence is approximately 20–25%, particularly during the first 6 mo after the discontinuation of the anticonvulsant. When the decision is made to discontinue the drug, the weaning process should occur for 3–6 mo, because abrupt withdrawal may cause status epilepticus.

CARBAMAZEPINE. This drug is effective for the management of

■ **TABLE 543–2 An Approach to the Child with a Suspected Convulsive Disorder**

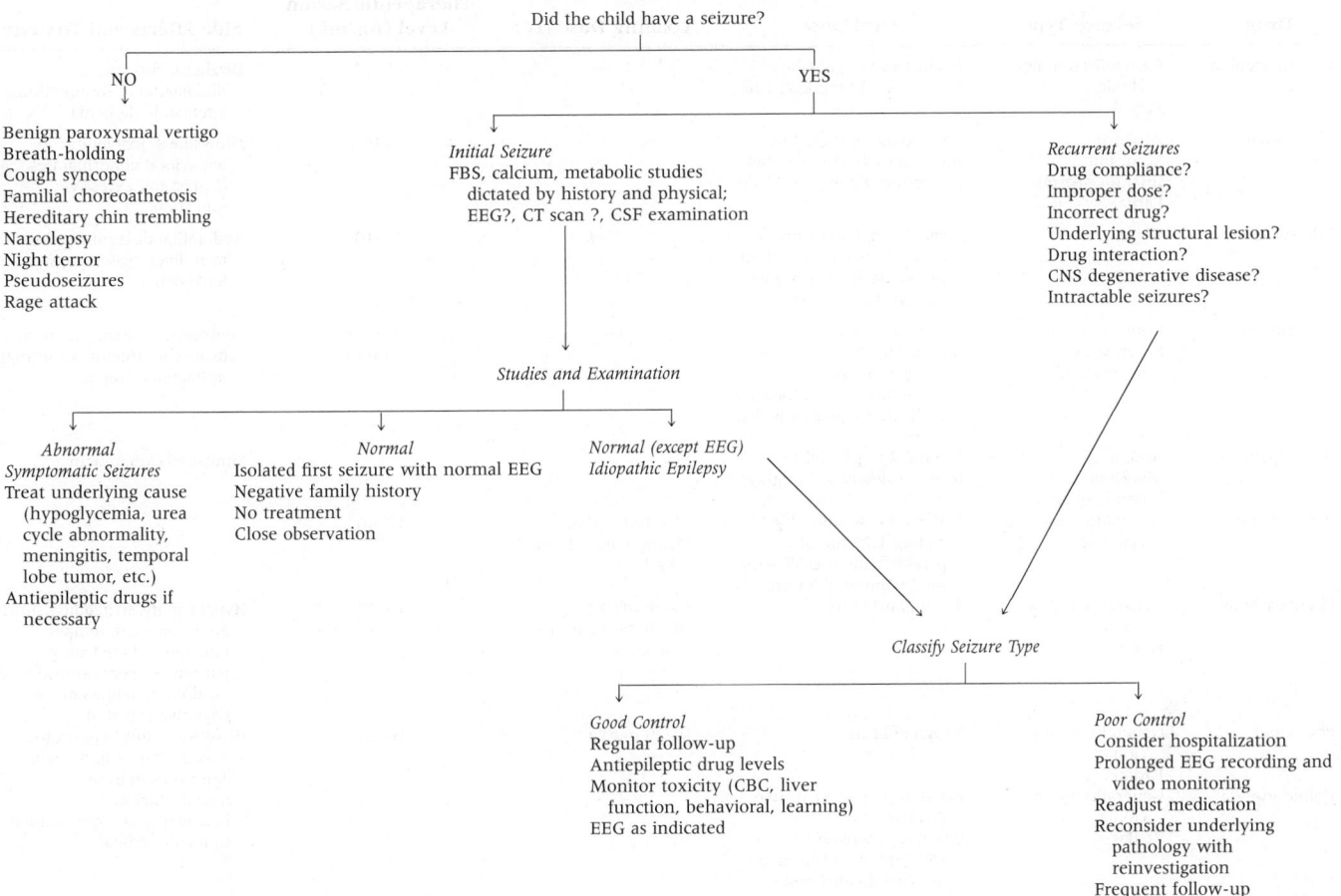

Did the child have a seizure?

- **NO**
  - Benign paroxysmal vertigo
  - Breath-holding
  - Cough syncope
  - Familial choreoathetosis
  - Hereditary chin trembling
  - Narcolepsy
  - Night terror
  - Pseudoseizures
  - Rage attack
- **YES**
  - *Initial Seizure*
    - FBS, calcium, metabolic studies dictated by history and physical; EEG?, CT scan ?, CSF examination
    - → *Studies and Examination*
      - *Abnormal* — *Symptomatic Seizures*: Treat underlying cause (hypoglycemia, urea cycle abnormality, meningitis, temporal lobe tumor, etc.); Antiepileptic drugs if necessary
      - *Normal*: Isolated first seizure with normal EEG; Negative family history; No treatment; Close observation
      - *Normal (except EEG)* — *Idiopathic Epilepsy* → *Classify Seizure Type*
  - *Recurrent Seizures*
    - Drug compliance?
    - Improper dose?
    - Incorrect drug?
    - Underlying structural lesion?
    - Drug interaction?
    - CNS degenerative disease?
    - Intractable seizures?
    - → *Classify Seizure Type*

Classify Seizure Type

- *Good Control*: Regular follow-up; Antiepileptic drug levels; Monitor toxicity (CBC, liver function, behavioral, learning); EEG as indicated
- *Poor Control*: Consider hospitalization; Prolonged EEG recording and video monitoring; Readjust medication; Reconsider underlying pathology with reinvestigation; Frequent follow-up

generalized tonic-clonic and partial seizures. Significant leukopenia (<1,000 neutrophils/mL^3) and hepatotoxicity may rarely develop, particularly during the initial 3–4 mo of therapy. Therefore, a complete blood count (CBC) and differential and an SGOT and SGPT should be obtained on a monthly basis during this period, although serious idiosyncratic drug reactions may develop despite normal liver function tests and routine bloodwork. Subsequent laboratory testing is determined by the presence of adverse symptoms or signs. The parents should be informed of untoward drug effects and instructed to report them immediately to the physician. Erythromycin should not be prescribed with carbamazepine because the two drugs compete for metabolism by the liver. The plasma concentration of carbamazepine is lowered by phenytoin, phenobarbital, and valproate. Carbamazepine 10, 11 epoxide, which is an active metabolite of carbamazepine, may produce toxicity despite therapeutic carbamazepine levels, particularly when sodium valproate is added to the drug regimen. Carbamazepine is supplied in 100- and 200-mg tablets and in a controlled release (CR) form, 200- and 400-mg tablets. The half-life is 8–20 hr, and the drug should be given two or three times daily.

GABAPENTIN. This anticonvulsant is used as an add-on drug for patients with refractory complex partial and secondarily generalized tonic-clonic seizures. The mechanism of action results from binding of the drug to neuronal membranes (glutamate synapses) and an increased brain GABA turnover. The drug is rapidly absorbed from the gastrointestinal tract, does not bind to plasma proteins, and is not metabolized. Gabapentin has no significant drug interactions and is relatively free of dose-related CNS adverse effects. Gabapentin is recommended for children 12 yr and over beginning with a dose of 300 mg/24 hr. The drug is increased by 300 mg every 3–5 days to a total dose of 900–1200 mg/24 hr, given in three equally divided doses. Adults can tolerate up to 2,400 mg/24 hr. The side effects include somnolence, dizziness, ataxia, headache, tremor, nausea and vomiting, nystagmus, and fatigue. Gabapentin is supplied in 100-mg, 300-mg, and 400-mg capsules.

PHENOBARBITAL AND PRIMIDONE. These are relatively safe anticonvulsants that are particularly useful for generalized tonic-clonic seizures. Unfortunately, approximately 25% of children undergo severe behavioral changes on these drugs. Neurologically abnormal children are at greater risk. Furthermore, there is evidence that phenobarbital may adversely affect the cognitive performance of children treated on a long-term basis. Sodium valproate interferes with the metabolism of phenobarbital, causing elevated phenobarbital plasma levels and toxicity despite the usual daily doses. Phenobarbital is supplied in an elixir (4 mg/mL) and in 15-, 30-, 60-, and 100-mg tablets. Primidone is prepared in a suspension, 50 mg/mL, and in 125- and 250-mg tablets. Phenobarbital is prescribed twice daily, and primidone is prescribed three times a day. Routine bloodwork is not indicated for these anticonvulsants.

PHENYTOIN. This drug may be used interchangeably with carbamazepine. Because of the long list of side effects, including rashes, Stevens-Johnson syndrome, lymphadenopathy, a lupus-like disease, gum hyperplasia, hirsutism, megaloblastic anemia, polyneuropathy, and rickets (especially with polytherapy), the drug has become less popular in the treatment of children. Phenytoin is supplied in 50-mg tablets, 30- and 100-

■ TABLE 543–3 Common Anticonvulsant Drugs

Drug	Seizure Type	Oral Dose	Loading Dose (IV)	Therapeutic Serum Level (μg/mL)	Side Effects and Toxicity
Carbamazepine	Generalized tonic-clonic Partial	Begin 10 mg/kg/24 hr Increase to 20 mg/kg/24 hr	—	8–12	Dizziness, drowsiness, diplopia, liver dysfunction, anemia, leukopenia
Clonazepam	Absence Myoclonic Infantile spasms Partial	Begin 0.05 mg/kg/24 hr Increase by 0.05 mg/kg/wk Maximum 0.2 mg/kg/24 hr	—	>0.013	Drowsiness, irritability, behavioral abnormalities, depression, excessive salivation
Ethosuximide	Absence	Begin 20 mg/kg/24 hr Increase to maximum of 40 mg/kg/24 hr or 1.5 g/24 hr, whichever is less	—	40–100	Abdominal discomfort, skin rash, liver dysfunction, leukopenia
Gabapentin	Complex partial Secondarily generalized	Begin 300 mg/24 hr Increase by 300 mg/24 hr every 3–5 days; maximum 900–1,200 mg/24 hr in 3 equally divided doses	—	Not necessary to monitor	Somnolence, dizziness, ataxia, headache, tremor, vomiting, nystagmus, fatigue
Nitrazepam	Absence Myoclonic Infantile spasms	Begin 0.2 mg/kg/24 hr Increase slowly to 1 mg/kg/24 hr	—		Similar to clonazepam
Paraldehyde	Generalized status epilepticus	Make a 5% solution by adding 1.75 mL of paraldehyde to D_5W with total volume of 35 mL	150–200 mg/kg Maintenance, 20 mg/kg/hr	10–40	
Phenobarbital	Generalized tonic-clonic Partial	3–5 mg/kg/24 hr	10–20 mg/kg 20–30 mg/kg in the neonate	15–40	Hyperactivity, irritability, short attention span, temper tantrums, altered sleep pattern, Stevens-Johnson syndrome, depression of cognitive function
Phenytoin	Generalized tonic-clonic Partial	5 mg/kg/24 hr	10–20 mg/kg	10–20	Hirsutism, gum hypertrophy, ataxia, skin rash, Stevens-Johnson syndrome
Primidone	Generalized tonic-clonic Partial	Begin 50 mg/24 hr in two divided doses Gradually increase to 150–500 mg/24 hr given in three divided doses	—	5–12	Aggressive behavior, personality changes, similar to phenobarbital
Sodium valproate	Generalized tonic-clonic Absence Myoclonic Partial	Begin 10 mg/kg/24 hr Increase by 5–10 mg/kg/wk Usual dose, 30–40 mg/kg/24 hr	—	50–100	Weight gain, alopecia, hepatotoxicity, tremor

mg capsules, and a suspension. The latter is not recommended, because phenytoin is immiscible in liquid and is more likely to produce erratic serum levels and toxicity.

SODIUM VALPROATE. This drug is useful for the management of many seizure types, including generalized tonic-clonic, absence, atypical absence, and myoclonic seizures. It rarely induces behavioral changes but is associated with mild gastrointestinal disturbances, alopecia, tremor, and hyperphagia. There are two rare, but serious, side effects of valproate: a Reye-like syndrome and irreversible hepatotoxicity. A small number of children develop progressive lethargy and coma with elevated serum ammonia and decreased levels of serum carnitine. Valproate may block the metabolism of carnitine, producing the altered state of consciousness in these patients. Discontinuation of valproate leads to recovery over several days. Another small group of patients, particularly children less than 2 yr of age with specific neurologic syndromes, who are managed with several anticonvulsants simultaneously, may develop an idiosyncratic hepatotoxic syndrome characterized by abdominal pain, anorexia, weight loss, and retching within a few weeks to months of beginning valproate therapy. These patients have normal liver function studies during the initial stages so that significant and persistent gastrointestinal symptoms are cause for alarm during the initial few months of valproate therapy. If reduction in the valproate dose does not provide immediate relief, the physician should discontinue the drug. These serious and sometimes lethal side effects do not tend to occur until after several months of symptom-free therapy. Valproate also may cause a decrease in serum-free carnitine levels by inhibition of plasmalemmal carnitine uptake. Some studies suggest that carnitine deficiency is a major cause of valproate hepatotoxicity and that supplementation with L-carnitine, 50–100 mg/kg/24 hr, may prevent this fatal complication. Until further data are available, it is recommended that L-carnitine supplementation be provided to those children at greatest risk for hepatotoxicity (see earlier). In older children on valproate therapy, L-carnitine supplementation should be administered if there are clinical symptoms suggestive of carnitine deficiency (weakness, lethargy, hypotonia) or there is a significant decrease in the serum-free carnitine levels measured on a periodic basis. Sodium valproate is available in a syrup, 50 mg/mL, 250- and 500-mg capsules, and 125-, 250-, and 500-mg tablets.

ADRENOCORTICOTROPIC HORMONE (ACTH). This is the preferred drug for the management of infantile spasms, although there is nonuniformity with regard to the dose and duration of therapy. Prednisone is equally effective. A common schedule includes ACTH, 20 units IM daily for 2 wk, and if no response occurs the dose is increased to 30 and then 40 units IM daily for an additional 4 wk. Unless there is complete seizure control, the ACTH is replaced with oral prednisone, 2 mg/kg/24 hr for 2 wk. If the seizures persist, prednisone is given for an additional 4 wk. The side effects of ACTH include hyperglycemia, hypertension, electrolyte abnormalities, gastrointestinal disturbances, infection, and transient brain shrinkage observed by CT scanning. ACTH and prednisone are equally effective for the treatment of cryptogenic and symptomatic seizures, and control can be expected in approximately 70% of patients. There is no relationship between the ease or degree of seizure control and ultimate neurologic and cognitive outcome. The response to medication is usually apparent within a few weeks of therapy, but one third of patients who respond will relapse when the ACTH or prednisone is discontinued.

KETOGENIC DIET. This treatment should be considered for the management of recalcitrant seizures, particularly for children with complex myoclonic epilepsy with associated tonic-clonic convulsions. The diet restricts the quantity of carbohydrate and protein, and most calories are provided as fat. Most children beyond the age of 2–3 yr will not tolerate this fatty unpalatable diet. Because the diet demands precise weighing of foodstuffs and is time consuming to prepare, it is not tolerated by all families. Some children respond to a liberalized ketogenic diet that substitutes medium-chain triglycerides for the high-fat content of the former diet. Although the mechanism of action of the ketogenic diet is unknown, there is some evidence that it has an effect on increasing the inhibitory neurotransmitter GABA.

SURGERY FOR EPILEPSY. Surgery should be considered for children with intractable seizures unresponsive to anticonvulsants. Until recently, surgery was reserved for adults with longstanding seizures with a focal onset. Studies have now shown that certain children, particularly those with focal seizures, are also candidates for surgery. Although the history and neurologic examination may suggest a focal onset of seizure activity, the EEG is critical in documenting the localization and extent of the epileptogenic discharges. Prolonged EEG recording with video monitoring, frequently necessary on more than one occasion, is essential for the precise localization of the epileptogenic area. It is often helpful to decrease or discontinue the anticonvulsant in the hospitalized patient to increase the probability of recording ictal and interictal epileptogenic activity. In those rare cases when the EEG with the use of sphenoidal or nasopharyngeal electrodes does not adequately localize the focus, the placement of subdural electrodes may provide invaluable information. The EEG studies are complemented by neuropsychologic testing, the WADA (intracarotid injection of amobarbital to establish the dominant hemisphere) test, single photon emission computed tomography (SPECT) or positron emission tomography (PET) scanning, and neuroimaging procedures including CT scanning and MRI. The results of surgery in children with a well-defined focus of epileptogenic activity supported by an identical structural lesion on CT scanning or MRI are extremely favorable and are comparable with the adult with similar pathology. Further refinement in electrophysiologic testing and neuroimaging will undoubtedly lead to even better surgical results in children with anticonvulsant-unresponsive epilepsy.

COUNSELING THE PARENTS. Most parents are initially frightened by the diagnosis of epilepsy and require support and accurate information. The physician should anticipate questions, including inquiries about the duration of the seizure disorder, side effects of medication and convulsions, etiology, social and academic repercussions, and parental guilt. Parents usually wish to know if restrictions should be placed on the child and whether the teacher should be informed. Others inquire about the genetic implications, including the risks for future children. The parents should be encouraged to treat the child as normally as possible. For most children with epilepsy, restriction of physical activity is unnecessary except that the child must be attended by a responsible adult while the child is bathing and swimming. The mechanism of the seizure and what epilepsy means should be explained, and the purpose and side effects of the specific anticonvulsant should be reviewed. Parents who understand the fundamental action and purpose of anticonvulsants and the need for a specific drug regimen are generally very compliant. Counseling should include first-aid measures to be used if the seizure recurs. Fortunately, most parents and children readily adapt to the seizure disorder and to the requirement for long-term anticonvulsants. Most children with epilepsy are well controlled on medication, have normal intelligence, and can be expected to lead normal lives. However, these children require careful monitoring as learning disabilities are more common in children with epilepsy than in the general population. Cooperation and understanding among the parent, physician, teacher, and child enhance the outlook for the patient with epilepsy.

Beaumanoir A: The Landau-Kleffner syndrome. *In:* Roger J, Dravet C, Bureau M, et al (eds): Epileptic Syndromes in Infancy, Childhood and Adolescence. London, John Libbey, 1985, pp 181–191.

Berkovic SF, Andermann F, Carpenter S, et al: Progessive myoclonus epilepsies: specific causes and diagnosis. N Engl J Med 315:296, 1986.

Bram TZ: Pathophysiology of massive infantile spasms: perspective on the putative role of the brain adrenal axis. Ann Neurol 33:231, 1993.

Bruni J, Sanders M, Anhut H, et al: Efficacy and safety of gabapentin (neurontin): a multicenter, placebo-controlled, double-blind study. Neurology 41(Suppl 1):330, 1991.

Camfield C, Camfield P, Gordon K, et al: Outcome of childhood epilepsy: A population-based study with a simple predictive scoring system for those treated with medication. J Pediatr 122:861, 1993.

Cross JH, Jackson GD, Neville BGR, et al: Early detection of abnormalities in partial epilepsy using magnetic resonance. Arch Dis Child 69:104, 1993.

Delgado-Escueta AV, Bacsal FE, Treiman DM: Complex partial seizures on closed circuit television and EEG: A study of 691 attacks in 79 patients. Ann Neurol 11:292, 1982.

Delgado-Escueta AV, Enrile-Bacsal FE: Juvenile myoclonic epilepsy of Janz. Neurology 34:285, 1984.

Dravet C, Bureau M, Roger J: Benign myoclonic epilepsy of infants. *In:* Roger J, Dravet C, Bureau M, et al (eds): Epileptic Syndromes in Infancy, Childhood and Adolescence. London, John Libbey, 1985, pp 68–72.

Duchowny MS: Complex partial seizures of infancy. Arch Neurol 44:911, 1987.

Engel JE Jr (ed): Surgical Treatment of the Epilepsies. New York, Raven Press, 1987.

Erba G, Browne TR: Atypical absence, myoclonic, atonic and tonic seizures and the "Lennox-Gastaut syndrome." *In:* Browne TR, Feldman RG (eds): Epilepsy, Diagnosis and Management. Boston, Little, Brown, 1983.

Farwell JR, Lee YJ, Hirtz DG, et al: Phenobarbital for febrile seizures: Effects on intelligence and on seizure recurrence. N Engl J Med 322:364, 1990.

Gale K: Mechanisms of seizure control mediated by γ-aminobutyric acid: role of the substantia nigra. Fed Proc 44:2414, 1985.

Holmes GL: Partial seizures in children. Pediatrics 77:725, 1986.

Hrachovy RA, Frost JD Jr, Kellaway P, et al: Double-blind study of ACTH vs prednisone therapy in infantile spasms. J Pediatr 103:641, 1983.

Jeavons PM, Bower BD: The natural history of infantile spasms. Arch Dis Child 36:17, 1961.

Lombroso CT: A prospective study of infantile spasms. Epilepsia 24:135, 1983.

Offringa M, Bossuyt PMM, Lubsen J, et al: Risk factors for seizure recurrence in children with febrile seizures: A pooled analysis of individual patient data from five studies. J Pediatr 124:574, 1994.

Rosman NP, Colton T, Labazzio J, et al: A controlled trial of diazepam administered during febrile illnesses to prevent reoccurrence of febrile seizures. N Engl J Med 329:79, 1993.

Sato S, Dreifuss FE, Penry JK: Prognostic factors in absence seizures. Neurology 26:788, 1976.

Tein I, DiMauro S, Xie Z-W, et al: Valproic acid impairs carnitine uptake in cultured human skin fibroblasts. An in vitro model for the pathogenesis of valproic acid-associated carnitine deficiency. Pediatr Res 34:281, 1993.

Thurston JH, Thurston DL, Hixon BB, et al: Prognosis in childhood epilepsy: Additional follow-up of 148 children 15–23 years after withdrawal of anticonvulsant therapy. N Engl J Med 306:831, 1982.

543.5 Neonatal Seizures

The neonate is at particular risk for the development of seizures because metabolic, toxic, structural, and infectious diseases are more likely to become manifest during this time than at any other period of life. Neonatal seizures are dissimilar from those in a child or adult because generalized tonic-clonic convulsions tend not to occur during the 1st mo of life. The arborization of axons and dendritic processes as well as myelination are incomplete in the neonatal brain. A seizure discharge therefore cannot readily be propagated throughout the neonatal brain to produce a generalized seizure. There are at least five seizure types that are recognizable in the newborn infant.

CLINICAL MANIFESTATIONS AND CLASSIFICATION. *Focal seizures* consist of rhythmic twitching of muscle groups, particularly the extremities and face. These seizures are often associated with localized structural lesions as well as with infections and subarachnoid hemorrhage. *Multifocal clonic* convulsions are similar to focal clonic seizures but differ in that multiple muscle groups are involved, frequently several simultaneously. *Tonic seizures* are characterized by rigid posturing of the extremities and trunk, and are sometimes associated with fixed deviation of the eyes. *Myoclonic seizures* are brief focal or generalized jerks of the extremities or body that tend to involve distal muscle groups. *Subtle seizures* consist of chewing motions, excessive salivation, and alterations in the respiratory rate including apnea, blinking, nystagmus, bicycling or pedaling movements, and changes in color.

Neonatal seizures may be difficult to recognize clinically, and some behaviors in the newborn that were considered previously to be convulsions are not substantiated by the EEG recording. Nonetheless, there are several clinical features that distinguish seizures from nonepileptic activity in the neonate. Autonomic changes such as tachycardia and elevation of the blood pressure are common with seizures but do not occur with nonepileptic events. Nonepileptic movements are suppressed by gentle restraint, but true seizures are not. Nonepileptic phenomena are enhanced by sensory stimuli that have no influence on seizures. Correct classification of neonatal seizures is important for the appropriate selection of anticonvulsant therapy. Recent studies utilizing polygraphic EEG recording with video monitoring have greatly enhanced the characterization of neonatal seizures and their medical management.

EEG CLASSIFICATION OF NEONATAL SEIZURES. Clinical Seizure with a Consistent EEG Event. In this category, a clinical seizure occurs in relationship to seizure activity recorded on the EEG and includes focal clonic, focal tonic, and some myoclonic seizures. These seizures are clearly epileptic and are likely to respond to an anticonvulsant.

Clinical Seizures with Inconsistent EEG Events. A neonate may have a clinical seizure without a corresponding seizure discharge. This is observed with all generalized tonic seizures and subtle seizures and with some myoclonic seizures. These infants tend to be neurologically depressed or comatose as a result of hypoxic-ischemic encephalopathy. Seizures in this category are likely to be of nonepileptic origin and may not require or respond to antiepileptics.

Electrical Seizures with Absent Clinical Seizures. Electrical seizures associated with a markedly abnormal background EEG may develop in the comatose infant who is not on anticonvulsants. Conversely, electrical seizures may persist in patients with focal tonic or clonic seizures without clinical signs following the introduction of an anticonvulsant.

ETIOLOGIC DIAGNOSIS. The most common cause of neonatal seizures, hypoxic-ischemic encephalopathy, is discussed in Chapter 84. There are many additional disorders that are likely to cause seizures, including metabolic, infectious, traumatic, structural, hemorrhagic, embolic, and maternal disturbances. Because seizures in the neonate may indicate a serious, life-threatening, and potentially reversible disease, it is imperative that a timely and organized approach to the investigation of neonatal seizures occur.

A careful neurologic examination of the infant may uncover the cause of the seizure disorder. An examination of the retina may show the presence of chorioretinitis, suggesting a congenital infection in which case TORCH titers of mother and infant are indicated. The *Aicardi syndrome,* which occurs exclusively in female infants, is associated with coloboma of the iris and retinal lacunae, refractory seizures, and absence of the corpus callosum. Inspection of the skin may show hypopigmented lesions characteristic of tuberous sclerosis or the typical crusted vesicular lesions of incontinentia pigmenti; both neurocutaneous syndromes are associated with generalized myoclonic seizures beginning early in life. An unusual body odor suggests an inborn error of metabolism.

Blood should be obtained for glucose, calcium, magnesium, electrolytes, and BUN. If hypoglycemia is a possibility, a serum Dextrostix is indicated so that treatment can be initiated immediately. See Chapter 93 for a discussion of the diagnosis and treatment of hypoglycemia. Hypocalcemia may occur in isolation or in association with hypomagnesemia. A lowered serum calcium is often associated with birth trauma or a CNS insult in the perinatal period. Additional causes include maternal diabetes, prematurity, the DiGeorge syndrome, and high phosphate feedings. See Chapters 56.9 and 92 for a full discussion. Hypomagnesemia (<1.5 mg/dL) is often associated with hypocalcemia and occurs particularly in infants of malnourished mothers. In this situation, the seizures are resistant to calcium therapy but respond to intramuscular magnesium, 0.2 mL/kg of a 50% solution of $MgSO_4$. See Chapter 92 for diagnosis and treatment of hypomagnesemia. The serum electrolytes may indicate significant hyponatremia (serum sodium <135 mEq/L) or hypernatremia (serum sodium >150 mEq/L) as a cause of the seizure disorder.

A *lumbar puncture* is indicated in virtually all neonates with seizures, unless the cause is obviously related to a metabolic disorder such as hypoglycemia or hypocalcemia secondary to feeding of high concentrations of phosphate. These latter infants are normally alert interictally and usually respond promptly to appropriate therapy. The CSF findings may indicate a bacterial meningitis or aseptic encephalitis (see Chapters 97 and 98). Prompt diagnosis and appropriate therapy improve the outcome for these infants. A bloody CSF indicates a traumatic tap or a subarachnoid/intraventricular bleed. Immediate centrifugation of the specimen may assist in the differentiation of the two disorders. A clear supernatant suggests a traumatic tap, and a xanthochromic color suggests a subarachnoid bleed. However, the mildly jaundiced normal infant may have a yellowish discoloration of the CSF that makes inspection of the supernatant less reliable in the newborn period.

Many *inborn errors of metabolism* cause generalized convulsions in the newborn period. As these conditions are often inherited in an autosomal recessive or X-linked recessive fashion, it is imperative that a careful family history be obtained to determine if siblings or close relatives developed seizures or expired at an early age. A serum ammonia is useful for the screening of suspected urea cycle abnormalities, such as ornithine transcarbamylase, arginosuccinic lysate, and carbamylphosphate synthetase deficiencies. Other than generalized clonic seizures, these infants present during the first few days of life with increasing lethargy progressing to coma, anorexia and vomiting, and a bulging fontanel. If the blood gases show an anion gap and a metabolic acidosis with hyperammonemia, urine organic acids should be immediately determined to investigate the possibility of methylmalonic or propionic acidemia. Maple syrup urine disease (MSUD), should be suspected when a metabolic acidosis occurs in association with generalized clonic seizures, vomiting, and muscle rigidity during the 1st wk of life. The result of a rapid screening test utilizing 2, 4-dinitrophenylhydrazine that identifies ketoderivatives in the urine is positive in MSUD. Additional metabolic causes of neonatal seizures include nonketotic hyperglycemia, a lethal condition characterized by markedly elevated plasma and CSF glycine levels, persistent generalized seizures, and lethargy rapidly leading to coma; ketotic hyperglycinemia in which seizures are associated with vomiting, fluid and electrolyte disturbances, and a metabolic acidosis; and Leigh disease suggested by elevated levels of serum and CSF lactate or an increased lactate/pyruvate ratio. A comprehensive description of the diagnosis and management of these metabolic diseases is discussed in Part X.

The unintentional *injection of a local anesthetic* into the fetus during labor can produce intense tonic seizures. These infants are often thought to have had a traumatic delivery because they are flaccid at birth, they have abnormal brain stem reflexes, and they show signs of respiratory depression that sometimes requires ventilation. Examination may show a needle puncture of the skin or a perforation or laceration of the scalp. An elevated serum anesthetic level confirms the diagnosis. The treatment consists of supportive measures and promotion of urine output by IV fluids with appropriate monitoring to prevent fluid overload.

Pyridoxine dependency, a rare disorder, must be considered when generalized clonic seizures begin shortly after birth with signs of fetal distress in utero. These seizures are particularly resistant to conventional anticonvulsants, such as phenobarbital or phenytoin. The history may suggest that similar seizures occurred in utero. Some cases of pyridoxine dependency are reported to begin later in infancy or in early childhood. This condition is inherited as an autosomal recessive. Although the precise biochemical defect is unknown, pyridoxine is essential for the synthesis of glutamic acid decarboxylase, which in turn is required for the synthesis of GABA. In these infants, large amounts of pyridoxine are required to maintain adequate production of GABA. When pyridoxine-dependent seizures are suspected, 100- to 200-mg of pyridoxine should be administered IV during the EEG, which should be promptly provided once the diagnosis is considered. The seizures will abruptly cease, and the EEG will normalize during the next few hours. In the future, measurement of CSF and plasma pyridoxal-5-phosphate may prove to be the more precise method of confirming the diagnosis of pyridoxine dependency. These children require lifelong supplementation of oral pyridoxine, 10 mg/day. Generally, the earlier the diagnosis and therapy with pyridoxine, the more favorable will be the outcome. Untreated children have persistent seizures and are uniformly severely mentally retarded (see also Chapter 43.7).

Drug withdrawal seizures can present in the newborn nursery but may take several weeks to develop because of prolonged excretion of the drug by the neonate. The incriminated drugs include barbiturates, benzodiazepines, heroin, and methadone. The infant may be jittery, irritable, and lethargic and may show myoclonus or frank clonic seizures. The mother may deny the use of drugs; a serum or urine analysis may identify the responsible agent (see Chapter 92).

Infants with severe *cytoarchitectural abnormalities* of the brain including lissencephaly, schizencephaly, neonatal adrenoleukodystrophy, and chromosome abnormalities are susceptible to severe seizures. The investigation of these infants may include a karyotype, CT scanning, MRI, and a long-chain fatty acid determination.

TREATMENT. Anticonvulsants should be utilized in the management of infants with seizures secondary to hypoxic-ischemic encephalopathy or an acute intracranial bleed (Chapters 84.7 and 85). The dose and administration of phenobarbital, diazepam, and other medications for the treatment of neonatal seizures are discussed in Chapter 84.7. The greater use of EEG recording in the infant with subtle seizures has identified a number of patients with abnormal movements unrelated to seizure discharges; anticonvulsants are not indicated for this group of neonates.

PROGNOSIS. This depends mainly on the primary cause of the disorder or the severity of the insult. In the case of the hypoglycemic infant of the diabetic mother or hypocalcemia associated with excessive phosphate feedings, the prognosis is excellent. Conversely, the child with intractable seizures due to severe hypoxic-ischemic encephalopathy or a cytoarchitectural abnormality of the brain will usually not respond to anticonvulsants and is susceptible to status epilepticus and early death. The challenge for the physician is to identify patients who will recover with prompt treatment and to avoid delays in diagnosis that could lead to severe irreversible neurologic damage.

Donn S, Grasela T, Goldstein G: Safety of a higher loading dose of phenobarbital in the term newborn. Pediatrics 75:1061, 1985.

Gilman JT, Gal P, Duchowny MS, et al: Rapid sequential phenobarbital treatment of neonatal seizures. Pediatrics 83:674, 1989.

Gospe SM, Olin KL, Keen CL: Reduced GABA synthesis in pyridoxine-dependent seizures. Lancet 343:1133, 1994.

Herzlinger RA, Krandall SR, Vaughan HG: Neonatal seizures associated with narcotic withdrawal. J Pediatr 91:683, 1977.

Hillman L, Hillman R, Dodson WE: Diagnosis, treatment and follow-up of neonatal mepivacaine intoxication secondary to paracervical and pudendal blocks during labor. J Pediatr 95:472, 1979.

Hunt AD, Stokes J, McCrory WW, et al: Pyridoxine dependency: Report of a case of intractable convulsions in an infant controlled by pyridoxine. Pediatrics 13:140, 1964.

Kellaway P, Mizrahi EM: Neonatal seizures. *In:* Luders H, Lesser RP (eds): Epilepsy, Electroclinical Syndromes. New York, Springer-Verlag, 1987, pp 13–47.

Koren G, Warwicke B, Rajchgot R, et al: Intravenous paraldehyde for seizure control in newborn infants. Neurology 36:108, 1986.

Legido A, Clancy RR, Berman P: Neurologic outcome after electroencephalographically proven neonatal seizures. Pediatrics 88:583, 1991.

Mizrahi E, Kellaway P: Characterizations and classification of neonatal seizures. Neurology 37:1837, 1987.

Painter MJ, Pippenger C, Wasterlain C, et al: Phenobarbital and phenytoin in neonatal seizures: Metabolism and tissue distribution. Neurology 31:1107, 1981.

Volpe JJ: Neonatal seizures: Current concepts and revised classification. Pediatrics 84:422, 1989.

543.6 Status Epilepticus

Status epilepticus is defined as a continuous convulsion lasting greater than 30 min or the occurrence of serial convulsions between which there is no return of consciousness. Status epilepticus may be classified as generalized (tonic-clonic, absence) or partial (simple, complex, or with secondary generalization). Generalized tonic-clonic seizures predominate in cases of status epilepticus. Status epilepticus is a medical emergency that requires an organized and skillful approach in order to minimize the associated mortality and morbidity.

ETIOLOGY. There are three major subtypes of status epilepticus in children: prolonged *febrile seizures, idiopathic status epilepticus* in which a seizure develops in the absence of an underlying CNS lesion or insult, and *symptomatic status epilepticus* when the seizure occurs in association with a longstanding neurologic disorder or a metabolic abnormality. A febrile seizure lasting for more than 30 min, particularly in a child less than 3 yr of age, is the most common cause of status epilepticus. The idiopathic group includes epileptic patients who have had sudden withdrawal of anticonvulsants (especially benzodiazepines and barbiturates) followed by status epilepticus. Epileptic children who are given anticonvulsants on an irregular basis or who are noncompliant are more likely to develop status epilepticus. Status epilepticus may also be the initial presentation of epilepsy. Sleep deprivation and an intercurrent infection tend to render epileptic patients more susceptible to status epilepticus. The mortality and morbidity among patients with prolonged febrile seizures and idiopathic status epilepticus are low. Status epilepticus owing to other causes has a much higher mortality and the cause of death is usually directly attributable to the underlying abnormality. Unlike those with idiopathic status epilepticus, many of these children have not previously had a convulsion. Severe anoxic encephalopathy presents with seizures during the first few days of life, and the ultimate prognosis relates partly to the ease in controlling the seizures. A prolonged convulsion may be the initial manifestation of encephalitis, and epilepsy may be a long-term complication of meningitis. Infants with congenital malformations of the brain (e.g., lissencephaly or schizencephaly) may have recurrent episodes of status epilepticus that are frequently refractory to anticonvulsants. Metabolic inborn errors of metabolism may present with status epilepticus in the newborn. These infants often have a progressive loss of consciousness associated with failure to thrive and excessive vomiting. Electrolyte abnormalities, hypocalcemia, hypoglycemia, drug intoxication, Reye syndrome, lead intoxication, extreme hyperpyrexia, and brain tumors, particularly in the frontal lobe, are additional causes of status epilepticus.

PATHOPHYSIOLOGY. The relationship between the neurologic outcome and the duration of status epilepticus is unknown in children and adults. There is some evidence that the period of status epilepticus that produces neuronal injury in a child is less than that for an adult. In the primate, pathologic changes can occur in the brain of the ventilated animal after 60 min of constant seizure activity when metabolic homeostasis is maintained. Thus, cell death may result from excessively increased metabolic demands by continually discharging neurons. The most vulnerable areas of the brain include the hippocampus, amygdala, cerebellum, middle cortical areas, and the thalamus. Characteristic acute pathologic changes consist of venous congestion, small petechial hemorrhages, and edema. Ischemic cellular changes are the earliest histologic finding, followed by neuronophagia, microglial proliferation, cell loss, and increased numbers of reactive astrocytes. Prolonged seizures are associated with lactic acidosis, an alteration in the blood-brain barrier, and elevation of intracranial pressure. A series of complex, poorly understood hormonal and biochemical changes ensues. Circulating levels of prolactin, adrenocorticotropic hormone, cortisol, glucagon, growth hormone, insulin, epinephrine, and cyclic nucleotides are elevated during status epilepticus in the animal. Neuronal concentrations of calcium, arachidonic acid, and prostaglandins rise and may promote cell death. Initially, the animal may be hyperglycemic, but ultimately hypoglycemia occurs. Inevitably, dysfunction of the autonomic nervous system develops, which may lead to hypotension and shock. Constant tonic-clonic muscle activity during a seizure may produce myoglobinuria and acute tubular necrosis.

Several investigations have shown significant increases in cerebral blood flow and metabolic rate during status epilepticus. In the animal, approximately 20 min of status epilepticus produces regional oxygen insufficiency, which promotes cell damage and necrosis. These studies have led to the concept of a critical period during status epilepticus when irreversible neuronal changes may develop. This *transitional period* varies between 20 and 60 min in the animal during constant seizure activity. Management of the child should be directed to supporting vital functions and to controlling the convulsions as expeditiously as possible, because the precise transitional period in humans is unknown.

TREATMENT. The *initial management* of the patient begins with an assessment of the respiratory and cardiovascular systems. The child should be transferred to an intensive care unit if possible. The oral airway is inspected for patency, and the pulse, temperature, respirations, and blood pressure are recorded. Excessive oral secretions are removed by gentle suction, and a properly fitting face mask attached to oxygen is applied. If the patient does not respond to oxygen by mask or is difficult to ventilate by an Ambu Bag, consideration should be given to intubation and assisted ventilation. An IV catheter is immediately inserted. If hypoglycemia is confirmed by Dextrostix, a rapid infusion of 5 mL/kg of 10% dextrose is provided. Blood is obtained for a CBC, electrolytes (including calcium and magnesium), glucose, creatinine, and anticonvulsant levels, if indicated. Blood and urine may be obtained for toxicology, keeping in mind that some drugs potentiate or precipitate status epilepticus (e.g., amphetamines, cocaine, phenothiazines, theophylline in toxic levels, and the tricyclic antidepressants). Arterial blood gases should be determined, and it is wise to maintain an arterial line for repeated examinations. Examination of the CSF is imperative if meningitis or encephalitis is considered, unless there is a contraindication for the procedure. In this case, appropriate antibiotics should be administered, followed by imaging studies, before the lumbar puncture is attempted. If the seizures are refractory to anticonvulsants, or the patient is paralyzed and is on a respirator, continuous EEG monitoring is important to follow the frequency of seizure discharges, their location, and the response to anticonvulsant therapy.

A physical and neurologic examination should be carried out concurrently to assess evidence of trauma; papilledema, a bulging anterior fontanel, or lateralizing neurologic signs suggesting increased intracranial pressure; manifestations of sepsis or meningitis; retinal hemorrhages that may indicate a subdural hematoma; Kussmaul breathing and dehydration suggestive of metabolic acidosis or irregular respirations signifying brain stem dysfunction; evidence of failure to thrive, a peculiar body odor, or abnormal hair pigmentation that suggests an inborn error of metabolism; and constriction or dilatation of pupils suggesting a toxin or drugs as the cause of the status epilepticus. A comprehensive examination should be undertaken once the seizures are under control. Further investigation of the patient including neuroradiologic studies depends on the physical and neurologic findings and on a precise history of the seizure type and frequency.

Drugs should always be delivered IV in the management of status epilepticus; the IM route is unreliable because some drugs are bound by muscle. One of the major problems in the management of status epilepticus is the inappropriate use of anticonvulsants. Too often an unsuitably low drug dose is given, and with lack of response, another antiepileptic is introduced immediately. Care should be given with regard to how the anticonvulsant is delivered. Phenytoin forms a precipitate in glucose solutions and is rendered ineffective. Other drugs interact with plastic containers or are altered by sunlight (e.g., paraldehyde). It is essential to have resuscitation equipment at the bedside and the ability to intubate and ventilate the patient immediately if respiratory depression should supervene.

Either *diazepam* or *lorazepam* may be used initially, because they are effective for the immediate control of prolonged tonic-clonic seizures in most children. Diazepam should be given IV directly into the vein (not the tubing) with a dose of 0.3 mg/kg and with a maximum dose of 10 mg at a rate no greater than 1 mg/min. Respiratory depression and hypotension can occur, especially if administered with a barbiturate. Diazepam is effective in the management of tonic-clonic status, but the drug has a short half-life so that the seizures will recur unless a longer acting anticonvulsant is administered simultaneously. Lorazepam is an equally effective short-term anticonvulsant, with a greater duration of action and decreased likelihood of producing hypotension and respiratory arrest. The recommended dose is 0.05–0.1 mg/kg administered slowly, IV. If an IV line cannot be established or the child is some distance from a medical center, rectal diazepam or lorazepam can be used safely. Undiluted diazepam is placed into the rectum by a syringe and a flexible tube at a dose of 0.3–0.5 mg/kg. The effective dose of rectal lorazepam is 0.05–0.1 mg/kg. Therapeutic serum levels occur within 5–10 min. Sublingual lorazepam may be used to treat children with serial seizures that tend to develop into status epilepticus while the children are at home.

The dose of sublingual lorazepam is 0.05–0.1 mg/kg. The tablet is placed under the patient's tongue and dissolves in a few seconds.

Following the administration of diazepam or lorazepam, several options are available for further management. If the convulsive activity ceases after diazepam or lorazepam therapy or if the seizures persist, *phenytoin* is given immediately. The loading dose of phenytoin is 15–20 mg/kg IV at the rate of 1 mg/kg/min. Phenytoin may be safely added to half-normal or normal saline but not to glucose solutions; the undiluted drug can cause pain, irritation, and phlebitis of the vein. An electrocardiogram tracing is recommended during the loading phase in order to identify arrhythmias, a rare complication in children. If the seizures do not recur, a maintenance dose of 5–8 mg/kg divided into two equal doses daily is begun 12–24 hr later. Serum phenytoin levels should be monitored as the maintenance dose varies considerably with age. Phenytoin is not always effective in controlling tonic-clonic status epilepticus, in which case an alternative drug is necessary. In some centers, *phenobarbital* is initiated before phenytoin. It is given in a loading dose of 10–15 mg/kg or in the neonate 20 mg/kg IV during 10–30 min. With control of the seizures, the maintenance dose is 3–5 mg/kg/24 hr divided into two equal doses.

If the status epilepticus is not controlled by the preceding strategy, the physician must make some important therapeutic decisions, because it is likely the *transitional period* has passed. The choices for further drug management include paraldehyde, a diazepam drip, lidocaine, pentobarbital coma, or general anesthesia. By this stage the patient is usually sedated and may show signs of respiratory depression, necessitating elective intubation and assisted ventilation.

Paraldehyde is an excellent anticonvulsant and is relatively safe for administration to children. A 5% solution of paraldehyde is prepared by adding 1.75 mL of paraldehyde (1 g/mL) to D_5W to a total volume of 35 mL. The loading dose is 150–200 mg/kg IV slowly for 15–20 min, and then seizure control is maintained with an infusion of 20 mg/kg/hr in a 5% concentration in a glass bottle, because the drug is incompatible with plastic. The IV drip rate may be lowered as the seizures and EEG improve. The drug should be freshly opened, because outdated paraldehyde can deteriorate to acetylaldehyde and acetic acid. Paraldehyde administered rectally or IM can produce tissue damage and sloughing, thus these routes should be reserved for exceptional circumstances.

A **diazepam constant infusion** may be considered rather than paraldehyde, particularly if the initial loading dose of diazepam briefly controlled the seizures. Diazepam is soluble in sterile water, normal saline, and Ringer lactate. A dilution of 0.04 mg/mL offers the greatest assurance of redissolution of diazepam and 24-hr stability. The suggested flow rate is 2–3 mg/hr, but the dose should be titrated against the patient's response and side effects.

If the status epilepticus persists following diazepam or lorazepam, and a trial of phenytoin, phenobarbital, and paraldehyde, serious consideration should be given to the induction of **pentobarbital coma.** In an intensive care setting, the patient is placed on a ventilator and a continuous EEG monitor. The initial IV loading dose of pentobarbital is 3–5 mg/kg followed by 2–3 mg/kg/hr to maintain the serum pentobarbital level between 25 and 40 μg/mL. A burst-suppression EEG pattern is maintained for a minimum of 48 hr, followed by cessation of the pentobarbital until the serum level falls to the therapeutic range. Pentobarbital coma requires careful monitoring by an experienced physician, because hypotension requiring pressor agents and electrolyte abnormalities are likely to occur.

General anesthesia is an alternative adjunct to the management of status epilepticus if conventional drug therapy is not effective or if pentobarbital coma is not an option. Several agents have been used successfully, including halothane and isoflurane. General anesthesia probably acts by reversing cerebral anoxia and the concomitant metabolic abnormalities, allowing the previously administered anticonvulsants to exert their effect. The major disadvantage of general anesthesia is that it must be administered in an operating room with anesthetic gas scavenging equipment for prolonged periods.

Sodium valproate has been an effective anticonvulsant in the management of several types of seizures. Because sodium valproate is not available parenterally, it must be given orally or rectally in patients with status epilepticus. Because vomiting and paralytic ileus are common in children with recurrent seizures, sodium valproate should be administered rectally during status epilepticus in order to achieve maximal absorption. Sodium valproate syrup (50 mg/mL) is diluted 1:1 with tap water and is given as a retention enema in a loading dose of 20 mg/kg. It may be considered in the management of status epilepticus in patients who do not respond to the conventional anticonvulsants and pentobarbital coma.

The use of anticonvulsant therapy following status epilepticus is controversial. There is little question that a long-term antiepileptic should be maintained in the child with a progressive neurologic disorder or with a history of recurrent seizures before the onset of status epilepticus. However, it is unlikely that a lengthy period of anticonvulsant treatment is necessary following an initial attack of idiopathic status epilepticus, particularly when a prolonged febrile seizure was the cause. Anticonvulsant therapy is maintained arbitrarily for 3 mo in this case and is discontinued if the child remains asymptomatic.

PROGNOSIS. The neurologic outcome following status epilepticus has improved significantly since the advent of modern pediatric intensive care units and the aggressive management of prolonged seizures. The mortality rate of status epilepticus is approximately 5% in most series. Most deaths occur in the symptomatic group, most of whom have a serious and life-threatening CNS disorder known before the onset of status epilepticus. In the absence of a progressive neurologic insult or metabolic disorder, the morbidity from status epilepticus is low. The fact that long-term sequelae such as hemiplegia, extrapyramidal syndromes, mental retardation, and epilepsy are more common in children less than 1 yr of age following status epilepticus is related to the fact that this group is more likely to have a premorbid underlying CNS disorder than the older child.

Aicardi J, Chevrie JJ: Convulsive status epilepticus in infants and children: A study of 239 cases. Epilepsia 11:187, 1970.

Aicardi J, Chevrie JJ: Consequences of status epilepticus in infants and children. Adv Neurol 34:115, 1983.

Cranford RE, Leppik IE, Patrick B, et al: Intravenous phenytoin in acute treatment of seizures. Neurology 29:1474, 1979.

Curless RG, Holzman BH, Ramsay RE: Paraldehyde therapy in childhood status epilepticus. Arch Neurol 40:477, 1983.

Delgado-Escueta AV, Bajorek JG: Status epilepticus: Mechanisms of brain damage and rational management. Epilepsia 23:S29, 1982.

Delgado-Escueta AV, Wasterlain CG, Treiman DM, et al: Management of status epilepticus. N Engl J Med 306:1337, 1982.

Dulac O, Aicardi J, Rey E, et al: Blood levels of diazepam after single rectal administration in infants and children. J Pediatr 93:1039, 1978.

Hauser AW: Status epilepticus, frequency, etiology and neurological sequelae. *In:* Delgado-Escueta AV, Wasterlain CG, Treiman DM, et al (eds): Status Epilepticus, Advances in Neurology, Vol 34. New York, Raven Press, 1983, pp 3–14.

Kreisman NR, Rosenthal M, LaManna JC, et al: Cerebral oxygenation during recurrent seizures. Adv Neurol 34:231, 1983.

Maytal J, Shinnar S, Moshe SL, et al: Low morbidity and mortality of status epilepticus in children. Pediatrics 83:323, 1989.

Walker JE, Homan RW, Vasko MR, et al: Lorazepam in status epilepticus. Ann Neurol 6:207, 1979.

Working Group on Status Epilepticus. Treatment of convulsive status epilepticus. JAMA 270:854, 1993.

Yager JY, Seshia SS: Sublingual lorazepam in childhood serial seizures. Am J Dis Child 142:931, 1988.

Young RSK, Ropper AH, Hawkes D, et al: Pentobarbital in refractory status epilepticus. Pediatr Pharmacol 3:63, 1983.

CHAPTER 544
Conditions That Mimic Seizures

Several conditions share features in common with epilepsy. Because these disorders may be associated with altered levels of consciousness, tonic or clonic movements, or cyanosis, they are often confused with epilepsy. These patients may be inappropriately placed on multiple anticonvulsants with no response and some risk; conditions that mimic epilepsy are refractory to antiepileptic drugs. The management of these children differs significantly from that of epilepsy.

BENIGN PAROXYSMAL VERTIGO

Benign paroxysmal vertigo (BPV) typically develops in the toddler and is relatively rare beyond 3 yr of age. The attacks develop suddenly and are associated with ataxia, causing the child to fall or refuse to walk or sit. Horizontal nystagmus may be evident during the duration of the attack. The child appears frightened and pale. Nausea and vomiting may be prominent. Consciousness and the ability to verbalize are not disturbed, and there is a lack of lethargy or drowsiness at the completion of the episode. The attacks vary in duration (seconds to minutes), frequency (daily to monthly), and intensity. A rotational sensation (vertigo) is verbalized by the older child with BPV. These children are susceptible to motion sickness and may develop migraine headaches several years later, suggesting a relationship between BPV and migraine. The neurologic evaluation characteristically has negative results, except for the finding of abnormal vestibular function detected by ice water caloric testing. Patients with clusters of attacks usually respond to dimenhydrinate, 5 mg/kg/24 hr with a maximum of 300 mg/24 hr PO, IM, IV, or per rectum.

NIGHT TERRORS

Night terrors are common, particularly in boys between 5 and 7 yr of age (Chapter 21.5). They occur in 1–3% of children and are usually short-lived. A night terror has a sudden onset, usually between midnight and 2.00 A.M. during stage 3 or 4 of slow-wave sleep. The child screams and appears frightened, with dilated pupils, tachycardia, and hyperventilation. There is little or no verbalization; the child may thrash violently, cannot be consoled, and is unaware of parents or surroundings. Sleep follows in a few minutes, and there is total amnesia the following morning. Approximately one third of children with night terrors experience somnambulism. An underlying emotional disorder should be explored in children with persistent and prolonged night terrors. A short course of diazepam or imipramine may be considered for treatment of protracted night terrors while the family dynamics are under investigation.

BREATH-HOLDING SPELLS

A breath-holding spell can be a frightening experience for the parent because the infant becomes lifeless and unresponsive owing to cerebral anoxia at the height of the attack. There are two major types of breath-holding spells: the more common cyanotic form and the pallid form. Also see Chapter 26.

CYANOTIC SPELLS. A cyanotic breath-holding spell is usually predictable and is always provoked by upsetting or scolding an infant. The episode is heralded by a brief, shrill cry followed by forced expiration and apnea. There is rapid onset of generalized cyanosis and a loss of consciousness that may be associated with repeated generalized clonic jerks, opisthotonus, and bradycardia. The interictal EEG is normal. A breath-holding spell can occur repeatedly within a few hours or it can recur sporadically, but it is always stereotyped. Breath-holding spells are rare prior to 6 mo of age; they peak at about 2 yr of age, and they abate by 5 yr of age. The management of breath-holding spells concentrates on the support and reassurance of the parents. Some parents feel that, whatever the physician recommends, they must splash cold water on the face, turn the child upside down, or initiate mouth-to-mouth resuscitation and even cardiopulmonary resuscitation. A thorough examination followed by an explanation of the mechanism of breath-holding spells is reassuring for most parents. The counseling session should emphasize the need for both parents to be consistent and not reinforce the child's behavior after the child recovers from the spell. This may be accomplished by placing the child safely in bed and by refusing to cuddle, play, or hold the child for a given period of time when recovery is complete.

PALLID SPELLS. These spells are much less common than cyanotic breath-holding spells, but they share several characteristics. Pallid spells are typically initiated by a painful experience, such as falling and striking the head or a sudden startle. The child stops breathing, rapidly loses consciousness, becomes pale and hypotonic, and may have a tonic seizure. Bradycardia with periods of asystole of longer than 2 sec may be recorded. The interictal EEG is normal. Pallid spells can in some cases be induced spontaneously in the laboratory by ocular compression that produces the oculocardiac reflex by afferent stimulation of the trigeminal nerve and by efferent inhibition of the heart by way of the vagus nerve. This procedure should not be attempted by an inexperienced physician, and appropriate resuscitation equipment should be readily available. Most children respond to conservative measures as outlined for cyanotic spells, but a trial of an anticholinergic, oral atropine sulfate 0.01 mg/kg/24 hr in divided doses with a maximum daily dose of 0.4 mg, which increases the heart rate by blocking the vagus nerve, may be considered in refractory cases. Atropine should not be prescribed during very hot weather as an episode of hyperpyrexia may be initiated.

SYNCOPE

SIMPLE SYNCOPE. Syncope follows an alteration in brain metabolism, the consequence of decreased cerebral blood flow, usually secondary to systemic hypotension. Decreased blood flow causes loss of consciousness, and the concomitant ischemia influences the higher cortical centers to release their inhibiting influence on the reticular formation within the brain stem. Neuronal discharges from the reticular formation then produce brief tonic contractions of the muscles of the face, trunk, and extremities in approximately 50% of patients with syncope. During a syncopal episode, the child may have fixed upward deviation of the eyes that can be confused with epilepsy. Simple syncope results from vasovagal stimulation and is precipitated by pain, fear, excitement, and extended periods of standing still, particularly in a warm environment. The EEG shows transient slowing during the attack but no seizure discharges. Simple syncope is uncommon prior to 10–12 yr of age but is quite prevalent in adolescent females. Tilt-table testing is an effective method of producing symptoms, including hypotension, in the majority of children with unexplained syncope. Most patients with positive tilt-table tests have vasovagal syncope, which if recurrent responds favorably to oral β-adrenergic blocking agents. Syncope can usually be differentiated from a seizure because of its short duration, associated symptoms of nausea and perspiration, and complete orientation following the event.

COUGH SYNCOPE. This is most common in asthmatic children. It often occurs shortly after the onset of sleep, and the coughing paroxysm abruptly awakens the child. The patient's face becomes plethoric, and the child perspires, becomes agitated, and frightened. Loss of consciousness is associated with generalized muscle flaccidity, vertical upward gaze, and clonic muscle contractions lasting for several seconds. Urinary incontinence is frequent. Recovery begins within seconds, and consciousness is usually restored a few minutes later. The child has no recollection of the attack except for the events surrounding the paroxysm of coughing. Coughing produces a marked increase in intrapleural pressure followed by a lowered venous return to the right side of the heart and an associated decrease in right ventricular output. Reduction of left ventricular filling follows, and a rapidly diminished cardiac output results in altered cerebral blood flow, cerebral hypoxia, and a loss of consciousness. The cornerstone of management for asthmatic children with cough syncope is an aggressive approach to the prevention of bronchoconstriction.

THE PROLONGED QT SYNDROME. The prolonged QT syndrome is characterized by sudden loss of consciousness during exercise or an emotional and stressful experience (see Chapter 388). Loss of consciousness in association with exercise or stress is rarely due to epilepsy, and in every case a cardiac cause must be considered. The onset of the condition is typically in late childhood or adolescence. During the period of syncope, a variety of cardiac arrhythmias are evident, particularly ventricular fibrillation. The child may recover within minutes or die during the event. The electrocardiogram may show prolongation of the QT interval, due to abnormal lengthening of the QT interval, especially during carefully monitored exercise. QT intervals corrected for heart rate of 0.48 sec or greater support the diagnosis. There are at least two varieties of the syndrome: those due to acquired heart disease (myocarditis, mitral valve prolapse, electrolyte abnormalities, drug induced) and two congenital forms. The QT syndrome may be inherited as an autosomal recessive trait that is associated with deafness or as autosomal dominant. Linkage studies in the latter indicate the genetic marker for the condition is located on the short arm of chromosome 11. All family members of an affected patient should have a 12 lead electrocardiogram. Further testing may include exercise tests or Holter monitoring. Beta blockers are usually effective and may be life-saving. Parents should be taught cardiopulmonary resuscitation, as exercise restriction and drug therapy may be ineffective for some children.

PAROXYSMAL KINESIGENIC CHOREOATHETOSIS

This disorder is characterized by a sudden onset of unilateral or occasionally bilateral choreoathetosis or dystonic posturing of a leg or an arm and associated facial grimacing and dysarthria. The condition is precipitated by sudden movement, particularly upon arising from a sitting position, or excitement and stress. The attacks rarely persist for longer than a minute and are never associated with loss of consciousness. The age of onset is typically between 8 and 14 yr, but the condition may begin as early as 2 yr. The child may have several attacks daily or they may be intermittent, occurring once or twice a month. The neurologic examination, EEG, and neuroimaging studies are normal, and neuropathologic studies in a few cases showed no abnormalities. Most reported cases are familial, suggestive of autosomal recessive inheritance. The attacks can be prevented by the use of anticonvulsants, particularly phenytoin. The attacks of paroxysmal kinesigenic choreoathetosis tend to diminish in frequency during adulthood, and the anticonvulsant can be successfully weaned at that time.

SHUDDERING ATTACKS

Shuddering attacks have their onset at 4–6 mo of age and may persist to 6–7 yr of age. They produce an interesting posture, with sudden flexion of the head and trunk and shuddering or shivering movements similar to what must occur if ice-cold water is poured down the back of an unsuspecting individual. These children may have 100 attacks/day followed by several symptom-free weeks. Shuddering attacks may be the childhood precursor of benign essential tremor, because examination of parents and relatives reveals a high incidence of that common condition.

BENIGN PAROXYSMAL TORTICOLLIS OF INFANCY

Infants with benign paroxysmal torticollis have recurrent attacks of head tilt associated with pallor, agitation, and vomiting with an onset between 2 and 8 mo of age. During the attack, the child resists passive head movement. There is no loss of consciousness, and spontaneous remission occurs by 2–3 yr of age. As with benign paroxysmal vertigo, abnormalities in vestibular function have been documented in these patients. Children with persistent torticollis should be investigated for abnormalities of the cervical vertebra, including dislocation or fracture, or a tumor located in the posterior fossa. Some infants with benign paroxysmal torticollis develop migraine headaches later in childhood.

HEREDITARY CHIN TREMBLING

Hereditary chin trembling may be confused with epilepsy due to repeated episodes of rapid 3/sec chin trembling movements. These brief attacks are precipitated by stress, anger, and frustration and are inherited as an autosomal dominant trait. The findings on the neurologic examination and EEG are normal.

NARCOLEPSY AND CATAPLEXY

See also Chapters 21.5 and 106. Narcolepsy is a disorder that rarely begins before adolescence and is characterized by paroxysmal attacks of irrepressible sleep, which is sometimes associated with transient loss of muscle tone (cataplexy). An EEG shows that the recurrent sleep attacks consist of rapid eye movement (REM) sleep. Patients with narcolepsy are easily aroused and become spontaneously alert, whereas a convulsion is followed by a deep sleep, postictal drowsiness, lethargy, and often a headache. Cataplexy is also occasionally confused with epilepsy. These patients experience sudden loss of muscle tone and fall to the floor because of laughter, stress, or frightening experiences. The cataplectic patient does not lose consciousness but lies without moving for a few minutes until normal body tone returns. Treatment consists of scheduled naps, amphetamines, methylphenidate, tricyclic antidepressants, and counseling with respect to occupational safety and driving.

RAGE ATTACKS OR EPISODIC DYSCONTROL SYNDROME

The *episodic dyscontrol syndrome,* a nonepileptic condition, can be confused with complex partial seizures. These patients develop sudden and recurrent attacks of violent physical behavior with minimal provocation. The attacks consist of kicking, scratching, biting, and shouting (including abusive and profane language). The child or adolescent cannot seem to control the behavior and may seem momentarily psychotic throughout the attack. The episode is followed by fatigue, amnesia, and sincere remorse. The routine EEG may show nonspecific abnormalities in patients with the rage syndrome. The EEG in such patients during the attack remains normal, which distinguishes this condition from complex partial seizures that always show an abnormal EEG during an attack.

MASTURBATION

Masturbation or self-stimulation behavior may occur in female infants between the ages of 2 mo and 3 yr. These children have repetitive stereotyped episodes of tonic posturing associated with copulatory movements, but without manual stimulation of the genitalia. The child suddenly becomes flushed and perspires, may grunt and breathe irregularly, but there is no loss of consciousness. The masturbatory activity has a sudden onset, usually persists for a few minutes (rarely hours), and tends to occur during periods of stress or boredom. The examination should include a search for evidence of sexual abuse or abnormalities of the perineum, but in most cases a cause will not be found. Treatment consists of reassurance that the self-stimulatory activity will subside by 3 yr of age and that no specific therapy is required.

PSEUDOSEIZURES

The diagnosis of a pseudoseizure should be made only after a thorough history and physical examination and exclusion of "true" seizures by prolonged EEG recording when indicated. Pseudoseizures occur typically between 10 and 18 yr of age and are more frequent among female patients. Pseudoseizures occur in many patients with a past history of epilepsy and in some with ongoing "true" seizures. A pseudoseizure may be quite realistic but frequently it is bizarre, with unusual postures, verbalizations, and uncharacteristic tonic or clonic movements. There are several distinguishing features of a pseudoseizure, including lack of cyanosis, normal reaction of the pupil to light, no loss of sphincter control, normal plantar responses, and the absence of tongue biting or injury during the attack. Many patients moan or cry during a pseudoseizure, and some patients can be persuaded to have an attack on request by the physician. Patients with pseudoseizures are likely to have a neurotic personality documented by formal psychologic testing. It is not unusual to find a patient on three or four anticonvulsants, which, of course, have no effect. The most reliable method of differentiating epilepsy from suspected pseudoseizures is to record an attack. The EEG shows an excess of muscle artifact during the pseudoseizure, but a normal background rhythm devoid of seizure discharges. Following true epileptic seizure there is a significant increase in serum prolactin, whereas there is no change from the baseline at the termination of a pseudoseizure.

Basser LS: Benign paroxysmal vertigo of childhood. Brain 87:141, 1964.

Fleisher DR, Morrison A: Masturbation mimicking abdominal pain or seizures in young girls. J Pediatr 116:810, 1990.

Grossman BJ: Trembling of the chin—an inheritable dominant character. Pediatrics 19:453, 1957.

Haslam RHA, Freigang B: Cough syncope mimicking epilepsy in asthmatic children. Can J Neurol Sci 12:45, 1985.

Kertesz A: Paroxysmal kinesigenic choreoathetosis. An entity within the paroxysmal choreoathetosis syndrome. Description of 10 cases, including 1 autopsied. Neurology 17:680, 1967.

Koenigsberger MR, Chutorian AM, Gold AP, et al: Benign paroxysmal vertigo of childhood. Neurology 20:1108, 1970.

Lombroso CT, Lerman P: Breath-holding spells (cyanotic and pallid infantile syncope). Pediatrics 39:563, 1967.

Mount LA, Reback S: Familial paroxysmal choreoathetosis. Arch Neurol Psychiatr 44:841, 1940.

O'Marcaigh AS, MacLellan-Tobert SG, Porter CJ: Tilt-table testing and oral metoprolol therapy in young patients with unexplained syncope. Pediatrics 93:278, 1994.

Pritchard PB, Wannamaker BB, Sagel J, et al: Serum prolactin and cortisol levels in evaluation of pseudoepileptic seizures. Ann Neurol 18:87, 1985.

Ruckman RN: Cardiac causes of syncope. Pediatr Rev 9:101, 1987.

Schneider S, Rice DR: Neurologic manifestations of childhood hysteria. J Pediatr 94:153, 1979.

Snyder CH: Paroxysmal torticollis in infancy. Am J Dis Child 117:458, 1969.

Vanasse M, Bedard P, Andermann F: Shuddering attacks in children: An early clinical manifestation of essential tremor. Neurology 26:1027, 1976.

Yoss R, Daly D: Narcolepsy in children. Pediatrics 25:1025, 1960.

Zarcone V: Narcolepsy. N Engl J Med 288:1156, 1973.

CHAPTER 545
Headaches

Headache is a common problem in pediatrics. The effect that headaches have on a child's academic performance, memory, personality, and interpersonal relationships, as well as school attendance, depends on their etiology, frequency, and intensity. A headache may occasionally indicate a severe underlying disorder (e.g., a brain tumor) and thus careful evaluation of children with recurrent, severe, or unconventional headaches is mandatory. Infants and children respond to a headache in unpredictable fashion. Most toddlers cannot communicate the characteristics of a headache, but rather they may become irritable and cranky, vomit, prefer a darkened room because of photophobia, or repeatedly rub their eyes and head. Children are poor historians when describing a headache and its associated symptoms. The most important causes of headache in children include migraine, increased intracranial pressure, and psychogenic or stress headaches. Refractive errors, strabismus, sinusitis, and malocclusion of the teeth are much less common causes of significant headaches in children.

545.1 Migraine

Migraine is defined as a recurrent headache with symptom-free intervals and at least three of the following symptoms or associated findings: abdominal pain, nausea or vomiting, throbbing headache, unilateral location, associated aura (visual, sensory, motor), relief following sleep, and a positive family history. It is the most important and frequent type of headache in the pediatric population. Most migraine headaches are not severe and are readily managed by conservative measures without requiring medical attention. The youngest child reported to develop migraine was 1 yr of age. The incidence of migraine among school-aged children between 7 and 15 yr of age was 4% in a comprehensive Swedish study. Girls are more likely to develop a migraine as adolescents, whereas males are in the slight majority among children under 10 yr old with migraine headaches. More than one half undergo spontaneous prolonged remission following the 10th birthday. The etiology of migraine headaches is unknown, but an inherited predisposition to vasomotor instability appears to be an important underlying factor. Hormonal changes, food allergies, personality traits characterized by high achievement, stress, bright flashing lights, and excessive sound have all been implicated. Increased levels of circulating serotonin and substance P, a vasodilating polypeptide, may act directly on the extracranial and intracranial vessels.

CLINICAL MANIFESTATIONS AND CLASSIFICATION. Migraine may be classified into subgroups, including common and classic migraine, migraine variants, cluster headaches, and complicated migraine. As cluster headaches rarely occur in children, they are not discussed here.

Common Migraine (migraine without aura). This migraine is not associated with an aura and is the most prevalent type of migraine in children. The headache is throbbing or pounding, and tends to be located in the bifrontal or temporal regions. It is often not hemicranial in children and is less intense compared with the migraine in an adult. The headache usually persists for 1–3 hr, although the pain may last for as long as 24 hr. A characteristic feature of childhood migraine is intense nausea and vomiting, which may be more bothersome than the headache. The vomiting may be associated with abdominal pain and fever, thus conditions such as appendicitis and a systemic infection may be erroneously confused with the primary diagnosis. Additional symptoms include extreme paleness, photophobia, light-headedness, and paresthesias of the hands and feet. A family history, particularly on the maternal side, is present in approximately 90% of children with common migraine. Thus, considerable caution should be exercised when making the diagnosis of a common migraine in the absence of a positive family history.

Classic Migraine (migraine with an aura). In this disorder an aura precedes the onset of the headache. Visual aurae are rarely present in children with migraine, but when they occur they may take the form of blurred vision, scotoma (an area of depressed vision within the visual field), photopsia (flashes of light), fortification spectra (brilliant white zig-zag lines), or irregular distortion of objects. Some patients also have vertigo and light-headedness during this stage of the headache. Sensory symptoms include perioral paresthesias and numbness of the hands and feet. Distortions of body image may predominate as a prelude to a classic migraine headache. Following the aura, a patient with classic migraine develops typical symptoms of a common migraine as described earlier.

Migraine Variants. These variants include cyclic vomiting, acute confusional states, and benign paroxysmal vertigo. The last condition is discussed in Chapter 544. *Cyclic vomiting* is characterized by recurrent, sometimes monthly bouts of severe vomiting that may be so intense that dehydration and electrolyte abnormalities occur, particularly in an infant. Initially, systemic symptoms such as fever, abdominal pain, and diarrhea are absent, but they may become prominent in association with excessive fluid losses secondary to vomiting. The vomiting may be protracted and persist for several days. The child may appear pale and frightened but does not lose consciousness. After a period of deep sleep, the child awakens and resumes normal play and eating habits as if the vomiting had not existed. Many children with cyclic vomiting have a positive family history of migraine, and, as they grow older and become verbal, they describe a typical migraine headache that leaves little doubt about the diagnosis and the association of the cyclic vomiting with the condition. Cyclic vomiting is treated with rectally administered antiemetics such as dimenhydrinate, 5 mg/kg/24 hr in four divided doses (maximum of 300 mg/24 hr) and careful attention to fluid replacement if the vomiting is excessive. Additional causes of cyclic vomiting include intermittent intestinal obstruction (e.g., malrotation, volvulus) and urea cycle defects.

Acute confusional states may be a manifestation of migraine. Migraine may present in a bizarre fashion, particularly in children, characterized by confusion, hyperactivity, disorientation, unresponsiveness, memory disturbances, vomiting, and lethargy. The neurologic examination shows defects of the sensorium, delayed responses to stimuli including touch and pain, and occasionally plantar extensor responses. The differential diagnosis includes toxic encephalopathy (particularly in an adolescent), encephalitis, acute psychosis, postictal state, petit mal (absence) status epilepticus, head trauma, and sepsis. The episode of acute confusion may persist for several hours and characteristically clears spontaneously following sleep; the patient has no recall of the confusional state. The diagnosis is usually made in retrospect as the patient or family recalls the onset of a severe headache or visual symptoms preceding the acute attack of confusion, and a family history of migraine is established. Acute confusional states as a component of migraine probably result from localized cerebral edema due to increased vascular permeability during the headache. The EEG shows regional areas of slowing (2–4 cps) during and shortly after the attack but routinely returns to normal within a few days.

Complicated Migraine. Complicated migraine refers to the development of neurologic signs during a headache that persist following the termination of the headache. The presence of neurologic signs in association with a headache suggests the possibility of an underlying structural lesion and requires a thorough investigation. There are three subsets of complicated migraine.

Brain stem signs predominate in patients with *basilar migraine,* owing to vasoconstriction of the basilar and posterior cerebral arteries. The major symptoms include vertigo, tinnitus, diplopia, blurred vision, scotoma, ataxia, and an occipital headache. The pupils may be dilated, and ptosis may be evident. Alterations in consciousness followed by a generalized seizure may result. After the attack there is a complete resolution of the neurologic symptoms and signs. There is a strongly positive family history for migraine in most of the children. Many develop classic migraine as adolescents or adults. Relatively minor head trauma may precipitate an episode of basilar migraine. The condition has been described in children of both sexes, with girls less than 4 yr of age at particular risk.

Ophthalmoplegic migraine is relatively rare in children. These patients develop a third-nerve palsy ipsilateral to the headache during the attack, owing to altered blood supply to the oculomotor nerve. The major differential diagnosis is a congenital aneurysm compressing the oculomotor nerve. *Amaurosis fugax,* acute, reversible, monocular blindness, may also be a variant of complicated migraine.

Hemiplegic migraine refers to the onset of unilateral sensory or motor signs during an episode of migraine. Hemisyndromes are more common in children than in adults and may be characterized by numbness of the face, arm, and leg, unilateral weakness, and aphasia. More than one attack is uncommon in the pediatric age group. The neurologic signs may be transient or may persist for days. It is unusual for a child to develop a completed stroke following a single episode. Hemiplegic migraine in the older child or adolescent has a relatively good prognosis, and often a positive family history of similar hemiplegic events is elicited. On the other hand, some children with migraine develop the syndrome of *alternating hemiplegia,* which has its onset during infancy. Acute hemiplegia may be the initial manifestation of migraine and may recur, affecting one side and then the other. Frequent episodes of vasoconstriction associated with ischemia may result in irreversible cerebral injury leading to mental retardation and epilepsy in this subgroup of children.

DIAGNOSIS AND DIFFERENTIAL DIAGNOSIS. A thorough history and physical examination suffice to establish the diagnosis in most cases. Basilar migraine may be confused with several conditions, including congenital malformations of the skull and cervical vertebrae, posterior fossa tumors, toxins and drugs, and metabolic abnormalities including Leigh disease and pyruvate decarboxylase deficiency. In children with hemiplegic migraine, an arteriovenous malformation, MELAS (mitochondrial myopathy, encephalopathy, lactic acidosis, and stroke), cerebral tumor, Todd paralysis, clotting disorders, hemoglobinopathies such as sickle cell disease, and metabolic conditions including homocystinuria should be considered. A lipid profile should be obtained in children with migraine and a positive family history of premature myocardial infarction or cerebrovascular accident. The organization of laboratory tests and radiologic studies depends on the constellation of symptoms and findings during the neurologic examination. A CT scan or MRI is indicated if the headache is associated with an unusual constellation of symptoms or signs or when increased intracranial pressure is suspected (Table 545–1).

TREATMENT. Migraine may be prevented or ameliorated by *avoiding certain initiating stimuli.* A few children can identify specific factors that uniformly result in a headache. The most common precipitators of migraine headaches are stress, fatigue, and anxiety. The child may be under undue stress because of difficulties at home or school, particularly when unrealistic pressures or demands are placed on the patient. Children who experience recurrent migraine headaches during the school year may have a learning disability or may have been placed in a too highly competitive classroom. Reassessment of the child's school placement and academic abilities may be the most important step in the management of the headache disorder. Some studies implicate certain foods as a cause of migraine, particularly nuts, chocolate, cola drinks, hot dogs, spicy meats, kippers, and Chinese food (monosodium glutamate). Elimination of the incriminating foodstuff is indicated if the history suggests a relationship between the ingestion of a particular food and the onset of headache. Avoidance of bright flashing lights, sun exposure, excessive physical exertion, mild head trauma, loud noises, hunger, fatigue, motion sickness, and drugs (including alcohol and oral contraceptives) is indicated when the history suggests a direct relationship. It is important to note that the frequency and severity of migraine headaches is reduced significantly in at least 50% of pediatric patients who undergo a careful history and neurologic examination followed by reassurance from the physician.

Management of an acute attack of migraine should include the use of *analgesics* and *antiemetics.* Most migraine headaches in children can be treated by the judicious use of *acetaminophen* or *ibuprofen,* particularly if the headaches are mild, infrequent, and of short duration. The *ergotamine preparations* (ergotamine tartrate) should be considered for older children and adolescents with severe, classic migraine headaches and are most efficacious during the early stages of the migraine attack. The usual dose is 1 mg, which may be administered orally, subcutaneously, or per rectum in the form of a suppository. A repeat dose may be given 30 min later. Ergotamine should not be prescribed for patients with hemiplegic episodes. The ergotamines are frequently ineffective in children because they must be used early in the evolution of the headache. Most children are either unaware of an aura or fail to communicate the onset of the headache to their parents. An antiemetic such as *dimenhydrinate,* 5 mg/kg/24 hr in four divided doses, is the mainstay of treatment when vomiting is the major symptom. The child usually prefers to rest in a quiet darkened room and typically awakens, refreshed and headache-free, several hours later after a deep sleep. *Sumatriptan,* a specific and selective 5-HT receptor agonist, is an effective drug in treating the acute phase of both classic and common migraine headaches in adults. The drug may be administered subcutaneously or orally, and the adverse effects, including hot flushes, nausea and vomiting, fatigue, and drowsiness, are usually minor and transient. Hypertension and coronary vasospasm have been reported in adults. The drug is not licensed at present for patients under 18 yr of age.

The decision to use *continuous daily medication* is based on the severity and frequency of the headaches and on the impact of the migraine on the child's daily activities, including school attendance and performance as well as participation in recreation. The use of prophylactic drugs should be considered if the child experiences more than 2–4 severe episodes monthly or is unable to attend school regularly (Table 545–2). Although few drugs have been subjected to well-designed clinical trials in children, propranolol, a β-adrenergic blocker, is the drug of choice in most centers. If a drug is effective, it is usually maintained for 1 yr, particularly during the school term.

Behavior management is an effective method for the treatment of migraine in some children and adolescents. Biofeedback and self-hypnosis are replacing pharmacologic treatment in some centers because of the undesirable side effects of drugs and the concern that some may produce chemical dependency. Biofeedback can be mastered by most children over 8 yr of age and has been effective in many clinical trials. Several studies of migrainous children show a significant decrease in frequency and no change in intensity of headaches in those treated by self-hypnosis compared with those taking the placebo or propranolol.

■ **TABLE 545–1 Indications for Neuroimaging a Child with Headaches***

Abnormal neurologic signs
Recent school failure, behavioral change, fall-off in linear growth rate
Headache awakens child during sleep; early morning headache, with increase in frequency and severity
Periodic headaches and seizures coincide, especially if seizure has a focal onset
Migraine and seizure occur in the same episode, and vascular symptoms precede the seizure (20–50% risk of tumor or arteriovenous malformation)
Cluster headaches in child; any child <5 or 6 yr whose principal complaint is a headache
Focal neurologic symptoms or signs developing during a headache (i.e., complicated migraine)
Focal neurologic symptoms or signs (except classic visual symptoms of migraine) develop during the aura, with fixed laterality; focal signs of the aura persisting or recurring in the headache phase
Visual graying out occurring at the peak of a headache instead of the aura
Brief cough headache in a child or adolescent

**Modified from Barlow CF: Headaches and Migraine in Childhood. Philadelphia, JB Lippincott, 1984, p 205.*

545.2 Organic Headaches

A headache may be the earliest symptom of increased intracranial pressure. The headache results from tension or traction of the cerebral blood vessels and dura, and occurs initially in a sporadic fashion, primarily in the early hours in the morning or shortly after the patient arises. The headache is diffuse and generalized and is more prominent over the frontal and occipital regions. Its onset may be insidious, and the pain is enhanced by any activity that raises the intracranial pressure (e.g., coughing, sneezing, or straining during a bowel movement). As the intracranial pressure increases, the child becomes lethargic and irritable, and the headache becomes constant. Early morning vomiting is often associated with increased intracranial pressure. Causes of organic headaches in children include brain tumors, particularly those located in the posterior fossa, hydrocephalus, meningitis and encephalitis, cerebral abscess, subdural hematoma, chronic lead poisoning, and pseudotumor cerebri. Additional causes of organic headaches in children that may not be associated with increased intracranial pressure include arteriovenous malformations, berry aneurysm, collagen vascular diseases affecting the CNS, hypertensive encephalopathy, acute subarachnoid hemorrhage, and stroke. The management of organic headaches depends on the cause. The initial step includes a thorough history and physical examination, including recording of the blood pressure and inspection of the eyegrounds. Ordering of laboratory tests and neuroradiologic procedures depends on the clues provided by the history and physical examination.

545.3 Tension or Stress Headaches

Stress or tension headaches are relatively uncommon in the pediatric age group, particularly before puberty, and are often

■ TABLE 545–2 Drugs for Migraine Prophylaxis

Drug	Dose	Side Effects	Contraindications
Propranolol	Children: begin 10 mg bid or tid, max 20 mg tid; adolescents: begin 10–20 mg tid, max 80 mg tid	Nausea, insomnia, fatigue, bradycardia, hypertension	Asthma, cardiac arrhythmias, depression, diabetes
Phenytoin	3–5 mg/kg/24 hr; adjust to maintain serum levels at 40–80 μmol/L	Hirsutism, gingival hyperplasia, ataxia, skin reaction, rarely hepatotoxicity	
Phenobarbital	2–5 mg/kg/24 hr; do not exceed serum level of 130 μmol/L	Hyperactivity, short attention span in 20% of children	Probable side effects in hyperactive or developmentally delayed child
Amitriptyline	Not approved for children; adolescents: 25–50 mg/24 hr	Dizziness, fatigue, urinary retention, constipation, weight gain, dry mouth	
Cyproheptadine	Children: 0.2–0.4 mg/kg/24 hr in 2–3 divided doses; adolescents: 4–10 mg/24 hr	Impaired learning, drowsiness, increased appetite, weight gain	
Methysergide	Not recommended for children under 10 yr old; adolescents: 2 mg bid or tid after meals. Do not use longer than 3 mo	Nausea, dizziness, drowsiness, retroperitoneal fibrosis with prolonged use	Restricted to patients with severe headache when other drug regimens have failed

difficult to differentiate from migraine headaches. The two are often associated in the same patient. Tension headaches infrequently appear in the morning hours but are most apparent during the school day, particularly coinciding with a test or similarly anxiety-provoking circumstance. Although these headaches can be continuous and persist for weeks, they tend to wax and wane and build in intensity during the day. The headache is described as hurting or aching but is rarely perceived as throbbing. Most tension headaches in children are distributed in the frontal region, but they may localize over the vertex or the occipital area. Unlike migraine or headaches associated with increased intracranial pressure, tension headaches are not, as a rule, associated with nausea and vomiting.

The *diagnosis* of tension headache is made by exclusion at the completion of the history and physical examination. Studies such as an EEG or a CT scan are rarely necessary. Management consists of a search for possible underlying emotional or stressful factors. Most children have considerable insight into the origin of tension headaches and, when given the opportunity, will share concerns and conflicts. A poor self-image, fear of school failure, and lack of self-confidence are common factors. Occasionally, a depressed child presents with severe headaches. These patients may also complain of sudden mood changes, weight loss, anorexia, disturbed sleep, fatigue, and withdrawal from social activities.

The *treatment* of tension headaches begins with reassurance and an explanation with regard to how stress may cause a headache. Anxiety and stress may unconsciously produce constant isometric contraction of the temporalis, masseter, or trapezius muscles, which leads to the characteristic, dull aching headache. Steps should be introduced to remove obvious anxiety-provoking situations. Acetaminophen and other mild analgesics are often all that are required to treat a tension headache. Sedatives and antidepressants are rarely necessary. Children with severe tension headaches may benefit from a brief hospitalization, particularly if an underlying depressive illness is under consideration. In the hospital setting, the child's interaction with other patients, nursing and medical staff, and family is observed while a plan is formulated for counseling or psychiatric intervention. In most cases, the child's headaches are considerably relieved during the period of observation. As with migraine headaches, biofeedback and self-hypnosis exercises are effective in the management of some patients with tension headaches.

Borge AIH, Nordhagen R, Moe B, et al: Prevalence and persistence of stomach ache and headache among children. Follow-up of a cohort of Norwegian children from 4 to 10 years of age. Acta Paediatr 83:433, 1994.

Ferrari MD: Sumatriptan in the treatment of migraine. Neurology 43(Suppl 3):S43–S47, 1993.

Forsythe WI, Gillies D, Sills MA: Propranolol in the treatment of childhood migraine. Dev Med Child Neurol 26:737, 1984.

Gascon G, Barlow C: Juvenile migraine, presenting as an acute confusional state. Pediatrics 45:628, 1970.

Glueck CJ, Bates SR: Migraine in children: Association with primary and familial dyslipoproteinemias. Pediatrics 77:316, 1986.

Igarashi M, May WN, Golden GS: Pharmacologic treatment of childhood migraine. J Pediatr 120:653, 1992.

Ling W, Oftedal G, Weinberg W: Depressive illness in childhood presenting as severe headache. Am J Dis Child 120:122, 1970.

Olness H, MacDonald JT, Uden DL: Comparison of self-hypnosis and propranolol in the treatment of juvenile classic migraine. Pediatrics 79:593, 1987.

Presnky AL, Sommer D: Diagnosis and treatment of migraine in children. Neurology 29:506, 1979.

Verret S, Steel JC: Alternating hemiplegia of childhood: A report of eight patients with complicated migraine beginning in infancy. Pediatrics 47:675, 1971.

CHAPTER 546

Neurocutaneous Syndromes

The neurocutaneous syndromes include a heterogeneous group of disorders characterized by abnormalities of both the integument and central nervous system (CNS). Although the etiology is unknown, most disorders are familial and believed to arise from a defect in the differentiation of the primitive ectoderm. Disorders classified as neurocutaneous syndromes include neurofibromatosis, tuberous sclerosis, Sturge-Weber disease, von Hippel-Lindau disease, ataxia telangiectasia (see Chapter 547.1), linear nevus syndrome, hypomelanosis of Ito (see Chapter 603), and incontinentia pigmenti (see Chapter 602).

546.1 Neurofibromatosis

Neurofibromatosis (NF) (von Recklinghausen disease) is a common autosomal dominant disorder affecting approximately 1 in 4,000 of the population. The condition is protean, as virtually every system and organ may be affected, and progressive in that distinctive features may be present at birth but the development of complications is delayed for decades. Neurofibromatosis is the consequence of an abnormality of neural crest differentiation and migration during the early stages of embryogenesis, possibly related to the influence of nerve or glial growth factor (see also chapter 602).

CLINICAL MANIFESTATIONS AND DIAGNOSIS. There are two distinct forms of neurofibromatosis. NF-1 is the most prevalent type of neurofibromatosis and is diagnosed if any two of the following signs are present: (1) *At least five café-au-lait spots over 5 mm in greatest diameter in prepubertal patients or at least six café-au-lait spots over 15 mm in postpubertal patients.* Café-au-lait spots are the hallmark of neurofibromatosis and are present in almost 100% of patients. They are present at birth but increase in size, number, and pigmentation, especially during the first few years of life. The spots are scattered throughout the body surface with predilection for the trunk and extremities and sparing of the face. (2) *Axillary or inguinal freckling* consists of multiple hyperpigmented areas 2–3 mm in diameter. (3) *Two or more iris Lisch nodules.* Lisch nodules are hamartomas located within the iris and are best identified with a slit lamp examination. They are present in more than 90% of patients with NF-1 but are not a component of NF-2. (4) *Two or more neurofibromas or one plexiform neurofibroma.* Neurofibromas typically involve the skin, but they may be situated along peripheral nerves and blood vessels and within viscera including the gastrointestinal tract. These cutaneous lesions appear characteristically during adolescence or pregnancy, suggesting a hormonal influence. They are usually small, rubbery lesions with a slight purplish discoloration of the overlying skin. Plexiform neurofibromas are usually evident at birth and result from diffuse thickening of nerve trunks that are frequently located in the orbital or temporal region of the face. The skin overlying a plexiform neurofibroma may be hyperpigmented to a greater degree than a café-au-lait spot. Plexiform neurofibromas may produce overgrowth of an extremity and a deformity of the corresponding bone. (5) *A distinctive osseous lesion.* Abnormalities of the skeleton are a common feature of neurofibromatosis. Kyphoscoliosis is reported in approximately 40% of patients. Dysplasia of the sphenoid wing causes a pulsating exophthalmos, whereas bowing of the tibula and fibula is often associated with pathologic fractures that have a propensity to develop pseudoarthroses. (6) *Optic gliomas* are present in approximately 15% of patients with NF-1. These relatively benign tumors consist of glial cells and a mucinous material. Most patients with optic gliomas are asymptomatic and have normal or near-normal vision, but approximately 20% have visual disturbances or evidence of precocious sexual development secondary to tumor invasion of the hypothalamus. Children rarely are aware of unilateral visual loss, thus diagnosis may be delayed. Patients with a unilateral optic glioma typically display an afferent pupillary defect. To test for this, each eye is alternatively stimulated by a bright light source (swinging flashlight test). The affected pupil dilates rather than constricts, whereas light in the unaffected eye causes both pupils to constrict equally. Patients with NF-1 and a plexiform neuroma of the eyelid have a high association with an ipsilateral optic glioma. The CT findings of an optic glioma include diffuse thickening, localized enlargement, or a distinct focal mass originating from the optic nerve or chiasm. (7) *A first-degree relative with NF-1 whose diagnosis was based on the aforementioned criteria.* The NF-1 gene is assigned to chromosome 17q11.2.

Children with NF-1 are susceptible to *neurologic complications.* Magnetic resonance imaging (MRI) studies in selected children have shown abnormal signals in the globus pallidus, thalamus, and internal capsule, which probably represent low-grade glioma or hamartoma that is not detected by computed tomography (CT) scanning. These findings may account for the high incidence of learning disabilities, attention deficit disorders, and abnormalities of speech among affected children. Complex partial and generalized tonic-clonic seizures are a frequent complication. Hydrocephalus is a rare manifestation secondary to aqueductal stenosis, whereas macrocephaly with normal-sized ventricles is a common finding. The cerebral vessels may be occluded owing to the neurofibromatosis, resulting in hemiparesis and intellectual deficits. Not surprisingly, *psychologic disturbances* are prevalent owing to the seriousness and uncertainty of the disease. *Malignant neoplasms* are also a significant problem in patients with NF-1. A neurofibroma occasionally differentiates into a neurofibrosarcoma or malignant schwannoma. The incidence of pheochromocytoma, rhabdomyosarcoma, leukemia, and Wilms tumor is higher than in the general population. However, tumors of the CNS (including optic gliomas, meningiomas of the brain and spinal cord, neurofibromas, astrocytomas, and neurilemmomas) account for significant morbidity and mortality because of their increased frequency in patients with NF-1.

NF-2 accounts for 10% of all cases of neurofibromatosis and may be diagnosed when one of the following is present: (1) *bilateral eighth nerve masses* consistent with acoustic neuromas as demonstrated by CT scanning or MRI. (2) A *parent, sibling, or child with NF-2* and either unilateral eighth nerve masses or any two of the following: neurofibroma, meningioma, glioma, schwannoma, or juvenile posterior subcapsular lenticular opacities. **Bilateral acoustic neuromas** are the most distinctive feature of NF-2. Symptoms of hearing loss, facial weakness, headache, or unsteadiness may appear during childhood, although signs of a cerebellopontine angle mass are more commonly present in the 2nd and 3rd decades of life. Although café-au-lait spots and skin neurofibromas are classic findings in NF-1, they are much less common in NF-2. Posterior subcapsular lens opacities are identified in approximately 50% of patients with NF-2. As with NF-1, CNS tumors, including schwann-cell and glial tumors, and meningiomas are common in patients with NF-2. Linkage analysis has shown that the gene for NF-2 is located near the center of the long arm of chromosome 22q1.11.

TREATMENT. As there is no specific treatment for neurofibromatosis, the management includes genetic counseling and early detection of treatable conditions or complications. The evaluation of a child with neurofibromatosis should include several baseline studies, such as an audiogram, auditory brain stem and visual evoked potentials, an electroencephalogram (EEG), psychologic testing (including studies predictive for learning disorders), a roentgenographic skeletal survey, and CT scanning or MRI of the brain and optic nerves. The asymptomatic patient should be re-examined annually with a neurologic assessment, including blood pressure, auditory and visual screening, and a thorough search for the complications of neurofibromatosis. A parent with neurofibromatosis has a 50% chance of transmitting the disease with each pregnancy. The type of neurofibromatosis (NF-1 and NF-2) "breeds true" for successive generations. Because approximately one half of all cases of neurofibromatosis result from fresh mutations, each parent should be carefully examined (including a search for Lisch nodules) before counseling for the risk of affected future pregnancies. Standard DNA diagnostic analysis is not practical for the prenatal diagnosis of the NF-1 gene because of the large size of the gene and the significant number of mutations. However, prenatal diagnosis is feasible if the mutation causing the condition is known in the affected parent. The majority of NF-2 cases are the result of a mutation. Examination of fetal DNA for the characteristic single-strand conformational polymorphism of an altered DNA sequence provides accurate prenatal testing. In familial cases, where affected and unaffected family members are available, linkage can be established, making prenatal diagnosis available with a certain degree of accuracy.

546.2 Tuberous Sclerosis

Tuberous sclerosis (TS) is inherited as an autosomal dominant trait with an estimated frequency of 1/30,000. The TS gene is located on chromosome 9q34, but at least one half of the cases are sporadic owing to new mutations. TS is an extremely heterogeneous disease with a wide clinical spectrum. The disease varies from severe mental retardation and incapacitating seizures to normal intelligence and a lack of seizures, often within the same family. As a rule, the younger the patient presents with symptoms and signs of TS, the greater will be the likelihood of mental retardation. The disease affects many organ systems other than the skin and brain, including the heart, kidney, eyes, lung, and bone.

PATHOLOGY. The characteristic brain lesions consist of tubers. Tubers are located in the convolutions of the cerebral hemispheres and are typically present in the subependymal region, where they undergo calcification and project into the ventricular cavity, producing a "candle-dripping" appearance. Tubers in the region of the foramen of Monro may cause obstruction of cerebrospinal fluid (CSF) flow and hydrocephalus. The microscopic appearance of the tuber consists of decreased numbers of neurons and a proliferation of astrocytes, and the presence of oddly shaped multinucleated giant neurons. MRI is useful for identification of the lesions. Generally, the greater the number of tubers, the more neurologically impaired will be the patient.

CLINICAL MANIFESTATIONS. TS may present during infancy with infantile spasms and a hypsarrhythmic EEG pattern. Careful examination of the skin on the trunk and extremities shows the typical hypopigmented skin lesions that have been likened to an ash leaf in more than 90% of cases in this age group. The visualization of the hypopigmented lesions is enhanced by the use of a Wood's ultraviolet lamp (see Chapter 595). The CT scan typically shows calcified tubers in the periventricular area, but these may not be apparent until 3–4 yr of age. The seizures may be difficult to control, and at a later age they may develop into myoclonic epilepsy. There is a high incidence of mental retardation in young patients with TS and infantile spasms.

During childhood, TS presents most often with a generalized seizure disorder and pathognomonic skin lesions. Sebaceous adenomas develop between 4 and 6 yr of age; they appear as tiny red nodules over the nose and cheeks, and are sometimes confused with acne. Later, they enlarge, coalesce, and assume a fleshy appearance. A **shagreen patch** is also characteristic of TS and consists of a roughened, raised lesion with an orange-peel consistency located primarily in the lumbosacral region. Subungual or periungual fibromas arise from the stratum lucidum of the finger and toe in many patients with TS during adolescence. Retinal lesions consist of two types: mulberry tumors that arise from the nerve head or round and flat gray-colored lesions (phakoma) in the region of the disk (Fig. 546–1). Brain tumors are much less common in TS compared with neurofibromatosis, but occasionally a tuber differentiates into a malignant astrocytoma. Approximately 50% of children with TS have rhabdomyomas of the heart, which may be detected in the fetus at risk by an echocardiogram. The rhabdomyomas may be multiple or located at the apex of the left ventricle and, although they can cause congestive heart failure and arrhythmias, they tend to slowly resolve spontaneously. The kidney is involved in most patients by hamartomas or polycystic disease, resulting in hematuria, pain, and, in some cases, renal failure. Angiomyolipomas may produce generalized cystic or fibrous pulmonary changes in the lung and lead to spontaneous pneumothorax.

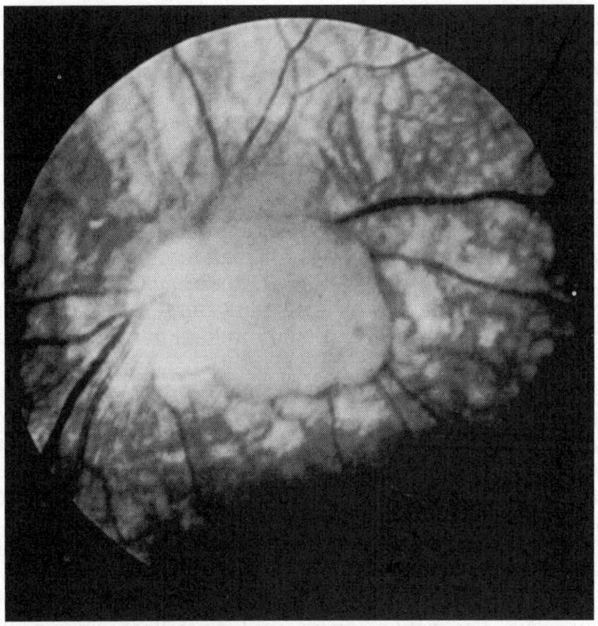

Figure 546–1. An astrocytoma of the retina (mulberry tumor) in a patient with tuberous sclerosis.

DIAGNOSIS. The diagnosis of TS relies on a high index of suspicion when assessing a child with infantile spasms. A careful search for the typical skin and retinal lesions should be completed in all patients with a seizure disorder. The head CT scan or MRI confirms the diagnosis in most cases.

TREATMENT. The management consists of seizure control and baseline studies, including renal ultrasound, an echocardiogram, and a chest roentgenogram with follow-up as indicated. Symptoms and signs of increased intracranial pressure suggest obstruction of the foramen of Monro by a tuber or malignant transformation of a tuber, and warrant immediate investigation and surgical intervention.

546.3 Sturge-Weber Disease

Sturge-Weber disease consists of a constellation of symptoms and signs including a facial nevus (port-wine stain), seizures, hemiparesis, intracranial calcifications, and, in many cases, mental retardation. It occurs sporadically with a frequency of approximately 1/50,000.

ETIOLOGY. The condition is thought to result from the anomalous development of the primordial vascular bed during the early stages of cerebral vascularization. At this stage the blood supply to the brain, meninges, and face is undergoing reorganization, while the primitive ectoderm in the region differentiates into the skin of the upper face and the occipital lobe of the cerebrum. The overlying leptomeninges are richly vascularized and the brain beneath becomes atrophic and calcified, particularly in the molecular layer of the cortex, in patients with Sturge-Weber disease.

CLINICAL MANIFESTATIONS. The facial nevus is present at birth and tends to be unilateral and always involves the upper face and eyelid. The nevus may also be evident over the lower face, trunk, and in the mucosa of the mouth and pharynx. Not all children with facial nevi have Sturge-Weber disease (Chapter 600). Buphthalmos and glaucoma of the ipsilateral eye are a common complication. Seizures develop in most patients during the 1st year of life. They are typically focal tonic-clonic and contralateral to the side of the facial nevus. The seizures tend to become refractory to anticonvulsants and are associated with a slowly progressive hemiparesis in many cases. Although neurodevelopment appears to be normal during the 1st year of life, mental retardation or severe learning disabilities are present in at least 50% during later childhood, probably the result of prolonged generalized seizures and increasing cerebral atrophy secondary to local hypoxia and multiple anticonvulsants.

DIAGNOSIS. The skull radiograph shows intracranial calcification in the occipitoparietal region in most patients. This characteristically assumes a serpentine or "railroad-track" appearance. The CT scan highlights the extent of the calcification that is usually associated with unilateral cortical atrophy and ipsilateral dilatation of the lateral ventricle (Fig. 546–2).

TREATMENT. The management of Sturge-Weber disease is multifaceted and somewhat controversial. Seizure frequency and the significant risk for mental retardation influence the treatment plan. For patients with well-controlled seizures and normal or near-normal development, the management is straightforward and conservative. However, there is increasing evidence that a hemispherectomy or lobectomy may prevent the development of mental retardation in the patient with recalcitrant seizures, particularly if the surgery is accomplished during the 1st year of life. Because of the risk of glaucoma, regular measurements of intraocular pressure with a tenonometer is indicated. The facial nevus is often a target for ridicule by classmates, leading to psychologic trauma. Flashlamp-pulsed laser therapy holds considerable promise for clearing of the port-wine stain. Finally, because of the high frequency of developmental disabilities, special educational facilities are frequently required.

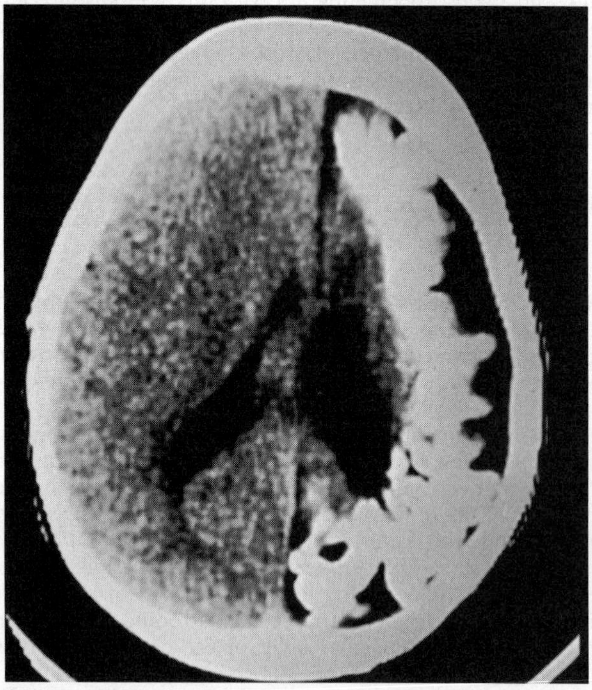

Figure 546–2. A CT scan of a patient with Sturge-Weber syndrome, showing unilateral calcification and atrophy of a cerebral hemisphere.

546.4 von Hippel-Lindau Disease

As with most of the neurocutaneous syndromes, von Hippel-Lindau disease affects multiple organs, including the cerebellum, spinal cord, medulla, retina, kidney, pancreas, and epididymis. von Hippel-Lindau disease is inherited as an autosomal dominant trait with variable penetrance and delayed expression. The gene for von Hippel-Lindau disease has been mapped to chromosome 3p25. The major neurologic features of the condition include cerebellar hemangioblastomas and retinal angiomata. Patients with cerebellar hemangioblastoma present in early adult life or beyond with symptoms and signs of increased intracranial pressure. A smaller number of patients have hemangioblastoma of the spinal cord, producing abnormalities of proprioception and disturbances of gait and bladder dysfunction. The CT scan typically shows a cystic cerebellar lesion with a vascular mural nodule. Total surgical removal of the tumor is curative. Approximately 25% of patients with cerebellar hemangioblastoma have retinal angiomata.

Retinal angiomata are characterized by small masses of thin-walled capillaries that are fed by large and tortuous arterioles and venules. They are usually located in the peripheral retina so that vision is unaffected. However, exudation in the region of the angiomata may lead to retinal detachment and visual loss. Retinal angiomata are treated with photocoagulation and cryocoagulation with good results. Cystic lesions of the kidney, pancreas, liver, and epididymis as well as pheochromocytoma are frequently associated with von Hippel-Lindau disease. Renal carcinoma is the most common cause of death. Regular follow-up and appropriate imaging studies are necessary to identify lesions that may be treated at an early stage.

546.5 Linear Nevus Syndrome

This sporadic condition is characterized by a facial nevus and neurodevelopmental abnormalities. The nevus is located on the forehead and nose, and tends to be midline in its distribution. It may be quite faint during infancy but later becomes hyperkeratotic with a yellow-brown appearance. More than one half of the patients have a seizure disorder and are mentally retarded. The seizures may be generalized myoclonic or focal motor. Most patients have normal CT studies, although hemimegalencephaly with hamartomatous changes has been reported. Focal neurologic signs including hemiparesis and homonymous hemianopia are more common in this group.

Alexander GL, Norman RM: The Sturge-Weber Syndrome. Bristol, England, John Wright, 1960.
Gutmann DH, Collins FS: Neurofibromatosis type 1: Beyond positional cloning. Arch Neurol 50:1185, 1993.
Hoffman HJ, Hendrick EB, Dennis M, et al: Hemispherectomy for Sturge-Weber syndrome. Childs Brain 5:233, 1979.
Hoffman KJ, Harris EL, Bryan RN, et al: Neurofibromatosis type 1: The cognitive phenotype. J Pediatr 124:51, 1994.
Horton WA, Wong V, Eldridge R: Von Hippel-Lindau disease: Clinical and pathological manifestations in nine families with 50 affected members. Arch Intern Med 136:769, 1976.
Hurst RW, Newman SA, Cail WS: Multifocal intracranial MR abnormalities in neurofibromatosis. AJNR 9:293, 1988.
Jozwiak S, Pedich M, Rajszys P, et al: Incidence of hepatic hamartomas in tuberous sclerosis. Arch Dis Child 67:1363, 1992.
Jozwiak S, Kawalec W, Dluzewska J, et al: Cardiac tumors in tuberous sclerosis: Their incidence and course. Eur J Pediatr 153:155, 1994.
Latif F, Tory K, Gmarra J, et al: Identification of the von Hippel-Landau disease tumor suppressor gene. Science 260:1317, 1993.
Listernick R, Charrow J: Neurofibromatosis type 1 in childhood. J Pediatr 116:845, 1990.

Listernick R, Charrow J, Greenwald MJ, et al: Optic gliomas in children with neurofibromatosis type 1. J Pediatr 114:788, 1989.
Lovejoy FH, Boyle LE: Linear nevus sebaceous syndrome: Report of two cases and a review of the literature. Pediatrics 52:382, 1973.
MacCollin M, Mohney T, Trofatter J, et al: DNA diagnosis of neurofibromatosis type 2: Altered coding sequence of the merlin tumor suppressor in an extended pedigree. JAMA 270:2316, 1993.
Martuza RL, Eldridge R: Neurofibromatosis 2 (bilateral acoustic neurofibromatosis). N Engl J Med 318:684, 1988.
Roach ES, Williams MD, Laster MD: Magnetic resonance imaging in tuberous sclerosis. Arch Neurol 44:301, 1987.
Seizinger BR, Martuza RL, Gusella JF: Loss of genes on chromosome 22 in tumorigenesis of human acoustic neuroma. Nature 322:644, 1986.
Tan OT, Sherwood K, Gilchrest BA: Treatment of children with port-wine stains using the flashlamp-pulsed tunable dye laser. N Engl J Med 320:416, 1989.

CHAPTER 547
Movement Disorders

Abnormalities of movement in children constitute a wide range of conditions with multiple causes. The type of movement disorder assists in the localization of the pathologic process, whereas the onset, age, and degree of the abnormal motor activity and associated neurologic findings help to classify the disorder and organize the investigation. Movement disorders are rarely limited to one form such as ataxia; the examination usually demonstrates additional abnormal movements such as tremor or chorea. This section highlights the major movement disorders in children and classifies the conditions based on the predominant motor disturbance.

547.1 Ataxias

Congenital anomalies of the posterior fossa, including the Dandy-Walker syndrome, the Chiari malformation, and encephalocele, are prominently associated with ataxia because of their destruction or replacement of the cerebellum (Chapter 542). **Agenesis of the cerebellar vermis** presents in infancy with generalized hypotonia and decreased deep tendon reflexes. Delayed motor milestones and truncal ataxia are typical. A familial variety (Joubert disease) is inherited as an autosomal recessive trait. These patients typically have abnormalities of respiration during infancy, characterized by alternating periods of hyperpnea and apnea. In addition to ataxia, mental retardation and abnormal eye movements have been described. MRI is the method of choice for investigating congenital abnormalities of the cerebellum, vermis, and related structures.

The major *infectious causes of ataxia* include cerebellar abscess, acute labyrinthitis, and acute cerebellar ataxia. **Acute cerebellar ataxia** occurs primarily in children 1–3 yr of age and is a diagnosis by exclusion. The condition often follows a viral illness, such as varicella, coxsackie, or echovirus infection, by 2–3 wk and is thought to represent an autoimmune response to the viral agent affecting the cerebellum (see Chapters 169, 209, and 213). The onset is sudden, and the truncal ataxia can be so severe that the child is unable to stand or sit. Vomiting may be present initially, but fever and nuchal rigidity are absent. Horizontal nystagmus is evident in approximately 50% of cases and, if the child is able to speak, dysarthria may be impressive. Examination of the cerebrospinal fluid (CSF) is typically normal at the onset of ataxia; however, a slight pleocytosis of lymphocytes (10–30/mm^3) is not unusual. Later in the course, the CSF protein undergoes a moderate elevation. The ataxia begins to improve in a few weeks but may persist for as long as 2 mo. The prognosis for complete recovery is excellent; however, a small number have long-term sequelae, including behavioral and speech disorders as well as ataxia and incoordination. **Acute labyrinthitis** may be difficult to differentiate from acute cerebellar ataxia in the toddler. The condition is associated with middle-ear infections and intense vertigo, vomiting, and abnormalities in labyrinthine function, particularly ice water caloric testing.

Toxic causes of ataxia include alcohol, thallium (which is used occasionally in the home as a pesticide), and the anticonvulsants, particularly phenytoin when serum levels reach or exceed 30 μg/mL (120 μmol/L).

Brain tumors, including tumors of the cerebellum and frontal lobe as well as neuroblastoma, may present with ataxia. Frontal lobe tumors may cause ataxia owing to the destruction of the association fibers connecting the frontal lobe with the cerebellum. Neuroblastoma may be associated with an encephalopathy characterized by progressive ataxia, myoclonic jerks, and opsoclonus (nonrhythmic horizontal and vertical oscillations of the eyes).

Several *metabolic disorders* are characterized by ataxia, including abetalipoproteinemia, arginosuccinic aciduria, and Hartnup disease. **Abetalipoproteinemia** (Bassen-Kornzweig disease) begins in childhood with steatorrhea and failure to thrive (see Chapter 72.4). A blood smear shows acanthocytosis and decreased serum levels of cholesterol and triglycerides; and the serum β-lipoproteins are absent. Neurologic signs become evident by late childhood and consist of ataxia, retinitis pigmentosa, peripheral neuritis, abnormalities in position and vibration sense, muscle weakness, and mental retardation. Vitamin E is undetectable in the serum of patients with neurologic symptoms.

Degenerative diseases of the central nervous system (CNS) represent an important group of ataxic disorders of childhood because of the genetic consequences and poor prognosis. **Ataxia telangiectasia,** an autosomal recessive condition, is the most common of the degenerative ataxias and is heralded by ataxia beginning at about 2 yr of age and progressing to loss of ambulation by adolescence (see Chapter 119). The gene responsible for ataxia telangiectasia has been assigned to chromosome 11q22.3–q23.1. Oculomotor apraxia, defined as having difficulty fixating smoothly on an object and therefore overshooting the target with lateral movement of the head followed by "re-fixating" the eyes, is a frequent finding, as is horizontal nystagmus. The telangiectasia becomes evident by mid-childhood and is found on the bulbar conjunctiva, over the bridge of the nose, and on the ears and exposed surfaces of the extremities. Examination of the skin shows a loss of elasticity. Abnormalities of immunologic function that lead to frequent sinopulmonary infections include decreased serum and secretory IgA as well as diminished IgG_2, IgG_4, and IgE levels in more than 50% of patients. Children with ataxia telangiectasia have a 50- to 100-fold greater chance of developing lymphoreticular tumors (lymphoma, leukemia, and Hodgkin disease) as well as brain tumors, compared with the normal population. Additional laboratory abnormalities include an increased incidence of chromosome breaks, particularly of chromosome 14, and elevated levels of α-fetoprotein. Death results from infection or tumor dissemination.

Friedreich ataxia is inherited as an autosomal recessive or dominant trait. The autosomal recessive disorder is most common and investigation of a large number of families has resulted in the assignment of the Friedreich ataxia locus to chromosome 9q13–q21.1. The onset of ataxia is somewhat later than in ataxia telangiectasia but occurs usually prior to

10 yr of age. The ataxia is slowly progressive and involves the lower extremities to a greater degree than the upper extremities. The Romberg test is positive; the deep tendon reflexes are absent (particularly the Achilles), and the plantar response is extensor. Patients develop a characteristic explosive, dysarthric speech, and nystagmus is present in most children. Although the patient may appear apathetic, the intelligence is preserved. There may be significant weakness of the distal musculature of the hands and feet. Typically, there is a marked loss of vibration and position sense owing to degeneration of the posterior columns and indistinct sensory changes in the distal extremities. Friedreich ataxia is also characterized by skeletal abnormalities, including high-arched feet (pes cavus) and hammer toes as well as progressive kyphoscoliosis. Electrophysiologic studies including visual, auditory brain stem, and somatosensory evoked potentials are often abnormal. Hypertrophic cardiomyopathy with progression to intractable congestive heart failure is the cause of death for most patients. Several forms of *spinocerebellar ataxia* are similar to Friedreich ataxia. **Roussy-Levy disease** has, in addition, atrophy of the muscles of the lower extremity with a similar pattern of wasting observed in Charcot-Marie-Tooth disease; the **Ramsay Hunt syndrome** has an associated myoclonic epilepsy.

The **olivopontocerebellar atrophies** (OPCA) include at least five familial subtypes with dominant inheritance that usually have the onset of ataxia, cranial nerve palsies, and abnormal sensory findings in the 2nd or 3rd decade. However, some cases have been described in children, particularly of Finnish ancestry, with rapidly progressive ataxia, nystagmus, dysarthria, and seizures. Recent classifications of the hereditary ataxias are based on biochemical analysis; aspartic acid and glutamic acid contents in the inferior olive and the Purkinje cell layer of the cerebellum are significantly decreased.

Rare forms of progressive cerebellar ataxia have been described in association with **vitamin E deficiency.** Additional degenerative ataxias include **Pelizaeus-Merzbacher disease,** neuronal ceroid lipofuscinoses, and late onset GM_2 gangliosidosis (see Chapter 548).

547.2 Chorea

Sydenham chorea is the most common acquired chorea of childhood and is the sole neurologic manifestation of rheumatic fever (Chapter 175). The pathogenesis of Sydenham chorea is probably an autoimmune response of the central nervous system to the streptococcus group A organism. The primary pathologic findings consist of vasculitis of the cortical arterioles with round cell infiltration of the gray and white matter in the surrounding area. The cerebral cortex, caudate nucleus, and subthalamic nuclei are most prominently involved. Chorea is likely the result of functional overactivity of the dopaminergic system. The three major features of Sydenham chorea include chorea, hypotonia, and emotional lability. The chorea is usually symmetric, although children may have the choreic movements limited to one side of the body. The movements, which are rapid and jerky, are prominent in the face, trunk, and distal extremities and dart from one muscle group to another, are increased by stress, and disappear during sleep. The onset may be abrupt, but typically the chorea has a slowly progressive course. Hypotonia may be a prominent sign and when combined with severe chorea the child may be incapable of feeding, dressing, or walking. The speech is often involved and is sometimes unintelligible. Periods of uncontrollable crying and extreme mood swings are characteristic, perhaps in part as the result of the motor handicap and feeling of helplessness. Several typical signs are associated with Sydenham chorea, including the "milkmaid's grip" (relaxing and tightening hand shake), the "choreic hand" (spooning of the extended hand by flexion at the wrist and extension of the fingers), "the darting tongue" (the tongue cannot be protruded for longer than a few seconds), and the "pronator sign" (the arms and palms turn outward when held above the head). Sydenham chorea may persist for several months and as long as 1–2 yr. About 20% of children experience a recurrence of chorea within 2 yr of the initial episode. Cases with minimal signs are treated conservatively with avoidance of stress as much as possible. Incapacitating chorea is managed with a trial of diazepam followed by phenothiazines or haloperidol if the former is unsuccessful. Although the phenothiazines and haloperidol are effective drugs in the treatment of Sydenham chorea, long-term use may be complicated by the development of another movement disorder, **tardive dyskinesia.** As patients with Sydenham chorea are at risk for the development of rheumatic carditis, particularly mitral stenosis, a regimen of daily penicillin prophylaxis should be instituted and maintained until adulthood. A much rarer cause of chorea during childhood, *paroxysmal kinesigenic choreoathetosis,* is discussed in Chapter 544.

Huntington disease is a progressive degenerative disorder of the CNS of unknown etiology that affects about 1:10,000 individuals and is inherited as an autosomal dominant trait. The gene is located on the tip of the long arm of chromosome 4p 16.3. The onset of symptoms of progressive chorea and presenile dementia occurs most typically between 35 and 55 yr of age. The disease is rare in the pediatric population; less than 1% of cases have the onset of symptoms prior to 10 yr of age. Rigidity and dystonia are the most common neurologic findings in the childhood patient. Chorea tends to involve proximal muscles, and the abnormal movements are often incorporated into semipurposeful acts in an attempt to mask the abnormality. Mental deterioration and behavioral problems are prominent in children. Generalized tonic-clonic seizures are common and are typically resistant to anticonvulsants. Cerebellar signs are present in 50%, and oculomotor apraxia occurs in approximately 20% of the cases. The course of the disease is more rapid in children, with an average duration of 8 yr until death compared with 14 yr in the adult. Computed tomography (CT) scanning, although nondiagnostic, shows the mean bifrontal to bicaudate ratio is decreased, indicating atrophy of the caudate nucleus and putamen. MRI shows hyperdensity of the putamen in adults with the akinetic-rigid form. There is no specific therapy for Huntington disease, but once the diagnosis is confirmed, the pediatrician should provide genetic counseling to the family so that risks for additional cases in future generations are understood. Molecular biologic testing (CAG trinucleotide repeat) is available but is inappropriate for children under the age of consent. Presymptomatic adult patients who test positive respond similarly to patients with cancer when the diagnosis is confirmed.

547.3 Dystonias

Dystonia is a slow, intermittent twisting motion that produces exaggerated turning and posture of the extremities and trunk. The principal causes of dystonia include perinatal asphyxia (see Chapters 81 and 84), dystonia musculorum deformans, drugs, Wilson disease (hepatolenticular degeneration), and Hallervorden-Spatz disease.

Dystonia musculorum deformans (DMD) is a slowly progressive disorder that typically begins during childhood. The etiology is unknown, but an abnormality of catecholamine metabolism within the CNS has been proposed. DMD is inherited as an autosomal dominant trait. One form occurs primarily in the Ashkenazi Jewish population, with an incidence of approximately 1:1,000. The gene has been mapped to chromosome 9q34. The initial manifestation of the disease during childhood is often unilateral posturing of the lower extremity, particularly the foot, which assumes an extended and rotated position causing tip-toe walking. Because the dystonic movement is initially intermittent and is aggravated by stress, patients are often labeled as hysterical. Ultimately, all four extremities and the axial musculature are affected as well as the muscles of the face and tongue so that speech and swallowing become impaired. Patients with generalized dystonia, including those with involvement of the muscles of swallowing, may respond to large doses of trihexphenidyl (Artane). The initial dose is 2 mg/24 hr and the drug is slowly increased to 60–80 mg/24 hr or until untoward side effects (urinary retention, mental confusion, or blurred vision) occur. Additional drugs that have been effective include carbamazepine, levodopa, bromocriptine, and diazepam.

Dopa-responsive dystonia (DRD), a variant of childhood-onset idiopathic torsion dystonia, is more common in females and typically presents at a mean age of 6.5 yr with dystonic posturing of a lower extremity. DRD responds remarkably to small daily doses (50–1,000 mg) of levodopa. The dystonia is diurnal, improving with sleep but becoming apparent and sometimes incapacitating during the daytime. Signs of Parkinson disease may ultimately become evident, including bradykinesia, tremors, and cogwheel rigidity. The disease is familial with an autosomal dominant inheritance.

Segmental dystonia, including writer's cramp, blepharospasm, and buccomandibular dystonia, is more common in the adult and tends to be limited to a specific group of muscles. Adults with segmental dystonia, particularly blepharospasm, may respond to local injections of botulism toxin, which holds promise for some children with generalized DMD. Cryothalamectomy with the placement of a lesion in the ventrolateral thalamus is reserved primarily for patients with extremity involvement.

Certain *drugs* are capable of producing an acute dystonic reaction in children. Therapeutic doses of phenytoin or carbamazepine may rarely cause progressive dystonia in children with epilepsy, particularly in those who have an underlying structural abnormality of the brain. Children may have an idiosyncratic reaction to the phenothiazines, characterized by acute dystonic posturing that is sometimes confused with encephalitis. IV diphenhydramine, 1–2 mg/kg/dose, may rapidly reverse the drug-related dystonia.

Wilson disease is a rare (incidence of 1:40,000 to 1:100,000 live births) autosomal recessive inborn error of copper transport characterized by cirrhosis of the liver and degenerative changes in the CNS, particularly the basal ganglia (see Chapter 303.2). The gene for Wilson disease has been mapped to chromosome 13q14.3. The precise etiology is unknown, but the basic mechanism relates to decreased excretion of biliary copper, owing partly to a lysosomal defect of the liver cells. The initial symptoms and signs in children under the age of 10 yr relate to acute or subacute hepatic failure that is frequently misinterpreted as infectious hepatitis. The neurologic manifestations of Wilson disease rarely appear before 10 yr of age, and the initial sign is often progressive dystonia. Tremors of the extremities develop, unilaterally at first, but eventually they become coarse, generalized, and incapacitating (the so-called "wing-beating" tremor). Signs of progressive basal ganglia destruction include drooling, a "fixed smile" owing to retraction of the upper lip, dysarthria, dysphonia, rigidity, contractures, dystonia, and choreoathetosis. The Kayser-Fleischer ring, which is best seen with the slit lamp, is pathognomonic and results from deposition of copper in Descemet membrane. In the untreated state, the patient typically becomes bedridden and demented, and dies in coma within a few years from the onset of the disease. The MRI or CT scan shows ventricular dilatation in advanced cases with atrophy of the cerebrum and lesions in the thalamus and basal ganglia (Fig. 547–1). The treatment of Wilson disease is discussed in Chapter 303.2.

Hallervorden-Spatz disease is a rare degenerative disorder inherited as an autosomal recessive trait. The condition begins usually during childhood and is characterized by progressive dystonia, rigidity, and choreoathetosis. Spasticity, extensor plantar responses, dysarthria, and intellectual deterioration become evident during adolescence, and death usually occurs by early adulthood. The CT scan shows lesions of the globus pallidus, and neuropathologic examination indicates an excessive accumulation of iron-containing pigments in the globus pallidus and substantia nigra.

Athetosis is most commonly associated with perinatal brain insults and is occasionally the major movement disorder of *phenothiazine idiosyncrasy.* Choreoathetosis may occur after hypothermic bypass surgery for congenital heart disease. Rigidity is associated with progressive destructive or neurodegenerative conditions, including Krabbe disease.

Tremor is an involuntary movement characterized by rhythmic oscillations of a part of the body, which may be more prominent during rest or with movement. **Jitteriness,** defined as rhythmic tremors of equal amplitude around a fixed axis, is the most common involuntary movement of healthy full-term infants. Jitteriness is most apparent when the infant is crying or being examined (e.g., Moro response) and is abnormal when the infant is awake and alert, and when the tremor persists beyond the second week of life. Organic causes of jitteriness include sepsis, intracranial hemorrhage, hypoxic encephalopathy, hypoglycemia, hypocalcemia, hypomagnesemia, prenatal exposure to maternal marijuana, and the narcotic abstinence syndrome. **Essential tremor** is a familial condition, inherited as an autosomal dominant. It may begin during childhood and is usually slowly progressive. The tremor has a

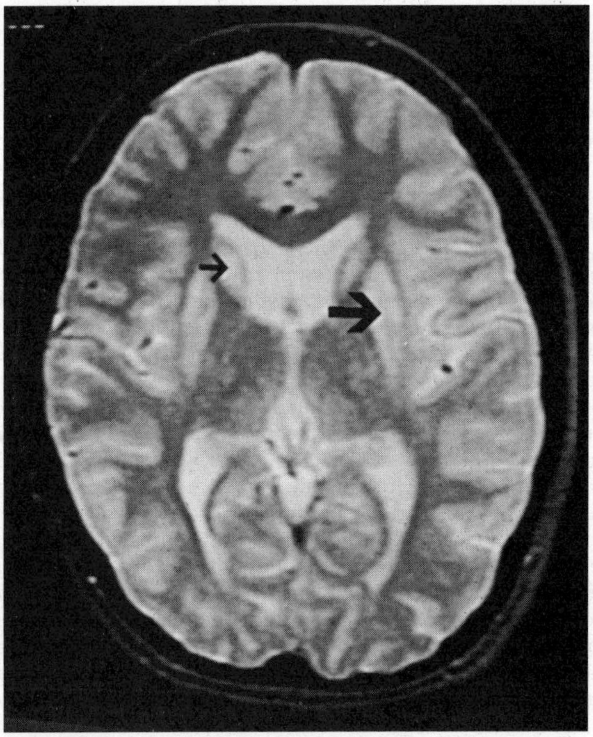

Figure 547–1. Wilson disease. MRI, T_2 image showing increased density of the caudate *(small arrow)* and the putamen *(large arrow)*.

frequency of 4–9 Hz, primarily affects the distal upper extremities, is typically postural, and commonly disappears with rest. If the tremor causes difficulty in writing or activities of daily living, a trial of propranolol hydrochloride or primidone usually provides a favorable response. **Primary writing tremor** only occurs during the action of writing and is characterized by a jerky tremor, often responsive to beta-blockers or anticholinergics. Drugs that can cause tremor include amphetamines, valproic acid, neuroleptics, tricyclic antidepressants, caffeine, and theophylline. Tremor may be the initial manifestation of a metabolic disorder, including hypoglycemia, thyrotoxicosis, neuroblastoma, and pheochromocytoma. Children recovering from a severe head injury may develop a proximal tremor that is enhanced by movement and responds to propranolol. Wilson disease often presents with a postural tremor associated with kinetic movement. These patients may also develop a "wing-beating" tremor of the shoulders when the upper arms are abducted and the elbows flexed. Hereditary dystonia-parkinsonism syndrome often displays a proximal tremor in addition to the characteristic dystonic movements.

547.4 Tics

Tics are spasmodic, involuntary, repetitive, stereotyped movements that are nonrhythmic, often exacerbated by stress, and may affect any muscle group. Tics can be classified into three subgroups: transient tics of childhood, chronic tics, and Gilles de la Tourette syndrome (TS). The **transient tic disorder** is the most common movement abnormality of childhood (see Chapter 22). The tics are more prevalent in boys, and there is often a positive family history. They consist of eyeblinking or facial movements and occasional throat-clearing noises. The disorder persists from weeks to less than a year and does not require drug therapy. The **chronic motor tic disorder** occurs in children and persists throughout adult life. The tics characteristically involve up to three muscle groups simultaneously and may occur throughout life. There is evidence that the gene for TS may manifest as simple transient tic of childhood and chronic motor tics, suggesting considerable overlap of these conditions.

Gilles de la Tourette syndrome is a life-long condition, with a prevalence of approximately 1:2,000, that has an onset between 2 and 21 yr of age. TS is probably inherited in most cases as autosomal dominant, and the gene has been mapped to chromosome 18q22.1. There are four components of TS, not all of which may be present in each patient: motor tics, vocal tics, obsessive-compulsive behavior, and attention deficit hyperactivity disorder (ADHD). These symptoms may wax and wane, and are always enhanced by stress and anxiety. TS is a life-long condition, and the ultimate prognosis can usually be determined by the severity of the symptoms during adolescence. Motor tics are associated with numerous fluctuating movements of the face, eyelids, neck, and shoulders. Ultimately, the tics are accompanied by vocalizations (vocal tics), including throat clearing, sniffling, barking, coprolalia (obscene words), echolalia (repetition of words addressed to the patient), palilalia (repetition of one's own words), and echokinesis (imitation of movement of others). The vocalizations are uncontrollable and frequently jeopardize the patient's social interaction with other children. Compulsive behavior, including touching, licking, repetitive thoughts, and motor actions, and a greater than 50% incidence of ADHD are common to TS.

Medication should be considered when the motor tics or vocalizations interfere significantly with the child's social and academic interactions, although behavior management and biofeedback programs have been successful for some patients. Several reports implicate stimulant medications (methylphenidate) as the cause of TS. All ADHD children treated with stimulant medication should be monitored closely for the onset of tics. The decision to continue the medication should be determined by the severity of the ADHD and tic disorder. Haloperidol, a dopamine-blocking agent, is effective in the management of approximately 50% of TS children. The initial dose is 0.25 mg/24 hr, and the drug is increased weekly by 0.25 mg to the usual dose range of 2–6 mg/24 hr, although some children can tolerate larger doses. Side effects include cognitive impairment, lethargy, fatigue, depression, restlessness, acute dystonic reactions, drug-induced parkinsonism, akathisia, and tardive dyskinesia syndromes, including tardive dystonia in children. Additional drugs that may prove useful include penfluridol, pimozide, and clonidine. Clonidine, an α_2-adrenergic agonist, is begun at a dose of 0.05 mg/24 hr and gradually increased to a maximum of 0.125–0.2 mg/24 hr. It may require several weeks of clonidine therapy to control the vocal and motor tics. The major side effects are lethargy, fatigue, and drowsiness. Because TS is a chronic disorder, associated with multiple social, behavioral, and learning problems, the pediatrician can play an important role in the multidisciplinary management as an advocate for the child.

Aron AM, Freeman JM, Carter S: The natural history of Sydenham's chorea. Am J Med 38:83, 1965.

Bebin EM, Bebin J, Currier RD, et al: Morphometric studies in dominant olivopontocerebellar atrophy: comparison of cell losses with amino acid decreases. Arch Neurol 47:188, 1990.

Boder E, Sedgwick RP: Ataxia-telangiectasia: A familial syndrome of progressive cerebellar ataxia, oculocutaneous telangiectasia and frequent pulmonary infection. Pediatrics 21:526, 1958.

Bray PF: Coincidence of neuroblastoma and acute cerebellar encephalopathy. J Pediatr 75:983, 1969.

Bull PC, Thomas GR, Rommens JM, et al: The Wilson disease gene is a putative copper transporting P-type ATPase similar to the Menkes gene. Nature Genet 5:327, 1993.

Chamberlain S, Farrall M, Shaw J, et al: Genetic recombination events which position the Friedreich ataxia locus proximal to the D9S15/D9S5 linkage group on chromosome 9q. Am J Hum Genet 52:99, 1993.

Curless RG, Katz DA, Perryman RA, et al: Choreoathetosis after surgery for congenital heart disease. J Pediatr 124:737, 1994.

Eldridge R: The torsion dystonia: Literature review and genetic and clinical studies. Neurology 20:1, 1970.

Fahn S: High dose anticholinergic therapy in dystonia. Neurology 33:1255, 1983.

Gatti RA: Candidates for the molecular defect in ataxia telangiectasia. Adv Neurol 61:127, 1993.

Golden GS: Tics and Tourette's: A continuum of symptoms? Ann Neurol 4:145, 1978.

Hansotia P, Cleeland CS, Chun RWM: Juvenile Huntington's chorea. Neurology 18:217, 1968.

Harding AE: Friedreich's ataxia: A clinical and genetic study of 90 families with an analysis of early diagnostic criteria and intrafamilial clustering of clinical features. Brain 104:589, 1981.

Joubert M, Eisenring JJ, Robb JP, et al: Familial agenesis of the cerebellar vermis. Neurology 19:813, 1969.

Konigsmark BW, Weiner LP: The olivopontocerebellar atrophies: A review. Medicine 49:227, 1970.

Martin JB: Molecular genetics in neurology. Ann Neurol 34:757, 1993.

Myers RH: Factors related to onset age of Huntington's disease. Am J Hum Genet 34:481, 1982.

Parker S, Zuckerman B, Bauchner H, et al: Jitteriness in full-term neonates: prevalence and correlates. Pediatrics 85:17, 1990.

Singer HS: Dopaminergic dysfunction in Tourette syndrome. Ann Neurol 12:361, 1982.

Suchowersky O: Gilles de la Tourette syndrome. Can J Neurol Sci 22:48, 1994.

Vakili S: Hallervorden-Spatz syndrome. Arch Neurol 34:729, 1977.

Van Caillie-Bertrand M, Degenhart HJ, Visso HKA, et al: Oral zinc sulphate for Wilson's disease. Arch Dis Child 60:656, 1985.

Weiss S, Carter S: Course and prognosis of acute cerebellar ataxia in children. Neurology 9:711, 1959.

CHAPTER 548
Encephalopathies

Encephalopathy is a term used to describe a generalized disorder of cerebral function that may be acute or chronic, progressive or static. The etiology of the encephalopathies in children includes infectious, toxic (e.g., carbon monoxide, drugs, lead), metabolic, and ischemic causes. Hypoxic-ischemic encephalopathy is discussed in Chapter 84.

548.1 Cerebral Palsy

See also Chapters 40 and 41.

Cerebral palsy (CP) is a static encephalopathy that may be defined as a nonprogressive disorder of posture and movement, often associated with epilepsy and abnormalities of speech, vision, and intellect resulting from a defect or lesion of the developing brain. CP is a common disorder, with an estimated prevalence of 2/1,000 population. The condition was first described almost 150 yr ago by Little, an orthopedic surgeon. He suggested that the primary causes included birth trauma and asphyxia, as well as prematurity, and that improved obstetrical care would significantly reduce the incidence of CP. During the last 2–3 decades, there have been considerable advances in obstetric and neonatal care, but, unfortunately, there has been virtually no change in the incidence of CP.

EPIDEMIOLOGY AND ETIOLOGY. The Collaborative Perinatal Project, in which approximately 45,000 children were regularly followed from pregnancy to the age of 7 yr, reported the prevalence rate of CP to be 4/1,000 live births. Birth asphyxia was an uncommon cause of CP; moreover, most high-risk pregnancies resulted in neurologically normal children. Although a cause for CP could not be identified in most cases, a substantial number of children with CP had congenital anomalies external to the central nervous system (CNS), which may have placed them at increased risk for developing asphyxia during the perinatal period. An Australian study comparing children with spastic CP with a group of matched controls had similar findings. Less than 10% of children with CP had evidence of intrapartum asphyxia. Although the increased survival of premature infants from improved perinatal care has resulted in more children with CP, the rate did not increase (see Chapter 82). These studies suggest that future developments aimed at enhancing perinatal care will have minimal impact on the incidence of CP and that research might be directed more profitably to the field of developmental biology in order to understand the pathogenesis of CP.

CLINICAL MANIFESTATIONS. CP may be classified by a description of the motor handicap in terms of physiologic, topographic, and etiologic categories and functional capacity (Table 548–1). The physiologic classification identifies the major motor abnormality, whereas the topographic taxonomy indicates the involved extremities. CP is also commonly associated with a spectrum of developmental disabilities, including mental retardation, epilepsy, and visual, hearing, speech, cognitive, and behavioral abnormalities. The motor handicap may be the least of the child's problems.

Infants with *spastic hemiplegia* have decreased spontaneous movements on the affected side and show hand preference at a very early age. The arm is often more involved than the leg, and difficulty in hand manipulation is obvious by 1 yr of age. Walking is usually delayed until 18–24 mo, and a circumductive gait is apparent. Examination of the extremities may show growth arrest, particularly in the hand and thumbnail, especially if the contralateral parietal lobe is abnormal, because extremity growth is influenced by this area of the brain. Spasticity is apparent in the affected extremities, particularly the ankle, causing an equinovarus deformity of the foot. The child often walks on tiptoes because of the increased tone, and the affected upper extremity assumes a dystonic posture when the child runs. Ankle clonus and a Babinski sign may be present; the deep tendon reflexes are increased; and weakness of the hand and foot dorsiflexors is evident. About one third of patients with spastic hemiplegia have a seizure disorder that usually develops during the first year or two, and approximately 25% have cognitive abnormalities including mental retardation. A computed tomography (CT) scan or magnetic resonance imaging (MRI) may show an atrophic cerebral hemisphere with a dilated lateral ventricle contralateral to the side of the affected extremities. Intrauterine thromboembolism with focal cerebral infarction may be one etiology; CT or MRI at birth in infants with focal seizures often demonstrates the area of infarction.

Spastic diplegia refers to bilateral spasticity of the legs. The first indication of spastic diplegia is often noted when the infant begins to crawl. The child uses the arms in a normal reciprocal fashion but tends to drag the legs behind more as a rudder (commando crawl) rather than using the normal four-stance crawling movement. If the spasticity is severe, the application of a diaper is difficult owing to excessive adduction of the hips. Examination of the child reveals spasticity in the legs with brisk reflexes, ankle clonus, and a bilateral Babinski sign. When the child is suspended by the axillae, a scissoring posture of the lower extremities is maintained. Walking is significantly delayed; the feet are held in a position of equinovarus; and the child walks on tiptoes. Severe spastic diplegia is characterized by disuse atrophy and impaired growth of the lower extremities and by disproportionate growth with normal development of the upper torso. The prognosis for normal intellectual development is excellent for these patients, and the likelihood of seizures is minimal. The most common neuropathologic finding is periventricular leukomalacia, particularly in the area where fibers innervating the legs course through the internal capsule. This lesion is noted among premature infants.

Spastic quadriplegia is the most severe form of CP because of marked motor impairment of all extremities and the high association with mental retardation and seizures. Swallowing difficulties are common owing to supranuclear bulbar palsies and often lead to aspiration pneumonia. At autopsy, the central white matter is disrupted by areas of necrotic degeneration that may coalesce into cystic cavities. Neurologic examination shows increased tone and spasticity in all extremities, decreased spontaneous movements, brisk reflexes, and plantar extensor responses. Flexion contractures of the knees and elbows are often present by late childhood. Associated developmental disabilities, including speech and visual abnormalities, are particularly prevalent in this group of children. Children with spastic quadriparesis often have evidence of athetosis and may be classified as mixed CP.

Athetoid CP is relatively rare, especially since the advent of aggressive management of hyperbilirubinemia and the prevention of kernicterus. These infants are characteristically hypotonic and have poor head control and marked head lag. Feeding may be difficult, and tongue thrust and drooling may be prominent. The athetoid movements may not become evident until 1 yr of age and tend to coincide with hypermyelination of the basal ganglia, a phenomenon called **status marmoratus.**

■ TABLE 548–1 Various Classification Systems for Cerebral Palsy*

Physiologic	Topographic	Etiologic	Functional
Spastic	Monoplegia	Prenatal (e.g., infection, metabolic, anoxia, toxic, genetic, infarction)	Class I—no limitation of activity
Athetoid	Paraplegia		
Rigid	Hemiplegia		Class II—slight to moderate limitation
Ataxic	Triplegia		
Tremor	Quadriplegia	Perinatal (e.g., anoxia)	Class III—moderate to great limitation
Atonic	Diplegia		
Mixed	Double hemiplegia	Postnatal (e.g., toxins, trauma, infection)	Class IV—no useful physical activity
Unclassified			

*Adapted from Minear WL: A classification of cerebral palsy. Pediatrics 18:841, 1956.

Speech is typically affected owing to involvement of the oropharyngeal muscles. Sentences are slurred, and voice modulation is impaired. Generally, upper motor neuron signs are not present, seizures are uncommon, and intellect is preserved in most patients.

DIAGNOSIS. A thorough history and physical examination should eliminate a progressive disorder of the CNS, including degenerative diseases, spinal cord tumor, or muscular dystrophy. Depending on the severity and the nature of the neurologic abnormalities, a baseline electroencephalogram (EEG) and CT scan may be indicated to determine the location and extent of structural lesions or associated congenital malformations. Additional studies may include tests of hearing and visual function. As CP is usually associated with a wide spectrum of developmental disorders, a multidisciplinary approach is most helpful in the assessment and management of such children.

TREATMENT. A team of physicians from various specialties as well as the occupational and physical therapists, speech pathologist, social worker, educator, and developmental psychologist provide important contributions to the management of the child. Parents should be taught how to handle their child in daily activities such as feeding, carrying, dressing, bathing, and playing in ways that will limit the effects of abnormal muscle tone. They also need to be instructed in the supervision of a series of exercises designed to prevent the development of contractures, especially a tight Achilles tendon. There is no proof that physical or occupational therapy will prevent the development of CP in the infant at risk or that it will correct the neurologic deficit, but there is ample evidence that therapy optimizes the development of the abnormal child. The child with spastic diplegia is treated initially with the assistance of adaptive equipment, such as walkers, poles, and standing frames. If the patient has marked spasticity of the lower extremities or if there is evidence of hip dislocation, consideration should be given to performing surgical soft-tissue procedures that reduce muscle spasm around the hip girdle, including an adductor tenotomy or psoas transfer and release. A rhizotomy procedure in which the roots of the spinal nerves are divided has produced considerable improvement in selected patients with severe spastic diplegia. A tight heel cord in a child with spastic hemiplegia may be treated surgically by tenotomy of the Achilles tendon. The quadriplegic patient is managed with motorized wheelchairs, special feeding devices, modified typewriters, and customized seating arrangements. Communication skills may be enhanced by the use of Bliss symbols, talking typewriters, and specially adapted computers including artificial intelligence computers to augment motor and language function. Significant behavior problems may substantially interfere with the development of a child with CP; their early identification and management are important, and the assistance of the psychologist or psychiatrist may be necessary. Learning and attention deficit disorders and mental retardation are assessed and managed by a psychologist and educator. Strabismus, nystagmus, and optic atrophy are common in children with CP; thus, an ophthalmologist should be included in the initial assessment. Lower urinary tract dysfunction should receive prompt assessment and treatment. Several drugs have been utilized to treat spasticity, including dantrolene sodium, the benzodiazepines, and baclofen. These medications are generally ineffective but should be considered if severe spasticity is not controlled by other measures. Intrathecal baclofen has been used successfully in selected children with severe spasticity. This experimental therapy requires a team approach and constant follow-up for complications of the infusion pumping mechanism and infection. Botulinum toxin is undergoing study for the management of spasticity in specific muscle groups, and the preliminary findings show a positive response in those patients studied. Occasionally, patients with incapacitating athetosis will respond to levodopa, and children with dystonia may benefit from carbamazepine or trihexyphenidyl.

548.2 Mitochondrial Encephalomyopathies

At least three associated disorders are characterized by cerebral disease and mitochondrial myopathy and are included in this section devoted to the encephalopathies. Leigh disease and Reye syndrome are discussed here because they result from disorders of mitochondrial function. Further discussion may be found in Chapters 72, 306, and 552.

MITOCHONDRIAL ENCEPHALOMYOPATHY, LACTIC ACIDOSIS, AND STROKE-LIKE EPISODES* (MELAS). Patients with MELAS may be normal for the first several years, but gradually they display delayed motor and cognitive developmental milestones. These children develop short stature and either a focal or generalized seizure disorder. Ultimately, the patient presents with an acute hemiparesis that can alternate from side to side. CT studies show basal ganglia calcification in some patients and lucent areas in the cerebral hemispheres. Serum lactate levels during an acute episode are elevated. Muscle biopsies usually, but not always, show ragged-red fibers. MELAS is a progressive disorder that has been reported in siblings. It is punctuated with episodes of hemiparesis, hemianopia, cortical blindness, and progressive dementia secondary to multiple strokes. The location of the lucent lesions noted on the CT scan is compatible with the acute neurologic deficit. Postmortem studies have demonstrated focal encephalomalacia, cortical microcystic liquefaction, and basal ganglia calcifications. The prognosis for patients with the full syndrome is dismal. Therapeutic trials have included corticosteroids and CoQ10. Lowering the serum lactate concentration with dichloroacetate in patients with severe lactic acidosis may result in marked clinical improvement. Most

*Written with the collaboration of Dr. Ingrid Tein.

patients will have a highly specific, although not exclusive, point mutation at nt 3243 in the $tRNA^{Leu}$ (UUR) gene of mtDNA, which has provided an important diagnostic tool. Biochemical studies of muscle have shown complex I deficiency in many patients; however, multiple defects of the respiratory chain, affecting complexes I, III, and especially complex IV, have also been documented.

MYOCLONUS EPILEPSY AND RAGGED-RED FIBERS (MERRF). Patients with MERRF may also be normal during the early years of development. However, all patients ultimately develop myoclonic epilepsy and progressive ataxia associated with dysarthria and nystagmus; a few have optic atrophy. Because some patients have abnormalities of deep sensation and pes cavus, the condition may be confused with Friedreich ataxia. Less common signs include dementia, hearing loss, peripheral neuropathy, and spasticity. Intellectual deterioration is slowly progressive in patients with MERRF. As with MELAS, a significant number of patients have a positive family history and short stature. Pathologic findings include elevated serum lactate levels, ragged-red fibers in muscle biopsies, marked loss and degeneration of neurons in the dentate nuclei and the inferior olivary complex with dropout of Purkinje cells and neurons of the red nucleus. The cerebral cortex and white matter are usually normal. Most patients will have a highly specific, although not exclusive, point mutation at nt 8344 in the $tRNA^{Lys}$ gene of mtDNA. There have been inconsistent results in biochemical studies of muscle, including defects of complex III; complexes II and IV; complexes I and IV; complexes I, III, and IV; or complex IV alone.

KEARNS-SAYRE SYNDROME (KSS). The criteria for KSS include a triad of (1) onset before age 20 yr, (2) progressive external ophthalmoplegia, and (3) pigmentary retinopathy. There must also be at least one of the following: heart block, cerebellar syndrome, or a cerebrospinal fluid protein above 100 mg/dL. Other nonspecific but common features include dementia, sensorineural hearing loss, and endocrine abnormalities, including short stature, diabetes mellitus, and hypoparathyroidism. The prognosis is poor despite placement of a pacemaker. Ragged-red fibers are found in muscle biopsies with a variable number of COX-negative fibers. Almost all patients have mtDNA deletions. These may be new mutations accounting for the sporadic nature of KSS.

GENETICS OF DISEASES CAUSED BY DEFECTS OF MITOCHONDRIAL DNA. Diseases caused by defects of mitochondrial DNA (mtDNA) include deletions and duplications as well as point mutations. In the group of deletions, patients have a single deletion in their mtDNA. This deletion is identical in all tissues in a given patient, although the number of deleted genomes varies from tissue to tissue *(heteroplasmy).* The three major clinical syndromes in the group of deletions and duplications, in which the inheritance tends to be sporadic, are Kearns-Sayre syndrome, progressive external ophthalmoplegia with ragged-red fibers, and Pearson marrow/pancreas syndrome.

In the group of point mutations, there are four maternally inherited diseases, which include *Leber hereditary optic neuroretinopathy,* MELAS, MERRF, and *ATPase 6 mutation syndrome.* In maternal inheritance, the transmission is maternal but both sexes are equally affected. The phenotypic expression of an mtDNA mutation will be dependent upon the relative proportions of mutant and wild-type genomes among the multiple copies of mtDNA in each cell. There is a minimum critical number of mutant genomes necessary for expression of the disease, and this is known as the *threshold effect.* The proportion of mutants may shift in daughter cells during cell division *(mitotic segregation),* and the phenotype may thereby change. The subsequent generations are affected by a pathologic mutation as in autosomal dominant diseases; however, the number of affected individuals in each generation should be higher than in autosomal dominant diseases. The threshold effect may vary from tissue to tissue depending upon the individual tissue vulnerability to oxidative impairment and may vary in the same tissue with time. The mitochondrial proliferation leading to the formation of ragged-red fibers appears to be triggered by an imbalance between the energy requirement and oxidation/phosphorylation efficiency of the muscle fiber.

LEIGH DISEASE (SUBACUTE NECROTIZING ENCEPHALOMYELOPATHY). There are at least three known genetically determined causes of Leigh disease: deficiency of the pyruvate dehydrogenase complex, deficiency of complex I, and deficiency of complex IV of the respiratory chain (see also Chapter 73). These defects may occur sporadically or be inherited by autosomal recessive transmission, as in the case of COX deficiency, or by x-linked transmission, as in PDH E_1 alpha deficiency. Most patients present during infancy with feeding and swallowing problems, vomiting, and failure to thrive. Delayed motor and language milestones may be evident, and generalized seizures, weakness, hypotonia, ataxia, tremor, pyramidal signs, and nystagmus are prominent findings. Intermittent respirations with associated sighing or sobbing are characteristic and suggest brain stem dysfunction. Some patients have external ophthalmoplegia, ptosis, optic atrophy, and decreased visual acuity. Abnormal results on CT scans consisting of bilaterally symmetric areas of low attenuation in the basal ganglia have been described in some patients. Pathologic changes consist of focal, symmetric areas of necrosis in the thalamus, basal ganglia, tegmental gray matter, periventricular and periaqueductal regions of the brain stem, and posterior columns of the spinal cord. Microscopically, these *spongiform* lesions show cystic cavitation with neuronal loss, demyelination, and vascular proliferation. Elevated serum lactate levels are the hallmark of Leigh disease. The overall outlook in Leigh disease is poor, but a few patients experience prolonged periods of remission.

REYE SYNDROME. This encephalopathy is associated with fatty degeneration of the viscera and a disorder of mitochondrial function (see Chapter 306).

548.3 Other Encephalopathies

ZELLWEGER SYNDROME (CEREBROHEPATORENAL SYNDROME [CHRS]). This rare, lethal disorder is inherited as an autosomal recessive trait. It represents the prototype of a group of peroxisomal disorders that have overlapping symptoms, signs, and biochemical abnormalities (see Chapter 72.2). Infants with Zellweger syndrome have dysmorphic facies consisting of frontal bossing and a large anterior fontanel. The occiput is flattened, and the external ears are abnormal. A high-arched palate, excessive skin folds of the neck, severe hypotonia, and areflexia are usually evident. Examination of the eyes reveals searching nystagmoid movements, bilateral cataracts, and optic atrophy. Generalized seizures become evident early in life, associated with severe global developmental delay and a significant bilateral hearing loss. Hepatomegaly is a prominent finding shortly after birth, often associated with a history of prolonged neonatal jaundice. Patients with Zellweger syndrome rarely survive beyond 1 yr of age.

ACQUIRED IMMUNODEFICIENCY SYNDROME (AIDS) ENCEPHALOPATHY. Encephalopathy is an unfortunate and common manifestation of infants and children with human immunodeficiency virus (HIV) infection (see Chapter 223). Neurologic signs in the congenitally infected patient may appear during early infancy or may be delayed to as late as 5 yr of age. The encephalopathy may have an acute onset with a relentless progressive course, but in some cases the process is either static or is characterized by insidious deterioration. The primary features of AIDS encephalopathy include an arrest in brain growth, evidence of developmental delay, and the evolution of neurologic signs.

LEAD ENCEPHALOPATHY. See Chapter 665.

BURN ENCEPHALOPATHY. An encephalopathy develops in approximately 5% of children with significant burns during the first several weeks of hospitalization (see also Chapter 60.5). There is no single cause of burn encephalopathy but rather a combination of factors that include anoxia (smoke inhalation, carbon monoxide poisoning, laryngospasm), electrolyte abnormalities, bacteremia and sepsis, cortical vein thrombosis, a concomitant head injury, cerebral edema, drug reactions, and emotional distress. Seizures are the most common clinical manifestation of burn encephalopathy, but altered states of consciousness, hallucinations, and coma may also occur. The management of burn encephalopathy is directed to a search for the underlying cause and treatment of hypoxemia, seizures, specific electrolyte abnormalities, or cerebral edema. The prognosis for complete neurologic recovery is generally excellent, particularly if seizures are the primary abnormality.

HYPERTENSIVE ENCEPHALOPATHY. Hypertensive encephalopathy is most commonly associated with renal disease in children, including acute glomerulonephritis, chronic pyelonephritis, and end-stage renal disease (see Chapters 404, 481.2). In some cases, hypertensive encephalopathy is the initial manifestation of underlying renal disease. Marked systemic hypertension produces vasoconstriction of the cerebral vessels, which leads to vascular permeability, causing areas of focal cerebral edema and hemorrhage. The onset may be acute, with seizures and coma, or more indolent, with headache, drowsiness and lethargy, nausea and vomiting, blurred vision, transient cortical blindness, and hemiparesis. Examination of the eyegrounds may be normal in children, but papilledema and retinal hemorrhages may occur. Treatment is directed to the restoration of a normotensive state and control of seizures with appropriate anticonvulsants.

RADIATION ENCEPHALOPATHY. Although techniques for administering radiation therapy to the brain have improved considerably and the incidence of serious side effects has decreased significantly, radiation encephalopathy remains an important complication. *Acute radiation encephalopathy* is most likely to develop in young patients who have received large daily doses. The excessive radiation injures vessel endothelium, resulting in enhanced vascular permeability, cerebral edema, and multiple hemorrhages. The child may suddenly become irritable and lethargic, complain of headache, or present with focal neurologic signs and seizures. The patient occasionally develops hemiparesis due to an infarct secondary to vascular occlusion of the cerebral vessels. Steroids are often beneficial in reducing the cerebral edema and reversing the neurologic signs. *Late radiation encephalopathy* develops months to years after the completion of therapy. It is rare in children. The condition is characterized by headaches and slowly progressive focal neurologic signs, including hemiparesis and seizures. Although the cause of late radiation encephalopathy is unknown, the CT scan shows cerebral atrophy and low-density lesions. Some children with acute lymphatic leukemia who are treated with a combination of intrathecal methotrexate and cranial irradiation develop neurologic signs months or years later, consisting of increasing lethargy, loss of cognitive abilities, dementia, and focal neurologic signs and seizures (see Chapter 448). The CT scan shows calcifications in the white matter, and the post mortem examination demonstrates a necrotizing encephalopathy. This devastating complication of the treatment of leukemia has prompted a re-evaluation of the use of cranial radiation in the management of these children.

Albright AL, Barron WB, Fasick MP, et al: Continuous intrathecal baclofen infusion for spasticity of cerebral origin. JAMA 270:2475, 1993.

Ciafaloni E, Ricci E, Shanske S, et al: MELAS: clinical features, biochemistry and molecular genetics. Ann Neurol 31:391, 1992.

Ens-Dokkum MH, Johnson A, Schreuder AM, et al: Comparison of mortality and rates of cerebral palsy in two populations of very low birthweight infants. Arch Dis Child 70:96, 1994.

Fukuhara N, Tokiguchi S, Shirakawa K, et al: Myoclonus epilepsy associated with ragged-red fibres (mitochondrial abnormalities): Disease entity or a syndrome? J Neurol Sci 47:117, 1980.

Gaffney G, Flavell V, Johnson A, et al: Cerebral palsy and neonatal encephalopathy. Arch Dis Child 70:195, 1994.

Goto Y, Itami N, Kajii N, et al: Renal tubular involvement mimicking Barter syndrome in a patient with Kearns-Sayre syndrome. J Pediatr 116:904, 1990.

Goto Y, Nonaka I, Horai S: A mutation in the $tRNA^{Leu(UUR)}$ gene associated with the MELAS subgroup of mitochondrial encephalomyopathies. Nature 348:651, 1990.

Karpati G, Carpenter S, Larbrisseau A, et al: The Kearns-Shy syndrome: A multisystem disease with mitochondrial abnormality demonstrated in skeletal muscle and skin. J Neurol Sci 19:133, 1973.

Kobayashi M, Morishita H, Sugiyama N, et al: Two cases of NADH-coenzyme Q reductase deficiency: relationship to MELAS syndrome. J Pediatr 110:223, 1987.

Koman LA, Mooney JF, Smith B, et al: Management of cerebral palsy with botulinum-A toxin: preliminary investigation. J Pediatr Orthop 13:489, 1993.

Kuban RCR, Leviton A: Cerebral palsy. N Engl J Med 330:188, 1994.

Mohnot D, Snead OC, Benton JW: Burn encephalopathy in children. Ann Neurol 12:42, 1982.

Monnens L, Heymans H: Peroxisomal disorders: Clinical characterization. J Inher Metab Dis 10 (Suppl 1):23, 1987.

Moraes CT, DiMauro S, Zeviani M, et al: Mitochondrial DNA deletions in progressive external ophthalmoplegia and Kearns-Sayre syndrome. N Engl J Med 320:1293, 1989.

Park TS, Owen AH: Surgical management of spastic diplegia in cerebral palsy. N Engl J Med 326:745, 1992.

Pavlakis SG, Phillips PC, Di Mauro S, et al: Mitochondrial myopathy, encephalopathy, lactic acidosis, and strokelike episodes: A distinctive clinical syndrome. Ann Neurol 16:481, 1984.

Peacock WJ, Staudt LA: Selective posterior rhizotomy: evolution of theory and practice. Pediatr Neurosurg 92:128, 1991.

Reed CJD, Borzyskowski: Lower urinary tract dysfunction in cerebral palsy. Arch Dis Child 68:739, 1993.

Robinson BH, Taylor J, Sherwood WG: The genetic heterogeneity of lactic acidosis: Occurrence of recognizable inborn errors of metabolism in a pediatric population with lactic acidosis. Pediatr Res 14:956, 1980.

Sheline GE: Irradiation injury of the human brain: A review of clinical experience. *In:* Gilbert HA, Kagan AR (eds): Radiation Damage to the Nervous System. New York, Raven Press, 1980.

Shoffner JM, Lott M, Lezza AMS, et al: Myoclonic epilepsy and ragged-red fiber disease (MERRF) is associated with a mitochondrial DNA $tRNA^{Lys}$ mutation. Cell 61:931, 1990.

Still JL, Cottom D: Severe hypertension in childhood. Arch Dis Child 42:34, 1967.

Wallace DC, Singh G, Lott MT, et al: Mitochondrial DNA mutation associated with Leber's hereditary optic neuropathy. Science 242:1427, 1988.

CHAPTER 549

Coma in Childhood

Coma is defined as a state of unconsciousness from which the child cannot be aroused by ordinary verbal, sensory, or physical stimuli. Coma is a medical emergency (see Chapter 60.2). Prompt diagnosis and appropriate management may be lifesaving. Treatment often precedes a thorough physical examination. The patient's airway and cardiorespiratory system must be examined immediately, and the vital signs must be recorded. If the patient is in shock or has had a cardiorespiratory arrest, the immediate management is directed to resuscitation and to the establishment of life support systems. Generally, a child with a Glasgow Coma Scale of seven or less should be intubated and placed on a respirator (see later). On the other hand, if the patient's vital signs and cardiovascular system are intact, attention may be directed to the history and physical examination.

The *history* may indicate the cause, but frequently the parent is unavailable or was not present at the onset of the coma. It is important to determine whether there has been a gradual change in personality and behavior or an abrupt loss of consciousness. The amount, type, and time of the last dose of insulin in the diabetic child is important to document. Because intoxication is a prominent cause of coma in the toddler and adolescent patient, a careful review of medications and their location at home should be completed. The discovery of the child in close proximity to the medicine cabinet or storage area or the finding of pills and empty medication containers is overwhelming evidence of drug-induced coma. If there is any doubt about the history, or if the clinical and laboratory findings do not support the history, a home visit may be invaluable. A toxic substance or spilled pills from an opened container may be found within the child's play area. An altered state of consciousness in the newborn period associated with vomiting, failure to thrive, and seizures suggests an inborn error of metabolism. The patient in status epilepticus or in a postictal state following an initial seizure, and the child with a history of chronic renal disease associated with hypertensive encephalopathy may present with coma. A child with severe pulmonary or heart disease or profound anemia may develop coma as a consequence of cerebral anoxia and ischemia. Rarely, brain tumors or cerebral abscess, particularly if there is rupture into the ventricular system, may produce sudden coma. These children may have a history of headache, vomiting, change in personality, or congenital heart disease. Acute subarachnoid hemorrhage secondary to a bleed from an arteriovenous malformation causes a sudden alteration in consciousness.

The child's level of consciousness and the response to stimuli should be carefully documented. A modification of the *Glasgow Coma Scale* in Table 59–5 is a useful tool for the grading of the degree of coma and the severity of the insult in infants and children. It is important to remember that the assessment of the verbal response is much different from that of the adult, and the child's developmental level must be kept in mind during the evaluation. A coma score of less than five is associated with a grave prognosis, whereas a score of five to eight may indicate a better prognosis in the child than in the adult.

The *physical examination* is helpful in distinguishing between a metabolic cause and structural cause for the coma. A slow, irregular pulse combined with systemic hypertension indicates increased intracranial pressure or hypertensive encephalopathy. The rate and rhythm of the respiratory pattern provide useful information about the etiology of the coma. Regular and deep hyperventilation (Kussmaul breathing) indicates metabolic acidosis; subdued and slow breathing suggests respiratory depression or sedation; and irregular, ataxic respiration suggests cerebellar herniation. Cherry-red discoloration of the face and cheeks is associated with carbon monoxide poisoning. A fruity breath is typical of diabetic ketoacidosis; a putrid odor indicates hepatic coma; and a sweet-smelling urine suggests maple syrup urine disease (see Chapter 71.6).

The examination should include a careful search for trauma and should test for the presence of nuchal rigidity. Cerebrospinal fluid (CSF) rhinorrhea, hematotympanum, and **Battle sign** (bruising over the mastoid) are suggestive of a basilar skull fracture. Nuchal rigidity may indicate meningitis, encephalitis, subarachnoid bleed, or herniation of the cerebellar tonsils. Pin-point *pupils* are associated with narcotics, barbiturate toxicity, organophosphates, and phencyclidine. Small and irregular pupils suggest a lesion in the pons, and dilated and unresponsive pupils are seen in the postictal state, with botulism, and with certain drugs, including glutethimide, amphetamine, atropine, cocaine, ethyl alcohol, and mydriatics. A unilaterally dilated and unresponsive pupil in the comatose child indicates herniation of the uncus of the ipsilateral temporal lobe. Check to ensure that a mydriatic was not the cause of the abnormal pupil. The integrity of the extraocular muscles may be tested by the doll's eye maneuver. The fundi must be examined for the presence of papilledema and retinal hemorrhages.

Brain stem function may be evaluated by *ice water* caloric testing (unless the tympanic membrane is ruptured) (see Chapter 541). The comatose child with an intact brain stem shows a fixed deviation of the eyes to the side of the stimulus, and the patient with irreversible coma has no response.

Focal neurologic signs may be difficult to elicit in the comatose patient. *Hemiparesis* may be demonstrated by passively flexing the legs and hips. The examiner suddenly releases the extremities. The hemiparetic leg will rapidly fall to an externally rotated position, whereas the normal limb will slowly slide back to the original posture. This maneuver should be carried out with the patient supine and on a flat surface. The quadriceps may be flattened, and the foot of the affected extremity is externally rotated owing to a decrease in muscle tone. Finally, the hemiparetic extremities may have altered reflexes, changes in muscle tone, and an extensor plantar reflex.

During the initial evaluation an *IV line* is established and blood is obtained for a complete blood count, electrolytes, calcium, phosphorus, glucose, creatinine, blood gases, liver function studies, prothrombin and partial thromboplastin, ammonium level, and a toxic screen. It is important to collect and store an additional 5 mL of heparinized blood that can be utilized later if a specific metabolic disease becomes apparent. Table 549–1 provides a framework to differentiate the various common causes of metabolic coma. If the initial Dextrostix suggests hypoglycemia, 2 mL/kg of 25% dextrose should be given IV. A *urinary catheter* is inserted; the urine volume is noted; and a sample is examined for glucose, ketones, and further studies as indicated. A *nasogastric tube* is placed in position, and the stomach is emptied with care to prevent aspiration, particularly if a toxin is suspected. The stomach contents may be analyzed in the laboratory for specific toxins. Structural causes of coma include concussion, contusion, subdural and epidural hematoma, cerebral edema, brain tumors, and cerebral abscess. The diagnosis and management of these conditions are discussed elsewhere in this section.

The principles of *treatment* include maintenance of the respiratory status, normalization of cardiovascular function, and correction of acid-base, fluid, and electrolyte abnormalities. IV fluids used for resuscitation and infusion should be carefully monitored as hyponatremia, which may aggravate a cerebral injury, is a common complication of IV therapy in the comatose patient. Seizures, increased intracranial pressure, and hyperthermia (or hypothermia) are managed appropriately. The primary goal of treatment is to identify the specific cause of the coma and to correct the problem in a safe and controlled fashion.

The use of **invasive intracranial pressure monitoring** should be considered for any infant or child with nontraumatic coma and suspected increase in intracranial pressure to assess cerebral perfusion and to anticipate shifts in brain tissue. Cerebral perfusion pressure is calculated as the difference between the mean arterial blood pressure and the mean intracranial pressure. Neurologic outcome is improved if the cerebral perfusion pressure can be maintained above 50 mm Hg. Poor neurologic outcome or death is associated with intracranial pressures above 50 mm Hg or cerebral perfusion pressures of less than 40 mm Hg. Intracranial pressure in the child may be monitored by the use of a subarachnoid screw, a subdural pressure transducer, or a fluid-filled intraventricular catheter. Raised intracranial pressure may be lowered by paralysis and sedation with pancuronium, phenobarbital, morphine, or diazepam, mechanical hyperventilation ($Paco_2$ lowered to 30–35 mm Hg), osmotherapy with IV mannitol or furosemide, or drainage of CSF through the ventricular catheter. Too aggressive hyperventilation may further compromise already ischemic areas of the brain. A decrease in cerebral perfusion pressure associated with a low systemic arterial pressure may be enhanced by infusions of colloid or dopamine.

■ TABLE 549–1 Coma in the Pediatric Population: Metabolic Coma

Etiology	Symptoms and Signs	Diagnosis
Intoxication		
Salicylism	Hyperventilation, dehydration, seizures	Metabolic acidosis, ketonuria, urine ferric chloride (burgundy color), increased serum salicylate
Barbiturates	Hypoventilation, decreased blood pressure, pin-point pupils	Increased serum phenobarbital level (>30 μg/mL)
Alcohol	Respiratory failure, seizures	Serum alcohol: coma = 300–500 mg/dL, >500 mg/dL may be lethal; hypoglycemia
Hyperglycemia		
Diabetes mellitus	Hyperventilation, fruity odor	Glycosuria, ketonuria, ketonemia, metabolic acidosis, hyperosmolality
Head injury	External evidence of trauma or focal signs	Glycosuria, no ketonemia or ketonuria
Hypoglycemia		
Insulin excess	Perspiration, pallor, seizures	Blood glucose <40 mg/dL
Salicylism	As above	—
Alcohol	As above	—
Inborn Errors	Vomiting, changes in tone, seizures	Metabolic acidosis, positive 2,4 dinitrophenyl-hydrazine, increased organic acids, increased amino acids, increased serum lactate
Electrolyte Abnormalities	Hypernatremia, hyponatremia, hypocalcemia, hypokalemia	Serum electrolytes, calcium and magnesium
Meningoencephalitis	Fever, nuchal rigidity, seizures	Examination of CSF; brain scan, EEG, and CT scan if herpes suspected
Encephalopathy		
Anoxic	Cardiac arrest, severe anemia/pulmonary disease	Pulseless, ECG, Hb, chest radiograph
Reye syndrome	Hyperpnea, apneic breathing, decerebrate posture, dilated pupils, seizures, combative	Increased serum ammonia, SGOT, SGPT, and prolonged PT, hyperaminoacidemia (lysine and glutamine), characteristic liver biopsy
Hypertensive	Renal disease, coarctation of the aorta, collagen vascular disease, pheochromocytoma	Increased blood pressure, retinal changes, decreased femoral pulses, neurofibromatosis?
Hemorrhagic shock (HSES)	Malaise, fever, vomiting and diarrhea, seizures, cyanosis	Metabolic acidosis, acute renal failure, increased liver enzymes, anemia, and DIC
Hemolytic-uremic syndrome (HUS)	Irritability, pallor, purpura, oliguria, seizures	Decreased Hb, decreased platelets, fragmented red blood cells, hematuria, renal failure, verotoxin-producing *Escherichia coli*
Lead	Vomiting, abdominal pain, ataxia, seizures	Blood lead greater than 100 μg/dL
Postseizure	Dilated pupils, Babinski, rapid return of consciousness	Medicalert bracelet?

The induction of pentobarbital coma and the use of steroids do not appear to influence the neurologic *prognosis* in the comatose child. The prediction of coma outcome during the acute illness depends in part on the etiology of the condition; diabetic ketoacidosis has a more favorable outlook than Reye syndrome, while trauma is more favorable than anoxia. However, certain physical signs provide some indication of outcome before inducing paralysis and placement on the respirator. These signs include severity of the coma (i.e., modified Glasgow score), eye movement, pupil reaction, hypotension, temperature, motor patterns, and the seizure type. The EEG is also useful to estimate the potential for neurologic recovery. For example, the reappearance of normal sleep spindles is an encouraging finding, even if associated with high-voltage slow waves that have no predictive value. EEG patterns associated with a poor prognosis include burst suppression, α-like activity, very low amplitude activity for age, and electrocerebral silence. Neurophysiologic studies have also been used to make a prognosis for comatose children, including brain stem auditory, visual, and somatosensory evoked potentials (SEPs). Generally, the absence of all wave forms in these three modalities is associated with death or severe neurologic residua. Somatosensory evoked potentials are the most sensitive and reliable method for the evaluation of neurologic outcome in the comatose child. If SEPs are recorded early during the course of coma and repeated within the first week, normal SEPs predict normal outcome in 93% of the cases and absent SEPs predict poor outcome in 100% of the cases; asymmetrical SEPs are typically associated with sequelae such as hemiparesis.

CHAPTER 550
Brain Death

See also Chapter 3.

The President's Commission for the Study of Ethical Problems in Medicine and Biomedical and Behavioral Research commented that "Death is defined as irreversible cessation of circulatory and respiratory functions or irreversible cessation of all functions of the entire brain, including the brain stem. A determination of death must be made in accordance with accepted medical standards." The criteria for establishing brain death are similar for adults and children; however, the period of observation may be longer in the latter. The diagnosis of brain death is established when the cause of coma is determined; the possibility for recovery of any brain function is excluded; and the cessation of all brain functions are documented for an appropriate period of observation or trial of therapy. The diagnosis of brain death is made primarily by clinical methods, irrespective of the age of the patient. The physical examination criteria are as follows: (1) the patient must be comatose, apneic, normothermic, and normotensive with absence of vocalization and volitional movement. Apnea is defined as an absence of spontaneous respirations despite an adequate carbon dioxide stimulus (i.e., 45–60 mm Hg). During apnea testing the patient is maintained on continuous positive airway pressure ventilation and is oxygenated with 100% oxygen. The confirmation of apnea is achieved when the patient fails to breathe spontaneously after 15 min or until the P_{CO_2} rises to 60 mm Hg. Apnea testing is reserved until the physical examination is completed and the diagnosis of brain death appears to be certain. (2) All brain stem responses must be absent. The pupils are midposition or fully dilated, and there is no direct or consensual pupillary response to a bright light. There is absence of spontaneous eye movements, including lack of a blink or eye movement to a loud noise (auriculo-ocular response), no response to ice water caloric stimulation (vestibulo-ocular), and no lateral eye movement with head turning (doll's eye maneuver). There is no corneal response, rooting reflex, gag, cough, or sucking reflexes. (3) Spontaneous movements (with the exception of spinal cord reflex withdrawal and myoclonus) must be absent, and there is generalized flaccidity. Laboratory studies are also performed to establish the cause of the coma and to specifically exclude a remedial condition, such as a toxic, metabolic, paralytic, or sedative cause.

Because the period of asphyxia or cause of coma may be unknown in the premature infant or newborn, a longer period of observation is required than in the older child or adult before a diagnosis of brain death is established. The diagnosis of brain death in these patients as well as in older children may be substantiated by an EEG, showing a period of electrocerebral silence utilizing standard techniques, or by the absence of carotid circulation at the base of the skull and the intracranial arterial circulation utilizing a cerebral radionuclide angiogram. Unfortunately, the correlation among the physical examination, EEG, and cerebral radionuclide angiogram is not absolute. Until more precise laboratory or imaging studies are developed, the diagnosis of brain death for all ages continues to be made on the basis of a careful physical examination with an appropriate period of observation to ensure that all the criteria discussed earlier have been met.

THE PERSISTENT VEGETATIVE STATE. The persistent vegetative state (PVS) is defined as a state of "wakefulness without awareness" or "permanent unconsciousness." Children may recover quickly and completely from coma, or slowly, with a gradual return of neurologic function. The term *PVS* is utilized when there is a lack of neurologic recovery over a period of at least 6 mo, with preservation of only autonomic nervous system vital functions, including cardiac action, blood pressure, and respiration. The eyes move spontaneously but there is inconsistent tracking. There is a lack of voluntary movement, but the child may withdraw from noxious stimuli. Cognitive function is absent. There is no language and the patient is unable to follow or comprehend commands. Sleep-wake cycles are present and brain stem reflexes, such as sucking, chewing, and swallowing, remain intact. The pupils react to light and the grasp; oculocephalic and tendon reflexes are usually present.

PVS may result from trauma, meningitis, asphyxia, aborted sudden infant death syndrome, near drowning, and congenital malformations of the brain. The diagnosis is established with relative certainty by the neurologic examination and assessment of higher cortical function in children beyond 2 yr of age. Because cognitive function is difficult to assess and language is not developed in the infant, a diagnosis of PVS is inaccurate and unreliable in patients less than 2 yr of age.

There is no test that is predictive of neurologic outcome. The EEG may show residual activity and neuroimaging studies indicate cortical atrophy. Pathologic examination of the PVS brain typically shows extensive damage of the forebrain structures with sparing of the brain stem. Treatment of PVS is supportive and includes adequate fluids and nutrition (frequently administered by gastrostomy), management of pain and discomfort (rarely apparent), and provision of a comfortable and nurturing environment. The physician should introduce the concept of "do not resuscitate" and review the prognosis and management with the family on a regular basis.

Ashwal S, Schneider S: Brain death in the newborn: Pediatrics 84:429, 1989.

Ashwal S, Bale JF, Coulter DL, et al: The persistent vegetative state in children: Report of the Child Neurology Society Ethics Committee. Ann Neurol 32:570, 1992.

Drake B, Ashwal S, Schneider S: Determination of cerebral death in the pediatric intensive care unit. Pediatrics 78:107, 1986.

Fois A, Malandrini F: Electroencephalographic findings in pediatric cases of coma. Clin Electroenceph 14:207, 1983.

Guidelines for the determination of brain death: Report of the medical consultants on the diagnosis of death to the President's Commission for the Study of Ethical Problems in Medicine and Biomedical and Behavioral Research. Neurology 32:395, 1982.

Johnston B, Seshia SS: Prediction of outcome in non-traumatic coma in childhood. Acta Neurol Scand 69:417, 1984.

Reilly PL, Simpson DA, Sprod R, et al: Assessing the conscious level in infants and young children: A paediatric version of the Glasgow Coma Scale. Childs Nerv Syst 4:30, 1988.

Tasker RC, Matthew DJ, Helms P, et al: Monitoring in non-traumatic coma. 1: Invasive intracranial measurements. Arch Dis Child 63:888, 1988.

CHAPTER 551
Head Injuries

Accidents are the major cause of morbidity and mortality in children beyond 1 yr of age, and head trauma is the injury most responsible for death. It is estimated that 100,000 children are hospitalized annually in the United States because of head injury, and 5–10% have long-term mental or physical handicaps as a result. Most head injuries involve an automobile accident; however, auto-bicycle and motorcycle accidents, falls, and nonaccidental trauma (e.g., child abuse) account for a significant number of head injuries in children. Injuries of males outnumber those of females by a ratio of 2:1. The degree of brain trauma depends on many variables, including age, velocity of the fall, whether the injury was a closed or open wound, and the use of protective head gear. It requires greater physical force to produce unconsciousness and brain trauma when the head is maintained in a fixed position compared with a freely moving skull at impact, which strongly supports the use of infant car seats and appropriate automobile seat belts and shoulder restraints.

SKULL FRACTURES. A skull fracture in association with head trauma does not necessarily imply injury to the underlying brain. Approximately one third of all children with a history of a head injury have radiologic evidence of a skull fracture, but most of these children are intact neurologically at the time of examination and remain free of sequelae. Conversely, approximately 50% of children who die of an acute brain injury have no evidence of a skull fracture. Furthermore, subdural hematoma occurs in twice as many injured children without a fracture compared with those with a skull fracture. Epidural hematoma is associated with a skull fracture in approximately 50% of cases. Finally, the location and type of skull fracture are rarely correlated with symptoms and physical findings. Thus, careful clinical appraisal and observation are more valuable in determining the extent of brain injury and the presence of neurologic complications than the finding of a skull fracture.

The most common skull fracture is *linear and nondepressed.* It does not, as a rule, interfere with the function and integrity of the brain; thus, the outcome in most cases is excellent. Serious consequences may result if the fracture traverses the groove of the meningeal vessels, the sagittal sinus, or the lambdoid suture. A **leptomeningeal cyst** is a rare and late complication of a linear skull fracture and is characterized by a slowly expanding pulsatile mass on the surface of the skull. The cyst is caused by the protrusion of the leptomeninges and traumatized brain through the interrupted dura and skull fracture and expansion by the propulsion of cerebrospinal fluid (CSF) into the cyst by the pulsating brain.

Basilar skull fractures are difficult to demonstrate by radiologic examination. Most frequently, the temporal bone is fractured, producing a bloody discharge from the middle ear (hematotympanum) or Battle sign a few days later (Fig. 551–1). Cranial nerve palsies may occur, particularly injury to the facial and auditory cranial nerves. Bilateral ecchymosis and swelling of the upper eyelids (**raccoon's eye sign**) suggests a basal anterior fossa fracture. Fracture of the sphenoid bone may damage the oculomotor, trochlear, and abducens nerves. CSF otorrhea or rhinorrhea may complicate a basilar skull fracture. Although CSF otorrhea usually does not persist beyond 24–48 hr, CSF rhinorrhea is less likely to arrest spontaneously. It may be difficult to distinguish CSF rhinorrhea from excessive nasal secretions. The fluid is clear in the former, tends to be profuse (particularly upon sitting), and tests positive for glucose using Dextrostix. If the rhinorrhea persists longer than 14 days, surgical repair of the defect is usually necessary. Bacterial meningitis, particularly *Streptococcus pneumoniae,* may complicate a basilar skull fracture because of the open defect between the nasopharynx or middle ear and the brain. The use of prophylactic antibiotics is controversial, but they are rarely used during the first week of CSF rhinorrhea because of the likelihood of spontaneous closure of the defect.

Depressed skull fractures must be treated surgically if a neurologic deficit results or a compound wound is present. Surgical treatment is necessary if the depression is greater than 3–5 mm.

There is no consensus about the guidelines for obtaining skull roentgenograms in the investigation of a pediatric head injury. National guidelines recommend that all children less than 5 yr of age with a history of head trauma undergo roentgenographic examination because of the unreliability of

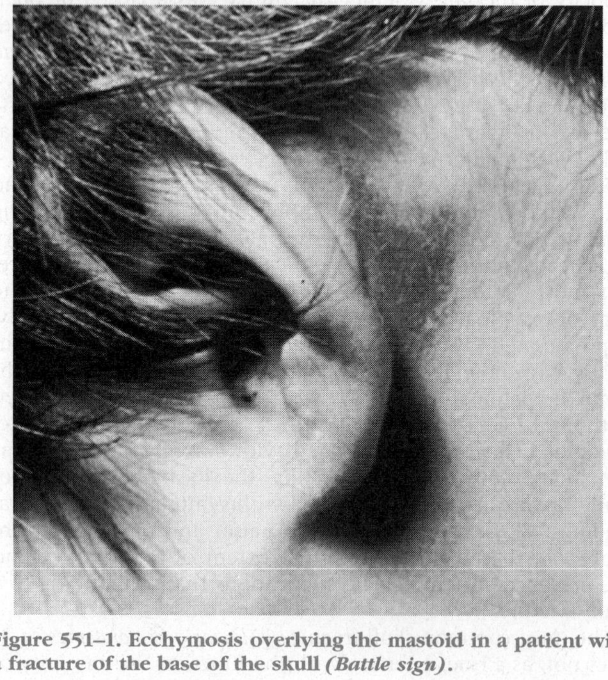

Figure 551–1. Ecchymosis overlying the mastoid in a patient with a fracture of the base of the skull *(Battle sign)*.

the history and neurologic examination in this age group. Unfortunately, the roentgenogram is usually ordered in a defensive, medicolegal-oriented atmosphere, and the negative results may add a false sense of security. A skull roentgenogram or a head computed tomography (CT) scan is indicated for a child with a cephalohematoma, prolonged unconsciousness, a penetrating scalp wound, palpable bony defects, focal neurologic signs including irregular pupils and hemiparesis, discharge from the nose or ear, a discolored tympanic membrane, blackened eyes, and symptoms and signs of increased intracranial pressure.

CONCUSSION. This is defined as a brief but variable and reversible alteration in the level of consciousness associated with transient paralysis of reflexes and amnesia for the events immediately surrounding the injury. The duration of retrograde and post-traumatic amnesia is a good indicator of the severity of the trauma. During the acute phase of concussion there is loss of tone, flaccidity and areflexia, dilatation of the pupils, and brief apnea. Cortical blindness may follow a concussion, probably as the result of localized cerebral edema in the region of the calcarine fissure. The child may appear irritable and restless, and the older child may deny blindness. The period of blindness is transient, and full recovery usually occurs within hours. The recovery phase of concussion is characterized by tachycardia, vomiting, pallor, lethargy, and confusion. Several mechanisms for the pathogenesis of concussion have been proposed, including shearing or stretching of the fibers within the white matter, temporary paralysis of nerve function, an alteration in neurotransmitter elaboration, and temporary changes in cerebral blood flow and oxygen consumption.

Although the outcome for children with concussion is uniformly excellent, it is sometimes difficult to determine which patients should be hospitalized for observation at the time of the accident. The following clinical manifestations are indicators for concern following concussion and justify hospitalization for monitoring and a period of frequent observation: (1) deterioration in the level of consciousness, (2) persistence of confusion and lethargy, (3) excessive and copious vomiting, (4) unwitnessed or uncertain history of trauma, (5) focal neurologic signs, (6) a seizure, and (7) any child with a confirmed skull fracture.

SUBDURAL HEMATOMA. A subdural hematoma is a collection of bloody fluid between the dura and cerebral mantle. It occurs as a consequence of the rupture of bridging cortical veins that drain the cerebral cortex. Although any form of head trauma may produce subdural hematoma, the physically abused infant who is repeatedly and forcedly shaken is particularly susceptible to this type of head injury. Large collections of blood that may be unilateral or bilateral interfere with normal cerebral function and may cause herniation of the brain. Inevitably, there is a degree of trauma to the underlying brain as a direct result of the initial injury. In the physically abused child there are often additional sites of trauma, including retinal hemorrhages and rib and extremity fractures.

Acutely, the subdural hematoma consists of dark red blood that changes to a straw-colored fluid owing to disintegration of the red blood cells. Within 1 wk of the injury, a subdural membrane begins to develop from the inner surface of the dura and eventually encapsulates the hematoma. The hematoma may gradually enlarge owing to the presence of a high concentration of albumin, which, by osmotic pressure, draws water across the subdural membrane. Repeated trauma can produce fresh bleeding into a chronic subdural hematoma. Infantile subdural hematoma presents during the first 6 mo of life, often with a focal or generalized convulsion. In addition, there is typically a history of poor feeding, failure to thrive, irritability, lethargy, vomiting, and fever. These common constitutional symptoms may have been present for some time and may have been overlooked. The examination may show a tense and bulging anterior fontanel and an enlarged head circumference. Frequently there is evidence of cerebral injury, because the infant is irritable with a shrill, high-pitched cry. The eyes may show a "setting-sun" position owing to increased intracranial pressure. Examination of the eyegrounds is critical because more than 50% show retinal or subhyaloid hemorrhages. The CT scan or magnetic resonance imaging (MRI) is invaluable in confirming the diagnosis (Fig. 551–2). Acute subdural hematomas produce a hyperdense image that may be indistinguishable from the surrounding bone, whereas chronic subdurals are hypodense and readily identified by the CT scan. A prothrombin and partial thromboplastin time are important to rule out the remote possibility of a coagulation disorder. An infant who is a suspected victim of physical abuse should be admitted to the hospital and should be evaluated thoroughly for evidence of additional injuries while the social and environmental factors are carefully investigated. Acute subdural hematomas may be associated with severe underlying brain injuries, including contusion and intracerebral hemorrhage. The prognosis for recovery is poor because of the cerebral insult rather than the presence of blood in the subdural space.

Chronic subdural hematomas are typically observed in the infant and the elderly adult, because these patients have a discrepancy between the size of the brain and the skull. The lesions tend to be bilateral in younger children and are characterized by increasing head circumference, headache, dullness, personality change, a focal convulsion, sudden loss of consciousness, and signs of increased intracranial pressure.

EPIDURAL HEMATOMA. An epidural hematoma results from bleeding into the extradural space from rupture of the middle meningeal artery or a tear in the dural veins owing to direct trauma to the region of the temporal bone. The hematoma enlarges rapidly because of arterial bleeding or more gradually if venous bleeding occurs; each is capable of causing compression of the temporal lobe and ultimately herniation of the uncus, which is life-threatening and demands immediate surgical intervention. After the injury, the child typically experiences a brief period of unconsciousness followed by a variable lucid interval from minutes to days, depending on the source of bleeding. As the hematoma impinges on the temporal lobe, the child undergoes progressive loss of consciousness associated with vomiting, a severe headache, and focal neurologic signs, including ipsilateral dilatation of the pupil followed by a complete third-nerve paresis, contralateral hemiparesis, and papilledema in approximately 20% of cases. The CT scan is the diagnostic test of choice, because a skull fracture is present in only one half of the cases. An epidural hematoma typically assumes a hyperdense biconcave image on the CT scan (Fig. 551–3). The prognosis for an epidural hematoma is excellent if the diagnosis is made early with prompt surgical evacuation, but there is significant mortality and morbidity in those cases in which treatment is delayed or when severe underlying brain injury accompanies the epidural hematoma.

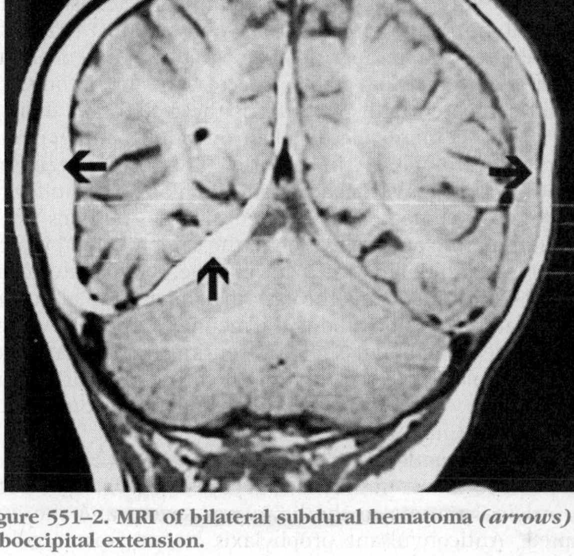

Figure 551–2. MRI of bilateral subdural hematoma *(arrows)* with suboccipital extension.

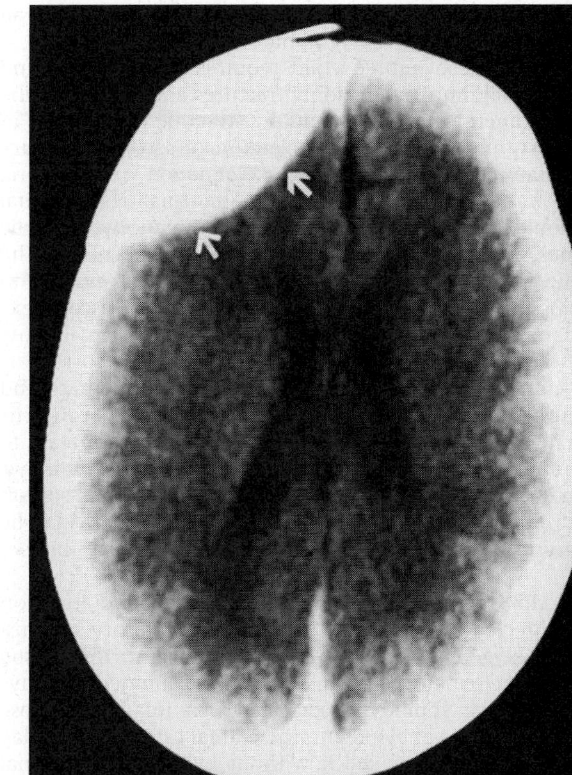

Figure 551–3. A CT scan of a frontal lobe epidural hematoma *(arrows)*. Note the minimal shift of the cerebral hemispheres.

SEVERE HEAD INJURIES. Major insults to the brain may result from contusion (particularly to the frontal lobes or inferolateral portion of the temporal lobes) a penetrating injury, the presence of an intracerebral hemorrhage, and diffuse axonal injury due to shear forces, all of which may produce cerebral edema. The incidence of space-occupying intracranial hematoma is less frequent in children than in adults, but the presence of diffuse cerebral swelling due to diffuse axonal injury is more frequent, particularly in a severe pediatric head injury. The clinical findings depend on the site and nature of the injury and on the degree of cerebral edema. The development of additional neurologic signs following admission to the hospital implies increased cerebral edema; an expanding intracerebral, subdural, or epidural hematoma; or compromised cerebral blood flow secondary to vasospasm. Initial signs associated with a poor prognosis include fixed and dilated pupils, apneic breathing, decorticate posturing, and a Glasgow Coma Scale score revised for children of less than 5. Some children are found to have cardiorespiratory arrest and hypotension at the site of an accident following a head injury, which is unrelated to acute blood loss. Cervical spine radiographs often show an injury to the high cervical spine, and postmortem examination shows intraparenchymal hemorrhage or laceration. Although this type of injury is uniformly fatal, it serves as a reminder to consider a spinal cord injury in every child with a severe head injury until appropriate radiographic studies are completed.

TREATMENT. A head-injured child requires identification and treatment of all injuries, including fractures and trauma to the pelvis, abdomen, and chest. Initially, treatment is aimed at resuscitation and then at the prevention of secondary injury by the maintenance of adequate oxygenation and cerebral blood flow and correction of metabolic abnormalities. The vital signs should be monitored and serial examination should be performed, including palpation of the scalp, inspection of the tympanic membranes, and a detailed neurologic evaluation (including pupillary reaction, eye movements, funduscopic examination, and a search for localizing signs). The Glasgow Coma Scale revised for children should be utilized to repeatedly document the level of consciousness in an accurate and reproducible fashion, avoiding ambiguous statements concerning the neurologic state and alerting the management team to deterioration in neurologic function. A minor head injury is sometimes difficult to distinguish from serious trauma, so that hospitalization and frequent observation for 24–48 hr may be necessary (see Concussion); a normal CT may reduce this period.

In the child with a major head injury, immediate attention must be directed to the cardiovascular and respiratory systems. Adequate oxygenation is essential to prevent further tissue damage. The circulatory system should be examined, and hypovolemic shock should be corrected. An infant may lose sufficient quantities of blood into the cranial cavity, which may cause severe anemia or shock without evidence of external bleeding. The cervical spine should be stabilized because there is an association between head trauma and neck injuries. When convenient and early in the course of management, a portable lateral neck roentgenogram should be obtained. Additional radiologic studies depend on the findings of the physical examination. A CT scan may readily identify correctable lesions, including subdural, epidural, and intracerebral hematomas as well as localized areas of cerebral edema and penetrating bony injuries. MRI is more reliable than a CT scan in the detection of posterior fossa hematomas but is difficult to undertake in the acute phase management of head injuries as the patient becomes inaccessible during the course of the study.

Cerebral edema is a major complication of head trauma and is the most common cause of death in the first few days after an accident. The management of cerebral edema and the concomitant increased intracranial pressure includes adequate oxygenation, elevation of the head of the bed to 30 degrees, and the judicious use of isotonic IV fluids. Inappropriate secretion of antidiuretic hormone may complicate acute head injury, in which case excessive fluid administration enhances the cerebral edema. Monitoring of the intracranial pressure is an important method of documenting the effectiveness of therapy (see Chapter 549). The role of ICP monitoring is threefold; (1) It has prognostic value in that pressures of greater than 30 mm Hg are rarely associated with intact survival; (2) it is used as a therapeutic guide, allowing one to institute methods of decreasing intracranial pressure; and (3) it is also an indicator of a sudden increase in pressure, which may be a reason for a repeat head CT scan and evacuation of a possible bleed. A number of patients with normal ICP ultimately die, and it has yet to be shown that aggressive management aimed at decreasing intracranial pressure is associated with improved outcome. Because an elevated P_{CO_2} causes vasodilation of the cerebral vessels and increases intracranial pressure, the patient is hyperventilated to maintain a P_{CO_2} in the region of 30–35 mm Hg. The use of hyperosmolar agents such as mannitol may be effective in controlling cerebral edema. Mannitol is given IV in a 20% solution at a dose of 1–1.5 g/kg. Subsequent pulses of mannitol of 0.25–0.5 g/kg are determined by the clinical state, intracranial pressure, and serum osmolarity, which should not be allowed to exceed 320 mOsm/L. Glucocorticoids, hypothermia, and barbiturate coma are no longer used in the management of serious head injury. In summary, intensive care management of severe head injuries is primarily supportive and designed to minimize secondary brain injuries.

The surgical management of head injuries includes the repair of depressed skull fractures, debridement of bony fragments within the cerebrum, evacuation of intracerebral hematomas producing a mass effect, removal of an epidural hematoma, and control of dural bleeding. Subdural hematomas of infancy may initially require percutaneous subdural taps if they are large or symptomatic. After bilateral subdural taps relieve the increased intracranial pressure, the child may be followed with repeated fontanel assessment, skull transillumination, head circumference measurements, and occasional CT scan to monitor the spontaneous resorption of the subdural hematoma over a period of weeks to months. Some children require repeated removal of the subdural collections because of recurrent symptoms and signs of increased intracranial pressure. Repeated subdural taps on alternate sides for several days may resolve the reaccumulation of subdural fluid and ameliorate the increased intracranial pressure. Rarely, a more aggressive surgical approach, including stripping of the membranes and the placement of a subdural-peritoneal shunt, is necessary to control subdural collections.

Seizures may complicate a head injury and can occur following relatively minor trauma. An immediate seizure (impact seizure) is often of short duration and of no prognostic significance. Seizures that develop within minutes or a few hours of head trauma are frequently brief and result from transient mechanical and neurochemical changes within the central nervous system. Most of these children will not have additional seizures and do not require anticonvulsants. Convulsions that develop within 24–48 hr of the injury are classified as early post-traumatic seizures and result from cerebral edema, petechial and hemorrhagic lesions, or a penetrating wound. Status epilepticus, which demands prompt management, may ensue. IV phenytoin is recommended, with a loading dose of 15–20 mg/kg followed by maintenance doses of 5–10 mg/kg/24 hr. Phenytoin is desirable in the acute stages of management because it does not alter the level of consciousness in a neurologically compromised patient. It is recommended that all children with a severe brain injury be placed on an anticonvulsant (phenytoin) to prevent secondary injury, which may result as a consequence of a generalized seizure.

PROGNOSIS. The most important determinant of neurologic and intellectual recovery in the head-injured child is the duration of coma. If the child survives the immediate consequences of the head injury and recovers from coma within 14 days, the likelihood of normal or near-normal cognitive and neuromotor function is extremely favorable. The reasons for optimism in the child compared with the adult is the contention that the former's brain is more "plastic" than the adult's and generally recovers more completely in a shorter time. However, infants less than 2 yr of age with major brain trauma have a uniformly poor prognosis compared with older children, perhaps as the result of immature autoregulation of the cerebral blood vessels, the greater susceptibility of the incompletely myelinated brain to irreversible injury, and the fact that open cranial sutures permit greater distortion among the meninges, cerebral vessels, and the underlying brain. The most sensitive and specific indicator of neurologic recovery during the acute and early stages of a head injury is an evaluation with somatosensory evoked potentials (see Chapters 549 and 550).

Late post-traumatic seizures tend to develop within 2 yr of the initial insult. Post-traumatic epilepsy is more likely to occur if the original trauma to the brain was severe and the dura disrupted. Anticonvulsant prophylaxis is not warranted for every head-injured child because the majority will not develop seizures. For patients who develop a seizure during hospitalization (excluding those with a brief seizure within a few hours of the accident), an anticonvulsant is prescribed for 2–3 mo. If the seizures recur, the drug is reinstituted for a more prolonged period. Post-traumatic seizures that result from localized glial scars may be unresponsive to anticonvulsants and require surgical extirpation in order to control the seizures.

With severe head injuries, a variety of persistent neurologic deficits may result, including hemiparesis, aphasia, cognitive disturbances, and behavioral disorders. Many studies have noted that children with personality disorders following serious head trauma had unusual behavioral traits prior to the injury that seemed to be enhanced by the accident. Abnormalities of short-term memory, specifically storage and retrieval of important information, is the most common cognitive sequela of significant head injury in children and adolescents. Children may show gradual recovery of neuropsychologic function up to 5 yr after an accident. Cognitive deficits may not be readily apparent during hospitalization. Neuropsychologic evaluation of the severely injured child, or the patient with an apparently mild injury who copes poorly at school following the accident, is an important method of identifying specific language, memory, or cognitive deficits that may be responsive to special education techniques.

The **post-traumatic syndrome** may occur in children following relatively minor head trauma (see Chapter 19). The essential features include hyperactivity, decreased attention span, temper outbursts, sleep disturbances, moodiness, and discipline problems. Occasionally, dizziness and headaches are also present. Treatment of the post-traumatic syndrome should include a thorough evaluation of the child to eliminate other causes, followed by reassurance and support; the condition improves spontaneously without specific intervention in most children.

Black P, Jeffries JJ, Blumer D, et al: The post-traumatic syndrome in children. *In*: Walker AE, Caveness WF, Critchley M (eds): The Late Effects of Head Injury. Springfield, IL, Charles C Thomas, 1969.
Bohn D, Armstrong D, Becker L, et al: Cervical spine injuries in children. J Trauma 30:463, 1990.
Bruce DA, Schut L, Bruno LA, et al: Outcome following severe head injuries in children. J Neurosurg 48:679, 1978.
Davis RL, Hughes M, Gublen KD, et al: The use of cranial CT scans in the triage of pediatric patients with mild head injury. Pediatrics 95:345, 1995.
Dershewitz RA, Kaye BA, Swisher CN: Treatment of children with post-traumatic transient loss of consciousness. Pediatrics 72:602, 1983.
Greenspan AI, Mackenzie EJ: Functional outcome after pediatric head injury. Pediatrics 94:425, 1994.
Klonoff H, Low MD, Clark C: Head injuries in children: A prospective 5 year follow-up. J Neurol Neurosurg Psychiatry 40:1211, 1977.
Kraus JF, Fife D, Conroy C: Pediatric brain injuries: The nature, clinical course and early outcomes in a defined United States population. Pediatrics 79:501, 1987.
Leonidas JC, Ting W, Binkiewicz A, et al: Mild head trauma in children: When is a roentgenogram necessary? Pediatrics 69:139, 1982.
Levin HS, Eisenberg HM: Neuropsychological outcome of head injury in children and adolescents. Childs Brain 5:281, 1979.
Lipton SA, Rosenberg PA: Excitatory amino acids as a final common pathway for neurologic disorders. N Engl J Med 330:613, 1994.
Mahoney WJ, D'Souza BJ, Haller JA, et al: Long-term outcome of children with severe head trauma and prolonged coma. Pediatrics 71:756, 1983.

CHAPTER 552
Neurodegenerative Disorders of Childhood

Neurodegenerative disorders of childhood encompass a large number of heterogeneous diseases that result from specific genetic and biochemical defects, chronic viral infections, and toxic substances and a significant group of conditions of unknown cause. Until recently, children with suspected neurodegenerative disorders were routinely subjected to brain and rectal biopsies, but with the advent of modern neuroimaging techniques and specific biochemical diagnostic tests, these invasive procedures are now rarely necessary. Nevertheless, the most important component of the investigation continues to be a thorough history and physical examination. The hallmark of a neurodegenerative disease is progressive deterioration of neurologic function with loss of speech, vision, hearing, or locomotion, often associated with seizures, feeding difficulties, and impairment of intellect. The age of onset, rate of progression, and the principal neurologic findings determine whether the disease is primarily affecting the white or gray matter. Upper motor neuron signs are prominent early in the former and convulsions, intellectual, and visual impairment in the latter. A precise history confirms regression of developmental milestones, and the neurologic examination localizes the process within the nervous system. Although the outcome is invariably fatal, and current therapeutic attempts have been unsuccessful, it is important to make the correct diagnosis so that genetic counseling may be offered and prevention strategies can be implemented. For all conditions in which the specific enzyme defect is known, prevention by prenatal diagnosis (chorionic villus sampling or amniocentesis) is possible. Carrier detection is also often possible by enzyme assay. Table 552–1 summarizes the heredity, biochemical defects, and specific diagnostic abnormality in the inherited neurodegerative disorders.

The inherited neurodegenerative disorders include the sphingolipidoses, neuronal ceroid lipofuscinoses, adrenoleukodystrophy, and sialidosis. The sphingolipidoses are characterized by the intracellular storage of a normal lipid component of the cell membrane owing to a defect in the catabolism of the compound. The sphingolipidoses are subclassified into six categories: Niemann-Pick disease, Gaucher disease, GM_1 gangliosidosis, GM_2 gangliosidosis, Krabbe disease, and metachromatic leukodystrophy. Niemann-Pick disease and Gaucher disease are discussed in Chapter 72.3. The spinocerebellar degenerative diseases (Friedreich ataxia, ataxia, telangiectasia, olivopontocerebellar atrophy, and abetalipoproteinemia) and degenerative disorders of the basal ganglia (Huntington disease, dystonia musculorum deformans, Wilson disease, and Hallervorden-Spatz disease) are included in Chapter 547. Finally, a miscellaneous group of degenerative diseases is discussed in this section, including multiple sclerosis, Pelizaeus-Merzbacher disease, Alexander disease, Canavan spongy degeneration, kinky hair disease, Rett syndrome, and subacute sclerosing panencephalitis.

552.1 Sphingolipidoses

GANGLIOSIDOSES
(See also Chapter 72.3)

Gangliosides are glycosphingolipids, normal constituents of the neuronal and synaptic membranes. The basic structure of GM_1 ganglioside consists of an oligosaccharide chain attached to a hydroxyl group of ceramide and sialic acid bound to galactose. The gangliosides are catabolized by sequential cleavage of the sugar molecules by specific exoglycosidases. Abnormalities in catabolism result in accumulation of the ganglioside within the cell. Defects in ganglioside degradation can be classified into two groups, the GM_1 gangliosidoses and the GM_2 gangliosidoses.

GM_1 GANGLIOSIDOSES. The three subtypes of GM_1 gangliosidoses

■ TABLE 552–1 Heredity and Biochemical Defects in the Neurodegenerative Disorders

Neurodegenerative Disorder	Mode of Inheritance	Biochemical Defect	Specimen for Analysis
Sphingolipidosis			
GM_1 gangliosidosis	AR*	β-Galactosidase	Serum, leukocytes, skin fibroblasts
GM_2 gangliosidosis			
Tay-Sachs disease	AR	Hexosaminidase A	Serum, leukocytes, skin fibroblasts
Sandhoff disease	AR	Hexosaminidase A and B	Serum, leukocytes, skin fibroblasts
Krabbe disease	AR	Galactocerebrosidase	Leukocytes and skin fibroblasts
Metachromatic leukodystrophy	AR	Arylsulfatase A	Leukocytes and skin fibroblasts
Neuronal Ceroid Lipofuscinoses	AR	?	EM† of skin biopsy
Adrenoleukodystrophy	XLR‡	VLCFA§ oxidation	Plasma, skin fibroblasts
Sialidosis	AR	Neuraminidase	Skin fibroblasts

*AR = autosomal recessive.
†EM = electron microscopy.
‡XLR = X-linked recessive.
§VLCFA = very long chain fatty acid.

are classified according to age at presentation: infantile (type 1), juvenile (type 2), and adult (type 3). The condition is inherited as an autosomal recessive trait and results from a marked deficiency of acid β-galactosidase. This enzyme may be assayed in leukocytes and cultured fibroblasts. The gene has been assigned to chromosome 3p14.2. Prenatal diagnosis is possible by the measurement of acid β-galactosidase in cultured amniotic cells.

Infantile GM_1 gangliosidosis presents at birth or during the neonatal period with anorexia, poor suck, and inadequate weight gain. Development is globally retarded, and generalized seizures are prominent. The phenotype is striking and shares many characteristics with Hurler syndrome. The facial features are coarse, the forehead is prominent, the nasal bridge is depressed, the tongue is large (macroglossia), and the gums are hypertrophied. Hepatosplenomegaly is present early in the course owing to accumulation of foamy histiocytes, and kyphoscoliosis is evident owing to anterior beaking of the vertebral bodies. The neurologic examination is dominated by apathy, progressive blindness, deafness, spastic quadriplegia, and decerebrate rigidity. A cherry red spot in the macular region is visualized in approximately 50% of cases. The **cherry red spot** is characterized by an opaque ring (sphingolipid-laden retinal ganglion cells) encircling the normal red-colored fovea (Fig. 552–1). Children rarely survive beyond 2–3 yr of age, and death is due to aspiration pneumonia.

Juvenile GM_1 gangliosidosis has a delayed onset beginning about 1 yr of age. The initial symptoms consist of incoordination, weakness, ataxia, and regression of language. Thereafter convulsions, spasticity, decerebrate rigidity, and blindness are the major findings. Unlike in the infantile type, coarse facial features and hepatosplenomegaly are usually absent. Radiographic examination of the lumbar vertebrae may show minor beaking. Children rarely survive beyond 10 yr of age. *Adult GM_1 gangliosidosis* is a slowly progressive disease consisting of spasticity, ataxia, dysarthria, and a gradual loss of cognitive function.

GM_2 GANGLIOSIDOSES. The GM_2 gangliosidoses comprise a heterogeneous group of autosomal recessive inherited disorders that consist of several subtypes, including Tay-Sachs disease (TSD), Sandhoff disease, juvenile GM_2 gangliosidosis, and adult GM_2 gangliosidosis. *TSD* is most prevalent in the Ashkenazi Jewish population and has a carrier rate of approximately 1/30. The gene for TSD maps to chromosome 15q23–q24. Affected infants appear normal until approximately 6 mo of age, except for a marked "startle" reaction to noise that is evident soon after birth. The affected child then begins to lag in developmental milestones, and by 1 yr of age the child loses the ability to stand, sit, and vocalize. Early hypotonia develops into progressive spasticity, and relentless deterioration follows, with convulsions, blindness, deafness, and cherry red spots in almost all patients (see Fig. 552–1). Macrocephaly becomes apparent by 1 yr of age and results from the 200- to 300-fold normal content of GM_2 ganglioside deposited within the brain. Few children live beyond 3–4 yr of age, and death is usually associated with aspiration or bronchopneumonia. A deficiency of the isoenzyme hexosaminidase A is found in tissues of patients with TSD. Mass screening for the prenatal diagnosis of TSD is a reliable and cost-effective method of prevention because the condition occurs in a defined population (Ashkenazi Jews). An accurate and inexpensive carrier detection test is available (serum or leukocyte hexosaminidase A), and the disease can be reliably diagnosed by chorionic villus sampling during the 1st trimester of pregnancy in couples at risk (heterozygote parents).

Sandhoff disease is very similar to TSD in the mode of presentation, including progressive loss of motor and language milestones beginning at 6 mo of age. Seizures, cherry red spots, macrocephaly, and doll-like facies are present in most patients; however, children with Sandhoff disease may also have splenomegaly. The visual evoked potentials (VEPs) are normal

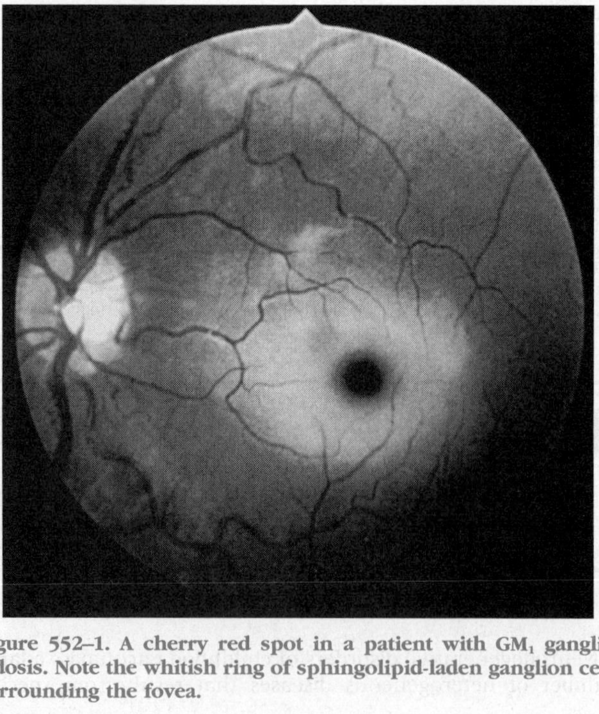

Figure 552–1. A cherry red spot in a patient with GM_1 gangliosidosis. Note the whitish ring of sphingolipid-laden ganglion cells surrounding the fovea.

early in the course of Sandhoff disease and TSD but become abnormal or absent as the disease progresses. The auditory brain stem responses (ABRs) show prolonged latencies. The diagnosis of Sandhoff disease is established by the finding of deficient levels of hexosaminidase A and B in serum and leukocytes. Children usually succumb by 3 yr of age. The gene for Sandhoff disease maps to chromosome 5q1.13.

Juvenile GM_2 gangliosidosis develops in midchildhood, initially with clumsiness followed by ataxia. Signs of spasticity, athetosis, loss of language, and seizures gradually develop. Progressive visual loss is associated with optic atrophy, but cherry red spots rarely occur in juvenile GM_2 gangliosidosis. A deficiency of hexosaminidase is variable (total deficiency to near normal) in these patients. Death occurs around 15 yr of age. *Adult GM_2 gangliosidosis* is characterized by a myriad of neurologic signs, including slowly progressive gait ataxia, spasticity, dystonia, proximal muscle atrophy, and dysarthria. Generally, visual acuity and intellectual function are unimpaired. Hexosaminidase A or A and B activity is reduced significantly in the serum and leukocytes.

KRABBE DISEASE (GLOBOID CELL LEUKODYSTROPHY). Krabbe disease (KD) is a rare autosomal recessive neurodegenerative disorder characterized by severe myelin loss and the presence of globoid bodies in the white matter. The gene for Krabbe disease is located on chromosome 14q21–q31. The disease results from a marked deficiency of the lysosomal enzyme galactocerebroside β-galactosidase, which cleaves a galactose moiety from the ceramide portion of galactocerebroside. KD is a disorder of myelin destruction rather than abnormal myelin formation. Normally, myelination begins during the 3rd trimester, corresponding with a rapid rise of galactocerebroside β-galactosidase activity in the brain. In patients with Krabbe disease, galactocerebroside cannot be metabolized during the normal turnover of myelin because of the deficiency of galactocerebroside β-galactosidase. When galactocerebroside is injected into the brains of experimental animals, a globoid cell reaction ensues. It has been postulated that a similar phenomenon occurs in humans; nonmetabolized galactocerebroside stimulates the formation of globoid cells that reflect the destruction of oligodendroglial cells. Because oligodendroglial cells are responsible for the elaboration of myelin, their loss results in myelin breakdown, thus producing additional galactocerebroside and causing a vicious circle of myelin destruction.

The symptoms of KD become evident during the first few months of life and include excessive irritability and crying, unexplained episodes of hyperpyrexia, feeding problems, vomiting, and failure to thrive. During the initial stages of KD, children are often treated for colic or "milk allergy" with frequent formula changes. Generalized seizures may appear early in the course of the disease. Alterations in body tone with rigidity and opisthotonus and visual inattentiveness owing to optic atrophy become apparent as the disease progresses. During the later stages of the illness, blindness, deafness, absent deep tendon reflexes, and decerebrate rigidity constitute the major physical findings. A non-enhanced computed tomography (CT) scan of the head may show symmetric increased densities in the caudate nuclei and thalami. Most patients expire by 2 yr of age.

A *late-onset KD* has been described beginning in childhood or during adolescence. These patients present with optic atrophy and cortical blindness, and their condition is often confused with the adrenoleukodystrophies. Slowly progressive gait disturbances, including spasticity and ataxia, are prominent. As with classic KD, globoid cells are abundant in the white matter, and leukocytes are deficient in galactocerebroside β-galactosidase. An examination of the cerebrospinal fluid (CSF) shows an elevated protein content, and the nerve conduction velocities are markedly delayed owing to segmental demyelination of the peripheral nerves. The VEPs decrease gradually in amplitude with no response in the late stages of the disease, and the ABRs are characterized by the presence of only waves I and II. CT scans and magnetic resonance imaging (MRI) studies highlight the marked decrease in white matter, especially of the cerebellum and centrum semiovale, with sparing of the subcortical u fibers. Prenatal diagnosis is possible by the assay of galactocerebroside β-galactosidase activity in chorionic villi or in cultured amniotic fluid cells.

METACHROMATIC LEUKODYSTROPHY (MLD). This disorder of myelin metabolism is inherited as an autosomal recessive trait and is characterized by a deficiency of arylsulfatase A activity. Several mutations in the gene encoding for arylsulfatase A have been identified. The gene is located on chromosome 22q13–13qter and DNA diagnosis is possible. The absence or deficiency of arylsulfatase A leads to the accumulation of cerebroside sulfate within the myelin sheath of the central nervous system (CNS) and peripheral nervous system owing to the inability to cleave sulfate from galactosyl-3-sulfate ceramide. The excessive cerebroside sulfate is thought to cause myelin breakdown and destruction of oligodendroglia. The prenatal diagnosis of MLD is made by the assay of arylsulfatase A in chorionic villi or cultured amniotic fluid cells. Cresyl violet applied to tissue specimens produces metachromatic staining of the sulfatide granules, giving the disease its name. Six disorders are included in the MLD group of diseases, classified by the age at onset and enzyme deficiency. Three conditions are briefly discussed: the classic or late infantile, juvenile, and adult leukodystrophy.

Late infantile MLD begins with the insidious onset of gait disturbance between 1 and 2 yr of age. Initially the child appears awkward and frequently falls, but gradually locomotion is impaired significantly and support is required in order to walk. The extremities are hypotonic, and the deep tendon reflexes are absent or diminished. Within the next several months the child can no longer stand, and a deterioration in intellectual function becomes apparent. The speech is slurred and dysarthric, and the child appears dull and apathetic. Visual fixation is diminished, nystagmus is present, and examination of the retina shows optic atrophy. Within 1 yr from the onset of the disease the child is unable to sit unsupported, and progressive decorticate postures develop. Feeding and swallowing are impaired owing to pseudobulbar palsies, and a feeding gastrostomy is required. The patient ultimately becomes stuporous and dies of aspiration or bronchopneumonia by 5–6 yr of age. Neurophysiologic evaluation shows progressive changes in the VEPs, ABRs, and the somatosensory evoked potentials (SSEPs), and the nerve conduction velocities (NCVs) of the peripheral nerves are significantly reduced. CT images of the brain indicate diffuse symmetric attenuation of the cerebellar and cerebral white matter, and examination of the CSF shows an elevated protein content. Bone marrow transplantation is a promising experimental therapy for the management of late infantile MLD. Favorable outcomes have been reported only in patients treated very early in the course of the disease. The total number of patients treated is relatively small and the follow-up too short to draw conclusions about the efficacy of bone marrow transplantation.

Juvenile MLD shares many features in common with late infantile MLD, but the onset of symptoms is delayed to 5–10 yr of age. Deterioration in school performance and alterations in personality may herald the onset of the disease. This is followed by incoordination of gait, urinary incontinence, and dysarthria. Muscle tone becomes increased, and ataxia, dystonia, or tremor may be present. During the terminal stages, generalized tonic-clonic convulsions are prominent and are difficult to control. The child rarely lives beyond midadolescence. *Adult MLD* occurs from the 2nd to 6th decade. Abnormalities in memory, psychiatric disturbances, and personality changes are prominent features. Slowly progressive neurologic signs, including spasticity, dystonia, optic atrophy, and generalized convulsions, lead eventually to a bedridden state characterized by decorticate postures and unresponsiveness.

552.2 Neuronal Ceroid Lipofuscinoses

Neuronal ceroid lipofuscinoses constitute the most common class of neurodegenerative diseases in children and consists of three disorders inherited as autosomal recessive traits. They are characterized by the storage of an autofluorescent substance within neurons and other tissues. *Infantile type (Haltia-Santavuori)* begins toward the end of the 1st year of life with myoclonic seizures, intellectual deterioration, and blindness. Optic atrophy and brownish discoloration of the macula are evident upon examination of the retina, and cerebellar ataxia is prominent. The electroretinogram (ERG) typically shows small amplitude or absent wave forms. Death occurs at approximately 10 yr of age. The gene defect causing the infantile form has been assigned to chromosome 1p32. *Late infantile (Jansky-Bielschowsky)* is the most common type of neuronal ceroid lipofuscinosis. The presenting manifestation is myoclonic seizures beginning between 2 and 4 yr of age in a previously normal child. Dementia and ataxia are combined with a progressive loss of visual acuity and microcephaly. An examination of the retina shows marked attenuation of vessels, peripheral black "bone spicule" pigmentary abnormalities, optic atrophy, and a subtle brown pigment in the macular region. The ERG is abnormal early in the course owing to the deposition of the abnormal storage substance within the rod and cone area of the retina. The VEP is characteristic and consists of markedly enlarged responses followed by absent wave forms with progression of the disease. The autofluorescent material is deposited in neurons, fibroblasts, and secretory cells. Electron microscopic examination of the storage material in skin or conjunctival biopsies typically shows curvilinear bodies or "fingerprint profiles." The gene for late infantile neuronal ceroid lipofuscinosis has not been localized. *Juvenile type (Spielmeyer-Vogt)* is characterized by progressive visual loss and intellectual impairment beginning between 5 and 10 yr of age. The funduscopic changes are similar to those for the late infantile type. The ERG is also abnormal early in the course of the disease, but in the juvenile type the VEP typically is characterized by small-amplitude waves and, later, absence of wave forms as the disease progresses. Myoclonic seizures are not as prominent as in the late infantile type of neuronal ceroid lipofuscinosis, but dystonic posturing is marked during the late stages of the disease. Elevated urine dolichol levels are a nonspecific finding. Ultrastructural abnormalities of skin biopsies are present in most cases. The gene for the juvenile form of neuronal ceroid lipofuscinosis is located on chromosome 16p12.1.

552.3 Adrenoleukodystrophy

(See Chapter 72.2)

The adrenoleukodystrophies consist of a group of CNS degenerative disorders that are often associated with adrenal cortical insufficiency, are inherited by X-linked recessive transmission, and are not responsive to any known treatments. *Classic adrenoleukodystrophy* (ALD) becomes symptomatic between 5 and 15 yr of age with evidence of academic deterioration, behavioral disturbances, and gait abnormalities. Generalized seizures are common in the early stages. Upper motor neuron signs include spastic quadriparesis and contractures, ataxia, and marked swallowing disturbances secondary to pseudobulbar palsy. These dominate the terminal stages of the illness. Hypoadrenalism is present in approximately 50% of cases, and adrenal insufficiency characterized by abnormal skin pigmentation (tanning without exposure to sun) may precede the onset of neurologic symptoms. CT scans and MRI studies of patients indicate periventricular demyelination beginning posteriorly, which advances progressively to the anterior regions of the cerebral white matter. ABRs, VEPs, and SSEPs may be normal initially but ultimately show prolonged latencies and abnormal wave forms. Death supervenes within 10 yr of the onset of the neurologic signs. The gene for classic adrenoleukodystrophy is located on Xq28.

Adrenomyeloneuropathy begins with a slowly progressive spastic paraparesis, urinary incontinence, and onset of impotence during the 3rd or 4th decade despite the fact that adrenal insufficiency may have been present since childhood. Cases of typical adrenoleukodystrophy have occurred in families in whom the propositus presented with adrenomyeloneuropathy. One of the most difficult problems in the management of X-linked ALD is the common observation that affected individuals in the same family may have quite different clinical courses. For example, families are encountered in which one affected male had severe classical ALD culminating in death by age 10 yr, another affected male (e.g., a brother) had late-onset adrenomyeloneuropathy, and a third has no symptoms at all. Counseling families with presymptomatic males is extraordinarily difficult because there is no reliable method to predict the clinical course.

Neonatal adrenoleukodystrophy is characterized by marked hypotonia, severe psychomotor retardation, and the early onset of seizures. It is inherited as an autosomal recessive condition. Visual inattention is secondary to optic atrophy. Adrenal function tests are normal, but adrenal atrophy is evident at post mortem. Correction of adrenal insufficiency is ineffective in halting neurologic deterioration.

552.4 Sialidosis

Sialidosis is inherited as an autosomal recessive trait and results from the accumulation of a sialic acid–oligosaccharide complex secondary to a deficiency in the lysosomal enzyme neuraminidase. The urinary excretion of sialic acid–containing oligosaccharides is increased significantly in affected patients. *Sialidosis type I*, the cherry red spot–myoclonus syndrome (CRSM), usually presents during the 2nd decade of life, when the patient complains of visual deterioration. Inspection of the retina shows a cherry red spot, but, unlike in patients with TSD, visual acuity declines slowly in individuals with CRSM. Myoclonus of the extremities is gradually progressive and often debilitating and eventually renders the patient non-ambulatory. The myoclonus is triggered by voluntary movement, touch, and sound and is not controlled with anticonvulsants. Generalized convulsions responsive to antiepileptic drugs have been reported in most patients. *Sialidosis type II* may be subdivided into an infantile and juvenile form, depending on the age at presentation. In addition to cherry red spots and myoclonus, these patients have somatic involvement, including coarse facial features, corneal clouding (rarely), and dysostosis multiplex, producing anterior beaking of the lumbar vertebrae. An examination of lymphocytes shows vacuoles in the cytoplasm; biopsy of the liver demonstrates cytoplasmic vacuoles in Kupffer cells; and membrane-bound vacuoles are found in

Schwann cell cytoplasm, all attesting to the multiorgan nature of sialidosis type II. There are no distinctive neuroimaging findings or abnormalities in electrophysiologic studies in this group of disorders. Patients with sialidosis have been reported to live beyond the 5th decade.

Some cases of what appears to be sialidosis type II are the result of combined deficiencies of β-galactosidase and α-neuraminidase due to deficiency of a "protective protein" that prevents the premature intracellular degradation of the two enzymes. Clinically, affected patients are indistinguishable from those with sialidosis type II, either the infantile or juvenile form, caused by isolated α-neuraminidase deficiency. The diagnosis may be missed if β-galactosidase testing is done and testing of α-neuraminidase activity in fibroblasts is not completed.

552.5 Miscellaneous Disorders

MULTIPLE SCLEROSIS

Multiple sclerosis (MS) is a chronic and remitting disorder characterized by multiple white matter lesions in the CNS separated by time and location. The condition is rare in the pediatric population, and onset prior to 10 yr of age occurs in 0.2–2% of all cases. There is a greater incidence of MS in females in the pediatric age group compared with adults. The etiology of MS is unknown, but interactive genetic, immunologic, and infectious factors are probably responsible. The most frequent presenting symptom is unilateral weakness or ataxia. Headache is an important early component of the disease and is often severe, prolonged, and generalized. Ill-defined paresthesias involving the lower extremities, distal portions of the hands and feet, and the face are common. Visual symptoms including diplopia, blurred vision, or sudden visual loss secondary to optic neuritis are also important early manifestations of MS. Vertigo, dysarthria, and sphincter disturbances are relatively uncommon. *Neuromyelitis optica (Devic disease)* is a variant of classic MS and consists of optic neuritis and transverse myelitis, which occur conjointly.

The pathology of MS consists of demyelination with the formation of plaques. There is no reliable laboratory test that unequivocally confirms the diagnosis of MS, except for an autopsy. MRI is the neuroimaging technique of choice; small plaques of 3–4 mm can be identified, particularly those located in the brain stem and spinal cord.

The treatment of MS is supportive, and particular attention is given to the management of a neurogenic bladder. There is no evidence that corticosteroids alter the long-term course of the disease, but they may expedite recovery following an acute attack. Studies indicate that interferon beta-1b given subcutaneously is effective in the treatment of MS by decreasing disease activity and disease burden, as shown by serial MRI scans in adults. The prognosis for childhood MS is similar to that in adults; recovery is often complete, and the progression of the disease tends to be slow with long periods of remission in most cases. Promising immunologic therapy is currently being investigated.

PELIZAEUS-MERZBACHER DISEASE

This disease consists of a group of disorders that are characterized by nystagmus and abnormalities of myelin. The classic form is inherited as an X-linked recessive trait and is recognized by nystagmus and roving eye movements with head-nodding during infancy. The gene is located on chromosome Xq22. Molecular diagnosis of Pelizaeus-Merzbacher disease is possible using mutation analysis. However, as with most X-linked diseases, the molecular diagnosis of Pelizaeus-Merzbacher disease is complex because almost every patient with the disease will have a different mutation. The child's developmental milestones are delayed, and ultimately ataxia, choreoathetosis, and spasticity develop. Optic atrophy and dysarthria are associated findings, and death occurs in the 2nd or 3rd decade. The major pathologic finding is a loss of myelin with intact axons, suggesting a defect in the function of oligodendroglia. Studies point to a genetic defect in the biosynthesis of proteolipid apoprotein, a protein that is concerned with the differentiation and maintenance of oligodendrocytes. The MRI scan shows a symmetric pattern of delayed myelination. Multimodal evoked potential studies demonstrate an interesting pattern early in the course, consisting of loss of waves III–V on the ABR. This finding is useful in the investigation of nystagmus in the male infant. VEPs show prolonged latencies, and SSEPs show absent cortical responses or delayed latencies.

ALEXANDER DISEASE

Alexander disease is a rare disorder that occurs sporadically and causes progressive macrocephaly during the 1st year of life. Pathologic examination of the brain features the deposition of eosinophilic hyaline bodies in a perivascular distribution throughout the brain and beneath the pia mater. Degeneration of white matter is most prominent in the frontal lobes, and a CT scan during this stage shows corresponding attenuation of the cerebral white matter. The child develops progressive loss of intellect, spasticity, and unresponsive seizures causing death by 5 yr of age.

CANAVAN SPONGY DEGENERATION

See Chapter 71.13.

MENKES DISEASE

Menkes disease (kinky hair disease) is a progressive neurodegenerative condition inherited as a sex-linked recessive trait. The gene is located on chromosome Xq12–q13. Symptoms begin during the first few months of life and include hypothermia, hypotonia, and generalized myoclonic seizures. The facies are distinctive, with chubby, rosy cheeks and kinky, colorless, friable hair. Microscopic examination of the hair shows several abnormalities, including trichorrhexis nodosa (fractures along the hair shaft) and pili torti (twisted hair). Feeding difficulties are prominent and lead to failure to thrive. Severe mental retardation and optic atrophy are constant features of the disease. Low serum copper and ceruloplasmin levels have been found consistently in patients with Menkes disease, and a defect in copper absorption and transport across the gut has been shown to be the cause of the condition. Neuropathologic changes include tortuous cerebral vessels secondary to defects in the intima, focal degeneration of the gray matter, and marked changes in the cerebellum with loss of the internal granule cell layer and necrosis of the Purkinje cells.

Death occurs by 3 yr of age in the untreated patient. Copper-histidine therapy has been shown to be effective in preventing neurologic deterioration in some patients with Menkes disease, particularly if treatment is begun during the neonatal period or, preferably, with the fetus. Copper is essential during the early stages of CNS development and its absence probably accounts for the neuropathologic changes. Copper-histidine is given subcutaneously in a dose of 50–150 μg elemental copper/kg/24 hr for the duration of the child's life. The serum copper and ceruloplasmin levels return to the normal range within 2–3 wk of commencing therapy. The *occipital horn syndrome*, a skeletal dysplasia caused by different mutations in the same gene as that involved in Menkes disease, is a relatively mild disease. The two diseases are often confused, as the biochemical abnormalities are identical. Resolution of the uncertainty about treatment of patients with Menkes disease will require careful genotype-phenotype correlation, along with further clinical trials of copper therapy.

RETT SYNDROME

Rett syndrome is a neurodegenerative disorder of unknown etiology that occurs exclusively in female children and has a prevalence of approximately 1/15,000 to 1/22,000. There are no biologic markers for the disease; the diagnosis is established by the history and clinical findings. The etiology of Rett syndrome is presumed to be the result of X-linked dominant inheritance, which is lethal to the male fetus. Development proceeds normally until 1 yr of age, when regression of language and motor milestones and acquired microcephaly become apparent. An ataxic gait or fine tremor of hand movements is an early neurologic finding. Most children develop peculiar sighing respirations with intermittent periods of apnea that may be associated with cyanosis. The hallmark of Rett syndrome is repetitive hand-wringing movements and a loss of purposeful and spontaneous use of the hands, which may not appear until 2–3 yr of age. Autistic behavior is a typical finding in all patients. Generalized tonic-clonic convulsions occur in the majority and are usually well controlled by anticonvulsants. Feeding disorders and poor weight gain are common. After the initial period of neurologic regression, the disease process appears to plateau, with a persistence of the autistic behavior. Death often occurs during adolescence or during the third decade. Cardiac arrhythmias may result in sudden, unexpected death. Postmortem studies show significantly reduced brain weight (60–80% of normal) with a decrease in the number of synapses, associated with a decrease in dendritic length and branching.

SUBACUTE SCLEROSING PANENCEPHALITIS

Subacute sclerosing panencephalitis (SSPE) is a rare, progressive slow-virus infection of the CNS caused by a measles-like virus (Chapter 206). The number of reported cases has decreased dramatically to 0.06 case/million population, paralleling the decline in reported measles cases. The initial clinical manifestations include personality changes, aggressive behavior, and impairment of cognitive function. Myoclonic seizures soon dominate the clinical picture. Later, generalized tonic-clonic convulsions, hypertonia, and choreoathetosis become evident followed by progressive bulbar palsy, hyperthermia, and decerebrate postures. Funduscopic examination early in the course of the disease reveals papilledema in approximately 20% of the cases. Optic atrophy, chorioretinitis, and macular pigmentation are observed in most patients. The *diagnosis* is established by the typical clinical course and one of the following: (1) measles antibody detected in the CSF, (2) a characteristic EEG consisting of bursts of high-voltage slow waves interspersed with a normal background in the early stages, and (3) typical histologic findings in the brain biopsy or postmortem specimen. *Treatment* with a series of antiviral agents has been attempted without success. Death occurs usually within 1–2 yr from the onset of symptoms.

Baram TZ, Goldman AM, Percy AK: Krabbe disease: Specific MRI and CT findings. Neurology 36:111, 1986.
Boustany RMN, Alroy J, Kolodny EH: Clinical classification of neuronal ceroid-lipofuscinosis subtypes. Am J Med Genet 5(Suppl):47, 1988.
Chelly J, Tumer Z, Tonnesen T, et al: Isolation of a candidate gene for Menkes disease that encodes a potential heavy metal binding protein. Nature Genet 3:14, 1993.
Danks DM, Campbell PE, Stevens BJ, et al: Menkes' kinky hair syndrome: An inherited defect in copper absorption with widespread effects. Pediatrics 50:188, 1972.
De Meirleir LJ, Taylor MJ, Logan WJ: Multimodal evoked potential studies in leukodystrophies of children. Can J Neurol Sci 15:26, 1988.
Duquette P, Murray TJ, Pleines J, et al: Multiple sclerosis in childhood: Clinical profile in 125 patients. J Pediatr 111:359, 1987.
Dyken PR, Cunningham SC, Ward LC: Changing character of subacute sclerosing panencephalitis in the United States. Pediatr Neurol 5:339, 1989.
Ebers GC, Bulman DE, Sadovnick AD, et al: A population-based study of multiple sclerosis in twins. N Engl J Med 315:1638, 1986.
Farrell DF, Swedberg K: Clinical and biochemical heterogeneity of globoid cell leukodystrophy. Ann Neurol 10:364, 1981.
Farrell K, Chuang S, Becker LE: Computed tomography in Alexander's disease. Ann Neurol 15:605, 1984.
Grover WD, Scrutton MC: Copper infusion therapy in trichopoliodystrophy. J Pediatr 86:216, 1975.
Hagberg B, Aicardi J, Dias K, et al: A progressive syndrome of autism, dementia, ataxia and loss of purposeful hand use in girls: Rett's syndrome: Report of 35 cases. Ann Neurol 14:471, 1983.
Jarvela I, Vesa J, Santavuori P, et al: Molecular genetics of neuronal ceroid lipofuscinoses Pediatr Res 32:645, 1992.
Johnson WG: The clinical spectrum of hexosaminidase deficiency disease. Neurology 31:1453, 1981.
Kelley RI, Datta NS, Dobyns WB, et al: Neonatal adrenoleukodystrophy: New cases, biochemical studies and differentiation from Zellweger and related peroxisomal polydystrophy syndromes. Am J Med Genet 23:869, 1986.
Koeppen AH, Ronca NA, Greenfield EA, et al: Defective biosynthesis of proteolipid protein in Pelizaeus-Merzbacher disease. Ann Neurol 21:159, 1987.
Kolodny EH: Metachromatic leukodystrophy and multiple sulfatase deficiency. *In*: Rosenberg RN, Prusiner SB, DiMauro S, et al (eds): The Molecular and Genetic Basis of Neurological Disease. Stoneham, MA, Butterworth-Heinemann, 1993, p 497.
Kozinetz CA, Skender ML, MacNaughton N, et al: Epidemiology of Rett syndrome: A population-based registry. Pediatrics 91:445, 1993.
Lowden JA, O'Brien JS: Sialidosis: A review of human neuraminidase deficiency. Am J Hum Genet 31:1, 1979.
MacFaul R, Cavanagh N, Lake BD, et al: Metachromatic leukodystrophy: Review of 38 cases. Arch Dis Child 57:168, 1982.
McKhann GM: Metachromatic leukodystrophy: Clinical and enzymatic parameters. Neuropediatrics 15(Suppl):4, 1984.
Mobley WC, White CL, Tennekoon G, et al: Neonatal adrenoleukodystrophy. Ann Neurol 12:204, 1982.
Moser HW, Moser AE, Singh I, et al: Adrenoleukodystrophy: Survey of 303 cases: Biochemistry, diagnosis, and therapy. Ann Neurol 16:628, 1984.
Neufeld EF: Lysosomal storage diseases. Annu Rev Biochem 60:259, 1991.
O'Brien JS: Beta-galactosidase deficiency; ganglioside sialidase deficiency. *In*: Scriver CR, Beaudet AL, Shy WS, Valle D (eds): The Metabolic Basis of Inherited Disease, 6th ed. New York, McGraw-Hill, 1989.
Paty DW, Li DKB, the UBC MS/MRI Study Group, et al: Interferon beta-lb is effective in relapsing-remitting multiple sclerosis. Neurology 43:662, 1993.
Percy AK: The inherited neurodegenerative disorders of childhood: Clinical assessment. J Child Neurol 2:82, 1987.
Percy AK: Second International Rett Syndrome Workshop and Symposium. J Child Neurol 8:97, 1993.
Rapin I, Goldfischer S, Katzman R, et al: The cherry-red spot myoclonus syndrome. Ann Neurol 3:234, 1978.
Sarkar B, Lingertat-Walsh K, Clarke JTR: Copper-histidine therapy for Menkes disease. J Pediatr 123:828, 1993.
Strautnieks S, Rutland P, Winter RM, et al: Pelizaeus-Merzbacher disease: detection of mutations Thr 181-Pro am Leu 223-Pro in the proteolipid protein gene, and prenatal diagnosis. Am J Hum Genet 51:871, 1992.
Tyler HR: Pelizaeus-Merzbacher disease. Arch Neurol Psychiatr 80:162, 1958.
Zeman W, Dyken P: Neuronal ceroid-lipofuscinosis (Batten's disease): Relationship to amaurotic family idiocy? Pediatrics 44:570, 1969.

CHAPTER 553

Acute Stroke Syndromes

Hemiplegia secondary to vascular disorders occurs in children with an incidence of 3–8/100,000. The pediatric causes of *stroke* are distinctive compared with adult causes. They include arterial and venous thrombosis, intracranial hemorrhage, embolism, and various miscellaneous conditions. The cause of stroke in children is established in approximately 50% of cases. As the mode of presentation of acute stroke syndromes is not uniform, a brief description of the most prevalent causes follows.

553.1 Arterial Thrombosis

Thrombosis of the internal carotid artery may result from blunt trauma due to a fall on a pencil or popsicle stick in the child's mouth. The injury produces a tear in the intima of the vessel wall, which may lead to the formation of a dissecting aneurysm. Cerebral symptoms result from the shedding of emboli from the thrombus. The onset of symptoms may be delayed up to 24 hr following the accident, with a stuttering but progressive flaccid hemiplegia, lethargy, and aphasia if the dominant hemisphere is involved. Focal motor seizures are a common complication. A *retropharyngeal abscess* may produce an identical clinical picture, but in this case the arterial thrombosis results from inflammation of the intima. A cerebral angiogram typically demonstrates occlusion of the internal carotid artery, and the computed tomography (CT) scan shows a hypodense lesion representing the area of infarction. *Cyanotic congenital heart disease* in children less than 2 yr of age may cause thrombosis of the middle cerebral artery. These patients are particularly vulnerable when the oxygen saturation is significantly decreased together with a viral illness or dehydration. The *collagen vascular diseases,* particularly lupus erythematosus and polyarteritis nodosa, frequently produce cerebral symptoms and signs, including hemiparesis due to arterial or venous thrombosis.

A series of occlusive vascular disorders, some of which are unique in children, are prominent causes of acute hemiplegia. *Basal arterial occlusion without telangiectasia* results from narrowing of the supraclinoid portion of the internal carotid artery or the proximal segments of the anterior and middle cerebral arteries. As these lesions tend to be congenital and collateral vessels develop, the prognosis for recovery is usually excellent. *Basal arterial occlusion with telangiectasia* or *moyamoya disease* has a characteristic angiogram (Fig. 553–1). The condition is more common in girls and often presents with severe headache and bilateral upper motor neuron signs. It may present with chorea. The prognosis for recovery is poor, with intermittent episodes of transient ischemic attacks coupled with progressive neurologic signs and severe disability. Surgical procedures have been designed to enhance cerebral blood flow (superficial temporal artery to middle cerebral artery shunt and laying the superficial temporal artery on the arachnoid membrane) with variable results. *Occlusion of distal arteries* is associated with diabetes mellitus, neurofibromatosis, sickle cell disease, and IV drug abuse. The patient presents with unilateral neurologic signs, and recovery is often complete owing to the small area of infarction. Patients with *thrombosis of small arteries,* including the perforating striate vessels, due to polyarteritis nodosa and homocystinuria, have a progressive debilitating course characterized by bilateral signs and a high mortality.

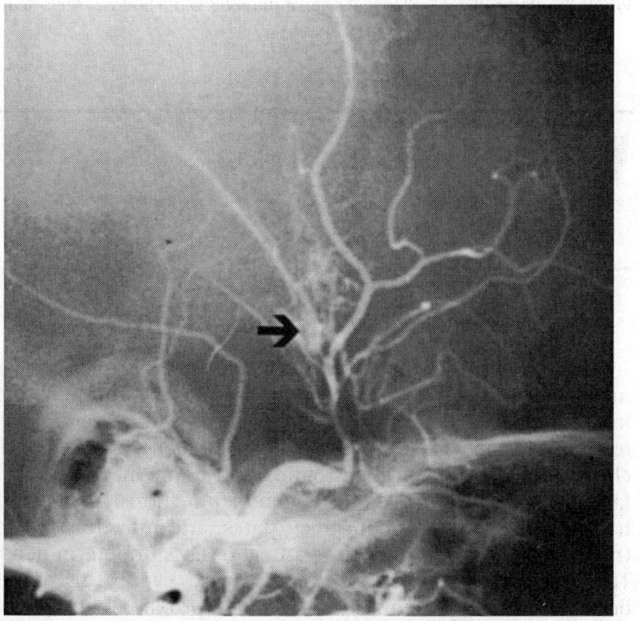

Figure 553–1. Cerebral angiogram showing idiopathic supraclinoid–internal carotid arteriopathy with classical Moyamoya collaterals *(arrow)*.

553.2 Venous Thrombosis/Embolism

Hemiplegia is a relatively common complication of *bacterial meningitis* due to thrombosis of the superficial cortical and deep penetrating veins. Additional infectious causes of stroke in children include *otitis media* and *mastoiditis* with involvement of the dural vessels, and retrograde orbital infections producing *cavernous sinus thrombosis. Severe dehydration* during infancy may cause thrombosis of the superior sagittal sinus and the superficial cortical veins due to hyperviscosity and sludging of blood. Conditions causing hypercoagulopathy, cyanotic congenital heart disease, and leukemic infiltrates of cerebral veins are additional causes of acute hemiplegia of childhood. Deficiencies of inhibitors of coagulation, including protein C, protein S, antithrombosis III, heparin cofactor II, and dysfunctional plasminogen or fibrinogen, are prominent causes of venous thrombosis. *Embolization* of cerebral vessels, although rare in children, may also produce acute hemiparesis. Cardiac causes include arrhythmias (particularly atrial fibrillation), myxoma, paradoxical emboli through a patent foramen ovale, and bacterial endocarditis that results in a mycotic aneurysm. Air emboli may complicate surgery, and fat emboli occur with fracture of long bones. Septic emboli may seed the cerebral vessels and evolve into an area of cerebritis leading to a cerebral abscess.

553.3 Intracranial Hemorrhage

Arteriovenous malformations result as a consequence of the failure of normal capillary bed development between arteries and veins during embryogenesis. Cavernous angiomas may be familial. The arteriovenous malformation produces abnormal shunting of blood, causing an expansion of vessels and a space-occupying effect or rupture of a vein and intracerebral bleeding. Arteriovenous malformations are typically located in the cerebral hemispheres, but they may be situated in the cerebellum, brain stem, or spinal cord. Although the malformation may remain asymptomatic throughout life, rupture and bleeding can occur at any age. Children with arteriovenous malformations frequently have a history of migraine-like headaches. Typical migraine alternates from one side of the head to the other, whereas headaches associated with an arteriovenous malformation classically remain on the same side. Auscultation of the skull is positive for a high-pitched bruit in approximately 50% of cases. Rupture of an arteriovenous malformation causes a severe headache, vomiting, nuchal rigidity due to subarachnoid bleeding, progressive hemiparesis, and a focal or generalized seizure. An **arteriovenous malformation of the**

vein of Galen during infancy can cause high-output congestive heart failure secondary to shunting of large volumes of blood or progressive hydrocephalus and increased intracranial pressure due to obstruction of the cerebrospinal fluid (CSF) pathways.

Cerebral aneurysms producing symptoms in children are relatively rare. In contrast to adults, aneurysms in children tend to be large and are located at the carotid bifurcation or on the anterior and posterior cerebral arteries rather than the circle of Willis. The aneurysmal dilatation results from a congenital weakness of the vessel, and in some cases a deficiency of type III collagen has been demonstrated. In children, there is an association between cerebral aneurysms and coarctation of the aorta and bilateral polycystic kidney disease. Although most ruptured aneurysms bleed into the subarachnoid space, causing an intense headache, nuchal rigidity, and coma, intracerebral hemorrhage and progressive hemiparesis also occur. Additional causes of intracerebral hematoma include hematologic disorders, particularly thrombocytopenic purpura and hemophilia. Finally, trauma can produce hemiparesis due to intracerebral bleeding or a subdural or epidural hematoma. A contrast CT scan or magnetic resonance imaging (MRI) with gadolinium is useful for the identification of large arteriovenous malformations; however, four-vessel cerebral angiography is the study of choice for the investigation of arteriovenous malformations and cerebral aneurysm.

553.4 Miscellaneous Causes of Stroke

Alternating hemiplegia of childhood is occasionally associated with migraine, but in most cases the etiology is unknown. It develops in infants between 2 and 18 mo of age and is characterized by intermittent episodes of hemiplegia alternating from one side of the body to the other. Rarely, both sides are involved during an attack. Choreoathetosis and dystonic movements are commonly observed in the hemiparetic extremity. Symptoms spontaneously regress with sleep but recur with awakening. The hemiplegia persists for minutes to weeks and then resolves spontaneously. The condition has a poor prognosis with progressive mental retardation and developmental disabilities. Neuroimaging and biochemical studies are negative. Several *metabolic diseases* are associated with strokelike episodes in children, including mitochondrial encephalomyolopathy (MELAS, see Chapter 548.2), ornithine transcarbamylase deficiency, pyruvate dehydrogenase deficiency, and homocystinuria. *Todd paralysis* may be confused initially with a stroke. The hemiparesis follows a focal seizure, but the weakness and neurologic signs disappear completely within 24 hr of the convulsion. Although the cause of Todd paralysis remains unknown, the hemiparesis probably results from an inhibitory phenomenon, possibly related to neurotransmitter dysfunction. Additional causes of hemiparesis include *cerebral tumor, encephalitis* (particularly herpes), *focal postviral encephalitis,* and *status epilepticus.* In some pediatric series of unexplained stroke, *lipid abnormalities,* including elevated triglycerides and low levels of high-density lipoprotein cholesterol, have been found in approximately 20% of the cases. The family histories of these children reveal an increased incidence of premature coronary heart disease and early ischemic cerebrovascular diseases. Screening of at-risk families will identify children who may benefit from long-term dietary management.

INVESTIGATION OF STROKES. The most critical component of the investigation is a thorough history and physical examination, searching for an underlying disease process; evidence of trauma; an infectious, metabolic, or hematologic disorder; neurocutaneous syndrome; increased intracranial pressure; or hydrocephalus. Appropriate tests for infectious diseases, metabolic disorders, and hematologic disorders are based on the results of the history and physical examination. An electroencephalogram (EEG) may be helpful in localizing the disease process but will rarely establish the diagnosis. A brain scan is extremely useful in cases of focal encephalitis, cerebritis, cerebral abscess, and infarction. A CT scan or MRI is mandatory in the investigation of children with acute hemiparesis. A cerebral angiogram is essential for those children in whom a CT scan or MRI is nondiagnostic. In these cases, a four-vessel cerebral angiogram should be planned. Electrocardiography and echocardiography may help to exclude intrinsic cardiac diseases or an arrhythmia as a cause of the stroke. Finally, a search for a lipid disorder is indicated in those cases of stroke with an unknown cause, particularly when a family history of premature cardiac or cerebrovascular disease is elicited.

Bourgeois M, Aicardi J, Goutières F: Alternating hemiplegia of childhood. J Pediatr 122:673, 1993.

Christodoulou J, Qureshi IA, McInnes RR, et al: Ornithine transcarbamylase deficiency presenting with strokelike episodes. J Pediatr 122:423, 1993.

David M, Andrew M: Venous thromboembolic complications in children. J Pediatr 123:337, 1993.

Glueck CJ, Daniels SR, Bates S, et al: Pediatric victims of unexplained stroke and their families: Familial lipid and lipoprotein abnormalities. Pediatrics 69:308, 1982.

Harwood-Nash DC, McDonald P, Argent W: Cerebral arterial disease in children: An angiographic study of 40 cases. Am J Roentgenol Radium Ther Nucl Med 111:672, 1971.

Kelly JJ, Mellinger JF, Sundt TM: Intracranial arteriovenous malformations in childhood. Ann Neurol 3:338, 1978.

Pitner SE: Carotid thrombosis due to intraoral trauma. N Engl J Med 274:764, 1966.

Schoenberg BS, Mellinger JF, Schoenberg DG: Cerebrovascular disease in infants and children: A study of incidence, clinical features and survival. Neurology 28:763, 1978.

Seeler RA, Royal JE, Powe L, et al: Moya-moya in children with sickle cell anemia and cerebrovascular occlusion. J Pediatr 93:808, 1978.

Shillito J Jr: Carotid arteritis: A cause of hemiplegia in childhood. J Neurosurg 21:540, 1964.

Thompson JR, Harwood-Nash DC, Fitz CR: Cerebral aneurysms in children. Am J Roentgenol 188:163, 1973.

Tomsick TA, Lukin RR, Chambers AA, et al: Neurofibromatosis and intracranial arterial occlusive disease. Neuroradiology 11:229, 1976.

Tyler HR, Clark DB: Cerebrovascular accidents in patients with congenital heart disease. Arch Neurol Psychiatry 77:483, 1957.

Watanabe K, Negoro T, Maehara M, et al: Moyamoya disease presenting with chorea. Pediatr Neurol 6:40, 1990.

Wisoff HS, Rothballer AB: Cerebral arterial thrombosis in children. Arch Neurol 4:258, 1961.

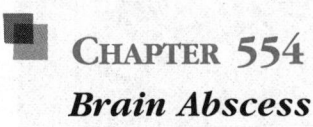

Chapter 554
Brain Abscess

Brain abscesses can occur in children of any age but are most common between 4 and 8 yr. The causes of brain abscess include embolization due to congenital heart disease with right to left shunts (especially tetralogy of Fallot), meningitis, chronic otitis media and mastoiditis, soft tissue infection of the face or scalp, orbital cellulitis, dental infections, penetrating head injuries, immunodeficiency states, and infection of ventriculo-peritoneal shunts. The pathogenesis is undetermined in 10–15% of cases. Cerebral abscesses are evenly distributed between the two hemispheres, and approximately 80% of cases are divided equally between the frontal, parietal, and temporal lobes. Brain abscesses in the occipital lobe, cerebellum, and brain stem comprise about 20% of the cases. Most brain abscesses are single, but 30% are multiple and may involve more than one lobe. An abscess in the frontal lobe is often caused by extension from sinusitis or orbital cellulitis, whereas abscesses located in the temporal lobe or cerebellum are frequently associated with chronic otitis media and mastoiditis. Abscesses resulting from penetrating injuries tend to be singular and caused by *Staphylococcus aureus,* whereas those resulting from septic emboli, congenital heart disease, or meningitis often have multiple causes.

ETIOLOGY. The responsible bacteria include *S. aureus,* streptococci (viridans, pneumococci, microaerophilic), anaerobic organisms (gram-positive cocci, *Bacteroides* spp, *Fusobacterium* spp, *Prevotella* spp, *Actinomyces* spp, and *Clostridium* spp), and gram-negative aerobic bacilli (enteric rods, *Proteus* spp, *Pseudomonas aeruginosa, Citrobacter diversus,* and *Haemophilus* spp). One organism will be cultured from the majority of abscesses (70%), two from 20%, and three or greater will be identified in 10% of cases. Abscesses associated with mucosal infections (sinusitis) frequently have anaerobic bacteria.

CLINICAL MANIFESTATIONS. The early stages of cerebritis and abscess formation are associated with nonspecific symptoms, including low-grade fever, headache, and lethargy. The significance of these symptoms is generally not recognized and an oral antibiotic is often prescribed with resultant transient relief. As the inflammatory process proceeds, vomiting, severe headache, seizures, papilledema, focal neurologic signs (hemiparesis), and coma may develop. A cerebellar abscess is characterized by nystagmus, ipsilateral ataxia and dysmetria, vomiting, and headache. If the abscess ruptures into the ventricular cavity, overwhelming shock and death usually ensue.

DIAGNOSIS. The white blood count can be normal or elevated, and the blood culture is positive in only 10%. Examination of the cerebrospinal fluid (CSF) shows variable results; the white blood cells and protein may be minimally elevated or normal. The glucose may be slightly low and CSF cultures are rarely positive. Because examination of the CSF is seldom useful and a lumbar puncture may cause herniation of the cerebellar tonsils, the procedure should not be undertaken in a child suspected of a brain abscess. The electroencephalogram (EEG) shows corresponding focal slowing, and the radionucleotide brain scan indicates an area of enhancement due to disruption of the blood-brain barrier in greater than 80% of cases. Computed tomography (CT) and magnetic resonance imaging (MRI) are the most reliable methods of demonstrating cerebritis and abscess formation. The CT findings of cerebritis are characterized by a parenchymal low-density lesion, and MRI T_2-weighted images indicate increased signal intensity. An abscess cavity shows a ring-enhancing lesion by contrast-CT, and the MRI also demonstrates an abscess capsule with gadolinium administration.

TREATMENT. The initial management of a brain abscess includes prompt diagnosis and the institution of an antibiotic regimen that is based upon the probable cause and most likely organism. In cases in which the cause is unknown, a combination of nafcillin or vancomycin with a third-generation cephalosporin and metronidazole is employed. The choice of antibiotics should be altered when the culture and sensitivity results become available. An abscess resulting from a penetrating injury, head trauma, or sinusitis should be treated with a combination of nafcillin or vancomycin, cefotaxime, and metronidazole, whereas the initial treatment of a lesion resulting from cyanotic heart disease is penicillin and metronidazole. Abscesses secondary to an infected ventriculo-peritoneal shunt may be initially treated with vancomycin and ceftazidime. When otitis media or mastoiditis is the likely cause, nafcillin or vancomycin in combination with ceftazidime and metronidazole is indicated. In those cases in which citrobacter meningitis (often in neonates) leads to abscess formation, a third-generation cephalosporin is used and an aminoglycoside is considered. In the immunocompromised patient, broad antibiotic coverage is employed, and amphotericin B therapy should be considered. The surgical management of brain abscesses has changed since the advent of CT. In the early stages of cerebritis or with multiple abscesses, antibiotics may be used alone. An encapsulated abscess, particularly if the lesion is causing a mass effect or increased intracranial pressure, should be treated by a combination of antibiotics and aspiration. Surgical excision of an abscess is rarely required, as the procedure may be associated with greater morbidity compared to aspiration of a cavity. Surgery is indicated if gas is present in the abscess, if it is multiloculated, if it is located in the posterior fossa, or if a fungus is identified. Associated infectious processes, such as mastoiditis, sinusitis, or a periorbital abscess, may require surgical drainage. The duration of antibiotic therapy depends on the organism and response to treatment, but usually requires 3–4 wk.

PROGNOSIS. The mortality of brain abscesses has decreased significantly to approximately 5–10% with the use of CT or MRI and prompt antibiotic and surgical management. Factors associated with high mortality at the time of admission include multiple abscesses, coma, and lack of CT facilities. Long-term sequelae occur in at least 50% of survivors and include hemiparesis, seizures, hydrocephalus, cranial nerve abnormalities, and behavior and learning problems.

Brook I: Aerobic and anaerobic bacteriology of intracranial abscesses. Pediatr Neurol 8:210, 1992.

Saez-Lloreus XJ, Umana NA, Odio CN, et al: Brain abscesses in infants and children. Pediatr Infect Dis J 8:449, 1989.

Sjolin J, Lilja A, Erikson N, et al: Treatment of brain abscess with cefotaxime and metronidazole: prospective study on 15 consecutive patients. Clin Infect Dis 17:857, 1993.

Smith RR: Neuroradiology of intracranial infection. Pediatr Neurosurg 18:92, 1992.

CHAPTER 555

Brain Tumors in Children

(See also Chapters 448 and 456)

Brain tumors are second only to leukemia as the most prevalent malignancy in childhood, and they account for the most common solid tumors in this age group. Brain tumors can present at any age, but each tends to have a peak age incidence. Metastatic brain tumors are common in the adult but are relatively rare in the child.

EPIDEMIOLOGY. Approximately two thirds of all intracranial tumors occurring in children between the ages of 2 and 12 yr are infratentorial (located in the posterior fossa). In adolescents and infants under the age of 2 yr, tumors occur with equal frequencies in the posterior fossa and in the supratentorial region.

PATHOLOGY AND PATHOGENESIS. There are two major histologic types of brain tumors in children, glial cell tumors and those of primitive neuroectodermal cell origin. Glial cell tumors are the most common and consist of a variety of cell types with variable prognoses, including the astrocytoma, ependymoma, and glioblastoma multiforme. Neuroectodermal tumors probably arise from a primitive, undifferentiated cell line and are prominent throughout the central nervous system (CNS), involving the cerebellum (medulloblastoma), cerebrum, spinal cord, and pineal gland (pineoblastoma) (see Chapter 456). Some tumors are unique because they originate from embryonic remnants, such as the craniopharyngioma, which arises from Rathke pouch; dermoid and epidermoid tumors originating from the invagination of epithelial cells during the closure of the neural tube; and the chordoma, which develops from traces of the embryonic notochord. The pathogenesis of brain tumors is complex because many factors influence their development. Conditions that result from abnormalities of neural crest development have a high association with tumors of the CNS. Both types of neurofibromatosis are associated with an increased incidence of specific brain tumors: optic glioma and low-grade astrocytoma in NF1 and acoustic neuroma and meningioma in NF II. Some patients who received radiation for scalp disorders during childhood develop cranial tumors years later, and occasionally, second brain tumors develop after radiation for the treatment of a primary brain tumor.

The evolution of brain tumors may involve sequential mutation or deletion of specific genes. For example, in gliomas deletion of 17p is found at high frequency in all grades of the tumor, while in high-grade glioma an additional loss of 9p occurs. In the case of glioblastoma multiforme, the most malignant variant, an addition or loss of a portion of chromosome 10 occurs in many tumors. Other tumors are associated with nonrandom chromosome loss: the meningioma with a portion of chromosome 22 and medulloblastoma with a segment of 17p, not related to the p53 tumor suppressor gene. A variety of growth factors appear to play prominent roles in the development and progression of brain tumors. An aberrant receptor site for epidermal growth factor (EGFR) has been demonstrated in gliomas, while alteration of platelet-derived growth factor receptor and increased expression of its ligand, platelet-derived growth factor, have been shown in meningiomas. The precise roles and relationship of the molecular oncogene events remain to be clarified.

CLINICAL MANIFESTATIONS. Brain tumors present in many ways depending on the location, type, and rate of growth of the tumor and the age of the child. Generally, there are two distinct patterns of presentation: symptoms and signs of increased intracranial pressure and focal neurologic signs. Tumors located within the posterior fossa primarily produce symptoms and signs of increased intracranial pressure due to obstruction of CSF pathways and the development of hydrocephalus. Supratentorial tumors are more likely to be associated with focal abnormalities, including long-tract signs and seizures.

Alterations in personality are often the first symptoms of a brain tumor, irrespective of its location. The child, beginning weeks or months prior to the discovery of the tumor, may have become lethargic, irritable, hyperactive, or forgetful or may perform poorly academically. It is not certain as to whether the behavioral changes result from increased intracranial pressure, the site of the lesion, or both. After the tumor has been removed and amelioration of the increased intracranial pressure occurs, there is usually a significant reversal of the behavioral problems.

Increased intracranial pressure is characterized by headache, vomiting, diplopia, and papilledema, and in the infant a bulging fontanel and increasing head size (macrocrania) develop. Initially, the *headache* tends to occur in the morning and is relieved with standing, as venous flow away from the head is enhanced in the upright position. The headache is described as dull, generalized, and steady, and may be intermittent and worsened by coughing or sneezing or during defecation. The headache is typically associated with *vomiting*, which often relieves the headache. Tumors that occupy the fourth ventricle are often associated with pernicious vomiting. Children who present with vomiting as the initial symptom of a brain tumor are frequently subjected to a series of gastrointestinal investigations. A thorough history and neurologic examination would obviate those tests in many cases. *Diplopia* is a common symptom of posterior fossa tumors. Children do not usually complain of double vision, because they seem to readily suppress the image of the affected eye. Examination of the eye movements shows strabismus owing to involvement of the abducens, oculomotor nerve, or, rarely, the trochlear nerve. Some children with diplopia compensate by tilting the head in an attempt to align the two images. *Head tilting* and *nuchal rigidity* may also indicate herniation of the cerebellar tonsils. In this situation, a lumbar puncture may enhance the herniation and result in death. *Nystagmus* is a prominent sign associated with posterior fossa tumors. Unilateral cerebellar tumors cause horizontal nystagmus, which is exaggerated upon looking to the side of the lesion. Tumors located in the posterior cerebellar vermis or fourth ventricle produce nystagmus in all directions of gaze. Brain stem tumors may result in horizontal, vertical, and rotatory nystagmus. *Papilledema* is the cardinal finding of increased intracranial pressure, but it is important to remember that in the infant, separation of the cranial sutures and bulging of the anterior fontanel may decompress the contents of the skull. The head may continue to accelerate in size without associated symptoms and signs of increased intracranial pressure. In this case, papilledema may be conspicuous by its absence. A rapid rise or prolonged increase in intracranial pressure may result in coma with alterations in the vital signs. Bradycardia, an irregular pulse, and systemic hypertension occur associated with alterations in the respiratory pattern. Initially, hyperventilation is noted, which, without intervention, progresses to ataxic and irregular breathing followed by respiratory arrest.

Supratentorial tumors may also be associated with symptoms and signs of increased intracranial pressure. However, focal neurologic signs including hemiparesis and complex partial seizures predominate, particularly with a temporal lobe tumor. The greatest oversight in the examination of a child with headache and vomiting is failure to examine the retina and optic nerve. *Obscuration of vision* characterized by blurring is a serious symptom that indicates marked vasoconstriction of cerebral vessels and impending cerebellar herniation. *Visual loss*, manifesting as clumsiness or, in the infant, developmental delay associated with roving eye movements or nystagmus, each is a feature of optic tract gliomas or of impingement of pituitary or suprasellar masses on the optic chiasm.

Ataxia is often associated with posterior fossa tumors, although it is interesting that some large tumors cause absolutely no abnormality of movement. Tumors of the cerebellar vermis characteristically cause truncal ataxia that is enhanced with sitting or standing, and involvement of the anterior cerebellum results in marked gait disturbances that are typically broad based. Tumors of a cerebellar hemisphere produce ipsilateral extremity ataxia and dysdiadochokinesia. The following sections highlight the pathology, management, and prognosis of the major brain tumors in the pediatric age group.

INFRATENTORIAL TUMORS. The *cerebellar astrocytoma* is the most common posterior fossa tumor of childhood and has the best prognosis. These neoplasms tend to be cystic and have a mural nodule of solid tumor; however, conversely, they can be solid with little or no cystic cavitation. Those tumors with cystic cavities are filled with a thickened xanthochromic fluid. Cerebellar astrocytomas may be midline involving the vermis or confined to a hemisphere, and, although usually of low grade, they are capable of invading the cerebellar peduncles (Fig. 555–1). The tumor causes hydrocephalus and symptoms and signs of increased intracranial pressure by obstructing the aqueduct of Sylvius or fourth ventricle. Histologically, the astrocytoma is characterized by protoplasmic and fibrillary astrocytes arranged in a radial fashion interspersed with Rosenthal fibers. The treatment is surgical resection, and the 5-yr survival is greater than 90%. Radiation therapy is reserved for patients with high-grade astrocytomas or in whom postop-

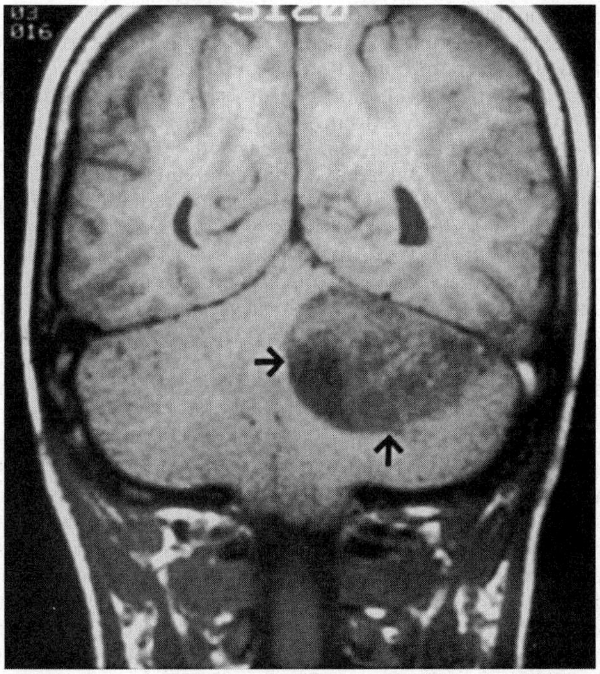

Figure 555–1. A coronal MRI scan of a large, primarily solid, cerebellar astrocytoma *(arrows)*.

erative tumor progression is evident by clinical and radiologic investigation.

The *medulloblastoma* is the next most common posterior fossa tumor in the pediatric age group and is the most prevalent brain tumor in children less than 7 yr of age. Although the site of origin of the medulloblastoma is unknown, in some cases it originates from the roof of the fourth ventricle and grows rapidly to fill the fourth ventricle or invade the adjacent cerebellar hemisphere. This tumor may spread over the cerebral convexities or along the CSF pathways and is capable of metastasizing to extracranial sites. Microscopically, the tumor is vascular and cellular, and is characterized by deeply staining nuclei with scant cytoplasm arranged in pseudorosettes. The prognosis and treatment depend on the age of the child and the size and dissemination of the tumor. All children with a diagnosis of medulloblastoma require neuroimaging of the neuraxis, preferably by MRI, or by CT myelography if MRI is not available. Children less than 2 yr of age have a poorer prognosis than older patients. All patients are treated with surgical extirpation, with irradiation for children greater than 4 yr, particularly those with small tumors and no evidence of dissemination, for whom the expected 5-yr survival rate is 70%. Irradiation is directed to the entire neuraxis because of the propensity for medulloblastomas to seed to remote sites. In children with tumor residual following surgery or with evidence of neuraxis dissemination, chemotherapy in addition to surgery and irradiation improves the survival to approximately 60%, significantly better than without chemotherapy. Chemotherapy agents used for the treatment of medulloblastoma include vincristine, cyclophosphamide, cisplatinum, and etoposide. In the very young patient, most centers follow surgery with chemotherapy and withhold radiation therapy to a later age when the brain is more tolerant of the effects of radiation.

Brain stem gliomas are the third most frequent posterior fossa tumor in children. These tumors are of two types: those that produce diffuse infiltration in the pons extending throughout the brain stem, which at postmortem examination are found to be anaplastic astrocytomas, and low-grade focal tumors in the midbrain and medulla (Fig. 555–2). The prognosis for the former is grave, while a focal brain stem tumor confined to the midbrain or the cervical medullary junction and the dorsally exophytic brain stem gliomas have excellent survival rates following surgery alone. The symptoms and signs result from invasion and destruction of cranial nerve nuclei and the pyramidal tracts. The most common cranial nerve symptoms include diplopia and facial weakness due to abducens and facial nerve involvement. Later, dysarthria, dysphagia, and dysphonia may result owing to infiltration of the cranial nuclei in the medulla. Pyramidal tract involvement is manifested by gait disturbances and the presence of generalized upper motor neuron signs. Changes in personality are particularly common with brain stem gliomas and include lethargy, irritability, and aggressive behavior.

Clinical manifestations of increased intracranial pressure including papilledema occur late (if at all) in the course, because the CSF pathways remain patent in most cases until the tumor has grown to a massive size.

The surgical treatment of brain stem gliomas is controversial. With newer radioimaging techniques, particularly MRI, the diagnosis is usually apparent and biopsy is unnecessary. If there is uncertainty following neuroimaging, a stereotactic biopsy is warranted. The primary treatment is irradiation, and although some brain stem gliomas are radiosensitive, the mean 5-yr survival is approximately 20%. In view of the very poor prognosis and response to radiotherapy, the role of hyperfractionated radiation therapy (smaller, more frequent doses ultimately resulting in a higher total dose) was investigated, and this radiotherapy mode was found not to be beneficial. Chemotherapy has not proven efficacious for the management of brain stem gliomas. Low-grade focal tumors of the midbrain or medulla have an excellent prognosis following radical excision. The patient is observed, and radiotherapy is withheld unless the residual tumor shows evidence of regrowth.

Ependymomas account for approximately 10% of childhood posterior fossa tumors. These lesions arise from within the fourth ventricle and cause hydrocephalus and signs of increased intracranial pressure due to obstruction of the CSF pathways. Aside from vomiting, headache, and diplopia, nuchal rigidity and torticollis may result owing to herniation of the cerebellar tonsils. Ataxia and focal neurologic signs are usually absent; however, papilledema is a consistent finding in the symptomatic child. The histologic picture consists of ro-

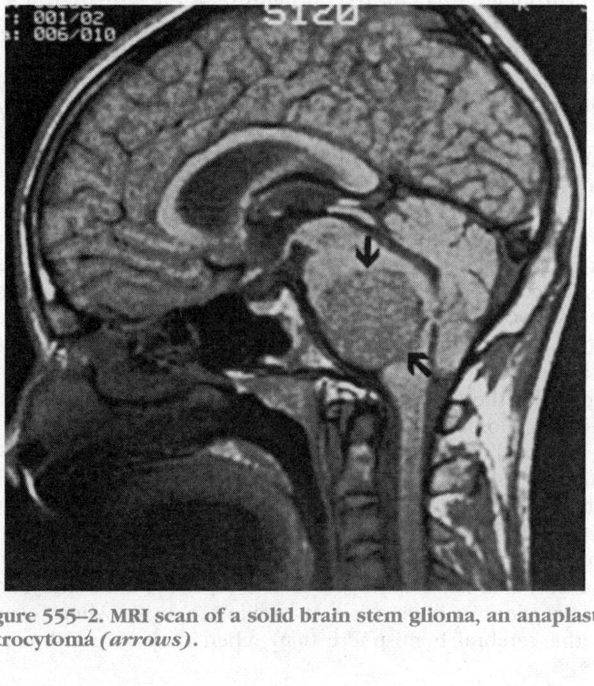

Figure 555–2. MRI scan of a solid brain stem glioma, an anaplastic astrocytoma *(arrows)*.

settes of ependymal cells with cilia protruding into the central cavity. Treatment includes surgical removal and radiation therapy to the tumor region, with a 5-yr survival approximating 50%. If the tumor histology reveals an aggressive anaplastic ependymoma, radiation should be delivered to the entire craniospinal region, because these tumors readily disseminate and are associated with a much less favorable prognosis.

Additional tumors that have a proclivity for the posterior fossa include several benign tumors, such as a choroid plexus papilloma of the fourth ventricle, dermoids, epidermoids, chordomas, and teratomas. Although generally nonmalignant, these lesions are capable of producing significant morbidity and death owing to their location, size, and possibility of obstructing the normal flow of CSF.

SUPRATENTORIAL TUMORS. The *craniopharyngioma* is one of the most common supratentorial tumors in children. The tumor may be confined to the sella turcica, or it can extend through the diaphragma sella and compress the optic nerve system, pons, or third ventricle, producing hydrocephalus. The tumor consists of solid and cystic areas that have a tendency to calcify. Approximately 90% of craniopharyngiomas show calcification on the plain skull roentgenogram or CT scan. Many children with craniopharyngioma are referred to endocrine clinics because of short stature due to pituitary-hypothalamic involvement. Pressure or injury to the optic chiasm typically produces bitemporal visual field defects, although most children are unaware of peripheral visual loss until the time of testing. Papilledema and symptoms of increased intracranial pressure are evident when hydrocephalus is prominent. The treatment is a craniotomy using a subfrontal approach. With complete or near-total removal, 60% of patients experience no further recurrence. The role of radiation therapy is still debated, but most centers favor radiation to the sellar region postoperatively only in those cases in which tumor removal is incomplete and recurrence occurs. Endocrine disorders, including diabetes insipidus, hypothyroidism, growth hormone, and adrenocortical deficiency, may develop postoperatively and warrant close follow-up. There is no effective chemotherapeutic agent.

Optic nerve gliomas present with decreased visual acuity and pallor of the disks. These tumors are primarily low-grade astrocytomas, and approximately 25% of patients have associated neurofibromatosis (see Chapter 546.1). Because the natural history of optic gliomas is variable, treatment is most often delayed until there is evidence of clinical or radiologic progression. Irradiation is effective in halting tumor growth and preserving vision but has major neurodevelopmental consequences in the young infant. The role of chemotherapy is undergoing experimental study. The glioma may invade the optic chiasm and hypothalamus, producing visual field defects or the **diencephalic syndrome**. These children are anorectic and emaciated, and have little or no subcutaneous tissue but normal linear growth. Their behavior is not in keeping with the nutritional state, because they are often hyperalert and euphoric. Approximately 25% have a coarse horizontal nystagmus. Conversely, tumor invasion of the hypothalamus can result in an insatiable appetite, obesity, diabetes insipidus, and hypogonadism. Resection of the optic glioma confined to an optic nerve produces blindness but prevents recurrence or extension through the chiasm, which may be the preferred therapy if the eye is already blind from tumor invasion. Optic chiasm gliomas with hypothalamic involvement may be treated with chemotherapy (carboplatinum and vincristine) in children less than 3 yr of age, and this may delay the requirement for radiation therapy. Radiotherapy in older patients with chiasmatic/hypothalamic gliomas results in an excellent prognosis, with 10-yr survival rates of almost 90%.

Astrocytoma and related glial tumors (ependymoma and oligodendrogliomas) have a less favorable prognosis when located in the cerebral hemisphere than when they are confined to the cerebellum. These patients may have a chronic history of complex partial epilepsy, particularly if the tumor is located within the temporal lobe. Neurologic examination frequently reveals subtle upper motor neuron signs or a contralateral growth arrest of the extremities. Surgical excision of a low-grade astrocytoma results in at least an 80% 5-yr survival. High-grade astrocytomas have a much greater mortality, with only a 30% survival following surgery and radiation therapy.

There are a series of *tumors peculiar to children that arise in the region of the pineal gland,* including varieties of germ cell tumors, pinealomas, pineoblastomas, and teratomas. These tumors are remarkably different in degrees of malignancy and invasion of surrounding structures. They may cause obstruction of the CSF pathways, resulting in macrocrania and hydrocephalus. Pressure by the tumor on the quadrigeminal plate produces the **Parinaud syndrome**, consisting of paralysis of conjugate upward movement of the eyes and poorly reactive pupils. There is no uniform agreement with regard to the management of pineal area tumors, because of the heterogeneity of the tumors and the variable response to radiotherapy. Most would concur that a tissue diagnosis is preferable before the initiation of therapy. Modern surgical techniques, including the use of the operating microscope, have significantly decreased the morbidity and mortality, and have allowed total resection of some tumors in the pineal region. The radiosensitive germinoma has a 5-yr survival greater than 75%. Some tumors (e.g., pinealomas) are resistant to radiation and are more likely to respond to chemotherapy (cisplatinum and etoposide), whereas others such as mature teratomas may be treated exclusively by surgery.

The *choroid plexus papilloma* produces slowly progressive hydrocephalus due to excessive production of CSF. The most common location is the lateral ventricle, followed by the third and fourth ventricles. These tumors arise from the choroid plexus epithelium and protrude into the ventricular cavity. The prognosis is excellent following surgical removal. Malignant choroid plexus carcinoma is extremely vascular and invasive. Cure requires complete resection, which may be facilitated by preoperative chemotherapy.

In *leukemia,* infiltrates may invade the leptomeninges, causing increased intracranial pressure due to infiltration of the pacchionian granulations, or may involve the brain parenchyma and, in combination with an acute hemorrhage, result in a mass lesion. Finally, cranial nerves, particularly the facial nerve, or peripheral nerves, such as the peroneal and sciatic nerves, may be invaded by leukemic infiltrates, resulting in weakness, pain, and sensory phenomena.

LABORATORY FINDINGS. MRI is the best technique for the delineation of brain tumors in children. Aside from the lack of ionizing radiation, the MRI study provides a superior image of the posterior fossa structures compared with a CT scan. Furthermore, the fine detail in MRI has identified cerebral tumors that are not visible with CT scanning. In addition, MRI is more accurate in defining the extent of an infiltrating tumor. Metastases to the spinal cord can be identified by noninvasive MRI enhanced with the contrast agent gadolinium; contrast myelography is a complementary study for small metastatic lesions in that region. Children with tumors of the sella turcica should undergo a series of baseline endocrine studies, including measurement of growth hormone, thyroid-stimulating hormone, adrenocorticotrophic hormone (ACTH), luteinizing hormone, follicle-stimulating hormone, antidiuretic hormone, and prolactin, as these hormones may require replacement if they are deficient. Germ cell tumors in the pineal gland are associated with elevated CSF human chorionic gonadotropin and α-fetoprotein levels. Monoclonal antibodies are proving helpful in differentiating medulloblastoma from CNS lymphoma antigens. CSF tumor cells may be examined at the time of surgery or as a component of routine follow-up. Positive

CSF cytology postoperatively is common, but the interpretation of the finding is not certain, because seeding and new growth may not occur.

PROGNOSIS. Neuropsychologic deficits, including changes in cognitive behavior, verbal performance, perceptual-motor function, and academic achievement, have been reported as frequent complications of cranial radiation therapy. Neurophysiologic abnormalities consisting of generalized slowing of the EEG and increased evoked potential latencies have also been noted. Following irradiation, CT scanning and MRI have shown a variety of lesions involving the cortex and myelin, including calcification, ventricular dilatation, white matter hypodensities, and cortical atrophy. Generally, the younger the patient, the greater will be the disability. However, there is little correlation between the site of the pathology as identified by imaging studies and the cognitive disorder. Abnormalities in linear growth and radiation-induced hypothyroidism are common after radiation therapy, secondary to growth hormone dysfunction. Baseline endocrine studies should be carried out on all newly diagnosed patients before the initiation of therapy. Second malignancies are rare after treatment of a primary brain tumor in children. Prospective studies by the age of the child and specific therapeutic regimens are required to better understand the consequences of cranial radiation therapy.

Newer therapeutic modalities, such as implantation of "radiation seeds" (brachytherapy) and the use of focal and focused radiation add promise for the treatment of brain tumors in children. The role of bone marrow transplantation to allow the use of higher concentrations of chemotherapeutic agents is under investigation. Molecular biologic studies are also likely to define the mechanisms of tumor behavior and provide a method for more effective therapy in the future.

Amacher AL: Craniopharyngioma: The controversy regarding radiotherapy. Childs Nerv Syst 6:57, 1980.
Bloom HJG, Glees J, Bell J, et al: The treatment and long-term prognosis of children with intracranial tumors; a study of 610 cases, 1950–1981. Int J Radiat Oncol Biol Phys 19:829, 1990.
Dowell RD Jr, Copeland DR: Cerebral pathology and neuropsychological effects. Am J Pediatr Hematol Oncol 9:68, 1987.
Duffner PK, Cohen ME, Myers MH, et al: Survival of children with brain tumors: SEER Program, 1973–1980. Neurology 36:597, 1986.
Duffner PK, Horowitz ME, Krischer JP, et al: Postoperative chemotherapy and delayed radiation in children less than three years of age with malignant brain tumors. N Engl J Med 328:1725, 1993.
Edwards MSB, Hudgins RJ, Wilson CB, et al: Pineal region tumors in children. J Neurosurg 68:689, 1988.
Epstein F, McCleary EL: Intrinsic brain-stem tumors of childhood: Surgical indications. J Neurosurg 64:11, 1986.
Finlay JL, Uteg R, Giese WL: Brain tumors in children. II: Advances in neurosurgery and radiation oncology. Am J Pediatr Hematol Oncol 9:256, 1987.
Hoffman JH: Benign brain stem gliomas in children. Prog Exp Tumor Res 30:154, 1987.
Horowitz ME, Mulhern RK, Kun LE, et al: Brain tumors in the very young child. Cancer 61:428, 1988.
Kadota RP, Allen JB, Hartman GA, et al: Brain tumors in children. J Pediatr 114:511, 1989.
Listernick R, Charrow J, Greenwald M, et al: Natural history of optic pathway tumors in children with neurofibromatosis type 1: A longitudinal study. J Pediatr 125:63, 1994.
Marsh WR, Laws ER Jr: Intracranial ependymomas. Progr Exp Tumor Res 30:175, 1987.
Packer RJ, Batnitzky S, Cohen ME: Magnetic resonance imaging in the evaluation of intracranial tumors of childhood. Cancer 56:1767, 1985.
Packer RJ, Sutton LN, Goldwein JW, et al: Improved survival with the use of adjuvant chemotherapy in the treatment of medulloblastoma. J Neurosurg 74:433, 1991.
Schmidek HH: The molecular genetics of nervous system tumors. J Neurosurg 67:1, 1987.
Shrieve DC, Wara WM, Edwards MSB, et al: Hyperfractionated radiation therapy for gliomas of the brainstem in children and in adults. Int J Radiat Oncol Biol Phys 24:599, 1992.
Sutton LN: Current management of low-grade astrocytomas of childhood. Pediatr Neurosci 13:98, 1987.
Tores CF, Rebsamen S, Silber JH, et al: Surveillance scanning of children with medulloblastoma. N Engl J Med 330:892, 1994.

CHAPTER 556
Pseudotumor Cerebri

Pseudotumor cerebri is a clinical syndrome that mimics brain tumors and is characterized by increased intracranial pressure with a normal cerebrospinal fluid (CSF) cell count and protein content, and normal ventricular size, anatomy, and position.

ETIOLOGY. There are many explanations for the development of pseudotumor cerebri, including alterations in CSF absorption and production, cerebral edema, abnormalities in vasomotor control and cerebral blood flow, and venous obstruction. The causes of pseudotumor are multiple and include *metabolic disorders* (galactosemia, hypoparathyroidism, pseudohypoparathyroidism, hypophosphatasia, prolonged corticosteroid therapy, possibly growth hormone treatment, hypervitaminosis A, vitamin A deficiency, Addison disease, obesity, menarche, oral contraceptives, and pregnancy), *infections* (roseola infantum, chronic otitis media and mastoiditis, Guillain-Barré syndrome), *drugs* (nalidixic acid, tetracycline), *hematologic disorders* (polycythemia, hemolytic and iron-deficiency anemia, Wiskott-Aldrich syndrome), and *obstruction of intracranial drainage by venous thrombosis* (lateral sinus or posterior sagittal sinus thrombosis, head injury, and obstruction of the superior vena cava).

CLINICAL MANIFESTATIONS. The most frequent symptom is headache, and although vomiting also occurs, it is rarely as persistent and pernicious as that associated with a posterior fossa tumor. Diplopia secondary to paralysis of the abducens nerve is a frequent complaint. Most patients are alert and lack constitutional symptoms. An examination of the infant is characterized by a bulging fontanel and a "cracked-pot sound" or Macewen sign (percussion of the skull produces a resonant sound) due to separation of the cranial sutures. Papilledema with an enlarged blind spot is the most consistent sign in the child beyond infancy. An inferior nasal defect may be detected on formal tangent screen testing. The presence of focal neurologic signs indicates a process other than pseudotumor cerebri.

TREATMENT. The prime goal in management should be the discovery and treatment of the underlying cause. Pseudotumor cerebri is mainly a self-limited condition, but optic atrophy and blindness are the most significant complications. Consideration should be given to treating sinus thrombosis with anticoagulation. For many patients, repeated follow-up and monitoring of the visual acuity are all that is required. Serial visual evoked potentials are useful if the visual acuity cannot be reliably documented. For others, the initial lumbar tap that follows a computed tomography (CT) scan is diagnostic and therapeutic. The spinal needle produces a small rent in the dura that allows CSF to escape the subarachnoid space, thus reducing the intracranial pressure. Occasionally, several additional lumbar taps and the removal of sufficient CSF to reduce the opening pressure by 50% lead to resolution of the process. Acetazolamide, 10–30 mg/kg/24 hr, and corticosteroids have been effective for some patients. Rarely, a lumboperitoneal shunt or subtemporal decompression is necessary if the aforementioned approaches are unsuccessful and optic nerve atrophy supervenes. Some centers are performing optic nerve sheath fenestration. Finally, any patient whose increased intracranial pressure proves to be refractory to treatment warrants consideration for repeat neuroradiologic studies. A slow-growing tumor or obstruction of a venous sinus may become evident at the time of reinvestigation.

Baker R, Baumann R, Buncic J: Idiopathic intracranial hypertension (pseudotumor cerebri) in pediatric patients. Pediatr Neurol 5:5, 1989.

Huckman MS: Computed tomography in the diagnosis of pseudotumor cerebri. Radiology 119:593, 1976.
Rush JA: Pseudotumor cerebri. Mayo Clin Proc 55:541, 1980.

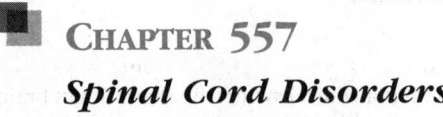

CHAPTER 557
Spinal Cord Disorders

557.1 Spinal Cord Tumors

In children, spinal cord tumors account for approximately 20% of neuraxial tumors and are classified according to anatomic position (Fig. 557–1). *Intramedullary tumors* arise within the substance of the cord and grow slowly by infiltration, usually in the cervical region. The most common intramedullary tumor is a low-grade astrocytoma, followed by an ependymoma. *Extramedullary, intradural tumors* tend to be benign and arise from neural crest tissue. Tumors in this area include neurofibroma, ganglioneuroma, and meningioma. *Extramedullary, extradural tumors* characteristically are metastatic lesions, particularly neuroblastoma, sarcoma, and lymphoma.

CLINICAL MANIFESTATIONS. Most children with spinal cord tumors present with a combination of gait disturbance, scoliosis, and back pain, depending on the locale of the tumor. Intramedullary gliomas are slow growing. Progressive difficulties in locomotion and sphincter disturbances are the earliest symptoms. Glial tumors in the cervical cord produce lower motor neuron signs in the upper extremities and upper motor neuron signs in the legs. Denervation of the intercostal muscles decreases chest wall movement and results in a weak cough. Loss of pain, temperature, and light touch sensation is evident in the lower extremities, and a cord level can be documented by light touch and pain sensation, the starch-iodine test, or somatosensory evoked potentials. With extramedullary tumors, the presenting symptom is often back pain. The child has difficulty in sleeping because of pain and maintains a tripod posture while attempting to assume the supine position. If the tumor is attached to a nerve root, segmental pain, paresthesia, and weakness will be evident. Extramedullary, extradural tumors have a propensity to cause an acute block of the cerebrospinal fluid (CSF) pathways owing to rapid growth within a confined space. Such children present with a flaccid paraplegia, urinary retention, and a patulous anus. Some extramedullary tumors produce the **Brown-Séquard syndrome** which consists of homolateral weakness, spasticity, and ataxia, with contralateral loss of pain and temperature sensation. Papilledema is observed in a few patients, usually in association with markedly elevated CSF protein levels that presumably interfere with normal CSF flow dynamics.

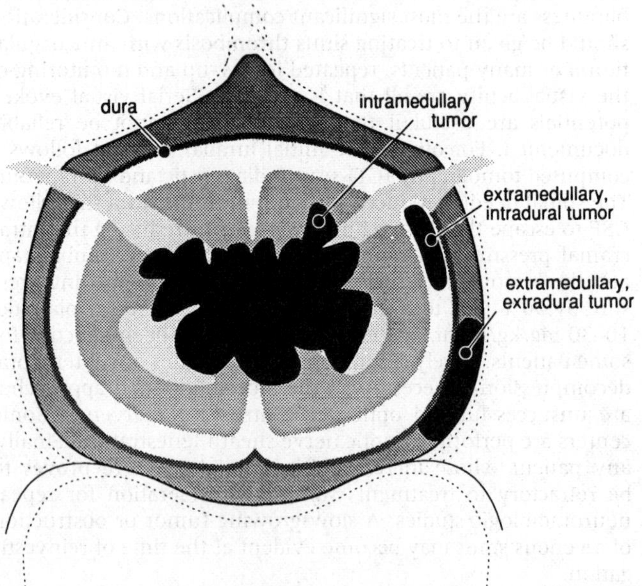

Figure 557–1. Diagram of the location of spinal cord tumors in children.

DIAGNOSIS. It is important to establish the diagnosis of a spinal cord tumor as early as possible, because the surgical management will be facilitated and irreversible damage to the cord will be prevented. In approximately 40% of the cases, routine roentgenograms show abnormalities including widening of the interpediculate distance, destruction or sclerosis of the adjacent vertebral bodies or pedicles, and widening of vertebral foramen on an oblique view in the case of a neurofibroma or ganglioneuroma. Magnetic resonance imaging (MRI) is the most important diagnostic test to establish the diagnosis. Intramedullary tumors produce a fusiform swelling of the cord, often with a complete block of the CSF. Neurofibroma tend to create a circular indentation of the cord, and extramedullary tumors show various degrees of blockage.

TREATMENT. With modern surgical techniques, many tumors can be totally and safely resected. Surgical removal of benign extramedullary tumors is associated with a good prognosis. For children with a primary neuroblastoma who present with a sudden onset of paraplegia secondary to metastases in the extradural space, immediate radiation therapy may circumvent the need for a laminectomy.

557.2 Spinal Cord Trauma
(See also Chapters 59 and 84)

Acute spinal cord injuries in children may result from indirect trauma due to hyperflexion, hyperextension, or vertical compression accidents; however, fracture dislocation of the vertebral column or epidural bleeding may also compromise spinal cord integrity secondary to a mass effect. As with the brain, the degree of injury to the spinal cord is variable and includes concussion, contusion, laceration, and transection. Recovery depends on the extent of the trauma as well as on the immediate and long-term management. Common causes of spinal cord injury include traumatic breech deliveries, physical abuse (as in the "shaken baby" syndrome), automobile and diving accidents, falls from playground equipment, and congenital defects such as the underlying vertebral abnormality in Down syndrome (DS).

DS individuals are susceptible to atlantoaxial instability owing to laxity of the transverse ligaments. Atlantoaxial instability has been defined as a distance greater than 4.5 mm between the odontoid process of the axis and the anterior arch of the atlas. Spinal cord compression (myelopathy) may be a consequence of atlantoaxial instability. Management should include the following: (a) lateral roentgenograms of the neck in the neutral, flexion, and extension positions should be obtained at 5–8 yr, 10–12 yr, and 18 yr in individuals with DS, as atlantoaxial instability can develop during periods of growth; (b) children with atlantoaxial instability should be advised not to participate in "risky" sports, such as tumbling, diving, and football; (c) radiographs of the neck should be obtained prior to operative procedures or therapeutic programs that involve active neck movement or manipulation; (d) parents and physicians should be made aware of the symptoms and signs of cord compression (neck pain, urinary and fecal incontinence, head tilt, gait abnormalities, ataxia, hyperreflexia, weakness, spasticity, and quadriplegia); and (e) there should be prompt investigation (neck radiographs, CT, MRI) followed by consideration for operative intervention in patients with signs of myelopathy.

A patient with *severe cord injury* presents with **spinal shock**, consisting of flaccidity, areflexia, and loss of sensation. This may persist for up to 4 wk and results from dysfunction of synaptic activity in the pathways caudal to the injury. Ultimately, reflex flexor movements develop, followed by extensor reflex activity associated with hyperactive deep tendon reflexes, spasticity, and an automatic bladder. *Fracture dislocations at the C5–C6 level* are the most common acute cause of spinal cord injuries and are characterized by a flaccid quadriparesis, loss of sphincter function, and a sensory level corresponding to the upper sternum. A transverse injury in the high cervical cord level (C1–C2) causes respiratory arrest and death in the absence of ventilatory support. Fractures in the low thoracic (T12–L1) region may produce the **conus medullaris syndrome**, which includes a loss of urinary and rectal sphincter control, flaccid weakness, and sensory disturbances of the legs. Spinal cord injury may occur in the absence of a vertebral fracture. A **central cord lesion** may result as a consequence of contusion and hemorrhage, and typically involves the upper extremities to a greater degree than the legs. There are lower motor neuron signs in the upper extremities and upper motor neuron signs in the legs, bladder dysfunction, and loss of sensation caudal to the lesion. There may be considerable recovery, particularly in the lower extremities.

Spinal cord injuries should be managed by stabilization and immobilization of the spine at the accident site using a cervical collar or sandbags. An adequate airway should be maintained, respiratory support should be provided, and shock should be treated with appropriate volume expanders. Following transportation, roentgenograms of the spine, including oblique views, should be obtained. Approximately 50% of children with severe cord injuries show no abnormality on the spine roentgenogram. Fracture dislocations are treated with traction, immobilization, and, if the injury is unstable, vertebral fusion. Laminectomy and inspection of the cord are reserved for the patient with progression of neurologic signs and appearance on CT or MRI scan that suggests an epidural or intraspinal hemorrhage. Additional therapeutic measures include management of bladder and gastrointestinal disturbances, nutritional and skin care, and a rigorous multidisciplinary rehabilitation program.

557.3 Tethered Cord

During fetal development the spinal cord occupies the entire length of the vertebral column, but due to differential growth the conus medullaris in the child ultimately assumes a position at the level of L1. Normal regression of the distal embryonic spinal cord produces a slender, threadlike filum terminale that is attached to the coccyx. A tethered cord results when a thickened ropelike filum terminale persists and anchors the conus at or below the L2 level. Neurologic signs may develop due to abnormal tension on the spinal cord, compromising blood supply, particularly during flexion and extension movements. Diastematomyelia may coexist with a tethered cord. Inspection of the back shows a midline skin lesion in approximately 70% of cases, such as a lipoma, cutaneous hemangioma, tuft of hair, hyperpigmentation, or a dermal pit. The clinical presentation varies, and signs may be evident at birth or may be delayed until adulthood. Infants may have asymmetric growth in a foot or leg associated with talipes cavus deformities and muscle wasting due to prolonged denervation. Abnormalities in bladder function with overflow incontinence, progressive scoliosis, and diffuse pain in the lower extremities are more common findings in the child. Plain roentgenograms of the lumbosacral spine demonstrate spina bifida in most cases. CT scanning with a small amount of metrizamide or MRI precisely outlines the level of the conus medullaris and the filum terminale. Surgical transection of the thickened filum terminale tends to halt the progression of neurologic signs and to prevent the development of dysfunction in the asymptomatic patient.

557.4 Diastematomyelia

Diastematomyelia refers to the division of the spinal cord into two halves by the projection of a fibrocartilaginous or bony septum originating from the posterior vertebral body and extending posteriorly. It represents a disorder of neural tube fusion with the persistence of mesodermal tissue from the primitive neurenteric canal acting as the septum. The defect involves the lumbar vertebrae (L1–L3) in approximately 50% of cases and tends to be associated with abnormalities of the vertebral bodies, including fusion defects, hemivertebra, hypoplasia, kyphoscoliosis, spina bifida, and myelomeningocele. A midline abnormality of the skin, such as a cutaneous hemangioma, provides a clue to the possibility of an underlying abnormality. The neurologic signs are thought to result from flexion and extension movements of the cord, which produce traction and additional trauma by the impaling septum. The clinical presentation of diastematomyelia varies, and in some cases the patient may remain asymptomatic. Most often unilateral foot abnormalities, including talipes equinovarus, claw toes, atrophy of the gastrocnemius, and loss of pain and temperature sensation, are apparent in the preschool child. A more progressive course may ensue, characterized by bilateral weakness and muscle atrophy in the lower extremities, absent ankle jerks, urinary incontinence, and low back pain. Plain roentgenograms of the vertebrae may not detect the septum due to lack of calcification, so that CT scanning or MRI is the study of choice. The treatment of symptomatic patients is excision of the bony spur or septum and lysis of the adjacent adhesions.

557.5 Syringomyelia

Syringomyelia may be defined as a cystic cavity within the spinal cord, which may communicate with the CSF pathways or remain localized and noncommunicating. *Syringobulbia* exists when the cystic cavity extends into the medulla. Although the pathogenesis of communicating syringomyelia is unknown, the prevailing hypothesis suggests a constriction of the central canal at the level of the foramen magnum during embryogenesis. CSF may pass caudad through the narrowed canal, especially during periods of increased intracranial pressure (e.g., sneezing, coughing), and produce dilatation of the central canal. Because of the constriction, CSF is prevented from flowing in a cephalic direction. Communicating syringomyelia is frequently associated with the Chiari type I malformation, whereas the noncommunicating syrinx is complicated by cord tumors, vascular accidents, trauma, and arachnoiditis.

Due to its slow evolution, syringomyelia rarely produces symptoms during childhood.

Interruption of the anterior white commissure at the level of the cervical cord disrupts the lateral spinothalamic tracts, causing an asymmetric loss of pain and temperature sensation in the upper extremities, with preservation of light touch (dissociation of sensation). Progressive enlargement of the cavity impinges on the anterior horn cells and corticospinal tracts, resulting in muscle wasting of the hands, absent deep tendon reflexes in the upper extremities, and upper motor neuron signs in the lower extremities. A rapidly progressive scoliosis may be the initial manifestation of syringomyelia. Trophic ulcers associated with vasomotor disturbances of the hands and arms indicate the loss of appreciation of pain. CT scanning with the intrathecal injection of metrizamide outlines an enlarged spinal cord in the region of the syrinx, and a delayed scan displays the contrast medium within the cavity. MRI is the study of choice. The management is surgical and depends on the site and etiology of the syringomyelia. Decompression of the foramen magnum and the upper cervical vertebrae is recommended when the syrinx is associated with a Chiari type I or II anomaly. Additional procedures include insertion of a tissue plug in the open end of the central canal, draining the cystic cavity into the subarachnoid space, and the percutaneous aspiration of the syrinx, which may result in marked improvement in neurologic function for prolonged periods.

557.6 Transverse Myelitis

Transverse myelitis is characterized by the abrupt onset of progressive weakness and sensory disturbances in the lower extremities. A history of a preceding viral infection accompanied by fever and malaise is documented in most cases. Several viruses have been implicated including the Epstein-Barr virus and herpes, influenza, rubella, mumps, and varicella viruses. At least three hypotheses have been proposed to explain the pathogenesis of transverse myelitis: cell-mediated autoimmune response, direct viral invasion of the spinal cord, and an autoimmune vasculitis. Pathologic examination of the cord shows marked softening and perivascular cuffing by lymphocytes, supporting an immunologic basis for the disorder.

Low back or abdominal pain and paresthesias of the legs are prominent symptoms in the early stages. The leg muscles are weak and flaccid, and a sensory level is present usually in the midthoracic region. Pain, temperature, and light touch sensation are affected, but joint position and vibration sense may be preserved. Sphincter disturbances are common, in which case catheterization of the bladder is necessary. Fever and nuchal rigidity are present early in most cases. The neurologic deficit evolves for 2–3 days and then plateaus, with flaccidity gradually changing to spasticity and with the concomitant development of upper motor neuron signs in the lower extremities. An examination of the CSF shows moderate lymphocyte pleocytosis and a normal or slightly elevated protein. CT scanning or MRI reveals mild fusiform swelling in the affected region. Spontaneous recovery occurs over a period of weeks or months and is complete in approximately 60% of cases. Residual deficits include bowel and bladder dysfunction and weakness in the lower extremities. Management is directed to bladder care and physiotherapy. There is no evidence that steroids influence the course or the outcome of transverse myelitis. The differential diagnosis includes meningitis, infectious polyneuropathy (Guillain-Barré syndrome), poliomyelitis, neuromyelitis optica (Devic disease), spinal cord neoplasm, epidural abscess, and a vascular malformation.

557.7 Arteriovenous Malformation

An arteriovenous malformation of the spinal cord consists of a collection of tortuous dilated veins that are usually located on the dorsal aspect of the thoracic cord. The malformation may cause neurologic symptoms by its mass effect on the cord or by the "steal" phenomenon, by which blood is shunted through the abnormal veins, bypassing the spinal cord, which produces transient and in some cases progressive loss of neurologic function. Occasionally, the patient presents with acute paraparesis and a sensory deficit due to a subarachnoid bleed from the malformation. More commonly, a gradual onset of gait abnormalities, low back pain, and bowel and bladder dysfunction is noted. The deep tendon reflexes are absent or reduced in the lower extremities, and the Babinski reflex is present. In approximately one third of cases, a midline cutaneous angioma overlies the arteriovenous malformation, and occasionally a spinal bruit may be auscultated. Roentgenograms of the spine may show erosion of the pedicles; however, contrast myelography and selective spinal angiography are required to delineate the blood supply and the extent of the malformation. The malformation is removed by surgical excision with the use of an operating microscope or is obliterated by embolization.

Cahan LD, Bentson JR: Considerations in the diagnosis and treatment of syringomyelia and Chiari malformation. J Neurosurg 57:24, 1982.

Cremers MJG, Bol E, deRoos F, et al: Risk of sports activities in children with Down's syndrome and atlantoaxial instability. Lancet 342:511, 1993.

De La Torre JC: Spinal cord injury: Review of basic and applied research. Spine 6:315, 1981.

DiJunno JF, Formal CS: Chronic spinal cord injury. N Engl J Med 330:550, 1994.

Haft H, Ransohoff J, Carter S: Spinal cord tumors in children. Pediatrics 23:1152, 1959.

Hendrick EB, Hoffman HJ, Humphreys RP: The tethered spinal cord. Clin Neurosurg 30:457, 1982.

Hilal S, Marton D, Pollack E: Diastematomyelia in children. Radiology 112:609, 1974.

McAtee-Smith J, Hebert AA, Rapini R, et al: Skin lesions of the spinal axis and spinal dysraphism. Arch Pediatr Adolesc Med 148:740, 1994.

Paine RS, Byers RK: Transverse myelopathy in childhood. Am J Dis Child 85:151, 1953.

Pueschel SM, Findley TW, Furia J, et al: Atlantoaxial instability in Down syndrome: Roentgenographic, neurologic and somatosensory evoked potential studies. J Pediatr 110:515, 1987.

Riche MC, Modenesi-Freitas J, Djindjian M, et al: Arteriovenous malformations (AVM) of the spinal cord in children: Review of 38 cases. Neuroradiology 22:171, 1982.

Scotti G, Musgrave MA, Harwood-Nash DC, et al: Diastematomyelia in children: Metrizamide and CT metrizamide myelography. AJR 135:1225, 1980.

PART XXVIII

Neuromuscular Disorders

Harvey B. Sarnat

The term *neuromuscular disease* refers to disorders of the motor unit and specifically excludes suprasegmental disorders, such as cerebral palsy, even though muscle tone, strength, function, and reflexes are influenced by cerebral disease. The *motor unit* consists of four components: (1) a motor neuron in the brain stem or ventral horn of the spinal cord; (2) its axon that, together with other axons, forms the peripheral nerve; (3) the neuromuscular junction; and (4) all muscle fibers innervated by a single motor neuron. The size of the motor unit varies among different muscles and with the precision of muscular function required. In large muscles, such as the glutei and quadriceps femoris, hundreds of muscle fibers are innervated by a single motor neuron; in small, finely tuned muscles, such as the stapedius or the extraocular muscles, a 1:1 ratio may prevail. The motor unit is influenced by suprasegmental or upper motor neuron control that alters properties of muscle tone, precision of movement, reciprocal inhibition of antagonistic muscles during movement, and sequencing of muscle contractions to achieve smooth, coordinated movements. Suprasegmental impulses also augment or inhibit the monosynaptic stretch reflex.

Diseases of the motor unit are common in children. These neuromuscular diseases may be genetically determined or nonhereditary, congenital or acquired, acute or chronic, and progressive or static. Because specific therapy is available for many diseases and because of genetic and prognostic implications, precise diagnosis is important; laboratory confirmation is required for most diseases because of overlapping clinical manifestations.

Many chromosomal loci have been identified with specific neuromuscular diseases as a result of genetic linkage analysis studies and the isolation and cloning of a few specific genes. In some cases, such as Duchenne muscular dystrophy, the genetic defect has been shown to be a deletion of nucleotide sequences and is associated with a defective protein product, *dystrophin*; in other cases, such as myotonic muscular dystrophy, the genetic defect is an expansion rather than a deletion in a codon (a set of three consecutive nucleotide repeats that encodes for a single amino acid), with many copies of a particular codon. Some diseases, such as nemaline rod myopathy and limb-girdle muscular dystrophy, present with autosomal dominant and autosomal recessive traits in different pedigrees; these different mendelian genotypes are different diseases despite many common phenotypic features and shared histopathologic findings in the muscle biopsy. Among the several clinically defined mitochondrial myopathies, specific mtDNA deletions and tRNA point mutations are recognized. The inheritance patterns and chromosomal and mitochondrial loci of common neuromuscular diseases affecting infants and children are summarized in Table 559–1. ■

CHAPTER 558

Evaluation and Investigation

CLINICAL MANIFESTATIONS. Examination of the neuromuscular system should always include an assessment of muscle bulk, tone, and strength. Tone and strength should not be confused: Passive tone is range of motion around a joint; active tone is physiologic resistance to movement. Head lag when an infant is pulled to a sitting position from supine is a sign of weakness, not of low tone. Hypotonia may be associated with normal strength or with weakness; enlarged muscles may be weak or strong; thin, wasted muscles may be weak or have unexpectedly normal strength. The distribution of these components is of diagnostic importance. In general, myopathies follow a proximal distribution of weakness and muscle wasting (with the notable exception of myotonic muscular dystrophy); neuropathies, by contrast, are generally distal in distribution (with the notable exception of juvenile spinal muscular atrophy). Involvement of the face, tongue, palate, and extraocular muscles provides an important distinction in the differential diagnosis. Tendon stretch reflexes are generally lost in neuropathies and in motor neuron diseases and are diminished but preserved in myopathies. A few specific clinical features are important in the diagnosis of some neuromuscular diseases. Fasciculations of muscle, which are often best seen in the tongue, are a sign of denervation. Sensory abnormalities indicate neuropathy. Fatigable weakness is characteristic of neuromuscular junctional disorders. Myotonia is specific for a few myopathies.

Some features do not distinguish myopathy from neuropathy. Muscle pain or myalgias are associated with acute disease of either myopathic or neurogenic origin. Acute dermatomyositis and acute polyneuropathy (Guillain-Barré syndrome) are both characterized by myalgias. Muscular dystrophies and spinal muscular atrophies are not associated with muscle pain. Myalgias also occur in several metabolic diseases of muscle and in ischemic myopathy. Contractures of muscles, whether present at birth or developing later in the course of an illness, occur in both myopathic and neurogenic diseases.

Male infants who are weak in late fetal life and in the neonatal period often have undescended testicles. The testicles are actively pulled into the scrotum from the anterior abdominal wall by a pair of cords that consist of smooth and striated muscle called the *gubernaculum* (Fig. 558–1). The gubernaculum is weakened in many congenital neuromuscular diseases, including spinal muscular atrophy, myotonic muscular dystrophy, and many congenital myopathies.

The thorax of infants with congenital neuromuscular disease often has a funnel shape, and the ribs are thin and radiolucent due to intercostal muscle weakness during intrauterine growth. This phenomenon is found characteristically in infantile spinal muscular atropy but also occurs in myotubular myopathy, neonatal myotonic dystrophy, and other disorders. Because of the small muscle mass, birth weight may be low for gestational age.

Generalized hypotonia and developmental delay are the most common presenting manifestations of neuromuscular

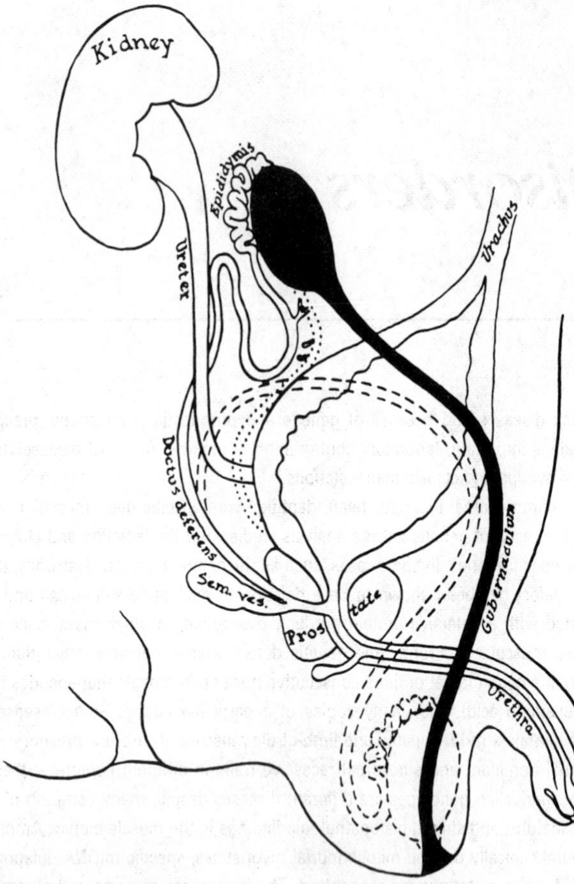

Figure 558–1. Undescended testes are common in male neonates with neuromuscular disease already symptomatic at birth, regardless of the etiology. The gubernaculum is a cylinder of striated muscle surrounding a core of smooth muscle that actively pulls the testicle into the scrotum in late gestation. Weakness of the gubernaculum in a generalized myopathy of fetal life prevents or delays the descent of the testis. Reproduced with permission from Sarnat HB, Sarnat MS: Disorders of muscle in the newborn. *In*: Moss AJ, Stern L (eds): Pediatrics Update, 4th ed. New York, Elsevier-North Holland, 1983.

disease in infants and young children. These features may also be expressions of neurologic disease, endocrine and systemic metabolic diseases, and Down syndrome, or they may be nonspecific neuromuscular expressions of malnutrition or chronic systemic illness. A prenatal history of decreased fetal movements and intrauterine growth retardation are often found in patients who are symptomatic at birth.

LABORATORY FINDINGS. Serum Enzymes. Several lysosomal enzymes are released by damaged or degenerating muscle fibers and may be measured in serum. The most useful of these is the creatine phosphokinase (CPK or CK), which is found in only three organs and may be separated into corresponding isozymes: MM for skeletal muscle, MB for cardiac muscle, and BB for brain. The serum CK is by no means a universal screening test for neuromuscular disease because many diseases of the motor unit may not be associated with elevated enzymes. However, the CK is characteristically elevated in certain diseases, such as Duchenne muscular dystrophy, and the magnitude of increase is characteristic for particular diseases.

Nerve Conduction Velocity (NCV). Motor and sensory nerve conduction may be measured electrophysiologically by using surface electrodes. Neuropathies of various types are detected by decreased conduction. The site of a traumatic nerve injury may also be localized. The nerve conduction at birth is about half of the mature value achieved by 2 yr of age. Tables are available for normal values at various ages in infancy, including for preterm infants. Because the NCV study measures only the fastest conducting fibers in a nerve, 80% of the total nerve fibers must be involved before slowing in conduction is detected.

Electromyography (EMG). EMG is less useful in pediatrics than in adult medicine, in part because of technical difficulties in recording young children and in part because the best results require patient cooperation for full relaxation and maximal voluntary contraction of a muscle. Most children are too frightened to provide such cooperation. EMG requires the insertion of a needle into the belly of a muscle and recording the electric potentials in various states of contraction. Characteristic patterns distinguish denervation from myopathic involvement. The specific type of myopathy is not usually definitively diagnosed, but certain specialized myopathic conditions, such as myotonia, may be demonstrated.

EMG combined with repetitive electrical stimulation of a motor nerve supplying a muscle to produce tetany is useful in demonstrating myasthenic decremental responses. Small muscles, such as the abductor digiti quinti of the hypothenar eminence, are used for such studies.

Muscle Biopsy. The muscle biopsy is the most important and specific diagnostic study of muscle. Not only are neurogenic and myopathic processes distinguished, but also the type of myopathy and specific enzymatic deficiencies may be determined. The vastus lateralis (quadriceps femoris) is the muscle that is most commonly sampled. The deltoid muscle should be avoided in most cases, because it normally has a 60–80% predominance of type I fibers, so that the distribution patterns of fiber types are difficult to recognize. Muscle biopsy is a simple outpatient procedure that may be performed under local anesthesia with or without femoral nerve block. Needle biopsies, advocated by some authors, require an incision in the skin similar to open biopsy, and numerous samples must be taken to do an adequate examination of the tissue; needle biopsies are as traumatic as open biopsies and provide inferior specimens.

Histochemical studies of frozen sections of the muscle are obligatory in all pediatric muscle biopsies, because many congenital and metabolic myopathies cannot be diagnosed from paraffin sections using conventional histologic stains. Immunohistochemistry is a useful supplement in some cases such as for the demonstration of dystrophin in suspected muscular dystrophy. A portion of the biopsy should be fixed for potential electron microscopy, but ultrastructure has additional diagnostic value only in selected cases. Muscle biopsy interpretation is complex and should be done by an experienced pathologist.

Nerve Biopsy. The most commonly sampled nerve is the sural nerve, which is a pure sensory nerve that supplies a small area of skin on the lateral surface of the foot. Whole or fascicular biopsies of this nerve may be taken. When the sural nerve is severed behind the lateral malleolus of the ankle, regeneration of the nerve occurs in more than 90% of cases, so that permanent sensory loss is not experienced. The sural nerve is often involved in many neuropathies that are clinically predominantly motor.

Electron microscopy should be performed on most nerve biopsies because the most important morphologic alterations cannot be appreciated at the resolution of the light microscope. Teased fiber preparations are sometimes useful in demonstrating segmental demyelination, axonal swellings, and other specific abnormalities, but this time-consuming procedure is not done routinely. Special stains may be applied to even ordinary frozen or paraffin sections of nerve biopsy to demonstrate myelin, axoplasm, and metabolic products.

Electrocardiography (ECG). Cardiac evaluation is important if myopathy is suspected, because of involvement of the heart in muscular dystrophies and in inflammatory and metabolic myopathies. The ECG often detects early cardiomyopathy or conduction defects that are clinically asymptomatic. Serial **pulmonary function tests** should be performed in muscular dystrophies and in other chronic or progressive diseases of the motor unit.

CHAPTER 559

Developmental Disorders of Muscle

A heterogeneous group of congenital neuromuscular disorders is sometimes known as the *congenital myopathies,* but in many of these disorders the assumption that the pathogenesis is primarily myopathic is unjustified. Most congenital myopathies are nonprogressive conditions, but some patients show slow clinical deterioration accompanied by additional changes in their muscle biopsy. Some of the diseases in the category of congenital myopathies are hereditary; others are sporadic. Although clinical features, including phenotype, may raise a strong suspicion of a congenital myopathy, the definitive diagnosis is determined by the histopathologic findings in the muscle biopsy. These morphologic and histochemical abnormalities differ considerably from those of the muscular dystrophies, spinal muscular atrophies, and neuropathies. Many are reminiscent of stages in the embryologic development of muscle and may represent aberrations of ontogenesis. To fully understand these disorders, a knowledge of classical embryology or morphogenesis must be supplemented with newly emerging data on the molecular genetic regulation of muscle development.

MYOGENIC REGULATORY GENES AND GENETIC LOCI OF INHERITED DISEASES OF MUSCLE (Table 559–1). A family of four myogenic regulatory genes shares encoding transcription factors of "basic helix-loop-helix" (bHLH) proteins associated with common DNA nucleotide sequences. These proto-oncogenes direct the differentiation of striated muscle from any undifferentiated mesodermal cell; some are so strongly expressed that they convert partially differentiated mesenchymal cells, such as fibroblasts or chondroblasts, into myoblasts. The earliest bHLH gene to program the differentiation of myoblasts is myogenic factor 5 *(myf-5).* The second gene, *myogenin,* promotes the fusion of myoblasts to form myotubes. *Herculin* (also known as *mrf-4* and *myf-6)* and *MyoD1* are the other two myogenic genes. In mice, *MyoD1* and *myf-5* may substitute their functions so that if either is deleted the muscle still develops normally, but the absence of both genes results in amyoplasia. Each of these four genes can activate the expression of at least one other and, under certain circumstances, can autoactivate as well. The expression of *myf-5* and of *herculin* is transient in early ontogenesis, but returns later in fetal life and persists into adult life. The human locus of the *MyoD1* gene is on chromosome 11, very near to the domain associated with embryonal rhabdomyosarcoma. The genes encoding *myf-5* and *herculin* are on chromosome 12 and that for *myogenin* is on chromosome 1. The precise role of the myogenic genes in developmental myopathies is not yet defined, but they are suspected of playing a role in pathogenesis.

559.1 Myotubular Myopathy

The term *myotubular myopathy* implies a maturational arrest of fetal muscle during the myotubular stage of development at 8–15 wk of gestation. It is based on the morphologic appearance of myofibers: A row of central nuclei lie within a core of cytoplasm; contractile myofibrils form a cylinder around this core (Fig. 559–1). Many challenge this interpretation and use the more neutral term *centronuclear myopathy* when referring to this myopathy. But this term is too nonspecific because internal nuclei occur in many unrelated myopathies.

PATHOGENESIS. Although the pathogenesis may be neurogenic, spinal motor neurons are normal in number and morphology.

■ **TABLE 559–1 Inheritance Patterns and Chromosomal or Mitochondrial Loci of Neuromuscular Diseases Affecting the Pediatric Age Group**

Disease	Transmission	Locus
Duchenne/Becker muscular dystrophy	XR	Xp21.2
Emery-Dreifuss muscular dystrophy	XR	Xq28
Myotonic muscular dystrophy (Steinert)	AD	19q13
Facio-scapulo-humeral muscular dystrophy	AD	4q35
Limb-girdle muscular dystrophy	AD	5q
Limb-girdle muscular dystrophy	AR	15q
Congenital muscular dystrophy (Fukuyama)	AR	8q31–33
Myotubular myopathy	XR	Xq28
Myotubular myopathy	AR	Unknown
Nemaline rod myopathy	AD	1q21–23
Nemaline rod myopathy	AR	Unknown
Congenital muscle fiber–type disproportion	AR	Unknown
Central core disease	AD	19q13.1
Myotonia congenita (Thomsen)	AD	7q35
Paramyotonia congenita	AD	17q13.1–13.3
Hyperkalemic periodic paralysis	AD	17q13.1–13.3
Hypokalemic periodic paralysis	AD	1q31–32
Glycogenosis II (Pompe; acid maltase deficiency)	AR	17q23
Glycogenosis V (McArdle; myophosphorylase deficiency)	AR	11q13
Muscle carnitine deficiency	AR	Unknown
Muscle carnitine palmityltransferase deficiency	AR	1p11–13
Spinal muscular atrophy (Werdnig-Hoffmann; Kugelberg-Welander)	AR	5q11–13
Familial dysautonomia (Riley-Day)	AR	9q31–33
Hereditary motor-sensory neuropathy (Charcot-Marie-Tooth; Déjerine-Sottas)	AD	17p11.2
Hereditary motor-sensory neuropathy (axonal type)	AD	1p35–36
Hereditary motor-sensory neuropathy (Charcot-Marie-Tooth-X)	XR	Xq13.1
Mitochondrial myopathy (Kearns-Sayre)	Maternal; sporadic	Single large mtDNA deletion
Mitochondrial myopathy (MERRF)	Maternal	tRNA point mutation at position 8344
Mitochondrial myopathy (MELAS)	Maternal	tRNA point mutation at positions 3243 and 3271

AD, autosomal dominant; AR, autosomal recessive; XR, X-linked recessive; MERRF, mitochondrial encephalomyopathy with ragged-red fibers; MELAS, mitochondrial encephalomyopathy with lactic acidosis and strokelike episodes; mtDNA, mitochondrial deoxyribonucleic acid; tRNA, transfer ribonucleic acid.

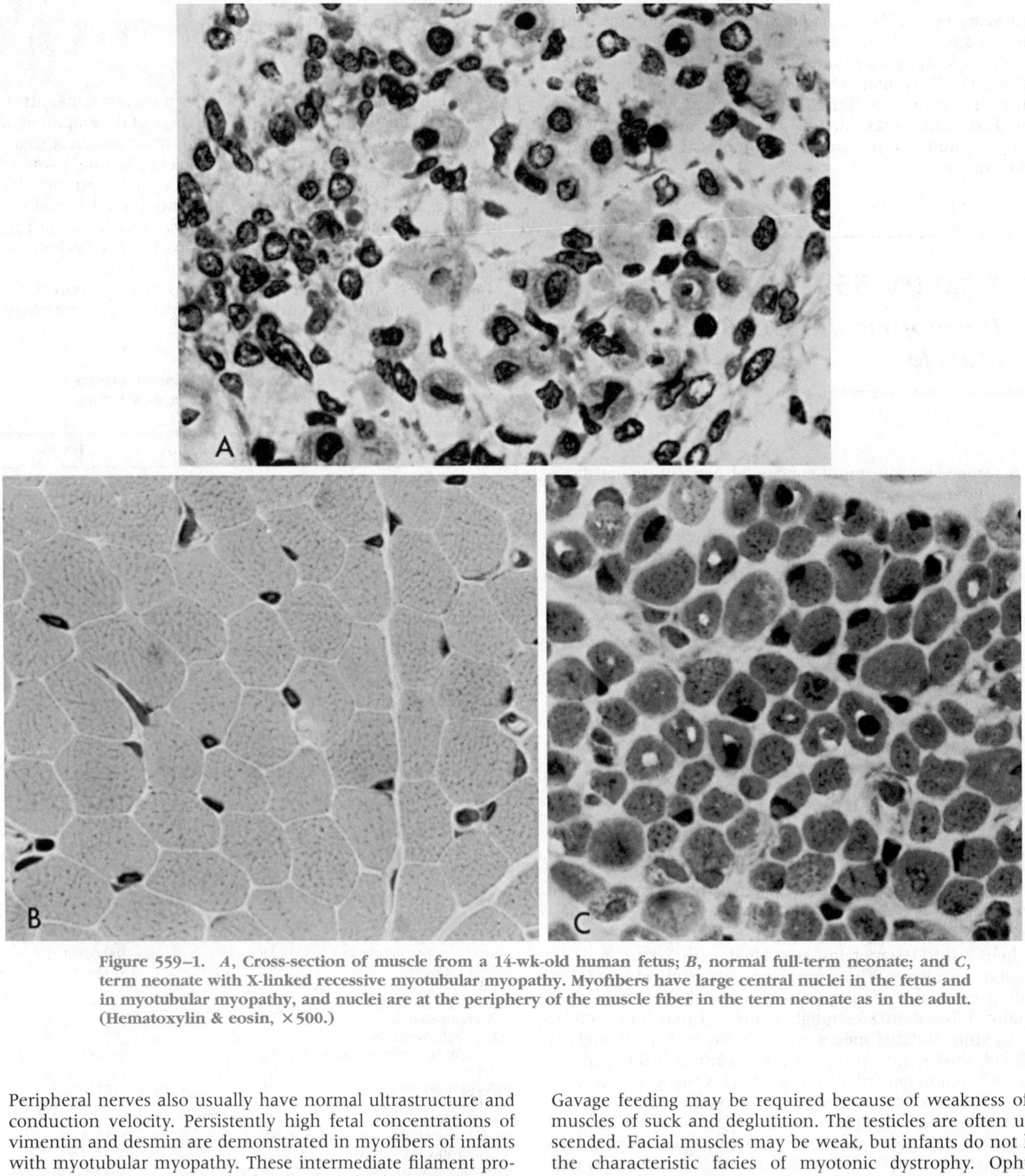

Figure 559–1. *A*, Cross-section of muscle from a 14-wk-old human fetus; *B*, normal full-term neonate; and *C*, term neonate with X-linked recessive myotubular myopathy. Myofibers have large central nuclei in the fetus and in myotubular myopathy, and nuclei are at the periphery of the muscle fiber in the term neonate as in the adult. (Hematoxylin & eosin, ×500.)

Peripheral nerves also usually have normal ultrastructure and conduction velocity. Persistently high fetal concentrations of vimentin and desmin are demonstrated in myofibers of infants with myotubular myopathy. These intermediate filament proteins serve as cytoskeletal elements in fetal myotubes, attaching nuclei and mitochondria to the sarcolemmal membranes to preserve their central positions. As intracellular organization changes with maturation, the nuclei move to the periphery and mitochondria are redistributed between myofibrils. At the same time, vimentin and desmin diminish. Vimentin disappears altogether by term and desmin remains only in trace amounts. Persistent fetal vimentin and desmin in muscle fibers may be the mechanism of "maturational arrest."

CLINICAL MANIFESTATIONS. Decreased fetal movements are perceived in late gestation. At birth, affected infants have a thin muscle mass involving axial, limb-girdle, and distal muscles; severe generalized hypotonia; and diffuse weakness. Respiratory efforts may be ineffective, requiring ventilatory support. Gavage feeding may be required because of weakness of the muscles of suck and deglutition. The testicles are often undescended. Facial muscles may be weak, but infants do not have the characteristic facies of myotonic dystrophy. Ophthalmoplegia is observed in a few cases. The palate may be high. The tongue is thin, but fasciculations are not seen. Tendon stretch reflexes are weak or absent. Myotubular myopathy is not associated with cardiomyopathy; mature cardiac muscle fibers normally have central nuclei. Congenital anomalies of the central nervous system or of other systems are not associated.

The original case described as "myotubular myopathy" in 1966 was an adolescent boy with mild weakness. Many subsequent cases of older children and adults with centronuclear myopathy and variable weakness have been reported, but their relation to the severe neonatal disease is uncertain.

LABORATORY FINDINGS. Serum CK is normal. The EMG does not show evidence of denervation and is usually normal or shows minimal nonspecific myopathic features in early infancy. Nerve conduction velocity may be slow but is usually normal. The electrocardiogram (ECG) is normal. Roentgenograms of the chest show no cardiomegaly, but the ribs may be thin.

DIAGNOSIS. The muscle biopsy is diagnostic at birth, even in premature infants. More than 90% of muscle fibers are small and have centrally placed, large vesicular nuclei in a single row. Spaces between nuclei are filled with sarcoplasm containing mitochondria. Histochemical stains for oxidative enzymatic activity and glycogen reveal a central distribution as in fetal myotubes. The cylinder of myofibrils shows mature histochemical differentiation with adenosine triphosphatase (ATPase) stains, however. The connective tissue of muscle, spindles, blood vessels, intramuscular nerves, and motor endplates are mature. Ultrastructural features in neonatal myotubular myopathy, other than those that define the disease, are also mature. Vimentin and desmin show strong immunoreactivity in muscle fibers in myotubular myopathy and no demonstrable activity in normal term neonatal muscle.

GENETICS. X-linked recessive inheritance is the most common trait; therefore, most patients are boys. The mothers of affected infants are clinically asymptomatic, but their muscle biopsy shows scattered small centronuclear fibers with increased vimentin and desmin. Autosomal dominant and autosomal recessive forms are also reported but are rarer.

Genetic linkage on the X chromosome has been localized to the Xq28 site, a different locus than the Xp21 gene of Duchenne and Becker muscular dystrophies. If persistent vimentin and desmin are primary defects, the genetics of this disease is probably complex, because synthesis of human vimentin is controlled by chromosome 10 (10p13), and synthesis of desmin is controlled by chromosome 2 (2q35). The defect is more probably in a muscle specific vimentin suppressor gene that normally stops vimentin synthesis in midgestation.

PROGNOSIS. About 75% of severely affected neonates die within the first few weeks or months of life. Survivors do not experience a progressive course but have major physical handicaps, rarely walk, and remain severely hypotonic.

559.2 Congenital Muscle Fiber-Type Disproportion (CMFTD)

This condition occurs as an isolated "congenital myopathy" but also develops in association with a variety of unrelated disorders that include nemaline rod disease, Krabbe disease (globoid cell leukodystrophy), cerebellar hypoplasia and certain other brain malformations (see later), fetal alcohol syndrome, some glycogenoses, Lowe syndrome, rigid spine syndrome, and some cases of myotonic muscular dystrophy.

PATHOGENESIS. The association of CMFTD with cerebellar hypoplasia (see later) suggests that the pathogenesis may be an abnormal suprasegmental influence on the developing motor unit during the stage of histochemical differentiation of muscle between 20 and 28 wk of gestation. Muscle fiber types and growth are determined by innervation and are mutable even in the adult. Although CMFTD does not actually correspond with any normal stage of development, it appears to be an embryologic disturbance of fiber type differentiation and growth. From an evolutionary perspective, CMFTD is the normal physiologic condition in small mammals such as rodents.

CLINICAL MANIFESTATIONS. As an isolated condition not associated with other diseases, CMFTD is a nonprogressive disorder present at birth. There is generalized hypotonia and weakness, but the weakness is usually not severe and respiratory distress and dysphagia are rare. Mild congenital contractures are often present. Poor head control and developmental delay for gross motor skills are common in infancy. Walking is usually delayed until 18–24 mo but is eventually achieved. Because of the hypotonia, subluxation of the hips may occur. Muscle bulk is reduced. The muscle wasting and hypotonia are proportionately greater than the weakness, and the child may be stronger than expected during examination.

The facies of children with CMFTD often raise the suspicion, especially if the child is referred for assessment of developmental delay and hypotonia. The head is dolichocephalic and facial weakness is present. The palate is usually high-arched. Thin muscles of the trunk and extremities give a thin, wasted appearance to the body habitus. Patients do not complain of myalgias. The clinical course is benign and nonprogressive.

LABORATORY FINDINGS. Serum CK, ECG, electromyogram (EMG), and nerve conduction velocity are all normal in simple CMFTD. If other diseases are associated, the laboratory investigation of those conditions will disclose the specific features.

DIAGNOSIS. CMFTD is diagnosed by a muscle biopsy that shows a disproportion in both size and relative ratios of histochemical fiber types: Type I fibers are uniformly small and type II fibers are hypertrophic; type I fibers are more numerous than those of type II. Degeneration of myofibers and other primary myopathic features are absent. The biopsy is diagnostic at birth.

GENETICS. Most cases of simple CMFTD are sporadic, although autosomal recessive inheritance is often suspected. A few autosomal dominantly transmitted cases have been described. CMFTD may also be associated with cerebellar hypoplasia.

TREATMENT. No drug therapy is available. Physiotherapy may be helpful for some patients in strengthening muscles that do not receive sufficient exercise in daily activities. Mild congenital contractures often respond well to gentle range of motion exercises and rarely require plaster casting or surgery.

559.3 Nemaline Rod Myopathy

Nemaline rods (derived from the Greek *nema*, meaning thread) are rod-shaped inclusion-like abnormal structures within muscle fibers. In histologic sections of muscle, they are difficult to demonstrate with conventional hematoxylin-eosin stain but are easily seen with special stains. They are not foreign inclusion bodies but rather consist of excessive Z-band material with a similar ultrastructure (Fig. 559–2). Chemically,

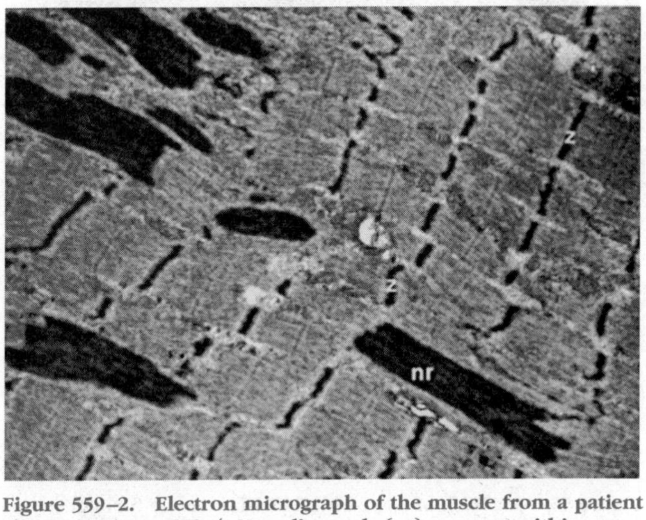

Figure 559–2. Electron micrograph of the muscle from a patient shown in Figure 559–4. Nemaline rods (nr) are seen within many myofibrils. They are identical in composition to the normal Z-bands (z) (×6,000).

the rods are mainly alpha-actinin. Nemaline rod formation may be an unusual reaction of muscle fibers to injury, because these rod structures have been found uncommonly in a variety of diseases. They are most abundant in the congenital myopathy known as nemaline rod disease.

CLINICAL MANIFESTATIONS. Severe infantile and juvenile forms of the disease are known. Patients resemble those with CMFTD, except that they are more severely affected. Generalized hypotonia, weakness including bulbar-innervated and respiratory muscles, and a very thin muscle mass are characteristic (Fig. 559–3). The head is dolichocephalic, and the palate high arched or even cleft. Muscles of the jaw may be too weak to hold it closed (Fig. 559–4). Infants may be severely weak at birth, and some die in the neonatal period. Survivors are confined to an electric wheelchair and are usually unable to overcome gravity. Both proximal and distal muscles are involved. Gastrostomy may be needed for chronic dysphagia. In the juvenile form, patients are ambulatory and are able to perform most tasks of daily living. Weakness is not usually progressive, but some patients have more difficulty over time or enter a phase of progressive weakness. Cardiomyopathy is an uncommon complication.

LABORATORY FINDINGS. Serum CK is normal. The muscle biopsy shows CMFTD or at least fiber type I predominance in addition to the nemaline rods. In some patients, uniform type I fibers are seen with few or no type II fibers. Focal myofibrillar degeneration and an increase in lysosomal enzymes have been found in a few severe cases associated with progressive symptoms.

GENETIC ASPECTS. Autosomal dominant and autosomal recessive forms of nemaline rod disease are well documented, and an X-linked dominant form in girls may occur. Autosomal dominant nemaline rod myopathy has been mapped to the 1q21-23 locus.

559.4 Central Core Disease

This autosomal dominant disease caused by an abnormal gene at the 19q13.1 locus is characterized pathologically by central cores within muscle fibers in which only amorphous, granular cytoplasm is found with an absence of myofibrils and organelles. Histochemical stains show a lack of enzymatic activities of all types within these cores. Clinically, infantile hypotonia, proximal weakness, muscle wasting, and involvement of facial muscles and neck flexors are the typical features. The course is nonprogressive, and the weakness is not usually severely disabling. Congenital dislocated hips and skeletal deformities are common. Scoliosis occurs even without much axial weakness.

Central core disease is consistently associated with **malignant hyperthermia**, and all patients should have special precautions with pretreatment by dantrolene, before an anesthetic agent is administered. The serum CK is normal in central core disease, except during crises of malignant hyperthermia.

Variants of central cores, called *minicores* and *multicores*, are described in some families. Some children with Prader-Willi syndrome have focal loss of myofilaments resembling early central cores.

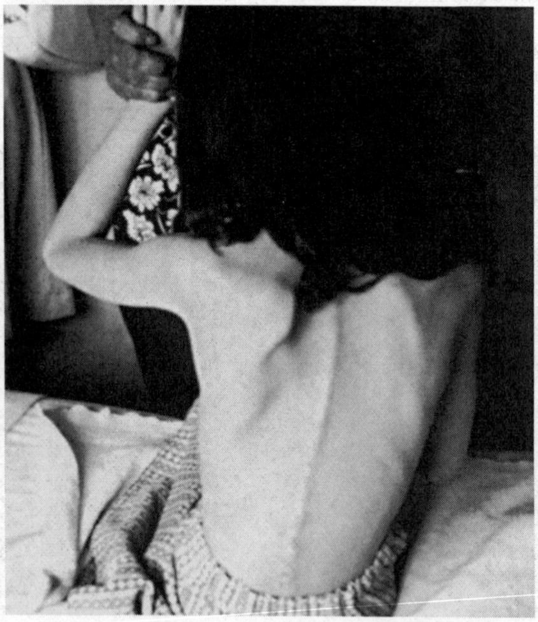

Figure 559–3. Back of 13-yr-old girl with juvenile form of nemaline rod disease. The paraspinal muscles are very thin, and winging of the scapulae is evident. The muscle mass of the extremities is also greatly reduced both proximally and distally.

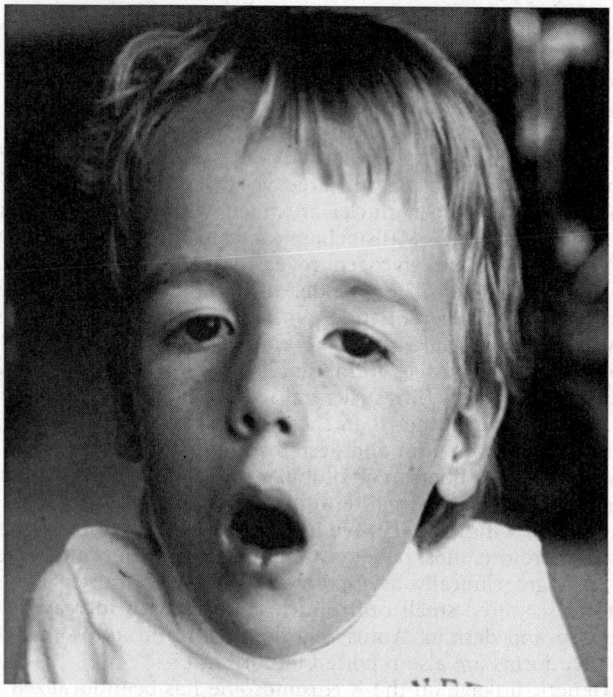

Figure 559–4. Infantile form of nemaline rod disease in a 6-yr-old boy. Facial weakness and generalized muscle wasting are severe. The head is dolichocephalic. The mouth is usually open because the masseters are too weak to lift the mandible against gravity for more than a few seconds.

559.5 Brain Malformations and Muscle Development

Infants with *cerebellar hypoplasia* are hypotonic and developmentally delayed. Muscle biopsy is sometimes performed to exclude a congenital myopathy. Such biopsies may show delayed maturation of muscle, fiber-type predominance, or CMFTD. Other malformations of the brain may also be associated with abnormal histochemical patterns, but supratentorial lesions are less likely than brain stem or cerebellar lesions to alter muscle development. Abnormal descending impulses along bulbospinal pathways probably alter discharge patterns of lower motor neurons that determine the histochemical differentiation of muscle. The corticospinal tract does not participate because it is not yet functional during this period of fetal life.

559.6 Amyoplasia

Congenital absence of individual muscles is common and is often asymmetric. One of the most common is the *palmaris longus* muscle of the ventral forearm, which is absent in one third of normal subjects and is compensated fully by other flexors of the wrist. Unilateral *absence of a sternocleidomastoid* muscle (SCM) is one cause of congenital torticollis. Absence of one *pectoralis major* muscle is part of the **Poland anomalad.**

When innervation does not develop, such as in the lower limbs in severe cases of *myelomeningocele,* muscles may fail to develop. In *sacral agenesis,* the abnormal somites that fail to form bony vertebrae may also fail to form muscles from the same defective mesodermal plate, a disorder of induction resulting in segmental amyoplasia. Skeletal muscles of the extremities fail to differentiate from embryonic myomeres if the long bones do not form. Absence of one long bone, such as the radius, is associated with variable aplasia or hypoplasia of associated muscles, such as the *carpi flexor radialis.*

Generalized amyoplasia due to defective myogenic regulatory genes is documented in mice and theoretical in humans but would result in spontaneous fetal loss. End-stage neurogenic atrophy of muscle is sometimes called *amyoplasia,* but this usage is semantically incorrect.

559.7 Muscular Dysgenesis

(Proteus Syndrome Myopathy)

The *Proteus syndrome* is a disturbance of cellular growth, involving ectodermal and mesodermal tissues. The etiology is unknown but it is not a mendelian trait. Clinically, it presents as asymmetric overgrowth of the extremities, verrucous cutaneous lesions, angiomas of various types, thickening of bones, hemimegalencephaly, and excessive growth of muscles without weakness. Histologically, the muscle is interpreted as a unique *muscular dysgenesis.* Abnormal zones are adjacent to zones of normal muscle formation and do not follow anatomic boundaries. It is suggested that the disorder may be due to abnormal paracrine growth factors. Historically the "elephant man," who was exploited for his grotesque features in late 19th century London and became a popular sensation, was long misdiagnosed as neurofibromatosis but is now recognized to have had Proteus syndrome.

559.8 Benign Congenital Hypotonia

Benign congenital hypotonia is not a disease but is a descriptive term for infants or children with nonprogressive hypotonia of unknown origin. The hypotonia is not usually associated with weakness or developmental delay, although some children acquire gross motor skills more slowly than normal. Tendon stretch reflexes are normal or hypoactive. There are no cranial nerve abnormalities. Intelligence is normal.

The diagnosis is one of exclusion, after laboratory studies including muscle biopsy and imaging of the brain with special attention to the cerebellum are normal.

The *prognosis* is generally good, and no specific therapy is required. Contractures do not develop. Hypotonia persists into adult life. The disorder is not always as "benign" as its name implies, because a common complication is recurrent dislocation of joints, especially the shoulders. Excessive motility of the spine may result in stretch injury, compression, or vascular compromise of nerve roots or of the spinal cord. These are particular hazards for patients who perform gymnastics or who become circus performers, because of agility of joints without weakness or pain.

559.9 Arthrogryposis

Arthrogryposis multiplex congenita is not a disease but is a descriptive term that signifies multiple congenital contractures. The etiologies encompass both neurogenic and primary myopathic diseases, but most cases, and indeed the most severe cases, are not due to neuromuscular disease. Myopathies that have a high incidence of either minor congenital contractures or extensive arthrogryposis include myotonic muscular dystrophy, many congenital myopathies, and intrauterine viral myositis. Neurogenic diseases causing arthrogryposis include infantile spinal muscular atrophy and the Pena-Shokeir and Marden-Walker syndromes (see later).

CHAPTER 560
Muscular Dystrophies

The term *dystrophy* means abnormal growth and is derived from the Greek *trophe* meaning nourishment. *Muscular dystrophy,* a term coined by Erb in 1891, implies much more than simply aberrant growth or nutrition of muscle fibers, however. A muscular dystrophy is distinguished from all other neuromuscular diseases by four obligatory criteria: (1) It is a primary myopathy; (2) there is a genetic basis for the disorder; (3) the course is progressive; (4) degeneration and death of muscle fibers occur at some stage in the disease. This definition excludes neurogenic diseases such as spinal muscular atrophy, nonhereditary myopathies such as dermatomyositis, nonprogressive and non-necrotizing congenital myopathies such as CMFTD, and nonprogressive inherited metabolic myopathies. Some metabolic myopathies may fulfill the definition of a progressive muscular dystrophy but are not traditionally classified as dystrophies. An example is muscle carnitine deficiency. Conversely, all muscular dystrophies might be reclassified eventually as metabolic myopathies once the biochemical defects are better defined.

Muscular dystrophies are a group of unrelated diseases, each transmitted by a different genetic trait and each differing in its clinical course and expression. Some are severe diseases at birth or lead to early death; others follow very slow progressive courses over many decades, may be compatible with normal longevity, or may not even become symptomatic until late adult life. Some categories of dystrophies, such as limb-girdle muscular dystrophy, are probably not homogeneous diseases but rather syndromes encompassing several unrelated myopathies. Relationships between the various muscular dystrophies are resolved by molecular genetics rather than by similarities or differences in clinical and histopathologic features.

560.1 Duchenne and Becker Muscular Dystrophies

Duchenne muscular dystrophy is the most common hereditary neuromuscular disease, affecting all races and ethnic groups. Its incidence is 1:3,600 liveborn male infants. This disease is inherited as an X-linked recessive trait. The abnormal gene is on the X-chromosome at the Xp21 locus and is one of the largest genes yet identified. Becker muscular dystrophy is the same fundamental disease as Duchenne dystrophy, with a genetic defect at the same locus, but clinically follows a milder and more protracted course.

Duchenne provided the first detailed description in 1861, in which he recognized most of the characteristic clinical features of the disease: hypertrophy of the calves, progressive weakness, intellectual impairment, and the proliferation of connective tissue in muscle. Not only did he study the histopathology of muscle at autopsy, but he also conceptualized the modern muscle biopsy by designing a harpoon-like biopsy needle to obtain muscle samples from living patients and a technique to minimize pain and bleeding.

CLINICAL MANIFESTATIONS. Male infants are only rarely symptomatic at birth or in early infancy, although some are already mildly hypotonic. Early gross motor skills, such as rolling over, sitting, and standing, are usually achieved at the appropriate ages or may be mildly delayed. Poor head control in infancy may be the first sign of weakness. Distinctive facies are not a feature, because facial muscle weakness is a late event. Walking is often accomplished at the normal age of about 12 mo, but hip girdle weakness may be seen in subtle form as early as the 2nd year. Toddlers may assume a lordotic posture when standing to compensate for gluteal weakness. An early **Gowers' sign** is often evident by 3 yr of age and is fully expressed by 5 or 6 yr of age (see Fig. 541–2). A **Trendelenburg gait,** or hip waddle, appears at this time.

The length of time that a patient remains ambulatory varies greatly. Some patients are confined to a wheelchair by 7 yr of age; most patients continue to walk with increasing difficulty until 10 yr of age without orthopedic intervention. With orthotic bracing, physiotherapy, and sometimes minor surgery (e.g., Achilles' tendon lengthening), most boys with Duchenne dystrophy are able to walk until 12 yr of age. Ambulation is important not only for postponing the psychological depression that accompanies the loss of an aspect of personal independence but also because scoliosis usually does not become a major complication as long as a patient remains ambulatory, even for as little as 1 hr/day; scoliosis becomes rapidly progressive after confinement to the wheelchair.

The relentless progression of weakness continues into the 2nd decade. The function of distal muscles is usually relatively well enough preserved, allowing the child to continue to use eating utensils, a pencil, and a computer keyboard. Respiratory muscle involvement is expressed as a weak and ineffective cough, frequent pulmonary infections, and decreasing respiratory reserve. Pharyngeal weakness may lead to episodes of aspiration, nasal regurgitation of liquids, and an airy or nasal voice quality. The function of the extraocular muscles remains well preserved. Incontinence due to anal and urethral sphincter weakness is an uncommon and very late event.

Contractures most often involve the ankles, knees, hips, and elbows. Scoliosis is common. The thoracic deformity further compromises pulmonary capacity and compresses the heart. Scoliosis is also uncomfortable or painful at times.

Enlargement of the calves **(pseudohypertrophy)** and wasting of thigh muscles is a classic feature. The enlargement is due to hypertrophy of some muscle fibers, infiltration of muscle by fat, and proliferation of collagen. After the calves, the next most common site of muscular hypertrophy is the tongue, followed by muscles of the forearm. Fasciculations of the tongue do not occur.

Unless ankle contractures are severe, ankle jerks remain well preserved until terminal stages. The knee jerks may be present until about 6 yr of age but are less brisk than the ankle jerks and are eventually lost. In the upper extremities, the brachioradialis reflex is usually stronger than the biceps or triceps brachii reflexes.

Cardiomyopathy is a constant feature of this disease. The severity of cardiac involvement does not necessarily correlate with the degree of skeletal muscle weakness. Some patients die early of severe cardiomyopathy while still ambulatory; others in terminal stages of the disease have well compensated cardiac function.

Intellectual impairment occurs in all patients, although only 20–30% have an intelligence quotient (IQ) less than 70. The majority have learning disabilities that still allow them to function in a regular classroom, particularly if remedial help is available. A few patients are profoundly mentally retarded, but there is no correlation with the severity of the myopathy. Epilepsy is slightly more common than in the general pediatric population.

The degenerative changes and fibrosis of muscle constitute a painless process. Myalgias and muscle spasms do not occur. Calcinosis of muscle is rare.

Death occurs usually at about 18 yr of age. The causes of death are respiratory failure in sleep, intractable congestive heart failure, pneumonia, or occasionally aspiration and airway obstruction.

In Becker muscular dystrophy, boys remain ambulatory until late adolescence or early adult life. Calf pseudohypertrophy, cardiomyopathy, and elevated serum CK are similar to Duchenne dystrophy. Learning disabilities are less frequent. The onset of weakness is later in Becker than in Duchenne disease. Death often occurs in the mid- to late 20s; fewer than half of patients are still alive by 40 yr of age, and these survivors are severely disabled.

LABORATORY FINDINGS. The serum CK is consistently greatly elevated in Duchenne muscular dystrophy, even in presymptomatic stages, including at birth. The usual serum concentration is 15,000–35,000 IU/L (normal <160 IU/L). A normal serum CK is incompatible with the diagnosis of Duchenne dystrophy, although in terminal stages of the disease the serum CK may be considerably lower than it was a few years earlier, because there is less muscle to degenerate. Other lysosomal enzymes present in muscle, such as aldolase and AST, are also increased but are less specific.

Cardiac assessment by electrocardiogram (ECG) and chest roentgenogram are essential and should be repeated periodically. After the diagnosis is established, the patient should be referred to a pediatric cardiologist for long-term cardiac care.

Electromyogram (EMG) shows characteristic myopathic features but is not specific for Duchenne muscular dystrophy. No evidence of denervation is found. Motor and sensory nerve conduction velocities are normal.

DIAGNOSIS. The muscle biopsy is diagnostic and shows characteristic changes (Figs. 560–1 and 560–2). Myopathic changes include endomysial connective tissue proliferation, scattered degenerating and regenerating myofibers, foci of mononuclear inflammatory cell infiltrates as a reaction to muscle fiber necrosis, mild architectural changes in still functional muscle fibers, and many dense fibers. These hypercontracted fibers

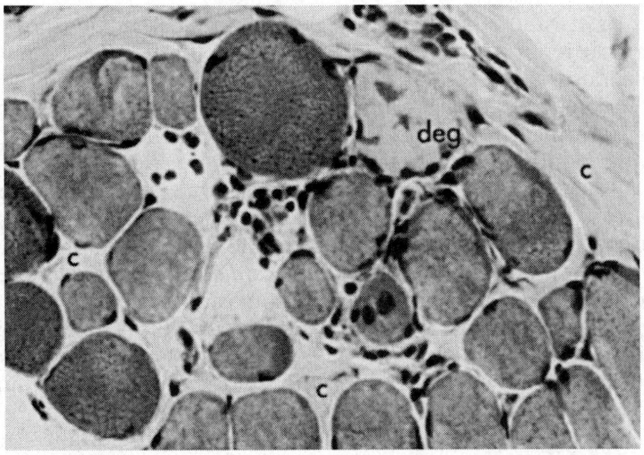

Figure 560–1. Muscle biopsy of 4-yr-old boy with Duchenne muscular dystrophy. Both atrophic and hypertrophic muscle fibers are seen, and some fibers are degenerating *(deg)*. Connective tissue (c) between muscle fibers is increased. (Hematoxylin & eosin, ×400.)

probably result from segmental necrosis at another level, allowing calcium to enter the site of breakdown of the sarcolemmal membrane and trigger a contraction of the whole length of the muscle fiber.

The decision of whether muscle biopsy should be performed to establish the diagnosis sometimes presents problems. If there is a family history of the disease, particularly in the case of an involved brother whose diagnosis has been confirmed, a patient with typical clinical features of Duchenne muscular dystrophy and high concentrations of serum CK probably does not need to undergo biopsy. A first case in a family, even if the clinical features are typical, should have the diagnosis confirmed to ensure that another myopathy is not masquerading as Duchenne dystrophy. The most common muscles sampled are the vastus lateralis (quadriceps femoris) and the gastrocnemius.

A specific molecular genetic diagnosis is now possible by demonstrating deficient or defective dystrophin by immunohistochemical staining of sections of muscle biopsy tissue or by DNA analysis from peripheral blood (see later). Confirmation of the diagnosis by one of these methods should be done in every case.

GENETIC ETIOLOGY AND PATHOGENESIS. Despite the X-linked recessive inheritance in Duchenne muscular dystrophy, about 30% of patients are new mutations and the mother is not a carrier. The female carrier state usually shows no muscle weakness or any clinical expression of the disease, but affected girls are occasionally encountered, usually having much milder weakness than boys. These symptomatic girls are explained by the Lyon hypothesis in which the normal X chromosome becomes inactivated and the one with the gene deletion is active (see Chapter 66). The full clinical picture of Duchenne dystrophy has occurred in several girls with Turner syndrome in whom the single X chromosome must have had the Xp21 gene deletion.

The asymptomatic carrier state is associated with elevated serum CK in 80% of cases. The level of increase is usually in the magnitude of hundreds or a few thousand but does not have the extreme values seen in affected males. Prepubertal girls who are Duchenne carriers also have increased serum CK, with highest levels at 8–12 yr of age. Approximately 20% of Duchenne carriers have normal serum CK. If the mother of an affected boy has a normal CK, it is unlikely that her daughter can be identified as a carrier by measuring CK. Muscle biopsy of suspected female carriers may detect an additional 10% in whom serum CK is not elevated; only a specific genetic diagnosis using PCR on peripheral blood is definitive.

Detection of the carrier state by serum CK or muscle biopsy will probably become obsolete because of recent discoveries in the molecular genetics of Duchenne muscular dystrophy. The Xp21 site of the Duchenne gene was previously recognized from translocations. The gene has more than 2,000 kilobases

Figure 560–2. Dystrophin is demonstrated by immunohistochemical reactivity in the muscle biopsies of *(A)* a normal term male neonate; *(B)* a 10-year-old boy with limb-girdle muscular dystrophy; *(C)* a 6-year-old boy with Duchenne muscular dystrophy; and *(D)* a 10-year-old boy with Becker muscular dystrophy. In the normal condition and also in non–X-linked muscular dystrophies in which dystrophin is not affected, the sacrolemmal membrane of every fiber is strongly stained, including atrophic and hypertrophic fibers. In Duchenne dystrophy, most myofibers express no detectable dystrophin, but a few scattered fibers known as "revertant fibers" show near-normal immunoreactivity. In Becker muscular dystrophy, the abnormal dystrophin molecule is expressed as thin, pale staining of the sarcolemma in which reactivity varies not only between myofibers but also along the circumference of individual fibers (X250).

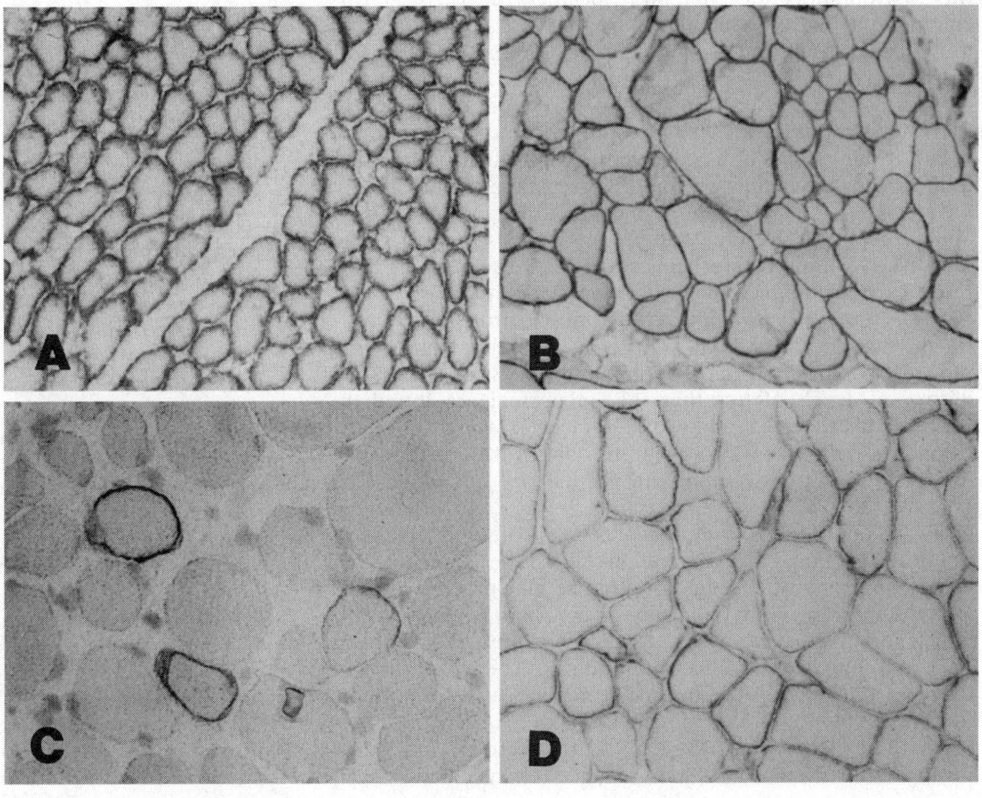

(kb) (2 million base pairs), but Duchenne DNA encompasses only 14 kb; less than 1% of the total genomic DNA is eventually transcribed into protein. Cloning of the breakpoint of the Xp21 gene has subsequently been accomplished, and the entire sequence of the gene has been mapped.

A 427 kD cytoskeletal protein known as *dystrophin* is encoded by a large gene at the Xp21.2 locus. This subsarcolemmal protein attaches to the sarcolemmal membrane overlying the A band and M band of the myofibrils and consists of four distinct regions or domains: the N-terminus contains 250 amino acids and is related to the N-actin binding site of alpha-actinin; the second domain is the largest, with 2,800 amino acids, and contains many repeats giving it a characteristic rod shape; a third cysteine-rich domain is related to the C-terminus of alpha-actinin; and the final C-terminus domain of 400 amino acids is unique to dystrophin and to a dystrophin-related protein encoded by chromosome 6. Dystrophin is first detected in developing human fetal muscle at 11 wk gestation. Dystrophin mRNA normally is detected in cardiac and smooth muscle as well as in skeletal muscle and brain. All of these tissues show various degrees of clinical involvement.

The dystrophin gene encodes a 14 kb mRNA of about 80 exons. The molecular defects in the dystrophinopathies are of various types: intragenic deletions, duplications, or point mutations of nucleotides. About 65% of patients have deletions and only 7% exhibit duplications. The site or size of the intragenic abnormality does not always correlate well with the phenotypic severity, though in both Duchenne and Becker forms the mutations are mainly near the middle of the gene, involving deletions of exons 46–51. Phenotypic or clinical variations are explained by the alteration of the translational reading frame of mRNA, which results in unstable, truncated dystrophin molecules and severe, classical Duchenne dystrophy; mutations that preserve the reading frame still permit the translation of coding sequences further downstream on the gene and produce a semifunctional dystrophin, expressed clinically as Becker muscular dystrophy. An even milder form of adult onset, formerly known as *quadriceps myopathy,* is also due to an abnormal dystrophin molecule. The clinical spectrum of the dystrophinopathies not only includes the classical Duchenne and Becker forms but ranges from a severe neonatal muscular dystrophy to asymptomatic children with persistent elevation of serum CK greater than 1,000 IU/l.

The absence of dystrophin leads to a secondary reduction in several dystrophin-associated glycoproteins in the sarcolemma, which results in loss of linkage to the extracellular matrix and renders the sarcolemma even more susceptible to necrosis.

Analysis of the dystrophin protein requires a muscle biopsy and is demonstrated by Western blot analysis or in tissue sections by immunohistochemical methods using either fluorescence or light microscopy of antidystrophin antisera (Fig. 560–2). In the Western blot method, muscle proteins are separated by molecular weight, transferred to nitrocellulose, and probed with antidystrophin antibodies. In classical Duchenne dystrophy, levels of less than 3% of normal are found; in Becker muscular dystrophy, the molecular weight of dystrophin is reduced to 20–90% of normal in 80% of patients, but in 15% the dystrophin is of normal size but reduced in quantity, and 5% have an abnormally large protein due to excessive duplications or repeats of codons. The demonstration of these deletions and duplications also can be made from blood samples by the lengthy Southern blot process of DNA analysis or by the more rapid polymerase chain reaction (PCR), which identifies as many as 98% of deletions by amplifying 18 exons but cannot detect duplications. The diagnosis can thus be confirmed at the molecular genetic level from either the muscle biopsy or from peripheral blood.

The same methods of DNA analysis from blood samples may be applied for carrier detection in female relatives at risk, such as sisters and cousins, and to determine whether the mother is a carrier or a new mutation occurred in the embryo. Prenatal diagnosis is possible as early as 12 wk gestation by sampling chorionic villi for DNA analysis by Southern blot or PCR, and is confirmed in aborted fetuses with Duchenne dystrophy by immunohistochemistry for dystrophin in muscle.

TREATMENT. There is presently neither a medical cure for this disease nor a method of slowing its progression. Nevertheless, much can be done to treat complications and to improve the quality of life of affected children. *Cardiac decompensation* often responds well to digoxin, at least in early stages. *Pulmonary infections* should be promptly treated. Patients should avoid contact with children who have obvious respiratory or other contagious illnesses. Immunizations for influenza virus and routine vaccinations are indicated.

Preservation of a good *nutritional state* is important. Duchenne muscular dystrophy is not a vitamin deficiency disease, and excessive doses of vitamins should be avoided. Adequate calcium intake is important to minimize osteoporosis in boys confined to the wheelchair, and fluoride supplements may also be given, particularly if the local drinking water is not fluoridated. Because sedentary children burn fewer calories than active children and because of depression as an additional factor, these children tend to eat excessively and gain weight. Obesity makes a patient with myopathy even less functional because part of the limited reserve muscle strength is dissipated in lifting the weight of excess subcutaneous adipose tissue. Dietary restrictions with supervision may be needed.

Physiotherapy delays but does not always prevent contractures. At times, contractures may actually be useful to functional rehabilitation. For example, if contractures prevent extension of the elbow beyond 90 degrees and the muscles of the upper limb no longer are strong enough to overcome gravity, the elbow contractures are functionally beneficial in fixing an otherwise flail arm and in allowing the patient to eat and write. The surgical correction of the elbow contracture may be technically feasible, but the result may be deleterious. Physiotherapy contributes little to muscle strengthening because the patient usually is already using his or her entire reserve for daily function, and exercise cannot further strengthen involved muscles. Excessive exercise may actually accelerate the process of muscle fiber degeneration.

The discovery of the dystrophin molecule, the gene encoding it, and the specific mutations in Duchenne and Becker muscular dystrophies raises the theoretical potential of a cure by molecular genetic engineering. One experimental approach is *myoblast transfer therapy.* Normal myoblasts from the muscle of a genetically close relative, usually the father, are cultured in vitro and then injected into dystrophic muscles with the expectation that they will form healthy myofibers with normal dystrophin to replace degenerating fibers. A major drawback is the requirement for immunosuppression to prevent rejection of the foreign cells. Another approach is the introduction by intramuscular injection of a recombinant dystrophin gene ligated to an appropriate promotor. A third promising strategy is the use of retroviruses, with viral DNA incorporating the deleted nucleotide sequences of the dystrophin gene that might be able to enter postmitotic muscle cells with the DNA insert. This method has had some success in the treatment of the *mdx* mouse model of Duchenne muscular dystrophy.

Other investigational treatment of human patients with Duchenne dystrophy involves the use of *prednisone or other steroids.* Glucocorticoids decrease the rate of apoptosis or programmed cell death of myotubes during ontogenesis and theoretically may decelerate the myofiber necrosis in muscular dystrophy. Strength usually improves initially, but the long-term complications of chronic steroid therapy, including considerable weight gain and osteoporosis, may offset this advantage or even result in greater weakness than might have occurred in the natural course of the disease.

560.2 Emery-Dreifuss Muscular Dystrophy

Emery-Dreifuss muscular dystrophy, also known as *scapuloperoneal* or *scapulohumeral muscular dystrophy,* is another X-linked recessive dystrophy, but the gene has not been isolated. Unlike Duchenne and Becker muscular dystrophies, it is rare. The locus is on the long arm, within the large Xq28 gene that includes other mutations that cause myotubular myopathy, neonatal adrenoleukodystrophy, and the Bloch-Sulzberger type of incontinentia pigmenti; it is far from the Duchenne muscular dystrophy gene on the short arm of the X chromosome.

Clinical manifestations begin in middle childhood, but many patients survive to late adult life because of the slow progression of its course. Hypertrophy of muscles does not occur. Contractures of elbows and ankles develop early, and muscle becomes wasted in a scapulohumeroperoneal distribution. Facial weakness does not occur, distinguishing this disease clinically from autosomal dominant scapulohumeral and scapuloperoneal syndromes of neurogenic origin. Myotonia is absent. Intellectual function is normal. Cardiomyopathy is severe and is often the cause of death. The serum CK is only mildly elevated, further distinguishing this disease from other X-linked recessive muscular dystrophies.

Nonspecific myofiber necrosis and endomysial fibrosis are seen in the muscle biopsy. Many centronuclear fibers and selective histochemical type I muscle fiber atrophy may cause confusion with myotonic dystrophy. Treatment should be supportive.

560.3 Myotonic Muscular Dystrophy

Myotonic dystrophy **(Steinert disease)** is the second most common muscular dystrophy in North America, Europe, and Australia, having an incidence of 1:30,000 general population. It is inherited as an autosomal dominant trait.

Myotonic dystrophy is an example of a genetic defect causing dysfunction in multiple organ systems. Not only is striated muscle severely affected, but smooth muscle of the alimentary tract and uterus is also involved; cardiac function is altered; and patients have multiple and variable endocrinopathies, immunologic deficiencies, cataracts, dysmorphic facies, intellectual impairment, and other neurologic abnormalities.

CLINICAL MANIFESTATIONS. In the usual clinical course, excluding the severe neonatal form, infants may appear almost normal at birth, or facial wasting and hypotonia may already be early expressions of the disease. The facial appearance is characteristic, consisting of an inverted V-shaped upper lip, thin cheeks, and scalloped, concave temporalis muscles (Fig. 560–3). The head may be narrow, and the palate is high and arched because the weak temporal and pterygoid muscles in late fetal life do not exert sufficient lateral forces on the developing head and face.

Weakness is mild in the first few years. Progressive wasting of distal muscles becomes increasingly evident, particularly involving intrinsic muscles of the hands. The thenar and hypothenar eminences are flattened, and the atrophic dorsal interossei leave deep grooves between the fingers. The dorsal forearm muscles and anterior compartment muscles of the lower legs also become wasted. The tongue is thin and atrophic. Wasting of the sternocleidomastoids gives the neck a long, thin, cylindrical contour. Eventually, proximal muscles also undergo atrophy, and scapular winging appears. Difficulty

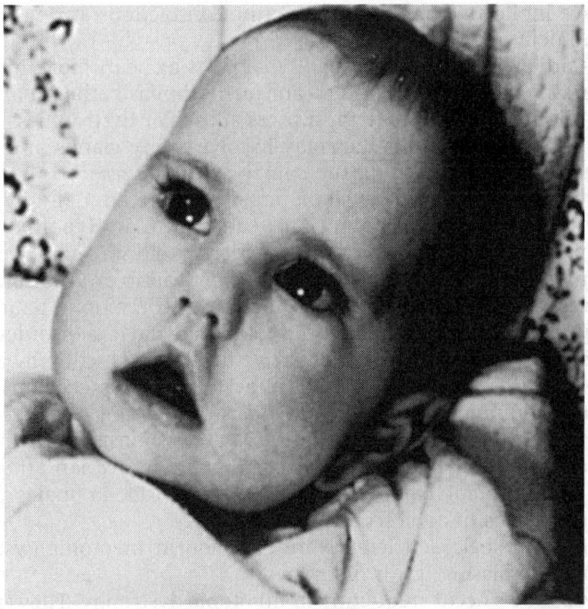

Figure 560–3. Facial weakness, inverted V-shaped upper lip, and loss of muscle mass in the temporal fossae are characteristic of myotonic muscular dystrophy, even in infancy, as seen in this 8-mo-old girl.

with climbing stairs and Gower sign are progressive. Tendon stretch reflexes are usually preserved.

The distal distribution of muscle wasting in myotonic dystrophy is an exception to the general rule of myopathies having proximal and neuropathies distal distribution patterns. The muscular atrophy and weakness in myotonic dystrophy are slowly progressive throughout childhood and adolescence and continue into adulthood. It is rare for patients with myotonic dystrophy to lose the ability to walk, however, even in late adult life, although splints or bracing may be required to stabilize the ankles.

Myotonia, a characteristic feature shared by few other myopathies, does not occur in infancy and is usually not clinically or even electromyographically evident until about 5 yr of age. Exceptional patients develop it as early as 3 yr of age. Myotonia is a very slow relaxation of muscle after contraction, regardless of whether that contraction was voluntary or was induced by a stretch reflex or electrical stimulation. During the physical examination, myotonia may be demonstrated by asking the patient to make tight fists and then to quickly open the hands. It may be induced by striking the thenar eminence with a rubber percussion hammer, and it may be detected by watching the involuntary drawing of the thumb across the palm. Myotonia may also be demonstrated in the tongue by pressing the edge of a wooden tongue blade against its dorsal surface and by observing a deep furrow that disappears slowly.

The severity of myotonia does not necessarily parallel the degree of weakness, and the weakest muscles often have only minimal myotonia. Myotonia is not a painful muscle spasm. Myalgias do not occur in myotonic dystrophy.

The speech of patients with myotonic dystrophy is often articulated poorly and is slurred because of the involvement of the muscles of the face, tongue, and pharynx. Difficulties with swallowing sometimes occur. Aspiration pneumonia is a risk in severely involved children. Incomplete external ophthalmoplegia may sometimes result from extraocular muscle weakness.

Smooth muscle involvement of the gastrointestinal tract results in slow gastric emptying, poor peristalsis, and constipation. Some patients have encopresis associated with anal sphincter weakness. Women with myotonic dystrophy may have ineffective or abnormal uterine contractions during labor and delivery.

Cardiac involvement usually manifests as heart block in the Purkinje conduction system and arrhythmias rather than as cardiomyopathy, unlike most other muscular dystrophies.

Endocrine abnormalities may involve many glands and appear at any time during the course of the disease, so that re-evaluation of endocrine status must be done annually in the first few years and every several years after that. Hypothyroidism is commonly associated; hyperthyroidism may occur rarely. Adrenocortical insufficiency may lead to an Addisonian crisis, even in infancy. Diabetes mellitus is common in patients with myotonic dystrophy; some children have a disorder of insulin release rather than defective insulin production by islet cells of the pancreas. Onset of puberty may be precocious or, more commonly, delayed. Testicular atrophy and testosterone deficiency are common in adults and are responsible for a high incidence of male infertility. A corresponding ovarian atrophy is rare. Frontal baldness is also characteristic in males and often begins in adolescence.

Immunologic deficiencies are common in myotonic dystrophy. The plasma IgG is often low.

Cataracts occur frequently in myotonic dystrophy. They may be congenital or they may begin at any time during childhood or adult life. Early cataracts are detected only by slit lamp examination, and periodic examination by an ophthalmologist is recommended. Visual evoked potentials are often abnormal in children with myotonic dystrophy and are unrelated to cataracts. They are not usually accompanied by visual impairment, however.

About half of the patients with myotonic dystrophy are intellectually impaired, but severe mental retardation is unusual. The remainder are of average or occasionally above average intelligence. Epilepsy is not common.

A **severe neonatal form of myotonic dystrophy** appears in a minority of involved infants born to mothers with myotonic dystrophy. Clubfoot deformities alone or more extensive congenital contractures of multiple joints may involve all extremities and even the cervical spine. Generalized hypotonia and weakness are present at birth. Some infants require gavage feeding or even ventilator support for respiratory muscle weakness or apnea. One or both leaves of the diaphragm may be nonfunctional. The abdomen becomes distended with gas in the stomach and intestine because of poor peristalsis due to smooth muscle weakness. The distention further compromises respiration. Inability to empty the rectum may compound the problem. About 75% of severely affected neonates die within the 1st year.

LABORATORY FINDINGS. The classic myotonic EMG is not found in infancy but may appear in toddlers or during the early school years. The serum CK and other serum enzymes from muscle may be normal or only mildly elevated in the hundreds (never the thousands).

An ECG should be performed annually in early childhood. Ultrasonic imaging of the abdomen may be indicated in affected infants to determine diaphragmatic function. Roentgenograms of the chest and abdomen and contrast studies of gastrointestinal motility may be needed.

Endocrine assessment should be undertaken to determine thyroid and adrenal cortical function and to verify carbohydrate metabolism (e.g., glucose tolerance test with serum insulin levels). Immunoglobulins should be examined, and more extensive immunologic studies should be performed if needed.

DIAGNOSIS. The muscle biopsy often shows many muscle fibers with central nuclei and selective atrophy of histochemical type I fibers, but degenerating fibers are usually few and widely scattered, and there is little or no fibrosis of muscle. Intrafusal fibers of muscle spindles are also abnormal. In young children with the common form of the disease, the biopsy may even appear normal or may at least not show myofiber necroses, which is a striking contrast with Duchenne muscular dystrophy. In the severe neonatal form of myotonic dystrophy, the muscle biopsy reveals maturational arrest in various stages of development. It is likely that the sarcolemmal membrane of muscle fibers not only has abnormal properties of electrical polarization but is also incapable of responding to trophic influences of the motor neuron. Muscle biopsy is not usually required for diagnosis, which in typical cases can be based on the clinical manifestations. It is recommended in severe neonatal cases because the biopsy may be of prognostic as well as of diagnostic value. Molecular genetic diagnosis from a blood sample and prenatal diagnosis are now possible.

GENETICS. The genetic defect in myotonic muscular dystrophy is on chromosome 19 at the 19q13 locus. It consists of an expansion of the gene rather than a deletion, with numerous repeats of the cytosine-thymine-guanine (CTG) codon. Rarely, the disease is associated with no detectable repeats, perhaps a spontaneous correction of a previous expansion but a phenomenon still incompletely understood. Both clinical and genetic expressivity may vary within a sibship or between an affected parent and child. In the severe neonatal form of the disease, the mother is the transmitting parent in 94% of cases, a fact not explained by increased male infertility alone. An additional maternal hormonal factor affecting the fetus had been suspected, but genetic analysis reveals that such infants usually have many more repeats of the CTG codon than do patients with the more typical form of the disease. This still does not explain why maternal DNA is less stable than paternal in this disease. Myotonic dystrophy often exhibits a pattern of *anticipation,* in which each successive generation has a tendency to be more severely involved than the previous generation.

TREATMENT. There is no specific medical treatment, but the cardiac, endocrine, gastrointestinal, and ocular complications can often be treated. Physiotherapy and orthopedic treatment of contractures in the neonatal form of the disease may be beneficial.

Myotonia may be diminished and function may be restored by drugs that raise the depolarization threshold of muscle membranes, such as phenytoin (PHT), carbamazepine (CBZ), procainamide, and quinidine sulfate. These drugs also have cardiotropic effects, thus cardiac evaluation is important before prescribing them. PHT and CBZ are used in doses similar to their use as anticonvulsants (see Chapter 543.4); serum concentrations of 40–80 μmol/L for PHT and 35–50 μmol/L for CBZ should be maintained. If the patient's disability is due mainly to weakness rather than to myotonia, these drugs will be of no value.

OTHER MYOTONIC SYNDROMES

Most patients with myotonia have myotonic dystrophy. However, myotonia is not specific for this disease and occurs in several rarer conditions.

Myotonic chondrodystrophy **(Schwartz-Jampel disease)** is a rare congenital disease characterized by generalized muscular hypertrophy and weakness. Dysmorphic phenotypical features and the roentgenographic appearance of long bones are reminiscent of Morquio disease (see Chapter 74), but abnormal mucopolysaccharides are not found. Dwarfism, joint abnormalities, and blepharophimosis are present. Several patients have been the products of consanguinity, suggesting autosomal recessive inheritance.

EMG reveals continuous electrical activity in muscle fibers closely resembling or identical to myotonia. Muscle biopsy reveals nonspecific myopathic features, which are minimal in some cases and pronounced in others. The sarcotubular system is dilated.

Myotonia congenita **(Thomsen disease)** was first described by Thomsen in 1876 in his own family. It is characterized by generalized muscular hypertrophy, so that affected children resemble body builders, but the large muscles are weak. Myotonia is prominent and may develop at 2–3 yr of age, earlier than in myotonic dystrophy. The disease is clinically stable and is apparently not progressive for many years. The muscle biopsy shows minimal pathologic changes, and the EMG demonstrates myotonia. Various families are described showing either autosomal dominant or recessive inheritance. Rarely, myotonic dystrophy and myotonia congenita coexist in the same family. Autosomal dominant myotonia congenita has been mapped to the 7q35 locus.

Paramyotonia is a temperature-related myotonia that is aggravated by cold and alleviated by warm external temperatures. Patients have difficulty when swimming in cold water or if they are dressed inadequately in cold weather. Paramyotonia congenita is a defect in a gene at the 17q13.1–13.3 locus, the identical locus identified in hyperkalemic periodic paralysis.

560.4 Limb-Girdle Muscular Dystrophy

This term encompasses a group of progressive hereditary myopathies that mainly affect muscles of the hip and shoulder girdles. Eventually, distal muscles also become atrophic and weak. Hypertrophy of the calves and ankle contractures develop in some forms (Fig. 560–4), causing potential confusion with Becker muscular dystrophy.

The initial symptoms and signs rarely appear before middle or late childhood or may be deferred until early adult life. Low back pain may be a presenting complaint because of the lordotic posture resulting from gluteal muscle weakness. Confinement to a wheelchair does not usually become obligatory until about 30 yr of age. The rate of progression varies from one pedigree to another but is uniform within a kindred. Although weakness of neck flexors and extensors is universal, facial, lingual, and other bulbar-innervated muscles rarely are clinically involved. As weakness and muscle wasting progress, tendon stretch reflexes become diminished. Cardiac involvement is unusual. Intellectual function is generally normal. The clinical differential diagnosis of limb-girdle muscular dystrophy includes juvenile spinal muscular atrophy **(Kugelberg-Welander disease)**, myasthenia gravis, and metabolic myopathies.

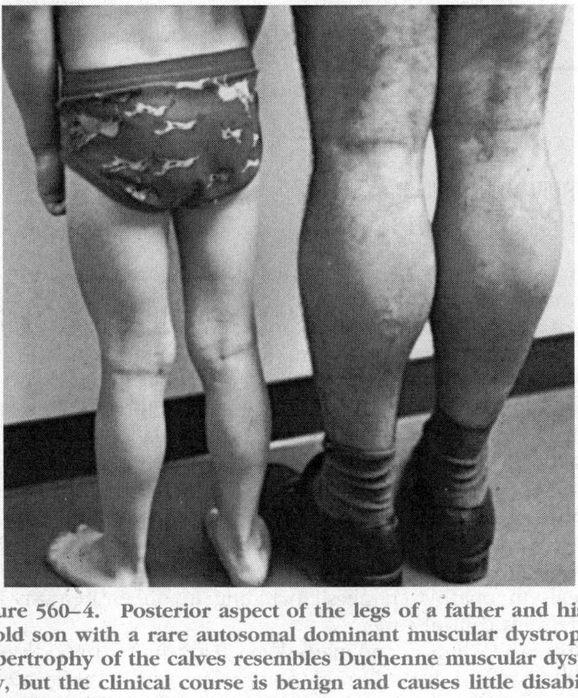

Figure 560–4. Posterior aspect of the legs of a father and his 6-yr-old son with a rare autosomal dominant muscular dystrophy. Hypertrophy of the calves resembles Duchenne muscular dystrophy, but the clinical course is benign and causes little disability throughout life.

Most cases of limb-girdle muscular dystrophy are of autosomal recessive inheritance, but some families express an autosomal dominant trait. The latter often follows a benign course with little functional impairment (see Fig. 560–4).

The EMG and muscle biopsy show confirmatory evidence of muscular dystrophy, but none of the findings are specific enough to make the definitive diagnosis without additional clinical criteria. Increased serum CK is usual, but the magnitude of elevation varies among families. The ECG is usually unaltered.

In the autosomal dominant form of limb-girdle muscular dystrophy, a genetic defect has been localized to the long arm of chromosome 5. In the autosomal recessive disease, it is on the long arm of chromosome 15.

560.5 Facioscapulohumeral Muscular Dystrophy

Facioscapulohumeral (FSH) muscular dystrophy, also known as **Landouzy-Déjerine disease,** is probably not a single disease entity but a group of diseases with similar clinical manifestations. Autosomal dominance is the rule, and the phenomenon of *anticipation* is often seen within several generations of a family, the succeeding more severely involved at an earlier age than the preceding. The genetic defect in autosomal dominant FSH muscular dystrophy is at the 4q35 locus.

CLINICAL MANIFESTATIONS. As the name implies, FSH dystrophy shows the earliest and most severe weakness in facial and shoulder girdle muscles. The facial weakness differs from that of myotonic dystrophy; rather than an inverted V-shaped upper lip, the mouth in FSH dystrophy is rounded and appears puckered because the upper and lower lips protrude. Inability to close the eyes completely in sleep is a common expression of upper facial weakness, and some patients have extraocular muscle weakness, although ophthalmoplegia is rarely complete. FSH dystrophy has been reported in association with Möbius syndrome on rare occasions. Pharyngeal and tongue weakness may be absent and are never as severe as the facial involvement. Hearing loss and retinal vasculopathy are associated features, particularly in cases of FSH dystrophy with early childhood onset of clinical myopathy.

Scapular winging is prominent, often even in infants. Flattening or even concavity of the deltoid contour is seen and the biceps and triceps brachii muscles are wasted and weak. Muscles of the hip girdles and thighs also eventually lose strength and undergo atrophy, and Gower sign and a Trendelenburg gait appear. Contractures are rare, however. Occasionally, finger and wrist weakness is the first symptom recognized by the patient with FSH muscular dystrophy. Weakness of the anterior tibial and peroneal muscles may lead to foot drop, but this complication usually occurs only in advanced cases with severe proximal weakness. Lumbar lordosis and kyphoscoliosis are common complications of axial muscle involvement. Calf hypertrophy is not a feature.

FSH muscular dystrophy may be a mild disease causing minimal disability in some cases. At times, clinical manifestations may not even be expressed in childhood and are delayed into middle adult life. Unlike most other muscular dystrophies, asymmetry of weakness is common.

LABORATORY FINDINGS. Serum CK and other enzymes vary greatly, ranging from normal or near-normal to elevations of several thousand. ECG should be performed, although the anticipated findings are usually normal. EMG reveals nonspecific myopathic muscle potentials.

DIAGNOSIS AND DIFFERENTIAL DIAGNOSIS. The muscle biopsy distinguishes more than one form of FSH, consistent with clinical evidence that several distinct diseases are embraced by the term *FSH dystrophy.* Muscle biopsy and EMG also distinguish the primary myopathy from a neurogenic disease with a similar distribution of muscular involvement. The general histopathologic findings in the muscle biopsy are extensive proliferation of connective tissue between muscle fibers, extreme variation in fiber size with many hypertrophic as well as atrophic myofibers, and scattered degenerating and regenerating fibers. An "inflammatory" type FSH muscular dystrophy is also distinguished, characterized by extensive lymphocytic infiltrates within muscle fascicles. Despite the resemblance of this form to true inflammatory myopathies, such as polymyositis, there is no evidence of autoimmune disease, and steroids and immunosuppressive drugs do not alter the clinical course. A precise histopathologic diagnosis, therefore, has important therapeutic implications. Mononuclear cell "inflammation" in a muscle biopsy of infants less than 2 yr of age is usually FSH dystrophy.

TREATMENT. Physiotherapy is of no value in regaining strength or in retarding progressive weakness or muscle wasting. Foot drop and scoliosis may be treated by orthopedic measures. Cosmetic improvement of the facial muscles of expression may be achieved by reconstructive surgery, which grafts a fascia lata to the zygomatic muscle and to the zygomatic head of the *quadratus labiae superioris* muscle.

560.6 Congenital Muscular Dystrophy

The term *congenital* muscular dystrophy is misleading because all muscular dystrophies are genetically determined, hence congenital, diseases. It is used to encompass several distinct diseases with a common characteristic of severe involvement at birth but that ironically usually follow a benign clinical course. Autosomal recessive inheritance is the rule in each.

CLINICAL MANIFESTATIONS. Infants often have contractures or arthrogryposis at birth and are diffusely hypotonic. The muscle mass is thin in the trunk and extremities. Head control is poor. Facial muscles may be mildly involved, but ophthalmoplegia, pharyngeal weakness, and a weak suck are not common. Tendon stretch reflexes may be hypoactive or absent. Arthrogryposis is common in all forms of congenital muscular dystrophy (see Chapter 559.8).

One form of congenital muscular dystrophy, the **Fukuyama type,** is the 2nd most common muscular dystrophy in Japan (following Duchenne dystrophy), but this disease has also been reported in children of Dutch, German, Scandinavian, and Turkish ethnic backgrounds and therefore is not limited to the Japanese. In the Fukuyama variety, severe cardiomyopathy and malformations of the brain usually accompany the skeletal muscle involvement. Signs and symptoms related to these organs are prominent: cardiomegaly and congestive failure, mental retardation, seizures, microcephaly, and failure to thrive. The genetic defect in Fukuyama congenital muscular dystrophy has been identified at the 8q31–33 locus in Japanese patients. The genetic relationship to non-Japanese congenital muscular dystrophies is not yet established.

Neurologic disease may accompany forms of congenital muscular dystrophy other than Fukuyama disease. Mental and neurologic status are the most variable features, and an apparently normal brain and normal intelligence do not preclude the diagnosis if other manifestations indicate this myopathy. The cerebral malformations that occur are not consistently of one type and vary from severe dysplasias (e.g., holoprosencephaly or lissencephaly) to milder conditions (e.g., agenesis of the corpus callosum, focal heterotopia of the cerebral cortex and subcortical white matter, and cerebellar hypoplasia). Congenital muscular dystrophy is a consistent association with cerebral dysgenesis in the **Walker-Warburg syndrome** and in **muscle-eye-brain disease of Santavuori.** The neuropathologic findings are those of neuroblast migratory abnormalities in the cerebral cortex, cerebellum, and brain stem.

LABORATORY FINDINGS. Serum CK is usually moderately elevated from several hundred to many thousand IU/L, but only marginal increases are sometimes found. EMG shows nonspecific myopathic features. Investigation of all forms of congenital muscular dystrophy should include cardiac assessment and an imaging study of the brain.

DIAGNOSIS. The muscle biopsy is diagnostic in the neonatal period or thereafter. An extensive proliferation of endomysial collagen envelops individual muscle fibers even at birth, also causing them to be rounded in cross-sectional contour by acting as a rigid sleeve, especially during contraction. The perimysial connective tissue and fat are also increased, and the fascicular organization of the muscle may be disrupted by the fibrosis. Tissue cultures of intramuscular fibroblasts exhibit increased collagen synthesis, but the structure of the collagen is normal. Muscle fibers vary in diameter, and many show central nuclei, myofibrillar splitting, and other cytoarchitectural alterations. Scattered degenerating and regenerating fibers are seen. No inflammation or abnormal inclusions are found.

Chapter 561

Endocrine Myopathies

THYROID MYOPATHIES

(See also Part XXVI, Section 2.)

Thyrotoxicosis causes proximal weakness and wasting accompanied by myopathic electromyogram (EMG) changes. Thyroxine binds to myofibrils, and an excess impairs contractile function. Hyperthyroidism may also induce myasthenia gravis and hypokalemic periodic paralysis (see later).

Hypothyroidism, whether congenital or acquired, consistently produces hypotonia and a proximal distribution of weakness. Although muscle wasting is most characteristic, one form of cretinism, the **Kocher-Debré-Sémélaigne syndrome,** is characterized by hypertrophy of weak muscles. The serum CK is elevated in hypothyroid myopathy and returns to normal after thyroid replacement therapy. The muscle biopsy reveals myopathic changes, including myofiber necrosis and sometimes central cores.

Both the clinical and pathologic features of hyperthyroid myopathy and hypothyroid myopathy resolve after appropriate treatment of the thyroid disorder.

HYPERPARATHYROIDISM

(See also Chapter 527.)

Most patients with primary hyperparathyroidism develop weakness, fatigability, and muscle wasting that are reversible after the removal of the parathyroid adenoma.

STEROID-INDUCED MYOPATHY

Both natural **Cushing's disease** and the iatrogenic **Cushing syndrome** from exogenous corticosteroid administration may cause progressive proximal weakness, increased serum CK, and a myopathic EMG and muscle biopsy (see Chapter 530). Myosin filaments may be selectively lost. Fluorinated steroids, such as dexamethasone, are the most likely to produce *steroid myopathy.* In patients with dermatomyositis or other myopathies treated with steroids, it is sometimes difficult to distinguish refractoriness of the disease from steroid-induced weakness, especially after the chronic administration of these drugs.

Hyperaldosteronism (Conn syndrome) is accompanied by episodic and reversible weakness similar to that of periodic paralysis (see later). The proximal myopathy may become irreversible in chronic cases. Elevated CK and even myoglobinuria sometimes occur during acute attacks.

CHAPTER 562
Metabolic Myopathies

562.1 Potassium-Related Periodic Paralysis

Episodic weakness or paralysis known as *periodic paralysis* is associated with transient alterations in serum potassium, usually hypokalemia but occasionally hyperkalemia. The disorder is inherited as an autosomal dominant trait. It is precipitated in some patients by hyperaldosteronism or hyperthyroidism, by amphotericin B, or by ingestion of licorice. The defective genes are at the 17q13.1–13.3 locus in hyperkalemic periodic paralysis, the same as in paramyotonia congenita, and at the 1q31–32 locus in hypokalemic periodic paralysis.

In childhood, periodic paralysis often occurs as an episodic event, the patient being unable to move after awakening and gradually recovering muscle strength during the next few minutes or hours. Muscles that remain active in sleep, such as the diaphragm and cardiac muscle, are not affected. Patients are normal between attacks, but in adult life the attacks become more frequent and the disorder causes progressive myopathy with permanent weakness even between attacks.

Alterations in serum potassium are seen only during acute episodes and are accompanied by T-wave changes in the ECG. The CK may be mildly elevated at those times. The muscle biopsy is often normal between attacks, but during an attack a vacuolar myopathy is demonstrated. The vacuoles are dilated sarcoplasmic reticulum and invaginations of the extracellular space into the cytoplasm, and they may be filled with glycogen. Hypoglycemia does not occur.

562.2 Malignant Hyperthermia

(See also Chapter 61.)

This syndrome is usually inherited as an autosomal dominant trait. It occurs in all patients with central core disease but is not limited to that particular myopathy. The defective gene is at the 19q13.1 locus in both central core disease and malignant hyperthermia without this specific myopathy. It occurs rarely in Duchenne and other muscular dystrophies, in a variety of other myopathies, and in an isolated syndrome not associated with other muscle disease. Affected children sometimes have peculiar facies. All ages are affected, including even a premature infant whose mother underwent general anesthesia for cesarean section.

Acute episodes are precipitated by exposure to general anesthetics and occasionally even to local anesthetic drugs. The patient suddenly develops extreme fever, rigidity of muscles, metabolic and respiratory acidosis, and the serum CK rises to as high as 35,000 IU/L. Myoglobinuria may result in tubular necrosis and acute renal failure.

The muscle biopsy during an episode of malignant hyperthermia or shortly afterward shows widely scattered necrosis of muscle fibers, known as *rhabdomyolysis.* Between attacks, the muscle biopsy is normal unless there is an underlying chronic myopathy.

It is important to recognize patients at risk for malignant hyperthermia because the attacks may be prevented by administering dantrolene sodium before an anesthetic is given. Identification of patients at risk, such as siblings of those who have experienced an episode, is done by the caffeine contracture test: A portion of fresh muscle biopsy tissue in a saline bath is attached to a strain gauge and exposed to caffeine and other drugs; an abnormal spasm is diagnostic.

562.3 Glycogenoses

(See also Chapters 73 and 548.)

Glycogenosis I **(von Gierke disease)** is not a true myopathy because the deficient liver enzyme, glucose-6-phosphatase, is not normally present in muscle. Nevertheless, children with this disease are hypotonic and mildly weak for uncertain reasons.

Glycogenosis II **(Pompe disease)** is an autosomal recessively inherited deficiency of the glycolytic lysosomal enzyme acid maltase. Two forms are described. The infantile form is a severe generalized myopathy and cardiomyopathy. Cardiomegaly and hepatomegaly are present, and patients are diffusely hypotonic and weak. The serum CK is greatly elevated. Muscle biopsy reveals a vacuolar myopathy with abnormal lysosomal enzymatic activity (Fig. 562–1). Death in infancy or early childhood is usual.

The late childhood or adult form of acid maltase deficiency is a much milder myopathy without cardiac or hepatic enlargement. It does not become clinically expressed until later childhood or early adult life, but the serum CK is greatly elevated and the muscle biopsy is diagnostic even in the presymptomatic stage.

The diagnosis of glycogenosis II is confirmed by quantitative assay of acid maltase activity in muscle or liver biopsy tissue.

Glycogenosis III **(Cori-Forbes disease),** deficiency of debrancher enzyme (amylo-1,6-glucosidase), is the most common of the glycogenoses, but also the least severe clinically. Hypotonia, weakness, hepatomegaly, and fasting hypoglycemia

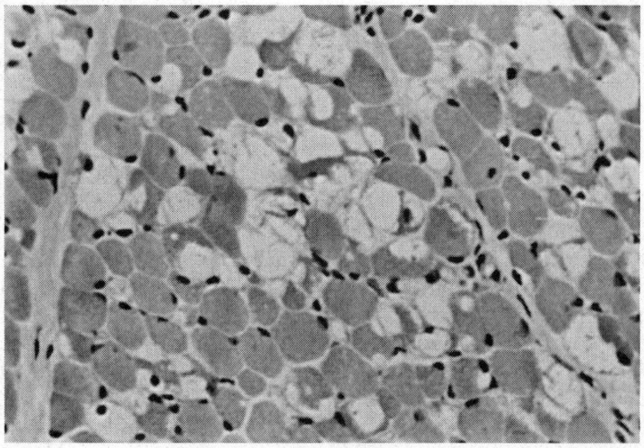

Figure 562–1. Muscle biopsy of 2-yr-old boy with glycogenosis II (Pompe disease; acid maltase deficiency). More than half of the myofibers have large vacuoles replacing contractile myofibrils and cytoplasmic organelles. Special stains show glycogen storage and abnormally strong activity of lysosomal enzymes. (Hematoxylin & eosin, ×250.)

in infancy are common, but these features often resolve spontaneously, and patients become asymptomatic in childhood and adult life. Others experience slowly progressive distal muscle wasting, hepatic cirrhosis, and heart failure. Minor myopathic findings including vacuolation of muscle fibers are found in the muscle biopsy.

Glycogenosis IV **(Andersen disease)** is a deficiency of brancher enzyme, resulting in the formation of an abnormal glycogen molecule, amylopectin, in the liver, reticuloendothelial cells, and skeletal and cardiac muscle. Hypotonia, generalized weakness, muscle wasting, and contractures are the usual signs of myopathic involvement. Most patients die before 4 yr of age because of hepatic or cardiac failure. A few children are described without neuromuscular manifestations.

Glycogenosis V **(McArdle disease)** is due to muscle phosphorylase deficiency, inherited as an autosomal recessive trait. Exercise intolerance is the cardinal clinical feature. Physical exertion results in cramps, weakness, and myoglobinuria, but strength is normal between attacks. The serum CK is elevated only during exercise. A characteristic clinical feature is lack of the normal rise in serum lactate during ischemic exercise, because of inability to convert pyruvate to lactate under anaerobic conditions in vivo. Myophosphorylase deficiency may be demonstrated histochemically and biochemically in the muscle biopsy.

A rare *neonatal form* of myophosphorylase deficiency causes feeding difficulties in early infancy, may be severe enough to result in neonatal death, or may follow a course of slowly progressive weakness resembling a muscular dystrophy.

The long-term prognosis is good. Patients must learn to moderate their physical activities, but they do not develop severe chronic myopathic handicaps or cardiac involvement.

Glycogenosis VII **(Tarui disease)** is muscle phosphofructokinase deficiency. Although rarer than glycogenosis V, the symptoms of exercise intolerance, clinical course, and inability to convert pyruvate to lactate are identical. The distinction is made by biochemical study of the muscle biopsy.

562.4 Mitochondrial Myopathies

(See also Chapter 548.2.)

Several diseases involving muscle, brain, and other organs are associated with structural and functional abnormalities of mitochondria, producing defects in aerobic cellular metabolism, the electron transport chain, and the Krebs cycle. The structural aberrations are best demonstrated by electron microscopy of the muscle biopsy, revealing abnormally shaped cristae and fusion of cristae to form *paracrystalline inclusions.* Histochemical study of sections of muscle biopsy reveal abnormal clumping of oxidative enzymatic activity, sometimes increased neutral lipids because of impaired lipid metabolism, and "ragged-red" muscle fibers with accumulations of membranous material beneath the muscle fiber membrane, best demonstrated by special stains. Several distinct mitochondrial diseases are identified.

The *Kearns-Sayre syndrome* is characterized by the triad of progressive external ophthalmoplegia, pigmentary degeneration of the retina, and onset before 20 yr of age. Heart block, cerebellar deficits, and high cerebrospinal fluid protein content are often associated. Visual evoked potentials are abnormal. Patients usually do not experience weakness of the trunk or extremities or dysphagia. Most cases are sporadic.

Chronic progressive external ophthalmoplegia may be isolated or accompanied by limb muscle weakness, dysphagia, and dysarthria. A few patients described as **ophthalmoplegia plus** have additional central nervous system (CNS) involvement. Autosomal dominant inheritance is found in some pedigrees, but most cases are sporadic.

Myoclonic epilepsy and ragged-red fibers (MERRF) and the *MELAS syndrome,* an acronym for *m*itochondrial myopathy, *e*ncephalopathy, *l*actic *a*cidosis, and *s*trokelike episodes, are other mitochondrial disorders affecting children. The latter is characterized by stunted growth, episodic vomiting, seizures, and recurrent cerebral insults causing hemiparesis, hemianopia or even cortical blindness, and dementia. The disease behaves as a degenerative disorder and children die within a few years.

Other "degenerative" diseases of the CNS that also involve myopathy with mitochondrial abnormalities include *Leigh's subacute necrotizing encephalopathy* (see Chapter 548.3) and *cerebrohepatorenal* **(Zellweger)** disease (see Chapter 72.2). Another recognized mitochondrial myopathy is *cytochrome-c-oxidase deficiency. Oculopharyngeal muscular dystrophy* also is fundamentally a mitochondrial myopathy. Many other rare diseases with only a few case reports are suspected of being mitochondrial disorders.

Mitochondrial DNA is distinct from the DNA of the cell nucleus and is inherited exclusively from the mother; mitochondria are present in the cytoplasm of the ovum but not in the head of the sperm, the only part that enters the ovum at the time of fertilization. The rate of mutation of mitochondrial DNA is 10 times higher than that of nuclear DNA. In the Kearns-Sayre syndrome, a single large mtDNA deletion has been identified; in the MERRF and MELAS syndrome of mitochondrial myopathy, point mutations occur in tRNA (see Table 559–1).

562.5 Lipid Myopathies

(See Chapter 72.)

Considered as a metabolic organ, the skeletal muscle is the most important site in the body for long-chain fatty acid metabolism because of its large mass and its rich density of mitochondria, where fatty acids are metabolized. Hereditary disorders of lipid metabolism that cause progressive myopathy are an important, relatively common, and often treatable group of muscle diseases.

Muscle carnitine deficiency is an autosomal recessive disease involving deficient transport of dietary carnitine across the intestinal mucosa. Carnitine, acquired from dietary sources and also synthesized in the liver and kidney from lysine and methionine, is the obligatory carrier of long- and medium-chain fatty acids into muscle mitochondria.

The clinical course is that of a progressive muscular dystrophy with generalized proximal myopathy and sometimes facial, pharyngeal, and cardiac involvement. Symptoms usually begin in late childhood or adolescence, or may be delayed until adult life. Progression is slow but may end in death.

Serum CK is mildly elevated. Muscle biopsy shows vacuoles filled with lipid within muscle fibers, in addition to nonspecific changes suggestive of a muscular dystrophy. Mitochondria may appear normal or abnormal. Carnitine measured in muscle biopsy tissue is reduced, but serum carnitine is normal.

Treatment stops the progression of the disease and may even restore lost strength if the disease is not too advanced. It consists of special diets low in long-chain fatty acids. Steroids may enhance fatty acid transport. Specific therapy with L-carnitine taken by mouth in large doses overcomes the intestinal barrier in some patients. Some patients also improve with supplementary riboflavin, and other patients seem to improve with propranolol.

Systemic carnitine deficiency is a disease of impaired renal and hepatic synthesis of carnitine rather than a primary myopathy. Patients with this autosomal recessive disease experience progressive proximal myopathy and show muscle biopsy changes similar to muscle carnitine deficiency. But the onset of weakness is earlier and may be evident at birth. Endocardial fibroelastosis also may occur. Episodes of acute hepatic encephalopathy resembling Reye syndrome may occur. Hypoglycemia and metabolic acidosis complicate acute episodes.

The concentration of carnitine is reduced in serum as well as in muscle and liver. A similar clinical syndrome may be a complication of the renal *Fanconi syndrome,* because of excessive urinary loss of carnitine or during chronic hemodialysis.

Treatment with L-carnitine improves the maintenance of blood glucose and serum carnitine levels but does not reverse the ketosis or acidosis or improve exercise capacity.

Muscle carnitine palmityltransferase (CPT) deficiency presents as episodes of rhabdomyolysis, coma, and elevated serum CK that may be indistinguishable from Reye syndrome. CPT transfers long-chain fatty acid-acyl-CoA residues to carnitine on the outer mitochondrial membrane for transport into the mitochondria. Exercise intolerance and myoglobinuria resemble glycogenoses V and VII (see earlier). Fasting hypoglycemia may also occur. Genetic transmission is autosomal recessive due to a defect on chromosome 1 at the 1p11–13 locus.

562.6 Vitamin E Deficiency Myopathy

Deficiency of vitamin E in experimental animals produces a progressive myopathy closely resembling a muscular dystrophy. Myopathy and neuropathy are recognized in humans who lack adequate intake of this antioxidant. Patients with malabsorption, on chronic dialysis, and premature infants who do not receive vitamin E supplements are particularly vulnerable.

CHAPTER 563

Disorders of Neuromuscular Transmission and of Motor Neurons

563.1 Myasthenia Gravis

Myasthenia gravis is a disease caused by immunologic neuromuscular blockade. The release of acetylcholine (ACh) into the synaptic cleft by the axonal terminal is normal, but the postsynaptic muscle membrane or *motor end-plate* is less responsive than normal. A decreased number of available ACh receptors is due to circulating receptor-binding antibodies. In most cases the disease is nonhereditary and is in the category of an autoimmune disorder. A rare familial myasthenia gravis is probably an autosomal recessive trait. Infants born to myasthenic mothers may have a transient neonatal myasthenic syndrome secondary to placentally transferred anti-ACh receptor antibodies.

CLINICAL MANIFESTATIONS. Ptosis and some degree of extraocular muscle weakness are the earliest and most constant signs in myasthenia gravis. Older children may complain of diplopia, and young children may hold open their eyes with their fingers or thumbs if the ptosis is severe enough to obstruct vision. The pupillary responses to light are preserved. Dysphagia and facial weakness are also common, and in early infancy feeding difficulties are often the cardinal sign of myasthenia. Poor head control due to weakness of the neck flexors also is prominent. Involvement may be limited to bulbar-innervated muscles, but the disease is systemic and weakness involves limb-girdle muscles and distal muscles of the hands in most cases. Fasciculations of muscle, myalgias, and sensory symptoms do not occur. Tendon stretch reflexes may be diminished but rarely are lost.

Rapid fatigue of muscles is a characteristic feature of myasthenia gravis that distinguishes it from most other neuromuscular diseases. Ptosis increases progressively as the patient is asked to sustain an upward gaze for 30–90 sec. Holding the head up from the surface of the examining table while lying supine is very difficult, and gravity cannot be overcome for more than a few seconds. Repetitive opening and closing of the fists produces rapid fatigue of hand muscles, and the patient cannot elevate the arms for more than 1–2 min because of fatigue of the deltoids. A careful history also discloses that the patient is more symptomatic late in the day or when tired. Dysphagia may interfere with eating, and the muscles of the jaw soon tire when the child chews.

If untreated, myasthenia gravis is usually progressive and may become life threatening because of respiratory muscle involvement and the risk of aspiration. Familial myasthenia gravis is usually not progressive.

Infants born to myasthenic mothers may have respiratory insufficiency, inability to suck or swallow, generalized hypotonia and weakness, and show little spontaneous motor activity for several days to weeks. Some require ventilatory support and feeding by gavage during this period. After the abnormal antibodies disappear, the infants have normal strength and are not at increased risk for developing myasthenia gravis in later childhood. The syndrome of **transient neonatal myasthenia gravis** is to be distinguished from a rare and often hereditary *congenital myasthenia gravis* not related to maternal myasthenia that is often permanent. An abnormality of the acetylcholine receptor channels, manifesting as high conductance and excessively fast closure, may be due to a point mutation in a subunit of the receptor affecting a single amino acid residue.

Myasthenia gravis is occasionally secondary to hypothyroidism, usually *Hashimoto thyroiditis*. Other collagen vascular diseases may also be associated. Thymomas are not found in myasthenia gravis in children as they are in adults, nor are oat cell carcinomas of the lung, which produce a myasthenic syndrome in adults.

LABORATORY FINDINGS AND DIAGNOSIS. Myasthenia gravis is one of the few neuromuscular diseases in which the electromyogram (EMG) is more specifically diagnostic than the muscle biopsy. A decremental response is seen in response to repetitive nerve stimulation; the muscle potentials diminish rapidly in amplitude until the muscle becomes refractory to further stimulation. Motor nerve conduction velocity remains normal. This unique EMG pattern is the electrophysiologic correlate of the fatigable weakness observed clinically and is reversed after a cholinesterase inhibitor is administered. A myasthenic decrement may be absent or difficult to demonstrate in muscles that are not involved clinically. This feature may be confusing in early cases or in patients showing only weakness of extraocular muscles.

Anti-ACh antibodies should be assayed in the serum but are not always demonstrated. Other serologic tests of autoimmune disease, such as antinuclear antibodies and abnormal immune complexes, should also be sought. A thyroid profile should always be examined. The serum CK is normal.

The heart is not involved, and the ECG remains normal. Roentgenograms of the chest often reveal an enlarged thymus, but the hypertrophy is not a *thymoma.* It may be further defined by tomography or by imaging of the anterior mediastinum.

The role of *muscle biopsy* in myasthenia gravis is controversial. It is not required in most cases, but about 17% of patients show inflammatory changes sometimes called **lymphorrhages** that are interpreted by some authors as a mixed myasthenia-polymyositis immune disorder. The muscle biopsy in myasthenia gravis shows nonspecific type II muscle fiber atrophy, similar to that seen with disuse atrophy, steroid effects on muscle, polymyalgia rheumatica, and many other conditions. The ultrastructure of motor end-plates shows simplification of the membrane folds.

A *clinical test for myasthenia gravis* is the administration of a short-acting cholinesterase inhibitor, usually edrophonium chloride. A small test dose is given intravenously (IV) initially to ensure that the patient is not allergic; if tolerated, the full dose of 0.2 mg/kg (maximum dose 10 mg) is given IV a few minutes later. Children weighing less than 30 kg should be given only 1–2 mg total dose. Within a few seconds, the ptosis and ophthalmoplegia improve, and fatigability of other muscles is greatly decreased. The effects only last 1–2 min, however. Edrophonium should not be given to young infants because cardiac arrhythmias may result. An alternative with fewer cardiogenic side effects is intramuscular (IM) neostigmine. If the initial test of 0.04 mg/kg is negative, the infant may be retested 4 hr later with 0.08 mg/kg. A maximal effect is seen in 20–40 min. Because of muscarinic side effects, such as abdominal distention, diarrhea, and profuse tracheal secretions, 0.01 mg/kg of atropine may be given just before the neostigmine.

TREATMENT. Some patients with mild myasthenia gravis require no treatment. *Cholinesterase-inhibiting drugs* are the primary therapeutic agents. Neostigmine methylsulfate (0.04 mg/kg) may be given IM every 4–6 hr, but most patients tolerate oral neostigmine bromide, 0.4 mg/kg every 4–6 hr. If dysphagia is a major problem, the drug should be given about 30 min before meals to improve swallowing. Pyridostigmine is an alternative; the dosage required is about four times greater than neostigmine, but it may be slightly longer acting. Overdoses of cholinesterase inhibitors produce cholinergic crises; atropine blocks the muscarinic effects but does not block the nicotinic effects that produce additional skeletal muscle weakness.

Because of the autoimmune basis of the disease, long-term *steroid treatment* with prednisone is often effective. *Thymectomy* should be considered and may provide a cure. Thymectomy is ineffective in congenital and familial forms of myasthenia gravis, however. Treatment of hypothyroidism usually abolishes an associated myasthenia.

Plasmapheresis is effective treatment in some children, particularly those who do not respond to steroids, but plasma exchange therapy may provide only temporary remission. Intravenous immunoglobulin (IVIG) is sometimes beneficial. Both plasmapheresis and IVIG appear to be most effective in patients with high circulating levels of antiacetylcholine receptor antibodies.

Neonates with transient maternally transmitted myasthenia gravis require cholinesterase inhibitors for only a few days or occasionally for a few weeks, especially to allow feeding. No other treatment is usually necessary.

COMPLICATIONS. Children with myasthenia gravis tolerate neuromuscular blocking drugs, such as succinylcholine and pancuronium, very poorly and may be paralyzed for weeks after a single dose. An anesthesiologist should carefully review myasthenic patients who require a surgical anesthetic. Also, certain antibiotics may potentiate myasthenia and should be avoided; these include the aminoglycosides (gentamicin, etc).

PROGNOSIS. This is difficult to predict. Some patients undergo spontaneous remission after a period of months or years; others have a permanent disease extending into adult life. Immunosuppression, thymectomy, and treatment of associated hypothyroidism may provide a cure.

OTHER CAUSES OF NEUROMUSCULAR BLOCKADE

Organophosphate chemicals, commonly used as insecticides, may cause a myasthenia-like syndrome in children exposed to these toxins (see Chapter 663).

Botulism results from ingestion of food containing the toxin of *Clostridium botulinum,* a gram-positive, spore-bearing, anaerobic bacillus (see Chapter 192). Honey is a common source of contamination. The incubation period is short, only a few hours, and symptoms begin with nausea, vomiting, and diarrhea. Cranial nerve involvement soon follows, with diplopia, dysphagia, weak suck, facial weakness, and absent gag reflex. Generalized hypotonia and weakness then develop and may progress to respiratory failure. Neuromuscular blockade is documented by EMG with repetitive nerve stimulation. Respiratory support may be required for days or weeks, until the toxin is cleared from the body. There is no specific antitoxin available. Guanidine, 35 mg/kg/24 hr, may be effective for extraocular and limb muscle weakness but not for respiratory muscle involvement.

Tick paralysis is a disorder of ACh release from axonal terminals due to a neurotoxin that blocks depolarization. It also affects large myelinated motor and sensory nerve fibers. This toxin is produced by the wood tick or dog tick, insects common in the Appalachian and Rocky Mountains of North America. The tick embeds its head into the skin, usually the scalp, and neurotoxin production is maximal about 5–6 days later. Motor symptoms include weakness, loss of coordination, and sometimes an ascending paralysis resembling the Guillain-Barré syndrome. Tendon reflexes are lost. Sensory symptoms of tingling paresthesias may occur in the face and extremities. The diagnosis is confirmed by EMG and nerve conduction studies and by identifying the tick. The tick must be removed completely, and the buried head not left beneath the skin of the scalp. The patient then recovers completely within hours or days.

563.2 Spinal Muscular Atrophies

Spinal muscular atrophies (SMA) are degenerative diseases of motor neurons that begin in fetal life and continue to be progressive in infancy and childhood. The progressive denervation of muscle is compensated in part by reinnervation from an adjacent motor unit, but giant motor units are thus created with subsequent atrophy of muscle fibers when the reinnervating motor neuron eventually becomes involved. Upper motor neurons remain normal.

SMA is classified into a severe infantile form, also known as **Werdnig-Hoffmann disease** or SMA type 1; a late infantile and more slowly progressive form, SMA type 2; and a more chronic or juvenile form, also called **Kugelberg-Welander disease** or SMA type 3. A variant of SMA, **Fazio-Londe disease,** is a progressive bulbar palsy resulting from motor neuron degeneration more in the brain stem than the spinal cord.

ETIOLOGY. The etiology of SMA is a pathologic continuation of a process of programmed cell death that is normal in embryonic life. A surplus of motor neuroblasts and other neurons is generated from primitive neuroectoderm, but only about half survive and mature to become neurons; the excess cells have a limited life cycle and degenerate. If the process that arrests physiologic cell death fails to intervene by a certain stage, neuronal death may continue in late fetal life and postnatally. The SMA gene arrests apoptosis (programmed cell death) of motor neuroblasts.

CLINICAL MANIFESTATIONS. Severe hypotonia, generalized weakness, thin muscle mass, absent tendon stretch reflexes, involvement of the tongue, face, and jaw muscles, and sparing of extraocular muscles and sphincters are the cardinal features of SMA type I. Infants who are symptomatic at birth may have respiratory distress and are unable to feed. Congenital contractures occur in about 10% of severely involved neonates. Infants lie flaccid with little movement, unable to overcome gravity. They lack head control. More than two thirds die by 2 yr of age, many early in infancy.

In type II SMA the infants are usually able to suck and swallow, and respiration is adequate in early infancy. They show progressive weakness, but many survive into the school years or beyond, though confined to an electric wheelchair and severely handicapped. Nasal speech and problems with deglutition develop later. Scoliosis becomes a major complication in many patients with long survival.

Kugelberg-Welander disease is the mildest SMA (type III), and patients may appear normal in infancy. The progressive weakness is proximal in distribution, particularly involving shoulder girdle muscles. Patients are ambulatory. Symptoms of bulbar muscle weakness are rare. Longevity may extend well into middle adult life.

Fasciculations are a specific clinical sign of denervation of muscle. In thin children, they may be seen in the deltoid, biceps brachii, and occasionally the quadriceps femoris, but the continuous involuntary wormlike movements may be masked by a thick pad of subcutaneous fat. Fasciculations are best observed in the tongue, where almost no subcutaneous connective tissue separates the muscular layer from the epithelium. If the intrinsic lingual muscles are contracted, such as in crying or when the tongue protrudes, fasciculations are more difficult to see than when the tongue is relaxed.

The outstretched fingers of children with SMA often show a characteristic tremor due to fasciculations and weakness. It should not be confused with a cerebellar tremor. Myalgias are not a feature of SMA.

The heart is not involved in SMA. Intelligence is normal, and children often appear brighter than their normal peers because the effort they cannot put into physical activities is redirected to intellectual development and they are often exposed to adult speech more than to juvenile language because of the social repercussions of the disease.

LABORATORY FINDINGS. The serum CK may be normal but more commonly is mildly elevated in the hundreds. Occasionally, a CK of several thousand is demonstrated. Motor nerve conduction studies are normal, an important feature distinguishing SMA from peripheral neuropathy. The EMG shows fibrillation potentials and other signs of denervation of muscle.

DIAGNOSIS. The muscle biopsy in SMA reveals a characteristic pattern of perinatal denervation that is unlike that of mature muscle. Groups of giant type I fibers are mixed with fascicles of severely atrophic fibers of both histochemical types (Fig. 563–1). In juvenile SMA, the pattern may be more similar to adult muscle that has undergone many cycles of denervation and reinnervation. Neurogenic changes in muscle also may be demonstrated by EMG, but the results are less definitive than by muscle biopsy in infancy.

Sural nerve biopsy sometimes shows mild sensory neuropathic changes, and sensory nerve conduction velocity may be slowed. At autopsy, mild degenerative changes are seen in sensory neurons of dorsal root ganglia and in somatosensory nuclei of the thalamus, but these alterations are not perceived clinically as sensory loss or paresthesias. The most pronounced neuropathologic lesions are the extensive neuronal degeneration and gliosis in the ventral horns of the spinal cord and brain stem motor nuclei, especially the hypoglossal nucleus.

GENETICS. Molecular genetic diagnosis by DNA probes in blood samples or in muscle biopsy or chorionic villi tissues are not yet available, but linkage analysis studies of some families are feasible. Most cases are inherited as an autosomal recessive trait, and the incidence of SMA is 1:25,000, affecting all ethnic groups. It is the second most common neuromuscular disease, following Duchenne muscular dystrophy. The genetic locus for all three of the common forms of SMA is on chromosome 5 at the 5q11–13 locus, proving that they are variants of the same

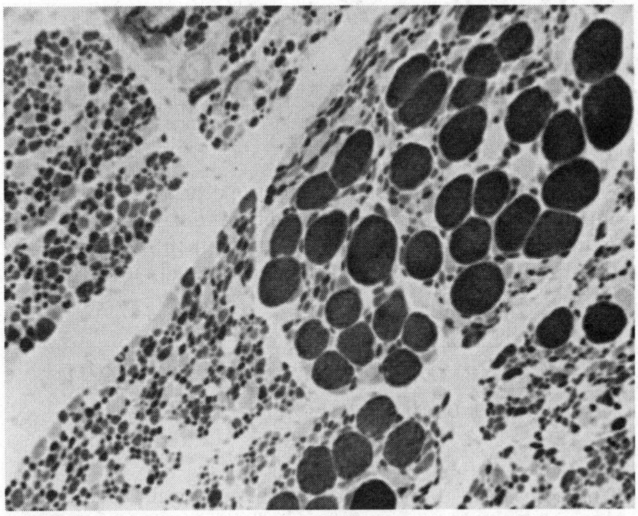

Figure 563–1. Muscle biopsy of neonate with infantile spinal muscular atrophy. Groups of giant type I (darkly stained) fibers are seen within muscle fascicles of severely atrophic fibers of both histochemical types. This is the characteristic pattern of perinatal denervation of muscle. Myofibrillar ATPase, preincubated at pH 4.6. (×400.)

disease rather than different diseases. A few families are described with autosomal dominant inheritance.

TREATMENT. There is no medical treatment to delay the progression. Supportive therapy includes orthopedic care with particular attention to scoliosis and joint contractures, mild physiotherapy, and mechanical aids for assisting the child to eat and to be as functionally independent as possible. Most children learn to use a computer keyboard with great skill but cannot use a pencil easily.

OTHER MOTOR NEURON DISEASES

Motor neuron diseases other than SMA are rare in children. *Poliomyelitis* used to be a major cause of chronic disability, but since the routine use of polio vaccine, this viral infection has now become rare (see Chapter 209). Other enteroviruses, such as Coxsackie and ECHO viruses, or the live polio vaccine virus, may also cause an acute infection of motor neurons with symptoms and signs similar to poliomyelitis, although usually milder. Serologic tests for specific antibodies and viral cultures of cerebrospinal fluid are diagnostic.

A juvenile form of *amyotrophic lateral sclerosis* is rare. Upper motor neuron loss as well as lower motor neuron loss is evident clinically, unlike SMA. The course is progressive and is ultimately fatal.

The **Pena-Shokeir** and **Marden-Walker syndromes** are progressive motor neuron degenerations associated with severe arthrogryposis and congenital anomalies of many organ systems. Pontocerebellar hypoplasias are progressive degenerative diseases of the CNS which begin in fetal life; one form also involves motor neuron degeneration resembling a spinal muscular atrophy.

Motor neurons become involved in several metabolic diseases of the nervous system, such as gangliosidosis (Tay-Sachs disease), ceroid-lipofuscinosis (Batten disease), and glycogenosis II (Pompe disease), but the signs of denervation may be minor or obscured by the more prominent involvement of other parts of the central nervous system or of muscle.

CHAPTER 564

Hereditary Motor-Sensory Neuropathies

The hereditary motor-sensory neuropathies (HMSN) are a group of progressive diseases of peripheral nerves. Motor components generally dominate the clinical picture, but sensory and autonomic involvement become expressed later.

564.1 Peroneal Muscular Atrophy

(Charcot-Marie-Tooth Disease; HMSN Type I)

This disease is the most common genetically determined neuropathy and has an overall prevalence of 3.8:100,000. It is transmitted as an autosomal dominant trait with 83% expressivity, and the 17p11.2 locus has been identified as the site of the abnormal gene. A much rarer X-linked HMSN type I results from a defect at the Xq13.1 locus, causing mutations in the gap junction protein *connexin-32.*

CLINICAL MANIFESTATIONS. Most patients are asymptomatic until late childhood or early adolescence, but young children sometimes show signs of gait disturbance as early as the 2nd year. The peroneal and tibial nerves are the earliest and most severely affected. The child is often described as being clumsy, falling easily, or tripping over her or his own feet. The onset of symptoms may be delayed until after the 5th decade.

Muscles of the anterior compartment of the lower legs become wasted, and the legs have a characteristic "storklike" contour. The muscular atrophy is accompanied by progressive weakness of dorsiflexion of the ankle and eventual foot drop. The process is bilateral but may be slightly asymmetric. Pes cavus deformities may develop because of denervation of intrinsic foot muscles, further destabilizing the gait. Atrophy of muscles of the forearms and hands is usually not as severe as that of the lower extremities, but in advanced cases contractures of the wrists and fingers produce a "claw hand." Proximal muscle weakness is a late manifestation and is usually mild. Axial muscles are not involved.

The disease is slowly progressive throughout life, but patients occasionally show accelerated deterioration of function over a few years. Most patients remain ambulatory and have a normal longevity, although orthotic appliances are required to stabilize the ankles.

Sensory involvement mainly affects large myelinated nerve fibers that convey proprioceptive information and vibratory sense, but the threshold for pain and temperature may also increase. Some children complain of tingling or burning sensations of the feet, but pain is rare. Because the muscle mass is reduced, the nerves are more vulnerable to trauma or compression. Autonomic manifestations may be expressed as poor vasomotor control with blotching or pallor of the skin of the feet and inappropriately cold feet.

Nerves often become palpably enlarged. Tendon stretch reflexes are lost distally. Cranial nerves are not clinically affected. Sphincter control remains well preserved. Autonomic neuropathy does not affect the heart, gastrointestinal tract, or bladder. Intelligence is normal.

The **Davidenkow syndrome** is a variant of HMSN type I with a scapuloperoneal distribution.

LABORATORY FINDINGS AND DIAGNOSIS. Motor and sensory nerve conduction velocities are greatly reduced, sometimes as slow as 20% of normal conduction time. Electromyogram (EMG) and muscle biopsy are not usually required for diagnosis, but they show evidence of many cycles of denervation and reinnervation. Serum CK is normal. Cerebrospinal fluid (CSF) protein may be elevated, but no cells appear in the CSF.

In uncertain cases, and particularly if the family history is negative, sural nerve biopsy is diagnostic. Large- and medium-sized myelinated fibers are reduced in number, collagen is increased, and characteristic *onion-bulb formations* of proliferated Schwann cell cytoplasm surround axons. This pathologic finding is called *interstitial hypertrophic neuropathy.* Extensive segmental demyelination and remyelination also occur.

TREATMENT. Stabilization of the ankle is a primary concern. In early stages, stiff boots that extend to midcalf often suffice, particularly when the patient walks on uneven surfaces such as ice and snow or stones. As the dorsiflexors of the ankles further weaken, lightweight plastic splints may be custom made to extend beneath the foot and around the back of the ankle. They are worn inside the socks and are not visible, reducing self-consciousness. External short leg braces may be required when foot drop becomes complete. Surgical fusion of the ankle may be considered in some cases.

The leg should be protected from traumatic injury. Compression neuropathy during sleep may be prevented by soft pillows beneath or between the lower legs in advanced cases. Burning paresthesias of the feet are not common but are often abolished by phenytoin or carbamazepine. No medical treatment is available to arrest or slow the progression.

In new cases, without a family history, both parents should be examined and nerve conduction studies should be performed.

564.2 Peroneal Muscular Atrophy, Axonal Type

(HMSN Type II)

This disease is clinically similar to HMSN type I, but the rate of progression is slower and the disability is less. EMG shows denervation of muscle. Sural nerve biopsy reveals axonal degeneration rather than demyelination and whorls of Schwann cell processes. The locus is on chromosome 1 at 1p35–36; hence, this is a different disease than HMSN type I, though both are transmitted as autosomal dominant traits.

564.3 Déjerine-Sottas Disease

(HMSN Type III)

This interstitial hypertrophic neuropathy of autosomal dominant transmission is similar to HMSN type I but is more severe. Symptoms develop in early infancy and are rapidly progressive. Pupillary abnormalities, such as lack of reaction to light or **Argyll-Robertson pupil** are common. Kyphoscoliosis and pes cavus deformities complicate about 35% of patients. Nerves become palpably enlarged at an early age.

The onion-bulb formations seen in the sural nerve biopsy are more pronounced. Hypomyelination also occurs.

The genetic locus of 17p11.2 is identical to that of HMSN type I or Charcot-Marie-Tooth disease. The clinical and pathologic differences are therefore only phenotypic variants of the same disease, analogous to the situation in Duchenne and Becker muscular dystrophies. An autosomal recessive form of Déjerine-Sottas disease also is described but is controversial.

564.4 Roussy-Lévy Syndrome

This syndrome is defined as a combination of HMSN type I and Friedreich ataxia.

564.5 Refsum Disease

(See Chapter 72.2)

This rare disease is due to an enzymatic block in α-oxidation of phytanic acid to pristanic acid. Phytanic acid is a branched-chain fatty acid that is derived mainly from dietary sources: spinach, nuts, and coffee. Phytanic acid is greatly elevated in plasma, CSF, and brain tissue. The CSF shows an albuminocytologic dissociation with a protein concentration of 100–600 mg/dL.

Clinical onset is usually between 4 and 7 yr of age, with intermittent motor and sensory neuropathy. Ataxia, progressive neurosensory hearing loss, retinitis pigmentosa and loss of night vision, ichthyosis, and liver dysfunction also develop in varying degrees. Motor and sensory nerve conduction velocities are delayed. Treatment is by dietary management and periodic plasma exchange.

564.6 Giant Axonal Neuropathy

This rare autosomal recessive disease with onset in early childhood is a progressive mixed peripheral neuropathy.

Ataxia and nystagmus also usually develop. Most affected children have been noted to have peculiar curly reddish hair. Focal axonal enlargements are seen in both the peripheral nervous system and the central nervous system (CNS), but the myelin sheath is intact. The disease is thought to be a disorder of neurofilament synthesis or organization.

564.7 Congenital Hypomyelinating Neuropathy

This disorder is a lack of normal myelination of motor and sensory peripheral nerves but not of CNS white matter. It is not a degeneration or loss of previously formed myelin, thus differentiating it from a leukodystrophy. Schwann cells are preserved and axons are normal. Cases in siblings suggest autosomal recessive inheritance.

The condition is present from birth; hypotonia and developmental delay are the hallmark clinical findings. Cranial nerves are inconsistently involved, and respiratory distress and dysphagia are rare complications. Tendon reflexes are absent. Arthrogryposis is present at birth in at least half the cases. It is uncertain whether the condition is progressive; myelination of nerves proceeds at a slow rate and remains incomplete.

Motor and sensory nerve conduction velocities are slow. The diagnosis is confirmed by sural nerve biopsy, which shows lack of myelination of large and small fibers, and sometimes interstitial hypertrophic reactive changes. Muscle biopsy may show mild neurogenic atrophy but not the characteristic alterations of spinal muscular atrophy. No inflammation is demonstrated in muscle or nerve.

564.8 Leukodystrophies

Several hereditary degenerative diseases of white matter of the CNS also cause peripheral neuropathy. The most important are *Krabbe's disease* (globoid cell leukodystrophy) and *metachromatic leukodystrophy* (see Chapter 552.5).

CHAPTER 565

Toxic Neuropathies

Many chemicals (organophosphates), toxins, and drugs are capable of causing peripheral neuropathy. *Heavy metals* are well-known neurotoxins. Lead poisoning, especially if chronic, causes mainly a motor neuropathy involving selective large nerves, such as the common peroneal, radial, or median nerves, a condition known as **mononeuritis multiplex** (see Chapter 665). Arsenic produces painful burning paresthesias as well as motor polyneuropathy.

Antimetabolic drugs, especially vincristine, produce polyneuropathies as complications of chemotherapy for neoplasms.

Chronic uremia is associated with toxic neuropathy and myopathy. The neuropathy is due to excessive levels of circulating parathormone. Reduction in serum parathyroid hormone is accompanied by clinical improvement and a return to normal of nerve conduction velocity.

CHAPTER 566

Autonomic Neuropathies

566.1 Familial Dysautonomia

Familial dysautonomia **(Riley-Day syndrome)** is an autosomal recessive disorder that is common in Eastern European Jews, among whom the incidence is 1:10,000–20,000 and the carrier state is estimated to be 1%. It is rare in other ethnic groups. The defective gene is at the 9q31-33 locus.

PATHOLOGY. This disease of the peripheral nervous system is characterized pathologically by a reduced number of small unmyelinated nerve fibers that carry pain, temperature, and taste sensations and that mediate autonomic functions. Large myelinated afferent nerve fibers that relay impulses from muscle spindles and Golgi tendon organs are also deficient. The degree of demonstrable anatomic change in peripheral and especially autonomic nerves is variable. Fungiform papillae of the tongue (taste buds) are absent or reduced in number.

CLINICAL MANIFESTATIONS. The disease is expressed in infancy by poor sucking and swallowing. Aspiration pneumonia may occur. Feeding difficulties remain a major symptom throughout childhood. Vomiting crises may occur. Excessive sweating and blotchy erythema of the skin are common, especially at mealtime or when the child is excited. Breath-holding spells followed by syncope are common in the first 5 yr. As the child becomes older, insensitivity to pain becomes evident and traumatic injuries are frequent. Corneal ulcerations are common. Newly erupting teeth cause tongue ulcerations. Walking is delayed, clumsy, or appears ataxic because of poor sensory feedback from muscle spindles. The "ataxia" is probably related more to deficient muscle spindle feedback and to vestibular nerve dysfunction than to cerebellar involvement. Tendon stretch reflexes are absent. Scoliosis is a serious complication in the majority of patients and usually is progressive. Overflow tearing with crying does not normally develop until 2–3 mo of age but fails to develop after that time or is severely reduced in children with familial dysautonomia.

About 40% of patients have generalized major motor seizures, some of which are associated with acute hypoxia during breath-holding, some with extreme fevers, but most without an apparent precipitating event. Intellectual function is usually impaired but is unrelated to epilepsy. Puberty is often delayed, especially in girls. Body temperature is poorly controlled, and hypothermia and extreme fevers both occur. Speech is often slurred or nasal.

After 3 yr of age, **autonomic crises** begin, usually with attacks of cyclic vomiting lasting 24–72 hr or even several days. Retching and vomiting occur every 15–20 min associated with hypertension, profuse sweating, blotching of the skin, apprehension, and irritability. Prominent gastric distention may occur, causing abdominal pain and even respiratory distress. Hematemesis may complicate pernicious vomiting.

LABORATORY FINDINGS. Electrocardiography discloses prolonged correcting QT intervals with lack of appropriate shortening with exercise, a reflection of the aberration in autonomic regulation of cardiac conduction. Chest roentgenograms show atelectasis and pulmonary changes resembling cystic fibrosis. Urinary vanillyl-mandelic acid (VMA) is decreased, and homovanillic acid (HVA) is increased. Plasma dopamine-β-hydroxylase (the enzyme that converts dopamine to epinephrine) is diminished. Sural nerve biopsy shows a decreased number of unmyelinated fibers. The electroencephalogram (EEG) is useful for evaluating seizures.

DIAGNOSIS. A slow IV infusion of norepinephrine produces an exaggerated pressor response. The hypotensive response to infusion of methacholine is increased. Intradermal injection of 1:1,000 histamine phosphate fails to produce a normal axon flare, and local pain is absent or diminished. Because normal infant skin reacts more intensely to histamine, a 1:10,000 dilution should be used. The instillation of 2.5% methacholine into the conjunctival sac produces miosis in patients with familial dysautonomia and no detectable effect on the normal pupil; this is a nonspecific sign of parasympathetic denervation from any cause, however. The methacholine is applied to only one eye in this test, with the other eye serving as a control; the pupils are compared at 5-min intervals for 20 min.

TREATMENT. Symptomatic treatment includes special attention to the respiratory and gastrointestinal systems, methylcellulose eye drops or topical ocular lubricants to replace tears and prevent corneal ulceration, orthopedic management of scoliosis and joint problems, and appropriate anticonvulsants for epilepsy. Chlorpromazine is an effective antiemetic and may be given as rectal suppositories during autonomic crises. It also reduces apprehension and lowers the blood pressure. Dehydration and electrolyte disturbances should be anticipated. Bethanechol may be an alternative drug for cyclic vomiting. It is also useful for enuresis, another common complication, and augments tear production. Protection from injuries is important because of the lack of pain as a protective mechanism. Scoliosis often requires surgical treatment.

PROGNOSIS. This is poor. Most patients die in childhood, usually of chronic pulmonary failure or aspiration.

566.2 Other Autonomic Neuropathies

MYENTERIC PLEXUS NEUROPATHIES

Aganglionic megacolon (Hirschsprung disease) is a failure of embryonic development of parasympathetic neurons in the submucosal and myenteric plexuses of segments of the colon and rectum. Nerves between the longitudinal and circular layers of smooth muscle of the gut wall are hypertrophic; ganglion cells are absent (see Chapter 278).

CONGENITAL INSENSITIVITY TO PAIN AND ANHIDROSIS

This hereditary disorder of uncertain genetic transmission affects boys much more frequently than girls and presents in early infancy. Patients have episodes of high fever related to warm environmental temperatures because they do not perspire. Frequent burns and traumatic injuries result from apparent lack of pain perception. Intelligence is normal. Nerve biopsy reveals an almost total absence of unmyelinated nerve fibers that convey impulses of pain, temperature, and autonomic functions.

REFLEX SYMPATHETIC DYSTROPHY

This disorder is a form of local causalgia, usually involving a hand or foot but not corresponding to the anatomic distribution of a peripheral nerve. A continuous burning pain and hyperesthesia are associated with vasomotor instability in the affected zone, resulting in increased skin temperature, erythema, and edema due to vasodilatation and hyperhydrosis. In the chronic state, atrophy of skin appendages, cool and clammy skin, and disuse atrophy of underlying muscle and bone occur. More than one extremity is occasionally involved. The pain is disabling and is exacerbated by the movement of an associated joint, though no objective signs of arthritis are seen; immobilization provides some relief. The most common preceding event is local trauma in the form of a contusion, laceration, sprain, or fracture days or weeks earlier.

Several theories of pathogenesis have been proposed to explain this phenomenon. The most widely accepted is reflexive overactivity of autonomic nerves in response to injury, and regional sympathetic blockade often affords temporary relief. Physiotherapy also is helpful. Some cases resolve spontaneously after weeks or months, but others continue to be symptomatic and require sympathectomy. A strong psychogenic component is suspected in some cases but is difficult to prove.

CHAPTER 567
Guillain-Barré Syndrome

The Guillain-Barré syndrome is a postinfectious polyneuropathy that causes demyelination in mainly motor but sometimes also sensory nerves. This syndrome affects people of all ages and is not hereditary. The disorder closely resembles experimental allergic polyneuritis in animals.

CLINICAL MANIFESTATIONS. The paralysis usually follows a nonspecific viral infection by about 10 days. The original infection may have caused only gastrointestinal (*Campylobacter* sp.) or upper respiratory tract symptoms. Weakness begins usually in the lower extremities and progressively involves the trunk, the upper limbs, and finally the bulbar muscles, a pattern formerly known as *Landry's ascending paralysis.* Proximal and distal muscles are involved relatively symmetrically, but asymmetry is found in 9% of patients. The onset is gradual and progresses over days or weeks. Particularly in cases with an abrupt onset, tenderness to palpation and pain in muscles is common in the initial stages. The child is irritable. Weakness may progress to inability or refusal to walk, and later to flaccid tetraplegia. Paresthesias occur in some cases.

Bulbar involvement occurs in about half of cases. Respiratory insufficiency may result. Dysphagia and facial weakness are often impending signs of respiratory failure. They interfere with eating and increase the risk of aspiration. Extraocular muscle involvement is rare, but in an uncommon variant, oculomotor and other cranial neuropathies are severe early in the course. The **Miller-Fisher syndrome** consists of acute external ophthalmoplegia, ataxia, and areflexia. Papilledema is found in some cases, although visual impairment is not clinically evident. Urinary incontinence or retention of urine is a complication in about 20% of cases but is usually transient.

Tendon reflexes are lost, usually early in the course, but are sometimes preserved until later, and this finding may be misleading in arriving at an early diagnosis.

The clinical course is usually benign, and spontaneous recovery begins within 2–3 wk. Most patients regain full muscular strength, although some are left with residual weakness. The tendon reflexes are usually the last function to recover. Improvement usually follows a gradient inverse to the direction of involvement, with recovery of bulbar function first and lower extremity weakness resolving last. Bulbar and respiratory muscle involvement may lead to death if the syndrome is not recognized and treated.

The autonomic nervous system may also be involved in some cases. Lability of blood pressure and cardiac rate, postural hypotension, episodes of profound bradycardia, and occasional asystole occur. Cardiovascular monitoring is important. A few patients require the insertion of a temporary venous cardiac pacemaker.

Occasional cases of acute Guillain-Barré syndrome are associated with *Mycoplasma pneumoniae* or *Campylobacter* spp. infections.

Chronic relapsing polyradiculoneuropathy and *chronic unremitting polyradiculoneuropathy* are chronic forms of Guillain-Barré syndrome that recur intermittently or do not improve for a period of months and years. About 7% of children with Guillain-Barré syndrome experience relapses. Patients are usually severely weak and may have a flaccid tetraplegia with or without bulbar and respiratory muscle involvement.

LABORATORY FINDINGS AND DIAGNOSIS. Cerebrospinal fluid (CSF) studies are essential for diagnosis. The CSF protein is elevated to more than twice the upper limit of normal, glucose is normal, and there is no pleocytosis. Fewer than 10 white cells/mm^3 are found. The results of bacterial cultures are negative, and viral cultures rarely isolate specific viruses. The dissociation between high CSF protein and a lack of cellular response in a patient with an acute or subacute polyneuropathy is diagnostic of the Guillain-Barré syndrome.

Motor nerve conduction velocities are greatly reduced, and sensory nerve conduction time also is often slow. The electromyogram shows evidence of acute denervation of muscle. Serum CK may be mildly elevated or normal. Muscle biopsy is not usually required for diagnosis; it is normal in early stages and shows evidence of denervation atrophy in chronic stages. Sural nerve biopsy shows segmental demyelination, focal inflammation, and wallerian degeneration but also is usually not required for diagnosis.

TREATMENT. Patients in early stages of this *acute* disease should be admitted to the hospital for observation, because the ascending paralysis may rapidly involve respiratory muscles during the next 24 hr. Patients with slow progression may simply be observed for stabilization and spontaneous remission without treatment. Rapidly progressive ascending paralysis is treated with plasma exchange therapy or with steroids and immunosuppressive drugs. Plasmapheresis may be the most effective treatment. Intravenous immunoglobulin (IVIG) is an alternative and has been widely used in the treatment of many autoimmune disorders. Supportive care, such as respiratory support, prevention of decubiti in children with flaccid tetraplegia, and treatment of secondary bacterial infections, is important.

Chronic relapsing polyradiculoneuropathy or unremitting chronic neuropathy is treated with plasma exchange, sometimes requiring as many as 10 exchanges daily. Remission in these cases may be sustained, but relapses may occur within days, weeks, or even after many months; relapses usually respond to another course of plasmapheresis. IVIG may be tried in the treatment of chronic or relapsing polyneuropathy as well as in the acute or subacute stages. Steroid and immunosuppressive drugs are an alternative, but their effectiveness is less predictable. High-dose "pulsed" methylprednisolone given IV is successful in some cases. The prognosis in chronic forms of the Guillain-Barré syndrome is more guarded than in the acute form, and many patients are left with major residual handicaps.

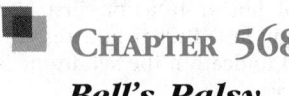

CHAPTER 568
Bell's Palsy

Bell's palsy is an acute unilateral facial nerve palsy that is not associated with other cranial neuropathies or brain stem dysfunction. It is a common disorder at all ages from infancy through adolescence and usually develops abruptly about 2 wk after a systemic viral infection. The preceding infection is due to the Epstein-Barr virus in about 20% of cases; Lyme disease (see Chapter 198), herpesvirus, and mumps virus are identified in many others. The disease is believed to be a postinfectious allergic or immune demyelinating facial neuritis rather than an active viral invasion of the nerve or of its motor neurons or origin. At times it is associated with hypertension.

CLINICAL MANIFESTATIONS. The upper and lower face is paretic, and the corner of the mouth droops. The patient is unable to close the eye on the involved side, and the patient may develop an exposure keratitis at night. Taste on the anterior two thirds of the tongue is lost on the involved side in about half of cases, which helps to establish the anatomic limits of the lesion proximal or distal to the chorda tympani branch of the facial nerve. Numbness and paresthesias do not occur.

TREATMENT. Protection of the cornea with methylcellulose eye drops or an ocular lubricant is especially important at night. Steroids do not induce remission and are not recommended. Surgical decompression of the facial canal, theoretically to provide more space for the swollen facial nerve, has not proved to be of value.

PROGNOSIS. The prognosis is excellent. More than 85% of cases recover spontaneously with no residual facial weakness; another 10% have mild facial weakness as a sequel; only 5% are left with permanent severe facial weakness. In chronic cases that do not recover within a few weeks, electrophysiologic examination of the facial nerve helps to determine the degree of neuropathy and regeneration. In chronic cases, other causes of facial neuropathy should be considered, including facial nerve tumors such as schwannomas and neurofibromas, infiltration of the facial nerve by leukemic cells or by a rhabdomyosarcoma of the middle ear, brain stem infarcts or tumors, and traumatic injury of the facial nerve.

FACIAL PALSY AT BIRTH. This is usually a compression neuropathy from forceps application during delivery and recovers spontaneously in a few days or weeks in most cases. Congenital Bell's palsy should not be diagnosed. *Congenital absence of the depressor angularis oris muscle* causes facial asymmetry, especially when the infant cries. It is not a facial nerve lesion but is a cosmetic defect that does not interfere with feeding.

GENERAL NEUROMUSCULAR

Brooke MH: A Clinician's View of Neuromuscular Disease, 2nd ed. Baltimore, Williams & Wilkins, 1986.
Dubowitz V: Color Atlas of Muscle Disorders in Childhood. Chicago, Year Book 1989.
Dubowitz V: The Floppy Infant, 2nd ed. Philadelphia, JB Lippincott, 1980.
Mastaglia FL, Walton J (eds): Skeletal Muscle Pathology, 2nd ed. Edinburgh, Churchill Livingstone, 1990.
Sarnat HB: Muscle Pathology and Histochemistry. Chicago, Am Soc Clin Pathol Press, 1983.
Walton J: Disorders of Voluntary Muscle, 4th ed. Edinburgh, Churchill Livingstone, 1981.

EMBRYOLOGY AND DEVELOPMENTAL DISORDERS OF MUSCLE

Barth PG, van Wijngaarden GK, Bethlem J: X-linked myotubular myopathy with fatal neonatal asphyxia. Neurology 25:531, 1975.
Fardeau M: Congenital myopathies. *In:* Mastaglia FL, Walton J (eds): Skeletal Muscle Pathology, 2nd ed. Edinburgh, Churchill Livingstone, 1991.
Iannaccone ST: Myogenes and myotubes. J Child Neurol 7:180, 1992.
Martinez BA, Lake BD: Childhood nemaline myopathy: A review of clinical presentation in relation to prognosis. Dev Med Child Neurol 29:815, 1987.
Miller JB: Myoblasts, myosins, MyoDs, and the diversification of muscle fibers. Neuromuscul Disord 1:7, 1991.
Sarnat HB: Cerebral dysgeneses and their influence on fetal muscle development. Brain Dev 8:495, 1986.
Sarnat HB: Myotubular myopathy: arrest in morphogenesis of myofibers associated with persistent fetal vimentin and desmin. Can J Neurol Sci 17:109, 1990.
Sarnat HB: Ontogenesis of striated muscle. *In:* Polin RA, Fox WW (eds): Neonatal and Fetal Medicine: Physiology and Pathophysiology. Orlando, FL, WB Saunders, 1991.
Sarnat HB: Vimentin and desmin in maturing skeletal muscle and developmental myopathies. Neurology 42:1616, 1992.
Sarnat HB: New insights into the pathogenesis of congenital myopathies. J Child Neurol 9:193, 1994.
Sarnat HB, Diadori P, Trevenen CL: Myopathy of the Proteus syndrome: Hypothesis of muscular dysgenesis. Neuromusc Disord 3:293, 1993.
Shimomura C, Nonaka I: Nemaline myopathy: Comparative muscle histochemistry in the severe neonatal, moderate congenital, and adult-onset forms. Pediatr Neurol 5:25, 1989.
Weintraub H: The MyoD family and myogenesis: redundancy, networks and thresholds. Cell 75:1241, 1993.

MUSCULAR DYSTROPHIES

Brook JD, McCurrach ME, Harley HG, et al: Molecular basis of myotonic dystrophy: expansion of a trinucleotide (CTG) repeat at the 3′ end of a transcript encoding a protein kinase family member. Cell 68:799, 1992.
Brouwer OF, Padberg GW, Wijmenga C, Frants RR: Facioscapulohumeral muscular dystrophy in early childhood. Arch Neurol 51:387, 1994.
Dubowitz V: Prednisone in Duchenne dystrophy. Neuromuscul Disord 1:161, 1991.
Egger J, Kendall BE, Erdohazi M, et al: Involvement of the central nervous system in congenital muscular dystrophies. Dev Med Child Neurol 25:32, 1983.
Engel AG: Gene therapy for Duchenne muscular dystrophy [editorial]. Ann Neurol 34:3, 1993.
Fukuyama Y, Osawa M, Suzuki H: Congenital progressive muscular dystrophy of the Fukuyama type: Clinical, genetic and pathological considerations. Brain Dev 3:1, 1981.
Höweler CJ, Busch HFM, Geraedts JPM, et al: Anticipation in myotonic dystrophy: Fact or fiction? Brain 112:779, 1989.
Karpati G, Ajdukovic D, Arnold D, et al: Myoblast transfer in Duchenne muscular dystrophy. Ann Neurol 34:8, 1993.
Koenig M, Beggs AH, Moyer M, et al: The molecular basis for Duchenne versus Becker muscular dystrophy: correlation of severity with type of deletion. Am J Hum Genet 45:498, 1989.
Love DR, Byth BC, Tinsley JM, et al: Dystrophin and dystrophin-related proteins: a review of protein and RNA studies. Neuromuscul Disord 3:5, 1993.
Miller G, Wessel HB: Diagnosis of dystrophinopathies: review for the clinician. Pediatr Neurol 9:3, 1993.
Sarnat HB, O'Connor T, Byrne PA: Clinical effects of myotonic dystrophy on pregnancy and the neonate. Arch Neurol 33:459, 1976.
Sarnat HB, Silbert SW: Maturational arrest of fetal muscle in neonatal myotonic dystrophy. Arch Neurol 33:466, 1976.
Thornton CA, Griggs RC, Moxley RT III: Myotonic dystrophy with no trinucleotide repeat expansion. Ann Neurol 35:269, 1994.
Tsilfidis C, MacKenzie AE, Mettler G, et al: Correlation between CTG trinucleotide repeat length and frequency of severe congenital myotonic dystrophy. Nature Genet 1:192, 1992.
Wijmenga C, Frants RR, Hewitt JE, et al: Molecular genetics of facioscapulohumeral muscular dystrophy. Neuromuscul Disord 3:487, 1993.

METABOLIC AND ENDOCRINE MYOPATHIES

DiMauro S, Bonilla E, Zeviani M, et al: Mitochondrial myopathies. J Inherit Metab Dis 10(Suppl 1):113, 1987.
Dimauro S, Hartlage PL: Fatal infantile form of muscle phosphorylase deficiency. Neurology 28:1124, 1978.
Lestienne P, Ponsot G: Kearns-Sayre syndrome with muscle mitochondrial DNA deletion. Lancet 1:885, 1988.
Lombes A, Bonilla E, DiMauro S: Mitochondrial encephalomyopathies. Rev Neurol 145:671, 1989.
Mastaglia FL, Ojeda VJ, Sarnat HB, et al: Myopathies associated with hypothyroidism. Aust NZ J Med 18:799, 1988.
Najjar SS: Muscular hypertrophy in hypothyroid children: The Kocher-Debré-Sémélaigne syndrome: A review of 23 cases. J Pediatr 85: 236, 1974.

Sarnat HB, Machin G, Darwish HZ, et al: Mitochondrial myopathy of cerebro-hepato-renal (Zellweger) syndrome. Can J Neurol Sci 10:170, 1983.

DISORDERS OF NEUROMUSCULAR TRANSMISSION

Afifi AK, Bell WE: Tests for juvenile myasthenia gravis: comparative diagnostic yield and prediction of outcome. J Child Neurol 8:403, 1993.
Engel AG, Uchitel OD, Walls TJ, et al. Newly recognized congenital myasthenic syndrome associated with high conductance and fast closure of the acetylcholine receptor channel. Ann Neurol 34:38, 1993.
Pickett J, Berg B, Chaplin E, et al: Syndrome of botulism in infancy: Clinical and electrophysiologic studies. N Engl J Med 295:770, 1976.

SPINAL MUSCULAR ATROPHIES

Gamstorp I, Sarnat HB (eds): Progressive Spinal Muscular Atrophies. New York, Raven Press, 1984.
Hageman G, Willemse J, van Ketel BA, et al: The heterogeneity of the Pena-Shokeir syndrome. Neuropediatrics 18:45, 1987.
Pearn JH, Gardner-Medwin D, Wilson J: A clinical study of chronic childhood spinal muscular atrophy: A review of 141 cases. J Neurol Sci 38:23, 1978.
Roy N, Mahedevan M, McLean M, et al: The gene for neuronal apoptosis inhibitory protein is partially deleted in individuals with spinal muscular atrophy. Cell 80:167, 1995.
Russman BS, Melchreit R, Drennan JC: Spinal muscular atrophy: The natural course of disease. Muscle Nerve 6:179, 1983.
Sees JN Jr, Towfighi J, Ladda RP: Marden-Walker syndrome: Neuropathologic findings. Pediatr Pathol, 1991.

HEREDITARY MOTOR-SENSORY NEUROPATHIES

Balestrini MR, Cavaletti G, D'Angelo A, et al: Infantile hereditary neuropathy with hypomyelination. Neuropediatrics 22:65, 1991.
Boylan KB, Ferriero DM, Greco CM, et al: Congenital hypomyelination neuropathy with arthrogryposis multiplex congenita. Ann Neurol 31:337, 1992.
Charnas L, Trapp B, Griffin J: Congenital absence of peripheral myelin. Neurology 38:966, 1988.
Buchtal F, Behse F: Peroneal muscular atrophy (PMA) and related disorders. I: Clinical manifestations as related to biopsy findings, nerve conduction, and electromyography. Brain 100:41, 1977.
Carpenter S, Karpati G, Andermann F: Giant axonal neuropathy: A clinically and morphologically distinct neurological disease. Arch Neurol 31:312, 1974.
Dyck PJ, Lambert EH: Lower motor and primary sensory neuron diseases with peroneal muscular atrophy. I: Neurologic, genetic, and electrophysiologic findings in various neuronal degenerations. Arch Neurol 18:619, 1968.
Pena SD: Giant axonal neuropathy: An inborn error of organization of intermediate filaments. Muscle Nerve 5:166, 1982.
Ronen GM, Lowry N, Wedge JH, et al: Hereditary motor-sensory neuropathy type I presenting as scapuloperoneal atrophy (Davidenkow syndrome): Electrophysiological and pathological studies. Can J Neurol Sci 13:264, 1986.

AUTONOMIC NEUROPATHIES

Axelrod FB, Gouge TH, Ginsburg HB, et al: Fundoplication and gastrostomy in familial dysautonomia. J Pediatr 118:388, 1991.
Axelrod FB, Nachtigal R, Dancis J: Familial dysautonomia: Diagnosis, pathogenesis and management. Adv Pediatr 21:75, 1974.
Blumenfeld A, Slaugenhaupt SA, Axelrod FB, et al: Localization of the gene for familial dysautonomia on chromosome 9 and definition of DNA markers for genetic diagnosis. Nature Genet 4:160, 1993.
Bonica JJ: Causalgia and other reflex sympathetic dystrophies. *In:* Bonica JJ (ed): The Management of Pain, 2nd ed. Philadelphia, Lea & Febiger, 1990, pp 220–243.
Glickstein JS, Schwartzman D, Friedman D, et al: Abnormalities of the corrected QT interval in familial dysautonomia: an indicator of autonomic dysfunction. J Pediatr 122:925, 1993.
Goebel HH, Veit S, Dyck PJ: Confirmation of virtual unmyelinated fiber absence in hereditary sensory neuropathy type IV. J Neuropathol Exp Neurol 39:670, 1980.

GUILLAIN-BARRÉ SYNDROME

D'Cruz OF, Shapiro ED, Spiegelman KN: Acute inflammatory demyelinating polyradiculoneuropathy (Guillain-Barré syndrome) after immunization with *Haemophilus influenzae* type b conjugate vaccine. J Pediatr 115:743, 1989.
Parry GJ: Guillain-Barré Syndrome. New York, Thieme Medical, 1993.
Maytal J, Eviatar L, Brunson SC: Use of demand pacemaker in children with Guillain-Barré syndrome and cardiac arrhythmias. Pediatr Neurol 5:303, 1989.
McKhann GM, Griffin JN, Cornblath DR, et al: Plasmapheresis and Guillain-Barré syndrome: Analysis of prognostic factors and the effects of plasmapheresis. Ann Neurol 23:347, 1988.
Shuaib A, Becker WJ: Variants of Guillain-Barré syndrome: Miller-Fisher syndrome, facial diplegia and multiple cranial nerve palsies. Can J Neurol Sci 14:611, 1987.
Thomas PK, Lascelles RG, Hallpike JF, et al: Recurrent and chronic relapsing Guillain-Barré polyneuritis. Brain 29:589, 1969.

PART XXIX

*Disorders of the Eye**

Leonard Nelson

CHAPTER 569

Growth and Development

At birth the eye of the normal full-term infant is approximately two thirds of adult size. Postnatal growth is maximal during the 1st yr, proceeds at a rapid but decelerating rate until the 3rd yr, and continues at a slower rate thereafter until puberty, after which little change occurs. In general, the anterior structures of the eye are relatively large at birth and thereafter grow proportionately less than the posterior structures. This growth pattern results in a progressive change in the shape of the globe; it becomes more nearly spherical.

In the infant the *sclera* is thin and translucent, with a bluish tinge. The *cornea* is relatively large in the newborn (averaging 10 mm) and attains adult size (nearly 12 mm) by the age of 2 yr or earlier. Its curvature tends to flatten with age, with progressive change in the refractive properties of the eye. The normal cornea is perfectly clear. In infants born prematurely there may be a transient opalescent haze. The anterior chamber in the newborn appears shallow, and the angle structures, so important to the maintenance of normal intraocular pressure, must undergo further differentiation after birth. The *iris*, typically light blue or gray at birth in whites, undergoes progressive change of color as the pigmentation of the stroma increases in the 1st 6 mo of life. The pupils of the newborn infant tend to be small and are often difficult to dilate. Often remnants of the pupillary membrane (anterior vascular capsule) are evident on ophthalmoscopic examination as cobweblike lines crossing the pupillary aperture, especially in preterm infants.

The *lens* of the newborn infant is more nearly spherical than that of the adult; its greater refractive power helps to compensate for the relative shortness of the young eye. The lens continues to grow throughout life; new fibers added to the periphery continually push older fibers toward the center of the lens. With age, the lens becomes progressively more dense and more resistant to change of shape during accommodation.

The *fundus* of the newborn eye is less pigmented than that of the adult; the choroidal vascular pattern is highly visible, and the retinal pigmentary pattern often has a fine "peppery" or mottled appearance. In some darkly pigmented infants, however, the fundus has a gray or opalescent sheen. In the newborn the macular landmarks, particularly the foveal light reflex, are less well defined and may not be readily apparent to ophthalmoscopic examination. The peripheral retina appears pale or grayish, and the peripheral retinal vasculature is immature, especially in the premature infant. The optic nervehead color varies from pink to slightly pale, sometimes grayish. Within 4–6 mo the appearance of the fundus more nearly approximates that of the mature eye.

Superficial retinal hemorrhages may be observed in many newborn infants. These are usually absorbed promptly and rarely leave any permanent effect. Conjunctival hemorrhages also may occur at birth and are resorbed spontaneously without consequence.

Remnants of the primitive hyaloid vascular system may also be seen as small tufts or wormlike structures projecting from the disk (Bergmeister papilla) or as a fine strand traversing the vitreous; in some cases only a small dot (Mittendorf dot) remains on the posterior aspect of the lens capsule.

As a rule, the infant eye is somewhat hyperopic (farsighted), but the refractive state at any time in life depends on the net effect of many factors, the principal ones being the size of the eye, the state of the lens, and the curvature of the cornea.

Newborn infants tend to keep their eyes closed much of the time, but the normal newborn can see, responds to changes in illumination, and can fixate points of contrast. The *visual acuity* in the newborn is estimated to be in the range of 20/400. One of the earliest responses to a formed visual stimulus is the infant's regard for the mother's face, evident especially during feeding. By 2 wk of age the infant shows more sustained interest in large objects, and by 8–10 wk of age the normal infant can follow an object through an arc of 180°. The acuity improves rapidly and may reach 20/30–20/20 by the age of 2–3 yr.

In many normal infants there may be imperfect coordination of the *eye movements* and *alignment* during the early days and weeks, but proper coordination should be achieved by 3–6 mo, usually sooner. Persistent deviation of an eye in an infant requires evaluation.

Tears often are not present with crying until after 1–3 mo.

Archer SM, Sondhi N, Helveston EM: Strabismus in infancy. Ophthalmology 96:133, 1989.

Friendly DS: Development of vision in infants and young children. Pediatr Clin North Am 40:693, 1993.

Gordon RA, Donzis PB: Refractive development of the human eye. Arch Ophthalmol 103:785, 1985.

Khodadoust AA, Ziai M, Biggs SL: Optic disc in normal newborns. Am J Ophthalmol 66:502, 1968.

Krishnamohan VK, Wheeler MB, Testa MA, et al: Correlation of postnatal regression of the anterior vascular capsule of the lens to gestational age. J Pediatr Ophthalmol Strab 19:28, 1982.

Roarty JD, Keltner JL: Normal pupil size and anisocoria in newborn infants. Arch Ophthalmol 108:94, 1990.

Robb RM: Increase in retinal surface area during infancy and childhood. J Pediatr Ophthalmol Strab 19:16, 1982.

Roth AM: Retinal vascular development in premature infants. Am J Ophthalmol 84:636, 1977.

Spieres A, Isenberg SJ, Inkelis SH: Characteristics of the iris in 100 neonates. J Pediatr Ophthalmol Strab 26:28, 1989.

*Modified from original by L. Martyn in 14th edition.

CHAPTER 570
Examination of the Eye

Examination of the eye should be a routine part of the periodic pediatric assessment beginning in the newborn period. Screening in schools and community programs can also be effective in detecting problems early. In 1992, the American Academy of Ophthalmology recommended preschool vision screening as a means of reducing preventable visual loss. Their recommended screening schedule is presented in Table 570–1. This testing should be done by primary providers during well-child visits. The child should be examined by an ophthalmologist whenever a significant ocular abnormality or vision defect is noted or even suspected. Ideally, every child should have a thorough ophthalmologic examination sometime in early childhood, preferably by the age of 3–4 yr; these are the crucial years for the detection and treatment of amblyopia, strabismus, high refractive errors, and many other significant disorders.

Basic examination, whether done by the pediatrician or ophthalmologist, must include evaluation of visual acuity and the visual fields, assessment of the pupils, ocular motility and alignment, a general external examination, and an ophthalmoscopic examination of the media and fundi. When indicated, biomicroscopy (slit lamp examination), cycloplegic refraction, and tonometry are performed by the ophthalmologist. In some cases special diagnostic procedures, such as ultrasonic examination, fluorescein angiography, electroretinography (ERG), or visual evoked response (VER) testing, are also indicated.

VISUAL ACUITY. Many tests of visual acuity exist. Which test is used depends on the child's age and ability to cooperate, as well as the clinician's preference and experience with each test. The most common visual acuity test in infants is an assessment of their ability to fixate and follow a target. If appropriate targets are used, this reflex can be demonstrated by about 6 wk of age. The test is performed by seating the child comfortably in the caretaker's lap. The object of visual interest, usually a bright-colored toy, is slowly moved to the right and to the left. The examiner observes whether the infant's eyes turn toward the object and follow its movements. The examiner can use a thumb to occlude one of the infant's eyes in order to test each eye separately. Although a sound-producing object might compromise the purity of the visual stimulus, in practice, toys that squeak or rattle heighten an infant's awareness and interest in the test.

Although test objects are often used, the human face is a better target. The examiner can exploit this by moving his or her face slowly in front of the infant's face. If the appropriate following movements are not elicited, the test should be repeated with the caretaker's face as the test stimulus.

An objective measurement of visual acuity is usually possible when children reach 2 1/2–3 yr of age. Children this age are tested using a schematic picture or other illiterate eye chart. Each eye should be tested separately. It is essential to prevent peeking. The examiner should hold the occluder in place and observe the child throughout the test. The child should be reassured and encouraged throughout the test, because many children are intimidated by the procedure and fear a "bad grade" or punishment for errors.

The E test, in which the child points in the direction of the letter, is the most widely used visual acuity test for preschool children. Right-left presentations are more confusing than up-down presentations. With pretest practice, this test can be performed by most children 3–4 yr of age.

An adult-type Snellen acuity chart can be used at about 5 or 6 yr if the child knows letters. An acuity of 20/40 is generally accepted as normal for 3-yr-old children. At age 4, 20/30 is typical. By age 5 or 6, most children attain 20/20 vision.

Optokinetic nystagmus (the response to a sequence of moving targets; "railroad" nystagmus) can also be used to assess vision; this can be calibrated by various-sized targets (stripes or dots) or a rotating drum at specified distances. The VER, an electrophysiologic method of evaluating the response to light and special visual stimuli, such as calibrated stripes or a checkerboard pattern, can also be used to study visual function in selected cases. Preferential looking tests are also used for the evaluation of vision in infants and children who cannot respond to standard acuity tests. This is a behavioral technique based on the observation that, given a choice, an infant prefers to look at patterned rather than unpatterned stimuli.

VISUAL FIELD ASSESSMENT. Like visual acuity testing, visual field assessment must be geared to the child's age and abilities. Formal visual field examination (perimetry and scotometry) can often be accomplished in the school-aged child. Often, however, the examiner must rely on confrontation techniques and finger counting in quadrants of the visual field. In many children only testing by attraction can be accomplished; the examiner observes the child's response to familiar objects brought into each of the four quadrants of the visual field of each eye in turn. The child's bottle, a favorite toy, and lollipops are particularly effective attention-getting items. Even such gross methods can often detect diagnostically significant field changes such as the bitemporal hemianopsia of a chiasmal lesion or the homonymous hemianopsia of a cerebral lesion.

COLOR VISION TESTING. This can be accomplished whenever the child is able to name or trace the test symbols; these may either be numbers or Xs, Os, triangles, or other symbols. Color vision testing is not frequently necessary in young children, but parents sometimes request it, particularly if the child seems

TABLE 570–1 Vision Screening Schedule for Infants and Children

Age	Screening Test	Findings Requiring Referral
Newborn to 3 months	Red reflex test	Opacity of the cornea, cataract, retinal detachment or disorder
	Corneal light reflex test	Ocular misalignment (strabismus)
	External examination	Structural defect
6–12 months	Red reflex test	As above
	Corneal light reflex test	As above
	Occlusion of each eye separately	Amblyopia if child resists occlusion unequally
	Fixation and following	Amblyopia if unable to do
3 years	Red reflex test	As above
	Corneal light reflex test	As above
	Visual acuity test	Refractive error, amblyopia
	Stereoacuity	Refractive error, amblyopia
5 years	Same as 3 yr	As above

From Catalano RA, Nelson LB: Pediatric Ophthalmology. A Text Atlas. Norwalk, CT, Appleton and Lange, 1994.

to be slow in learning colors. Defective color vision is not uncommon in males but is rare in females. Occasionally, there is achromatopsia, a total color vision defect with subnormal visual acuity, nystagmus, and photophobia. A change in color discrimination can be a sign of optic nerve or retinal disease.

PUPILLARY EXAMINATION. This includes evaluation of both the direct and consensual reactions to light, the reaction on near gaze, and the response to reduced illumination, noting the size and symmetry of the pupils under all conditions. Special care must be taken to differentiate the reaction to light from the reaction to near gaze; the natural tendency of a child is to look directly at the approaching light, inducing the near gaze reflex when one is attempting to test only the reaction to light; accordingly, every effort must be made to control fixation. The swinging flashlight test is especially useful for detecting unilateral or asymmetric prechiasmatic afferent defects in children (see Marcus Gunn pupil, Chapter 573).

OCULAR MOTILITY. This is tested by having the child follow an object into the various positions of gaze. Movements of each eye individually (ductions) and of the two eyes together (versions, conjugate movements, and convergence) are assessed. Alignment is judged by the symmetry of the corneal light reflexes and by the response to alternate occlusion of each eye (see cover tests for strabismus, Chapter 574).

EXTERNAL EXAMINATION. This begins with general inspection in good illumination, noting size, shape, and symmetry of the orbits, position and movement of the lids, and the position and symmetry of the globes. Viewing the eyes and lids from above aids in detection of orbital asymmetry, lid masses, proptosis (exophthalmos), and abnormal pulsations. Palpation is also important in detection of orbital and lid masses.

The lacrimal apparatus is assessed by looking for evidence of tear deficiency, overflow of tears (epiphora), and erythema and swelling in the region of the tear sac or gland. The sac is massaged to check for reflux when obstruction is suspected. The presence and position of the puncta are also checked.

The lids and conjunctiva are specifically examined for focal lesions, foreign bodies, and inflammatory signs; loss and maldirection of lashes should also be noted. When necessary, the lids can be everted in the following manner: (1) instruct the patient to look down; (2) grasp the lashes of the patient's upper lid between the thumb and index finger of one hand; (3) place a probe, a cotton-tipped applicator, or the thumb of the other hand at the upper margin of the tarsal plate; and (4) pulling the lid down and outward, evert it over the probe, using the instrument as a fulcrum. Skill at eversion of the lid should be acquired. Foreign bodies commonly lodge in the concavity just above the lid margin and are exposed only by fully everting the lid.

The anterior segment of the eye is then evaluated with oblique focal illumination, noting luster and clarity of the cornea, depth and clarity of the anterior chamber, and features of the iris. Transillumination of the anterior segment aids in detecting opacities and in demonstrating atrophy or hypopigmentation of the iris; these latter signs are important when ocular albinism is suspected. When necessary, fluorescein dye can be used to aid in the diagnosis of abrasions, ulcerations, and foreign bodies.

BIOMICROSCOPY (SLIT LAMP EXAMINATION). This provides a highly magnified view of the various structures of the eye and an optical section through the media of the eye—that is, the cornea, aqueous humor, lens, and vitreous. Lesions can be not only identified but also localized as to their depth within the eye, and the resolution is sufficient to allow detection even of individual inflammatory cells in the aqueous and vitreous. With the addition of special lenses and prisms, the angle of the anterior chamber and regions of the fundus also can be examined with the slit lamp. Biomicroscopy is often crucial in trauma and in examining for iritis. It is also helpful in the diagnosis of many metabolic diseases of childhood.

FUNDUS EXAMINATION (OPHTHALMOSCOPY). This is best done with the pupil dilated unless there are neurologic or other contraindications. Tropicamide (Mydriacyl), 0.5–1%, and phenylephrine (Neo-Synephrine), 2.5%, are recommended as mydriatics of short duration. These are safe for most children, but the possibility of adverse systemic effects must be recognized. For very small infants more dilute preparations may be advisable. Beginning with posterior landmarks, the disk and the macula, the four quadrants are systematically examined by following each of the major vessel groups to the periphery. More of the fundus can be seen if the child is directed to look up, down, right, and left. Even with care, only a limited amount of the fundus can be seen with the direct or handheld ophthalmoscope. For examination of the far periphery the indirect ophthalmoscope is used, and full dilation of the pupil is essential.

It should be noted that, before the retina is examined, the ophthalmoscope is used to examine the clarity of the media. With a high plus lens (+8 or +10) in place, the ophthalmoscope can also be used for examination of external lesions and foreign bodies, because it provides magnification and good illumination.

REFRACTION. This determines the refractive state of the eye, that is, the degree of nearsightedness, farsightedness, or astigmatism. Retinoscopy provides an objective determination of the amount of correction needed and can be done at any age. In young children it is best done with cycloplegia. Subjective refinement of refraction involves asking the patient for preferences in the strength and axis of corrective lenses; it can be accomplished in many school-aged children. Refraction and determination of visual acuity with appropriate corrective lenses in place are essential steps in deciding whether or not the patient has a visual defect or amblyopia.

TONOMETRY. This measures intraocular pressure; it is usually done by the indentation method with the Schiotz gauge or by the applanation method with the slit lamp. Alternative methods are pneumatic and electronic tonometry. When accurate measurement of the pressure is necessary in a child who cannot cooperate, it may be done with sedation or general anesthesia. A gross estimate of pressure can be made by palpating the globe with the index fingers placed side by side on the upper lid above the tarsal plate.

American Academy of Ophthalmology: Preferred practice pattern: Comprehensive pediatric eye evaluation. San Francisco, American Academy of Ophthalmology, 1992.

Fulton A: Screening preschool children to detect visual and ocular disorders. Arch Ophthalmol 110:1553, 1992.

Isenberg S, Everett S, Parelhoff E: A comparison of mydriatic eyedrops in low-weight infants. Ophthalmology 91:278, 1984.

Isenberg SJ: Clinical application of the pupil examination in neonates. J Pediatr 118:650, 1991.

Nelson LB: Pediatric Ophthalmongy. Philadelphia, WB Saunders, 1984.

Reinecke RD: Screening 3-year olds for visual problems: Are we gaining or falling behind? Arch Ophthalmol 105:1497, 1987.

Sokol S, Hansen VC, Moskowitz A, et al: Evoked potentials and preferential looking estimates of visual acuity in pediatric patients. Ophthalmology 90:552, 1983.

Sturner RA, Green JA, Funk S, et al: A developmental approach to preschool vision screening. J Pediatr Ophthalmol Strab 18:61, 1981.

Teller DY, McDonald MA, Preston KI, et al: Assessment of visual acuity in infants and children: The acuity card procedure. Dev Med Child Neurol 28:779, 1986.

CHAPTER 571
Abnormalities of Refraction and Accommodation

When parallel rays of light come to focus on the retina with the eye in a state of rest (nonaccommodating), emmetropia exists. Such an ideal optical state is not uncommon, but more often the opposite condition, ametropia, exists. Three principal types occur: hyperopia (farsightedness), myopia (nearsightedness), and astigmatism. The majority of children are physiologically hyperopic at birth, but a significant number, especially those born prematurely, are myopic, and there is often some degree of astigmatism. With growth, the refractive state tends to change and should be evaluated periodically.

Measurement of the refractive state of the eye (refraction) can be accomplished objectively and subjectively. The objective method involves focusing a beam of light from a retinoscope onto the patient's retina through lenses of various powers placed in front of the eye. This method is precise and can be carried out at any age, because it requires no response from the patient. In infants and children it is best done after the instillation of eye drops that produce *mydriasis* (dilatation of the pupil) and *cycloplegia* (relaxation of accommodation); those used most commonly are tropicamide (Mydriacyl), cyclopentolate (Cyclogyl), homatropine hydrobromide, and atropine sulfate. The subjective method involves placing various lenses in front of the eye and having the patient report which lenses provide the clearest image of the letters on the chart. This method depends on the patient's ability to discriminate and communicate, but it can be used for some children and can be helpful in determining the best refractive correction for many youngsters who are developmentally capable of these tasks.

HYPEROPIA

If parallel rays of light come to focus posterior to the retina with the eye in a state of rest (nonaccommodating), hyperopia or farsightedness exists. This may result because the anteroposterior diameter of the eye is too short, because the refractive power of the cornea or lens is less than normal, or because the lens is dislocated posteriorly.

In hyperopia, accommodation is used to bring objects into focus for both far and near gaze. If the accommodative effort required is not too great, the child has clear vision and is comfortable for both distant and close work. In high degrees of hyperopia requiring greater accommodative effort, vision may be blurred, and the child may complain of "eye strain," headaches, or fatigue. Squinting, eye rubbing, lid inflammation, and lack of interest in reading are also frequent manifestations. There may be associated esotropia (convergent strabismus, accommodative esotropia, Chapter 574). Convex lenses (spectacles or contact lenses) of sufficient strength to provide clear vision and comfort are prescribed when indicated.

MYOPIA

In myopia parallel rays of light come to focus anterior to the retina. This may result because the anteroposterior diameter of the eye is too long, because the refractive power of the cornea or lens is greater than normal, or because the lens is dislocated forward. The principal symptom is blurred vision for distant objects. The far point of clear vision varies inversely with the degree of myopia; as the myopia increases, the far point of clear vision comes closer. With myopia of 1 diopter, for example, the far point of clear focus is 1 m from the eye; with myopia of 3 diopters, the far point of clear vision is only 1/3 m from the eye. Thus, myopic children tend to hold objects and reading matter close, prefer to be close to the blackboard, and may be uninterested in distant activities. Frowning and squinting are common, because the visual acuity is improved when the lid aperture is reduced; the effect is similar to that achieved by closing or "stopping down" the aperture of the diaphragm of a camera.

Myopia is infrequent in infants and preschool children. It is more common in preterm infants and in infants with retinopathy of prematurity. Also, there is a hereditary tendency to myopia, and children of myopic parents should be examined at an early age. The incidence of myopia increases during the school years, especially during the preteen and teen years. The degree of myopia also tends to increase with age during the growing years.

Concave lenses (spectacles or contact lenses) of appropriate strength to provide clear vision and comfort are prescribed. Changes are usually needed periodically, sometimes in 1–2 yr, sometimes every few months. Some practitioners advocate the use of cycloplegic agents and bifocals in an effort to retard the progression of myopia, but the value of such treatment is controversial.

In most cases myopia is not a result of pathologic alteration of the eye and is referred to as simple or physiologic myopia. Some children, however, may have pathologic myopia, a rare condition caused by a pathologically abnormal axial length of the eye; this is usually associated with thinning of the sclera, choroid, and retina, and often with some degree of uncorrectable visual impairment. Myopia may also occur as the result of other ocular abnormalities, such as keratoconus, ectopia lentis, and glaucoma, and is also a major feature of Stickler syndrome.

ASTIGMATISM

In astigmatism there is a difference in the refractive power of the various meridians of the eye. Most cases are caused by irregularity in the curvature of the cornea; some astigmatism results from changes in the lens. Mild degrees of astigmatism are very common and may produce no symptoms. With greater degrees there may be distortion of vision. In an effort to achieve a clearer image, the person with astigmatism uses accommodation or frowns or squints to obtain a pinhole effect. Symptoms include "eye strain," headache, and fatigue. Eye rubbing and lid hyperemia, indifference to schoolwork, and holding reading matter close are common manifestations in childhood. Cylindric or spherocylindric lenses are used to provide optical correction when indicated. Glasses may be needed constantly or only part time, depending on the degree of astigmatism and the severity of the attendant symptoms. In some cases, contact lenses are used.

Infants and children with corneal irregularity resulting from injury, periorbital and eyelid hemangiomas, and ptosis are at increased risk for astigmatism and attendant amblyopia.

ANISOMETROPIA

When the refractive state of one eye is significantly different from the refractive state of the other eye, anisometropia exists. Uncorrected, this may lead to amblyopia, or "lazy eye." Early detection and correction are essential if normal visual development in both eyes is to be achieved.

ACCOMMODATION

During accommodation the ciliary muscle contracts, the suspensory fibers of the lens relax, and the lens assumes a more rounded shape to bring rays of light into focus on the retina. The amplitude of accommodation is greatest during childhood and gradually diminishes with age. The physiologic decrease in accommodative ability that occurs with age is called presbyopia.

Disorders of accommodation in children are relatively rare. Premature presbyopia is occasionally seen in youngsters. The most common cause of paralysis of accommodation in children is the intentional or inadvertent use of cycloplegic substances, topically or systemically; included are all the anticholinergic drugs and poisons, as well as plants and plant substances having these effects. Neurogenic causes of accommodative paralysis include lesions affecting the oculomotor nerve (3rd cranial nerve) in any part of its course. Differential diagnosis includes tumors, degenerative diseases, vascular lesions, trauma, and infectious diseases. Impairment of accommodation may occur in botulism, diphtheria, Wilson disease, diabetes mellitus, and syphilis, and after some viral illnesses. Rarely, inability to accommodate is caused by a congenital defect of the ciliary muscle. An apparent defect in accommodation may be psychogenic in origin; it is not uncommon for a child to feign inability to read when it can be demonstrated that visual acuity and ability to focus are normal.

Brodstein RS, Brodstein DE, Olson RJ, et al: The treatment of myopia with atropine and bifocals: A long-term prospective study. Ophthalmology 91:1373, 1984.

Catalano RA, Nelson LB: Pediatric Ophthalmology: A Text Atlas. Norwalk, CT, Appleton and Lange, 1994.

Curtin BJ: The etiology of myopia. *In*: Curtin BJ (ed): The Myopias: Basic Science and Clinical Management. Philadelphia, Harper and Row, 1985, pp 113–124.

Fulton AB, Dobson V, Salem D, et al: Cycloplegic refractions in infants and young children. Am J Ophthalmol 90:239, 1980.

Gordon RA, Donzia PB: Refractive development of the human eye. Arch Ophthalmol 103:785, 1985.

Mäntyjärvi MI: Changes in refraction in schoolchildren. Arch Ophthalmol 103:790, 1985.

Nelson LB: Pediatric Ophthalmology. Philadelphia, WB Saunders, 1984.

Slataper FJ: Age norms of refraction and vision. Arch Ophthalmol 43:466, 1950.

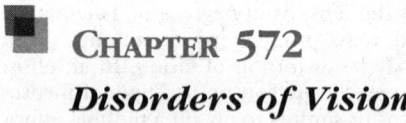

CHAPTER 572
Disorders of Vision

AMBLYOPIA

Amblyopia is subnormal visual acuity in one or both eyes despite correction of any significant refractive error. The term may embrace various vision defects of organic or nonorganic origin (e.g., organic amblyopia designates vision loss directly attributable to trauma or to an organic lesion or disease of the eye or visual pathways), but the term is preferentially used to denote a specific developmental disorder of visual function arising from sensory stimulation deprivation or abnormal binocular interaction (i.e., malalignment or strabismus). In the latter sense amblyopia is familiarly known as "lazy eye."

Under normal conditions the development of visual acuity proceeds rapidly in infancy and early childhood. Anything that interferes with the formation of a clear retinal image during this early developmental period can produce *sensory deprivation amblyopia*. For example, during a critical developmental period in early life, a cataract can interfere with retinal stimulation to such a degree that even after the cataract is successfully removed and the aphakic refractive error is corrected with glasses or a contact lens that provides a clear retinal image, vision may be relatively poor. Similarly, uncorrected anisometropia in the young child can lead to amblyopia; in this condition the eye with the more normal refractive state and clearer retinal image is used for definitive seeing and the eye with the greater refractive error and blurred retinal image becomes amblyopic from sensory deprivation or disuse. Even the child with an abnormally high refractive error in both eyes may develop some degree of bilateral amblyopia because of retinal blur during the critical period of development.

In children with strabismus there is a tendency to suppress or "tune out" the image of the deviating eye as a sensory adaptation to avoid diplopia. If allowed to persist untreated in the young child, such suppression can result in amblyopia.

Susceptibility to amblyopia is greatest within the 1st 2–3 yr of life and especially in the 1st months of life, but risk of amblyopia lasts until full visual potential and stability have been achieved, generally by the age of 9.

The *diagnosis* of amblyopia is confirmed when a complete ophthalmologic examination reveals reduced acuity that is unexplained by an organic abnormality. If the history and ophthalmologic examination do not support the diagnosis of amblyopia in a child with poor vision, consideration must be given to other etiologies (i.e., neurologic, psychologic). Amblyopia is usually asymptomatic and detected only by screening programs. Screening is easier in older children but amblyopia is more resistent to treatment in that age group. Amblyopia is reversed more rapidly in younger children whose visual system is less mature, although screening is more difficult. The key to the successful treatment of amblyopia is early detection and prompt intervention. Treatment of amblyopia involves the following: (1) providing the clearest possible retinal image (e.g., by correction of refractive error, removal of cataract); and (2) stimulation or forced use of the amblyopic eye. The latter is accomplished by occlusion therapy, often referred to as "patching"; the better eye is covered to force use of the amblyopic eye. In many cases best results are achieved with complete and constant occlusion throughout the waking hours by the use of adhesive eye "patches"; in some cases part-time occlusion is sufficient or preferred. Occluders placed on spectacles allow peeking, and the adjustable headband type of cloth or plastic occluder is too easily removed by the child. In selected cases an opaque contact lens or a contact lens of sufficiently high power to blur the vision in the better eye is used. In certain cases cycloplegic drops are used to blur the image in the better eye. Most children and their families tolerate occlusion therapy well. In some cases the child resists therapy because of the severity of the vision defect, the cosmetic blemish of the patching, or related psychologic disturbances. The goals of treatment must be thoroughly understood and the treatment carefully supervised. Close monitoring of occlusion therapy is essential, especially in the very young, to avoid deprivation amblyopia in the occluded eye. Also, many families need reassurance and support throughout the trying course of treatment.

AMAUROSIS

The term *amaurosis* refers to partial or total loss of vision; it is usually reserved for profound impairment, blindness, or near blindness. When amaurosis exists from birth, primary consideration in differential diagnosis must be given to developmental malformations, damage consequent to gestational or perinatal infection, anoxia or hypoxia, perinatal trauma, and the genetically determined diseases that can affect the eye itself or the visual pathways. In certain cases the reason for the amaurosis can be readily determined by objective ophthalmic examination; examples are severe microphthalmia, corneal opacification, dense cataracts, chorioretinal scars, macular defects, retinal dysplasia, and severe optic nerve hypoplasia. In some cases there is intrinsic retinal disease that may not be apparent on initial ophthalmoscopic examination; an example is Leber congenital retinal amaurosis. In this retinal dystrophy the fundus may appear normal or near normal for some time before ophthalmoscopically appreciable signs of retinal degeneration (e.g., pigmentary deposits, arteriolar attenuation, optic disk pallor) develop; in such cases electroretinography is important in diagnosis, because the electroretinographic response in this condition is markedly reduced or absent. In many cases of amaurosis the defect lies not in the eye or optic nerve but in the brain, requiring neurologic and neuroradiologic evaluation, including computed tomography or magnetic resonance imaging.

Amaurosis that develops in a child who once had useful vision has different implications. In the absence of obvious ocular disease (e.g., cataract, chorioretinitis, retinoblastoma, retinitis pigmentosa) consideration must be given to many neurologic and systemic disorders that can affect the visual pathways. Amaurosis of rather rapid onset may indicate an encephalopathy (such as might occur with hypertension), infectious or parainfectious processes, vasculitis, migraine, leukemia, toxins, or trauma. It may be caused by acute demyelinating disease affecting the optic nerves, chiasm, or cerebrum. In some cases precipitous loss of vision is the result of increased intracranial pressure, a rapidly progressive hydrocephalus, or dysfunction of a shunt. More slowly progressive visual loss suggests tumor or neurodegenerative disease. Gliomas of the optic nerve and chiasm and craniopharyngiomas are primary diagnostic considerations in children who show progressive loss of vision.

Manifestations of impairment of vision vary with the age and abilities of the child, the mode of onset, and the laterality and severity of the deficit. The 1st clue to amaurosis in an infant may be nystagmus or strabismus, the vision defect itself passing undetected for some time. Timidity, clumsiness, or behavioral change may be the initial clues in the very young. Deterioration in school progress and indifference to school activities are common signs in the older child. School-aged children often try to hide their disability and, in the case of very slowly progressive disorders, may not themselves realize the severity of the problem; some detect and promptly report small changes in their vision.

Any evidence of loss of vision requires prompt and thorough ophthalmic evaluation. More often than not, the complete delineation of childhood amaurosis and its etiology requires extensive investigation involving neurologic evaluation, electrophysiologic tests, neuroradiologic procedures, and sometimes metabolic and genetic studies. Furthermore, there may be attendant special educational, social, and emotional needs to be met.

NYCTALOPIA

Nyctalopia or "night blindness" refers to vision that is defective in reduced illumination. It generally implies impairment in function of the rods, particularly in dark adaptation time and perceptual threshold. *Stationary congenital night blindness* may occur as an autosomal dominant, autosomal recessive, or X-linked recessive condition. It may be associated with myopia and disk anomaly. *Progressive night blindness* usually indicates primary or secondary retinal, choroidal, or vitrioretinal degeneration (see Chapter 581); it occurs also in vitamin A deficiency or as the result of retinotoxic drugs such as quinine.

DIPLOPIA

Diplopia or "double vision" is most frequently the result of malalignment of the visual axes, that is, displacement or deviation of the eye. It is common in heterophoria, in heterotropia of recent onset (particularly when caused by acquired nerve palsy), and in proptosis. Because in such cases occluding one eye relieves the diplopia, affected children commonly squint, cover one eye with a hand, or assume abnormal head postures (a face turn or head tilt) to alleviate the bothersome sensation. These mannerisms, especially in preverbal children, are important clues to diplopia. The onset of diplopia in any child warrants prompt evaluation; it may signal the onset of a serious problem such as increased intracranial pressure, a brain tumor, an orbital mass, or myasthenia gravis.

Monocular diplopia results from dislocation of the lens or some defect in the media or macula.

PSYCHOGENIC DISTURBANCES

Vision problems of psychogenic origin are not uncommon in school-aged children. Both conversion reactions and willful feigning are encountered. The usual manifestation is a report of reduced visual acuity in one or both eyes. Another common manifestation is constriction of the visual field. In some cases the symptom is diplopia or polyopia.

Important clues to the diagnosis are inappropriate affect, excessive grimacing, inconsistency in performance, and suggestibility. Thorough ophthalmologic examination is essential to differentiate organic from functional visual disorders.

As a rule, affected children do well with reassurance and positive suggestion. In some cases psychiatric care is indicated. In all cases the approach must be supportive and nonpunitive.

DYSLEXIA

The term *dyslexia* is used to describe a specific reading disability that is attributable to a primary or developmental defect in the higher cortical processing of graphic symbols. It is to be differentiated from reading retardation that may be secondary to other causes (e.g., intellectual impairment, maturational delay, cultural or educational deprivation, emotional disturbances, organic brain disease, or sensory defects) and from acquired word blindness (alexia) occurring as the result of a lesion in the dominant cerebral hemisphere.

Neither dyslexia nor the often associated symptoms such as letter or word reversal and so-called mirror writing are caused by any defect in the eye or visual acuity per se, nor are they attributable to a defect in ocular motility or binocular alignment, but ophthalmologic evaluation of the child with a reading problem is recommended for several reasons: (1) such assessment is of value in differential diagnosis; (2) correction of any concurrent ocular problems such as a refractive error, amblyopia, or strabismus ensures the best possible visual function for the child's education; and (3) the ophthalmologist can be of help in counseling the patient and family.

The approach to treatment is remedial instruction. Treatment directed to the eyes themselves cannot be expected to correct developmental dyslexia.

American Academy of Ophthalmology: Policy Statement: Learning Disabilities, Dyslexia, and Vision. San Francisco, American Academy of Ophthalmology, 1992.

Barnet AB, Manson JI, Wilmer E: Acute cerebral blindness in childhood. Six cases studied clinically and electrophysiologically. Neurology 30:1147, 1970.

Catalano RA, Simon JW, Krohel GB, et al: Functional visual loss in children. Ophthalmology 93:385, 1986.

Duffy FH, Burchfield JL, Snodgrass SR: The pharmacology of amblyopia. Ophthalmology 86:489, 1978.

Francois J: Diagnosis of blindness in the infant. Ann Ophthalmol 2:533, 1970.

Flynn JT: Amblyopia revisited. J Pediatr Ophthalmol Strab 28:171, 1991.

Hittner HM, Borda RP, Justice J Jr: X-linked recessive congenital stationary night blindness, myopia, and tilted discs. J Pediatr Ophthalmol 18:15, 1981.

Ingram RM, Walker C, Wilson JM, et al: Prediction of amblyopia and squint by means of refraction at age 1 year. Br J Ophthalmol 70:12, 1986.

Jastrzebski GR, Hoyt CS, Marg E: Stimulus deprivation amblyopia in children: Sensitivity, plasticity, and elasticity (SPE). Arch Ophthalmol 102:1030, 1984.

Kushner BJ: Functional amblyopia associated with organic ocular lesions. Am J Ophthalmol 91:39, 1981.

Mäntyjärvi MI: The amblyopic schoolgirl syndrome. J Pediatr Ophthalmol Strab 18:30, 1981.

Mellor DH, Fields AR: Dissociated visual development: Electrodiagnostic studies in infants who are "slow to see." Dev Med Child Neurol 22:327, 1980.

Stager DR: Amblyopia and the pediatrician. Pediatr Ann 8:91, 1977.

Tongue AC: Low vision examination in children with visual impairment. J Pediatr Ophthalmol Strab 17:175, 1980.

Von Noorden GK: Amblyopia: A multidisciplinary approach. Invest Ophthalmol Vis Sci 26:1704, 1985.

Von Noorden GK, Milane JB: Penalization in the treatment of amblyopia. Am J Ophthalmol 88:511, 1979.

CHAPTER 573
Abnormalities of Pupil and Iris

ANIRIDIA

Aniridia is a rare, bilateral, condition occurring in 1 in 64,000–96,000 live births. Three genetic types exist. The first (AN 1) is an isolated defect of the eye. The second (AN 2) is associated with Wilms tumor, genitourinary anomalies, and mental retardation. The third (AN 3) is associated with cerebellar ataxia, congenital cataracts, and mental retardation. Both AN 1 and AN 2 are inherited as autosomal dominant conditions. AN 1 is associated with a deletion on the short arm of chromosome 2 and AN 2 with a deletion on the short arm of chromosome 11. AN 3 is an autosomal recessive disorder. One third of all cases occur sporadically; 25% of these patients develop Wilms' tumor.

The term *aniridia* is a misnomer, as at least a small rudimentary iris invariably exists (Fig. 573–1). The cornea may be small, and occasionally a cellular infiltrate (pannus) develops in the superficial layers of the peripheral cornea. Clinically this appears as a gray opacification. Cataracts occur in 50–85% of individuals. In addition to cataract formation, the ocular lens can also dislocate.

Macular hypoplasia occurs in both AN 1 and AN 2 and is believed to be responsible for the associated findings of visual reduction, nystagmus, and optic nerve hypoplasia. Glaucoma occurs in as many as 75% of individuals with aniridia; it is unusual in the neonatal period. Children with aniridia are typically photophobic and have reduced vision to 20/200 or worse.

Wilms' tumor usually presents before the 3rd birthday. Therefore, these children should be screened using renal ultrasound every 3–6 mo, until approximately age 5.

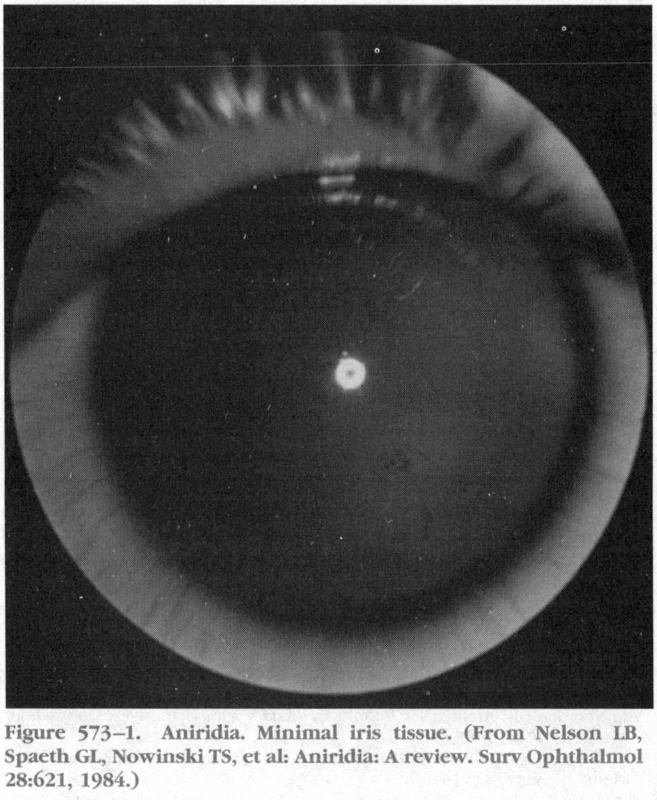

Figure 573–1. Aniridia. Minimal iris tissue. (From Nelson LB, Spaeth GL, Nowinski TS, et al: Aniridia: A review. Surv Ophthalmol 28:621, 1984.)

COLOBOMA OF THE IRIS

Coloboma is a developmental defect that may take the form of a defect in a sector of the iris, a hole in the substance of the iris, or a notch in the pupillary margin. Simple colobomata are frequently transmitted as an autosomal dominant characteristic and may occur alone or be associated with other anomalies. An iris coloboma may be part of an extensive coloboma involving the fundus and optic nerve as a result of malclosure of the embryonic fissure.

MICROCORIA

Absence or malformation of the dilator pupillae muscle may result in an abnormally small pupil that is difficult to dilate, a condition referred to as congenital miosis, or microcoria. Both sporadic and hereditary cases (autosomal dominant and autosomal recessive) occur. They may be associated with other anomalies of the anterior segment.

CONGENITAL MYDRIASIS

In this disorder the pupils appear dilated, do not constrict significantly to light or near gaze, and respond minimally to miotic agents. The iris is otherwise normal, and the affected child is usually healthy. The basis for the abnormality is not clear, though a defect of the iris musculature must be considered. There is evidence for autosomal dominant and possibly X-linked dominant transmission.

This congenital condition should be differentiated from aniridia or other structural abnormalities of the iris, from the fixed dilated pupil of neurologic disease, and from pharmacologic mydriasis.

DYSCORIA AND CORECTOPIA

Dyscoria is abnormal shape of the pupil, and corectopia is abnormal pupillary position. They may occur together or independently as congenital anomalies. Corectopia may be associated with dislocation of the lens. Distortion and displacement of the pupil are frequently the result of trauma and are important signs of prolapse of the iris in perforating injuries of the eye; they may also be seen with tears of the iris, with segmental iridoplegia, and with synechiae (adhesions of iris to lens or cornea).

ANISOCORIA

This is inequality of the pupils. As a general rule, if the inequality is more pronounced in the presence of bright focal illumination or on near gaze, the larger pupil is abnormal, whereas if the anisocoria is worse in reduced illumination, the smaller pupil is abnormal. Neurologic causes of anisocoria (parasympathetic or sympathetic lesions) must be differentiated from local causes such as synechiae (adhesions), congenital iris defects (colobomata, aniridia), and pharmacologic effects. Simple central anisocoria may occur in otherwise healthy individuals.

DILATED FIXED PUPIL

Differential diagnosis of the dilated unreactive pupil includes internal ophthalmoplegia caused by a central or peripheral lesion, the Hutchinson pupil of transtentorial herniation, tonic pupil, pharmacologic blockade, and iridoplegia secondary to ocular trauma.

The most common cause of a dilated unreactive pupil is the purposeful or accidental instillation of a cycloplegic agent, particularly atropine and related substances. Internal ophthalmoplegia may occur with central lesions, and in children the possibility of pinealoma must be considered. The "blown pupil" of transtentorial herniation, as occurs with subdural hematoma and increasing intracranial pressure, is generally unilateral, and usually the patient is obviously ill. The pilocarpine test can help differentiate neurologic iridoplegia from pharmacologic blockade. In the case of neurologic iridoplegia the dilated pupil constricts within minutes after the instillation of 1 or 2 drops of 0.5–1% pilocarpine; if the pupil has been dilated with atropine, the pilocarpine has no effect. Because pilocarpine is a long-acting drug, this test is not to be used in acute situations in which pupillary signs must be carefully monitored.

TONIC PUPIL

This is typically a large pupil that reacts poorly to light (the reaction may be very slow or essentially nil), reacts poorly and slowly to accommodation, and redilates in a slow, tonic manner. The features of tonic pupil are explained by cholinergic supersensitivity of the sphincter following peripheral (postganglionic) denervation and imperfect reinnervation. A distinctive feature of the tonic pupil is its sensitivity to dilute cholinergic agents, such as 0.125% pilocarpine. The condition is usually unilateral.

Tonic pupil may develop after the acute stage of a partial or complete iridoplegia. It can be seen after trauma to the eye or orbit and may occur in association with toxic or infectious conditions. In those in the pediatric age group, tonic pupil is uncommon. Infectious processes (primarily viral syndromes) and trauma are the primary causes. Features of tonic pupil may also be seen in infants and children with familial dysautonomia (Riley-Day syndrome), although the significance of these findings has been questioned. Tonic pupil has also been reported in young children with Charcot-Marie-Tooth disease. The occurrence of tonic pupil in association with decreased deep tendon reflexes in young women is referred to as *Adie syndrome.*

MARCUS GUNN PUPIL

The Marcus Gunn pupil sign indicates an asymmetric, prechiasmatic, afferent conduction defect. It is best demonstrated by the swinging flashlight test; this allows comparison of the direct and consensual pupillary responses in both eyes. With the patient fixing on a distant target (to control accommodation) a bright focal light is directed alternately into each eye in turn. In the presence of an afferent lesion, both the direct response to light in the affected eye and the consensual response in the fellow eye are subnormal. Swinging the light to the better or normal eye causes both pupils to react (constrict) normally. Swinging the light back to the affected eye causes both pupils to redilate to some degree, reflecting the defective conduction. This is a very sensitive and useful test for detecting and confirming optic nerve and retinal disease. A relative afferent defect may be found in some children with amblyopia.

HORNER SYNDROME

The principal signs of oculosympathetic paresis (Horner syndrome) are homolateral miosis, mild ptosis, and apparent enophthalmos with slight elevation of the lower lid. There may also be decrease in facial sweating, increased amplitude of accommodation, and transient decrease in intraocular pressure. If paralysis of the ocular sympathetic fibers occurs before the age of 2 yr, there may be heterochromia iridis with hypopigmentation of the iris on the affected side.

Oculosympathetic paralysis may be caused by a lesion in the midbrain, brain stem, upper spinal cord, neck, middle fossa, or orbit. Congenital oculosympathetic paresis resulting from birth trauma, often as part of Klumke brachial palsy, is common, although the ocular signs, particularly the anisocoria, may pass undetected for years. Horner syndrome is also seen in some children following thoracic surgery, as for congenital heart disease. Congenital Horner syndrome may occur in association with vertebral anomalies and with enterogenous cysts. In some infants and children, Horner syndrome is the presenting sign of tumor in the mediastinal or cervical region, particularly neuroblastoma. Rare causes of Horner syndrome, such as vascular lesions, also occur in the pediatric age group. In some cases, no etiology for the Horner syndrome can be identified. Occasionally, the condition is familial.

When the etiology of Horner syndrome is in question, investigative procedures should be implemented, including chest radiography, computed tomography, magnetic resonance imaging of the head and neck, and 24-hr urinary catecholamine assay. Sometimes examining old photographs and old records can be helpful in establishing the age of onset of the Horner syndrome.

The cocaine test is useful in the diagnosis of oculosympathetic paralysis; a normal pupil dilates within 20–45 min after instillation of 1 or 2 drops of 4% cocaine, whereas the miotic pupil of an oculosympathetic paresis dilates poorly, if at all, to cocaine. In some cases there is denervation supersensitivity to dilute phenylephrine; 1 or 2 drops of a 1% solution dilates the affected but not the normal pupil. Furthermore, the instillation of 1% hydroxyamphetamine hydrobromide dilates the pupil only if the postganglionic sympathetic neuron is intact.

PARADOXIC PUPIL REACTION

Some children exhibit paradoxic constriction of the pupils to darkness. There is an initial brisk constriction of the pupils when the light is turned off, followed by slow redilation of the pupils. The response to direct light stimulation and the near response are normal. The mechanism is not clear, but paradoxic constriction of the pupils in reduced light can be a sign of retinal or optic nerve abnormalities. The phenomenon has been observed in children with congenital stationary night blindness, albinism, retinitis pigmentosa, Leber congenital retinal amaurosis, and Best disease. It has also been observed in those with optic nerve anomalies, optic neuritis, optic atrophy, and possibly amblyopia.

PERSISTENT PUPILLARY MEMBRANE

Involution of the pupillary membrane and anterior vascular capsule of the lens is usually completed prior to birth. It is not uncommon, however, to see some remnants of the pupillary membrane in newborns, particularly in premature infants. These fine, weblike strands or vascular arcades are arranged in a radiating or spokelike pattern in the pupil and can be visualized with the ophthalmoscope. The remnants tend to atrophy in time and usually present no problem. In some cases, however, significant remnants remain, sometimes forming a dense band that traverses and distorts the pupil, a broad sheath of tissue that may be firmly attached to the anterior lens capsule, or an opaque hyperplastic membrane that obscures the pupil and interferes with vision. Rarely, there is patency of the vascular elements; hyphema resulting from rupture of persistent vessels may occur.

Intervention must be considered to minimize amblyopia in infants with extensive persistent pupillary membrane of sufficient degree to interfere with vision in the early months of life. In some cases mydriatics and occlusion therapy may be effective, but in others surgery may be needed to provide an adequate pupillary aperture.

HETEROCHROMIA

In heterochromia the two irides are of different color (heterochromia iridum), or a portion of an iris differs in color from the remainder (heterochromia iridis). Simple heterochromia may occur as an autosomal dominant characteristic. Congenital heterochromia is also a feature of Waardenburg syndrome, an autosomal dominant condition characterized principally by lateral displacement of the inner canthi and puncta, pigmentary disturbances (usually a median white forelock and patches of hypopigmentation of the skin), and defective hearing. Change in the color of the iris may occur as the result of trauma, hemorrhage, intraocular inflammation (iridocyclitis, uveitis), intraocular tumor (especially retinoblastoma), intraocular foreign body, glaucoma, iris atrophy, oculosympathetic palsy (Horner syndrome), or melanosis oculi.

OTHER IRIS LESIONS

Discrete nodules of the iris, referred to as Lisch nodules, may be seen in patients with neurofibromatosis. The lesions vary from slightly elevated pigmented areas to distinct ball-like excrescences. Slit lamp examination may aid in the diagnosis of neurofibromatosis.

In leukemia there may be infiltration of the iris, sometimes with hypopyon, an accumulation of white cells in the anterior chamber, which may herald relapse or involvement of the central nervous system.

The lesion of juvenile xanthogranuloma (nevoxanthoendothelioma) may occur in the eye as a yellowish fleshy mass or plaque of the iris. Spontaneous hyphema (blood in the anterior chamber), glaucoma, or a red eye with signs of uveitis may be associated. A search for the skin lesions of xanthogranuloma (see also Chapter 72) should be made in any infant or young child with spontaneous hyphema. In many cases the ocular lesion responds to topical corticosteroid therapy.

LEUKOCORIA

This term describes any white pupillary reflex, or so-called cat's eye reflex. Primary diagnostic considerations in any child with leukocoria are cataract, persistent hyperplastic primary vitreous, cicatricial retinopathy of prematurity, retinal detachment and retinoschisis, larval granulomatosis, and retinoblastoma (Fig. 573–2). Also to be considered are endophthalmitis, organized vitreous hemorrhage, leukemic ophthalmopathy, exudative retinopathy (as in Coats disease), and a few rare conditions such as medulloepithelioma, massive retinal gliosis, the retinal pseudotumor of Norrie disease, the so-called pseudoglioma of the Bloch-Sulzberger syndrome, retinal dysplasia, and the retinal lesions of the phakomatoses. A white reflex may also be seen with fundus coloboma, large atrophic chorioretinal scars, and ectopic medullation of retinal nerve fibers. Leukocoria is an indication for prompt and thorough evaluation.

Often the diagnosis can be made by direct examination of the eye by ophthalmoscopy and biomicroscopy. Ultrasonographic and radiologic examinations are often helpful. In some cases the final diagnosis rests with the pathologist.

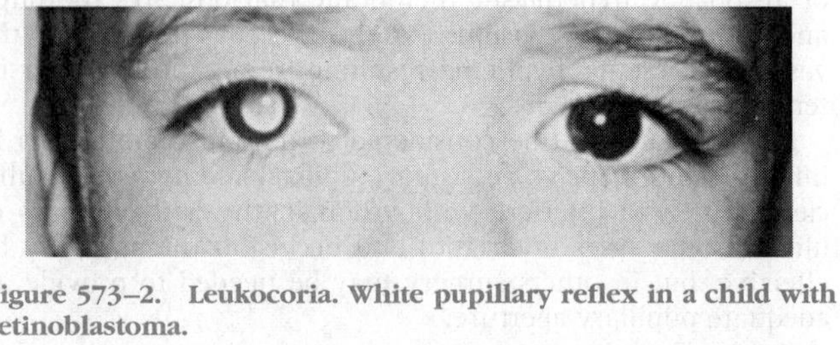

Figure 573–2. Leukocoria. White pupillary reflex in a child with retinoblastoma.

Francois J: Differential diagnosis of leukokoria in children. Ann Ophthalmol 10:1375, 1978.

Frank JW, Kushner BJ, France TD: Paradoxic pupillary phenomenon: A review of patients with pupillary constriction to darkness. Arch Ophthalmol 106:1564, 1988.

Greenwald MJ, Folk ER: Afferent pupillary defects in amblyopia. J Pediatr Ophthalmol Strab 20:63, 1983.

Hersh JH, Douglas C, Houston J, et al: Familial iridoplagia. J Pediatr Ophthalmol Strab 24:49, 1982.

Jaffe N, Cassady JR, Filler RM, et al: Heterochromia and Horner syndrome associated with cervical and mediastinal neuroblastoma. J Pediatr 87:75, 1975.

Krishnamohan VK, Wheeler MD, Testa MA, et al: Correlation of postnatal regression of the anterior vesicular capsule of the lens to gestational age. J Pediatr Ophthalmol Strab 19:28, 1982.

Lewis RA, Riccardi VM: Von Recklinghausen neurofibromatosis: Incidence of iris hamartomata. Ophthalmology 88:348, 1981.

Lowenfeld IE: "Simple, central" anisocoria: A common condition seldom recognized. Trans Am Acad Ophthalmol Otolaryngol 83:832, 1977.

Maloney WF, Younge BR, Moyer NJ: Evaluation of the causes and accuracy of pharmacologic localization in Horner's syndrome. Am J Ophthalmol 90:394, 1980.

Miller RW, Fraumeni JF, Manning MD: Association of Wilms' tumor with aniridia, hemihypertrophy and other congenital malformations. N Engl J Med 270:922, 1964.

Nelson CB, Shields JA: The white pupil (leukokoria). *In:* Kelley VC (ed): Practice of Pediatrics. Philadelphia, Harper and Row, 1987.

Nelson LB, Spaeth GL, Nowenski TS, et al: Aniridia. A review. Surv Ophthalmol 28:621, 1984.

Schachat AP, Jabs DA, Graham ML, et al: Leukemic iris infiltration. J Pediatr Ophthalmol Strab 25:135, 1988.

Thompson HS: Segmental palsy of the iris sphincter in Adie's syndrome. Arch Ophthalmol 96:1615, 1978.

Thompson HS, Newsome DA, Loewenfeld IE: The fixed dilated pupil: Sudden iridoplegia or mydriatic drops? A simple diagnostic test. Arch Ophthalmol 86:21, 1971.

Woodruff G, Buncic JR, Morin JD: Horner syndrome in children. J Pediatr Ophthalmol Strab 25:40, 1988.

CHAPTER 574

Disorders of Eye Movement and Alignment

STRABISMUS

Strabismus, or misalignment of the eyes, is a common condition, affecting approximately 4% of children younger than 6 yr of age. It is an important ocular disorder that can disable sight in one eye and have significant psychological effects. Early detection and treatment of strabismus is essential to prevent permanent visual impairment. Of children with strabismus, 30–50% will develop secondary visual loss, or amblyopia. Restoration of proper alignment of the visual axis must occur at an early stage of visual development to allow these children a chance to develop normal binocular vision.

DEFINITIONS. The word *strabismus,* derived from the Greek word *strabismos,* means to squint or to look obliquely. Many terms are employed in discussing strabismus; unless they are used correctly and uniformly, confusion and misunderstanding may ensue.

Orthophoria is the ideal condition of ocular balance. It implies that the oculomotor apparatus is in perfect equilibrium so that the eyes remain coordinated and aligned in all positions of gaze and at all distances. Even when fusion is interrupted, as by occlusion of one eye, the true orthophoric individual maintains perfect alignment. In reality, orthophoria is seldom encountered, and the vast majority of individuals have a small latent deviation (heterophoria).

Heterophoria is a latent tendency to malalignment: the eye deviates only under certain conditions, such as fatigue, illness, or stress, or tests that interfere with maintainance of normal fusion (such as covering one eye). If the amount of heterophoria is large, it may give rise to bothersome symptoms, such as transient diplopia (double vision), headaches, or asthenopia (eye strain). Some degree of heterophoria is found in almost all normal individuals; however, it is usually asymptomatic.

Heterotrobia is a misalignment of the eyes that is manifest at all times. It occurs because of an inability of the fusional mechanism to control the deviation. Tropias can be alternating, involving both eyes, or unilateral. In an alternating tropia, there is no preference for fixation of either eye, and both eyes drift at an equal rate. Vision usually develops normally in both eyes because each eye is used in turn. A unilateral tropia indicates a more serious situation because only one eye is constantly malaligned. The undeviated eye becomes the preferred eye, resulting in loss of vision or amblyopia of the deviated eye.

It is common in ocular misalignments to describe the type of deviation present because this indicates different etiologies and treatments of the strabismus. The prefixes *eso-*, *exo-*, *hyper-*, and *hypo-* are added to the terms *-phoria* and *-tropia* to further delineate the type of deviation. *Esophorias* of *esotropias* indicate an inward of convergent deviation of the eyes, commonly known as *crossed eyes*. *Exophorias* and *exotropias* refer to divergent or outward turning of the eyes, *wall-eyed* being the lay term. Hyperdeviations and hypodeviations designate upward or downward deviations of an eye.

DIAGNOSIS OF STRABISMUS. Many techniques are used to assess ocular alignment and movement of the eyes to aid in the diagnosis of strabismic disorders. Pediatricians should be knowledgeable and skilled at the two used most often: the corneal light reflex tests and cover tests. In a child with strabismus or any other ocular disorder, assessment of visual acuity is mandatory. Decreased vision in one eye requires evaluation for ocular deviation or other ocular abnormalities, which may be difficult to discern on a quick screening evaluation.

Corneal light reflex tests are perhaps the most rapid and easily performed diagnostic tests for strabismus. They are particularly useful in children who are uncooperative and in those who have poor ocular fixation. To perform the Hirschberg corneal reflex test, the examiner projects a light source onto the cornea of both eyes simultaneously as the child looks straight ahead. Comparison should then be made of the placement of the corneal light reflex in each eye. In straight eyes, the light reflection appears symmetrical, in the center of both pupils, or at the same point on each cornea. If strabismus is present, the reflected light is asymmetric and appears off center in one eye. The Krimsky method of the corneal reflex test uses prisms placed over one or both eyes to align the light reflections. The amount of prism needed to align the reflections is used to quantitate the degree of the deviation of the eye.

Cover tests for strabismus require the child's attention and cooperation, good eye movement capability, and ability to fixate the vision on the macula of each eye. However, if any of these are lacking the results of these tests may not be valid. These tests consist of the cover-uncover test and the alternate-cover test. To perform the cover-uncover test, the child should look at an object in the distance, preferably 20 ft away. An eye chart is commonly used for fixation in children older than 3 yr of age. For younger children, a brightly colored or noise-making toy helps hold their attention for the test. As the child looks at the distant object, the examiner covers one eye and watches for movement of the uncovered eye. If no movement occurs, there is no apparent misalignment of that eye. After testing one eye, the same procedure is repeated on the other eye. When performing the alternate-cover test, the examiner rapidly covers and uncovers each eye, shifting back and forth from one eye to another like a windshield wiper. If the child has any ocular deviation, the eye rapidly moves as the cover is shifted to the other eye. Both the cover-uncover test and the alternate-cover test should be performed at both distance and near fixation, with and without glasses. The cover-uncover test differentiates tropias, or manifest deviations, from latent deviations, called *phorias*.

CLINICAL TYPES OF STRABISMUS. The etiologic classification of strabismus is complex and knowledge of the causative types must be distinguished; these are nonparalytic and paralytic types.

Nonparalytic Strabismus. Nonparalytic strabismus is the most common type. There is usually no defect of the individual extraocular muscles. The amount of deviation is constant, or relatively constant, in the various directions of gaze.

ESODEVIATIONS. Esodeviations are the most common type of ocular misalignment in children and represent well over 50% of all ocular deviations.

Pseudostrabismus (pseudoesotropia) is one of the most common reasons a pediatric ophthalmologist is asked to evaluate an infant. This condition is characterized by the false appearance of strabismus when the visual axes are aligned accurately. This appearance may be caused by a flat, broad nasal bridge; prominent epicanthal folds; and/or a narrow interpupillary distance. The observer may see less white sclera nasally than would be expected, which creates the impression that the eye is turned in toward the nose, especially when the child is gazing to either side. Pseudoesotropia can be differentiated from a true misalignment of the eyes when the corneal light reflex is centered in both eyes and when the cover-uncover test shows no refixation movement.

Documented presence of *esotropia* prior to 6 mo of age is the general definition of infantile or congenital esotropia. The deviation is quite large and constant. Owing to the large deviation, cross-fixation is frequently encountered. This is a condition in which the child looks to the right with the left eye and to the left with the right eye. With cross-fixation there is a reluctance to turn each eye away from the nose (abduction); this condition simulates a 6th nerve palsy. Abduction can be demonstrated by the doll's head maneuver or by patching one eye for a short period of time.

With time, it is common to see the development of vertical deviations in children with infantile esotropia. One form of vertical deviation occurs due to overaction of the inferior oblique muscles. When this occurs, side gaze produces an upshoot of the eye closest to the nose. Dissociated vertical deviation also develops in children with infantile esotropia. In this type of deviation, one eye drifts up slowly with no movement of the other eye. Nystagmus also can occur and may be rotary, horizontal, or even latent, appearing only on occlusion of one eye.

The treatment of congenital esotropia consists of the improvement of poor vision in one eye with patching therapy. Glasses should be used to correct any significant farsightedness. Most pediatric ophthalmologists prefer to operate before the child is 2 yr old, because the visual system is still pliable enough to allow better binocular vision to develop postsurgically.

The image entering a hyperopic (farsighted) eye is blurred. If the amount of hyperopia is not significant, the blurred image can be sharpened by accommodating (focusing of the lens of the eye). Accommodation is closely linked with convergence (eyes turning inward). If a child's hyperopic refractive error is large, or if the amount of convergence that occurs in response to each unit of accommodative effort is great, esotropia may develop. This type of esodeviation is called *accommodative esotropia.*

Accommodative esotropia occurs between 6 mo and 7 yr at an average age of 2.5 yr. The deviation may be intermittent at the start but can become constant. One eye may be used habitually for fixation, causing poor vision (amblyopia) in the other.

Treatment of accommodative esotropia requires spectacle correction for the full amount of hyperopic error (Fig. 574–1). These glasses reduce the need for accommodation and thus reduce the stimulus for excessive convergence. Sometimes the full hyperopic correction straightens the eye position at distance fixation but leaves a residual deviation at near fixation. Bifocals can be useful in the control of this residual esotropia. Some children with an acquired esotropia may have a residual amount of crossing that cannot be controlled with glasses alone. If the residual deviation is significant, eye muscle surgery may be indicated.

EXODEVIATIONS. Exodeviations are the second most common type of misalignment. The divergent deviation may be intermittent or constant.

Intermittent exotropia is the most common exodeviation in childhood. It is characterized by an outward drift of one eye, which usually occurs when a child is fixating at distance. The deviation is generally more frequent with fatigue or illness. Exposure to bright light may cause reflex closure of the exotropic eye. Because the eyes initially can be kept straight most of the time, visual acuity tends to be good in both eyes and binocular vision is normal.

The age of onset of intermittent exotropia varies but is often between age 6 mo and 4 yr. The decision to perform eye muscle surgery is based on the amount and frequency of the deviation. If the deviation is small and infrequent, it is reasonable just to observe the child. If the exotropia is large or increasing in frequency, surgery is indicated.

Constant exotropia may rarely be congenital. Exotropia also may be associated with neurologic disease or abnormalities of the bony orbit, as in Crouzon syndrome. It also may result from deterioration of an intermittent exotropia or from overcorrection after surgery for esotropia. If poor vision exists in one eye, occlusion therapy should be instituted. If the deviation is cosmetically significant, eye muscle surgery can be performed after reliable and consistent measurements.

Paralytic Strabismus. When an eye muscle is paretic or palsied, a characteristic muscle imbalance occurs whereby the deviation of the eye varies according to the direction of gaze. Recent onset of a paretic muscle can be suggested by the symptom of double vision that increases in one direction, the findings of an ocular deviation that increases in the field of action of the paretic muscle, and an increase in the deviation when the child fixates with the paretic eye. It is important to differentiate an extraocular muscle paresis or palsy from a comitant deviation because noncomitant forms of strabismus are often associated with trauma, systemic disorders, or neurologic abnormalities.

THIRD NERVE PALSY. In the pediatric population, 3rd nerve palsies are usually congenital. The congenital form is often associated with a developmental anomaly or birth trauma. Acquired 3rd nerve palsies in children can be an ominous sign and may indicate a neurologic abnormality such as an intracranial neoplasm or an aneurysm. Other less serious causes include inflammatory or infectious lesion, head trauma, postviral syndromes, and migraines.

A 3rd nerve palsy, whether congenital or acquired, usually results in an exotropia. In this situation, the exotropia is associated with a hypotropia, or downward deviation of the affected eye, as well as a complete or partial ptosis of the upper lid. This characteristic deviation results from the action of the remaining unopposed muscles, the lateral rectus muscle and the superior oblique muscle. If the internal branch of the 3rd nerve is involved, pupillary dilation may be noted as well. Eye movements are usually limited nasally, in elevation and in depression. In addition, clinical findings and treatment may be complicated in congenital and traumatic cases of 3rd nerve palsy due to misdirection of regenerating nerve fibers, referred to as *aberrant regeneration.* This results in anomalous and paradoxic eyelid, eye and pupil movement such as elevation of the eyelid, constriction of the pupil, or depression of the globe on attempted medial gaze.

FOURTH NERVE PALSY. These palsies can be congenital or acquired. Because the 4th nerve has the longest intracranial course, it is susceptible to head trauma. In children, however, 4th nerve palsies are more frequently congenital than traumatic. The palsied 4th nerve results in weakness in the superior oblique muscle, which causes an upward deviation of the eye, a hypertropia. Typically, children present with a head tilt to the shoulder opposite the affected eye. This position is assumed to minimize the deviation and the associated double vision. Because this head tilt maintains the child's ocular alignment, amblyopia is uncommon. Because no abnormality exists in the neck muscles, attempts to correct the head tilt by exercises and neck muscle surgery are ineffective. Recognition of a superior oblique paresis can be difficult because the deviation of the head and the eye may be minimal. When the deviations are significant, eye muscle surgery can be performed to improve the ocular alignment and eliminate the head tilt.

SIXTH NERVE PALSY. These palsies produce markedly crossed eyes with limited ability to move the afflicted eye laterally. Frequently, children present with a head turn toward the palsied muscle, which helps preserve binocular vision. The esotropia is largest when the eye is moved toward the affected muscle.

Congenital 6th nerve palsies are rare. Decreased lateral gaze in infants is often associated with other disorders, such as congenital esotropia or Duane retraction syndrome. In neonates, a transient 6th nerve paresis can occur, which usually clears spontaneously by 6 wk of age. It is believed that increased intracranial pressure associated with labor and delivery is the contributing factor. A benign 6th nerve palsy, which is painless and acquired, can be noted in infancy and older children. This is frequently preceded by a febrile illness or upper respiratory infection and may be recurrent. Complete resolution of the palsy is usually seen.

Acquired 6th nerve palsies in childhood are often an ominous sign because the 6th nerve is susceptible to increased intracranial pressure associated with hydrocephalous and in-

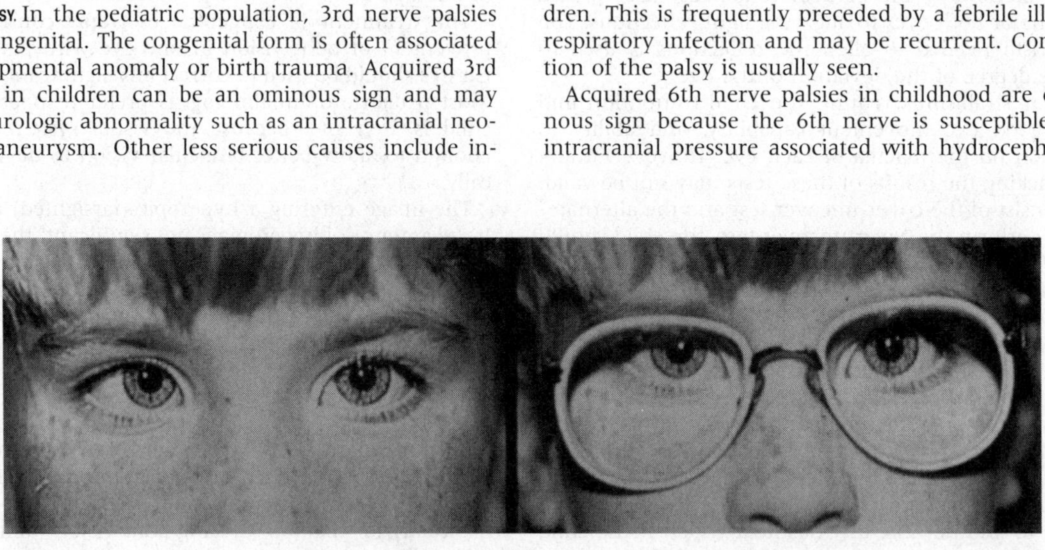

Figure 574–1. Accommodative esotropia; control of deviation with corrective lenses.

tracranial tumors. Other etiologies of 6th nerve defects in children include trauma, vascular malformations, meningitis, and Gradenigo syndrome. In this syndrome, otitis media precipitates a mastoiditis with associated petrositis and edema of the dura. These events result in pinching the 6th nerve against the petrosphenoidal ligament as the nerve passes between the ligament and the dura on its intracranial course. The 6th nerve palsy resolves with antibiotic treatment.

STRABISMUS SYNDROMES. There are special types of strabismus that have unusual clinical features. Most of these disorders are caused by structural anomalies of the extraocular muscles or adjacent tissues.

Double Elevator Palsy. A monocular elevation deficit in both abduction and adduction is referred to as a double elevator palsy. It may represent a paresis of both elevators, the superior rectus and inferior oblique muscles, or a possible restriction to elevation from a fibrotic inferior rectus muscle. When the child fixates with the nonparetic eye, the paretic eye is hypotropic and the ipsilateral upper eyelid may be ptotic. Fixation with the paretic eye causes a hypertropia of the nonparetic eye and a disappearance of the ptosis.

DUANE SYNDROME

This congenital disorder of ocular motility is characterized by retraction of the globe on adduction. This is attributed to anomalous innervation, which results in cocontraction of the medial and lateral rectus muscles on attempted adduction of the affected eye. Within the spectrum of Duane syndrome patients may exhibit impairment of abduction, impairment of adduction, or upshoot or downshoot of the involved eye on adduction. They may have esotropia, exotropia, or relatively straight eyes. Many exhibit compensatory posturing for the defect in horizontal eye movement. Some develop amblyopia. Surgery to improve ocular motility and alignment can be helpful in selected cases.

Duane syndrome usually occurs sporadically. Sometimes it is inherited as an autosomal dominant condition. It usually occurs as an isolated condition but may occur in association with various other ocular and systemic anomalies.

MÖBIUS SYNDROME

The distinctive features of Möbius syndrome are congenital facial paresis and abduction weakness. The facial palsy is commonly bilateral, frequently asymmetric, and often incomplete, tending to spare the lower face and platysma. Ectropion, epiphora, and exposure keratopathy may develop. The abduction defect may be unilateral or bilateral. It is usually complete, and esotropia is common. The etiology is unknown. Whether the primary defect is maldevelopment of cranial nerve nuclei, hypoplasia of the muscles, or a combination of central and peripheral factors is unclear. Gestational factors such as trauma, illness, and intake of various drugs, particularly thalidomide, have been implicated. Some familial cases have been reported. Associated developmental defects may include ptosis, palatal and lingual palsy, hearing loss, pectoral and lingual muscle defects, micrognathia, syndactyly, supernumerary digits, or the absence of hands, feet, fingers, or toes. Surgical correction of the esotropia is indicated in selected cases, and any attendant amblyopia should be treated.

BROWN SYNDROME

In this syndrome elevation of the eye in the adducted position is restricted or absent. Often, there is an associated downward deviation of the affected eye in adduction. There may be a compensatory tilt of the head. Various causes have been described. Some cases have been attributed to structural abnormalities such as a tight superior oblique tendon, congenital shortening or thickening of the superior oblique tendon sheath, or connective tissue trabeculae between the superior oblique tendon and the trochlea. Sometimes no anatomic abnormality is found.

Acquired Brown syndrome may follow trauma to the orbit involving the region of the trochlea or sinus surgery. It may also occur with inflammatory processes, particularly sinusitis and juvenile rheumatoid arthritis.

Acquired inflammatory Brown syndrome may respond to treatment with steroids. Surgery may be helpful for children with true congenital Brown syndrome.

PARINAUD SYNDROME

This eponym designates a palsy of vertical gaze, isolated or associated with pupillary or nuclear oculomotor (cranial nerve III) paresis. It indicates a lesion affecting the mesencephalic tegmentum. The ophthalmic signs of midbrain disease include vertical gaze palsy, dissociation of the pupillary responses to light and to near focus, general pupillomotor paralysis, corectopia, dyscoria, accommodative disturbances, pathologic lid retraction, ptosis, extraocular muscle paresis, and convergence paralysis. In some cases there are spasms of convergence, convergent retraction nystagmus, and vertical nystagmus, particularly on attempted vertical gaze. Combinations of these signs are referred to as the Koerber-Salus-Elschnig or sylvian aqueduct syndrome.

A principal cause of vertical gaze palsy and associated mesencephalic signs in children is tumor of the pineal gland or 3rd ventricle. Differential diagnosis includes trauma and demyelinating disease. In children with hydrocephalus, impairment of vertical gaze and pathologic lid retraction are referred to as the *setting sun sign.* A transient supranuclear disorder of gaze is sometimes seen in healthy neonates.

CONGENITAL OCULAR MOTOR APRAXIA

This congenital disorder of conjugate gaze is characterized by a defect in voluntary horizontal gaze, compensatory jerking movement of the head, and retention of slow pursuit and reflexive eye movements. Additional features are absence of the fast (refixation) phase of optokinetic nystagmus and obligate contraversive deviation of the eyes on rotation of the body. Typically, the affected child is unable to look quickly to either side voluntarily in response to command or in response to an eccentrically presented object but may, however, be able to follow a slowly moving target to either side. To compensate for the defect in purposive lateral eye movements, the child jerks the head to bring the eyes into the desired position and may also blink repetitively in an attempt to change fixation. The signs tend to become less conspicuous with age.

The pathogenesis of congenital ocular motor apraxia is unknown. It may be a result of delayed myelination of the ocular motor pathways. Structural abnormalities of the central nervous system have been found in a few patients, including agenesis of the corpus callosum and cerebellar vermis, porencephaly, hamartoma of the foramen of Monro, and macrocephaly. Many children with congenital ocular motor apraxia show delayed motor and cognitive development.

A disorder of eye movement resembling congenital ocular motor apraxia may occur in patients with certain metabolic neurodegenerative diseases (particularly Gaucher disease) or with ataxia-telangiectasia, or as a sign of brain tumor.

NYSTAGMUS

Nystagmus (rhythmic oscillations of one or both eyes) may be caused by an abnormality in any one of the three basic mechanisms that regulate position and movement of the eyes: the fixation, conjugate gaze, or vestibular mechanisms. In addition, physiologic nystagmus may be elicited by appropriate stimuli.

Congenital pendular nystagmus is commonly associated with ocular and visual defects; it typically occurs with albinism, aniridia, achromatopsia, congenital cataracts, congenital macular lesions, congenital optic atrophy, and high refractive errors. In some instances pendular nystagmus occurs as a dominant or X-linked characteristic without obvious ocular abnormalities. There may be associated rhythmic movements of the head.

Congenital jerky nystagmus is characterized by horizontal jerky oscillations with gaze preponderance; the nystagmus is coarser in one direction of gaze than in the other, with the jerk toward the direction of gaze. There is usually a point of reversal or a null point in which the nystagmus lessens and in which position vision is best; compensatory posturing, turning of the head to bring the eyes into the position of least nystagmus, is characteristic. The cause of congenital jerky nystagmus is unkown; in some instances it is familial.

Acquired nystagmus requires prompt and thorough evaluation. Worrisome pathologic types are the gaze-paretic or gaze-evoked oscillations of cerebellar, brain stem, or cerebral disease.

Nystagmus retractorius or *convergent nystagmus* is repetitive jerking of the eyes into the orbit or toward each other. It is usually seen with vertical gaze palsy as a feature of the Parinaud or Koerber-Salus-Elschnig (sylvian aqueduct) syndrome. The causal condition may be neoplastic, vascular, or inflammatory. In children nystagmus retractorius suggests particularly the presence of pinealoma or hydrocephalus.

Spasmus nutans is a special type of acquired nystagmus in childhood (see also Chapter 547). In its complete form it is characterized by the triad of pendular nystagmus, head nodding, and torticollis. The nystagmus is characteristically very fine, very rapid, horizontal, and pendular; it is often asymmetric, sometimes unilateral. Signs usually develop within the 1st yr or two of life. Components of the triad may develop at varying times. In many cases the condition is benign and self-limited, usually lasting a few months, sometimes years. The cause of this classic type of spasmus nutans, which resolves spontaneously, is unknown. Many children exhibiting signs resembling those of spasmus nutans have underlying brain tumors, particularly hypothalamic and chiasmal optic gliomas. Appropriate neurologic and neuroradiologic evaluation and careful monitoring of infants and children with nystagmus is therefore recommended.

OTHER ABNORMAL EYE MOVEMENTS

To be differentiated from true nystagmus are certain special types of abnormal eye movements, particularly opsoclonus, ocular dysmetria, and flutter.

Opsoclonus

Opsoclonus and ataxic conjugate movements are terms that describe spontaneous, nonrhythmic, multidirectional, chaotic movements of the eyes. The eyes appear to be in agitation, with bursts of conjugate movement of varying amplitude in varying directions. Opsoclonus is most often associated with encephalitis. It may be the first sign of neuroblastoma.

Ocular Motor Dysmetria

This is analogous to dysmetria of the limbs. There is lack of precision in performing movements of refixation, characterized by an overshoot (or undershoot) of the eyes with several corrective to-and-fro oscillations on looking from one point to another. Ocular motor dysmetria is a sign of cerebellar or cerebellar pathway disease.

Flutter-Like Oscillations

These intermittent to-and-fro horizontal oscillations of the eyes may occur spontaneously or on change of fixation. They are characteristic of cerebellar disease.

Anthony JH, Ouvrier RA, Wise G: Spasmus nutans: A mistaken identity. Arch Neurol 37:373, 1980.

Baker JD, Parks MM: Early-onset accommodative esotropia. Am J Ophthalmol 90:11, 1980.

Bixenman WW, von Noorden GK: Benign recurrent VI nerve palsy in childhood. J Pediatr Ophthalmol Strab 18:29, 1981.

Catalano RA: Nystagmus. *In*: Nelson LB, Calhoun JH, Harley RD (eds): Pediatric Ophthalmology, 3rd ed. Philadelphia, WB Saunders, 1991.

Catalano RA, Nelson LB: Pediatric Opthalmology: A Text Atlas. Norwalk, CT, Appleton and Lange, 1994.

Chan CC, Sogg RL, Steinman L: Isolated oculomotor palsy after measles immunization. Am J Ophthalmol 89:446, 1980.

Cogan DG: Heredity of congenital ocular motor apraxia. Trans Am Acad Ophthalmol Otolaryngol 76:60, 1972.

DeRespinis PA, Caputo AR, Wagner RS, Guo S: Duane's retraction syndrome. Surv Ophthalmol 38:257, 1993.

Harley RD: Paralytic strabismus in children: Etiologic incidence and management of the third, fourth and sixth nerve palsies. Ophthalmology 87:24, 1980.

Hoyt CS, Mousel DK, Weber AA: Transient supranuclear disturbance of gaze in healthy neonates. Am J Ophthalmol 89:708, 1980.

Ing M: Early surgical alignment for congenital esotropia. Ophthalmology 90:132, 1983.

Kushner BJ: Ocular causes of abnormal head postures. Ophthalmology 86:2115, 1979.

Lavery MA, O'Neill JF, Chau FC, et al: Acquired nystagmus in early childhood: A presenting sign of intracranial tumor. Ophthalmology 91:425, 1984.

Miller MT, Ray V, Owens P, et al: Möbius and Möbius-like syndromes (TTV-OFM, OMLH). J Pediatr Ophthalmol Strab 26:176, 1989.

Miller NR: Solitary oculomotor nerve palsy in children. Am J Ophthalmol 83:106, 1977.

Mohindra I, Zwann J, Held R, et al: Development of acuity and stereopsis in infants with esotropia. Ophthalmology 92:691, 1985.

Morre RT, Morin JD: Bilateral acquired inflammatory Brown's syndrome. J Pediatr Ophthalmol Strab 22:26, 1985.

Nelson LB, Wagner RS, Simon JW, Harley RD: Congenital esotropia. Surv Ophthalmol 31:363, 1987.

Norton EWD, Cogan DG: Spasmus nutans: A clinical study of twenty cases followed two years or more since onset. Arch Ophthalmol 52:442, 1954.

Rappaport L, Urlon D, Strand K, et al: Concurrence of congenital oculomotor apraxia and other motor problems: An expanded syndrome. Dev Med Child Neurol 29:85, 1987.

Richard JM, Parks M: Intermittent exotropia: Surgical results in different age groups. Ophthalmology 90:1172, 1983.

Shetty T, Rosman NP: Opsoclonus in hydrocephalus. Arch Ophthalmol 88:585, 1972.

Smith JL, Walsh FB: Opsoclonus—ataxic conjugate movements of the eye. Arch Ophthalmol 64:244, 1960.

Smith JL, Ziepes I, Gay AJ, et al: Nystagmus retractorius. Arch Ophthalmol 62:864, 1959.

Summers CG, MacDonald JT, Wirtschafter JD: Oculomotor apraxia associated with intracranial lipoma. J Pediatr Ophthalmol Strab 24:267, 1987.

Wang FM, Wertenbaker C, Behrens MM, et al: Acquired Brown's syndrome in children with juvenile rheumatoid arthritis. Ophthalmology 91:23, 1984.

Wilson ME, Eustis HS, Parks MM: Brown's syndrome. Surv Ophthalmol 34:153, 1989.

Zaret CR, Behrens MM, Eggers HM: Congenital ocular motor apraxia and brain stem tumor. Arch Ophthalmol 98:328, 1980.

CHAPTER 575

Abnormalities of the Lids

PTOSIS

Blepharoptosis exists when the upper eyelid droops below its normal level. Congenital ptosis is usually a result of faulty development of the levator muscle or its innervating branch of the 3rd nerve. There may be associated involvement of the superior rectus muscle and attendant impairment in elevation of the eye. The condition may be familial, transmitted as a dominant trait. Congenital ptosis can be corrected surgically; the age at which surgery is done depends on its degree, its cosmetic and functional severity, the presence or absence of compensatory posturing, the wishes of the parents, and the discretion of the surgeon. Ptosis of sufficient degree to interfere with visual development requires early correction to prevent amblyopia. Correction of mild ptosis for purely cosmetic reasons is often deferred until age 3–4 yr. Children with ptosis may have associated anisometropia and/or strabismus, which may lead to amblyopia. Early evaluation and treatment of these problems are indicated in all children with ptosis.

Congenital ptosis occurs with a large number of syndromes. In the Marcus Gunn jaw winking syndrome of aberrant innervation, there is abnormal synkinesis of lid and jaw movements; paradoxic elevation of the ptotic lid occurs as the child sucks, chews, or cries. In the congenital fibrosis syndrome, a hereditary condition, ptosis is associated with paralysis or "fibrosis" of other extraocular muscles. Minimal ptosis occurs in the Horner syndrome (oculosympathetic palsy). In the Sturge-Weber syndrome, ptosis is often secondary to hemangiomatous involvement of the upper lid, and in von Recklinghausen syndrome there may be ptosis resulting from plexiform neuroma of the upper lid.

Differential diagnosis of acquired ptosis in childhood includes myasthenia gravis, botulism, progressive external ophthalmoplegia, progressive intracranial lesions affecting the 3rd nerve, and inflammation or tumors affecting the levator, the orbit, or lid. Ptosis may also result from trauma. Aberrant regeneration of injured 3rd nerve fibers may produce paradoxic lid and eye movements.

EPICANTHAL FOLDS

These vertical or oblique folds of skin extend on either side of the bridge of the nose from the brow or lid area, covering the inner canthal region. They are present to some degree in most young children and become less apparent with age. The folds may be sufficiently broad to cover the medial aspect of the eye, making the eyes appear crossed (pseudoesotropia).

Epicanthal folds are a common feature of many syndromes, including chromosomal aberrations (particularly the trisomies) or disorders of single genes.

LAGOPHTHALMOS

This exists when complete closure of the lids over the globe is difficult or impossible. It may be paralytic, because of a facial palsy involving the orbicularis muscle, or spastic, as in thyrotoxicosis. It may be structural when retraction or shortening of the lids results from scarring or atrophy consequent to injury (e.g., burns) or disease. Infants with collodion membrane may have temporary lagophthalmos caused by the restrictive effect of the membrane on the lids. Lagophthalmos may accompany proptosis or buphthalmos when the lids, although normal, cannot effectively cover the enlarged or protuberant eye. A degree of physiologic lagophthalmos may occur normally during sleep, but functional lagophthalmos in the unconscious or debilitated patient can be a problem.

When lagophthalmos exists, exposure of the eye may lead to drying, infection, corneal ulceration, or perforation of the cornea; the result may be loss of vision, even loss of the eye. In lagophthalmos protection of the eye by artificial tear preparations, ophthalmic ointment, or moisture chambers is essential. Gauze pads are to be avoided, because the gauze may abrade the cornea. In some cases surgical closure of the lids (tarsorrhaphy) may be necessary for long-term protection of the eye.

LID RETRACTION

Pathologic retraction of the lid may be myogenic or neurogenic. Myogenic retraction of the upper lid occurs in thyrotoxicosis, in which it is associated with three classic signs: a staring appearance (Dalrymple sign), infrequent blinking (Stellwag sign), and lag of the upper lid on downward gaze (von Graefe sign).

Neurogenic retraction of the lids may occur in conditions affecting the anterior mesencephalon. Lid retraction is a feature of the syndrome of the sylvian aqueduct. In children it is commonly a sign of hydrocephalus. It may occur with meningitis.

Paradoxic retraction of the lid is a feature of the Marcus Gunn jaw winking syndrome. Paradoxic lid retraction may also occur during recovery from a 3rd nerve palsy as a result of aberrant regeneration or misdirection of oculomotor fibers.

To be differentiated from pathologic lid retractions are simple staring and the physiologic or reflexive lid retraction ("eye popping") that occurs in infants in response to a sudden reduction in illumination or as a startle reaction.

ENTROPION AND ECTROPION

Entropion is inversion of the lid margin, which may cause discomfort and corneal damage because of the inward turning of the lashes (trichiasis). A principal cause is scarring secondary to inflammation such as occurs in trachoma or as a sequela of Stevens-Johnson syndrome. There is also a rare congenital form. Surgical correction is effective in many cases.

Ectropion is eversion of the lid margin; it may lead to overflow of tears (epiphora) and subsequent maceration of the skin of the lid, to inflammation of exposed conjunctiva, or to superficial exposure keratopathy. Common causes are scarring consequent to inflammation, burns, or trauma, or weakness of the orbicularis muscle as a result of facial palsy; these forms may be corrected surgically. Protection of the cornea is essential. Eversion of the lids may occur during delivery; this can resolve with conservative management.

Ectropion is also seen in certain children who have faulty development of the lateral canthal ligament; this may occur in Down syndrome.

BLEPHAROSPASM

This spastic or repetitive closure of the lids may be caused by irritative disease of the cornea, conjunctiva, or facial nerve, fatigue or uncorrected refractive error, or common tic. Thorough ophthalmic examination for pathologic causes, such as trichiasis, keratitis, conjunctivitis, or foreign body, is indicated. Local injection of botulinum toxin may give relief.

BLEPHARITIS

This inflammation of the lid margins is characterized by erythema and crusting or scaling; the usual symptoms are irritation, burning, and itching. The condition is commonly bilateral and chronic or recurrent. There are two main types, staphylococcal and seborrheic. In *staphylococcal blepharitis* ulceration of the lid margin is common, the lashes tend to fall out, and there is often associated conjunctivitis and superficial keratitis. In *seborrheic blepharitis* the scales tend to be greasy, the lid margins are less red, and ulceration usually does not occur. The blepharitis is often of mixed type.

Thorough daily cleansing of the lid margins with a cloth or moistened cotton applicator to remove scales and crusts is important in the treatment of both forms of blepharitis. Staphylococcal blepharitis is treated with antistaphylococcal antibiotic or sulfonamide ophthalmic ointment applied directly to the lid margins daily at bedtime. When seborrhea exists, concurrent treatment of the scalp is important.

Pediculosis of the eyelashes may produce the clinical picture of blepharitis. The lice can be smothered with opthalmic-grade petrolatum ointment applied to the lid margin and lashes. Nits should be mechanically removed from the lashes.

HORDEOLUM

Infection of the glands of the lid may be acute or subacute; there is tender focal swelling and redness. The usual agent is *Staphylococcus aureus*.

When the meibomian glands are involved, the lesion is referred to as an *internal hordeolum*; the abscess tends to be large and may point through either the skin or conjunctival surface. When the infection involves the glands of Zeis or Moll, the abscess tends to be smaller and more superficial and points at the lid margin; it is then referred to as an *external hordeolum* or *stye*.

As with abscesses elsewhere, treatment is frequent, warm compresses and, if necessary, surgical incision and drainage. In addition, topical antibiotic or sulfonamide preparations are often used. Untreated, the infection may progress to cellulitis of the lid or orbit, requiring the use of systemic antibiotics. Recurrence is common, possibly by reinfection through contaminated hands. Itching resulting from an underlying allergy is a common contributory factor. Recurrent styes in children may also signal an immunologic defect.

CHALAZION

Chalazion is granulomatous inflammation of a meibomian gland characterized by a firm, nontender nodule in the upper or lower lid. This lesion tends to be chronic and differs from internal hordeolum in the absence of acute inflammatory signs. When a chalazion is large enough to distort vision (it may cause astigmatism by exerting pressure on the globe) or to be a cosmetic blemish, excision is advised. In some cases chalazion subsides spontaneously.

COLOBOMA OF THE EYELID

This cleftlike deformity may vary from a small indentation or notch of the free margin of the lid to a large defect involving almost the entire lid. If the gap is extensive, xerosis, ulceration, and corneal opacities may result from exposure. Early surgical correction of the lid defect is recommended. Other deformities frequently associated with lid colobomata include dermoid cysts or dermolipomata on the globe; often, they occur in a position corresponding to the site of the lid defect. Lid colobomata may also be associated with extensive facial malformation, as in mandibulofacial dysostosis (Franceschetti or Treacher Collins syndrome).

TUMORS OF THE LID

A number of lid tumors arise from surface structures (the epithelium and sebaceous glands). Nevi may appear in early childhood; most are junctional. Compound nevi tend to develop in the prepubertal years, dermal nevi at puberty. Malignant epithelial tumors (basal cell carcinoma and squamous cell carcinoma) are rare in children, but the basal cell nevus syndrome and the malignant lesions of xeroderma pigmentosum and of the Rothmund-Thomson syndrome may develop in childhood. Adenoma sebaceum (vascular fibroma) may also occur in the lids, with or without cutaneous lesions elsewhere; these usually appear in infancy and regress spontaneously by the age of 1–2 yr.

Other lid tumors arise from deeper structures (the neural, vascular, and connective tissues). Hemangiomas are especially common. Most tend to regress spontaneously, although they may show alarmingly rapid growth in infancy. In many cases the best management of such hemangiomas is patient observation, allowing spontaneous regression to occur (see Chapter 600). In the case of a rapidly expanding lesion that threatens to obstruct vision and produce sensory deprivation amblyopia, corticosteroid treatment should be considered.

Nevus flammeus (port wine stain), a noninvoluting hemangioma, occurs as an isolated lesion or in association with other signs of Sturge-Weber syndrome. Affected patients should be examined for glaucoma.

Lymphangiomas of the lid appear as firm masses at or soon after birth and tend to enlarge slowly during the growing years. Associated conjunctival involvement, appearing as a clear, cystic, sinuous conjunctival mass, may provide a clue to the diagnosis. In some cases there is also orbital involvement. The treatment is surgical excision.

Plexiform neuromas of the lids occur in children with neurofibromatosis, often with ptosis as the first sign.

The lids may also be involved by other tumors, such as retinoblastoma, neuroblastoma, and rhabdomyosarcoma of the orbit; these conditions are discussed elsewhere.

Crawford JS: Congenital eyelid anomalies in children. J Pediatr Ophthalmol Strab 21:140, 1984.
Crawford JS, Iliff CE, Stasier OG: Symposium on congenital ptosis. J Pediatr Ophthalmol Strab 19:245, 1982.
Johnson CC: Epicanthus and epiblepharon. Arch Ophthalmol 96:1030, 1978.
Kushner BJ: Intralesional corticosteroid injection for infantile adnexal hemangioma. Am J Ophthalmol 93:496, 1982.
Masaki S: Congenital bilateral facial paralysis. Arch Otolaryngol 94:260, 1971.
McCully JP, Dougherty JM, Deneau DG: Classification of chronic blepharitis. Ophthalmology 89:1173, 1982.
Merriam WW, Ellis FD, Helveston EM: Congenital blepharoptosis, anisometropia, and amblyopia. Am J Ophthalmol 89:401, 1980.
Moainie R, Kopelowitz N, Rosenfeld W, et al: Congenital eversion of the eyelids: A report of two cases treated with conservative management. J Pediatr Ophthalmol Strab 19:326, 1982.
Pićo G: Congenital ectropion and distichiasis. Etiologic and hereditary factors. A report of cases and review of the literature. Am J Ophthalmol 47:363, 1959.
Pratt SG, Beyer CK, Johnson CC: The Marcus Gunn phenomenon: A review of 71 cases. Ophthalmology 91:27, 1984.
Stigmar G, Crawford JS, Ward CM, et al: Ophthalmic sequelae of infantile hemangiomas of the eyelid and orbit. Am J Ophthalmol 85:806, 1978.
Zak TA: Congenital primary upper eyelid entropion. J Pediatr Ophthalmol Strab 21:69, 1984.

CHAPTER 576
Disorders of the Lacrimal System

DACRYOSTENOSIS AND DACRYOCYSTITIS

The tear film, which bathes the eye, is actually a complex structure composed of three layers. The outermost layer is an oily layer, produced largely from the sebaceous meibomian glands of the eyelid. The bulk of the tear film, the middle aqueous layer, is produced by the main lacrimal gland and accessory lacrimal glands. The innermost layer is a mucin layer produced by goblet cells that are scattered over the conjunctiva. Tears drain medially into the punctal openings of the lid margin and flow through the canaliculi into the lacrimal sac and then through the nasolacrimal duct into the nose.

Congenital nasolacrimal duct obstruction (CNLDO), or dacryostenosis, is the most common disorder of the lacrimal system, occurring in up to 5% of newborn infants. It is usually caused by an incomplete canalization of the nasolacrimal duct with a residual membrane at the lower end of the nasolacrimal duct, where the duct enters the nasal cavity.

Signs may appear days or weeks after birth and are often aggravated by upper respiratory infection or by exposure to cold or wind. The usual manifestations of nasolacrimal obstruction are "tearing," ranging in degree from a "wetness" of the eye (an increase in the tear lake, "pooling," or "puddling") to frank overflow of tears (epiphora), accumulation of mucoid or mucopurulent discharge (often described by the parents as "matter"), and crusting. There may be erythema or maceration of the skin because of irritation and rubbing produced by dripping of tears and discharge. In many cases reflux of clear fluid or mucopurulent discharge can be elicited by massaging the nasolacrimal sac, proving obstruction to outflow.

Infants with CNLDO may develop acute infection and inflammation of the nasolacrimal sac (dacryocystitis), inflammation of the surrounding tissues (pericystitis), or even periobital cellulitis. With dacryocystitis the sac area is swollen, red, and tender, and there may be systemic signs of infection such as fever and irritability.

The primary treatment of uncomplicated nasolacrimal obstruction is a regimen of nasolacrimal massage, usually two to three times a day, accompanied by cleansing of the lids with warm water. Topical antibiotics are used for significant mucopurulent drainage. In most cases, the problem resolves with conservative management by the age of 1 yr, if not earlier. If symptoms persist beyond 1 yr of age, then a probing is indicated. A small percentage of children do not respond to the first probing. Most pediatric ophthalmologists will repeat simple probing once or twice before proceeding to the placement of tubes or more extensive reconstructive surgery (such as dacryocystorhinostomy).

Acute dacryocystitis or cellulitis requires prompt treatment with antibiotics. In such cases some form of definitive surgical intervention is usually indicated.

A mucocele is an unusual presentation of a nonpatent nasolacrimal sac that is obstructed both proximally and distally. Mucoceles can be seen at birth or shortly after birth as a bluish subcutaneous mass just below the medial canthal tendon. Initial treatment should include warm compresses and gentle massage of the lacrimal sac. At the earliest sign of inflammation, a probing should be performed.

It should be noted that not all tearing in infants and children is caused by nasolacrimal obstruction. Tearing may also be a sign of glaucoma, intraocular inflammation, or external irritation, such as that from a corneal abrasion or foreign body.

DACRYOADENITIS

Dacryoadenitis, or inflammation of the lacrimal gland, is uncommon in childhood. It may occur with mumps (in which case it is usually acute and bilateral, subsiding in a few days or weeks), or with infectious mononucleosis. Chronic dacryoadenitis is associated with certain systemic diseases, particularly sarcoidosis, tuberculosis, and syphilis. Some systemic diseases may produce enlargement of the lacrimal and salivary glands (Mikulicz syndrome).

ALACRIMA AND "DRY EYE"

Marked deficiency of tears may occur as an isolated unilateral or bilateral congenital defect or in association with other nervous system anomalies, such as aplasia of cranial nerve nuclei. It occurs congenitally in familial dysautonomia (Riley-Day syndrome) and in the anhidrotic type of ectodermal dysplasia; it may occur with glucocorticoid deficiency, sometimes in association with swallowing dysfunction. Tear deficiency may be a sign of Sjögren syndrome, in which it is sometimes associated with salivary gland enlargement and with arthritis. Deficiency of tears may also follow inflammation; it is not uncommon after Stevens-Johnson syndrome. Drying of the eye, corneal ulceration, and scarring may result. Preventive care includes the frequent instillation of an artificial tear preparation. In some cases occlusion of the lacrimal puncta is helpful. In severe cases tarsorrhaphy may be necessary to protect the cornea.

Caccamise WC, Townes PL: Congenital absence of the lacrymal puncta associated with alacrima and aptyalism. Am J Ophthalmol 89:62, 1980.

Cachoun JH: Disorders of the lacrimal apparatus in infancy and childhood. *In*: Nelson LB, Calhoun JH, Harley RD (eds): Pediatric Ophthalmology, 3rd ed. Philadelphia, WB Saunders, 1991.

Christian CJ, Nelson LB: Lacrimal system disorders in infants and children. Ophthalmol Clin North Am 3:239, 1990.

Geffner ME, Lippe BM, Kaplan SA, et al: Selective ACTH insensitivity, achalasia, and alacrima: A multisystem disorder presenting in childhood. Pediatr Res 17:532, 1983.

El-Mansoury J, Calhoun JH, Nelson LB, et al: Results of late probing for congenital nasolacrimal duct obstruction. Ophthalmology 93:1052, 1986.

Goldberg MF, Payne JW, Brunt PW: Ophthalmologic studies of familial dysautonomia. Arch Ophthalmol 80:732, 1966.

Manson AM, Cheng KP, Mumma JV, et al: Congenital dacryocele. Ophthalmology 98:1744, 1991.

Mondino BJ, Brown SI: Hereditary congenital alacrima. Arch Ophthalmol 94:1478, 1976.

Nelson LB, Calhoun JH, Menduke H: Medical management of congenital nasolacrimal duct obstruction. Ophthalmology 92:1187, 1985.

Paul TO: Medical management of congenital nasolacrymal duct obstruction. J Pediatr Ophthalmol Strab 22:68, 1985.

Weinstein GS, Biglan AW, Patterson JH: Congenital lacrimal sac mucoceles. Am J Ophthalmol 94:106, 1982.

CHAPTER 577

Disorders of the Conjuctiva

CONJUNCTIVITIS

The conjunctiva reacts to a wide range of bacterial and viral agents, allergens, irritants, toxins, and systemic diseases. Conjunctivitis is common in childhood and may be infectious or noninfectious.

OPHTHALMIA NEONATORUM

Ophthalmia neonatorium is a form of conjunctivitis occurring in infants less than 4 wk of age. It is the most common eye disease of newborns. There have been many different etiologic agents implicated that differ greatly in their virulence and clinical courses. For instance, silver nitrate instillation may result in a mild self-limited conjunctivitis, whereas *Neisseria gonorrhoeae* and *Pseudomonas* are capable of causing corneal perforation, blindness, and death. The relative frequency with which each etiologic agent causes conjunctivitis in newborns is dependent on frequencies of maternal infections, prophylactic measures, if any, circumstances during labor and delivery, and postdelivery exposures to microorganisms.

EPIDEMIOLOGY. Conjunctivitis during the neonatal period is usually acquired during vaginal delivery and reflects the sexually transmitted diseases prevalent in the community. In 1880, 10% of European children developed gonococcal conjunctivitis at birth. Ophthalmia neonatorum was the leading cause of blindness during that period. The epidemiology of this condition changed dramatically in 1881, when Crede reported that 2% silver nitrate solution instilled in the eyes of newborns reduced the incidence of gonococcal ophthalmia from 10% to 0.3%.

During the 20th century, the spectrum of organisms causing ophthalmia neonatorum changed significantly. The incidence of gonococcal ophthalmia neonatorum decreased in industrialized countries secondary to the widespread use of silver nitrate prophylaxis and the prenatal screening and treatment of maternal gonorrhea. Presently, gonococcal ophthalmia neonatorum has an incidence of 0.3%/1,000 live births in the United States. In comparison, *Chlamydia trachomatis* has become the most common organism causing ophthalmia neonatorum in the United States, with an incidence of 8.2/1,000 births.

CLINICAL MANIFESTATIONS. The clinical manifestations of the various forms of ophthalmia neonatorum are not specific enough to allow an accurate diagnosis. Although the timing and character of the signs are somewhat typical for each cause of this condition, there is considerable overlap and the physician should not rely solely on clinical findings. Regardless of its etiology, ophthalmia neonatorum is characterized by redness and chemosis (swelling) of the conjunctiva, edema of the eyelids, and discharge, which may be purulent.

Ophthalmia neonatorum is a potentially blinding condition. The infection may also have associated systemic manifestations that require treatment. Therefore, any newborn infant who develops signs of conjunctivitis needs a prompt and comprehensive workup in order to determine the etiologic agent causing the infection and the appropriate treatment necessary.

The onset of inflammation caused by silver nitrate drops usually occurs within 6–12 hr after birth, with clearing by 24–48 hr. The usual incubation period for conjunctivitis due to *N. gonorrhoeae* is 2–5 days and for that due to *C. trachomatis*, 5–14 days. Gonococcal infection may be present at birth or delayed beyond 5 days of life owing to partial suppression by ocular prophylaxis. Gonococcal conjunctivitis may also begin in infancy following inoculation by the contaminated fingers of adults. The time of onset of disease with other bacteria is highly variable.

Gonococcal conjunctivitis begins with mild inflammation and a serosanguineous discharge. Within 24 hr the discharge becomes thick and purulent, and tense edema of the eyelids with marked chemosis occurs. If proper treatment is delayed, the infection may spread to involve the deeper layers of the conjunctivae and the cornea. Complications include corneal ulceration and perforation, iridocyclitis, anterior synechiae, and rarely panophthalmitis. Conjunctivitis caused by *C. trachomatis* (inclusion blennorrhea) may vary from mild inflammation to severe swelling of the eyelids with copious purulent discharge. The process involves mainly the tarsal conjunctivae; the corneas are rarely affected. Conjunctivitis due to *Staphylococcus aureus* or other organisms is similar to that produced by *C. trachomatis*. Conjunctivitis due to *Pseudomonas aeruginosa* is uncommon, is acquired in the nursery, and is a potentially serious process. It is characterized by the appearance on day 5–18 of edema, erythema of the lids, purulent discharge, pannus formation, endophthalmitis, sepsis, shock, and death.

DIAGNOSIS. Conjunctivitis appearing after 48 hr should be evaluated for a possibly infectious cause. Gram stain of the purulent discharge should be performed and the material cultured. If a viral etiology is suspected, a swab should be submitted in tissue culture media for virus isolation. In chlamydial conjunctivitis the diagnosis is made by examining Giemsa-stained epithelial cells scraped from the tarsal conjunctivae for the characteristic intracytoplasmic inclusions, by isolating the organisms from a conjunctival swab using special tissue culture techniques, by immunofluorescent staining of conjunctival scrapings for chlamydial inclusions, or by tests for chlamydial antigen. The differential diagnosis includes dacrocystitis, caused by congenital lacrimal duct obstruction with lacrimal sac distention (dacrocystocele).

TREATMENT. Treatment of the infant in whom gonococcal ophthalmia is suspected and the Gram stain shows the characteristic intracellular gram-negative diplococci should be initiated immediately with ceftriaxone, 25–50 mg/kg/day for 7 days. Single-dose therapy also has been reported to be effective. In addition, the eye should be irrigated initially with saline every 10–30 min, gradually increasing to 2-hr intervals, until the purulent discharge has cleared. An alternate regimen includes a single dose of kanamycin (75–150 mg intramuscularly) with gentamicin eye ointment applied for 3 days. Inclusion blennorrhea is treated with oral erythromycin for 2 wk. This cures conjunctivitis and may prevent subsequent chlamydial pneumonia. *Pseudomonas* neonatal conjunctivitis is treated with systemic antibiotics, including an aminoglycoside, plus local saline irrigation and gentamicin ophthalmic ointment. Staphylococcal conjunctivitis is treated with parenteral methicillin and local saline irrigation.

PROGNOSIS AND PREVENTION. Prior to the institution of topical ophthalmic prophylaxis at birth, gonococcal ophthalmia was a common cause of blindness or permanent eye damage. If properly applied, this form of prophylaxis is highly effective unless infection is present at birth. Drops of 0.5% erythromycin or 1% silver nitrate are instilled directly into the open eyes at birth using wax or plastic single-dose containers. Saline irrigation after silver nitrate application is unnecessary. Silver nitrate is ineffective against active infection.

Identification of maternal gonococcal infection and appropriate treatment has become a standard element of routine prenatal care. An infant born to a woman who has untreated gonococcal infection should receive a single dose of ceftriaxone, 50 mg/kg (maximum 125 mg) intravenously or intramuscularly, in addition to topical prophylaxis. Dosage should be reduced for premature infants. Penicillin (50,000 units) should be used if the mother's gonococcal isolate is known to be penicillin sensitive.

Neither silver nitrate nor topical antibiotics are effective for prophylaxis for chlamydial ophthalmia. Furthermore, topical prophylaxis does not prevent the afebrile pneumonia that occurs in 10–20% of infants exposed to *C. trachomatis*. Although chlamydial conjunctivitis is often a self-limiting disease, chlamydial pneumonia may have serious consequences. Treatment of colonized pregnant women with erythromycin may prevent neonatal disease.

Hammerschlag MR, Cummings C, Roblin PM, et al: Efficacy of neonatal ocular prophylaxis for the prevention of chlamydial and gonococcal conjunctivitis. N Engl J Med 320:769, 1989.
Hammerschlag MR: Neonatal ocular prophylaxis. Pediatr Infect Dis J 7:81, 1988.
O'Hara MA: Ophthalmia Neonatorum. Pediatr Clin North Am 40:715, 1993.
Schacter J: Why we need a program for the control of *Chlamydia trachomatis*. N Engl J Med 320:802, 1989.
Schnall BM, Nelson LB: Ophthalmia neonatorum. Sem Ophthalmol 5:107, 1990.

Acute Purulent Conjunctivitis

This is characterized by more or less generalized conjunctival hyperemia, edema, mucopurulent exudate, and various degrees of ocular discomfort. It is usually a result of bacterial infection. The most frequent causes are *Haemophilus influenzae*, pneumococci, staphylococci, and streptococci. Conjunctival smear and culture are helpful in differentiating specific types. These common forms of acute purulent conjunctivitis usually respond well to warm compresses and frequent topical instillation of antibiotic drops. Brazilian purpuric fever due to *Haemophilis aegyptius* manifests conjunctivitis and sepsis. Unfortunately, however, *Neisseria gonorrhoeae* and *Chlamydia* are emerging as common causes of acute purulent conjunctivitis in children beyond the newborn period, especially in adolescents. These infections require specific testing and treatment.

Ophthalmia neonatorum is acute conjunctivitis in the newborn infant. Any of the common bacterial conjunctivitides can occur in the newborn period, but emphasis in differential diagnosis must be given to recognition of gonococcal and chlamydial infections. To be differentiated from the infectious types of ophthalmia neonatorum is the chemical conjunctivitis caused by the prophylactic use of silver nitrate. This usually develops 12–24 hr after instillation and lasts only 24–48 hr; no treatment is needed.

Viral Conjunctivitis

This is generally characterized by a watery discharge. Often, there are follicular changes (small aggregates of lymphocytes) in the palpebral conjunctiva. Conjunctivitis resulting from adenovirus infection is relatively common, sometimes with corneal involvement (see later). Outbreaks of conjunctivitis caused by enterovirus are also seen; this type may be hemorrhagic.

Conjunctivitides are commonly associated with such systemic viral infections as the childhood exanthems, particularly measles. These are self-limited.

Epidemic Keratoconjunctivitis

This is caused by adenovirus type 8 and is transmitted by direct contact. Initially there is a sensation of a foreign body beneath the lids with itching and burning. Edema and photophobia develop rapidly, and large oval follicles appear within the conjunctiva. Preauricular adenopathy and a pseudomembrane on the conjunctival surface occur frequently. Subepithelial corneal infiltrates may develop and may cause blurring of vision; these usually disappear but may reduce visual acuity permanently. Corneal complications are less common in children than in adults. Children may have associated upper respiratory infection. No specific therapy is available. Emphasis must be placed on prevention of spread of the disease.

Membranous and Pseudomembranous Conjunctivitis

These types can be seen in a number of diseases. The classic membranous conjunctivitis is that of diphtheria, accompanied by a fibrin-rich exudate that forms on the conjunctival surface and permeates the epithelium; the membrane is removed with difficulty and leaves raw bleeding areas. In pseudomembranous conjunctivitis the layer of fibrin-rich exudate is superficial and can often be stripped easily, leaving the surface smooth. This type occurs with many bacterial and viral infections, including staphylococcal, pneumococcal, streptococcal, or chlamydial conjunctivitis, and in epidemic keratoconjunctivitis. It is seen also in vernal conjunctivitis and in Stevens-Johnson disease.

Allergic Conjunctivitis

This is usually accompanied by intense itching, tearing, and conjunctival edema. It is commonly seasonal. Cold compresses and decongestant drops give symptomatic relief. Topical cromalyn sodium also may help. In selected cases, topical corticosteroids are used under an ophthalmologist's supervision.

Vernal Conjunctivitis

This usually begins in the prepubertal years and may recur for many years. Atopy appears to play a role in its origin, but the pathogenesis is uncertain. Extreme itching and tearing are the usual complaints. Large, flattened, cobblestone-like papillary lesions of the palpebral conjunctivae are characteristic. A stringy exudate and a milky conjunctival pseudomembrane are frequently present. There may be small elevated lesions of the bulbar conjunctiva adjacent to the limbus (limbal form). Smear of the conjunctival exudate reveals many eosinophils. Topical corticosteroid therapy and cold compresses afford some relief. Cromolyn sodium drops may help.

Chemical Conjunctivitis

This can result when an irritating substance enters the conjunctival sac (as in the acute but benign conjunctivitis caused by silver nitrate in the newborn). Other common offenders are household cleaning substances, sprays, smoke, smog, and industrial pollutants.

Alkalis tend to linger in the conjunctival tissues and continue to inflict damage over a period of hours or days. Acids precipitate the proteins in tissues and so produce their effect immediately. In either case prompt, thorough, and copious irrigation is crucial. Extensive tissue damage, even loss of the eye, can result, especially if the offending agent is an alkali.

OTHER CONJUNCTIVAL DISORDERS

Subconjunctival hemorrhage is manifested by bright or dark red patches in the bulbar conjunctiva and may result from injury or inflammation. It may occasionally result from severe sneezing or coughing or be a manifestation of a blood dyscrasia.

Pingueculum is a yellowish-white, slightly elevated mass on the bulbar conjunctiva, usually in the interpalpebral region. It represents elastic and hyaline degenerative changes of the conjunctiva. No treatment is required except for cosmetic reasons, in which case simple excision suffices.

Pterygium is a fleshy triangular conjunctival lesion that may encroach on the cornea. It typically occurs in the nasal interpalpebral region. The pathologic findings are similar to those of a pingueculum. Irritation such as exposure to dust or wind is thought to aggravate the lesion. Removal is suggested when the lesion encroaches far onto the cornea.

Dermoid cyst and *dermolipoma* are benign lesions, clinically similar in appearance. They are smooth, elevated, round to oval lesions of various sizes. The color varies from yellowish-white to a fleshy pink. The most frequent site is the upper outer quadrant of the globe; they also commonly occur near or straddle the limbus. The dermolipoma is composed of adipose and connective tissue. Dermoid cysts may also contain glandular tissue, hair follicles, and hair shafts. Excision for cosmetic reasons is feasible.

Conjunctival nevus is a small, slightly elevated lesion that may vary in pigmentation from pale salmon to dark brown. It is usually benign, but careful observation for progressive growth or changes suggestive of malignancy is advised.

Symblepharon is a cicatricial adhesion between the conjunctiva of the lid and the globe; the lower lid is usually affected. It follows operation or injuries, especially burns from lye, acids, or molten metals. It is a serious complication of Stevens-Johnson syndrome. It may interfere with motion of the eyeball and cause diplopia. The adhesions should be separated and the raw surfaces kept from uniting during healing. Grafts of oral mucous membrane may be necessary.

Arstikaitis MJ: Ocular aftermath of Stevens-Johnson syndrome. Arch Ophthalmol 90:376, 1973.

Brook I: Anaerobic and aerobic bacterial flora of acute conjunctivitis in children. Arch Ophthalmol 98:833, 1980.

Catalano RA, Nelson LB: Conjunctivitis. *In*: Dershervitz RA (ed): Ambulatory Pediatric Care, 2nd ed. Philadelphia, JB Lippincott, 1992.

Clark SW, Culbertson WW, Forster RK: Clinical findings and results of treatment in an outbreak of acute hemorrhagic conjunctivitis in southern Florida. Am J Ophthalmol 99:45, 1983.

Fischer MC: Conjunctivitis in children. Pediatr Clin North Am 34:1447, 1987.

Foster CS: Evaluation of topical cromolyn sodium in the treatment of vernal conjunctivitis. Ophthalmology 95:194, 1988.

Gigliotti F, Williams WT, Hayden FG, et al: Etiology of acute conjunctivitis in children. J Pediatr 98:531, 1981.
Howard GM: The Stevens-Johnson syndrome. Am J Ophthalmol 55:893, 1963.
Isenberg SJ, Apt L, Yoshimora R, et al: Bacterial flora of the conjunctiva at birth. J Pediatr Ophthalmol Strab 23:284, 1986.
Knopf HLS, Hierholzer JC: Clinical and immunologic responses in patients with viral keratoconjunctivitis. Am J Ophthalmol 80:661, 1975.
Matobu A: Ocular viral infections. Pediatr Infect Dis 3:358, 1984.

CHAPTER 578

Abnormalities of the Cornea

MEGALOCORNEA

This denotes a developmental anomaly in which the diameter of the cornea is greater than 13 mm. The condition is nonprogressive, although there is often a high refractive error. Vision in adults is threatened by a high incidence of glaucoma, lens subluxation, and the early development of cataracts. These complications rarely present in childhood. Megalocornea is often familial and may be associated with other developmental abnormalities.

Pathologic corneal enlargement caused by glaucoma is to be differentiated from this anomaly. Any progressive increase in the size of the cornea, especially when accompanied by photophobia, lacrimation, or haziness of the cornea, requires prompt ophthalmologic evaluation.

MICROCORNEA

Microcornea, or anterior microphthalmia, describes an abnormally small cornea in an otherwise relatively normal eye. It may be familial, transmission being dominant more often than recessive. More commonly, a small cornea is just one feature of an otherwise developmentally abnormal or microphthalmic eye; associated defects include colobomata, microphakia, congenital cataract, glaucoma, and aniridia.

KERATOCONUS

Keratoconus is a disease of unclear pathogenesis characterized by progressive thinning and bulging of the central cornea, which becomes cone shaped. Although familial cases are known, most cases are sporadic. Eye rubbing and contact lens wear have been implicated as pathogenic, but the evidence to support this is equivocal. An increased incidence occurs in individuals with atopy, Down syndrome, Marfan syndrome, and retinitis pigmentosa.

Most cases are bilateral, but the eyes may be very asymmetrically involved. The disorder usually presents and progresses rapidly during adolescence; progression slows and stabilizes when the individual reaches full growth. Signs of keratoconus include Munson's sign (bulging of the lower eyelid upon looking downward) and the presence of a Fleischer's ring (a deposit of iron in the epithelium at the base of the cone). Corneal transplantation is indicated if satisfactory visual acuity cannot be attained with the use of hard contact lenses.

SCLEROCORNEA

In sclerocornea the normal translucent cornea is replaced by "scleral-like" tissue. Instead of a clearly demarcated cornea, white, feathery, often ill-defined and vascularized tissue develops in the peripheral cornea, appearing to blend with and extend from the sclera. The central cornea is usually clearer, but rare cases of total replacement of the cornea with sclera have been reported. Potentially coexisting abnormalities include a shallow anterior chamber, iris abnormalities, and microphthalmus. Associated skeletal, chromosomal, and central nervous system anomalies have been reported, but there are no invariable systemic findings. In generalized sclerocornea, early keratoplasty should be considered in an effort to provide vision.

DENDRITIC KERATITIS

Infection of the eye with the virus of herpes simplex produces a characteristic lesion of the corneal epithelium, referred to as a dendrite; it has a branching treelike pattern that can be demonstrated by fluorescein staining. The acute episode is accompanied by pain, photophobia, tearing, blepharospasm, and conjunctival infection. Specific treatment is 5-iodo-2′-deoxyuridine (IDU) in the form of drops or ointment, or topical vidarabine or trifluridine. In addition, a cycloplegic agent such as cyclogel is useful to relieve pain from spasm of the ciliary muscle. Recurrent infection and deep stromal involvement can lead to corneal scarring.

It has been clearly demonstrated that the topical use of corticosteroids causes exacerbation of superficial herpetic disease of the eye; eyedrops combining steroids and antibiotics are, therefore, to be avoided in treatment of "red eye" unless there are clear-cut indications for their use and close supervision during therapy.

Infants born to mothers infected with herpes simplex should be examined carefully for signs of ocular involvement. Intravenous acyclovir is required for treatment of ocular herpes in the newborn.

CORNEAL ULCERS

In corneal ulcers, the usual signs and symptoms are focal or diffuse corneal haze, hyperemia, lid edema, pain, photophobia, tearing, and blepharospasm. Often, there is hypopyon (pus in the anterior chamber).

Corneal ulcers require prompt treatment. They result most frequently from traumatic lesions that become secondarily infected. Many organisms are capable of infecting the cornea. One of the most troublesome is *Pseudomonas aeruginosa*; it can rapidly destroy stromal tissue and lead to corneal perforation. *Neisseria gonorrhoeae* also is particularly damaging to the cornea. Indolent ulcers may be caused by fungi, often in association with the use of contact lenses. In each case scrapings of the cornea must be studied in an effort to identify the infectious agent and to determine the best therapy. Generally, both systemic and local treatment are needed to save the eye. Perforation or scarring resulting from corneal ulceration is an important cause of blindness throughout the world and is estimated to be responsible for 10% of blindness in the United States.

Unexplained corneal ulcers in infants and young children should raise the question of a sensory defect, as in Riley-Day or Goldenhar-Gorlin syndrome, or of a metabolic disorder such as tyrosinemia.

PHLYCTENULES

These are small, yellowish, slightly elevated lesions usually located at the corneal limbus; they may encroach on the cornea and extend centrally. Often, there is a small corneal ulcer at the head of the advancing lesion, with a fascicle of blood vessels behind the head of the lesion. Phlyctenular keratoconjunctivitis was once thought to represent hypersensitivity to tuberculin proteins, but the cause is not really known. Staphylococcal infections may be associated with phlyctenular changes. There is strong evidence for an immunologic factor. The condition usually responds to topical corticosteroid therapy, sometimes leaving superficial stromal pannus and scarring.

INTERSTITIAL KERATITIS

This denotes inflammation of the corneal stroma. The most common cause is syphilis, interstitial keratitis being one of the characteristic late manifestations of congenital syphilis. The deep inflammation produces pain, photophobia, tearing, circumcorneal injection, and corneal haze. Corneal vascularization and opacities develop and generally remain as permanent stigmata of the disease.

Cogan syndrome is a nonluetic interstitial keratitis associated with hearing loss and vestibular symptoms. Both the corneal changes and the auditory involvement may respond to corticosteroids.

Less frequently, interstitial keratitis is caused by other infectious diseases, such as tuberculosis or leprosy.

PETERS ANOMALY

In this condition maldevelopment of the anterior segment of the eye may affect the cornea, anterior chamber angle, and iris. The terms *mesodermal dysgenesis, anterior cleavage syndrome,* and others describe these defects and various combinations thereof.

Peters anomaly consists of a congenital corneal opacity (leukoma) with corresponding defects in the posterior corneal stroma, Descemet membrane, and endothelium, often with associated iridocorneal or lenticulocorneal adhesions. The condition is usually bilateral. It is generally sporadic, but recessive and dominant inheritances have been suggested.

Other anomalies within the spectrum of anterior chamber cleavage syndrome are abnormalities of the peripheral cornea and angle, including a prominent, anteriorly displaced ring of Schwalbe, Axenfeld anomaly (fine iris strands that cross the chamber to the displaced ring of Schwalbe), or Rieger anomaly. There may be associated glaucoma or lens abnormalities.

CORNEAL MANIFESTATIONS OF SYSTEMIC DISEASE

Several metabolic diseases produce distinctive corneal changes in childhood. Refractile polychromatic crystals are deposited throughout the cornea in cystinosis. Corneal deposits producing various degrees of corneal haze also occur in certain of the mucopolysaccharidoses, particularly MPS IH (Hurler), MPS IS (Scheie), MPS I H/S (Hurler-Scheie compound), MPS IV (Morquio), MPS VI (Maroteaux-Lamy), and sometimes MPS VII (Sly). Corneal deposits may develop in patients with GM_1 (generalized) gangliosidosis. In Fabry disease fine opacities radiating in a whorl or fanlike pattern occur, and corneal changes can be important in identifying the carrier state. A spray-like pattern of corneal opacities may also be seen in the Bloch-Sulzberger syndrome. In Wilson disease the distinctive corneal sign is the Kayser-Fleischer ring, a golden brown ring in the peripheral cornea resulting from changes in Descemet membrane. Pigmented corneal rings may develop in neonates with cholestatic liver disease. Corneal changes may occur in autoimmune hypoparathyroidism, and band keratopathy in patients with hypercalcemia. Transient keratitis may occur with rubeola, sometimes with rubella.

Beauchamp GR, Gillette TE, Friendly DS: Phlyctenular keratoconjunctivitis. J Pediatr Ophthalmol Strab 18:22, 1981.
Boger WP III, Peterson RA, Robb RM: Keratoconus and acute hydrops in mentally retarded patients with congenital rubella syndrome. Am J Ophthalmol 91:231, 1981.
Burns RB: Soluble tyrosine aminotransferase deficiency: An unusual cause of corneal ulcers. Am J Ophthalmol 73:400, 1972.
Cobo LM, Haynes BF: Early corneal findings in Cogan's syndrome. Ophthalmology 91:903, 1984.
Deckard PS, Bergstrom TJ: Rubeola keratitis. Ophthalmology 88:810, 1981.
Dunn LL, Annable WL, Kliegman RM: Pigmented corneal rings in neonates with liver disease. J Pediatr 110:771, 1987.
Elliott JH, Feman SS, O'Day DM, et al: Hereditary sclerocornea. Arch Ophthalmol 103:676, 1985.
Goldberg MF: A review of selected inherited corneal dystrophies associated with systemic disease. Birth Defects: Original Article Series VII:13, 1971.
Goldberg MF, Payne JW, Brunt PW: Ophthalmologic studies of familial dysautonomia. Arch Ophthalmol 80:732, 1966.
Hutchison DS, Smith RE, Haughton PB: Congenital herpetic keratitis. Arch Ophthalmol 93:70, 1975.
Kraft SP, Judisch GF, Grayson DM: Megalocornea: A clinical and echographic study of an autosomal dominant pedigree. J Pediatr Ophthalmol Strab 21:190, 1984.
Laibson PR, Waring GO: Diseases of the cornea. *In*: Nelson LB, Calhoun JH, Harley RD (eds): Pediatric Ophthalmology, 3rd ed. Philadelphia, WB Saunders, 1991.
Mohandessan MM, Romano PE: Neuroparalytic keratitis in Goldenhar-Gorlin syndrome. Am J Ophthalmol 85:111, 1978.
Schanzlin DJ, Goldberg DB, Brown SI: Transplantation of congenitally opaque corneas. Ophthalmology 87:1253, 1980.
Stieglitz LM, Kind HP, Kazden JJ, et al: Keratitis with hypoparathyroidism. Am J Ophthalmol 84:467, 1972.
Stone DL, Kenyon KR, Green WR, et al: Congenital central corneal leukoma (Peters' anomaly). Am J Ophthalmol 81:173, 1976.
Tso MOM, Fine BS, Thorpe HE: Kayser-Fleischer ring and associated cataract in Wilson's disease. Am J Ophthalmol 79:479, 1975.

CHAPTER 579
Abnormalities of the Lens

CATARACTS

A cataract is any opacity of the lens. Some are clinically insignificant, others significantly affect visual function, and many signify associated ocular or systemic disease.

DIFFERENTIAL DIAGNOSIS. The differential diagnosis of cataracts in infants and children includes a wide range of developmental disorders, infectious and inflammatory processes, metabolic diseases, and toxic and traumatic insults. Cataracts may also develop secondary to intraocular processes, such as retinopathy of prematurity, persistent hyperplastic primary vitreous, retinal detachment, retinitis pigmentosa, and uveitis.

Developmental Variants. Early developmental processes may lead to various congenital lens opacities. Not uncommon are discrete dots or white plaquelike opacities of the lens capsule, sometimes with involvement of the contiguous subcapsular region. Small opacities of the posterior capsule may be associated with persistent remnants of the primitive hyaloid vascular system (the common Mittendorf dot), whereas those of the anterior capsule may be associated with persistent strands of the pupillary membrane or vascular sheath of the lens. Congenital cataracts of this type are usually stationary and rarely interfere with vision; in some cases, however, progression occurs.

Prematurity. A special type of lens change seen in some preterm newborns is the so-called cataract of prematurity. The appearance is of a cluster of tiny vacuoles in the distribution of the Y sutures of the lens. They can be visualized with the ophthalmoscope and are best seen with the pupil well dilated. The pathogenesis is unclear. In most cases the opacities disappear spontaneously, often within a few weeks.

Mendelian Inheritance. Many cataracts are hereditary, unassociated with other disease. The most common mode of inheritance is autosomal dominant. Penetrance and expressivity vary. Autosomal recessive inheritance occurs less frequently; it is sometimes found in populations with high rates of consanguinity. X-linked inheritance of cataracts unassociated with disease is relatively rare, whereas cataracts occurring in association with X-linked disease, such as Lowe syndrome, Alport syndrome, and Fabry disease, are not uncommon.

Congenital Infection Syndrome. Frequently, cataracts in infants and children are the result of prenatal infection. Lens opacity may occur in any of the major congenital infection syndromes (e.g., toxoplasmosis, cytomegalovirus infection, syphilis, rubella, perinatal herpes simplex virus infection). Cataracts attributed to other maternal infections, including measles, poliomyelitis, influenza, varicella-zoster, and vaccinia, have also been reported.

Metabolic Disorders. Cataracts are a prominent manifestation of many metabolic diseases, particularly certain disorders of carbohydrate, amino acid, calcium, and copper metabolism. A primary consideration in any infant with cataracts is the possibility of galactosemia (see Chapter 73). In classic infantile galactosemia, galactose-1-phosphate uridyl transferase deficiency, the cataract is typically of the zonular type, with haziness or opacification of one or more of the perinuclear layers of the lens; often, haziness or clouding of the nucleus also occurs. In its early stages the cataract generally has a distinctive "oil droplet" appearance and is best detected with the pupil fully dilated. There may be progression to complete opacification of the lens within weeks. With early treatment (galactose-free diet) the lens changes may be reversible.

In galactokinase deficiency, cataracts may be the sole or presenting clinical manifestation. The cataracts are usually zonular and may appear in the 1st months or years of life, or later in childhood.

In children with juvenile-onset diabetes mellitus, lens changes are uncommon. Some, however, develop snowflake-like white opacities and vacuoles of the lens. Others develop cataracts that may progress and mature rapidly, sometimes in a matter of hours or days, especially during adolescence. An antecedent event may be the sudden development of myopia caused by changes in the optical density of the lens.

Congenital lens opacities may be seen in children of diabetic and prediabetic mothers. Hypoglycemia in the neonate can also be associated with early development of cataracts. Another disorder of carbohydrate metabolism associated with the development of cataracts is ketotic hypoglycemia of childhood.

An association between cataracts and hypocalcemia is well established. Various lens opacities may be seen in patients with hypoparathyroidism.

A metabolic disorder of major importance in the differential diagnosis of cataracts in infants and children is the oculocerebral renal syndrome of Lowe. Affected male children frequently have dense bilateral cataracts at birth, often in association with glaucoma and miotic pupils. Punctate lens opacities are frequently present in heterozygous females.

The distinctive sunflower cataract of Wilson disease is not commonly seen in children. Various lens opacities may be seen in children with certain of the sphingolipidoses, mucopolysaccharidoses and mucolipidoses, particularly Niemann-Pick disease, mucosulfatidosis, Fabry disease, and aspartyl-glycosaminuria.

Miscellaneous Disorders. The list of multisystem syndromes and diseases associated with lens opacities of various types is long. The clinical features of some of the major disorders are presented in Table 579–1.

Chromosomal Defects. Lens opacities of various types may occur in association with chromosomal defects, including 13-, 18-, and 21-trisomy; Turner syndrome; and a number of deletion (e.g., 11p13, 18p, 18q) and duplication syndromes (e.g., 3q, 20p, 10q).

Drugs, Toxic Agents, and Trauma. Of the various drugs and toxic agents that may produce cataracts, corticosteroids are of major importance in the pediatric age group. Steroid-related cataracts characteristically are posterior subcapsular lens opacities. The incidence and severity vary. The relative significance of dose, duration of treatment, and individual susceptibility is controversial, and the pathogenesis of steroid-induced cataracts is unclear. The effect on vision depends on the extent and density of the opacity. In many cases, the acuity is only minimally or moderately impaired. Reversibility of steroid-induced cataracts may occur in some cases. All children being treated with long-term steroids should have periodic eye examinations.

Trauma to the eye is a major cause of cataracts in children. Opacification of the lens may result from contusion or penetrating injury. Cataracts are an important manifestation of child abuse. Other physical agents, such as radiation, can also damage the lens and produce cataracts.

MANAGEMENT PRINCIPLES. The treatment of cataracts that significantly interfere with vision includes the following: (1) surgical removal of lens material to provide an optically clear visual axis; (2) correction of the resultant aphakic refractive error with spectacles, contact lenses, or, in selected cases, intraocular lens implantation or refractive corneal surgery; and (3) correction of any associated sensory deprivation amblyopia. Treatment of the amblyopia may be the most demanding and difficult step in the visual rehabilitation of infants or children with cataracts.

PROGNOSIS. Prognosis depends on many factors, including the nature of the cataract, age of onset, age of intervention, duration and severity of any attendant amblyopia, and presence of any associated ocular abnormalities (e.g., microphthalmia, retinal lesions, optic atrophy, glaucoma, nystagmus, strabismus). In addition, secondary conditions and complications may develop in children who have had cataract surgery, including inflammatory sequelae, secondary membranes, glaucoma, retinal detachment, and changes in the axial length of the eye. All these factors and possibilities should be considered in planning treatment. The ultimate management decision should rest jointly with the ophthalmologist, pediatrician, and family.

ECTOPIA LENTIS

Normally, the lens is suspended in place behind the iris diaphragm by the zonular fibers of the ciliary body. Abnormalities of the suspensory system resulting from a developmental defect, disease, or trauma may result in instability or displacement of the lens. Displacement of the lens is classified as luxation (dislocation—complete displacement of the lens) or as subluxation (partial displacement—shifting or tilting of the lens). Symptoms include blurring of vision, which is often the result of refractive changes such as myopia, astigmatism, or aphakic hyperopia. Some patients experience diplopia. An important sign of displacement is iridodeneses, a tremulousness of the iris caused by the loss of its usual support. Also, the anterior chamber may appear deeper than normal. Sometimes the equatorial region ("edge") of the displaced lens may be visible in the pupillary aperture. On ophthalmoscopy this may appear as a black crescent. Also, the difference between the phakic and aphakic portions can be appreciated when focusing on the fundus.

DIFFERENTIAL DIAGNOSIS. A major cause of lens displacement is trauma. Displacement may occur as the result of ocular disease, such as uveitis, intraocular tumor, congenital glaucoma, high myopia, megalocornea, or aniridia, or in association with cataract. Also important in the differential diagnosis of lens displacement in children are the hereditable forms of ectopia lentis and those associated with systemic disease.

Displacement of the lens occurring as a hereditable ocular condition unassociated with systemic abnormalities is referred

■ TABLE 579–1 Clinical Features of Ocular Changes in Developmental Pediatric Syndromes

- CNS anomalies
  - Anencephaly (see Chapter 542)
    - Optic nerve aplasia or hypoplasia
  - Holoprosencephaly (see Chapter 542)
    - Hypotelorism; in extreme form, cyclopia; in some cases, iris coloboma
- Cyclopia
  - A single eye of variable complexity, usually accompanied by a proboscis-like structure on the forehead; often associated with holoprosencephaly; sometimes fusion of both eyes with duplication of lenses, corneas, and other structures; rosette formation in the retina; optic nerve rudimentary or absent; orbit diamond-shaped
  - Arnold-Chiari malformation (see Chapter 542)
    - Nystagmus, usually vertical, often downbeat; ocular motor palsies with diplopia; sometimes skew deviation
  - Dandy-Walker syndrome (see Chapter 542)
    - Ophthalmic manifestations of increased intracranial pressure
- Septo-optic dysplasia (deMorsier syndrome)
  - Malformation of anterior midline structures (agenesis of septum pellucidum, primitive optic ventricle, with hypoplasia of optic nerves, chiasm, and infundibulum); sometimes associated endocrine abnormalities; vision defects, strabismus, nystagmus; in some cases, other anomalies of eyes
- Craniostenosis syndromes (see Chapter 542)
  - Apert syndrome (acrocephalosyndactyly)
    - Orbits shallow, eyes protuberant (proptosis) and widely spaced; antimongoloid slant of palpebral fissures; ocular motor abnormalities (strabismus, partial ophthalmoplegia, nystagmus); papilledema; optic atrophy; cataracts; sometimes dislocated lenses; occasionally iris and fundus colobomata
  - Carpenter syndrome (acrocephalopolysyndactyly)
    - Orbits shallow; lateral displacement of medial canthi; epicanthus; antimongoloid slant of palpebral fissures; optic atrophy; microcornea and corneal opacities in some cases
  - Crouzon syndrome (dysostosis craniofacialis)
    - Eyes protuberant (proptosis) and widely spaced; luxation of globe may occur; antimongoloid slant of palpebral fissures; strabismus; papilledema; optic atrophy; vision loss; cataracts in some patients
  - Kleeblattschädel syndrome (cloverleaf skull)
    - Shallow orbits with proptosis; high risk of corneal ulceration
- Miscellaneous craniofacial defects and syndromes
  - Frontonasal dysplasia (median cleft-face syndrome)
    - Hypertelorism (radiographic interorbital distance 2 SD above normal for age); in some cases, anophthalmia, microphthalmia, epibulbar dermoids, lid colobomata, congenital cataracts
  - Opitz syndrome
    - Hypertelorism, particularly associated with hypospadias; antimongoloid slant of palpebral fissures; epicanthus; strabismus
  - Waardenburg syndrome
    - Lateral displacement of medial canthi and inferior puncta; heterochromia iridis, total or partial; in some cases both irides completely blue (isochromia); fundus pigmentary changes in some cases
  - Oculodentodigital dysplasia (Meyer-Schwickerath syndrome)
    - Hypotelorism, microphthalmos, microcornea, dental anomalies and enamel hypoplasia, camptodactyly, syndactyly, and other skeletal defects; persistent pupillary membrane; glaucoma
  - Hallermann-Streiff syndrome (dyscephalia oculomandibulofacialis)
    - Microphthalmos, cataract, sparse eyebrows and lashes, blue sclerae, nystagmus
  - Pierre Robin syndrome
    - Congenital glaucoma; retinal detachment; strabismus
  - Treacher Collins syndrome (mandibulofacial dysostosis; Franceschetti-Klein syndrome)
    - Antimongoloid slant of palpebral fissures; underdevelopment of supraorbital ridges, colobomata of lower eyelids and in some cases of iris or choroid
  - Goldenhar syndrome (oculoauriculovertebral dysplasia)
    - Antimongoloid slant of palpebral fissures; colobomata of eyelid, upper lid more commonly involved than lower; hypoplasia or coloboma of iris; hypertelorism; sometimes microphthalmos
- Chromosomal abnormalities
  - 21-Trisomy (Down syndrome; see Chapter 67)
    - Mongoloid slant of palpebral fissures; epicanthus; dacryostenosis; blepharitis; Brushfield spots of iris; peripheral thinning of iris stroma; keratoconus and corneal hydrops; cataracts; high refractive errors; strabismus; nystagmus; increased vessels at disk
  - 18-Trisomy (Edwards syndrome; see Chapter 67)
    - Ptosis; short palpebral fissures; epicanthus; hypoplastic supraorbital ridges; microphthalmia; corneal opacities; anisocoria; cataracts; fundus and disk colobomata; retinal hypopigmentation
  - 13-Trisomy (Patau syndrome; see Chapter 67)
    - Microphthalmos; anophthalmos; cyclopia in some cases; dysgenesis of anterior segment (iris hypoplasia, iris adhesions, chamber angle abnormalities); corneal opacities; congenital glaucoma; cataracts; persistent hyperplastic primary vitreous; retinal dysplasia; colobomata of iris, ciliary body, fundus; intraocular cartilage, optic nerve hypoplasia
  - 9-Trisomy
    - Antimongoloid slant of palpebral fissures; deeply set eyes; corectopia; strabismus
  - 8-Trisomy
    - Dysmorphic skull; strabismus
  - Syndrome 45X (Turner, and mosaic variants; see Chapter 67)
    - Ptosis; epicanthus; blue sclerae; defective color vision; cataracts; strabismus; nystagmus
  - 47,XXY; 48,XXXY; 49,XXXXY (Klinefelter) syndromes (see Chapters 517 and 535)
    - Hypertelorism; epicanthus; Brushfield spots of iris; myopia; strabismus
  - Partial deletion short arm chromosome 4 (4p −) (see Chapter 67)
    - Ptosis; hypertelorism; epicanthus; colobomata
  - Partial deletion short arm chromosome 5 (5p −) (cri-du-chat syndrome; see Chapter 67)
    - Antimongoloid slant of palpebral fissures; hypertelorism; epicanthus; strabismus
  - Partial deletion short arm chromosome 9 (9p −) (see Chapter 67)
    - Mongoloid slant of palpebral fissures; epicanthus; arched brows
  - Partial deletion long arm chromosome 13 (13q −)
    - Ptosis; epicanthus; hypertelorism; microphthalmos; colobomata; retinoblastoma
  - Partial deletion long arm chromosome 18 (18q −) (see Chapter 67)
    - Horizontal palpebral fissures; epicanthus; deeply set eyes; optic disk pallor; tapetoretinal degeneration; nystagmus
  - Partial deletion, long arm chromosome 21 (21q −)
    - Downward slanting palpebral fissures
  - Partial deletion long arm chromosome 22 (22q −)
    - Ptosis; epicanthus
  - Extrachromosomal material (cat-eye syndrome)
    - Antimongoloid slant of palpebral fissures; epicanthus; hypertelorism; microphthalmos; colobomata of iris, fundus, optic nerve; macular defects; pale disks; cataracts; strabismus; nystagmus
- Disorders of amino acid metabolism
  - Albinism*
    - Defect in the formation of melanin; several forms:
      - (1) *Oculocutaneous albinism, tyrosinase negative;* generalized hypopigmentation; iris blue or gray; generalized hypopigmentation of eye; typical pink or orange reflex; fundus bright, with increased choroidal vascular pattern; macula/fovea poorly defined (hypoplastic); photophobia; nystagmus; subnormal vision; often high refractive error
      - (2) *Oculocutaneous albinism, tyrosinase positive;* pigmentation may increase with age; iris blue, yellow, or brownish; color increasing with age; photophobia; nystagmus; subnormal vision, which may improve with age
      - (3) *Amish* or *yellow* mutant; generalized albinism in which a yellowish pigment is produced instead of melanin, providing some skin and hair color
      - (4) *Hermansky-Pudlak syndrome;* tyrosine negative albinism associated with a hemorrhagic diathesis; iris blue-gray to brown; photophobia; nystagmus; slight to moderate vision defect
      - (5) *Cross syndrome;* tyrosine positive; a syndrome of hypopigmentation, gingival fibromatosis, spasticity, athetoid movements, and microphthalmos; iris blue-gray, microphthalmos; cataracts; severe vision defect; nystagmus
      - (6) *Ocular albinsim;* pigment deficiency limited to the eye; generalized ocular hypopigmentation; macular hypoplasia; nystagmus (in blacks, fundus tessellated)
  - Alcaptonuria (see Chapter 71.5)
    - Black discoloration of sclera, most noticeable at insertion of extraocular muscles
  - Tyrosinemia (Richner-Hanhart syndrome; see Chapter 71.2)
    - Corneal ulceration, "herpetiform"
  - Cystinosis (see Chapter 71.4)
    - Accumulation of refractile crystals in cornea (best seen with slit lamp, but corneal haze may be detected grossly); photophobia; pigmentary retinopathy; fundi generally hypopigmented, with fine to coarse spotty pigmentation, most marked peripherally; vision usually normal to nearly normal
  - Homocystinemia, type I (see Chapter 71.4)
    - Ectopia lentis; cataract; secondary glaucoma; peripheral cystic degeneration of retina
  - Sulfite oxidase deficiency (see Chapter 71.5)
    - Subluxation of lens; spherophakia; strabismus
  - Hartnup disease (see Chapter 71.5)
    - Photophobia; nystagmus; strabismus
  - Maple syrup urine disease (see Chapter 71.6)
    - Strabismus, varying with condition of child
- The mucopolysaccharidoses (MPS)
  - Hurler syndrome (MPS IH; α-L-iduronidase deficiency; see Chapter 74)

**To be differentiated from these forms of albinism is the Chédiak-Higashi syndrome in which the defect is in the morphology of the melanosomes, not in the formation of melanin. Ocular signs include hypopigmentation of iris and fundus, photophobia, nystagmus, and papilledema with lymphocytic infiltration of optic nerve.*

Table continued on following page

■ **TABLE 579–1 Clinical Features of Ocular Changes in Developmental Pediatric Syndromes** *Continued*

Hypertelorism, prominent eyes; puffy lids; heavy brows; deposition of MPS and attendant cellular changes throughout most regions of eye, particularly the conjunctiva, cornea, sclera, iris, ciliary body, retina, and optic nerve; characteristic corneal clouding, clinically evident early in life, and progressing to dense milky "ground-glass" haze, often with associated photophobia; progressive retinal degeneration with pigmentary dispersion and clumping, arteriolar attenuation and disk pallor, and reduced ERG; optic atrophy; vision loss, principally because of corneal, retinal, and optic nerve changes; hydrocephalus and cerebral changes; glaucoma in some cases

Scheie syndrome (MPS IS; α-L-iduronidase deficiency; see Chapter 74)
Progressive corneal clouding, diffuse but sometimes more dense peripherally than centrally; progressive retinal degeneration; visual symptoms, field loss, and night blindness often commencing in 2nd or 3rd decade; glaucoma in some cases

Hurler-Scheie Compound (MPS IH/S; α-L-iduronidase deficiency; see Chapter 74)
Corneal clouding, diffuse and progressive; glaucoma in some cases; vision loss because of corneal clouding or optic nerve effects of arachnoid cysts

Hunter syndrome (MPS II; iduronosulfate sulfatase deficiency)
Phenotypically similar to MPS IH; both mild and severe forms occur; progressive retinal degeneration with pigmentary changes, arteriolar attenuation, optic atrophy, vision, loss, reduced ERG; corneas macroscopically (clinically) clear, but microscopic corneal changes documented; papilledema secondary to hydrocephalus in some cases

Sanfillippo syndrome (MPS III; type A [heparin sulfate sulfatase deficiency], B [*N*-acetyl-α-D-glucosaminidase deficiency], and C [acetyl-Co A:α-glucosaminide *N*-acetyl transferase deficiency])
Retinal changes in some patients—arteriolar narrowing; reduced ERG; corneas clinically clear but some microscopic changes reported

Morquio syndrome (MPS IV; galactosamine-6-sulfate sulfatase deficiency in classic form, β-galactosidase deficiency reported in variants; see Chapter 74)
Fine corneal clouding in many patients; slowly, progressive; often not clinically apparent for several years

Maroteaux-Lamy syndrome (MPS VI; arylsulfatase-B deficiency; see Chapter 74)
Diffuse corneal clouding, usually evident within 1st few yr of life; tortuosity of retinal vessels in some patients; papilledema and 6th nerve paresis in some patients with hydrocephalus

Sly syndrome (MPS VII; β-D-glucuronidase deficiency)
Some diversity of phenotype; corneas clear or cloudy; corneal haze of either fine or coarse type

Di Ferrenti syndrome (MPS VIII; *N*-acetylglucosamine-6-sulfate sulfatase deficiency)
Short stature; mild dysostosis multiplex; odontoid hypoplasia; hepatosplenomegaly; mental retardation; ophthalmologic abnormalities not yet described

The sphingolipidoses

Generalized gangliosidosis (GM_1 gangliosidosis type 1; β-galactosidase deficiency; see Chapter 552.1)
Diffuse corneal clouding (MPS accumulation); macular cherry red spot of retinal ganglioside accumulation; retinal vascular tortuosity and retinal hemorrhages; optic atrophy; vision loss, nystagmus, strabismus

Juvenile GM_1 gangliosidosis (GM_1 gangliosidosis type 2; β-galactosidase deficiency; see Chapter 552.1)
Corneas clinically clear; histologic changes of retinal ganglioside storage without clinically obvious signs; optic atrophy and vision loss; nystagmus and strabismus

Tay-Sachs disease (GM_2 gangliosidosis type 1; hexosaminidase A deficiency; see Chapter 552)
Macular cherry red spot; optic atrophy (demyelination and degeneration of optic nerves, chiasm, and tracts); progressive loss of vision, caused by ocular and cerebral abnormalities; sequential deterioration of eye movements

Sandhoff variant (GM_2 gangliosidosis type 2; hexosaminidase A and B deficiency; see Chapter 552)
Macular cherry red spot; optic atrophy and progressive loss of vision; corneas clinically clear or slightly opalescent; histologic evidence of storage cytosomes in cornea

Juvenile GM_2 gangliosidosis (GM_2 gangliosidosis type 3; partial deficiency of hexosaminidase; see Chapter 552)
Retinal pigmentary degeneration; macular changes (cherry red spot type) in some cases; optic atrophy; blindness later in course of disease

Krabbe globoid cell leukodystrophy (galactosyl ceramide lipidosis; galactosylceramide β-galactosidase deficiency)
Cortical blindness and optic atrophy caused by degenerative changes in brain and visual pathways; nystagmus; strabismus

Gaucher disease (glycosyl ceramide lipidosis; glucosyl ceramide β-glucosidase deficiency; see Chapter 552)
Paralytic strabismus caused by brain stem and cranial nerve involvement in neuronopathic forms; nystagmus; macular changes (grayness) in some cases; retinal hemorrhages secondary to anemia, thrombocytopenia; discrete white spots in or on retina reported in juvenile form; pingueculae (wedge-shaped conjunctival lesions) in chronic non-neuronopathic form; possibly corneal clouding

Niemann-Pick disease (sphingomyelin lipidoses; sphingomyelinase deficiency; see Chapter 552)
Grayish macular haze in classic infantile neuronopathic form (type A), and in subacute neurovisceral or juvenile form (type C); corneal clouding, lens opacities in some cases (type A); vertical gaze palsy in some patients

Fabry disease (glycosphingolipid lipidosis; α-galactosidase A deficiency; see Chapter 552)
Corneal dystrophy related to epithelial lipid deposits (radiating lines/whorls in affected males and in carrier females); aneurysmal dilatation and tortuosity of conjunctival and retinal vessels; renovascular signs of renal hypertension; papilledema; orbital and lid edema; cataracts (spokelike posterior cortical lens opacities—anterior lens opacities in some cases)

Farber disease (ceramide lipidosis; ceramidase deficiency; see Chapter 552)
Cherry red-like spot; grayish posterior pole; retinal pigmentary mottling; granulomata in and around eye

Ceroid lipofuscinoses (see also Chapters 72.3 and 552.2)

Infantile (Finnish variant; unsaturated fatty acid lipidosis)
Microcephaly; marked atrophy of brain; loss of vision; granular inclusions; ataxia; myoclonus; profound dementia, decorticate state; onset 1–2 yr; death by 10 yr

Late infantile (Jansky-Bielschowsky)
Intellectual deterioration, seizures, ataxia; pigmentary retinal degeneration, in some cases, predominantly macular; ERG abnormal; optic atrophy; inclusions of curvilinear type; onset 2–4 yr; death by 10 yr

Juvenile (Batten-Mayou-Spielmeyer-Vogt)
Intellectual deterioration, seizures, ataxis, progressive loss of motor function; pigmentary retinal degeneration, resembling retinitis pigmentosa, with progressive loss of vision; in some cases predominantly macular degeneration; ERG abnormal; optic atrophy as a late manifestation; mixed inclusion bodies including curvilinear and fingerprint types, and lipofuscin in brain; onset 5–8 yr, sometimes later; death in teens or 20s

Late juvenile or adult (Kufs)
Behavior disturbances and intellectual impairment; ataxia, spasticity, myoclonic seizures; vision and fundi usually normal; macular degeneration in some cases; mostly lipofuscin in brain; onset in childhood, adolescence, or eary adult life

Cherry red spot myoclonus syndrome
Macular cherry red spot; vision loss; intention myoclonus; variable inclusions in brain; light inclusions in hepatocytes and Kupffer cells; onset in childhood; survival to adulthood

Leukodystrophies (see also Chapters 552.3 and 564.8)

Metachromatic leukodystrophy (arylsulfatase A deficiency)
Retinal degeneration resembling retinitis pigmentosa; in some cases, early macular involvement (macular grayness with accentuation of central red spot); optic atrophy; vision loss; strabismus and nystagmus

Pelizaeus-Merzbacher syndrome
"Eye-rolling" (rhythmic eye movements) noted soon after birth, sometimes with rotary movements of the head; optic atrophy as a late manifestation

Canavan disease
Vacuolization of ganglion cell layer of retina reportedly detectable with slit lamp; retinal pigmentary changes; optic atrophy; blindness early in course; ERG normal; VER reduced; strabismus, roving eye movements, and nystagmus

Demyelinating scleroses (see Chapter 552.5)

Schilder disease (encephalitis periaxialis diffusa)
Involvement of visual pathways, producing retrobulbar neuritis, optic atrophy, central scotomas, chiasmal syndromes, homonymous field defects; disorders of cortical gaze functions; nystagmus

Multiple sclerosis
Optic neuritis (episodic loss of vision, typically a central scotoma, unilateral more often than bilateral, often with retrobulbar pain); other visual pathway lesions (various field defects); internuclear ophthalmoplegia; supranuclear gaze palsies; nystagmus; sheathing of peripheral retinal vessels in some cases

Neuromyelitis optica (Devick disease)
Optic neuritis (usually papillitis with visible disc edema), with resultant optic atrophy; other visual pathway lesions (various visual field defects); in some cases extraocular muscle palsies, conjugate gaze palsies, nystagmus, pupil abnormalities

Hamartomatoses and phakomatoses

Tuberous sclerosis (Bourneville disease; see Chapter 546.2)
Retinal phakomata (glial hamartomas, ranging from small flat or slightly elevated white or yellowish lesions to large elevated refractile yellowish multinodular or cystic masses often likened to an unripe mulberry); fibroangioma of the lids; in some, papilledema or optic atrophy, vision defects, pupil or ocular motor signs related to CNS changes (tumors, hydrocephalus); occasionally iris or pigmentary changes

Neurofibromatosis (von Recklinghausen syndrome; see Chapter 546.1)
Plexiform neuromas of eyelids, often producing ptosis; episcleral and conjunctival neurofibromas; prominent corneal nerves; Lisch iris nodules; uveal hypercellularity; glaucoma (related to angle anomalies, uveal hypercellularity, neovascularization, or synechiae); hamartomas (phakomata) of disk and retina; fundus pigmentary changes likened to

■ TABLE 579–1 Clinical Features of Ocular Changes in Developmental Pediatric Syndromes *Continued*

café-au-lait spots; optic gliomas and vision loss (presenting with proptosis, strabismus, nystagmus if intraorbital—with signs of increased intracranial pressure, hydrocephalus, or diencephalic syndrome when intracranial); orbital asymmetry; orbital wall defects; pulsatile exophthalmos, intraorbital neurofibromas, with proptosis

- Angiomatosis of the retina and cerebellum (von Hippel-Lindau disease; see Chapter 546.4)
  - Retinal hemangioblastoma (reddish or yellowish globular mass with paired vessels coursing to and from the lesion, sometimes likened to a toy balloon in the fundus); may lead to hemorrhage, exudates, retinal detachment
- Encephalofacial angiomatosis (Sturge-Weber syndrome; see Chapter 546)
  - Lid and conjunctival involvement of facial nevus flammeus; choroidal hemangioma; dilated and tortuous retinal vessels; glaucoma, congenital or later in infancy or childhood (related to possible angle anomalies, vascular lesion, or hypersecretion); visual field defects associated with CNS lesions; hemianopsia in some cases)
- Angiomatosis of mid-brain and retina (Wyburn-Mason syndrome)
  - Extensive vascular malformations involving principally the midbrain and eye; angiomatosis of the retina; vessels dilated and tortuous; angiomatosis affecting optic nerve and orbit

Neurocutaneous syndromes

- Ataxia-telangiectasia (Louis-Barr syndrome; see Chapter 547.1)
  - Telangiectasias of bulbar conjunctivae, usually by the age of 4–6 yr; apraxic disorder of conjugate eye movements; horizontal and vertical gaze performed in halting dyssynergic fashion; difficulty in maintaining eccentric gaze; sometimes convergence defect; nystagmus
- Sjögren-Larsson syndrome (see Chapter 608)
  - Chorioretinal lesions; discrete defects in retinal pigment epithelium of unknown etiology; circumscribed symmetric lesions of varying size in and about the macula in approximately 25% of cases
- Incontinentia pigmenti (Bloch-Sulzberger syndrome; see Chapter 602)
  - Intraocular retrolental masses ("pseudogliomas") and membranes, apparently secondary to an underlying retinal vascular disorder characterized by aneurysmal dilatation, abnormal arteriovenous connections, and vasoproliferative changes; sometimes intraocular hemorrhage and inflammation; microphthalmos; corneal opacities; cataracts; optic atrophy
- Linear nevus sebaceus of Jadassohn (see Chapter 602)
  - Coloboma of the eyelids, iris, and fundus; corectopia; epibulbar lipodermoids; orbital teratomas; proptosis; aberrant lacrimal gland; corneal vascularization; ocular motor palsies; nystagmus; defective vision
- Xerodermic idiocy of de Sanctis and Cacchione (see Chapter 606)
  - Atrophy of eyelids; loss of cilia, ectropion, entropion, symblepharon, ankyloblepharon; drying and infection of conjunctiva; ulceration of cornea; iritis; photophobia
- Klippel-Trenaunay-Weber syndrome (see Chapter 600)
  - Conjunctival telangiectasia; choroidal hemangioma; iris coloboma; heterochromia; glaucoma; strabismus

Special neurobiothrophies

- Subacute sclerosing panencephalitis (Dawson disease; Van Bogaert disease; see Chapter 206)
  - Focal retinitis (edema, hemorrhage, pigmentary changes), with chorioretinal scarring (usually macular or paramacular, usually bilateral)—may precede other neurologic manifestations; papilledema; optic atrophy; visual symptoms of retinal and optic nerve involvement; field defects of cerebral involvement; nystagmus; extraocular muscle palsies; ptosis
- Subacute necrotizing encephalomyopathy (Leigh disease; see Chapter 548.2)
  - Abnormal eye movements (bizarre rolling eye movements, disconjugate eye movements, horizontal and vertical nystagmus, saccadic ocular movements); extraocular muscle palsies (sometimes complete external ophthalmoplegia); blepharoptosis; progressive optic atrophy and vision loss; sometimes retinal changes (diminished macular reflex); afferent and efferent pupil defects
- Hepatolenticular degeneration (Wilson disease; see Chapter 303.2)
  - Kayser-Fleischer ring of cornea (copper deposition in periphery of Descemet membrane, particularly in deepest zone adjacent to endothelium, seen as granules of golden, greenish, grayish, or brown hue); Sonnenblumenkatarakt ("sunflower" cataract); occasionally ocular motor abnormalities (jerky oscillations of eyes, involuntary upward deviation of eyes, or paresis of upward gaze); accommodation sometimes affected; in some cases, optic neuritis secondary to penicillamine therapy
- Trichopoliodystrophy (Menkes disease; kinky hair disease; see Chapter 552.5)
  - Decrease in retinal ganglion cells, thinning of retinal nerve fiber layer, and partial atrophy of optic nerve; progressive vision loss; abnormal ERG; microcysts of pigment epithelium of iris
- Abetalipoproteinemia (acanthocytosis; Bassen-Kornzweig disease; see Chapter 70)
  - Pigmentary retinal degeneration with progressive impairment of visual function (pigment dispersion, arteriolar attenuation, disk pallor, impaired dark adaptation); cataracts, ptosis, and ocular motor abnormalities; in some cases, progressive exotropia, paresis of medial recti, and dissociated nystagmus on lateral gaze
- Heredopathia atactica polyneuritiformis (Refsum syndrome; phytanic acid α-hydrolase deficiency; see Chapters 72.2 and 564)
  - Pigmentary retinal degeneration (pigmentary clumping, arteriolar attenuation, optic atrophy, progressive impairment of night vision and visual field); ERG abnormal; sometimes vitreous opacities, cataracts, cornea guttata, miosis; ophthalmoparesis; nystagmus
- Familial dysautonomia (Riley-Day syndrome; see Chapter 566)
  - Depressed or absent corneal sensation, with corneal ulceration and scarring common; defective lacrimation; tortuosity of retinal vessels; tonic pupil in some cases; myopia and exotropia common
- Congenital familial sensory neuropathy with anhidrosis (Pinsky-DiGeorge syndrome; see Chapter 566)
  - Defective corneal sensation, with defective lacrimation; corneal ulceration and scarring may result

Disorders of connective tissues, bones, and joints

- Arachnodactyly (Marfan syndrome; see Chapter 646)
  - Ectopia lentis (lens dislocation, usually upward) and iridodonesis (tremulous iris); microphakia, spherophakia; cataract; myopia; glaucoma; retinal changes; degeneration, detachment
- Cutis hyperelastica (Ehlers-Danlos syndrome; see Chapter 609)
  - Epicanthus; blue sclera; keratoconus; subluxation of lens; retinal detachment
- Pseudoxanthoma elasticum (see Chapter 609)
  - Angioid streaks (breaks in Bruch membrane appearing as dark lines in the fundus radiating from the disk); tendency to retinal hemorrhage
- Osteogenesis imperfecta (see Chapter 643)
  - Blue sclera; prominent eyes; in some cases, megalocornea, keratoconus, corneal opacities
- Polyostotic fibrous dysplasia (McCune-Albright syndrome; see Part XXVI, Sec. 5)
  - Thickening of bones of orbit
- Osteopetrosis (Albers-Schönberg disease; "marble bones"; see Chapter 643)
  - Vision loss and extraocular muscle palsies, caused by bony overgrowth of cranial foramina; in some cases, retinal degeneration, optic atrophy
- Chondrodystrophia calcificans congenita (Conradi syndrome; see Part XXVII, Sec. 2)
  - Cataract, optic atropy; hypertelorism
- Spondyloepiphyseal dysplasia congenita (see Part XXXII, Sec. 2)
  - Myopia; retinal detachment; cataract; buphthalmos
- Spondyloepiphyseal dysplasia variants (see Part XXXII, Sec. 2)
  - Punctate corneal dystrophy without impairment of vision
- Hereditary onchyo-osteodysplasia (nail-patella syndrome)
  - Dark "cloverleaf" pigmentation of iris; cataract; microphakia; microcornea; keratoconus; ptosis
- Progressive arthro-ophthalmopathy (Stickler syndrome)
  - Pain and stiffness of joints with bony enlargement; kyphosis, cleft palate; Pierre Robin anomaly; deafness; progressive myopia; retinal detachment; glaucoma

Dermatologic disorders

- Focal dermal hypoplasia (Goltz syndrome; see Chapter 598)
  - Nystagmus; strabismus; microphthalmos; coloboma
- Hypohidrotic (anhidrotic) ectodermal dysplasia (see Chapter 598)
  - Deficiency of tears, leading to keratopathy, photophobia; stenosis of the lacrimal puncta; cataracts; lashes and brows sparse
- Dyskeratosis congenita (see Chapter 598)
  - Bullous conjunctivitis, with minimal scarring of cornea; chronic blepharitis; loss of lashes and ectropion; keratinization of lacrimal puncta
- Ichthyosis (see Chapter 608)
  - Conjunctivitis, ectropion, and corneal erosions in lamellar and sex-linked forms; cataracts in congenital and vulgaris forms
- Basal cell nevus syndrome (see Chapter 620)
  - Prominent supraorbital ridges; hypertelorism or dystopia canthorum; cataracts; coloboma; vision defects; strabismus
- Juvenile xanthogranuloma (nevoxanthoendothelioma; see Chapter 620)
  - Xanthogranuloma in ocular tissues, as infiltrates in orbit, iris, episclera, ciliary body; presenting signs may be proptosis, heterochromia, spontaneous hyphema, uveitis, glaucoma
- Poikiloderma congenitale (Rothmund-Thomson syndrome; see Chapter 606)
  - Sparse eyebrows and eyelashes; cataracts (onset 2–7 yr); corneal dystrophy
- Bloom syndrome (see Chapter 606)
  - Conjunctivitis; conjunctival telangiectasias; drusen at posterior pole of fundus

Syndromes of multiple developmental abnormalities

- Cornelia de Lange syndrome
  - Microbrachycephaly, short neck, low hair line, anteverted nares, micrognathism, and low-set ears; physical and mental retardation; limb defects including micromelia phocomelia, oligodactyly, polydactyly; cardiac and urogenital anomalies; synophrys (confluent eyebrows) and long curly eyelashes; ptosis; epicanthus; microphthalmos with eccentric pupils; corneal opacities; optic atrophy; strabismus
- Fraser syndrome
  - Facial, genitourinary, skeletal anomalies (including lateral cleft of nostril, ear deformity, renal agenesis, hydronephrosis, hypospadias, cryptorchidism, syndactyly); cerebral defects, meningoencephalocele;

Table continued on following page

■ **TABLE 579–1 Clinical Features of Ocular Changes in Developmental Pediatric Syndromes** *Continued*

cryptophthalmos (eye hidden, fused lids—absence of palpebral fissure), sometimes with symblepharon (adhesion of lid to globe); microphthalmos in some cases; flat supraorbital ridge

Rieger syndrome

Various dental and limb anomalies; occasionally intellectual retardation, muscular dystrophy, and myotonic dystrophy; dysplasia of anterior segment of the eye; posterior embryotoxon (prominence and anterior displacement of Schwalbe line), often with bands of iris tissue attached (Axenfeld syndrome); iris hypoplasia; glaucoma; cataracts; ectopia lentis; colobomata; micro- or megalocornea; strabismus; ptosis; optic atrophy

Peter syndrome

Skeletal anomalies; developmental defects of the gastrointestinal tract and central nervous system; hydrocephalus and mental retardation; central defect of Descemet membrane, with central corneal leukoma, shallow anterior chamber, peripheral anterior synechia; cataracts

Lenz syndrome

Microcephaly, mental retardation; short stature, digital anomalies, and dental defects; colobomatous microphthalmos; blepharoptosis; nystagmus; strabismus

Meckel syndrome (Meckel-Gruber syndrome)

Microcephaly, occipital encephalocele, or anencephaly; polycystic kidneys; polydactyly; congenital heart disease; genital abnormalities; microphthalmos, anophthalmos, cryptophthalmos; sclerocornea; partial aniridia; cataract; retinal dysplasia; optic nerve hypoplasia

Otopalatodigital syndrome (Rubinstein-Taybi syndrome)

Intellectual and growth retardation; abnormally broad thumbs and broad great toes; characteristic facies with hypoplasia of maxilla and mandible, beaked nose, posterior rotation of ears; hypertrichosis; cryptorchidism; cardiac and renal anomalies; hypertelorism, with epicanthus, ptosis, and antimongoloid slant of palpebral fissures; cataract, colobomata, strabismus

Seckel syndrome

Growth retardation with small head circumference and characteristic face, narrow with beaklike nose ("bird head"); micrognathia and apparent prominence of maxilla; sometimes musculoskeletal and genitourinary anomalies; hypertelorism, with antimongoloid slant of palpebral fissures, prominent eyes; strabismus

Freeman-Sheldon syndrome

Syndrome characterized by masklike face with small pursed mouth, "whistling face"; ulnar deviation of the hand and fingers; talipes equinovarus; deep-set eyes; epicanthus, blepharophimosis, ptosis; strabismus

Aicardi syndrome

Agenesis of the corpus callosum, with cortical heterotopia; seizures; mental retardation; costovertebral anomalies; multiple discrete chorioretinal defects of varying size; sometimes microphthalmos

Wildervanck syndrome

Association of the Klippel-Feil malformation with congenital deafness and *Duane syndrome*, unilateral or bilateral (congenital defect in abduction with retraction of the globe or attempted adduction of the affected eye); epibulbar dermoid cysts

Falls-Kertesz syndrome

Pterygium coli; later onset of lymphedema of lower extremities; distichiasis of all four lids; partial ectropion of lower lids

Kartagener syndrome (see Chapter 364)

Pigmentary retinal disorder; cataracts

Miscellaneous multisystem disorders

Oculocerebrorenal syndrome (Lowe syndrome; see Chapter 634)

Congenital cataracts in affected males; fine lens opacities in carrier females; glaucoma; rarely, microphthalmos

Cerebrohepatorenal syndrome (Zellweger syndrome) (congenital adrenoleukodystrophy)

Profound hypotonia, growth retardation, and failure to thrive; hepatomegaly, jaundice, hypoprothrombinemia; renal cortical cysts; characteristic facies; flat profile; accumulation of iron in various organs; mild hypertelorism, flat supraorbital ridges, and epicanthal folds, cataracts; glaucoma (also, nonglaucomatous corneal haze); vitreous opacities; optic nerve hypoplasia; retinal pigmentary disorder (fundi generally hypopigmented with fine to coarse spotty pigmentation, most marked peripherally)

Laurence-Moon-Biedl syndrome (see Chapter 535.2)

Pleomorphic pigmentary retinal degeneration (retinitis pigmentosa type, with prominent macular involvement in some cases), with progressive vision impairment

Prader-Willi syndrome

Hypotonia, hypomentia, hypogonadism, and obesity, with tendency to diabetes mellitus; strabismus

Cockayne syndrome (see Chapter 606)

Pigmentary retinal degeneration; optic atrophy, cataracts; photophobia

Werner syndrome

Syndrome of premature aging; in the 2nd decade, with cessation of growth, graying of the hair, alopecia, scleroderma-like changes of the skin, atherosclerosis, and diabetes mellitus; hypogonadism, increased risk of neoplasia; cataracts, juvenile onset; pigmentary retinal degeneration ("retinitis pigmentosa"); macular degeneration; glaucoma

Asphyxiating thoracic dysplasia (Jeune syndrome; see Chapter 374)

Pigmentary retinal degeneration; with progressive vision impairment in some cases

Alstrom disease

Nerve deafness, diabetes mellitus, and obesity in childhood; pigmentary retinal degeneration; cataracts

Renal-retinal dystrophy

Interstitial nephritis; progressive pigmentary retinal degeneration, with attenuation of arterioles, reduced ERG, optic atrophy, and loss of vision

Usher syndrome

Nerve deafness; pigmentary retinal degeneration ("retinitis pigmentosa"); cataracts

Norrie disease

A syndrome of retinal malformation, mental retardation, and deafness; congenital retinal pseudoglioma; persistent hyperplastic primary vitreous, with vision loss; degenerative changes with phthisis bulbi; corneal opacities; cataracts

Congenital infection syndromes

Congenital rubella (see Chapter 97.5)

Ophthalmic sequelae, both teratogenic and inflammatory; bilateral or unilateral effects; persistence of virus in the eye for months or years; microphthalmia; cataract (usually a dense pearly nuclear opacity with relatively clearer cortical rim); iris hypoplasia, atrophy synechiae (pupils often difficult to dilate); congenital glaucoma; transient nonglaucomatous corneal clouding in the newborn; retinopathy (pigmentary mottling "salt and pepper," focal or generalized, without loss of function); acute maculopathy (submacular neovascularization) as a delayed complication later in childhood in some cases, with attendant vision impairment; optic atrophy; vision defects and ocular motor abnormalities (nystagmus, strabismus) related not only to ocular involvement but also to effects of encephalomyelitis

Congenital cytomegalovirus infection (see Chapter 97.1)

Chorioretinitis (single or multifocal atrophic and pigmented fundus lesions, more often peripheral than macular—sometimes perivascular retinal exudates and hemorrhages); anterior uveitis, conjunctivitis, and corneal clouding; optic atrophy; optic nerve hypoplasia; coloboma; microphthalmos; vision defects with strabismus, nystagmus

Congenital toxoplasmosis (see Chapter 244.8)

Retinochoroditis (retinitis, with secondary choroiditis; often with exudate into vitreous in early stages, resulting in single or multifocal atrophic and pigmented scars); often large macular lesions; satellite lesions and recurrent inflammation common in later years caused by persistence of organism in eye; vision loss, optic atrophy, retinal detachment, cataract, and glaucoma common; attendant oculomotor abnormalities (strabismus, nystagmus) attributed to ocular and/or CNS involvement; congenital anomalies of eye (e.g., microphthalmos)

Congenital syphilis (see Chapter 201.1)

Perivascular infiltration by *T. pallidum*, with inflammation in the cornea, uvea, retina, and optic nerve; persistence of the organism in the eye for years; interstitial keratitis, usually appearing after age 5 or 6 yr (iridocyclitis and intense photophobia in acute phase, vascularization and corneal opacification later, with decreased vision); retinopathy ("salt and pepper" pigmentary changes, frequently with arteriolar attenuation and disk pallor); retinal periphlebitis, sometimes with vascular occlusion; exudative uveitis in some cases; phthisis may result; disk edema; optic atrophy

---

to as simple ectopia lentis. Usually simple ectopia lentis is transmitted as an autosomal dominant condition. The lens is generally displaced upward and temporally. The ectopia may be present at birth or appear later in life.

Another form of hereditable dislocation is ectopia lentis et pupillae. In this condition there is displacement of both the lens and pupil, usually in opposite directions. This condition is generally bilateral, with one eye being almost a mirror image of the other. Ectopia lentis et pupillae is a recessive condition, although variable expression with some intermingling with simple ectopia lentis has been reported.

Systemic disorders associated with displacement of the lens include Marfan syndrome, homocystinuria, Weill-Marchesani syndrome, and sulfite oxidase deficiency. Ectopia lentis occurs in approximately 80% of patients with Marfan syndrome, and in about 50% of patients the ectopia is evident by the age of 5 yr. In most cases the lens is displaced superiorly and temporally; it is almost always bilateral and relatively symmetric. In homocystinuria the lens is usually displaced inferiorly and somewhat nasally. It occurs early in life and is often evident by 5 yr of age. In Weill-Marchesani syndrome the displacement of the lens is often downward and forward, and the lens tends to be small and round.

Ectopia lentis is also associated occasionally with other conditions, including Ehler-Danlos, Sturge-Weber, Crouzon, or Klippel-Feil syndrome; oxycephaly; and mandibulofacial dysostosis. A syndrome of dominantly inherited blepharoptosis, high myopia, and ectopia lentis has also been described.

TREATMENT AND PROGNOSIS. Displacement of the lens often results only in optical problems; in other cases, however, more serious complications may develop, such as glaucoma, uveitis, retinal detachment, or cataract. Management must be individualized according to the type of displacement, its etiology, and the presence of any complicating ocular or systemic conditions. For many patients optical correction by spectacles or contact lenses can be provided. Sometimes manipulation of the iris diaphragm with mydriatic or myotic drops may help improve vision. In selected cases the best treatment is surgical removal of the lens. In many children treatment of any associated amblyopia must be instituted early. In addition, for the child with ectopia lentis, safety precautions should be taken to prevent injury to the eye.

MICROSPHEROPHAKIA

The term *microspherophakia* refers to a small, round lens that may occur as an isolated anomaly (probably autosomal recessive) or in association with other ocular abnormalities, such as ectopia lentis, myopia, or retinal detachment (possibly autosomal dominant). Microspherophakia may also occur in association with various systemic disorders, including Marfan syndrome, Marchesani syndrome, Alport syndrome, mandibulofacial dysostosis, and Klinefelter syndrome.

POSTERIOR LENTICONUS

This unusual anomaly is characterized by a circumscribed round or oval bulge of the posterior lens capsule and cortex, restricted to the 2- to 7-mm central (axial) region. In the early stages, by the red reflex test, this may look like an oil droplet. It occurs in infants and young children and it tends to increase with age. Usually the lens material within and surrounding the capsular bulge eventually becomes opacified. Lenticonus usually occurs as an isolated ocular anomaly. It is generally unilateral but may be bilateral. It is believed to be sporadic, although autosomal dominant heredity has been suggested in some cases. Occasionally, it is a feature of a systemic disorder such as Alport syndrome. The infant or child with lenticonus may require lens surgery for progressive cataract, optical correction, amblyopia treatment, and care of secondary conditions, such as strabismus.

Alden ER, Kalina RE, Hodson WA: Transient cataracts in low-birth-weight infants. J Pediatr 82:314, 1973.
Bateman JB, Spence MA, Marazita ML, et al: Genetic linkage analysis of autosomal dominant congenital cataracts. Am J Ophthalmol 101:218, 1986.
Birch EE, Stager DR: Prevalence of good visual acuity following surgery for congenital unilateral cataract. Arch Ophthalmol 106:40, 1988.
Calhoun JH: Cataracts and lens anomalies in children. *In:* Nelson LB, Calhoun JH, Harley RD (eds): Pediatric Ophthalmology, 3rd ed. Philadelphia, WB Saunders, 1991.
Casper DS, Simon JW, Nelson LB, et al: Familial simple ectopia lentis. A case study. J Pediatr Ophthalmol Strab 22:227, 1985.
Chrousos GA, Parks MM, O'Neill JF: Incidence of chronic glaucoma, retinal detachment and secondary membrane surgery in pediatric aphakic patients. Ophthalmology 91:1238, 1984.
Cotlier E: Congenital varicella cataract. Am J Ophthalmol 86:627, 1978.
Cross HE: Ectopia lentis et pupillae. Am J Ophthalmol 88:381, 1979.
Cross HE, Jensen AD: Ocular manifestations in the Marfan syndrome and homocystinuria. Am J Ophthalmol 75:405, 1973.
Forman AR, Loreto JA, Tina LU: Reversibility of corticosteroid-associated cataracts in children with the nephrotic syndrome. Am J Ophthalmol 84:75, 1977.
Francois J: Late results of congenital cataract surgery. Ophthalmology 86:1586, 1979.
Gelbart SS, Hoyt CS, Jastrebski G, et al: Long-term visual results in bilateral congenital catarats. Am J Ophthalmol 93:615, 1982.
Gillum WN, Anderson RL: Dominantly inherited blepharoptosis, high myopia, and ectopia lentis. Arch Ophthalmol 100:282, 1982.
Goldberg MF: Clinical manifestations of ectopia lentis et pupillae in 16 patients. Ophthalmology 95:1080, 1988.
Hiles DA: Intraocular lens implantation in children with monocular cataracts, 1974–1983. Ophthalmology 91:1231, 1984.
Jaafar MS, Robb RM: Congenital anterior polar cataract: A review of 63 cases. Ophthalmology 91:249, 1984.
Jensen AD, Cross HE, Paton D: Ocular complications in the Weill-Marchesani syndrome. Am J Ophthalmol 77:261, 1975.
Khalil M, Saheb N: Posterior lenticonus. Ophthalmology 91:1429, 1984.
Kirkam TH: Mandibulofacial dysostosis with ectopia lentis. Am J Ophthalmol 70:947, 1979.
Kohn BA: The differential diagnosis of cataracts in infancy and childhood. Am J Dis Child 130:184, 1976.
Levin AV, Edmonds SA, Nelson LB, et al: Extended-wear contact lenses for the treatment of pediatric aphakia. Ophthalmology 95:1107, 1988.
Maumenee IH: Classification of heredity cataracts in children by linkage analysis. Ophthalmology 86:1554, 1979.
Morgan KS, McDonald MB, Hiles DA, et al: The nationwide study of epikeratophakia for aphakia in older children. Ophthalmology 95:526, 1988.
Morgan KS, McDonald MB, Hiles DA, et al: The nationwide study of epikeratophakia for aphakia in children. Am J Ophthalmol 103:366, 1989.
Nelson LB: Diagnosis and management of congenital and developmental cataracts. Sem Ophthalmol 5:154, 1990.
Nelson LB, Maumenee IH: Ectopia lentis. Surv Ophthalmol 27:143, 1982.
Nelson LB, Calhoun JH, Simon JW, et al: Progression of congenital anterior polar cataracts in childhood. Arch Ophthalmol 103:1842, 1985.
Parks MM: Visual results in aphakic children. Am J Ophthalmol 94:441, 1982.
Rasoby R, Ben Ezra D: Congenital and traumatic cataracts: The effect on ocular axial length. Arch Ophthalmol 106:1066, 1988.
Schimke RN, McKusick VA, Huang T, et al: Homocystinuria: Studies of 28 families with 38 affected members. JAMA 193:87, 1965.
Seetner AA, Crawford JS: Surgical correction of lens dislocation in children. Am J Ophthalmol 91:106, 1981.
Smith T, Holland MG, Woody NC: Ocular manifestations of familial hyperlysinemia. Trans Am Acad Ophthalmol Otolaryngol 75:355, 1971.
Townes PL: Ectopia lentis et pupillae. Arch Ophthalmol 94:1126, 1976.
Wets B, Milot JA, Polomeno RC, et al: Cataracts and ketotic hypoglycemia. Ophthalmology 89:999, 1982.

CHAPTER 580

Disorders of the Uveal Tract

UVEITIS

(Iritis, Cyclitis, Chorioretinitis)

The uveal tract (the inner vascular coat of the eye, consisting of the iris, ciliary body, and choroid) is subject to inflammatory involvement in a number of systemic diseases, both infectious and noninfectious, and in response to exogenous factors, including trauma and toxic agents. Inflammation may affect any one portion of the uveal tract preferentially or all parts together.

Iritis may occur alone or in conjunction with inflammation of the ciliary body as iridocyclitis or in association with pars planitis. Pain, photophobia, and lacrimation are the characteristic symptoms of acute anterior uveitis, but the inflammation may develop insidiously without disturbing symptoms. Signs of anterior uveitis include conjunctival hyperemia, particularly in the perilimbal region (ciliary flush), cells and protein ("flare") in the aqueous humor, inflammatory deposits on the posterior surface of the cornea (keratic precipitates, or "KP"), congestion of the iris, and sometimes neovascularization of the iris. In more chronic cases there may be degenerative changes of the cornea (band keratopathy), lenticular opacities (cataract), and impairment of vision. The etiology of anterior uveitis is often obscure; primary considerations in children are rheumatoid disease, particularly pauciarticular rheumatoid arthritis, Kawasaki disease, and sarcoidosis. Iritis may be secondary to corneal disease, such as herpetic keratitis or a bacterial or fungal corneal ulcer, or to a corneal abrasion or foreign body. Traumatic iritis and iridocyclitis are especially common in children.

Choroiditis, inflammation of the posterior portion of the uveal tract, invariably also involves the retina; when both are obviously affected, the term *chorioretinitis* is used (Fig. 580–1). The causes of posterior uveitis are numerous; the more common are toxoplasmosis, histoplasmosis, cytomegalic inclusion disease, sarcoidosis, syphilis, tuberculosis, and toxocariasis. Depending on the etiology, the inflammatory signs may be diffuse or focal. Often there is vitreous reaction as well. With many types the result is atrophic chorioretinal scarring demarcated by pigmentation, often with visual impairment. Secondary complications include retinal detachment, glaucoma, or phthisis.

Panophthalmitis is inflammation involving all parts of the eye. It is frequently suppurative, most often as a result of a perforating injury or of septicemia. It produces severe pain, marked congestion of the eye, inflammation of the adjacent orbital tissues and eyelids, and loss of vision. In many cases the eye is lost despite intensive treatment of the infection and inflammation. Enucleation of the eye or evisceration of the orbit may be necessary.

Sympathetic ophthalmia is a rare type of inflammatory response that affects both eyes following perforating injury of one eye. It may occur weeks or even months after the injury. A hypersensitivity phenomenon is the most probable cause. Loss of vision may result.

TREATMENT. The various forms of intraocular inflammation are treated according to their etiologic factors. When infection is proven or suspected, appropriate antimicrobial therapy is used. Often, systemic and ocular treatment are required. In some cases subconjunctival or intravitreal injection of antibiotics is indicated. Prevention or reduction of inflammatory sequelae is also important in the treatment of these conditions; in selected cases, topical or systemic corticosteroids are used. Cycloplegic agents, particularly atropine, are also used to reduce inflammation and to prevent adhesion of the iris to the lens, especially in anterior uveitis.

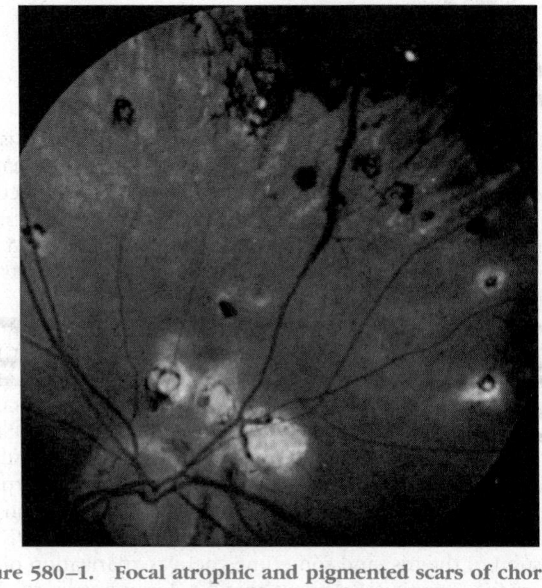

Figure 580–1. Focal atrophic and pigmented scars of chorioretinitis.

Burke MJ, Rennebohm RM: Eye involvement in Kawasaki disease. J Pediatr Ophthalmol Strab 18:7, 1981.

Cochereau-Massin I, LeHoang P, Lautier-Frau M, et al: Efficacy and tolerance of intravitreal ganciclovir in cytomegalovirus retinitis in acquired immune deficiency syndrome. Ophthalmology 98:1348, 1991.

Contreras F, Pereda J: Congenital syphilis of the eye with lens involvement. Arch Ophthalmol 96:1052, 1978.

Giles CL: Uveitis in children. *In*: Nelson LB, Calhoun JH, Harley RD (eds): Pediatric Ophthalmology, 3rd ed. Philadelphia, WB Saunders, 1991.

Hart WM, Reed AB, Freedman HL, et al: Cytomegalovirus in juvenile iridocyclitis. Am J Ophthalmol 86:329, 1978.

Kanski JJ: Anterior uveitis in juvenile rheumatoid arthritis. Arch Ophthalmol 96:1794, 1977.

Kanski JJ: Juvenile arthritis and uveitis. Surv Ophthalmol 34:253, 1990.

Kimura SJ: Uveitis in children: Analysis of 274 cases. Trans Am Ophthalmol Soc 62:171, 1964.

Lonn LL: Neonatal cytomegalic inclusion disease chorioretinitis. Arch Ophthalmol 88:434, 1972.

Lou P, Kazdan J, Basu PK: Ocular toxoplasmosis in three consecutive siblings. Arch Ophthalmol 96:613, 1978.

Makkey TA, Azar A: Sympathetic ophthalmia: A long-term follow-up. Arch Ophthalmol 96:257, 1978.

Molk R: Ocular toxocariasis: A review of the literature. Ann Ophthalmol 15:216, 1983.

Regillo CD, Shields CL, Shields JA, et al: Ocular tuberculosis. JAMA 266:1490, 1991.

Ryan SJ, Hardy PH, Hardy JM, et al: Persistence of virulent *Treponema pallidum* despite penicillin therapy in congenital syphilis. Am J Ophthalmol 73:258, 1972.

Smith ME, Zimmerman LE, Harley RD: Ocular involvement in congenital cytomegalic inclusion disease. Arch Ophthalmol 76:696, 1966.

Stern GA, Romano PE: Congenital ocular toxoplasmosis: Possible occurrence in siblings. Arch Ophthalmol 96:615, 1978.

Wilkinson CP, Welch RB: Intraocular toxocara. Am J Ophthalmol 71:921, 1971.

Winterkorn JMS: Lyme disease: Neurologic and ophthalmologic manifestations. Surv Ophthalmol 35:191, 1990.

CHAPTER 581

Disorders of the Retina and Vitreous

RETINOPATHY OF PREMATURITY

This retinal angiopathy occurs primarily but not exclusively in preterm infants (see Chapter 82.2). It may be active (early stages) or chronic (late stages). Clinical manifestations range from mild or transient changes of the peripheral retina to severe progressive vasoproliferation, cicatrization, and potentially blinding retinal detachment. Retinopathy of prematurity (ROP) refers to all stages of the disease and its sequelae. Retrolental fibroplasia (RLF), the term previously used for this disease, described only the cicatricial stages.

PATHOGENESIS. Beginning at 16 wk of gestation, retinal angiogenesis normally proceeds from the optic disk to the periphery, reaching the outer rim of the retina (ora serrata) nasally at about 36 wk and temporally by approximately 40 wk. Injury to the process can result in various pathologic and clinical changes. The 1st observation in the acute or active phase is cessation of vasculogenesis. Rather than a gradual transition from vascularized to avascular retina, there is an abrupt termination of the vessels, marked by a line in the retina. The line may then grow into a ridge composed of mesenchymal and endothelial cells. Cell division and differentiation may later resume, and vascularization of the retina may proceed. Alternatively, there may be progression to an abnormal proliferation of vessels out of the plane of the retina, into the vitreous, and over the surface of the retina, the ciliary body, and the equator of the lens. Cicatrization and traction on the retina may follow, leading to detachment.

The factors that cause ROP and determine its outcome are not fully known, but prematurity and the degree of retinal immaturity at birth are major factors. Hyperoxia is also a major factor, but other problems, such as respiratory distress, apnea, bradycardia, heart disease, infection, hypoxia, hypercarbia, acidosis, anemia, and the need for transfusion, may be contributory factors. Generally, the lower the birthweight and the sicker the infant, the greater the risk for ROP.

CLASSIFICATION. The currently used international classification of ROP (ICROP) describes the location, extent, and severity of the disease. To delineate location the retina is divided into three concentric zones, centered on the optic disk. Zone I, the posterior or inner zone, extends twice the disk-macular distance, or 30 degrees in all directions from the optic disk. Zone II, the middle zone, extends from the outer edge of zone I to the ora serrata nasally and to the anatomic equator temporally. Zone III, the outer zone, is the residual crescent that extends from the outer border of zone II to the ora serrata temporally; this area of the retina is vascularized last and is most frequently involved with ROP.

The extent of involvement is described by the number of circumferential clock hours involved. In the right eye 3 o'clock is nasal and 9 o'clock is temporal, whereas in the left eye 3 o'clock is temporal and 9 o'clock is nasal.

The phases and severity of the disease process are classified into five stages. Stage 1 is characterized by a demarcation line that separates vascularized from avascular retina (Fig. 581–1*A*). This line lies within the plane of the retina and appears relatively flat and white. There is often abnormal branching or arcading of the retinal vessels that lead into the line. Stage 2 is characterized by a ridge—the demarcation line has grown, acquiring height, width, and volume, and extending up and out of the plane of the retina. It may change from white to pink. Vessels may leave the plane of the retina to enter the ridge. Stage 3 is characterized by the presence of a ridge and by the development of extraretinal fibrovascular tissue. Stage 4 is characterized by subtotal retinal detachment caused by traction from the proliferating tissue in the vitreous or on the retina. Stage 4 is subdivided into two phases: (1) subtotal retinal detachment not involving the macula; and (2) subtotal retinal detachment involving the macula. Stage 5 is total retinal detachment.

When signs of vascular decompensation accompany the active stages of ROP, the term *plus* disease is used. These signs include dilatation and tortuosity of the retinal vessels, engorgement of the iris, pupillary rigidity, and vitreous haze.

CLINICAL COURSE AND PROGNOSIS. In more than 90% of infants the course is one of spontaneous arrest and regression of the usually asymmetric disease process, with little or no residual effects or visual disability. In less than 10% of infants there is progression toward severe disease, with significant extraretinal vasoproliferation, cicatrization, detachment of the retina, and impairment of vision.

Some children with arrested or regressed ROP are left with demarcation lines, undervascularization of the peripheral retina, or abnormal branching, tortuosity, or straightening of the retinal vessels. Some are left with retinal pigmentary changes, dragging of the retina (so-called "dragged disk"), ectopia of the macula, retinal folds, or retinal breaks (Fig. 581–1*B*). Others proceed to total retinal detachment, which commonly assumes a funnel-like configuration. The clinical picture is often that of a retrolental membrane, producing leukocoria (a white or cat's eye reflex in the pupil). Some patients develop cataract, glaucoma, and signs of inflammation. The end stage is often a painful blind eye or a degenerated phthisical eye. The spectrum of ROP also includes myopia, which is often progressive and of significant degree in infancy. There may also be an increased incidence of anisometropia, strabismus, amblyopia, and nystagmus.

DIAGNOSIS. Systematic ophthalmologic examination of infants at risk is recommended. Guidelines vary and are changing but generally include infants weighing less than 2,000 g at birth, especially those weighing less than 1,500 g, those born before 33 wk gestational age, and those requiring supplemental oxygen. Some studies suggest that the optimal time for initial examination is from 7–9 wk, whereas others suggest 4–7 wk. ROP is diagnosed most often at 32–44 wk postconception. The examination can be stressful to the fragile preterm infant and the dilating drops can have untoward side effects, so discretion must be used in timing the eye examination and the infant must be carefully monitored during and after the examination. Follow-up is based on the initial findings and risk factors.

TREATMENT. In selected cases, cryotherapy to the avascular retina has been shown to reduce the more severe complications of progressive ROP to some extent. Also, advances in vitreoretinal surgical techniques have led to some success in reattaching the retina in infants with total retinal detachment (stage 5 ROP), but the visual results are often disappointing.

PREVENTION. Prevention of ROP ultimately depends on the prevention of premature birth and its attendant problems. Despite advances in technology and the meticulous care given to high-risk infants in modern nurseries, ROP continues to occur. Oxygen alone is neither sufficient nor necessary to produce ROP, and no safe level of oxygen has yet been deter-

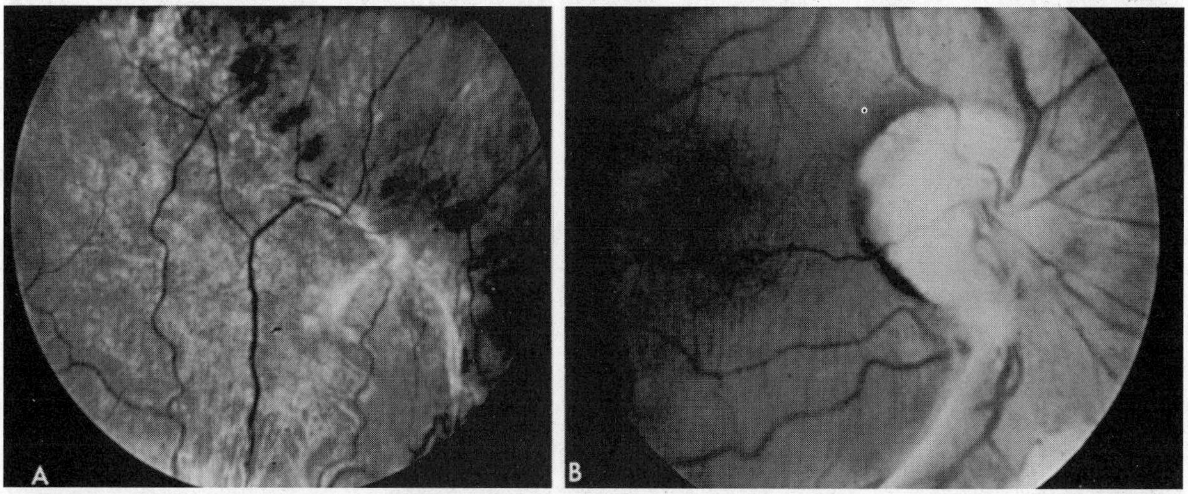

Figure 581–1. *A*, Developing retinopathy of prematurity in the temporal periphery. *B*, "Dragged disk" phenomenon in cicatricial retinopathy of prematurity.

mined. Each infant must be treated with whatever is necessary to sustain life and neurologic function. Some investigators have suggested the use of supplemental vitamin E for its antioxidant properties in infants at risk for ROP. Its efficacy has not been proven, however, and at certain dosage levels it may produce untoward side effects (see Chapter 82), but maintaining a sufficient vitamin E level is prudent.

PERSISTENT HYPERPLASTIC PRIMARY VITREOUS

Persistent hyperplastic primary vitreous (PHPV) refers to a spectrum of manifestations caused by the persistence of various portions of the fetal hyaloid vascular system and associated fibrovascular tissue.

During development of the eye, the hyaloid artery extends from the optic disk to the posterior aspect of the lens; it sends branches into the vitreous (vasa hyaloidea propria) and ramifies to form the posterior portion of the vascular capsule of the lens (tunica vasculosa lentis). The posterior portion of the hyaloid system normally regresses by the 7th fetal mo and the anterior portion by the 8th fetal mo. Small remnants of the system, such as a tuft of tissue at the disk (Bergmeister papilla) or a tag of tissue on the posterior capsule of the lens (Mittendorf dot), are common findings in healthy persons. More extensive remnants and associated complications constitute PHPV. Two major forms are described, anterior PHPV and posterior PHPV. Variability is great, and mixed or intermediate forms occur.

The usual manifestation of anterior PHPV is the presence of a vascularized plaque of tissue on the back surface of the lens in an eye that is microphthalmic or slightly smaller than normal. The condition is usually unilateral and may occur in infants with no other abnormalities and no history of prematurity. The fibrovascular tissue tends to undergo gradual contracture. The ciliary processes characteristically become elongated and the anterior chamber may become shallow. The lens usually is smaller than normal. The lens may be clear, but often it becomes cataractous and may swell or absorb fluid. Large or anomalous vessels of the iris may be present. There may be abnormalities of the anterior chamber angle. In time, the cornea may become cloudy.

Anterior PHPV is usually noted in the 1st weeks or months of life. The most frequent presenting signs are leukocoria (white or cat's eye reflex), strabismus, or nystagmus. The course is usually progressive and ill fated. Major complications are spontaneous intraocular hemorrhage, swelling of the lens caused by rupture of the posterior capsule, and glaucoma. The eye may eventually deteriorate. In selected cases, surgery can be done in an effort to prevent complications, to preserve the eye and a reasonably good cosmetic appearance, and, in some cases, to salvage vision. Surgical treatment usually involves aspirating the lens and excising the abnormal tissue. If useful vision is to be attained, refractive correction and aggressive amblyopia therapy are required, but the visual results tend to be disappointing.

In some cases the affected eye is enucleated, because the differential diagnosis between this white mass and that of retinoblastoma can be difficult. Ultrasound and computed tomography are valuable aids in the differential diagnosis.

The spectrum of posterior PHPV includes fibroglial veils around the disk and macula, vitreous membranes and stalks containing hyaloid artery remnants projecting from the disk, and meridional retinal folds. Traction detachment of the retina may occur. Vision may be impaired, but the eye is usually retained.

RETINOBLASTOMA

Retinoblastoma (Fig. 581–2) is the most common primary malignant intraocular tumor of childhood (see also Chapter 455). It occurs in approximately 1 in 18,000 infants; 250–300 new cases are diagnosed in the United States annually. Hereditary and nonhereditary patterns of transmission occur; there is no sex or race predilection. The tumor occurs bilaterally in 25–35% of cases. The average age at diagnosis for bilateral tumors is 12 mo; unilateral cases are diagnosed, on average, at 21 mo. Occasionally, the tumor is discovered at birth, during adolescence, or even in adulthood.

The clinical manifestations of retinoblastoma vary depending on the stage at which the tumor is detected. The initial sign in the majority of patients is a white pupillary reflex (leukocoria). Leukocoria results because of the reflection of light off the white tumor. The second most frequent initial sign of retinoblastoma is strabismus. Less frequent presenting signs include pseudohypopyon (tumor cells layered inferiorly in front of the iris), caused by tumor seeding in the anterior chamber of the eye; hyphema (blood layered in front of the iris), secondary to iris neovascularization; vitreous hemorrhage; or signs of orbital cellulitis. On examination the tumor appears as a white mass, sometimes small and relatively flat, sometimes large and pro-

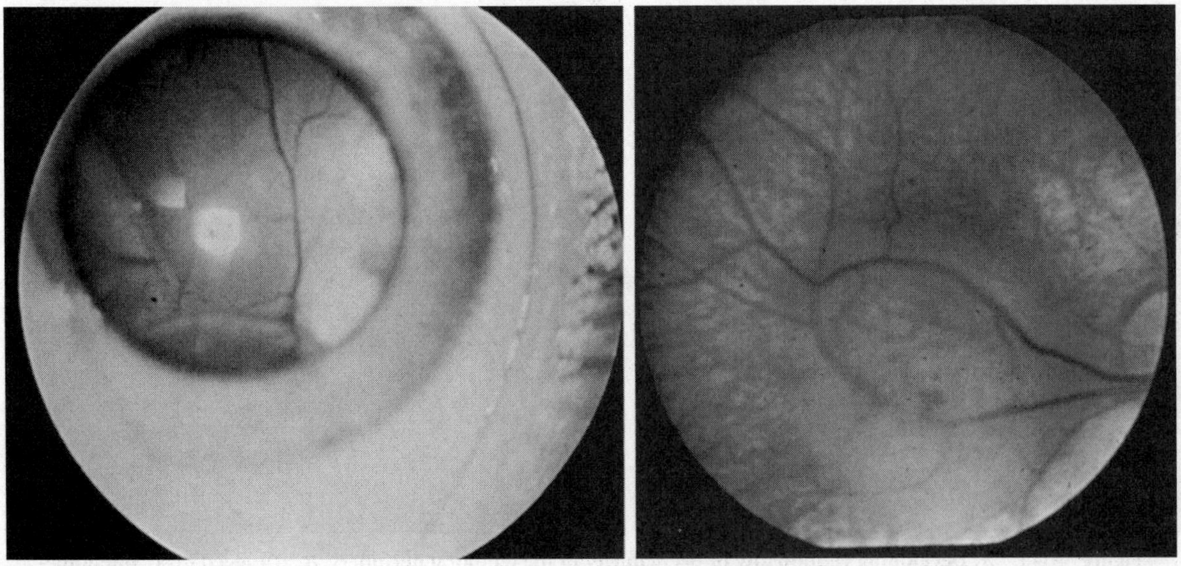

Figure 581–2. Retinoblastoma.

tuberant. It may appear nodular. Vitreous haze or tumor seeding may be evident.

The retinoblastoma gene is a recessive suppressor gene located on chromosome 13 at the 13 q 14 segment, and some affected children have other systemic features of the 13 q deletion syndrome.

The prognosis for patients with retinoblastoma is directly related to the size and extension of the tumor. Most tumors that are confined to the eye can be cured; the prognosis is poor when orbital or optic nerve extension has occurred. The suspicion of retinoblastoma requires prompt referral to an ophthalmologist.

RETINITIS PIGMENTOSA

This progressive retinal degeneration is characterized by pigmentary changes, arteriolar attenuation, usually some degree of optic atrophy, and progressive impairment of visual function. Dispersion and aggregation of the retinal pigment produce various ophthalmoscopically visible changes, ranging from granularity or mottling of the retinal pigment pattern to distinctive focal pigment aggregates with the configuration of bone spicules (Fig. 581–3).

Impairment of night vision or dark adaptation is often the 1st symptom. Progressive loss of peripheral vision, often in the form of an expanding ring scotoma or concentric contraction of the field, is usual. There may be loss of central vision. Retinal function, as measured by electroretinography (ERG), is characteristically reduced. Manifestations commonly begin in childhood. The disorder may be autosomal recessive, autosomal dominant, or sex linked.

A special form of retinitis pigmentosa is Leber congenital retinal amaurosis, in which the retinal changes tend to be pleomorphic, with varying degrees of pigment disorder, arteriolar attenuation, and optic atrophy. Vision impairment is usually evident soon after birth, and the ERG is abnormal early.

To be differentiated from retinitis pigmentosa are clinically similar, secondary, pigmentary retinal degenerations that occur in a wide variety of metabolic diseases, neurodegenerative processes, and multifaceted syndromes. Examples include the progressive retinal changes of the mucopolysaccharidoses (particularly the syndromes of Hurler, Hunter, Scheie, and Sanfilippo) and certain of the late-onset gangliosidoses (the syndromes of Batten-Mayou, Spielmeyer-Vogt, and Jansky-Bielschowsky), the retinal manifestations of abetalipoproteinemia (Bassen-Kornzweig syndrome), the progressive retinal degeneration that is associated with progressive external ophthalmoplegia (Kearns-Sayre syndrome), and the retinitis pigmentosa–like changes in the Laurence-Moon and Bardet-Biedl syndrome. There is also a high association of retinitis pigmentosa and hearing loss, as in Usher syndrome.

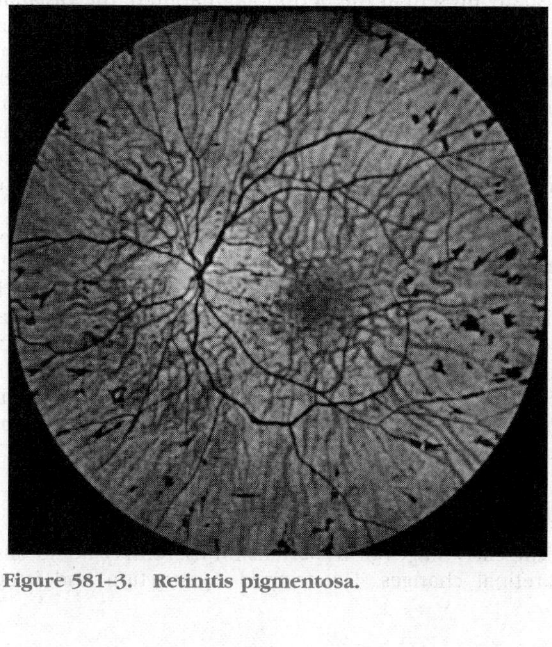

Figure 581–3. Retinitis pigmentosa.

STARGARDT DISEASE

(Fundus Flavimaculatus)

This autosomal recessive retinal disorder is characterized by slowly progressive bilateral macular degeneration and vision impairment. It usually appears at 8–14 yr of age, and affected children are often initially misdiagnosed as having functional visual loss. The foveal reflex becomes obtunded or appears grayish, pigment spots develop in the macular area, and eventually macular depigmentation and chorioretinal atrophy occur. Macular hemorrhages also may develop. In some patients there are also white or yellow spots beyond the macula or pigmentary changes in the periphery; for such patients the term *fundus flavimaculatus* is used. Central visual acuity is reduced, often to 20/200, but total loss of vision does not occur. ERG findings vary. The condition is not associated with CNS abnormalities and is to be differentiated from the macular changes of many progressive metabolic neurodegenerative diseases.

BEST VITELLIFORM DEGENERATION

This macular dystrophy is characterized by a distinctive yellow or orange discoid subretinal lesion in the macula, resembling the intact yolk of a fried egg. Diagnosis is usually made between 3 and 15 yr of age, with a mean age of presentation of 6 yr. Vision is usually normal at this stage. The condition may be progressive; the yolklike lesion may eventually degenerate ("scramble") and result in pigmentation, chorioretinal atrophy, and vision impairment. The condition is almost always bilateral. There is no association with systemic abnormalities. Inheritance is usually autosomal dominant.

In vitelliform macular degeneration the electroretinographic response is normal. The electro-oculogram, however, is abnormal in affected patients and carriers, and is therefore a useful test in diagnosis and in genetic counseling.

CHERRY RED SPOT

Because of the special histologic features of the macula, certain pathologic processes affecting the retina produce an ophthalmoscopically visible sign referred to as a cherry red spot, a bright to dull red spot at the center of the macula surrounded and accentuated by a grayish-white or yellowish halo. The halo is the result of loss of transparency of the multilayered ganglion cell ring as a result of edema, lipid accumulation, or both. The sign occurs typically in certain sphingolipidoses, principally in Tay-Sachs disease (GM_2 type 1), in the Sandhoff variant (GM_2 type 2), and in generalized gangliosidosis (GM_1 type 1). Similar but less distinctive macular changes occur in some cases of metachromatic leukodystrophy (sulfatide lipidosis), in some forms of neuronopathic Niemann-Pick disease, and in certain mucolipidoses. To be differentiated from the cherry red spot of neurodegenerative disease is the cherry red spot that characteristically occurs as the result of retinal ischemia secondary to vasospasm, ocular contusion, or occlusion of the central retinal artery.

PHAKOMATA

These are the herald lesions of the hamartomatous disorders. In Bourneville disease (tuberous sclerosis) the distinctive ocular lesion is a refractile, yellowish, multinodular cystic lesion arising from the disk or retina; the appearance of this typical lesion is often compared to that of an unripe mulberry (Fig. 581–4). Equally characteristic and more common in tuberous sclerosis are flatter, yellow to whitish retinal lesions, varying in size from minute dots to large lesions approaching the size of the disk. These lesions are benign astrocytic proliferations. Rarely, similar retinal phakomata occur in von Recklinghausen disease (neurofibromatosis). In von Hippel-Lindau disease (angiomatosis of the retina and cerebellum) the distinctive fundus lesion is a hemangioblastoma; this vascular lesion usually appears as a reddish globular mass with large paired arteries and veins passing to and from the lesion. In Sturge-Weber syndrome (encephalofacial angiomatosis) the fundus abnormality is a choroidal hemangioma; the hemangioma may impart a dark color to the affected area of the fundus, but the lesion is best seen with fluorescein angiography.

RETINOSCHISIS

Congenital hereditary retinoschisis, also referred to as *juvenile X-linked retinoschisis,* is a bilateral vitreoretinal dystrophy that appears early in life, often in infancy. It is characterized by a splitting of the retina into inner and outer layers. The usual ophthalmoscopic finding in affected males is an elevation of the inner layer of the retina, most commonly in the inferotemporal quadrant of the fundus, often with round or oval holes visible in the inner layer. Schisis of the fovea is virtually pathognomonic and is found in almost 100% of patients. Ophthalmoscopically this appears in early stages as small, fine striae in the internal limiting membrane that radiate outward in a petaloid or spokewheel configuration. In some cases frank retinal detachment or vitreous hemorrhage occurs.

Vision impairment varies from mild to severe; visual acuity may worsen with age, but good vision is often retained.

Carrier females are asymptomatic, but linkage studies may be useful to help detect carriers.

RETINAL DETACHMENT

A retinal detachment is a separation of the outer layers of the retina from the underlying retinal pigment epithelium. The detachment can occur as a congenital anomaly, but more commonly arises secondary to other ocular abnormalities or trauma. Three types of detachment are described, each of which may occur in children. Rhegmatogenous detachments result from a break in the retina that allows fluid to enter the subretinal space. In children, these are usually the result of trauma (such as child abuse) but may occur secondary to myopia or retinopathy of prematurity, or following congenital cataract surgery. Tractional retinal detachments result when vitreoretinal membranes pull on the retina. They can occur in diabetes, sickle-cell disease, and retinopathy of prematurity. Exudative retinal detachments result when exudation exceeds absorption. This can be seen in Coats disease, retinoblastoma, and ocular inflammation.

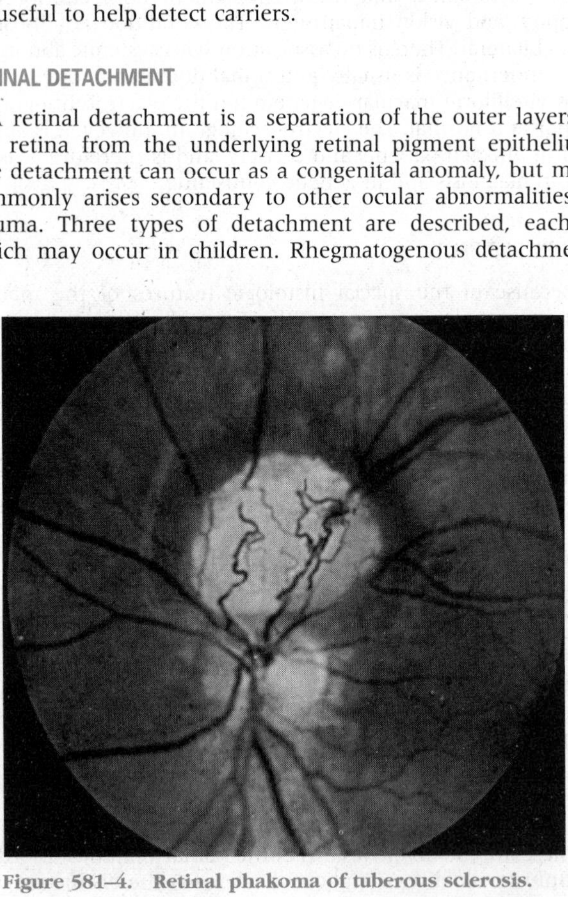

Figure 581–4. Retinal phakoma of tuberous sclerosis.

The presenting sign of retinal detachment in an infant or child may be loss of vision, secondary strabismus and/or nystagmus, or leukocoria (white pupillary reflex). In addition to direct examination of the eye, special diagnostic studies such as ultrasonography and neuroimaging (computed tomography, magnetic resonance imaging) may be necessary to establish the etiology of the detachment and the appropriate treatment. Prompt care is essential if vision is to be salvaged.

COATS DISEASE

This exudative retinopathy of obscure etiology is characterized by telangiectasis of retinal vessels with leakage of plasma to form intraretinal and subretinal exudates, and by retinal hemorrhages and detachment. The condition is usually unilateral. It affects predominantly boys, usually appearing in the 1st decade. The condition is nonfamilial and for the most part occurs in otherwise healthy children. The most frequent presenting signs are blurring of vision, leukocoria, and strabismus. Rubeosis of the iris, glaucoma, and cataract may develop. Treatment with photocoagulation or cryotherapy may be helpful.

FAMILIAL EXUDATIVE VITREORETINOPATHY

This progressive retinovascular disorder is of unknown etiology, but clinical and angiographic findings suggest an aberration of vascular development. A significant finding in most cases is avascularity of the peripheral temporal retina, with abrupt cessation of the retinal capillary network in the region of the equator. The avascular zone often has a wedge- or V-shaped pattern in the temporal meridian. There may be glial proliferation or well-marked retinochoroidal atrophy in the avascular zone. Excessive branching of retinal arteries and veins, dilatation of the capillaries, arteriovenous shunt formation, neovascularization, and leakage from retinal vessels of the farthest vascularized retina occur. Vitreoretinal adhesions are usually present at the peripheral margin of the vascularized retina. Traction, retinal dragging and temporal displacement of the macula, falciform retinal folds, and retinal detachment are common. Intraretinal or subretinal exudation, retinal hemorrhage, and recurrent vitreous hemorrhages may develop. Patients may also develop cataracts and glaucoma. Vision impairment of varying severity occurs. The condition is usually bilateral. Familial exudative retinopathy (FEV) is an autosomal dominant condition; sporadic cases have been reported.

The findings in FEV may resemble those of retinopathy of prematurity in the cicatricial stages but, unlike ROP, the neovascularization of FEV seems to develop years after birth and in most patients with FEV there is no history of prematurity, oxygen therapy, prenatal or postnatal injury or infection, or developmental abnormalities.

FEV is also to be differentiated from Coats disease, angiomatosis of retina, peripheral uveitis, and other disorders of the posterior segment.

HYPERTENSIVE RETINOPATHY

In the early stages of hypertension there may be no observable retinal changes. Generalized constriction and irregular narrowing of the arterioles are usually the 1st signs in the fundus. Other alterations include retinal edema, flame-shaped hemorrhages, "cotton-wool patches," and papilledema (Fig. 581–5). These changes are reversible if the disease can be controlled in the early stages, but in longstanding hypertension, irreversible changes may occur. Thickening of the vessel wall may produce a silver- or copper-wire appearance.

Hypertensive retinal changes in the child should alert the physician to renal disease, pheochromocytoma, collagen disease, and cardiovascular disorders, particularly coarctation of the aorta.

DIABETIC RETINOPATHY

The retinal changes of diabetes mellitus are classified as simple or nonproliferative (early) or proliferative (more advanced).

Nonproliferative diabetic retinopathy is characterized by retinal microaneurysms, venous dilatation, and retinal hemorrhages and exudates. The microaneurysms appear as tiny red dots. The hemorrhages may be of both the dot and blot type, representing deep intraretinal bleeding, and the splinter or flame-shaped type, involving the superficial nerve fiber layer. The exudates tend to be deep and to appear waxy. There may also be superficial nerve fiber infarcts called cytoid bodies or cotton-wool spots, and retinal edema. These signs may wax and wane. They are seen primarily in the posterior pole, around the disc and macula, well within the range of direct ophthalmoscopy.

Proliferative retinopathy, the more serious form, is characterized by neovascularization and proliferation of fibrovascular tissue on the retina, extending into the vitreous. The vision-threatening complications of proliferative diabetic retinopathy are retinal and vitreous hemorrhages, cicatrization, traction, and retinal detachment. Rubeosis of the iris and secondary glaucoma may develop.

Diabetic retinopathy involves the alteration and nonperfusion of retinal capillaries, retinal ischemia, and neovascularization, but its pathogenesis is not yet completely understood, either as to location of the primary pathogenetic mechanism (retinal vessels versus surrounding neuronal or glial tissue) or to the specific biochemical factors involved. The precise relationship between control of blood glucose and the genesis or progression of retinopathy remains unsettled, but data suggest that the better the degree of long-term metabolic control, the lower the risk of diabetic retinopathy.

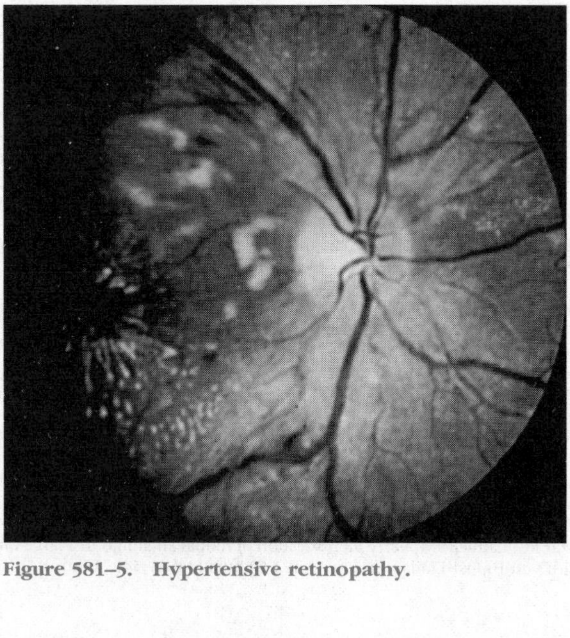

Figure 581–5. Hypertensive retinopathy.

Clinically, the prevalence and course of retinopathy relate to the patient's age and to duration of disease. Detectable microvascular changes are rare in prepubertal children, with the prevalence of retinopathy increasing significantly after puberty, especially after the age of 15 yr. The incidence of retinopathy is low during the 1st 5 yr of disease and increases progressively thereafter, with the incidence of proliferative retinopathy becoming substantial after 10 yr and with increased risk of visual impairment after 15 yr or more. Periodic ophthalmologic evaluation is recommended for all patients with diabetes mellitus.

In addition to retinopathy, patients with juvenile-onset diabetes may develop optic neuropathy, characterized by swelling of the disk and blurring of vision. Patients with diabetes may also develop cataracts, even at an early age, sometimes with rapid progression.

It is also prudent to check the color vision of children and their caregivers who must interpret the results of color-dependent glucose strip tests.

Advances in ocular therapy, such as retinal photocoagulation and vitrectomy, offer hope in reducing visual morbidity in some patients with diabetes. The value of technologic advances, such as insulin infusion pumps and pancreatic transplants, in the prevention of ocular complications is under investigation (see Part XXVI, Section 6).

SUBACUTE BACTERIAL ENDOCARDITIS

At some time during the course of the disease, retinopathy is present in approximately 40% of cases of subacute bacterial endocarditis. The lesions include hemorrhages, hemorrhages with white centers (Roth spots), papilledema, and, rarely, embolic occlusion of the central retinal artery.

BLOOD DISORDERS

In primary and secondary anemias, retinopathy in the form of hemorrhages and cotton-wool patches may occur. Vision can be affected if hemorrhage occurs in the macular area. The hemorrhages may be light and feathery, or dense and preretinal. In polycythemia vera, the retinal veins are dark, dilated, and tortuous. Retinal hemorrhages, retinal edema, and papilledema may be observed. In leukemia the veins are characteristically dilated, with sausage-shaped constrictions; hemorrhages, particularly white-centered hemorrhages and exudates, are common during the acute stage. In the sickling disorders, fundus changes include vascular tortuosity, arterial and venous occlusions, "salmon patches," refractile deposits, pigmented lesions, arteriolar-venous anastomoses, and neovascularization (with "sea-fan" formations), sometimes leading to vitreous hemorrhage and retinal detachment.

TRAUMA-RELATED RETINOPATHY

Retinal changes may occur in patients who suffer trauma to other parts of the body. The occurrence of retinal hemorrhages in infants who have been physically abused is well documented (see Chapter 38). Retinal, subretinal, subhyaloid, and vitreous hemorrhages have been described. Often there are no signs of direct trauma to the eye, periocular region, or head. Such cases may result from violent shaking of the infant, and permanent retinal damage may result.

Retinal, subhyaloid, and vitreous hemorrhages are common in patients with traumatic and nontraumatic subarachnoid hemorrhage, an association referred to as Terson syndrome.

In patients with head or chest trauma, a traumatic retinal angiopathy known as Purtscher retinopathy may occur. This is characterized by retinal hemorrhage, cotton-wool spots, sometimes disk swelling, and decreased vision. The pathogenesis is unclear, but there is evidence for arteriolar obstruction in this condition.

Retinal hemorrhages and cotton-wool spots may also be seen after bone fractures or pelvic surgery, probably as the result of fat embolism.

MEDULLATED NERVE FIBERS

Myelination of the optic nerve fibers normally terminates at the level of the disk, but in some individuals ectopic medullation extends to nerve fibers of the retina. The condition is most commonly seen adjacent to the disk, although more peripheral areas of the retina may be involved. The characteristic ophthalmoscopic picture is a focal white patch with a feathered edge or brush-stroke appearance. Because the macula is generally unaffected, the visual prognosis is good. A relative or absolute visual field defect corresponding to areas of ectopic medullation is usually the only associated ocular abnormality. Extensive unilateral involvement, however, has been associated with ipsilateral myopia, amblyopia, and strabismus. If unilateral high myopia and amblyopia are present, appropriate optical correction and occlusion therapy should be instituted. For unknown reasons, the disorder is more commonly encountered in patients with craniofacial dysostoris, oxycephaly, neurofibromatosis, and Down syndrome.

COLOBOMA OF THE FUNDUS

The term *coloboma* describes a defect such as a gap, notch, fissure, or hole. The typical fundus coloboma is a result of malclosure of the embryonic fissure, which leaves a gap in the retina, retinal pigment epithelium, and choroid, thus baring the underlying sclera. The defect may be extensive, involving the ciliary body, iris, and even lens, or it may be localized to one or more portions of the fissure. The usual appearance is of a well-circumscribed, wedge-shaped white area extending inferonasally below the disk, sometimes involving or engulfing the disk. In some cases there is ectasia or cyst formation in the area of the defect. Less extensive colobomatous defects may appear as only single or multiple focal "punched-out" chorioretinal defects or anomalous pigmentation of the fundus in the line of the embryonic fissure. Colobomata may occur in one or both eyes. Usually a visual field defect corresponds to the chorioretinal defect. Visual acuity may be impaired, particularly if the defect involves the disk or macula.

Fundus colobomata may occur in isolation as sporadic defects or inherited as a dominant or recessive condition, or may be associated with such abnormalities as microphthalmia, glioneuroma of the eye, cyclopia, or an encephaly. They occur in children with various chromosomal disorders, including 13-trisomy, 18-trisomy, triploidy, cat-eye syndrome, and 4p-. Ocular colobomata also occur in many multisystem disorders, including the CHARGE* association, Joubert, Aicardi, Meckel, Warburg, and Rubinstein-Taybi, linear sebaceous nevus, Goldenhar, Lenz microphthalmia syndromes, and Goltz focal dermal hypoplasia. Colobomata of the optic nerve in particular may be associated with basal encephalocele and serous detachment of the retina. Ocular colobomata have also been associated with congenital infection, including cytomegalovirus infection, and with the maternal use of thalidomide and lysergic acid diethylamide (LSD).

Aaby AA, Kushner BJ: Acquired and progressive myelinated nerve fibers. Arch Ophthalmol 103:542, 1985.
Barr CC, Glaser JS, Blankenship G: Acute disc swelling in juvenile diabetes: Clinical profile and natural history of 12 cases. Arch Ophthalmol 98:2185, 1980.

*C = coloboma; H = heart disease; A = atresia choanae; R = retarded growth and development and/or CNS anomalies; G = genetic anomalies and/or hypogonadism; E = ear anomalies and/or deafness.

Bateman JB, Riedner E, Levin LS, et al: Heterogeneity of retinal degeneration and hearing impairment syndromes. Am J Ophthalmol 90:755, 1980.
Berson EL, Rosner B, Siminoff E: Risk factors for genetic typing and detection in retinitis pigmentosa. Am J Ophthalmol 89:763, 1980.
Boldrey EE, Egbert P, Gass DM, et al: The histopathology of familial exudative vitreoretinopathy: A report of two cases. Arch Ophthalmol 103:238, 1985.
Burns RP, Lourien EW, Cibis AB: Juvenile sex-linked retinoschisis: Clinical and genetic studies. Trans Am Acad Ophthalmol Otolaryngol 75:1011, 1971.
Chang M, McLean IW, Merritt JC: Coats' disease: A study of 62 histologically confirmed cases. J Pediatr Ophthalmol Strab 21:163, 1984.
Cotlier E: Café-au-lait spots of the fundus in neurofibromatosis. Arch Ophthalmol 95:1990, 1977.
CRYD-ROP group: Multicenter trial of cryotherapy for retinopathy of prematurity: three month outcome. Arch Ophthalmol 108:195, 1990.
Doft BH, Kingsley LA, Orchard TJ, et al: The association between long-term diabetic control and early retinopathy. Ophthalmology 91:763, 1984.
Duane TD, Osher RH, Green WR: White-centered hemorrhages: Their significance. Ophthalmology 87:66, 1980.
Eagle RC, Lucier AC, Bernardino VB Jr, et al: Retinal pigment epithelial abnormalities in fundus flavimaculatus. Ophthalmology 87:1189, 1980.
Fishman GA: Retinitis pigmentosa: Genetic percentages. Arch Ophthalmol 96:822, 1978.
Frank RN: On the pathogenesis of diabetic retinopathy. Ophthalmology 91:626, 1984.
Frank RN, Hoffman WH, Podgor MJ, et al: Retinopathy in juvenile-onset diabetes of short duration. Ophthalmology 87:1, 1980.
Gallie BL, Phillips RA: Retinoblastoma: A model of oncogenesis. Ophthalmology 91:666, 1984.
Goldberg MF, Mafee M: Computed tomography for diagnosis of persistent hyperplastic primary vitreous (PHPV). Ophthalmology 90:442, 1983.
Hardwig P, Robertson DM: Von Hippel-Lindau disease: A familial, often lethal, multi-system phakomatosis. Ophthalmology 91:263, 1984.
Jackson RL, Ide CH, Guthrie RA, et al: Retinopathy in adolescents and young adults with onset of insulin-dependent diabetes in childhood. Ophthalmology 89:7, 1982.
Juan Verdaguer T: Juvenile retinal detachment. Am J Ophthalmol 93:145, 1982.
Kline R, Klein BEK, Moss SE, et al: The Wisconsin epidemiologic study of diabetic retinopathy: II. Prevalence and risk of diabetic retinopathy when age at diagnosis is less than 30 years. Arch Ophthalmol 102:520, 1984.
Knobloch WH, Layer JM: Clefting syndromes associated with retinal detachment. Am J Ophthalmol 73:517, 1972.
Kushner BJ: Strabismus and amblyopia associated with regressed retinopathy of prematurity. Arch Ophthalmol 100:256, 1982.
Kushner BJ, Sondheimer S: Medical treatment of glaucoma associated with cicatricial retinopathy of prematurity. Am J Ophthalmol 94:313, 1982.
Laverda AM, Saia OS, Drigo P, et al: Chorioretinal coloboma and Joubert syndrome: A nonrandom association. J Pediatr 105:282, 1984.
Mann E, Kut LJ, Lee CB: Rheumatogenous retinal detachment in infancy. Arch Ophthalmol 95:1774, 1971.
Matthews JD, Weiter JJ, Kolodny EH: Macular halos associated with Niemann-Pick type B disease. Ophthalmology 93:933, 1986.
McNamara JA, Tasman W, Brown GC, et al: Laser photocoagulation for stage 3+ retinopathy of prematurity. Ophthalmology 98:576, 1991.
Miyakulo H, Hashimoto K, Miyakulo S: Retinal vascular pattern in familial exudative vitreoretinopathy. Ophthalmology 91:1524, 1984.
Mohler CW, Fine SL: Long-term evaluation of patients with Best's vitelliform dystrophy. Ophthalmology 88:688, 1981.
Noble KG, Carr RE: Leber's congenital amaurosis: A retrospective study of 33 cases and a histopathological study of one case. Arch Ophthalmol 96:818, 1978.
Noble KG, Carr RE: Stargardt's disease and fundus flavimaculatus. Arch Ophthalmol 97:1281, 1979.
Nyboer JH, Robertson DM, Gomez MR: Retinal lesions in tuberous sclerosis. Arch Ophthalmol 94:1277, 1976.
Pagon RA: Ocular coloboma. Surv Ophthalmol 25:223, 1981.
Pagon RA, Graham JM, Zonana J, et al: Coloboma, congenital heart disease, and choanal atresia with multiple anomalies: CHARGE association. J Pediatr 99:223, 1981.
Palmer EA, Flynn JT, Hardy RJ, et al: Incidence and early course of retinopathy of prematurity. Ophthalmology 98:1628, 1991.
Phelps DL: Retinopathy of prematurity. Pediatr Clin North Am 40:705, 1993.
Pruett RC, Schepens CI: Posterior hyperplastic primary vitreous. Am J Ophthalmol 69:535, 1970.
Quinn GE, Dobson V, Pepka MX, et al: Development of myopia in infants with birthweights less than 1251 grams. Ophthalmology 99:329, 1992.
Ridgeway EW, Jaffe N, Walton DS: Leukemic ophthalmopathy in children. Cancer 38:1744, 1976.
Ridley ME, Shields JA, Brown GC, et al: Coats' disease: Evaluation of management. Ophthalmology 89:1381, 1982.
Riley FC, Campbell RJ: Double phakomatosis. Arch Ophthalmology 97:518, 1979.
Romayananda N, Goldberg MF, Green WR: Histopathology of sickle cell retinopathy. Ophthalmology 77:652, 1973.
Rosenthal AR: Ocular manifestations of leukemia. Ophthalmology 90:899, 1983.
Salazar FG, Lamiell JM: Early identification of retinal angiomas in a large kindred with von Hippel-Lindau disease. Am J Ophthalmol 89:540, 1980.

Schaffer DB, Palmer EA, Plotsky DF, et al: Prognostic factors in the natural course of retinopathy of prematurity (ROP). Ophthalmology 100:230, 1993.
Shields JA, Augsburger JJ: Current approaches to the diagnosis and management of retinoblastoma. Surv Ophthalmol 25:347, 1981.
Shields JA, Shields CL: Intraocular Tumors. A Text and Atlas. Philadelphia, WB Saunders, 1992.
Shields CL, Shields JA: Genetics of retinoblastoma. *In*: Tasman WS, Jaeger EA (eds): Duane's Foundation of Clinical Ophthalmology. Philadelphia, JB Lippincott, 1991.
Stark WJ, Lindsey PS, Fagadau WR, et al: Persistent hyperplastic primary vitreous: Surgical treatment. Ophthalmology 90:452, 1983.
Stein MR, Gay AJ: Acute chorioretinal infarction in sickle cell trait. Arch Ophthalmol 84:485, 1970.
Straatsma BR, Foos RY, Heckenlively JR, et al: Myelinated retinal nerve fibers. Am J Ophthalmol 91:25, 1981.
Tasman W: Late complications of retrolental fibroplasia. Ophthalmology 86:1724, 1979.
The Committee for the Classification of Retinopathy of Prematurity: An international classification of retinopathy of prematurity. Arch Ophthalmol 102:1130, 1984.
The International Committee for the Classification of the Late Stages of Retinopathy of Prematurity: An international classification of retinopathy of prematurity. II: The classification of retinal detachment. Arch Ophthalmol 105:906, 1987.
Topilow HW, Ackerman AL, Wang FM: The treatment of advanced retinopathy of prematurity by cryotherapy and scleral buckling surgery. Ophthalmology 92:379, 1985.
Trese MT: Surgical results of stage V retrolental fibroplasia and timing of surgical repair. Ophthalmology 91:461, 1984.
Tso MOM, Jampol LM: Pathophysiology of hypertensive retinopathy. Ophthalmology 89:1132, 1982.
Walsh JB: Hypertensive retinopathy: Description, classification and prognosis. Ophthalmology 89:1127, 1982.
Yassur Y, Nissenkorn I, Ben-Sira I, et al: Autosomal dominant inheritance of retinoschisis. Am J Ophthalmol 94:338, 1982.

CHAPTER 582
Abnormalities of the Optic Nerve

OPTIC NERVE HYPOPLASIA

This developmental deficiency of optic nerve fibers has been attributed to primary failure in the differentiation of retinal ganglion cells or their axons. Alternatively, it may result from prenatal degeneration of the ganglion cell axons. In typical cases the nerve head is small and pale, with a pale or pigmented peripapillary halo or "double ring sign." This anomaly is associated with defects of vision and of visual fields of varying severity, ranging from blindness to normal or near-normal vision in the affected eye. Hypoplasia may be unilateral or bilateral, with clinical findings varying with the severity and laterality of the condition. Unilateral or asymmetric hypoplasia commonly presents as deviation (heterotropia, strabismus) of the more severely affected eye; the deviation usually develops early in life, but often the underlying visual defect is not suspected or detected until a later age. When there is bilateral hypoplasia of relatively severe degree, the defect in vision is usually appreciated early, and there is often obvious strabismus or secondary nystagmus. Mild hypoplasia may be unrecognized for years.

Optic nerve hypoplasia may occur alone or with other developmental abnormalities, including microphthalmia, anencephaly, hydrocephalus, and encephalocele. Optic nerve hypoplasia is a principal feature of septo-optic dysplasia of de Morsier, a developmental disorder characterized by the association of anomalies of the midline structures of the brain with hypoplasia of the optic nerves, optic chiasm, and optic tracts; typically, there is agenesis of the septum pellucidum, partial or complete agenesis of the corpus callosum, and malformation of the fornix, with a large chiasmatic cistern. There may be hypothalamic abnormalities and endocrine defects, ranging from panhypopituitarism to isolated deficiency of growth hormone, hypothyroidism, diabetes insipidus, or diabetes mellitus. Neonatal hypoglycemia and seizures are important presenting signs in affected infants. The condition does not appear to be familial, although it has occurred in siblings. There is no regularly associated chromosomal defect, although it may be present in infants with chromosomal aberrations such as 13-trisomy. Optic nerve hypoplasia is common in patients with albinism and aniridia. It may occur with somewhat increased frequency in infants of diabetic mothers. Optic nerve hypoplasia has been associated with the maternal use of dilantin, quinine, LSD, and alcohol during pregnancy.

OPTIC NERVE APLASIA

This very rare congenital anomaly is characterized by the absence of the optic nerves, retinal ganglion cells, and retinal blood vessels, with attendant blindness and absence of the pupillary reaction to light in the affected eye. It may occur as an isolated anomaly or in association with gross maldevelopment of the globe, malformation of the brain, or other developmental defects. The pathogenesis of this disorder is unknown. A number of teratogenic agents have been implicated, including maternal diabetes, fetal alcohol syndrome, maternal drug abuse, and intrauterine cytomegalovirus infection.

MORNING GLORY DISK ANOMALY

This term describes a congenital malformation of the optic nerve characterized by an enlarged, excavated, funnel-shaped disk with an elevated rim, resembling the flower for which it is named. There often is whitish tissue in the funnel, the abnormal vessel pattern involves multiple branches emerging radially, and there is usually pigmentary mottling of the peripapillary region. Most cases are unilateral. The visual acuity usually ranges from 20/200 to hand motion. Contralateral eyes can have ocular abnormalities, including microphthalmos, microcornea, anterior cleavage syndrome, and duane retraction syndrome. Detachment of the retina may occur. The anomaly may be associated with developmental midline defects, including cleft lip and palate, agenesis of the corpus callosum, hypertelorism, and encephalocele.

TILTED DISK

In this congenital anomaly the vertical axis of the optic disk is directed obliquely, so a that the upper temporal portion of the nerve head is more prominent and anterior to the lower nasal portion of the disk, and the retinal vessels emerge from the upper temporal portion of the disk rather than from the nasal side. Often there is a peripapillary crescent or conus. There may be associated visual field defects and myopic astigmatism. Clinical recognition of the tilted disk syndrome is important to avoid confusion of its disk and visual field signs with those of papilledema and intracranial tumor.

DRUSEN OF THE OPTIC NERVE

These globular, acellular bodies are thought to arise from axoplasmic derivatives of disintegrating nerve fibers. Drusen may be buried within the optic nerve, producing elevation of the optic nerve head (which can be confused with papilledema), or they may be partially or completely exposed, appearing as refractile bodies at the surface of the disk. Visual field defects and spontaneous peripapillary nerve fiber layer hemorrhages may occur in association with drusen. Drusen may occur as an autosomal dominant condition. They have also been observed in children, with various neurologic disorders, including primary megalencephaly, seizures, learning disorders, mental retardation, schizophrenia, tuberous sclerosis, Down syndrome, and intracranial tumors.

PAPILLEDEMA

The term *papilledema* ("choked disk") can be applied to swelling of the nerve head of diverse etiologies, but it preferentially denotes the disk changes of increased intracranial pressure, including edematous blurring of the disk margins, fullness or elevation of the nervehead, partial or complete obliteration of the disk cup, capillary congestion and hyperemia of the nerve head, generalized engorgement of the veins, loss of spontaneous venous pulsation, nerve fiber layer hemorrhages around the disk, and peripapillary exudates. In some cases there may be edema extending into the macula, producing a fan- or star-shaped figure. In addition, there may be concentric peripapillary retinal wrinkling. There may be transient obscuration of vision, lasting seconds. Normally, when the intracranial pressure is relieved, the papilledema resolves and the disk returns to a normal or nearly normal appearance within 6–8 wk. Sustained chronic papilledema or longstanding unrelieved increased intracranial pressure may, however, lead to permanent nerve fiber damage, atrophic changes of the disk, macular scarring, and impairment of vision. In cases of impending or progressive vision loss caused by papilledema in patients with benign intracranial hypertension, decompression of the optic nerve by slitting the sheath may preserve vision.

The sequence of events as increased intracranial pressure leads to papilledema is probably as follows: elevation of intracranial subarachnoid cerebrospinal fluid pressure, elevation of cerebrospinal fluid pressure in the sheath of the optic nerve, elevation of tissue pressure in the optic nerve, stasis of axoplasmic flow and swelling of the nerve fibers in the optic nervehead, and secondary vascular changes and the characteristic ophthalmoscopic signs of venous stasis. Associated neurophthalmic signs of increased intracranial pressure in infants and children include abducent palsy and attendant esotropia, lid retraction, paresis of upward gaze, tonic downward deviation of the eyes, and convergent nystagmus.

The common causes of increased intracranial pressure and choked disk in childhood are intracranial tumors and obstructive hydrocephalus, intracranial hemorrhage, the cerebral edema of trauma, meningoencephalitis and toxic encephalopathy, and certain metabolic diseases. Whatever the etiology, the disk signs of increased intracranial pressure in early childhood may be modified by the distensibility of the young skull. In the absence of conditions associated with early closure of sutures and early obliteration of the fontanel (craniosynostosis, Crouzon, and Apert syndromes), infants with increased intracranial pressure usually do not develop papilledema.

To be differentiated from true papilledema are certain structural changes of the disk ("pseudopapilledema," "pseudoneuritis," drusen, and medullated fibers), with which it may be confused, and the disk swelling of hypertension and diabetes mellitus.

Papilledema is a neurological emergency. It can be accompanied by other signs of increased intracranial pressure, including headaches, nausea, and vomiting. Neuroimaging should be performed; if no intracranial masses are detected, a lumbar puncture should follow.

OPTIC NEURITIS

This term is used to describe any inflammation, demyelinization, or degeneration of the optic nerve with attendant impairment of function. The process is usually acute, with rapidly progressive loss of vision. It may be unilateral or bilateral. Pain on movement of the globe or pain on palpation of the globe may precede or accompany the onset of visual symptoms.

When the retrobulbar portion of the nerve is affected without ophthalmoscopically visible signs of inflammation at the disk, the term *retrobulbar neuritis* is applied. When there is ophthalmoscopically visible evidence of inflammation of the nervehead, the term *papillitis* or *intraocular optic neuritis* is used. When there is involvement of both the retina and papilla, the term *optic neuroretinitis* is used.

In childhood, optic neuritis rarely occurs as an isolated condition but is usually a manifestation of a neurologic or systemic disease. It may occur with bacterial meningitis or with viral infection (often accompanying encephalomyelitis following an exanthem). It may signify one of the many demyelinizing diseases of childhood. It may be the first manifestation of disseminated sclerosis. Alternatively, the cause may be an exogenous toxin or drug; optic neuritis may develop, for example, with lead poisoning or as a complication of long-term, high-dose treatment with chloramphenicol or vincristine therapy. Extensive pediatric neurologic and ophthalmic investigation, including neuroradiologic and electrophysiologic studies, is usually required.

In most cases of acute optic neuritis there is some improvement in vision beginning within 1–4 wk after onset, and vision may improve to normal or near normal within weeks or months. In some cases there is permanent impairment of vision. The course varies with etiology. Treatment of optic neuritis with high doses of systemic corticosteroids may sometimes be helpful in reducing inflammation and improving vision.

LEBER OPTIC NEUROPATHY

This maternally (mitochondrial DNA) inherited disorder may manifest in childhood, and affects males and females. Early signs include peripapillary telangiectatic microangiopathy, disk swelling, and sudden or gradual decrease in vision. One eye is usually affected before the other. In time there is usually progressive optic atrophy and vision loss. There may be associated electrocardiographic abnormalities.

OPTIC ATROPHY

This denotes degeneration of optic nerve axons, with attendant loss of function. The ophthalmoscopic signs of optic atrophy are pallor of the disk and loss of substance of the nerve head, sometimes with enlargement of the disk cup. The associated vision defect varies with the nature and site of the primary disease or lesion.

Optic atrophy is the common expression of a wide variety of congenital or acquired pathologic processes. The cause may be traumatic, inflammatory, degenerative, neoplastic, or vascular; intracranial tumors and hydrocephalus are principal causes of optic atrophy in children. In some cases, progressive optic atrophy is hereditary. Dominantly inherited infantile optic atrophy is a relatively mild heredodegenerative type that tends to progress through childhood and adolescence. Autosomal recessively inherited congenital optic atrophy is a rare condition that is evident at birth or develops at a very early age; the visual defect is usually profound. Behr optic atrophy is a hereditary type associated with hypertonia of the extremities, increased deep tendon reflexes, mild cerebellar ataxia, some degree of mental deficiency, and possibly external ophthalmoplegia. This disorder afflicts principally males from 3–11 yr of age. Some forms of heredodegenerative optic atrophy are associated with sensorineural hearing loss, as may occur in some children with juvenile-onset (insulin-dependent) diabetes mellitus. In the absence of an obvious cause, optic atrophy in an infant or child warrants extensive etiologic investigation.

OPTIC GLIOMA

The most frequent tumor of the optic nerve in childhood is optic glioma. This neuroglial tumor may develop in the intraorbital, intracanalicular, or intracranial portion of the nerve; often the chiasm is involved.

Histologically, optic glioma is usually a benign lesion; its deleterious effects vary with its location and growth pattern. Rarely, it may show malignant characteristics. The principal manifestations of intraorbital optic glioma are unilateral loss of vision, proptosis, and deviation of the eye; there may be optic atrophy or congestion of the optic nerve head. With chiasmal gliomas there may be defects of vision and visual fields (often bitemporal hemianopsia), increased intracranial pressure, papilledema or optic atrophy, hypothalamic dysfunction, pituitary dysfunction, and, sometimes, nystagmus, and/or strabismus.

Optic glioma occurs with increased frequency in patients with neurofibromatosis.

The natural clinical course of optic glioma often involves relatively slow, often self-limited progression; there may, however, be relentless progression to death. In some cases the course is rapidly progressive to death.

Management of optic glioma is controversial. When the tumor is confined to the intraorbital, intracanalicular, or prechiasmal portion of the nerve, resection is often done, especially when there is unsightly proptosis with complete or nearly complete loss of vision of the affected eye. When the chiasm is involved, surgery is not advocated, although surgical intervention to control secondary hydrocephalus and increased intracranial pressure, or to obtain biopsy material, may be necessary. Radiation may alter growth of the tumor. Chemotherapy is under trial.

Barr CC, Glaser JS, Blankenship G: Acute disc swelling in juvenile diabetes: Clinical profile and natural history of 12 cases. Arch Ophthalmol 98:2185, 1980.
Beck RW: The neuritis treatment trial. Arch Ophthalmol 106:1051, 1988.
Blanco R, Salvador F, Galan A, et al: Aplasia of the optic nerve: Report of three cases. J Pediatr Ophthalmol Strab 29:228, 1992.
Brown GC, Tasmon W: Congenital Anomalies of the Optic Disc. New York, Grune & Stratton, 1983.
Costin G, Murgpree AL: Hypothalamic-pituitary function in children with optic nerve hypoplasia. Am J Dis Child 139:249, 1985.
Danoff BF, Kramer S, Thompson N: The radiotherapeutic management of optic nerve gliomas in children. J Radiat Oncol Biol Phys 6:45, 1980.
Flickinger JC, Torres C, Deutsch M: Management of low-grade gliomas of the optic nerve and chiasm. Cancer 61:635, 1988.
Haik BG, Greenstein SH, Smith ME, et al: Retinal detachment in the morning glory anomaly. Ophthalmology 91:1638, 1984.
Hayreh SS: Optic disc edema in raised intracranial pressure: V. Pathogenesis. Arch Ophthalmol 95:1553, 1977.
Hayreh SS: Optic disc edema in raised intracranial pressure: VI. Associated visual disturbances and their pathogenesis. Arch Ophthalmol 95:1566, 1977.
Hoover DL, Robb RM, Petersen RA: Optic disc drusen and primary megalencephaly in children. J Pediatr Ophthalmol Strab 26:81, 1989.
Hotchkiss ML, Green WR: Optic nerve aplasia and hypoplasia. J Pediatr Ophthalmol Strab 16:225, 1979.
Hoyt CS: Autosomal dominant optic atrophy: A spectrum of disability. Ophthalmology 87:245, 1980.
Imes RK, Hoyt WF: Childhood chiasmal gliomas: Update on the fate of patients in the 1969 San Francisco study. Br J Ophthalmol 70:179, 1986.
Kazarian EL, Gager WE: Optic neuritis complicating measles, mumps and rubella vaccination. Am J Ophthalmol 86:544, 1978.
Kennedy C, Carter S: Relation of optic neuritis to multiple sclerosis in children. Pediatrics 28:377, 1961.
Kim RY, Hoyt WF, Lessell S, et al: Superior segmental optic hypoplasia: A sign of maternal diabetes. Arch Ophthalmol 107:1312, 1989.
Koenig SB, Naidich TP, Lissner G: The morning glory syndrome associated with sphenoidal encephalocele. Ophthalmology 89:1368, 1982.
Layman PR, Anderson DR, Flynn JT: Frequent occurrence of hypoplastic optic discs in patients with aniridia. Am J Ophthalmol 77:513, 1974.
Lessell S, Rosman P: Juvenile diabetes mellitus and optic atrophy. Arch Neurol 34:759, 1977.
Lewis RA, Gerson LP, Axelson KA, et al: Von Recklinghausen neurofibromatosis: II. Incidence of optic gliomata. Ophthalmology 91:929, 1984.
Margalith D, Jan JE, McCormick AQ, et al: Clinical spectrum of congenital optic nerve hypoplasia: Review of 51 patients. Dev Med Child Neurol 26:311, 1984.
Margalith D, Tse WJ, Jan JE: Congenital optic nerve hypoplasia with hypothalamic-pituitary dysplasia: A review of 16 cases. Am J Dis Child 139:361, 1985.
McLeod AR: Acute blindness in childhood optic glioma caused by hematoma. J Pediatr Ophthalmol Strab 20:31, 1983.
Nikoskelainen EK, Savontaus M-L, Wanne OP, et al: Leber's hereditary optic neuropathy, a maternally inherited disease: A genealogic study in four pedigrees. Arch Ophthalmol 105:665, 1987.
O'Dwyer JA, Newton TH, Hoyt WF: Radiologic features of septo-optic dysplasia: deMorsier syndrome. AJNR 1:443, 1980.
Packer RJ, Savino PJ, Bilaniuk LT, et al: Chiasmatic gliomas of childhood: A reappraisal of natural history and effectiveness of cranial irradiation. Child's Brain 10:393, 1983.
Petersen RA, Walton DS: Optic nerve hypoplasia with good visual acuity and visual field defects: A study of children of diabetic mothers. Arch Ophthalmol 95:254, 1977.
Repka MX, Miller NR: Optic atrophy in children. Am J Ophthalmol 106:191, 1988.
Rosenberg MA, Savino PJ, Glaser JS: A clinical analysis of pseudopapilledema. I: Population, laterality, acuity, refractive error, ophthalmoscopic characteristics, and coincident disease. Arch Ophthalmol 97:65, 1979.
Rosenstock JG, Packer RJ, Bilaniuk L, et al: Chiasmatic optic glioma treated with chemotherapy: A preliminary report. J Neurosurg 63:862, 1985.
Rush JA, Younge BR, Campbell RJ, et al: Optic glioma: Long-term follow-up of 85 histopathologically verified cases. Ophthalmology 89:1213, 1982.
Schwartz JF, Chutorian AM, Evans RA, et al: Optic atrophy in childhood. Pediatrics 34:670, 1964.
Selbst RG, Selhorst JB, Harbison JW, et al: Parainfectious optic neuritis: Report and review following varicella. Arch Neurol 40:347, 1983.
Sergott RC, Savino PJ, Bosley TM: Modified optic nerve sheath decompression provides long-term visual improvement for pseudotumor cerebri. Arch Ophthalmol 106:1384, 1988.
Singh G, Lott MT, Wallace DC: A mitochondrial DNA mutation as a cause of Leber's hereditary optic neusopathy. N Engl J Med 320:1300, 1989.
Skarf B, Hoyt CS: Optic nerve hypoplasia in children: Association with anomalies of the endocrine and CNS. Arch Ophthalmol 102:62, 1984.
Traboulsi EI, O'Neill JE: The spectrum in the morphology of the so-called "morning glory disc anomaly." J Pediatr Ophthalmol Strab 25:93, 1988.
Weiss AH, Beck RW: Neuroretinitis in childhood. J Pediatr Ophthalmol Strab 26:198, 1989.
Weiter JJ, McClean IW, Zimmerman IE: Aplasia of the optic nerve and disc. Am J Ophthalmol 83:569, 1977.

CHAPTER 583

Childhood Glaucoma

Glaucoma is a general term used to indicate damage to the optic nerve caused by, or related to, elevated pressure within the eye. It is classified according to the age of the affected individual at presentation and the association of other ocular or systemic conditions. Glaucoma that begins within the first 3 yr of life is called infantile (congenital); that which begins between the ages of 3 and 30 yr is called juvenile.

Primary glaucoma indicates that the etiology is an isolated anomaly of the drainage apparatus of the eye (trabecular meshwork). More than 50% of infantile glaucoma is primary. Secondary glaucoma indicates that other ocular or systemic abnormalities are associated, even if a similar developmental defect of the trabecular meshwork is also present. Primary infantile glaucoma occurs with an incidence of only 0.03%. A general ophthalmologist may see only one case every 5 yr, and the pediatrician only one case every 10 yr.

CLINICAL MANIFESTATIONS. The symptoms of infantile glaucoma include the classic triad of epiphora (tearing), photophobia (sensitivity to light), and blepharospasm (eyelid squeezing). Each of these can be attributed to corneal irritation. Only about one third of affected infants, however, demonstrate the classic symptom complex. Parents are just as likely to notice signs. These include corneal edema, corneal and ocular enlargement, conjunctival injection, and visual impairment.

Under 3 mo of age the cornea is very sensitive to elevated

intraocular pressure. Corneal signs, including edema and breaks in the endothelial basement membrane (Descemet membrane), are present in more than 90% of affected infants. Haziness of the cornea confirms edema, and a sudden increase in haziness suggests that breaks in Descemet membrane (Haab striae) have occurred. The latter are visible as horizontal, edematous lines that cross or curve around the central cornea. They rarely occur beyond 3 yr of age or in corneas less than 12.0 mm in diameter. Older infants, with a gradual and moderate rise in intraocular pressure, may have only mild corneal edema.

Until approximately 3 yr of age, the cornea and sclera of the eye can be distended by elevated intraocular pressure. Glaucoma is suggested by a corneal diameter of greater than 12.0 mm in an infant. With longstanding glaucoma, enlargement of the entire globe or buphthalmos ("ox eye") can occur.

Other signs, especially cupping of the optic nerve head, are detected by ocular examination. The optic nerve of the infant is easily distended by excessive pressure. Deep, central cupping readily occurs and may regress with normalization of pressure.

In some infants and children with early-onset glaucoma there is more extensive maldevelopment of the anterior segment of the eye. Mesodermal dysgenesis, anterior cleavage syndrome, or various eponyms are used to describe these defects. One type, Peters anomaly, is characterized by the presence of a central corneal opacity (leukoma) with corresponding defects in the posterior corneal stroma, Descemet membrane, and endothelium, often with associated iridocorneal or lenticulocorneal adhesions. The condition is usually bilateral, although often asymmetric. It is generally sporadic, but recessive and dominant inheritance patterns have been suggested. Other anomalies within the spectrum of anterior chamber cleavage syndromes are anterior embryotoxon (prominent anteriorly displaced ring of Schwalbe), Axenfeld anomaly (presence of fine iris strands crossing the anterior chamber, attaching to the displaced ring of Schwalbe), and Rieger anomaly (anteriorly displaced ring of Schwalbe and iris adhesions, iris hypoplasia, and dyscoria). Within the spectrum there may be associated cataracts and various other abnormalities. Chromosomal defects have been found in some patients.

Other ocular anomalies that may be associated with glaucoma in infants and children are aniridia, cataract, spherophakia, and ectopia lentis. Glaucoma may also develop secondary to persistent hyperplastic primary vitreous (PHPV) or retinopathy of prematurity (ROP).

Trauma, intraocular hemorrhage, ocular inflammatory disease, and intraocular tumor are also important causes of glaucoma in the pediatric population.

Systemic disorders associated with glaucoma in infants and children are Sturge-Weber syndrome, von Recklinghausen disease, Lowe syndrome, Marfan syndrome, congenital rubella, a number of chromosomal syndromes, and juvenile xanthogranuloma.

TREATMENT. The treatment of congenital and infantile glaucoma is primarily surgical; surgery should be performed as early as the child's general medical condition allows. Procedures used to reduce and control ocular tension are goniotomy, goniopuncture, trabeculotomy, trabeculectomy and, in some cases, cyclocryotherapy. Frequently, multiple surgical procedures are required. In many cases, even after surgery, long-term medical therapy is also required. The prognosis for vision depends on normalization of intraocular pressure and prevention of optic nerve damage. In addition to control of ocular pressure, attention must be directed to the correction of associated refractive errors and the treatment of amblyopia. In some children there are also complicating factors, such as cataracts, corneal opacities, and retinal and optic nerve abnormalities, that affect visual outcome.

Barsoum-Homsy M, Chevrette L: Incidence and prognosis of childhood glaucoma: A study of 63 cases. Ophthalmology 93:1323, 1986.

Bardelli AM, Hadjistilianou T: Congenital glaucoma associated with other abnormalities in 150 cases. Glaucoma 9:10, 1987.

Boger WP III, Walton DS: Timolol in uncontrolled childhood glaucomas. Ophthalmology 88:253, 1981.

Catalono RA, Nelson LB: Pediatric Ophthalmology: A Text Atlas. Norwalk, CT, Appleton & Lange, 1994.

Cibis GW, Tripathi RC, Tripathi BJ: Glaucoma in Sturge-Weber syndrome. Ophthalmology 91:1061, 1984.

Cohen SMZ, Brown FR, Martyn L, et al: Ocular histopathologic and biochemical studies of the cerebrohepatorenal syndrome (Zellweger's syndrome) and its relationship to neonatal adrenoleukodystophy. Am J Ophthalmol 96:488, 1983.

Ginsberg J, Bove KE, Fogelson MH: Pathological features of the eye in the oculocerebrorenal (Lowe) syndrome. J Pediatr Ophthalmol Strab 18:16, 1981.

Heckenlively JR, Isenberg SJ, Fox LE: The Reiger syndrome: A heritable disorder associated with glaucoma. Genet Clin Johns Hopkins Hosp 151:351, 1982.

Kivlin JD, Fineman RM, Crandall AS, et al: Peter's anomaly as a consequence of genetic and nongenetic syndromes. Arch Ophthalmol 104:61, 1986.

Kushner BJ, Sondheiner S: Medical treatment of glaucoma associated with cicatricial retinopathy of prematurity. Am J Ophthalmol 94:313, 1982.

McMahon CD, Hetherington J Jr, Hoskins HD, et al: Timolol and pediatric glaucomas. Ophthalmology 88:249, 1981.

McPherson SD Jr, Berry DP: Goniotomy vs external trabeculotomy for developmental glaucoma. Am J Ophthalmol 95:427, 1983.

Quigley HA: Childhood glaucoma: Results with trabeculotomy and study of reversible cupping. Ophthalmology 89:219, 1982.

Robin AL, Quigley HA, Pollack IP, et al: An analysis of visual acuity, visual fields, and disc cupping in childhood glaucoma. Am J Ophthalmol 88:847, 1979.

Seidman DJ, Nelson LB, Calhoun JH, et al: Signs and symptoms in the presentation of primary infantile glaucoma. Pediatrics 77:399, 1986.

Stern JH, Catalono RA: Current status of diagnostic and therapeutic measures in infantile glaucoma. Semin Ophthalmol 5:166, 1990.

Zimmerman L: Ocular lesions of juvenile xanthogranuloma (nevoxanthoendothelioma). Trans Am Acad Ophthalmol Otolaryngol 69:412, 1965.

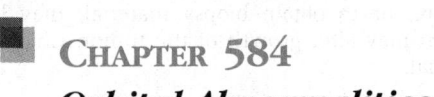

CHAPTER 584
Orbital Abnormalities

HYPERTELORISM AND HYPOTELORISM

Hypertelorism refers to wide separation of the eyes or an increased interorbital distance, which may occur as a morphogenetic variant, a primary deformity, or a secondary phenomenon in association with developmental abnormalities, such as frontal meningocele or encephalocele or the persistence of a facial cleft. There is often associated strabismus, generally exotropia, and sometimes optic atrophy.

Hypotelorism refers to narrowness of the interorbital distance, which may occur as a morphogenetic variant alone or in association with other anomalies, such as epicanthus, holoprosencephaly, or secondary to a cranial dystrophy, such as scaphocephaly.

EXOPHTHALMUS AND ENOPHTHALMUS

Protrusion of the eye is referred to as exophthalmos or proptosis. It may be caused by shallowness of the orbits, as in many craniofacial malformations, or by increased tissue mass within the orbit, as with neoplastic, vascular, and inflammatory disorders. Ocular complications include exposure keratopathy, ocular motor disturbances, and optic atrophy with loss of vision.

Posterior displacement or sinking of the eye back into the orbit is referred to as enophthalmos. This may occur with orbital fracture or with atrophy of orbital tissue. It is a feature of Horner syndrome.

ORBITAL CELLULITIS

Orbital cellulitis refers to a condition involving inflammation of the tissues of the orbit, with proptosis, limitation of movement of the eye, edema of the conjunctiva (chemosis), and inflammation and swelling of the eyelids. There is often some discomfort, usually with general symptoms of toxicity, fever, and leukocytosis.

In general, orbital cellulitis may follow direct infection of the orbit from a wound, metastatic deposition of organisms during bacteremia, or direct extension or venous spread of infection from contiguous sites such as the lids, conjunctiva, globe, lacrimal gland, nasolacrimal sac, or paranasal sinuses. In some cases primary or metastatic tumor in the orbit can produce the clinical picture of orbital cellulitis.

The most common cause of orbital cellulitis in children is paranasal sinusitis, with the most frequent pathogenic organisms being *Haemophilus influenzae, Staphylococcus aureus*, group A beta-hemolytic streptococci, and *Streptococcus pneumoniae*.

The orbital inflammatory manifestations of paranasal sinusitis vary with the location and extent of involvement. Stage 1 is swelling of the lids—the edema of impaired venous drainage or the reactive inflammation of underlying periostitis; in this stage the infection is still confined to the sinus. The 2nd stage is subperiosteal abscess, a collection of pus between the periosteum and the wall of the orbit, often with localized tenderness, displacement of the globe, and some limitation of eye movement. The 3rd stage is true orbital cellulitis, diffuse inflammation of the tissues within the orbit, with proptosis and impairment of ocular motility. The 4th stage is orbital abscess, resulting from localization of infection in the orbit or from extension of a subperiosteal abscess through the periosteum.

The potential for complications is great. Involvement of the optic nerve may result in loss of vision. Extension of infection from the orbit into the cranial cavity may lead to cavernous sinus thrombosis or meningitis or to epidural, subdural, or brain abscess.

Orbital cellulitis must be recognized promptly and treated aggressively. Hospitalization and systemic antibiotic therapy are usually indicated. In some cases surgical intervention is necessary to drain infected sinuses or a subperiosteal or orbital abscess.

PERIORBITAL CELLULITIS

Inflammation of the lids and periorbital tissues without signs of true orbital involvement (such as proptosis or limitation of eye movement) is generally referred to as periorbital or preseptal cellulitis. This is common in young children and may be caused by trauma, or by an infected wound, or by abscess of the lid or periorbital region (e.g., pyoderma, hordeolum, conjunctivitis, dacryocystitis, insect bite). It may be associated with respiratory infection or bacteremia, often with *H. influenzae*, streptococcus, or pneumococcus. What initially appears to be periorbital or preseptal cellulitis may be the 1st sign of sinusitis that may progress to true orbital cellulitis. Prompt antibiotic therapy and careful monitoring for signs of progression are essential.

TUMORS OF THE ORBIT

Various tumors occur in and about the orbit in childhood. Among benign tumors, the most common are vascular lesions (principally hemangiomas) and dermoids. Among malignant neoplasms, rhabdomyosarcoma, lymphosarcoma, and metastatic neuroblastoma are the most frequent. Optic gliomata and retinoblastomas that extend into the orbit also occur.

The effects of orbital tumors vary with their locations and growth patterns. The principal signs are proptosis, resistance to retroplacement of the eye, and impairment of eye movement. There may be a palpable mass. Other significant signs are ptosis, optic nerve head congestion, optic atrophy, and loss of vision. Bruit and visible pulsation of the globe are important clues to vascular lesions.

The differential diagnosis of orbital tumors is difficult; ultrasonography, magnetic resonance imaging, and computed tomography may be particularly helpful. Pseudotumor of the orbit also must be considered in children with signs of a mass lesion.

Haik BG, Jakobiec FA, Ellsworth RM, et al: Capillary hemangioma of the lids and orbit: An analysis of the clinical features and therapeutic results in 101 cases. Ophthalmology 86:760, 1979.
Hawkins DB, Clark RW: Orbital involvement in acute sinusitis: Lessons from 24 childhood patients. Clin Pediatr 16:464, 1977.
Mottow LS, Jakobiec FA: Idiopathic inflammatory orbital pseudotumor in childhood. Arch Ophthalmol 96:1410, 1978.
Pollard ZF, Calhoun J: Deep orbital dermoid with draining sinus. Am J Ophthalmol 79:310, 1975.
Porterfield JF: Orbital tumors in children: A report of 214 cases. Int Ophthalmol Clin 2:319, 1962.
Shields JA: Diagnosis and Management of Orbital Tumors. Philadelphia, WB Saunders, 1989.
Shields JA, Bakewell B, Augsberger JJ, et al: Space-occupying orbital masses in children: A review of 250 consecutive biopsies. Ophthalmology 93:379, 1988.
Smith TF, O'Day D, Wright PF: Clinical implications of preseptal (periorbital) cellulitis in childhood. Pediatrics 62:1006, 1978.
Weiss A, Friendly D, Eglin K, et al: Bacterial periorbital cellulitis in childhood. Ophthalmology 90:195, 1983.

CHAPTER 585
Injuries to the Eye

About one third of all blindness in children results from trauma, usually avoidable. Children and adolescents account for a disproportionate number of episodes of ocular trauma. Boys aged 11–15 yr are the most vulnerable; their injuries outnumber those in girls by a ratio of about 4:1. The majority of injuries are related to sports, toy darts, other projectiles, sticks, stones, and air-powered BB guns. The latter cause particularly devastating ocular and orbital injuries.

ECCHYMOSES AND SWELLING OF THE EYELIDS

These are common after blunt trauma. Hemorrhage into the lids and periorbital region (the "black eye" or "shiner") is usually of no consequence and absorbs spontaneously, but it should prompt careful examination of the eye for deeper, more serious injury, such as intraocular hemorrhage or rupture of the globe.

LACERATIONS OF THE EYELIDS

These require careful management. Horizontal laceration of the upper lid may involve the levator, the tarsal plate, or the orbital septum. Faulty repair can result in ptosis, distortion of the lid, or herniation of orbital fat. Lacerations involving the lid margins require meticulous surgical apposition to prevent notching, eversion, or inversion of the margin or misdirection of the lashes that might lead to epiphora (tear overflow) and chronic irritation. Lacerations situated near the medial canthus may involve the punctum, canaliculi, or nasolacrimal duct and require the attention of an experienced ophthalmic surgeon. In all cases of lid laceration, examination of the globe for perforating injury is mandatory.

SUPERFICIAL ABRASIONS OF THE CORNEA

When the corneal epithelium is scratched, abraded, or denuded, it exposes the underlying epithelial basement layer and superficial corneal nerves. This is accompanied by pain, tearing, photophobia, and decreased vision. Corneal abrasions are detected by instilling fluorescein dye and inspecting the cornea using a blue-filtered light. The slit lamp is ideal for this examination, but a handheld Wood lamp is adequate for young children.

The treatment of a corneal abrasion is directed at promoting healing and relieving pain. Very small abrasions can be treated with frequent applications of a topical antibiotic ointment four times daily. Larger abrasions require a semipressure patch to immobilize the eyelids and protect the healing epithelium from the constant trauma of repeated blinking. The patch should not be removed for 24 hr, even to instill antibiotics. A topical cycloplegic agent (such as cyclopentolate hydrochloride 1%) can relieve the pain from ciliary spasm in patients with large abrasions.

FOREIGN BODY ON OR IN THE CORNEA OR CONJUNCTIVA

This usually produces acute discomfort, lacrimation, and inflammation. Most foreign bodies can be detected by examination in good light with the aid of magnification; the direct ophthalmoscope set on a high plus lens (+10 or +12) is helpful. In many cases slit lamp examination is necessary, especially if the particle is deep or metallic. Some conjunctival foreign bodies tend to lodge under the upper eyelid, producing the sensation of corneal foreign body as they come into contact with the globe on eyelid movement; eversion of the lid may be necessary to detect such foreign particles. If a foreign body is suspected but not found, further examination is indicated. If the history suggests injury with a high-velocity particle, roentgenographic examination of the eye may be needed to explore the possibility of intraocular foreign body.

Removal of a foreign body can be facilitated by the instillation of a drop of topical anesthetic. Many foreign bodies can be removed by irrigating or by gently wiping them away with a moistened cotton-tipped applicator. Embedded foreign bodies should be handled by an ophthalmologist. Removal of corneal foreign bodies may leave epithelial defects, which are treated as corneal abrasions. Metallic foreign bodies may cause rust to form in the corneal tissues; examination by an ophthalmologist a day or two after removal of a foreign body is recommended, because a rust ring would require further treatment (curettage).

LACERATIONS AND PERFORATING WOUNDS OF THE CORNEA OR SCLERA

These require immediate referral to an ophthalmologist and prompt surgical repair if the eye and vision are to be saved. Important clues to perforating injury of the eye are collapse of the anterior chamber, distortion and displacement of the pupil, and protrusion of dark tissue (uvea) into the wound. Emergency treatment consists of protecting the injured eye from further damage by applying a sterile bandage and a rigid eye shield. If these medical supplies are not on hand, an adequate eye shield can be fashioned from a plastic or styrofoam cup or from a piece of cardboard bent into a box or cone shape. Manipulation should be kept to a minimum, and no medication should be instilled except under the direction of an ophthalmologist.

HYPHEMA

This is the presence of blood in the anterior chamber of the eye. It may occur with either a blunt or perforating injury. Hyphema appears as a bright or dark red fluid level between the cornea and iris or as a diffuse murkiness of the aqueous humor. Children with hyphema have pain and may be somnolent. The treatment of hyphema usually includes bed rest, with the head elevated 30–45 degrees to promote settling and resorption of the blood. In some cases topical mydriatics, miotics, steroids, or oral aminocaproic acid are used. In some cases secondary bleeding occurs 3–5 days after the initial hemorrhage, increasing the risk of sequelae. The blood in the anterior chamber may produce elevation of intraocular pressure and blood staining of the cornea. These complications may affect vision. In such cases surgical evacuation of the clot and irrigation of the anterior chamber may be necessary.

OTHER INJURIES

Chemical Injuries

Chemical burns of the cornea and adnexal tissue are among the most urgent of ocular emergencies. Alkali burns are usually more destructive than acid burns because they react with fats to form soaps, which damage cell membranes, allowing further penetration of the alkali into the eye. Acids generally cause less severe, more localized tissue damage. The corneal epithelium offers moderate protection against weak acids, and little damage is seen unless the pH is 2.5 or less. Most stronger acids precipitate tissue proteins, creating a physical barrier against their further penetration.

Mild acid or alkali burns are characterized by conjunctival injection and swelling and mild corneal epithelial erosions. The corneal stroma may be mildly edematous, and the anterior chamber may have mild to moderate cell and flare. With strong acids the cornea and conjunctiva rapidly become white and opaque. The corneal epithelium may slough, leaving a relatively clear stroma; this appearance may initially mask the severity of the burn. Severe alkali burns are characterized by corneal opacification.

Emergency treatment of a chemical burn begins with copious immediate irrigation with water or saline. Local débridement and removal of foreign particles should be performed while still irrigating. If the nature of the chemical injury is unknown, the use of pH paper is helpful in determining whether the agent was basic or acidic. Irrigation should continue for at least 30 min or until 2 L of irrigant has been instilled in mild cases, and 2–4 hr or until 10 L of irrigant has been instilled in severe cases. At the end of irrigation, the pH should be within a normal range (7.3–7.7). The pH should be checked again approximately 30 min after irrigation to ensure that it has not changed.

Fractures

The term *direct orbital floor fracture* describes a floor fracture associated with an orbital rim fracture. The term *indirect orbital floor fracture* describes an isolated floor fracture and is more commonly known as a "blowout fracture." Floor fractures are common when objects larger than the orbital opening, such as a ball, fist, or the dashboard of an automobile, impact the orbit, particularly the inferior lateral orbit.

The most obvious clinical sign of an orbital floor fracture is a limitation of upward gaze. Additional signs include lower eyelid ecchymosis, nosebleed, orbital emphysema, and hypesthesia of the ipsilateral cheek and upper lip. The latter results from disruption of the infraorbital nerve as it transverses the orbital floor.

The best imaging techniques to visualize orbital fractures are plain-film radiography and computed tomography. The Waters view best demonstrates the orbital floor and maxillary sinus.

Therapeutic measures for children with accute orbital fractures include antibiotic prophylaxis, nasal decongestants, and

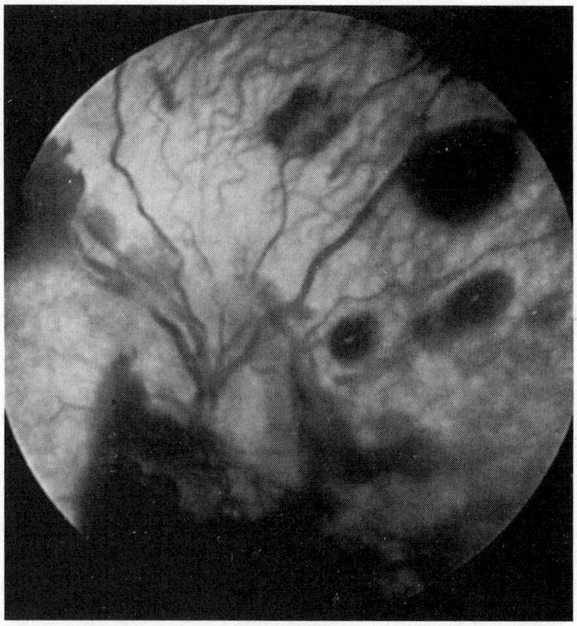

Figure 585–1. Retinal hemorrhages in the abused child with subdural hematoma.

ice packs. If entrapment of the extraocular muscles (resulting in restriction of movement of the eye and diplopia) and herniation of orbital fat or of the eye itself (resulting in enophthalmos) occur, then surgical repair may be necessary.

Penetrating Wounds of the Orbit

These demand careful evaluation for possible damage to the eye, the optic nerve, or the brain. Examination should include investigation for retained foreign body. Orbital hemorrhage and infection are common with penetrating wounds of the orbit; such injuries must be treated as emergencies.

Child Abuse

This is a major cause of injuries to the eye and orbital region. The manifestations are numerous and may play a prominent role in the recognition of this syndrome. The possibility of nonaccidental trauma must be considered in any child with ecchymosis or laceration of the lids, hemorrhage in or about the eye, cataract or dislocated lens, retinal detachment, or fracture of the orbit (Fig. 585–1).

Sports-Related Ocular Injuries and Their Prevention

Although sports injuries occur in all age groups, far more children and adolescents participate in high-risk sports than adults. The greater number of participating children, their athletic immaturity, and the increased likelihood of their using inadequate or improper eye protection account for their disproportionate share of sports-related eye injuries.

The sports with the highest risk of eye injury are those in which no eye protection can be worn, including boxing, wrestling, and martial arts. High-risk sports include those that use a rapidly moving ball or puck, bat, stick, racquet, or arrow (baseball, hockey, lacrosse, racquet sports, and archery) or involve aggressive body contact (football and basketball). Related to both risk and frequency of participation, the highest percentage of eye injuries are seen in basketball and baseball.

Protective eyewear, designed for a specific activity, is available for most sports. For basketball, racquet sports, and other recreational activities that do not require a helmet or face mask, molded polycarbonate sports goggles that are secured to the head by an elastic strap are suggested. For hockey, football, lacrosse, and baseball (batter), specific helmets with polycarbonate faceshields and guards are available. Children should also wear sports goggles under the helmets. For baseball, goggles and helmets should be worn for batting, catching, and baserunning; goggles alone are usually sufficient for other positions.

Catalono RA: Eye injuries and prevention. Pediatr Clin North Am 40:827, 1993.
Emery JM, von Noorden GK, Schlernitzauer DA: Orbital floor fractures: Long-term follow-up of cases with and without surgical repair. Trans Am Acad Ophthalmol Otolaryngol 75:802, 1971.
Friendly DS: Ocular manifestations of physical child abuse. Trans Am Acad Ophthalmol Otolaryngol 75:318, 1971.
Grin TR, Nelson LB, Jeffers JB: Eye injuries in childhood. Pediatrics 80:13, 1987.
Hofman RF, Paul TO, Pentelei-Molner J: The management of corneal birth trauma. J Pediatr Ophthalmol Strab 18:45, 1981.
Lavrich JB, Goldberg DS, Nelson LB, et al: Visual outcome of severe eye injuries during the amblyopiagenic years. Binocular Vis 9:39, 1994.
Levin AV: Ocular manifestations of child abuse. Ophthalmol Clin North Am 3:249, 1990.
Nelson LB, Wilson TW, Jeffers JB: Eye injuries in childhood: Demography, etiology and prevention. Pediatrics 84:438, 1989.
Pfister RR: Chemical injuries of the eye. Ophthalmology 90:1246, 1983.
Vinger PF: Sports eye injuries: A preventable disease. Ophthalmology 88:108, 1981.
Wilson FM: Traumatic hyphema: Pathogenesis and management. Ophthalmology 87:910, 1980.

PART XXX

The Ear*

James E. Arnold

Diseases and disorders of the ear are among the most frequently encountered morbid conditions of childhood. The ability to recognize their presence, the adequate knowledge of the most efficacious treatment, and the skills to prevent complications and sequelae are imperative for every physician caring for children. ■

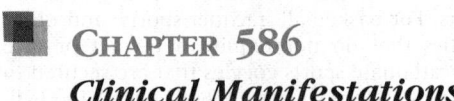

CHAPTER 586
Clinical Manifestations

Eight prominent signs and symptoms are associated primarily with diseases of the ear and temporal bone:

OTALGIA. This is most commonly associated with inflammation of the external and middle ear, but it may also arise from involvement of the temporomandibular joint, teeth, or pharynx. In young infants, pulling at the ear or general irritability, especially when either is associated with fever, may be the only sign of ear pain.

PURULENT OTORRHEA. This is a sign of otitis externa, otitis media with perforation of the tympanic membrane, or both. Bloody discharge may be associated with acute or chronic inflammation, trauma, neoplasm, or blood dyscrasias. Clear drainage suggests either a perforation of the drum with a serous middle ear effusion or a cerebrospinal fluid otorrhea draining through a defect in the external auditory canal or through the tympanic membrane from the middle ear.

HEARING LOSS. This results from disease of either the external or middle ear (conductive hearing loss) or from pathology in the inner ear, retrocochlea, or central auditory pathways (sensorineural hearing loss).

SWELLING. Swelling about the ear is most commonly the result of inflammation (e.g., external otitis, perichondritis, mastoiditis), trauma (hematoma) or, on rare occasions, neoplasm.

VERTIGO. This is not a common complaint in children, but may sometimes be present. *Vertigo*, a specific type of dizziness, is defined as any hallucination or illusion of motion; *dizziness* refers to any altered orientation in space. The most frequent cause is eustachian tube-middle-ear disease, but vertigo may also be caused by labyrinthitis, perilymphatic fistula between the inner and middle ear from a congenital defect, trauma, or cholesteatoma, vestibular neuronitis, benign paroxysmal positional vertigo, Menière disease, or disease of the central nervous system. Older children may describe a feeling of spinning or turning, whereas younger children may manifest the disequilibrium only by falling, stumbling, or clumsiness.

NYSTAGMUS. Unidirectional, horizontal, or jerk nystagmus, usually associated with vertigo, is vestibular in origin.

TINNITUS. Although infrequently described by children, tinnitus is common, especially in patients with eustachian tube-middle-ear disease or with conductive or sensorineural hearing loss.

FACIAL PARALYSIS. This is an infrequent but frightening condition for both child and parents. When resulting from disease within the temporal bone in children, it most commonly occurs as a complication of acute or chronic otitis media, but it may also be idiopathic (Bell's palsy) or be the result of temporal bone fracture or neoplasm; on rare occasions it may be caused by herpes zoster oticus. Other conditions associated with ear disease may also be present (e.g., symptoms of upper respiratory allergy associated with otitis media).

PHYSICAL EXAMINATION. Adequately examining the entire child, paying special attention to the head and neck, can reveal a condition that may predispose to or be associated with ear disease. The facial appearance and the character of speech may be important clues to an abnormality of the ear. Many of the craniofacial anomalies, such as mandibulofacial dysostosis (Treacher Collins syndrome) and 21-trisomy (Down syndrome), are associated with disorders of the ear. Mouth breathing and hyponasality may indicate intranasal or postnasal obstruction; hypernasality is a sign of velopharyngeal insufficiency. Examining the oropharyngeal cavity may uncover an overt cleft palate or a submucous cleft, both of which predispose to otitis media with effusion. A bifid uvula may also be associated with middle-ear disease. Examination may reveal posterior nasal or pharyngeal inflammation and discharge. Polyposis, severe deviation of the nasal septum, or a nasopharyngeal tumor may be associated with otitis media.

The *position* of the patient for examination of the ear, nose, and throat depends on the patient's age, ability to cooperate, clinical setting, and preference of the examiner. The evaluation of an infant is best performed on an examining table. The presence of a parent or assistant is necessary to restrain the baby, because undue movement usually prevents an adequate evaluation (Fig. 586–1). Some clinicians prefer to place the infant prone on the table, whereas others prefer the patient to be supine. Use of the examining table is also desirable for older infants who are uncooperative or when a tympanocentesis or myringotomy is performed without general anesthesia. Infants and young children who are only apprehensive and not struggling actively can be evaluated adequately while sitting on the parent's lap. When necessary, the child may be restrained firmly on a adult's lap if the parent holds the child's wrists over the abdomen with one hand and holds the patient's head against the adult's chest with the other hand. If necessary, the child's legs can be held between the adult's thighs. Some infants can be examined by placing the child's head on the parent's knee. Cooperative children sitting in a chair or on the edge of an examination table can usually be evaluated successfully. The examiner should hold the otoscope with the hand or finger placed firmly against the child's head or face,

*Modified from sections in the 14th edition by Charles D. Bluestone and Robert J. Nozza.

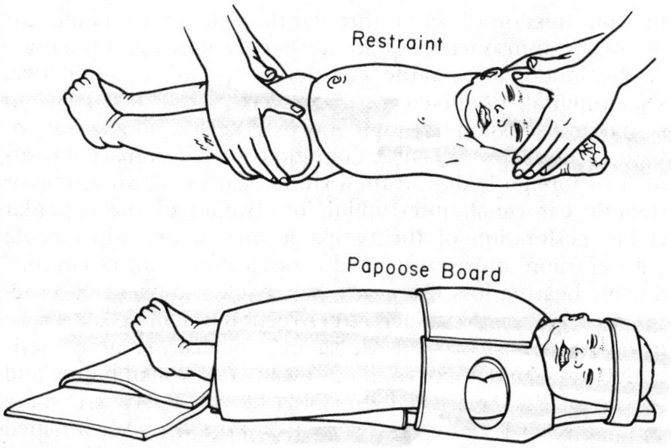

Figure 586–1. Methods of restraining an infant for examination and for procedures such as tympanocentesis or myringotomy. (From Bluestone CD, Klein JO: Otitis Media in Infants and Children. Philadelphia, WB Saunders, 1988.)

so that the otoscope moves with the head rather than cause trauma (pain) to the ear canal if the child moves suddenly. Pulling up and out on the pinna usually straightens the ear canal enough to allow exposure of the tympanic membrane. In the young infant, the tragus must be moved forward and out of the way.

Examining the ear itself is the most critical assessment. The auricle and external auditory meatus should be examined first, because the presence or absence of signs of infection in these areas may aid later in the differential diagnosis or evaluation of complications of otitis media. For instance, eczematoid external otitis may result from acute otitis media with discharge, or inflammation of the postauricular area may indicate a periosteitis or subperiosteal abscess extending from the mastoid air cells.

Next, the otoscopic examination, the most important part of physical assessment, is undertaken. However, before adequate visualization of the external canal and tympanic membrane is possible, obstructing cerumen must be removed from the canal. **Removal of cerumen** can usually be accomplished by use of an otoscope with a surgical head and a wire loop or a blunt cerumen curette, or by irrigating the ear canal *gently* with warm water. Instillation of hydrogen peroxide (3% solution) in the ear canal for 2–3 min softens cerumen and may facilitate removal with subsequent irrigation. Use of some commercial preparations (e.g., triethanolamine polypeptide oleate-condensate [Cerumenex]) may cause dermatitis of the external canal. These materials may be of value, however, if used infrequently and under the physician's supervision. The absence of cerumen and inflammation of the ear canal indicate external otitis. The external canal of the newborn is filled with vernix caseosa, which disappears shortly after birth.

The tympanic membrane and its mobility are properly assessed by using the pneumatic otoscope; assessing the light reflex is of limited value. The normal tympanic membrane is in the neutral position; a drum that is bulging is a condition that may be caused by increased middle-ear air pressure, by an effusion within the middle ear, or by both; the visualization of the malleus handle and short process is obscured by a bulging drum. Retraction of the tympanic membrane usually indicates the presence of middle-ear negative pressure, but it may also result from previous disease and subsequent fixation of the ossicles and ligaments. When retraction is present, the short process of the malleus is prominent and the long process is foreshortened.

The normal tympanic membrane has a "ground-glass" appearance; a blue or yellow color usually indicates a middle-ear effusion. A red membrane alone may not indicate pathology, because the blood vessels of the drum head may be engorged as the result of crying, sneezing, or blowing the nose. The normal tympanic membrane is also translucent, allowing the observer to look through it to visualize the middle-ear landmarks—incudostapedial joint, promontory, round window niche, and frequently the chorda tympani nerve. If a middle-ear effusion is present medial to a translucent drum, an air-fluid level or bubbles of air mixed with the fluid may be visible. Inability to visualize the middle-ear structures indicates opacification of the drum, usually caused by thickening of the tympanic membrane, a middle-ear effusion, or both.

Normal and abnormal middle-ear pressure are reflected in the pattern of **tympanic membrane mobility** when positive and then negative pressure are applied to the external canal using a pneumatic otoscope with a rubber ring around the tip of the end of the ear speculum to obtain a better seal in the external auditory canal. Normal middle-ear pressure is reflected by the neutral position of the tympanic membrane as well as by its response to both positive and negative pressures.

The eardrum may be retracted, usually because negative middle-ear pressure is present. The compliant membrane is maximally retracted by even moderate negative middle-ear pressure and hence cannot visibly be deflected inward further with applied positive pressure in the ear canal. Negative pressure produced by releasing the rubber bulb of the pneumatic otoscope, however, causes a return of the eardrum toward the neutral position if a negative pressure equivalent to that in the middle ear can be created by releasing the rubber bulb, a condition that occurs when air, with or without an effusion, is present in the middle ear. When the middle ear pressure is even lower, there may be only slight outward mobility of the tympanic membrane because of the limited negative pressure that can be exerted through the otoscopes that are currently available. When assessing the mobility of the tympanic membrane in which a negative pressure is present within the middle ear, return of the tympanic membrane to the resting retracted position after the application of applied negative external canal pressure should not be confused with movement to applied positive pressure. This "rebound" of the eardrum after applied negative pressure may lead the examiner to conclude erroneously that the tympanic membrane is mobile to both positive and negative pressures and that, therefore,

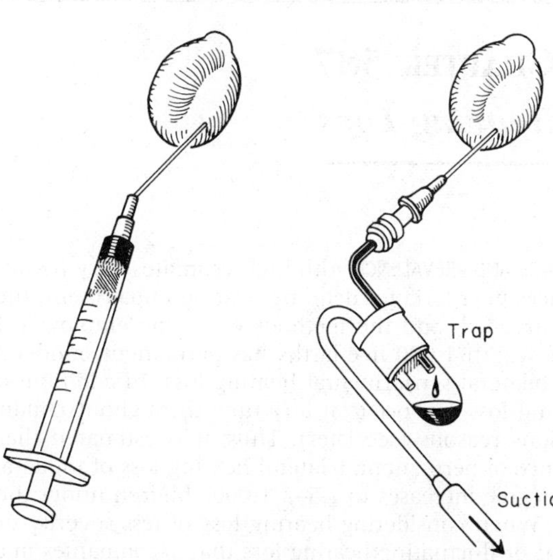

Figure 586–2. Tympanocentesis can be performed by employing a needle attached to a tuberculin syringe *(left)* or by using an Alden-Senturia collection trap (Storz Instrument Co., St. Louis). (From Bluestone CD, Klein JO: Otitis Media in Infants and Children. Philadelphia, WB Saunders, 1988.)

the middle-ear pressure is ambient. If the eardrum is severely retracted with extremely high negative middle-ear pressure or in the presence of a middle-ear effusion or both, the examiner is not able to produce significant outward movement.

The tympanic membrane that exhibits fullness moves to applied positive pressure but not to applied negative pressure if the pressure within the middle ear is positive and air, with or without an effusion, is present. In such an instance, the tympanic membrane is stretched laterally to the point of maximal compliance and does not visibly move outward any farther to the applied negative pressure but moves inward to applied positive pressure as long as some air is present within the middle ear-mastoid air cell system. A full tympanic membrane and positive middle-ear pressure without a middle-ear effusion are frequently seen in neonates and in young infants who are crying during the otoscopic examination; in older infants and children, the same situation may be encountered when the nose is obstructed. However, in the initial stage of acute otitis media, the tympanic membrane may be full, with the characteristic findings of pneumatic otoscopy described before, because air is usually present within the middle ear. When the middle ear-mastoid air cell system is filled with an effusion and little or no air is present, the mobility of the bulging tympanic membrane is severely decreased or absent to both applied positive and negative pressures.

Aspiration of the middle ear is the definitive method of verifying the presence and type of a middle-ear effusion. Diagnostic tympanocentesis is performed by inserting, through the inferior portion of the tympanic membrane, an 18-gauge spinal needle attached to a syringe or a collection trap (Fig. 586–2). Alcohol cleansing and culturing of the ear canal should precede tympanocentesis and culture of the middle-ear aspirate. The canal culture helps to determine whether cultured organisms are contaminants from the external canal or pathogens from the middle ear.

Roentgenographic assessment of the ear and temporal bone is frequently helpful. When the tympanic membrane is not intact (as a result of perforation or insertion of a tympanostomy tube), *assessment of the ventilatory function of the eustachian tube* by pressure-flow studies may be an additional diagnostic aid. *Assessment of labyrinthine function* is essential in the evaluation of a child with a vestibular disorder (Chapter 591).

CHAPTER 587
Hearing Loss

INCIDENCE AND PREVALENCE. Although estimates vary because of differences in criteria for defining hearing impairment, the age group surveyed, and the methods of testing employed, from 0.5–1 newborn/1,000 live births has permanent, moderate to severe, bilateral sensorineural hearing loss. In addition, onset of hearing loss can occur at any time throughout childhood, for various reasons (see later). Thus, it is estimated that the prevalence of permanent, bilateral hearing loss of moderate to severe degree increases to 1.5–2/1,000 children under the age of 6 yr. When considering hearing loss of less severity or the transient or fluctuating hearing loss that accompanies middle-ear disease, so common in young children, the number of children with hearing loss at any given point in time increases substantially.

TYPES. Hearing loss can be peripheral or central in origin. Peripheral hearing loss is commonly caused by dysfunction in the transmission of sound through the external or middle ear or by the transduction of sound energy into neural activity at the inner ear and the 8th nerve. It can be conductive, sensorineural, or mixed. *Conductive hearing loss* occurs when sound transmission through the external or middle ear, or both, is physically impeded. Conditions such as impacted cerumen or foreign bodies in the external ear canal, an atretic or stenotic ear canal, interruption or fixation of the ossicular chain, perforation of the tympanic membrane, otitis media with effusion, otosclerosis, and cholesteatoma can cause conductive hearing loss. Damage to or maldevelopment of structures in the inner ear, such as destruction of hair cells because of noise, disease, or ototoxic agents, cochlear agenesis, perilymphatic fistula of the round or oval window membrane, and lesions of the acoustic division of the 8th nerve are some conditions that cause *sensorineural hearing loss*. A combined conductive and sensorineural hearing loss is considered a *mixed hearing loss*.

Auditory deficits originating along the central auditory nervous system pathways, from the proximal 8th nerve to the cortex, are generally considered central hearing losses. Tumors, demyelinating disease, seizures, and various syndromes (e.g., Landau syndrome), can cause hearing deficits in the presence of normal outer, middle, and inner ears. Other forms of central auditory deficits, known as central auditory processing disorders, include those that make it difficult for normal hearing children to listen selectively to noise, to combine information from the two ears properly to process speech when it is slightly degraded, and to integrate auditory information that is delivered faster than at a slow rate. Often no organic cause can be identified for such problems, but they can be quantified. They often manifest as poor attention or academic achievement, or as behavior problems in school. Strategies for coping with such disorders are available, and identification and documentation of the central auditory processing disorder is often valuable because parents and teachers are made aware of a valid reason for the child's poor attention or behavior, so adjustments can be made.

ETIOLOGY. The etiology of hearing impairment can be divided into four categories. Hearing impairment can be caused prior to or during birth (congenital), can occur at some time after birth (postnatal), can be caused by genetic factors or may be acquired in another, nongenetic fashion. It is estimated that about 50% of cases of childhood hearing impairment of moderate to profound degree are genetically determined.

Genetic–Congenital Hearing Impairment. These disorders may be associated with other abnormalities or may be part of a syndrome. Hearing impairment occurs along with abnormalities of the external ear and eye and with disorders of the metabolic, musculoskeletal, integumentary, renal, and nervous systems. Pendred, Usher, and Waardenburg syndrome account for a large proportion of the sensorineural hearing impairments in this category. Chromosomal abnormalities such as 13–15-trisomy, 18-trisomy, and 21-trisomy can also be accompanied by hearing impairment. Agenesis or malformation of cochlear structures, including the Scheibe, Bing-Siebermann, Mondini, and Michel anomalies, are also genetic causes of congenital sensorineural hearing impairment.

Conductive hearing loss can also be genetically determined. Conditions, diseases, or syndromes that include craniofacial abnormalities are often associated with conductive hearing loss, and possibly also with sensorineural hearing loss. Pierre Robin, Treacher Collins, Klippel-Feil, and Crouzon syndromes and osteogenesis imperfecta are often associated with hearing loss. Congenital anomalies causing conductive hearing loss include malformations of the middle-ear structures and atresia of the external auditory canal.

A child with a parent having familial deafness is at risk for hearing impairment. Familial deafness can be dominant, recessive, or X-linked. Familial hearing impairment of the autosomal recessive type accounts for 70–80% of genetic-congenital sensorineural hearing impairment; X-linked disorders account for 1–3%. Whereas children with an easily identified syndrome or with anomalies of the outer ear may be identified as being at risk for hearing loss and monitored adequately, deafness of autosomal recessive genetic origin is often difficult to identify.

Genetic-Postnatal. Some genetically determined causes of hearing impairment do not express themselves until after birth. Familial hearing impairment can be of late onset with no other signs. Alport, Alstrom, and von Recklinghausen diseases and Hunter-Hurler syndrome are genetically determined hearing impairments with late onset in childhood.

Nongenetic-Congenital. Early in pregnancy the embryo is vulnerable to the effects of toxic modalities and substances. In the 1st trimester, ototoxic drugs (e.g., streptomycin, quinine, thalidomide), radiation, and infection (e.g., rubella, cytomegalovirus [CMV]) can damage the developing ear. Table 587–1 lists factors that place a newborn at risk for hearing impairment, including the genetic factors described in the previous chapter. Congenital CMV warrants special attention because it is associated with hearing loss in its symptomatic and asymptomatic forms, and the hearing loss may be progressive. Some children with congenital CMV have lost residual hearing suddenly at 4–5 yr of age. Persistent pulmonary hypertension of the newborn (PPHN) may also place newborns at risk for hearing impairment. All these factors account for about 50% of cases of moderate to profound sensorineural hearing impairment in neonates.

Nongenetic-Postnatal. Many of the risk factors mentioned in the preceding section (and in Table 587–1) can also affect the child after birth. Viral and bacterial infections can damage the inner ear. Some infections in children that are associated with sudden deafness include cryptococcal meningitis, measles, and mumps. Bacterial meningitis (especially pneumococcus and *H. influenzae*) is a major cause of childhood acquired hearing impairment (see also Chapter 169.1). Hearing loss in childhood can also be caused by ototoxic medications (e.g., aminoglycosides, platinum), noise exposure, head trauma, otitis media, vascular insults, lesions of the cranium, and various toxic substances.

EFFECTS OF HEARING IMPAIRMENT. These depend on the nature and degree of the hearing loss and on the individual characteristics of the child. Hearing loss may be unilateral or bilateral, conductive, sensorineural, or mixed, mild, moderate, severe, or profound, of sudden or gradual onset, stable, progressive, or fluctuating, and selective in the region of the acoustic spectrum affected (or it can affect most of the audible spectrum). Factors such as intelligence, medical or physical condition (including accompanying syndromes), family support, age at onset, age at time of identification, and promptness of intervention also affect the impact of hearing loss on a child.

Most hearing-impaired children have some usable hearing—only 6% of those in the hearing-impaired population have profound hearing loss. In general, hearing loss very early in life can affect the development of speech and language, social and emotional development, behavior, attention, and academic achievement. Some hearing-impaired children are misdiagnosed because they have sufficient hearing to respond to environmental sounds, can learn some language, and have some speech but, when challenged in the classroom, cannot perform to full potential.

Even a mild or unilateral hearing loss may have a detrimental effect on the development of a young child and on school performance. Children with such hearing impairments have greater difficulty when listening conditions are unfavorable (e.g., when there is background noise and poor acoustics), such as may occur in the classroom. Unfortunately, the fact that schools are auditory-verbal environments is not appreciated by those who minimize the impact of hearing impairment on learning. Hearing loss should be considered in any child with below-par performance, poor behavior, or inattention in school (Table 587–2).

Children with moderate, severe, or profound hearing impairment and/or those with other handicapping conditions are often educated in classes or schools for exceptional children. The auditory management and choices regarding modes of communication and education for children with hearing handicaps must be individualized, because these children are not a homogeneous group. A team approach to individual case management is essential, because each child and family unit represents unique needs and abilities.

HEARING SCREENING. Because hearing impairment can have a major impact on the development of a child, and because the earlier the impairment is identified the better the prognosis, early identification through screening programs is widely advocated. Many medical centers have such programs. Some use the high-risk register criteria (see Table 587–1) to decide which infants to screen, some screen all infants who require intensive care, and some do both. Screening methods include observing behavioral responses to uncalibrated noise-makers, using automated systems such as the Crib-o-gram or the auditory response cradle (in which movement of the infant in response to sound is recorded by motion sensors), and carrying out evoked potentials and otoacoustic emissions testing. The auditory brain stem response (ABR) test, an auditory evoked electrophysiologic response that correlates highly with hearing, also has been used successfully and cost-effectively to screen newborns.

Many children who are congenitally hearing impaired are not identified by the high-risk register or do not spend time in intensive care units. Such infants are not routinely screened at birth, although many centers advocate screening all newborns. Furthermore, many children become hearing impaired after the neonatal period (see earlier). It is not until children are in school (or possibly in preschool) that formal hearing screening efforts are made. Consequently, the primary care physician or pediatrician should be alert to the signs and symptoms of childhood hearing impairment, so that those with hearing impairment who are not screened formally can be identified as early as possible.

Identification of Hearing Impairment. The impact of hearing impair-

■ **TABLE 587–1 Risk Factors That Identify Neonates At-risk for Sensorineural Hearing Impairment***

Family history of congenital or delayed onset childhood sensorineural impairment
Congenital infection known or suspected to be associated with sensorineural hearing impairment, such as toxoplasmosis, syphilis, rubella, cytomegalovirus, and herpes
Craniofacial anomalies including morphologic abnormalities of the pinna and ear canal, absent philtrum, low hairline
Birth weight less than 1,500 g (~3.3 lb)
Hyperbilirubinemia at a level exceeding indication for exchange transfusion
Ototoxic medications including but not limited to the aminoglycosides used for more than 5 days (e.g., gentamicin, tobramycin, kanamycin, streptomycin) and loop diuretics used in combination with aminoglycosides
Bacterial meningitis
Severe depression at birth, which may include infants with Apgar scores of 0–3 at 5 min or those who fail to initiate spontaneous respiration by 10 min or those with hypotonia persisting to 2 hr of age
Prolonged mechanical ventilation for a duration equal to or greater than 10 days (e.g., persistent pulmonary hypertension)
Stigmata or other findings associated with a syndrome known to include sensorineural hearing loss (e.g., Waardenburg syndrome or Usher syndrome)

**From the Joint Committee on Infant Hearing (1991) and Position Statement. ASHA 33:3, 1990.*

■ **TABLE 587–2 Hearing Handicap as a Function of Average Hearing Threshold Level of the Better Ear***

Average Threshold Level (dB) at 500–2,000 Hz (ANSI)†	Description	Common Causes	What Can Be Heard Without Amplification	Degree of Handicap (if not treated in 1st yr of life)	Probable Needs
0–15	Normal range		All speech sounds	None	None
16–25	Slight hearing loss	Serous otitis, perforation, monomeric membrane, sensorineural loss, tympanosclerosis	Vowel sounds heard clearly, may miss unvoiced consonant sounds	Possible mild or transitory auditory dysfunction Difficulty in perceiving some speech sounds	Consideration of need for hearing aid Lip reading Auditory training Speech therapy Preferential seating Appropriate surgery
26–40	Mild	Serous otitis, perforation, tympanosclerosis, monomeric membrane, sensorineural loss	Hears only some of speech sounds, the louder voiced sounds	Auditory learning dysfunction Mild language retardation Mild speech problems Inattention	Hearing aid Lip reading Auditory training Speech therapy Appropriate surgery
41–65	Moderate hearing loss	Chronic otitis, middle ear anomaly, sensorineural loss	Misses most speech sounds at normal conversational level	Speech problems Language retardation Learning dysfunction Inattention	All of the above, plus consideration of special classroom situation
66–95	Severe hearing loss	Sensorineural loss or mixed loss, caused by sensorineural loss plus middle ear disease	Hears no speech sound of normal conversations	Severe speech problems Language retardation Learning dysfunction Inattention	All of the above; probable assignment to special classes
96+	Profound hearing loss	Sensorineural loss or mixed	Hears no speech or other sounds	Severe speech problems Language retardation Learning dysfunction Inattention	All of the above; probable assignment to special classes

*From Northern JL, Downs MP: Hearing in Children, 3rd ed. © 1984, The Williams & Wilkins Co., Baltimore.
†ANSI = American National Standards Institute.

ment is greatest on the infant who has yet to develop language; therefore, identification, diagnosis, description, and habilitation should be done as soon as possible. In general, infants with a prenatal or perinatal history that puts them at risk (see Table 587–1) or those who have failed a formal hearing screening, should be followed closely by a clinical audiologist experienced in the evaluation and management of hearing-impaired children until a reliable assessment of auditory function has been obtained. The pediatrician and family physician are important in encouraging families to cooperate with the follow-up plan. Infants born at risk but who have not been screened as neonates should have a hearing screening by 3 mo of age, carried out by a pediatric audiologist. Most infants, however, are born at facilities that do not have hearing screening programs.

Hearing-impaired infants who are born at risk and/or screened for hearing loss in a neonatal hearing screening program comprise only a portion of those in the pediatric hearing-impaired population. Those who are congenitally deaf because of autosomal recessive inheritance or silent TORCH infection are often not identified until the 2nd or 3rd year of life. Usually, the more severe the hearing loss, the earlier the age at identification, but, identification occurs later than the age necessary for an optimal outcome. Normal hearing children have developed a great deal of language by 3 yr of age. Parental concern regarding hearing and any delayed development of speech and language should alert the practitioner; often, parental concern precedes formal identification and diagnosis of hearing impairment by 6 mo-1 yr. Primary care physicians are uniquely able to respond to the concerns of parents and to monitor the development of speech and language. Table 587–3 presents guidelines for screening language development in young children and Table 587–4 provides guidelines for identifying children with abnormal auditory behavior. Failure to fulfill these criteria should be reason for referral for an audiologic evaluation.

Clinical Audiologic Evaluation. The importance of identification and diagnosis of hearing loss is widely understood, but what is not so well understood is the ability of a pediatric audiologist to obtain information on the hearing of infants and young children in a diagnostic setting. Even the youngest infants can be evaluated for auditory function. When hearing impairment is suspected in the young child, reliable and valid estimates of auditory function can be obtained. Successful management strategies for hearing-impaired children rely on prompt identification and ongoing assessment to define the dimensions of auditory function. Cooperation among the pediatrician and those specializing in such areas as audiology, speech and language pathology, education, and child development is necessary to optimize auditory-verbal development. Management of the hearing-impaired child includes the consideration (and often fitting) of an amplification device; the monitoring hearing and auditory skills, counseling parents and families, advising teachers, and dealing with public agencies.

AUDIOMETRY. The goal of the audiologic evaluation can vary as a function of the age or developmental level of the child, the reason for the evaluation, and the child's otologic condition and/or history. The audiogram provides the fundamental de-

■ **TABLE 587–3 Criteria for Referral for Audiologic Assessment***

Age (mo)	Referral Guidelines for Children with "Speech" Delay
12	No differentiated babbling or vocal imitation
18	No use of single words
24	Single-word vocabulary of ≤10 words
30	Fewer than 100 words; no evidence of two-word combinations; unintelligible
36	Fewer than 200 words; no use of telegraphic sentences, clarity <50%
48	Fewer than 600 words; no use of simple sentences; clarity ≤80%

From Matkin ND: Early recognition and referral of hearing-impaired children. Pediatr Rev 6:151, 1984. Reproduced by permission of Pediatrics.

■ **TABLE 587–4 Guidelines for Referral of Children Suspected of Hearing Loss***

Age (mo)	Normal Development
0–4	Should startle to loud sounds, quiet to mother's voice, momentarily cease activity when sound is presented at a conversational level
5–6	Should correctly localize to sound presented in a horizontal plane, begin to imitate sounds in own speech repertoire or at least reciprocally vocalize with an adult
7–12	Should correctly localize to sound presented in any plane Should respond to name, even when spoken quietly
13–15	Should point toward an unexpected sound or to familiar objects or persons when asked
16–18	Should follow simple directions without gestural or other visual cues; can be trained to reach toward an interesting toy at midline when a sound is presented
19–24	Should point to body parts when asked; by 21–24 mo, can be trained to perform play audiometry

From Matkin ND: Early recognition and referral of hearing-impaired children. Pediatr Rev 6:151, 1984. Reproduced by permission of Pediatrics.

scription of hearing sensitivity (Fig. 587–1). Hearing thresholds are assessed as a function of frequency using pure tones (sine waves) at octave intervals from 250–8,000 Hz. Typically, earphones are used and hearing is assessed independently for each ear. Air-conducted signals are presented through earphones (or loudspeakers) and are used to provide information regarding the sensitivity of the auditory system. To begin, the differential diagnosis of hearing loss, these same test sounds can be delivered to the ear through an oscillator that is placed on the head, usually on the mastoid. Such signals are considered bone-conducted signals, because the bones of the skull are vibrated and sound energy is transmitted directly to the inner ear, essentially bypassing the outer and middle ears. In the normal ear, the air and bone conduction thresholds are the same; they are also the same in those with sensorineural hearing loss. In those with conductive hearing loss, however, there is a difference between the air and bone conduction thresholds. This is called the air-bone gap; it indicates the amount of hearing loss attributable to dysfunction in the outer and/or middle ear. When there is mixed hearing loss, both the bone and air conduction thresholds are abnormal, and there is an air-bone gap.

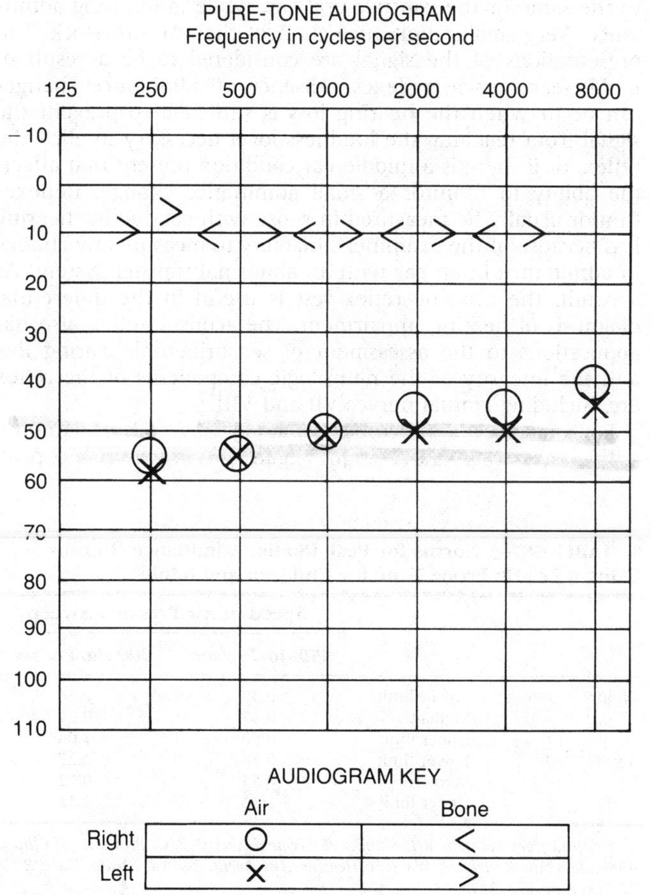

Figure 587–1. Audiogram demonstrating a bilateral conductive hearing loss.

Speech Recognition Threshold. Another measure useful in describing auditory function is the speech recognition threshold (SRT), which is the lowest intensity level at which a score of approximately 50% correct is obtained on a task of recognizing spondee words. Spondee words are two-syllable words or phrases that have equal stress on each syllable (e.g., baseball, hot dog, pancake). The listener must be familiar with all the words in order for a valid test result to be obtained. The SRT should correspond with the average of pure-tone thresholds at 500, 1,000, and 2,000 Hz, the pure-tone average (PTA). The SRT is relevant because much of the rationale for assessing hearing in children involves determining the adequacy for development and use of speech and language. It also serves to check the validity of the evaluation, because children with nonorganic hearing loss (i.e., malingerers) often have a large discrepancy between the PTA and SRT. Audiometric configuration, however, can also affect the SRT-PTA relationship and should be considered before assessing the possibility of malingering.

The basic battery of hearing tests concludes with an assessment of the child's ability to understand monosyllabic words when presented at a comfortable listening level. Performance on such word intelligibility tests assists in the differential diagnosis of hearing impairment, and also provides a measure of how well a child performs when speech is presented at loudness levels similar to those encountered in the environment.

Play Audiometry. For children at or above the developmental level of a 5- or 6-yr-old, conventional test methods can be used. For children from 2½–5 yr old, a technique called play audiometry can be used. Responses in play audiometry are usually conditioned motor activities associated with a game, such as dropping blocks in a bucket, placing rings on a peg, stringing beads, or completing a puzzle. The technique can be used to obtain a reliable audiogram of the preschool child. For those who will not or cannot repeat words clearly for the SRT and word intelligibility tasks, pictures can be used with a pointing response.

Visual Reinforcement Audiometry. For those between the ages of about 5–6 mo and 2½ yr, visual reinforcement audiometry (VRA) is commonly used. The technique incorporates a head-turning response with the activation of an animated (mechanical) toy reinforcer. If infants are properly conditioned, VRA can provide reliable estimates of hearing sensitivity for tones and speech sounds. In most applications of VRA sounds are presented by loudspeaker(s) in a sound field, so no ear-specific information is obtained. Often, however, assessment of the infant is designed to rule out hearing loss that would affect the development of speech and language. Normal sound field response levels of infants indicate sufficient hearing for this purpose in spite of the possibility of different hearing levels in the two ears.

Behavioral Observation Audiometry. For those below 5 mo of age, behavioral hearing assessment is limited to unconditioned, reflexive responses to complex (i.e., not frequency-specific) test sounds, such as noise, speech, or music presented using calibrated signals from a loudspeaker or uncalibrated noisemakers. Response levels can vary widely within and across infants, and usually do not represent a good estimate of sensitivity. Behavioral observation audiometry (BOA), as this technique is called, is used primarily as a screening device.

Assessment of a child with suspected hearing loss is not complete until pure-tone hearing thresholds and SRTs have been obtained in each ear (i.e., until a reliable audiogram has been obtained). Estimates of hearing responsivity obtained using BOA or VRA in a sound field (loudspeakers) cannot be used satisfactorily to describe hearing in both ears.

ACOUSTIC IMMITTANCE TESTING. This is a standard part of the clinical audiologic test battery and includes tympanometry. Acoustic immittance testing is a useful, objective assessment technique that provides information about the status of the middle ear. It is helpful in the diagnosis and management of otitis media with effusion, one of the leading causes of mild to moderate hearing loss in young children. Tympanometry may also be performed by physicians.

Tympanometry. This technique provides a graph of the ability of the middle ear to transmit sound energy (admittance, or compliance) or impede sound energy (impedance) as a function of air pressure in the external ear canal. Because most immittance test instruments measure acoustic admittance, the term "admittance" is used here. In general, the principles apply to whatever units of measure are used.

A probe is inserted into the entrance of the external ear canal so that an airtight seal is obtained. The probe varies air pressure, presents a tone, and measures sound pressure level in the ear canal through the probe assembly. The sound pressure measured in the ear canal relative to the known intensity of the probe signal is used to estimate the acoustic admittance of the ear canal and middle-ear system. Admittance can be expressed in a unit called a millimho (mmho) or as a volume of air (in mL) with equivalent acoustic admittance. The test is done so that an estimate of the volume of air enclosed between the probe tip and tympanic membrane can be made. The acoustic admittance of this volume of air is deducted from the overall admittance measure to obtain a measure of the admittance of the middle-ear system alone. Estimating ear canal volume also has some diagnostic benefit, because an abnormally large value is consistent with the presence of an opening in the tympanic membrane (perforation or tube).

With the elimination of the admittance of the air mass in the external auditory canal, it is assumed that the remaining admittance measure accurately reflects the admittance of the entire middle-ear system. Its value is largely controlled by the dynamics of the tympanic membrane. Abnormalities of the tympanic membrane can dictate the shape of tympanograms and thus obscure abnormalities that lie beyond the tympanic membrane. In addition, the frequency of the probe tone, the speed and direction of the air pressure change, and the air pressure at which the tympanogram is initiated are all factors that can influence the outcome of the tympanometric assessment.

When air pressure in the ear canal is equal to that in the middle ear, the middle-ear system is functioning optimally. Therefore, the ear canal pressure at which there is the greatest flow of energy (admittance) should be a reasonable estimate of the air pressure in the middle-ear space. This pressure is determined by finding the admittance maximum (peak) on the tympanogram and obtaining its value on the x axis. The value on the y axis at the tympanogram peak is an estimate of peak admittance. This peak measure is sometimes referred to as static acoustic admittance, even though it is estimated from a dynamic measure (Fig. 587–2). Table 587–5 presents the norms for peak admittance based on admittance tympanometry for normal adults and children.

Acoustic Reflex Test. This is also part of the immittance test battery. With a properly functioning middle-ear system, admittance at the tympanic membrane changes on activation of the stapedius and tensor tympani muscles. In healthy ears, the stapedial reflex occurs following exposure to loud sounds. Admittance instruments are designed to present reflex activating signals (pure tones of various frequencies or noise), either to the same or the contralateral ear, while monitoring admittance. Very small admittance changes that are time-locked to presentations of the signal are considered to be a result of middle-ear muscle reflexes. Absence of admittance changes can occur when the hearing loss is sufficient to prevent the signal from reaching the loudness level necessary to elicit the reflex, or if there is a middle-ear condition present that affects the ability to monitor a small admittance change. Reflexes cannot usually be measured in those with conductive hearing loss because of the examiner's inability to measure any change in admittance in an ear with an abnormal transfer system. As a result, the acoustic reflex test is useful in the differential diagnosis of hearing impairment. The acoustic reflex also has applications to the assessment of sensorineural hearing loss and the integrity of the neurologic components of the reflex arc, including cranial nerves VII and VIII.

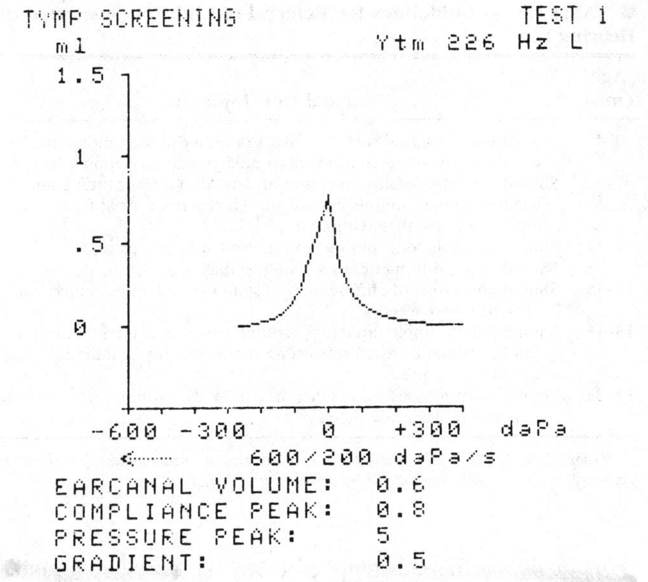

Figure 587–2. **Admittance tympanogram of a normal ear of a 7-yr-old child. Ear canal volume, compliance peak (i.e., peak admittance in mL using the y-axis scale), and tympanometric peak pressure and gradient are all within normal limits. For this instrument, the gradient can range from 0 to 1.0, and the sharpest peaks get the highest values.**

Tympanometry in Otitis Media with Effusion. Often, children with otitis media have high negative tympanometric peak

■ TABLE 587–5 Norms for Peak (Static) Admittance (in mL) Using a 226-Hz Probe Tone for Children and Adults*

		Speed of Air Pressure Sweep	
		≤50 *da/Pa/sec*†	**200 *da/Pa/sec*‡**
Children (3–5 yr)	Lower limit	0.30	0.36
	Median	0.55	0.61
	Upper limit	0.90	1.06
Adults	Lower limit	0.56	0.27
	Median	0.85	0.72
	Upper limit	1.36	1.38

**Adapted from Margolis RH, Shanks JE: Tympanometry: Basic Principles of Clinical Application.* In: *Rintelman WS (ed): Hearing Assessment, 2nd ed. Austin, TX, PRO-ED, 1991, pp 179–245.*

†Ear canal volume measurement based on admittance at lowest tail of tympanogram.

‡Ear canal measurement based on admittance at lowest tail of tympanogram for children and at +200 da/Pa for adults.

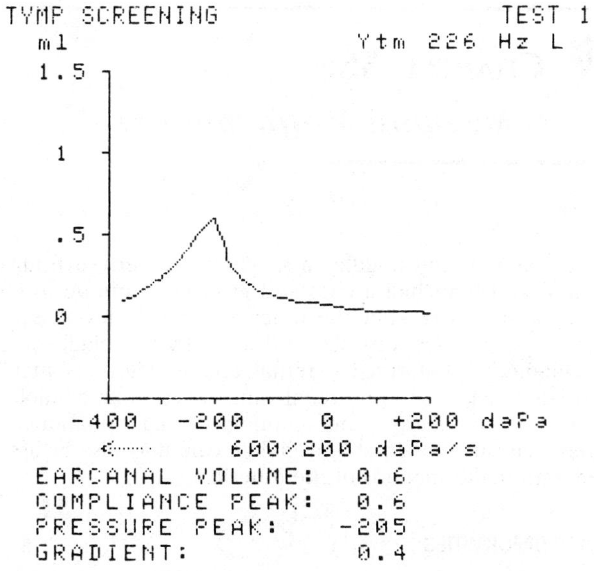

Figure 587–3. Admittance tympanogram of the same ear as that shown in Figure 587–2, only 2 wk earlier. On this occasion, tympanometric peak pressure is abnormal. Whereas the other variables are in the normal range, peak admittance and gradient are both slightly reduced relative to the values shown in Figure 587–2.

pressure (Fig. 587–3) and/or reduced peak admittance values. However, in regard to the diagnosis of middle-ear effusion, the tympanometric measure that has the greatest sensitivity and specificity is the tympanogram shape, rather than its peak pressure (poor predictive value) or peak admittance (fair predictive value). This shape is sometimes referred to as the tympanometric gradient or tympanometric width; it quantifies the degree of roundness or "peakedness" of the tympanogram. Generally, the more rounded the peak (or, ultimately, an absent peak), the higher the probability that an effusion is present (Fig. 587–4). Some instruments compute gradient automatically, whereas others do not. Various ways to compute this gradient can be used so, until the measure becomes standardized, the individual characteristics of the instrument used must be known and applied accordingly.

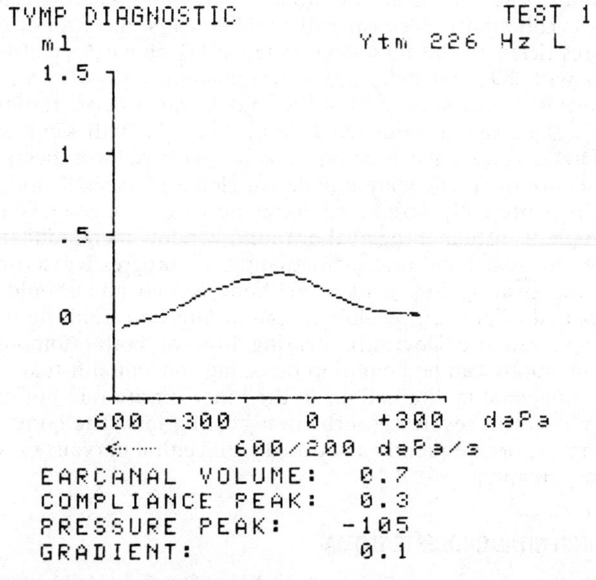

Figure 587–4. Admittance tympanogram of the left ear of a 4-yr-old child with middle-ear effusion. Note that the peak admittance and gradient are both very low, whereas the tympanometric peak pressure is grossly within normal limits.

AUDITORY BRAIN STEM RESPONSE. The ABR test is used for neonatal newborn hearing screening, and it is also important in the diagnosis of auditory dysfunction and of disorders of the auditory nervous system. The ABR is a far-field recording of minute electrical discharges from multiple neurons. The stimulus, therefore, must be able to cause the simultaneous discharge of the large numbers of neurons involved. Stimuli with very rapid onset, such as clicks or tone bursts, must be used. Unfortunately, the rapid onset required to create a measurable ABR also causes energy to be spread in the frequency domain, reducing the frequency-specificity of the response.

The ABR is not affected by sedation or general anesthesia. Infants and children from about 6 mo–4 yr of age are routinely sedated to avoid problems related to the electrical interference caused by muscle activity during testing. Also, ABR testing can be done in the operating room when a child is anesthetized for another procedure.

The ABR is recorded as five to seven waves. Waves I, III, and V can be obtained consistently in all age groups. Waves II and IV appear less consistently, between and within subjects. The latency of each wave (i.e., time of occurrence of the wave peak following stimulus onset) increases and the amplitude decreases with reductions in stimulus intensity or loudness. There is developmental change in the latency of the various waves; latency decreases with increasing age, with the earliest waves reaching mature latency values earlier in life than the later waves.

The ABR commonly has two major uses in the pediatric setting: (1) it is used as an audiometric test, providing information regarding the ability of the peripheral auditory system to transmit information to the auditory nerve and beyond; (2) it is used in the differential diagnosis or monitoring of central nervous system pathology. For the audiometric approach, a search is conducted for the minimum stimulus intensity that yields an observable ABR. Plotting latency versus intensity for various waves also aids in the differential diagnosis of hearing impairment. A major advantage of auditory assessment using the ABR is that ear-specific threshold estimates on infants or otherwise difficult-to-test patients can be obtained. ABR thresholds using click stimuli are correlated best with behavioral hearing thresholds in the higher frequencies (1,000/4,000 Hz). Measurement of the responsivity of the peripheral auditory system to low-frequency stimuli requires different stimuli (tone bursts or filtered clicks) or the use of masking, neither of which isolates the low-frequency region of the cochlea in all cases. ABR responses for low frequencies should be interpreted by those knowledgeable and experienced in ABR testing.

The ABR test does not assess "hearing." It reflects auditory neuronal electric responses that can be correlated to behavioral hearing thresholds, but a normal ABR only suggests that the auditory system, up to the level of the midbrain, is responsive to the stimulus used. Conversely, a failure to elicit an ABR indicates an impairment of the system's synchronous response, but does not necessarily mean that there is no "hearing." Sometimes the behavioral response to sound is normal but no ABR can be elicited (e.g., neurologic demyelinating disease). The ABR may be used to infer whether and at what level of the auditory system an impairment exists. Hearing losses that are sudden, progressive, or unilateral are indications for ABR testing. Although it is commonly believed that the different waves of the ABR reflect activity in increasingly rostral levels of the auditory system, the neural generators of the response have not been determined precisely. Each ABR wave beyond the earliest waves is probably the result of neural firing at multiple levels of the system, and each level of the system probably contributes to multiple ABR waves.

For the neurologic application, typically high intensity click stimuli are used. The morphology of the response and wave and interwave latencies are examined in respect to age appropriate forms. Delayed or missing waves in the ABR often have diagnostic significance.

The ABR and other electrical responses are extremely complex and difficult to interpret. A number of factors, including instrumentation design and settings, environment, degree and configuration of hearing loss, and patient characteristics may influence the quality of the recording. Therefore, testing and interpretation of electrophysiologic activity should be done by trained professionals to avoid the risk that unreliable and/or erroneous conclusions will affect patient care.

OTOACOUSTIC EMISSIONS (OAEs). During normal hearing these emissions originate from sensitive amplifying processes in the cochlea. They travel from the cochlea through the middle ear to the external auditory canal, where they can be detected using miniature microphones. Transient evoked otoacoustic emission (TEOAE) may be used to check the integrity of the cochlea. In the neonatal period, registration of OAEs can be accomplished during natural sleep and TEOAEs can be used as screening tests in infants and children for hearing at the 30dB HL level. They are less time-consuming and elaborate than ABR and are more sensitive than behavioral tests. TEOAEs are reduced or absent owing to various dysfunctions in the inner ear. However, they are absent in patients with more than 30 dB HL hearing loss and, thus, cannot be used to determine hearing threshold. Diseases such as otitis media reduce the transfer of TEOAEs and may wrongly indicate a cochlear hearing disorder.

TREATMENT. Once a hearing loss is identified, a full developmental and speech and language evaluation is needed. Parental counseling as well as involvement in all stages of the evaluation and eventual habilitation or rehabilitation is mandatory. A conductive hearing loss may often be corrected through treatment of a middle ear effusion or surgical correction of the abnormal sound-conducting mechanism. Children with sensorineural hearing loss should be evaluated for possible hearing aid use. Audiologists with special experience and training in working with children are required. Hearing aids may be fitted for children as young or younger than 6 mo. In these children, repeat audiologic testing is needed to more reliably identify the degree of hearing loss and fine-tune the use of hearing aids. There is ongoing controversy as to the best educational approach to children with significant hearing loss. Since we live in a predominantly speaking world, some have advocated only an auditory and oral approach to hearing habilitation. As these children often are slow to develop communication skills, a total communication approach has also been advocated; this blends the use of sign language, lip-reading, hearing aids, and speaking as appropriate for each individual child. The appropriate program for each child will vary with the patient, family, and resources available. The use of a cochlear implant in children with severe to profound hearing loss and little or no help from conventional hearing aids has been shown to improve the development of communication skills. This is currently approved for use in the United States in children aged 2 yr and older. Some members of the hearing-impaired community object to its use in children who have no decision in the matter and who may develop excellent communication abilities using more conventional habilitation strategies.

CHAPTER 588
Congenital Malformations

The external and middle ears, which are derived from the 1st and 2nd branchial arches and grooves, continue to grow throughout puberty, but the inner ear, which develops from the otocyst, reaches adult size and shape by the middle of fetal development. Malformed external and middle ears may be associated with serious renal anomalies, mandibulofacial dysostosis, and many other craniofacial malformations. Severely deformed external and middle ears may also be associated with malformations of the inner ear.

MINOR DEFORMITIES

Severe malformations of the external ear are rare, but minor deformities are common. A pit-like cutaneous depression just in front of the helix and above the tragus may represent a cyst or an epidermis-lined fistulous tract; these are common but do not require surgical removal unless they become recurrently infected. Accessory skin tags on narrow pedicles may be removed by ligation but, if the pedicle is broad-based or contains cartilage, the defect should be corrected surgically. The unusually prominent or "lop" ear results from lack of bending of the cartilage that creates the antihelix; it may be improved cosmetically by otoplasty after the auricle has developed sufficiently (at about the age of 5 yr). Microtia includes cases of rudimentary auricles that, in addition to being abnormally small in size, are often more anterior and inferior in placement than normal auricles. Rarely, the auricle may be totally absent (anotia).

CONGENITAL STENOSIS
(Atresia of the External Auditory Canal)

This may be associated with malformation of the auricle and middle ear. Audiometric, tympanometric, and roentgenographic assessments are essential in diagnosing and managing these conditions. Reconstructive middle-ear surgery for atresia is restricted to the following patients: (1) above 5 yr of age; (2) with bilateral deformities or unilateral lesions in which there is a deformity only of the middle-ear ossicles, resulting in a significant conductive hearing loss; (3) with significant bilateral conductive hearing loss; (4) with roentgenographic evidence of an adequate middle-ear cleft and mastoid; and (5) with a normally positioned facial nerve. A congenital perilymphatic fistula of the oval or round window membrane may present as a rapid-onset, fluctuating, or progressive sensorineural hearing loss with or without vertigo and should be repaired to prevent possible spread of infection from the middle ear to the labyrinth, hearing loss, or both. Computed tomography can be helpful in detecting congenital fistula.

Congenital malformations of the inner ear are rare but usually result in severe sensorineural hearing loss. The bony deformities are frequently associated with central nervous system malformations.

CONGENITAL CHOLESTEATOMA

This is a congenital rest of epithelial tissue trapped behind the developing tympanic membrane that may appear as a white, cyst-like structure medial to or within an intact tympanic membrane. It is unrelated to infections of the middle ear. This white mass behind the eardrum is usually in the anteriosuperior quadrant of the middle ear. It should be suspected when deep retraction pockets, keratin debris, chronic drainage, aural granulation tissue, or a mass behind the tympanic membrane are present. As a result, erosion of the ossicles of the middle ear, pressure on the facial nerve, erosion into the inner ear, or exposure of the dura may occur. Besides acting as a benign tumor, the keratinatous debris of a cholesteatoma is a perfect culture medium and may become a focus of infection for severe chronic otitis. Cholesteatoma should be removed surgically.

CHAPTER 589
External Otitis

In the infant, the outer two thirds of the ear canal is cartilaginous and the inner third is bony, whereas in the older child and adult only the outer third is cartilaginous. The highly viscid secretions of the sebaceous glands and the watery, pigmented secretions of the apocrine glands in the outer portion of the canal combine with exfoliated surface cells of the skin to form a protective, waxy, water-repellent coating. The normal flora of the external canal consists of *Staphylococcus epidermidis, Corynebacterium* (diphtheroids), *Micrococcus* sp., and occasionally *S. aureus* and *Streptococcus viridans.* Excessive wetness (swimming, bathing, or increased environmental humidity) or dryness (previous infection, dematoses, or insufficient cerumen) and trauma (digital or foreign body) make the skin of the canal vulnerable to infection by endogenous bacteria or virulent exogenous bacteria.

ETIOLOGY. External otitis is most commonly caused by *Pseudomonas aeruginosa, Enterobacter aerogenes, Proteus mirabilis, Klebsiella pneumoniae,* streptococci, *S. epidermidis,* and fungi such as *Candida* and *Aspergillus.* The condition known as "swimmer's ear" results from the loss of protective cerumen and chronic irritation and maceration from excessive moisture in the canal; *Pseudomonas* sp. is the most commonly isolated bacterium. Herpesvirus hominis and varicella-zoster may also cause external otitis.

CLINICAL MANIFESTATIONS. The predominant symptom is ear pain, accentuated by manipulation of the pinna and especially by pressure on the tragus. The severity of the pain and tenderness may be disproportionate to the degree of inflammation, because the skin of the external ear canal is attached to the perichondrium and periosteum. Itching is a frequent precursor of pain and is usually characteristic of chronic inflammation of the canal. Conductive hearing loss may occur as a result of edema of the skin and tympanic membrane, serous or purulent secretions, or the progressive meatal skin thickening associated with longstanding external otitis. Edema of the canal, erythema, and greenish otorrhea are prominent signs of the acute disease.

Frequently, the canal is so tender and swollen that the entire ear canal and tympanic membrane cannot be adequately visualized, in which instance complete otoscopic examination should be delayed until the acute swelling subsides. If the tympanic membrane can be visualized, it may be either normal or opaque in appearance and the mobility of the drum may be normal or, when the drum is thickened, reduced in response to positive and negative pressure.

Periauricular edema and fever often result from a combined infection with *Pseudomonas* sp. and *S. pyogenes* or from *S. aureus.* When there is such secondary infection, lymphadenitis, with tender nodes anterior to the tragus or in the postauricular region, may also occur.

DIFFERENTIAL DIAGNOSIS. Diffuse external otitis may be confused with furunculosis, otitis media, and mastoiditis. A furuncle usually causes a localized swelling of the canal limited to one quadrant, whereas external otitis is associated with concentric swelling. In otitis media the eardrum may be perforated, severely retracted, or bulging and immobile, and hearing is usually impaired. Pain on manipulation of the auricle and lymphadenitis are not features of middle-ear disease. In some patients with external otitis, the periauricular edema is so extensive that the auricle is pushed forward, creating a condition that may be confused with acute mastoiditis and a subperiosteal abscess; however, in mastoiditis the postauricular fold is obliterated, whereas in external otitis the fold is maintained. When the edema over the mastoid process is a result of mastoiditis, there is also usually a history of otitis media and hearing loss, and tenderness is noted over the mastoid antrum or tip and not on movement of the auricle as in external otitis. Sagging of the posterior external canal wall may also occur with acute mastoiditis.

TREATMENT. Topical otic preparations containing neomycin (active against gram-positive organisms and also against some gram-negative organisms, notably *Proteus* sp.) with either colistin or polymyxin (active against gram-negative bacilli, notably *Pseudomonas* sp.) and corticosteroids are effective in treating most forms of acute diffuse external otitis. If canal edema is marked, a cotton or selvedged-gauze wick should be inserted into the outer third of the ear canal and the medication applied to the wick as frequently as possible for 24–48 hr; the wick can be removed after these applications and the otic medication instilled 3–4 times a day. Acetic acid preparations (2%), with or without corticosteroids, or half-strength Burow solution (aluminum acetate, 1:20) are probably equally effective. When the pain is severe, analgesics (e.g., salicylates, codeine) and dry heat may be necessary.

As the inflammatory process subsides, cleaning the canal with cotton-tipped applicators or, more effectively, irrigating with 2% acetic acid to remove the debris enhances the effectiveness of the topical medications. In subacute and chronic infections, periodic cleansing of the canal is essential. In severe, acute, diffuse external otitis associated with fever and lymphadenitis from which bacteria have been cultured, oral and, on occasion, parenteral antibiotics are indicated; the choice of drug depends on the antibiotic susceptibility of the organism. A fungal infection (otomycosis) of the external auditory canal may be treated by applying metacresol acetate. Preventing external otitis may be necessary for individuals susceptible to recurrences, especially children who swim frequently. The most effective prophylaxis is instillation of dilute alcohol or acetic acid immediately following swimming or bathing.

Furunculosis. This is caused by *S. aureus* and is seen only in the hair-containing outer third of the ear canal. It is treated with incision and drainage and systemic penicillin or one of the penicillinase-resistant penicillins, depending on the antibiotic susceptibility of the organism.

Acute Cellulitis. Acute cellulitis of the auricle and external auditory canal is usually caused by *S. pyogenes,* occasionally by *S. aureus.* The skin is red, hot, and indurated, without a sharply defined border. Fever may be present with little or no exudate in the canal. Parenteral administration of penicillin G or a penicillinase-resistant penicillin is the therapy of choice.

Dermatoses. Various dermatoses (e.g., seborrheic, contact, infectious eczematoid, atopic, or neurodermatoid) are common causes of inflammation of the external canal and can be precursors of acute diffuse external otitis caused by scratching and the introduction of infecting organisms.

Seborrheic dermatitis is characterized by greasy scales that flake and crumble as they are detached from the epidermis; associated changes in the scalp, forehead, cheeks, brow, postauricular areas, and the concha are usual.

Contact dermatitis may be caused by topical otic medications such as neomycin, polymyxin, and colistin, which may produce erythema, vesiculation, edema, and weeping. Poison ivy, oak, and sumac may also produce contact dermatitis.

Infectious eczematoid dermatitis is caused by a purulent infection of the external canal, middle ear, or mastoid; the purulent drainage infects the skin of the canal, auricle, or both. The lesion is weeping, erythematous, or crusted.

Atopic dermatitis occurs in children with familial or personal histories of allergy; the auricle, particularly the postauricular fold, becomes thickened, scaly, and excoriated.

Neurodermatitis is recognized by the intense itching and erythematous, thickened epidermis localized to the concha and orifice of the meatus. Treatment of these dermatoses depends on the type but should include application of the aural medication described for external otitis, elimination of the source of infection or contactant when identified, and management of any underlying dermatologic problem.

Herpes Simplex. This may appear as vesicles on the auricle and lips, which eventually become encrusted and dry up, and may be confused with impetigo. Topical application of a 10% solution of carbamide peroxide in anhydrous glycerol is symptomatically helpful.

Herpes Zoster Oticus (Ramsay Hunt Syndrome). This is a vesicular eruption on the posterior canal wall accompanied by facial paralysis. Spontaneous recovery is usual.

Bullous Myringitis. This is commonly associated with an acute upper respiratory infection. The ear is very painful, and there are hemorrhagic or serous blebs on the membrane. The disease is difficult to differentiate from acute otitis media, because early in the course of acute otitis the drum may appear to have bullae. The organisms involved are probably the same as those causing acute otitis media. Treatment consists of antibiotic therapy of the type generally used for acute otitis media. Incision of the bullae, although not necessary, promptly relieves the pain.

CHAPTER 590
Otitis Media and its Complications

Inflammation of the middle ear, otitis media, is the most prevalent disease of childhood after respiratory tract infections. There are an estimated 25 million yearly visits to pediatricians related to otitis media; it is the most common diagnosis for children in the United States and the second most common in medicine overall. Over the past 2 decades there has been a dramatic increase in the number of visits to the pediatrician for otitis. This probably reflects a combination of factors ranging from a true change in disease pattern with more children in child care and increased awareness by the examining pediatrician, to improved technical capabilities including improved illumination with the use of halogen bulbs in otoscopes and the use of sensitive tests such as tympanograms to identify abnormal tympanic membrane motion. Correct diagnosis and treatment of otitis media are important not only because it is such a common illness but also because it is occasionally followed by significant complications such as intracranial spread of infection with meningitis or a brain abscess and acute inflammation of the middle ear followed by persistent middle ear effusion over a variable time. The latter can cause a significant conductive hearing loss, which may adversely affect speech and language development. Acute otitis media is usually suppurative or purulent, but serous effusions may also have an acute onset. There are many terms for otitis media with effusion, including serous, secretory, catarrhal, mucoid, nonsuppurative, and allergic otitis media.

EPIDEMIOLOGY. Nearly 85% of children have at least one episode of acute otitis media by 3 yr of age, and 50% of children will have two or more episodes. Infants and young children are at highest risk for otitis media; incidence rates are 15–20%, with peaks occurring from 6–36 mo and 4–6 yr of age. Children who develop otitis media in the 1st year of life have an increased risk of recurrent acute or chronic disease. After the 1st episode, about 40% of children have a middle-ear effusion that persists for 4 wk and 10% have an effusion that is still present at 3 mo. The incidence of the disease tends to decrease as a function of age after the age of 6 yr. The incidence is high in males, lower socioeconomic groups, Alaskan natives, native Americans, and children with cleft palate and other craniofacial anomalies, and is higher in whites than in blacks. The incidence is also increased in winter and early spring.

PATHOGENESIS. The high incidence of acute and recurrent otitis media in children probably reflects a combination of factors, with eustachian tube dysfunction and the child's susceptibility to recurrent upper respiratory infections being of most importance. The eustachian tube opens into the anterior middle ear space and connects that structure with the nasopharynx. It is lined by respiratory epithelium and surrounded for a short distance near the middle ear by bone, but for most of its length it is surrounded by cartilage. The child's eustachian tube is different from the adult's in that it is more horizontal and its opening, the torus tubarius, is likely to have numerous lymphoid follicles surrounding it. Also in a child, adenoids may fill the nasopharynx, mechanically blocking the nose and eustachian tube orifice or acting as a focus of infection that may contribute to edema and eustachian tube dysfunction. The eustachian tube is normally closed at rest and opens with swallowing by action of the tensor veli palatini, which runs from the skull base and inserts laterally into the soft palate. The eustachian tube protects the middle ear from nasopharyngeal secretions, provides drainage into the nasopharynx of secretions produced within the middle ear, and permits equilibration of air pressure with atmospheric pressure in the middle ear. Mechanical or functional obstruction of the eustachian tube can result in middle-ear effusion. Intrinsic mechanical obstruction can result from infection or allergy and extrinsic obstruction from obstructive adenoids or nasopharyngeal tumors. Persistent collapse of the eustachian tube during swallowing can result in functional obstruction related to decreased tubal stiffness, and inefficient active opening mechanism, or both. Functional obstruction is common in infants and younger children because the amount and stiffness of the cartilage support of the tube are less than that in older children and adults. Since the eustachian tube is intimately involved with muscles attached to the soft palate and since it is part of the skull base, patients with anomalies in these areas, such as cleft palate patients and children with Down syndrome, have a much higher incidence of eustachian tube dysfunction and chronic otitis media with effusion.

Eustachian tube obstruction results in negative middle-ear pressure and, if persistent, in a sterile transudative middle-ear effusion. Drainage of the effusion is inhibited by impaired mucociliary transport and by sustained negative pressure. When the eustachian tube is not totally obstructed mechanically, contamination of the middle-ear space from nasopharyngeal secretions may occur by reflux (especially when the tympanic membrane has a perforation or when a tympanostomy tube is present), by aspiration (from high negative middle-ear pressure), or by insufflation during crying, nose blowing, sneezing, and swallowing when the nose is obstructed. Rapid alterations in ambient pressure or barotrauma during deep water diving or flying can also result in acute middle-ear effusion that may be hemorrhagic. Infants and young children have a shorter eustachian tube than older children and adults, which makes them more susceptible to reflux of nasopharyngeal secretions into the middle-ear space and to the development of acute otitis media.

Young children suffer an increased frequency of viral upper respiratory tract infections. These infections probably lead to edema of the eustachian tube mucosa, causing increased eustachian tube dysfunction. Reactive enlargement of lymphoid tissue, such as the adenoids or tissue at the eustachian tube orifice, may also mechanically block tube function and provide a site of inflammation. The presence of viral infection has been shown to increase bacterial adhesion in nasopharyngeal tissue. There has been a significant increase in the number of children in child care centers in the United States in the past 2 decades, and children in these centers are prone to increased upper respiratory infections. This may account in part for the parallel increase in middle ear problems seen during this time. Elevated levels of cotinine, a metabolite of nicotine, also have been correlated with an increased incidence of both otitis media with effusion and acute otitis media in children, indicating that passive exposure to cigarette smoke increases ear problems, probably by acting as an irritant to respiratory epithelium and having an adverse effect on ciliary motion and mucociliary clearance. Children with well-documented allergies appear to have approximately the same incidence of recurrent ear problems as those without allergies. However, on an individual basis, allergic factors probably do play a part in at least some children's recurrent ear infections.

Young children have an immature, developing immune system, which is probably another factor leading to a high incidence of otitis in this age group; however, studies assaying quantitative immunoglobulin levels and IgG subclass levels have shown no differences between children with and without recurrent ear infections. Trials of prophylactic intravenous immunoglobulin in children with recurrent otitis media have shown conflicting results. There does appear to be an increased incidence of humoral immune problems affecting respiratory epithelium in children who have failed prophylactic antibiotics or ventilation tube placement and who have had recurrent infections involving the sinonasal or the lower respiratory tract.

590.1 Acute Otitis Media

CLINICAL MANIFESTATIONS. In the usual course, a child suffering an upper respiratory infection for several days suddenly develops otalgia, fever, generalized discomfort, and hearing loss. Fever occurs in approximately one third to one half of these patients. In infants, the symptoms may be less localizing and include irritability, diarrhea, vomiting, or malaise. Examination with the pneumatic otoscope reveals a hyperemic, opaque, bulging tympanic membrane of poor mobility; purulent otorrhea may be present, but earache and fever are not invariably present (Fig. 590–1). Children with diminished or absent mobility and opacification of the tympanic membrane should be suspected of having bacterial otitis media with effusion. Any child with a fever without a focus must also be evaluated for a middle-ear infection (Chapter 167).

DIAGNOSIS. The diagnosis of otitis is based on visualization of

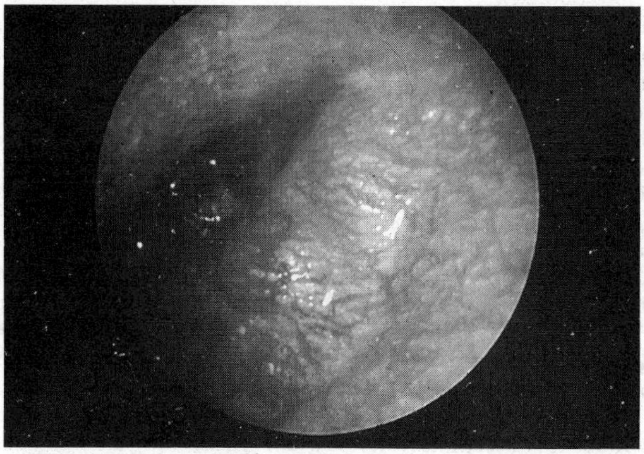

Figure 590–1. Acute left otitis media. See also color section.

the tympanic membrane. In some children who have small ear canals or large amounts of cerumen or who are very uncooperative, this may be a difficult undertaking. The outer portion of the ear canal has cushioning soft tissue, cartilage, and skin adnexal structures including modified sweat glands that produce cerumen. The skin of the inner half of the ear canal is a very thin squamous epithelium overlying periosteum and bone and is exquisitely sensitive to touch. The epithelium of the ear canal has a unique migratory function, growing from the tympanic membrane and medial external auditory canal laterally so there is a natural, built-in cleansing function. Although it is important to have an unobstructed view of the tympanic membrane, home use of cotton swabs or instruments such as bobby pins will often push wax farther into the ear canal, with the potential of traumatizing the canal or the eardrum itself. Physicians examining the ear should try to manipulate only the less sensitive outer portion of the ear canal, if possible. Cerumen should be gently cleaned by using a fine wire loop through the open or operating head of an otoscope. Gentle syringe irrigation of the ear canal and use of commercial cerumen-loosening products may be helpful. Commercial products for removing wax should not be used if there is a question of a tympanic membrane perforation and should not be left in the ear of a young child longer than a few minutes before the ear is irrigated (see Chapter 586). When the diagnosis of acute otitis media is doubtful or identification of the causative agent is desirable, aspiration of the middle ear should be performed. Tympanocentesis should also be considered in the following: for seriously ill children or those who appear toxic; for children who respond unsatisfactorily to antibiotic therapy; for an onset of otitis media in a patient receiving antibiotic agents; for patients who develop suppurative intratemporal or intracranial complications; and for otitis in the newborn, the very young infant, or the immunologically deficient patient, in each of whom unusual organisms may cause infection.

DIFFERENTIAL DIAGNOSIS. A red tympanic membrane is associated with an infectious process; however, a normal eardrum can turn red in a crying child, just as his or her cheeks turn red. An eardrum immobile on pneumatic otoscopy indicates the presence of significant negative pressure or fluid. A retracted tympanic membrane may move better with negative pressure. Potential structural damage to the eardrum should also be identified. Focal thickening of the eardrum that is associated with chronic infections and prior ventilation tube placement is called *tympanosclerosis*. This is a hyaline degeneration of the middle fibrous layer of the tympanic membrane that may be calcified. If there has been a prior perforation or ventilation tube placement, the tympanic membrane may heal without this normal middle fibrous layer. The resulting thinned portion of the eardrum is prone to retraction when negative middle ear pressure is present. The most superior portion of the tympanic membrane is called the pars flaccida. In this location, the collagen bundles are less well organized, and the eardrum is more prone to retraction. Deep retraction pockets may lead to squamous epithelium within the middle ear and mastoid cavities, causing a *cholesteatoma* that may grow in size by the enzymatic activity of the skin tissues and by accumulation of squamous debris within the cholesteatoma.

TREATMENT. Therapy depends on the bacterial cause of the disease and on the results of antibacterial susceptibility testing. The most common infecting organism for acute otitis media is *Streptococcus pneumoniae*. The next two major pathogens are untypable *Haemophilus influenzae* and *Moraxella catarrhalis*. A variety of other bacteria account for the remaining small percentage of infections (Fig. 590–2). These may include both gram-positive and gram-negative bacteria. In neonates over 2 wk old, *S. pneumoniae* and *H. influenzae* continue to be the most common infecting organisms. However, in infants less than 2 wk old or in those still hospitalized, gram-negative bacteria, *Staphylococcus aureus*, and group B *Streptococcus* become more common.

Oral amoxicillin is the initial antibiotic of choice when the causative organism is unknown because it is usually effective against the most commonly encountered bacteria. It is administered: 40 mg/kg/24 hr tid for 10 days. However, nearly all *M. catarrhalis* and 25% of *H. influenzae* are resistant to amoxicillin. In addition, increasing incidence of penicillin resistance has been noted in *S. pneumoniae*, and multiply resistant *S. pneumoniae* have been identified worldwide. There also is a concern for the increasing incidence of the multiply resistant *S. pneumoniae* associated with frequent use of antibiotics in children in close physical contact, such as in child care centers. Therefore, for patients who have recently taken amoxicillin or who live in areas with a high incidence of β-lactamase–mediated resistance, there are a variety of other antibiotics available to treat acute otitis media in children. These agents vary in efficacy for each bacterium as well as in taste and expense (Table 590–1). If otitis media does not appear to be responding to an antibiotic, it is reasonable to switch to another class of drug. If there is clinical deterioration or if a resistant organism is likely (immunosuppressed patient, multiple prior antibiotics), a tympanocentesis should be performed to identify the infecting organism (see Chapter 586). When a resistant organism is cultured from a middle-ear aspirate or from otorrhea, or when the patient fails to improve clinically after initial amoxicillin treatment (probably because of an ampicillin-resistant bacterium) and if a tympanocentesis or myringotomy is not performed, the initial antimicrobial agent should be changed. Appropriate choices may be erythromycin (50 mg/kg/24 hr) combined with a sulfonamide (100 mg/kg/24 hr of triple sulfonamides or 150 mg/kg/24 hr of sulfisoxazole) qid, trimethoprim-sulfamethoxazole (8 and 40 mg/kg/24 hr) bid, cefaclor (40 mg/kg/24) tid, amoxicillin-clavulanate (40 mg/kg/24) tid, cefuroxime axetil (125–250 mg/24 hr) bid, or cefixime (8 mg/kg/24 hr) once daily or bid. If the patient is allergic to the penicillins, the combination of oral erythromycin and triple sulfonamides or sulfisoxazole is an alternative. Combined trimethoprim-sulfamethoxazole can also be given initially to penicillin-sensitive individuals, but its effectiveness in treating acute otitis media caused by *Staphylococcus pyogenes* or resistant strains of *S. pneumoniae* is uncertain. Sulfonamide combinations have a high rate of adverse side effects, which on rare occasion have been serious and even fatal. The administration of cefaclor has been associated with a serum sickness-type reaction.

Additional supportive therapy, including analgesics, antipyretics, and local heat, is usually helpful. Meperidine hydrochloride may also be required for sedation. An oral decongestant (e.g., pseudoephedrine hydrochloride) may relieve some nasal congestion and antihistamines may help patients with known or suspected nasal allergy. The efficacy of antihistamines and decongestants in the treatment of acute otitis media, however, is not established.

In patients with unusually severe earache, myringotomy may be performed initially to provide immediate relief. When therapeutic drainage is required, a myringotomy knife should be used and the incision made large enough to allow for adequate drainage of the middle ear.

If the patient's clinical manifestations of acute infection increase during the 1st 24 hr despite antimicrobial therapy a concurrent infection such as meningitis or a suppurative complication of otitis media should be suspected. The child should be re-examined and tympanocentesis and myringotomy performed. Similarly, if the patient continues to have appreciable pain, fever, or both after 24–48 hr, tympanocentesis and myringotomy should be performed as diagnostic and therapeutic procedures; identification of the organism(s) is recommended at this stage but, when a diagnostic aspiration is not performed, antimicrobials effective against resistant organisms prevalent in the community should be administered.

All patients should be re-evaluated approximately 2 wk after the institution of treatment, at which time there should be some otoscopic evidence of resolution, such as a decrease in

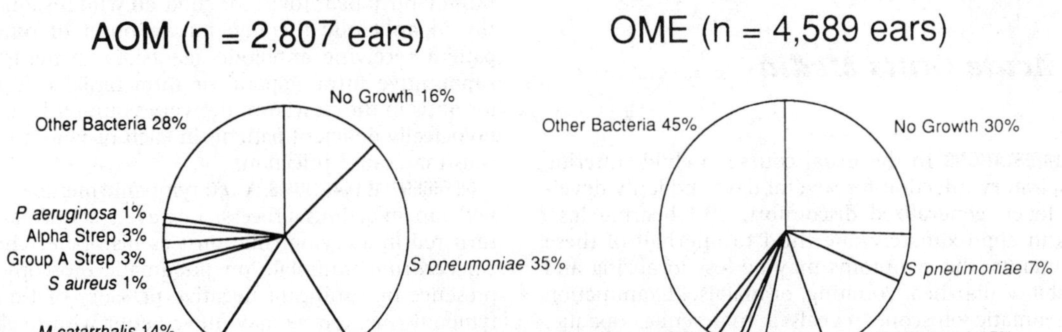

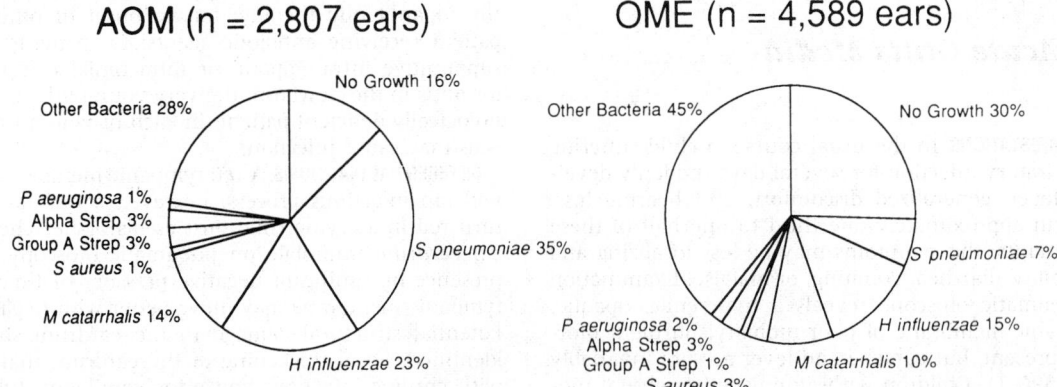

Figure 590–2. Comparison of distribution of isolates in 2807 effusions from patients with acute otitis media and 4589 effusions from patients with otitis media with effusion at the Pittsburgh Otitis Media Research Center between 1980 and 1989. *AOM*, acute otitis media; *OME*, otitis media with effusion. (Total percentages are greater than 100% because of multiple organisms.) (From Bluestone CD, Klein JO: Otitis Media in Infants and Children, 2nd ed. WB Saunders, Philadelphia, 1995.)

■ **TABLE 590–1 Features of Commonly Used Oral Antibiotics for Acute Otitis Media**

	Susceptibility				
	Streptococcus pneumoniae[1]	***Haemophilus influenzae***[2]	***Moraxella catarrhalis***[2]	***Dosage***	***Palatability***[3]
Amoxicillin	+++	−	−	TID	++++
Amoxicillin-clavulanate	+++	+++	+++	TID	++
Ceclor	+++	+	+++	BID/TID	+++
Cefuroxime axetil	++	+++	+++	BID	+
Cefixime	+	+++	+++	QD	++++
Cefpodoxime Proxetil	++	+++	+	BID	++
Cefprozil	+++	+++	+++	BID	+++
Loracarbef	++	++	+++	BID	++++
Trimethoprim-sulfamethoxazole	++	+++	+++	BID	++
Clarithromycin[4]	++	++	++	BID	+

[1]*Does not include pencillin-resistant strains.*
[2]*For penicillinase-producing strains (*H.flu 25%, M.cat. >80%*).*
[3]*Personal reports from patients and parents.*
[4]*The primary metabolite is most effective against* H. influenzae.

inflammation and return of mobility of the tympanic membrane. Periodic follow-up is indicated for patients who have had recurrent episodes. If the middle-ear fluid is persistent, the patient should be treated as described in the next section.

590.2 Persistent Middle-Ear Effusion

If the middle-ear effusion persists after the initial 10–14 days of antimicrobial therapy for acute otitis media, one or more of the following options have been advocated for use during the next, subacute phase, but none of these have been demonstrated to be effective in randomized, controlled trials: (1) a course of an antimicrobial different from the initial agent (the new antimicrobial agent may be effective against an organism resistant to the previous one); (2) a topical or systemic nasal decongestant, antihistamine, or combination of these drugs; (3) systemic corticosteroids; and (4) eustachian tube-middle-ear-inflation. Many clinicians do not treat children who have asymptomatic (except for hearing loss) middle-ear effusion still present after 2 wk, but rather re-examine the child 6 wk later—that is, 2 mo after the initial visit—at which time most patients are effusion-free. Treatment with another antimicrobial, such as cefaclor, trimethoprim-sulfamethoxazole, erythromycin-sulfisoxazole, amoxicillin-clavulanate, cefuroxime axetil, or cefixime, which are effective against resistant bacteria, may be indicated if the child has any signs or symptoms of persistent infection, such as otalgia, or if such organisms have been isolated from subacute effusions in the community.

590.3 Recurrent Acute Otitis Media

Some children develop recurrent acute episodes of otitis media with almost every respiratory tract infection, have more or less dramatic symptoms, respond well to therapy, and have fewer episodes with advancing age. Others have persistent middle-ear effusion and suffer recurrent episodes of acute otitis media superimposed on the chronic disorder. The child with recurrent acute otitis media that completely clears between episodes may be managed as previously outlined, but if the bouts are frequent and close together, further evaluation similar to that described below for patients having chronic otitis media with effusion is indicated. In many of these children the underlying cause is not evident, but prophylactic antibiotics (a daily dose of amoxicillin, 20 mg/kg/24 hr, or sulfonamides, 50 mg/kg/24 hr) may be effective in some children when administered over a period of several months, usually through the winter. Myringotomy and ventilating tubes may also be effective but should be reserved for patients in whom antimicrobial prophylaxis following an etiologic diagnosis of the organisms in the effusion fails to prevent recurrent acute otitis media with hearing loss or in whom chemoprophylaxis is not desirable because of allergy to the penicillins or the sulfonamides. The preventive efficacies of antimicrobial chemoprophylaxis and myringotomy with tympanotomy tube insertion have been demonstrated in clinical trials. Adenoidectomy is usually of no benefit for the prevention of recurrent acute otitis media. However, immunization with the polyvalent pneumococcal vaccine may be effective when administered to patients above 2 yr of age.

590.4 Otitis Media with Effusion

Otitis media with effusion is a middle-ear effusion lacking the clinical manifestations of acute infection, such as otalgia and fever. It follows successfully treated acute otitis media and clears by 3 mo in 90% of children after the first episode of otitis media. The duration (not the severity) of the effusion can be divided into acute (less than 3 wk), subacute (3 wk-3 mo), and chronic (greater than 3 mo). The effusions may be serous (thin), mucoid (thick), and purulent.

CLINICAL MANIFESTATIONS. Frequently, either a retracted or convex tympanic membrane is seen. The membrane is usually opaque but, when it is translucent, an air-fluid level or air bubbles may be seen and an amber or sometimes bluish fluid may be apparent in the middle ear (Fig. 590–3). The mobility of the eardrum is almost always impaired. Occasionally, even when there is little effusion, the tympanic membrane is retracted and its mobility impaired, usually because of negative middle-ear air pressure; when extreme, this is termed "atelectasis of the tympanic membrane." There is no associated erythema unless the child is crying vigorously and the tympanic membrane has turned pink, in which case a differentiation

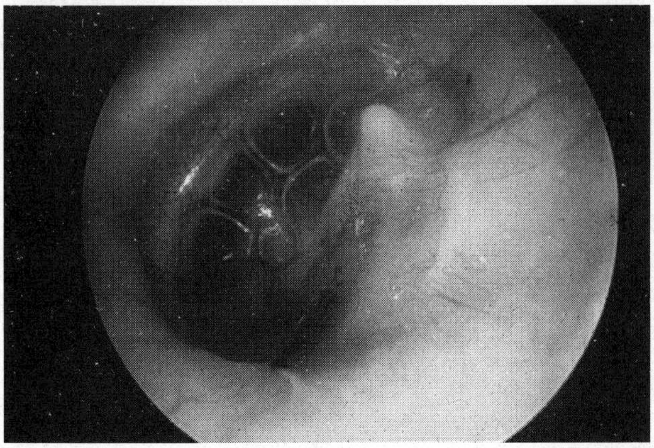

Figure 590–3. Otitis media with effusion of left ear. Retracted ear drum, prominent short process of malleus, and air bubbles seen anteriorly through the tympanic membrane. See also color section.

from acute otitis media may be difficult. The auditory acuity is usually decreased and, although systemic symptoms are generally absent, there may be behavioral disturbances resulting from the child's inability to communicate adequately. A feeling of fullness in the ear, tinnitus, and even vertigo may be present. Some patients, even with thick middle-ear effusions, can hear fairly well; tympanometry is more reliable than audiometry.

TREATMENT. Treatment may not be indicated, because little is known about the possible complications and sequelae associated with this condition or its treatments, and because most of these effusions usually resolve spontaneously with observation and control of environmental risk factors. However, although the significance of hearing loss is uncertain, such a loss may impair cognitive and language development and result in disturbances in psychosocial adjustment. Because of these uncertainties, some clinicians believe treatment is indicated under certain conditions. For example, treatment may be indicated for a child with bilateral chronic middle-ear effusions and a marked hearing loss, although treatment may not be necessary for a child having a unilateral, asymptomatic otitis media with effusion and only a mild hearing loss, without serious secondary changes in the tympanic membrane. In addition to conductive or sensorineural hearing loss, other conditions to be considered in deciding whether to treat and which therapy to use include the following: (1) occurrence of otitis media with effusion in young infants who are unable to communicate about their symptoms and may have suppurative disease; (2) an associated purulent upper respiratory tract infection; (3) vertigo; (4) alterations of the tympanic membrane such as severe atelectasis, especially a deep retraction pocket in the posterosuperior quadrant, the pars flaccida, or both; (5) middle-ear changes such as adhesive otitis or ossicular involvement; (6) when the effusion persists for 3 mo or longer; and (7) when the episodes frequently recur, resulting in an accumulation of an excessive amount of effusion over many months.

One of the most popular treatments for otitis media with effusion, an orally administered combination of a decongestant and antihistamine, has been shown to be ineffective in infants and children with acute, subacute and chronic otitis media with effusion. The efficacy of topical intranasal and systemic corticosteroid therapy is unproven, and the risks of corticosteroid therapy generally outweigh the possible benefits. However, even though the efficacy of immunotherapy and allergy control has not been established for children with evidence of upper respiratory allergy, this method of management seems reasonable for those who have frequent recurrent otitis media with effusion. Inflation of the eustachian tube, using the method of Politzer or employing the Valsalva maneuver, is also ineffective in children with chronic otitis media with effusion.

Either observation or a trial of antibiotics and control of environmental risk factors are indicated treatment options for children with acute or subacute effusions (Fig. 590–4). Because bacteria similar to those found in acute otitis media have been isolated from a significant proportion of middle-ear aspirates in children with otitis media with effusion, the antibiotic chosen and duration of treatment should be the same as that recommended for acute otitis media (see Fig. 590–2). In clinical trials, both amoxicillin and amoxicillin-clavulanate have been shown to be significantly more effective than placebo; recommended treatment is for 10–30 days in therapeutic doses. The efficacy of other antimicrobial agents for the treatment of this stage of otitis media has not been demonstrated adequately in clinical trials.

If the effusion persists for 3 mo or longer (chronic), or if there have been frequent recurrences of episodes of acute otitis media, the patient requires further evaluation for hearing loss, respiratory allergy, adenoid tissue obstructing the nose and nasopharynx, and immunologic disorder (if other organs are involved), or abnormalities such as submucous cleft palate or a tumor of the nasopharynx. If none of these conditions is present, further observation or antibiotic therapy and control of environmental risk factors are appropriate alternatives. If there is significant hearing loss myringotomy with insertion of tympanostomy tubes is an additional option, after a trial of antibiotics. Effusion persisting for 4–6 mo, following an adequate course of antibiotics, with significant hearing loss (especially bilateral) is an indication for myringotomy and insertion of tympanostomy tubes (Fig. 590–4). The rationale for this procedure is to improve middle ear ventilation. It is the most frequent surgical procedure performed on children in the United States.

Myringotomy and the insertion of ventilation tubes may also be helpful in patients with atelectasis of the tympanic membrane when pain, hearing loss, vertigo, or tinnitus is present. Ventilation tubes may prevent permanent structural damage and cholesteatoma if a deep retraction pocket develops in the posterosuperior quadrant or in the attic (pars flaccida) portion of the tympanic membrane. The efficacy of ventilation tubes in these various circumstances, however, is not proven. Furthermore, troublesome otorrhea occasionally develops after the insertion of tubes and can usually be treated successfully with ear drops containing neomycin, polymyxin, or colistin with hydrocortisone. If otitis media occurs, it should be treated with systemic antibiotics. Because these medications may be ototoxic, some physicians use systemic antibiotics without the aural drops. Myringotomy with aspiration of the middle-ear effusion may be appropriate in those children in whom the procedure can be performed without the aid of a general anesthetic. A second myringotomy may be indicated if the effusion is still present soon after the myringotomy incision heals (i.e., if the disease is persistent).

Adenoidectomy for chronic otitis media with effusion may benefit some children, but others spontaneously improve, and still other patients have persistent disease despite adenoid or tonsil surgery. Because the effectiveness of adenoidectomy for chronic otitis media with effusion apparently is not related to adenoid size, the selection of children who might benefit from adenoidectomy at present must be related to the potential benefits weighed against the costs and potential risks. For children who have recurrent or chronic otitis media with effusion and who had had one or more myringotomy and tympanostomy tube operations in the past, adenoidectomy may be a reasonable option. The presence of upper airway obstruction, recurrent acute or chronic adenoiditis, or both conditions are

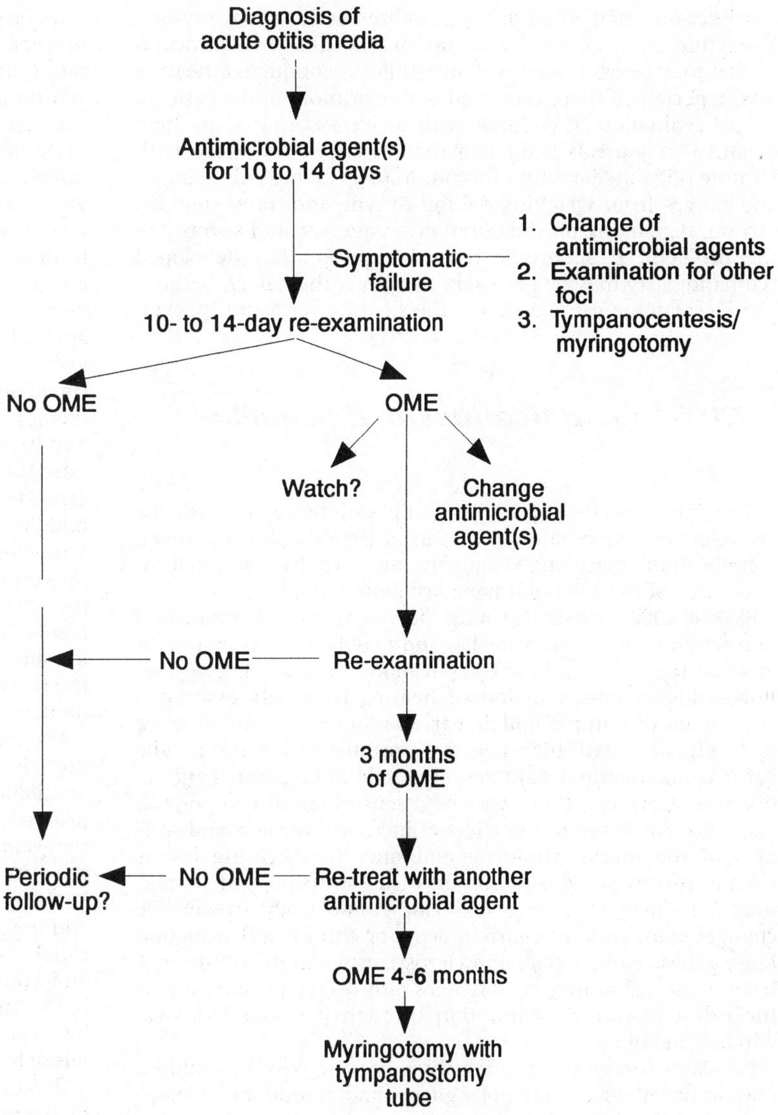

Figure 590–4. Recommended management plan for children with acute otitis media. Otitis media with effusion (OME). (Modified from Bluestone CD, Klein JO.: Otitis Media in Infants and Children, 2nd ed. WB Saunders, Philadelphia, 1995.)

also more compelling indications in the consideration of adenoidectomy for children who have chronic otitis media with effusion.

590.5 Atelectasis of the Tympanic Membrane–Middle Ear and High Negative Pressure

Atelectasis of the tympanic membrane may be acute or chronic, generalized or localized, and mild or severe. The tympanic membrane may be retracted or collapsed. High negative pressure may be present or absent. When middle-ear effusion is also present the clinical picture is the same as when acute or chronic otitis media is present. In such cases it is not unusual to visualize a severely retracted malleus through the otoscope in association with a tympanic membrane that is full or even bulging in the posterior portion. The malleus is retracted by concurrent high negative middle-ear pressure, chronic inflammation of the tensor tympani muscle or the malleolar ligaments, or both, whereas the hydrostatic pressure of the effusion (not completely filling the middle ear-mastoid air cell system) results in bulging of the most compliant (floppy) portion of the pars tensa, the posterosuperior and posteroinferior quadrants. Frequently an effusion is evident by the presence of an air-fluid level or bubbles behind a severely retracted tympanic membrane.

There may not be specific otologic symptoms with or without effusion. The child may have a severely retracted translucent tympanic membrane with evidence of high negative pressure by pneumatic otoscopy (immobile to applied positive pressure and decreased or absent mobility to applied negative pressure) or a high negative middle-ear pressure tracing on the tympanogram. The otoscopist can look through the tympanic membrane and see that there is no effusion present. Some children with such an otoscopic (and tympanometric) examination may not have any complaint, whereas others may have a feeling of fullness in the ear, otalgia, tinnitus, hearing loss, and even vertigo. The condition may be self-limited and in some it may be physiologic because of temporary eustachian tube obstruction. In others, however, especially those with symptoms, the condition is pathologic and should be managed in a manner similar to that employed when an effusion is present.

When there is localized atelectasis or a retraction pocket, especially in the pars flaccida or posterosuperior portion of the pars tensa of the tympanic membrane, the condition may be more serious than when only generalized atelectasis is present. The child may be totally asymptomatic but the retraction pocket may be associated with a significant conductive hearing loss, especially if there is erosion of one or more of the ossicles.

The evaluation of children with atelectasis caused by high negative pressure is similar to that described for those with chronic otitis media with effusion. Management is also similar and ranges from watchful waiting to tympanostomy tube insertion, depending on the duration, frequency, and severity of the problem. If a chronic retraction pocket has developed tympanoplasty may be necessary to correct the defect, because a cholesteatoma can develop at the site of a retraction pocket.

590.6 Complications and Sequelae

The intracranial suppurative complications of otitis media are relatively uncommon except in neglected cases. However, complications occurring within the aural cavity and adjacent structures of the temporal bone are more common.

HEARING LOSS. This is the most prevalent complication, and morbid outcome of otitis media, and may be caused by one or more of the intratemporal complications. To a varying degree, fluctuating or persistent loss of hearing is usually associated with acute or chronic middle-ear effusions or, in the absence of an effusion, with high negative pressure within the middle ear. The audiogram usually reveals a mild to moderate conductive loss. However, there may be a sensorineural component, generally attributed to the effect of increased tension and stiffness of the round window membrane. This hearing loss is usually reversible with resolution of the effusion, but permanent conductive hearing loss can result from irreversible changes secondary to recurrent acute or chronic inflammation (e.g., adhesive otitis, tympanosclerosis, ossicular discontinuity). Irreparable sensorineural loss may also occur, presumably as the result of spread of infection through the round or oval window membrane.

Persistent or episodic conductive hearing loss in children may impair their cognitive, language, and emotional development, but the degree and duration of the hearing loss required to produce such deficits are unknown. The accumulated results of many studies suggest that children do suffer such long-term effects from otitis media early in life. The scientific evidence, however, remains incomplete. Some experts are skeptical about the available data and have concluded that no causal link can be established between early, recurrent, middle-ear effusion and language delay or learning problems. Several studies, however, have shown an association between early otitis media and later deficits. Prolonged durations of middle-ear effusions, which are associated with significant loss of hearing, may be detrimental to the child's ability to develop speech and language optimally when the otitis media occurs early in life.

PERFORATION. Perforation of the tympanic membrane most frequently occurs when the central portion of the eardrum spontaneously ruptures during an episode of acute otitis media. In addition, a large number of temporary perforations are created by the surgical treatment of otitis media with tympanostomy tubes. Over 1 million tympanostomy tubes are inserted annually for the treatment of recurrent acute otitis media and otitis media with effusion, and approximately two thirds of these children develop otorrhea once or more while the tubes are in place and patent. The organisms most frequently cultured from the aural discharge, which occurs through a perforation by tympanostomy tube when acute otitis media is present, are the same as those cultured from acute middle-ear effusions when a tympanocentesis was performed (e.g., *S. pneumoniae, H. influenzae* and *M. catarrhalis*). *S. pyogenes*, when present and untreated, has been associated with acute, spontaneous perforation of the tympanic membrane.

Antimicrobial therapy for patients with acute perforation of the eardrum is the same as that for acute otitis media when a perforation is not present. When an aural discharge is present, however, it may be desirable to culture the drainage. The antimicrobial regimen can then be adjusted according to the results of the Gram stain, culture, and antibiotic susceptibility testing. The patient may also benefit from otic drops instilled into the external canal. Ototopical medication is usually beneficial when infectious eczmatoid external otitis is present. The application of an antibiotic-cortisone otic medication whenever a discharge is present has been advocated by many clinicians, despite the possibility of ototoxicity, because the topical medication may treat or prevent an external canal infection and hasten the resolution of the middle-ear infection. In addition, the ototopical drops may prevent bacteria in the external canal (e.g., staphylococci and *Pseudomonas*) from entering the middle ear and causing a chronic infection. Healing of the tympanic membrane frequently follows cessation of the suppurative process in the middle ear, but the perforated tympanic membrane may remain open after an episode of acute otitis media. When the perforation is present with no signs of healing and there are no signs of otitis media for several months, the perforation is considered to be chronic and possibly permanent.

The management of noninfected chronic perforations in children is difficult and controversial. The perforation provides ventilation and drainage of the middle ear, but the physiologic protective function of the eustachian tube and middle-ear system is impaired. The middle ear and mastoid air cells no longer have an air cushion to prevent nasopharyngeal secretions from entering the ear, which can result in reflux otitis media. In addition, the middle ear may be infected from the external canal, especially when swimming and bathing. Many infants and young children may benefit by the open tympanic membrane but, for patients over 5 yr of age, the perforation should be evaluated for repair (i.e., tympanoplasty) to restore the eustachian tube-middle-ear air cushion.

If otorrhea persists despite adequate antimicrobial therapy, or if the drainage seems to be coming from an apparent posterosuperior or attic (pars flaccida) defect, a cholestratoma should be suspected. Aural polyps, which appear as red, friable masses, may protrude through one of these defects, indicating the presence of a cholesteatoma.

CHRONIC SUPPURATIVE OTITIS MEDIA WITH MASTOIDITIS. In this stage of ear disease there is chronic infection of the middle ear and mastoid (mastoiditis), a nonintact tympanic membrane (because of perforation or tympanostomy tube), and discharge (otorrhea). It develops from a chronic bacterial infection, but the bacteria that caused the initial episode of acute otitis media with perforation are usually not those that are isolated from the chronic discharge. The most common bacterial species isolated are *P. aeruginosa* and *S. aureus*. The most common anaerobic species isolated are *Bacteroides, Peptostreptococcus*, and *Peptococcus*. Thus, the antimicrobial therapy recommended for acute otitis media is not effective for most cases of chronic suppurative otitis media. Tympanomastoid surgery is indicated when cholesteatoma is present.

The medical treatment of chronic suppurative otitis media without cholesteatoma is directed toward eliminating the infection from the middle ear and mastoid. Antimicrobial agents should be selected for effectiveness against the cultured organisms. Because of the high prevalence of *P. aeruginosa*, suspensions that contain polymyxin B, neomycin, and hydrocortisone (Cortisporin), or neomycin, polymyxin E, and hydrocortisone (ColyMycin), have been recommended, but their potential ototoxicity limits their usefulness. In children, orally administered antibiotics are usually not effective unless an organism is seen on Gram stain or is cultured from the discharge that is susceptible to a specific antibiotic, such as *S. aureus*, pneumococcus, or *H. influenzae*. Ciprofloxacin, a new oral antimicrobial agent with activity against most organisms that cause chronic suppurative disease (including *Pseudomonas*), may be effective, but this drug is *not* indicated for patients below the age of 17 yr.

Because of concern over the toxicity of the ototopical agents, patients and parents should be informed of their potential danger if they are used. If a topical antibiotic medication is used, the patient should return to the outpatient facility daily so that the discharge can be thoroughly aspirated. The discharge rapidly improves with this type of treatment, usually within 1–2 wk.

As an alternative, it is recommended that children be given a parenteral β-lactam antipseudomonal drug, such as ticarcillin. The middle ear is aspirated daily. In most children, the middle ear is free of discharge and the signs of otitis media greatly improved or absent within 7–10 days.

When the discharge fails to respond to intensive medical therapy, surgery on the middle ear and mastoid is indicated. In a study of 36 pediatric patients with chronic suppurative otitis media, in which all received parenteral antimicrobial therapy and daily aural cleansing, 32 children (89%) had their initial infection resolved with medical therapy alone and 4 (11%) required tympanomastoidectomy.

If the infection is eliminated using these methods, prevention of recurrence is usually achieved by the following: (1) prophylactic antimicrobial therapy; (2) removal of the tympanostomy tube; or (3) surgical repair of the tympanic membrane defect. The appropriate choice depends on the age of the patient and the function of the eustachian tube.

ACQUIRED CHOLESTEATOMA. This sac-like structure within the middle ear is lined by keratinized, stratified, squamous epithelium and contains desquamated epithelium or keratin. White, shiny, greasy debris accompanied by a foul-smelling discharge may be observed. Tympanomastoid surgery is indicated but if it is delayed, the disease can invade and destroy other structures of the temporal bone and spread to the intracranial cavity. A retraction pocket is a deformity of the tympanic membrane that is usually caused by persistent or fluctuating high negative middle-ear pressure, and can progress into cholesteatoma.

MASTOIDITIS. Mastoiditis is classified into acute and chronic forms. Acute mastoiditis is further subdivided into pathologic stages, which are the basis for management. In almost every child with acute otitis media the mastoid air cells are also inflamed; thus, acute mastoiditis is a natural extension and part of the pathologic process of the acute middle-ear infection. No specific signs or symptoms of the mastoid infection are present in this most common stage of acute mastoiditis. The hearing loss, otalgia, and fever are primarily the result of the acute infection within the middle ear. CT scans of the mastoid area are usually interpreted as "cloudy mastoids," which is indicative of the general inflammation. No mastoid osteitis is evident on the CT scan. The process is usually reversible because the middle-ear-mastoid effusion resolves, either as a natural process or as a result of treatment of the acute infection. If resolution of the infection does not occur at this stage, one or more of the following conditions may develop: (1) acute mastoiditis with periosteitis; (2) acute mastoid osteitis (with or without a subperiosteal abscess); or (3) chronic mastoiditis.

Acute Mastoiditis With Periosteitis. This occurs when the infection within the mastoid air cells spreads to the periosteum covering the mastoid process, causing periosteitis. The condition should not be confused with the presence of a subperiosteal abscess, because the management of the latter condition requires incision and drainage of the abscess and a complete simple (cortical) mastoidectomy; the former, however, usually responds to immediate but less aggressive surgical intervention.

When acute mastoiditis with periosteitis occurs in the absence of roentgenographic evidence of osteitis of the mastoid, management consists of hospitalization, immediate tympanocentesis (for aspiration and microbiologic assessment of the middle-ear-mastoid effusion), and myringotomy for drainage of the system. The insertion of a tympanostomy tube is desirable and enhances drainage over a longer period than myringotomy alone. Parenteral antimicrobial agents should be administered as described in the section on acute mastoid osteitis (see later).

Resolution of the periosteal involvement should occur within 24–48 hr after the tympanic membrane has been opened for drainage and appropriate antimicrobial therapy has begun. Surgical drainage of the mastoid—complete simple mastoidectomy—should be performed if the symptoms of the acute infection, such as fever and otalgia, persist, if the postauricular involvement does not progressively improve, or if a subperiosteal abscess develops.

Failure to institute immediate treatment at this stage may result in the development of acute mastoid osteitis with or without a subperiosteal abscess or, more dangerous to the child, a suppurative intratemporal or intracranial complication such as lateral sinus thrombosis, extradural abscess, or meningitis.

ACUTE MASTOID OSTEITIS (ACUTE COALESCENT MASTOIDITIS, ACUTE SURGICAL MASTOIDITIS). This occurs when the infection within the mastoid progresses, causing destruction of the bony trabeculae that separate the mastoid cells and coalescence of the cells. A mastoid empyema is present. The primary clinical manifestations include swelling, redness, and tenderness to touch over the mastoid bone. The pinna is displaced outward and downward, and swelling or sagging of the posterosuperior canal wall may also be present. A purulent discharge may issue through a perforation in the tympanic membrane. Ear drainage may be persistent and the ear canal filled with pus and debris. Alternatively, there may be a nipple-like protrusion at the site of the tympanic membrane perforation. A fluctuant subperiosteal abscess or even a drainage fistula from the mastoid to the postauricular area may be present. The patient may be toxic and febrile, with systemic signs of acute illness. In the subacute disease, fever may be prolonged and low grade, with occasional temperature spikes. When no clinical signs of extension of pus from the mastoid are evident, CT scans of the mastoids must be obtained to rule out the presence of an acute mastoid osteitis. Any infant or child with a fever of unknown origin also may require CT scans of the mastoids to eliminate the possibility that the fever is caused by acute mastoid osteitis (without otitis media).

The diagnosis should be suspected on the basis of clinical signs. CT scans of the mastoid area may reveal one or more of the following: (1) haziness, distortion, or destruction of the mastoid outline; (2) fuzziness of the shadows of cellular walls as a result of demineralization, atrophy, and/or ischemia of the bony septa; (3) a decrease in the density and cloudiness of the areas of pneumatization because of inflammatory swelling of the air cells; and (4) in longstanding cases, a chronic osteoblastic inflammatory reaction that may obliterate the cellular structure. Small abscess cavities in sclerotic bone may be confused with pneumatic cells. CT scans may also be helpful in ruling out the coexistence of other suppurative intratemporal or intracranial complications of otitis media.

Antimicrobial agents are the mainstay of treatment of acute disease. If the case is otherwise uncomplicated (i.e., there was no prior infection), *S. pneumoniae* or *H. influenzae* is probably responsible, and a 2nd- or 3rd-generation cephalosporin should be used (see Chapters 175 and 176). A complete, simple ("cortical") mastoidectomy should also be performed, especially when the mastoid empyema has extended outside the mastoid bone. The procedure should be considered an emergency, but the timing of the operation must depend on the status of the child. Failure to control infection during the acute stage of mastoid osteitis may lead to a chronic infection within the mastoid bone or to a suppurative complication.

Chronic Mastoiditis. Chronic mastoiditis is invariably associated with chronic suppurative otitis media. The mastoid may be poorly pneumatized or sclerotic. The chronic infection should be controlled by medical treatment, but when extensive granulation tissue and osteitis in the mastoid are present, mastoidectomy is usually necessary to eliminate the chronic mastoid osteitis, especially if a cholesteatoma is present.

PETROSITIS. This may result from acute or chronic infections of the pneumatized apical and perilabyrinthine cells of the temporal bone. The triad of otitis media, paralysis of the external rectus muscle, and pain in the homolateral orbit or retroorbital area with headache constitutes petrous apicitis, i.e., Gradenigo syndrome.

ADHESIVE OTITIS. This is the result of healing following chronic inflammation of the middle ear. The mucous membrane is thickened by proliferation of fibrous tissue, which frequently impairs the movement of the ossicles and results in an irreversible conductive hearing loss.

TYMPANOSCLEROSIS. This is a complication of chronic middle-ear inflammation characterized by whitish plaques in the tympanic membrane and nodular deposits in the submucosal layers of the middle ear. There is hyalinization with deposition of calcium and phosphate crystals and conductive hearing loss may result from the ossicles embedding in the deposits. Prevention is the only successful means of controlling this disease and adhesive otitis media.

OSSICULAR DISCONTINUITY. This is the result of rarefying osteitis secondary to chronic middle-ear inflammation. The long process of the incus is commonly involved, but the crural arch of the stapes, the body of the incus, or the manubrium of the malleus may also be eroded. The conductive hearing loss that frequently results can be corrected surgically.

FACIAL PARALYSIS. This may occur during an episode of acute otitis media because of exposure of the facial nerve from a congenital bony dehiscence within the middle ear. When it occurs as an isolated complication, a myringotomy should be performed and parenteral antibiotics administered. The paralysis usually improves rapidly without further surgery (i.e., facial nerve decompression). Mastoidectomy is not indicated unless mastoid osteitis is present. However, immediate surgical intervention is indicated when a facial paralysis develops in a child who has chronic suppurative otitis media with or without cholesteatoma.

SUPPURATIVE LABYRINTHITIS. This may occur during an episode of acute otitis media from the direct invasion of bacteria through the round or oval windows. When chronic otitis media is present the infection may penetrate the windows or enter through a fistula of the bony horizontal semicircular canal. There may be vertigo, nystagmus, tinnitus, hearing loss, nausea, and vomiting. Treatment consists of intensive parenteral antibiotic therapy, but labyrinthectomy may be indicated to prevent spread to the intracranial cavity.

CHOLESTEROL GRANULOMA. Cholesterol granuloma is a sequela of chronic otitis media with effusion. It has been described as "idiopathic hemotympanum," because the tympanic membrane appears to be dark blue. The treatment of choice is middle-ear and mastoid surgery.

NECK ABSCESS. Neck muscles such as the sternocleidomastoid and posterior belly of the digastric attach to the mastoid tip, and occasionally, a mastoid infection will break through deep to these muscles and present as an abscess in the neck called a *Bezold's abscess*. In all cases of cervical infection, it is important to visualize the tympanic membrane and to consider the possible role of otitis media and mastoiditis.

INFECTIOUS ECZEMATOID DERMATITIS. This may be associated with an infection of the external auditory canal (see Chapter 589), or may occur secondary to a discharge from the middle ear and mastoid. Management should be directed toward resolving the middle ear-mastoid infection.

INTRACRANIAL SUPPURATIVE COMPLICATIONS. The incidence of suppurative intracranial complications of otitis media has declined because of the use of antimicrobial agents. They now occur most often in association with chronic suppurative otitis media and mastoiditis, with or without cholesteatoma. The middle-ear and mastoid air cells are adjacent to important structures, including the dura of the posterior and middle cranial fossa, the sigmoid venous sinus of the brain, and the inner ear. Suppuration in the middle ear or mastoid, or both, may spread to these structures through progressive thromboplebitis, bony erosion, or direct extension, resulting in meningitis, extradural abscess, subdural empyema, focal encephalitis, brain abscess, lateral (sigmoid) sinus thrombosis, and otic hydrocephalus. Multiple complications frequently depend on the route of infection. For example, a patient may have meningitis, lateral sinus thrombosis, and a cerebellar abscess.

Any child with acute or chronic otitis media who develops one or more of the following signs or symptoms, especially while receiving medical treatment, should be suspected of having a suppurative intracranial complication: persistent headache, lethargy, malaise, irritability, change in personality, severe otalgia, persistent or recurrent fever, nausea, and vomiting. Fever is rarely present in children with chronic suppurative otitis media; when present, it should suggest an impending intracranial complication. The following are definitive clinical manifestations requiring an intensive search for an intracranial complication: stiff neck, focal seizures, ataxia, blurred vision, papilledema, diplopia, hemiplegia, aphasia, dysdiadochokinesia, intention tremor, dysmetria, and hemianopsia. Conversely, children with intracranial infection, such as meningitis or a brain abscess, should have middle-ear-mastoid disease ruled out as the origin of, or concomitant with, the central nervous system disease.

The diagnosis of intracranial complications is greatly improved by the use of CT scanning, but, when unavailable, arteriography should be used. Magnetic resonance imaging (MRI) also provides excellent definition of intracranial suppuration and its consequences (e.g., edema, thrombosis, hydrocephalus), but it does not provide the bony detail needed to evaluate the mastoid.

MENINGITIS. Meningitis may occur because of the following: (1) direct invasion, in which a suppurative focus in the middle ear or mastoid spreads through the dura and extends to the pia-arachnoid, causing generalized meningitis; (2) suppuration in an adjacent area, such as a subdural abscess, brain abscess, or lateral sinus thrombophlebitis, which causes the meninges to become inflamed, and (3) concurrent infection, in which otitis media arises by contiguous spread from an infectious focus in the upper respiratory tract, and meningitis results from invasion of the blood from the upper respiratory focus. The latter is the most common route. The infections are simultaneous, but meningitis does not arise from the middle-ear infection. See Chapter 169.1.

EXTRADURAL ABSCESS. Extradural (epidural) abscess usually results from the destruction of bone adjacent to dura by cholesteatoma, infection, or both. This occurs when granulation tissue and purulent material collect between the lateral aspect of the dura and adjacent temporal bone. Dural granulation tissue within a bony defect is more common than an actual accumulation of pus. When an abscess is present a dural sinus thrombosis or, less commonly, a subdural or brain abscess, may also be present. If extensive bony destruction has occurred because of acute mastoid osteitis (acute coalescent mastoiditis), an extradural abscess may develop in the area of the sigmoid dural sinus.

Clinical manifestations may include severe earache, low-grade fever, and headache in the temporal region with deep local throbbing pain. There may be no signs or symptoms. An asymptomatic extradural abscess may be found in patients undergoing elective mastoidectomy for cholesteatoma. When otorrhea occurs, it is characteristically profuse, creamy, and pulsatile. Compression of the ipsilateral jugular vein may increase the rate of discharge and the degree of pulsation. Usually, there is no accompanying fever (but malaise and anorexia may be observed), no neurologic signs, the intracranial pressure is normal, and it is difficult to detect any displacement of the brain. The cerebrospinal fluid cell count and pressure are normal unless meningitis is also present. CT scanning may reveal a large extradural abscess.

The *treatment* of extradural abscess consists of surgical drainage. A mastoidectomy is performed, enough bone is removed so that the dura of the middle and posterior fossae may be inspected directly, the extradural abscess is identified and removed (and sometimes a drain is also inserted), and the otologic procedure that can provide optimal exteriorization of the diseased area is completed by removing all the granulation tissue until normal dura is found.

SUBDURAL EMPYEMA. A subdural empyema is a collection of purulent material within the potential space between the dura externally and arachnoid membrane internally. It may develop as a direct extension of infection or, more rarely, by thrombophlebitis through venous channels. It is a rare complication of otitis media and mastoiditis (see also Chapter 169.1).

Children with subdural empyema are extremely toxic and febrile. There are usually the signs and symptoms of a locally expanding intracranial mass. Severe headache in the temporoparietal area is usually present. Central nervous system findings may include seizures, hemiplegia, dysmetria, belligerent behavior, somnolence, stupor, deviation of the eyes, dysphagia, sensory deficits, stiff neck, and a positive Kernig sign. Hemiplegia and jacksonian epilepsy in a child with suppurative disease of the middle ear and mastoid usually indicate a subdural empyema. CT scanning is often diagnostic. The peripheral white blood cell count is high and there is a predominance of polymorphonuclear leukocytes. The cerebrospinal fluid glucose concentration is normal and no microorganisms are seen on smear or culture of the cerebrospinal fluid.

Treatment of subdural empyema includes intensive intravenous antimicrobial therapy, anticonvulsants, and neurosurgical drainage of the empyema through burr holes or craniectomy. Corticosteroids are occasionally needed to diminish severe edema. Mastoid surgery to locate and drain the source of infection is usually delayed until after neurosurgical intervention has yielded some improvement in neurologic status. The condition has a high mortality rate, and more than 50% of children who recover have some residual neurologic deficit.

FOCAL OTITIC ENCEPHALITIS. Edematous and inflamed focal areas of brain may occur as a complication of acute or chronic otitis media or of the other suppurative complications of these disorders. The signs and symptoms of this focal otic encephalitis may be similar to those of a brain abscess or subdural empyema, except that the suppuration within the brain is absent. Ataxia, nystagmus, vomiting, and giddiness suggest a possible focus within the cerebellum, whereas drowsiness, disorientation, restlessness, seizures, and coma suggest a cerebral focus. At both sites, headache may be present. CT and/or needle aspiration may be necessary to eliminate the presence of an abscess. If an abscess is not present, the focal encephalitis should be treated by administering antimicrobial agents and by carrying out an appropriate otologic surgical procedure to remove the source of infection as soon as possible. Failure to control the source of the infection within the temporal bone, as well as the focal encephalitis, may result in the development of a brain abscess. Anticonvulsive medication is given when there is cerebral involvement.

OTOGENIC BRAIN ABSCESS (also see Chapter 554). Otogenic abscess of the brain may result directly from acute or chronic middle-ear and mastoid infection (with or without cholesteatoma) or may follow the development of an adjacent infection, such as lateral sinus thrombophlebitis, petrositis, or meningitis. The dura overlying the infected mastoid is invaded along vascular pathways or by adherence of the dura to underlying infected bone. Chronic otitis media or mastoiditis (with or without cholesteatoma) may lead to erosion of the tegmen tympani by pressure necrosis and perforation of the bone, with resultant inflammation of the dura and invasion by pathogenic organisms. An extradural abscess occurs with subsequent infiltration of the dura and spreads to the subdural space. A localized subdural abscess or leptomeningitis ensues. Invasion of brain tissue follows. The abscess is located closest to the primary source of infection. Thus, temporal lobe abscesses occur following invasion through the tegmen tympani or petrous bone. Cerebellar abscesses occur when the infectious focus is the posterior surface of the petrous bone or thrombophlebitis of the lateral sinus. The former occurs more frequently than the latter, and multiple abscesses are not uncommon.

Signs and symptoms of invasion of the central nervous system usually occur about 1 mo after an episode of acute otitis media or an acute exacerbation of chronic otitis media. Most children are febrile, although systemic signs, including fever and chills, vary and may be absent. Signs of a generalized central nervous system infection include severe headache, vomiting, drowsiness, seizures, irritability, personality change, altered levels of consciousness, anorexia and weight loss, and meningismus. Temporal lobe abscesses are associated with seizures in some children, may be associated with visual field deficits (e.g., optic radiation involvement), or may be silent. Cerebellar abscesses cause vertigo, nystagmus, ataxia, dysmetria, and symptoms of hydrocephalus. There may be persistent purulent ear drainage, suggesting the primary site of infection. See Chapter 554 for treatment.

LATERAL SINUS THROMBOSIS. Lateral and sigmoid sinus thrombosis or thrombophlebitis arises from inflammation in the adjacent mastoid. The superior and petrosal dural sinuses are also intimately associated with the temporal bone, but are rarely affected. The mastoid infection in contact with the sinus walls produces inflammation of the adventitia followed by penetration of the venous wall. Formation of a thrombus occurs after the infection has spread to the intima. The mural thrombus may become infected and propagate, occluding the lumen. Embolization of septic thrombi or extension of infection into the tributary vessels may cause further disease. This complication is still common in children, and can be caused by both acute and chronic otitis media and mastoiditis.

The clinical signs of lateral sinus thrombosis include the following: (1) general—fever, headache, and malaise (with the formation of the infectious mural thrombus, the patient may have spiking fever and chills); (2) central nervous system—headache, papilledema, signs of increased intracranial pressure, altered states of consciousness, and seizures; (3) metastatic disease caused by infected thrombi and septic infarcts—pneumonia, septic infarcts, empyema, bone and joint infection, and, less commonly, thyroiditis, endocarditis, ophthalmitis, and abscess of the kidney; (4) spread to skin and soft tissues—cellulitis or abscess; and (5) signs of intracranial complications, including meningitis, cavernous sinus thrombosis, and brain abscess.

CT and MRI are invaluable in making the diagnosis, and their use should precede a lumbar puncture. Variations in cerebrospinal fluid pressure can occur, so demonstration by the Queckenstedt test is contraindicated because of the risk of herniation. In some cases, there is leakage of red cells and subsequent xanthochromia may occur.

Treatment includes the use of antimicrobial agents and surgery. The administration of anticoagulant medication is controversial because of the risks of releasing septic emboli or causing uncontrollable hemorrhage in the mastoid. The sinus should be uncovered and any perisinuous abscesses drained. The lateral sinus should be opened and the thrombus removed if there is septic thrombophlebitis.

OTITIC HYDROCEPHALUS. Otic hydrocephalus is a syndrome of increased intracranial pressure without other abnormalities of the cerebrospinal fluid, complicating acute otitis media. The pathogenesis is unknown, but, because the ventricles are not dilated, the term "benign intracranial hypertension" may also be appropriate. The disease is frequently associated with lateral sinus thrombosis. Symptoms include a headache that is often intractable, blurring of vision, nausea, vomiting, and diplopia. Signs include a draining ear, abducens paralysis of one or both lateral rectus muscles, and papilledema.

CT should be performed prior to lumbar puncture to prevent brain herniation. The cerebrospinal fluid pressure is sometimes above 300 mm H_2O, and the ventricles are of normal or small size. Although usually benign, otic hydrocephalus may proceed to loss of vision secondary to optic atrophy (see Chapter 542.11).

Treatment includes the use of antimicrobial agents, mastoidectomy, normalization of intracranial pressure by medications (e.g., acetazolamide, furosemide), repeated lumbar punctures, or a lumboperitoneal shunt. An aggressive approach is warranted because of the possibility of optic atrophy.

CHAPTER 591

Inner Ear and Diseases of the Bony Labyrinth

The inner ear may be affected by viral or bacterial infections. Congenital rubella, cytomegalovirus, and mumps are causes of severe sensorineural deafness.

Labyrinthitis may be a complication of acute or chronic otitis media and mastoiditis but may also follow bacterial meningitis as a result of organisms entering the labyrinth through the internal auditory meatus, endolymphatic duct, vascular channel, or perilymphatic duct. Clinical manifestations may include vertigo, disequilibrium, deep seated pain, nausea, vomiting, and sensorineural hearing loss. Acute suppurative labyrinthitis requires intensive antimicrobial therapy, and may, in the absence of meningitis, require otologic surgery. Chronic labyrinthitis, most commonly caused by a cholesteatoma also requires surgery.

Otosclerosis, an autosomal dominant disease, can cause a fixation of the stapes, resulting in progressive hearing loss in older children and teenagers. A hearing aid may be necessary. Corrective surgery is more successful and permanent in adults than in children.

Osteogenesis imperfecta may involve both the middle and inner ears. If the hearing loss is severe enough, a hearing aid is a preferable alternative to surgical correction of the fixed stapes, because the disease is progressive.

Osteoporosis may involve the middle ear, resulting in a moderate to severe hearing loss. A hearing aid may be necessary for rehabilitation.

CHAPTER 592

Traumatic Injuries of the Ear and Temporal Bone

AURICLE AND EXTERNAL AUDITORY CANAL

Hematoma, or accumulation of blood between the perichondrium and the cartilage, may follow trauma to the pinna. Immediate needle aspiration or, when the hematoma is extensive, incision and drainage and a pressure dressing are necessary to prevent perichondritis, which can result in a cauliflower ear deformity.

Frostbite of the auricle should be managed by rapidly rewarming the exposed pinna with warm irrigation or warm compresses.

Foreign bodies in the external canal are common in childhood. These can usually be removed without general anesthesia if the child is informed of the procedure (if old enough to understand it), if the child is properly restrained, when an adequate headlight or surgical head otoscope is used for visualizing the object, and when an alligator forceps, wire loop, or blunt cerumen curet is used, depending on the shape of the object. Irrigation is sometimes helpful. General anesthesia and the otomicroscope are necessary for the removal of more difficult foreign bodies, especially those deeply embedded in the canal just lateral to the tympanic membrane. Following removal of the external canal foreign body, the tympanic membrane should be carefully inspected for possible traumatic perforation or for a pre-existing middle-ear effusion. If the foreign body has resulted in acute inflammation of the canal, treatment as described for acute diffuse external otitis should be instituted.

TYMPANIC MEMBRANE AND MIDDLE EAR

Traumatic perforation of the tympanic membrane usually occurs as the result of a sudden external compression (e.g., a slap) or penetration by a foreign object (e.g., a stick or cotton-tipped applicator). The perforation may be linear or stellate and is most frequently in the anterior portion of the pars tensa when it is caused by compression; it may be in any quadrant of the tympanic membrane when caused by a foreign object. Spontaneous healing usually occurs but, if the drum does not heal within 2–3 mo, tympanoplastic surgery is indicated. Systemic antibiotics and topical otic medications are not required unless suppurative otorrhea is present. However, otorrhea may occur at any time during periods of upper respiratory tract infection, because the middle-ear air cushion is lost, permitting reflux of nasopharyngeal secretions into the middle-ear cavity. Perforations resulting from penetrating foreign bodies are less likely to heal than those caused by compression. Implantation of epithelium from a traumatic perforation can result in a cholesteatoma. Immediate surgical exploration is indicated if the injury is accompanied by one or more of the following: vertigo, nystagmus, severe tinnitus, moderate to severe hearing loss, or cerebrospinal fluid otorrhea. Exploratory tympanotomy is necessary to inspect the ossicles, especially the stapes, that may have been dislocated.

Perilymphatic fistula may occur following sudden barotrauma or increase in cerebrospinal fluid pressure. This condition is probably more common than generally appreciated and should always be suspected in a child who develops a sudden or fluctuating sensorineural hearing loss, vertigo, or both, following physical exertion, deep water diving, flying in an airplane, playing a wind instrument, or any other activity that suddenly increases the pressures within the middle ear or the intracranial-labyrinthine system. Characteristically, the leak is at the oval or the round window, which may be congenitally abnormal; immediate repair of the fistula is essential, because the hearing loss may become irreversible.

TEMPORAL BONE FRACTURES

Children are particularly prone to basilar skull fractures, which usually involve the temporal bone. Most temporal bone fractures are longitudinal and are commonly manifested by the following: bleeding from a laceration of the external canal and tympanic membrane or, if the drum is intact, a hemotympanum; conductive hearing loss resulting from the laceration of the tympanic membrane, hemotympanum, or ossicular injury; delayed onset of facial paralysis (which usually improves spontaneously); and temporary cerebrospinal fluid otorrhea. Transverse fractures of the temporal bone have a graver prognosis than longitudinal fractures and are associated with the following: immediate facial paralysis, which may not improve without surgical intervention; severe sensorineural hearing loss, vertigo, nystagmus, tinnitus, nausea, and vomiting associated with complete loss of cochlear and vestibular function; hemotympanum and, rarely, external canal bleeding; and cerebrospinal otorrhea, seen either in the external auditory canal or behind the tympanic membrane, which may come through the nose via the eustachian tube.

Vigorous removal of external auditory canal blood clots, tympanocentesis, and application of otic preparations are not indicated, but prophylactic parenteral administration of antibiotics when cerebrospinal otorrhea is present has been advocated. Surgical intervention is reserved for children who require tympanoplastic repair of the perforated tympanic membrane (that fails to heal spontaneously), who have suffered dislocation of the ossicular chain, or who need decompression of the facial nerve. Sensorineural hearing loss can also occur following a blow to the head without an obvious fracture of the temporal bone (labyrinthine concussion).

ACOUSTIC TRAUMA

This results from exposure to high-intensity sound (e.g., fireworks, gunfire, rock music) and is manifested by a depression at 4,000 Hz on the audiometric examination. The loss is usually temporary but may become permanent if the noise exposure is chronic. Avoiding chronic exposure to loud noise and protecting the ear against unavoidable exposure are preventive measures.

CHAPTER 593

Tumors of the Ear and Temporal Bone

Benign tumors of the external canal include osteoma and monostotic and polyostotic fibrous dysplasia. Osteomas present as bony masses in the canal and require removal only if hearing is impaired or external otitis results.

Eosinophilic granuloma of the middle ear should be suspected when there are otalgia, otorrhea, hearing loss, and roentgenographic findings of a sharply delineated destructive lesion of the temporal bone.

Rhabdomyosarcoma originating in the middle ear should be considered when there is bleeding from the ear or otorrhea associated with paralysis of the facial nerve.

Non-Hodgkin lymphoma and leukemia may also present in the middle ear. Although primary neoplasms of the middle ear are relatively uncommon, the initial signs and symptoms of the more common nasopharyngeal neoplasms (e.g., angiofibroma, rhabdomyosarcoma, epidermoid carcinoma) may be associated with the insidious onset of a chronic otitis media with effusion (see Part XXII).

GENERAL REFERENCES

American Academy of Otolaryngology—Head and Neck Surgery Subcommittee on cochlear implants. Status of cochlear implantation in children. J Pediatr 118:1, 1991.

American Academy of Pediatrics: Joint Committee on Infant Hearing [Position statement 1994]. Pediatrics 95:152, 1995.

American Academy of Pediatrics: Managing otitis medias with effusion in young children. Pediatrics 94:766, 1994.

Arola M, Ziegler T, Ruuskanen O: Respiratory virus infection as a cause of prolonged symptoms in acute otitis media. J Pediatr 116:697, 1990.

Bergstrom L: Infectious agents that deafen. *In*: Bess FH (ed): Hearing Impairment in Children. Parkton, MD, York Press, 1988.

Bess FH (ed): Hearing Impairment in children. Parkton, MD, York Press, 1988.

Bluestone CD, Klein JO: Otitis Media in Infants and Children. Philadelphia, WB Saunders, 1995.

Bluestone CD, Klein JO: Intracranial suppurative complications of otitis media and mastoiditis. *In*: Bluestone CD, Stool SE (eds): Pediatric Otolaryngology, 2nd ed. Philadelphia, WB Saunders, 1990, pp 537–546.

Bluestone CD, Klein JO: Intratemporal complications and sequelae of otitis media. *In*: Bluestone CD, Stool SE (eds): Pediatric Otolaryngology, 2nd ed. Philadelphia, WB Saunders, 1990, pp 487–536.

Bluestone CD, Klein JO: Otitis media, atelectasis, and eustachian tube dysfunction. *In*: Bluestone CD, Stool SE (eds): Pediatric Otolaryngology, 2nd ed. Philadelphia, WB Saunders, 1990, pp 320–486.

Brookhouser PE, Moeller MP: Choosing the appropriate habilitative track for the newly identified hearing-impaired child. Ann Otol Rhinol Laryngol 95:51, 1986.

Carlin SA, Marchant CD, Shurin PA, et al: Host factors and early therapeutic response in acute otitis media. J Pediatr 118:178, 1991.

Clinical Practice Guideline No. 12: Otitis media with effusion in young children. U.S. Dept of HHS, Public Health Services. Agency for Health Care Policy and Research, 1994. Publication No. 94–0622, Rockville, MD.

Glasscock ME, McKennan KX, Levine SC: Differential diagnosis of sensorineural hearing loss in children. *In*: Bess FH (ed): Hearing Impairment in Children. Parkton, MD, York Press, 1988, pp 1–14.

Konigsmark BW, Gorlin RJ: Genetic and Metabolic Deafness. Philadelphia, WB Saunders, 1976.

Mancuso AA, Hanafee WN: Computed Tomography and Magnetic Resonance Imaging of the Head and Neck, 2nd ed. Baltimore, Williams & Wilkins, 1985.

Margolis RH, Heller JW: Screening tympanometry: Criteria for medical referral. Audiology 25:197, 1987.

Matkin ND: Early recognition and referral of hearing-impaired children. Pediatr Rev 6:151, 1984.

Matkin ND: Re-evaluating our approach to evaluation: Demographics are changing—are we? *In*: Bess FH (ed): Hearing Impairment in Children. Parkton, MD: York Press, 1988, pp 101–11.

Nozza RJ, Fria TJ: The assessment of hearing and middle ear function in children. *In*: Bluestone CD, Stool SE (eds): Pediatric Otolaryngology, 2nd ed. Philadelphia, WB Saunders, 1990, pp 125–153.

Rubin IL, Crocker AC: Developmental Disabilities. Lea & Febiger, 1989, Philadelphia.

Shapiro GG, Virant FS, Furukawa CT, et al: Immunologic defects in patients with refractory sinusitis. Pediatrics 87:311, 1991.

Shaver KA. Genetic causes of childhood deafness. *In*: Bess FH (ed): Hearing impairment in children. Parkton, MD, York Press, 1988, pp 15–32.

Vignaud J, Jardin C, Rosen L: The Ear—Diagnostic Imaging. New York, Masson Publishing USA, 1986.

SPECIAL REFERENCES

Berman S, Roark R, Luckey D: Theoretical cost effectiveness of management options for children with persistent middle ear effusions. Pediatrics 93:353, 1994.

Bluestone CD: Otitis media and congenital perilymphatic fistula as a cause of sensorineural hearing loss in children. Pediatr Infect Dis J 7:S141, 1988.

Breiman RF, Butler JC, Tenover FC, et al: Emergence of drug-resistant pneumococcal infections in the United States. JAMA 271:1831, 1994.

Chan KH, Bluestone CD: Lack of efficacy of middle-ear inflation: Treatment of otitis media with effusion in children. Otolaryngol Head Neck Surg 100:317, 1989.

Chan KH, Mandel EM, Rockette HE, et al: A comparative study of amoxicillin-clavulanate and amoxicillin. Arch Otolaryngol 114:142, 1988.

Eilers RE, Oller DK: Infant vocalizations and early diagnosis of severe hearing impairment. J Pediatr 124:199, 1994.

Fria TJ, Cantekin EI, Eichler JA: Hearing acuity of children with otitis media with effusion. Arch Otolaryngol 111:10, 1985.

Gates GA, Avery CA, Prihoda TJ, et al: Effectiveness of adenoidectomy and tympanostomy tubes in the treatment of chronic otitis media with effusion. N Engl J Med 317:1444, 1987.

Hayden GF, Schwartz RH: Characteristics of earache among children with acute otitis media. Am J Dis Child 139:721, 1985.

Hough JVD, Stuart WD: Middle ear injuries in skull trauma. Laryngoscope 78:899, 1968.

Isaacson G, Rosenfeld RM: Care of the child with tympanostomy tubes: A visual guide for the pediatrician. Pediatrics 93:924, 1994.

Kaleida PH, Bluestone CD, Rockette HE, et al: Amoxicillin-clavulanate potassium comparison with cefaclor for acute otitis media in infants and children. Pediatr Infect Dis J 6:265, 1987.

Kaleida PH, Casselbrant ML, Rockette HE, et al: Amoxicillin or myringotomy or both for acute otitis media: results of a randomized clinical trial. Pediatrics 87:466, 1991.

Kenna MA, Bluestone CD, Fall P, et al: Cefixime vs. cefaclor in the treatment of acute otitis media in infants and children. Pediatr Infect Dis J 6:992, 1987.

Kenna M, Bluestone CD, Reilly J: Medical management of chronic suppurative otitis media without cholesteatoma in children. Laryngoscope 96:146, 1986.

Kleinman LC, Kosecoff J, Dubois RW, et al: The medical appropriateness of tympanostomy tubes proposed for children younger than 16 years in the United States. JAMA 271:1250, 1994.

Mandel EM, Rockette HE, Bluestone CD, et al: Efficacy of amoxicillin with and without decongestant-antihistamine for otitis media with effusion in children. N Engl J Med 316:432, 1987.

Mandel EM, Rockette HE, Bluestone CD, et al: Myringotomy with and without tympanostomy tubes for chronic otitis media with effusion. Arch Otolaryngol Head Neck Surg 115:1217, 1989.

Maniglia AJ, Goodwin WJ, Arnold JE, et al: Intracranial abscesses secondary to nasal, sinus and orbital infections in adults and children. Arch Otolaryngol Head Neck Surg 115:1424, 1989.

Odio CM, Kusmiesz H, Shelton S, et al: Comparative treatment trial of augmentin versus cefaclor for acute otitis media with effusion. Pediatrics 75:819, 1985.

Paradise JL, Bluestone CD, Rogers KD, et al: Efficacy of adenoidectomy for recurrent otitis media: Results from parallel random and nonrandom trials. Pediatr Res 21:286A, 1987.

Reichler MR, Allphin A, Breiman R, et al: The spread of multiply resistant *Streptococcus pneumoniae* at a day care center in Ohio. J Infect Dis 166:1346, 1992.

Rosenfeld RM, Vertress JE, Carr J, et al: Clinical efficacy of antimicrobial drugs for acute otitis media: Metaanalysis of 5400 children from thirty-three randomized trials. J Pediatr 124:355, 1994.

Samuel J, Fernandes CMC, Steinberg JL: Intracranial otogenic complications: A persisting problem. Laryngoscope 96:272, 1986.

Shurin PA, Rehmus JM, Johnson CE, et al: Bacterial polysaccharide immune globulin for prophylaxis of acute otitis media in high-risk children. J Pediatr 123:801, 1993.

Teele DW, Klein JO, Rosner BA: Otitis media with effusion during the first three years of life and development of speech and language. Pediatrics 74:282, 1984.

The Medical Letter: Drugs for Treatment of Acute Otitis Media in Children. Vol 36, issue 917, March 4, 1994.

Zorowka PG: Otoacoustic emissions: A new method to diagnose hearing impairment in children. Eur J Pediatr 152:626, 1993.

PART XXXI

The Skin*

CHAPTER 594
Morphology of the Skin

Gary L. Darmstadt and Al Lane

EPIDERMIS. The mature epidermis is a stratified epithelial tissue composed predominantly of *keratinocytes.* The lowest keratinocyte layer, the basal cell layer, is constantly renewing the epidermis by mitotic division of the basal cells. Recent evidence suggests that keratinocyte stem cells originate from hair follicles. Individual keratinocytes mature through a process of epidermal differentiation that results in the barrier portion of the epidermis, the stratum corneum. When composed of mature, differentiated keratinocytes, the stratum corneum is 10–50 μm thick. Damage to the stratum corneum increases skin permeability and may increase the potential for systemic toxicity to topically applied medications or chemicals.

The continuous renewal of the surface keratinocytes of the epidermis normally proceeds in an orderly fashion as the cells of the basal cell layer move upward to the stratum corneum. The total life span from mitotic division of the basal cell until loss from the stratum corneum is approximately 28 days. In hyperproliferative diseases, the movement of the cells is more rapid. The newly arrived keratinocytes in the stratum corneum are not fully differentiated and form a defective barrier. Keratinocytes are joined together by attachment plaques, the desmosomes. Cytoplasmic tonofibrils project to the desmosome and aid in cell attachment. Autoantibodies to various desmosomal adhesion molecules cause acantholysis (detachment of joined keratinocytes with bullae formation).

In addition to keratinocytes, the epidermis contains three additional cell types. The *melanocytes* are pigment-forming cells, which are responsible for skin color. Melanocytes produce melanosomes containing melanin. Epidermal melanocytes are derived from the neural crest and migrate to the skin during embryonic life. They reside in the interfollicular epidermis and in the hair follicles and increase in number in the epidermis by mitosis or migration of additional cells into the epidermis. *Merkel cells* are nerve-associated epidermal cells that may be important in the sensation of touch and in skin development. *Langerhans cells* are dendritic cells of the mononuclear phagocyte system. They contain a specific organelle, the Birbeck granule. These cells are derived from bone marrow and participate in immune reactions in the skin, playing an active role in antigen presentation and processing.

DERMIS. The dermis forms a tough, pliable, fibrous supporting structure between the epidermis and the subcutaneous fat. It consists of collagen and elastic and reticulin fibers embedded in an amorphous ground substance; it contains blood vessels, lymphatics, neural structures, eccrine and apocrine sweat glands, hair follicles, sebaceous glands, and smooth muscle. Morphologically, the dermis can be divided into two layers: the superficial papillary layer that interdigitates with the rete ridges of the epidermis and the deeper reticular layer that lies beneath the papillary dermis. The papillary layer is less dense and more cellular, whereas the reticular layer appears more compact because of the coarse network of interlaced collagen and elastic fibers.

The junction of the epidermis and dermis is the *basement membrane zone.* This complex structure is the result of contributions from both epidermal and mesenchymal cells. The dermoepidermal junction extends from the basal cell plasma membrane to the uppermost region of the dermis. Ultrastructurally, the basement membrane appears as a trilaminar structure, consisting of a *lamina lucida* immediately adjacent to the basal cell plasma membrane, a central *lamina densa,* and the *subbasal lamina* on the dermal side of the lamina densa. Several structures within this zone act to anchor the epidermis to the dermis. The plasma membrane of basal cells contains electron-dense plates known as hemidesmosomes; tonofilaments course within basal cells to insert at these sites. Anchoring filaments originate in the plasma membrane, primarily near the hemidesmosomes, and insert into the lamina densa. Anchoring fibrils, composed predominantly of type VII collagen, extend from the lamina densa into the uppermost dermis where they insert into anchoring plaques. The composition of the basement membrane is the subject of intensive investigation; primary components identified to date include type IV collagen, laminin, heparin sulfate, and nidogen/entactin. Molecular defects in basement membrane components have been shown to underlie several of the blistering diseases (see Chapter 604).

The predominant dermal cell is a spindle-shaped *fibroblast* that is responsible for the synthesis of collagen, elastic fibers, and mucopolysaccharides. Phagocytic histiocytes, mast cells, and motile leukocytes are also present. The gelatinous ground substance serves as a supporting medium for the fibrillar and cellular components and as a storage place for a substantial portion of body water. Nutrients are supplied to both epidermis and dermis by the dermal blood vessels.

SUBCUTANEOUS TISSUE. Panniculus, or subcutaneous tissue, consists of fat cells and fibrous septa that divide it into lobules and anchor it to the underlying fascia and periosteum. Blood vessels and nerves are also present in this layer, which serves as a storage depot for lipid, an insulator to conserve body heat, and a protective cushion against trauma.

APPENDAGEAL STRUCTURES. These structures are derived from aggregates of epidermal cells that become specialized during early embryonic development. Small buds (primary epithelial germs) appear during the 3rd fetal mo and give rise to hair follicles, sebaceous and apocrine glands, and the attachment bulges for the arrector pili muscles. Eccrine sweat glands are derived from separate epidermal downgrowths that arise during the 2nd fetal mo and are completely formed by the 5th mo. Formation of nails is initiated during the 3rd intrauterine mo.

HAIR FOLLICLES. The hair follicle is the most prominent structure in the pilary complex, which includes the sebaceous

*Modified from N. Esterly, 14th edition.

gland, the arrector pili muscle, and, in areas such as the axillae, an apocrine gland. Hair follicles are distributed throughout the skin, except in the palms, soles, lips, and glans penis; if destroyed, they cannot regenerate. Individual follicles extend from the surface of the epidermis to the deep dermis, where the matrix cells with the dermal papilla form a bulbous hair root. The growing hair consists of a bulb and a matrix from which the keratinized hair shaft is generated; the shaft consists of an inner medulla, a cortex, and an outer cuticular layer.

Human hair growth is cyclical, with alternate periods of growth (anagen) and rest (telogen). The length of the anagen phase varies from months to years. At birth, all hairs are in the anagen phase. Subsequent generative activity lacks synchrony, so that an overall random pattern of growth and shedding prevails. Scalp hair usually grows about 1 cm/mo.

The types of hair are fetal lanugo, terminal, and vellus. *Lanugo* hair is thin and short; this hair is shed before term and is replaced by vellus hair by 36–40 wk of gestation. *Terminal hair* is long and coarse and is found on the scalp, beard, eyebrows, eyelashes, axillary, and pubic areas. *Vellus hair* is short, soft, and frequently unpigmented and is distributed over the rest of the body. During puberty, androgenic hormone stimulation causes pubic, axillary, and beard hair to change from vellus hair to terminal hair.

SEBACEOUS GLANDS. These glands occur in all areas except the palms of the hands and soles and dorsa of the feet, but they are most numerous on the face, upper chest, and back. Their ducts open into the hair follicles except on the lips, prepuce, and labia minora, where they emerge directly onto the mucosal surface. These holocrine glands are saccular structures that are often branched and lobulated and consist of a proliferative basal layer of small flat cells peripheral to the central mass of lipidized cells. The latter cells disintegrate as they move toward the duct and form the lipid secretion known as sebum, which consists of cellular debris, triglycerides, phospholipids, and cholesterol esters. Sebaceous glands depend on hormonal stimulation and are activated by androgens at puberty. Fetal sebaceous glands are stimulated by maternal androgens, and their lipid secretion, together with desquamated stratum corneum cells, constitutes the vernix caseosa.

APROCRINE GLANDS. The apocrine glands are located in the axillae, areolae, perianal and genital areas, and the periumbilical region. These large, coiled, tubular structures continuously secrete an odorless milky fluid that is discharged in response to adrenergic stimuli, usually the result of emotional stress. Bacterial decomposition of apocrine sweat accounts for the unpleasant odor associated with perspiration. Apocrine glands remain dormant until puberty when they enlarge and secretion begins in response to androgenic activity. The secretory coil of the gland consists of a single layer of cells enclosed by a layer of contractile myoepithelial cells. The duct is lined with a double layer of cuboidal cells and opens into the pilosebaceous complex. Although apocrine glands do not function in thermoregulation, they are involved in certain disease processes.

ECCRINE SWEAT GLANDS. These glands are distributed over the entire body surface, including the palms and soles, where they are most abundant. Those on the hairy skin respond to thermal stimuli and serve to regulate body temperature by delivering water to the skin surface for evaporation; in contrast, sweat glands on the palms and soles respond mainly to psychophysiologic stimuli.

Each eccrine gland consists of a secretory coil located in the reticular dermis or subcutaneous fat and a secretory duct that opens onto the skin surface. Sweat pores can be identified on the epidermal ridges of the palm and fingers with a magnifying lens but are not readily visualized elsewhere. Two types of cells compose the single-layered secretory coil: small dark cells and large clear cells; these rest on a layer of contractile myoepithelial cells and a basement membrane. The glands are supplied by sympathetic nerve fibers, but the pharmacologic mediator of sweating is acetylcholine rather than epinephrine. Sweat consists of water, sodium, potassium, calcium, chloride, phosphorus, lactate, and small quantities of iron, glucose, and protein. The composition varies with the rate of sweating but is always hypotonic in normal children.

NAILS. Nails are specialized protective epidermal structures that form convex, translucent, tight-fitting plates on the distal dorsal surfaces of the fingers and toes. The nail plate, which is derived from a metabolically active matrix of multiplying cells situated beneath the posterior nail fold, grows forward at the rate of approximately 1 cm every 3 mo. The nail plate is bounded by the lateral and posterior nail folds; a thin eponychium (the cuticle) protrudes from the posterior fold over a crescent-shaped white area called the lunula. The pink color reflects the underlying vascular bed.

Goldsmith LA: Physiology, Biochemistry, and Molecular Biology of the Skin, 2nd ed. New York, Oxford University, 1991.

CHAPTER 595
Evaluation of the Patient

Al Lane and Gary L. Darmstadt

HISTORY AND PHYSICAL EXAMINATION. Although many skin disorders are recognized easily by simple inspection, a painstaking history and physical examination are often necessary for accurate assessment. In all cases, the entire body surface, mucous membranes, conjunctiva, hair, and nails should be examined thoroughly under adequate illumination. The color, turgor, texture, temperature, and moisture of the skin and the growth, texture, caliber, and luster of the hair and nails should be noted. Skin lesions should be palpated, inspected, and classified on the bases of morphology, size, color, texture, firmness, configuration, location, and distribution. One must also decide whether the changes are those of the primary lesion itself or whether the clinical pattern has been altered by a secondary factor such as infection, trauma, or therapy.

Primary lesions are classified as macules, papules, nodules, tumors, vesicles, bullae, pustules, wheals, and cysts. A *macule* represents an alteration in skin color but cannot be felt. When larger than 1 cm, the term *patch* is used. *Papules* are palpable solid lesions smaller than 0.5–1 cm, whereas *nodules* are larger in diameter. *Tumors* are usually larger than nodules and vary considerably in mobility and consistency. *Vesicles* are raised, fluid-filled lesions less than 0.5 cm in diameter; when larger, they are called *bullae*. *Pustules* contain purulent material. *Wheals* are flat-topped, palpable lesions of variable size and configuration that represent dermal collections of edema fluid. *Cysts* are circumscribed, thick-walled lesions that are located deep in the skin; are covered by a normal epidermis; and contain fluid or semisolid material. Aggregations of papules and pustules are referred to as *plaques*.

Secondary lesions represent what has happened to the skin over time. Primary lesions may change into secondary lesions, or no primary lesion may have existed. Primary lesions are usually more helpful for diagnostic purposes than secondary lesions. Secondary lesions include scales, ulcers, excoriations, fissures, crusts, and scars. *Scales* consist of compressed layers of stratum corneum cells that are retained on the skin surface. *Ulcers* are excavations of necrotic or traumatized tissue. Ulcer-

■ TABLE 595–1 Immunofluorescent Findings in Immune-Mediated Cutaneous Diseases

Disease	Involved Skin	Uninvolved Skin	Direct IF	Indirect IF	Other Antibodies
Dermatitis herpetiformis	Negative	Positive	Granular IgA ± C in papillary dermis	None	IgA antireticulum in 20–70%. Antigliadin antibodies with celiac disease
Bullous pemphigoid	Positive	Positive	Linear IgG and C band in BMZ, occasionally IgM, IgA, IgE	IgG to BMZ in 70%	None
Pemphigus (all variants)	Positive	Positive	IgG in intercellular spaces of epidermis between keratinocytes	IgG to intercellular space	None
Pemphigus foliaceus	Positive	Positive	IgG to desmosomal glycoprotein, desmoglein$_1$	Same as direct IF	None
Herpes gestationis	Positive	Positive	C3 at BMZ, occasionally IgG	IgG anti-BMZ	None
Linear IgA bullous dermatosis (chronic bullous dermatosis of childhood)	Positive	Positive	Linear IgA at BMZ, occasionally C	Low titer, rare IgA, anti-BMZ	None
Discoid lupus erythematosus	Positive	Negative	Linear IgG, IgM, IgA, and C3 and BMZ (lupus band)	None	ANA negative
Systemic lupus erythematosus	Positive	Variable; exposed to sun, 30–50%; nonexposed, 10–30%	Linear IgG, IgM, C3 at BMZ (lupus band)	None	ANA Anti Ro (SSA) Anti-RNP Anti-DNA Anti-Sm
Henoch-Schönlein purpura	Positive	Negative	IgA around vessel walls	None	IgA rheumatoid factor, occasionally

C = complement; IF = immunofluorescent findings; Ig = immunoglobulin; ANA = antinuclear antibody; BMZ = basement membrane zone at the dermoepidermal junction.

ated lesions inflicted by scratching are often linear or angular in configuration and are called *excoriations*. *Fissures* are caused by splitting or cracking; they occur usually in diseased skin. *Crusts* consist of matted, retained accumulations of blood, serum, pus, and epithelial debris on the surface of a weeping lesion. *Scars* are end-stage lesions that can be thin, depressed and atrophic, raised and hypertrophic, or flat and pliable; they are composed of fibrous connective tissue. *Lichenification* is a thickening of skin with accentuation of normal skin lines that is caused by chronic irritation (rubbing, scratching) or inflammation.

If the diagnosis is not clear after a thorough examination, one or more diagnostic procedures may be indicated. Besides those discussed here, others are identified in appropriate subsections (e.g., scrapings of scabies lesions and smears, cultures of vesicles and pustules for detection of virus or bacteria).

BIOPSY OF SKIN. Biopsy of skin by excision is rarely required for diagnosis in children. *Punch biopsy* is a simple, relatively painless procedure and usually provides adequate tissue for examination if the appropriate lesion is sampled. A fresh but well-developed lesion should be selected for removal. The selection of primary lesions is extremely important to obtain an accurate diagnosis. The site of the biopsy should have relatively low risk for damage to underlying dermal structures. Lidocaine (Xylocaine) 1 or 2%, with or without epinephrine, should be injected intradermally with a 27- or 30-gauge needle after cleansing of the site. A punch, 3 or 4 mm in diameter, is pressed firmly against the skin and rotated until it sinks to the proper depth. All three layers (epidermis, dermis, subcutis) should be contained in the plug. The plug should be lifted gently with forceps or extracted with a needle and separated from the underlying tissue with an iris scissors. Bleeding abates with firm pressure and with suturing. The biopsy specimen should be placed in 10% formaldehyde solution (Formalin) for appropriate processing.

WOOD LAMP. The Wood lamp transmits ultraviolet light mainly in a wavelength of 365 nm. The examination, which is performed in a darkened room, is useful in certain superficial fungal infections of the scalp. Blue-green fluorescence is detectable at the base of each infected hair shaft in ectothrix and in some endothrix infections. Scales and crusts may appear pale yellow, but this is not evidence of a fungal infection. Dermatophyte lesions of the skin (tinea corporis) do not fluoresce; macules of tinea versicolor, however, have a golden fluorescence under the Wood lamp. *Erythrasma*, an intertriginous infection due to *Corynebacterium minutissimum* may fluoresce pink-orange, whereas *Pseudomonas aeruginosa* has a yellow-green color under a Wood lamp. Discrete areas of altered pigment can often be visualized more clearly by use of a Wood lamp, particularly if the pigmentary change is epidermal. Hyperpigmented lesions appear darker and hypopigmented lesions, lighter than the surrounding skin.

KOH PREPARATION. This provides a rapid and reliable method for the detection of fungal elements of both yeasts and dermatophytes. Scaly lesions should be scraped at the active border for optimal recovery of mycelia and spores. Vesicles should be unroofed, and the blister top should be clipped and placed on a slide for examination. In tinea capitis, infected hairs must be plucked from the follicle; scales from the scalp do not usually contain mycelia. A few drops of 20% potassium hydroxide are added to the specimen, which is then gently heated over an alcohol lamp until it begins to bubble. As an alternative to heating, DMSO can be included in the potassium hydroxide solution. The preparation is examined under low-intensity light for fungal elements.

TZANCK SMEAR. This is useful in the diagnosis of some viral infections (herpes simplex, varicella, herpes zoster, eczema herpeticum) and for the detection of acantholytic cells in pemphigus. An intact, fresh blister should be ruptured and drained of fluid. The base of the blister is then vigorously scraped with a dull-edged instrument; the material is smeared on a clear glass slide and air dried. Staining with Giemsa stain is preferable, but Wright stain is acceptable. Balloon cells and multinucleated giant cells are diagnostic of herpesvirus infection; acantholytic epidermal cells are characteristic of pemphigus.

The *direct fluorescent assay* is more sensitive and specific. The keratinocytes are scraped from the base of the blister as above. The laboratory stains the slide with labeled antibodies specific for varicella-zoster virus or herpes simplex virus. Observations of the slide with a fluorescence microscope documents the presence of the specific virus within the cells.

IMMUNOFLUORESCENCE STUDIES. Immunofluorescence studies of skin can be used to detect tissue-fixed antibodies to skin components and complement; characteristic staining patterns are specific for certain skin disorders. Serum can be used for the identification of circulating antibodies. Skin biopsies for direct immunofluorescence preparations should be obtained from involved sites except in those diseases for which paralesional skin or uninvolved skin is required (Table 595–1). A punch biopsy is obtained, and the tissue is placed in a special transport medium or immediately frozen in liquid nitrogen for transport or storage. Thin cryostat sections of the specimen are incubated with fluorescein-conjugated antibodies to the specific antigens.

Serum of patients can be examined by indirect immunofluorescence techniques using sections of normal human skin, guinea pig lip, or monkey esophagus as substrate. The substrate is incubated with fresh or thawed frozen serum and then with fluorescein-conjugated antihuman globulin. If the serum contains antibody to epithelial components, its specific staining pattern can be seen on fluorescence microscopy. By serial dilution, the titer of circulating antibody can be estimated.

Gately LE, Nesbitt LT: Update on immunofluorescent testing in bullous diseases and lupus erythematosus. Dermatol Clin 12:133, 1994.

CHAPTER 596

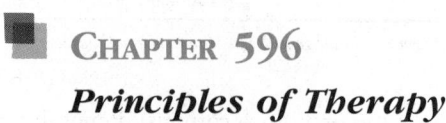

Principles of Therapy

Al Lane and Gary L. Darmstadt

Dermatologic therapy is a mixture of art and science in which the nuances often determine the success of management. Competent skin care requires a specific diagnosis, knowledge of the natural course of the disease, and an appreciation of primary vs secondary lesions. If the diagnosis is uncertain, it is better to err on the side of less rather than more aggressive treatment. Even when the diagnosis is clear, an acute dermatitis may require gentle and bland therapy initially.

In the use of topical medication, consideration of vehicle is as important as the specific therapeutic agent. Acute weeping lesions respond best to wet compresses, followed by lotions or creams. For dry, thickened, scaly skin, an ointment base is more effective. Gels and solutions are most useful for the scalp and other hairy areas. The site of involvement is of considerable importance because the most desirable vehicle may not be cosmetically or functionally appropriate, such as an ointment on the face or hands. The patient's preference should also play a role in the choice of vehicle because compliance is poor if the medication is not acceptable to the patient.

Most *lotions* are mixtures of water and oil that pour. After the water evaporates, the small amount of oil covers the skin. Some *shake lotions* are a suspension of water and insoluble powder; as the water evaporates, cooling the skin, a thin film of powder covers the skin. *Creams* are emulsions of oil and water that are viscous and do not pour (more oil than in lotions). *Ointments* have oils and a small amount of water or no water at all; they feel greasy, lubricate dry skin, trap water, and may be occlusive. Ointments without water usually require no preservatives because microorganisms require water to survive.

Therapy should be kept as simple as possible, and specific written instructions with regard to the frequency and duration of application should be provided. Drug combinations in a single vehicle may exacerbate a dermatitis and cause diagnostic confusion. The physician should become familiar with one or two preparations in each category and should learn to use them appropriately. Careless prescribing of nonspecific proprietary medications that may contain sensitizing agents should be avoided. Certain preparations such as topical antihistamines and sensitizing anesthetics are never indicated.

WET DRESSINGS. These dressings decrease pruritus, burning, and stinging sensations; they are indicated for any acutely inflamed moist or oozing dermatitis. Although a variety of astringent and antiseptic substances may be added to the solution, tap water compresses are just as effective.

Open Wet Dressings. These dressings cool and dry the skin by evaporation and cleanse by removal of crusts and exudate that cause further irritation if permitted to remain. The solution should be cool or tepid and consist of tap water, isotonic saline, or aluminum acetate (Burow solution) in a 1:20 or 1:40 dilution. Potassium permanganate is messy and offers no advantage. Boric acid can be toxic if absorbed and should *never* be used for compresses. Dressings of multiple layers of Kerlix, gauze, or soft cotton material should be saturated with the solution and remoistened as often as necessary. Compresses should be applied for 10–20 min at least every 4 hr and should be continued usually for 24–48 hr.

Closed Wet Dressings. These dressings are indicated for abscesses. The solution should be warm, and the dressings should be covered with plastic to prevent evaporation. Closed wet dressings, if prolonged, cause maceration because they prevent evaporation and heat loss.

BATH OILS, COLLOIDS, SOAPS. *Bath oil* has little benefit in the treatment of children. The bath oil offers little moisturizing effect while increasing the risk of injury during the bath. The bath oil may lubricate the surface of the bathtub, causing the adult or child to fall when they step into the tub. Tar bath solutions (Balnetar, Zetar) can be prescribed and may be helpful for psoriasis and atopic dermatitis. *Colloids* such as starch powder or colloidal oatmeal (Aveeno) are soothing and antipruritic for some patients when added to the bath water. Oilated Aveeno contains mineral oil and lanolin derivatives for lubrication if the skin is dry. These can also lubricate the bathtub surface. Ordinary toilet *soaps* may be irritating and drying if patients have dry skin or dermatitis. Examples of soaps that are usually not harmful to skin are Dove, Lowila, Aveeno, Neutrogena, Basis, Alpha Keri, and Oilatum. When skin is acutely inflamed, avoidance of soap is advised. Some patients find that lipid-free cleansers containing cetyl alcohol (Cetaphil) are soothing.

LUBRICANTS. Lubricants, such as lotions, creams, and ointments, can be used as emollients for dry skin and as vehicles for topical agents such as corticosteroids and keratolytics. In general, ointments are the most effective emollients. Numerous commercial preparations are available in addition to standard items, such as petrolatum, cold cream, stearin-lanolin cream, and hydrophilic ointment. Some patients do not tolerate ointments, and some may be sensitized to a component of the lubricant; some preservatives of creams (most commonly parabens) are sensitizers. Useful lubricating lotions include Lubriderm, Nutraderm, and Nivea. Creams include Eucerin, Neutrogena, Nutraderm, Purpose, Vanicream, and Complex 15. Aquaphor is a cosmetically acceptable alternative to petrolatum. These preparations can be applied several times a day if necessary. Maximal effect is achieved when they are applied *immediately* to damp skin after a bath or shower. Sarna lotion contains menthol and camphor in an emollient vehicle for control of pruritus and dryness.

SHAMPOOS. Special shampoos containing sulfur, salicylic acid, antiseptics, and selenium sulfide (Selsun, Exsel) are useful for conditions in which there is scaling of the scalp. Most shampoos also contain surfactants and detergents. Shampoos with sulfur or salicylic acid include Ionil, Sebulex, Fostex, and Vanseb. Those with only antiseptic agents include DHS-Zinc, Danex, and Head and Shoulders. Tar-containing shampoos such as T-Gel, Ionil-T, Sebutone, and Polytar are useful for psoriasis and severe seborrheic dermatitis. In general, they can be used as frequently as necessary to control scaling, but use should be limited to avoid irritation. Patients should be instructed to leave the lathered shampoo in contact with the scalp for 5–10 min.

SHAKE LOTIONS. These lotions are useful antipruritic agents; they consist of a suspension of powder in a liquid vehicle. A water-dispersible oil may be added for lubrication. Calamine lotion is acceptable but tends to cake on the skin. A prototype lotion is zinc oxide 20 g, talc 20 g, glycerin 20 g, Alpha Keri 5 g, and water to make 120 g. These preparations can be used effectively in combination with wet dressings for exudative dermatitis. Cooling occurs as the lotion evaporates and moisture is absorbed by the powder deposited on the skin.

POWDERS. Powders are hygroscopic and serve as absorptive agents in areas of excessive moisture. When dry, powders decrease friction between two surfaces. They are most useful in the intertriginous areas and between the toes, where maceration and abrasion may result from friction on movement. Coarse powders may cake; therefore, they should be of fine particle size and inert unless medication has been incorporated in the formulation. Zeasorb is a bland, finely milled, general purpose powder that can be applied to any area of the body.

PASTES. These contain a fine powder in an ointment vehicle and are not often prescribed in current dermatologic therapy; in certain situations, however, they can be used effectively to protect vulnerable or damaged skin. For example, a stiff zinc oxide paste is bland and inert and can be applied to the diaper area to prevent further irritation due to diaper dermatitis. Zinc paste should be applied in a thick layer completely obscuring the skin and is removed more easily with mineral oil than with soap and water.

KERATOLYTIC AGENTS. *Urea-containing agents* are hydrophilic; they hydrate the stratum corneum and make the skin more pliable. In addition, because urea dissolves hydrogen bonds and epidermal keratin, it is effective in treatment of scaling disorders. Concentrations of 10–25% are available in several commercial lotions and creams (Carmol 20, Carmol 10, Nutraplus, Aquacare HP), which can be applied once or twice daily as tolerated. *Salicylic acid* is an effective keratolytic agent and can be incorporated into a variety of vehicles in concentrations up to 6% to be applied two to three times daily. Salicylic acid preparations should not be used in the treatment of small infants or on large surface areas or denuded skin; percutaneous absorption may result in salicylism. The *α-hydroxy acids,* particularly *lactic acid* and *glycolic acid,* are available in commercial preparations (Lacticare, LacHydrin, Aqua Glycolic) or can be incorporated in an ointment vehicle such as petrolatum or Aquaphor in concentrations up to 5%. Eucerin Plus Creme contains both urea and lactic acid. The α-hydroxy acid preparations are useful for the treatment of keratinizing disorders and may be applied once or twice daily. Some patients complain of burning; in this case, the frequency of application should be decreased.

TAR COMPOUNDS. Tars are obtained from bituminous coal, shales, petrolatum (coal tars), and wood. They are antipruritic and astringent and appear to promote normal keratinization. They may be useful for chronic eczema and psoriasis, and their efficacy may be increased if the affected area is exposed to ultraviolet (UV) light after the tar has been removed. *Tars should not be used in acute inflammatory lesions.* Tars are often messy and unacceptable because they may stain and they have an odor. Tars may be incorporated into shampoos, bath oils, lotions, and ointments. A useful preparation for pediatric patients is liquor carbonis detergens (LCD) 2–5% in a cream or ointment vehicle. Tar gels (Psorigel, Estargel, Aquatar) and tar in a light body oil (T-Derm) are relatively pleasant cosmetic preparations that cause minimum staining of skin and fabrics. Tars can also be incorporated into a vehicle with a topical corticosteroid. The frequency of application varies from one to three times daily, according to tolerance. Many children refuse to use tar preparations because of their odor and staining characteristics.

ANTIFUNGAL AGENTS. These agents are now available as powders, lotions, creams, and ointments for the treatment of dermatophyte and yeast infections. Nystatin (Mycostatin) and amphotericin B (Fungizone) are specific for *Candida* and are ineffective in other fungal disorders. Tolnaftate (Tinactin) is effective against dermatophytes and is not effective for yeast. The spectrum for haloprogin (Halotex) includes the dermatophytes, *Pityrosporum orbiculare* and *Candida albicans.* The imidazoles, miconazole (Monistat-Derm), clotrimazole (Lotrimin), econazole (Spectazole), and ketoconazole (Nizoral) have a spectrum similar to that of haloprogin. They should be applied one to two times a day for most fungal infections. All these agents have low sensitizing potential; however, additives such as preservatives and stabilizers in the vehicles may cause allergic contact dermatitis. Whitfield ointment (6% benzoic acid and 3% salicylic acid) is a potent keratolytic agent that has also been used for the treatment of dermatophyte infections. Irritant reactions are common.

TOPICAL ANTIBIOTICS. Topical antibiotics have been used to treat local cutaneous infections for many years, although their efficacy, with the exception of mupirocin, has been questioned. Ointments are the preferred vehicle, and combinations with other topical agents, such as corticosteroids, are in general inadvisable. Whenever possible, the etiologic agent should be identified and treated specifically. Antibiotics in wide use as systemic preparations should be avoided because of the risk of sensitization. The sensitizing potential of certain other antibiotics (e.g., neomycin, nitrofurazone [Furacin]) should be kept in mind. Mupirocin (Bactroban) appears to be the most effective topical agent currently available and has been documented to be as effective as oral erythromycin in treatment of impetigo. Polysporin and bacitracin are not as effective as mupirocin or oral antibiotics.

TOPICAL CORTICOSTEROIDS. Topical corticosteroids are potent anti-inflammatory agents and effective antipruritic agents. Successful therapeutic results have been achieved in a wide variety of skin conditions. In general, corticosteroids fall into two classes: nonfluorinated preparations, such as hydrocortisone (Hytone), desonide (Tridesilon, Des Owen), hydrocortisone butyrate (Locoid), and mometasone furoate (Elocon), and fluorinated compounds including triamcinolone (Kenalog, Aristocort), flurandrenolide (Cordran), fluocinolone (Synalar), betamethasone (Valisone, Benisone, Flurobate), and amcinonide (Cyclocort). The nonfluorinated steroids are usually of lesser potency and may cause fewer local and systemic side effects, whereas fluorinated steroids are potentially more harmful, particularly with long-term use. Other fluorinated compounds, for example, fluorocinonide (Lidex), halcinonide (Halog), betamethasone dipropionate (Diprolene), and clobetasol propionate (Temovate), are extremely potent and should be prescribed with care. Some of these compounds are formulated in several strengths based on their clinical efficacy and vasoconstrictive ability. The physician using topical steroids should become familiar with several preparations and be familiar with the potency of the preparations used.

Virtually all corticosteroids can be obtained in a variety of vehicles, including creams, ointments, solutions, gels, and aerosols. Absorption is enhanced by an ointment or gel vehicle, but the selection of the vehicle should be based on the type of disorder and the site of involvement. Frequency of application should be determined by the potency of the preparation and the severity of the eruption. In general, the application of a *thin film* two times daily suffices. Adverse local effects include cutaneous atrophy, striae, telangiectasia, hypopigmentation, and increased hair growth.

In selected circumstances, corticosteroids may be administered by intralesional injection (acne cysts, keloids, psoriatic plaques, alopecia areata, persistent insect bite reactions). This method of administration should be used only by physicians who are experienced with this technique of dermatologic therapy.

SUNSCREENS. Sunscreens are of two general types: those that reflect all wavelengths of UV and visible spectrums, such as zinc oxide and titanium dioxide; and a heterogeneous group of chemicals that selectively absorb energy of various wavelengths within the UV spectrum. Some sunscreens permit tanning without burning; others prevent both. In addition to the spectrum of light that is blocked, other factors to be considered include cosmetic acceptance, sensitizing potential, retention on skin while swimming or sweating, required frequency of application, and cost. Effective opaque total barrier agents are A-Fil, zinc oxide ointment, Covermark, Dermablend, and RVPaque. Para-aminobenzoic acid (PABA)–ethanol (Pabanol, PreSun) and cinnamate-benzophenone combinations (Maxafil, Solbar, Uval) effectively prevent transmission of UVB and at least some UVA wavelengths. PABA esters (Eclipse, Pabafilm, Sundown) afford partial protection. Lip protectants that absorb in the UVB range (Sunstick, RVPaba lipstick, Blistik, PreSun) are also available for patients with photo-induced lip disorders such as recurrent herpesvirus infections. Sunscreens are designated by sun protection factor (SPF). The SPF is defined as the amount of time to develop a mild sunburn with the sunscreen compared with the amount of time without the sunscreen. A minimum SPF factor of 15 is required in most fair-skinned individuals to prevent sunburn. The higher the SPF, the better the protection is against UVB rays. Examples of sunscreens offering maximal protection are Supershade, Photoplex, and Total Eclipse. The efficacy of these agents depends on careful attention to instructions for use. PABA-containing sunscreens should be applied at least 30 min before sun exposure to permit penetration of the epidermis. Most patients with photosensitivity eruptions require protection by agents that absorb UVB wavelengths; patients with porphyria, phototoxic eruptions, and some types of solar urticaria require agents with a broader spectrum of prevention (see Chapter 606).

Sunscreens do not give complete protection against all harmful UV light. Sun avoidance is also important during the times when the sun is more intense, such as during midday. Clothing and hats also offer additional sun protection.

Morelli JG, Weston WL: Soaps and shampoos in pediatric practice. Pediatrics 80:634, 1987.

Nilsson EJ, Henning CG, Magnusson J: Topical corticosteroids and *Staphylococcus aureus* in atopic dermatitis. J Am Acad Dermatol 27:29, 1992.

Yohn JJ, Weston WL: Topical glucocorticosteroids. Curr Probl Dermatol 2:33, 1990.

CHAPTER 597
Diseases of the Neonate

Gary L. Darmstadt and Al Lane

Minor evanescent lesions of the newborn infant, particularly when florid, may cause undue concern. Most of the entities described in this chapter are relatively common, benign, and transient; they do not require therapy.

SEBACEOUS HYPERPLASIA. Minute, profuse, yellow-white papules are frequently found on the forehead, nose, upper lip, and cheeks of the term infant; they represent hyperplastic sebaceous glands. These tiny papules diminish gradually in size and disappear entirely within the first few weeks of life.

MILIA. The milium is a superficial epidermal inclusion cyst that contains laminated keratinized material. The lesion is a firm papule, 1–2 mm in diameter, and pearly, opalescent white. Milia may occur at any age but, in the neonate, are most frequently scattered over the face and gingivas and on the midline of the palate, where they are called *Epstein pearls*. Milia exfoliate spontaneously in most infants and may be ignored; those that appear in scars or sites of trauma in older children may be gently unroofed and "shelled out" with a fine-gauge needle.

SUCKING BLISTERS. Solitary or scattered superficial bullae on the upper limbs of infants at birth are presumed to be induced by vigorous sucking on the affected part in utero. Common sites are the radial aspect of the forearm, thumb, and index finger. These bullae resolve rapidly without sequelae. These lesions should be distinguished from sucking pads (calluses), which are found on the lips in the first few months and represent combined intracellular edema and hyperkeratosis. The diagnosis can be confirmed by observing the neonate suck the affected area.

CUTIS MARMORATA. When the newborn infant is exposed to low environmental temperatures, an evanescent, lacy, reticulated red or blue cutaneous vascular pattern appears over most of the body surface. This vascular change represents an accentuated physiologic vasomotor response that disappears with increasing age, although it is sometimes discernible even in older children. Persistent and pronounced cutis marmorata occurs in de Lange, Down, and trisomy 18 syndromes. Cutis marmorata telangiectatica congenita is clinically similar, but the lesions are more intense and are persistent.

HARLEQUIN COLOR CHANGE. This rare but dramatic vascular event occurs in the immediate newborn period and is most common in infants of low birthweight. It probably reflects an imbalance in the autonomic vascular regulatory mechanism. When the infant is placed on his or her side, the body is bisected longitudinally into a pale upper half and a deep red dependent half. The color change lasts only for a few minutes and occasionally affects only a portion of the trunk or face. The pattern may be reversed by changing the infant's position. Muscular activity causes generalized flushing and obliterates the color differential. Multiple episodes may occur but do not indicate permanent autonomic imbalance.

SALMON PATCH (NEVUS SIMPLEX). Salmon patches are small, pale pink, ill-defined, flat vascular lesions that occur most commonly on the glabella, eyelids, upper lip, and nuchal area of 30–40% of normal newborn infants. These lesions, which represent localized vascular ectasia, persist for several months and may become more visible during crying or changes in environmental temperature. Most lesions on the face eventually fade and disappear completely, but those on the posterior neck and occipital area often persist. When they become covered with hair, they are not noticeable. The facial lesions should not be confused with a port-wine stain, which is a permanent lesion. The salmon patch is usually symmetric with lesions on both eyelids or both sides of midline. Port-wine stains are often larger, unilateral, and usually end along the midline (see Chapter 600).

MONGOLIAN SPOTS. These blue or slate-gray macular lesions have variably defined margins; they occur most commonly in the presacral area but may be found over the posterior thighs, legs, back, and shoulders. They may be solitary or multiple and often involve large areas. More than 80% of black, Asian, and East Indian infants have these lesions, whereas the incidence in white infants is less than 10%. The peculiar hue of these macules is due to the dermal location of melanin-containing melanocytes that are presumed to have been arrested

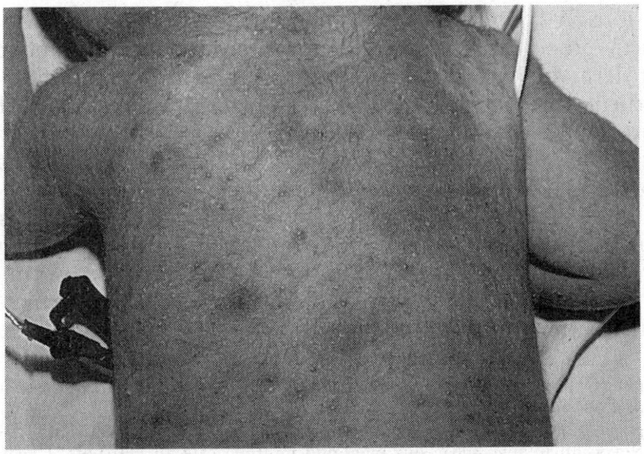

Figure 597–1. Erythema toxicum on the trunk of a newborn infant. See also color section.

in their migration from neural crest to epidermis. Mongolian spots usually fade during the first few years of life but occasionally persist. Malignant degeneration does not occur. Widespread multiple lesions, particularly those in unusual sites, are unlikely to disappear. The characteristic appearance and congenital onset distinguish these spots from the bruises of child abuse.

ERYTHEMA TOXICUM. This benign, self-limited, evanescent eruption occurs in approximately 50% of full-term infants; preterm infants are affected less commonly. The lesions are firm, yellow-white, 1- to 2-mm papules or pustules with a surrounding erythematous flare (Fig. 597–1 [color plate section]). At times, splotchy erythema is the only manifestation. Lesions may be sparse or numerous and clustered in several sites or widely dispersed over much of the body surface. Palms and soles are usually spared. Peak incidence occurs on the 2nd day of life, but new lesions may erupt during the 1st few days as the rash waxes and wanes. Occasionally onset may be delayed for a few days to weeks in premature infants. The pustules form below the stratum corneum or deeper in the epidermis and represent collections of eosinophils that also accumulate around the upper portion of the pilosebaceous follicle. The eosinophils can be demonstrated in Wright-stained smears of the intralesional contents. Cultures are sterile.

The cause of erythema toxicum is unknown. The lesions can mimic pyoderma, candidosis, herpes simplex, transient neonatal pustular melanosis, and miliaria but can be differentiated by the characteristic infiltrate of eosinophils and the absence of organisms on a stained smear. The course is brief, and no therapy is required. Incontinentia pigmenti and eosinophilic pustular folliculitis also have eosinophilic infiltration but can be distinguished by their distribution, histologic type, and chronicity.

TRANSIENT NEONATAL PUSTULAR MELANOSIS. Pustular melanosis, which is more common in black than in white infants, is a transient, benign, self-limited dermatosis of unknown cause that is characterized by three types of lesions: (1) evanescent superficial pustules; (2) ruptured pustules with a collarette of fine scale, at times with a central hyperpigmented macule; and (3) hyperpigmented macules (Fig. 597–2). Lesions are present at birth, and one or all types of lesions may be found in a profuse or sparse distribution. Pustules represent the early phase of the disorder and macules, the late phase. The pustular phase rarely lasts more than 2–3 days; hyperpigmented macules may persist for as long as 3 mo. Sites of predilection are the anterior neck, forehead, and lower back, although the scalp, trunk, limbs, palms, and soles may be affected.

Biopsies of tissue during the active phase show an intracorneal or subcorneal pustule filled with polymorphonuclear leukocytes, debris, and an occasional eosinophil. The macules are characterized only by increased melanization of epidermal cells. Cultures and smears can be used to distinguish these pustules from those of erythema toxicum and pyoderma because they do not contain bacteria or dense aggregates of eosinophils. No therapy is required.

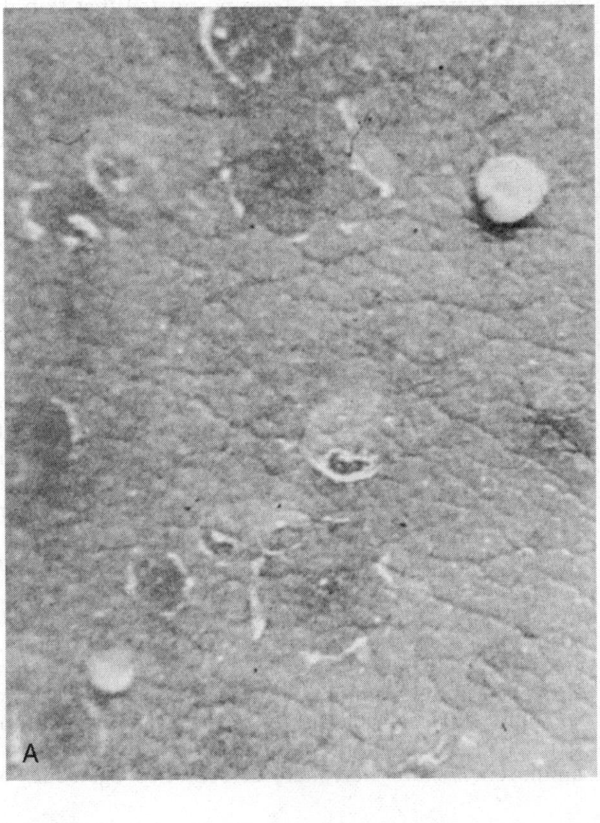

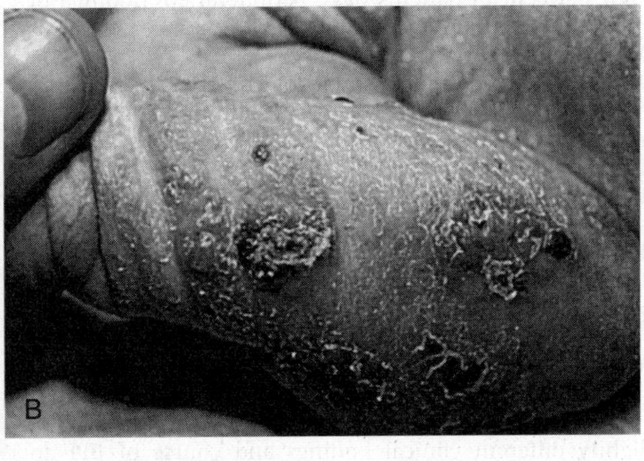

Figure 597–2. ***A* and *B*, Transient neonatal pustular melanosis showing pustules, rings of scales, and hyperpigmented macules.**

INFANTILE ACROPUSTULOSIS. Infantile acropustulosis generally has its onset at 2–10 mo of age; lesions are occasionally noted at birth. Black males have a predisposition for this eruption, but infants of both sexes and all races may be affected. The cause is unknown.

The lesions are initially discrete, erythematous papules that become vesiculopustular within 24 hr and subsequently crust before healing. They are intensely pruritic, and a fresh outbreak is usually accompanied by fretfulness and irritability. Preferred sites are the palms of the hands and soles and sides of the feet, where the lesions may develop in profusion. A less dense eruption may be found on the dorsum of the hands and feet, ankles, and wrists. Pustules may occasionally occur elsewhere on the body. Each episode lasts 7–14 days, during which time pustules continue to appear in crops. After a 2- to 4-wk remission, a new outbreak follows. This cyclic pattern continues for about 2 yr; permanent resolution is often preceded by longer intervals of remission between periods of activity. Infants with acropustulosis are otherwise well.

Wright-stained smears of intralesional contents show masses of neutrophils or, occasionally, a predominance of eosinophils. Histologically, well-circumscribed, subcorneal, neutrophilic pustules, with or without eosinophils, are noted.

The *differential diagnosis* in the neonate includes transient neonatal pustular melanosis, erythema toxicum, milia, cutaneous candidosis, and staphylococcal pustulosis. In the older infant and toddler, additional diagnostic considerations include scabies; dyshidrotic eczema; pustular psoriasis; subcorneal pustular dermatosis; and hand, foot, and mouth disease. A therapeutic trial of a scabicide is warranted in equivocal cases.

Therapy is directed at minimizing discomfort for the infant. Topical corticosteroid preparations or oral antihistamines decrease the severity of the pruritus and irritability of the infant. Dapsone 2 mg/kg/24 hr divided twice daily has been effective orally but has potentially serious side effects and should be used only with caution.

EOSINOPHILIC PUSTULAR FOLLICULITIS. This was first described by Ofuji, et al. in 1970 as recurrent crops of pruritic, coalescing, follicular papulopustules on the face, trunk, and extremities. Fifty-four per cent of patients have peripheral eosinophilia of more than 5% and about one third (32%) have leukocytosis (> 10,000/mm^3).

Infants with eosinophilic pustular folliculitis (EPF) make up less than 10% of all cases reported. The clinical and histologic appearance of this disorder in infants closely resembles that found in immunocompetent adults, with minor exceptions. In infants, the lesions are most prominent on the scalp, although they also occur on the trunk and extremities. Also, the classic annular and polycyclic appearance with centrifugal enlargement, as described by Ofugi, et al., is not seen in infants. Histopathologically, adults have an eosinophilic infiltrate that invades sebaceous glands and the outer root sheath of hair follicles, often leading to spongiosis in the outer root sheath. The eosinophilic infiltrate in most infants, however, is perifollicular, without spongiosis in the outer root sheath. Because of the slightly different clinical findings and course of EPF in immunocompetent adults compared with infants or patients with acquired immunodeficiency syndrome, it has been proposed recently that EPF should be subclassified into classic (Japanese), human immunodeficiency virus–related, and infantile forms. The differential diagnosis includes erythema toxicum neonatorum, infantile acropustulosis, localized pustular psoriasis, pustular folliculitis, and transient neonatal pustular melanosis.

The pathogenesis of EPF is linked epidemiologically to sebaceous gland activity because lesions appear most commonly in association with hair follicles in areas of the body with a high density of sebaceous glands. Most theories on the pathogenesis of EPF invoke immunologic mechanisms in the initiation of lesions. A cyclo-oxygenase–generated metabolite with chemotactic properties; an exaggerated response to skin saprophytes or dermatophytes, leading to eosinophilic infiltration and destruction of the follicle; or autoantibodies directed against the intercellular substance of the lower epidermis or the cytoplasm of basal cells of the epidermis and the outer sheath of hair follicles have been proposed to be etiologic in EPF.

Response of EPF to therapy has been variable, and no one specific treatment is the therapy of choice. In general, antimicrobials and medicated shampoos have been ineffective; mid-potency topical corticosteroids have been modestly effective in the treatment of scalp lesions in infants.

Alper JC, Holmes LB: The incidence and significance of birthmarks in a cohort of 4,641 newborns. Pediatr Dermatol 1:58, 1983.
Alper J, Holmes LB, Mihm MC: Birthmarks with serious medical significance: Nevocellular nevi, sebaceous nevi, and multiple café au lait spots. J Pediatr 95:696, 1979.
Darmstadt GL, Tunnessen WW, Sweren RJ: Eosinophilic pustular folliculitis. Pediatrics 89:1095, 1992.
Jacobs AH, Walton RG: The incidence of birthmarks in the neonate. Pediatrics 58:281, 1976.
Jennings JL, Burrows WM: Infantile acropustulosis. J Am Acad Dermatol 9:733, 1983.
Lucky AW, Esterly NB, Heskel N, et al: Eosinophilic pustular folliculitis in infancy. Pediatr Dermatol 1:202, 1984.

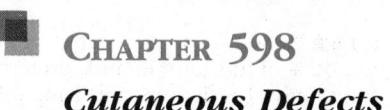

CHAPTER 598
Cutaneous Defects

Gary L. Darmstadt and Al Lane

SKIN DIMPLES. Cutaneous depressions over bony prominences and in the sacral area, at times associated with pits and creases, may occur in normal children and in association with dysmorphologic syndromes. It has been postulated that skin dimples develop in utero as a result of interposition of tissue between a sharp bony point and the uterine wall, which leads to decreased subcutaneous tissue formation. A rare benign autosomal dominant anomaly presents with dimples near the acromion bilaterally in association with deletion of the long arm of chromosome 18. Dimples tend to occur over the patella in congenital rubella, over the lateral aspects of the knees and elbows in prune-belly syndrome, on the pretibial surface in camptomelic dwarfs, and in the shape of an H on the chin in whistling-face syndrome. Sacral dimples occur as part of multiple syndromes, including Bloom syndrome, Smith-Lemli-Opitz syndrome, 4p deletion syndrome, spina bifida occulta, and diastomyelia.

REDUNDANT SKIN. Loose folds of skin must be differentiated from a congenital defect of elastic tissue or collagen such as cutis laxa, Ehlers-Danlos syndrome, or pseudoxanthoma elasticum. Redundant skin over the posterior neck is common in Turner, Noonan, Down, and the Klippel-Feil syndromes; more generalized folds of skin occur in infants with trisomy 18 and short-limbed dwarfism.

AMNIOTIC CONSTRICTION BANDS. Partial or complete constriction bands that produce defects in extremities and digits are found in 1:10,000–1:45,000 otherwise normal infants. Constrictive tissue bands are caused by primary amniotic rupture, with subsequent entanglement of fetal parts, particularly limbs, in shriveled fibrotic amniotic strands. This event is probably sporadic with negligible risk of recurrence. Formation of constrictive tissue bands is associated with abdominal trauma, amniocentesis, and hereditary defects of collagen such as Ehlers-Danlos syndrome or osteogenesis imperfecta. Constriction bands on the limbs may be removed by plastic surgical procedures.

Adhesive bands involve the craniofacial area and are associated with severe defects such as encephalocele and facial clefts. Adhesive bands result from broad fusion between disrupted fetal parts and an intact amniotic membrane. The craniofacial defects do not appear to be caused by constrictive amniotic bands but result from a vascular disruption sequence with or without cephaloamniotic adhesion.

The *limb-body wall complex* (LBWC) involves vascular disruption early in development, affecting several embryonic structures, including at least two of the following three characteristics: exencephaly or encephalocele with facial clefts, thoraco- and/or abdominoschisis, and limb defects. Amniotic rupture may be the cause of embryonic vascular disruption, leading to the LBWC; the LBWC, however, has been reported in the absence of amniotic rupture.

PREAURICULAR SINUSES AND PITS. Pits and sinus tracts anterior to the pinna may be the result of imperfect fusion of the tubercles of the first and second branchial arches. These anomalies may be unilateral or bilateral, may be familial, are more common in females and blacks, and at times are associated with other anomalies of the ears and face. Preauricular pits are present in branchio-otorenal dysplasia, an autosomal dominant disorder that consists of external ear malformations, branchial fistulas, hearing loss, and renal anomalies. When the tracts become chronically infected, retention cysts may form and drain intermittently; such lesions may require excision.

ACCESSORY TRAGI. An accessory tragus typically appears as a single, pedunculated, flesh-colored papule in the preauricular region anterior to the tragus. Less commonly, accessory tragi are multiple, unilateral or bilateral and may be located in the preauricular area, on the cheek along the line of the mandible, or on the lateral neck anterior to the sternocleidomastoid muscle. In contrast to the rest of the pinna, which develops from the second branchial arch, the tragus and accessory tragi derive from the first branchial arch. Accessory tragi may occur as isolated defects or in chromosomal first branchial arch syndromes that include anomalies of the ears and face such as cleft lip, cleft palate, and mandibular hypoplasia. Accessory tragus is consistently found in *oculoauriculovertebral syndrome (Goldenhar syndrome)*. Surgical excision is appropriate.

BRANCHIAL CLEFT AND THYROGLOSSAL CYSTS AND SINUSES. Cysts and sinuses in the neck may be formed along the course of the first, second, third, or fourth branchial clefts as a result of improper closure during embryonic life. Second branchial cleft cysts are the most common. The lesions may be unilateral or bilateral (2–3%) and may open onto the cutaneous surface or drain into the pharynx. Secondary infection is an indication for systemic antibiotic therapy. These anomalies may be inherited as autosomal dominant traits.

Thyroglossal cysts and fistulas are similar defects located in or near the midline of the neck; they may extend to the base of the tongue. A pathognomonic sign is vertical motion of the mass with swallowing and tongue protrusion. Cysts in the tongue base may also be differentiated from an undescended lingual thyroid by radionuclide scanning. Unlike branchial cysts, a thyroglossal duct cyst often appears after an upper respiratory infection.

SUPERNUMERARY NIPPLES. Solitary or multiple accessory nipples may occur in a unilateral or bilateral distribution along a line from the anterior axillary fold to the inguinal area. They are more common in black (3.5%) than white (0.6%) children. Accessory nipples may or may not have an areola and may be mistaken for congenital nevi. They may be excised for cosmetic reasons. Rarely, they undergo malignant change. Renal or urinary tract anomalies may occur in children with this finding.

APLASIA CUTIS CONGENITA (CONGENITAL ABSENCE OF SKIN). Developmental absence of skin is usually noted on the scalp as multiple or solitary (70%), noninflammatory, well-demarcated, oval or circular 1- to 2-cm ulcers. The appearance of lesions varies, depending on when they occurred during intrauterine development. Those that form early in gestation may heal before delivery and appear as an atrophic, fibrotic scar with associated alopecia, whereas more recent defects may present as an ulceration. Most occur at the vertex just lateral to the midline, but similar defects may also occur on the face, trunk, and limbs, where they are often symmetric. The depth of the ulcer varies. Only the epidermis and upper dermis may be involved, resulting in minimal scarring or hair loss, or the defect may extend to the deep dermis, subcutaneous tissue, and, rarely, to the periosteum, skull, and dura.

There is no unifying theory that can account for all lesions of aplasia cutis congenita. *Diagnosis* is made on the basis of physical findings indicative of in utero disruption of skin development. Lesions are sometimes mistakenly attributed to scalp electrodes or obstetric trauma. Rather, they appear to be due to a variety of factors, including genetic factors, teratogens, compromised vasculature to the skin, and trauma.

Although most individuals with aplasia cutis congenita have no other abnormalities, these lesions may be associated with isolated physical anomalies or with a number of malformation syndromes. Scalp lesions may be seen in association with distal limb reduction anomalies, generally with autosomal dominant inheritance, or sporadically in association with epidermal and organoid nevi. Aplasia cutis congenita may also be found in association with an overt or underlying embryologic malformation, such as meningomyelocele, gastroschisis, omphalocele, or spinal dysraphism. Aplasia cutis congenita in association with fetus papyraceus is apparently due to ischemic or thrombotic events in the placenta and fetus. Blistering or skin fragility and/or absence or deformity of nails in association with aplasia cutis congenita is a well-recognized presentation of epidermolysis bullosa. Maternal ingestion of the teratogen methimazole or intrauterine herpes simplex virus or varicella-zoster virus infection may also be associated with lesions of aplasia cutis congenita. Finally, aplasia cutis congenita may also occur in the setting of a malformation syndrome such as several of the ectodermal dysplasias, trisomy 13 or 14, deletion of the short arm of chromosome 4, Johanson-Blizzard syndrome, focal facial dermal dysplasia, or focal dermal hypoplasia.

Major *complications* are hemorrhage, secondary local infection, and meningitis. If the defect is small, recovery is uneventful with gradual epithelialization and formation of a hairless atrophic scar over a period of several weeks (Fig. 598–1). Small bony defects usually close spontaneously during the 1st yr of life. Large or multiple scalp defects may require excision and primary closure, if feasible; rotation of a flap to fill the defect; or the use of tissue expanders. Truncal and limb defects, despite large size, usually epithelialize and form atrophic scars, which can later be revised, if necessary.

FOCAL FACIAL DERMAL DYSPLASIA (BITEMPORAL APLASIA CUTIS CONGENITA, ECTODERMAL DYSPLASIA OF THE FACE). This rare disorder is characterized by congenital atrophic, scarlike lesions on the temples. Autosomal dominant and autosomal recessive inheritance have been documented in affected kindreds; both subgroups of patients lack associated facial anomalies. A third category of patients have a constellation of facial anomalies in association with temporal scarlike defects, including periorbital puffiness; upward slanting, laterally deficient eyebrows; absence of, or multiple rows of eyelashes; abnormalities of the nose, including flattening of the nasal bridge, bulbous nasal tip, and a nasal septum that extends below the nasal alae; and increased mobility of the skin and connective tissue of the upper lip. Growth and development is generally normal.

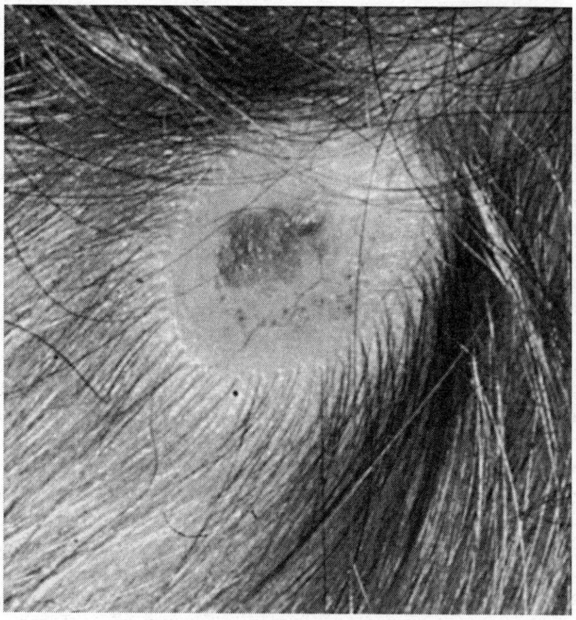

Figure 598–1. Healing solitary lesion of aplasia cutis congenita.

FOCAL DERMAL HYPOPLASIA (GOLTZ SYNDROME). This rare congenital mesoectodermal disorder is characterized by dysplasia of connective tissue in the skin and skeleton. It presents with multiple soft, tan papillomas. Other cutaneous findings include linear atrophic lesions; reticulated hypopigmentation and hyperpigmentation; telangiectasias; congenital absence of skin; angiofibromas presenting as verrucous excrescences; and papillomas of the lips, tongue, circumoral region, vulva, anus and the inguinal, axillary, and periumbilical areas. Partial alopecia, sweating disorders, and dystrophic nails are additional less common ectodermal anomalies. The most frequent skeletal defects include syndactyly, clinodactyly, polydactyly, and scoliosis. Osteopathia striata are fine, parallel, vertical stripes noted on radiographs in the metaphyses on long bones; these are highly characteristic, but not pathognomonic, of focal dermal hypoplasia. There are many ocular abnormalities, the most common of which are colobomas, strabismus, nystagmus, and microphthalmia. Small stature, dental defects, soft tissue anomalies, and peculiar dermatoglyphic patterns are also common. Mental deficiency occurs occasionally.

This familial disorder occurs principally in girls. It has been postulated that an X-linked dominant gene, lethal in hemizygous males, may account for the sex distribution. The linear pattern of skin and bone lesions may be due to random X-inactivation in females. Cases of father-daughter transmission, evidence for an autosomal locus 9q32-qter, and the unusually high (10%) proportion of males with the disorder, however, argue against X-linked dominance with lethality in males. Affected males may have an early half chromatid mutation or autosomal dominant inheritance affecting the germ line.

The primary defect has been hypothesized by some to be a deficiency of collagen caused by a fibroblastic defect. Others suggest that the cutaneous defects represent heterotopic proliferations of fatty nevi within the dermis, resulting from dysplasia, not hypoplasia, followed by herniation of subcutaneous fat.

This disorder is often confused with incontinentia pigmenti because of the sex predilection for females, the linear distribution of skin lesions, and the initial inflammatory phase, which are features of both disorders. The cutaneous lesions may also superficially resemble epidermal nevi. *Treatment* should be directed at amelioration of specific anomalies; genetic counseling is advisable.

DYSKERATOSIS CONGENITA (ZINSSER-ENGMAN-COLE SYNDROME). This rare familial syndrome consists classically of the triad of reticulated hyperpigmentation of the skin, dystrophic nails, and mucous membrane leukoplakia. It usually affects males and is inherited most often in an X-linked recessive fashion, although autosomal recessive or dominant inheritance has been reported. Onset occurs during childhood, most commonly as nail dystrophy, at age 5–13 yr. The nails become atrophic and ridged longitudinally, and there is considerable loss of the nail plate. Skin changes usually appear 2–3 yr after onset of nail changes and consist of reticulated gray-brown pigmentation, atrophy, and telangiectasia, especially on the neck, face, and chest. Hyperhidrosis and hyperkeratosis of the palms and soles, acrocyanosis, and occasional bullae on the hands and feet are also characteristic. Blepharitis, ectropion, and excessive tearing as a result of atresia of the lacrimal ducts are occasional manifestations. Vesiculobullous lesions may occur on the oral mucous membranes and result in ulceration, formation of epithelial tags, atrophic changes of the tongue, and oral leukokeratosis. Oral leukokeratosis generally presents after the 3rd decade of life and may give rise to squamous cell carcinoma. Similar changes have been noted in the urethral and anal mucosae. The scalp hair, eyebrows, and lashes may become sparse. Hypoplastic anemia, at times of the Fanconi variety, may present at age 10 yr or older, in up to 50% of patients. Impaired cell-mediated immunity and other T-cell abnormalities have also been noted. The primary causes of death are infections, including *Pneumocystis carinii,* and carcinoma. In one large series, 12% of patients had tumors, most commonly oral and anal squamous cell carcinoma, pancreatic adenocarcinoma, or Hodgkin disease. The *differential diagnosis* includes the ectodermal dysplasias, pachyonychia congenita, poikilodermas, epidermolysis bullosa, keratoderma of the palms and soles, and lichen sclerosus et atrophicus. The abnormalities noted in skin biopsies are those of poikiloderma.

Treatment includes biopsy of leukoplakic sites to identify malignancies. Etretinate may cause regression of leukoplakia, and orally administered β-carotene has some utility for treatment of leukoplakia and as a preventive agent for oral cancer. Aplastic anemia may be treated by administration of androgens or granulocyte-macrophage colony-stimulating factor or bone marrow transplantation.

CUTIS VERTICIS GYRATA. This bizarre alteration of the scalp, which is more common in males, may be present from birth or develop during adolescence. The scalp is characterized by convoluted elevated folds, 1–2 cm in thickness, usually in the fronto-occipital axis. Unlike the lax skin of other disorders, the convolutions cannot generally be flattened by traction. Primary cutis gyrata is often associated with mental retardation, ocular defects, abnormal size and shape of the head, seizures, and spasticity. Secondary cutis gyrata may be due to chronic inflammatory diseases; tumors; nevi; acromegaly; and pachydermoperiostosis, a syndrome characterized by hypertrophy of the skin and bones.

Drachtman RA, Alter BP: Dyskeratosis congenita: Clinical and genetic heterogeneity. Am J Pediatr Hematol Oncol 14:297, 1992.

Frieden IJ: Aplasia cutis congenita: A clinical review and proposal for classification. J Am Acad Dermatol 14:646, 1986.

Howell JB, Freeman RG: Cutaneous defects of focal dermal hypoplasia: An ectomesodermal dysplasia syndrome. J Cutan Pathol 16:237, 1989.

Kowalski DC, Fenske NA: The focal facial dermal dysplasias: Report of a kindred and proposed new classification. J Am Acad Dermatol 27:575, 1992.

Mann M, Weintraub R, Hashimoto K: Focal dermal hypoplasia with an initial inflammatory phase. Pediatr Dermatol 7:278, 1990.

Moerman P, Fryns JP, Vandenberghe K, et al: Constrictive amniotic bands, amniotic adhesions, and limb-body wall complex: Discrete disruption sequences with pathogenetic overlap. Am J Med Genet 42:470, 1992.

Sebben JE: The accessory tragus—no ordinary skin tag. J Dermatol Surg Oncol 15:304, 1989.

Spencer JM, Schreiderman PI, Grossman ME: Bilateral skin dimples on the shoulders. Pediatr Dermatol 10:16, 1993.

CHAPTER 599
Ectodermal Dysplasias

Gary L. Darmstadt and Al Lane

The term ectodermal dysplasia is used to designate a heterogeneous group of disorders characterized by a constellation of findings involving a primary defect of the teeth, skin, and appendageal structures, including hair, nails, and eccrine and sebaceous glands. Disturbances in tissue derived from embryologic layers other than ectoderm are not uncommon. The most recent clinical classification distinguished 121 ectodermal dysplasias with all possible modes of inheritance. Many of the syndromes have overlapping features and are distinguished by the presence or absence of a single defect.

HYPOHIDROTIC (ANHIDROTIC) ECTODERMAL DYSPLASIA. This syndrome manifests as a triad of defects: partial or complete absence of sweat glands, anomalous dentition, and hypotrichosis. It is usually inherited as an X-linked recessive trait, with full expression only in males; however, an autosomal recessive mode of inheritance may be operative in some families.

Heterozygotic females may have no or variable *clinical manifestations*, including dental defects, sparse hair, and reduced sweating; because of random X-inactivation, they are mosaics of functionally normal and abnormal cells. Affected children, unable to sweat, may experience episodes of high fever in warm environments and may be mistakenly considered to have fever of unknown origin. This is particularly the case in infancy when the facial changes are not easily appreciated. The typical facies is characterized by frontal bossing; malar hypoplasia; a flattened nasal bridge; recessed columella; thick, everted lips; wrinkled, hyperpigmented periorbital skin; and prominent, low-set ears (Fig. 599–1). The skin over the entire body is dry, finely wrinkled, and hypopigmented, often with a prominent venous pattern. Extensive peeling of the skin is a clinical clue to diagnosis in the newborn period. The paucity of sebaceous glands may account for the dry skin. The hair is sparse, unruly, and lightly pigmented, and eyebrows and lashes are sparse or absent. Anodontia or hypodontia with widely spaced, conical teeth is a consistent feature (see Fig. 599–1). Less commonly, stenotic lacrimal puncta, corneal opacity, cataracts, hypoplastic or absent mammary glands, and conductive hearing loss have been observed. The incidence of atopic diseases in these children is relatively high. Poor development of mucous glands in the respiratory and gastrointestinal tract may result in increased susceptibility to respiratory infection, purulent rhinitis, dysphonia, dysphagia, and diarrhea. Sexual development is usually normal. Approximately 30% of males die during the first 2 yr of life of hyperpyrexia or respiratory infection.

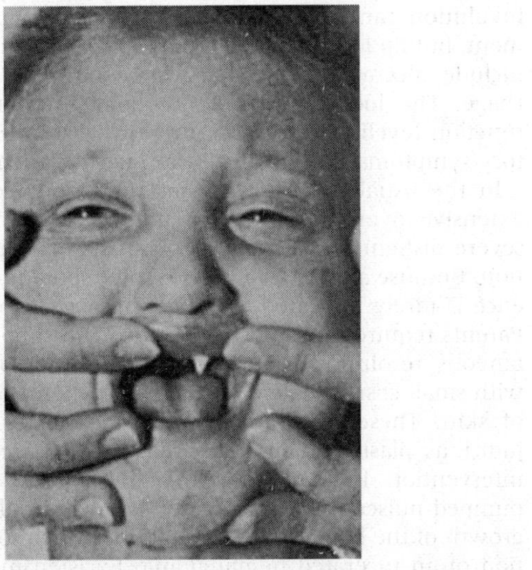

Figure 599–1. Hypohidrotic ectodermal dysplasia is characterized by pointed ears, wispy hair, periorbital hyperpigmentation, midfacial hypoplasia, and pegged teeth.

The sweating deficit is a reflection of hypoplasia or absence of eccrine glands; this may be *diagnosed* by skin biopsy. The palmar skin is an appropriate site for biopsy. Reduction or absence of sweating can be documented by pilocarpine iontophoresis or by topical application of o-phthalaldehyde to the palmar skin. Sweat pores are not visible in the palmar ridges in affected children and are decreased in number in carrier females. Application of a 2% solution of iodine in alcohol to the back, followed by application of a suspension of corn starch in castor oil also allows highlighting of sweat glands by the appearance of a black dot; this test may be useful for detection of female carriers. Linkage analysis has been used for prenatal and early neonatal diagnosis.

Treatment of these children includes protecting them from exposure to high ambient temperatures. Early dental evaluation is necessary so that prostheses can be provided for cosmetic reasons and for adequate nutrition. The use of artificial tears prevents damage to the cornea in patients with defective lacrimation. Alopecia may necessitate the wearing of a wig to improve appearance.

HIDROTIC ECTODERMAL DYSPLASIA (CLOUSTON TYPE). Dystrophic, hypoplastic, or absent nails; sparse hair; and hyperkeratosis of the palms and soles are the salient features of this autosomal dominant disorder. The dentition is usually normal, although small teeth and numerous caries are occasionally found. Sweating is always normal. Absence of eyebrows and lashes and hyperpigmentation over the knees, elbows, and knuckles have been noted in some affected individuals.

EEC SYNDROME. Ectrodactyly (split hand and foot), ectodermal dysplasia, cleft lip and palate, and tear duct abnormalities constitute the EEC syndrome, which is probably inherited as an autosomal dominant trait of low penetrance and variable expressivity. The ectodermal dysplasia consists of dry, poorly pigmented skin; light-colored, wispy, sparse scalp hair and eyebrows; and absence of lashes. Decreased numbers of hair follicles and sebaceous glands have been demonstrated by biopsy. Clinical expression of the EEC syndrome is variable; any one of these signs may be absent, except the ectodermal signs. Associated defects include anomalies of the hands and feet, nail hypoplasia, granulomatous perlèche frequently complicated by candidosis, defective dentition, deafness, ocular abnormalities (blepharophimosis, strabismus), and abnormalities of the urinary tract.

Clarke A, Burn J: Sweat testing to identify female carriers of X linked hypohidrotic ectodermal dysplasia. J Med Genet 28:330, 1991.

Clarke A, Phillips DIM, Brown R, et al: Clinical aspects of X-linked hypohidrotic ectodermal dysplasia. Arch Dis Child 62:989, 1987.

Freire-Maia N, Pinheiro M: Ectodermal dysplasias. Some recollections and a classification. *In:* Salinas CF, Opitz JM, Paul NW (eds): Recent Advances in Ectodermal Dysplasias, Vol 24. New York, Alan R. Liss, 1988, p. 3.

Rodini ESO, Richieri-Costa A: EEC syndrome: report on 20 new patients, clinical and genetic considerations. Am J Med Genet 37:42, 1990.

Zonana J: Hypohidrotic (anhidrotic) ectodermal dysplasia: Molecular genetic research and its clinical application. Semin Dermatol 12:241, 1993.

CHAPTER 600
Vascular Disorders

Al Lane and Gary L. Darmstadt

Developmental vascular anomalies may occur as isolated defects or as part of a syndrome. They can be separated into two major categories: hemangiomas and malformations. Hemangiomas are proliferative lesions of vascular endothelium that predictably enlarge and then spontaneously involute. Hemangiomas are the most common tumor of infancy; with rare exceptions, they occur sporadically and without a genetic basis. Cutaneous hemangiomas are superficial (capillary) in approximately 60% of patients and are deep (cavernous) in 15% of patients; they have both a superficial and a deep component (mixed) in approximately 20% of patients. Malformations are derived from capillaries, veins, arteries, or lymphatics or any combination thereof. Malformations do not regress but usually enlarge over time.

PORT-WINE STAIN (NEVUS FLAMMEUS, PORT-WINE NEVUS). Port-wine stains are always present at birth. They consist of mature dilated dermal capillaries and represent a permanent developmental defect. The lesions are macular, sharply circumscribed, pink to purple, and tremendously varied in size (Fig. 600–1). The head and neck region is the most common site of predilection, and most lesions are unilateral. The mucous membranes can be involved. As the child matures into adulthood, the port-wine stain may become darker in color, pebbly in consistency, and may occasionally develop elevated areas that bleed spontaneously.

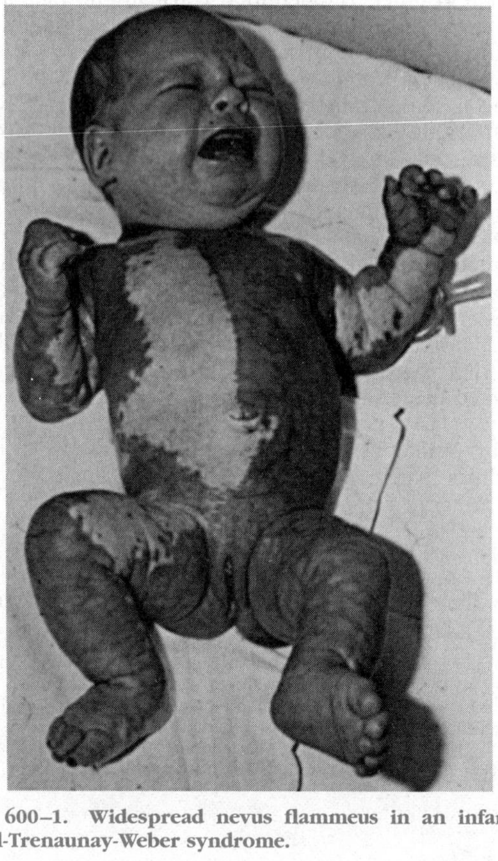

Figure 600–1. Widespread nevus flammeus in an infant with Klippel-Trenaunay-Weber syndrome.

True port-wine stains should be distinguished from the common salmon patch of the neonate, which is, in contrast, a relatively transient lesion (see Chapter 597). Stretching the skin horizontally or placing firm pressure on a glass slide over the involved skin decreases the red color of both lesions and is not diagnostic. When the port-wine stain is localized to the trigeminal area of the face, specifically around the eyelids, the diagnosis of *Sturge-Weber syndrome* (glaucoma, leptomeningeal venous angioma, seizures, hemiparesis contralateral to the facial lesion, intracranial calcification) must be considered (see Chapter 546.3). Early screening for glaucoma is important to prevent additional damage to the eye. Port-wine stains also occur as a component of *Klippel-Trenaunay-Weber syndrome* and with moderate frequency in other syndromes, including the *Rubinstein-Taybi, Cobb* (spinal arteriovenous malformation, port-wine stain), *Beckwith-Wiedemann,* and *trisomy 13* syndromes. In the absence of associated anomalies, morbidity from these lesions may include a poor self-image, hypertrophy of underlying structures, and traumatic bleeding.

The most effective treatment for port-wine stains is the flashlamp-pumped–pulsed dye laser. This therapy is targeted at the lesion and avoids thermal injury to the surrounding normal tissue. After such treatment, the texture and pigmentation of the skin is generally normal without scarring. Therapy can begin in infancy when the surface area of involvement is smaller and the response seems to be better. Other therapies including masking with cosmetics (Covermark, Dermablend), cryosurgery, excision, grafting, and tattooing.

CAPILLARY HEMANGIOMA (STRAWBERRY NEVUS). So-called strawberry hemangiomas are bright red, protuberant, compressible, sharply demarcated lesions that may occur on any area of the body. Although sometimes present at birth, more often, they appear within the first 2 mo, heralded by an erythematous mark or an area of pallor, which subsequently develops a fine telangiectatic pattern before the phase of expansion. Girls are affected more often than boys. Favored sites are the face, scalp, back, and anterior chest; lesions may be solitary or multiple. Most superficial hemangiomas undergo a phase of rapid expansion, followed by a stationary period, and finally by spontaneous involution. Regression may be anticipated when the lesion develops blanched or pale gray areas that indicate fibrosis. The course of a particular lesion is unpredictable, but approximately 60% of these lesions involute completely by the age of 5 yr, with 90–95% by the age of 9 yr. Spontaneous involution cannot be correlated with size or site of involvement, but lip lesions seem to persist most often. Complications include ulceration, secondary infection, and, rarely, hemorrhage. The location of a lesion may interfere with a vital function (eyelid with vision, urethra with urination). Respiratory symptoms should suggest a tracheobronchial lesion.

In the usual patient who has no serious complications or extensive overgrowth that results in tissue destruction and severe disfigurement, *treatment* consists of expectant observation. Because almost all lesions resolve spontaneously, interference is rarely indicated and may, in fact, cause further harm. Parents require repeated reassurance and support. After spontaneous resolution, approximately 10% of patients are left with small cosmetic defects, such as puckering or discoloration of skin. These defects can be eliminated or minimized by judicious plastic repair if desired. In the rare case in which intervention is required, early therapy by the flashlamp-pumped-pulsed dye laser may be beneficial in decreasing growth of the hemangioma and in inducing more rapid resolution of an ulcerated hemangioma. Excision may be advisable in lesions that have remained large for several years; the extent of scarring anticipated should influence the final decision. Radiation can be hazardous and should be considered only in life-threatening situations, such as the Kasabach-Merritt syndrome (see later). Elastic bandages may reduce the amount of tissue distortion resulting from rapid growth, but they are appropriate only in selected patients with large hemangiomas. Systemic or intralesional administration of corticosteroids and interferon alpha (IFN-α) may be indicated for infants at risk for serious sequelae from exceptionally large or rapidly growing hemangiomas in vital areas (see later).

CAVERNOUS HEMANGIOMAS. These are more deeply situated lesions and, therefore, appear more diffuse and ill-defined than capillary hemangiomas. The lesions are cystic, firm, or compressible, and the overlying skin may appear normal in color or have a bluish hue. Mixed hemangiomas consist of a deep component with a superimposed capillary hemangioma (Fig. 600–2). Cavernous hemangiomas progress from a growth phase to a stationary phase to a period of involution. These lesions are as likely to regress as capillary hemangiomas, and the outcome cannot be predicted from size or site of involvement. A course of expectant observation should be followed in most cases. If involvement of underlying structures is suspected, appropriate radiologic studies should be performed for elucidation. Rarely, these lesions impinge on vital structures, interfere with functions such as vision or feeding, cause grotesque disfigurement because of rapid growth, or are associated with life-threatening complications such as thrombocytopenia and hemorrhage (see Kasabach-Merritt syndrome).

If *treatment* becomes necessary, a course of prednisone (2–4 mg/kg/24 hr) is effective in some infants. Termination of growth and sometimes regression may be evident after approximately 4 wk of therapy. When a response is obtained, the dosage should be decreased gradually. Alternate-day corticosteroid therapy has also been administered with success. Intralesional corticosteroid injection with the patient anesthetized can also induce rapid involution of a localized hemangioma. IFN-α therapy may also be effective.

Cavernous hemangiomas are associated with macrocephaly and pseudopapilledema in a rare autosomal dominant syndrome and occur with variable frequency in I cell and *Gorham disease* (cavernous hemangiomas, disappearing bones).

KASABACH-MERRITT SYNDROME. This syndrome is a combination of a rapidly enlarging hemangioma, thrombocytopenia, and an acute or chronic consumption coagulopathy. The *clinical manifestations* are usually evident during early infancy, but occasionally the onset is later. The hemangioma is often present at birth and characteristically is solitary and large, although multiple and small hemangiomas have also been associated with this syndrome. The vascular lesion is usually cutaneous and is only rarely located in viscera. The associated platelet defect may lead to precipitous hemorrhage accompanied by ecchymoses, petechiae, and a rapid increase in size of the hemangioma. Severe anemia as a result of hemorrhage or microangiopathic hemolysis may ensue. The platelet count is depressed, but the bone marrow contains increased numbers of normal or immature megakaryocytes. The thrombocytopenia has been attributed to sequestration or increased destruction of platelets within the hemangioma. Hypofibrinogenemia and decreased levels of consumable clotting factors are relatively common (see Chapter 438).

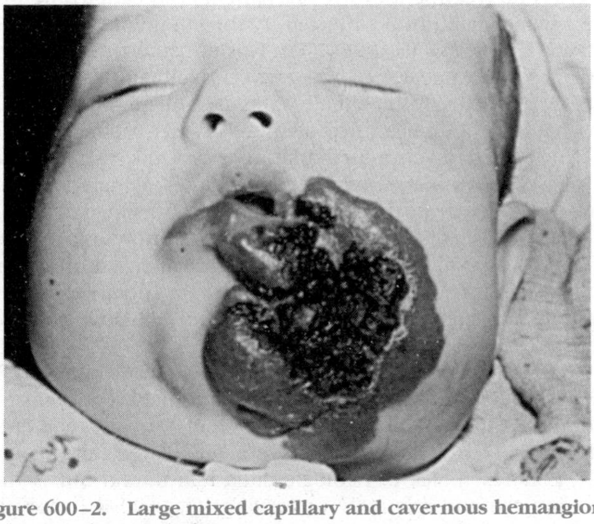

Figure 600–2. Large mixed capillary and cavernous hemangioma with central crusted ulcer.

Treatment includes the management of thrombocytopenia, anemia, and consumptive coagulopathy by administering platelets and by transfusion of red blood cells and fresh frozen plasma. Heparinization is controversial but has benefitted some patients when combined with transfusions. Arteriovenous shunts in large lesions may produce high-output heart failure requiring digitalization (see Chapter 403). Treatment of these lesions includes systemic steroids, embolization, radiation therapy, aminocaproic acid (inhibits fibrinolysis), and recombinant IFN-α, which may inhibit proliferation of endothelial and smooth muscle cells. The mortality rate is 20–30%.

DISSEMINATED HEMANGIOMATOSIS. This is a serious condition in which multiple hemangiomas are widely distributed. On the skin, there are usually numerous small, red, or purple papular hemangiomas, but infrequently they may be sparse or absent. The internal hemangiomas may involve any of the viscera; the liver, gastrointestinal tract, central nervous system, and lung are the most common sites. Ultrasound and computed tomographic (CT) scanning are indicated to determine the extent of visceral or neural involvement. The disorder is often fatal because of high-output cardiac failure, visceral hemorrhage, obstruction of the respiratory tract, or compression of central neural tissue. In some cases, systemic corticosteroid therapy alone or in combination with IFN-α, surgery, or irradiation has been life saving. Multiple cutaneous hemangiomas may occur in the absence of visceral involvement (benign neonatal hemangiomatosis); spontaneous regression of the lesions without complications is probable in such cases. Multiple hemangiomas may also occur in several rare syndromes, such as macrocephaly combined with pseudopapilledema or with lipomas.

BLUE RUBBER BLEB NEVUS. This syndrome consists of multiple cavernous hemangiomas of the skin, mucous membranes, and gastrointestinal tract. Typical lesions are blue-purple and rubbery in consistency; they vary in size from a few millimeters to a few centimeters in diameter. They are sometimes painful or tender. Large disfiguring hemangiomas and irregular blue marks may also occur. The lesions, which can rarely be located in the liver, spleen, and central nervous system in addition to the skin and gastrointestinal tract, do not involute spontaneously. Recurrent gastrointestinal hemorrhage may lead to severe anemia. Palliation can be achieved by excision of involved bowel. Cutaneous angiomas have been removed successfully by laser therapy.

PYOGENIC GRANULOMA (LOBULAR CAPILLARY HEMANGIOMA, TELANGIECTATIC GRANULOMA). A pyogenic granuloma is a small, red, glistening, sessile or pedunculated papule that often has a discernible epithelial collarette (Fig. 600–3). The surface may be weeping and crusted or completely epithelialized. Pyogenic granulomas initially grow rapidly, may ulcerate, and bleed easily when traumatized because they consist of exuberant granulation tissue. They are relatively common in children, particularly on the face, arms, and hands. Those located on a finger or hand may appear as a subcutaneous nodule. Lesions that develop on the oral mucosa during pregnancy are called *granuloma gravidarum.* Pyogenic granulomas generally arise at sites of injury, but often a history of trauma cannot be elicited. Clinically, they resemble and are often indistinguishable from small hemangiomas. Microscopically, an early lesion resembles an early capillary hemangioma. Collarette formation at the base of the tumor and edema of the stroma may allow differentiation from a capillary hemangioma.

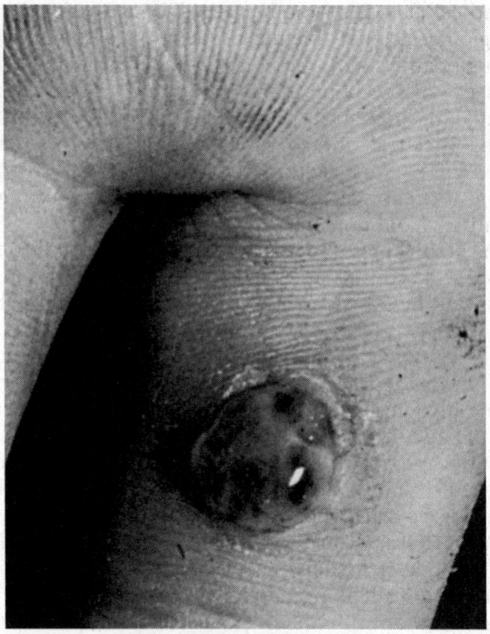

Figure 600–3. Pyogenic granuloma with a moist surface and epithelial collarette at the base.

Pyogenic granulomas are benign but a nuisance because they bleed easily with trauma and may recur if incompletely removed. Numerous satellite papules have developed after incomplete removal of pyogenic granulomas from the back, particularly in the interscapular region. Small lesions may regress after cauterization with silver nitrate; larger lesions require excision and electrodesiccation of the base of the granuloma.

MAFFUCCI SYNDROME. The association of cavernous hemangiomas, phlebectasias, lymphangiomas, and lymphangiectasias with nodular echondromas in the metaphyseal or diaphyseal portion of long bones is known as Maffucci syndrome. Onset occurs during childhood. Bone lesions may produce limb deformities and pathologic fractures. Chondrosarcoma or angiosarcoma may become a complication (see Chapters 453 and 454).

KLIPPEL-TRENAUNAY-WEBER SYNDROME. A port-wine stain in combination with bony and soft tissue hypertrophy and venous varicosities constitutes the triad of defects of this nonheritable disorder. The anomaly is present at birth and usually involves a lower limb but may involve more than one and portions of the trunk or face (see Fig. 600–1). Enlargement of the soft tissues may be gradual and may involve the entire extremity, a portion of it, or selected digits. In addition to venous varicosities, lymphatic abnormalities may be present, arteriovenous fistulas can develop, and bruits may be audible in the affected part. This disorder can be confused with Maffucci syndrome or, if the surface hemangioma is minimal, with Milroy disease. Pain, limb swelling, and cellulitis may occur. Thrombophlebitis, dislocations of joints, gangrene of the affected extremity, congestive heart failure, hematuria secondary to urinary tract hemangiomas, rectal bleeding from lesions of the gastrointestinal tract, pulmonary lesions, and malformations of the lymphatic vessels are infrequent complications. Arteriograms, venograms, and CT or magnetic resonance imaging scans may delineate the extent of the anomaly, but surgical correction or palliation is often difficult. The indications for radiologic studies of viscera and bones are best determined by clinical evaluation. Supportive care includes compression bandages for varicosities; surgical treatment may help carefully selected patients. Leg-length differences should be treated with orthotic devices to prevent the development of spinal deformities. Eventually, corrective bone surgery may be needed to treat significant leg-length discrepancy.

HEREDITARY HEMORRHAGIC TELANGIECTASIA (OSLER-WEBER-RENDU DISEASE). This disorder is inherited as an autosomal dominant trait. Affected children may experience recurrent epistaxis before detection of the characteristic skin and mucous membrane lesions. The mucocutaneous lesions, which usually develop at puberty, are 1–4 mm, sharply demarcated, red to purple macules, papules, or spider-like projections, each composed of a tightly woven mat of tortuous telangiectatic vessels. The nasal mucosa, lips, and tongue are usually involved; less commonly, cutaneous lesions occur on the face, ears, palms, and nail beds. Vascular ectasias may also arise in the conjunctivae, larynx, pharynx, gastrointestinal tract, bladder, vagina, bronchi, brain, and liver.

Massive hemorrhage is the most serious complication and may result in severe anemia. Bleeding may occur from the nose, mouth, gastrointestinal tract, genitourinary tract, and lungs. Persons with hereditary hemorrhagic telangiectasia have normal levels of clotting factors and an intact clotting mechanism. In the absence of serious complications, life span is normal. Local lesions may be ablated temporarily with chemical cautery or electrocoagulation. More drastic surgical measures may be required for lesions in critical sites such as the lung or gastrointestinal tract. Anemia should be treated with iron.

SPIDER ANGIOMAS. The vascular spider (nevus araneus) consists of a central feeder artery with multiple dilated radiating vessels and a surrounding erythematous flush, varying from a few millimeters to several centimeters in diameter. Pressure over the central vessel causes blanching; pulsations visible in larger nevi are evidence for the arterial source of the lesion. Spider angiomas are associated with conditions in which there are increased levels of circulating estrogens, such as cirrhosis and pregnancy, but they also occur in up to 15% of normal preschool-aged children and 45% of school-aged ones. Sites of predilection in children are the dorsum of the hand, forearm, face, and ears. Angiomas can be obliterated by application of liquid nitrogen, electrocoagulation, or pulsed dye laser; they may also regress spontaneously.

GENERALIZED ESSENTIAL TELANGIECTASIA. A rare and presumably nevoid anomaly of unknown cause, essential telangiectasia may have its onset in childhood or adulthood. Mild expression consists of patchy retiform telangiectases, particularly on the limbs, with occasional progression to involve large areas of the body surface. The condition must be distinguished from the secondary telangiectasias of connective tissue diseases, xeroderma pigmentosum, poikiloderma, and ataxia-telangiectasia. There is no treatment; however, patients can be reassured that their health will not be affected by the cutaneous disorder.

UNILATERAL NEVOID TELANGIECTASIA. This unusual entity is characterized by the appearance of telangiectasia in a unilateral distribution, particularly in females at onset of menses or during pregnancy. The appearance of these lesions usually coincides with elevated levels of circulating estrogens, whatever the cause. When initiated by pregnancy, the telangiectasia may fade or disappear postpartum.

HEREDITARY BENIGN TELANGIECTASIA. This rare disorder is inherited as an autosomal dominant trait and develops during childhood. The face, upper trunk, and arms are the areas of predilection. The condition is progressive but remains limited to the skin.

CUTIS MARMORATA TELANGIECTATICA CONGENITA (CONGENITAL GENERALIZED PHLEBECTASIA). This benign vascular anomaly represents dilatation of superficial capillaries and veins and is apparent at birth. Involved areas of skin have a reticulated red or purple hue that resembles physiologic cutis marmorata but is more pronounced and relatively unvarying (Fig. 600–4 [color plate section]). The lesions may be restricted to a single limb and a

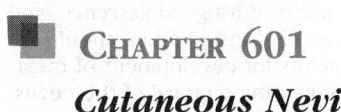

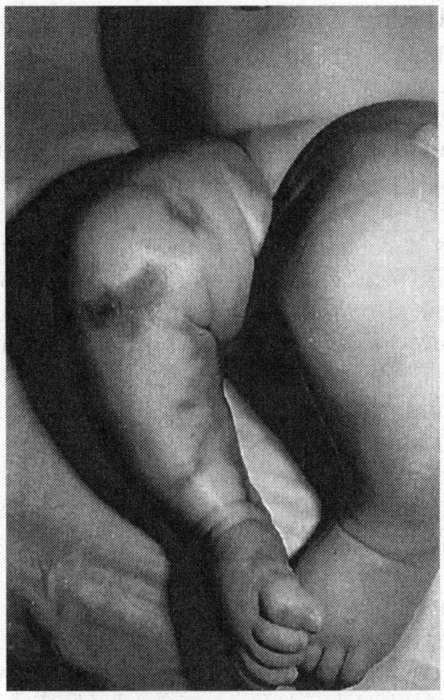

Figure 600–4. Marbled pattern of cutis marmorata telangiectatica congenita on the right leg. See also color section.

portion of the trunk or may be more widespread. Port-wine stain may also be associated. The lesions become more pronounced during changes in environmental temperature, physical activity, or crying. In some cases, the underlying subcutaneous tissue is underdeveloped, and ulceration may occur within the reticulated bands. Rarely, defective growth of bone and other congenital abnormalities may be present. No specific therapy is indicated; the expected course is one of gradual improvement, with partial or complete resolution by adolescence.

ATAXIA-TELANGIECTASIA (see Chapter 119.12). This disorder *(Louis-Bar syndrome)* is transmitted as an autosomal recessive trait. The characteristic telangiectasias develop at about 3 yr of age, first on the bulbar conjunctivae and later on the nasal bridge, malar areas, external ears, hard palate, upper anterior chest, and antecubital and popliteal fossae. Additional cutaneous stigmata include café au lait spots, premature graying of the hair, and sclerodermatous changes.

ANGIOKERATOMAS. Several forms of angiokeratomas have been described, but some do not occur during childhood or adolescence. Angiokeratomas look like flat hemangiomas with a verrucous irregular surface. *Angiokeratoma of Mibelli,* probably transmitted in an autosomal dominant pattern, is characterized by 1- to 8-mm red, purple, or black scaly, verrucous, occasionally crusted papules and nodules that appear on the dorsum of the fingers and toes and on the knees and the elbows. Less commonly, palms, soles, and ears may be affected. In many patients, onset has followed frostbite or chilblains. These nodules bleed freely after injury and may involute in response to trauma. *Angiokeratoma circumscriptum* is a rare solitary lesion that presents as a plaque of blue-red papules or nodules with a verrucous surface. These usually develop during infancy and early childhood, and they increase in size at adolescence. The lower limb is the site of predilection. They may be effectively eradicated by cryotherapy, fulguration, or excision.

ANGIOKERATOMA CORPORIS DIFFUSUM (FABRY DISEASE) (see Chapter 72). This inborn error of glycolipid metabolism is an X-linked recessive disorder that is fully penetrant in males and is of variable penetrance in carrier females. The skin lesions have their onset before puberty and occur in profusion over the genitalia, hips, buttocks, and thighs and in the umbilical and inguinal regions. They consist of 0.1- to 3-mm red to blue-black papules that may have a hyperkeratotic surface. Telangiectasias are seen in the mucosa and conjunctiva. On light microscopy, these angiokeratomas appear as blood-filled, dilated, endothelial-lined vascular spaces. Granular lipid deposits are demonstrable in dermal macrophages, fibrocytes, and endothelial cells.

Additional *clinical manifestations* include recurrent episodes of fever and agonizing pain, cyanosis and flushing of the acral limb areas, paresthesias of the hands and feet, corneal opacities detectable by slit-lamp examination, and hypohidrosis. Renal and cardiac involvement are the usual causes of death. The biochemical defect is a deficiency of the lysosomal enzyme α-galactosidase, with accumulation of ceramide trihexoside in tissues and excretion in urine. There is no specific therapy. Similar cutaneous lesions have also been described in another lysosomal enzyme disorder, α-L-fucosidase deficiency, and in sialidosis, a storage disease with neuraminidase deficiency.

NEVUS ANEMICUS. Although present at birth, nevus anemicus may not be detectable until early childhood. The nevus consists of solitary or multiple, sharply delineated, pale macules that are most often on the trunk but may also occur on the neck or limbs. These nevi may simulate plaques of vitiligo, leukoderma, or nevoid pigmentary defects, but they can be readily distinguished by their response to firm stroking. Stroking evokes an erythematous line and flare in normal surrounding skin, but the skin of a nevus anemicus does not redden. Although the cutaneous vasculature appears normal histologically, the blood vessels within the nevus do not respond to injection of vasodilators. It has been postulated that the persistent pallor may represent a sustained localized adrenergic vasoconstriction.

LYMPHANGIOMAS (see Chapter 461.3).

Enjolras O, Riche MC, Merland JJ, et al: Management of alarming hemangiomas in infancy: A review of 25 cases. Pediatrics 85:491, 1990.

Ezekowitz RAB, Mulliken JB, Folkman J: Interferon alfa-2a therapy for life-threatening hemangiomas of infancy. N Engl J Med 326:1456, 1992.

Garden J, Bakus A, Paller A: Treatment of cutaneous hemangiomas by the flashlamp-pumped pulsed dye laser: Prospective analysis. J Pediatr 120:555, 1992.

Mulliken JB, Young AE: Vascular Birthmarks: Hemangiomas and Malformations. Philadelphia, WB Saunders, 1988.

Patice SJ, Wiss K, Mulliken JB: Pyogenic granuloma (lobular capillary hemangioma): a clinicopathologic study of 178 cases. Pediatr Dermatol 8:267, 1991.

Picascia DD, Esterly NB: Cutis marmorata telangectatica congenita: A report of 22 cases. J Am Acad Dermatol 20:1098, 1989.

Strauss RP, Resnick SD: Pulsed dye laser therapy for port-wine stains in children: Psychosocial and ethical issues. J Pediatr 122:505, 1993.

Takahashi K, Mulliken JB, Kozakewich HPW, et al: Cellular markers that distinguish phases of hemangioma during infancy and childhood. J Clin Invest 93:2357, 1994.

Tallman B, Tan OT, Morelli JG, et al: Location of port-wine stains and the likelihood of ophthalmic and/or central nervous system complications. Pediatrics 87:323, 1991.

CHAPTER 601

Cutaneous Nevi

Gary L. Darmstadt and Al Lane

Nevus skin lesions are characterized histopathologically by collections of well-differentiated cell types normally found in the skin. Vascular nevi (hemangiomas) are described in Chapter 600. Melanocytic nevi are subdivided into two broad categories: those that appear after birth, or acquired nevi, and those that are present at birth, the congenital nevi.

ACQUIRED MELANOCYTIC NEVUS. Melanocytic nevi are a benign cluster of melanocytic nevus cells that arise as a result of proliferation of melanocytes at the epidermal-dermal junction. Nevus cells may have the same origin as and are probably identical to melanocytes. An alternative, less popular theory is that nevus cells are of dual origin, with superficially located cells arising from melanocytes *(melanocytic nevus)* and cells in the deeper layers arising from Schwann cells *(neuroid nevus)*.

Epidemiology. The number of acquired melanocytic nevi increases gradually during childhood, sharply at adolescence, and more slowly in early adulthood; reaches a plateau in number during the third or fourth decade; and then slowly decreases thereafter. The mean number of melanocytic nevi in an adult is 25 to 35. The greater the number of nevi present, the greater the risk for development of melanoma. Sun exposure during childhood, particularly intermittent, intense exposure of an individual with light skin and a propensity to burn and freckle rather than tan, is an important determinant of the number of melanocytic nevi that develop. Increased numbers of nevi are also associated with immunosuppression and administration of chemotherapy.

Clinical Manifestations. Nevocellular nevi have a well-defined life history and are classified as junctional, compound, or dermal in accordance with the location of the nevus cells in the skin. In childhood, more than 90% of nevi are junctional; melanocyte proliferation occurs at the junction of the epidermis and dermis to form nests of cells. *Junctional nevi* appear anywhere on the body in varying shades of brown; they are relatively small, discrete, flat, and variable in shape. The melanized nevus cells are cuboidal or epithelioid in configuration and occur in nests on the epidermal side of the basement membrane. Although some nevi, particularly those on the palms, soles, and genitalia, remain junctional throughout life, most become compound as melanocytes migrate into the papillary dermis to form nests at both the epidermal-dermal junction and within the dermis. If the junctional melanocytes stop proliferating, nests of melanocytes remain only within the dermis, forming an intradermal nevus. With maturation, *compound* and *intradermal nevi* may become raised, dome-shaped, verrucous, or pedunculated. Slightly elevated lesions are usually compound. Distinctly elevated lesions are usually intradermal. With age, the dermal melanocytic nests regress, and the nevi gradually disappear.

Prognosis and Treatment. Acquired pigmented nevi are benign, but a very small percentage undergo malignant transformation. Suspicious changes such as rapid increase in size; development of satellite lesions; variegation of color, particularly with shades of red, brown, gray, black, and blue; pigmentary incontinence; notching or irregularity of the borders; and changes in texture such as scaling, erosion, ulceration, induration, or regional lymphadenopathy are indications for excision and histopathologic evaluation. Most of these changes are due to irritation, infection, or maturation; darkening and gradual increase in size and elevation normally occur during adolescence and should not be cause for concern. Consideration should be given to the presence of risk factors for development of melanoma and the parent's wishes regarding removal of the nevus. If doubt remains about the benign nature of a nevus, excision is a safe and simple outpatient procedure that may be justified to allay anxiety.

ATYPICAL MELANOCYTIC NEVUS. Atypical nevocellular nevi occur in both a familial, melanoma-prone setting and as a sporadic event. *Familial mole-melanoma syndrome* is an autosomal dominant trait that affects an estimated 32,000 Americans. Only 2% of all pediatric melanomas occur in individuals with this syndrome, and 10% of those with the syndrome have a melanoma develop before age 20 yr. Risk for development of melanoma is essentially 100% in individuals with *familial dysplastic nevus syndrome* and two family members who have had melanomas. The term *atypical mole syndrome* has been proposed for those individuals without an autosomal dominant familial history of melanoma but with more than 50 nevi, some of which are atypical. The lifetime risk of melanoma associated with dysplastic nevi in this context is estimated to be 5–10%.

Atypical nevi tend to be large (5–15 mm) and round to oval. They have irregular margins, variegated color, and elevation of a portion of the lesion. These nevi are most common on the posterior trunk, suggesting that intermittent, intense sun exposure plays a role in their genesis. They may also occur, however, in sun-protected areas such as the breasts, buttocks, and scalp. Atypical nevi do not usually develop until puberty, although scalp lesions may be present earlier. Histopathologically, atypical nevi demonstrate disordered proliferation of atypical intraepidermal melanocytes, lymphocytic infiltration, fibroplasia, and angiogenesis. It may be helpful to obtain histopathologic documentation of dysplastic change by biopsy to identify these individuals. It is prudent to excise borderline atypical nevi in immunocompromised children or in those treated with x-ray irradiation or chemotherapeutic agents. Although chemotherapy has been associated with the development of a greater number of melanocytic nevi, it has not yet been directly linked to increased risk for development of melanoma. The threshold for removal of clinically atypical nevi is also lower at sites that are difficult to follow, such as the scalp. Children with atypical nevi should have a complete skin examination every 6–12 mo. Parents must be counseled regarding the importance of sun protection and avoidance and instructed to look for early signs of melanoma on a regular basis, approximately every 3–4 mo.

CONGENITAL MELANOCYTIC NEVUS. Congenital melanocytic nevi are present in approximately 1% of newborn infants. These nevi have been categorized by size: giant congenital nevi are more than 20 cm in diameter (adult size), small congenital nevi are less than 2 cm in diameter, and intermediate nevi are in between in size. Histopathologically, congenital nevi are characterized by the presence of nevus cells in the lower reticular dermis; between collagen bundles; surrounding cutaneous appendages, nerves, and vessels in the lower dermis; and, occasionally, extending to the subcuticular fat. Identification is often uncertain, however, as they may have the histologic features of ordinary junctional, compound, or intradermal nevi. Some nevi that were not present at birth display histopathologic features of congenital nevi. Furthermore, congenital nevi may be difficult to distinguish clinically from other types of pigmented lesions, adding to the difficulty that parents may have in identifying nevi that were present at birth. The clinical differential diagnosis includes mongolian spots, café au lait spots, smooth muscle hamartoma, and dermal melanocytosis (nevi of Ota and Ito).

Sites of predilection of *small congenital nevi* are the lower trunk, upper back, shoulders, chest, and proximal limbs. The lesions may be flat, elevated, verrucous, or nodular and may be various shades of brown, blue, or black. Given the difficulty in identifying small congenital nevi with certainty, data regarding their malignant potential is controversial. Based on historical criteria, it is estimated that approximately 15% of melanomas arise within small congenital nevi. With histopathologic criteria, a congenital nevus has been found in association with approximately 3–8% of melanomas. Removal of all small congenital nevi is not warranted, particularly in view of the fact that development of melanoma in a small congenital nevus is an exceedingly rare event before puberty. A number of factors must be weighed in the decision of whether or not to remove a nevus, including its location and ability to be followed clinically, the potential for scarring, the presence of other risk factors for melanoma, and the presence of atypical clinical features.

Giant congenital pigmented nevi ($<$ 1:20,000 births) occur most commonly on the posterior trunk but may also appear on the head or the extremities. These nevi are of special significance because of their association with leptomeningeal melanocytosis and their predisposition for development of malignant melanoma. Leptomeningeal involvement occurs most often when the nevus is located on the head or midline on the trunk. Nevus cells within the leptomeninges and brain parenchyma may cause increased intracranial pressure, hydrocephalus, seizures, retardation, and motor deficits and may result in melanoma. Malignancy can be identified by careful cytologic examination of the cerebrospinal fluid for melanin-containing cells. Asymptomatic leptomeningeal melanosis was noted recently on magnetic resonance imaging (MRI) scans of approximately one third of individuals with a giant congenital nevus. The overall incidence of malignant melanoma arising in a giant congenital nevus is estimated to be approximately 5–10%, and approximately 3% of all melanomas arise within a giant congenital nevus. Approximately one half of all melanomas that arise within a giant congenital nevus do so by age 5 yr. The mortality rate is approximately 45%. Management of giant congenital nevi remains controversial and should involve the parents, pediatrician, dermatologist, and plastic surgeon. If the nevus lies over the head or spine, an MRI scan may allow detection of neural melanosis; its presence makes the gross removal of a nevus from the skin a futile effort. In the absence of neural melanosis, early excision and repair aided by tissue expanders or grafting may reduce the burden of nevus cells and thus the potential for development of melanoma, but at the cost of multiple potentially disfiguring surgeries. Even then, nevus cells deep within subcutaneous tissues may evade excision. Random biopsies of the nevus are not helpful, but biopsy of newly expanding nodules is indicated. Follow-up is recommended every 6 mo for 5 yr and every 12 mo thereafter. Serial photographs of the nevus may aid in detecting changes.

MELANOMA. Malignant melanoma accounts for 1–3% of all pediatric malignancies and is the most common cancer in young adults aged 25–29 yr. Melanoma develops primarily in white individuals, on the head and trunk in males and on the extremities in females. Risk factors for development of melanoma include the presence of the familial atypical mole-melanoma syndrome or xeroderma pigmentosum; increased number of melanocytic nevi, either acquired nevi, giant congenital nevus, or atypical nevi; fair complexion; excessive sun exposure, especially intense sunlight intermittently; a personal or family (i.e., first-degree relative) history of a previous melanoma; and immunosuppression. Less than 5% of childhood melanomas develop within giant congenital nevi or in those with the familial atypical mole-melanoma syndrome. Approximately 30–50% of the time, melanoma develops at a site where there was no apparent nevus. The mortality rate from melanoma is related primarily to tumor thickness and the level of invasion into the skin. The overall mortality rate reaches approximately 40%, regardless of whether it arises in a child or adult. Given the lack of effective therapy for melanoma, prevention and early detection are the most effective measures. Avoidance of intense midday sun exposure between 10 A.M. to 3 P.M.; use of protective clothing such as a hat, long sleeves, and pants; and use of sunscreen should be stressed.

HALO NEVUS (LEUKODERMA ACQUISITUM CENTRIFUGUM). Halo nevi occur primarily in children and young adults, most commonly on the back (Fig. 601–1). Development of the halo may coincide with puberty or pregnancy. Frequently, several pigmented nevi develop a halo simultaneously. Subsequent disappearance of the central nevus over several months is the usual outcome, and the depigmented area may or may not become repigmented. Excision and histopathologic examination of the lesion is indicated only when the nature of the central lesion is in question. Occasionally, an acquired melanocytic nevus develops a peripheral zone of depigmentation over a period of days to weeks. Histopathologically, there is a dense inflammatory infiltrate of lymphocytes and histiocytes in addition to the nevus cells. The pale halo reflects disappearance of the melanocytes. This phenomenon is associated with congenital nevi, blue nevi, Spitz nevi, dysplastic nevi, neurofibromas, primary and secondary malignant melanoma, and occasionally with poliosis, Vogt-Koyanagi-Harada syndrome, and pernicious anemia. Patients with vitiligo have an increased incidence of halo nevi. Individuals with halo nevi have circulating antibodies against the cytoplasm of malignant melanoma cells, and their lymphocytes display enhanced killing of melanoma cells in culture.

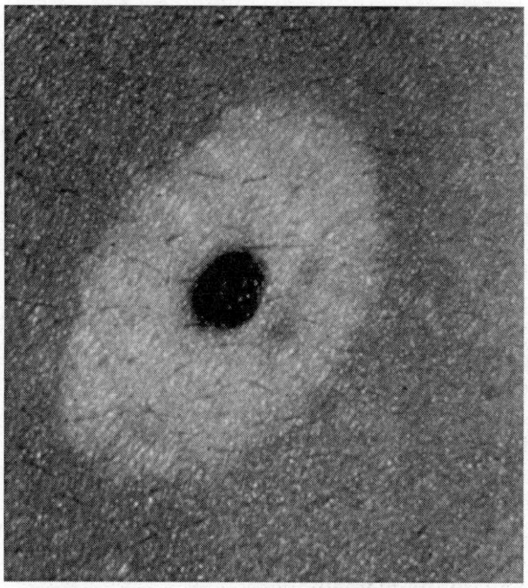

Figure 601–1. Well-developed halo nevus.

SPITZ NEVUS (SPINDLE AND EPITHELIOID CELL NEVUS). Spitz nevus presents most commonly during the first 2 decades of life as a pink to red, smooth, dome-shaped, firm, hairless papule on the face, shoulder, or upper limb. Most are less than 1 cm in diameter, but they can achieve a size of 3 cm. Rarely, they occur as multiple grouped lesions. Visually similar lesions include pyogenic granuloma, hemangioma, nevocellular nevus, juvenile xanthogranuloma, and basal cell carcinoma, but histologically these entities are distinguishable. Spitz nevus may be difficult to distinguish histopathologically from malignant melanoma because nuclear atypia is a common feature, particularly after local recurrence of the nevus. Local recurrence after excision may occur up to 5% of the time. If there is clinical suspicion that a nevus may be a melanoma, then an excisional biopsy of the entire lesion is recommended. If the margins of excision of a Spitz nevus are positive, a re-excision of the site is prudent to avoid difficulties in histopathologic interpretation of the lesion in the future.

ZOSTERIFORM LENTIGINOUS NEVUS (AGMINATED LENTIGENES). This nevus is a unilateral, linear, bandlike collection of multiple 2–10-mm brown or black macules on the face, trunk, or limbs. The nevus may be present at birth or may develop during childhood. Histopathologically, there are increased numbers of melanocytes in elongated rete ridges of the epidermis.

NEVUS SPILUS (SPECKLED LENTIGINOUS NEVUS). This nevus is a flat, brown patch, within which are darker, flat or raised, brown melanocytic elements. These nevi vary considerably in size and can occur anywhere on the body. Nevus spilus is rare at birth and is commonly acquired during late infancy or early childhood. Dark elements within the nevus are usually present initially and tend to increase in number gradually over time. The darker macules represent nevus cells in a junctional or dermal location; the patch has increased numbers of melanocytes in a lentiginous epidermal pattern. The malignant potential of these nevi is uncertain; nevus spilus is found more commonly in individuals with melanoma compared with matched controls. The nevi need not be excised, however, unless atypical features or recent clinical changes are noted.

NEVUS OF OTA. Nevus of Ota is more common in females and in Asian and black patients. This nevus consists of a permanent patch composed of blue, black, and brown, partially confluent macules. The intensity of pigmentation may vary from day to day, and enlargement and darkening may occur with time. Occasionally, some areas of the nevus are raised. The macular nevi resemble mongolian spots in color and occur unilaterally in the areas supplied by the 1st and 2nd divisions of the trigeminal nerve. Nevus of Ota differs from a mongolian spot, not only by its distribution, but also by having a speckled rather than a uniform appearance. It also has a greater concentration of elongated, dendritic dermal melanocytes located in the upper rather than the lower portion of the dermis. Nevus of Ota is sometimes present at birth; in other cases, it may arise during the 1st or 2nd decade of life. Patchy involvement of the conjunctiva, hard palate, pharynx, nasal mucosa, buccal mucosa, or tympanic membrane occurs in some patients. Malignant change is exceedingly rare. Laser therapy may effectively decrease the pigmentation.

Nevus of Ito is localized to the supraclavicular, scapular, and deltoid regions. This nevus tends to be more diffuse in its distribution and less mottled than the nevus of Ota. The only available treatment is masking with cosmetics or laser therapy.

BLUE NEVI. The *common blue nevus* is a solitary, asymptomatic, smooth, dome-shaped, blue to blue-gray papule less than 10 mm in diameter on the dorsal hands and feet. Rarely, common blue nevi form large plaques. The nevus is nearly always acquired, often during childhood, and more commonly in females. Microscopically, it is characterized by groups of intensely pigmented, spindle-shaped melanocytes in the dermis. This nevus is benign.

The *cellular blue nevus* is typically 1–3 cm in diameter and occurs most frequently on the buttocks and in the sacrococcygeal area. In addition to collections of deeply pigmented dermal dendritic melanocytes, cellular islands composed of large spindle-shaped cells are noted in the dermis and may extend into the subcutaneous fat. The cellular blue nevus has a low but definite incidence of malignant transformation, and therefore excision is the treatment of choice. A *combined nevus* is the association of a blue nevus with an overlying melanocytic nevus.

The blue-gray color that is characteristic of these nevi is an optical effect caused by dermal melanin. Longer wavelengths of visible light penetrate to the deep dermis and are absorbed there by melanin; shorter-wavelength blue light cannot penetrate deeply but instead is reflected back to the observer.

ACHROMIC NEVUS (NEVUS DEPIGMENTOSUS). These nevi are usually present at birth; they are localized macular hypopigmented patches or streaks, often with bizarre, irregular borders. They can resemble hypomelanosis of Ito clinically, except that they are more localized and often unilateral. Small lesions may also resemble the white leaf macules of tuberous sclerosis. They appear to represent a focal defect in transfer of melanosomes to keratinocytes.

EPIDERMAL NEVI. These may be visible at birth or may develop within the first months or years of life. They affect both sexes equally and usually occur sporadically. Epidermal nevi are hamartomatous lesions characterized by hyperplasia of the epidermis and/or adnexal structures in a focal area of the skin. Proliferation of nevocellular nevus cells is not present in these lesions.

Epidermal nevi are classified into a number of variants, depending on the morphology and extent of the nevus and the epidermal structure that is predominant. An epidermal nevus may appear initially as a discolored, slightly scaly patch that, with maturation, becomes more linear, thickened, verrucous, and hyperpigmented. Systematized refers to a diffuse or extensive distribution of lesions, and ichthyosis hystrix indicates that the distribution is extensive and bilateral. Morphologic types include pigmented papillomas, often in a linear distribution; unilateral hyperkeratotic streaks involving a limb and perhaps a portion of the trunk; velvety hyperpigmented plaques; and whorled or marbled hyperkeratotic lesions in localized plaques (Fig. 601–2) or over extensive areas of the body along Blaschko lines. An inflammatory linear verrucous variant is markedly pruritic and tends to become erythematous, scaling, and crusted.

The histologic pattern evolves as the lesion matures, but epidermal hyperplasia of some degree is apparent in all stages of development. One or another dermal appendage may predominate in a particular lesion. These nevi must be distinguished from lichen striatus, lymphangioma circumscriptum, shagreen patch of tuberous sclerosis, congenital hairy nevi, linear porokeratosis, linear lichen planus, linear psoriasis, the verrucous stage of incontinentia pigmenti, and nevus sebaceous (Jadassohn). Keratolytic agents such as retinoic acid or salicylic acid may be moderately effective in reducing scaling and controlling pruritus, but definitive *treatment* requires full-thickness excision; recurrence is usual if more superficial removal is attempted. Alternatively, the nevus may be left intact. Rarely, basal cell carcinoma or squamous cell carcinoma have developed in a verrucous epidermal nevus that shows sudden growth, nodularity, or erosions.

Epidermal nevi are occasionally associated with other abnormalities of the skin and soft tissues; eyes; and nervous, cardiovascular, musculoskeletal, and urogenital systems. In these instances, referred to as *epidermal nevus syndrome,* a mosaic phenotype is expressed. This syndrome, however, is not a distinct clinical entity. The well-established syndromes that involve a type of epidermal nevus and distinct birth defects include the sebaceous nevus, Proteus, and CHILD (congenital hemidysplasia with ichthyosiform erythroderma and limb defects) syndromes.

Nevus Sebaceous (Jadassohn). This is a relatively small, sharply demarcated, oval or linear, yellow-orange, elevated plaque that is usually devoid of hair and occurs on the head and neck of infants. They may occur occasionally on the trunk. Although characterized histopathologically by an abundance of sebaceous glands, all elements of the skin are represented. It is frequently flat and inconspicuous in early childhood. With maturity, usually during adolescence, the lesions become verrucous and studded with large rubbery nodules. The changing clinical appearance reflects the histologic pattern, which is characterized by a variable degree of hyperkeratosis, hyperplasia of the epidermis, malformed hair follicles, and often a

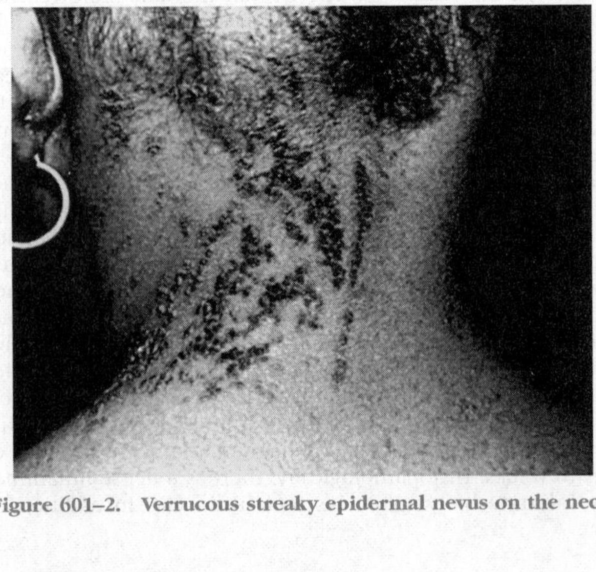

Figure 601–2. Verrucous streaky epidermal nevus on the neck.

profusion of sebaceous glands and the presence of ectopic apocrine glands. It is believed that these nevi form from pleuripotential primary epithelial germ cells, which can dedifferentiate into various epithelial tumors. Consequently, during adulthood, these nevi are frequently complicated by secondary malignancies and benign adnexal tumors, most commonly basal cell carcinoma or syringocystadenoma papilliferum. Diagnosis can be established by biopsy; the treatment of choice is total excision before adolescence. Sebaceous nevi associated with central nervous system, skeletal, and ocular defects represent a variant of the epidermal nevus syndrome.

Becker Nevus (Becker Melanosis). This form of epidermal nevus develops predominantly in males, during childhood or adolescence, initially as a hyperpigmented patch. The lesion commonly develops hypertrichosis, limited to the area of hyperpigmentation, and evolves into a unilateral, slightly thickened, irregular, hyperpigmented plaque. The most common sites are the upper torso and upper arm. Histopathologically, the nevus shows an increased number of basal melanocytes and variable epidermal hyperplasia. Commonly, Becker melanosis is associated with a smooth muscle hamartoma, which may appear as slight perifollicular papular elevations or slight induration. Stroking such a lesion may induce smooth muscle contraction and make the hairs stand up. Androgen sensitivity may play a role in the development of Becker melanosis. The nevus is benign, has no risk for malignant change, and is very rarely associated with other anomalies.

NEVUS COMEDONICUS. This is an uncommon organoid nevus of epithelial origin that consists of linear plaques of plugged follicles that simulate comedones; they may be present at birth or appear during childhood. The horny plugs represent keratinous debris within dilated, malformed pilosebaceous follicles. The lesions are most often unilateral and may develop at any site. Rarely, they are associated with other congenital malformations, including skeletal defects, cerebral anomalies, and cataracts. Although often asymptomatic, some individuals experience recurrent inflammation, resulting in cyst formation, fistulas, and scarring. There is no effective treatment except full-thickness excision; palliation of larger lesions may be achieved by regular applications of a retinoic acid preparation.

CONNECTIVE TISSUE NEVUS. This is a hamartoma of collagen, elastin, and/or glycosaminoglycans of the dermal extracellular matrix. It may occur as a solitary defect or as a manifestation of an associated disorder. These nevi may occur at any site but are most common on the back, buttocks, arms, and thighs. They are skin-colored, ivory, or yellow plaques, 2–15 cm in diameter, composed of multiple tiny papules or grouped nodules that are frequently difficult to appreciate visually because of the subtle color changes. The plaques have a rubbery or cobblestone consistency on palpation. Biopsy findings are variable and include increased amounts and/or degeneration or fragmentation of dermal collagen, elastic tissue, or ground substance. Similar lesions occurring with tuberous sclerosis are called shagreen patches; however, shagreen patches consist only of excessive amounts of collagen. The association of multiple small papular connective tissue nevi with osteopoikilosis is called *dermatofibrosis lenticularis disseminata* (Buschke-Ollendorf syndrome).

SMOOTH MUSCLE HAMARTOMA. This hamartoma is a developmental anomaly resulting from hyperplasia of the smooth muscle (arrector pili) associated with hair follicles. It is usually evident at birth or shortly thereafter as a flesh-colored or lightly pigmented plaque with overlying hypertrichosis on the trunk or limbs. Transient elevation or a rippling movement of the lesion, caused by contraction of the muscle bundles, can sometimes be elicited by stroking the surface. Smooth muscle hamartoma can be mistaken for congenital pigmented nevus, but the distinction is important because it has no risk for malignant melanoma and need not be removed.

Ackerman AB, Milde P: Naming acquired melanocytic nevi. Common and dysplastic, normal and atypical, or Unna, Miescher, Spitz, and Clark? Am J Dermatopathol 14:447, 1992.

Arons MS, Hurwitz S: Congenital nevocellular nevus: a review of the treatment controversy and a report of 46 cases. Plast Reconstr Surg 72:355, 1983.

Casso EM, Grin-Jorgensen CM, Grant-Kels JM: Spitz nevi. J Am Acad Dermatol 27:901, 1992.

Ceballos PI, Ruiz-Maldonado R, Mihm MC: Melanoma in children. N Engl J Med 332:656, 1995.

Frieden IJ, Williams ML, Barkovich AJ: Giant congenital melanocytic nevi: Brain magnetic resonance findings in neurologically asymptomatic children. J Am Acad Dermatol 31:423, 1994.

Gallagher RP, McClean DI, Yang CP, et al: Anatomic distribution of acquired melanocytic nevi in white children. Arch Dermatol 125:466, 1990.

Gallagher RP, McClean DI, Yang CP, et al: Suntan, sunburn, and pigmentation factors and the frequency of acquired melanocytic nevi in children. Arch Dermatol 126:770, 1990.

Green MH, Clark WH, Tucker MA, et al: Acquired precursors of cutaneous malignant melanoma. (The familial dysplastic nevus syndrome.) N Engl J Med 312:91, 1985.

Happle R: How many epidermal nevus syndromes exist? A clinicogenetic classification. J Am Acad Dermatol 25:550, 1991.

Illig L, Weidner F, Hundeiker M, et al: Congenital nevi ≤ 10 cm as precursors to melanoma: 52 cases, a review and a new concept. Arch Dermatol 121:1274, 1985.

Jacobs AH, Walton RG: The incidence of birthmarks in the neonate. Pediatrics 58:281, 1976.

Kaplan EN: The risk of malignancy in large congenital nevi. Plast Reconstr Surg 53:421, 1974.

Marghoob AA, Orlow SJ, Kopf AW: Syndromes associated with melanocytic nevi. J Am Acad Dermatol 29:373, 1993.

Mehregan AH, Mehregan DA: Malignant melanoma in childhood. Cancer 71:4096, 1993.

Rhodes AR: Congenital nevi: should these be excised? JAMA 262:1696, 1989.

Rhodes AR, Melski JW: Small congenital nevocellular nevi and the risk of cutaneous melanoma. J Pediatr 100:219, 1982.

Rothman KF, Esterly N: Dysplastic nevi in children. Pediatr Dermatol 7:218, 1990.

Shpall S, Frieden I, Chesney M, et al: Risk of malignant transformation of congenital melanocytic nevi in blacks. Pediatr Dermatol 11:204, 1994.

Swenen RJ: Management of congenital nevocytic nevi: A survey of current practices. J Am Acad Dermatol 11:629, 1984.

Tucker MA, Clarke WH, Fraser MC, et al: Dysplastic nevi on the scalp of prepubertal children from melanoma-prone families. J Pediatr 103:65, 1983.

Walter SD, Marrett LF, Hertzman C, et al: The association of cutaneous malignant melanoma with the use of sunbeds and sunlamps. Am J Epidemiol 131:232, 1990.

Weinstock MA, Colditz GA, Willett WC: Nonfamilial cutaneous melanoma incidence in women associated with sun exposure before 20 years of age. Pediatrics 84:199, 1989.

Williams ML, Pennella R: Melanoma, melanocytic nevi, and other melanoma risk factors in children. J Pediatr 124:833, 1994.

Williams ML, Sagebiel RS, Vasconez LO: Special symposium. The management of congenital nevocytic nevi. Pediatr Dermatol 2:143, 1984.

CHAPTER 602

Hyperpigmented Lesions

Gary L. Darmstadt and Al Lane

DISORDERS OF PIGMENT. Alterations in skin color may be generalized or localized and may result from a variety of defects, ranging from absence of melanocytes and defective melanization of melanosomes to overproduction of melanin and increased numbers of melanocytic cells. Some of these aberrations are induced by hormones (hyperpigmentation of Addison disease); others represent focal developmental defects (white spots of tuberous sclerosis); still others may be nonspecific and the result of cutaneous inflammation (postinflammatory hypopigmentation or hyperpigmentation).

EPHELIDES OR FRECKLES. These are light or dark brown macules usually less than 3 mm in diameter, with a poorly defined margin, that occur in sun-exposed areas, such as the face, upper back, arms, and hands. They are induced by exposure to sun, particularly during the summer, and may fade or disappear during the winter. They are more common in fair-haired individuals, appear first during the preschool years, and are determined by an autosomal dominant gene. Histologically, they are marked by increased melanin pigment in epidermal basal cells, which have more numerous and larger dendritic processes than the melanocytes of the surrounding paler skin. Freckles have been identified as a risk factor for melanoma independent of melanocytic nevi.

LENTIGINES. Lentigines, often mistaken for freckles or junctional nevi, are small (<3 cm), round, dark brown macules that can appear anywhere on the body; are unrelated to sun exposure; and remain permanently. Histologically, they have elongated, club-shaped, epidermal rete ridges with increased numbers of melanocytes and dense epidermal deposits of melanin. No nests of melanocytes are found. The lesions are benign and, when few, may be viewed as a normal occurrence.

Lentigines may increase in number and darken excessively in Addison's disease and during pregnancy. *Lentiginosis profusa* involves innumerable small, pigmented macules that are present at birth or appear during childhood. There are no associated abnormalities, and mucous membranes are spared. *LAMB syndrome* consists of lentigines of the face and vulva, atrial myxoma, mucocutaneous myxomas, and blue nevi. The *multiple lentigines (LEOPARD) syndrome* is an autosomal dominant entity consisting of a generalized, symmetric distribution of lentigines in association with electrocardiogram abnormalities, ocular hypertelorism, pulmonary stenosis, abnormal genitalia (cryptochidism, hypogonadism, hypospadius), growth retardation, and sensorineural deafness. Other features include hypertrophic obstructive cardiomyopathy and pectus excavatum or carinatum.

The *Peutz-Jeghers syndrome* is characterized by melanotic macules on the lips and mucous membranes and by gastrointestinal polyposis. It is inherited as an autosomal dominant trait. Onset is noted during infancy and early childhood when pigmented macules appear on the lips and buccal mucosa. The macules are usually a few millimeters in size but may be as large as 1–2 cm. Macules also appear occasionally on the palate, gums, tongue, and vaginal mucosa. Cutaneous lesions may develop on the nose, hands, feet; around the mouth, eyes, and umbilicus; and as longitudinal bands or diffuse hyperpigmentation of the nails. Pigmented macules often fade from the lips and skin during puberty and adulthood but generally do not disappear from mucosal surfaces. Buccal mucosal macules are the most constant feature of the disorder; in some families, however, occasional members may be affected only with the pigmentary changes. Indistinguishable pigmentary changes beginning in adult life also occur sporadically in individuals without intestinal involvement.

Polyposis usually involves the jejunum and ileum but may also occur in the stomach, duodenum, colon, and rectum. Episodic abdominal pain, diarrhea, melena, and intussusception are frequent complications. Patients have a significantly increased risk of gastrointestinal tract and nongastrointestinal tract tumors at a young age. Gastrointestinal cancer has been reported in approximately 2–3% of patients; the lifetime relative risk of gastrointestinal malignancy is 13. The relative risk of nongastrointestinal tract malignancies is 9, including ovarian, cervical, and testicular tumors. Peutz-Jeghers syndrome must be differentiated from other syndromes associated with multiple lentigines (*Laugier-Hunziker syndrome*), from ordinary freckling, from *Gardner syndrome,* and from *Cronkhite-Canada syndrome,* a disorder characterized by gastrointestinal polyposis; alopecia; onychodystrophy; and diffuse pigmentation of the palms, volar aspects of the fingers, and dorsal hands. Treatment of Peutz-Jeghers melanotic macules has been successful, in some cases, with carbon dioxide, ruby, or argon lasers.

CAFÉ AU LAIT SPOTS. These are uniformly hyperpigmented, sharply demarcated, macular lesions, the hues of which vary with the normal degree of pigmentation of the individual: they are tan or light brown in white individuals and may be dark brown in black children. Café au lait spots vary tremendously in size and may be large, covering a significant portion of the trunk or limb. Generally, the borders are smooth, but some have an exceedingly irregular border. The lesions are characterized by increased numbers of melanocytes and melanin in the epidermis but lack the clubbed rete ridges that typify lentigines. One to three café au lait spots are common in normal children; approximately 10% of normal children have café au lait macules. They may be present at birth or develop during childhood.

Large, often asymmetric café au lait spots with irregular borders are characteristic of patients with *McCune-Albright syndrome* (see Chapter 517.5). This disorder includes polyostotic fibrous dysplasia of bone, leading to pathologic fractures; precocious puberty; and multiple hyperfunctional endocrinopathies. The macular hyperpigmentation may be present at birth or develop late in childhood. Cutaneous pigmentation is most extensive on the side showing the most severe bone involvement. The full syndrome with precocious puberty occurs only in girls. A mutation in the gene for the α-subunit of G_s, the G protein that stimulates cyclic adenosine monophosphate formation, occurs in these patients.

Neurofibromatosis Type 1 (von Recklinghausen disease). The café au lait spot is the most familiar cutaneous hallmark of this autosomal dominant neurocutaneous syndrome (see Chapter 546.1). These lesions also occur with certain other disorders, including other types of neurofibromatosis (Table 602–1). Included in the criteria for this diagnosis is the presence of five or more café au lait spots more than 5 mm in diameter in prepubertal patients or six or more café au lait spots more than 15 mm in diameter in postpubertal children.

INCONTINENTIA PIGMENTI (BLOCH-SULZBERGER DISEASE). This rare, heritable, multisystem ectodermal disorder features dermatologic, dental, and ocular abnormalities. The phenotype is produced by functional mosaicism caused by random X-inactivation of an X-linked dominant gene that is lethal in males. The paucity of affected males, the occurrence of female-to-female transmission, and an increased frequency of spontaneous abortions in carrier females supports this supposition. The gene is linked to the Xq28 region.

Cutaneous Manifestations. There are four phases, not all of which may occur in a given patient. The *first phase* is evident at birth or during the first few weeks of life and consists of erythematous, linear streaks and plaques of vesicles that are most pronounced on the limbs and circumferentially on the trunk. The lesions may be confused with those of herpes simplex, bullous impetigo, or mastocytosis, but the linear configuration is unique. Histopathologically, epidermal edema and eosinophil-filled intraepidermal vesicles are present. Eosinophils also infiltrate the adjacent epidermis and dermis. Blood eosinophilia up to 65% is also common. The first stage generally resolves by 4 mo of age, but mild, short-lived recurrences of blisters may develop during febrile illnesses of childhood. In the *second phase,* as blisters on the distal limbs resolve, they become dry and hyperkeratotic, forming verrucous plaques. The verrucous plaques rarely affect the trunk or face and

■ **TABLE 602–1 Disorders with Café au Lait Spots**

Neurofibromatosis	Tuberous sclerosis
McCune-Albright syndrome	Bloom syndrome
Russell-Silver syndrome	Epidermal nevus syndrome
Multiple lentigines	Gaucher disease
Ataxia telangiectasia	Chédiak-Higashi syndrome
Fanconi anemia	

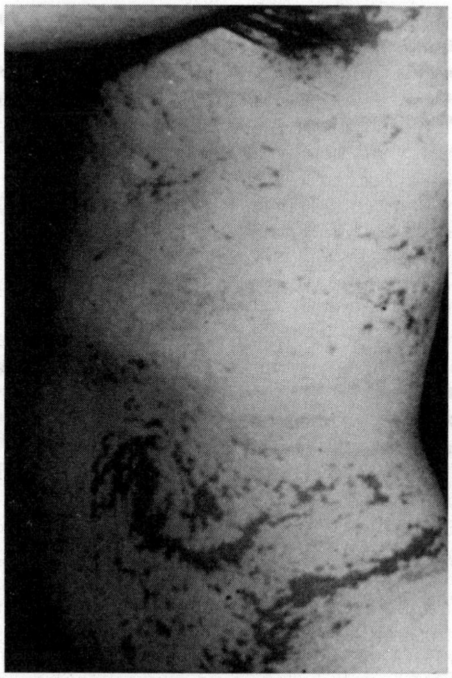

Figure 602–1. Whorled macular hyperpigmentation of incontinentia pigmenti.

generally involute within 6 mo. Epidermal hyperplasia, hyperkeratosis, and papillomatosis are characteristic. The *third* or *pigmentary stage* is the hallmark of incontinentia pigmenti. It generally develops over weeks to months and may overlap the earlier phases, be evident at birth, or, more commonly, begin to appear within the first few weeks of life. Hyperpigmentation is more often apparent on the trunk than the limbs and is distributed in macular whorls, reticulated patches, flecks, and linear streaks that follow Blaschko lines. The axillae and groin are invariably affected. The sites of involvement are not necessarily those of the preceding vesicular and warty lesions. The pigmented lesions, once present, persist throughout childhood (Fig. 602–1B). They generally begin to fade by early adolescence, however, and often have disappeared by age 16 yr. Occasionally, the pigmentation remains permanently, particularly in the groin. The lesion, histopathologically, shows vacuolar degeneration of the epidermal basal cells and melanin in melanophages of the upper dermis as a result of incontinence of pigment. In the *fourth stage*, hypopigmented, hairless, anhidrotic patches or streaks occur as a late manifestation of incontinentia pigmenti; they may develop, however, before the hyperpigmentation of stage three has resolved. The lesions develop mainly on the flexor aspect of the lower legs and less often on the arms and trunk.

Although skin lesions may constitute the only manifestation, approximately 80% of affected children have other defects. Alopecia, which may be scarring and patchy or diffuse, is most common on the vertex and occurs in up to 40% of patients. Hair may be lusterless, wiry, and coarse. Dental anomalies, which are present in up to 80% of patients and are persistent throughout life, consist of late dentition, hypodontia, conical teeth, and impaction. Central nervous system manifestations, including motor and cognitive developmental retardation, seizures, microcephaly, spasticity, and paralysis are found in up to one third of affected children. Ocular anomalies, such as neovascularization, microphthalmos, strabismus, optic nerve atrophy, cataracts, or retrolenticular masses occur in more than 30% of children. Nonetheless, greater than 90% of patients have normal vision. Less common abnormalities include dystrophy of nails (ridging, pitting) and skeletal defects.

Diagnosis of incontinentia pigmenti is made on clinical grounds, although major and minor criteria have been established to aid in diagnosis. Wood lamp examination may be useful in older children and adolescents to highlight pigmentary abnormalities.

Treatment. The choice of investigative studies and the plan of management depend on the occurrence of particular noncutaneous abnormalities because the skin lesions are benign. The high incidence of associated major anomalies warrants genetic counseling.

POSTINFLAMMATORY PIGMENTARY CHANGES. Either hyperpigmentation or hypopigmentation can occur as a result of cutaneous inflammation. Alteration in pigmentation usually follows a severe inflammatory reaction but may result from mild dermatitis. Dark-skinned children are more likely to show these changes than fair-skinned ones. Although altered pigmentation may persist for weeks to months, patients can be reassured that these lesions are usually temporary. These changes must be distinguished from nevoid lesions and diseases manifested by pigmentary alterations such as vitiligo.

Crowe FW, Schull WJ: Diagnostic significance of café-au-lait spot in neurofibromatosis. Arch Intern Med 91:758, 1953.

Hizawa K, Iida M, Matsumoto T, et al: Neoplastic transformation arising in Peutz-Jeghers polyposis. Dis Colon Rectum 36:953, 1993.

Landy SJ, Donnai D: Incontinentia pigmenti (Bloch-Sulzberger syndrome). J Med Genet 30:53, 1993.

NIH Consensus Development Conference. Neurofibromatosis. Arch Neurol 45:575, 1988.

Osterlind A, Tucker MA, Hou-Jensen K, et al: The Danish case-control study of cutaneous malignant melanoma. I. Importance of host factors. Int J Cancer 42:200, 1988.

Riccardi VM: Neurofibromatosis: clinical heterogeneity. Curr Probl Cancer 7:1, 1982.

Spigelman AD, Murday V, Phillips RKS: Cancer and the Peutz-Jeghers syndrome. Gut 30:1588, 1989.

CHAPTER 603
Hypopigmented Lesions

Gary L. Darmstadt and Al Lane

ALBINISM. There are several types of congenital oculocutaneous albinism that consist of partial or complete failure of melanin production in the skin, hair, and eyes. The various forms of albinism, including nine autosomal recessive and one rare autosomal dominant variants, may be distinguished by clinical manifestations, morphology of the melanosomes, and the hair bulb incubation test, in which hair bulbs are plucked and incubated with tyrosine to determine whether tyrosinase is present. Tyrosinase is the copper-containing enzyme that catalyzes at least three steps in melanin biosynthesis (see Chapter 71.2). Tyrosinase-positive variants, which are characterized by darkening of the hair bulb on incubation with tyrosine, are most common.

Ocular albinism, which involves only the eyes, presents in two X-linked forms, one autosomal dominant form, and one autosomal recessive form. Two of these types are associated with deafness. Female carriers of the X-linked types may show irregular retinal pigmentation.

Tyrosinase-negative or type 1 oculocutaneous albinism is characterized by greatly reduced or absent tyrosinase activity. Type 1A albinism, the most severe form, is characterized by a lack of visible pigment in hair, skin, and eyes. This manifests as photophobia, nystagmus, defective visual acuity, white hair, and white skin. The irises are blue-gray in oblique light and prominent pink in reflected light. Type 1B or yellow mutant albinism presents at birth with white hair, pink skin, and gray eyes. This type is particularly prevalent in Amish communities. Progressively, however, the hair becomes yellow-red, the skin tans lightly on exposure to the sun, and the irises may accumulate some brown pigment, with a resultant improvement in visual acuity. Photophobia and nystagmus are present but are mild. Numerous different allelic mutations in the tyrosinase gene account for types 1A and 1B albinism. In whites, no single mutant tyrosinase allele accounts for a significant fraction of the total, complicating molecular approaches to carrier detection and prenatal diagnosis.

The phenotype of *tyrosinase-positive or type II albinism* ranges from nearly normal to closely resembling type 1 albinism. Little or no melanin is present at birth, but pigment, particularly red-yellow pigment, may accumulate rapidly during childhood to produce a straw-colored or light brown skin color in whites. There is also progressive improvement in visual acuity and nystagmus with aging. Blacks may have a yellow-brown skin color, dark-brown freckles in sun-exposed areas, and brown coloration of the irises. The defect in type 2 albinism has been mapped to chromosome 15 and may involve a tyrosine-specific transport protein.

The *Hermansky-Pudlak syndrome* is tyrosinase-positive albinism, with variable pigmentation, in association with a platelet storage pool deficiency and a hemorrhagic diathesis. Additional features include the accumulation of a ceroid-like pigment in cells of the reticuloendothelial system, pulmonary fibrosis, granulomatous colitis, and lupus nephritis.

The *Cross-McKusick-Breen syndrome* consists of tyrosinase-positive albinism with microphthalmia, retardation, spasticity, and athetosis.

Because of the absence of normal protection by adequate amounts of epidermal melanin, persons with albinism are predisposed to develop actinic keratoses and cutaneous carcinoma secondary to skin damage by ultraviolet light. Protection with a broad-spectrum sunscreen preparation (see Chapter 606) should be provided during exposure to sunlight.

PARTIAL ALBINISM (PIEBALDISM). This congenital autosomal dominant disorder is characterized by sharply demarcated amelanotic patches that occur most frequently on the forehead, anterior scalp (producing a white forelock), ventral trunk, elbows, and knees. Islands of normal pigmentation may be present within the amelanotic areas. The plaques are the result of a permanent localized absence of melanocytes and melanosomes or reduced numbers of abnormally large melanocytes. Piebaldism results from mutations in the *KIT* proto-oncogene, which encodes the cellular transmembrane tyrosinase kinase for mast/stem cell growth factor. The pattern of depigmentation is thought to stem from defective melanocyte proliferation or migration from the neural crest during development. Piebaldism must be differentiated from vitiligo, which may be progressive and is not usually congenital; nevus depigmentosus; and Waardenburg syndrome.

WAARDENBURG SYNDROME. This congenital syndrome is characterized by lateral displacement of the medial canthi with dystopia canthorum (99%), broad nasal root (80%), heterochromic irises (25%), congenital deafness (20%), a white forelock (17%), and cutaneous hypopigmentation. A few patients have skin changes identical to piebaldism. Premature graying may develop in the 3rd decade. Waardenburg syndrome is inherited as an autosomal dominant trait with variable penetrance.

CHÉDIAK-HIGASHI SYNDROME (see Chapter 119).

TUBEROUS SCLEROSIS (see Chapter 546.2). This disorder is a multisystemic disorder affecting primarily tissues derived from ectoderm but also involving organs of mesodermal and endodermal origin, particularly the eye, kidney, and heart. The classic clinical triad is skin lesions in association with epilepsy and mental retardation.

Etiology and Epidemiology. This is an autosomal dominant condition with variable expression; the defect has been mapped to chromosome 9. Approximately one half of cases are due to new mutations. The most reliable early cutaneous sign is the white- or ash-leaf macule, which presents at birth or in early infancy, often years before other signs of the disease. Ash-leaf macules also appear in 2–3 per 1,000 normal newborns. They are sharply demarcated, pale, 0.5–3-cm lesions that often assume the shape of a mountain ash leaflet.

Clinical Manifestations. Single or multiple ash-leaf lesions are most often found on the trunk (Fig. 603–1A) but also occur on the face and limbs. Small, confetti-like hypopigmented macules are also present in some instances, reflecting inadequate melanization of the melanosomes in melanocytes. *Adenoma sebaceum* is the most commonly recognized cutaneous marker of tuberous sclerosis; the lesions appear on the face during middle to late childhood or adolescence in approximately 80% of patients. These red-brown or flesh-colored, smooth, glistening, telangiectatic 1–10-mm papules may extend from the nasolabial folds to the cheeks and chin (Fig. 603–1B). The presence of telangiectasias and the lack of comedones and pustules help to distinguish this eruption from acne vulgaris. The term adenoma sebaceum is a misnomer because these growths are angiofibromas rather than tumors of the sebaceous glands. Similar fibromatous nodules may be scattered on the forehead, trunk, and limbs. Large, skin-colored, irregularly thickened plaques with an orange peel or cobblestone texture *(shagreen patch)* may occur in the lumbosacral area. At puberty, firm, flesh-colored *periungual fibromas* (Fig. 603–1C) emerge on the nail folds of some children; gingival fibromas may also occur, unassociated with the administration of anticonvulsant medications. Café au lait spots occur with increased frequency but are not as numerous as in neurofibromatosis. Mental deficiency occurs in 60–70%, nearly all of whom have epilepsy. Epilepsy is also present in approximately 70% of those patients without mental retardation. Epilepsy begins in infancy or early childhood and is often progressively more severe. Cardiac rhabdomyomas are present in approximately one half of infants but regress in most cases; mechanical obstruction is a potential complication. Rarely, the presenting sign of tuberous sclerosis is hematuria, caused by a renal angiomyolipoma, which occurs exclusively in this condition. Seventy-five per cent of patients with tuberous sclerosis die before the age of 25 yr, most commonly as a complication of epilepsy, of intercurrent infection, or occasionally from cardiac failure or pulmonary fibrosis.

HYPOMELANOSIS OF ITO (INCONTINENTIA PIGMENTI ACHROMIANS). This congenital skin disorder affects children of both sexes and is frequently associated with defects in several organ systems. There is no evidence for genetic transmission; 40% of patients have chromosomal mosaicism, and 60% have X-chromosome abnormalities. One of the genetic forms of hypomelanosis of Ito involves a mutation at Xp11, as is also found in some sporadic patients with incontinentia pigmenti; this raises the possibility that these two disorders may represent allelic forms or a contiguous gene syndrome. Given the current state of understanding of hypomelanosis of Ito, the diagnosis is descriptive rather than definitive.

The skin lesions of hypomelanosis of Ito are generally present at birth but may be acquired within the first 2 yrs of life. The lesions are similar to a negative image of that present in incontinentia pigmenti, consisting of bizarre, patterned, hypopigmented macules arranged in sharply demarcated whorls, streaks, and patches over the body surface that follow the lines of Blaschko (Fig. 603–2). The palms, soles, and mucous membranes are spared. The hypopigmentation remains unchanged throughout childhood but fades during adulthood. The degree of depigmentation varies from hypopigmented to achromic. Neither inflammatory nor vesicular lesions precede

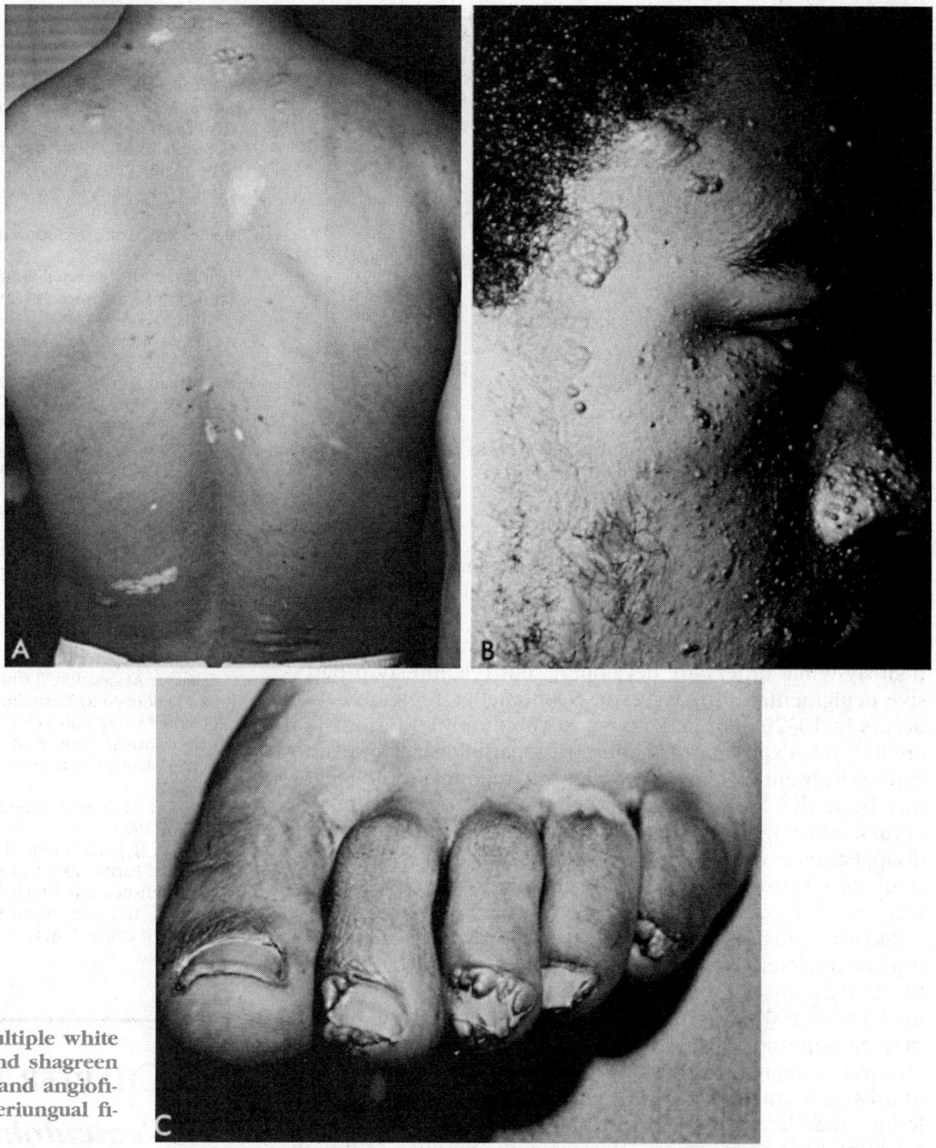

Figure 603–1. Tuberous sclerosis. *A*, Multiple white leaf macules, small papular fibromas, and shagreen patch on lower back. *B*, Angiofibromas and angiofibromatous plaques on the temple. *C*, Periungual fibromas.

the development of the pigmentary changes as in incontinentia pigmenti. Histopathologic changes in the hypopigmented areas include fewer and smaller melanocytes and a decreased number of melanin granules in the basal cell layer than normal. Inflammatory cells or pigment incontinence are lacking.

The most commonly associated abnormalities involve the nervous system, including mental retardation (70%), seizures (40%), microcephaly (25%), and muscular hypotonia (15%). The musculoskeletal system is the second most frequently involved system, including scoliosis and thoracic and limb deformities. Minor ophthalmologic defects (strabismus, nystagmus) are present in 25% of patients, and 10% have cardiac defects. The differential diagnosis includes systemitized nevus depigmentosus, which is a stable leukoderma not associated with systemic manifestations. Differentiation from incontinentia pigmenti, particularly the hypopigmented fourth stage, is critical for genetic counseling because incontinentia pigmenti, unlike hypomelanosis of Ito, is inherited.

VITILIGO. Approximately one half of cases of this acquired pigmentary defect present before age 20 yr. The lesions are sharply circumscribed, depigmented macules that vary in size and shape.

Epidemiology and Etiology. Although no clear-cut pattern of genetic transmission is established, 30–40% of patients have a positive family history. Associated abnormalities include uveitis and premature graying of hair. *Vogt-Koyanagi syndrome* presents with vitiligo, uveitis, and premature graying of hair but also involves the central nervous system. Vitiligo is more prevalent in patients with thyroid disease (hypo- or hyperthyroidism), adrenal insufficiency, pernicious anemia, and diabetes mellitus. The cause of vitiligo is unknown, but trauma appears to play a role in induction of the lesions. The most popular theory on the pathogenesis of vitiligo is an autoimmune mechanism, based on the finding that organ-specific autoantibodies to thyroid, gastroparietal, and adrenal tissue are found more frequently in the serum of patients with vitiligo than in the general population. Alternatively a neurogenic theory purports that a compound, which is released at peripheral nerve endings in the skin, may inhibit melanogenesis, and a self-destruct theory suggests that melanocytes destroy themselves due to a defective protective mechanism that normally would remove toxic melanin precursors.

Clinical Manifestations. Areas of predilection are normally relatively hyperpigmented, such as the face, particularly around the eyes or mouth, the axillae, the inguinal region and genitalia, and the areolae. Sites that are subjected frequently to trauma and friction are also likely to be affected, including the hands and feet, elbows, knees, and ankles (Fig. 603–3). When

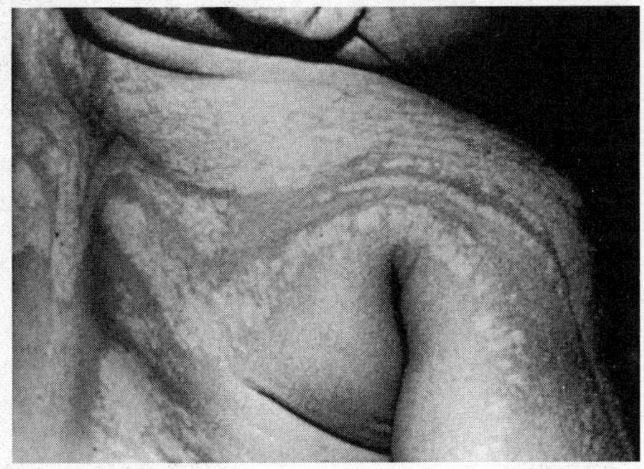

Figure 603–2. Marbled hypopigmented streaks of hypomelanosis of Ito (incontinentia pigmenti achromians).

the scalp or brow is affected, the hair may lose pigment. The distribution of involvement is generally symmetric but occasionally is unilateral or dermatomal.

The course of vitiligo varies; some lesions may remit spontaneously while others are developing, but relentlessly progressive depigmentation may occur. Spontaneous repigmentation occurs in 10–20% of patients, most commonly in lesions that are in a sun-exposed distribution. Histopathologically, melanocytes are absent from involved sites and repopulate the epidermis from the hair follicle epithelium when repigmentation occurs. Although the diagnosis is usually made clinically, the disappearance of melanocytes can be confirmed by DOPA stains or electron microscopy of specimens obtained from depigmented skin.

Treatment. This usually involves administration of oral or topical psoralen compounds in conjunction with exposure to sunlight or an ultraviolet light source. Repigmentation may be partial or complete, but many months of therapy may be required. High-potency topical steroids are sometimes effective in repigmenting small areas of vitiligo or early lesions in areas not amenable to phototherapy such as the lips. Small lesions may be camouflaged by application of a specially prepared makeup (Covermark, Dermablend). Because of the absence of melanin, vitiliginous skin burns readily on sun exposure and should be protected at all times with an appropriate sunscreen.

Bologna J, Pawelek JM: Biology of hypopigmentation. J Am Acad Dermatol 19:217, 1988.

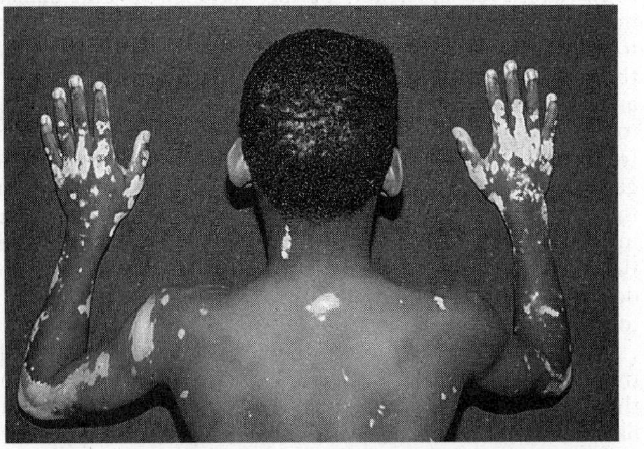

Figure 603–3. Multiple, sharply demarcated, symmetric, depigmented areas of vitiligo.

Cui J, Arita Y, Bystryn JC: Cytolytic antibodies to melanocytes in vitiligo. J Invest Dermatol 100:812, 1993.
da-Silva EO: Waardenburg I syndrome: A clinical and genetic study of two large Brazilian kindreds, and literature review. Am J Med Genet 40:65, 1991.
Glover M, Brett EM, Atherton DJ: Hypomelanosis of Ito: Spectrum of the disease. J Pediatr 115:75, 1989.
Gorski JL, Burright EN: The molecular genetics of incontinentia pigmenti. Semin Dermatol 12:255, 1993.
Grimes PE: Vitiligo: An overview of therapeutic approaches. Dermatol Clin 11:325, 1993.
Halder RM, Grimes PE, Cowan CA, et al: Childhood vitiligo. J Am Acad Dermatol 16:948, 1987.
Janniger CK: Childhood vitiligo. Cutis 51:25, 1993.
Janniger CK, Schwartz RA: Tuberous sclerosis: Recent advances for the clinician. Cutis 51:167, 1993.
Kuster W, Happle R: Neurocutaneous disorders in children. Curr Opin Pediatr 5:436, 1993.
Monoghan HP, Krafchik BP, MacGregor DL, et al: Tuberous sclerosis complex in children. Am J Dis Child 135:912, 1981.
Mosher DB, Fitzpatrick TB: Piebaldism. Arch Dermatol 124:364, 1988.
Naughton GK, Reggiardo D, Bystryn J-C: Correlation between vitiligo antibodies and extent of depigmentation in vitiligo. J Am Acad Dermatol 15:978, 1986.
Nordlund JJ, Halder RM, Grimes P: Management of vitiligo. Dermatol Clin 11:27, 1993.
Northrup H, Wheless JW, Bertin, et al: Variability of expression in tuberous sclerosis. J Med Genet 30:41, 1993.
Pinto FJ, Bolognia JL: Disorders of hypopigmentation in children. Pediatr Clin North Am 38:991, 1991.
Roach ES, Smith M, Huttenlocher P, et al: Diagnostic criteria: Tuberous sclerosis complex. Report of the Diagnostic Criteria Committee of the National Tuberous Sclerosis Association. J Child Neurol 7:221, 1992.
Ruiz-Maldonado R, Toussaint S, Tamayo L, et al: Hypomelanosis of Ito: Diagnostic criteria and report of 41 cases. Pediatr Dermatol 9:1, 1992.
Schwartz MF Jr, Esterly NB, Fretzin DF, et al: Hypomelanosis of Ito (incontinentia pigmenti achromians): A neurocutaneous syndrome. J Pediatr 90:236, 1977.
Spritz RA: Molecular genetics of oculocutaneous albinism. Semin Dermatol 12:167, 1993.
Sybert VP: Hypomelanosis of Ito. Pediatr Dermatol 7:74, 1990.
Thibaut H, Parizel PM, Van Goethem J, et al: Tuberous sclerosis: CT and MRI characteristics. Eur J Radiol 16:176, 1993.
Winship I, Young K, Martell P, et al: Piebaldism: An autonomous autosomal dominant entity. Clin Genet 39:330, 1991.

CHAPTER 604

Vesiculobullous Disorders

Gary L. Darmstadt and Al Lane

Many diseases are characterized by vesiculobullous lesions; they vary considerably in cause, age of occurrence, and pattern. Some of them (varicella) are discussed in other chapters; some are described in other chapters of this part because the vesicobullous lesions represent only a transient stage of the disease (incontinentia pigmenti, mastocytosis). The morphology of the blister often provides a visual clue to the location of the lesion within the skin. Blisters localized to the epidermal layers are thin walled, relatively flaccid, and tend to rupture easily. Subepidermal blisters are tense, thick walled, and more durable. Biopsies of blisters can be diagnostic because the level of cleavage within the skin and associated findings such as the nature of the inflammatory infiltrate are constant and characteristic for a particular disorder. Other diagnostic procedures such as immunofluorescence and electron microscopy can often distinguish vesiculobullous disorders that have nearly identical histopathologic findings (Table 604–1).

ERYTHEMA MULTIFORME (see Chapter 142). This acute, sometimes recurrent vesiculobullous disorder has numerous manifestations on the skin, mucous membranes, and occasionally

■ TABLE 604–1 Sites of Blister Formation and Diagnostic Studies for the Vesiculobullous Disorders

Disorder	Blister Cleavage Site	Cutaneous Diagnostic Studies
Acrodermatitis enteropathica	IE	—
Bullous impetigo	GL	Smear, culture
Bullous pemphigoid	SE (junctional)	Direct and indirect immunofluorescence studies
Candidosis	SC	KOH preparation, culture
Chronic bullous dermatosis of childhood	SE	Direct immunofluorescence studies
Dermatitis herpetiformis	SE	Direct immunofluorescence studies
Dermatophytosis	IE	KOH preparation, culture
Dyshidrotic eczema	IE	—
EB simplex	IE	Electron microscopy; immunofluorescence mapping
Hands and feet	IE	Electron microscopy; immunofluorescence mapping
Junctional EB (lethalis)	SE (junctional)	Electron microscopy; immunofluorescence mapping
Recessive dystrophic EB	SE	Electron microscopy; immunofluorescence mapping
Dominant dystrophic EB	SE	Electron microscopy; immunofluorescence mapping
Epidermolytic hyperkeratosis	IE	—
Erythema multiforme	SE	—
Erythema toxicum	SC, IE	Smear for eosinophils
Incontinentia pigmenti	IE	Smear for eosinophils
Insect bites	IE	—
Mastocytosis	SE	Smear for mast cells
Miliaria crystallina	IC	—
Pachyonychia congenita	IC	—
Pemphigus foliaceus	GL	Direct and indirect immunofluorescence studies Tzanck smear
Pemphigus vulgaris	SB	Direct and indirect immunofluorescence studies Tzanck smear
Pseudomonas infection	IE, SE	Smear, culture
Scabies	IE	Scraping
Staphylococcal scalded skin syndrome	GL	Frozen section biopsy
Syphilis	SE	Dark-field preparation
Toxic epidermal necrolysis (Lyell)	SE	Frozen section biopsy
Transient neonatal pustular melanosis	SC, IE	Smear for cells
Viral blisters	IE	Tzanck smear for herpesvirus infections

GL = granular layer; IC = intracorneal; IE = intraepidermal; SB = suprabasal; SC = subcorneal; SE = subepidermal; EB = epidermolysis bullosa; KOH = potassium hydroxide.

in internal organs. The eruption occurs most commonly between the ages of 10–30 yr and is usually asymptomatic, although pruritus or a burning sensation may be present. The pathogenesis of eythema multiforme is unknown but is generally regarded as a hypersensitivity reaction triggered by drugs, infections, and exposure to toxic substances (Table 604–2); the etiologic agents that have been documented most conclusively are infection with herpes simplex virus or *Mycoplasma pneumoniae*. Approximately 20% of cases, however, have no identifiable cause.

Clinical Manifestations. Lesions of erythema multiforme may begin as erythematous macules and evolve into papules, vesicles, bullae, urticarial plaques, or patches of confluent erythema. The center of the lesion may be vesicular, purpuric, or necrotic. Iris or target lesions, pathognomonic for erythema multiforme, have a dusky center, an inner pale ring, and an erythematous outer border. *Erythema multiforme minor* is characterized by symmetric crops of skin lesions of diverse morphology, primarily on the extensor surfaces of the arms and legs, often including the palms and soles, with relative sparing of the mucous membranes and trunk. Prodromal symptoms are generally absent. *Stevens-Johnson syndrome* (erythema multiforme major) is a serious systemic disorder in which at least two mucous membranes and the skin are involved. Purulent conjunctivitis and uveitis usually develop, and cutaneous lesions tend to rupture, leaving denuded skin that may result in significant fluid loss, anemia, and a high risk for bacterial superinfection and sepsis. The eruption may be preceded by a nonspecific upper respiratory infection and may be accompanied by fever, chills, malaise, and weakness. Complete healing may take 4–6 wk; skin lesions heal with hypopigmentation or hyperpigmentation but without scarring. Esophageal stricture or visual impairment from corneal scarring may complicate eythema multiforme major. Approximately 25% of all cases of erythema multiforme are confined to the oral mucosa, with a predilection for the vermilion border of the lips and the buccal mucosa, generally sparing the gingiva. Most patients experience a single episode of erythema multiforme. Recurrence may be triggered by drugs or, most commonly, by infection with herpes simplex virus. In these instances, viral DNA can be detected in skin lesions by polymerase chain reaction.

The *differential diagnosis* of erythema multiforme includes bullous pemphigoid, pemphigus, linear IgA dermatosis, graft versus host disease, bullous drug eruption, urticaria, viral infections such as herpes simplex, Reiter disease, Kawasaki disease, Behçet disease, allergic vasculitis, erythema annulare centrifugum, and periarteritis nodosa. Erythema multiforme

■ TABLE 604–2 Potential Causes of Erythema Multiforme

Infectious Agents	**Anticonvulsants**
Herpes simplex 1,2*	Phenytoin
Mycoplasma pneumoniae	Phenobarbital
Mycobacterium tuberculosis	Carbamazepine
Group A streptococci	Aspirin
Hepatitis B	**Other**
Epstein-Barr virus	Radiation therapy
Francisella tularensis	Captopril
Yersinia	Etoposide
Enteroviruses	Non-steroidal anti-inflammatory agents, e.g., phenylbutazone
Histoplasma	Sunlight
Coccidioides	Pregnancy
Neoplasia	
Leukemia	
Lymphoma	
Antibiotics	
Penicillin	
Sulfonamides	
Isoniazid	
Tetracyclines	

*Recurrent erythema multiforme.
Drug reactions occur 1–3 wk after exposure.

that primarily involves the oral mucosa may be confused with a handful of other conditions, including bullous pemphigoid, pemphigus vulgaris, vesiculobullous or erosive lichen planus, Behçet syndrome, recurrent aphthous stomatitis, and primary herpetic gingivostomatitis. Histopathologic examination of early skin lesions of erythema multiforme shows slight intercellular edema, rare dyskeratotic keratinocytes, basal vacuolization in the epidermis and a perivascular lymphohistiocytic infiltrate, and edema in the upper dermis. More mature lesions show an accentuation of these characteristics and the development of lymphocytic exocytosis and an intense perivascular, interstitial mononuclear infiltrate.

Treatment. Management of Stevens-Johnson syndrome is supportive and symptomatic. Ophthalmologic consultation is mandatory because ocular sequelae such as corneal scarring can lead to loss of vision. Oral lesions should be managed with mouthwashes and glycerin swabs. Vaginal lesions should be observed closely and treated to prevent vaginal stricture or fusion. Topical anesthetics (diphenhydramine, dyclonine, and viscous lidocaine) may provide relief from pain, particularly when applied before eating. Denuded skin lesions can be cleansed with saline or Burow solution compresses. Antibiotic therapy is appropriate for secondary bacterial infection. Frequent recurrences of herpes-associated erythema multiforme may warrant prophylactic acyclovir. Treatment may require intensive care admission; intravenous fluids; nutritional support; sheepskin or air-fluid bedding; daily saline or Burow solution compresses; paraffin gauze or hydrogel dressing to denuded areas; saline compresses to the eyelids, lips, or nose; analgesics; and urinary catheterization (when needed). A daily examination for infection and ocular lesions, which constitute the major cause of long-term morbidity, is essential. Systemic antibiotics are indicated for urinary or cutaneous infections and for suspected bacteremia because infection is the leading cause of death. Prophylactic systemic antibiotics, systemic corticosteroids, and extensive debridement are not necessary.

TOXIC EPIDERMAL NECROLYSIS (LYELL SYNDROME)

Epidemiology and Etiology. The pathogenesis of toxic epidermal necrolysis is not proved but appears to involve a hypersensitivity phenomenon that results in damage primarily to the basal cell layer of the epidermis. This condition is triggered by many of the same factors that are responsible for erythema multiforme, including drugs such as the sulfonamides, amoxicillin, phenobarbital, hydantoin, butazones, allopurinol, and aspirin; infections; vaccinations such as diphtheria, poliomyelitis, and measles; radiotherapy; and malignancies such as lymphoma and leukemia. Goldstein et al. defined toxic epidermal necrolysis by (1) widespread blister formation and morbilliform or confluent erythema, associated with skin tenderness; (2) absence of target lesions; (3) sudden onset and generalization within 24–48 hr; and (4) histologic findings of full-thickness epidermal necrosis and a minimal-to-absent dermal infiltrate. These criteria categorize toxic epidermal necrolysis as a separate entity from erythema multiforme; many authors, however, believe that toxic epidermal necrolysis represents the most severe form of the spectrum of erythema multiforme. This condition is exceedingly rare in infants less than 6-mo old; only three such cases have been documented.

Clinical Manifestations. The prodrome consists of fever, malaise, localized skin tenderness, and diffuse erythema. Inflammation of the eyelids, conjunctivae, mouth, and genitalia may precede skin lesions. Flaccid bullae may develop, although this is not a prominent feature. Characteristically, full-thickness epidermis is lost in large sheets. *Nikolsky sign* (denudation of the skin with gentle tangential pressure) is present but only in the areas of erythema. Conjunctivitis and oral lesions are usually not as severe as in Stevens-Johnson syndrome. Healing takes place over 14 or more days. Scarring, particularly of the eyes, may result in corneal opacity. The course may be relentlessly progressive, complicated by severe dehydration, electrolyte imbalance, shock, and secondary localized infection and septicemia. Loss of nails and hair may also occur. The differential diagnosis includes staphylococcal scalded skin syndrome, in which the blister cleavage plane is intraepidermal; graft versus host disease; chemical burns; drug eruptions; and pemphigus.

Treatment. Appreciation of the specific etiologic factor is crucial, particularly when the disorder is drug induced its administration must be discontinued. Management is similar to that for severe burns and may be best accomplished in a burn unit. It may include strict reverse isolation, meticulous fluid and electrolyte therapy, use of an air-fluid bed, and daily cultures. Systemic antibiotic therapy is indicated when secondary infection is evident or suspected. Skin care consists of cleansing with isotonic saline or Burow solution and applications of mupirocin ointment. Biologic or hydrogel dressings alleviate pain and reduce fluid loss. Narcotics are often required for pain relief. Mouth and eye care may be necessary, such as for erythema multiforme major. Early high-dose systemic corticosteroids are not of proved benefit. The mortality rate is approximately 25% in drug-induced cases and 50% in idiopathic cases.

EPIDERMOLYSIS BULLOSA. Diseases categorized under this general term are a heterogeneous group of congenital, hereditary blistering disorders. They differ in severity and prognosis, clinical and histologic features, and inheritance patterns (Table 604–3) but are all characterized by induction of blisters by trauma and exacerbation of blistering in warm weather. The disorders can be categorized under three major headings: epidermolysis bullosa simplex, junctional epidermolysis bullosa, and dystrophic epidermolysis bullosa.

Epidermolysis bullosa simplex. This is a nonscarring, autosomal dominant disorder. The defect in all types of epidermolysis

■ **TABLE 604–3 Characteristics of Epidermolysis Bullosa**

Type	Predominant Inheritance	Level of Blister Formation	Features
Simplex (epidermolytic)	Autosomal dominant	Superficial; basal cell layer; above hemidesmosomes	4 variants; usually congenital onset; hands and feet involved; minimal mucosal lesions; no scarring
Junctional (lethalis)	Autosomal recessive	Lamina lucida, between bullous pemphigoid antigen and laminin; absence or rare hemidesmosomes	2 variants; localized or progressive; congenital; heals with scarring; pyloric atresia; mucosal lesions; dysplastic teeth; loss of nails
Recessive dystrophic (dermolytic)	Autosomal recessive	Deep in dermis below the lamina densa; excessive production of abnormal dermal collagenase; absent anchoring fibrils	2 congenital variants; mitten scarring of the hands and feet; marked deformities; mucosal lesions produce esophageal stricture or gastrointestinal perforation; varied clinical course; risk for aggressive squamous cell cancer of the skin, tongue, esophagus
Dominant dystrophic (dermolytic)	Autosomal dominant	Deep in dermis below the lamina densa, below type IV collagen layer, sparse anchoring fibrils	2 variants; hyperkeratotic lesions; variable severity; risk for squamous cell cancer

bullosa simplex is in the central α-helical coil of keratin 5 or 14, which makes up intermediate filaments of the basal keratinocytes. Keratin 5 and 14 genes are located on chromosomes 17q and 12q, respectively. The intraepidermal bullae result from cytolysis of the basal cells.

Blisters are usually present at birth or during the neonatal period. Sites of predilection are the hands, feet, elbows, knees, legs, and scalp. Intraoral lesions are minimal, nails rarely become dystrophic and usually regrow even when they are shed, and dentition is normal. Bullae heal with minimal-to-no scar or milia formation. Secondary infection is the only serious complication. The propensity to blister decreases with age, and the long-term prognosis is good. Blisters should be drained by puncturing, but the blister top should be left intact to protect the underlying skin. Erosions may be covered with mupirocin if there is evidence of infection, and a semi-permeable dressing. Genetic counseling should be offered to families of affected children.

Epidermolysis bullosa simplex of hands and feet (Weber-Cockayne type) often presents when the child begins to walk; onset may be delayed, however, until puberty or early adulthood when heavy shoes are worn or the feet are subjected to increased trauma. Bullae are usually restricted to the hands and feet; rarely, they occur elsewhere such as the dorsal arms and the shins. The disorder ranges from mildly incapacitating to crippling at times of severe exacerbations. *Generalized epidermolysis bullosa simplex* (Köbner type) is characterized at birth or during early infancy with blisters on the occiput, back, and legs and in childhood with blisters on the hands, feet, and other friction points. The *herpetiformis (Dowling-Meara) variant of epidermolysis bullosa simplex* is characterized by grouped blisters. During infancy, blistering may be severe and extensive; may involve mucous membranes; and may result in shedding of nails, formation of milia, and mild pigmentary changes, without scarring. After the first few months of life, warm temperatures do not appear to exacerbate blistering. Hyperkeratosis and hyperhidrosis of the palms and soles may develop, but generally, the condition improves with age.

Junctional epidermolysis bullosa. *Epidermolysis bullosa lethalis* (Herlitz type) is an autosomal recessive condition that is life threatening; serious morbidity and disfigurement can be predicted from the complications. The infant is usually blistered at birth or develops lesions during the neonatal period, particularly on the perioral area, scalp, legs, diaper area, and thorax. In contrast to other variants of epidermolysis bullosa, sparing of the hands and feet is striking, with the exception of the distal digits and the nail plates; these are dystrophic or permanently lost. Mucous membrane involvement may be severe and ulceration of the respiratory, gastrointestinal, and genitourinary epithelium has been documented in many affected children, although less frequently than in severe, recessive dystrophic epidermolysis bullosa. Healing is delayed, and vegetating granulomas may persist for a long time. Large, moist, erosive plaques may provide a portal of entry for bacteria, and septicemia is a frequent cause of death. Mild atrophy may be seen in areas of recurrent blistering. Defective dentition with early loss of teeth as a result of rampant caries is characteristic. Growth retardation and recalcitrant anemia are almost invariable. In addition to infection, cachexia and circulatory failure are common causes of death. Most patients die within the first 3 yr of life.

A subepidermal blister is found on light microscopic examination, and electron microscopy demonstrates a cleavage plane in the lamina lucida, between the plasma membranes of the basal cells and the basal lamina. Absent or greatly reduced anchoring filaments are seen on electron micrographs. Mutations in laminin, K-laminin, and kalinin/nicein of the lamina lucida are under investigation as the protein involved in the pathogenesis of the disease. Absence of kalinin in amniocytes has been shown to be a prenatal marker for the Herlitz type of junctional epidermolysis bullosa.

Generalized atrophic benign epidermolysis bullosa, a milder autosomal recessive variant, presents with blistering at birth, is also nonscarring, and is characterized by identical histologic changes as the Herlitz type. It may be impossible to distinguish from the Herlitz variety for up to 2–3 yr. Pattern baldness with significant scalp atrophy is a prominent feature. The course is compatible with normal growth and life span.

Treatment for junctional epidermolysis bullosa is supportive, including genetic counseling for the family. An adequate caloric diet and supplemental iron should be provided. Infections should be treated promptly with antibiotics. Transfusions of packed red blood cells may be required.

Dystrophic epidermolysis bullosa. *Dominant dystrophic epidermolysis bullosa* occur sporadically in some cases, although an autosomal dominant mode of transmission has been documented in many families. Blisters may be present at birth and are often limited to the hands, feet, and sacrum. The lesions heal promptly with the formation of soft, wrinkled scars; milia; and alterations in pigmentation. The general health is unimpaired; in many cases, the blistering process is rather mild, causing little restriction of activity and unimpaired growth and development. Mucous membrane involvement tends to be minimal, but nail loss is common.

The *Cockayne-Touraine variant* of dominant dystrophic epidermolysis bullosa presents during infancy or early childhood with blisters predominantly on the extremities. The *albopapuloid Pasini form* presents during adolescence with blistering that may be widespread, but occurs predominantly on the hands, feet, elbows, and knees, and with flesh-colored papules called albopapuloid lesions on the trunk. The blister is subepidermal in both variants, with separation beneath the basement membrane. On electron microscopy, anchoring fibrils, a major component of which is type VII collagen, are abnormal and decreased in number over the entire skin in the Pasini type but only in areas of blister predilection in the Cockayne-Touraine variant. The type VII collagen gene, located on the short arm of chromosome 3, is the major candidate gene for dystrophic epidermolysis bullosa.

Recessive dystrophic epidermolysis bullosa is probably the most incapacitating form of epidermolysis bullosa, although the clinical spectrum is wide. Some have blisters, scarring, and milia formation primarily on the hands, feet, elbows, and knees. Others have extensive erosions and blister formation at birth that seriously impede the care and feeding of the infant. Mucous membrane lesions are common and may cause severe nutritional deprivation, even in older children, whose growth may be retarded. During childhood, esophageal erosions and strictures, scarring of the buccal mucosa, flexion contractures of joints secondary to scarring of the integument, development of cutaneous carcinomas, and the development of digital fusion (Fig. 604–1) may significantly limit the quality of life. The subepidermal bullae are located beneath the basement membrane, where there is an absence of anchoring fibrils.

Although the skin becomes less sensitive to trauma with aging, the progressive and permanent deformities complicate management, and the overall prognosis is poor. Foods that traumatize the buccal or esophageal mucosa should be avoided. If esophageal scarring develops, a semi-liquid diet and esophageal dilatations may be required. Alternatively, stricture excision or colonic interposition may be needed to relieve esophageal obstruction. In infants, severe oropharyngeal involvement may necessitate the use of special feeding devices such as a button gastrostomy tube. Continuous iron therapy for anemia; intermittent antibiotic therapy for secondary infections, which are a common cause of death; and periodic plastic procedures for release of digits may reduce morbidity.

PEMPHIGUS. Pemphigus occurs during childhood as pemphigus vulgaris or pemphigus foliaceus.

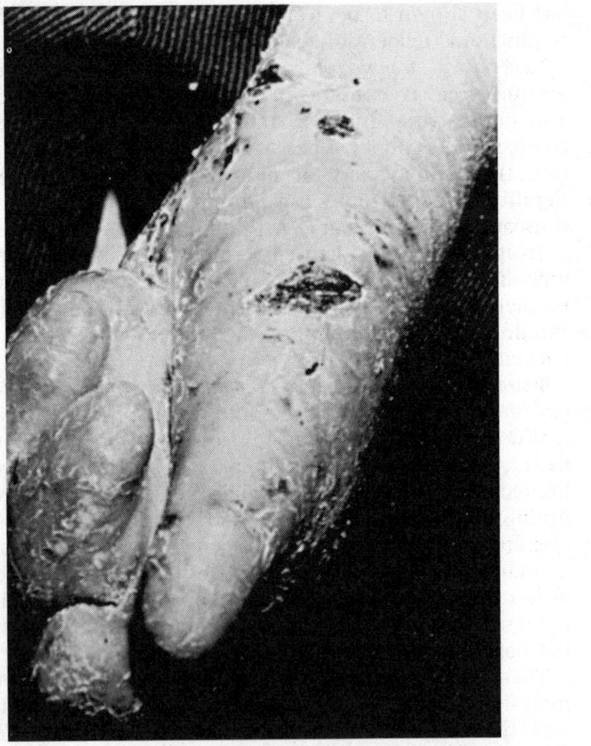

Figure 604–1. Mitten-hand deformity of recessive dystrophic epidermolysis bullosa.

Pemphigus Vulgaris. This usually first appears as painful oral ulcers, which may be the only evidence of the disease for weeks or months. Subsequently, large, flaccid bullae emerge on nonerythematous skin, most commonly on the face, trunk, pressure points, groin, and axillae. Nikolsky sign is present. The lesions rupture and enlarge peripherally, producing painful, raw, denuded areas that have little tendency to heal. When healing occurs, it is without scarring, but hyperpigmentation is common. Malodorous verrucous and granulomatous lesions may develop at sites of ruptured bullae, particularly in the skin folds; as this becomes more pronounced, the condition may be more properly referred to as pemphigus vegetans.

Biopsy is best performed of a fresh, small blister, which reveals a suprabasal (intraepidermal) blister containing loose, acantholytic epidermal cells that have lost their intercellular bridges and thus their contact with one another. IgG antibody to epidermal intercellular substance produces a characteristic pattern on direct immunofluorescence preparations of both involved and uninvolved skin of essentially all patients (Table 604–4). Serum IgG antibody titers to the epidermal intercellular substance correlate with the clinical course of many patients; thus, serial determinations may have predictive value. Pemphigus antibodies are pathogenic. The antigen recognized by pemphigus vulgaris antibodies is a 130-kD glycoprotein that is complexed with plakoglobin, a plaque protein of desmosomes. The pemphigus vulgaris antigen is a member of the desmoglein subfamily of the cadherin cell adhesion molecules.

Neonatal pemphigus vulgaris develops in utero as a result of placental transfer of maternal antibodies from women who have active pemphigus vulgaris, although it may occur when the mother is in remission. High antepartum maternal titers of pemphigus vulgaris antibodies and increased maternal disease activity correlate with a poor fetal outcome, including demise.

The *differential diagnosis* includes erythema multiforme, bullous pemphigoid, Stevens-Johnson syndrome, and toxic epidermal necrolysis. Because the course may rapidly lead to debility, malnutrition, and death, prompt diagnosis is essential. The disease is best treated initially with high-dose systemic corticosteroid therapy. Azathioprine, cyclophosphamide, methotrexate, and gold therapy have all been useful in maintenance regimens.

Pemphigus Foliaceus. This is extremely rare. It is characterized by intraepidermal blistering; the site of cleavage, however, is high in the epidermis rather than suprabasal as in pemphigus vulgaris. The superficial blisters rupture quickly, leaving erosions surrounded by erythema that heal with crusting and scaling. Nikolsky sign is present. Focal lesions are usually localized to the scalp, face, neck, and upper trunk. Mucous membrane lesions are minimal or absent. Pruritus, pain, and a burning sensation are frequent complaints. When generalized, the eruption may resemble exfoliative dermatitis or any of the chronic blistering disorders, but localized erythematous

■ TABLE 604–4 Immunofluorescent Findings in Immune-Mediated Cutaneous Diseases

Disease	Involved Skin	Uninvolved Skin	Direct IF	Indirect IF	Other Antibodies
Dermatitis herpetiformis	Negative	Positive	Granular IgA ± C in papillary dermis	None	IgA antireticulum in 20–70%. Antigliadin antibodies with celiac disease
Bullous pemphigoid	Positive	Positive	Linear IgG and C band in BMZ, occasionally IgM, IgA, IgE	IgG to BMZ in 70%	None
Pemphigus (all variants)	Positive	Positive	IgG in intercellular spaces of epidermis between keratinocytes	IgG to intercellular space	None
Pemphigus foliaceus	Positive	Positive	IgG to desmosomal glycoprotein, desmoglein	Same as direct IF	None
Herpes gestationis	Positive	Positive	C3 at BMZ, occasionally IgG	IgG anti-BMZ	None
Linear IgA bullous dermatosis (chronic bullous dermatosis of childhood)	Positive	Positive	Linear IgA at BMZ, occasionally C	Low titer, rare IgA, anti-BMZ	None
Discoid lupus erythematosus	Positive	Negative	Linear IgG, IgM, IgA, and C3 at BMZ (lupus band)	None	ANA negative
Systemic lupus erythematosus	Positive	Variable; exposed to sun, 30–50%; nonexposed, 10–30%	Linear IgG, IgM, C3 at BMZ (lupus band)	None	ANA Anti Ro (SSA) Anti-RNP Anti-DNA Anti-Sm
Henoch-Schönlein purpura	Positive	Negative	IgA around vessel walls	None	IgA rheumatoid factor, occasionally

C = complement; IF = immunofluorescent findings; Ig = immunoglobulin; ANA = antinuclear antibody; BMZ = basement membrane zone at the dermoepidermal junction.

plaques simulate seborrheic dermatitis, psoriasis, impetigo, eczema, or lupus erythematosus. The clinical course varies but is generally more benign than that of pemphigus vulgaris. *Fogo selvagem,* which is edemic in certain areas of Brazil, is identical clinically, histopathologically, and immunologically to pemphigus foliaceus.

An intraepidermal acantholytic bulla high in the epidermis is diagnostic; it is imperative, however, to select an early lesion for biopsy. Tissue-bound and circulating intercellular epidermal antibodies bind to a 50-kD portion of the 160-kD desmosomal glycoprotein, desmoglein I (see Table 604–4). Long-term remission is usual after suppression of the disease by systemic corticosteroid therapy. Dapsone or a topical corticosteroid preparation are occasionally sufficient.

BULLOUS PEMPHIGOID. Bullous pemphigoid rarely occurs in children but must be considered in the differential diagnosis of any chronic blistering disorder.

Clinical Manifestations. Typically, the blisters arise in crops on a normal, erythematous, eczematous, or urticarial base. Bullae appear predominantly on the flexural aspects of the extremities, in the axillae, and on the groin and central abdomen. Infants have involvement of the palms, soles, and face more frequently than older children. Individual lesions vary greatly in size, are tense, and are filled with serous fluid that may become hemorrhagic or turbid. Oral lesions occur less frequently (50%) and are less severe than in pemphigus vulgaris but are found more commonly in children than in adults with bullous pemphigoid. Pruritus, a burning sensation, and subcutaneous edema may accompany the eruption, but constitutional symptoms are not prominent.

Diagnosis and Differential Diagnoses. Biopsy should be taken from an early bulla arising on an erythematous base. A subepidermal bulla and a dermal inflammatory infiltrate, predominantly of eosinophils, can be identified histopathologically. In sections of a blister or perilesional skin, a band of Ig (usually IgG) and C3 can be demonstrated in the basement membrane zone by direct immunofluorescence (see Table 604–4). Indirect immunofluorescence studies of serum are positive in approximately 70% of cases for IgG antibodies to the basement membrane zone; the titers, however, do not correlate well with the clinical course. The differential diagnosis includes bullous erythema multiforme, pemphigus, linear IgA dermatosis, bullous drug eruption, dermatitis herpetiformis, herpes simplex infection, and bullous impetigo, which can be differentiated by histologic examination, immunofluorescence studies, and cultures. The large, tense bullae of bullous pemphigoid can generally be distinguished from the smaller, flaccid bullae of pemphigus vulgaris. The major targets for bullous pemphigoid autoantibodies are proteins of molecular weight 230 and 180 kD. The 230-kD protein is part of the hemidesmosome, whereas the 180-kD antigen localizes to both the hemidesmosome and the upper lamina lucida and is a transmembrane collagenous protein.

Treatment. Bullous pemphigoid can be successfully suppressed with systemic corticosteroid therapy alone or in combination with azathioprine, sulfapyridine, or dapsone. Ultimately, the condition usually remits permanently.

DERMATITIS HERPETIFORMIS. This is seen most commonly in children 2–7 yr of age. It is characterized by symmetric, grouped, small, tense, erythematous, stinging, intensely pruritic papules and vesicles. The eruption is pleomorphic, including erythematous, urticarial, papular, vesicular, and bullous lesions. Sites of predilection are the knees, elbows, shoulders, buttocks, and scalp; mucous membranes are usually spared. Hemorrhagic lesions may develop on the palms and soles. When pruritus is severe, excoriations may be the only visible sign.

Etiology. This is unknown; however, an association with gluten-sensitive enteropathy is found in 75–90% of patients. Aggressive gluten challenge generally unmasks the condition in the remainder of patients with dermatitis herpetiformis (see Chapter 286.8). Subepidermal blisters composed predominantly of neutrophils are found in dermal papillae on skin biopsy, and IgA and C3 can be detected in the dermal papillary tips of normal and perilesional skin in the sublamina densa region of the dermoepidermal junction by immunofluorescence studies. The frequent finding of immune complexes and autoimmune antibodies in serum, and the association with histocompatibility antigen HLA-B8 in approximately 85% of patients suggests an immune mechanism. An antibody to smooth muscle endomysium is found in 70% of patients with dermatitis herpetiformis–associated gluten-sensitive enteropathy. Antibody titers correlate with the severity of intestinal disease; they decline rapidly on institution of a gluten-free diet. Enteric infection with adenovirus type 12 or 40 may increase the risk of developing gluten-sensitive enteropathy and dermatitis herpetiformis in genetically susceptible individuals.

Treatment. Dermatitis herpetiformis may mimic other chronic blistering diseases and may also resemble scabies, papular urticaria, insect bites, contact dermatitis, and papular eczema. The most effective treatment is oral administration of sulfapyridine or dapsone. These drugs provide immediate relief from the intense pruritus but must be used with caution because of possible serious side effects. Local antipruritic measures may also be useful. Jejunal biopsy is indicated to diagnose gluten-sensitive enteropathy because cutaneous manifestations may precede malabsorption. Enteropathy responds to a gluten-free diet more rapidly than skin lesions.

LINEAR IgA DERMATOSIS (CHRONIC BULLOUS DERMATOSIS OF CHILDHOOD). This rare dermatosis is most common in the 1st decade of life, with a peak incidence during the preschool years. The eruption consists of multiple large, tense bullae filled with clear or hemorrhagic fluid that develop on a normal or erythematous, urticarial base. Areas of predilection are the genitalia and buttocks, the perioral region, and the scalp. Sausage-shaped bullae may be arranged in an annular or rosette-like fashion around a central crust (Fig. 604–2). Erythematous plaques with gyrate margins bordered by intact bullae may develop over larger

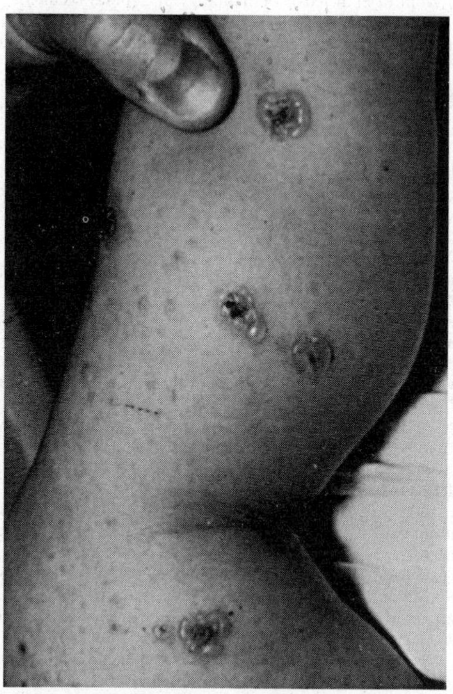

Figure 604–2. Rosette-like blisters around a central crust typical of linear IgA dermatosis (chronic bullous dermatosis of childhood).

areas. Pruritus may be absent or very intense, and systemic signs or symptoms are absent. Gluten-sensitive enteropathy is not present, but there is a strong association with HLA-B8.

Etiology. The cause of the eruption is unknown. Histologic examination shows a subepidermal bulla infiltrated with a mixture of inflammatory cells. Neutrophilic abscesses may be noted in the dermal papillary tips, indistinguishable from those of dermatitis herpetiformis. The infiltrate may also be largely eosinophilic, resembling bullous pemphigoid. Therefore, direct immunofluorescence studies are required for a definitive *diagnosis;* lesional or perilesional skin demonstrates linear deposition of IgA and sometimes C3 at the dermoepidermal junction (see Table 604–4). Indirect immunofluorescence studies are sometimes positive for circulating antibodies. Immunoelectron microscopy has localized the immunoreactants to the sublamina densa, although a combined sublamina densa and lamina lucida pattern has also been seen. The linear IgA bullous dermatosis antigen has a molecular weight of 285 kD. The eruption can be distinguished by histopathologic and immunofluorescence studies from pemphigus, bullous pemphigoid, dermatitis herpetiformis, and erythema multiforme. Gram stain and culture exclude the diagnosis of bullous impetigo, with which dermatitis herpetiformis is often confused on initial presentation. The lack of bullous formation in response to trauma differentiates epidermolysis bullosa.

Treatment. Many patients respond favorably to oral sulfapyridine or dapsone. During therapy with sulfapyridine, attention should be paid to maintaining urinary output and alkalinization to avoid crystal formation within the renal parenchyma. Hematologic and biochemical studies must be obtained at regular intervals during treatment with either drug to avoid serious side effects. Children who do not respond to either of these drugs may benefit from oral therapy with a corticosteroid or a combination of these drugs. The usual course is 2–4 yr, although some children have persistent or recurrent disease; there are no long-term sequelae.

Anhalt GJ, Labib RS, Voorhees JJ, et al: Induction of pemphigus in neonatal mice by passive transfer of IgG from patients with disease. N Engl J Med 306:1189, 1982.
Bauer EA, Briggaman RA: Hereditary epidermolysis bullosa. *In:* Fitzpatrick TB, Eisen AZ, Wolff K, et al (eds): Dermatology in General Medicine, 4th ed. New York, McGraw-Hill, 1993, p 654.
Castillo G: Chronic bullous disease of childhood: linear IgA dermatosis of childhood. Dermatol Clin 1:231, 1983.
DEBRA Workshop Participants: Pathogenesis, clinical features, and management of nondermatologic complications of epidermolysis bullosa. Arch Dermatol 124:705, 1988.
Eichenfield LF, Honig P: Blistering disorders in childhood. Pediatr Clin North Am 38:959, 1991.
Fine JD: Epidermolysis bullosa: clinical aspects, pathology, and recent advances in research. Int J Dermatol 25:143, 1986.
Ginsberg CM: Stevens-Johnson syndrome in children. Pediatr Infect Dis J 1:155, 1982.
Goldstein SM, Wintroub BW, Elias PM, et al: Toxic epidermal necrolysis: unmuddying the waters. Arch Derm 123:1153, 1987.
Goodyear HM, Abrahamson EL, Harper JI: Childhood pemphigus foliaceus. Clin Exp Dermatol 16:229, 1991.
Halebian PH, Corder VJ, Madden MR, et al: Improved burn center survival of patients with toxic epidermal necrolysis managed without corticosteroids. Ann Surg 204:503, 1986.
Lin A, Carter D: Epidermolysis bullosa: when the skin falls apart. J Pediatr 114:349, 1989.
Marinkovich MP: The molecular genetics of basement membrane diseases. Arch Dermatol 129:1557, 1993.
Nemeth AJ, Klein AD, Gould EW, et al: Childhood bullous pemphigoid: clinical and immunologic features, treatment, and prognosis. Arch Dermatol 127: 378, 1991.
Oranje AP, van Joost T: Pemphigoid in children. Pediatr Dermatol 6:267, 1989.
Patterson R, Miller M, Kaplan M, et al: Effectiveness of early therapy with corticosteroids in Stevens-Johnson syndrome: experience with 41 cases and a hypothesis regarding pathogenesis. Ann Allergy 73:27, 1994.
Prendiville J, Hebert A, Greenwald M, et al: Management of Stevens-Johnson syndrome and toxic epidermal necrolysis in children. J Pediatr 115:881, 1989.
Rabinowitz LG, Esterly NB: Inflammatory bullous diseases in children. Dermatol Clin 11:565, 1993.
Revuz J, Penso D, Roujeau J-C, et al: Toxic epidermal necrolysis: clinical findings and prognostic factors in 87 patients. Arch Dermatol 123:1160, 1987.
Revuz J, Roujeau J-C, Guillaume J-C, et al: Treatment of toxic epidermal necrolysis: Creteil experience. Arch Dermatol 123:1156, 1987.
Sahn EE: Vesiculopustular lesions of neonates and infants. Curr Opin Pediatr 6:442, 1994.
Weston WL, Brice SL, Jester JD, et al: Herpes simplex virus in childhood erythema multiforme. Pediatrics 89:32, 1992.

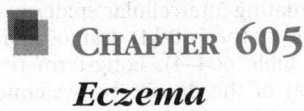

CHAPTER 605
Eczema

Al Lane and Gary L. Darmstadt

Eczema is a generic term used to designate a particular type of reaction pattern in the skin, which includes exudation, lichenification, and pruritus. Acute eczematous lesions are characterized by erythema, weeping, oozing, and the formation of microvesicles within the epidermis. Chronic lesions are generally thickened, dry, and scaly with coarse skin markings (lichenification) and altered pigmentation. Many types of eczema occur in children, of which the most common is atopic dermatitis (see Chapter 138); however, seborrheic dermatitis, allergic and irritant contact dermatitis, nummular eczema, and dyshidrosis are also relatively common childhood eczemas. Pyoderma may become eczematized from scratching, as may insect bites, papular urticaria, dermatophytosis, and a variety of dermatoses. Atopic skin is sensitive to many factors that increase pruritus, such as soap, wool, cool air, and food allergens.

Once the diagnosis of eczema has been established, it is important to classify the eruption more specifically for proper management. Pertinent historical data often provide the clue. In some instances, the subsequent course and character of the eruption permit classification. Histologic changes are relatively nonspecific, but all types of eczematous dermatitis are characterized by intraepidermal edema known as spongiosis.

CONTACT DERMATITIS. This form of eczema can be subdivided into irritant dermatitis, resulting from nonspecific injury to the skin, and allergic contact dermatitis, in which the mechanism is a delayed hypersensitivity reaction. Irritant dermatitis is more frequent in children, particularly during the early years of life.

Irritant contact dermatitis can result from prolonged or repetitive contact with a variety of substances that include saliva, citrus juices, bubble bath, detergents, abrasive materials, strong soaps, and proprietary medications. Saliva is probably one of the most common offenders; it may cause dermatitis on the face and in the neck folds of the drooling infant or retarded child. Older children who habitually lick their lips because of dryness may develop a striking, sharply demarcated perioral rash (Fig. 605–1A). Among the exogenous irritants, citrus juices, proprietary medications, and bubble bath preparations are relatively common; bubble bath dermatitis is a cause of severe pruritus. Excessive accumulation of sweat and moisture as a result of wearing occlusive shoes may also be responsible for irritant dermatitis.

Clinically, irritant contact dermatitis may be indistinguishable from atopic dermatitis or allergic contact dermatitis. A detailed history and consideration of the sites of involvement, the age of the child, and contactants usually provide clues to the etiologic agent. The propensity to develop irritant dermatitis varies considerably among children, and some may respond to minimal injury in this fashion. In general, all irritant contact dermatitis clears after removal of the stimulus and after temporary treatment with a topical corticosteroid preparation.

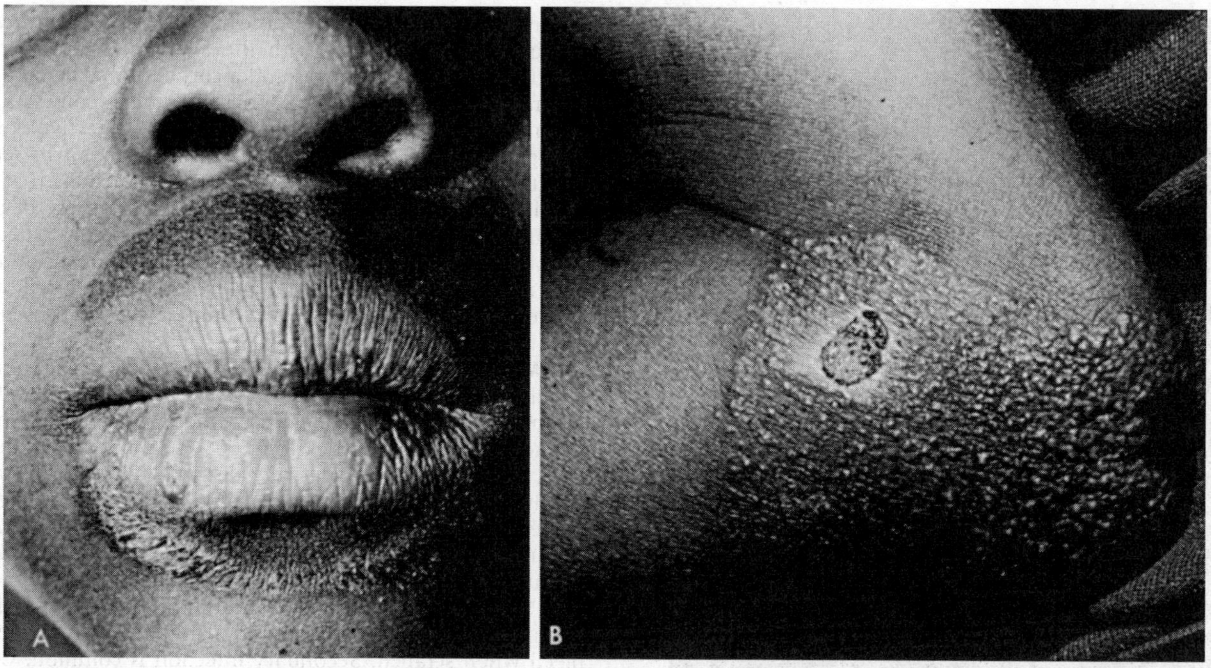

Figure 605–1. *A*, Perioral irritant contact dermatitis from lip licking. *B*, Allergic contact dermatitis to Merthiolate spray. Note the sharp angular border of vesicular eruption.

Education of patient and parents as to the causes of contact dermatitis is crucial to successful therapy.

Diaper dermatitis can be regarded as the prototype of irritant contact dermatitis. As a reaction to overhydration of the skin, friction, maceration, and prolonged contact with urine and feces, retained diaper soaps, and topical preparations, the skin of the diaper area may become erythematous and scaly, often with papulovesicular or bullous lesions, fissures, and erosions. The eruption can be patchy or confluent, but the genitocrural folds are often spared. Chronic hypertrophic, flat-topped papules, and infiltrative nodules may simulate syphilitic lesions. Secondary infection with bacteria and yeasts is common; discomfort may be marked because of intense inflammation. Such conditions as allergic contact dermatitis, seborrheic dermatitis, candidosis, atopic dermatitis, and rare disorders such as histiocytosis X and acrodermatitis enteropathica should be considered when the eruption is persistent or recalcitrant to simple therapeutic measures.

Diaper dermatitis often responds to simple measures; however, some infants seem predisposed to diaper dermatitis, and management may be difficult. The damaging effects of overhydration of the skin and prolonged contact with feces and ammoniac urine can be obviated by frequent changing of diapers and meticulous washing of the genitalia with warm water and mild soap. Disposable diapers containing a superabsorbent material may help to maintain a relatively dry environment. Frequent applications of a bland protective topical agent (petrolatum or zinc oxide paste) after thorough gentle cleansing may suffice to prevent dermatitis. When the aforementioned measures are not sufficient to promote healing, a light application of 0.5–1% topical hydrocortisone ointment after each diaper change for a limited time is often effective. Before initiation of such therapy, the possibility of candidal infection should considered. Candidal infection can be identified by red-pink tender skin that has multiple 1–2-mm pustules and papules at the periphery of the dermatitis. Treatment with a topical anticandidal agent may be helpful. For infants requiring additional protection, zinc oxide paste can be applied, after the steroid and topical antifungal, as a thick covering. Secondary complications can result from prolonged use of corticosteroids, especially fluorinated compounds.

Juvenile plantar dermatosis is a common form of irritant contact dermatitis occurring mainly in prepubertal children. The dermatitis characteristically involves the weight-bearing surfaces, is painful rather than pruritic, and causes a glazed appearance of the plantar skin. Fissuring may become extensive, producing considerable discomfort. The dermatitis results from alternating excessive hydration and rapid moisture loss, which causes chapping of the skin and cracking of the stratum corneum. Affected children often have hyperhidrosis, wear occlusive synthetic footwear, and subject their feet to rapid drying without moisturization. Immediate application of a thick emollient when socks and shoes are removed or immediately after swimming usually prevents this condition.

Allergic contact dermatitis is a T-cell–mediated hypersensitivity reaction that is provoked by application of an antigen to the skin surface. The antigen penetrates the skin, where it is conjugated with a cutaneous protein, and the hapten-protein complex is transported to the regional lymph nodes by antigen-presenting Langerhans cells. A primary immunologic response occurs locally in the nodes and becomes generalized, presumably because of dissemination of sensitized T cells. Sensitization requires several days and, when followed by a fresh antigenic challenge, becomes manifest as allergic contact dermatitis. Generalized distribution may also occur if enough antigen finds its way into the circulation. Once sensitization has occurred, each new antigenic challenge may provoke an inflammatory reaction within 8–12 hr; sensitization to a particular antigen usually persists for many years.

Acute allergic contact dermatitis is an erythematous, intensely pruritic, eczematous dermatitis, which, if severe, may be edematous and vesiculobullous. The chronic condition has the features of a long-standing eczema: lichenification, scaling, fissuring, and pigmentary change. The distribution of the eruption often provides a clue to the diagnosis. Volatile sensitizers usually affect exposed areas, such as face and arms. Jewelry, topical agents, shoes, clothing, and plants cause dermatitis at points of contact.

Rhus dermatitis (poison ivy, poison sumac, poison oak) is often vesiculobullous and may be distinguished by linear streaks of vesicles where the plant leaves have brushed against the skin. Contrary to popular opinion, fluid from ruptured

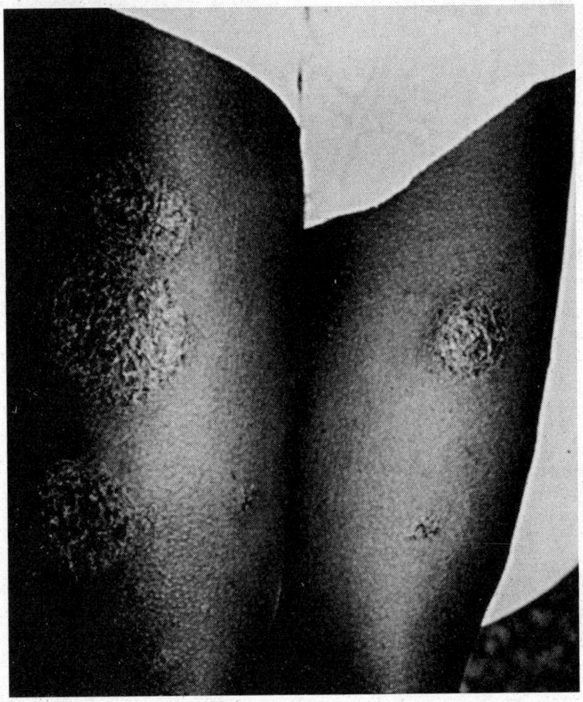

Figure 605–2. Multiple hyperpigmented scaly plaques of nummular eczema.

cutaneous vesicles does not spread the eruption; however, antigen retained on the skin, under the fingernails, and on clothing initiates new plaques of dermatitis if they are not removed by washing with soap and water. Antigen may also be carried by animals on their fur. The saplike allergen (oleoresin) is present on live or dead leaves, and sensitization to one plant produces cross-reactions with the others.

Nickel dermatitis usually develops from contact with jewelry or metal closures on clothing and is seen most frequently on the earlobes, such as when nickel-containing posts rather than nonmetallic materials or stainless steel are used to keep a pierced tract open. Some children are exquisitely sensitive to nickel, with even the trace amounts found in gold jewelry provoking eruptions.

Shoe dermatitis typically affects the dorsum of the feet and toes, sparing the interdigital spaces; it is usually symmetric. Other forms of allergic contact dermatitis, in contrast to irritant dermatitis, rarely involve the palms and soles. Common allergens are the antioxidants and accelerators in shoe rubber and the chromium salts in tanned leather or shoe dyes. These substances are often leached out by excessive sweating.

Wearing apparel contains a number of sensitizers, including dyes, mordants, fabric finishes, fibers, resins, and cleaning solutions. Dye may be poorly fixed to clothing and leached out with sweating, as are the partially cured formaldehyde resins. The elastic in garments is also a frequent cause of clothing dermatitis.

Topical medications and cosmetics may be unsuspected as allergens, particularly if the medication is being used for a preexisting dermatitis. The most common offenders are neomycin, thimerosal (Merthiolate) (Fig. 605–1*B*), topical antihistamines (Caladryl), anesthetics (dibucaine [Nupercainal] and cyclomethycaine [Surfacaine]), preservatives (parabens), and ethylenediamine, a stabilizer present in many medications. All types of cosmetics can cause facial dermatitis; involvement of the eyelids is characteristic for nail polish sensitivity.

Contact dermatitis can be confused with other types of eczema, dermatophytoses, and vesiculobullous diseases. Patch testing may clarify the situation but should be performed only by an experienced person. The essential principle in *treatment* is elimination of contact with the allergen. Acute dermatitis responds to cool compresses and a corticosteroid agent applied several times daily. Chronic dermatitis often requires a more potent fluorinated steroid ointment with protective covering at night. An antihistamine may be used orally for its sedative effect. Massive acute bullous reactions or reactions that cause swelling around the eyes or genitalia such as those of poison ivy are best treated by a 2-wk tapering course of oral corticosteroid therapy. Facial lesions often require a 3-wk course of systemic steroids. If secondary infection has occurred, appropriate systemic antibiotic therapy should be given. Desensitization therapy is rarely indicated.

NUMMULAR ECZEMA. This disorder is unusual in children and unrelated to other types of eczema. The eczematous plaques are more or less coin shaped. Common sites are the extensor surfaces of the extremities (Fig. 605–2), buttocks, and shoulders. The plaques are relatively discrete, boggy, vesicular, severely pruritic, and exudative; when chronic, they often become thickened and lichenified. The cause is unknown. Most frequently, these lesions are mistaken for tinea corporis, but plaques of nummular eczema are distinguished by the lack of a raised, sharply circumscribed border, the lack of fungal organisms on a KOH preparation, and they often weep or bleed when scraped. Secondary infection is common. Control of pruritus is usually achieved with a fluorinated corticosteroid preparation. Sedation with an antihistamine is helpful, particularly at night. Antibiotics are indicated for secondary infection.

PITYRIASIS ALBA. This occurs mainly in children; the lesions are hypopigmented, round or oval, macular or slightly elevated patches with fine adherent scale (Fig. 605–3 [color plate section]). They may be mildly erythematous and relatively well defined but lack a sharply marginated border. Lesions occur on the face, neck, upper trunk, and proximal arms. Itching is minimal or absent. The cause is unknown, but the eruption appears to be exacerbated by dryness and is often regarded as a mild form of eczema. Pityriasis alba is frequently misdiagnosed as tinea versicolor or corporis, each of which can be readily excluded by performing a KOH examination of surface scale. The lesions wax and wane but eventually disappear. Application of a lubricant may ameliorate the condition; if pruritus is troublesome, a topical 1% hydrocortisone preparation applied three to four times daily may be more effective. Normal pigmentation returns in weeks to months.

LICHEN SIMPLEX CHRONICUS. This lesion is characterized by a chronic pruritic, eczematous, circumscribed, solitary plaque that is usually lichenified and hyperpigmented. The most common sites are the posterior neck, dorsum of the feet, wrists, and ankles. Trauma from rubbing and scratching accounts for persistence of the plaque, although the initiating event may be a transient lesion, such as an insect bite. Pruritus must be

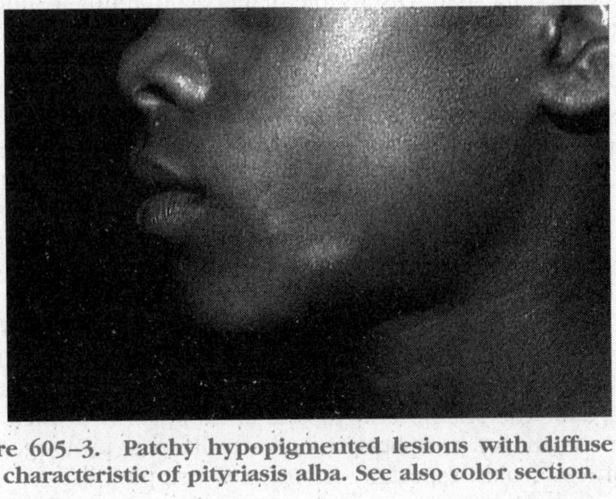

Figure 605–3. Patchy hypopigmented lesions with diffuse borders characteristic of pityriasis alba. See also color section.

controlled to permit healing. A topical fluorinated corticosteroid preparation is often helpful, but constant irritation to the skin must be avoided. A covering to prevent scratching may be necessary.

DYSHIDROTIC ECZEMA (DYSHIDROSIS, POMPHOLYX). This is a recurrent, sometimes seasonal, blistering disorder of the hands and feet; it occurs in all age groups but is uncommon in infancy. The pathogenesis is not known; there does not appear to be a genetic factor, although an increased incidence of atopy has been recorded in patients and their relatives. The disease is characterized by recurrent crops of intensely pruritic, small vesicles on the hands and feet. Sites of predilection are the palms, soles, and lateral aspects of the fingers and toes. Primary lesions are noninflammatory and filled with clear fluid, which, unlike sweat, has a physiologic pH and contains protein. Larger vesicobullae may occur, and maceration and secondary infection are frequent because of scratching (Fig. 605–4). The chronic phase is characterized by thickened, fissured plaques that may cause considerable discomfort. Hyperhidrosis is common in many patients, but the association may be fortuitous. The diagnosis is made clinically. The disorder may be confused with allergic contact dermatitis, which usually affects the dorsal rather than the volar surfaces, and with dermatophytosis, which can be distinguished by a KOH preparation of the roof of a vesicle and by appropriate cultures.

Dyshidrotic eczema responds to wet dressings, followed by a topical corticosteroid preparation during the acute phase. Control of the chronic stage is difficult; lubricants containing mild keratolytic agents in conjunction with a potent topical fluorinated corticosteroid preparation may be indicated. Secondary bacterial infection should be treated systemically with an appropriate antibiotic. Patients should be told to expect recurrence and should protect their hands and feet from the damaging effects of excessive sweating, chemicals, harsh soaps, and adverse weather.

SEBORRHEIC DERMATITIS. This is a chronic inflammatory disease that occurs at all ages; in the pediatric age group, it is most common during infancy and adolescence, paralleling the distribution, size, and activity of the sebaceous glands. The cause is unknown, as is the role of the sebaceous gland in this disease. A generalized eruption with features of seborrheic dermatitis is extremely common in human immunodeficiency virus-infected children and adolescents.

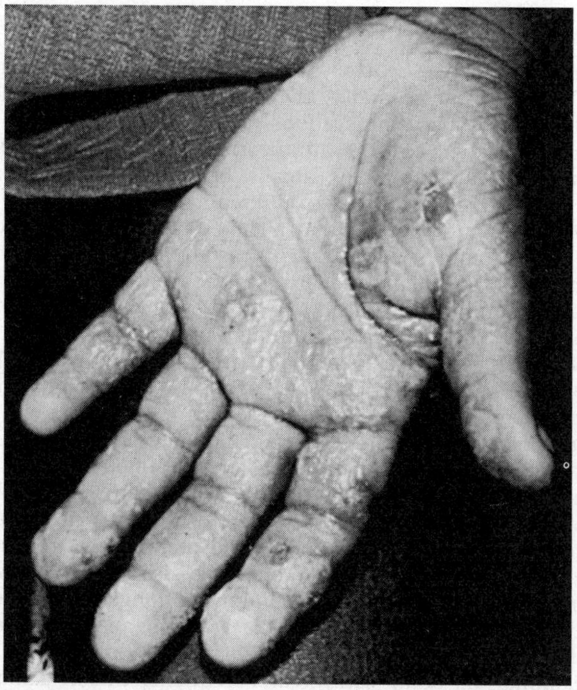

Figure 605–4. Vesicular palmar lesions of dyshidrotic eczema that have become secondarily infected.

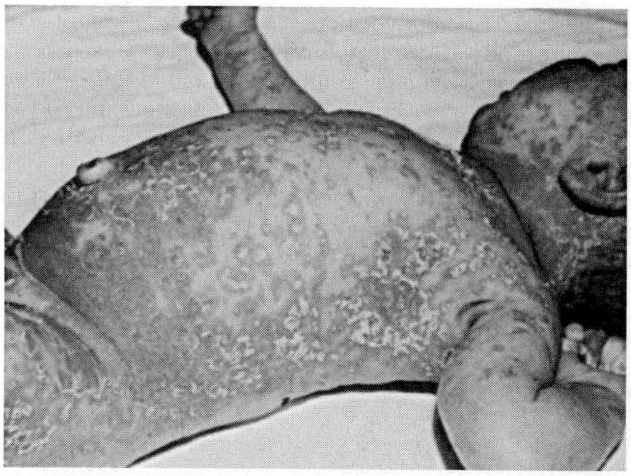

Figure 605–5. Widespread seborrheic dermatitis in an infant.

Clinical Manifestations. The disorder may begin within the 1st mo of life and may be most troublesome during the 1st yr. Diffuse or focal scaling and crusting of the scalp, sometimes called *cradle cap,* may be the initial and at times the only manifestation. A greasy, scaly, erythematous papular dermatitis, which is usually nonpruritic, may involve the face, neck, retroauricular areas, axillae, and diaper area. The dermatitis may be patchy and focal or may spread to involve almost the entire body (Fig. 605–5). Postinflammatory pigmentary changes are common, particularly in black infants. When the scaling becomes pronounced, the condition may resemble psoriasis and, at times, can be distinguished only with difficulty. The possibility of coexistent atopic dermatitis must be considered when there is an acute weeping dermatitis with pruritus. An intractable seborrhea-like dermatitis with chronic diarrhea and failure to thrive *(Leiner disease)* may reflect dysfunction of the immune system. A chronic seborrhea-like pattern, which responds poorly to treatment, may also result from cutaneous histiocytic infiltrates in infants with Langerhans cell histiocytosis X. Seborrheic dermatitis is a common cutaneous manifestation of acquired immunodeficiency syndrome among young adults and is characterized by thick, greasy scales in the scalp and large hyperkeratotic erythematous plaques on the face, chest, and genitalia.

During adolescence, seborrheic dermatitis is more localized and may be confined to the scalp and intertriginous areas. There may also be marginal blepharitis and involvement of the external auditory canal. Scalp changes may vary from diffuse, brawny scaling to focal areas of thick, oily, yellow crusts with underlying erythema. Loss of hair is not uncommon, and pruritus may be absent to marked. When the dermatitis is severe, erythema and scaling may occur at the frontal hairline, at the medial aspects of the eyebrows, and in the nasolabial and retroauricular folds. Red, scaly plaques may appear in the axillae, inguinal region, gluteal cleft, and umbilicus. On the extremities, seborrheic plaques may be more eczematous and less erythematous and demarcated.

Etiology. Seborrheic dermatitis is a condition that is reactivated in some patients by stressful situations, poor hygiene, and excessive perspiration. *Pityrosporum ovale (Malassezia ovalis)* has also been implicated as a causative agent. The *differential diagnosis* includes psoriasis, atopic dermatitis, dermatophytosis, and candidosis. Secondary bacterial infections and superimposed candidosis are not uncommon.

Treatment. Scalp lesions should be controlled with an antiseborrheic shampoo (selenium sulfide, sulfur, salicylic acid, zinc pyrithion, tar), used daily if necessary. Inflamed lesions usually respond promptly to topical corticosteroid therapy given two to four times daily. Topical antifungal agents effective against *Pityrosporum* have also been advocated as therapy. Wet compresses should be applied to the moist or fissured lesions before application of the steroid ointment. Many patients require the continued use of an antiseborrheic shampoo for control. Response to therapy is usually rapid unless there are complicating factors or the diagnosis is in error.

Fergusson DM, Horwood J, Shannon FT: Early solid feeding and recurrent childhood eczema: A 10-year longitudinal study. Pediatrics 86:541, 1990.
Podmore P, Burrows D, Eady DJ, et al: Seborrheic eczema—a disease entity or a clinical variant of atopic eczema? Br J Dermatol 115:341, 1986.

CHAPTER 606

Photosensitivity

Gary L. Darmstadt and Al Lane

Photosensitivity denotes a qualitatively or quantitatively abnormal cutaneous reaction to sunlight or artificial light.

ACUTE SUNBURN REACTION. The most common photosensitive reaction seen in children is acute sunburn. Sunburn is caused mainly by ultraviolet (UV)B radiation (290–320-nm wavelength). Sunlight contains many-fold more UVA (320–400 nm) than UVB radiation but UVA must be encountered in much larger quantities than UVB radiation to produce sunburn.

Pathophysiology and Clinical Manifestations. Transmitted radiation below 300 nm is largely absorbed in the epidermis, whereas that above 300 nm is mostly transmitted to the dermis after variable epidermal melanin absorption. Children vary in susceptibility to UV radiation, depending on their skin type (amount of pigment) (Table 606–1). Immediate pigment darkening is due to UVA radiation–induced photo-oxidative darkening of existing melanin and its transfer from melanocytes to keratinocytes. This effect generally lasts for a few hours, and like a UVA-induced tanning salon tan, is not photoprotective. UVB-induced effects appear 6–12 hr after initial exposure and reach a peak in 24 hr. Effects include redness, tenderness, edema, and blistering. The vasodilatation seen in UVB-induced erythema is mediated by prostaglandins E_2 and F_2. Delayed melanogenesis as a result of UVB radiation begins in 2–3 days and lasts several days to a few weeks. Manufacture of new melanin in melanocytes, transfer of melanin from melanocytes to keratinocytes, increase in size and arborization of melanocytes, and activation of quiescent melanocytes produces delayed melanogenesis. This effect reduces skin sensitivity to development of erythema by approximately two- to three-fold. Additional effects and possible complications of sun exposure include increased thickness of the stratum corneum, recurrence or exacerbation of herpes simplex labialis, lupus erythematosus, and multiple other conditions, as outlined in Table 606–2.

■ TABLE 606–1 Sun-Reactive Skin Types

Type	Demographics	Sunburn, Tanning History
I	Red hair, freckles, Celtic origin	Always burns easily; no tanning
II	Fair skin, fair-haired, blue-eyed, white	Usually burns; minimal tanning
III	Darker skinned white	Sometimes burns, gradual light brown tan
IV	Mediterranean background	Minimal to no burning, always tans
V	Middle eastern white, Mexican	Rarely burns, tans profusely dark brown
VI	Blacks	Never burns, pigmented black

■ TABLE 606–2 Cutaneous Reactions to Sunlight

Sunburn

Photoallergic Drug Eruptions

Systemic drugs include tetracyclines (declomycin), psoralens, chlorthiazides, sulfonamides, barbiturates, griseofulvin, thiazides, quinidine, phenothiazines
Topical agents include coal tar derivatives, furocoumarins (plants), psoralens, halogenated salicylanilides (soaps), perfume oils (e.g., oil of bergamot)

Phototoxic Drug Eruptions

High doses of agents causing photoallergic eruptions such as nalidixic acid, 5-fluorouracil, psoralens, furosemide, nonsteroidal anti-inflammatory agents (naproxen, piroxicam)

Genetic Disorder with Photosensitivity

Xeroderma pigmentosum
Bloom syndrome
Cockayne syndrome
Rothmund-Thomson syndrome

Inborn Errors of Metabolism

Porphyrias
Hartnup disease
Pellagra

Infectious Diseases Associated with Photosensitivity

Recurrent herpes simplex infection
Lymphogranuloma venereum
Viral exanthems (accentuated photodistribution)

Skin Disease Exacerbated or Precipitated by Light

Lichen planus
Darier disease
Lupus erythematosus
Dermatomyositis
Scleroderma
Solar urticaria
Polymorphous light eruptions (?)
Hydroa aestivale and vacciniforme (?)
Granuloma annulare
Psoriasis
Erythema multiforme
Sarcoid
Atopic dermatitis
Hailey-Hailey disease
Pemphigus
Acne rosacea
Bullous pemphigoid

Deficient Protection Due to Lack of Pigment

Vitiligo
Oculocutaneous albinism
Partial albinism
Phenylketonuria
Chédiak-Higashi syndrome
Piebaldism

Treatment. Acute severe sunburn should be managed with cool tap water compresses; topical corticosteroids may diminish inflammation and pain, and oral prostaglandin inhibitors such as aspirin and indomethacin may decrease erythema and pain. Proprietary preparations containing topical anesthetics are relatively ineffective and potentially hazardous because of their propensity to cause contact dermatitis. A bland emollient is effective in the desquamative phase.

Prognosis and Prevention of Sequelae. The long-term sequelae of chronic and intense sun exposure are not often seen in children, but most individuals receive more than 50% of their lifetime UV dose by age 20 yr. Therefore, pediatricians play a pivotal role in educating patients and their parents regarding the harmful effects, potential malignancy risks, and irreversible skin damage that result from unduly prolonged exposure to the sun and tanning lights. Premature aging, senile elastosis, actinic keratoses, squamous and basal cell carcinomas, and melanomas all occur with greater frequency in sun-damaged skin. In particular, blistering sunburns in childhood and adolescence significantly increase the risk for development of *ma-*

lignant melanoma. Protection is enhanced by a wide variety of sunscreen agents. Physical opaque sunscreens (zinc oxide, titanium dioxide) block ultraviolet light, whereas chemical sunscreens (para-aminobenzoic acid [PABA], PABA esters, salicylates, benzophenones, dibenzoylmethanes, cinnamates) absorb damaging radiation. The benzophenones and dibenzoylmethanes provide protection in both the UVA and UVB ranges. Children with skin types I to III (see Table 606–1) require sunscreens with a sun protection factor (SPF) of at least 15. SPF is defined as the minimal dose of sunlight required to produce cutaneous erythema after applying a sunscreen, divided by the dose required with no sunscreen on. Protective clothing (hats) and avoidance of sun exposure between 10:00 A.M. and 2:00 P.M. are additional prudent practices.

PHOTOSENSITIVE REACTIONS. Photosensitizers in combination with a particular wavelength of light cause dermatitis that can be classified as a phototoxic or a photoallergic reaction. Contact of the skin with the photosensitizer may occur externally, internally by enteral or parenteral administration, or by host synthesis of photosensitizers in response to an administered drug.

Photoallergic reactions occur only in a small percentage of persons exposed to photosensitizers and light and require a time interval for sensitization to take place. Thereafter, dermatitis appears within approximately 24 hr of re-exposure to the photosensitizer and light. Photoallergic dermatitis is a T-cell–mediated delayed hypersensitivity reaction in which the drug, acting as a hapten, may combine with a skin protein to form the antigenic substance. Photoallergic reactions vary in morphology and may occur on partially covered and on light-exposed skin. Some of the important classes of drugs and chemicals responsible for photosensitivity reactions are listed in Table 606–2.

Phototoxic reactions occur in all individuals who accumulate adequate amounts of a photosensitizing drug or chemical within the skin. Prior sensitization is not required. Dermatitis develops within hours after exposure to radiation in the range of 285–450 nm. The eruption is confined to light-exposed areas and often resembles an exaggerated sunburn, but it may be urticarial or bullous. It results in postinflammatory hyperpigmentation. All the drugs that cause photoallergic reactions may also cause a phototoxic dermatitis, if given in sufficiently high doses. Several additional drugs and contactants cause phototoxic reactions, notably the plant-derived furocoumarins (see Table 606–2). Differentiation from contact dermatitis as a result of poison ivy or oak may be difficult, but itching is prominent in contact dermatitis. In phytophotodermatitis, burning is prominent and is confined to sun-exposed areas, sparing the upper eyelids, beneath the nose and chin, and the retroauricular areas.

Although photodermatitis caused by drugs or chemicals may be diagnosed by photopatch testing, facilities for this diagnostic procedure are not widely available. A high index of suspicion combined with an appreciation of the distribution pattern of the eruption and a history of application or ingestion of a known photosensitizing agent are all that is required to make a diagnosis. Discontinuation of the offending medication or avoidance of sun exposure, oral administration of an antihistamine, and application of a topical corticosteroid to alleviate pruritus are appropriate therapeutic measures. Severe reactions may necessitate systemic corticosteroid therapy for a brief time.

PORPHYRIAS (see Chapter 76). Porphyrias are acquired or inborn abnormalities of specific enzymes in the heme biosynthetic pathway; they are diverse in their clinical manifestations. Two in particular occur in children and have photosensitivity as a consistent feature. Signs and symptoms may be negligible during the winter, when sun exposure is minimal.

Congenital erythropoietic porphyria (Günther disease) is a rare autosomal recessive disorder caused by a deficiency of uroporphyrinogen III cosynthase. This condition presents within the first few months of life with exquisite sensitivity to light, which may induce repeated severe bullous eruptions that result in mutilating scars. Hyperpigmentation, hyperkeratosis, vesiculation, and fragility of skin develops in light-exposed areas. Hirsutism in areas of mild involvement, scarring alopecia in severely affected areas, pink to red urine, brown teeth, hemolytic anemia, splenomegaly, and increased amounts of uroporphyrin I in urine, plasma, and erythrocytes and of coproporphyrin I in feces are additional characteristic manifestations. Urine from affected patients fluoresces reddish-pink under a Wood light.

Erythropoietic protoporphyria is inherited as an autosomal dominant trait. It is due to decreased activity of ferrochelatase, which converts protoporphyrin to heme. Photosensitivity becomes apparent in early childhood and is manifested by pain, tingling, and a burning sensation within approximately 30 min of sun exposure, followed by erythema, edema, urticaria, and, rarely, vesicles on light-exposed areas. Nail changes consist of opacification of the nail plate, onycholysis, pain, and tenderness. Mild systemic symptoms of malaise, chills, and fever may accompany the acute skin reaction. Recurrent sun exposure produces a chronic eczematous dermatitis with thickened, lichenified skin, especially over the finger joints, and persistent violaceous erythema, ulcers, and pitted or linear, crusted atrophic scars on the face and rims of the ears. Pigmentation, hypertrichosis, skin fragility, and mutilation are uncommon. Liver disease is generally mild. Symptoms often improve spontaneously after age 10–11 yr.

The wavelengths of light mainly responsible for eliciting cutaneous reactions in porphyria are in the region of 400 nm. Window glass, which transmits wavelengths greater than 320 nm, is not protective, and artificial lights of the proper wavelength may be pathogenic. Patients must avoid direct sunlight, wear protective clothing, and use a sunscreen agent that effectively blocks wavelengths in the region of 400 nm. The administration of β-carotene (Solatene) quenches the fluorescence of the porphyrin molecule by imparting a yellow color to the skin; its effectiveness in reducing photosensitivity in patients with protoporphyria has onset within 1–3 mo and is variable.

COLLOID MILIUM. This is a rare, asymptomatic disorder that occurs on the face (nose, upper lip, upper cheeks) and may extend to the dorsum of the hands and the neck as a profuse eruption of ivory to yellow, firm, tiny, grouped papules. Lesions appear before puberty on otherwise normal skin, unlike the adult variant that develops on sun-damaged skin. Onset may follow an acute sunburn or chronic sun exposure. Most cases reach maximal severity within approximately 3 yr and remain unchanged thereafter, although the condition may remit spontaneously after puberty. Histopathologic changes include well-circumscribed accumulations of fissured eosinophilic material, primarily in the upper dermis in contact with the epidermis. Basal cells, which are transformed into these colloid bodies, appear to be abnormally susceptible to degeneration after actinic exposure.

HYDROA VACCINIFORME. This vesicobullous disorder is more common in boys than girls, begins in early childhood, but may remit at puberty. The peak incidence is in the spring and summer. Erythematous, pruritic macules develop symmetrically within hours of sun exposure over the ears, nose, lips, cheeks, and dorsa of the hands and forearms. Lesions progress to stinging tender papules and hemorrhagic vesicles and bullae. Severe lesions of hydroa vacciniforme resemble the vesicles of chickenpox; they become umbilicated, ulcerated, and crusted and heal with pitted scars and telangiectasias. Fever and malaise are noted occasionally during the acute phase. Histopathologically, lesions show intraepidermal multilocular vesicles, leading to focal epidermal and dermal necrosis. Early on, there is a dermal perivascular mononuclear cell infiltrate that later surrounds areas of necrosis. This eruption should be distinguished from erythropoietic protoporphyria, which rarely shows vesicles. Pathogenesis of hydroa vacciniforme is unknown, but typical lesions have been reproduced with repeated doses of UVA light. A topical corticosteroid may be useful for the inflammatory phase of the eruption. Prophylactic broad-spectrum sunscreens may also be helpful, as may low-dose courses of UVB or psoralen with UVA (PUVA) therapy. β-Carotene and antimalarial agents are sometimes beneficial.

ACTINIC PRURIGO. This is a chronic familial photodermatitis that is inherited as an autosomal dominant trait among the Native Americans of North and South America. The first episode generally occurs in early childhood several hours to 2 days after intense sun exposure. Most patients are female and are sensitive to UVA radiation. Lesions are intensely pruritic, erythematous papules on the face, lower lip, distal extremities, and, in severe cases, buttocks. Facial lesions may heal with minute, pitted, or linear scarring. Lesions often become chronic, without periods of total clearing, merging into eczematous plaques that lichenify and may become secondarily infected. Associated features that distinguish this disorder from other photoeruptions and atopic dermatitis include cheilitis, conjunctivitis, and traumatic alopecia of the outer half of the eyebrows. Actinic prurigo is a chronic condition that generally persists into adult life, although it may improve spontaneously in the late teenage years. Topical corticosteroids palliate the pruritus and inflammation. Antimalarials and β-carotene afford little to no protection, but broad-spectrum sunscreens such as butyl methoxydibenzoylmethane may be helpful. Thalidomide also has been found to be an effective treatment in the Native American population.

SOLAR URTICARIA. This is a rare disorder induced by UV or visible irradiation. Primary solar urticaria is probably mediated by allergic type 1 hypersensitivity to a cutaneous or circulating irradiation-induced allergen, leading to mast cell degranulation and histamine release. This reaction occurs within 5–10 min of sun exposure, fades within 1–2 hr, and is characterized by widespread severe wheal formation, which may lead to faintness, headache, nausea, syncope, or bronchospasm. H_1-blocking antihistamines may be useful to prevent or abate the eruption. Secondary solar urticaria is due to photosensitization to exogenous chemicals or systemic drugs and may rarely be a presenting sign of erythropoietic protoporphyria. Treatment consists of avoidance of the photosentizing wavelength of light and/or the drug.

POLYMORPHOUS LIGHT ERUPTION. Polymorphous light eruption develops most commonly in females who are younger than 30 yr of age. The first eruption typically appears after prolonged sun exposure during the spring or summer. Onset of the eruption is delayed by hours to days after sun exposure and lasts for hours to sometimes weeks. Areas of involvement tend to be symmetric and are characteristic for a given patient, including some, but not all, of the exposed or lightly covered skin on the face, neck, upper chest, and distal extremities. Lesions have various morphologies but most commonly are pruritic, 2–5-mm grouped erythematous papules or papulovesicles or edematous plaques that are more than 5 cm in diameter. Most cases involve sensitivity to UVA radiation, although some are UVB induced. Therapeutic approaches include sun avoidance, broad-spectrum sunscreens, topical or systemic corticosteroids, β-carotene, nicotinamide, antimalarials, or prophylactic UVB or PUVA phototherapy.

COCKAYNE SYNDROME. Onset of this autosomal recessive disorder is characterized by the appearance, at approximately 1 yr of age, of facial erythema in a butterfly distribution after sun exposure, followed by loss of adipose tissue and development of thin, atrophic, hyperpigmented skin, particularly over the face. Associated features include dwarfism; mental retardation; large, protuberant ears; long limbs; disproportionately large hands and feet, which are sometimes cool and cyanotic; pinched nose; carious teeth; unsteady gait with tremor; limitation of joint mobility; progressive deafness; cataracts; retinal degeneration; optic atrophy; decreased sweating and tearing; and premature graying of the hair. Diffuse extensive demyelination of the peripheral and central nervous systems ensues, and patients generally die before the 3rd decade from atheromatous vascular disease. Photosensitivity is due to deficient rates of repair of UV-induced damage, specifically within actively transcribing regions of DNA. The syndrome is distinguished from progeria (see Chapter 659) by photosensitivity and the ocular abnormalities.

XERODERMA PIGMENTOSUM. This is a rare autosomal recessive disorder that results from a defect in nucleotide excision repair. Ten complementation groups have been recognized, based on each group's separate defect in the ability to repair damaged DNA. The wavelength of light that induces the DNA damage ranges from 280–340 nm. Skin changes are first noted during infancy or early childhood in sun-exposed areas such as the face, neck, hands, and arms; lesions may occur, however, at other sites, including the scalp. The skin lesions consist of erythema, scaling, bullae, crusting, ephelides, telangiectasia, keratoses, basal and squamous cell carcinomas, and malignant melanomas. Ocular manifestations include photophobia, lacrimation, blepharitis, symblepharon, keratitis, corneal opacities, tumors of the lids, and possible eventual blindness. Neurologic abnormalities such as mental deterioration and sensorineural deafness may develop in approximately 20% of patients. Some patients with xeroderma pigmentosum have the clinical phenotype of Cockayne syndrome, suggesting that these two disorders may represent an overlapping spectrum of excision-repair defects. The association of xeroderma pigmentosum with microcephaly, mental retardation, dwarfism, and hypogonadism is known as *De Sanctis-Cacchione syndrome.*

This disease is a serious, mutilating disorder, and the life span is often brief. Affected families should have genetic counseling. The disorder is detectable in cells cultured from amniotic fluid. Affected children should be totally protected from sun exposure; protective clothing, eyeglasses, and opaque broad-spectrum sunscreens should be used even for mildly affected children. Light from unshielded fluorescent bulbs and sunlight passing through glass windows are also harmful. Early detection and removal of malignancies is mandatory. Grafting of skin from nonlight-exposed areas may be helpful, as is the use of topical antimitotic agents such as 5-fluorouracil.

ROTHMUND-THOMSON SYNDROME. This syndrome is also known as *poikiloderma congenitale* because of the striking skin changes; it is inherited as an autosomal recessive trait, although a preponderance of affected females has been reported. Skin changes are noted as early as 3 mo of age. Plaques of erythema and edema appear on the cheeks, forehead, ears, neck, dorsal hands, extensor arms, and buttocks and are replaced gradually by reticulated, atrophic, hyperpigmented, telangiectatic plaques. Light sensitivity is present in many cases, and exposure to the sun may provoke formation of bullae. Areas of involvement, however, are not strictly photodistributed. Short stature; frontal bossing; saddle nose; prognathism; small hands and feet; sparse eyebrows, eyelashes, pubic and axillary hair; sparse, fine, prematurely gray hair or alopecia; dystrophic nails; defective dentition; bony defects; and hypogenitalism are common. Cataracts commonly become apparent at 2–7 yr of age. Most patients have normal mental development and life expectancy. Keratoses and later squamous cell carcinomas may develop on exposed skin. In addition, the incidence of noncutaneous malignancies, particularly osteosarcoma, is higher than in the general population.

HARTNUP DISEASE (see Chapter 71.5). This is a rare inborn error of metabolism with autosomal recessive inheritance. Neutral amino acids, including tryptophan, are not transported across the brush border epithelium of the intestine and kidney, resulting in deficiency of synthesis of nicotinamide and causing a photoinduced pellagra-like syndrome. The urine contains increased amounts of monoamine monocarboxylic amino acids. Cutaneous signs, which precede neurologic manifestations, initially develop during the early months of life when an eczematous, occasionally vesicobullous, eruption is noted on the face and extremities in a glove-and-stocking photodistribution. Hyperpigmentation and hyperkeratosis may supervene and are intensified by further exposure to sunlight. Episodic flares may be precipitated by febrile illness, sun exposure, emotional stress, and poor nutrition. In most cases, mental development is normal, but some patients display emotional instability and episodic cerebellar ataxia. Neurologic symptoms are fully reversible. Administration of nicotinamide and protection from sunlight result in improvement of both cutaneous and neurologic manifestations. Neomycin may also be beneficial in abating neurologic symptoms by reducing the intestinal bacterial flora and minimizing formation of indole and indican.

BLOOM SYNDROME. The defect in Bloom syndrome is inherited in an autosomal recessive manner on chromosome 15. Erythema and telangiectasia develop during infancy in a butterfly distribution on the face after exposure to sunlight. A bullous eruption on the lips and telangiectatic erythema on the hands and forearms may develop. Café au lait spots, ichthyosis, acanthosis nigricans, and hypertrichosis are less constant cutaneous manifestations. Pre- and postnatal short stature and a distinctive facies consisting of a prominent nose and ears and a small, narrow face are generally found. Defective dentition, pilonidal cysts, sacral dimples, syndactyly, polydactyly, clinodactyly of the fifth fingers, shortened lower extremities, and club feet are additional inconstant features. Intellect is normal. Patients frequently have low levels of IgA, IgM, and IgG and are susceptible to infections. They are sensitive to UV radiation, and their rate of chromosomal breaks and sister chromatid exchanges is markedly increased. Affected children have an unusual tendency to develop lymphoreticular malignancies.

Council on Scientific Affairs: Harmful effects of ultraviolet radiation. JAMA 262:380, 1989.
Elder GH: Molecular genetics of disorders of haem biosynthesis. J Clin Pathol 46:977, 1993.
Holzle E, Plewig G, von Kries R, et al: Polymorphous light eruption. J Invest Dermatol 88:32s, 1987.
Jung EG: The red face: photogenodermatoses. Clin Dermatol 11:275, 1993.
Kraemer KW, Slor H: Xeroderma pigmentosum. Clin Dermatol 3:33, 1985.
Lane PR, Hogan DJ, Martel MJ, et al: Actinic prurigo: clinical features and prognosis. J Am Acad Dermatol 26:683, 1992.
O'Donovan A, Davies AA, Moggs, et al: XPG endonuclease makes the 3′ incision in human DNA nucleotide excision repair. Nature 371:432, 1994.
Oliphant JA, Forster JL, McBride CM: The use of commercial tanning facilities by suburban Minnesota adolescents. Public Health Briefs 84:476, 1994.
Poh-Fitzpatrick MB, Ramsay CA, Frain-Bell W, et al: Photodermatoses in infants and children. Pediatr Dermatol 5:189, 1988.
Schmidt H, Knitker G, Thomson K, et al: Erythropoietic protoporphyria: a clinical study based on 29 cases in 14 families. Arch Dermatol 110:58, 1974.
Soter NA: Acute effects of ultraviolet radiation on the skin. Semin Dermatol 9:11, 1990.
Vennos EM, Collins M, James WD: Rothmund-Thomson syndrome: review of the world literature. J Am Acad Dermatol 27:750, 1992.

CHAPTER 607

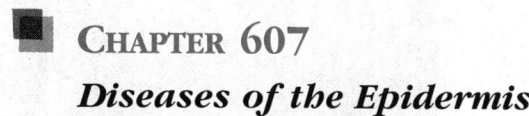

Diseases of the Epidermis

Gary L. Darmstadt and Al Lane

PSORIASIS. This common, chronic skin disorder is first evident in approximately one third of affected individuals within the first 2 decades of life. When the onset occurs during childhood, about 50% have a positive family history of the disease, and girls are more frequently affected. The mode of transmission is unknown; a multifactorial type of inheritance has been proposed. There is an association with histocompatibility antigens (HLA)-BW17, -B13, -B16, and -BW37, but the most significant association is with -CW6. These HLA types are not associated with the pustular form of the disease. The pathogenesis is also unknown; epidermal turnover time, however, is distinctly accelerated compared with that of normal epidermis.

Clinical Manifestations. The lesions consist of erythematous papules that coalesce to form plaques with sharply demarcated, irregular borders. If they are unaltered by treatment, a thick silvery or yellow-white scale (resembling mica) develops; removal of it may result in pinpoint bleeding (Auspitz sign). The *Köbner,* or isomorphic, *response* in which new lesions appear at sites of trauma is a valuable diagnostic feature. Lesions may occur anywhere, but preferred sites are the scalp, knees (Fig. 607–1A), elbows, umbilicus, and genitalia. Scalp lesions may be confused with seborrheic dermatitis or tinea capitis. Small, raindrop-like lesions on the face are moderately common. Nail involvement, a valuable diagnostic sign, is characterized by pitting of the nail plate (Fig. 607–1B), detachment of the plate (onycholysis), and accumulation of subungual debris.

Age is an important factor in determining the clinical pattern. Psoriasis is rare in the neonate but may be severe and recalcitrant and pose a diagnostic problem. The initial lesions may involve the diaper area and mimic seborrheic dermatitis, eczematous diaper dermatitis, perianal streptococcal disease, or candidosis. Biopsy or prolonged observation may be required for definitive diagnosis. Other rare forms include psoriatic erythroderma, localized or generalized pustular psoriasis, and linear psoriasis. Hospitalization may be required for severe forms of the disease. *Guttate psoriasis,* a variant that occurs predominantly in children, is characterized by an explosive eruption of profuse, small, oval or round lesions that morphologically are identical to the larger plaques of psoriasis (Fig. 607–1C). Sites of predilection are the trunk, face, and proximal portions of the limbs. The onset frequently follows a recent streptococcal respiratory infection; a culture of the throat and serologic titers should be obtained. Guttate psoriasis has also been observed after perianal streptococcal infection, viral infections, sunburn, and withdrawal of systemic corticosteroid therapy. Recent evidence suggests that psoriatic skin lesions may be induced, in a genetically susceptible host, by $CD4^+$ T-cells which were initially activated by streptococcal pyrogenic exotoxins acting as superantigens. The source of the streptococcal antigens can be the throat or the skin. Some of the superantigen-activated T-cells recognize streptococcal M-protein in the skin, and also appear to have cross reactivity with an abnormal keratin which has homology with streptococcal M protein. The autoreactive T-cells may be responsible for the formation and maintenance of psoriatic skin lesions. The lesions may be confused with viral exanthems and guttate parapsoriasis (see later).

Diagnosis. This is based on the clinical manifestations. The differential diagnosis includes Reiter syndrome, which, in con-

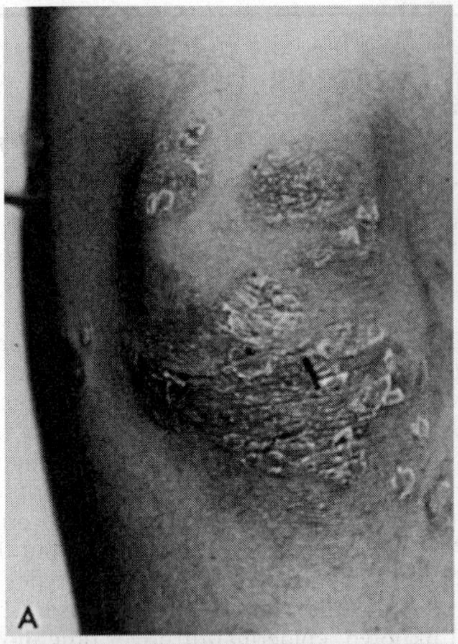

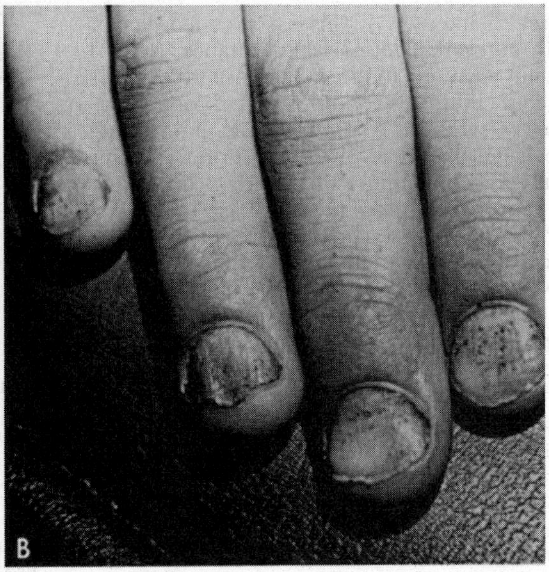

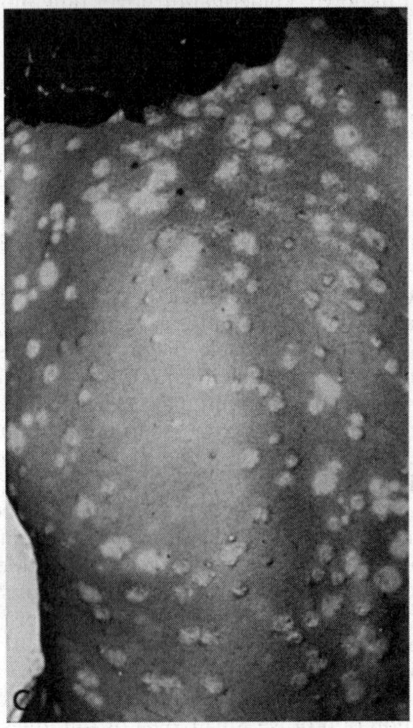

Figure 607–1. *A,* Chronic psoriatic plaques on the knee. *B,* Psoriatic nail changes of pitting and dystrophy. *C,* Guttate psoriasis in widespread distribution over the trunk.

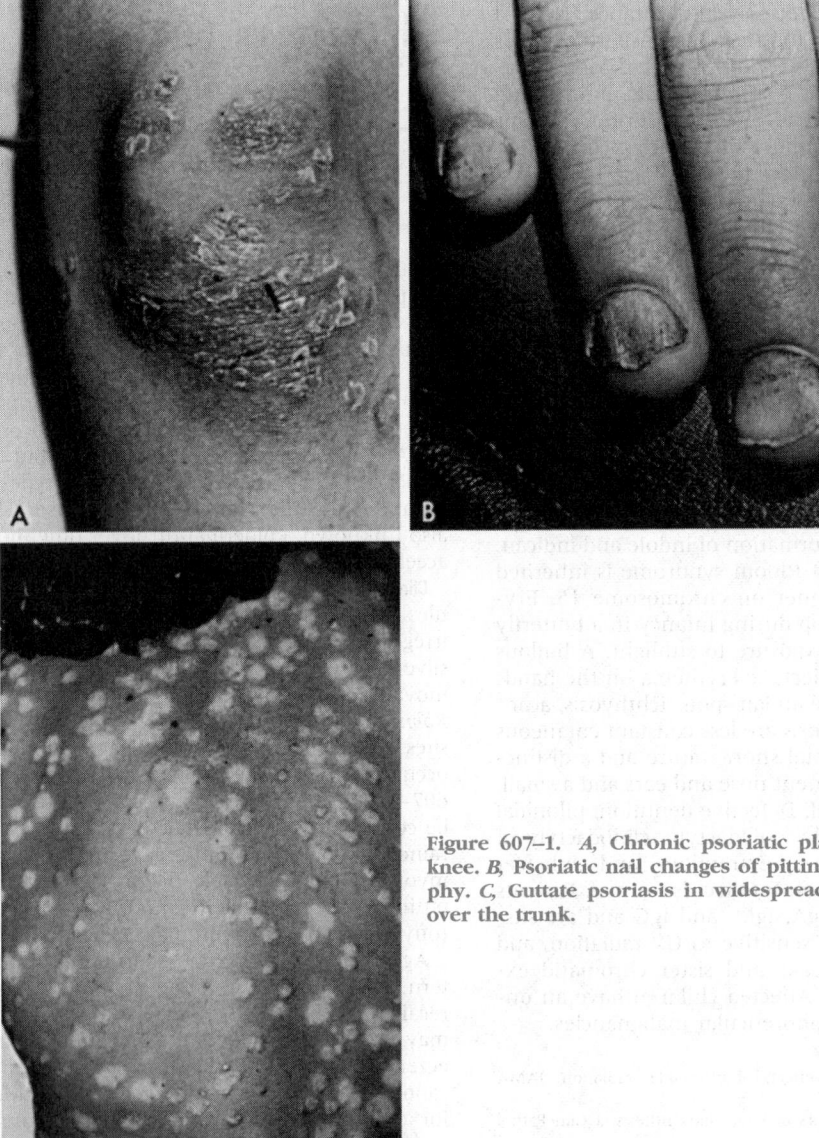

trast to psoriasis, involves mucous membranes, and pityriasis rubra pilaris.

Treatment. The therapeutic approach varies with the age of the child, type of psoriasis, sites of involvement, and extent of the disease. Therapy is mainly palliative and should not be overly aggressive. Physical and chemical trauma to the skin should be avoided as much as possible (see the Köbner response, earlier).

Tar preparations may be used in the form of an emulsion added to the daily bath, gel preparations, or ointments such as crude coal tar (1–5%) and liquor carbonis detergens (5–15%) in petrolatum alone or in conjunction with ultraviolet (UV)B light or natural sunlight. Occasionally, sunlight has an adverse rather than a beneficial effect, and the use of tar preparations may have to be decreased during the summer to avoid phototoxic reactions. Salicylic acid ointment (1–3%) may provide an alternative for removal of scale, but extensive application may result in toxicity, particularly in small children. Topical corticosteroid preparations are effective during the first several weeks of therapy for an individual lesion and then their effectiveness decreases. Topical corticosteroids must be used with caution. Fluorinated compounds produce cutaneous atrophy if applied excessively or if occluded with polyethylene film for prolonged periods. The least potent but effective preparation should be applied one to two times daily as adrenal suppression can occur. The topical vitamin D analog, calcipotriene, may also be effective for limited lesions. Calcipotriene can burn and sting, which limits its usefulness in children. In addition, several weeks of therapy are necessary before benefit is seen. For scalp lesions, applications of a phenol and saline solution (Baker P & S) followed by a tar shampoo are effective in the removal of scales. A corticosteroid in a lotion or gel base may be applied when the scaling is diminished. Rarely, the more severe forms of psoriasis may require systemic therapy.

The use of psoralens and UV light (PUVA) is effective in severe psoriasis in adults, but the safety of PUVA has not been established for children. Methotrexate and oral retinoids (in combination with PUVA) are utilized for the rare severe and generalized forms of psoriasis. The retinoid etretinate is useful in severe disorders, has a half-life of several years, and may have serious side effects; dermatologic consultation is essential when its use is being considered. Psoriasis in infants and acute guttate psoriasis may flare with vigorous treatment and should be managed conservatively. Nail lesions are usually recalcitrant to therapy.

Prognosis. This is best for children with limited disease. Psoriasis is characterized by remissions and exacerbations; if present during adolescence, it is a lifelong disease. Arthritis may be an extracutaneous complication.

PITYRIASIS LICHENOIDES. This has historically encompassed pityriasis lichenoides et varioliformis acuta (PLEVA, Mucha-Habermann disease), which tends to develop acutely, and pityriasis lichenoides chronica (PLC), which follows a chronic course. The designation of pityriasis lichenoides as acute or chronic may more properly refer to morphologic appearance of the lesions, which is often hemorrhagic or necrotic in PLEVA, than the duration of the disease. In a series of 89 pediatric cases, no correlation was found between the type of lesion at the onset of the eruption and the duration of the disease. Many patients have both acute and chronic lesions simultaneously, and transition of lesions from one form into another occurs occasionally. There is a correlation between the distribution of lesions and the duration of disease follows: (1) disease characterized by diffusely distributed lesions may resolve relatively quickly (mean disease duration 11 mo); (2) centrally distributed lesions on the trunk, neck, and/or proximal extremities are intermediate in duration; and (3) disease located peripherally or acrally usually persists the longest (mean 31 mo). Pityriasis lichenoides most commonly presents in the 2nd and 3rd decades; approximately one third of cases present before age 20 yr.

Clinical Manifestations. PLC presents with generalized, multiple, asymptomatic 3–5-mm brown-red papules that are covered by a grayish mica-like scale. A useful clinical sign is the easy detachment of the adherent scale, revealing a shining surface. Lesions may be asymptomatic or may cause minimal pruritus and occasionally become infiltrated, vesicular, hemorrhagic, and crusted. Individual papules become flat and brownish over 2–6 wk, ultimately leaving a hyperpigmented or hypopigmented macule. Scarring is unusual. Lesions are most common on the trunk and extremities and generally spare the face, palmoplantar surfaces, scalp, and mucous membranes. The eruption persists for months to years and is characterized by polymorphous lesions in various stages of evolution. PLC histologically shows a parakeratotic, thickened corneal layer; epidermal spongiosis; a superficial perivascular infiltrate of macrophages and predominantly CD8+ lymphocytes, which may extend into the epidermis; and small numbers of extravasated erythrocytes in the papillary dermis.

PLEVA presents with an abrupt eruption of multiple papules that have a vesiculopustular and then a purpuric center, are covered by a dark adherent crust, and are surrounded by an erythematous halo. Constitutional symptoms of fever, malaise, headache, and arthralgias may be present for 2–3 days after the initial outbreak. Lesions are distributed diffusely on the trunk and extremities, as in PLC. Individual lesions heal within a few weeks, sometimes leaving a varioliform scar, and successive crops of papules produce the characteristic polymorphous appearance of the eruption. The condition is generally self-limited from several weeks to months. The histopathologic changes of PLEVA reflect its more severe nature compared with PLC. Intercellular and intracellular edema in the epidermis may lead to degeneration of keratinocytes. A dense perivascular mononuclear cell infiltrate that extends upward into the epidermis and downward into the reticular dermis, endothelial cell swelling, and extravasation of erythrocytes into the epidermis and dermis are additional characteristic features. Severe changes of vasculitis are exceptional. Differential diagnosis includes guttate psoriasis, pityriasis rosea, drug eruptions, secondary syphilis, viral exanthems, and lichen planus. The chronicity of pityriasis lichenoides helps to exclude pityriasis rosea, viral exanthems, and some drug eruptions. A skin biopsy helps to exclude other differential diagnoses.

A rare form of PLEVA has been described that presents with fever and ulceronecrotic plaques up to 1 cm in diameter, which are most common on the anterior trunk and flexors of the proximal upper extremities. Arthritis and superinfection of cutaneous lesions with *Staphylococcus aureus* may also develop. The ulceronecrotic lesions appear within papules of PLEVA and heal with hypopigmented scarring in a few weeks. Leukocytoclastic vasculitis is occasionally seen histopathologically. The eruption may resemble erythema multiforme, but it generally spares the mucous membranes.

Etiology. The cause of pityriasis lichenoides in unknown, but sporadic outbreaks have led to an unsuccessful search for an infectious agent, despite the fact that human-to-human transmission has not been documented. Nevertheless, a popular hypothesis is that pityriasis lichenoides is a hypersensitivity reaction to an infectious organism. Cell-mediated mechanisms appear to be important in the pathogenesis because most infiltrating cells are cytotoxic-suppressor cells. Clonal gene rearrangement studies of the T-cell receptor and immunohistologic studies have led to the suggestion that PLEVA may be a T-cell lymphoproliferative process. The condition in two children with PLEVA was reported recently to evolve into cutaneous T-cell lymphoma. It has been postulated that the relatively greater proportion of cytotoxic-suppressor cells than helper-inducer T cells in lesions of PLEVA compared with those of lymphomatoid papulosis or T-cell lymphoma reflects the more effective host response in PLEVA.

Treatment. In general, pityriasis lichenoides should be considered a benign condition that does not alter the health of the child. A lubricant to remove excessive scaling may be all that is necessary if the patient is asymptomatic. The most appropriate treatment includes erythromycin (30–50 mg/kg/24 hr for 2 mo) in combination with natural sunlight. If this regimen is effective, erythromycin should then be tapered slowly over several months. The rare febrile ulceronecrotic form may be controlled effectively by systemic corticosteroids. Additional modalities that have been effective in some adult patients, but are rarely appropriate for children, include PUVA, tetracycline, dapsone, and methotrexate.

KERATOSIS PILARIS. This moderately common papular eruption may vary in extent from sparse lesions over the extensor aspects of the limbs to involvement of most of the body surface. The lesions may resemble gooseflesh; they are noninflammatory, scaly, follicular papules that do not coalesce. Irritation of the follicular plugs occasionally causes folliculitis. Because the lesions are associated with and accentuated by dry skin, they are often more prominent during the winter. They are more frequent in patients with atopic dermatitis and are most common during childhood and early adulthood, tending to subside during the 3rd decade of life. Mild or localized eruptions respond to lubrication with a bland emollient; more pronounced or widespread lesions require regular applications of a 10–25% urea cream, an α-hydroxy acid preparation such as lactic acid in an emollient, or topical retinoic acid. Therapy usually improves the condition but does not cure it.

LICHEN SPINULOSUS. This uncommon disorder occurs principally in children and more frequently in boys. The cause is unknown. The lesions consist of sharply circumscribed irregular plaques of spiny, keratinous projections that protrude from the orifices of the pilosebaceous canals (Fig. 607–2). Plaques may occur anywhere on the body and are often distributed symmetrically on the trunk, elbows, knees, and extensor surfaces of the limbs. Although sometimes erythematous, the lesions

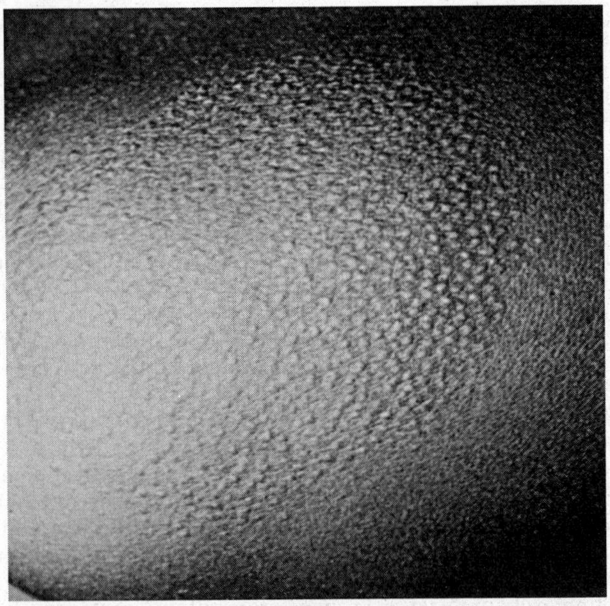

Figure 607–2. Sharply circumscribed plaque of follicular papules characteristic of lichen spinulosus.

are usually skin colored. They are readily palpable and represent keratotic follicular plugs. Lichen spinulosus is easily differentiated from keratosis pilaris because the latter lesions are never grouped to form plaques. More commonly, it is confused with papular eczema.

Treatment is usually unnecessary. For patients who regard the eruption as a cosmetic defect, keratolytic agents such as salicylic acid ointment (3–7%), urea-containing lubricants (10–25%), and retinoic acid preparations are often effective in flattening the projections. The plaques usually disappear spontaneously after several months or years.

PITYRIASIS ROSEA. This benign, common eruption occurs most frequently in children and young adults. Although a prodrome of fever, malaise, arthralgia, and pharyngitis may precede the eruption, children rarely complain of such symptoms. The cause of pityriasis rosea is unknown; a viral agent is suspected.

Clinical Manifestations. A *herald patch,* a solitary, round or oval lesion that may occur anywhere on the body and is often but not always identifiable by its large size, usually precedes the generalized eruption. Herald patches vary from 1–10 cm in diameter; they are annular in configuration; and they have a raised border with fine, adherent scales. Approximately 5–10 days after the appearance of the herald patch, a widespread, symmetric eruption becomes evident involving mainly the trunk and proximal limbs (Fig. 607–3). When the disease is extensive, the face, scalp, and distal limbs may be involved, or, in the inverse form of pityriasis rosea, only those sites may be affected. Lesions may appear in crops for several days. Typical lesions are oval or round, less than 1 cm in diameter, slightly raised, and pink to brown. The developed lesion is covered by a fine scale that gives the skin a crinkly appearance; some lesions clear centrally, producing a collarette of scale that is attached only at the periphery. Papular, vesicular, urticarial, hemorrhagic, and large annular lesions are unusual variants. The long axis of each lesion is usually aligned with the cutaneous cleavage lines, a feature that creates the so-called Christmas tree pattern on the back. Actually, conformation to skin lines is often more discernible in the anterior and posterior axillary folds and supraclavicular areas. Duration of the eruption varies from 2–12 wk. The lesions may be asymptomatic or mildly to severely pruritic.

Diagnosis. This is clinical. The herald patch may be mistaken for tinea corporis, a pitfall that can be avoided if a potassium hydroxide preparation is obtained. The generalized eruption resembles a number of other diseases; of these, secondary syphilis is the most important. Drug eruptions, viral exanthems, guttate psoriasis, pityriasis lichenoides chronica, and eczema can also be confused with pityriasis rosea.

Treatment. Therapy is unnecessary for the asymptomatic patient. If scaling is prominent, a bland emollient may suffice. Pruritus may be suppressed by a lubricating lotion containing menthol and camphor or by an oral antihistamine for sedation, particularly at night, when itching may be troublesome. Occasionally, a nonfluorinated topical corticosteroid preparation may be necessary to alleviate pruritus. After the eruption has resolved, postinflammatory hypopigmentation or hyperpigmentation may be pronounced, particularly in black patients; these changes disappear during subsequent weeks to months.

PITYRIASIS RUBRA PILARIS. This rare chronic dermatosis often has an insidious onset with diffuse scaling and erythema of the scalp, which is indistinguishable from seborrheic dermatitis, and with thick hyperkeratosis of the palms and soles. The characteristic primary lesion is a firm, dome-shaped, tiny, acuminate papule, which is pink to red and has a central keratotic plug pierced by a vellus hair. Masses of these papules coalesce to form large, erythematous, sharply demarcated orangish plaques, within which islands of normal skin can be distinguished, creating a bizarre effect. Typical papules on the dorsum of the proximal phalanges are readily palpated. Gray plaques or papules resembling lichen planus may be found in the oral cavity. Dystrophic changes in the nails may occur and mimic those of psoriasis. In advanced stages, marked hyperkeratosis of the scalp and face may cause alopecia and ectropion. Differential diagnosis includes ichthyosis, seborrheic dermatitis, keratoderma of the palms and soles, and psoriasis.

Etiology. The cause is unknown. A genetic form with autosomal dominant transmission may account for some cases in childhood, but most appear to be sporadic. Attempts to link the disease with a defect in vitamin A metabolism have not been definitive. Skin biopsy may help to differentiate this condition from psoriasis and seborrheic dermatitis, which it resembles most closely.

Treatment. The numerous therapeutic regimens recommended are difficult to evaluate because the disease has a capricious course with exacerbations and remissions. Oral and topical retinoids and viatmin A have been used most frequently.

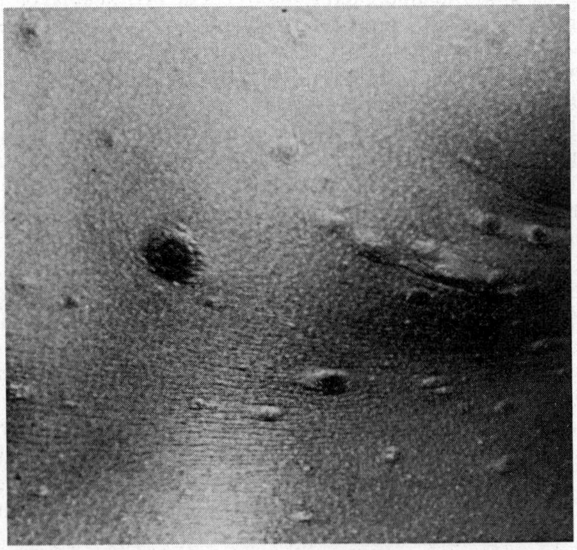

Figure 607–3. Ovoid, maculopapular lesions of pityriasis rosea. Note the distribution along the skin lines and the herald patch on the chest.

When vitamin A or synthetic retinoids are administered orally, the child should be observed carefully for signs of toxicity (see Psoriasis, Treatment). In childhood, the *prognosis* for eventual resolution is relatively good.

DARIER DISEASE (KERATOSIS FOLLICULARIS). This rare genetic disorder is inherited as an autosomal dominant trait. Onset occurs usually during late childhood. Typical lesions are small, firm, skin-colored papules that are not always follicular in location. Eventually, the lesions acquire yellow, malodorous crusts; coalesce to form large, gray-brown, vegetative plaques; and usually involve the face, neck, shoulders, chest, back, and limb flexures in a symmetric distribution. Papules, fissures, crusts, and ulcers may appear on the mucous membranes of the lips, tongue, buccal mucosa, pharynx, larynx, and vulva. Hyperkeratosis of the palms and soles and nail dystrophy with subungual hyperkeratosis are variable features. Severe pruritus, secondary infection, offensive odor, and aggravation of the dermatosis on exposure to sunlight may occur. Darier disease is most likely to be confused with seborrheic dermatitis or juvenile flat warts. Histologic changes are diagnostic: hyperkeratosis, intraepidermal separation with formation of suprabasal clefts, and dyskeratotic epidermal cells are characteristic features.

Treatment is nonspecific. Some patients have responded to large oral doses of vitamin A or to topical retinoic acid, with or without occlusive dressings. Secondary infection may require local cleansing and systemically administered antibiotics. Affected individuals usually suffer more during the summer.

LICHEN NITIDUS. This chronic, benign, papular eruption is characterized by minute (1–2 mm), flat-topped, shiny, firm papules of uniform size, which are most often skin colored but may be pink or red. In black individuals, they are usually hypopigmented. Sites of predilection are the genitalia, abdomen, chest, forearms, wrists, and inner aspects of the thighs. The lesions may be sparse or numerous and form large plaques; careful examination usually discloses linear papules in a line of scratch (Köbner phenomenon), a valuable clue to the diagnosis because it occurs in only a few diseases (Fig. 607–4). Lichen nitidus occurs in all age groups. The cause is unknown. Patients are usually asymptomatic and constitutionally well. The lesions may be confused with and rarely coexist with those of lichen planus.

Widespread keratosis pilaris can also be confused with lichen nitidus, but the follicular localization of the papules and the absence of the Köbner phenomenon in the former distinguishes them. Verruca plana (flat warts), if small and uniform in size, may occasionally resemble lichen nitidus. Although the diagnosis can be made clinically, a biopsy is occasionally indicated. Histopathologically, the lichen nitidus papule consists of sharply circumscribed nests of lymphocytes and histiocytes in the upper dermis enclosed by clawlike epidermal rete ridges. The course of lichen nitidus takes months to years, but the lesions eventually involute completely. There is no effective therapy.

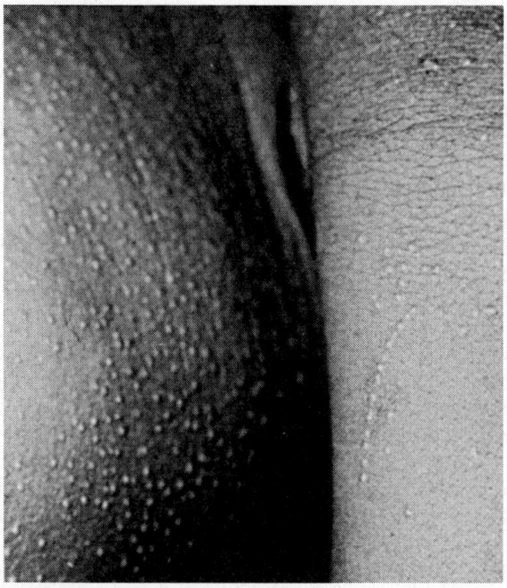

Figure 607–4. Tiny flat-topped papules of lichen nitidus on the arm and trunk. Note the Köbner response on the arm (papules in a line of scratch).

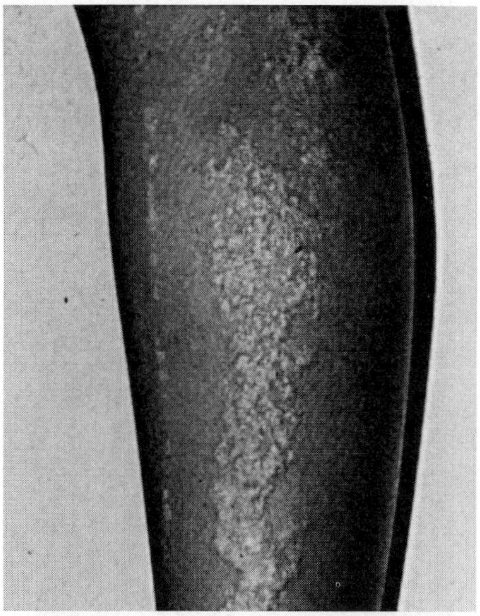

Figure 607–5. Multiple linear plaques and streaks of lichen striatus.

LICHEN STRIATUS. This benign, self-limited eruption consists of a continuous or discontinuous linear band of papules in a zosteriform distribution. The primary lesion is a flat-topped, red to violaceous papule covered with fine scale. Aggregates of these papules form multiple bands or plaques (Fig. 607–5). In black patients, the lesions may be hypopigmented. The cause and explanation for the linear distribution are unknown. The eruption evolves over a period of days or weeks in an otherwise healthy child, remains stationary for weeks to months, and finally remits without sequelae. Symptoms are usually absent; some children complain of itching. Nail dystrophy may occur when the eruption involves the posterior nail fold and matrix.

Lichen striatus is confused occasionally with other disorders. The initial plaque may resemble papular eczema or lichen nitidus until the linear configuration becomes apparent. Linear lichen planus and linear psoriasis are usually associated with typical individual lesions elsewhere on the body. Linear epidermal nevi are permanent lesions that often become more hyperkeratotic and hyperpigmented than those of lichen striatus. A lubricating lotion containing menthol and camphor or a mild corticosteroid preparation provides sufficient relief when pruritus is a problem.

LICHEN PLANUS. This is a rare disorder in the young child and uncommon in the older one. The primary lesion is a violaceous, sharply demarcated, polygonal papule with fine lines or thin white scales on the surface; papules may coalesce to form large plaques. The papules are intensely pruritic, and additional ones are often induced by scratching (Köbner phenomenon) so that lines of them are often detected (Fig. 607–6). Sites of predilection are the flexor surfaces of the wrists, forearms, and inner aspects of the thighs. Characteristic lesions

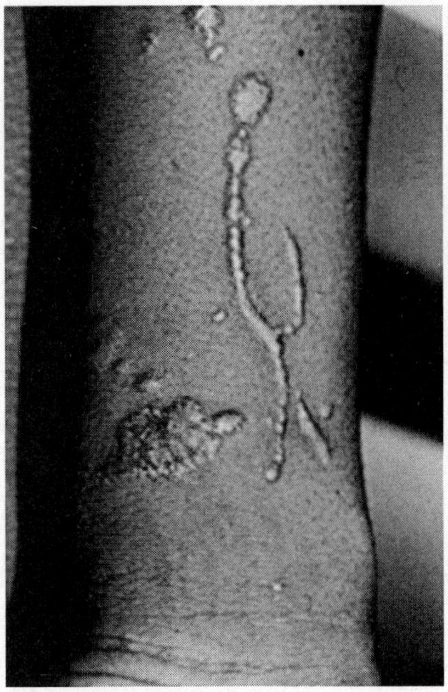

Figure 607–6. Violaceous polygonal papules of lichen planus. Note the striking Köbner response.

of mucous membranes consist of pinhead-sized, white papules that coalesce to form reticulated and lacy patterns on the oral mucosa and sometimes on the lips and tongue.

Acute eruptive lichen planus is probably the most common form in children. The lesions erupt in an explosive fashion, much like a viral exanthem, and spread to involve most of the body surface. Hypertrophic, linear, bullous, atrophic, annular, follicular, erosive, and ulcerative forms of lichen planus may also occur. Nail involvement may develop in the chronic forms but is rarely evident in children (see Chapter 613). The disorder may persist for months to years, but the acute eruptive form is most likely to involute permanently. Frequently, intense hyperpigmentation persists for a long time after the resolution of lesions. The histopathologic findings of lichen planus are specific, and a biopsy is indicated if the diagnosis is unclear.

Treatment is directed at alleviation of the intense pruritus and amelioration of the skin lesions. Oral antihistamines and/or tranquilizers are often helpful. The skin lesions respond best to regular applications of a topical corticosteroid preparation. Rarely, systemic corticosteroid therapy is necessary to gain control of widespread, intractable lesions.

POROKERATOSIS. This rare, chronic, progressive disease is inherited as an autosomal dominant trait. Several forms have been delineated: solitary plaques, linear porokeratosis, hyperkeratotic lesions of the palms and soles, disseminated eruptive lesions, and superficial actinic porokeratosis. The last form, probably induced by excessive sun exposure, occurs more commonly in adult females. Other types of porokeratosis are more common in males and begin during childhood. Sites of predilection are the limbs, face, neck, and genitalia. The primary lesion is a small, keratotic papule that enlarges peripherally so that the center becomes depressed, with the edge forming an elevated wall or collar. The configuration of the plaque may be round, oval, or gyrate; its elevated border is split by a thin groove from which minute cornified projections protrude. The enclosed central area is yellow, gray, or tan and sclerotic, smooth, and dry, whereas the hyperkeratotic border is a darker gray, brown, or black.

The differential diagnosis includes warts, epidermal nevi, lichen planus, granuloma annulare, and elastosis perforans serpiginosa. A skin biopsy discloses the characteristic cornoid lamella (plug of stratum corneum cells with retained nuclei), which is responsible for the invariable linear ridge of the lesion. The disease is slowly progressive but relatively asymptomatic. Lesions are sometimes responsive to applications of liquid nitrogen or occasionally may be surgically excised. Topical agents such as retinoic acid and 5-fluorouracil may be effective in some patients.

PAPULAR ACRODERMATITIS OF CHILDHOOD (GIANOTTI-CROSTI SYNDROME). This distinctive eruption is occasionally associated with malaise and low-grade fever but few other constitutional symptoms. The incidence peaks in early childhood. Occurrences are usually sporadic, but epidemics have been recorded. The skin lesion is a monomorphous, usually nonpruritic, dusky or coppery red, flat-topped, firm papule ranging in size from 1–5 mm. The papules appear in crops and may become profuse but remain discrete, forming a symmetric eruption on the face, buttocks, and limbs, including the palms and soles. The papules often have the appearance of vesicles; when opened, however, no fluid is obtained. The papules sometimes become hemorrhagic. Lines of papules (Köbner phenomenon) may be noted on the extremities. The trunk is relatively spared, as are the scalp and mucous membranes. Generalized lymphadenopathy and hepatomegaly (in those with hepatitis B viremia) constitute the only other abnormal physical findings. The eruption resolves spontaneously in about 15–60 days. Lymphadenopathy and hepatomegaly, if present, may persist for several months. This eruption in Italy was initially associated with primary liver infection by hepatitis B virus and surface antigenemia. Elevation of serum transaminase and alkaline phosphatase values without concomitant hyperbilirubinemia was usual. Skin biopsy was characterized by a perivascular mononuclear cell infiltrate and capillary endothelial swelling.

Generally, the disease is benign and is not associated with hepatitis in the United States. This eruption has been seen in children infected with Epstein-Barr virus, coxsackievirus A16, parainfluenza virus, and other viral infections. Papular acrodermatitis can be confused with lichen planus, erythema multiforme, histiocytosis X, and Henoch-Schönlein purpura.

ACANTHOSIS NIGRICANS. This is characterized by hyperpigmented, velvety, hyperkeratotic plaques that are most often localized to the neck, axillae, inframammary areas, groin, inner thighs, and anogenital region. The histologic changes are those of papillomatosis and hyperkeratosis rather than acanthosis or excessive pigment formation. Acanthosis nigricans has classically been associated with obesity; drugs such as nicotinic acid; endocrinopathies, including diabetes mellitus, Addison disease, Cushing syndrome, acromegaly, hypo- and hyperthyroidism, Stein-Leventhal syndrome, and hyperandrogenic or hypogonadal syndromes; many different syndromes such as Bloom, Crouzon, or Rud syndromes, Wilson disease, lipoatrophic diabetes, partial lipodystrophy, and leprechaunism; and malignancies, usually an adult with an abdominal adenocarcinoma. Occasionally, it may be familial with autosomal dominant inheritance. Acanthosis nigricans is found in 7% of children and is nearly always associated with obesity; this form is termed pseudoacanthosis nigricans.

The skin lesions appear to be a manifestation of insulin resistance. The clinical severity and histopathologic features of acanthosis nigricans correlate positively with the degree of hyperinsulinism. It has been hypothesized that insulin resistance, with compensatory hyperinsulinism, leads to insulin binding to and activation of insulin-like growth factor receptors, promoting epidermal growth. In the malignant form, tumor-secreted growth factors, and hyperinsulinemia could be pathogenic.

This skin disorder is extremely difficult to treat but may be improved by palliation of the underlying disorder, weight loss in the case of pseudoacanthosis nigricans, reduction in insulin resistance, and topical or oral retinoids.

CORTICOSTEROID-INDUCED ATROPHY. Both topical and systemic corticosteroid treatment can result in cutaneous atrophy. This is particularly common when a potent topical corticosteroid is applied under occlusion or to the intertriginous areas for a prolonged period. Affected skin is thin, fragile, smooth, and semi-transparent, with telangiectasias and loss of normal skin markings. Histopathologically, one sees thinning of the stratum corneum and malpighii. Spaces between dermal collagen and elastic fibers are small, producing a more compact but thin dermis. The mechanism involves inhibition of synthesis of collagen type I, noncollagenous proteins, and total protein content of the skin; progressive reduction of dermal proteoglycans and glycosaminoglycans; and possibly prolonged vasoconstriction-induced ischemia. Retinoids applied topically restore these steroid-induced biochemical changes in the dermal connective tissue of the hairless mouse, without abrogating the beneficial anti-inflammatory effects.

Caputo R, Gelmetti C, Ermacora E, et al: Gianotti-Crosti syndrome: A retrospective analysis of 308 cases. J Am Acad Dermatol 26:207, 1992.
Farber EM, Muller RH, Jacobs AH, et al: Infantile psoriasis: A follow-up study. Pediatr Dermatol 3:237, 1986.
Forston JS, Schroeter AL, Esterly NB: Cutaneous T-cell lymphoma (parapsoriasis en plaque). An association with pityriasis lichenoides et varioliformis acuta in young children. Arch Dermatol 126:1449, 1990.
Gelmetti C, Rigoni C, Alessi E, et al: Pityriasis lichenoides in children: A long term follow-up of eighty-nine cases. J Am Acad Dermatol 23:473, 1990.
Luberti AA, Rabinowitz LG, Verrereli KO: Severe febrile Mucha-Habermann's disease in children: Case report and review of the literature. Pediatr Dermatol 8:51, 1991.
Rogers M: Pityriasis lichenoides and lymphomatoid papulosis. Semin Dermatol 11:73, 1992.
Taieb A, Youbi E, Grosshans E, et al: Lichen striatus: A Blaschko linear acquired inflammatory skin eruption. J Am Acad Dermatol 25:637, 1991.
Truhan AP, Herbert AA, Esterly NB: Pityriasis lichenoides in children: Therapeutic response to erythromycin. J Am Acad Dermatol 15:66, 1986.
Valdimarsson H, Baker BS, Jonsdottir I, et al: Psoriasis: A T-cell mediated autoimmune disease induced by streptococcal superantigens? Immunol Today 16:145, 1995.

CHAPTER 608

Disorders of Keratinization

Gary L. Darmstadt and Al Lane

DISORDERS OF CORNIFICATION. Disorders of cornification, also known as the ichthyoses, are a primary group of inherited conditions that are characterized clinically by patterns of scaling and histopathologically by hyperkeratosis. They are usually distinguishable on the basis of inheritance patterns, clinical features, associated defects, and histopathologic changes. Because some of these conditions cause disfigurement and considerable psychosocial stress, early diagnosis is helpful to predict probable course and prognosis and to provide supportive management for the patient and family.

HARLEQUIN FETUS. This rare keratinizing disorder probably represents several genotypes with similar *clinical manifestations.* At birth, markedly thickened, ridged, and cracked skin forms horny plates over the entire body, disfiguring the facial features and constricting the digits. Severe ectropion and chemosis obscure the orbits, the nose and ears are flattened, and the lips are everted and gaping. Nails and hair may be absent. Joint mobility is restricted, and the hands and feet appear fixed and ischemic. The affected neonate has respiratory difficulty and a poor suck and is subject to severe cutaneous infection. Most die within the 1st days to weeks of life, but patients occasionally survive beyond infancy and are afflicted with severe ichthyosis. Ectropion and eclabium resolve, and the cracked, horny plated skin is replaced by large, thin scales with surrounding erythema.

Nearly all cases have autosomal recessive inheritance, but some cases may represent new dominant mutations. Common morphologic abnormalities include hyperkeratosis, accumulation of lipid droplets within corneocytes, and absence of normal lamellar granules. One type has an altered catalytic subunit of 2A protein phosphorylase, which is encoded on chromosome 11. The basic defect of all types is suggested to be an abnormality of lamellar granules, which play an important role in desquamation.

Initial treatment includes a high fluid intake to avoid dehydration from transepidermal water loss and use of a humidified heated incubator, emulsifying ointments, and oral retinoids such as etretinate. Prenatal diagnosis has been accomplished by fetoscopy, fetal skin biopsy, and recently microscopic examination of cells from amniotic fluid taken at the 17th and 21st wk of gestation.

COLLODION BABY. These infants are covered at birth by a thick, taut membrane resembling oiled parchment or collodion, which is subsequently shed. The condition is usually a manifestation of congenital ichthyosiform erythroderma or lamellar ichthyosis; like the harlequin fetus, the collodion baby appears to be one phenotype for several genotypes. Infrequently, an affected infant has normal skin after the membrane is shed. Affected neonates have ectropion, flattening of the ears and nose, and fixation of the lips in an O-shaped configuration (Fig. 608–1). Hair may be absent or may perforate the horny covering. The membrane cracks with initial respiratory efforts and, shortly after birth, begins to desquamate in large sheets. Complete shedding may take several weeks, and occasionally a new membrane may form in localized areas.

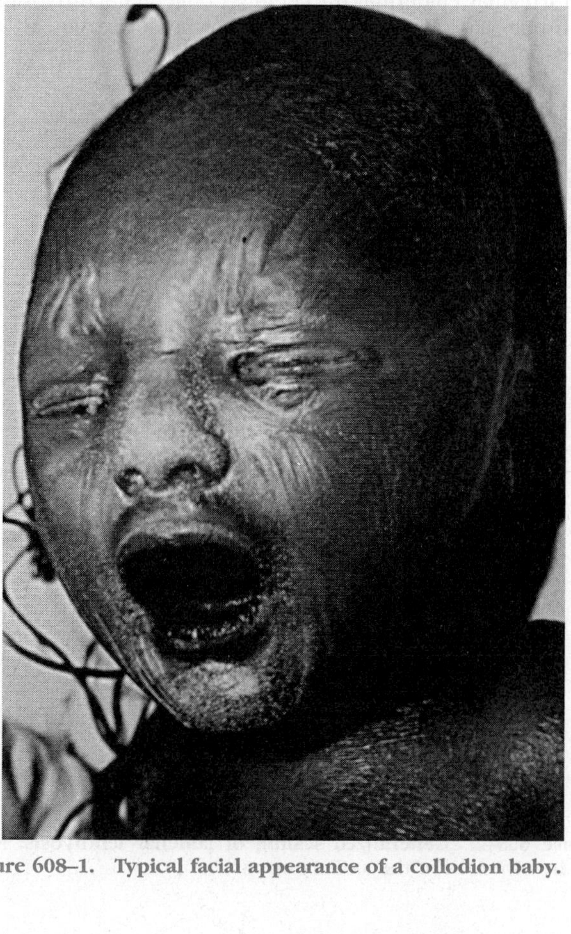

Figure 608–1. Typical facial appearance of a collodion baby.

Neonatal morbidity and deaths may be due to cutaneous infection, aspiration pneumonia (squamous material), hypothermia, or hypernatremic dehydration from excessive transcutaneous fluid losses as a result of increased skin permeability. The outcome is uncertain, and accurate prognosis is impossible with respect to the subsequent development of ichthyosis. Treatment with a high-humidity environment and application of nonocclusive lubricants may facilitate shedding of the membrane.

LAMELLAR ICHTHYOSIS AND CONGENITAL ICHTHYOSIFORM ERYTHRODERMA (NONBULLOUS CONGENITAL ICHTHYOSIFORM ERYTHRODERMA). There are two major forms of autosomal recessively inherited ichthyosis. Both forms are present soon or shortly after birth and are the most common forms of ichthyosis to present as collodion babies.

After shedding of the collodion membrane, *lamellar ichthyosis* evolves into large, quadilateral scales that are free at the edges and adherent at the center. Scaling is often pronounced and involves the entire body surface, including flexural surfaces. The face is often markedly involved, including ectropion and crumpled, small ears. The palms and soles are generally hyperkeratotic (Fig. 608–2). The hair may be sparse and fine, but the teeth and mucosal surfaces are normal. In contrast to congenital ichthyosiform erythroderma, there is little erythema.

In *congenital ichthyosiform erythroderma,* erythroderma tends to be persistent, and scales, although they are generalized, are finer and whiter than in lamellar ichthyosis. Erythema decreases in later life and may disappear in middle age, whereas scaling persists and may even worsen with age. Hyperkeratosis is particularly noticeable around the knees, elbows, and ankles. Palms and soles are uniformly hyperkeratotic. Some patients have sparse hair; cicatricial alopecia and nail dystrophy are found occasionally.

On histopathologic examination, lamellar ichthyosis is characterized by a markedly thickened stratum corneum and mild irregular epidermal thickening. Congenital ichthyosiform erythroderma has more epidermal thickening with parakeratosis but less hyperkeratosis and hypergranulosis than in lamellar ichthyosis. In congenital ichthyosisform erythroderma, there is a marked increase in the rate of epidermal cell production, considerably greater than the slightly increased rate observed in patients with lamellar ichthyosis.

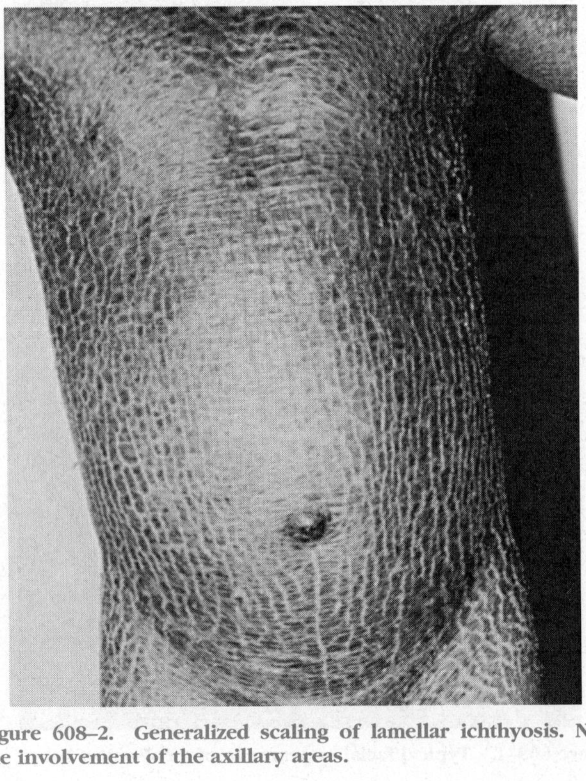

Figure 608–2. Generalized scaling of lamellar ichthyosis. Note the involvement of the axillary areas.

Pruritus may be severe and responds minimally to antipruritic therapy. The unattractive appearance of the child and the malodor from bacterial colonization of macerated scales may create serious psychologic problems. Effective *treatment* includes prolonged baths with bath oil to remove excessive scales. Restriction of bathing, on the erroneous premise that accentuation of dryness will occur, only promotes malodor and accumulation of keratinous debris and contributes to pruritus and discomfort. A high-humidity environment in winter and air conditioning in summer reduce discomfort. Generous and frequent applications of emollients and keratolytic agents such as lactic or glycolic acid (5%), urea (10–25%), and retinoic acid (0.1% cream) may lessen the scaling to some extent. Oral retinoids have a beneficial effect in these conditions but do not alter the underlying defect and, therefore, must be administered indefinitely. The long-term risks of these compounds (e.g., teratogenic effects and toxicity to bone) limit their usefulness. Ectropion requires ophthalmologic care and, at times, plastic procedures. Genetic counseling should be provided.

ICHTHYOSIS VULGARIS. This autosomal dominant ichthyosis is the most common of the disorders of keratinization, with an incidence of approximately 1 in 300 live births. Onset generally occurs sometime after birth during the 1st yr of life and, in most cases, is trivial, consisting only of slight roughening of the skin surface. Scaling is most prominent on the extensor aspects of the extremities, particularly the legs and back. Flexural surfaces are spared, and the abdomen and face are relatively uninvolved. Keratosis pilaris, particularly on the upper arms and thighs, accentuated markings and hyperkeratosis on the palms and soles, and atopy are relatively common. Scaling is most pronounced during the winter months and may abate completely during warm weather. The condition may improve and even disappear with age. There is no accompanying disorder of hair, teeth, mucosal surfaces, or other organ systems.

The histopathologic changes differ from those of other types of ichthyosis in that the hyperkeratosis is associated with a decreased or absent granular layer. Abnormally small and crumbly keratohyalin granules are found in epidermal cells on electron microscopy. The rate of epidermal proliferation is normal; rather, the hyperkeratosis is due to defective desquamation. Profilaggrin, which plays a role in desmosome dissolution, is deficient.

Scaling may be diminished by use of a bath oil and daily applications of an emollient or a lubricant containing urea, salicylic acid, or an α-hydroxy acid, such as lactic acid.

X-LINKED ICHTHYOSIS. X-linked ichthyosis often presents at birth and is largely limited to males, although female carriers may display some *clinical manifestations* of the disorder. Scaling is most pronounced on the sides of the neck, lower face, preauricular areas, anterior trunk, and the limbs, particularly the legs. The elbow and knee flexures are generally spared but may be mildly involved. The palms and soles may be slightly thickened but are also usually spared. The condition gradually worsens in severity and extent. Keratosis pilaris is not present, and there is no increased incidence of atopy. Deep corneal opacities that do not interfere with vision develop during late childhood or adolescence and are a useful marker for the disease because they may also be present in carrier females. Cryptorchidism occurs in approximately 25% of affected males, although this may reflect an association with Kallmann syndrome, which also involves a deletion on the short arm of the X-chromosome. Histologic changes include hyperkeratosis of the stratum corneum, a well-developed granular layer, and a hyperplastic epidermis.

Like ichthyosis vulgaris, the rate of epidermal proliferation is normal, and the hyperkeratosis is due to retention of corneocytes and delayed dissolution of the desmosomal disks. X-linked ichthyosis, however, involves a deficiency of steroid sulfatase, which hydrolyzes cholesterol sulfate and other sulfated steroids to cholesterol; cholesterol sulfate accumulates in the stratum corneum and plasma and may cause hyperkeratosis by inhibiting desmosomal proteolysis. Elevated cholesterol sulfate levels can be demonstrated in the serum, erythrocyte membranes, and epidermal cells and scales of affected males. Reduced enzyme activity can be detected in fibroblasts, keratinocytes, and leukocytes and, prenatally, in amniocytes or chorionic villus cells. In affected families, an affected male can be detected by restriction enzyme analysis of cultured chorionic villus cells or amniocytes or by in situ hybridization, which identifies steroid sulfatase deletions prenatally in chorionic villus cells. A placental steroid sulfatase deficiency in carrier mothers results in low urinary and serum estriol values, prolonged labor, and insensitivity of the uterus to oxytocin and prostaglandins. The gene for steroid sulfatase is located on the short arm of the X chromosome. Correction of steroid sulfatase deficiency was accomplished recently by gene transfer into tissue-cultured keratinocytes.

Hydration by bathing with bath oil and daily application of emollients and a urea-containing lubricant are usually effective *treatments.* Glycolic or lactic acid (5%) in an emollient base and propylene glycol 40–60% in water with occlusion overnight are alternative forms of therapy.

EPIDERMOLYTIC HYPERKERATOSIS (BULLOUS CONGENITAL ICHTHYOSIFORM ERYTHRODERMA). Approximately one half of cases of epidermolytic hyperkeratosis are sporadic, and the other half are autosomal dominantly inherited. The *clinical manifestations* are characterized by the onset at birth of generalized erythroderma and severe hyperkeratosis. The scales are small, hard, and verrucous; distinctive, parallel hyperkeratotic ridges develop over the joint flexures, including the axillary, popliteal, and antecubital fossae, and on the neck and hips. Although erythema becomes less prominent after infancy, the hyperkeratosis persists throughout adult life. Recurrent blistering may be widespread in the neonate and may cause diagnostic confusion with other blistering disorders. Blistering becomes accentuated at sites of trauma such as the knees, elbows, and lower limbs but is not problematic after age 7–8 yr. The palms and soles may be thickened, but the hair, nails, mucosa, and sweat glands are normal. Secondary bacterial infection is common and requires appropriate antibiotic therapy. Severely affected patients may have crumpled ears and ectropion.

The histopathologic pattern is *diagnostic* and consists of hyperkeratosis, a markedly thickened granular layer with an increased number of keratohyalin granules, clear spaces around nuclei, and indistinct cellular boundaries of cells in the upper epidermis. On electron microscopic examination, keratin intermediate filaments are clumped, and many desmosomes are attached to only one keratinocyte instead of connecting neighboring keratinocytes. Epidermolytic hyperkeratosis has been shown to be due to defects in either keratin 1 or 10. These keratins are required to form the keratin intermediate filaments in cells of the suprabasilar layers of the epidermis. Localized forms of the disease may resemble epidermal nevi (ichthyosis hystrix) or keratoderma of the palms and soles but share the distinctive histopathologic changes of epidermolytic hyperkeratosis. Prenatal diagnosis for affected families is now possible by examination of DNA extracts from chorionic villus cells or amniocytes, provided that the specific mutation in the affected parent is known.

Treatment is difficult. Morbidity is increased in the neonatal period as a result of prematurity, sepsis, and fluid and electrolyte imbalance. Bacterial colonization of macerated scales produces a distinctive malodor that can be controlled somewhat by use of an antibacterial cleanser. Keratolytic agents are often poorly tolerated. Genetic counseling should be provided.

ICHTHYOSIS LINEARIS CIRCUMFLEXA. This rare autosomal recessive disorder presents at birth or in the first few months of life with generalized erythema and scaling. The trunk and limbs have diffuse erythema and superimposed migratory, polycyclic, and serpiginous hyperkeratotic lesions, some with a distinctive double-edged margin of scale. Lichenification or hyperkeratosis tends to persist in the antecubital and popliteal fossae. The face and scalp may remain erythematous and scaling. Multiple hair shaft deformities, most notably trichorrhexis invaginata, have been described in more than one half of patients. This type of ichthyosis is characteristic of patients with the Netherton syndrome (see later). Nonspecific psoriasiform changes are found on histopathologic examination.

ERYTHROKERATODERMA VARIABILIS. This is an autosomal dominant disorder, with genetic linkage to the Rh blood group, which usually presents in the early months of life but may not become apparent until childhood or adulthood. It is characterized by sharply demarcated hyperkeratotic plaques with geographic borders that develop in areas of normal skin or within discrete erythematous patches. The areas of erythema resolve, change shape or size, or migrate. The distribution is generalized but sparse; sites of predilection are the face, buttocks, axillae, and extensor surfaces of the limbs. The palms and soles may be thickened, but hair, teeth, and nails are normal. Histopathologic changes include hyperkeratosis, papillomatosis, and irregular hyperplasia of the epidermis.

Symmetric progressive erythrokeratoderma is an autosomal dominant disorder that presents in childhood with large, fixed, geographic and symmetric fine, scaling, hyperkeratotic, erythematous plaques primarily on the extremities, buttocks, face, ankles, and wrists. Palmoplantar keratoderma is also present. The primary distinguishing feature from erythrokeratoderma variabilis is the lack of variable erythema, as seen in the latter condition. These two conditions may be manifestations of the same disorder.

ICHTHYOSIFORM DERMATOSES. Several syndromes that include ichthyosis as a constant feature have been established as rare but distinct entities.

Sjögren-Larsson Syndrome. This is an autosomal recessive inborn error of metabolism and consists of ichthyosis of the lamellar or congenital ichthyosiform erythroderma types, occasionally with onset as a collodion baby. The ichthyosis is generalized but is accentuated on the flexures and the lower abdomen. A degenerative defect of retinal pigment epithelium has been detected in 20–30% of affected individuals. Glistening dots in the foveal area are a cardinal ophthalmologic sign. Motor and speech developmental delays are usually noted before 1 yr of age, and spastic diplegia or tetraplegia, epilepsy, and mental retardation generally become evident within the first 3 yr of life. Some patients may walk with the aid of braces, but most are confined to a wheelchair. The primary defect is an abnormality of fatty alcohol oxidation as a result of a deficiency of fatty aldehyde dehydrogenase, a component of the fatty alcohol–nicotinamide adenine dinucleotide oxidoreductase enzyme complex. This deficiency can be demonstrated in cultured skin fibroblasts of affected patients and carriers and, prenatally, in cultured chorionic villus cells and amniocytes from affected fetuses.

Netherton Syndrome. This is an autosomal recessive disorder characterized by ichthyosis (usually ichthyosis linearis circumflexa but, occasionally, the lamellar or congenital ichthyosiform erythroderma types), trichorrhexis invaginata, and other hair shaft anomalies such as pili torti or trichorrhexis nodosa, and atopic diathesis (see Chapter 612). The ichthyosis is present in the first 10 days of life and may be especially marked around the eyes, mouth, and perineal area. The erythroderma often is intensified after infection. Infants may suffer from failure to thrive and marked hypernatremia. Scalp hair is sparse, short, and fractures easily; eyebrows, eyelashes, and body hair are also abnormal. The most frequent allergic manifestations are urticaria, angioedema, atopic dermatitis, and asthma. Some patients are mentally retarded. The characteristic hair abnormality is seen on electron microscopy as invagination of the distal end of the hair shaft into the proximal end.

Refsum syndrome (see Chapter 72.2). This is a multisystem disorder, which is inherited as an autosomal recessive trait and becomes symptomatic during the 2nd or 3rd decade of life. The ichthyosis may be generalized, is relatively mild, and resembles ichthyosis vulgaris. The ichthyosis may also be localized to the palms and soles. Chronic polyneuritis with progressive paralysis and ataxia, atypical retinitis pigmentosa, anosmia, deafness, bony abnormalities, and electrocardiographic changes are the most characteristic features. This condition is diagnosed by lipid analysis of the blood or skin, which shows elevated phytanic acid levels. Dietary avoidance of phytanic acid–containing green vegetables and dairy products produces clinical improvement.

Chondrodysplasia punctata (see Chapter 72.2). This includes several genetically heterogeneous disorders: *Conradi-Hunermann syndrome,* inherited as an autosomal dominant trait; *rhizomelic dwarfism,* transmitted as an autosomal recessive trait; and an *X-linked dominant* form affecting females only. Approximately 25% of patients with the recessive or dominant types have cutaneous lesions, ranging from severe, generalized erythema and scaling to mild hyperkeratosis. Rhizomelic chondrodysplasia punctata is associated with cataracts, hypertelorism, optic nerve atrophy, disproportionate shortening of the proximal extremities, severe psychomotor retardation, failure to thrive, and spasticity; most patients die during infancy. Multiple dysfunctional peroxisomal enzymes are found in patients with rhizomelic chondrodysplasia, producing defects in plasmalogen synthesis, decreased phytanic acid oxidation, and failure to process the enzyme 3-ketoacyl-coenzyme A thiolase. Patients with the X-linked dominant form have a distinctive ichthyosiform eruption at birth. Thick, yellow, tightly adherent keratinized plaques are distributed in a whorled pattern over the entire body, which may be intensely erythematous. The histologic changes include hyperkeratosis that penetrates to the depths of the hair follicles. The eruption disappears completely during the first few weeks to months of life and may be superseded by a follicular atrophoderma and patchy alopecia.

Additional features in all variants include cataracts with or without optic atrophy; an abnormal facies with saddle nose, frontal bossing, and hypertelorism; and cardiovascular and central nervous system abnormalities. The pathognomonic defect, termed chondrodysplasia punctata, is stippled epiphyses in the cartilaginous skeleton. This defect disappears by approximately age 3–4 yr.

Rud Syndrome. This consists of mental retardation, epilepsy, ichthyosis (type uncertain), and sexual infantilism. Associated defects of the skeleton, eyes, dentition, and hearing have also been reported.

A number of other rare syndromes with ichthyosis as a consistent feature include the following: ichthyosis with keratitis and deafness (KID syndrome); ichthyosis with defective hair having a banded pattern under polarized light and a low sulfur content (trichothiodystrophy), hypogonadism, and mental and growth retardation (Tay syndrome); multiple sulfatase deficiency; neutral lipid storage disease with ichthyosis (Chanarin-Dorfman syndrome); and CHILD syndrome (congenital hemidysplasia with ichthyosiform erythroderma and limb defects).

KERATODERMA OF PALMS AND SOLES (KERATOSIS PALMARIS ET PLANTARIS). Excessive hyperkeratosis of the palms and soles may occur as a manifestation of a focal or generalized congenital hereditary skin disorder or may result from such chronic skin diseases as psoriasis, eczema, pityriasis rubra pilaris, lupus erythematosus, or Reiter disease. The names of individual disorders have been based on descriptive titles, modes of inheritance, histopathologic findings, and biochemical defects.

Diffuse Hyperkeratosis of Palms and Soles (Unna-Thost syndrome, Tylosis). This is an autosomal dominant disorder that presents in the first few months of life with sharply demarcated hyperkeratotic scaling plaques over the palms and soles, without extension to the wrists. Hyperhidrosis is usually present, but hair, teeth, and nails are usually normal. Striate and punctate forms have also been described.

Epidermolytic Hyperkeratosis. This type of hyperkeratosis, which is localized to the palms and soles, is an autosomal dominant defect with clinical findings identical to those of the Unna-Thost type. There is no hyperhidrosis, however, and affected areas may blister. Histopathologic changes are characteristic.

Mal de Meleda (Keratoderma Palmoplantaris Transgrediens). This is a rare, progressive autosomal recessive condition characterized by erythema and thick scales on the palms; fingers; soles; and flexor aspects of the wrists, knees, and elbows. Hyperhidrosis, nail thickening or koilonychia, and eczema may also occur.

Mutilating Keratoderma (Vohwinkel Syndrome). This is a progressive autosomal dominant disease with honeycombed hyperkeratosis of palms and soles, sparing the arches; starfish-like and linear keratoses on the dorsum of the hands, fingers, feet, and knees; and ainhum-like constriction of the digits that sometimes leads to autoamputation. This disorder may be associated with alopecia, deafness, spastic paraplegia, and myopathy.

Papillon-Lefèvre Syndrome. This is an autosomal recessive erythematous hyperkeratosis of the palms and soles that sometimes extends to the dorsal hands and feet, elbows, and knees. This syndrome is characterized by periodontal inflammation, leading to loss of teeth by age 4–5 yr if untreated; a tendency to frequent pyogenic skin infections; nail dystrophy, including transverse nail grooves; hyperhidrosis; and ectopic calcification of the dura.

Keratoderma of palms and soles also occurs as a feature of ichthyosis and ectodermal dysplasia. *Richner-Hanhart syndrome* is an autosomal recessive palmoplantar keratoderma with corneal ulcers, progressive mental impairment, and a deficiency of tyrosine aminotransferase, which leads to tyrosinemia. *Pachyonychia congenita (Jadassohn-Lewandowski syndrome)* is transmitted as an autosomal dominant trait with variable expressivity. The nail dystrophy is the most striking feature and may be present at birth or develop early in life. The nails are thickened and tubular, projecting upward at the free edge to form a conical roof over a mass of subungual keratotic debris. Repeated paronychial inflammation may result in shedding of the nails. The feature that is seen most consistently among patients with this condition is keratoderma of the palms and soles. Associated features include follicular hyperkeratosis, especially of the elbows and knees, hyperhidrosis of the palms and soles, oral leukokeratosis, and bullae and erosions on the palms and soles. Some patients have shown a selective cell-mediated defect in recognition and processing of *Candida.* Surgical removal of the nails and excision of the nail matrix have been helpful in some patients.

Patients with palmoplantar hyperhidrosis may have macerated plaques that become secondarily infected and malodorous. Morbidity is lessened if the hyperkeratosis can be controlled by *treatment*; however, only mild palliation is achieved with applications of lubricants, keratolytic agents (urea, salicylic acid, lactic acid), and retinoic acid. Etretinate or excision and split-skin grafting have been successful in patients with extreme hyperkeratosis and painful fissuring.

Bale SJ, Doyle SZ: The genetics of ichthyosis: A primer for epidemiologists. J Invest Dermatol 102:495, 1994.
DiGiovanna JJ, Bale SJ: Epidermolytic hyperkeratosis: Applied molecular genetics. J Invest Dermatol 102:390, 1994.
Jackson SM, Williams ML, Feingold KR, et al: Pathobiology of the stratum corneum. West J Med 158:279, 1993.

Kousseff BG: Collodion baby, sign of Tay syndrome. Pediatrics 87:571, 1991.
Lavrijsen AP, Oestmann E, Hermans J, et al: Barrier function parameters in various keratinization disorders: Transepidermal water loss and vascular response to hexyl nicotinate. Br J Dermatol 129:547, 1993.
Paller AS: Laboratory tests for ichthyosis. Dermatol Clin 12:99, 1994.
Proksch E, Holleran WM, Menon GK, et al: Barrier function regulates epidermal lipid and DNA synthesis. Br J Dermatol 128:473, 1993.
Rabinowitz LG, Esterly NB: Atopic dermatitis and ichthyosis vulgaris. Pediatr Rev 15:220, 1994.
Rand RE, Baden HP: The ichthyoses—a review. J Am Acad Dermatol 8:285, 1983.
Rizzo WB: Sjögren-Larsson syndrome. Semin Dermatol 12:210, 1993.
Rizzo WB, Dammaum AL, Craft DA, et al: Sjögren-Larsson syndrome: inherited defect in the fatty alcohol cycle. J Pediatr 115:228, 1989.
Williams ML: Ichthyosis: Mechanisms of disease. Pediatr Dermatol 9:365, 1992.
Williams ML, Elias PM: From basket weave to barrier. Unifying concepts for the pathogenesis of the diseases of cornification. Arch Dermatol 129:626, 1993.

CHAPTER 609
Diseases of the Dermis

Gary L. Darmstadt and Al Lane

KELOID. A keloid is a sharply demarcated, benign, dense growth of connective tissue that forms in the dermis after trauma. The lesions are firm, raised, pink, and rubbery; they may be tender or pruritic. Sites of predilection are the face, earlobes, neck, shoulders, upper trunk, sternum, and lower legs. Keloids are usually induced by trauma and commonly follow ear piercing, burns, scalds, and surgical procedures. Certain individuals, especially blacks, seem predisposed to keloid formation. In some cases, a familial tendency (recessive or dominant inheritance) or the presence of foreign material in the wound appear to play a pathogenic role. Keloids are a rare feature of Ehlers-Danlos syndrome, Rubinstein-Taybi syndrome, and pachydermoperiostosis. In both keloids and hypertophic scars, new collagen forms over a much longer period than in wounds that heal normally. Histopathologically, a keloid consists of whorled and interlaced hyalinized collagen fibers.

Keloids should be differentiated from hypertrophic scars, which remain confined to the site of injury and gradually involute over time. Young keloids may diminish in size if injected intralesionally at 4-wk intervals with triamcinolone suspension (10 mg/mL). At times, a more concentrated suspension is required. Large or old keloids may require surgical excision followed by intralesional injections of corticosteroid. The risk of recurrence at the same site argues against surgical excision alone. Placement of topical silicon gel sheeting over the keloid for several hours per day for several weeks may help some patients.

STRIAE CUTIS DISTENSAE. These thinned, depressed, erythematous bands of atrophic skin eventually become silvery, opalescent, and smooth. They occur most frequently in areas that have been subject to distention, such as the lower back, buttocks, thighs, breasts, abdomen, and shoulders. The most frequent causes are rapid growth, pregnancy, obesity, Cushing disease, or prolonged corticosteroid therapy. Adolescent striae tend to become less conspicuous with time. Histopathologically, striae distensae resemble scars.

GRANULOMA ANNULARE. This is a common dermatosis that occurs predominantly in children and young adults. Typical lesions begin as erythematous, firm, smooth papules; they gradually enlarge to form annular plaques with a papular border and a normal, slightly atrophic or discolored central area (Fig. 609–1) up to several centimeters in size. Lesions may occur anywhere on the body, but mucous membranes are spared. Favored sites include the dorsum of the hands and feet. *Annular lesions* are often mistaken for tinea corporis because of the elevated advancing border; they differ in that they are not scaly. *Papular lesions,* another variant, may simulate rheumatoid nodules, particularly when grouped on the fingers and elbows. The disseminated papular form, which is provoked by light in some cases, is rare in children. *Subcutaneous granuloma annulare* is especially common in children; it tends to develop on the scalp and limbs, particularly in the pretibial area. These lesions are firm, usually nontender, skin-colored nodules. *Perforating granuloma annulare* is characterized by the development of a yellowish center in some of the superficial papular lesions as a result of transepidermal elimination of altered collagen.

A biopsy is occasionally required for diagnosis. The lesions consist of a granuloma with a central area of necrotic collagen; mucin deposition; and a peripheral palisading infiltrate of lymphocytes, histiocytes, and foreign body giant cells. The pattern resembles that of necrobiosis lipoidica and rheumatoid nodule (see Chapter 148), but subtle histologic differences usually permit differentiation. The cause of granuloma annulare is unknown. Affected children are usually healthy. Some cases of granuloma annulare, particularly the generalized form, may be associated with diabetes mellitus. The eruption persists for months to years, but spontaneous resolution without residual change is usual; 75% of lesions clear within 2 yr. Application of a potent topical corticosteroid preparation or intralesional injections of corticosteroid may hasten involution, but nonintervention is acceptable.

NECROBIOSIS LIPOIDICA. This rare disorder presents as erythematous papules that evolve into irregularly shaped, sharply demarcated, yellow, sclerotic plaques with central telangiectasia and a violaceous border. Scaling, crusting, and ulceration are frequent. Lesions develop most commonly on the shins. Slow extension of a given lesion over the years is usual, but long periods of quiescence or complete healing with scarring may occur.

Histopathologically, poorly defined areas of necrobiotic collagen are seen throughout, but primarily low in the dermis, associated with mucin deposition. Surrounding the necrobiotic, disordered areas of collagen is a palisading lymphohistiocytic granulomatous infiltrate. Some lesions are more characterisically granulomatous, with limited necrobiosis of collagen. Necrobiosis lipoidica must be differentiated clinically from xan-

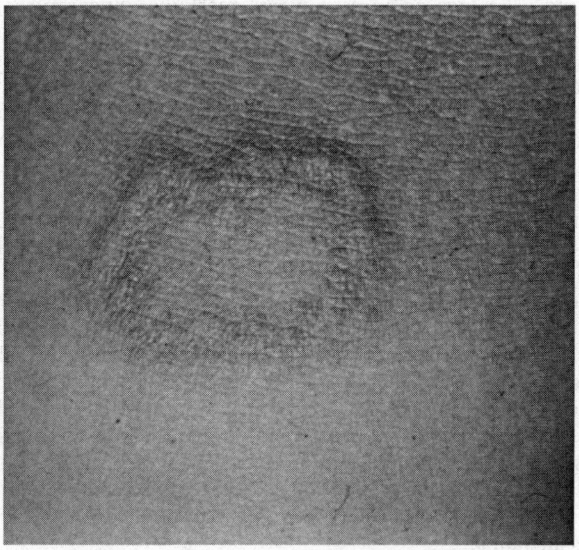

Figure 609–1. Annular lesion with a raised papular border and depressed center, characteristic of granuloma annulare.

thomas, morphea, granuloma annulare, and pretibial myxedema. Fifty to 75% of patients have diabetes mellitus; necrobiosis lipoidica occurs in 0.3% of all diabetic patients. The lesions persist despite good control of the diabetes but may improve minimally after applications of high-potency topical steroids or local injection of a corticosteroid.

LICHEN SCLEROSUS ET ATROPHICUS. This presents initially with ivory-colored, shiny, indurated papules, often with a violaceous halo. The surface shows prominent dilated pilosebaceous or sweat duct orifices that often contain yellow or brown horny plugs. The papules coalesce to form irregular plaques of variable size, which may develop hemorrhagic bullae in their margins. In the latter stages, atrophy results in a depressed plaque with a wrinkled surface. This disorder occurs more commonly in girls than boys. Sites of predilection in girls are the vulvar, perianal, and perineal skin. Extensive involvement may produce a sclerotic, atrophic plaque of hourglass configuration; shrinkage of the labia and stenosis of the introitus may result. Vaginal discharge precedes vulvar lesions in approximately 20% of patients. In boys, the prepuce and glans penis are often involved, usually in association with phimosis; most boys with the disorder were not circumcised early in life. Sites elsewhere on the body that are most commonly involved include the upper trunk, the neck, in the axillae, on the flexor wrists, and around the umbilicus and the eyes. Pruritus may be severe.

In children, this disorder is most frequently confused with focal scleroderma (morphea) (see Chapter 154), with which it may coexist. In the genital area, it may be mistakenly attributed to sexual abuse. Biopsy is diagnostic, revealing hyperkeratosis with follicular plugging, hydropic degeneration of basal cells, a bandlike dermal lymphocytic infiltrate, homogenized collagen, and thinned elastic fibers in the upper dermis. The lesions may involute spontaneously, usually before or at the time of menarche; involution is more likely to occur in those in whom the disorder developed at a younger age. Leukoplakia and squamous cell carcinoma may rarely develop. Potent topical corticosteroids may provide relief from pruritus, and produce clearing of lesions, including those in the genital area. Topical progesterone 1% and testosterone 2% preparations have also been used for genital lesions.

SCLEREDEMA (SCLEREDEMA ADULTORUM, SCLEREDEMA OF BUSCHKE). Approximately 30% of cases of scleredema develop before the age of 10 yr. Onset is sudden, with brawny edema of the face and neck that spreads rapidly to involve the thorax and arms in a "sweater" distribution; the abdomen and legs are usually spared. The face acquires a waxy, masklike appearance; the involved areas feel indurated and woody, are nonpitting, and are not sharply demarcated from normal skin. The overlying skin is normal in color and is not atrophic. Systemic involvement, which is uncommon, is marked by thickening of the tongue; dysarthria; dysphagia; restriction of eye and joint movements; and pleural, pericardial, and peritoneal effusions. Electrocardiographic changes may also be observed.

In 65–90% of cases, the disease follows an infection such as tonsillitis, pharyngitis, influenza, scarlet fever, measles, mumps, impetigo, or cellulitis after an interval of days or weeks; most cases follow a streptococcal infection. Onset may be heralded by a prodrome of fever, arthralgia, myalgia, and malaise. Onset in diabetic patients may occur insidiously. Laboratory data are not helpful. Some cases, however, are associated with immunoglobulin (Ig)G or IgA paraproteinemia. Skin biopsy demonstrates an increase in dermal thickness as a result of swelling and homogenization of the collagen bundles, which are separated by large interfibrous spaces. Increased amounts of mucopolysaccharides in the dermis can be identified by special stains.

The active phase of the disease persists for 2–8 wk; spontaneous and complete resolution usually occurs in 6 mo to 2 yr. Recurrent attacks are unusual. The disorder must be differentiated from scleroderma, morphea, myxedema, trichinosis, dermatomyositis, sclerema neonatorum, and subcutaneous fat necrosis. There is no specific therapy.

LIPOID PROTEINOSIS (URBACH-WIETHE DISEASE). This autosomal recessive disorder consists of infiltration of hyaline material into skin, oral cavity, larynx, and internal organs. It may be noted initially in early infancy as hoarseness. Skin lesions appear during childhood and consist of yellowish papules and nodules that may coalesce to form plaques on the face, forearms, neck, genitalia, dorsum of the fingers, and scalp, where they result in patchy alopecia. Similar deposits are found on the lips, undersurface of the tongue, fauces, uvula, epiglottis, and vocal cords. The tongue becomes enlarged and feels firm on palpation; the patient may be unable to protrude the tongue. Translucent nodules along the margins of the eyelids, causing thickening of the eyelids, are the most characteristic clinical manifestation. Hypertrophic, hyperkeratotic nodules occur at sites of friction such as the elbows and knees; the palms may be diffusely thickened. The disease progresses until early adult life, but the prognosis is good. Involvement of the larynx can lead to respiratory compromise, particularly in infancy, necessitating tracheostomy. Associated anomalies include dental abnormalities, epilepsy, and recurrent parotitis as a result of infiltrates in the Stensen duct; virtually any organ can be involved. There is no specific treatment.

The distinctive histologic pattern includes dilatation of dermal blood vessels and infiltration of homogeneous eosinophilic extracellular hyaline material along capillary walls and around sweat glands. Hyaline material in homogeneous bundles, diffusely arranged in the upper dermis, produces a thickened dermis. The infiltrates appear to contain both lipid and mucopolysaccharide substances. Symmetric ossification lateral to the sella turcica in the medial temporal region, identifiable roentgenographically, is pathognomonic but is not always present. The biochemical defect is unknown but may represent a lysosomal storage disorder caused by single or multiple enzyme defects. Alterations in the distribution of collagens I, III, IV, and V have also been described.

MACULAR ATROPHY (ANETODERMA). Anetoderma is characterized by circumscribed areas of slack skin associated with loss of dermal substance. This disorder may have no associated underlying disease (primary macular atrophy) or may develop after an inflammatory skin condition (secondary macular atrophy) such as syphilis, lupus erythematosus, acne, varicella, leprosy, urticaria pigmentosa, or *Staphylococcus epidermidis* folliculitis. Lesions vary from 0.5–1 cm in diameter and, if inflammatory, may initially be erythematous. Subsequently, they become thin, wrinkled, and blue-white or hypopigmented. The lesions often protrude as small outpouchings that, on palpation, may be readily indented into the subcutaneous tissue because of the dermal atrophy. Sites of predilection include the trunk, thighs, upper arms, and less commonly the neck and face. Lesions remain unchanged for life; new lesions often continue to develop for years. There is no effective therapy, although some authors have reported benefit from penicillin or pentoxifylline.

All types of macular atrophy show focal loss of elastic tissue on histopathologic examination, a change that is not recognizable unless special stains are used. The elastolysis may be due to release of elastase from inflammatory cells, such as macrophages, in contact with elastic fibers. Lesions of anetoderma occasionally resemble morphea, lichen sclerosus et atrophicus, focal dermal hypoplasia, atrophic scars, or end-stage lesions of chronic bullous dermatoses.

CUTIS LAXA (DERMATOMEGALY, GENERALIZED ELASTOLYSIS). Cutis laxa is a congenital, autosomal recessive or autosomal dominant disorder. A newborn infant may appear prematurely aged. When onset appears to occur during childhood or adulthood, the disorder is termed *acquired cutis laxa.* Cutis laxa has developed after a febrile illness, inflammatory skin diseases such as lupus erythematosus or erythema multiforme, amyloidosis, urticaria, angioedema, hypersensitivity reactions to penicillin, and in infants born to women who were taking penicillamine.

Clinical Manifestations. There may be widespread folds of lax skin, or changes may be mild and limited in extent, resembling anetoderma. Patients with severe cutis laxa have characteristic facial features, including an aged appearance with sagging jowls ("bloodhound" appearance), a hooked nose with everted nostrils, a short columella, a long upper lip, and everted lower eyelids. The skin is also lax elsewhere on the body and may resemble an ill-fitting suit (Fig. 609–2). Hyperelasticity and hypermobility of the joints are not present as they are in the Ehlers-Danlos syndrome. Many infants have a hoarse cry, probably as a result of laxity of the vocal cords. Tensile strength of the skin is normal. Histologically, elastic tissue is reduced throughout the dermis, with fragmentation, distention, and clumping of the elastic fibers.

The dominant form of cutis laxa may develop at any age and is generally benign and mainly of cosmetic significance. When it presents in infancy, it may be associated with intrauterine growth retardation, ligamentous laxity, and delayed closure of fontanels. Affected males may be impotent, have infantile genitalia, and scanty body hair. Pulmonary emphysema and mild cardiovascular manifestations may also occur. In contrast, those with the more common recessive form of the disease are susceptible to severe complications, such as multiple hernias, rectal prolapse, diaphragmatic atony, diverticula of the gastrointestinal and genitourinary tracts, cor pulmonale, emphysema, pneumothoraces, peripheral pulmonary artery stenosis, and aortic dilatation. Characteristic facial features include downward slanting palpebral fissures; a broad, flat nose; and large ears. Skeletal anomalies, dental caries, growth retardation, and developmental delay also occur. Such patients often have a shortened life span.

The *pathogenesis* of cutis laxa is not well known. Abnormalities that have been described include excessive enzymatic destruction of elastin, decreased elastase inhibitor levels, and decreased elastin messenger RNA levels in fibroblasts.

EHLERS-DANLOS SYNDROME. This is a group of genetically heterogeneous connective tissue disorders. Affected children appear normal at birth, but skin hyperelasticity, fragility of the skin and blood vessels, and joint hypermobility develop. The essential defect is a quantitative deficiency of collagen. Ehlers-Danlos syndrome has been classified into 10 clinical forms.

I. Gravis Type. This autosomal dominant disorder is characterized by premature birth caused by rupture of membranes, skin hyperelasticity and fragility, easy bruising, generalized and severe joint hypermobility, scoliosis, and mitral valve prolapse. Insignificant lacerations may form gaping wounds that leave broad, atrophic, papyraceous scars. Additional cutaneous manifestations include molluscoid pseudotumors over pressure points from accumulations of connective tissue. Life expectancy is not reduced.

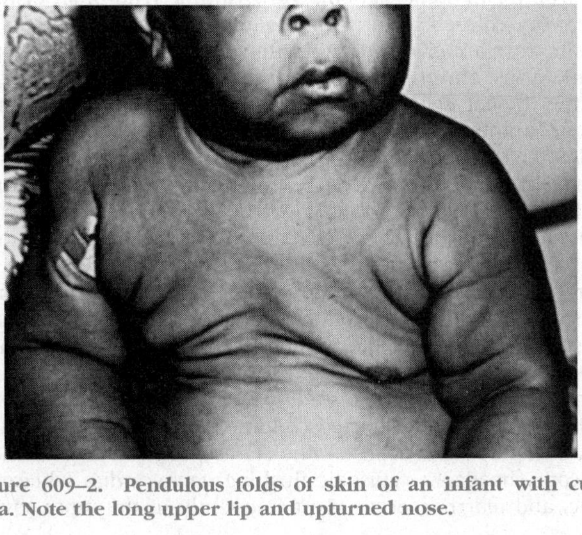

Figure 609–2. Pendulous folds of skin of an infant with cutis laxa. Note the long upper lip and upturned nose.

II. Mitis Type. This autosomal dominant form is characterized by mild skin and joint manifestations, the latter limited to hands and feet. The incidence of premature birth is not increased.

III. Benign, Hypermobile Type. This disorder has autosomal dominant inheritance and manifests as generalized severe joint hypermobility and minimal skin manifestations. Osteoarthritis may develop prematurely.

IV. Ecchymotic (Sack) Type. This form may have autosomal dominant or autosomal recessive inheritance and shows the most pronounced dermal thinning of all; consequently, the underlying venous network is prominent. The skin has minimal hyperextensibility and the joints are not hypermobile, except perhaps during childhood. Premature birth; extensive ecchymoses from trauma; a high incidence of keloids; rupture of the bowel, especially the colon; uterine rupture during pregnancy; rupture of the great vessels; dissecting aortic aneurysm; and stroke all contribute to the increased morbidity and shortened lifespan. Patients should be advised to avoid becoming pregnant, avoid activities such as trumpet playing that raise intracranial pressure as a result of a Valsalva maneuver, and minimize trauma to the skin. Defects that have been identified in affected patients include multiple deletions, exon skipping, or point mutations in the *COL3A1* gene of collagen III.

V. X-Linked Type. This is characterized by minimal joint hypermobility and skin hyperelasticity and moderate bruising, skin fragility, and scarring. The lifespan is normal. Lysyl oxidase was deficient in one family with this disorder.

VI. Autosomal Recessive Ocular Type. These patients have joint hyperextensibility, hypotonia, kyphoscoliosis, fragile cornea, keratoconus, skin hyperelasticity, and fragile bones. There is a mutation affecting a collagen structural protein. Patients lack lysyl hydroxylase, a crucial enzyme in collagen biosynthesis that catalyzes the formation of hydroxylysine, which cross-links collagen. Prenatal diagnosis is available by measuring lysyl hydroxylase activity in amniocytes. The diagnosis can also be confirmed by detecting decreased lysyl hydroxylase activity in cultured dermal fibroblasts. This form may respond to oral ascorbic acid.

VII. Arthrochalasis Multiplex Congenita. The A type is an autosomal recessive disorder characterized by short stature, marked joint hyperextensibility and dislocation, and moderate hyperelasticity and bruisability of skin. The defect is a failure of cleavage of the aminoterminal propeptide of type I procollagen chains by procollagen N-proteinase caused by a mutation in the *COL1A1* gene that results in loss of the procollagen N-proteinase cleavage site. The B type, possibly autosomal dominant, is characterized by skin hyperelasticity and marked joint hypermobility. Mutations in the *COL1A2* gene cause loss of the N-proteinase cleavage site in the pro-α_2 (I) collagen chain. The type C disorder, known as dermatosparaxis, includes premature rupture of membranes, delayed closure of fontanels; skin fragility and laxity; easy bruisability; growth retardation; short limbs; umbilical hernia; and characteristic facies with micrognathia, jowls, and prominent, puffy eyelids. This disorder is due to a lack of N-proteinase activity.

VIII. Periodontitis Type. This autosomal dominant disorder has mild skin hyperelasticity, small joint hypermobility, bruisability, moderate cutaneous fragility, abnormal scarring, and severe periodontitis, leading to premature loss of teeth and alveolar bone. The proportion of type III collagen is reduced.

IX. X-Linked Recessive Skeletal Type. This form is characterized by occipital exostoses; widening and bowing of long bones at tendinous and ligamentous insertion sites; short, broad clavicles; mild skin hyperelasticity; bladder diverticula with spontaneous rupture; inguinal hernias; and chronic diarrhea. Defective copper transport results in low serum copper and ceruloplasm levels and diminished lysyl oxidase activity, an important copper-dependent enzyme required for collagen cross-linking. Menke's disease and X-linked cutis laxa also have altered copper metabolism and defective collagen fibril formation; these may be examples of type IX Ehlers-Danlos syndrome.

X. Dysfibronectinemic Type. This autosomal recessive disorder is characterized by fibronectin-correctable failure of platelet aggregation, easy bruisability, joint hypermobility, and skin hyperextensibility.

Differential Diagnosis. Ehlers-Danlos syndrome has been confused with cutis laxa, but the features of the two disorders differ considerably. The skin of patients with cutis laxa hangs in redundant folds, whereas the skin in Ehlers-Danlos syndrome is hyperextensible and snaps back into place when stretched. Because of the marked skin fragility in Ehlers-Danlos syndrome, minor trauma results in ecchymoses, bleeding, and poor healing with atrophic cigarette-paper scars, which are most prominent on the forehead, lower legs, and over pressure points. Surgical procedures are fraught with risk; dehiscence of wounds is common.

PSEUDOXANTHOMA ELASTICUM. This is a disorder of elastic tissue that primarily affects the dermis, retina, and cardiovascular system.

Clinical Manifestations. Onset of skin manifestations often occurs during childhood, but the changes produced by early lesions are subtle and may not be recognized. The characteristic pebbly "plucked chicken skin" cutaneous lesions are asymptomatic, 1–2-mm yellow papules that are arranged in a linear or reticulated pattern or in confluent plaques. Preferred sites are the flexural neck, axillary and inguinal folds, umbilicus, thighs, and antecubital and popliteal fossae. As the lesions become more pronounced, the skin acquires a velvety texture and droops in lax, inelastic folds. The face is usually spared. Mucous membrane lesions may involve the lips, buccal cavity, rectum, and vagina. Involvement of the connective tissue of the media and intima of blood vessels, Bruch membrane of the eye, and endocardium or pericardium may result in visual disturbances; angioid streaks in Bruch membrane; intermittent claudication; cerebral and coronary occlusion; hypertension; and hemorrhage from the gastrointestinal tract, uterus, or mucosal surfaces. Affected women have an increased risk of miscarriage in the first trimester. Arterial involvement generally presents in adulthood, but claudication and angina have occurred in early childhood. There is no effective *treatment*, although laser therapy may help to prevent retinal hemorrhage.

Pathology and Pathogenesis. Histopathologic examination shows fragmented, swollen, and clumped elastic fibers in the middle and lower third of the dermis. The fibers stain positively for calcium. Collagen in the vicinity of the altered elastic fibers is reduced in amount and is split into small fibers. Aberrant calcification of the elastic fibers of the internal elastic lamina of arteries leads to narrowing of vessel lumina. It is hypothesized that an abnormal glycosaminoglycan is secreted by fibroblasts and deposited on the surface of elastic fibers, leading to fragmentation and calcification of the coated fibers. Candidate genes for pseudoxanthoma elasticum include the genes encoding elastin; the fibrillins, which form a microfibrillar coating around elastin; and lysyl oxidase, which catalyzes formation of the desmosines, the covalent interchain cross-links that stabilize elastin polypeptides into its fibrillar structure. There are two autosomal dominant and two autosomal recessive forms of the disease. However, all affected patients tend to merge into a single classic phenotype involving the skin, eyes, and cardiovascular system, with considerable variability in expression of the disorder, particularly in the vascular and ophthalmologic complications.

ELASTOSIS PERFORANS SERPIGINOSA. This is an unusual skin disorder in which 1–3-mm, skin-colored, keratotic, firm papules tend to cluster in arcuate and annular patterns on the posterolateral neck and limbs and, occasionally, on the face and trunk. Onset usually occurs during childhood or adolescence. Histopathologically, a papule consists of a circumscribed area of epidermal hyperplasia that communicates with the underlying dermis by a narrow channel. Elastotic material is extruded from the channel. There is a great increase in the amount and size of elastic fibers in the upper dermis, particularly in the dermal papillae. The primary abnormality is probably in the dermal elastin, which provokes a cellular response that ultimately leads to the extrusion of the abnormal elastic tissue. Approximately one third of cases occur in association with osteogenesis imperfecta, Marfan syndrome, pseudoxanthoma elasticum, Ehlers-Danlos syndrome, Rothmund-Thomson syndrome, and Down syndrome. It has also occurred in association with penicillamine therapy. Differential diagnosis includes tinea corporis, perforating granuloma annulare, reactive perforating collagenosis, lichen planus, creeping eruption, and porokeratosis of Mibelli. Treatment is ineffective; however, the lesions are asymptomatic and disappear spontaneously.

REACTIVE PERFORATING COLLAGENOSIS. This usually presents in early childhood with small papules on the dorsal hands and forearms, elbows, knees, and sometimes face and trunk. The condition is often familial and may be inherited in an autosomal recessive pattern. Over a period of several weeks, the papules increase in size to 5–10 mm, become umbilicated, and develop a keratotic plug in the center. Individual lesions resolve spontaneously in 2–4 mo, leaving a hypopigmented macule or scar. Lesions may recur in crops; may undergo a linear Köbner reaction; and may form in response to cold temperatures or superficial trauma such as abrasions, insect bites, and acne lesions. Histopathologically, collagen in the papillary dermis is engulfed within a cup-shaped perforation in the epidermis. The central crater contains pyknotic inflammatory cells and keratinous debris. The process appears to represent transepidermal elimination of altered collagen. Topical retinoic acid may reduce the number of lesions.

XANTHOMAS. See Chapter 72.4.

FABRY DISEASE. See Chapter 72.3.

MUCOPOLYSACCHARIDOSES. See Chapter 71.13. In several of these disorders, thick, inelastic, rough skin, particularly on the extremities, and generalized hirsutism are characteristic but nonspecific features. Telangiectasias on the face, forearms, trunk, and legs have been observed in the Scheie and Morquio syndromes. In some patients with Hunter syndrome, distinctive ivory-colored, firm papulonodules with a corrugated surface texture are grouped into symmetric plaques on the upper trunk, arms, and thighs. Onset of these unusual lesions occurs during the 1st decade of life, and spontaneous disappearance has been noted.

MASTOCYTOSIS. Mastocytosis encompasses a spectrum of disorders that range from solitary cutaneous nodules to diffuse infiltration of skin associated with involvement of other organs. All the disorders are characterized by aggregates of mast cells in the dermis. Mast cell growth factor, which can be secreted by keratinocytes, stimulates the proliferation of mast cells and increases the production of melanin by melanocytes. Mastocytosis may be due to altered cutaneous metabolism of mast cell growth factor and, thus, may represent a hyperplastic rather than a neoplastic disorder.

Clinical Manifestations. Affected children can have intense pruritus. Systemic signs of histamine release, such as hypotension, syncope, headache, episodic flushing, tachycardia, wheezing, colic, and diarrhea occur most frequently in the more severe types of mastocytosis. The local and systemic manifestations of the disease are due, at least partially, to release of histamine and heparin from mast cell granules; although heparin is present in significant amounts in mast cells, coagulation disturbances occur only rarely. The vasodilator prostaglandin D_2, or its metabolite, appears to exacerbate the flushing response.

Mastocytomas are solitary lesions 1–5 cm in diameter. Lesions may be present at birth or arise during early infancy at any site; the wrist, neck, and trunk are sites of predilection. The lesions may present as recurrent, evanescent wheals or bullae; in time, however, an infiltrated, rubbery, pink, yellow, or tan plaque develops at the site of whealing or blistering (Fig. 609–3*A*). The surface acquires a pebbly, orange peel–like texture, and hyperpigmentation may become prominent. Stroking or trauma to the nodule may result in urtication (Darier sign) as a result of local histamine release; rarely, systemic signs of histamine release become apparent. The differential diagnosis includes recurrent bullous impetigo, nevi, and juvenile xanthogranuloma. Mastocytomas usually involute spontaneously during early childhood; troublesome lesions can be excised and do not recur. Only rarely do multiple cutaneous lesions develop.

Urticaria pigmentosa is the most common form of mastocytosis and occurs primarily in infants and children. Lesions may be present at birth but more often erupt in crops during the first several months to 2 yr of age. In some cases, early bullous or urticarial lesions fade, only to recur at the same site, ultimately becoming fixed and hyperpigmented; in others, the initial lesions are hyperpigmented. Vesiculation usually abates by 2 yr of age. Individual lesions range in size from a few millimeters to several centimeters and may be macular, papular, or nodular; they range in color from yellow-tan to chocolate brown and often have ill-defined borders (Fig. 609–3*B*). Larger nodular lesions, like mastocytomas, may have a characteristic orange peel texture (Fig. 609–3*C*). Lesions of urticaria pigmentosa may be sparse or numerous and are often symmetrically distributed. Palms, soles, and face are sometimes spared, as are the mucous membranes. The rapid appearance of erythema and whealing in response to vigorous stroking of a lesion can usually be elicited; dermographism of intervening normal skin is also common. Urticaria pigmentosa can be confused with drug eruptions, postinflammatory pigmentary change, juvenile xanthogranuloma, pigmented nevi, ephelides, xanthomas, chronic urticaria, insect bites, and bullous impetigo.

Prognosis. This is good; spontaneous involution occurs in about 50% of patients by puberty; another 25% have partial resolution by adulthood. The incidence of systemic manifestations is very low.

Diffuse Cutaneous Mastocytosis. This varient is characterized by dif-

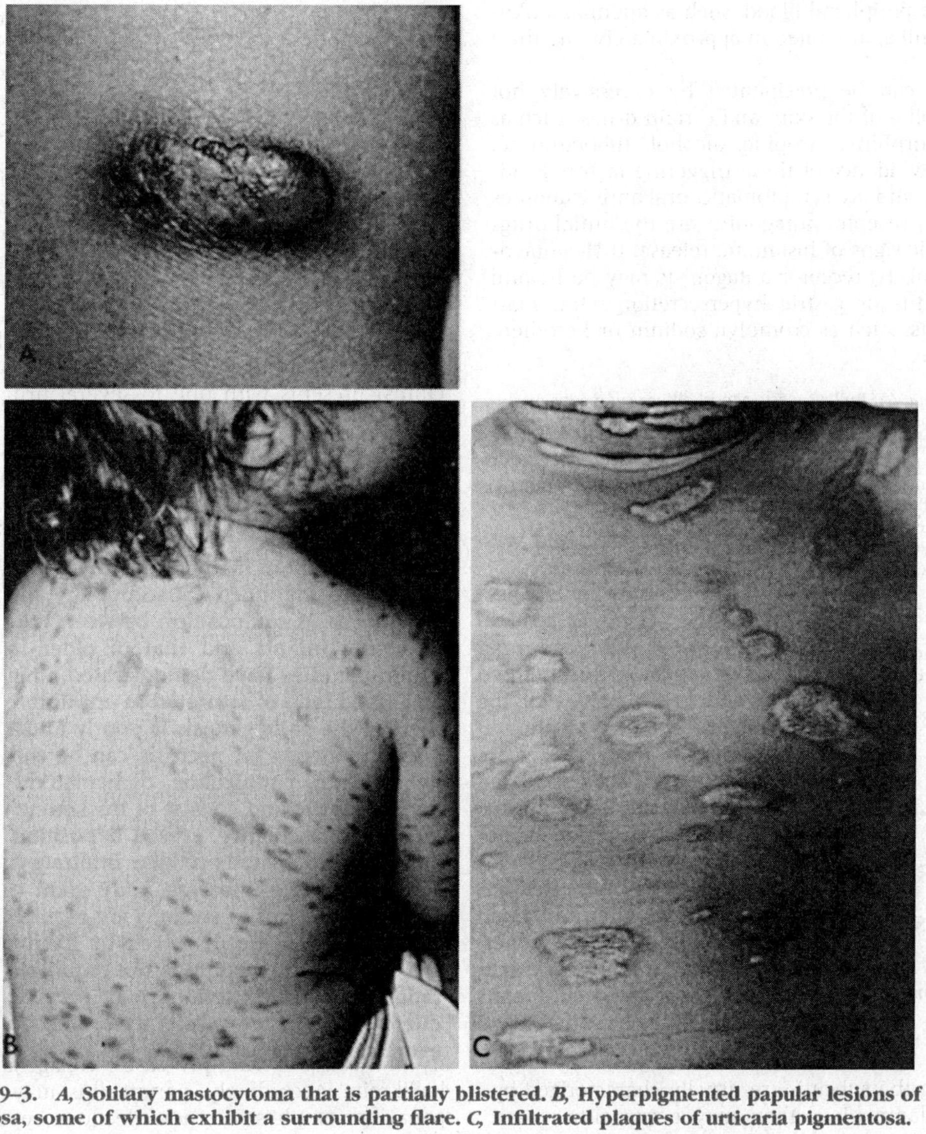

Figure 609–3. ***A,* Solitary mastocytoma that is partially blistered. *B,* Hyperpigmented papular lesions of urticaria pigmentosa, some of which exhibit a surrounding flare. *C,* Infiltrated plaques of urticaria pigmentosa.**

fuse involvement of the skin rather than discrete hyperpigmented lesions. Affected patients are usually normal at birth and develop features of the disorder after the first few months of life. Rarely, the condition may present with intense generalized pruritus in the absence of visible skin changes. The skin usually appears thickened and pink to yellow and may have a doughy feel and a texture resembling an orange peel. Surface changes are accentuated in flexural areas. Recurrent bullae, intractable pruritus, and flushing attacks are common, as is systemic involvement.

Telangiectasia macularis eruptiva perstans is another variant that consists of telangiectatic hyperpigmented macules that are usually localized to the trunk. These lesions do not urticate when stroked. This form of the disease is seen in adolescents and adults primarily.

Systemic Mastocytosis. In this disorder, there is an abnormal increase in the number of mast cells in other than cutaneous tissues. It occurs in approximately 5–10% of patients with mastocytosis and is more common in adults than in children. Bone lesions may be silent but are detectable radiologically as osteoporotic or osteosclerotic areas, principally in the axial skeleton. Gastrointestinal tract involvement may produce diarrhea and steatorrhea. Mucosal infiltrates may be detectable by barium studies or by small bowel biopsy. Peptic ulcers also occur. Hepatosplenomegaly as a result of mast cell infiltrates and fibrosis has been described, as has mast cell proliferation in lymph nodes, kidneys, periadrenal fat, and bone marrow. Abnormalities in the peripheral blood, such as anemia, leukocytosis, and eosinophilia, are noted in approximately one third of patients.

Treatment. Flushing can be precipitated by excessively hot baths, vigorous rubbing of the skin, and certain drugs, such as codeine, aspirin, morphine, atropine, alcohol, tubocurarine, and polymyxin B. Avoidance of these triggering factors is advisable. For patients who are symptomatic, oral antihistamines may be palliative. H_1 receptor antagonists are the initial drugs of choice for systemic signs of histamine release. If H_1 antagonists are unsuccessful, H_2 receptor antagonists may be helpful in controlling pruritus or gastric hypersecretion. Oral mast cell–stabilizing agents, such as cromolyn sodium or ketotifen, may also be effective.

Golitz LE, Weston WL, Lane AT: Bullous mastocytosis: diffuse cutaneous mastocytosis with extensive blisters mimicking scalded skin syndrome or erythema multiforme. Pediatr Dermatol 1:288, 1984.
Hacker SM, Ramos-Caro FA, Beers BB, et al: Juvenile pseudoxanthoma elasticum: recognition and management. Pediatr Dermatol 10:19, 1993.
Helm KF, Gibson LE, Muller SA: Lichen sclerosus et atrophicus in children and young adults. Pediatr Dermatol 8:97, 1991.
Lebwohl M, Neldner K, Pope M, et al: Classification of pseudoxanthoma elasticum: Report of a consensus conference. J Am Acad Dermatol 30:103, 1994.
Lucky AW, Prose NS, Bove K, et al: Papular umbilicated granuloma annulare. A report of four pediatric cases. Arch Dermatol 128:1375, 1992.
Mulbauer JE: Granuloma annulare. J Am Acad Dermatol 3:217, 1980.
Murray JC: Keloids and hypertrophic scars. Clin Dermatol 12:27, 1994.
Tilstra DJ, Byers PH: Molecular basis of hereditary disorders of connective tissue. Annu Rev Med 45:149, 1994.
Yeowell HN, Pinnell SR: The Ehlers-Danlos syndromes. Semin Dermatol 12:229, 1993.

CHAPTER 610
Diseases of Subcutaneous Tissue

Gary L. Darmstadt and Al Lane

Diseases involving the subcutis are usually characterized by necrosis and/or inflammation; they may occur either as a primary event or as a secondary response to a variety of stimuli or disease processes. Unfortunately, these disorders cannot all be distinguished by their histopathologic changes, which may merely reflect the stage of the lesion at the time of biopsy. The principal diagnostic criteria are the appearance and distribution of the lesions, associated symptoms, laboratory studies, and an appreciation of the natural history and exogenous provocative factors of these conditions.

CORTICOSTEROID-INDUCED ATROPHY. The injection of a corticosteroid intradermally can produce deep atrophy accompanied by surface pigmentary changes and telangiectasia. These changes occur approximately 2 wk after injection and may last for months. The deltoid area is most susceptible to this complication (see Chapter 607).

PANNICULITIS. Inflammation of fibrofatty subcutaneous tissue may primarily involve the fat lobule or, alternatively, the fibrous septum that compartmentalizes the fatty lobules. Lobular panniculitis that spares the subcutaneous vasculature includes poststeroid panniculitis, lupus erythematosus profundus, pancreatic panniculitis, α_1-antitrypsin deficiency, subcutaneous fat necrosis of the newborn, sclerema neonatorum, cold panniculitis, subcutaneous sarcoidosis, and factitial panniculitis. Lobar panniculitis with vasculitis occurs in erythema induratum and occasionally as a feature of Crohn disease (see Chapter 283.2). Inflammation predominantly within the septum, sparing the vasculature, may be seen in erythema nodosum (see Chapter 156), necrobiosis lipoidica, scleroderma (see Chapter 154), and subcutaneous granuloma annulare (see Chapter 609). Septal panniculitis that includes inflammation of the vessels is found primarily in leukocytoclastic vasculitis and polyarteritis nodosa (see Chapter 152).

Poststeroid panniculitis has been observed in children who received high-dose corticosteroids orally for relatively short periods, usually for rheumatic fever. Within 1–2 wk after discontinuation of the drug, multiple subcutaneous nodules may appear on the cheeks, trunk, and arms. Nodules range in size from 0.5–4 cm, are erythematous or skin colored, and may be pruritic. The mechanism of the inflammatory reaction in the fat is unknown. Treatment is unnecessary because the lesions remit spontaneously over a period of months without scarring.

Lupus erythematosus profundus (lupus erythematosus panniculitis) presents with one to several firm, well-defined, 1 to several centimeter in diameter plaques or nodules most commonly on the face, buttocks, or proximal extremities. This condition may occur in patients with systemic or discoid lupus erythematosus and may precede or follow the development of other cutaneous lesions. The overlying skin is usually normal but may be erythematous, atrophic, poikilodermatous, or hyperkeratotic. Lesions may be painful and may ulcerate. On healing, a shallow depression generally remains; rarely, soft, pink areas of anetoderma may result. The histopathologic changes are distinctive and may allow one to make the diagnosis in the absence of other cutaneous lesions of lupus erythematosus. The lupus band and antinuclear antibody test results are usually positive. Nodules tend to be persistent but may respond to antimalarials, oral or intralesional corticosteroids, or in debilitating cases, immunosuppressive agents such as azathioprine or cyclophosphamide. Avoidance of sun exposure and trauma is also important.

α_1-*Antitrypsin deficiency* may present with cellulitis-like areas or red, tender nodules on the trunk or proximal extremities. (see Chapter 303.6). Nodules tend to ulcerate spontaneously and discharge an oily, yellow fluid. Trauma is an inciting factor in some patients. Affected individuals have severe homozygous deficiency or rarely a partial deficiency of the protease inhibitor α_1-antitrypsin, which inhibits trypsin activity and the activity of elastase, serine proteases, collagenase, factor VIII, and kallikrein. Accordingly, panniculitis may be associated with panacinar emphysema, noninfectious hepatitis, cirrhosis, persistent cutaneous vasculitis, cold-contact urticaria, or acquired angioedema. Diagnosis can be substantiated by a decreased level of serum α_1-antitrypsin activity, although, because the protein behaves as an acute-phase reactant, the level may be elevated spuriously during an acute attack of pancreatitis. Some patients respond to dapsone or infusion of random-donor–derived α_1-protease inhibitor concentrate.

Pancreatic panniculitis presents most commonly on the pretibial regions, thighs, or buttocks as tender, erythematous nodules that may be fluctuant and occasionally discharge a yellowish, oily substance. It presents most often in alcoholic males but may also occur in patients with pancreatitis as a result of cholelithiasis or abdominal trauma, with rupture of a pancreatic pseudocyst, with pancreatic ductal adenocarcinoma, or with pancreatic acinar cell carcinoma. Associated features may include arthropathy and synovitis, particularly in the ankles; eosinophilia; polyserositis; and painful osteolytic bone lesions with medullary necrosis. Microscopic changes consist of multiple foci of fat necrosis that contain ghost cells with thick, shadowy walls and no nuclei. A polymorphous inflammatory infiltrate surrounds the areas of fat necrosis. Pathogenesis of the panniculitis appears to be multifactorial, involving liberation of the lipolytic enzymes lipase, trypsin, and amylase into the circulation, causing adipocyte membrane damage and intracellular lipolysis. There is no correlation, however, between the occurrence of pancreatitis and the serum concentration of pancreatic enzymes.

Subcutaneous fat necrosis is an inflammatory disorder of adipose tissue that occurs primarily in the first 4 wk of life in full-term or post-term infants. Affected infants generally have a history of perinatal asphyxia or a difficult labor and delivery. Typical lesions are asymptomatic, rubbery to firm, erythematous to violaceous plaques or nodules on the cheeks, buttocks, back, thighs, or upper arms (Fig. 610–1 [color plate section]). Lesions may be focal or extensive and are generally asymptomatic, although they may be tender during the acute phase. Histopathologic changes are diagnostic and consist of necrosis of fat; a granulomatous cellular infiltrate composed of lymphocytes, histiocytes, multinucleated giant cells, and fibroblasts; and radially arranged clefts of crystalline triglyceride within fat cells and multinucleated giant cells. Calcium deposits are commonly found in areas of fat necrosis. Subcutaneous fat necrosis in the infant may be due to ischemic injury under various circumstances such as maternal pre-eclampsia, birth trauma, asphyxia, and prolonged hypothermia; in many of the affected infants, however, no provocative factors are identified. Susceptibility has been attributed to differences in composition between the subcutaneous tissue of young infants and that of older infants, children, and adults. Neonatal fat solidifies at a relatively high temperature because of its relatively greater concentration of high-melting-point saturated fatty acids such as palmitic and stearic acids.

Uncomplicated lesions involute spontaneously within weeks to months, usually without scarring or atrophy. Occasionally, calcium deposition may occur within areas of fat necrosis, and this may sometimes result in rupture and drainage of liquid material. A rare but potentially life-threatening complication is *hypercalcemia*. This presents at 1–6 mo of age with lethargy, poor feeding, vomiting, failure to thrive, irritability, seizures, shortening of the QT interval, or renal failure. The origin of the hypercalcemia is unknown but is postulated to involve excess bone resorption through elevated levels of prostaglandin E or increased intestinal calcium uptake by unregulated extrarenal production of 1,25-dihydroxyvitamin D by macrophages in the granulomatous infiltrate. Subcutaneous fat necrosis can be confused with sclerema neonatorum, panniculitis, cellulitis, or hematoma. Because the lesions are self-limited, therapy is not required for uncomplicated cases. Needle aspiration of fluctuant lesions may prevent rupture and subsequent scarring. Treatment of hypercalcemia is aimed at enhancing renal calcium excretion by hydration and furosemide administration and at limiting dietary calcium and vitamin D intake. Reduction of intestinal calcium absorption and alteration of vitamin D metabolism may be accomplished by administration of corticosteroids.

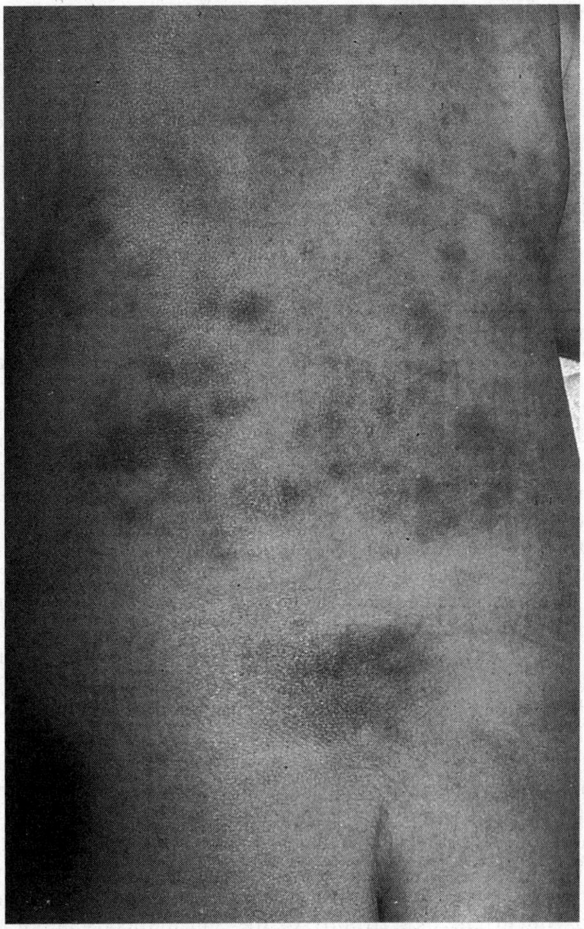

Figure 610–1. Red-purple nodular infiltration of skin of back caused by subcutaneous fat necrosis. See also color section.

Sclerema neonatorum is an uncommon disorder of adipose tissue that presents abruptly in preterm, gravely ill infants as diffuse, yellowish-white woody induration of the skin. Affected skin becomes stony in consistency, cold, and nonpitting. The face assumes a masklike expression, and joint mobility may be compromised because of inflexibility of the skin. Histopathologic changes in sclerema neonatorum consist of an increase in the size of fat cells and an increase in the width of the fibrous connective tissue septa. In contrast to subcutaneous fat necrosis, with which it is most apt to be confused, fat necrosis, inflammation, giant cells, and calcium crystals are generally absent. Sclerema neonatorum almost always is associated with serious illness, such as sepsis, congenital heart disease, multiple congenital anomalies, or hypothermia. The appearance of sclerema in a sick infant should be regarded as an ominous prognostic sign. The outcome depends on the response of the underlying disorder to treatment.

Cold panniculitis may result in localized lesions in infants after prolonged cold exposure, especially on the cheeks, or after prolonged application of a cold object such as an ice cube, ice bag, or popsicle to any area of the skin. Erythematous to bluish, indurated, ill-defined plaques or nodules arise within hours to a couple days of exposure, persist for 2–3 wk, and heal without residua. Recurrence of the lesions is common, however, stressing the importance of parental education in managing these patients. Histopathologic examination reveals an infiltrate of lymphoid and histiocytic cells around blood vessels at the dermal-subdermal junction; by the 3rd day, some of the fat cells in the subcutis may have ruptured and coalesced into cystic structures. Cold panniculitis may be confused with facial cellulitis caused by *Haemophilus influenzae* type b. Unlike buccal cellulitis, however, the area may be cold to the touch, and the patient is afebrile. Frost bite is painful and histopathologically involves the epidermis, dermis, and subcutaneous fat. The pathogenic mechanism of cold panniculitis may be similar to that of subcutaneous fat necrosis, involving an increased propensity of fat to solidify in infants compared with that in older children and adults as a result of the higher percentage of saturated fatty acids in the subcutaneous fat of infants.

Factitial panniculitis results from the subcutaneous injection by self or proxy of a foreign substance, the most common types of which include organic materials such as milk or feces; drugs such as the opiates or pentazocine; oily materials such as mineral oil or paraffin; and the synthetic polymer povidone. Indurated plaques, ulcers, or nodules that liquefy and drain may be noted clinically. The histopathologic picture is variable, depending on the injected substance, but may include the presence of birefringent crystals, oil cysts surrounded by fibrosis and inflammation, and an acute inflammatory reaction with fat necrosis. Vessels are characteristically spared.

LIPODYSTROPHY. Several rare conditions are associated with loss of fatty tissue in a partial or generalized distribution.

Partial lipodystrophy occurs more commonly in females than in males and generally begins on the face during the 1st decade of life. There is gradual symmetric loss of subcutaneous tissue over the face, upper trunk, and arms, resulting in a cadaverous facies and marked disproportion between the upper and lower halves of the body (Weir-Mitchell type). In some cases, there is a concurrent hypertrophy of the subcutaneous fat of the lower part of the body (Laignel-Lavastine and Viard types); others have hemilipodystrophy involving one half of the face or body. Loss of adipose tissue is not preceded by an inflammatory phase, and histopathologic examination reveals only absence of subcutaneous fat. Some patients have had hypocomplementemia (i.e., low C3) and associated renal disease, particularly progressive membranous mesangiocapillary glomerulonephritis, disordered glucose metabolism, or abnormal serum lipid profiles. The cause of the disorder is not understood, and there is no effective treatment.

Congenital generalized lipodystrophy (Seip-Lawrence syndrome) is a progressive multisystem disorder inherited as an autosomal recessive trait. The earliest manifestation is generalized loss of subcutaneous and visceral fat; it may be evident at birth or may occur during infancy. Associated cutaneous changes include prominent superficial veins, hirsutism, abundant and curly scalp hair, and acanthosis nigricans. Accelerated skeletal growth, resulting in tall stature; enlarged joints, especially of the hands and feet; accelerated muscle growth, resulting in a protuberant abdomen; precocious enlargement of the genitalia; and mental deficiency and hemiplegia are seen commonly. Abnormalities of carbohydrate homeostasis, insulin production, and growth hormone appear to be age dependent, generally developing after age 10 yr. Hyperlipidemia, hyperinsulinism, and insulin-resistant nonketotic diabetes mellitus develop gradually and are reflected by increasing hepatomegaly caused by fatty infiltration and cirrhosis. Serum levels of growth hormone may be normal, but its secretion in response to stimuli may be disturbed. Hypothalamic releasing factors that are not ordinarily found in plasma have been identified in affected patients and suggest a lack of hypothalamic regulation. Pimozide, a selective dopamine blocker, may be helpful in restoring fat. Control of the diabetes with insulin is difficult to achieve and does not affect the course of the lipodystrophy. Dietary fat reduction, however, has been shown to improve lipoprotein metabolism, reduce carbohydrate intolerance, and decrease insulin requirements.

Localized lipoatrophy is an idiopathic condition that presents as annular atrophy at the ankles, a bandlike semicircular depression 2–4 cm in diameter on the thighs or, rarely, on the abdomen and upper groin as a centrifugally spreading, bluish, depressed plaque with an erythematous margin. It occurs predominantly in Japanese children.

Insulin lipoatrophy usually occurs approximately 6 mo to 2 yr after initiation of relatively high doses of insulin. A dimple or well-circumscribed depression at the site of injection is typically seen, although loss of fat may extend beyond the site of injection, leading to an extensive, depressed plaque. Biopsy reveals a marked decrease or absence of subcutaneous tissue, without inflammation or fibrosis. In some patients, hypertrophy occurs clinically. In these cases, the mid-dermal collagen is replaced by hypertrophic fat cells on histopathologic sections. The mechanism of insulin lipoatrophy may be due to cross-reaction of insulin antibodies with fat cells, as the incidence of this condition has decreased since the implementation of widespread use of highly purified insulins. Lesions may also be prevented by frequent alteration of injection sites.

Aronson IK, Zeitz HJ, Variakojis D: Panniculitis in childhood. Pediatr Dermatol 5:216, 1988.
Koransky JS, Esterly NB: Lupus panniculitis (profundus). J Pediatr 98:241, 1981.
Senior B, Gellis SS: The syndromes of total lipodystrophy and of partial lipodystrophy. Pediatrics 33:593, 1964.
Silverman RA, Newman AJ, LeVine MJ: Post-steroid panniculitis; a case report. Pediatr Dermatol 5:92, 1988.

CHAPTER 611

Disorders of the Sweat Glands

Gary L. Darmstadt and Al Lane

Eccrine glands are found over nearly the entire skin surface and are the primary means, through evaporation of the water in sweat, for cooling the body. These glands have no anatomic relationship to hair follicles and secrete a relatively large amount of odorless aqueous sweat. In contrast, apocrine glands are limited in distribution to the axillae, anogenital skin, mammary glands, ceruminous glands of the ear, Moll glands in the eyelid, and selected areas of the face and scalp. The apocrine gland duct enters the pilosebaceous follicle at the level of the infundibulum and secretes a small amount of a complex, viscous fluid that, on alteration by microorganisms, produces a distinctive body odor. Some disorders of these two sweat glands are similar pathogenetically, whereas others are unique to a given gland.

ANHIDROSIS. *Neuropathic anhidrosis* results from a disturbance in the neural pathway from the control center in the brain to the peripheral efferent nerve fibers that activate sweating. Disorders in this category, which are characterized by generalized anhidrosis, include tumors of the hypothalamus and damage to the floor of the third ventricle. Pontine or medullary lesions may produce anhidrosis of the ipsilateral face or neck and ipsilateral or contralateral anhidrosis of the rest of the body. Peripheral or segmental neuropathies, caused by leprosy, amyloidosis, diabetes mellitus, alcoholic neuritis, or syringomyelia, may be associated with anhidrosis of the innervated skin. A variety of autonomic disorders are also associated with altered eccrine sweat gland function.

■ **TABLE 611–1 Causes of Hyperhidrosis**

Cortical	***Vasomotor***
Emotional	Cold injury
Familial dysautonomia	Raynaud phenomenon
Congenital ichthyosiform erythroderma	Rheumatoid arthritis
Epidermolysis bullosa	***Neurologic***
Nail-patella syndrome	Abscess
Jadassohn-Lewandowsky syndrome	Familial dysautonomia
Pachyonychia congenita	Postencephalitic
Palmoplantar keratoderma	Tumor
Hypothalamic	***Miscellaneous***
Drugs	Chédiak-Higashi syndrome
Antipyretics	Compensatory
Emetics	Phenylketonuria
Insulin	Pheochromocytoma
Meperidine	Vitiligo
Exercise	**Medullary**
Infection	Physiologic gustatory sweating
Defervescence	Encephalitis
Chronic illness	Granulosis rubra nasi
Metabolic	Syringomyelia
Debility	Thoracic sympathetic trunk injury
Diabetes mellitus	**Spinal**
Hyperpituitarism	Cord transection
Hyperthyroidism	Syringomyelia
Hypoglycemia	**Changes in Blood Flow**
Obesity	Maffucci syndrome
Porphyria	Arteriovenous fistula
Pregnancy	Klippel-Trenaunay syndrome
Rickets	Glomus tumor
Infantile scurvy	Blue rubber bleb nevus syndrome
Cardiovascular	
Heart failure	
Shock	

At the *level of the sweat gland,* drugs such as the anticholinergics atropine and scopolamine may paralyze the sweat glands. Acute intoxication with barbiturates or diazepam has produced necrosis of sweat glands, resulting in anhidrosis with or without erythema and bullae. Eccrine glands are largely absent throughout the skin or present in a localized area of patients with anhidrotic ectodermal dysplasia and localized congenital absence of sweat glands, respectively. Infiltrative or destructive disorders that may produce atrophy of sweat glands by pressure or scarring include scleroderma, acrodermatitis chronica atrophicans, radiodermatitis, burns, Sjögren disease, multiple myeloma, and lymphoma. Obstruction of sweat glands may occur in miliaria and in a number of inflammatory and hyperkeratotic disorders such as the ichthyoses, psoriasis, lichen planus, pemphigus, porokeratosis, atopic dermatitis, and seborrheic dermatitis. Occlusion of the sweat pore may also occur with the topical agents aluminum and zirconium salts, formaldehyde, or glutaraldehyde.

A wide variety of *disorders that are associated with anhidrosis by unknown mechanisms* include dehydration; toxic overdose with lead, arsenic, thallium, fluorine, or morphine; uremia; cirrhosis; endocrine disorders such as Addison disease, diabetes mellitus, diabetes insipidus, or hyperthyroidism; and inherited conditions such as Fabry disease, Franceschetti-Jadassohn syndrome, which combines features of incontinentia pigmenti and anhidrotic ectodermal dysplasia, and familial anhidrosis with neurolabyrinthitis.

Whereas anhidrosis may be complete, in many cases, what appears clinically to be anhidrosis is actually *hypohidrosis* caused by anhidrosis of many but not all eccrine glands. Compensatory, localized *hyperhidrosis* of the remaining functional sweat glands may occur, particularly in diabetes mellitus and miliaria. The primary complication of anhidrosis is hyperthermia, seen primarily in anhidrotic ectodermal dysplasia or in the otherwise normal preterm or full-term *neonate* who has immature eccrine glands.

HYPERHIDROSIS. The numerous disorders that may be associated with increased production of eccrine sweat may also be classified into those with neural mechanisms involving an abnormality in the pathway from the neural regulatory centers to the sweat gland and those that are non-neurally mediated by direct effects on the sweat gland (Table 611–1). Excessive sweating of the palms and soles in response to emotional stimuli (volar hyperhidrosis) may respond to 10% glutaraldehyde soaks, 20% aluminum chloride in anhydrous ethanol applied under occlusion for several hours, iontophoretic therapy with anticholinergics, or in severe, refractory cases, cervicothoracic or lumbar sympathectomy. Axillary hyperhidrosis does not respond to topical glutaraldehyde or salts of aluminum, zirconium, or zinc. Aluminum chloride (Drysol) applied to the axillae at bedtime under occlusion, aided, if necessary, by oral administration of an anticholinergic agent such as glycopyrrolate (Robinul), may produce a prompt and significant reduction in sweating. Cervicothoracic sympathectomy or selective surgical removal of the most highly sudoriferous eccrine glands in the axillae may be effective in refractory cases.

MILIARIA. This results from retention of sweat in occluded eccrine sweat ducts as a result of a keratinous plug in the sweat duct. Retrograde pressure may result in rupture of the duct and leakage of sweat into the epidermis and/or the dermis. The eruption is most often induced by hot, humid weather, but it may also be caused by high fever. Infants who are dressed too warmly may develop this eruption indoors even during the winter.

In *miliaria crystallina,* asymptomatic, noninflammatory, pinpoint clear vesicles may erupt suddenly in profusion over large areas of the body surface, leaving brawny desquamation on healing (Fig. 611–1). The clarity of the fluid, superficiality of the vesicles, and absence of inflammation permit differentiation from other blistering disorders. This type of miliaria occurs most frequently in newborn infants because of the relative immaturity and delayed patency of the sweat duct and the tendency for infants to be nursed in relatively warm, humid conditions. It may also occur in older patients with hyperpyrexia. Histopathologically, an intracorneal or subcorneal vesicle is seen in communication with the sweat duct.

Miliaria rubra is a less superficial eruption characterized by erythematous, minute papulovesicles that may impart a prickling sensation. The lesions are usually localized to sites of

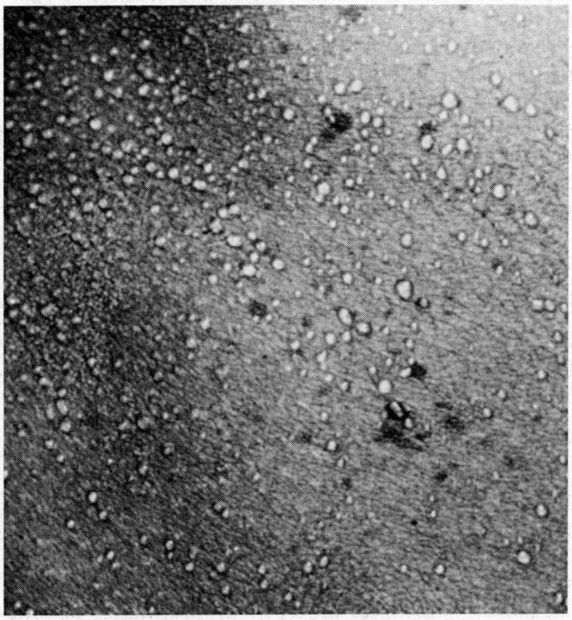

Figure 611–1. Superficial clear vesicles of miliaria crystallina in a patient with hyperpyrexia and lymphoma.

occlusion or to flexural areas, such as the neck, groin, and axillae, where friction may play a role in their pathogenesis. Involved skin may become macerated and eroded. This lesion may be confused with or superimposed on other diaper area eruptions, including candidosis and folliculitis; lesions of miliaria rubra, however, are extrafollicular. Histopathologically, one sees focal areas of spongiosis and spongiotic vesicle formation in close proximity to sweat ducts that generally contain a keratinous plug. The keratinous plug does not form, however, until the later stages of the disease and therefore does not appear to be the primary cause of sweat duct obstruction. The initial obstruction is postulated to be due to swelling of the ductal epidermal cells, perhaps from imbibition of water. Miliaria rubra is generally reversible. Supplemental vitamin C may help to restore normal sweating in refractory cases. Prophylactic use of antibacterial agents may prevent development of miliaria rubra. Repeated attacks of miliaria rubra may lead to *miliaria profunda,* which is due to rupture of the sweat duct deeper in the skin at the level of the dermoepidermal junction. Severe, extensive miliaria rubra or miliaria profunda may result in disturbance of heat regulation. Lesions of miliaria rubra may become infected, particularly in malnourished or debilitated infants, leading to development of periporitis staphylogenes, which involves extension of the process from the sweat duct into the sweat gland.

All forms of miliaria respond dramatically to cooling the patient by regulation of environmental temperatures and by removal of excessive clothing and, in patients with fever, to administration of antipyretics. Topical agents are usually ineffective and may exacerbate the eruption.

GRANULOSIS RUBRA NASI. This autosomal dominant or recessive condition presents between the ages of 6 mo and 16 yr, most commonly in early childhood, with diffuse erythema of the tip of the nose, which subsequently may extend to involve the cheeks, upper lip, and chin. Beads of sweat, minute red papules, and sometimes vesicles appear at sweat duct orifices. The nose may be pruritic and feels cold to the touch. Hyperhidrosis of the palms and soles and poor peripheral circulation may be associated findings. The differential diagnosis includes lupus vulgaris, lupus erythematosus, acne rosacea, and perioral dermatitis. The condition generally remits spontaneously at puberty but occasionally persists indefinitely. There is no effective therapy.

BROMHIDROSIS. The excessive odor that characterizes bromhidrosis may result from alteration of either apocrine or eccrine sweat. Apocrine bromhidrosis develops after puberty as a result of the formation of short-chain fatty acids and ammonia by the action of anaerobic diphtheroids on axillary apocrine sweat. Treatments that may be helpful include cleansing with germicidal soaps; topical application of aluminum, zirconium, or zinc salts or gentamicin cream, all of which have antibacterial action; and axillary shaving. Eccrine bromhidrosis is caused by microbiologic degradation of stratum corneum that has become softened by excessive eccrine sweat. The soles of the feet and the intertriginous areas are the primary affected sites. Hyperhidrosis, warm weather, obesity, intertrigo, and diabetes mellitus are predisposing factors. In addition to local measures, oral anticholinergic drugs such as propantheline (Pro-Banthine) may decrease eccrine sweating but do not alter apocrine gland secretion. Topical aluminum chloride preparations such as Drysol are particularly useful for plantar eccrine bromhidrosis.

HIDRADENITIS SUPPURATIVA. This is a chronic, inflammatory, suppurative disorder of the apocrine glands in the axillae; anogenital area; and, occasionally, the scalp, posterior aspect of the ears, female breasts, and around the umbilicus. Onset of *clinical manifestations,* sometimes preceded by pruritus or discomfort, usually occurs during puberty or early adulthood. Solitary or multiple painful, erythematous nodules, deep abscesses, and contracted scars are sharply confined to areas of skin containing apocrine glands. When the disease is severe and chronic, sinus tracts, ulcers, and thick, linear fibrotic bands develop. Hidradenitis suppurativa tends to persist for many years, punctuated by relapses and partial remissions. Complications include cellulitis, ulceration, and burrowing abscesses that may perforate adjacent structures, forming fistulas to the urethra, bladder, rectum, or peritoneum. Episodic inflammatory arthritis develops in some patients. A minority of patients have the follicular occlusion triad, which includes acne and perifolliculitis capitis. Early lesions are often mistaken for infected epidermal cysts, furuncles, scrofuloderma, actinomycosis, cat-scratch disease, granuloma inguinale, or lymphogranuloma venereum. Sharp localization to areas of the body that bear appocrine glands, however, should suggest hidradenitis. When involvement is limited to the anogenital region, the condition may be difficult to distinguish from, and may coexist with, Crohn disease.

Histopathologically, early lesions are characterized by a keratinous plug in the apocrine duct or hair follicle orifice, and cystic distention of the follicle. The process generally, but not necessarily, extends into the apocrine gland. Later changes include inflammation within and around apocrine glands and the presence of groups of cocci within apocrine glands and in the adjacent dermis. Skin appendages may become obliterated by scarring. The disease is probably initiated by plugging of apocrine gland ducts with keratinous debris. Bacterial infection, particularly with *Staphylococcus aureus, Streptococcus milleri, Escherichia coli,* and possibly anaerobic streptococci, appears to be important in the progressive dilatation below the obstruction, leading to rupture of the duct, inflammation, sinus tract formation, and destructive scarring. Pathogenesis of hidradenitis suppurativa is controversial, but it appears to be an androgen-dependent condition.

Patients should be counseled to avoid tight-fitting clothes, as occlusion may exacerbate the condition. *Treatment* with topical antibiotic agents such as chlorhexidine, erythromycin, or clindamycin or with topical retinoids may be effective in early, indolent disease. Systemic antibiotics, chosen on the basis of bacterial culture (usually staphylococcal and streptococcal pathogens) and sensitivity tests, should be administered in the acute phase. Empirical therapy may be initiated with tetracycline, doxycycline, or minocycline if the patient is 8 yr or older; clindamycin or cephalosporins are also effective. Some patients require long-term treatment with tetracycline or erythromycin. Intralesional triamcinolone acetonide (5–10 mg/mL) is often helpful in early disease. The addition of prednisone, 40–60 mg/day for 7–10 days, tapering gradually as inflammation subsides, to the regimen of patients who respond poorly to antibiotics may decrease fibrosis and scarring. Oral contraceptive agents, which contain a high estrogen : progesterone ratio and low androgenicity of the progesterone, or oral retinoids may be helpful in some patients. Warm compresses encourage spontaneous rupture of abscesses; those that are "pointing" should be incised and drained. Ultimately, surgical measures may be required for control or cure.

FOX-FORDYCE DISEASE. This disease is most common in females and presents during puberty or the 3rd decade of life with pruritus in the axillae and, occasionally, in the anogenital region and around the breasts. Pruritus is exacerbated by emotional stress and stimuli that induce apocrine sweating. Skin-colored to slightly hyperpigmented dome-shaped follicular papules develop in the pruritic areas. Histopathologically, one sees keratinous plugging of the distal apocrine duct, rupture of the intraepidermal portion of the apocrine duct, paraductal microvesicle formation, and paraductal acanthosis. The condition generally remits during pregnancy, particularly in the third trimester. Oral contraceptive pills and topical corticosteroids or retinoic acid may help some patients.

Barth JH, Kealey T: Androgen metabolism by isolated human axillary apocrine glands in hidradenitis suppurativa. Br J Dermatol 125:304, 1991.
Holzle E, Kligman AM: The pathogenesis of miliaria rubra. Br J Dermatol 99:117, 1978.
Jackman PJH: Body odor—the role of skin bacteria. Semin Dermatol 1:143, 1982.
Sato K, Kang WH, Saga K, et al: Biology of sweat glands and their disorders. J Am Acad Dermatol 20:537, 1989.

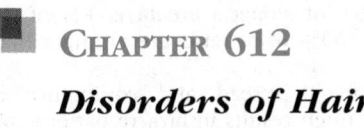

CHAPTER 612

Disorders of Hair

Gary L. Darmstadt and Al Lane

Disorders of hair in infants and children may be due to intrinsic disturbances of hair growth, underlying biochemical or metabolic defects, inflammatory dermatoses, or structural anomalies of the hair shaft. Excessive and abnormal hair growth is referred to as hypertrichosis or hirsutism. Hypertrichosis is excessive hair growth at inappropriate locations; hirsutism is an androgen-dependent male pattern of hair growth in women. Hypotrichosis is deficient hair growth, and hair loss, partial or complete, is called alopecia. Alopecia may be classified as nonscarring or scarring; the latter type is rare in children and, if present, is most often due to prolonged or untreated inflammatory conditions such as pyoderma or tinea capitis.

HYPERTRICHOSIS

Hypertrichosis is rare in children and may be localized or generalized and permanent or transient. Hypertrichosis has many causes, some of which are listed in Table 612–1.

■ TABLE 612–1 Causes of and Conditions Associated with Hypertrichosis

Intrinsic Factors
Racial and familial forms such as hairy ears, hairy elbows, intraphalangeal hair, or generalized hirsutism
Extrinsic Factors
Local trauma
Malnutrition
Anorexia nervosa
Long-standing inflammatory dermatoses
Drugs
Diazoxide, phenytoin, corticosteroids, Cortisporin, cyclosporine, androgens, anabolic agents, hexachlorobenzene, minoxidil, psoralens, penicillamine, streptomycin
Hamartomas or Nevi
Congenital pigmented nevocytic nevus, nevus pilosus, Becker nevus, congenital smooth muscle hamartoma, fawn-tail nevus asssociated with diastematomyelia
Endocrine Disorders
Virilizing ovarian tumors, Cushing syndrome, acromegaly, hyperthyroidism, hypothyroidism, congenital adrenal hyperplasia, adrenal tumors, gonadal dysgenesis, male pseudohermaphroditism, nonendocrine hormone–secreting tumors, polycystic ovary syndrome
Congenital and Genetic Disorders
Hypertrichosis lanuginosa, mucopolysaccharidosis, leprechaunism, congenital generalized lipodystrophy, de Lange syndrome, craniofacial dysostosis, trisomy 18, Rubinstein-Taybi syndrome, Bloom syndrome, congenital hemihypertrophy, gingival fibromatosis with hypertrichosis, porphyrias, dystrophic epidermolysis bullosa, Winchester syndrome, lipoatrophic diabetes (Lawrence-Seip syndrome), fetal hydantoin syndrome, fetal alcohol syndrome

■ TABLE 612–2 Disorders Associated with Alopecia and Hypotrichosis

Congenital total alopecia: isolated autosomal recessive abnormality, progeria, hidrotic ectodermal dysplasia, Moynahan syndrome, atrichia with keratin cysts, Baraitser syndrome
Congenital localized alopecia: aplasia cutis, alopecia triangularis, epidermal nevus, hair follicle hamartoma, facial hemiatrophy (Romberg syndrome)
Hereditary hypotrichosis: hypotrichosis with keratosis pilaris, Marie-Unna hypotrichosis, phenylketonuria, arginosuccinic aciduria, hyperlysinemia, homocystinuria, orotic aciduria, Menkes kinky hair syndrome, Cockayne, Rothmund-Thomson, dyskeratosis congenita, Seckel, cartilage-hair hypoplasia, Conradi syndrome, trichorhinophalangeal, pachyonychia congenita, Hallermann-Streiff, Treacher Collins, oculodentodigital, orofaciodigital, incontinentia pigmenti, focal dermal hypoplasia, keratosis follicularis, epidermolysis bullosa, ectodermal dysplasias, ichthyoses
Diffuse alopecia of endocrine origin: hypopituitarism, hypothyroidism, hypoparathyroidism, hyperthyroidism, diabetes mellitus
Alopecia of nutritional origin: marasmus, kwashiorkor, iron deficiency, zinc deficiency (acrodermatitis enteropathica), gluten-sensitive enteropathy, essential fatty acid deficiency
Disturbances of the hair cycle: telogen effluvium
Toxic alopecia: anagen effluvium
Autoimmune alopecia: alopecia areata
Traumatic alopecia: traction alopecia, trichotillomania
Cicatricial alopecia: lupus erythematosus, lichen planus pilaris, pseudopelade, scleroderma, dermatomyositis, infection (kerion, favus, tuberculosis, syphilis, folliculitis, leishmaniasis, herpes zoster, varicella), acne keloidalis, follicular mucinosis, cicatricial pemphigoid, lichen sclerosus et atrophicus, sarcoidosis
Trichodystrophies: trichorrhexis nodosa, monilethrix, trichorrhexis invaginata, pili torti, woolly hair syndrome, trichoschisis, pili annulati

HYPOTRICHOSIS AND ALOPECIA

Some of the disorders associated with hypotrichosis and alopecia are listed in Table 612–2. True alopecia is only rarely congenital; it is more often related to an inflammatory dermatosis, mechanical factors, drug ingestion, infection, endocrinopathy, nutritional disturbance, or disturbance of the hair cycle. Any inflammatory condition of the scalp, such as atopic dermatitis or seborrheic dermatitis, if severe enough, may result in partial alopecia. In all these disorders, hair growth returns to normal if the underlying condition is treated successfully unless there has been permanent damage to the hair follicle.

TELOGEN EFFLUVIUM. Telogen effluvium presents with sudden loss of large amounts of hair, often with brushing, combing, and washing of hair. Diffuse loss of scalp hair occurs from the premature conversion of growing, or anagen hairs, which normally constitute 80–90% of hairs, to resting, or telogen hairs. Hair loss is noted 6 wk to 3 mo after the precipitating cause, which may include childbirth; a febrile episode; surgery; acute blood loss, including blood donation; sudden severe weight loss; discontinuation of high-dose corticosteroids or oral contraceptives; and psychiatric stress. Telogen effluvium also accounts for the loss of hair by infants during the first few months of life; friction from bedsheets, particularly in infants with pruritic, atopic skin, may exacerbate the problem. There is no inflammatory reaction; the hair follicles remain intact, and telogen bulbs can be demonstrated microscopically on shed hairs. Because more than 50% of the scalp hair is rarely involved, alopecia is usually not severe. Parents should be reassured that normal hair growth will return in approximately 6 mo.

TOXIC ALOPECIA (Anagen Effluvium). Anagen effluvium is an acute, severe, diffuse inhibition of growth of anagen follicles, resulting in loss of greater than 80–90% of scalp hair. Hairs become dystrophic, and the hair shaft breaks at the narrowed segment. Loss is diffuse, rapid (1–3 wk after treatment), and temporary, as regrowth occurs after the offending agent is discontinued. Causes of anagen effluvium include radiation; cancer chemotherapeutic agents such as antimetabolites, alkylating agents, and mitotic inhibitors; thallium; thiouracil; heparin; the coumarins; boric acid; and hypervitaminosis A.

TRACTION ALOPECIA (Marginal or Traumatic Alopecia). Traction alopecia is due to trauma to hair follicles by tight braids or "ponytails," headbands, rubber bands, curlers, and rollers (Fig. 612–1A). Broken hairs and inflammatory follicular papules in circumscribed patches at the scalp margins are characteristic and may be subtended by regional lymphadenopathy. Children and parents must be encouraged to avoid devices that cause trauma to the hair and, if necessary, to alter the hair style. Otherwise, scarring of hair follicles may occur.

TRICHOTILLOMANIA. Compulsive pulling, twisting, and breaking of hair produces irregular areas of incomplete hair loss, most often on the crown and in the occipital and parietal areas of the scalp (Fig. 612–1B). Occasionally, eyebrows, eyelashes, and body hair are traumatized. Some plaques of alopecia may have a linear outline. The hairs remaining within the areas of loss are of varying lengths and are typically blunt tipped because of breakage. The scalp is normal in appearance, although chronic folliculitis may also occur. Trichophagy, resulting in trichobezoars, may complicate this disorder. The lifetime occurrence is 3% in girls and 1% in boys.

The *diagnosis* of trichotillomania is often difficult and may require biopsy confirmation. The revised third edition of the *Diagnostic and Statistical Manual of Mental Disorders* diagnostic criteria include visible hair loss attributable to pulling; mounting tension preceding hair pulling; gratification or release of tension after hair pulling; and absence of hair pulling attributable to hallucinations, delusions, or an inflammatory skin condition. Histologic changes include coexistent normal and damaged follicles, perifollicular hemorrhage, atrophy of some follicles, and catagen transformation of hair. In late stages, perifollicular fibrosis may occur. Long-term repeated trauma may result in irreversible damage and permanent alopecia. Tinea capitis and alopecia areata must be considered in the differential diagnosis.

Trichotillomania is closely related to, and may be an expression of, obsessive-compulsive disorder in some children; in others, it is a benign habit disorder. *Treatment* of concurrent thumb sucking may be effective in the latter children. When trichotillomania occurs secondary to obsessive-compulsive disorder, clomipramine, fluoxetine, or trazodone may be helpful, particularly when combined with behavioral interventions.

ALOPECIA AREATA. Alopecia areata is characterized by rapid and complete loss of hair in round or oval patches on the scalp (Fig. 612–1C) and on other body sites. In *alopecia totalis,* all the scalp hair is lost; *alopecia universalis* involves all body and scalp hair. The lifetime incidence of alopecia areata is 1% of the population; approximately 60% of patients are younger than 20 yr of age.

Clinical Manifestations. Peripheral spread and confluence of plaques of alopecia areata often results in bizarre patterns. At the margin of active patches, the hairs can often be extracted with gentle traction and, on examination, demonstrate an attenuated or catagen bulb at the termination of a tapered, poorly pigmented shaft (i.e., exclamation hair). The skin within the plaques of hair loss is normal in appearance. A perifollicular infiltrate of inflammatory round cells is found in biopsy specimens from active areas. In the chronic stages, the number of telogen hairs is increased, the diameter of hair fibers is reduced, and trichodystrophies such as trichorrhexis nodosa and trichomalacia may be found. Alopecia areata is associated with atopy; nail changes such as pits, ridges, opacification, serration of the free nail edge, dystrophy, and a red lunula; cataracts or lens opacification; and autoimmune diseases such as Hashimoto thyroiditis, Addison disease, pernicious anemia, ulcerative colitis, myasthenia gravis, collagen-vascular diseases, and vitiligo. An increased incidence of alopecia areata has been reported in patients with Down syndrome (5–10%).

Etiology. The cause of alopecia areata is unknown. Emotional factors and stress have been suggested as triggering factors, but

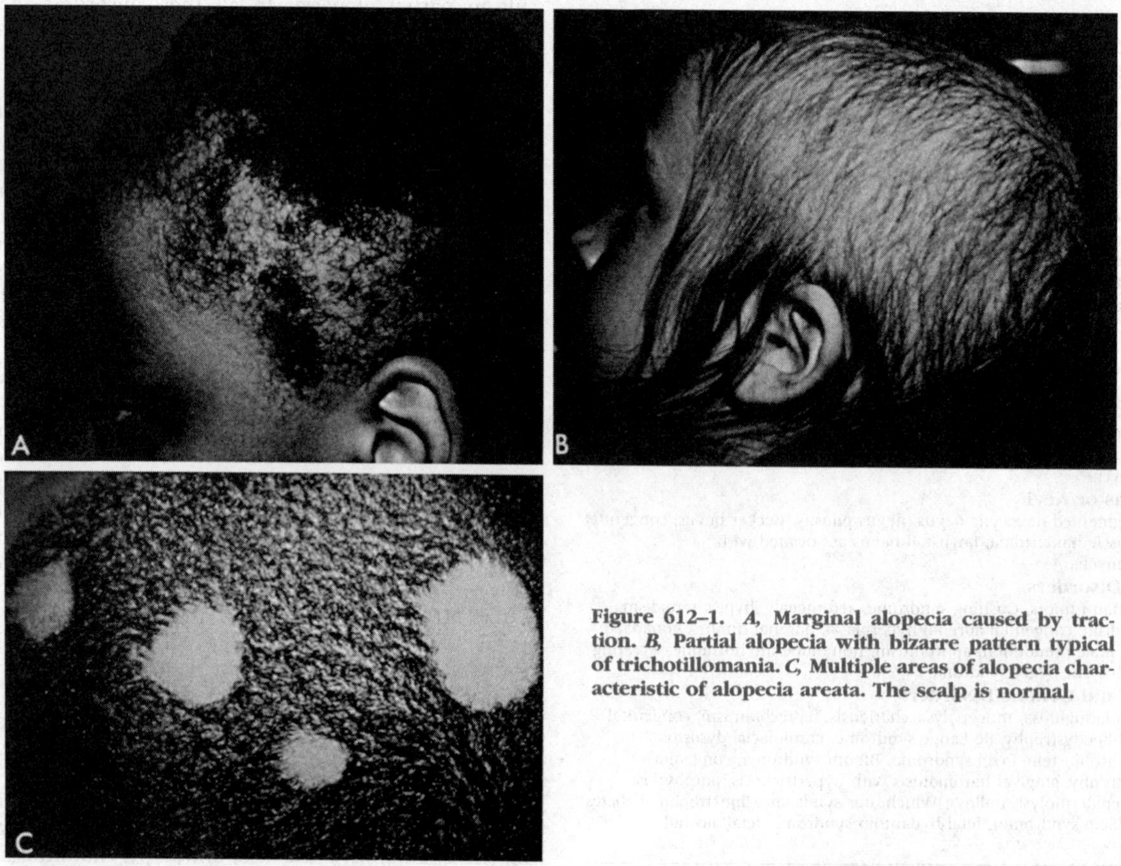

Figure 612–1. *A,* Marginal alopecia caused by traction. *B,* Partial alopecia with bizarre pattern typical of trichotillomania. *C,* Multiple areas of alopecia characteristic of alopecia areata. The scalp is normal.

supportive evidence is tenuous. About 25% of patients have a family history of alopecia areata; inheritance is thought to be autosomal dominant with variable penetrance. The infrequent but striking association with autoimmune diseases has suggested an autoimmune pathogenesis. Some patients have serum antibodies to thyroglobulin, parietal cells, and adrenal gland, and autoantibodies to hair follicle antigens has been demonstrated recently.

Differential Diagnosis and Prognosis. Tinea capitis, seborrheic dermatitis, trichotillomania, traumatic alopecia, and lupus erythematosus should be considered. The course is unpredictable, but spontaneous resolution within 6–12 mo is usual, particularly when relatively small, stable patches of alopecia are present. Recurrences, however, are common. In general, onset at a young age, extensive or prolonged hair loss, multiple episodes, and associated atrophy are poor prognostic signs. Alopecia universalis, totalis, and *ophiasis,* a type of alopecia areata in which hair loss is circumferential, are also less likely to resolve.

Treatment. This is difficult to evaluate because the course is erratic and unpredictable. The use of high-potency topical, fluorinated corticosteroids with occlusion at night is effective in some patients. Intradermal injections of steroid may also stimulate hair growth locally, but this mode of treatment is impractical in young children or in those with extensive hair loss. Systemic corticosteroid therapy has, on occasion, been associated with good results; however, the permanence of cure is questionable, and the side effects are a serious deterrent. Additional therapies that are sometimes effective include short-contact anthralin, topical minoxidil, and contact sensitization with squaric acid dibutylester or diphencyprone. Psoralen and ultraviolet A phototherapy may also be effective but has limited applicability in children. In general, parents and patients can be reassured that spontaneous remission usually occurs. New hair growth may initially be of finer caliber and lighter color, but replacement by normal terminal hair can be expected.

STRUCTURAL DEFECTS OF HAIR

Structural defects of the hair shaft may be congenital, reflect known biochemical aberrations, or relate to damaging grooming practices. All the defects can be demonstrated by microscopic examination of affected hairs, particularly by scanning and transmission electron microscopy.

TRICHORRHEXIS NODOSA. This is the most common of all hair shaft abnormalities. The hair is dry, brittle, and lusterless, with ends that appear like a paint brush and grayish-white nodes on the hair shaft. Microscopically, the nodes have the appearance of two interlocking brushes. The defect results from a fracture of the hair shaft at the nodal points caused by disruption of the cells in the hair cortex. Trichorrhexis nodosa has been noted as an isolated congenital defect in some families, has been observed in some infants with argininosuccinic aciduria, and may occur in Netherton syndrome or in association with ectodermal dysplasia and other hair shaft abnormalities such as pili annulati.

Acquired Trichorrhexis Nodosa. This, the most common cause of hair breakage, occurs in two forms. *Proximal defects* are found most frequently in black children, whose complaint is not of alopecia but of failure of their hair to grow. The hair is short, and longitudinal splits, knots, and whitish nodules can be demonstrated in hair mounts. Easy breakage is demonstrated by gentle traction on the hair shafts. A history of other affected family members may be obtained. The problem is thought to be caused by a combination of genetic predisposition and the cumulative mechanical trauma of rough combing and brushing, hair-straightening procedures, and "permanents." The patient must be cautioned to avoid damaging grooming techniques. A soft, natural-bristle brush and a wide-toothed comb should be used. The condition is self-limited, with resolution in 2–4 yr if the patient avoids damaging practices. *Distal trichorrhexis nodosa* is seen more frequently in white and Asian children. The distal portion of the hair shaft is thinned, ragged, and faded; white specks, sometimes mistaken for nits, may be noted along the shaft. Hair mounts reveal the paintbrush defect and the sites of excessive fragility and breakage. Localized areas of the moustache or beard may also be affected. Avoidance of traumatic grooming, regular trimming of affected ends, and the use of cream rinses to lessen tangling ameliorates this condition.

PILI TORTI. This is the second most common trichodystrophy, and it presents at age 3 mo to 2 yr with spangled, brittle, coarse hair of different lengths over the entire scalp or with circumscribed alopecia. There is a structural defect in which the hair shaft is grooved and flattened at irregular intervals and is twisted on its axis in varying degrees. Minor twists that occur in normal hair should not be misconstrued as pili torti. Curvature of the hair follicle apparently leads to the flattening and rotation of the hair shaft. Most cases of classic, isolated pili torti of early onset have autosomal dominant inheritance. Autosomal recessive forms have been described, however, and many cases are sporadic. Keratosis pilaris, nail dystrophy, and corneal opacity develop in some patients. Syndromes in which the hair shaft abnormalities of pili torti are seen in association with other cutaneous and systemic abnormalities include Menkes kinky hair, Bazex, Bjornstad, Crandall, and Rapp-Hodgkin ectodermal dysplasia syndrome and trichothiodystrophy. It has also occurred in children treated with retinoids.

MONILETHRIX. This rare defect of the hair shaft is inherited as an autosomal dominant trait with variable age of onset, severity, and course. The hair appears dry, lusterless, and brittle, and it fractures spontaneously or with mild trauma. Eyebrows, lashes, body and sexual hair, and scalp hair may be affected. Monilethrix may be present at birth, but the hair is usually normal at birth and is replaced over the first few months of life by abnormal hairs; the condition sometimes is first apparent in childhood. Follicular papules may appear on the nape of the neck and the occiput and, occasionally, over the entire scalp. Short, fragile beaded hairs that emerge from the horny follicular plugs give a distinctive appearance. Keratosis pilaris and koilonychia of fingernails and toenails may also be present. Microscopically, a distinctive, regular beading pattern of the hair shaft is evident, characterized by elliptical nodes that are separated by narrower internodes. Not all hairs have nodes, and both normal and beaded hairs may break. Treatment is generally ineffective, although topical minoxidil and oral etretinate have helped some patients. Spontaneous improvement may occur at puberty, during pregnancy, and with use of oral contraceptive pills.

TRICHOTHIODYSTROPHY. Hair in trichothiodystrophy is sparse, short, brittle, and uneven and may involve the scalp hair, eyebrows, or eyelashes. Microscopically, the hair is flattened, folded, and variable in diameter; has longitudinal grooving; and has nodal swellings that resemble those of trichorrhexis nodosa. Under the polarizing microscope, distinctive alternating dark and light bands are seen. The abnormal hair has a cystine content that is less than 50% of normal because of a major reduction and altered composition of constituent high-sulfur matrix proteins. Trichothiodystrophy may occur as an isolated finding or in association with various syndrome complexes that include intellectual impairment, short stature, ichthyosis, nail dystrophy, dental caries, cataracts, decreased fertility, neurologic abnormalities, bony abnormalities, and immunodeficiency. Some patients are photosensitive and have impaired DNA repair mechanisms, similar to that seen in group D xeroderma pigmentosum; the incidence of skin cancers, however, is not increased. Patients with trichothiodystrophy tend to resemble one another, with a receding chin, protruding ears, raspy voice, and sociable, outgoing personality. *Tri-*

choschisis, a fracture perpendicular to the hair shaft, is characteristic of the many syndromes that are associated with trichothiodystrophy. Perpendicular breakage of the hair shaft has also been described in association with other hair abnormalities, particularly monilethrix.

TRICHORRHEXIS INVAGINATA (Bamboo Hair). Short, sparse, fragile hair without apparent growth is characteristic of this condition, which is found only in association with Netherton syndrome (see Chapter 608). The distal portion of the hair is invaginated into the cuplike proximal portion, forming a fragile nodal swelling. The abnormality is thought to result from a transient defect in keratinization of the inner root sheath. The abnormality may be identified in body and scalp hair and seems to abate as the child matures.

MENKES KINKY HAIR SYNDROME (Trichopoliodystrophy). Males with this sex-linked recessive trait are born to an unaffected mother after a normal pregnancy. Neonatal problems include hypothermia, hypotonia, poor feeding, and failure to thrive. Hair is normal at birth but is replaced by short, brittle, light-colored hair that may have features of trichorrhexis nodosa, pili torti, or monilethrix. The skin is hypopigmented, the cheeks typically appear plump, and the nasal bridge is depressed. Heterozygotes may have loss of skin pigmentation. Progressive psychomotor retardation is noted in early infancy. The disorder has been localized by linkage analysis to chromosome Xq13.3 and is due to a maldistribution of copper in the body.

PILI ANNULATI. Pili annulati is characterized by alternate light and dark bands of the hair shaft. When one is viewing the hair under the light microscope, the region that appeared bright in reflected light instead appears dark in the transmitted light as a result of focal aggregates of abnormal air-filled cavities within the hair shaft. The hair is not fragile. The defect may be autosomal dominant or sporadic. *Pseudopili annulati* is a variant of normal blond hair; an optical effect caused by the refraction and reflection of light from the partially twisted and flattened shaft creates the impression of banding.

WOOLLY HAIR DISEASE. This disorder presents at birth with peculiarly tight, curly, abnormal hair in a nonblack person. It becomes worse in childhood and ameliorates in adulthood. An autosomal dominant form, evident at birth or in infancy, consists of excessively curly, fragile hair. An autosomal recessive type includes scalp hair that is brittle, has a bleached appearance, and is markedly reduced in diameter; body hair is short and pale. Woolly hair nevus, a sporadic form, involves only a circumscribed portion of the scalp hair. The affected hair is fine, tightly curled, light colored, and grows poorly. It may be associated with a pigmented or epidermal nevus in another site of the body or with ocular defects.

UNCOMBABLE HAIR SYNDROME (Spun Glass Hair). The hair of patients with this syndrome appears disorderly, is often silvery-blond, and may break because of repeated, futile efforts to control it. The condition is probably autosomal dominant in inheritance, is usually first noticed in the first 3 yr of life, and may spontaneously improve in childhood. Eyebrows and eyelashes are normal. A longitudinal depression along the hair shaft is a constant feature, and most hair follicles and shafts are triangular. The shape of the hair varies along its length, however, preventing the hairs from lying flat.

Birnbaum PS, Baden HP: Heritable disorders of hair. Dermatol Clin 5:137, 1987.

Custer R, Dietz PE, Geller J, et al: Impulse control disorders not elsewhere classified. *In*: Spitzer RL, Williams JBW (eds): Diagnostic and Statistical Manual of Mental Disorders, 3rd ed. Washington, DC, American Psychiatric Association, 1987, pp 321–328.

Dawber R: Self-induced hair loss. Semin Dermatol 4:53, 1985.

Headington JT: Telogen effluvium. New concepts and review. Arch Dermatol 129:356, 1993.

Price VH: Trichothiodystrophy: update. Pediatr Dermatol 9:369, 1992.

Thiers BH, Bergfeld WF, Fiedler-Weiss VC, et al: Alopecia areata symposium. Pediatr Dermatol 4:136, 1987.

Tobin DJ, Orentreich N, Fenton DA, et al: Antibodies to hair follicles in alopecia areata. J Invest Dermatol 102:721, 1994.

Verbov J: Hair loss in children. Arch Dis Child 68:702, 1993.

CHAPTER 613
Disorders of the Nails

Gary L. Darmstadt and Al Lane

Nail abnormalities in children may be manifestations of generalized skin disease, skin disease localized to the periungual region, systemic disease, drugs, trauma, or localized bacterial and fungal infections. Nail anomalies are also common in certain congenital disorders (Table 613–1).

Anonychia is absence of the nail plate, usually the result of a congenital disorder or trauma. It may be an isolated finding or may be associated with malformations of the digits. *Koilonychia* is flattening and concavity of the nail plate with loss of normal contour, producing a spoon-shaped nail. Koilonychia occurs as an autosomal dominant trait or in association with hypochromic anemia, Plummer-Vinson syndrome, and hemochromatosis. The nail plate is relatively thin during the first 1–2 yr of life and, consequently, may be spoon shaped in otherwise normal children.

Leukonychia is a white opacity of the nail plate that may involve the entire plate or may be punctate or striate. The nail plate itself remains smooth and undamaged. Leukonychia can be traumatic or associated with infections such as leprosy and tuberculosis, dermatoses such as lichen planus and Darier disease, malignancies such as Hodgkin disease, anemia, and arsenic poisoning (Mees lines). Leukonychia of all nail surfaces is an uncommon hereditary trait that may be associated with congenital epidermal cysts and deafness. Paired parallel white bands that do not change position with growth of the nail, and thus reflect a change in the nail bed, are associated with hypoalbuminemia and are called Muehrcke lines. When the proximal portion of the nail is white and the distal 20–50% of the nail is red, pink, or brown, the condition is called half-and-half nails or Lindsay nails; this is seen most commonly in patients with renal disease but may occur as a normal variant. White nails of cirrhosis or Terry nails are characterized by a white ground-glass appearance of the entire or the proximal end of the nail and a normal pink color of the distal 1–2 mm of the nail; this is associated with hypoalbuminemia.

Onycholysis indicates separation of the nail plate from the distal nail bed. Common causes are trauma, chronic exposure to moisture, hyperhidrosis, cosmetics, psoriasis, fungal infection (distal onycholysis), atopic or contact dermatitis, porphyria, drugs (bleomycin, vincristine, retinoid agents, indomethacin, thorazine), and drug-induced phototoxicity from tetracycline, doxycycline, or chloramphenicol. *Beau lines* are transverse grooves in the nail plate that represent a temporary

■ **TABLE 613–1 Congenital Disease with Nail Defects**

Large nails: Pachyonychia congenita, Rubinstein-Taybi syndrome, hemihypertrophy

Small or absent nails: Ectodermal dysplasias, nail-patella, dyskeratosis congenita, focal dermal hypoplasia, cartilage-hair hypoplasia, Ellis–van Creveld, Larsen, epidermolysis bullosa, incontinentia pigmenti, Rothmund-Thomson, Turner, popliteal web, trisomy 13, trisomy 18, Apert, Gorlin-Pindborg, long arm 21 deletion, otopalatodigital, fetal alcohol, fetal hydantoin, elfin facies, anonychia, acrodermatitis enteropathica disruption of formation of the nail plate. The line(s) first appear a few weeks after the event that caused the disruption in nail growth. A single transverse ridge appears at the proximal nail fold in most 4–6-wk-old infants and works its way distally as the nail grows; this line may reflect metabolic changes after delivery. At other ages, Beau lines are usually indicative of periodic trauma or episodic shutdown of the nail matrix secondary to a systemic disease such as measles, mumps, pneumonia, or zinc deficiency.

Nail changes may be particularly associated with a variety of other diseases. Nail changes of *psoriasis* most characteristically include pitting, onycholysis, yellow-brown discoloration, and thickening. Nail changes in *lichen planus* include violaceous papules in the proximal nail fold and nail bed, leukonychia, longitudinal ridging, thinning of the entire nail plate, and *pterygium* formation, which is abnormal adherence of the cuticle to the nail plate or, if the plate is destroyed focally, to the nail bed. *Reiter disease* may include painless erythematous induration of the base of the nail fold; subungual parakeratotic scaling; and thickening, opacification, or ridging of the nail plate. *Dermatitis* that involves the nail folds may produce dystrophy, roughening, and course pitting of the nails. Nail changes are more common in atopic dermatitis than in other forms of dermatitis that affect the hands. *Darier disease* includes white streaks that extend longitudinally and cross the lunula. Where the streak meets the distal end of the nail, a V-shaped notch may be present. Total leukonychia may also occur. Transverse rows of fine pits are characteristic of *alopecia areata*. In severe cases, the entire nail surface may be rough. *Acrodermatitis enteropathica* may include tranverse grooves (Beau lines) and nail dystrophy as a result of periungual dermatitis.

Twenty nail dystrophy is characterized by longitudinal ridging, fragility, thinning, distal notching, and opalescent discoloration of all the nails. There are no associated skin or systemic diseases and no other ectodermal defects. Its occasional association with alopecia areata has led some authors to suggest that twenty nail dystrophy may reflect an abnormal immunologic response to the nail matrix, whereas histopathologic studies have suggested that it may be a manifestation of lichen planus or spongiotic (eczematous) inflammation of the nail matrix. The disorder must be differentiated from fungal infections, psoriasis, nail changes of alopecia areata, and nail dystrophy secondary to eczema. Eczema and fungal infections rarely produce changes of all the nails simultaneously. The disorder is self-limited and eventually remits.

Black pigmentation of an entire nail plate or linear bands of pigmentation (melanonychia striata) are common in black (90%) and Asian (10–20%) individuals but are unusual in whites (less than 1%). Most often, the pigment is melanin, which is produced by melanocytes of a junctional nevus in the nail matrix and nail bed and is of no consequence. Extension or alteration in the pigment should be evaluated by biopsy because of the possibility of malignant change. A characteristic bluish-black to greenish coloration of the nail may be caused by *Pseudomonas* infection, particularly in association with onycholysis or chronic paronychia. The coloration is due to subungual debris and pyocyanin pigment from the bacterial organisms.

Splinter hemorrhages most often result from minor trauma but may also be associated with subacute bacterial endocarditis, vasculitis, severe rheumatoid arthritis, peptic ulcer disease, hypertension, chronic glomerulonephritis, cirrhosis, scurvy, trichinosis, malignant neoplasms, and psoriasis.

Clubbing of the nails (hippocratic nails) is characterized by swelling of the distal digit, an increase in the angle between the nail plate and the proximal nail fold (Lovibond angle) to greater than 180 degrees, and a spongy feeling when one pushes down and away from the interphalangeal joint because of an increase in fibrovascular tissue between the matrix and the phalanx. The pathogenesis is not known, but altered prostaglandin metabolism has been described. Nail clubbing is seen in association with diseases of numerous organ systems, including pulmonary, cardiovascular, gastrointestinal, and hepatic systems, and in healthy individuals as an idiopathic finding.

Habit tic deformity consists of a depression down the center of the nail with numerous horizontal ridges extending across the nail from it. Usually, one or both thumbs are involved as a result of chronic rubbing and picking at the nail with an adjacent finger.

Fungal infection of the nails has been classified into four types. *White superficial onychomycosis* presents with diffuse or speckled white discoloration of the surface of the toenails. It is caused primarily by *Trichophyton mentagrophytes* and involves invasion of the nail plate. The organism may be scraped off the nail plate with a blade, but treatment is best accomplished by the addition of a topical azole antifungal agent. *Distal subungual onychomycosis* presents with foci of onycholysis under the distal nail plate or along the lateral nail groove, followed by development of hyperkeratosis and yellow-brown discoloration. The process extends proximally, resulting in nail plate thickening, crumbling, and separation from the nail bed. *T. rubrum* and *T. mentagrophytes* are most common on toenails; fingernail disease is almost exclusively due to *T. rubrum*, which may be associated with superficial scaling of the plantar surface of the feet and usually of one hand. These dermatophytes are found most readily at the most proximal area of the nail bed or adjacent ventral portion of the nail plates that are involved. Topical therapies alone are ineffective in most cases, but nail evulsion in combination with topical antifungal agents may be effective. Oral griseofulvin, ketoconazole, or the newer agents terbinafine or itraconazole may also be effective but require several months of use. The risks, most concerning of which is hepatic toxicity, and costs of oral therapy must be weighed carefully against the benefits of treatment for a condition that generally causes only cosmetic problems.

Proximal white subungual onychomycosis occurs when the organism, generally *T. rubrum, T. megninii, T. schoenleinii,* or *Epidermophyton floccosum,* enters the nail through the proximal nail fold, producing yellow-white portions of the undersurface of the nail plate. The surface of the nail is unaffected. This occurs almost exclusively in immunocompromised patients and is a well-recognized manifestation of acquired immunodeficiency syndrome (AIDS).

Candidal onychomycosis involves the entire nail plate in patients with chronic mucocutaneous candidiasis. It is also commonly seen in patients with AIDS. The organism, generally *Candida albicans,* enters distally or along the lateral nail folds; rapidly involves the entire thickness of the nail plate; and produces thickening, crumbling, and deformity of the plate. Topical azole antifungal agents may be sufficient for treatment of candidal onychomycosis in the immunocompetent host, but oral antifungal agents are necessary for treatment of those with immune deficiencies.

Paronychial inflammation may be acute or chronic and generally involves one or two nail folds on the fingers. Acute paronychia presents with erythema, warmth, edema, and tenderness of the proximal nail fold, most commonly as a result of pathogenic staphylococci or streptococci. Warm soaks and oral antibiotics such as clindamycin or amoxicillin plus clavulanic acid are generally effective; incision and drainage may be necessary in some cases. Development of chronic paronychia is favored by prolonged immersion in water, such as occurs in finger or thumb sucking; exposure to irritating solutions; nail fold trauma; or diseases including Raynaud phenomenon, collagen-vascular diseases, or diabetes. Swelling of the proximal nail fold is followed by separation of the nail fold from the underlying nail plate and suppuration. Foreign material, embedded in the dermis of the nail fold, becomes a nidus for inflammation and infection with *Candida* species and mixed bacterial flora. A combination of attention to predisposing factors; meticulous drying of the hands, including use of 4% thymol solution; and long-term antifungal, antibacterial, and topical anti-inflammatory agents may be required for successful treatment of chronic paronychia. The primary chancre of syphilis also may present on the finger as a relatively nontender paronychia.

Ingrown nails occur when the lateral edge of the nail, including spicules that have separated from the nail plate, penetrates the soft tissue of the lateral nail fold. Erythema, edema, and pain, most often involving the lateral great toes, are noted acutely; recurrent episodes may lead to formation of granulation tissue. Predisposing factors include compression of the side of the toe from poorly fitting shoes, particularly if the great toes are abnormally long and the lateral nail folds are prominent, and improper cutting of the nail in a curvilinear manner rather than straight across. Management includes proper fitting of shoes; allowing the nail to grow out beyond the free edge before cutting it straight across; warm water soaks; oral antibiotics if there is cellulitis of the lateral nail fold; and, in severe, recurrent cases, application of silver nitrate to granulation tissue, nail avulsion, or excision of the lateral aspect of the nail followed by matricectomy.

Tumors in the paronychial area include pyogenic granulomas, mucous cysts, subungual exostoses, and junctional nevi. Periungual fibromas that appear during late childhood should suggest a diagnosis of tuberous sclerosis.

Nail-patella syndrome is an autosomal dominant disorder in which the nails are 30–50% their normal size and often have triangular or pyramidal lunulas. The thumbnails are always involved, although in some cases only the ulnar half of the nail may be affected or may be missing. The nails, from the index finger to the little finger, are progressively less damaged. The patella is also smaller than usual, which may lead to knee instability. Bony spines arising from the posterior aspect of the iliac bones, overextension of joints, skin laxity, hyperhidrosis, and renal anomalies may also be present.

Pachyonychia congenita (see Chapter 608).

Yellow nail syndrome presents with thickened, excessively curved, slow-growing, yellow nails without lunulas. All nails are affected in most cases. Associated systemic disease includes bronchiectasis, recurrent bronchitis, chylothorax, and focal edema of the limbs and face. Deficient lymphatic drainage, due to hypoplastic lymphatic vessels, is believed to lead to the manifestations of this syndrome.

Barth JH, Dawber RPR: Diseases of the nails in children. Pediatr Dermatol 12:275, 1987.
DeCoste SD, Imber MJ, Baden HP: Yellow nail syndrome. J Am Acad Dermatol 22:608, 1990.
Hazelrigg DE, Duncan C, Jarrett M: Twenty-nail dystrophy of childhood. Arch Dermatol 113:73, 1977.
Juhlin L, Baran R. *In*: Baran R, Dawber RPR (eds): Diseases of the Nails and Their Management. Oxford, Blackwell Scientific Publications, 1984, p 303.
Peluso AM, Tosti A, Piraccini BM, et al: Lichen planus limited to the nails in childhood: Case report and literature review. Pediatr Dermatol 10:36, 1993.
Stone OJ, Mullins JF: Chronic paronychia in childhood. Clin Pediatr 7:104, 1968.
Turano AF: Beau's lines in infancy. Pediatrics 41:996, 1968.

CHAPTER 614
Disorders of the Mucous Membranes

Gary L. Darmstadt and Al Lane

The mucous membranes may be involved in developmental disorders, infections, acute and chronic skin diseases, genodermatoses, and benign and malignant tumors. Some of the more common and distinctive diseases specific to mucous membranes are presented in this chapter.

CHEILITIS. Inflammation of the lips (cheilitis) and angles of the mouth (angular cheilitis or perlèche) are most commonly due to dryness, chapping, and lip licking; excessive salivation and drooling, particularly in children with neurologic deficits, may also cause chronic irritation. Lesions of oral thrush may occasionally extend to the angles of the mouth. Protection can be provided by frequent applications of a bland ointment such as petrolatum. Candidosis should be treated with an appropriate antifungal agent, and contact dermatitis of the perioral skin should be treated with a mild topical corticosteroid preparation and an emollient.

FORDYCE SPOTS. These are asymptomatic, minute, yellow-white papules on the vermilion border of the lips and buccal mucosa. They are ectopic sebaceous glands, may be found in otherwise normal individuals, and require no therapy.

MUCOCELE. Mucous retention cysts are painless, bluish, fluctuant, tense, 2–10-mm papules on the lips, tongue, palate, or buccal mucosa. Traumatic severance of the duct of a minor salivary gland leads to submucosal retention of mucous secretion. Those on the floor of the mouth are known as *ranulas* when the submaxillary or sublingual salivary ducts are involved. Fluctuations in size are usual, and the lesions may disappear temporarily after traumatic rupture. Mucoceles must be excised to prevent recurrence.

APHTHOUS STOMATITIS (Canker Sores). Solitary or multiple painful ulcerations occur on the labial, buccal, or lingual mucosa and on the sublingual, palatal, or gingival mucosa. Lesions may present initially as erythematous, indurated papules that erode rapidly to form sharply circumscribed, necrotic ulcers with a gray fibrinous exudate and an erythematous halo. Minor aphthous ulcers are 2–10 mm in diameter and heal spontaneously in 7–10 days. Major aphthous ulcers are greater than 10 mm in diameter and take 10–30 days to heal. A third type of aphthous ulceration is herpetiform in appearance, presenting with a few to multiple grouped 1–2-mm lesions that tend to coalesce into plaques that heal over 7–10 days. Approximately one third of patients with recurrent aphthous stomatitis have a family history of the disorder.

The *etiology* of aphthous stomatitis is probably multifactorial; the condition probably represents an oral manifestation of a number of conditions. Altered local regulation of the cell-mediated immune system, after activation and accumulation of cytotoxic T cells, may contribute to the localized mucosal breakdown. Predisposing factors include trauma, emotional stress, low serum iron or ferritin levels, deficiency of vitamin B_{12} or folate, malabsorption in association with celiac or Crohn disease, menstruation accompanied by a fall in progestogens during the luteal phase, food hypersensitivity, and allergic or toxic drug reactions. It is a common misconception that aphthous stomatitis is a manifestation of herpes simplex virus infection. Recurrent herpes infections remain localized to the lips and rarely cross the mucocutaneous junction; involvement of the oral mucosa occurs only in primary infections.

Treatment of aphthous stomatitis is palliative at best. Use of 0.2% aqueous chlorhexidine gluconate mouthwash helps to maintain oral hygiene. Relief of pain, particularly before eating, may be achieved by use of a topical anesthetic such as viscous lidocaine (Xylocaine) or an oral rinse with a solution of elixir of diphenhydramine, viscous lidocaine, and 0.5% dyclonine hydrochloride. A topical corticosteroid in a mucosal adhering agent (0.1% triamcinolone in Orabase) may help to reduce inflammation, and topical tetracycline mouthwash may also hasten healing. In severe, debilitating cases, systemic therapy with corticosteroids, colchicine, or dapsone may be helpful.

COWDEN SYNDROME (Multiple Hamartoma Syndrome). This is an autosomal dominant condition that usually presents during the 2nd or 3rd decade with smooth, pink or whitish papules on the palatal, gingival, buccal, and labial mucosae. These benign fibromas may coalesce into a cobblestoned appearance. Multiple flesh-colored papules also develop on the face, particularly around the mouth, nose, and ears; these papules are trichilemmomas, a benign neoplasm of the hair follicle. Associated findings may include acral keratotic papules, thyroid goiter, gastrointestinal polyps, fibrocystic breast nodules, and carcinoma of the breast or thyroid.

EPSTEIN PEARLS (Gingival Cysts of the Newborn). These are white keratin-containing cysts on the palatal or alveolar mucosa of approximately 80% of neonates. They cause no symptoms and are generally shed within a few weeks.

GEOGRAPHIC TONGUE (Benign Migratory Glossitis). This consists of single or multiple sharply demarcated, irregular, smooth red plaques on the dorsum of the tongue caused by transient atrophy of the filiform papillae and the surface epithelium, often with elevated, gray margins composed of intervening filiform papillae that are increased in thickness. Symptoms of mild burning or irritation may occasionally be bothersome. Onset is rapid, and the pattern may change over hours to days. Geographic tongue is associated with scrotal tongue in nearly 50% of patients. Some patients have atopy; some feel that the condition is exacerbated by stress or by hot or spicy foods; and some have anemia, diabetes mellitus, Reiter disease, seborrheic dermatitis, or pustular psoriasis. Geographic tongue may be an oral manifestation of pustular psoriasis, with which it shares histologic features. No therapy other than reassurance is necessary.

SCROTAL (FISSURED) TONGUE. Approximately 1% of infants and 2.5% of children have many folds with deep grooves on the dorsal tongue that impart a pebbled or wrinkled appearance. Some cases are congenital, caused by incomplete fusion of the two halves of the tongue; others develop in association with infection, trauma, malnutrition, or low vitamin A levels. Many patients with fissured tongue also have geographic tongue. Food particles and debris may become trapped in the fissures, resulting in irritation, inflammation, and halitosis. Careful cleansing with a mouth rinse and soft-bristled toothbrush is recommended.

BLACK HAIRY TONGUE. This is a dark coating on the dorsum of the tongue caused by hyperplasia and elongation of the filiform papillae; overgrowth of chromogenic bacteria and fungi and entrapped pigmented residues that adsorb to microbial plaque and desquamating keratin may contribute to the dark coloration. Changes often begin posteriorly and extend anteriorly on the dorsum of the tongue. The condition is most common in adults but may also present during adolescence. Poor oral hygiene and bacterial overgrowth, treatment with systemic antibiotics such as tetracycline (which promotes the growth of *Candida* species), and smoking are predisposing factors. Improved oral hygiene and brushing with a soft-bristled toothbrush may be all that are necessary for treatment. The filiform hyperplasia may also be decreased with topical keratolytic agents such as trichloroacetic acid, urea, or podophyllin.

ORAL HAIRY LEUKOPLAKIA. This occurs in approximately 25% of patients with acquired immunodeficiency syndrome but is rare in the pediatric population. It presents as a white thickening and accentuation of the normal vertical folds of the lateral margins of the tongue. The mucosa is white and irregularly thickened but remains soft. Spread may occur occasionally to the ventral tongue, floor of the mouth, tonsillar pillars, and pharynx. The plaques have no malignant potential. The disorder occurs predominantly in human immunodeficiency virus–infected patients but may also be found in individuals who are immunosuppressed for other reasons, such as organ transplantation or leukemia and chemotherapy. The condition is generally asymptomatic and does not require therapy. Resolution of the plaques may be hastened, however, by use of topical or systemic antifungal agents, especially if *Candida* infection plays a secondary role; antiviral agents such as acyclovir; or local application of 0.1% vitamin A acid twice daily.

VINCENT GINGIVITIS (Acute Necrotizing Ulcerative Gingivitis, Fusospirochetal Gingivitis, Trench Mouth). This disorder presents with punched-out ulceration, necrosis, and bleeding of interdental papillae. A grayish-white pseudomembrane may cover the ulcerations. Lesions may spread to involve the buccal mucosa, lips, tongue, tonsils, and pharynx and may be associated with dental pain, a bad taste, low-grade fever, and lymphadenopathy. It presents most commonly during the 2nd or 3rd decade, particularly in the context of poor dental hygiene, scurvy, or pellagra. A synergistic association between fusospirochetal organisms *(Fusobacterium nucleatum)* and *Borrelia vincenti* has been proposed to contribute to the pathogenesis.

Noma is a severe form of fusospirillary gangrenous stomatitis that presents primarily in malnourished children 2–5 yr of age who have had a preceding illness such as measles, scarlet fever, tuberculosis, malignancy, or immunodeficiency. It presents as a painful, red, indurated papule on the alveolar margin, followed by ulceration and mutilating gangrenous destruction of tissue in the oronasal region. The process may also involve the scalp, neck, shoulders, perineum, and vulva. *Noma neonatorum* presents in the 1st mo of life with gangrenous lesions of the lips, nose, mouth, and anal regions. Affected infants are usually small for gestational age, malnourished, premature, and frequently ill, particularly with *Pseudomonas aeruginosa* sepsis. Care consists of nutritional support, conservative débridement of necrotic soft tissues, empirical broad-spectrum antibiotics such as penicillin and metronidazole, and in the case of noma neonatorum, antipseudomonal antibiotics.

Herbert AA, Berg JH: Oral mucous membrane diseases of childhood: I. Mucositis and xerostomia. II. Recurrent aphthous stomatitis. III. Herpetic stomatitis. Semin Dermatol 11:80, 1992.

Itin PH, Bircher AJ, Litzisdorf Y, et al: Oral hairy leukoplakia in a child: Confirmation of the clinical diagnosis by ultrastructural examination of exfoliative cytologic specimens. Dermatology 189:167, 1994.

Prose NS: Mucocutaneous disease in pediatric human immunodeficiency virus infection. Pediatr Clin North Am 38:977, 1991.

Sigal MJ, Mock D: Symptomatic benign migratory glossitis: Report of two cases and literature review. Pediatr Dent 14:392, 1992.

CHAPTER 615

Cutaneous Bacterial Infections

Gary L. Darmstadt and Al Lane

Skin complaints or findings are noted in 20–30% of children who attend general pediatric clinics. Bacterial skin infection is the single most common diagnosis among those with skin problems, accounting for 17% of all clinic visits. The most common bacterial skin infection of children is impetigo, which makes up approximately 10% of all skin problems.

IMPETIGO (see Chapter 174)

CLINICAL MANIFESTATIONS. Nonbullous Impetigo. There are two classic forms of impetigo: nonbullous and bullous. Nonbullous impetigo accounts for more than 70% of cases. Lesions typically begin on skin of the face or extremities that has been traumatized. The most common lesions that precede nonbullous impetigo include chickenpox, insect bites, abrasions, lacerations, and burns. A tiny vesicle or pustule forms initially (Fig. 615–1*A*) and rapidly develops into a honey-colored crusted plaque that is generally less than 2 cm in diameter (Fig. 615–1*B*). The infection may be spread to other parts of the body by the fingers, clothing, and towels. Lesions are associated with little to no pain or surrounding erythema, and constitutional symptoms are generally absent. Pruritus occurs occasionally, regional adenopathy is found in up to 90% of cases, and leukocytosis is present in approximately 50% of patients. Without treatment, most cases resolve spontaneously without scarring within approximately 2 wk. The differential diagnosis of nonbullous impetigo includes viral (herpes simplex, varicella zoster), fungal (tinea corporis, kerion), and parasitic infections (scabies, pediculosis capitis), all of which may become impetiginized.

Staphylococcus aureus is the predominant organism of nonbullous impetigo in the United States; group A β-hemolytic streptococci (GABHS) are implicated in the development of some lesions. Staphylococci generally spread from the nose to normal skin and then infect the skin. In contrast, the skin becomes colonized with GABHS an average of 10 days before development of impetigo. GABHS then colonize the nasopharynx an average of 2–3 wk after the appearance of lesions of impetigo. The skin serves as the source for acquisition of GABHS in the respiratory tract and the probable primary source for spread of impetigo. Lesions of nonbullous impetigo that grow staphylococci in culture cannot be distinguished clinically from those that grow pure cultures of GABHS. Whereas *S. aureus* can be cultured from lesions of impetigo on children of all ages, GABHS is most commonly cultured from children of preschool age and is unusual before 2 yr of age, except in highly endemic areas. The staphylococcal types that cause nonbullous impetigo are variable but are not generally from phage group 2, the group that is associated with scalded skin and toxic shock syndromes. Several serotypes of GABHS, termed "impetigo strains," are found most frequently in lesions of nonbullous impetigo and are different from those that cause pharyngitis.

Bullous Impetigo. This is mainly an infection of infants and young children. Bullous impetigo is always caused by coagulase-positive *S. aureus;* approximately 80% are from phage group 2, among which 60% are type 71, and most of the remainder are types 3A, 3B, 3C, and 55. Flaccid, transparent bullae develop most commonly on skin of the face, buttocks, trunk, perineum, and extremities; neonatal bullous impetigo can begin in the diaper area. Rupture of bullae occurs easily, leaving a narrow rim of scale at the edge of a shallow, moist erosion. Surrounding erythema and regional adenopathy are generally absent. Unlike those of nonbullous impetigo, lesions of bullous impetigo are a manifestation of localized staphylococcal scalded skin syndrome and develop on intact skin.

DIAGNOSIS. Cultures of fluid from an intact blister should yield the causative agent; when the patient appears ill, blood cultures should also be obtained. On histopathologic examination, lesions of bullous impetigo show vesicle formation in the subcorneal or granular region, neutrophils and occasionally acantholytic cells within the blister, spongiosis, edema of the papillary dermis, and a mixed infiltrate of lymphocytes and neutrophils around blood vessels of the superficial plexus. Unless staphylococci can be cultured from the bullae or, less commonly, can be seen on Gram stain, it may be impossible to differentiate bullous impetigo from pemphigus foliaceous or subcorneal pustular dermatosis histopathologically. Nonbullous impetigo has histopathologic findings similar to those of the bullous variant, except that blister formation is slight.

The *differential diagnosis* of bullous impetigo in the neonate includes epidermolysis bullosa, bullous mastocytosis, herpetic infection, and early scalded skin syndrome. In older children, allergic contact dermatitis, burns, erythema multiforme, chronic bullous dermatosis of childhood, pemphigus, and bullous pemphigoid must be considered, particularly if the lesions do not respond to therapy.

COMPLICATIONS. Potential but rare complications of either nonbullous or bullous impetigo include osteomyelitis, septic arthritis, pneumonia, and septicemia; positive blood cultures are rare. Cellulitis has been reported in approximately 10% of patients with nonbullous impetigo but rarely follows the bullous form. Lymphangitis, suppurative lymphadenitis, guttate psoriasis, and scarlet fever may follow streptococcal disease occasionally. There is no correlation between number of lesions and clinical involvement of the lymphatics or development of cellulitis in association with streptococcal impetigo.

Infection with nephritogenic strains of GABHS may result in acute poststreptococcal glomerulonephritis. The clinical character of impetigo lesions is not different between those that lead to poststreptococcal glomerulonephritis and those that do not. The most commonly affected age group is school-aged children 3–7 yr old. The latent period from onset of impetigo to development of poststreptococcal glomerulonephritis averages 18–21 days, which is longer than the 10-day latency period after pharyngitis. Poststreptococcal glomerulo-

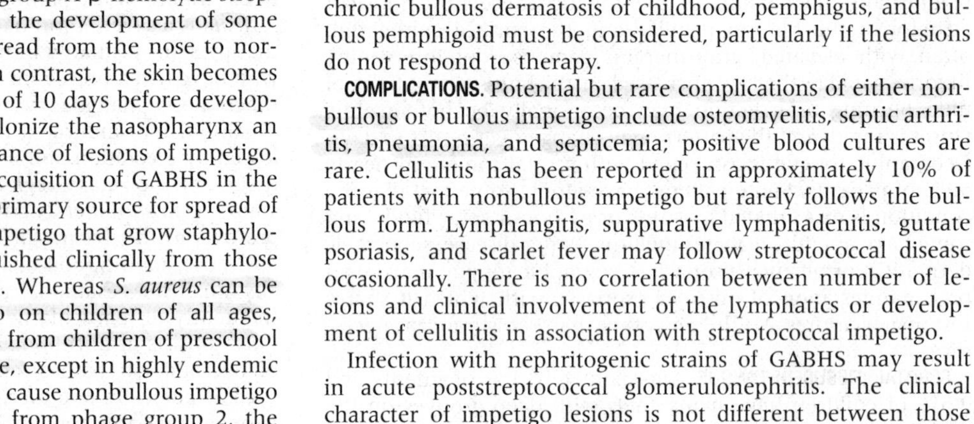

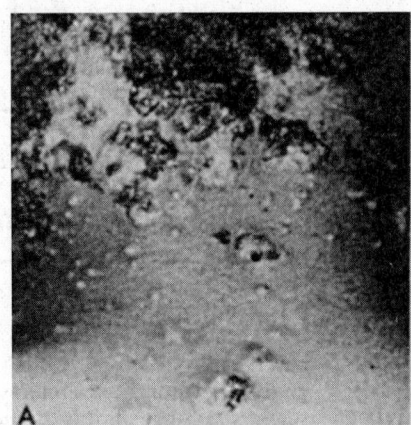

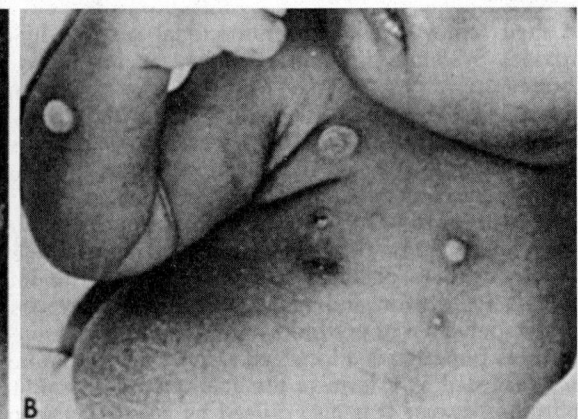

Figure 615–1. *A,* Multiple crusted and oozing lesions of streptococcal impetigo. *B,* Multiple tense and flaccid blisters of bullous impetigo on the trunk and arm of an infant.

nephritis occurs epidemically after either pharyngeal or skin infection. Impetigo-associated epidemics are caused by M groups 2, 49, 53, 55, 56, 57, and 60. Strains of GABHS that are associated with endemic impetigo in the United States have little or no nephritogenic potential. Acute rheumatic fever does not occur as a result of impetigo.

TREATMENT. Topical or systemic antibiotic treatment is superior to placebo or cleansing with 3% hexachlorophene soap. Furthermore, cleansing with 3% hexachlorophene soap adds little to no benefit over systemic antibiotics alone. Mupirocin is an ointment that is bactericidal by reversible inhibition of bacterial isoleucyl-transfer RNA synthetase. Applied topically three times daily for 7–10 days, it is equal to or greater in effectiveness, with fewer side effects, than oral erythromycin ethylsuccinate, 30–50 mg/kg/24 hr for 7–10 days, for treatment of impetigo in children. Rare instances of bacterial resistance to mupirocin have been reported, but most patients were treated irregularly and/or prophylactically for more than 2 wk.

In patients with widespread involvement; lesions near the mouth, where topical medication may be licked off; or evidence of deep involvement, including cellulitis, furunculosis, abscess formation, or suppurative lymphadenitis, systemic therapy with a β-lactamase–resistant oral antibiotic should be prescribed. In areas without a high prevalence of *S. aureus* resistance to erythromycin, erythromycin ethylsuccinate (40 mg/kg/24 hr divided three to four times daily for 7 days) or erythromycin estolate (30 mg/kg/24 hr divided three to four times daily) is the preferred oral therapy. If there is widespread erythromycin resistance in the community, alternative oral antibiotics that have been shown to be effective in children for treatment of impetigo include dicloxacillin; amoxicillin plus clavulanic acid; clindamycin; and a cephalosporin such as cephalexin, cefaclor, cefadroxil, cefprozil, or cefpodoxime. The choice among these various agents may be guided primarily by issues of cost, local availability, and compliance. The macrolide clarithromycin may be advantageous primarily in instances of intolerance to erythromycin but will not provide cure rates superior to those of erythromycin. There is no evidence to suggest that a 10-day course of therapy is superior to a 7-day one. If a satisfactory clinical response is not achieved within 7 days, however, a culture should be taken by swabbing beneath the lifted edge of a crusted lesion. If a resistant organism is detected, an appropriate antibiotic should be given for an additional 7 days.

STAPHYLOCOCCAL SCALDED SKIN SYNDROME

(Ritter Disease)

CLINICAL MANIFESTATIONS. Staphylococcal scalded skin syndrome occurs predominantly in infants and children under 5 yr of age and includes a range of disease from localized bullous impetigo to generalized cutaneous involvement with systemic illness. Onset of the rash may be preceded by malaise, fever, irritability, and exquisite tenderness of the skin. Scarlatiniform erythema develops diffusely and is accentuated in flexural and periorificial areas. The conjunctivae are inflamed and occasionally become purulent. The brightly erythematous skin may rapidly acquire a wrinkled appearance, and in severe cases sterile, flaccid blisters and erosions develop diffusely. Characteristically, circumoral erythema is prominent, as is radial crusting and fissuring around the eyes, mouth, and nose. At this stage, areas of epidermis may separate in response to gentle shear force (Nikolsky sign). As large sheets of epidermis peel away, moist, glistening, denuded areas become apparent, initially in the flexures and subsequently over much of the body surface (Fig. 615–2 [color plate section]). This may lead to secondary cutaneous infection, sepsis, and fluid and electrolyte disturbances. The desquamative phase begins after 2–5 days of cutaneous erythema; healing occurs without scarring in 10–14 days. There may be pharyngitis, conjunctivitis, and superficial erosions of the lips, but intraoral mucosal surfaces are spared. Although some patients appear ill, many are reasonably comfortable except for the marked skin tenderness.

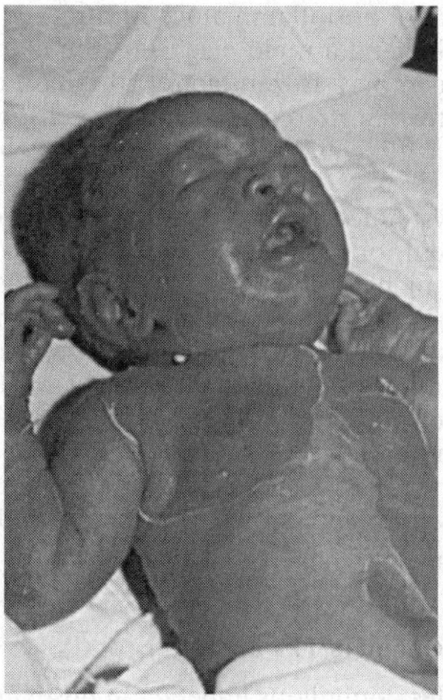

Figure 615–2. Infant with staphylococcal scalded skin syndrome. See also color section.

A presumed abortive form of the disease presents with diffuse, scarlatiniform, tender erythroderma, which is accentuated in the flexural areas, but does not progress to blister formation. In these patients, the Nikolsky sign may be absent. Although the exanthem is similar to that of streptococcal scarlet fever, strawberry tongue and palatal petechiae are absent. Staphylococcal scalded skin syndrome may be mistaken for a number of other blistering and exfoliating disorders, including bullous impetigo, epidermolysis bullosa, epidermolytic hyperkeratosis, pemphigus, drug eruption, erythema multiforme, and drug-induced toxic epidermal necrolysis. Toxic epidermal necrolysis can often be distinguished by a history of drug ingestion, presence of the Nikolsky sign only at sites of erythema, absence of perioral crusting, full-thickness epidermal necrosis, and a blister cleavage plane in the lowermost epidermis.

ETIOLOGY AND PATHOGENESIS. Staphylococcal scalded skin syndrome is caused predominantly by phage group 2 staphylococci, particularly strains 71 and 55, which are present at localized sites of infection. Foci of infection include the nasopharynx and, less commonly, the umbilicus, urinary tract, a superficial abrasion, conjunctivae, and blood. The clinical manifestations of staphylococcal scalded skin syndrome are mediated by hematogenous spread, in the absence of specific antitoxin antibody, of staphylococcal epidermolytic or exfoliative toxins A or B. The toxins have reproduced the disease in both animal models and human volunteers. Decreased renal clearance of the toxins may account for the fact that the disease is most common in infants and young children. Epidermolytic toxin A is heat stable and is encoded by bacterial chromosomal genes; epidermolytic toxin B is heat labile and is encoded on a 37.5-kilobase plasmid. Histopathologically, the site of blister cleavage is subcorneal through the granular layer. The epidermolytic toxins appear to produce the granular layer split by binding to desmoglein I within desmosomes. There is evidence that the toxins are members of the trypsin-like serine protease family and may exert their action through proteolysis.

DIAGNOSIS. Intact bullae are consistently sterile, unlike those of bullous impetigo, but cultures should be obtained from all suspected sites of localized infection and from the blood to identify the source for elaboration of the epidermolytic toxins. The subcorneal, granular layer split can be identified on skin biopsy; absence of an inflammatory infiltrate is characteristic. In cases that demand a rapid diagnosis, the exfoliated corneal layer can be seen on a frozen biopsy specimen of the desquamating epidermis. Scattered acantholytic cells, which are evident in the cleftlike bullae, can also be seen in a Tzanck preparation.

TREATMENT. Systemic therapy, either orally, in cases of localized involvement, or parenterally, with a semi-synthetic penicillinase-resistant penicillin, should be prescribed because the staphylococci are usually penicillin resistant. The skin should be gently moistened and cleansed with Burow solution, Dakin solution, or isotonic saline. Application of an emollient provides lubrication and decreases discomfort. Topical antibiotics are unnecessary. Recovery is usually rapid, but complications such as excessive fluid loss, electrolyte imbalance, faulty temperature regulation, pneumonia, septicemia, and cellulitis may cause increased morbidity.

ECTHYMA (see Chapters 175 and 184)

This resembles nonbullous impetigo in onset and appearance but gradually evolves into a deeper, more chronic infection. The initial lesion is a vesicle or vesiculopustule with an erythematous base that erodes through the epidermis into the dermis to form an ulcer with elevated margins. The ulcer becomes obscured by a dry, heaped-up, tightly adherent crust that contributes to the persistence of the infection and scar formation. Lesions may be spread by autoinoculation, may be as large as 4 cm, and occur most frequently on the legs. Predisposing factors include pruritic lesions, such as insect bites, scabies, or pediculosis, which are subject to frequent scratching; poor hygiene; and malnutrition. Complications include lymphangitis, cellulitis, and rarely poststreptococcal glomerulonephritis. The causative agent is usually GABHS; *S. aureus* is also cultured from most lesions but is probably a secondary pathogen. Crusts should be softened with warm compresses and removed with an antibacterial soap. Systemic antibiotic therapy, as for impetigo, is indicated; almost all lesions are responsive to treatment with penicillin.

Ecthyma gangrenosa is a necrotic ulcer covered with a gray-black eschar. It is usually a sign of *Pseudomonas aeruginosa* sepsis and usually occurs in immunosuppressed patients. Ecthyma gangrenosum occurs in up to 6% of patients with systemic *P. aeruginosa* infection but can also occur as a primary cutaneous infection by inoculation. The lesion begins as a red or purpuric macule that vesiculates and then ulcerates; there is a surrounding rim of pink to violaceous skin. The punched-out ulcer develops raised edges with a dense, black, depressed, crusted center. Lesions may be single or multiple; patients with bacteremia commonly have lesions in apocrine areas. Clinically similar lesions may also develop as a result of infection with other agents such as *S. aureus, Aeromonas hydrophila, Enterobacter* species, *Proteus* species, *Pseudomonas cepacia, Serratia marcescens, Aspergillus* species, Mucorales, *Escherichia coli,* and *Candida* species. Histopathologic examination reveals bacterial invasion of the adventitia and media of dermal veins but not arteries; the intima and lumina are spared. Blood cultures and skin biopsy for culture should be obtained, and empirical broad-spectrum, systemic therapy that includes coverage for *Pseudomonas* should be initiated as soon as possible.

BLASTOMYCOSIS-LIKE PYODERMA

(Pyoderma Vegetans)

This is an exuberant cutaneous reaction to bacterial infection, primarily in children who are malnourished and immunosuppressed. The organisms isolated most commonly from lesions are *S. aureus* and GABHS, but several other organisms have been associated with these lesions, including *P. aeruginosa, Proteus mirabilis,* diphtheroids, *Bacillus* species and *Clostridium perfringens.* Hyperplastic, crusted plaques on the extremities are characteristic, sometimes forming from the coalescence of multiple, pinpoint, purulent, crusted abscesses. Ulceration and sinus tract formation may develop, and additional lesions may appear at sites distant from the site of inoculation. Regional lymphadenopathy is common, but fever is not. Histopathologic examination reveals pseudoepitheliomatous hyperplasia and abscesses composed of neutrophils and/or eosinophils; giant cells are usually lacking. The differential diagnosis includes deep fungal infection, particularly blastomycosis and tuberculous and atypical mycobacterial infection. Underlying immunodeficiency should be ruled out, and the selection of antibiotics should be guided by susceptibility testing because the response to antibiotics is often poor.

BLISTERING DISTAL DACTYLITIS

This is a superficial blistering infection of the volar fat pad on the distal portion of the finger or thumb. More than one finger may be involved, as may the volar surfaces of the proximal phalanges, palms, and toes. Blisters are filled with a watery purulent fluid that contains polymorphonuclear leukocytes and chains of gram-positive cocci. There is usually no preceding history of trauma, and systemic symptoms are generally absent. Poststreptococcal glomerulonephritis has not occurred after blistering distal dactylitis. The infection is caused most commonly by GABHS but has also occurred as a result of infection with group B β-hemolytic streptococci and *S. aureus.* If left untreated, blisters may continue to enlarge and extend to the paronychial area. The infection responds to incision and drainage and a 10-day course of systemic penicillin or erythromycin therapy.

PERIANAL DERMATITIS

This presents most commonly in boys (70% of cases) between the ages of 6 mo and 10 yr as perianal dermatitis (90% of cases) and pruritus (80% of cases). The incidence of perianal dermatitis is not known precisely but ranges from 1 in 2,000 to 1 in 218 patient visits. The rash is superficial, erythematous, well marginated, nonindurated, and confluent from the anus outward. Acutely (<6-wk duration), the rash tends to be bright red, moist, and tender to touch. At this stage, a white pseudomembrane may be present. As the rash becomes more chronic, the perianal eruption may consist of painful fissures, a dried mucoid discharge, and little erythema or of psoriasiform plaques with yellow,. peripheral crust. In girls, the perianal rash may be associated with vulvovaginitis; the penis may be involved in boys. Approximately 50% of patients have rectal pain, most commonly described as burning inside the anus during defecation, and 33% have blood-streaked stools. Fecal retention is a frequent behavioral response to the infection. Patients have presented with guttate psoriasis. Although local induration or edema may occur, constitutional symptoms of fever, headache, and malaise are absent, suggesting that subcutaneous involvement, as in cellulitis, is absent. Familial spread of perianal dermatitis is common, particularly when family members bathe together or use the same water.

The *differential diagnosis* of perianal dermatitis includes psoriasis, seborrheic dermatitis, candidosis, pinworm infestation, sexual abuse, and inflammatory bowel disease. Differentiation from these other conditions can be accomplished by culturing a moderate to heavy growth of GABHS on 5% sheep blood agar; *E. coli* is frequently also isolated in these cultures. Perianal dermatitis may also be caused by *S. aureus.* Children with asymptomatic perianal colonization have light growth of GABHS on blood agar. Direct antigen studies for GABHS are also very sensitive (89%) but may be falsely negative early in the course of the disease. Acute and convalescent sera for antistreptolysin O or anti-DNase B are not helpful in making the diagnosis. The index case and family members should be cultured initially, and follow-up cultures to document bacteriologic cure after a course of treatment are also recommended.

Treatment with a single 10-day course of oral penicillin produces resolution of the dermatitis and symptoms in most patients; however, recurrence rates of 40–50% have been reported, emphasizing the need for close follow-up, including repeat culture. Erythromycin estolate and ethylsuccinate are excellent alternative treatments for those who are allergic to penicillin, who have not responded to a course of penicillin, or who are infected with *S. aureus.* Clindamycin has also been used successfully to treat recurrent perianal dermatitis. Mupirocin has been used in conjunction with oral antibiotics to treat recurrences but has not been evaluated as a single-drug therapy.

ERYSIPELAS (see Chapter 175)

FOLLICULITIS

This superficial infection of the hair follicle is most often caused by *S. aureus* (Bockhart impetigo); coagulase-negative staphylococci are the cause occasionally. The lesions are typically small, discrete, dome-shaped pustules with an erythematous base, located at the ostium of the pilosebaceous canals. Hair growth is unimpaired, and the lesions heal without scarring. Favored sites include the scalp, buttocks, and extremities. Poor hygiene, maceration, and drainage from wounds and abscesses can be provocative factors. Folliculitis can also occur as a result of tar therapy or occlusive wraps; the moist environment encourages bacterial proliferation. In human immunodeficiency virus (HIV)–infected patients, *S. aureus* may produce confluent erythematous patches with satellite pustules in intertriginous areas and violaceous plaques composed of superficial follicular pustules in the scalp, axillae or groin.

The causative organism of folliculitis can be identified by Gram stain and culture of purulent material from the follicular orifice. *Treatment* for folliculitis includes topical antibiotic cleansers such as chlorhexidine or hexachlorophene. Topical antibiotic therapy is usually all that is required for mild cases, but more severe cases may require use of penicillinase-resistant systemic antibiotics such as dicloxacillin or cephalexin. In chronic recurrent folliculitis, daily application of a benzoyl peroxide lotion or gel may facilitate resolution.

Folliculitis caused by gram-negative organisms occurs primarily in patients with acne vulgaris who have been treated long term with broad-spectrum systemic antibiotics. A superficial pustular form, caused by *Klebsiella, Enterobacter, E. coli,* or *P. aeruginosa,* occurs around the nose and spreads to the cheeks and chin. A deeper, nodular form of folliculitis on the face and trunk is caused by *Proteus.* Culture of infected follicles is necessary to establish the diagnosis. Treatment consists of incision and drainage of the deeper, larger cysts; topical neomycin or bacitracin; or selection of an oral antibiotic based on the sensitivity profile of the pathogenic organism. For severe, recalcitrant cases, 13-*cis*-retinoic acid, 1 mg/kg/24 hr, is helpful but should be administered only by experienced physicians because of side effects.

Sycosis barbae is a deeper, more severe, recurrent, inflammatory form of folliculitis caused by *S. aureus* that involves the entire depth of the follicle. Erythematous, follicular papules and pustules develop on the chin, upper lip, and angle of the jaw, primarily in young black males. Papules may coalesce into plaques, and healing may occur with scarring. Affected individuals frequently are found to be *S. aureus* carriers. Treatment with warm saline compresses and topical antibiotics such as mupirocin generally clears the infection. More extensive, recalcitrant cases may require therapy with β-lactamase–resistant systemic antibiotics and elimination of *S. aureus* from sites of carriage.

Hot tub folliculitis is attributable to *P. aeruginosa,* predominantly serotype O-11. The lesions are pruritic papules and pustules or deeply erythematous to violaceous nodules that develop 8–48 hr after exposure and are most dense in areas covered by a bathing suit. Patients occasionally develop fever, malaise, and lymphadenopathy. The organism is readily cultured from pus. The eruption usually resolves spontaneously within 1–2 wk, often leaving postinflammatory hyperpigmentation, but sometimes topical agents with antipseudomonal activity, such as potassium permanganate and gentamicin cream, are necessary. Consideration should be given to use of systemic antibiotics (e.g., ciprofloxacin) in patients with constitutional symptoms.

FURUNCLES AND CARBUNCLES

These follicular lesions may originate from a preceding folliculitis or may arise initially as a deep-seated, tender, erythematous, perifollicular nodule. Although lesions are initially indurated, central necrosis and suppuration follow, leading to rupture and discharge of a central core of necrotic tissue and destruction of the follicle. Healing occurs with scar formation. Sites of predilection are hair-bearing areas on the face, neck, axillae, buttocks, and groin. Pain may be intense if the lesion is situated in an area where the skin is relatively fixed, such as in the external auditory canal or over the nasal cartilages. Patients with furuncles usually have no constitutional symptoms; occasionally, however, bacteremia may ensue. Rarely, lesions on the upper lip or cheek may lead to cavernous sinus thrombosis. Infection of a group of contiguous follicles, with multiple drainage points, accompanied by inflammatory changes in surrounding connective tissue is termed a carbuncle. Carbuncles may be accompanied by fever, leukocytosis, and bacteremia.

ETIOLOGY. The causative agent is almost always *S. aureus,* which penetrates abraded perifollicular skin. Conditions predisposing to furuncle formation include obesity, hyperhidrosis, maceration, friction, and pre-existing dermatitis. Furunculosis is also more common in individuals with low serum iron levels, diabetes, malnutrition, HIV infection, or other immunodeficiency states. Recurrent furunculosis is frequently associated with carriage of *S. aureus* in the nares, axillae, or perineum or close contact with someone such as a family member who is a carrier. Other bacteria or fungi may occasionally cause furuncles or carbuncles; therefore, Gram stain and culture of the pus are indicated.

TREATMENT. This should include regular bathing with antimicrobial soaps and use of loose-fitting clothing, which will minimize predisposing factors for furuncle formation. Frequent application of a hot, moist compress may facilitate drainage of lesions. Large lesions may be drained by a small incision. Carbuncles and large or multiple furuncles should be treated with systemic penicillinase-resistant antibiotics such as cloxacillin orally or oxacillin parenterally. The penicillin-allergic patient can be treated with a cephalosporin, clindamycin, or erythromycin. Treatment of recurrent cases has been successful by colonization of the individual with a less virulent strain of *S. aureus* such as 502A. The carriage state may be eliminated temporarily by application of mupirocin ointment for 5 days to the anterior nares. Attention to personal hygiene, use of an antibacterial soap, low-dose oral antistaphylococcal penicillin or clindamycin, and frequent handwashing may also be beneficial.

PITTED KERATOLYSIS

Pitted keratolysis occurs most frequently in humid tropical and subtropical climates, particularly in those whose feet are moist for prolonged periods, for example, as a result of hyperhidrosis, prolonged wearing of boots, or immersion in water. The lesions consist of 1–7-mm irregularly shaped, superficial erosions of the horny layer on the soles, particularly at weight-bearing sites. Brownish discoloration of involved areas may be apparent. The condition is nearly always asymptomatic but frequently is malodorous. A rare, painful variant manifests as thinned, erythematous to violaceous plaques in addition to the typical pitted lesions. The most likely etiologic agent is a species of *Corynebacterium.* Actinomycetes, dermatophili, and micrococci have also been isolated from lesions. Avoidance of moisture and maceration produces slow, spontaneous resolution of the infection. Therapeutic regimens that have been effective include topical application of 2% buffered glutaraldehyde, 20% formaldehyde solution (Formalin) in Aquaphor; erythromycin, clindamycin, and the imidazoles.

ERYTHRASMA

This is a benign chronic superficial infection caused by *Corynebacterium minutissimum.* Predisposing factors include heat, humidity, obesity, skin maceration, and poor hygiene. Approximately 20% of healthy individuals have involvement of the toe webs. Other frequently affected sites are moist intertriginous areas such as the groin and axillae; the inframammary and perianal regions are involved occasionally. Sharply demarcated, irregularly bordered, brownish-red, slightly scaly patches are characteristic of the disease. Mild pruritus is the only constant symptom. *C. minutissimum* is a complex of related organisms that produce porphyrins that fluoresce a brilliant coral-red color under ultraviolet light. The diagnosis is readily made, and erythrasma is differentiated from dermatophyte infection and from tinea versicolor by Wood lamp examination. Bathing within 20 hr of the Wood lamp examination, however, may remove the water-soluble porphyrins. Staining of skin scrapings with methylene blue or Gram stain reveals the pleomorphic, filamentous coccobacillary forms.

Most cases represent colonization, are asymptomatic, and require no therapy. Effective *treatment* can be achieved with topical erythromycin, clindamycin, miconazole, or Whitfield ointment, or a 10–14-day course of oral erythromycin. Recurrence may be inhibited by frequent use of an antibacterial soap or an astringent such as 10–20% aluminum chloride in anhydrous ethyl alcohol.

ERYSIPELOID

This is a rare cutaneous infection caused by inoculation of *Erysipelothrix rhusiopathiae* from contaminated animals, birds, fish, or their products. The localized cutaneous form is most common, characterized by well-demarcated, diamond-shaped, erythematous to violaceous patches at sites of inoculation. Local symptoms are generally not severe, constitutional symptoms are rare, and the lesions resolve spontaneously after weeks but can recur at the same site or develop elsewhere weeks to months later. The diffuse cutaneous form presents with lesions at several areas of the body in addition to the site of inoculation; it is also self-limited. The systemic form, caused by hematogenous spread, is accompanied by constitutional symptoms and may include endocarditis, septic arthritis, cerebral infarct and abscess, meningitis, and pulmonary effusion. Diagnosis is confirmed by skin biopsy, which reveals the gram-positive organisms, and culture. The treatment of choice is parenteral erythromycin or penicillin.

TUBERCULOSIS OF THE SKIN (see Chapters 199 and 200)

Cutaneous tuberculosis infection occurs worldwide, particularly in association with HIV infection, malnutrition, and poor hygiene. The type of cutaneous lesion that develops depends on virulence properties of the causative organism, the general health and immune responsiveness of the host, and the mode of introduction of the bacteria into the skin. Primary cutaneous tuberculosis is rare in the United States but occurs with the greatest frequency in infants and children; the overall incidence of cutaneous tuberculosis among those with all forms of tuberculosis in the United States is approximately 1–2%. All forms of cutaneous disease are caused by *Mycobacterium tuberculosis,* by *M. bovis,* and occasionally by the bacillus Calmette-Guérin (BCG), an attenuated form of *M. bovis;* the manifestations caused by a given organism are indistinguishable from one another. After invasion of the skin, mycobacteria either multiply intracellularly within macrophages, leading to progressive disease, or are controlled by the host immune reaction.

A primary lesion, a *tuberculous chancre,* results when *M. tuberculosis* or *M. bovis* gains access to the skin or mucous membranes through trauma. Sites of predilection are the face, lower extremities, and genitalia. The initial lesion develops 2–4 wk after introduction of the organism into the damaged tissue. A red-brown papule gradually enlarges to form a shallow, firm, sharply demarcated ulcer; satellite abscesses may be present. Some lesions acquire a crust resembling impetigo, and others become heaped-up and verrucous at the margins. The primary lesion occurs in one third of cases as a painless ulcer on the conjunctiva, gingiva, or palate and occasionally as a painless acute paronychia. Painless regional adenopathy appears approximately 3–8 wk after inoculation and may be accompanied by lymphangitis, lymphadenitis, or perforation of the skin surface, forming scrofuloderma. Erythema nodosum develops in approximately 10% of cases. Untreated lesions heal with scarring within approximately 12 mo but may reactivate, may form lupus vulgaris, or rarely may progress to the acute miliary form.

M. tuberculosis or *M. bovis* can be cultured from the skin lesion and local lymph nodes, but acid-fast staining of histologic sections, particularly of a well-controlled infection, often does not reveal the organism. Clinically, the differential diagnosis is broad, including a syphilitic chancre; deep fungal or atypical mycobacterial infection; leprosy; tularemia; cat-scratch disease; sporotrichosis; nocardiosis; leishmaniasis; reaction to foreign substances such as zirconium, beryllium, silk or nylon sutures, talc, or starch; papular acne rosacea; and lupus miliaris disseminatum faciei. Spontaneous healing with scarring coincides with acquisition of immunity, at which time the skin lesions and infected nodes may become calcified. Antituberculous therapy is indicated (see Chapter 199).

Direct cutaneous inoculation of the tubercle bacillus into a previously infected individual with a moderate to high degree of immunity initially produces a small papule with surrounding inflammation. *Tuberculosis verrucosa cutis* (warty tuberculosis) forms when the papule becomes hyperkeratotic and warty, and several adjacent papules coalesce or a single papule expands peripherally to form a brownish-red to violaceous, exudative, crusted, verrucous plaque. Irregular extension of the margins of the plaque produces a serpiginous border. Children have the lesion most commonly on the lower extremities after trauma and contact with infected material such as sputum or soil. Regional lymph nodes are involved only rarely. Spontaneous healing with atrophic scarring takes place slowly, over months to years; healing is also gradual with antituberculous therapy.

Lupus vulgaris is a rare, chronic, progressive form of cutaneous tuberculosis that develops in individuals with a moderate to high degree of tuberculin sensitivity induced by previous infection. The incidence is greater in cool, moist climates, particularly in females. Lupus vulgaris develops as a result of direct extension from underlying joints or lymph nodes;

through lymphatic or hematogenous spread; or rarely, by cutaneous inoculation with BCG vaccine. It most commonly follows cervical adenitis or pulmonary tuberculosis. Approximately 33% of cases are preceded by scrofuloderma, and 90% of cases present on the head and neck, most commonly on the nose or cheek; involvement of the trunk is uncommon. A typical solitary lesion consists of a brownish-red, soft papule that has an apple-jelly color when examined by diascopy. Expansion of the papule peripherally, or occasionally the coalescence of several papules, forms an irregular lesion of variable size and form. One or several lesions may develop, including nodules or plaques that are flat and serpiginous, hypertrophic and verrucous, or edematous in appearance. Spontaneous healing occurs centrally, and lesions characteristically reappear within the area of atrophy. Chronicity is characteristic, and persistence and progression of plaques over many years is common. Lymphadenitis is present in 40% of those with lupus vulgaris, and 10–20% have infection of the lungs, bones, or joints. Vegetative masses and ulceration involving the nasal, buccal, or conjunctival mucosa; the palate; the gingiva; or the oropharynx may cause extensive deformities. Squamous cell carcinoma, with a relatively high metastatic potential, may develop, usually after several years of the disease. After a temporary impairment in immunity, particularly after measles infection (i.e., *lupus exanthematicus*), multiple lesions may form at distant sites as a result of hematogenous spread from a latent focus of infection. The histopathologic changes are those of a tuberculoid granuloma without caseation, and organisms are extremely difficult to demonstrate. The differential diagnosis includes sarcoidosis, leprosy, atypical mycobacterial infection, blastomycosis, chromoblastomycosis, actinomycosis, leishmaniasis, tertiary syphilis, leprosy, hypertrophic lichen planus, psoriasis, lupus erythematosus, lymphocytoma, and Bowen disease. Small lesions can be excised; antituberculous drug therapy usually halts further spread and induces involution.

Scrofuloderma results from enlargement, cold abscess formation, and breakdown of a lymph node, most frequently in a cervical chain, with extension to the overlying skin. Linear or serpiginous ulcers and dissecting fistulas and subcutaneous tracts studded with soft nodules may develop. Spontaneous healing may take years, eventuating in cordlike keloidal scars; lupus vulgaris may also develop. Scrofuloderma of a cervical lymph node often originates in the larynx and was linked in the past to ingestion of milk containing *M. bovis.* Lesions may also originate from an underlying infected joint, tendon, bone, or epididymis. The differential diagnosis includes syphilitic gumma, deep fungal infections, actinomycosis, and hidradenitis suppurativa. The course is indolent, and constitutional symptoms are typically absent. Antituberculous therapy is usually effective.

Orificial tuberculosis presents on the mucous membranes and periorificial skin after autoinoculation of mycobacteria from sites of progressive infection; it is a sign of advanced internal disease and carries a poor prognosis. Lesions appear as yellowish or red, painful nodules that form punched-out ulcers with inflammation and edema of the surrounding mucosa. Treatment consists of identification of the source of infection and initiation of antituberculous therapy.

Miliary tuberculosis (hematogenous primary tuberculosis) rarely presents cutaneously, most commonly in infants and in individuals who are immunosuppressed after chemotherapy or infection with measles or HIV. The eruption consists of crops of symmetrically distributed, minute, erythematous to purpuric macules, papules, or vesicles. The lesions may ulcerate, drain, crust, and form sinus tracts or may form subcutaneous gummas, especially in malnourished children with impaired immunity. Constitutional signs and symptoms are common, and a leukemoid reaction or aplastic anemia may develop. Tubercle bacilli are readily identified in an active lesion. A fulminant course should be anticipated, and aggressive antituberculous therapy is indicated.

Single or multiple *metastatic tuberculous abscesses* (tuberculous gummas) may develop on the extremities and trunk by hematogenous spread from a primary focus of infection during a period of decreased immunity, particularly in malnourished and immunosuppressed children. The fluctuant, nontender, erythematous subcutaneous nodules may ulcerate and form fistulas.

Vaccination with BCG characteristically produces a papule approximately 2 wk after vaccination. The papule expands in size, typically ulcerates within 2–4 mo, and heals slowly with scarring. In approximately 1–2 per million vaccinations, a complication caused specifically by the BCG organism occurs, including regional lymphadenitis, lupus vulgaris, scrofuloderma, and subcutaneous abscess formation.

Tuberculids are skin reactions that exhibit tuberculoid features histologically but do not contain detectable mycobacteria. The lesions appear in a host who usually has moderate to strong tuberculin reactivity, has a history of previous tuberculosis of other organs, and usually but not always shows a therapeutic response to antituberculous therapy. The cause of tuberculids is poorly understood. Most patients are in good health with no clear focus of disease at the time of the eruption. The most commonly observed tuberculid is the *papulonecrotic tuberculid.* Recurrent crops of symmetrically distributed, asymptomatic, firm, sterile, dusky-red papules appear on the extensor aspects of the limbs, the dorsum of the hands and feet, and the buttocks. The papules may undergo central ulceration and eventually heal, leaving sharply delineated, circular, depressed scars. The duration of the eruption is variable, but disappearance usually occurs promptly following treatment of the primary infection. *Lichen scrofulosorum,* another form of tuberculid, is characterized by asymptomatic, grouped, pinhead-sized, often follicular, pink or red papules that form discoid plaques, mainly on the trunk. Healing occurs without scarring.

Atypical mycobacterial infection may cause cutaneous lesions in children. *M. marinum* is found in salt and freshwater and diseased fish; in the United States, it is most commonly acquired from tropical fish tanks and swimming pools. Traumatic abrasion of the skin serves as a portal of entry for the organism. Approximately 3 wk after inoculation, a single reddish papule develops and enlarges slowly to form a violaceous nodule or occasionally a warty plaque. The lesion occasionally breaks down to form a crusted ulcer or a suppurating abscess. Sporotrichoid erythematous nodules along lymphatics may also suppurate and drain. Lesions are most common on the elbows, knees, and feet of swimmers and the hands and fingers in aquarium-acquired infection. Systemic signs and symptoms are absent; regional lymph nodes occasionally become slightly enlarged but do not break down. Rarely, the infection becomes disseminated, particularly in an immunosuppressed host. A biopsy specimen of a fully developed lesion demonstrates a granulomatous infiltrate with tuberculoid architecture; intracellular organisms can usually be identified within the histiocytes with appropriate stains. The most effective antituberculous regimens include tetracycline, minocycline, and rifampin plus ethambutol. Application of heat to the affected site may be a useful adjunctive therapy. Spontaneous healing with scarring can be expected within several months to 2 years (see Chapter 200).

M. kansasii primarily causes pulmonary disease; skin disease is rare, often occurring in an immunocompromised host. Most commonly, sporotrichoid nodules develop after inoculation of traumatized skin. Lesions may develop into ulcerated, crusted, or verrucous plaques. The organism is relatively sensitive to antituberculous medications, which should be chosen on the basis of susceptibility testing.

M. scrofulaceum causes cervical lymphadenitis (scrofuloderma) in young children, typically in the submandibular region. Nodes enlarge over several weeks, ulcerate, and drain. The local reaction is nontender and circumscribed, constitutional symptoms are absent, and there generally is no evidence of lung or other organ involvement. Other atypical mycobacteria may cause a similar presentation, including *M. avium* complex, *M. kansasii,* and *M. fortuitum.* Treatment is accomplished by excision and antituberculous drugs (see Chapter 200).

M. ulcerans causes a painless, subcutaneous nodule after inoculation of abraded skin. Most infections occur in children in tropical rain forests. The nodule usually ulcerates, develops undermined edges, and may spread over large areas, most commonly on an extremity. Local necrosis of subcutaneous fat, producing a septal panniculitis, is characteristic. Ulcers persist for months to years before healing spontaneously with scarring and sometimes with lymphedema. Constitutional symptoms and lymphadenopathy are absent. Diagnosis is made by culturing the organism at 32–33° C. Treatment of choice is early excision of the lesion. Local heat therapy and oral chemotherapy may benefit some patients.

M. avium complex, composed of more than 20 subtypes, most commonly causes chronic pulmonary infection; cervical lymphadenitis and osteomyelitis occur occasionally; and papules or purulent leg ulcers occur rarely by primary inoculation. Skin lesions may be an early sign of disseminated infection; the lesions may take various forms, including erythematous papules, pustules, nodules, abscesses, ulcers, panniculitis, and sporotrichoid spread along lymphatics. For treatment, see Chapters 200 and 223.

M. fortuitum complex is composed of two organisms: *M. fortuitum* and *M. chelonei.* These organisms cause disease in an immunocompetent host principally by primary cutaneous inoculation after traumatic injury, injection, or surgery. A nodule, abscess, or cellulitis develops 4–6 wk after inoculation. In an immunocompromised host, multiple subcutaneous nodules may form that break down and drain. Treatment is based on identification and susceptibility testing of the organism.

Amon RB, Dimond RL: Toxic epidermal necrolysis; rapid differentiation between staphylococcal and drug-induced disease. Arch Dermatol 111:1433, 1975.

Amren DP, Anderson AS, Wannamaker LW: Perianal cellulitis associated with group A streptococci. Am J Dis Child 112:546, 1966.

Anthony BF, Kaplan EL, Wannamaker LW, et al: Attack rates of acute nephritis after type 49 streptococcal infection of the skin and of the respiratory tract. J Clin Invest 48:1697, 1969.

Barnett BO, Frieden IJ: Streptococcal skin diseases in children. Semin Dermatol 11:3, 1992.

Beyt BE Jr, Ortbals DW, Santa Cruz DJ: Cutaneous mycobacteriosis: Analysis of 34 cases with a new classification of the disease. Medicine (Baltimore) 60:95, 1980.

Cochran RJ, Rosen T, Landers T: Topical treatment for erythrasma. Int J Dermatol 20:562, 1981.

Dajani AS, Ferrier P, Wannamaker LW: Natural history of impetigo II. Etiologic agents and bacterial interactions. J Clin Invest 51:2863, 1972.

Darmstadt GL, Lane AT: Impetigo: an overview. Pediatr Dermatol 11:293, 1994.

Derrick CW, Reilly KM, Stallworth P, et al: Erythromycin in the treatment of streptococcal infections. Pediatr Infect Dis 5:172, 1986.

Dillon HC Jr: Impetigo contagiosa: Suppurative and non-suppurative complications. I. Clinical, bacteriologic, and epidemiologic characteristics of impetigo. Am J Dis Child 115:530, 1968.

Dillon HC Jr, Reeves MSA: Streptococcal immune responses in nephritis after skin infection. Am J Med 56:333, 1974.

Doebbeling BN, Breneman DL, Neu HC, et al: Elimination of *Staphylococcus aureus* nasal carriage in health care workers: Analysis of six clinical trials with calcium mupirocin ointment. Clin Infect Dis 17:466, 1993.

Eady EA, Cove JH: Topical antibiotic therapy: Current status and future prospects. Drugs Exp Clin Res 16:423, 1990.

Elias PM, Levy W: Bullous impetigo. Occurrence of localized scalded skin syndrome in an adult. Arch Dermatol 112:856, 1976.

Ferrieri P, Dajani AS, Wannamaker LW, et al: Natural history of impetigo I. Site sequence of acquisition and familial patterns of spread of cutaneous streptococci. J Clin Invest 51:2851, 1972.

Gart GS, Forstall GJ, Tomecki KJ: Mycobacterial skin disease: Approaches to therapy. Semin Dermatol 12:352, 1993.

Hayden GF: Skin diseases encountered in a pediatric clinic. Am J Dis Child 139:36, 1985.

Hedstrom SA: Treatment and prevention of recurrent staphylococcal furunculosis: clinical and bacteriologic follow up. Scand J Infect Dis 17:55, 1985.

Iseman MD, Sbarbaro JA: Consensus statements. Arch Intern Med 145:630, 1985.

Katz AR, Morens DM: Severe streptococcal infections in historical perspective. Clin Infect Dis 14:298, 1992.

Leyden JJ: Review of mupirocin ointment in the treatment of impetigo. Clin Pediatr 31:549, 1992.

Lillibridge CB, Melish ME, Glasgow LA: Site of action of exfoliative toxin in the staphylococcal scalded skin syndrome. Pediatrics 50:723, 1972.

Lyell A: The staphylococcal scalded skin syndrome in historical perspective: Emergence of dermopathic strains of *Staphylococcus aureus* and discovery of the epidermolytic toxin. J Am Acad Dermatol 9:285, 1983.

McCray MK, Esterly NB: Cutaneous eruptions in congenital tuberculosis. Arch Dermatol 117:460, 1981.

Melish ME, Glasgow LA: Staphylococcal scalded skin syndrome: The expanded clinical syndrome. J Pediatr 78:958, 1971.

Rice TD, Duggan AK, DeAngelis C: Cost-effectiveness of erythromycin versus mupirocin for the treatment of impetigo in children. Pediatrics 89:210, 1992.

Strauss WB, Maibach HI, Shinefield HR: Bacterial interference treatment of recurrent furunculosis. JAMA 208:861, 1969.

Tunnessen WW Jr: A survey of skin disorders seen in pediatric general and dermatology clinics. Pediatr Dermatol 1:219, 1984.

Tunnessen WW Jr: Practical aspects of bacterial skin infections in children. Pediatr Dermatol 2:255, 1985.

CHAPTER 616
Cutaneous Fungal Infections

Gary L. Darmstadt and Al Lane

TINEA VERSICOLOR

This common, innocuous, chronic fungal infection of the stratum corneum is caused by the dimorphic yeast *Malassezia furfur.* The synonyms *Pityrosporum ovale* and *P. orbiculare* were used previously to identify the causal organism.

ETIOLOGY. *M. furfur* is part of the normal flora, predominantly in the yeast form, and is found, particularly, in areas of skin that are rich in sebum production. Proliferation of filamentous forms occurs in the disease state. Predisposing factors include a warm, humid environment, excessive sweating, occlusion, high plasma cortisol levels, immunosuppression, malnourishment, and genetically determined susceptibility. The disease is most prevalent in adolescents and young adults.

CLINICAL MANIFESTATIONS. The lesions vary widely in color: in whites, they are typically reddish-brown, whereas in blacks they may be either hypopigmented or hyperpigmented. The characteristic macules are covered with a fine scale; they often begin in a perifollicular location, enlarge, and merge to form confluent patches, most commonly on the neck, upper chest, back, and upper arms (Fig. 616–1*A*). Facial lesions are not unusual in adolescents, and lesions occasionally appear on the forearms, dorsum of the hands, and pubis. There may be little or no pruritus. Involved areas do not tan after sun exposure. A papulopustular perifollicular variant of the disorder may occur on the back, chest, and sometimes the extremities.

DIAGNOSIS. Examination with a Wood lamp discloses a yellowish-gold fluorescence. A potassium hydroxide (KOH) preparation of scrapings is diagnostic, demonstrating groups of thick-walled spores and myriad short, thick, angular hyphae, resembling "spaghetti and meatballs" (Fig. 616–1*B*). Skin biopsy, including culture and special stains for fungi (e.g., periodic acid–Schiff), are often necessary to make the diagnosis in cases of primarily follicular involvement; organisms and keratinous debris can be seen within dilated follicular ostia.

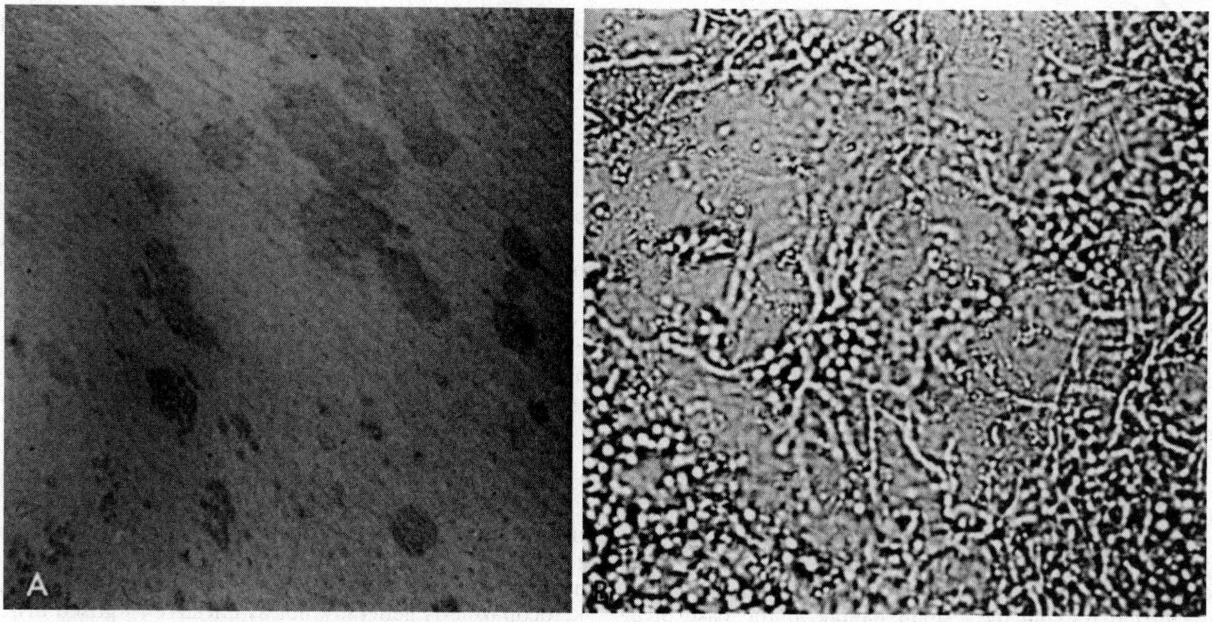

Figure 616–1. *A,* Hyperpigmented, sharply demarcated macules of varying sizes on the upper trunk characteristic of tinea versicolor. *B,* KOH preparation of *Malassezia furfur* demonstrating short, thick hyphae and clusters of spores.

Tinea versicolor must be distinguished from dermatophyte infections, seborrheic dermatitis, pityriasis alba, and secondary syphilis. Nonscaling pigmentary disorders, such as postinflammatory pigmentary change, may be mimicked if the patient has removed the scales by scrubbing. Disseminated candidiasis must be differentiated from *M. furfur* folliculitis.

TREATMENT. Many therapeutic agents can be used to treat this disease successfully; however, the causative agent, a normal human saprophyte, is not eradicated from the skin, and the disorder recurs in predisposed individuals. Appropriate topical therapy may include one of the following: a selenium sulfide suspension applied for 5–10 min each day for 2 wk; 25% sodium hyposulfite or thiosulfate lotion applied twice daily for 2–4 wk; lotions, ointments, or creams containing 3–6% salicylic acid twice daily for 2–4 wk; or miconazole, clotrimazole, ketoconazole, or terbinafine cream twice daily for 2–4 wk. Recurrent episodes continue to respond promptly to these agents. Oral therapy may be more convenient and may be achieved successfully with ketoconazole or fluconazole, 400 mg, repeated in 1 wk, or itraconazole, 200 mg/24 hr for 5–7 days.

DERMATOPHYTOSES

Dermatophytoses are caused by a group of closely related filamentous fungi with a propensity for invading the stratum corneum, hair, and nails. The three principal genera responsible for infections are *Trichophyton, Microsporum,* and *Epidermophyton.*

ETIOLOGY. *Trichophyton* species cause lesions of all keratinized tissue, including skin, nails, and hair; *T. rubrum* is the most common dermatophyte pathogen overall. *Microsporum* species principally invade the hair, and the *Epidermophyton* species invade the intertriginous skin. Dermatophyte infections are designated by the word tinea followed by the Latin word for the anatomic site of involvement. The dermatophytes are also classified according to source and natural habitat. Fungi acquired from the soil are called *geophilic;* they infect humans sporadically, inciting an inflammatory reaction. Dermatophytes that are acquired from animals are *zoophilic;* transmission may be through direct contact or indirectly by infected animal hair or clothing. The infected animal is frequently asymptomatic. Dermatophytes acquired from humans are referred to as *anthropophilic;* these infestations range from chronic, low-grade to acute, inflammatory disease. *Epidermophyton* infections are transmitted only by humans, but various species of *Trichophyton* and *Microsporum* can be acquired from both human and nonhuman sources.

EPIDEMIOLOGY. Host defense has an important influence on the severity of the infection. Disease tends to be more severe in individuals with diabetes mellitus, lymphoid malignancies, immunosuppression, and states with high plasma cortisol levels, such as Cushing syndrome. Some dermatophytes, most notably the zoophilic species, tend to elicit more severe, suppurative inflammation in humans. Some degree of resistance to reinfection is acquired by most infected persons and may be associated with a delayed hypersensitivity response. No relationship has been demonstrated, however, between antibody levels and resistance to infection. The frequency and severity of infection are also affected by the geographic locale, the genetic susceptibility of the host, and the virulence of the strain of dermatophyte. Additional local factors that predispose to infection include trauma to the skin, hydration of the skin with maceration, occlusion, and elevated temperature.

Occasionally, a secondary skin eruption referred to as a *dermatophytid* or *"id" reaction* appears in sensitized individuals and has been attributed to circulating fungal antigens derived from the primary infection. The eruption occurs most frequently on the fingers, hands, and arms and is characterized by grouped papules and vesicles and, occasionally, by sterile pustules. Symmetric urticarial lesions and a more generalized maculopapular eruption can also occur. Id reactions are most often associated with tinea pedis but also occur with tinea capitis; in the latter case, a generalized papulovesicular follicular eruption may occur.

DIAGNOSIS. The important diagnostic procedures for the various dermatophyte diseases include examination of infected hairs with a Wood lamp, microscopic examination of KOH preparations of infected material, and identification of the etiologic agent by culture. Hairs infected with common *Microsporum* species fluoresce a bright blue-green; most *Trichophyton*-infected hairs do not fluoresce.

CLINICAL MANIFESTATIONS. *Tinea capitis* is a dermatophyte infection of the scalp most often caused by *Trichophyton tonsurans,* occasionally by *Microsporum canis,* and much less commonly by other *Microsporum* and *Trichophyton* species. It is particularly common in black and Hispanic children aged 4–14 yr. In *Microsporum* and some *Trichophyton* infections, the spores are distributed in a sheathlike fashion around the hair shaft (ectothrix infection), whereas *T. tonsurans* produces an infection within the hair shaft (endothrix). Endothrix infections may continue past the anagen phase of hair growth into telogen and are more chronic than infections with ectothrix organisms that persist only during the anagen phase. *T. tonsurans* is an anthropophilic species acquired most often by contact with infected hairs and epithelial cells that are on such surfaces as theater seats, hats, and combs. Dermatophyte spores may also be airborne within the immediate environment, and high carriage rates have been demonstrated in noninfected schoolmates and household members. *M. canis* is a zoophilic species that is acquired from cats and dogs.

The *clinical presentation* of tinea capitis varies with the infecting organism. The pattern produced by *M. audouinii,* the most common cause of tinea capitis in the 1940s and 1950s, is characterized initially by a small papule at the base of a hair follicle. The infection spreads peripherally, forming an erythematous and scaly circular plaque *(ringworm)* within which the infected hairs become brittle and broken. Multiple, confluent patches of alopecia develop, and the patient may complain of severe pruritus. *M. audouinii* infection is no longer common in the United States. Endothrix infections such as those caused by *T. tonsurans* create a pattern known as "black-dot ringworm," characterized initially by multiple, small, circular patches of alopecia in which hairs are broken off close to the hair follicle. Another clinical variant presents with diffuse scaling with minimal hair loss secondary to traction; it strongly resembles seborrheic dermatitis, psoriasis, or atopic dermatitis. *T. tonsurans* may also produce a chronic and more diffuse alopecia (Fig. 616–2*A*). A severe inflammatory response produces elevated, boggy granulomatous masses *(kerions),* which are often studded with sterile pustules (Fig. 616–2*B*). Fever, pain, and regional adenopathy are common, and permanent scarring and alopecia may result. The zoophilic organism *M. canis* or the geophilic organism *M. gypseum* may also cause kerion formation. *Favus,* a chronic form of tinea capitis that is rare in the United States, is caused by the fungus *T. schoenleinii.* Favus starts as yellowish-red papules at the opening of hair follicles. The papules expand and coalesce to form cup-shaped, yellowish, crusted patches that fluoresce dull green under the Wood lamp.

Tinea capitis can be confused with seborrheic dermatitis, psoriasis, alopecia areata, trichotillomania, and certain dystrophic hair disorders. When inflammation is pronounced, as in kerion, primary or secondary bacterial infection must also be considered. In adolescents, the patchy, moth-eaten type of alopecia associated with secondary syphilis may resemble tinea capitis. After prolonged tinea capitis has produced scarring, discoid lupus erythematosus and lichen planopilaris must also be considered in the differential diagnosis.

Microscopic examination of a KOH preparation of infected hair from the active border of a lesion discloses tiny spores surrounding the hair shaft in *Microsporum* infections and chains of spores within the hair shaft in *T. tonsurans* infections. Fungal elements are usually not seen in scales. A specific etiologic *diagnosis* of tinea capitis may be obtained by planting broken off infected hairs on Sabouraud medium with antibiotics; such identification may require 2 wk or more.

Oral administration of griseofulvin microcrystalline (15 mg/kg/24 hr) is the recommended *treatment* for all forms of tinea capitis; it may be necessary for 8–12 wk and should be terminated only after fungal culture is negative. Adverse reactions to griseofulvin are rare but include nausea, vomiting, headache, blood dyscrasias, phototoxicity, and hepatotoxicity. Oral ketoconazole is generally not as effective as griseofulvin, particularly for infections caused by *M. canis.* Ketoconazole is useful in instances of griseofulvin resistance, intolerance, or allergy. Uncontrolled studies indicate that itraconazole, 100 mg/24 hr for 30 days, may be an effective alternative treatment. Topical therapy alone is ineffective; it may be an important adjunct because it may decrease the shedding of spores. For this purpose, vigorous shampooing with a 2.5% selenium sulfide or zinc pyrithione preparation is helpful. It is not necessary to shave the scalp.

Tinea corporis, infection of the glabrous skin, excluding the palms, soles, and groin, can be caused by most of the dermatophyte species, although *T. rubrum* and *T. mentagrophytes* are the most prevalent etiologic organisms. In children, infections with *M. canis* are also frequent. Tinea corporis can be acquired by direct contact with infected persons or by contact with infected scales or hairs deposited on environmental surfaces. *M. canis* infections are usually acquired from infected pets. Not infrequently, a single dermatophyte lesion is responsible for dissemination.

The most typical *clinical lesion* begins as a dry, mildly erythematous, elevated, scaly papule or plaque and spreads centrifugally as it clears centrally to form the characteristic annular lesion responsible for the designation "ringworm" (Fig. 616–3). At times, plaques with advancing borders may spread over large areas. Grouped pustules are another variant. Most lesions clear spontaneously within several months, but some may

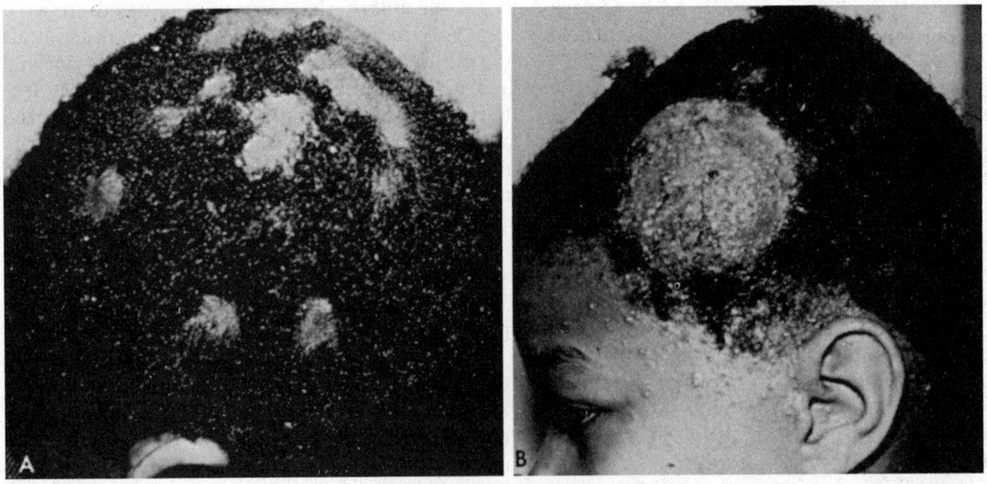

Figure 616–2. *A,* Patchy alopecia associated with tinea capitis. *B,* Elevated, boggy granuloma with multiple pustules (kerion) caused by inflammatory tinea capitis.

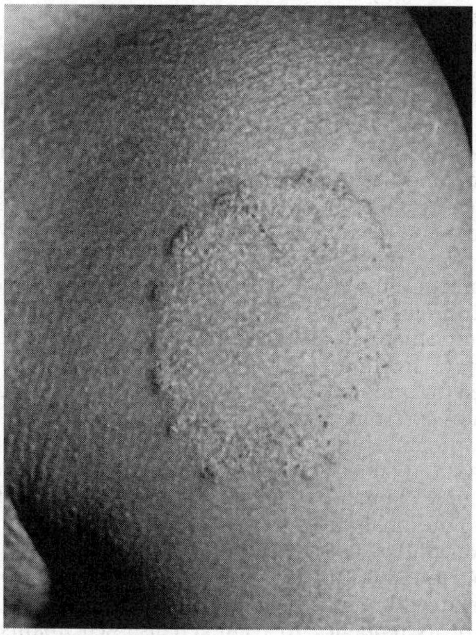

Figure 616–3. Circinate lesion of tinea corporis on the shoulder. Note the active papular border, scaling, and relative clearing centrally.

become chronic. Central clearing does not always occur, and differences in host response may result in wide variability in the clinical appearance, for example, granulomatous lesions called *Majocchi granuloma* and the kerion-like lesions referred to as *tinea profunda*.

Many skin lesions, both infectious and noninfectious, must be differentiated from the lesions of tinea corporis. Those most frequently confused are granuloma annulare, nummular eczema, pityriasis rosea, psoriasis, seborrheic dermatitis, erythema chronicum migrans, and tinea versicolor. Microscopic examination of KOH wet mount preparations and cultures should always be obtained when fungal infection is considered. Tinea corporis usually does not fluoresce with a Wood lamp.

Tinea corporis usually responds to *treatment* with one of the topical antifungal agents (miconazole, clotrimazole, econazole, terbinafine, naftifine) twice daily for 2–4 wk. In unusually severe or extensive disease, a course of therapy with oral griseofulvin microcrystalline may be required for several weeks. Itraconazole has produced excellent results in many cases with a 1–2-wk course of oral therapy.

Tinea cruris, infection of the groin, occurs most often in adolescent males and is usually caused by the anthropophilic species, *Epidermophyton floccosum* or *T. rubrum,* but occasionally by the zoophilic species *T. mentagrophytes.*

The initial *clinical lesion* is a small, raised, scaly, erythematous patch on the inner aspect of the thigh that spreads peripherally, often developing multiple tiny vesicles at the advancing margin. It eventually forms bilateral, irregular, sharply bordered patches with hyperpigmented, scaly centers. In some cases, particularly in infections with *T. mentagrophytes,* the inflammatory reaction is more intense and the infection may spread beyond the crural region. The penis is usually not involved in the infection, which can be important in differentiating this condition from candidosis. Pruritus may be severe initially but abates as the inflammatory reaction subsides. Bacterial superinfection may alter the clinical appearance, and erythrasma or candidosis may coexist. Tinea cruris is more prevalent in obese persons and in those who perspire excessively and wear tight-fitting clothing.

The *diagnosis* is confirmed by culture and by demonstrating septate hyphae on a KOH preparation of epidermal scrapings. Tinea cruris must be differentiated from intertrigo, allergic contact dermatitis, candidosis, and erythrasma. Bacterial superinfection must be excluded when there is a severe inflammatory reaction.

The patient should be advised to wear loose cotton underwear. Topical *treatment* with an imidazole is recommended for severe infection, especially because these agents are effective in mixed candidal-dermatophytic infections. Pure dermatophytic infection may also be treated with tolnaftate.

Tinea pedis (athlete's foot), infection of the toe webs and soles of the feet, is uncommon in young children but occurs with some frequency in preadolescent and adolescent males. The usual etiologic agents are *T. rubrum, T. mentagrophytes,* and *E. floccosum.*

Most commonly, the lateral toe webs (third to fourth and fourth to fifth interdigital spaces) and the subdigital crevice are fissured with maceration and peeling of the surrounding skin. Severe tenderness, itching, and a persistent, foul odor are characteristic. These lesions may become chronic. This type of infection may involve overgrowth by bacterial flora, including *Micrococcus sedantarius, Brevibacterium epidermidis,* and gram-negative organisms. Less commonly, a chronic, diffuse hyperkeratosis of the sole of the foot occurs with only mild erythema. In many cases, two feet and one hand are involved. This type of infection is more refractory to treatment and tends to recur. An inflammatory, vesicular type of reaction may occur with *T. mentagrophytes* infection; this type is most common in young children. These lesions involve any area of the foot, including the dorsal surface, and are usually circumscribed. The initial papules progress to vesicles and bullae that may become pustular (Fig. 616–4). A number of factors, such as occlusive footwear and warm, humid weather, predispose to infection. The disease may be transmitted in shower facilities and swimming pool areas.

Tinea pedis must be differentiated from simple maceration and peeling of the interdigital spaces, which is common in children. Infection with *Candida albicans* and a variety of bacterial organisms (erythrasma) may cause confusion or may coexist with primary tinea pedis. Contact dermatitis, dyshidrotic eczema, and atopic dermatitis also simulate tinea pedis. Fungal mycelia can be seen on microscopic examination of a KOH preparation or by culture; the fourth toe web provides a high yield of infected scales; a blister top can also be used.

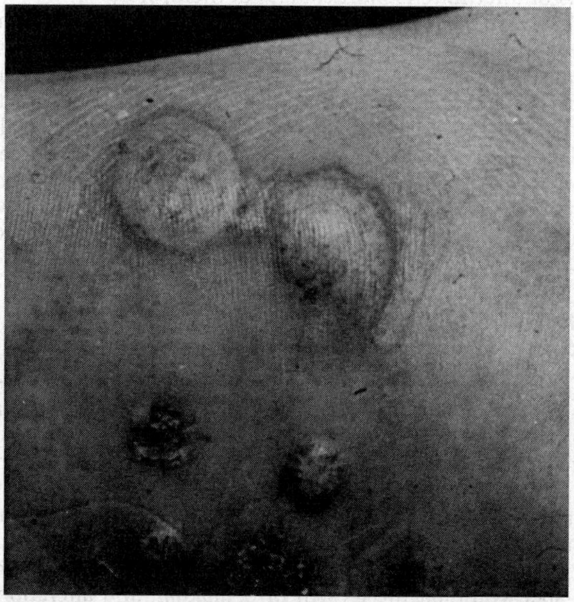

Figure 616–4. Multiple inflammatory bullae of tinea pedis.

Treatment for mild infections includes simple measures such as avoidance of occlusive footwear, careful drying between the toes after bathing, and the use of an absorbent antifungal powder such as zinc undecylenate. Topical therapy with clotrimazole, miconazole, or econazole is curative in most cases; each of these agents is also effective against candidal infection. Tolnaftate can be used in uncomplicated dermatophyte infections. Several weeks of therapy may be necessary, and low-grade, chronic infections, particularly those caused by *T. rubrum,* may be refractory. In such patients, oral griseofulvin therapy may effect a cure, but recurrences are common.

Tinea unguium is a dermatophyte infection of the nail plate; it occurs most often in patients with tinea pedis, but it may occur as a primary infection. It can be caused by a number of dermatophytes, of which *T. rubrum* and *T. mentagrophytes* are the most common.

The most superficial form of tinea unguium is often due to *T. mentagrophytes;* it is manifested by irregular, single or multiple white patches on the surface of the nail unassociated with paronychial inflammation or deep infection. *T. rubrum* generally causes a more invasive, subungual infection that is initiated at the lateral distal margins of the nail and is often preceded by mild paronychia. The middle and ventral layers of the nail plate, and perhaps the naid bed, are the sites of infection. The nail initially develops a yellowish discoloration and slowly becomes thickened, brittle, and loosened from the nail bed. In advanced infection, the nail may turn dark brown to black and may crack or break off.

Tinea unguium must be differentiated from a variety of dystrophic nail disorders. Changes due to trauma, psoriasis, lichen planus, and eczema can all be confused with tinea unguium. Nails infected with *C. albicans* have several distinguishing features, most prominently the presence of pronounced paronychial swelling. Thin shavings taken from the infected nail, preferably from the deeper areas, should be examined microscopically with KOH and cultured. Repeated attempts may be required to demonstrate the fungus.

Results of therapy for tinea unguium are frequently disappointing. Prolonged therapy with griseofulvin and the application of topical fungistatic agents to the nail bed may be effective in some cases. Griseofulvin therapy may be required for more than 1 yr and should be reserved for especially severe disease in patients who are motivated to obtain a cure. The long half-life of itraconazole in the nail has led to promising trials of intermittent short courses of therapy.

Tinea nigra palmaris is a rare but distinctive superficial fungal infection that occurs principally in children and adolescents. It is caused by the dimorphic fungus *Exophiala werneckii,* which imparts a gray-black color to the affected palm. The characteristic lesion is a well-defined hyperpigmented macule; scaling and erythema are rare, and the lesions are asymptomatic. Tinea nigra is often mistaken for a junctional nevus, melanoma, or staining of the skin by contactants. Treatment with Whitfield ointment, undecylenic acid ointment, miconazole, or tincture of iodine is most successful.

CANDIDAL INFECTIONS

(Candidosis, Candidiasis, and Moniliasis) (see Chapter 229)

The dimorphic yeasts of the genus *Candida* are ubiquitous in the environment, but *C. albicans* is the one that usually causes candidosis in children. This yeast is not part of the normal skin flora, but it is a frequent transient on skin and may colonize the human alimentary tract and the vagina as a saprophytic organism. Certain environmental conditions, notably elevated temperature and humidity, are associated with an increased frequency of isolation of *C. albicans* from the skin. Many bacterial species inhibit the growth of *C. albicans,* and alteration of normal flora by the use of antibiotics may promote overgrowth of the yeast.

ORAL CANDIDOSIS (Thrush) (see Chapters 98.6 and 229)

VAGINAL CANDIDOSIS (see Chapters 229 and 503). *C. albicans* is an inhabitant of the adult female vagina in 5–10% of women, and vaginal candidosis is not uncommon in adolescent girls. A number of factors can predispose to this infection, including antibiotic therapy, corticosteroid therapy, diabetes mellitus, pregnancy, and the use of oral contraceptives. The infection is manifested by cheesy white plaques on an erythematous vaginal mucosa and by a thick white-yellow discharge. The disease may be relatively mild or may produce pronounced inflammation and scaling of the external genitalia and surrounding skin with progression to vesiculation and ulceration. Patients often complain of severe itching and burning in the vaginal area. Before treatment is initiated, the diagnosis should be confirmed by culture. The infection may be eradicated by insertion of nystatin or imidazole vaginal tablets, suppositories, creams, or foam. If these products are ineffective, the addition of oral nystatin tablets, one to two tablets three times daily for 14 days, may eliminate or decrease the candidal population in the gastrointestinal tract.

CONGENITAL CUTANEOUS CANDIDOSIS (see Chapter 98.6)

CANDIDAL DIAPER DERMATITIS. This is a ubiquitous problem in infants and, although relatively benign, is often frustrating because of its tendency to recur. Predisposed infants usually carry *C. albicans* in their intestinal tract, and the warm, moist, occluded skin of the diaper area provides an optimal environment for its growth. Usually, a seborrheic, atopic, or primary irritant contact dermatitis provides a portal of entry for the yeast.

The primary *clinical manifestation* consists of an intensely erythematous, confluent plaque with a scalloped border and a sharply demarcated edge. It is formed by the confluence of numerous papules and vesiculopustules; satellite pustules, those that stud the contiguous skin, are a hallmark of localized candidal infections. Usually, the perianal skin, inguinal folds, perineum, and lower abdomen are involved (Fig. 616–5 [color plate section]). In males, the entire scrotum and penis may be involved with an erosive balanitis of the perimeatal skin; in females, the lesions may be found on the vaginal mucosa and labia. In some infants, the process is generalized, with erythematous lesions distant from the diaper area; in some cases, the generalized process may represent a fungal id (hypersensitivity) reaction.

The *differential diagnosis* includes other eruptions of the diaper area that may coexist with candidal infection. For this reason, it is important to establish a diagnosis by a KOH preparation or culture.

Treatment consists of applications of an anticandidal agent (nystatin, miconazole, clotrimazole, ketoconazole) with each diaper change or four times daily. Ointments are better tolerated than creams; lotions and creams may cause a burning

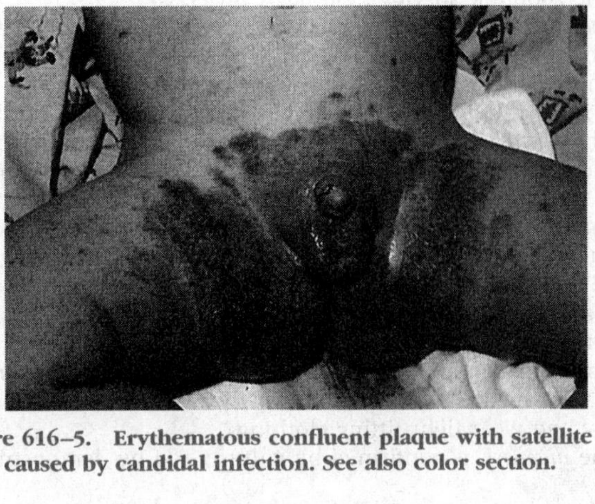

Figure 616–5. Erythematous confluent plaque with satellite pustules caused by candidal infection. See also color section.

sensation when applied to irritated skin, and powder may cake and cause erosion from friction during movement. The combination of a corticosteroid and an antifungal agent is justified if inflammation is severe but may confuse the situation if the diagnosis is not firmly established. Corticosteroid should not be continued for more than a few days. Protection of the diaper area by an application of thick zinc oxide paste overlying the anticandidal preparation may be helpful; the paste is more easily removed with mineral oil than with soap and water. *Fungal id reactions* gradually abate with successful treatment of the diaper dermatitis or may be treated with a mild corticosteroid preparation. When recurrences of diaper candidosis are frequent, it may be helpful to prescribe a course of oral anticandidal therapy to decrease the yeast population in the gastrointestinal tract. Some infants seem to be receptive hosts for *C. albicans* and may reacquire the organism from a colonized adult.

INTERTRIGINOUS CANDIDOSIS. This occurs most often in the axillae and groin, under the breasts, under pendulous abdominal fat folds, in the umbilicus, and in the gluteal cleft. Typical lesions are large, confluent areas of moist, denuded, erythematous skin with an irregular, macerated, scaly border. Satellite lesions are characteristic and consist of small vesicles or pustules on an erythematous base. With time, intertriginous candidal lesions may become lichenified, dry, scaly plaques. The lesions develop on skin subjected to irritation and maceration. Candidal superinfection is more likely to occur under conditions that lead to excessive perspiration, especially in obese children and in those with underlying disorders, such as diabetes mellitus. A similar condition, *interdigital candidosis,* commonly occurs in individuals whose hands are constantly immersed in water; fissures occur between the fingers and have red, denuded centers, with an overhanging, white epithelial fringe. Similar lesions between the toes may be secondary to occlusive footgear. Treatment is the same as for other candidal infections.

PERIANAL CANDIDOSIS. Perianal dermatitis develops at sites of skin irritation due to occlusion, constant moisture, poor hygiene, anal fissures, and pruritus from pinworm infestation. It may become superinfected with *C. albicans,* especially in children who are receiving oral antibiotic or corticosteroid medication. The involved skin becomes erythematous, macerated, and excoriated, and the lesions are identical to those of candidal intertrigo or candidal diaper rash. Application of a topical antifungal agent in conjunction with improved hygiene is usually effective. Underlying disorders such as pinworm infection must also be treated (see Chapter 245.5).

CANDIDAL PARONYCHIA AND ONYCHIA (see Chapter 613)

CANDIDAL GRANULOMA. This is a rare response to an invasive candidal infection of skin. The lesions appear as crusted, verrucous plaques and hornlike projections on the scalp, face, and distal limbs. Affected patients may have single or multiple defects in immune mechanisms and are often refractory to topical therapy. A systemic anticandidal agent may be required for palliation or eradication of the infection.

Allen H, Honig P, Leyden J, et al: Selenium sulfide: Adjunctive therapy for tinea capitis. Pediatrics 69:81, 1982.
Aly R: Ecology and epidemiology of dermatophyte infections. J Am Acad Dermatol 31:S21, 1994.
Baley J, Silverman R: Systemic candidiasis: Cutaneous manifestations in low birth weight infants. Pediatrics 82:211, 1988.
DeCastro P, Jorizzo JL: Cutaneous aspects of candidosis. Semin Dermatol 4:165, 1985.
Degreef HJ, DeDoncker PRG: Current therapy of dermatophytosis. J Am Acad Dermatol 31:S25, 1994.
DeVroey C: Epidemiology of ringworm (dermatophytosis). Semin Dermatol 4:185, 1985.
Elewski B: Tinea capitis: Itraconazole in *Trichophyton tonsurans* infection. J Am Acad Dermatol 31:65, 1994.
Faergemann J: Pityrosporum infections. J Am Acad Dermatol 31:S18, 1994.
Frieden IJ, Howard R: Tinea capitis: Epidemiology, diagnosis, treatment, and control. J Am Acad Dermatol 31:S42, 1994.
Hubbard TW, de Triquet JM: Brush-culture method for diagnosing tinea capitis. Pediatrics 90:416, 1992.
Jacobs AH, O'Connell BM: Tinea in tiny tots. Am J Dis Child 140:1034, 1986.
Kaaman T, Torssander J: Dermatophytid—a misdiagnosed entity? Acta Derm Venereol (Stockh) 63:404, 1983.
Krowchuk DP, Lucky AW, Primmer SI: Current status of the identification and management of tinea capitis. Pediatrics 72:625, 1983.
Leyden JJ: The role of bacteria in the signs and symptoms of interdigital "athlete's foot" infections. Dermatol Clin 2:81, 1984.
Odom R: Pathophysiology of dermatophyte infections. J Am Acad Dermatol 5:S2, 1993.
Philpot CM, Shuttleworth D: Dermatophyte onychomycosis in children. Clin Exp Dermatol 14:203, 1989.
Rezabek GH, Friedman AD: Superficial fungal infections of the skin. Diagnosis and current treatment recommendations. Drugs 43:674, 1992.
Rosenthal JR: Pediatric fungal infections from head to toe: What's new? Curr Opin Pediatr 6:435, 1994.
Svejgaard E: Immunologic investigations of dermatophytes and dermatophytosis. Semin Dermatol 4:201, 1985.
Zienicke HC, Korting HC, Lukacs K, et al: Dermatophytosis in children and adolescents: Epidemiological, clinical, and microbiological aspects changing with age. J Dermatol 18:438, 1991.

CHAPTER 617
Cutaneous Viral Infections

Gary L. Darmstadt and Al Lane

WART
(Verruca)

Human papillomaviruses (HPV) cause a spectrum of disease from warts to squamous cell carcinoma of the skin and mucous membranes, including the larynx (see Chapter 224). The incidence of all types of warts is highest in children and adolescents. HPV is spread by direct contact and autoinoculation, but transmission by fomites can occur. The clinical manifestations of infection develop 1 mo or longer after inoculation and depend on the HPV type, of which more than 70 are recognized; the size of the inoculum; the immune status of the host; and the anatomic site.

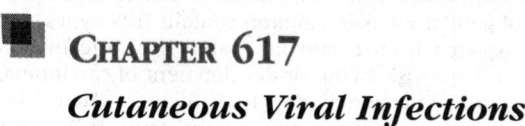

CLINICAL MANIFESTATIONS. Cutaneous warts develop in 5–10% of children. *Common warts (verruca vulgaris),* caused by HPV types 2 and 4, occur most frequently on the fingers, dorsum of the hands, paronychial areas, face, knees, and elbows. They are well-circumscribed papules with a roughened, keratotic, irregular surface. When the surface is pared away, multiple black dots representing thrombosed dermal capillary loops are often visible. Periungual warts are often painful and may spread beneath the nail plate, separating it from the nail bed. *Plantar warts,* although similar to the common wart, are caused by HPV type 1 and are usually flush with the surface of the sole because of the constant pressure from weight bearing; they may be painful. Similar lesions (palmar) can also occur on the palms. They are sharply demarcated, often with a ring of thick callus. The surface keratotic material must sometimes be removed before the boundaries of the wart can be appreciated; in contrast to calluses, warts obliterate normal skin markings. Several contiguous warts may fuse to form a large plaque, the so-called *mosaic wart. Flat warts (verruca plana),* caused by HPV types 3 and 10, are slightly elevated, minimally hyperkeratotic papules that usually remain less than 3 mm in size and vary in color from pink to brown. They may occur in profusion on the face, arms, dorsum of the hands, and knees. The distribution of multiple lesions along a line of cutaneous trauma is a helpful diagnostic feature. Lesions may be disseminated in the beard area by shaving and from the hairline onto the scalp by combing the hair. *Epidermodysplasia verruciformis,* caused primarily by HPV types 5 and 8, presents with multiple, diffuse verrucous papules. Approximately 25% of cases are familial, occurring by autosomal recessive or X-linked inheritance, and 3–10% of patients have HPV-associated squamous cell carcinoma on sun-exposed skin.

Genital HPV infection occurs in nearly 40% of sexually active adolescents, most commonly as a result of infection with HPV types 6, 11, 16, and 18. *Condylomata acuminata (mucous membrane warts)* are moist, fleshy, papillomatous lesions that occur on the perianal mucosa (Fig. 617–1), labia, vaginal introitus, and perineal raphe and on the shaft, corona, and glans penis. They may occasionally obstruct the urethral meatus or the vaginal introitus. Because they are located in intertriginous areas, they may become moist and friable. When untreated, condylomata proliferate and become confluent, at times forming large cauliflower-like masses. Lesions can also occur on the lips, gingivae, tongue, and conjunctivae. Genital warts in children may occur as a consequence of sexual abuse; after inoculation during birth through an infected birth canal; or from incidental spread from cutaneous warts. A significant proportion of genital warts in children contain HPV types that are usually isolated from cutaneous warts. HPV infection of the cervix is a major risk factor for development of carcinoma, particularly if the infection is due to HPV types 16 or 18. *Laryngeal (respiratory) papillomas* contain the same HPV types as in anogenital papillomas. Transmission is believed to occur from mothers with genital HPV infection to neonates who aspirate infectious virus during birth.

PATHOLOGY. The various types of warts differ in minor ways but share the basic changes of hyperplasia of the epidermal cells and vacuolization of the spinous keratinocytes, which may contain basophilic intranuclear inclusions (viral particles). Parakeratosis, papillomatosis, and eosinophilic cytoplasmic inclusions, thought to represent altered keratohyalin, are additional variable histologic changes. Individuals with impaired cell-mediated immunity are particularly susceptible to HPV infection. Antibodies occur in response to infection but appear to have little protective effect.

DIFFERENTIAL DIAGNOSIS. Common warts are most often confused with molluscum contagiosum. Plantar and palmar warts may be difficult to distinguish from punctate keratoses, corns, and calluses. Juvenile flat warts mimic lichen planus, lichen nitidus, angiofibromas, syringomas, milia, and acne. Condylomata acuminata may resemble condylomata lata of secondary syphilis.

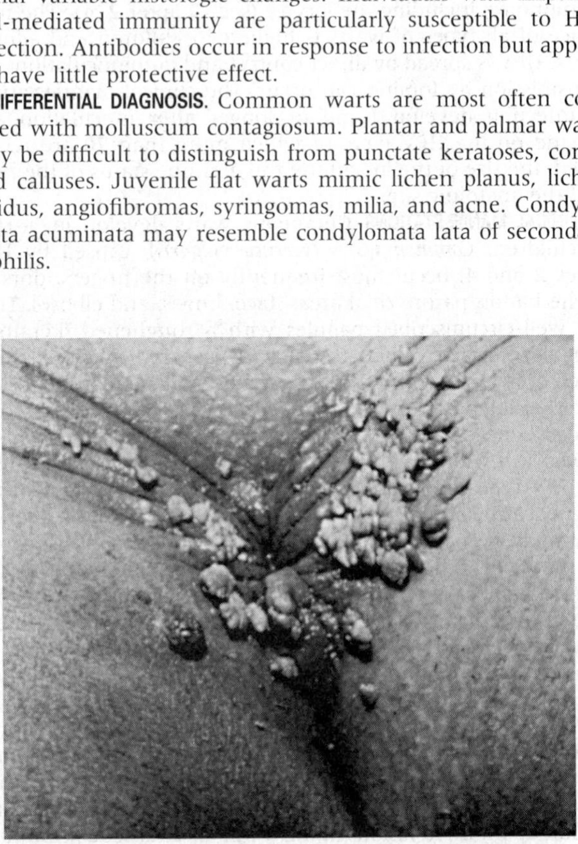

Figure 617–1. Condylomata acuminata in the perianal area of a toddler.

TREATMENT. A variety of therapeutic measures are effective in the treatment of warts. More than 50% of warts disappear spontaneously within 2 yr, but failure to treat incurs the risk of spread to other sites. Warts are epidermal lesions and do not produce scarring unless they are managed surgically or treated in an overly aggressive fashion. Hyperkeratotic lesions (common, plantar, and palmar warts) are more responsive to therapy if the excess keratotic debris is gently pared with a scalpel until thrombosed capillaries are apparent; further paring induces bleeding. Treatment is most successful when done regularly and frequently.

Common warts can be destroyed by applications of liquid nitrogen or cantharidin or by light electrodesiccation and curettage. Daily applications of 10–17% lactic acid and 10–17% salicylic acid in flexible collodion is a slow but painless method of removal that is effective in some patients. Plantar and palmar warts may be treated with salicylic and lactic acids in collodion or 40% salicylic acid plasters. After prolonged soaking in lukewarm water, keratotic debris can be removed by an emery board or pumice stone. Occlusive taping for several days may also be effective. Condylomata respond best to weekly applications of 25% podophyllin in tincture of benzoin; the medication should be left on the warts for 4–6 hr and then removed by bathing. Condylomata localized to keratinized sites (e.g., buttocks) may not respond to podophyllin. Resistant lesions can usually be eradicated by weekly freezing with liquid nitrogen or by treatment with a carbon dioxide laser. Although intralesional injection of 1 million units of interferon alpha or beta three times weekly for 3–4 wk appears to be effective against condylomata, this is not recommended because of a low incidence of effectiveness, high toxicity rate, and high cost. With all types of therapy, care should be taken to protect the surrounding normal skin from irritation.

MOLLUSCUM CONTAGIOSUM

The poxvirus that causes molluscum contagiosum is a large double-stranded DNA virus that replicates in the cytoplasm of host epithelial cells. There are three types that cannot be differentiated on the basis of clinical appearance, location of lesions, or patient age or sex. Type 1 virus causes most infections. The disease is acquired by direct contact with an infected person or from fomites and is spread by autoinoculation. School-age children who are otherwise well and individuals who are immunosuppressed are affected most commonly. The incubation period is estimated to be 2 wk or longer.

CLINICAL MANIFESTATIONS. Discrete, pearly, skin-colored, dome-shaped, smooth papules vary in size from 1–5 mm. Typically, they have a central umbilication from which a plug of cheesy material can be expressed (Fig. 617–2). The papules may occur anywhere on the body, but the face, eyelids, neck, axillae, and thighs are sites of predilection. They may be found in clusters on the genitalia or in the groin of adolescents and may be associated with other venereal diseases in sexually active individuals. Lesions commonly involve the genital area in children but in most cases are not acquired by sexual transmission; a search should be undertaken, however, for other signs of sexual abuse. Lesions on the eyelid margin can produce unilateral conjunctivitis; rarely, lesions may appear on the conjunctiva or cornea. Mild surrounding erythema or an eczematous dermatitis may accompany the papules. Lesions on patients with acquired immunodeficiency syndrome (AIDS) tend to be large and numerous, particularly on the face; exuberant lesions may also be found in children with leukemia and other immunodeficiencies.

DIFFERENTIAL DIAGNOSIS. This includes trichoepithelioma, basal cell carcinoma, ectopic sebaceous glands, syringoma, hidrocystoma, keratoacanthoma, and warty dyskeratoma. In individuals with AIDS, cryptococcosis may be indistinguishable clinically from molluscum contagiosum.

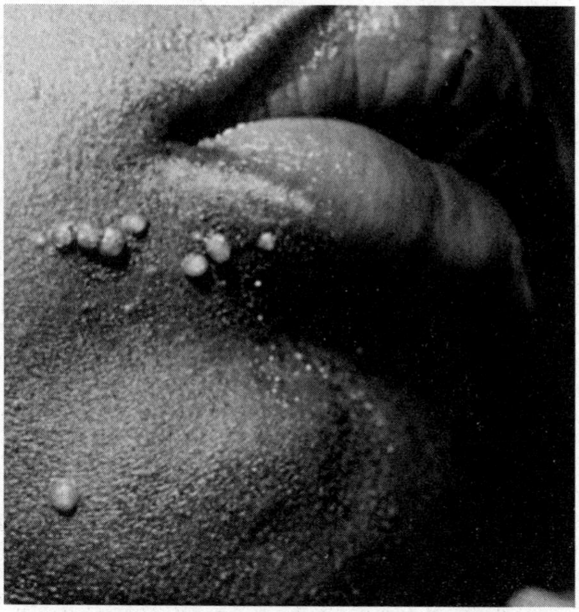

Figure 617–2. Grouped papules of molluscum contagiosum on the face.

PATHOLOGY AND DIAGNOSIS. The epidermis is hyperplastic and hypertrophied, extending into the underlying dermis and projecting above the skin surface. The molluscum papule consists of a lobulated adhesive mass of virus-infected epidermal cells. Eosinophilic viral inclusion bodies (Henderson-Patterson or molluscum bodies) become more prominent as the cells move upward from the basal layer to the stratum corneum. The central plug of material, which is composed of virus-laden cells, may be shelled out from a lesion (see Treatment) and examined under the microscope with 10% potassium hydroxide or Wright or Giemsa stain. The rounded, cup-shaped mass of homogeneous cells, often with identifiable lobules, is diagnostic. Specific antibody against molluscum contagiosum virus is detectable in most infected individuals but is of uncertain immunologic significance. Cell-mediated immunity is thought to be important in host defense.

TREATMENT. Molluscum contagiosum is a self-limited disease; the average attack lasts 6–9 mo. However, lesions can persist for years, can spread to distant sites, and may be transmitted to others. Affected patients should be advised to avoid shared baths and towels until the infection is clear. Infection may spread rapidly and produce hundreds of lesions in children with atopic dermatitis or immunodeficiency. A brief, 6–9-sec application of liquid nitrogen is very effective and, in most instances, is the treatment of choice. The papules can also be destroyed by expressing the plug with a needle, a sharp curette, or a comedo extractor. Cantharidin 0.9% may be applied to each lesion without occlusion and frequently causes enough inflammation to facilitate spontaneous extrusion of the plug. Occasionally, treatment of a few lesions is followed by resolution of the others. Molluscum is an epidermal disease and should not be overtreated so that scarring results. A lesion-free period of 4 mo can be regarded as a cure.

Beutner KR: Cutaneous viral infections. Pediatr Ann 22:247, 1993.
Epstein WL: Molluscum contagiosum. Semin Dermatol 11:184, 1992.
Gissmann L: Papillomaviruses and their association with cancer in animals and man. Cancer Surv 3:161, 1984.
Kipping HF: Molluscum dermatitis. Arch Dermatol 103:106, 1971.
Pauly CR, Artis WM, Jones HE: Atopic dermatitis, impaired cellular immunity, and molluscum contagiosum. Arch Dermatol 114:391, 1978.
Pfister H: Biology and biochemistry of papillomaviruses. Rev Physiol Biochem Pharmacol 99:111, 1983.
Porter CD, Blake NW, Cream JJ, et al: Molluscum contagiosum virus. Mol Cell Biol Hum Dis Series 1:233, 1992.
Rock B, Naghashfar Z, Barnett N, et al: Genital tract papillomavirus infections in children. Arch Dermatol 122:1129, 1986.
Schachner L, Hankin DE: Assessing child abuse in childhood condyloma acuminatum. J Am Acad Dermatol 12:157, 1985.
Weston WL, Lane AT: Should molluscum be treated? Pediatrics 65:865, 1980.

CHAPTER 618
Arthropod Bites and Infestations

Gary L. Darmstadt and Al Lane

ARTHROPOD BITES

Arthropod bites are a common affliction of children and occasionally pose a problem in diagnosis. The patient may be unaware of the source of the lesions or deny being bitten, making interpretation of the eruption difficult. In these cases, knowledge of the habits, life cycle, and clinical signs of the more common arthropod pests of humans may help lead to a correct diagnosis. The principal classes of arthropods that cause skin injury to humans are listed in Table 618–1. Some of the important dermatoses caused by arthropod bites and infestations are covered in this chapter; others are discussed in chapters addressing infectious organisms (see Part XVII).

CLINICAL MANIFESTATIONS. The type of reaction that occurs after an arthropod bite depends on the species of insect and the age group and reactivity of the human host. Arthropods may cause injury to the host by a variety of mechanisms, including mechanical trauma, such as the lacerating bite of a tsetse fly; invasion of host tissues, as in myiasis; contact dermatitis, as seen with repeated exposure to cockroach antigens; granulomatous reaction to retained mouth parts; transmission of systemic disease; injection of irritant cytotoxic or pharmacologically active substances, such as hyaluronidase, proteases, peptidases, and phospholipases in sting venom; and induction of anaphylaxis. Most reactions to arthropod bites, however, depend on antibody formation to antigenic substances in saliva or venom. The type of reaction is determined primarily by the degree of previous exposure to the same or a related species of arthropod. When someone is bitten for the first time, no reaction develops. An immediate petechial reaction is occasionally seen, however, in newborn babies after a mosquito bite. After repeated bites, sensitivity develops, producing a pruritic papule approximately 24 hr after the bite; this is the most common reaction seen in young children. With prolonged, repeated exposure, a wheal develops within minutes after a bite, followed 24 hr later by papule formation; this combination of reactions is seen commonly in older children. By adolescence or adulthood, only a wheal may form, unac-

■ TABLE 618–1 Arthropods That Cause Human Skin Disease

Class Arachnida (four pairs of legs): mites, spiders, ticks
Class Chilopoda: centipedes
Class Diplopoda: millipedes
Class Insecta (three pairs of legs):
Order Diptera: mosquitoes, flies
Order Siphonaptera: fleas
Order Hymenoptera: ants, bees, wasps
Order Anoplura: lice
Order Hemiptera: bedbugs, kissing bugs
Order Coleoptera: beetles
Order Lepidoptera: butterflies, moths

companied by the delayed papular reaction. Thus, adults may be unaffected in the same household as affected children. Ultimately, as the person becomes insensitive to the bite, there is no reaction at all. This stage of nonreactivity is maintained only as long as the individual continues to be bitten regularly. Individuals in whom papular urticaria develops are in the transitional phase between development of primarily a delayed, papular reaction and development of an immediate urticarial reaction.

Arthropod bites may occur as solitary, multiple, or profuse lesions, depending on the feeding habits of the perpetrator. For example, fleas tend to sample their host multiple times within a small, localized area, whereas mosquitoes tend to attack a host at more randomly scattered sites. *Delayed hypersensitivity reactions* to insect bites, the predominant lesions in the young and uninitiated, are characterized by firm, persistent papules that may become hyperpigmented and are often excoriated and crusted. Pruritus may be mild or severe, transient or persistent. A central punctum is usually visible but may disappear as the lesion ages or is scratched. The *immediate hypersensitivity reaction* is characterized by an erythematous, evanescent wheal. If edema is marked, the wheal may be surmounted by a tiny vesicle. Certain beetles produce bullous lesions through the action of cantharidin, and hemorrhagic nodules and ulcers may be caused by a variety of insects, including beetles and spiders. Bites on the lower extremities are more apt to be severe or persistent or become bullous than those located elsewhere. Complications of arthropod bites include development of impetigo, folliculitis, cellulitis, lymphangitis, and severe anaphylactic hypersensitivity reactions, particularly after the bite of certain Hymenoptera. The histopathologic changes are variable, depending on the arthropod, the age of the lesion, and the reactivity of the host. Acute urticarial lesions tend to show central vesiculation in which eosinophils are numerous. Papules most commonly show dermal edema and a mixed, superficial and deep perivascular inflammatory infiltrate, often including a number of eosinophils. At times, however, the dermal cellular infiltrate is so dense that a lymphoma is suspected. Retained mouth parts may stimulate a foreign body type of granulomatous reaction.

Papular urticaria occurs principally in the 1st decade of life, during the warmer months of the year. The most common culprits are species of fleas, mites, bedbugs, gnats, mosquitoes, chiggers, and animal lice. Individuals with papular urticaria have predominantly transitional lesions in various stages of evolution between delayed-onset papules and immediate-onset wheals. The most characteristic lesion is an edematous, red-brown papule; an individual lesion frequently starts as a wheal that in turn is replaced by a papule. A given bite may incite an id reaction at distant sites of quiescent bites in the form of erythematous macules, papules, and/or urticarial plaques. The disorder is characterized by a temporary arrest at a transitional phase; after a season or two, however, the reaction progresses from a transitional to a primarily immediate hypersensitivity urticarial reaction.

One of the most commonly encountered arthropod bites is that due to human, cat, or dog *fleas* (family Pulicidae). Eggs, which are generally laid in dusty areas and cracks between floorboards, give rise to larvae that then form cocoons. The cocoon stage can persist for up to 1 yr, and the animal emerges in response to vibrations from footsteps, accounting for the assaults that frequently befall the new owners of a recently reopened dwelling. Adult dog fleas can live without a blood meal for approximately 60 days. Attacks from fleas are more likely to occur when the fleas do not have access to their usual host; for example, cat or dog fleas are more voracious and problematic when one visits an area frequented by the pet than when the pet is encountered directly. Flea bites tend to be grouped in lines or irregular clusters. Fleas are often not seen on the body of a pet; diagnosis of flea bites, however, is aided by examination of debris from the animal's bedding material. The debris is collected by shaking the bedding into a plastic bag and examining the contents for fleas, eggs, larvae, or feces.

TREATMENT. This is directed at alleviation of pruritus by oral antihistamines; cool compresses; and soothing lotions such as calamine, to which 0.25% menthol and 0.5% phenol can be added. Topical corticosteroid creams are rarely effective, and topical antihistamines are potent sensitizers and have no role in the treatment of insect bite reactions. A short course of systemic steroids may be helpful if multiple, severe reactions occur, particularly around the eyes. Insect repellents containing diethyl-meta-toluamide (DEET) may afford moderate protection against mosquitoes, fleas, flies, chiggers, and ticks but are relatively ineffective against wasps, bees, and hornets. DEET must be applied to exposed skin and clothing to be effective. The most effective protection against mosquitoes, the human body louse, and other blood-feeding arthropods is use of DEET and permethrin-impregnated clothing; these measures are not effective, however, against the phlebotomine sand fly, which transmits leishmaniasis. Advocates of treatment with B-complex vitamins or thiamine hydrochloride maintain that these agents impart an offensive odor to sweat, warding off mosquitoes; this claim has not been substantiated by clinical trials.

An effort should be made to identify and eradicate the etiologic agent. Pets should be carefully inspected; crawl spaces, eaves, and other sites of the house or outbuildings frequented by animals and birds should be decontaminated; and baseboard crevices, mattresses, rugs, furniture, and animal sleeping quarters should be decontaminated. Agents that are effective for ridding the home of fleas include chlorophenothane (DDT), chlordane, lindane, pyrethroids, and organic thiocyanates. Flea-infested pets may be treated with powders containing rotenone, pyrethroids, malathion, or methoxychlor.

INFESTATIONS

SCABIES. Scabies is caused by burrowing and release of toxic or antigenic substances by the female mite *Sarcoptes scabiei* var. *hominis*. The most important factor that determines spread of scabies is the extent and duration of physical contact with an affected individual; the children and sexual partner of an affected individual are most at risk. Scabies is transmitted only rarely by fomites because the isolated mite dies within 2–3 days.

Clinical Manifestations. In an immunocompetent host, scabies is frequently heralded by intense pruritus, particularly at night. The first sign of the infestation often consists of 1–2-mm red papules, some of which are excoriated, crusted, or scaling. Threadlike burrows are the classic lesion of scabies but may not be seen in infants. In infants, bullae and pustules are relatively common; the eruption may also include wheals, papules, vesicles, and a superimposed eczematous dermatitis; and the palms, soles (Fig. 618–1B), face, and scalp are often affected. In older children and adolescents, the clinical pattern is similar to that in adults, in whom preferred sites are the interdigital spaces, wrist flexors, anterior axillary folds, ankles, buttocks, umbilicus and belt line, groin, genitalia in men, and areolae in women (Fig. 618–1A); the head, neck, palms and soles are generally spared. Red-brown nodules, most often located in covered areas such as the axillae, groin, and genitalia, predominate in the less common variant called nodular scabies. Untreated, scabies may lead to eczematous dermatitis, impetigo, ecthyma, folliculitis, furunculosis, cellulitis, lymphangitis, and id reaction. Children have been reported to develop glomerulonephritis as a result of streptococcal impetiginization of scabies lesions. In some tropical areas, scabies is the predominant underlying cause of pyoderma. A latent pe-

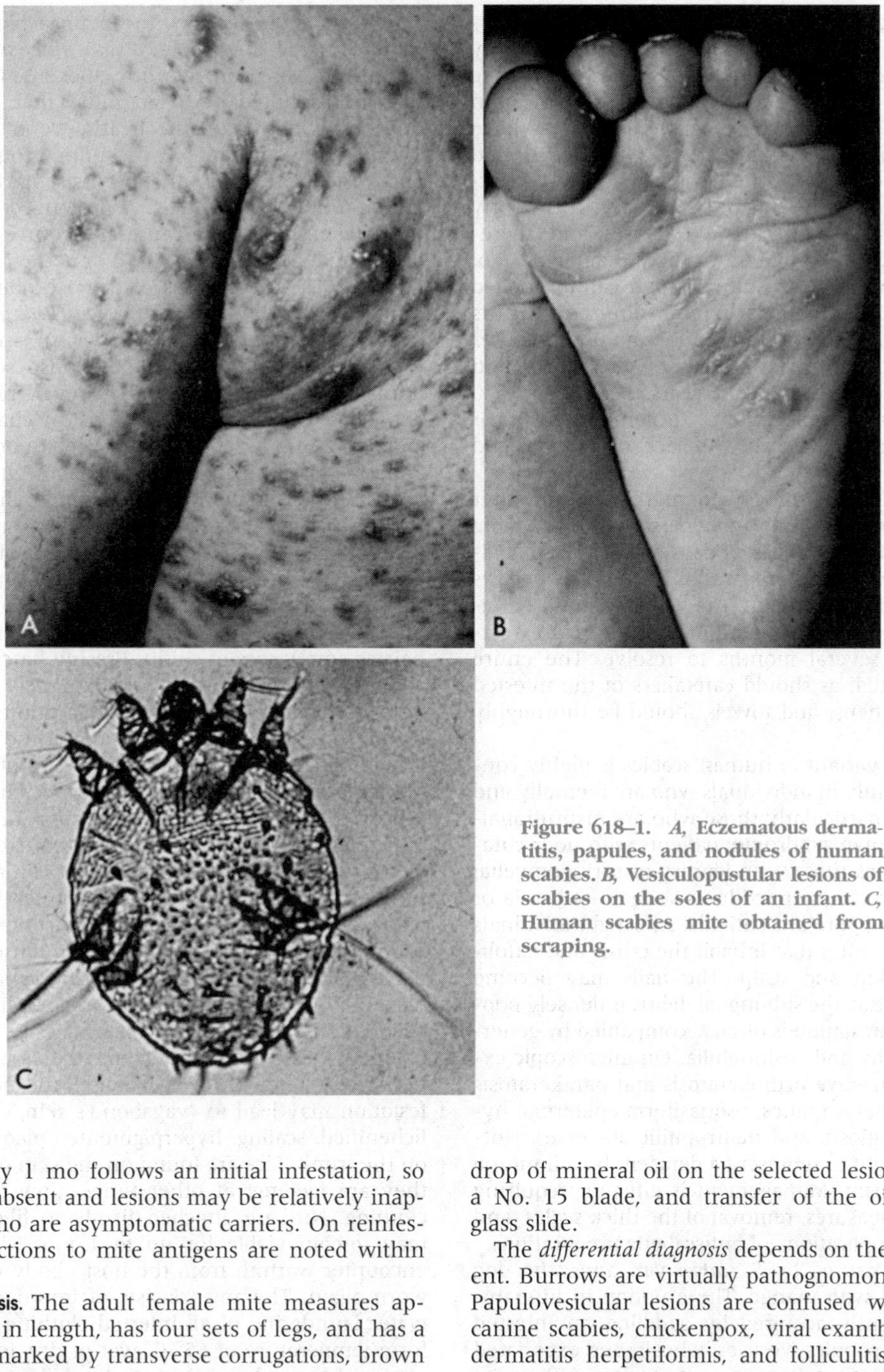

Figure 618–1. *A,* Eczematous dermatitis, papules, and nodules of human scabies. *B,* Vesiculopustular lesions of scabies on the soles of an infant. *C,* Human scabies mite obtained from scraping.

riod of approximately 1 mo follows an initial infestation, so that itching may be absent and lesions may be relatively inapparent in contacts who are asymptomatic carriers. On reinfestation, however, reactions to mite antigens are noted within hours.

Etiology and Pathogenesis. The adult female mite measures approximately 0.4 mm in length, has four sets of legs, and has a hemispherical body marked by transverse corrugations, brown spines, and bristles on the dorsal surface. The male mite is approximately one half her size and is similar in configuration. After impregnation on the skin surface, the gravid female exudes a keratolytic substance and burrows into the stratum corneum, often forming a shallow well within 30 min. She gradually extends this tract by 0.5–5 mm/24 hr along the boundary with the stratum granulosum. She deposits one to three oval eggs and numerous brown fecal pellets (scybala) daily. When egg laying is completed, in 4–5 wk, she dies within the burrow. The eggs hatch in 3–5 days, releasing larvae that move to the skin surface to molt into nymphs. Maturity is achieved in about 2–3 wk. Mating occurs, and the gravid female invades the skin to complete the life cycle.

Diagnosis. This can often be made clinically but can be confirmed by microscopic identification of mites (Fig. 618–1C), ova, and scybala in epithelial debris. Scrapings are most often positive when obtained from burrows, eczematous lesions, or fresh papules. The most reliable method is application of a drop of mineral oil on the selected lesion, scraping of it with a No. 15 blade, and transfer of the oil and scrapings to a glass slide.

The *differential diagnosis* depends on the types of lesions present. Burrows are virtually pathognomonic for human scabies. Papulovesicular lesions are confused with papular urticaria, canine scabies, chickenpox, viral exanthems, drug eruptions, dermatitis herpetiformis, and folliculitis. Eczematous lesions may mimic atopic dermatitis and seborrheic dermatitis, and the less common bullous disorders of childhood may be suspected in the infant with predominantly bullous lesions. Nodular scabies is frequently misdiagnosed as urticaria pigmentosa and histiocytosis X. The histopathologic appearance of nodular scabies, consisting of a deep, dense, perivascular infiltrate of lymphocytes, histiocytes, plasma cells, and atypical mononuclear cells, may mimic malignant lymphoid neoplasms.

Treatment. Application of 1% lindane cream or lotion to the entire body from the neck down, with particular attention to intensely involved areas, is standard therapy. Scabies is frequently found above the neck in infants, however, also necessitating treatment of the scalp. The medication is left on the skin for 8–12 hr; if necessary, it may be reapplied in 1 wk for another 8–12-hr period. The vulnerability of small infants to percutaneous absorption of this potentially neurotoxic substance dictates caution in prescribing it for them. Signs of toxicity include nausea, vomiting, weakness, tremors, irritability, disorientation, seizures, and respiratory compromise. Systemic absorption and toxicity of lindane can be minimized by not applying the medication to warm, moist skin; not repeating an application within 7 days; and not using the medication on children who are underweight or malnourished or have extensive areas of inflamed, denuded, or secondarily infected skin. Permethrin 5% cream (Elimite) is a slightly more effective scabicide than lindane but is more expensive. It is poorly absorbed, rapidly metabolized by tissue esterases, and, therefore, of very low toxicity. For infants younger than age 2 mo, alternative therapy includes 6% sulfur in petrolatum applied for three consecutive 24-hr periods. Topical sulfur ointment is messy, is malodorous, stains clothing, and commonly causes irritant dermatitis. No controlled studies of its efficacy and safety have been published in recent years. Permethrin 5% cream is a better alternative for infants. Crotamiton cream or lotion is not recommended because of lack of efficacy and toxicity data.

Transmission of mites is unlikely more than 24 hr after treatment. Pruritus, which is due to hypersensitivity to mite antigens, may persist for a number of days and may be alleviated by a topical corticosteroid preparation. If pruritus persists for more than 2 wk after treatment, the patient should be reexamined for mites. Nodules are extremely resistant to treatment and may take several months to resolve. The entire family should be treated, as should caretakers of the infested child. Clothing, bed linens, and towels should be thoroughly laundered.

Norwegian Scabies. This variant of human scabies is highly contagious and occurs mainly in individuals who are mentally and physically debilitated, particularly those who are institutionalized and those with Down syndrome; patients with poor cutaneous sensation, such as those with leprosy or syringomyelia; patients who have severe systemic illness such as leukemia or diabetes; and immunosuppressed patients. Affected individuals are infested by myriad mites that inhabit the crusts and exfoliating scales of the skin and scalp. The nails may become thickened and dystrophic; the subungual debris is densely populated by mites. The infestation is often accompanied by generalized lymphadenopathy and eosinophilia. On microscopic examination, one sees massive orthokeratosis and parakeratosis with numerous interspersed mites, psoriasiform epidermal hyperplasia, foci of spongiosis, and neutrophilic abscesses. Norwegian scabies is thought to represent a deficient host immune response to the organism. Management is difficult, requiring scrupulous isolation measures, removal of the thick scales, and repeated but careful applications of antiscabetic preparations.

Canine Scabies. This is caused by *S. scabiei* var. *canis*, the dog mite that is associated with mange. The eruption in humans, which is most frequently acquired by cuddling an infested puppy, consists of tiny papules, vesicles, wheals, and excoriated eczematous plaques. Burrows are not present because the mite infrequently inhabits human stratum corneum. The rash is pruritic and has a predilection for the arms, chest, and abdomen, the usual sites of contact with dogs. Onset is sudden and usually follows exposure by 1–10 days, possibly resulting from development of a hypersensitivity reaction to mite antigens. Recovery of mites or ova from scrapings of human skin is rare. The disease is self-limited because humans are not a suitable host; bathing and changing clothes are generally sufficient. Removal or treatment of the infested animal, however, is also necessary. Symptomatic therapy for itching is helpful. In rare cases in which mites are demonstrated in scrapings from the affected child, they can be eradicated by the same measures applicable to human scabies.

Other mites that occasionally bite humans include the *chigger* or harvest mite *(Eutrombicula alfreddugesi)*, which prefers to live on grass, shrubs, vines, and stems of grain. Larvae have hooked mouth parts, which allow the chigger to attach to the skin, but not to burrow, to obtain a blood meal, most commonly on the lower legs. *Avian mites* may affect those who come into close contact with chickens. Occasionally, humans may be assaulted by avian mites that have infested a nest outside a window, an attic, heating vents, or an air conditioner. The dermatitis is variable, including grouped papules, wheals, and vesicular lesions on the wrists, neck, breasts, umbilicus, and anterior axillary folds. A prolonged investigation is often undertaken before the cause and source of the dermatitis are discovered.

PEDICULOSIS. Three types of lice are obligate parasites of the human host: body or clothing lice (*Pediculus humanus corporis*), head lice (*Pediculus humanus capitis*), and pubic or crab lice (*Pthirus pubis*). Only the body louse serves as a vector of human disease (typhus, trench fever, relapsing fever). Body and head lice have similar physical characteristics; they are about 2–4 mm in length. Pubic lice are only 1–2 mm in length and are greater in width than length, giving them a crablike appearance. Female lice live for approximately 1 mo and deposit 3–10 eggs daily on the human host; body lice, however, generally lay eggs in or near the seams of clothing. The ova or nits are glued to hairs or fibers of clothing but not directly on the body. Ova hatch in 1–2 wk and require another week to mature; once the eggs hatch, the nits remain attached to the hair as empty sacs of chitin. Freshly hatched larvae die unless a meal is obtained within approximately 24 hr and every few days thereafter. Both nymphs and adult lice feed on human blood, injecting their salivary juices into the host and depositing their fecal matter on the skin. Symptoms of infestation do not appear immediately but develop as the individual becomes sensitized. *The hallmark of all types of pediculosis is pruritus.*

Pediculosis corporis is rare in children except under conditions of poor hygiene, especially in colder climates when the opportunity to change clothes on a regular basis is lacking. The parasite is transmitted mainly on contaminated clothing or bedding. The primary lesion is an intensely pruritic small red macule or papule with a central hemorrhagic punctum located on the shoulders, trunk, or buttocks. Additional lesions include excoriations, wheals, and eczematous, secondarily infected plaques. Massive infestation may be associated with constitutional symptoms of fever, malaise, and headache. Chronic infestation may lead to "vagabond's skin," which is manifest as lichenified, scaling, hyperpigmented plaques, most commonly on the trunk. Lice are found on the skin only transiently when they are feeding; at other times, they inhabit the seams of clothing. Nits are attached firmly to fibers in the cloth and may remain viable for up to 1 mo. Nits hatch when they encounter warmth from the host's body when the clothes are worn again. Therapy consists of improved hygiene and hot-water laundering of all infested clothing and bedding; a uniform temperature of 65° C, wet or dry, for 15–30 min kills all eggs and lice. Alternatively, eggs will hatch and nymphs will starve if clothing is stored for 2 wk at 75–85° F. For people who are unable to change clothes, the clothes may be dusted while inside out with 10% lindane powder; the effect lasts for approximately 1 mo. Lindane lotion or permethrin cream applied for 8–12 hr can be used to eradicate any eggs and lice that happen to be on body hair.

Pediculosis capitis is an intensely pruritic infestation of lice in the scalp hair. Head-to-head contact is the most important mode of transmission. In summer months in many areas of the United States and in the tropics at all times of the year, shared combs, brushes, or towels play a more important role in louse transmission. Transculent 0.5-mm eggs are laid near the proximal portion of the hair shaft and become adherent to one side of the hair shaft. A nit cannot be moved along or knocked off the hair shaft with the fingers. Secondary pyoderma, after trauma from scratching, may result in matting together of the hair, and cervical and occipital lymphadenopa-

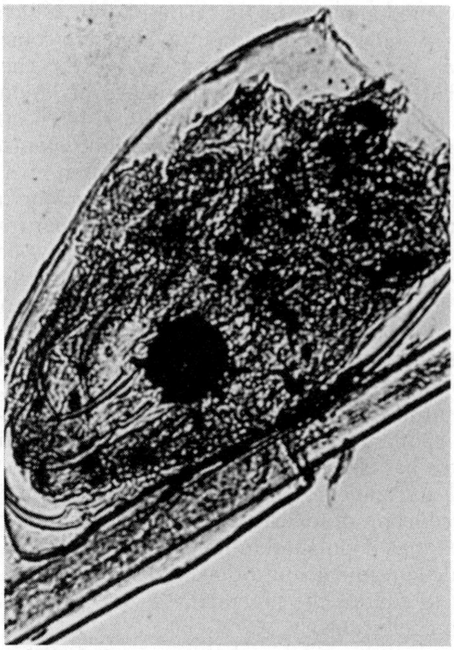

Figure 618–2. Intact nit on a human hair.

thy. Hair loss does not result from pediculosis but may accompany the secondary pyoderma. Head lice are a major cause of multiple pyodermas of the scalp, particularly in tropical environments. Lice are not always visible, but nits are detectable on the hairs, most commonly in the occipital region and above the ears, rarely on beard or pubic hair. Dermatitis may also be noted on the neck and pinnae. An id reaction, consisting of eythematous patches and plaques, may develop, particularly on the trunk. For unknown reasons, head lice infrequently infest blacks.

Brushing and combing of the hair regularly helps to reduce the number of lice and eggs and helps to minimize the severity of the infestion. The *treatment* of choice is permethrin 1% cream rinse (NIX) applied for 10 min with a repeat application in 7–10 days. Alternative treatments include natural pyrethrin shampoos (RID; A-200 Pyrinate liquid, shampoo, or gel; R & C shampoo; Barc; Paratrol; Paranit; Triple X) and 1% lindane shampoo (Kwell) for 10 min with a repeat application in 7–10 days. All household members should be treated at the same time. Nits can be removed with a fine-toothed comb after a 1:1 vinegar:water rinse or, if tenacious, after application of a creme rinse containing 8% formic acid, which dissolves the chitin attaching the nits to the hair shafts. Clothing and bed linens should be laundered in very hot water or dry-cleaned; brushes and combs should be discarded or coated with a pediculicide for 15 min and then thoroughly cleaned in boiling water.

Pediculosis pubis is transmitted by skin-to-skin or sexual contact with an infested individual; the chance of acquiring the louse by one sexual exposure is approximately 95%. The infestation is usually encountered in adolescents, although small children may occasionally acquire pubic lice on the eyelashes. Patients experience moderate to severe pruritus and may develop a secondary pyoderma from scratching. Excoriations tend to be shallower and the incidence of secondary infection is lower than in pediculosis corporis. Maculae ceruleae are steel-gray spots, usually less than 1 cm in diameter, which may appear in the pubic area and on the chest, abdomen, and thighs. Oval, translucent nits, which are firmly attached to the hair shafts, may be visible to the naked eye or may be readily identified by a hand lens or by microscopic examination (Fig. 618–2). Grittiness, as a result of adherent nits, may sometimes be detected when the fingers are run through infested hair. Adult lice are difficult to detect because of their lower level of activity and smaller, translucent body size compared with head or body lice. Because the pubic louse may occasionally wander or be transferred to other sites on fomites, terminal hair on the trunk, thighs, axillary region, beard area, and eyelashes should be examined for nits. The coexistence of other venereal diseases should be considered.

Treatment by a 10-min application of a pyrethrin preparation is usually effective. Retreatment may be required in 7–10 days. The shampoo form of lindane, which requires a 10-min application time, is an alternative choice, but lindane cream and lotion are no longer recommended for treatment of pubic lice. Infestation of eyelashes is eradicated by petrolatum applied three to five times/24 hr for 8–10 days. A less safe but effective alternative is 0.25% physostigmine ophthalmic ointment applied twice daily for 3 days. Clothing, towels, and bed linens may be contaminated with nit-bearing hairs and should be thoroughly laundered or dry-cleaned.

SEABATHER'S ERUPTION. Seabather's eruption is a severely pruritic dermatosis of inflammatory papules that develops within approximately 12 hr of bathing in salt water, primarily on body sites that were covered by a bathing suit. The eruption has been described primarily in waters of Florida and the Caribbean. Lesions, which may include pustules, vesicles, and urticarial plaques, are more numerous in those individuals who keep their bathing suit on for an extended period after leaving the water. The eruption may be accompanied by systemic symptoms of fatigue, malaise, fever, chills, nausea, and headache; approximately 40% of children younger than age 16 yr had fever in one large series. Duration of the pruritus and skin eruption is 1–2 wk. Histopathologically, lesions consist of a superficial and deep perivascular and interstitial infiltrate of lymphocytes, eosinophils, and neutrophils. The eruption appears to be due to an allergic hypersensitivity reaction to venom from larvae of the thimble jellyfish *(Linuche unguiculata)*. Treatment is largely symptomatic; potent topical corticosteroids have been shown to provide relief to some patients.

DeFelice J, Wagner D: Head Lice Outbreaks and Their Impact on the Community—A Public Health Perspective. World Health Communications Symposium, Ft. Lauderdale, FL, 1985.

Ginsberg CM, Lowry W: Absorption of gamma benzene hexachloride following application of Kwell shampoo. Pediatr Dermatol 1:74, 1983.

Green MS: Epidemiology of scabies. Epidemiol Rev 11:126, 1989.

Gurevitch AW: Scabies and lice. Pediatr Clin North Am 32:987, 1985.

Honig PJ: Arthropod bites, stings, and infestations: Their prevention and treatment. Pediatr Dermatol 3:189, 1986.

Meinking TL, Taplin D, Kalter DC, et al: Comparative efficacy of treatments for pediculosis capitis infestations. Arch Dermatol 122:267, 1986.

Rasmussen JE: Pediculosis and the pediatrician. Pediatr Dermatol 2:74, 1984.

Reisman RE: Natural history of insect sting allergy: Relationship of severity of symptoms of initial sting anaphylaxis to re-sting reactions. J Allergy Clin Immunol 90:335, 1992.

Taplin D, Meinking TL, Castillero PM, et al: Permethrin 1% cream rinse (Nix) for treatment of *Pediculus humanus* var *capitis* infestation. Pediatr Dermatol 3:344, 1986.

Taplin D, Meinking TL, Porcelain SL, et al: Permethrin 5% dermal cream: A new treatment for scabies. J Am Acad Dermatol 15:995, 1986.

CHAPTER 619
Acne

Gary L. Darmstadt and Al Lane

ACNE VULGARIS

Acne, particularly the comedonal form, occurs in approximately 80% of adolescents.

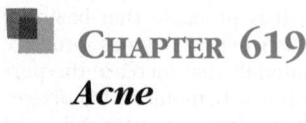

PATHOGENESIS. Lesions of acne vulgaris develop in sebaceous follicles, which consist of a large, multilobular sebaceous gland that drains its products into the follicular canal. The initial lesion of acne is a *comedo,* which is a dilated epithelium-lined follicular sac filled with lamellated keratinous material, lipid, and bacteria. An open comedo, known as a blackhead, has a patulous pilosebaceous orifice that permits visualization of the plug. An open comedo less commonly becomes inflammatory than a closed comedo or whitehead, which has only a pinpoint opening. An inflammatory papule or nodule develops from a comedo that has ruptured and extruded its follicular contents into the subadjacent dermis, inducing a neutrophilic inflammatory response. If the inflammatory reaction is close to the surface, a papule or pustule develops; if the inflammatory infiltrate develops deeper in the dermis, a nodule forms. Suppuration and an occasional giant cell reaction to the keratin and hair are the cause of nodulocystic lesions; these are not true cysts but liquefied masses of inflammatory debris.

The primary pathogenetic alterations in acne are (1) abnormal keratinization of the follicular epithelium, resulting in impaction of keratinized cells within the follicular lumen; (2) increased sebaceous gland production of sebum; (3) proliferation of *Propionibacterium acnes* within the follicle; and (4) inflammation. At puberty, the sebaceous gland enlarges and sebum production increases in response to the increased activities of androgens of primarily adrenal origin. Comedonal acne, particularly of the central face, is frequently the first sign of pubertal maturation. The prevalence and severity of acne correlate with pubertal development and amount of sebum production. Initiation of acne in prepubertal children aged 7–10 yr has been shown to correlate significantly with the amount of wax esters in skin surface lipids and the concentration of serum dehydroepiandrosterone sulfate (DHEA-S), which is an androgenic steroid secreted primarily by the adrenal gland. DHEA-S levels are not elevated, however, in the serum of many individuals with acne. DHEA-S may act locally, however, to stimulate sebum production by the sebaceous gland after being metabolized in hair follicle dermal papillae and sebaceous glands by 5α-reductase to more potent androgens such as 5α-dihydrotestosterone. Other sex steroid hormones such as testosterone and estradiol may also play a role in enhancing sebum production. A significant number of women with acne (25–50%), particularly those with relatively mild papulopustular acne, note that their acne flares approximately 1 wk before menstruation. The pathogenesis of this phenomenon is unknown.

Freshly formed sebum consists of a mixture of triglycerides, wax esters, squalene, and sterol esters. Normal follicular bacteria produce lipases that hydrolyze sebum triglycerides to free fatty acids; those of medium chain length (C8 to C14) may be provocative factors in initiating an inflammatory reaction. Sebum also provides a favorable substrate for proliferation of bacteria. Sebaceous follicles are colonized by organisms of three types: an anaerobic diphtheroid, *P. acnes*; coagulase-negative *Staphylococcus epidermidis*; and a dimorphic yeast, *Pityrosporum ovale.* Each of these organisms possesses lipolytic enzymes; however, *P. acnes* appears to be largely responsible for the formation of free fatty acids. It is probable that bacterial proteases, hyaluronidases, and hydrolytic enzymes produce biologically active extracellular materials that increase the permeability of the follicular epithelium. Chemotactic factors released by the intrafollicular bacteria attract neutrophils and monocytes. Lysosomal enzymes from the neutrophils, released in the process of phagocytizing the bacteria, further disrupt the integrity of the follicular wall and intensify the inflammatory reaction.

CLINICAL MANIFESTATIONS. Acne vulgaris is characterized by four basic types of lesions: open and closed comedones, papules, pustules, and nodulocystic lesions. One or more types of lesions may predominate; in its mildest form, which is often seen early in adolescence, lesions are limited to comedones on the central face. Lesions may also involve the chest, upper back, and deltoid areas. A predominance of lesions on the forehead, particularly closed comedones, is often attributable to prolonged use of greasy hair preparations (pomade acne). Marked involvement on the trunk is most often seen in males. Lesions often heal with temporary postinflammatory erythema and hyperpigmentation; pitted, atrophic, or hypertrophic scars may be interspersed, depending on the severity, depth, and chronicity of the process. Diagnosis of acne is rarely difficult, although flat warts, folliculitis, and other types of acne may be confused with acne vulgaris.

TREATMENT. There is no evidence that early treatment, with the exception of isotretinoin, alters the course of acne. Acne can be controlled and severe scarring prevented, however, by judicious maintenance therapy that is continued until the disease process has abated spontaneously. Therapy must be individualized and aimed at preventing microcomedo formation through reduction of follicular hyperkeratosis, sebum production, the *P. acnes* population in follicular orifices, and free fatty acid production. Initial control takes at least 4–8 wk. It is also important to address the potentially severe emotional impact of acne on adolescents.

Diet. There is little evidence that ingestion of particular foods can trigger acne flares. When a patient is convinced, however, that certain dietary items exacerbate acne, it is prudent to omit those foods; it is unnecessary, however, to impose unwarranted dietary restrictions.

Climate. Climate appears to influence acne in that improvement frequently occurs during summer and flares are more common during winter. Remission during summer may relate, in part, to the relative absence of stress. Emotional tension and fatigue seem to exacerbate acne in many individuals; the mechanism is unclear but has been proposed to relate to an increased adrenocortical response.

Cleansing. Cleansing with soap and water removes surface lipid and renders the skin less oily in appearance, but there is no evidence that surface lipid plays a role in generating acne lesions. Only superficial drying and peeling are achieved by cleansing, and almost any mild soap or astringent is adequate. Repetitive cleansing can be harmful because it irritates and chaps the skin. Cleansing agents that contain abrasives and keratolytic agents, such as sulfur, resorcinol, and salicylic acid, may temporarily remove sebum from the skin surface; exert a mild drying and peeling effect; and suppress lesions to a limited degree; they do not, however, prevent microcomedones from forming. There is no evidence that preparations containing alcohol or hexachlorophene decrease acne because surface bacteria are not involved in the pathogenesis. Greasy cosmetic and hair preparations must be discontinued because they exacerbate pre-existing acne and cause further plugging of follicular pores. Manipulation and squeezing of facial lesions only ruptures intact lesions and provokes a localized inflammatory reaction.

Topical Therapy. The most effective topical preparations, particularly for comedones and papulopustular acne, include the benzoyl peroxide gels, retinoic acid, and topical antibiotics. *Benzoyl peroxide* is an organic peroxide and oxidizing agent that dries and peels the skin, inhibits triglyceride hydrolysis and production of free fatty acids, is bacteriostatic for *P. acnes,* and causes follicular desquamation, disimpacting the follicle. Preparations are available in concentrations of 2.5%, 5%, and 10% prescription gels and 5% and 10% over-the-counter lotions. Benzoyl peroxide should be applied as a thin film, initially every other day, advancing over 2–3 wk to once-daily use as tolerated; the incidence of irritant or allergic contact dermatitis is 1%. Water-based gels are less irritating than alcohol-based ones, particularly for patients with atopic dermatitis or otherwise sensitive skin. Over-the-counter lotions are less effective than prescription gels.

Tretinoin (Retin-A), a derivative of retinoic acid, is the single most effective agent for treatment of comedonal acne. It affects keratinization in the sebaceous follicle by increasing turnover of epidermal cells and by decreasing the cohesiveness of the squamous cells; it thus aids in elimination of the keratinous plug. Erythema and peeling may be expected, particularly on initiation of therapy, and pustular flares from rupture of microcomedones are common. Flares may be minimized by starting treatment with benzoyl peroxide 2–3 wk before tretinoin. It may be applied once daily, 30 min after washing, in the form best tolerated (0.025% cream, 0.05% cream, 0.1% cream, 0.01% gel, 0.025% gel, and 0.05% liquid in increasing order of potency). Typically, 0.025% cream is prescribed initially; the strength of the formulation is increased sequentially until adequate control, without undue irritation, is achieved. Optimal results are not seen for 3–6 mo. Increased sensitivity to sunlight may occur, necessitating use of a sunscreen.

Topical antibiotics for use in patients with acne include clindamycin and erythromycin; they may be applied once or twice daily. Although not as effective as orally administered antibiotics or benzoyl peroxide, they serve as a useful therapeutic adjunct by inhibiting growth of *P. acnes*. The effectiveness of a topical antibiotic is enhanced by the concurrent use of benzoyl peroxide or tretinoin. Use of topical erythromycin or clindamycin has occasionally resulted in the emergence of resistant bacteria.

All topical preparations must be used for 4–8 wk before their effectiveness can be assessed. They may be used alone but frequently are more effective when used together. A popular and effective combination is use of benzoyl peroxide gel in the morning and tretinoin at night.

Systemic Therapy. *Antibiotics*, especially tetracycline and its derivatives, are indicated for treatment of patients who cannot tolerate or have not responded to topical medications, who have moderately to severe inflammatory papulopustular and nodulocystic acne, and who have a propensity for scarring. The tetracyclines act by inhibiting bacterial lipases, causing a reduction in the concentration of free fatty acids; suppressing the normal follicular flora, mainly *P. acnes*; and inhibiting neutrophil chemotaxis and follicular inflammation. Tetracycline, minocycline, and doxycycline were recently shown to suppress granuloma formation, perhaps by inhibition of protein kinase C, an important membrane signal transducer. For most adolescent patients, therapy may be initiated with 1 g/24 hr, divided twice daily, for at least 6 wk, followed by a gradual decrease to the minimal effective dosage. The drugs are best administered in combination with topical benzoyl peroxide or tretinoin but not topical antibiotics. Tetracycline absorption is inhibited by food, milk, iron supplements, aluminum hydroxide gel, and calcium-magnesium salts. It should be taken on an empty stomach 1 hr before or 2 hr after meals. Side effects of tetracycline include vaginal candidosis, particularly in those who take tetracycline concurrently with oral contraceptives; gastrointestinal irritation; phototoxic reactions, including onycholysis and brown discoloration of nails; esophageal ulceration; inhibition of fetal skeletal growth; and staining of growing teeth, precluding its use during pregnancy and in those younger than age 9 yr. Oral antibiotics may decrease the effectiveness of oral contraceptive pills. Alternatives to tetracycline include erythromycin, minocycline, doxycycline, clindamycin, and, occasionally, trimethoprim-sulfamethoxazole. A possible complication of prolonged systemic antibiotic use is proliferation of gram-negative organisms, particularly *Enterobacter, Klebsiella, Escherichia coli,* or *Pseudomonas aeruginosa,* producing severe, refractory folliculitis.

Women with acne who have hormonal abnormalities, are unresponsive to antibiotic therapy, or are not candidates for isotretinoin therapy should be considered for a trial of *hormonal therapy.* An effective combination is an antiandrogen such as cyproterone acetate or spironolactone, given on days 5–15 of the menstrual cycle, and ethinyl estradiol, a synthetic estrogen used in oral contraceptives that is a potent inhibitor of sebum production, given on days 5–26. Topically applied antiandrogens without systemic side effects are currently under investigation.

Isotretinoin (13-*cis*-retinoic acid, Accutane) is indicated for moderate to severe nodulocystic acne that has not responded to conventional therapy or has recurred quickly after several successful courses of conventional therapy; for severe, scarring acne such as acne conglobata and acne fulminans; and for acne that is associated with severe psychologic disturbance. The recommended dosage is approximately 0.5–1.0 mg/kg/24 hr; younger male patients and those with primarily truncal lesions tend to require dosages at the upper end of this range. Four months of therapy is required for most patients; a standard course in the United States lasts 16–20 wk. At the end of one course of isotretinoin, approximately 30% are cured, 35% need conventional topical and/or oral medications to maintain adequate control, and 25% have relapses and need an additional course of isotretinoin. Dosages below 0.5 mg/kg/24 hr, or a cumulative dose of less than 120 mg/kg, are associated with a significantly higher rate of treatment failure and relapse. If the disease process is not in remission 2 mo after the first course of isotretinoin, a second course should be considered. Isotretinoin reduces sebum excretion by 80% within 1 mo, converts sebaceous units to epithelial buds, decreases the population of *P. acnes,* decreases ductal cornification, and inhibits neutrophil chemotaxis and thus decreases the inflammatory response. Isotretinoin therapy does not alter gonadal or adrenal functions but induces a significant local decrease in 5α-dihydrotestosterone formation in the skin.

There are many side effects of isotretinoin use. It is teratogenic and is contraindicated in pregnancy; pregnancy should be avoided for 1 mo after discontinuation of therapy. Two or three forms of birth control are required, as are monthly pregnancy tests. Most patients experience cheilitis, xerosis, periodic epistaxis, and blepharoconjunctivitis. Increased serum triglyceride and cholesterol levels are also common; it is important to rule out pre-existent liver disease and hyperlipidemia before initiating therapy and to check the triglyceride response 4 wk after commencing therapy. Less common but significant side effects include arthralgias, myalgias, depression, temporary thinning of the hair, paronychia, increased susceptibility to sunburn, formation of pyogenic granulomas, and colonization of the skin with *Staphylococcus aureus*, leading to impetigo, secondarily infected dermatitis, and scalp folliculitis. Rarely, hyperostotic lesions of the spine develop after more than one course of isotretinoin. Concomitant use of tetracycline and isotretinoin is contraindicated because either drug, but particularly when used together, can cause benign intracranial hypertension.

Surgical Therapy. Intralesional injection of low-dose (3 mg/mL) midpotency glucocorticoids (e.g., triamcinolone) with a 30-gauge needle on a tuberculin syringe may hasten the healing of individual, painful nodulocystic lesions. Dermabrasion to minimize scarring should be considered only after the active process is quiescent.

DRUG-INDUCED ACNE

Pubertal and postpubertal patients who are receiving systemic corticosteroid therapy or potent topical steroids are predisposed to steroid-induced acne. This monomorphous folliculitis occurs primarily on the face, neck, chest (Fig. 619–1A), shoulders, upper back, arms, and, rarely, the scalp. Onset follows the initiation of steroid therapy by about 2 wk. The lesions are small, erythematous papules or pustules that may

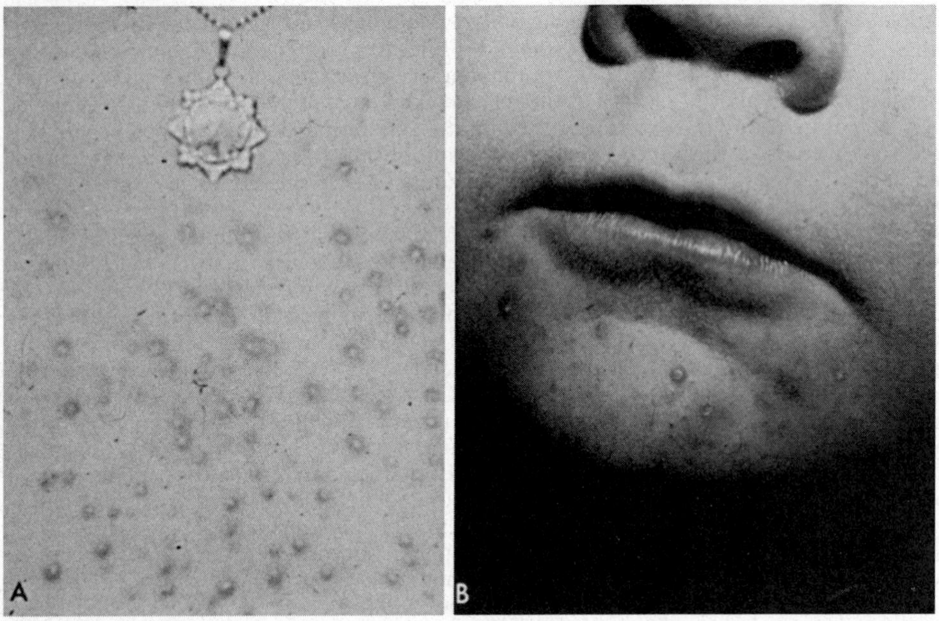

Figure 619–1. *A*, Monomorphous papular eruption of steroid acne. *B*, Acne in a male infant.

erupt in profusion and are all in the same stage of development. Comedones may occur subsequently, but nodulocystic lesions and scarring are rare. Pruritus is occasional. The steroid appears to induce focal degeneration of the follicular epithelium, which incites a localized neutrophilic inflammatory response. Although steroid acne is relatively refractory if the medication is continued, the eruption may respond to use of tretinoin and a benzoyl peroxide gel. A prepubertal child with severe acne should be examined for endocrine disorders such as congenital adrenal hyperplasia. Studies of adrenal function are indicated in appropriate patients (see Chapter 529).

Other drugs that can induce acneiform lesions in susceptible individuals include isoniazid, phenytoin, phenobarbital, trimethadione, lithium carbonate, androgens (anabolic steroids), and vitamin B_{12}.

HALOGEN ACNE

Administration of medications containing iodides or bromides or, rarely, ingestion of massive amounts of vitamin-mineral preparations or iodine-containing "health foods" such as kelp may induce halogen acne. The lesions are often very inflammatory. Discontinuation of the provocative agent and appropriate topical preparations usually achieve reasonable therapeutic results.

CHLORACNE

Chloracne is due to external contact with, inhalation of, or ingestion of halogenated aromatic hydrocarbons, including polyhalogenated biphenyls, polyhalogenated naphthalenes (e.g., Halowax, which may be a component of wood preservatives and sealing compounds), and dioxins. Lesions are primarily comedonal; inflammatory lesions are infrequent but may include papules, pustules, nodules, and cysts. Healing occurs with atrophic or hypertrophic scarring. The face, postauricular regions, neck, axillae, genitals, and chest are involved most commonly. The nose is often spared. In cases of severe exposure, associated findings may include hepatitis, production of porphyrins, bullae formation on sun-exposed skin, hyperpigmentation, hypertrichosis, and palmar and plantar hyperhidrosis. Topical or oral retinoids may be effective; benzoyl peroxide and antibiotics are generally ineffective.

NEONATAL ACNE

Approximately 20% of normal neonates develop at least a few comedones within the 1st mo of life. Closed comedones predominate on the cheeks and forehead (see Fig. 619–1B); open comedones and papulopustules occur occasionally. The cause of neonatal acne is unknown but has been attributed to placental transfer of maternal androgens, hyperactive neonatal adrenal glands, and a hypersensitive neonatal end-organ response to androgenic hormones. Placental transfer of maternally ingested lithium and hydantoin may also cause acne in the neonate. The hypertrophic sebaceous glands involute spontaneously over a few months, as does the acne. If desired, the lesions can be treated effectively with topical tretinoin and/or benzoyl peroxide.

INFANTILE ACNE

Infantile acne usually presents at 3–6 mo of life, more commonly in boys than girls. Acne lesions are more numerous, pleomorphic, severe, and persistent than in neonatal acne. Open and closed comedones predominate on the face; papules and pustules occur frequently, but only occasionally do nodulocystic lesions develop. Pitted scarring is rare. The course may be relatively brief, or the lesions may persist for many months, although the eruption generally resolves by age 3 yr. Use of topical benzoyl peroxide gel and tretinoin usually clears the eruption within a few weeks; oral erythromycin is necessary occasionally. There is often a history of severe acne in one or both parents, and the child is at risk for development of severe acne in adolescence. A child with refractory acne warrants a search for an abnormal source of androgens such as a virilizing tumor or congenital adrenal hyperplasia.

TROPICAL ACNE

A severe form of acne occurs in tropical climates and is believed to be due to the intense heat and humidity; hydration of the pilosebaceous duct pore may accentuate blockage of the duct. Affected individuals tend to have an antecedent history of adolescent acne that is quiescent at the time of the eruption. Lesions occur mainly on the entire back, chest, buttocks, and thighs, with a predominance of suppurating papules and nodules. Secondary infection with *S. aureus* may be a complication.

The eruption is refractory to acne therapy if the environmental factors are not eliminated.

ACNE CONGLOBATA

Acne conglobata is a chronic, progressive inflammatory disease that occurs mainly in adult males, more commonly in whites than in blacks, but may begin during adolescence. There usually, but not always, is a history of pre-existing acne vulgaris. The principal lesion is the nodule, although one often finds a mixture of comedones with multiple pores, papules, pustules, nodules, cysts, abscesses, and subcutaneous dissection with formation of multichanneled sinus tracts. Severe scarring is characteristic. The face is relatively spared, but, in addition to the back and chest, the buttocks, abdomen, arms, and thighs may be involved. Constitutional symptoms and anemia may accompany the inflammatory process. Coagulase-positive staphylococci and β-hemolytic streptococci are frequently cultured from lesions but do not appear to be involved primarily in the pathogenesis. Acne conglobata occasionally occurs in association with hidradenitis suppurativa and dissecting cellulitis of the scalp (as the follicular occlusion triad) and may be complicated by erosive arthritis and ankylosing spondyloarthritis. Endocrinologic studies are not revealing. Routine acne therapy is generally ineffective. Systemic therapy with a corticosteroid or sulfone may be required to suppress the intense inflammatory activity. Isotretinoin is the most effective form of therapy for some patients but may produce a flare after its initiation. Consequently, corticosteroids are often started before isotretinoin.

ACNE FULMINANS

(Acute Febrile Ulcerative Acne)

Acne fulminans is characterized by abrupt onset of extensive, inflammatory, tender ulcerative acneiform lesions on the back and chest of male teenagers. The distinctive feature is the tendency for large nodules to form exudative, necrotic, ulcerated, crusted plaques. Lesions often spare the face and heal with scarring. A preceding history of mild papulopustular or nodular acne is noted in most patients. Constitutional symptoms and signs are common, including fever, debilitation, arthralgias, myalgias, weight loss, and leukocytosis. Blood cultures are sterile. Lesions of erythema nodosum sometimes develop on the shins. Osteolytic bone lesions may develop in the clavicle, sternum, and epiphyseal growth plates; affected bones appear normal or have slight sclerosis or thickening on healing. Salicylates may be helpful for the myalgias, arthralgias, and fever. Corticosteroids (1.0 mg/kg of prednisone) are started first; then approximately 1 wk later, isotretinoin (0.5 mg/kg) is added and continued for as long as inflammatory lesions persist, generally 3–4 mo. Dapsone may be effective if isotretinoin cannot be used. The corticosteroids are tapered over approximately 6 wk. Antibiotics are not indicated unless there is evidence of secondary infection. Compared with acne conglobata, acne fulminans presents in younger patients, is more explosive in onset, more commonly has associated constitutional symptoms and ulcerated crusted lesions, and less commonly has multiheaded comedones or involves the face.

Feibleman CE, Rasmussen JE: Gram-negative acne. Cutis 25:194, 1980.
Hurwitz S: Acne vulgaris: Pathogenesis and management. Pediatr Rev 15:47, 1994.
Karvonen SL: Acne fulminans: report of clinical findings and treatment of twenty-four patients. J Am Acad Dermatol 28:572, 1993.
Layton AM, Knaggs H, Taylor J, et al: Isotretinoin for acne vulgaris—10 years later: a safe and successful treatment. Br J Dermatol 129:292, 1993.
Lever L, Marks R: Current views on the aetiology, pathogenesis and treatment of acne vulgaris. Drugs 39:681, 1990.
London BM, Lookingbill DP: Frequency of pregnancy in acne patients taking oral antibiotics and oral contraceptives. Arch Dermatol 130:392, 1994.
Pochi PE: The pathogenesis and treatment of acne. Annu Rev Med 41:187, 1990.
Stainforth JM, Layton AM, Taylor JP, et al: Isotretinoin for the treatment of acne vulgaris: which factors may predict the need for more than one course? Br J Dermatol 129:297, 1993.
Stewart ME, Downing DT, Cook JS, et al: Sebaceous gland activity and serum dehydroepiandrosterone sulfate levels in boys and girls. Arch Dermatol 128:1345, 1992.

CHAPTER 620
Tumors of the Skin

Gary L. Darmstadt and Al Lane

See also Chapter 460.

EPIDERMAL INCLUSION CYST (Epidermoid Cyst). These are sharply circumscribed, dome-shaped, firm, freely movable, skin-colored nodules, often with a central dimple or punctum that is a plugged, dilated pore of a pilosebaceous follicle. Epidermoid cysts form most frequently on the face, neck, chest, or upper back and may periodically become inflamed and infected secondarily, particularly in association with acne vulgaris. The cyst wall may also rupture and induce an inflammatory reaction in the dermis. The wall of the cyst is derived from the follicular infundibulum; a mass of layered keratinized material that may have a cheesy consistency fills the cavity. Epidermoid cysts may arise from occlusion of pilosebaceous follicles, from implantation of epidermal cells into the dermis as the result of an injury that penetrates the epidermis, and from rests of epidermal cells. Multiple epidermoid cysts may be present in *Gardner syndrome* and the *nevoid basal cell carcinoma syndrome.* Excision of the cysts with removal of the entire sac and its contents is indicated. A fluctuant, infected cyst should first be incised, drained, and packed, and the patient should receive an antibiotic that covers against *Staphylococcus aureus.* After the inflammation subsides, the cyst should be removed.

MILIUM. This is a pearly-white or yellowish, firm, 1–2-mm subepidermal keratin cyst. Milia in newborns is discussed in Chapter 597. Secondary milia occur in association with subepidermal blistering diseases, chronic corticosteroid-induced atrophy, 5-fluorouracil therapy, or after dermabrasion. They are retention cysts caused by hyperproliferation of injured epithelium and are indistinguishable histopathologically from primary milia; those that develop after blistering usually arise from the eccrine sweat duct, but they may develop from the hair follicle, sebaceous duct, or epidermis. A milium body differs from an epidermoid cyst only in its small size.

PILAR CYST (Trichilemmal Cyst). This is clinically indistinguishable from an epidermoid cyst. It presents as a smooth, firm, mobile nodule, predominantly on the scalp. These cysts occasionally develop on the face, neck, or trunk. The cyst may become inflamed and, occasionally, may suppurate and ulcerate. The cyst wall is composed of epithelial cells with indistinct intercellular bridges. The peripheral cell layer of the wall shows a palisade arrangement, which is not seen in an epidermoid cyst. There is no granular layer present, the cyst cavity contains homogeneous eosinophilic keratinous material, and foci of calcification are seen in 25% of cases. The propensity to develop pilar cysts is inherited in an autosomal dominant manner; more than one cyst generally develops. Multiple pilar and epidermoid cysts, desmoid tumors, fibromas, lipomas, or osteomas may be associated with colonic polyposis or adenocarcinoma in Gardner syndrome. Pilar cysts shell out easily from the dermis.

PILOMATRICOMA. This is a benign tumor that presents as a 3–30-mm, firm, solitary, deep dermal or subcutaneous tumor on the head, neck, or upper extremities. The overlying epidermis is usually normal; the tumor may occasionally be located more superficially, however, imparting a blue-red coloration to the overlying skin. Pilomatricomas may enlarge rapidly as a result of inflammation or hemorrhage and, occasionally, perforate the epidermis. Patients with both pilomatricoma and myotonic dystrophy are more likely to have multiple tumors and to have familial occurrence; in general, however, pilomatricomas are not hereditary. Histopathologically, irregularly shaped islands of epithelial cells are embedded in a cellular stroma. Calcium deposits are found in 75% of tumors.

TRICHOEPITHELIOMA. This is a smooth, round, firm, skin-colored 2–8-mm papule that is derived from immature hair follicles. Trichoepitheliomas generally occur singly on the face during childhood or early adulthood. Multiple trichoepitheliomas *(epithelioma adenoides cysticum)* are inherited autosomal dominantly, appear in childhood or at puberty, and gradually increase in number on the nasofacial folds, nose, forehead, and upper lip, and, occasionally, on the scalp, neck, and upper trunk. Microscopically, these benign tumors are characterized by horn cysts composed of a fully keratinized center surrounded by basophilic cells in an adenoid network. Surgical excision is the therapy.

ERUPTIVE VELLUS HAIR CYSTS. These are asymptomatic, follicular, skin-colored, soft 1–3-mm papules on the chest. They may become crusted or umbilicated. Abnormal vellus hair follicles become occluded at the level of the infundibulum, resulting in retention of hairs within an epithelial-lined cystic dilatation of the proximal part of the follicle. Most cases are chronic, but spontaneous regression has been reported.

STEATOCYSTOMA MULTIPLEX. This condition usually presents in adolescence or early adulthood with multiple soft to firm cystic nodules that are adherent to the underlying skin and are a few millimeters to 3 cm in diameter. When punctured, the cysts may drain oily or cheesy material. Sites of predilection include the sternal region, axillae, arms, and scrotal skin. The multiply folded cyst wall is lined on the luminal side with a thick, homogeneous, eosinophilic horny layer and lacks a granular layer. Flattened sebaceous gland lobules are often visible in the cyst wall, and lanugo hairs may be present in the cystic cavity.

SYRINGOMA. These benign tumors are soft, small, skin-colored or yellowish-brown papules that develop on the face, particularly in the periorbital regions. Other sites of predilection include the axillae and umbilical and pubic areas. They often develop during puberty and are more frequent in females. Eruptive syringomas (eruptive hidradenoma) develop in crops over the anterior trunk during childhood or adolescence. A syringoma is derived from an intraepidermal sweat gland duct. They are of cosmetic significance only. Sparse lesions may be excised, but they are often too numerous to remove.

INFANTILE DIGITAL FIBROMA. This is a firm, smooth, erythematous or skin-colored nodule on the dorsal or lateral surfaces of the distal phalanges of the fingers and toes. More than 80% of tumors present in infancy; they may be present at birth. Lesions may be solitary or multiple and may present as "kissing" tumors on opposing digits. Generally, they are asymptomatic, but flexion deformity of the digits may occur. Clinically, the lesions resemble a fibroma, leiomyoma, angiofibroma, acquired digital fibrokeratoma, accessory digit, or mucous cyst. The diagnosis is confirmed by finding numerous spindle-shaped fibroblasts that contain small, dense, round eosinophilic cytoplasmic inclusion bodies composed of collections of actin microfilaments. A viral cause has been postulated. Local recurrence after simple excision of this tumor has been reported in 75% of patients. Because the tumor does not metastasize and may regress spontaneously within 2–3 yr, a course of expectant observation is advised. If functional impairment or flexion deformity of the digit becomes apparent, prompt full excision of the tumor is indicated.

DERMATOFIBROMA (Histiocytoma). These benign dermal tumors may be pedunculated, nodular, or flat and are usually well circumscribed and firm but occasionally feel soft on palpation. The overlying skin is usually hyperpigmented, may be shiny or keratotic, and dimples when the tumor is pinched. Dermatofibromas range in size from 0.5–10 mm, arise most frequently on the limbs, and are usually asymptomatic but may occasionally be pruritic. They are composed of fibroblasts, young and mature collagen, capillaries, and histiocytes in varying proportions, forming a nodule in the dermis that has poorly defined edges. The cause of these tumors is unknown, but trauma such as an insect bite or folliculitis appears to induce reactive fibroplasia. The differential diagnosis includes epidermal inclusion cyst, juvenile xanthogranuloma, hypertrophic scar, and neurofibroma. Dermatofibromas may be excised or left intact according to the patient's preference; they usually persist indefinitely but occasionally involute spontaneously.

JUVENILE XANTHOGRANULOMA. These are firm, dome-shaped, yellow, pink, or orange papules or nodules that vary in size from a few millimeters to approximately 4 cm in diameter. They usually present at birth or within the first several months of life; occasionally, they first appear in late childhood and, rarely, in adulthood. They are 10 times more common in white than in black individuals. Sites of predilection are the scalp, face, and upper trunk, where they may erupt in profusion or remain as solitary lesions. Nodular lesions may appear on the oral mucosa. Mature lesions are characterized histopathologically by a dermal infiltrate of lipid-laden histiocytes, admixed inflammatory cells, and Touton giant cells. The lesions may clinically resemble papulonodular urticaria pigmentosa, dermatofibromas, or xanthomas of hyperlipoproteinemia but can be distinguished from these entities histopathologically.

Affected infants are nearly always otherwise normal, and blood lipid values are not elevated. Café au lait macules are found on 20% of patients with juvenile xanthogranuloma. Xanthogranulomatous infiltrates occur occasionally in ocular tissues. This may result in glaucoma, hyphema, uveitis, heterochromia iridis, iritis, or sudden proptosis. There appears to be an association among juvenile xanthogranuloma, neurofibromatosis, and childhood leukemia, most frequently juvenile chronic myelogenous leukemia. There is no need to remove these benign lesions because most of them regress spontaneously during the first few years. Residual pigmentation and atrophy, but not scarring, may result.

LIPOMA. These benign collections of fatty tissue appear on the trunk, neck, and proximal limbs. They are soft, compressible, lobulated, subcutaneous masses that are movable against the overlying skin. Multiple lesions may occur occasionally, as in Gardner syndrome. Atrophy, calcification, liquefaction, or xanthomatous change may sometimes complicate their course. A lipoma is composed of normal fat cells and surrounded by a thin connective tissue capsule. They represent a cosmetic defect and may be surgically excised. Multiple lipomas, identical to those that occur singly, are inherited in an autosomal dominant fashion and often appear by the 3rd decade in patients with *familial multiple lipomatosis*. Lipomas may appear intra-abdominally, intramuscularly, and subcutaneously. *Congenital lipomatosis* presents during the first few months of life as large subcutaneous fatty masses on the chest, with extension into skeletal muscle. Congenital lipomatosis can also be a manifestation of Proteus syndrome. *Angiolipomas* usually present as multiple, painful, subcutaneous nodules on the arms and trunk.

BASAL CELL EPITHELIOMA (Basal Cell Carcinoma). Basal cell carcinoma is rare in children in the absence of a predisposing condition, such as nevoid basal cell carcinoma syndrome, xeroderma pigmentosum, nevus sebaceus of Jadassohn, arsenic intake, or exposure to irradiation. The lesions are pink, pearly, telangiectatic, smooth papules that enlarge slowly and may bleed or ulcerate. Sites of predilection are the face, scalp, and upper back. The differential diagnosis includes pyogenic granuloma, nevocellular nevus, epidermal inclusion cyst, closed comedo, dermatofibroma, and adnexal tumor. Depending on the site of occurrence and associated disease of the host, electrodesiccation and curettage or simple excision is usually curative. When the tumor is recurrent, larger than 2 cm in diameter, located on problematic anatomic areas such as the midface or ears, or is an aggressive histopathologic type, Mohs microscopically controlled surgery may be the most appropriate treatment.

NEVOID BASAL CELL CARCINOMA SYNDROME (Basal Cell Nevus Syndrome, Gorlin Syndrome). This autosomal dominant syndrome, which has been mapped to chromosome 9q22.3–9q31, includes a wide spectrum of defects involving the skin, eyes, central nervous and endocrine systems, and bones. The predominant features are early-onset basal cell carcinomas and mandibular cysts. Approximately 20% of those in whom a basal cell carcinoma develops before age 19 yr have this syndrome. Basal cell carcinomas appear between puberty and age 35 yr, erupting in crops of tumors that vary in size, color, and number and may be difficult to distinguish from other types of skin lesions. Sites of predilection are the periorbital skin, nose, malar areas, and upper lip, but the lesions can develop on the trunk and limbs and are not restricted to sun-exposed areas. Ulceration, bleeding, crusting, and local invasion can occur. Small milia, epidermal cysts, pigmented lesions, hirsutism, and palmar and plantar pits are additional cutaneous findings.

The facies of patients with this syndrome is characterized by temporoparietal bossing, prominent supraorbital ridges, a broad nasal root, ocular hypertelorism or dystopia canthorum, and prognathism. Keratinized cysts (odontogenic keratocysts) in the maxilla and mandible occur in most patients. They range in size from a few millimeters to several centimeters; may result in maldevelopment of the teeth; and cause pain, swelling of the jaw, facial deformity, bone erosion, pathologic fractures, and suppurating sinus tracts. Osseous defects such as anomalous rib development, spina bifida, kyphoscoliosis, and brachymetacarpalism occur in two thirds of patients, and ocular abnormalities including cataracts, glaucoma, coloboma, strabismus, and blindness occur in approximately one fourth. Some males have hypogonadism, with absent or undescended testes. Kidney malformations have also been reported. Neurologic manifestations include calcification of the falx, seizures, mental retardation, partial agenesis of the corpus callosum, hydrocephalus, and nerve deafness. There is increased incidence of medulloblastoma, ameloblastoma of the oval cavity, fibrosarcoma of the jaw, teratoma, cystadenoma, cardiac fibroma, and ovarian fibroma.

The *treatment* of these patients requires participation of various specialists according to individual clinical problems. Basal cell carcinomas should not be treated with irradiation. Most of the basal cell carcinomas have a clinically benign course, and it is often impossible to remove them all; those with an aggressive growth pattern and those on the central face, however, should be removed promptly. Oral retinoids have been shown to be helpful in preventing the development of new tumors in some patients. Genetic counseling is also indicated.

MUCOSAL NEUROMA SYNDROME (Sippel Syndrome). Mucosal neuroma syndrome is inherited as an autosomal dominant trait and is easily recognized by characteristic physical features. An asthenic or marfanoid habitus is accompanied by scoliosis, pectus excavatum, pes cavus, and muscular hypotonia. Patients have thick, patulous lips and soft tissue prognathism simulating acromegaly. Multiple mucosal neuromas or neurofibromas appear as pink, pedunculated or sessile nodules on the anterior third of the tongue, at the commissures of the lips, and on the buccal mucosa and palpebral conjunctiva. A variety of ophthalmologic defects and intestinal ganglioneuromatosis with recurrent diarrhea are additional common findings. There is a high incidence of medullary thyroid carcinoma associated with high calcitonin levels, pheochromocytoma, and hyperparathyroidism. Periodic screening tests for the associated malignant tumors are mandatory.

Cerio R, Jones EW: Histiocytoma cutis: a tumour of dermal dendrocytes (dermal dendrocytoma). Br J Dermatol 120:197, 1989.
Coskey RJ, Dalrey KW: Recurring digital fibrous tumor of childhood: Review of the literature. J Pediatr Orthop 6:612, 1986.
Evans DGR, Ladusans EJ, Riommer S, et al: Complications of the nevoid basal cell carcinoma syndrome: Results of a population based study. J Med Genet 30:460, 1993.
Milstone EG, Helwig EB: Basal carcinoma in children. Arch Dermatol 108:523, 1973.
Roper SR, Spraker MK: Cutaneous histiocytosis syndromes. Pediatr Dermatol 3:19, 1985.
Rotte JJ, de Vaan GA, Koopman RJ: Juvenile xanthogranuloma and acute leukemia: A case report. Med Pediatr Oncol 23:57, 1994.
Taaffe, Wyatt EH, Bury HPR, et al: Pilomatricoma (Malherbe): A clinical and histopathologic survey of 78 cases. Int J Dermatol 27:477, 1988.

CHAPTER 621
Nutritional Dermatoses

Gary L. Darmstadt and Al Lane

ACRODERMATITIS ENTEROPATHICA. This is a rare, autosomal recessive disorder caused by an inability to absorb sufficient zinc from the diet. Initial signs and symptoms usually occur during the first few months of life, often after weaning from breast to cow's milk. The cutaneous eruption consists of vesiculobullous, eczematous, dry, scaly, or psoriasiform skin lesions symmetrically distributed in the perioral, acral, and perineal areas and on the cheeks, knees, and elbows (Fig. 621–1). The hair often has a peculiar reddish tint, and alopecia of some degree is characteristic. Ocular manifestations include photophobia, conjunctivitis, blepharitis, and corneal dystrophy, detectable by slit-lamp examination. Associated manifestations include chronic diarrhea, stomatitis, glossitis, paronychia, nail dystrophy, growth retardation, irritability, delayed wound healing, intercurrent bacterial infections, and superinfection with *Candida albicans*. Lymphocyte function and free radical scavenging are impaired. Without treatment, the course is chronic and intermittent but often relentlessly progressive. When the disease is less severe, only growth retardation and delayed development may be apparent.

The *diagnosis* is established by the constellation of clinical findings and detection of a low plasma zinc concentration. Histopathologic changes in the skin are nonspecific and include parakeratosis and pallor of the upper epidermis. The variety of manifestations of the syndrome may be due to the fact that zinc plays a role in multiple metabolic pathways, including those of copper, protein, essential fatty acids, and prostaglandins, and zinc is incorporated into many zinc metalloenzymes.

Oral therapy with zinc compounds is the *treatment* of choice. Optimal doses range from 50 mg of zinc sulfate, acetate, or gluconate daily for infants up to 150 mg/24 hr for children; plasma zinc levels should be monitored, however, to individualize the dosage. Zinc therapy rapidly abolishes the manifestations of the disease. A syndrome resembling acrodermatitis enteropathica has been observed in patients with secondary zinc deficiency caused by long-term total parenteral nutrition without supplemental zinc, or chronic malabsorption syndromes. A rash similar to that of acrodermatitis enteropathica has also been reported in infants fed breast milk that is low in

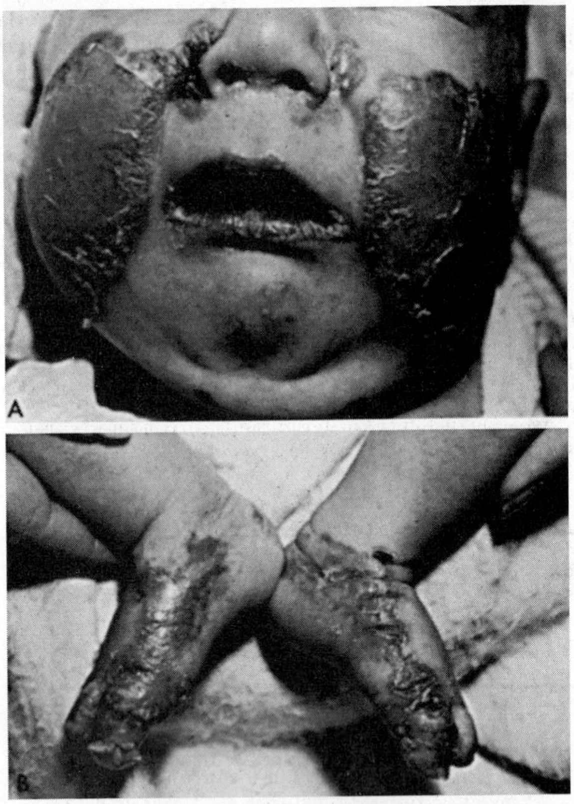

Figure 621–1. *A*, Psoriasiform facial lesions of zinc deficiency dermatitis. *B*, Similar lesions on the feet with secondary nail dystrophy.

zinc and in those with maple syrup urine disease, organic aciduria, methylmalonic acidemia, biotinidase deficiency, essential fatty acid deficiency, severe protein malnutrition (e.g., kwashiorkor), and cystic fibrosis.

ESSENTIAL FATTY ACID DEFICIENCY. This causes a generalized, scaly dermatitis composed of thickened, erythematous, desquamating plaques. The eruption has been induced experimentally in animals fed a fat-free diet and has been observed in patients with chronic, severe malabsorption such as in short-gut syndrome and in those sustained on a fat-free diet or fat-free parenteral alimentation. Linoleic (18:2 n-6) and arachidonic (20:4 n-6) acids are deficient, and an abnormal metabolite, 5,8,11-eicosatrienoic acid (20:3 n-9), is present in the plasma. Additional manifestations of essential fatty acid deficiency include alopecia, thrombocytopenia, and failure to thrive. The horny layer of the skin is cracked microscopically, the barrier function of the skin is disturbed, and transepidermal water loss is increased. Topical application of linoleic acid, which is present in sunflower seed oil, may ameliorate the clinical and biochemical skin manifestations. Appropriate nutrition should be provided.

KWASHIORKOR. Severe protein and essential amino acid deprivation in association with adequate caloric intake can lead to kwashiorkor, particularly at the time of weaning to a diet that consists primarily of corn, rice, or beans (see Chapter 45.3). Cutaneous erythema develops first and, in mild cases in white children, progresses to fine desquamation along natural skin lines and on the shins, outer thighs, and back. In dark-skinned children, characteristic early findings include circumoral pallor, cutaneous depigmentation, and development of purple patches. As the disease advances, well-marginated, slightly raised, purplish, waxy plaques appear, particularly in the diaper area and at sites of pressure such as the elbows, knees, ankles, and on the trunk. In severe cases, erosions and linear fissures develop. Sun-exposed skin is relatively spared, as are the feet and dorsal hands. Nails are thin and soft, and hair is sparse, thin, and depigmented, sometimes displaying a flag sign of alternating light and dark bands that reflect alternating periods of adequate and inadequate nutrition. The cutaneous manifestations may closely resemble those of acrodermatitis enteropathica. The serum zinc level is often deficient, and in some cases, skin lesions of kwashiorkor heal more rapidly when zinc is applied topically.

CYSTIC FIBROSIS (see Chapter 363). Five to 10% of patients with cystic fibrosis develop protein-calorie malnutrition. Rash in infants with cystic fibrosis and malnutrition is rare but may appear by 6 mo of age. The initial eruption consists of erythematous, scaling papules and progresses within 1–3 mo to extensive, desquamating plaques. The rash is accentuated around the mouth and perineum and on the extremities (lower > upper). Alopecia may be present, but mucous membranes and nails are uninvolved.

PELLAGRA (see Chapter 45.3). This presents with edema, erythema, and burning of sun-exposed skin on the face, neck, and dorsal hands, forearms, and feet. Lesions of pellagra may also be provoked by burns, pressure, friction, and inflammation. The eruption on the face frequently follows a "butterfly" distribution, and the dermatitis encircling the neck has been termed "Casal necklace." Blisters and scales develop, and the skin increasingly becomes dry, rough, thickened, cracked, and hyperpigmented. Skin infections may be unusually severe. Pellagra develops in those with insufficient dietary intake or absorption of niacin and/or tryptophan. Administration of isoniazid, 6-mercaptopurine, or 5-fluorouracil may also produce pellagra. Nicotinamide supplementation and sun avoidance are the mainstays of therapy.

SCURVY (Vitamin C or Ascorbic Acid Deficiency) (see Chapter 45.3). This presents initially with follicular hyperkeratosis and coiling of hair on the upper arms, back, buttocks, and lower extremities. Perifollicular erythema and hemorrhage, particularly on the legs, advancing to involve large areas of hemorrhage; swollen, erythematous gums; stomatitis; and subperiosteal hematomas are also seen. The best method for confirmation of a clinical diagnosis of scurvy is a trial of vitamin C supplementation.

VITAMIN A DEFICIENCY (see Chapter 45.3). This deficiency presents initially with impairment of visual adaptation to the dark. Cutaneous changes include xerosis and hyperkeratosis and hyperplasia of the epidermis, particularly the lining of hair follicles and sebaceous glands. In severe cases, desquamation may be prominent.

Darmstadt GL, Schmidt CP, Wechsler DS, et al: Dermatitis as a presenting sign of cystic fibrosis. Arch Dermatol 128:1358, 1992.

Hansen AE, Wiese HF, Boelsche AN, et al: Role of linoleic acid in infant nutrition. Pediatrics 31:171, 1963.

Hansen RC, Lemen R, Revsin B: Cystic fibrosis manifesting with acrodermatitis enteropathica-like eruption. Arch Dermatol 119:51, 1983.

Hendricks WM: Pellagra and pellagra-like dermatoses: Etiology, differential diagnosis, dermatopathology, and treatment. Semin Dermatol 10:282, 1991.

Krieger I, Evans GW: Acrodermatitis enteropathica without hypozincemia: Therapeutic effect of a pancreatic enzyme preparation due to a zinc-binding ligand. J Pediatr 96:32, 1980.

Neldner KH, Hambidge KM: Zinc deficiency of acrodermatitis enteropathica. N Engl J Med 292:879, 1975.

PART XXXII

Bone and Joint Disorders

SECTION 1

Orthopedic Problems

George H. Thompson ▪ *Peter V. Scoles*

Musculoskeletal disorders in children and adolescents are common, and the pediatrician is usually the first physician consulted. Many of these disorders can be managed safely and effectively by the pediatrician provided an accurate diagnosis can be established. The differential diagnosis of pediatric musculoskeletal disorders is extensive and involves all diagnostic categories: congenital, developmental, acquired, infectious, neuromuscular, neoplastic, as well as psychogenic. This chapter provides basic information relevant to the more common disorders and emphasizes the pediatrician's role in making an accurate diagnosis. Neoplasms (benign and malignant), infections (osteomyelitis and septic arthritis), and neuromuscular disorders (cerebral palsy, myelodysplasia, and muscular dystrophy) are presented in other chapters.

Before beginning on the evaluation of the child with an orthopedic problem, it is important to have a basic understanding of the effects of in utero positioning, the mechanism in which normal musculoskeletal growth occurs, and the relationships among growth, neurologic maturation, and normal developmental milestones.

IN UTERO POSITIONING. In the newborn, the imprint of the in utero positioning may be evident and confused as an abnormality. In utero positioning produces joint and muscle contractures and affects the torsional alignment of the long bones, especially the lower extremities. Normal full-term newborns have 20–30 degree hip and knee flexion contractures. These resolve by 4–6 mo of age. The newborn hip externally rotates in extension 80–90 degrees and has limited internal rotation to 0–10 degrees. The lower leg frequently has inward rotation (internal tibial torsion), and the feet are supinated from their medial borders, being wrapped against the posterolateral aspect of the opposite thigh. The top leg in the in utero position may show more changes than the bottom leg. The face may also be distorted, whereas the spine and upper extremities are less affected by the in utero position. The effects of in utero positioning, therefore, are physiologic in origin but may produce parental concerns. The child may be 3–4 yr old before the effects of the in utero position completely resolve.

GROWTH AND DEVELOPMENT. Each of the individual components of the skeletal system grow by different mechanisms. The long bones of the extremities (humerus, radius-ulna, femur, and tibia-fibula) have growth or physeal plates at each end. Each will contribute a varying proportion to the longitudinal growth of the individual bone as well as the extremity through a process termed *endochondral ossification.* The ends of each long bone are composed of the epiphyses. These are covered by articular cartilage and form the associated joints. The epiphyses are initially almost entirely cartilaginous and then become progressively more ossified with time. The articular cartilage also has growth potential, which contributes to the growth of the epiphysis. The perichondrial ring, which surrounds the physeal plates, as well as the perichondrium around the epiphyses and periosteum, which surrounds the metaphysis and diaphyseal regions of the bone, contributes to apositional or circumferential growth.

Bones without physeal plates, such as the pelvis, scapulae, carpals, and tarsal bones, grow by apositional bone growth from their surrounding perichondrium and periosteum. Other bones, such as the metacarpals, metatarsals, phalanges, and spine, grow by a combination of both apositional and endochondral ossification.

Trauma, infections, nutritional deficiencies (rickets), regional soft tissue processes, inborn errors of metabolism (mucopolysaccharidosis, mucolipidosis, Gaucher disease, and disorders of cartilage and cartilage synthesis), and other metabolic processes may affect each of these growth processes, producing a distinct alteration in the particular growth function.

DEVELOPMENTAL MILESTONES. Neurologic maturation, marked by the passage of motor milestones at regular intervals, is important for normal musculoskeletal development. The milestones for locomotion include independent sitting at 6 mo of age, crawling at 9 mo, walking without assistance at 12–15 mo, and running at 18 mo (see Chapter 11). There is a distinct relationship between skeletal form and gross motor function. Any process that produces a neurologic abnormality may secondarily cause a delay in developmental milestones and an alteration of normal skeletal growth. ▪

CHAPTER 622

Evaluation of the Child

The key to an accurate diagnosis in a child with musculoskeletal disorder is a careful history, a thorough physical examination, appropriate radiographic imaging, and occasionally laboratory testing. A glossary of common orthopedic terminology is provided in Table 622–1.

HISTORY. The history of the musculoskeletal complaint is often the most important part of the evaluation. This is usually obtained from the parents or guardian, but the child, if old enough and cooperative, can also give useful information. The chief complaint is established first. This may include pain, deformity, joint stiffness, gait disturbance (limp, toe walking, in-toeing, and out-toeing), swelling, or generalized muscle weakness. One must ascertain location and duration of symptoms; antecedent factors such as fever, trauma, radiation of pain, and neurologic symptoms; factors aggravating or alleviating the symptoms; and previous evaluations or treatment.

In children who do not have an acute injury or disorder, the medical history may also be important in guiding the pediatrician to the correct diagnosis. The prenatal or pregnancy history should be obtained (see Chapters 79, 80, and 81). This includes maternal diseases or illnesses, vaginal bleeding, ingestion of toxic substance or medications, and trauma. The birth history should determine the length of pregnancy, dura-

■ **TABLE 622–1 Glossary of Orthopedic Terminology**

Term	Definition
Abduction	Movement away from the midline
Adduction	Movement toward and possibly across the midline
Anteversion	Increased angulation of the femoral head and neck with respect to the knee in the frontal plane
Apophysis	Bone growth center that is not a growth plate or physis and that has a strong muscle insertion (e.g., greater trochanter of femur)
Arthroplasty	Surgical reconstruction of a joint
Arthrotomy	Surgical incision into a joint
Calcaneus	Dorsiflexion of hindfoot
Cavovarus	High longitudinal or medial arch of foot with plantar-flexed supinated forefoot and hindfoot varus
Cavus	High longitudinal arch of the foot (usually plantar-flexed forefoot)
Dislocation	Complete loss of contact between two joint surfaces
Equinus	Plantar flexion of the forefoot, hindfoot, or entire foot
Extension	Means to straighten; is the reverse of flexion
External or lateral rotation	Outward rotation away from the midline
Flexion	Means to bend
Internal or medial rotation	Inward rotation, toward the midline
Subluxation	Incomplete loss of contact between two joint surfaces
Valgum	Angulation of a bone or joint in which the apex is toward the midline; genu valgum results in knock-knee because the angulation of the knee is toward the midline
Varum	Angulation of a bone or joint away from the midline; genu varum results in bowleg because the angulation is away from the midline

tion of labor, type of difficulty, if any, with delivery, birth presentation, birthweight, and the Apgar ratings (see Chapters 82, 83, and 84). The condition of the child during the neonatal period is also important (see Chapter 83). In older infants and young children, the presence and delay of developmental milestones for posture, locomotion, dexterity, social activities, and speech are also important.

PHYSICAL EXAMINATION. Physical examination of a child with a musculoskeletal disorder must be thorough. It includes the careful evaluation of the musculoskeletal and neurologic systems followed by an appropriate general physical examination. Many common musculoskeletal disorders can be diagnosed by the history and physical examination alone. The examination of the musculoskeletal system includes four parts: observation, palpation, assessment of joint range of motion, and gait assessment in ambulatory children.

Observation. The first part of the musculoskeletal examination begins with inspection of the body. This must be accomplished by observing the child undressed. If the child can stand, then posture, truncal alignment, and symmetry of the extremities can be evaluated. The skin is assessed for cutaneous lesions. The presence of café au lait spots may be indicative of neurofibromatosis, whereas a maculopapular rash may indicate juvenile rheumatoid arthritis. Infants or young children may be examined on their parent's lap, where they feel more secure and are more likely to be cooperative.

Palpation. The involved joint or area of the extremity or trunk that is of concern should be palpated for tenderness, masses, soft tissue swelling, and increased warmth. Abnormal joints should also be palpated for effusion, synovial thickening, increased warmth, and areas of increased tenderness.

Joint Range of Motion. The range of motion of the involved joint or joints should be assessed and recorded. If the opposite joint is normal, this range should also be recorded for comparison purposes. It must be remembered that the range of motion of joints changes from infancy through childhood and into adolescence.

Gait Assessment. Gait disturbances are one of the most common parental concerns in children. It is, therefore, important to have a thorough understanding of the development of normal gait. Human gait is dynamic, complex, and repetitive. The gait cycle is the time between right heel strike followed by left toe-off, left heel strike, and right toe-off and ends with right heel strike. The five events describe one gait cycle and include two phases: stance and swing. The stance phase is the period of time during which one of the two feet are on the ground. The swing phase is the portion of the gait cycle during which a limb is being advanced forward without ground contact.

Neurologic maturation is necessary for the development of gait and the normal progression of developmental milestones. The normal 1-yr-old child has a wide-based stance and rapid cadence with short steps, the elbows are flexed, and reciprocal arm motion is not present. Foot strike occurs without initial heel strike. A 2-yr-old child will show increased velocity and step length and diminished cadence compared with a 1-yr-old. Most of the adult gait patterns are present in children by 3 yr of age with changes of velocity, stride, and cadence continuing to 7 yr. The gait characteristics of a 7-yr-old child are similar to those of an adult.

Common gait disturbances include limp (antalgic and Trendelenburg), torsional variations (in-toeing and out-toeing), and toe walking. In evaluating gait disturbance, it is important to observe the child walking and running. The child must be sufficiently undressed to allow visualization of the lower extremities and trunk during ambulation.

LIMPING. Limping is categorized into either painful (antalgic) or nonpainful (Trendelenburg gait) on the basis of the length of the stance phase. In a painful gait, the stance phase is shortened as the child decreases the time spent on the painful extremity. In a nonpainful gait, which is indicative of underlying proximal muscle weakness or hip instability, the stance phase is equal between the involved and uninvolved side, but the child will lean or shift the center of gravity over the involved extremity for balance. If the disorder is bilateral, it will produce a waddling gait. The differential diagnosis of limping is extensive. The vast majority of causes involve the lower extremity, but it must be remembered that spinal disorders, especially spinal cord or peripheral nerve disorders, can also produce limping and difficulty walking. Painful gaits are predominantly a result of trauma, infection, neoplasia, and rheumatologic disorders. Trendelenburg gaits are generally due to congenital, developmental, or muscular disorders. Thus, antalgic gaits are acute processes, whereas Trendelenburg gaits are chronic. The differential diagnosis of limping is presented in Table 622–2 and causes according to age in Table 622–3.

TORSIONAL VARIATIONS. Torsional variations, in-toeing and out-toeing, are the most common gait disturbances that cause parents to seek advice from their pediatrician (see Chapter 624). Many do not require treatment because they are physiologic in origin and will improve and resolve with normal growth and development. However, they produce significant anxiety and require that the pediatrician have a clear understanding of the cause and natural history to reassure the family appropriately. The common causes of in-toeing and out-toeing are presented in Table 622–4. It is important to realize that the presence of in-toeing and out-toeing does not imply an abnormality of the foot but rather only the direction in which the foot is pointing during ambulation. The causes for torsional variations can occur from proximal (hip) to distal (foot) in the involved extremity. Some of the causes, such as clubfoot, are obvious, whereas others can be subtle.

TOE WALKING. Toe walking or equinus gait is one of the least common causes of gait disturbances. It can be a normal finding in children up to 3 yr of age. Persistent toe walking thereafter or acquired toe walking at a later age is considered abnormal and requires careful evaluation. The common causes of unilat-

■ TABLE 622–2 Differential Diagnosis of Limping

Antalgic	Trendelenburg
Congenital	***Developmental***
Tarsal coalition	DDH
Acquired	Leg length discrepancy
LCPD	***Neuromuscular***
SCFE	Cerebral palsy
Trauma	
Sprains, strains, contusions	
Fractures	
Occult	
Toddler's fracture	
Neoplasia	
Benign	
Unicameral bone cyst	
Osteoid osteoma	
Malignant	
Osteogenic sarcoma	
Ewing sarcoma	
Leukemia	
Spinal cord tumors	
Infectious	
Septic arthritis	
Osteomyelitis	
Acute	
Subacute	
Diskitis	
Rheumatologic	
Hip monoarticular synovitis	

LCPD = Legg-Calvé-Perthes disease; SCFE = slipped capital femoral epiphysis; DDH = developmental dysplasia of the hip.

From Thompson GH: Gait disturbances. In: *Kliegman RM, Nieder ML, Super DM (eds): Practical Strategies of Pediatric Diagnosis and Therapy. Philadelphia, WB Saunders, in press.*

■ TABLE 622–3 Common Causes of Limping According to Age

Age	Antalgic	Trendelenburg	Leg Length Discrepancy
Toddler	Infection	Hip dislocation (DDH)	⊖
(1–3 yr)	Septic arthritis	Neuromuscular disease	
	Hip	Cerebral palsy	
	Knee		
	Osteomyelitis		
	Diskitis		
	Occult trauma		
	Toddler's fracture		
	Neoplasia		
Childhood	Infection	Hip dislocation (DDH)	⊕
(4–10 yr)	Septic arthritis	Neuromuscular disease	
	Hip	Cerebral palsy	
	Knee		
	Osteomyelitis		
	Diskitis		
	Transient synovitis, hip		
	LCPD		
	Rheumatologic disorder		
	JRA		
	Trauma		
	Neoplasia		
Adolescence	SCFE		⊕
(11 + yr)	Rheumatologic disorder		
	JRA		
	Trauma		

LCPD = Legg-Calvé-Perthes disease; JRA = juvenile rheumatoid arthritis; SCFE = slipped capital femoral epiphysis; DDH = developmental dysplasia of the hip; ⊖ = absent; ⊕ = present.

From Thompson GH: Gait disturbances. In: *Kliegman RM, Nieder ML, Super DM (eds): Practical Strategies of Pediatric Diagnosis and Therapy. Philadelphia, WB Saunders, in press.*

eral and bilateral toe walking are listed in Table 622–5. The differential diagnosis for persistent or acquired toe walking include (1) neuromuscular disorders, such as cerebral palsy, Duchenne muscular dystrophy, or spinal cord abnormalities, (2) congenital tendo-Achilles contracture, (3) leg length discrepancy, and (4) habit.

Neurologic Evaluation. After the musculoskeletal examination, a careful neurologic evaluation must be performed. This should include muscle strength testing, sensory assessment, and evaluation of deep tendon and pathologic reflexes such as Babinski. The pertinent negative and positive findings should be recorded for future reference. Part of the neurologic evaluation should also include assessment of the spine. This includes the presence of deformity such as scoliosis or kyphosis as well as spinal mobility. The child's ability to forward flex and reverse the normal lumbar lordosis is a sign of normal mobility. Areas of tenderness and muscle spasm are determined by palpation.

RADIOGRAPHIC ASSESSMENT. Radiography is the principal method for the evaluation of the pediatric musculoskeletal system. This can include routine radiographs as well as special procedures such as technetium bone scan, computed tomography (CT), magnetic resonance imaging (MRI), and ultrasonography.

Routine Radiography. This is the first step in the evaluation of most pediatric musculoskeletal disorders. Routine radiographs consist of anteroposterior and lateral views of the involved joint, bone, or area. Comparison views of the opposite side, if uninvolved, may be helpful in difficult situations but are usually not necessary or ordered routinely. The type of radiographs for each anatomic area are discussed in the sections on specific disorders.

Technetium Bone Scans. These are particularly useful in assessing for occult lesions when routine radiographs are normal. Common indications for bone scans include (1) early septic arthritis or osteomyelitis; (2) tumors such as osteoid osteomas; (3) metastatic lesions; (4) occult fractures such as the toddler fracture of the tibia; and (5) inflammatory disorders. Unfortunately, the radiation levels are high, and these scans should be obtained only when necessary.

Computed Tomography (CT). Coronal and axial cross-section studies with CT can be beneficial in evaluating complex disorders of the spine, pelvis, and feet. It allows visualization of the bone anatomy and the relationship of bones to contiguous structures, which routine radiographs do not.

Magnetic Resonance Imaging (MRI). This avoids ionizing radiation and is presumed not to produce biologically harmful effects. It produces excellent anatomic images of the musculoskeletal system, including the spinal cord and brain. It is especially useful for soft tissue lesions, allowing distinction between different muscles or muscle groups. Cartilage structures can be visualized and even different forms distinguished; articular cartilage of the knee can be distinguished from the fibrocartilage of the meniscus. MRI can be very helpful in visualizing joints that are unossified, such as may occur in the shoulders, elbows, and hips of young infants. MRI can also distinguish physiologic changes that occur in the bone marrow with respect to age and disease such as avascular necrosis. In children MRI can be very useful in the evaluation of (1) avascular necrosis of bone, especially the capital femoral epiphysis or femoral head; (2) bone and soft tissue neoplasms; (3) intra-articular abnormalities of the knee joint; and (4) assessment of intraspinal pathology.

■ TABLE 622–4 Common Causes of In-Toeing and Out-Toeing

In-Toeing	Out-Toeing
Internal femoral torsion	External femoral torsion
Internal tibial torsion	External tibial torsion
Metatarsus adductus	Calcaneovalgus feet
Talipes equinovarus (Clubfoot)	Hypermobile pes planus

From Thompson GH: Pediatric orthopedics (spine, hips, lower extremities, and feet). In: *Marcus RE (ed): Orthopedics. Los Angeles, Practice Management Information Corporation, 1991, pp 209–300.*

■ **TABLE 622–5 Common Causes of Toe Walking (Equinus Gait)**

Unilateral	Bilateral
Neuromuscular disorder	Neuromuscular disorder
Cerebral palsy (hemiplegia)	Cerebral palsy (diplegia)
Leg length discrepancy	Duchenne muscular dystrophy
Hip dislocation (DDH)	Congenital tendo-Achilles contracture
	Habitual

DDH = Developmental dysplasia of the hip.
From Thompson GH: Gait disturbances. In: *Kliegman RM, Nieder ML, Super DM (eds): Practical Strategies of Pediatric Diagnosis and Therapy. Philadelphia, WB Saunders, in press.*

Ultrasonography. Ultrasound evaluation is being increasingly used in pediatric orthopedics. As with MRI scans, it has no ionizing radiation, no contrast material to be administered, and no biologically harmful effects and can be repeated as often as necessary. The equipment is portable but relatively expensive. Scans can be obtained in any plane. The disadvantages of ultrasonography include the following: bone is not penetrated by sound waves, (2) static images are difficult to interpret, and (3) the results are very heavily operator dependent. The major indications for ultrasonography are (1) obstetric studies of the extremities and spine; (2) developmental dysplasia of the hip; (3) joint effusions; (4) occult neonatal spinal dysraphism; (5) foreign bodies in soft tissues; and (6) popliteal cysts of the knee.

LABORATORY STUDIES. Occasionally, hematologic tests are necessary in the evaluation of the pediatric musculoskeletal system. These may include a complete blood count, erythrocyte sedimentation rate, and C-reactive protein for infectious disorders, such as septic arthritis or osteomyelitis. Rheumatoid factor, antinuclear antibodies, and human leukocyte antigen B27 are necessary for children with suspected rheumatologic disorders. Creatine phosphokinase, aldolase, serum glutamic-oxaloacetic transaminase, and dystrophin testing are indicated in children with suspected disorders of striated muscle such as Duchenne or Becker muscular dystrophy.

TALKING WITH PARENTS. Talking effectively with parents of children with musculoskeletal problems is critically important as well as challenging. Many problems are normal or physiologic variations, will resolve with growth and development, and require only observation. This is particularly true in torsional variations of the lower extremities, which can produce significant anxiety in parents and grandparents. Establishing a strong rapport with the family is an important component in the patient-family-physician relationship. Active treatment is indicated when the disorder has the potential to produce disability and the treatment is effective in altering the natural history. In many instances, the treatment may not significantly improve the child's condition initially, but by altering the natural history, problems in adult life, such as degenerative osteoarthritis, will be avoided.

Several steps are helpful in establishing a working relationship with parents. The diagnosis should be accurate and accompanied by a clear explanation of the cause and natural history of the disorder. Treatment options, including observation, should be discussed along with the expected results, both short term and long term. If observation is recommended, a follow-up evaluation should be performed to document resolution and give the family additional reassurance.

Finally, not all physiologic conditions resolve. A small percentage of these disorders may persist into adolescence. These may require treatment if problems as an adult are to be avoided. The longer a problem persists, the greater is the chance that the problem will not resolve and may require treatment.

Forero N, Okamura LA, Larson MA: Normal ranges of hip motion in neonates. J Pediatr Orthop 9:391, 1989.
Hall TR, Kangarloo H: Magnetic resonance imaging of the musculoskeletal system in children. Clin Orthop 244:119, 1989.
Harcke HT, Grissom LE, Finkelstein MS: Evaluation of the musculoskeletal system with sonography. AJR 150:1253, 1988.
Harcke HT, Kumar SJ: Current concepts review: The role of ultrasound in the diagnosis and management of congenital dislocation and dysplasia of the hip. J Bone Joint Surg 73A:622, 1991.
Jones ET: Use of computed axial tomography in pediatric orthopaedics. J Pediatr Orthop 1:329, 1981.
Scoles PV (ed): Pediatric Orthopedics in Clinical Practice, 2nd ed. Chicago, Year Book Medical Publishers, 1988.
Sutherland DH, Olsten R, Cooper L, et al: The development of gait. J Bone Joint Surg 62A:336, 1980.
Thompson GH: Gait disturbances. *In*: Kliegman RM, Nieder ML, Super DM (eds): Practical Strategies in Pediatric Diagnosis and Therapy. Philadelphia, WB Saunders, in press.

CHAPTER 623
The Foot and Toes

The foot and toes are important in stance and locomotion. Abnormalities affecting the foot can produce pain and abnormal shoe wear and can have an adverse effect on function. The foot articulates with the lower end of the tibia. The ankle joint is a box joint, which allows foot dorsiflexion and plantar flexion with essentially no rotation. The talus articulates with the distal end of the tibia. Support is achieved through the medial malleolus of the tibia and the lateral malleolus of the distal fibula. The foot is divided into three regions: hindfoot, midfoot, and forefoot. The toes are a portion of the forefoot.

The hindfoot is composed of the talus and calcaneus. The latter forms the heel. The joint between these two bones is the talocalcaneal or subtalar joint. This joint has a gliding and rotatory motion, which allows for inversion and eversion of the hindfoot. This is important for walking on uneven ground.

The midfoot is composed of the navicular bone, the cuboid bone, and the three cuneiform bones. The midfoot and hindfoot articulate through the transverse tarsal joint (calcaneocuboid and talonavicular joints). This joint is important for midfoot rotation and for walking on uneven ground. Deformity or malalignment of subtalar, talonavicular, or calcaneocuboid joints can have a significant effect on the alignment and function of the foot and produces abnormal stress on the ankle joint.

The forefoot is composed of the metatarsals and toes. The first metatarsal is unique because it has a single physeal plate that is located proximally. The lateral four metatarsals have a single physis located distally. The great toe is composed of proximal and distal phalanges and a single interphalangeal joint. The lateral four toes have proximal, middle, and distal phalanges that articulate through a proximal interphalangeal joint and a distal interphalangeal joint. All phalanges have their physeal plates located proximally. Normal function of the foot and toes requires a coordinated action between the extrinsic muscles of the calf and intrinsic muscles of the foot.

FOOT DISORDERS

The most common pediatric foot disorders include (1) metatarsus adductus, (2) calcaneovalgus feet, (3) talipes equinovarus (clubfoot), (4) congenital vertical talus, (5) hypermobile pes planus, (6) tarsal coalition, (7) cavus feet, (8) osteochondroses, and (9) puncture wounds of the foot.

623.1 Metatarsus Adductus

Congenital metatarsus adductus is a common problem among infants and young children. It is also known as metatarsus varus if the forefoot is supinated as well as adducted. It occurs equally in males and females and is bilateral in approximately 50% of patients. There are hereditary tendencies; it tends to be more common in first-born than in later children as a result of increased molding effect from the primigravida uterus and abdominal wall. There is also an association with hip dysplasia. Approximately 10% of children with metatarsus adductus will have acetabular dysplasia. Thus, careful clinical examination of the hips is necessary in any child with metatarsus adductus. Pelvic radiographs are obtained in suggestive cases.

CLINICAL MANIFESTATIONS. Clinically, the forefoot is adducted and occasionally supinated. The hindfoot and midfoot are normal. The lateral border of the foot is convex, and the base of the fifth metatarsal appears prominent (Fig. 623–1). The medial border of the foot is concave. There is usually an increased interval between the first and second toes, with the great toe being held in a greater varus position. Ankle dorsiflexion and plantar flexion are normal. Forefoot mobility can vary from flexible to rigid. This is assessed by stabilizing the hindfoot and midfoot in a neutral position with one hand and applying pressure over the first metatarsal head with the other. In the walking child with an uncorrected metatarsus adductus deformity, an in-toe gait and abnormal shoe wear may occur.

RADIOGRAPHIC EVALUATION. Radiographs of the foot are not routinely necessary in metatarsus adductus because they do not demonstrate forefoot mobility. Anteroposterior (AP) and lateral weightbearing or simulated weightbearing radiographs may be obtained when necessary. The AP radiographs will demonstrate adduction of the metatarsals at the tarsometatarsal articulation and an increased intermetatarsal angle between the first and second metatarsals. The lateral four metatarsals appear to have increased closeness and occasionally overlap at their base. The hindfoot and midfoot are normal.

TREATMENT. The treatment of metatarsus adductus is predominantly nonoperative. There are limited indications for surgery.

Nonoperative. Most children with metatarsus adductus deformities undergo conservative treatment. The feet may be classified into three groups depending on forefoot flexibility. Type I feet are flexible and actively and passively overcorrect into mild abduction. Voluntary correction can be elicited by stimulating the peroneal musculature by stroking the lateral border of the foot. These feet usually require no treatment. Type II feet correct to the neutral position both passively and actively. These feet may benefit from an orthosis or corrective shoes such as straight or reverse last shoes. These are worn full time (22 hr/day), and the condition is re-evaluated in 4–6 wk. If improvement is seen, the treatment can be continued. If no improvement occurs, then serial plaster casts are necessary. Type III feet are rigid and do not correct to neutral. These feet are treated with serial casts. The best results are obtained when casting is initiated before 8 mo of age. Once correction has been achieved, orthoses or corrective shoes may be used for an additional 1–2 mo to maintain correction. Mild hallux varus, the "searching toe," may persist for several years after conservative correction and may be of concern to the parents. However, this will eventually disappear with growth and the wearing of shoes.

Operative. Metatarsus adductus deformities in children 4 yr of age and older require surgical intervention. Children 4–6 yr of age may benefit from a soft tissue release. Serial casting is performed until forefoot correction has been obtained. This usually requires 2–3 mo. Children 6 yr of age or older require base of the metatarsal osteotomies or other osseous procedures to achieve satisfactory correction.

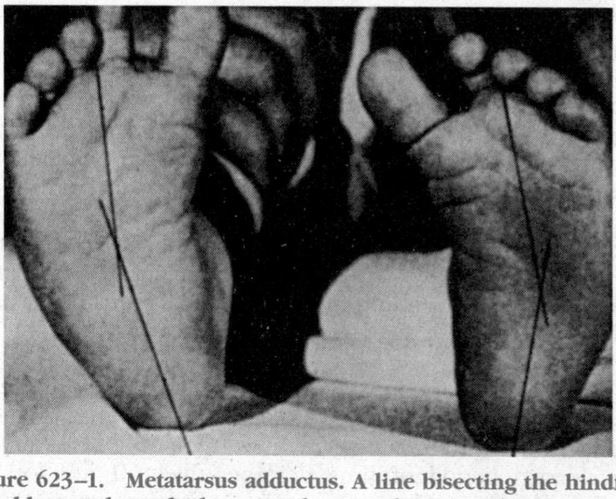

Figure 623–1. Metatarsus adductus. A line bisecting the hindfoot should pass through the second toe or between the second and third toes.

623.2 Calcaneovalgus Feet

The calcaneovalgus foot is a relatively common finding in the newborn and is secondary to in utero positioning. This condition is manifested by a hyperdorsiflexed foot with forefoot abduction and increased heel valgus. It is almost always associated with external tibial torsion. It usually occurs unilaterally but occasionally may be bilateral. In utero, the plantar surface of the foot was against the wall of the uterus, forcing it into a hyperdorsiflexed, abducted, and externally rotated position. The position also produces the external tibial torsion. When these two conditions are combined with the normal newborn increased external rotation of the hip (tight posterior capsule), it results in a lower extremity that appears excessively externally rotated.

CLINICAL MANIFESTATIONS. The infant typically presents with an out-toe position of the involved extremity. The dorsum of the foot can easily be brought into contact with the anterior aspect of the tibia; the forefoot will be abducted, and the heel will be in valgus. This should not be confused with the neonatal maturity classification of Dubowitz (see Chapter 82). External tibial torsion (20–50 degrees) is a common associated finding. Ankle motion will show normal or almost normal plantar flexion.

Three conditions must be distinguished from the calcaneovalgus foot: (1) congenital vertical talus, (2) posteromedial bow of the tibia, and (3) neuromuscular abnormalities with paralysis of the gastrocnemius muscle. The differentiation can usually be made clinically during the physical examination.

RADIOGRAPHIC EVALUATION. AP and lateral simulated weightbearing radiographs of the feet may be necessary to differentiate between the calcaneovalgus foot and a congenital vertical talus. In a calcaneovalgus foot, either the radiographs are normal or there may be increased hindfoot valgus and forefoot abduction. If a posteromedial bow of the tibia is suspected, then AP and lateral radiographs of the tibia and fibula will be necessary.

TREATMENT. The typical calcaneovalgus foot requires no treatment. The hyperdorsiflexion of the foot will resolve during the first 6 mo of life. The external tibial torsion, however, will persist and follow the same natural history as internal tibial torsion. Spontaneous improvement will not occur until the child begins to pull to stand and walk independently. It will take approximately 6–12 mo thereafter for complete correction to occur. The majority of infants with calcaneovalgus feet and external tibial torsion will have normally aligned feet and lower extremities by 2 yr of age.

623.3 Talipes Equinovarus (Clubfoot)

A clubfoot represents a deformity not only of the foot but of the entire lower leg. It can be classified into three groups: (1) congenital, (2) teratologic, and (3) positional. The congenital clubfoot is usually an isolated abnormality, whereas the teratologic form is associated with a neuromuscular disorder such as myelodysplasia, arthrogryposis multiplex congenita, or a syndrome complex. The congenital form has also been called idiopathic or neurogenic on the basis of possible causes. The positional clubfoot is a normal foot that has been held in a deformed position in utero.

The *cause* of clubfoot is unknown. There are inheritance factors, and these are currently considered multifactorial with a major influence from a single autosomal dominant gene. Recent biopsy studies of the extrinsic muscles of the calf have indicated a probable neuromuscular cause. There are fiber-type disproportions and increased neuromuscular junctions within these muscles. Electron microscopy abnormalities are also present. These findings are in contrast to previous etiologic theories in which deformity of the talus was believed to be the primary abnormality. Although the talus is certainly deformed with medial deviation of the head and neck, this is currently considered to be a secondary deformity.

CLINICAL MANIFESTATIONS. The congenital form of clubfoot, which constitutes approximately 75% of all cases, is characterized by (1) the absence of other congenital abnormalities, (2) variable rigidity of the foot, (3) mild calf atrophy, and (4) mild hypoplasia of the tibia, fibula, and bones of the foot. It occurs more commonly in males (2:1) and is bilateral in 50% of cases. The probability for the deformity to occur at random is approximately 1:1,000 births, but within involved families the probability is approximately 3% for subsequent siblings and 20–30% for offspring of involved parents.

Examination of the infant clubfoot demonstrates hindfoot equinus, hindfoot and midfoot varus, forefoot adduction, and variable rigidity. All of these findings are secondary to the medial dislocation of the talonavicular joint. In the older child, the calf and foot atrophy are more obvious than in the infant regardless of how well corrected or functional the foot is. These findings are due to the etiologic aspects of clubfoot, not the method of treatment.

RADIOGRAPHIC EVALUATION. AP and lateral standing or simulated weightbearing radiographs are used in the assessment of clubfeet. Non-weightbearing radiographs are useless. Multiple different radiographic measurements can be made. The navicular bone, which is the primary site of deformity, does not ossify until 3 yr in the female and 4 yr in the male. This necessitates line measurements to determine the position of the unossified navicular bone and the overall alignment of the foot.

TREATMENT. Nonoperative. Conservative methods of treatment include taping and use of malleable splints and serial plaster casts. Taping and malleable splints are particularly useful in premature infants until they obtain an appropriate size for casting. Serial plaster casts are the major method of nonoperative treatment. Before the cast is applied, the foot is gently manipulated toward the corrected position. The cast is then applied and changed at 1- to 2-wk intervals. Complete correction, both clinically and radiographically, should be achieved by 3 mo of age. If this is accomplished, then holding casts are used for an additional 3–6 mo followed by orthoses or corrective shoes until the child is walking well. Failure to achieve clinical and radiographic correction by 3 mo of age is an indication for surgical treatment. Further attempts at conservative management may result in articular damage and a midfoot breech (rocker-bottom deformity).

Operative. The current method of surgical treatment is a complete soft tissue release. This is usually performed between 6 and 12 mo of age. Satisfactory long-term results can be expected in 80–90% of cases. Feet with unsatisfactory results that require additional treatment are usually secondary to extrinsic muscle imbalance rather than incomplete correction. The use of tendon transfers and bone procedures, including arthrodeses (fusions), are primarily for salvage of recurrent or incompletely corrected feet. Centralization of the tibialis anterior tendon has been particularly beneficial in young children with a dynamic pes varus, the most common residual abnormality. Triple arthrodeses are indicated in painful, deformed feet in adolescence.

623.4 Congenital Vertical Talus

Congenital vertical talus is an uncommon foot deformity with causes similar to those of talipes equinovarus. It must be distinguished from a calcaneovalgus foot, which is a much more common deformity. Typically, a congenital vertical talus is a rigid rocker-bottom deformity. The majority of involved infants will have an underlying disorder such as teratologic malformation (myelodysplasia and arthrogryposis multiplex congenita) or a syndrome such as trisomy 18.

CLINICAL MANIFESTATIONS. The clinical characteristic of a congenital vertical talus is a rocker-bottom foot. There is hindfoot equinovalgus, a convex plantar surface, forefoot abduction and dorsiflexion, and rigidity. A careful physical examination must be performed on all children to assess for an underlying disorder or syndrome.

RADIOGRAPHIC EVALUATION. Radiographic evaluation of a congenital vertical talus consists of an AP and lateral simulated weightbearing radiograph of the feet as well as a maximum plantar flexed lateral film. This typically will reveal the vertically oriented talus, the dorsal displacement of the midfoot on the hindfoot, hindfoot valgus, and mobility.

TREATMENT. As in clubfeet, nonoperative treatment is the initial method of management. However, the vast majority of children with a congenital vertical talus will require surgical correction.

Nonoperative. Serial casting after manipulation of the feet is performed beginning at birth. The forefoot is manipulated into equinus in an attempt to reduce the navicular bone on to the head of the talus. However, the success rate with nonoperative treatment is exceedingly low.

Operative. The operative management of congenital vertical talus is predominantly through an extensive or complete soft tissue release performed as a one-stage or two-stage procedure. Occasionally, in severe deformities, a naviculectomy may be necessary to realign the midfoot and hindfoot adequately. Fortunately, this is rarely necessary. In older children with persistent hindfoot valgus and pronation, a subtalar arthrodesis or a triple arthrodesis may be necessary to realign the foot and provide stability.

The goals of treatment of congenital vertical talus are pessimistic and include a plantigrade, pain-free foot that is able to wear shoes. Orthotic management is frequently necessary for a prolonged period of time postoperatively, if not for life, because of associated muscle weakness resulting from an underlying disorder.

623.5 Hypermobile Pes Planus (Flexible Flatfeet)

Hypermobile flatfeet or pronated feet are common sources of concern of parents. In general, these children are asymptomatic and have no functional limitations. Flatfeet are common in neonates and toddlers because of an associated laxity in the bone-ligament complexes of the feet and fat in the area of the medial longitudinal arch. These children usually demonstrate significant improvement by 6 yr of age. In the older child, flexible flatfeet are usually secondary to generalized ligamentous laxity, an autosomal dominant condition. Almost all children and adolescents with flexible flatfeet will be asymptomatic.

CLINICAL MANIFESTATIONS. In the non-weightbearing position in the older child with a flexible flatfoot, the normal medial longitudinal arch is present, but in the weightbearing position, the foot becomes pronated with varying degrees of pes planus and heel valgus. Instead of weightbearing over the lateral column of the foot, weight is shifted medially, producing pronation. Subtalar motion will be normal or slightly increased. Loss of subtalar motion indicates a rigid flatfoot. Common causes of rigid flatfeet include a tendo-Achilles contracture, tarsal coalitions, neuromuscular abnormalities (cerebral palsy), and familial trait.

RADIOGRAPHIC EVALUATION. Routine radiographs of asymptomatic flexible flatfeet are usually not indicated. AP and lateral weightbearing radiographs are obtained if there is rigidity or symptoms. On the AP radiograph, there will be excessive heel valgus. The lateral view shows distortion of the normal straight line relationship between the long axis of the talus and the first metatarsal with either a sag of the talonavicular or naviculocuneiform joint, resulting in flattening of the normal medial longitudinal arch.

TREATMENT. The treatment of flexible flatfeet is conservative. Affected children do not predictably have symptoms. Therefore, modified shoes and orthoses do not significantly alter the clinical or radiographic appearance of the feet. It should be emphasized that the diagnosis of flexible flatfeet is usually not possible until after 6 yr of age. Treatment is indicated for abnormal shoe wear or symptoms not attributable to other causes. Feet that are symptomatic with vigorous physical activities usually respond readily to the use of a commercially available medial longitudinal arch support. Custom-made supports are much more expensive and, in most cases, not any more effective.

623.6 Tarsal Coalition

Tarsal coalition, also known as peroneal spastic flatfoot, is a relatively common foot disorder characterized by a painful, rigid flatfoot deformity and peroneal (lateral calf) muscle spasm but without true spasticity. It represents a congenital fusion or failure of segmentation between two or more tarsal bones. However, any condition that alters the normal gliding and rotatory motion of the subtalar joint may produce the clinical appearance of a tarsal coalition. Thus, congenital malformations, arthritis or inflammatory disorders, infection, neoplasms, and trauma can be possible causes.

The most common tarsal coalitions occur at the medial talocalcaneal (subtalar) facet and between the calcaneus and navicular (calcaneonavicular) tarsal bones. Coalitions can be fibrous, cartilaginous, or osseous. Tarsal coalition occurs in approximately 1% in the general population, and it appears to be inherited as a unifactorial autosomal dominant trait with nearly full penetrance. Approximately 60% of calcaneonavicular and 50% of the medial-facet talocalcaneal coalitions are bilateral.

CLINICAL MANIFESTATIONS. The onset of symptoms usually occurs during the 2nd decade of life. Although mild limitation of subtalar motion and the flatfoot may have been present since early childhood, the onset of symptoms will vary with the age at which the fibrous or cartilaginous bar begins to ossify and further decrease motion. The talonavicular coalition ossifies between 3 and 5 yr of age, the calcaneonavicular coalition between 8 and 12 yr, and the medial facet talocalcaneal coalition between 12 and 16 yr. The pain is typically felt laterally in the hindfoot and radiates proximally along the lateral malleolus and distal fibula (peroneal muscle spasm). Symptoms are frequently aggravated by sports or walking on uneven ground. Clinically, the foot is flat or pronated both in the weightbearing and the non-weightbearing positions. Subtalar and transverse tarsal joint motion is diminished or absent, and attempts at motion may produce pain.

RADIOGRAPHIC EVALUATION. The diagnosis of a tarsal coalition is confirmed radiographically. AP and lateral weightbearing radiographs and an oblique radiograph of the foot should be ordered initially. Beaking of the anterior aspect of the talus on the lateral view is suspicious for a tarsal coalition. The oblique view will demonstrate a calcaneonavicular coalition. Axial views through the hindfoot can be useful in the diagnosis of the medial facet talocalcaneal coalition. However, computed tomography is the procedure of choice in the evaluation of coalitions, especially those involving the subtalar joint.

TREATMENT. The treatment of symptomatic tarsal coalitions varies according to the type of coalition, age of the patient, extent of the coalition, presence or absence of degenerative osteoarthritis, and degree of disability. The treatment may be nonoperative or operative. Nonoperative treatment may consist of cast immobilization, shoe inserts, or orthotics. Operative management consists of excision of the coalition and interposition of muscle (calcaneonavicular) and fat or split flexor hallucis longus tendon (medial facet talocalcaneal) to prevent hematoma formation and reossification of the coalition (Fig. 623–2). Resections are very effective in relieving pain, improving subtalar motion, and allowing resumption of normal activities. However, if degenerative osteoarthritis is present, a triple arthrodesis may be necessary.

623.7 Cavus Feet

Cavus feet represent an exaggeration in the medial longitudinal arch associated with hindfoot varus and occasionally adduction of the forefoot. When the latter occurs, the deformity is called a cavovarus deformity. This type of deformity appears most commonly during middle childhood years. Both idiopathic and neuromuscular types may be seen. In either case, a cavovarus foot is usually a progressive deformity leading to considerable compromise of foot function. These deformities tend to be rigid. The most important aspect of the evaluation of a patient with a cavovarus foot is to establish an accurate diagnosis. Possible causes include spinal cord disease and peripheral neuropathies, such as Charcot-Marie-Tooth disease.

TREATMENT. Aggressive treatment is usually necessary for moderate to severe cavus feet. This usually involves reconstructive surgery. Special shoes and shoe modifications are not helpful from a therapeutic standpoint but sometimes may be warranted to provide relief from abnormal pressure during weighbearing. Surgical correction by soft tissue balancing and occasionally by osseous procedures are usually necessary.

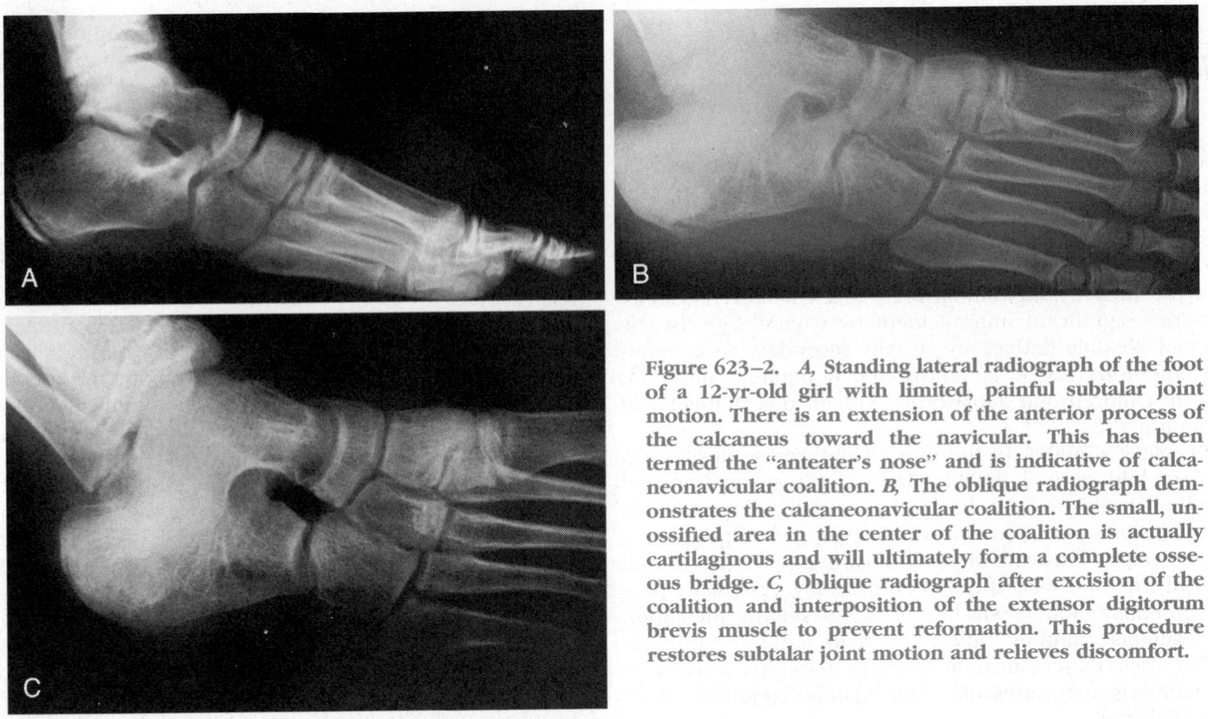

Figure 623–2. *A*, Standing lateral radiograph of the foot of a 12-yr-old girl with limited, painful subtalar joint motion. There is an extension of the anterior process of the calcaneus toward the navicular. This has been termed the "anteater's nose" and is indicative of calcaneonavicular coalition. *B*, The oblique radiograph demonstrates the calcaneonavicular coalition. The small, unossified area in the center of the coalition is actually cartilaginous and will ultimately form a complete osseous bridge. *C*, Oblique radiograph after excision of the coalition and interposition of the extensor digitorum brevis muscle to prevent reformation. This procedure restores subtalar joint motion and relieves discomfort.

623.8 Osteochondroses

Osteochondroses are pathologic processes that involve infarction, revascularization, resorption, and replacement of the affected bone. These are commonly termed *idiopathic avascular necrosis.* Both the tarsal navicular (*Köhler disease*) and the head or epiphysis of the second metatarsal (*Freiberg disease*) may sustain avascular necrosis. These conditions are relatively uncommon and both produce pain, especially with activities. Symptomatic treatment is based on the severity of the child's complaint. Occasionally, a short leg cast and non-weightbearing with crutches may be helpful in relieving symptoms.

As the older child enters the period of pubescent growth spurt, the fibrocartilaginous insertion of major muscle groups to bone is vulnerable to microfracture, resulting in inflammatory and healing responses. The usual site of microfractures in the foot is the attachment of the tendo-Achilles (heel cord) to the posterior aspect of the calcaneus. This produces another osteochondrosis: *Sever disease,* which is a common cause of heel pain. Symptoms wax and wane depending on the level of activity, and until skeletal maturity is achieved, the usual residual manifestation, if any, is bony enlargement at the tendon insertion site secondary to overgrowth during the healing response. Treatment is again symptomatic and includes the use of an anti-inflammatory agent and heel cord stretching.

623.9 Puncture Wounds of the Foot

For most of these injuries, extensively cleansing the wound, ensuring prophylaxis for tetanus, and administering a broad-spectrum oral antibiotic are all that is needed. When infection occurs despite these measures, *Pseudomonas aeruginosa* and *Staphylococcus aureus* are the usual offending organisms. In *Pseudomonas* osteomyelitis, the puncture usually injured the bone or joint. This is most common when the puncture wound is through the sole of a sneaker. The heat and perspiration and the material within the sneakers tend to promote the growth of this organism. Treatment of established infections includes wound debridement to remove necrotic tissue. Broad-spectrum antibiotics are administered, including methicillin and gentamicin, pending the outcome of the cultures. Subsequent antibiotic treatment is based on the results of these tests. After surgery, further microbial therapy is continued for 10–14 days.

623.10 Toe Deformities

Common toe deformities in children and adolescents include (1) adolescent bunions, (2) curly toes, (3) overlapping fifth toe, (4) polydactyly, (5) syndactyly, (6) hammer toe, (7) mallet toe, (8) claw toes, (9) annular bands (constriction rings), (10) subungual exostosis, and (11) ingrown toenail.

ADOLESCENT BUNIONS

Adolescent bunions are a common pediatric foot deformity. They are more common in girls (3:1), and there is frequently a positive family history. There are both intrinsic and extrinsic factors associated with this deformity. The intrinsic factors include metatarsus primus varus, oblique first metatarsal–medial cuneiform articulation, short first metatarsal, and pes planus. Extrinsic factors include abnormal shoe wear (narrow toe box with an elevated heel) and an underlying neurologic disorder, such as cerebral palsy.

CLINICAL MANIFESTATIONS. An adolescent presenting with bunions requires careful evaluation. It must be determined whether it is the symptoms, the deformity, or both that are of concern to the patient and the family. If pain is present, it must be ascertained whether this is due to activities and whether it produces functional limitation. It is also important to know what type of shoes are being worn when symptoms are present. When evaluating the foot, weightbearing alignment, walking alignment, mobility of the first metatarsophalangeal joint, presence or absence of callous formation, and preferred shoe style must be determined.

RADIOGRAPHIC EVALUATION. AP and lateral weightbearing radiographs of the feet are necessary in the assessment of adolescent bunions. This will allow measurement of the (1) intermetatarsal angle, (2) hallux valgus angle, (3) alignment of the first metatarsal–medial cuneiform joint, and (4) pes planus. The normal intermetatarsal angle between the long axes of the first and second metatarsals is 10 degrees or less, and the normal hallux valgus angle is 25 degrees or less. A short first metatarsal can be diagnosed from these radiographs.

TREATMENT. Nonoperative. Conservative management of adolescent bunions consists primarily of shoe modifications. It is important that footwear accommodate the width of the forefoot. Adolescents should be discouraged from wearing narrow-toed shoes with elevated heels. In the presence of a pes planus, an orthotic to restore the medial longitudinal arch may be beneficial.

Operative. The indications for surgical correction include an intermetatarsal angle between 12 and 18 degrees and failure of nonoperative management. The major indication for surgical treatment is symptoms, not cosmesis. Surgery rarely restores the foot to a completely normal appearance but is very effective in narrowing the width of the forefoot, correcting the hallux valgus, improving weightbearing alignment, and relieving symptoms. Surgery typically consists of a combination of a soft tissue and bone procedure. The osseous procedures are numerous and can be performed on the first metatarsal and medial cuneiform or both.

CURLY TOES

The most common lesser toe deformity of childhood is curly toes. These represent a flexion deformity at the proximal interphalangeal joint with lateral rotation and varus alignment of the toe (Fig. 623–3). The fourth and fifth toes are the most commonly involved. Occasionally, the second and third toes will be involved. The disorder is usually familial, bilateral, symmetric, and asymptomatic. The condition is secondary to short, tight flexor digitorum longus and flexor digitorum brevis tendons. The tightness in these tendons can be demonstrated by dorsiflexing the foot, which will increase the curling of the toes. Plantar flexion usually results in improvement. Radiographic evaluation of curly toe deformities is not necessary.

TREATMENT. In infants and young children, curly toe deformities should be observed because 25–50% will resolve spontaneously. Taping or splinting is ineffective. At 3–4 yr of age, an open tenotomy of the toe flexor tendons can be performed. In older children and adolescents, a proximal interphalangeal joint fusion may be necessary.

OVERLAPPING FIFTH TOE

This is a relatively common condition in which the fifth toe is adducted and overriding the fourth toe. It can result in abnormal shoe wear and pain in approximately 50% of patients.

Examination of the fifth toe will show an extensor digitorum longus contracture. There will also be a dorsal metatarsophalangeal joint contracture. The fifth toe will be adducted, extended, and laterally rotated. The toe may be able to be realigned passively but will not maintain the corrected position. Radiographs are not necessary in the evaluation of an overlapping fifth toe.

TREATMENT. Nonoperative treatment is ineffective for this deformity. It can be corrected surgically. The most common procedure consists of a racket-shaped incision around the base of the toe. The extensor digitorum longus tendon is released along with the dorsal joint contracture. This allows the toe to flex into its normal position.

POLYDACTYLY

This is a relatively common deformity. It usually involves the fifth toe. It occurs in approximately 2 per 1,000 births. Approximately 30% will have a positive family history. It is important to assess for other deformities such as polydactyly of the hand and syndactyly of adjacent toes. Duplication of the great toe is also possible. There may be associated metatarsal abnormalities.

AP and lateral weightbearing radiographs of both feet are obtained in the management of children with polydactyly. This will demonstrate whether the duplication is articulated or rudimentary and whether there are metatarsal abnormalities.

TREATMENT. Nonoperative management of polydactyly is not indicated. Rudimentary-type digits can be ligated at birth and allowed to autoamputate. Those that are articulated require excision at approximately 1 yr of age. The guidelines in polydactyly are to save the digit with best axial alignment, resect the projecting symptomatic toe, repair the capsule, balance the soft tissues, and shave any metatarsal prominences.

SYNDACTYLY

This is a relatively common lesser toe condition. Cases of syndactyly are almost always asymptomatic and there may be a positive familial history. These can be classified into *zygosyndactyly* and *polysyndactyly.* In zygosyndactyly, there is complete or incomplete webbing. This usually occurs between the second and third toes. In polysyndactyly, there may be a duplication of the fifth toe, with a syndactyly between the fourth and fifth toes. Synostosis of the lateral metatarsals is common.

TREATMENT. Zygosyndactyly does not require treatment, but the polysyndactyly may because of the associated anomalies.

HAMMER TOE

A hammer toe is similar to a curly toe except there is no malrotation of the involved toe. There is a flexion deformity

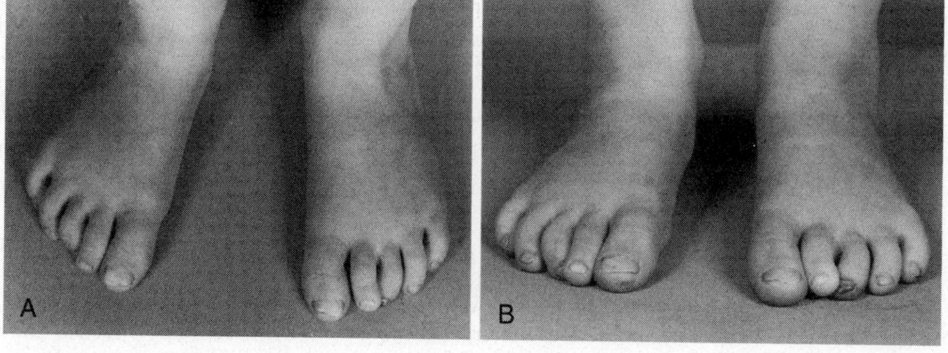

Figure 623–3. *A,* **Bilateral curly toe deformities in a 4-yr-old. There is flexion and varus rotation of the lateral three toes.** *B,* **The frontal view better demonstrates the curling of the toes, especially the third toes.**

at the proximal interphalangeal joint, and the metatarsophalangeal joint is extended. The metatarsal head may appear depressed. It is usually symmetric and bilateral, with the second toe most commonly involved. The major problems with this deformity are painful calluses over the proximal phalangeal joint.

TREATMENT. Passive stretching and taping may be helpful in infants and young children. However, the majority will require surgical correction of the contracted flexor digitorum longus and flexor digitorum brevis tendons. Occasionally, tendon transfers are required.

MALLET TOE

Mallet toe is a flexion deformity at the distal interphalangeal joint. It may become symptomatic in adolescents as a result of a dorsal callosity or perhaps from nail bed irritation.

TREATMENT. Nonoperative treatment is usually ineffective. Correction is usually obtained by the release of the flexor digitorum longus tendon. Occasionally, in the adolescent, a distal interphalangeal joint fusion may be necessary.

CLAW TOE

Claw toes represent an extension contracture with dorsal subluxation of the metatarsophalangeal joint in association with flexion deformities of both the proximal and distal interphalangeal joints. These can occur idiopathically, but the majority will be associated with a pes cavus deformity and will be secondary to an underlying neurologic disorder such as Charcot-Marie-Tooth disease. These deformities are complex and require very careful assessment to determine the underlying cause.

TREATMENT. Claw toes are treated surgically, usually with soft tissue rebalancing and, occasionally, fusions of the proximal interphalangeal joint.

ANNULAR BANDS

Annular bands or constriction rings are relatively common disorders that involve the toes and fingers. They may consist of simple constriction rings or rings with deformity of the distal part of the toe with swelling and lymphedema. Occasionally, the rings may be deep enough to have produced an amputation. Sometimes there will be an associated syndactyly with the adjacent toe.

TREATMENT. The treatment of annular or constriction bands is predominantly observation. If there are deep rings with swelling and lymphedema, surgery may be necessary to relieve the congestion.

SUBUNGUAL EXOSTOSES

This is an uncommon problem that primarily involves the great toe. It may simulate an ingrown toenail. On physical examination there is a palpable mass beneath the toenail. The toe may appear irritated and similar to an infection; however, palpation will reveal a mass rather than granulation tissue. Radiographs of the toe will demonstrate the exostosis of the distal phalanx.

TREATMENT. Nonoperative treatment is ineffective. Subungual exostoses are managed by partial excision of the nail bed and removal of the underlying exostosis.

INGROWN TOENAIL

Ingrown toenails are relatively common in infants and young children and later in adolescents. These typically involve the medial and lateral borders of the great toe.

TABLE 623–1 Differential Diagnosis of Foot Pain by Age

0–6 yr	6–12 yr	12–20 yr
Poor-fitting shoes	Poor-fitting shoes	Poor-fitting shoes
Foreign body	Sever disease	Stress fracture
Fracture	Enthesopathy (JRA)	Foreign body
Osteomyelitis	Foreign body	Ingrown toenail
Leukemia	Accessory navicular	Metatarsalgia
Puncture wound	Tarsal coalition	Plantar fasciitis
Drawing of blood	Ewing sarcoma	Osteochondroses
	Hypermobile flatfoot	Freiberg
	Trauma (sprains)	Köhler
	Puncture wound	Achilles tendinitis
		Trauma (sprains)
		Plantar warts

JRA = juvenile rheumatoid arthritis.

TREATMENT. Conservative treatment is usually effective. This consists of appropriate shoe modification, warm soaks, antibiotics, elevation of the nail edge, and proper nail-cutting techniques. If this fails, surgery with wedge section of the involved border, including the nail matrix, is usually effective.

623.11 Painful Foot

The causes of a painful foot can usually be determined from history and physical examination. The common causes are listed in Table 623–1. The specific treatment depends on the diagnosis and occasionally on the age of the child or adolescent.

623.12 Shoes

Clothing is worn for comfort, to enhance appearance, and for protection. Shoes should be selected on the same basis. Shoes are not corrective, and the foot does not need support for normal activities. The foot requires mobility to function normally. It has been demonstrated that populations that are predominantly barefoot have better feet than those that wear shoes. The best shoes for children are those that simulate the bare foot. They should be flexible, flat, and nonconstricting and made of material that breathes. Shoes do not have to be expensive.

Because overuse foot symptoms are common, especially in the athletic adolescent, shock-absorbing shoes are a good choice. The thick-cushioned sole absorbs some of the shock of impact and thereby decreases discomfort.

Shoe modifications are sometimes appropriate for a specific problem. A lift may be prescribed if the limb is short, and a shoe insert may be helpful for the stiff and deformed foot or to distribute the weight load more evenly over the sole.

METATARSUS ADDUCTUS

Crawford AH, Gabriel KR: Foot and ankle problems. Orthop Clin North Am 18:649, 1987.

Farsetti P, Weinstein SL, Ponseti IV: The long-term functional and radiographic outcomes of untreated and non-operatively treated metatarsus adductus. J Bone Joint Surg 76A:257, 1994.

CALCANEOVALGUS FOOT

Gibson DA: Torsional variations in the lower limbs of children. Appl Ther 8:236, 1966.

Meehan P: Other conditions of the foot. *In:* Morrissy RT (ed): Lovell and Winter's Pediatric Orthopaedics. Philadelphia, JB Lippincott, 1990, pp 997–998.

CONGENITAL TALIPES EQUINOVARUS (CLUBFOOT)

Cowell HR, Wein BK: Current concepts review: Genetic aspects of clubfoot. J Bone Joint Surg 62A:1381, 1980.
Handelsman J, Badalamente MA: Neuromuscular studies in clubfoot. J Pediatr Orthop 1:23, 1981.
Herzenberg JE, Carroll NC, Christofersen MR, et al: Clubfoot analysis with three-dimensional computer modeling. J Pediatr Orthop 8:257, 1988.
Howard CB, Benson MKD: Clubfoot: Its pathological anatomy. J Pediatr Orthop 13:654, 1993.
Ponseti IV: Current concepts review: Treatment of congenital club foot. J Bone Joint Surg 74A:448, 1992.
Thompson GH, Simons GW III: Congenital talipes equinovarus (clubfeet) and metatarsus adductus. *In:* Drennan JC (ed): The Child's Foot and Ankle. New York, Raven Press, 1992, pp 97–133.

CONGENITAL VERTICAL TALUS

Drennan JC: Congenital vertical talus. *In:* Drennan JC (ed): The Child's Foot and Ankle. New York, Raven Press, 1992, pp 155–168.

HYPERMOBILE FLATFOOT

Staheli LT, Chew DE, Corbet M: The longitudinal arch: A survey of 882 feet in normal children and adults. J Bone Joint Surg 69A:426, 1987.
Wenger DR, Mauldin D, Speck G, et al: Corrective shoes and inserts as treatment for a flexible flatfoot in infants and children. J Bone Joint Surg 71A:800, 1989.

TARSAL COALITION

Gonzalez PK, Kumar SJ: Calcaneonavicular coalition treated by resection and interposition of the extensor digitorum brevis muscle. J Bone Joint Surg 72A:71, 1990.
Herzenberg JE, Goldner JL, Martinez S, et al: Computerized tomography of talocalcaneal tarsal coalitions: A clinical and anatomic study. Foot Ankle 6:273, 1986.
Kumar SJ, Guille JT, Couto JC: Osseous and non-osseous coalition of the middle facet of the talocalcaneal joint. J Bone Joint Surg 74A:529, 1992.
Leonard MA: The inheritance of tarsal coalition and its relationship to spastic flat foot. J Bone Joint Surg 56B:520, 1974.
Thompson GH, Cooperman DR: Peroneal spastic flatfoot. *In:* Gould JS (ed): Operative Foot Surgery. Philadelphia, WB Saunders 1993, pp 858–877.

ADOLESCENT BUNIONS

Koop SE: Adolescent hallux valgus. *In:* Drennan JC (ed): The Child's Foot and Ankle. New York, Raven Press, 1992, pp 417–423.
Meehan PL: Adolescent bunion. *In:* Morrissy RT (ed): Lovell and Winter's Pediatric Orthopaedics. Philadelphia, JB Lippincott, 1990, pp 983–990.
Scranton PE, Zuckerman JD: Bunion surgery in adolescents—Results of surgical treatment. J Pediatr Orthop 4:39, 1984.

CURLY TOES

Hamer AJ, Stanley D, Smith TW: Surgery for curly toe deformity: A double-blind, randomized, prospective trial. J Bone Joint Surg 75B:662, 1993.
Ross ERS, Menelaus MB: Open flexor tenotomy for hammer and curly toes in children. J Bone Joint Surg 66B:770, 1984.

OVERLAPPING FIFTH TOE

Black GB, Grogan DP, Bobechko WP: Butler arthroplasty for correction of the adducted fifth toe: A retrospective study of 36 operations between 1968 and 1982. J Pediatr Orthop 5:439, 1985.
DeBoeck H: Butler's operation for congenital overriding of the fifth toe: Retrospective 1–7 year study of 23 cases. Acta Orthop Scand 64:343, 1993.
Paton RW: V-Y plasty for correction of varus fifth toe. J Pediatr Orthop 10:248, 1990.

POLYDACTYLY

Crawford AH, Gabriel KR: Foot and ankle problems. Orthop Clin North Am 18:649, 1987.
Mubarak SJ, O'Brien TJ, Davids JR: Metatarsal epiphyseal bracket: Treatment by central physiolysis. J Pediatr Orthop 13:5, 1993.
Nogami H: Polydactyly and polysyndactyly of the fifth toe. Clin Orthop 204:216, 1986.
Phelps DA, Grogan DP: Polydactyly of the foot. J Pediatr Orthop 5:446, 1985.
Venn-Watson EA: Problems in polydactyly of the foot. Orthop Clin North Am 7:909, 1976.

SYNDACTYLY

Meehan PL: Other conditions of the foot. *In:* Morrissy RT (ed): Lovell and Winter's Pediatric Orthopaedics. Philadelphia, JB Lippincott, 1990, pp 991–1021.

HAMMER TOE

Newman RJ, Fitton JM: An evaluation of operative procedures in the treatment of hammer toe. Acta Orthop Scand 50:709, 1979.
Ross ERS, Menelaus MB: Open flexor tenotomy for hammer toes and curly toes in childhood. J Bone Joint Surg 66B:770, 1984.

MALLET TOE

Tachdjian MO: Pediatric orthopaedics. Philadelphia, WB Saunders, 1992, pp 2670–2671.

CLAW TOES

Coughlin MJ, Mann RA: Lesser toe deformities. *In:* Mann RA (ed): Surgery of the Foot. St. Louis, CV Mosby, 1986, pp 132–148.
Myerson MS, Shereff MJ: The pathological anatomy of claw and hammer toes. J Bone Joint Surg 71A:45, 1989.

ANNULAR BANDS

Greene WB: One-stage release of congenital circumferential constriction bands. J Bone Joint Surg 75A:650, 1993.
Tada K, Yanenobu K, Swanson A: Congenital constriction band syndrome. J Pediatr Orthop 4:726, 1984.

SUBUNGUAL EXOSTOSES

Landon G, Johnson K, Dahlin DC: Subungual exostoses. J Bone Joint Surg 61A:256, 1979.

INGROWN TOENAILS

Grieg JD, Anderson JH, Ireland AJ et al: The surgical treatment of ingrown toenails. J Bone Joint Surg 73B:131, 1991.

CHAPTER 624
Torsional and Angular Deformities

Torsional and angular deformities or variations of the femur and tibia in infants and young children are extremely common. Many will be physiologic in origin, whereas others may be congenital or acquired. It is important to be able to distinguish those that are physiologic and that will resolve with normal growth and development from those that require treatment.

624.1 Normal Developmental Alignment

Before a discussion of torsional and angular deformities, it is important to have an understanding of the effects of in utero positioning on the developing lower extremities. In the typical in utero position, the hips are flexed, abducted, and externally rotated; the knees are flexed and the lower legs are internally rotated; and the feet are in slight equinus, supinated, and in contact with the posterolateral aspect of the opposite thigh. The combination of external rotation of the hip and internal rotation of the lower leg produces a bowed appearance of the lower extremities when the child begins to ambulate. This is not true bowing but rather a torsional combination. Physiologic bowing resolves with 6–12 mo of independent ambulation.

Physiologic genu valgum or knock-knees is seen between 3 and 4 yr of age. This is true genu valgum and not the result of a torsional combination. This, too, resolves with growth, with the normal adult knee alignment obtained between 5 and 8 yr of age. The mean tibiofemoral angle at birth is 15 degrees of varus (Fig. 624–1). This decreases to approximately 10 degrees by 1 yr of age. Neutral alignment occurs between 18 and 20 mo of age. The maximum valgus of 12 degrees occurs at 3–4 yr of age. The values are similar for boys and girls. By 7 yr the valgus alignment corrects to that of a normal adult (8 degrees in women; 7 degrees in men). Overall, 95% of developmental physiologic genu varum and genu valgum cases resolve with growth. This is also true for children with more pronounced physiologic varus or valgus, although some may not completely correct until adolescence.

TORSIONAL PROFILE

The torsional profile can be very beneficial in the diagnosing and monitoring of children with torsional variations (Fig. 624–2). The profile includes (1) foot progression angle; (2) hip rotation in extension; (3) thigh-foot angle; and (4) shape of the foot.

Foot Progression Angle

The foot progression angle represents the long axis of the foot with respect to the direction in which the child is walking (Fig. 624–3). Inward rotation is given a negative value and outward rotation a positive value. A normal foot progression angle in children and adolescence is 10 degrees (range, −3–20 degrees). The foot progression angle serves only to define whether there is an in-toeing or out-toeing gait. The latter is considered abnormal when this angle exceeds 20 degrees.

Hip Rotation

Hip rotation in extension is assessed with the child prone, the thighs together, and the knees flexed 90 degrees (Fig. 624–4). In this position the hip is in neutral alignment. As the lower leg is rotated outwardly, this produces internal rotation of the hip, whereas inward rotation produces external rotation. This is due to the anatomic shape of the proximal femur. The femoral neck normally has a 135 degree angle with the femoral shaft. Typically, there is 15 degrees of anterior angulation between the axis representing the femoral neck and the transcondylar axis of the distal femur. This angulation is also known as femoral version. By 1 yr of age there is approximately 45 degrees of internal and external rotation. Hip rotation should be symmetric. Asymmetric rotation may be indicative of a hip disorder, and radiographs of the pelvis will be necessary.

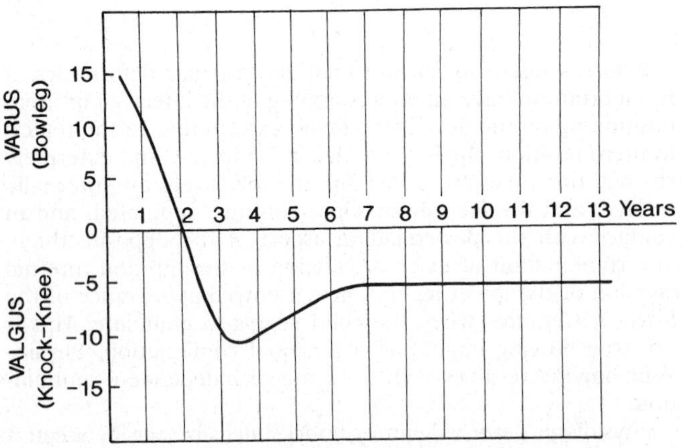

Figure 624–1. Graph demonstrating the normal development of the tibiofemoral or knee angle during growth. (Adapted from Salenius P, Vankka E: The development of the tibiofemoral angle in children. J Bone Joint Surg 57A:259, 1975.)

Thigh-Foot Angle

With the child in the prone position for assessment of hip rotation, the long axis of the foot in the simulated weightbearing position can be compared with the long axis of the thigh (Fig. 624–5). Inward rotation is given a negative value, whereas outward rotation is given a positive value. Inward rotation is indicative of internal tibial torsion, whereas outward rotation represents external tibial torsion. Infants have a mean angle of −5 degrees (range, −35 to 40 degrees) as a consequence of normal in utero position. In middle childhood through adult life, the mean thigh-foot angle is 10 degrees (range, −5 to 30 degrees).

Foot Shape

With the child still in the prone position, the shape of the foot is easily assessed (Fig. 624–6). This position is very helpful in the assessment of metatarsus adductus or a calcaneovalgus foot. The mobility of the ankle and subtalar can also be evaluated with the child in this position.

TORSIONAL DEFORMITIES

The common causes of in-toeing and out-toeing are presented in Table 622–4.

IN-TOE GAIT

The common lower extremity causes of an in-toe gait include internal femoral torsion and internal tibial torsion.

624.2 Internal Femoral Torsion

Internal femoral torsion is the most common cause of in-toeing in children 2 yr of age or older. It occurs more commonly in girls than boys (2:1). The majority of children with this condition have generalized ligamentous laxity. The cause of femoral torsion is controversial. Some believe that it is congenital as a result of persistent infantile femoral anteversion, whereas others believe it is acquired secondary to abnormal sitting habits.

CLINICAL MANIFESTATIONS. Clinical features of internal femoral torsion demonstrate that the entire lower leg is inwardly rotated during gait. Characteristically, there will be 80–90 degrees of internal rotation of the hip in the prone position (torsional profile). External rotation, as a consequence, is limited to 0 to 10 degrees (Fig. 624–7). There will be features of generalized ligamentous laxity including elbow and finger hyperextension, thumb hyperabduction, knee recurvatum, and hypermobile pes planus. Affected children commonly sit in the "television" or "W" style position. It is believed that this position allows the lower leg to act as a lever, thereby producing torsional changes in the "biologically plastic" femora. This condition is also called femoral anteversion, implying an abnormality of the proximal femur. However, the torsion actually occurs throughout the femoral shaft and results in a change in the normal alignment between the hip and the knee.

RADIOGRAPHIC EVALUATION. Radiographic evaluation of internal femoral torsion is not routinely necessary, although a variety of radiographic techniques to measure femoral torsion have been described. Computed tomography and ultrasonography can assess the relationship between the proximal and distal femur. These studies are rarely indicated because the clinical measurements are equally accurate.

TREATMENT. The treatment of internal femoral torsion is pre-

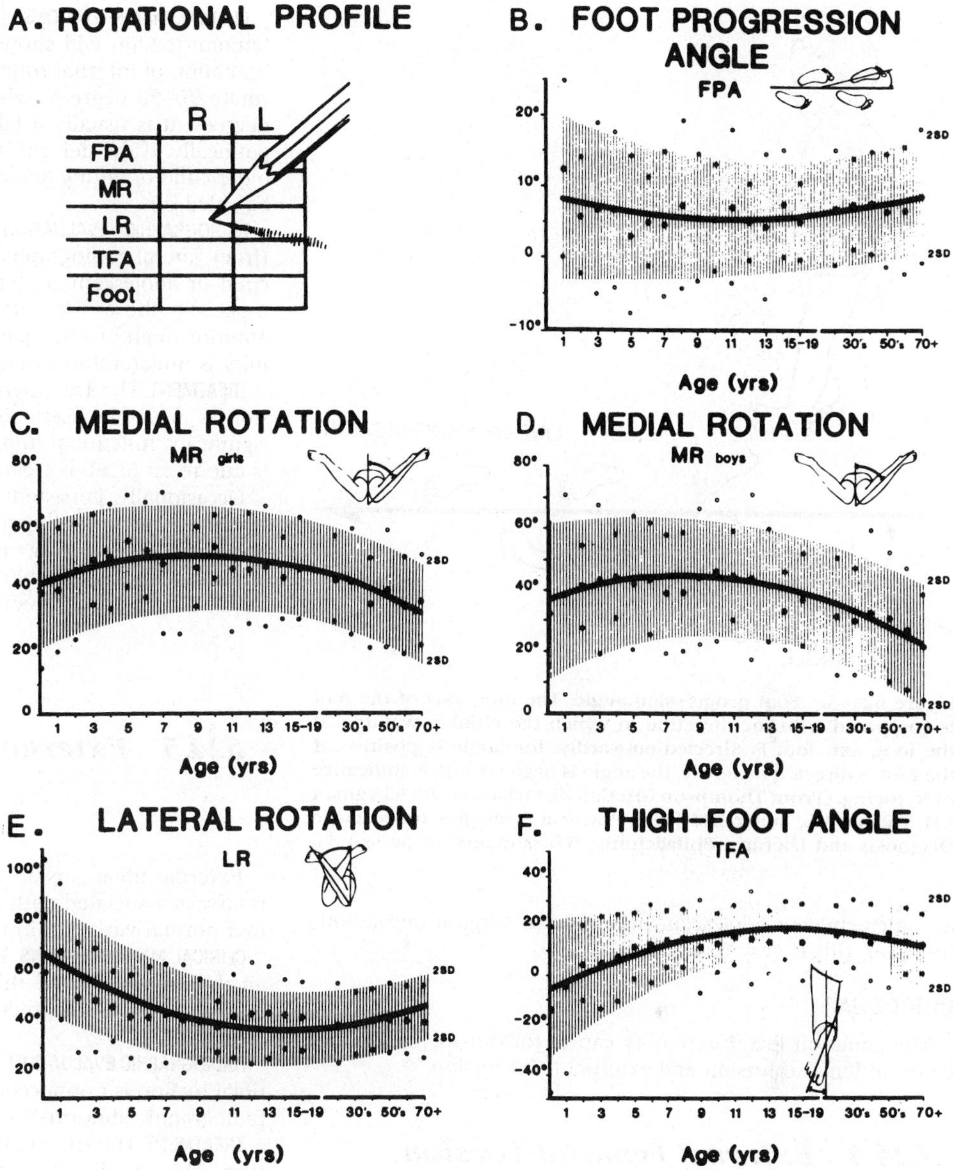

Figure 624–2. Range of normal values by age and sex with respect to the alignment of the lower extremity. *A*, Torsional profile. *B*, Foot progression angle (FPA) to determine the degree of in-toeing and out-toeing during ambulation. *C* and *D*, Medial (MR) or internal rotation of the hips in girls (*D*) and boys (*C*). *E*, Lateral (LR) or external rotation of the hips. *F*, Thigh-foot angle (TFA) to determine the degree of tibial torsion. Internal or medial tibial torsion is present if the angle is more than 20–30 degrees (From Staheli LT: Torsional deformities. Pediatr Clin North Am 33:1373, 1986.)

dominantly by observation. Correction of abnormal sitting habits will usually allow the torsion to resolve with normal growth and development. However, it will take 1–3 yr for complete correction to occur, depending on the age of the child when the sitting habits are corrected. The correction of sitting habits can be very difficult in preschool-age children and usually does not occur until they reach school age. The use of nighttime orthoses or daytime twister cables are of no value and may produce a compensatory external tibial torsion. The combination of internal femoral and compensatory external tibial torsion produces a pathologic genu valgum deformity. This can result in patellofemoral malalignment with patella subluxation or dislocation and pain.

Children 10 yr of age or older may not have enough remaining musculoskeletal growth for spontaneous correction to occur, and surgical intervention may be necessary. The procedures advocated include proximal femoral varus derotation osteotomy and simple derotation osteotomy of either the proximal or the distal femur. Sufficient derotation is performed to allow for equal internal and external hip rotation postoperatively.

624.3 Internal Tibial Torsion

Internal tibial torsion is the most common cause of in-toeing in children younger than 2 yr and is secondary to normal in utero positioning. This condition is commonly seen during the 2nd year of life and may be associated with metatarsus adductus.

CLINICAL MANIFESTATIONS. The degree of tibial torsion can be measured by the prone thigh-foot angle (torsional profile).

RADIOGRAPHIC EVALUATION. Radiographic assessment is of no value in this predominantly clinical disorder.

TREATMENT. Treatment of internal tibial torsion is also by observation. This is a physiologic condition, and spontaneous resolution with normal growth and development can be anticipated. However, significant improvement usually does not occur until the child begins to pull to stand and walk independently. Thereafter, it takes 6–12 mo and occasionally longer for complete correction to occur. Night splints are of no value and should be avoided. Persistent internal tibial torsion in

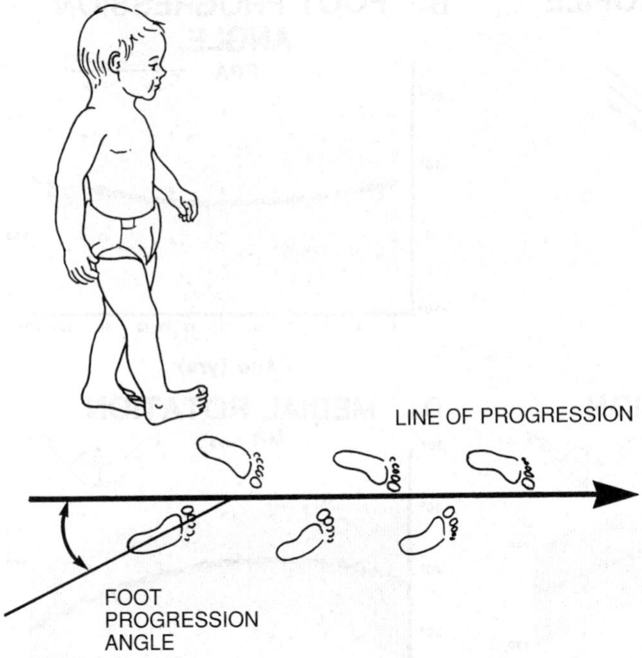

Figure 624–3. Foot progression angle. The long axis of the foot is compared with the direction in which the child is walking. If the long axis foot is directed outwardly, the angle is positive. If the foot is directed inwardly, the angle is negative and is indicative of in-toeing. (From Thompson GH: Gait disturbances. *In:* Kliegman RM, Nieder ML, Super DM [eds]: Practical Strategies in Pediatric Diagnosis and Therapy. Philadelphia, WB Saunders, in press.)

an older child or adolescent may require surgical derotation; however, this is very rare.

OUT-TOE GAIT

The common lower extremity causes for out-toeing include external femoral torsion and external tibial torsion.

624.4 External Femoral Torsion

External femoral torsion, also known as femoral retroversion, is an uncommon disorder unless associated with a slipped capital femoral epiphysis (SCFE).

CLINICAL MANIFESTATIONS. The clinical examination of external femoral torsion will show excessive hip external rotation and limitation of internal rotation. Typically, the hip will externally rotate 70–90 degrees, whereas internal rotation is only 0–20 degrees. It is usually a bilateral disorder when it occurs idiopathically. If the deformity is unilateral, especially in an obese older child or young adolescent, the presence of an SCFE must be ruled out.

RADIOGRAPHIC EVALUATION. Anteroposterior and Lauenstein (frog) lateral radiographs of the pelvis are necessary in any child or adolescent presenting with external femoral torsion, especially those who are obese or who have nontraumatic anterior thigh or knee pain (referred pain) or when the deformity is unilateral to assess for a possible SCFE.

TREATMENT. The treatment of idiopathic external femoral torsion is usually observation because it ordinarily causes no significant functional impairment. A femoral retroversion that is due to an SCFE is treated surgically.

Occasionally, persistent femoral retroversion after SCFE can produce functional impairment such as a severe out-toe gait and difficulty opposing one's knees in the sitting position. The latter can be very disabling to adolescent females. Should this occur, a derotation osteotomy will be beneficial.

624.5 External Tibial Torsion

External tibial torsion is a relatively common disorder and is always associated with a calcaneovalgus foot. It is secondary to a normal variation in in utero positioning.

CLINICAL MANIFESTATIONS. External tibial torsion is indicated by an abnormally positive thigh-foot angle (torsional profile). This is typically 30–50 degrees. There will be a calcaneovalgus foot (Fig. 624–8).

RADIOGRAPHIC EVALUATION. Radiographic assessment for external tibial torsion is not necessary because there is no demonstrable radiographic abnormality.

TREATMENT. The treatment of external tibial torsion is observation. This condition will follow the same clinical course as internal tibial torsion. Significant improvement does not occur during the 1st year of life. However, with the onset of independent ambulation, spontaneous improvement will begin to occur and is typically complete by 2–3 yr of age.

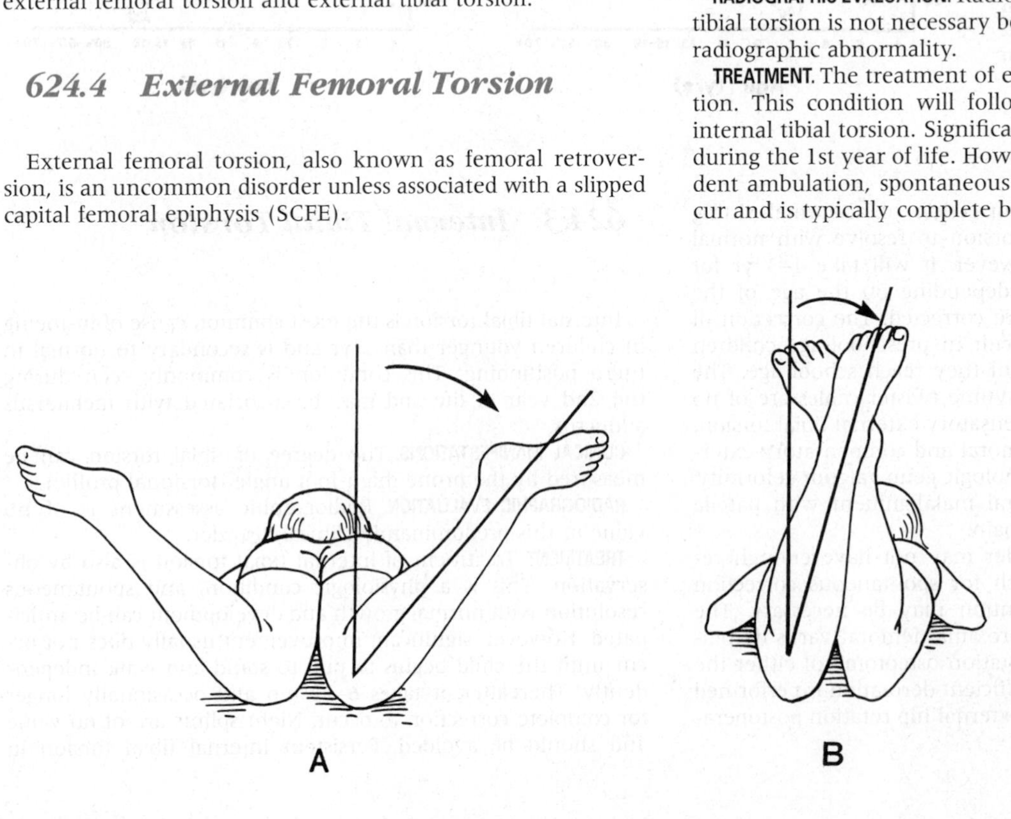

Figure 624–4. Hip rotation in extension. This is measured with the child in the prone position and the knee flexed 90 degrees. The lower leg is vertically oriented. This is considered the neutral position. On outward rotation (*A*), the leg produces internal hip rotation, and on inward rotation (*B*), the leg produces external hip rotation. (From Thompson GH: Gait disturbances. *In:* Kliegman RM, Nieder ML, Super DM [eds]: Practical Strategies in Pediatric Diagnosis and Therapy. Philadelphia, WB Saunders, in press.)

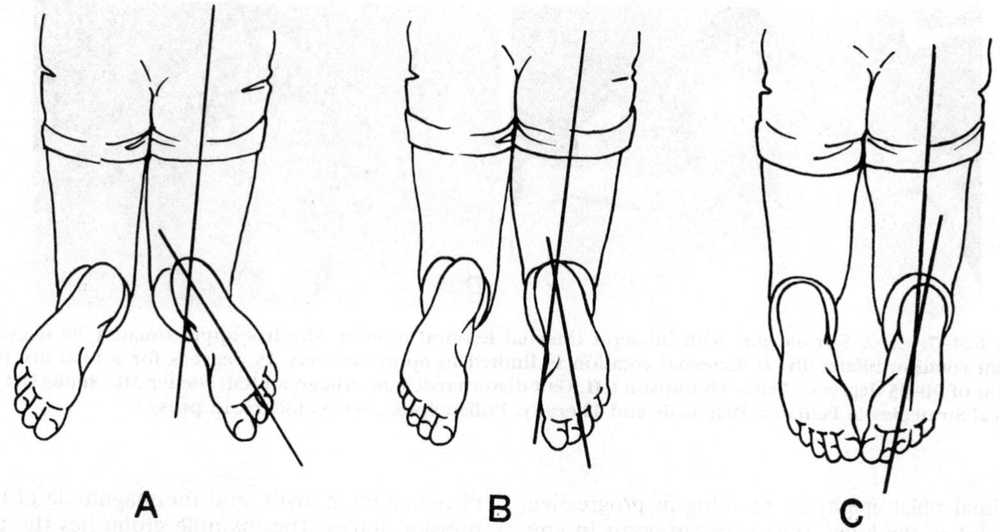

Figure 624–5. Thigh-foot angle. With the child in the prone position and the knees flexed and approximated, the long axis of the foot can be compared with the long axis of the thigh. The long axis of the foot bisects the heel and the second toe or lies between the second and third toes. External tibial torsion (*A*) produces excessive outward rotation. Normal alignment (*B*) is characterized by slight external rotation. Internal tibial torsion produces inward rotation of the foot and is a negative angle (*C*). (From Thompson GH: Gait disturbances. *In:* Kliegman RM, Nieder ML, Super DM [eds]: Practical Strategies in Pediatric Diagnosis and Therapy. Philadelphia, WB Saunders, in press.)

ANGULAR DEFORMITIES

624.6 Genu Varum (Bowlegs)

The classification of genu varum is presented in Table 624–1. Physiologic genu varum and tibia vara (Blount disease) are the most common disorders.

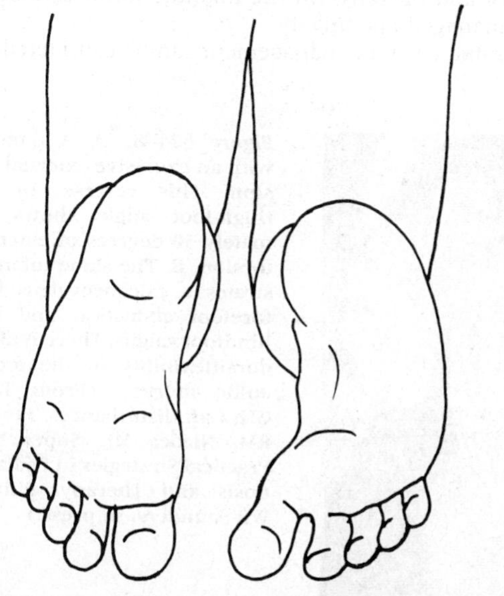

Figure 624–6. Foot shape. Using the same position for measurement of the thigh-foot angle, the shape of the foot can also be evaluated. In this illustration, the left foot has normal alignment, whereas the right foot demonstrates metatarsus adductus. (From Thompson GH: Gait disturbances. *In:* Kliegman RM, Nieder ML, Super DM [eds]: Practical Strategies in Pediatric Diagnosis and Therapy. Philadelphia, WB Saunders, in press.)

Physiologic Genu Varum

Physiologic bowlegs is a common torsional combination that is secondary to normal in utero positioning (Fig. 624–9). The tight posterior hip capsule results in an external rotation contracture. When it is combined with internal tibial torsion, it gives the clinical appearance of a bowleg deformity. Because it is physiologic, spontaneous resolution with normal growth and development can be anticipated. Significant improvement does occur during the 1st year of life. By 2 yr of age, the majority of children have straight or neutrally aligned lower extremities.

Tibia Vara

Idiopathic tibia vara, or Blount disease, is an uncommon disorder characterized by abnormal growth of the medial as-

■ **TABLE 624–1 Classification of Genu Varum (Bowlegs)**

Physiologic
Asymmetric Growth
Tibia vara (Blount disease)
Infantile
Juvenile
Adolescent
Focal fibrocartilaginous
Dysplasia
Physeal Injury
Trauma
Infection
Tumor
Metabolic Disorders
Vitamin D deficiency (nutritional rickets)
Vitamin D–resistant rickets
Hypophosphatasia
Skeletal Dysplasia
Metaphyseal dysplasia
Achondroplasia
Enchondromatosis

Modified from Thompson GH: Angular deformities of the lower extremities. In *Chapman MW (ed): Operative Orthopedics, 2nd ed. Philadelphia, JB Lippincott, 1993, pp 3131–3164.*

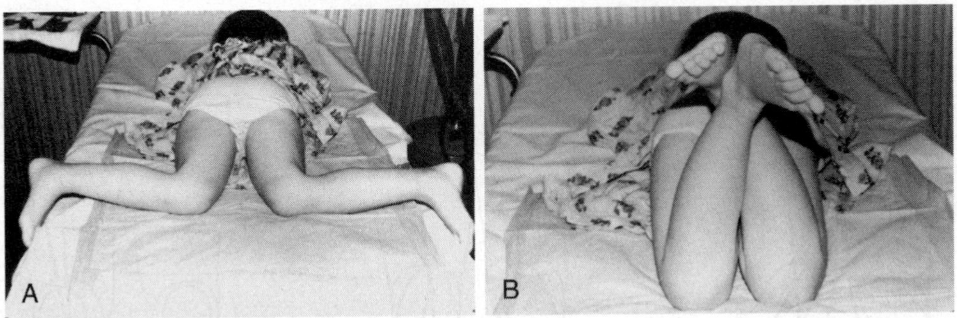

Figure 624–7. *A*, A 5-yr-old girl with bilateral internal femoral torsion. She has approximately 80 degrees of internal rotation bilaterally. *B*, External rotation is limited to approximately 15 degrees for a total arc of hip rotation of 90–95 degrees. (From Thompson GH: Gait disturbances. *In:* Kliegman RM, Nieder ML, Super DM [eds]: Practical Strategies in Pediatric Diagnosis and Therapy. Philadelphia, WB Saunders, in press.)

pect of the proximal tibial epiphysis, resulting in progressive varus angulation below the knee. Tibia vara can occur in any age group in a growing child and is classified as infantile (1–3 yr), juvenile (4–10 yr), and adolescent (11 yr or older). The juvenile and adolescent forms are commonly combined as late-onset tibia vara. All three groups share relatively common clinical characteristics, whereas the radiographic changes in the late-onset groups are less pronounced than in the infantile form. Although the exact cause of tibia vara remains unknown, it appears to be secondary to growth suppression from increased compressive forces across the medial aspect of the knee.

CLINICAL MANIFESTATIONS. The infantile form of tibia vara is the most common, and its characteristics include female and black predominance, marked obesity, approximately 80% bilateral involvement, a prominent medial metaphyseal beak, internal tibial torsion, and leg length discrepancy. The characteristics of the juvenile and adolescent forms (late-onset) include male and black predominance, marked obesity, normal or above normal height, approximately 50% bilateral involvement, slowly progressive genu varum deformity, pain rather than deformity as the primary initial complaint, no palpable proximal medial metaphyseal beak, minimal internal tibial torsion, mild medial collateral ligament laxity, and mild lower extremity length discrepancy. The differences between the three groups appear to be primarily due to age at onset, the amount of remaining growth, and the magnitude of the medial compression forces. The infantile group has the potential for the greatest deformity, and the adolescent group has the least.

RADIOGRAPHIC EVALUATION. Children with tibia vara are usually assessed radiographically from an anteroposterior standing radiograph of both lower extremities and a lateral radiograph of the involved extremity. Positioning the child in weightbearing stance allows maximum presentation of the clinical deformity. Fragmentation with a protuberant step deformity and beaking of the proximal medial tibial metaphysis are the major features of the infantile group. The changes in the proximal medial tibial metaphysis are less conspicuous in the late-onset forms, which are characterized by wedging of the medial portion of the epiphysis, a mild posteromedial articular depression, a serpiginous cephalad curved physis, and mild or no fragmentation or beaking of the proximal medial metaphysis (Fig. 624–10).

Occasionally, arthrography, magnetic resonance imaging, or tomography may be necessary to assess the meniscus, the articular surface of the proximal tibia, or the integrity of the proximal tibial physis. These are usually reserved for the more severe deformities.

TREATMENT. The management of tibia vara may be both nonoperative and operative in the infantile form. Late-onset tibia vara is managed operatively.

Nonoperative. Orthotic management can be considered for chil-

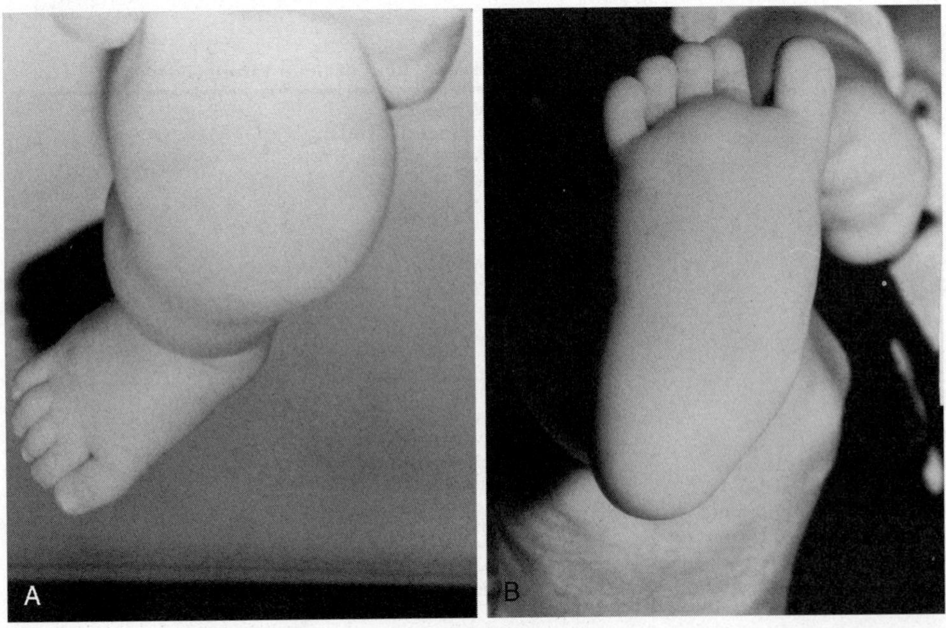

Figure 624–8. *A*, A 6-mo-old girl with an excessive external tibial torsion. This reverse, or anterior, thigh-foot angle shows approximately 50 degrees of external tibial torsion. *B*, The same infant demonstrates a calcaneovalgus foot with forefoot abduction and increased hindfoot valgus. There is also hyperdorsiflexibility of the foot in the ankle mortise. (From Thompson GH: Gait disturbances. *In:* Kliegman RM, Nieder ML, Super DM [eds]: Practical Strategies in Pediatric Diagnosis and Therapy. Philadelphia, WB Saunders, in press.)

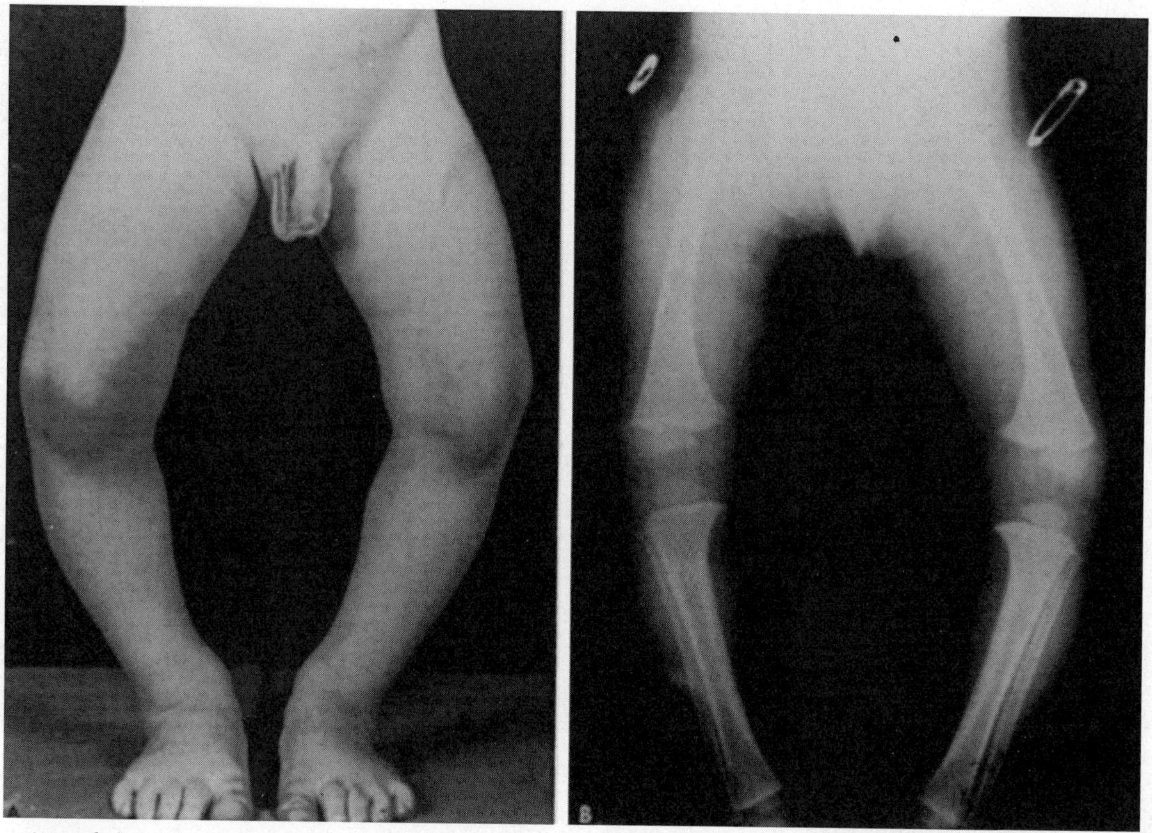

Figure 624–9. Infant with bilateral genu varum at 18 mo of age. This resolved spontaneously before 7 yr of age. *A,* Clinical photograph. *B,* Standing anteroposterior radiograph of the lower extremities (From Tachdjian MO: Pediatric Orthopedics, 2nd ed. Philadelphia, WB Saunders, 1990.)

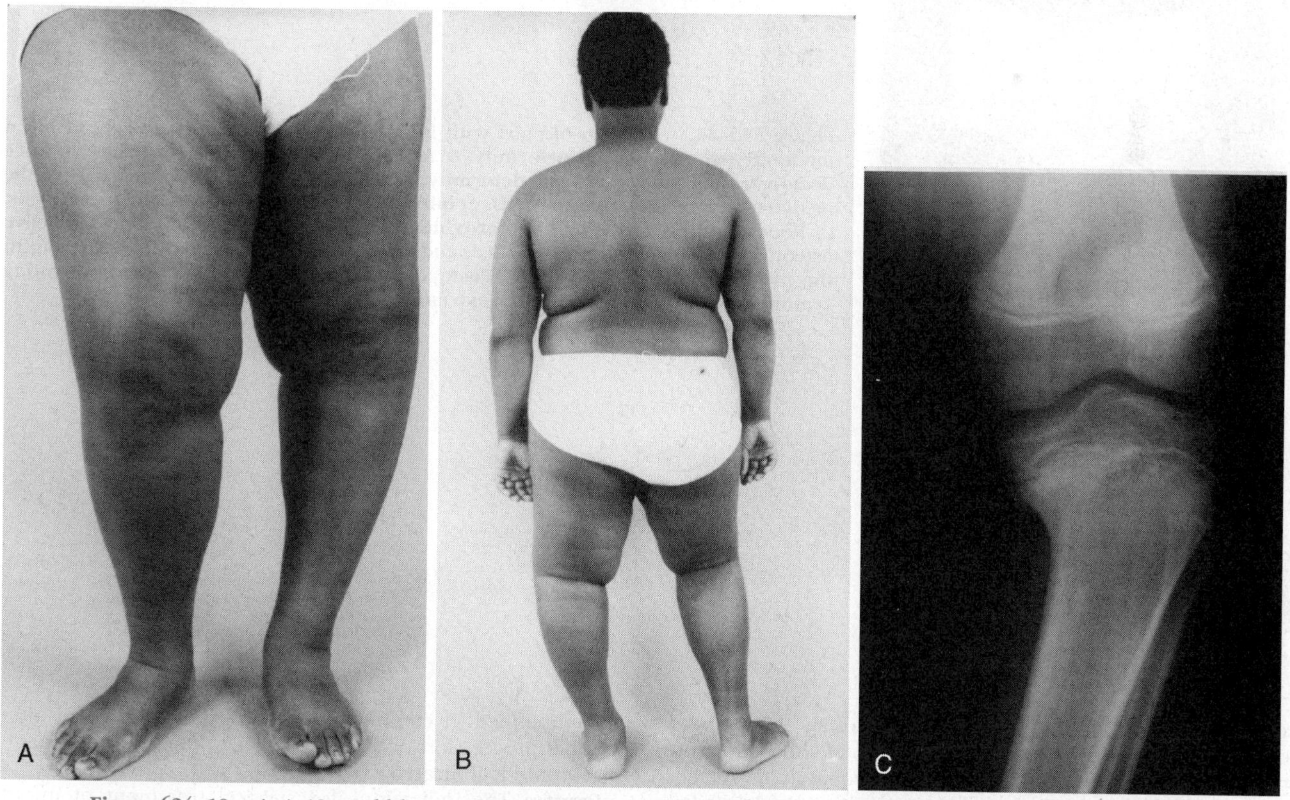

Figure 624–10. *A,* A 13-yr-old boy with late-onset, or adolescent, tibia vara. There is marked obesity and mild genu varum deformity of the left knee. *B,* Posterior view of the same child. *C,* Standing anteroposterior radiograph of the left knee demonstrating the tibia vara deformity but with less obvious changes than in the infantile form. The medial aspect of the proximal tibial epiphysis is narrow and the growth plate is irregular. The typical metaphyseal "beaking" is not present.

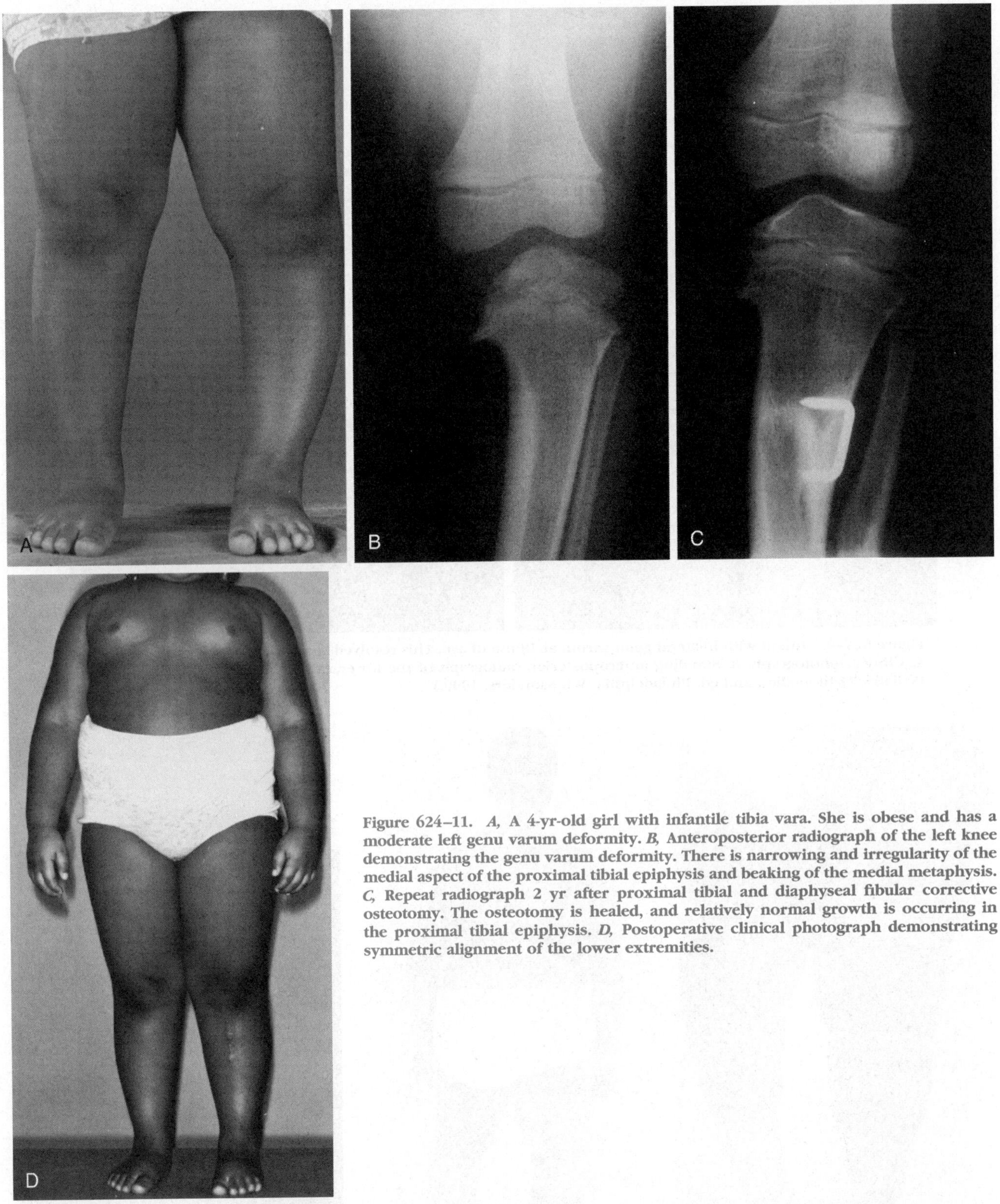

Figure 624–11. *A,* A 4-yr-old girl with infantile tibia vara. She is obese and has a moderate left genu varum deformity. *B,* Anteroposterior radiograph of the left knee demonstrating the genu varum deformity. There is narrowing and irregularity of the medial aspect of the proximal tibial epiphysis and beaking of the medial metaphysis. *C,* Repeat radiograph 2 yr after proximal tibial and diaphyseal fibular corrective osteotomy. The osteotomy is healed, and relatively normal growth is occurring in the proximal tibial epiphysis. *D,* Postoperative clinical photograph demonstrating symmetric alignment of the lower extremities.

dren with infantile tibia vara who are 3 yr of age or younger with mild deformities. In approximately 50% of children meeting these criteria, the deformity may be adequately corrected. A knee-ankle-foot orthosis should be used with a single medial upright, without a knee hinge. Pads and straps should be placed over the distal femur and proximal tibia to apply a valgus force. The orthosis should be worn 22–23 hr each day. A maximum trial of 1 yr of orthotic management is currently recommended. If complete correction is not obtained after 1 yr or if progression occurs during this time, then a corrective osteotomy is indicated.

Operative. The indications for surgical treatment of infantile tibia vara include age of 4 yr or more, failure of orthotic management, and more severe deformities. Proximal tibial valgus osteotomy and associated fibular diaphyseal osteotomy are usually the procedures of choice (Fig. 624–11). In late-onset tibia vara, correction is also necessary to restore the mechanical axis of the knee. The same surgical options as presented for older children with infantile tibia vara are applicable in these age groups. A proximal tibial valgus osteotomy and diaphyseal fibular osteotomy are the most common procedures.

624.7 Genu Valgum (Knock-Knees)

The classification of genu valgum is presented in Table 624–2. Fortunately, the pathologic causes, with the exception of post-traumatic disorders, are relatively uncommon. As the spontaneous correction of physiologic bowlegs continues, there is typically an overcorrection, of variable degree, into mild genu valgum, or knock-knees. This physiologic angular variation, or genu valgum, is commonly seen between 3 and 5 yr of age. It is a true angular deformity that resolves spontaneously, with the normal knee alignment being obtained between 5 and 8 yr. Rarely is a knock-knee orthosis indicated. Surgery may be required in adolescence for a persistent deformity. Options include medial physeal stapling, medial hemiepiphysiodesis, and corrective osteotomy.

624.8 Congenital Angular Deformities of the Tibia and Fibula

The differential diagnosis of congenital angular deformities of the lower leg (Table 624–3) include posteromedial angulation, which is a benign process, and anterolateral angulation, which is a pathologic process.

CONGENITAL POSTEROMEDIAL TIBIAL ANGULATION (BOWING). This is an uncommon angular deformity that involves the distal one third of the tibia and fibula. There is a posteromedial bowing in association with a calcaneovalgus foot. The clinical appearance can be very dramatic. The diagnosis is confirmed radiographically. This will show the posteromedial angulation without other osseous abnormalities. A significant portion of the calcaneovalgus foot is due to the position of the distal tibia and ankle.

The *cause* of the congenital posteromedial bowing is unknown. The natural history is characterized by spontaneous resolution by 3–5 yr of age. However, there will be residual shortening in the tibia and fibula. The fibula is usually slightly shorter than the tibia. The mean growth inhibition is 12–13% (range, 5–27%). The mean leg length discrepancy at maturity is 4 cm (3–7 cm).

The *treatment* of congenital posteromedial bowing of the tibia and fibula is observation. All components of the deformity with the exception of leg length inequality will resolve with growth and development. The child should have periodic radiographic measurements to determine the degree of discrepancy and to predict the maximum discrepancy at maturity. This will also allow information regarding the appropriate age for surgical intervention. Operative intervention for a defect other than leg length discrepancy is rarely indicated. A corrective osteotomy may be necessary in patients with severe deformity that is not improving with growth and development. Patients with discrepancies greater than 5 cm may be candidates for lengthening.

CONGENITAL ANTEROLATERAL TIBIAL ANGULATION (BOWING). This type of bowing is associated with an underlying pathologic disorder (see Table 624–3). The diagnosis is made radiographically. *Congenital fibular hemimelia* represents a congenital absence of the fibula and usually the lateral portion of the foot, especially the fourth and fifth rays. *Congenital tibial hemimelia* represents a congenital absence of the tibia, either partial or total. Surgical reconstruction of these deformities is difficult, and most defects require amputation to achieve satisfactory function. *Congenital pseudoarthrosis* of the tibia is usually associated with neurofibromatosis. It represents a defect in the tibia that predisposes to pathologic fracture, which will not heal. A variety of surgical techniques, including intramedullary rodding, electrical stimulation, and vascularized fibular transplants, have been used with varying success in this very complex problem.

■ TABLE 624–2 Classification of Genu Valgum (Knock-Knees)

Physiologic
Asymmetric Growth
- Tibia valga
- Physeal injury
- Trauma following fracture of the proximal tibial metaphysis
- Infection
- Tumor

Metabolic Disorders
- Renal osteodystrophy

Skeletal Dysplasia
- Kniest syndrome

Congenital Abnormalities
- Congenital dislocation of the patella

Neuromuscular Disorders
- Cerebral palsy
- Myelodysplasia

From Thompson GH: Angular deformities of the lower extremities. In *Chapman MW (ed): Operative Orthopedics, 2nd ed. Philadelphia, JB Lippincott, 1993, pp 3131–3164.*

■ TABLE 624–3 Differential Diagnosis of Congenital Angular Deformities of the Tibia and Fibula

Posteromedial Angulation
Anterolateral Angulation
- Congenital pseudoarthrosis of the tibia
- Congenital longitudinal deficiency of the tibia (paraxial tibial hemimelia)
- Congenital longitudinal deficiency of the fibula (paraxial fibular hemimelia)

Modified from Thompson GH: Angular deformities of the lower extremities. In *Chapman MW (ed): Operative Orthopedics, 2nd ed. Philadelphia, JB Lippincott, 1993, pp 3131–3164.*

TORSIONAL MALALIGNMENT

Medial Tibial and Femoral Torsion

Ruwe PA, Gage JR, Ozonoff MB, et al: Clinical determination of femoral anteversion: A comparison of established techniques. J Bone Joint Surg 74A:820, 1992.

Staheli LT, Corbett M, Wyss C, et al: Lower extremity rotational problems in children: Normal values to guide management. J Bone Joint Surg 67A:39, 1985.

Staheli LT: Rotational problems of the lower extremities. Orthop Clin North Am 18:503, 1987.

Staheli LT: Instructional course lecture: Rotational problems in children. J Bone Joint Surg 75A:939, 1993.

Svenvingsen S, Terjesen T, Auflein M, et al: Hip rotation and in-toeing gait: A study of normal subjects from four years until adult age. Clin Orthop 251:177, 1990.

ANGULAR DEFORMITIES

Physiologic Genu Varum and Genu Valgum

Kling TF Jr: Angular deformities of the lower limbs in children. Orthop Clin North Am 18:513, 1987.

Levine AM, Drennan JC: Physiological bowing and tibia vara: The metaphyseal angle in the measurement of bowleg deformities. J Bone Joint Surg 64A:1158, 1982.

Salenius P, Vankka E: The development of the tibio-femoral angle in children. J Bone Joint Surg 57A:259, 1975.

Thompson GH: Angular deformities of the lower extremities in children. *In:* Chapman MW (ed): Operative Orthopedics, 2nd ed. Philadelphia, JB Lippincott, 1993, pp 3131–3164.

Vankka E, Salenius P: Spontaneous correction of severe tibiofemoral deformity in growing children. Acta Orthop Scand 53:567, 1982.

Tibia Vara

Henderson RC, Kemp GJ, Greene WB: Adolescent tibia vara: Alternatives for operative treatment. J Bone Joint Surg 74A:342, 1992.
Johnston CE II: Infantile tibia vara. Clin Orthop 255:13, 1990.
Langenskiold A: Tibia vara: A critical review. Clin Orthop 264:195, 1989.
Loder RT, Johnston CE II: Infantile tibia vara. J Pediatr Orthop 7:639, 1987.
Schoenecker PL, Meade WC, Pierron RL, et al: Blount's disease: A retrospective review and recommendations for treatment. J Pediatr Orthop 5:181, 1985.
Thompson GH, Carter JR: Late-onset tibia vara (Blount's disease): Current concepts. Clin Orthop 255:24, 1990.
Greene WB: Instructional course lecture: Infantile tibia vara. J Bone Joint Surg 75A:130, 1993.
Henderson RC, Kemp GJ, Hayes PRL: Prevalence of late-onset tibia vara. J Pediatr Orthop 13:255, 1993.
Feldman MD, Schoenecker PL: Use of metaphyseal-diaphyseal angle in the evaluation of bowed-legs. J Bone Joint Surg 75A:1602, 1993.

Congenital Posteromedial Tibial Bowing

Hofmann A, Wenger DR: Posteromedial bowing of the tibia: Progression of discrepancy in leg lengths. J Bone Joint Surg 63A:384, 1981.
Pappas AM: Congenital posteromedial bowing of the tibia and fibula. J Pediatr Orthop 4:525, 1984.

CHAPTER 625
Leg Length Discrepancy

Leg length discrepancies are common in childhood, and many factors must be evaluated before management decisions can be made.

ETIOLOGY. The cause of leg length discrepancy is extensive, and the more common causes are presented in Table 625–1.

CLINICAL MANIFESTATIONS AND DIAGNOSIS. Signs and symptoms associated with leg length discrepancy usually are related to the underlying cause. Approximately 65% of the growth of the entire lower extremity comes from the distal femoral (37%) and proximal tibial (28%) physes. Thus, growth disturbances about the knee can have the most adverse effect on leg length. Determination of the *skeletal, or bone, age* allows for a relatively accurate assessment of remaining growth. The *Gruelich and Pyle Atlas* (1950) remains the standard by which bone age is determined from an anteroposterior radiograph of the left hand and wrist. It is possible to estimate the *ultimate discrepancy at maturity* using growth remaining tables such as the Moseley straight-line graph (Fig. 625–1) and the Green-Anderson table.

■ **TABLE 625–1 Common Causes of Leg Length Discrepancies**

Congenital	**Infectious**
Proximal femoral focal deficiency	Pyogenic osteomyelitis with physeal damage
Coxa vara	**Trauma**
Hemiatrophy-hemihypertrophy (anisomelia)	Physeal injury with premature closure
Development dysplasia of the hip	Overgrowth
Developmental	Malunion (shortening)
Legg-Calvé-Perthes disease	**Tumor**
Neuromuscular	Physeal destruction
Polio	Radiation-induced physeal injury
Cerebral palsy (hemiplegia)	Overgrowth

Modified from Thompson GH: Gait disturbances. In: *Kliegman RM, Nieder ML, Super DM (eds): Practical Strategies of Pediatric Diagnosis and Therapy. Philadelphia, WB Saunders, in press.*

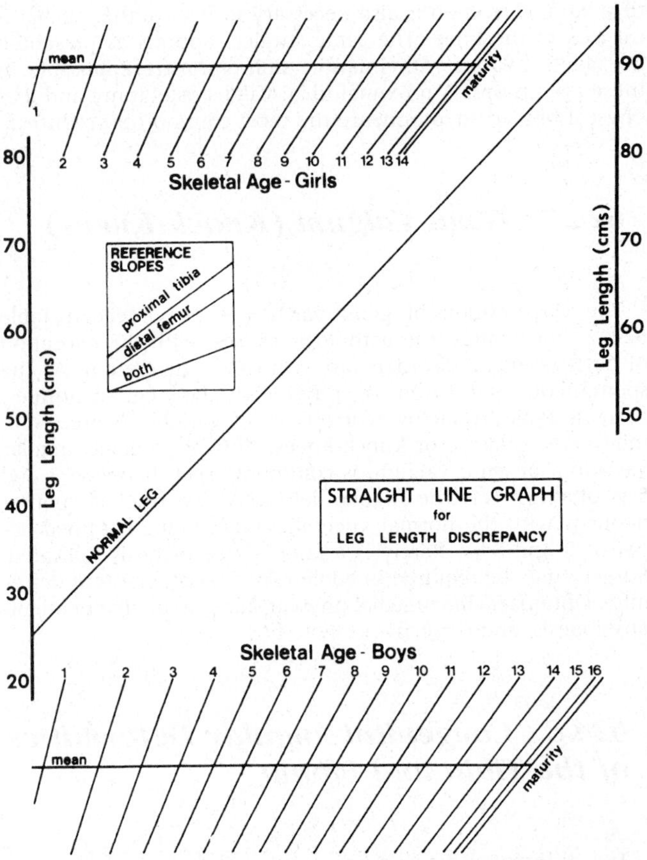

Figure 625–1. **The Moseley straight-line graph for the assessment of leg length inequalities. This allows simultaneous correlation of the normal leg, short leg, and bone age of the child. It will accurately predict lengths of each extremity at skeletal maturity. The reference slopes are used as a guide in determining when appropriate treatment should be performed.**

The former, the most commonly used today, utilizes scanographic and bone age data to determine the ultimate discrepancy. It can also be used to follow the response of treatment. The clinical methods available are less accurate than the radiographic techniques, but they are useful. The most common clinical measurement is leveling the pelvis. Blocks of various thickness may be placed beneath the foot on the involved side until the iliac crests are level. The thickness indicates the amount of discrepancy.

Adult sitting height is approximately 52% of total height in the male and 53% in the female. Thus, two times the predicted length of the normal leg at maturity gives a close approximation of the *anticipated adult height.* This height plays an important role in determining equalization. Lengthening procedures are more applicable in predicted short adults, whereas shortening procedures are generally used for predicted normal height or taller individuals. In either case, acceptable body proportions must be maintained.

Children with *neuromuscular disorders* such as spastic hemiplegia benefit from 1–2 cm of shortening on the involved side to improve the swing phase of gait and increased toe clearance. Only extremities that are neurologically normal should be considered for complete equalization of leg lengths.

Angular deformities and limitation of motion are important considerations in children with unequal leg lengths. This is especially true when lengthening procedures are being considered. A child with a dysplastic acetabulum may subsequently experience a hip dislocation if femoral lengthening is attempted. Thus, any significant angular deformities or joint abnormalities should be corrected either before or simultaneously with leg length equalization.

RADIOGRAPHIC EVALUATION. Radiographic evaluations are the most accurate methods of assessing leg lengths. Four different types of radiographic techniques are available. The *teleoroentgenogram* is a single exposure of both lower extremities. Its primary indication is for young children, usually younger than 5 yr. There is a small amount of magnification error present, but it has the advantage of demonstrating any associated angular deformity. The *orthoroentgenogram* consists of three separate, slightly overlapping exposures of the hips, knees, and ankles on a long cassette. Bone length is measured directly on the radiograph. There is less magnification, and it is relatively accurate and will demonstrate angular deformities. The *scanogram* is a simple, accurate method of assessment. It consists of three narrow exposures of the hips, knees, and ankles on a standard cassette with a radiographic ruler laying next to the extremity. Thus, minimal magnification is present, and accurate measurements can be made. However, angular deformities cannot be fully visualized and, if present, can lead to errors in measurement. *Computed tomography* is the most accurate technique and will also show angular deformity.

TREATMENT. The psychological status of the child as well as the parents is an important consideration in treatment selection. Some equalization techniques are simple and safe, whereas others, especially lengthening procedures, are complex with high complication rates and require strict cooperation by the child and parents. Discrepancies of greater than 2 cm at skeletal maturity usually require treatment because these often cause the patient to limp. Equalization can be achieved by nonsurgical and surgical methods. In general, the goals are to maintain adult height (5′6″ in males, 5′0″ in females) and adequate body proportions. Shortening procedures are preferred, and lengthening procedures should be used cautiously.

Orthotics and Prosthetics. Orthotic devices are generally indicated for discrepancies between 2–3 cm in skeletally mature individuals. A heel lift is frequently all that is necessary to provide the patient with a normal gait. Because of normal pelvic rotation during the gait cycle, complete equalization is not necessary. The smallest lift that will allow the patient to walk without a limp is all that is necessary. Prostheses are necessary for severe discrepancies or uncorrectable deformities.

Extremity-Shortening Procedures. Three procedures are used to shorten the longer extremity. *Epiphysiodesis* is indicated in children who have 5 cm or less predicted discrepancy at maturity, have adequate remaining growth for satisfactory correction, and have a predicted relatively normal, corrected adult height. It requires accurate timing to achieve equalization of the leg lengths at maturity. The disadvantages of epiphysiodesis include shortened stature, surgery on the unaffected extremity, the possibility of an angular growth deformity, and the irreversibility of the procedure itself. Percutaneous epiphysiodesis under fluoroscopic control currently is the most popular technique. This is an outpatient procedure that is effective and has a low complication rate. *Epiphyseal stapling* is performed to slow the rate of physeal growth. Three staples inserted extraperiosteally on each side of the physis are required to retard growth adequately. Once equalization has been achieved, the staples are removed, allowing normal growth to resume. Stapling on one side of the physis can be used to correct angular deformities about the knee. *Bone resection* is indicated for ultimate discrepancies of 5–6 cm in adults or adolescents who have inadequate remaining growth to undergo an epiphysiodesis. The femur can be shortened up to 6 cm and the tibia-fibula, up to 3 cm before irreversible muscle weakness occurs.

Extremity-Lengthening Procedures. The advantages of lengthening are equalization of significant leg length discrepancies; maintenance of ultimate adult height; preservation of normal body proportions; surgery on the affected limb; correction of existing angular deformities; and elimination of orthoses. The disadvantages are that they are technically difficult to perform and have a significant complication rate. Common complications include pin tract infection, wound infection, hypertension, hip and knee subluxation, ankle equinus, loss of correction, delayed union, metal failure, and fatigue fractures after metal removal. ***Transiliac, or pelvic lengthening, osteotomies*** can provide a gain of up to 3 cm in length. They are generally reserved for those individuals with mild discrepancies who have ipsilateral shortening with acetabular dysplasia, an asymmetric pelvis, or possibly decompensated scoliosis. The callotasis technique allows for progressive *lengthening of the femur or tibia*. An osteotomy is performed after application of an external fixator lengthening system. There is no initial lengthening. After 7–10 days, lengthening is begun at 1.0 mm/day (0.25 mm every 6 hr). This allows elongation of the forming callus. Significant lengthening of the bone can be achieved with this technique. Once the desired length has been achieved, the callus is allowed to consolidate. The lengthening device is removed after consolidation. The entire process requires approximately 1.0 mo per centimeter lengthened. The advantages of this procedure over previous lengthening techniques is that it requires only one procedure, allows greater lengthening, and has a lower complication rate. Occasionally, *a combination of a transiliac, femoral, or tibial diaphyseal lengthening and possibly leg-shortening procedures* such as epiphysiodesis is necessary to equalize leg lengths. The combination of femoral diaphyseal lengthening and contralateral epiphysiodeses is very useful for discrepancies of 8–10 cm when a single lengthening is insufficient for complete correction.

Aaron A, Weinstein D, Thickman D, et al: Comparison of orthoroentgenography and computed tomography in the measurement of limb-length discrepancy. J Bone Joint Surg 74A:897, 1992.

Anderson M, Green WT, Messner M: Growth and predictions of growth in the lower extremities. J Bone Joint Surg 45A:1, 1963.

Barry K, McManus F, O'Brien T: Leg lengthening by the transiliac method. J Bone Joint Surg 74B:275, 1992.

Canale ST, Russell TA, Holcomb RL: Percutaneous epiphysiodesis: Experimental study and preliminary clinical results. J Pediatr Orthop 6:150, 1986.

Gruelich WW, Pyle SI: Radiographic Atlas of Skeletal Development of the Hand and Wrist, 2nd ed. Stanford, CA, Stanford University Press, 1959.

Huurman WW, Jacobsen FS, Anderson JC, et al: Limb-length discrepancy measured with computerized axial tomographic equipment. J Bone Joint Surg 69A:699, 1987.

Millis MR, Hall JE: Transiliac lengthening of the lower extremity: A modified innominate osteotomy for the treatment of postural imbalance. J Bone Joint Surg 61A:1182, 1979.

Moseley CF: A straight line graph for leg-length discrepancies. J Bone Joint Surg 59A:174, 1977.

Moseley CF: Leg length discrepancy. Orthop Clin North Am 18:529, 1987.

Paley D: Current techniques of limb lengthening. J Pediatr Orthop 8:73, 1988.

Shapiro F: Developmental patterns in lower extremity length discrepancies. J Bone Joint Surg 64A:639, 1982.

Timberlake RW, Bowen JR, Guille JT, et al: Prospective evaluation of 53 consecutive percutaneous epiphysiodeses of the distal femur and proximal tibia and fibula. J Pediatr Orthop 11:350, 1991.

Velazquez RJ, Bell DF, Armstrong PF, et al: Complications of use of the Ilizarov technique in the correction of limb deformities in children. J Bone Joint Surg 75A:1148, 1993.

CHAPTER 626

The Knee

The knee joint is unique because the tibiofemoral articulation is constrained only by soft tissues rather than by geometric fit. The distal femur is cam shaped, allowing it to have a gliding, hinged motion. The major constraints of the knee are the medial and lateral collateral ligaments, the anterior and posterior cruciate ligaments, and the medial and lateral menisci. Weight is transmitted through both the articular cartilage and the menisci. A second important area of the knee is the patellofemoral joint. It is the common site of problems, especially in adolescence.

Pain about the knee is one of the most common presenting complaints in older children and adolescents. This may be insidious in onset or the result of trauma. *Accumulation of fluid* (effusion) in the knee is indicative of an abnormal intra-articular process. Fluid accumulating after injury is usually blood (hemarthrosis) and is indicative of a potentially serious injury to one or more of the ligaments or menisci. Recurrent effusions may indicate a chronic internal derangement such as a meniscal tear. Unexplained accumulation of fluid may occur with arthritis (septic, viral, postinfectious, juvenile rheumatoid arthritis, or systemic lupus erythematosus) and with overactivity. Occasionally, this fluid requires aspiration to relieve discomfort as well as to help establish the diagnosis. The presence of fat globules in the blood aspirated from a hemarthrosis may be indicative of an occult fracture. The presence of purulent material indicates septic arthritis or osteomyelitis.

PEDIATRIC KNEE DISORDERS

Common pediatric knee problems include (1) discoid lateral meniscus, (2) popliteal cyst, (3) osteochondritis dissecans, and (4) Osgood-Schlatter disease. Overuse syndromes, ligament injuries, and meniscal tears also occur in children and adolescents and are discussed in the chapter on sports medicine (see Chapter 633).

626.1 Discoid Lateral Meniscus

CLINICAL MANIFESTATIONS AND DIAGNOSIS. Each meniscus is semilunar or "C" shaped, but occasionally the lateral meniscus persists as a solid disc of cartilage, and this is referred to as a discoid lateral meniscus. The normal meniscus is attached about its periphery and glides anteriorly and posteriorly with knee motion, but a discoid meniscus is less mobile and may be torn. Occasionally, there will be no peripheral attachment about the posterolateral aspect of the meniscus, which may allow it to displace anteriorly with knee flexion, producing a loud click or clunk. A tear or anterior displacement is most likely to occur in late childhood or early adolescence (11–15 yr). Physical examination may show a mild effusion and a positive McMurray test in which the displacement of the meniscus is both palpable and audible. Anteroposterior radiograph of the knee may show only widening of the lateral aspect of the knee joint. Magnetic resonance imaging (MRI) or arthrography are required for definitive diagnosis.

TREATMENT. The treatment of discoid menisci is to excise tears and reshape the meniscus arthroscopically. Peripheral detachments may be repaired and the body reshaped.

626.2 Popliteal Cyst

Popliteal cyst (Baker cyst) is commonly seen during the middle childhood years. There is distention of the gastrocnemius and semimembranous bursa along the posterior aspect of the knee by synovial fluid from a tendon sheath or the knee joint. Knee radiographs will be normal. The diagnosis may be confirmed by ultrasonography or aspiration. *Treatment* is by observation, especially in children 10 yr of age and younger, because resolution over several years usually occurs. The only indications for surgical excision are the presence of symptoms or progressive enlargement.

626.3 Osteochondritis Dissecans

Osteochondritis dissecans commonly involves the knee and occurs when an area of bone adjacent to the articular cartilage becomes avascular and ultimately separates from the underlying bone. The exact cause is unknown, but trauma from the adjacent tibial spines is commonly implicated. The lateral portion of the medial femoral condyle is the most common site.

CLINICAL MANIFESTATIONS AND DIAGNOSIS. The child or adolescent typically presents with a vague knee pain. Occasionally, a mild effusion may be present. With the knee fully flexed, it is possible to palpate directly the involved area on the articular cartilage of the medial femoral condyle. This is usually tender.

Anteroposterior, lateral, and tunnel radiographs of the knee are necessary to establish the diagnosis and to follow the disease process. In younger children, the overlying articular cartilage usually remains intact. As revascularization occurs, the bone will heal spontaneously. With increasing age, the risk increases for articular cartilage fracture and separation of the bony fragment, producing a loose body. MRI is helpful in determining the integrity of the articular cartilage.

TREATMENT. In children 11 yr of age and younger, the treatment is primarily by observation. Periodic radiographs and occasionally MRI scans may be necessary to assess the degree of healing. In adolescents, 13 yr of age and older, especially those with suspected loose body, arthroscopic surgical intervention may be necessary. This may consist of (1) excision of the loose body, (2) replacement and internal fixation, or (3) drilling of an intact lesion to promote revascularization and healing.

626.4 Osgood-Schlatter Disease

The patellar tendon inserts into the tibia tubercle, which is an extension of the proximal tibial epiphysis. This area is vulnerable to microfracture during late childhood or adolescence, especially in those individuals who are athletic, producing Osgood-Schlatter disease. It is most common in males. The natural history is almost always benign. Physical examination will demonstrate swelling, tenderness, and increased prominence of the tibia tubercle. Radiographs are usually necessary to rule out other lesions. Rest, restriction of activities, and, occasionally, a knee immobilizer may be necessary, combined with an isometric exercise program. Anti-inflammatory medications are usually not beneficial. Complete resolution of symptoms through physiologic healing (physeal closure) of the tibia tubercle usually will require 12–24 mo.

PATELLOFEMORAL DISORDERS

The patellofemoral joint depends on balance among the restraining ligaments, muscle forces, and the articular anatomy of the patellofemoral groove. The patella has a "V"-shaped bottom that guides it through the matching groove (trochlea) in the distal femur. The force of the muscles pulling through the quadriceps mechanism and the patellar tendon does not act in a straight line because the patellar tendon inclines in a slightly lateral direction with respect to the line of the quadriceps. This lateral movement, coupled with the movement of the restraining ligaments, tends to move the patella in a lateral direction. The vastus medialis muscle is necessary to counteract the laterally acting forces. An abnormality of any one or a group of these factors may make the patellofemoral joint function abnormally. The usual clinical manifestation is knee pain that is aggravated by vigorous activities.

626.5 Idiopathic Adolescent Anterior Knee Pain Syndrome

This common patellofemoral disorder was previously known as *chondromalacia patellae*. The term was used to describe a deranged patellar articular surface. However, there is now evidence to indicate that the articular surface is normal. The cause of the knee pain, which commonly occurs in early adolescence, is unknown.

CLINICAL MANIFESTATIONS AND DIAGNOSIS. The anterior peripatellar knee pain is poorly localized. Symptoms are usually produced by vigorous physical activities, such as running. Typically, there is no history of injury. The child does not complain of locking, giving way, or recurrent effusion. Gait, range of motion, alignment of the lower extremity, knee stability, patellar tracking, and areas of focal tenderness should be evaluated. The presence of patellofemoral crepitation is common in normal individuals and does not indicate underlying knee disease. Routine radiographs, including anteroposterior, lateral, and tunnel views, are not particularly helpful in evaluating the cause of adolescent anterior knee pain. They may eliminate other sources of pain.

TREATMENT. The treatment is predominantly conservative and may include flexibility exercises, strengthening exercises (isometric quadriceps), contrast therapies (ice and heat), orthoses, and medications (aspirin and nonsteroidal anti-inflammatory medications). About 70–90% success can be anticipated. Only rarely will arthroscopic evaluation of the knee and patellofemoral joint be necessary.

626.6 Patellar Subluxation and Dislocation

Patellar maltracking is usually due to a congenital deficiency within the patellofemoral joint. This can consist of a high-riding patella (patella alta), genu valgum, hypoplasia of the lateral femoral condyle, and ligamentous laxity. Traumatic patellar subluxation and dislocation can occur as a result of a direct blow to the patella along its medial aspect, but this is uncommon.

CLINICAL MANIFESTATIONS AND DIAGNOSIS. Examination of a child with a maltracking patella that is predisposed to dislocation will usually show terminal subluxation of the patella when the knee is brought into full extension. There may be tenderness to palpation over the inferior surface of the lateral facet of the patella. Attempting to displace the patella laterally will yield a subjective feeling of subluxation, resulting in the patient grabbing the examiner's hand. This has been termed the *apprehension sign*. After an acute dislocation, there may be a hemarthrosis from capsular tearing or an osteochondral fracture.

Radiographs are necessary in the evaluation of patellar subluxation or after an acute dislocation. These should include anteroposterior, lateral, and skyline tangential views of the patella to assess for an osteochondral fracture from the lateral femoral condyle or inferior surface of the patella.

TREATMENT. The majority of children presenting with acute patellar dislocation can be treated nonoperatively. This normally consists of immobilization with the knee in extension for approximately 6 wk. However, the patient is started on isometric, straight leg–raising exercises as soon as possible. Once the immobilization is discontinued, the isometric exercise program should be continued until the knee is fully rehabilitated. Using this method, approximately 75% of patients will not have recurrent dislocations.

In patellar subluxation, the cause should be determined. If it is due to dynamic muscle imbalance, then a specific muscle rehabilitation program, such as strengthening the vastus medialis, may be successful.

In children and adolescents with recurrent dislocations or failure of conservative management for patellar subluxation, operative stabilization may be necessary. Depending on the disease, this may consist of an arthroscopic lateral release and, occasionally, a soft tissue reconstruction. The latter can be performed either proximally or distally depending on the age of the patient and the nature of the disease.

Cash JD, Hughston JC: Treatment of acute patellar dislocation. Am J Sports Med 16:244, 1988.

Dickhaut SC, Delee JC: The discoid lateral meniscus syndrome. J Bone Joint Surg 64A:1068, 1982.

Dinham JM: Popliteal cysts in children: The case against surgery. J Bone Joint Surg 57B:69, 1975.

Krause BPL, Williams JPR, Caterall A: The natural history of Osgood-Schlatter's disease. J Pediatr Orthop 10:65, 1990.

Sandow MJ, Goodfellow JW: The natural history of anterior knee pain in adolescents. J Bone Joint Surg 67B:36, 1985.

Stanitski CL: Instructional course lecture: Anterior knee pain syndromes in the adolescent. J Bone Joint Surg 75A:1407, 1993.

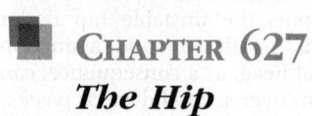

CHAPTER 627
The Hip

The hip is a ball-and-socket (femoral head and acetabulum, respectively) joint that allows for geometric motion, including flexion, extension, abduction, adduction, and internal and external rotation. The bulk of the femoral head is composed of the capital femoral epiphysis (CFE). The femoral head and acetabulum have a trophic relationship and are interdependent for normal growth and development. When this relationship is interrupted, abnormal hip development follows. Muscle balance and activity related to appropriate gross motor function are essential to the normal development of the hip.

The blood supply to the CFE is quite unique. The retinacular vessels lie on the surface of the femoral neck but are intracapsular. They enter the epiphysis from the periphery. This makes the blood supply vulnerable to damage from septic arthritis, trauma, and other vascular insults. If the blood supply is lost, avascular necrosis or osteonecrosis may occur. This can result in deformity, either acutely or as a consequence to abnormal growth and development, and predisposes to abnormal hip function and degenerative osteoarthritis as an adult.

627.1 Developmental (Congenital) Dysplasia of the Hip

Developmental dysplasia of the hip (DDH) usually occurs in the neonatal period. The hips at birth are rarely dislocated but rather "dislocatable." Dislocations tend to occur after delivery and, thus, are postnatal in origin, although the exact time when dislocations occur is controversial. Because they are not truly congenital in origin, the term *development dysplasia of the hip* is now recommended. DDH is classified into two major groups: typical, in a neurologically normal infant, and teratologic, in which there is an underlying neuromuscular disorder such as myelodysplasia, arthrogryposis multiplex congenita, or a syndrome complex. Teratologic dislocations occur in utero and are therefore truly congenital. This discussion will concentrate only on typical DDH, the most common form.

ETIOLOGY. The cause of DDH is multifactorial, having both physiologic and mechanical factors. The positive family history (20%) and the generalized ligamentous laxity are related etiologic factors. The majority of children with DDH have generalized ligamentous laxity, and this can predispose to hip instability. Maternal estrogens and other hormones associated with pelvic relaxation result in further, although temporary, relaxation of the newborn hip joint. There is also a 9:1 female predominance.

Approximately 60% of children with typical DDH are first-born, and 30–50% developed in the breech position. The frank breech position with the hips flexed and the knees extended is the position of highest risk. The breech position results in extreme hip flexion and limitation of hip motion. Increased hip flexion results in stretching of the already lax capsule and ligament teres. It also produces posterior uncoverage of the femoral head. Decreased hip motion leads to a lack of normal development of the cartilaginous acetabulum.

There is also an association of congenital muscular torticollis (14–20%) and metatarsus adductus (1–10%) with DDH. The presence of either condition requires a careful examination of the hips.

Postnatal factors are also important determinants. Maintaining the hips in the position of adduction and extension may lead to dislocation. This puts the unstable hip under pressure because of the normal hip flexion and abduction contractures. An unstable femoral head, as a consequence, can be displaced from the acetabulum over several days or weeks.

PATHOANATOMY. Because hips are not dislocated at birth, the components of the hip joint, excluding the hip capsule and ligamentum teres, are relatively normal. There may be some variations in the shape of the cartilaginous acetabulum, especially if the child developed in a breech position. If a dislocation is allowed to occur, then acetabular dysplasia and maldirection, excessive femoral anteversion (torsion), and hip muscle contractures will develop.

CLINICAL MANIFESTATIONS. The Barlow test is the most important maneuver in examining the newborn hip. This provocative test to dislocate an unstable hip is performed by stabilizing the pelvis with one hand and then flexing and adducting the opposite hip and applying a posterior force (Fig. 627–1). If the hip is dislocatable, it is usually readily felt. After release of the posterior force, the hip will usually spontaneously relocate. It has been estimated that only 1 in 100 newborn infants have clinically unstable hips (subluxation or dislocation), whereas only one in 800 to 1,000 of these infants eventually experience a true dislocation. The Ortolani test is a maneuver to reduce a recently dislocated hip. It is most likely to be positive in infants who are 1–2 mo of age because adequate time must have passed for the true dislocation to have occurred. In performing this test, the thigh is flexed and abducted, and the femoral head is lifted anteriorly into the acetabulum (see Fig. 627–1). If reduction is possible, the relocation will be felt as a "clunk," not a "click." After 2 mo of age, manual reduction of a dislocated hip is usually not possible because of the development of soft tissue contractures.

Limitation of hip abduction is indicative of soft tissue contractures and may indicate DDH. Conversely, hip abduction contractures may indicate dysplasia of the contralateral hip. An asymmetric number of thigh skinfolds and apparent shortening of an extremity, uneven knee levels, when the supine infant's feet are placed together on the examining table with the hips and knees flexed (Galeazzi sign) indicate DDH with

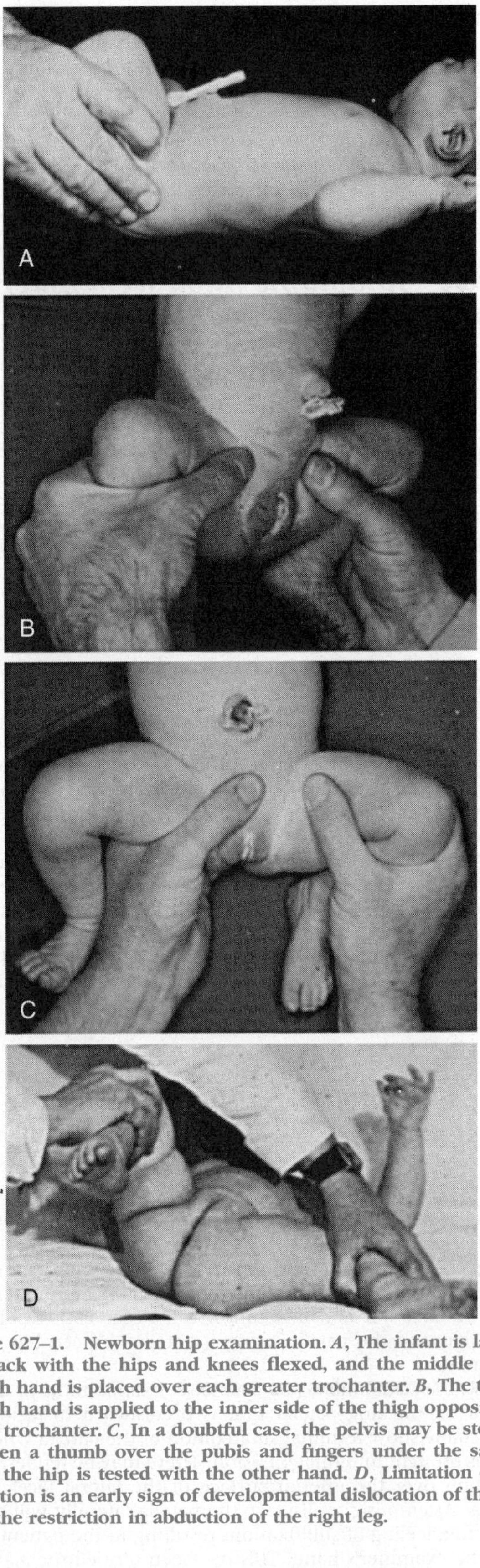

Figure 627–1. Newborn hip examination. *A*, The infant is laid on her back with the hips and knees flexed, and the middle finger of each hand is placed over each greater trochanter. *B*, The thumb of each hand is applied to the inner side of the thigh opposite the lesser trochanter. *C*, In a doubtful case, the pelvis may be steadied between a thumb over the pubis and fingers under the sacrum while the hip is tested with the other hand. *D*, Limitation of hip abduction is an early sign of developmental dislocation of the hip. Note the restriction in abduction of the right leg.

proximal displacement of the femoral head. Absent normal knee flexion contracture also occurs.

A common concern is the presence of *hip clicks* in infants. Hip clicks per se are usually not pathologic and are secondary to (1) breaking the surface tension across the hip joint, (2) snapping of gluteal tendons, (3) patellofemoral motion, or (4) femorotibial (knee) rotation.

In older or walking children, complaints of limping, waddling, increased lumbar lordosis, toe walking, and leg-length discrepancy may indicate an unrecognized DDH.

RADIOGRAPHIC EVALUATION. Hip stability as well as acetabular development may accurately be assessed by ultrasonography. Radiographic evaluation in older infants and children includes anteroposterior and Lauenstein (frog) lateral radiographs of the pelvis. The ossific nucleus of the femoral head does not appear until 3–7 mo of age, and it may be further delayed in DDH. Line measurements are usually made to determine the relationship of the femoral head to the acetabulum (acetabular index, quadrant assessment, Shenton line, and the center edge angle of Wiberg) (Fig. 627–2). Arthrography, computed tomography, and magnetic resonance imaging (MRI) scans may be beneficial in difficult cases, especially in those involving older infants and children.

TREATMENT. The treatment of DDH should be individualized and depends on the patient's age and whether the hip is subluxated or dislocated.

Birth. When an unstable hip is recognized at birth, maintenance of the hip in the position of flexion and abduction ("human" position) for 1–2 mo is usually sufficient. This position maintains reduction of the femoral head and allows for tightening of the ligamentous structures as well as for stimulation of normal growth and development. Methods that can be used to maintain the hip in this position include Pavlik harness, Frejka splint, and a variety of abduction orthoses. Double and triple diapers, although controversial, are commonly used in infants with dislocatable hips because the latter devices usually do not fit satisfactorily. Treatment is continued until there is clinical stability of the hip and ultrasonographic or radiographic measurements are normal.

Age of 1–6 Mos. During this age, a true dislocation may develop. As a consequence, treatment is directed toward reduction of the femoral head into the acetabulum. The Pavlik harness is the major mode of treatment in this age group. The harness attempts to place the hips in the human position by flexing them more than 90 degrees (preferably 100–110 degrees) and maintaining relatively full but gentle abduction (50–70 degrees). This redirects the femoral head toward the acetabulum. Usually, spontaneous relocation of the femoral head will occur within 3–4 wk. The Pavlik harness is approximately 95% successful in dysplastic or subluxated hips and 80% successful in true dislocations. If reduction is achieved, the harness is continued until radiographic parameters have returned to normal. If a spontaneous reduction does not occur, then a surgical closed reduction is indicated. This consists of (1) preliminary skin traction for 1–3 wk to bring the femoral head opposite the acetabulum, (2) percutaneous adductor tenotomy, (3) closed reduction, (4) arthrogram to assess the concentricity of the reduction, and (5) application of a hip spica cast in the "human" position. Treatment is continued until the radiographic parameters are within normal limits.

Age of 6–18 Mo. In the older infant, surgical closed reduction is the major method of treatment. If the reduced hip shows significant residual instability, an open reduction may be indicated. This can be through a medial or anterior approach.

Age of 18 Mo–8 Yr. After 18 mo of age, the progressive deformities are so severe that open reduction followed by pelvic (innominate) osteotomy, femoral osteotomy, or both are necessary to realign the hip. A femoral shortening derotation osteotomy is performed concomitantly if the reduction is tight, if there is excessive femoral anteversion, or if the child is 3 or 4 yr of age or older. Postoperatively, a hip spica cast is worn for 6–8 wk to allow for healing. Thereafter, the child may be permitted

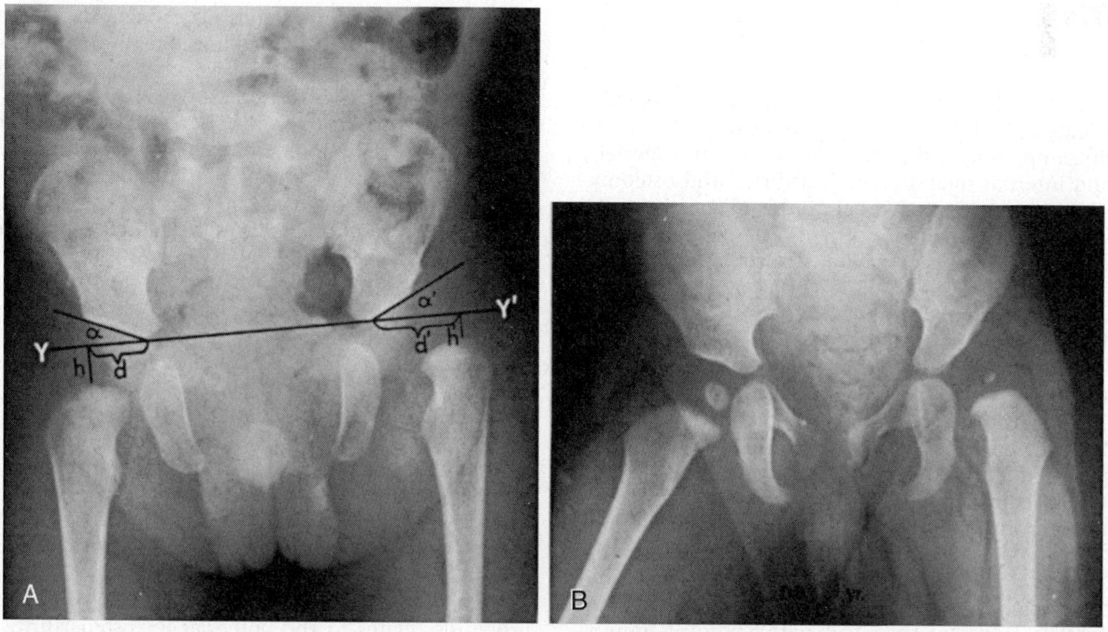

Figure 627–2. Pelvic radiographs demonstrating development dysplasia of the left hip. *A*, The Hilgenreiner method for identification of dysplasia of the hip before ossification of the capital femoral epiphysis; *a'* is greater than *a*, indicating greater obliquity of the acetabular roof. *d'* is greater than *d*, indicating lateral displacement of the femur. *h* is greater than *h'*, indicating cephalad displacement of the femur. These relationships indicate dysplasia of the patient's left hip. *B*, Developmental dislocation of the left hip. The bony roof of the left acetabulum is quite oblique, and there is the beginning of a false acetabulum above its most lateral aspect. The left femur is displaced laterally and superiorly. The ossification center of the left capital femoral epiphysis is smaller than that of the right.

to return to full activities gradually. Implanted metal is removed shortly after healing to prevent incorporation into the growing bone. Eighteen months of age is not an arbitrary age for these procedures. It has been demonstrated that approximately 25% of children who have a closed reduction performed between 9 and 12 mo of age, 50% who have one between 12 and 18 mos, and 75% who have one between 18 and 36 mos will have residual acetabular dysplasia requiring a pelvic or femoral osteotomy at a later date.

COMPLICATIONS. The most important and severe complication of DDH is avascular necrosis of the CFE. This is an iatrogenic complication; reduction of the femoral head under pressure produces cartilaginous compression, and this can result in occlusion of the intra-articular, extraosseous epiphyseal vessels and produce CFE infarction, either partial or total. Revascularization follows, but abnormal growth and development may occur, especially if the physis is severely damaged. The hip is very vulnerable to this complication before the development of the ossific nucleus (4–6 mo). The management outlined previously is designed to minimize this complication; with appropriate use of these treatments, the incidence of avascular necrosis will be approximately 5–15%. Other potential complications in DDH include redislocation, residual subluxation or acetabular dysplasia, and postoperative complications such as wound infections.

SEPTIC ARTHRITIS AND OSTEOMYELITIS

See Chapter 172 for a full discussion. Diagnosis of septic arthritis and osteomyelitis is made by hip aspiration (arthrocentesis). This can be technically difficult and must always be done under a fluoroscopic control. If no fluid is obtained from the hip joint, an arthrogram should be performed, documenting that the hip joint has been entered.

627.2 Transient Monoarticular Synovitis

Transient synovitis of the hip is one of the more common causes of limping in a normal child. It is characterized by acute onset of pain, limp, and mild restriction of motion, especially abduction and internal rotation. Septic arthritis and osteomyelitis of the hip must be excluded before this diagnosis can be confirmed. The cause remains uncertain, but possibilities include (1) active or recent systemic viral syndrome, (2) trauma, and (3) allergic hypersensitivity. Biopsy specimens from the hip joint have demonstrated synovial hypertrophy secondary to nonspecific inflammatory reaction.

CLINICAL MANIFESTATIONS. Transient monoarticular synovitis can occur in all age groups, but the mean age of onset is 6 yrs; it occurs predominantly in the 3- to 8-yr age range. Approximately 70% of affected children will have had a nonspecific upper respiratory tract infection 7–14 days before the onset of symptoms. There is usually an acute onset of symptoms with pain felt in the groin, anterior thigh, or knee; nontraumatic anterior thigh or knee pain may be referred from the hip. These children are usually ambulatory, and the hip is not held flexed, abducted, and laterally rotated unless a significant effusion is present. However, they walk with a painful, limping gait. They are usually afebrile or have a low-grade fever (temperature less than 38° C).

Laboratory values are usually within normal limits, but occasionally a slight elevation in the erythrocyte sedimentation rate may be seen. Arthrocentesis is negative, although a synovial effusion from 1–3 mL is not uncommon.

RADIOGRAPHIC EVALUATION. Anteroposterior and Lauenstein (frog) lateral radiographs of the pelvis should be obtained and are usually normal. Ultrasonography of the hip may demonstrate a hip joint effusion. Technetium bone scan or MRI may be of value in ruling out the presence of other lesions, such as infection or early Legg-Calvé-Perthes disease (LCPD). Transient monoarticular synovitis is a diagnosis of exclusion.

TREATMENT. Treatment for monoarticular synovitis of the hip is conservative. Bed rest and non-weightbearing until the pain resolves followed by limited activities thereafter are the treatments of choice. Most children are maintained on bed rest for approximately 7 days. They are then maintained on limited activities for 1–2 additional weeks. This sometimes is difficult because children want to return to normal activities when their symptoms resolve. However, if the child is allowed to return to normal activities too early, then exacerbation of symptoms may occur.

627.3 Legg-Calvé-Perthes Disease

LCPD is idiopathic osteonecrosis or avascular necrosis of the CFE, and the associated complications thereof, occurring in an immature, growing child. This osteochondrosis is caused by an interruption of the CFE blood supply. It is primarily a disorder affecting males (4–5:1) and is bilateral in approximately 20% of children. Children with LCPD also often have delayed bone ages, disproportionate growth, and mild short stature.

CLINICAL MANIFESTATIONS. The clinical onset of LCPD typically is between the ages of 2 and 12 yr (mean, 7 yr). Most children present with mild or intermittent pain in the anterior thigh and a limp. The classic presentation has been described as a "painless limp." The pertinent early physical findings include antalgic gait; muscle spasm with mild restriction of motion, especially abduction and internal rotation; proximal thigh atrophy; and mild shortness of stature.

RADIOGRAPHIC EVALUATION: DIAGNOSIS AND PROGNOSIS. Anteroposterior and Lauenstein (frog) lateral radiographs of the pelvis should be obtained to establish the diagnosis. The radiographic characteristics can be divided into five distinct stages representing a continuum of the disease process: (1) cessation of CFE growth, (2) subchondral fracture, (3) resorption (fragmentation), (4) reossification, and (5) healed or residual stage.

There are three radiographic classification systems of the extent of CFE involvement. Catterall developed a four-group classification on the basis of the appearance of the CFE at maximum resorption. Although this classification has been helpful in retrospective analysis of results, it has limited prognostic value because it is difficult to apply in the earliest phases of the disease process. Salter-Thompson used two groups and Herring and colleagues, three groups, depending on involvement or extent of involvement of the lateral portion of the CFE. When intact, this area acts as a supporting column or pillar that shields the involved portion of the CFE from compression, which can produce collapse, deformity, and possible extrusion. Involvement results in a poorer prognosis.

The short-term prognosis relates to the femoral head deformity at the completion of the healing stage. Adverse risk factors include older age at clinical onset, extensive CFE involvement, femoral head containment, reduced range of hip motion, and premature growth plate closure. The long-term prognosis relates to the potential for osteoarthritis of the hip in adulthood. Older children with significant residual femoral head deformity are at risk for degenerative arthritis. The incidence is essentially 100% in children who are 10 yr of age or older at onset and who have residual femoral head deformity. This compares with a negligible risk in children who are 5 yr of age and younger at onset and 38% when onset occurs between 6 and 9 yr of age.

Two radiographic techniques evaluate the sphericity of the femoral head at the completion of the disease process, which correlates with the risk for degenerative osteoarthritis as an adult. In the Mose circle criteria, a transparent template with concentric circles is placed over the anteroposterior and Lauenstein lateral radiographs. If the variation of sphericity of the femoral head in the two views is 0–2 mm, the result is good; 2–3 mm, fair; and 3 mm or more, poor. Stulberg and colleagues' five-group classification is based on the shape of the femoral head and congruency with the acetabulum: class I, a spherical femoral head that is equal in size to the opposite uninvolved hip; class II, a spherical femoral head with coxa magna; class III, nonspherical femoral head with a congruent acetabulum; class IV, a flat femoral head with abnormalities of the femoral neck and acetabulum; and class V, a flat femoral head with a normal acetabulum. Classes I and II are spherical congruent hips, class III a nonspherical congruent hip, and classes IV and V incongruent hips.

TREATMENT. LCPD is a local, self-healing disorder. Prevention of femoral head deformity and secondary osteoarthritis are the only justifications for treatment. The treatment goals are (1) elimination of hip irritability, (2) restoration and maintenance of a good range of hip motion, (3) prevention of CFE collapse, extrusion, or subluxation, and (4) attainment of a spherical femoral head at healing. Current treatment methods use the concept of containment (i.e., the femoral head is contained within the acetabulum so that the latter acts as a mold for the reossifying CFE. This may be accomplished by nonsurgical and surgical techniques. The currently accepted forms of management are now discussed.

Observation. Expectant observation is appropriate for all children younger than 6 yr at clinical onset regardless of the extent of CFE involvement. However, these children must be monitored closely, both clinically and radiographically.

Intermittent Symptomatic Treatment. Temporary or periodic treatment with bed rest or abduction stretching exercises to maintain mobility can be used in conjunction with observation. Recurrent episodes of hip irritability with a temporary decrease in motion commonly occur during the phases of subchondral fracture and fragmentation, and the child may benefit from symptomatic treatment.

Definitive Early Treatment. Nonsurgical or surgical containment of the femoral head in the course of the disease is indicated when (1) the age at clinical onset is 6 yr or older (possibly 5 yr in girls), (2) the lateral column or pillar of the CFE is involved, or (3) there is a loss of containment, as manifested by extrusion of the femoral head on anteroposterior radiograph.

NONSURGICAL CONTAINMENT. Abduction casts (Petrie) or orthoses are commonly used to contain the femoral head within the acetabulum. Containment is continued only until there is early radiographic subchondral reossification. Because this usually occurs 12–17 mo after clinical onset, nonsurgical containment methods can be limited to 18 mo or less with no adverse effect on the outcome. Currently, the Atlanta Scottish Rite Hospital orthosis is the most widely used because it allows reciprocal motion and ambulation without crutches or external support. The success of nonsurgical containment has recently been challenged on the grounds that it does not alter the natural history of untreated LCPD.

SURGICAL CONTAINMENT. The selection of pelvic or femoral osteotomy for surgical containment is based on the philosophy and technical expertise of the surgeon. The results of surgical containment appear to be better than those of nonsurgical containment; approximately 85% will have Stulberg class I, II, or III.

Late Surgical Management for Deformity. If significant femoral head deformity prevents reduction of the femoral head into the acetabulum, an alternative method must be considered. Several surgical procedures at least partially correct the various existing deformities, thereby alleviating the associated symptoms.

627.4 Slipped Capital Femoral Epiphysis

Slipped capital femoral epiphysis (SCFE) is the most common adolescent hip disorder. Its cause is unknown, but an endocrine basis has been suggested because SCFE is frequently accompanied by abnormalities of growth. Sex hormones and growth hormone alter the rate of proliferation of the cartilage cells in the CFE physes and the rate of skeletal growth. SCFE typically occurs in adolescents who are either obese and have delayed skeletal maturation or in tall, thin individuals who have had a recent growth spurt. In obese adolescents, a low level of sex hormones has been postulated, whereas in tall, thin individuals, an overabundance of growth hormone is implicated. SCFE can also occur as a complication of an underlying endocrine disorder such as hypothyroidism, pituitary disorders, pseudohypoparathyroidism, and others. When a slip occurs before puberty (10 yr of age or younger), a hormonal abnormality or systemic disorder should be suspected.

RADIOGRAPHIC EVALUATION. Anteroposterior and Lauenstein (frog) lateral radiographs of the pelvis are used for assessment of SCFE (Fig. 627–3). Both hips must be evaluated and compared. The earliest sign of SCFE is widening of the growth plate without slippage, a preslip condition. As slippage occurs, the CFE stays in the acetabulum and the femoral neck rotates predominantly anteriorly (although occasionally superiorly), resulting in a varus retroverted femoral head and neck. The degree of slippage between the CFE and the femoral neck can be classified as mild (0–33%), moderate (34–50%), and severe (greater than 50%) by radiographic measurement techniques.

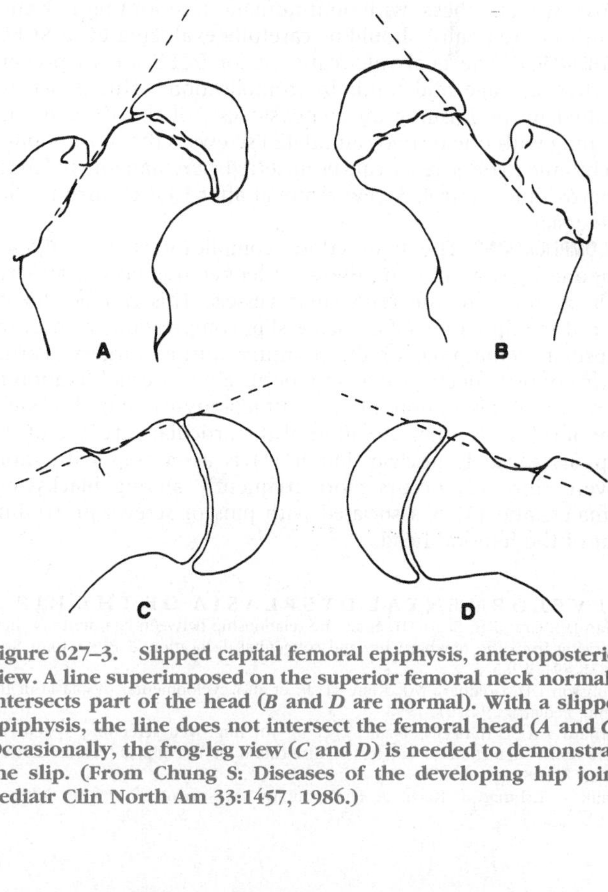

Figure 627–3. Slipped capital femoral epiphysis, anteroposterior view. A line superimposed on the superior femoral neck normally intersects part of the head (*B* and *D* are normal). With a slipped epiphysis, the line does not intersect the femoral head (*A* and *C*). Occasionally, the frog-leg view (*C* and *D*) is needed to demonstrate the slip. (From Chung S: Diseases of the developing hip joint. Pediatr Clin North Am 33:1457, 1986.)

DIAGNOSTIC CLASSIFICATION. SCFE is ranked in four distinct clinical groups, as discussed next.

Preslip. The physis is wide, but slippage has not occurred. There may be mild discomfort, but the physical examination is usually normal. Preslips are frequently seen in the opposite hip of an adolescent with a previous SCFE.

Acute SCFE. In acute SCFE, there are no or only mild antecedent symptoms such as pain or limp for less than 3-wk duration. Slippage occurs suddenly, with or without significant trauma, and the pain is so severe that the child is usually unable to stand or bear weight even with external support on the involved extremity. An acute SCFE is unstable.

Acute-on-Chronic SCFE. In the acute-on-chronic SCFE, the epiphysis slips acutely on an existing chronic slip. These adolescents have had previous symptoms (pain, limp, out-toe gait) for several months or longer. This, too, is unstable and so painful that the child is unable to stand or bear weight on the involved side.

Chronic SCFE. This is the most common type. There is usually a history of the previously described symptoms for several months. The symptoms typically worsen as the slip progresses. However, because there is continuity between the femoral neck and CFE, the symptoms are not severe, and the child is able to walk with a mildly antalgic, externally rotated gait. A chronic SCFE is stable.

CLINICAL MANIFESTATIONS. The physical findings in SCFE depend on the degree of slippage and the classification. In the acute or acute-on-chronic unstable SCFE, the physical examination is limited as a result of pain with any attempted hip motion. In a chronic, stable SCFE, the patient will have an antalgic gait, and the affected extremity is externally rotated. Hip range of motion will demonstrate a lack of internal rotation and increased external rotation. Also, as the hip is flexed, it will become progressively externally rotated. Limitation of flexion and abduction may also be present because of a varus deformity of the proximal femur. Twenty per cent of patients will complain of only knee pain, although they will have decreased hip rotation on physical examination. Adolescents, especially those who are obese, with nontraumatic anterior thigh or knee pain (referred pain) should be carefully evaluated for a SCFE.

TREATMENT. The goals of treatment for SCFE are to prevent further slippage and minimize complications. This is accomplished by performing an epiphysiodesis of the CFE. In situ pinning with one or two cannulated screws is the most popular technique. The screws can be inserted percutaneously under fluoroscopic control. Screw removal after CFE closure is controversial.

COMPLICATIONS. The two serious complications in SCFE are osteonecrosis and chondrolysis. Osteonecrosis occurs as a result of injury to the retinacular vessels. This can be due to forced manipulation of an acute slip, compression from intracapsular hematoma, or direct injury during surgery. Partial forms of osteonecrosis may also occur after internal fixation as a result of disruption of the intraepiphyseal blood vessels. Chondrolysis is a degeneration of the articular cartilage of the hip. Its cause is unclear, but it (1) is associated with more severe slips, (2) occurs more frequently among blacks and females, and (3) is associated with pins or screws protruding out of the femoral head.

DEVELOPMENTAL DYSPLASIA OF THE HIP

Allan DB, Gray RH, Scott TD, et al: The relationship between ligamentous clicks arising from the newborn hip and congenital dislocation. J Bone Joint Surg 67B:491, 1985.

Aronsson DD, Goldberg MJ, Kling TF Jr, et al: Developmental dysplasia of the hip. Pediatrics 94:201, 1994.

Bernard AA, O'Hara JN, Bazin S, et al: An improved screening system for the early detection of congenital dislocation of the hip. J Pediatr Orthop 7:277, 1987.

Bialik V, Tishman J, Katzir J, et al: Clinical assessment of hip instability in the newborn by an orthopaedic surgeon and a pediatrician. Pediatr Orthop 6:703, 1986.

DeRosa GP, Feller N: Treatment of congenital dislocation of the hip: Management before walking age. Clin Orthop 225:77, 1987.

Gabuzda GM, Renshaw TS: Current concept review: Reduction of congenital dislocation of the hip. J Bone Joint Surg 74A:624, 1992.

Grill F, Bensahel H, Canadell J, et al: The Pavlik harness in the treatment of the congenitally dislocating hip: Report on a multicenter study of the European Pediatric Orthopaedic Society. J Pediatr Orthop 8:1, 1988.

Harcke HT, Kumar SJ: Current concepts review: The role of ultrasound in the diagnosis and management of congenital dislocation and dysplasia of the hip. J Bone Joint Surg 73A:622, 1991.

Hensinger RD: Congenital dislocation of the hip: Treatment in infancy to walking age. Orthop Clin North Am 18:597, 1987.

Hummer CD, MacEwen GD: The coexistence of torticollis and congenital dislocation of the hip. J Bone Joint Surg 54A:1255, 1972.

Keret D, MacEwen GD: Growth disturbance of the proximal part of the femur after treatment for congenital dislocation of the hip. J Bone Joint Surg 73A:410, 1991.

Viere RG, Birch JG, Herring JA, et al: Use of the Pavlik harness in congenital dislocation of the hip: An analysis of failures of treatment. J Bone Joint Surg 72A:238, 1990.

TRANSIENT MONOARTICULAR SYNOVITIS

Hauseisen DC, Weiner DS, Weiner SD: The characterization of "transient synovitis of the hip" in children. J Pediatr Orthop 6:11, 1986.

Landin LA, Danielsson LG, Wattsgard C: Transient synovitis of the hip—Its incidence, epidemiology and relation to Perthes disease. J Bone Joint Surg 69B:238, 1987.

LEGG-CALVÉ-PERTHES DISEASE

Bos CFA, Bloem JL, Bloem RM: Sequential magnetic resonance imaging in Perthes disease. J Bone Joint Surg 73B:219, 1991.

Catterall A: The natural history of Perthes disease. J Bone Joint Surg 53B:37, 1971.

Herring JA, Neustadt JB, Williams JJ, et al: The lateral pillar classification of Legg-Calvé-Perthes disease. J Pediatr Orthop 12:143, 1992.

Herring JA, Williams JJ, Neustadt JN, et al: Evolution of femoral head deformity during the healing phase of Legg-Calvé-Perthes disease. J Pediatr Orthop 13:41, 1993.

Inoue A, Freeman MAR, Vernon-Roberts B, et al: The pathogenesis of Perthes disease. J Bone Joint Surg 58B:453, 1976.

Lovell WW, MacEwen GD, Stewart WR, et al: Legg-Perthes disease in girls. J Bone Joint Surg 64B:637, 1982.

McAndrews MP, Weinstein SL: A long-term follow-up of Legg-Calvé-Perthes disease. J Bone Joint Surg 66A:860, 1984.

Meehan PL, Angel D, Nelson JM: The Scottish Rite abduction orthosis for the treatment of Legg-Perthes disease. J Bone Joint Surg 74A:2, 1992.

Pinto MR, Peterson HA, Berquist TH: Magnetic resonance imaging in early diagnosis of Legg-Calvé-Perthes disease. J Pediatr Orthop 9:19, 1989.

Stulberg SD, Cooperman DR, Wallensten R: The natural history of Legg-Calvé-Perthes disease. J Bone Joint Surg 63A:1095, 1981.

Thompson GH, Salter RG: Legg-Calvé-Perthes disease: Current concepts and controversies. Orthop Clin North Am 18:617, 1987.

Thompson GH, Westin GW: Legg-Calvé-Perthes disease: Results of discontinuing treatment in the early reossification phase. Clin Orthop 139:70, 1979.

Wenger DR, Ward TW, Herring JA: Current concepts review: Legg-Calvé-Perthes disease. J Bone Joint Surg 73A:778, 1991.

SLIPPED CAPITAL FEMORAL EPIPHYSIS

Aronson DD, Carlson WE: Slipped capital femoral epiphysis: A prospective study of fixation with a single screw. J Bone Joint Surg 74A:810, 1992.

Betz R, Steel HH, Emper WD, et al: Treatment of slipped capital femoral epiphysis: Spica cast immobilization. J Bone Joint Surg 72A:587, 1990.

Busch MT, Morrissey RT: Slipped capital femoral epiphysis. Orthop Clin North Am 18:637, 1987.

Carney BT, Weinstein SL, Noble J: Long-term follow-up of slipped capital femoral epiphysis. J Bone Joint Surg 73A:677, 1991.

Cooperman DR, Charles LM, Pathria M, et al: Post-mortem description of slipped capital femoral epiphysis. J Bone Joint Surg 74B:595, 1992.

Ingram AJ, Clarke MS, Clarke CS Jr, et al: Chondrolysis complicating slipped capital femoral epiphysis. Clin Orthop 165:99, 1982.

Loder RT, Richards BS, Shapiro PS, et al: Acute slipped capital femoral epiphysis: The importance of physeal stability. J Bone Joint Surg 75A:1134, 1993.

Mann DC, Weddington J, Richton S: Hormonal studies in patients with slipped capital femoral epiphysis without evidence of endocrinopathy. J Pediatr Orthop 8:543, 1988.

Siegel DB, Kasser JR, Sponseller P, et al: Slipped capital femoral epiphysis: A quantitative analysis of motion, gait, and femoral remodeling after in situ fixation. J Bone Joint Surg 73A:659, 1991.

Wells D, King JD, Roe TF, et al: Review of slipped capital femoral epiphysis associated with endocrine disease. J Pediatr Orthop 13:610, 1993.

CHAPTER 628
The Spine

Abnormalities in the vertebral column are among the most common nontraumatic pediatric musculoskeletal problems. They may be present at birth or may develop during childhood or adolescence. Some of these disorders worsen with growth and may lead to unacceptable appearance, alterations in pulmonary function, and early degenerative osteoarthritis of the spine. A simplified classification of the common spinal abnormalities is presented in Table 628–1.

Seven cervical, 12 thoracic, and 5 lumbar vertebrae plus the sacrum form the spinal column. The nerves exit below their respective vertebrae except in the cervical spine, where they exit above. This accounts for the presence of eight cervical nerves. The C-7 nerve root exits above the seventh cervical vertebrae and the C-8 nerve root exits below. In the anteroposterior (AP), or frontal, plane, the vertebral bodies are stacked squarely one on the other, with little or no deviation from vertical alignment. The vertebral endplates are parallel and the intervertebral discs are symmetric in height. In the lateral, or sagittal, plane, the spine has normal curvatures that provide balance and stability. The cervical and lumbar spine are lordotic; the thoracic spine and sacrum are kyphotic. The magnitude of lordosis and kyphosis varies with age as well as among individuals of the same age. Children normally have less cervical lordosis and more lumbar lordosis than adults or adolescents; flexible increases in thoracic kyphosis are common in adolescents.

TABLE 628–1 Classification of Spinal Deformities

Scoliosis
- ***Idiopathic***
  - Infantile
  - Juvenile
  - Adolescent
- ***Congenital***
  - Failure of formation
    - Wedge vertebrae
    - Hemivertebrae
  - Failure of segmentation
    - Unilateral bar
    - Bilateral bar
  - Mixed
- ***Neuromuscular***
  - Neuropathic diseases
    - Upper motor neuron
      - Cerebral palsy
      - Spinocerebellar degeneration (Friedreich ataxia, Charcot-Marie-Tooth disease)
      - Syringomyelia
      - Spinal cord tumor
      - Spinal cord trauma
    - Lower motor neuron
      - Poliomyelitis
      - Spinal muscular atrophy
    - Myopathic diseases
      - Duchenne muscular dystrophy
      - Arthrogryposis
      - Other muscular dystrophies
- ***Syndromes***
  - Neurofibromatosis
  - Marfan syndrome
- ***Compensatory***
  - Leg-length discrepancy

Kyphosis
- ***Postural Round Back***
- ***Scheuermann Disease***
- ***Congenital Kyphosis***

Adapted from the Terminology Committee, Scoliosis Research Society: A glossary of scoliosis terms. Spine 1:57, 1976.

SCOLIOSIS

Alterations in normal spinal alignment that occur in the AP or frontal plane are termed *scoliosis*. The majority of scoliotic deformities are idiopathic (of unknown causation). Others, however, can be congenital, associated with a neuromuscular disorder or syndrome, or compensatory from a leg-length discrepancy or intraspinal abnormality.

628.1 Idiopathic Scoliosis

ETIOLOGY AND EPIDEMIOLOGY. Idiopathic scoliosis is the most common form of scoliosis. It occurs in healthy, neurologically normal children, but its exact cause is unknown. The incidence is only slightly greater in girls than in boys, but scoliosis is more likely to progress and require treatment in girls than in boys. This suggests that hormonal factors are important. Hereditary tendencies also occur because approximately 20% of children with scoliosis have other family members with the same condition. Both autosomal and multifactorial traits have been suggested. Although the daughters of affected mothers are more likely than other children to experience scoliosis, the magnitude of curvature in an affected individual is not related to the magnitude of curvature in relatives. Involved children also tend to show subtle changes in proprioception and vibratory sensation. This suggests abnormalities of spinal cord posterior-column function. Cerebellar dysfunction may also cause spinal imbalance.

Idiopathic scoliosis can be divided into three groups on the basis of age at onset: infantile, birth–3 yr; juvenile, 4–10 yr; and adolescent, 11 yr and older. Adolescent scoliosis is the most common form and accounts for approximately 80% of idiopathic scoliosis. Infantile scoliosis is very rare in the United States but more common in England. The majority of these patients are male, and most curves are convex toward the left rather than the right as in other varieties of scoliosis. Although many infantile curves regress spontaneously, others progress and are difficult to treat effectively. Juvenile scoliosis is not common, but in many children with the diagnosis of adolescent scoliosis onset actually occurred when they were juveniles, but it was not diagnosed until later.

CLINICAL MANIFESTATIONS. A complete physical examination is required for any child or adolescent with scoliosis because the deformity may be indicative of an underlying disease process. Idiopathic scoliosis is usually a painless disorder. Any child with scoliosis and back pain requires a careful neurologic examination for neuromuscular or intraspinal disorders. With left thoracic curves and back pain there is an increased incidence of intraspinal disease such as a tumor. These children should be evaluated by magnetic resonance imaging (MRI). Because of the possibility of associated disease, special attention also should be given to the skin (hairy patches, nevi, lipomas, café au lait spots), the extremities (skeletal dysplasia), and heart (murmurs from Marfan syndrome).

The back is examined with the patient in the standing position and viewed from behind. The shoulders and waist are evaluated for symmetry. The levelness of the pelvis is assessed first. Leg-length discrepancies result in pelvic obliquity that can produce the clinical appearance of scoliosis. When the pelvis is level or has been leveled with blocks, the spine is examined for asymmetry, deformity, and areas of tenderness. The patient's palms are then brought together, and the patient is asked to bend forward with the hands directed between the feet. This maintains balance and symmetry of the trunk. Tangential view of the spine while standing behind (thoracic area) and in front (lumbar area) allows the pediatrician to determine the symmetry of the back. The presence of a hump or asymmetry is the hallmark of a scoliotic deformity (Fig. 628–1). The corresponding area opposite the hump is typically depressed. These "humps and valleys" are due to spinal rotation. Scoliosis represents a rotational malalignment of one vertebra on another. This results in rib rotation when the curve is in the thoracic area and paravertebral muscle rotation when in the lumbar region. On the convexity of the curve, the ribs are rotated posteriorly (hump), and in the concavity of the curvature, they are rotated anteriorly (valley). This rotation will also produce distortion anteriorly such as rib prominence or breast asymmetry.

When the trunk is viewed from the side with the patient in the forward flexed position, the degree of *kyphosis* can be evaluated. Normally, there is a smooth gradual mild kyphosis or round back in the thoracic region and reversal of lumbar lordosis. A sharp, abrupt, or accentuated forward angulation in the thoracic or thoracolumbar region is indicative of a kyphotic deformity.

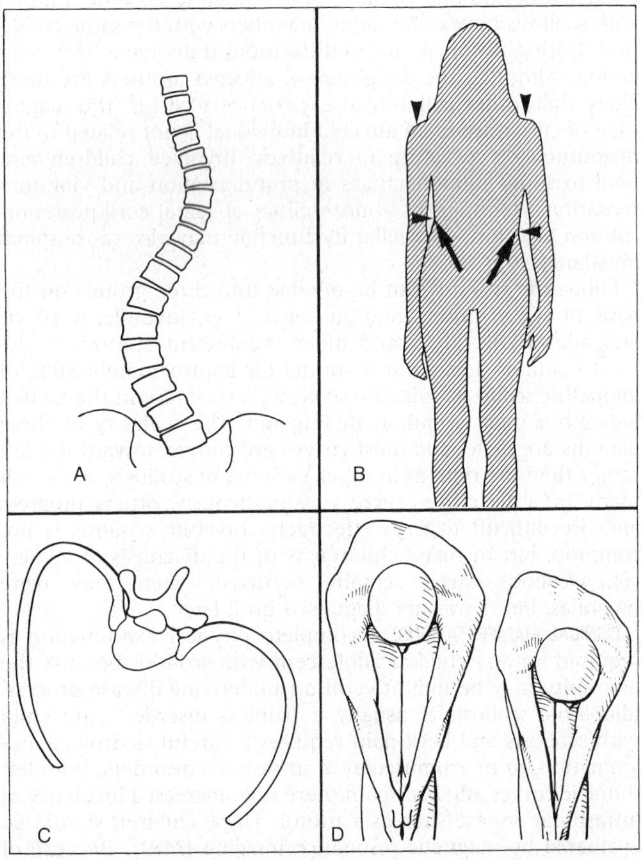

Figure 628–1. Structural changes in idiopathic scoliosis. *A*, As curvature increases, alterations in body configuration develop in both the primary and compensatory curve regions. *B*, Asymmetry of shoulder height, waistline, and the elbow-to-flank distance are common findings. *C*, Vertebral rotation and associated posterior displacement of the ribs on the convex side of the curve are responsible for the characteristic deformity of the chest wall in scoliosis patients. *D*, In the school screening examination for scoliosis, the patient bends forward at the waist. Rib asymmetry of even a small degree is obvious. (From Scolies PV: Spinal deformity in childhood and adolescence. *In*: Behrman RE, Vaughn VC III [eds]: Nelson Textbook of Pediatrics, Update 5. Philadelphia, WB Saunders, 1989.)

RADIOGRAPHIC EVALUATION. Posteroanterior (PA) and lateral standing radiographs of the entire spine are obtained for assessment of scoliosis, kyphosis, lordosis, congenital malformations, and if the iliac crests are visible, the skeletal maturity of the patient. The degree of curvature is measured from the most tilted or end vertebra of the curve superiorly and inferiorly, using the Cobb method. In this method, a line is drawn across the proximal endplate of the superior end vertebra and the distal endplate of the inferior end vertebra, and perpendicular lines are erected. The angle at the intersection of the perpendicular lines determines the degree of curvature. Other radiographic procedures that may occasionally be necessary in the evaluation of spinal deformities include computed tomography, MRI, myelography, and tomography. The decision for these procedures is based on the differential diagnosis.

TREATMENT. Treatment of idiopathic scoliosis is based on curve progression and the age of the patient. No treatment is necessary for nonprogressive deformities. The risk for curve progression varies according to sex, age, menarchal status, curve location, and curve magnitude. Although the female:male ratio in idiopathic adolescent scoliosis is approximately 1:1, the risk for curve progession is much higher for females. Premenarchal girls with curves of more than 20 degrees have a significantly higher risk for progression than girls 1–2 yr after menarche with similar curves. The risk of progression in premenarchal girls with curves of greater than 20 degrees is approximately 70%; the risk is even higher if the curve is greater than 30 degrees. Curves of less than 25 degrees are observed and reevaluated radiographically at 4- to 6-mo intervals. They need only a single standing PA radiograph of the spine.

The treatment of progressive idiopathic adolescent scoliosis is orthotic or surgical. Exercises alone are ineffective. Progressive curves between 25 and 45 degrees in a skeletally immature patient are managed by orthoses. Curves greater than 45 degrees require surgery. In orthotic management, the apex of the curve is important. When the apical vertebra is at the eighth thoracic vertebra or higher, a Milwaukee brace, a cervicothoracolumbar spinal orthosis is necessary to control the upper thoracic and cervical spine. When the apex is below this level, a molded plastic thoracolumbar spinal orthosis (TLSO) may be used. Orthoses are 60–75% effective in controlling curve progression. They do not provide permanent correction of the deformity.

If surgery is necessary, a variety of techniques may be used, but most generally involve a posterior spinal fusion and some type of segmental spinal instrumentation (Fig. 628–2). Harrington, Cotrel-Dubousset, Texas Scottish Rite Hospital, and Isola instrumentation are commonly used for idiopathic deformities. Occasionally, anterior spinal fusion and instrumentation may be indicated, especially in thoracolumbar and lumbar curves.

628.2 Congenital Scoliosis

Abnormalities of vertebral development during the first trimester of pregnancy often result in structural deformities of the spine that are evident at birth or become obvious in early childhood. Congenital scoliosis can be classified as (1) partial or complete failure of vertebral formation (wedge vertebrae or hemivertebrae); (2) partial or complete failure of segmentation (unsegmented bars); or (3) mixed. They may occur as an isolated deformity or in combination with other organ system malformations that are differentiating at the same time as the spine.

Congenital genitourinary malformations occur in 20% of children with congenital scoliosis. Unilateral renal agenesis is

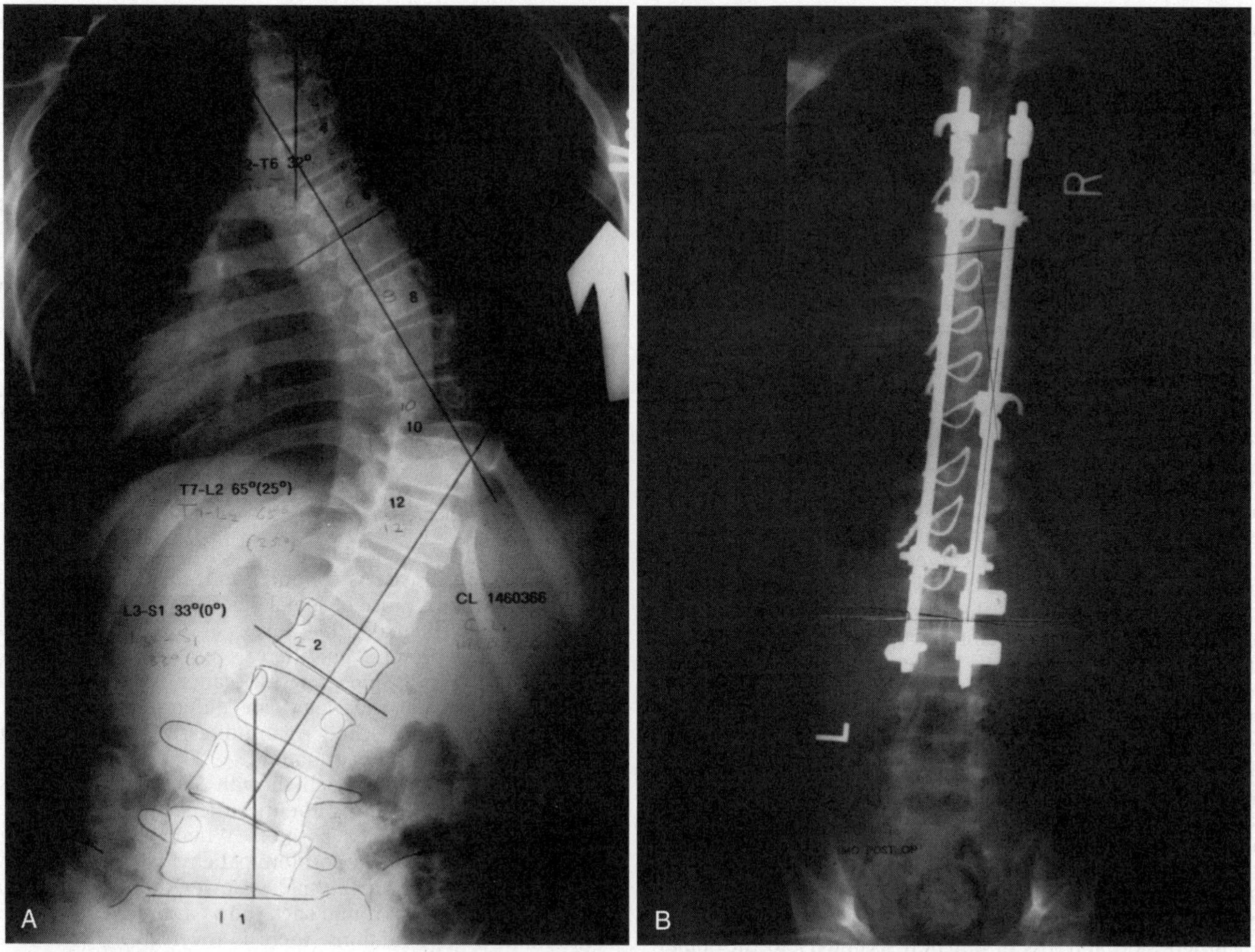

Figure 628–2. *A*, Preoperative standing posteroanterior radiograph of a 13-year-old girl with a severe right thoracic section. Note the Cobb measurement technique. The numbers in parentheses indicate the degree of correction of the deformity on side-bending radiographs. *B*, Postoperative radiograph demonstrating a selective right thoracolumbar fusion and instrumentation from T-3 to L-2. Note the spontaneous improvement in the compensatory left lumbar curve after correction of the structural right thoracolumbar curve.

the most common abnormality. Duplication of ureters, horseshoe kidney, and genital anomalies also occur. Approximately 2% of children with associated genitourinary abnormalities will have a silent, obstructive uropathy. Renal ultrasonography should be performed in all children with congenital scoliosis to assess for possible genitourinary problems. Other procedures such intravenous pyelography or MRI may be necessary if the ultrasonogram is abnormal. Congenital heart disease occurs in 10–15% of children having congenital scoliosis.

Spinal dysraphism is a general term for coexistent vertebral and spinal cord defects; it occurs in about 20% of children having congenital scoliosis. Spina bifida occulta is the most common and benign defect, whereas myelomeningocele is the most severe. Other lesions include intradural and extradural lipomas, cysts and teratomas, and spinal cord tethers. These abnormalities are frequently associated with cutaneous lesions of the back such as hairy patches, skin dimples, hemangiomas, and abnormalities of the feet and lower extremities such as cavus feet, calf atrophy, asymmetric foot size, and neurologic changes. MRI is the procedure of choice for evaluating possible spinal dysraphism.

Congenital scoliosis also occurs in association with syndromes. Approximately, one third of children with Klippel-Feil syndrome, failure of segmentation of two or more cervical vertebra, will have renal anomalies, congenital heart disease, congenital elevation of the scapula (Sprengel deformity), and hearing impairment. The VATER association includes vertebral anomalies, imperforate anus, tracheoesophageal fistula, and radial (clubhand) and renal abnormalities.

The risk for progression of spinal deformity in a child with congenital scoliosis is variable depending on the growth potential of the malformed vertebra. Defects such as block vertebra have little growth potential and usually do not cause significant spinal deformity. Hemivertebrae may or may not cause significant deformity, depending on location and their potential for growth. Unilateral unsegmented bars almost always produce progressive deformities. Overall, approximately 25% of patients with congenital scoliosis will not demonstrate curve progression and do not require treatment. However, 75% of patients will demonstrate some progression, and approximately 50% will require treatment. If progression occurs, it almost always continues until the cessation of growth. Rapid progression can be expected during periods of rapid growth before 2 and after 10 yr of age.

Early diagnosis and prompt treatment of progressive curves are the most essential elements in the care of congenital spinal deformity. Orthotic treatment is of limited value because these curves tend to be rigid. Combined anterior and posterior spinal fusion across the area of the deformity is required to halt progression and counteract the strong forces of growth. Instrumentation is rarely necessary and increases the risk of injury to the spinal cord. It is a serious mistake to defer treatment of progressive spinal curvatures while awaiting further spinal growth.

628.3 Neuromuscular Scoliosis, Syndromes, and Compensatory Scoliosis

Progressive spinal deformity is a common and potentially serious abnormality associated with many neuromuscular disorders of childhood. The more common disorders include cerebral palsy, Duchenne muscular dystrophy, spinal muscular atrophy, myelodysplasia, and arthrogryposis multiplex congenita. Progression is usually continuous once scoliosis begins. The magnitude of the deformity depends on the severity of involvement, the pattern of weakness, and whether the disease process is progressive. In nonambulatory patients, the curves tend to be long and sweeping, produce pelvic obliquity, involve the cervical spine, and alter pulmonary functions, producing respiratory problems. As these curves progress, sitting balance can be lost and affected individuals must use their arms to support an upright position, thus further increasing their disability. It is, therefore, important that spinal evaluation be part of the periodic examination of children with a neuromuscular disorder. Ambulatory patients have a much lower incidence of spinal deformity than the nonambulatory or more severely involved patients.

The standing or sitting forward bending test can be used for assessing the symmetry of spinal alignment. Any asymmetry is an indication for radiographic evaluation. This should include PA and lateral standing radiographs of the entire spine. If the child or adolescent cannot stand, then a sitting or supine (AP) radiograph may be necessary.

The goal of treatment of neuromuscular scoliosis is to prevent progression and loss of function secondary to the spinal deformity. Nonambulatory patients are usually most comfortable, are more independent, and have better respiratory function when they are able to sit erect without external support. Orthotic management or bracing is usually not effective in neuromuscular scoliosis. It may be effective in certain cases, particularly young children, in slowing the rate of curve progression, allowing further spinal growth, and delaying surgical intervention. Surgery will be necessary in most cases. The current instrumentation systems, especially the Luque rod system, are sufficiently strong and distribute the corrective forces such that postoperative immobilization is usually not necessary and the patient may be out of bed immediately after surgery.

SYNDROMES. Children with certain syndromes are also at increased risk for spinal deformities. Common syndromes include neurofibromatosis and Marfan syndrome. These children require careful periodic evaluation and prompt referral for orthopedic evaluation at the first sign of a spinal deformity.

COMPENSATORY SCOLIOSIS. Adolescents with a leg-length discrepancy may have a positive screening examination for scoliosis (Chapter 625). With a pelvic obliquity, the patients will stand erect and curve their spines in the opposite direction in order to stand erect. The magnitude of the leg-length discrepancy can be measured radiographically. It is important to distinguish between a structural and a compensatory spinal deformity. Any child with a lower extremity inequality should be referred for orthopedic evaluation.

628.4 Kyphosis

Kyphosis refers to a round-back deformity or to an increased angulation in the thoracic or thoracolumbar spine in the sagittal plane. Kyphotic deformities can be postural, idiopathic, or congenital in origin. Idiopathic kyphosis is termed Scheuermann disease.

POSTURAL KYPHOSIS
(Round-Back)

Postural kyphosis is secondary to bad posture. It is a common concern of parents. Postural kyphosis is diagnosed by the ability of the adolescent to correct the round-back appearance voluntarily in both the standing and prone position. Radiographically, no vertebral abnormalities are present. There may be some increase in the normal kyphosis of the thoracic region, but a supine hyperextension film will show complete correction. The child should be responsible for correcting posture; active orthopedic treatment is not indicated. Orthopedic referral is not necessary for postural kyphosis.

SCHEUERMANN DISEASE
(Idiopathic Kyphosis)

Scheuermann disease is common and second only to idiopathic scoliosis as a cause of spinal deformity. It occurs equally among males and females. Its cause is also unknown. Hereditary factors are present, but there is no definite pattern of inheritance. Kyphosis appearing in infants or young children is usually congenital in origin. The differentiation between postural kyphosis and Scheuermann disease is determined by clinical and radiographic evaluation.

CLINICAL MANIFESTATIONS. A patient with Scheuermann disease cannot correct the kyphosis in either the standing position or the prone, hyperextended position. When viewed from the side in the forward flexed position, patients will usually show an abrupt angulation in the mid to lower thoracic region. A patient with a postural round back shows a smooth, symmetric contour. In both conditions, there is reversal of the normal lumbar lordosis. Approximately 50% of patients with Scheuermann disease will have apical back pain, especially those patients with thoracolumbar kyphosis. A careful neurologic evaluation is indicated.

RADIOGRAPHIC EVALUATION. Radiographic assessment for kyphosis includes PA and lateral standing radiographs of the entire spine (Fig. 628–3). The classic findings of Scheuermann kyphosis include (1) narrowing of disc space; (2) loss of the normal anterior height of the involved vertebra, producing wedging of 5 degrees or more in three or more vertebrae; (3) irregularities of the endplates; and (4) Schmorl nodes. The supine, hyperextension radiographs will demonstrate the degree of flexibility.

TREATMENT. Treatment is similar to scoliosis and is dependent on the age of the patient, the degree of deformity, and the presence or absence of pain in the apical region. Nonoperative treatment consists of either corrective plaster casts or an orthosis. Thoracic kyphosis usually requires a Milwaukee brace; in patients with thoracolumbar kyphosis, an underarm hyperextension TLSO can be used. Compared with scoliosis, permanent correction of the kyphotic deformity usually can be achieved with nonoperative management. Surgical treatment of Scheuermann disease is rarely necessary. It is indicated only for those patients who have completed growth, who have a significant deformity, or who have chronic pain in the apical region. When these indications occur, both anterior and posterior spinal fusions are usually necessary. The anterior procedure consists of excision of the discs in the apical area of the curvature. This provides increased spinal flexibility and places the arthrodesis under compression. The latter minimizes the risk for pseudarthrosis. The correction of the deformity is achieved posteriorly with some form of instrumentation (Harrington, Luque, Cotrel-Dubousset, or Isola compression).

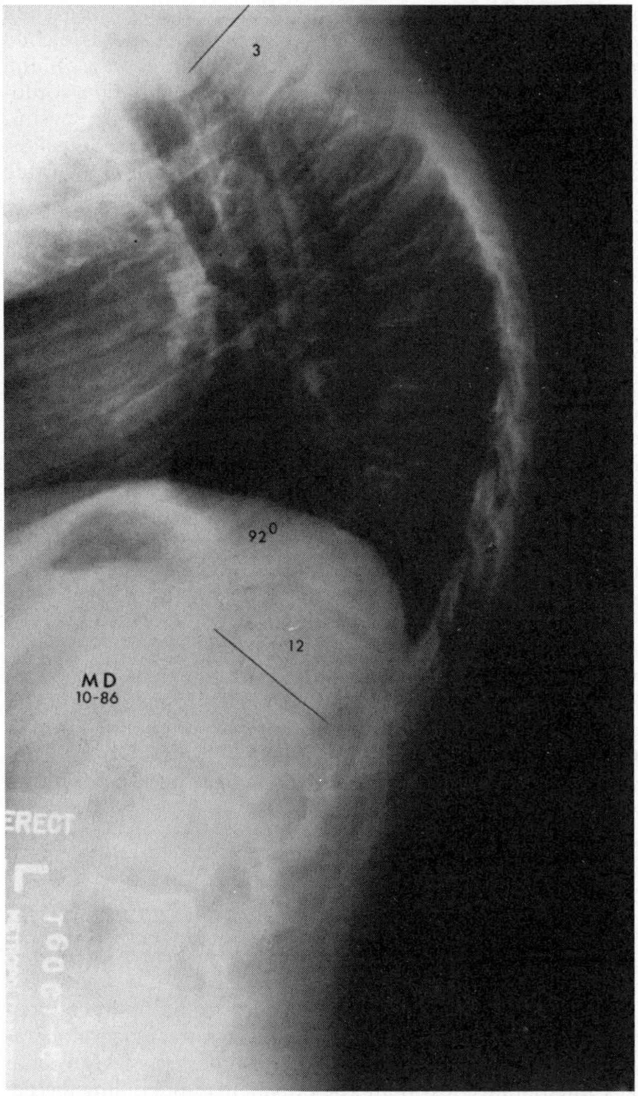

Figure 628–3. Standing lateral radiograph of a 14-year-old boy with severe Scheuermann kyphosis. This measures 92 degrees between T-3 and T-12. Note the wedging of the vertebrae at T-6, T-7, T-8, and T-9. The normal thoracic kyphosis is 40 degrees or less.

CONGENITAL KYPHOSIS

Congenital kyphosis, or kyphotic deformity, is due to vertebral malformations. There are two basic types: (1) congenital failure of formation of all or part of the vertebral body but with preservation of the posterior elements and (2) failure of anterior segmentation of the spine (anterior unsegmented bar). The more severe deformities are usually recognized at birth and rapidly progress thereafter. The less obvious deformities may not appear until years later. Once the progression begins, it does not cease until the end of growth and a progressive deformity in the thoracic spine may result in paraplegia. The latter is usually associated with the failure of vertebral body formation. Treatment of congenital scoliosis, when necessary, is operative. Orthotic management is ineffective.

628.5 Back Pain in Children

Back pain in children is unusual and should be viewed with concern. In contrast to adults, in whom back pain is frequently mechanical or psychologic in origin, back pain in children is frequently due to organic causes, especially in the preadolescent. Back pain lasting more than a few days requires careful investigation. It has been reported that approximately 85% of children with back pain lasting more than 2 mo will have a specific diagnosable lesion: 33% post-traumatic (occult fracture, spondylolysis); 33% developmental (kyphosis, scoliosis); and 18% infection or tumor. Only in the remaining 15% will the diagnosis be nonspecific.

CLINICAL MANIFESTATIONS. When confronted with a child with back pain, a careful history and physical evaluation are mandatory. The history includes the onset and duration of symptoms; antecedent factors; general health; family history; location, character, and radiation of pain; and neurologic symptoms such as muscle weakness, sensory changes, and bowel or bladder dysfunction. Physical examination includes a complete musculoskeletal and neurologic evaluation. Spinal alignment, mobility, muscle spasm, and areas of tenderness are evaluated and recorded. The danger signs in childhood back pain include (1) persistent or increasing pain; (2) systemic symptoms such as fever, malaise, or weight loss; (3) neurologic symptoms or findings; (4) bowel or bladder dysfunction; (5) young age, especially less than 4 yr (suspect tumor); and (6) painful left thoracic spinal curvatures.

RADIOGRAPHIC AND LABORATORY EVALUATION. Plain radiographs are the first diagnostic procedure to use in the evaluation of pediatric back pain, usually PA and lateral standing radiographs of the spine with right and left oblique views of the involved area. However, MRI or bone scans may be necessary, depending on the location of the pain and the differential diagnoses. Laboratory studies such as complete blood count, erythrocyte sedimentation rate (ESR), and tests for the juvenile forms of arthritis (juvenile rheumatoid arthritis and ankylosing spondylitis) may be necessary in certain cases (see Chapter 146). Cerebrospinal fluid should be evaluated if myelography is performed.

DIFFERENTIAL DIAGNOSIS. The differential diagnosis in pediatric back pain is extensive and is presented in Table 628–2.

628.6 Spondylolysis and Spondylolisthesis

Spondylolysis is a defect in the pars interarticularis without forward slippage of one vertebra on another. Spondylolisthesis refers to the forward slippage or displacement of one vertebra in relation to another. It is the most common cause of adolescent low back pain. Isthmic spondylolisthesis is the most common type, occurring in approximately 5% of the general population. The lesions are not present at birth but occur in 5% of affected children by 6 yr of age. Children involved in certain sports, such as gymnastics, have a higher incidence of spondylolysis. This has been attributed to repetitive hyperextension stresses. Spondylolisthesis is classified according to the degree of slippage of one vertebra on the other: grade 1, less than 25%; grade 2, 25–50%; grade 3, 50–75% grade 4, 75–100%; grade 5, complete displacement. The most common location for spondylolisthesis is the fifth lumbar vertebra on the sacrum (L-5–S-1).

CLINICAL MANIFESTATIONS. Physical examination for spondylolysis or spondylolisthesis is similar to that for any disorder of the spine and includes general spinal alignment, posture, presence or absence of scoliosis or kyphosis, and areas of tenderness. A palpable "step-off" at the lumbosacral area, and a vertically oriented sacrum, are indicative of severe spondylolisthesis. Complete neurologic examination should also be per-

■ **TABLE 628–2 Differential Diagnosis of Back Pain**

Inflammatory Diseases
Diskitis (common before 6 yr)
Vertebral osteomyelitis (pyogenic, tuberculous)
Spinal epidural abscess
Pyelonephritis
Pancreatitis

Rheumatologic Diseases
Pauciarticular juvenile rheumatoid arthritis
Reiter syndrome
Ankylosing spondylitis
Psoriatic arthritis

Developmental Diseases
Spondylolysis (common in adolescents)
Spondylolisthesis (common in adolescents)
Scheuermann syndrome (common in adolescents)
Scoliosis (especially left thoracic)

Mechanical Trauma and Abnormalities
Hip-pelvic anomalies
Herniated disc
Overuse syndromes (common with athletic training and in gymnasts and dancers)
Vertebral stress fractures
Upper cervical spine instability

Neoplastic Diseases
Primary vertebral tumors (e.g., osteogenic sarcoma)
Metastatic tumor (e.g., neuroblastoma)
Primary spinal tumor (e.g., neuroblastoma, lipoma)
Malignancy of bone marrow (e.g., acute lymphocytic leukemia, lymphoma)
Benign tumors (e.g., eosinophilic granuloma, osteoid osteoma)

Other
After lumbar puncture
Conversion reaction
Juvenile osteoporosis

formed because nerve root involvement can occur, especially with severe displacement.

RADIOLOGIC EVALUATION. This should include standing PA and lateral view radiographs of the entire spine with oblique radiograph of the lumbar spine. MRI may be required in patients with neurologic signs or symptoms.

TREATMENT. Treatment of spondylolysis is rarely required. Children and adolescents with asymptomatic spondylolysis require periodic evaluation during growth to assess for possible slippage. Painful spondylolysis may benefit from orthotic management. If this does not relieve pain, then surgical intervention with an in situ posterior spinal fusion may be required.

Adolescents with spondylolisthesis may require treatment. This depends on several factors, including (1) age of the patient; (2) type of defect; (3) degree of the slippage; and (4) associated malalignment in the involved area. Grade 1 spondylolisthesis usually does not require treatment unless there is chronic pain. Conservative management may be tried initially; if this fails, then surgical intervention may be necessary. Grade 2 usually requires a spinal fusion because of the high risk for further progression. Grades 3 and 4 spondylolisthesis almost always require fusion to prevent further deformity.

628.7 Disc Space Infection

A benign, self-limiting inflammation or infection of an intervertebral disc space or a vertebral endplate is usually regarded as an osteomyelitis of the vertebral endplates that secondarily invades the disc without producing an acute osteomyelitis of the vertebral body. Others, however, consider this disorder to be an inflammatory response secondary to trauma or other causes.

CLINICAL MANIFESTATIONS. Children may present with back pain or abdominal or pelvic pain. The physical findings in a child with a disc space infection are usually characteristic. The child maintains the spine in a straight, stiff, or splinted position and will refuse to flex the lumbar spine. The normal lumbar lordosis is reversed, and there may be paravertebral muscle spasms. However, in comparison with other forms of osteomyelitis, there are a few systemic symptoms such as fever or an elevated white cell count. The ESR is usually elevated.

RADIOGRAPHIC EVALUATION. The radiographic features vary according to the interval between the onset of symptoms and the diagnosis. AP, lateral, and oblique radiographs of the lumbar spine or thoracic spine, depending on the location of symptoms, are usually necessary to make the diagnosis. Characteristically, there is narrowing of the disc space with irregularity of the adjacent vertebral body endplates. Lateral tomograms are occasionally necessary to demonstrate the abnormalities. In very early cases, technetium bone scan or MRI may be helpful because these may be positive before routine radiographic changes are present.

TREATMENT. The treatment of disc space infection in children is usually antibiotic therapy. When a causative organism is identified, it is most commonly *Staphylococcus aureus.* Blood cultures may be helpful in identifying the organism. Aspiration needle biopsy of the spine is reserved for children who do not respond to initial treatment with antistaphylococcal antibiotics. Immobilization of the spine is used on a symptomatic basis. However, most children's symptoms rapidly resolve with intravenous antibiotics. See Chapter 172 for recommended antibiotic therapy for osteomyelitis. Intravenous antibiotics are continued for 1–2 wk and are followed by oral antibiotics for an additional 4 wk.

628.8 Intervertebral Disc Herniation

Intervertebral disc rupture is much less common in children than in adults. Because most patients are treated nonoperatively, the absolute incidence of the disorder is not known. In the United States, less than 1% of patients undergoing discectomy are younger than 16 yr. The frequency of symptomatic intervertebral disc herniation is more common in Asiatic populations than in whites, perhaps because of the smaller size of the spinal canal.

CLINICAL MANIFESTATIONS. Symptoms of intervertebral disc herniation in adolescents are similar to those in adults. The majority of affected patients report back pain and most have sciatic pain. About one third complain of decreased sensation or paresthesia in the lower extremities. On physical examination, lumbar muscle spasm, scoliosis, and a decreased range of lumbar motion are common findings. A positive straight leg–raising test is present in most patients. Abnormal reflex patterns and lower extremity weakness are much less likely to be present in young patients than in adults. A history of trauma is occasionally present, and patients tend to be taller and slightly heavier than their peers. A positive family history for intervertebral disc disease is frequently present.

RADIOGRAPHIC EVALUATION. Radiographs often show loss of lumbar lordosis and lumbar scoliosis. Loss of intervertebral disc height is rarely noted on plain films. MRI is currently the study of choice for localization of the lesion.

TREATMENT. Most symptoms respond to be bed rest followed by gradual resumption of activities. When sciatic pain, loss of reflexes, or weakness persist, surgical excision of the intervertebral disc is indicated. Fusion is not necessary unless there is accompanying evidence of spinal instability. Good results can be expected about 75% of the time. The incidence of recurrent symptoms requiring repeat surgery is about 25%.

628.9 Tumors

Back pain may be the presenting complaint in children who have a tumor involving the vertebral column or the spinal cord. Other associated symptoms may include weakness of the lower extremities, scoliosis, and sphincter disturbances. Both benign and malignant tumors may occur; most are benign (see Chapter 454). Common benign tumors include osteoid osteomas, osteoblastoma, solitary bone cysts, and eosinophilic granuloma. Malignant tumors may be osseous (osteogenic or Ewing sarcoma), neurogenic (neuroblastoma), or metastatic. Routine radiographs are usually normal, and special studies such as technetium bone scans or MRI are necessary for localization and diagnosis. The treatment of tumors of the spinal column is usually surgical. Fusions will be necessary if there is instability. Adjuvant therapy will be necessary for a malignant tumor.

IDIOPATHIC SCOLIOSIS

Bradford DS, Lonstein JE, Ogilvie JW, et al: Moe's Textbook of Scoliosis and Other Spinal Deformities, 2nd ed. Philadelphia, WB Saunders, 1987, pp 191–233.
Bunnell WP: The natural history of idiopathic scoliosis. Clin Orthop 229:20, 1988.
Ceballas T, Ferrer-Torrelles M, Castillo F, et al: Prognosis in infantile idiopathic scoliosis. J Bone Joint Surg 62A:863, 1980.
Figueiredo UM, James JIP: Juvenile idiopathic scoliosis. J Bone Joint Surg 61B:36, 1979.
Lonstein JE: Natural history and school screening for scoliosis. Orthop Clin North Am 19:227, 1988.
Lonstein JE, Carlson JM: The prediction of curve progression in untreated idiopathic scoliosis during growth. J Bone Joint Surg 66A:1061, 1984.
MacEwen GD, Bunnell WP, Sriram K: Acute neurologic complications in the treatment of scoliosis (a report of the Scoliosis Research Society). J Bone Joint Surg 57A:404, 1975.
MacLean WE Jr, Green NE, Pierre CB, et al: Stress and coping with scoliosis: Psychological effects on adolescents and their families. J Pediatr Orthop 9:257, 1989.
Nottage W, Waugh TR, McMaster WC: Radiation exposure during scoliosis screening radiology. Spine 6:456, 1981.
Renshaw TS: Screening school children for scoliosis. Clin Orthop 229:26, 1988.
Scoles PV, Salvagno R, Villalba D, et al: Relationship of iliac crest maturation to skeletal and chronological age. J Pediatr Orthop 8:639, 1988.
Winter RB, Lonstein JE, Drogt J, et al: The effectiveness of bracing in the nonoperative treatment of idiopathic scoliosis. Spine 11:790, 1986.
Wyatt MP, Barrack RL, Mubarak SJ, et al: Vibratory response in idiopathic scoliosis. J Bone Joint Surg 68B:714, 1986.

CONGENITAL SCOLIOSIS

McMaster MJ: Occult intraspinal anomalies and congenital scoliosis. J Bone Joint Surg 66A:588, 1984.
McMaster MJ, Ohtsuka K: The natural history of congenital scoliosis: A study of 251 patients. J Bone Joint Surg 68B:588, 1986.
Winter RB: Congenital Deformities of the Spine. New York, Thieme-Stratton, 1983.
Winter RB, Haven JJ, Moe JH, et al: Diastematomyelia and congenital spine deformities. J Bone Joint Surg 56A:27, 1974.
Winter RB, Moe JH, Eilers VE: Congenital scoliosis—A study of 234 patients treated and untreated. J Bone Joint Surg 50A:1, 1968.

NEUROMUSCULAR SCOLIOSIS

Cambridge W, Drennan JC: Scoliosis associated with Duchenne muscular dystrophy. J Pediatr Orthop 7:436, 1987.
Ferguson RI, Allen BL Jr: Consideration in the treatment of cerebral palsy patients with spinal deformities. Orthop Clin North Am 19:419, 1988.
Kalamchi A, Thompson GH: Congenital anomalies of the spine. *In*: Dee R, Mango E, Hurst LC (eds): Principles of Orthopaedic Practice. New York, McGraw-Hill, 1989, pp 839–860.
Nash CL: Spinal deformities. *In*: Thompson GH, Rubin IL, Bilenker RM (eds): Comprehensive Management of Cerebral Palsy. New York, Grune & Stratton, 1983, pp 257–272.
Piggott H: The natural history of scoliosis in myelodysplasia. J Bone Joint Surg 62B:54, 1980.
Smith AD, Koreska J, Moseley CF: Progression of scoliosis in Duchenne muscular dystrophy. J Bone Joint Surg 71A:1066, 1989.

KYPHOSIS—SCHEUERMANN AND CONGENITAL

Lonstein JE, Winter RB, Moe JH, et al: Spinal cord compression due to spine deformity. Reconstr Surg Traumatol 13:58, 1972.
Lowe TG: Current concepts review: Scheuermann disease. J Bone Joint Surg 72-A:940, 1990.
Sachs B, Bradford D, Winter R, et al: Scheuermann's kyphosis: Follow-up of Milwaukee brace treatment. J Bone Joint Surg 69A:50, 1987.
Winter RB, Moe JH, Wang JF: Congenital kyphosis: Its natural history and treatment as observed in a study of 130 patients. J Bone Joint Surg 55A:223, 1973.

SPONDYLOLYSIS AND SPONDYLOLISTHESIS

Bell DF, Ehrlich MG, Zaleski D: Brace treatment for symptomatic spondylolisthesis. Clin Orthop 236:192, 1988.
Hensinger RN: Current concepts review: Spondylolysis and spondylolisthesis in children and adolescents. J Bone Joint Surg 71A:1098, 1989.
Pizzutillo PD, Hummer CD III: Nonoperative treatment of painful adolescent spondylolysis or spondylolisthesis. J Pediatr Orthop 9:538, 1989.
Saraste H: Long-term clinical and radiographical follow-up of spondylolysis and spondylolisthesis. J Pediatr Orthop 7:631, 1987.
Seitsalo S, Österman K, Hyvärinen H, et al: Severe spondylolisthesis in children and adolescents. J Bone Joint Surg 72B:259, 1990.

DISC SPACE INFECTION

Crawford AH, Kucharzyk DW, Ruda R, et al: Diskitis in Children. Clin Orthop 266:70, 1991.
Scoles PV, Quinn TP: Intervertebral discitis in children and adolescents. Clin Orthop 162:31, 1982.
Szaly E, Green N, Heller R: Magnetic resonance imaging in the diagnosis of childhood discitis. J Pediatr Orthop 7:164, 1987.
Wenger DR, Bobechko WP, Gilday DL: The spectrum of intervertebral disc-space infection in children. J Bone Joint Surg 60A:100, 1978.

BACK PAIN

Conrad EM III, Olszewski AD, Berger M, et al: Pediatric spine tumors with spinal cord compromise. J Pediatr Orthop 12:454, 1992.
Delamarter RB, Sachs BL, Thompson GH, et al: Primary neoplasms of the thoracic and lumbar spine: An analysis of 29 conservative cases. Clin Orthop 256:87, 1990.
King HA: Evaluating the child with back pain. Pediatr Clin North Am 33:1489, 1986.
Thompson GH: Back pain in children. J Bone Joint Surg 75A:928, 1993.

CHAPTER 629
The Neck

Nonosseous abnormalities of the neck are relatively common in children. These are predominantly soft tissue, congenital, and neurologic in origin.

629.1 Torticollis

Torticollis means twisted, or wry, neck. It refers to the head being tipped to one side with the occiput rotated toward the shoulder and the chin rotated in the opposite direction and elevated. The differential diagnosis of torticollis is extensive and is presented in Table 629–1. However, the more common causes are muscular torticollis, rotatory fixation, congenital anomalies, and posterior fossa tumor.

Muscular torticollis is the most common type and usually occurs at birth from a suspected injury to the sternocleidomastoid muscle. Large infants who have had difficult vertex deliveries are at special risk. Stretching of the neck during delivery results in tearing and bleeding within the sternocleidomastoid muscle. The blood is contained within its own fascial compartment, resulting in increased pressure. The increased pressure further damages the muscle, resulting in an area of ischemia

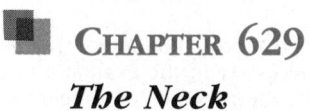

■ TABLE 629–1 Differential Diagnosis of Torticollis

Nonosseous
Muscular Torticollis
Sandifer Syndrome
Gastroesophageal reflux
Neurogenic
Posterior fossa (cerebellar) tumors
Spinal cord tumors
Osseous
Congenital Cervical Spine Malformations
Occipitocervical invagination
Atlas malformation
Congenital cervical scoliosis
Rotatory Fixation (C1–C2)
Trauma
Upper respiratory infection
Cervical adenitis

that secondarily becomes replaced by fibrous tissue, contracts, and produces torticollis. Congenital anomalies are usually malformations of the atlas or congenital cervical scoliosis. *Rotatory fixation* occurs between the first and second cervical vertebrae, usually after a minor injury or upper respiratory infection, and results in soft tissue impingement. As a consequence, motion is restricted and painful. The neck was normal before this acute episode. Older children who have a slow, insidious onset of torticollis should be suspected of having a *posterior fossa tumor* or other neurologic abnormality.

CLINICAL MANIFESTATIONS. Children with a torticollis have the head held in the characteristic position. In muscular torticollis, there will frequently be a palpable mass in the inferior aspect of the sternocleidomastoid muscle, which represents the contracted area of fibrous tissue. In rotatory fixation and acquired forms of torticollis, this mass will not be present. The range of motion may be limited because of pain. The neurologic evaluation will be normal in muscular torticollis and rotatory fixation, but there may be subtle neurologic abnormalities with a posterior fossa tumor.

RADIOGRAPHIC EVALUATION. Anteroposterior and lateral radiographs of the cervical spine are necessary in the evaluation of a child with torticollis to rule out the presence of congenital malformations. Dynamic computed tomography (CT) will usually establish the diagnosis of rotatory fixation. In this procedure, the scan is performed with the head rotated to the involved side and then maximally rotated to the opposite side. Sections between the first and second cervical vertebrae will show no change in the relationship with rotation, thereby confirming the fixed alignment. In children with suspected posterior fossa tumor or other neurologic abnormalities, a magnetic resonance image will usually be diagnostic.

TREATMENT. The treatment of torticollis is dependent on an accurate diagnosis. In muscular torticollis, passive stretching will usually be effective in restoring range of motion of the neck in infants. If the deformity persists after 1 yr of age, then a release or lengthening of the sternocleidomastoid muscle will be necessary. In rotatory fixation, gentle halter traction for 1 or 2 days will usually allow slow resolution to the soft tissue impingement between the first and second cervical vertebrae. Once this occurs, the range of motion will typically return to normal. However, if rotatory fixation persists more than 1 mo, the associated scarring may prevent spontaneous resolution. Because of the persistent deformity, the child will subsequently experience significant facial asymmetry (plagiocephaly). In these children a surgical realignment and posterior spinal fusion between C-1 and C-2 may be indicated. If the deformity is due to a posterior fossa tumor, this will be treated surgically as well as with adjunctive therapy depending on the diagnosis.

Canale ST, Griffin DW, Hubbard CN: Congenital muscular torticollis: Long-term follow-up. J Bone Joint Surg 64A:810, 1982.
Davids J, Wenger D, Mubarak S: Congenital muscular torticollis: Sequela of intrauterine or perinatal compartment syndrome. J Pediatr Orthop 13:141, 1993.
Phillips W, Hensinger R: The management of rotary atlanto-axial subluxation in children. J Bone Joint Surg 71A:664, 1989.

629.2 Klippel-Feil Syndrome*

This rare malformation is due to a congenital fusion of two or more cervical vertebrae (congenital synostosis) and is also called brevicollis (short neck). There is a low hairline, limited neck motion, a short neck, and other anomalies of the urinary (agenesis, horseshoe kidney), genital (absent vagina, ovarian agenesis), cardiovascular (ventricular septal defect, patent ductus arteriosus, coarctation of aorta), pulmonary, and nervous systems (synkinesis, deafness, spinal cord compression, ptosis, seventh nerve palsy). Other common problems include scoliosis or kyphosis, torticollis (resulting from bone anomalies or sternocleidomastoid contractures), pterygium colli (webbing of each side of the neck), Sprengel deformity, cervical ribs, short trachea, syndactyly, hypoplastic thumbs, supernumerary digits, and unilateral hypoplasia of the pectoralis major muscle. The latter is *Poland anomaly* if it is associated with syndactyly and hypoplasia of the nipple and areola.

Roentgenography confirms the diagnosis and identifies other lesions, such as hemivertebrae, cervical ribs, and platybasia. The differential diagnosis includes bilateral Sprengel deformity, occipitalization of C-1, and acquired postinflammatory (diskitis, rheumatoid arthritis) or post-traumatic fusion. Treatment is by observation.

Hensinger R, Lang J, MacEwen G: Klippel-Feil syndrome: A constellation of associated anomalies. J Bone Joint Surg 56A:246, 1974.

629.3 Atlantoaxial Instability*

Atlantoaxial or atlanto-occipital instability may be due to congenital anomalies or trauma or may occur spontaneously in association with inflammatory processes of the retropharyngeal, neck, or pharyngeal spaces or with rheumatoid arthritis of the joint space. Instability may produce spinal cord injury and neurologic signs.

Congenital anomalies of the odontoid process include aplasia, hypoplasia (occasionally familial), and a separate odontoid process. The latter may also be post-traumatic. There may be localized pain, limited motion, transient neurologic manifestations, or quadriplegia owing to cord compression. Children with trisomy 21 have atlantoaxial instability owing to laxity of the transverse ligament and abnormal odontoid process development (dysplasia, hypoplasia). Odontoid hypoplasia is also noted in children with skeletal dysplasias (osteochondrodystrophies). The latter inborn errors of metabolism include mucopolysaccharidosis (particularly Morquio disease), spondyloepiphyseal dysplasias, achondroplasia, pseudoachondroplasia, and multiple epiphyseal dysplasia.

Clinical manifestations of cord compression may not be evident during infancy but may occur spontaneously between 5 and 15 yr of age or after episodes of minor trauma. The older child complains of paresthesias of the upper extremities and manifests sleep apnea, neck pain, torticollis, distal muscle weakness, gait disturbances and later, bowel or bladder dysfunction, spasticity, or quadriplegia.

*From L.T. Staheli, 14th edition.

Anteroposterior and lateral roentgenographs and then, if determined to be safe, flexion and extension lateral positions confirms the diagnosis and identifies the distance of displacement of the anterior arch of the atlas (C-1) from the odontoid process of the axis (C-2) and anomalies of the odontoid itself. The distance between the posterior margin of the atlas anterior arch and the front of the vertical odontoid process (atlanto-odontoid interval) is less than 4.5 mm in children and 2.5 mm in adults. The distance between the posterior margin of the axis (C-2) body and the posterior atlas arch (anteroposterior canal diameter) helps to determine the risk for cord compression, which is unusual if the distance is more than 18 mm. Open-mouth anteroposterior roentgenograms may be needed to visualize rotary displacement. CT scanning and magnetic resonance imaging may delineate bone abnormalities and cord involvement, respectively.

Treatment of an unstable atlantoaxial or atlanto-occipital joint may require a posterior fusion of the upper cervical spine. Inflammation-related subluxation may be managed with reduction under general anesthesia and cast fixation or reduction with dorsally directed traction. Halo brace reduction and immobilization for approximately 3 mo may permit healing. If this method is unsuccessful, fusion is indicated.

Fielding JW, Hensinger RN, Hawkins RJ: Os odontoideum. J Bone Joint Surg 62A:376, 1980.
Georgopoulos G, Pizzutillo PD, Lee MS: Occipito-atlantal instability in children: A report of five cases and review of the literature. J Bone Joint Surg 69A:429, 1987.
Hensinger RN: Congenital anomalies of the cervical spine. Clin Orthop 264:16, 1991.
Locke GR, Gardner JI, Van Epps EF: Atlas-dens interval (ADI) in children: A survey based on 200 normal cervical spines. Am J Roentgenol 97:135, 1966.
Paeschal SM, Scola FH, Tapper TB, Pezzulo JC: Skeletal anomalies of the upper cervical spine in children with Down syndrome. J Pediatr Orthop 10:607, 1990.
Spierings ELH: The management of os odontoideum: Analysis of 37 cases. J Bone Joint Surg 64B:422, 1982.

CHAPTER 630
The Upper Limb

Upper limb disorders, with the exception of fractures, are less common in children and adolescents than those involving the other areas of the musculoskeletal system.

SHOULDER

The shoulder joint is composed of the relatively small glenoid fossa, which articulates with a proportionally larger hemispherical humeral head. The stability of the shoulder joint is provided by muscular and tendinous (rotator cuff) attachments. The shoulder has a relatively large range of motion because of this small articular surface and large muscle mass. Shoulder motion is a combination of glenohumeral and scapulothoracic motion.

630.1 Sprengel Deformity

Failure of the scapula to descend to its normal location is termed *Sprengel deformity.* The scapula is located at an abnormally high position with respect to the child's neck and thorax. This abnormality occurs with varying degrees of severity. Webbing of the skin between the neck and scapula and a low posterior hairline may be associated findings. In the severe form, a bone (omovertebral) may connect the scapula with the cervical spine and prevent scapulothoracic movement. There may also be associated muscle anomalies that further limit strength and stability of the shoulder girdle. In severe cases, the scapula is very high, producing a significant cosmetic deformity with markedly limited shoulder range of motion, particularly forward flexion and abduction. In the mild form, the scapula is slightly high riding with less than normal motion. A Klippel-Feil anomaly, congenital fusion of one or more of the cervical spine vertebra, may also occur with Sprengel deformity.

TREATMENT. The best outcome in severe Sprengel deformity is achieved by surgically repositioning or, occasionally, partially resecting the scapula. An osteotomy of the clavicle is frequently necessary to bring the scapula to a more normal position. This improves the cosmetic appearance and will increase shoulder motion, especially abduction.

630.2 Shoulder Dislocation

Traumatic dislocation of the shoulder is uncommon in childhood but increases in frequency during adolescence. Anterior dislocation is the most common type. It usually occurs when the shoulder is forced into an abduction and external rotation. In young children, a Salter-Harris type II epiphyseal fracture is more likely to occur. Once a traumatic dislocation has occurred, there is damage to the anterior capsule and the associated musculature that may predispose to recurrent dislocation. The younger individuals are at the time of the initial dislocation, the more likely they are to experience recurrent dislocations.

TREATMENT. Closed reduction and immobilization in a shoulder immobilizer followed by rehabilitation for 3–6 wk is recommended for the first dislocation. However, some favor early reconstruction rather than instituting conservative treatment because of the risk for recurrent dislocations.

ELBOW

The elbow joint is composed of three bones: the distal humerus and the proximal radius and ulna. There are three articulations: the radiohumeral, the ulnohumeral, and the proximal radioulnar. There are anterior and posterior indentations on the distal surface of the humerus: the anterior coronoid and the posterior olecranon fossa. These accept the coronoid and olecranon processes of the proximal ulna. It allows the elbow to flex 150 degrees and extend to neutral. The proximal radius is a relatively flat, circular structure that allows pronation and supination of the forearm to occur, with approximately 90 degrees of motion at each. Abnormalities involving the elbow typically produce pain and loss of motion.

630.3 Nursemaid's Elbow

The radial head is not as bulbous in infants and young children as in older children. During early childhood, the annular ligament that passes around the neck of the proximal radius just below the radial head provides stability between the radius and ulna. When longitudinal traction is applied to the upper extremity with the elbow in extension, the annular ligament can slide over the radial head and become partially entrapped in the radiohumeral joint (Fig. 630–1). This is known as nursemaid's elbow or subluxation of the radial head. It represents a soft tissue interposition in the elbow joint. The subluxation of the annular ligament is initiated by either a jerk on the arm when the child falls with the hand being held by a parent or when the child is forcibly lifted by the hand. It may also occur if the child falls and holds onto an object for support but allows longitudinal traction to be applied across the elbow. The hand typically is held in a pronated position, and the child may refuse to use the hand and may cry when the elbow is moved.

TREATMENT. Rotating the hand and forearm to a supinated position with pressure over the radial head usually reduces the annular ligament and restores full, normal use of the extremity. With reduction of the annular ligament, there will be a palpable "click" felt along the lateral aspect of the elbow. Radiographs are usually not necessary to make the diagnosis. In a child sent for radiographic evaluation before reducing the annular ligament, this may inadvertently occur during positioning for radiographs.

The parents should be educated about the mechanism of injury and encouraged to avoid lifting the child or holding him or her up by the hands or forearm. Once a subluxation has occurred, there is a propensity for recurrent episodes. Usually, there is sufficient development of the radial head to prevent subluxation of the annular ligament by 4 yr of age.

630.4 Panner Disease

Panner disease is an osteochondrosis that involves the ossific nucleus of the capitellum, the lateral aspect of the distal humeral epiphysis. This disorder is most common in adolescence and occurs predominantly in those engaged in sport activities that involve throwing. The adolescents complain of pain and may have crepitation and loss of motion, particularly pronation and supination.

The diagnosis can usually be made from anteroposterior and lateral radiographs of the elbow. Occasionally, oblique radiographs may be beneficial. Additional radiographic studies such as magnetic resonance imaging may be helpful in identifying the extent of the lesion and determining whether the overlying articular cartilage is intact or disrupted.

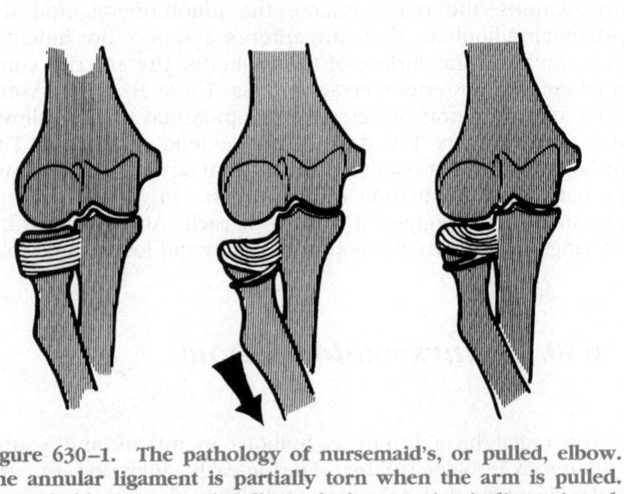

Figure 630–1. The pathology of nursemaid's, or pulled, elbow. The annular ligament is partially torn when the arm is pulled. The radial head moves distally, and when traction is discontinued, the ligament is carried into the joint. (From Rang M: Children's Fractures, 2nd ed. Philadelphia, JB Lippincott, 1983, p 193.)

TREATMENT. The treatment is usually conservative with restriction of activities. If the overlying articular cartilage is disrupted and joint fluid gets beneath the lesion, it may ultimately become a loose body. A loose osteocartilaginous fragment may be excised through an arthrotomy or arthroscopy. Occasionally, it is possible to repair the lesion by drilling it to allow for ingrowth of new blood vessels or by internal fixation with absorbable pins, which may allow the lesions to heal.

WRIST

The wrist is the articulation between the hand and the distal radius and ulna. The proximal row of carpal bones (scaphoid, lunate, and hamate) comprises the articular surface of the hand. Anatomically, the distal radius has a 25 degree ulnar tilt and 12 degree volar angulation. The distal ulna is relatively flat, with the exception of the ulnar styloid, and has a small, triangle-shaped meniscus between its articulation with the hamate. There are three articulations: radiocarpal, ulnocarpal, and radioulnar. The wrist is not a common site for pediatric musculoskeletal disorders with the exceptions of fractures involving the distal radius and ulna.

630.5 Ganglion

A synovial fluid–filled cyst about the wrist, a ganglion, is relatively common in childhood. The usual site is the dorsum of the wrist near the radiocarpal joint; a common second site is over the volar radial aspect of the wrist. The disease is a defect in one of the joint capsules, which allows herniation of the synovium through the defect. If the synovium is ruptured, the fluid may be pumped into the soft tissues through the action of wrist motion; the fluid is subsequently walled off by reactive fibrous tissue.

TREATMENT. In children, ganglia are benign and tend to disappear over time. If a ganglion is sufficiently large, causes pain, or interferes with normal tendon functioning, aspiration of the cyst is sometimes helpful. Surgical excision of the cyst accompanied by removal of the tract that extends into the joint is curative.

630.6 Radial Clubhand

Absence of the radius, either total or partial, results in radial deviation of the hand and abnormal function. The ulna is usually hypoplastic as well as bowed, contributing to the shortness and deformity of the forearm and hand. This is an uncommon disorder but may be associated with a variety of other syndromes such as VATER (vertebral defects, anal atresia, tracheoesophageal fistula with esophageal atresia and radial and renal anomalies) or the Holt-Oram syndrome. Any child with a radial clubhand requires a very careful evaluation for other disorders. The diagnosis is usually evident on physical examination, but radiographs will show whether the radius is completely absent or whether there is a proximal remnant. Congenital absence of the thumb is a common accompaniment.

TREATMENT. The treatment of radial clubhand in infancy begins with serial casting or splinting in an attempt to center the carpus on the end of the ulna. Usually, a surgical procedure is ultimately necessary to centralize the hand adequately, provide stability, and place it into a position to maximize function. If the thumb is absent, a pollicization of the index finger can be performed to improve hand function.

HAND AND FINGERS

The hand and fingers are composed of the carpal and metacarpal bones proximally and the phalanges distally. The thumb has two phalanges (proximal and distal), whereas the fingers have three phalanges (proximal, middle, and distal). Thus, the thumb has an interphalangeal (IP) joint, and the fingers have proximal (PIP) and distal interphalangeal (DIP) joints. The thumb and fingers articulate with the metacarpals at the metacarpophalangeal joints. The hand has a delicate balance between the intrinsic muscle system, a powerful extrinsic muscle system, fine sensory innervation, and specialized skin to allow it to be a highly mobile, sensitive, delicate yet powerful appendage. Thumb and finger disorders, other than trauma, are relatively uncommon. When present, they tend to be due to congenital rather than developmental abnormalities.

630.7 Polydactyly

Extra digits, or polydactyly, occur as both simple and complex deformities. Skin tags and digit remnants are typically seen near the metacarpophalangeal joint of the small finger or the thumb. They do not have palpable bone in the base or possess voluntary motion and may simply be ligated or excised in the newborn period. Complex varieties require formal amputation, which is usually performed at approximately 1 yr of age. Syndromes in which polydactyly commonly occurs are listed in Table 630–1.

630.8 Syndactyly

Syndactyly also occurs in both simple and complex patterns. There should be concern about sharing of common important structures between the digits such as the neurovascular bundle. There is also a tethering effect on the growth of the affected digits. Referral for delineation of specific disease and development of treatment strategies is indicated when the condition is recognized. Syndromes associated with syndactyly are presented in Table 630–2.

630.9 Congenital Trigger Thumb and Finger

A thickening in the tendon of the flexor hallucis longus (thumb) or the flexor digitorum longus (fingers) just below the first pulley of the digit may result in a triggering phenomenon. Each finger has a series of pulleys that prevent the tendons from bowstringing when flexed. This nodule may slide through the first pulley with a snapping, popping, or triggering sensation; this may or may not be painful. As the nodule enlarges because of the stimulation from triggering, it may ultimately be unable to pass beneath the pulley, resulting in a fixed flexion deformity of the IP joint of the thumb or the PIP and DIP joints of the fingers. The nodule is typically palpable in the palm just proximal to the skin crease of the metacarpophalangeal joint. This is a clinical diagnosis and radiographs are not helpful.

TREATMENT. The treatment of a congenital trigger thumb or finger is a release of the first pulley. The normal excursion of the tendon will not allow the nodule to reach the next pulley. The release of the pulley will not cause bowstringing of the tendon.

■ TABLE 630–1 Syndromes Associated with Polydactyly

Carpenter syndrome
Ellis–van Creveld syndrome
Meckel-Gruber syndrome
Polysyndactyly
Trisomy 13
Orofaciodigital syndrome
Rubinstein-Taybi syndrome

■ TABLE 630–2 Syndromes Associated with Syndactyly

Apert syndrome
Carpenter syndrome
de Lange syndrome
Holt-Oram syndrome
Orofaciodigital syndrome
Polysyndactyly
Trisomy 21
Fetal Hydantoin syndrome
Laurence-Moon-Biedl syndrome
Fanconi pancytopenia
Trisomy 13
Trisomy 18

Bora FW: The Pediatric Upper Extremity: Diagnosis and Management. Philadelphia, WB Saunders, 1986.
Satku K, Ganesh B: Ganglia in children. J Pediatr Orthop 5:13, 1985.
Wagner KT, Lyne ED: Adolescent traumatic dislocations of the shoulder with an open epiphysis. J Pediatr Orthop 3:61, 1983.

CHAPTER 631
Arthrogryposis

Arthrogryposis multiplex congenita (AMC) refers to a symptom complex characterized by multiple joint contractures present at birth. The involved muscles are replaced partially or completely by fat and fibrous tissue. However, it is not a single disease because there are approximately 150 different syndromes occurring with multiple congenital contractures that have been loosely categorized as arthrogryposis. Some infants with arthrogryposis have maternal antibodies to the fetal antigens expressed on the acetylcholine receptor. Although most children who have this disorder survive, some die in infancy as a result of involvement of respiratory muscles. The major form of AMC is called amyoplasia. This refers to the classic syndrome in which there is involvement of the upper and lower extremities. Amyoplasia accounts for approximately 40% of children who have multiple congenital contractures.

631.1 Amyoplasia

The cause of amyoplasia is unknown, but children with this disorder have a decreased number of anterior horn cells in the spinal cord, suggesting a neuropathic cause. However, other studies have shown that the disorder may be myopathic in origin. In the latter instance, diminution of in utero movement may be the final common pathway leading to contractures.

Every child presenting with multiple joint contractures should have a complete musculoskeletal evaluation.

CLINICAL MANIFESTATIONS. The distribution of involvement of multiple joint contractures is variable. The classic presentation involves the upper and lower extremities. The lower extremities are typically more involved than the upper extremities. Involvement of all four extremities is quadrimelic involvement. It is also possible that only the lower extremities or upper extremities (bimelic) may be involved. It is unusual to see only one extremity or a portion of one extremity involved.

The clinical features may include (1) adduction, internal rotation contractures of the shoulders; (2) fixed flexion or extension contractures of the elbow; (3) rigid volar flexion—ulnar deviation or dorsiflexion—radial deviation contractures of the wrists; (4) thumb and palm deformity; (5) rigid interphalangeal joints of the thumb and fingers; (6) flexion, abduction, external rotation hip contractures with dislocation of one or both hips; (7) fixed extension or flexion contractures of the knees; and (8) severe rigid bilateral clubfeet.

RADIOGRAPHIC AND LABORATORY EVALUATION. Radiographs should be obtained of the involved joints in all children presenting with multiple joint contractures. Screening radiographs of the spine and pelvis are almost always necessary for evaluation of possible spinal deformity and underlying hip dysplasia. Routine laboratory studies are usually not helpful in evaluating amyoplasia. If an underlying syndrome is suspected, such as congenital muscular dystrophy, then creatine phosphokinase, molecular genetic, or chromosomal studies may be helpful.

TREATMENT. Correction of orthopedic deformities may be beneficial in maximizing walking or other functions. Each child must be individualized with respect to potential rehabilitation and the possible treatment.

Physical Therapy. Physical therapy with passive range of motion exercises can be very beneficial in improving range of motion of involved joints. However, it rarely will completely correct the existing contractures. Splinting (daytime, nighttime, or both) of the extremities may also improve joint range of motion. This is particularly useful in the hands and wrists. Postoperative splinting is important in maintaining alignment and preventing recurrence.

Serial Casting. Serial casting can be helpful in further correcting soft tissue contractures after physical therapy has reached its maximum benefit. Serial casting is particularly useful in knee flexion contractures and in clubfeet. Casts are changed at weekly intervals, followed by a gentle manipulation of the involved area.

Orthoses. Orthotics can be beneficial in providing joint stability as well as maintaining alignment after satisfactory correction of contractures. The type of orthosis will depend on the individual child's particular needs. This may be include ankle-foot orthosis if there is only ankle and foot involvement, a knee-ankle-foot orthosis if there is concomitant knee involvement, and a hip-knee-ankle-foot orthosis if there is involvement of all the joints of the lower extremities. Should scoliosis develop, a spinal orthosis such as a thoracolumbar spinal orthosis may be tried; it may slow the rate of progression and delay surgical intervention.

Fracture Management. Perinatal fractures commonly occur in children with arthrogryposis. These should be suspected if there is localized deformity, soft tissue swelling, erythema, or irritability. Rigid joints and hypotonia contribute to the increased incidence of fractures. These typically involve the shafts as well as the epiphyseal regions and should be managed with appropriate immobilization until adequate healing has occurred. It is important that radiographs be obtained in all children suspected of having a fracture before initiating any physical therapy.

Surgery. Surgery is usually necessary to achieve maximum correction of soft tissue contractures and joint deformities; to reduce and stabilize dislocated hips; to correct clubfoot deformities; and to partially correct and stabilize spinal deformities.

UPPER EXTREMITIES. Surgical treatment of upper extremity deformities depends on the type and degree of contracture as well as the motor capabilities and functional needs of the patient. A child's compensatory or adaptive functioning of the upper extremities can be remarkable, and it is essential not to diminish function for cosmesis inadvertently. Internal rotation contractures of the shoulder can be treated by soft tissue releases and proximal humeral derotation osteotomies at a level proximal to the deltoid insertion. Extension contractures of the elbow may benefit from posterior capsulotomy and triceps tenotomy or lengthening to allow restoration of passive or active flexion. Active flexion can be partially restored with a transfer of the pectoralis muscle and its neurovascular bundle. Wrist deformities may be managed by tendon transfers, proximal row carpectomy, or shortening dorsal wedge radial osteotomies.

LOWER EXTREMITIES. Most infants with clubfoot will not respond completely to passive stretching or serial casting. Complete soft tissue releases are usually required. Occasionally, excision of the talus or talar decancellation may also be required to achieve a plantigrade foot.

Knee flexion contractures that are unresponsive to serial casting may benefit by a lengthening of the hamstring in association with a posterior knee capsulotomy. If this fails to correct the deformity to within 15–20 degrees of neutral, then an extension osteotomy of the distal femur may be required. The value of walking with the knee extended is extremely beneficial. A recurrent flexion deformity may occur after an extension osteotomy if it is done before adolescence. Knee extension contractures may also require treatment, especially if the child or adolescent cannot sit comfortably because of the extended position. Lengthening of the quadriceps mechanism may be beneficial.

Hip contractures may be improved by soft tissue releases. Occasionally, extension derotation osteotomies of the proximal femur may be helpful in completing the correction of the flexion, abduction, or external rotation contractures. Controversy exists as to whether bilateral dislocations of the hip should be reduced. If there is a unilateral dislocation, then treatment is usually necessary to prevent lower extremity length inequality, pelvic obliquity, and possible scoliosis. Open reduction is accompanied by soft tissue releases, shortening derotation varus osteotomies of the proximal femurs, and pelvic osteotomies.

SCOLIOSIS. Scoliosis is common in children with amyoplasia. The age at onset and patterns of deformity are variable. Orthotic management is usually effective only in slowing the rate of progression. In the majority of children, progression will slowly occur, and they ultimately will require surgical intervention. Because of the associated soft tissue contractures, it is important that these curves not be allowed to become too severe because only partial correction will be obtained. Most children can be satisfactorily managed by a posterior spinal fusion and some type of segmental spinal instrumentation.

Banker BQ: Arthrogryposis multiplex congenita. *In*: Engel AG, Banker BQ (eds): Myology: Basic and Clinical. New York, McGraw-Hill, 1986, pp 2109–2150.

Daher YH, Lonstein JE, Winter RB, et al: Spinal deformities in patients with arthrogryposis: A review of 16 patients. Spine 10:609, 1985.

Diamond LS, Alegado R: Perinatal fractures in arthrogryposis multiplex congenita. J Pediatr Orthop 1:189, 1981.

Sarwark JF, MacEwen GD, Scott CI Jr: Current concepts review: Amyoplasia (a common form of arthrogryposis). J Bone Joint Surg 72A:465, 1990.

Shapiro F, Specht L: Current concepts review: The diagnosis and orthopaedic treatment of childhood spinal muscular atrophy, peripheral neuropathy, Friedreich ataxia and arthrogryposis. J Bone Joint Surg 75A:1699, 1993.

Sodergard J, Ryoppy S: The knee in arthrogryposis multiplex congenita. J Pediatr Orthop 10:177, 1990.

Staheli LT, Chew DE, Elliott JS, et al: Management of hip dislocations in children with arthrogryposis. J Pediatr Orthop 7:681, 1987.
Thompson GH: Arthrogryposis multiplex congenita. Clin Orthop 194:2, 1985.

CHAPTER 632
Common Fractures

Fractures in children have been estimated to account for 10–15% of all childhood injuries. The skeletal system of children has anatomic, biomechanical, and physiologic differences from that of adults. This results in different fracture patterns, including epiphyseal fractures, problems of diagnosis, and management techniques.

The anatomic differences in the pediatric skeletal system include the presence of preosseous cartilage, physes, and a thicker, stronger, more osteogenic periosteum that produces callus more rapidly and in greater amounts. Biomechanically, the pediatric skeletal system can absorb more energy before deformation and fracture than adult bone. This has been attributed to lower mineral content and the greater porosity of young bone. The increased porosity is due to larger, more abundant haversian canals. This results in a lower modulus of elasticity and lower bending strength. As maturation occurs, the porosity decreases and the cortical bone becomes thicker and stronger.

Ligaments frequently insert into epiphyses. As a consequence, traumatic forces applied to an extremity may be transmitted to the physes. The strength of the physes is enhanced by interdigitating mamillary bodies and the perichondrial ring. However, the physes are still not as strong biomechanically as the metaphyseal or diaphyseal bone. The physis is most resistant to traction and least resistant to torsional forces. Thus, the majority of injuries to the physes are secondary to rotational and angular forces.

The thick periosteum of a child's bones is a major determinant in whether a fracture becomes displaced. The thick periosteum may also act as an impediment to closed reduction, because of the hinging phenomenon, or it may help stabilize a fracture after reduction.

FRACTURE REMODELING. Remodeling occurs by a combination of periosteal resorption and new bone formation. Thus, anatomic alignment in certain pediatric fractures is not always necessary. The major factors affecting fracture remodeling include the child's age, proximity of the fracture to a joint, and relationship of a residual deformity to the plane of the joint axis of motion. The amount of remaining growth provides the basis for remodeling: the younger the child, the greater is the remodeling potential. Fractures adjacent to a physis undergo the greatest amount of remodeling, provided the deformity is in the plane of axis of motion for that joint. Fracture remodeling will be less effective in displaced intra-articular fractures, diaphyseal fractures, malrotation, and deformity not in the plane of joint axis of motion.

OVERGROWTH. Overgrowth, especially in long bones such as the femur, is due to physeal stimulation from the hyperemia associated with fracture healing. Femoral fractures in children younger than 10 yr frequently overgrow 1–3 cm. This is the reason for bayonet apposition of bone to compensate for the overgrowth that will occur over the next 1–2 yr. After 10 yr of age, overgrowth is less of a problem and anatomic alignment is recommended.

PROGRESSIVE DEFORMITY. Injuries to the physes can result in complete or partial closure. As a consequence, angular deformity, shortening, or both can occur. The magnitude depends on the physis involved and the amount of remaining growth.

RAPID HEALING. Fractures in children heal faster than those in adults. This is due to children's growth potential and thicker, more metabolically active periosteum. As children approach adolescence and maturity, the rate of healing slows and becomes similar to that of an adults.

632.1 Pediatric Fracture Patterns

These patterns result, in part, from the anatomic, biomechanical, and physiologic characteristics of a child's skeletal system. The majority of pediatric patients can be managed by closed methods.

COMPLETE. Complete fractures are the most common type and occur when both sides of the bone are fractured. These fractures may be classified as spiral, transverse, oblique, or comminuted, depending on the direction of the fracture lines. Comminuted fractures are unusual in children.

BUCKLE, OR TORUS, FRACTURE. Compression of bone produces a buckle or torus fracture. These fractures typically occur in the metaphyseal areas in young children, especially in the distal radius. They are inherently stable and heal in 2–3 wk with simple immobilization.

GREENSTICK. When a bone is angulated beyond the limits of plastic deformation, a greenstick fracture may occur. This represents bone failure on the tension side and a plastic or bend deformity on the compression side. The energy was insufficient to result in a complete fracture.

PLASTIC DEFORMATION, OR BEND, FRACTURES. Traumatic bowing or bend deformities are due to plastic deformation of bone. The bone was angulated beyond its limit of plastic deformation, but the energy was insufficient to produce a fracture. Thus, no fracture line is visible radiographically. It is most commonly seen in the ulna and occasionally the fibula.

EPIPHYSEAL FRACTURES. Salter and Harris classified epiphyseal injuries into five groups: (1) type I, separation through the physis, usually through the zones of hypertrophic and degenerating cartilage cell columns; (2) type II, a fracture through a portion of the physis but extending through the metaphyses; (3) type III, a fracture through a portion of the physis extending through the epiphysis and into the joint; (4) type IV, a fracture across the metaphysis, physis, and epiphysis; and (5) type V, a crush injury to the physis (Fig. 632–1). This classification allows generalized prognostic information regarding the risk for premature physeal closure and the indications for treatment. Types III and IV epiphyseal fractures require anatomic alignment because of displacement of both the physis and the articular surface. Type V fractures are usually recognized in retrospect as a consequence of premature physeal closure. Types I and II fractures usually can be managed by closed reduction techniques and do not require perfect alignment. A major exception is type II fractures of the distal femur. Fractures in this location have a poor prognosis unless almost anatomic alignment is obtained by either closed or open methods.

632.2 Clavicular Fractures

Fractures involving the junction of the middle and lateral aspects of the clavicle are very common. These can be the result of birth injuries in newborns but are more typically the

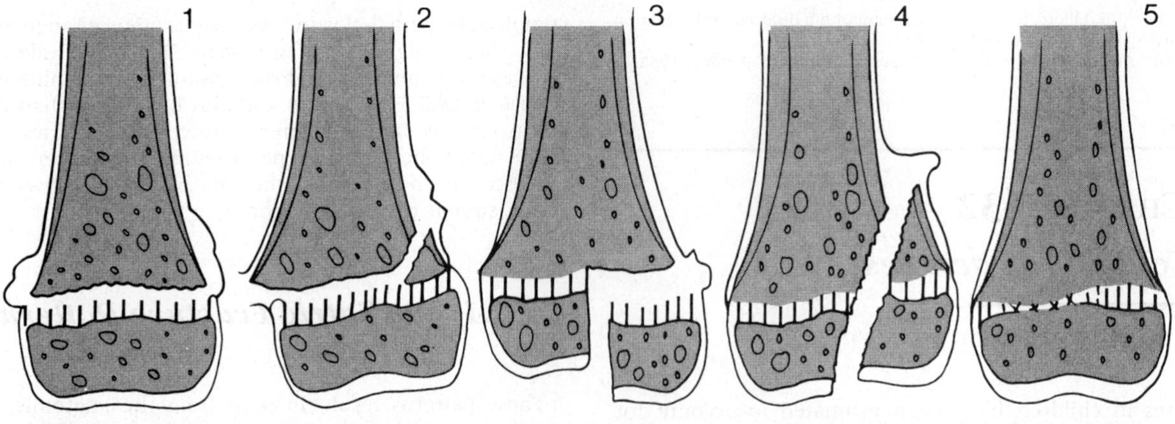

Figure 632–1. The types of growth plate injury as classified by Salter and Harris. (From Salter RB, Harris WR: Injuries involving the epiphyseal plate. J Bone Joint Surg 45A:587, 1963.)

result of a fall on the outstretched arm or a direct blow to the clavicle. These are rarely associated with a neurovascular injury. Diagnosis is easily made by physical and radiographic evaluation. Anteroposterior radiograph of the clavicle and, occasionally, a cephalic view will demonstrate the fracture. Typically, the fracture fragments are displaced and overlap 1–2 cm.

TREATMENT. The treatment of most clavicle fractures consists of an application of a figure-of-eight clavicle strap. This will extend the shoulders and minimize the amount of overlap of the fracture fragments. Rarely is anatomic alignment achieved, but this is not necessary. The fractures heal rapidly, usually in 3–6 wk. Commonly, a palpable mass of callus may be visible in thin children. This will remodel satisfactorily in 6–12 mo.

632.3 Proximal Humerus Fractures

Salter-Harris type II fractures of the proximal humerus commonly occur in children and are due to a backward fall on the involved extremity with the elbow extended. Neurovascular injuries rarely occur. Diagnosis is made from anteroposterior and lateral radiographs of the shoulder or humerus.

TREATMENT. The treatment of these fractures is usually simple immobilization. Occasionally, a closed reduction may be necessary. A significant amount of deformity can be accepted because of the remodeling potential of this region; 80% of the growth of the humerus occurs from the proximal humeral epiphysis. A sling and swath and, occasionally, a coaptation splint may be necessary to provide satisfactory immobilization and comfort. In severely displaced fractures, closed reduction with immobilization may be necessary.

632.4 Distal Radius and Ulna Fractures

Torus, or buckle, fractures of the distal radial metaphysis are among the most common fractures of childhood. These are usually the result of a simple fall on the hand with the wrist in dorsiflexion. This is an impacted fracture, and there is minimal soft tissue swelling or hemorrhage. It is not uncommon for a child to present 1–2 days later because the initial injury was felt to be only a sprain or contusion. The clinical characteristics are very nonspecific, with usually only mild tenderness to palpation directly over the fracture. Diagnosis is confirmed by anteroposterior and lateral radiographs of the wrist.

TREATMENT. Treatment of torus fractures of the distal radius and ulna is by a short-arm cast. Fractures are typically healed in 3–4 wk.

632.5 Phalangeal Fractures

Phalangeal fractures in children are usually the result of a direct blow to the finger. They are typically trapped in doors or struck by another object. If the distal phalanx is involved, there may be a subungual hematoma, which can be quite painful. This will require drainage. If the nail bed is avulsed or partially detached in association with a fracture, this is an open fracture and should be treated aggressively with irrigation, tetanus prophylaxis, and appropriate antibiotics. Occasionally, physeal involvement, especially Salter-Harris type II epiphyseal fracture, may occur. Anteroposterior and lateral radiographs of the digit will confirm the fracture.

TREATMENT. The treatment of phalangeal fractures is usually by splint immobilization. Rarely is a closed reduction necessary. However, if there is angulation or malrotation, this may need to be performed.

632.6 Toddler Fracture

Toddler fractures represent a spiral fracture of the distal one third of the tibia. These are usually the results of simple falls while running or playing. They may also occur when stepping on an object on the floor. These occur in children between 2–4 yr and, occasionally, up to 6 yr of age. Clinical features include pain, refusal to walk, minimal soft tissue swelling, a slight increase in warmth to palpation over the fracture, and pain with palpation. These fractures may not be visible radiographically on anteroposterior and lateral radiographs of the tibia. Occasionally, oblique radiographs may reveal the fractures. The fracture can be detected by a technetium bone scan, but this is rarely necessary.

TREATMENT. Application of a long-leg cast in suspected cases will relieve symptoms. Within 1–2 wk there will be radiographic evidence of subperiosteal new bone formation. These fractures are usually healed within 3–4 wk.

632.7 Lateral Malleolar Fractures

A Salter-Harris type I separation of the distal fibular epiphysis is very common in childhood. These fractures usually appear as ankle sprains. However, it must be remembered that ligaments are stronger than bone and that the epiphysis is more likely to separate than a ligament is to tear. Children will present with soft tissue swelling and pain over the lateral malleolus. Careful palpation will reveal that the bone is the site of greatest tenderness rather than the area over one of the three lateral ligaments. Anteroposterior, lateral, and mortise radiographs of the ankle will typically be normal. The diagnosis can be confirmed by stress radiographs, but this is rarely necessary.

TREATMENT. Distal fibular epiphyseal separations require immobilization in a short-leg cast for 4–6 wk. Treatment will be the same as for a severe ankle sprain. This is why stress radiographs are rarely necessary. Follow-up radiographs show subperiosteal new bone formation in the metaphyseal region of the distal fibula.

632.8 Metatarsal Fractures

Fractures of the metatarsal shaft are usually the result of direct trauma to the dorsum of the foot. Children present with a history of injury followed by soft tissue swelling and, sometimes ecchymosis. There is tenderness to palpation directly over the fracture. Diagnosis is obtained by anteroposterior and lateral radiographs of the foot.

Fractures of the tuberosity of the fifth metatarsal are also quite common. This has been termed *dancer's fracture*. It is an apophyseal avulsion from overpull of the peroneus brevis tendon. It typically occurs with the foot in an inverted position and the peroneal muscles contracting to realign the foot. The swelling, ecchymosis, and tenderness are limited to the tuberosity of the fifth metatarsal. Contraction of the peroneal musculature will also increase discomfort. The diagnosis is confirmed radiographically.

TREATMENT. Metatarsal fractures are treated by a short-leg cast for 4–6 wk. Weight bearing is allowed as tolerated. The one exception is the fifth metatarsal diaphyseal shaft fracture. This has an increased incidence of nonunion and should be treated by non-weightbearing until there is radiographic evidence of early union.

632.9 Toe Phalangeal Fractures

Fractures of the lesser toes are very common and are usually secondary to direct blows. They commonly occur when the child is barefoot. The toes will be swollen, ecchymotic, and tender. There may be a mild deformity. Diagnosis is made radiographically.

TREATMENT. The lesser toes usually do not require closed reduction unless significantly displaced. If necessary, reduction can usually be accomplished with longitudinal traction on the toe. Casting is usually not necessary. "Buddy" taping of the fractured toe to an adjacent stable toe will usually provide satisfactory alignment and relief of symptoms. Crutches may be beneficial for several days until the soft tissue swelling and discomfort decreases.

632.10 Operative Treatment

Certain pediatric fractures have better prognoses if the fractures are reduced, by either open or closed techniques, and then internally or externally stabilized (Table 632–1). Approximately 4–5% of pediatric fractures require surgery. The common indications for operative stabilization in children and adolescents with open physes include (1) displaced epiphyseal fractures, (2) displaced intra-articular fractures, (3) unstable fractures, (4) fractures in the multiply injured child, and (5) open fractures.

The principles of surgical management of pediatric fractures are distinctly different from those of mature adolescents and adults. Multiple closed reductions of an epiphyseal fracture are contraindicated because they may cause repetitive damage to the germinal cells of the physis. Anatomic alignment at surgery is mandatory, especially for displaced intra-articular and epiphyseal fractures. When internal fixation is used, it should be simple; (use of Kirschner wires, for example, which can be removed as soon as the fracture is healed.) Rigid fixation to allow immobilization of the extremity is usually not the goal but rather stability sufficient to maintain anatomic alignment with supplemental immobilization, usually a plaster cast. Last, external fixators, when used, are removed as soon as possible and cast immobilization is substituted. The latter is indicated when soft tissue problems have been corrected, when the fracture is stable, or both.

SURGICAL TECHNIQUES. Three basic surgical techniques are used in the management of pediatric fractures. *Open reduction and internal fixation* may be required for displaced epiphyseal fractures, especially Salter-Harris types III and IV fractures, intra-articular fractures, and unstable fractures, such as those involving the forearm diaphysis, spine, and ipsilateral fractures of the femur and tibia (floating knee). Other indications include neurovascular injuries requiring repair and, occasionally, open fractures of the femur and tibia. *Closed reduction and internal fixation* is indicated for specific displaced epiphyseal, intra-articular, and unstable metaphyseal and diaphyseal fractures. Common indications include supracondylar fractures of the distal humerus, phalangeal, and femoral neck fractures. Anatomic alignment must be attained by a closed reduction before this method can be used. Failure to obtain anatomic alignment is an indication for an open reduction.

The indications for *external fixation* in pediatric fractures in-

■ TABLE 632–1 Common Indications for Operative Stabilization

Indication	Location
Displaced epiphyseal fractures (usually Salter-Harris types III and IV)	Lateral condyle Radial head Phalanx Distal femur Proximal tibia Distal tibia
Displaced intra-articular fractures	Radial neck Olecranon Femoral neck Patella
Unstable fractures	Distal humerus (supracondylar) Radius-ulna diaphysis Phalanx Spine
Multiply injured child (especially with associated head and neurologic injury)	Femoral diaphysis Tibial diaphysis Pelvis Spine
Open fractures	Upper and lower extremities Severe soft tissue injury

Adapted from Thompson GH, Wilber JH, Marcus RE: Internal fixation of fractures in children and adolescents: A comparative analysis. Clin Orthop 188:10–20, 1984.

clude (1) severe grade II and grade III open fractures; (2) fractures associated with severe burn; (3) fractures with bone or extensive soft tissue loss that may require reconstructive procedures, such as free vascularized grafts, skin grafts, or other; (4) fractures requiring distractions such as those with significant bone loss; (5) unstable pelvic fractures; (6) fractures in children with associated head injuries and spasticity; and (7) fractures associated with vascular or nerve repairs or reconstruction. The advantages of external fixation include rigid mobilization of the fractures, separation of the management of the fractured limb and associated wounds, and patient mobilization for treatment of other injuries and transportation for diagnostic and therapeutic procedures. The majority of complications with external fixation are pin tract infections and refracture after pin removal.

Cramer KG, Limbird TJ, Green NE: Open fractures of the diaphysis of the lower extremity in children. J Bone Joint Surg 74A:218, 1992.
Green NE, Swiontkowski MF (eds): Skeletal Trauma in Children, Vol 3. Philadelphia, WB Saunders, 1994.
Gustilo RB, Merkow RL, Templeman D: Current concepts review: The management of open fractures. J Bone Joint Surg 72A:299, 1990.
Loder RT: Pediatric polytrauma: Orthopaedic care in hospital course. J Orthop Trauma 1:48, 1987.
Mabrey JD, Fitch RD: Plastic deformation in pediatric fractures: Mechanism and treatment. J Pediatr Orthop 9:310, 1989.
Rockwood CA Jr, Wilkens KE, King RE: *In*: Fractures in Children, 3rd ed. Philadelphia, JB Lippincott, 1990.
Salter RB, Harris WR: Injuries involving the epiphyseal plate. J Bone Joint Surg 45A:587, 1963.
Scoles PV: Pediatric Orthopaedics in Clinic Practice, 2nd ed. Chicago, Year Book, 1988.
Staheli LT: Fundamentals of Pediatric Orthopedics. New York, Raven Press, 1992.
Thompson GH: Nailing children's fractures. Perspective Orthop Surg 2:40, 1991.
Thompson GH, Wilber JH: Fracture management in the multiply injured child. *In*: Marcus RE (ed): Trauma in Children. Rockville, MD, Aspen Publishers, 1986, pp 99–146.
Tolo VT: External fixation in multiply injured children. Orthop Clin North Am 21:393, 1990.

CHAPTER 633
*Sports Medicine**

Participation in sports is important for normal development because it fosters physical fitness and overall health, provides opportunities for psychosocial development (team work, peer relations), improves decision-making abilities, and promotes self-confidence. Sports activity also provides the child with an enjoyable experience as well as an opportunity to learn some skills that can be continued throughout life. Play is sometimes referred to as the "occupation" of the child. The role of physicians is to provide health services, counseling, instruction, and rehabilitation. Physicians need to avoid unnecessary restriction of a child's play and sports activities while trying to prevent injury. Restrictions of activity should be (1) made when the need is definite; (2) made for only the shortest necessary period; and (3) tailored to the child's specific requirements. Alternatives are often appropriate. For example, swimming is often a good substitute for contact sports. The most stressful activities are those that involve competition or body contact and are supervised or promoted by adults. It is prudent to tell parents that children should be allowed normal activity when parents impose restrictions that are too stringent and confining. Alternately, parents and coaches may push the child too far (see Overuse Injuries).

*Modified from L. T. Staheli, 14th edition.

PREPARTICIPATION HEALTH EXAMINATION. The goal of this evaluation is to determine specific conditions that place the child at risk for injury or death during participation in sports. In addition, residual abnormalities of earlier athletic activity may become evident. Furthermore, because the preparticipation examination may be the only contact an adolescent athlete has with the health care provider, it provides an opportunity to perform a general health evaluation. The preparticipation examination should be performed every 3–4 yr or with changes in the level of competition (change to high school or college).

Areas of concern include *orthopedic* (knee or ankle injury, subluxing patella, chondromalacia patella, cervical spine disease, scoliosis), *cardiovascular* (heart murmur, hypertension, arrhythmia, current or repaired congenital heart disease), *pulmonary* (chronic versus exercise-induced asthma, obstructive lung disease), *anatomic* (organomegaly, absence of one of paired organs; e.g., eye, kidney, testis), *ocular* (poor vision, anisocoria), *hematologic* (sickle cell or other anemias, hemorrhagic disease), *cutaneous* (contagious infection including staphylococcal, streptococcal, herpes simplex), and *neurologic* (mental retardation, repeated head injury and concussions, seizures, syncope) problems.

Sudden death during sports may occur owing to cardiac disease such as hypertrophic or other cardiomyopathies, coronary artery disease (single or anomalous vessels, atherosclerosis), congenital heart disease (aortic stenosis), and ruptured aorta in Marfan syndrome. In many cases the underlying heart disease is not suspected, and sudden death is the first sign of heart disease. A chest roentgenogram, electrocardiogram, and echocardiogram are not recommended for screening but are indicated if there is concern about heart disease on the basis of history and physical examination.

Disqualifications and limitations for sports participation among various medical conditions are noted in Table 633–1. Classification of sports activities is further delineated in Table 633–2. Students have a legal right to participate in a sport, despite a disqualifying condition. Physicians must, nonetheless, provide complete information about the risks associated with participation in sports.

The *psychologic assessment* should determine attitudes and behaviors that would suggest the risk for burnout and overuse injuries. Burnout may be prevented by keeping sports fun, by having a proper perspective with regard to winning and losing, and by taking time out from practice and competition. Pain is often reduced by rest, rehabilitation, and avoiding a premature return to participation.

Sports injuries in young children are predominantly due to fractures, contusions, and overuse syndromes. Ligamentous injuries, especially about the knee, are very uncommon in children because the physes are weaker than the ligament and will usually separate before a ligament will tear. Thus, Salter-Harris type I injury should always be considered when there is apparent injury about a joint in which the initial radiographs are normal. Stress radiographs may be necessary to reveal the physeal separation. In adolescence, however, sports-related injuries become more similar to those of adults. Contusions, sprains, and fractures still occur, but ligament injuries about the knee increase in frequency as well as severity.

633.1 Overuse Syndromes

Overuse syndromes result from unresolved submaximum stress in previously normal tissues. Normal physiologic adaptation occurs in response to use, and a reasonable amount of

■ **TABLE 633–1 Medical Conditions and Sports Participation**

Condition	May Participate?
Atlantoaxial instability (instability of the joint between cervical vertebrae 1 and 2) *Explanation:* Athlete needs evaluation to assess risk of spinal cord injury during sports participation.	Qualified Yes
Bleeding disorder *Explanation:* Athlete needs evaluation.	Qualified Yes
Cardiovascular diseases	
Carditis (inflammation of the heart) *Explanation:* Carditis may result in sudden death with exertion.	No
Hypertension (high blood pressure) *Explanation:* Those with significant essential (unexplained) hypertension should avoid weight and power lifting, body building, and strength training. Those with secondary hypertension (hypertension caused by a previously identified disease), or severe essential hypertension, need evaluation.	Qualified Yes
Congenital heart disease (structural heart defects present at birth) *Explanation:* Those with mild forms may participate fully; those with moderate or severe forms, or who have undergone surgery, need evaluation.	Qualified Yes
Dysrhythmia (irregular heart rhythm) *Explanation:* Athlete needs evaluation because some types require therapy or make certain sports dangerous, or both.	Qualified Yes
Mitral valve prolapse (abnormal heart valve) *Explanation:* Those with symptoms (chest pain, symptoms of possible dysrhythmia) or evidence of mitral regurgitation (leaking) on physical examination need evaluation. All others may participate fully.	Qualified Yes
Heart murmur *Explanation:* If the murmur is innocent (does not indicate heart disease), full participation is permitted. Otherwise the athlete needs evaluation (see congenital heart disease and mitral valve prolapse above).	Qualified Yes
Cerebral palsy *Explanation:* Athlete needs evaluation.	Qualified Yes
Diabetes mellitus *Explanation:* All sports can be played with proper attention to diet, hydration, and insulin therapy. Particular attention is needed for activities that last 30 minutes or more.	Yes
Diarrhea *Explanation:* Unless disease is mild, no participation is permitted, because diarrhea may increase the risk of dehydration and heat illness. See "Fever" below.	Qualified No
Eating disorders Anorexia nervosa Bulimia nervosa *Explanation:* These patients need both medical and psychiatric assessment before participation.	Qualified Yes
Eyes Functionally one-eyed athlete Loss of an eye Detached retina Previous eye surgery or serious eye injury *Explanation:* A functionally one-eyed athlete has a best corrected visual acuity of <20/40 in the worse eye. These athletes would suffer significant disability if the better eye was seriously injured as would those with loss of an eye. Some athletes who have previously undergone eye surgery or had a serious eye injury may have an increased risk of injury because of weakened eye tissue. Availability of eye guards approved by the American Society for Testing Materials (ASTM) and other protective equipment may allow participation in most sports, but this must be judged on an individual basis.	Qualified Yes
Fever *Explanation:* Fever can increase cardiopulmonary effort, reduce maximum exercise capacity, make heat illness more likely, and increase orthostatic hypotension during exercise. Fever may rarely accompany myocarditis or other infections that may make exercise dangerous.	No
Heat illness, history of *Explanation:* Because of the increased likelihood of recurrence, the athlete needs individual assessment to determine the presence of predisposing conditions and to arrange a prevention strategy.	Qualified Yes
HIV infection *Explanation:* Because of the apparent minimal risk to others, all sports may be played that the state of health allows. In all athletes, skin lesions should be properly covered, and athletic personnel should use universal precautions when handling blood or body fluids with visible blood.	Yes

Table continued on following page

stress is essential for normal soft tissue function. When this systemic response is overwhelmed and an adequate time frame for stress resolution is not provided, overuse injuries occur. These are uncommon in childhood but may be seen in adolescence. The shoulder, elbow, and knee are common areas for overuse injuries, but any body area can be involved. The symptoms are typically activity-related pain that is relieved by rest. Training factors, particularly training abuses, are the most common sources of overuse. The approach to overuse syndromes is fivefold: (1) factor identification, (2) factor modification, (3) pain control, (4) progressive rehabilitation, and (5) maintenance.

633.2 Throwing Injuries

Older children who engage in throwing sports, such as baseball, are at risk for traumatic *epiphysiolysis of the proximal humeral epiphysis.* This disorder is a fatigue separation or fracture through the physis. It heals with rest and avoidance of repetitive throwing activities. Pain about the shoulder is the usual presenting complaint. It is the most severe expression of the overuse syndromes.

The elbow is especially vulnerable to throwing injuries in the

■ **TABLE 633–1 Medical Conditions and Sports Participation** *(Continued)*

Condition	May Participate?
Kidney: absence of one *Explanation:* Athlete needs individual assessment for collision/contact and limited contact sports.	Qualified Yes
Liver: enlarged *Explanation:* If the liver is acutely enlarged, participation should be avoided because of risk of rupture. If the liver is chronically enlarged, individual assessment is needed before collision/contact or limited contact sports are played.	Qualified Yes
Malignancy *Explanation:* Athlete needs individual assessment.	Qualified Yes
Musculoskeletal disorders *Explanation:* Athlete needs individual assessment.	Qualified Yes
Neurologic History of serious head or spine trauma, severe or repeated concussions, or craniotomy. *Explanation:* Athlete needs individual assessment for collision/contact or limited contact sports, and also for noncontact sports if there are deficits in judgment or cognition. Recent research supports a conservative approach to management of concussion.	Qualified Yes
Convulsive disorder, well controlled *Explanation:* Risk of convulsion during participation is minimal	Yes
Convulsive disorder, poorly controlled *Explanation:* Athlete needs individual assessment for collision/contact or limited contact sports. Avoid the following noncontact sports: archery, riflery, swimming, weight or power lifting, strength training, or sports involving heights. In these sports, occurrence of a convulsion may be a risk to self or others.	Qualified Yes
Obesity *Explanation:* Because of the risk of heat illness, obese persons need careful acclimatization and hydration.	Qualified Yes
Organ transplant recipient *Explanation:* Athlete needs individual assessment.	Qualified Yes
Ovary: absence of one *Explanation:* Risk of severe injury to the remaining ovary is minimal.	Yes
Respiratory Pulmonary compromise including cystic fibrosis *Explanation:* Athlete needs individual assessment, but generally all sports may be played if oxygenation remains satisfactory during a graded exercise test. Patients with cystic fibrosis need acclimatization and good hydration to reduce the risk of heat illness.	Qualified Yes
Asthma *Explanation:* With proper medication and education, only athletes with the most severe asthma will have to modify their participation.	Yes
Acute upper respiratory infection *Explanation:* Upper respiratory obstruction may affect pulmonary function. Athlete needs individual assessment for all but mild disease. See "Fever" above.	Qualified Yes
Sickle cell disease *Explanation:* Athlete needs individual assessment. In general, if status of the illness permits, all but high exertion, collision/contact sports may be played. Overheating, dehydration, and chilling must be avoided.	Qualified Yes
Sickle cell trait *Explanation:* It is unlikely that individuals with sickle cell trait (AS) have an increased risk of sudden death or other medical problems during athletic participation except under the most extreme conditions of heat, humidity, and possibly increased altitude. These individuals, like all athletes, should be carefully conditioned, acclimatized, and hydrated to reduce any possible risk.	Yes
Skin: boils, herpes simplex, impetigo, scabies, molluscum contagiosum *Explanation:* While the patient is contagious, participation in gymnastics with mats, martial arts, wrestling, or other collision/contact or limited contact sports is not allowed. Herpes simplex virus probably is not transmitted via mats.	Qualified Yes
Spleen, enlarged *Explanation:* Patients with acutely enlarged spleens should avoid all sports because of risk of rupture. Those with chronically enlarged spleens need individual assessment before playing collision/contact or limited contact sports.	Qualified Yes
Testicle: absent or undescended *Explanation:* Certain sports may require a protective cup.	Yes

This table is designed to be understood by medical and nonmedical personnel. In the "Explanation" section, "needs evaluation" means that a physician with appropriate knowledge and experience should assess the safety of a given sport for an athlete with the listed medical condition. Unless otherwise noted, this is because of the variability of the severity of the disease or of the risk of injury among specific sports, or both.

HIV = human immunodeficiency virus; AS = sickle cell trait.

Modified from Committee on Sports Medicine and Fitness, American Academy of Pediatrics: Medical conditions affecting sports participation. Pediatrics 1994; 94:757–758.

immature child. The most common pathologic factors result from abnormal compressive forces acting across the lateral side of the elbow or radiohumeral articulation. In addition to **Panner disease** (see Chapter 630.4), the epiphysis of the radial head may become asymmetric compared with the opposite side or may become fragmented. Some irregularities in the shape of the cartilaginous radial head are usually present. Additionally, there may be irregularity of the ossified portion of the capitellum. Before the problem becomes established or severe, the child or adolescent complains of pain about the elbow, which is generally worse after throwing than during times of rest. Clinical examination will show early loss of motion, especially supination.

TREATMENT. Children who have more advanced lesions generally have high emotional involvement in their particular sport, most commonly baseball, and nonparticipation is a difficult option for them to accept. Avoidance of pitching until the symptoms have resolved and the elbow motion becomes normal is the best solution. Often, switching the baseball player to another position allows the child to avoid pitching. Behind

■ **TABLE 633–2 Classification of Sports by Contact**

Contact/Collision	Limited Contact	Noncontact
Basketball	Baseball	Archery
Boxing*	Bicycling	Badminton
Diving	Cheerleading	Body building
Field hockey	Canoeing/kayaking	Bowling
Football	(white water)	Canoeing/kayaking
Flag	Fencing	(flat water)
Tackle	Field	Crew/rowing
Ice hockey	High jump	Curling
Lacrosse	Pole vault	Dancing
Martial arts	Floor hockey	Field
Rodeo	Gymnastics	Discus
Rugby	Handball	Javelin
Ski jumping	Horseback riding	Shot put
Soccer	Racquetball	Golf
Team handball	Skating	Orienteering
Water polo	Ice	Power lifting
Wrestling	Inline	Race walking
	Roller	Riflery
	Skiing	Rope jumping
	Cross-country	Running
	Downhill	Sailing
	Water	Scuba diving
	Softball	Strength training
	Squash	Swimming
	Ultimate Frisbee	Table tennis
	Volleyball	Tennis
	Windsurfing/surfing	Track
		Weight lifting

**Participation not recommended.*
From Committee on Sports Medicine and Fitness, American Academy of Pediatrics: Medical conditions affecting sports participation. Am Acad Pediatr 94:757, 1994.

such highly motivated youngsters is usually an overzealous parent or coach who is also in need of appropriate counseling.

633.3 Knee Problems

Medial and lateral collateral knee ligament injuries are very uncommon in children. The ligaments are stronger than the physes, and it is more common to have a Salter-Harris type I or type II fracture. The Salter-Harris type I fracture may be seen on normal radiographs. Stress views may be necessary to demonstrate the instability of the injured epiphysis.

An epiphyseal fracture requires immobilization for approximately 6 wk to allow for adequate healing of the distal femoral or proximal tibial epiphysis. If a true ligamentous injury occurs, there is a period of initial immobilization followed by mobilization in a protective knee orthosis.

Anterior cruciate ligament injuries are uncommon in childhood. There is an increasing incidence, however, as the child approaches adolescence. The ligament can be torn either within its substance or at one of its bony attachments proximally or distally. There is an increased incidence of these injuries with tibial eminence fractures. Clinical findings include a hemarthrosis and ligamentous instability. Routine anteroposterior lateral radiographs of the knee will usually be normal. A magnetic resonance image (MRI) is necessary to confirm the tear of the ligament.

The treatment of anterior cruciate ligaments is predominantly nonoperative in skeletally immature children. There is an initial period of immobilization to allow for resolution of the acute injury. Range-of-motion exercises are then instituted. Once full range of motion and strength have been regained, children may be allowed to return to normal activities. If they continue to be involved with sports, an orthosis may be beneficial to prevent additional stress to the involved ligaments. If this fails, then extra-articular surgery may be used as a temporizing method of management until they are close to skeletal maturity when the more standard adult reconstructions can be performed.

Posterior cruciate ligament injuries are rare in children. When this type of injury occurs, it is usually associated with an osteochondral fracture of the medial femoral condyle. Anteroposterior and lateral radiographs are necessary to demonstrate this fracture. An MRI may be required to demonstrate a tear within the substance of the posterior cruciate ligament. The treatment of posterior cruciate ligament injuries includes repair of the osteochondral fracture, if present. If the ligament is torn within its substance, a reconstruction is performed at maturity.

Meniscal injuries in children younger than 12 yr are uncommon. When they occur they are usually sports related. Peripheral detachments are common. Discoid meniscus should also be considered in a young child presenting with meniscus-type symptoms. These symptoms include locking, giving way, and recurrent effusions. They may have tenderness to palpation over the joint line where the meniscus has been torn or detached. There may be a positive McMurray test. Anteroposterior and lateral radiographs of the knee in a child with a meniscal tear will usually be normal. Increased widening of the joint space may be suggestive of a discoid meniscus. An MRI or arthrography may demonstrate the meniscal detachment or tear.

The treatment of meniscal injuries in children is usually operative. Repair of peripheral tears is advocated so that the function of the menisci is not sacrificed. This can be performed arthroscopically. If the meniscus is torn within its substance, a partial meniscectomy is performed. It is important to avoid total meniscectomy because the menisci play an important role in the biomechanics of the knee.

633.4 Stress Fractures

Stress (fatigue) fractures are caused by chronic repetitive muscular action on a bony insertion site or by repeated direct trauma (march fracture), usually occurring in poorly trained patients engaged in physical activities. This common overuse syndrome produces local dissolution of bone and should be distinguished from conditions in which a physiologic force acts on a site with abnormal elastic resistance (osteogenesis imperfecta, osteopetrosis, rickets, scurvy, Cushing syndrome, hyperparathyroidism, disuse, immobilization, inflammatory lesions).

Stress fractures occur in typical locations associated with specific activities: first metatarsal sesamoid—standing; metatarsal shaft—marching, running, ballet; tarsal navicular—running, high-impact aerobics; distal fibula and proximal diaphysis of the tibia—running; patella—hurdling; neck and shaft of the femur—ballet, gymnastics, running; pelvic ischial pubic rami—bowling, gymnastics; lumbar vertebral pars interarticularis—ballet, weightlifting; ribs—coughing, golf; and coronoid ulnar process and distal humerus—throwing a ball.

Clinical manifestations include limp, gradual onset of pain that is increased with activity and relieved with rest, point tenderness, distal atrophy, and local swelling. There is no fever or abnormality of the complete blood count or erythrocyte sedimentation rate. Roentgenographic findings may be normal or demonstrate a radiolucent zone without periosteal reaction, focal sclerosis, and callus formation. Bone scans or ultrasonography may be needed to identify the lesion if the results of plain roentgenograms are negative. The differential diagnosis includes osteoid osteoma, acute or chronic osteomyelitis, bone tumors, leukemia, and rickets.

Treatment includes rest, casting for complete fractures, and subsequent rehabilitation to correct muscle imbalance or anatomic variations. See Chapter 622.

SOFT TISSUE INJURIES. Most sports-related injuries are not skeletal injuries but rather are injuries of the ligaments (sprains) and muscle-tendon units (strains). Additional injuries include muscle contusions and lacerations.

Musculotendinous strains also known as pulls, tears, or ruptures are an indirect injury caused by excessive stretch from an antagonistic muscle group, external objects, gravity, or active muscle contraction. Muscle strains may occur rapidly with a single contraction and are classified as grade I (mild, microscopic muscle tear, intact fascia, local tenderness, minimal swelling, or ecchymosis), grade II (moderate, larger number of muscle fibers torn, fascia involved, a "pop" felt by athlete, small defect palpated), or grade III (severe, complete rupture, a palpable defect, severe pain, marked ecchymosis or hematoma formation, loss of function). The greater the size of the disruption (palpable defect) and the greater the ecchymosis, the more likely it is to be a grade III strain. Grade III tendon injuries do not bleed (tendons are relatively avascular), but a palpable defect is present before the onset of edema and swelling. Avulsion fractures from the point of bony tendinous insertion may occur instead of a muscle strain. Such lesions are common in muscles originating at the pelvis or femur and include rectus femoris, gluteus, sartorius, iliopsoas, adductor longus, and hamstrings.

Treatment of muscle strains includes ice and compression immediately after the injury, nonsteroidal anti-inflammatory agents for pain, very short periods of immobilization (1–2 days rest), and subsequent strengthening (passive range-of-motion and active stretching exercises during rehabilitation). To avoid reinjury, the child should not return to active participation in sports until strength training returns the muscle to normal function. Prevention of strains may be possible by warming up and stretching.

Ligamentous sprains are likely to occur in forceful activities, such as football or wrestling. Sites include the knee, ankle, wrist, shoulder, or elbow. Sprains are graded on the basis of loss of stability: grade I demonstrates overstretching, microscopic tearing without instability; grade II involves partial tearing and instability; grade III includes marked ligamentous laxity, maximal instability, and discontinuous ligaments. Grade III (severe sprains) is associated with pain, a snapping or popping sound, hemorrhage, markedly diffuse swelling that develops rapidly, immediate disability, and loss of function. The patient often has instability. Fractures or dislocations usually produce more immediate pain than a sprain; however, the nature of the pain does not always distinguish a fracture from a sprain. Treatment of sprains includes immediate anti-inflammatory therapy (see strains), protection from tension-producing injuries during the healing phase, and occasionally casting or surgery (arthroscopic or open) for grade III sprains.

Muscle contusions are common in contact sports. There is local pain, disability, swelling, hematoma formation, and potential for subsequent connective tissue scar formation. The quadriceps muscle is the most common site of contusion that is graded as grade I (mild, local tenderness, normal gait, knee range of motion greater than 90 degrees); grade II (moderate, more tenderness and swelling, limp, inability to do deep leg bends, range of motion less than 90 degrees); and grade III (severe, cannot walk unassisted, marked swelling and tenderness, range of motion less than 45 degrees).

Treatment includes ice, elevation, compression, and nonsteroidal anti-inflammatory agents during the acute phase, followed by range-of-motion, stretching, and strengthening exercises. Massage is not recommended, and the serious nature of the injury should not be made trivial, because **myositis ossificans** is a common sequela to grade II–III contusions. The ossification of the intramuscular hematoma occurs mainly in adolescent patients, appears 2–4 wk after the injury, increases in size until 6 mo later, and manifests as continued pain and stiffness. Surgical excision is usually not indicated unless pain persists for more than 1 yr.

633.5 Specific Sports and Associated Injuries

GYMNASTICS. Competitive female gymnasts often begin the sport at 6 yr of age, achieve high-level competition at 16 yr of age, and retire at 18–20 yr of age. A similar activity pattern occurs in males at 9, 22, and 24–26 yr of age. In addition to mechanical or traumatic injuries, female gymnasts have delayed menarche and often have eating disorders.

Common problems include traumatic and overuse injuries, such as ankle sprain and wrist and spine injuries. The incidence of injury increases with the level of skill and is most common in the floor exercise. Wrist pain may be due to chronic upper extremity weightbearing with distal radial physeal trauma. Ligamentous laxity may predispose to elbow or shoulder dislocation and ankle sprains. Spine problems include acute traumatic or overuse injuries such as pars interarticularis injury, resulting in spondylolysis and spondylolisthesis. Therapy includes rest, immobilization, nonsteroidal anti-inflammatory agents, and, if pain persists, MRI or arthroscopic examination to rule out intra-articular tears, loose bodies, or ligamentous instability. Prevention includes wrist strengthening, flexibility exercises, and an ulnar variance brace.

SWIMMING. Shoulder injury is the most common overuse injury of competitive swimmers. *Swimmer shoulder* is rotation cuff tendinitis of the supraspinatus or biceps and manifests as shoulder pain and tenderness of the supraspinatus tendon. The onset may be insidious. Supraspinatus tendinitis produces pain with active abduction between 60 and 100 degrees, whereas biceps tendinitis is demonstrated by resisting flexion of a straight supinated arm. Treatment includes ice, modification of stroke technique, rest, stretching, muscle strengthening, physiotherapy, and nonsteroidal anti-inflammatory agents. Prevention includes avoiding overwork, proper technique, and strengthening and stretching exercises.

BASEBALL. Throwing injuries of the elbow and shoulder (especially among pitchers) are the most common baseball injuries. See Chapter 633.2.

BALLET. This very demanding activity is associated with delayed menarche and eating disorders in female dancers. Foot problems include metatarsal stress fractures, subungual hematomas, callus, sesamoiditis, bunion formation, proximal phalangeal epiphysitis, and accessory navicular pain syndrome. Ankle problems include inversion sprains, anterior and posterior impingement syndromes, and osteochondritis dessicans of the talus. Leg problems include shin splints, tibial or fibular stress fracture, and compartment syndromes (see Running). Knee problems include Osgood-Schlatter disease, excessive recurvatum owing to lax ligaments (pseudo-genu varum), osteochondritis dessicans, and patellar malalignment (subluxation dislocation) owing to lax ligaments (see Chapter 633.3). Hip problems include the medial **snapping hip syndrome** caused by iliopsoas tendon riding over the anterior hip capsule, tendinitis (pyriformis, iliopsoas, rectus femoris), and subclinical slipped capital femoral epiphysis, usually seen in male dancers. Spine problems include associated Scheuermann disease in males, idiopathic scoliosis in females, and purposeful excessive lumbar lordosis.

WRESTLING. Wrestlers have great fluctuations in weight to meet weight-matched competition standards. Such fluctuations are associated with fasting, dehydration, and then binging.

Wrestling holds may produce injury by various torques or forces applied to the extremities and spine; wrestling throws with subsequent falls may produce concussions, neck strain, or spinal cord injury. "Stingers" and "burners" are neurogenic pain syndromes seen with traumatic stretching or pinching of the bracheal plexus (see Football). Severe electric-like pain starts with impact and radiates from the shoulders to the fingertips. There is numbness, weakness (predominantly of the abductor deltoid muscles), and tenderness over the paraspinous and trapezius muscles, lasting a few seconds to 5 min. Treatment includes ice, nonsteroidal anti-inflammatory agents, strengthening exercises, and, if severe, oral steroids, cervical collar for 24–48 hr, and transcutaneous electrical nerve stimulation.

Shoulder subluxation is common but does not usually present with only pain and weakness. Patients are usually aware of their shoulders slipping in and out. See Chapter 630.2. Hand injuries are usually not severe and include recurrent metacarpophalangeal and proximal interphalangeal sprains. Treatment of hand injuries includes splinting and taping.

Knee injuries are common and potentially serious and include prepatellar bursitis, medial and lateral sprains, and medial and lateral meniscus tears. See Chapter 633.3. Prepatellar bursitis is the most common knee problem, is caused by a traumatic forceful impact to the mat or chronic trauma, and demonstrates swelling over the knee and no limitation of motion except full flexion. Treatment includes protective neoprene knee sleeves, nonsteroidal anti-inflammatory agents, steroid application, aspiration of effusions, and bursectomy after the third recurrence.

Dermatologic problems include herpes simplex (herpes gladiatorum), impetigo, staphylococcus furunculosis or folliculitis, superficial fungal infections, and contact dermatitis.

FOOTBALL. Football injuries are common, in part owing to the popularity of the sport. Fortunately, most injuries are minor because the incidence of serious injuries has been reduced by prohibition of clipping blocks and "spearing" or head-butting tackling, improvement of techniques, equipment (pads, shoes with wider, more, shorter cleats, helmet), pre-season conditioning (strength and flexibility training), ankle taping, proper rehabilitation of injuries, and playing on grass rather than artificial surfaces.

Head and neck football injuries include concussion, neck sprain, and brachial plexus trauma ("stinger," "burner," see Wrestling) and often are unreported because athletes expect these problems. "Burners" represent a brachial plexus neurapraxia, possibly owing to lateral neck bending, manifesting without neck pain but with painful arm dysesthesia and deltoid muscle weakness. They are usually transient with immediate recovery. Cervical collars (neck rolls) may reduce the risks of this injury.

Lumbar spine injury manifest as low back pain probably represents spondylolysis. Shoulder trauma includes instability, rotator cuff, and tendinitis injury to the proximal humerus, shaft, and clavicular articulation. Rest, immobilization, and nonsteroidal anti-inflammatory agents may be effective therapies for mild shoulder injuries. Repeated shoulder subluxation requires strengthening exercises, bracing, and possible surgical stabilization in the off-season.

Contusions to the arm and thigh muscles are common, may produce knee effusions, and are at risk for the development of **myositis ossificans.**

Knee injuries are common reasons why a player seeks medical attention and include anterior cruciate (ACL), posterior cruciate (PCL), and collateral ligament tears. See Chapter 633.3. Functional hinged-knee bracing for ACL injuries reduces the number of "giving-out" episodes and may improve performance. PCL injuries are usually isolated and respond to routine rehabilitation, whereas medial collateral ligament sprains are common, cause temporary disability, and may be rehabilitated with a brace.

Ankle sprains are frequent problems among football players and may be prevented by ankle taping or by reusable straps and supports. **Turf toe,** an injury to the first metatarsophalangeal joint (usually of the great toe), is caused by forceful dorsiflexion while playing on artificial turf in soft, lightweight, flexible shoes. Treatment of turf toe includes ice, nonsteroidal anti-inflammatory agents, compression, and rest. Corticosteroid injections are not beneficial.

HOCKEY. Hockey is a collision sport associated with injuries caused by the puck and the stick, producing contusions, lacerations, or concussions or by the players' bodies, the ice, and the boards, producing fractures, sprains, or concussions. The risk for injury is reduced by proper equipment (helmets with face masks) and rules regarding dangerous body contact (checking from behind, high sticking).

Specific hockey injuries include ankle sprains (dorsiflexion, eversion, and external rotation in contrast to usual sprain of inversion in other sports), hip adductor strain, and various shoulder injuries from body contact. The latter include acromioclavicular sprain, dislocation, and clavicular fractures.

BASKETBALL AND VOLLEYBALL. Common physical activities of these two sports include shooting, jumping, pivoting, running, and sudden stopping, which increase the risks for ankle, knee, and finger injury.

Knee overuse injuries include patellar tendinitis ("jumper knee"), traction apophysitis (Osgood-Schlatter disease), physeal fractures of the distal femur and proximal tibia, fracture of the patella, and ligament sprains (medial collateral with or without anterior cruciate ligaments).

Ankle sprain is the most common injury and is usually caused by inversion with plantar flexion placing the lateral ligaments at high tension. An avulsion fracture of the base of the fifth metatarsal at the insertion of the peroneus brevis tendon is another sequela of inversion ankle injuries. **Achilles tendinitis** is overuse injury, which may be exacerbated by rubbing of the tendon over high-top shoes. Foot pain may be due to retrocalcaneal bursitis, posterior tibial tendinitis, accessory tarsal navicular, calcaneal periostitis, plantar fasciitis, stress fracture of the tarsal navicular, Jones stress fracture of the fifth metatarsal, sesamoiditis, blisters, subungual hematoma, and paronychia.

RUNNING. Running problems are due to either overuse (chronic repetitive motion) injury exacerbated by muscle imbalance, minor skeletal deformity, or poor flexibility or overload trauma from repeated poorly absorbed foot impact that ranges from three to eight times the child's body weight. Most problems are seen as the child increases the distance or intensity of training. Minor variations (e.g., malalignment) in anatomy, which do not cause problems at rest, predispose to injury at specific sites (patellofemoral stress, overpronation). Muscle fatigue, environmental temperature, and running surface (grass vs unyielding concrete) also contribute to injuries. Prevention of injuries is possible by using good-quality running shoes without excessive sole wear, stretching, muscle-strengthening exercises, varying the running surface, cross-training (bicycling, swimming), and rest.

Iliac crest apophysitis produces pelvic pain and is probably caused by repeated microscopic stress fractures. Stress fractures may occur on the femoral neck, inferior pubic rami, subtrochanteric area, proximal femoral shaft, proximal tibia, fibula, navicular, metatarsal, sesamoid, and calcaneal apophysitis.

Muscle strains frequently affect the hamstrings followed by the quadriceps, adductors, soleus, and gastrocnemius muscles. Tendinitis involving the tendon and its sheath is commonly seen in the Achilles tendon followed by the posterior tibial, peroneal, iliopsoas, and proximal hamstring tendons. Achilles tendinitis develops chronically; initially may get better during a run; manifests tenderness and crepitance if acute and nodularity if chronic; and must be distinguished from a retrocalcaneal bursitis. Treatment includes temporary abstinence from running (begin cross-training), a ½-in heel lift, heel cord stretching, and nonsteroidal anti-inflammatory agents. Steroid injection is not needed.

Anterior knee pain is usually due to patellofemoral stress syndrome (runners' knee), which results from excessive dynamic, usually lateral, motion of the patellar tendon in relationship to the femoral intracondylar groove. Chondromalacia patellae may develop. Treatment includes stretching, quadriceps-strengthening exercises, and foot orthotics. Posterior knee pain is caused by gastrocnemius strain, whereas posteromedial pain is due to proximal tibial stress fractures or semimembranosus tendinitis and lateral knee pain may be due to iliotibial band syndrome and popliteus tendinitis. **Iliotibial band syndrome** may be a combination of a bursitis and tendinitis owing to mechanical friction of the band (an extension of the tensor fasciae latae) and the lateral femoral epicondyle.

Shin splints is a descriptive term for pain over the anterior tibia and should be distinguished from tibial stress fractures and chronic compartment syndromes. Shin splints may be due to chronic fatigue tearing of collagenous fibers that connect muscle to bone. Bone scans may show diffuse uptake compared with the more focal area noted with stress fractures. Shin splints have diffuse areas of tibial tenderness involving bone and muscle, whereas stress fractures demonstrate point tenderness. Shin splints usually occur in new runners with overpronation. Treatment includes running on soft surfaces, shoe orthotics, nonsteroidal anti-inflammatory agents, and rest (or cross-training).

Compartment syndromes involving the anterior, lateral, deep posterior, or superficial posterior may be induced by running, and they produce local pain confined to the muscle (not to the bone). During exercise muscles gradually expand and if entrapped in unyielding fascia will result eventually in increased intracompartment pressure. Pain usually prevents further training, thus limiting the risk of permanent nerve damage.

Plantar fasciitis is an inflammation of the supporting structure of the longitudinal arch owing to repetitive cyclic loading with foot strike. Pain increases with running and is located on the medial aspect of the heel. Treatment is similar to that for shin splints.

SOCCER. Injuries in soccer include abrasions, contusions, muscle strains, and ligament sprains (ankle, knee) owing partly to body-to-body contact, falls, running, and the kicking or heading motion.

Hip problems include the "hip pointer" (iliac crest contusion), iliac crest apophysitis, and chronic groin pain (muscle strain, hernia, osteitis pubis). Femoral neck stress fractures, slipped femoral capital epiphysis, and avulsion fractures of the pelvis or femur may also cause hip pain.

Knee problems include injuries to the medial collateral ligament, anterior collateral ligament, and the menisci. Additional problems are similar to those in the section on running.

TENNIS. Common areas of injury in tennis include muscle and tendon problems of the elbow, shoulder, back, and abdomen. The risk for injury is increased by personal physical deficiencies (muscle imbalance, malalignment), prior injury, and poor technique. Acute injuries include ankle sprains, abdominal or leg muscle strains, and knee problems (patellofemoral syndrome, menisci); overuse injuries include tendinitis (shoulder, elbow, patellar, Achilles, plantar fascia) and apophysitis (elbow, knee, or calcis).

Shoulder tendinitis is caused by rotation cuff and biceps tendon inflammation. Subluxation of the glenohumeral joint may also be present.

Lateral tennis elbow tendinitis produces pain on backhand shots and tenderness over the extensor brevis origin. Medial elbow tendinitis manifests pain at the medial epicondyle with wrist flexion and forearm pronation. Medial epicondylar apophysitis is noted in young tennis players and may be associated with ulnar nerve dysfunction if there is an avulsion fracture. Olecranon apophysitis is similar to Osgood-Schlatter disease and manifests pain at the olecranon with elbow extension.

Wrist problems include dorsal ganglion, radiocarpal joint capsular (impingement) synovitis, and degenerative attrition (tears) of the triangular fibrocartilage.

Basic treatment includes rest, nonsteroidal anti-inflammatory agents, ice, compression (acute phase), rehabilitation, learning proper mechanics, protective counterforce bracing (elbow, wrist), strengthening exercises, and gradual return to tennis. Surgery is rarely needed but is indicated for rotator cuff tendinitis (subluxation), patellofemoral or meniscal injury, and capitellar osteochondritis.

SKIING. Injuries are related to falls (contusion, lacerations) and ski-specific mechanisms. Overall injuries have declined owing partly to better equipment (boots, bindings, poles) and slope conditions.

Thumb injuries resulting from falls with the thumb in abduction and hyperextension produce a sprain of the ulnar collateral ligament (skier thumb). Complete tears with a 45 degree joint opening require surgical intervention, whereas smaller degrees may be treated with a thumb spica cast for 4 wk. A Salter-Harris type III fracture may also be present, and if the epiphyseal fracture is displaced it requires open reduction and internal fixation.

Lower extremity injuries include ankle sprains (less common in good boots), fractures (often spiral) of the tibia ("boot top") and ankle, and ACL sprains with or without tibial eminence fracture. Hemarthrosis is present in severe ACL sprain. Treatment of ACL sprains includes bracing, intra-articular reconstruction, and closed or open anatomic reduction of a tibial eminence fracture fragment.

Committee on Sports Medicine and Fitness: Cardiac dysrhythmias and sports. Pediatrics 95:786, 1995.
Micheli LJ: Overuse injuries in children's sports: The growth factor. Orthop Clin North Am 14:337, 1983.
Sullivan JA: Ligament injuries of the knee in children. Clin Orthop 225:44, 1990.
Sullivan JA, Grana WA (eds): The Pediatric Athlete. Park Ridge, IL, American Academy of Orthopaedic Surgeons, 1988.
Wiley JJ, Baxter MP: Tibial spine fractures in children. Clin Orthop 255:54, 1990.

SECTION 2

Genetic Skeletal Dysplasias*

Bryan D. Hall

CHAPTER 634

Diagnosis and Assessment

Skeletal dysplasia infers generalized involvement of epiphyses, metaphyses, or diaphyses, which is usually associated with disproportionate short stature before and/or after birth. Individuals with disproportionate shortness have a dwarfing condition, while proportionately short persons have nanism or, if severely short, are termed midgets in lay terms. Except for some phenocopies produced by drugs (e.g., warfarin) or vitamin deficiencies (e.g., vitamin K), all skeletal dysplasias appear to have a genetic basis. As a group or category of disorders, skeletal dysplasias are common, occurring with a birth prevalence of 1 in 4,100. There is a high rate of stillborns (23%) and early postnatal death (32%), indicating an acute need for correct diagnosis and appropriate intervention strategies. Many skeletal dysplasias can be diagnosed in the early prenatal period by ultrasonography, biochemical assays, and molecular techniques, indicating the potential for effective obstetric management and informed parental decisionmaking. Because almost half of the children born with a skeletal dysplasia survive beyond the neonatal period and have the potential for a relatively normal life span, the long-term medical and social problems need specialized attention to minimize unnecessary adverse effects.

An immediate or early accurate diagnosis is critical for individuals with skeletal dysplasias in order to optimally handle the numerous inherent ramifications (Table 634–1). This section focuses on categorization and diagnosis of skeletal dysplasias with discussion of associated complications, therapies, and genetic issues where pertinent. Because the skeletal radiographs are pathognomic for each skeletal dysplasia, emphasis will be placed on categorizing the sum of the radiologic abnormalities. The same will be done for associated anomalies when present (Table 634–2). No attempt will be made in the discussion or tables to be all inclusive because there are over 300 known bone dysplasias. In some cases the discussion and tables represent the most common situations and entities, while in other instances they are just good examples.

RECOGNITION OF DISPROPORTION AND SHORTNESS. Except for lethal neonatal bone dysplasias, the early recognition of disproportion may not be as obvious as it would seem. Generally, the term *disproportion* infers a discrepancy in limb length to trunk length or vice versa. In bone dysplasia segments of the limb often may be shorter than other segments of the same limb. For instance, if the proximal limb (e.g., humerus, femur) is more shortened, this is called *rhizomelia.* If the middle portion of the limb (e.g., radius/ulna, tibia/fibula) is shorter, then the descriptive term would be *mesomelia.* When the distal limb (e.g., hands, feet) is more involved than its companion segments, the term *acromelia* is used. Some disproportionate dwarfing conditions are known as rhizomelic, mesomelic, or acromelic forms. Asymmetric limb shortening can occasionally be seen, particularly in the rhizomelic form of chondrodysplasia punctata and in multiple exostosis.

Disproportional shortening of the limbs can be suspected if the limbs, when extended down the lateral side of the trunk,

*Modified from David O. Sillence in 14th edition.

TABLE 634–1 Major Problems Associated with Skeletal Dysplasias

Problem	Example
Lethality*	Thanatophoric dysplasia
Associated anomalies†	Ellis–van Creveld syndrome
Short stature	Spondyloepiphyseal dysp. congenita
Cervical spine dislocations	Larsen syndrome
Severe limb bowing	Metaphyseal dysp. type Schmid
Spine curvatures	Metatrophic dysplasia
Club feet	Diastrophic dysplasia
Fractures	Osteogenesis imperfecta
Pneumonias/aspirations	Camptomelic dysplasia
Hydrocephalus	Achondroplasia
Joint problems (hips, knees)	Most skeletal dysplasias
Hearing loss	Common (greatest with cleft palate)
Myopia/cataracts	Stickler syndrome
Immune deficiency‡	Cartilage-hair hypoplasia
Mental retardation	Hypochondroplasia (some)
Sudden infant death syndrome	Achondroplasia
Poor body image	Variable, but common to all
Sex reversal	Camptomelic dysplasia

dysp., dysplasia.
**Mostly due to severely reduced size of thorax.*
†See Table 634–2.
‡At least four additional disorders, all involving the metaphyses, can have immunodeficiency.

TABLE 634–2 Associated Anomalies in Skeletal Dysplasias

Anomaly	Example
Heart defects	Ellis–van Creveld syndrome
Polydactyly	Short rib-polydactyly, Majewski type
Cleft palate	Diastrophic dysplasia
Ear cysts	Diastrophic dysplasia
Hydrocephalus	Achondroplasia
Encephalocele	Dyssegmental dysplasia
Hemivertebrae	Dyssegmental dysplasia
Micrognathia	Campomelic dysplasia
Nail dysplasia	Ellis–van Creveld syndrome
Conical teeth/oliogodontia	Ellis–van Creveld syndrome
Multiple oral frenulae	Ellis–van Creveld syndrome
Dentinogenesis imperfecta	Osteogenesis imperfecta
Pretibial skin dimples	Camptomelic dysplasia
Cataracts/retinal detachment	Stickler syndrome
Intestinal atresia	Saldino-Noonan
Renal cysts	Saldino-Noonan
Campodactyly	Diastrophic dysplasia
Craniosynostosis	Thanatophoric dysplasia
Ichthyosis	Chondrodystrophica punctata
Hitchhiker thumb	Diastrophic dysplasia
Facial hemangioma	Many severe dwarfing conditions
Sparse scalp hair	Cartilage-hair hypoplasia
Hypertelorism	Robinow syndrome
Hypoplastic nasal bridge	Acrodysostosis
Clavicular agenesis	Cleidocranial dysplasia
Genital hypoplasia	Robinow syndrome
Tail	Metatropic dysplasia
Omphalocele	Beemer-Langer
Blue sclera	Osteogenesis imperfecta

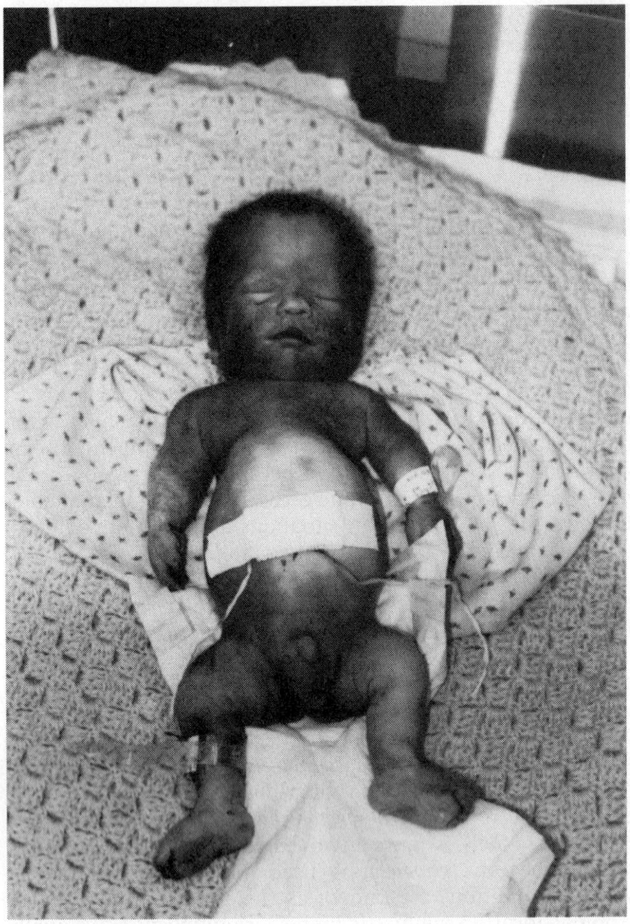

Figure 634–1. Stillborn with thanatophoric dysplasia. Limbs are very short with upper limbs extending only two thirds of the way down the abdomen. The chest is hypoplastic, making the abdomen look protuberant. The head is relatively large.

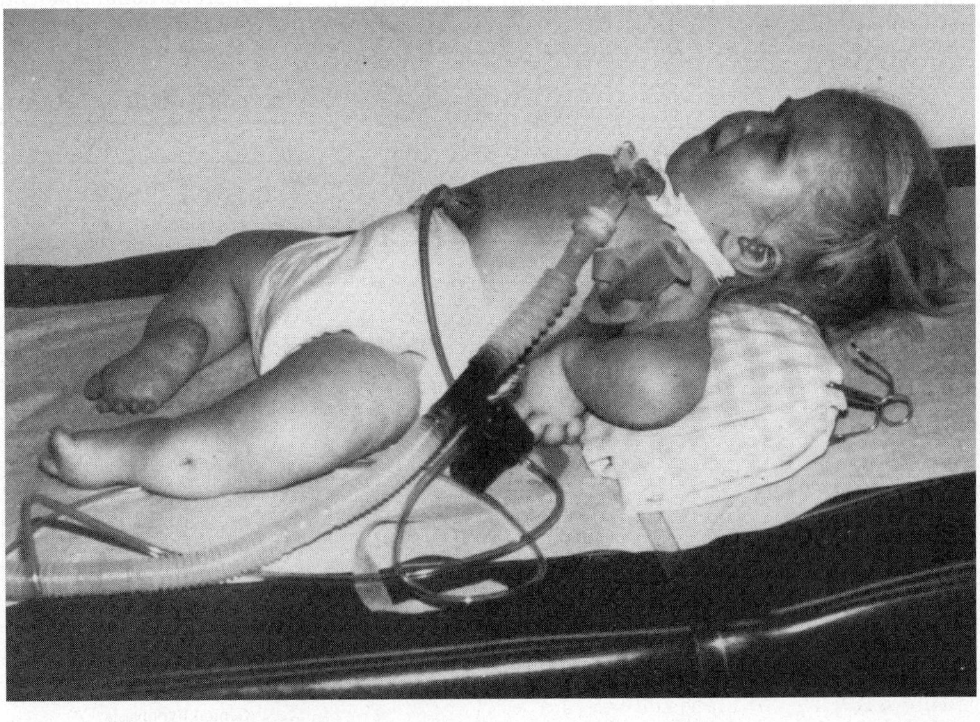

Figure 634–2. Long-term survivor with camptomelic dysplasia who is on a respirator because of dislocation of hypoplastic cervical vertebrae. She has a flat face, micrognathia, and bowed short limbs. The pretibial skin dimple is located at the sharpest convexity of the bowed tibia.

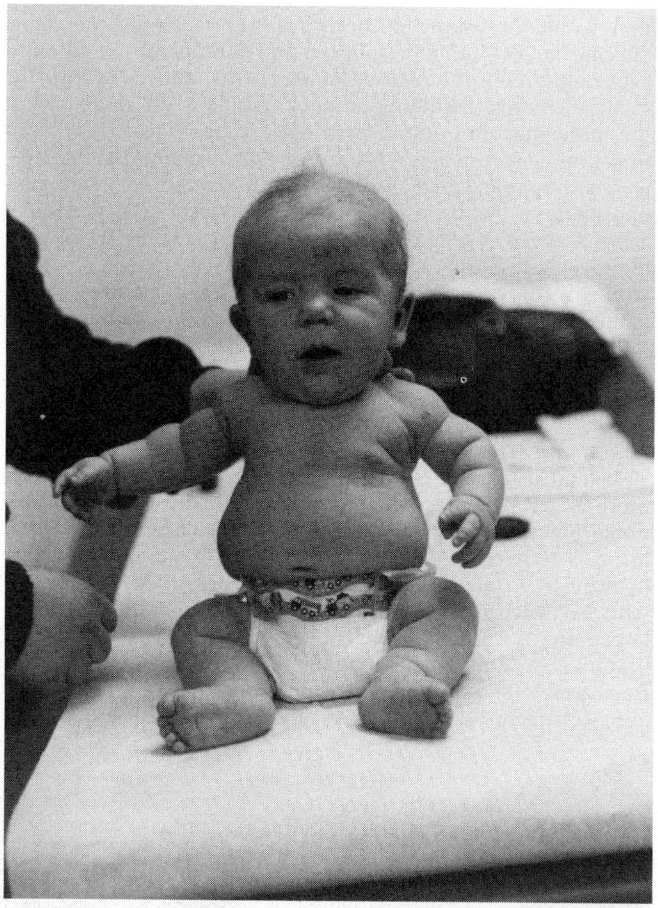

Figure 634–3. Infant with achondroplasia. The cranium is large and the forehead prominent. The nasal bridge is moderately flat and the chest is small compared with the abdomen. Note medial arm and forearm creases, which reflect bowing at the sharpest concavity of the limbs.

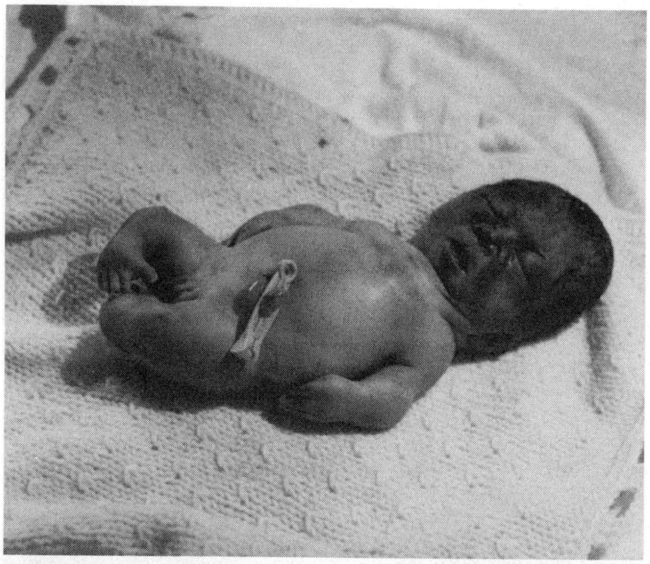

Figure 634–4. Stillborn with dyssegmental dysplasia. Besides the very short, bowed limbs, small chest, micrognathia, and redundant neck skin, note the single raised prominences on each knee. These are caused by fibular points secondary to greater than 90 degree bending.

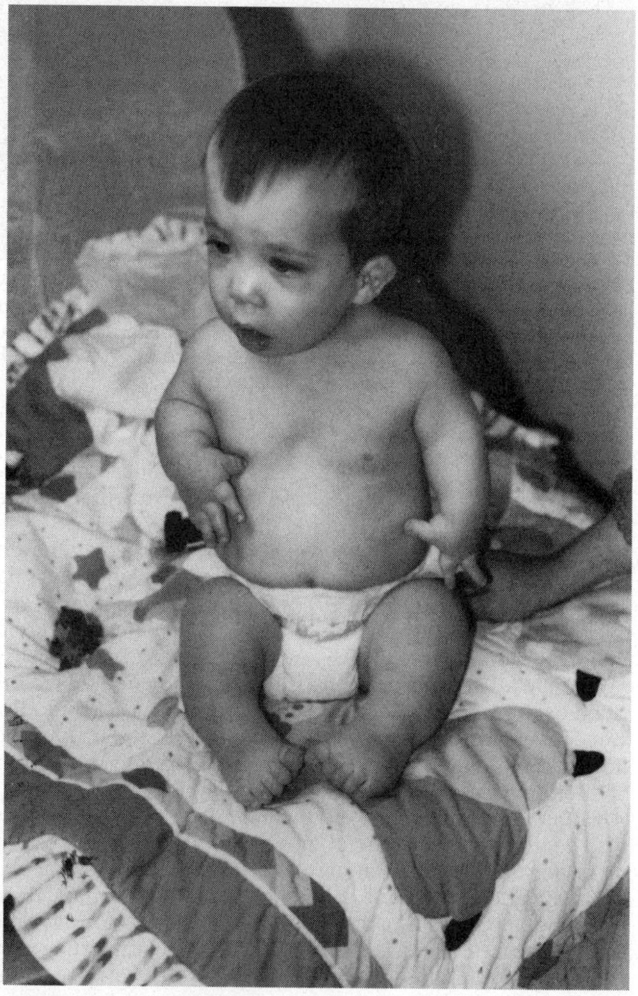

Figure 634–5. Toddler with diastrophic dysplasia. Note the left ear with multiple cystic swellings. These are only found in diastrophic dysplasia and can be congenital or develop in the first 3 mo of life. The low-placed "hitchhiker" thumbs are typical for this disorder.

do not reach midpelvis in infancy or the upper thigh after infancy (Fig. 634–1). Fat or edematous infants may artificially look disproportionate because their limbs are pushed laterally and upward by the extra upper arm and axillary bulk. If the trunk is short, the chest often appears small and/or the abdomen appears relatively protuberant (Fig. 634–1). Disproportion normally infers reduced body length or height; however, absolute measurements may not be less than the 3rd percentile for a number of months or years after birth despite the presence of disproportion. Additionally, in some bone dysplasias both the trunk and limbs are abnormally short. This usually occurs in the more severe disorders in terms of severe shortness or lethality. When the spine is disproportionate and the limbs normal or only mildly short, the upper limbs may extend well down the thigh.

ADDITIONAL FEATURES. Once disproportion has been established, the next step is to identify additional features. These features may be in the form of secondary effects of the bone dysplasia, such as bowing, medial skin creases on bowed limbs, skin dimples in the pretibial region (Fig. 634–2), club feet, macrocephaly/prominent forehead (Fig. 634–3), large anterior fontanel, craniotabes, joint prominence, protuberances around the joints (Fig. 634–4), restricted/excessive joint movement, dislocation, fractures, and clinodactyly or camptodactyly. If the child with skeletal dysplasia has only secondary effects (deformations), then he or she is considered to have a *pure skeletal dysplasia*. Excellent examples would be achondroplasia (see Fig. 634–3) and hypochondroplasia.

Primary defects (e.g., anomalies) can also be particularly

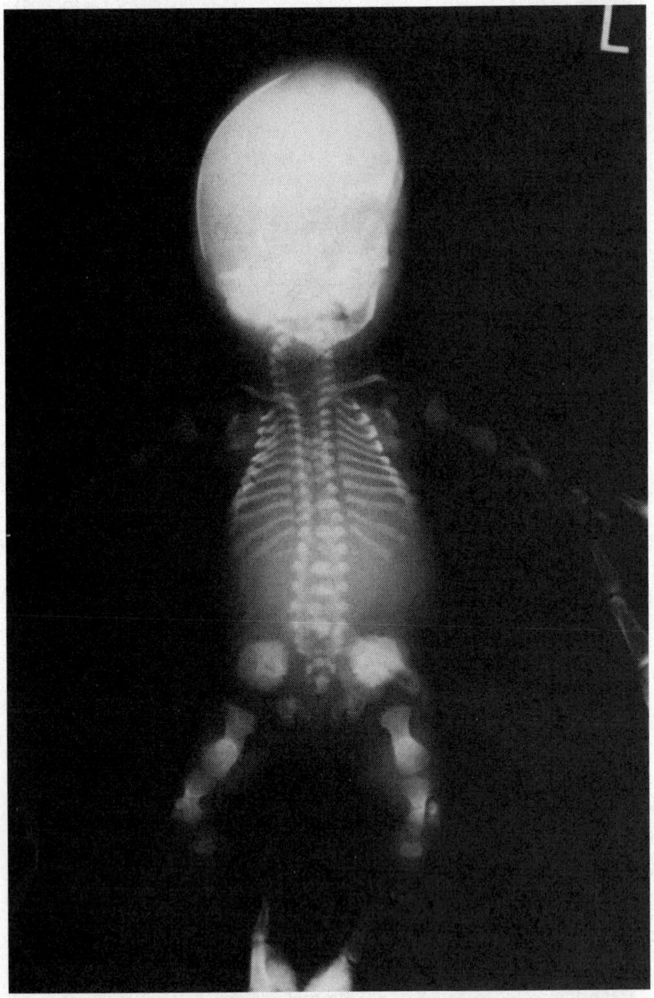

Figure 634–6. Radiograph of stillborn in Figure 634–4 with dyssegmental dysplasia. Note irregular massive dyssegmentation of vertebral bodies, which is typical for this disorder. The fibulae are sharply angulated, and all long bones are short with wide metaphyses. The iliac bones are almost square.

useful to recognize because their pattern and uniqueness should immediately raise the possibility of a particular skeletal dysplasia. Good examples would be cystic ears (Fig. 634–5), cleft palate, polydactyly, hemivertebrae (Fig. 634–6), and encephalocele. The combination of a generalized skeletal dysplasia with anomalies is categorized as a *skeletal dysplasia/multiple congenital anomaly* (SD/MCA) syndrome. When mental retardation is present along with the anomalies and skeletal dysplasia (SD/MCA/MR), this further narrows the differential diagnosis. Good examples of SD/MCA are diastrophic dysplasia and Ellis–van Creveld syndrome, while SD/MCA/MR disorders are typified by camptomelic dysplasia (see Fig. 634–2) and some forms of chondrodysplasia punctata.

HISTORY. The family history, including the patient's history, may be the single most useful source of information in evaluating a person with skeletal dysplasia. The earlier it is obtained in the diagnostic sequence, the more useful it becomes. However, the appropriate family members are often not available at the time the child is seen. This is particularly true when the neonate presents with a lethal form of dwarfism and is transferred to a tertiary center. Nevertheless, tenacious pursuit of the available facts is important, because almost all skeletal dysplasias have a genetic basis. The most pertinent question to ask is whether there are relatives with the same type of shortness and/or features as those of propositus. A follow-up question would be asking if there are "short" family members. Specific details should be solicited and photographs at different ages requested if the relative cannot be examined. Eventually, medical records (including autopsy results) and radiographs of the individuals in question will need to be reviewed. It is not uncommon for inexperienced physicians to confuse thanatophoric dysplasia (see Fig. 634–1) with achondroplasia, hypophosphatasia with osteogenesis imperfecta (Fig. 634–7), achondrogenesis (Fig. 634–8) with a macerated fetus with hydrocephalus, and campomelic dysplasia (see Fig. 634–2) with arthrogryposis (see Chapter 631). The diagnosis in the relatives should be verified by examination and radiographs.

Fetal loss, stillbirths, and other abnormal pregnancy outcomes may be cryptic clues to some type of skeletal dysplasia. The presence or absence of consanguinity should be established, as many skeletal dysplasias are autosomal recessive in inheritance. The pregnancy history may raise the suspicion of a skeletal dysplasia. Polyhydramnios, increased or decreased uterine size, and decreased fetal activity are frequent gestational events in skeletal dysplasias, particularly in the lethal forms. Polyhydramnios may or may not be accompanied by hydrops (see Chapter 80). Often, polyhydramnios is associated with excessive maternal weight gain and a paradoxically enlarged uterus in the presence of a small fetus. Without polyhydramnios, a small uterus may accurately reflect a small fetus. Decreased fetal movement may be secondary to a small uterus, joint contractures, dislocations, and/or fractures. Drug expo-

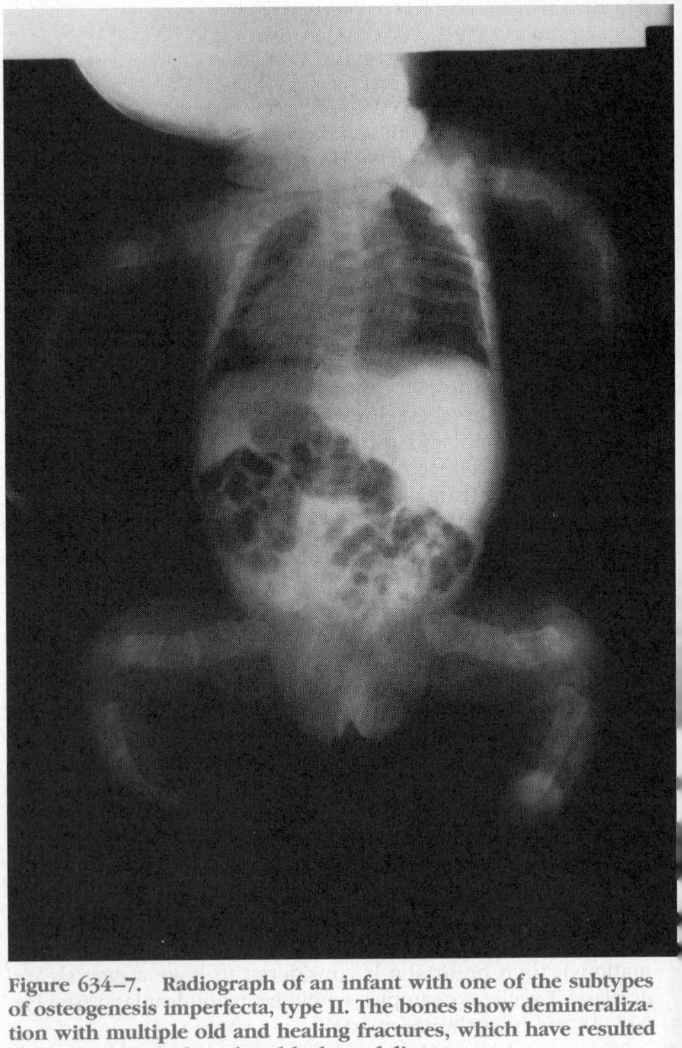

Figure 634–7. Radiograph of an infant with one of the subtypes of osteogenesis imperfecta, type II. The bones show demineralization with multiple old and healing fractures, which have resulted in bones that are broad and lack modeling.

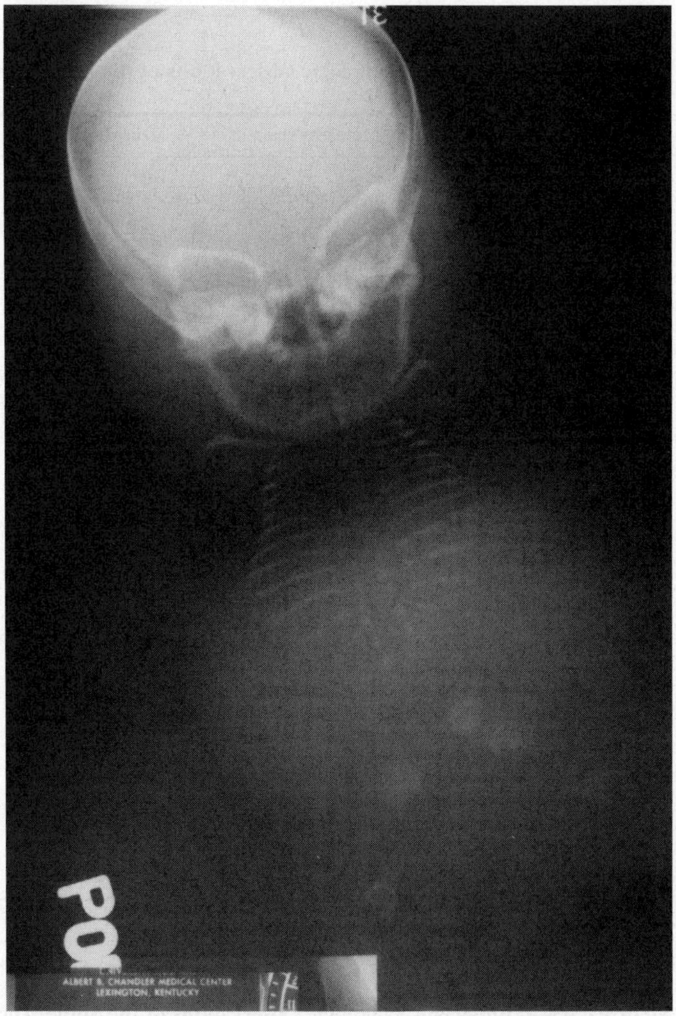

Figure 634–8. Stillborn with achondrogenesis whose radiographs show no ossification of vertebral bodies, which is almost pathognomonic for the various forms of this lethal disorder. Note small chest with reasonably formed ribs, extreme long bone shortening, and hypoplastic iliac bones.

sure in the mother is important to document because maternal warfarin (Coumadin) intake can result in clinical and osseous findings typical of chondrodysplasia punctata.

GENETICS AND ETIOLOGY. Pedigree analysis has established inheritance patterns for most skeletal dysplasias except those sporadic lethal cases that probably represent new dominant mutations. Gonadal mosaicism for a dominant gene (e.g., achondroplasia) has resulted in a normal parent having multiple offspring with a dominant skeletal dysplasia. This complicates genetic counseling and working out the genetics of rare skeletal dysplasias. The gene for diastrophic dysplasia is localized to the distal end of the long arm of chromosome 5, achondroplasia on the short arm of chromosome 4, and multiple epiphyseal dysplasia on the pericentromeric region of chromosome 19. Two X-linked disorders (X-linked recessive chondrodysplasia punctata Xp22.31 and Christian syndrome Xq27-qter) have also been localized.

How genes cause osseous abnormalities prenatally and/or postnatally is not well understood. Osteogenesis imperfecta

■ TABLE 634–3 Categorical Designation of Bone Dysplasias with General Involvement

Area Involved	Categorical Designation	Additional Area	Expanded Designation
Epiphyses	Epiphyseal dysplasia (multiple)*	Spine	Spondyloepiphyseal dysplasia
Metaphyses	Metaphyseal dysplasia	Spine	Spondylo-metaphyseal dysplasia
		Cranium	Craniometaphyseal dysplasia
		Forehead	Frontometaphyseal dysplasia
Diaphyses	Diaphyseal dysplasia	Spine	Spondylodiaphyseal dysplasia
		Cranium	Craniodiaphyseal dysplasia
Spine	Spondylo (brachyolmia)	Epiphyses† + metaphyses	Spondylo-epimetaphyseal dysplasia
		Metaphyses† + epiphyses	Spondylometaepiphyseal dysplasia

*Often called multiple epiphyseal dysplasia.
†Used first if it is more severely involved than other physes.

■ TABLE 634–4 Categorical Designation of More Localized* Features Found in Bone Dysplasias

Area Involved	Categorical Designation	Terms Used
Hand/foot only	Acro-	Acromelia, peripheral dysostosis
Hand/foot plus	Acro-	Acrodysostosis, acromicric, acromesomelia
Middle limb segment	Meso-	Mesomelia
Proximal limb segment	Rhizo-	Rhizomelia

*While terms are created based on localized areas of involvement, most patients will have more distant osseous involvement, necessitating expanding the categorical terms to fit the specific pattern.

■ TABLE 634–5 Important Radiologic Observations of the Epiphyses, Metaphyses, Diaphyses, Long Bones, and Hands in Skeletal Dysplasias

Epiphyses	Metaphyses	Diaphyses	Long Bones	Hands
Presence/absence	*Width*	*Width*	*Width*	*Carpals*
Size	Increased (flared)	Increased	Increased (broad)	Number
Small	*Configuration*	Decreased	Decreased (thin)	Increased
Large	Irregular border	*Cortex*	*Length*	Decreased
Configuration	Cupped	Thickened	Decreased	Bone age
Flat	Spurs (lateral)		Total bone	Fusions
Irregular	Hooks		Localized	*Metacarpals*
Hypoplastic	*Angulation*		(e.g., short femoral	Number
Ossification	Medial		neck)	Length
Sclerotic	(as in distal		*Bowing*	Width
Stippled	radius)		Specific bones	Configuration
Coned (digits)	*Growths*		Location	*Phalanges*
	Exostosis		Degree	Presence
	Hemangiomas		*Shortest segment*	Increased number
	Enchondromatosis		Humerus/femur	Polydactyly
			rhizomelia	Decreased number
			Radius/ulna mesomelia	Oligodactyly
			Tibia/fibula mesomelia	Length
			Hands/feet acromelia	Decreased
			Ossification	Brachydactyly
			Decreased (fractures)	Wide/short
			Increased (hyperostosis)	*Configuration*
			Anomalies	Epiphyses
			Cysts	Flat
			Absent bone	Coned
			Deficiencies	Metaphyses
			Tubulation	Wide
			Overtubulated	Cupped
			Undertubulated	Overall phalanx
				Square
				Bullet shape
				Tubular
				Fusions
				Joint symphalangism

■ TABLE 634–6 Important Radiologic Observations of the Spine, Thorax, Pelvis, and Skull in Skeletal Dysplasias

Spine	Thorax	Pelvis	Skull	Miscellaneous
Length	*Size*	*Configuration*	*Size*	*Clavicle*
Normal	Small	Square	Large	Absent
Short	Short	Narrow	Small	Hypoplastic
Curvature	*Configuration*	*Ilium*	*Configuration*	Straight
Scoliosis	Triangular	Wings	Scaphocephaly	*Scapulae*
Kyphosis	Tubular	Flared	Dolicocephaly	Absent
Lordosis	Flared lower costal margin	Base	Acrocephaly	Hypoplastic
Vertebrae	Prominent	Short	Brachycephaly	*Mandible*
Size	Pectus carinatum	Narrow	*Fontanels*	Small
Hypoplastic	Pectus excavatum	Acetabulum	Open	Large
Height	*Ribs*	Irregular	Widely	Prognathic
Short (platy)	Short	Flat	Closed	Cysts
Tall	Broad	Hypoplastic	Synostosis	*Joints*
Configuration	Hypoplastic	Borders	*Ossification*	Dislocations
Triangular	Thin	Irregular	Increased	Contractures
Ovoid	Ends	Horns	Hyperostosis	
Square	Cupped	*Pubic bones*	Decreased	
Rectangular	Wide	Hypoplastic	Thin calvarium	
Margins	Ossification	Widely spaced	Wormian bones	
Beaked	Decreased		*Calvarial defects*	
Concave	Increased		Lacunae	
Convex	Fractures		Parietal foramina	
Humped	Absent		Localized agenesis	
Segmentation	Bifid			
Hemivertebra				
Dys-segmentation				
Clefts (coronal)				
Ossification				
Reduced				
Dense				
Pedicles				
Present				
Spacing				

■ **TABLE 634–7 Diagnostic Worksheet for Skeletal Dysplasias**

Step I:	Family, gestational, and patient history (information may enter worksheet sequence at any point)
Step II:	Recognition of reduced length/height (some skeletal dysplasias may not show this initially)
Step III:	Recognition of disproportion
Step IV:	Which body areas are short? (limbs, trunk, both)
Step V:	Specific body segments short? (limbs = proximal, middle, distal; trunk = thorax, neck, entire trunk)
Step VI:	Associated anomalies?
Step VII:	Radiologic features A. Categorical designation Physes Spine Other body areas B. Descriptors (localized) Physes Spine Other body areas
Step VIII:	Overall categorization Plus descriptor pattern Plus anomalies if present
Step IX:	Pattern recognition (match)

(OI), particularly lethal type II forms, has been shown to have defects in the structure of type I collagen, with specific amino acid substitutions documented. Type II collagen abnormalities have been found in some instances of spondyloepiphyseal dysplasia congenita, achondrogenesis type II, hypochondrogenesis, Stickler syndrome, and Kniest dysplasia. Prenatal diagnosis has been accomplished in a few instances.

RADIOLOGIC FEATURES. If the patient is disproportionately short and no anomalies are present, it is tentatively assumed that the child represents a *pure bone dysplasia*. This assumption could change if radiologic studies show internal anomalies as in dyssegmental dysplasia when no cleft palate is present (see Fig. 634–6). When external anomalies such as cleft lip or polydactyly are noted, then the child would be categorized as having a *skeletal dysplasia/multiple congenital anomaly syndrome*.

The radiologic films should be reviewed to determine whether the epiphyses, metaphyses, or diaphyses are primarily involved. Table 634–3 illustrates the categorical designation for each physeal area affected. If additional osseous body areas such as the spine, cranium, or forehead (fronto-) are involved, then an expanded designation can be applied. The spine is included with the physeal areas and as an additional area because it is often associated with both. More localized abnormalities of the limbs, such as the hand, forearm, or arm, are designated as listed in Table 634–4. Very rare combinations, such as spondylocostal and spondylocarportarsal, cannot be listed in this scheme and may be more closely related to bone dysostoses.

There are a multitude of descriptors for abnormalities of the physes, long bones, hands, spine, thorax, pelvis, and skull. A reasonable representation of these are listed in Tables 634–5 and 634–6. These descriptors, when combined with accurate categorization, represent the finesse factor toward the ultimate diagnosis because their individual defects and combined pattern identify a unique set of features.

DIAGNOSIS. Table 634–7 presents a worksheet for the sequential approach to the diagnosis of skeletal dysplasias. Pediatricians should be able to accurately document items in steps I–VII including step VII A (categorical designation). Step VII B (descriptors), describing the subtleties of radiologic abnormalities, usually requires consultation with a radiologist. It is suggested that physicians, once at step VII B, note the osseous defects in their own terminology and go on to step VIII, which is the final overall categorization. The categorical designation (e.g., spondyloepiphyseal dysplasia) arrived at in step VII A can be used to search literature sources for a differential diagnosis.* Diagnosticians can then compare the descriptors (step VII B) noted in their patients with ones found in disorders under the same categoric designation. If anomalies are present, this frequently makes the ultimate diagnosis easier. Step IX represents pattern recognition as determined from the overall categorization plus descriptor pattern and anomalies, if any. This is the point at which the final match or diagnosis may be determined. Bone dysplasias can vary in severity and do frequently change with age, which complicates the diagnostic process. Nevertheless, the osseous pattern is usually pathognomonic for each bone dysplasia, making the radiologic features very helpful.

*Books that are particularly useful in helping to diagnose skeletal dysplasias are indicated under Resources in the reference list. There is also a computer diagnostic program from the Murdoch Institute in Parkville, Australia, called OSSUM that is specifically designed for skeletal dysplasias. All cases of skeletal dysplasias without a secure diagnosis should be reviewed by a specialist in skeletal dysplasias.

CHAPTER 635
Pseudoachondroplasia

Figure 635–1 is a worksheet that illustrates the above-mentioned approach (see Chapter 634) in a patient who had carried the diagnosis of Morquio syndrome throughout his life. There are four types of pseudoachondroplasia, which are usually classified as spondylometa-epiphyseal dysplasia. The patient's pattern best fits type 3 pseudoachondroplasia, which is an autosomal dominantly inherited form described by Maroteaux and Lamy. The diagnosis is based on spine abnormalities of platyspondyly (flat vertebral bodies) and vertebral body anterior beaking/tonguing (Fig. 635–2), short bowed limbs with very wide metaphyses and poorly formed epiphyses (Fig. 635–3), severe generalized brachydactyly with ballooning of distal metacarpals (Fig. 635–4), short ilial base and thick ribs in the presence of bowed limbs, very short stature, and the absence of anomalies.

It should be noted that the diagnostic term *pseudoachondroplasia* does not represent a categorical designation. The name originated solely because of its peripheral similarity to achondroplasia, which is actually a spondylometaphyseal dysplasia. Many skeletal dysplasias have names that offer little explanation of what the specific osseous findings are (e.g., Dyggve-Melchior-Clausen) or what categorical designation they represent (e.g., hypochondrogenesis, achondrogenesis, diastrophic dysplasia). Some names attempt to define which bones are involved, such as omodysplasia (omo = humerus), or characteristics of bone, such as opsimodysplasia (opsimos = late/delayed maturation). Although crude sounding, snail-like pelvis (schneckenbecken dysplasia), boomerang radius/femur (boomerang dysplasia), and wrenchlike proximal femur (Desbuquois syndrome, Fig. 635–5) can be very specific descriptive features that quickly lead to a diagnosis. The diagnostician will have to deal with these permutations of nosology. Nevertheless, the ultimate diagnoses are best served by accurately categorizing the patient and then making comparisons using whatever descriptors, anomalies, or other idiosyncrasies may be present.

Family history: Negative

Presence of reduced length/height noted: Height, 117 cm

Recognition of association with disproportion: Positive

<u>Body area with greatest shortness</u>

Long bones (limbs) ------------------ + + + +

Hands ------------------ + + +

Trunk (spine) ------------------ +

<u>Shortest body area with a relatively shorter portion</u>

Long bones: proximal + + +, middle segments + + +

Hands: phalanges + + + +, metacarpals (−), carpals (−)

Trunk: thorax +, neck + +, lumbar region + + +

Identification of any secondary effects: Negative
(deformations)

Identification of any primary defects: Negative
(malformations)

General categorization based on clinical and radiologic findings:

<u>Pure skeletal dysplasia</u>

Roentgenographic examination of entire skeleton:

Epiphyses, metaphyses, and spine involved

* *Final categorization: spondylo-meta-epiphyseal dysplasia*

Diagnosis (presumptive): pseudoachondroplastic dysplasia, **Type III*

*Dr. Bryan D. Hall's suggested diagnosis.

Figure 635–1. Worksheet for unknown skeletal dysplasia. (Provided by Drs. deKremer, Concel, and Guelbart, Cordoba, Argentina.)

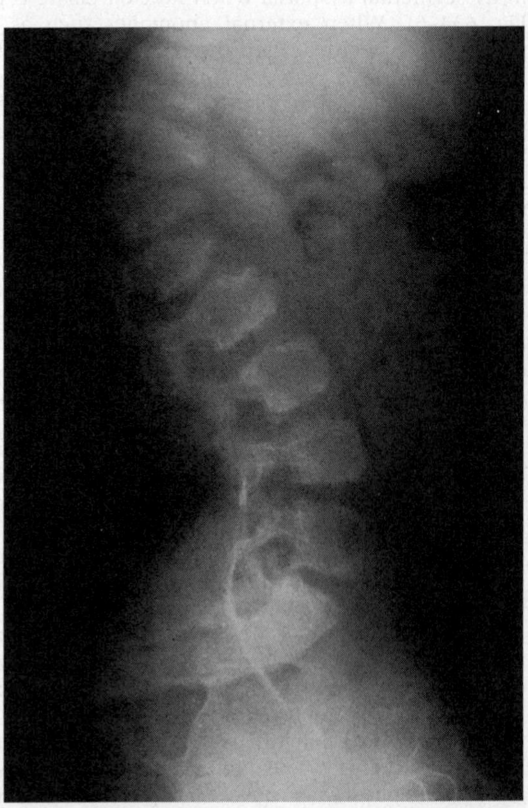

Figure 635–2. Lateral thoracolumbar spine radiograph of Argentinian patient showing central protrusion (tonguing) of the anterior aspect of upper lumbar and lower thoracic vertebrae in pseudoachondroplasia. Note reduced vertebral heights (platyspondyly) and secondary lordosis.

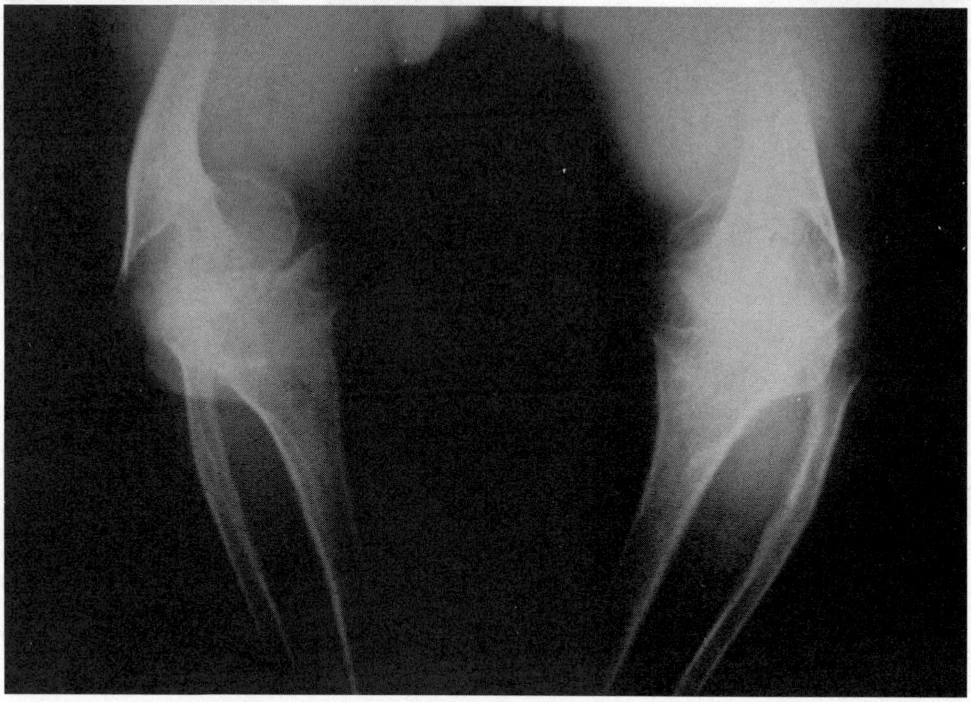

Figure 635–3. Lower extremity radiograph of Argentinian patient with pseudoachondroplasia showing large metaphyses, poorly formed epiphyses, and marked bowing of the long bones.

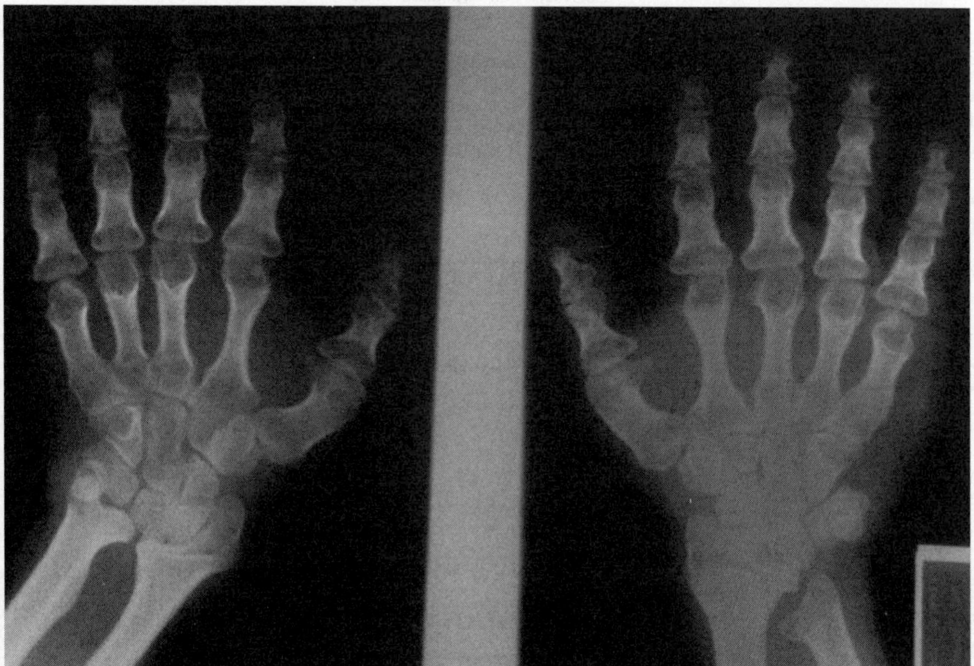

Figure 635–4. Radiograph of the hands of the Argentinian patient with pseudoachondroplasia showing shortening of all phalanges (brachydactyly) plus balloon expansion of distal metacarpal metaphyses. All metacarpal bones are short (brachymetacarpy). Note wide distal radius and ulnar metaphyses with secondary diagonal angulation, which tends to make the wrist joints prominent.

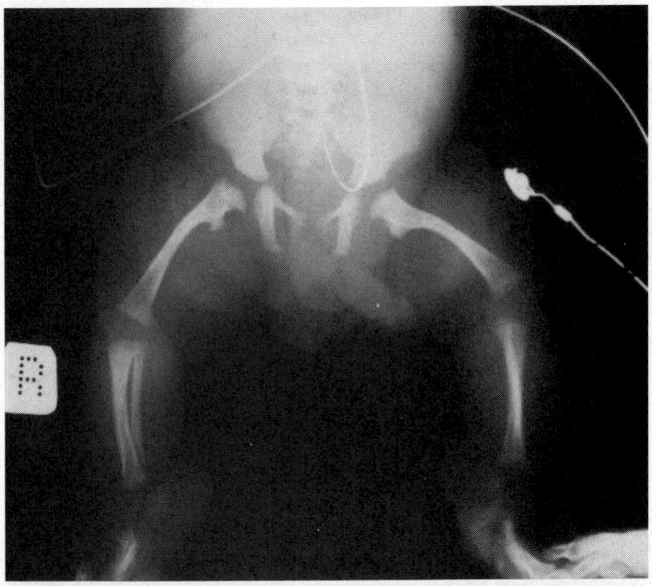

Figure 635–5. Radiograph of newborn with Desbuquois syndrome, a lethal autosomal recessive disorder. Note unique wrenchlike configuration of proximal femurs.

CHAPTER 636

Lethal and Nonlethal Bone Dysplasias

A problem in using the categorical approach exclusively is that some of the "always" or "usually" lethal bone dysplasias (Table 636–1) have such severe distortion of all their physeal areas that no accurate categorization using the epiphyses, metaphyses, or diaphyses is possible. In such instances, more attention is directed to the general bone configuration, the degree of involvement, and what areas are not involved.

Bone dysplasias that are recognizable at birth but are not generally lethal (Table 636–2) can ordinarily be more accurately categorized. For other bone dysplasias (Table 636–3), the disproportion and reduced length/height is not present or recognized until later in life, and radiographs may not be abnormal or specific. This is particularly a problem for some of the storage disorders such as the mucopolysaccharidoses (see Chapter 74). It is beneficial to repeat a skeletal survey every 6 mo during the 1st yr of life, yearly between 1–3 yr, and every 3 yr thereafter until puberty is completed in any patient who has a skeletal dysplasia that is unrecognized. Changes seen over time allow for better categorization, often through clarification of descriptors that could not be accurately identified earlier.

■ **TABLE 636–1 Lethal Neonatal Dwarfism**

Always/Usually Fatal*
Achondrogenesis
Thanatophoric dwarfism
Short rib-polydactyly, Majewski type
Short rib-polydactyly, Saldino-Noonan type
Homozygous achondroplasia
Osteopetrosis (congenital form)
Camptomelic dysplasia
Dys-segmental dysplasia, Silverman-Handmaker type
Osteogenesis imperfecta, type II
Hypophosphatasia (congenital form)
Chondrodysplasia punctata (rhizomelic form)
Often Fatal
Thoracic dystrophy (Jeune syndrome)
Occasionally Fatal
Ellis–van Creveld syndrome
Diastrophic dysplasia
Metatropic dwarfism
Kniest dysplasia

**A few prolonged survivors have been reported in most of these disorders.*

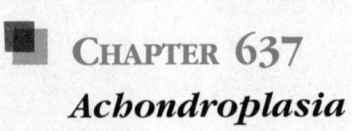

■ **TABLE 636–2 Usually Nonlethal Dwarfing Conditions Recognizable at Birth or Within First Few Months of Life**

Most Common
Achondroplasia
Hypochondroplasia
Osteogenesis imperfecta (types I, III, IV)
Spondyloepiphyseal dysplasia congenita
Diastrophic dysplasia
Ellis–van Creveld syndrome
Less Common
Chondrodysplasia punctata (some forms)
Kniest dysplasia (not severe congenital forms)
Metatrophic dysplasia
Langer mesomelic dysplasia

■ **TABLE 636–3 Late Onset/Recognized Dwarfing Conditions**

Predominantly Epiphyseal Abnormalities
Multiple epiphyseal dysplasia, Fairbank type
Multiple epiphyseal dysplasia, Ribbing type
Miscellaneous multiple epiphyseal disorders
Predominantly Metaphyseal Abnormalities
Metaphyseal dysplasia, Schmid type
Metaphyseal dysplasia, Jansen type
Cartilage-hair hypoplasia
Hypophosphatasia (nonlethal forms)
Vitamin D–resistant rickets
Predominantly Spine Abnormalities
Spondyloepiphyseal dysplasia tarda
Pseudoachondroplasia
Spondylometaphyseal dysplasia, Kozlowski type
Predominant Involvement of Single Geographic Sites
Dyschondrosteosis of Leri-Weil (Madelung deformity)
Pseudo-/pseudo-pseudohypoparathyroidism
Acrodysostosis
Peripheral dysostosis
Abnormal (Increased) Bone Density Disorders
Craniometaphyseal dysplasia
Craniodiaphyseal dysplasia
Osteopetrosis (later onset forms)
Pyknodysostosis
Storage Disorders
Mucopolysaccharidoses

CHAPTER 637

Achondroplasia

The classic or prototypic dwarfing condition is achondroplasia with an incidence of 1 in 15,000 to 1 in 27,000. It is a pure skeletal dysplasia inherited in an autosomal dominant fashion (Fig. 637–1) representing a spondylometaphyseal dysplasia.

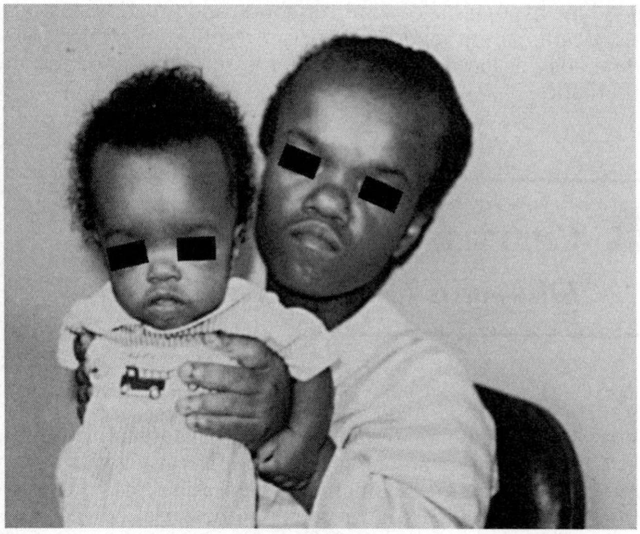

Figure 637–1. Mother and infant son with achondroplasia. Particularly note macrocephaly with a wide, prominent forehead and a flat nasal bridge. The mother's relative prognathic mandible is typical for individuals with achondroplasia as they get older. A flat midface accentuates the prognathism.

CLINICAL MANIFESTATIONS. The trunk and limbs are short. The limbs are bowed and the proximal limb segment is shorter (rhizomelia). The cranium is usually greater than the 97th percentile in circumference with frontal bossing, and the nasal bridge is flat. There is usually moderate brachydactyly with wide hands and resembling a trident consisting of the thumb, the 2nd and 3rd digits, and the 4th and 5th digits, with a wedge-shaped gap separating the 3rd and 4th fingers. The trident appearance is usually lost in late childhood or adolescence, with the hand remaining short and broad. The elbows may be limited in extension and pronation. A lumbar gibbus is common in infancy, but after the 1st yr this almost always disappears and is replaced frequently by a straight back, invariably with a prominent lumbar lordosis.

Achondroplastic infants are often hypotonic with delayed motor development. Normal neuromuscular tone is usually gained by 2–3 yr of age. Joint laxity, particularly in the interphalangeal joints, may persist throughout childhood. In the absence of hydrocephalus, mental and motor development are usually normal. A Denver developmental profile has been compiled for monitoring developmental progress in achondroplasia.

The head is large throughout life, with prominent frontal bossing, hypoplasia of the maxilla, and relative mandibular prognathism. Specific growth curves for achondroplasia have been developed, which are particularly valuable in monitoring the rapid growth in head size in infancy because hydrocephalus may complicate achondroplasia.

Dental malocclusion with anterior open bite is common and should be managed by an orthodontist who is familiar with the problem of achondroplasia. High frequencies of recurrent otitis media and chronic serous otitis media are found in these children and lead to a high incidence of conductive hearing loss in adulthood if not recognized and treated in childhood. Sleep apnea owing to obstructive or central apnea should be sought for, investigated, and treated if present. Sudden infant or early childhood death has been reported in some cases secondary to cervical cord compression due to a small foramen magnum.

ROENTGENOGRAPHIC MANIFESTATIONS. Roentgenograms show a short pelvis with broad iliac wings, horizontal acetabular roofs, and narrow, deep sacrosciatic notches. The vertebral interpedicular distance diminishes from L1 to L5, in contrast to the normal caudal widening; this is a distinctive feature of achondroplasia, although it may not be apparent in the newborn. The disk spaces are increased at the expense of the vertebral bodies, and the spinal canal is narrowed. There may be anterior tonguing and wedging of a lower thoracic or upper lumbar vertebra. There is posterior scalloping of the lumbar vertebrae; the pedicles appear short on lateral view. The base of the skull is shortened, and the foramen magnum is small and irregular. The cranium is large relative to the face, with frontal prominence and maxillary hypoplasia. The long bones are decreased in length, particularly in proximal limb segments, and appear rather wide and squat. The metaphyses have some flaring and may appear V-shaped (circumflex sign). There is relative overgrowth of the fibulas. The short tubular bones of the hands and feet are shorter and wider than normal; the shortening is greatest in the phalanges. The chest has a decreased anterioposterior diameter, with anterior cupping of the ribs.

TREATMENT. Achondroplasia may be complicated by *hydrocephalus,* which results from obstruction of the foramen magnum, and by lumbar cord and nerve root compression syndromes, dental malocclusion, hearing impairment from repeated otitis media, and strabismus (resulting from craniofacial dysmorphism). *Bowing of the legs* and persistent *kyphosis* may also require attention. Besides the prompt recognition and appropriate treatment of these problems, management during childhood will be concerned mainly with the social and psychologic effects of severe short stature and unusual appearance, and with genetic counseling. Prompt and appropriate therapy is particularly necessary for each episode of *acute otitis media.* Hydrocephalus is not common but must be recognized as early as possible. There is some evidence that physiotherapy and bracing during childhood can ameliorate the complications of prolonged infantile kyphosis or of the severe lordosis that may aggravate lumbar stenosis in adult life. Osteotomies may be indicated just prior to or during adolescence to correct severe progressive leg bowing.

PROGNOSIS. Except for the rare patient with hydrocephalus or with severe complications of cervical or lumbar spinal cord compression, the life span in achondroplasia is normal. The mean adult height in achondroplasia is about 131.5 cm (51.8 in) in men and 125 cm (49.2 in) in women.

CHAPTER 638

Thanatophoric Dysplasia

This "always" lethal neonatal dwarfing condition (see Fig. 634–1) has had a few survivors beyond the 1st yr of life. It is the most common (1 in 16,000 births) of the lethal dwarfing conditions. The head is large compared to the body, which often causes diagnostic confusion with achondroplasia. Moderately short bowed limbs, a severely small thorax, a mildly flat nasal bridge, and brachydactyly are also characteristic. The radiologic features include wafer-thin vertebral bodies (e.g., severe platyspondyly), a banana-like contour to the femoral head, metaphyseal flaring, marginal spicules, cupping, and square hypoplastic iliac bones with acetabular spurs (Fig. 638–1). An occasional patient has had multiple congenital suture fusions resulting in a kleeblattschadel (cloverleaf) skull contour. The genetics are not completely understood; a few sibling pairs exist among mostly sporadic cases.

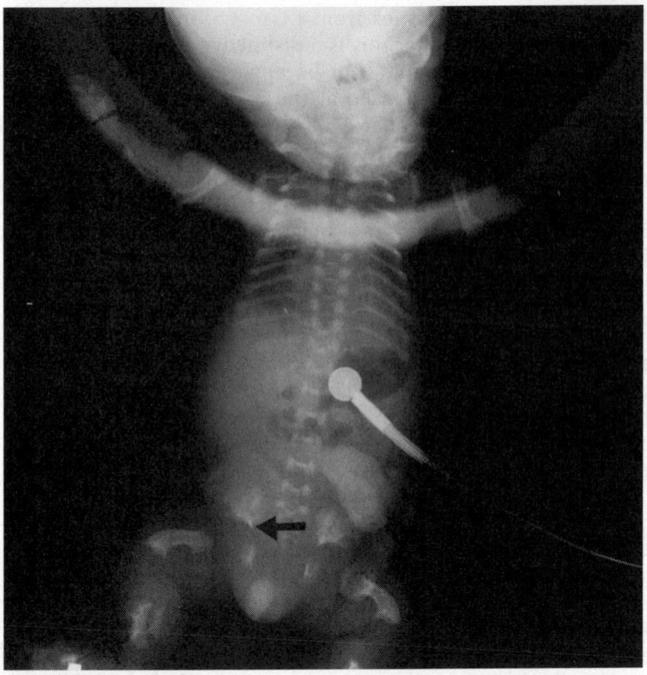

Figure 638–1. Neonatal radiograph of a child with thanatophoric dysplasia. Note medial acetabular spurs *(black arrow)*, hypoplastic iliac bones, bowed femora with rounded protrusion of proximal femurs, hypoplastic thorax, and wafer-thin vertebral bodies.

CHAPTER 639
Diastrophic Dysplasia

The term *diastrophic* means twisted, for example, scoliosis, a condition that occurs after infancy in patients with diastrophic dysplasia. At birth these infants are not generally in respiratory distress. They have short bowed limbs with club feet, knee contractures, low-set thumbs, and clino-camptodactyly (see Fig. 634–5). The majority have ear cysts at birth or within the first 3 mo of life. In about 85% of children the pinnae of the ears become acutely inflamed and swollen during the first 2–5 wk of life and remain thickened, firm, and irregular (cauliflower ear). With time, the ear lesions calcify and may ossify. The palate is broad and high arched; cleft palate occurs in approximately 30% of cases. Laryngomalacia may lead to respiratory distress. Midline frontal hemangiomas are common. Micrognathia and a high prominent forehead typify the facial features. Some patients may have pretibial skin dimples and joint dislocations.

The hips are normal at birth, but hip and knee dislocations frequently develop on weight bearing. Both stiff joints and loose joints may occur in the same patient, with subluxations and dislocations as well as contractures. Progressive scoliosis may develop during the 1st yr of life. Kyphosis may begin at adolescence and lead to respiratory difficulty in adults. The head and skull are normal. Some cases involving milder features of diastrophic dysplasia have been termed *diastrophic variant.*

Radiologically, there are short bowed long bones with greater shortening of the radius and ulna, short 1st metacarpals with abnormally formed carpal and phalangeal bones, wide metaphyses, delayed ossification of the epiphyses, platyspondyly, hypoplastic cervical vertebrae, and progressive scoliosis. Death, paresis, and paralysis can result from cervical vertebral body dislocation. This disorder is autosomal recessive in inheritance.

CHAPTER 640
Ellis–van Creveld Syndrome

This skeletal dysplasia/multiple congenital anomaly disorder has a high frequency among the Amish of Pennsylvania, Ohio, and West Virginia. It is inherited as an autosomal recessive disorder. These patients have four limb postaxial polydactyly, nail dysplasia, oligodontia with conical teeth, multiple gingival frenulae (Fig. 640–1), a tubular shaped trunk, and a 40% incidence of congenital heart defects (septal defects or single ventricle). Radiologically, they have a generalized metaphyseal disorder with wide metaphyses, short bowed limbs, square iliac bones with a short ilial base, medial acetabular spurs, a mildly small thorax, brachydactyly that is greater for fingers 2 and 3, and coned epiphyses. This disorder is often clinically and radiologically confused with thoracic dystrophy of Juene. Some patients with Ellis-van Creveld syndrome die from their heart defect and a few from respiratory difficulties.

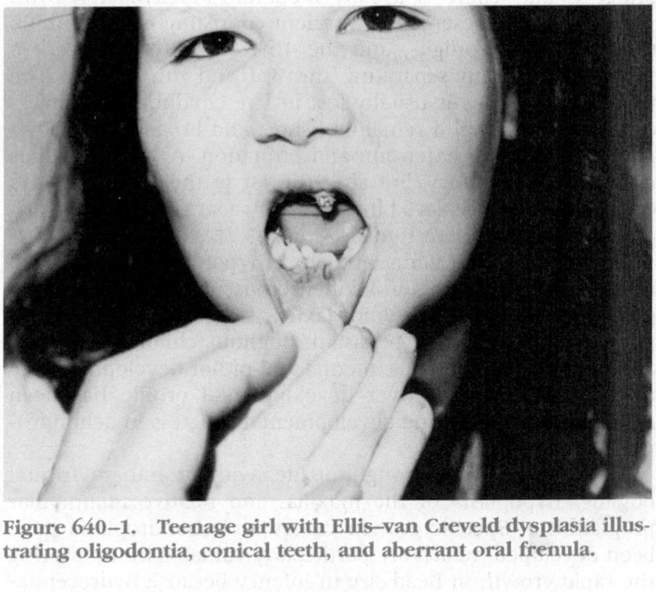

Figure 640–1. Teenage girl with Ellis–van Creveld dysplasia illustrating oligodontia, conical teeth, and aberrant oral frenula.

CHAPTER 641
Camptomelic Dysplasia

Camptomelia means bent or bowed limb. When dysplasia is added to the term camptomelia, it becomes a specific, usually lethal, disorder having sharp angulations of the tibiae with pretibial skin dimples at the apex of the bowed tibiae (see Fig.

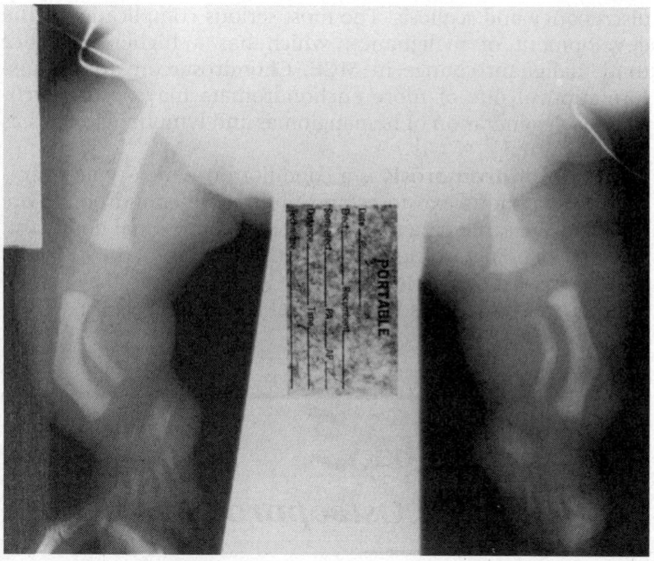

Figure 641–1. Radiograph of the lower extremities of a child with camptomelic dysplasia. Note gently bowed femurs, which are not particularly wide as compared with the thick sharply bowed tibiae and fibulae.

634–2). Other long bones are also slender and bent at their midpoints. The fingers are short (e.g., brachydactyly) plus there is frequently a cleft palate in addition to micrognathia and a prominent forehead. The chest is not small and these children do not die from a hypoplastic thorax, but severe respiratory distress usually leads to an early death. Radiologically, the femur is short and gently bowed, while the short, thick tibias are sharply angulated near their midportions (Fig. 641–1). Vertically, narrow iliac bones, absent thoracic pedicles, hypoplastic/absent scapulae, and hypoplastic cervical vertebrae round out the very specific osseous pattern. These children often die of aspiration and pneumonia but can also die from cervical vertebral body dislocation after prolonged survival. They are mentally retarded and can have anatomic brain anomalies. Many congenital anomalies are associated with this disorder, and camptomelia occurs in many other skeletal dysplasias and malformations. Inheritance was thought to be autosomal recessive; however, autosomal dominant inheritance may be more common.

CHAPTER 642

Osteochondrodysplasias with Anarchic Development of Cartilaginous or Fibrous Tissue

These form a group of disorders in which development of abnormally placed cartilage or fibrous elements leads to skeletal deformity during growth, with relative hyperplasia or hypoplasia of skeletal elements. Two subgroups can be distinguished according to whether the anarchic proliferation involves cartilage or fibrous tissue: those involving cartilage include dysplasia epiphysealis hemimelica, multiple cartilaginous exostoses, Langer-Giedion syndrome (multiple cartilaginous exostoses–peripheral dysplasia), multiple enchondromatosis (Ollier), enchondromatosis with hemangioma (Maffucci), and metachondromatosis. Those involving fibrous tissue include fibrous dysplasia (Jaffe-Lichtenstein), fibrous dysplasia with skin pigmentation and precocious puberty (McCune-Albright), cherubism, and neurofibromatosis.

Abnormally situated growths of osteocartilaginous tissue may be localized to the epiphyses, the metaphyses, or the diaphyses of the long bones. Dysplasia epiphysealis hemimelica or tarsomegaly affects the skeleton of only one portion of the lower extremity. Cartilage may develop within bone (i.e., as an enchondroma) or on the surface of bone, commonly at the edge of the metaphyses (i.e., as exostosis or enchondroma).

In **dysplasia epiphysealis hemimelica (Trevor disease)** there is asymmetric overgrowth of the epiphyses, tarsal centers, and, rarely, carpal centers. All cases have been sporadic, and there is a male predominance. Because there may be involvement of an entire epiphysis rather than half, the term *unilateral epiphyseal dysplasia* has been suggested as an alternative name.

This condition is usually recognized in the first years of life because of foot or knee deformity, a limp, or a painful gait. Usually, there is a medial or lateral firm swelling at the knee or tibiotarsal joint, with minimal loss of length in the involved leg. Roentgenographically, fragmentation and excessive growth of the involved epiphysis are seen, which commonly involves only one part of the epiphysis. Simultaneous involvement of several epiphyses is common, especially of the foot and the knee. The talus, distal femoral, and distal tibial epiphyses are the most common sites of disease. Lesions of the upper extremities are rare.

Multiple cartilaginous exostoses (MCE) are bony projections found near the ends of the tubular bones and ribs, the vertebral bodies, the scapulas, and the iliac crest. Roentgenographically, these tumors appear to originate at the borders of metaphyses and sometimes along the shafts (diaphyses) of the long bones. They are distinct from enchondromata (chondromata), which arise within the metaphyses and sometimes the diaphyses and which appear to be expanding within the metaphyses into the epiphyses. Inheritance is autosomal dominant with high penetrance but widely variable expression. It is generally believed that the pathogenesis involves proliferation of normal cartilage at the borders of the metaphyses, along the diaphyses, or alongside the cartilaginous borders of the vertebrae and scapulas. The center of the tumor becomes ossified and its medullary cavity may communicate with the marrow space of the shaft of the affected bone.

The tumors may undergo rapid growth during infancy but are rarely detected roentgenographically prior to 3 yr of age, when they appear as bony projections from the affected bones, which have a normal pattern of ossification. Exostoses at the ends of the long bones point away from the epiphyses. Involvement of metacarpals and phalanges frequently occurs, but the exostoses are small and rarely deform the fingers. Exostoses of the shaft of the humerus characteristically occur at the junction of the upper and middle thirds on the medial surface. The exostoses are not only unsightly but disturbing to the growth of long bones, producing deformation and sometimes compression of nerves and blood vessels. Severe deformity of the distal ulna is often associated with an asymmetric growth disturbance, dislocation of the radial head, and ulnar deviation of the hand. Involvement of the lower limbs may lead to coxa valga, genu valgum, or obliquity of the distal tibial epiphyses and limb length discrepancy. Final adult height tends to be in the normal range, but mild skeletal disproportion may occur because limb involvement (often asymmetric) is much greater than spinal involvement. Malignant degeneration may occur, but rarely, if ever, in childhood.

Surgical treatment is indicated for cosmetically deforming lesions or those producing neurovascular complications. Wherever possible, surgery should be delayed until the end of growth because of the high chance of regression of the lesions.

MCE—peripheral dysplasia (Langer-Giedion syndrome), also known as trichorhinophalangeal syndrome type II, is characterized by predominantly acromelic or acromesomelic short stature of postnatal onset, facial appearance similar to that in the trichorhinophalangeal syndrome (see earlier), mild microcephaly of postnatal onset, and multiple cartilaginous exostoses. All reported cases have been sporadic. The characteristic facies includes large, poorly developed, laterally protruding ears, sparse scalp hair with thick eyebrows, a large bulbous nose with a thick prominent septum, a simple prominent elongated philtrum, and a relatively recessed chin. Redundant or loose skinfolds and hyperextensibility of skin and ligaments in infancy may lead to confusion with the Ehlers-Danlos syndromes.

Roentgenographically, two types of lesions are apparent: (1) multiple exostoses with all the possibilities for skeletal deformity produced by MCE alone, and (2) abnormalities in metacarpal and proximal phalanges consisting of cone-shaped epiphyses (see TRP syndrome), widening with lack of normal funnelization, and a hooklike, often asymmetric, projection of the metaphyses. Cytogenetic studies commonly show a deletion involving band 8q 24.

Enchondromata arise within bone, usually within areas of endochondral ossification. Single enchondromata of bone are not uncommon and may be incidentally detected. They may, on the other hand, produce local pain because of intramedullary expansion. *Multiple enchondromata* (Ollier disease) have widespread involvement of the skeleton, including the hands; they are detected because of bone pain or deformity. Virtually all cases have been sporadic. Roentgenographically, the lesions may be detectable in early infancy as clear, homogeneous, oval lesions with axes parallel to the longitudinal axis of the bone.

Patients present because of growth disturbance, which may be asymmetric, leading to limp, or because of swelling of the fingers and toes in infancy. The tumors may produce visible or palpable swelling, particularly in the hands or the growing ends of the long bones; they are somewhat elastic and may limit mobility of neighboring joints. Phalangeal chondromas may lead to severe deformation of the fingers.

The effect of enchondromata on growth is usually much more serious than that of exostoses, and the prognosis is more serious than in MCE. Asymmetric growth disturbance is more severe. Involvement of distal ulna and radius may produce a severe deformation at the wrist leading to ulnar deviation of the hand. Malignant change is uncommon in childhood but has a higher frequency in adults. Pain and rapid growth in size or radiologic evidence of endosteal erosion may indicate malignant change.

Surgical intervention is indicated for lesions causing local symptoms or for growth plate deformation leading to marked limb asymmetry. Radionuclide scanning may be useful in investigating large enchondromata at risk of malignant change.

In **enchondromatosis with hemangiomatosis** *(Maffucci syndrome)* multiple enchondromata and hemangiomata of bone and overlying skin develop during childhood. The majority of affected persons are normal at birth; the lesions develop during infancy. All reported cases have been sporadic. The cutaneous lesions are usually cavernous or capillary hemangiomas, with or without lymphangiomas. Their distribution in skin appears to be independent of skeletal lesions; they may be found also in mucous membranes and intra-abdominal viscera. The skeletal lesions are typical enchondromata, involving metaphyses throughout the body; in some cases unilateral deformity predominates.

Maffucci syndrome produces a severe, cosmetically unsightly, and often painful deformation of the skeleton. Neither the hemangiomata nor the enchondromata are amenable to surgical intervention except for palliation. The lesions lead to short stature or, if predominantly unilateral, to leg length discrepancy and scoliosis. The most serious complication is the development of malignancy, which has a higher incidence than malignant change in MCE. Chondrosarcomatous transformation of one or more enchondromata may occur; sarcomatous degeneration of hemangiomas and lymphangiomas has been reported.

Metachondromatosis is a condition in which typical multiple cartilaginous exostoses and multiple enchondromata are found in the same patient. Inheritance is autosomal dominant. Affected patients are normal at birth; in infancy they acquire lesions in digits and long bones. Short stature may occur, although most patients have normal stature.

CHAPTER 643
Inherited Osteoporoses

Osteopenia (insufficiency of bone) is a roentgenographic feature of many inherited or acquired disorders of childhood; it results from reduced production or increased breakdown of bone, or both. Osteoporosis (the clinical syndrome resulting from osteopenia) is characterized by susceptibility to fractures and particularly to crush fractures of vertebrae. Osteogenesis imperfecta is the most prevalent of the osteoporosis syndromes in childhood and is characterized by fractures and skeletal deformities. Some of the affected die in the newborn period with extreme fragility of bone and numerous fractures (osteogenesis imperfecta congenita); others manifest bone fragility in life and live a normal life span (osteogenesis imperfecta tarda). At least four genetic syndromes account for variability in osteogenesis imperfecta. Serum alkaline phosphatase activity is normal or elevated in all forms.

643.1 Osteogenesis Imperfecta Type I (OI Type I)

This is characterized by osteoporosis and excessive bone fragility, distinctly blue sclerae, and presenile conductive hearing loss in adolescents and adults. Inheritance is autosomal dominant. This most common variety of osteogenesis imperfecta has an incidence of about 1/30,000 live births.

The sclerae are generally of a deep blue-black hue. Fractures result from minimal trauma, but not all accidental trauma produces fractures. About 10% of affected infants have a few fractures at birth. Occurrence of neonatal fractures does not predict more deformity, more handicap, or a greater number of fractures than in other patients who have their first fractures after 1 yr of age. Deformities of the limbs in OI type I are largely the result of fractures, but bowing, particularly of the lower limbs, is common. Other deformities, such as genu valgum and flat feet with metatarsus varus, are also common. About 20% of affected adults have progressive kyphoscoliosis, which may be severe. Kyphosis alone is common in older adults but is rarely seen in children. There is usually excessive hyperlaxity of ligaments, particularly at the small joints of the hands, feet, and knees, but this feature is less marked in adults. There is usually mild short stature; body proportions depend on the relative involvement of limbs or spine. During adolescence there is a marked spontaneous reduction in the frequency of fractures.

Hearing impairment affects most patients by the 5th decade; it is rare, however, before the end of the 1st decade.

Hereditary opalescent dentin (dentinogenesis imperfecta) is observed in some families with this trait. It produces distinctively yellow (or sometimes gray-blue) transparent teeth, which are frequently prematurely eroded or broken. These teeth have short roots and constricted coronoradicular junctions. Opalescent dentin distinguishes a subgroup of patients with OI type I from a subgroup with normal teeth.

Roentgenographic studies in OI type I show generalized osteopenia, evidence of previous fractures, and normal callus formation at the site of recent fractures. Deformities are usually the result of angulation at the site of previous fractures, but bowing of the femora, tibia, and fibula occurs as well as deformity in the bones of the feet, particularly metatarsus varus. Severe osteoporosis of the spine and codfish vertebrae are occasionally seen; kyphoscoliosis is not usually observed in childhood.

Studies of collagen synthesized by cultured skin fibroblasts show a reduction in type I procollagen synthesis. There is a substitution for a residue other than glycine in the triple helix of α(I).

643.2 Osteogenesis Imperfecta Type II (OI Type II)

This lethal syndrome is characterized by low birthweight and length, and typical roentgenographic findings of crumpled long bones and beaded ribs. Autosomal recessive inheritance occurs in a small proportion of cases, with the majority of instances representing new autosomal dominant mutations. The condition affects about 1 infant in 60,000 live births.

Approximately 50% are stillborn, and the remainder die soon after birth of respiratory insufficiency owing to a defective thoracic cage. The skull is soft, and there are multiple palpable bone islands. The face may show beaking of the nose and apparent hypotelorism, and the limbs are extremely short, bent, and deformed. The thighs are broad and fixed at right angles to the trunk (Fig. 643–1). The skin is thin and fragile, and may be torn during delivery.

Roentgenograms show multiple fractures of the ribs, which are often continuously beaded, and a crumpled (accordion-like) appearance of the long bones (especially the femora). There is diffuse osteopenia in the face and skull, and multiple bone islands in the vault.

A number of distinct biochemical defects have been discovered predominantly in the α_1(I) chains of type I collagen that have the common effect of a marked reduction in the synthesis of type I collagen, the principal collagen of bone. These are mainly point mutations leading to substitution of an amino acid such as cysteine or arginine for glycine with disruption of triple helix formation.

643.3 Osteogenesis Imperfecta Type III (OI Type III)

This syndrome is characteristically manifested in the newborn or young infant by severe bone fragility and multiple fractures, which lead to progressive skeletal deformity (Fig. 643–2). The sclerae may be blue at birth and become less blue with age. Inheritance is autosomal recessive; clinical variability suggests genetic heterogeneity.

Very few patients with OI type III reach adult life. Infants generally have normal birthweight and often normal birth length, but the latter may be reduced by deformities of the lower limbs. Fractures are present in most cases at birth and occur frequently during childhood. Kyphoscoliosis develops during childhood and progresses into adolescence. Skull de-

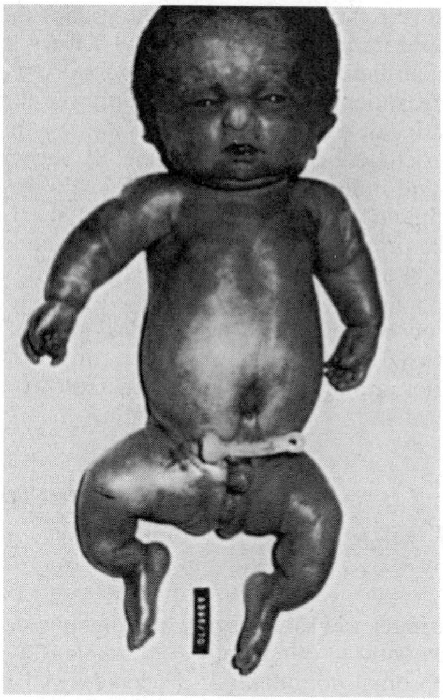

Figure 643–1. Osteogenesis imperfecta type II (lethal crumpled bone variety) with broad thighs and angulation deformities of the limbs.

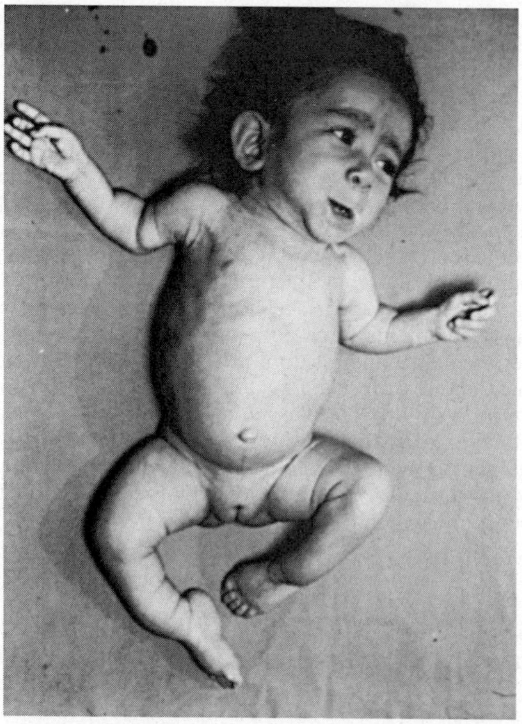

Figure 643–2. Osteogenesis imperfecta type III showing less shortening of the limbs but angulation deformities of the legs.

formity is severe, with temporal bulging contributing to the triangular appearance of the head. Final stature is very short. Hearing impairment has not been reported. A considerable proportion of patients succumb to cardiorespiratory complications in infancy or childhood.

Skeletal roentgenograms in OI type III show generalized osteopenia and multiple fractures, without the beading of the ribs or crumpling of long bones seen in OI type II. Osteopenia appears to be progressive, with platyspondyly and codfish vertebrae. The skull shows osteopenia and multiple wormian bones.

Collagen gene and protein biochemical studies in one case showed the α_2(I) chain of type I collagen could not be incorporated into the normal helix. Bone contained α_1(I) trimers.

643.4 Osteogenesis Imperfecta Type IV (OI Type IV)

This syndrome is characterized by osteoporosis leading to bone fragility without other features of classic OI type I. Inheritance is autosomal dominant. The sclerae in OI type IV may be bluish at birth but may become less blue as the patient matures. Hearing impairment is less common, but opalescent dentin has been observed in some families, suggesting heterogeneity within this group.

Patients with OI type IV have variable ages of onset of fractures, ranging from birth to adult life, and variable deformity of long bones and spine. Significant bowing of the lower limbs at birth may be the only feature of this syndrome, and progressive deformity of the long bones and spine has been reported without fractures. In several patients bowing has lessened with age. Like those with OI type I, patients with OI type IV show spontaneous improvement with puberty, few fractures showing up in adolescents and adults. Most patients, however, have short stature. Roentgenographically, there is generalized osteopenia. Multiple fractures may be observed at birth and occur throughout life, but these patients have less osteopenia and fewer fractures than infants with recessive varieties of osteogenesis imperfecta. There are a variety of point mutations and small deletions in the α_2(I) chain and, rarely, point mutations in the α_1(I) chain.

MANAGEMENT OF OSTEOGENESIS IMPERFECTA. For OI type II, no therapeutic intervention is effective. For other forms of OI careful nursing of the newborn on a firm mattress or pillows may prevent excessive fractures. Beyond the newborn period the mainstay of management is an aggressive orthopedic regimen aimed at prompt splinting of fractures and correction of deformities arising from fractures and from the progressive bowing or bending of the skeleton. Therapeutic regimens, including supplements of calcium or fluoride, of vitamin C, or magnesium oxide, and calcitonin therapy, have shown no clear benefit. Genetic counseling for affected families should aim at primary prevention. Reliable prenatal diagnosis is not available for all types of osteogenesis imperfecta, but some severely affected fetuses with OI type II may be confidently recognized prenatally through a combination of ultrasound, roentgenographic, and biochemical studies.

643.5 Osteoporosis with Pseudogliomatosis and Blindness

This rare autosomal recessive syndrome is characterized by generalized osteoporosis leading to fractures and deformities of long bones and spine. Ocular pseudogliomas, which may be mistaken for retinoblastoma, develop in infancy. Mild mental retardation has been observed in several of those affected but may be unrelated.

CHAPTER 644

Osteopetrosis, Pyknodysostosis, Dysosteosclerosis, and Cortical Hyperostosis

These conditions are characterized by a generalized increase in skeletal density. Individually, they are distinguished by their mode of inheritance, age of onset, and pattern of skeletal involvement. At least nine forms of **osteopetrosis** ("marble bone disease") have been described with overlapping spectra of clinical and roentgenographic features. A form with manifestations in the newborn and a progressive course leading to death at an early age is called *osteopetrosis with precocious manifestations.* A usually milder disorder with delayed manifestations is known as *osteopetrosis tarda* or *Albers-Schönberg disease.* Intermediate forms occur and include a type of osteopetrosis with renal tubular acidosis and cerebral calcification.

OSTEOPETROSIS WITH PRECOCIOUS MANIFESTATIONS. This form is most frequently discovered during the first months of life; it may appear as failure to thrive, malignant hypocalcemia, anemia with thrombocytopenia, or severe, perhaps overwhelming infection. Inheritance is generally autosomal recessive, but some cases may show autosomal dominant inheritance.

Rarely, fractures lead to medical attention. Hyperostosis may crowd the marrow cavity, with anemia and extramedullary hematopoiesis, hepatosplenomegaly, and thrombocytopenia. Anemia results from excessive hemolysis. A defect in macrophage killing of bacteria may account for recurrent and sometimes overwhelming infection. Bony encroachment on the optic foramina may lead to optic atrophy and blindness, in some cases detectable at birth. Hypocalcemia is not uncommon, and serum phosphorus may be low. Serum alkaline phosphatase activity is elevated. Roentgenographically, the diagnostic findings are a generalized increase in bone density, with defective metaphyseal modeling and a "bone in bone" appearance most marked in the vertebral bodies. Diffuse hyperostosis leads to loss of demarcation between the cortex and the medullary cavity. Irregular condensation of bone at the metaphyses may produce the appearance of parallel plates of dense bone at the ends of the long bones. The base of the skull is dense, having normal to increased density of the vault and markedly increased density in the orbital margins.

Treatment is aimed at decreasing or arresting progressive hyperostosis, correcting anemia and thrombocytopenia, and treating infections promptly and vigorously; a regimen of oral cellulose phosphate, prednisone, and low-calcium diet has been reported effective in some but not all patients. The prednisone arrests the progress of anemia and thrombocytopenia. Long-term treatment with recombinant human interferon gamma may also be beneficial. Neurosurgical unroofing of the optic foramina is useful in selected cases. Bone marrow transplantation with appropriately HLA-matched donor marrow has been curative in several patients. Generally, the prognosis for survival is poor, and death in the first few months or years from anemia, bleeding, or overwhelming infection is not uncommon.

OSTEOPETROSIS WITH RENAL TUBULAR ACIDOSIS. This important entity is usually recognized because of failure to thrive in the 1st yr of life. Electrolyte investigation shows a metabolic acidosis. Intracerebral calcification may be found on a roentgenogram. Inheritance is autosomal recessive, and a defect in the enzyme carbonic anhydrase II can be shown in red blood cells.

OSTEOPETROSIS TARDA (ALBERS-SCHÖNBERG DISEASE). This condition presents in childhood, adolescence, or young adult life because of fractures (about 10% of patients), mild craniofacial disproportion, mild anemia, complications arising from neurologic involvement, or osteitis with osteonecrosis (usually of the mandible). Increased bone density may be discovered incidentally on a roentgenographic study made for some other problem. Most cases represent autosomal dominant inheritance, a few autosomal recessive.

Skeletal roentgenograms show generalized increase in density of cortical bone, with a club-shaped appearance of the long bones due to defective metaphyseal modeling. More than 50% of patients have longitudinal and transverse dense striations at the ends of the long bones. The vertebrae show alternating lucent and dense bands. The base of the skull is dense and thickened, but the face and vault are less affected.

Management should be directed at recognition and treatment of complications, with frequent testing of visual fields and acuity and periodic roentgenograms of the optic foramina. Transfusion may be required for anemia, and splenectomy may be useful in some patients.

PYKNODYSOSTOSIS. This autosomal recessive disorder is characterized by postnatal onset of short-limbed short stature and generalized hyperostosis. A disproportionately large skull, frontal and occipital bossing, and a wide anterior fontanelle may bring the patient to the physician's attention. The hands and feet are short and broad, and the nails may be deformed and brittle. The sclerae are often blue; this evidence combined with a tendency to fractures may lead to confusion with osteogenesis imperfecta.

Roentgenographically, there is a generalized increase in bone density without metaphyseal striation. The distal phalanges are characteristically hypoplastic or aplastic. The skull has wide sutures and wormian bones; the face has a small mandible with an obtuse mandibular angle.

DYSOSTEOSCLEROSIS. This rare autosomal recessive disorder is characterized by generalized increase in bone density and short stature of postnatal onset. Dysosteosclerosis differs from osteopetrosis and pyknodysostosis in showing platyspondyly with superior and inferior irregularity of vertebral ossification. Developmental defects of the teeth are common, with delayed eruption of primary dentition, severe hypodontia, and early loss of the teeth. Secondary dentition may fail to erupt. Other complications (fractures, visual and hearing loss, and recurrent infections of mandible and paranasal sinuses) are similar to those of osteopetrosis.

INFANTILE CORTICAL HYPEROSTOSIS (CAFFEY DISEASE). This condition of unknown cause must be differentiated from hyperphosphatasia with osteoectasia (see Chapter 656). The disorder is usually recognized in the first 3 mo of life. The course is febrile, with marked swelling of soft tissues over the face and jaws, and progressive cortical thickening of long bones and flat bones. Alkaline phosphatase activity is usually mildly increased. The condition has exacerbations and remissions with spontaneous regression after several years. Corticosteroids can relieve symptoms during exacerbations.

CHAPTER 645

Treatment

Most of the myriad of problems (see Table 634–1) confronting individuals with skeletal dysplasias are treated in relatively standard fashion. Evaluation and treatment of cervical vertebral body hypoplasia and/or dislocation is particularly important. Early evaluation and intervention are should be done by experienced orthopedists and neurosurgeons. Spondyloepiphyseal dysplasia (SED) disorders such as Morquio syndrome and SED congenita are at increased risk of cervical vertebral body dislocations, as are the skeletal dysplasia/multiple congenital anomaly disorders of diastrophic dysplasia (see Fig. 634–5), camptomelic dysplasia (see Fig. 634–2), and Larsen syndrome. Long bone stretching of the lower extremities has been successful in adding significant height to individuals with achondroplasia, although it does require multiple surgeries and long-term commitment (see Chapter 637). Growth hormone has been used in a few individuals with skeletal dysplasias (e.g., hypochondroplasia) with some success, although it remains experimental. Bone marrow transplant may be curative or ameliorative for some metabolic skeletal dysplasias such as osteopetrosis or Hurler syndrome (see Chapter 74).

GENERAL

Chen H: Skeletal dysplasias and mental retardation. *In:* Papadatos CJ, Bartsocas CS (eds): Skeletal Dysplasias. Progress in Clinical and Biological Research, Vol 104. New York, Alan R. Liss, 1982.

Erik PA Jr, Hauge M: Congenital generalized bone dysplasias: A clinical, radiological and epidemiological survey. J Med Genet 27:37, 1989.

Hall BD, Spranger J: Congenital bowing of the long bones. Eur J Pediatr 133:131, 1980.

Hall BD: Approach to skeletal dysplasia. Pediatr Clin North Am Med Genet II 39:279, 1992.

Van Der Harten HJ, Brons JTJ, Dijkstra PF, et al: Some variants of lethal neonatal short-limbed platyspondylic dysplasia: A radiological ultrasonographic, neurological and histopathological study of 22 cases. Clin Dysmorphol 2:1, 1993.

Whyte M: Chipping away at marble-bone disease. N Engl J Med 332:1639, 1995.

Wynne-Davies R (Skeletal Dysplasia Group): Instability of the upper cervical spine. Arch Dis Child 64:283, 1989.

FREQUENCY

Anderson PE: Prevalence of lethal osteochondrodysplasias in Denmark. Am J Med Genet 32:484, 1989.

Camerh G, Mastroiacovo P: Birth prevalence of skeletal dysplasias in the Italian multicentric monitoring system for birth defects. *In:* Papadatos CJ, Bartsocas CS (eds): Skeletal Dysplasias. Progress in Clinical and Biological Research, Vol. 104. New York, Alan R. Liss, 1982.

Oriol, IM, Castilla EE, Barbosa-Neto JG: The birth prevalence rates for the skeletal dysplasias. J Med Genet 23:328, 1986.

GROWTH

Appan S, Laurent S, Chapman M, et al: Growth and growth hormone therapy in hypochondroplasia. Acta Paediatr Scand 79:796, 1990.

Horton WA, Hall JG, Scott CI, et al: Growth curves for height for diastrophic dysplasia, spondyloepiphyseal dysplasia congenita, and pseudoachondroplasia. Am J Dis Child 136:316, 1982.

MOLECULAR/GENE STUDIES

Cole WG, Patterson E, Bonadio J, et al: The clinicopathological features of three babies with lethal osteogenesis imperfecta resulting from the substitution of glycine by valine in the pro α_1 (I) chain of type I procollagen. J Med Genet 29:112, 1992.

Cole WG, Hall RK, Rogers JG: The clinical features of spondyloepiphyseal dysplasia congenita resulting from the substitution of glycine 997 by serine in the α (II) chain of type II collagen. J Med Genet 30:27, 1993.

Diab M, Wu J-J, Shapiro F, Eyre D: Abnormality of type IX collagen in a patient with diastrophic dysplasia. Am J Med Genet 49:402, 1994.

Dlouhy SR, Christian JC, Haines JL, et al: Localization of the gene for a syndrome of X-linked skeletal dysplasia and mental retardation to Xq27-qter. Hum Genet 75:136, 1987.

Hastbacka J, Salonen R, Laurila P, et al: Prenatal diagnosis of diastrophic dysplasia with polymorphic DNA markers. J Med Genet 30:265, 1993.

Oehlmann R, Summerville GP, Yeh G, et al: Genetic linkage mapping of multiple epiphyseal dysplasia to the pericentromeric region of chromosome 19. Am J Hum Genet 54:3, 1994.
Spranger J, WinterPacht A, Zabel B: The type II collagenopathies: A spectrum of chondrodysplasias. Eur J Pediatr 153:56, 1994.
Velinov M, Slaugenhaupt SA, Stoilov I, et al: The gene for achondroplasia maps to the telomer region of chromosome 4p. Nature Genet 6:314, 1994.
Wulfsberg EA, Curtis J, Jayne CH: Chondrodysplasia punctata: A boy with X-linked recessive chondrodysplasia punctata due to an inherited X-Y translocation with a current classification of these disorders. Am J Med Genet 43:823, 1992.

NOSOLOGY

Spranger J: Radiologic nosology of bone dysplasias. Am J Med Genet 34:96, 1989.
Spranger J: International classification of osteochondrodysplasias (The International Working Group on Constitutional Diseases of Bone). Eur J Pediatr 151:407, 1992.

RESOURCES

Buyse ML: Birth Defects Encyclopedia. Cambridge, MA, Blackwell, 1990.
Cremin BJ, Beighton P: Bone Dysplasias of Infancy. Berlin, Springer-Verlag, 1978.
Gorlin RJ, Cohen MM Jr, Levin LS: Syndromes of the Head and Neck, 3rd ed. New York, Oxford University Press, 1990.
Jones KL: Smith's Recognizable Patterns of Human Malformation, 4th ed. Philadelphia, WB Saunders, 1988.
Maroteaux P: Bone Disorders of Children. Oxford Monographs on Medical Genetics, No. 23. Oxford, Oxford University Press, 1992.
Rubin P: Dynamic Classification of Bone Dysplasias. Chicago, Year Book Medical, 1964.
Spranger JW, Langer LO, Wiedemann H-R: Bone Dysplasias: An Atlas of Constitutional Disorders of Skeletal Development. Philadelphia, WB Saunders, 1974.
Taybi H, Lachman RS: Radiology of Syndromes, Metabolic Disorders and Skeletal Dysplasias, 3rd ed. Chicago, Year Book Medical, 1990.
Winter RM, Baraitser M: Multiple Congenital Anomalies. A Diagnostic Compendium. London, Chapman and Hall, 1991.
Wynne-Davies R, Fairbank TJ: Atlas of Skeletal Dysplasias. London, Churchill, 1985.

CHAPTER 646
Marfan Syndrome

Luther K. Robinson

The Marfan syndrome is an autosomal dominantly inherited disorder with nearly complete penetrance but variable expressivity. The disorder has an incidence of 1 in 10,000 people; 15–30% of cases are sporadic owing to a new mutation.

PATHOGENESIS. This is related to mutations of fibrillin, a 350 kD protein that is the major component of extracellular microfibrils and that contributes to the structural integrity of the connective tissue. The *FBN1* locus resides on the long arm of chromosome 15. Over 20 mutations are known; these appear to be unique to a given affected family. The relatively even distribution of mutations throughout the *FBN1* gene likely contribute to the phenotypic variability of the disorder. Diagnosis is based on clinical features, some of which are growth dependent.

CLINICAL MANIFESTATIONS. Diagnosis is based on the overall pattern of malformation; the features occurring in isolation are rather nonspecific. Tallness and slimness of stature may be present at birth and persist postnatally. Diminished subcutaneous fat may suggest failure to thrive in early infancy. Hypotonia and ligamentous laxity may predispose to motor delays; cognitive performance, however, usually is normal.

The neonatal or infantile form of the Marfan syndrome is more severe than cases observed in older children and may have clinical similarity to congenital contractural arachnodactyly, with joint dislocations, flexion contractures, large pliant ears, iridodonesis, megalocornea, aortic valve dilatation, and mitral valve prolapse being the most commonly observed features.

Older patients often have a long, thin face with narrowness of the maxilla and dental crowding. Ocular abnormalities reflect the connective tissue defect and include ectopia lentis, blue sclerae, and myopia. Slit lamp examination as early as infancy may disclose lens dislocation, which may be congenital. Iridodonesis is a helpful clinical sign, but suspected cases of the Marfan syndrome should have ophthalmologic evaluations that include slit lamp examinations, even in the absence of a gross ocular abnormality.

A wide range of skeletal malformations has been reported. The limbs are long and thin (dolichostenomelia), and the arm span is substantially greater than the length. The distance from the pubis to heel (lower segment) is increased and contributes to a diminished upper segment to lower segment ratio (Fig. 646–1). Hand findings are somewhat nonspecific and include long, thin fingers (arachnodactyly) that are hyperextensible. The thumb may be adducted across the narrow palm, the *Steinberg sign.* The wrist sign, in which the thumb and 5th finger appreciably overlap when encircling the thin wrist, is another feature.

Long, gracile ribs may contribute to abnormalities of the anterior thorax as either sternal depression (pectus excavatum) or prominence (pectus carinatum, "pigeon breast"). Scoliosis can be a problem among older children and adolescents.

The connective tissue defect may contribute to increased distensibility of lung parenchyma and increase the risks of spontaneous pneumothorax or formation of pulmonary blebs.

Progressive cardiovascular defects contribute to the substantial morbidity of the Marfan syndrome. Echocardiography has permitted the early detection of patients with an increased risk of cardiac complications. As in adults, progressive aortic root dilatation, with or without auscultatory evidence of aortic

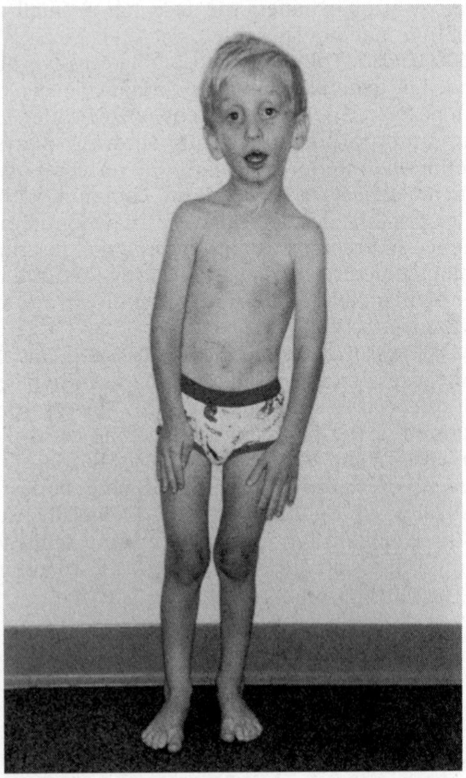

Figure 646–1. Note the elongated facies, droopy lids, apparent dolichostenomelia, and mild scoliosis.

disease, occurs in 80–100% of cases and may be congenital. In contrast to adults, frank aortic regurgitation is less common in children, perhaps because the amount and duration of distension required to cause aortic dysfunction does not manifest until later life. Mitral valve prolapse (MVP) occurs as frequently as aortic dilatation. It, too, tends to be progressive in nature in contrast to the more static lesion of idiopathic MVP, and it is the most common cause of morbidity in children with the Marfan syndrome.

DIAGNOSIS. Diagnosis of the Marfan syndrome is based upon clinical criteria. In general, the diagnosis of a sporadic, or fresh mutation, case requires that major manifestations of the disorder are present, whereas in cases in which a 1st degree relative is unequivocally affected, milder manifestations with at least one major malformation are supportive of the diagnosis. Tall stature with an abnormally low upper segment to lower segment ratio is the most consistent presenting feature. Echocardiography should demonstrate at least aortic root dilatation for age. Other abnormalities, such as mitral valve prolapse, mitral regurgitation, or aortic regurgitation, are supportive findings. A slit lamp examination is indicated in all suspected cases.

There should be documentation of a negative urinary cyanide nitroprusside test or specific amino acid studies to exclude cystathionine synthase deficiency (homocystinuria). Other conditions that should be excluded include the Stickler syndrome, idiopathic mitral valve prolapse syndrome, the congenital contractural arachnodactyly syndrome, and isolated cystic medial necrosis of the aorta (Erdheim syndrome). Molecular genetic studies may be applicable to pedigrees with multiple affected family members.

TREATMENT. Therapy focuses on prevention of complications and genetic counseling. In view of the potential complexity of management required by some affected individuals, periodic referral to a multidisciplinary center with experience in the Marfan syndrome is advisable.

The pediatrician should work in concert with pediatric subspecialists to coordinate a rational approach to expectant monitoring and treatment of potential complications. Yearly evaluations for such problems as scoliosis, cardiac valvular disease, or ophthalmologic problems are imperative. Physical therapy may improve neuromuscular tone in infancy. Moderate nontraumatic physical activity, such as swimming or bicycling, should be encouraged as tolerated. Maximal exertion should be discouraged because of the stresses that increased cardiac output place on the aorta.

Affected patients should receive bacterial endocarditis prophylaxis before dental or other invasive surgical procedures.

Recent evidence indicates that β-adrenergic blockade with agents such as propanolol or atenolol improves survival with respect to catastrophic cardiac events and aortic dilatation. Acute aortic dissection may be managed by composite graft.

Optimal management of the pregnant adolescent with the Marfan syndrome is not established. The risk that pregnancy will worsen cardiovascular abnormalities is of concern. Although data are lacking, it is reasonable to consider that young women with aortic regurgitation avoid pregnancy. Those with mild aortic dilatation should be monitored echocardiographically at regular intervals. Though β-adrenergic blockers have not been shown to be teratogenic, the prenatally exposed offspring of women with the Marfan syndrome who are treated with β-antagonists should be monitored in the neonatal period for such drug-induced problems as hypotension, bradycardia, or hypoglycemia.

PROGNOSIS. Longevity in the Marfan syndrome is diminished in comparison with population norms, primarily because of the increased risk of cardiovascular complications. Dilatation of the aortic root and ascending aorta is progressive and may lead to aneurysm formation and increased risk of aortic dissection. These and other concerns pose not only medical problems but also psychologic stresses for the affected child and the parents, particularly during adolescence. Awareness of these issues and referral for support services may facilitate a positive perspective toward this condition.

GENETIC COUNSELING. The heritable nature of the Marfan syndrome makes recurrence risk (genetic) counseling mandatory. As noted previously, approximately 15–30% of cases are the first affected individuals in their families. Fathers of these sporadic cases have been, on average, 7–10 years older than fathers in the general population. This paternal age effect suggests that these cases represent new dominant mutations with minimal recurrence risks to the future offspring of the normal parents. Each child of an affected individual, however, has a 50% risk of inheriting the number 15 chromosome with the Marfan mutation and thus being affected. Recurrence risk counseling is best accomplished by professionals with expertise in the issues surrounding this chronic debilitating disorder.

Aoyama T, Francke U, Dietz HC, et al: Quantitative differences in biosynthesis and extracellular deposition of fibrillin in cultured fibroblasts distinguish five groups of Marfan syndrome patients and suggest distinct pathogenic mechanisms. J Clin Invest 94:130, 1994.

Beighton P, dePaepe A, Danks D, et al: International nosology of heritable disorders of connective tissue, Berlin, 1986. Am J Med Genet 29:581, 1988.

Dietz HC, McIntosh I, Sakai LY, et al: Four novel *FBN1* mutations: Significance for mutant transcript level and EGF-like domain calcium binding in the pathogenesis of Marfan syndrome. Genomics 17:468, 1993.

Franke U, Furthmayr H: Genes and gene products involved in Marfan syndrome. Semin Thorac Cardiovasc Surg 5:3, 1993.

Gross DM, Robinson LK, Smith LT, et al: Severe perinatal Marfan syndrome. Pediatrics 84:83, 1989.

Pereira L, Lesran O, Ramirez F, et al: A molecular approach to the stratification of cardiovascular risk in families with Marfan's syndrome. N Engl J Med 331:148, 1994.

Pyeritz RE, McKusick VA: The Marfan syndrome: Diagnosis and management. N Engl J Med 300:772, 1979.

Pyeritz RE: Maternal and fetal complications of pregnancy in the Marfan syndrome. Am J Med 71:784, 1981.

Shores J, Berger KR, Murphy EA, et al: Progression of aortic dilatation and the benefit of long-term β-adrenergic blockade in Marfan's syndrome. N Engl J Med 330:1335, 1994.

Sisk HE, Zahka KG, Pyeritz RE: The Marfan syndrome in early childhood: Analysis of 15 patients diagnosed at less than 4 years of age. Am J Cardiol 52:353, 1983.

SECTION 3

Metabolic Bone Disease

Russell W. Chesney

Bone is a dynamic organ capable of rapid turnover, weight bearing, and withstanding the stresses of a variety of physical activities. It is constantly being formed (modeling) and reformed (remodeling). It is the major body reservoir for calcium, phosphorus, and magnesium. Disorders that affect this organ and the process of mineralization are designated *metabolic bone diseases*.

Since bone growth and turnover rates are high during childhood, many clinical features of metabolic bone diseases are more prominent in children than in adults. Advances in our knowledge of bone metabolism, the process of mineralization, interactions of the vitamin D–PTH–endocrine axis, and metabolism of vitamin D to active compounds have led to improved treatment of metabolic bone diseases.

The human skeleton consists of a protein matrix, largely comprised of a collagen-containing protein, osteoid, on which is deposited a crystalline mineral phase. Although collagen-containing osteoid comprises 90% of bone protein, other proteins are present, including osteocalcin, which contains gamma-carboxyglutamic acid. Synthesis of osteocalcin is vitamin K and vitamin D dependent and, in high bone turnover states, serum osteocalcin values are often elevated.

The microfibrillar matrix of osteoid permits deposition of highly organized calcium phosphate crystals, including hydroxyapatite [$C_{10}(PO_4)_6 \cdot 6H_2O$] and octacalcium phosphate [$Ca_8(H_2PO_4)_6 \cdot 5H_2O$], plus less organized amorphous calcium phosphate, calcium carbonate, sodium, magnesium, and citrate. Hydroxyapatite is deep within bone matrix, whereas amorphous calcium phosphate coats the surface of newly formed or remodeled bone.

Bone growth occurs in children by the process of calcification of the cartilage cells present at the ends of bone. In accord with the prevailing extracellular fluid calcium and phosphate concentrations, mineral is deposited in those chondrocytes or cartilage cells set to undergo mineralization. The main function of the vitamin D–PTH–endocrine axis is to maintain the extracellular fluid calcium and phosphate concentrations at appropriate levels to permit mineralization.

Other hormones also appear to regulate the growth and mineralization of cartilage, including growth hormone acting through insulin-like growth factors, thyroid hormones, insulin, and androgens, and estrogens during the pubertal growth spurt. By contrast, supraphysiologic concentrations of glucocorticoids impair cartilage function and bone growth, and augment bone resorption. ■

CHAPTER 647

Bone and Vitamin D Metabolism

See also Chapters 43.6, 43.7, and 50.

Rates of bone formation are coordinated with alterations in mineral metabolism at both the intestine and kidney. Inadequate dietary intake or intestinal absorption of calcium causes a fall in serum calcium and its ionized fraction. This serves as the signal for PTH synthesis and secretion, resulting in greater bone resorption to raise serum calcium, enhanced distal tubular reabsorption of calcium, and higher rates of synthesis by the kidney of 1,25-dihydroxy vitamin D (1,25[OH]$_2$D or calcitriol), the most active metabolite of vitamin D (Fig. 647–1). Calcium homeostasis thus is controlled at the intestine, because the availability of 1,25(OH)$_2$D will ultimately determine the fraction of ingested calcium that is absorbed.

By contrast, phosphate homeostasis is regulated by the kidney, because intestinal phosphate absorption is nearly complete and renal excretion determines the serum level. Excessive intestinal phosphate absorption causes a fall in serum ionized calcium and a rise in PTH secretion, resulting in phosphaturia, thus lowering serum phosphate and permitting calcium to rise. Hypophosphatemia blocks PTH secretion and promotes renal 1,25(OH)$_2$D synthesis. This latter compound also promotes greater intestinal phosphate absorption.

An understanding of the metabolism of vitamin D is necessary to appreciate rickets (see Fig. 647–1). The skin contains 7-dehydrocholesterol, which is converted to vitamin D$_3$ by ultraviolet radiation; other inactive vitamin D sterols are also produced. Reduced skin exposure ultraviolet light (from smog or clothing) results in rickets (see Chapters 43.6 and 43.7). Vitamin D$_3$ is then transported in the blood stream to the liver by a vitamin D binding protein (DBP); DBP binds all forms of vitamin D. The plasma concentration of free or nonbound vitamin D is much lower than the level of DBP-bound vitamin D metabolities.

Vitamin D also can enter the metabolic pathway by ingestion of dietary vitamin D$_2$ (ergocalciferol) or vitamin D$_3$ (cholecalciferol), both of which are absorbed from the intestine along with other fat-soluble vitamins because of the action of bile salts. After absorption, ingested vitamin D is transported by chylomicrons to the liver where, along with skin-derived vitamin D$_3$, it is converted to 25-hydroxy vitamin D (25[OH]D) by the action of an hepatic microsomal enzyme requiring oxygen, NADPH, and magnesium to hydroxylate vitamin D at the 25th carbon atom. The 25(OH)D is next transported by DBP to the kidney, where it undergoes further metabolism. 25(OH)D is the main circulating vitamin D metabolite in humans at a concentration of 20–80 ng/mL (Table 647–1). Because its synthesis is weakly regulated by feedback, its plasma level rises in summer and falls in winter. High vitamin D intake raises the plasma level of 25(OH)D to many times above normal, but the parent vitamin D itself is absorbed by adipose tissue.

In the kidney, the 25(OH)D undergoes further hydroxylation, depending on the prevailing serum concentration of calcium, phosphate, and PTH. If calcium or phosphate is reduced

■ **TABLE 647–1 Vitamin D Metabolite Values in Plasma of Normal Healthy Subjects**

Metabolite	Plasma Value
Vitamin D$_2$	1–2 ng/mL
Vitamin D$_3$	1–2 ng/mL
25 (OH)D$_2$	4–10 ng/mL
25 (OH)D$_3$	12–40 ng/mL
Total 25 (OH)D	15–50 ng/mL
24, 25 (OH)$_2$D	1–4 ng/mL
1, 25 (OH)$_2$D	
Infancy	70–100 pg/mL
Childhood	30–50 pg/mL
Adolescence	40–80 pg/mL
Adulthood	20–35 pg/mL

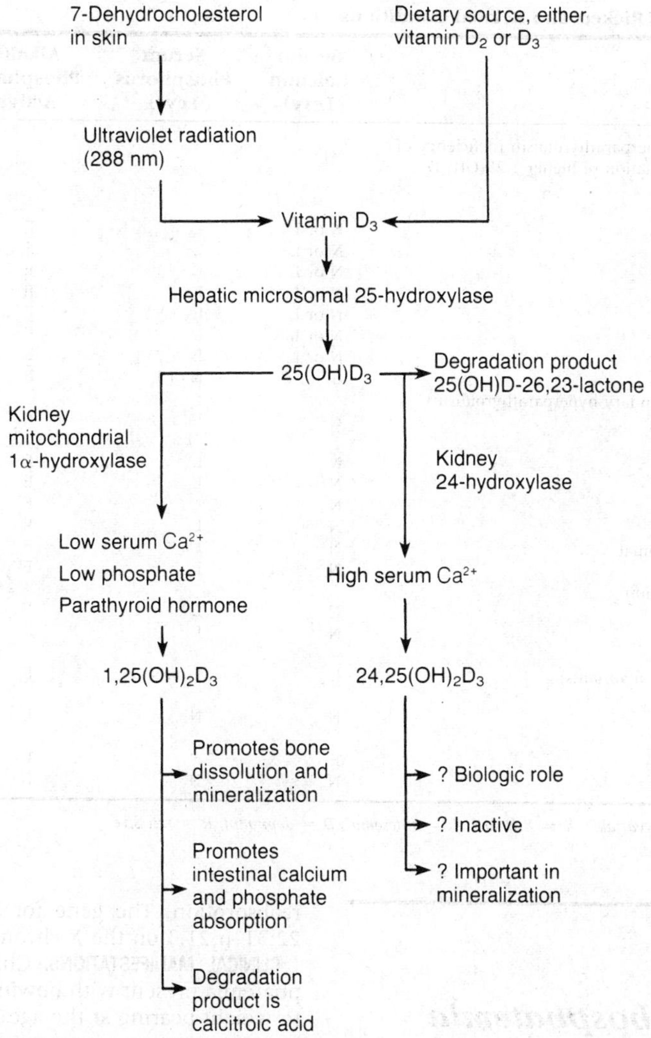

Figure 647–1. The metabolic pathway of vitamin D, indicating its conversion to the hormone $1,25(OH)_2D_3$ and to $24,25(OH)_2D_3$. Vitamin D_2 (ergosterol) of plant origin appears to undergo similar metabolic steps.

or PTH is elevated, the enzyme 25(OH)D-1α-hydroxylase is activated and $1,25(OH)_2D$ is formed (see Fig. 647–1). This metabolite circulates at a level that is only 0.1% of the level of 25(OH)D (see Table 647–1) and acts on the intestine to increase the active transport of calcium and stimulate phosphate absorption. Because 1α-hydroxylase is a mitochondrial enzyme that is tightly feedback regulated, the synthesis of $1,25(OH)_2D$ declines after serum calcium or phosphate values return to normal. Excessive $1,25(OH)_2D$ is converted to an inactive metabolite. In the presence of normal or elevated serum calcium or phosphate concentrations, the renal 25(OH)D-24-hydroxylase is activated, producing 24,25-dihydroxy vitamin D ($24,25[OH]_2D$), which is a pathway for the removal of excess vitamin D, because the serum levels of $24,25(OH)_2D$ (1–5 ng/mL) become higher after ingestion of large amounts of vitamin D. Although hypervitaminosis D and production of inactive metabolites can occur after oral dosing (see Chapter 43.7), extensive skin exposure to sunlight does not usually produce toxic levels of $25(OH)D_3$, suggesting natural regulation of the production of this metabolite in cutaneous tissue.

Serum $1,25(OH)_2D$ levels are higher in children than in adults, are not as subject to seasonal variability, and peak in the 1st yr of life and again during the adolescent growth spurt. These values must be interpreted in light of the prevailing serum calcium, phosphate, and PTH values, and also with regard to the entire vitamin D metabolite profile.

Mineral deficiency prevents the normal process of bone mineral deposition. If mineral deficiency occurs at the growth plate, growth slows and bone age is retarded—a condition called *rickets.* Poor mineralization of trabecular bone resulting in a greater proportion of unmineralized osteoid is the condition of *osteomalacia.* Rickets is found only in growing children prior to fusion of the epiphyses, whereas osteomalacia is present at all ages. All patients with rickets have osteomalacia, but not all patients with osteomalacia have rickets. These conditions should not be confused with *osteoporosis,* a condition of equal loss of bone volume and mineral, caused in childhood by glucocorticoid administration, found in Turner and Klinefelter syndromes, or as an idiopathic condition.

Rickets may be classified as calcium-deficient or phosphate-deficient rickets. Because both calcium and phosphate ions comprise bone mineral, the insufficiency of either type in the extracellular fluid that bathes the mineralizing surface of bone results in rickets and osteomalacia. The two types of rickets are distinguishable by their clinical manifestations (Table 647–2).

■ TABLE 647–2 Clinical Variants of Rickets and Related Conditions

Type	Serum Calcium Level	Serum Phosphorus Level	Alkaline Phosphatase Activity	Urine Concentration of Amino Acids	Genetics
I. Calcium deficiency with secondary hyperparathyroidism (deficiency of vitamin D; low 25(OH)D and no stimulation of higher $1,25(OH)_2D$ values)					
1. Lack of vitamin D					
a. Lack of exposure to sunlight	N or L	L	E	E	
b. Dietary deficiency of vitamin D	N or L	L	E	E	
c. Congenital	N or L	L	E	E	
2. Malabsorption of vitamin D	N or L	L	E	E	
3. Hepatic disease	N or L	L	E	E	
4. Anticonvulsive drugs	N or L	L	E	E	
5. Renal osteodystrophy	N or L	E	E	V	
6. Vitamin D–dependent type I	L	N or L	E	E	AR
II. Primary phosphate deficiency (no secondary hyperparathyroidism)					
1. Genetic primary hypophosphatemia	N	L	E	N	XD
2. Fanconi syndromes					
a. Cystinosis	N	L	E	E	AR
b. Tyrosinosis	N	L	E	E	AR
c. Lowe syndrome	N	L	E	E	XR
d. Acquired	N	L	E	E	
3. Renal tubular acidosis, type II proximal	N	L	E	N	
4. Oncogenic hypophosphatemia	N	L	E	N	
5. Phosphate deficiency or malabsorption					
a. Parenteral hyperalimentation	N	L	E	N	
b. Low phosphate intake	N	L	E	N	
III. End-organ resistance to $1,25(OH)_2D_3$					
1. Vitamin D–dependent type II (several variants)	L	L or N	E	E	AR
IV. Related conditions resembling rickets					
1. Hypophosphatasia	N	N	L	Phosphoethanolamine elevated	AR
2. Metaphyseal dysostosis					
a. Jansen type	E	N	E	N	AD
b. Schmidt type	N	N	N	N	AD

N = normal; L = low; E = elevated; V = variable; X = X-linked; A = autosomal; D = dominant; R = recessive.

CHAPTER 648

Familial Hypophosphatemia

(Vitamin D–Resistant Rickets, X-Linked Hypophosphatemia)

The most commonly encountered non-nutritional form of rickets is familial hypophosphatemia. The usual mode of inheritance is X-linked dominant, indicating that some mothers of affected children exhibit clinical evidence of disease such as bowing or short stature, whereas others manifest only fasting hypophosphatemia. Autosomal recessive and sporadic forms have also been reported.

PATHOGENESIS. Pathogenic mechanisms involve defects in the proximal tubular reabsorption of phosphate and in the conversion of 25(OH)D to $1,25(OH)_2D$. The latter defect is evidenced by low-normal serum $1,25(OH)_2D$ levels despite hypophosphatemia and by the finding that further phosphate depletion of subjects with familial hypophosphatemia does not stimulate $1,25(OH)_2D$ synthesis as it does in normal subjects. Both a renal tubular reabsorption defect and reduced $1,25(OH)_2D$ synthesis are found in an animal model of this disease. In addition, oral phosphate supplementation alone cannot completely heal bone disease; the correction of osteomalacia requires $1,25(OH)_2D$ therapy. The activity of the Na^+–-dependent phosphate transporter in the renal proximal tubule is reduced, resulting in excessive urinary phosphate excretion; this transporter protein is encoded on chromosome 5. Because the disorder has an X-linked inheritance pattern, the abnormal gene must represent a "nuisance" for a protein regulating phosphate reabsorption. The gene for this disorder is confined to X p 22.31–p 21.3 on the X chromosome.

CLINICAL MANIFESTATIONS. Children with familial hypophosphatemia present with bowing of the lower extremities related to weight bearing at the age of walking. Tetany is not present, and the profound myopathy, rachitic rosary, and Harrison groove (pectus deformity) characteristic of calcium-deficient rickets are not evident. These children develop a waddling gait, smooth (rather than angular) bowing of the lower extremities, coxa vara, genu varus, genu valgum, and short stature. The adult height of untreated patients is 130–165 cm.

Pulp deformities and a lesion called *intraglobular dentin* are characteristic tooth abnormalities, although enamel defects are found only occasionally. By contrast, calcium-deficient rickets usually results in enamel defects. Periapical infections are found in both forms of rickets. Therapy of metabolic bone disease does not correct the defect in intraglobular dentin in this condition.

Roentgenographic findings include metaphyseal widening and fraying, and coarse-appearing trabecular bone. Cupping of the metaphysis occurs at the proximal and distal tibia, and at the distal femur, radius, and ulna.

LABORATORY FINDINGS. There is a normal or slightly reduced serum calcium level (9–9.4 mg/dL; 2.24–2.34 mM/L), a moderately reduced serum phosphate level (1.5–3 mg/dL; 0.48–0.96 mM/L), elevated alkaline phosphatase activity, and no evidence of secondary hyperparathyroidism. Urinary phosphate excretion is large, despite hypophosphatemia, indicating a defect in renal tubular phosphate reabsorption. This disorder is typical of pure phosphate-deficient rickets since aminoaciduria, glucosuria, bicarbonaturia, and kaliuria are never found. In potential obligate heterozygotes, who later develop disease, serum phosphate levels may remain normal for the first several months of life. The first laboratory abnormality is often a rise in serum alkaline phosphatase activity. The serum phosphate level probably remains normal for several months, because the glomerular filtration rate is quite low in neonates. Parathyroid hyperplasia with elevated serum parathyroid hormone (PTH) values is occasionally found, usually in sporadic cases.

TREATMENT. Oral phosphate supplements coupled with a vitamin D analog to offset the secondary hyperparathyroidism that may accompany an oral phosphate load is the preferred treatment. Oral phosphate is usually given every 4 hr for at least 5 times a day, because urinary excretion is constant and patients quickly become hypophosphatemic. Young children should receive 0.5–1 g/24 hr, whereas older children require 1–4 g/24 hr. Phosphate can be given as Joulie solution (dibasic sodium phosphate, 136 g/L, and phosphoric acid, 58.8 g/L), which contains 30.4 mg of phosphate/mL. Thus, a 5 mL dose given every 4 hr, 5 times daily, provides 760 mg of phosphate. A capsule form of phosphate (Neutraphos) provides 250 mg of phosphorous per capsule. Patient compliance is readily assessed because almost all of this dose is excreted in a 24-hr urine collection. The main side effect of oral phosphate therapy is diarrhea, which often improves spontaneously.

Providing a vitamin D analog is important for complete bone healing and prevention of secondary hyperparathyroidism. Classically, vitamin D_2 was used at 2,000 IU/kg/24 hr, but more recently, dihydrotachysterol at a dosage of 0.02 mg/kg/24 hr or $1,25(OH)_2D$ at 50–65 ng/kg/24 hr has been effectively used.

Familial hypophosphatemia was previously treated with 50,000–200,000 IU/24 hr (1.25–10 mg) of vitamin D_2, but this caused hypervitaminosis D with nephrocalcinosis, hypercalcemia, and permanent renal damage.

The term *vitamin D–resistant rickets* was used in the past to describe rickets in which patients failed to respond to a dose of vitamin D that would cure vitamin D deficiency. If appropriate doses of vitamin D or any of its metabolites fail to heal rickets, and if serum phosphate is not reduced, metaphyseal dysplasia should be considered (see Chapter 634).

With early diagnosis and good compliance, the bowing deformities can be minimized, and an adult height above 170 cm may be achievable. However, the influence of therapy on final height is controversial, because most patients remain short while in other studies good growth patterns are evident. Corrective osteotomies should always be deferred until rickets appears healed roentgenographically and until the serum alkaline phosphatase level is in the normal range. Surgery prior to bone healing may be followed by redevelopment of deformity and bowing. In some patients, aggressive medical management may obviate the need for surgical intervention. Patients undergoing osteotomy should stop taking all vitamin D preparations before surgery and should not start them again until they are again ambulating to avoid immobilization hypercalcemia. Because $1,25(OH)_2D$ has such a short half-life, it can be stopped just prior to surgery, whereas vitamin D_2 should be discontinued at least 1 mo before surgery. An additional advantage of $1,25(OH)_2D$ therapy is that it augments intestinal phosphate absorption and may improve phosphate balance. However, $1,25(OH)_2D$ should not be used without concomitant oral phosphate.

Certain patients have hypophosphatemia and hyperphosphaturia but no roentgenographic evidence of rickets. This condition, inherited as an autosomal dominant disorder, has been called *hypophosphatemic bone disease.* The serum concentrations of $1,25(OH)_2D$ are normal, and the renal tubular phosphate excretion defect is not as marked as in familial hypophosphatemic rickets. Short stature is not as prominent. Oral phosphate and $1,25(OH)_2D$ have been used to treat this disorder.

Chapter 649
Vitamin D–Dependent Rickets
(Pseudovitamin D Deficiency, Hypocalcemic Vitamin D Resistant Rickets)

Vitamin D–dependent rickets appears at age 3–6 mo in children who have been receiving dosages of vitamin D (400–600 IU/24 hr) that ordinarily prevent rickets. Serum calcium and phosphate levels are low, and alkaline phosphatase activity is elevated. This condition is a calcium-deficient form of rickets because patients have secondary hyperparathyroidism, aminoaciduria, glucosuria, renal tubular bicarbonate wasting, and renal tubular acidosis. These children also develop dental enamel hypoplasia. While the rickets and biochemical features of this autosomal recessive disorder can be treated with a massive dosage of vitamin D_2 (200,000–1 million IU/24 hr), the use of relatively low-dose $1,25(OH)_2D$ at 1–2 μg/24 hr will heal this disorder. The current hypothesis to account for these findings is that the enzyme activity of $25(OH)D\text{-}1\alpha$-hydroxylase is deficient or greatly reduced. As evidence of this hypothesis, the serum levels of $1,25(OH)_2D$ are low, despite hypocalcemia, hypophosphatemia, and elevated parathyroid hormone (PTH) levels.

Some patients with vitamin D–dependent rickets fail to reverse their rickets after treatment either with high-dose vitamin D_2 or $1,25(OH)_2D$ at 1–2 μg/24 hr. Hypocalcemia, hypophosphatemia, aminoaciduria, and rickets persist in the presence of extremely high circulating levels of $1,25(OH)_2D$, usually above 180 pg/mL. Patients with hereditary $1,25\text{-}(OH)_2D_3$–resistant rickets have (1) reduced or absent $1,25\text{-}(OH)_2D_3$ binding to the human vitamin D nuclear receptor; (2) decreased affinity of this receptor for DNA so that transcription cannot occur; or (3) defective nuclear translocation or retention. An abnormal gene product is produced by the vitamin D receptor gene in these patients. A single amino acid substitution in an important DNA-binding site in the receptor may cause this disorder, thus preventing the binding of $1,25(OH)_2D$ and its receptor to the nucleus. Mis-sense mutations of the DNA binding or the steroid ($1,25\text{-}[OH]_2D_3$) of the vitamin D receptor have been found. This form of the disease, which is particularly prevalent among children of 1st-cousin marriages, is termed *vitamin D dependency, type II,* or hereditary resistance to $1,25(OH)_2D$. Some patients have short stature and alopecia totalis. Rickets can sometimes be reversed by administration of 15–30 μg/24 hr of $1,25(OH)_2D$, but absent hair does not regrow.

Chapter 650
Hepatic Rickets

Rickets is not uncommon in children with hepatic disorders, particularly in extrahepatic biliary atresia, where failure of bile salt secretion prevents adequate absorption of vitamin D and other fat-soluble vitamins. Rickets may also occur in neonatal hepatitis and following hepatocellular damage induced by total parenteral nutrition. Although it was initially thought that hepatic disease would impair 25-hydroxylation and thus reduce serum 25(OH)D levels, it is now believed that reduced absorption of vitamin D accounts for rickets. The usual findings of nutritional rickets are seen—reduced serum 25(OH)D values, hypocalcemia, roentgenographic evidence, and elevated serum alkaline phosphatase activity (bone and hepatic isoenzyme levels are raised). Because rickets mainly relates to vitamin D malabsorption, this form can be treated with high enough doses to overcome malabsorption. Thus, 4,000–10,000 IU of vitamin D_2 (100–250 μg), 50 μg of 25(OH)D, or 0.2 μg/kg of $1,25(OH)_2D$ should be given daily, along with oral calcium. Calcium supplements are particularly indicated in infants having ascites who are receiving loop diuretics, such as furosemide, which result in excessive urinary calcium losses.

CHAPTER 651

Rickets Associated with Anticonvulsant Therapy

A small group of children receiving chronic anticonvulsant therapy will present with calcium-deficient rickets, despite apparently adequate vitamin D intake. This condition is more common after the combination of phenobarbital and phenytoin, but it has been associated with almost all anticonvulsant drugs. Affected patients have reduced serum levels of 25(OH)D and may have normal levels of $1,25(OH)_2D$. Because these anticonvulsants induce hepatic cytochrome P-450 hydroxylation enzyme activities, 25(OH)D is readily converted to more polar, inactive metabolites, thus accounting for lower serum 25(OH)D concentrations. However, this condition is much more complex because many patients have a low intake of dairy products, which represent the major dietary source of calcium, and very poor exposure to sunlight. This condition is more common in institutionalized children. Thus, the relatively normal serum $1,25(OH)_2D$ values are actually subnormal in relation to the degree of hypocalcemia, hypophosphatemia, and secondary hyperparathyroidism.

In children receiving chronic anticonvulsant therapy, the serum values of calcium, phosphate, and alkaline phosphatase activity should be evaluated periodically. This form of rickets usually can be prevented by providing an extra 500–1,000 IU of vitamin D_2 each day and by ensuring that the dietary intake of calcium is adequate.

CHAPTER 652

Oncogenous Rickets

(Primary Hypophosphatemic Rickets Associated with Tumor)

Rickets associated with a tumor of mesenchymal origin that resolves upon removal of the tumor has been described in more than 90 cases. These tumors, which cause a phosphate-deficient form of rickets, are mostly benign, may become apparent only years after the development of rickets, and may be located in sites difficult to detect, such as the small bones of the hands and feet, abdominal sheath, nasal antrum, and pharynx. This syndrome is also associated with the epidermal nevus syndrome, neurofibromatosis (von Recklinghausen disease), and linear nevus syndrome.

In addition to hypophosphatemia and hyperphosphaturia, glycinemia and glycinuria are sometimes found in this form of rickets. Evidence suggests that these tumors elaborate a still-unidentified substance, which causes phosphaturia and impairs the conversion of 25(OH)D to $1,25(OH)_2D$. Serum 25(OH)D levels are normal, and serum $1,25(OH)_2D$ levels are low but rapidly rise to normal after tumor excision. Hypophosphatemia in this syndrome may be caused by ectopic production by tumor cells of a heat-labile factor with a molecular weight of 8,000–25,000 kD, which inhibits renal tubular reabsorption of phosphate. This surgery also cures the bone pain and myopathy, which, if untreated, may confine the child to a wheelchair. Children with acquired or late-appearing hypophosphatemic rickets should undergo bone roentgenographic examination and/or bone scan to search for tumors. If a tumor cannot be removed or is metastatic, treatment with $1,25(OH)_2D$ and oral phosphate is often beneficial.

CHAPTER 653

Hypophosphatasia (see Chapter 647)

Hypophosphatasia is an autosomal recessive disorder that roentgenographically resembles rickets and is defined by low serum alkaline phosphatase activity. Hypophosphatasia is now recognized to be an inborn error of metabolism in which there is deficient activity of the tissue-nonspecific (liver/bone/kidney) alkaline phosphatase. Single point mutations of the gene for alkaline phosphatase prevent the expression of the activity of this enzyme in vitro and indicate the necessity of this enzyme for normal skeletal mineralization. Activity of the intestinal and placental enzyme is normal. There is considerable heterogeneity in the severity of the disease. Some cases appear at birth, and diagnosis has even been made in utero by roentgenographic examination of the fetus. The disease may appear in a lethal neonatal or perinatal form (*congenital lethal hypophosphatasia*), a severe infantile form, or a milder form occurring in childhood or late adolescence (*hypophosphatasia tarda*). The lethal form is characterized by a moth-eaten appearance at the ends of the long bones, by severe deficiency of ossification throughout the skeleton, and by marked shortening of the long bones. Patients with the mild disease may present with bowing of the legs and variable statural shortening. Because calcium accumulation by mature chondrocytes does not occur, patients may appear to have rickets, and in the neonatal and infantile form they may have hypercalcemia.

Unusual clinical manifestations include wormian bones in the calvarium, poor calcification of the frontal, parietal, and occipital bones, and premature loss of deciduous or permanent teeth owing to hypoplasia of dental cementum. Because of the hypercalcemia in the infantile form, nephrocalcinosis is also found. In the childhood form, bone pain, frequent fractures, and milder skeletal deformities are evident, as well as premature tooth loss. The metaphyseal defect consists of irregular ossification, punched-out areas, and metaphyseal cupping.

In hypophosphatasia, large quantities of phosphoethanolamine are found in the urine because this compound cannot be degraded in the absence of adequate alkaline phosphatase activity. Plasma inorganic pyrophosphate and pyridoxal-5-phosphate are also elevated for the same reason. Although no satisfactory therapy has been found, infusion of plasma rich in alkaline phosphatase activity has been helpful in healing bone in short-term studies. The clinical course of this condition often improves spontaneously as the child matures, although early death from renal failure or flail chest leading to pneumonia may also occur in the severe infantile form of the disorder. Rare patients presenting identical clinical and roentgenographic patterns have normal serum alkaline phosphatase activities. Their disease has been labeled *pseudohypophosphatasia* and may represent the presence of a mutant alkaline phosphatase isozyme that reacts to artificial substrates in an alkaline environment (i.e., in a test tube) but not in vivo with natural substrates.

CHAPTER 654

Primary Chondrodystrophy

(Metaphyseal Dysplasia)

In this condition bowing of the legs, short stature, and a waddling gait appear in the absence of abnormalities of serum calcium, phosphate, alkaline phosphatase activity, or vitamin D metabolites. Metaphyseal chondrodysplasia (*Jansen type*) is typified by cupped and ragged metaphyses, which develop mottled calcification at the distal ends of bone over time. Hypercalcemia, with serum values of 13–15 mg/dL may occur. The spine may also be deformed by the irregular growth of vertebrae. The *Schmid type* of metaphyseal chondrodysplasia is less severe, although the roentgenographic appearance of the knees and extreme bowing of the lower limbs resemble signs seen in patients with familial hypophosphatemia. It is associated with defects in collagen type X. The hip abnormalities are more debilitating, however. Patients with both types of metaphyseal chondrodysplasia have lifelong short stature.

Metaphyseal dysotosis, or *Pyle disease,* results from defects in endochondral bone formation and metaphyseal modeling. The long ends of bones are splayed, resulting in an "Erlenmeyer flask" defect. Short stature is not present, and serum chemical levels are normal. Leonine features develop if the facial bones are involved.

No effective forms of treatment are available for the chondrodystrophies or the dysostosis.

CHAPTER 655

Idiopathic Hypercalcemia

Medical attention was initially drawn to hypercalcemia shortly after World War II ended, when excessive quantities of vitamin D were used to enrich food for infants in England. Although many infants were exposed to high levels of vitamin D, only a few developed hypercalcemia, failure to thrive, nephrolithiasis, and decline in renal function. These infants had roentgenographic evidence of osteosclerosis and dense bones at the metaphyses. This disorder disappeared with reduction in the vitamin D content of milk. Subsequently, at least three separate forms of hypercalcemia of unknown origin have been described.

Williams syndrome, or the elfin facies syndrome, consists of a constellation of manifestations, of which hypercalcemia is an infrequent finding. The characteristic facial features include a small mandible, prominent maxilla, and upturned nose. The upper lip has a Cupid's bow curve. Small peglike teeth with numerous caries are common. Feeding problems and failure to thrive during the 1st yr of life are usual. Mild mental retardation and an unusual "cocktail party patter" personality are typical. The types of cardiac lesions found separately or together include supravalvular aortic stenosis, peripheral pulmonary stenosis, hypoplasia of the aorta, and atrial or ventricular septal defects. In hypercalcemic patients, nephrocalcinosis and sclerotic long bones are sometimes evident.

Williams syndrome is sporadic, and some children have hypervitaminosis D without evidence of increased maternal or infantile vitamin D intake. In most cases, the circulating values for vitamin D metabolites are normal. Patients with this disorder slowly excrete an infused calcium load and have evidence for increased production of 25(OH)D from vitamin D. Impaired calcitonin secretion to an infused calcium load has also been reported. Treatment is directed at cardiac, social, and educational problems.

Children may also have mild *idiopathic hypercalcemia,* which is usually transient. Phenotypic features of Williams syndrome are not found. These patients have hypercalciuria and sometimes nephrocalcinosis, possibly resembling the English infants who received excessive vitamin D after World War II. However, no evidence for abnormalities in vitamin D metabolism has been found.

Familial hypocalciuric hypercalcemia is an autosomal dominant condition in which affected children have asymptomatic hypercalcemia without hypercalciuria. Pancreatitis may occur in some families and, in a few kindreds, neonates may present with life-threatening parathyroid hyperplasia. Instead of serum calcium levels of 12–15 mg/dL, typically found in the parent, these infants have levels exceeding 18 mg/dL. All these children have had mild parathyroid hyperplasia despite hypercalcemia, indicating that the parathyroid gland does not respond appropriately to the signal of hypercalcemia. Vitamin D metabolism is normal. Only the infants with serious hyperparathyroidism require treatment—an emergency parathyroidectomy. Although serum magnesium is elevated, it is not a serious concern.

CHAPTER 656

Hyperphosphatasia

Excessive elevation of the bone isozyme of alkaline phosphatase in serum and significant growth failure characterize hyperphosphatasia. Osteoid proliferation in the subperiosteal portion of bone results in separation of the periosteum from the bone cortex. Bowing and thickening of the diaphyses are common, along with osteopenia. The disease usually has its onset by 2–3 yr of age, when painful deformity developing in the extremities leads to abnormal gait and sometimes fractures. Other common findings include pectus carinatum, kyphoscoliosis, and rib fraying. The skull is large and the cranium is thickened (widened diplöe) and may be deformed. Roentgenographically, the bony texture is variable; dense areas (showing a teased cotton-wool appearance) are interspersed with radiolucent areas and general demineralization. Long bones appear cylindric, lose metaphyseal modeling, and contain pseudocysts showing a dense bony halo.

In this autosomal recessive disorder, serum levels of both calcium and phosphate are normal, whereas urinary leucine amino acid peptidase activity and serum acid phosphatase are increased. This disorder is often called *juvenile Paget disease* because, as in adult-onset Paget disease, calcitonin may reduce the rapid bone turnover found in this disorder; in children the disorder is more generalized and symmetric.

Transient hyperphosphatasia occurs between 2 mo and 2 yr of age, has no associated manifestations other than some mild gastrointestinal symptoms, and is usually detected during routine (screening) laboratory evaluation for some unrelated complaint. Both liver and bone isoenzyme fractions are elevated; however, there are no other manifestations of hepatic or bone dysfunction. The etiology is unknown. Resolution usually occurs within 4–6 mo.

Familial hyperphosphatemia, an autosomal dominant trait, is another benign condition that is distinguished from the transient infantile form by persistent and asymptomatic elevations of serum alkaline phosphatase levels.

Cai Q, Hodgson SF, Kao PC, et al: Inhibition of phosphate transport by a tumor product in a patient with oncogenic osteomalacia. N Engl J Med 230:1645, 1994.

Casella SJ, Reiner BJ, Chen TC, et al: A possible genetic defect in 25-hydroxylation as a cause of rickets. J Pediatr 124:929, 1994.

Chesney RW: Requirements and upper limits of vitamin D intake in the term neonate, infant, and older child. J Pediatr 116:159, 1990.

Chesney RW, Kaplan BS, Phelps M, et al: Renal tubular acidosis does not alter the circulating values of calcitriol ($1,25(OH)_2$-vitamin D). J Pediatr 104:51, 1984.

Chesney RW, DeLuca HF, Gertner JM, et al: Circulating levels of vitamin D metabolites in children with the Williams syndrome. N Engl J Med 313:888, 1985.

Culler FL, Jones KL, Deftos LJ: Impaired calcitonin secretion in patients with Williams syndrome. J Pediatr 107:720, 1985.

Econs MJ, Presner MK: Tumor-induced osteomalacia—unveiling a new hormone. N Engl J Med 330:1679, 1994.

Eil C, Lieberman UA, Rosen JF, et al: Cellular defect in hereditary vitamin D-dependent rickets type II: Defective nuclear uptake of 1,25-dihydroxyvitamin D in cultured skin fibroblasts. N Engl J Med 304:1588, 1981.

Hanna JD, Niimi K, Chan JC: X-linked hypophosphatemic rickets: Genetic and clinical correlates. Am J Dis Child 145:865, 1991.

Harrison HE, Harrison HC: Disorders of Calcium and Phosphate Metabolism in Childhood and Adolescence. Philadelphia, WB Saunders, 1979.

Hughes MR, Malloy PJ, O'Malley BW, et al: Genetic defects of the 1,25 dihydroxyvitamin D_3 receptor. J Recept Res 11:699, 1991.

Markowitz ME, Rosen JF, Smith C, et al: 1,25-dihydroxyvitamin D_3-related hypoparathyroidism: 35 patient years in 10 children. J Clin Endocrinol Metab 55:727, 1982.

Opshaug O, Maurseth K, Howlid H, et al: Vitamin D metabolism in hypophosphatasia: Case report. Acta Paediatr Scand 71:517, 1982.

Rosen JF, Chesney RW: Circulating calcitriol concentrations in health and disease of infancy and childhood J Pediatr 103:1, 1983.

Scriver CR, Reade T, Halal F, et al: Autosomal hypophosphatemic bone disease responds to $1,25(OH)_2D_3$. Arch Dis Child 56:203, 1981.

Verge CF, Cowell CT, Howard NJ, et al: Growth in children with X-linked hypophosphatemic rickets. Acta Pediatr Suppl 388:70, 1993.

Warman ML et al: A type X collagen mutation causes Schmid metaphyseal chondrodysplasia. Nature Genet 5:79, 1993.

Weiss MJ, Cole DE, Ray K, et al: First identification of a gene defect for hypophosphatasia: Evidence that alkaline phosphatase acts in skeletal mineralization. Connect Tissue Res 21:99, 1990.

PART XXXIII

Unclassified Diseases

CHAPTER 657

Sudden Infant Death Syndrome

Carl E. Hunt

Sudden infant death syndrome (SIDS) is defined as the sudden death of any infant or young child that is unexpected by history and unexplained by a thorough postmortem examination, which includes a complete autopsy, investigation of the scene of death, and review of the medical history. An autopsy is required in all sudden and unexpected infant deaths because the history and death scene investigation are not sufficient to exclude many of the other congenital and acquired causes (Fig. 657–1).

SIDS is the most common cause of postneonatal infant death in developed countries, generally accounting for 40–50% of infant deaths between 1 mo and 1 yr of age. In the United States, the SIDS rate is 1.3/1,000 live births; at least 6,000 deaths occur each year. SIDS is rare before 1 mo of age, the peak incidence is 2–4 mo, and 95% of all SIDS cases have occurred by 6 mo of age.

SIDS has been recognized since biblical times. Despite extensive efforts, however, the causes of SIDS remain unknown. There is no accurate method for prospective identification, and there is no proven strategy for intervention. A brain stem developmental abnormality or maturational delay related to neuroregulation of cardiorespiratory control, sleep-wake regulation, and circadian rhythmicity appears to be the most compelling and comprehensive hypothesis.

PATHOLOGY. The autopsy findings in victims of SIDS have not been of sufficient specificity and sensitivity to explain the disease. Mild pulmonary edema and diffuse intrathoracic petechias have been observed. Evidence (tissue markers) of chronic asphyxia occurs in nearly 66% of SIDS cases.

Brain stem abnormalities in victims of SIDS include focal astrogliosis, persistent dendritic spines, and hypomyelination. The primary area of persisting brain stem dendritic spines is in the magnocellular nucleus of the reticular formation and dor-

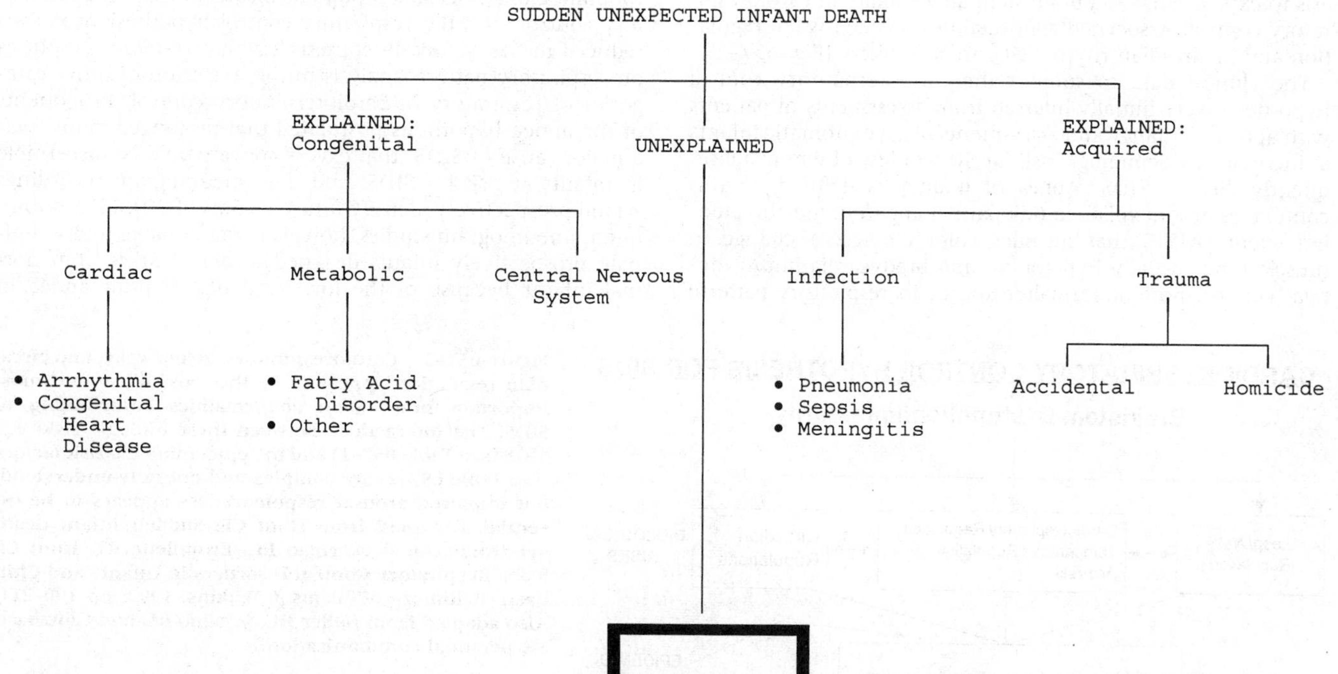

Figure 657–1. Differential diagnosis of sudden, unexpected death during infancy. An autopsy is necessary to exclude important but clinically undiagnosed congenital and acquired abnormalities. Death caused by infection may not be exclusively an acquired explanation; an immune deficit has also been postulated to be present in SIDS victims. (Adapted from Hunt CE: Apnea and SIDS. *In*: Kliegman RM, Nieder ML, Super DM [eds]: Practical Strategies in Pediatric Diagnosis and Therapy. Philadelphia, WB Saunders, in press.)

sal and solitary nuclei of the vagal nerve. Significant increases in the number of reactive astrocytes in the medulla have also been observed; the location of these increases is not confined to areas related to respiratory neuroregulation. Substance P, a neuropeptide transmitter found in selected primary sensory neurons of the central nervous system, is present in increased amounts in the pons of SIDS cases. A small subset of victims of SIDS has hypoplasia of the arcuate nucleus; this region is a site of cardiorespiratory control in the ventral medulla and is integrated with other regions that regulate arousal, autonomic, and chemosensory function. The various morphologic abnormalities identified in victims of SIDS thus include delayed neuronal maturation of medullary catecholaminergic neurons and increased activity in afferent neurons, providing pathophysiologic support of abnormalities in neural cardiorespiratory control and sleep-wake mechanisms.

Other postmortem observations are consistent with a response to chronic asphyxia. Infants with SIDS have both prenatal and postnatal growth retardation and elevated blood cortisol levels. Elevated levels of hypoxanthine in vitreous humor have been reported in such infants compared with control infants, and death thus appears in most cases to be preceded by a relatively long period of tissue hypoxia. Because adenosine, a precursor of hypoxanthine, is a respiratory inhibitor, these observations also indicate a potentially important interaction between asphyxia and hypoventilation; in response to asphyxia from any cause, the secondary acceleration of adenosine monophosphate catabolism and adenosine accumulation stimulates and then perpetuates hypoventilation.

PATHOPHYSIOLOGY. The postmortem findings are directly related to abnormal brain stem development and chronic asphyxia. The asphyxic changes are either secondary to the underlying abnormality that caused the impaired brain stem development or are the result of the brain stem dysfunction. Based on postmortem data and the functional abnormalities present in infants at increased risk for SIDS, the most compelling hypothesis to explain SIDS is a brain stem abnormality in cardiorespiratory control. Associated abnormalities in sleep-wake regulation and in circadian rhythmicity are also likely (Fig. 657–2).

The clinical data to support the cardiorespiratory control hypothesis were initially inferred from assessments of patients with apnea of infancy and assessments of asymptomatic infants at increased epidemiologic risk for SIDS, a few of whom subsequently died of SIDS. Apnea of infancy is defined, in this context, as an unexplained (idiopathic) apparent life-threatening event (ALTE) that includes color change, a change in muscle tone (usually hypotonia), and bradycardia and/or apnea. One or more abnormalities occur in respiratory pattern;

■ **TABLE 657–1 Biologic Risk Factors**

Biologic markers or risk factors associated with sudden infant death syndrome.
Interaction(s) with one or more epidemiologic risk factors (Table 657–2) are likely to be important, but such interactions are complex and not well understood.

- Family history of sudden infant death syndrome
- Apnea of infancy
- Prematurity
- Deficient brain stem control
  - Arousal/gasping
  - Ventilatory responsiveness
  - Respiratory pattern
  - Cardiac control
  - Temperature regulation
  - Other autonomic deficit(s)
- Hypothetical
  - Metabolic
  - Infectious
  - Immune

chemoreceptor sensitivity; and control of heart rate, cardiorespiratory interaction, or asphyxic arousal responsiveness (Table 657–1). Studies of apnea of infancy episodes associated with recurrent cyanotic episodes and rapid-onset severe hypoxemia also suggest interactions among central sympathetic activity, brain stem respiratory and vasomotor control, and respiratory tract reflexes. Whether related to delayed maturation or to a congenital defect, there are complex interactions between various categories of brain stem function. The peripheral chemoreceptors may also be involved.

Respiratory Pattern. Respiratory pattern abnormalities have been observed in infants at risk for SIDS and in a few infants who later died of SIDS. These abnormalities include prolonged apnea, excess brief apneas, and periodic breathing. Because apnea was the most visible manifestation of an abnormal respiratory pattern and the easiest to assess as a clinical marker for a respiratory control deficit, cardiorespiratory recordings (pneumograms) became a popular means of assessing respiratory control, and the respiratory control hypothesis was thus reduced to the "apnea hypothesis," with a resultant emphasis on respiratory pattern analysis to the exclusion of other categories of respiratory or cardiorespiratory control. Proponents of the apnea hypothesis postulated that prolonged apnea was a major cause of SIDS, that excess apnea would be discernible in infants at risk for SIDS, and that pneumogram recordings would prospectively identify future victims of SIDS. The subsequent pneumogram studies, however, were unable to discriminate prospectively infants destined to die of SIDS from normal infants because of the low incidence of prior apnea in

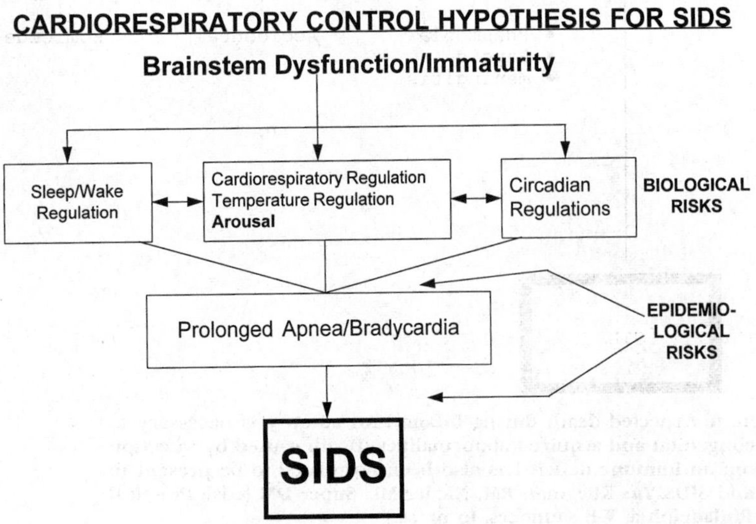

Figure 657–2. Cardiorespiratory, sleep/wake, and circadian regulation appear to be the most likely and most important brain stem abnormalities contributing to SIDS. The interactions between these biologic risks for SIDS (see Table 657–1) and the epidemiologic risk factors (see Table 657–2) are complex and not fully understood, but impaired arousal responsiveness appears to be essential. (Adapted from Hunt CE: Sudden infant death syndrome. *In*: Beckerman RC, Brouillette RT, Hunt CE [eds]: Respiratory Control Disorders in Infants and Children. Baltimore, Williams & Wilkins, 1992, pp 190–211. Also adapted from Heller HC, Ariagno RL, and Glotzbach SF, personal communication.)

victims of SIDS and the occurrence of respiratory pattern "abnormalities" in infants without any subsequent morbidity or mortality from an ALTE or SIDS. Respiratory pattern abnormalities are only one category of cardiorespiratory control, however, and probably one of the less important categories (see Fig. 657–1 and Table 657–1).

Chemoreceptor Sensitivity. Some infants at increased risk for SIDS have diminished ventilatory responsiveness to hypercarbia and/or to hypoxia. Such assessments, however, are costly and time consuming, and the overlap between normal and at-risk infants is such that one cannot prospectively distinguish normal infants from those who will later die of SIDS.

Arousal Responses. Respiratory pattern abnormalities and diminished ventilatory responsiveness are not inherently life threatening. A deficiency in arousal responsiveness, however, could be life threatening because the infant has thereby been rendered incapable of responding effectively to progressive sleep-related asphyxia, regardless of its cause (see Fig. 657–2 and Table 657–1). Asymptomatic infants at increased epidemiologic risk for SIDS and patients with apnea of infancy and diminished ventilatory responsiveness to hypercarbia and/or hypoxia generally also have an abnormality in hypercarbic and/or hypoxic arousal responsiveness. A deficit in arousal responsiveness may be a necessary prerequisite for SIDS to occur but insufficient in itself to cause SIDS in the absence of other biologic and/or epidemiologic risk factor(s) (Table 657–2).

Hypoxic and hypercapnic arousal responses correlate with the occurrence and severity of recurrent symptoms in patients with apnea of infancy (see Chapter 87.2). All infants arouse to hypercarbia during quiet sleep, but normal infants arouse at a significantly lower Pco_2 level than do those with apnea of infancy. All normal infants, but only about 33% of those with

■ **TABLE 657–2 Epidemiologic Factors Associated with Increased Risk for Sudden Infant Death Syndrome**

There is substantial uncertainty as to which factors are causal, independent risks. The extent and importance of interactions with biologic risk factors (Table 657–1) are not fully understood.

Maternal and Antenatal Risk Factors
- Intrauterine hypoxia
- Fetal growth retardation
- Urinary tract infection
- Smoking
- Anemia
- Drug exposure (e.g., cocaine, heroin)
- Nutritional deficiency
- Less prenatal care
- Low socioeconomic status
- Decreased age, education
- Increased placental weight
- Increased parity
- Shorter interpregnancy interval

Neonatal Risk Factors
- Growth failure
- Asphyxia
- Prematurity

Postneonatal Risk Factors
- Male
- Age (peak 2–4 mo)
- Bottle feeding
- Thermal stress
- Noncentral heating
- Co-sleeping
- Recent (febrile) illness
- Smoking exposure
- Soft sleeping surface, e.g., natural fiber mattress
- Swaddling
- No pacifier
- Prone sleep position

Other Risk Factors
- Geographic factors
- Colder season and climate
- Race/ethnicity (e.g., black, Native American, Gypsy, Maori, Hawaiian, Filipino)

apnea of infancy, arouse to mild hypoxia during quiet sleep. Furthermore, patients with apnea of infancy without hypoxic arousal responsiveness have a significantly higher incidence of subsequent apneas than do those with intact hypoxic arousal response, and the proportion of infants with intact hypoxic arousal responsiveness significantly decreases as the severity of the most severe subsequent apnea increases.

A relationship exists between arousal and age; only 10–15% of normal infants older than 9 wk of age and most infants younger than 9 wks of age arouse in response to mild hypoxia. These data thus suggest that, as normal infants mature, their ability to arouse in response to hypoxia diminishes by 2–3 mo of age. Siblings of victims of SIDS and patients with apnea of infancy also have a relative inability to awaken from sleep that is most evident around 2–3 mo of age. Unfortunately, current methods for assessing arousal responsiveness are cumbersome and time consuming and do not prospectively identify infants destined to die of SIDS with sufficient accuracy to be clinically useful.

Victims of SIDS may also have deficient autoresuscitation (gasping) as a complement to the asphyxic arousal response deficit. A failure of autoresuscitation in victims of SIDS is presumably the final and most devastating physiologic failure.

Temperature Regulation. Increased body and/or environmental temperature is associated with SIDS. There are complex interactions among temperature regulation, respiratory pattern, chemoreceptor sensitivity, cardiac control, and arousal/gasping (Table 657–1). The increased sleep-related sweating that occurs in some patients with apnea of infancy may be caused by alveolar hypoventilation and secondary asphyxia or by autonomic dysfunction and, thus, be indicative of an even more generalized deficiency in brain stem function; sweating, however, may also be an indication of overheating.

Cardiac Control. A small percentage of cases of SIDS has been attributed to a prolonged Q-T interval (see Chapter 388). The ability to shorten Q-T interval as heart rate increases is impaired in some SIDS cases, which suggests that relatively prolonged cardiac repolarization may predispose such infants to ventricular arrhythmias. Infants with SIDS have higher heart rates in all sleep-waking states and diminished heart rate variability during wakefulness. Computer analysis of respiratory sinus arrhythmia in infants who later died of SIDS has also revealed significantly lower heart rate variation across all sleep-waking cycles. Even in early infancy, therefore, future victims of SIDS differ in the extent to which cardiac and respiratory activity are coupled. Part of the decreased heart rate variability, and the increased heart rate, observed in infants who later died of SIDS may be related to decreased vagal tone. This could be related to vagal neuropathy, to brain stem damage in areas responsible for parasympathetic control of the heart, or to other factors. Furthermore, because the greatest reduction in all types of heart rate variability occurs while the infant is awake, these reductions may be related to the reduced motility retrospectively reported in victims of SIDS. Reduced motility has also been observed in infants at increased risk for SIDS.

Home monitors with memory capability have recorded some terminal episodes. In most instances, there has been sudden and rapid progression of severe bradycardia, too rapid to be explained by progressive desaturation from prolonged central apnea, thus providing some confirmation of an abnormality in autonomic control of heart rate variability. Obstructive apnea and/or hypoxemia may, in some instances, be the precipitating mechanism for the severe bradycardia. Current home monitoring technology, however, does not permit detection of obstructive apnea because breath detection is based on respiratory effort (by thoracic impedance) rather than breath volume or air flow. These systems can include oxygen saturation measurements, but the pulse oximeter is so sensitive to movement artifact that it is impractical to document isolated desaturation as a precursor of the severe bradycardia that causes the terminal event in infants with SIDS.

EPIDEMIOLOGY. No epidemiologic differences are sufficiently sensitive and specific to permit prospective identification of victims of SIDS (see Table 657–2). The prenatal epidemiologic risk factors for SIDS are generally identical to those for prematurity, and the prenatal and postnatal risk factors for SIDS overlap considerably with non-SIDS risks for infant death. It is not possible to determine the relative importance of each individual risk factor or to quantify the effect of multiple risks that occur in combination. Some of these factors are likely surrogates for more fundamental risk factors, and some are probably duplicative.

The increased SIDS risk associated with numerous obstetric factors suggests that the in utero environment of future victims of SIDS is suboptimal. Maternal smoking during pregnancy doubles the risk for SIDS; infants of smoking mothers also appear to die at a younger age. The risk of death is progressively greater as daily cigarette exposure increases and as the degree of maternal anemia worsens. Fetal ischemia caused by vasoconstriction is thought to be the mechanism by which maternal smoking predisposes to SIDS. However, the number of postneonatal regular care visits and immunizations are also significantly less in victims of SIDS than in normal infants, suggesting that postneonatal care is also suboptimal.

SIDS is associated with illnesses in the last 2 wk of life and an increased frequency of doctor's office visits in the preceding week, especially for gastrointestinal illness and a droopy or listless appearance during the last 24 hr before death. Future victims of SIDS have also been observed to have repeated fatigue during feedings and profuse sweating during sleep, consistent with abnormal temperature regulation (see Table 657–1 and Fig. 657–2) or a febrile illness in the days and/or weeks preceding death. The cause of feeding-related fatigue is unclear, except insofar as it is secondary to intercurrent respiratory infection.

Sleeping Position. Prone sleep position is a significant risk factor for SIDS. The frequency of SIDS is more than threefold greater when the predominant sleep position is prone (on the stomach) than when it is supine (on the back). Population-based intervention programs to reduce prone sleeping have resulted in substantial declines in the prevalence of prone sleeping and substantial reductions in SIDS rates of 50% or more. Countries that have achieved prone prevalence rates of 3–10% have SIDS frequency rates as low as 0.4–0.5/1,000 live births, significantly less than the 1.3/1,000 SIDS incidence still present in the United States where the prone sleeping prevalence is about 40%. These dramatic results have not been associated with increases in non-SIDS infant deaths or with any decreases in the incidence of other important epidemiologic risk factors. A comprehensive professional and public educational/intervention campaign has now been initiated in the United States to establish supine or side sleeping as the preferred infant sleep position.

The mechanism(s) for the epidemiologic association between decreased prone sleeping prevalence and the decreased risk for SIDS is unknown. However, there may be an interaction between prone sleeping and impaired cardiorespiratory control, especially impaired ventilatory and arousal responsiveness. To the extent that an inadequate arousal/gasping response is necessary for SIDS to occur, face-down sleeping could increase the likelihood of airway occlusion or rebreathing to which the infant has reduced capacity for perception and response. This could facilitate the development of fatal asphyxia. Sleeping on a very soft surface such as a natural fiber mattress might increase the potential risk of face-down sleeping if an intrinsic deficit in arousal/gasping responsiveness exists; swaddling could add to this risk if the swaddling interferes with ability to maintain or return to a face-to-the-side position. Alternatively, many investigators attribute the risk of prone sleeping to thermal stress, hypothesizing that face-down sleeping causes a significant degree of thermal stress, and this could further compromise infants with deficient cardiorespiratory control. There, thus, may be links between epidemiologic risk factors such as soft bedding, prone sleep position, and thermal stress, and biologic risk factors such as cardiorespiratory control deficits (ventilatory and arousal abnormalities) and temperature/metabolic regulation deficits. Prone position might also be a surrogate for one or more epidemiologic risk factors that are less amenable to intervention (see Table 657–2).

Risk Groups (Table 657–3). Patients with apnea of infancy are at increased risk for SIDS, but no data are available regarding the extent, if any, to which home intervention might decrease this risk. The risk of SIDS increases significantly as the number of ALTEs increases.

The risk of SIDS also is increased in subsequent siblings of prior victims of SIDS, although the magnitude of the risk varies among countries. However, because the non-SIDS infant mortality rates in subsequent siblings of victims of SIDS are also increased, the phenomenon of increased mortality rates in subsequent siblings of victims of SIDS may not indicate any genetic or hereditary predisposition for SIDS per se. Nevertheless, some clinical data in subsequent siblings indicate differences in cardiorespiratory control compared with control infants. There is a tendency in subsequent siblings, once asleep, to remain asleep longer than controls. Also, subsequent siblings in active sleep tend to proceed into quiet sleep instead of awakening. Although a small number of families with more than two SIDS deaths in siblings have later been identified as examples of fatal child abuse (filicide), estimates indicate that more than 90% of all sudden and unexpected infant deaths are caused by SIDS. A familial metabolic disorder also needs to be considered in families with multiple unexplained infant deaths. SIDS risk has also been studied in prior rather than subsequent siblings, and SIDS rates 10 times greater than in control infants have been observed. The SIDS risk in surviving twins is also increased compared with siblings in general.

Several studies have documented an increased risk of SIDS in preterm infants. The incidence is inversely proportional to birthweight. There are no data indicating that the presence or

■ **TABLE 657–3 Estimated Incidence of Sudden Infant Death Syndrome in Infant Groups at Increased Epidemiologic Risk**

Risk Group	Incidence/1,000 Live Births*
Apnea of Infancy	
No further episodes	0–60
Further episodes	8–280
Siblings	
Single occurrence	10–20
Multiple occurrences	185
Twins	10
Preterm Infants	
<2,000-g birthweight	8
<1,500-g birthweight	10
Racial	
Blacks†	2.0–5.2
Native Americans‡	2.3
Prenatal Drug Exposure	
Heroin/methadone	20–30
Cocaine	12–30

**Among all live births in the United States, the incidence is 1.3/1,000 live births; Per 1,000 live births unless otherwise indicated.*

†Relative risk compared with whites is 1.7–5.2.

‡Relative risk compared with whites is 2.9–3.5.

(Adapted from Hunt CE: Sudden infant death syndrome. In: *Beckerman RC, Brouillette RT, Hunt CE (eds): Respiratory Control Disorders in Infants and Children. Baltimore, Williams & Wilkins, 1992, pp 190–211.)*

severity of apnea of prematurity or any other complication(s) of prematurity has any effect on SIDS risk except insofar as it is associated with the postconceptional age at birth.

All studies of SIDS incidence have shown significantly higher rates in black than in white infants, independent of any other factors such as low birthweight, young maternal age, or high parity. Native Americans have a birthweight-specific SIDS rate that is in the same general range as that of black infants. SIDS rates in other racial groups in the United States do not differ from those in white infants, but assimilation of foreign born into the United States culture may be associated with increased rates to levels comparable to those observed in blacks and Native Americans. Some ethnic groups in other countries may have increased SIDS rates, including Gypsy, Maori, Hawaiian, and Filipino groups.

Infants with prenatal drug exposure also have an increased risk of SIDS (see Table 657–3).

PROSPECTIVE IDENTIFICATION. A major objective of SIDS research has been to develop a screening test capable of accurately identifying those infants destined to die of SIDS. Such a test should have a negligible false-negative rate and an acceptable false-positive rate (see Chapter 2). Prospective pneumogram and polysomnographic screening studies, focused on respiratory and cardiorespiratory pattern abnormalities, have not had sufficient sensitivity and specificity to be useful for prospective identification of future victims of SIDS. New home monitoring technologies utilizing event recordings can now include respiratory pattern, heart rate and electrocardiogram, and oxygenation. However, currently, it is not known whether such monitoring will be useful in predicting the risk of SIDS.

Home Monitors. The apnea hypothesis led to the hope that home electronic surveillance would reduce the risk for SIDS. Although respiratory pattern abnormalities do not appear to be a critical component of the cardiorespiratory control abnormality, home monitoring could still be effective if bradycardia and/or desaturation were occurring sufficiently early so as to be responsive to intervention. A major problem related to determining the efficacy of home monitoring is uncertainty as to the extent of monitor use. Anecdotal postmortem interviews with parents of victims of SIDS who died with a monitor in the home suggest that 50% or more of such families were not utilizing the home monitor at the time death occurred. Experiences with documented monitoring indicate that less than 10% of monitor alarms are related to physiologic events; movement, a loose lead, or other nonsignificant alarms may thus easily lead to parental frustration and noncompliance. If early detection and resolution of excessive false alarms can be accomplished technically and this improves parental compliance, then it can be determined whether home electronic surveillance has any effective clinical role in preventing SIDS.

Medications. No medication is effective in preventing SIDS, although caffeine and theophylline administered for apnea of prematurity and infancy has improved the respiratory pattern and reduced the incidence of apnea in these groups. Although the effects of methylxanthines in infants with impaired asphyxic arousal responsiveness have not been systematically studied, caffeine decreases the auditory arousal threshold in young adults.

GENERAL

Brooks JC: Unraveling the mysteries of sudden infant death syndrome. Curr Opin Pediatr 5:266, 1993.

Hunt CE: Sudden infant death syndrome. *In*: Beckerman RC, Brouillette RT, Hunt CE (eds): Respiratory Control Disorders in Infants and Children. Baltimore, Williams & Wilkins, 1992, pp 190–211.

Hunt CE: Sudden infant death syndrome. J Neonatol 1:25, 1994.

Hunt CE: Apnea and SIDS. *In*: Kliegman RM, Nieder ML, Super DM (eds): Practical Strategies in Pediatric Diagnosis and Therapy. Philadelphia, WB Saunders, in press.

PATHOLOGY

Kinney HC, Filiano JJ, Harper RM: The neuropathology of sudden infant death syndrome. A review. J. Neuropathol Exp Neurol 51:115, 1992.

Rognum TO, Saugstad OD: Hypoxanthine levels in the vitreous humor: Postmortem evidence of hypoxia in most cases of SIDS. Pediatrics 87:306, 1991.

PATHOPHYSIOLOGY

Bolton DPG, Taylor BJ, Campbell AJ, et al: Rebreathing expired gases from bedding: A cause of cot death? Arch Dis Child 69:187, 1993.

Chiodini BA, Thach B: Impaired ventilation in infants sleeping facedown: Potential significance for sudden infant death syndrome. J Pediatr 123:686, 1993.

Hunt CE: The cardiorespiratory control hypothesis for SIDS. *In*: Hunt CE (ed): Clinics in Perinatology: Apnea and SIDS. Philadelphia, WB Saunders, 1992, pp 757–772.

Kemp JS, Kowalski RM, Burch PM, et al: Unintentional suffocation by rebreathing: A death scene and physiologic investigation of a possible cause of sudden infant death. J Pediatr 122:874, 1993.

Meny RG, Carroll JL, Carbone MT, et al: Cardiorespiratory recordings from infants dying suddenly and unexpectedly at home. Pediatrics 93:44, 1994.

Poets CF, Samuels MP, Noyes JP, et al: Home event recordings of oxygenation, breathing movements, and heart rate and rhythm in infants with recurrent life-threatening events. J Pediatr 123:693, 1993.

Riordan LL, Kelly DH, Shannon DC: Slow weight gain is associated with increased periodic breathing in health infants. Pediatr Pulmonol 17:22, 1994.

Schechtman VL, Harper RM: Minute-by-minute association of heart rate variation with basal heart rate in developing infants. Sleep 16:23, 1993.

Schechtman VL, Harper RK, Harper RM: Development of heart rate dynamics during sleep-waking states in normal infants. Pediatr Res 34:618, 1993.

Thrane PS, Rognum TO, Brandtzaef P: Up-regulated epithelial expression of HLA-DR and secretory component in salivary glands: Reflection of mucosal immunostimulation in sudden infant death syndrome. Pediatr Res 35:625, 1994.

EPIDEMIOLOGY AND PREVENTION

deJonge GA, Burgmeijer JF, Engelberts AC, et al: Sleeping position for infants and cot death in Netherlands 1985–91. Arch Dis Child 69:660, 1993.

Ford RPK, Taylor BJ, Mitchell EA, et al: Breastfeeding and the risk of sudden infant death syndrome. Int J Epidemiol 22:885, 1993.

Green A: Biochemical screening in newborn siblings of cases of SIDS. Arch Dis Child 68:793, 1993.

Hoffman HJ, Hillman LS: Epidemiology of the sudden infant death syndrome: Maternal, neonatal, and postneonatal risk factors. Clin Perinatol 19:717, 1992.

Hunt CE: Infant sleeping position and SIDS risk (editorial). Pediatrics 94:105, 1994.

Kahn A, Groswasser J, Sottiaux M, et al: Prone or supine body position and sleep characteristics in infants. Pediatrics 91:1112, 1993.

Kattwinkel J, Brooks J, Myerberg D: Infant sleep position and SIDS in the U.S.: Joint Commentary from the AAP and selected agencies of the federal government. Pediatrics 93:820, 1994.

Kilkenny M, Lumley J: Ethnic differences in the incidence of the sudden infant death syndrome (SIDS) in Victoria, Australia 1985–1989. Paediatr Perinat Epidemiol 8:27, 1994.

Ponsonby A-L, Dwyer T, Gibbons LE, et al: Factors potentiating the risk of sudden infant death syndrome associated with the prone position. N Engl J Med 329:377, 1993.

Scragg R, Mitchell EA, Taylor BJ, et al: Bed sharing, smoking, and alcohol in the sudden infant death syndrome. BMJ 307:1312, 1993.

Tuohy PG, Counsell AM, Geddis DC: Sociodemographic factors associated with sleeping position and location. Arch Dis Child 69:664, 1993.

Willinger M, Hoffman HJ, Hartford RB: Infant sleep position and risk for sudden infant death syndrome: Report of meeting held January 13 and 14, 1994. National Institutes of Health, Bethesda, MD. Pediatrics 93:814, 1994.

CHAPTER 658
Sarcoidosis

Margaret W. Leigh

Sarcoidosis, a chronic, multisystem, granulomatous disease of unknown etiology, occurs most frequently in young adults but can occur during childhood. The initial clinical presentation is extremely variable, depending on the organ systems involved, but in most pediatric cases includes weight loss, cough, fatigue, bone and joint pain, and anemia. Definitive diagnosis requires demonstration of the characteristic noncaseating, granulomatous lesions in an appropriate biopsy. The

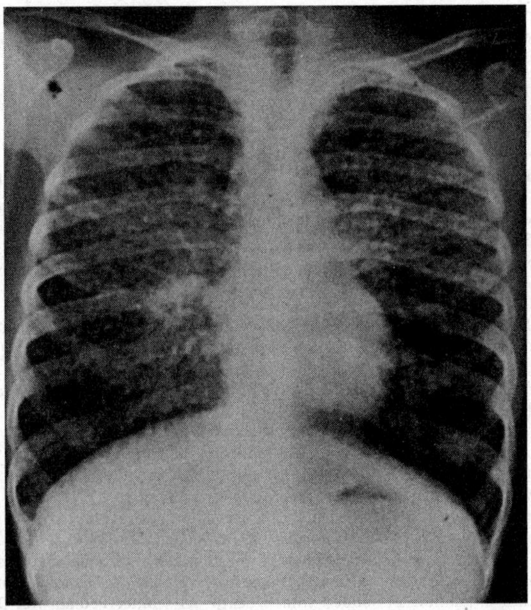

Figure 658–1. Sarcoidosis in a white 10-yr-old girl. There are widely disseminated peribronchial infiltrations, multiple small nodular densities, overaeration of the lungs, and hilar adenopathy.

granulomas in sarcoidosis resemble those caused by microbial agents (e.g., mycobacteria and fungi) or by hypersensitivity to organic agents. These similarities have led to the speculation that microbes or organic dusts may be inciting agents. However, despite extensive studies, the etiology remains obscure.

Epidemiologic studies indicate that sarcoidosis is particularly prevalent in the southeastern United States and occurs more frequently in blacks than in whites. Familial clustering of this disease has been observed and suggests a genetic predisposition; however, the mode of inheritance is unclear.

The granulomatous lesions of sarcoidosis may occur in almost any organ of the body. Typically, the granulomas are not necrotic and contain epithelioid cells, macrophages, and giant cells in the center surrounded by a mixture of monocytes, lymphocytes, and fibroblasts. Activated lymphocytes and macrophages within the granulomas release a variety of mediators, such as interleukin-1, interleukin-2, interferon, and other cytokines, that are thought to promote and maintain granulomatous lesions. During active disease, lymphocytes in and around the granulomas are predominantly helper T lymphocytes; as the lesions resolve, the T lymphocytes decrease in number and shift to predominantly suppressor cells. These lesions usually heal with complete preservation of the parenchyma; however, in approximately 20% of the lesions, fibroblasts proliferate at the periphery of the granuloma and may produce fibrotic scar tissue.

The lung is the most frequently affected organ; pulmonary involvement is variable in its extent and characteristics. Parenchymal infiltrates, miliary nodules, and hilar and paratracheal lymphadenopathy (Fig. 658–1) occur. Pulmonary function tests primarily show restrictive changes. Peripheral lymphadenopathy, eye changes consisting of uveitis or iritis, skin lesions, and hepatic involvement occur frequently. The clinical manifestations of sarcoidosis in the older child are different from those of the very young, which consist of a maculopapular erythematous rash, uveitis, and arthritis; pulmonary changes are minimal. The arthritis, which can be confused with rheumatoid arthritis, produces large, painless, boggy synovial effusions of the tendon sheaths; there is little limitation of motion.

There are no specific diagnostic tests. An elevated erythrocyte sedimentation rate, hyperproteinemia, hypercalcemia, hypercalciuria, eosinophilia, and an elevated angiotensin-converting enzyme level are common. The Kveim test, consisting of intradermal injection of material from a sarcoid lesion and observation for the formation of a granuloma several weeks later, is used infrequently for diagnosis because of difficulty in obtaining a standardized test material and reports of varying sensitivity and specificity of the test. Biopsy of tissue from affected areas is the most valuable diagnostic measure. Significant eye disease and renal damage from hypercalciuria can occur without symptoms; therefore, all patients with sarcoidosis should be evaluated at the initial presentation and monitored at regular intervals for evidence of ocular disease and hypercalciuria.

Because of its protean manifestations, the differential diagnosis of sarcoidosis is extremely broad; it includes tuberculosis, the various pulmonary mycoses, lymphoma, Crohn disease, and inflammatory ocular lesions such as phlyctenular conjunctivitis.

Treatment is symptomatic and supportive. Adrenal corticosteroids may suppress the acute manifestations, especially the inflammatory ocular lesions, progressive pulmonary disease, and the hypercalcemia/hypercalciuria. Pulmonary function tests are useful in following the progress of lung involvement, and angiotensin-converting enzyme levels have been shown to correlate with disease activity.

The prognosis and natural history of sarcoidosis in children are uncertain. Spontaneous recovery may occur after a prolonged illness of several months to several years, or the condition may be very chronic, involving progressive lung disease. Eye involvement may lead to blindness.

Hetherington S: Sarcoidosis in young children. Am J Dis Child 136:13, 1982.
Marcille R, McCarty M, Barton JW, et al: Long-term outcome of pediatric sarcoidosis with emphasis on pulmonary status. Chest 102:1444, 1992.
Pattishall EN, Kendig EL: Sarcoidosis. *In*: Chernick V (ed): Kendig's Disorders of the Respiratory Tract in Children, 5th ed. Philadelphia, WB Saunders, 1990, p 769.
Pattishall EN, Strope GL, Denny FW: Pulmonary function in children with sarcoidosis. Am Rev Respir Dis 133:94, 1986.
Pattishall EN, Strope GL, Spinola SM, et al: Childhood sarcoidosis. J Pediatr 108:169, 1986.
Thomas PD, Hunninghake GW: Current concepts of the pathogenesis of sarcoidosis. Am Rev Respir Dis 135:747, 1987.

CHAPTER 659
Progeria

Franklin L. DeBusk and W. Ted Brown

The progeria syndrome, first reported in 1886 by Hutchinson and Gilford in England, has now been described more than 100 times in the medical literature. Although the incidence is only approximately 1 in 8 million, the condition has been of considerable interest because of its striking features, which resemble, to some degree, accelerated aging. The disease is presumed to be due to a genetic mutation, although parent-to-child transmission has not been observed. As a result of severe failure to thrive, the children do not become sexually mature and reproduce. Although two sets of identical twins have been noted, no examples of recurrence of classic progeria among siblings have been documented. Paternal age is significantly increased, but there is no increase in consanguinity, features associated with dominant mutations and autosomal

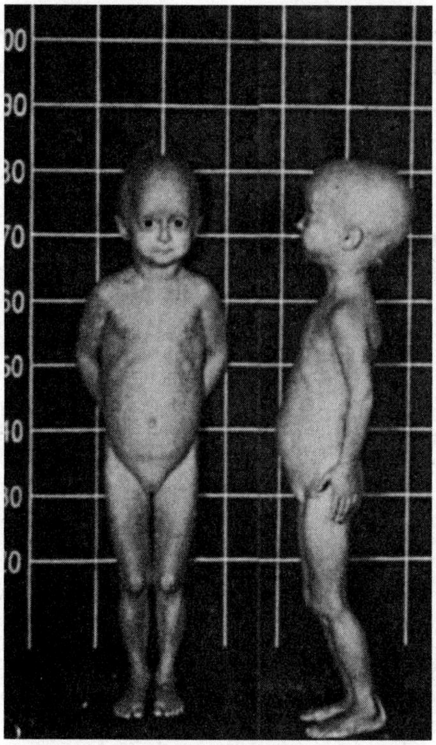
Figure 659–1. A 4.5-yr-old girl with height age of 1.75 yr and bone age of 4 yr. (From Wilkins L: Diagnosis and Treatment of Endocrine Disorders in Childhood and Adolescence, 3rd ed. Charles C Thomas, Springfield, IL, 1965.)

recessive inheritance, respectively. Therefore, each child with progeria most likely represents a new sporadic dominant mutation. The molecular basis of such mutations is unknown.

Children with progeria are usually considered to be normal in early infancy, but manifestations such as "scleroderma," midfacial cyanosis, and "sculpted nose" may suggest the existence of the syndrome at birth. Profound growth failure occurs during the 1st yr of life. The characteristic facies, alopecia, loss of subcutaneous fat, abnormal posture, stiffness of joints, and bone and skin changes usually become apparent during the 2nd yr of life (Fig. 659–1). Motor and mental development are normal. The clinical manifestations almost always present include short stature; weight distinctly low for height; failure to complete sexual maturation; diminished subcutaneous fat; head disproportionately large for face; micrognathia; prominent scalp veins; generalized alopecia; prominent eyes; delayed and abnormal dentition; pyriform thorax; short, dystrophic clavicles; "horse-riding" stance; wide-based shuffling gait; and coxa valga, thin limbs, and prominent, stiff joints.

Features frequently present are skin that is thin, taut, dry, wrinkled, and brown-spotted in various areas; "sclerodermatous" skin over lower abdomen, proximal thighs, and buttocks; prominent superficial veins; loss of eyebrows and eyelashes; persistently patent anterior fontanel; "sculpted," beaked nasal tip; faint nasolabial cyanosis; thin lips; protruding ears; absence of ear lobules; thin, high-pitched voice; dystrophic nails; progressive radiolucency of the terminal phalanges and distal clavicles (acro-osteolysis); and wormian bones of skull.

Variable degrees of insulin resistance, occasionally insulin-dependent diabetes mellitus, abnormalities of collagen, increased metabolic rate, and inconsistent abnormalities of serum cholesterol and other lipids are found, but there are no demonstrable abnormalities of thyroid, parathyroid, pituitary, or adrenal function. Twenty-four-hour growth hormone levels are normal, but reduced levels of insulin-like growth factor I have been noted. Dramatically increased levels of hyaluronic acid occur in the urine of such patients. Variable decrease of DNA repair has also been observed.

Children with progeria usually have severe atherosclerosis, and death occurs as a result of complications of cardiac or cerebral vascular disease between 6 and 19 yr, with a median life span of approximately 13 yr. Cataracts and tumors have infrequently been noted, and many changes associated with normal aging in adults such as presbycusis, presbyopia, arcus senilis, osteoarthritis, senile personality changes, or brain changes of Alzheimer disease are not found.

No specific treatment for this condition exists, but physiotherapy may be effective in preventing contractures. There are now support groups for the families of children with progeria, and a Progeria Registry exists to help define the incidence and genetic basis of the disorder better.

Brown WT: Progeria: A human-disease model of accelerated aging. Am J Clin Nutr 55:122S, 1992.
DeBusk FL: The Hutchinson-Gilford progeria syndrome. J Pediatr 80:697, 1972.
Wang S, Nishigori C, Yagi T, Takebi H: Reduced DNA repair in progeria cells and effects of gamma-ray irradiation on UV-induced unscheduled DNA synthesis in normal and progeria cells. Mutat Res 256:59, 1991.

CHAPTER 660
Histiocytosis Syndromes of Childhood

Stephan Ladisch

The childhood histiocytoses constitute a diverse group of disorders, which, although rare in occurrence, may be severe in their clinical expression. These disorders are grouped together because they have in common a prominent proliferation/accumulation of cells of the monocyte-macrophage system of bone marrow origin. Sometimes difficult to distinguish clinically, accurate diagnosis is nevertheless essential for facilitating progress in treatment. To this end, a systematic classification of the childhood histiocytoses has been developed (Table 660–1). This diagnostic classification rests on histiopathologic findings, and, therefore, a thorough, comprehensive evaluation of a biopsy specimen obtained at the time of diagnosis is essential. This evaluation includes studies (electron microscopy, immunostaining) that may require special sample processing.

CLASSIFICATION AND PATHOLOGY. Three classes of childhood histiocytosis are recognized, based on histiopathologic findings. The most well-known childhood histiocytosis, previously known as histiocytosis X, constitutes class I and includes the clinical entities of eosinophilic granuloma, Hand-Schüller-Christian disease, and Letterer-Siwe disease. The name Langerhans cell histiocytosis (LCH) has been applied to the class I histiocytoses. The normal Langerhans cell is an antigen-presenting cell of the skin. The hallmark of LCH in all forms is the presence of cells of the monocyte lineage containing the characteristic electron microscopic findings of a Langerhans cell. This is the Birbeck granule, a tennis racket–shaped bilamellar granule, which when seen in the cytoplasm of lesional cells in LCH is diagnostic of the disease. Alternatively, the definitive diagnosis of LCH can be made by demonstrating CD1-positivity of lesional cells. The lesions may contain various proportions of

■ TABLE 660–1 Classification of the Childhood Histiocytoses

Class I	Class II	Class III
	DISEASES	
Langerhans cell histiocytosis	Familial erythrophagocytic lymphohistiocytosis (FEL) Infection-associated hemophagocytic syndrome (IAHS)	Malignant histiocytosis Acute monocytic leukemia
	CELLULAR CHARACTERISTICS OF THE LESIONS	
Langerhans cells with Birbeck granules	Morphologically normal reactive macrophages with prominent erythrophagocytosis	Neoplastic proliferation of cells with characteristics of monocytes/macrophages or their precursors
	TREATMENT	
Local therapy for isolated lesions; chemotherapy for disseminated disease	Chemotherapy; allogeneic bone marrow transplantation (experimental)	Antineoplastic chemotherapy, including anthracyclines

these Langerhans granule-containing cells, lymphocytes, and eosinophils.

In contrast to a prominence of an antigen-presenting cell (the Langerhans cell) in the class I histiocytoses, the class II histiocytoses are characterized by accumulation of antigen-processing cells, i.e., macrophages. With the characteristic morphology of normal macrophages by light microscopy, these phagocytic cells lack the two markers (Birbeck granules and CD1 positivity) characteristic of the cells found in LCH. The two major diseases among the class II histiocytoses have indistinguishable pathologic findings. One is *familial erythrophagocytic lymphohistiocytosis* (FEL, which is the only inherited form of histiocytosis and is autosomal recessive). The other is the *infection-associated hemophagocytic syndrome* (IAHS). Both diseases are characterized by disseminated lesions that involve multiple organ systems. The lesions are characterized by infiltration of the involved organ with activated phagocytic macrophages and lymphocytes, leading to the term lymphohistiocytosis.

The mixed cellular lesions of both the class I and class II histiocytoses suggest that these may be disorders of immune regulation, resulting either from an unusual and unidentified antigenic stimulation or an abnormal and somehow defective cellular immune response. In contrast, the class III histiocytoses are unequivocal malignancies of cells of monocyte-macrophage lineage. By this definition, acute monocytic leukemia and true malignant histiocytosis are included among the class III histiocytoses. These malignancies are considered elsewhere (see Chapter 449). The existence of neoplasms of Langerhans cells is controversial.

CLASS I HISTIOCYTOSES

CLINICAL MANIFESTATIONS. LCH has an extremely variable presentation. The skeleton is involved in 80% of patients and may be the only affected site in the child older than 5 yr of age. Bone lesions may be single or multiple and are seen most commonly in the skull (Fig. 660–1). They may be asymptomatic or associated with pain and local swelling. Involvement of the spine may result in collapse of the vertebral body, which can be seen roentgenographically, and may cause secondary compression of the spinal cord. In flat and long bones, osteolytic lesions with sharp borders occur, and no evidence exists of reactive new bone formation. Lesions that involve weight-bearing long bones may result in pathologic fractures. Chronically draining, infected ears are commonly associated with destruction in the mastoid area. Bony destruction of the mandible and maxilla may result in teeth that, on roentgenograms, appear to be free floating. With response to therapy, there may be complete healing.

Skin involvement occurs in about 50% of patients at some time during their course (usually, a seborrheic dermatitis of the scalp). The lesions may spread to involve the back, palms, and soles. The exanthem may be petechial or hemorrhagic, even in the absence of thrombocytopenia. Localized or disseminated lymphadenopathy is present in approximately 33% of patients. Hepatosplenomegaly occurs in approximately 20%. Various degrees of hepatic malfunction may occur, including jaundice and ascites.

Exophthalmos, when present, is often bilateral and is caused by retro-orbital accumulation of granulomatous tissue. Gingival mucous membranes may be involved with infiltrative lesions that appear superficially like candidiasis. In 10–15% of patients, pulmonary infiltrates are found on roentgenogram. The lesions may vary from diffuse fibrosis and disseminated nodular infiltrates to diffuse cystic changes. Rarely, pneumothorax may be a complication. If the lungs are severely involved, tachypnea and progressive respiratory failure may result.

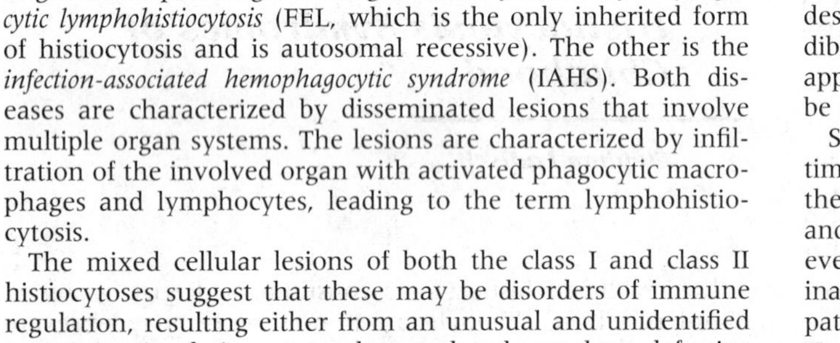

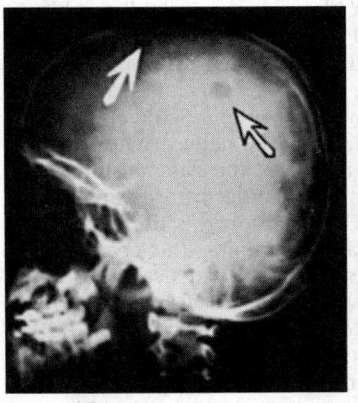

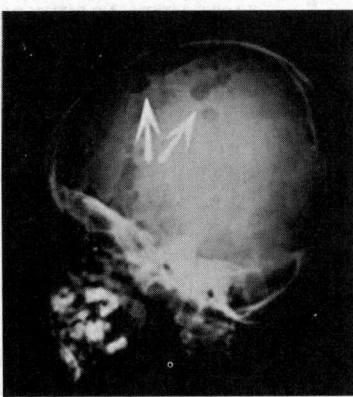

Figure 660–1. Two skull roentgenograms from patients with LCH. The patient on the left was over 2 yr of age and had involvement limited to isolated bone lesions. She had a good recovery. The patient on the right was under 2 yr of age and had extensive bone disease, febrile course, anemia, severe skin eruption, generalized adenopathy, hepatosplenomegaly, pulmonary infiltration, and a fatal outcome despite antitumor chemotherapy. These patients represent opposite ends of the clinical spectrum of LCH.

Pituitary dysfunction or hypothalamic involvement may result in growth retardation. In addition, there may be diabetes insipidus; patients suspected of having LCH should demonstrate the ability to concentrate their urine before going to the operating room for a biopsy. Rarely, panhypopituitarism may occur. Other symptomatic involvement of the central nervous system (CNS) is uncommon but may be serious; histiocytes can sometimes be demonstrated in the cerebrospinal fluid when neurologic disease is present.

Patients who are affected more severely may have systemic manifestations, including fever, weight loss, malaise, irritability, and failure to thrive. Bone marrow involvement may cause anemia and thrombocytopenia.

After tissue biopsy, which is diagnostic and easiest to perform on skin or bone lesions, a thorough clinical and laboratory evaluation should be undertaken. This should include a series of studies in all patients (complete blood count, liver function tests, coagulation studies, skeletal survey, chest roentgenogram, measurement of urine osmolality). In addition, detailed evaluation of any organ system that has been shown to be involved by physical examination or by these studies should be performed to establish the extent of disease before initiation of treatment.

TREATMENT AND PROGNOSIS. The clinical course of single-system disease (usually, bone, lymph node, or skin) is generally benign with a high chance of spontaneous remission. Therefore, treatment should be minimal and should be directed to arresting the progression of a lesion (such as a bone lesion) that could result in permanent damage before it resolves spontaneously. Curettage or low-dose local radiation therapy (5–6 Gy) may accomplish this goal. Multisystem disease, in contrast, should be treated with systemic chemotherapy. Several different regimens have been proposed, but a central element is the inclusion of either vinblastine or etoposide. Treatment including the latter agent has recently been shown to be very effective in LCH. The response rate to therapy, contrary to previous opinion, may be high, especially if the diagnosis is accurately and expeditiously ascertained. Experimental therapies, suggested only for unresponsive disease (frequently very young children with multisystem disease), include allogeneic bone marrow transplantation, immunosuppressive therapy with cyclosporine/antithymocyte globulin, and possibly certain new agents, such as 2-chlorodeoxyadenosine.

CLASS II HISTIOCYTOSES

CLINICAL MANIFESTATIONS. The major forms of class II histiocytosis, FEL and IAHS, have a remarkably similar presentation, consisting of a generalized disease process, most often with fever, weight loss, and irritability. FEL is also characterized by severe immunodeficiency. Affected children are usually younger than 4 yr old (always in FEL); children may present with IAHS at an older age. Physical examination frequently reveals hepatosplenomegaly, symptoms of CNS involvement (with an aseptic meningitis, the cerebrospinal fluid cells are the same phagocytic macrophages as found in the peripheral blood or bone marrow). As in the class I histiocytoses, the *diagnosis rests on the pathologic findings*. Associated laboratory findings in both forms of class II histiocytosis include hyperlipidemia, hypofibrinoginemia, elevated hepatic enzymes, extremely elevated levels of circulating soluble interleukin-2 receptors released by the activated lymphocytes, and sometimes cytopenias. There is no absolute clinical or laboratory distinction that can be made between FEL and IAHS. Without a genetic marker for FEL at the present time, the distinction can definitively be made only by a positive family history for other affected children in FEL.

TREATMENT AND PROGNOSIS. The diagnostic distinction between FEL and IAHS can sometimes be made by the acute onset of IAHS in the face of a documented infection. In this case, treatment of the underlying infection, coupled with supportive care, is critical. If the diagnosis is made in a setting of iatrogenic immunodeficiency, immunosuppressive treatment should be withdrawn, and supportive care should be instituted along with specific therapy for underlying infection. When FEL is diagnosed or suspected and when an infection cannot be documented, therapy currently includes etoposide or immunosuppressive therapy. Nevertheless, no curative chemotherapy therapy for FEL has been found, and the disease is almost uniformly fatal. Recently, allogeneic bone marrow transplantation was shown to be possibly effective in curing some patients with FEL.

In contrast, in IAHS, when an infection can be documented and effectively treated, the prognosis is good without any other specific treatment. However, when a treatable infection cannot be documented (as is the case in most patients presumed to have IAHS), etoposide is also recommended. It is theorized that, by its cytotoxic effect on macrophages, etoposide interrupts the hemophagocytic process and the accumulation of macrophages, both of which contribute to the pathogenesis of IAHS. A broad spectrum of infectious agents, viruses, fungi, protozoa, and bacteria, may trigger IAHS, usually in the setting of immunodeficiency. Therefore, a thorough evaluation for infection should be undertaken in immunodeficient patients with hemophagocytosis. Rarely, the same syndrome may be seen in conjunction with a neoplasm (e.g., leukemia); in this case, treatment of the underlying disease causes resolution of the hemophagocytosis.

EXPERIMENTAL THERAPY

The histiocytoses are rare but frequently fatal. Consequently, they are the subject of intense study with respect to cause, pathogenesis, and treatment. The very recent findings of clonality among the lesional cells in some cases of LCH has raised the issue of a malignant etiologic factor. This is not yet resolved because benign clonal proliferations of lymphocytes, for example, are well known. On the other hand, the fatal outcome in some forms of LCH has accelerated the search for new therapies, including studies of the use of etoposide. Despite evidence of a (low) risk of leukemogenicity of etoposide used in combination with other agents, the data suggest that the use of this effective drug in the childhood histiocytoses not be curtailed, pending the results of further study. Continued careful diagnosis and the entry of patients into international, randomized studies should continue to improve the treatment of the childhood histiocytoses.

Broadbent V, Gadner H, Komp D, Ladisch S: Histiocytosis syndromes in children II. Approach to the clinical and laboratory evaluation of children with Langerhans-cell histiocytosis. Med Pediatr Oncol 17:492, 1989.

Gadner H, Heitger A, Grois N, et al: A treatment strategy for disseminated Langerhans cell histiocytosis. Med Pediatr Oncol 23:72, 1994.

Henter J, Elender G: Familial hemophagocytic lymphohistiocytosis. Acta Paediatr 80:269, 1991.

Ladisch S, Gadner H, Arico M, et al: LCH-I: A randomized trial of etoposide vs. vinblastine in disseminated Langerhans cell histiocytosis. Med Pediatr Oncol 23:107, 1994.

Lahey ME: Histiocytosis X: An analysis of prognostic factors. J Pediatr 87:184, 1975.

Willman CL, Busque L, Griffith BB, et al: Langerhans cell histiocytosis (histiocytosis X)—a clonal proliferative disease. N Engl J Med 331:154, 1994.

Writing Group of the Histiocyte Society: Histiocytosis syndromes in childhood. Lancet 1:208, 1987.

Yu R, Chu CE, Bulewa L, et al: Langerhans cell histiocytosis: A clonal proliferation of Langerhans cells. Lancet 343:767, 1994.

CHAPTER 661
Chronic Fatigue Syndrome

Hal B. Jenson

Numerous terms (e.g., chronic mononucleosis, chronic Epstein-Barr virus infection, immune dysfunction syndrome) have been applied to the syndrome of easy fatigability associated with mild to debilitating somatic symptoms. This syndrome was formally defined by the Centers for Disease Control and Prevention (CDC) in 1988 as chronic fatigue syndrome because it is fatigue that is the principal and invariable physical symptom. Chronic fatigue syndrome is neither a new disease nor the result of enhanced appreciation of previously unrecognized clinical illness. It is an *illness* that is the subjective experience of symptoms that encompass a variety of clinical conditions of organic, psychologic, and mixed causes. No evidence exists that this is a single *disease* with an identifiable etiologic agent or characteristic physiologic or pathologic abnormalities, although the differential diagnosis includes many infectious and noninfectious diseases. Current understanding of this condition is derived largely from studies in adults, and to a lesser extent in adolescents; little information is available about the existence of chronic fatigue syndrome in young children. Although chronic fatigue syndrome is not recognized to be an infectious disease, it is frequently purported to be associated with various infectious agents and shares various epidemiologic and clinical manifestations with many recognized infectious illnesses.

EPIDEMIOLOGY. Chronic fatigue is a common presenting symptom of adolescents and adults; it can be disabling. Approximately 20% of adults in primary care clinics or in surveys complain of chronic fatigue; the incidence in children is unknown. Most patients are white, 20–50 yr of age, well educated, high achievers, and in above-average income brackets. These epidemiologic observations may be artifactual because assertive individuals may be less likely to accept being told by their physician that there is nothing physically wrong and more likely to insist on referral to medical specialists. Women constitute 75% of patients. Prevalence rates vary significantly, but chronic fatigue syndrome is seen in all patient populations. The overall incidence in the general population is estimated to range from 0.002–1%. Most cases of chronic fatigue syndrome are sporadic and are not associated with secondary cases.

PATHOGENESIS. The cause of chronic fatigue syndrome is unknown, and the hypothesis that infection with replication of a known or new virus is the primary cause of the symptoms in most cases of chronic fatigue syndrome is unsubstantiated. However, most patients diagnosed with chronic fatigue syndrome give a history of a viral-like illness as the inciting event, including Epstein-Barr virus, influenza virus, varicella, rubella, or nonspecific symptoms of sore throat, fever, myalgia, and/or diarrhea. In many cases, the clinical symptoms of depression, such as fatigue, lack of energy and interest, and inability to concentrate, merge with or are intensified by the weakness often found during convalescence from a systemic infectious disease, resulting in disabling fatigue. Persistent fatigue after an otherwise uncomplicated primary infection is well recognized with many acute infections, especially Epstein-Barr and influenza viruses. Symptoms of fatigue and exhaustion may last for months to a few years and may be accompanied by signs of depression. Several studies of convalescence after acute systemic infection support the view that symptomatic recovery is critically dependent on the emotional state and attitude of the individual. Individuals with a propensity to become depressed are more likely to respond to acute infection with depression-like symptoms than are individuals who do not have such a vulnerability.

Approximately 80% of patients with chronic fatigue syndrome include psychologic or neuropsychiatric difficulties among their principal complaints. Up to 25% of patients meet the criteria for major (nonendogenous) depression at the time of initial diagnosis, and up to 50% of patients have a psychiatric diagnosis (usually major depression) accompanying their somatic complaints during the course of their illness.

Several diverse and sometimes conflicting in vitro immunologic abnormalities (e.g., hypo- or hypergammaglobulinemia, immunoglobulin subclass deficiencies, elevated levels of circulating immune complexes, mild increased helper/suppressor lymphocyte ratios, natural killer cell dysfunction, monocyte dysfunction) have been reported in patients diagnosed with chronic fatigue syndrome. A history of food, inhalant, or drug allergy is reported by approximately 67% of patients. However, such abnormalities do not occur in most individuals diagnosed with chronic fatigue syndrome, the magnitude of the abnormalities described is small, and the degree of immune aberrations do not correlate with the severity of clinical symptoms.

CLINICAL MANIFESTATIONS. The symptoms of the chronic fatigue syndrome are protean, with a spectrum of gradation from subtle to debilitating. Although the perception of fatigue is subjective and undoubtedly varies from individual to individual, fatigue as a symptom should not be dismissed as a minor ailment. The syndrome is characterized by multiple somatic complaints of at least 6 mo to several years' duration associated with significant impairment (below 50% of normal) of: the work or school schedule; activities of daily living; exercise tolerance; and interpersonal relationships. Fatigue is generally manifest as lassitude, tiredness, weakness, intolerance to exertion and easy fatigability, significant sleeping during the day, and general malaise. Nocturnal sleeping is not usually changed and does not differ from that in unaffected individuals. This fatigue is characteristically accompanied by myalgias and low-grade fever in 50–95% of cases. Headache and sore throat are common. A multitude of other symptoms (chest palpitations, visual blurring, nausea, dizziness, arthralgias, paresthesias, dry eyes and mouth, diarrhea, cough, night sweats, lymphadenopathy, rash) have been reported in 30–60% of cases. Emphasis on one particular symptom other than the constitutional symptoms of malaise and fatigability is somewhat uncommon and should prompt further investigation. Weight loss is also uncommon in chronic fatigue syndrome.

Most patients diagnosed with chronic fatigue syndrome relate an abrupt onset to their symptoms, often as part of an initial viral-like illness characterized by low-grade fever accompanied by sore throat and cough. Less frequently, the initial symptoms indicate gastrointestinal tract involvement with nausea and diarrhea. Myalgia is common after either set of initial symptoms.

Symptoms in children appear to be similar to those in adolescents and adults, and school absenteeism is a major problem. In a small retrospective study of 23 patients with a median age of 14 yr and a median duration of symptoms of 6 mo, 67% missed 2 wk or more of school, and 33% required a home tutor.

Abnormal physical examination findings are conspicuously absent and provide reassurance to both the patient and the physician.

DIAGNOSIS. The CDC operational definition for chronic fatigue syndrome is presented in Table 661–1. The diagnosis of chronic fatigue syndrome is a diagnosis of exclusion. Prior instances of depression, anxiety, or panic disorder do not exclude a current diagnosis of chronic fatigue syndrome, but coexistent major depression or other psychologic illnesses are considered exclu-

■ **TABLE 661–1 Summary of the Centers for Disease Control and Prevention: Case Definition of Chronic Fatigue Syndrome**

A case of chronic fatigue syndrome must fulfill both major criteria and the following minor criteria: either 6 or more of the 11 symptom criteria plus 2 or more of the physical criteria or 8 or more of the symptom criteria.

Major Criteria

Fatigue of at least 6 mo duration. New onset of persistent or relapsing debilitating fatigue or easy fatigability in a person with no previous history of similar symptoms that does not resolve with bed rest and is severe enough to reduce or impair average daily activity below 50% of the patient's premorbid activity level for a period of at least 6 mo.

Exclusion of other causes of chronic fatigue. Other clinical conditions that may produce similar symptoms must be excluded by thorough evaluation based on history, physical examination, and appropriate laboratory investigations. These conditions include malignancy; autoimmune disease; infections; chronic psychiatric disease; neuromuscular disease; endocrine disease; drug dependency; or other known or defined chronic pulmonary, cardiac, gastrointestinal, hepatic, renal, or hematologic disease.

Minor Criteria

Symptom criteria: The symptoms must have begun at or after the time of onset of increased fatigability and must have persisted or occurred over a period of at least 6 mo.

- Mild fever (oral temperature 37.6–38.6° C if measured by the patient).
- Sore throat.
- Painful cervical or axillary lymph nodes.
- Unexplained, generalized muscle weakness.
- Myalgia.
- Prolonged (greater than 24 hr) generalized fatigue after levels of exercise that would have been easily tolerated in the patient's premorbid state.
- Generalized headaches (of a type, severity, or pattern that is different from headaches the patient may have had in the premorbid state).
- Migratory arthralgia, without swelling or erythema.
- Neuropsychologic complaints (photophobia, transient scotomata, forgetfulness, excessive irritability, confusion, difficulty thinking, inability to concentrate, depression).
- Sleep disturbance (hypersomnia or insomnia).
- Description of the main symptom complex as initially developing over a few hours to a few days.

Physical criteria: These two must be documented by a physician on at least two occasions, at least 1 mo apart.

- Low-grade fever (oral temperature 37.6–38.6° C).
- Nonexudative pharyngitis.
- Palpable or tender cervical or axillary lymph nodes (less than 2 cm in diameter).

sion criteria. Most patients, including children, with chronic fatigue syndrome attribute their symptoms to physical rather than psychologic causes.

Fibromyalgia (fibrositis) is a relatively common rheumatic syndrome characterized by symptoms of chronic fatigue syndrome but with widespread musculoskeletal *pain* in addition to multiple specific tender point sites (see Chapter 148). Fibromyalgia may represent a subset of patients with chronic fatigue syndrome characterized by heightened musculoskeletal symptoms.

Although evaluation of each patient should be individualized, the initial laboratory evaluation should be limited to general tests to provide reassurance of the lack of significant organic dysfunction, including a complete blood count with leukocyte differential, erythrocyte sedimentation rate, electrolyte and blood urea nitrogen levels, creatinine concentration, serum alanine transaminase and aspartate transaminase measurements, thyroid function tests, and urinalysis. Further tests should be directed primarily toward excluding treatable diseases with the same symptoms as chronic fatigue syndrome.

Diagnostic evaluation for chronic fatigue should include psychologic evaluation for depression or anxiety disorders, which should precede exhaustive searches for organic causes.

TREATMENT. Development of definitive treatment for chronic fatigue syndrome awaits delineation of the causes of the symptoms. No specific therapeutic agents are recommended. Therapy should be directed toward emotional support for the patient and family, relief of symptoms, and minimizing unnecessary and misleading diagnostic and therapeutic tests. This may include a combination of restoration of a normal sleep pattern; rehabilitation strategies, including exercise for fatigue; and optimism. Psychologic or psychiatric intervention may be a principal part of supportive treatment.

Patients with severe limitation of activity should be started on a schedule of graded remobilization and physical therapy. Complete bed rest only perpetuates immobility; rapid remobilization, for whatever reason, may not be tolerated. Return to school should also be initiated gradually but systematically. The patient and the family should clearly understand that there is no evidence that activity will harm patients with chronic fatigue syndrome. Continued empathy and support by the treating physician is important in maintaining a physician-patient relationship conducive to identification and resolution of both organic and psychologic illness. Periodic medical reevaluation approximately every 3 mo is warranted for early detection of other identifiable causes of chronic fatigue, especially with development of new symptoms.

PROGNOSIS. Chronic fatigue syndrome is an illness of prolonged duration with significant morbidity but almost no deaths. Most adult patients never return to their preillness level of activity, but about 20% of patients return to their previous state of health for periods of at least 1 yr without any specific medical intervention. Some of these patients, however, subsequently have relapses. Approximately 60% of patients—adults, adolescents, and children—report gradual but marked improvement in symptoms over a period of 2–3 yr without specific therapy, although some patients appear to have no improvement or occasionally deteriorate. The eventual clinical course is unpredictable. Patients should be instructed that their symptoms will likely wax and wane.

Carter BD, Edwards JF, Kronenberger WG, et al: Case control study of chronic fatigue in pediatric patients. Pediatrics 95:179, 1995.

Fukuda K, Straus SE, Hickie I, et al: The chronic fatigue syndrome: A comprehensive approach to its definition and study. Ann Intern Med 121:953, 1994.

Gold D, Bowden R, Sixbey J, et al: Chronic fatigue. A prospective clinical and virologic study. *JAMA* 264:48, 1990.

Klimas NG, Salvato FR, Morgan R, et al: Immunologic abnormalities in chronic fatigue syndrome. *J Clin Microbiol* 28:1403, 1990.

Klonoff DC: Chronic fatigue syndrome. *Clin Infect Dis* 15:812, 1992.

Kruesi MJP, Dale J, Straus SE: Psychiatric diagnoses in patients who have chronic fatigue syndrome. *J Clin Psychiatry* 50:53, 1989.

Smith MS, Mitchell J, Corey L, et al: Chronic fatigue in adolescents. *Pediatrics* 88:195, 1991.

Part XXXIV

Environmental Health Hazards

Chapter 662

Radiation Injury

Robert W. Miller and Deborah P. Merke

The possibility of untoward biologic effects of radiation is of special interest in pediatrics since these effects may be most serious in growing tissues. Ionizing radiation produces injury in the same manner regardless of the type of particle or ray emitted. The variation is quantitative rather than qualitative. Absorption of energy may cause molecules in the path of the radiation to become ionized. In attaining stability these molecules may form substances that alter biochemical processes within the cell or its environment. These effects on cellular structures result in the deaths of persons exposed to ionizing radiation, the death of certain cancer cells treated with roentgen rays, genetic mutations, and the production of cancer as a late effect of exposures to radiation.

Susceptibility of tissues to roentgen rays is generally greater in rapidly mitosing and in undifferentiated cells. Because of an abundance of this type of tissue in the abdomen, a patient is more likely to have radiation sickness from roentgen therapy to this region than from comparable exposure elsewhere.

DOSAGE FACTORS. Radiation absorption increases with the volume of the child's body exposed, with prolongation of exposure, or with an increase in amperage or voltage. Absorption decreases in relation to the effectiveness of filters used and with an increase in distance between the patient and the source.

Adverse acute effects of roentgen rays are diminished when the total dose is administered in several exposures separated by sufficient time for recovery from the subclinical effects of each. Repeated exposures may produce pathologic effects not manifested until years later. Some of the chemical changes produced in cells by roentgen rays are irreversible and may lie dormant until aging, infection, hormonal alterations, or further exposure to toxic agents activates them.

The infant may be more susceptible to the effects of roentgen rays than the adult. Moreover, even if there are no essential differences in susceptibility, the infant's longer life span provides more time for such changes to develop.

Radioactivity is measured in a dose unit called the Becquerel defined as 1 disintegration/sec. More appropriately, its absorbed dose, the Gray, is the energy deposited into tissue (1 J/kg). Roentgens are converted to Grays by dividing the former by 100.

EARLY EFFECTS OF IRRADIATION. Exposure of the entire body to 100 roentgens (1–2 Gy) usually produces illness in humans. A dose of about 350 roentgens (3–6 Gy) will cause death in 50% of exposed persons. Higher doses can be tolerated if only a part of the body is exposed. Death results within hours to days when the entire body is exposed to the overwhelming dosage of an atomic bomb.

Symptoms of radiation sickness, which vary with the exposure, are malaise, fever, nausea, vomiting, and diarrhea. Leukopenia develops rapidly, and in more severe instances thrombocytopenia may appear within 1 wk. When the initial symptoms are not severe, they are followed by a temporary period of well-being. Epilation begins about 2 wk after the exposure. The leukopenia increases susceptibility to infection, and the low platelet count predisposes to hemorrhage. When autopsy does not reveal the cause of death, one can only assume that the radiation injury was responsible for lethal "cytochemical changes." If the patient survives for 6 wk, death is not likely from these effects of radiation. Bone marrow transplantation and granulocyte-macrophage colony-stimulating factors may be indicated for severe pancytopenia.

Only a small percentage of deaths caused by an atomic explosion can be attributed to radiation effects alone; thermal and blast injuries account for most of them. Traumatic injuries do not heal effectively in persons with radiation sickness.

Clinical observation of the effects of radiation on children with genetic disease has led to a new understanding of molecular biology. Children with ataxia-telangiectasia are markedly predisposed to lymphoma, and when treated for it with the usual doses of radiotherapy, they sometimes suffer severe reactions (see Chapter 119.12). These patients have defective repair of DNA after damage by γ-radiation, analogous to defective repair of DNA damage by ultraviolet light (UV) in xeroderma pigmentosum (see Chapter 606). The defects in repair after γ-radiation or UV damage are enzyme mediated and nonoverlapping. Another interaction involving genetics, neoplasia, and radiosensitivity may occur in the heritable (usually bilateral) form of retinoblastoma. For example, radiogenic tumors of the orbit occur more frequently and after a shorter latent period than in patients with nonheritable cancers given similar doses of radiotherapy.

LATE EFFECTS OF IRRADIATION. Within the decade following the detonations of the atomic bombs in Japan, there was a significant rise in the incidence of leukemia in proportion to exposure to the explosions. An increase in leukemia rates has been observed at doses as low as 20–49 rad (1 rad equals 1 cGy) among Hiroshima survivors of all ages. Children 10 yr of age at the time of the bombing were more susceptible to leukemogenesis than were older persons. When girls (younger than 10 yr of age) exposed to 50 rad or more reached the usual age for breast cancer (i.e., 35–45 yr), the frequency of this neoplasm was increased and now exceeds that for females who were older when exposed.

A committee of the National Academy of Sciences has reported that new dosimetry concerning exposures to the atomic bombs lowers the doses that produce late effects by about two thirds. The new dosimetry is based on re-evaluation of the physical effects of the bomb, such as effects on roof tiles and buttons, and revisions in mathematical modeling of the dose-response relationships (i.e., the shape of the curve).

In Great Britain and in the United States, in utero exposures to diagnostic radiation have been reported to increase the relative risk of death from cancer before 10 yr of age by about 50%. No such effect was found among children exposed in utero to the atomic bomb.

Among persons exposed in utero to radiation from the Hiroshima atomic bomb (beginning at 10–19 rad) before the 18th wk of gestation, small head circumference occurred excessively. The effect increased in frequency and severity with increasing dose. Mental retardation occurred in those exposed to doses of 60 rad or more and affected the majority exposed in the 8–15th wk of gestation to 150 rad or more. Because of the catastrophic effects of the bomb, the observations at low doses may not apply directly to medical radiology. This question might be clarified by studying the head size of Soviet children exposed in utero at less than 18 wk of gestational age to radiation from the nuclear reactor accident at Chernobyl.

Complex chromosomal abnormalities were still found in the peripheral lymphocytes of atomic bomb survivors more than 35 yr after exposure, including those who were in utero, but not among persons conceived after the explosion. On the basis of animal experimentation, there is no doubt that point mutations occurred, but no effect could be demonstrated among the 75,000 first-generation offspring examined.

Small opacities of the posterior capsule of the lens have developed in 85% of those who epilated soon after the bomb explosion; the lesions are asymptomatic (≥ 150 rad). Only 10 of the thousands of survivors have grade III or IV radiation-induced cataracts.

Thyroid disease has occurred in children in the Marshall Islands who were exposed to fallout from nuclear weapons tests in the South Pacific in 1954. Two children, who were 1 yr old when exposed to a thyroid dose of 5,000 rad, developed severe hypofunction. Older persons developed less marked hypothyroidism, benign tumors, and, in a few instances, thyroid cancer. At Chernobyl, several hundred cases of childhood thyroid cancers were attributed to radioiodines in fallout in the Ukraine and Belarus. Thyroid disorders may be prevented by immediate ingestion of potassium iodide after an acute exposure.

Therapeutic doses of partial-body radiation may predispose to cancer. This is indicated by reports of a greater incidence of leukemia among adults treated for ankylosing spondylitis and of thyroid tumors among persons treated in early infancy for thymic enlargement. That repeated small doses of radiation to the entire body may predispose to leukemia is indicated by the increased occurrence of this disease among radiologists in the past.

Effects of exposure of parts of the body include temporary sterility, dermatitis, bone and skin tumors, and developmental defects of teeth. Arrest in bone growth may occur in children who received cancericidal doses of roentgen rays.

LOW-DOSE EFFECTS. In general, the lowest radiation dose that produces a measurable effect is 20+ rad for leukemia, breast cancer, somatic cell mutations, and long-lasting chromosomal aberrations. Exceptions are small head size after exposure to the atomic bomb in Japan in fetuses younger than 18 wk of gestational age to 10–19 rad and thyroid cancer in Israeli children treated with x-ray epilation for tinea capitis (the average thyroid dose was 9 rad). A small cluster of leukemia and lymphoma in children near the Sellafield nuclear facility in England was ascribed to paternal exposure there in the 6 mo before conception of the child. Expert re-evaluation of the study has led to the conclusion that paternal exposure was not to blame.

Increased mortality rates from leukemia have been reported in children in southwestern Utah and in military participants on maneuvers at the test site. The exposures were presumably low. In addition, controversial claims have been made that atomic energy workers in decades past now have increased cancer rates. The findings are not in accord with expectation based on a linear or quadratic extrapolation from effects at high or intermediate levels, as among Japanese atomic bomb survivors. The question about low-level effects is unlikely to be solved by further epidemiologic studies because the number of exposed persons needed for study far exceeds the number available. Judgments will probably eventually be based on a knowledge of the fundamental biology of radiation carcinogenesis.

PREVENTIVE MEASURES. Exposures to ionizing radiation should be limited to situations in which commensurate benefits are expected (Table 662–1). The average whole-body exposure of the general population, based on the genetically significant dose, should not exceed 100 mrem/yr, according to the National Council on Radiation Protection and Measurements.

It is thought that radiation changes within somatic cells are incompletely additive throughout life. The pediatrician should limit as much as possible the exposure of patients (and self) to the emanations of roentgen ray machines and radioisotopes but should not refrain from using them for essential diagnostic and therapeutic procedures. The patient's gonads should be shielded whenever possible.

Roentgen therapy should never be used except when the indications are unmistakable or the risk justified, as, for example, in the treatment of malignant tumors. Great care must be exercised to avoid unnecessary damage to osseous growth centers and tooth buds.

INDOOR RADON. Radon gas comes from radioactive decay prod-

■ **TABLE 662–1 Examples of Radiation Doses Received in Various Medical and Nonmedical Activities**

Type of Radiation	Dose (Rad, Rem; Very Approximate)*	Length of Exposure	Where Received
Medical			
Chest film, newborn	0.004	Milliseconds	Skin entrance dose; exit dose lower
Computed tomography, contiguous slices,	2–5	Seconds	Scanned volume
child	0.5	Seconds	Skin entrance dose; exit dose much lower
Lateral series of lumbosacral spine, adult	10–100	Hour	Skin entrance dose; exit dose much lower
Cardiac catheterization	7,000	Weeks	Tumor and adjacent structures
Curative radiotherapy			
Nonmedical			
Natural background at sea level	0.08	Year	Whole body
Some professional jet pilots and flight crews, from cosmic rays	1	Year	Whole body
Residents of certain areas of India with radioactive soil	3	Year	Whole body
Radiation workers, current permitted dose	5	Permitted/year	Radiation badge (usually worn on neck)
Dose at which 50% of population dies, nuclear warfare	350	Minutes	Whole body

To convert to Gray, divide by 100.

ucts of ubiquitous naturally occurring uranium deposits in the soil. The decay products emit α-radiation, which, when inhaled, raise the rate of lung cancer among uranium miners; the rate is higher if miners smoke cigarettes. Radon enters houses through cracks in the foundation, porous cinderblocks, and granite walls. By extrapolation downward from the doses that induce lung cancer in miners, it is estimated that 18,000 lung cancer deaths may occur annually in the United States as a result of indoor radon. Epidemiologic studies, however, have not convincingly demonstrated an association between lung cancer and indoor radon levels. The inability of residential studies to detect an increased risk may be due to the very low expected increase and the difficulty in measuring exposures in previous homes. Another consideration is that lung cancer among miners may be partially due to concomitant exposures, such as arsenic, silica, and diesel and blasting fuels.

The Environmental Protection Agency has issued a guideline that recommends that houses be tested; if the level is 4+ pCi/L, repairs should be made to seal out the radon. Pediatricians should be aware of this information so they can advise families and point out that primary or secondary cigarette smoke interacts with radiation exposure to multiply the risk of lung cancer decades hence.

ELECTROMAGNETIC FIELDS. It has been hypothesized that extremely low-frequency electromagnetic fields (EMF) are carcinogenic. These fields are created by electric charges in the alternating current (60 Hz) supplied to households in the United States. An investigator, seeking a cause of cancer in Denver children, was impressed by the proximity of several of their homes to high-voltage power lines. In an epidemiologic study, these lines were classified by their electrical wiring configurations (high current or not), which they termed *wiring codes*. It has since been shown that wiring codes account for only 15% of the EMF variation among homes, even less for persons who spend much of the day elsewhere. The lay press alarmed the public by reporting clusters of childhood leukemia or brain tumors near power lines. After a plethora of epidemiologic studies based on direct measurements of EMF produced discrepant results, expert committees in Great Britain and the United States independently came to the conclusion that there is no convincing evidence from human, animal, or cellular studies that EMF is related to the development of cancer. The Environmental Protection Agency, in a widely distributed draft report, declared EMF a possible carcinogen in 1990, but the final report in 1992 deemed the evidence insufficient to support this conclusion. EMF can affect animal behavior, so there may be noncarcinogenic effects of unknown clinical significance in humans.

Committee on the Biological Effects of Ionizing Radiations: Health Effects of Exposures to Low Levels of Ionizing Radiation. Washington, DC, National Academy Press, 1990.
Doll R, Evans HJ, Darby SC: Paternal exposure is not to blame. Nature 367:678, 1994.
Mettler FA Jr, Upton AC: Medical Effects of Ionizing Radiation, 2nd ed. Philadelphia, W. B. Saunders, 1995, p 430.
Miller RW: Effects of prenatal exposure to ionizing radiation. Health Phys 59:57, 1990.
Miller RW: Cerebral effects and cancer after intrauterine exposure to the atomic bomb. *In*: Poznanski AK (ed): Radiation Protection in Medicine. Proceedings of the Twenty-Eigth Annual Meeting of the National Council on Radiation Protection and Measurements. Bethesda, National Council on Radiation Protection and Measurement, 1993.
Neel JV, Schull WJ (eds): The Children of Atomic Bomb Survivors. A Genetic Study. Washington, DC, National Academy Press, 1991.
Nygaard OF, Sinclair WK, Lett JT (eds): Effects of low dose and low dose rate radiation. Adv Radiat Biol 16:1–324, 1992.
Oak Ridge Associated Universities Panel: Health Effects of Low Frequency Electric and Magnetic Fields. Publication no. ORAU 92/F9, Washington, DC, US Government Printing Office, 1992.
Report of an Advisory Committee on Non-Ionising Radiation: Electromagnetic Fields and the Risk of Cancer. Documents of the NCRB, Vol 3. National Radiological Protection Board, Chilton, Didcot, Oxford, England, 1992, p 1.
Sagan LA (ed): Extremely-low-frequency electromagnetic fields: Issues in biological effects and public health. *In* Proceedings 16 (the Thirtieth Annual Meeting) of the National Council on Radiation Protection and Measurements. Bethesda, National Council on Radiation Protection and Measurement, 1995.
United Nations Scientific Committee on the Effects of Atomic Radiation: Sources and effects of ionizing radiation. New York, United Nations, 1993.

CHAPTER 663
Chemical Pollutants

Robert W. Miller

As chemicals increasingly permeate our environment, there is a need to consider the special exposures and vulnerability of the fetus and child. Each pediatrician should be alert for evidence of new environmental effects on children's health.

INTRAUTERINE EFFECTS

METHYLMERCURY. In the mid 1950s methylmercury caused the first epidemic of congenital cerebral palsy attributable to intrauterine exposures to a chemical pollutant (see Chapter 664). It was associated with severe, sometimes fatal, neurologic disorders in the population at large and was traced to contamination of fish by waste dumped into Minamata Bay, Japan, by a factory that made vinyl plastics. Similar episodes have occurred in Alamogordo, New Mexico, and Iraq due to grain treated prior to planting with a methylmercury-containing fungicide that was mistakenly used for animal feed or baking.

POLYCHLORINATED BIPHENYLS (PCBs). In 1968, in Kyushu, Japan, there was an epidemic of chloracne, and women who were pregnant at the time gave birth to infants who were small for gestational age and had, among other findings, dark skin that cleared with time. The outbreak was traced to contamination of cooking oil by PCBs, a heat-transfer agent, through pinhole erosions in pipes during the manufacture of the oil. PCBs from factory waste have now been found in major waterways of the United States and other countries. In Taiwan an episode virtually identical to that in Kyushu occurred. Comprehensive health examinations were made of about 100 children who were conceived after their mothers were exposed to PCBs. The children, from 1 mo to 7 yr of age, had an increased frequency of defects of the skin, hair, and nails, 11 were born with teeth. They were exposed in utero to PCBs that had been stored in their mothers' fat. Compounds similar to PCBs, *polybrominated biphenyls (PBBs)*, were accidentally mixed with animal feed in Michigan and widely distributed within the state. Animals became ill and died, but no fetal effects or overt illnesses have been found in human beings.

DIOXIN AND RELATED COMPOUNDS. In 1976 a runaway reaction in a factory in Seveso, Italy, spewed a chemical cloud of dioxin, a potent animal teratogen, downwind over farms and homes. Many animals died, and 2 wk later about 40 exposed children developed chloracne. No human teratogenesis has been found among the abortuses or liveborn children of Seveso women exposed early in pregnancy. The highest exposures yet known occurred among children of Seveso, several of whom had blood levels up to 56,000 parts per trillion 2 wk after exposure, as compared with less than 20 parts per trillion among unexposed persons. In Missouri, horse arenas and roads were sprayed with waste oil to which dioxin had been added; about 60 horses died, and foals were born malformed. Transient illness, but not chloracne, occurred in one arena owner and her two children.

Families that live near toxic waste dumps worry about adverse health effects on their children. The 82 chemicals deposited decades ago into the Love Canal near Niagara Falls are not known to have produced an excess of illness among the thousands of children who attended the school built on top of this mixture. A study of birth defects among infants whose residences were near one of 590 waste sites in New York State suggests a 12% increase in the (total) malformation rate. The Centers for Disease Control and Prevention developed a large battery of tests (Priority Toxicant Reference Range Study) to measure urine or blood levels of chemicals (or their metabolites) from patients living near toxic waste sites.

Ground troops thought to have been exposed in Vietnam to the spraying of dioxin-containing Agent Orange were found to have no increase in their blood levels of dioxin compared with men who had never been to Vietnam. Air Force personnel involved in the spraying did have elevated blood levels.

Eleven of 15 children in a Hungarian village were born with birth defects after their mothers had eaten fish from ponds on fish farms; the fish had been treated with trichlorfon, an insecticide that slowly releases a potent anticholinesterase. The malformations were of diverse types but included three sets of twins. Down syndrome was concordant in one pair, discordant in another, and also affected one singleton. The origin of nondysjunction was identifiable in two cases, both of which showed an error in maternal meiosis II instead of meiosis I, as is usual, which supports an environmental influence.

CIGARETTE SMOKE. On the average, the birthweight of infants whose mothers smoke heavily during pregnancy is 200 g less than normal, and perinatal morbidity is increased when medical care is inadequate (see Chapters 80 and 81.1).

TRANSPLACENTAL CARCINOGENESIS. The discovery that cancer of the cervix or vagina occurs in women after intrauterine exposure to diethylstilbestrol raises the possibility that other chemicals, including pollutants, may also be transplacental carcinogens. Four children have now been reported with fetal hydantoin syndrome and neuroblastoma, suggesting that phenytoin is a transplacental carcinogen. Among other possible carcinogens is benzene, which causes leukemia after heavy occupational exposures.

LACTATIONAL EFFECTS

Because of chemical pollution, new questions are being raised about the safety of breast feeding. PCBs, PBBs, dioxin, and certain pesticides are stored in fat and are not readily cleared from the body except in the fat of breast milk. Japanese infants whose mothers were exposed post partum to PCB-contaminated cooking oil were exposed to high levels in their mothers' milk while nursing. Elsewhere, samples of breast milk have rarely shown high levels of these chemicals. When unusual exposures occur, however, before advice on breast feeding is given, the milk should be tested (e.g., for dioxin in Seveso, for PBBs in Michigan, or for PCBs in upper New York State). No general recommendation against breast feeding should be made because of its many benefits. Cow's milk may also contain these chemicals, but tests are routinely made to determine that the milk sold commercially does not exceed limits set by federal regulation. Game fish have also been contaminated from PCB-polluted waters.

EFFECTS OF OTHER EXPOSURES

ASBESTOS. Although asbestos is a naturally occurring chemical, its capacity to induce cancer is related to its physical properties. Long, thin fibers are carcinogens, whereas short, thick ones are not. The latent period from exposure until the development of mesothelioma is usually more than 30 yr. Exposure in childhood may thus induce cancer in adulthood. Asbestos dust brought home on a father's work clothes was implicated as the cause of mesothelioma in his daughter (onset at 34 yr), as well as in his wife.

Bronchogenic carcinoma is induced by exposure to asbestos, especially among cigarette smokers; the risk is about 5 times greater than it is in cigarette smokers not exposed to asbestos and 54 times greater than in persons exposed to neither. From 1947–1973, asbestos fibers were sprayed on new schoolroom ceilings in the United States; about 10,000 schools were treated. With time the asbestos frayed, and fibers floated through the schoolrooms. In theory the exposure could increase the frequencies of mesothelioma and bronchogenic carcinoma. As yet, no increases have been observed in young adults, but sufficient time may not yet have passed to allow for both deterioration of asbestos and the latent period. Asbestos in schools is being removed, sealed with plastic, or contained by dropped ceilings. The interaction between asbestos exposure and the use of cigarettes in causing lung cancer adds to the reasons for urging young persons not to smoke.

WATER. About 200 chemicals have been found in small amounts in various water supplies. Some are known to cause human cancer after heavy occupational exposure, but the claim that regional increases in cancer mortality rates are attributable to chemicals in the water supply is not generally accepted. Fluoride, added to water or naturally occurring, is not associated with human cancer but may produce *fluorosis.* The latter is characterized acutely by salivation, emesis, diarrhea, and abdominal pain. Hypocalcemia, hyperkalemia, paresthesias, and ventricular arrhythmias may ensue.

AIR. Major air pollutants generated by fossil fuel consumption are sulfur oxides, carbon monoxide, photochemical oxidants (especially ozone), and nitrogen oxides. The most common respiratory diseases associated with these pollutants are asthma, chronic bronchitis, and emphysema. Automotive exhausts add lead to the atmosphere and, in enclosed spaces, can cause intense pollution with carbon monoxide to which children have been especially susceptible, as in underground garages or at skating rinks where gasoline-powered vehicles were used to scrape the ice. Some industries have caused specific diseases in neighboring residential areas through air pollution with asbestos, beryllium, lead, methylmercury, or dioxin. There is an increased mortality rate from lung cancer among persons living in counties with arsenic-emitting smelters or petrochemical industries.

WORK CLOTHES. Illnesses in the child are at times traceable to a parent's work clothes; toxicity from lead, beryllium, organophosphate pesticides, and asbestos has occurred. Pediatricians, in considering the origins of noninfectious diseases, should ask about parental occupation, unusual household exposures, and neighborhood factories. A growing number of studies have found an association between childhood cancer or birth defects and exposure of the father to chemicals or radiation before conception of the child. These occurrences may be due to chance and cannot be explained by mendelian genetics.

FOOD. In addition to the foregoing chemical pollutants that may enter the food chain, many other chemicals are intentionally added to food to improve appearance, taste, texture, or preservation. Evaluation of the safety of these chemicals is difficult because of problems in measuring exposures and in separating them from the effects of the myriad of variables that may confound interpretation of the alleged untoward effects.

Chen YC, Guo YL, Hsu CC, et al: Cognitive development of yu-cheng ("oil disease") children prenatally exposed to heat-degraded PCBs. JAMA 268:3323, 1992.

Chen YC, Yu ML, Rogan WJ, et al: A 6-year follow up of behavior and activity disorders in the Taiwan yu-cheng children. Am J Public Health 64:415, 1994.

Chisolm JJ Jr: Fouling one's own nest. Pediatrics 62:614, 1978.

Committee on Pesticides in the Diets of Infants and Children, National Research Council: Pesticides in the Diets of Infants and Children. Washington, DC, National Academy Press, 1993.

Czeizel AW, Elek C, Gundy S, et al: Environmental trichlorfon and cluster of congenital abnormalities. Lancet 341:539, 1993.
Geschwind SA, Stolwijik JAJ, Bracken M, et al: Risk of congenital malformations associated with proximity to hazardous waste sites. Am J Epidemiol 135:1197, 1992.
Gessner B, Beller M, Middaugh J, et al: Acute fluoride poisoning from a public water system. N Engl J Med 330:95, 1994.
Guzelian PS, Henry CJ, Olin SS (eds): Similarities and Differences between Children and Adults: Implications for Risk Assessment. Washington, DC, ILSI Press, 1992.
Miller RW: Frequency and environmental epidemiology of childhood cancer. *In*: Pizzo PA, Poplack D (eds): Principles and Practice of Pediatric Oncology. New York, JB Lippincott, 1989.
Mocarelli P, Needham LL, Marocchi A, et al: Serum concentrations of 2,3,7,8-tetrachlorodibenzo-p-dioxin and test results from selected residents of Seveso, Italy. J Toxicol Environ Health 32:357, 1991.
Mossman BT, Gee BL: Asbestos-related diseases. N Engl J Med 320:1721, 1989.
Needham LL: Experiences and progress report of Priority Toxicant Reference Range Study. Environ Health Perspect, in press.
Public Health Service: Report on fluoride benefits and risks. MMWR Morb Mortal Wkly Rep 40:(RR-7)1, 1991.

CHAPTER 664
Mercury Exposure and Intoxication

George H. Lambert

Mercury is the second most common cause of heavy metal poisoning, and it can result in a wide range of organ dysfunction, including irreversible brain damage and even death. The signs and symptoms of mercury poisoning are frequently not recognized to be caused by mercury, delaying effective therapeutic intervention. This occurs even though some of the clinical findings, such as acrodynia, are pathognomonic for mercury poisoning. When a nonoccupational exposure to mercury occurs, children are frequently the most highly exposed subjects. The developing human in utero and child are more susceptible to mercury toxicity than any other age group.

Mercury has been widely used in industry and medicine, despite its known toxicities for at least 3,000 yr. It has been used as a vermifuge, cathartic, diuretic, antiseptic, antisyphilitic, antipyretic, antiphlogistic, and antiparasitic, in addition to many other uses. As more effective agents were discovered and the toxic effects of mercury became better understood, the use of mercury in pharmaceutics has almost disappeared, while the use of mercury in the work place has been increasing. The toxic effects of mercury exposure in the work place have long been recognized and occupational health measures to decrease exposure have been implemented since the time of Christ.

EPIDEMIOLOGY. Mercury is an element that exists in three states (Table 664–1): elemental mercury (Hg^0), inorganic mercury salts (Hg^{1+} and Hg^{2+}), and organic mercury (e.g., methyl, phenyl, alkyl). *Elemental mercury* is a silver-grey liquid at room temperatures and readily vaporizes when heated. It is commonly called quicksilver and is used in thermometers, barometers, batteries, and electrical instruments. There are numerous *mercurous salts* (Hg^{1+}). The best known is mercurous chloride or calomel, which was used in teething powder, diaper powders, and ointments, and in other medications until the 1940s, when it was shown to be toxic. Mercuric salts (Hg^{2+}) inhibit bacterial and fungal growth and are found in pesticides, disinfectants, antiseptics, pigments, dry batteries, and explosives. Both salts readily disassociate in the body to form ions.

Organic mercury compounds are used in diuretics, antiseptics, insecticides, pesticides, and in the processing of wood, plastics, and paper. Hg^{2+} can be methylated to form organic mercury. Methyl mercury readily passes through cellular membranes and across the placenta, and is therefore the most toxic form of mercury.

Any mercury compound in the environment has the potential to be methylated to methyl mercury by microorganisms found in the soil or water. Methyl mercury in water rapidly accumulates in fish and other aquatic organisms. The higher the organism is on the aquatic food chain, the higher the mercury body burden. A large predator fish at the top of the food chain can have mercury at levels that are 100,000 times higher than the water.

Atmospheric mercury comes from off-gasing of mercury from soils and surface waters, and combustion of fossil fuels. Atmospheric mercury is increased by landfills containing elemental mercury products and the use of mercury-containing paints, fungicides, and pesticides. Mercury in the water comes from mercury in the rocks, industrial effluents, and runoff from landfills containing mercury products. Industrial processes that can have mercury-containing effluents include chlorine and caustic soda production, mining and metallurgy, electroplating, chemical and textile manufacturing, paper and pharmaceutical manufacturing, and leather tanning. Although not common, elevated mercury levels have been found in certain drinking water supplies.

The main source of mercury exposure to the general population is methyl mercury from the diet, primarily from fish. Predacious fish (e.g., Northern Pike from fresh waters and swordfish from oceans) can have 50 times the mercury concentration of other fish. The U.S. Food and Drug Administration is responsible for ensuring that commercial fish contain less mercury than 1 part per million. Some states require lower fish mercury levels (0.05 ppm) and issue fish advisories that recommend fish from certain freshwater lakes and streams or certain fish types not be eaten. The advisories also recommend a maximal number of freshwater fish meals that should be eaten per month. In recognition of the increased sensitivity of the fetus and pregnant females and children to mercury toxicity, many states recommend that children and pregnant females should more severely limit their freshwater fish intake to less than the intake advised for nonpregnant adults. The states that currently have fish advisories are listed in Table 664–2. Physicians (and parents) should be aware of the relevant fish advisories in their own and surrounding states and should ascertain if their patients may be consuming contaminated freshwater fish. The fish advisories are usually available from the state's department of public health.

Mercury-containing paint is another source of exposure to the general population. Up until 1991 about 30% of latex paints contained mercury; since September 1991 no paint can contain mercury. However, many people may keep old cans of paint so there may be a risk of mercury exposure from old paint for many years. Elemental mercury is found in several other products, including thermometers, barometers, and batteries. Elemental mercury has also been used in folk remedies by Asian and Mexican populations for chronic stomach pain and by Latin Americans and Caribbean natives in occult practices. Small amounts of mercurials are used as preservatives in some eye drops and ointments, nasal sprays and vaccines, and as antiseptics and diuretics. Elemental mercury is also used as a weight in Miller–Abbott gastrointestinal tubes.

Silver dental amalgams can be 50% elemental mercury by weight. Chewing releases trace amounts of mercury vapor, which is then partially absorbed. The amount of mercury absorbed by this route is less than 1% of the daily mercury vapor considered safe in the work place, does not pose a credible risk, and amalgams should not be replaced in an effort to reduce mercury exposure.

In mercury exposures to the general population, children

■ TABLE 664–1 Forms of Mercury

Form	State	Source	Absorption	Half-Life	Primary Effects	Secondary Effects
Elemental						
Liquid*	Hg^0	Thermometers, barometers	Dermal contact: minimally absorbed Ingestion: poorly absorbed	60 days	Toxicity rare†	
Vapor*	Hg^0	Industrial	Inhalation: 80% absorbed Percutaneous: minimally absorbed		Lungs, skin, eyes, gingiva	Central nervous system, kidneys
Inorganic Salts						
Mercurous	Hg^{1+}	Medicines, antiseptics	Ingestion: about 10% absorbed Dermal contact: lethal doses can be absorbed by animals	40 days	Kidneys, gastrointestinal tract	Central nervous system
Mercuric	Hg^{2+}					
Organic						
Methyl mercury*	CH_3Hg^-	Fish	Ingestion: 100% absorbed Inhalation: readily absorbed	70 days	Central nervous system	
Phenyl mercury	$C_6H_5Hg^-$	Fungicides, bactericides	Ingestion: 80–100% absorbed Dermal contact: same as salts		Kidneys	Central nervous system

**Crosses the blood-brain barrier.*
†Liquid elemental mercury is poorly absorbed through the intestinal tract (0.01%) or dermally; systemic toxicity is rare.

frequently have the highest body burden because of the combination of the physical chemical properties of elemental mercury and the characteristics of children. For example, elemental mercury can exist as a vapor that is heavier than air and settles near the floor. Children will inhale the air with the highest mercury content and Hg can be absorbed through the lungs. In addition, children inhale more air on a weight basis because they have higher minute volume respiration based on body weight than an adult. So the child, as compared with the adult, will inhale more air with a higher concentration of mercury, resulting in higher body burdens of mercury. Children during play or normal activity may also accidentally ingest or inhale dirt or dust contaminated with mercury by putting their hands or play objects into their mouths, or may frequently be fascinated by the unique properties of elemental mercury and play with this heavy metal in its liquid form.

PATHOPHYSIOLOGY. Organic, inorganic, and elemental mercury (liquid and vapor) can all be absorbed transcutaneously to a degree that results in toxic effects. Elemental mercury inhaled as a vapor is about 80% absorbed and diffuses rapidly across the placenta and blood-brain barrier. Dissolved mercury vapor is oxidized to Hg^{2+} by hydrogen peroxide catalase in the plasma, red blood cells, and tissue. Elemental mercury is poorly absorbed from the gastrointestinal tract, with less than 0.01% being absorbed. One case report indicated that a young adolescent ingested 204 g of elemental mercury without overt signs of toxicity. The half-life of mercury in the tissues is about 60 days, with most of the excretion being in the urine. Salivary secretion and sweat contribute to some mercury excretion.

Mercury salt is absorbed from the gastrointestinal tract at about 10%. Mercuric salts are more soluble than mercurous salts and therefore produce more toxicities. Mercuric and mercurous ions cross the blood-brain barrier to a much less extent than elemental mercury and their biologic half-lives are about 40 days.

Organic mercury is easily absorbed by inhalation, dermal contact, and ingestion. Methyl mercury distributes to all tissue and concentrates more in the blood and brain than other forms of mercury. Most is found bound to red blood cells, where it is slowly metabolized to mercury ions. Methyl mercury is about 90% excreted into the bile, with the remainder being excreted into the urine. The half-life of methyl mercury is 70 days. Phenyl mercury is less well absorbed than methyl mercury and is rapidly metabolized to Hg^{2+}; effects are similar to the mercury salts, and it is primarily excreted in urine.

Children and the developing fetus have increased susceptibility to mercury-induced toxicity. Mercury vapor can cause more severe respiratory complications in children than in adults, and the onset of symptoms after exposure occurs more rapidly in children. The most dramatic evidence for increased susceptibility of the developing human to mercury toxicity is when a pregnant female is exposed to high levels of methyl mercury. One instance involved humans ingesting methyl mercury–contaminated fish from Minamata Bay in Japan and another involved humans consuming bread made with methyl mercury fungicide–contaminated flour in Iraq. When pregnant females consumed the contaminated food products, the offspring had severe and irreversible central and peripheral neurological disease, while the mothers were less affected neurologically. The signs and symptoms of methyl mercury intoxication are now referred to as Minamata disease.

The central nervous system (CNS) and kidney are the primary organs affected by mercury. The form of mercury, durations of exposure, and route of the exposure are the determining factors of the toxic effects. The CNS effects are seen primarily in chronic exposure to methyl mercury and elemental mercury vapor. Both forms readily cross the blood-brain barrier and can result in permanent brain damage. Elemental mercury causes intention tremors, erethism, and gingivitis. Erethism is a constellation of psychological and emotional disturbances. Methyl mercury–induced effects may not be apparent until months after the exposure. There is a loss of myelinated fibers with a relative increase in small-sized fibers. The peripheral autonomic nerves are also altered with loss of unmyelinated fibers and autonomic dysfunction, such as lower skin temperature and lower amounts of sweating. Motor and

■ TABLE 664–2 Fish Consumption: States With Fish Consumption Advisories

Alabama	Illinois*†	New Hampshire*†	Pennsylvania
Arizona	Kentucky	New Jersey*†	Rhode Island
Arkansas	Louisiana*†	New Mexico*†	South Carolina*†
California	Maine	New York*†	Tennessee
Colorado	Massachusetts*†	North Carolina*†	Texas
Connecticut*†	Michigan	North Dakota*†	Vermont*†
Florida	Minnesota	Oklahoma	Virginia*†
Georgia*†	Nebraska*†	Oregon*†	Wisconsin*†
Idaho	Nevada*†		

**Special precautions for pregnant females.*
†Special precautions for children.

sensory nerve conduction velocity is delayed, with the sensory nerves being more severely affected. The fetal brain can be severely damaged by methyl mercury poisoning. There is evidence of abnormal neuronal migration and cell division. Peripheral neuropathy is not a cardinal finding in the congenital form.

The kidneys may be affected by mercury salts and phenyl mercury accumulating in the renal tissue, resulting in increased permeability of the tubular epithelium. Exposure to mercury vapor or salts can also result in dose-dependent proteinuria or nephrotic syndrome; acute tubular necrosis and renal failure; and dysuria, hyperchloremia, urinary anion gap, and decreased creatinine clearance. A single dose of about 1 g of mercuric chloride will cause death by acute renal failure. The mechanism is by direct renal damage to kidney cells and indirect effects of cardiovascular collapse. Repeated exposure to low doses affects the immune system by causing overproduction of a variety of antibodies that collect at the glomerulus and damage the filtration process; a nephrotic syndrome can ensue.

The respiratory, gastrointestinal, and cardiovascular systems can also be affected. The respiratory system can be affected by acute inhalation of mercury vapor, resulting in pulmonary tissue damage and respiratory failure, and in the most severe cases this may even lead to death. The lung damage may be in part irreversible. Gastritis, necrotizing ulceration of the intestinal mucosa, stomatitis, nausea, vomiting, and diarrhea can be seen in mercury salt ingestion. Gingivitis, stomatitis, burning sensation in the oropharynx, nausea, and vomiting can be seen after inhalation of elemental mercury. Cardiovascular collapse has been observed in inorganic mercury salt ingestion and can lead to death. Hypertension and hypotension have been observed in individuals who have been exposed to elemental mercury.

The specific toxic mechanism of action of mercury on organ and cellular function is unknown. Mercury ions can alter the structure and function of enzymes and other proteins by binding to their sulfhydryl, amine, and phosphoryl groups.

CLINICAL MANIFESTATIONS. Mercury poisoning can cause a wide range of signs and symptoms. This array of frequently nonspecific signs and symptoms and the fact that overt mercury toxicity is somewhat rare makes the etiological diagnosis difficult to identify. The clinician should maintain a high index of suspicion. Evidence of nervous system and renal dysfunction should be carefully sought, as well as evidence of recent behavioral changes or altered developmental milestone achievements.

Clinical evaluation of patients suspected of mercury toxicity includes a detailed history to identify any sources of mercury exposure. Consideration should be given to occupation of all household members, the source and amount of fish consumption, hobbies of all family members and children's friends, recent use of latex paints or other household repair items that contain mercury such as caulk, use of folk remedies, a school project using mercury, playing with elemental mercury, and exposure to some mascaras, hair wave fixatives, and skin lighteners sold outside the United States that may contain mercury.

The signs and symptoms of *acute exposure* are dependent upon the form of mercury and the duration of exposure (see earlier). Acute exposure to elemental mercury vapor may result in rapid onset of cough, dyspnea, chest pain, nausea, vomiting, diarrhea, fever, a metallic taste in the mouth, stomatitis, colitis, nephrotic syndrome, and salivation. Interstitial pneumonitis, necrotizing bronchiolitis, and pulmonary edema may then develop. Children less than 30 mo of age may be particularly susceptible to mercury toxicity, and the onset of respiratory failure may be rapid. Conjunctivitis with erythematous and pruritic rash has also been reported. Elemental mercury when ingested is not well absorbed and presents little risk. Skin contact with elemental mercury can cause a papular rash.

Acute exposure to mercury salts can present in a few hours, with nausea, vomiting, bloody diarrhea, severe abdominal pain and tenesmus, intestinal wall necrosis, which can cause fibrosis, and stenosis, which can lead to hematemesis and cardiovascular collapse, and rapidly to death. Protein, casts, and red blood cells can appear in the urine, with diminished urine output secondary to acute tubular necrosis. Death due to uremia may occur. The acute lethal dose for an adult is 1–4 g. No data are available for children.

Acute exposure to methyl mercury is well documented in the two widespread poisonings in Iran and Japan. The signs and symptoms are nonspecific and may not be apparent for months. The symptoms are ataxia, paresthesia, malaise, blurred vision, and impaired hearing, smell, and taste. The exposed fetus can have severe neurologic damage, including mental retardation, cerebral palsy, microcephaly, ataxia, deafness, constriction of visual fields, blindness, and dysphasia. Computed tomography (CT) changes are apparent.

Chronic exposure to high levels of elemental mercury vapor results in peripheral nervous system and CNS effects. At low doses the body metabolizes the mercury to mercuric salts, which do not cross the blood-brain barrier. At high doses the elemental mercury reaches the brain, resulting in psychological changes, insomnia, loss of appetite, emotional instability, irritability, headaches, and short-term memory loss. Peripheral nervous system effects include tremors (which are characteristic of mercury exposure) and distal paresthesia, motor and sensory conduction delay, and limb weakness.

Acrodynia is a rare syndrome, usually seen in children after exposure to elemental mercury, mercury salts, and phenyl mercury. The syndrome is characterized by pruritus, paresthesia, generalized pain, pink rash, and peeling hands, nose, and feet.

Chronic exposure to mercury salts can result in irritability, colitis, chronic renal failure, gingivitis, stomatitis, and salivation. These findings have been reported in individuals chronically ingesting laxatives containing mercury.

Methyl mercury chronic exposure can result in malaise; tunnel and blurred vision; loss of hearing, taste, and smell; paresthesia; ataxia; tremors; incoordination; depression; insomnia; memory loss; dysarthria; and dementia. Peripheral neuropathy is one of the cardinal signs of Minamata disease and includes perioral dysesthesia and sensory impairment of the glove-and-stocking type. Deep tendon reflexes can be greatly decreased or absent, but in up to 40% of the subjects the deep tendon reflexes may be exaggerated. Cerebellar ataxia, akinesia, and subjective complaints of numbness, tingling sensations, and hyperesthesia are also common. The subjects can have gait disturbances with elements of weakness, ataxia, rigidity, and/or spasticity. The mental deterioration can be from mild memory loss to severe dementia. Diffuse changes in the occipital lobe, cerebellum, and cerebrum are seen on CT scan. The effects may not be apparent for months after the exposure. Chronic exposure results in permanent CNS damage, with the developing human at greatest risk.

LABORATORY DATA. Blood is used to determine acute mercury exposure because the half-life of mercury in blood is short. Urine tests provide the best estimate of the current body burden of chronic mercury exposure. However, because hair grows at a rate of 1 cm/mo, the exposure to mercury over time also can be estimated by measuring the mercury in long strains of hair.

Blood samples must be collected in a heparinized container and refrigerated. Normal adult blood mercury levels are usually < 1.5 μg/dL (0.07 μmol/L), and 5 μg/dL (0.25 μmol/L) or greater is considered the toxic threshold in adults. The toxic threshold for mercury in infants, children, and pregnant females is not known but is most likely less than the adult.

A 24 hr urine sample collected in an acid-washed container

■ **TABLE 664–3 Correlation of Urinary Mercury Concentration and Effects**

Urinary Mercury Concentration	Signs and Symptoms
<20 μg/L (<100 nmol/L)	None
20–100 μg/L (100–499 nmol/L)	Decreased response on tests for nerve conduction, brain wave activity, and verbal skills Early indication of tremor on testing
100–500 μg/L (499–2,493 nmol/L)	Irritability, depression, memory loss, minor tremor, and other nervous system disturbances Early signs of disturbed kidney function
500–1,000 μg/L (2,493–4,985 nmol/L)	Kidney inflammation Swollen gums to gingivitis Significant tremor and nervous system disturbances

is the optimal sample, but a 1st morning void may provide reasonable accuracy if the sample is adjusted for concentration of urine by using urine creatinine or specific gravity. The range of urinary mercury that is toxic to the infant or child is not known; however, the range of urinary mercury that can be associated with adverse effects in adults is listed in Table 664–3. Children and infants probably will manifest symptoms at lower urinary mercury levels.

Urine or blood measurements in subjects who have chronic mercury exposure may not correlate with signs and symptoms of mercury toxicity because the mercury may be in a relatively unexchangeable tissue compartment. In addition, some signs and symptoms of mercury poisoning are irreversible, and the current body burdens of mercury may not be representative of past mercury exposures.

TREATMENT. This is initially based on stopping the exposure and then increasing the clearance of the mercury from the body. Most of the experience is from adults occupationally exposed to mercury. The mainstay of treatment is chelation with substrates that contain sulfhydryl groups. The sulfhydryl group binds the mercury to facilitate its excretion in urine and stool. Chelation for methyl mercury poisoning is not efficacious. Once the diagnosis is established, the local poison control facility should be contacted and care coordinated with physicians who are familiar with the use of the chelators and the necessary support and follow-up of these poisoned patients.

Chelation therapy should be used in subjects who are symptomatic from mercury poisoning or have toxic blood or urine concentrations. The blood and urine concentrations that are toxic to the child are not known, but they probably are lower than those described for the adult. Chelation therapy removes only a very small percent of the total body burden of mercury, and the efficacy of chelation in chronic elemental exposure has been questioned because of the relatively unexchangeable tissue stores. Chelation in acute exposures is most effective when given as soon as possible after the exposure and should be given by 3 hr after the ingestion of mercury salts.

The most effective chelators presently available in the United States are 2,3-dimercaptosuccinic acid, dimercaprol (BAL), 2,3-dimercaptopropane-1-sulfonate, penicillamine, and N-acetylpenicillamine. Although only labeled for lead chelation and with limited experience in children, 2-3-dimercaptosuccinic acid appears to be the chelator of choice in subjects who can ingest oral medications. 2,3-Dimercaptosuccinic acid is the most efficacious mercury chelator and the chelator with the least amount of adverse effects. In addition, 2,3-dimercaptosuccinic acid, along with penicillamine, are given orally, while BAL must be given by deep intramuscular injection. 2,3-dimercaptopropane-sulfonate may be efficacious as 2, 3-dimercaptosuccinic acid but is only available on an investigational new drug (IND)–based protocol. If the subject cannot take oral medications, the chelator of choice is BAL.

Chelation therapy should be given for several days and then stopped several days, and repeated. This intermittent therapy should be repeated until the patients are symptom-free or the remaining mercury-induced toxic effects are felt to be irreversible. Urinary mercury levels are useful to follow the progress of mercury chelation. The recommended dose of 2,3-dimercaptosuccinic acid is 10 mg/kg/dose or 350 mg/m^2 orally administered every 8 hr for 5 days, then administered every 12 hr for an additional 14 days. For patients who need repeated courses of therapy, a minimum of 2 wk between courses is recommended. Adverse drug reactions include vomiting, nausea, diarrhea, appetite loss, and transient elevations of serum aminotransferases. Hemolysis in patients with glucose-6-phosphate dehydrogenase deficiencies have been reported, and this drug's use should be avoided in these patients.

Dimercaprol (BAL in oil) is used to chelate inorganic mercury. BAL is contraindicated to chelate methyl mercury because it (and potentially other chelators) increases the brain concentration of methyl mercury and the patient can become more symptomatic. BAL should be effective in chelating phenyl mercury because it is rapidly oxidized to Hg^{2+}. In some cases, oral penicillamine has been used as an adjunct to BAL or as an alternative to BAL. BAL recommended therapeutic regimen is 3–5 mg/kg IM every 4 hr on days 1 and 2; 2.5–3 mg/kg every 6 hr on days 3 and 4; and 2.5–3 mg/kg every 12 hr for 1 wk. Some authors recommend that the total dose of BAL should not exceed 24 mg/kg. The course can be repeated after a 5 day period of no therapy. Adverse drug reactions occur in about 50% of the subjects receiving BAL. These reactions include a marked increase in blood pressure; tachycardia; nausea and vomiting; headache; a burning sensation in the lips, mouth, and throat; and a feeling of constriction in the throat, chest, or hands.

In addition to chelation, patients need supportive care. Patients with significant inhalation of elemental mercury vapor may need supplemental oxygen and to be observed for respiratory failure. Elemental mercury ingestion usually is not toxic, but rarely the patient may require surgery to remove entrapped mercury in the appendix or intestine.

After ingestion of inorganic mercury, the mercury can be removed from the gastrointestinal tract by emesis, catharsis, or lavage. It is most important to keep the patient well hydrated and to reduce the concentration of mercury in the kidneys. Chelation therapy should be initiated as soon as possible. With a potentially lethal ingestion, peritoneal dialysis or hemodialysis should be considered to enhance mercury clearance and to prevent renal failure. Inorganic mercury poisoning results in renal dysfunction; serum electrolytes, blood urea nitrogen, and serum creatinine should be monitored. The liver profile and blood pressure also need to be followed.

Mercury decontamination of the environment will most likely be required. Vacuum cleaning may further disperse the mercury in the air. State departments of health should be useful in helping to clean up a contaminated site. Unfortunately there are no guidelines for the cleanup of a home and no guidelines as to what mercury levels are safe to reoccupy the residence.

Chapter 665
Lead Poisoning

Sergio Piomelli

EPIDEMIOLOGY. Lead is a nonessential metal. Lead in the body is unnatural and reflects contamination of the human internal milieu. An average blood lead level near 0 was found in an "unacculturated" population, the Yanomamo Indians living at the remote source of the Orinoco River. In a study of children and adults living near the Himalayas, the average blood lead level was found to be 3 μg/dL; this very low level could be explained by the combustion of heating materials in huts without chimneys.

In the United States, the penetration of lead in the environment has been pervasive, primarily through vehicular emissions and lead paint in old deteriorated housing. In the 1970s, lead poisoning was a common and devastating illness, particularly for inner-city children. Lead encephalopathy was common, and thousands of children suffered marked brain damage.

The situation has profoundly changed, primarily because of the progressive elimination of lead in gasoline. According to the III National Health and Nutritional Examination Survey, the average blood lead level of the entire United States population decreased from 12.2 μg/dL in 1980 to 3.2 μg/dL in 1991. In 1991, the prevalence of children age 1–5 yr with blood lead levels of 15 μg/dL or more was 8.9% and that of children with blood lead levels of 20 μg/dL or more (the level at which the Centers for Disease Control and Prevention (CDC) recommend medical intervention) was 1.1%. These figures refer to the entire nation; great differences in the percentages between different socioeconomic groups persist. The situation has further improved in 1994. For instance, in the author's urban pediatric clinic, the average blood lead level has declined from 5.2 μg/dL in 1991 to 3.2 μg/dL in 1994. The estimates of the prevalence of blood lead levels of 10 μg/dL or more in children age 1–5 yr, range from 2–9%. The percentage of children with blood lead level of 15 μg/dL or more is now much lower than these values, and the percentage of children with blood lead level of 20 μg/dL or more is now less than 1%. There is, however, great variability within the United States and within each city itself. The prevalence of elevated blood lead levels is much higher in children living in pre-World War II dilapidated housing; it is almost nonexistent among those living in recent housing.

The decline in the average blood lead level has been accompanied by a decrease in the frequency and severity of clinical lead intoxication. Lead encephalopathy has almost disappeared; most children tested by the current screening programs have blood lead levels well below 10 μg/dL. These remarkable results reflect primarily the effect of the reduction of vehicular lead emissions mandated by the Clean Air Act and demonstrate the effectiveness and importance of prevention. Nonetheless, many primarily urban children have an excessive body burden of lead and suffer some degree of unnecessary neuropsychologic damage. Lead poisoning continues to be a public health problem.

The major source for children in the United States is the lead-containing paint present in most dwellings built before World War II; this is most dangerous when the paint is deteriorating. Lead-containing dust is taken up by the smallest children through respiration and through their normal hand-to-mouth activities. When lead-laden homes are renovated, lead dust raises a particularly serious risk; children should always be removed from the premises during such renovations. Although airborne and dust-laden lead are continuous sources of low-level exposure, other nonpaint sources may provide an intense exposure that may result in a rapid accumulation of a very toxic level of lead, provoking severe and acute lead poisoning. Acidic fruit juices stored in poorly glazed ceramic vessels, lead dust carried home by lead industry workers, fumes from burning batteries, some Asian cosmetics, and some Mexican folk medicines all have resulted in sporadic cases of lead poisoning in children. Sniffing of leaded gasoline by teenagers and older children can be another unsuspected cause of lead poisoning.

PATHOPHYSIOLOGY. The high toxicity of lead results from its avidity for the sulfhydryl (SH) group of proteins. Lead irreversibly binds to the SH group of a protein and thus impairs its function. Certain metabolic effects of lead can be detected even at minimal levels of exposure. The enzyme δ-aminolevulinic acid dehydratase, which catalyzes the formation of the porphobilinogen ring, a key step of the heme synthetic pathway, is progressively inhibited by lead in an exponential manner, without any threshold. Its inactivation can be reversed "in vitro" by removal of the lead with SH reagents. The loss of activity of the δ-aminolevulinic acid dehydratase is a continuously progressing phenomenon. However, at very low levels of lead exposure, the impact of a partial inactivation of this enzyme is probably negligible, because the potential enzyme activity is largely in excess of the needs of heme synthesis. At higher levels of exposure, on the other hand, the nearly complete inactivation of the enzyme results in serious clinical consequences because it leads to a substantial accumulation of δ-aminolevulinic acid, which is neurotoxic.

Another enzyme in the heme synthesis chain that is severely damaged by lead is ferrochelatase, the enzyme that catalyzes the culminating step of heme synthesis, the insertion of iron into the protoporphyrin IX ring. The result of an ineffective ferrochelatase is an accumulation of protoporphyrin in erythrocytes. This, because of its fluorescence, is easily detected and permits a rapid and accurate measurement of the erythrocyte protoporphyrin (EP). EP is a useful adjunct in the detection of childhood lead poisoning because it reflects the biochemical effects of lead and also detects iron deficiency.

The accumulation of protoporphyrin is not only of diagnostic value; it also sheds light on the pathogenesis of certain symptoms of lead poisoning. For instance, a defect in the heme-containing cytochrome P450 underlies the failure of the alcohol dehydrogenase system in workers of the lead industry that results in very prolonged hangovers (the Monday morning colic). Organotypic neural tissue cultures exposed to lead demyelinate and accumulate fluorescent porphyrins; these effects can be prevented by the addition of heme to the system. Thus, the abnormalities of heme synthesis induced by lead underlie and parallel the neurologic abnormalities.

CLINICAL MANIFESTATIONS. There is no precise direct correlation between blood lead level and clinical manifestations. Children with blood lead levels greater than 100 μg/dL may occasionally appear clinically well, and children with blood lead level 30–35 μg/dL may be symptomatic. The probability of severe symptoms increases with the increase in exposure to lead, and it is greater the higher the blood lead level is.

The most serious manifestation of lead poisoning is acute encephalopathy. This may appear without a prodrome or may be preceded by behavioral changes and/or lead colic, characterized by occasional vomiting, intermittent abdominal pain, and constipation. Encephalopathy includes persistent vomiting, ataxia, seizures, papilledema, impaired consciousness, and coma. If it is necessary for the diagnosis, a spinal tap may be carefully performed: This usually reveals mild pleocytosis, modest hyperproteinemia, and increased pressure. Peripheral neuropathy, which is common in adults, is rarely seen in children, except for those with sickle cell disease. The symptoms of childhood lead poisoning in the absence of clear signs of encephalopathy are usually non-specific and vague. Abdominal colic, behavioral abnormalities, attention disorders, hyperactivity, or severe unexplained retardation should lead one to suspect clinical lead poisoning.

Lead encephalopathy rarely occurs at blood lead levels below 100 μg/dL. However, children with elevated blood lead levels, even well below 100 μg/dL, may present with a constellation of neurologic symptoms. These can be obvious at higher blood level (hyperactivity, anorexia, decreased play activity). At lower levels, the neurologic abnormalities become progressively less obvious. Neurobehavioral abnormalities, demonstrated at low levels of lead exposure by epidemiologic studies, include lower intelligence and poor school performance. Peak blood lead levels in the affected children were approximately 35 μg/dL. Similar neurobehavioral abnormalities have been shown at even lower levels of lead exposure. Needleman in 1989 demonstrated significant neurobehavioral abnormalities when comparing two groups of children: one with high and the other with low lead in their deciduous teeth dentine. The validity of that study, that some had contested, was confirmed by a rigorous analysis by the National Research Council. The effect of lead on children's intelligence has been the object of several recent studies. All of those results have been critically reviewed in two independent "meta-analyses." Despite different and sometimes opposing criteria, both came to the same conclusions: an increase of blood lead from 10 μg/dL to 20 μg/dL results in an average decrease in I. Q. of approximately 2 points, which some consider a trivial effect. The current techniques for the detection of neurobehavioral abnormalities are much less sensitive than those used to detect biochemical abnormalities. Subtle abnormalities detectable only on large cohorts with sophisticated statistics may have potential but undetermined physiologic relevance, as is the case of the demonstrable, but not physiologically relevant, partial inactivation of the δ-aminolevulinic acid dehydratase.

DIAGNOSIS. Of critical importance in the diagnosis is an accurate environmental history, particularly of exposure to lead-containing paint. History of pica, when present, is strongly suggestive; however, pica is not a prerequisite for lead poisoning. Children, with a normal rate of hand-to-mouth activity, ingest substantial amounts of lead from household dust when deteriorating lead-containing paint is present. Large radiopaque flakes of paint, when present on abdominal radiologic examination, are a clear indicator of pica. However, lead poisoning results mostly from ingestion of dust. The large flakes of paint themselves pass essentially untouched through the intestine into the stool.

Environmental investigation should involve not only the child's own home but also other locations where the child spends considerable time, such as the grandmother's or baby sitter's residence. It is also important to consider the other nonpaint sources of exposure (see above). When the diagnosis of lead poisoning is established, technicians from the local Department of Health should be immediately dispatched to examine the involved homes.

Unless the symptoms of lead poisoning are clearly evident, in most cases, the diagnosis needs to be established by blood lead testing. Lead poisoning is often diagnosed through a screening program in children who are essentially asymptomatic. Blood lead levels should preferably be measured on a venous blood sample. However, pragmatic considerations often make this difficult, particularly in large clinics and screening sites, when the number of children to be tested is very large. In these situations, lead can be measured from blood samples obtained by finger puncture. If the finger puncture technique is impeccably executed by experienced technicians, the percentage of contaminated samples can be kept at less than 10%. The result of an elevated blood lead level obtained by finger puncture should never be used as the only criterion to initiate therapy. In an asymptomatic child, therapy should be delayed until the result of a confirmatory venous blood lead level is available. If the child has symptoms of lead poisoning and a venous blood lead level cannot be rapidly obtained, supportive evidence should be used, such as measuring erythrocyte porphyrins, an abdominal film to search for lead, and radiography of the long bones to look for *"lead lines."* None of these tests is, *per se,* diagnostic of lead poisoning, but each can, in critical situations, provide useful supportive information.

Measurements of blood lead levels are difficult and cumbersome. They are rarely available in hospital laboratories. Most large cities and all state laboratories provide blood lead analysis. Even in the best laboratories, however, the accuracy is only ±2 μg/dL, and often it is ±4 μg/dL. Such a margin of error is acceptable when the blood lead level is high (≥30 μg/dL). But, when the blood lead level is low (≤15 μg/dL), the uncertainty creates difficulties in classification. Blood lead levels between 10 and 14 μg/dL should be confirmed before classifying a child on a single measurement as having "lead poisoning" according to the 1991 CDC definition.

Elevation of the EP level is an indication of alterations of the process of heme synthesis. It reflects either iron deficiency or lead poisoning. The EP level is most markedly elevated when both iron deficiency and lead poisoning coexist, a frequent occurrence, particularly in children from low socioeconomic levels in urban areas. Measurements of EP were used extensively to screen children in the 1970s when the frequency of elevated blood lead levels was very high. The EP level was then a very useful test to detect the most severe cases of lead poisoning, as it is 100% positive when the blood lead is 55 μg/dL or more. However, at lower blood lead levels, the frequency of positive results declines; at blood lead level of 32 μg/dL, only 50% of the children tested have positive results, and only a few children test positive when the blood lead level is 20 μg/dL or less. Because the current screening programs are directed at detecting lower blood lead levels, EP levels cannot be used anymore as primary screening tools. This test remains useful to diagnose iron deficiency, to assess the biochemical damage of lead, and to provide supportive evidence in symptomatic children, when measurements of blood lead levels are not promptly available. EP measurements are also useful in follow-up of the effectiveness of long-term therapy. The EP level promptly rises within 24–48 hr of exposure, but because it is incorporated into the hemoglobin molecule itself, it persists for the entire red cell life span of 120 days. Thus, for children in treatment, a slow but progressive decline of the EP level reflects the elimination of lead from the body.

DEFINITION AND CLASSIFICATION OF LEAD POISONING. The natural blood lead level is 0 μg/dL, and any exposure to lead results in some biochemical damage that becomes continuously progressive with increasing levels. Thus, in a very precise sense, we all have *lead poisoning.* In practice, however, it is necessary to choose a threshold blood lead value below which the adverse effects of lead are "trivial" (i.e., physiologically irrelevant). The choice is always somewhat arbitrary, and this leads to further controversy.

In 1991, the CDC's expert panel defined all children with blood lead level of 10 μg/dL or more as having *"lead poisoning."* This unqualified definition gives equal importance to a blood lead level of 12 μg/dL as to one of 75 μg/dL or more. In the forthcoming revision of the CDC document, a gradation system will be made, and children with blood lead levels of 10–19 μg/dL will be defined as having *"mild lead poisoning."* The classification based on blood lead level proposed by CDC (Table 665–1) is useful to provide management guidelines and to help large programs establish priorities. However, it does not replace sound clinical judgment in managing the individual child.

■ TABLE 665–1 Centers for Disease Control and Prevention 1991 Classification and Recommendations

Blood Lead Level (μg/dL)		Action Recommended
0–9	No immediate concern	
≥10		"Lead poisoning"
10–14	Environmental survey	If found in too many children, survey the community
15–19	Environmental survey	Education about lead exposure
20–24	Remove from lead source	Bring to medical attention
25–54	Remove from lead source	EDTA test: if positive, 25–44 EDTA; 45–54 EDTA or DMSA
55–69	Remove from lead source	Treat with EDTA or DMSA
≥70 or symptomatic	Emergency hospitalization	Treat with BAL and EDTA
	Always return the child to a clean house	

EDTA = edetate calcium-disodium; DMSA = succimer; BAL = dimercaprol.

TREATMENT. Removing the Source of Lead Exposure. The most important aspect of therapy is to remove the child from the source of exposure to lead. In most cases, this is the only necessary action; only in more severe cases is treatment indicated. The removal from the source, however, must be complete and exhaustive. Often, in the case of poor urban children, there is more than one source; in addition to the child's own home, the grandmother or the baby sitter's home may be equally contaminated. It is essential that children should be removed from their own homes to another safer home that has been appropriately inspected by Health Department technicians. Similarly, while the child's home is being repaired, the child should stay out of it day and night. Repairs should be followed by cleaning with a high-efficiency particle accumulator (HEPA) vacuum cleaner, and the areas should be scrubbed with high-phosphate detergent two or three times, followed by HEPA vacuum cleaning again, before the child is allowed to return. Treatment of more severe cases requires chelation therapy.

Symptomatic Children and Children with Blood Lead Levels of More than 70 μg/dL. In symptomatic children, regardless of blood lead level, the treatment is always given in a hospital. Children with blood lead levels of 70 μg/dL or more, even if asymptomatic, should also be considered medical emergencies and immediately hospitalized for treatment. Treatment should consist of dimercaprol (BAL, 75 mg/m^2 every 4 hr; total daily dose of 450 mg/m^2), followed by edetate calcium-disodium (EDTA) (1,500 mg/m^2/24 hr by continuous infusion). It is important to start with BAL and to initiate the EDTA only 3–4 hr later. EDTA also binds zinc and renders even more complete the paralysis of the δ-aminolevulinic acid dehydratase (a zinc-dependent enzyme); this, in turn, results in a burst of δ-aminolevulinic acid in the blood, which may induce convulsions. Treatment should be continued for 5 days; the BAL may be suspended as soon as the blood lead level falls below 60 μg/dL. Repeated courses of treatment may be necessary in these children until the blood lead level returns to a safe range (≤ 20 μg/dL).

Management of the Encephalopathy. Management of these critically ill patients consists of controlling convulsions (if present), establishing a urine flow, and administering the same chelation therapy as above. A careful control of fluids is necessary to avoid aggravating the increased intracranial pressure. Intravenous EDTA, at the dosage recommended above, can be safely fitted into a controlled fluid administration. See Chapter 60.2 for management of increased intracranial pressure.

Asymptomatic Children with Blood Lead Levels of 45–69 μg/dL. Asymptomatic children with blood lead levels of 45–69 μg/dL almost always should be treated. The treatment may consist of EDTA alone (1,000 mg/m^2/24 hr intravenously, in a 24-hr infusion or in a short—20–30-min—infusion) for 5 consecutive days. EDTA is best given intravenously; when the intravenous route is not possible, EDTA may be given intramuscularly. Intramuscular EDTA is extremely painful, and the pain is only partially alleviated if the drug is mixed with procaine. EDTA can be administered again, if necessary, after a 2-day interval.

An alternative therapy consists of Succimer (DMSA *[Chemet]*). DMSA can be given orally, has minimal side effects, and appears to be an excellent chelator. However, outpatient *DMSA should never be used unless there is absolute certainty that the child's environment is perfectly clean.* DMSA is administered for 5 days at a dose of 350 mg/m^2 every 8 hr for 5 consecutive days, followed by 2 wk more of therapy at reduced frequency (350 mg/m^2 every 12 hr) for a total of 19 days. Additional courses may be given, if needed, after a 2 wk interval. Repeated courses of treatment may be necessary in these children to bring the blood lead into a safe range (≤ 20 μg/dL).

Asymptomatic Children with Blood Lead Levels of 20–45 μg/dL. When the blood lead level is in this range, it is preferable to perform an EDTA-provocative chelation test to ascertain the usefulness of treatment. This test consists of the administration of EDTA (500 mg/m^2), preferably intravenously, in 5% dextrose, over 30 min, followed by a urinary collection of 8 hr duration. The urinary excretion of lead is measured, and the results are expressed as the following ratio:

$$\frac{\text{Lead excreted } (\mu g)}{\text{EDTA given (mg)}}$$

A ratio greater than 0.7 is considered an abnormal (positive) provocative test result and suggests that treatment will be effective and, thus, is indicated. If the results of the EDTA provocative chelation test suggest treatment, only EDTA is administered because, at these blood lead levels, the use of DMSA is not approved by the Food and Drug Administration. EDTA should be given at a dose of 1,000 mg/m^2/24 hr, preferably on an outpatient basis.

Asymptomatic Children with Blood Lead Levels of 10–19 μg/dL. At these levels, no treatment or medical intervention is necessary; only general education is recommended. A high frequency of children with blood lead levels in this range in a given community suggests the possible presence of environmental lead contamination.

PREVENTION AND SCREENING. Today, the major source of lead remains old house paint. Lead poisoning will not completely disappear until the current housing stock is completely repaired and made lead free. This would represent a substantial cost, but it is the responsibility of a civilized society. In *"Strategic Plan for Elimination of Childhood Lead Poisoning,"* the CDC indicated the need and the cost effectiveness of eliminating lead from the homes where children live. However, in 1991, the CDC chose to emphasize the alternative approach of recommending universal screening by blood lead measurement, whether children live in a contaminated community or not. Screening should occur at 10–14 mo of age and again at approximately 2 yr of age. This approach has been widely criticized in the pediatric community. Screening would be better directed to those communities where old housing stock is in poor condition; these are the only communities in the United States where a significant amount of lead paint is still present.

Annest JL, Pirkle JL, Maguk D, et al: Chronological trend in blood lead level between 1976 and 1980. N Engl J Med 308:1373, 1983.
Binder S, Matte T: Childhood lead poisoning: the impact of prevention. JAMA 269:1679, 1993.
Centers for Disease Control, Risk Management Subcommittee: Strategic Plan for Elimination of Childhood Lead Poisoning. Bethesda, US Department Of Health and Human Services, 1991.
Centers for Disease Control: Preventing Lead Poisoning in Young Children. Bethesda, US Department of Health and Human Services, 1991.
Fowler BA (ed): National Research Council, Board on Environmental Studies and Toxicology: *Measuring Lead Exposure in Infants, Children and Other Sensitive Populations.* Washington, DC, National Academy Press, 1993.
Harvey B: Should blood lead screening recommendation be revised? Pediatrics 93:201, 1994.
Hernberg S, Nikkanen J: Enzyme inhibition by lead under normal urban conditions. Lancet 1:63, 1970.
Hoekelman RA: A lead balloon. Pediatr Ann 21:335, 1992.
National Academy of Sciences, National Research Council: Measuring Lead Exposure in Infants, Children and Other Sensitive Populations. Washington, DC, National Academy Press, 1993.
Needleman HL, Gunnoe C, Leviton A, et al: Deficits in psychologic and classroom performance of children with elevated dentine lead levels. N Engl J Med 300:689, 1979.
Oski FA: Lead poisoning—what are the facts? Contemp Pediatr 10:145, 1993.
Patterson CC: Contaminated and natural lead environment of man. Arch Environ Health 11:344, 1985.
Pirkle JL, Brody DJ, Gunter EW, et al: The decline in blood lead levels in the United States. The National Health and Nutritional Examination Surveys (NHANES). JAMA 272:294, 1994.
Piomelli S: Childhood lead poisoning in the '90's. Pediatrics 93:508, 1994.
Piomelli S, Rosen JF, Chisolm JJ, et al: Management of childhood lead poisoning. J Pediatr 105:523, 1984.
Pocock S, Smith M, Baghurst P: Environmental lead and children's intelligence: a systemic review of the epidemiologic evidence. B M J 309:1189, 1994.
Schwartz J: Low-level lead exposure and children's I.Q.: A meta-analysis and search for a threshold. Env Res 56:42, 1994.

CHAPTER 666

Chemical and Drug Poisoning

Barry H. Rumack

666.1 Principles of Management

From 1985–1989, 3,810,405 poisoning exposures to children younger than age 6 yr were reported to the American Association of Poison Control Centers (AAPCC). During the same time 6,116,635 total cases were reported. Generally, children younger than age 6 yr encounter poisons accidentally or as a result of abuse. Cases 6–12 yr of age are rarer, representing 3.2% of the 1992 total. Cases 13–19 yr of age were 2.4% in 1992 and are primarily intentional or occupational and are not similar to the unintentional cases seen in the younger-than-age-6 population. Children in this younger age group tend to put virtually anything in their mouth. Most (92.1%) occur in the home, with more than 93% involving a single substance. Sixty percent of cases were related to nonpharmaceutical and 40%, to pharmaceutical products. Ingestion accounted for 75.4% of all cases in 1992 with dermal at 7.7%, ophthalmic at 6.3%, and inhalation at 6.1%. Bites and stings were 3.6%, with all others at 1%.

The AAPCC data likely represent some skewing of cases away from reports of suicide with heavier emphasis on accidental cases, owing to the kinds of questions referred to a poison center. Many suicidal patients are taken directly to an emergency facility, which may or may not report to or request consultation from a poison information center. The peak age of suicide attempts for children is 13–17 yr (see Chapters 25 and 104). Thus, pediatricians have to contend with two major groups of children in regard to poisoning: (1) those age 6 and younger exposed to plants, household products, medications, and so on and (2) the adolescent exposed most frequently to medications. Once the diagnosis of poisoning or potential poisoning is entertained, the pediatrician should follow a specific management plan to ensure optimum care.

MANAGEMENT PLAN FOR POISONING AND OVERDOSE

Initial contact with a poisoned patient will usually be over the telephone. The following data should be obtained at the time of initial contact:

Phone Number. Getting the caller's telephone number is necessary in case the phone contact is accidentally broken and to permit follow-up calls.

Address. This may be crucial if emergency equipment needs to be dispatched or if the person on the phone becomes hysterical or develops lethargy, convulsions, and so on.

Evaluation of Severity. Although many callers may begin with a description of symptoms or signs such as a convulsion, it is vital to evaluate the current status of the patient in terms of immediate danger, potential danger, and no danger. Further history may be necessary to evaluate an asymptomatic patient.

Weight and Age. This permits estimation of potential toxicity.

Time of Ingestion. This permits interpretation of onset of symptoms or signs as well as evaluation of laboratory data and other prognostic information.

Past Medical History. Brief information should be elicited to determine the usual health status of the patient as a basis for interpreting signs. It will also suggest interactions of chronic medications or allergies with the current ingestion.

Type of Exposure. Product names and ingredients should be obtained from labels or from the POISINDEX System.

Amount of Exposure. How many tablets or how much fluid has been consumed should be estimated. Tablets or fluid remaining in the container should be counted or measured.

Route of Exposure. It should be determined if the exposure was by ingestion, inhalation, local application to the eyes or skin, or parenteral.

Caller's Relationship to Victim. It is important to determine if the call is from a baby sitter, friend, relative, or stranger and who gives permission to treat the patient.

Such basic information should be a standard procedure in every office or clinic where such cases may be reported. Written records should be kept of each event. It may be acceptable practice either to see the patient or to treat and observe the patient at home, depending on the exposure and patient's condition. If treatment is at home, then follow-up calls *must* be made at approximately 0.5, 1, and 4 hr after exposure. Any change in the patient's condition may warrant a change in the decision to treat at home. Since as many as half the histories obtained from poisoned patients will have an error of some magnitude, the physician must be ready to change treatment or disposition decisions in light of changes in onset of symptoms or new history. Diphenoxylate-atropine combination (Lomotil) is an example of a drug for which even careful follow-up may be inadequate. Because of the idiosyncratic nature of its ingestion, *all* children consuming this drug younger than age 6 yr *must* be hospitalized and monitored for 24 hr; delayed onset of coma for 8–12 hr requires that these patients receive intensive medical observation.

Initial Medical Care

If after telephone consultation or direct primary evaluation the decision is made to have the patient seen by others, transportation appropriate to the patient's condition should be arranged. The site of initial medical contact should also be considered in relation to the exposure history. For example, if it is expected that respiratory support will be required, then paramedic transport to a well-equipped emergency facility is mandatory. Once the decision is made, then the receiving personnel should be notified so that proper preparation can be made, including notification of the poison center if that has not yet been done. Before transport, all product containers thought likely to be related to the exposure should be gathered up and brought with the patient. If the patient has vomited spontaneously or by induction with syrup of ipecac, this emesis should be saved and brought with the patient.

Once the patient has arrived in the appropriate medical care setting, initial attention should focus on life support, with primary emphasis on cardiorespiratory care. Shock, arrhythmias, and convulsions must be dealt with as in the case of any other critically ill patient (see Chapter 60). There are few poisons for which there is an antidote. Except for the poisons listed below, specific treatment directed at the poison can be delayed until the physician is satisfied that the patient's condition is stable. The following poisons require simultaneous use of an antagonist and life support measures.

CARBON MONOXIDE. Oxygen (100%) should be administered as early as possible to reduce the concentration of carbon monoxide in the blood and increase oxygen transport to tissues. Symptomatic patients or those with high levels may be candidates for hyperbaric oxygen therapy (see Chapter 60).

CYANIDE. Oxygen should be supplied immediately, followed by specific antidotal treatment. Although the antidote that is available in the United States is not ideal, appropriate doses should be administered to a symptomatic patient with cyanide poisoning. The antidote kit contains the following: (1) amyl nitrite inhalers, which may be broken under the patient's nose for 30 sec of each minute while the sodium nitrite solution is being readied; (2) sodium nitrite 3% solution, which should be administered at a dose of 0.33 mL/kg (10 mg/kg) to a maximum dose of 10 mL/patient with normal hemoglobin; and (3) sodium thiosulfate 25% solution, which should be administered next at a dose of 1.65 mL/kg to a maximum dose of the entire ampule. These agents produce methemoglobin, which may help remove cyanide by competition for the cytochrome. An alternative antidote, a hydroxocobalamin-thiosulfate mixture, is available outside the United States; it should be given in doses of 4–10 g. Hydroxocobalamin alone cannot be given in sufficient quantity to be effective.

OPIATES AND RELATED POISONS. Naloxone in sufficient doses is very effective in treating these poisonings. A minimum dose of 0.4 mg can be given to any patient, regardless of age or weight. If there is failure of response, up to 2.0 mg should be administered rapidly intravenously to larger children and adolescents. This may be repeated as necessary. Newborns to infants 6 mo of age should be given a dose of 0.2 mg/kg.

SUBSTANCES PRODUCING METHEMOGLOBINEMIA. Although relatively uncommon, exposure to aniline dyes, nitrobenzene, azo compounds, and nitrites may produce methemoglobinemia that is unresponsive to oxygen administration. The diagnosis is suggested by comparing a drop of the patient's blood with that of the physician. If there is at least 20% methemoglobinemia, the patient's blood will be relatively brown when dried on a sheet of filter paper; the color would be red at a lower percentage of methemoglobin. Methylene blue at a dose of 0.1–0.2 mL/kg (1–2 mg/kg) in a 1% solution is therapeutic. If two doses are unsuccessful, exchange transfusion may be required.

CHOLINERGIC AGENTS. Children exposed to organophosphate insecticides and carbamates may develop salivation, lacrimation, urination, defecation, and fasciculations. Atropine at a dose of 0.05 mg/kg to a maximum initial dose of 2–5 mg should be administered while the patient is being decontaminated with soap and water. Repeated doses of atropine may be necessary if the patient is unresponsive. In severe cases or when the cholinesterase level falls to 25% of normal or lower, pralidoxime, a cholinesterase regenerator, may be indicated. The dosage is 25–50 mg/kg given over 30 min intravenously every 8–12 hr in young children, to a maximum of 1 g/dose in older children.

OTHER "ANTIDOTES." These are not generally required immediately and may be administered after the diagnosis is confirmed (e.g., ethanol for ethylene glycol or methanol poisoning or *N*-acetyl cysteine (NAC) for acetaminophen overdose).

Preventing Absorption

The goal of therapy is to reduce the amount of the poison taken up by the body. In some cases, this may be preventative (e.g., a child who ingested something just prior to calling the physician may have absorbed very little). In other cases, it may be desirable to reduce further absorption (e.g., oral activated charcoal following oral or intravenous theophylline overdosage). Before using any of these techniques, their safety should be evaluated for the particular child.

EMESIS. In 1983, 13.4% of poison exposures were treated with ipecac, and this has gradually dropped to 4.0% in 1992. It is a procedure that should be abandoned in children and probably adults, except in rare instances. Administration of syrup of ipecac, 15–30 mL, followed by a clear liquid such as water results in vomiting in over 95% of children younger than age 5 yr. Ipecac dosing in children 6–12 mo of age should be 10 mL; it should not be used in children younger than 6 mo of age. The airway may be protected by positioning the patient on the left side with the head down (spanking position). Emesis should not be induced if the patient is comatose, is convulsing, has ingested strong acids or bases, or when there is a significant risk of aspiration. Data in adolescents and adults have brought into question whether emesis affects outcome; it produces only an average of 8–30% recovery of ingested material. The initial emesis should be saved for diagnostic analysis.

LAVAGE. Except in unusual circumstances lavage is unnecessary in children. It may be useful with drugs that decrease gastric motility or form bezoars not adsorbed by charcoal. Outcome in an adult study was positively affected only if the procedure was done within 1 hr. Complications in adults have included esophageal perforation. It is probably unsafe in young children in whom there may be airway obstruction and in whom cuffed endotracheal tubes cannot be used.

CHARCOAL. In 1983, 4% of cases were treated with this agent and, in 1991, 7%; this demonstrates a growing trend in the use of activated charcoal. The administration of a good grade of activated charcoal (*not* burned toast or universal antidote) may be the most effective and safest procedure to prevent absorption. Charcoal is capable of adsorbing almost all drugs and many other chemicals. It should be given as a water slurry with a minimum dose of 15–30 g in a child and 30–100 g in an adolescent. Repeat doses may be given every 2–6 hr accompanied by a cathartic for the first dose. The procedure should be terminated with the first charcoal stool. Charcoal is ineffective in heavy metal or volatile hydrocarbon poisoning.

CATHARTIC. Sorbitol (maximum 1 g/kg), magnesium sulfate (maximum 250 mg/kg), sodium citrate (maximum 250 mg/kg), or phosphosoda (maximum 250 mg/kg) can be used to hasten emptying of the gastrointestinal tract once the ingested material has passed through the stomach. These agents should be used cautiously in young children. They may be useful in older children following administration of activated charcoal, especially for agents that delay bowel motility or hydrocarbons with the potential for systemic toxicity. Whole bowel irrigation with colonic lavage solution (Colyte, GoLYTELY) has been used successfully (especially with retained, agglutinated iron pills) but is still considered controversial in children.

Enhancing Excretion

FORCED DIURESIS. Forced diuresis is an overused technique for treating poisoned children. It has little general use, and its administration is even questionable in phenobarbital and salicylate ingestion, since alkalinization without diuresis may be just as effective. Acid diuresis is contraindicated for agents such as amphetamines, phencyclidine, and so on, owing to aggravation of renal problems with myoglobinuria and methemoglobinemia.

HEMODIALYSIS. Hemodialysis is now used rarely and selectively. Many drugs have very large volumes of distribution so that even if there is good clearance by dialysis, total-body removal may be extremely small. For example, after a digoxin or tricyclic antidepressant overdose, only a small percentage of the drug can be removed by dialysis. The major indications for hemodialysis are severe salicylate intoxication unresponsive to standard care, poisoning with methanol and ethylene glycol with blood levels above 20 mg/dL and acidosis, and symptomatic theophylline overdoses with blood levels at 60–100 μg/dL or higher.

HEMOPERFUSION OVER ACTIVATED CHARCOAL OR RESIN. Hemoperfusion over activated charcoal or resin may be helpful in some situations when there is a small volume of distribution and the agent is well adsorbed. It may be valuable in theophylline, salicylate, and paraquat poisoning of patients who have not responded well to other forms of therapy. It is not recommended for poisonings with tricyclic antidepressants, acetaminophen, digoxin, and so on, since it does not remove substantial amounts of total-body load or change the clinical outcome.

Laboratory Evaluation

In some cases (e.g., poisoning with salicylates, acetaminophen, iron, methanol, and ethylene glycol), the laboratory provides data sufficient to change the treatment plan. In other instances (e.g., opiates, in which there is definitive treatment unrelated to levels, and cyanide, in which it would be too late if the physician waited for laboratory assistance), the laboratory data may be helpful but will not likely change treatment. "Drug screens" are generally not helpful. The best way to use the laboratory is to discuss the case with the technologist and provide appropriate samples and clinical data so that specific analysis can be interpreted. There is little use in doing certain portions of the screen if it is already known what the patient has consumed and that symptoms are consistent with its toxicity. If a "toxic screen" is obtained, it is important to know the specific drugs that are included in the test.

Dine MS, McGovern ME: Intentional poisoning of children: An overlooked category of child abuse. Pediatrics 70:32, 1982.
Ellenhorn MJ, Barceloux DG: Medical Toxicology: Diagnosis and Treatment in Human Poisonings. New York, Elsevier, 1988.
Goldfrank LR: Goldfrank's Toxicologic Emergencies. Norwalk, CT, Appleton-Century-Crofts, 1990.
Litovitz TL, Holm KC, Clancy C, et al: 1992 Annual Report of the American Association of Poison Control Centers Toxic Exposure Surveillance System. Am J Emerg Med 11:494, 1993.
Litovitz TL, Manoguerra A: Comparison of pediatric poisoning hazards: An analysis of 3.8 million exposure incidents. A report from the American Association of Poison Control Centers. Pediatrics 89:999, 1992.
Merigian KS: Prospective evaluation of gastric emptying in the self poisoned patient. Am J Emerg Med 8:479, 1990.
Rumack BH: Poisoning. *In*: Hathway WE, Groothuis JR, Hay WW Jr, et al (eds): Current Pediatric Diagnosis & Treatment. Appleton & Lange, Norwalk, CT, 1993.
Rumack BH, Hess AJ (eds): Poisindex. Denver, 1995.
Vale JA: Reviews in medicine: Clinical toxicology. Postgrad Med J 69:19, 1993.

666.2 Acetaminophen

Acetaminophen has become the most widely used analgesic antipyretic, owing, in part, to the finding of a relationship between Reye syndrome and salicylates. Consequently, acetaminophen is more available for accidental or intentional use by young children and adolescents in the home. There are significant differences in the degree of toxicity that may occur in children younger than age 6 yr and in the older child.

PATHOPHYSIOLOGY. Acetaminophen is primarily metabolized to the sulfate or glucuronide (94%), and the shift from sulfate to glucuronide predominance between ages 9 and 12 yr parallels the change in degree of toxicity at these ages. A small amount of acetaminophen is excreted unchanged, and the remaining approximately 4% is metabolized by cytochrome P450 and glutathione to the mercapturic acid conjugate. This latter pathway produces the toxicity of acetaminophen; when hepatic stores of glutathione are depleted to less than 70% of normal, the highly reactive intermediate metabolites combine with hepatic macromolecules and produce cellular damage.

Although therapeutic peak plasma levels of acetaminophen usually occur at 1–2 hr when hepatic function is normal, measurement prior to 4 hr cannot be used to determine the severity of an overdose because full absorption may not yet have occurred. If there is pre-existing hepatic disease or if the therapeutic half-life is measured after the onset of hepatotoxicity, then the half-life may be extended to 4 hr or more. Because the half-life primarily reflects the sulfate and glucuronide pathways and not the toxic metabolite, it does not relate to the degree of toxicity.

CLINICAL AND LABORATORY MANIFESTATIONS. If untreated, patients who have overdosed pass through four stages of toxicity (Table 666–1). Without a history of ingestion or high index of suspicion, the pediatrician may not diagnose the ingestion. If there is a history of acetaminophen ingestion, the plasma level should be assessed at 4 hr or more after ingestion. Interpretation of this level should be plotted on the nomogram (Fig. 666–1) to determine whether antidotal treatment is indicated. Concomitant ethanol ingestion may produce hepatoxicity at lower than usual levels. Aspartate (AST) and alanine transaminase (ALT) tests, bilirubin level, and prothrombin time should be followed daily in all patients with levels in the toxic range on the nomogram. In adults, renal damage and failure is associated with chronic ingestion, suggesting the need to monitor renal function in some children.

TREATMENT. Therapy for patients with potentially toxic plasma levels of acetaminophen as determined from the nomogram is most effective if oral NAC (Mucomyst) is administered prior to 16 hr postingestion. Institution of NAC may be beneficial with initiation up to 36 hr after ingestion. The mode of administration should be as an initial loading dose of 140 mg/kg. Follow-up doses of 70 mg/kg should be given at 4-hr intervals for 17 additional doses (3 days). The drug should be diluted to a 5%

■ **TABLE 666–1 Stages in the Clinical Course of Acetaminophen Toxicity**

Stage	Time Following Ingestion	Characteristics
I	½–24 hr	Anorexia, nausea, vomiting, malaise, pallor, diaphoresis
II	24–48 hr	Resolution of above; upper quadrant abdominal pain and tenderness; elevated bilirubin, prothrombin time, hepatic enzymes; oliguria
III	72–96 hr	Peak liver function abnormalities; anorexia, nausea, vomiting, malaise may reappear
IV	4 days–2 wk	Resolution of hepatic dysfunction

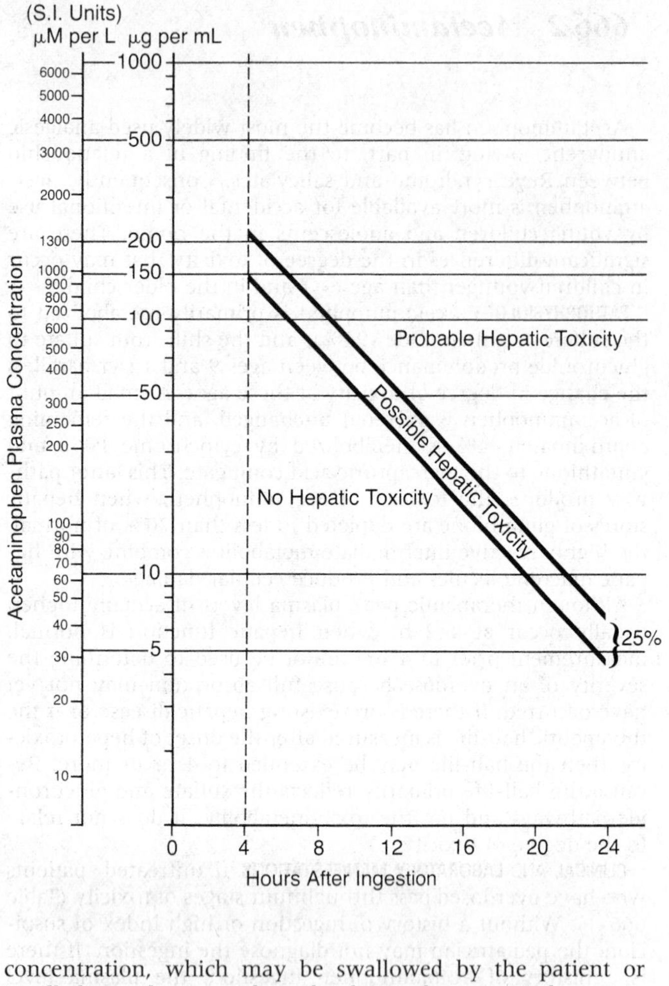

Figure 666–1. **Rumack-Matthew nomogram for acetaminophen poisoning. Semilogarithmic plot of plasma acetaminophen levels versus time.** ***Cautions for the use of this chart*****: (1) The time coordinates refer to time after** ***ingestion*****. (2) Serum levels drawn before 4 hr may not represent peak levels. (3) The graph should be used only in relation to a single acute ingestion. (4) The lower** ***solid line*** **25% below the standard nomogram is included to allow for possible errors in acetaminophen plasma assays and estimated time from ingestion of an overdose. (From Rumack BH, Hess AJ (eds): Poisindex. Denver, 1995. Adapted from Rumack BH, Matthew H: Acetaminophen poisoning and toxicity. Pediatrics 55:871, 1975.)**

concentration, which may be swallowed by the patient or instilled into the stomach or duodenum by gastric tube.

Intravenous use of NAC should be done after an experimental 48-hr protocol similar to the oral protocol, except not utilizing the last day. The oral form is not an approved nonpyrogenic form.

PROGNOSIS. Children younger than age 6 yr are unlikely to develop significant toxicity following ingestion of even relatively large doses of acetaminophen. In a large series, 55 of 417 children developed potentially toxic plasma levels following ingestion, but only 3 of the 417 developed AST peaks of greater than 1,000 IU/L, which is considered a toxic response. In two other series totaling 2,787 cases, no patients had toxic plasma levels, and only 35 were hospitalized. Nevertheless, at this time children with a significant ingestion should have the plasma level measured and receive treatment with the antidote if the level falls within the toxic range on the nomogram. Adolescents have a higher incidence (23.2%) of toxic plasma levels following ingestion than children, and 29% of those with toxic levels are likely to develop AST of greater than 1,000 IU/L. Even after a serious case of hepatotoxicity, the mortality rate is well under 0.5%. Patients who recover have no sequelae when followed at 3–12 mo after the acute toxicity. Severely affected patients may require liver transplantation.

Lauterburg BH, Vaishnav Y, Stillwell WG, et al: The effects of age and glutathione depletion on hepatic glutathione turnover in vivo determined by acetaminophen probe analysis. J Pharmacol Exp Ther 213:54, 1980.
Mancini RE, Sonaware BR, Yaffe SJ: Developmental susceptibility to acetaminophen toxicity. Res Commun Chem Pathol Pharmacol 27:603, 1980.
Miller RP, Roberts RJ, Fisher LJ: Acetaminophen elimination kinetics in neonates, children, and adults. Clin Pharmacol Ther 19:284, 1976.
Peterson RG, Rumack BH: Age as a variable in acetaminophen overdose. Arch Intern Med 141:390, 1981.
Rumack BH: Acetaminophen overdose in young children. Am J Dis Child 138:428, 1984.
Rumack BH, Matthew H: Acetaminophen poisoning and toxicity. Pediatrics 55:871, 1975.
Rumack BH, Peterson RG: Acetaminophen overdose: Incidence, diagnosis and management in 416 patients. Pediatrics 62:898, 1978.
Smilkstein MJ, Bronstein AC, Linden C, et al: Acetaminophen overdose: A 48-hour intravenous N-acetylcysteine treatment protocol. Ann Emerg Med 20:1058, 1991.
Smilkstein MJ, Knapp GL, Kulig KW, et al: Efficacy of oral N-acetylcysteine in the treatment of acetaminophen overdose. N Engl J Med 319:1557, 1988.

666.3 Salicylates

The incidence of ingestion of salicylates has gradually dropped as the use of acetaminophen has increased. Toxicity related to salicylates must be considered in therapeutic situations as well as when there has been an overdose.

PATHOPHARMACOLOGY. Understanding the pharmacokinetics of salicylates permits a clearer evaluation of the plasma levels of salicylate and other laboratory data. The usual half-life of salicylate is 1–2 hr. This may be extended to 25–30 hr once the urine becomes acidic and ion excretion becomes limited. The normal volume of distribution of salicylate is 0.15 L/kg, but with significant toxicity this may increase to 0.3–0.4 L/kg as protein binding is saturated and central nervous system and other distribution occurs. In cases of chronic toxicity, the metabolism of salicylates plays an insignificant role, urine excretion becomes minimal, and further doses add to the accumulated pool of drug in the patient.

Ionization of salicylate is related to the absorption and excretion of salicylate. In an alkaline state (e.g., urine of pH 7), this weak acid (pK approximately 3.0) is mostly ionized. Thus, it does not cross cell membranes very well and stays in the glomerular filtrate, permitting the drug to be excreted. As the urine pH becomes acid, less and less of the drug is ionized, reabsorption from glomerular filtrate occurs, and excretion decreases. Therapy directed at changing urine pH, therefore, affects urine excretion. In some circumstances, patients with various illnesses (e.g., juvenile rheumatoid arthritis) who are doing well on aspirin will suddenly develop problems after dietary changes. A large increase in use of orange juice, for example, will enhance excretion and reduce the plasma salicylate level, perhaps exacerbating the basic disease. Conversely, large ingestions of cranberry juice may acidify the urine, decrease excretion of salicylate, and raise plasma levels to toxic ranges.

CLINICAL MANIFESTATIONS. Young infants may have few signs of toxicity other than dehydration or hyperpnea. Temperature elevation may occur, leading to increased dosages of salicylates in a patient with salicylate toxicity. Older children demonstrate hyperpnea, vomiting, and progressive lethargy as the drug is distributed throughout the central nervous system (CNS). Tinnitus and sudden deafness may occur early in patients with salicylate toxicity. In adolescents, salicylate level measurement is required to distinguish hyperpnea from the "hyperventilation syndrome."

Although a large number of complex metabolic phenomena are involved following a salicylate ingestion, the clinically important relationships can be easily summarized.

Phase 1. Salicylates directly stimulate the respiratory center following absorption. The increased respiratory rate results in respiratory alkalosis and obligate alkaluria as a compensatory mechanism. Both K^+ and Na^+ are lost along with bicarbonate in the urine. This phase may last for as long as 12 hr after ingestion in an adolescent and may be totally missed in a young infant.

Phase 2. When sufficient K^+ has been lost to deplete the kidney of this ion, an exchange of K^+ for H^+ occurs, and the urine becomes relatively acid. The hypokalemia is initially limited to renal tissue and is not reflected either in serum K^+ or on the electrocardiogram. This "paradoxical aciduria" occurs in the presence of a continued respiratory alkalosis. As this phase progresses, hypokalemia is reflected throughout the rest of the body. This phase may begin within hours after ingestion in a young child and may last as long as 12–24 hr in an adolescent.

Phase 3. Eventually dehydration, hypokalemia, and progressive accumulation of lactic acid and other metabolic acids predominate over the respiratory alkalosis. The patient's rapid breathing is in response to the acidosis rather than to primary respiratory center drive. The plasma level of salicylate is generally higher than in phase 1 or 2 because of inability to excrete salicylate in an acid urine and because of continued absorption from the intestine. Uncoupling of oxidative phosphorylation and other metabolic activity contribute a small amount to this phenomenon. The patient is acidotic, with an even more acid urine. This phase may begin 4–6 hr after ingestion in a young infant or 24 hr or more after ingestion in an adolescent. This is also the presentation of chronic salicylate poisoning following repeated therapeutic dosing in the face of dehydration.

The more severe cases may develop pulmonary edema or hemorrhage, although both of these complications are rare. Hyperglycemia or hypoglycemia has also been observed. Virtually all seriously poisoned patients will be more than 5% dehydrated, usually 10% or more.

LABORATORY DATA. Following a single acute ingestion of salicylate, plasma level should be measured 6 hr or more after ingestion and plotted on the nomogram (Fig. 666–2). Levels observed before 6 hr may not reflect peak levels. The nomogram cannot be used when the drug has accumulated over several ingestions, because patients with chronic salicylate toxicity may have very low levels in relation to the severity of their illness, owing to a three- to fourfold increase in the volume of distribution. Levels in chronic toxicity may be in the therapeutic range of 10–20 mL/dL.

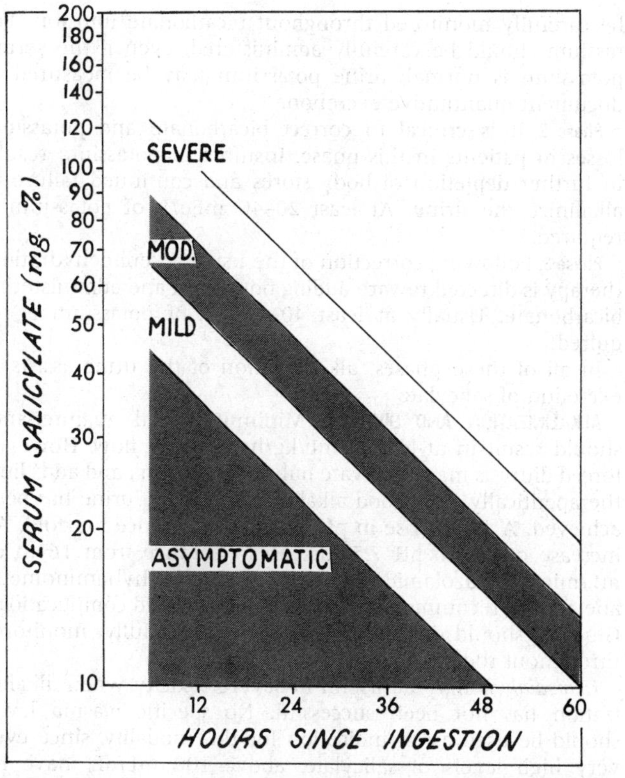

Figure 666–2. Nomogram relating serum salicylate concentration and expected severity of intoxication at varying intervals following the ingestion of a single dose of salicylate. (From Done AK: Salicylate intoxication: Significance of measurements of salicylate in blood in cases of acute ingestion. Pediatrics 26:800, 1960.)

In all patients with salicylate poisoning serious enough to be hospitalized, the plasma levels should be plotted on semilog paper against time. Although the concept of half-life is not precisely correct in salicylate overdoses, calculation of this value from these plots is important. By seeing whether the apparent half-life decreases with therapy, the success of that therapy can be monitored. As long as the relative half-life is greater than 10–15 hr, treatment is not optional.

Urine pH and volume should be measured hourly in all seriously poisoned children. Plasma pH should be checked at regular intervals. K^+ and other electrolytes are critical to calculating replacement fluid therapy; serum K^+ will lag behind the K^+ status of the kidney. Prothrombin time should also be measured in all severely poisoned patients. Arterial blood gas measurements, as well as other ancillary laboratory measures required for the general support of the patient, should be performed. Hepatotoxicity from salicylate in severe, chronic cases will be demonstrated by AST, ALT, bilirubin, and prothrombin abnormalities. Ferric chloride or Phenistix only indicate presence of the drug and should not be substituted for salicylate measurements. Neither of these tests will detect unhydrolyzed asprin (acetylsalicylic acid) in tablets or vomitus.

TREATMENT. Dehydration and electrolyte abnormalities should be corrected after initiating activated charcoal, emesis, and other general acute measures.

Phase 1. If dehydration and electrolyte losses have occurred for several hours, the patient may have a relative depletion of body bicarbonate, which requires treatment. Failure to administer sufficient bicarbonate, *even in the presence of an alkaline plasma*, may result in progression to phase 2. Plasma pH should be carefully monitored throughout bicarbonate infusion. Potassium should be carefully administered, even if the serum potassium is normal; urine potassium may be measured to document quantitative excretion.

Phase 2. It is critical to correct bicarbonate and potassium losses in patients in this phase. Insufficient potassium results in further depletion of body stores and continued failure to alkalinize the urine. At least 20–40 mEq/L of potassium is required.

Phase 3. Following correction of the usual severe dehydration, therapy is directed toward adding potassium and administering bicarbonate. Usually at least 40 mEq/L of potassium is required.

In all of these phases, alkalinization of the urine assists in excretion of salicylate.

ALKALINIZATION AND DIURESIS. Minimum fluid maintenance should result in at least 2 mL/kg/hr of urine flow. However, forced diuresis may aggravate pulmonary edema and adds little therapeutically once good alkalinization of the urine has been achieved. A 1-unit rise in pH increases clearance fourfold. An increase of 6.5 to pH 7.5 increases clearance from 16 to 64 mL/min. Acetazolamide and tris(hydroxymethyl)aminomethane are not recommended because of associated complications. Glucose should be administered and carefully monitored throughout the course of treatment.

Hemodialysis may be useful in severe toxicity when alkalinization has not been successful. No specific plasma levels should be used as an indication for this modality, since even very high levels of salicylate, above 100 mL/dL, have responded to alkalinization. *Peritoneal dialysis* is almost totally useless, even with addition of albumin. *Charcoal hemoperfusion* may be a useful adjunct; however, it is easier to correct fluid and electrolyte problems with hemodialysis.

Anderson RJ, Potts DE, Gabow PA, et al: Unrecognized adult salicylate intoxication. Ann Intern Med 85:745, 1976.
Done AK: Salicylate intoxication: Significance of measurements of salicylates in blood in cases of acute ingestion. Pediatrics 26:800, 1960.
Gaudreault P, Temple AR, Lovejoy FH: The relative severity of acute versus chronic salicylate poisoning in children. A clinical comparison. Pediatrics 70:566, 1982.
Jacobsen D, Wiik-Larsen, Bredesen JE: Haemodialysis or hemoperfusion in severe salicylate poisoning. Hum Toxicol 7:161, 1988.
Levy G, Yaffe SJ: Relationship between dose and apparent volume of distribution of salicylate in children. Pediatrics 54:713, 1974.
Prescott LF, Balali-Mood M, Critchley JA, et al: Diuresis or urinary alkalinization for salicylate poisoning? BMJ 285:1381, 1982.
Snodgrass W, Rumack BH, Peterson RG: Salicylate toxicity following therapeutic doses in young children. Clin Toxicol 18:247, 1981.
Temple AR: Acute and chronic effects of aspirin toxicity and their treatment. Arch Intern Med 141:364, 1981.

666.4 Hydrocarbons

Accidental ingestion of products containing hydrocarbons involves an extremely wide array of chemical substances, and many factors are involved in determining whether a particular exposure will produce systemic or local toxicity. The following general classification of hydrocarbons relates to acute exposure and lists only representative examples.

1. High likelihood of systemic toxicity following ingestion.
   Halogenated and aliphatic hydrocarbons
   - Trichloroethane
   - Trichlorethylene
   - Carbon tetrachloride
   - Methylene chloride

   Aromatic
   - Benzene
   - Hydrocarbons with additives
   - Heavy metals
   - Insecticides
   - Herbicides
   - Nitrobenzene
   - Aniline
2. Systemic and local toxicity unlikely.
   - Toluene
   - Xylene
   - Petroleum ether (benzene)
   - Petroleum naphtha ("lighter fluid")
   - VM & P naphtha ("paint thinner")
   - Mineral spirits (Stoddard solvent, white spirit, mineral turpentine, petroleum spirits)
   - Turpentine
3. Local toxicity (e.g., aspiration) highly likely after ingestion. Systemic toxicity unlikely.
   - Mineral seal oil
   - Signal oil
   - Furniture polish mixtures
   - Gasoline
   - Kerosene
   - Charcoal lighter fluid
4. Generally nontoxic after ingestion in over 95% of cases.
   - Asphalt or tar
   - Lubricants (motor oil, transmission oil, cutting oil, household oil and heavy grease)
   - Mineral or liquid petrolatum

PATHOPHYSIOLOGY. Once absorbed through ingestion, inhalation, or dermal routes, hydrocarbons can produce many kinds of *systemic toxicity*. The most common is CNS depression related to the anesthetic properties of certain hydrocarbons. Because most commercial products are mixtures or impure distillates, it is not possible to be precise about each product. In most cases, even following ingestion of hazardous hydrocarbons, the blood concentration may remain low enough to avoid CNS depression. Myocardial sensitization may follow ingestion of halogenated or nonhalogenated hydrocarbons. Hepatic toxicity, while usually related to carbon tetrachloride, is associated with many substances. Primary respiratory irritation with chemical pneumonitis, as well as irritation of the gastrointestinal tract, may occur. Renal and hematologic toxicity is usually related to long-term exposure. In some instances when there is high concentration of a hydrocarbon in the atmosphere, inhaling oxygen-poor air may produce anoxia or other findings not related to the toxicity of the actual hydrocarbon. Methylene chloride, found in most paint strippers, is an example of a substance that is metabolized after absorption to another substance, carbon monoxide, which produces systemic toxicity. Nitrobenzene or aniline-related compounds produce methemoglobinemia.

Volatile substance abuse from a wide range of compounds, including adhesives, propellants, refrigerants, correcting fluids, and volatile nitrites, is increasing in number. Sudden death from cardiac arrest is the major risk, but chronic pulmonary, renal, neurologic, and other complications are seen.

Local toxicity includes defatting of skin, irritation of mucous membranes, and most importantly, **aspiration pneumonitis** (see Chapter 340.2). Furniture polishes are the most common products containing mineral seal oil, the most notorious of the substances producing aspiration pneumonitis. During the act of swallowing, the very small amount of this substance that passes into the pulmonary tree is all that is required to produce significant pneumonitis. The chemical has very low viscosity and consequently is capable of spreading to involve large surface areas of the lung after only 0.1–0.2 mL is inhaled. Interstitial inflammation, hyperemia (sometimes with hemorrhage), and alveolar necrosis result.

CLINICAL MANIFESTATIONS. Aspiration pneumonia is characterized by coughing, which usually is the first clinical finding. Chest roentgenograms may be unremarkable for as long as 8–12 hr after aspiration. Most commonly, however, infiltrates will be seen by 2–3 hr after ingestion. Fever occurs later and may persist for as long as 10 days after ingestion. Accompanying leukocytosis may be misleading, since in most cases of aspiration pneumonitis, no bacteria are present in the lung. Later in the course of this illness, after resolution of most clinical findings and 2–3 wk after exposure, pneumatoceles may appear on the chest roentgenogram.

Older children, adolescents, and adults may be involved in solvent abuse. Symptoms of CNS depression, congestive heart failure, headache, vertigo, ataxis, euphoria, and renal and hepatic damage may be seen acutely. White matter changes have been reported in chronic abusers.

TREATMENT. Emesis, once thought to be useful, is of no benefit. Instillation of vegetable oils or mineral oil into the stomach in an attempt to prevent absorption is contraindicated. Similarly, corticosteroids should be avoided, since they do not provide any benefit and may be harmful. Antibiotics should not be given prophylactically. Fever and leukocytosis usually result from the pyrogenic effect of the agent; bacterial pneumonia occurs in only a small percentage of cases.

Anas N, Nanasonthi V, Ginsburg CM: Criteria for hospitalizing children who have ingested products containing hydrocarbons. JAMA 246:840, 1981.
Banner W, Walson PD: Systemic toxicity following gasoline aspiration. Am J Emerg Med 3:292, 1983.
Dice WH, Ward G, Kelley J: Pulmonary toxicity following gastrointestinal ingestion of kerosene. Ann Emerg Med 11:138, 1982.
Flanagan RJ, Ruprah M, Meredith TJ, et al: An introduction to the clinical toxicology of volatile substances. Drug Safety 5:359, 1990.
Kulig K, Rumack BH: Hydrocarbon ingestion. Curr Topics Emerg Med 3:1, 1981.
Rosenberg NL, Kleinschmidt-DeMaster BK, Davis KA, et al: Toluene abuse causes diffuse central nervous system white matter changes. Ann Neurol 23:611, 1988.
Rumack BH, Hess AJ (eds): Poisindex. Denver, 1995.
Travner P, Harrison DJ, Bell GM: Acute renal failure due to interstitial nephritis induced by "glue-sniffing" with subsequent recovery. Scot Med J 33:2116, 1988.

666.5 Iron

Iron poisoning occurs frequently in childhood, related partially to the prevalence of iron-containing tablets in many homes and to the resemblance of many iron tablets to candy. Although iron poisoning rarely results in death, prompt action may be life saving. The severity of iron poisoning is related to the amount of elemental iron absorbed. Death has been reported after ingestion of as little as 650 mg of elemental iron, an amount contained in only 10 iron sulfate tablets. Absorption of 60 mg/kg is probably necessary for development of significant iron poisoning.

CLINICAL MANIFESTATIONS. The diagnosis of iron poisoning is usually made by history. Roentgenographic confirmation is often possible, because undisintegrated iron tablets are radiopaque.

Five phases may be observed with serious iron poisoning:

1. The local irritative effects of iron on the gastrointestinal mucosa have their onset 30 min–2 hr after ingestion and usually subside after 6–12 hr. They are the result of local necrosis and hemorrhage at the sites of iron contact. Nausea, vomiting, diarrhea, abdominal pain, hematemesis, and bloody diarrhea result. Severe hypotension may also occur.
2. The next phase of 2–6 hr is seen as a period of apparent recovery. The patient appears better, which may lead the physician to a false sense of security. During this time iron accumulates in mitochondria and various organs.
3. About 12 hr after ingestion the cellular damage produced by the iron produces manifestations. Hypoglycemia and a metabolic acidosis may occur, attributable to an impairment of electron transport by the damaged mitochondrial membranes. Lactic and citric acids accumulate owing to development of anaerobic metabolism and interference with the Krebs cycle.
4. After apparent recovery, 2–4 days after ingestion, severe hepatic necrosis with elevation of AST and ALT levels, and abnormalities of bilirubin and prothrombin may occur.
5. There may be scarring and stenosis of the pyloric area 2–4 wk after ingestion as a result of the local irritative action during the first phase. This stenosis may be symptomatic and occasionally requires surgical intervention.

Not all patients demonstrate the phases in easily discernible increments. Most children with a history of ingestion develop few, if any, signs or symptoms, but they should be followed for 4–6 hr before being considered free of toxicity.

LABORATORY FINDINGS. The measurement of free iron in the serum is the best way to determine the potential for toxicity. This should be done by assessing levels of total serum iron and of total serum iron-binding capacity; if the total iron exceeds the iron-binding capacity, then free iron exists. Toxicity is unlikely unless there is at least 50 mg/kg or more of free iron. Total iron levels in excess of 350 mg/kg, regardless of iron-binding capacity, may also be toxic. An expression of symptomatic toxicity must take precedence over any laboratory data, which should only be used as a guide. Usually, levels of serum iron greater than 300 mg/kg will be seen in patients who have diarrhea, vomiting, leukocytosis, hyperglycemia, and positive abdominal roentgenograms. Vomiting has some correlation with high toxicity, and its absence has some correlation with low toxicity.

TREATMENT. Induced emesis is of little value and lavage is not helpful. Whole-bowel lavage with colonic lavage solution (Colyte, Golytely) may be of benefit, if tablets are agglutinated or obstructive. Whereas 250-mg/kg oral dose of a saline cathartic may be helpful, activated charcoal is of little value. Emergency gastrotomy to remove tablets has occasionally been done; however, this should be reserved for very rare cases.

Oral bicarbonate (2%) or dilute phosphosoda (1:4) forms a less soluble complex, but clinical benefits are questionable. Oral deferoxamine is expensive, may increase absorption, and is generally not used by this route in treating an acute overdose.

Supportive care for hypotension and the other severe problems associated with phases 1 and 3 should be instituted as for any other life-threatening illness (see Chapter 60). If there is free serum iron level of greater than 50 mg/dL, if the total iron level is greater than 350 mg/dL, or if the patient is symptomatic, then *parenteral deferoxamine* should be given. In severe cases, 10–15 mg/kg/hr for up to 24 hr may be given intravenously. For less severe cases, 90 mg/kg up to a 1 g/dose may be given intramuscularly every 8 hr for three doses. The total dose should not exceed 6.0 g intravenously or intramuscularly. Once the deferoxamine-iron chelate is achieved, the complex will be excreted, imparting a reddish (vin rosé) color to the urine. Although some believe that administering deferoxamine in this way can be used to predict serum free iron by evaluating urine color, at best this gives an indication of presence but not severity. The use of chelation in renal failure requires hemodialysis to remove the complex.

Boehnert M, Lacouture PG, Guttmacher A, et al: Massive iron overdose treated with high-dose deferoxamine infusion (abstr). Vet Hum Toxicol 28:291, 1985.
Czajka PA, Conrad JD, Duffy JP: Iron poisoning: An in vitro comparison of bicarbonate and phosphate lavage solutions. J Pediatr 98:491, 1981.
Fischer DS, Parkman R, Finch SC: Acute iron poisoning in children. JAMA 218:1179, 1971.
Gleason WA Jr, deMello DE, deCastro FJ, et al: Acute hepatic failure in severe iron poisoning. J Pediatr 38:140, 1979.
Helfer RE, Rodgerson DO: The effect of deferoxamine on the determination of serum iron and iron-binding capacity. J Pediatr 68:804, 1966.
Knasel AL, Collins-Barrow MD: Applicability of early indicators of iron toxicity. J Natl Med Assoc 78:1037, 1986.

Schauben JL, Augenstein WL, Cox J, et al: Iron poisoning: Report of three cases and a review of therapeutic intervention. J Emerg Med 8:309, 1990.
Yatscoff RW, Wayne EA, Tenenbein M: An objective criterion for the cessation of deferoxamine therapy in the acutely iron poisoned patient. J Toxicol Clin Toxicol 29:1, 1991.

666.6 Cyclic Antidepressants

This group of drugs includes the tricyclics and a variety of associated agents primarily used as antidepressants. Table 666–2 lists these agents by structural classification as well as by relative toxicity. The mortality rate from all of these agents is estimated to be 7–12%. If exposures involving only accidental ingestion reported to poison centers in children younger than 5 yr old are considered, then the mortality rate is lower.

PATHOPHYSIOLOGY. Cyclic antidepressants, notably the tricyclics, are structurally similar to the phenothiazines and have similar anticholinergic, adrenergic, and α-blocking properties. Following absorption, these agents are extensively bound to plasma proteins and also bind to tissue and cellular sites, including the mitochondria. The blood/tissue ratio varies from 1:10 to 1:30, which explains the ineffectiveness of forced diuresis and dialysis techniques in removal of the drug. They block the neuronal reuptake of norepinephrine, 5-hydroxytryptamine, serotonin, or dopamine. Therapeutic doses, initially, may cause drowsiness and difficulty concentrating and thinking; dulling of depressive ideation may explain the efficacy of these agents in depressive disorders. Hallucinations, excitement, and confusion have occurred in a small percentage of patients during antidepressant therapy. These agents also have a slight α-adrenergic blocking effect. Trazodone inhibits the neuronal uptake of serotonin and has antiserotonin and α-adrenergic blocking properties.

■ **TABLE 666–2 Cyclic Antidepressants**

Generic	Trade Name	Structural Classification	CNS Toxicity	CV Toxicity
Amitriptyline	Elavil Amitid Endep Amitril	Tricyclic	++++	++++
Amoxapine*	Asendin	Tricyclic	++++	+
Clomipramine	Anafranil	Tricyclic	++++	++++
Desipramine	Norpramin Pertofrane	Tricyclic	++++	++++
Doxepin	Adapin Sinequan	Tricyclic	++++	++++
Imipramine	Tofranil Presamine SK-Pramine Janimine	Tricyclic	++++	++++
Loxapine	Loxitane	Tricyclic	++++	+
Maprotiline†	Ludiomil	Tetracyclic	++++	++++
Mianserin	INV‡	Tetracyclic	?	?
Nortriptyline	Aventyl Pamelor	Tricyclic	++++	++++
Protriptyline	Vivactil	Tricyclic	++++	++++
Trazodone	Desyrel	Miscellaneous¶	+	+
Trimipramine	Surmontil	Tricyclic	++++	++++
Viloxazine	INV§	Bicyclic	?	?
Zimeldine	INV§	Bicyclic	?	?

**Amoxapine is structurally similar to loxapine, an antipsychotic agent, and appears to have similar toxicity. Amoxapine is an active metabolite of loxapine.*

†Available evidence suggests that maprotiline may have less cardiovascular toxicity when compared with the tricyclic antidepressants.

‡Investigational or newly released drug; tetracyclic antidepressant toxicity to be determined.

§Investigational or newly released drug; bicyclic antidepressant toxicity to be determined.

¶This agent has a unique dual bicyclic structure.

Combination products: *Combination products containing tricyclic antidepressants include Limbitrol (amitriptyline and chlordiazepoxide); Etrafon, Perphenyline, Triavil, and Triptazine (amitriptyline and perphenazine).*

(From Rumack BH, Hess AJ (eds): Poisindex. Denver, 1995.)

CLINICAL MANIFESTATIONS. The initial presentation is the onset of the anticholinergic syndrome including tachycardia, pupillary dilatation, dryness of mucous membranes, urinary retention, hallucinations, and flushing. Although hypertension also may initially occur, hypotension rapidly develops and is a serious sign. Convulsions, coma, and major arrhythmias ensue as tissue saturation occurs. Cardiac findings include quinidine-like effects such as slowing of myocardial conduction, multifocal premature ventricular contractions, ventricular tachycardia, flutter, and fibrillation. In addition to widening of the QRS complex, QT prolongation occurs with T wave flattening or inversion, ST segment depression, right bundle branch block, and complete heart block.

CNS toxicity includes manifestations of depression, lethargy, and hallucinations. Choreoathetosis and myoclonus have been reported and must be differentiated from generalized seizures. Coma, when it occurs, has a mean duration of 6.4 hr but may last for longer than 24 hr.

A withdrawal syndrome in neonates delivered of patients who have been taking tricyclics has occurred, with tachypnea, irritability, and restlessness lasting the 1st mo of life. Amoxapine differs from other tricyclics; there is significantly greater incidence of seizures and coma. Cardiovascular toxicity is less prominent, and seizures and coma may be associated with normal QRS complexes.

Loxapine is similar to its metabolite amoxapine in having a greater incidence of CNS toxicity and a lesser incidence of cardiovascular toxicity.

Exposure to the tetracyclics appears to be associated with a higher incidence of cardiovascular effects than does exposure to the tricyclics. Bicyclics are similar to tetracyclics but additionally appear to cause less anticholinergic toxicity. Trazodone, which has a uniquely different structure appears to result in little CNS or cardiovascular toxicity.

Children should be observed and their electrocardiogram monitored for at least 6 hr. If any tissue manifestations (such as a QRS interval longer than 0.12 or an altered mental status) are present, then patients should be monitored for 24 hr. Catastrophic deterioration has been observed in patients who at first appear mildly, if at all, poisoned and whose condition then rapidly becomes seriously toxic. Only completely asymptomatic children should be discharged after 6 hr. Others should be admitted to intensive care units and monitored for at least 24 hr.

LABORATORY FINDINGS. Laboratory tests may be helpful in establishing the type of agent ingested. However, because these agents have extremely high volumes of distribution, blood level measurements may not be helpful in establishing severity. The observation of signs and symptoms is extremely helpful and should be relied on when laboratory test results are negative.

TREATMENT. Following general life support measures, efforts should be made to *prevent absorption*. Emesis should be avoided in children showing clinical manifestations because of the danger of aspiration from vomiting following onset of coma. Activated charcoal should be administered at a dose of 50–100 g in adolescents and 15–30 g in younger children. Repeated doses of activated charcoal should be given to all symptomatic children at a dose of 10–20 g every 2–6 hr. Obtunded patients may have this agent administered through a small-bore nasogastric tube. Multiple-dose charcoal will remove drug being re-excreted in the gastrointestinal tract. Single-dose *cathartics* such as sorbitol, magnesium, or sodium sulfate should be administered.

Although there is controversy as to which *antiarrhythmic drugs* should be given and in what order, the following is generally accepted. Sodium bicarbonate should be administered in doses sufficient to achieve a pH of 7.45–7.55. This is superior to artificial hyperventilation. Phenytoin, once regarded as a key drug, should now only be considered if sodium bicarbonate and lidocaine are ineffective. Its use prophylactically has been abandoned. Children with ventricular arrhythmias should have their acidosis corrected immediately with bicarbonate followed by lidocaine at a loading dose of 1 mg/kg/dose and by appropriate maintenance doses thereafter. Lidocaine is utilized if arrhythmias develop despite alkalinization or if arrhythmias already exist. It should not be used with torsades de pointes. Isoproterenol may be useful in this particular arrhythmia, but the data are incomplete. Quinidine and procainamide should not be used. Bretylium tosylate should not be used in hypotensive patients or in those with fixed cardiac output. Physostigmine should be used only rarely. It is an exceptionally dangerous agent, especially if given rapidly. It is most useful in supraventricular arrhythmias.

Patients with *seizures* should be primarily treated with diazepam at a dose of up to 10 mg intravenously in an adolescent or 0.1–0.3 mg/kg, up to 10 mg, in a child. Phenytoin should then be given. Physostigmine may be used for myoclonic seizures, psychosis, or choreoathetosis but is not very effective for generalized seizures.

Hypotension may respond to norepinephrine but usually does not respond to dopamine. Severe hypotension is very serious and may require fluids and an intra-aortic balloon. *Hypertension* usually responds to physostigmine. Patients who have a seriously deteriorating course may have such a significant degree of tissue loading that they cannot be saved. Although hemodialysis and charcoal hemoperfusion have been attempted, these procedures are rarely helpful in such overdoses.

Albertson TE, Derlet RW, Foulke GE, et al: Superiority of activated charcoal alone compared with ipecac and activated charcoal in the treatment of acute toxic ingestions. Ann Emerg Med 18:56, 1989.
Callaham M, Kassel D: Epidemiology of fatal tricyclic antidepressant ingestion: Implications for management. Ann Emerg Med 14:1, 1985.
Callaham M, Schumaker H, Pentel P: Phenytoin prophylaxis of cardiotoxicity in experimental amitriptyline poisoning. J Pharmacol Exp Ther 245:216, 1988.
Ellison DW, Pentel PR: Clinical features and consequences of seizures due to cyclic antidepressant overdose. Am J Emerg Med 7:5, 1989.
Krishel S, Jackimczyk K: Cyclic antidepressants, lithium, and neuroleptic agents: Pharmacology and toxicology. Emerg Med Clin North Am 9:53, 1991.
Kulig K, Rumack BH, Sullivan JB, et al: Amoxapine overdose: Coma and seizures without cardiotoxic effects. JAMA 248:1092, 1982.
Molloy DW, Penner SB, Rabson J, et al: Use of sodium bicarbonate to treat tricyclic antidepressant-induced arrhythmias in a patient with alkalosis. Can Med Assoc J 130:1457, 1984.
Rumack BH, Hess AJ (eds): Poisindex. Denver, 1995.
Shannon MW, Merola J, Lovejoy FH Jr: Hypotension in severe tricyclic antidepressant overdose. Am J Emerg Med 6:439, 1988.
Slovis CM, Murray LM, Segar D: Emergency management of cyclic antidepressant overdose: An effective and organized approach. Emerg Med Rep 14:115, 1993.

666.7 Alkalis and Acids

The incidence of severe injury from this variety of ingestions has dropped dramatically following the removal from the market of liquid corrosive drain cleaners. These agents had the tenacious capacity to coat the esophagus and produce major tissue destruction.

PATHOPHYSIOLOGY. *Alkaline agents* tend to produce liquefaction necrosis (e.g., when the strong base binds to the fats and oils in the tissue and produces a soap [saponification]). Tablets such as Clinitest tend to lodge at about the level of the aortic arch in the esophagus and produce circumferential burns. Crystalline drain cleaners may produce a small streaklike burn; they result in circumferential burns in only 15% of all cases. Solutions of greater than 4% NaOH may produce very widespread circumferential burns. Linear streak burns usually do not constrict and form obstructions, but circumferential burns are likely to develop esophageal strictures, which may become totally occlusive. Alkaline agents in the crystal form may spare the mouth and hypopharynx as they travel across these areas on the saliva. Once in the esophagus, they may then produce damage. Common household bleach (5.4% or less), while producing hyperemia, is less likely to produce burns.

Two other sources of alkaline irritation include *disc batteries* and *automatic dishwasher detergents*. Complications may occur when disc batteries lodge in the esophagus, gastrointestinal tract, nose, or ears. Localized tissue necrosis with possible tracheoesophageal fistula or burns may occur due to leaking contents. Most automatic dishwasher compounds have a pH of from 10.5 to 12.5. Actual burn development depends on several factors, including free alkalinity, composition, formulation, viscosity, and concentration.

Strong acid agents, such as sulfuric, nitric, or hydrochloric acid, are frequently concentrated at the pyloric end of the stomach, resulting in scarification and eventually stricture formation. They may also seriously damage the esophagus and other areas of the stomach, leading to necrosis and perforation.

CLINICAL MANIFESTATIONS. When burns of the esophagus or hypopharynx have occurred, swallowing is likely to be impeded, and consequently the child may drool excessively. Burns on lips and tongue may be seen. No correlation exists between oral and esophageal burns; either can exist without the other. Pain and difficulty swallowing may be encountered. Occasionally, when the diagnosis has been missed, the patient will present with esophageal strictures and vomiting.

TREATMENT (see Chapter 270). If the patient can swallow safely, milk or water should be administered, 1–2 cups in the first few minutes after ingestion. Following this, the child should be kept from having anything orally. Esophagoscopy with a flexible endoscope should be performed 12–24 hr after ingestion to determine whether a circumferential burn exists. Performing this procedure earlier may be of less value, since the full extent of the burns may not be apparent. If there are significant burns, the patient should remain on clear liquids to avoid possible esophageal perforation. At 2–3 wk after injury, patients may develop strictures, necessitating a feeding gastrostomy. Endoscopic dilation and a colonic interposition or a gastric tube may then be necessary as a more definitive procedure.

Administering acids (such as fruit juice) to children who have consumed bases and bases to children after acid ingestion is contraindicated, since an exothermic reaction may occur and aggravate the injury. Surgical evaluation in significant cases is mandatory.

Ferguson MK, Miglore M, Staszak YM, et al: Early evaluation and therapy for caustic esophageal injury. Am J Surg 157:116, 1989.
French RJ, Tabb HG, Rutledge LJ: Esophageal stenosis produced by ingestion of bleach. South Med J 63:1140, 1970.
Gaudreault P, Parent M, McGuigan MA: Predictability of esophageal injury from signs and symptoms: A study of 378 children. Pediatrics 71:761, 1983.
Haller JA, Andrews HG, White JJ, et al: Pathophysiology and management of acute corrosive burns of the esophagus. J Pediatr Surg 6:578, 1971.
Leape LL, Ashcraft KW, Scarpelli DG, et al: Hazard to health—liquid lye. N Engl J Med 284:578, 1971.
Linden CH, Buner JM, Kulig K, et al: Acid ingestion: Toxicity following systemic absorption. Vet Hum Toxicol 25:282, 1983.
Maull KI, Osmand AP, Maull CD: Liquid caustic ingestions: An in vitro study of the effects of buffer, neutralization, and dilation. Ann Emerg Med 14:1160, 1985.
Penner GE: Acid ingestion: Toxicology and treatment. Ann Emerg Med 9:374, 1980.

Pense SC, Wood WJ, Stempel TK, et al: Tracheoesophageal fistula secondary to muriatic acid ingestion. Burns 14:35, 1988.
Spitz L, Lakhoo K: Caustic ingestion. Arch Dis Child 68:157, 1993.

666.8 Nonsteroidal Anti-Inflammatory Drugs

The anti-inflammatory agents ibuprofen and naproxen sodium, which have become available over the counter, are likely to be involved in progressively more accidental and intentional overdoses because of wider distribution.

IBUPROFEN

Use of the agents in this group have increased over the past 10 yr. There are five classes of these agents with the most widely available examples listed for each:

Acetic acids: diclofenac, ketorolac.
Fenamic acids: meclofenamate, mefenamic acid.
Oxicams: piroxicam.
Propionic acids: naproxen sodium, ibuprofen, oxaprozin, flurbiprofen.
Naphthylalkanone: nabumetone.

Toxicity after overdose of these agents is rare, occurring in less than 0.5% of cases reported to the AAPCC national database.

Most data in the literature is related to ibuprofen, which is the most widely available nonsteroidal anti-inflammatory drug (NSAID).

PATHOPHYSIOLOGY. Peak plasma levels occur after 1-1½ hr. The volume of distribution is 0.11–0.13 L/kg, which is similar to that seen with salicylates. Only about 10% of the drug is excreted unchanged; the rest is metabolized in the liver. About 90% of a therapeutic dose of ibuprofen is bound to protein, and its half-life is about 2 hr.

LABORATORY FINDINGS. The drug can be measured in plasma; levels of 20–30 μg/mL at 2 hr are therapeutic. Levels in the 70–100-μg/mL range 2 hr after ingestion are not associated with symptoms, but mild symptoms of gastrointestinal upset and lethargy occur at 3 hr in the range of 80–200 μg/mL. Seriously toxic findings have been seen at a 2-hr level of 360 μg/mL, but levels as high as 704 μg/mL have been seen without toxicity. Elevated blood urea nitrogen and creatinine levels and urine protein have been seen after large overdose.

CLINICAL MANIFESTATIONS. Gastrointestinal disorders including nausea, epigastric pain, and upper gastrointestinal tract bleeding have been reported. Renal failure and toxicity have been noted in adults and children with marked increase in serum potassium and creatinine and blood urea nitrogen levels. Hypotension has occurred but is rare. Nystagmus, diplopia, headache, tinnitus, and transient deafness have all been reported.

The most serious and rare problems with this drug are lethargy, coma, seizures, and transient apnea. Although not reported in adults or adolescents, children 1–1½ yr of age have developed apnea following ingestion of 2.8–7.6 g. Lethargy and drowsiness are common and occur in pediatric patients following ingestion of 120–230 mg/kg. Acid-base disturbances are not common. Acidosis is seen especially in younger children. Anaphylactoid reactions have been reported with circulatory collapse, angioedema, and pruritus.

TREATMENT. Respiratory and cardiovascular support should be given immediately. Emesis is of little benefit, but activated charcoal should be administered. Ingested amounts of less than 100 mg/kg are not likely to produce toxicity; however, as in any ingestion, the history should be cautiously interpreted. Hypotension should be treated. Although the manufacturer recommends alkaline diuresis, this is unlikely to be beneficial because of 90% protein binding. Hemodialysis and charcoal hemoperfusion in severe cases may be of benefit because of the small volume of distribution.

In general, good supportive care of coma or apnea until the drug is metabolized should permit resolution of the overdose in 24 hr. Children with a history of ingestion should be observed at least 6 hr to be certain that apnea and CNS depression do not occur.

OTHER NSAIDS

Mefenamic acid overdoses manifest seizures in 33% of cases, a rare finding in other NSAIDS. Propionic class members are more likely to produce metabolic acidosis, respiratory depression, and coma.

Barry WS, Meinzinger MM, Howse CR: Ibuprofen overdose and exposure in utero: Results from a postmarketing voluntary reporting system. Am J Med 77:35, 1984.
Court H, Streete P, Volans GN: Acute poisoning with ibuprofen. Hum Toxicol 2:381, 1983.
Hall AH, Rumack BH: Treatment of patients with ibuprofen overdose. Ann Emerg Med 17:185, 1988.
Hall AH, Smolinske SC, Conrad FL, et al: Ibuprofen overdose: 126 cases. Ann Emerg Med 15:1308, 1986.
Hall AH, Smolinske SC, Kulig KW, et al: Ibuprofen overdose: A prospective study. West J Med 148:653, 1988.
Katona BG, Wigley FM, Walters JK, et al: Aseptic meningitis from over-the-counter ibuprofen. Lancet 1:59, 1988.
Poirier TI: Reversible renal failure associated with ibuprofen: Case report and review of the literature. DICP 18:27, 1984.
Rumack BH, Hess AJ (eds): Poisindex. Denver, 1995.
Smolinske SC, Hall AH, Vandenberg SA, et al: Toxic effects of nonsteroidal anti-inflammatory drugs in overdose: An overview of recent evidence on clinical effects and dose-response relationships. Drug Safety 5:252, 1990.

666.9 Plants

Ingestion or exposure to plants both inside the home and outside in backyards and fields is one of the most common accidental poisoning problems. Table 666–3 lists the 20 most frequent exposures in young children. Fortunately, most plant ingestions result in little or no toxicity, and those children

■ **TABLE 666–3 Frequency of Plant Exposures by Plant Type**

Botanical Name	Common Name	Frequency
Capsicum annuum	Pepper	3,923
Dieffenbachia spp.	Dumbcane	3,653
Euphorbia pulcherrima	Poinsettia	3,087
Ilex spp.	Holly	2,943
Philodendron spp.	Philodendron	2,155
Crassula spp.	Jade plant	2,086
Spathiphyllum spp.	Peace lily	1,988
Phytolacca americana	Pokeweed, inkberry	1,676
Epipremnum aureum	Pothos, devil's ivy	1,646
Brassaia and *Schefflera* spp.	Umbrella tree	1,600
Saintpaulia spp.	African violet	1,347
Toxicodendron radicans	Poison ivy	1,312
Pyracantha spp.	Fire thorn	1,215
Taxus spp.	Yew	1,125
Rhododendron spp.	Rhododendron, azalea	1,031
Chrysanthemum spp.	Chrysanthemum	941
Eucalyptus globulus	Eucalyptus	905
Hedera helix	English ivy	898
Chlorophytum comosum	Spider plant	878
Solanum dulcamara	Climbing nightshade	844

(From Litovitz TL, Holm KC, Clancy C, et al: 1992 annual report of the American Association of Poison Control Centers toxic exposure surveillance system. Am J Emerg Med 11:494, 1993.)

developing clinical manifestations usually can be dealt with symptomatically. The following are some of the common groups, their major findings, and treatment.

ARUM FAMILY. Examples are dieffenbachia, caladium, and philodendron. In this family, the entire plant contains various concentrations of calcium oxalate crystals. The most common problems occur in the oropharynx and include irritation of the lips, tongue, and mucous membrane. Intense pain and swelling may be seen. Washing of the affected area may be helpful, along with ice chips to chew and relieve pain. Corticosteroids may be helpful in very serious cases. Systemic toxicity is extremely rare.

ANTICHOLINERGIC (ATROPINE AND RELATED) FAMILY. Examples are jimson weed, deadly nightshade, and potato. All parts of these plants, especially the green portions, contain solanaceous (atropinic) alkaloids. Findings include tachycardia, dryness, flushing, hypertension, delirium, hallucinations, thirst, and, in some cases, coma and convulsions. If the syndrome is very severe, physostigmine may be used in doses similar to that with the cyclic antidepressants. If the findings are mild, then the patient should receive no treatment but be carefully observed.

CASTOR BEAN AND JEQUIRITY BEAN. These plants contain toxalbumins: ricin in castor bean and abrin in jequirity bean. Severe, crampy diarrhea along with nausea, vomiting, CNS depression, shock, and convulsions may occur. Hemolytic anemia may occur with ricin, whereas renal failure is more common with abrin. There is no specific treatment. Children should be managed symptomatically, and urine flow should be monitored. Activated charcoal should be administered.

FOXGLOVE. These plants contain the classic cardiac glycoside digitalis. Substantial similarity to overdose with any of the digitalis glycosides exists. Bradycardia with nausea and vomiting are seen as heart block gradually progresses. Fab fragments (Digibind) are effective in treatment. Potassium levels should be monitored. Treatment by phenytoin loading should be considered, as well as administration of activated charcoal to prevent further absorption.

OLEANDER. Oleander contains cardiac glycosides somewhat different from those of foxglove. In addition to local irritation, patients exhibit nausea, vomiting, diarrhea, and, in severe cases, atrioventricular block, with ST segment depression and severe bradycardia. It is unknown whether Fab fragments (Digibind) will help. Potassium levels should be carefully followed. Phenytoin or atropine may be useful, as well as oral activated charcoal.

HEMLOCK. Poison hemlock contains the alkaloid coniine, which initially produces hyperactivity followed by CNS depression and respiratory failure. There is no specific treatment. Activated charcoal should be administered soon after ingestion, and respirations should be monitored. The intoxication is similar to that of nicotine.

Water hemlock contains the agent cicutoxin, which is likely to cause the rapid onset of hyperactivity, leading to convulsions within 30 min. Abdominal pain, emesis, and salivation are usually seen. Dilatation of the pupils is usual after onset of major signs. There is no specific treatment. Control of seizures with diazepam and administration of activated charcoal, if the patient can swallow, may be helpful. Supportive care should be provided.

Antman EM, Wenger TL, Butler VP Jr, et al: Treatment of 150 cases of life-threatening digitalis intoxication with digitoxin-specific Fab antibody fragments. Circulation 81:1744, 1990.

Challoner KR, McCarron MM: Castor bean intoxication. Ann Emerg Med 19:1177, 1991.

Frohne D, Pfander HJ: A Color Atlas of Poisonous Plants. London, Wolfe Publishing, 1984.

Fuller TC, McClintock E: Poisonous Plants of California. Berkeley, University of California Press, 1986.

Guharoy SR, Barajas M: Atropine intoxication from the ingestion and smoking of jimson weed *(Datura stramonium)*. Vet Hum Toxicol 33:588, 1991.

Hardin JW, Arena JM: Human Poisoning from Native and Cultivated Plants. Durham, NC, Duke University Press, 1974.

Iwu MM: Handbook of African Medicinal Plants. Boca Raton, FL, CRC Press, 1993.

Kingsbury JM: Poisonous Plants of the United States and Canada. Englewood Cliffs, NJ, Prentice-Hall, 1964.

Lampe KF, McConn MA: AMA Handbook of Poisonous and Injurious Plants. Chicago, American Medical Association, 1985.

Maxwell LS: Florida's Poisonous Plants, Snakes, Insects. Tampa, Lewis S. Maxwell, 1986.

McIntire MS, Guest JR, Porterfield JF: Philodendron—an infant death. J Toxicol Clin Toxicol 28:177, 1990.

Mulligan GA, Munro DB: Poisonous Plants of Canada. Ottawa, Canadian Government Publishing Centre, 1990.

Rumack BH, Hess AJ (eds): Poisindex. Denver, 1995.

Westbrooks RG, Preacher JW: Poisonous Plants of Eastern North America. Columbia, University of South Carolina Press, 1986.

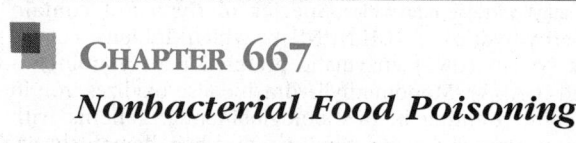

CHAPTER 667
Nonbacterial Food Poisoning

Stephen C. Aronoff

MUSHROOM POISONING

The consumption of wild mushrooms, a favorite pastime in Europe, is increasingly popular in the United States, with concomitant increases in fatal cases of mushroom poisoning.

There are four clinical syndromes and seven classes of toxins associated with wild mushroom poisoning. The clinical syndromes are divided according to the predominant system involved and the rapidity of onset of symptoms. The toxins produced by wild mushrooms are categorized as follows: cyclopeptides, monomethylhydrazine, muscarine, coprine, ibotenic acid, psilocybin, and unknown.

GASTROINTESTINAL—DELAYED ONSET. Amanita Poisoning. Poisoning from species of *Amanita* and *Galerina* account for 95% of the fatalities from mushroom intoxication, although the mortality rate for this group is 5–10%. Most species produce two classes of cyclopeptide toxins: (1) phalloidins, which are heptapeptides believed to be responsible for the early symptoms of *Amanita* poisoning; and (2) amanitotoxin, which is an octapeptide that inhibits RNA polymerase and subsequent production of messenger RNA. Cells with high turnover rates, such as those in the gastrointestinal mucosa, kidney, and liver, are the most severely affected.

Histopathologically, *Amanita* poisoning causes cellular necrosis, which may occur throughout the gastrointestinal tract, the most heavily exposed site. Acute yellow atrophy of the liver and necrosis of the proximal renal tubules are found in lethal cases.

The clinical course produced by poisoning with *Amanita* or *Galerina* species is biphasic, after an initial 6–12-hr latent period. Six to 24 hr following ingestion, patients develop nausea, vomiting, and severe abdominal pain. Profuse, watery diarrhea follows shortly thereafter and may last for 12–24 hr. During this time, as much as 9 L of fluid may be lost. Twenty-four to 48 hr after poisoning, jaundice, hypertransaminasemia (peaking at 72–96 hr), renal failure, and coma are noted. Death occurs 4–7 days after the ingestion. A prothrombin time less than 10% of control is a poor prognostic factor.

The treatment of *Amanita* poisoning is both supportive and specific. Fluid loss during the early course of the illness is profound, requiring aggressive therapy for correction of this loss in patients with severe diarrhea. In the late phase of the disease, management of renal and hepatic failure is also necessary.

Specific therapy for *Amanita* poisoning is designed to remove the toxin rapidly and to block binding at its target site. Because amanitotoxin may be recovered from the duodenum up to 36 hr after ingestion, aspiration of duodenal contents will significantly decrease toxin load. Forced diuresis should be avoided, since this increases renal exposure.

Although cytochrome C protects mice from lethal doses of amanitotoxin, clinical trials with this agent have failed to demonstrate any benefit. Intravenous penicillin G (250 mg/kg/24 hr) administered as a continuous infusion combined with silibinin, the water-soluble form of the flavolignone silymarin, in an intravenous dosage of 20–50 mg/kg/24 hr act synergistically to inhibit binding of both toxins and to interrupt enterohepatic recirculation of amanitotoxin. Orthotopic liver transplantation is recommended for children in whom severe hepatic failure develops.

Monomethylhydrazine Intoxication. Species of *Gyromitra* contain monomethylhydrazine (CH_3NHNH_2), which inhibits central nervous system (CNS) enzymatic production of γ-aminobutyric acid (GABA). Monomethylhydrazine also oxidizes iron in hemoglobin, resulting in methemoglobinemia. Patients with *Gyromitra* poisoning develop vomiting, diarrhea, hematochezia, and abdominal pain within 6–24 hr of ingestion of the toxin. Symptoms of CNS depression and seizures develop later in the clinical course. Hemolysis and methemoglobinemia are potential life-threatening complications of monomethylhydrazine poisoning. Severe methemoglobinemia may require dialysis.

Hypovolemia from gastrointestinal fluid losses and seizures require supportive intervention. Pyridoxal phosphate, the coenzyme that catalyzes the production of GABA, can reverse the effects of monomethylhydrazine when administered in high dosages. Pyridoxine hydrochloride (25 mg/kg) is administered intravenously at a frequency dependent on clinical improvement. Parenteral administration of methylene blue is indicated if the methemoglobin concentration exceeds 30%. Blood transfusions may be required for significant hemolysis.

AUTONOMIC NERVOUS SYSTEM—RAPID ONSET. Muscarine Poisoning. Mushrooms of the genera *Inocybe* and, to a lesser degree, *Clitocybe* contain muscarine or muscarine-related compounds. These quaternary ammonium derivatives bind to postsynaptic receptors, producing an exaggerated cholinergic response.

The clinical syndrome is characterized by the following hypercholinergic response: the onset of symptoms is rapid (30 min–2 hr after consumption) and consists of diaphoresis, excessive lacrimation, salivation, miosis, urinary and fecal incontinence, and vomiting. Respiratory distress caused by bronchospasm and increased bronchopulmonary secretions is the most serious complication. The symptoms subside spontaneously within 6–24 hr.

Atropine sulfate, the specific antidote, is administered intravenously (0.1 mg/kg). This is repeated until the pulmonary symptoms resolve or the patient becomes overtly tachycardic.

Coprine Ingestion. *Coprinus atramentarius* and *Clitocybe clavipes* contain coprine. Like disulfiram (Antabuse), coprine inhibits the metabolism of acetaldehyde following ethanol ingestion. The clinical symptomatology results from accumulation of acetaldehyde.

Coprine intoxication becomes apparent after ethanol ingestion and may occur up to 5 days after consuming the mushroom. Hyperemia of the face and trunk, tingling of the hands, metallic taste, tachycardia, and vomiting occur acutely. Hypotension may result from intense peripheral vasodilatation.

The syndrome is typically self-limited and lasts only several hours. No specific antidote is available. If hypotension is severe, vascular re-expansion with isotonic parenteral solutions may be required. Small oral doses of propranolol have also been suggested.

CENTRAL NERVOUS SYSTEM—RAPID ONSET. Ibotenic Acid and Muscimol Intoxication. Although *Amanita muscaria* and *A. pantherina* may contain muscarine (see earlier), the toxins responsible for the CNS symptoms following ingestion of these mushrooms are muscimol and ibotenic acid. Muscimol, a hallucinogen, and ibotenic acid, an insecticide, have anticholinergic effects. One-half to 3 hr after ingestion, CNS symptoms appear; obtundation, alternating lethargy and agitation, and occasionally seizures are seen. Nausea and vomiting are uncommon. If large amounts of muscarine are contained in the mushroom, symptoms of cholinergic crisis may also occur.

Specific therapy must be carefully selected. If an exaggerated cholinergic response is observed, atropine should be administered. Because ingestions of *A. muscaria* are frequently associated with anticholinergic findings, the acetylcholinesterase inhibitor physostigmine is used to reverse the delirium and coma. Seizures can be controlled with diazepam. Early treatment with ipecac (if the patient is conscious) and close observation are all that is required in most cases.

Indole Intoxication. Mushrooms belonging to the genus *Psilocybe* ("magic mushrooms") contain psilocybin and psilocin, two psychotropic compounds. Within 30 min after ingestion, patients develop euphoria and hallucinations, often accompanied by tachycardia and mydriasis. Fever and seizures have also been observed in children with psilocybin poisoning. These symptoms are short-lived, usually lasting 6 hr after consumption of the mushroom. Severely agitated patients may respond to diazepam.

GASTROINTESTINAL—RAPID ONSET. Many mushrooms from a variety of genera produce local gastrointestinal symptoms. The causative toxins are diverse and largely unknown.

Within 1 hr of ingestion, patients develop acute abdominal pain, nausea, vomiting, and diarrhea. Symptoms may last from hours to days, depending on the species.

Treatment is mainly supportive. Patients with large fluid losses may require parenteral fluid therapy. It is imperative to differentiate ingestion of mushrooms of this class from ingestions of *Amanita* and *Galerina* species containing cyclopeptide toxins (see earlier).

SOLANINE POISONING

Solanine is a mixture of several related toxins found in "greened" and sprouted potatoes. Potatoes exposed to light and allowed to sprout produce a number of alkaloidal glycosides containing the cholesterol derivative solanidine. Two of these glycosides, α-solanine and α-chaconine, are found in highest concentration in the peels of greened potatoes and in the sprouts. The solanine alkaloids bind to serum cholinesterase, suggesting a possible pathophysiologic mechanism.

Clinical manifestations of solanine intoxication occur within 7–19 hr after ingestion. The most common symptoms are vomiting and diarrhea; in more severe instances of poisoning, fever, generalized abdominal pain, coma, and hypovolemic shock occur.

Treatment of solanine poisoning is largely supportive. In the most severe cases, symptoms resolve within 11 days. Atropine treatment has not been evaluated.

SEAFOOD POISONING

CIGUATERA FISH POISONING. Major outbreaks of ciguatera fish poisoning have been reported in Florida, Hawaii, and the Virgin Islands; however, with modern methods of transportation, the illness now occurs worldwide. Grouper is the most frequently identified source of the toxin, followed by snapper, kingfish, amberjack, dolphin, and barracuda.

The source of this poisoning is the dinoflagellate *Gambierdiscus toxicus*, a microscopic organism found in the food chain along coral reefs, which contains high concentrations of ciguatoxin and maitotoxin. After ingestion of the organism by small fish, the toxin is absorbed and concentrated in fish flesh and musculature. Larger fish consume the smaller fish, and again the toxin is absorbed from the gastrointestinal tract and concentrated in the musculature.

Ciguatoxin, a lipid with a molecular weight of approximately 1,100 Daltons, increases the sodium permeability of excitable membranes. This action is inhibited by calcium and tetrodotoxin.

The onset of symptoms following ingestion of fish containing ciguatoxin is rapid, usually occurring within 2–30 hr. The illness is often biphasic. The earliest symptoms are diarrhea, vomiting, and abdominal pain; the second phase includes myalgias and circumoral or extremity dysesthesias. The dysesthesia is characterized by reversal of hot and cold sensation. Tachycardia, bradycardia, and hypotension occur infrequently.

Treatment of ciguatera fish poisoning is supportive. Gastric lavage is recommended to remove any remaining toxin. Intravenous fluids may be required for severe diarrhea, and parenteral administration of calcium can be used to treat hypotension. In a few patients with coma, mannitol has successfully reversed the neurologic manifestations of intoxication. However, further studies are needed before a blanket recommendation for mannitol therapy can be made. Most cases are self-limited; symptoms may last up to 3 wk.

SCOMBROID (PSEUDOALLERGIC) FISH POISONING. Epidemics have been associated with the ingestion of members of the Scombresocidae or Scombridae families, notably albacore, mackerel, tuna, bonita, and kingfish. Nonscombroid fish and marine mammals, such as mahi-mahi (dolphin) and bluefish, have also been linked to outbreaks of poisoning.

The "scombrotoxin," either histamine or the product of the action of the toxin on fish flesh, is responsible for the clinical syndrome. Histidine is found in high concentrations in the flesh of scombroid fish; the action of bacterial decarboxylases during putrification converts the histidine to histamine. Fish containing more than 20 mg of histamine per 100 g of flesh are toxic. In patients receiving isoniazid, a potent histaminase blocker, ingestion of fish flesh containing lower concentrations of histamine may be toxic.

The onset of clinical illness is acute and occurs within 10 min–2 hr following ingestion. The most common symptoms include diarrhea, flushing, diaphoresis, urticaria, nausea, and headache. Abdominal pain, tachycardia, oral burning, dizziness, respiratory distress, and facial swelling also occur. The illness is usually self-limited, terminating within 8–10 hr.

Treatment is mainly supportive. Gastric lavage decreases continued absorption of histamine. With severe diarrhea, fluid replacement may be necessary. Antihistamines have been variably successful. Four patients with severe toxicity treated with cimetidine (a histamine blocker) responded rapidly. Since data are limited, cimetidine or ranitidine should be reserved for severe cases.

PARALYTIC SHELLFISH POISONING. Filter-feeding mollusks, such as the black mussel and sea scallop, may become contaminated during dinoflagellate blooms or "red tides." The dinoflagellate *Ptychodiscus brevis* is often responsible for these "red tides" and contains several potent neurotoxins. Saxitoxin is the most important of the neurotoxins responsible for paralytic shellfish poisoning. This toxin prevents nerve conduction by inhibiting the sodium-potassium pump. Although six other toxins have been isolated from contaminated scallops, these toxins may be bioconverted to less toxic structures.

The onset of clinical symptoms of paralytic shellfish poisoning occurs rapidly, 30 min–2 hr after ingestion. Abdominal pain and nausea are common. Paresthesias are common and occur circumorally, in a stocking-glove distribution, or both. Vertigo, ataxia, and the sensation of floating occur less commonly. Hot-cold reversal in temperature sensation is not unusual. In severe cases, respiratory failure due to diaphragmatic paralysis may result.

There is no known antidote for paralytic shellfish poisoning. Supportive care, including mechanical ventilation, may be needed. Although the symptoms are usually self-limited and short-lived, weakness and malaise may persist for weeks following ingestion.

MUSHROOM POISONING

Benjamin DR: Mushroom poisoning in infants and children: The *Amanita pantherina/muscaria* group. Clin Toxicol 30:13, 1992.
Editorial: Mushroom poisoning. Lancet 2:351, 1980.
Hanrahan JP, Gordon MA: Mushroom poisoning: Case reports and a review of therapy. JAMA 251:1057, 1984.
Klein AS, Hart J, Brems JJ, et al: *Amanita* poisoning: Treatment and the role of liver transplantation. Am J Med 86:187, 1989.
Litten W: The most poisonous mushrooms. Sci Am 232:90, 1975.
McCormick DJ, Avbel AJ, Biggons RB: Nonlethal mushroom poisoning. Ann Intern Med 90:332, 1979.
McDonald A: Mushrooms and madness: Hallucinogenic mushrooms and some psychopharmacological implications. Can J Psychiatry 25:586, 1980.
Mitchell DH: *Amanita* mushroom poisoning. Annu Rev Med 31:51, 1980.
Rumack BH, Spoerke DG (eds): POISINDEX System®: A Computerized Poison Information System, Vol 68. Denver, CO, Micromedex, Inc, 1991.

SOLANINE POISONING

Editorial: Potato poisoning. Lancet 2:681, 1979.
McMillan M, Thompson JC: An outbreak of suspected solanine poisoning in school boys: Examination of criteria of solanine poisoning. Q J Med 48:227, 1979.

CIGUATERA FISH POISONING

Lawrence DN, Enriquez MB, Lumish RM, et al: Ciguatera fish poisoning in Miami. JAMA 244:254, 1980.
Morris JG, Lewin P, Hargrett NT, et al: Clinical features of ciguatera fish poisoning. Arch Intern Med 142:1090, 1982.
Palafox NA, Jain LG, Pinano AZ, et al: Successful treatment of ciguatera fish poisoning with intravenous mannitol. JAMA 259:2740, 1988.
Withers NW: Ciguatera fish poisoning. Ann Rev Med 33:97, 1982.

SCOMBROID FISH POISONING

Blakesley ML: Scombroid poisoning: Prompt resolution of symptoms with cimetidine. Ann Emerg Med 12:104, 1983.
Gilbert RJ, Hobbs G, Murray CK, et al: Scombrotoxic fish poisoning: Features of the first 50 incidents to be reported in Britain (1976–9). BMJ 281:71, 1980.
Hughes JM, Potter ME: Scombroid fish poisoning: From pathogenesis to prevention. N Engl J Med 324:766, 1991.
Morrow JD, Margolies GR, Rowland J, et al: Evidence that histamine is the causative toxin of scombroid fish poisoning. N Engl J Med 324:716, 1991.

PARALYTIC SHELLFISH POISONING

Hughes JM, Merson MH: Fish and shellfish poisoning. N Engl J Med 295:1117, 1976.
Morris PD, Campbell DS, Taylor TJ, et al: Clinical and epidemiological features of neurotoxic shellfish poisoning in North Carolina. Am J Public Health 81:471, 1991.
Popkiss MEE, Horstman DA, Harpur D: Paralytic shellfish poisoning: A report of 17 cases in Cape Town. S Afr Med J 55:1017, 1979.
Shimizu Y, Yoshioka M: Transformation of paralytic shellfish toxins as demonstrated in scallop homogenates. Science 212:547, 1981.

CHAPTER 668
Envenomations

Kenneth H. Webb

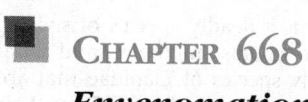

There are thousands of animal species that can cause human envenomation. The venoms produced are complex, species-specific mixtures of polypeptides, proteolytic enzymes, toxins, and vasoactive substances, which are both toxic and antigenic. As symptoms of envenomation may be venom- or immunoglobulin (Ig)E-mediated, the severity of symptoms relates either to the potency and concentration of the venom or the allergen sensitivity of the victim. Children are at special risk for severe envenomation reactions because of their small size and the relatively high serum concentrations of venom that they endure.

ANTIVENINS. For every venom capable of invoking an immune response, there is a potential antivenin. Antivenins are animal-derived Igs that work by direct binding and neutralization of the antigens contained in the venom. Antivenins are especially effective if administered shortly after envenomation, often leading to dramatic diminution of symptoms within 1–3 hr.

Because antivenins are concentrates of animal serum, both immediate and delayed hypersensitivity reactions are common and may themselves be life threatening. The decision to use an antivenin should be made as quickly as possible and should be based on both the known potency of the venom and the clinical severity of the victim. There are only three Food and Drug Administration (FDA)–approved, commercially available antivenin preparations in the United States,* but antivenins to the venom of other species are often available through local zoologic societies or poison control centers.

Antivenin should be given only in the intensive care setting with resuscitation equipment and epinephrine at the bedside. Skin testing with 0.02 mL of a 1:10 dilution of antivenin should be performed before intravenous infusion of any antivenin. A negative skin test is reassuring but does not guarantee safety. Conversely, a positive skin test does not preclude use of the antivenin; if antivenin is still believed to be necessary, a desensitization protocol should be followed. Antihistamines and epinephrine are effective both prophylactically and in the treatment of immediate hypersensitivity reactions.

Serum sickness has been documented in up to 50% of patients who receive antivenin. Serum sickness results from the deposition of antibody-antigen complexes on endothelial surfaces. Symptoms commonly occur 7–21 days after administration of the antivenin and may last days or weeks. Symptoms include fever, malaise, lymphadenopathy, morbilliform or urticarial rash, and arthralgia. In severe cases, arthritis, nephritis, vasculitis, and neuropathy may occur. Antihistamines and corticosteroids are used to treat this syndrome.

SNAKEBITES

Although there are greater than 3,500 known species of snakes in the world, only 200 are poisonous to humans. All poisonous species are members of four families: the Colubridae, the Elapidae, the Hydrophidae, and the Viperidae (true vipers). An important subfamily of the true vipers are the Crotalidae (pit vipers), which account for greater than 95% of all poisonous snakebites in the United States. Pit vipers may be identified by their large triangular heads and identifiable pit between the eyes and nose. Members of the pit viper family include rattlesnakes, cottonmouths (water moccasins), and copperheads.

The Elapidae are among the most deadly species of snakes. Members of this family include cobras, mambas, and coral snakes. Coral snakes are the only species of Elapidae that are native to the United States; they may be identified by their wide black and red circumferential bands that are separated by narrower yellow bands ("red on yellow, kill a fellow; red on black, venom lack").

The Hydrophidae are poisonous sea snakes. They are probably the most abundant reptiles on earth, inhabiting tropical waters throughout the world.

EPIDEMIOLOGY. There are approximately 300,000 poisonous snakebites in the world each year. Approximately 10% of these bites result in death; most of these are due to cobra bites in Southeast Asia. There are approximately 7,000 poisonous snakebites in the United States each year, more than 50% of which involve individuals younger than 20 yr of age. Most poisonous snakebites in the United States are due to pit vipers; less than 0.2% of these result in death.

PATHOGENESIS. Snake venom is a complex mixture of polypeptides, proteolytic enzymes, and toxins, the composition of which is largely species specific. Venoms produced by the Elapidae and the Hydrophidae are primarily neurotoxic; they act by blocking neuronal transmission at the neuromuscular junction. Death from envenomation by these snakes is typically due to respiratory depression. Venoms produced by the Crotalidae are primarily cytolytic, causing cellular necrosis, vascular leak, hemolysis, and coagulopathy. Death from envenomation by the Crotalidae is typically due to hemorrhage, shock, or renal failure.

CLINICAL MANIFESTATIONS. Approximately 20% of all poisonous snakebites result in no envenomation. In the remainder, the severity of the envenomation depends on many variables: those related to the victim (age, general health, size), those related to the snake (species, condition of venom glands and fangs), those related to the bite (number, location, depth, amount of venom injected), and those related to the promptness and effectiveness of initial therapy.

Pit viper bites usually occur on the extremities, causing burning pain and swelling at the site within minutes. As the venom spreads to the body through the lymphatics, there is advancing edema and ecchymosis of the involved extremity with marked regional lymphadenopathy. In severe cases, local signs include formation of bullae and tissue necrosis of the involved extremity. Systemic symptoms include nausea and vomiting; diaphoresis; numbness or tingling around the mouth, scalp, and digits; and muscle fasciculations. In the most severe cases, there is generalized edema, shock, cardiac arrhythmias, and death. Complex clotting abnormalities are common in pit viper envenomations. They are due to species-specific components of the venom, which may lead to sequestration of platelets, activation of proteins in the coagulation cascade, and/or activation of fibrinolytic proteins. The severity of crotalid envenomations is commonly graded on a four-point scale (Table 668–1).

Bites of the Elapidae and the Hydrophidae may be minimally painful (as with the eastern coral snake and most species of Hydrophidae) or painful and necrotic (as with the cobra). As the venom of both families is primarily neurotoxic, systemic symptoms include drowsiness, cranial nerve palsies, motor weakness, and paralysis. In more severe cases, symptoms may progress to seizures, coma, and death by respiratory depression.

LABORATORY DATA. Because of the dramatic cytolytic and hemorrhagic consequences of crotalid envenomations, baseline and serial laboratory measurements are critical to their management. Initial blood tests should include type and cross-match; complete blood and platelet counts; prothrombin and partial thromboplastin times; fibrinogen and fibrin degradation products; and blood urea nitrogen, creatinine, and creatinine phosphokinase levels. Many of these studies should be repeated frequently, with the interval depending on the severity of the envenomation and the instability of the patient's condition.

■ **TABLE 668–1 Envenomation Severity**

Grade 0	No envenomation
Grade 1	Minimal envenomation (local swelling and pain without progression)
Grade 2	Moderate envenomation (swelling, pain, or ecchymosis progressing beyond the site of injury; mild systemic or laboratory manifestations)
Grade 3	Severe envenomation (marked local response, severe systemic findings, and significant alteration in laboratory findings)

*Antivenin (Crotalidae) polyvalent, Wyeth-Ayerst Laboratories; Antivenin *(Micruris fulvius)*, Wyeth-Ayerst Laboratories; and Antivenom *(Latrodectus mactans)*, Merck, Sharp, and Dohme.

TREATMENT. A working knowledge of the species of snakes endemic to one's geographic location is critical in the optimal management of snakebites. One must know which snakes are poisonous and whether envenomation has occurred. Nonpoisonous snakes account for greater than 80% of the 45,000 snakebites in the United States each year. In general, these bites do not leave distinct fang punctures and do not cause a great deal of local pain or swelling. No therapy is necessary.

In the emergency care of envenomations, it should be remembered that venom gains access to the circulation primarily by way of the lymphatics. First aid maneuvers should attempt to impede local lymphatic flow. The patient should be placed at rest with local pressure and immobilization of the involved extremity. Pressure at the site of envenomation causes collapse of the microcirculation. Immobilization of the extremity decreases the muscular contractions that promote lymphatic flow. A tourniquet should be placed proximal to the site(s) of envenomation and tightened such that only the superficial venous and lymphatic drainage is impaired. As a test of optimal tightness, one should be able to insert a finger gently beneath the tourniquet. The arterial blood supply to the extremity should not be compromised because ischemia may exacerbate the severity of the local tissue reaction.

If initiated within minutes of envenomation, a commercial venom suction device* may recover 20–30% of the venom inoculum. Such devices should be left on continuous suction for approximately 30 min. They are ineffective if their application is delayed. Direct application of ice has been shown to do more harm than good; the same may be said of traditional cruciate incision and oral suction of the venom.

On presentation to the emergency room, the victim should be monitored closely, and large-bore intravenous access should be established. Initial blood and urine samples should be sent for analysis. Vital signs, circumference of the affected extremity, urine output, and fluid intake should be monitored frequently. Isotonic solutions should be administered in an effort to combat shock. Fresh frozen plasma, cryoprecipitate, and platelet infusions should be used as necessary to correct coagulopathy. Appropriate tetanus prophylaxis should be given. A broad-spectrum antibiotic should be started. Narcotics should be used in an effort to control pain.

The decision to use antivenin should be based on the severity or rapid progression of the symptoms. Antivenin is most effective if administered within 4 hr of the bite; it is of questionable value if delayed by more than 12 hr. There are two snake antivenin preparations commercially available in the United States: antivenin (Crotalidae) polyvalent, which is effective for most pit viper bites, and antivenin *(Micrurus fulvius)*, which is effective for bites caused by the North American coral snake. For bites from other species, antivenin may be obtained from the local zoologic society or poison control center.

COMPLICATIONS. Complications of snakebites include compartment syndrome and tissue necrosis. Compartment syndrome can be prevented by the use of serial examinations and manometry devices. Clinically, compartment syndrome can be remembered by the six P's: pain out of context to injury, pressure (swollen limb), paresthesia, pulses absent, pain with passive stretch, and paresis. Treatment is surgical exposure of the affected compartments.

ARACHNID ENVENOMATIONS

There are more than 20,000 species of spiders in the world; all but two are venomous. Most spiders are not particularly dangerous to humans, lacking either potent venom or fangs capable of penetrating human skin. Most of the morbidity caused by poisonous spider bites in the United States are attributable to two genera: *Latrodectus* and *Loxosceles*.

*Extractor, Sawyer Products.

Latrodectism

Although commonly known as "black widows," only three of the five species of *Latrodectus* found in the United States are actually black, and only one *(L. mactans)* has the well-known orange hourglass marking on the ventral surface of its abdomen. Females of this species have a body that can measure 1.5 cm in length and a leg span that can measure 4–5 cm. Males of this species are approximately 30% the size of females and pose no threat to humans because their fangs are too short to penetrate the skin.

Members of this genus are found throughout the United States and are most common in the South. Black widows are trapper spiders who live in dark, rarely disturbed areas such as woodpiles, sheds, privies, and garages. They are shy and nonaggressive unless trapped against the skin.

CLINICAL MANIFESTATIONS. The venom of the black widow is an extremely potent neurotoxin that leads to continuous release of acetylcholine and norepinephrine at the presynaptic junction. The bite may be moderately painful or go completely unnoticed. Symptoms of envenomation begin locally with the development of a pruritic wheal. Symptoms progress to muscle cramps and spasm at the site of the bite, which may be associated with pain and fasciculations. Muscle spasm may spread to the rest of the body in less than 1 hr. Associated symptoms include severe abdominal pain, diaphoresis, hypertension, nausea, and vomiting. In severe cases, symptoms may progress to shock, coma, respiratory arrest, and death.

Because painful abdominal muscle contractions are the prominent feature of latrodectism, *differential diagnosis* includes acute abdomen, renal colic, opiate withdrawal, and tetanus.

TREATMENT. This begins with maintenance of the airway, breathing, and circulation. The wound should be cleansed thoroughly, and appropriate tetanus prophylaxis should be given. Narcotics should be given for pain and benzodiazepines for muscle relaxation. Antihypertensive medications should be given if hypertension does not respond to pain relief and muscle relaxation. Calcium infusions have traditionally been used in the relief of muscle spasms, but there is controversy about their effectiveness.

There is a commercially available antivenin for *L. mactans* envenomations, which should be used in severe cases. The dose is one vial, which may be repeated if necessary. Administration typically leads to improvement of pain, spasm, and hypertension within 1 hr.

Necrotic Arachnidism

Although there are many species of spider the bites of which lead to tissue necrosis, species in the *Loxosceles* genus are the most common cause in the United States. Also known as the "fiddleback spider" because of a brown violin-shaped marking on the cephalothorax, there are 12 species in this genus. Six species have bites that may cause tissue necrosis. *L. reclusa*, the brown recluse spider, is the species most commonly found in the United States.

The brown recluse spider is ubiquitous in the United States. It is especially common in the South and Midwest. Its body can measure 1.2 cm and its leg span can extend 4–5 cm. This spider is a nocturnal hunter who can live for months without food or water. It lives in dark, rarely disturbed areas such as woodpiles, under rocks, and in closets or basements. It is typically nonaggressive except when attacked or trapped.

CLINICAL MANIFESTATIONS. The venom of *L. reclusa* is a complex mixture of cytotoxins, of which sphingomyelinase D seems to be the most important. The clinical course after a bite by *L. reclusa* is fairly predictable. The bite itself may be moderately painful but often goes unnoticed. Within 30–60 min after the bite, there is burning and pruritus at the site of the bite. After becoming erythematous, indurated, and painful, a hemorrhagic blister is formed at the bite within days. As the blister sloughs, it leaves a necrotic, enlarging ulcer. These ulcers can grow to 15 cm in size and seem to be especially prominent when involving skin overlying areas of high fat content, such as the thighs and buttocks.

Systemic symptoms include fever and chills; nausea and vomiting; a generalized, scarlatiniform rash; and arthralgias. Hemolysis, disseminated intravascular coagulation, and renal failure may complicate the clinical course and may be life threatening, especially in small children.

Differential diagnosis includes the bites and stings of other insects and those rashes that are characteristically associated with blisters; rhus dermatitis, herpes simplex, toxic epidermal necrolysis, and Stevens-Johnson syndrome.

TREATMENT. Therapy is controversial. Accepted mainstays of therapy include appropriate tetanus prophylaxis and frequent cleansing and dressing of the wound. Antihistamines should be used in the treatment of pruritus. Analgesics should be used as necessary. The use of steroids and excision of the bite is controversial. Dapsone, an antibiotic used in the therapy of leprosy and dermatitis herpetiformis, has been used by some. Use of this drug is contraindicated in patients with glucose-6-phosphate dehydrogenase deficiency. An antivenin is under development.

Scorpion Bites

Unlike spiders that deliver their venom by a bite, scorpions deliver their venom by a stinger located on the final segment of a curved, six-segment tail. There are more than 2,000 species of scorpions worldwide; important genera include the *Buthus* in India and Israel, *Androctonus* in Africa, and *Tityus* in Trinidad. The only scorpion of medical importance in the United States is *Centruroides exilicauda (C. sculpturatus)*, which is found primarily in the southwestern United States.

CLINICAL MANIFESTATIONS. Generally shy by nature, scorpions sting only when disturbed or in self-defense. The sting is usually painful. Although the composition of the venom varies by species, the venom of *C. exilicauda* is a potent neurotoxin that causes depolarization of the presynaptic membrane with resultant release of acetylcholine. Both the sympathetic and parasympathetic nervous systems may be affected. Mild envenomations may cause local pain, paresthesia, and perioral numbness. Symptoms of more significant envenomation include agitation, tachypnea, tachycardia, hypertension, blurred vision, and hypersalivation. Muscle twitching, contractions, and nystagmus are common and may resemble seizures, although the patient is usually alert and responsive throughout the attack. Severe envenomations may result in confusion, convulsions, or coma.

There are also symptoms of envenomation that are more species specific. Envenomation by *Tityus trinitatis* is the most common cause of pancreatitis in Trinidad. Envenomation by *Buthus (Leiurus) quinquestriatus* may also cause pancreatitis and is well known to cause life-threatening myocardial ischemia.

TREATMENT. Therapy of scorpion envenomation begins with immobilization of the extremity in an effort to delay the spread of the venom. Local application of ice or lidocaine may be used in relief of pain. Both α- and β-adrenergic antagonists should be used to control sympathetic effects. Afterload reduction with either nifedipine or an angiotensin-converting enzyme inhibitor should be considered, especially after envenomation by *L. quinquestriatus*.

In the United States, there is an antivenin for stings caused by *C. exilicauda*. Produced from goat serum at Arizona State University, the produce is not approved by the FDA but should be considered in cases of severe envenomation. After administration, symptoms decrease within 1–3 hr. Serum sickness reactions have been described in as many as 58% of patients receiving the antivenin.

HYMENOPTERA ENVENOMATIONS

Bees, wasps, and ants are members of the order Hymenoptera. In the United States, stings from Hymenoptera are usually caused by honeybees, bumblebees, paper wasps, yellowjackets, and fire ants. Each of these insects has a stinger located at the caudal end of the abdomen through which the venom is inoculated. Stings caused by flying Hymenoptera are usually single unless a swarm is encountered.

Hymenoptera venoms are a complex mixture of protein toxins, enzymes, and vasoactive compounds. The venom is not very potent, and most severe reactions are due to immediate hypersensitivity reactions and anaphylaxis. In the unsensitized victim, stings usually result in local pain, erythema, and edema, which resolves in a few hours. The stinger should be removed by gentle scraping. No treatment is necessary, although cold compresses and analgesics may provide symptomatic relief. A topical paste of unseasoned meat tenderizer (papain) may denature the protein elements of bee and wasp venom, leading to rapid pain relief.

In moderately sensitized victims, stings may result in hives, edema, rhinitis, conjunctivitis, and wheezing. Treatment should include antihistamines and systemic corticosteroids in addition to that provided for the unsensitized victim.

In the most severe allergic reactions, urticaria, angioedema, bronchospasm, and shock may result, usually within 15–30 min of the sting. Continuous maintenance of the airway, breathing, and circulation is crucial in these patients because they may deteriorate rapidly. The patient should be given supplemental oxygen by mask, with use of endotracheal intubation or cricothyroidotomy if necessary. Aqueous epinephrine (1:1,000) should be administered subcutaneously at a dose of 0.01 mL/kg in an effort to limit airway edema. This dosage may be repeated every 20–30 min as necessary. If the patient does not respond to this therapy, an intravenous epinephrine drip should be used, with a starting dose of 0.1 μg/kg/min. Intravenous corticosteroids may be beneficial in severe allergic reactions.

Venom immunotherapy should be considered for all children who have had a life-threatening reaction. Greater than 95% of patients will be protected by immunotherapy, with lifelong protection conferred after 3–5 yr of treatment (see Chapter 143).

MARINE ENVENOMATIONS

Stingrays

The stingray accounts for more human envenomations than any other marine vertebrate. They are usually found in tropical and subtropical waters, generally staying in the shallow intertidal areas used by humans for recreation. Stingrays are shy by nature, stinging with their whiplike tails only when disturbed or frightened. Because the stinging spines found on their tails are retroserated, they commonly cause a jagged laceration and envenomation.

Stingray envenomation is intensely painful; pain may last for 2 days. Minor punctures may resemble cellulitis; in more severe envenomations, there may be marked tissue destruction and necrosis. Systemic manifestations include vomiting, edema, limb paralysis, hypotension, bradycardia, and seizures.

Treatment begins with thorough cleaning and débridement of the wound. Appropriate tetanus prophylaxis should be given. Superinfection with aerobic and anaerobic organisms, including *Vibrio* species, is common; antibiotic prophylaxis should be considered. Because the toxins are heat labile, immersion in hot water is a mainstay of therapy, limiting pain while denaturing the protein elements of the venom. Additional analgesia should be provided as necessary.

Scorpionfish

Members of the family Scorpaenidae include zebrafish (lionfish), scorpionfish, and stonefish, all of which have venomous spines that become erect on stimulation. The most dangerous of these, the stonefish, has a venom as potent as that of the cobra. Envenomation by the Scorpaenidae causes immediate pain, which may last for hours or days. There may be intense local tissue destruction in which superinfections are common. Systemic manifestations include vomiting, abdominal pain, headache, delirium, seizures, and cardiorespiratory failure. Therapy is similar as that for stingray envenomations. There is a stonefish antivenin available;* it should be used in severe envenomations by any of these species.

Coelenterate Envenomations

Members of the phylum Cnidaria are common to the oceans of the world. Cnidarian species all share a common anatomic feature: miniscule capsules (cnidae) that contain a highly folded tubule that everts on contact, thereby injecting the venom. Medically important species include fire coral, anemones, box jellyfish, and Portuguese man-of-war.

Envenomation causes an immediate stinging sensation, which may be associated with paresthesias, pruritus, and local edema. In more severe envenomations, systemic signs may be life threatening and include nausea, vomiting, abdominal pain, myalgias and arthralgias, headache, paralysis, seizures, coma, and cardiorespiratory collapse. Most lethal envenomations have been attributed to the Pacific box jellyfish, *Chironex fleckeri*, which is indigenous to the waters off Australia, and the Atlantic Portuguese man-of-war, *Physalia physalis*.

Treatment of these envenomations begins in the ocean; the wounds should be rinsed in seawater because fresh water may lyse venom-producing cells (nematocysts), leading to further envenomation. A number of household solvents have been used in irrigation of these stings; acetic acid (vinegar), rubbing alcohol, or baking soda are good inhibitors of nematocyst discharge. Visible tentacle fragments should be removed with forceps; microscopic fragments may be removed by a gentle shaving of the affected area. Antihistamines and corticosteroids are indicated in the presence of extensive swelling and urticaria.

Seabather's Eruption

Seabather's eruption is an intensely pruritic, vesicular or maculopapular eruption that primarily affects the skin surfaces covered by swimwear. It is caused by exposure to the larvae of at least two species of the phylum Cnidaria: the sea anemone, *Edwardsiella lineata*, and the thimble jellyfish, *Linuche unguiculata*. The larvae of *E. lineata* are the principal cause of seabather's eruption in ocean waters of the northeastern United States. The larvae of *L. unguiculata* are the principal cause of seabather's eruption in Florida and the Caribbean.

Epidemics of seabather's eruption occur during summer months in which there are large quantities of larvae in the water. An intensely pruritic rash begins within 4–24 hr of exposure and may persist for days or weeks. Associated symptoms may include fever, chills, headache, malaise, conjunctivitis, and urethritis. Antihistamines are the mainstay of treatment, although corticosteroids, applied either topically or systemically, may be beneficial in severe cases.

ANTIVENINS

Sutherland SK: Antivenom use in Australia. Med J Aust 157:734, 1992.

SNAKEBITES

Christopher DG, Rodning CB: Crotalidae envenomation. South Med J 79:159, 1986.

*Commonwealth Serum Laboratories, Melbourne, Australia.

Simon TL, Grace TG: Envenomation coagulopathy in wounds from pit vipers. N Engl J Med 305:443, 1981.

Snyder CC, Pickins JE, Knowles RP, et al: A definitive study of snakebite. J Fla Med Assoc 55:330, 1968.

ARACHNID AND INSECT ENVENOMATIONS

Clark RF, Wethern-Kestner S, Vance MV, et al: Clinical presentation and treatment of black widow spider envenomation: A review of 163 cases. Ann Emerg Med 21:782, 1992.

King LE, Rees RS: Dapsone treatment of a brown recluse bite. JAMA 250:648, 1983.

Reisman R: Insect stings. N Engl J Med 331:523, 1994.

Sofer S, Shahak E, Gueron M: Scorpion envenomation and antivenom therapy. J Pediatr 124:973, 1994.

MARINE ENVENOMATIONS

Auerbach PS: Marine envenomations. N Engl J Med 325:486, 1991.

CHAPTER 669
Mammalian Bites

Stephen C. Aronoff

In the United States, 1–3.5 million emergency department visits occur each year as a result of mammalian bite injuries. Over 80% of these episodes are due to dog bites, 6% to cat bites, and 1–3% to human bites. Ten per cent of bite injuries require surgical closure, and 1–2% result in hospitalization.

EPIDEMIOLOGY. Most animal bites follow provocation and are to the hand. Ferrets may attack the face of infants without provocation. Closed-fist injuries (lacerations over the 3rd and 4th metacarpal following a blow to the mouth) are the most common form of human bite. Rat bites occur typically on the lower extremities.

CLINICAL MANIFESTATIONS. The diagnosis of a mammalian bite is usually straightforward and requires a compatible history and evidence of cutaneous injury. Crush injuries may accompany dog and human bites, while severe damage to facial cartilage may follow ferret bites in young infants. Cat bites are typically deep punctures, while rat and squirrel bites tend to be superficial. Bites to the hand, especially closed-fist injuries, may damage tendons, tendon compartments, deep fascia, bone, and/or joint capsules.

Infectious Complications (see Chapters 193 and 227 for discussions of tetanus and rabies). Because of the numerous bacterial species in mammalian oral cavities and on the victim's skin, contamination of bite injuries is universal; wound infections, cellulitis, and lymphangitis appearing 24–36 hr after the injury are the most common precipitating causes for hospitalization of bite injuries. Four per cent of dog bites, 35% of cat bites, and almost all closed-fist injuries become infected locally. The etiologies of infections following mammalian bites are polymicrobial and consist of mixed anaerobic and aerobic bacteria. In one study, an average of three different bacterial species was isolated from infected dog bites while a mean of five different species was recovered from infected human bites. In general, anaerobic bacteria are recovered from over half of all bite victims with infected wounds. *Pasteurella multocida* is a common pathogen in infected dog and cat bites, while viridans streptococci, *Staphylococcus aureus*, and *Bacteroides* species are likely to be recovered from infected human bites. Approximately half of the bites inflicted by monkeys become infected; the bacterial etiology of these infections parallels those of human bites. Bites that occur in fresh water (e.g., domestic piranha) may become infected with *Aeromonas hydrophila*.

Besides wound infections, osteomyelitis, septic arthritis, abscesses, and bacterial tenosynovitis uncommonly follow mammalian bites. In immunoincompetent patients, bacteremia and meningitis may follow mammalian bites; *P. multocida* meningitis and sepsis is particularly important in this patient population following dog or cat bites.

Noninfectious Complications. Significant cosmetic and functional damage may accompany severe bites. Although rare, hemorrhagic shock may occur following attacks by "pack" animals such as stray dogs. Finally, psychologic stress and subsequent fear of animals may be a consequence of animal bites.

PREVENTION. Children's interactions with pets should be closely supervised to prevent the animal from becoming provoked by the child. Dogs should not be permitted to run free. Stray animals should be reported promptly to local authorities. Ferrets should not be kept as pets in families with small children. It is illegal to keep ferrets as pets in California, Georgia, and New Hampshire.

TREATMENT. Most bite wounds can be managed in an ambulatory setting. Hospitalization is recommended for patients with (1) extensive injury that may require operative repair or grafts; (2) injury to or breach of tendon, joint capsule, bone, or facial cartilage; (3) extensive local infection; (4) infection that developed during prophylaxis; and (5) anticipated poor compliance.

Aside from tetanus and rabies prophylaxis, the preliminary care for mammalian bites requires cleansing, high-pressure irrigation, and débridement. Because of the high risk for infection, physical scrubbing rather than passive soaking with povidone-iodine solution is recommended for initial decontamination. Additional cleansing is achieved by high-pressure saline irrigation using a large syringe (or Waterpik) and a large-bore needle. Under local anesthesia, devitalized tissue is removed, and the wound is explored for injury to underlying structures such as bone, joint capsules, tendons, or cartilage. For noncomplicated bites, reirrigation is recommended following exploration.

Whether severe mammalian bites should be sutured initially is controversial. Because of the relatively low incidence of infection, clean, recent (< 8 hr old), adequately decontaminated dog bites may be closed initially using tape or suture with a low risk of subsequent infection (3%). Noninfected, fresh (< 12 hr old) mammalian bites of the hands or face may be closed primarily, if needed, but must be followed closely; sutures should be removed at the earliest sign of infection. Closed-fist injuries are particularly susceptible to infection. Other wounds that require closure should be thoroughly decontaminated, irrigated, and débrided; packed with gauze; and re-evaluated 4–7 days later for possible infection.

Aerobic and anaerobic bacterial cultures followed by antimicrobial therapy are indicated for the treatment of infected bite wounds. Since most of these infections have a polymicrobial etiology, initial therapy should be broad. For superficial infections, orally administered amoxicillin-clavulanate (Augmentin; 50 mg/kg/24 hr in three doses) is sufficiently broad and effective; erythromycin (40 mg/kg/24 hr in four doses) is an alternative in penicillin-allergic patients. Therapy may be changed after culture results are known. Severe infections require hospitalization and parenteral antimicrobial therapy. Ampicillin-sulbactam (Unasyn; 25–50 mg ampicillin/kg/dose every 6 hr) has an identical spectrum of activity to amoxicillin-clavulanate and may be used initially. Cefoxitin (30–40 mg/kg/24 hr every 6 hr) is another option. Since clindamycin (30–40 mg/kg/24 hr in four doses) is active against most anaerobes, *S. aureus*, and aerobic streptococci but not against *P. multocida*, this agent should be used initially for the treatment of infected human bites in penicillin-allergic and nonallergic patients. Because a significant minority of *P. multocida* and *Bacteroides* species isolates are resistant to oxacillin (100 mg/kg/24 hr in six doses), oxacillin plus penicillin (100,000 U/kg/24 hr in six doses) and cefoxitin alone are additional options for empiric therapy. Erythromycin or minocycline are alternatives for the penicillin-allergic patient.

Little comparative data are available addressing the efficacy of prophylactic antibiotic use. Accepted indications for prophylaxis include (1) any cat, human, or monkey bite; (2) wounds planned for delayed closure; (3) any bites of the hands or face; (4) bites that have not or cannot be adequately débrided; and (5) victims who are infants, diabetic, or immunocompromised. Oral administration of amoxicillin-clavulanate, erythromycin, or minocycline (in older patients; 4 mg/kg/24 hr in two doses) for 3 days should be adequate prophylaxis in these cases.

Brook I: Microbiology of human and animal bite wounds in children. Pediatr Infect Dis J 6:29, 1987.
Feder HM, Shanley JD, Barbera JA: Review of 59 patients hospitalized with animal bites. Pediatr Infect Dis J 6:24, 1987.
Gershman K, Sacks J, Wright J: Which dogs bite? A case-control study of risk factors. Pediatrics 93:913, 1994.
Goldstein EJC, Citron DM, Wield B, et al: Bacteriology of human and animal bite wounds. J Clin Microbiol 8:667, 1978.
Paisley JW, Lauer BA: Severe facial injuries to infants due to unprovoked attacks by pet ferrets. JAMA 259:2005, 1988.
Revord ME, Goldfarb J, Shurin SB: *Aeromonas hydrophila* wound infection in a patient with cyclic neutropenia following a piranha bite. Pediatr Infect Dis J 7:70, 1988.
Trott A: Care of mammalian bites. Pediatr Infect Dis J 6:8, 1987.

PART XXXV

Laboratory Medicine and Reference Tables

CHAPTER 670

Laboratory Testing and Reference Values (Table 670–2) in Infants and Children

John F. Nicholson and Michael A. Pesce

Also see Chapters 2 and 5.

For a number of reasons—genetic heterogeneity, biologic and environmental variability, and inhomogeneity of subclinical health status—normal values for many laboratory tests do not show a gaussian bell-shaped curve of distribution. As a result, the population mean and standard deviation (SD) are frequently less useful than the range of normal values, generally given as the 95% normal range, that is, the range of values obtained in testing a normal population minus the lowest 2.5% and the highest 2.5%. As shown in Table 670–1, serum sodium, which is tightly controlled physiologically, has a distribution that is essentially gaussian in a large group of children. This is indicated by the fact that the mean value ± 2 SD gives a range very close to that actually observed in 95% of the children. On the other hand, serum creatine kinase, which is subject to diverse influences and is not actively controlled, does not show a gaussian distribution, as evidenced by the lack of agreement between the range actually observed and that predicted by the mean value ± 2 SD.

A refinement of referencing that is used with increasing frequency is reporting the value obtained together with the percentile of normal values into which the value obtained falls. This method is useful when one is testing for risk factors such as in determination of serum cholesterol.

A further modification that is necessary for many tests performed in infants and children is calculating the age-related adjustment of the normal range. Both age adjustment and the use of percentiles are illustrated in the normal values for serum cholesterol in Table 670–2.

A final modification needed for reporting normal ranges is referencing to the Tanner stage of sexual maturation, which is most useful in assessing pituitary and gonadal function.

ACCURACY AND PRECISION OF LABORATORY TESTS. An important consideration in interpreting the results of a laboratory test is the technical accuracy of the test. Because of improvements in methods of analysis and elimination of analytic interferences, the accuracy of most tests is limited primarily by their precision. Accuracy is a measure of the nearness of the test result to the actual value, whereas precision is a measure of the reproducibility of a result. No test can be more accurate than it is precise. Analysis of precision by repetitive measurements of a single sample gives rise to a gaussian distribution with a meaningful mean and SD. The estimate of precision generally used is the coefficient of variation (CV):

$$CV = SD/mean \times 100\ (\%)$$

The CV is not likely to be constant over the full range of values obtained in clinical testing but ordinarily is about 5% in the normal range. The CV is generally not reported but is always known by the laboratory. It is particularly important in assessing the significance of changes in laboratory results. For example, a common situation is the need to assess hepatotoxicity incurred as a result of administration of a therapeutic drug and reflected in the serum alanine aminotransferase (ALT) value. If serum ALT increases from 25 U/L to 40 U/L, is the change significant? The CV for ALT is 7%. Using the value obtained plus or minus 2 × CV to express the extremes of imprecision, it can be seen that a value of 25 is unlikely to reflect an actual concentration of greater than 29 U/L, and a value of 40 U/L is unlikely to reflect an actual concentration of less than 34 U/L. Therefore, the change in the value as obtained by testing is likely to reflect a real change in circulating ALT levels, and continued monitoring of ALT is indicated even though both values for ALT are within normal limits. "Likely" in this case is only a probability. Inherent biologic variability is such that the results of two successive tests may suggest a trend that will disappear on further testing.

The precision of a test may also be indicated by providing confidence limits for a given result. Ordinarily, 95% confidence limits are used, indicating that it is 95% certain that the value obtained lies between the two limits reported. Confidence limits are calculated using the mean and SD of replicate determinations:

$$95\%\ \text{Confidence limits} = mean \pm t \times SD$$

where t is a constant derived from the number of replications. In most cases t = 2.

PREDICTIVE VALUE OF LABORATORY TESTS. Predictive value (PV) theory deals with the usefulness of tests as defined by their

TABLE 670–1 Gaussian and Nongaussian Laboratory Values in 458 Normal School Children Aged 7–14 Yr

	Serum Sodium (mM/L)	Serum Creatine Kinase (U/L)
Mean	141	68
SD*	1.7	34
Mean ± 2 SD	138–144	0–136
Actual 95%range	137–144	24–162

**SD= standard deviation.*

sensitivity (ability to detect a disease) and specificity (ability to define absence of a disease).

Sensitivity = No. positive by test/no. with disease × 100
Specificity = No. negative by test/no. without disease × 100

The PV of a positive test = true +/total + × 100, and the PV of a negative test = true −/total − × 100, where total + is the sum of true + and false +, and total − is the sum of true − and false −. The problems addressed by the theory are false-negative and false-positive tests; these are major considerations in interpreting screening tests in general and neonatal screening tests specifically.

Testing for human immunodeficiency virus (HIV) seroreactivity serves to illustrate some of these considerations. If it is assumed that approximately 1,000,000 of 250,000,000 residents of the United States are infected with HIV (prevalence = 0.4%.) and that 90% of those infected show appropriate antibodies, we can consider the usefulness of a simple test with 99% sensitivity and 99.5% specificity. If the total population of the United States were screened, it would be possible to identify most of those infected with HIV.

$$1{,}000{,}000 \times 0.9 \times 0.99 = 891{,}000\ (89.1\%)$$

There will be 109,000 false-negative test results. Even with a 99.5% specificity, the number of false-positive test results would be larger than the number of true-positive results.

$$249{,}000{,}000 \times 0.005 = 1{,}245{,}000$$

There will be 247,755,000 true-negative results.

$$\text{PV of + test} = \frac{891{,}000}{891{,}000 + 1{,}245{,}000} \times 100 = 42\%$$

$$\text{PV of − test} = \frac{247{,}755{,}000}{247{,}755{,}000 + 109{,}000} \times 100 = > 99.9\%$$

Given the high cost associated with follow-up of false-positive test results, the anguish produced by a false-positive result, and the limited effectiveness of current treatment, it is easy to see why universal screening for HIV seropositivity has received a low priority.

By contrast, we can consider the screening of 100,000 individuals from groups at increased risk for HIV in whom the overall prevalence of disease is 10%, all other considerations being unchanged.

$$\text{True-positive results} = 0.9 \times 0.99 \times 10{,}000 = 8{,}910$$

$$\text{False-positive results} = 0.005 \times 90{,}000 = 450$$

$$\text{False-negative results} = 10{,}000 - 8{,}910 = 1{,}090$$

$$\text{PV of positive result} = \frac{8{,}910}{8{,}910 + 450} \times 100 = 95\%$$

$$\text{PV of negative result} = \frac{89{,}550}{89{,}550 + 1{,}090} \times 100 = 99\%$$

It is clear from these two hypothetical testing strategies that the diagnostic efficiency of testing is heavily dependent on the prevalence of the disease being tested for, even if the test is a superior one like the test for HIV antibodies.

NEONATAL SCREENING TESTS. Most neonatal screening tests are more problematic in a theoretical sense than would be the case with widespread screening for HIV. First, almost all the diseases detected in neonatal screening programs have a very low prevalence, and second, the tests are, for the most part, quantitative rather than qualitative. In general, the strategy is to use the initial screening test to separate a highly suspect group of patients from normal infants (i.e., to increase the prevalence) and then to follow this suspect group aggressively. This strategy is illustrated by a scheme used in screening newborns for congenital hypothyroidism, the prevalence of which is 25/100,000 liveborn infants. The initial test performed is for thyroxine in whole blood, and infants with the lowest 10% of test results are considered suspect. If all infants with hypothyroidism were in the suspect group, the prevalence of disease in this group would be 250/100,000 infants. The original samples obtained from the suspect group are retested for thyroxine and then tested for thyroid-stimulating hormone. This second round of testing results in an even more highly suspect group comprising 0.1% of the infants screened and having a prevalence of hypothyroidism of 25,000/100,000 subjects. This final group is aggressively pursued for further testing and treatment. Even with a 1,000-fold increase in prevalence, 75% of the population aggressively tested is euthyroid. The justifications advanced for the program are that treatment is easy and effective and that the alternative, long-term custodial care, is both unsatisfactory and expensive.

TESTING IN DIFFERENTIAL DIAGNOSIS. The use of laboratory tests in differential diagnosis will satisfy predictive value theory because a correct differential diagnosis should result in a relatively high prevalence of the disease under consideration. An example of testing in differential diagnosis is the measurement of urinary vanillylmandelic acid (VMA) for diagnosis of neuroblastoma. Galen and Gambino pointed out that a simple spot test for VMA was not useful in general screening programs because of the low prevalence of neuroblastoma (3/100,000) and the low sensitivity of the test (69%). Even though the specificity of urinary VMA was 99.6%, testing of 100,000 children would produce 2 true-positive test results, 400 false-positive results, and 1 false-negative result. The predictive value of a positive test in this setting is 0.5%, and the predictive value of a negative test is 99.99%, not much different from the assumption that neuroblastoma is not present at all. However, testing for urinary VMA in a 3-yr-old child with an abdominal mass gives a useful result because the prevalence of neuroblastoma is at least 50% in 3-yr-old children with abdominal masses. If 100 such children are tested and the prevalence of neuroblastoma in the group is assumed to be 50%, satisfactory predictive values are obtained.

$$\text{PV of positive test} = \frac{0.69 \times 50}{0.69 \times 50 + 0.004 \times 50} \times 100 = 99\%$$

$$\text{PV of negative test} = \frac{0.996 \times 50}{0.996 \times 50 + 0.31 \times 50} \times 100 = 76\%$$

Here a test with a low sensitivity is quite powerful in differential diagnosis because the predictive value of a positive result is almost 100% in the setting of high prevalence.

PROBLEMS IN LABORATORY TESTING FOR DIFFERENTIAL DIAGNOSIS: SEROLOGIC TESTS FOR LYME DISEASE. Lyme disease, the consequence of tick-borne infection by *Borrelia burgdorferi*, has various manifestations in both early and late stages of infection (see Chapter 198). One manifestation—*erythema chronicum migrans*—occurs early, although not in all patients, and is considered pathognomonic. Direct demonstration of the organism is difficult, but serologic tests for Lyme disease are not reliably positive in young patients presenting early with erythema chronicum migrans. These tests become positive after some weeks of infection and remain positive for years. In an older population being evaluated for late-stage Lyme disease, some individuals will have recovered from either clinical or subclinical Lyme disease, and some will have active Lyme disease, with both groups having true-positive serologic test results. Of those individuals without Lyme disease, some will have true-negative serologic test results, but a significant percentage will have antibodies to other organisms that cross-react with *B. burgdorferi* antigens. This set of circumstances gives rise to a number of problems. First, the protean nature of Lyme disease makes it difficult to ensure a high prevalence of disease in subjects to be tested. Second, the most appropriate antibodies to be detected are imperfectly defined, leading to a wide variety of entry tests with varying rates of false positivity and false negativity. Third, the natural history of the infection and the difficulty of demonstrating the causative organism directly combine to make the laboratory diagnosis of early Lyme disease difficult because of poor sensitivity of the serologic tests to early Lyme disease. Fourth, in the diagnosis of late-stage Lyme disease in older subjects, the laboratory diagnosis is plagued by misleading positive (either false-positive or true-positive but not clinically relevant) results of the entry test, typically an enzyme-linked immunosorbent assay, that uses whole *B. burgdorferi* organisms. A review of 788 patients referred to a specialty clinic with the diagnosis of Lyme disease revealed that 180 patients had been correctly diagnosed, 156 patients had true seropositivity without active Lyme disease, and 452 had never had Lyme disease, even though 45% of them were seropositive by at least one test before referral. Use of a more specific Western blot technique that allows definition of the actual bacterial antigens to which antibodies are directed is helpful in identifying false-positive results of the entry tests. However, routine use of the Western blot technique as the entry test would be prohibitively expensive.

RISK FACTORS AND PREDICTIVE VALUE. When a given laboratory value within the spectrum of the reference range is considered a risk factor, it is generally true that, in the absence of clinical manifestations, the value has no predictive worth as an indicator of disease and has little worth in predicting the likelihood of future disease in any individual case.

Galen RS, Gambino SR: Beyond Normality. New York, Academic Press, 1975.
Novogroder M: Neonatal screening for hypothyroidism. Pediatr Clin North Am 27:881, 1980.
Steere AC, Taylor E, McHugh GL, et al: The overdiagnosis of Lyme disease. JAMA 269:1812, 1993.

■ **TABLE 670–2 Reference Ranges for Laboratory Tests**

Prefixes Denoting Decimal Factors

Prefix	*Symbol*	*Factor*
mega	M	10^{6}
kilo	k	10^{3}
hecto	h	10^{2}
deka	da	10^{1}
deci	d	10^{-1}
centi	c	10^{-2}
milli	m	10^{-3}
micro	μ	10^{-6}
nano	n	10^{-9}
pico	p	10^{-12}
femto	f	10^{-15}

To conserve space, the following common abbreviations are used.

Abbreviations

Ab	absorbance
AI	angiotensin I
AU	arbitrary unit
cAMP	cyclic adenosine 3′,5′ monophosphate
cap	capillary
CH^{50}	dilution required to lyse 50% of indicator RBC; indicates complement activity
CHF	congestive heart failure
CKBB	brain isoenzyme of creatine kinase
CKMB	heart isoenzyme of creatine kinase
CNS	central nervous system
conc.	concentration
Cr.	creatinine
d	diem, day, days
F	female
g	gram
hr	hour, hours
Hb	hemoglobin
HbCO	carboxyhemoglobin
Hgb	hemoglobin
hpf	high-power field
HPLC	high-performance liquid chromatography
IFA	indirect fluorescent antibody
IU	International Unit of hormone activity
L	liter
M	male
MCV	mean corpuscular volume
mEq/L	milliequivalents per liter
min	minute, minutes
mm^3	cubic millimeter; equivalent to microliter (μL)
mm Hg	millimeters of mercury
mo	month, months
mol	mole
mOsm	milliosmole
MW	relative molecular weight
Na	sodium

Symbols

>	greater than
≥	greater than or equal to
<	less than
≤	less than or equal to
±	plus/minus
≃	approximately equal to

Abbreviations for Specimens

S	serum
P	plasma
(H)	heparin
(LiH)	lithium heparin
(E)	EDTA
(C)	citrate
(O)	oxalate
W	whole blood
U	urine
F	feces
CSF	cerebrospinal fluid
AF	amniotic fluid
(NaC)	sodium citrate
(NH_4H)	ammonium heparinate

Key to Comments

30°, 37°	temperature of enzymatic analysis (Celsius)
a	atomic absorption
b	optical density
c	colorimetry
d	Ektachem, proprietary analytic system of Johnson & Johnson Clinical Diagnostics, Inc.
e	enzyme-amplified immunoassay
f	values in older females higher than those in older males
g	electrophoresis
h	gas chromatography
i	radioimmunoassay
l	fluorescence-activated cell sorting
m	values obtained are significantly method dependent

Table continued on following page

■ **TABLE 670–2 Reference Ranges for Laboratory Tests** *(Continued)*

Abbreviations

nm	nanometer (wavelength)
Pa	pascal
pc	postprandial
RBC	red blood cell(s); erythrocyte(s)
RIA	radioimmunoassay
RID	radial immunodiffusion
RT	room temperature
s	second, seconds
SD	standard deviation
std.	standard
therap.	therapeutic
U	International Unit of enzyme activity
V	volume
WBC	white blood cell(s)
WHO	World Health Organization
wk	week, weeks
yr	year, years

Key to Comments

n	nephelometry
o	borate affinity chromatography
p	high-performance liquid chromatography
q	cation-exchange chromatography
r	radial immunodiffusion
s	values in older males higher than those in older females
v	fluorometric method
w	ion-selective electrode
x	fluorescence polarization
z	enzymatic assay

Sources

Colombo JP, Peheim E, Kretschmer R, et al: Plasma ammonia concentrations in newborns and children. Clin Chim Acta 138:283, 1984.

De Schepper J, Derde MP, Goubert P, et al: Reference values for fructosamine concentrations in children's sera: Influence of protein concentration, age and sex. Clin Chem 34:2444, 1988.

Denny T, Yogev R, Gelman, R et al: Lymphocyte subsets in healthy children during the first five years of life. JAMA 267:1484, 1992.

Dickinson JC, Hamilton PB: The free amino acids of human spinal fluid determined by ion exchange chromatography. J Neurochem 13:1179, 1966.

Endocrine Sciences, Tarzana, CA.

Gibson LE, de Sant'Agnese PA, Schwachman H: Procedure for the quantitative iontophoretic sweat test for cystic fibrosis. Rockville, MD, Cystic Fibrosis Foundation, 1985, pp 1–4.

Gillard BK, Simbala JA, Goodglick L: Reference intervals for amylase isoenzymes in serum and plasma of infants and children. Clin Chem 29:1119, 1983.

Hoffman G, Aramari S, Blum–Hoffman E, et al; Quantitative analysis for organic acids in biological samples: Batch isolation followed by gas chromatographic–mass spectometric analysis. Clin Chem 35:587, 1989.

Jedeikin R, Makela SK, Shennan AT, et al: Creatinine kinase isoenzymes in serum from cord blood and the blood of healthy full-term infants during the first three postnatal days. Clin Chem 28:317, 1982.

Jung D, Lun L, Zinsmeyer J, et al: The concentration of hypoxanthine and lactate in the blood of healthy and hypoxic newborns. J Perinat Med 13:43, 1985.

Knight JA, Haymond RE: γ-Glutamyltransferase and alkaline phosphatase activities compared in serum of normal children and children with liver disease. Clin Chem 27:48, 1981.

Koren G, Butt W, Rajchgot P, et al: Intravenous paraldehyde for seizure control in neonates. Neurology 36:108, 1986.

Lockitch G, Halstead AC, Albersheim S, et al: Age and sex specific pediatric reference intervals for biochemistry analyses as measured on the Ektachem-700 analyzer. Clin Chem 34:1622, 1988*a*.

Lockitch G, Halstead AC, Quigley G, et al: Age and sex specific pediatric reference intervals: Study design and methods illustrated by measurement of serum proteins with the Behring LN nephelometer. Clin Chem 34:1618, 1988*b*.

Lockitch G, Halstead AC, Wadsworth L, et al: Age and sex specific pediatric reference intervals and correlations for zinc, copper, selenium, iron, vitamins A and E, and related proteins. Clin Chem 34:1625, 1988*c*.

Mayo Clinic Laboratories, Rochester, MN, 1989.

Meites S (ed): Pediatric Clinical Chemistry, Reference (Normal) Values, 3rd ed. Washington, DC, Clinical Chemistry, 1989.

Nichols Institute Reference Laboratories, San Juan Capistrano, CA.

Pesce MA, Boudorian S: Clinical significance of plasma galactose and erythrocyte galactose-1-phosphate measurements in transferase-deficient galactosemia and in individuals with below-normal transferase activity. Clin Chem 28:301, 1982.

Rosenthal P, Pesce MA: Long-term monitoring of D-lactic acidosis in a child. J Pediatr Gastroenterol Nutr 4:674, 1985.

Sherry B, Jack RM, Weber A, et al: Reference interval for prealbumin for children two to 36 months old. Clin Chem 34:1878, 1988.

Taylor WJ, Caviness MHD: A Textbook for the Clinical Application of Therapeutic Drug Monitoring. Irving, TX, Abbott Laboratories, Diagnostic Division, 1986.

TDM Serum Sample Guide. Palo Alto, CA, Syva Company, 1986.

Unten SK, Hokama Y: Enzyme immunoassay for C-reactive protein analysis. J Clin Lab Anal 1:205, 1987.

Usmani SS, Cavaliere T, Casatelli J, et al: Plasma ammonia levels in very low birth weight preterm infants. J Pediatr 123:797, 1993.

Visnapu LA, Karlson LK, Dubinsky EJ, et al: Pediatric reference ranges for serum aldolase. Am J Clin Pathol 91:476, 1989.

■ **TABLE 670–2 Reference Ranges for Laboratory Tests** *(Continued)*

Test	Specimen	Reference Range		Factor	Reference Range (SI)	Comments
Acetaminophen. See end of table under Drugs						
Acetone						
Semiquantitative	S, P(O)	Negative (<3 mg/dL)			Negative (<0.5 mmol/L)	
Quantitative		0.3–2.0 mg/dL		× 0.1722	0.05–0.34 mmol/L	
Semiquantitative	U	Negative			Negative	
Activated partial thromboplastin time (APTT)	P(C)	25–35 s Infant: <90 s			25–35 s Infant: <90 s	
Adrenocorticotropic hormone (ACTH)	P(H)	Cord blood	130–160 pg/mL	× 1	130–160 μg/L	
		1–7 d postnatal	100–140 pg/mL		100–140 μg/L	
		Adult				
		0800 hr	25–100 pg/mL		25–100 μg/L	
		1800 hr	<50 pg/mL		<50 μg/L	
Alanine aminotransferase (ALT, SGPT)	S	0–5 d	6–50 U/L	× 1	6–50 U/L	37° s d (Lockitch, et al., *a*)
		1–19 yr	5–45 U/L		5–45 U/L	
Albumin	P	Premature 1 d	1.8–3.0 g/dL	× 10	18–30 g/L	c (Meites)
		Full-term <6 d	2.5–3.4 g/dL		25–34 g/L	
		<5 yr	3.9–5.0 g/dL		39–50 g/L	
		5–19 yr	4.0–5.3 g/dL		40–53 g/L	
	U	4–16 yr	3.35–15.3 mg/ 24 hr/1.73 m²			e (Meites)
	CSF	10–30 mg/dL			100–300 mg/L	
Aldolase	S	10–24 mo	3.4–11.8 U/L	× 1	3.4–11.8 U/L	z (Visnapu, et al.)
		25 mo–16 yr	1.2–8.8 U/L		1.2–8.8 U/L	
Aldosterone	S, P(H,E)	Ad lib Na intake				(Endocrine Sciences)
		Premature infants, supine				
		26–28 wk	5–635 ng/dL	× 0.0277	0.14–17.6 nmol/L	

■ **TABLE 670–2 Reference Ranges for Laboratory Tests** *(Continued)*

Test	Specimen	Reference Range		Factor	Reference Range (SI)	Comments
		31–35 wk	19–141 ng/dL		0.53–3.9 nmol/L	
		Full-term infants, supine				
		3 d	7–184 ng/dL		0.19–5.1 nmol/L	
		1 wk	5–175 ng/dL		0.14–4.8 nmol/L	
		1–12 mo	5–90 ng/dL		0.14–2.5 nmol/L	
		Children, supine				
		1–2 yr	7–54 ng/dL		0.19–1.5 nmol/L	
		2–10 yr	3–35 ng/dL		0.1–0.97 nmol/L	
		10–15 yr	2–22 ng/dL		0.1–0.6 nmol/L	
		Adults, supine	3–16 ng/dl		0.1–0.4 nmol/L	
		Children, upright				
		2–10 yr	5–80 ng/dL		0.14–2.2 nmol/L	
		10–15 yr	4–48 ng/dL		0.11–1.3 nmol/L	
		Adults, upright	7–30 ng/dL		0.19–0.83 nmol/L	
	U	Ad lib Na intake				
		Newborn 1–3 d	20–140 µg/g Cr.	× 0.3139	6.28–43.94 nmol/mmol Cr.	
			0.5–5 µg/24 hr	× 2.775	1.39–13.88 nmol/d	
		Prepubertal 4–10 yr	4–22 µg/g Cr.	× 0.3139	1.26–6.91 nmol/mmol Cr.	
			1–8 µg/24 hr	× 2.775	2.78–22.20 nmol/d	
		Adults	1.5–20 µg/g Cr.	× 0.3139	0.47–6.28 nmol/mmol Cr.	
			3–19 µg/24 hr	× 2.775	8.32–52.72 nmol/d	
Alkaline phosphatase, leukocyte. See Neutrophil alkaline phosphate						
Alkaline phosphate, serum. See Phosphatase, alkaline						
Amino acids in CSF	CSF					q (Dickinson, et al.)
Taurine			6.3 ± 1.8 µmol/L	× 1	6.3 ± 1.8 µmol/L	
Aspartic acid			0.9 ± 0.5 µmol/L		0.9 ± 0.5 µmol/L	
Threonine			25.0 ± 10.0 µmol/L		25.0 ± 10.0 µmol/L	
Serine + asparagine			38.0 ± 23.0 µmol/L		38.0 ± 23.0 µmol/L	
Glutamine			509.0 ± 144.0 µmol/L		509.0 ± 144.0 µmol/L	
Proline			0.6 ± — µmol/L		0.6 ± — µmol/L	
Glutamic acid			7.0 ± 4.9 µmol/L		7.0 ± 4.9 µmol/L	
Glycine			6.6 ± 1.8 µmol/L		6.6 ± 1.8 µmol/L	
Alanine			23.0 ± 9.4 µmol/L		23.0 ± 9.4 µmol/L	
Valine			14.0 ± 5.5 µmol/L		14.0 ± 5.5 µmol/L	
Half cystine			0.2 ± — µmol/L		0.2 ± — µmol/L	
Methionine			2.6 ± 1.6 µmol/L		2.6 ± 1.6 µmol/L	
Isoleucine			4.4 ± 1.3 µmol/L		4.4 ± 1.3 µmol/L	
Leucine			11.0 ± 3.6 µmol/L		11.0 ± 3.6 µmol/L	
Tyrosine			9.1 ± 5.0 µmol/L		9.1 ± 5.0 µmol/L	
Phenylalanine			9.2 ± 5.8 µmol/L		9.2 ± 5.8 µmol/L	
Ornithine			5.7 ± 1.8 µmol/L		5.7 ± 1.8 µmol/L	
Lysine			19.0 ± 6.6 µmol/L		19.0 ± 6.6 µmol/L	
Histidine			13.0 ± 4.4 µmol/L		13.0 ± 4.4 µmol/L	
Arginine			20.0 ± 5.8 µmol/L		20.0 ± 5.8 µmol/L	
Amino acids, plasma	P(H)					q (Nichols Institute)

Test	*0–30 d*	*>1 mo–16 yr*	*>16 yr*	Factor
Phosphoserine	0–30	0–12	3–7 µmol/L	× 1
Taurine	74–216	22–192	27–168 µmol/L	
Aspartic acid	0–17	5–59	0–24 µmol/L	
Hydroxyproline	20–70	0–40	0–40 µmol/L	
Threonine	114–335	73–160	79–193 µmol/L	
Serine	94–243	90–226	73–167 µmol/L	
Asparagine	20–58	28–246	14–104 µmol/L	
Glutamic acid	0–50	0–210	0–88 µmol/L	
Glutamine	538–958	52–669	415–964 µmol/L	
Proline	107–177	67–238	102–336 µmol/L	
Glycine	224–514	89–360	120–554 µmol/L	
Alanine	236–410	142–484	210–661 µmol/L	
Citrulline	8–28	1–55	12–55 µmol/L	
2-Aminobutyric acid	6–29	0–42	3–38 µmol/L	
Valine	80–246	110–271	141–317 µmol/L	
Cysteine	70–167	0–106	16–167 µmol/L	
Methionine	9–41	0–90	6–40 µmol/L	
Isoleucine	27–53	34–85	36–98 µmol/L	
Leucine	46–109	55–165	75–175 µmol/L	
Tyrosine	42–99	29–86	21–87 µmol/L	
Phenylalanine	42–110	22–98	37–88 µmol/L	
Homocystine	0–0	0–0	0–0 µmol/L	
Tryptophan	17–71	24–79	20–95 µmol/L	
Ornithine	49–151	15–143	30–106 µmol/L	
Lysine	114–269	68–266	83–238 µmol/L	
1-Methylhistidine	0–27	0–27	0–27 µmol/L	
Histidine	49–114	52–124	31–107 µmol/L	
3-Methylhistidine	0–10	0–6	0–4 µmol/L	
Arginine	22–88	6–187	36–145 µmol/L	

Test	Specimen	Reference Range	Factor	Reference Range (SI)	Comments
Amino acids, urine	U				q (Nichols Institute)

Table continued on following page

■ **TABLE 670–2 Reference Ranges for Laboratory Tests** *(Continued)*

Test	Specimen	Reference Range		Factor	Reference Range (SI)	Comments
		0–30 d (μmol/g creatinine)	**>1 mo (μmol/g creatinine)**		**0–30 d (mmol/mol creatinine)**	**>1 mo (mmol/mol creatinine)**
Phosphoserine		0–53	0–35	× 0.1131	0–6.0	0–4.0
Taurine		1,521–6,922	0–1,450		172–783	0–164
Phosphoethanolamine		0–23	23–203		0–2.6	2.6–23
Aspartic acid		78–172	0–82		8.8–19.5	0–9.3
Hydroxyproline		210–2,413	0–210		23.7–273	0–23.7
Threonine		99–509	27–265		11.2–57.6	3.1–30
Serine		80–1,096	86–566		9.1–124	9.7–64
Asparagine		0–438	0–107		0–49.5	0–12.1
Glutamic acid		34–363	0–80		3.8–41.1	0–9
Glutamine		256–1,096	168–849		29–124	9.7–64
Sarcosine		93–850	93–850		10.5–96.1	10.5–96.1
Proline		74–537	0–57		8.4–60.7	0–6.4
Glycine		1,423–7,143	0–2,953		161–808	0–334
Alanine		403–715	68–534		45.6–80.9	7.7–60.4
Citrulline		9–212	8–106		1.0–24	0.9–12
2-Aminobutyric acid		354–1,061	44–221		40–120	5–25
Valine		18–314	7–50		2.0–35.5	0.8–5.6
Cysteine		226–812	5–177		25.8–91.9	0.6–20
Methionine		15–71	6–111		1.7–8	0.7–12.5
Homocitrulline		0–266	0–266		0–30.1	0–30.1
Cystathionine		27–111	3–23		3.1–12.5	0.3–2.6
Isoleucine		43–179	0–65		4.9–20.2	0–7.3
Leucine		17–72	15–57		1.9–8.1	1.7–6.5
Tyrosine		27–97	19–145		3–11	2.2–16.4
Phenylalanine		39–156	17–102		4.4–17.7	1.9–11.5
β-Alanine		0–1,202	0–1,202		0–136	0–136
		0–30 d (μmol/g creatinine)	**>1 mo (μmol/g creatinine)**		**0–30 d (mmol/mol creatinine)**	**>1 mo (mmol/mol creatinine)**
3-Aminoisobutyric acid		0–111	0–111		0–12.5	0–12.5
4-Aminoisobutyric acid		0–2,643	0–2,643		0–299	0–299
Homocystine		0–0	0–0		0–0	0–0
Argininosuccinic acid		0–9	0–7		0–1.0	0–0.8
Ethanolamine		840–3,492	57–308		95–395	6.5–34.8
Tryptophan		0–106	0–106		0–12	0–12
Hydroxylysine		0–106	0–106		0–12	0–12
Ornithine		34–156	1–44		3.9–17.7	0.1–5.0
Lysine		74–1,282	0–548		8.4–145.0	0–62.0
1-Methylhistidine		72–425	0–691		8.1–48.1	0–78.2
Histidine		148–721	0–1,353		16.7–81.6	0–153.0
3-Methylhistidine		115–401	19–413		13–45.4	2.1–46.7
Anserine		0–561	0–561		0–63.5	0–63.5
Carnosine		0–127	0–127		0–14.4	0–14.4
Arginine		50–73	8–32		5.6–8.3	0.9–3.6
Aminolevulinic acid (ALA)	S	15–23 μg/dL (lower in child)		× 0.076	1.1–1.8 μmol/L	
	U	1.3–7.0 mg/24 hr		× 7.626	9.9–53.4 μmol/d	
Ammonia nitrogen	S, P(LiH)	Newborn	90–150 μg N/dL	× 0.714	64–107 μmol/L	z q
		0–2 wk	79–129 μg/N/dL		56–92 μmol/L	
		>1 mo	29–70 μg N/dL		21–50 μmol/L	
		Thereafter	15–45 μg N/dL		11–32 μmol/L	
		1–90 d	59–202 μg N/dL	× 0.714	42–144 μmol/L	
		3 mo–3 yr	48–195 μg N/dL		34–139 μmol/L	
	U		500–1,200 mg N/ 24 hr	× 0.0714	36–86 mmol/d	
Amniotic fluid analysis (Ab 450 nm)	AF	28 wk 0–0.048 A			0–0.048 A	
		40 wk 0–0.02 A			0–0.02 A	
Amphetamine. See end of table under Drugs						
Amylase	S	1–19 yr	35–127 U/L	× 1	35–127 U/L	c (Meites)
Pancreatic isoenzymes	S, P(H)	Cord blood 8 mo	0–34%	× 0.01	0–0.34 fraction of total	(Gillard, et al.)
		9 mo–4 yr	5–56%		0.05–0.56 fraction of total	
		5–19 yr	23–59%		0.23–0.59 fraction of total	
Androstenedione	S	M				(Endocrine Sciences)
		Tanner 1 <9.8 yr	8–50 ng/dL	× 0.03479	0.28–1.74 nmol/L	
		Tanner 2 9.8–14.5 yr	31–65 ng/dL		1.08–2.26 nmol/L	
		Tanner 3 10.7–15.4 yr	50–100 ng/dL		1.74–3.48 nmol/L	
		Tanner 4 11.8–16.2 yr	48–140 ng/dL		1.67–4.87 nmol/L	
		Tanner 5 12.8–17.3 yr	65–210 ng/dL		2.26–7.30 nmol/L	
		Adult	75–205 ng/dL		2.61–7.13 nmol/L	
		F				
		Tanner 1 <9.2 yr	8–50 ng/dL		0.28–1.74 nmol/L	
		Tanner 2 9.2–13.7 yr	42–100 ng/dL		1.46–3.48 nmol/L	
		Tanner 3 10.0–14.4 yr	80–190 ng/dL		2.78–6.61 nmol/L	
		Tanner 4 10.7–15.6 yr	77–225 ng/dL		2.68–7.83 nmol/L	
		Tanner 5 11.8–18.6 yr	80–240 ng/dL		2.78–8.35 nmol/L	
		Adult Follicular	85–275 ng/dL		2.96–9.57 nmol/L	
		Luteal	85–275 ng/dL		2.96–9.57 nmol/L	

■ **TABLE 670–2 Reference Ranges for Laboratory Tests** *(Continued)*

Test	Specimen	Reference Range		Factor	Reference Range (SI)		Comments
Anion gap (Na − (Cl + CO_2))	P(H)	7–16 mmol/L			7–16 mmol/L		
Antideoxyribonuclease B titer (Anti-DNAse titer)	S	≤170 units			≤170 units		
Antidiuretic hormone (hADH, vasopressin)	P(E)	***Plasma Osmolarity***	***Plasma ADH***		***Plasma ADH***		
		270–280 mOsm/kg	<1.5 pg/mL	× 1	<1.5 ng/L		
		280–285 mOsm/kg	<2.5 pg/mL		<2.5 ng/L		
		285–290 mOsm/kg	1–5 pg/mL		1–5 ng/L		
		290–295 mOsm/kg	2–7 pg/mL		2–7 ng/L		
		295–300 mOsm/kg	4–12 pg/mL		4–12 ng/L		
Antistreptolysin-O titer (ASO titer)	S	≤166 Todd units 170–330 Todd units in school-aged children					
α_1-Antitrypsin	S	0–5 d	143–440 mg/dL	× 0.01	1.43–4.40 g/L		n (Lockitch, et al.)
		1–9 yr	147–245 mg/dL		1.47–2.45 g/L		
		9–19 yr	152–317 mg/dL		1.52–3.17 g/L		
	F	<1 yr					r (Meites)
		breast milk	<4.4 mg/g solid				
		formula	<2.9 mg/g solid				
		6 mo–44 yr					
		cow milk, regular diet	<1.7 mg/g solid				
Ascorbic acid. See Vitamin C							
Aspartate aminotransferase (AST, SGOT)	S	0–5 d	35–140 U/L	× 1	35–140 U/L		37° s (Lockitch, et al., *b*)
		1–9 yr	15–55 U/L		15–55 U/L		
		10–19 yr	5–45 U/L		5–45 U/L		
Base excess	W(H)	Newborn	(−10)–(−2) mmol/L		(−10)–(−2) mmol/L		
		Infant	(−7)–(−1) mmol/L		(−7)–(−1) mmol/L		
		Child	(−4)–(+2) mmol/L		(−4)–(+2) mmol/L		
		Thereafter	(−3)–(+3) mmol/L		(−3)–(+3) mmol/L		
Bicarbonate	S, P	Arterial	21–28 mmol/L		21–28 mmol/L		
		Venous	22–29 mmol/L		22–29 mmol/L		
Bile acids, total	S, fasting	0.3–2.3 μg/mL		× 1	0.3–2.3 mg/L		
	S, 2-hr pc	1.8–3.2 μg/mL			1.8–3.2 mg/L		
	F	120–225 mg/24 hr		× 1	120–225 mg/24 hr		
Bilirubin	S, P	***Premature***	***Full-Term***		***Premature***	***Full-Term***	
Total	S	Cord blood <2.0 mg/dL	<2.0 mg/dL	× 17.10	<34 μmol/L	<34 μmol/L	
		0–1 d <8.0 mg/dL	<6.0 mg/dL		<137 μmol/L	<103 μmol/L	
		1–2 d <12.0 mg/dL	<8.0 mg/dL		<205 μmol/L	<137 μmol/L	
		2–5 d <16.0 mg/dL	<12.0 mg/dL		<274 μmol/L	<205 μmol/L	
		>5 d <2.0 mg/dL	0.2–1.0 mg/dL		<34 μmol/L	3.4–17.1 μmol/L	
	U	Negative			Negative		
	AF	28 wk <0.075 mg/dL (or Ab450 <0.048)		× 17.10	<1.3 μmol/L (or Ab450 <0.048)		
		40 wk <0.025 mg/dL (or Ab450 <0.02)			<0.43 μmol/L (or Ab450 <0.02)		
Conjugated	S	0–0.2 mg/dL		× 17.10	0–3.4 μmol/L		
Bleeding time (BBT)							
Ivy		Normal 2–7 min Borderline 7–11 min			Normal 2–7 min Borderline 7–11 min		
Simplate (G–D)		2.75–8 min			2.75–8 min		
Blood volume	W(H)	M 52–83 mL/kg F 50–75 mL/kg		× 0.001	M 0.052–0.083 L/kg F 0.050–0.075 L/kg		
Brucellosis, agglutinins	S	≤1:8		×1	≤1:8		
C-peptide	P	0.5–2 μg/L (fasting)		× 1	0.5–2 μg/L (fasting)		i (Nichols Institute)
C-reactive protein	S	Cord blood	52–1,330 ng/mL	×1	52–1,330 μg/L		e (Unten and Hokana)
		2–12 yr	67–1,800 ng/mL		67–1,800 μg/L		
CSF. See Cerebrospinal fluid							
Calcitonin	S, P(H,E)	Children	<25–70 pg/mL	× 0.28	<7–19.6 pmol/L		(Endocrine Sciences)
		Adults	<25–150 pg/mL		<7–42 pmol/L		
		Higher in newborn infants					
Calcium, ionized (Ca)	S, P(H), W(H)	Cord blood	5.0–6.0 mg/dL	× 0.25	1.25–1.50 mmol/L		
		Newborn					
		3–24 hr	4.3–5.1 mg/dL		1.07–1.27 mmol/L		
		24–48 hr	4.0–4.7 mg/dL		1.00–1.17 mmol/L		
		Thereafter	4.8–4.92 mg/dL, or		1.12–1.23 mmol/L		
			2.24–2.46 mEq/L	× 0.5	1.12–1.23 mmol/L		
Calcium, total	S	Cord blood	9.0–11.5 mg/dL	× 0.25	2.25–2.88 mmol/L		
		Newborn					
		3–24 hr	9.0–10.6 mg/dL		2.3–2.65 mmol/L		
		24–48 hr	7.0–12.0 mg/dL		1.75–3.0 mmol/L		
		4–7 d	9.0–10.9 mg/dL		2.25–2.73 mmol/L		
		Child	8.8–10.8 mg/dL		2.2–2.70 mmol/L		
		Thereafter	8.4–10.2 mg/dL		2.1–2.55 mmol/L		
	U	Ca in diet					
		Ca-free	5–40 mg/24 hr	× 0.025	0.13–1.0 mmol/24 hr		
		Low to average	50–150 mg/24 hr		1.25–3.8 mmol/24 hr		

Table continued on following page

■ **TABLE 670–2 Reference Ranges for Laboratory Tests** *(Continued)*

Test	Specimen		Reference Range	Factor	Reference Range (SI)	Comments
		Average (20 mmol/24 hr)	100–300 mg/24 hr		2.5–7.5 mmol/24 hr	
	CSF		2.1–2.7 mEq/L or	× 0.50	1.05–1.35 mmol/L	
			4.2–5.4 mg/dl	× 0.25	1.05–1.35 mmol/L	
	F	Average	0.64 g/24 hr	× 25	16 mmol/24 hr	
Carbamazepine. See end of table under Drugs						
Carbon dioxide	W(H)	Newborn	27–40 mm Hg	× 0.1333	3.6–5.3 kPa	
		Infant	27–41 mm Hg		3.6–5.5 kPa	
Partial pressure (P_{CO_2})		Thereafter				
		M	35–48 mm Hg		4.7–6.4 kPa	
		F	32–45 mm Hg		4.3–6.0 kPa	
Total (tco_2)	S, P(H)	Cord blood	14–22 mmol/L	× 1	14–22 mmol/L	
		Premature	14–27 mmol/L		14–27 mmol/L	
		Newborn	13–22 mmol/L		13–22 mmol/L	
		Infant	20–28 mmol/L		20–28 mmol/L	
		Child	20–28 mmol/L		20–28 mmol/L	
		Thereafter	23–30 mmol/L		23–30 mmol/L	
Carbon monoxide	W(E)	Nonsmokers	<2% HbCO	× 0.01	HbCO fraction <0.02	
		Smokers	<10%		<0.10	
		Lethal	>50%		>0.5	
Carboxyhemoglobin. See Carbon monoxide						
β-Carotene	S	Infant	20–70 μg/dL	× 0.0186	0.37–1.30 μmol/L	
		Child	40–130 μg/dL		0.74–2.42 μmol/L	
		Thereafter	60–200 μg/dL		1.12–3.72 μmol/L	
Catecholamines, fractionated	P(E)	Norepinephrine				
		Supine	100–400 pg/mL	× 5.911	591–2,364 pmol/L	
		Standing	300–900 pg/mL		1,773–5,320 pmol/L	
		Epinephrine				
		Supine	<70 pg/mL	× 5.458	<382 pmol/L	
		Standing	<100 pg/mL		<546 pmol/L	
		Dopamine (no postural change)	<30 pg/mL	× 6.528	<196 pmol/L	
	U	Norepinephrine				
		0–1 yr	0–10 μg/24 hr	× 5.911	0–59 nmol/24 hr	
		1–2 yr	0–17 μg/24 hr		0–100 nmol/24 hr	
		2–4 yr	4–29 μg/24 hr		24–171 nmol/24 hr	
		4–7 yr	8–45 μg/24 hr		47–266 nmol/24 hr	
		7–10 yr	13–65 μg/24 hr		77–384 nmol/24 hr	
		Thereafter	15–80 μg/24 hr		87–473 nmol/24 hr	
		Epinephrine				
		0–1 yr	0–2.5 μg/24 hr	× 5.458	0–13.6 nmol/24 hr	
		1–2 yr	0–3.5 μg/24 hr		0–19.1 nmol/24 hr	
		2–4 yr	0–6.0 μg/24 hr		0–32.7 nmol/24 hr	
		4–7 yr	0.2–10 μg/24 hr		1.1–55 nmol/24 hr	
		7–10 yr	0.5–14 μg/24 hr		2.7–76 nmol/24 hr	
		Thereafter	0.5–20 μg/24 hr		2.7–109 nmol/24 hr	
		Fractionated Dopamine				
		0–1 yr	0–85 μg/24 hr	× 6.528	0–555 nmol/24 hr	
		1–2 yr	10–140 μg/24 hr		65–914 nmol/24 hr	
		2–4 yr	40–260 μg/24 hr		261–1,697 nmol/24 hr	
		Thereafter	65–400 μg/24 hr		424–2,611 nmol/24 hr	
Catecholamines, total, free	U	0–1 yr	10–15 μg/24 hr	× 1	10–15 μg/24 hr	
		1–5 yr	15–40 μg/24 hr		15–40 μg/24 hr	
		6–15 yr	20–80 μg/24 hr		20–80 μg/24 hr	
		Thereafter	30–100 μg/24 hr		30–100 μg/24 hr	
Cerebrospinal fluid						
Pressure	CSF	70–180 mm water			70–180 mm water	
Volume	CSF	Child	60–100 mL	× 0.001	0.06–0.10 L	
		Adult	100–160 mL		0.1–0.16 L	
Ceruloplasmin	S	0–5 d	5–26 mg/dL	× 10	50–260 mg/L	n f (Lockitch, et al., *b*)
		1–19 yr	20–46 mg/dL		200–460 mg/L	
Chloral hydrate. See end of table under Drugs						
Chloride	S, P(H)	Cord blood	96–104 mmol/L	× 1	96–104 mmol/L	
		Newborn	97–110 mmol/L		97–110 mmol/L	
		Thereafter	98–106 mmol/L		98–106 mmol/L	
	CSF		118–132 mmol/L	× 1	118–132 mmol/L	
	U	Infant	2–10 mmol/24 hr	× 1	2–10 mmol/24 hr	
		Child	15–40 mmol/24 hr		15–40 mmol/24 hr	
		Thereafter	110–250 mmol/24 hr (varies greatly with Cl intake)		110–250 mmol/24 hr	
	Sweat	Normal	<40 mmol/L	× 1	<40 mmol/L	(Gibson, et al.)
		Borderline	45–60 mmol/L		45–60 mmol/L	
		Cystic fibrosis	>60 mmol/L		>60 mmol/L	
Cholesterol, total	S	1–3 yr	45–182 mg/dL	× 0.0259	1.15–4.70 mmol/L	z (Lockitch, et al., *a*)
		4–6 yr	109–189 mg/dL		2.80–4.80 mmol/L	
	S			× 0.0259		(Mayo Clinic Laboratories)

■ **TABLE 670–2 Reference Ranges for Laboratory Tests** *(Continued)*

Test	Specimen	Reference Range	Factor	Reference Range (SI)	Comments
		Percentiles 5 / 75 / 95		*Percentiles* 5 / 75 / 95	
		M		M	
		6–9 yr 126 172 191 mg/dL		6–9 yr 3.26 4.45 4.94 mmol/L	
		10–14 yr 130 179 204 mg/dL		10–14 yr 3.36 4.63 5.28 mmol/L	
		15–19 yr 114 167 198 mg/dL		15–19 yr 2.95 4.32 5.12 mmol/L	
		Percentiles 5 / 75 / 95		*Percentiles* 5 / 75 / 95	
		F		F	
		6–9 yr 122 173 209 mg/dL		6–9 yr 3.16 4.47 5.41 mmol/L	
		10–14 yr 124 174 217 mg/dL		10–14 yr 3.21 4.50 5.61 mmol/L	
		15–19 yr 125 175 212 mg/dL		15–19 yr 3.23 4.53 5.48 mmol/L	
Chorionic gonadotropin β-subunit (β-hCG)	S, P(E)	Child, male, nonpregnant female <5.0 IU/L	× 1.0	<5.0 IU/mL	
		F (postconception) >5.0 mU/mL		>5.0 IU/L	
		7–10 d >100 mU/mL		>100 IU/L	
		30 d >2,000 mU/mL		>2,000 IU/L	
		40 d 50,000–100,000 mU/mL		50,000–100,000 IU/L	
		10 wk 1000–2000 mU/mL		1000–2000 IU/L	
		>10 wk			
		Trophoblastic disease >100,000		>100,000 IU/L	
Clotting time, Lee-White, 37° C	W	Glass tubes 5–8 min (5–15 min at RT)		Glass tubes 5–8 min (5–15 min at RT)	
		Silicone tubes about 30 min prolonged		Silicone tubes about 30 min prolonged	
Coagulation factor assays	P(C)				
Factor I. See Fibrinogen					
Factor II		0.5–1.5 U/mL or 60–150% of normal	× 1	0.5–1.5 kU/L 60–150 AU	
Factor IV. See Calcium					
Factor V		0.5–2.0 U/mL or 60–150% of normal	× 1	0.5–2.0 kU/L 60–150 AU	
Factor VII		65–135% of normal	× 1	65–135 AU	
Factor VIII		60–145% of normal	× 1	60–145 AU	
Factor VIII antigen		50–200% of normal	× 1	50–200 AU	
Factor IX		60–140% of normal	× 1	60–140 AU	
Factor X		60–130% of normal	× 1	60–130 AU	
Factor XI		65–135% of normal	× 1	65–135 AU	
Factor XII		65–150% of normal	× 1	65–150 AU	
Factor XII (fibrin-stabilizing factor, FSF)	W(C,O)	Minimal hemostatic level 0.02–0.05 U/mL or	× 1,000	20–50 U/L or	
		1–2% of normal	× 1	1–2 AU	
Complement components					
Total hemolytic complement activity	P(E)	75–160 U/mL of plasma CH_{50}	× 1	75–160 IU/mL of plasma CH_{50}	
Total complement decay rate (functional)	P(E)	~10–20%	× 0.01	~0.10–0.20 (fraction of decay rate)	
		Deficiency >50%		0.50 (fraction of decay rate)	
Classical pathway components					
C1q	S	Cord blood 1.0–14.9 mg/dL	× 10	10–149 mg/L	
		1 mo 2.2–6.2 mg/dL		22–62 mg/L	
		6 mo 1.2–7.6 mg/dL		12–76 mg/L	
		Adult 5.1–7.9 mg/dL		51–79 mg/L	
C1r	S	2.5–3.8 mg/dL	× 10	25–38 mg/L	
C1s (C1 esterase)	S	2.5–3.8 mg/dL	× 10	25–38 mg/L	
C2	S	Cord blood 1.6–2.8 mg/dL	× 10	16–28 mg/L	
		1 mo 1.9–3.9 mg/dL		19–39 mg/L	
		6 mo 2.4–3.6 mg/dL		24–36 mg/L	
		Adult 1.6–4.0 mg/dL		16–40 mg/L	
C3	S	Cord blood 57–116 mg/dL	× 10	570–1,160 mg/L	n (Meites)
		1–3 mo 53–131 mg/dL		530–1,310 mg/L	
		3 mo–1 yr 62–180 mg/dL		620–1,800 mg/L	
		1–10 yr 77–195 mg/dL		770–1,950 mg/L	
		Adult 83–177 mg/dL		830–1,770 mg/L	
C4	S	Cord blood 7–23 mg/dL	× 10	70–230 mg/L	n (Meites)
		1–3 mo 7–27 mg/dL		70–270 mg/L	
		3 mo–10 yr 7–40 mg/dL		70–400 mg/L	
		Adult 15–45 mg/dL		150–450 mg/L	
C5	S	Cord blood 3.4–6.2 mg/dL	× 10	34–62 mg/L	
		1 mo 2.3–6.3 mg/dL		23–63 mg/L	
		6 mo 2.4–6.4 mg/dL		24–64 mg/L	
		Adult 3.8–9.0 mg/dL		38–90 mg/L	
C6	S	Cord blood 1.0–4.2 mg/dL	× 10	10–42 mg/L	
		1 mo 2.2–5.2 mg/dL		22–52 mg/L	
		6 mo 3.7–7.1 mg/dL		37–71 mg/L	
		Adult 4.0–7.2 mg/dL		40–72 mg/L	
C7	S	4.9–7.0 mg/dL	× 10	49–70 mg/L	
C8	S	4.3–6.3 mg/dL	× 10	43–63 mg/L	

Table continued on following page

■ **TABLE 670–2 Reference Ranges for Laboratory Tests** *(Continued)*

Test	Specimen		Reference Range	Factor	Reference Range (SI)	Comments
C9	S		4.7–6.9 mg/dL	× 10	47–69 mg/L	
Alternative pathway components						
C4 binding protein	S		18.0–32.0 mg/dL	× 10	180–320 mg/L	
Factor B (C3 proactivator)	P(E)	Cord blood	7.8–15.8 mg/dL	× 10	78–158 mg/L	
RID		1 mo	6.2–28.6 mg/dL		62–286 mg/L	
		6 mo	16.9–29.3 mg/dL		169–293 mg/L	
		Adult	14.7–33.5 mg/dL		147–335 mg/L	
Nephelometry	S	Newborn	14–33 mg/dL	× 10	140–330 mg/L	
		Adult	20–45 mg/dL		200–450 mg/L	
Properdin	S	Cord blood	1.3–1.7 mg/dL	× 10	13–17 mg/L	
		1 mo	0.6–2.2 mg/dL		6–22 mg/L	
		6 mo	1.3–2.5 mg/dL		13–25 mg/L	
		Adult	2.0–3.6 mg/dL		20–36 mg/L	
Regulatory protein b1H-globulin (C3b inactivator-accelerator)	S	Cord blood	26–42 mg/dL	× 10	260–420 mg/L	
		1 mo	24–56 mg/dL		240–560 mg/L	
		6 mo	33–61 mg/dL		330–610 mg/L	
		Adult	40–72 mg/dL		400–720 mg/L	
C1 inhibitor (esterase inhibitor)	P(E)		17.4–24.0 mg/dL	× 10	174–240 mg/L	
Complement decay rate (functional)	S	<20% decay rate		× 0.01	<0.20 (fraction of decay rate)	
					>0.50 (fraction of decay rate)	
		Deficiency >50% decay rate				
C3b inactivator (KAF)	S	Cord blood	1.8–2.6 mg/dL	× 10	18–26 mg/L	
		1 mo	1.5–3.9 mg/dL		15–39 mg/L	
		6 mo	2.3–4.3 mg/dL		23–43 mg/L	
		Adult	2.6–5.4 mg/dL		26–54 mg/L	
S protein	S		41.8–60.0 mg/dL	× 10	418–600 mg/L	
Copper	S	0–5 d	9–46 μg/dL	× 0.157	1.4–7.2 μmol/L	f a (Lockitch, et al., c)
		1–9 yr	80–150 μg/dL		12.6–23.6 μmol/L	
		10–14 yr	80–121 μg/dL		12.6–19.0 μmol/L	
		15–19 yr	64–160 μg/dL		11.3–25.2 μmol/L	
	U	5–18 yr	0.36–7.56 mg/mol Cr.	× 15.7	6–119 μmol/mol Cr.	
Coproporphyrin	U	34–234 μg/24 hr		× 1.5	51–351 nmol/24 hr	
	F (24-hr)	<30 μg/g dry wt		× 1.5	<45 nmol/g dry wt	
		400–1,200 μg/24 hr			600–1,800 nmol/24 hr	
Corticobinding globulin (CBG). See Transcortin						
Cortisol	S, P(H)	Newborn	1–24 μg/dL	× 27.59	28–662 nmol/L	
		Adults				
		0800 hr	5–23 μg/dL		138–635 nmol/L	
		1600 hr	3–15 μg/dL		82–413 nmol/L	
		2000 hr	≤50% of 0800 h	× 0.01	Fraction of 0800 hr ≤0.50	
Cortisol, free	U	Child	2–27 μg/24 hr	× 2.759	5.5–74 nmol/24 hr	
		Adolescent	5–55 μg/24 hr		14–152 nmol/24 hr	
		Adult	10–100 μg/24 hr		27–276 nmol/24 hr	
Creatine kinase	S	Cord blood	70–380 U/L	× 1	70–380 U/L	30° s (Jedeikin, et al.)
		5–8 hr	214–1,175 U/L		214–1,175 U/L	
		24–33 hr	130–1,200 U/L		130–1,200 U/L	
		72–100 hr	87–725 U/L		87–725 U/L	
		Adult	5–130 U/L		5–130 U/L	
Creatine kinase isoenzymes	S		*CKMB* / *CKBB*			
		Cord blood	0.3–3.1% / 0.3–10.5%			
		5–8 hr	1.7–7.9% / 3.6–13.4%			
		24–33 hr	1.8–5.0% / 2.3–8.6%			
		72–100 hr	1.4–5.4% / 5.1–13.3%			
		Adult	0–2% / 0			
Creatinine plasma						
Jaffe, kinetic, or enzymatic	S, P	Cord blood	0.6–1.2 mg/dL	× 88.4	53–106 μmol/L	
		Newborn	0.3–1.0 mg/dL		27–88 μmol/L	
		Infant	0.2–0.4 mg/dL		18–35 μmol/L	
		Child	0.3–0.7 mg/dL		27–62 μmol/L	
		Adolescent	0.5–1.0 mg/dL		44–88 μmol/L	
		Adult				
		M	0.6–1.2 mg/dL		53–106 μmol/L	
		F	0.5–1.1 mg/dL		44–97 μmol/L	
Jaffe, manual	S, P		0.8–1.5 mg/dL	× 88.4	70–133 μmol/L	
	AF	After 37-wk gestation	>2.0 mg/dL	× 88.4	>180 μmol/L	
Creatinine, urinary	U	Premature	8.1–15.0 mg/kg/24 hr	× 8.84	72–133 μmol/kg/24 hr	m d (Meites)
		Full-term	10.4–19.7 mg/kg/24 hr		92–174 μmol/kg/24 hr	
		1.5–7 yr	10–15 mg/kg/24 hr		88–133 μmol/kg/24 hr	
		7–15 yr	5.2–41 mg/kg/24 hr		46–362 μmol/kg/24 hr	
Creatinine clearance (endogenous)	S, P, and U	Newborn	40–65 mL/min/1.73 m^2			
		<40 yr				
		M	97–137 mL/min/1.73 m^2			
		F	88–128 mL/min/1.73 m^2			
		Decreases	~6.5 mL/min/decade			
Cyclic AMP	P(E)	M	5.6–10.9 ng/mL	× 3.04	17–33 nmol/L	

■ **TABLE 670–2 Reference Ranges for Laboratory Tests** *(Continued)*

Test	Specimen	Reference Range	Factor	Reference Range (SI)	Comments
		F 3.6–8.9 ng/mL		11–27 nmol/L	
	U	<3.3 mg/24 h or	× 3040	<10,000 nmol/24 hr	
		<1.64 mg/g Cr.		<6,000 nmol cAMP/g Cr.	
Dehydroepiandrosterone	S	M			(Endocrine Sciences)
		Tanner 1 <9.8 yr 31–345 ng/dL	× 0.0347	1.07–11.96 nmol/L	
		Tanner 2 9.8–14.5 yr 110–495 ng/dL		3.81–17.16 nmol/L	
		Tanner 3 10.7–15.4 yr 170–585 ng/dL		5.89–20.28 nmol/L	
		Tanner 4 11.8–16.2 yr 160–640 ng/dL		5.55–22.19 nmol/L	
		Tanner 5 12.8–17.3 yr 250–900 ng/dL		8.67–31.21 nmol/L	
		Adult 160–800 ng/dL		5.55–27.74 nmol/L	
		F			
		Tanner 1 <9.2 yr 31–345 ng/dL	× 0.0347	1.07–11.96 nmol/L	
		Tanner 2 9.2–13.7 yr 150–570 ng/dL		5.20–19.76 nmol/L	
		Tanner 3 10.0–14.4 yr 200–600 ng/dL		6.93–20.80 nmol/L	
		Tanner 4 10.7–15.6 yr 200–780 ng/dL		6.93–24.27 nmol/L	
		Tanner 5 11.8–18.6 yr 215–850 ng/dL		7.45–29.47 nmol/L	
		Adult Follicular 160–800 ng/dL		5.55–27.74 nmol/L	
		Luteal 160–800 ng/dL		5.55–27.74 nmol/L	
Dehydroepiandrosterone sulfate (DHEA sulfate) (DHEA-S)		M			(Endocrine Sciences)
		Tanner 1 <9.8 yr 13–83 μg/dL	× 0.026	0.34–2.16 μmol/L	
		Tanner 2 9.8–14.5 yr 42–109 μg/dL		1.09–2.83 μmol/L	
		Tanner 3 10.7–15.4 yr 48–200 μg/dL		1.25–5.20 μmol/L	
		Tanner 4 11.8–16.2 yr 102–385 μg/dL		2.65–10.01 μmol/L	
		Tanner 5 12.8–17.3 yr 120–370 μg/dL		3.12–9.62 μmol/L	
		Adult 180–450 μg/dL		4.68–11.70 μmol/L	
		F			
		Tanner 1 <9.2 yr 19–114 μg/dL		0.49–2.96 μmol/L	
		Tanner 2 9.2–13.7 yr 34–129 μg/dL		0.88–3.35 μmol/L	
		Tanner 3 10.0–14.4 yr 32–326 μg/dL		0.83–8.48 μmol/L	
		Tanner 4 10.7–15.6 yr 58–260 μg/dL		1.51–6.76 μmol/L	
		Tanner 5 11.8–18.6 yr 44–248 μg/dL		1.14–6.45 μmol/L	
		Adult 60–255 μg/dL		1.56–6.63 μmol/L	
Diazepam. See end of table under Drugs					
Differential count. See Leukocyte differential count					
Digitoxin. See end of table under Drugs					
Digoxin. See end of table under Drugs					
Dihydrotestosterone (DHT)	S	M			(Endocrine Sciences)
		Tanner 1 <9.8 yr <3 ng/dL	× 0.03443	<0.10 nmol/L	
		Tanner 2 9.8–14.5 yr 3–17 ng/dL		0.10–0.59 nmol/L	
		Tanner 3 10.7–15.4 yr 8–33 ng/dL		0.28–1.14 nmol/L	
		Tanner 4 11.8–16.2 yr 22–52 ng/dL		0.76–1.79 nmol/L	
		Tanner 5 12.8–17.3 yr 24–65 ng/dL		0.83–2.24 nmol/L	
		Adult 30–85 ng/dL		1.03–2.93 nmol/L	
		F			
		Tanner 1 <9.2 yr <3 ng/dL		<0.10 nmol/L	
		Tanner 2 9.2–13.7 yr 5–12 ng/dL		0.17–0.41 nmol/L	
		Tanner 3 10.0–14.4 yr 7–19 ng/dL		0.24–0.65 nmol/L	
		Tanner 4 10.7–15.6 yr 4–13 ng/dL		0.14–0.45 nmol/L	
		Tanner 5 11.8–18.6 yr 3–18 ng/dL		0.10–0.62 nmol/L	
		Adult Follicular 4–22 ng/dL		0.14–0.76 nmol/L	
		Luteal 4–22 ng/dL		0.14–0.76 nmol/L	
Diphenylhydantoin. See end of table under Drugs					
Disaccharide absorption test	S	Change in glucose from fasting value	× 0.055	Change in glucose from fasting value	
		Normal >30 mg/dL		>1.67 mmol/L	
		Inconclusive 20–30 mg/dL		1.11–1.67 mmol/L	
		Abnormal <20 mg/dL		<1.11 mmol/L	
Dithionite tube test. See Sickle cell tests					
Electrophoresis, Hemoglobin. See Hemoglobin electrophoresis					
Eosinophil count	W(E,H) capillary	50–350 cells/mm³ (μL)	× 10^6	50–350 × 10^6 cells/L	
Epinephrine. See Catecholamines, fractionated					
Erythrocyte count RBC count)	W(E)	***Millions of cells/mm³ (μL)***		***× 10^{12} cells/L***	
		Cord blood 3.9–5.5	× 1	3.9–5.5	
		1–3 d (capillary) 4.0–6.6		4.0–6.6	
		1 wk 3.9–6.3		3.9–6.3	
		2 wk 3.6–6.2		3.6–6.2	
		1 mo 3.0–5.4		3.0–5.4	
		2 mo 2.7–4.9		2.7–4.9	
		3–6 mo 3.1–4.5		3.1–4.5	

Table continued on following page

■ **TABLE 670–2 Reference Ranges for Laboratory Tests** *(Continued)*

Test	Specimen	Reference Range	Factor	Reference Range (SI)	Comments
		0.5–2 yr 3.7–5.3		3.7–5.3	
		2–6 yr 3.9–5.3		3.9–5.3	
		6–12 yr 4.0–5.2		4.0–5.2	
		12–18 yr			
		M 4.5–5.3		4.5–5.3	
		F 4.1–5.1		4.1–5.1	
		18–49 yr			
		M 4.5–5.9		4.5–5.9	
		F 4.0–5.2		4.0–5.2	
Erythrocyte sedimentation rate (ESR)	W(E)				
Westergren, modified		Child 0–10 mm/hr		0–10 mm/hr	
		Adult			
		M < 50 yr 0–15 mm/hr		0–15 mm/hr	
		F < 50 yr 0–20 mm/hr		0–20 mm/hr	
Wintrobe		Child 0–13 mm/hr		0–13 mm/hr	
		Adult			
		M 0–9 mm/hr		0–9 mm/hr	
		F 0–20 mm/hr		0–20 mm/hr	
ZETA		41–54%		41–54 AU	
Erythropoietin RIA	S	<5–20 mU/mL	× 1	<5–20 U/L	
Hemagglutination		25–125 mU/mL		25–125 U/L	
Bioassay		5–18 mU/mL		5–18 U/L	
Estradiol	S	M	× 36.71		(Endocrine Sciences)
		Tanner 1 <9.8 yr 0.5–1.1 ng/dL		18–40 pmol/L	
		Tanner 2 9.8–14.5 yr 0.5–1.6 ng/dL		18–59 pmol/L	
		Tanner 3 10.7–15.4 yr 0.5–2.5 ng/dL		18–92 pmol/L	
		Tanner 4 11.8–16.2 yr 1.0–3.6 ng/dL		37–132 pmol/L	
		Tanner 5 12.8–17.3 yr 1.0–3.6 ng/dL		37–132 pmol/L	
		Adult 0.8–3.5 ng/dL		29–128 pmol/L	
		F			
		Tanner 1 <9.2 yr 0.5–2.0 ng/dL		18–73 pmol/L	
		Tanner 2 9.2–13.7 yr 1.0–2.4 ng/dL		37–88 pmol/L	
		Tanner 3 10.0–14.4 yr 0.7–6.0 ng/dL		26–220 pmol/L	
		Tanner 4 10.7–15.6 yr 2.1–8.5 ng/dL		77–312 pmol/L	
		Tanner 5 11.8–18.6 yr 3.4–17 ng/dL		125–624 pmol/L	
		Adult Follicular 3–10 ng/dL		110–367 pmol/L	
		Luteal 7–30 ng/dL		257–1,100 pmol/L	
Estradiol, urinary	U	Adult M 0–6 µg/24 hr	× 3.671	0–22 nmol/24 hr	
		Adult F			
		Follicular 0–3 µg/24 hr		0–11 nmol/24 hr	
		Ovulatory peak 4–14 µg/24 hr		15–51 nmol/24 hr	
		Luteal 4–10 µg/24 hr		15–37 nmol/24 hr	
Estriol (E_3), free	S	***Wk of Gestation***			
		25 3.5–10.0 µg/L	× 3.47	12.1–34.7 nmol/L	
		28 4.0–12.5 µg/L		13.9–43.4 nmol/L	
		30 4.5–14.0 µg/L		15.6–48.6 nmol/L	
		32 5.0–16.0 µg/L		17.4–55.5 nmol/L	
		34 5.5–18.5 µg/L		19.1–64.2 nmol/L	
		36 7.0–25.0 µg/L		24.3–86.8 nmol/L	
		37 8.0–28.0 µg/L		27.8–97.2 nmol/L	
		38 9.0–32.0 µg/L		31.2–111.0 nmol/L	
		39 10.0–34.0 µg/L		34.7–118.0 nmol/L	
		40–41 10.5–25.0 µg/L		36.4–86.8 nmol/L	
	AF	***Wk of Pregnancy***			
		16–20 1.0–3.2 ng/mL (95% range)	× 3.47	3.5–11.1 nmol/L (95% range)	
		20–24 2.1–7.8 ng/mL (95% range)		7.3–27.1 nmol/L (95% range)	
		24–28 2.1–7.8 ng/mL (95% range)		7.3–27.1 nmol/L (95% range)	
		28–32 4.0–13.6 ng/mL (95% range)		13.9–47.2 nmol/L (95% range)	
		32–36 3.6–15.5 ng/mL (95% range)		12.5–53.8 nmol/L (95% range)	
		36–38 4.6–18.0 ng/mL (95% range)		16.0–62.5 nmol/L (95% range)	
		38–40 5.4–19.8 ng/mL (95% range)		18.7–68.7 nmol/L (95% range)	
Estriol (E_3), total	S	***Pregnancy (wk)***			
		24–28 30–170 ng/mL	× 3.47	104–590 nmol/L	
		28–32 40–220 ng/mL		140–760 nmol/L	
		32–36 60–280 ng/mL		208–970 nmol/L	
		36–40 80–350 ng/mL		280–1,210 nmol/L	
		Adult M and non-pregnant F <2 ng/mL		<7 nmol/L	
	U	***Pregnancy (wk)***			
		30 6–18 mg/24 hr	× 3.47	21–62 µmol/24 hr	
		35 9–28 mg/24 hr		31–97 µmol/24 hr	
		40 13–42 mg/24 hr		45–146 µmol/24 hr	
		Decrease of >40% of previous value suggests fetus at risk		Fraction of previous value of <0.60 suggests fetus at risk	

■ **TABLE 670–2 Reference Ranges for Laboratory Tests** *(Continued)*

Test	Specimen	Reference Range		Factor	Reference Range (SI)	Comments
Estrogens, total	S	Child	<30 pg/mL	× 1	<30 ng/L	
		M	40–115 pg/mL		40–115 ng/L	
		F cycle (days)				
		1–10 d	61–394 pg/mL		61–394 ng/L	
		11–20 d	122–437 pg/mL		122–437 ng/L	
		21–30 d	156–350 pg/mL		156–350 ng/L	
		Prepubertal	≤40 pg/mL		≤40 ng/L	
	U (24 hr)	Child	<10 μg/24 hr	× 1	<10 μg/24 hr	
		Adult (M)	5–25 μg/24 hr		5–25 μg/24 hr	
		F				
		Preovulation	5–25 μg/24 hr		5–25 μg/24 hr	
		Ovulation	28–100 μg/24 hr		28–100 μg/24 hr	
		Luteal peak	22–80 μg/24 hr		22–80 μg/24 hr	
		Pregnancy	<45,000 μg/24 hr		<45,000 μg/24 hr	
		Postmenopausal	<10 μg/24 hr		<10 μg/24 hr	
Ethanol. See end of table under Drugs						
Ethosuximide. See end of table under Drugs						
Fat, fecal	F (72 hr)	Infant, breast-fed	<1 g/24 hr	× 1	<1 g/24 hr	
		0–6 yr	<2 g/24 hr		<2 g/24 hr	
		Adult				
		Normal diet	<7 g/24 hr		<7 g/24 hr	
		Fat-free diet	<4 g/24 hr		<4 g/24 hr	
		Coefficient of Fat Absorption (%)			***Absorbed Fraction***	
		Infant		× 0.01		
		Breast-fed	>93		>0.93	
		Formula-fed	>83		>0.83	
		>1 yr	≥95		≥0.95	
Free fatty acids	S	Premature 10–55 d	0.15–0.71 mmol/L	× 1	0.15–0.71 mmol/L	(Meites)
Ferric chloride test	U	Negative			Negative	
Ferritin	S	Newborn	25–200 ng/mL	× 1	25–200 μg/L	
		1 mo	200–600 ng/mL		200–600 μg/L	
		2–5 mo	50–200 ng/mL		50–200 μg/L	
		6 mo–15 yr	7–140 ng/mL		7–140 μg/L	
		Adult				
		M	15–200 ng/mL		15–200 μg/L	
		F	12–150 ng/mL		12–150 μg/L	
α-Fetoprotein (AFP)	S maternal	***Pregnancy (wk)***	***Median***		***Median***	
		15	34 ng/mL	× 1	34 μg/L	
		16	38 ng/mL		38 μg/L	
		17	44 ng/mL		44 μg/L	
		18	49 ng/mL		49 μg/L	
		19	56.5 ng/mL		56.5 μg/L	
		20	66 ng/mL		66 μg/L	
	AF		***Mean***			
		15	13.5 ± 3.42 μg/mL			
		16	11.7 ± 3.38 μg/mL			
		17	10.3 ± 3.03 μg/mL			
		18	9.5 ± 3.22 μg/mL			
		19	7.1 ± 2.86 μg/mL			
		20	5.0 ± 2.45 μg/mL			
Fibrin degradation products						
Agglutination (Thrombo-Wellco test)	W; special tube thrombin and proteolytic inhibitors		<10 μg/mL	× 1	<10 mg/L	
	U: 2 mL in special tube (see above)		<0.25 μg/mL	× 1	<0.25 mg/L	
Fibrinogen	P(NaCl)	Newborn	125–300 mg/dL	× 0.01	1.25–3.00 g/L	
		Adult	200–400 mg/dL		2.00–4.00 g/L	
Folate	S	Newborn	7.0–32 ng/mL	× 2.265	15.9–72.4 nmol/L	
		Thereafter	1.8–9 ng/mL		4.1–20.4 nmol/L	
	W(E)		150–450 ng/mL RBCs		340–1,020 nmol/L cells	
Follicle-stimulating hormone (FSH)	S	M				
		Tanner 1 <9.8 yr	0.26–3.0 mIU/mL	× 1	0.26–3.0 U/L	
		Tanner 2 9.8–14.5 yr	1.8–3.2 mIU/mL		1.8–3.2 U/L	
		Tanner 3 10.7–15.4 yr	1.2–5.8 mIU/mL		1.2–5.8 U/L	
		Tanner 4 11.8–16.2 yr	2.0–9.2 mIU/mL		2.0–9.2 U/L	
		Tanner 5 12.8–17.3 yr	2.6–11.0 mIU/mL		2.6–11.0 U/L	
		Adult	2.0–9.2 mIU/mL		2.0–9.2 U/L	
		F				
		Tanner 1 <9.2 yr	1.0–4.2 mIU/mL		1.0–4.2 U/L	
		Tanner 2 9.2–13.7 yr	1.0–10.8 mIU/mL		1.0–10.8 U/L	
		Tanner 3 10.0–14.4 yr	1.5–12.8 mIU/mL		1.5–12.8 U/L	
		Tanner 4 10.7–15.6 yr	1.5–11.7 mIU/mL		1.5–11.7 U/L	
		Tanner 5 11.8–18.6 yr	1.0–9.2 mIU/mL		1.0–9.2 U/L	

Table continued on following page

■ **TABLE 670–2 Reference Ranges for Laboratory Tests** *(Continued)*

Test	Specimen	Reference Range		Factor	Reference Range (SI)	Comments
		Adult				
		Follicular	1.8–11.2 mIU/mL		1.8–11.2 U/L	
		Midcycle	6–35 mIU/mL		6–35 U/L	
		Luteal	1.8–11.2 mIU/mL		1.8–11.2 U/L	
Fructosamine	S	0–3 yr	1.56–2.27 mmol/L	× 1	1.56–2.27 mmol/L	c (De Schepper, et al.)
		3–6 yr	1.73–2.34 mmol/L		1.73–2.34 mmol/L	
		6–9 yr	1.82–2.56 mmol/L		1.82–2.56 mmol/L	
		9–15 yr	2.02–2.63 mmol/L		2.02–2.63 mmol/L	
Galactose	S	Newborn	0–20 mg/dL	× 0.0555	0–1.11 mmol/L	
	P	5 mo–17 yr	0.0–0.5 mg/dL		0.0–0.03 mmol/L	z (Pesce and Boudorian)
	U	Newborn	≤60 mg/dL	× 0.0555	≤3.33 mmol/L	
		Thereafter	14 mg/24 hr	× 0.00555	<0.08 mmol/24 hr	
Galactose-1-PO_4	W(H)	5 mo–17 yr	0–44 μg/g Hgb	× 0.0038	0–0.17 μmol/g Hgb	v (Pesce and Boudorian)
Galactose-1-PO_4 uridylyltransferase	W(H)	18–26 U/g Hgb		× 1	18–26 U/g Hgb	(Pesce and Boudorian)
Gastrin	S(fasting)	Children	<10–125 pg/mL	× 1	<10–125 ng/L	m (Dickinson and Hamilton)
Glucagon	S	Neonate (1–7 d)	210–1,500 pg/mL	× 1	210–1,500 ng/L	(Endocrine Sciences)
		Children and adults	25–250 pg/mL		25–250 ng/L	
Glucose	S	Cord blood	45–96 mg/dL	× 0.0555	2.5–5.3 mmol/L	
		Newborn				
		1 d	40–60 mg/dL		2.2–3.3 mmol/L	
		>1 d	50–90 mg/dL		2.8–5.0 mmol/L	
		Child	60–100 mg/dL		3.3–5.5 mmol/L	
		Adult	70–105 mg/dL		3.9–5.8 mmol/L	
	W (H)	Adult	65–95 mg/dL		3.6–5.3 mmol/L	
	CSF	Adult	40–70 mg/dL		2.2–3.9 mmol/L	
Quantitative, enzymatic	U	<0.5 g/24 hr		× 5.55	<2.8 mmol/24 hr	
Qualitative	U	Negative			Negative	
Glucose, 2 hr pc	S	<120 mg/dL		× 0.0555	<6.7 mmol/L	
		(For diabetes, see Glucose tolerance test, oral)				
Glucose-6-phosphate dehydrogenase in erythrocytes	W(E,H,C)					
Bishop, modified		Adult			Adult	
		3.4–8.0 U/g Hb		× 0.0645	0.22–0.52 mU/mol Hb	
		98.6–232 U/10^{12} RBC		× 10^{-3}	0.10–0.23 nU/10^6 RBC	
		1.16–2.72 U/mL RBC		× 1	1.16–2.72 kU/L RBC	
		Newborn: 50% higher			Newborn: 50% higher	
Glucose tolerance test (GTT), oral	S		Normal / Diabetic		Normal / Diabetic	
Adult dose: 75 g		Fasting	70–105 mg/dL / >115 mg/dL	× 0.0555	3.9–5.8 mmol/L / >6.4 mmol/L	
Child dose: 1.75 g/kg of ideal weight up to maximum of 75 g		60 min	120–170 mg/dL / ≥200 mg/dL		6.7–9.4 mmol/L / ≥11 mmol/L	
		90 min	100–140 mg/dL / ≥200 mg/dL		5.6–7.8 mmol/L / ≥11 mmol/L	
		120 min	70–120 mg/dL / ≥140 mg/dL		3.9–6.7 mmol/L / ≥7.8 mmol/L	
γ-Glutamyltranspeptidase (GGT, GGTP)	S	Cord blood	37–193 U/L	× 1	37–193 U/L	37° s (Knight and Haymond)
		0–1 mo	13–147 U/L		13–147 U/L	
		1–2 mo	12–123 U/L		12–123 U/L	
		2–4 mo	8–90 U/L		8–90 U/L	
		4 mo–10 yr	5–32 U/L		5–32 U/L	
		10–15 yr	5–24 U/L		5–24 U/L	
Growth hormone (hGH, somatotropin)	S, P(E,H)	Newborn				(Endocrine Sciences)
		1 d	5–53 ng/mL	× 1	5–53 μg/L	
		1 wk	5–27 ng/mL		5–27 μg/L	
		1–12 mo	2–10 ng/mL		2–10 μg/L	
	Fasting, at rest	Child	<0.7–6 ng/mL		<0.7–6 μg/L	
		Adult	<0.7–6 ng/mL		<0.7–6 μg/L	
Ham's test. See Acidified serum test						
Haptoglobin (Hp)	S					
RID		30–175 mg/dL		× 10	300–1750 mg/L	
Sephadex		40–180 mg Hb bound/dL of serum			400–1800 mgHb bound/L of serum	
Nephelometry		Newborn	5–48 mg/dL	× 10	50–480 mg/L	
		Thereafter	25–175 mg/dL		250–1750 mg/L	
HDL cholesterol	S	1–13 yr	35–84 mg/dL	× 0.0259	0.9–2.15 mmol/L	f m (Meites)
		14–19 yr	35–65 mg/dL		0.90–1.65 mmol/L	
Hematocrit (HCT, Hct)	W(E)		***Per cent Packed Red Cells (Vol Red Cells/Vol Whole Blood Cells × 100)***		***Volume Fraction (Vol Red Cells/ Vol Whole Blood)***	
Calculated from MCV and RBC (electronic displacement or laser)		1 d (capillary)	48–69%	× 0.01	0.48–0.69	
		2 d	48–75%		0.48–0.75	
		3 d	44–72%		0.44–0.72	
		2 mo	28–42%		0.28–0.42	
		6–12 yr	35–45%		0.35–0.45	
		12–18 yr				
		M	37–49%		0.37–0.49	
		F	36–46%		0.36–0.46	
		18–49 yr				
		M	41–53%		0.41–0.53	
		F	36–46%		0.36–0.46	

■ **TABLE 670–2 Reference Ranges for Laboratory Tests** *(Continued)*

Test	Specimen	Reference Range	Factor	Reference Range (SI)	Comments
Hemoglobin (Hb)	W(E)	1–3 d (capillary) 14.5–22.5 g/dL	× 0.155	2.25–3.49 mmol/L	MW Hgb = 64,500
		2 mo 9.0–14.0 g/dL		1.40–2.17 mmol/L	
		6–12 yr 11.5–15.5 g/dL		1.78–2.40 mmol/L	
		12–18 yr			
		M 13.0–16.0 g/dL		2.02–2.48 mmol/L	
		F 12.0–16.0 g/dL		1.86–2.48 mmol/L	
		18–49 yr			
		M 13.5–17.5 g/dL		2.09–2.27 mmol/L	
		F 12.0–16.0 g/dL		1.86–2.48 mmol/L	
	P(H)	<10 mg/dL	× 0.155	<1.55 μmol/L	
		<3 mg/dL with butterfly set-up and 18-g needle		<0.47 μmol/L with butterfly set-up and 18-g needle	
	U	Negative		Negative	
		Per cent of Total Hemoglobin		*Fraction of Total Hemoglobin*	
Glycohemoglobin	W(H)	1–5 yr 2.1–7.7%	× 0.01	1–5 yr 0.021–0.077	
Hemoglobin A1c		5–16 yr 3.0–6.2%		5–16 yr 0.030–0.062	q (Meites)
Total glycohemoglobin	W(H)	4–16 yr 6.0–10.0%		4–16 yr 0.060–0.100	o (Meites)
Hemoglobin A	W(E,C,H)	>95%	× 0.01	Fraction of hemoglobin >0.95	
Hemoglobin A_2 (HbA_2)	W(E,O)	Adult: 1.5–3.5% (2 SD)		0.015–0.035 (2 SD) mass fraction	
		Lower in infants <1 yr			
Hemoglobin electrophoresis	W(H,E,C)	HbA >95%	× 0.01	HbA >0.95 mass fraction	
		HbA_2 1.5–3.5%		HbA_2 0.015–.035 mass fraction	
		HbF <2%		HbF <0.02 mass fraction	
Hemoglobin F	W(E)				
Alkali denaturation		1 d 63–92 %HbF	× 0.01	0.62–0.92 mass fraction	
		5 d 65–88 %HbF		0.65–0.88 mass fraction	
		3 wk 55–85 %HbF		0.55–0.85 mass fraction	
		6–9 wk 31–75 %HbF		0.31–0.75 mass fraction	
		3–4 mo <2–59 %HbF		<0.02–0.59 mass fraction	
		6 mo <2–9 %HbF		<0.02–0.09 mass fraction	
		Adult <2 %HbF		<0.02 mass fraction	
Hemoglobin H (HbH)	W(H,E,C)				
Isopropanol precipitation		No precipitation at 40 min		No precipitation at 40 min	
Homovanillic acid	U (24-hr)	0–1 yr <32.2 mg/g creatinine	× 0.62	<20 mmol/mol creatinine	p (Meites)
		2–4 yr <22 mg/g creatinine		<14 mmol/mol creatinine	
		5–19 yr <14 mg/g creatinine		<8 mmol/mol creatinine	
17-Hydroxycorticosteroids (17-OHCS)	U	0–1 yr 0.5–1.0 mg/24 hr	× 2.76	1.4–2.8 μmol/24 hr	(Conversion based on hydrocortisone MW 362)
		Child 1.0–5.6 mg/24 hr		2.8–15.5 μmol/24 hr	
		Adult			
		M 3.0–10.0 mg/24 hr		8.2–27.6 μmol/24 hr	
		F 2.0–8.0 mg/24 hr or 3–7 mg/g creatinine	× 3.12	5.5–22 μmol/24 hr or 0.9–2.5 mmol/mol creatinine	
5-Hydroxyindoleacetic acid (5-HIAA)					
Qualitative	U	Negative		Negative	
Quantitative	U	2–8 mg/24 hr	× 5.230	10.5–42 μmol/24 hr	
17-Hydroxyprogesterone (17-OHP)	S	Premature infants			
		26–28 wk, day 4 124–841 ng/dL	× 0.03029	3.76–25.5 nmol/L	
		31–35 wk, day 4 26–568 ng/dL		0.79–17.2 nmol/L	(Endocrine Sciences)
		Full-term infants			
		3 d 7–77 ng/dL		0.2–2.33 nmol/L	
		1–12 mo			
		Male			
		Peak values between 30 and 60 d 40–200 ng/dL		Peak values of 1.21–6.1 nmol/L between 30 and 60 d	
		Female 13–106 ng/dL		0.39–3.21 nmol/L	
		M			
		Tanner 1 <9.8 yr 3–90 ng/dL		0.09–2.73 nmol/L	
		Tanner 2 9.8–14.5 yr 5–115 ng/dL		0.15–3.48 nmol/L	
		Tanner 3 10.7–15.4 yr 10–138 ng/dL		0.30–4.18 nmol/L	
		Tanner 4 11.8–16.2 yr 29–180 ng/dL		0.88–5.45 nmol/L	
		Tanner 5 12.8–17.3 yr 24–175 ng/dL		0.73–5.30 nmol/L	
		Adult 27–199 ng/dL		0.82–6.03 nmol/L	
		F			
		Tanner 1 <9.2 yr 3–82 ng/dL		0.09–2.48 nmol/L	
		Tanner 2 9.2–13.7 yr 11–98 ng/dL		0.33–2.97 nmol/L	
		Tanner 3 10.0–14.4 yr 11–155 ng/dL		0.33–4.69 nmol/L	
		Tanner 4 10.7–15.6 yr 18–230 ng/dL		0.55–6.97 nmol/L	
		Tanner 5 11.8–18.6 yr 20–265 ng/dL		0.61–8.03 nmol/L	
		Adult Follicular 15–70 ng/dL		0.45–2.12 nmol/L	
		Luteal 35–290 ng/dL		1.06–8.78 nmol/L	
Hydroxyproline, free and bound	U	3 d 33–112 μmol/24 hr	× 1	33–112 μmol/24 hr	c (Meites)
		10 d 148–225 μmol/24 hr		148–225 μmol/24 hr	
		20 d 229–310 μmol/24 hr		229–310 μmol/24 hr	
Hypoxanthine	W	12–36 hr 2.7–11.2 μmol/L	× 1	2.7–11.2 μmol/L	(Jung, et al.)
		3 d 1.3–7.9 μmol/L		1.3–7.9 μmol/L	

Table continued on following page

■ **TABLE 670–2 Reference Ranges for Laboratory Tests** *(Continued)*

Test	Specimen		Reference Range	Factor	Reference Range (SI)	Comments
		5 d	0.6–5.7 µmol/L		0.6–5.7 µmol/L	
	CSF	0–1 mo	1.8–5.5 µmol/L		1.8–5.5 µmol/L	(Meites)
Immunoglobulin A (IgA)	S	Cord blood	1.4–3.6 mg/dL	× 10	14–36 mg/L	n (Meites)
		1–3 mo	1.3–53 mg/dL		13–530 mg/L	
		4–6 mo	4.4–84 mg/dL		44–840 mg/L	
		7 mo–1 yr	11–106 mg/dL		110–1,060 mg/L	
		2–5 yr	14–159 mg/dL		140–1,590 mg/L	
		6–10 yr	33–236 mg/dL		330–2,360 mg/L	
		Adult	70–312 mg/dL		700–3,120 mg/L	
Immunoglobulin D (IgD)	S	Newborn	None detected	× 10	None detected	
		Thereafter	0–8 mg/dL		0–80 mg/L	
Immunoglobulin E (IgE)	S	M	0–230 IU/mL	× 1	0–230 kIU/L	
		F	0–170 IU/mL		0–170 kIU/L	
Immunoglobulin G (IgG)	S	Cord blood	636–1,606 mg/dL	× 0.01	6.36–16.06 g/L	n (Meites)
		1 mo	251–906 mg/dL		2.51–9.06 g/L	
		2–4 mo	176–601 mg/dL		1.76–6.01 g/L	
		5–12 mo	172–1,069 mg/dL		1.72–10.69 g/L	
		1–5 yr	345–1,236 mg/dL		3.45–12.36 g/L	
		6–10 yr	608–1,572 mg/dL		6.08–15.72 g/L	
		Adult	639–1,349 mg/dL		6.39–13.49 g/L	
Subclasses	S			× 10		(Mayo Clinic)

	IgG1	IgG2	IgG3	IgG4	IgG1	IgG2	IgG3	IgG4
Cord	435–1,084 mg/dL	143–453 mg/dL	27–146 mg/dL	1–47 mg/dL	4,350–10,840 g/L	1,430–4,530 g/L	70–1,460 g/L	10–470 g/L
1–7 d	381–937 mg/dL	117–382 mg/dL	21–115 mg/dL	1–44 mg/dL	3,810–9,370 g/L	1,170–3,820 g/L	10–1,150 g/L	10–440 g/L
8–14 d	327–790 mg/dL	92–310 mg/dL	16–85 mg/dL	1–40 mg/dL	3,270–7,900 g/L	920–3,100 g/L	160–850 g/L	10–400 g/L
3–4 wk	218–496 mg/dL	40–167 mg/dL	4–23 mg/dL	1–33 mg/dL	2,180–4,960 g/L	400–1,670 g/L	40–230 g/L	10–330 g/L
2 mo	194–480 mg/dL	35–164 mg/dL	4–36 mg/dL	1–30 mg/dL	1,940–4,800 g/L	350–1,640 g/L	40–360 g/L	10–300 g/L
3 mo	167–447 mg/dL	28–157 mg/dL	4–52 mg/dL	1–24 mg/dL	1,670–4,470 g/L	280–1,570 g/L	40–520 g/L	10–240 g/L
4 mo	143–394 mg/dL	23–147 mg/dL	4–65 mg/dL	1–14 mg/dL	1,430–3,940 g/L	230–1,470 g/L	40–650 g/L	10–140 g/L
5 mo	158–392 mg/dL	24–132 mg/dL	6–68 mg/dL	1–13 mg/dL	1,580–3,920 g/L	240–1,320 g/L	60–680 g/L	10–130 g/L
6 mo	175–390 mg/dL	24–115 mg/dL	8–72 mg/dL	1–11 mg/dL	1,750–3,900 g/L	240–1,150 g/L	80–720 g/L	10–110 g/L
7 mo	190–388 mg/dL	25–100 mg/dL	10–75 mg/dL	1–10 mg/dL	1,900–3,880 g/L	250–1,000 g/L	100–750 g/L	10–100 g/L
8 mo	200–417 mg/dL	26–123 mg/dL	10–76 mg/dL	1–16 mg/dL	2,000–4,170 g/L	260–1,230 g/L	100–760 g/L	10–160 g/L
9 mo	211–450 mg/dL	26–149 mg/dL	10–77 mg/dL	1–22 mg/dL	2,110–4,500 g/L	260–1,490 g/L	100–770 g/L	10–220 g/L
10–12 mo	241–543 mg/dL	28–221 mg/dL	10–80 mg/dL	1–39 mg/dL	2,410–5,430 g/L	280–2,210 g/L	100–800 g/L	10–390 g/L
13–20 mo	281–692 mg/dL	30–343 mg/dL	10–88 mg/dL	1–68 mg/dL	2,810–6,920 g/L	300–3,430 g/L	100–880 g/L	10–680 g/L
21 mo–<3 yr	310–729 mg/dL	46–387 mg/dL	10–96 mg/dL	1–77 mg/dL	3,100–7,290 g/L	460–3,870 g/L	100–960 g/L	10–770 g/L
3 yr	348–773 mg/dL	72–441 mg/dL	10–105 mg/dL	1–87 mg/dL	3,480–7,730 g/L	720–4,410 g/L	100–1,050 g/L	10–870 g/L
4 yr	370–804 mg/dL	88–455 mg/dL	11–108 mg/dL	1–97 mg/dL	3,700–8,040 g/L	880–4,550 g/L	110–1,080 g/L	10–970 g/L
5 yr	375–835 mg/dL	94–468 mg/dL	12–111 mg/dL	1–106 mg/dL	3,750–8,350 g/L	940–4,680 g/L	120–1,110 g/L	10–1,060 g/L
6 yr	380–866 mg/dL	100–481 mg/dL	14–115 mg/dL	1–115 mg/dL	3,800–8,660 g/L	1,000–4,810 g/L	140–1,150 g/L	10–1,150 g/L
7 yr	385–896 mg/dL	105–494 mg/dL	16–118 mg/dL	1–124 mg/dL	3,850–8,960 g/L	1,050–4,940 g/L	160–1,180 g/L	10–1,240 g/L
8 yr	390–927 mg/dL	111–507 mg/dL	18–122 mg/dL	1–133 mg/dL	3,900–9,270 g/L	1,110–5,070 g/L	180–1,220 g/L	10–1,330 g/L
9 yr	395–958 mg/dL	117–520 mg/dL	19–125 mg/dL	1–142 mg/dL	3,950–9,580 g/L	1,170–5,200 g/L	190–1,250 g/L	10–1,420 g/L
10 yr	400–989 mg/dL	123–534 mg/dL	21–129 mg/dL	1–151 mg/dL	4,000–9,890 g/L	1,230–5,340 g/L	210–1,290 g/L	10–1,510 g/L
11 yr	405–1,020 mg/dL	128–547 mg/dL	23–132 mg/dL	1–160 mg/dL	4,050–10,200 g/L	1,280–5,470 g/L	230–1,320 g/L	10–1,600 g/L
12 yr	410–1,051 mg/dL	134–560 mg/dL	25–136 mg/dL	1–169 mg/dL	4,100–10,510 g/L	1,340–5,600 g/L	250–1,360 g/L	10–1,690 g/L
13 yr	415–1,081 mg/dL	140–573 mg/dL	27–139 mg/dL	1–178 mg/dL	4,150–10,810 g/L	1,400–5,730 g/L	270–1,390 g/L	10–1,780 g/L
14 yr	419–1,102 mg/dL	145–582 mg/dL	28–141 mg/dL	1–184 mg/dL	4,190–11,020 g/L	1,450–5,820 g/L	280–1,410 g/L	10–1,840 g/L
≥15 yr	423–1,112 mg/dL	149–586 mg/dL	29–142 mg/dL	1–187 mg/dL	4,230–11,120 g/L	1,490–5,860 g/L	290–1,420 g/L	10–1,870 g/L

Test	Specimen		Reference Range	Factor	Reference Range (SI)	Comments
Immunoglobulin M (IgM)	S	Cord blood	6.3–25 mg/dL	× 10	63–250 mg/L	n (Meites)
		1–4 mo	17–105 mg/dL		170–1,050 mg/L	
		5–9 mo	33–126 mg/dL		300–1,260 mg/L	
		10 mo–1 yr	41–173 mg/dL		410–1,730 mg/L	
		2–8 yr	43–207 mg/dL		430–2,070 mg/L	
		9–10 yr	52–242 mg/dL		520–2,420 mg/L	
		Adult	56–352 mg/dL		560–3,520 mg/L	
Insulin (12-hr fasting)	S	Newborn	3–20 µU/mL	× 1.0	3–20 mU/L	
		Thereafter	7–24 µU/mL		7–24 mU/L	
Insulin with oral glucose tolerance test	S		Insulin			
		0 min	7–24 µU/mL	× 1	7–24 mU/L	
		30 min	25–231 µU/mL		25–231 mU/L	
		60 min	18–276 µU/mL		18–276 mU/L	
		120 min	16–166 µU/mL		16–166 mU/L	
		180 min	4–38 µU/mL		4–38 mU/L	
Insulin-like growth factor I (IGFI/Somatomedin C)	S	M		× 0.1307		(Endocrine Sciences)
		1–2 yr	31–160 ng/mL		4.05–21.96 nmol/L	
		3–4 yr	45–230 ng/mL		5.88–30.07 nmol/L	
		5–6 yr	51–288 ng/mL		6.67–37.65 nmol/L	
		7–8 yr	158–385 ng/mL		20.66–50.33 nmol/L	
		9–10 yr	136–308 ng/mL		17.78–40.27 nmol/L	
		11–12 yr	180–440 ng/mL		23.53–57.52 nmol/L	
		13–14 yr	220–616 ng/mL		28.76–80.53 nmol/L	
		15–16 yr	200–836 ng/mL		26.15–109.30 nmol/L	
		17–18 yr	286–627 ng/mL		37.39–81.97 nmol/L	
		19–20 yr	339–418 ng/mL		44.32–54.65 nmol/L	
		21–25 yr	202–433 ng/mL		26.4 –56.61 nmol/L	
		Puberty M	***Mean ± SD***		***Mean ± SD***	
		Tanner 1	215 ± 71 ng/mL		28.11 ± 9.28 nmol/L	
		Tanner 2	320 ± 137 ng/mL		41.84 ± 17.91 nmol/L	
		Tanner 3	475 ± 176 ng/mL		62.10 ± 23.01 nmol/L	
		Tanner 4	500 ± 135 ng/mL		65.37 ± 17.65 nmol/L	

■ **TABLE 670–2 Reference Ranges for Laboratory Tests** *(Continued)*

Test	Specimen	Reference Range			Factor	Reference Range (SI)		Comments
		Tanner 5	490 ± 120 ng/mL			64.06 ± 15.69 nmol/L		
		F						
		1–2 yr	11–206 ng/mL			1.43–26.93 nmol/L		
		3–4 yr	75–320 ng/mL			9.81–41.84 nmol/L		
		5–6 yr	70–288 ng/mL			9.15–37.65 nmol/L		
		7–8 yr	125–396 ng/mL			16.34–51.77 nmol/L		
		9–10 yr	123–330 ng/mL			16.08–43.14 nmol/L		
		11–12 yr	191–462 ng/mL			24.97–60.40 nmol/L		
		13–14 yr	286–660 ng/mL			37.39–87.33 nmol/L		
		15–16 yr	242–660 ng/mL			31.64–87.33 nmol/L		
		17–18 yr	240–506 ng/mL			31.38–66.15 nmol/L		
		19–20 yr	242–550 ng/mL			31.64–71.90 nmol/L		
		21–25 yr	231–453 ng/mL			30.19–59.21 nmol/L		
		Puberty F	***Mean ± SD***			***Mean ± SD***		
		Tanner 1	255 ± 83 ng/mL			33.34 ± 10.85 nmol/L		
		Tanner 2	410 ± 84 ng/mL			53.60 ± 10.98 nmol/L		
		Tanner 3	492 ± 180 ng/mL			64.32 ± 23.53 nmol/L		
		Tanner 4	505 ± 155 ng/mL			66.02 ± 20.26 nmol/L		
		Adult	(26–85 yr) 135–449 ng/mL)			17.65–58.70 nmol/L		
Insulin-like growth factor II	S	Prepubertal	334–642 ng/mL		× 0.1333	44.53–85.60 nmol/L		(Endocrine Sciences)
		Pubertal	245–737 ng/mL			32.67–98.27 nmol/L		
		Adults	288–736 ng/mL			38.40–98.13 nmol/L		
Iron	S	Newborn	100–250 μg/dL		× 0.179	17.90–44.75 μmol/L		
		Infant	40–100 μgdL			7.16–17.90 μmol/L		
		Child	50–120 μg/dL			8.95–21.48 μmol/L		
		Thereafter						
		M	50–160 μg/dL			8.95–28.64 μmol/L		
		F	40–150 μg/dL			7.16–26.85 μmol/L		
		Intoxicated child	280–2,550 μg/dL			50.12–456.5 μmol/L		
		Fatally poisoned child	>1,800 μ/dL			>322.2 μmol/L		
Iron-binding capacity, total (TIBC)	S	Infant	100–400 μg/dL		× 0.179	17.90–71.60 μmol/L		
		Thereafter	250–400 μg/dL			44.75–71.60 μmol/L		
17-Ketogenic steroids (17-KGS)	U	0–1 yr	<1.0 mg/24 hr		× 3.467	<3.5 μmol/24 hr		Conversion based on dehydroepiandrosterone, MW 288
		1–10 yr	<5 mg/24 hr			<17 μmol/24 hr		
		11–14 yr	<12 mg/24 hr			<42 μmol/24 hr		
		Thereafter						
		M	5–23 mg/24 hr			17–80 μmol/24 hr		
		F	3–15 mg/24 hr			10–52 μmol/24 hr		
Ketone bodies								
Qualitative	S	Negative				Negative		
	U	Negative				Negative		
Quantitative	S	0.5–3.0 mg/dL			× 10	5–30 mg/L		
17-Ketosteroid (17-KS), total	U	14 d–2 yr	<1 mg/24 hr		× 3.467	<3.5 μmol/24 hr		
		2–6 yr	<2 mg/24 hr			< 7 μmol/24 hr		
		6–10 yr	1–4 mg/24 hr			3.5–14 μmol/24 hr		Zimmerman reaction Conversion based on dehydroepiandrosterone, MW 288
		10–12 yr	1–6 mg/24 hr			3.5–21 μmol/24 hr		
		12–14 yr	3–10 mg/24 hr			10–35 μmol/24 hr		
		14–16 yr	5–12 mg/24 hr			17–42 μmol/24 hr		
		Thereafter						
		M: 18–30 yr	9–22 mg/24 hr			31–76 μmol/24 hr		
		>30 yr	8–20 mg/24 hr			28–70 μmol/24 hr		
		F, decreases with age	6–15 mg/24 hr			21–52 μmol/24 hr		
LDL-cholesterol (LDLC)	S, P(E)							
			M (mg/dL)	***F (mg/dL)***		***M (mmol/L)***	***F (mmol/L)***	
		Cord blood	10–50	10–50	× 0.0259	0.26–1.30	0.26–1.30	
		1–9 yr	60–140	60–150		1.55–3.63	1.55–3.89	
		10–19 yr	50–170	50–170		1.30–4.40	1.30–4.40	
		20–29 yr	60–175	60–160		1.55–4.53	1.55–4.14	
		30–39 yr	80–190	70–170		2.07–4.92	1.81–4.40	
		40–49 yr	90–205	80–190		2.33–5.31	2.07–4.92	
		Recommended (desirable) range for adults	<130 mg/dL			1.68–4.53 mmol/L		
Lactate								
L(+)-lactate	W(H)	Venous	0.5–2.2 mmol/L			0.5–2.2 mmol/L		
		Arterial	0.5–1.6 mmol/L			0.5–1.6 mmol/L		
		Inpatients						
		Venous	0.9–1.7 mmol/L			0.9–1.7 mmol/L		
		Arterial	<1.25 mmol/L			<1.25 mmol/L		
D(−)-lactate	P(H)	6 mo–3 yr	0.0–0.3 mmol/L		× 1	0.0–0.3 mmol/L		z (Rosenthal and Pesce)
Lactate dehydrogenase (LD)	S	<1 yr	170–580 U/L		× 1	170–580 U/L		37° m (Meites)
		1–9 yr	150–500 U/L			150–500 U/L		
		10–19 yr	120–330 U/L			120–330 U/L		

Table continued on following page

■ **TABLE 670–2 Reference Ranges for Laboratory Tests** *(Continued)*

Test	Specimen	Reference Range	Factor	Reference Range (SI)	Comments
Isoenzymes	S	***Percentage of Total Activity***			
		1–6 yr / **7–19 yr**			
		LD1 20–38 / 20–35			
		LD2 27–38 / 31–38			
		LD3 16–26 / 19–28			
		LD4 5–16 / 7–13			
		LD5 3–13 / 5–12			
Lead	W(H)	Child <10 µg/dL	× 0.0483	<0.48 µmol/L	
		Adult <40 µg/dL		<1.93 µmol/L	
		Acceptable for industrial exposure <60 µg/dL		<2.90 µmol/L	
		Toxic ≥100 µg/dL		≥4.83 µmol/L	
	U (24-hr)	<80 µg/dL	× 0.00483	<0.39 µmol/L	
Lecithin/sphingomyelin (L/S) ratio	AF	2.0–5.0 indicates probable fetal lung maturity (>3.0 IDM)		2.0–5.0 indicates probable fetal lung maturity	
Lecithin phosphorus	AF	>0.10 mg/dL indicates probably adequate fetal lung maturity	× 0.03229	>0.032 mmol/L indicates probably adequate fetal lung maturity	
Leukocyte count (WBC)	W(E)	***× 1,000 cells/mm³ (µL)***		***× 10⁹ cells/L***	
		Birth 9.0–30.0		9.0–30.0	
		24 hr 9.4–34.0		9.4–34.0	
		1 mo 5.0–19.5		5.0–19.5	
		1–3 yr 6.0–17.5		6.0–17.5	
		4–7 yr 5.5–15.5		5.5–15.5	
		8–13 yr 4.5–13.5		4.5–13.5	
		Adult 4.5–11.0		4.5–11.0	
Cell count	CSF	Premature 0–25 mononuclear cells/µL	× 10⁶	0–25 × 10⁶ cells/L	
		0–10 polymorphonuclear cells/µL		0–10 × 10⁶ cells/L	
		0–1,000 RBC/µL		0–1,000 × 10⁶ cells/L	
		Newborn 0–20 mononuclear cells/µL		0–20 × 10⁶ cells/L	
		0–10 polymorphonuclear cells/µL		0–10 × 10⁶ cells/L	
		0–800 RBC/µL		0–800 × 10⁶ cells/L	
		Neonate 0–5 mononuclear cells/µL		0–5 × 10⁶ cells/L	
		0–10 polymorphonuclear cells/µL		0–10 × 10⁶ cells/L	
		0–50 RBC/µL		0–50 × 10⁶ cells/L	
				0–5 cells/L	
		Thereafter 0–5 mononuclear cells/µL (numbers of cells in very young infants are greater than those in the CSF of older individuals without substantial implications for growth and development in most instances)			
Leukocyte differential	W(E)				
Myelocytes		0	× 0.01	0	
Neutrophils—"bands"		3–5%		0.03–0.05 no. fraction	
Neutrophils—"segs"		54–62%		0.54–062 no. fraction	
Lymphocytes		25–33%		0.25–0.33 no. fraction	
Monocytes		3–7%		0.03–0.07 no. fraction	
Eosinophils		1–3%		0.01–0.03 no. fraction	
Basophils		0–0.75%		0–0.0075 no. fraction	
Leukocyte differential	Specimen	***Cells/mm³ (µL)***			
Myelocytes		0	× 1	0 × 10⁶ cells/L	
Neutrophils—"bands"		150–400		150–400 × 10⁶ cells/L	
Neutrophils—"segs"		3,000–5,800		3,000–5,800 × 10⁶ cells/L	
Lymphocytes		1,500–3,000		1,500–3,000 × 10⁶ cells/L	
Monocytes		285–500		285–500 × 10⁶ cells/L	
Eosinophils		50–250		50–250 × 10⁶ cells/L	
Basophils		15–50		15–50 × 10⁶ cells/L	
Lymphocytes	CSF	62% ± 34%	× 0.01	0.62 ± 0.34 no. fraction	
Monocytes		36% ± 20%		0.36 ± 0.20 no. fraction	
Neutrophils		2% ± 5%		0.02 ± 0.05 no. fraction	
Histiocytes		0–rare		0–rare	
Ependymal cells		0–rare		0–rare	
Eosinophils		0–rare		0–rare	
Lipase	S	1–4 yr 18–95 U/L	× 1	18–95 U/L	37° (Meites)
		5–14 yr 21–128 U/L		21–128 U/L	
		15–19 yr 28–149 U/L		28–149 U/L	
Lipoprotein electrophoresis	S	Distinct β band; negligible chylomicron and pre-β bands			
Lithium. See end of table under Drugs					
Long-acting thyroid-stimulating hormone (LATS)	S	Undetectable		Undetectable	
Luteinizing hormone (LH)	S	M			(Endocrine Sciences)
		Tanner 1 <9.8 yr 0.02–0.3 mIU/mL	× 1	0.02–0.3 U/L	
		Tanner 2 9.8–14.5 yr 0.2–4.9 mIU/mL		0.2–4.9 U/L	

■ **TABLE 670–2 Reference Ranges for Laboratory Tests** *(Continued)*

Test	Specimen	Reference Range			Factor	Reference Range (SI)	Comments
		Tanner 3	10.7–15.4 yr	0.2–5.0 mIU/mL		0.2–5.0 U/L	Referred to WHO second International Standard
		Tanner 4–5	11.8–17.3 yr	0.4–7.0 mIU/mL		0.4–7.0 U/L	
		Adult		1.5–9 mIU/mL		1.5–9 U/L	
		F					
		Tanner 1	<9.2 yr	0.02–0.18 mIU/mL		0.02–0.18 U/L	
		Tanner 2	9.2–13.7 yr	0.02–4.7 mIU/mL		0.02–4.7 U/L	
		Tanner 3	10.0–14.4 yr	0.10–12.0 mIU/mL		0.10–12.0 U/L	
		Tanner 4–5	10.7–15.6 yr	0.4–11.7 mIU/mL		0.4–11.7 U/L	
		Adult					
		Follicular		2–9 mIU/mL		2–9 U/L	
		Midcycle		18–49 mIU/mL		18–49 U/L	
		Luteal		2–11 mIU/mL		2–11 U/L	

Test	Specimen		Age: 2–3 mo	4–8 mo	12–23 mo	24–59 mo	Comments
Lymphocyte subsets	W(E)						(Denny, et al.)
		Median lymphocytes, total	5.68×10^9/L	5.99×10^9/L	5.16×10^9/L	4.06×10^9/L	
		5th–95th percentiles	2.92–8.84	3.61–8.84	2.18–8.27	2.40–5.81	
		Median CD3$^+$ lymphocytes	4.03×10^9/L	4.27×10^9/L	3.33×10^9/L	3.04×10^9/L	
		5th–95th percentiles	2.07–6.54	2.28–6.45	1.46–5.44	1.16–4.23	
		Median CD4$^+$ lymphocytes	2.83×10^9/L	2.95×10^9/L	2.07×10^9/L	$1{,}80 \times 10^9$/L	
		5th–95th percentiles	1.46–5.11	1.69–4.60	1.02–3.60	0.90–2.86	
		Median CD8$^+$ lymphocytes	1.41×10^9/L	1.45×10^9/L	1.32×10^9/L	1.18×10^9/L	
		5th–95th percentiles	0.65–2.45	0.72–2.49	0.57–2.23	0.63–1.91	
		Median % lymphocytes	66	64	59	50	
		5th–95 percentiles	55–78	45–79	44–72	38–64	
		Median % CD3$^+$ lymphocytes	72	71	66	72	
		5th–95th percentiles	60–87	57–84	53–81	62–80	
		Median % CD4$^+$ lymphocytes	52	49	43	42	
		5th–95th percentiles	41–64	36–61	31–54	35–51	
		Median % CD8$^+$ lymphocytes	25	24	25	30	
		5th–95th percentiles	16–35	16–34	16–38	22–38	

Test	Specimen	Reference Range		Factor	Reference Range (SI)	Comments
Lysergic acid diethylamide. See end of table under Drugs						
Magnesium	P(H)	0–6 d	1.2–2.6 mg/dL	× 0.411	0.48–1.05 mmol/L	d (Meites)
		7 d–2 yr	1.6–2.6 mg/dL		0.65–1.05 mmol/L	
	U (24-hr)	2–14 yr	1.5–2.3 mg/dL		0.60–0.95 mmol/L	
		1–6 mo				
		Breast-fed	0.04–1.55 mmol/L	× 1	0.04–1.55 mmol/L	
		Formula-fed	0.04–1.40 mmol/L		0.04–1.55 mmol/L	
Mean corpuscular hemoglobin concentration (MCHC)	W(E)	Birth	31–37 pg/cell	× 0.0155	0.48–0.57 fmol/cell	
		1–3 d (capillary)	31–37 pg/cell		0.48–0.57 fmol/cell	
		1 wk–1 mo	28–40 pg/cell		0.43–0.62 fmol/cell	
		2 mo	26–34 pg/cell		0.40–0.53 fmol/cell	
		3–6 mo	25–35 pg/cell		0.39–0.54 fmol/cell	
		0.5–2 yr	23–31 pg/cell		0.36–0.48 fmol/cell	
		2–6 yr	24–30 pg/cell		0.37–0.47 fmol/cell	
		6–12 yr	25–33 pg/cell		0.39–0.51 fmol/cell	
		12–18 yr	25–35 pg/cell		0.39–0.54 fmol/cell	
		18–49 yr	26–34 pg/cell		0.40–0.53 fmol/cell	
Mean corpuscular hemoglobin	W(E)		***Percentage Hb/cell or g Hb/dL RBC***		***mmol Hb/L RBC***	
		Birth	30–36	× 0.155	4.65–5.58	
		1–3 d (capillary)	29–37		4.50–5.74	
		1–2 wk	28–38		4.34–5.89	
		1–2 mo	29–37		4.50–5.74	
		3 mo–2 yr	30–36		4.65–5.58	
		2–18 yr	31–37		4.81–5.74	
		>18 yr	31–37		4.81–5.74	
Mean corpuscular volume (MCV)	W(E)	1–3 d (capillary)	95–121 μm^3	× 1	95–121 fL	
		0.5–2 yr	70–86 μm^3		70–86 fL	
		6–12 yr	77–95 μm^3		77–95 fL	
		12–18 yr				
		M	78–98 μm^3		78–98 fL	
		F	78–102 μm^3		78–102 fL	
		18–49 yr				
		M	80–100 μm^3		80–100 fL	
		F	80–100 μm^3		80–100 fL	
Metanephrines, total	U (24-hr)	<1 yr	<15.9 μmol/g creatinine	× 0.1131	<1.80 mmol/mol creatinine	(Meites)
		1–2 yr	<14.8 μmol/g creatinine		<1.67 mmol/mol creatinine	

Table continued on following page

■ **TABLE 670–2 Reference Ranges for Laboratory Tests** *(Continued)*

Test	Specimen	Reference Range	Factor	Reference Range (SI)	Comments
		3–4 yr <12.8 μmol/g creatinine		<1.45 mmol/mol creatinine	
		5–8 yr <11.7 μmol/g creatinine		<1.32 mmol/mol creatinine	
		9–13 yr <10.5 μmol/g creatinine		<1.19 mmol/mol creatinine	
Methemoglobin (MetHb)	W(E,H,C)	0.06–0.24 g/dL or	×155	9.3–37.2 μmol/L	
		0.78 ± 0.37% of total Hb	× 0.01	0.0078 ± 0.0037 (mass fraction)	
Methylmalonic acid	U	6–12 wk 0–57 mg/g creatinine	× 0.9579	0–55 mmol/mol creatinine	h (Meites)
Microsomal antibodies, thyroid. See Thyroid microsomal antibodies					
Mucopolysaccharides	U	<2 yr <50 μg/g creatinine	× 0.1131	<5.7 mg/mmol creatinine	(Meites)
		2–4 yr <25 μg/g creatinine		<2.8 mg/mmol creatinine	
		4–15 yr <20 μg/g creatinine		<2.3 mg/mmol creatinine	
Myoglobin	S	6–85 ng/mL	× 1	6–85 μg/L	
	U	Negative		Negative	
Niacin (nicotinic acid)	U	0.3–1.5 mg/24 hr	× 8.113	2.43–12.17 μmol/24 hr	
Occult blood	F	Negative (<2 mL blood/24 hr in ~100–200 g stool)		Negative	
	U	Negative		Negative	
Organic acids	U	Adult			(Hoffman, et al.)
Lactic		115–407 μM/g creatinine	× 0.1132	13–46 mmol/mol creatinine	
2-Hydroxyisobutyric		Not detected		Not detected	
Glycolic		159–486 μM/g creatinine		18–55 mmol/mol creatinine	
3-Hydroxybutyric		Not detected–18 μM/g creatinine		Not detected–2.0 mmol/mol creatinine	
3-Hydroxyisobutyric		36–168 μM/g creatinine		4.1–19 mmol/mol creatinine	
2-Hydroxyisovaleric		Not detected		Not detected	
3-Hydroxyisovaleric		61–221 μM/g creatinine		6.9–25 mmol/mol creatinine	
Methylmalonic		Not detected		Not detected	
4-Hydroxybutyric		2.7–51 μM/g creatinine		0.3–5.8 mmol/mol creatinine	
Ethylmalonic		3.5–37 μMg creatinine		0.4–4.2 mmol/mol creatinine	
Succinic		4.4–141 μM/g creatinine		0.5–16 mmol/mol creatinine	
Fumaric		1.8–7 μM/g creatinine		0.2–0.8 mmol/mol creatinine	
Glutaric		5.3–23 μM/g creatinine		0.6–2.6 mmol/mol creatinine	
3-Methylgutaric		Not detected		Not detected	
Adipic		7–309 μM/g creatinine		0.8–35 mmol/mol creatinine	
Pyruvic		23–70 μM/g creatinine		2.6–7.9 mmol/mol creatinine	
Pyroglutamic		8–577 μM/g creatinine		0.9–63 mmol/mol creatinine	
2-Oxoisovaleric		Not detected		Not detected	
Acetoacetic		Not detected		Not detected	
Mevalonic		0.5–1.9 μM/g creatinine		0.06–0.22 mmol/mol creatinine	
2-Hydroxyglutaric		7–460 μM/g creatinine		0.8–52 mmol/mol creatinine	
3-Hydroxy-3-methylglutaric		Not detected–88		Not detected–10 mmol/mol creatinine	
p-Hydroxyphenylacetic		31–195 μM/g creatinine		3.5–22 mmol/mol creatinine	
2-Oxoisocaproic		Not detected		Not detected	
Suberic		Not detected–26 μM/g creatinine		Not detected–2.9 mmol/mol creatinine	
Orotic		Not detected		Not detected	
cis-Aconitic		24–389 μM/g creatinine		2.7–44 mmol/mol creatinine	
Homovanillic		8–49 μM/g creatinine		0.9–5.5 mmol/mol creatinine	
Azeleic		11–137 μM/g creatinine		1.3–5.5 mmol/mol creatinine	
Isocitric		318–743 μM/g creatinine		36–84 mmol/mol creatinine	
Citric		619–1,998 μM/g creatinine		70–226 mmol/mol creatinine	
Sebacic		Not detected		Not detected	
4-Hydroxyphenyl lactic		1.8–23 μM/g creatinine		0.2–2.6	
2-Oxoglutaric		35–654 μM/g creatinine		4–74 mmol/mol creatinine	
5-Hydroxyindoleacetic		Not detected–64 μM/g creatinine		Not detected–7.2 mmol/mol creatinine	
Succinylacetone		Not detected		Not detected	
Orotic acid	U	0–20.1 mg/g creatinine	× 0.7247	0–4.16 mmol/mol creatinine	c m (Meites)
Osmolality	S	Child and adult 275–295 mOsm/kg H_2O			
	U	50–1,400 mOsm/kg H_2O, depending on fluid intake. After 12 hr of fluid restriction, normal range is >850 mOsm/kg H_2O			
	U (24-hr)	300–900 mOsm/kg H_2O			
Osmotic fragility test (RBC fragility) pH 7.4, 20° C	W(H)				

NaCl	*Per cent Hemolysis*		*NaCl*	*Hemolyzed Fraction*
0.30 g/dL	97–100	× 0.01	3.0 g/L	0.97–1.00
0.35 g/dL	90–99	(Hemolyzed	3.5 g/L	0.90–0.99
0.40 g/dL	50–95	fraction)	4.0 g/L	0.50–0.95
0.45 g/dL	5–45		4.5 g/L	0.05–0.45
0.50 g/dL	0–6		5.0 g/L	0.00–0.06
0.55 g/dL	0		5.5 g/L	0.00

■ **TABLE 670–2 Reference Ranges for Laboratory Tests** *(Continued)*

Test	Specimen	Reference Range	Factor	Reference Range (SI)	Comments
Sterile incubation at 37° C		*NaCl* — *Per cent Hemolysis*		*NaCl* — *Hemolyzed Fraction*	
		0.20 g/dL — 95–100	× 0.01 (Hemolyzed fraction)	2.0 g/L — 0.95–1.00	
		0.30 g/dL — 85–100		3.0 g/L — 0.85–1.00	
		0.35 g/dL — 75–100		3.5 g/L — 0.75–1.00	
		0.40 g/dL — 65–100		4.0 g/L — 0.65–1.00	
		0.45 g/dL — 55–95		4.5 g/L — 0.55–0.95	
		0.50 g/dL — 40–85		5.0 g/L — 0.40–0.85	
		0.55 g/dL — 15–70		5.5 g/L — 0.15–0.70	
		0.60 g/dL — 0–40		6.0 g/L — 0.00–0.40	
		0.65 g/dL — 0–10		6.5 g/L — 0.00–0.10	
		0.70 g/dL — 0–5		7.0 g/L — 0.00–0.05	
		0.85 g/dL — 0		8.5 g/L — 0.00	
Oxygen, partial pressure of (Po_2)	W(H), arterial	Birth 8–24 mm Hg	× 0.133	1.1–3.2 kPa	
		5–10 min 33–75 mm Hg		4.4–10.0 kPa	
		30 min 31–85 mm Hg		4.1–11.3 kPa	
		>1 hr 55–80 mm Hg		7.3–10.6 kPa	
		1 d 54–95 mm Hg		7.2–12.6 kPa	
		Thereafter (decreases with age) 83–108 mm Hg		11–14.4 kPa	
Oxygen saturation	W(H), arterial	Newborn 85–90%	× 0.01	0.85–0.90 Saturated fraction	
		Thereafter 95–99%		0.95–0.99 Saturated fraction	
Po_2. See Oxygen, Partial pressure of					
Po_2 at half saturation (Po_2 [0.5] or P_{50})	W(H), arterial	25–29 mm Hg	× 0.133	3.3–3.9 kPa	
Paraldehyde. See end of table under Drugs					
Parathyroid hormone	S				
C-terminal (mid-molecule)		1–16 yr 51–217 pg/mL	× 0.1053	5.4–22.8 pmol/L	m (Nichols Institute)
Intact (IRMA)		1–18 yr 1–43 pg/mL		0.1–4.5 pmol/L	
Intact N-terminal specific		2–13 yr 14–21 pg/mL		1.5–2.2 pmol/L	
Partial thromboplastin time (PTT)	W(NaCl)				
Nonactivated		60–85 s (Platelin)		60–85 s	
Activated		25–35 s (differs with method)		25–35 s	
pH	W(H), arterial			*H^+* **Concentration**	
		Premature (48 hr) 7.35–7.50		31–44 nmol/L	
		Birth, full-term 7.11–7.36		43–77 nmol/L	
		5–10 min 7.09–7.30		50–81 nmol/L	
		30 min 7.21–7.38		41–61 nmol/L	
		>1 hr 7.26–7.49		32–54 nmol/L	
		1 d 7.29–7.45		35–51 nmol/L	
		Thereafter 7.35–7.45		35–44 nmol/L	
		Must be corrected for body temperature			
	U	Newborn/neonate 5–7		0.1–10 μmol/L	
		Thereafter (average 6) 4.5–8		0.01–32 μmol/L (average 1.0 μmol/L)	
	F	7.0–7.5		31–100 nmol/L	
Phenacetin. See end of table under Drugs					
Phenobarbital. See end of table under Drugs					
Phensuximide. See end of table under Drugs					
Phenylalanine	S	Premature 2.0–7.5 mg/dL	× 60.54	120–450 μmol/L	
		Newborn 1.2–3.4 mg/dL		70–210 μmol/L	
		Thereafter 0.8–1.8 mg/dL		50–110 μmol/L	
	U	10 d–2 wk 1–2 mg/24 hr	× 6.054	6–12 μmol/24 hr	
		3–12 yr 4–18 mg/24 hr		24–110 μmol/24 hr	
		Thereafter trace–17 mg/24 hr		trace–103 μmol/24 hr	
Phenylpyruvic acid, qualitative	U	Negative by $FeCl_3$ test		Negative by $FeCl_3$ test	
Phenytoin. See end of table under Drugs					
Phosphatase, acid Prostatic (RIA)	S	<3.0 ng/mL	× 1	<3.0 μg/L	
Roy Brower and Hayden 37° C		0.11–0.60 U/L		0.11–0.60 U/L	
Phosphatase, alkaline	S	1–9 yr 145–420 U/L	× 1	1–9 yr 145–420 U/L	37° C m d (Lockitch, et al., *a*)
		10–11 yr 130–560 U/L		10–11 yr 130–560 U/L	
		M — *F*		*M* — *F*	
		12–13 yr 200–495 U/L — 105–420 U/L		12–13 yr 200–495 U/L — 105–420 U/L	
		14–15 yr 130–525 U/L — 70–230 U/L		14–15 yr 130–525 U/L — 70–230 U/L	
		16–19 yr 65–260 U/L — 50–130 U/L		16–19 yr 65–260 U/L — 50–130 U/L	
Phospholipids, total	S, P(E)	Newborn 75–170 mg/dL	× 0.01	0.75–1.70 g/L	
		Infant 100–275 mg/dL		1.00–2.75 g/L	
		Child 180–295 mg/dL		1.80–2.95 g/L	

Table continued on following page

■ **TABLE 670–2 Reference Ranges for Laboratory Tests** *(Continued)*

Test	Specimen	Reference Range	Factor	Reference Range (SI)	Comments
		Adult 125–275 mg/dL		1.25–2.75 g/L	
Phosphorus, inorganic	S, P(H)	0–5 d 4.8–8.2 mg/dL	× 0.3229	1.55–2.65 mmol/L	d (Meites)
		1–3 yr 3.8–6.5 mg/dL		1.25–2.10 mmol/L	
		4–11 yr 3.7–5.6 mg/dL		1.20–1.80 mmol/L	
		12–15 yr 2.9–5.4 mg/dL		0.95–1.75 mmol/L	
		16–19 yr 2.7–4.7 mg/dL		0.90–1.50 mmol/L	
Plasma volume	P(H)	M 25–43 mL/kg	× 0.001	M 0.025–0.043 L/kg	
		F 28–45 mL/kg		F 0.028–0.045 L/kg	
Platelet count (thrombocyte count)	W(E)	Newborn 84–478 × 10^3/mm³ (μL) (after 1 wk same as adult)	× 10^6	84–478 × 10^9/L	
		Adult 150–400 × 10^3/mm³ (μL)		150–400 × 10^9/L	
Porphobilinogen (PBG)					
Quantitative	U	0–2.0 mg/24 hr	× 4.42	0–8.8 μmol/24 hr	
Qualitative	U	Negative		Negative	
Potassium	S	<2 mo 3.0–7.0 mmol/L	× 1	3.0–7.0 mmol/L	w (Meites) Increased by hemolysis. Serum values systematically higher than plasma values
		2–12 mo 3.5–6.0 mmol/L		3.5–6.0 mmol/L	
		>12 mo 3.5–5.0 mmol/L		3.5–5.0 mmol/L	
	P(H)			3.5–4.5 mmol/L	
	U (24-hr)	2.5–125 mmol/L (varies with diet)		2.5–125 mmol/L (varies with diet)	
Prealbumin (transthyretin)	P	2–6 mo 142–330 mg/L	× 1	142–330 mg/L	n (Sherry, et al.)
		6–12 mo 120–274 mg/L		120–274 mg/L	
		1–3 yr 108–259 mg/L		108–259 mg/L	
Pregnanetriol	U	2 wk–2 yr 0.02–0.2 mg/24 hr	× 2.972	0.06–0.6 μmol/24 hr	
		2–5 yr <0.5 mg/24 hr		<1.5 μmol/24 hr	
		5–15 yr <1.5 mg/24 hr		<4.5 μmol/24 hr	
		>15 yr <2.0 mg/24 hr		<5.9 μmol/24 hr	
Primidone. See end of table under Drugs					
Progesterone	S	M			(Endocrine Sciences)
		Tanner 1 <9.8 yr <10–33 ng/dL	× 0.03180	<0.32–1.05 nmol/L	
		Tanner 2 9.8–14.5 yr <10–33 ng/dL		<0.32–1.05 nmol/L	
		Tanner 3 10.7–15.4 yr <10–48 ng/dL		<0.32–1.53 nmol/L	
		Tanner 4 11.8–16.2 yr 10–108 ng/dL		0.32–3.43 nmol/L	
		Tanner 5 12.8–17.3 yr 21–82 ng/dL		0.67–2.61 nmol/L	
		Adult 13–97 ng/dL		0.41–3.08 nmol/L	
		F			
		Tanner 1 <9.2 yr <10–33 ng/dL		<0.32–1.05 nmol/L	
		Tanner 2 9.2–13.7 yr <10–55 ng/dL		<0.32–1.75 nmol/L	
		Tanner 3 10.0–14.4 yr 10–450 ng/dL		0.32–14.31 nmol/L	
		Tanner 4 10.7–15.6 yr 10–1,300 ng/dL		<0.32–41.34 nmol/L	
		Tanner 5 11.8–18.6 yr 10–950 ng/dL		<0.32–30.21 nmol/L	
		Adult Follicular 15–70 ng/dL		0.48–2.23 nmol/L	
		Luteal 200–2,500 ng/dL		6.36–79.50 nmol/L	
Prolactin	S	M 3–18 ng/mL	× 0.0426	M 0.13–0.77 nmol/L	(Endocrine Sciences)
		F 3–24 ng/mL		F 0.13–1.02 nmol/L	
		Higher in newborn infants		Higher in newborn infants	
Propranolol. See end of table under Drugs					
Protein					
Total	S	Premature 4.3–7.6 g/dL	× 10	43–76 g/L	
		Newborn 4.6–7.4 g/dL		46–74 g/L	
		1–7 yr 6.1–7.9 g/dL	× 10	61–79 g/L	(Meites)
		8–12 yr 6.4–8.1 g/dL		64–81 g/L	
		13–19 yr 6.6–8.2 g/dL		66–82 g/L	
Electrophoresis	S				
Albumin		Premature 3.0–4.2 g/dL		30–42 g/L	
		Newborn 3.6–5.4 g/dL		36–54 g/L	
		Infant 4.0–5.0 g/dL		40–50 g/L	
		Thereafter 3.5–5.0 g/dL		35–50 g/L	
α_1-Globulin		Premature 0.1–0.5 g/dL		1–5 g/L	
		Newborn 0.1–0.3 g/dL		1–3 g/L	
		Infant 0.2–0.4 g/dL		2–4 g/L	
		Thereafter 0.2–0.3 g/dL		2–3 g/L	
α_2-Globulin		Premature 0.3–0.7 g/dL		3–7 g/L	
		Newborn 0.3–0.5 g/dL		3–5 g/L	
		Infant 0.5–0.8 g/dL		5–8 g/L	
		Thereafter 0.4–1.0 g/dL		4–10 g/L	
β-Globulin		Premature 0.3–1.2 g/dL		3–12 g/L	
		Newborn 0.2–0.6 g/dL		2–6 g/L	
		Infant 0.5–0.8 g/dL		5–8 g/L	
		Thereafter 0.5–1.1 g/dL		5–11 g/L	
γ-Globulin		Premature 0.3–1.4 g/dL		3–4 g/L	
		Newborn 0.2–1.0 g/dL		2–10 g/L	
		Infant 0.3–1.2 g/dL		3–12 g/L	
		Thereafter 0.7–1.2 g/dL (higher in blacks)		7–12 g/L	

■ **TABLE 670–2 Reference Ranges for Laboratory Tests** *(Continued)*

Test	Specimen	Reference Range	Factor	Reference Range (SI)	Comments
Protein	U (24-hr)	1–14 mg/dL		10–140 mg/L	
Total urinary		50–80 mg/24 hr (at rest)		50–80 mg/24 hr (at rest)	
		< 250 mg/24 hr after intense exercise		<250 mg/24 hr after intense exercise	
Electrophoresis		***Average Total Protein***		***Fraction of Total Protein***	
Albumin		37.9%	× 0.01	0.379	
α_1-Globulin		27.3%		0.273	
α_2-Globulin		19.5%		0.195	
β-Globulin		8.8%		0.088	
γ-Globulin		3.3%		0.033	
Protein					
Total protein (column)	CSF	Lumbar 8–32 mg/dL	× 10	80–320 mg/L	
Turbidimetry		Lumbar			
		Premature 40–300 mg/dL		400–3,000 mg/dL	
		Newborn 45–120 mg/dL		450–1,200 mg/L	
		Child 10–20 mg/dL		100–200 mg/L	
		Adolescent 15–20 mg/dL		150–200 mg/L	
		Thereafter 15–45 mg/dL		150–450 mg/L	
Electrophoresis		Prealbumin 2–7% of total	× 0.01	0.02–0.07 fraction of total	
		Albumin 56–76% of total		0.56–0.76 fraction of total	
		α_1-Globulin 2–7% of total		0.02–0.07 fraction of total	
		α_2-Globulin 4–12% of total		0.04–0.12 fraction of total	
		β-Globulin 8–18% of total		0.08–0.18 fraction of total	
		γ-Globulin 3–12% of total		0.03–0.12 fraction of total	
Prothrombin time (PT)					
One-stage (quick)	W(NaC)	In general, 11–15 s (varies with type of thromboplastin)		11–15 s	
		Newborn: prolonged by 2–3 s		Newborn: prolonged by 2–3 s	
Two-stage modified (Ware and Seegers)	W(NaC)	18–22 s		18–22 s	
Quinidine. See end of table under Drugs					
RBC count. See Erythrocyte count					
RBC fragility. See Osmotic fragility					
Red cell volume	W(H)	M 20–36 mL/kg	× 0.001	0.020–0.036 L/kg	
		F 19–31 mL/kg		0.019–0.031 L/kg	
Renin (renin activity, plasma; PRA)	P(E)	0–3 yr <16.6 ng/mL/hr	× 1	<16.6 μg/L/hr	
		3–6 yr <6.7 ng/mL/hr		<6.7 ng/L/hr	
		6–9 yr <4.4 ng/mL/hr		<4.4 μg/L/hr	
		9–12 yr <5.9 ng/mL/hr		<5.9 μg/L/hr	
		12–15 yr <4.2 ng/mL/hr		<4.2 μg/L/hr	
		15–18 yr <4.3 ng/mL/hr		<4.3 μg/L/hr	
		Normal sodium diet			
		Supine 0.2–2.5 ng/mL/hr		0.2–2.5 μg/L/hr	
		Upright 0.3–4.3 ng/mL/hr		0.3–4.3 μg/L/hr	
		Low sodium diet			
		Upright 2.9–24 ng/mL/hr		2.9–24 μg/L/hr	
Reticulocyte count	W (E,H,O)	Adults 0.5–1.5% of erythrocytes, or	× 0.01	0.005–0.015 number fraction	
		25,000–75,000/mm³ (μL)	× 10^6	25,000–75,000 × 10^6/L	
	W (capillary)	1 d 0.4–6.0%	× 0.01	0.004–0.060 number fraction	
		7 d <0.1–1.3%		<0.001–0.013 number fraction	
		1–4 wk <1.0–1.2%		<0.001–0.012 number fraction	
		5–6 wk <0.1–2.4%		<0.001–0.024 number fraction	
		7–8 wk 0.1–2.9%		0.001–0.029 number fraction	
		9–10 wk <0.1–2.6%		<0.001–0.026 number fraction	
		11–12 wk 0.1–1.3%		0.001–0.013 number fraction	
Retinol-binding protein (RBP)	S	0–5 d 0.8–4.5 mg/dL	× 10	8–45 mg/L	n (Lockitch, et al., *b*)
		1–9 yr 1.0–7.8 mg/dL		10–78 mg/L	
		10–13 yr 1.3–9.9 mg/dL		13–99 mg/L	
		14–19 yr 3.0–9.2 mg/dL		30–92 mg/L	
Reverse triiodothyronine (rT_3)	S	1–5 yr 15–71 ng/dL	× 0.0154	0.23–1.1 nmol/L	
		5–10 yr 17–79 ng/dL		0.26–1.2 nmol/L	
		10–15 yr 19–88 ng/dL		0.29–1.36 nmol/L	
		Adults 30–80 ng/dL		0.46–1.23 nmol/L	
Riboflavin (vitamin B_2)	U	1–3 yr 500–900 μg/g creatinine	× 0.3	150–270 μmol/mol creatinine	
		4–6 yr 300–600 μg/g creatinine		90–180 μmol/mol creatinine	
		7–9 yr 270–500 μg/g creatinine		81–150 μmol/mol creatinine	
		10–15 yr 200–400 μg/g creatinine		60–1200 μmol/mol creatinine	
		Adult 80–269 μg/g creatinine		24–81 μmol/mol creatinine	
Salicylate. See end of table under Drugs					
Sediment	U				
Casts		Hyaline seen occasionally (0–1)/hpf		Hyaline seen occasionally (0–1)/hpf	
		RBC Not seen		RBC Not seen	
		WBC Not seen		WBC Not seen	
		Tubular epithelial Not seen		Tubular epithelial Not seen	
		Transitional and squamous epithelial Not seen		Transitional and squamous epithelial Not seen	

Table continued on following page

■ **TABLE 670–2 Reference Ranges for Laboratory Tests** *(Continued)*

Test	Specimen	Reference Range	Factor	Reference Range (SI)	Comments
Cells		RBC 0–2/hpf		RBC 0–2/hpf	
		WBC		WBC 0–3/hpf	
		M 0–3/hpf		M 0–3/hpf	
		F and children 0–5/hpf		F and children 0–5/hpf	
		Epithelial (more frequent in newborn) Few		Epithelial (more frequent in newborn) Few	
		Bacterial, no organism/oil immersion		Bacterial, no organism/oil immersion	
		Field unspun		Field unspun	
		Spun <20 organisms/hpf		Spun <20 organisms/hpf	
Sedimentation rate. See Erythrocyte sedimentation rate					
Selenium	S	0–5 d 5.7–9.4 µg/dL	× 0.127	0.72–1.20 µmol/L	a (Lockitch, et al., *c*)
		1–9 yr 9.6–16.1 µg/dL		1.22–2.05 µmol/L	
		10–19 yr 10.3–18.5 µg/dL		1.31–2.35 µmol/L	
Sickle cell tests					
Sodium metabisulfite	W(E,H,O)	Negative			
Dithionite test	W(E,H,O)	Negative			
Sodium	S,P(LiH, NH_4H)	Newborn 134–146 mmol/L	× 1	134–146 mmol/L	
		Infant 139–146 mmol/L		139–146 mmol/L	
		Child 138–145 mmol/L		138–146 mmol/L	
		Thereafter 136–146 mmol/L		136–148 mmol/L	
	U (24-hr)	(depending on diet) 40–220 mmol		40–220 mmol	
	Sweat	Normal <40 mmol/L	× 1	<40 mmol/L	(Gibson, et al.)
		Indeterminate 45–60 mmol/L		45–60 mmol/L	
		Cystic fibrosis >60 mmol/L		>60 mmol/L	
Somatomedin C. See Insulin-like growth factor I					
Specific gravity	U	Adult 1.002–1.030		1.002–1.030	
		After 12-hr fluid restriction >1.025		>1.025	
	U (24-hr)	1.015–1.025			
Sucrose hemolysis and sugar-water tests for paroxysmal nocturnal hemoglobinuria (PNH)	W(C,O)	≤5% lysis	× 0.01	Lysed fraction ≤0.05	
		6–10% lysis, questionable		0.06–0.10, questionable	
T_3. See Triiodothyronine					
T_4. See Thyroxine					
Testosterone	S	M	× 3.4670		(Endocrine Sciences)
		Tanner 1 <9.8 yr <3–10 ng/mL		<10–35 nmol/L	
		Tanner 2 9.8–14.5 yr 18–150 ng/mL		62–520 nmol/L	
		Tanner 3 10.7–15.4 yr 100–320 ng/mL		347–1,110 nmol/L	
		Tanner 4 11.8–16.2 yr 200–620 ng/mL		693–2,150 nmol/L	
		Tanner 5 12.8–17.3 yr 350–970 ng/mL		1,214–3,363 nmol/L	
		Adult 350–1,030 ng/mL		1,214–3,571 nmol/L	
		F			
		Tanner 1 <9.2 yr <3–10 ng/dL		<10–35 nmol/L	
		Tanner 2 9.2–13.7 yr 7–28 ng/mL		24–97 nmol/L	
		Tanner 3 10.0–14.4 yr 15–35 ng/mL		52–121 nmol/L	
		Tanner 4 10.7–15.6 yr 13–32 ng/mL		45–111 nmol/L	
		Tanner 5 11.8–18.6 yr 20–38 ng/mL		69–132 nmol/L	
		Adult 10–55 ng/mL		35–191 nmol/L	
Free	S	M ***pg/mL*** ***% Free***		***pmol/L*** ***Fraction Free***	(Endocrine Sciences)
		5–22 2.0–4.4%		17–76 0.02–0.044	
		1–15 d 1.5–31 0.9–1.7%		5.2–107 0.009–0.017	
		1–3 mo 3.3–18 0.4–0.8%		11.4–62 0.004–0.008	
		3–5 mo 0.7–14 0.4–1.1%		2.4–49 0.004–0.011	
		5–7 mo 0.4–4.8 0.4–1.0%		1.4–16.6 0.004–0.011	
		1–10 yr 0.15–0.6 0.4–0.9%		0.5–2.1 0.004–0.009	
		Puberty Not defined		Not defined	
		Adult 52–280 1.5–3.2%		180–971 0.015–0.032	
		F ***% Free***		***pmol/L*** ***Fraction Free***	(Endocrine Sciences)
		4–16 2.0–3.9%		13.9–55 0.02–0.039	
		1–15 d 0.5–2.5 0.8–1.5%		1.7–8.7 0.008–0.015	
		1–3 mo 0.1–1.3 0.4–1.1%		0.3–4.5 0.004–0.011	
		3–5 mo 0.3–1.1 0.5–1.0%		1.1–3.8 0.005–0.01	
		5–7 mo 0.2–0.6 0.5–0.8%		0.7–2.1 0.005–0.008	
		1–10 yr 0.15–0.6 0.4–0.9%		0.5–2.1 0.004–0.009	
		Puberty Not defined		Not defined	
		Adult 1.1–6.3 0.8–1.4		3.8–21.8 0.005–0.008	
Theophylline. See end of table under Drugs					
Thiamine (vitamin B_1)	S	0–2.0 µg/dL	× 37.68	0.0–75.4 nmol/L	
	U (acidified with HCl)	1–3 yr 176–200 µg/g creatinine	× 0.426	75–85 µmol/mol	
		4–6 yr 121–400 µg/g creatinine		52–170 µmol/mol	
		7–9 yr 181–350 µg/g creatinine		77–149 µmol/mol	
		10–12 yr 181–300 µg/g creatinine		77–128 µmol/mol	
		13–15 yr 151–250 µg/g creatinine		64–107 µmol/mol	
		Thereafter 66–129 µg/g creatinine		28–55 µmol/mol	
Thrombin time	W(NaC)	Control time ± 2 s when control is 9–13 s		Control time ± 2 s when control is 9–13 s	

■ TABLE 670–2 Reference Ranges for Laboratory Tests *(Continued)*

Test	Specimen	Reference Range			Factor	Reference Range (SI)		Comments
Thromboplastin time, activated. See Activated partial thromboplastin time (APTT)								
Thyroglobulin (Tg)	S	<50 ng/mL (higher in newborn infants)			× 1	<50 μg/L		
Thyroid microsomal antibodies	S	Nondetectable (hemagglutination) or <1:10 (IFA)				Nondetectable (hemagglutination) or <1:10 (IFA)		
Thyroid thyroglobulin tanned RBC agglutination test	S	Children ≤1:4 dilution				≤1:4 dilution		
		Thereafter ≤1:10 dilution				≤1:10 dilution		
Thyroid-stimulating hormone (hTSH)	S, P(H)	Cord blood	3–12 μU/mL		× 1	3–12 mU/L		
		Newborn	3–18 μU/mL			3–18 mU/L		
		Thereafter	2–10 μU/mL			2–10 mU/L		
Thyroid uptake of radioactive iodine	Activity over thyroid gland	2 hr	<6%		× 0.01	2 hr	<0.06	
		6 hr	3–20%			6 hr	0.03–0.20	
		24 hr	8–30%			24 hr	0.08–0.30	
Thyroid uptake of $^{99m}TcO_4$	Activity over thyroid gland	After 24 hr	0.4–3.0%		× 0.01	Fractional uptake, 0.004–0.03		
Thyrotropin-releasing hormone (hTRH)	P	5–60 pg/mL			× 1	5–60 ng/L		
Thyroxine-binding globulin (TBG)	S		*Range*			*Range*		
		Cord blood	1.4–9.4 mg/dL		× 10	14–94 mg/L		
		1–4 wk	1.0–9.0 mg/dL			10–90 mg/L		
		1–12 mo	2.0–7.6 mg/dL			20–76 mg/L		
		1–5 yr	2.9–5.4 mg/dL			29–54 mg/L		
		5–10 yr	2.5–5.0 mg/dL			25–50 mg/L		
		10–15 yr	2.1–4.6 mg/dL			21–46 mg/L		
		Adult	1.5–3.4 mg/dL			15–34 mg/L		
Thyroxine								
Total	S	Full-term infants			× 12.8700			(Endocrine Sciences)
		1–3 d	8.2–19.9 μg/dL			106–256 nmol/L		
		1 wk	6.0–15.9 μg/dL			77–205 nmol/L		
		1–12 mo	6.1–14.9 μg/dL			79–192 nmol/L		
		Prepubertal children						
		1–3 yr	6.8–13.5 μg/dL			88–174 nmol/L		
		3–10 yr	5.5–12.8 μg/dL			71–165 nmol/L		
		Pubertal children and adults	4.2–13.0 μg/dL			54–167 nmol/L		
Free	S	Newborn infants			× 12.87			(Endocrine Sciences)
		3 d	2.0–4.9 ng/dL			26–631 pmol/L		
		Infants						
		1–12 mo	0.9–2.6 ng/dL			12–33 pmol/L		
		Prepubertal children	0.8–2.2 ng/dL			10–28 pmol/L		
		Pubertal children and adults	0.8–2.3 ng/dL			10–30 pmol/L		
Thyroxine, total	W	Newborn screen (filter paper)	6.2–22 μg/dL					
Tourniquet test		<5–10 petechiae in 2.5-cm circle on forearm (halfway between systolic and diastolic); pressure maintained for 5 min				<5–10 petechiae in 2.5-cm circle on forearm (halfway between systolic and diastolic); pressure maintained for 5 min		
		0–8 petechiae in 6-cm circle (50 mm Hg for 15 min)				0–8 petechiae in 6-cm circle (50 mm Hg for 15 min)		
		10–20 petechiae in 5-cm circle (80 mm Hg)				10–20 petechiae in 5-cm circle (80 mm Hg)		
Transcortin	S	M	1.5–2.0 mg/dL		× 10	15–20 mg/L		
		F						
		Follicular	1.7–2.0 mg/dL			17–20 mg/L		
		Luteal	1.6–2.1 mg/dL			16–21 mg/L		
		Postmenopausal	1.7–2.5 mg/dL			17–25 mg/L		
		Pregnancy						
		21–28 wk	4.7–5.4 mg/dL			47–54 mg/L		
		33–40 wk	5.5–7.0 mg/dL			55–70 mg/L		
Transferrin (siderophilin)	S	1–3 yr	218–347 mg/dL		× 0.01	2.18–3.47 g/L		n (Lockitch, et al., *c*)
		4–9 yr	208–378 mg/dL			2.08–3.78 g/L		
		10–19 yr	224–444 mg/dL			2.24–4.44 g/L		
Triglycerides	S after ≥12-hr fast		*M (mg/dL)*	*F (mg/dL)*		*M (g/L)*	*F (g/L)*	
		Cord blood	10–98	10–98	× 0.01	0.10–0.98	0.10–0.98	
		0–5 yr	30–86	32–99		0.30–0.86	0.32–0.99	
		6–11 yr	31–108	35–114		0.31–1.08	0.35–1.14	
		12–15 yr	36–138	41–138		0.36–1.38	0.41–1.38	
		16–19 yr	40–163	40–128		0.40–1.63	0.40–1.28	
		20–29 yr	44–185	40–128		0.44–1.85	0.40–1.28	
		Adults: Recommended (desirable) levels				Adults: Recommended (desirable) levels		
		M	40–160 mg/dL			M	0.40–1.60 g/L	
		F	35–135 mg/dL			F	0.35–1.35 g/L	
Triidothyronine								
Free	S	Cord blood	20–240 pg/dL		× 0.01536	0.3–3.7 pmol/L		

Table continued on following page

■ **TABLE 670–2 Reference Ranges for Laboratory Tests** *(Continued)*

Test	Specimen	Reference Range		Factor	Reference Range (SI)	Comments
		1–3 d	200–610 pg/dL		3.1–9.4 pmol/L	
		6 wk	240–560 pg/dL		3.7–8.6 pmol/L	
		Adult (20–50 yr)	230–660 pg/dL		3.5–10.0 pmol/L	
Resin uptake test (T_3RU)	S	Newborn	26–36%	× 0.01	0.26–0.36 fractional uptake	
		Thereafter	26–35%		0.26–0.35 fractional uptake	
Total triiodothyronine (T_3)	S	Cord blood	30–70 ng/dL	× 0.0154	0.46–1.08 nmol/L	
		Newborn	75–260 ng/dL		1.16–4.00 nmol/L	
		1–5 yr	100–260 ng/dL		1.54–4.00 nmol/L	
		5–10 yr	90–240 ng/dL		1.39–3.70 nmol/L	
		10–15 yr	80–210 ng/dL		1.23–3.23 nmol/L	
		Thereafter	115–190 ng/dL		1.77–2.93 nmol/L	
Tyrosine	S	Premature	7.0–24.0 mg/dL	× 0.0552	0.39–1.32 mmol/L	
		Newborn	1.6–3.7 mg/dL		0.088–0.20 mmol/L	
		Adult	0.8–1.3 mg/dL		0.044–0.07 mmol/L	
Urea nitrogen	S, P	Cord blood	21–40 mg/dL	× 0.357	7.5–14.3 mmol urea/L	
		Premature (1 wk)	3–25 mg/dL		1.1–9 mmol urea/L	
		Newborn	3–12 mg/dL		1.1–4.3 mmol urea/L	
		Infant/child	5–18 mg/dL		1.8–6.4 mmol urea/L	
		Thereafter	7–18 mg/dL		2.5–6.4 mmol urea/L	
Uric acid	S	1–5 yr	1.7–5.8 mg/dL	× 59.48	100–350 μmol/L	z (Meites)
		6–11 yr	2.2–6.6 mg/dL		130–390 μmol/L	
		12–19 yr				
		M	3.0–7.7 mg/dL		180–460 μmol/L	
		F	2.7–5.7 mg/dL		160–340 μmul/L	
Urinary sediment. See Sediment						
Urine, volume	U (24-hr)	Newborn	50–300 mL/24 hr	× 0.001	0.050–0.300 L/24 hr	
		Infant	350–550 mL/24 hr		0.350–0.550 L/24 hr	
		Child	500–1,000 mL/24 hr		0.500–1.000 L/24 hr	
		Adolescent	700–1,400 mL/24 hr		0.700–1.400 L/24 hr	
		Thereafter				
		M	800–1,800 mL/24 hr		0.800–1.800 L/24 hr	
		F	600–1,600 mL/24 hr (varies with intake and other factors)		0.600–1.600 L/24 hr	
Valproic acid. See end of table under Drugs						
Vanillylmandelic acid (VMA)	U	0–1 yr	<18.8 mg/g creatinine	× 0.5709	<11 mmol/mol creatinine	p (Meites)
		2–4 yr	<11.0 mg/g creatinine		<6 mmol/mol creatinine	
		5–19 yr	<8.0 mg/g creatinine		<5 mmol/mol creatinine	
Vitamin A (retinol)	S	1–6 yr	20–43 μg/dL	× 0.0349	0.7–1.5 μmol/L	p (Lockitch, et al., *c*)
		7–12 yr	25–48 μg/dL		0.9–1.7 μmol/L	
		13–19 yr	26–72 μg/dL		0.9–2.5 μmol/L	
Vitamin B_1. See Thiamine						
Vitamin B_2. See Riboflavin						
Vitamin B_6	P(E)	3.6–18 ng/mL		× 4.046	14.6–72.8 nmol/L	
Vitamin B_{12}	S	Newborn	175–800 pg/mL	× 0.738	129–590 pmol/L	
		Thereafter	140–700 pg/mL		103–157 pmol/L	
Vitamin C	P(O,H,E)		0.6–2.0 mg/dL	× 56.78	34–113 μmol/L	
Vitamin D_2, 25-hydroxy	P(H)	Summer	15–80 ng/mL	× 2.496	37–200 nmol/L	
		Winter	14–42 ng/mL		35–105 nmol/L	
Vitamin D_3, 1,25-dihydroxy (calcitriol)	S		25–45 pg/mL	× 2.4	60–108 pmol/L	
Vitamin E (tocopherol)	S	1–6 yr	3.0–9.0 mg/L	× 2.32	7–21 μmol/L	p (Lockitch, et al., *c*)
		7–19 yr	4.4–10.4 mg/L		10–24 μmol/L	
WBC. See Leukocytes						
Xylose absorption test (0.5g/kg in H_2O to a maximum of 25 g)	S	Child (1 hr)	>20 mg/dL	× 0.0667	>1.33 mmol/L	
		Adult (2 hr)	>25 mg/dL		>1.67 mmol/L	
	U (5-hr)	Child 16–33% of ingested dose		× 0.01	0.16–0.33 (fraction ingested dose)	
		Adult				
		5-g dose	>1.2 g/5 hr	× 6.66	>8.00 mmol/5 hr	
		25-g dose	>4.0 g/5 hr		>26.64 mmol/5 hr	
	S	70–150 μg/dL		× 0.153	10.7–22.9 μmol/L	
Zinc	S	1–19 yr	64–118 μg/dL	× 0.1530	9.8–18.1 μmol/L	a (Lockitch, et al., *c*)
	U	5–18 yr	10.1–95.9 mg/mol creatinine	× 0.0153	0.15–1.47 mmol/mol creatinine	

Drugs	Specimen	Reference Range: Peak Therapeutic (μg/mL)	Peak Toxic (μg/mL)	Trough Therapeutic (μg/mL)	Trough Toxic (μg/mL)	Factor	Reference Range: SI Peak Therapeutic (μmol/mL)	SI Peak Toxic (μmol/mL)	SI Trough Therapeutic (μmol/mL)	SI Trough Toxic (μmol/mL)	Comments
Antibiotics											
Amikacin	S	20–25	>30	1–4	>8	× 1.708	34–43	>51	1.7–6.8	>14	x e (Taylor and Caviness)
Chloramphenicol	S	10–20	>25			× 3.095	31–62	>77			e (Taylor and Caviness)
Gentamicin	S	6–10	>12	0.5–2.0	>2.0	× 2.064	12–21	>25	1.0–4.1	>4.1	e x (Taylor and Caviness)
Netilmicin	S	6–10	>12	0.5–2.0	>2	× 2.103	13–21	>25	1.1–4.2	>4.2	e x (Taylor and Caviness)

■ **TABLE 670–2 Reference Ranges for Laboratory Tests** *(Continued)*

Test	Specimen	Reference Range				Factor	Reference Range (SI)				Comments
Tobramycin	S	6–10	>12	0.5–2.0	>2	× 2.139	13–21	>26	1.1–4.3	>4.3	e x (Taylor and Caviness)
Vancomycin	S	30–40	>60	5–10	>20	× 0.303	9.1–12.1	>18.2	1.5–3.0	>6.1	e x (Syva Co.)

Other Drugs	Specimen	Reference Range		Factor	Reference Range (SI)	Comments
Acetaminophen	S, P(H,E)	Therap. conc.	10–30 μg/mL	× 6.62	66–200 μmol/L	xz
		Toxic conc.	>200 μg/mL		>1,300 μmol/L	
Amphetamine	S, P(H,E)	Therap. conc.	20–30 ng/mL	× 7.396	150–220 nmol/L	
		Toxic conc.	>200 ng/mL		>1,500 nmol/L	
Amitriptyline (includes nortriptyline)	S	Therap. conc.	100–250 ng/mL	× 1	Therap. conc. 100–250 μg/L	(Syva Co.)
Nortriptyline (only)		Therap. conc.	50–150 ng/mL	× 1	Therap. conc. 50–150 μg/L	
Caffeine	S, P	Therap. conc. for neonatal apnea	5–20 μg/mL	× 5.150	26–103 μmol/L	e (Syva Co.)
Carbamazepine	S, P(H,E) at trough	Therap. conc.	8–12 μg/mL	× 4.233	34–51 μmol/L	ex (Syva Co.)
		Toxic conc.	>15 μg/mL		>63 μmol/L	
Chloral hydrate	S	As trichloroethanol				
		Therap. conc.	2–12 μg/mL	× 6.694	13–80 μmol/L	
		Toxic conc.	>20 μg/mL		>134 μmol/L	
Diazepam	S, P(H,E) at trough	Therap. conc.	100–1,000 ng/mL	× 3.512	350–3,500 nmol/L	
		Toxic conc.	>5,000 ng/mL		>17,500 nmol/L	
Digitoxin	S, P(H,E) (6-hr post)	Therap. conc.	20–35 ng/mL	× 1.307	26–46 nmol/L	x
		Toxic conc.	>45 ng/mL		>59 nmol/L	
Digoxin	S, P(H,E) (12-hr post)	Therap. conc.				
		CHF	0.8–1.5 ng/mL	× 1.281	1.0–1.9 nmol/L	xe
		Arrhythmias	1.5–2.0 ng/mL		1.9–2.6 nmol/L	
		Toxic conc.				
		Child	>2.5 ng/mL		>3.2 nmol/L	
		Adult	>3.0 ng/mL		>3.8 nmol/L	
Diphenylhydantoin	See Phenytoin					
Doxepin (includes desmethyldoxepine)	S, P	Therap. conc.	110–250 ng/mL	× 1	110–250 μg/L	(Syva Co.)
Ethanol	W(O), S	Toxic conc.	50–100 mg/dL	× 0.2171	11–22 mmol/L	
		CNS depression	>100 mg/dL		>22 mmol/L	
Ethosuximide	S, P(H,E) at trough	Therap. conc.	40–100 μg/mL	× 7.084	280–700 μmol/L	xe
		Toxic conc.	>150 μg/mL		>1,060 μmol/L	
Imipramine (includes desipramine)	S	Therap. conc.	150–250 ng/mL	× 1	150–250 μg/L	e (Syva Co.)
Lithium	S, P(not LiH)	12 hr after dose				
		Therap. conc.	0.6–1.2 mmol/L	× 1	Therap. conc. 0.6–1.2 mmol/L	
		Toxic conc.	>2 mmol/L		Toxic conc. >2 mmol/L	
Lysergic acid diethylamide		After hallucinogenic dose			After hallucinogenic dose	
	P(E)		0.005–0.009 μg/mL	× 3089	15.5–27.8 nmol/L	
	U		0.001–0.050 μg/mL		3.1–155 nmol/L	
Methotrexate	S, P	After high-dose therapy			After high-dose therapy	e
		Toxic	>5 μmol/L at 24 hr	× 1	Toxic >5 μmol/L at 24 hr	
		Toxic	>1 μmol/L at 48 hr		Toxic >1 μmol/L at 48 hr	
Paraldehyde	S, P(H,E)	Sedative	10–100 μg/mL	× 7.567	75–750 μmol/L	(Koren, et al.)
		Anticonvulsant	100–200 μg/mL		>750–1,500 μmol/L	
		Toxic	>200 μg/mL		>1,500 μmol/L	
		Lethal	>500 μg/mL		>3,750 μmol/L	
Phenacetin	P(E)	Therap. conc.	1–20 μg/mL	× 5.580	5.6–110 μmol/L	
		Toxic conc.	50–250 μg/mL		280–1,400 μmol/L	
Phenobarbital	S, P(H,E) at trough	Therap. conc.	15–40 μg/mL	× 4.306	65–170 μmol/L	xe
		Toxic conc.				
		Slowness, ataxia, nystagmus	35–80 μg/mL		150–345 μmol/L	
		Coma				
		With reflexes	65–117 μg/mL		280–504 μmol/L	
		Without reflexes	>100 μg/mL		>430 μmol/L	
Phensuximide (both parent and *N*-desmethyl metabolite)	S, P(H,E)	Therap. conc.	40–60 μg/mL	× 5.71	228–343 μmol/L	
Phenytoin	S, P(H,E)	Therap. conc.	10–20 μg/mL	× 3.964	40–80 μmol/L	
Primidone	S, P(H,E) at trough	Therap. conc.	5–12 μg/mL	× 4.582	23–55 μmol/L	(Taylor and Caviness)
		Toxic conc.	>15 μg/mL		>69 μmol/L	
		Toxic (neonatal)	>20 μg/mL		>92 μmol/L	
Procainamide	S, P(H,E)	Therap conc.	4–10 μg/mL	× 4.25	17–42 μmol/L	
		Toxic conc. (also consider conc. of metabolite *N*-acetylprocainamide [NAPA])	>10–12 μg/mL		42–51 μmol/L	

Table continued on following page

■ TABLE 670–2 Reference Ranges for Laboratory Tests *(Continued)*

Test	Specimen	Reference Range		Factor	Reference Range (SI)	Comments
Propranolol	S, P(H,E) at trough	Therap. conc.	50–100 ng/mL	× 3.856	190–380 nmol/L	
Quinidine	S, P(H,E)	Therap. conc.	2–5 μg/mL	× 3.083	6.2–15.5 μmol/L	
		Toxic conc.	>6 μg/mL		>18.5 μmol/L	
Salicylate	S, P(H,E) at trough	Therap. conc.	15–30 mg/dL	× 0.0724	1.1–2.2 mmol/L	
		Toxic conc.	>30 mg/dL		>2.2 mmol/L	
Theophylline	S, P(H,E)	Therap conc., bronchodilator	10–20 μg/mL	× 5.550	56–110 μmol/L	xz
		Premature apnea	5–10 μg/mL		28–56 μmol/L	
		Toxic conc.	>20 μg/mL		>110 μmol/L	
Valproic acid	S, P(H,E) at trough	Therap. conc.	50–100 μg/mL	× 6.934	350–700 μmol/L	
		Toxic conc.	>100 μg/mL		>700 μmol/L	

■ TABLE 670–3 Drug Dosages (Drugs Listed Alphabetically by Generic Name) (See Related conversion Table 670–4 and Figs. 670–1 and 670–2)

KEY:

NB	newborn (birth to end of 1st mo)	†	available as generic preparation
IN	infant (1–12 mo)	‡	available also under other brand name(s)
CH	child (1–12 yr)		
AD	adult		
caps	capsules	g	gram
div	divided	mg	milligram = 10^{-3} g
D/W	dextrose in water	μg	microgram = 10^{-6} g (sometimes abbreviated mcg)
IM	intramuscular		
inj	injection	ng	nanogram = 10^{-9} g
IV	intravenous	kg	kilogram = 10^3 g
LO	linguo-occlusal	mL	milliliter = 10^{-3} liter ≃ cm^3 = cc (cubic centimeter)
ointm	ointment		
PO	per os, oral	℞	prescription
PR	per rectum	Q	every (as in Q 4 hr)
prn	pro re nata, when necessary	max	maximum daily dose
SC	subcutaneous	US	United States
SL	sublingual	CNS	central nervous system
sol	solution	G-6-PD	glucose-6-phosphate
suppos	suppositories	GI	gastrointestinal
susp	suspension		
tabl	tablets		

Adapted from Table 27–3 in the 14th edition by S. Cohen.

Acetaminophen, paracetamol, APAP, NAPAP
℞ antipyretic, analgesic: IN, CH = PO, PR: 60 mg/kg/24 hr, div, every 4–6 hr, prn
†, LIQUIPRIN, TYLENOL, ‡; tabl, caps, caplet, drops, suppository, liquid preparations
Caution: Massive overdose may cause hepatic necrosis through formation of a toxic metabolite. Lesser overdoses frequently cause reversible jaundice (see Chapter 666.2).

Acetazolamide, carbonic anhydrase inhibitor
℞ as adjunct in the treatment of glaucoma, short-term diuresis, convulsive disorders (ketotic effect): CH = PO: 8–30 mg/kg/24 hr, div, every 6–8 hr
†, DIAMOX; tabl

Acetylcysteine (*N*-acetylcysteine), mucolytic agent; detoxifying agent in acetaminophen overdose
℞ to loosen tenacious bronchial secretions by local application to the bronchial tree with nebulizer: 3–5 mL 20% sol diluted with equal volume of sterile water or saline, or 6–10 mL of 10% sol, every 6–8 hr; or by direct instillation: 1–2 mL of 10% or 20% sol every 1–4 hr
℞ in acetaminophen overdose: IN, CH, AD = PO: 140 mg/kg/1st dose, followed by 70 mg/kg/dose every 4 hr for a total of 72 hr; IV dose (investigational in US): 150 mg/kg in 200 mL of 5% D/W over 15 min, followed by 50 mg/kg in 500 mL of 5% D/W over 4 hr, followed by 100 mg/kg in 1,000 mL of 5% D/W over 16 hr; or 140 mg/kg loading dose, followed by 70 mg/kg Q 4 hr × 12 doses.
MUCOMYST; vials 10% (100 mg/mL) or 20% (200 mg/mL)

Acetylsalicylic acid, ASA, Aspirin
℞ antipyretic, analgesic, anti-inflammatory: IN, CH = PO: 30–65 mg/kg/24 hr, div, every 4–6 hr, prn. This dosage corresponds to 27–58 mg salicylate sodium/kg/24 hr, or 20–50 mg salicylic acid/kg/24 hr
℞ antirheumatic: CH = PO: 65–130 mg/kg/24 hr, div, every 4–6 hr
†, BUFFERIN, ‡: tabl; also contained in many combination products
Caution: Acute or chronic overdose may cause life-threatening poisoning syndrome (see Chapter 666). Use in children <16 yr with varicella or flulike illnesses is associated with Reye syndrome (see Chapter 666.3)

ACTH, adrenocorticotropic hormone
℞ for infantile spasms: IM: 24–40 units every 12 hr, or 2.5–4.0 units/kg every 12 hr. Observe for hypertension, use with caution in presence of congestive heart failure, acute psychosis, ocular herpes
CORTICOTROPIN, CORTROSYN, ACTHAR; inj: 10 units/mL, 20 units/mL, 40 units/mL vials

Actinomycin D, see Dactinomycin

Activated charcoal, adsorbent for treatment of oral drug overdose; may also enhance drug elimination (theophylline, phenobarbital)
PO: 10 times (by weight) estimated quantity of drug ingested or 0.25–1 g/kg orally; may repeat every 4 hr when necessary
Commercial ready-to-use suspensions may contain sorbitol, which induces osmotic diarrhea in some patients
Multiple products, consider continuous nasogastric administration

Acyclovir, antiviral agent against herpes simplex and varicella-zoster virus by selective inhibition of viral DNA synthesis
℞ in clinical herpes simplex infection in neonates: NB = IV (over 60 min): 10 mg/kg/dose every 8 hr, for 10–14 days
Dosing interval should be increased to 24 hr if renal function is less than 25% of normal
℞ in immunocompromised individuals with herpes simplex or varicella-zoster virus infection: CH = IV (over 60 min): 7.5 mg/kg per dose every 8 hr for 7 days. PO: 7.5–20 mg/kg per dose administered 4–5 times per day. AD = IV (over 60 min); PO: 800 mg 5 times per day for 7–10 days.
℞ mucocutaneous herpes simplex virus (HSV) infection: CH = IV (over 60 min) 5 mg/kg per dose every 8 hr for 7 days; HSV encephalitis: 10 mg/kg per dose every 8 hr for 10–14 days; varicella-zoster infection: 5 mg/kg per dose every 8 hr for 7 days.
℞ IV prophylaxis in bone marrow transplant recipients: HSV seropositive 4.5–5 mg/kg every 8–12 hr; CMV seropositive 15 mg/kg per dose every 8 hr; in markedly symptomatic patients, consider ganciclovir.
℞ in severe first episode of herpes genitalis: CH, AD = LO: 5% ointm
Caution: Acyclovir dosing should be adjusted for patients with renal insufficiency, i.e., glomerular filtration rates <50 mL/min in patients >6 mo of age.
ZOVIRAX; inj, ointm, caps, susp, tabl

■ TABLE 670–3 Drug Dosages (Drugs Listed Alphabetically by Generic Name) *(Continued)*

Adenosine, an endogenous nucleoside used in the treatment of paroxysmal supraventricular tachycardia. Slows conduction through atrioventricular node; clinical effects are rapid and very brief, adenosine half-life ($t_{1/2}$) <10 sec.
℞ for supraventricular tachycardia, CH = IV (rapid bolus infusion): 0.1 mg/kg, if no effect within 2 min administer 0.2 mg/kg/dose, maximum single dose 12 mg. AD = IV (rapid bolus injection): 6 mg, if not effective within 2 min administer 12-mg dose.

Albuterol, catecholamine analog; β-adrenergic receptor agonist with preferential effect on β_2-adrenergic receptors
℞ bronchodilator: CH = PO: 0.1–0.2 mg/kg, div, every 8 hr; 6–12 yr, 2 mg 3–4 times/24 hr; nebulization 0.01–0.05 mL/kg of 5 mg/mL solution Q 4–6 hr. AD = PO 2–4 mg per dose 3–4 times a day. In status asthmaticus, may use continuous administration by aerosol; monitor heart rate, serum potassium level. See Bronchodilator aerosols below.
VENTOLIN, PROVENTIL; tab, liquid, inhalation

Allopurinol, analog of hypoxanthine; inhibitor of xanthine oxidase and thereby of the terminal steps of uric acid biosynthesis
℞ against hyperuricemia and urate deposition in tissues and kidneys, especially in patients receiving antineoplastic chemotherapy: CH = PO: 10 mg/kg/24 hr, div or in single daily dose. AD = PO 300 mg daily.
Note that allopurinol and its metabolite alloxanthine (oxypurinol) inhibit xanthine oxidase, and that reduced glomerular filtration requires lowering the dose to compensate for delayed excretion. A high urine output should be established—with a neutral or slightly alkaline urine pH—to allow for excretion of uric acid precursors.
Caution: If azathioprine or mercaptopurine, each of which is metabolized by xanthine oxidase, is to be given concomitantly with allopurinol, the dosage of azathioprine or mercaptopurine should be reduced substantially (to ¼–⅓ of usual dosage).
†, ZYLOPRIM; tabl

Alprostadil, prostaglandin E_1 for the temporary maintenance of ductus arteriosus patency until surgery can be performed. NB, IN = continuous IV infusion, 0.05–0.1 μg/kg/min increased until desired therapeutic response, then reduce dose to lowest effective dose, usually 0.01–0.4 μg/kg/min.
Note: Apnea may occur in as many as 10–12% of neonates with congenital heart disease who receive the drug, particularly in infants weighing <2 kg.
PROSTN VR, inj.

Aluminum hydroxide, antacid
℞ for treatment of peptic ulcer: CH = PO: 5–15 mL/dose every 3–6 hr, or 1 and 3 hr after meals and at bedtime
℞ for prophylaxis of gastrointestinal bleeding:
IN = PO (by nasogastric tube): 2–5 mL every 1–2 hr
CH = PO (by nasogastric tube): 5–15 mL every 1–2 hr
℞ against hyperphosphatemia: IN, CH = PO: 50–150 mg/kg/24 hr, div. every 4–6 hr
Note: May cause constipation, aluminum toxicity, phosphorus depletion. Inhibits gastric emptying. Interferes with absorption of tetracyclines
†, AMPHOJEL; susp (320 mg/5 mL), tabl (300 mg, 600 mg), gel liquid (600 mg/5 mL)

Aluminum hydroxide and **magnesium hydroxide,** antacid
Note: Magnesium-containing antacids are laxative. In renal failure, magnesium and aluminum may be retained. Interferes with absorption of tetracyclines
℞ for treatment of peptic ulcer: same as for aluminum hydroxide alone.
†, MAALOX, ‡; susp, tabl

Amantadine, antiviral drug used for prophylaxis and treatment of influenza A infections; also used as adjunctive treatment of Parkinson disease. CH <8 yr of age = PO, 5–9 mg/kg/24 hr, div Q 12 hr, max 200 mg/24 hr. CH >8 yr and AD = PO 100–200 mg/24 hr, div Q 12–24 hr, max dose 200 mg/24 hr.
Caution: anticholinergic effects may predominate, may cause CNS stimulation. Reduce dose in renal disease.
†SYMMETREL, caps, sol

Amikacin sulfate, antimicrobial aminoglycoside effective primarily against gram-negative microorganisms.
NB <7 days: <28 wk = IM, IV (over 20–30 min): 7.5 mg/kg once daily; 28–34 wk, 7.5 mg/kg every 18 hr; >34 wk, 7.5 mg/kg every 12 hr
NB >7 days: <28 wk, 7.5 mg/kg every 18 hr; 28–34 wk, 7.5 mg/kg every 12 hr; >34 wk, 7.5 mg/kg every 8 hr
IN, CH = IM, IV 15–25 mg/kg/24 hr. AD = IM, IV 15 mg/kg/24 hr Q 12 hr.
AMIKIN, inj.
Serum concentrations should be monitored; therapeutic peak concentration 25–35 mg/L, trough concentration <10 mg/L (see Table 670–2).

Aminophylline, See Theophylline.

Aminosalicylate sodium, para-aminosalicylate sodium, PAS sodium; structural analog of para-aminobenzoic acid with weak bacteriostatic activity against *Mycobacterium tuberculosis,* used only in combination with other antituberculous agents
℞ as adjunct to isoniazid therapy: CH = PO: 200–300 mg/kg/24 hr, div, every 4–6 hr
†, PAMISYL-Sodium, PARASAL-Sodium, ‡; tabl, caps
Note: Frequent nausea, vomiting, diarrhea, abdominal pain, and poor acceptance by patients restrict the usefulness of this substance. 1 g of aminosalicylate sodium contains 4.7 mEq Na^+.

Amiodarone, antiarrhythmic, category class III; used for the treatment of ventricular arrhythmias, usually reserved for use in the management of life-threatening arrhythmias unresponsive to more conventional antiarrhythmic drugs. CH = PO loading dose 10–15 mg/kg/24 hr div in 1–2 doses for 10–14 days, dose should then be reduced to ~5 mg/kg/24 hr.
Caution: amiodarone may increase the plasma concentrations of digoxin and other cardiac glycosides, flecainide, phenytoin, procainamide, quinidine, and warfarin. Concurrent amiodarone with β-receptor antagonists, digoxin, or calcium channel antagonists may cause clinically significant bradycardia.
CORDARONE, tabl

Amitriptyline, cyclic (tricyclic) antidepressant used for the treatment of various forms of depression, select cases of ADHD and enuresis.
℞ for depression, hyperactivity: CH = PO: 1 mg/kg/24 hr div 1–2 doses; may gradually increase dose to 1.5 mg/kg/24 hr. AD = PO 30–100+ mg/24 hr div 1–2 doses.
Note: use with caution in patients with cardiac conduction abnormalities or cardiac disease. Initial therapy usually accompanied by marked sedation as predominant symptom of anticholinergic effects. Overdose may be associated with serious and fatal cardiac arrhythmia.
ELAVIL, ENDEP, tabl, inj.

Ammonium chloride, urinary acidifying drug most often used as a source of chloride ion in the treatment of hypochloremia.
℞ for hypochloremia, may calculate body chloride deficit and replace slowly; alternatively, IN, CH = IV, PO, 75 mg/kg/24 hr div 3–6 doses, AD = IV, 1.5 g per dose every 6 hr, PO, 2–3 g every 4–6 h.
Note: close monitoring or serum chloride and blood pH should guide therapy. Use with caution in patients with liver disease.
tabl, inj.

Amobarbital, central nervous system depressant of barbiturate class with intermediate duration of action. Tolerance to its hypnotic effect may develop on continued use. Initially, hypnotic effect lasts 3–8 hr
℞ for sedation: IN, CH = PO, IM: 1–2 mg/kg/24 hr, div, every 6 hr
℞ for sleep: IN, CH = PO, IM: 2–3 mg/kg/dose, repeat prn after 12–24 hr
†, AMYTAL: tabl, elixir; amobarbital sodium, ‡, AMYTAL sodium: inj, caps

Amoxicillin, acid-resistant ampicillin congener
IN, CH = PO: 20–50 mg/kg/24 hr, div, every 8 hr
†, AMOXIL, LAROTID, ‡; caps, oral susp, pediatric drops

Amoxicillin + clavulanic acid, combination of a β-lactam antibiotic with a β-lactamase (penicillinase) inhibitor. The addition of clavulanic acid extends the activity of amoxicillin from group A and other streptococci, *Streptococcus pneumoniae,* many strains of *Escherichia coli,* and *Proteus mirabilis,* non–β-lactamase-producing strains of staphylococci, *Neisseria gonorrhoeae,* and *Haemophilus influenzae* to include β-lactamase–producing strains of *H. influenzae, E. coli, P. mirabilis,* as well as *Klebsiella pneumoniae, Staphylococcus aureus* (but not methicillin-resistant strains), *Moraxella catarrhalis, Bacteroides fragilis,* and *Legionella pneumophila. Pseudomonas aeruginosa,* many strains of *Serratia,* and *Enterobacter* are resistant.
℞ for otitis media, sinusitis, lower respiratory tract, skin, soft tissue, and urinary tract infections: CH = PO: amoxicillin 20–40 mg/kg/24 hr + clavulanic acid 5–10 mg/kg/24 hr, div, every 8 hr; AD = PO 250–500 mg Q 8 hr: maximum 2 g/24 hr.
Note: may cause diarrhea, abdominal pain, urticaria, and other rashes, due possibly to clavulanic acid alone. Amoxicillin is available as single component.
AUGMENTIN; tabl of 2 strengths: 250 mg amoxicillin + 125 mg clavulanic acid, and 500 mg amoxicillin + 125 mg clavulanic acid; oral susp with amoxicillin 125 mg + clavulanic acid 31.25 mg/5 mL, or amoxicillin 250 mg + clavulanic acid 62.5 mg/5 mL

Amphotericin B, antifungal agent of the "polyene" type (nystatin, another example); insoluble in water, unstable below pH 4, should be given IV. Effective through binding to sterol components of the membrane of sensitive fungi, thereby altering its permeability; interference with renal function of patients seems an extension of the mode of action of this drug, demanding caution and continued monitoring during amphotericin B therapy.
Owing to potential toxicity for a variety of biologic functions, amphotericin B should be used only in progressive and potentially fatal infections with fungi sensitive to it.
Use as solution of amphotericin B at concentration of 0.1 mg/mL in 5% dextrose (all other drugs, including antimicrobial agents, and electrolytes must be kept away from the colloidal suspension of amphotericin B).

Table continued on following page

■ **TABLE 670–3 Drug Dosages (Drugs Listed Alphabetically by Generic Name)** *(Continued)*

See Chapters 229 to 236 for dose and administration. Optimal dose and duration of therapy not clearly determined.
Available as lyophilized powder containing sodium deoxycholate as emulsifier. Colloidal suspension prepared by adding required volume of sterile water and shaking appropriately, subsequently diluted in 5% sterile D/W to a final concentration of amphotericin B of 0.1 mg/mL, for slow IV administration.
FUNGIZONE IV; inj

Ampicillin, acid-resistant penicillin congener effective against many gram-positive and gram-negative organisms. Drug is effectively destroyed by β-lactamase.
NB <7 days: <2,000 g = IV (over 15–30 min), IM: 50 mg/kg/24 hr, div, every 12 hr; >2,000 g, div, every 8 hr
NB >7 days: <2,000 g = IV (over 15–30 min), IM: 100 mg/kg/24 hr, div, every 8 hr; >2,000 g, div, every 6 hr
℞ for septicemia: IV: 100–200 mg/kg/24 hr, div, every 4 hr; IN, CH = PO: 50–100 mg/kg/24 hr, div, every 4–6 hr
℞ for meningitis: IV (over 15–30 min) 200–400 mg/kg/24 hr, div, every 4 hr (usual maximum: 12 g/24 hr)
Other infections: 100–200 mg/kg/24 hr, div, every 4–6 hr
Ampicillin sodium, for injection, OMNIPEN-N, PENBRITIN-S, ‡; inj ampicillin trihydrate, †, OMNIPEN, PENBRITIN, ‡; caps, oral susp, pediatric drops

Ampicillin/sulbactam, combination of a β-lactam antibiotic with a β-lactamase (penicillinase) inhibitor. The addition of sulbactam extends the activity of ampicillin to include β-lactamase–producing strains of *H. influenzae, E. coli, P. mirabilis, K. pneumoniae, S. aureus* (but not methicillin-resistant strains), *M. catarrhalis B. fragilis,* and *L. pneumophila* (see Amoxicillin + clavulanic acid, above)
℞ for systemic infections: IN, CH = IV 100–200 mg/kg/24 hr div every 4–6 hr. AD = IV 3–8 g/24 hr div 3–4 doses.
Note: dose adjustment necessary in patients with renal dysfunction, glomerular filtration rates <30 mL/min.
UNASYN, inj

Amrinone lactate, adrenergic agonist used in the treatment of low-output cardiac disease. Positive inotropic effect due to drug's ability to augment intracellular cyclic adenosine monophosphate (cAMP) concentrations by inhibiting myocardial cAMP phosphodiesterase. Drug may also possess additional systemic and pulmonary vasodilating effects.
℞ as an adjunct for the treatment of congestive heart failure, pulmonary hypertension: NB = IV loading dose (over 2–3 min) 0.75 mg/kg, then 3–5 μg/kg/min continuous IV infusion; CH, AD = IV loading dose (over 2–3 min) 0.75 mg, then 5–10 μg/kg/min continuous IV infusion.
Note: monitor patients closely for drug-associated hypotension, thrombocytopenia, and hepatotoxicity. Ventricular and/or supraventricular arrhythmias may be related to infusion rate and respond to dose reduction.
INOCOR, inj.

Antihemophilic factor, human, used for the management of factor VIII deficiency, hemophilia A disease.
℞ as replacement therapy, individualize dose to patient requirements based on clotting studies; 20–50 units/kg/dose administered every 12–24 hr as needed. The following formula can be used to approximate the increase in plasma antihemophilic factor: Units required = body weight (kg) × 0.5 × desired increase in factor VIII (i.e., percent of normal), inj.

ARA-C, see Cytarabine

Arginine hydrochloride, amino acid used as a source of hydrogen ion in the treatment of alkalosis and as a test of pituitary function.
℞ for growth hormone reserve test CH = IV (over 30 min) 500 mg/kg. AD = IV (over 30 min) 30 g (300 mL of a 10% solution).
℞ for metabolic alkalosis: dose can be calculated from the following formula; arginine dose (g) = weight (kg) × 0.1 [patient serum bicarbonate concentration (HCO_3) in mEq/L minus 24]. Administer ½–⅔ of dose and re-evaluate patient need.
R-GENE, inj. (10% solution; 0.475 mEq chloride/mL).

Astemizole, antihistamine used for the symptomatic treatment of perennial and seasonal allergic rhinitis and other allergic symptoms. Competitive antagonist of the classic histamine H_1 receptor associated with less sedation than earlier antihistamines (e.g., diphenhydramine) due to preferential antagonism of peripheral rather than peripheral and central H_1 receptors.
℞ for allergic symptoms: CH: <6 yr of age = PO 0.2 mg/kg once daily; CH: 6–12 yr of age = PO 5 mg/day; CH: >12 yr and AD = PO 10–30 mg/day once daily.
Note: concurrent ciprofloxacin, cimetidine, disulfiram, erythromycin, and ketoconazole may reduce hepatic metabolism of astemizole, leading to accumulation and cardiac toxicity. Reduced dose necessary in patients with liver disease.
Caution: excessive dosing or drug interactions may result in serious, life-threatening cardiac arrhythmias.
HISMANAL, tabl.

Atenolol, synthetic, relatively selective β_1-(cardioselective) adrenoreceptor blocking agent that possesses no membrane-stabilizing or intrinsic sympathomimetic effects. β_1-Antagonist properties are relative, and at higher doses atenolol inhibits β_2-adrenoreceptors, which are chiefly located in the bronchial and vascular musculature.
IN, CH = PO: 1.0–1.3 mg/kg/24 hr, once daily or div, every 12 hr: AD = PO 50–100 mg/dose daily
TENORMIN; inj, tabl

Atropine sulfate, *dl*-hyoscyamine; anticholinergic agent used mainly in premedication for anesthesia, as antiarrhythmic agent and as antispasmodic. Dosage varies according to indications and sensitivity of patients. On the average for IN, CH = SC, PO (IV): 0.01–0.02 mg/kg/dose, to be repeated prn after 2 hr until desired effect is obtained or adverse effects preclude further increase; for continued
℞ PO: 0.04 mg/kg 24 hr, div, every 6 hr, preferably with meals. Much higher doses may be necessary in the management of insecticide (acetylcholinesterase inhibitor) intoxication. Drug may be administered intratracheally; IN, CH = intratracheal 0.02 mg/kg/dose, minimum dose 0.1 mg, maximum dose 0.5 mg in children and 1 mg in adolescents.
Note: for intratracheal administration, atropine dose should be diluted to 1–2 mL total volume in normal saline.
℞ for bronchospasm, 0.025–0.05 mg/kg/dose inhalation administered every 4–6 hr.
℞ ophthalmic, 1–2 drops 1% solution before procedure.
†; inj, tabl
Caution: As for Belladonna, below.

Azathioprine, an imidazolyl derivative of 6-mercaptopurine and immunosuppressive antimetabolite. The drug is cleaved in the body to mercaptopurine. Both compounds are pharmacologically active.
CH = PO, IV 3–5 mg/kg/24 hr once daily. Maintenance dose usually 1–3 mg/kg/24 hr administered once daily.
Note: Limited experience for treatment of children with rheumatoid arthritis. The primary metabolic pathway for azathioprine is via xanthine oxidase, which is inhibited by allopurinol. Patients receiving concurrent allopurinol should have azathioprine dose reduced to approximately ⅓–¼ the usual dose.
IMURAN; inj, tabl

Azithromycin, macrolide antibiotic indicated for the treatment of mild to moderate upper and lower respiratory tract infections and infections of the skin caused by susceptible bacteria, *Chlamydia trachomatis, H. influenzae, M. catarrhalis, M. pneumoniae, S. aureus, Streptococcus pneumoniae.* Less gastrointestinal distress than associated with erythromycin.
CH = PO, 10 mg/kg day 1 followed by 5 mg/kg/day administered once daily for 5 days. AD = 500 mg day 1 followed by 250 mg once daily for 5 days.
Caution: coadministration with aluminum- and/or magnesium-containing antacids may decrease azithromycin peak serum concentrations by 25%.
ZITHROMAX, caps.

AZT, see Zidovudine

Aztreonam, monobactam antibiotic that possesses a unique monocyclic β-lactam nucleus that is effective against a wide spectrum of gram-negative aerobic pathogens.
NB <7 days old: <2,000 g: 60 mg/kg/24 hr, div, every 12 hr; >2,000 g: 90 mg/kg/24 hr, div, every 8 hr; >7 days old: <2,000 g: 90 mg/kg/24 hr, div, every 8 hr; <2,000 g, 120 mg/kg/24 hr, every 6 hr; NB administration is IV for 15–20 min or IM
IN, CH = IV (over 3–5 min), IM: 90–120 mg/kg/24 hr, div, every 6–8 hr; AD = IM, IV 1–2 g per dose Q 6–8 hr; max 8 g/24 hr.
AZACTAM; inj

Bacampicillin, inactive prodrug that is hydrolyzed to ampicillin. Drug effect, mechanism of action, and clinical indications are identical for ampicillin in the treatment of mild to moderate infections caused by ampicillin-susceptible bacteria.
℞ for mild to moderate ampicillin-susceptible infections, CH = PO 25–50 mg/kg/24 hr, div 2–3 doses. AD = PO 400–800 mg administered every 12 hr.
SPECTROBID, powder for susp 125 mg/5 mL (equivalent to 87.5 mg ampicillin/5 ml), tbl.

Baclofen, central-acting skeletal muscle relaxant used in the symptomatic treatment of spasticity. Inhibits transmission of mono- and polysynaptic reflexes at the level of the spinal chord by a mechanism(s) unknown. CH = PO, 10–15 mg/24 hr, div every 8 hr. Dose may be titrated upward by 5–15 mg/24 hr every 3–5 days to a total daily dose of 40 mg/kg/24 hr. In CH >8 yr of age, dose may approach 60 mg/24 hr. AD = PO, 5 mg 3 times daily, dose titrated upward to a usual maximum of 80 mg/24 hr.
Note: muscle relaxation may not be observed for 3–5 days after starting therapy with maximal effects observed after 5–10 days.
LIORESAL, tabl.

Beclomethasone dipropionate, chlorinated synthetic corticosteroid
℞ for topical treatment to the bronchial tissues in long-term, steroid-dependent asthma. Delivered from metered-dose aerosol unit, releasing approximately 50 μg of beclomethasone by activation of the dispenser unit: CH (6–12 yr): 1–2 inhalations every 6–8 hr. AD = 2 inhalations Q 6–8 hr.

■ TABLE 670–3 Drug Dosages (Drugs Listed Alphabetically by Generic Name) *(Continued)*

℞ for seasonal/perennial rhinitis, nasal polyposis: CH, AD = 1–2 nasal inhalations each nostril Q 8–12 hr.
Effect usually apparent within 1–4 wk after beginning of steroid inhalations
Note: Avoid use with active wheezing
Caution: On transfer from systemic steroid therapy for asthma to inhalation therapy, adrenocortical competency of the patient must be watched and supported, if indicated, since inhalation therapy does not contribute to systemic corticosteroid supply.
VANCERIL, BECLOVENT, inhaler; BECONASE, VANCENASE, nasal spray, inhaler

Belladonna tincture, aqueous-alcoholic extract of belladonna leaves; anticholinergic preparation; used chiefly as antispasmodic
Contains the equivalent of approximately 0.3 mg of atropine sulfate/mL. Usual dose: 1 drop/4.5 kg (10 lb) body weight 15–30 min before meals, 3 times/day
Caution: Erythematous skin, persistently dilated pupils, and tachycardia are indications for discontinuing, then lowering dose. Extreme hypersensitivity may exist in patients with Down syndrome.

Benzoyl peroxide, for topical use only in the treatment of mild to moderate acne. Free radical oxygen releaser oxidizes bacterial proteins in sebaceous glands, decreasing number of anaerobic bacteria. CH, AD = topical application, apply sparingly 1–3 times daily. Amount applied, duration of exposure, and strength of preparation increased as tolerated.
Caution: overly aggressive application can cause serious dermal irritation, contact dermatitis, erythema.
BENOXYL, CLEARASIL, LOROXIDE, OXY-5, PanOxy, VANOXIDE, creams, gels, lotions, soaps

Benztropine mesylate, anticholinergic agent used for the treatment of drug-induced extrapyramidal effects and acute dystonic reactions, as an adjunct in the treatment of Parkinson disease. CH (>3 yr of age) = PO, IM, IV, 0.02–0.05 mg/kg/dose every 8–12 hr. AD = PO, IM, IV, 1–4 mg/dose administered every 12–24 hr.
Note: adverse effects result of anticholinergic activity. Effective in reversing phenothiazine-associated dystonic effects.
COGENTIN, inj, tabl.

Beractant, bovine (natural) lung surfactant used in the prevention or treatment of respiratory distress syndrome (RDS) in premature infants, prophylactic therapy, rescue therapy for acute respiratory distress syndrome (ARDS) in mechanically ventilated patients.
℞ for RDS, ARDS in CH, AD = intratracheal instillation, 4 ml/kg. Up to as many as 4 doses may be administered at 6-hr intervals over the first 48 hr of treatment. Insufficient data are available addressing the potential efficacy and safety of additional doses administered more frequently.
Note: suction patient before intratracheal instillation. Administer each dose as 1-ml/kg aliquots instilled over 2–3 sec per patient's tolerance. Each 1/4 dose is administered with patient in a different position, e.g., downward inclination of the head turned to the right, then turned to the left, etc.
SURVANTA, intratracheal susp.

Betamethasone, long-acting anti-inflammatory corticosteroid with little to no sodium retention potential. CH = IM, 0.0175–0.2 mg base/kg/24 hr div every 6–12 hr; PO 0.0175–0.25 mg/kg/24 hr div every 6–8 hr. AD = IM 0.6–9 mg/24 hr div every 12–24 hr; PO, 2–5 mg/24 hr div every 12–24 hr.
Note: for more information on steroid medications, see Corticosteroids.
CELESTONE, VALISONE, inj, syrup, tabl, topical cream, gel, lotion, ointm.

Bethanechol chloride, chloinergic agent used in the treatment of neurogenic bladder, nonobstructive urinary retention, and gastroesophageal reflux disease. Stimulates cholinergic receptors present in smooth muscle, enhancing urinary bladder tone, gastrointestinal and ureteral peristaltic activity.
℞ urinary retention, abdominal distention. CH = PO 0.6 mg/kg/24 hr div every 6–8 hr. AD = PO 10–50 mg administered 2–4 times daily.
℞ for gastroesophageal reflux disease. CH = PO 0.1–0.2 mg/kg/dose 30 min–1 hr before each meal, maximum 4 doses per 24 hr. SC 0.12–0.2 mg/kg/24 hr div every 6–8 hr.
DUVOID, URECHOLINE, inj, tabl.

Bisacodyl, cathartic, structurally related to phenolphthalein
℞ laxative: PO: 0.3 mg/kg/dose, 6–8 hr before desired large bowel action. CH (>12 yr), AD = PO 10 mg once daily.
Note: tablets are enteric coated and should be swallowed whole, with the added precaution of avoiding oral antacids or milk within at least 1 hr of ingestion.
DULCOLAX; tabl, suppos

Bretylium tosylate, antiarrhythmic class III agent used in the treatment of ventricular arrhythmias, venticular fibrillation unresponsive to more conventional agents. Bretylium stimulates an initial release of norepinephrine from peripheral nerve terminals, then inhibits further release by postganglionic neurons. Patients usually undergo defibrillation/cardioversion before and after bretylium doses. CH = IM 2.5 mg/kg as a single dose. CH, AD IV (over 0.5–5 min) 5 mg/kg per dose given as needed every 10–20 min to a maximum dose of 30 mg/kg. Maintenance therapy, 5 mg/kg/dose administered every 6–8 hr.
Caution: hypotension occurs commonly.
BRETYLOL, inj.

Brompheniramine maleate, alkylamine; antihistamine with mild anticholinergic and mild sedative effects.
℞ antiallergic effect: CH = PO: 0.5 mg/kg/24 hr, div, every 6 hr
†, DIMETANE; elixir, tabl, inj

Bronchodilator aerosols
℞ in acute asthmatic attack, provided effective inhalation is possible (e.g., in early stages of attack or with assisted ventilation [IPPB] or as continuous nebulization). Effectiveness of a delivered dose depends on microdispersion in the aerosol generated from different types of nebulizers, breathing mechanics, and patient minute ventilation. Onset of effect usually occurs within 2–5 min after inhalation of aerosol. Risk of self-overuse or overdosage in children is high with aerosol preparations, particularly in emergency situations. These limitations apply to all bronchodilator aerosols (epinephrine, racemic epinephrine, isoproterenol, metaproterenol, isoetharine, albuterol), some of which can be dispensed from "metered" nebulization nozzles, and products for use in adults. Patients and their families should be warned against over-self-medication from the home aerosol preparations. Nevertheless, aerosol/nebulization of selective β_2-agonist bronchodilating drugs can be a safe, highly effective means of reversing acute airways bronchoconstriction.

Bumetanide, saluretic with a duration of action of approximately 2 hr when administered IV. Bumetanide inhibits sodium reabsorption in the ascending limb of the loop of Henle ("loop diuretic"), inhibits chloride and sodium reabsorption, and interferes with concentration of urine. One milligram of bumetanide possesses a diuretic potency equivalent to approximately 40 mg of furosemide.
IN, CH = PO, IV, IM: 0.01–0.02 mg/kg/dose; if needed may be repeated at intervals of 6–12 hr AD = PO, IV (over 1–2 min) IM 0.5–2 mg dose every 12–24 hr.
BUMEX; tabl, inj

Caffeine, CNS stimulant and vasoconstrictor of cerebral vessels
℞ against vascular headache and as an analeptic: CH = PO: 10 mg/kg/24 hr, div, every 4–6 hr; single dose usually 2–3 mg/kg/dose.
℞ against neonatal apnea; loading dose 10 mg/kg followed by maintenance therapy 2.5–5 mg/kg/24 hr, div, every 12–24 hr
Note: Above dosages should be doubled if citrated caffeine preparation is used. Serum concentrations may be monitored; therapeutic concentrations are 8–20 mg/L. In newborn, because caffeine elimination is markedly diminished compared with adult (including parturient women), transplacentally acquired blood concentrations of caffeine are maintained within a possibly effective range for several days after delivery. Danger of toxic manifestations owing to accumulation exists if additional caffeine is administered without appropriate dose adjustment.

Calcitriol, 1,25-dihydroxycholecalciferol used in the treatment of hypocalcemia associated with chronic renal failure, vitamin D–deficient rickets and hypoparathyroidism.
℞ for hypocalcemia: IN (premature) = PO 1 μg/24 hr for 5 days, IV (over 1–2 min) 0.05 μg/kg/24 hr for 5–10 days.
℞ for hypocalcemia and renal failure: titrate to desired effect, CH = PO 0.25–2 μg/24 hr with hemodialysis; 0.014–0.041 μg/kg/24 hr not undergoing hemodialysis; IV 0.01–0.05 μg/kg administered 3 times weekly while undergoing hemodialysis. AD = PO 0.25 μg/24 hr 3 times weekly, IV 0.5 μg 3 times weekly.
CALCIJEX, ROCALTROL; inj., caps

Calcium salts: Elemental content of calcium per gram of salt preparation

Calcium Preparation	*mg of Calcium/g*	*mEq/g of Calcium*
Calcium acetate	253	12.7
Calcium carbonate	400	20
Calcium chloride	270	13.5
Calcium glubionate	64	3.3
Calcium gluceptate	82	4.1
Calcium gluconate	92	4.6
Calcium lactate	130	6.5
Calcium phosphate dibasic anhydrous	290	14.5
Calcium phosphate dibasic dihydrate	230	11.5

Calcium gluconate $[CH_2OH(CHOH)_4COO]_2Ca{\cdot}H_2O$
1 g equivalent to 92 mg elemental calcium or to 4.6 mEq Ca^{2+}. Solution "10%" contains 100 mg/mL of calcium gluconate. This concentration equivalent to elemental calcium, 8.9 mg/mL, or Ca^{2+} 0.45 mEq/mL.
℞ to compensate for manifestations of hypocalcemia (tetany, seizures, myocardial insufficiency, hypoparathyroidism). Urgency and severity of clinical situation dictate dose and route of administration: IN, CH = IV (infused slowly, with monitoring of heart for bradycardia, arrest): "10%" calcium gluconate solution: 1–2 mL/kg/dose, equivalent to Ca 0.45–0.90

Table continued on following page

■ **TABLE 670–3 Drug Dosages (Drugs Listed Alphabetically by Generic Name)** *(Continued)*

mEq/kg/dose, repeat prn after 6 hr. Daily dose needed might be as high as Ca 2.7 mEq/kg/24 hr.

Caution: Do not use any calcium preparation for intramuscular injection because of risk of sterile abscess formation. Extravascular leakage may cause local necrosis.

IN, CH = PO: calcium gluconate 500 mg/kg/24 hr, equivalent to elemental calcium 45 mg/kg/24 hr or Ca^{2+} 2.3 mEq/kg/24 hr, div, every 4–8 hr

Note: Concomitant oral intake of phosphate exerts a major influence on the amount of calcium made available for absorption in the intestine.

†, powder, tabl

Calcium lactate $[CH_3CHOHCOO]_2Ca{\cdot}5H_2O$

1 g of Ca lactate equivalent to 130 mg elemental calcium or to 6.49 mEq Ca^{2+}.

IN, CH = PO: 500 mg/kg/24 hr, equivalent to elemental calcium 65 mg/kg/24 hr or Ca^{2+} 3.2 mEq/kg/24/hr, div every 4–8 hr

Note: Concomitant oral intake of phosphate exerts major influence on amount of calcium available for absorption in intestine. To ensure appropriate absorption in neonatal transient hypoparathyroidism, a calcium/phosphorus ratio of 4:1 (by weight, corresponding to 3:1 on molar basis) should be achieved in the feeding. This would require 10 g of calcium lactate powder added to a daily formula containing 500 mL of whole cow's milk.

†, powder, tabl

Captopril, competitive inhibitor of angiotensin I–converting enzyme, antihypertensive agent, congestive heart failure

℞ for cardiovascular response: NB = PO: 0.1–0.4 mg/kg/dose administered every 6–24 hr; IN = PO: 0.5–0.6 mg/kg/24 hr div, every 6–12 hr; CH = PO: 0.15 mg/kg every 4–8 hr. Dose may be slowly increased to desired effect; max pediatric dose 6 mg/kg/24 hr. AD = PO 6.25–12.5 mg/dose Q 8–12 hr, usual AD max 450 mg/24 hr.

Note: May cause renal impairment, neutropenia, immunodeficiency, rashes, disturbances of taste. Adjust dose with renal failure.

CAPOTEN; tabl

Carbamazepine, anticonvulsant agent; structurally related to tricyclic antidepressants

IN, CH = PO: initially 5–10 mg/kg/24 hr, div, every 8–12 hr; to be increased progessively, if needed, to 20 mg/kg/24 hr, div, every 12 hr or as a single daily dose, if tolerated. Usual mainteance dose range 20–30 mg/kg/24 hr CH (>12 yr), AD = PO initially 200 mg every 24 hr, titrated as needed, max 800–1200 mg/24 hr.

Note: Carbamazepine is a potent inducer of hepatic microsomal metabolizing enzymes that may stimulate the metabolism of numerous other drugs metabolized via the liver.

TEGRETOL; tabl, chew tabl, susp

Carbenicillin disodium, semisynthetic penicillin susceptible to destruction by penicillinase

℞ for systemic use: NB = IV (over 15–30 min), IM: initial dose 100 mg/kg, followed by maintenance therapy according to the following criteria:
≤12,000 g + ≤7 days old: 225 mg/kg/24 hr, div, every 8 hr
≤2,000 g + >7 days old: 400 mg/kg/24 hr, div, every 6 hr
>2,000 g + ≤7 days old: 300 mg/kg/24 hr, div, every 6 hr
>2,000 g + >7 days old: 400 mg/kg/24 hr, div, every 6 hr

IN, CH = IV (over 15–30 min), IM: 400–600 mg/kg/24 hr, div, every 4 hr (IV) or every 6 hr (IM). IM injection is painful.

GEOPEN; inj; 1 g carbenicillin disodium contains 5.3 mEq Na^+

℞ for treatment of urinary tract infection only: CH = PO: 30–50 mg/kg/24 hr, div, every 6 hr carbenicillin indanyl sodium

GEOCILLIN; tabl

Carbinoxamine maleate, ethanolamine; antihistamine with mild anticholinergic effect and low incidence of sedation and drowsiness

℞ antiallergic effect: IN, CH = PO: 0.6 mg/kg/24 hr, div, every 6 hr

RONDEC; liquid tabl, oral drops; component of many combination products

Cascara sagrada aromatic fluid extract; contains anthraquinones as active ingredients

℞ laxative: IN = PO: 1–2 mL/dose; CH = PO: 2–8 mL/dose

Cephalosporins, semisynthetic derivative of 7-amino cephalosporanic acid, structurally related to penicillins

a. **First-generation cephalosporins:** active against most gram-positive cocci (excluding enterococci and methicillin-resistant *S. aureus*), some strains of *E. coli, K. pneumoniae,* and *P. mirabilis*

Note: First-generation drugs do not cross the blood-brain barrier and thus are ineffective for treatment of infections within the central nervous system.

Cefadroxil: relatively resistant against β-lactamases; absorption appears unaffected by food intake; minimal inhibitory concentrations for *E. coli, P. mirabilis, Klebsiella* species may be maintained in urine for about 20 hr after single dose

℞ CH = PO: 30 mg/kg/24 hr, div, every 12 hr

DURICEF, ULTRACEF; caps, powder for oral susp

Cefazolin sodium: NB = IV (over 15–30 min), IM: 40 mg/kg/24 hr, div, every 12 hr; IN, CH = IV (over 15–30 min), IM: 50–100 mg/kg/24 hr, div, every 6 hr

ANCEF, KEFZOL; inj

Cephalexin: IN, CH = PO: 25–100 mg/kg/24 hr, div, every 6 hr

KEFLEX; inj

Cephalothin: NB = IV (over 15–30 min), IM: ≤ 7 days old: 40 mg/kg/24 hr, div, every 12 hr; >7 days old: 60 mg/kg/24 hr, div, every 8 hr; IN, CH = IV: 80–160 mg/kg/24 hr, div, every 4 hr

KEFLIN; inj

Cephapirin sodium: CH = IV, IM: 40–80 mg/kg 24 hr, div, every 6 hr

CEFADYL; inj

Cephradine: CH = PO: 50–100 mg/kg/24 hr, div, every 6 hr; IV, IM: 50–100–300 mg/kg/24 hr, div, every 6 hr

ANSPOR, VELOSEF; caps, oral susp, inj

b. **Second-generation cephalosporins:** more active against gram-negative bacteria such as *H. influenzae* type b, *N. gonorrhoeae,* and enteric gram-negative bacilli

Note: Some second-generation cephalosporins cross the blood-brain barrier and may be effective for treatment of bacterial meningitis. See later.

Cefaclor: effective against some β-lactamase–producing ampicillin-resistant strains of *H. influenzae;* absorption not affected by food intake.

℞ for treatment of otitis media and infections of the upper and lower respiratory tracts, urinary tract, skin, and soft tissues with susceptible organisms: IN, CH = PO: 20–40 mg/kg/24 hr, div, every 8 hr

Note: may cause serum sickness

CECLOR: powder for oral susp, caps

Cefamandole: IN, CH =IV, IM: 50–150 mg/kg/24 hr, div, every 4–6 hr

Note: May cause rash, neutropenia, and bleeding. Adjust dose with renal disease. Cefamandole does not effectively cross into the central nervous system and should not be used in the treatment of bacterial meningitis.

MANDOL; vials, plastic bags, inj

Cefoxitin: IN (>3 mo old), CH = IV, IM: 80–160 mg/kg/24 hr, div, every 4–6 hr

MEFOXIN; vials, infusion bottles, inj

Cefuroxime: IN (>3 mo old), CH: IV, IM: 50–100 mg/kg/24 hr, div, every 6–8 hr

℞ in bacterial meningitis: IN, CH = IV: 200–240 mg/kg/24 hr, div, every 6–8 hr

ZINACEF, vials, infusion bottles, inj; tabs

LORACARBEF see Loracarbef

c. **Third-generation cephalosporins:** less active against gram-positive cocci than older cephalosporins but more active against most strains of enteric gram-negative bacilli (except *Clostridium difficile*), moderately active against *P. aeruginosa (ceftazidine),* highly active against *H. influenzae* and *N. gonorrhoeae.*

Ceftriaxone sodium: biliary and renal excretion.

℞ for misc. infection: 50–75 mg/kg/12–24 hr (not to exceed 2 g) divided every 12 hr; meningitis 80–100 mg/kg/24 hr (not to exceed 4 g) divided every 12 hr.

Cefotaxime sodium: NB <7 days old IV, IM 100 mg/kg/24 hr, div, every 12 hr; >7 days old, 150 mg/kg/24 hr, div, every 8 hr; IN, CH = IV, IM: 100–200 mg/kg/24 hr, div, every 6–8 hr

℞ in bacterial meningitis: 200 mg/kg/24 hr, div, every 6 hr

Note: May cause hypersensitivity reactions in penicillin-sensitive patients. Adjust dose in patients with renal failure.

CLAFORAN; vials, inj

Cefpodoxime proxetil: renally eliminated. IN, CH = PO: 10 mg/kg/24 hr, div Q 12 h. CH >12 yr, AD = PO: 200–800 mg/24 hr, div Q 12 h.

VANTIN, tabl, susp.

Ceftazidime: possesses antipseudomonal activity

NB = IV, IM: <7 days <2,000 g, 100 mg/kg/24 hr, div, every 12 hr; >2,000 g, 100 mg/kg/24 hr, div, every 8 hr; >7 days, 100–150 mg/kg/24 hr, div, every 8 hr

IN, CH = IV, IM: 100–150 mg/kg/24 hr, div, every 8 hr (meningitis, 150 mg/kg/24 hr, div, every 8 hr)

FORTAZ; TAZIDIME; inj

Ceftibuten: active against broad spectrum of pathogens; inactive against infections caused by group B streptococci, staphylococci, enterococci, *Listeria* spp., *Bacteroides* spp., and *Clostridium* spp. Renally eliminated CH = PO 9 mg/kg/24 hr Q 24 h.

Ceftizoxime: not metabolized, excreted unchanged by the kidneys. IN, CH = IM, IV 100–200 mg/kg/24 hr Q 4–6 hr

CEFIZOX; vials, inj

Cefixime: orally available agent against many gram-positive and gram-negative organisms; possesses no antistaphylococcal or antipseudomonal activity

IN, CH = PO: 8 mg/kg/24 hr, div every 12–24 hr (max 400 mg/24 hr)

SUPRAX; liquid, tabl

Charcoal, see Activated charcoal

Chloral hydrate, trichloro derivative of acetaldehyde; tolerance to its hypnotic effect may develop

℞ for sedation: IN, CH = PO: 25 mg/kg/24 hr, div, every 6–8 hr

℞ for sleep: IN, CH = PO, (PR): 25–75 mg/kg/dose (maximum total daily dose: 1.5–2.0 g/24/hr)

†, NOCTEC, SOMNOS, ‡; syrup, suppos, caps

Chlorambucil, antineoplastic agent that interferes with DNA replication and

■ **TABLE 670–3 Drug Dosages (Drugs Listed Alphabetically by Generic Name)** *(Continued)*

RNA transcription. Used for the treatment of certain leukemias, lymphomas, and the nephrotic syndrome unresponsive to more conventional therapy.
℞ in anticancer and nephrotic syndrome: CH, AD = PO 0.1–0.2 mg/kg/24 hr every 12–24 hr. Daily dose is often titrated based on blood counts.
Caution: bone marrow suppression dose limiting.
Leukeran; tab

Chloramphenicol, derivative of dichloracetic acid combined to a structure containing a nitrobenzene ring
NB = IV (over 15–30 min), PO:
≤14 days old, regardless of weight: 25 mg/kg/24 hr, div, every 12 hr
15–30 days old and ≤2,000 g: 25 mg/kg/24 hr, div, every 4 hr
15–30 days old and >2,000 g: 50 mg/kg/24 hr, div, every 4 hr
IN, CH = PO: 50–100 mg/kg/24 hr, div, every 6 hr; IV (over 15–30 min): 100 mg/kg/24 hr, div, every 4 hr
Caution: Newborn infants are susceptible to development of high blood levels and gray-baby syndrome on usual doses; therefore, careful monitoring (of blood levels, if available) is mandatory. Dose-duration–related suppression of erythrocyte production is reversible; weekly hematocrit or hemoglobin and reticulocyte count are mandatory. Idiosyncratic aplastic anemia occasionally occurs without warning and may be fatal. Use only when specifically indicated. Monitor serum concentrations; in NB may be desirable to quantitate succinate concentration.
CHLOROMYCETIN, caps; chloramphenicol palmitate, CHLOROMYCETIN palmitate; oral susp chloramphenicol sodium succinate, CHLOROMYCETIN sodium succinate; inj

Chloroquine, a 4-aminoquinoline antimalarial agent; drug of choice for the treatment of attacks of malaria caused by *Plasmodium vivax, P. ovale, P. malariae,* and susceptible strains of *P. falciparum.* Not advised for use in treatment of juvenile rheumatoid arthritis.
℞ for oral treatment of uncomplicated attacks (excluding those caused by chloroquine-resistant *P. falciparum*):
Chloroquine disphosphate: CH = PO:
first day: 25 mg/kg/first 24 hr (equivalent to base: 15 mg/kg/first 24 hr), div in initial dose of 16.5 mg/kg (equivalent to base 10 mg/kg) and subsequent dose of 8.5 mg/kg (equivalent to base 5 mg/kg) 6 hr later;
second and third days: 8.5 mg/kg/24 hr (equivalent to base 5 mg/kg/24 hr), as single daily dose
℞ for intramuscular treatment of severe illness (excluding malaria caused by chloroquine-resistant *P. falciparum*):
Chloroquine dihydrochloride: CH = IM: 6 mg/kg/dose (equivalent to base 5 mg/kg/dose), every 12 hr, until clinical response is obtained and treatment can be completed by the oral route
℞ for clinical prophylaxis of malaria (prevention of clinical manifestations from infection with any of the *Plasmodium* species):
Chloroquine diphosphate: CH = PO: 8.5 mg/kg/dose (equivalent to base 5 mg/kg/dose) once every 7 days, beginning 2 wk before entering the malarious area and continuing for 8 wk after return. For eradication of *P. vivax* and *P. ovale,* treatment for 14 days with primaquine should be considered on leaving malarious area.
Caution: Irreversible retinal damage may occur with prolonged use; frequent ophthalmologic examination necessary to detect early changes.
Note: Chloroquine does *not* cause hemolysis in individuals with G-6-PD deficiency
chloroquine diphosphate, ARALEN diphosphate, RESOCHIN diphosphate, tabl; chloroqine dihydrochloride, ARALEN dihydrochloride, inj; (1 mg chloroquine base is equivalent to 1.65 mg chloroquine diphosphate or 1.2 mg chloroquine dihydrochloride)

Chlorothiazide, saluretic, thiazide diuretic, inhibiting sodium reabsorption and interfering with dilution of urine
IN, CH = PO: 20–40 mg/kg/24 hr, div, every 12 hr IV (3–5 min) = 2–8 mg/kg/24 hr Q 12 hr AD = PO 500–1000 mg/24 hr Q 12–24 hr. Often co-administered with a loop diuretic (given 30 min before loop agent) for synergism in difficult-to-treat patients.
†, DIURIL; tabl, oral susp, inj

Chlorpheniramine maleate, alkylamine; antihistamine with anticholinergic and mild sedative effects
℞ antiallergic effect: CH = PO: 0.35 mg/kg/24 hr, div, every 6 hr
†, CHLORTRIMETON, ‡; tabl, syrup, inj

Chlorpromazine, phenothiazine with aliphatic side chain
℞ for sedation: CH = PO: 2 mg/kg/24 hr, div, every 4–6 hr, prn; IM, slow IV: 2 mg/kg/24 hr; maximum single IV dose 0.5 mg/kg
†, THORAZINE; chlorpromazine hydrochloride, THORAZINE hydrochloride; tabl, syrup, inj, suppos
Caution: Overdose may produce parkinsonian syndrome and acute dystonic reactions. Diphenhydramine or benztropine may be antidotal

Chlortetracycline, see Tetracyclines

Chlorthalidone, nonthiazide saluretic with protracted duration of action
CH = PO: 1–2 mg/kg/24 hr, as single dose
†, HYGROTON; tabl

Cholestyramine, ion-exchange resin for treatment of cholestatic jaundice, hyperlipidemia, diarrhea or pruritus secondary to bile salt abnormalities
Toxicity includes constipation; vitamin A, D, and K deficiencies; and altered medication absorption (digoxin, phenobarbital, propranolol, thiazides)
CH = PO: 240 mg/kg/24 hr, div, every 8–12 hr with meals; AD = PO: 9–16 g/24 hr Q 6–8 hr, max 32 g/24 hr
QUESTRAN, CHOLYBAR; 4-g packets, 378-g tins, 4 g cholestyramine per 9 g Questran, chewable bars

Cimetidine, H_2-receptor antagonist competitively inhibits secretion of gastric acid.
℞ for treatment of duodenal and gastric ulcers and for relief of symptoms caused by gastroesophageal reflux: compatible with concomitant treatment with oral antacids (which should be administered at frequent intervals and in adequate doses) or other therapeutic modalities.
NB = PO, IM, IV (15–20 min) 5–10 mg/kg/24 hr Q 8–12 hr;
IN, CH = IV, PO: 20–40 mg/kg/24 hr, div, every 4–6 hr
Note: Cimetidine may compete with hepatic metabolism of other hepatically metabolized drugs. Many possible drug interactions. May cause gynecomastia, rash, and neutropenia. Reduce dose in renal insufficiency.
TAGAMET; tabl, inj, syrup

Ciprofloxacin hydrochloride, see Fluoroquinolones.

Cisplatin, antineoplastic agent that inhibits DNA synthesis. Commonly used as a component of treatment regimens for metastatic testicular cancer, osteosarcoma, neuroblastoma. Contains platinum. Dosage usually directed by specific tumor-directed treatment protocol. Dose should be adjusted in patients with renal disease. Nephrotoxic drug that may increase incidence of renal toxicity when coadministered with other nephrotoxic agents, e.g., aminoglycosides, amphotericin B.
PLATINOL, inj.

Clarithromycin, macrolide antibiotic indicated for the treatment of mild to moderate upper and lower respiratory tract infections and infections of the skin structure caused by susceptible bacteria, *C. trachomatis, H. influenzae, M. catarrhalis, M. pneumoniae, S. aureus, S. pneumoniae, Legionella* spp. Less gastrointestinal distress than associated with erythromycin. CH = PO 15 mg/kg/24 hr div, every 12 hr. AD = PO 500–1000 mg/24 hr div, every 12 hr.
Note: dose adjustment is necessary with renal disease, creatinine clearance <30 mL/min. May interfere with the hepatic metabolism of certain drugs, e.g., carbamazepine, theophylline.
BIAXIN, tabl

Clindamycin, semisynthetic derivative of lincomycin. Effective for susceptible streptococci, *S. aureus, Bacteroides* spp.
NB <7 days <2,000 g, 10 mg/kg/24 hr, div, every 12 hr; <2,000 g, 15 mg/kg/24 hr, div, every 8 hr; <7 days >2,000 g, 15 mg/kg/24 hr, div, every 8 hr; >2,000 g, 20 mg/kg/24 hr, div, every 6 hr
IN, CH: 20–45 mg/kg/24 hr, div, every 6–8 hr
Can be applied topically for acne.
Note: Therapy may be associated with the development of pseudomembranous colitis.
clindamycin hydrochloride, CLEOCIN hydrochloride; caps clindamycin palmitrate hydrochloride, CLEOCIN pediatric; oral susp clindamycin phosphate, CLEOCIN phosphate; inj

Clonazepam, benzodiazepine with selective anticonvulsant effect
CH = PO: start with 0.01–0.05 mg/kg/24 hr, div, every 8 hr, and progressively increase up to 0.3 mg/kg/24 hr, div, every 8 hr, if needed.
AD = PO initial dose 1.5 mg/24 hr Q 8–12 hr. Max 20 mg/24 hr.
Caution: Concomitant use of clonazepam and valproate sodium may lead to petit mal status.
KLONOPIN; tabl

Clonidine, central acting α_2-receptor agonist antihypertensive. Stimulation of central α_2-receptors, an inhibitory neuron, reduces sympathetic outflow, decreasing vessel tone and heart rate. Effective in the management of hypertension and other cardiovascular diseases.
CH = PO 5–10 μg/kg/24 hr div, every 8–12 hr, dose titrated upward to desired effect. Usual maximum 25 μg/kg/ to 0.9 mg/24 hr. AD = PO 0.2–1.2 mg/24 hr div, every 6–12 hr. Usual max 2.4 mg/24 hr. Transdermal patch formulation available for once-weekly application.
Caution: Rebound hypertension has been observed after abrupt discontinuation of clonidine; should taper dose downward over 5–7 days before stopping drug. β-receptor antagonists may potentiate bradycardia and increase rebound effect.
CATAPRES, tabl; CATAPRES-TTS (transdermal)., tabl, transdermal patch 1, 2, or 3 mg equivalent to 0.1, 0.2, or 0.3 mg of clonidine/24 hr for 7-day duration.

Cloxacillin sodium monohydrate, penicillinase-resistant penicillin. Effective against penicillin-resistant *S. aureus.*

Table continued on following page

■ **TABLE 670–3 Drug Dosages (Drugs Listed Alphabetically by Generic Name)** *(Continued)*

IN, CH = PO: 50–100 mg/kg/24 hr, div, every 6 hr (expressed in terms of the base) CH = Max 4 g/24 hr. AD = PO 1–2 g/24 hr Q 6 hr.
TEGOPEN, CLOXAPEN; caps, oral susp

Cocaine hydrochloride, topical anesthetic with great abuse potential and local vasoconstrictor. Cocaine inhibits initiation and conduction of nerve impulses.
℞ local anesthesia; apply lowest dose to obtain desired effect.

Codeine phosphate or sulfate, narcotic analgesic
℞ as antitussive: CH = 1–1.5 mg/kg/24 hr, div, every 4 hr, prn
℞ against moderately severe pain; CH = PO: 4 mg/kg/24 hr, div, every 4–6 hr, prn; SC: 3 mg/kg/24 hr, div, every 4–6 hr, prn
Note: Additive respiratory depression with other respiratory depressants. Effects reversed with naloxone.
†; tabl, oral susp, inj; mostly in combination with other drugs

Colfosceril palmitate, synthetic lung surfactant used in the prevention or treatment of respiratory distress syndrome (RDS) in premature infants, prophylactic therapy, as rescue therapy for acute respiratory distress syndrome (ARDS) in mechanically ventilated patients.
℞ for RDS, ARDS in CH = intratracheal instillation, 5 ml/kg. Up to 2–3 doses may be administered at 12-hr intervals over first 24 hr. Insufficient data are available addressing the potential efficacy and safety of additional doses administered more frequently.
Note: suction patient before intratracheal instillation. Administer dose as two 2.5-ml aliquots instilled over 2–3 sec positioning the infant's head; instillation to the right, then to the left.
EXOSURF, intratracheal susp.

Colistin sodium methanesulfonate, colistimethate sodium, and colistin sulfate, polymyxin E; polypeptide antimicrobial agent with cationic detergent activity
℞ inhibition of gastrointestinal flora, justified only in selected cases (gastroenteritis with susceptible organism): IN, CH = PO (colistin sulfate): 5–15 mg/kg/24 hr, div, every 8 hr
℞ for systemic infection IM, IV (by slow infusion): 3–5 mg/kg/24 hr, div, every 8 hr
Caution: against pathogen overgrowth; monitor for nephrotoxicity and ototoxicity.
colistimethate sodium, COLY-MYCIN N, inj; colistin sulfate, COLY-MYCIN S, oral susp

Corticosteroids
℞ for physiologic replacement: *cortisone:* PO: 1 mg/kg/24 hr, div, every 8 hr; IM: 0.5 mg/kg/24 hr, every 24 hr. (*Note:* "Increased demand" under stressful situation; e.g., in children with congenital adrenogenital syndrome, receiving replacement therapy, for stressful situation in which 2 mg/kg/24 hr of cortisol may be safer)
℞ for use in pharmacologic doses (leukemia, lymphoma, nephrosis, rheumatic carditis, certain types of tuberculosis, immunologic reactions, and other types of autoimmune disease): adjust dosage to the specific situation.
Cortisone: PO: 10 mg/kg/24 hr, div, every 6–8 hr; IM: 3–6 mg/kg/24 hr, div, every 12 hr
Prednisone: PO: 2 mg/kg/24 hr, div, every 6–8 hr (or analog in equally effective dosage; see following table)
(For continued treatment after initial response, adjust dosage, frequency of administration, and duration of treatment according to type of disease and side effects to be avoided.)
℞ in status asthmaticus refractory to other types of treatment: methylprednisolone 2–4 mg/kg/24 hr, div, every 4–6 hr
℞ in endotoxin shock: methylprednisolone 2–4 mg/kg/24 hr, div, every 4–6 hr

Relative Potencies of Corticosteroids

Drug	Anti-inflammatory Effect (mg)	Sodium-Retaining Effect (mg)
Hydrocortisone (cortisol)	100	100
Cortisone	80	80
Prednisolone	20	100
Prednisone	20	100
Methylprednisolone	16	0
Triamcinolone	16	0
Dexamethasone	2	0
Desoxycorticosterone	0	2

dexamethasone, DECADRON, GAMMACORTEN, ‡; tabl, elixir
dexamethasone sodium phosphate, DECADRON phosphate; inj
hydrocortisone, †, CORTEF, HYDROCORTONE, ‡; tabl, oral susp
hydrocortisone sodium phosphate, † HYDROCORTONE phosphate; inj
hydrocortisone sodium succinate, †, SOLU-CORTEF; inj
methylprednisolone, MEDROL; tabl
methylprednisolone sodium succinate, SOLU-MEDROL; inj
prednisone, †, DELTASONE, METICORTEN, ‡; tabl
prednisolone, †, DELTA-CORTEF, METICORTELONE, ‡; tabl
triamcinolone, ARISTOCORT, KENACORT; tabl, syrup
Caution: May inhibit clinical signs of infection.

Cortisone, see Corticosteroids

Co-trimoxazole, See Sulfonamides.

Cromolyn sodium
℞ for topical prophylaxis of bronchial asthma, allergic rhinitis: not useful in the treatment of acute asthmatic attack because it is not a bronchodilator. CH (≥5 yr) = inhalation of 20 mg every 6 hr; nebulize contents of one ampule (2 ml) every 6–8 hr; aerosol inhaler, 1–2 puffs 4 times daily. Oral capsule used in food allergy, inflammatory bowel disease, CH = PO 400 mg/24 hr Q 6 hr 15–20 min before meals, AD = PO 800 mg/24 hr Q 6 hr. Max 1,600 mg/24 hr
AARANE, INTAL; inhalation with Spinhaler, sol, nasal spray, ophthalmic drops

Cyclizine hydrochloride, antihistamine, antiemetic, and anticholinergic agent
℞ for prevention and relief of symptoms of motion sickness: CH (6–10 yr) = PO: 3 mg/kg/24 hr, div, every 8 hr. The 1st dose should be taken about 20 min before departure.
MAREZINE; tabl; cyclizine lactate for IM inj

Cyclophosphamide, antineoplastic drug that interferes with DNA synthesis, used in the treatment of leukemias, lymphomas, neuroblastoma, the nephrotic syndrome, systemic lupus erythematosus (SLE), and severe rheumatoid arthritis.
℞ in neoplastic disorders, see specific protocol-directed dose guidelines.
℞ in SLE in CH, AD = PO, IV 15–25 mg/kg administered once monthly, dose and dose interval titrated to desired effect and patient tolerance.
℞ in nephrotic syndrome in CH, AD = PO, IV 2–3 mg/kg/24 hr administered once daily titrated to response.
Caution: Causes bone marrow suppression. Hemorrhagic cystitis associated with prolonged and/or high-dose therapy. Encourage patients to maintain adequate hydration. Mesna may be antidote for hemorrhagic cystitis. Potential drug interactions with allopurinol, barbiturates, chloramphenicol, phenothiazines.
CYTOXAN, NEOSAR; inj, tabl.

Cycloserine, antitubercular drug useful in a multidrug combination regimen for the treatment of pulmonary or extrapulmonary tuberculosis. Inhibits cell wall synthesis of susceptible mycobacterium.
CH = PO 10–20 mg/kg/24 hr, div every 12 hr. Usual max 1,000 mg/24 hr. AD = PO initial dose 500 mg/24 hr div every 12 hr, increased as tolerated to 1,000 mg/24 hr div every 12 hr.
Note: may cause vitamine B_{12} and folate deficiency. May interfere with hepatic metabolism of phenytoin. Neurotoxic effects (e.g., confusion, drowsiness, dizziness, psychosis, seizures, and tremor) may be reversed with pyridoxine.
SEROMYCIN, caps.

Cyclosporine, cyclic polypeptide immunosuppressant agent produced as a metabolite from a fungus. Cyclosporine is a potent immunosuppressive drug that prolongs survival of transplants involving skin, heart, kidney, pancreas, bone marrow, and lung. The drugs's mechanism of action remains to be elucidated but appears to include inhibition of T-cell–dependent B cell activation, expansion of unprimed T helper and cytotoxic T cell subsets, clonal expansion of aloe-reactive cells, and induction of γ-interferon secretion.
IN, CH = PO: 14–18 mg/kg daily and tapered downward to a maintenance dose approximately 5–10 mg/kg/24 hr, div, every 12–24 hr. The oral absorption of cyclosporine is highly variable. IV (slow infusion over 2–6 hr or continuous 24 hr): 2–6 mg/kg/24 hr, div, every 12–24 hr.
Note: Renal function must be monitored closely. Dosage frequently adjusted to obtain desired trough blood concentration, which is dependent on type of assay used for cyclosporine determination and organ transplanted. Oral absorption enhanced by water-soluble vitamin E (d-α-tocopheryl-polyethylene-glycol).
SANDIMMUNE; oral sol, inj

Cyproheptadine hydrochloride, piperidine; serotonin and histamine antagonist with mild anticholinergic and mild sedative effects
℞ antiallergic effect: CH = PO: 0.25–0.5 mg/kg/24 hr, div, every 4–6 hr; AD = PO 12 mg/24 hr Q 8 hr. Max 0.5 mg/kg/24 hr.
†, PERIACTIN; tabl, syrup

Cytarabine (ARA-C), antineoplastic agent that inhibits DNA synthesis; specific for S phase of the cell cycle. Dose dependent on type of cancer and protocol regimen used. Administered in high-dose continuous-infusion regimens, intermittent doses, and intrathecally.
CYTOSAR, inj.

Dactinomycin (actinomycin D), an antineoplastic agent useful in the

■ **TABLE 670–3 Drug Dosages (Drugs Listed Alphabetically by Generic Name)** *(Continued)*

treatment of neuroblastoma, rhabdomyosarcoma, testicular carcinoma, Wilms tumor. Most often combined with other agents. Dose dependent on type of cancer and protocol regimen used.
COSMEGEN. inj.

Dantrolene sodium, antispasmodic used in the management of chronic muscle spasticity resulting from upper motoneuron disorders (e.g., spinal cord injury, cerebral palsy, multiple sclerosis). Dantrium works directly on skeletal muscle; it disassociates the excitation-contraction coupling, probably by interfering with the release of calcium from the sarcoplasmic reticulum. Common medication used in conjunction with other drugs in structured therapeutic environments.
CH = PO: 1 mg/kg/24 hr, div, every 12 hr, increasing to a maximum 3 mg/kg/24 hr, given 2–4 times daily to max of 400 mg/24 hr. AD = PO 25 mg/24 hr increasing by 25 mg/24 hr to total <400 mg/24 hr Q 6–12 hr
℞ in malignant hyperthermal crisis: IV (rapid infusion): 1 mg/kg repeated immediately until signs of malignant hyperthermia resolve, up to a total dose of 10 mg/kg; maintenance 4–8 mg/kg/24 hr (IV/PO), div, every 6 hr, for 1–3 days.
Caution: Use may be associated with hepatotoxicity
DANTRIUM; caps, IV

Deferoxamine, chelating agent for treatment of iron intoxication. May be used for aluminum toxicity. May cause hypotension; contraindicated in renal failure or acute anuria unless concomitant hemodialysis is used.
CH = IV: 10–15 mg/kg/hr infusion IM 250 mg/kg/24 hr Q 8 hr. Max 6 g/24 hr. Similar doses used for chronic iron overload; may be administered as continuous SC infusion.
DESFERAL; 500 mg/vial inj

Demeclocycline, see Tetracyclines

Desipramine, cyclic (tricyclic) antidepressant used in the treatment of various forms of depression, select cases of ADHD (see **Methylphenidate**), and enuresis.
℞ for depression CH (6–12 yr of age) = PO 1–5 mg/kg/24 hr (10–30 mg/24 hr) div every 12–24 hr, titrated upward to desired effect to usual maximum of 5 mg/kg/24 hr. CH (>12 yr), AD = PO 50–75 mg/24 hr titrated upward to desired effect to 100–200 mg/24 hr.
Note: use with caution in patients with cardiac conduction abnormalities or cardiac disease. Initiation of therapy usually accompanied by marked sedation.
NORPRAMIN, PERTOFRANE; cap, tabl.

Desmopressin acetate, synthetic analog of vasopressin indicated as replacement therapy in the management of central diabetes insipidus. Toxicities include headache, abdominal cramping, and excessive water retention.
Nasal insufflation: 5–30 μg/24 hr divided every 12–24 hr. Dose determined by patient response.
DDAVP; inj; nasal insufflation

Dexamethasone, see Corticosteroids

Dextroamphetamine sulfate, noncatecholamine sympathomimetic amphetamine agent for ADHD
See **Methylphenidate:** drug treatment not recommended below age of 3 yr or in nonstructured therapeutic situation. CH (above 3 yr) = PO: initiate treatment with 2.5 mg/dose given at onset of daytime activities and again 4–6 hr later. If needed, increase at weekly intervals by increments of 2.5 mg/dose and adjust respective size of separate doses according to response. Daily dose should not exceed 1 mg/kg/24 hr.
℞ in narcolepsy: PO: proceed for dosage as in minimal brain dysfunction. End points: control of symptoms, maximal dose.
To avoid insomnia do not administer closer than 6 hr before bedtime.
Caution: against diversion of CNS stimulants from legitimate use in patient to misuse in adults. Do not use in patients receiving monoamine oxidase inhibitors.
Caution: Severe mental depression may follow withdrawal. Overdose may produce extreme restlessness and psychotic behavior.
†, DEXEDRINE; tabl, caps, oral sol

Dextromethorphan hydrobromide, D-isomer of a codeine analog, and probably free of addictive effects
℞ antitussive agent: IN, CH = PO: 1 mg/kg/24 hr, div, every 6–8 hr
†, ROMILAR; syrup; contained in many combination products

Diazepam, benzodiazepine with anxiolytic and muscle-relaxant effects
℞ in status epilepticus: NB, IN, CH = IV (slowly, as controlled "push" injection): 0.1–0.5 mg/kg/dose; may be repeated at 3–5 min intervals; may administer IM if IV not possible (efficacy may be diminished). Too rapid IV bolus may precipitate respiratory failure. Flumazenil, a benzodiazepine antagonist, can reverse sedation but may not reverse respiratory depression.
℞ for symptomatic relief of anxiety, sedation, muscle relaxation: IN, CH = PO: 0.1–0.3 mg/kg/24 hr, div, every 4–8 hr; dosage adjusted according to clinical response.
Caution: Confusion and prolonged extreme drowsiness may follow overdose or concurrent ingestion of alcohol in any form.
†, VALIUM; tabl, inj, caps, oral sol

Diazoxide, nondiuretic benzothiazide derivative with several prominent actions: (1) relaxation of smooth muscles in the peripheral arterioles after IV injection only; (2) hyperglycemic effect (beginning 1 hr after administration and lasting for approximately 8 hr) through inhibition of release of insulin; (3) retention of sodium and concomitantly of water; (4) hyperuricemic effect
℞ for emergency reduction of hypertension: CH, AD = IV (injection within 30 sec of calculated amount of undiluted diazoxide solution into a peripheral vein): 1–3 mg/kg/dose not to exceed 150 mg per dose, may administer as timed infusion. If 1st injection fails to elicit adequate response within 30 min, administer a 2nd complementary dose. Repeat as needed Q 5–15 min. Subsequent doses Q 4–24 hr or by continuous IV infusion. Hypotensive effect usually lasts 2–12 hr. As soon as possible, switch to oral regimen with alternative antihypertensive medication.
℞ for hyperinsulinemic hypoglycemia: NB, IN = PO: 8–15 mg/kg/24 hr, div, every 8–12 hr; CH = PO: 3–8 mg/kg/24 hr, div, every 8–12 hr. Slow dosage titration is necessary for optimal response.
Note: Diazoxide is ineffective against hypertension due to pheochromocytoma. A concurrently administered thiazide diuretic (which characteristically exerts a diuretic response) may potentiate the antihypertensive, hyperglycemic, and hyperuricemic effects of diazoxide.
Caution: hypotensive circulatory failure (responding to catecholamine such as norepinephrine), congestive heart failure (responding to plasma volume depletion by saluretic), and hyperosmolar coma in patients with diabetes mellitus (responding to insulin) may occur.
HYPERSTAT, inj; PROGLYCEM, cap, susp

Dicloxacillin, sodium monohydrate, penicillinase-resistant penicillin; effective against *S. aureus*
IN, CH = PO: 12.5–50 mg/kg/24 hr, div, every 6 hr. Doses as high as 100 mg/kg/24 hr have been used for osteoarticular infections. AD = PO 500–2,000 mg/24 hr Q 6 hr.
DYNAPEN, DYCILL, PATHOCIL; caps, oral susp

Dicyclomine hydrochloride, anticholinergic agent used primarily as a gastrointestinal antispasmodic, adjunctive therapy in the irritable bowel syndrome.
IN (>6 mo of age) = PO 5 mg/dose administered 3–4 times daily. CH = PO 10 mg/dose 3–4 times daily, AD = PO 40 mg/dose 3–4 times daily. Dose titrated to desired effect and patient tolerance. Use associated with classic anticholinergic side effects, e.g., blurred vision, dry mouth, sedation, urinary retention.
ANTISPAS, BENTYL, BYCLOMINE; caps, syrup, tabl

Digoxin, cardiac glycoside with rapid onset of action and half-life of approximately 48 hr
℞ for digitalization: 0.5 × digitalizing dose initially, 0.25 × digitalizing dose 8 and 16 hr later.
Digitalizing dose: NB = IV, IM: 0.010–0.030 mg/kg div in fractions, or PO: 0.040 mg/kg, div in fractions.
IN = IV, IM 0.030–0.040 mg/kg div in fractions, or PO: 0.050 mg/kg, in fractions
CH = IV, IM, PO: 0.010–0.015 mg/kg in fractions
℞ for maintenance: begin maintenance dosage 24 hr after 1st fraction of digitalizing dose. NB = PO: 0.005–0.010 mg/kg/24 hr, div, every 12 hr. IN, CH = PO: 0.002–0.005 mg/kg/24 hr, div, every 12 hr
Note: Digitalizing and maintenance doses must be adjusted to clinical condition and response of the patient. Systemic absorption from IM administration may be erratic and unpredictable. Serum digoxin concentrations may be monitored to assist in therapy. Caution is needed in interpreting serum digoxin concentrations in patients <6 mo of age due to the presence of immunoreactive digoxin-like substances (consult pharmacology or clinical pathology textbooks).
Caution: Fatal arrhythmia may follow overdose. Antacids, cholestyramine, kaolin pectin, and metoclopramide decrease digoxin absorption. Amiodarone, erythromycin, indomethacin, propafenone, and verapamil may increase digoxin levels.
†, LANOXIN; tabl, elixir, inj, caps
Digoxin immune Fab, antigen-binding fragments (Fab) derived from specific antidigoxin antibodies in sheep, used in the treatment of digoxin overdose or intoxication. Digoxin Fab antibodies bind digoxin, rendering drug unavailable to bind to their site of action. The Fab fragment-digoxin complex will accumulate in blood, may be easily quantitated, and is excreted slowly by the kidney. Fab fragment-digoxin complex is not pharmacologically active. Dose of digoxin immune Fab is dependent on amount of digoxin reversal desired. More specific information about dose, intervals, and monitoring should be obtained from a clinical pharmacy or pharmacology service or a poison control center.

Dihydrotachysterol, vitamin D congener used in the management of hypocalcemia usually associated with chronic renal disease.

Table continued on following page

■ TABLE 670–3 Drug Dosages (Drugs Listed Alphabetically by Generic Name) *(Continued)*

℞ for hypoparathyroidism: NB = PO 0.05–1 mg/24 hr, IN, CH = PO initially 1–5 mg/24 hr for 5 days with dose reduction (e.g., 0.5–1.5 mg/24 hr). Doses are titrated to response. Older CH, AD = PO 0.75–2.5 mg/24 hr for 5 days with dose reduction.
℞ renal osteodystrophy in: CH = PO 0.1–0.5 mg/24 hr. AD = PO 0.1–0.6 mg/24 hr.

Dimenhydrinate, chlorotheophylline salt of diphenhydramine
℞ for the prevention and treatment of motion sickness: CH = PO: 5 mg/kg/24 hr, div, every 6 hr. Max 400 mg/24 hr. AD = PO 300–400 mg/24 hr Q 4–6 hr.
†, DRAMAMINE; tabl, oral susp, suppos

Dimercaprol in oil, metal-chelating agent used in the treatment of arsenic, gold, mercury, and lead poisoning
℞ in the treatment of heavy metal poisoning depending on severity of intoxication. Doses range from 12 to 24 mg/kg/24 hr, div, every 4 hr via IM injection.
BAL in oil; IM inj

Diphenhydramine hydrochloride; ethanolamine; antihistamine with mild anticholinergic, sedative, antiemetic, and antitussive effects
℞ antiallergic effect; sometimes used as sedative. IN, CH = PO, IM, IV: 5 mg/kg/24 hr, div, every 6–8 hr
Caution: topical diphenhydramine may be absorbed, resulting in toxicity
†, BENADRYL; caps, elixir, inj

Diphenoxylate hydrochloride + atropine sulfate, opiate analog (diphenoxylate) combined with an anticholinergic (atropine) used as short-term adjunctive therapy in the management of diarrhea. Need for routine use of this drug in infants and children is questionable.
℞ for symptomatic short-term use as an antidiarrheal; CH = PO: 0.3–0.4 mg/kg/24 hr, div, every 4–12 hr
†, LOMOTIL; tabl; liquid

Dipyridamole, originally released as a coronary vasodilator for the treatment of angina, subsequently found to be effective antiplatelet agent. Primary use as antiplatelet drug to maintain patency after surgical grafting, for postoperative prophylaxis, and in combination with other medications, e.g., aspirin as prophylaxis against thromboembolic events.
CH = PO 3–6 mg/kg/24 hr div every 8 hr. AD = PO 75–400 mg/24 hr div every 6–8 hr.
Note: adverse effects mostly associated with vasodilatation, e.g., flushing, syncope.
PERSANTINE; inj., tabl.

Disopyramide phosphate, antiarrhythmic, class Ia, used in the management of ventricular dysrhythmias. Primarily used to suppress and/or prevent unifocal and multifocal ventricular premature contractions (PVCs), coupled PVCs, paroxysmal ventricular tachycardia.
℞ for ventricular dysrhythmias IN = PO <1 yr of age 10–30 mg/kg/24 hr div every 6 hr; 1–4 yr of age 10–20 mg/kg/24 hr div every 6 hr; 4–12 yr of age, 10–15 mg/kg/24 hr div every 6 hr; >12 yr of age, 6–15 mg/kg/24 hr div every 6 hr. AD: 100–150 mg/dose every 6 hr or timed-release preparation every 12 hr.
Caution: drug decreases myocardial contractility and, thus, may precipitate congestive heart failure. Use associated with hypotension, hypocalcemia, hypercholesterolemia, hypertriglyceridemia, cholestasis. Dose must be adjusted in patients with renal disease.
NORPACE; caps, sustained-release caps.

Dobutamine, β-adrenergic inotropic agent used for short-term treatment of cardiac failure due to depressed cardiac contractility. Heart rate, blood pressure, and cardiac electrical activity should be monitored during infusion. Do not mix with sodium bicarbonate.
IV: 0.0025–0.020 mg/kg/min constant infusion, depending on patient response.
DOBUTREX; 250-mg vials for injection

Docusate sodium (Dioctyl sodium sulfosuccinate), wetting agent, emulsifier, demulcent
℞ as stool softener: IN, CH = PO: 5 mg/kg/24 hr, div, with meals
†, COLACE, DOXINATE, ‡; caps, oral sol, syrup

Dopamine, α- and β-adrenergic as well as dopaminergic agent (positive inotropic effect on heart)
℞ to increase cardiac output and improve organ perfusion: IV infusion (into large vein): Example: to prepare a solution containing 0.400 mg/mL, mix 100 mg of dopamine HCl in 250 mL of 5% D/W or appropriate electrolyte solution with pH below 7.0 (do not include bicarbonate!), and infuse at rate adjusted to response in patient, beginning with 0.002–0.005 mg/kg/min and increasing by increments of 0.005 mg/kg/min if needed up to 0.020 mg/kg/min. In case of extravasation causing peripheral ischemia, use phentolamine (REGITINE) for local infiltration.
INTROPIN; inj

Dornase alfa, recombinant human deoxyribonuclease I (rhDNase), is an enzyme that selectively cleaves DNA. Mucokinetic drug useful in reducing sputum viscoelasticity by hydrolyzing sputum DNA. High concentrations of extracellular DNA, mostly from destroyed leukocytes (e.g., infection, irritation), accumulate in respiratory secretions, which is an important variable responsible for increasing the purulence of pulmonary secretions. Nebulized dose titrated to effect, usual starting dose 2.5 mg of DNase nebulized once to twice daily. Adverse effects include voice alteration, laryngitis, and conjunctivitis.
PULMOZYME, inhaled sol.

Doxapram hydrochloride, central nervous system and respiratory stimulant. May stimulate respiration via central effect and/or reflex stimulation of carotid, aortic, or other peripheral chemoreceptors.
℞ for neonatal apnea: NB = IV initial loading dose 2.5–3 mg/kg followed by continuous IV infusion of 1 mg/kg/hr with dose titrated downward to lowest dose that achieves desired effect.
Note: some commercial doxapram preparations contain benzyl alcohol and with continuous IV infusion may precipitate toxicity (e.g., "gasping syndrome").
Caution: use may be associated with hypertension, tachycardia, central nervous system stimulation, irritability, seizures, and hyperreflexia.
DOPAM; inj.

Doxorubicin hydrochloride, antineoplastic agent useful as a component of specific treatment protocols for lymphomas, leukemias, neuroblastoma, osteosarcoma. Dose dependent on specific protocol.
Note: use may be associated with transient, reversible cardiotoxic effects to congestive heart failure. Patients may have red/orange color to urine for up to 48 hr after receiving the drug. Dose should be reduced in patients with liver disease.
ADRIAMYCIN; inj.

Doxycycline, see Tetracyclines

Dronabinol, Δ-9-tetrahydrocannabinol (Δ-9-THC), is used as adjunctive therapy in the treatment of nausea and vomiting associated with cancer chemotherapy, most often in patients who have failed to respond adequately to conventional antiemetic treatment. Dronabinol therapy may be associated with disturbing psychotomimetic reactions.
CH = PO: 5 mg/m^2 beginning 1–3 hr before chemotherapy and every 2–4 hr thereafter. Dose may be increased as necessary to control emesis (usually 2.5 mg/m^2 dose).
Note: Dronabinol may have profound effects on mental status; patient should be cautioned.
MARINOL; gelatin caps

Edetate calcium disodium (EDTA), a heavy metal–chelating agent with greatest affinity for lead. Used in the diagnosis and treatment of lead poisoning. EDTA-lead chelate excreted from the body via the kidney. Drug has affinity for calcium, which is the reason for administering the drug as the calcium (disodium) salt.
℞ for lead poisoning. Many regimens have been suggested; CH = IM, IV (over 1 hr to continuous 24-hr infusion); 50–75 mg/kg/24 hr div every 4–6 hr or by continuous IV infusion.
℞ as a diagnostic test for lead body burden. CH = IM, IV 500 mg/m^2 and collect all urine excreted over the next 8–24 hr to determine EDTA:lead ratio.
Note: Painful on IM injection. For comfort, may add 1 mL of 1% lidocaine with each 1 mL of EDTA injection. Dose must be adjusted for patients with renal disease.

Edrophonium chloride, cholinesterase inhibitor with short duration of action
℞ for myasthenia in NB of myasthenic mother = IV (slowly) or IM: 0.2 mg/kg/dose. Symptoms should be relieved almost immediately. Continue cholinesterase-inhibiting treatment, if indicated, PO with pyridostigmine.
℞ for differential diagnosis of myasthenic crisis, or as adjunct treatment to carotid massage in supraventricular tachycardia: NB, IN, CH = IV: 0.05 mg/kg/dose, and watch for effect after 15–30 s, *or* IM: 0.1 mg/kg/dose, and expect effect after 2–10 min
If edrophonium test is given during "cholinergic crisis," weakness of affected muscles, including respiratory muscles, will worsen or not improve. Ventilation should be assisted, if needed, and bradycardia can be influenced by atropine. If recovery from weakness occurs, continuation of cholinesterase inhibition is indicated using inhibitors with longer duration of action, such as pyridostigmine, neostigmine, ambenonium. Their dosage must be individually titrated and adjusted.
Manifestations of overdosage with cholinesterase-inhibiting medication: increase in muscle weakness and worsening of respiratory difficulty and dysphagia after each dose of drug; fasciculations of muscles; excessive salivation, increase in bronchial secretion; vomiting, diarrhea, pallor, sweating, bradycardia.
Caution: Administration during cholinergic crisis may cause paralysis of respiratory muscles. Use only when ventilatory assistance is available.
TENSILON; inj

Enalapril/enalaprilat, angiotensin-converting enzyme (ACE) inhibitor used in the treatment of hypertension and/or congestive heart failure. Prevents conversion of angiotensin I to angiotensin II, a potent vasoconstrictor; also promotes accumulation of vasodilatory bradykinin. Enalapril is an inactive prodrug that is converted to active enalaprilat by the liver.
IN, CH = PO 0.1 mg/kg/24 hr div every 12–24 hr. Dose may be increased to

■ TABLE 670–3 Drug Dosages (Drugs Listed Alphabetically by Generic Name) *(Continued)*

desired effect over the next 2 wk to a total of 0.5 mg/kg/24 hr. IN, CH = IV (over 5 min) 5–10 μg/dose administered every 8–24 hr.
Note: IV formulation is active drug, not prodrug, which explains markedly reduced dose requirements. Caution in using ACE inhibitors in patients whose renal function is dependent on renin-angiotensin system. Slowly initiate therapy in patients with renal artery stenosis, hypovolemic and/or hyponatremic patients.
VASOTEC; inj, tabl.

Ephedrine, phenylethylamine (direct and indirect sympathomimetic)
℞ for treatment of asthma in subacute stage; tolerance develops. CH = PO: 3 mg/kg/24 hr, div, every 4–6 hr. Contained in many antiasthma preparations; should be replaced with more selectively active drug
Caution: Acute overdose may produce seizures and coma.
Ephedrine hydrochloride; ephedrine sulfate; caps, tabl, syrup

Epinephrine, catecholamine (α- and β-adrenergic agonist)
℞ bronchodilator (β_2 stimulatory effect), in acute asthma attack: IN, CH = SC: 0.01 mg/kg/dose, repeat prn every 20 min, 2 times
Note: With epinephrine solution 1:1,000 this corresponds to 0.01 mL/kg/dose.
Caution: Cardiac arrhythmia or acute hypertension may follow overdose.

Epinephrine, racemic.
℞ for inhalation treatment of acute spasmodic croup.
Inhalation: 0.25–0.5 mL of 2.25% solution diluted in 3 mL of saline given via nebulizer.
VAPONEPHRINE; inhalation 2.25% sol

Epoetin alfa, recombinant human erythropoietin used to stimulate erythropoiesis in the treatment of anemia due to chronic renal failure, prematurity, severe drug-induced anemia, and as an adjuvant to autoharvesting before surgery.
℞ in anemia of prematurity: NB = SC, IV (over 1–3 min) 25–100 units/kg/dose administered 3 times weekly.
℞ in anemia of chronic renal failure, drug induced: CH, AD = SC, IV dose to desired effect 25–100 units/kg 3 times weekly. Higher doses may be used initially followed by dose reduction. Iron therapy is beneficial for optimum effect.
EPOGEN, PROCRIT; inj.

Ergotamine, adrenergic blocking agent as well as direct vasoconstrictor of vessels to the brain and serotonin antagonist
℞ against acute attack of vascular headache (migraine): older child and adolescent = IM, SC (in acute attack): 0.25–0.50 mg/dose, in single application. Minimal effective dose should be established for each patient by titration of the amount required to control headaches in that patient. Older child and adolescent = SL, PO (at 1st symptoms of attack): 1 mg/dose; if no improvement within 30 min, repeat same dose once.
Note: Signs of therapeutic overdosage: nausea, vomiting, diarrhea, tingling of hands and feet, weakness, muscle pain.
ergotamine tartrate: CYNERGEN, inj, tabl; ergotamine tartrate + caffeine: CAFERGOT, tabl, suppos; dehydroergotamine mesylate: D.H.E. 45, inj

Erythromycin, macrolide antimicrobial agent
IN, CH = PO: 30–50 mg/kg/24 hr for estolate, ethylsuccinate salts, 20–40 mg/kg/24 hr for stearate salt, div, every 6 hr; IV: 15–20 mg/kg/24 hr, div, every 6 hr
Caution: erythromycin may interfere with hepatic metabolism of other drugs (astemizole, carbamazepine, cyclosporine, terfenadine, theophylline), leading to toxicity.
erythromycin, †, ILOTYCIN, ‡: tabl; erythromycin estolate, ILOSONE: tabl; oral susp erythromycin ethylsuccinate, PEDIAMYCIN, EES, ‡: tabl, oral susp, drops, erythromycin gluceptate, ILOTYCIN gluceptate IV; inj: erythromycin lactobionate, ERYTHROCIN lactobionate: IV, inj; erythromycin stearate, ERYTHROCIN stearate, ‡: tabl

Esmolol hydrochloride, short-acting parenterally administered nonspecific β_2-receptor antagonist used in the treatment of hypertension and as an antiarrhythmic in the treatment of supraventricular tachycardia. Dose is titrated to desired response and patient tolerance.
CH = IV (over 1–2 min and by continuous IV infusion) 100–500 μg/kg load followed by 200–300 μg/kg/min infusion dosed to effective heart rate. Infusion rate may be increased by 50–100 μg/kg/min every 5–10 min to effect.
Caution: use may be associated with severe hypotension and bradycardia. Use very cautiously in patients with reactive airways disease.
BREVIBLOC; inj.

Ethacrynic acid, saluretic, inhibiting chloride and sodium reabsorption and interfering mainly with concentration of urine
CH = PO: approximately 1 mg/kg/dose, as single daily dose. Adjust according to effect, and repeat prn on alternate days; dosage in infants and children not firmly established (PO, IV)
EDECRIN, tabl; ethacrynate sodium, IV; sodium EDECRIN, inj (IV only)

Ethambutol hydrochloride, antituberculous agent used concomitantly with other agents
℞ in the treatment of tuberculosis as part of multiple drug regimen. Conditions for safe use in children not firmly established. In adults: 15–25 mg/kg/24 hr, as single daily dose, for course of treatment or retreatment. *Because of rare side effects of optic neuritis and decreased visual acuity,* eye examinations are indicated before inception of treatment and at monthly intervals thereafter.
MYAMBUTOL; tabl

Ethosuximide, anticonvulsant agent of the succinimide type.
CH = PO: 15–40 mg/kg/24 hr, div, every 12–24 hr
ZARONTIN; caps, syrup

Fentanyl, fentanyl citrate, potent narcotic analgesic, addictive. A fentanyl dose of 0.1 mg possesses an approximate equivalent analgesic activity to 10 mg of morphine or 75 mg of meperidine.
℞ against severe pain; NB, IN, CH = IV, IM: 0.5–5 μg/kg/dose every 1–4 hr; may be administered as a continuous intravenous infusion: 1–5 μg/kg/hr. Transdermal patch formulation may be used to provide continuous 24-hr administration in patients currently receiving the drug in whom the hourly fentanyl requirement has been determined. Note fentanyl effects are reversible with naloxone. inj, transdermal patch system equivalent to 25 (10 cm^2), 50 (20 cm^2), 75 (30 cm^2), and 100 (40 cm^2) μg/hr release characteristics.

Filgrastim, granulocyte colony-stimulating factor that stimulates the production and maturation of neutrophils used to reduce periods of neutropenia from various causes, e.g., antineoplastic drug therapy.
CH, AD = SC, IV (over 15–30 min) 5–10 μg/kg/24 hr administered once daily. Dose and duration titrated to absolute neutrophil count. Note therapy may be associated with medullary bone pain (up to 24% of patients), which may be dose related and is often localized to the lower back, posterior iliac crests, and sternum.
NEUPOGEN; inj.

Flecainide acetate, class Ic antiarrhythmic used in the prevention or treatment of ventricular arrhythmias, i.e., sustained ventricular tachycardia. Slows conduction in cardiac tissue, moderate negative inotropic effects.
CH = PO 3–6 mg/kg/24 hr div every 8 hr; dose adjusted upward to desired effect and tolerance to 11 mg/kg/24 hr.
Note: dose adjustment necessary in patients with renal disease. Flecainide may cause increased serum digoxin concentrations; amiodarone and cimetidine may increase serum flecainide concentrations. Suggested therapeutic serum flecainide concentrations 0.2–1 mg/L (0.4–2 μmol/L)
TAMBOCOR; tabl

Fluconazole, synthetic broad-spectrum *bis*-triazole antifungal drug. Selective inhibitor of fungal cytochrome P_{450} sterol C-14 α-demethylation; limited data in pediatrics available.
℞ for the treatment of fungal infections: CH = PO, IV (over 1–2 min): 3–6 mg/kg/24 hr, div, every 12–24 hr. Higher doses (10–12 mg/kg/24 hr) have been used in immunocompromised patients.
Caution: possible drug interactions with warfarin, phenytoin, cyclosporine, and rifampin. Dose adjustment necessary in patients with renal dysfunction.
DIFLUCAN; tabl, inj

Flucytosine, fluorinated pyrimidine antifungal agent. Mechanism of drug action remains to be elucidated but may be a result of competitive inhibition of fungal cell purine and pyrimidine metabolism or may be due to intracellular metabolism to 5-fluorouracil. Flucytosine is used in combination with other antifungal agents.
℞ in combination with other antifungal agents: IN, CH = PO: 50–150 mg/kg/24 hr, div, every 6–8 hr.
Note: May cause bone marrow suppression. Therapeutic serum levels < 100–150 mg/L. Adjust dose with renal dysfunction.
ANCOBON: caps

Flumazenil, competitive antagonist of the γ-aminobutyric acid–benzodiazepine receptor complex, specific in reversing effects of benzodiazepines only. May not reverse respiratory depressant effect of benzodiazepines. Limited data in pediatrics.
℞ for reversal of conscious sedation/anesthesia: CH = IV (over 1–2 min or as a continuous infusion) 0.01 mg/kg/dose (maximum dose 0.2 mg) followed by 0.005 mg/kg (maximum dose 0.2 mg) every minute, as needed, to a maximum dose of 1 mg.
℞ for benzodiazepine overdose: 0.01–0.02 mg/kg/dose (maximum dose 0.125–0.2 mg/kg) repeated as needed or administered by continuous infusion with dose titrated to desired effect.
Caution: flumazenil may precipitate seizures in benzodiazepine-dependent (addicted) patients.
ROMAZICON; inj.

Fluroquinolones, antimicrobial agents that inhibit the action of microbial DNA gyrase (topoisomerase 2). Drugs in this class include ciprofloxacin, enoxacin, norfloxacin, ofloxacin, and so on. Many of these drugs possess potent activity against a wide range of pathogens, including *P. aeruginosa,* and are available for oral administration. The use of these drugs in pediatrics, primarily for the treatment of children with cystic fibrosis, has been limited owing to concern about possible fluroquinolone-induced joint

Table continued on following page

■ **TABLE 670–3 Drug Dosages (Drugs Listed Alphabetically by Generic Name)** *(Continued)*

damage. Toxicity studies in animals have shown destructive lesions of growing cartilage following administration of these agents. Reports of arthropathy in teenage patients with cystic fibrosis have appeared in the literature, suggesting caution in the use of this class of compounds in patients whose skeletal growth is incomplete.

Ciprofloxacin: CH = PO 20–30 mg/kg/24 hr div every 8–12 hr. Usual maximum dose 1.5 g/24 hr. IV (over 60 min) 4–15 mg/kg/24 hr div every 8–12 hr. Dose should be adjusted in patients with creatinine clearance <20 mL/min.

Fluoxetine hydrochloride, serotonin antagonist used in the treatment of various forms of depression. Selectively inhibits neuronal serotonin reuptake in CNS with little to no effect on norepinephrine or dopamine. Peak drug effect may not be observed for 3–4 wk into therapy.

CH = PO 10–20 mg/24 hr div every 12–24 hr. Dose is titrated to patient response. AD = PO 20 mg/24 hr div every 12–24 hr, increasing as needed to a usual maximum of 80 mg/24 hr.

Note: metabolized in the liver to an active metabolite (norfluoxetine) with prolonged elimination half-life that may contribute to minor side effects of sedation, fatigue.

PROZAC; caps, liquid.

Foscarnet, antiviral agent mostly used for the treatment of infections due to cytomegalovirus and the treatment of acyclovir-resistant herpes simplex and herpes zoster infections.

CH, AD = IV (slow IV infusion ≤ 1 hr): Initial therapy (induction) 180 mg/kg/24 hr div, every 8 hr for 14–21 days. Maintenance therapy 90–120 mg/kg/24 hr div every 8–24 hr.

Caution: IV infusion rate should not exceed 60 mg/kg/dose over 1 hr. Use may be associated with peripheral neuropathy, renal dysfunction. Dose must be adjusted in patients with decreased renal function.

FOSCAVIR; inj.

Furosemide, saluretic with a duration of action of about 2 hr when given IV; inhibits chloride and sodium reabsorption and interferes with concentration of urine

IN, CH = PO: start with 2 mg/kg/dose; if needed, increase progressively to 3–6 mg/kg/dose, at intervals of 6–8 hr. IV: start with 1 mg/kg/dose; if needed, increase progressively to 6 mg/kg/dose, with an interval of at least 2 hr between doses

Note: may be ototoxic, particularly with other ototoxins (aminoglycosides, vancomycin).

LASIX; tabl, oral sol, inj

Ganciclovir, antiviral agent used for prophylaxis and treatment of cytomegalovirus infections.

CH, AD = IV (slow IV infusion ≥ 1 hr): Initial therapy (induction) 10 mg/kg/24 hr, div every 8–12 hr for 14–21 days. Maintenance therapy 5–6 mg/kg/24 hr, div, every 12–24 hr for 5 days/wk.

Note: dose adjustment necessary in patients with decreased renal function.

CYTOVENE; inj.

Gentamicin sulfate, antimicrobial aminoglycoside

NB = IV (30–60 min), IM: <7 days, <34 wk <1,500 g, 3 mg/kg every 24 hr; <34 wk >1,500 g, 2.5 mg/kg every 18 hr; >34 wk >1,500 g, 2.5 mg/kg/every 12 hr; >7 days and term NB, 5 mg/kg/24 hr, div, every 12 hr.

IN, CH = IM, IV (30–60 min): 5–7.5 mg/kg/24 hr, div, every 6–8 hr

Serum concentrations should be monitored, therapeutic peak concentration 5–10 mg/L, trough <2 mg/L (see Table 670–2). Dosage and interval may require modification for treatment of patients with cystic fibrosis.

Caution: Ototoxic, nephrotoxic.

GARAMYCIN; inj

Glucagon, natural hormone that promotes hepatic glycogenolysis and gluconeogenesis, leading to increases in blood glucose concentrations; positive inotropic and chronotropic effects, which may be beneficial in the treatment of severe intoxications with β-receptor antagonists.

℞ in hypoglycemia, insulin shock: NB = IM, SC, IV 0.3 mg/kg/dose (maximum dose 1 mg). CH = IM, SC, IV 0.025–0.1 mg/kg/dose (maximum dose 1 mg). AD = IM, SC, IV 0.5–1 mg/dose. Repeated doses administered as needed.

Note: 1 unit = 1 mg.

Glycopyrrolate, anticholinergic agent orally administered as a gastrointestinal antispasmodic and via IM, IV, or aerosol to control excessive respiratory secretions.

℞ for control of respiratory secretions: CH = PO 160–400 μg/kg/24 hr div every 6–8 hr; IM, IV (over 20–30 min) 15–40 μg/kg/24 hr div every 6–8 hr.

℞ for reversal of neuromuscular blockade: CH, AD = IV 0.2 mg of glycopyrrolate for every 1 mg of neostigmine or 5 mg of pyridostigmine administered.

ROBINUL; inj, tabl.

Granisetron hydrochloride, competitive antagonist of the serotonin-3 receptor. Primarily used for the treatment of nausea and vomiting for the management of chemotherapy-associated nausea and vomiting.

℞ for emesis, CH, AD = IV (over 5 min) 10 μg/kg once daily.

Note: devoid of sedative and dystonic effects observed with other antiemetics.

KYTRIL, inj.

Griseofulvin, antifungal agent

℞ against deep-seated mycotic infections (skin, hair, nails) with organisms of the species *Microsporum, Trichophyton, Epidermophyton:* CH = PO (microcrystalline): 10–15 mg/kg/24 hr for 4–6 wk (4–6 mo for fingernails, 6–12 mo for toenails)

Note: "Ultramicrosize" form is an ultramicrocrystalline suspension for which 125 mg is biologically equivalent to 250 mg of a "microsize" preparation. The daily dose of an ultramicrosize preparation is reduced to 5–8 mg/kg/24 hr and offers comparable efficacy without additional advantages.

Griseofulvin, microcrystalline, †, FULVICIN-U/F, GRIFULVIN V, ‡; tabl, oral susp griseofulvin, ultramicrocrystalline GRIS-PEG; tabl

Haloperidol, butyrophenone; antipsychotic drug that competitively blocks postsynaptic dopamine receptors in the mesolimbic system. Used in the treatment of psychosis, Tourette disorder, and severe behavioral problems.

CH = PO 0.05 mg/kg/24 hr div 8–12 hr. Dose is slowly increased to desired effect and as tolerated. Usual AD maximum dose is 30 mg/24 hr with some patients requiring as much as 100+ mg/24 hr.

Note: IM formulation should not be administered IV. Extrapyramidal and acute oculogyric effects similar to those with phenothiazines are observed and can be reversed with benztropine or diphenhydramine.

HALDOL; inj, tabl, concentrated liquid.

Heparin, anticoagulant that potentiates the activity of antithrombin III, inactivating thrombin and activated clotting factors IX, X, XI, and XII; also stimulates lipoprotein lipase activity.

℞ for flushing IV lines, 1–10-unit/mL solutions used sparingly as needed.

℞ in thromboembolic disorders 50–100 units/kg/dose administered every 4–6 hr based on achieving desired prolongation of patient's clotting time. Dose requirement determined by monitoring prothrombin time, activated partial thromboplastin time, and/or INR. Continuous infusion may be associated with less risk/incidence of bleeding; IV 50–100-units/kg loading dose followed by continuous IV infusion of 15–25 units/kg/hr. Infusion rate increased by 2–5 units/kg/hr every 6–8 hr to desired effect. Inj.

Note: Some preparations contain benzyl alcohol. Use may be associated with thrombocytopenia.

Caution: important drug interactions include medications with antithrombotic/antiplatelet effects and those that may potentiate the risk of hemorrhage, e.g., streptokinase, urokinase, aspirin, dipyridamole, and nonsteroidal anti-inflammatory drugs (ibuprofen, ketorolac).

Hyaluronidase, primarily used as an adjunctive agent in the treatment of extravasation. Increases the permeability of connective tissue by hydrolyzing hyaluronic acid, the primary adhesive affording resistance to fluid diffusion through tissue.

℞ in IV extravasation: IN, CH = inject 0.2-mL aliquots of a 15-unit/mL solution SC or intradermally into the leading edge of the extravasation site.

Note: hypersensitivity reactions may occur.

WYDASE; inj.

Hydralazine hydrochloride, phthalazine derivative; causes relaxation of vascular smooth muscles, especially of arterioles

℞ as antihypertensive in long-term treatment: CH = PO: initially 0.75 mg/kg/24 hr, div, every 6 hr; increase progressively until desired response or daily maximum dose of 7.5 mg/kg/24 hr is reached

℞ for emergency reduction of hypertension: IV (immediate onset of action), IM (onset of action after 15–20 min): 0.15 mg/kg/dose; repeat prn every 30–90 min up to daily dose of 1.7–3.6 mg/kg/24 hr; switch to oral administration if conditions permit

Note: Hydralazine may produce sodium retention and usually increases plasma renin activity.

Caution: May induce lupus erythematosus–like syndrome; frequency related to dosage.

†, APRESOLINE, ‡; tabl, inj

Hydrochlorothiazide, saluretic thiazide, inhibiting sodium reabsorption and interfering with dilution of urine

IN, CH = PO: 2–3.5 mg/kg/24 hr, div, every 12 hr

†, ESIDRIX, HYDRODIURIL, ‡; tabl

Hydroxyzine hydrochloride, neuroleptic agent of the piperazine type, with sedative and antihistamine effects

℞ for sedation or antihistamine effect: CH = PO: 2 mg/kg/24 hr, div, every 6–8 hr, prn

ATARAX: tabl, syrup; VISTARIL IM: inj (IM); hydroxyzine pamoate, VISTARIL; caps, oral susp

Ibuprofen, nonsteroidal anti-inflammatory agent of the propionic acid class that possesses analgesic and antipyretic activities. The drug's mechanism of action remains to be described but may involve prostaglandin synthetase inhibition. Pharmacologic effect appears to be equivalent to that of equipotent doses of acetaminophen or aspirin.

℞ as antipyretic or for mild analgesia. CH = PO: 10–15 mg/kg/dose at intervals of 4–6 hr; max 40–60 mg/kg/24 hr

■ **TABLE 670–3 Drug Dosages (Drugs Listed Alphabetically by Generic Name)** *(Continued)*

℞ for juvenile rheumatoid arthritis, CH = PO: 30–70 mg/kg/24 hr, div, every 4–6 hr

Note: complete scope of associated adverse reactions in infants and children remains to be described. Adverse effects appear to be similar to those associated with aspirin administration, including gastritis, platelet dysfunction, and possible compromise in renal function. Drug should be used cautiously in patients with renal insufficiency.

†, ADVIL, MEDIPRIN, MOTRIN, NUPRIN; tabs, caps, susp

Imipenem/Cilastatin, β-lactam, carbapenem antibiotic that possesses a broad spectrum of antibacterial activity, including gram-positive and gram-negative aerobic and anaerobic pathogens. Cilastatin is an antibacterially inactive compound, which competitively antagonizes the dihydropeptidase I enzyme present in the brush border of the proximal renal tubule; this enzyme metabolizes imipenem to an inactive compound.

NB = IM, IV (over 30–60 min) 0–4 wk < 1,200 g; 20 mg/kg/dose administered every 18–24 hr. By postnatal age: <7 days, >1,200 g 40 mg/kg/24 hr div every 12 hr; 1,200–2,000 g ,40 mg/kg/24 hr div every 12 hr; >2,000 g, 60 mg/kg/24 hr div every 8 hr. CH = IM, IV 60–100 mg/kg/24 hr div every 6 hr; AD = IM, IV 2–4 g/24 hr div every 8–12 hr.

Note: dose adjustment necessary in patients with renal dysfunction (creatinine clearance < 50 mL/min).

Caution: Seizures, particularly in patients receiving high doses and possibly in those patients with CNS infections.

PRIMAXIN; inj

Imipramine hydrochloride, tricyclic antidepressant used for depression and enuresis

℞ against enuresis, as adjunct therapy to proper medical and educational approach, after age 4 yr: CH (after age 4 yr) = PO: 10–25 mg/24 hr, to be given in single dose before bedtime; if response unsatisfactory, dose may be increased slowly to 100 mg/24 hr. Do not exceed 2.5 mg/kg/24 hr

℞ for depression: CH = PO 1.5 mg/kg/24 hr Q 8–12 hr. Increase 1 mg/kg/24 hr to max 3.5–5 mg/kg/24 hr.

†, JANIMINE, TOFRANIL; tabl, cap, inj

Indomethacin, nonsteroidal anti-inflammatory agent used in the treatment of inflammatory disorders and for pharmacologic management of patent ductus arteriosus in premature infants.

℞ as anti-inflammatory: CH = PO: 1–3 mg/kg/24 hr, div, every 6–8 hr

℞ for closure of ductus arteriosus: IN = IV: < 48 hr, 0.2 mg/kg for 1 dose, then 2 doses of 0.1 mg/kg; 2–7 days of age, 3 doses of 0.2 mg/kg; >7 days of age, 0.2 mg/kg once, then 2 doses of 0.25 mg/kg

Note: May cause GI irritation and bleeding and decreased glomerular filtration rate.

INDOCIN; PO, inj

Ipecac, emetic agent used in the adjunctive management of poisoning or intoxication. Active ingredient emetidine produces local gastric irritation and central effect, resulting in emesis, which usually occurs within 15–35 min of drug administration.

℞ to induce vomiting:

IN >8 mo of age, CH = PO: 15–30 mL/dose: if no effect occurs same dose may be repeated in 30 min

IN <8 mo of age = PO: 1 mL/kg single dose

Note: Children usually vomit 3–5 times within 1 hr of receiving ipecac. Ipecac should be available in all households with young infants and children but should not be administered except on the advice of a physician or a poison control center.

Ipratropium bromide, anticholinergic aerosol used as a bronchodilator in the treatment of reversible airways disease.

IN = nebulize 250 μg per dose 3 times/24 hr. CH (> 3 yr of age): 1–2 inhalations (18 μg per actuation) 3 times/24 hr (usual max 6 inhalations/24 hr). CH (>14 yr of age), AD = 2 inhalations 4 times/24 hr (usual max 12 inhalations/24 hr).

Note: may cause usual anticholinergic side effects, blurred vision, dry mouth, sedation.

ATROVENT; inhaler

Iron preparations

℞ Daily maintenance iron requirement: elemental iron: PO: 0.5–1 mg/kg/24 hr, in single dose or divided

℞ In iron-deficiency anemia, as elemental iron: PO: 6 mg/kg/24 hr, div, with meals

Note: Iron supply at this dosage level ought to be continued for 2–3 mo to compensate for the deficits in erythrocytes and iron stores. Only iron in the ferrous form (Fe^{2+}) is absorbed from the gastrointestinal tract. The content of elemental iron in different preparations varies. The percentage of dry weight as elemental iron of ferrous choline citrate is 20; ferrous fumarate, 33; ferrous gluconate, 12; ferrous lactate, 19; ferrous sulfate, 20; and iron-dextran complex (ferric hydroxide), 2.

Dose calculation for parenteral iron administration: elemental Fe deficit = 2.5 mg/kg × deficit of hemoglobin concentration (in g/dL) in blood. (The deficit of the hemoglobin concentration is obtained as the difference between the measured and the desirable values, expressed in g/dL.) When iron has to be supplied by the parenteral route, deep IM injection is preferable to IV administration. In either case, a test dose of approximately 25 mg of elemental Fe in the form of the dextran complex should precede the administration of the total dose. If the total dose is large, it should be divided in separate daily doses of which none should exceed 5 mg/kg/24 hr of elemental iron.

Note: An additional 20–30% of the calculated deficit is needed to restore the tissue iron reserves.

Caution: Acute overdose may lead to shock, CNS depression, death (see Chapter 666.5).

Isoniazid, INH, isonicotinic acid hydrazide; tuberculostatic agent

℞ in the treatment of active tuberculosis, in combination with other antituberculous drugs: IN, CH = PO, IM: 10–20 mg/kg/24 hr, div, every 8–12 hr; max: 500 mg/24 hr. AD = PO, IM: 5–10 mg/kg/24 hr, div, every 8–12 hr; max: 300 mg/24 hr

℞ for prophylaxis of complications in recent conversion to positive tuberculin reaction (primary tuberculosis), or after suspected exposure: IN, CH = PO: 5–10 mg/kg/24 hr, as single dose, or div, every 12 hr; max: 300 mg/24 hr

Note: "Slow" acetylators (homozygous) need only about 0.20–0.50 of this dose to reach therapeutically effective plasma concentrations achieved by "rapid" acetylators (homozygous and heterozygous). Higher than necessary plasma concentrations of unmetabolized isoniazid seem not to be associated with risk of isoniazid hepatotoxicity.

Caution: Formation of toxic metabolite in some patients may lead to hepatic necrosis with usual doses (rare under 20 yr of age).

†, INH; tabl, syrup, inj

Isoproterenol hydrochloride, β-adrenergic agent

℞ to overcome atrioventricular block: IV infusion: Example: to prepare a solution containing 0.004 mg/mL, mix 1 mg of isoproterenol in 250 mL of 5% D/W or appropriate electrolyte solution and infuse at rate adjusted to response in patient (beginning with approximately 0.0001–0.0002 mg/kg/min)

†, ISUPREL; inj

Isotretinoin, 13-cis-retinoic acid, used in the treatment of severe recalcitrant cystic acne.

CH, AD = 0.5–2 mg/kg/24 hr div, every 12 hr for 15–20 wk. Actual duration of therapy dependent on patient response, usually to < 70% of initial lesions.

Caution: approximate 20% teratogenesis. Contrainidicated in patients who are pregnant or intend to become pregnant during therapy.

ACCUTANE; caps

Kanamycin sulfate, antimicrobial aminoglycoside

NB = IM, IV (over 20–30 min):
≤2,000 g and ≤7 days old: 15 mg/kg/24 hr, div, every 12 hr
≤2,000 g and >7 days old: 20 mg/kg/24 hr, div, every 12 hr
>2,000 g and ≤7 days old: 20 mg/kg/24 hr, div, every 12 hr
>2,000 g and >7 days old: 30 mg/kg/24 hr, div, every 8 hr

IN, CH = IM, IV (over 20–30 min): 15–30 mg/kg/24 hr, div, every 8–12 hr. Usual duration of therapy: 7–10 days; not indicated in long-term therapy because of ototoxic hazard.

Caution: Ototoxic, nephrotoxic.

KANTREX; inj

Ketamine, dissociative anesthetic agent used in general anesthesia or for short-term sedation before bedside surgical procedures and/or dressing changes.

CH = IV (≤ 0.5 mg/kg/min): Induction 0.5–2 mg/kg; lower doses may be used for minor procedures 0.5–1 mg/kg. IM dose 3–7 mg/kg. AD = IM 3–8 mg/kg; IV 1–4.5 mg/kg.

Caution: increases respiratory secretions in many patients requiring atropine (0.01 mg/kg) co-administration. Postanesthetic emergence reaction may manifest as vivid dreams, hallucinations, and/or delirium in approximately 15% of patients. Contraindicated in patients with increased intracranial or intraocular pressure.

KETALAR; inj

Ketoconazole, imidazole antifungal agent used for prophylaxis and treatment of a variety of mild to moderate fungal infections. Is not effective against infections arising within the CNS as the drug does not penetrate the blood-brain barrier.

CH = PO 5–10 mg/kg/24 hr div every 12–24 hr. Usual max 800 mg/24 hr. AD = PO 200–400 mg/24 hr administered once daily.

Note: gastric acidity is necessary for best oral absorption; thus, avoid drug administration with antacids or H_2 receptor antagonists. Numerous potential drug interactions, including ketoconazole-induced increases in serum drug concentrations of astemizole, cyclosporine, phenytoin, terfenadine, theophylline, warfarin. Use may be associated with hepatotoxicity.

NIZORAL; tabl, susp, topical cream/shampoo

Ketorolac tromethamine, nonsteroidal anti-inflammatory drug (NSAID) available for oral or parenteral administration. Possesses analgesic and antipyretic activities. Mechanism of action most likely inhibition of prostaglandin synthesis via antagonism of cyclo-oxygenase activity.

Table continued on following page

■ **TABLE 670–3 Drug Dosages (Drugs Listed Alphabetically by Generic Name)** *(Continued)*

CH = PO, IM 2 mg/kg/24 hr div every 6 hr. Many centers have administered the IM formulation via the IV route over 15–20 min.
Note: As with all NSAIDs, the use of these drugs may be associated with gastritis, reversible antiplatelet activity, and possible compromised renal function. Drug should be used cautiously in NB and other patients with decreased renal function.
TORADOL; inj, tabl

Labetalol hydrochloride, combined α- and β-receptor antagonist useful in the treatment of hypertension. Contraindicated in cardiogenic shock, uncompensated congestive heart failure, and lung disease.
CH = PO 3–4 mg/kg/24 hr div every 8–12 hr. IV = 0.3–1 mg/kg/dose; may be administered via continuous IV infusion; starting doses have ranged from 0.4–1 mg/kg/hr. Doses are titrated to desired effect and patient tolerance, i.e., blood pressure, heart rate.
NORMODYNE, TRANDATE; inj, tabl

Lactulose, nonabsorbed sugar that is degraded by colonic bacteria to lactic and acetic acids, resulting in an acid pH and ammonium ion (NH_4^-) trapping. Effective in decreasing systemic ammonia concentrations in patients with impaired hepatic function, e.g., hepatic encephalopathy.
IN = PO 2.5–10 mL/24 hr div every 6–8 hr. CH = PO 40–90 mL/24 hr div every 6–8 hr. Doses are adjusted to produce 2–3 loose stools/24 hr. May be administered as an enema.
CEPHULAC, ENULOSE; syrup

Leucovorin calcium, reduced form of folic acid, which is readily incorporated into purine and thymidine synthesis. Unlike folic acid, does not require enzyme reduction. Most often used for "rescue" therapy with high-dose methotrexate antineoplastic regimens to reverse methotrexate effect.
℞ for megaloblastic anemia in congenital dihydrofolate reductase deficiency: IM, PO = 3–6 mg/24 hr.
℞ for methotrexate rescue therapy: PO, IV 0.3 mg/kg/dose every 6 hr. Doses are often adjusted based on serum methotrexate concentration and/or specific protocol.
WELLCOVORIN; inj, tabl, powder for sol

Levocarnitine, endogenous dietary mineral required in energy metabolism, for the treatment of primary carnitine deficiency.
CH = PO 50–100 mg/kg/24 hr div every 8–12 hr. Usual max 3 g/24 hr. Dose is titrated to patient need and tolerance (abdominal cramps, body odor). CH, AD = IV (over 2–3 min) 50 mg/kg/24 hr div every 4–6 hr.
CARNITOR, VITACARN; inj, caps, tabl, liquid

Lidocaine hydrochloride, anesthetic agent used systemically for its antiarrhythmic effects; delayed slow diastolic depolarization, diminished automaticity. Does not affect normal conduction but seemingly improves conduction velocity in damaged areas of myocardium. In therapeutic doses does not depress myocardial contractility or atrioventricular conduction.
℞ for ventricular tachyarrhythmia; IN, CH = IV loading dose: 1 mg/kg/dose may be repeated every 5–10 min to desired effect until total dose of 5 mg/kg has been administered. Maintenance therapy administered by continuous infusion: 20–50 μg/kg/min (maximum dose 4 mg/min)
Caution: Excessive depression of cardiac conductivity may occur; electrocardiographic monitoring is indicated during treatment. Monitoring of serum lidocaine concentrations may also assist in therapy; seizurogenic metabolite of lidocaine may accumulate in patients with compromised renal function.
†, XYLOCAINE hydrochloride; IV, inj

Lincomycin hydrochloride, antimicrobial macrolide
CH = PO: 30–60 mg/kg/24 hr, div, every 8 hr. IM, IV (over 1–4 hr, as 10 mg/mL sol): 10–20 mg/kg/24 hr, div, every 8–12 hr
LINCOCIN; caps, syrup, inj

Lithium, cation effective in the treatment of acute manic episodes, bipolar disorders, and depression.
CH = PO 15–60 mg/kg/24 hr div every 6–8 hr. AD = PO 900–1,200 mg/24 hr div every 6–8 hr. Usual max 2.4 g/24 hr. Serum lithium concentrations correlate well with efficacy and toxicity. Target serum lithium concentrations 0.6–1.5 mEqg/L (0.6–1.5 mmol/L). Toxic effects observed with serum concentrations > 2 mEqg/L (2 mmol/L).
Body lithium elimination influenced by sodium intake and excretion (e.g., diuretics).
ESKALITH, LITHOBID, LITHOTABS; caps, tabl, syrup, controlled-release tabl

Loperamide, synthetic antidiarrheal agent used as short-term adjunctive therapy in the management of diarrhea. Drug slows intestinal motility thus affecting water and electrolyte movement through the bowel. Decreased peristaltic activity of the bowel results from a direct effect of loperamide on the circular and longitudinal muscles of the intestinal wall. Need for routine use of this drug in infants and children is questionable.
CH = PO: 0.4–1.5 mg/kg/24 hr, div, every 6–12 hr
IMODIUM; caps, liquid

Loracarbef, a synthetic β-lactam antibiotic of the carbapenem class. Spectrum of antibacterial activity very similar to cefaclor and other second-generation orally administered cephalosporins. Adverse effects similar to orally administered cephalosporins, although, unlike cefaclor, serum sickness reactions have not, thus far, been described with loracarbef.
IN, CH = PO 15–30 mg/kg/24 hr div Q 12 h; AD = PO 200–800 mg/24 hr div Q 12 h. Dose adjustment in moderate to severe renal dysfunction.
LORABID, caps, susp

Lorazepam, benzodiazepine that possesses antianxiety and sedative effects. Most experience with use of this drug in children is limited to its use as an alternative agent in the treatment of status epilepticus.
℞ for the treatment of status epilepticus: IN, CH = IV (slowly, as controlled "push" injection): 0.05 mg/kg/dose, which may be repeated every 15–20 min for 2 doses; may administer IM if IV not possible (efficacy may be diminished)
℞ for sedation: IN, CH = PO 0.05 mg/kg/dose Q 4–8 hr prn
†, ATIVAN; inj, tabs

Magnesium hydroxide, $Mg(OH)_2$
℞ as cathartic: PO: < 2 yr, 0.5 mL/kg dose; 2–5 yr, 5–15 mL/kg/24 hr; 6–12 yr, 15–30 mL/24 hr > 12 yr, 30–60 mL/24 hr given daily
Milk of magnesia, susp, "8%" containing $Mg(OH)_2$ 80 mg/mL

Magnesium sulfate, $MgSO_4 \cdot 7H_2O$, Epsom salt; 1 g of the salt is equivalent to 98.6 mg of elemental Mg or to 8.11 mEq of Mg^{2+}
℞ as cathartic: PO ($MgSO_4 \cdot 7H_2O$): 250 mg/kg/dose
℞ in hypomagnesemia: IM (in solution containing $MgSO_4 \cdot 7H_2O$ 500 mg/mL, equivalent to Mg^{2+} 4 mEq/mL, also labeled "50%"): $MgSO_4 \cdot 7H_2O$ 100 mg/kg/dose, equivalent to Mg^{2+} 0.8 mEq/kg/dose, repeat every 4–6 hr
IV (in solution containing $MgSO_4 \cdot 7H_2O$ 100 mg/mL, equivalent to Mg^{2+} 0.08 mEq/mL, also labeled "10%"): Infuse slowly $MgSO_4 \cdot 7H_2O$ up to 100 mg/kg/dose, equivalent to Mg^{2+} 0.08 mEq/kg/dose
†; crystalline salt, sterile sol for inj available as 50%, 25%, and 10%

Mannitol, osmotic diuretic
℞ test dose for oliguria: CH = IV: 0.2 g/kg/dose, injected within 3–5 min
℞ in cerebral edema: CH = IV (over 3–5 min): 0.25–1 g/kg/dose, injected as 15–25% sol over 30–60 min; target serum osmolality = 300–310 mOsmol/L

Mebendazole, anthelmintic agent that blocks glucose uptake by the susceptible parasites and interferes with their survival
℞ against pinworms (*Enterobius vermicularis*; cure rate 90–100%): CH = PO: 100 mg/dose; as single dose; against whipworms (*Trichuris trichiura*, cure rate 61–75%), roundworms (*Ascaris lumbricoides*, cure rate 91–100%), and hookworms (*Ancylostoma duodenale, Necator americanus*, cure rate 96%): alternative method = PO: 200 mg/24 hr, div, every 12 hr, for 3 consecutive days. If patient is not free of parasites 3 wk after treatment a 2nd course is indicated
Note: Not extensively studied in children under 2 yr of age.
VERMOX; chewable tabl

Meclizine hydrochloride, antihistamine used in the prevention and treatment of motion sickness and vertigo.
℞ for motion sickness: CH (>12 yr of age), AD = PO 25–50 mg 1 hr before event; dose may be repeated every 12–24 hr.
℞ for vertigo: 25–100 mg/24 hr.
ANTIVERT, BONINE, VERGON; caps, chewable tabl, tabl

Meperidine hydrochloride, synthetic narcotic analgesic agent; addictive
℞ against severe pain: IN, CH = PO, SC, IM, IV (over 5–10 min); 6–9 mg/kg/24 hr, div, prn every 4–6 hr (maximum single dose 100 mg)
†, DEMEROL hydrochloride, ‡; tabl, elixir, inj
Caution: May produce respiratory depression, seizures (metabolite normeperidine accumulates with renal insufficiency), coma in some sensitive patients. Naloxone is antidote.

Mephenytoin, anticonvulsant for the treatment of tonic-clonic and partial seizures uncontrolled by more conventional agents.
CH = PO 3–15 mg/kg/24 hr div every 8 hr. Usual maintenance dose 100–400 mg/24 hr; usual max AD 800 mg/24 hr. Therapy may be guided by serum concentration monitoring, 25–40 mg/L may be therapeutic.
MESANTOIN; tabl

Mercaptopurine (6-MP), antineoplastic antimetabolite that interferes with DNA and RNA synthesis via altered purine metabolism. Dose usually based on specific chemotherapy protocol.
CH = PO induction 2.5–5 mg/kg/24 hr and maintenance 1.5–2.5 mg/kg/24 hr administered once daily.
PURINETHOL; tabl

Mesna, used for the prevention of cyclophosphamide- and ifosfamide-associated hemorrhagic cystitis. Mesna (sodium-2-mercaptoethane sulfonate) binds to and detoxifies acreolin, the urotoxic metabolite of ifosfamide/cyclophosphamide.
CH, AD = IV 20% w/w of ifosfamide or cyclophosphamide dose administered before and at 4 and 8 hr after ifosfamide and at 3, 6, 9, and 12 hr after cyclophosphamide dose. Some have administered mesna dose orally.
MESNEX; inj

Metaproterenol sulfate, catecholamine analog; β-adrenergic receptor agonist with relatively selective effect on β_2-adrenergic receptors.

■ **TABLE 670–3 Drug Dosages (Drugs Listed Alphabetically by Generic Name)** *(Continued)*

℞ bronchodilator: IN, CH (<6 yr of age) = PO: 1.3–2.6 mg/kg/24 hr, div, every 6–8 hr; >6 yr of age: 10–20 mg/dose administered 3–4 times daily. Inhalation: CH >12 yr, AD = 2–3 inhalations Q 3–4 hr
†, ALUPENT; METAPREL; syrup, tabl, inhalation

Methacycline, see Tetracyclines

Methadone hydrochloride, narcotic analgesic with prolonged duration of effect; addictive. Frequently used as a component of a narcotic detoxification program. Approximate equianalgesic dose; 10 mg of methadone is approximately equivalent to 10 mg of morphine and 75–100 mg of meperidine.
℞ for analgesia CH = PO, IM 0.7 mg/kg/24 hr initially div every 4–8 hr but may administer less frequently (e.g., every 12–24 hr) as tolerated. IV 0.1 mg/kg/dose as needed.
Caution: drug has prolonged elimination half-life of approximately 12–30 hr. Drug can accumulate with repeated doses, increasing risk of toxicity. Naloxone reverses opiate effects.
DOLOPHINE; inj, liquid, tabl

Methenamine mandelate, urinary antibacterial agent effective in a nonspecific manner against microorganisms by liberating formaldehyde on decomposing in urine at pH below 5.5
℞ for prevention of bacterial growth in urine, provided pH is sufficiently low: CH = PO: initially 100 mg/kg/24 hr, div, every 6 hr, followed by 50 mg/kg/24 hr, div, every 6 hr
Note: Should not be used (and is useless) when urine acidification is contraindicated or not attainable (as in infections with urea-splitting bacteria). If situation permits, acidification of urine below pH 5.5 might be implemented by adjusting acid load or intake.
†, MANDELAMINE, tabl, oral susp: methenamine hippurate, HI-PREX, tabl

Methicillin sodium, semi-synthetic penicillinase-resistant penicillin
NB = IM, IV (over 15–30 min): according to the following criteria:
≤2,000 g and ≤14 days old: 50 mg/kg/24 hr, div, every 12 hr
≤2,000 g and 15–30 days old: 75 mg/kg/24 hr, div, every 8 hr
>2,000 g and ≤14 days old: 75 mg/kg/24 hr, div, every 8 hr
>2,000 g and 15–30 days old: 100 mg/kg/24 hr, div, every 6 hr
IN, CH = IV (over 15–30 min), IM: 200–400 mg/kg/24 hr, div, every 4 hr (IV) or every 6 hr (IM)
Caution: may produce interstitial nephritis.
Note: adjust dose with severe renal dysfunction (creatinine clearance <10 mL/min)
CELBENIN, STAPHCILLIN; inj

Methimazole, antithyroid drug that inhibits the synthesis of thyroid hormones by interfering with iodine oxygenation in the thyroid gland.
CH = PO initial dose 0.4 mg/kg/24 hr decreased to 0.2 mg/kg/24 hr div every 8 hr, depending on patient response, as determined by thyroid function studies.
Caution: rare hepatotoxic reaction.
Note: dose adjustment necessary in patients with decreased renal function, creatinine clearance < 50 mL/min.
TAPAZOLE; tabl

Methsuximide, anticonvulsant used as an adjunct in the treatment of absence and partial complex seizures.
CH = PO 10–15 mg/kg/24 hr div every 6–8 hr. Dose increased to effect, usual max 30 mg/kg/24 hr.
CELONTIN; caps

Methyldopa, antihypertensive agent, inhibitor of aromatic amino acid decarboxylase, and precursor of α-methylnorepinephrine. Probably lowers arterial blood pressure by stimulation of central inhibitory α-adrenergic receptors, false neurotransmission, or reduction of plasma renin activity
℞ as antihypertensive in long-term treatment: CH = PO: initially 10 mg/kg/24 hr, div, every 6–12 hr; decrease or increase the dose progressively at intervals of 2 days until adequate response achieved; maximum daily dosage: 65 mg/kg/24 hr
℞ for hypertensive crisis: CH = IV: 20–40 mg/kg/24 hr, div, every 6 hr
Caution: Positive direct Coombs test develops in 10–20% of patients on prolonged treatment, usually between 6 and 12 mo of continued administration. Positive indirect Coombs test, fever, and liver dysfunction occur less frequently. If evidence of hemolysis or liver dysfunction is present, methyldopa should be discontinued and not reinstituted.
ALDOMET; tabl

Methylphenidate hydrochloride, piperidine derivative structurally related to amphetamine; CNS stimulant with more prominent effects on mental than on motor activities
℞ in attention deficit hyperactivity disorder (ADHD): drug treatment of ADHD not recommended below the age of 3 yr or in nonstructured therapeutic situation. CH (over 3 yr) = PO: initiate treatment with 5-mg dose given at the onset of daytime activities and again 4–6 hr later; if needed, increase the dose at weekly intervals by increments of 5 mg/dose and adjust the size of the respective doses (early morning and midday) according to the response of the patient; daily dose usually should not exceed 2 mg/kg/24 hr. To avoid insomnia do not administer closer than 6 hr before bedtime. Once effective dose is identified, time-release tablet may be used with or without prompt-release tablet.
Caution: Reduction of growth rate and weight gain may accompany prolonged use. Chronic abuse can lead to tolerance.
℞ in narcolepsy: PO: proceed for dosage adjustment as in ADHD, with correction of the abnormal symptomatology as the end point.
RITALIN; tabl, time-release tabl

Metoclopramide hydrochloride, gastrointestinal prokinetic agent that increases lower esophageal sphincter pressure and rate of gastric emptying and augments gastrointestinal peristaltic activity. Use of this drug for the treatment of symptomatic gastroesophageal reflux in infants and children remains controversial. Drug is also used for the treatment of diabetic gastroparesis and as an adjunctive measure facilitating small bowel intubation when the tube does not pass the pylorus with conventional maneuvers. High-dose metoclopramide therapy has been shown to be an effective aid in the adjunctive management of nausea and vomiting associated with cancer chemotherapy.
℞ for gastroesosphageal reflux or gastrointestinal dismotility: CH = PO: 0.1 mg/kg/dose administered 4 times a day
℞ for prevention of chemotherapy-induced emesis: 2–3 mg/kg/dose administered before and after chemotherapeutic drug; timing of dose and actual regimen are dependent upon the specific chemotherapeutic agent administered.
Caution: Metoclopramide possesses dopamine receptor antagonist activity; thus, acute dystonic reactions may occur and are relatively frequent with high-dose therapy. Diphenhydramine may be used to treat metoclopramide (or phenothiazine)–induced acute dystonic reaction. It may be appropriate to co-administer diphenhydramine with high-dose metoclopramide to prevent dystonic reactions in patients receiving this therapy for nausea and vomiting associated with cancer chemotherapy.
†, REGLAN; tabs, syrup, inj

Metolazone, saluretic, inhibiting sodium reabsorption, and interfering with dilution of urine. A quinazoline diuretic with pharmacologic properties similar to those of thiazide diuretics. Dosage is titrated to effect in the management of edema as an antihypertensive agent.
CH = PO: 0.2–0.4 mg/kg/24 hr, div, every 12–24 hr
DIULO, *ZAROXOLYN,* tabl

Metoprolol tartrate, a relatively selective β_1-adrenoreceptor antagonist, used in the treatment of hypertension and other cardiovascular disorders.
CH = PO: 1–5 mg/kg/24 hr, div, every 12 hr, dose adjusted to patient response.
Caution: Experience with the use of this drug in children is limited. Despite relatively selective β_1-adrenoreceptive antagonism, it should be used cautiously in patients with bronchospastic disorders.
LOPRESSOR; tabl, inj

Metronidazole hydrochloride, synthetic antibacterial agent highly active against most obligate anaerobes, including *Bacteroides* species, such as *B. fragilis,* and *Clostridium* and *Peptostreptococcus* species. The drug is also effective in the treatment of amebiasis, *giardiasis* and *trichomoniasis*
℞ for amebiasis: CH = PO: 35–50 mg/kg/24 hr, div, every 8 hr
℞ for the treatment of anaerobic infections: IV
NB <2,000 g, 15 mg/kg/24 hr, div, every 12 hr
NB >2,000 g, <7 days: 15 mg/kg/24 hr, div, every 8 hr
NB >2,000 g, >7 days: 30 mg/kg/24 hr, div, every 8 hr
CH = PO, IV (slow over 30–60 min) 30 mg/kg/24 hr Q 6 hr
℞ for giardiasis: CH = PO: 15 mg/kg/day, div, every 8 hr
℞ for *Trichomonas* vaginitis: CH = PO: 15 mg/kg/24 hr, div, every 8 hr, for 7 days.
Topical therapy: Apply and rub in thin film twice daily to affected area. May be administered as vaginal suppositories.
Caution: Patient should not ingest alcohol for 24 hr after receiving a dose of this drug (disulfiram-type reaction). Drug interactions possible; may prolong anticoagulant effect of warfarin-type anticoagulants.
†, FLAGYL; tabs, inj

Mexiletine, class Ib antiarrhythmic used for the management of serious ventricular arrhythmias; suppression of premature ventricular contractions. Structurally related to lidocaine.
CH = PO 4–15 mg/kg/24 hr div every 8 hr.
Note: dose adjustment necessary in patients with renal dysfunction. Contraindicated in patients with second- or third-degree block or cardiogenic shock.
MEXITIL; tabl

Mezlocillin sodium, semi-synthetic penicillin susceptible to destruction by penicillinase.
℞ for systemic use: NB = IV (over 15–30 min), IM when IV not possible: <7 days, 150 mg/kg/24 hr, div, every 12 hr; >7 days, 225 mg/kg/24 hr, div, every 8 hr; IN, CH: 200–300 mg/kg/24 hr, div, every 4–6 hr
Note: Each gram of drug contains 1.85 mEq of sodium; IM injection is painful.
MEZLIN; inj

Table continued on following page

■ TABLE 670–3 Drug Dosages (Drugs Listed Alphabetically by Generic Name) *(Continued)*

Miconazole, synthetic antifungal imidazole derivative effective against systemic infections with *Coccidioides immitis, Candida albicans, Cryptococcus neoformans, Paracoccidioides brasiliensis.* IV infusion alone is inadequate for the treatment of fungal meningitis and urinary bladder infection; intrathecal administration and bladder instillation must also be carried out.
℞ for treatment of proven coccidioidomycosis, candidiasis, cryptococcosis, or paracoccidioidomycosis: CH = IV (after dilution with isotonic saline or 5% D/W and over 30–60 min): 20–40 mg/kg/24 hr, div, every 8 hr, until clinical and laboratory tests no longer indicate activity of fungal infection. Dose may vary with type of fungus involved. Topical application for skin/vaginal fungal infections
MONISTAT IV; ampules for IV inj, cream, vag. suppos.

Midazolam hydrochloride, benzodiazepine with rapid onset and short duration of action. Useful for conscious sedation preprocedures or for mechanical ventilation and as an initial acute-acting anticonvulsant.
℞ for preoperative sedation: CH = PO 0.4–0.5 mg/kg; IM 0.07–0.1 mg/kg 30–45 min presurgery. Intranasal 0.2 mg/kg; IV (over 2–3 min) 0.035 mg/kg/dose.
℞ for conscious sedation: CH = IV 0.05–0.2 mg/kg loading dose followed by 0.1–0.2 mg/kg/hr dose titrated to desired effect.
Caution: Abrupt discontinuation after long-term continuous administration may precipitate benzodiazepine withdrawal. Too rapid IV infusion may precipitate respiratory depression. Sedative and skeletal muscle effects are reversible with flumazenil.
VERSED; inj

Mineral oil, indigestible liquid hydrocarbon with limited absorbability; lubricant
℞ mild laxative: PO: 0.5 mL/kg/dose; AD = PO 15–45 mL/24 hr Q 8–24 hr
†, liquid petrolatum; plain liquid or emulsion

Minocycline, see Tetracyclines

Minoxidil, direct-acting peripheral vasodilator
℞ in severely hypertensive patients who do not adequately respond to maximum therapeutic doses of a diuretic and 2 other antihypertensive agents. Usually a β-adrenergic blocking agent has to be given concomitantly to prevent tachycardia and increased myocardial workload, as well as a diuretic such as hydrochlorothiazide, chlorthalidone, or furosemide to prevent serious fluid retention.
CH = PO: initial dosage 0.2 mg/kg/24 hr as single dose; thereafter dosage may be increased stepwise to 0.25–1.0 mg/kg/24 hr under careful titration of the size and frequency of administration of the doses according to the individual needs of the patient. Therapy is usually associated with extensive hirsutism.
LONITEN; tabl

Morphine sulfate, narcotic analgesic agent; addictive
℞ against severe pain: NB = SC, IM, IV (over 5 min or continuous infusion) 0.01 mg/kg/dose or per hour if continuous. IN, CH = SC, IM, IV 0.1–0.2 mg/kg/dose Q 2–4 hr prn; PO (tabl or sol) = 0.2–0.5 mg/kg/dose Q 4–6 hr; sustained-release tabl = 0.3–0.6 mg/kg/dose Q 12 hr. CH >12 yr, AD = IM, IV 3–8 mg/dose Q 3–6 hr prn.
Caution: Overdose produces severe respiratory depression, hypothermia, coma. Naloxone antidotal.
†, inj

Mupirocin, topical antibacterial ointment that inhibits bacterial protein synthesis by reversibly binding to bacterial isoleucyl transfer-RNA synthetase. Antibacterial spectrum of activity limited to gram-positive organisms only, including methicillin-resistant and β-lactamase–producing strains of staphylococci. No drug is absorbed systemically following topical administration. Mupirocin has been used in surgical dressings, as a prophylactic agent in the care of venous catheter access sites, and in topical management of impetigo.
℞ for topical application: applied to affected skin area every 8 hr
BACTROBAN; oint

Nafcillin sodium, semi-synthetic penicillinase-resistant penicillin
NB = IM, IV (over 15–30 min):
<2,000 g <7 days of age: 50 mg/kg/24 hr, div, every 12 hr
<2,000 g >7 days of age: 75 mg/kg/24 hr, div, every 8 hr
>2,000 g <7 days of age: 50 mg/kg/24 hr, div, every 8 hr
>2,000 g >7 days of age: 75 mg/kg/24 hr, div, every 6 hr
IN, CH: 100–200 mg/kg/24 hr, div, every 4–6 hr
†, UNIPEN, NAFCIL; caps, tabl, oral susp, inj

Nalidixic acid, antimicrobial agent effective against a selected group of gram-negative bacteria, apparently by inhibiting DNA synthesis
℞ for treatment of selected cases of urinary tract infection, when infective organisms can be shown to be sensitive: IN (>3 mo), CH = PO: 55 mg/kg/24 hr, div, every 6 hr, for 10–14 days
Note: If prolonged treatment is indicated, daily dose should be reduced to 33 mg/kg/24 hr, div, every 6 hr, and periodic evaluation for adverse side effects should be made. Resistance of initially sensitive micro-organisms develops in about 25% of infections and can occur within 48 hr. If resistance is suspected, a therapeutic alternative must be chosen. Action of nalidixic acid is antagonized by nitrofurantoin.
Caution: Even therapeutic doses may cause increased intracranial pressure, toxic psychosis, seizures in some patients.
NegGram; oral susp, caplets

Naloxone hydrochloride, opioid antagonist; nonaddictive
℞ in respiratory depression due to opioids: NB, IN, CH = IV, IM, SC: 0.01–0.1 mg/kg/dose, to be repeated prn after 2–3 min up to 3 times. After satisfactory response the dose must be repeated every 1–2 hr, as long as opioid depression persists. May require frequent repetitive doses or administration as a continuous IV infusion, depending on the elimination characteristics of the specific opioid agonist.
NARCAN, NARCAN neonatal; inj

Naproxen, nonsteroidal anti-inflammatory agent of the arylacetic acid group that possesses antipyretic and analgesic activities. Experience with this drug in children has been mostly limited to use in the treatment of juvenile rheumatoid arthritis.
℞ for rheumatoid arthritis: CH = PO: 10 mg/kg/24 hr, div, every 12 hr
NAPROSYN, ANAPROX; tabl

Neomycin sulfate, nonabsorbable antimicrobial aminoglycoside
℞ for inhibition of gastrointestinal flora; justified only in selected cases (danger of hyperammonemia, enterocolitis with pathogenic *E. coli*): IN, CH = PO: 50–100 mg/kg/24 hr, div, every 6–8 hr
Caution: Possible overgrowth of abnormal organisms.
†, MYCIFRADIN sulfate, ‡; oral susp, tabl

Neostigmine, competitive acetylcholinesterase inhibitor used to intensify and prolong the effects of acetylcholine.
℞ for myasthenia gravis diagnosis: CH = IM 0.025–0.04 mg/kg. AD = IM 0.022 mg/kg as single doses. Treatment CH = SC, IM, IV (over 5–10 min) 0.01–0.04 mg/kg/dose administered every 2–4 hr titrated to patient response.
℞ for reversal: of anesthetic nondepolarizing neuromuscular blockade: IN = IV 0.025–0.1 mg/kg/dose; CH = IV 0.025–0.08 mg/kg/dose; AD = IV 0.5–2.5 mg/dose.
Caution: use cautiously in patients with bradycardia, cardiac dysrhythmias, asthma, peptic ulcer disease.
Note: does not penetrate into the CNS.

Netilmicin sulfate, antimicrobial aminoglycoside.
NB = IM, IV (slowly over 30–60 min): <7 days of age, 5 mg/kg/24 hr, div, every 12 hr; >7 days of age, 7.5 mg/kg/24 hr, div, every 8 hr. IN, CH = IM, IV (slowly over 30–60 min): 7.5 mg/kg/24 hr, div, every 8 hr.
Serum concentrations may be monitored; therapeutic peak concentration is 5–10 mg/L, trough is <2 mg/L (see Table 670–2)

Niclosamide, anthelmintic agent useful particularly against cestodes, which under the effect of the drug become susceptible to the proteolytic action of intestinal secretions
℞ against *Diphyllobothrium latum* (fish tapeworm) and *Taenia saginata* (beef tapeworm): CH = PO: 40 mg/kg, as single dose; AD = PO: 2,000 mg, as single dose
℞ against *T. solium* (pork tapeworm): same dose as for fish and beef tapeworms. Since viability of ova contained in the segments is not affected by the drug and there is risk of cysticercosis with *T. solium* if ova spill out of digested segments, it is mandatory to give an adequate purge 1 hr after niclosamide administration to clear the bowel of all dead segments before they can be digested
℞ against *Hymenolepis nana* (dwarf tapeworm): CH = PO: 40 mg/kg/24 hr, as single daily dose, for 7 consecutive days. AD = PO: 2,000 mg/24 hr, as single daily dose, for 7 consecutive days
Note: Niclosamide tablets must be thoroughly chewed before being swallowed or finely ground and mixed with some liquid before they are ingested to be fully effective. Niclosamide is available in the US from the Parasitic Disease Drug Service, Bureau of Epidemiology, Centers for Disease Control and Prevention, Atlanta, GA 30333.
NICOLIDE; tabl

Nifedipine, calcium channel antagonist used in the treatment of hypertension or hypertrophic cardiomyopathy
℞ for hypertensive emergencies: CH = PO: 0.25–0.5 mg/kg/dose, administered every 6–8 hr. Contents of gelatin capsule may be placed sublingually for immediate onset of activity.
℞ hypertrophic cardiomyopathy, IN, CH = PO: 0.6–0.9 mg/kg/24 hr Q 6–8 hr. AD = PO: 30–60 mg/24 hr.
Caution: may cause severe hypotension, flushing, tachycardia, and palpitations.
ADALAT, PROCARDIA, liquid-filled gelatin caps, sustained-release tabl

Nitrofurantoin, nitrofuran-substituted hydantoin; antimicrobial agent effective against selected organisms, by interfering with enzyme systems of the microorganisms
℞ in the treatment of urinary tract infections, when infecting organisms are shown to be sensitive or likely to respond by clinical experience: IN (>3 mo), CH = PO: 5–7 mg/kg/24 hr, div, every 6 hr (with meals to minimize gastric upset), for 10–14 days. Repeated treatment courses with nitrofurantoin should be separated by "rest" periods. For long-term

■ **TABLE 670–3 Drug Dosages (Drugs Listed Alphabetically by Generic Name)** *(Continued)*

suppressive therapy dosage should be reduced, possibly to as low as 2 mg/kg/24 hr, div, every 6 hr
Note: Because of rapid elimination by the kidneys, bacteriostatic concentrations are achieved only in urine. Better antibacterial activity is obtained in acid urine.
Caution: Hemolysis occurs in G-6-PD–deficient individuals and in newborns because of insufficient detoxification capabilities. Nitrofurantoin should not be given to pregnant women at term or to women who breast feed.
†, FURADANTIN, MICRODANTIN, ‡; oral susp, tabl, caps

Nitroprusside, sodium nitrosylpentacyanoferrate, $Na_2Fe(CN)_5 \cdot NO \cdot 2H_2O$; vasodilator by direct action on smooth muscles of blood vessels; effect appears almost immediately and ends promptly, 1–10 min after stopping of administration of nitroprusside
℞ for emergency reduction of hypertension: IV infusion: Example: to prepare a solution of nitroprusside containing 0.1 mg/mL, dissolve 50 mg mg nitroprusside first in 2–3 mL 5% dextrose in water, and transfer this amount to 500 mL 5% dextrose water,* and start continuous infusion using a microdrip regulator or an infusion pump that allows precise measurement of flow; begin with infusion rate of 0.003 mg/kg/min (equivalent to 0.03 mL/kg/min of solution containing 0.1 mg/mL nitroprusside), and decrease or increase dosage according to response, for which there exists a wide dosage range (0.0005–0.008 mg/kg/min)
*Only 5% D/W should be used to prepare nitroprusside solution, and no other drug should be added. To prevent decomposition of nitroprusside by exposure to light, protect infusion bottle and possibly tubing from light; for instance, by wrapping in aluminum foil (optional).
Caution: Fall in arterial blood pressure is dose dependent, with risk of hypotensive circulatory failure on overdosage if careful monitoring of blood pressure does not lead to prompt adjustment of infusion rate.
Note: In patients receiving concomitant antihypertensive medications, a smaller dosage of nitroprusside is required for comparable reduction of hypertension. Thiocyanate metabolite may accumulate, causing toxicity (cyanosis, metabolic acidosis, seizures) after prolonged therapy or with existing renal dysfunction. Sodium thiosulfate antidote.
NIPRIDE; powder for preparation of solution prior to inj

Nystatin, antifungal agent; 1 mg = 2,000 units; seems to be active by altering permeability of cell membrane of yeasts
℞ for topical treatment of candidosis of the buccal cavity (thrush) and the gastrointestinal tract. Very poorly absorbed. In oral candidosis, spread nystatin suspension into recesses of mouth: NB (<2,000 g) = PO: 200,000–400,000 units/24 hr, div, every 4–6 hr. NB (>2,000 g), IN = PO: 400,000–800,000 units/24 hr, div, every 4–6 hr. CH = PO: 800,000–2,000,000 units/24 hr, div, every 4–6 hr
†, MYCOSTATIN, NILSTAT; oral susp, tabl

Octreotide acetate, somatostatin analog. Limited data available in pediatrics.
℞ vasoactive intestinal peptide–secreting tumors: AD = 200–300 μg/24 hr div every 6–12 hr.
℞ secretory diarrhea: only preliminary data and doses highly variable, titrated to response, e.g., 0.0003–0.0005 mg/kg
IV SQ every 4–8 hr.
SANDOSTATIN, inj

Ondansetron, competitive antagonist of the serotonin-3 receptor. Primarily used for the management of nausea and vomiting associated with cancer chemotherapy. Is effective for nausea and vomiting due to many causes, e.g., anesthesia, drug toxicity.
℞ for emesis: IV (over 15 min) 0.15 mg/kg/dose 30 min before and 4 and 8 hr after chemotherapy; alternatively, administer IV as 0.45-mg/kg single dose per 24 hr. Some clinicians have administered as a continuous 24-hr infusion for patients refractory to other intermittent dosing. CH = PO 4–8 mg/dose before stimulus as needed.
Note: devoid of sedative and dystonic effects observed with other antiemetics. Oral dosing often used for less severe stimulus to nausea and vomiting.
ZOFRAN; inj, tabl

Oxacillin sodium, semi-synthetic penicillinase-resistant penicillin
NB = IM, IV (over 10–15 min): <2,000 g, <7 days of age, 50 mg/kg/24 hr, div, every 12 hr; >7 days of age, 100 mg/kg/24 hr, div, every 8 hr; >2,000 g, <7 days of age, 75 mg/kg/24 hr, div, every 8 hr; >7 days of age, 150 mg/kg/24 hr, div, every 6–8 hr; IN, CH = PO, IM, IV: 50–200 mg/kg/24 hr, div, every 4–6 hr
BACTOCILL, PROSTAPHLIN; caps, oral susp, inj

Pancrelipase, pancreatic enzyme supplement containing lipase, amylase, and protease. Different amounts of these enzymes are found in the many different drug products available.
℞ for pancreatic enzyme replacement: IN, CH, AD = PO dose titrated to effect and patient tolerance (primarily stooling characteristics).
Note: high doses may produce intestinal strictures
COTAZYME, PANCREASE, VIOKASE; caps, tabl, powder

Pancuronium bromide, nondepolarizing neuromuscular blocking agent used during surgery to facilitate endotracheal intubation and mechanical ventilation.
IN, CH, AD = IV 0.04–0.1 mg/kg/dose as needed.
Note: dose adjustment necessary in patients with renal dysfunction. Support respiration.
PAVULON; inj

Paraldehyde, cyclic ether compound that decomposes to acetaldehyde on exposure to light and air; rapidly acting hypnotic agent
℞ in status epilepticus: CH = IM (injection remote from nerves because of risk of damage): 0.15 g/kg/dose, corresponding to 0.15 mL/kg/dose of paraldehyde solution containing 1 g/mL; occasionally 1 additional dose may be given after 30 min, prn
Note: Use glass syringe because paraldehyde reacts with plastic equipment. When given IV, injection should be slow, and paraldehyde solution should be diluted with isotonic sodium chloride solution to lessen risk of thrombophlebitis. IV use is not reccommended.
℞ to calm agitation: CH = PO, IM (PR, diluted in equal amount of olive oil): 0.15 mL/kg/dose, to be repeated prn after 4–6 hr
Caution: Before use, make sure that drug is not decomposed (acetaldehyde, acetic acid). Avoid IM administration if possible
†, PARAL; liquid for inj, oral use (risk of gastric irritation), and rectal use

Paregoric, camphorated tincture of opium. Used for the temporary treatment of diarrhea and as a component of neonatal opiate withdrawal program.
℞ for neonatal withdrawal; 3–6 drops administered every 3–6 hr as needed. Dose titrated to desired effect. CH = PO 0.25–0.5 mL/kg administered every 6–24 hr. AD = PO 5–10 mL administered every 6–24 hr.
Note: each 5 mL of paregoric contains 2 mg of morphine equivalent, 0.02 mL of anise oil, 20 mg of benzoic acid, 20 mg of camphor, 0.2 mL of glycerin, and alcohol. Final alcohol content is 45%.

Pemoline, an oxazolidone; structurally different from amphetamine and methylphenidate; CNS stimulant with minimal sympathomimetic effects
℞ in ADHD: drug treatment of ADHD not recommended below the age of 3 yr or in nonstructured therapeutic situation: CH (so far insufficient data have been accumulated in children below the age of 6 yr to assess efficacy and safety in this age group) = PO: initiate treatment with approximately 1 mg/kg/24 hr, as single dose each morning. If needed, increase dosage at weekly intervals by increments of 0.5 mg/kg/24 hr. On this schedule of titration of dose therapeutic response may not become evident until 4th wk of continued administration. Daily dose should not exceed 3 mg/kg/24 hr
Note: Insomnia, anorexia, and weight loss have been observed. The degree of reduced growth pattern on continued treatment is not yet established. Drug treatment of ADHD should be discontinued at appropriate intervals to observe behavior of the patient and assess indication for further treatment.
CYLERT; tabl

Penicillamine, metal-chelating agent with therapeutic affinity for copper and lead.
℞ for rheumatoid arthritis: CH = PO 3 mg/kg/24 hr (usually <250 mg total dose/24 hr) div every 12 hr for 3 mo with dose increase to 6 mg/kg/24 hr (max 600 mg/24 hr) as tolerated. AD = PO 125–250 mg/24 hr increased up to 1–1.5 g/24 hr.
℞ for Wilson disease: IN, CH = PO 20 mg/kg/24 hr div every 6–12 hr. Dose titrated to urinary copper excretion (>1 mg/24 hr).
℞ for cystinuria: CH = PO 30 mg/kg/24 hr div every 6 hr; usual max 4 g/24 hr.
℞ for lead poisoning: CH = PO 25–40 mg/kg/24 hr div every 6–8 hr.
Note: possible allergic reactions. Do not use in penicillin-allergic patients. Consider concurrent pyridoxine supplementation during therapy. Monitor for iron-deficiency anemia and nephrotic-like syndrome.
CUPRIMINE, DEPEN; cap, tabl

Penicillin G, benzylpenicillin; potassium penicillin G (1 mg = 1,595 units); sodium penicillin G (1 mg = 1,667 units). One million units of these salts of penicillin contain 1.68 mEq of either K^+ or Na^-; in other terms, 1 g contains 2.7 K^- or 2.8 mEq of either Na^-.
NB = IV (over 15–30 min) IM:
<2,000 g, 50,000 units/kg/24 hr, div, every 12 hr
℞ for meningitis: 100,000 units/kg/24 hr, div, every 12 hr
>2,000 g, 75,000 units/kg/24 hr, div, every 8 hr
℞ for meningitis: 150,000–200,000 units/kg/24 hr, div every 8 hr
IN, CH = PO, IM, IV (15–30 min): 100,000–250,000 units/kg/24 hr, div, every 4–6 hr
℞ for meningitis: 200,000–300,000 units/kg/24 hr, div, every 4 hr
(The higher doses should be chosen for meningitis caused by group B streptococci.)
IN, CH = PO, IM, IV (over 15–30 min): 25,000–50,000 units/kg/24 hr, equivalent to 15.5–31 mg/kg/24 hr, div, every 4–6 hr; if given PO, administer penicillin G 0.5 hr before or 2 hr after the meal.
℞ in severe infections: IV: 200,000–400,000 units/kg/24 hr, equivalent to 125–250 mg/kg/24 hr, as continuous drip infusion or div, every 2–4 hr
℞ for prophylaxis of rheumatic fever: PO: 200,000 units/dose, equivalent to 125 mg/dose, twice daily, spaced from meals (see Chapter 175.1)

Table continued on following page

■ **TABLE 670–3 Drug Dosages (Drugs Listed Alphabetically by Generic Name)** *(Continued)*

Penicillin G benzathine, for injection: combination of 1 mole of dibenzylethylenediamine with 2 moles of penicillin G; 1 mg = 1,211 units
℞ for prophylaxis of rheumatic fever: CH = IM: 600,000–1,200,000 units, equivalent to 500–1,000 mg penicillin G, once a month
†, BICILLIN L-A, PERMAPEN, ‡; susp for inj
†, PENTIDS, PFIZERPEN G, ‡, tabl, caps, oral susp, inj (IV)

Penicillin G procaine, for injection; combination of penicillin G with procaine, mole for mole (1 mg = 1,009 units)
NB = IM: 50,000 units/kg/24 hr, equivalent to 50 mg/kg/24 hr, in single daily dose. IN, CH = IM: 25,000–50,000 units/kg/24 hr, equivalent to 25–50 mg/kg/24 hr, in single daily dose
†, CRYSTICILLIN, DURACILLIN A.S., ‡; susp for IM inj

Penicillin V, phenoxymethyl penicillin, acid-resistant penicillin; 1 mg = 1695 units
IN, CH = PO: 25,000–50,000 units/kg/24 hr, equivalent to 15–30 mg/kg/24 hr, div, every 6–8 hr.
Note: 400,000 units = 250 mg (approx).
†, PEN-VEE K, VEETIDS, ‡; tabl, oral susp, drops

Pentamidine isethionate, antimicrobial effective against *Pneumocystis carinii.*
℞ for *P. carinii* pneumonia: CH = IM (deep), IV (over 60 min) 4 mg/kg/24 hr once daily for 10–14 days. Prophylaxis: IM, IV 4 mg/kg once weekly to once monthly. Inhalation: CH (<5 yr of age) 8 mg/kg/aerosol dose. CH (>5 yr of age) 300 mg/dose.
Note: inhalation may cause airway irritation, bronchospasm. May cause liver and renal abnormalities and thrombocytopenia.
NebuPent, PENTAM-300; inhalation, inj

Pentazocine hydrochloride, narcotic analgesic of the benzomorphan type; addictive
℞ against severe pain: Clinical experience in children under 12 yr of age is limited. AD = PO: 50 mg/dose, to be repeated prn after 3–4 hr; IM, SC (pentazocine lactate); 30 mg/dose, to be repeated prn after 4 hr
Caution: As for *morphine,* above.
FORTRAL, TALWIN; tabl (hydrochloride); inj (lactate)

Pentobarbital, CNS depressant of barbiturate class with short duration of action; tolerance to hypnotic effect may develop on continued use; initially, hypnotic effect of 3–5 hr
℞ for sedation hynosis: IN, CH = PO, IM: 2–6 mg/kg/24 hr, div, every 6 hr or single dose for hypnosis. Doses may be given PR.
℞ for pentobarbital coma; 5–15 mg/kg loading dose IV (over 1–2 hr); then 1–5 mg/kg/hr infusion to maintain burst suppression on EEG
Note: monitor respirations
†, NEMBUTAL elixir, pentobarbital sodium, †, NEMBUTAL sodium; inj, caps, suppos

Phenazopyridine hydrochloride, urinary anesthetic for possible symptomatic relief of urinary burning, itching associated with urologic procedures or urinary tract infection.
CH = PO 12 mg/kg/24 hr div every 8 hr. AD = PO 100–200 mg/dose every 6–8 hr.
PYRIDIUM, tabl

Phenobarbital, central nervous system depressant of barbiturate class with long duration of action; initially, hypnotic effect of 8–12 hr; tolerance to hypnotic effect may develop on continued use
℞ for sedation: IN, CH = PO, IM: 2–3 mg/kg/24 hr, div, every 8–12 hr
℞ for sleep: IN, CH = PO, IM: 2–3 mg/kg/dose, repeat prn after 12–24 hr
℞ as anticonvulsant: Status IV (rate <1 mg/kg/min or 50 mg/min for patients weighing >60 kg). Loading dose NB = 15–20 mg/kg in single or div dose; IN, CH, AD = 15–18 mg/kg in single or div dose. Maintenance dosing NB = PO, IV 3–4 mg/kg/24 hr div every 12–24 hr; IN, CH 5–8 mg/kg/24 hr div every 12–24 hr. CH (>12 yr of age), AD = PO, IV 1–3 mg/kg/24 hr.
℞ hyperbilirubinemia: CH (<8 yr of age) = PO 3–8 mg/kg/24 hr div every 8–12 hr.
Note: dosing may be guided by serum concentration monitoring, therapeutic values 15–40 mg/L.
Caution: All barbiturates, including phenobarbital, are respiratory depressants. Serum concentrations should be monitored.
†, LUMINAL, elixir, tabl; phenobarbital sodium, †, LUMINAL sodium, inj

Phenolphthalein, laxative acting primarily on the colon
CH = PO: 1 mg/kg/dose
†, tabl, oral susp; component of several preparations

Phenoxybenzamine hydrochloride, α-adrenergic receptor antagonist used primarily for the symptomatic treatment of pheochromocytoma-associated episodes of hypertension. The bioavailability of phenoxybenzamine from capsules appears to range between 20 and 30%.
℞ in the treatment of pheochromocytoma: 1–2 mg/kg/24 hr, div, every 6–12 hr, titrated to clinical effect.
DIBENZYLINE, caps

Phenylephrine hydrochloride, catecholamine with exclusively α-adrenergic action; peripheral vasoconstrictor
℞ to increase blood pressure in orthostatic hypotension, or
℞ to trigger vagal reflex in response to blood pressure increase, in the treatment of atrial tachyarrhythmia: PO: 1 mg/kg/24 hr, div, every 4 hr; SC, IM: 0.1 mg/kg/dose, repeat prn by monitoring response
Caution: With regard to hypertensive state and peripheral ischemia.
†, NEO-SYNEPHRINE hydrochloride; inj, elixir; also available as nose drops for local decongestant effect

Phenytoin, diphenylhydantoin; anticonvulsant agent; effective also in certain types of cardiac arrhythmias; antiarrhythmic effects similar to those of lidocaine: delayed slow diastolic depolarization, diminished automaticity; may facilitate conduction in damaged myocardial areas; does not depress myocardial activity
℞ as anticonvulsant. Status IV (rate <1–3 mg/kg/min or 50 mg/min), PO loading dose NB = 15–20 mg/kg in single or div dose; IN, CH, AD = 15–18 mg/kg in single or div dose. Maintenance dosing IV, PO = NB 5 mg/kg/24 hr div every 8–12 hr; IN, CH 5–10 mg/kg/24 hr div every 8–12 hr; CH (>12 yr of age) 5 mg/kg/24 hr div every 12 hr.
℞ for arrhythmias. CH, AD = IV 1.25 mg/kg IV (over 1–3 min) every 5 min as needed up to total loading dose of 15 mg/kg.
Note: anticonvulsant effects may be guided by monitoring serum phenytoin concentrations, therapeutic 10–20 mg/L.
Note: Phenytoin disposition is most often characterized by nonlinear (Michaelis-Menten) pharmacokinetics. Phenytoin is highly protein bound (>90%) and may be associated with protein binding displacement interaction; therapy is associated with unpredictable effects upon the activity of hepatic drug-metabolizing enzymes. Caution should be used in generic substitution because all generic preparations may not be bioequivalent.
Caution: Imbalance in phenytoin protein binding reflected by abnormally low but therapeutic free serum phenytoin concentrations in patients with renal dysfunction and critically ill with acute head trauma.
†, DILANTIN; oral susp; phenytoin sodium, †, DILANTIN sodium; caps, inj

Physostigmine salicylate, competitive acetylcholinesterase inhibitor intensifying and prolonging the effects of acetylcholine. Unlike neostigmine, which has peripheral-only effects, physostigmine crosses into the CNS, prolonging both the central and peripheral effects of acetylcholine.
℞ for reversal of anticholinergic toxicity. should be attempted only by experienced individuals, for unusual patients, with close monitoring and the ability to resuscitate. IV (0.5 mg/min or less) 0.01–0.03 mg/kg/dose; may repeat in 15–20 min.
Caution: use cautiously in patients with bradycardia, cardiac dysrhythmias, asthma, peptic ulcer disease.
ANTILIUM; inj, ophthalmic oint, sol

Phytonadione, vitamin K_1
℞ for hemorrhagic disease of the newborn. SC, IM, IV (over 15–30 min): Prophylaxis: 0.5–1 mg within 1 hr of birth; may repeat if needed in 6–8 hr. Treatment: 1–2 mg/dose/24 hr.
℞ for warfarin-type anticoagulant toxicity: IN = IV, PO 1–2 mg/dose as needed; CH, AD = PO, IV 2.5–10 mg/dose as needed. Doses titrated to patient response with monitoring of coagulation studies.
Note: too rapid IV administration associated with hypotension and flushing.
AQUAMEPHYTON, MEPHYTON; inj, tabl

Piperacillin sodium, semi-synthetic broad-spectrum aminobenzylpenicillin. Each gram of piperacillin contains 1.85 mEq of sodium: The drug is not absorbed when administered orally and is available only for parenteral administration.
℞ NB = IM, IV (over 15–30 min) <7 days 150 mg/kg/24 hr div every 8 hr; >7 days, 200 mg/kg/24 hr div every 6 hr. IN, CH = IM, IV 200–300 mg/kg/24 hr div every 4–8 hr. Usual max 24 g/24 hr. Dose adjustment necessary for patients with renal dysfunction, creatinine clearance <50 mL/min
PIPRACIL; inj

Piperacillin/tazobactam, semi-synthetic broad-spectrum penicillin combined with tazobactam, a β-lactamase inhibitor. Added spectrum of antibacterial activity includes β-lactamase-positive *S. aureus* and *H. influenzae.* Limited data in pediatrics. IN, CH = IV (over 15–30 min) 240–300 mg/kg/24 hr div every 6–8 hr. Dose adjustment necessary in patients with renal dysfunction, <50 ml/min.

Piperazine citrate, anthelmintic.
℞ for pinworms: CH, AD = PO 65 mg/kg/24 hr as a single dose for 7 days. In severe infestations, may repeat course after 1-wk interval. Usual max 2.5 g/24 hr.
℞ for roundworms: CH = PO 75 mg/kg/24 hr as a single dose for 2 days. Usual maximum 3.5 g/24 hr.
Note: most often used as an alternative to first-line agents, e.g., mebendazole, pyrantel.

Pralidoxime chloride, 2-PAM acetylcholinesterase reactivator.
℞ for acetylcholinesterase inhibitor insecticide poisoning (most often used in conjunction with atropine). CH = IM, IV (over 15–30 min) 20–50 mg/kg/dose repeated in 1–2 hr, with monitoring of muscle weakness response. May be administered as continuous IV infusion.

■ **TABLE 670–3 Drug Dosages (Drugs Listed Alphabetically by Generic Name)** *(Continued)*

Note: dose adjustment necessary in patients with renal dysfunction. 2-PAM overdose may potentiate insecticide toxicity.
PROTOPAM; inj

Praziquantel, anthelmintic.
℞ for schistosomiasis. CH, AD = PO 40–60 mg/kg/24 hr div every 8–12 hr for 1 day of therapy.
℞ for fluke infestation. CH, AD = PO 75 mg/kg/24 hr div every 8 hr for 1–2 days.
℞ for cysticercosis. CH, AD = PO 50 mg/kg/24 hr div every 8 hr for 14 days.
℞ for tapeworms. CH, AD = PO 10–20 mg/kg as a single dose. *H. nana* infestations: 25 mg/kg single dose.
Note: therapy may be associated with dizziness, drowsiness, vertigo.
BILTRICIDE; tabl

Prazosin hydrochloride, competitive inhibitor of postsynaptic α-adrenergic receptors.
℞ hypertension. CH = PO 0.1 mg/kg/24 hr div every 6 hr. May require initial test dose of 0.005 mg to assess patient initial response. AD = PO 1 mg/dose administered every 8–12 hr.
MINIPRESS; caps

Primaquine, 8-aminoquinoline antimalarial agent, used for prophylaxis against *Plasmodium vivax, P. ovale,* and *P. malariae* and for "radical" cure of infections due to *P. vivax* and *P. ovale*
IN, CH = PO: 0.55 mg/kg/24 hr (equivalent to 0.3 mg/kg/24 hr of base), as single daily dose, for 14 days
Note: Degree of intravascular hemolysis in individuals with G-6-PD deficiency is related to dosage and particular variant of the deficiency
Primaquine diphosphate; tabl

Primidone, a deoxybarbiturate that is partially metabolized to phenobarbital; anticonvulsant agent
℞ for long-term therapy of selected types of convulsive disorder: NB = PO 12–20 mg/kg/24 hr Q 6–12 hr; CH <8 yr = PO 10–25 mg/kg/24 hr Q 8–12 hr; CH >8 yr, AD = PO 125–1,500 mg/24 hr div to patient response and tolerance. Max 2 g/24 hr.
Note: Serum concentration monitoring should include evaluation of both PEMA and phenobarbital (see Table 670–2).
MYSOLINE; oral susp, tabl

Probenecid, competitive inhibitor of tubular secretion and reabsorption of organic acids
℞ for uricosuric action (aspirin antagonizes this effect), or
℞ in conjunction with penicillin G or V, or ampicillin, methicillin, oxacillin, cloxacillin, nafcillin, and many cephalosporins to achieve longer persistence of therapeutic blood and tissue concentrations of the antimicrobial agent. CH = PO: initial dose of 25 mg/kg, followed by 40 mg/kg/24 hr, div, every 6 hr
BENEMID; tabl

Procainamide hydrochloride, antiarrhythmic agent with general cardiodepressant effects; diminished myocardial excitability (decreased threshold potential, prolonged refractory period), reduced conduction velocity, diminished automaticity; decreases myocardial contractility; effects similar to those of quinidine
℞ titrated to patient response: CH = PO 15–50 mg/kg/24 hr div every 3–6 hr; IM 20–30 mg/kg/24 hr div every 4–6 hr; IV (>5 min and slower for loading dose, e.g., 25–30 min): Loading dose 3–6 mg/kg, usual maximum single dose 100 mg repeated as needed until total load of 15 mg/kg achieved. Maintenance dosing by continuous IV infusion 20–80 μg/kg/min.
Note: too rapid IV infusion often associated with hypotension.
Serum concentration should be monitored for both procainamide and its active metabolite *N*-acetyl procainamide (see Table 670–2).
†, PRONESTYL; tabl, caps, inj

Prochlorperazine, piperazine-type phenothiazine with antiemetic effect
℞ for sedation/antiemetic: CH (over 2 yr old) = PO suppos. 0.4 mg/kg/24 hr, div, every 6–8 hr, prn. IM: 0.1–0.15 mg/kg/24 hr, div, every 8–12 hr, prn
Caution: May produce parkinsonian syndrome and acute dystonic reaction. Diphenhydramine and benztropine may be antidotal. Other antiemetic agents may be more desirable for use in children.
†, COMPAZINE edisylate; oral liquid, syrup, inj, suppos

Promethazine hydrochloride, phenothiazine with aliphatic side chain that affords antihistaminic activity.
℞ for sedation, prevention or treatment of motion sickness, and as antihistaminic: CH = PO: 1 mg/kg/24 hr, divided into half dose at bedtime and quarter doses every 6 hr of the remaining daytime
℞ as antiemetic: CH = PO, IM, IV (slow), suppos 0.25–1 mg/kg/dose Q 4–6 hr.
†, PHENERGAN; syrup, tabl, suppos

Propantheline bromide, antispasmodic synthetic antimuscarinic agent as well as partial ganglionic blocking drug
℞ as adjunctive therapy against spasms in the gastrointestinal tract: CH = PO: 1.5 mg/kg/24 hr, div, every 6 hr, with meals, if applicable. IM: 0.8 mg/kg/24 hr, div, every 6 hr
†, PRO-BANTHINE; tabl, inj

Propoxyphene hydrochloride, and propoxyphene napsylate; opioid analgesic with less dependence liability than seen with codeine
℞ for mild to moderately severe pain: CH = PO: 2–3 mg/kg/24 hr, div, every 6 hr
propoxyphene hydrochloride, †, DARVON, ‡, caps; propoxyphene napsylate, DARVON-N, oral susp, tabl

Propranolol hydrochloride, β-adrenergic blocking agent (β_1 and β_2); racemic mixture of D- and L-propranolol, of which only L form has adrenergic blocking activity
℞ against selected forms of supraventricular and ventricular tachycardia: IN, CH = IV: 0.01–0.10 mg/kg/dose, given slowly; repeat every 6–8 hr prn. PO: 0.5–4.0 mg/kg/24 hr, div, every 6–8 hr
℞ as antihypertensive in long-term therapy: CH = PO: initially 1 mg/kg/24 hr, div, every 6 hr, and progressive increase of dosage, if needed to achieve adequate response, up to 5 mg/kg/24 hr, div, every 6 hr. Combination with diuretic or other hypertensive is indicated because propranolol blocks physiologic compensatory mechanisms such as adrenergic inotropic and chronotropic responses, as well as renin activity
℞ for prevention of migraine attack in severe cases and to combat the manifestations of thyrotoxicosis: propranolol requirements vary widely from patient to patient because of individual differences in severity of underlying disease, endogenous sympathetic neuronal activity, sensitivity of β-adrenergic receptors to blockade, degree of protein binding, hepatic blood flow. For comparable effect, oral dose should be 6–10 times higher than intravenous dose in spite of good absorption from the gut because of inactivation of important fraction of propranolol in liver after entrance through portal vein (i.e., first-pass effect).
Measures in case of exaggerated response: against bradycardia, atropine; if no response, isoproterenol, *cautiously;* against cardiac failure, digitalization and diuretics; against hypotension, epinephrine; against bronchospasm, isoproterenol, theophylline (aminophylline)
†, INDERAL; tabl, inj

Propylthiouracil (PTU), antithyroid that inhibits thyroid hormone synthesis by interfering with iodine incorporation.
℞ for hyperthyroidism. NB = PO 5–10 mg/kg/24 hr div every 8 hr; CH = PO 5–7 mg/kg/24 hr div every 8 hr.
Note: dose adjustment necessary in patients with renal dysfunction, creatinine clearance <50 mL/min

Protamine sulfate, protamines are low molecular weight basic proteins that bind tightly to heparin in vitro, thus neutralizing its anticoagulant effect. Protamine is used to reverse the effects of heparin. Protamine 1 mg is capable of binding to and thus neutralizing approximately 100 units of heparin. The dose of protamine to be administered is based on the expected amount of heparin remaining in the body, as determined by the heparin elimination half-life.
Caution: Protamine dose should be calculated cautiously because excess protamine may cause anticoagulation.
PROTAMINE, inj

Pseudoephedrine hydrochloride, indirectly acting sympathomimetic
℞ as nasal decongestant by systemic route: CH = PO: 4 mg/kg/24 hr, div, every 6 hr
†, SUDAFED, ‡; syrup, caps; contained in many combination products

Pyrantel pamoate, anthelmintic agent effective by means of neuromuscular paralysis of the parasite
℞ against pinworms *(E. vermicularis), A. lumbricoides,* and hookworms *(N. americanus, A. duodenale)*: pyrantel pamoate has not been extensively studied in infants and children below 2 yr of age; hence, particular attention should be given to children of this age; group during treatment of parasitic infestation with pyrantel. CH = PO: 11 mg/kg/dose, as single dose and without regard to food intake or time of day; purging not necessary prior to, during, or after therapy
Note: In pinworm infestation, in which possibility of reinfection with eggs from the host exists, a 2nd treatment 2–3 wk after the 1st might be indicated.
ANTIMINTH; oral susp

Pyrazinamide, antitubercular drug used in combination with other agents.
CH = PO 15–40 mg/kg/24 hr div every 12–24 hr. Usual maximum dose 2 g/24 hr. AD = PO 15–30 mg/kg/24 hr not to exceed 2 g/24 hr.
Note: use may be associated with hepatotoxicity, particularly with doses >30 mg/kg/24 hr.
tabl

Pyridostigmine bromide, cholinesterase inhibitor
℞ for diagnosis of myasthenia gravis: see Edrophonium chloride
℞ in myasthenia gravis: NB, IN, CH = IM: 0.1 mg/kg/dose, and continue with PO medication. PO: frequency of dosage and size of dose must be

Table continued on following page

■ **TABLE 670–3 Drug Dosages (Drugs Listed Alphabetically by Generic Name)** *(Continued)*

adjusted individually to provide optimum compensation during cycle of daily activities; average effective dose: 7 mg/kg/24 hr, div, every 4–5 hr
℞ for reversal of nondepolarizing muscle relaxants (tubocurarine, gallamine, pancuronium): IV (preceded by IV injection of atropine to prevent excessive secretions and bradycardia): 0.15 mg/kg/dose, and watch for recovery, which ought to occur after 15–30 min; assure appropriate ventilation until complete recovery
Caution: As for Edrophonium chloride.
MESTINON; tabl, syrup, inj

Pyrimethamine, inhibitor of dihydrofolate reductase, antimalarial agent; for use in treatment of toxoplasmosis
℞ for clinical prophylaxis of malaria, especially effective against *P. falciparum:* IN, CH = PO: 0.5–0.75 mg/kg/dose, once every 7 days. Begin prophylaxis 2 wk before entering malarious area and continue for 8 wk after leaving. To eradicate *P. vivax* and *P. ovale* infections, treatment for 14 days with primaquine should be considered immediately on leaving malarious area while pyrimethamine prophylaxis is still in effect (see Chapter 244.7)
Note: Hematologic abnormalities (anemia, thrombocytopenia, leukopenia) secondary to folic and folinic acid depletion can be prevented or reversed by IM administration of folinic acid (leucovorin) without affecting the efficacy of pyrimethamine.
DARAPRIM; tabl

Quinacrine hydrochloride, mepacrine hydrochloride; acridine derivative formerly used as antimalarial agent and against infestation with tapeworms, presently regarded as drug of choice against giardiasis
℞ against *Giardia lamblia (Lamblia intestinalis):* CH = PO: 6 mg/kg/24 hr, div, every 8 hr, for 5 consecutive days; max 300 mg/24 hr
℞ against dwarf tapeworm: CH (4–8 yr of age) PO = 200 mg first dose, then 100 mg once daily. CH (8–10 yr of age) 300 mg first dose 100 mg twice daily for 3 days. CH (11–14 yr of age) 400 mg first dose, 100 mg thrice daily for 3 days.
℞ against tapeworm (beef, pork, fish): CH (5–10 yr of age) = PO 100 mg administered every 10 min for 4 doses. CH (11–14 yr of age) 200 mg every 10 min for 4 doses.
℞ for malaria suppression: CH (<8 yr of age) 50 mg/24 hr for 1–3 mo. CH (>8 yr of age), AD = PO 100 mg/24 hr for 1–3 mo.
Note: sodium bicarbonate administration may decrease quinacrine-associated nausea and vomiting.
ATABRINE; tabl

Quinidine gluconate, quinidine sulfate, and quinidine polygalacturonatel; alkaloid with general cardiodepressant effects: diminished myocardial excitablity (decrease in threshold potential), reduced conduction velocity (widening of QRS complex, possibility of atrioventricular block), increased refractory period, diminished automaticity, especially in ectopic sites; depresses myocardial contractility with risk of congestive heart failure if myocardial damage present
℞ against atrial tachycardia (usually after digitalization), or ventricular tachyarrhythmia: IN, CH = 2 mg/kg test dose PO, IM (IV) to exclude idiosyncrasy. For treatment: PO (quinidine sulfate): 15–60 mg/kg/24 hr, div, every 5–6 hr. IV, IM (quinidine gluconate): 2–10 mg/kg/dose, prn every 3–6 hr
Caution: Overdose may lead to cardiac arrest.
quinidine gluconate, QUINAGLUTE; tabl, inj quinidine sulfate, †, QUINDEX, ‡; tabl quinidine polygalacturonate. CARDIOQUIN; tabl

Quinine sulfate, antimalarial.
℞ for chloroquine-resistant malaria: CH = PO 25 mg/kg/24 hr div every 8 hr for 3–7 days.
℞ for babesiosis: CH = PO 25 mg/kg/24 hr div every 8 hr for 7 days. Usual maximum dose 650 mg.
℞ for leg cramps: AD = PO 200–300 mg at bedtime.
Note: use cautiously in patients with cardiac disease as quinine possesses some quinidine-like activity.

Quinolone, see Fluroquinolone.

Ranitidine hydrochloride, H_2-receptor antagonist that competitively inhibits secretion of gastric acid
℞ for treatment of duodenal and gastric ulcers, for relief of symptoms caused by gastroesophageal reflux and prophylaxis against stress ulcers in critically ill children; compatible with concomitant treatment with oral antacids (which should be administered at frequent intervals and in adequate doses) or other therapeutic modalities. NB, IN, CH = IV: 1–3 mg/kg/24 hr, div, every 6–12 hr; PO: 2–6 mg/kg/24 hr, div, every 8–12 hr
Ranitidine may be administered as a continuous 24-hr infusion. Ranitidine dosage is often titrated to effect (i.e., measurement of hydrogen ion excretion (pH) of gastric aspirate).
ZANTAC; tabl; inj

Ribavirin, synthetic nucleoside antiviral drug. Ribavirin possesses antiviral inhibitory activity in vitro against respiratory syncytial virus (RSV), influenza virus, and herpes simplex virus. Various protocols exist for the use of this compound; the drug is usually reserved for use in the treatment of severe lower respiratory tract infections due to RSV. Ribavirin is administered by continuous aerosolization for 12–18 hr daily for 3–7 days. Aerosol solution is usually prepared in sterile water, without preservatives, to a final concentration of 20 mg/ml.
VIRAZOLE; aerosol

Rifabutin, antitubercular agent, most often used in the treatment of *Mycobacterium avium* complex (MAC) infection in patients with advanced human immunodeficiency disease. Limited data in pediatrics.
℞ for MAC prophylaxis 5 mg/kg/24 hr div every 8–12 hr.
Note: possible drug interactions with corticosteroids, cyclosporine, dapsone, opioid analgesics, oral contraceptives, quinidine, and warfarin. Should not be administered to patients with active tuberculosis as may promote cross-resistance with rifampin. May cause liver disease.
MYCOBUTIN; caps

Rifampin, synthetic antimicrobial and antimycobacterial agent, interfering with RNA polymerase of infecting organisms
℞ in treatment of tuberculosis, in conjunction with at least 1 other antituberculous agent (isoniazid), and
℞ in carriers of *Neisseria meningitidis* resistant to penicillin and sulfonamide; treatment course of 4 consecutive days (possibility of rapid emergence of resistance): IN, CH = PO: 10–20 mg/kg/24 hr, in single daily dose (1 hr before or 2 hr after meal); maximum daily dose: 600 mg (= adult dose)
Note: Rifampin is a potent inducer of hepatic drug-metabolizing enzymes that may reduce the activity of a number of medications, including anticoagulants, corticosteroids, cyclosporine, cardiac glycoside drugs, oral contraceptives, and opioid analgesics. Rifampin administration may cause the urine, feces, saliva, sputum, sweat, and tears to turn red-orange color. Permanent discoloration of soft contact lenses may occur.
RIFADIN, RIMACTANE; caps, inj

Salicylate sodium
℞ antipyretic, analgesic, anti-inflammatory: CH, adolescents = PO: 25–50 mg/kg/24 hr, div, every 4–6 hr, prn
℞ antirheumatic: CH, adolescents = PO: 50–100 mg/kg/24 hr, div, every 6 hr
Caution: See Chapter 267 (Reye Syndrome)
†, tabl

Salmeterol xinafoate, selective β_2-receptor agonist useful in the treatment of reversible airways disease. Long-acting bronchodilator, approximately 12+ hr; slower onset of effect, approximately 10–20 min. Inhalation dose titrated to effect.
Note: not for use in acute asthma attack.
SEREVENT, inhaler

Sargramostim, granulocyte-macrophage colony-stimulating factor. Stimulates the proliferation, differentiation, and activity of neutrophils, eosinophils, monocytes, and macrophages.
℞ to reduce/reverse marrow suppression: CH = SC, IV (over 2 hr) 3–15 μg/kg/24 hr, once daily for 14–21 days. AD = SC, IV 7.5 μg/kg/24 hr once daily for 14–21 days.
Note: therapy may be accompanied by bone pain and "first-dose" reaction, i.e., fever, hypotension, tachycardia, rigors, dyspnea, flushing, vomiting.
LEUKINE, PROKINE; inj

Scopolamine methylbromide, also methscopolamine bromide, an antimuscarinic agent and quaternary ammonium compound that essentially lacks the central nervous system actions (sedation or excitement, amnesia, euphoria, hallucinations, unexpected behavior) of scopolamine
℞ as adjunctive therapy in the treatment of spasms in the gastrointestinal and urinary tracts: CH = PO: 0.15 mg/kg/24 hr, div, every 6 hr; SC, IM: 0.01 mg/kg/dose, repeat prn every 6–8 hr
Caution: As for Belladonna.
PAMINE; tabl, inj

Secobarbital, central nervous system depressant of the barbiturate class with a short duration of action; tolerance to the hypnotic effect may develop on continued use; initially, hypnotic effect of 3–5 hr
℞ for sedation: IN, CH = PO, IM: 2–5 mg/kg/24 hr, div, every 6–8 hr
℞ for sleep: IN, CH = PO, IM: 3–6 mg/kg/dose, repeat prn after 12–24 hr
†, SECONAL elixir secobarbital sodium, †, SECONAL Sodium; inj, caps, suppos

Senna, contains anthraquinones, sennosides A and B, which stimulate the intramural nerve plexuses of the colon
℞ as laxative: CH (syrup) = PO: 0.15 mL/kg/dose; to be repeated only once per wk, if indicated, to avoid interfering with normal bowel motility and not inducing laxative dependence. Max 5–10 ml/24 hr.
℞ CH (tabl) 10–20 mg/kg/dose daily.
†; syrup, tabl

Simethicone, antiflatulent available as an individual agent and as an ingredient in many antacid preparations. Frequently used for symptomatic relief of the symptoms associated with excessive gas in the digestive tract (i.e., conditions such as colic, lactose intolerance, or air swallowing). Dosage is titrated to clinical effect and patient tolerance.
†, MYLICON, drops, tabl, liquid

Sodium polystyrene sulfonate, ion-exchange resin that removes potassium in exchange for sodium.

■ **TABLE 670–3 Drug Dosages (Drugs Listed Alphabetically by Generic Name)** *(Continued)*

℞ for hyperkalemia: CH = PO 4 g/kg/24 hr div every 6 hr; PR 4–12 g/kg/24 hr div every 2–6 hr. Dose is titrated to desired target serum potassium concentration. AD = PO 15 g administered 1–4 times daily.
Note: may cause nausea, vomiting, contipation. Will interfere with cation-donating antacids, e.g., calcium carbonate, magnesium hydroxide.
KAYEXALATE; powder, susp

Sodium sulfate, $Na_2SO_4 \cdot 10H_2O$, Glauber salt; 1 g of salt traps about 30 mL of water to make the solution isosmotic
℞ as salinic cathartic: CH = PO: 300 mg/kg/dose
†, crystalline substance to be dissolved in a liquid for PO administration

Sodium thiosulfate, cyanide and cisplatin antidote; topical antifungal agent.
℞ nitroprusside (cyanide) antidote: 1 g of sodium thiosulfate for every 100 mg of nitroprusside (may be mixed in same IV infusion container and administered simultaneously).
℞ cisplatin antidote: AD = IV 12 g administered over 6 hr; may be administered before or with cisplatin dosing.

Spironolactone, aldosterone antagonist and potassium-sparing diuretic, which interferes with sodium reabsorption
℞ as diuretic in selected cases (with normal renal function), most effective in combination with a potassium-wasting diuretic: CH = PO: 1.5–3 mg/kg/24 hr, div, every 6–12 hr
Note: Monitoring of serum concentration of potassium, of potassium intake, and of renal function is indicated during treatment with spironolactone.
†; ALDACTONE; tabl

Streptomycin sulfate, antimicrobial aminoglycoside
Caution: Because this drug when administered in large doses and/or for long periods can damage the 8th cranial nerve in adults, children, and transplacentally in fetuses, its indications are stringently selective today.
℞ in tuberculous meningitis and progressive tuberculosis, in association with isoniazid and other antituberculous medication: CH = IM: 20–40 mg/kg/24 hr, div, every 12 hr, for 2–3 mo; max regardless of weight: 1 g/24 hr. See Table 670–2.
†; susp, inj

Succimer, orally administered chelating agent.
℞ for lead poisoning: CH = PO 30 mg/kg/24 hr div every 8 hr for 5 days decreased to 10 mg/kg/24 hr div every 12 hr for 14 days.
Note: therapy may be associated with skin rash, nausea, vomiting, elevations of liver enzymes, unpleasant sufurous odor to urine and/or breath, flu-like symptoms.
CHEMET; caps

Sucralfate, antiulcer agent that forms a complex (pastelike substance) when combined with gastric acid, which adheres to damaged mucosa. Useful in the treatment of gastric ulcer disease and for prophylaxis against stress ulcers in critically ill patients.
℞ CH = PO 40–80 mg/kg/24 hr div every 6 hr. AD = PO 1 g administered 4 times daily.
Note: aluminum ion may accumulate in patients with severe renal disease.
CARAFATE; tabl, susp

Sulfasalazine, 5-aminosalicylic acid derivative with antiinflammatory properties.
℞ for ulcerative colitis: CH = PO moderate to severe ulcerative colitis 40–75 mg/kg/24 hr div every 4–6 hr. Usual max 6 g/24 hr. Maintenance therapy CH = PO 30–50 mg/kg/24 hr div every 4–8 hr.
Note: may cause orange-yellow discoloration of skin, urine; may stain contact lenses. Contraindicated in patients allergic to aspirin or sulfa.
AZULFIDINE; tabl

Sulfonamides, analogs of para-aminobenzoic acid, interfering with the synthesis of tetrahydrofolic acid in sensitive bacteria
Sulfadiazine, sulfisoxazole, and *trisulfapyrimidines:* IN, CH = PO: initial dose 75 mg/kg/1st dose, followed by 120–150 mg/kg/24 hr, div, every 4–6 hr. IV (over 30 min), SC: 100–110 mg/kg/24 hr, div, every 4–6 hr
Sulfadiazine, †; tabl sulfadiazine sodium, †; inj sulfisoxazole, †, GANTRISIN; tabl sulfisoxazole acetyl, GANTRISIN acetyl; oral susp, syrup sulfisoxazole diolamine, GANTRISIN diolamine; inj trisulfapyrimidines (equal parts of sulfadiazine, sulfamerazine, and sulfamethazine), †, ‡; tabl, oral susp
Sulfamethoxazole: IN, CH = PO: initial dose 50–60 mg/kg/1st dose, followed by 50–60 mg/kg/24 hr, div, every 12 hr
GANTANOL; oral susp, tabl
Trimethoprim-sulfamethoxazole (combination): IN (>2 mo old), CH = PO: 6–12 mg trimethoprim (TMP) + 30–60 mg sulfamethoxazole (SMX)/kg/24 hr, div, every 12 hr
℞ in severe urinary tract or *Shigella* infection: CH = PO, IV: 8–10 mg TMP + 40–60 mg SMX/kg/24 hr, div, every 6–8 hr
℞ against *P. carinii:* CH = PO, IV: 15–20 mg TMP + 75–100 mg SMX/kg/24 hr, div, every 6–8 hr
Caution: Do not use in infants less than 2 mo old. Reduce dose in severe renal insufficiency. May cause bone marrow depression.
BACTRIM, SEPTRA; susp: 40 mg TMP + 200 mg SMX/5 mL; tabl: double strength 80 mg TMP + 400 mg SMX/tabl or 160 mg TMP + 800 mg SMX/tabl; ampule: 80 mg TMP + 400 mg SMX/5 mL

Terbutaline sulfate, catecholamine; β-adrenergic receptor agonist with preferential effect on β_2-adrenergic receptors
℞ for bronchodilator: CH (<12 yr of age) = PO 0.15 mg/kg/24 hr div every 8 hr; SC = 0.005–0.01 mg/kg/dose. Usual maximum SC dose 0.4 mg. CH (>12 yr of age), AD = PO 2.5–5 mg/dose administered every 6–8 hr; SC = 0.25 mg/dose. Dose is slowly titrated upward to desired response and patient tolerance.
℞ for status asthmaticus. Limited experience with continuous IV infusion: 10–20 μg/kg load (over 3–5 min) followed by 1–3 μg/kg/min continuous infusion. Dose adjusted as to effect on heart rate, blood pressure, and respiratory rate.
Note: therapy may be associated with tachycardia, hypotension, tremors, nausea, tinnitus.
BRETHINE, BRICANYL; tabl, inj, aerosol

Terfenadine, antihistamine used for the symptomatic treatment of perennial and seasonal allergic rhinitis and other allergic symptoms. Competitive antagonist of the classic histamine H_1 receptor, associated with less sedation than earlier antihistamines (e.g., diphenhydramine) due to preferential antagonism of peripheral rather than peripheral and central H_1 receptors.
CH (3–6 yr of age) = PO 30 mg/24 hr div every 12 hr; CH (6–12 yr of age) = PO 60 mg/24 hr div every 12 hr. CH (>12 yr of age), AD = PO 120 mg/24 hr div every 12 hr.
Caution: careful use in patients with cardiac disease; drug interactions with erythromycin, ketoconazole, itraconazole. Therapy has been associated with severe, life-threatening cardiac dysrhythmias.
SELDANE; tabl

Tetracyclines, a group of derivatives of polycyclic naphthacenecarboxamide
Chlortetracycline hydrochloride: CH = PO: 25–50 mg/kg/24 hr, div, every 6 hr
AUREOMYCIN; caps, inj (IV)
Demeclocycline and *demeclocycline hydrochloride:* CH = PO: 7–13 mg/kg/24 hr, div, every 6–12 hr
DECLOMYCIN; pediatric drops, syrup; DECLOMYCIN hydrochloride; caps, tabl
Doxycycline monohydrate and *doxycycline hyclate:* CH = PO: 5 mg/kg/24 hr, div, every 12 hr
†, VIBRAMYCIN monohydrate; oral susp; †, VIBRAMYCIN hyclate; caps, inj (IV)
Methacycline hydrochloride: CH = PO: 7–13 mg/kg/24 hr, div, every 6–12 hr
RONDOMYCIN; caps, syrup
Minocycline hydrochloride: CH = PO, IV: initial dose 4 mg/kg, followed by 4 mg/kg/24 hr, div, every 12 hr
MINOCIN, VECTRIN; caps, syrup, inj (IV)
Oxytetracycline, oxytetracycline hydrochloride, oxytetracycline calcium: same dosage as tetracycline hydrochloride, below
TERRAMYCIN: tabl, inj (IM); TERRAMYCIN hydrochloride: †, caps, inj (IV, IM); TERRAMYCIN calcium: pediatric drops, syrup
Tetracycline hydrochloride: CH = PO: 25–50 mg/kg/24 hr, div, every 8 hr; IM (often very painful): 15–25 mg/kg/24 hr, div, every 8–12 hr; IV: 10–20 mg/kg/24 hr, div, every 12 hr
†, ACHROMYCIN V, PANMYCIN, ‡; caps, inj (IV, IM); sol for IM inj contains local anesthetic. Pediatric drops, oral susp, and syrup prepared with tetracycline base
Note: Tetracyclines have limited indications in infancy and childhood because of their accumulation in bone and teeth and their potential to interfere with growth. Their use should be avoided insofar as possible until formation of dental enamel is complete in most permanent teeth (at about 8 yr), to avoid unsightly discolored, pitted teeth. Tetracyclines may cause increased intracranial pressure in infants (pseudotumor cerebri).

Theophylline, methylxanthine; commonly used in acute and chronic management of reversible airways disease (asthma), neonatal apnea, bronchopulmonary dysplasia, among others. Cellular mechanism of action originally believed to be a result of phosphodiesterase inhibition; however, pharmacologic effect is most likely a result of adenosine receptor antagonism.
℞ in neonatal apnea: IV, PO: initial loading dose 5 mg/kg followed by maintenance therapy depending upon age; preterm NB (<36 wk): 1–2 mg/kg/24 hr, div, every 8–12 hr; term infants (>36 wk): 2–4 mg/kg/24 hr, div, every 8–12 hr
℞ in status asthmaticus: initial loading dose IV: 4–7 mg/kg/dose, infused over 20–30 min, followed by maintenance IV: 20 mg/kg/24 hr, div, every 4–6 hr, or by continuous IV drip; switch to PO maintenance as soon as possible. Daily theophylline dose adjustment necessary relative to patient age and hepatic and cardiac function.
℞ oral maintenance: PO: 20–25 mg/kg/24 hr, div, every 6 hr; as conditions permit, taper to lowest effective dosage, usually around 15–20 mg/kg/24 hr, div, every 6 hr. Time-release theophylline preparations permit extension of the dosage interval (i.e., administration every 8–12 hr).
Note: theophylline content in the following formulations: theophylline (anhydrous), 100%; aminophylline, 85%; theophylline monoethan-

Table continued on following page

■ **TABLE 670–3 Drug Dosages (Drugs Listed Alphabetically by Generic Name)** *(Continued)*

olamine, 75%; dihydroxypropyltheophylline, 70%; oxtriphylline, choline salt, 64%; theophylline sodium glycinate, 50%; theophylline calcium salicylate, 48%. Serum concentration should be monitored; therapeutic range for neonatal apnea, 7–13 mg/L; in the management of bronchospasm, 10–20 mg/L

Caution: Circulatory collapse, seizures, coma may result from acute or chronic overdose.

†, ELIXOPHYLLIN elixir, ELIXICON oral susp, SLOPHYLLIN caps, oral susp, SOMOPHYLLIN caps, ‡: component of many combination products aminophylline, †, SOMOPHYLLIN oral liquid, ‡; inj, oral preparations

Ticarcillin disodium, semi-synthetic penicillin susceptible to penicillinase; each gram of drug contains 5.2 mEq of sodium.

NB = IV (over 20–30 min), IM: <7 days: <2,000 g, 150 mg/kg/24 hr, div, every 12 hr; >2,000 g, 225 mg/kg/24 hr, div, every 8 hr; >7 days: <2,000 g, 225 mg/kg/24 hr, div, every 8 hr; >2,000 g, 300 mg/kg/24 hr, div, every 8 hr

IN, CH = IV (over 20–30 min), IM: 200–300 mg/kg/24 hr, div, every 4–6 hr. IM injection is painful.

TICAR; IV and IM inj

Ticarcillin + clavulanic acid, combination of a β-lactam antibiotic (ticarcillin) with a β-lactamase (penicillinase) inhibitor (clavulanic acid). The addition of clavulanic acid extends the activity of ticarcillin to include β-lactamase–producing strains of *H. influenzae* and other drug-resistant pathogens. Doses administered as either IM or IV are the same as those for ticarcillin disodium noted above.

Tobramycin sulfate, antimicrobial aminoglycoside

NB = IV (30–60 min), IM: <7 days: <34 wk <1,500 g, 3 mg/kg every 24 hr; <34 wk >1,500 g, 2.5 mg/kg every 18 hr; >34 wk >1,500 g, 2.5 mg/kg every 12 hr; >7 days and term NB, 5 mg/kg/24 hr, div, every 12 hr

IN, CH = IV (30–60 min), IM: 5–7.5 mg/kg/24 hr, div, every 6–8 hr. Serum concentration should be monitored; therapeutic peak concentration 5–10 mg/L, trough <2 mg/L (see Table 670–2). Dosage and interval may require modification for the treatment of patients with cystic fibrosis.

Caution: Ototoxic; nephrotoxic.

†, NEBCIN; inj

Tolmentin sodium, nonsteroidal anti-inflammatory agent of the indole class that possesses analgesic and antipyretic activities. The drug's mechanism of action remains to be described but may involve prostaglandin synthetase inhibition. The drug is most often used in the treatment of juvenile rheumatoid arthritis.

℞ for juvenile rheumatoid arthritis: CH = PO: 15–30 mg/kg/24 hr

TOLMECTIN; tabl

Triamterene, potassium-sparing diuretic; inhibits the reabsorption of Na^+ in exchange for K^+ and H^+; its effect is potentiated by concomitant use of diuretics that act more proximally

CH = PO: 2–4 mg/kg/24 hr, div, every 12 hr (after meals).

Note: For maintenance, dosage must be adjusted to needs of individual patient; in conjunction with other diuretics dosage usually can be decreased.

Caution: Because of the risk of hyperkalemia, serum potassium concentrations and potassium intake should be monitored.

DYRENIUM; caps

Trimethadione, oxazolidinedione; anticonvulsant agent

℞ as an adjunct in the treatment of convulsive disorders: CH = PO: 20 mg/kg/24 hr, div, every 8 hr; if needed, dosage can be progressively adjusted to 40 mg/kg/24 hr, div, every 8 hr

Note: The methylated metabolite of trimethadione accumulates progressively in the body and is partially responsible for anticonvulsant effect.

TRIDIONE; tabl, caps, oral susp

Trimethoprim, see Sulfonamides

Tripelennamine hydrochloride, an ethylenediamine with antihistaminic, mild cholinergic, and slight sedative effects

℞ antiallergic effect: CH = PO: 5 mg/kg/24 hr, div, every 6 hr

†, PBZ hydrochloride, tabl; tripelennamine citrate, PBZ citrate, elixir

Valproic acid, valproate, carboxylic acid; (dipropylacetic acid); antiepileptic agent chemically unrelated to other antiseizure medications. Mechanism of anticonvulsant activity remains unknown but may be associated with increasing brain concentrations of γ-aminobutyric acid. Valproate may be used as monotherapy or in combination with other anticonvulsants in the treatment of a wide range of seizure disorders.

℞ for treatment of seizures: CH = PO: 15 mg/kg/24 hr, div, every 8–12 hr; if needed, dosage may be increased, generally on a weekly basis, in increments of 5–10 mg/kg/24 hr up to a max recommended 30–60 mg/kg/24 hr, div, every 8–12 hr

Caution: Valproate is highly protein bound (>90%) and may be associated with drug-protein displacement interactions. Valproate may retard hepatic drug-metabolizing enzymes, slowing the metabolism of and thus leading to increases in serum concentrations of other drugs, most notably other anticonvulsant agents. Fatal hepatic dysfunction has been reported in patients receiving valproate. Patients at primary risk for this fatal drug-induced toxicity appear to be children ≤2 yr of age who are receiving valproate concurrently with other anticonvulsant agents. Thus, valproate should be used with extreme caution in children under the age of 2 yr. Serum concentrations may be monitored, therapeutic range 50–100 mg/L

†, DEPAKENE; caps, syrup; divalproex, DEPAKOTE; enteric-coated tabs

Vancomycin, complex glycopeptide that inhibits synthesis of cell wall in gram-positive bacteria and is effective against methicillin-resistant staphylococci; in oral application effective in pseudomembranous colitis caused by toxin-producing bacteria such as *C. difficile* and *S. aureus;* excreted mainly by kidneys

NB = IV (slow over 1+ hr) <7 days, <1,200 g, 15 mg/kg/24 hr administered once daily; <7 days, >1,200 g, 30 mg/kg/24 hr div every 12 hr; >7 days, <1,200 g, 15 mg/kg/24 hr administered once daily; >7 days, >1,200 g, 30–45 mg/kg/24 hr div every 8–12 hr. IN, CH (<12 yr of age) 45–60 mg/kg/24 hr div every 6–8 hr. AD = IV 0.5 g every 6 hr to 1 g every 12 hr.

℞ for *C. difficile*–associated pseudomembranous colitis in CH = PO 40–50 mg/kg/24 hr div, every 6–8 hr.

Caution: combined administration with an aminoglycoside enhances nephrotoxic potential of both drugs.

Note: Reduced dosage in renal insufficiency. Therapy may be associated with ototoxicity and renal impairment, skin rashes ("red man" syndrome), and hematologic side effects. Serum concentration should be monitored, therapeutic peak concentration 30–40 mg/L, trough 5–10 mg/L (see Table 670–2).

†, VANCOCIN; inj

Vasopressin, ADH, antidiuretic hormone.

℞ for diabetes insipidus: CH = SC, IM 2.5–10 units administered 2–4 times daily. AD = SC, IM 5–10 units 2–4 times daily. Dose is highly variable and titrated to desired serum and urine sodium and osmolality.

℞ for bleeding esophageal varices: Cl = continuous IV infusion 0.01 unit/kg/min titrated to response.

Verapamil, calcium channel blocker. Toxic effects include allergic reactions, urticaria, bronchospasm, hypotension, decreased cardiac output, and asystole. Cardiac monitoring should be used during administration.

IN = IV: 0.1–0.2 mg/kg infused over 2 min

CH = IV: 0.1–0.3 mg/kg infused over 2 min

Maintenance dose = 1–2 mg/kg every 8 hr

CALAN, ISOPTIN; IV 2.5 mg/kg-vial inj; PO tabs: 80, 120 mg

Vidarabine, antiviral agent used for treatment of neonatal herpes simplex infections.

℞ for herpes simplex NB-IV (over 12–24 hr) 15–30 mg/kg/24 hr once daily

℞ for herpes simplex encephalitis: CH, AD = IV (over 12 hr) 15 mg/kg/24 hr once daily.

℞ for herpes zoster, varicella-zoster infection: CH, AD = IV (over 12 hr) 10 mg/kg/24 hr once daily.

Note: May rarely cause hepatic and hematologic toxicity. Reduce dose with renal dysfunction (creatinine clearance <10 mL/min).

VIRA-A; 200 mg/mL-vial inj

Zidovudine, AZT, thymidine analog antiviral agent that interferes with the human immunodeficiency virus (HIV) RNA-dependent DNA polymerases, interfering with viral replication.

CH (3 mo–12 yr) = PO 12–22 mg/kg/24 hr div every 6 hr; usual maximum single dose 200 mg; IV (over 1 hr) 12 mg/kg/24 hr div every 6 hr or by continuous IV infusion CH 0.5–1.8 mg/kg/hr. (>12 yr of age) AD = PO 500 mg/24 hr (asymptomatic infection) to 1,200 mg/24 hr for symptomatic HIV infection. IV 6–12 mg/kg/24 hr div, every 4 hr.

Note: potential drug interactions; acyclovir, ganciclovir, cimetidine, indomethacin. Monitor blood counts closely. Adjust dose in the presence of renal dysfunction.

RETROVIR, caps, inj

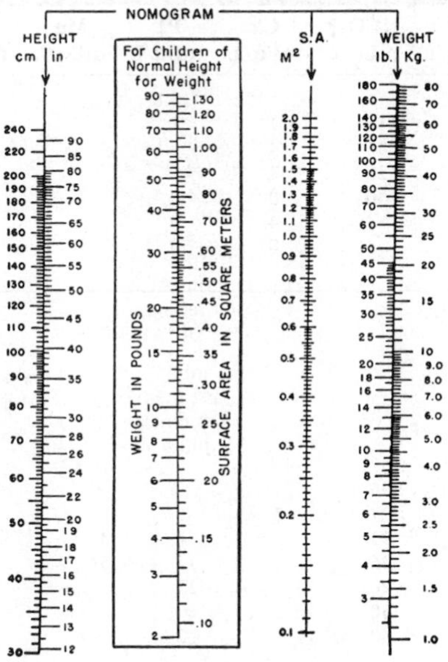

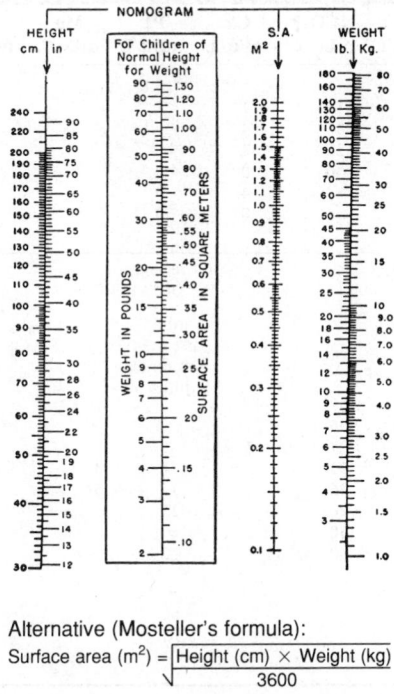

Alternative (Mosteller's formula):

$$\text{Surface area (m}^2\text{)} = \sqrt{\frac{\text{Height (cm)} \times \text{Weight (kg)}}{3600}}$$

Figure 670–1. Nomogram for estimation of surface area. The surface area is indicated where a straight line that connects the height and weight levels intersects the surface area column; or if the patient is roughly of average size, from the weight alone *(enclosed area)*. (Nomogram modified from data of E. Boyd by C.D. West.) (See also Briars G, Bailey B: Surface area estimation: pocket calculator v nomogram. Arch Dis Child 70:246, 1994.)

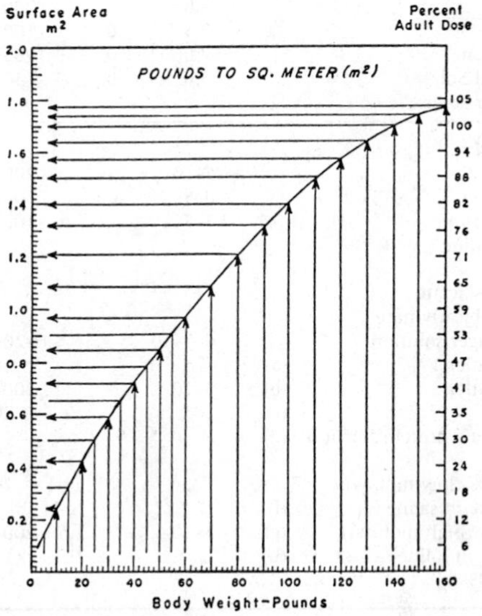

Figure 670–2. Relations between body weight in pounds, body surface area, and adult dosage. The surface area values correspond with those set forth by Crawford and associates (1950). Note that the 100% adult dose is for a patient weighing about 140 lb and having a surface area of about 1.7 m². (From Talbot NB, et al: Metabolic Homeostasis—A Syllabus for Those Concerned with the Care of Patients. Cambridge, Harvard University Press, 1959.)

■ **TABLE 670–4 Conversion of Apothecary's Measures to Metric Equivalents**

1 grain = 64 mg
60 minims = 1 fl dram = 3.7 mL
1 mL = 16.22 minims

■ **TABLE 670–5 Composition of Commonly Used Oral and Parenteral Solutions (Raymond Adelman and Michael Solhaug) (see related conversion Tables 670–6 to 670–8)**

Fluid	CHO g/dL	Prot*	Calories per L	Na mEq/L	K mEq/L	Cl mEq/L	HCO_3† mEq/L	Ca mEq/L	P‡ mEq/L	Mg mEq/L	Osm§ mOsm/kgH_2O
Oral											
Apple juice¶	11.9	0.1	480	0.4	26			3	4.5		700
Coca-Cola¶	10.9		435	4.3	0.1		13.4				656
Ginger ale¶	9.0		360	3.5	0.1		3.6				565
Grape juice¶	16.6	0.2	672	0.4	30		32				1027
Grapefruit juice¶ (canned, sugar added)	17.8	0.6	736	0.2	35			6.5			591
Milk	4.9	3.5	670	22	36	28	30	60	54		260**
Orange juice¶	10.4	0.7	444	0.2	49		50				654
Pepsi-Cola	12.0		480	6.5	0.8		7.3				—
Pineapple juice (canned)¶	13.5	0.4	556	0.2	38			7.5	9		783
Prune juice¶	19	0.4	776	0.9	60			7	20		—
Root beer¶				3.5	3.9						588
Seven-Up¶	8.0		320	7.5	0.2			0.3			564
Tomato juice (canned, salted)¶	4.3		172	100	59	150	10	3	18		592

Table continued on following page

■ **TABLE 670–5 Composition of Commonly Used Oral and Parenteral Solutions (Raymond Adelman and Michael Solhaug)** *Continued*
(see related conversion Tables 670-6 to 670-8)

Fluid		CHO g/dL	Prot*	Calories per L	Na mEq/L	K mEq/L	Cl mEq/L	HCO_3† mEq/L	Ca mEq/L	P‡ mEq/L	Mg mEq/L	Osm§ mOsm/kgH_2O
Gatorade		5.9		250	21	2.5	17			6.8		377
Hydra-lyte		2.5		100	84	10	59	15	<1	<1		300
Lytren		7.0		280	30	25	25	36	4	5	4	267 **
Pedialyte		5.0		200	30	20	30	28	4		4	387
Rehydrate		2.5	0	100	75	25	65	30	0	0	0	305
Resol Solution		2.0	0	83	50	20	50	34	4	5	4	269
Ricelyte Oral Sol. (rice syrup solids)		3.0	0	140	50	25	45	34	0	0	0	200
Parenteral												
CHO†† in H_2O		5–10		200–400								266–532
Isotonic saline		0–5		0–200	154		154					292–558
½ isotonic saline		2.5–5		100–200	77		77					280–415
3% (M/2) saline					513		513					969
5% saline					855		855					1616
M/6 sodium lactate					167			167				
5% sodium bicarbonate					595			595				
Lactated Ringer solution		0–5–10		0–200–400	130	4	109	28	3			261–531–801
Modified Butler 1	(a)	5		200	25	20	22	23		3	3	360
Modified Butler 2	(b)	5–10		200–400	56	25	49	26		12	5	423–719**
Talbot	(c)	5		200	40	35	40	20		15		409
Human plasma protein fraction	(d)		5		130	2	50	50				
Blood‡‡			3		95	4	50	40		2	1–2	
Dextran 10% (low mol. wt.)	(e)	5		200								
Dextran 10% in saline	(f)				154		154					
Dextran 6% (high mol. wt)	(g)	5–10		200–400								
Dextran 6% in saline	(h)				154		154					
Mannitol 20%§§												

Available Additives

Glucose 50%	0.5 g/mL
Sodium chloride	2.5 and 5 mEq/mL
Sodium acetate	2 and 4 mEq/mL
Sodium lactate	5 mEq/mL
Sodium bicarbonate	0.5 (4.2%) mEq/mL and 0.9 (7.5%) mEq/mL, 1 mEq/mL (8.4%)
Potassium acetate	2 and 4 mEq/mL
Potassium chloride	2 and 3 mEq/mL
Potassium phosphate	4.4 mEq/mL of potassium and 3 mM/ml phosphate
Calcium gluconate 10%	9.3 mg (0.465 mEq/mL) elemental calcium
Calcium chloride 10%	27.3 mg (1.4 mEq/mL) elemental calcium
Ammonium chloride	5 mEq/mL
Magnesium sulfate	0.8 mEq/mL, 1 mEq/mL, and 4 mEq/mL available as the 10%, 12.5%, and 50% solutions

Selected Commercial Preparations in the United States
(possible slight variations in composition from values in Table)

(A, Abbott; B, Baxter; C, Cutter; M, McGaw; P, Pharmacia)

(a)	Ionosol MB in D5W (A); Isolyte P with 5% Dextrose (M)
(b)	Ionosol B in D5W (A); Electrolyte #2 with 10% Invert Sugar (C,M); 10% Travert in Electrolyte #2 (B)
(c)	Ionosol T in D5W (A); Isolyte M (M)
(d)	Plasmatein (A); Plasmanate (C)
(e)(f)	LMD 10% (A); Dextran 40 (C,M); Rheomacrodex (P); Gentran 40 (B)
(g)(h)	Dextran 70 (A); Macrodex (P); Gentran 75 in 10% Travert (B)

**Protein or amino acid equivalent.*
†Actual or potential bicarbonate, such as acetate, lactate, citrate.
‡Calculated according to valence of 1.8.
*§Osmolality except for values shown,** which are osmolarity (in mOsm/L).*
¶Composition varies slightly depending on source.
***See § above.*
††Glucose (dextrose, fructose or invert sugar).
‡‡Red cell contents not included in calculations.
§§Also available: mannitol 5%, 10%, 15%, and 20%.
(Sources: Bowes Church Food Values of Portions Commonly Used, Pennington, Jean A.T. editor, 16th ed. JB Lippincott, Philadelphia 1994; Facts and Comparisons, Olin BR, editor, JB Lippincott, St. Louis, 1993; Murray BN, Peterson LJ: Unpublished observations. Additional Values in Wendland BE, Arbus GS: Can Med Assoc J 121:564, 1979.)

■ TABLE 670–6 Method for Conversion of Milligrams to Milliequivalents per Liter (or to Millimoles per Liter)

Mg = milligrams   mL = milliliter
g = grams   1 mL = 1.000027 cc
dL = deciliter = 100 mL

$$\text{mEq/L (milliequivalents per liter)} = \frac{\text{mg/L}}{\text{equivalent weight}}$$

$$\text{Equivalent weight} = \frac{\text{atomic weight}}{\text{valence of element}}$$

For example: A sample of blood serum contains 10 mg of Ca in 1 dL (100 mL).

The valence of Ca is 2, and the atomic weight is 40. The equivalent weight of Ca is therefore 40 ÷ 2, or 20. The milliequivalents of Ca per liter are 10 (mg/dL) × 10 (dL/L) ÷ 20, or 5 milliequivalents per liter.

$$\text{mM/L (millimoles per liter)} = \frac{\text{mg/L}}{\text{molecular weight}}$$

Vol. % (volumes per cent) = mM/L × 2.24 for a gas whose properties approach that of an ideal gas, such as oxygen or nitrogen. For carbon dioxide, the factor is 2.226.

■ TABLE 670–7 Factors for Conversion of Concentration Expressed in Milliequivalents per Liter to Milligrams per Deciliter (100 mL), and Vice Versa, for Common Ions That Occur in Physiologic Solutions

Element or Radical	mEq/L to mg/dL		mg/dL to mEq/L	
Sodium	1	2.30	1	0.4348
Potassium	1	3.91	1	0.2558
Calcium	1	2.005	1	0.4988
Magnesium	1	1.215	1	0.8230
Chloride	1	3.55	1	0.2817
Bicarbonate (HCO_3)	1	6.1	1	0.1639
Phosphorus valence 1	1	3.10	1	0.3226
Phosphorus valence 1.8	1	1.72	1	0.5814
Sulfur valence 2	1	1.60	1	0.625

Example: to convert milliequivalents of magnesium per liter to milligrams per deciliter (100 mL), multiply by the factor 1.215.

To convert milligrams of potassium per deciliter (100 mL) to milliequivalents per liter, multiply by the factor 0.2558.

■ TABLE 670–8 Milliequivalents and Milligrams of Cations and Anions Present in a Millimole of Salts Commonly Used in Physiologic Solutions

Salt	mg/mmole salt	Cation	mEq/mmole salt	mg/mmole salt	Anion	mEq/mmole salt	mg/mmole salt
Sodium chloride (NaCl)	58.5	Na^+	1	23.0	Cl^-	1	35.5
Potassium chloride (KCl)	74.6	K^+	1	39.1	Cl^-	1	35.5
Sodium bicarbonate ($NaHCO_3$)	84.0	Na^+	1	23.0	HCO_3^-	1	61.0
Sodium lactate ($CH_3CHOHCOONa$)	112.0	Na^+	1	23.0	Lactate$^-$	1	89.0
Potassium phosphate (K_2HPO_4) dibasic	174.2	K^+	2	78.2	HPO_4^{2-}	2	96.0
Potassium phosphate (KH_2PO_4) monobasic	136.1	K^+	1	39.1	$H_2PO_4^-$	1	97.0
Calcium chloride, anhydrous ($CaCl_2$)	111.0	Ca^{2+}	2	40.0	Cl_2^{2-}	2	71.0
Calcium chloride dihydrate ($CaCl_2 \cdot 2H_2O$)	147.0	Ca^{2+}	2	40.0	Cl_2^{2-}	2	71.0
Magnesium chloride, anhydrous ($MgCl_2$)	95.2	Mg^{2+}	2	24.3	Cl_2^{2-}	2	71.0
Magnesium chloride hexahydrate ($MgCl_2 \cdot 6H_2O$)	203.3	Mg^{2+}	2	24.3	Cl_2^{2-}	2	71.0
Ammonium chloride (NH_4Cl)	53.5	NH_4^+	1	18.0	Cl^-	1	35.5

■ TABLE 670–9 Food Composition for Short Method of Dietary Analysis (Lewis A. Barness and John S. Curran)*

Food and Approximate Measure	Weight *g*	Food Energy *kcal*	Protein *g*	Fat *g*	Carbohydrate *g*	Calcium *mg*	Iron *mg*	Vitamin A *IU*	Thiamine *mg*	Riboflavin *mg*	Niacin *mg*	Ascorbic Acid *mg*
Milk, Cheese, Cream; Related Products												
Cheese: blue, cheddar (1 cu in, 17 g), cheddar process (1 oz), Swiss (1 oz)	30	105	6	9	1	165	0.2	345	0.01	0.12	Trace	0
cottage (from skim) creamed (½ c)	115	120	16	5	3	105	0.4	190	0.04	0.28	0.1	0
Cream: half-and-half (cream and milk) (2 tbsp)	30	40	1	4	2	30	Trace	145	0.01	0.04	Trace	Trace
For light whipping add 1 pat butter												
Milk: whole (3.5% fat) (1 c)	245	160	9	9	12	285	0.1	350	0.08	0.42	0.1	2
fluid, nonfat (skim) and buttermilk (from skim)	245	90	9	Trace	13	300	Trace	—	0.10	0.44	0.2	2
milk beverage (1 c): cocoa, chocolate drink made with skim milk. For malted milk add 4 tbsp half-and-half (270 g)	245	210	8	8	26	280	0.6	300	0.09	0.43	0.3	Trace
milk desserts, custard (1 c) 248 g, ice cream (8 fl oz) 142 g		290	8	17	29	210	0.4	785	0.07	0.34	0.1	1
cornstarch pudding (248 g), ice milk (1 c) 187 g		280	9	10	40	290	0.1	390	0.08	0.41	0.3	2
White sauce, med (½ c)	130	215	5	16	12	150	0.2	610	0.06	0.22	0.3	Trace
Egg: 1 Large	50	80	6	6	Trace	25	1.2	590	0.06	0.15	Trace	0
Meat, Poultry, Fish, Shellfish, Related Products												
Beef, lamb, veal: lean and fat, cooked, inc. corned beef (3 oz) (all cuts)	85	245	22	16	0	10	2.9	25	0.06	0.19	4.2	0
lean only, cooked; dried beef (2+ oz) (all cuts)	65	140	20	5	0	10	2.4	10	0.05	0.16	3.4	0
Beef, relatively fat, such as steak and rib, cooked (3 oz)	85	350	18	30	0	10	2.4	60	0.05	0.14	3.5	0
Liver: beef, fried (2 oz)	55	130	15	6	3	5	5.0	30,280	0.15	2.37	9.4	15
Pork, lean and fat, cooked (3 oz) (all cuts)	85	325	20	24	0	10	2.6	0	0.62	0.20	4.2	0
lean only, cooked (2+ oz) (all cuts)	60	150	18	8	0	5	2.2	0	0.57	0.19	3.2	0
ham, light cure, lean and fat, roasted (3 oz)	85	245	18	19	0	10	2.2	0	0.40	0.16	3.1	0

Table continued on following page

■ TABLE 670–9 Food Composition for Short Method of Dietary Analysis (Lewis A. Barness and John S. Curran)* *(Continued)*

Food and Approximate Measure	Weight *g*	Food Energy *kcal*	Protein *g*	Fat *g*	Carbohydrate *g*	Calcium *mg*	Iron *mg*	Vitamin A *IU*	Thiamine *mg*	Riboflavin *mg*	Niacin *mg*	Ascorbic Acid *mg*
Luncheon meats: bologna (2 sl), pork sausage, cooked (2 oz), frankfurter (1), bacon, broiled or fried crisp (3 sl)		185	9	16	—	5	1.3	—	0.21	0.12	1.7	0
Poultry												
chicken: flesh only, broiled (3 oz)	85	115	20	3	0	10	1.4	80	0.05	0.16	7.4	0
fried (2+ oz)	75	170	24	6	1	10	1.6	85	0.05	0.23	8.3	0
turkey, light and dark, roasted (3 oz)	85	160	27	5	0	—	1.5	—	0.03	0.15	6.5	0
Fish and shellfish												
salmon (3 oz) (canned)	85	130	17	5	0	165	0.7	60	0.03	0.16	6.8	0
fish sticks, breaded, cooked (3–4)	75	130	13	7	5	10	0.3	—	0.03	0.05	1.2	0
mackerel, halibut, cooked	85	175	19	10	0	10	0.8	515	0.08	0.15	6.8	0
bluefish, haddock, herring, perch, shad, cooked (tuna canned in oil, 20 g)	85	160	19	8	2	20	1.0	60	0.06	0.11	4.4	0
clams, canned; crab meat, canned; lobster; oyster, raw; scallop; shrimp, canned	85	75	14	1	2	65	2.5	65	0.10	0.08	1.5	0
Mature Dry Beans and Peas, Nuts, Peanuts, Related Products												
Beans: white with pork and tomato, canned (1 c)	260	320	16	7	50	140	4.7	340	0.20	0.08	1.5	5
red (128 g), lima (96 g), cowpeas (125 g), cooked (½ c)		125	8	—	25	35	2.5	5	0.13	0.06	0.7	—
Nuts: almonds (12), cashews (8), peanuts (1 tbsp), peanut butter (1 tbsp), pecans (12), English walnuts (2 tbsp), coconut (¼ c)	15	95	3	8	4	15	0.5	5	0.05	0.04	0.9	—
Vegetables and Vegetable Products												
Asparagus, cooked, cut spears (⅔ c)	115	25	3	Trace	4	25	0.7	1,055	0.19	0.20	1.6	30
Beans: green (½ c) cooked 60 g; canned 120 g		15	1	Trace	3	30	0.4	340	0.04	0.06	0.3	8
Lima, immature, cooked (½ c)	80	90	6	1	16	40	2.0	225	0.14	0.08	1.0	14
Broccoli spears, cooked (⅔ c)	100	25	3	Trace	4	90	0.8	2,500	0.09	0.20	0.8	90
Brussels sprouts, cooked (⅔ c)	85	30	3	Trace	5	30	1.0	450	0.07	0.12	0.7	75
Cabbage (110 g); cauliflower, cooked (80 g); and sauerkraut, canned (150 mg) (reduce ascorbic acid value by one third for kraut) (⅔ c)		20	1	Trace	4	35	0.5	80	0.05	0.05	0.3	37
Carrots, cooked (⅔ c)	95	30	1	Trace	7	30	0.6	10,145	0.05	0.05	0.5	6
Corn, 1 ear, cooked (140 g); canned (130 g) (½ c)		75	2	Trace	18	5	0.4	315	0.06	0.06	1.1	6
Leafy greens: collards (125 g), dandelions (120 g), kale (75 g), mustard (95 g), spinach (120 g), turnip (100 g cooked, 150 g canned) (⅔ c cooked and canned) (reduce ascorbic acid one half for canned)		30	3	Trace	5	175	1.8	8,570	0.11	0.18	0.8	45
Peas, green (½ c)	80	60	4	1	10	20	1.4	430	0.22	0.09	1.8	16
Potatoes, baked, boiled (100 g), 10 pc. French fried (55 g) (for fried, add 1 tbsp cooking oil)		85	3	Trace	30	10	0.7	Trace	0.08	0.04	1.5	16
Pumpkin, canned (½ c)	115	40	1	1	9	30	0.5	7,295	0.03	0.06	0.6	6
Squash, winter, canned (½ c)	100	65	2	1	16	30	0.8	4,305	0.05	0.14	0.7	14
Sweet potato, canned (½ c)	110	120	2	—	27	25	0.8	8,500	0.05	0.05	0.7	15
Tomato, 1 raw, ⅔ c canned, ⅔ c juice	150	35	2	Trace	7	14	0.8	1,350	0.10	0.06	1.0	29
Tomato catsup (2 tbsp)	35	30	1	Trace	8	10	0.2	480	0.04	0.02	0.6	6
Other, cooked (beets, mushrooms, onions, turnips) (½ c)	95	25	1	—	5	20	0.5	15	0.02	0.10	0.7	7
Other, commonly served raw, cabbage (½ c, 50 g), celery (3 sm stalks, 40 g), cucumber (¼ med, 50 g), green pepper (½, 30 g), radishes (5, 40 g)		10	Trace	Trace	2	15	0.3	100	0.03	0.03	0.2	20
carrots, raw (½ carrot)	25	10	Trace	Trace	2	10	0.2	2,750	0.02	0.02	0.2	2
lettuce leaves (2 lg)	50	10	1	Trace	2	34	0.7	950	0.03	0.04	0.2	9
Fruits and Fruit Products												
Cantaloupe (½ med)	385	60	1	Trace	14	25	0.8	6,540	0.08	0.06	1.2	63
Citrus and strawberries: orange (1), grapefruit (½), juice (½ c), strawberries (½ c), lemon (1), tangerine (1)		50	1	—	13	25	0.4	165	0.08	0.03	0.3	55
Yellow, fresh: apricots (3), peach (2 med); canned fruit and juice (½ c) or dried, cooked, unsweetened: apricot, peaches (½ c)		85	—	—	22	10	1.1	1,005	0.01	0.05	1.0	5
Other, dried: dates, pitted (4), figs (2), raisins (¼ c)	40	120	1	—	31	35	1.4	20	0.04	0.04	0.5	—
Other, fresh apple (1), banana (1), figs (3), pear (1)		80	—	—	21	15	0.5	140	0.04	0.03	0.2	6

■ **TABLE 670–9 Food Composition for Short Method of Dietary Analysis (Lewis A. Barness and John S. Curran)*** *(Continued)*

Food and Approximate Measure	Weight *g*	Food Energy *kcal*	Protein *g*	Fat *g*	Carbo-hydrate *g*	Calcium *mg*	Iron *mg*	Vitamin A *IU*	Thiamine *mg*	Ribo-flavin *mg*	Niacin *mg*	Ascorbic Acid *mg*
Grain Products												
Enriched and whole grain: bread (1 sl, 23 g), biscuit (½), cooked cereals (½ c), prepared cereals (1 oz), Graham crackers (2 lg), macaroni, noodles, spaghetti (½ c, cooked), pancake (1, 27 g), roll (½), waffle (½, 38 g)		65	2	1	16	20	0.6	10	0.09	0.05	0.7	—
Unenriched bread (1 sl, 23 g), cooked cereal (½ c), macaroni, noodles, spaghetti (½ c), popcorn (½ c), pretzel sticks, small (15), roll (½)		65	2	1	16	10	0.3	5	0.02	0.02	0.3	—
Desserts												
Cake, plain (1 pc), doughnut (1). For iced cake or doughnut add value for sugar (1 tbsp). For chocolate cake add chocolate (30 g)	45	145	2	5	24	30	0.4	65	0.02	0.05	0.2	—
Cookies, plain (1)	25	120	1	5	18	10	0.2	20	0.01	0.01	0.1	—
Pie crust, single crust (1/7 shell)	20	95	1	6	8	3	0.3	0	0.04	0.03	0.3	—
Flour, white, enriched (1 tbsp)	7	25	1	Trace	5	1	0.2	0	0.03	0.02	0.2	0
Fats and Oils												
Butter, margarine (1 pat, ½ tbsp)	7	50	Trace	6	Trace	1	0	230	—	—	—	—
Fats and oils, cooking (1 tbsp), French dressing (2 tbsp)	14	125	0	14	0	0	0	0	0	0	0	0
Salad dressings, mayonnaise type (1 tbsp)	15	80	Trace	9	1	2	0.1	45	Trace	Trace	Trace	0
Sugars, Sweets												
Candy, plain (½ oz), jam and jelly (1 tbsp), syrup (1 tbsp), gelatin dessert, plain (½ c), beverages, carbonated (1 c)		60	0	0	14	3	0.1	Trace	Trace	Trace	Trace	Trace
Chocolate fudge (1 oz), chocolate syrup (3 tbsp)		125	1	2	30	15	0.6	10	Trace	0.02	0.1	Trace
Molasses (1 tbsp), caramel (½ oz)		40	Trace	Trace	8	20	0.3	Trace	Trace	Trace	Trace	Trace
Sugar (1 tbsp)	12	45	0	0	12	0	Trace	0	0	0	0	0
Miscellaneous												
Chocolate, bitter (1 oz)	30	145	3	15	8	20	1.9	20	0.01	0.07	0.4	0
Sherbet (½ c)	96	130	1	1	30	15	Trace	55	0.01	0.03	Trace	2
Soups												
Bean, pea (green) (1 c)		150	7	4	22	50	1.6	495	0.09	0.06	1.0	4
Noodle, beef, chicken (1 c)		65	4	2	7	10	0.7	50	0.03	0.04	0.9	Trace
Clam chowder, minestrone, tomato, vegetable (1 c)		90	3	2	14	25	0.9	1, 880	0.05	0.04	1.1	3

**See related conversion Tables 670–6 to 670–8.*
(From Wilson ED, Fisher KH, Fuqua ME: Principles of Nutrition, 2nd ed. New York, John Wiley & Sons, 1965, pp 528–533.)

■ **TABLE 670–10 Nutritive Value of Baby Foods (Per Serving)***

Food	Serving *g*	Energy *kcal*	Protein *g*	Fat *g*	Carbo-hydrate *g*	Sodium *mg*	Calcium *mg*	Iron *mg*	Vitamin A *IU*	Thiamine *mg*	Ribo-flavin *mg*	Niacin *mg*	Ascorbic Acid *mg*
Cereals													
Barley	2.4	9	0.3	0.1	1.8	1	19	1.1		0.07	0.07	0.9	0
High protein	2.4	9	0.9	0.1	1.1	1	17	1.8		0.06	0.07	0.8	0
Mixed	2.4	9	0.3	0.1	1.8	1	18	1.5		0.06	0.07	0.8	0
Oatmeal	2.4	10	0.3	0.2	1.7	1	18	1.8		0.07	0.06	0.9	0
Rice	2.4	9	0.2	0.1	1.9	1	20	1.8		0.06	0.05	0.8	0
Dinners, Jar													
Beef and egg noodle	213	122	5.4	4.0	15.7	37	18	0.9	1,400	0.06	0.08	1.2	3
Chicken and noodles, jr.	213	109	4.1	3.0	16.1	36	36	0.8	1,900	0.06	0.07	1.1	3
Macaroni and ham, jr.	213	127	6.8	2.9	18.0	101	159	0.8	1,100	0.12	0.21	1.7	5
Turkey and rice, jr.	213	104	3.8	2.9	15.3	33	50	0.6	2,200	0.02	0.06	0.6	3
Spaghetti, tomato, beef, jr.	213	135	5.4	2.7	21.6	42	39	1.1	1,500	0.14	0.15	2.3	5
Fruits													
Applesauce, jr.	213	79	0.1	0.0	21.9	5	10	0.4	20	0.03	0.06	0.1	81
Applesauce, apricots, jr.	220	104	0.5	0.5	27.3	6	13	0.6	745	0.03	0.07	0.3	39
Bananas, tapioca, jr.	220	147	0.8	0.4	39.1	21	17	0.7	100	0.03	0.04	0.5	57
Peaches	220	157	1.3	0.4	41.6	10	11	0.6	400	0.03	0.07	1.4	42
Pears	213	93	0.6	0.2	24.7	4	18	0.5	70	0.03	0.06	0.4	47
Meats, Poultry													
Beef	99	105	14.3	4.9	0	65	8	1.6	100	0.01	0.16	3.3	2
Chicken	99	148	14.6	9.5	0	50	54	1.0	200	0.01	0.16	3.4	2
Ham	99	123	14.9	6.6	0	66	5	1.0	30	0.14	0.19	2.8	2
Lamb	99	111	15.0	5.2	2.5	73	7	1.6	30	0.02	0.20	3.2	2
Turkey	99	128	15.2	7.0	0	72	28	1.3	600	0.02	0.25	3.4	2
Egg Yolks	94	191	9.4	16.3	0.9	37	72	2.6	1,200	0.07	0.25	1.45	1

Table continued on following page

■ **TABLE 670–10 Nutritive Value of Baby Foods (Per Serving)** *(Continued)*

Food	Serving *g*	Energy *kcal*	Protein *g*	Fat *g*	Carbo-hydrate *g*	Sodium *mg*	Calcium *mg*	Iron *mg*	Vitamin A *IU*	Thiamine *mg*	Ribo-flavin *mg*	Niacin *mg*	Ascorbic Acid *mg*
Vegetables													
Beans	206	51	2.5	0.3	11.8	3	133	2.2	900	0.04	0.21	0.7	17
Beets	128	43	1.7	0.1	9.8	106	18	0.4	40	0.01	0.06	0.2	4
Carrots	213	67	1.7	0.4	15.4	104	49	0.8	25,000	0.05	0.09	1.1	12
Mixed	213	88	3.1	0.8	17.4	77	24	0.9	9,000	0.06	0.07	1.4	5
Peas	213	113	7.0	1.1	19.0	15	34	1.9	700	0.15	0.13	2.0	9
Squash	213	51	1.8	0.4	12.0	3	50	0.7	4,000	0.02	0.14	0.8	17
Sweet potatoes	220	113	2.4	0.3	30.7	49	35	0.8	15,000	0.06	0.08	0.8	21

**See related conversion Tables 670–6 to 670–8.*
(Data from Pennington JAT (ed): Bowes and Church's Food Values of Portions Commonly Used, 15th ed. New York, Harper & Row, 1989.)

■ **TABLE 670–11 Equivalent Temperature Readings (Celsius and Fahrenheit)***

C	F	C	F	C	F	C	F
0	32.0	37.2	99	39.2	102.6	41.2	106.2
20	68.0	37.4	99.3	39.4	102.9	41.4	106.5
30	86.0	37.6	99.7	39.6	103.3	41.6	106.9
31	87.8	37.8	100.1	39.8	103.7	41.8	107.2
32	89.6	38.0	100.4	40.0	104	42	107.6
33	91.4	38.2	100.8	40.2	104.4	43	109.4
34	93.2	38.4	101.2	40.4	104.7	44	111.2
35	95.0	38.6	101.5	40.6	105.1	100	212
36	96.8	38.8	101.8	40.8	105.4		
37	98.6	39.0	102.2	41.0	105.8		

**To convert Celsius (centigrade) readings to Fahrenheit, multiply by 1.8 and add 32. To convert Fahrenheit readings to Celsius, subtract 32 and divide by 1.8.*

INDEX

Note: Page numbers in *italics* indicate illustrations; page numbers followed by t indicate tables.

ISBN 0-7216-5578-5

90071

9 780721 655789